PART XII
DISEASES OF THE LIVER, GALLBLADDER, AND BILE DUCTS 752

PART XIII
HEMATOLOGIC DISEASES 817

PART XIV
ONCOLOGY 1004

PART XV
METABOLIC DISEASES 1078
   Disorders of Carbohydrate Metabolism 1080
   Disorders of Lipid Metabolism 1086
   Inborn Errors of Amino Acid Metabolism 1099
   Inherited Disorders of Connective Tissue 1118
   Disorders of Porphyrins and Metals 1124

PART XVI
NUTRITIONAL DISEASES 1139

PART XVII
ENDOCRINE AND REPRODUCTIVE DISEASES 1176

PART XVIII
DISEASES OF BONE AND BONE MINERAL METABOLISM 1351

PART XIX
DISEASES OF THE IMMUNE SYSTEM 1393

PART XX
MUSCULOSKELETAL AND CONNECTIVE TISSUE DISEASES 1440

(Continued inside back cover)

CECIL
TEXTBOOK
OF
MEDICINE

The Consulting Editors

ENDOCRINOLOGY
METABOLISM

GORDON N. GILL, M.D.

Professor of Medicine
Co-Director, Division of Endocrinology and Metabolism
University of California, San Diego
La Jolla, California

RENAL DISEASES

JUHA P. KOKKO, M.D., Ph.D.

Asa G. Candler Professor and Chairman of Medicine
Emory University School of Medicine
Atlanta, Georgia

INFECTIOUS DISEASES
HIV AND ASSOCIATED DISORDERS

GERALD L. MANDELL, M.D.

Owen R. Cheatham Professor of Sciences
Professor of Internal Medicine
Chief, Infectious Diseases
University of Virginia Health Sciences Center
Charlottesville, Virginia

GASTROINTESTINAL DISEASES
DISEASES OF THE LIVER, GALLBLADDER, AND BILE DUCTS

ROBERT K. OCKNER, M.D.

Professor of Medicine
Director, Liver Center
University of California, San Francisco
San Francisco, California

CARDIOVASCULAR DISEASES
RESPIRATORY DISEASES
CRITICAL CARE MEDICINE

THOMAS WOODWARD SMITH, M.D.

Professor of Medicine
Harvard Medical School
Chief, Cardiovascular Division
Brigham and Women's Hospital
Boston, Massachusetts

CECIL
TEXTBOOK
OF
MEDICINE

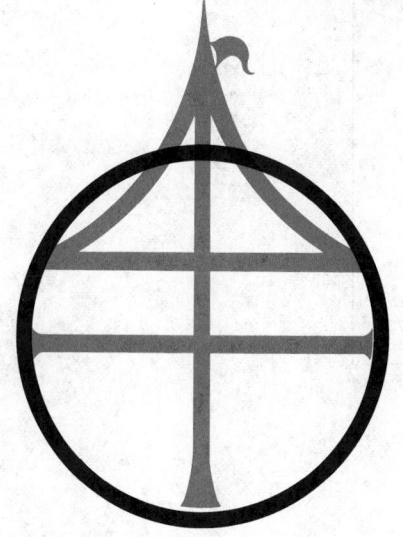

Edited by

J. CLAUDE BENNETT, M.D.

President, University of Alabama at Birmingham
Birmingham, Alabama;
Formerly Spencer Professor of Medicine
and Chairman, Department of Medicine
University of Alabama School of Medicine
Birmingham, Alabama

FRED PLUM, M.D.

Anne Parrish Titzell Professor of Neurology and Neuroscience
Chairman, Department of Neurology and Neuroscience
Cornell University Medical College;
Neurologist-in-Chief
The New York Hospital-Cornell Medical Center
New York, New York

W.B. SAUNDERS COMPANY

A Division of Harcourt Brace & Company

PHILADELPHIA • LONDON • TORONTO • MONTREAL • SYDNEY • TOKYO

W. B. SAUNDERS COMPANY
A Division of Harcourt Brace & Company

The Curtis Center
Independence Square West
Philadelphia, PA 19106

Library of Congress Cataloging-in-Publication Data

Cecil textbook of medicine / edited by J. Claude Bennett, Fred Plum.—20th ed.

    p.   cm.

  Includes bibliographical references and index.

  ISBN 0–7216–3561–X (single v.).—ISBN 0–7216–3574–1 (v. 1).—ISBN 0–7216–3575–X (v. 2).—
ISBN 0–7216–3573–3 (set)

  1. Internal medicine. I. Cecil, Russell L. (Russell La Fayette), 1881–1965. II. Bennett, J. Claude.
III. Plum, Fred, IV. Title: Textbook of medicine.
  [DNLM: 1.   Medicine. WB 100 C3888 1996]

RC46.C423   1996
616—dc20

DNLM/DLC   94–43773

ISBN 0–7216–3574–1   Volume 1
ISBN 0–7216–3575–X   Volume 2
ISBN 0–7216–3573–3   Set (Vols 1 & 2)
ISBN 0–7216–3561–X   Single volume

CECIL TEXTBOOK OF MEDICINE

Last digit is the print number: 9   8   7   6   5   4   3   2

DOSAGE NOTICE

Every effort has been made by the authors, the editors, and the publisher of this book to ensure that dosage recommendations are precise and in agreement with the standards of practice accepted at the time of publication.

However, dosage schedules are changed from time to time in the light of accumulating clinical experience and continuing laboratory studies. This is most likely to occur in the case of recently introduced products.

We urge, therefore, that you check the package information data for the manufacturer's recommended dosage to be certain that changes have not been made in the recommended dose or in the contraindications for administration. In addition, there are some quite serious situations in which drug therapy must be individualized and expert judgment advises the use of a higher dosage or administration by a different route than is included in the manufacturer's recommendations. Throughout the text examples of such instances are indicated by a footnote.

THE EDITORS

ALSO ASSOCIATED WITH THE CECIL TEXTBOOK OF MEDICINE

Review of General Internal Medicine: A Self-Assessment Manual, 6th Edition, 1996

Editors: J. Allen D. Cooper, Jr., M.D., Peter G. Pappas, M.D.

The sixth edition of this self-assessment book contains approximately 1200 questions covering all the specialty areas of internal medicine. The answers are linked to this edition of the Cecil Textbook of Medicine, to the Cecil Essentials of Medicine, and to other readily available sources.

Bennett & Plum: Cecil Textbook of Medicine, 20th Edition—CD-ROM

Available in IBM or MAC versions.

Available from W. B. Saunders Company
The Curtis Center
Independence Square West
Philadelphia, PA 19106

Material in the chapters listed below is in the public domain:

Chapter 10	Vaccination/Immunization
Chapter 136.4	The Thalassemias
Chapter 157	The Epidemiology of Cancer
Chapter 163	Oncologic Emergencies
Chapter 164	Approach to the Patient with Metastatic Cancer, Primary Site Unknown
Chapter 209.1	The Testis
Chapter 211	Mineral and Bone Homeostasis
Chapter 214	The Parathyroid Glands, Hypercalcemia, and Hypocalcemia
Chapter 231	Mastocytosis
Chapter 266	The Compromised Host
Chapter 277	Rheumatic Fever
Chapter 342	Retroviruses Other Than HIV
Chapter 343	Enteroviruses
Chapter 344	Viral Gastroenteritis
Chapter 349	Coccidioidomycosis
Chapter 362	Epidemiology of HIV Infection and AIDS
Chapter 371	Treatment of HIV Infection and AIDS
Chapter 376	American Trypanosomiasis (Chagas' Disease)

CONTRIBUTORS

JUDITH C. AHRONHEIM, M.D.

Associate Professor of Medicine and of Geriatrics and Adult Development, and Medicine, Mount Sinai School of Medicine of the City University of New York. Attending Physician, Department of Geriatrics and Adult Development, Mount Sinai Medical Center, New York, New York

8   *Special Problems in the Geriatric Patient*

ALLEN C. ALFREY, M.D.

Professor of Medicine, University of Colorado Health Sciences Center Medical School. Chief, Renal Section, Denver Veterans Affairs Hospital, Denver, Colorado

191   *Disorders of Magnesium Metabolism*

NANCY B. ALLEN, M.D.

Associate Professor of Medicine, Division of Rheumatology, Allergy, and Immunology, Duke University Medical Center, Durham, North Carolina

245   *Wegener's Granulomatosis*

ROBERT H. ALLEN, M.D.

Cleo Meador and George Ryland Scott Professor of Hematology, Director, Division of Hematology, Department of Medicine, University of Colorado Health Sciences Center School of Medicine, Denver, Colorado

133   *Megaloblastic Anemias*

JOSEPH S. ALPERT, M.D.

Robert S. and Irene P. Flinn Professor of Medicine, University of Arizona College of Medicine. Head, Department of Medicine, University of Arizona Health Science Center, Tucson, Arizona

38   *Pulmonary Hypertension*

KARL E. ANDERSON, M.D.

Professor of Preventive Medicine and Community Health, Internal Medicine, and Pharmacology and Toxicology, University of Texas Medical Branch at Galveston. Full-time Active Staff, University of Texas Medical Branch Hospitals, Galveston, Texas

187   *The Porphyrias*

HANS C. ANDERSSON, M.D.

Assistant Professor of Pediatrics, Tulane University School of Medicine. Clinical Biochemical/Molecular Geneticist, Human Genetics Program/Hayward Genetics Center, Tulane University Medical Center, New Orleans, Louisiana

182   *The Mucopolysaccharidoses*

MICHAEL A. APICELLA, M.D.

Professor and Head, Department of Microbiology, University of Iowa College of Medicine, Iowa City, Iowa

281   *Meningococcal Infections*

GERALD B. APPEL, M.D.

Professor of Clinical Medicine, Columbia University College of Physicians and Surgeons. Director of Clinical Nephrology, Columbia-Presbyterian Medical Center, New York, New York

79   *Glomerular Disorders*

FREDERICK R. APPELBAUM, M.D.

Professor of Medicine, University of Washington School of Medicine. Director, Clinical Research Division, Fred Hutchinson Cancer Research Center, Seattle, Washington

143   *The Acute Leukemias*

GORDON L. ARCHER, M.D.

Professor of Medicine, Microbiology and Immunology, and Chairman, Division of Infectious Diseases, Department of Medicine, Medical College of Virginia, Virginia Commonwealth University, Richmond, Virginia

279   *Staphylococcal Infections*

FRANK C. ARNETT, M.D.

George S. Bruce, Jr., Professor in Arthritis and Other Rheumatic Diseases, and Professor of Internal Medicine, and of Pathology and Laboratory Medicine, University of Texas Medical School at Houston. Chief, Rheumatology Services, Hermann Hospital and Lyndon B. Johnson Hospital, Houston, Texas

237   *Rheumatoid Arthritis*

WILLIAM J. ARNOLD, M.D.

Clinical Professor of Medicine, University of Chicago Pritzker School of Medicine, Chicago. Chairman and Program Director, Department of Medicine, Lutheran General Hospital, Park Ridge, Illinois

236   *Specialized Procedures in the Management of Patients with Rheumatic Diseases*

ALEJANDRO C. ARROLIGA, M.D.

Director, Pulmonary and Critical Care Fellowship Program, The Cleveland Clinic Foundation, Cleveland, Ohio

52   *Chronic Airways Diseases;*   53   *Localized Abnormalities of Lung Aeration*

DENNIS A. AUSIELLO, M.D.

Professor of Medicine, Harvard Medical School. Chief, Renal Unit, Massachusetts General Hospital, Boston, Massachusetts

200   *Endorphins/Opioid Peptides, Prostaglandins, and Natriuretic Hormones*

GROVER C. BAGBY, Jr., M.D.

Professor of Medicine and of Molecular and Medical Genetics and Head, Division of Hematology/Oncology, Oregon Health Sciences University. Acting Head, Section of Hematology/Oncology, Veterans Affairs Medical Center, Portland, Oregon

140   *Disorders of Neutrophil Production*

WILLIAM P. BALDUS, M.D.

Professor of Internal Medicine, Mayo Medical School. Consultant, Mayo Clinic and Mayo Foundation, Rochester, Minnesota

189 *Iron Overload (Hemochromatosis)*

EUGENE V. BALL, M.D.

Professor of Medicine, Division of Clinical Immunology and Rheumatology, Department of Medicine, University of Alabama School of Medicine, Birmingham, Alabama

249 *Behçet's Disease;* 256 *Systemic Diseases in Which Arthritis Is a Feature;* 257 *Miscellaneous Forms of Arthritis;* 258 *Nonarticular Rheumatism;* 259 *Articular Tumors;* 260 *Erythromelalgia*

ROBERT W. BALOH, M.D.

Professor of Neurology and Head and Neck Surgery, University of California, Los Angeles, UCLA School of Medicine, Los Angeles, California

403 *The Special Senses*

MURRAY G. BARON, M.D.

Professor and Associate Chairman of Radiology, Department of Radiology, Emory University School of Medicine, Atlanta, Georgia

33 *Specialized Diagnostic Procedures*

ROBERT B. BARON, M.D.

Associate Professor of Clinical Medicine, University of California, San Francisco, School of Medicine. Vice Chief, Division of General Internal Medicine, Director, Primary Care Internal Medicine Residency Program, and of Continuing Medical Education, University of California San Francisco Medical Center, San Francisco, California

194 *Protein-Energy Malnutrition*

WILLIAM H. BARRY, M.D.

Nora Eccles Harrison Professor of Cardiology, Department of Medicine, University of Utah School of Medicine, Salt Lake City, Utah

33 *Specialized Diagnostic Procedures*

BRUCE A. BARSHOP, M.D., Ph.D.

Assistant Professor of Pediatrics, University of California, San Diego, School of Medicine, La Jolla, California

180 *Homocystinuria*

JOHN A. BARTLETT, M.D.

Assistant Professor of Medicine, Duke University Medical Center, Durham, North Carolina

372 *Management and Counseling for Persons with HIV Infection*

JOHN G. BARTLETT, M.D.

Professor of Medicine, Johns Hopkins University School of Medicine. Chief, Division of Infectious Diseases, Johns Hopkins University Hospital, Baltimore, Maryland

56 *Lung Abscess;* 288 *Botulism;* 289 *Tetanus;* 366 *Gastrointestinal Manifestations of AIDS*

NATHAN M. BASS, M.D., Ph.D.

Associate Professor, Department of Medicine, University of California, San Francisco School of Medicine. Attending Physician, University of California San Francisco Hospitals and Clinics, San Francisco, California

118 *Toxic and Drug-Induced Liver Disease*

STEPHEN B. BAYLIN, M.D.

Professor of Oncology and Medicine, The Oncology Center, Johns Hopkins University School of Medicine. Active Staff in Medicine, Johns Hopkins Hospital, Baltimore, Maryland

159 *Endocrine Manifestations of Tumors: "Ectopic" Hormone Production*

PAUL E. BENDHEIM, M.D.

Visiting Professor, Department of Neurobiology, Weizmann Institute of Science, Rehovat, Israel

428 *Slow Virus Infections of the Nervous System*

J. CLAUDE BENNETT, M.D.

President, University of Alabama at Birmingham, Professor of Medicine, University of Alabama at Birmingham School of Medicine. Rheumatologist, Department of Medicine, University of Alabama Hospital, Birmingham, Alabama

1 *Medicine As a Learned and Humane Profession;* 221 *Approach to the Patient with Immune Disease*

NEAL L. BENOWITZ, M.D.

Professor of Medicine, Psychiatry and Pharmacy and Chief, Division of Clinical Pharmacology and Experimental Therapeutics, University of California, San Francisco, School of Medicine. Staff Physician, San Francisco General Hospital Medical Center, San Francisco, California

9 *Principles of Preventive Health Care*

EDWARD J. BENZ, Jr., M.D.

Osler Professor of Medicine, and Director, Department of Medicine, and Professor of Molecular Biology and Genetics, Johns Hopkins University School of Medicine, Physician-in-Chief, Johns Hopkins Hospital, Baltimore, Maryland

136 *Hemoglobin and Hemoglobinopathies*

JAY BERNSTEIN, M.D.

Director, Research Institute, and Associate Medical Director, William Beaumont Hospital, Royal Oak. Clinical Professor of Pathology, Wayne State University School of Medicine, Detroit, Michigan

90 *Anomalies of the Urinary Tract*

JOSEPH R. BERTINO, M.D.

American Cancer Society Professor of Pharmacology and Medicine, Cornell University School of Medicine. Chairman, Program of Molecular Pharmacology and Therapeutics, and Attending Physician, Department of Medicine, Memorial Sloan-Kettering Cancer Center, New York, New York

162 *Principles of Cancer Therapy*

BRUCE BEUTLER, M.D.

Associate Professor and Associate Investigator, University of Texas Southwestern Medical Center at Dallas Southwestern Medical School, and Howard Hughes Medical Institute, Dallas, Texas

264 *The Pathogenesis of Fever*

STEVEN M. BEUTLER, M.D.

Voluntary Assistant Clinical Professor of Medicine, University of California School of Medicine, Irvine. Director, Division of Infectious Diseases, San Bernardino County Medical Center, and Chief of Staff, St. Bernardine Medical Center, San Bernardino, California

264 *The Pathogenesis of Fever*

J. THOMAS BIGGER, Jr., M.D.

Professor of Medicine and of Pharmacology, Columbia University College of Physicians and Surgeons. Director, Arrhythmia Service, Presbyterian Hospital in the City of New York, New York, New York

35 *Cardiac Arrhythmias*

ALAN L. BISNO, M.D.

Professor of Medicine, University of Miami School of Medicine. Chief, Medical Service, Miami Veterans Administration Medical Center, and Attending Physician, Jackson Memorial Hospital, Miami, Florida

277 *Rheumatic Fever*

BRUCE R. BISTRIAN, M.D., M.P.H., Ph.D.

Professor of Medicine, Harvard Medical School. Chief, Division of Clinical Nutrition, New England Deaconess Hospital, Boston, Massachusetts

193 *Nutritional Assessment*

GERALD G. BLACKWELL, M.D.

Assistant Professor of Medicine, Division of Cardiovascular Diseases and Clinical Director, Cardiovascular MRI, University of Alabama School of Medicine, Birmingham, Alabama

33   *Specialized Diagnostic Procedures*

WILLIAM A. BLATTNER, M.D.

Chief, Viral Epidemiology Branch, National Cancer Institute, National Institutes of Health, Bethesda, Maryland

342   *Retroviruses Other Than HIV*

WILLIAM J. BLOT, Ph.D.

Chief Executive Officer, International Epidemiology Institute, Rockville, Maryland

157   *The Epidemiology of Cancer*

ROGER C. BONE, M.D.

President, Chief Executive Officer, and Professor of Medicine, Medical College of Ohio, Toledo, Ohio

57   *Bronchiectasis;*   58   *Cystic Fibrosis*

JAMES R. BONNER, M.D.

Professor of Medicine, Division of Developmental and Clinical Immunology, University of Alabama School of Medicine, Birmingham, Alabama

230   *Drug Allergy*

DENNIS W. BOULWARE, M.D.

Professor of Medicine, University of Alabama School of Medicine, Birmingham, Alabama

255   *The Painful Shoulder*

ROBERT C. BOURGE, M.D.

Professor, Departments of Medicine (Cardiovascular Diseases), of Radiology (Nuclear Medicine), and of Surgery (Transplantation), The University of Alabama School of Medicine. Medical Director of Cardiac Transplantation and of the Advanced Heart Failure Clinic, The University of Alabama Hospital and The Kirklin Clinic, Birmingham, Alabama

48   *Cardiac Transplantation*

LAURENCE A. BOXER, M.D.

Professor and Director, Division of Pediatric Hematology/Oncology, University of Michigan Medical School. Professor and Director, Division of Pediatric Hematology/Oncology, C. S. Mott Children's Hospital, Ann Arbor, Michigan

139   *Function of Neutrophils and Mononuclear Phagocytes*

LAWRENCE J. BRANDT, M.D.

Professor of Medicine, Albert Einstein College of Medicine. Director, Division of Gastroenterology, Moses Campus of Montefiore Medical Center, Bronx, New York

105   *Vascular Disorders of the Intestine*

BARRY D. BRAUSE, M.D.

Clinical Associate Professor of Medicine, Cornell University Medical College. Associate Attending Physician, New York Hospital and The Hospital for Special Surgery, New York, New York

283   *Osteomyelitis*

CHARLES B. BRENDLER, M.D.

Professor and Chief of Urology, University of Chicago, Pritzker School of Medicine, Chicago, Illinois

209   *Endocrinologic Diseases Unique to Men*

WILLIAM J. BRITT, M.D.

Professor of Pediatrics and Microbiology, University of Alabama School of Medicine. Scientist, University of Alabama Comprehensive Cancer Center and AIDS Center, Birmingham, Alabama

340   *Infections Associated with Human Cytomegalovirus*

SAMUEL BRODER, M.D.

Director, National Cancer Institute, National Institutes of Health, Bethesda, Maryland

371   *Treatment of HIV Infection and AIDS*

PHILIP A. BRUNELL, M.D.

Professor of Pediatrics, University of California, Los Angeles, UCLA School of Medicine. Vice Chair and Chief of Infectious Diseases, Department of Pediatrics, Cedars Sinai Medical Center, Los Angeles, California

334   *Measles;*   335   *Rubella (German Measles);*   336   *Varicella (Chickenpox, Shingles)*

ROBERT C. BRUNHAM, M.D., F.R.C.P.C.

Head, Department of Medical Microbiology and Section of Infectious Diseases, University of Manitoba Faculty of Medicine. Director, Department of Clinical Microbiology, Health Sciences Centre, Winnipeg, Manitoba, Canada

323   *Diseases Caused by Chlamydiae*

REBECCA H. BUCKLEY, M.D.

J. Buren Sidbury Professor of Pediatrics and Professor of Immunology, Duke University School of Medicine. Chief, Division of Allergy and Immunology, Duke University Medical Center, Durham, North Carolina

223   *Primary Immunodeficiency Diseases*

WARD E. BULLOCK, M.D.

Dean, School of Medicine, and Professor, Department of Medicine, University of Connecticut School of Medicine. Attending Physician, John Dempsey Hospital, Farmington, Connecticut

306   *Actinomycosis;*   307   *Nocardiosis*

THOMAS BUTLER, M.D.

Professor of Internal Medicine and of Microbiology and Immunology, Texas Tech University Health Sciences Center School of Medicine. Chief of Infectious Diseases and Attending Physician, University Medical Center, Lubbock, Texas

292   *Typhoid Fever;*   294   *Shigellosis*

PETER H. BYERS, M.D.

Professor, Departments of Pathology and Medicine (Medical Genetics), University of Washington School of Medicine, Seattle, Washington

183   *The Marfan Syndrome;*   184   *Ehlers-Danlos Syndrome;*
185   *Osteogenesis Imperfecta*

STEPHEN D. CEDERBAUM, M.D.

Professor of Psychiatry and Pediatrics/Medical Genetics, University of California, Los Angeles, UCLA School of Medicine. Attending Physician, University of California Los Angeles Medical Center; Consultant in Metabolic Disorders, Kaiser Permanente Clinics of Southern California, Los Angeles, California

178   *Diseases of the Urea Cycle*

BARTOLOME R. CELLI, M.D.

Associate Professor of Medicine, Tufts University School of Medicine. Chief, Division of Pulmonary and Critical Care Medicine, St. Elizabeth's Medical Center, Boston, Massachusetts

63   *Diseases of the Diaphragm, Chest Wall, Pleura, and Mediastinum*

JOHN P. CELLO, M.D.

Professor of Medicine and Surgery, University of California, San Francisco, School of Medicine. Chief of Gastroenterology, Hepatology and Clinical Nutrition, San Francisco General Hospital Medical Center, San Francisco, California

95 *Gastrointestinal Hemorrhage*

RUSSELL W. CHESNEY, M.D.

Le Bonheur Professor and Chairman of Pediatrics, University of Tennessee, Memphis, College of Medicine. Vice President for Academic Affairs, Le Bonheur Children's Medical Center, Memphis, Tennessee

82 *Specific Renal Tubular Disorders*

SANDY F. S. CHUN, M.D.

Staff Physician, Department of Medicine, Kaiser Hospital, Santa Clara, California

356 *Mucormycosis*

C. GLENN COBBS, M.D.

Professor of Medicine, University of Alabama School of Medicine. Chief, Medical Service, Department of Veterans Affairs Medical Center, Birmingham, Alabama

310 *Bartonellosis*

GENE D. COHEN, M.D., Ph.D.

Director, Center on Aging, Health and Humanities, George Washington University School of Medicine and Health Sciences, Washington, D.C.

7 *Neuropsychiatric Aspects of Aging*

LAWRENCE S. COHEN, M.D.

Ebenezer K. Hunt Professor of Medicine and Deputy Dean, Yale University School of Medicine. Attending Physician, Yale–New Haven Medical Center, New Haven, Connecticut

45 *Diseases of the Aorta*

SIDNEY COHEN, M.D.

Richard Laylord Evans Professor and Chairman, Department of Medicine, Temple University School of Medicine. Assistant Vice President for the Health Sciences Center, Temple University Hospital, Philadelphia, Pennsylvania

97 *Diseases of the Esophagus*

LAWRENCE H. COHN, M.D.

Professor of Surgery, Harvard Medical School. Chief of Cardiac Surgery, Brigham and Women's Hospital, Boston, Massachusetts

41 *Disorders of the Coronary Arteries*

ZANVIL A. COHN, M.D.†

Professor and Senior Physician, Laboratory of Cellular Physiology and Immunology, and Vice-President for Medical Affairs, The Rockefeller University, New York, New York

313 *Leprosy (Hansen's Disease)*

ROBERT M. CONRY, M.D.

Assistant Professor of Hematology and Oncology, University of Alabama School of Medicine. Attending Staff, University of Alabama Hospital, Birmingham, Alabama

208 *Endocrinologic Diseases Unique to Women*

DENNIS L. COOPER, M.D.

Associate Professor of Medicine, Section of Medical Oncology, Yale School of Medicine, New Haven, Connecticut

158 *Systemic Secretions of Cancer Cells and Their Effects*

---

† Dr. Cohn is deceased.

MAX D. COOPER, M.D.

Professor of Medicine, Pediatrics and Microbiology, University of Alabama School of Medicine. Investigator, Howard Hughes Medical Institute, Birmingham, Alabama

232 *Diseases of the Thymus*

JAMES D. CRAPO, M.D.

Professor of Medicine and Pathology; Chief, Division of Pulmonary and Critical Care Medicine, Duke University School of Medicine, Durham, North Carolina

50 *Respiratory Structure and Function*

DAVID T. CURIEL, M.D.

Director, Gene Therapy Program, University of Alabama School of Medicine, Birmingham, Alabama

25 *Gene Therapy*

JAMES W. CURRAN, M.D., M.P.H.

Associate Director for HIV/AIDS, Centers for Disease Control and Prevention, Atlanta, Georgia

362 *Epidemiology of HIV Infection and AIDS*

JOHN J. CURTIS, M.D.

Professor of Medicine and of Surgery, Division of Nephrology, University of Alabama School of Medicine. Staff Physician, University of Alabama Hospital, Birmingham, Alabama

78 *Treatment of Irreversible Renal Failure*

JOHN J. CUSH, M.D.

Assistant Professor of Internal Medicine, University of Texas Southwestern Medical Center at Dallas, Dallas, Texas

238 *The Spondylarthropathies*

DAVID C. DALE, M.D.

Professor of Medicine, University of Washington School of Medicine. Attending Physician, University of Washington Medical Center, Seattle, Washington

263 *The Febrile Patient*

ANTONIO R. DAMASIO, M.D., Ph.D.

M. W. Van Allen Professor and Head, Department of Neurology, University of Iowa College of Medicine, Iowa City, Iowa. Adjunct Professor, The Salk Institute for Biological Studies, La Jolla, California

398 *Diagnosis of Regional Cerebral Dysfunction;* 399 *Disturbances of Memory and Language;* 400 *Alzheimer's Disease and Related Dementias*

TROY E. DANIELS, D.D.S., M.S.

Professor of Stomatology, School of Dentistry, and Professor of Pathology, University of California, San Francisco, School of Medicine, San Francisco, California

96 *Diseases of the Mouth and Salivary Glands*

BESS DAWSON-HUGHES, M.D.

Associate Professor of Medicine, Division of Endocrinology, Tufts University School of Medicine. Chief, Calcium and Bone Metabolism Laboratory, The Jean Mayer USDA Human Nutrition Research Center on Aging at Tufts University, Boston, Massachusetts

212 *Vitamin D*

SUSAN C. DAY, M.D., M.P.H.

Adjunct Associate Professor of Medicine, University of Pennsylvania School of Medicine. Vice President, General Internal Medicine, American Board of Internal Medicine, Philadelphia, Pennsylvania

15 *The Domain of the Generalist Physician*

HAILE T. DEBAS, M.D.

Maurice Galante Distinguished Professor of Surgery and Dean, University of California, San Francisco, School of Medicine, San Francisco, California

99   *Peptic Ulcer*

MICHAEL DECK, M.B., B.S., F.R.A.C.R., F.R.C.K.

Professor of Radiology, Cornell University Medical College. Attending Radiologist, New York Hospital, New York, New York

392   *Neurology: Clinical Study of the Patient*

LEONARD J. DEFTOS, M.D., J.D.

Professor of Medicine, University of California, San Diego, School of Medicine, San Diego. Staff Physician and Head of Endocrine Research Laboratory, Department of Veterans Affairs Medical Center, La Jolla, California

215   *Calcitonin and Medullary Thyroid Carcinoma*

MICHAEL W. DeGREGORIO, Ph.D.

Associate Professor of Medicine, Division of Hematology and Oncology, Department of Internal Medicine, University of California, Davis School of Medicine. Associate Director of Experimental Therapeutics, University of California Davis Cancer Center, Davis, California

165   *Molecular Mechanisms of Drug Resistance*

ANDREW DEISS, M.D.

Professor of Internal Medicine, University of Utah School of Medicine. Associate Chief of Staff for Research and Development, Veterans Affairs Medical Center, Salt Lake City, Utah

188   *Wilson's Disease*

RICHARD D. deSHAZO, M.D.

Director, Division of Allergy-Immunology, Professor of Medicine and Pediatrics, and Chairman, Department of Internal Medicine, University of South Alabama College of Medicine, Mobile, Alabama

225   *Allergic Rhinitis;*   228   *Immune Complex Diseases*

ROBERT J. DESNICK, M.D., Ph.D.

Arthur J. and Nellie Z. Cohen Professor of Pediatrics and Genetics and Professor and Chairman of Human Genetics, Mount Sinai School of Medicine, New York, New York

174   *Lysosomal Storage Diseases*

IVAN DIAMOND, M.D., Ph.D.

Professor and Vice Chair, Department of Neurology, and Professor of Pediatrics and Pharmacology, University of California, San Francisco, School of Medicine. Director, Ernest Gallo Clinic and Research Center, San Francisco, California

11   *Alcoholism and Alcohol Abuse*

ROBERT B. DIASIO, M.D.

Newman H. Waters Professor of Clinical Pharmacology and Professor of Medicine and Pharmacology/Toxicology, and Chairman, Department of Pharmacology and Toxicology, University of Alabama School of Medicine, Birmingham, Alabama

16   *Principles of Drug Therapy*

WOLFGANG H. DILLMANN, M.D.

Professor of Medicine, University of California, San Diego, School of Medicine, San Diego, California

203   *The Thyroid*

EUGENE P. DiMAGNO, M.D.

Professor of Medicine, Mayo Medical School. Consultant, Division of Gastroenterology, Department of Internal Medicine, and Director, Gastroenterology Research Unit, Mayo Clinic, Rochester, Minnesota

108   *Carcinoma of the Pancreas*

CHARLES A. DINARELLO, M.D.

Professor of Medicine and Pediatrics, Tufts University School of Medicine. Staff Physician, New England Medical Center, Boston, Massachusetts

265   *The Acute Phase Response*

WILLIAM E. DISMUKES, M.D.

Professor and Vice Chairman, Department of Medicine, and Director, Division of Infectious Diseases, University of Alabama School of Medicine. Attending Physician, University of Alabama Hospital, Birmingham, Alabama

347   *Introduction to the Mycoses;*   348   *Histoplasmosis;*
350   *Blastomycosis;*   351   *Paracoccidioidomycosis;*
352   *Cryptococcosis;*   353   *Sporotrichosis;*   354   *Candidiasis*

R. GORDON DOUGLAS, Jr., M.D.

Adjunct Professor of Medicine, Cornell University Medical College, New York, New York. President, Merck Vaccine Division, Merck and Company, Inc., Whitehouse Station, New Jersey

326   *Introduction to Viral Diseases;*   346   *Other Arthropod-Borne Viruses*

JEFFREY M. DRAZEN, M.D.

Parker R. Francis Professor of Medicine, Harvard Medical School. Chief, Respiratory Division, Brigham and Women's Hospital, Boston, Massachusetts

51   *Asthma*

MARC K. DREZNER, M.D.

Professor of Medicine and Chief, Division of Endocrinology, Metabolism and Nutrition, and Director, Sarah W. Stedman Nutrition Center, Duke University School of Medicine, Durham, North Carolina

213   *Osteomalacia and Rickets*

DOUGLAS A. DROSSMAN, M.D.

Professor of Medicine and Psychiatry, University of North Carolina at Chapel Hill School of Medicine. Attending Physician, University of North Carolina Hospitals, Chapel Hill, North Carolina

195   *The Eating Disorders*

THOMAS D. DuBOSE, Jr., M.D.

Professor of Internal Medicine, Physiology and Cell Biology, University of Texas, Houston Medical School, Houston, Texas

85   *Vascular Disorders of the Kidney*

THOMAS P. DUFFY, M.D.

Professor of Medicine, Yale University School of Medicine. Attending Physician, Yale–New Haven Hospital, New Haven, Connecticut

131   *Normochromic, Normocytic Anemias;*   132   *Microcytic and Hypochromic Anemias*

RICHARD J. DUMA, M.D., Ph.D.

Clinical Professor of Medicine and Infectious Diseases, Medical College of Virginia, Virginia Commonwealth University, Richmond, Virginia. Executive Director, National Foundation for Infectious Diseases, Bethesda, Maryland

271   *Pneumococcal Pneumonia*

HERBERT L. DuPONT, M.D.

Mary W. Kelsey Professor of Medical Sciences, University of Texas Medical School and School of Public Health. Chief, Internal Medicine Service and H. Irving Schweppe, MD, Chair in Internal Medicine, St. Luke's Episcopal Hospital, Houston, Texas

291   *Introduction to Enteric Infections*

PAUL H. EDELSTEIN, M.D.

Professor of Pathology and Laboratory Medicine, University of Pennsylvania School of Medicine. Director of Clinical Microbiology and Attending Physician in Infectious Diseases, Hospital of the University of Pennsylvania, Philadelphia, Pennsylvania

275 *Legionellosis*

RONALD J. ELIN, M.D., Ph.D.

Clinical Professor of Pathology, Uniformed Services University of the Health Sciences, F. Edward Hebert School of Medicine. Chief, Clinical Pathology Department, National Institutes of Health, Bethesda, Maryland

477 *Reference Intervals and Laboratory Values*

LOUIS J. ELSAS II, M.D.

Professor of Pediatrics, and Associated Professor of Biochemistry and of Medicine, Emory University School of Medicine. Director, Division of Medical Genetics, Henrietta Egleston Children's Hospital at Emory University Hospital, Grady Memorial Hospital, Atlanta, Georgia

24 *Inborn Errors of Metabolism;* 168 *Approach to the Patient with Metabolic Disease;* 179 *Branched-Chain Aminoacidurias*

STEPHEN H. EMBURY, M.D.

Professor of Medicine, University of California, San Francisco, School of Medicine. Chief, Hematology Division, San Francisco General Hospital, San Francisco, California

137 *Sickle Cell Anemia and Associated Hemoglobinopathies*

EDWARD A. EMMETT, M.B., B.S., M.S.

Professor, University of Sydney. Chief Executive Officer, National Occupational Health & Safety Commission, Sydney, Australia

476 *Occupational Diseases of the Skin*

ANDREW G. ENGEL, M.D.

Professor of Neuroscience, Mayo Medical School. Consultant, Mayo Clinic, Rochester, Minnesota

453–459 *Diseases of Muscle (Myopathies) and Neuromuscular Junction*

MARC S. ERNSTOFF, M.D.

Associate Professor of Medicine, Dartmouth Medical School. Director, Clinical Therapeutics Research Program, Norris Cotton Cancer Center, Lebanon, New Hampshire

158 *Systemic Secretions of Cancer Cells and Their Effects*

LUIS R. ESPINOZA, M.D.

Professor and Chief, Section of Rheumatology, Louisiana State University School of Medicine, New Orleans, Louisiana

239 *Infectious Arthritis*

VIRGIL F. FAIRBANKS, M.D.

Professor of Internal Medicine and of Laboratory Medicine and Pathology, Mayo Medical School. Consultant, Mayo Clinic and Mayo Foundation, Rochester, Minnesota

189 *Iron Overload (Hemochromatosis)*

DOUGLAS V. FALLER, Ph.D., M.D.

Professor of Medicine, Biochemistry, Pediatrics, Microbiology, Pathology, and Laboratory Medicine; Director, Cancer Research Center, and Vice Chairman, Division of Medicine, Boston University School of Medicine, Boston, Massachusetts

150 *Diseases of Lymph Nodes and Spleen*

BARRY L. FANBURG, M.D.

Professor of Medicine, Tufts University School of Medicine. Chief, Pulmonary and Critical Care Division, New England Medical Center, Boston, Massachusetts

61 *Sarcoidosis*

ROBERT FEKETY, M.D.

Professor of Internal Medicine, Division of Infectious Diseases, Department of Internal Medicine, University of Michigan Medical School. Infectious Diseases Service, University of Michigan Hospitals, Ann Arbor, Michigan

287 *Pseudomembranous Colitis*

DAVID W. FERGUSON, M.D.

Professor of Medicine, Uniformed Services University of the Health Sciences. Director, Cardiology Training Programs, National Naval Medical Center, Bethesda, Maryland

69 *Cardiogenic Shock*

THOMAS F. FERRIS, M.D.

Nesbitt Professor and Chairman, Department of Medicine, University of Minnesota School of Medicine, Minneapolis, Minnesota

86 *Hypertension and Renal Disease in Pregnancy*

CALEB E. FINCH, Ph.D.

Professor of Gerontology and Biological Sciences, Ethel P. Andrus Gerontology Center, University of Southern California, Los Angeles, School of Medicine, Los Angeles, California

5 *Biology of Aging*

JOEL S. FINKELSTEIN, M.D.

Assistant Professor of Medicine, Harvard Medical School. Assistant in Medicine, Massachusetts General Hospital, Boston, Massachusetts

217 *Osteoporosis*

GARRET A. FITZGERALD, M.D.

Professor of Medicine and Pharmacology, Robinette Professor of Cardiovascular Medicine, and Director, Center for Experimental Therapeutics, University of Pennsylvania, School of Medicine, Philadelphia, Pennsylvania

200 *Endorphins/Opioid Peptides, Prostaglandins, and Natriuretic Hormones*

SUZANNE W. FLETCHER, M.D., M.Sc.

Professor, Department of Ambulatory Care and Prevention, Harvard Medical School. Senior Physician, Brigham and Women's Hospital, and Physician, Harvard Community Health Plan, Boston, Massachusetts

14 *Clinical Decision Making*

JEFFREY S. FLIER, M.D.

Professor of Medicine, Harvard Medical School. Chief, Division of Endocrinology, Beth Israel Hospital, Boston, Massachusetts

206 *Hypoglycemia/Pancreatic Islet Cell Disorders*

KATHLEEN M. FOLEY, M.D.

Professor of Neurology, Neuroscience and Clinical Pharmacology, Cornell University Medical College. Chief, Pain Service, Memorial Sloan-Kettering Cancer Center, New York, New York

17 *Pain*

JAY W. FOX, Ph.D.

Professor of Microbiology, University of Virginia School of Medicine. Director, Biomolecular Research Facility, University of Virginia Health Sciences Center, Charlottesville, Virginia

391 *Venoms and Poisons from Marine Organisms*

MICHAEL M. FRANK, M.D.

Samuel L. Katz Professor of Pediatrics and Professor of Medicine and Immunology, Duke University School of Medicine. Chairman, Department of Pediatrics, Duke University Medical Center, Durham, North Carolina

224 *Urticaria and Angioedema*

WILLIAM T. FRIEDEWALD, M.D.

Clinical Professor of Medicine and of Public Health, College of Physicians and Surgeons of Columbia University. Professional Staff, The Presbyterian Hospital in the City of New York, New York, New York

31 *Epidemiology of Cardiovascular Diseases*

SCOTT L. FRIEDMAN, M.D.

Associate Professor of Medicine, University of California, School of Medicine. Attending Physician and Gastroenterologist, San Francisco General Hospital, San Francisco, California

122 *Cirrhosis of the Liver and its Major Sequelae*

PATRICIA A GABOW, M.D.

Professor of Medicine, University of Colorado Health Sciences Center School of Medicine. Chief Executive Officer, Denver Health and Hospitals, Denver, Colorado

89 *Cystic Diseases of the Kidney*

JOHN N. GALGIANI, M.D.

Professor of Internal Medicine, University of Arizona College of Medicine. Chief, Section of Infectious Diseases, Veterans Affairs Medical Center, Tucson, Arizona

349 *Coccidioidomycosis*

MARC B. GARNICK, M.D.

Associate Professor of Medicine, Harvard Medical School, Boston, Massachusetts

91 *Tumors of the Kidney, Ureter, and Bladder*

RENATE E. GAY, M.D.

Research Associate Professor of Medicine, University of Alabama School of Medicine, Birmingham, Alabama

234 *Connective Tissue Structure and Function*

STEFFEN GAY, M.D.

Professor of Medicine, The University of Alabama School of Medicine, Birmingham, Alabama

234 *Connective Tissue Structure and Function*

GORDON N. GILL, M.D.

Professor of Medicine and Co-Director, Division of Endocrinology and Metabolism, and Associate Chair for Scientific Affairs, University of California, San Diego, School of Medicine, La Jolla, California

199 *Principles of Endocrinology*

JOHN W. GITTINGER, Jr., M.D.

Professor of Ophthalmology and Neurology and Chair, Department of Ophthalmology, University of Massachusetts Medical School. Chief of Ophthalmology, University of Massachusetts Medical Center, Worcester, Massachusetts

460–470 *Eye Diseases*

JOHN W. GNANN, Jr., M.D.

Associate Professor of Medicine, University of Alabama School of Medicine, Birmingham, Alabama

338 *Mumps*

NORA GOLDSCHLAGER, M.D.

Professor of Clinical Medicine, University of California, San Francisco, School of Medicine. Associate Chief, Cardiology Division and Director, Coronary Care Unit, San Francisco General Hospital Medical Center, San Francisco, California

33 *Specialized Diagnostic Procedures*

ELLIE J. C. GOLDSTEIN, M.D.

Clinical Professor of Medicine, University of California, Los Angeles, School of Medicine, Los Angeles. Director, R. M. Alden Research Laboratory, Santa Monica Hospital Medical Center, Santa Monica, California

290 *Diseases Caused by Non–Spore-Forming Anaerobic Bacteria*

CLEON W. GOODWIN, M.D.

Johnson and Johnson Distinguished Associate Professor of Surgery, Cornell University Medical College. Director, Burn Center, The New York Hospital–Cornell Medical Center, New York, New York

13 *Principles of Occupational and Environmental Medicine*

DUNCAN A. GORDON, M.D.

Professor of Medicine, University of Toronto Faculty of Medicine. Senior Rheumatologist, The Toronto Hospital Arthritis Centre, Toronto, Ontario, Canada

233 *Approach to the Patient with Musculoskeletal Disease*

DAVID Y. GRAHAM, M.D.

Professor of Medicine and Molecular Virology, Baylor College of Medicine. Chief, Digestive Disease Section, Veterans Affairs Medical Center, Houston, Texas

99 *Peptic Ulcer*

HARRY L. GREENE, M.D.

Clinical Professor of Pediatrics, Vanderbilt University School of Medicine, Nashville, Tennessee, and Indiana University School of Medicine, Indianapolis, Indiana

170 *Glycogen Storage Diseases;* 171 *Fructose Intolerance*

WILLIAM B. GREENOUGH III, M.D.

Professor of Medicine and of International Health, Johns Hopkins University Schools of Medicine and Hygiene and Public Health. Division of Geriatric Medicine, Johns Hopkins Bayview Medical Center and Johns Hopkins Geriatric Center, Baltimore, Maryland

296 *Cholera*

JOHN W. GRIFFIN, M.D.

Professor of Neuroscience and Director, Department of Neurology, Johns Hopkins University. Active Staff, Johns Hopkins Hospital, Baltimore, Maryland

445–452 *Diseases of the Peripheral Nervous System*

JEROME E. GROOPMAN, M.D.

Professor of Medicine, Harvard Medical School. Chief, Division of Hematology/Oncology, Deaconess Hospital, Boston, Massachusetts

369 *Hematology/Oncology in AIDS*

RICHARD L. GUERRANT, M.D.

Thomas H. Hunter Professor of International Medicine, Chief, Division of Geographic and International Medicine, and Director, Office of International Health, University of Virginia School of Medicine. Attending Physician, and Professor of Medicine, University of Virginia Hospital, Charlottesville, Virginia

295 Campylobacter *Enteritis;* 297 *Enteric* Escherichia coli *Infections*

LESTER M. HADDAD, M.D.

Clinical Associate Professor of Family Medicine, Medical University of South Carolina. Attending Emergency Physician, Charleston Memorial Hospital, Charleston, South Carolina

72 *Acute Poisoning*

STEPHEN M. HAHN, M.D.

Senior Investigator, Radiation Oncology Branch, Clinical Pharmacology Branch, National Cancer Institute, National Institutes of Health, Bethesda, Maryland

163 *Oncologic Emergencies*

JUDITH G. HALL, M.D., M.Sc., F.A.A.P., F.A.B.M.G., F.R.C.P., F.C.C.M.G.

Professor of Pediatrics, University of British Columbia. Head, Department of Pediatrics, British Columbia Children's Hospital, Vancouver, British Columbia, Canada

27 *Congenital Anomalies*

STEPHEN B. HANAUER, M.D.

Professor of Medicine and Clinical Pharmacology, University of Chicago Pritzker School of Medicine. Co-Director, Inflammatory Bowel Disease Research Center, University of Chicago Medical Center, Chicago, Illinois

104 *Inflammatory Bowel Disease*

IAIN R. B. HARDY, M.B.Ch.B., M.P.H.

Medical Epidemiologist, National Immunization Program, Centers for Disease Control and Prevention, Atlanta, Georgia

285 *Diphtheria*

LAURENCE A. HARKER, M.D.

Blomeyer Professor of Medicine and Director, Division of Hematology and Oncology, Emory University School of Medicine, Atlanta, Georgia

20 *Antithrombotic Therapy*

FREDERICK G. HAYDEN, M.D.

Professor of Internal Medicine and Pathology, University of Virginia School of Medicine. Staff Physician and Associate Director of Clinical Microbiology (Virology), University of Virginia Health Sciences Center, Charlottesville, Virginia

332 *Influenza*

LOUIS W. HECK, M.D.

Associate Professor of Medicine, Department of Medicine, University of Alabama School of Medicine, Birmingham, Alabama

248 *The Amyloid Diseases*

DOUGLAS C. HEIMBURGER, M.D.

Associate Professor and Director, Division of Clinical Nutrition, Departments of Nutrition Sciences and Medicine, University of Alabama School of Medicine. Staff Physician, University of Alabama Hospital and Birmingham Veterans Affairs Medical Center; Chief, Nutrition Section, University of Alabama Veterans Affairs Medical Center, Birmingham, Alabama

192 *Nutrition's Interface with Health and Disease*

DONALD A. HENDERSON, M.D., M.P.H.

University Distinguished Professor, Johns Hopkins University, Baltimore, Maryland. Senior Science Advisor, Department of Health and Human Services, Washington, D.C.

337 *Variola and Vaccinia*

J. OWEN HENDLEY, M.D.

Professor of Pediatrics, University of Virginia School of Medicine. Head, Division of Pediatric Infectious Diseases, University of Virginia Health Sciences Center, Charlottesville, Virginia

328 *The Common Cold*

MICHAEL S. HERSHFIELD, M.D.

Professor of Medicine, Duke University Medical Center, Durham, North Carolina

181 *Disorders of Purine and Pyrimidine Metabolism;*   251 *Gout and Uric Acid Metabolism*

HOBY HETHERINGTON, Ph.D.

Associate Professor of Medicine, Division of Cardiovascular Diseases, University of Alabama School of Medicine, Birmingham, Alabama

22 *Overview of Imaging Techniques for the Future*

DOUGLAS M. HEUMAN, M.D.

Associate Professor of Medicine, Medical College of Virginia, Virginia Commonwealth University, Richmond, Virginia

126 *Diseases of the Gallbladder and Bile Ducts*

MARTIN F. HEYWORTH, M.D.

Professor of Medicine, University of North Dakota School of Medicine. Chief, Medical Service, Department of Veterans Affairs Medical Center, Fargo, North Dakota

109 *Food Poisoning*

RICHARD E. HILLMAN, M.D.

Professor of Child Health and of Biochemistry, University of Missouri School of Medicine. Medical Director and Associate Chairman of the Child Health Medical Service, Children's Hospital at University Hospital and Clinics, Columbia, Missouri

172 *Primary Hyperoxaluria*

MARC C. HOCHBERG, M.D., M.P.H.

Professor of Medicine, Epidemiology and Preventive Medicine, University of Maryland School of Medicine, Baltimore, Maryland

242 *Sjögren's Syndrome*

EDWARD W. HOOK III, M.D.

Professor of Medicine and Epidemiology, Division of Infectious Diseases, University of Alabama School of Medicine. Medical Director, Sexually Transmitted Disease Control Program, Jefferson County Health Department, Birmingham, Alabama

316 *Granuloma Inguinale (Donovanosis);*   317 *Chancroid;*
318 *Syphilis;*   319 *Nonsyphilitic Treponematoses*

PHILIP C. HOPEWELL, M.D.

Professor of Medicine, University of California, San Francisco, School of Medicine. Chief, Division of Pulmonary and Critical Care Medicine, San Francisco General Hospital, San Francisco, California

365 *Pulmonary Manifestations of HIV Infection*

RICHARD B. HORNICK, M.D.

Clinical Professor of Internal Medicine, University of Florida School of Medicine, Gainesville. Vice President of Medical Education, Orlando Regional Healthcare System, Orlando, Florida

301 *Tularemia;*   324 *Rickettsial Diseases*

THOMAS H. HOSTETTER, M.D.

Professor of Medicine, University of Minnesota School of Medicine. Director, Division of Renal Diseases and Hypertension, University of Minnesota Hospitals and Clinics, Minneapolis, Minnesota

83 *Diabetes and the Kidney*

DAVID S. HOWELL, M.D.

Professor of Medicine, University of Miami School of Medicine. Attending Physician, Jackson Memorial Hospital and University of Miami Clinics, and Medical Research Scientist, Veterans Affairs Medical Center, Miami, Florida

405 *Disorders of Sensation*

KEITH HRUSKA, M.D.

Ira M. Lang Professor of Medicine, Washington University School of Medicine. Director, Renal Division, Jewish Hospital of St. Louis, St. Louis, Missouri

88 *Renal Calculi (Nephrolithiasis)*

GENE G. HUNDER, M.D.

Professor of Medicine, Mayo Medical School. Chairman, Division of Rheumatology, Department of Internal Medicine, Mayo Clinic, Rochester, Minnesota

246 *Polymyalgia Rheumatica and Giant Cell Arteritis*

DANIEL C. IHDE, M.D.

Professor of Medicine and Director, Division of Medical Oncology, Washington University, School of Medicine. Medical Oncologist-in-Chief, Barnes and Jewish Hospitals, St. Louis, Missouri

164 *Approach to the Patient with Metastatic Cancer, Primary Site Unknown*

ROBERT W. IKE, M.D.

Assistant Professor, Department of Internal Medicine, Division of Rheumatology, University of Michigan Medical School, Ann Arbor, Michigan

236 *Specialized Procedures in the Management of Patients with Rheumatic Diseases*

MICHAEL D. ISEMAN, M.D.

Professor of Medicine, Division of Pulmonary Medicine and Infectious Diseases, University of Colorado Health Science Center School of Medicine. The Beno Chair in Mycobacterial Diseases, National Jewish Center for Immunology and Respiratory Medicine, Denver, Colorado

311 *Tuberculosis*

JON I. ISENBERG, M.D.

Professor of Medicine, University of California, San Diego, School of Medicine, La Jolla, California

99 *Peptic Ulcer*

MARK A. JACOBSON, M.D.

Associate Professor of Medicine in Residence, University of California, San Francisco, School of Medicine. Attending Physician, San Francisco General Hospital, San Francisco, California

368 *Ophthalmologic Manifestations of AIDS*

J. LARRY JAMESON, M.D., Ph.D.

Kettering Professor of Medicine and Chief of Endocrinology, Metabolism, and Molecular Medicine, Northwestern University Medical School. Attending Physician and Chief, Section of Endocrinology and Metabolism, Northwestern Memorial Hospital, Consultant, Endocrinology and Metabolism, Veterans Administration Lakeside Hospital, Chicago, Illinois

202 *The Pituitary*

JOSEPH JANKOVIC, M.D.

Professor of Neurology and Director, Parkinson's Disease Center and Movement Disorder Clinic, Department of Neurology, Baylor College of Medicine. Senior Attending Physician, The Methodist Hospital, Houston, Texas

407–412 *The Extrapyramidal Disorders*

ROBERT T. JENSEN, M.D.

Digestive Diseases Branch, National Institute of Diabetes and Digestive and Kidney Diseases, National Institutes of Health, Bethesda, Maryland

99 *Peptic Ulcer*

WALDEMAR G. JOHANSON, Jr., M.D., M.P.H.

Professor and Chairman, University of Medicine and Dentistry of New Jersey–New Jersey Medical School. Physician-in-Chief, University of Medicine and Dentistry of New Jersey–University Hospital, Newark, New Jersey

55 *Overview of Pneumonia;* 273 *Pneumonia Caused by Aerobic Gram-Negative Bacilli;* 274 *Aspiration Pneumonia*

RICHARD B. JOHNSTON, Jr., M.D.

Adjunct Professor and Chief, Section of Immunology, Department of Pediatrics, Yale University School of Medicine, New Haven, Connecticut. Medical Director, March of Dimes Birth Defects Foundation, White Plains, New York

284 *Whooping Cough (Pertussis)*

HOWARD W. JONES III, M.D.

Professor of Obstetrics and Gynecology and Director, Department of Gynecology and Oncology, Vanderbilt University School of Medicine, Nashville, Tennessee

208 *Endocrinologic Diseases Unique to Women*

KENNETH LYONS JONES, M.D.

Professor of Pediatrics, University of California, San Diego, School of Medicine, La Jolla. Staff Physician, University of California San Diego Medical Center, San Diego, California

28 *Hereditary Syndromes Involving Multiple Organ Systems*

NATHALIE JOSSO, M.D.

Biology Department, Ecole Normale Supérieure. Research Director, Institut de la Santé et de la Recherche Médicale, Montrouge, France

207 *Disorders of Sexual Differentiation*

JOHN A. KANIS, M.D.

Professor of Human Metabolism and Clinical Biochemistry, University of Sheffield Medical School. Director, WHO Collaborating Unit for Metabolic Bone Diseases, Hallamshire Hospital, Sheffield, United Kingdom

218 *Paget's Disease of Bone (Osteitis Deformans)*

PHILIP W. KANTOFF, M.D.

Assistant Professor of Medicine, Harvard Medical School. Director, Geniturinary Oncology, Dana-Farber Cancer Institute, Brigham and Women's Hospital, Boston, Massachusetts

91 *Tumors of the Kidney, Ureter, and Bladder*

ALBERT Z. KAPIKIAN, M.D.

Head, Epidemiology Section, Laboratory of Infectious Diseases, National Institute of Allergy and Infectious Diseases, National Institutes of Health, Bethesda, Maryland

344 *Viral Gastroenteritis*

ALLEN P. KAPLAN, M.D.

Professor of Medicine, State University of New York at Stony Brook Health Sciences Center School of Medicine, Stony Brook, New York

226 *Anaphylaxis*

GILLA KAPLAN, Ph.D.

Associate Professor of Medicine, Laboratory of Cellular Physiology and Immunology, The Rockefeller University, New York, New York

313 *Leprosy (Hansen's Disease)*

ADOLF W. KARCHMER, M.D.

Professor of Medicine, Harvard Medical School. Chief, Division of Infectious Diseases, New England Deaconess Hospital, Boston, Massachusetts

270 *Antibacterial Therapy*

PAUL KATZ, M.D.

Professor of Medicine and of Microbiology and Immunology, Georgetown University School of Medicine and Health Sciences. Vice Chairman, Department of Medicine and Chief, Division of Rheumatology, Immunology and Allergy, Georgetown University Medical Center, Washington, D.C.

18 *Glucocorticosteroids in Relation to Inflammatory Disease*

DONALD KAYE, M.D.

Klinghoffer Professor and Chairman, Department of Medicine, Medical College of Pennsylvania and Hahnemann University School of Medicine. President and Chief Executive Officer, Medical College of Pennsylvania and Hahnemann University Hospital System, Philadelphia, Pennsylvania

293 Salmonella *Infections Other Than Typhoid Fever*

JAMES W. KAZURA, M.D.

Professor of Medicine and International Health, Case Western Reserve University School of Medicine. Staff Physician, University Hospitals of Cleveland, Cleveland, Ohio

387 *Nematode Infections*

MICHAEL J. KEATING, M.B., B.S.

Associate Vice President for Clinical Investigations and Professor of Medicine, University of Texas M. D. Anderson Cancer Center, Houston, Texas

142 *The Chronic Leukemias*

CATARINA I. KIEFE, Ph.D., M.D.

Associate Professor of Medicine, University of Alabama School of Medicine; Associate Professor of Biostatistics, University of Alabama School of Public Health. Staff Physician, University of Alabama Hospital and Birmingham Veterans Administration Medical Center; Scholar, Lister Hill Center for Health Policy Research, University of Alabama, Birmingham, Alabama

14 *Clinical Decision Making*

ELLIOTT D. KIEFF, M.D., Ph.D.

Harriet Ryan Albee Professor of Medicine, Microbiology and Molecular Genetics, Harvard University Medical School. Director, Infectious Diseases, Brigham and Women's Hospital, Boston, Massachusetts

341 *Infectious Mononucleosis: Epstein-Barr Virus Infection*

CHARLES H. KING, M.D.

Associate Clinical Professor of Medicine, Case Western Reserve University School of Medicine, Cleveland, Ohio

384 *Cestode Infections*

SAULO KLAHR, M.D.

Simon Professor of Medicine and Co-Chairman, Department of Medicine, Washington University School of Medicine. Physician-in-Chief, Jewish Hospital of St. Louis, St. Louis, Missouri

81 *Obstructive Uropathy*

JUHA P. KOKKO, M.D. Ph.D.

Asa G. Candler Professor and Chairman of Medicine, Emory University School of Medicine. Chief of Medicine, Emory University Hospital, Atlanta, Georgia

73 *Approach to the Patient with Renal Disease;*   75 *Disorders of Fluid Volume, Electrolyte, and Acid-Base Balance*

DIANE M. KOMP

Professor of Pediatrics, Yale University School of Medicine. Attending Physician, Yale-New Haven Hospital, New Haven, Connecticut

147 *Langerhans Cell (Eosinophilic) Granulomatosis*

HERMES A. KONTOS, M.D., Ph.D.

Professor of Internal Medicine and Dean, School of Medicine, Virginia Commonwealth University Medical College of Virginia, Richmond, Virginia

46 *Vascular Diseases of the Limbs*

GUENTER J. KREJS, M.D.

Professor and Chairman, Department of Medicine, Karl Franzens University, Graz, Austria

102 *Diarrhea*

WILLIAM L. KRINSKY, M.D., Ph.D.

Associate Clinical Professor, Department of Epidemiology and Public Health, Yale University School of Medicine. Faculty Affiliate, Division of Entomology, Peabody Museum of Natural History, Yale University, New Haven, Connecticut

389 *Arthropods and Leeches*

DONALD J. KROGSTAD, M.D.

Henderson Professor and Chair, Departments of Tropical Medicine and of Parasitology, and Professor of Medicine, Tulane University School of Medicine. Staff Physician, Tulane Medical Center Hospital, Charity Hospital, and Veterans Administration Medical Center, New Orleans, Louisiana

374 *Malaria*

HENRY M. KRONENBERG, M.D.

Professor of Medicine, Harvard Medical School. Chief, Endocrine Unit, Massachusetts General Hospital, Boston, Massachusetts

210 *Multiple-Organ Syndromes*

CALVIN M. KUNIN, A.B., M.D.

Pomerene Professor of Internal Medicine, The Ohio State University School of Medicine. Attending Physician, The Ohio State University Hospitals, Columbus, Ohio

84 *Urinary Tract Infections and Pyelonephritis*

ROBERT C. KURTZ, M.D.

Professor of Clinical Medicine, Cornell University Medical College. Attending Physician and Member, Gastroenterology and Nutrition Service, Memorial Sloan-Kettering Cancer Center, New York, New York

100 *Neoplasms of the Stomach*

ROBERT A. KYLE, M.D.

Consultant, Division of Hematology and Internal Medicine, Mayo Clinic and Mayo Foundation; Professor of Medicine and of Laboratory Medicine, Mayo Medical School, Rochester, Minnesota

149 *Plasma Cell Disorders*

PHILIP J. LANDRIGAN, M.D., M.Sc.

Ethel H. Wise Professor and Chairman, Department of Community Medicine, Mount Sinai School of Medicine of the City University of New York, New York, New York

13 *Principles of Occupational and Environmental Medicine*

ROBERT B. LAYZER, M.D.

Professor of Neurology, University of California, San Francisco, School of Medicine, San Francisco, California

413–417 *Degenerative Diseases of the Nervous System*

GERALD S. LAZARUS, M.D.

Professor of Dermatology and Biochemistry and Dean, School of Medicine, University of California, Davis, School of Medicine, Davis, California

250 *Panniculitis and Disorders of the Subcutaneous Fat*

E. CARWILE LeROY, M.D.

Professor of Medicine, and Director, Division of Rheumatology and Immunology, Medical University of South Carolina, Charleston, South Carolina

241 *Systemic Sclerosis (Scleroderma)*

BERNARD LEVIN, M.B.Ch.B. (RAND), F.A.C.P.

Professor of Medicine, University of Texas Medical School at Houston. Vice President for Cancer Prevention, and Betty B. Marcus Chair in Cancer Prevention, University of Texas M. D. Anderson Cancer Center, Houston, Texas

106 *Neoplasms of the Large and Small Intestines*

STUART LEVIN, M.D.

James R. Lowenstine Professor, Department of Internal Medicine, Rush Medical College. Chairman, Department of Internal Medicine; Vice Dean, Rush Medical College; and Associate Vice President, Office of Medical Affairs, Rush-Presbyterian-St. Luke's Medical Center, Chicago, Illinois

325 *Zoonoses*

MATTHEW E. LEVISON, M.D.

Professor of Medicine and Chief, Division of Infectious Diseases, Medical College of Pennsylvania, Philadelphia, Pennsylvania

278 *Infective Endocarditis*

BRIAN J. LEWIS, M.D.

Clinical Professor of Medicine, University of California, San Francisco, School of Medicine. Staff Oncologist, The Permanente Medical Group, San Francisco, California

208 *Endocrinologic Diseases Unique to Women*

ALFRED J. LEWY, M.D., Ph.D.

Professor of Psychiatry, Ophthalmology, and Pharmacology, Oregon Health Sciences University School of Medicine, Portland, Oregon

201 *Neuroendocrinology*

LAWRENCE M. LICHTENSTEIN, M.D. Ph.D.

Professor of Medicine and Director, Johns Hopkins Asthma and Allergy Center, Baltimore, Maryland

227 *Insect Sting Allergy*

JOHN LINDENBAUM, M.D.

Professor of Medicine and Associate Chairman, Department of Medicine, Columbia University College of Physicians and Surgeons. Attending Physician and Associate Director, Medical Service, Presbyterian Hospital in the City of New York, New York, New York

129 *An Approach to the Anemias*

PETER E. LIPSKY, M.D.

Professor of Internal Medicine and Microbiology, and Director, Rheumatic Diseases Division and Harold C. Simmons Arthritis Research Center, University of Texas Southwestern Medical Center, Dallas, Texas

238 *The Spondylarthropathies*

EDISON T. LIU, M.D.

Professor of Medicine, Epidemiology, and Biochemistry, University of North Carolina at Chapel Hill School of Medicine, Chapel Hill, North Carolina

156 *Oncogenes and Suppressor Genes: Genetic Control of Cancer*

D. LYNN LORIAUX

Professor of Medicine and Chairman, Department of Medicine, and Head, Division of Endocrinology, Oregon Health Sciences University, Portland, Oregon

204 *The Adrenal Gland*

JOHN M. LUCE, M.D.

Professor of Medicine and Anesthesia, University of California, San Francisco, School of Medicine. Associate Director, Medical-Surgical Intensive Care Unit, San Francisco General Hospital Medical Center, San Francisco, California

67 *Approach to the Patient in a Critical Care Setting;*
68 *Respiratory Aspects of Critical Care Medicine*

MICHAEL R. LUCEY, M.D., F.R.C.P.I.

Associate Professor of Internal Medicine, University of Pennsylvania School of Medicine. Director, Hepatology, and Medical Director, Liver Transplant Program, Hospital of the University of Pennsylvania, Philadelphia, Pennsylvania

111 *Diseases of the Peritoneum, Mesentery, and Omentum*

SAMUEL E. LUX, M.D.

Professor of Pediatrics, Harvard Medical School. Chief, Division of Hematology/Oncology, Children's Hospital, Boston, Massachusetts

134 *Hereditary Defects in the Membrane or Metabolism of the Red Cell*

WILLIS C. MADDREY, M.D.

Professor of Internal Medicine and Executive Vice-President for Clinical Affairs, University of Texas Southwestern Medical Center at Dallas, Dallas, Texas

120 *Parasitic, Bacterial, Fungal, and Granulomatous Liver Diseases*

R. ELLEN MAGENIS, M.D.

Professor, Child Development Rehabilitation Center, Department of Molecular and Medical Genetics and of Pediatrics, Oregon Health Sciences University. Staff Physician, University Hospitals, Portland, Oregon

26 *Chromosomes and Their Disorders*

JACQUELYN J. MAHER, M.D.

Assistant Professor of Medicine, University of California, San Francisco, School of Medicine. Attending Physician, San Francisco General Hospital, San Francisco, California

121 *Inherited, Infiltrative, and Metabolic Disorders Involving the Liver*

ADEL A. F. MAHMOUD, M.D., Ph.D.

John H. Hord Professor and Chairman, Department of Medicine, Case Western Reserve University School of Medicine. Physician-in-Chief, University Hospitals of Cleveland, Cleveland, Ohio

373 *Introduction to Protozoan and Helminthic Diseases;*
385 *Schistosomiasis (Bilharziasis);* 386 *Liver, Intestinal, and Lung Fluke Infections*

STEPHEN E. MALAWISTA, M.D.

Professor of Medicine, Department of Internal Medicine, Yale University School of Medicine. Consultant in Medicine, Yale-New Haven Medical Center, New Haven, and West Haven Veterans Administration Medical Center, West Haven, Connecticut

321 *Lyme Disease*

GERALD L. MANDELL, M.D.

Professor of Internal Medicine and Owen R. Cheatham Professor of Sciences, University of Virginia School of Medicine. Chief, Infectious Diseases, University of Virginia Health Sciences Center, Charlottesville, Virginia

262 *Introduction to Microbial Disease;* 269 *Introduction to Bacterial Disease;* 359 *Introduction to HIV and Associated Disorders*

DOUGLAS J. MARCHANT, M.D.

Professor Emeritus of Surgery and of Obstetrics and Gynecology, Tufts University School of Medicine, Boston, Massachusetts. Adjunct Professor of Brown University School of Medicine. Director, Breast Health Center, Women and Infants Hospital, Providence, Rhode Island

208 *Endocrinologic Diseases Unique to Women*

LAWRENCE F. MARSHALL, M.D.

Professor of Surgery, University of California, San Diego, School of Medicine. Chief of Neurosurgical Services, University of California, San Diego Medical Center, San Diego, California

437, 438 *Injury to the Head and Spinal Cord*

MANUEL MARTINEZ-MALDONADO, M.D.

Professor and Vice Chairman, Department of Medicine, Emory University School of Medicine, Atlanta. Chief, Medical Service, Atlanta Department of Veterans Affairs Medical Center, Decatur, Georgia

87 *Hereditary Chronic Nephropathies*

STEPHEN J. MARX, M.D.

Chief, Genetics and Endocrinology Section, National Institute of Diabetes and Digestive and Kidney Diseases, National Institutes of Health, Bethesda, Maryland

211 *Mineral and Bone Homeostasis*

JOEL B. MASON, M.D.

Assistant Professor of Medicine and Nutrition, Tufts University School of Medicine, and the Jean Mayer USDA Human Nutrition Research Center on Aging at Tufts University. Staff, Divisions of Gastroenterology and Clinical Nutrition, and Director, Adult Nutrition Support Service, New England Medical Center, Boston, Massachusetts

192   *Nutrition's Interface with Health and Disease*

ALVIN M. MATSUMOTO, M.D.

Associate Professor of Medicine, Division of Gerontology and Geriatric Medicine, University of Washington School of Medicine. Chief of Gerontology, Associate Director, Geriatric Research, Education and Clinical Center, and Associate Chief of Staff for Geriatrics and Extended Care, Department of Veterans Affairs Medical Center, Seattle, Washington

209   *Endocrinologic Diseases Unique to Men*

RICHARD A. MATTHAY, M.D.

Boehringer Ingelheim Professor and Associate Director, Pulmonary and Critical Care Section, Yale University School of Medicine, New Haven, Connecticut

52   *Chronic Airways Diseases;*   53   *Localized Abnormalities of Lung Aeration*

JAMES R. McARTHUR, M.D.

Professor of Medicine, Hematology, University of Washington School of Medicine. Director, American Society of Hematology Slide Bank, Seattle, Washington

Hematology Color Plates

MARGARET M. McGOVERN, M.D., Ph.D.

Assistant Professor of Human Genetics and Pediatrics, Mount Sinai School of Medicine. Attending Staff, Mount Sinai Hospital, New York, New York

174   *Lysosomal Storage Diseases*

T. DWIGHT McKINNEY, M.D.

Professor of Medicine, Indiana University School of Medicine. Executive Director, Clinical Pharmacology, Eli Lilly and Company, Indianapolis, Indiana

80   *Tubulointerstitial Diseases and Toxic Nephropathies*

ELIZABETH McLOUGHLIN, Sc.D.

Associate Adjunct Professor, Department of Surgery, University of California, San Francisco, School of Medicine. Director, San Francisco Injury Center for Research and Prevention, San Francisco General Hospital Medical Center, San Francisco, California

9   *Principles of Preventive Health Care*

M. MOLLY McMAHON, M.D.

Consultant, Division of Endocrinology, Metabolism, and Internal Medicine, Mayo Clinic and Mayo Foundation, Rochester, Minnesota

198   *Parenteral Nutrition*

KENNETH R. MEEHAN, M.D.

Assistant Professor of Medicine, Georgetown University School of Medicine. Attending Staff, Georgetown University Medical Center, Washington, D.C.

158   *Systemic Secretions of Cancer Cells and Their Effects*

JAY E. MENITOVE, M.D.

Professor of Internal Medicine, University of Cincinnati College of Medicine. Deputy Director, Medical Services, Hoxworth Blood Center, Cincinnati, Ohio

138   *Blood Transfusion*

ROBERT MESSING, M.D.

Associate Professor of Neurology, Department of Neurology, University of California, San Francisco, School of Medicine. Associate Professor of Neurology, Moffitt-Long Hospitals, San Francisco General Hospital, and San Francisco Veterans Administration Medical Center, San Francisco, California

406   *Nutritional Disorders of the Nervous System*

DEAN D. METCALFE, M.D.

Head, Allergic Diseases Section, Laboratory of Clinical Investigation, National Institute of Allergy and Infectious Diseases, National Institutes of Health, Bethesda, Maryland

231   *Mastocytosis*

DONALD M. MILLER, M.D., Ph.D.

Professor of Internal Medicine, University of Alabama School of Medicine. Director, Hematology Oncology, University of Alabama Hospital, Birmingham, Alabama

167   *The Future of Oncology*

YORK E. MILLER, M.D.

Professor of Pulmonary Sciences, of Critical Care Medicine and of Medical Oncology, Department of Medicine, University of Colorado Health Sciences Center, School of Medicine. Assistant Chief, Respiratory Department, Veterans Affairs Medical Center, Denver, Colorado

62   *Pulmonary Neoplasms*

WILLIAM E. MITCH, M.D.

E. Garland Herndon Professor of Medicine, Emory University School of Medicine. Director of Nephrology, Emory University School of Medicine, Atlanta, Georgia

76   *Acute Renal Failure*

BEVERLY S. MITCHELL, M.D.

Professor of Medicine and Pharmacology, and Chief, Division of Hematology/Oncology, University of North Carolina at Chapel Hill School of Medicine, Chapel Hill, North Carolina

181   *Disorders of Purine and Pyrimidine Metabolism*

MARK E. MOLITCH, M.D.

Professor of Medicine, Center for Endocrinology, Metabolism and Molecular Medicine, Northwestern University Medical School. Attending Physician, Northwestern Memorial Hospital, Chicago, Illinois

201   *Neuroendocrinology*

J. GLENN MORRIS, Jr., M.D., M.P.H.&T.M.

Professor of Medicine and of Epidemiology and Preventive Medicine, University of Maryland School of Medicine. Chief, Infectious Diseases Service, Veterans Affairs Medical Center, Baltimore, Maryland

300   Yersinia *Infections*

DEANE F. MOSHER, M.D.

Professor of Medicine and Head, Section of Hematology, University of Wisconsin Medical School, Madison, Wisconsin

153   *Disorders of Blood Coagulation*

BALFOUR M. MOUNT, C.M., O.Q., M.D., F.R.C.S.(C)

Professor of Surgery/Palliative Care and Director, Division of Palliative Care Medicine, Department of Oncology, McGill University Faculty of Medicine. Director, Royal Victoria Hospital Palliative Care Service, Montreal, Quebec, Canada

3   *Care of Dying Patients and Their Families*

JAMES M. MOUNTZ, M.D., Ph.D.

Associate Professor of Radiology, Division of Nuclear Medicine, and Director of Neuro-Nuclear Imaging, Division of Nuclear Medicine, University of Alabama School of Medicine, Birmingham, Alabama

22   *Overview of Imaging Techniques for the Future*

MAURICE A. MUFSON, M.D.

Professor and Chairman, Department of Medicine, Marshall University School of Medicine. Associate Chief of Staff for Research and Development, Veterans Administration Medical Center; Active Staff, St. Mary's Hospital and Cabell Huntington Hospital, Huntington, West Virginia

329 *Viral Pharyngitis, Laryngitis, Croup, and Bronchitis*

DAVID G. NATHAN, M.D.

Robert A. Stranahan Professor of Pediatrics, Harvard Medical School. Physician-in-Chief, Children's Hospital, Boston, Massachusetts

127 *Approach to the Patient with Hematologic Disease;*
128 *Hemolytic Disorders: Introduction*

FRANKLIN A. NEVA, M.D.

Acting Scientific Director, Institute of Allergy and Infectious Diseases, National Institutes of Health, Bethesda, Maryland

376 *American Trypanosomiasis (Chagas' Disease)*

MARIA I. NEW, M.D.

Professor of Pediatrics and Harold and Percy Uris Professor of Pediatric Endocrinology and Metabolism, Cornell University Medical College. Chairman, Department of Pediatrics, and Chief, Pediatric Endocrinology, New York Hospital-Cornell Medical Center, New York, New York

207 *Disorders of Sexual Differentiation*

ARTHUR W. NIENHUIS, M.D.

St. Jude Professor of Pediatrics and Medicine, University of Tennessee, Memphis, School of Medicine. Director, Department of Hematology/Oncology, St. Jude Children's Research Hospital, Memphis, Tennessee

136 *Hemoglobin and Hemoglobinopathies*

JOHN A. OATES, M.D.

The Thomas F. Frist, Sr, Professor and Chairman, Department of Medicine, Vanderbilt University School of Medicine, Nashville, Tennessee

210 *Multiple-Organ Syndromes*

ALBERT OBERMAN, M.D., M.P.H.

Professor and Director, Division of Preventive Medicine, Department of Medicine, University of Alabama School of Medicine, Birmingham, Alabama

9 *Principles of Preventive Health Care*

CHARLES P. O'BRIEN, M.D., Ph.D.

Professor and Vice-Chairman, Department of Psychiatry, University of Pennsylvania School of Medicine. Chief of Psychiatry, Veterans Administration Medical Center, Philadelphia, Pennsylvania

12 *Drug Abuse and Dependence*

ROBERT K. OCKNER, M.D.

Professor of Medicine and Director, Liver Center, University of California, San Francisco, School of Medicine, San Francisco, California

92 *Introduction to Gastrointestinal Diseases;* 113 *Clinical Approach to Liver Disease;* 117 *Acute Viral Hepatitis;* 119 *Chronic Hepatitis*

DANIEL T. O'CONNOR, M.D.

Professor of Medicine, University of California, San Diego, School of Medicine. Chief, Hypertension, Department of Veterans Affairs Medical Center, San Diego, California

204 *The Adrenal Gland*

GILBERT S. OMENN, M.D., Ph.D.

Professor and Dean, School of Public Health and Community Medicine, University of Washington School of Medicine. Attending Staff, University of Washington Medical Center, Seattle, Washington

155 *Cancer Prevention*

SUZANNE OPARIL, M.D.

Professor of Medicine, University of Alabama School of Medicine. Director, Vascular Biology and Hypertension Program, Division of Cardiovascular Disease, University of Alabama Hospital, Birmingham, Alabama

37 *Arterial Hypertension*

WALTER A. ORENSTEIN, M.D.

Director, National Immunization Program, Centers for Disease Control and Prevention, Atlanta, Georgia

10 *Vaccination/Immunization*

SUSAN L. ORLOFF, M.D.

Clinical Instructor, Transplantation, Department of Surgery, University of California, San Francisco, School of Medicine, San Francisco, California

99 *Peptic Ulcer*

ERIC A. OTTESEN, M.D.

Filariasis Control, Division of Control of Tropical Diseases, World Health Organization, Geneva, Switzerland

388 *Filariasis*

MICHAEL N. OXMAN, M.D.

Professor of Medicine and Pathology, University of California, San Diego, School of Medicine. Infectious Diseases Section, Department of Veterans Affairs Medical Center, San Diego, California

343 *Enteroviruses*

FRANK PARKER, M.D.

Professor of Dermatology, Oregon Health Sciences University, Portland, Oregon

161 *Cutaneous Manifestations of Internal Malignancy;*
471–475 *Skin Diseases*

HENRY P. PARKMAN, M.D.

Assistant Professor of Medicine, Temple University School of Medicine. Director, GI Motility Laboratory, Temple University Hospital, Philadelphia, Pennsylvania

97 *Diseases of the Esophagus*

JOSEPH E. PARRILLO, M.D.

James B. Herrick Professor of Medicine, Rush Medical College. Chief, Sections of Cardiology and Critical Care Medicine, and Medical Director, Rush Heart Institute, Rush-Presbyterian-St. Luke's Medical Center, Chicago, Illinois

70 *Shock Syndromes Related to Sepsis*

STEPHEN G. PAUKER, M.D.

Professor of Medicine, Tufts University School of Medicine. Chief, Division of Clinical Decision Making, New England Medical Center, Boston, Massachusetts

14 *Clinical Decision Making*

RICHARD D. PEARSON, M.D.

Professor of Medicine and Pathology, Division of Geographic and International Medicine, Departments of Internal Medicine and Pathology, University of Virginia School of Medicine, Charlottesville, Virginia

268 *Advice to Travelers;* 377 *Leishmaniasis;* 382 *Other Protozoan Diseases*

TIMOTHY A. PEDLEY, M.D.

Professor and Vice Chairman, Department of Neurology, College of Physicians and Surgeons of Columbia University. Director, Comprehensive Epilepsy Center, and Associate Director, Neurology Service, The Neurological Institute, Columbia Presbyterian Medical Center, New York, New York

433 *The Epilepsies*

NEAL S. PENNEYS, M.D. Ph.D.

Professor of Medicine and Director of Dermatology, Saint Louis University School of Medicine, Saint Louis, Missouri

367 *Cutaneous Signs of AIDS*

EDITH A. PEREZ, M.D.

Associate Professor of Medicine, Mayo Clinic, Rochester, Minnesota

165 *Molecular Mechanisms of Drug Resistance*

JOSEPH K. PERLOFF, M.D.

Streisand/American Heart Association Professor of Medicine and Pediatrics, University of California, Los Angeles, UCLA School of Medicine, Los Angeles, California

39 *Congenital Heart Disease in Adults*

WILLIAM A. PETRI, Jr., M.D., Ph.D.

Associate Professor of Medicine, Microbiology and Pathology, University of Virginia School of Medicine. Attending Physician and Associate Director of Clinical Microbiology, University of Virginia Health Sciences Center, Charlottesville, Virginia

320 *Relapsing Fever;* 322 *Leptospirosis*

JAMES M. PHANG, M.D.

Chief, Laboratory of Nutritional and Molecular Regulation, Division of Cancer Prevention and Control, National Cancer Institute–Frederick Cancer Research and Development Center, Frederick, Maryland

177 *The Hyperprolinemias and Hydroxyprolinemia*

CLAUDE A. PIANTADOSI, M.D.

Professor of Medicine and Director, F. G. Hall Center for Hypobaric and Hyperbaric Medicine, Duke University Medical Center. Attending Physician, Department of Medicine, Duke University Medical Center, Durham, North Carolina

54 *Interstitial Lung Disease*

F. XAVIER PI-SUNYER, M.D.

Professor of Medicine, Columbia College of Physicians and Surgeons. Director, Division of Endocrinology, Diabetes, and Nutrition, St. Luke's–Roosevelt Hospital Center, New York, New York

196 *Obesity*

PHILIP A. PIZZO, M.D.

Professor of Pediatrics, Uniformed Services University for the Health Sciences. Chief of Pediatrics and Head, Infectious Disease Section, National Cancer Institute, National Institutes of Health, Bethesda, Maryland

266 *The Compromised Host*

FRED PLUM, M.D.

Anne Parrish Titzell Professor and Chairman, Department of Neurology and Neuroscience, Cornell University Medical College. Neurologist-in-Chief, New York Hospital–Cornell Medical Center, New York, New York

1 *Medicine as a Learned and Humane Profession;* 6 *Neurologic Problems Associated with Aging;* 392 *Clinical Study of the Patient;* 393 *Disturbances of Consciousness and Arousal;* 394 *Sustained Impairments of Consciousness;* 395 *Brain Death;* 396 *Brief Loss of Consciousness;* 397 *Disorders of Sleep and Arousal;* 404 *Disorders of Motor Function*

RICHARD L. POPP, M.D.

Professor of Medicine, Cardiovascular Medicine Division, Department of Medicine, Stanford University School of Medicine, Stanford, California

33 *Specialized Diagnostic Procedures*

CAROL S. PORTLOCK, M.D.

Associate Professor of Clinical Medicine, Cornell University Medical College. Associate Attending Physician, Memorial Sloan-Kettering Cancer Center, New York, New York

144 *Introduction to Neoplasms of the Immune System;* 145 *Non-Hodgkin's Lymphomas;* 146 *Hodgkin's Disease*

JEROME B. POSNER, M.D.

Professor of Neurology, Cornell University Medical College. Chairman, Department of Neurology, Memorial Sloan-Kettering Cancer Center, New York, New York

160 *Nonmetastatic Effects of Cancer on the Nervous System;* 392 *Clinical Study of the Patient;* 405 *Disorders of Sensation;* 439–444 *Mechanical Lesions of Nerve Roots and Spinal Cord*

MICHAEL PRATT, M.D., M.P.H.

Physical Activity Coordinator and Medical Epidemiologist, Division of Chronic Disease Control and Community Intervention, National Center for Chronic Disease Prevention and Health Promotion, Centers for Disease Control and Prevention, Atlanta, Georgia

9 *Principles of Preventive Health Care*

LAUREL C. PREHEIM, M.D.

Professor of Medicine and of Medical Microbiology, Creighton University School of Medicine, and University of Nebraska College of Medicine. Chief, Section of Infectious Diseases, Creighton University School of Medicine, University of Nebraska Medical Center, and Omaha Veterans Affairs Medical Center, Omaha, Nebraska

312 *Other Mycobacterioses*

RICHARD W. PRICE, M.D.

Professor of Neurology, University of Minnesota Medical School. Attending Neurologist, University Hospital and Clinic, Minneapolis, Minnesota

364 *Neurologic Complications of HIV-1 Infection;* 423–428 *Viral Infections of the Nervous System*

WILLIAM A. PULSINELLI, M.D., Ph.D.

Semmes-Murphey Professor and Chairman, Department of Neurology, University of Tennessee, Memphis College of Medicine, Memphis, Tennessee

418–420 *Cerebrovascular Diseases*

THOMAS C. QUINN, M.D.

Professor of Medicine, Johns Hopkins University School of Medicine, Baltimore. Senior Investigator, National Institute of Allergy and Infectious Diseases, National Institutes of Health, Bethesda, Maryland

375 *African Trypanosomiasis (Sleeping Sickness)*

CHARLES E. RACKLEY, M.D.

Professor of Medicine, Georgetown University School of Medicine and Health Sciences. Attending Physician, Division of Cardiology, Georgetown University Medical Center, Washington, D.C.

42 *Valvular Heart Disease*

JEFFREY M. RANK, M.D.

Associate Professor of Medicine, Gastroenterology and Hepatology, University of Minnesota Medical School, Minneapolis, Minnesota

94 *Gastrointestinal Endoscopy*

JOEL RAPPEPORT, M.D.

Professor of Medicine and Pediatrics, Yale School of Medicine. Attending Physician, Yale–New Haven Hospital, New Haven, Connecticut

151 *Bone Marrow Transplantation*

JONATHAN I. RAVDIN, M.D.

Professor and Vice Chairman, Department of Medicine, and Professor of International Health, Case Western Reserve University School of Medicine. Chief of Medicine, Cleveland Department of Veterans Affairs Medical Center, Cleveland, Ohio

381 *Amebiasis*

ROBERT W. REBAR, M.D.

Professor and Director, Department of Obstetrics and Gynecology, University of Cincinnati College of Medicine. Chief of Obstetrics and Gynecology, University of Cincinnati Hospital, Cincinnati, Ohio

208 *Endocrinologic Diseases Unique to Women*

ANNETTE C. REBOLI, M.D.

Assistant Professor of Medicine, Division of Infectious Diseases, Medical College of Pennsylvania and Hahnemann University School of Medicine, Philadelphia, Pennsylvania

305 *Erysipeloid*

DAVID A. RELMAN, M.D.

Assistant Professor of Medicine, and of Microbiology and Immunology, Stanford University School of Medicine, Stanford. Staff Physician, Department of Veterans Affairs Medical Center, Palo Alto, California

309 *Cat Scratch Disease and Bacillary Angiomatosis*

JACK S. REMINGTON, M.D.

Professor of Medicine, Division of Infectious Diseases, Department of Medicine and Geographic Medicine, Stanford University School of Medicine, Stanford. Marcus A. Krupp Research Chair and Chairman, Department of Immunology and Infectious Diseases, Research Institute, Palo Alto Medical Foundation, Palo Alto, California

378 *Toxoplasmosis*

RICHARD K. RIEGELMAN, M.D., Ph.D.

Associate Dean for Public Health Programs, George Washington University School of Medicine and Health Sciences. Attending Physician, George Washington University Hospital, Washington, D.C.

9 *Principles of Preventive Health Care*

ROGER S. RITTMASTER, M.D.

Professor of Medicine, Dalhousie University Faculty of Medicine. Active Staff, Queen Elizabeth II Health Sciences Center, Halifax, Nova Scotia, Canada

208 *Endocrinologic Diseases Unique to Women*

NORMAN W. RIZK, M.D.

Director of Clinical Programs and Associate Professor of Medicine, Division of Pulmonary and Critical Care Medicine, Stanford University School of Medicine, Stanford, California

66 *Lung Transplantation*

JOHN P. ROBERTS, M.D., F.A.C.S.

Associate Professor of Surgery, University of California San Francisco, School of Medicine, San Francisco, California

124 *Liver Transplantation*

WILLIAM O. ROBERTSON, M.D.

Professor of Pediatrics, University of Washington School of Medicine. Medical Director, Washington Poison Center, Seattle, Washington

13 *Principles of Occupational and Environmental Medicine*

ALAN G. ROBINSON, M.D.

Vice Provost and Executive Associate Dean, University of California, Los Angeles, UCLA School of Medicine, Los Angeles, California

202 *The Pituitary*

WILLIAM J. ROGERS, M.D.

Professor of Medicine, University of Alabama at Birmingham School of Medicine. Director, Coronary Care Unit, University of Alabama Hospital, Birmingham, Alabama

41 *Disorders of the Coronary Arteries*

JOHN L. ROMBEAU, M.D.

Professor of Surgery, University of Pennsylvania School of Medicine. Attending Staff, Hospital of the University of Pennsylvania, Philadelphia, Pennsylvania

197 *Enteral Nutrition*

DANIEL I. ROSENTHAL, M.D.

Associate Professor of Radiology, Harvard University Medical School. Associate Radiologist-in-Chief, Massachusetts General Hospital, Boston, Massachusetts

220 *Bone Tumors*

LANNY J. ROSENWASSER, M.D.

Professor of Medicine and Co-Director, Allergy and Clinical Immunology Division, Department of Medicine, University of Colorado Health Science Center School of Medicine. Senior Faculty Member and Head, Allergy and Clinical Immunology, National Jewish Center for Immunology and Respiratory Medicine, Denver, Colorado

243 *The Vasculitic Syndromes;* 244 *Polyarteritis Nodosa Group*

JOHN ROSS, Jr., M.D.

Professor of Medicine, University of California, San Diego, School of Medicine, La Jolla. Attending Physician, University of California San Diego Medical Center, San Diego, California

32 *Cardiac Function and Circulatory Control*

RUSSELL ROSS, Ph.D., D.D.S.

Professor, Department of Pathology and Adjunct Professor, Department of Biochemistry, University of Washington School of Medicine. Director, Center for Vascular Biology, University of Washington Medical Center, Seattle, Washington

40 *Atherosclerosis*

RICHARD A. RUDICK, M.D.

Professor of Neurology, Ohio State University College of Medicine, Columbus. Director, Mellen Center for Multiple Sclerosis Treatment and Research, Cleveland Clinic Foundation, Cleveland, Ohio

429–431 *Neurologic Disorders Associated with Altered Immunity or Unexplained Host-Parasite Alterations;* 432 *The Demyelinating Diseases*

MICHAEL S. SAAG, M.D.

Associate Professor of Medicine, University of Alabama School of Medicine. Director, University of Alabama AIDS Outpatient Clinic, Division of Infectious Disease, Birmingham, Alabama

357 *Mycetoma;* 358 *Dematiaceous Fungal Infections;*
363 *Prevention of HIV Infection;* 370 *Renal, Cardiac, Endocrine, and Rheumatologic Manifestations of HIV Infection*

R. BRADLEY SACK, M.D., Sc.D.

Professor of International Health and Medicine, Johns Hopkins University School of Hygiene and Public Health, Baltimore, Maryland

298 *The Diarrhea of Travelers*

ROBERT A. SALATA, M.D.

Associate Professor of Medicine and Associate Chief and Clinical Program Director, Division of Infectious Disease, Case Western Reserve University School of Medicine. Attending Physician and Consultant Hospital Epidemiologist, University Hospitals of Cleveland, Cleveland, Ohio

308 *Brucellosis*

SYDNEY E. SALMON, M.D.

Regents Professor of Medicine, University of Arizona College of Medicine. Director, Arizona Cancer Center, Tucson, Arizona

162 *Principles of Cancer Therapy*

JONATHAN M. SAMET, M.D.

Professor and Chairman, Department of Epidemiology, Johns Hopkins University School of Hygiene and Public Health, Baltimore, Maryland

54 *Interstitial Lung Disease*

JAY P. SANFORD, M.D.

Professor of Internal Medicine, University of Texas Southwestern Health Sciences Center, Dallas, Texas. Dean Emeritus, F. Edward Hebert School of Medicine, Uniformed Services University of the Health Sciences, Bethesda, Maryland

390 *Snake Bites*

CLIFFORD B. SAPER, M.D., Ph.D.

James Jackson Putnam Professor of Neurology and Neuroscience, Harvard Medical School. Chairman of Neurology, Beth Israel Hospital, Boston, Massachusetts

402 *Autonomic Disorders and Their Management*

FRED R. SATTLER, M.D.

Professor of Medicine, Section of Infectious Diseases, University of Southern California School of Medicine. Staff Physician, Los Angeles County—University of Southern California Medical Center, Los Angeles, California

383 Pneumocystis carinii *Pneumonia*

DAVID T. SCADDEN, M.D.

Assistant Professor of Medicine, Harvard Medical School. Director, AIDS Hematology/Oncology Research Unit, Deaconess Hospital, Boston, Massachusetts

369 *Hematology/Oncology in AIDS*

WILLIAM SCHAFFNER, M.D.

Professor and Chairman, Department of Preventive Medicine, and Professor of Medicine (Infectious Diseases), Vanderbilt University School of Medicine. Hospital Epidemiologist, Vanderbilt University Medical Center, Nashville, Tennessee

267 *Prevention and Control of Hospital-Acquired Infections*

BRUCE F. SCHARSCHMIDT, M.D.

Professor of Medicine and Director, Gastroenterology Division, University of California San Francisco School of Medicine. Attending Physician, Moffitt-Long Hospitals, University of California, San Francisco Medical Center, San Francisco, California

115 *Bilirubin Metabolism, Hyperbilirubinemia, and Approach to the Jaundiced Patient;* 123 *Acute and Chronic Hepatic Failure and Hepatic Encephalopathy;* 125 *Hepatic Tumors*

STEPHEN C. SCHIMPFF, M.D.

Professor of Medicine, Oncology and Pharmacology, University of Maryland School of Medicine. Executive Vice President, University of Maryland Medical System, Baltimore, Maryland

303 *Diseases Caused by Pseudomonads*

DAVID SCHLOSSBERG, M.D.

Professor of Medicine, Medical College of Pennsylvania. Director, Department of Medicine, and Head, Infectious Disease Division, Episcopal Hospital, Philadelphia, Pennsylvania

272 *Mycoplasmal Infection*

EDWARD L. SCHNEIDER, M.D.

Professor of Gerontology and Medicine, Ethel P. Andrus Gerontology Center, University of Southern California, Los Angeles, School of Medicine, Los Angeles. Scientific Advisor, Buck Center for Research on Aging, Marin, California

5 *Biology of Aging*

THOMAS J. SCHNITZER, M.D., Ph.D.

Willard L. Wood Professor of Medicine, Professor of Internal Medicine, and Director, Sections of Rheumatology and Geriatric Medicine, Rush Medical College of Rush University. Medical Director, Johnston R. Bowman Health Center for the Elderly, Senior Attending Physician, Rush-Presbyterian-St. Luke's Medical Center, Chicago, Illinois

254 *Osteoarthritis (Degenerative Bone Disease)*

ALAN D. SCHREIBER, M.D.

Assistant Dean for Research and Research Training and Professor of Medicine, University of Pennsylvania School of Medicine, Philadelphia, Pennsylvania

135 *Autoimmune Hemolytic Anemia*

THEODORE R. SCHROCK, M.D.

Professor and Interim Chairman, Department of Surgery, University of California San Francisco, San Francisco, California

110 *Diseases of the Rectum and Anus*

HARRY W. SCHROEDER, Jr., M.D., Ph.D., F.A.C.M.G.

Associate Professor, Division of Developmental and Clinical Immunology, Departments of Medicine and Microbiology, University of Alabama School of Medicine, Birmingham, Alabama

23 *Human Heredity*

H. RALPH SCHUMACHER, Jr., M.D.

Professor of Medicine, University of Pennsylvania School of Medicine. Director, Arthritis-Immunology Center, Veterans Administration Medical Center, Philadelphia, Pennsylvania

252 *Other Crystal Deposition Arthropathies;* 253 *Relapsing Polychondritis;* 261 *Multifocal Fibrosclerosis*

PETER H. SCHUR, M.D.

Professor of Medicine, Harvard Medical School. Senior Physician, Brigham and Women's Hospital, Boston, Massachusetts

240 *Systemic Lupus Erythematosus*

BENJAMIN D. SCHWARTZ, M.D., Ph.D.

Professor of Clinical Medicine, Washington University School of Medicine. Senior Director, Immunology, G. D. Scarle/Monsanto; Attending Physician, Barnes Hospital and Jewish Hospital, St. Louis, Missouri

229 *The Major Histocompatibility Complex and Disease Susceptibility*

CHARLES R. SCRIVER, M.D.C.M.

Professor of Biology, Human Genetics and Pediatrics, McGill University Faculty of Medicine. Director, DeBelle Laboratory for Biochemical Genetics, McGill University–Montreal Children's Hospital Research Institute, Montreal, Quebec, Canada

175 *Hyperaminoaciduria;* 176 *The Hyperphenylalaninemias and Alkaptonuria*

MARGRETTA R. SEASHORE, M.D.

Professor of Human Genetics and Pediatrics, Yale University School of Medicine. Attending Physician, Yale–New Haven Hospital, New Haven, Connecticut

29 *Genetic Counseling*

STANTON SEGAL, M.D., F.A.C.P.

Professor of Pediatrics and of Medicine, University of Pennsylvania School of Medicine. Director, Division of Biochemical Development and Molecular Diseases and Senior Physician, Children's Hospital of Philadelphia; Attending Physician in Medicine, Hospital of the University of Pennsylvania, Philadelphia, Pennsylvania

169 *Galactosemia*

ROBERT M. SENIOR, M.D.

Dorothy R. and Hubert C. Moog Professor of Pulmonary Diseases in Medicine, Washington University School of Medicine. Director, Respiratory and Critical Care Division, Department of Medicine, Jewish Hospital of St. Louis, St. Louis, Missouri

59 *Pulmonary Embolism;*   60 *Fat Embolism Syndrome*

RALPH SHABETAI, M.D., F.A.C.C.

Professor of Medicine, University of California, San Diego, School of Medicine. Chief of Cardiology, San Diego Veterans Affairs Medical Center, San Diego, California

44 *Diseases of the Pericardium*

EMMANUEL SHAPIRA, M.D., Ph.D.

Karen Gore Chair in Human Genetics and Professor of Pediatrics and Biochemistry, Tulane University School of Medicine. Director, Human Genetics Program, Hayward Genetics Center, Tulane University Medical Center, New Orleans, Louisiana

182 *The Mucopolysaccharidoses*

CHARLES L. SHAPIRO, M.D.

Instructor in Medicine, Harvard Medical School. Attending Staff, Dana-Farber Cancer Institute, Boston, Massachusetts

91 *Tumors of the Kidney, Ureter, and Bladder*

GEORGE M. SHAW, M.D., Ph.D.

Professor of Medicine, University of Alabama at Birmingham School of Medicine. Oncology Physician, University of Alabama Hospital and University of Alabama Health Services Foundation-Kirklin Clinic, Birmingham, Alabama

361 *Biology of Human Immunodeficiency Viruses*

ROBERT S. SHERWIN, M.D.

Professor of Medicine and Director, Diabetes Endocrinology Research Center, Yale University School of Medicine. Attending Physician, Yale-New Haven Hospital, New Haven, Connecticut

205 *Diabetes Mellitus*

ROBERT E. SHOPE, M.D.

Professor of Pathology, Center for Tropical Diseases, Department of Pathology, University of Texas Medical Branch, Galveston, Texas

345 *Introduction to Hemorrhagic Fever Viruses*

JONAS A. SHULMAN, M.D.

Professor of Medicine and Executive Assistant. Dean of Medical Education and Student Affairs, Emory University School of Medicine, Atlanta, Georgia

302 *Anthrax*

MARC SHUMAN, M.D.

Professor of Medicine, University of California, San Francisco, School of Medicine. Chief of Hematology, San Francisco. Moffit–Long Hospital and University of California Medical Center, San Francisco, California

152 *Hemorrhagic Disorders: Abnormalities of Platelet and Vascular Function*

MARK SIEGLER, M.D.

Professor of Medicine and Director, MacLean Center for Clinical Medical Ethics, University of Chicago Pritzker School of Medicine. Attending Physician, University of Chicago Hospitals, Chicago, Illinois

2 *Clinical Ethics in the Practice of Medicine*

MURRAY N. SILVERSTEIN, M.D., Ph.D.

Professor of Medicine, Mayo Medical School. Consultant in Hematology and Internal Medicine, Mayo Clinic and Mayo Foundation, Rochester, Minnesota

141 *Proliferative Disorders of the Hematologic System*

MICHAEL S. SIMBERKOFF, M.D.

Associate Professor of Medicine, New York University School of Medicine. Chief, Infectious Diseases Section, New York Veterans Affairs Medical Center, New York, New York

282 *Infections Caused by* Haemophilus *Species*

ROGER P. SIMON, M.D.

Professor and Chairman, Department of Neurology, University of Pittsburgh School of Medicine, Pittsburgh, Pennsylvania

421, 422 *Infections and Inflammatory Disorders of the Nervous System*

JOSEPH V. SIMONE, M.D.

Professor of Pediatrics, Cornell Medical College. Physician in Chief, Benno C. Schmidt Chair of Clinical Oncology, Memorial Sloan-Kettering Cancer Center, New York, New York

154 *Oncology: Introduction*

PETER A. SINGER, M.D., M.P.H., F.R.C.P.C.

Associate Professor of Medicine and Associate Director, Centre for Bioethics, University of Toronto Faculty of Medicine. Staff Physician, Toronto Hospital, Toronto, Ontario, Canada

2 *Clinical Ethics in the Practice of Medicine*

EDUARDO SLATOPOLSKY, M.D.

Joseph Friedman Professor of Renal Diseases in Medicine, Washington University School of Medicine. Director, Chromalloy American Kidney Center, Attending Physician, Barnes Hospital at Washington University Medical Center, St. Louis, Missouri

216 *Renal Osteodystrophy*

THOMAS WOODWARD SMITH, M.D.

Professor of Medicine, Harvard Medical School. Chief, Cardiovascular Division, Brigham and Women's Hospital, Boston, Massachusetts

30 *Approach to the Patient with Cardiovascular Disease;*   34 *Heart Failure*

WILLIAM J. SNAPE, Jr., M.D.

Clinical Professor of Medicine, University of California, Irvine School of Medicine, Irvine. Director, Gastrointestinal Motility Center, Long Beach Memorial Medical Center, Long Beach, California

101 *Disorders of Gastrointestinal Motility*

ROSEMARY SOAVE, M.D.

Associate Professor of Medicine and Public Health, Cornell University Medical College. Associate Attending Physician, New York Hospital-Cornell Medical Center, New York, New York

379 *Cryptosporidiosis*

BURTON E. SOBEL, M.D.

Amidon Professor and Chairman, Department of Medicine, University of Vermont College of Medicine. Physician-in-Chief, Medical Center Hospital of Vermont, Burlington, Vermont

41 *Disorders of the Coronary Arteries*

KONRAD H. SOERGEL, M.D.

Professor of Medicine and Physiology, Division of Gastroenterology, Medical College of Wisconsin, Milwaukee, Wisconsin

107 *Pancreatitis*

ANDREW H. SOLL, M.D.

Professor of Medicine, University of California, Los Angeles, UCLA School of Medicine. Chief, Gastroenterology Section, West Lost Angeles Veterans Affairs Medical Center, Los Angeles, California

98 *Gastritis;* 99 *Peptic Ulcer*

ANASTACIO de QUEIROZ SOUSA, M.D.

Professor of Medicine, Núcleo de Medicina Tropical, Universidade Federal do Ceará, Fortaleza, Ceará, Brazil

377 *Leishmaniasis*

P. FREDERICK SPARLING, M.D.

Chair, Department of Medicine, J. Herbert Bate Professor of Medicine, Microbiology and Immunology, University of North Carolina at Chapel Hill School of Medicine. Chief, Medical Service, University of North Carolina Hospitals, Chapel Hill, North Carolina

314 *Introduction to Sexually Transmitted Diseases and Common Syndromes;* 315 *Gonococcal Infections*

ALLEN M. SPIEGEL, M.D.

Scientific Director, National Institute of Diabetes and Digestive and Kidney Diseases, National Institutes of Health, Bethesda, Maryland

214 *The Parathyroid Glands, Hypercalcemia, and Hypocalcemia*

ALAN M. STAMM, M.D.

Associate Professor of Medicine, University of Alabama School of Medicine. Attending Physician, University of Alabama Hospital, Birmingham, Alabama

304 *Listeriosis*

DANIEL STEINBERG, M.D., Ph.D.

Professor of Medicine, Department of Medicine, University of California, San Diego, School of Medicine, La Jolla, California

173 *The Hypolipoproteinemias*

GARY D. STEINBERG, M.D.

Assistant Professor of Surgery (Urology), University of Chicago Pritzker School of Medicine, Chicago, Illinois

209 *Endocrinologic Diseases Unique to Men*

DAVID A. STEVENS, M.D.

Professor of Medicine and Associate Chief, Division of Infectious Diseases and Geographic Medicine, Stanford University Medical School, Stanford. Chief, Division of Infectious Diseases, Department of Medicine, Santa Clara Valley Medical Center, San Jose, California

355 *Aspergillosis;* 356 *Mucormycosis*

DAVID P. STEVENS, M.D.

Vice Dean and Scott R. Inkley Professor of General Internal Medicine, Case Western Reserve University School of Medicine, Cleveland, Ohio

380 *Giardiasis*

DENNIS L. STEVENS, M.D., Ph.D.

Professor of Medicine, University of Washington School of Medicine. Seattle, Washington. Chief, Infectious Disease Section, Veterans Affairs Medical Center, Boise, Idaho

276 *Streptococcal Infections;* 286 *Clostridial Myonecrosis and Other Clostridial Diseases*

LYNNE WARNER STEVENSON, M.D.

Associate Professor of Medicine, Harvard Medical School. Clinical Director, Cardiomyopathy and Transplant Program, Brigham and Women's Hospital, Boston, Massachusetts

43 *Diseases of the Myocardium*

KINGMAN P. STROHL, M.D.

Professor of Medicine, Case Western Reserve University School of Medicine. Staff Physician, Division of Pulmonary and Critical Care Medicine, University Hospitals of Cleveland and Veterans Administration Medical Center, Cleveland, Ohio

64 *Upper Airway Diseases*

CARLOS S. SUBAUSTE, M.D.

Research Associate, Department of Immunology and Infectious Diseases, Research Institute, Palo Alto Medical Foundation, and Consultant in Infectious Diseases, Palo Alto Veterans Affairs Medical Center, Palo Alto, California

378 *Toxoplasmosis*

WADI N. SUKI, M.D.

Professor of Medicine and of Molecular Physiology and Biophysics, Baylor College of Medicine. Chief, Renal Service, The Methodist Hospital, Houston, Texas

190 *Phosphorus Deficiency and Hypophosphatemia*

WARREN R. SUMMER, M.D.

Howard A. Buechner Professor of Pulmonary Medicine, Louisiana State University School of Medicine. Section Chief, Pulmonary/Critical Care Medicine, Ochsner Institute, New Orleans, Louisiana

65 *Respiratory Failure*

MORTON N. SWARTZ, M.D.

Professor of Medicine, Harvard Medical School. Chief, Jackson Firm of Medical Service, Emeritus Chief, Infectious Disease Unit, Massachusetts General Hospital, Boston, Massachusetts

280 *Bacterial Meningitis*

AYALEW TEFFERI, M.D.

Assistant Professor of Medicine, Mayo Medical School. Consultant in Hematology and Internal Medicine, Mayo Clinic and Mayo Foundation, Rochester, Minnesota

141 *Proliferative Disorders of the Hematologic System*

C. CRAIG TISHER, M.D.

Professor of Medicine and Pathology, and Chief, Division of Nephrology, Hypertension and Transplantation, University of Florida College of Medicine. Attending Physician, Shands Hospital of the University of Florida, Gainesville, Florida

74 *Structure and Function of the Kidneys*

GALEN B. TOEWS, M.D.

Professor of Internal Medicine, University of Michigan Medical School. Chief, Division of Pulmonary and Critical Care Medicine, University of Michigan Medical Center, Ann Arbor, Michigan

54 *Interstitial Lung Disease*

PHILLIP P. TOSKES, M.D.

Professor of Medicine and Associate Chairman for Clinical Affairs, University of Florida College of Medicine. Director, Division of Gastroenterology, Hepatology and Nutrition, Shands Hospital at the University of Florida, Gainesville, Florida

103 *Malabsorption*

JOHN J. TREANOR, M.D.

Associate Professor of Medicine, Infectious Disease Unit, University of Rochester, School of Medicine and Dentistry, Rochester, New York

333 *Adenovirus Diseases*

GARY J. TUCKER, M.D.

Professor and Chairman, University of Washington School of Medicine, Seattle, Washington

401 *Psychiatric Disorders in Medical Practice*

GERARD M. TURINO, M.D.

John H. Keating, Sr. Professor of Medicine, Columbia University College of Physicians and Surgeons. Director Emeritus, Department of Medicine, St. Luke's–Roosevelt Hospital Center, New York, New York

49 *Approach to the Patient with Respiratory Disease*

JOUNI UITTO, M.D., Ph.D.

Professor of Dermatology and of Biochemistry and Molecular Biology, and Chairman, Department of Dermatology, Jefferson Medical College of Thomas Jefferson University, Philadelphia, Pennsylvania

186 *Pseudoxanthoma Elasticum*

ARTHUR C. UPTON, M.D.

Clinical Professor of Pathology and Radiology, University of New Mexico School of Medicine, Albuquerque, New Mexico. Professor Emeritus, Department of Environmental Medicine, New York University School of Medicine, New York, New York

13 *Principles of Occupational and Environmental Medicine*

MARGOT I. VAN ALLEN, M.D., M.Sc., F.A.A.P., F.A.B.M.G., F.R.C.P., F.C.C.M.G.

Clinical Associate Professor of Medical Genetics, University of British Columbia. Department of Medical Genetics, Provincial Medical Genetics Program, British Columbia Children's Hospital, Vancouver, British Columbia, Canada

27 *Congenital Anomalies*

JACK A. VENNES, M.D.

Professor of Medicine, Gastroenterology and Hepatology, University of Minnesota Medical School, Minneapolis, Minnesota

94 *Gastrointestinal Endoscopy*

NICHOLAS A. VICK, M.D.

Professor of Neurology, Northwestern University School of Medicine. Head, Division of Neurology, Evanston Hospital, Evanston, Illinois

434–436 *Intracranial Tumors and States of Altered Intracranial Pressure*

JONATHAN D. VICTOR, M.D.

Professor of Neurology and Neuroscience, Cornell University Medical College. Attending Neurologist, New York Hospital-Cornell Medical Center, New York, New York

392 *Neurology: Clinical Study of the Patient*

Z. RENO VLAHCEVIC, M.D.

Charles Caravati Professor of Medicine, Medical College of Virginia, Virginia Commonwealth University, Richmond, Virginia

126 *Diseases of the Gallbladder and Bile Ducts*

JOHN E. VOLANAKIS, M.D.

Anna Louis Waters Professor of Medicine in Rheumatology, University of Alabama School of Medicine, Birmingham, Alabama

222 *Complement*

BRUCE D. WALKER, M.D.

Associate Professor of Medicine, Harvard Medical School. Director, AIDS Research Program, Massachusetts General Hospital, Boston, Massachusetts

360 *Immunology Related to AIDS*

SUSAN D. WALL, M.D.

Associate Professor of Radiology, University of California, San Francisco, School of Medicine. Assistant Chief of Radiology, San Francisco Veterans Administration Medical Center, San Francisco, California

93 *Diagnostic Imaging Procedures in Gastroenterology*

EDWARD E. WALSH, M.D.

Associate Professor of Medicine and Pediatrics, University of Rochester School of Medicine and Dentistry. Attending Physician, Rochester General Hospital, Rochester, New York

330 *Respiratory Syncytial Virus;*   331 *Parainfluenza Viral Disease*

DAVID G. WARNOCK, M.D.

Professor of Medicine and Physiology, University of Alabama School of Medicine. Director, Division of Nephrology and Nephrology Research and Training Center, and Staff Physician, Veterans Administration Medical Center, Birmingham, Alabama

77 *Chronic Renal Failure*

STANLEY J. WATSON, Ph.D., M.D.

Professor of Psychiatry; Associate Chair of Research, and Associate Director and Research Scientist, Mental Health Research Institute, University of Michigan, Ann Arbor, Michigan

200 *Endorphins/Opioid Peptides, Prostaglandins, and Natriuretic Hormones*

ROLAND L. WEINSIER, M.D., M.P.H.

Professor and Chair, Department of Nutrition Sciences, University of Alabama School of Medicine, Birmingham, Alabama

9 *Principles of Preventive Health Care*

RICHARD A. WEISIGER, M.D., Ph.D.

Professor of Medicine, University of California, San Francisco, School of Medicine, San Francisco, California

114 *Hepatic Metabolism in Liver Disease;*   116 *Laboratory Tests in Liver Disease*

GERALD WEISSMANN, M.D.

Professor of Medicine, Division of Rheumatology, New York University Medical Center, New York, New York

19 *NSAID's: Aspirin and Aspirin-Like Drugs;*   235 *Tissue Injury in Rheumatic Diseases*

PETER F. WELLER, M.D., F.A.C.P.

Associate Professor of Medicine, Department of Medicine, Harvard Medical School. Associate Physician, Department of Medicine, Beth Israel Hospital, Boston, Massachusetts

148 *Eosinophilic Syndromes*

JOHN E. WENNBERG, M.D., M.P.H.

Professor of Medicine and of Community and Family Medicine and Director, Center for the Evaluative Clinical Sciences, Dartmouth Medical School, Hanover, New Hampshire

4 *Social and Economic Issues in Medicine*

RICHARD J. WHITLEY, M.D.

Professor of Pediatrics, and of Microbiology, and of Medicine, University of Alabama School of Medicine. Loeb Eminent Scholar Chair in Pediatrics, University of Alabama Children's Hospital, Birmingham, Alabama

327 *Antiviral Therapy (Non-AIDS);*   339 *Herpes Simplex Virus Infections*

MICHAEL P. WHYTE, M.D.

Professor of Medicine and Pediatrics, Washington University School of Medicine. Medical Director, Metabolic Research Unit, Shriners Hospital for Crippled Children, St. Louis, Missouri

219 *Osteonecrosis, Osteosclerosis, and Other Disorders of Bone*

VALERIE J. WIEBE, P.D.

Pharmacist, University of California, Davis, School of Medicine, Davis, California

166 *Treatment of Neoplastic Disease During Pregnancy*

C. MEL WILCOX, M.D.

Associate Professor of Medicine, University of Alabama School of Medicine. Attending Physician, University Hospital, Birmingham, Alabama

112 *Miscellaneous Inflammatory Diseases of the Intestine*

SIDNEY J. WINAWER, M.D.

Professor of Medicine, Cornell University Medical College. Chief, Gastroenterology and Nutrition Service, Memorial Sloan-Kettering Cancer Center, New York, New York

100 *Neoplasms of the Stomach*

JOSEPH L. WITZTUM, M.D.

Professor of Medicine, Department of Medicine, University of California, San Diego, School of Medicine, La Jolla, California

173 *The Hypolipoproteinemias*

ROBERT L. WORTMANN, M.D.

Professor and Chairman, Department of Medicine, East Carolina University School of Medicine. Chief of Medicine, Pitt County Memorial Hospital, Greensville, North Carolina

247 *Idiopathic Inflammatory Myopathies*

DANIEL G. WRIGHT, M.D.

Professor of Medicine, Boston University School of Medicine. Chief, Section of Hematology and Oncology, Boston University Medical Center and Boston City Hospital, Boston, Massachusetts

139 *Function of Neutrophils and Mononuclear Phagocytes*

ALBERT W. WU, M.D., M.P.H.

Assistant Professor of Medicine and of Health Policy and Management, School of Hygiene and Public Health, School of Medicine, Johns Hopkins University. Attending Physician, Johns Hopkins Hospital, Baltimore, Maryland

21 *Principles of Outcome Assessment*

JOSHUA WYNNE, M.D.

Professor of Medicine and Chief of Cardiology, Wayne State University School of Medicine. Chief, Section of Cardiology, Harper Hospital, Detroit, Michigan

47 *Miscellaneous Conditions of the Heart: Tumor, Trauma, and Systemic Disease*

JOACHIM YAHALOM, M.D.

Associate Professor, Cornell University Medical College. Associate Member, Memorial Sloan-Kettering Cancer Center, New York, New York

146 *Hodgkin's Disease*

ROBERT YARCHOAN, M.D.

Head, Retroviral Diseases Section, and Attending Physician, Medicine Branch, National Cancer Institute, National Institutes of Health, Bethesda, Maryland

371 *Treatment of HIV Infection and AIDS*

ERNEST YODER, M.D.

Director of Curriculum Development and Associate Professor of Medicine, Wayne State University School of Medicine. Director of Medical Education, and Vice Chief of Internal Medicine, Grace Hospital, Detroit, Michigan

71 *Disorders Due to Heat and Cold*

NEAL S. YOUNG, M.D.

Chief, Hematology Branch, National Heart, Lung, and Blood Institute, Bethesda, Maryland

130 *Aplastic Anemia and Related Bone Marrow Failure Syndromes*

BARRY L. ZARET, M.D.

Robert W. Berliner Professor of Medicine, Professor of Diagnostic Radiology, Chief, Section of Cardiovascular Medicine, and Associate Chair for Clinical Affairs, Department of Internal Medicine, Yale University School of Medicine. Chief of Cardiology, Yale–New Haven Hospital, New Haven, Connecticut

33 *Specialized Diagnostic Procedures*

ELIZABETH J. ZIEGLER, M.D.

Professor of Medicine, University of California, San Diego, School of Medicine, La Jolla. Attending Physician, University of California San Diego Medical Center, San Diego, California

299 *Extraintestinal Infections Caused by Enteric Bacteria*

DOUGLAS P. ZIPES, M.D.

Distinguished Professor of Medicine, Pharmacology and Toxicology, Indiana University School of Medicine. Senior Research Associate, Krannert Institute of Cardiology, Indianapolis, Indiana

36 *Sudden Cardiac Death*

PREFACE

In this edition of *Cecil Textbook of Medicine,* Albert Wu (see Chapter 21, "Principles of Outcome Assessment") reminds us that health was defined by the World Health Organization in 1948 as "a state of complete physical, mental, and social well being, and not merely the absence of disease and infirmity." This is the tone that we think is important to be set for this 20th edition of the *Cecil* textbook because the responsibilities of physicians and the knowledge base for physicians in training must include disciplines beyond the ordinary understanding of disease processes, pathogenesis, treatment, and outcomes. This knowledge base must include an understanding of the psychosocial basis of disease, the influence of the environment, and the role of prevention as a lifelong commitment. More and more as internal medicine gains and expands because of extraordinary technologic developments, it requires the physician to come back to the roots of medicine. As Roger Bulger has said, the three entities—"preventing, curing, and caring, but perhaps the greatest of these is caring"—can always be remembered and expressed in every patient encounter.

Cecil Textbook of Medicine has enjoyed a worldwide reputation for excellence since it was first published in 1927 by Russell Cecil. Cecil's ability to bring together clinical manifestations of disease with its basic biological sciences, as well as treatment and outcomes, was most significant. In the *Cecil* textbook the emphasis on basic pathophysiology, pharmacology, and more recently molecular biology has been heightened as relationships lead to better understanding of the clinical manifestations of disease and its treatment. Cecil believed that, to obtain this intellectual integration, one should assemble the most expert authors so that all information be not only informative but authoritative. He also thought that each disease topic should be presented in its entirety so that everything one needed to know about a given disease was present in one place under one heading.

Since the early editions of *Cecil,* the policy of the Editors has been to continually rotate authors so that an author participates in the endeavor through three edition cycles and then rotates off. This means that for every new edition at least one third of the book comprises new authors incorporating a fresh approach to their topics. We would like to take this opportunity to express our appreciation to those authors who "retired" after service in the writing of the 19th edition and also to welcome those authors new to the 20th edition. Many of these authors not only are covering full topics with new information but also have written about an entirely new topic or new areas not covered in previous *Cecil* editions. Although James Wyngaarden and H. (Holly) Lloyd Smith have now retired from *Cecil,* their spirit, talents, and enthusiasm are still evident in this 20th edition. They continue to be valuable advisors and critics for *Cecil Textbook of Medicine,* and it is our hope that they will remain so.

Several of our Consulting Editors have also rotated off, including Thomas E. Andreoli, John F. Murray, and David G. Nathan. With us for another edition are Gerald L. Mandell, Robert K. Ockner, and Thomas W. Smith, and we welcome our new Consulting Editors Juha P. Kokko and Gordon N. Gill. This group has been enormously helpful to us in constructing the full textbook, selecting authors, and reviewing selected manuscripts. The Editors, however, take full responsibility for the book as well as its integration from topic to topic. We believe that all the authors involved in writing this 20th edition have met the high standards set by their predecessors and that this has resulted in an extremely comprehensive and useful textbook.

This edition continues the two-color presentation of figures and charts that has been the standard in both the 18th and 19th editions. With the 20th edition we are also pleased that we will have a companion CD-ROM version of the text available.

Many new chapters have been added to Cecil 20. These include *Social and Economic Issues in Medicine* by John Wennberg (Ethics part, Chapter 4); *Biology of Aging* by Caleb Finch and Edward

L. Schneider, and the *Neuropsychiatric Aspects of Aging* by Gene Cohen (Aging part, Chapters 5 and 7). The part on Preventive Health has been significantly reorganized and now includes Chapter 13, *Principles of Occupational and Environmental Medicine,* a subsection of which covers common poisons, which was once a stand-alone chapter. *Clinical Decision Making—Fundamental Statistics* by Catarina Kiefe, *The Domain of the Generalist Physician,* by Susan Day, *Antithrombotic Therapy* by Laurence Harker, and *Principles of Outcome Assessment* by Albert Wu have been added to the Evaluation part (Chapters 14.3, 15, 20, and 21). *Cardiac Transplantation* by Robert Bourge and *Cardiovascular Magnetic Resonance Imaging* by Gerald Blackwell have been added to the Cardiovascular section (Chapters 48 and 33.5). *Upper Airway Diseases* by Kingman Strohl and *Lung Transplantation* by Norman Rizk have been added to the Respiratory section (Chapters 64 and 65). The Critical Care part now includes a separate chapter on *Respiratory Aspects of Critical Care Medicine* by John Luce (Chapter 68). *Cancer Prevention* by Gilbert Omenn, *Molecular Mechanisms of Drug Resistance* by Michael DeGregorio and Edith Perez, *Treatment of Neoplastic Disease During Pregnancy* by Valerie Wiebe, and *The Future of Oncology* by Donald Miller have been added to the Oncology part (Chapters 155, 165, 166, and 167). Pneumocystis carinii *Pneumonia* (Chapter 383) by Fred Sattler is now a separate chapter once again and is presented under Protozoa/Metazoa rather than being a major part of the Pulmonary section in the HIV part. Under the Infectious Diseases part, an effort has been made to aggregate groups of organisms and their diseases, e.g., Rickettsial Diseases (Chapter 324), the Herpes Group of Viruses (Chapters 339–341), Enteric Viral Infections (Chapters 343–344), and the Hemorrhagic Fever Viruses (Chapters 345–346). This has allowed considerable condensation of topic headings from previous editions. Great effort has been made at cross-referencing sections and topics in the Neurology part to other sections of the textbook. Color plates have been increased to 20, consisting of 171 illustrations.

We feel a great sense of camaraderie as well as gratitude toward the 415 contributors who have written the 477 chapters for the 20th edition. Special appreciation is extended particularly to editorial assistance in Birmingham (Dvora Aksler Konstant) and also to editorial assistance in New York (Maureen O'Connor). We have been most fortunate to have them handling the manuscripts, polishing the language, and keeping the flow of paper work at a manageable level. Without them the very large task of compiling the 20th edition of *Cecil Textbook of Medicine* would have been a near impossibility. At W.B. Saunders, Les Hoeltzel, Lorraine Kilmer, Frank Polizzano, and Edna Dick have been especially supportive and helpful to us in organizing, editing, and developing graphics. Darlene Pedersen was the person responsible overall at W.B. Saunders Company for the 20th edition, and she provided constant encouragement, stimulation, and an eloquently good sense of humor. She is indeed a good friend.

J. CLAUDE BENNETT, M.D.
FRED PLUM, M.D.

CONTENTS

PART I
MEDICINE AS A LEARNED AND HUMANE PROFESSION...1

PART II
SOCIAL AND ETHICAL ISSUES IN MEDICINE...4

PART III
AGING AND GERIATRIC MEDICINE..12

PART IV
PREVENTIVE HEALTH CARE...26

PART V
PRINCIPLES OF EVALUATION AND MANAGEMENT..75

PART VI
PRINCIPLES OF HUMAN GENETICS...134

PART VII
CARDIOVASCULAR DISEASES..166

PART VIII
RESPIRATORY DISEASES...368

PART IX
CRITICAL CARE MEDICINE...464

PART X
RENAL DISEASES...511

PART XI
GASTROINTESTINAL DISEASES..627

PART XII
DISEASES OF THE LIVER, GALLBLADDER, AND BILE DUCTS..752

PART XIII
HEMATOLOGIC DISEASES...817

PART XIV
ONCOLOGY..1004

PART XV
METABOLIC DISEASES..1078

PART XVI
NUTRITIONAL DISEASES..1139

PART XVII
ENDOCRINE AND REPRODUCTIVE DISEASES..1176

PART XVIII
DISEASES OF BONE AND BONE MINERAL METABOLISM...1351

PART XIX
DISEASES OF THE IMMUNE SYSTEM...1393

PART XX
MUSCULOSKELETAL AND CONNECTIVE TISSUE DISEASES...1440

PART XXI
INFECTIOUS DISEASES...1531

PART XXII
HIV AND THE ACQUIRED IMMUNODEFICIENCY SYNDROME..1837

PART XXIII
DISEASES OF PROTOZOA AND METAZOA...1892

PART XXIV
NEUROLOGY...1957

PART XXV
EYE DISEASES...2174

PART XXVI
SKIN DISEASES...2184

PART XXVII
LABORATORY REFERENCE INTERVALS AND VALUES...2223

(Detailed Table of Contents begins on the following page)

PART I MEDICINE AS A LEARNED AND HUMANE PROFESSION

1 MEDICINE AS A LEARNED AND HUMANE PROFESSION, *J. Claude Bennett and Fred Plum* 1

PART II SOCIAL AND ETHICAL ISSUES IN MEDICINE

2 CLINICAL ETHICS IN THE PRACTICE OF MEDICINE, *Peter A. Singer and Mark Siegler* 4
3 CARE OF DYING PATIENTS AND THEIR FAMILIES, *Balfour M. Mount* 6
4 SOCIAL AND ECONOMIC ISSUES IN MEDICINE, *John E. Wennberg* 9

PART III AGING AND GERIATRIC MEDICINE

5 BIOLOGY OF AGING, *Caleb E. Finch and Edward L. Schneider* 12
6 NEUROLOGIC PROBLEMS ASSOCIATED WITH AGING, *Fred Plum* 16
7 NEUROPSYCHIATRIC ASPECTS OF AGING, *Gene D. Cohen* 17
8 SPECIAL PROBLEMS IN THE GERIATRIC PATIENT, *Judith C. Ahronheim* ... 21

PART IV PREVENTIVE HEALTH CARE

9 PRINCIPLES OF PREVENTIVE HEALTH CARE, *Albert Oberman* 26
  9.1 The Preventive Health Examination, *Richard K. Riegelman* 27
  9.2 Diet, *Roland L. Weinsier* 29
  9.3 Exercise, *Michael Pratt* 31
  9.4 Tobacco, *Neal L. Benowitz* 33
  9.5 Violence and Injury, *Elizabeth McLoughlin* 36
10 VACCINATION/IMMUNIZATION, *Walter A. Orenstein* 40
11 ALCOHOLISM AND ALCOHOL ABUSE, *Ivan Diamond* 47
12 DRUG ABUSE AND DEPENDENCE, *Charles P. O'Brien* 49
13 PRINCIPLES OF OCCUPATIONAL AND ENVIRONMENTAL MEDICINE, *Philip J. Landrigan* 56
  13.1 Radiation Injury, *Arthur C. Upton* 59
  13.2 Electrical Injury, *Cleon W. Goodwin* 64
  13.3 Chronic Poisoning: Trace Metals and Others, *William O. Robertson* 67

PART V PRINCIPLES OF EVALUATION AND MANAGEMENT

14 CLINICAL DECISION MAKING 75
  14.1 Approach to the Patient, *Suzanne W. Fletcher* 75
  14.2 Clinical Decision Making: Handling and Analyzing Clinical Data, *Stephen G. Pauker* 78
  14.3 Fundamental Statistics, *Catarina I. Kiefe* 83
15 THE DOMAIN OF THE GENERALIST PHYSICIAN, *Susan C. Day* 85
16 PRINCIPLES OF DRUG THERAPY, *Robert B. Diasio* 89

Problems of Overarching Importance Which Transcend Organ Systems
17 PAIN, *Kathleen M. Foley* 100
18 GLUCOCORTICOSTEROIDS IN RELATION TO INFLAMMATORY DISEASE, *Paul Katz* 108
19 NSAID'S: ASPIRIN AND ASPIRIN-LIKE DRUGS, *Gerald Weissmann* 111
20 ANTITHROMBOTIC THERAPY, *Laurence A. Harker* 115
21 PRINCIPLES OF OUTCOME ASSESSMENT, *Albert W. Wu* 122
22 OVERVIEW OF IMAGING TECHNIQUES FOR THE FUTURE, *James M. Mountz and Hoby Hetherington* 126

PART VI PRINCIPLES OF HUMAN GENETICS

23 HUMAN HEREDITY, *Harry W. Schroeder, Jr.* 134
24 INBORN ERRORS OF METABOLISM, *Louis J. Elsas II* 142
25 GENE THERAPY, *David T. Curiel* 147
26 CHROMOSOMES AND THEIR DISORDERS, *R. Ellen Magenis* 150
27 CONGENITAL ANOMALIES, *Margot I. Van Allen and Judith G. Hall* ... 157
28 HEREDITARY SYNDROMES INVOLVING MULTIPLE ORGAN SYSTEMS, *Kenneth Lyons Jones* 160
29 GENETIC COUNSELING, *Margretta R. Seashore* 162

PART VII CARDIOVASCULAR DISEASES

30 APPROACH TO THE PATIENT WITH CARDIOVASCULAR DISEASE, *Thomas Woodward Smith* 166
31 EPIDEMIOLOGY OF CARDIOVASCULAR DISEASES, *William T. Friedewald* .. 170
32 CARDIAC FUNCTION AND CIRCULATORY CONTROL, *John Ross, Jr.* 174
33 SPECIALIZED DIAGNOSTIC PROCEDURES 181
  33.1 Radiology of the Heart, *Murray G. Baron* 181
  33.2 Electrocardiography, *Nora Goldschlager* 188
  33.3 Echocardiography, *Richard L. Popp* 194
  33.4 Nuclear Cardiology, *Barry L. Zaret* 199
  33.5 Cardiovascular Magnetic Resonance Imaging, *Gerald G. Blackwell* 202
  33.6 Cardiac Catheterization and Angiography, *William H. Barry* 208
34 HEART FAILURE, *Thomas Woodward Smith* 211
35 CARDIAC ARRHYTHMIAS, *J. Thomas Bigger, Jr.* 231
36 SUDDEN CARDIAC DEATH, *Douglas P. Zipes* 253
37 ARTERIAL HYPERTENSION, *Suzanne Oparil* 256
38 PULMONARY HYPERTENSION, *Joseph S. Alpert* 271
39 CONGENITAL HEART DISEASE IN ADULTS, *Joseph K. Perloff* 277
40 ATHEROSCLEROSIS, *Russell Ross* 291
41 DISORDERS OF THE CORONARY ARTERIES 296
  41.1 Angina Pectoris, *William J. Rogers* 296
  41.2 Acute Myocardial Infarction, *Burton E. Sobel* 301
  41.3 Surgical Treatment of Coronary Artery Disease, *Lawrence H. Cohn* 316
42 VALVULAR HEART DISEASE, *Charles E. Rackley* 319
43 DISEASES OF THE MYOCARDIUM, *Lynne Warner Stevenson* 327
44 DISEASES OF THE PERICARDIUM, *Ralph Shabetai* 336
45 DISEASES OF THE AORTA, *Lawrence S. Cohen* 342
46 VASCULAR DISEASES OF THE LIMBS, *Hermes A. Kontos* 346
47 MISCELLANEOUS CONDITIONS OF THE HEART: TUMOR, TRAUMA, AND SYSTEMIC DISEASE, *Joshua Wynne* 357
48 CARDIAC TRANSPLANTATION, *Robert C. Bourge* 360

PART VIII RESPIRATORY DISEASES

49 APPROACH TO THE PATIENT WITH RESPIRATORY DISEASE, *Gerard M. Turino* 368
50 RESPIRATORY STRUCTURE AND FUNCTION, *James D. Crapo* 371
51 ASTHMA, *Jeffrey M. Drazen* 376
52 CHRONIC AIRWAYS DISEASES, *Richard A. Matthay and Alejandro C. Arroliga* 381
53 LOCALIZED ABNORMALITIES OF LUNG AERATION, *Richard A. Matthay and Alejandro C. Arroliga* 389
54 INTERSTITIAL LUNG DISEASE, *Galen B. Toews* 390
  54.1 Occupational Pulmonary Disorders, *Jonathan M. Samet* 399
  54.2 Physical, Chemical, and Aspiration Injuries of the Lung, *Claude A. Piantadosi* 403
55 OVERVIEW OF PNEUMONIA, *Waldemar G. Johanson, Jr.* 411
56 LUNG ABSCESS, *John G. Bartlett* 413
57 BRONCHIECTASIS, *Roger C. Bone* 416
58 CYSTIC FIBROSIS, *Roger C. Bone* 419
59 PULMONARY EMBOLISM, *Robert M. Senior* 422
60 FAT EMBOLISM SYNDROME, *Robert M. Senior* 430
61 SARCOIDOSIS, *Barry L. Fanburg* 431
62 PULMONARY NEOPLASMS, *York E. Miller* 436
63 DISEASES OF THE DIAPHRAGM, CHEST WALL, PLEURA, AND MEDIASTINUM, *Bartolome R. Celli* 442
64 UPPER AIRWAY DISEASES, *Kingman P. Strohl* 449
65 RESPIRATORY FAILURE, *Warren R. Summer* 452
66 LUNG TRANSPLANTATION, *Norman W. Rizk* 459

PART IX CRITICAL CARE MEDICINE

67 APPROACH TO THE PATIENT IN A CRITICAL CARE SETTING, *John M. Luce* . 464
68 RESPIRATORY ASPECTS OF CRITICAL CARE MEDICINE, *John M. Luce* 466
69 CARDIOGENIC SHOCK, *David W. Ferguson* 477
70 SHOCK SYNDROMES RELATED TO SEPSIS, *Joseph E. Parrillo* 496
71 DISORDERS DUE TO HEAT AND COLD, *Ernest Yoder* 501
72 ACUTE POISONING, *Lester M. Haddad* 503

PART X   RENAL DISEASES

73 APPROACH TO THE PATIENT WITH RENAL DISEASE, *Juha P. Kokko* 511
74 STRUCTURE AND FUNCTION OF THE KIDNEYS, *C. Craig Tisher* 517
75 DISORDERS OF FLUID VOLUME, ELECTROLYTE, AND ACID-BASE BALANCE,
    Juha P. Kokko 525
    75.1   Volume Disorders 525
    75.2   Osmolality Disturbances 532
    75.3   Disturbances in Potassium Balance 538
    75.4   Disturbances in Acid-Base Balance 543
76 ACUTE RENAL FAILURE, *William E. Mitch* 552
77 CHRONIC RENAL FAILURE, *David G. Warnock* 556
78 TREATMENT OF IRREVERSIBLE RENAL FAILURE, *John J. Curtis* 563
    78.1   Dialysis 563
    78.2   Renal Transplantation 568
79 GLOMERULAR DISORDERS, *Gerald B. Appel* .. 572
80 TUBULOINTERSTITIAL DISEASES AND TOXIC NEPHROPATHIES,
    T. Dwight McKinney 580
81 OBSTRUCTIVE UROPATHY, *Saulo Klahr* 589
82 SPECIFIC RENAL TUBULAR DISORDERS, *Russell W. Chesney* 594
83 DIABETES AND THE KIDNEY, *Thomas H. Hostetter* 599
84 URINARY TRACT INFECTIONS AND PYELONEPHRITIS, *Calvin M. Kunin* .. 602
85 VASCULAR DISORDERS OF THE KIDNEY, *Thomas D. DuBose, Jr.* 606
86 HYPERTENSION AND RENAL DISEASE IN PREGNANCY, *Thomas F. Ferris* . 609
87 HEREDITARY CHRONIC NEPHROPATHIES, *Manuel Martinez-Maldonado* 611
88 RENAL CALCULI (*Nephrolithiasis*), *Keith Hruska* 613
89 CYSTIC DISEASES OF THE KIDNEY, *Patricia A. Gabow* 617
90 ANOMALIES OF THE URINARY TRACT, *Jay Bernstein* 621
91 TUMORS OF THE KIDNEY, URETER, AND BLADDER, *Charles L. Shapiro,*
    Marc B. Garnick, and Philip W. Kantoff 623

PART XI   GASTROINTESTINAL DISEASES

92 INTRODUCTION TO GASTROINTESTINAL DISEASES, *Robert K. Ockner* 627
93 DIAGNOSTIC IMAGING PROCEDURES IN GASTROENTEROLOGY,
    Susan D. Wall 630
94 GASTROINTESTINAL ENDOSCOPY, *Jeffrey M. Rank and Jack A. Vennes* 636
95 GASTROINTESTINAL HEMORRHAGE, *John P. Cello* 642
96 DISEASES OF THE MOUTH AND SALIVARY GLANDS, *Troy E. Daniels* 645
97 DISEASES OF THE ESOPHAGUS, *Sidney Cohen and Henry P. Parkman* 650
98 GASTRITIS, *Andrew H. Soll* 659
99 PEPTIC ULCER 662
    99.1   Pathophysiology, *Andrew H. Soll* 662
    99.2   Epidemiology, Clinical Manifestations, and Diagnosis,
            Jon I. Isenberg and Andrew H. Soll 664
    99.3   Medical Therapy, *David Y. Graham* 667
    99.4   Surgical Therapy, *Haile T. Debas and Susan L. Orloff* 669
    99.5   Complications, *David Y. Graham* 672
    99.6   Zollinger-Ellison Syndrome, *Robert T. Jensen* 674
100 NEOPLASMS OF THE STOMACH, *Robert C. Kurtz and*
     Sidney J. Winawer 676
101 DISORDERS OF GASTROINTESTINAL MOTILITY, *William J. Snape, Jr.* 680
102 DIARRHEA, *Guenter J. Krejs* 689
103 MALABSORPTION, *Phillip P. Toskes* 695
104 INFLAMMATORY BOWEL DISEASE, *Stephen B. Hanauer* 707
105 VASCULAR DISORDERS OF THE INTESTINE, *Lawrence J. Brandt* 715
106 NEOPLASMS OF THE LARGE AND SMALL INTESTINES, *Bernard Levin* 721
     Neoplasms of the Large Intestine 721
     Neoplasms of the Small Bowel 728
107 PANCREATITIS, *Konrad H. Soergel* 729
108 CARCINOMA OF THE PANCREAS, *Eugene P. DiMagno* 736
109 FOOD POISONING, *Martin F. Heyworth* 738
110 DISEASES OF THE RECTUM AND ANUS, *Theodore R. Schrock* 740
111 DISEASES OF THE PERITONEUM, MESENTERY, AND OMENTUM,
     Michael R. Lucey 743
112 MISCELLANEOUS INFLAMMATORY DISEASES OF THE INTESTINE,
     C. Mel Wilcox 748

PART XII   DISEASES OF THE LIVER, GALLBLADDER, AND BILE DUCTS

113 CLINICAL APPROACH TO LIVER DISEASE, *Robert K. Ockner* 752
114 HEPATIC METABOLISM IN LIVER DISEASE, *Richard A. Weisiger* 753
115 BILIRUBIN METABOLISM, HYPERBILIRUBINEMIA, AND APPROACH
     TO THE JAUNDICED PATIENT, *Bruce F. Scharschmidt* 755

116 LABORATORY TESTS IN LIVER DISEASE, *Richard A. Weisiger* 759
117 ACUTE VIRAL HEPATITIS, *Robert K. Ockner* 762
118 TOXIC AND DRUG-INDUCED LIVER DISEASE, *Nathan M. Bass* 772
119 CHRONIC HEPATITIS, *Robert K. Ockner* 776
120 PARASITIC, BACTERIAL, FUNGAL, AND GRANULOMATOUS LIVER DISEASES,
     Willis C. Maddrey 781
121 INHERITED, INFILTRATIVE, AND METABOLIC DISORDERS
     INVOLVING THE LIVER, *Jacquelyn J. Maher* 785
122 CIRRHOSIS OF THE LIVER AND ITS MAJOR SEQUELAE, *Scott L. Friedman* 788
123 ACUTE AND CHRONIC HEPATIC FAILURE AND HEPATIC ENCEPHALOPATHY,
     Bruce F. Scharschmidt 797
124 LIVER TRANSPLANTATION, *John P. Roberts* 800
125 HEPATIC TUMORS, *Bruce F. Scharschmidt* 802
126 DISEASES OF THE GALLBLADDER AND BILE DUCTS, *Z. Reno Vlahcevic*
     and Douglas M. Heuman 805

PART XIII   HEMATOLOGIC DISEASES

127 APPROACH TO THE PATIENT WITH HEMATOLOGIC DISEASE,
     David G. Nathan 817
128 HEMOLYTIC DISORDERS: INTRODUCTION, *David G. Nathan* 821
129 AN APPROACH TO THE ANEMIAS, *John Lindenbaum* 823
130 APLASTIC ANEMIA AND RELATED BONE MARROW FAILURE SYNDROMES,
     Neal S. Young 831
131 NORMOCHROMIC, NORMOCYTIC ANEMIAS, *Thomas P. Duffy* 837
132 MICROCYTIC AND HYPOCHROMIC ANEMIAS, *Thomas P. Duffy* 839
133 MEGALOBLASTIC ANEMIAS, *Robert H. Allen* 843
134 HEREDITARY DEFECTS IN THE MEMBRANE OR METABOLISM
     OF THE RED CELL, *Samuel E. Lux* 851
135 AUTOIMMUNE HEMOLYTIC ANEMIA, *Alan D. Schreiber* 859
136 HEMOGLOBIN AND HEMOGLOBINOPATHIES, ... 868
     136.1   Structure, Function, and Synthesis of the Human Hemoglobins,
              Edward J. Benz, Jr. 868
     136.2   Classification and Basic Pathophysiology
              of the Hemoglobinopathies, *Edward J. Benz, Jr.* 872
     136.3   Hemoglobinopathies with Altered Solubility or Oxygen Affinity,
              Edward J. Benz, Jr. 873
     136.4   The Thalassemias, *Arthur W. Nienhuis and*
              Edward J. Benz, Jr. 877
137 SICKLE CELL ANEMIA AND ASSOCIATED HEMOGLOBINOPATHIES,
     Stephen H. Embury 882
138 BLOOD TRANSFUSION, *Jay E. Menitove* 893
139 FUNCTION OF NEUTROPHILS AND MONONUCLEAR PHAGOCYTES,
     Laurence A. Boxer 897
     139.1   Disorders of Neutrophil Function, *Laurence A. Boxer* 902
     139.2   Familial Mediterranean Fever, *Daniel G. Wright* 907
140 DISORDERS OF NEUTROPHIL PRODUCTION, *Grover C. Bagby, Jr.* 908
     140.1   Leukopenia 908
     140.2   Leukocytosis and Leukemoid Reactions 915
141 PROLIFERATIVE DISORDERS OF THE HEMATOLOGIC SYSTEM 920
     141.1   Erythrocytosis and Polycythemia Vera, *Murray N. Silverstein*
              and Ayalew Tefferi. 920
     141.2   Chronic Myeloproliferative Diseases, *Ayalew Tefferi and*
              Murray N. Silverstein 922
142 THE CHRONIC LEUKEMIAS, *Michael J. Keating* 925
143 THE ACUTE LEUKEMIAS, *Frederick R. Appelbaum* 936
144 INTRODUCTION TO NEOPLASMS OF THE IMMUNE SYSTEM,
     Carol S. Portlock 941
145 NON-HODGKIN'S LYMPHOMAS, *Carol S. Portlock* 942
146 HODGKIN'S DISEASE, *Carol S. Portlock and Joachim Yahalom* 947
147 LANGERHANS CELL (EOSINOPHILIC) GRANULOMATOSIS, *Diane M. Komp* . 955
148 EOSINOPHILIC SYNDROMES, *Peter F. Weller* 956
149 PLASMA CELL DISORDERS, *Robert A. Kyle* 958
150 DISEASES OF LYMPH NODES AND SPLEEN, *Douglas V. Faller* 968
151 BONE MARROW TRANSPLANTATION, *Joel Rappeport* 974
152 HEMORRHAGIC DISORDERS: ABNORMALITIES OF PLATELET AND
     VASCULAR FUNCTION, *Marc Shuman* 977
153 DISORDERS OF BLOOD COAGULATION, *Deane F. Mosher* 987

PART XIV   ONCOLOGY

154 INTRODUCTION, *Joseph V. Simone* 1004
155 CANCER PREVENTION, *Gilbert S. Omenn* 1008
156 ONCOGENES AND SUPPRESSOR GENES: GENETIC CONTROL OF CANCER,
     Edison T. Liu 1011

157 THE EPIDEMIOLOGY OF CANCER, William J. Blot 1013
158 SYSTEMIC SECRETIONS OF CANCER CELLS AND THEIR EFFECTS 1017
    158.1 Paraneoplastic Syndromes, Kenneth R. Meehan and
           Marc S. Ernstoff 1017
    158.2 Tumor Markers, Dennis L. Cooper 1021
159 ENDOCRINE MANIFESTATIONS OF TUMORS: "ECTOPIC"
    HORMONE PRODUCTION, Stephen B. Baylin 1024
160 NONMETASTATIC EFFECTS OF CANCER ON THE NERVOUS SYSTEM,
    Jerome B. Posner 1027
161 CUTANEOUS MANIFESTATIONS OF INTERNAL MALIGNANCY, Frank Parker .1030
162 PRINCIPLES OF CANCER THERAPY, Sydney E. Salmon and
    Joseph R. Bertino 1036
163 ONCOLOGIC EMERGENCIES, Stephen M. Hahn 1049
164 APPROACH TO THE PATIENT WITH METASTATIC CANCER,
    PRIMARY SITE UNKNOWN, Daniel C. Ihde 1054
165 MOLECULAR MECHANISMS OF DRUG RESISTANCE,
    Michael W. DeGregorio and Edith A. Perez 1056
166 TREATMENT OF NEOPLASTIC DISEASE DURING PREGNANCY,
    Valerie J. Wiebe 1060
167 THE FUTURE OF ONCOLOGY, Donald M. Miller 1071

PART XV METABOLIC DISEASES

168 APPROACH TO THE PATIENT WITH METABOLIC DISEASE,
    Louis J. Elsas II 1078

Disorders of Carbohydrate Metabolism

169 GALACTOSEMIA, Stanton Segal 1080
170 GLYCOGEN STORAGE DISEASES, Harry L. Greene 1082
171 FRUCTOSE INTOLERANCE, Harry L. Greene 1083
172 PRIMARY HYPEROXALURIA, Richard E. Hillman 1085

Disorders of Lipid Metabolism 1086

173 THE HYPERLIPOPROTEINEMIAS Joseph L. Witztum and
    Daniel Steinberg 1086
174 LYSOSOMAL STORAGE DISEASES, Margaret M. McGovern and
    Robert J. Desnick 1095

Inborn Errors of Amino Acid Metabolism

175 HYPERAMINOACIDURIA (With a Classification of the Inborn and
    Developmental Errors of Amino Acid Metabolism),
    Charles R. Scriver 1099
176 THE HYPERPHENYLALANINEMIAS AND ALKAPTONURIA,
    Charles R. Scriver 1105
177 THE HYPERPROLINEMIAS AND HYDROXYPROLINEMIA, James M. Phang ..1109
178 DISEASES OF THE UREA CYCLE, Stephen D. Cederbaum 1109
179 BRANCHED-CHAIN AMINOACIDURIAS, Louis J. Elsas II 1111
180 HOMOCYSTINURIA, Bruce A. Barshop 1112
181 DISORDERS OF PURINE AND PYRIMIDINE METABOLISM,
    Beverly S. Mitchell and Michael S. Hershfield 1114

Inherited Disorders of Connective Tissue

182 THE MUCOPOLYSACCHARIDOSES, Hans C. Andersson and
    Emmanuel Shapira 1118
183 THE MARFAN SYNDROME, Peter H. Byers 1119
184 EHLERS-DANLOS SYNDROME, Peter H. Byers 1120
185 OSTEOGENESIS IMPERFECTA, Peter H. Byers 1122
186 PSEUDOXANTHOMA ELASTICUM, Jouni Uitto 1123

Disorders of Porphyrins and Metals

187 THE PORPHYRIAS, Karl E. Anderson 1124
188 WILSON'S DISEASE, Andrew Deiss 1131
189 IRON OVERLOAD (Hemochromatosis), Virgil F. Fairbanks and
    William P. Baldus 1132
190 PHOSPHORUS DEFICIENCY AND HYPOPHOSPHATEMIA, Wadi N. Suki 1135
191 DISORDERS OF MAGNESIUM METABOLISM, Allen C. Alfrey 1137

PART XVI NUTRITIONAL DISEASES

192 NUTRITION'S INTERFACE WITH HEALTH AND DISEASE 1139
    192.1 Introduction, Douglas C. Heimburger 1139
    192.2 Consequences of Altered Micronutrient Status, Joel B. Mason .1144
193 NUTRITIONAL ASSESSMENT, Bruce R. Bistrian 1151
194 PROTEIN-ENERGY MALNUTRITION, Robert B. Baron 1154
195 THE EATING DISORDERS, Douglas A. Drossman 1158
196 OBESITY, F. Xavier Pi-Sunyer 1161
197 ENTERAL NUTRITION, John L. Rombeau 1168
198 PARENTERAL NUTRITION, M. Molly McMahon 1171

PART XVII ENDOCRINE AND REPRODUCTIVE
           DISEASES

199 PRINCIPLES OF ENDOCRINOLOGY, Gordon N. Gill 1176
200 ENDORPHINS/OPIOID PEPTIDES, PROSTAGLANDINS,
    AND NATRIURETIC HORMONES 1186
    200.1 The Endorphin Family of Opioid Peptides: Biochemistry, Anatomy,
           and Physiology, Stanley J. Watson 1186
    200.2 Prostaglandins and Related Compounds,
           Garret A. FitzGerald 1187
    200.3 Natriuretic Hormones, Dennis A. Ausiello 1194
201 NEUROENDOCRINOLOGY 1197
    201.1 The Neuroendocrine System, Mark E. Molitch 1197
    201.2 The Pineal Gland, Alfred J. Lewy 1204
202 THE PITUITARY 1205
    202.1 Anterior Pituitary, J. Larry Jameson 1205
    202.2 Posterior Pituitary, Alan G. Robinson 1221
203 THE THYROID, Wolfgang H. Dillmann 1227
204 THE ADRENAL GLAND 1245
    204.1 Adrenal Cortex, D. Lynn Loriaux 1245
    204.2 Adrenal Medulla, Daniel T. O'Connor 1253
205 DIABETES MELLITUS, Robert S. Sherwin 1258
206 HYPOGLYCEMIA/PANCREATIC ISLET CELL DISORDERS, Jeffrey S. Flier ...1278
    206.1 Hypoglycemia 1278
    206.2 Islet Cell Tumors 1282
207 DISORDERS OF SEXUAL DIFFERENTIATION, Maria I. New and
    Nathalie Josso 1284
208 ENDOCRINOLOGIC DISEASES UNIQUE TO WOMEN 1293
    208.1 The Ovaries, Robert W. Rebar 1293
    208.2 Ovarian Carcinoma, Howard W. Jones, III 1313
    208.3 Hirsutism, Roger S. Rittmaster 1315
    208.4 Nonmalignant Diseases of the Breast, Douglas J. Marchant ..1317
    208.5 Breast Cancer, Brian J. Lewis and Robert M. Conry 1320
209 ENDOCRINOLOGIC DISEASES UNIQUE TO MEN 1325
    209.1 The Testis, Alvin M. Matsumoto 1325
    209.2 Diseases of the Prostate, Gary D. Steinberg and
           Charles B. Brendler 1341
210 MULTIPLE-ORGAN SYNDROMES 1345
    210.1 Polyglandular Disorders, Henry M. Kronenberg 1345
    210.2 Carcinoid Syndrome, John A. Oates 1348

PART XVIII DISEASES OF BONE AND BONE
            MINERAL METABOLISM

211 MINERAL AND BONE HOMEOSTASIS, Stephen J. Marx 1351
212 VITAMIN D, Bess Dawson-Hughes 1357
213 OSTEOMALACIA AND RICKETS, Marc K. Drezner 1359
214 THE PARATHYROID GLANDS, HYPERCALCEMIA, AND HYPOCALCEMIA,
    Allen M. Spiegel 1365
215 CALCITONIN AND MEDULLARY THYROID CARCINOMA, Leonard J. Deftos .1373
216 RENAL OSTEODYSTROPHY, Eduardo Slatopolsky 1375
217 OSTEOPOROSIS, Joel S. Finkelstein 1379
218 PAGET'S DISEASE OF BONE (Osteitis Deformans), John A. Kanis 1384
219 OSTEONECROSIS, OSTEOSCLEROSIS, AND OTHER DISORDERS OF BONE,
    Michael P. Whyte 1387
220 BONE TUMORS, Daniel I. Rosenthal 1391

PART XIX DISEASES OF THE IMMUNE SYSTEM

221 APPROACH TO THE PATIENT WITH IMMUNE DISEASE, J. Claude Bennett .1393
222 COMPLEMENT, John E. Volanakis 1398
223 PRIMARY IMMUNODEFICIENCY DISEASES, Rebecca H. Buckley 1401
224 URTICARIA AND ANGIOEDEMA, Michael M. Frank 1408
225 ALLERGIC RHINITIS, Richard D. deShazo 1413
226 ANAPHYLAXIS, Allen P. Kaplan 1417
227 INSECT STING ALLERGY, Lawrence M. Lichtenstein 1420
228 IMMUNE COMPLEX DISEASES, Richard D. deShazo 1421
229 THE MAJOR HISTOCOMPATIBILITY COMPLEX AND DISEASE SUSCEPTIBILITY,
    Benjamin D. Schwartz 1424
230 DRUG ALLERGY, James R. Bonner 1432
231 MASTOCYTOSIS, Dean D. Metcalfe 1435
232 DISEASES OF THE THYMUS, Max D. Cooper 1437

PART XX MUSCULOSKELETAL AND CONNECTIVE TISSUE DISEASES

233 APPROACH TO THE PATIENT WITH MUSCULOSKELETAL DISEASE, *Duncan A. Gordon* 1440
234 CONNECTIVE TISSUE STRUCTURE AND FUNCTION, *Steffen Gay and Renate E. Gay* 1443
235 TISSUE INJURY IN RHEUMATIC DISEASES, *Gerald Weissmann* 1448
236 SPECIALIZED PROCEDURES IN THE MANAGEMENT OF PATIENTS WITH RHEUMATIC DISEASES, *Robert W. Ike and William J. Arnold* 1455
237 RHEUMATOID ARTHRITIS, *Frank C. Arnett* 1459
238 THE SPONDYLARTHROPATHIES, *John J. Cush and Peter E. Lipsky* 1466
239 INFECTIOUS ARTHRITIS, *Luis R. Espinoza* 1473
240 SYSTEMIC LUPUS ERYTHEMATOSUS, *Peter H. Schur* 1475
241 SYSTEMIC SCLEROSIS *(Scleroderma)*, *E. Carwile LeRoy* 1483
242 SJÖGREN'S SYNDROME, *Marc C. Hochberg* 1488
243 THE VASCULITIC SYNDROMES, *Lanny J. Rosenwasser* 1490
244 POLYARTERITIS NODOSA GROUP, *Lanny J. Rosenwasser* 1492
245 WEGENER'S GRANULOMATOSIS, *Nancy B. Allen* 1495
246 POLYMYALGIA RHEUMATICA AND GIANT CELL ARTERITIS, *Gene G. Hunder* 1498
247 IDIOPATHIC INFLAMMATORY MYOPATHIES, *Robert L. Wortmann* 1500
248 THE AMYLOID DISEASES, *Louis W. Heck* 1504
249 BEHÇET'S DISEASE, *Eugene V. Ball* 1506
250 PANNICULITIS AND DISORDERS OF THE SUBCUTANEOUS FAT, *Gerald S. Lazarus* 1507
251 GOUT AND URIC ACID METABOLISM, *Michael S. Hershfield* 1508
252 OTHER CRYSTAL DEPOSITION ARTHROPATHIES, *H. Ralph Schumacher, Jr.* 1515
253 RELAPSING POLYCHONDRITIS, *H. Ralph Schumacher, Jr.* 1517
254 OSTEOARTHRITIS *(Degenerative Bone Disease)*, *Thomas J. Schnitzer* ... 1517
255 THE PAINFUL SHOULDER, *Dennis W. Boulware* 1521
256 SYSTEMIC DISEASES IN WHICH ARTHRITIS IS A FEATURE, *Eugene V. Ball* 1525
257 MISCELLANEOUS FORMS OF ARTHRITIS, *Eugene V. Ball* 1526
258 NONARTICULAR RHEUMATISM, *Eugene V. Ball* 1527
259 ARTICULAR TUMORS, *Eugene V. Ball* 1528
260 ERYTHROMELALGIA, *Eugene V. Ball* 1528
261 MULTIFOCAL FIBROSCLEROSIS, *H. Ralph Schumacher, Jr.* 1529

PART XXI INFECTIOUS DISEASES

Introduction
262 INTRODUCTION TO MICROBIAL DISEASE, *Gerald L. Mandell* 1531
263 THE FEBRILE PATIENT, *David C. Dale* 1532
264 THE PATHOGENESIS OF FEVER, *Bruce Beutler and Steven M. Beutler* 1533
265 THE ACUTE PHASE RESPONSE, *Charles A. Dinarello* 1535
266 THE COMPROMISED HOST, *Philip A. Pizzo* 1537
267 PREVENTION AND CONTROL OF HOSPITAL-ACQUIRED INFECTIONS, *William Schaffner* 1548
268 ADVICE TO TRAVELERS, *Richard D. Pearson* 1553

Bacterial Diseases
269 INTRODUCTION TO BACTERIAL DISEASE, *Gerald L. Mandell* 1556
270 ANTIBACTERIAL THERAPY, *Adolf W. Karchmer* 1558
271 PNEUMOCOCCAL PNEUMONIA, *Richard J. Duma.* 1569
272 MYCOPLASMAL INFECTION, *David Schlossberg* 1576
273 PNEUMONIA CAUSED BY AEROBIC GRAM-NEGATIVE BACILLI, *Waldemar G. Johanson, Jr.* 1579
274 ASPIRATION PNEUMONIA, *Waldemar G. Johanson, Jr.* 1581
275 LEGIONELLOSIS, *Paul H. Edelstein* 1583
276 STREPTOCOCCAL INFECTIONS, *Dennis L. Stevens* 1585
277 RHEUMATIC FEVER, *Alan L. Bisno* 1590
278 INFECTIVE ENDOCARDITIS, *Matthew E. Levison* 1596
279 STAPHYLOCOCCAL INFECTIONS, *Gordon L. Archer* 1605

Bacterial Meningitis
280 BACTERIAL MENINGITIS, *Morton N. Swartz* 1610
281 MENINGOCOCCAL INFECTIONS, *Michael A. Apicella* 1618
282 INFECTIONS CAUSED BY *HAEMOPHILUS* SPECIES, *Michael S. Simberkoff* 1622

Osteomyelitis
283 OSTEOMYELITIS, *Barry D. Brause* 1625

Whooping Cough
284 WHOOPING COUGH *(Pertussis)*, *Richard B. Johnston, Jr.* 1627

Diphtheria
285 DIPHTHERIA, *Iain R. B. Hardy* 1629

Clostridial Disease
286 CLOSTRIDIAL MYONECROSIS AND OTHER CLOSTRIDIAL DISEASES, *Dennis L. Stevens* 1630
287 PSEUDOMEMBRANOUS COLITIS, *Robert Fekety* 1633
288 BOTULISM, *John G. Bartlett* 1635
289 TETANUS, *John G. Bartlett* 1636

Anaerobic Bacteria
290 DISEASES CAUSED BY NON–SPORE-FORMING ANAEROBIC BACTERIA, *Ellie J. C. Goldstein* 1638

Enteric Infections
291 INTRODUCTION TO ENTERIC INFECTIONS, *Herbert L. DuPont* 1641
292 TYPHOID FEVER, *Thomas Butler* 1642
293 *SALMONELLA* INFECTIONS OTHER THAN TYPHOID FEVER, *Donald Kaye* 1644
294 SHIGELLOSIS, *Thomas Butler* 1647
295 *CAMPYLOBACTER* ENTERITIS, *Richard L. Guerrant* 1649
296 CHOLERA, *William B. Greenough, III* 1652
297 ENTERIC *ESCHERICHIA COLI* INFECTIONS, *Richard L. Guerrant* 1654
298 THE DIARRHEA OF TRAVELERS, *R. Bradley Sack* 1657
299 EXTRAINTESTINAL INFECTIONS CAUSED BY ENTERIC BACTERIA, *Elizabeth J. Ziegler* 1659

Other Bacterial Infections
300 *YERSINIA* INFECTIONS, *J. Glenn Morris, Jr.* 1661
301 TULAREMIA, *Richard B. Hornick* 1662
302 ANTHRAX, *Jonas A. Shulman* 1664
303 DISEASES CAUSED BY PSEUDOMONADS, *Stephen C. Schimpff* 1667
304 LISTERIOSIS, *Alan M. Stamm* 1672
305 ERYSIPELOID, *Annette C. Reboli* 1673
306 ACTINOMYCOSIS, *Ward E. Bullock* 1674
307 NOCARDIOSIS, *Ward E. Bullock* 1676
308 BRUCELLOSIS, *Robert A. Salata* 1678
309 CAT SCRATCH DISEASE AND BACILLARY ANGIOMATOSIS, *David A. Relman* 1680
310 BARTONELLOSIS, *C. Glenn Cobbs* 1682

Diseases Due to Mycobacteria
311 TUBERCULOSIS, *Michael D. Iseman* 1683
312 OTHER MYCOBACTERIOSES, *Laurel C. Preheim* 1690
313 LEPROSY *(Hansen's Disease)*, *Gilla Kaplan and Zanvil A. Cohn* 1691

Sexually Transmitted Diseases
314 INTRODUCTION TO SEXUALLY TRANSMITTED DISEASES AND COMMON SYNDROMES, *P. Frederick Sparling* 1696
315 GONOCOCCAL INFECTIONS, *P. Frederick Sparling* 1700
316 GRANULOMA INGUINALE *(Donovanosis)*, *Edward W. Hook III* 1703
317 CHANCROID, *Edward W. Hook III* 1704
318 SYPHILIS, *Edward W. Hook III* 1705

Spirochetal Diseases Other Than Syphilis
319 NONSYPHILITIC TREPONEMATOSES, *Edward W. Hook III* 1714
320 RELAPSING FEVER, *William A. Petri, Jr.* 1715
321 LYME DISEASE, *Stephen E. Malawista* 1715
322 LEPTOSPIROSIS, *William A. Petri, Jr.* 1720
323 DISEASES CAUSED BY CHLAMYDIAE, *Robert C. Brunham* 1721
324 RICKETTSIAL DISEASES, *Richard B. Hornick* 1726
    Introduction 1726
    324.1 The Typhus Group 1726
    324.2 Rocky Mountain Spotted Fever 1730
    324.3 Other Tick-borne Rickettsioses 1732
    324.4 Rickettsialpox 1733
    324.5 Scrub Typhus 1734
    324.6 Q Fever 1735
325 ZOONOSES, *Stuart Levin* 1737

Viral Diseases
326 INTRODUCTION TO VIRAL DISEASES, *R. Gordon Douglas, Jr.* 1739
327 ANTIVIRAL THERAPY *(Non-AIDS)*, *Richard J. Whitley* 1742

Viral Infections of the Respiratory Tract
328 THE COMMON COLD, *J. Owen Hendley* 1747
329 VIRAL PHARYNGITIS, LARYNGITIS, CROUP, AND BRONCHITIS, *Maurice A. Mufson* 1749
330 RESPIRATORY SYNCYTIAL VIRUS, *Edward E. Walsh* 1751
331 PARAINFLUENZA VIRAL DISEASE, *Edward E. Walsh* 1752
332 INFLUENZA, *Frederick G. Hayden* 1753
333 ADENOVIRUS DISEASES, *John J. Treanor* 1757

Exanthems and Mumps

334 MEASLES, *Philip A. Brunell* 1759
335 RUBELLA *(German Measles), Philip A. Brunell* 1761
336 VARICELLA *(Chickenpox, Shingles), Philip A. Brunell* 1763
337 VARIOLA AND VACCINIA, *Donald A. Henderson* 1765
338 MUMPS, *John W. Gnann, Jr.* 1768

The Herpes Group of Viruses

339 HERPES SIMPLEX VIRUS INFECTIONS, *Richard J. Whitley* 1770
340 INFECTIONS ASSOCIATED WITH HUMAN CYTOMEGALOVIRUS,
      William J. Britt 1774
341 INFECTIOUS MONONUCLEOSIS: EPSTEIN-BARR VIRUS INFECTION,
      Elliott D. Kieff 1776

Retroviruses

342 RETROVIRUSES OTHER THAN HIV, *William A. Blattner* 1779

Enteric Viral Infections

343 ENTEROVIRUSES, *Michael N. Oxman* 1783
344 VIRAL GASTROENTERITIS, *Albert Z. Kapikian* 1793

Hemorrhagic Fever Viruses

345 INTRODUCTION TO HEMORRHAGIC FEVER VIRUSES, *Robert E. Shope* 1797
      345.1 Yellow Fever 1798
      345.2 Hemorrhagic Fever Caused by Dengue Viruses 1800
      345.3 Tick-Borne Flavivirus Diseases: Kyasanur Forest Disease and
              Omsk Hemorrhagic Fever 1801
      345.4 Crimean-Congo Hemorrhagic Fever 1802
      345.5 Hemorrhagic Diseases Caused by Arenaviruses *(Argentine,
              Bolivian, Venezuelan, and Brazilian Hemorrhagic Fevers and
              Lassa Fever)* 1802
      345.6 African-Hemorrhagic Fever *(Marburg-Ebola Disease)* 1803
      345.7 Hemorrhagic Fever with Renal Syndrome 1804
      345.8 Hantavirus Pulmonary Syndrome 1804
346 OTHER ARTHROPOD-BORNE VIRUSES, *R. Gordon Douglas, Jr.* 1805

The Mycoses

347 INTRODUCTION TO THE MYCOSES, *William E. Dismukes* 1815
348 HISTOPLASMOSIS, *William E. Dismukes* 1816
349 COCCIDIOIDOMYCOSIS, *John N. Galgiani* 1819
350 BLASTOMYCOSIS, *William E. Dismukes* 1821
351 PARACOCCIDIOIDOMYCOSIS, *William E. Dismukes* 1822
352 CRYPTOCOCCOSIS, *William E. Dismukes* 1823
353 SPOROTRICHOSIS, *William E. Dismukes* 1826
354 CANDIDIASIS, *William E. Dismukes* 1827
355 ASPERGILLOSIS, *David A. Stevens* 1830
356 MUCORMYCOSIS, *Sandy F. S. Chun and David A. Stevens* 1832
357 MYCETOMA, *Michael S. Saag* 1834
358 DEMATIACEOUS FUNGAL INFECTIONS, *Michael S. Saag* 1836

**PART XXII HIV AND THE ACQUIRED
                   IMMUNODEFICIENCY SYNDROME**

359 INTRODUCTION TO HIV AND ASSOCIATED DISORDERS,
      Gerald L. Mandell 1837
360 IMMUNOLOGY RELATED TO AIDS, *Bruce D. Walker* 1837
361 BIOLOGY OF HUMAN IMMUNODEFICIENCY VIRUSES,
      George M. Shaw 1841
362 EPIDEMIOLOGY OF HIV INFECTION AND AIDS, *James W. Curran* 1846
363 PREVENTION OF HIV INFECTION, *Michael S. Saag* 1851
364 NEUROLOGIC COMPLICATIONS OF HIV-1 INFECTION,
      Richard W. Price 1855
365 PULMONARY MANIFESTATIONS OF HIV INFECTION,
      Philip C. Hopewell 1858
366 GASTROINTESTINAL MANIFESTATIONS OF AIDS, *John G. Bartlett* 1866
367 CUTANEOUS SIGNS OF AIDS, *Neal S. Penneys* 1868
368 OPHTHALMOLOGIC MANIFESTATIONS OF AIDS, *Mark A. Jacobson* 1868
369 HEMATOLOGY/ONCOLOGY IN AIDS, *David T. Scadden and
      Jerome E. Groopman* 1870
370 RENAL, CARDIAC, ENDOCRINE, AND RHEUMATOLOGIC MANIFESTATIONS
      OF HIV INFECTION, *Michael S. Saag* 1875
371 TREATMENT OF HIV INFECTION AND AIDS, *Robert Yarchoan and
      Samuel Broder* 1880
372 MANAGEMENT AND COUNSELING FOR PERSONS WITH HIV INFECTION,
      John A. Bartlett 1888

**PART XXIII DISEASES OF PROTOZOA AND
                    METAZOA**

373 INTRODUCTION TO PROTOZOAN AND HELMINTHIC DISEASES,
      Adel A. F. Mahmoud 1892

Protozoan Diseases

374 MALARIA, *Donald J. Krogstad* 1893
375 AFRICAN TRYPANOSOMIASIS *(Sleeping Sickness), Thomas C. Quinn* 1896
376 AMERICAN TRYPANOSOMIASIS *(Chagas' Disease), Franklin A. Neva* 1899
377 LEISHMANIASIS, *Richard D. Pearson and
      Anastacio de Queiroz Sousa* 1903
378 TOXOPLASMOSIS, *Carlos S. Subauste and Jack S. Remington* 1907
379 CRYPTOSPORIDIOSIS, *Rosemary Soave* 1910
380 GIARDIASIS, *David P. Stevens* 1912
381 AMEBIASIS, *Jonathan I. Ravdin* 1913
382 OTHER PROTOZOAN DISEASES, *Richard D. Pearson* 1915
383 *PNEUMOCYSTIS CARINII* PNEUMONIA, *Fred R. Sattler* 1917

Helminthic Diseases

384 CESTODE INFECTIONS, *Charles H. King* 1922
385 SCHISTOSOMIASIS *(Bilharziasis), Adel A. F. Mahmoud* 1927
386 LIVER, INTESTINAL, AND LUNG FLUKE INFECTIONS, *Adel A. F. Mahmoud* 1931
387 NEMATODE INFECTIONS, *James W. Kazura* 1934
388 FILARIASIS, *Eric A. Ottesen* 1939
      388.1 Introduction 1939
      388.2 Lymphatic Filariasis 1940
      388.3 Tropical Eosinophilia 1942
      388.4 Onchocerciasis (River Blindness) 1942
      388.5 Loiasis 1943
      388.6 Dracunculiasis 1944
      388.7 Other Filarial Infections 1944
389 ARTHROPODS AND LEECHES, *William L. Krinsky* 1945
390 SNAKE BITES, *Jay P. Sanford* 1951
391 VENOMS AND POISONS FROM MARINE ORGANISMS, *Jay W. Fox* 1953

PART XXIV NEUROLOGY

Section One   Principles of Clinical Neurologic Diagnosis

392 CLINICAL STUDY OF THE PATIENT 1957
      392.1 Approach to the Patient, *Fred Plum and Jerome B. Posner* .. 1957
      392.2 Clinical Diagnosis, *Fred Plum and Jerome B. Posner* 1958
      392.3 The Neurologic History, *Jerome B. Posner* 1958
      392.4 The Neurologic Examination, *Fred Plum* 1959
      392.5 Neurologic Diagnostic Procedures, *Jonathan D. Victor* 1959
      392.6 Radiologic Imaging Procedures, *Michael Deck* 1962

Section Two   Disorders of Cerebral Function

393 DISTURBANCES OF CONSCIOUSNESS AND AROUSAL, *Fred Plum* 1969
394 SUSTAINED IMPAIRMENTS OF CONSCIOUSNESS, *Fred Plum* 1970
395 BRAIN DEATH, *Fred Plum* 1978
396 BRIEF LOSS OF CONSCIOUSNESS, *Fred Plum* 1979
      396.1 Syncope 1979
      396.2 Nonsyncopal Causes of Brief Alterations of Consciousness 1981
397 DISORDERS OF SLEEP AND AROUSAL, *Fred Plum* 1982
398 DIAGNOSIS OF REGIONAL CEREBRAL DYSFUNCTION,
      Antonio R. Damasio 1985
399 DISTURBANCES OF MEMORY AND LANGUAGE, *Antonio R. Damasio* 1988
400 ALZHEIMER'S DISEASE AND RELATED DEMENTIAS, *Antonio R. Damasio* .1992
401 PSYCHIATRIC DISORDERS IN MEDICAL PRACTICE, *Gary J. Tucker* 1996

**Section Three   Pathophysiology and Management
                        of Major Neurologic Symptoms**

402 AUTONOMIC DISORDERS AND THEIR MANAGEMENT, *Clifford B. Saper* ... 2007
403 THE SPECIAL SENSES, *Robert W. Baloh* 2014
      403.1 Smell and Taste 2014
      403.2 Neuro-ophthalmology 2015
      403.3 Hearing and Equilibrium 2021
404 DISORDERS OF MOTOR FUNCTION, *Fred Plum* 2027
      404.1 Weakness, Asthenia, and Fatigue 2027
      404.2 Ataxia and Related Gait Disorders 2028
405 DISORDERS OF SENSATION, *Jerome B. Posner* 2030
      405.1 Major Sensory Symptoms 2030
      405.2 Headache and Other Head Pain 2031
      405.3 Some Specific Pain Syndromes 2036
      405.4 The Painful Back, *David S. Howell* 2037
406 NUTRITIONAL DISORDERS OF THE NERVOUS SYSTEM, *Robert Messing* ...2039

Section Four   The Extrapyramidal Disorders, *Joseph Jankovic*
407   INTRODUCTION 2042
408   PARKINSONISM 2044
409   TREMORS 2047
410   DYSTONIAS 2047
411   CHOREAS, ATHETOSIS, AND BALLISM 2048
412   TICS, MYOCLONUS, AND STEREOTYPIES 2049

Section Five   Degenerative Diseases of the Nervous System,
           Robert B. Layzer
413   HEREDITARY CEREBELLAR ATAXIAS AND RELATED DISORDERS 2051
414   HEREDITARY SPASTIC PARAPLEGIAS 2052
415   HEREDITARY AND ACQUIRED INTRINSIC MOTOR NEURON DISEASES 2052
416   SYRINGOMYELIA 2055
417   THE PHAKOMATOSES 2056

Section Six   Cerebrovascular Diseases, *William A. Pulsinelli*
418   CEREBROVASCULAR DISEASES—PRINCIPLES 2057
419   ISCHEMIC CEREBROVASCULAR DISEASE 2063
      419.1   Focal Ischemia 2063
      419.2   Diffuse Ischemia 2073
420   ISCHEMIC CEREBROVASCULAR DISEASE 2073
      420.1   Aneurysmal Subarachnoid Hemorrhage 2073
      420.2   Hemorrhage from Vascular Malformations 2076
      420.3   Focal Cerebral Hemorrhage 2077
      420.4   Hypertensive Encephalopathy 2080

Section Seven   Infections and Inflammatory Disorders
           of the Nervous System, *Roger P. Simon*
421   PARAMENINGEAL INFECTIONS 2080
422   NEUROSYPHILIS 2085

Section Eight   Viral Infections of the Nervous System
423   INTRODUCTION, *Richard W. Price* 2087
424   ACUTE VIRAL MENINGITIS AND ENCEPHALITIS, *Richard W. Price* .. 2088
425   POLIOMYELITIS, *Richard W. Price* 2091
426   HERPESVIRUS INFECTIONS OF THE NERVOUS SYSTEM, *Richard W. Price* . 2092
      426.1   Herpes Simplex Encephalitis (HSE) 2092
      426.2   Neurologic Complications of Genital Herpes 2093
      426.3   Neurologic Complications of Varicella-Zoster Virus Infections ... 2093
      426.4   Neurologic Complications of Cytomegalovirus and Epstein-Barr
              Virus Infections 2095
427   RABIES, *Richard W. Price* 2095
428   SLOW VIRUS INFECTIONS OF THE NERVOUS SYSTEM, *Richard W. Price* .. 2097
      428.1   Introduction 2097
      428.2   Human Immunodeficiency Virus Infection and the AIDS
              Dementia Complex 2097
      428.3   Human T Cell Lymphotropic Virus Type I-Associated Myelopathy
              and Tropical Spastic Paraparesis 2099
      428.4   Subacute Sclerosing Panencephalitis and Progressive
              Rubella Panencephalitis 2100
      428.5   Progressive Multifocal Leukoencephalopathy 2101
      428.6   Creutzfeldt-Jakob Disease, *Paul E. Bendheim* 2102

Section Nine   Neurologic Disorders Associated with
           Altered Immunity or Unexplained Host-Parasite
           Alterations, *Richard A. Rudick*
429   CENTRAL NERVOUS SYSTEM COMPLICATIONS OF VIRAL INFECTIONS
      AND VACCINES 2103
430   REYE SYNDROME 2105
431   NEUROLOGIC COMPLICATIONS IN THE IMMUNOLOGICALLY
      COMPROMISED HOST 2105

Section Ten   The Demyelinating Diseases *Richard A. Rudick*
432   MULTIPLE SCLEROSIS AND RELATED CONDITIONS 2106

Section Eleven   The Epilepsies *Timothy A. Pedley*
433   THE EPILEPSIES 2113

Section Twelve   Intracranial Tumors and States
           of Altered Intracranial Pressure, *Nicholas A. Vick*
434   INTRACRANIAL TUMORS 2125
435   SPECIFIC TYPES OF BRAIN TUMORS AND THEIR MANAGEMENT 2130
436   DISORDERS OF INTRACRANIAL PRESSURE 2132

Section Thirteen   Injury to the Head and Spinal Cord,
           Lawrence F. Marshall
437   HEAD INJURY 2135
438   SPINAL CORD INJURY 2139

Section Fourteen   Mechanical Lesions of Nerve Roots and Spinal Cord,
           Jerome B. Posner
439   ANATOMY, PHYSIOLOGY, AND DIFFERENTIAL DIAGNOSIS 2141
440   INTERVERTEBRAL DISC DISEASE 2144
441   NEOPLASMS OF THE SPINAL CANAL 2146
442   INFLAMMATORY DISEASES COMPRESSING THE SPINAL CORD 2148
443   VASCULAR DISORDERS COMPRESSING THE SPINAL CORD 2148
444   CONGENITAL ANOMALIES OF THE CRANIOVERTEBRAL JUNCTION, SPINE AND
      SPINAL CORD 2149

Section Fifteen   Diseases of the Peripheral Nervous System,
           John W. Griffin
445   ANATOMY AND BASIC TERMINOLOGY 2150
446   PATHOPHYSIOLOGY OF PERIPHERAL NEUROPATHIES 2150
447   IMMUNE-MEDIATED NEUROPATHIES 2151
448   HEREDITARY NEUROPATHIES 2153
449   METABOLIC NEUROPATHIES 2154
450   TOXIC NEUROPATHIES 2156
451   NEUROPATHIES ASSOCIATED WITH INFECTIOUS DISEASES 2156
452   ENTRAPMENT AND COMPRESSIVE NEUROPATHIES 2157

Section Sixteen   Diseases of Muscle (Myopathies) and Neuromuscular
           Junction, *Andrew G. Engel*
453   GENERAL APPROACH TO MUSCLE DISEASES 2158
454   MUSCULAR DYSTROPHIES 2161
455   MORPHOLOGICALLY DISTINCT CONGENITAL MYOPATHIES 2163
456   INFLAMMATORY MYOPATHIES 2163
457   METABOLIC MYOPATHIES 2165
458   MISCELLANEOUS MYOPATHIES 2170
459   DISORDERS OF NEUROMUSCULAR TRANSMISSION 2171

PART XXV   EYE DISEASES, *John W. Gittinger, Jr.*
460   VISUAL LOSS 2174
461   CATARACT 2175
462   GLAUCOMA 2175
463   DISC SWELLING AND OPTIC ATROPHY 2177
464   UVEITIS 2178
465   OCULAR INFECTIONS 2179
466   ORBITAL DISEASE AND TUMORS 2180
467   INTRAOCULAR TUMORS 2180
468   EPISCLERITIS, SCLERITIS, AND THE DRY EYE 2181
469   OCULAR VASCULAR DISEASE 2181
470   THE EYE AND MEDICATIONS 2183

PART XXVI   SKIN DISEASES
471   INTRODUCTION, *Frank Parker* 2184
472   STRUCTURE AND FUNCTION OF SKIN, *Frank Parker* 2184
473   EXAMINATION OF THE SKIN AND AN APPROACH
      TO DIAGNOSING SKIN DISEASES, *Frank Parker* 2190
474   PRINCIPLES OF THERAPY, *Frank Parker* 2193
475   SKIN DISEASES OF GENERAL IMPORTANCE, *Frank Parker* 2197
476   OCCUPATIONAL DISEASES OF THE SKIN, *Edward A. Emmett* 2220

PART XXVII   LABORATORY REFERENCE INTERVALS
           AND VALUES
477   REFERENCE INTERVALS AND LABORATORY VALUES, *Ronald J. Elin* .. 2223

INDEX I

COLOR PLATES

GASTROINTESTINAL DISEASES

Plate 1   (between pages 646 and 647)

GASTROINTESTINAL AND CARDIOVASCULAR DISEASES

Plate 2   (between pages 646 and 647)

CARDIOVASCULAR AND RHEUMATOLOGIC DISEASES

Plate 3   (between pages 646 and 647)

RENAL DISEASES

Plate 4   (between pages 646 and 647)

HEMATOLOGIC DISEASES

Plates 5–8   (between pages 838 and 839)

INFECTIOUS AND PROTOZOAN DISEASES

Plate 9   (between pages 1814 and 1815)

INFECTIOUS, MUSCULOSKELETAL, AND PROTOZOAN DISEASES

Plate 10   (between pages 1814 and 1815)

INFECTIOUS DISEASES AND HIV

Plate 11   (between pages 1814 and 1815)

HIV AND ASSOCIATED DISORDERS

Plate 12   (between pages 1814 and 1815)

EYE DISEASES

Plates 13 and 14   (between pages 2198 and 2199)

SKIN DISEASES

Plates 15–20   (between pages 2198 and 2199)

The following codes refer to the approximate magnification of the hematology color photomicrographs.

(L.P.) = Low-power magnification (dry)

(H.P.) = High-power magnification (dry)

(L.O.) = Low oil immersion magnification ($\sim 800-1000 \times$)

(H.O.) = High oil immersion magnification ($\sim 1500 \times$)

(V.H.O.) = Very high oil magnification (significantly in excess of $1500 \times$)

HIGHLIGHTED TABLES

The tables listed below contain important information about administering medications, their possible interactions, and necessary precautions as well as immunization information. Highlighted tables are indicated in the text by a check mark.

PART III AGING AND GERIATRIC MEDICINE

CHAPTER 7
NEUROPSYCHIATRIC ASPECTS OF AGING
Table 7–4   Dosage and Relative Side Effects of Selected Antidepressants in Elderly Patients, p. 20

PART IV PREVENTIVE HEALTH CARE

CHAPTER 10
VACCINATION/IMMUNIZATION
Table 10–1   Passive Immunization for Adults, p. 41
Table 10–2   Selected Immunizing Agents Indicated for Adults, p. 42

PART V PRINCIPLES OF EVALUATION AND MANAGEMENT

CHAPTER 16
PRINCIPLES OF DRUG THERAPY
Table 16–1   Pharmacokinetic Parameters for Some Commonly Used Drugs, p. 91
Table 16–2   Adjustment of Drug Dosage in Renal Failure, p. 94
Table 16–5   Adverse Drug Reactions, p. 98

PART VII CARDIOVASCULAR DISEASES

CHAPTER 35
CARDIAC ARRHYTHMIAS
Table 35–6   Emergency Treatment of Cardiac Arrhythmias, p. 237
Table 35–11   Adverse Effects of Antiarrhythmic Drugs, p. 247

PART IX CRITICAL CARE MEDICINE

CHAPTER 72
ACUTE POISONING
Table 72–1   Common Emergency Antidotes, p. 504

PART XIX DISEASES OF THE IMMUNE SYSTEM

CHAPTER 230
DRUG ALLERGY
Table 230–4 β-Lactam Desensitization, p. 1435

PART XXI INFECTIOUS DISEASES

CHAPTER 268
ADVICE TO TRAVELERS
Table 268–1   Immunization of International Travelers, p. 1554
Table 268–2   Chemoprophylaxis for Malaria, p. 1555
CHAPTER 270
ANTIBACTERIAL THERAPY
Table 270–3   Dosage, Pharmacologic Factors, and Adjustment in Renal and Hepatic Failure, p. 1562
Table 270–4   Important Antibiotic-Drug Interactions, p. 1563
Table 270–5   Antibacterial Drugs of Choice for Infections Caused by Selected Bacteria, p. 1564
Table 270–6   Activity of Major Antibiotics Against Selected Organisms, p. 1566
Table 270–7   Untoward Effects of Antimicrobial Agents, p. 1568

CHAPTER 278
INFECTIVE ENDOCARDITIS
Table 278–8   Antibiotic Therapy (Adult Doses), p. 1603
Table 278–11   Prophylactic Regimens for Bacterial Endocarditis, p. 1604

PART XXII   HIV AND THE ACQUIRED IMMUNODEFICIENCY SYNDROME

CHAPTER 371
TREATMENT OF HIV INFECTION AND AIDS
Table 371–3   Selected Antiretroviral Drugs (Experimental and Approved) for the Therapy of AIDS, p. 1885
Table 371–4   Recommendations for Antiretroviral Therapy of HIV-Infected Adults for a 1993 State-of-the-Art Conference, p. 1887

PART XVII   LABORATORY REFERENCE INTERVALS AND VALUES

CHAPTER 477
REFERENCE INTERVALS AND LABORATORY VALUES, p. 2223

CECIL
TEXTBOOK
OF
MEDICINE

PART I

MEDICINE AS A LEARNED AND HUMANE PROFESSION

1 MEDICINE AS A LEARNED AND HUMANE PROFESSION

J. Claude Bennett and
Fred Plum

Becoming a physician has meaning far beyond completing medical school and residency. It is the entry to a way of life, the one characteristic common to every true profession. It may sound old-fashioned, but the learned professions are really "callings" from which the members cannot separate their lives. There are no part-time professionals; having accepted such a calling, one is bound to live it or to leave it. This does not mean that a physician cannot be a good spouse, a good parent, or a good citizen of his/her community; it just means that the spouse, parent, and citizen is always a physician as well.

The paragraphs that follow stress the scientific infrastructure of medicine as one of the keys to the profession. We then discuss the physician as scientist, the physician as caregiver, and the melding of these roles in the physician as professional. The environment in which the physician carries out his/her role and responsibilities is discussed in the final section dealing with systems of patient care as they are evolving at the close of the twentieth century.

THE SCIENTIFIC INFRASTRUCTURE OF MEDICINE

Medicine is not a science, but a profession that encompasses medical science learning as well as personal, humanistic, and professional attributes. Nonetheless, the delivery of Western medicine depends totally on science and the scientific method. Since Flexner issued his famous report on the subject in 1910, American medical education has strived to develop a strong scientific base as an integral part of medical education at every level: premedical, medical, residency, and continuing medical education. Biomedical science is fundamental to understanding disease, making diagnoses, applying new therapies, and appreciating the complexities and opportunities of new technologies. The process of becoming a physician and being committed to lifelong learning requires that one possess the scientific base not only to acquire and appreciate new knowledge but to see new ways for applying it to patient care as well. The physician must be able to understand reports of current research in the medical literature in order to grasp and evaluate the newest and latest approaches, no matter how complicated the field may become. That is why this textbook of medicine strongly emphasizes how things work, how they go amiss when pathologic processes ensue, and what effect a given therapy can be expected to have in correcting abnormalities. We seek to create in our readers a yearning for a greater depth of understanding and a continuing commitment to stay at the frontier of scientific knowledge throughout their professional lives.

Medicine has advanced to an outstanding degree in the past half century. (The 100 years from 1850 to 1950 were characterized—with the important exceptions of the discovery of penicillin, sulfon-

amides, and insulin—by the application of chemistry and physics to biologic materials, e.g., blood and urine, or to the body, e.g., roentgenography and sphygmomanometry, and by the empirical use of medicinal chemicals.) The advances of the last 50 years have come at the most fundamental levels of science and have reflected the general explosion in scientific knowledge worldwide. Much of this explosion has been stimulated by the strong influence of the American National Institutes of Health (NIH) and their programs of intramural research and extramural research support. Thanks to the NIH and a variety of public philanthropies, since World War II universities throughout the nation have become deeply engaged in biomedical science at levels that long precede applications to specific disease. What has come from these basic discoveries, however, has been the very substance of new technologies to understand and cure disease.

True understanding of disease processes depends on levels of scientific knowledge which are just being discovered. For example, when one learns how proteins are synthesized, fold into their native conformation, and express their various physical properties, one gains an understanding of why erythrocytes sickle when the β-chain of hemoglobin undergoes a Glu to Val change at amino acid number 6. One becomes able to understand the deposition of protein casts in multiple myeloma; the complexities of amyloid formation and how it influences organ function; the nature of protein aggregation as a fundamental process of Alzheimer's disease; and the importance of protein-protein interaction in transmitting messages across cell membranes, within the cytoplasm, and to the nucleus of cells. Once a student understands the way G-proteins function,* he/she understands how membrane transport events take place and messages transfer from the outside to the inside of cells. Furthermore, he/she gains an understanding of how microbial toxins operate, hormones influence cell action, and cells respond to external stimuli and are regulated in their response. When a student has knowledge of the basic processes of DNA synthesis, mutation, and somatic alteration of gene expression, he/she is in a position to understand inherited diseases as well as those that have their fundamental processes expressed in a continuous pattern of somatic alteration within a given individual. Understanding such pathogenetic processes and events is the essential first step in being able to identify and apply appropriate therapeutic maneuvers. Fundamental science is crucial as a knowledge base for any member of our profession. Fortunately, for a physician studying and learning in this complex environment, medical science has become so fundamental that understanding of a few fundamental and critical processes can provide insights into a whole variety of diseases.

A list of major clinical achievements in any particular branch of medicine reveals that more than 60% of the enabling discoveries arise from the category of very basic science and that these discoveries were made without any particular notion of how they might be applied to human disease. Our repertoire of breakthroughs in infectious diseases, the regulation of blood pressure, fundamental immunology, fundamental genetics, and metabolic regulation by hormones represents milestones in the course of medical history that

---

* The 1994 Nobel Prize for Physiology or Medicine was awarded to Alfred Gilman and Martin Rodbell for their discoveries relating to G-proteins.

now provide the tools to help unravel the intricacies of human disease. In spite of unbelievable successes, many diseases remain for which we still have no absolute answers. These include cancer, Alzheimer's disease, autoimmune diseases such as rheumatoid arthritis and lupus erythematosus, psychiatric diseases including manic-depressive psychosis and schizophrenia, and many others. Nonetheless, the clues now being ferreted out at the molecular level anticipate solutions of even these disorders, realistically filling our future expectations with excitement and anticipation.

The scientific infrastructure that we appreciate today is the springboard for the future in which most of the readers of *Cecil Textbook of Medicine,* 20th edition, will practice. Throughout most of the recorded history of medicine, diagnoses and therapies have not been based on scientific fact, and the degree of certainty with which physicians worked was inexact, if not totally flawed. But this has entirely changed: By 150 years ago things were beginning to change and by the 20 years spanning the turn of the century, the first fundamental lights began to illuminate the "golden age of microbiology." During this period, Pasteur, working in Paris, and Robert Koch, working in Berlin, began to unravel the intricacies of infectious diseases. To define microorganisms, to understand how they cause infection and transmit diseases, and to understand the host response represented a real turning point and forever established the scientific method as the basis for understanding and treating disease. It is an amazing experience to read the scientific papers from Paris and Berlin at that time because in a relatively short period those two schools of thought set us on a pathway from which medicine can never depart—that of demanding precision, of requiring experimental proof, and of building confidence by accumulating irrefutable data.

Today's medicine is more than intuition and common sense. It is precision based on a century or more of refining definitions of disease in highly specific terms. We now experience these "golden ages" in more rapid order: the discovery of antibiotics less than 60 years ago; an understanding of immunology in molecular terms within the last 30 years; and now in genetics, not just knowledge at the molecular level but understanding how to manipulate genes for the immediate benefit of mankind.

We are indeed in the age of molecular-biophysical medicine, an influence that permeates and unifies all of the traditional disciplines of medicine. Whether one is talking about inborn errors of metabolism, neurotransmitters, cytokines, oncogenes, or hormone regulation, all are being defined with exquisite detail at the molecular level. Programs aimed toward the goal of the human genome project—to totally sequence the DNA within the entire genome by the end of the century—are moving forward with accelerating speed. The ability to define every gene, its product, and its role and explicit function has become a shared international goal.

This pattern of attaining scientific knowledge, beginning with a sick patient and moving in a reductionist process to individual molecules and fundamental biochemical processes, should not be allowed to lessen our appreciation for the other contributors to the human condition. Advances in molecular and structural biology and the wonders of immunology and genetics must not allow us to neglect the many aspects of human psychology, anthropology, and sociology that influence the world in which we live and that play such a major role in morbidity and eventual mortality. According to the National Center for Health Statistics, behavioral causes—including alcohol, drugs, violence, suicide, smoking, and excessive aggression—generate more than half the cost to the nation for health care. We are only just beginning to grasp the impact of these factors on our nation and the world. In our joy—and sometimes arrogant pride—over achievements in molecular medicine, we must also humbly realize that the sciences that analyze human or population behavior and attempt to improve it, and the way society is structured, are indispensable to the future of medicine and must be incorporated into the discipline of our profession.

THE PHYSICIAN AS A SCIENTIST

Physicians must be trained as scientists if they are to use scientific medicine correctly. This involves understanding and applying the thinking patterns of the scientific method, developing an inquiring mind, knowing how to design experiments and obtain data, learning how to analyze the correctness and specificity of those data, and sensing how to evaluate it so as to ask questions and provide truthful answers within defined limits of precision. Biomedical science becomes the working instrument for the physician who by definition practices an analytic profession. Most of these learned skills extend to the management of individual cases at the bedside, i.e., how to gather data, how to synthesize it, how to interpret it to make a full diagnostic story, and how to bring collective wisdom together in the design and execution of appropriate therapy. A central tenet of all sciences is to constantly ask, "Could my conclusion be wrong?" The rigors of the scientific method also provide the physician with learning skills and a process of analysis that are indispensable to dealing with individual patients as well as providing the opportunity to contribute to medical progress and the improvement of care.

Every physician must delight in learning the new, correcting the old, and perfecting the future. Much of what medicine now accomplishes depends on large-scale testing of procedures, interventions, vaccines, and new drugs. The fact that many such studies must be conducted in large populations, through a multicenter approach, provides an opportunity for every physician to participate in clinical investigation in some way at some time in his/her professional career. Indeed, this step is essential for the future of medicine and for physicians to move forward together as a profession.

The goal of every patient-physician interaction is to reduce uncertainty (Ludo Baghuis, Philips Medical Systems. Best, The Netherlands, Personal communication, June 1992). When this goal is approached in a rigorous scientific manner, which does not mean coldly or impersonally, over time the results become reproducible and generalizable. New information, new techniques, and new technology can be brought into the process and their contribution evaluated in the conceptualization of the scientific method now popularly known as continuous quality improvement. Through such constant commitment to advancing the frontiers of medicine, physicians improve health, discover true cures, devise new ways of delivering care, and reduce ultimate health costs.

THE PHYSICIAN AS CAREGIVER

Being both professional and caring is an acquired skill. A physician can diagnose and prescribe in a technically correct and scientific, but insensitive, way. The patient may be made better, even cured, but still feel unsatisfied with the interaction. In these cases, patients are likely to ask the questions: Does my physician really care? Does what happens to me matter to him/her? Does my doctor show sensitivity and compassion beyond mere technical ability? Patients want to be listened to and understood. They want their physicians to be interested in them as individuals seeking relief from pain and uncertainty. They want to sense that they can safely share their deepest thoughts and their most heartfelt confidences with their physicians. In short, they want to value him/her as a trusted friend. Patients also expect to be kept informed while they are receiving competent professional service. As a caregiver, it is this sharing of oneself that is so very important.

To some it may seem odd to talk about caring as a learned skill, but it is just that. In studying to be a physician, one must learn both compassion and caring. Easy, supportive interaction with patients and others less fortunate is a skill that comes readily for some and with great difficulty for others. In learning how to demonstrate compassion, Kahlil Gibran taught us: "You give but little when you give of your possessions—it is when you give of yourself that you truly give" *(The Prophet).* The giving of oneself with ease, with grace, and with meaning is, for most persons, an acquired skill. Sometimes a deep sense of awakening within is required in order to release the innate sensitivity and compassion that perhaps have not been expressed since childhood. Nevertheless, these traits remain imperatives if our aim is to become the "complete physician."

When patients seek medical attention, they entrust their doctors with their very lives. The physician must earn such complete trust. Technical abilities and skilled treatment of disease alone do not suffice. Patients must believe that their physicians care about them as people, not just as patients. Physicians, in turn, must understand that they do far better as professionals if they err on the side of being human with their patients. Dag Hammarskjöld reminds us of "the humility that comes from others having faith in you." Without that touch of humility, physicians may be unable to understand and accept the trust that patients place in us. The physician must be willing to answer the patient's need and also willing to undertake a long-term commitment to the patient's care. This commitment continues beyond a single insightful diagnosis or the completion of a procedure. The patient still needs care when the data come back from the clinical laboratory, the radiology department, the cardiac catheterization laboratory, or surgical pathology laboratory. The patient continues to need help with understanding his/her disease, with family interactions, and in finding a caring ear when he/she suffers most. He/she often needs help with obtaining necessary additional medical help from specialists or consultants and personal help in dealing with processes involving families and personal situations. Many patients need a link to community or social support systems. A particularly difficult time comes as we deal with patients who become old, frail, dependent, crippled, or cognitively impaired. These are the circumstances from which the most sensitive among us truly learn what it means to give of ourselves. Sometimes we may find once again that our parents are the best teachers.

THE PHYSICIAN AS A PROFESSIONAL

To help orient our professional compass, the American Board of Internal Medicine recently promulgated a definition of "professionalism":

> Definition: Professionalism in internal medicine comprises those attributes and behaviors that serve to maintain the interest of the patient above one's own self-interest.
> - A commitment to the highest standards of excellence in the practice of medicine and in the generation and dissemination of knowledge.
> - A commitment to the attitudes and behaviors which sustain the interests and welfare of patients.
> - A commitment to be responsive to the health needs of society.
> Professionalism aspires to altruism, accountability, excellence, duty, service, honor, integrity and respect for others.

The interest of the patient lies above self-interest, providing an indispensable attribute, not only of medicine, but of all professions. It has to do with our personal behaviors transcending our technical abilities, our scientific knowledge, and even our attitudes of compassion and caring. What it means is that we offer to others a special sensitivity—whether they be physician colleagues, students, residents, nonphysician caregivers, patients, or their families. To remain professionals, a dignity and an understanding must permeate all of our interactions—all of our thinking, teaching, learning, and listening.

SYSTEMS OF PATIENT CARE FOR THE 1990's AND BEYOND

Students of medicine learn by didactics, observation, and directed participation. As they pass into residency, the avenues of participation become an increasingly independent course of training. In this intellectual experience of growing independence young physicians learn how to analyze information, organize it, render compassionate and considered care, and deal with their professional colleagues as well as with patients and their families. This historical independence of thought and action makes it difficult for many physicians who will be entering practice in the future to understand that the evolving changes in the health care delivery system will unavoidably affect that perceived level of independence.

The virtually anonymous third-party payers of the past have now emerged as aggressive, prudent purchasers who are highly competitive with other payers. Patient care in the mass is becoming a big business, at least as it relates to insurers, managed care organizations, and groups of employers. Each of these have virtual control of large blocks of "covered lives" (patients) and have enormous influence over whether, when, and which physicians and hospitals deliver services. The system has been evolving over the past several years because of the perceived complexity of health care delivery, the increasing costs ascribed to technology and professional subspecialization, and the sheer size of the fraction of gross national product dedicated to health care. American businesses, large and small, realize the need to exert some sort of cost brake on the health care delivery system. The federal Medicare program of health insurance for persons over age 65 and the federal and state government Medicaid programs of health insurance for defined categories of low-income people have grown as entitlement programs, adding to the

federal deficit and the limitations of budgetary flexibility. Additionally, because this country contains large numbers of uninsured and relatively poor, underinsured people, the government must respond by developing a mechanism for universal coverage and easier access to health care. Since about 1990, these pressures—read as challenges by some and as opportunities by others—have resulted in rapid development of "integrated health care delivery systems." James E. Lewis has indicated that such systems will have several shared characteristics: (1) Each patient will be treated in the most cost-effective appropriate setting; (2) physicians will be salaried; (3) the system organization will contract directly with employers and other managed care organizations; (4) care will be capitated; i.e., the system organization will be responsible for blocks of patients while bearing much of the financial risk; (5) the system organization will decide how to deploy revenues; (6) the organizational goal will be to minimize resource utilization while maintaining satisfaction of the subscriber population; and (7) there will be a greater emphasis on health education and prevention. Lewis, as well as others, anticipates that teams of physicians and other health professionals will be responsible for the health of panels of subscribers.

The above major changes in medical care organization will produce enormous stresses, and the perturbations will extend from the practice of medicine into the academic environment. Without doubt the educational process for physicians and the correlative tendency to de-emphasize subspecialty training and emphasize generalist training will have major effects on residency programs. We anticipate even greater stresses at the level of the individual physician in terms of knowledge base, stature among the health professions, and caring for patients. We trust, however, that these vast changes will produce a healthier nation, providing all citizens easier access to excellent health care.

Advances in medical science and increased individual responsibility for health-promoting behavior are both necessary for a fair, equitable, and cost-effective health care system that provides a level of quality acceptable to the American public. Advances in medical science are central to achieving high quality at acceptable costs. It follows that integrated health care delivery systems will seek out proven technology in order to maintain their competitive position. Physicians in those organizations will have to be continuously educated in order to provide the best professional advice regarding the adoption of new technologic advances, including not only their safety and efficacy but estimating its effect on medical outcomes, patient satisfaction, and cost-effectiveness. From the standpoint of the physician as professional, the future is, in a sense, a return to the past where the physician and the patient were not insulated from economic realities and psychosocial contexts. High technology and high caring are not antithetical; they go together.

Even though these economic and social changes are coming about in rather turbulent fashion, the future stands out clearly. The practice of medicine will continue to be an exciting career pursuit and an honored profession, providing its deliverers a rewarding opportunity to help others. The number of clinical specialists will necessarily decline, but those who remain will continue to generate innovative ideas and new therapies. The great diagnosticians will be the ones who also have the greatest access to the newest and most comprehensive therapies. It is comprehensive medicine toward which we must strive rather than generalist medicine or subspecialist medicine; it is doing whatever is necessary to treat all aspects of the patient's *dis*-ease. Whether it be in the intricacies of gene therapy or in behavior modification to treat substance abuse, "comprehensive" means being able to care for individuals in the best way with the greatest depth of knowledge. For physicians of the next century, this pursuit will be professionally and personally satisfying and will be welcomed by them as well as by the society as a whole.

American Board of Internal Medicine Committee on Evaluation of Clinical Competence: Project Professionalism. Philadelphia, ABIM, 1994.
Lewis JE: Academic departments of internal medicine in the 1990's. Am J Med 97:i-vi, 1994.

PART II

SOCIAL AND ETHICAL ISSUES IN MEDICINE

2 CLINICAL ETHICS IN THE PRACTICE OF MEDICINE

Peter A. Singer and Mark Siegler

Clinical ethics is a practical discipline that contributes to improving patient care. It focuses on the central importance of patient preferences and choices in the physician-patient relationship and on the moral obligations of physicians, such as the need for honesty, competence, compassion, and respect for the patient. Clinical ethics teaches physicians about a wide range of specifically ethical issues—informed consent, orders not to resuscitate, end-of-life decisions, advance directives, and third-party constraints on the autonomy of both patients and physicians—that arise with increasing frequency in the practice of modern medicine. Although these issues have been analyzed and seemingly resolved at a theoretical level, few physicians are comfortable with them in practice. This chapter offers guidance about the following ethical issues that arise frequently in the practice of internal medicine: (1) decision making by competent patients, (2) substitute decision making (including advance directives), (3) end-of-life decisions, (4) futility, and (5) clinical-ethical concerns in an era of health care reform.

DECISION MAKING BY COMPETENT PATIENTS

During the past generation, the relationship between patients and physicians has become more equal. Most clinical decisions are now reached by a process of shared decision making in which physicians provide information and guidance that allow competent adult patients to make their own decisions based on their personal preferences, values, and goals. Competent adult patients have an ethical and legal right to accept or refuse medical care, including life-sustaining treatments, recommended by physicians. Patients are in control of their own health care. In general, patients accept their physician's recommendations because physician and patient share the same goal—improving the patient's health status—and because patients usually trust and have confidence in both the physician's technical abilities and his/her concerns for the patient as an individual.

INFORMED CONSENT. The clinical-ethical process of shared decision making is mirrored by the legal doctrine of informed consent. Informed consent is defined as voluntary acceptance by a competent patient of a plan for medical care after the physician adequately discloses the proposed plan, its risks and benefits, and alternative approaches. The informed consent process applies not only to invasive surgical procedures but to every clinical decision. Moreover, the legal and ethical standards of informed consent are not satisfied merely by obtaining the patient's signature on a consent form but require a process of effective communication and education between the physician and patient. If the patient has decision-making capacity (see later), the physician should seek consent from the patient; if the patient lacks decision-making capacity, the physi-

cian should seek consent from the appropriate substitute decision maker. The best way for young physicians to learn how to obtain informed consent from patients is by observing a clinician who is recognized for skill in negotiating the consent process.

The patient's right to participate in treatment decisions is well recognized in law, philosophy, public policy, and clinical practice. Perhaps the clearest *legal* statement of this right was enunciated in 1914 by Justice Cardozo: "Every human being of adult years and sound mind has the right to determine what shall be done with his own body." The *philosophical* right of patients to control their own medical care is based on the principle of individual autonomy. In the 1980's, a Presidential commission clearly stated that respect for patient preferences should be the basis of *public policy* in medical ethics. Moreover, evidence from *clinical* research indicates that empowering patients to participate in their own health care may lead to improved functional outcomes in several chronic diseases.

DISCLOSURE AND TRUTH TELLING. For the purposes of informed consent, disclosure must include proposed diagnostic tests and treatments, their risks and benefits, and possible alternative approaches. Although standards for disclosure may vary from one jurisdiction to another, the physician should disclose all the information that a reasonable person in the patient's situation would want or need to know before making a decision. This usually includes information about risks that are either highly likely to occur or less likely but very serious when they do occur (e.g., death or permanent disability). Although a subjective standard of disclosure based on an individual patient's personal view is a difficult clinical standard to achieve, physicians should try to know their patients well enough to tailor disclosure to a patient's particular situation.

Another aspect of disclosure separate from the need to obtain informed consent involves telling patients the truth about unfavorable diagnoses such as metastatic cancer and their prognoses. In the United States, the current medical standard is to be honest with patients and not to conceal bad news. The patient's right to know an unfavorable diagnosis, even if no further tests or treatment is proposed, is grounded in the ethical principle of respect for persons and in the implied promise by physicians to be truthful in their relationships with a patient. Of course, the real clinical skill in "telling the truth" or delivering bad news to a patient involves determining exactly what the "truth" is in a particular case and then deciding how and when it should be imparted in a sensitive way that does not destroy the patient's hope.

COMPETENCY AND DECISION-MAKING CAPACITY. Decision-making capacity (DMC), a clinical concept, is one of the central ethical issues in clinical patient care. (Competency is the parallel legal concept.) Patients who have been determined to have DMC should make their own health care decisions (based on the principle of autonomy), whereas patients determined to lack DMC should be protected from making bad and sometimes irreversible decisions (based on the principle of beneficence). DMC is a dynamic state and may change quickly, as when a patient is admitted stuporous, hypotensive, and with sepsis, and lacks DMC, but 6 hours later, after appropriate treatment, is sitting in bed, conversing normally, and has regained DMC. Moreover, DMC is decision specific. For example, patients with substantial cognitive impairment may retain DMC to decide whether they wish to accept a recommended elective cholecystectomy.

DMC requires that a patient have the ability to communicate and understand information and appreciate the consequences of a particular decision. Unfortunately, no valid and widely accepted clinical measures exist to assess DMC. Physicians should assess DMC by asking patients if they understand and appreciate their medical problem and the risks and benefits of the proposed treatment and why they have chosen to accept or reject it. In practice, physicians often assess DMC by means of a sliding scale that varies with the likelihood and seriousness of the risks and benefits. Thus, a low level of DMC is often clinically acceptable if a patient elects a proposed life-saving treatment that has low risks and a high probability of benefit, whereas clinicians might require a higher standard of DMC if the patient refuses the same treatment.

Who should decide about DMC? In practice, the physician or health care team responsible for the patient should determine whether a patient retains or has lost DMC. When doubt exists, consulting a psychiatrist, hospital attorney, or clinical ethicist may be helpful. In cases of irremediable conflict and if clinical circumstances permit, the ultimate judge of a patient's competency is a court. Often, physicians must make decisions without the benefit of a judicial determination, relying on clinical judgment and assistance from consultants to reach the best and most ethical determination.

SUBSTITUTE DECISION MAKING

American legal theory accords incompetent patients the same rights as competent patients to consent to or refuse diagnostic tests and treatment. In practice, however, patients who lack DMC cannot exercise this right. To address this paradox and to facilitate reaching decisions for the many patients who lack DMC, substitute decision makers are permitted to make health care decisions for the patient lacking DMC. The overall goal of substitute decision making is to approximate the decisions the patient would make if he/she were still capable of making a decision. Substitute decision making policies raise two questions: Who should make decisions for the patient who lacks DMC, and by what standards should the decision be made?

The most appropriate person to make substitute decisions is someone designated by the patient while still competent, either orally or through a written proxy advance directive (see below). Other substitute decision makers, in their usual order of priority, include a spouse, adult child, parent, brother or sister, and any other relative or concerned friend. In some jurisdictions, a public official may serve as substitute decision maker for a patient who has no other decision maker available. More than 25 states have now passed health surrogate laws that permit a substitute decision maker to be appointed without going to court when a patient lacks DMC and has no formal advance directive.

The standards for making substitute decisions for patients without DMC are the following (in decreasing order of priority): explicit patient preferences, values and beliefs, and best interests. Patient preferences are prior expressions by the patient, while competent, that apply to the actual decision that needs to be made, such as whether the patient wants mechanical ventilation in the late stages of amyotrophic lateral sclerosis. Sometimes patients record their specific preferences in an instruction advance directive (see below). Values and beliefs are less specific than explicit preferences, but they allow the substitute decision maker to guess what the patient might have decided based on other past choices of the patient and his/her general approach to life. Best interests, which are "objective" estimates of the benefits and burdens of treatment to the patient, are invoked only when the patient's preferences and values are unknown.

ADVANCE DIRECTIVES. An advance directive (sometimes called a "living will") is a written document containing a person's preferences about life-sustaining treatment and about a proxy decision maker. The person completes the advance directive when competent, and the directive takes effect if the person becomes incompetent. The two types of advance directives are proxy directives, which state *whom* a person wants to make treatment decisions on his/her behalf, and instruction directives, which state *what* treatment the person would or would not want in various situations. (By far the best-studied and most widely used form of advance directive is the order not to resuscitate, i.e., DNR order, written to withhold a specific intervention, cardiopulmonary resuscitation, from a person who experiences a specific medical event, cardiorespiratory arrest.) At present, advance directives are recognized legally in every state,

and the federal Patient Self-Determination Act (PSDA) requires health care facilities to inquire whether patients have an advance directive and to inform patients of their rights under state law to complete an advance directive. Although public opinion polls indicate strong support for advance directives and although many different advance directive forms are available, relatively few Americans have filled out such directives. The development and evaluation of advance directives, including efforts to encourage their use, are areas of active empirical research.

END-OF-LIFE DECISIONS

With the possible exception of informed consent, no issue in clinical ethics has been as thoroughly analyzed as end-of-life decisions. Nevertheless, the spectrum of end-of-life decisions remains confusing for clinicians and the public. Three distinct practices can be delineated: decisions to forego life-sustaining treatment, euthanasia/physician-assisted suicide, and palliative care.

The right of patients to refuse medical interventions also applies to life-sustaining treatment such as cardiopulmonary resuscitation, mechanical ventilation, dialysis, and artificial nutrition and hydration, even if such a decision results in the patient's death. A patient's decision to not initiate (withhold) or to discontinue (withdraw) life-sustaining treatment is not considered the moral or legal equivalent of suicide, and physician participation in such an action is not the equivalent of physician-assisted suicide. These decisions may be made by the patient or substitute decision maker and are legally and ethically permissible when clinicians follow appropriate procedures, as outlined in the previous discussions of decision making by competent patients and substitute decision making. Clinicians must understand that such actions do not place them at legal risk and often reflect the best standards of clinical practice.

In contrast to foregoing life-sustaining treatment, euthanasia and assisted suicide are legally prohibited in almost every legal system in the world. Euthanasia can be defined as an action that leads directly to the death of a patient, e.g., an injection of potassium chloride. Assisted suicide can be defined as providing patients with medical means that the patient uses to commit suicide, e.g., the prescription of a large amount of barbiturates to a patient who then uses the drugs to commit suicide.

Recent cases of physician-assisted suicide reported in the medical literature and by the media and several legislative initiatives to legalize it have placed the issues of physician-assisted suicide and euthanasia high on the public policy agenda. The main arguments supporting physician-assisted suicide and euthanasia are based on respect for patient freedom of choice and the claimed right of individuals to enlist physician assistance to end their pain and suffering by either action. The main arguments opposing these practices include respect for human life, protection of vulnerable patients, and fear of abuse. Both proponents and opponents of physician-assisted suicide and euthanasia appeal to the role-related responsibility of being a physician to support their arguments. Even if assisted suicide and euthanasia receive legal sanction in selected jurisdictions, physicians will still be confronted with the fundamental issue of whether such practices are ethical in a medical context.

A third practice in the spectrum of end-of-life decisions is the provision of palliative care. Palliative care is ethically and legally permissible, even mandatory, and is an essential component of quality clinical care of the dying. A practical problem for physicians, however, is to distinguish palliative care from euthanasia. We suggest that if a physician's actions meet all of the following three criteria, they represent appropriate palliative care: (1) subjective or objective evidence indicates that the terminally ill patient is experiencing pain; (2) the physician's therapeutic response is commensurate with the level of the patient's pain and an ongoing feedback loop between the patient's symptoms and signs and the physician's therapeutic response is evident; and (3) the physician's intention is to relieve pain and not to kill the patient (the physician's actions do not cause an immediate death, as by administering a clearly lethal dose of a drug).

FUTILITY

Futile treatments offer absolutely no possibility of changing the patient's health status or achieving any medical goals. In such cases, the physician's responsibility to the patient and substitute decision maker changes: The physician is not required to offer a futile therapy. (Of course, the physician is obligated to provide care and counseling under these circumstances.) Unfortunately, ambiguity in determining futility arises from disagreements about both the goals of therapy and the probability of attaining the goals (e.g., 0.1%, 1%, 10%) which should be considered futile. Little agreement exists currently about who has the right to decide what interventions should be called futile. Usually, a physician describes a treatment as futile either because the probability of success is very low or because the quality of life (the goal of treatment) achievable is regarded by the physician as unacceptable. The classic example of low probability of success is the use of CPR in a patient with metastatic cancer. In these cases, the core issue is usually the patient's fear of death, and this should be addressed directly. If patient and physician continue to disagree about whether CPR should be given, the physician should either provide CPR or find the patient another doctor. If the futility discussion is about quality of life, the best judge of quality of life is the patient or substitute decision maker. Sometimes physicians are uncomfortable with providing care that they describe as futile because they consider the limited benefits or low probability of success to be a waste of scarce health care resources. Such rationing decisions should not be conflated with futility but should be addressed explicitly at the level of policy guidelines. Ad hoc attempts to ration at the bedside are often clinically and ethically unsound.

CLINICAL-ETHICAL CONCERNS IN AN ERA OF HEALTH REFORM

Two forces are driving health reform: escalating and seemingly uncontrollable health costs and the substantial number of people in America who lack health insurance, limiting their access to beneficial health services. The goals of American health reform—to provide universal access to high-quality and cost-effective health care—are laudable and ethically unproblematic. The strategies for achieving these goals include reducing administrative costs, using outcome data to rationalize services and develop clinical guidelines, and encouraging patients and physicians to participate in managed care organizations, in which a primary care physician supervises the patient's overall care. Successful efforts at cost containment may also require restricting services with marginal benefits, rationing potentially beneficial services, and limiting both patient and physician freedom to make individual clinical decisions. Many of these strategies for achieving health reform will place enormous stress on the doctor-patient relationship.

Our recommendations for maintaining the ethical integrity of medical practice and for improving patient outcomes are to emphasize the following approaches: a patient-centered approach to medicine that encourages freedom of personal choice; a maximization of patient and physician autonomy even within complex bureaucratic systems like managed care organizations and health alliances; reinforcing the centrality and importance of the doctor-patient relationship; and encouraging a focus on patients' rights when developing clinical guidelines and appeal mechanisms for the large number of clinical and administrative decisions that, despite outcomes research, will continue to be made in the face of substantial uncertainty.

CONCLUSIONS

Scientific and technologic developments in medicine have created unprecedented ethical dilemmas for physicians. The coming revolution in molecular medicine will generate additional ethical problems. In the last decade, clinical ethics has emerged as a new and useful component of medical practice by emphasizing that technical and ethical concerns are inseparable in the practice of medicine. Clinical ethics focuses on the continuing centrality of the doctor-patient relationship and on how patients and physicians work within existing administrative and political structures to reach mutual agreement on clinical decisions affecting the patient. In addition, clinical ethics offers a language of discourse that broadens the medical model from one that is narrowly technical to one that takes serious account of individual patient preferences. The language and content of clinical ethics have been adopted not only by patients, physicians, nurses, other health care providers, and medical educators but also by health economists, hospital administrators, policy developers, and judges. In this regard, ethical considerations in

medicine are likely to remain an important component of medical education, clinical practice, biomedical research, and the political evolution of our health care system.

Almost 2500 years ago, Plato recognized that good clinical medicine is a marriage of scientific knowledge and human care. In Book IV of *The Laws,* he described the excellent physician as one who ". . . treats disease by going into things thoroughly from the beginning in a scientific way and takes the patient and family into confidence. Thus he learns something from the sufferer . . . . He does not give prescriptions until he has won the patient's support, and when he has done so, he steadfastly aims at providing complete restoration to health by persuading the sufferer into compliance . . . ." The best clinical medicine and patient outcomes are achieved when patient and physician have established a relationship in which technical and personal aspects of care are integrated. The practice of ethical medicine in the twenty-first century will require nothing more but demand nothing less.

Appelbaum PS, Grisso T: Assessing patients' capacities to consent to treatment. N Engl J Med 319:1635, 1988. *A review of the four factors to consider in assessing patients' decision-making capacity.*

Danis M, Southerland L, Garrett JM, et al.: A prospective study of advance directives for life-sustaining care. N Engl J Med 324:882, 1991. *Empirical study examines the effect of advance directives on clinical care.*

Emanuel LL, Barry M, Stoeckle JD, et al.: Advance directives for medical care—a case for greater use. N Engl J Med 324:889, 1991. *Empirical study examines the process of completion of advance directives.*

Epstein AM: Changes in the delivery of care under comprehensive health care reform. N Engl J Med 329:1672, 1993. *An optimistic perspective that envisions that health reform will ". . . empower physicians . . . and enrich the patient relationship."*

Jonsen AR, Siegler M, Winslade WJ: Clinical Ethics: A Practical Approach to Ethical Decisions in Clinical Medicine. 3rd ed. New York, Pergamon Press, 1990. *A practical guide to help clinicians deal with ethical problems that occur frequently in medical practice.*

Menikoff JA, Sachs GA, Siegler M: Beyond advance directives: Health care surrogate laws. N Engl J Med 327:1165, 1992. *Health care surrogate laws to enable decisions to be reached for incompetent patients may meet the needs of the large majority of patients who choose not to complete advance directives.*

Paris JJ, Schreiber MD, Statter M, et al.: Beyond autonomy—physicians' refusal to use life-prolonging extracorporeal membrane oxygenation. N Engl J Med 329:354, 1993. *Patient rights are not absolute and on occasion may be overridden by clinical factors, including especially bad prognoses.*

Quill TE, Cassel CK, Meier DE: Care of the hopelessly ill. Proposed clinical criteria for physician-assisted suicide. N Engl J Med 327:1380, 1992. *Argues for legalization of physician-assisted suicide but not voluntary euthanasia; proposes clinical criteria to guide practice of assisted suicide if legalized.*

Singer PA, Siegler M: Elective use of life-sustaining treatments. *In* Stollerman GH (ed): Advances in Internal Medicine, Vol. 36. Chicago, Year Book, 1991. *Reviews empirical studies about decisions to forego life-sustaining treatment.*

3 CARE OF DYING PATIENTS AND THEIR FAMILIES
Balfour M. Mount

Death calls into question our competence, our unconscious premises regarding the omniscience of modern medical science, and the nature of our role as caregivers. It raises questions concerning meaning, life, death, and immortality. It may undermine communication with our patients and their family members, resulting in increased isolation and despair. It is the time when it is erroneously said that "nothing more can be done," yet it is a time to relieve suffering and develop individually tailored support programs. The physician has an unparalleled opportunity to act as a catalyst to enable comfort, communication, integration, and healing.

DEFINITION AND GOALS OF PALLIATIVE CARE

Palliative care aims to improve the quality of life when treatment aimed at cure and prolonging life is no longer a realistic objective. It offers services designed to address the physical, psychological, social, and spiritual needs of dying patients and their families. Its goals are to relieve suffering, to attain patient comfort without iatrogenic somnolence or change in affect, to assist patient and family in making the most of decreasing resources, and to support those involved in a search for meaning.

Attentive control of pain and other symptoms and detailed consideration of psychosocial and spiritual issues should characterize care from the time of diagnosis. When neglected until the late stages of disease, problems in these domains tend to become entrenched, interactive, and increasingly difficult to control. Vigilant prophylaxis of symptoms and attention to the nonphysical factors contributing to suffering lead to enhanced quality of life and diminished drug requirements. Ch. 17 provides a detailed review of pain and its management.

Table 3–1 offers guidelines for controlling symptoms. Because symptoms may change rapidly, frequent re-evaluation is an essential component of effective care of the dying. Norms of care are redefined in this setting. Only investigations which may lead to a treatment that will improve quality of life are considered. Blood pressure, pulse, and temperature are not routinely monitored, whereas the frequency of bowel movements is!

Attention to detail is required for planning both assessment and care. For one very weak patient, using a bedside commode or a bedpan and simply accepting occasional incontinence of urine and stool enabled conservation of scant energy reserves for eagerly anticipated daily visits with his family. Bowel care for the equally weak, fiercely independent man in the next bed involved planned nonintervention while he laboriously struggled unaided to the toilet some 15 feet from his bed. A gentle offer of assistance was given ("When you wish, just let us know"), and a discussion of his need for autonomy was held with family members. Thus, radically different approaches to the details of bowel care were used for two dying men with divergent needs.

Competent care of the dying involves compulsive care of skin, mouth, and eyes; adapting activities of daily living, furniture, and utensils to accommodate progressive weakness (a favorite chair raised on blocks, a padded and raised toilet seat, a spoon with a padded handle to accommodate a weak grip); clean smooth sheets; quiet music, flowers, and a few cherished belongings; the reassuring glow of soft lighting at night; and the reliable availability of both skilled nursing and an interested physician.

Fears and misunderstandings about existing or anticipated symptoms and the effects of medication are common. Involve the patient and family in both planning and providing care. Clear explanations of symptoms and treatment options give reassurance that "the doctor understands what's going on" and "there is a plan."

COMMUNICATION ISSUES

Giving bad news is always difficult. The physician should bring to discussions of prognosis not a set of fixed rules concerning whether "to tell" or "not to tell," but an openness to examining with the patient the reality at hand. Communication that is insensitive in the interest of "telling all" or evasive, falsely optimistic, or otherwise misleading in the interest of "protecting" the patient generally risks seriously undermining long-range physician credibility.

TABLE 3–1. GUIDELINES FOR SYMPTOM CONTROL

1. "Nothing matters more than the bowels" (Saunders). Daily assessment needed.
2. Control of one symptom improves control of all symptoms.
3. Most symptoms are caused by multiple factors. Psychological distress may augment all symptoms.
4. "Assessment must precede treatment" (Twycross).
5. Rule out correctable factors underlying each symptom.
6. Clarify who is bothered by symptom: patient, family, or staff.
7. Give simple explanation for each symptom to patient and family. Diagrams helpful.
8. Consider anticipated prognosis, functional status, and the patient's goals in determining appropriate treatment.
9. Discuss treatment options with patient and family and involve them in treatment planning where practical.
10. Determine what was helpful in the past.
11. Use a total-care approach employing nondrug, environmental, and other supportive measures.
12. If needed, use combinations of pharmacologic agents when differing mechanisms of action and toxicity permit.
13. Prescribe drugs prophylactically in individually optimized, regular doses for persistent symptoms.
14. Never say "Nothing more can be done." Consult or refer if comfort is not achieved.

Studies suggest that the majority of patients with a serious illness sense the possibility of death, whether or not they have been told. Fears are usually diminished if they can be named.

Integrating "bad news" is usually a process, not an event. Grave tidings are often repressed and simply "not heard" at the first airing. The physician should follow the pace of disclosure set by the patient, being sensitive to all forms of communication: plain language ("I fear I may be dying"), symbolic language ("I keep dreaming of a long tunnel with a candle at the end and I am afraid someone is going to blow the candle out"), and nonverbal communication (depressed facial expression, excessive muscle tension). It has been estimated that 80% of communication is nonverbal. The absence of questions does not mean that questions do not exist for the patient. The physician who says "I never tell patients they have cancer unless they ask me" risks leaving the responsibility of broaching the most sensitive and awesome questions to the one who is most vulnerable, the patient.

Discussions should be positive yet reality oriented. "Am I dying? How long do I have?" may be responded to by, "I don't know how long any of us have to live. If you are asking if it is serious enough to warrant getting your affairs in order, I would say yes, get your house in order. While you're doing that, you and I will deal with the medical problems you're experiencing."

Discussions focused on the goals of treatment minimize uncertainty and foster confidence. Involving the family in these discussions facilitates their subsequent mutual support. Sitting together, patient, family, and doctor examine what is still possible rather than what has been lost.

"There are only three aims we can have in treating any illness, Bill—to cure, to prolong life, and to improve the quality of life. We are not going to be able to cure your tumor, in the sense of making it go away permanently. But, you know, there are many medical problems we can't cure—including diabetes, arthritis, and most types of heart disease—yet many people with these conditions live meaningful lives, sometimes for longer periods than we expect.

"So 'cure' isn't an option. What about the next goal, 'to prolong life'? You could undergo surgery, but there is no sense putting you through something that wouldn't be helpful." (Surgery is often used as the first example, since it presents a concrete, easily grasped image of futility.) "With treatments as they now stand, the same would be said for chemotherapy, radiotherapy, and immunotherapy." (The phrasing focuses on the limitations of current therapy, not the hopelessness of the illness.)

"Does this mean nothing can be done?" (thus naming the worst fear). "Not at all! It simply means we are at the third goal—that of focusing on the quality of life. How can we make the best of this? Let's examine that. If I understand you, the three complaints you have right now are your backache, that cough, and your loss of appetite. Let's see what we can do about each of these. . . . "

The patient and family are left with a clear understanding that the issue is not "to treat or not to treat," but an appropriate shifting in therapeutic goals by a physician who is interested, involved, and undaunted by the specter of this illness. Hope is contagious. Hope is a way through, not a way out.

Specific estimates of survival should never be given because they are based on data relevant to populations of patients with the same illness, not to the patient in question. No matter how carefully phrased, such pronouncements always unsheathe a sword of Damocles that heightens anxiety and drains ability to live fully in the moment. "I have only 2 more months."

Accepting the present reality, including the increasing weakness, dependence, uncertain future, and impending loss, frees the patient to choose from available options. Acceptance of that kind is not born out of despair and resignation. It is the transcendent alternative to denial. It is a path to meaning which is possible even in the face of physical deterioration and advancing disease.

FAMILY AS THE UNIT OF CARE

Terminal illness is a pressure cooker of family stress. Grief, fear, anger, and guilt abound. Longstanding interpersonal tensions tend to be accentuated. Brief family meetings to discuss treatment plans and identify problems and fears are a time-efficient tool highly effective in preventing impending crises, clarifying misunderstandings, and building bridges of mutual support.

Table 3–2 presents a checklist of areas of inquiry useful in family assessment. Ensure that children and the elderly are informed and involved. Their exclusion often leaves them ill-prepared for loss.

The bereaved are a high-risk population with an increased incidence of impaired function, medical illness, psychological distress, and even death. Some who have been found to have an increased risk of bereavement morbidity are listed in Table 3–3. Referral to programs offering bereavement support may be beneficial.

DYING AT HOME

Death has been moved from the home to the institution in industrial nations, and family members often feel ill-prepared to care for dying loved ones. With careful planning, family education, mobilization of community resources, and continuing support, however, both family and patient may benefit from experiencing this last time together in the home.

Home care of the dying begins with careful home assessment performed by an experienced home care team able to direct the family to needed community resources and to recommend modifications in living arrangements and furnishings to simplify care. "You will find it much easier if you rent a hospital bed. They are inexpensive. Try placing it in the living room where she can be quiet, close to the family, and able to see the children passing in the street."

"She is weaker now. You will need a handrail and small bench for the bath tub and a walker. I think you would find a commode for the bedside helpful as well."

An effective palliative home care program implies the involvement of a team. Regularly scheduled nursing visits are supplemented by emergency visits as required. A trusted physician is essential to consult in the home and collaborate with community-based nurses when the need arises. A social worker, occupational therapist, chaplain, and volunteers may all play a role. Simple, clear routines for medications and treatments are established. A sense of order and safety is fostered by round-the-clock availability of telephone consultation with experienced staff who are aware of recent changes in the patient's condition and medications. Brief respite admissions before family exhaustion sets in may serve to prolong capability of home care.

A sensitive discussion with the family about what to do when their loved one dies may promote a sense of confidence and preparedness. Acknowledgment of a job well done ("You certainly have done well to keep her at home this long") helps to allay feelings of inadequacy and guilt should admission to the hospital become necessary.

AS DEATH APPROACHES

During the final weeks or days of a terminal illness, frequent changes in clinical status may occur. Eventualities such as the need for parenteral or rectal medications should be foreseen and planned for. Common crises include progressive weakness, inability to swallow and aspiration of oral intake, inability or refusal to take medications, changing levels of consciousness and orientation, restlessness, and urinary or fecal incontinence. Careful planning and prompt response to the request for emergency assistance can avoid unnecessary hospital admission.

Decreasing requirements for most medications are encountered as

TABLE 3–2. FAMILY ASSESSMENT ISSUES

1. Identity of nuclear family, extended family, and social network.
2. Characteristics of family system: roles, relationships, communication patterns.
3. Presence of concurrent life crises.
4. History of coping with past crises.
5. Values and beliefs about death.
6. Response to current illness: changes in roles and relationships.
7. Family resources: physical, emotional, financial, social, spiritual.
8. Immediate family needs.
9. Long-range family needs.

TABLE 3–3. SELECTED BEREAVEMENT RISK INDICATORS

1. Parental grief.
2. Social isolation.
3. Timid, dependent personality; poorly developed coping skills.
4. Short preparation time (duration of illness).
5. Ambivalent or charged relationship with deceased.
6. Concurrent life crisis.
7. Pining and clinging in final illness.
8. Grief expression repressed by cultural or family norms.
9. Disenfranchised grief: mistress, lover, divorceé, loss of a secret relationship.

death approaches. Individualized reductions in dose can prolong an alert, interactive, comfortable state, often to the moment of death.

Noisy upper airway secretions ("death rattle") are troubling to the family, who will need reassurance, but they are generally not troubling to the patient. They may be reduced by early intervention with hyoscine 0.4 mg given subcutaneously at intervals of 2 to 4 hours as needed.

Questions and fears the patient and family have about death should be gently explored. The will, funeral arrangements, and a "life review" may be discussed as a means of completing unfinished business and facilitating closure.

Encourage family members, including the young, the elderly, and those from out of town, to visit earlier rather than later. Assess bereavement risks and arrange follow-up support if indicated.

Decathexis, a protective "separating off" or "turning in" by the patient, is sometimes seen as death approaches. A simple explanation may reassure the concerned family that this is not depression or rejection but a normal protective mechanism. "He doesn't need you to say much now, but your presence will help."

Take premonitions of death seriously, and watch for the need for family members to give their lingering loved one permission to die. "It's all right, John. You can let go. You've taken care of everything. We'll miss you, but thanks to you we'll be O.K."

AT THE TIME OF DEATH

The hours that surround the death of a family member are charged with meaning for the bereaved and are usually remembered for years to come. Caregivers may use this to therapeutic advantage by establishing guidelines for patient and family care that facilitate subsequent grief work.

Endeavor to have someone sitting at the bedside of the imminently dying person. If the bedside companion is a family member, be sensitive to his/her need either for support or for time to be alone with the loved one. Encourage available family members to view the body before it has been moved to the funeral home. Seeing the body facilitates acceptance of the fact of death.

When family members arrive they need support and quiet hospitality, including a handkerchief, a cup of tea, a listening ear. Acknowledge the support given by the bereaved to the deceased during the illness.

Allow sufficient time with the body for active grieving. It may be helpful for a caregiver to unobtrusively touch the body, indicating that there is nothing frightening about physical contact with the body—an experience that may be highly effective in promoting closure.

Discuss whether the family wishes to have an autopsy. Many find the documentation of reality that it provides helpful in the months and years to come.

When death occurs in a hospital, ask the family if they would prefer to collect and pack their loved one's personal effects, particularly if a child has died. A memento of the event such as a lock of hair or a picture may be an aid to bereavement, especially in parental grief.

Respect cultural differences in the expression of acute grief. Certain cultural groups may be extremely vocal and demonstrative in their grieving. Wails, screams, fainting attacks, and other dramatic gestures have therapeutic value for many and may be followed in a remarkably short period of time by a sense of composure and evident relief.

Acknowledge the mystery of death without offering "answers" concerning the unknowable. Honor religious rites and prayers meaningful to the bereaved.

The presence at the death or funeral service of the physician who was involved during the illness assists review of the illness, emphasizes the value of the deceased, underscores respect for the family, and assists the physician's own grief work.

THE PHYSICIAN AND DEATH

In caring for the dying, physicians are challenged in each dimension of their personhood. William James termed death "the worm at the core of man's pretensions to happiness," while La Rochefouchauld observed: "Death and the sun are not to be looked at steadily." What do we do with our accumulated losses as caregivers? How do we establish a new balance in our emotional economy when an important investment has been lost? At what cost? To whom? Do our professional encounters with death leave a need for thicker defensive shells, emotional distancing, intellectualization, and acting out? The risk is minimized if we accept relief of suffering as our mandate rather than the narrower goal of fighting disease and if we attend to our own physical, psychosocial, and spiritual needs. Indeed, confrontation with death may foster insight and enrich life. It has been said that to live is to suffer and to survive is to find meaning in the suffering; that having a "why" to live can enable living with any "how"; that our last freedom, when all others have been stripped away, is the ability to choose our response in a given set of circumstances. It is a privilege to be able to assist our patients in their growing toward an understanding of the truth of these observations. It is a source of personal growth when we recognize their truth ourselves.

Cassel E: The nature of suffering and the goals of medicine. N Engl J Med 306:639, 1982. *A classic examination of the components of personhood and their impact on the experience of illness.*

Doyle D, Hanks GWC, MacDonald N: Oxford Textbook of Palliative Medicine. New York, Oxford Medical Publications, 1993. *A comprehensive review of palliative care issues.*

Frankl V: Man's Search for Meaning. New York, Simon and Schuster, 1963. *A psychiatrist and Auschwitz survivor reflects on motivation, meaning, and quality of life. Moving. Insightful. A classic.*

Saunders C: The Management of Terminal Malignant Disease. 2nd ed. Baltimore, Edward Arnold, 1984. *The principles and practice of palliative medicine by the pioneering founder of the modern hospice movement.*

Twycross RG, Lack SA: Therapeutics in Terminal Cancer. 2nd ed. New York, Churchill Livingstone, 1990. *A useful and authoritative guide to caring for patients with advanced cancer. Pragmatic. Organized for easy reference at the bedside.*

Walsh TD: Symptom Control. Cambridge, Mass., Blackwell Scientific Publications, 1989. *Detailed consideration of symptom control from angina to xerostomia, with additional chapters on ten specific areas of clinical concern.*

Worden JW: Grief Counselling and Grief Therapy. A Handbook for the Mental Health Practitioner. New York, Springer Publishing, 1982. *Mechanisms of grief and approaches to helping the bereaved accomplish the "tasks of mourning." Lucid and informative. An excellent resource for the general physician.*

4   SOCIAL AND ECONOMIC ISSUES IN MEDICINE

John E. Wennberg

There is a great deal about medical practice that you will not find in this edition of *Cecil Textbook of Medicine.* You will look in vain for guidelines about whether and when to hospitalize patients with a broad variety of medical conditions. You will not find conclusive evidence on the efficacy of many common surgical procedures or information about how patients actually value the outcomes of interventions that physicians are likely to recommend.

In the absence of this information, and relying on a traditional model of decision making, which assumes that the physician is able to act as the rational agent for the patient in choosing between treatment options, the medical system has developed as an economy of supplier-induced demand, in which the availability of hospital beds, physicians, and other local resources determines the pattern of care.

Experts in economics have long held that the market for medical care differs from that for most goods and services, because a competitive market assumes that the consumer is informed about availability, price, and market competition. Patients, by contrast, simply do not have enough information to choose their own care—and

patients' widespread use of insurance means that the price of care does not closely modulate the decision to use it. In this market, the traditional remedy is to rely on professionals to control demand and for patients to delegate decision making to their physicians. The tacit agreement between patient and physician is that professionals, in fulfilling their ethical roles, prescribe only needed care. Physicians are also assumed to serve conscientiously as agents for society, ensuring that the supply of resources is adequate—but only adequate—to meet a rational level of demand. While the physician's understood role as decision-making agent for both patient and society can be compromised by unethically inducing use for self-serving reasons, it has also been assumed that such activity is controlled by agencies, such as the Medicare program's Professional Review Organization, that patrol the market to discipline those who depart from the central consensus about what works and what patients need.

It is increasingly apparent, however, that the foundation of much of medical care is not an evidence-based professional consensus about effectiveness and value. The decision to use care, such as hospitalization for a patient with pneumonia, is often driven by availability, not explicit theory. Even when theories of care are explicit—as in treating conditions such as angina pectoris or benign prostatic hypertrophy (BPH) (for which treatment options can range from surgery to drugs or watchful waiting)—the outcomes are often not well understood. Further, physicians are imperfect agents; their own preferences for treatments or outcomes often become entangled with and overpower those of the patient.

FLAWS IN THE SCIENTIFIC AND ETHICAL BASIS OF CLINICAL DECISION MAKING

For a number of conditions, such as those in Table 4–1, medical theories of efficacy and professional discourse are well organized; opinions are strongly held concerning appropriate treatment, even when experts disagree. Often, disagreements cannot be resolved by appeal to evidence because adequate outcomes studies have not been performed. In a market where patients rely on the profession to prescribe treatments, the existence of diverse professional opinions about the value of options invites supplier-induced demand. In fee-for-service markets where provider income and the financial stability of institutions depend on the level of utilization, it becomes inevitable.

The marked variation in the rates of surgery for BPH found in studies conducted in the state of Maine in the early 1980's exposed the lack of consensus about how patients with BPH should be treated. Rates of surgery for BPH ranged between 15% of men undergoing surgery by age 85 in one town and 50% in another, quite similar community. The rates were physician-specific and attributable to the fact that among Maine's urologists, there were at least two widely held and opposing theories about the benefits associated with surgery for BPH. The physicians differed in their assumptions about the nature of the underlying illness, as well as the benefits to be derived from surgery. Some believed in a preventive theory: Operate early to avoid later complications, including premature death. Others were more optimistic about untreated BPH. They argued for the quality-of-life theory: Surgery benefits most men by reducing symptoms and improving the quality of life.

The unresolved competition between the prevention and the quality-of-life theories reflected indeterminacy rooted in poor clinical science. The outcomes research we undertook showed that the preventive theory was incorrect; early surgery appears to lead to a slight *decrease* in life expectancy, because for most men BPH does not progress to life-threatening obstruction, and the small operative mortality risk reduces life expectancy slightly. Moreover, the studies showed that urine flow, the standard used to determine the urologists' estimate of the need for (and the success of) surgery, was an extremely poor indicator of how patients themselves valued their preoperative conditions and their surgical outcomes. What *did* matter to patients was the degree to which their symptoms bothered them (which was not necessarily related to symptom severity) and the possible negative outcomes of surgery, such as impotence and incontinence.

When patients are offered an active role in choosing treatment through shared decision making, the link between supply and utilization can be broken. When patients enrolled in two separate prepaid group practices were informed about their options for treatment of BPH through an interactive videodisc program, with information specific to their own clinical situations, most elected conservative treatment. Among those with severe symptoms, only one in five chose surgery, and the per capita rates of surgery declined about 50%.

THE THRESHOLD EFFECT FOR INTERVENTION

Medical practice occurs within a context of available supply that is only rarely known to the participants—physicians generally have no idea how many beds per capita are available in their communities. The exception is the prepaid group practice model, exemplified by Kaiser-Permanente and the Group Health Cooperative of Puget Sound. The administrators of these classic-model HMO's know the number of people enrolled in their health plans and use population-based health planning to determine the per capita numbers of beds they provide and health workers they hire. Classic HMO's typically use about 150 hospital beds per 100,000 enrollees and employ physicians according to specialty-specific population-based ratios. Population-based planning is essential because HMO's receive a fixed amount of money for each enrollee for whom they agree to provide all "necessary" care. A fixed budget requires controlling resources, which is accomplished by setting limits on supply.

In fee-for-service markets, by contrast, neither administrators nor health care providers know the size of the population their organizations serve. Private sector, population-based health planning that relates supply to consumption is virtually nonexistent. Populations do not "enroll"; there are no fixed budgets; revenues are generated by providing services.

The lack of information on the quantity of local resources and the actuarial costs of local consumption supports a dynamic of market growth that is not closely constrained by the size or the health care needs of the population. An institution's growth is determined by its own perceived needs and its assumed roles in the community and the region. Size is influenced by such nonmedical factors as competition, prestige, or the expansion of professional staff to meet the critical mass required to ensure night and weekend coverage. And, as most residents are aware, the decision about how many subspecialty fellows to train is less a function of how many are needed in a community than of the needs (and desires) of the fellowship directors in these disciplines.

Increasingly, the tools of epidemiology, applied to the study of supply and utilization in local health care markets, make it possible to compare resource allocation and utilization rates among communities (and in some cases between individual hospitals) as if they were the closed and countable populations of enrollees in classic HMO's. These studies reveal remarkable differences in the per capita supply of resources, even among demographically similar markets. The studies also show that variations in supply affect the threshold for clinical decision making. The effect of supply of beds on the decision for hospitalization provides a cogent example. For example, although some of Boston's beds (and some of New Haven's) are used to care for people who live outside the city, the net effect is a higher level of local investment: 3.8 beds per 1000 residents of Boston and only 2.6 beds per 1000 people living in New Haven (1989) (Table 4–1).

The differential in population-based availability of hospital resources exercises a diffuse effect on the admission threshold for most conditions. A few "demand-driven" conditions, such as myocardial infarction and hip fracture, are unaffected by the available supply of resources. (For these, virtually all physicians, regardless of the context of supply, agree on the need to hospitalize the patient.) The increments of beds and other resources in high-resource communities are used for patients with "supply-sensitive" conditions such as pneumonia, congestive heart failure, and bronchitis, which in low-rate markets are more often treated on an outpatient basis. For such conditions, hospitalization rates for people living in Boston are typically 60% higher than for residents of New Haven. Capacity and utilization vary substantially from hospital to hospital even within these cities. Patients with myocardial infarctions or strokes who are discharged from St. Raphael's Hospital in New Haven experience a 24% higher probability for readmission than patients admitted to Yale–New Haven Hospital for the same conditions. Using the same benchmark, Bostonians discharged from the Massachusetts General Hospital experience a 50% higher and those from University Hospital a 92% higher readmission rate.

The threshold effect is not scaled simply on the severity of illness. As capacity increases, populations who are very sick as well as those who are not so sick receive more hospital care. A strong linear relationship exists between capacity and level of investment in terminal care. Yet more is not better in the dimension of life expectancy: Residents of Boston and New Haven experience the same population-based mortality rates. The effects of supply on decision making are subliminal, as neither administrators, clinicians, nor patients are directly aware of the supply context of local practice. The impact is primarily on the problem-solving tasks of medicine—the care of sick people with conditions about which medical theory is weak and evidence that one course of action is better than another is unproven.

REMEDIES

Dealing effectively with the problem of supplier-induced demand and the need for shared decision making between physicians and patients requires substantial changes in science policy, the doctor-patient relationship, and the mechanisms for limiting capacity.

FIND OUT WHAT WORKS. Biomedical science creates the fundamental understanding of the mechanisms of disease at the cellular and molecular levels and is a fruitful source of clinical theory and practice technologies for intervening in the lives of patients. But its mission as a branch of applied biology does not emphasize evaluating medical theories or communicating about options. It is the job of the evaluative sciences to conduct technology assessments and outcomes research to estimate the probabilities for outcomes that matter to patients and to elucidate the importance of patient preferences in choosing treatment. Although some progress has been made, a federal science policy adequate to ensure the orderly evaluation of relevant treatment theories and the education of health professionals in evaluative sciences is not yet in place.

FIND OUT WHAT PATIENTS WANT. The success of the biomedical revolution greatly increases medical options and by doing so exacerbates the problem of choice in medicine. Although the assumption that physicians can make vicarious decisions that reflect the patient's true preferences may seem naive, throughout most of the history of Western medicine it did not make much difference

TABLE 4–1. RATIOS OF BOSTON TO NEW HAVEN UTILIZATION RATES AND NUMBER OF EXCESS HOSPITAL BEDS BY TYPE OF SERVICE

Type of Service	Boston/New Haven Ratio			Excess Boston Beds
	Discharges/1000	Length of Stay	Days/1000	
All cases	1.34	1.07	1.44	739
Adult medical cases	1.49	1.09	1.64	527
Demand-driven conditions	1.06	1.11	1.17	
Supply-sensitive conditions	1.56	1.11	1.74	
Pediatric medical cases	1.47	1.16	1.70	35
Surgical cases				
Minor	1.38	1.17	1.61	89
Major	1.00	1.13	1.13	88

Adapted from Wennberg JE, Freeman JL, Culp WJ: Are hospital services rationed in New Haven or over-utilized in Boston? Lancet 1:1185, 1987.

because there was not much to choose from. Biomedicine and technology have changed the medical landscape; for many conditions, there are now a number of options that carry different sets of risks and benefits. Rational choice among them depends on learning how to communicate medical options in ways that enable patients to choose among effective treatments according to their own preferences. Although emphasis on the ethical and legal requirements for physicians to share decision making with patients is now greater, and it is asserted in Ch. 2 that a fundamental change in the doctor-patient relationship has already taken place, the striking variations in rates of surgery among communities and the association between capacity and the intensity of investment in terminal care are reminders that supplier-induced demand remains a powerful force in medical markets. Successfully implementing shared decision making requires practice environments in which the choices patients make are not in conflict with the financial interests of health care organizations, employers, or individual providers. Creating such an environment is one of the great challenges of health care reform, because breaking the link between supply and utilization creates a market in which demand emanates from patients, resulting in different per capita rates of consumption and different demands for resources.

LIMIT CAPACITY. Stability in health care markets also requires that capacity be limited in some reasonable way. Many believe that practice guidelines will discipline the decisions of physicians to bring utilization and supply into equilibrium on the basis of medical efficacy. But the evidence from Boston and New Haven indicates otherwise. The extraordinary variations in hospitalization rates among some of the nation's most prestigious teaching hospitals suggest that the rules have no firm scientific basis; some form of population-based planning is required.

Arrow K: Uncertainty and the welfare economics of medical care. Am Econ Rev 53:941, 1963. *A classic presentation of rational agency theory by a Nobel laureate in economics.*

Katz J: The Silent World of Doctor and Patient. London, Collier Macmillan, 1984. *An excellent review of the history of the doctor-patient relationship and the difficulty of establishing shared decision making.*

Wennberg JE: Innovation and the policies of limits in a changing health care economy. *In* Gelijns AC (ed.): Medical Innovations at the Crossroads. Vol. 3, Modern Methods of Clinical Investigation. Washington, DC, National Academy Press, 1992, p 9. *Further discussion of the problem of professional uncertainty and supplier-induced demand in medicine.*

Wennberg JE, Gittelsohn A: Variations in medical care among small areas. Sci Am 246:120, 1982. *Discussion of small area variations and supplier-induced demand.*

PART III

AGING AND GERIATRIC MEDICINE

5 BIOLOGY OF AGING
*Caleb E. Finch and
Edward L. Schneider*

THE LONGEVITY REVOLUTION

A remarkable new phenomenon is occurring throughout the world: Older ages are becoming far more common. In most countries, the fastest-growing age group is the oldest. This is a fact even in countries like Mexico, where the age group 15 and younger is twice as big and where the life expectancy at birth is about 5 years less than in the United States or Canada. In the United States since 1950, the age group 65 years and older has grown from 8% to 13% of the general population. By 2020, it is predicted to further increase by 50%, so that a total of 50 million will live to be at least 65 years of age (Fig. 5–1).

Although these demographic trends are relatively recent, surely many in the ancient world enjoyed long lives through good fortune in their access to good food and clean water and in respite from epidemics of disease and warfare. From the days of the Roman Empire, we have, for example, Pliny's praise of the healthy nature of his summer home in Apennines:

> Hence the number of elderly people living there—you can see the grandfathers and great grandfathers of people . . . and hear stories and tales of the past . . . a visit here is like a return to another age.

These lifespans contrast with the 30-year life expectancy at birth in the Roman upper class.

The maximum lifespan is always a fascinating number. *The Guiness Book of World Records* recognizes Shigichio Izumi as living 120 years. This record appears to be more reliable than those of the notorious supercentenarians who lived high in the Andes and Caucasus mountains; unfortunately, their birth dates were eventually found to be inaccurate.

The key to maximum lifespan concerns how mortality rates change at later ages. During most of the adult lifespan, the mortality rate accelerates according to the Gompertz equation, such that graphs of the log of the mortality rate for each year give a straight line when plotted against the age. As a rule, the mortality rate doubles every 8 years throughout the world after puberty. However, new evidence hints that at advanced ages of 100 years or more, the acceleration of mortality rates slows considerably. If so, then those already reaching advanced ages could soon achieve new record lifespans.

ARE DISEASE AND DISABILITY INEVITABLE DURING AGING?

We do not fully understand the powerful historical trend for increasing survival to later ages. It seems unlikely that all of the improvements can be attributed to the success of medical interventions and improved public health. Obviously, the decline of infant and maternal mortality played a major role in the observed increase of life expectancy at birth during this century. However, the increases of life expectancy at *middle age* preceded the introduction of antibiotics and other major life-saving interventions. At least some groups in the United States seem also to be aging with greater health, as judged by the declining rates of death from cardiovascular disease in the last decades. Lifestyle choices such as smoking, diet, and exercise certainly have a role, but other factors may be found.

Major differences exist between populations in age-related diseases and changes that implicate environmental factors. Breast cancer, for example, has a 10-fold higher incidence in Japanese women who live in California versus Japan; this difference is found at all ages from puberty through menopause. Within the same country, many differences can be seen. Even brain functions are subject to environmental influences, as suggested by the progressive improvement of scores on intelligence tests in different birth cohorts when tested at later ages. These examples imply that the outcomes of aging are subject to a great many environmental influences. Biologists

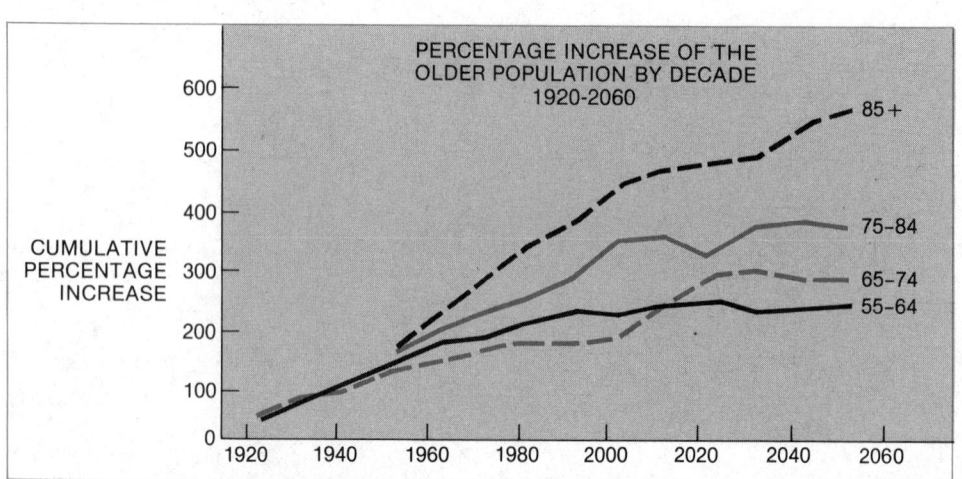

FIGURE 5–1. Past and projected increases in the elderly by decade. (From Bureau of the Census, Current Population Reports, Series P-25, No. 952, 1984.)

refer to these environmentally influenced differences as *plasticity in the aging processes.*

Alzheimer's disease (AD) shows both hereditary and environmental influences. Overall, the risk increases steadily with age and afflicts about 35% of those over 85 years (Ch. 400). AD is not a new disease but is becoming increasingly prominent because of the increased numbers of individuals who are surviving to the eighth, ninth, and tenth decades. Genetic risk factors for AD are identified on at least three different chromosomes: 14, 19, and 21. The recently found association with AD on chromosome 19 implicates the blood protein apolipoprotein E (apoE). The apoE $\epsilon4$ allele, when present in two copies (homozygotes), is associated with a high risk of AD but also of atherosclerosis, with sequelae of stroke and heart attacks. The other genes on chromosomes 14 and 21 are dominant, and only one copy of the allele suffices to cause inevitable AD. On the other hand, there are environmental influences on AD, among which is the surprising finding that higher education in several countries is associated with lower risk of AD. Although education could be a proxy for environmental effects, the mental demands of higher education could generate a greater synaptic reserve that could slow the loss of function during AD. Many studies of AD show strong correlations between synaptic density and the extent of cognitive impairment.

The trends for increased survival to later ages lead to fundamental questions about the biology of aging, particularly about genetic control over the lifespan. The next section considers this question, with examples of species whose lifespans are rigidly programmed as well as those that are not.

MYTHS OF AGING: EVERYTHING DECLINES WITH AGING

Many fears about aging are related to the myth that everything declines with aging. In fact, a number of important physiologic variables do decline with aging and are discussed in the next section. Early studies of human aging did indeed show a universal decline in a number of physiologic functions with aging. Nathan Shock's pioneering studies of human performance at different ages resulted in a famous diagram, reproduced in many textbooks since 1961, that shows uniform decline with age in many functions. We caution that these early studies were cross-sectional, with subjects of very different backgrounds at different ages (the young were laboratory workers and normal volunteers for comparison with nursing home patients).

Shock also established longitudinal studies of the same measurements with normal volunteers who were tested over a period of years (the Baltimore Longitudinal Study). The outcome was very different from the initial cross-sectional study. Many of the variables that were thought to change with aging such as crystallized intelligence or cardiac output were found to be relatively stable with aging. Longitudinal measurements of other characteristics revealed that some individuals had rapid declines with aging, others had moderate declines with aging, and still others had no change. Figure 5–2 shows the example of kidney function as assayed by creatinine clearance. Exactly how performance changes with age depends on the particular function being examined, as well as on the genetics and lifestyle of the individual.

SOME PHYSIOLOGIC AGING CHANGES CAN BE REVERSED OR SLOWED

Maximum aerobic exercise capacity declines with aging and is probably responsible for the retirement of star athletes. Marathon times become progressively longer with advancing age, even in devoted athletes. Nonetheless, older individuals who exercise can raise their maximum aerobic capacity to the level of young sedentary individuals. Skeletal muscles, even in the very old, show remarkable capacity for regaining strength with proper exercise. Regular exercise programs can also slow down age-related bone loss and thus partially protect against hip and other fractures in the elderly. Exercise also can improve cardiac performance as well as diminish the risk of hypertensive disease.

HETEROGENEITY OF AGING: DIVERSITY OF CLINICAL PRESENTATION

Even genetically identical mice experience heterogeneity in their physiologic responses to aging. In aging humans, the interplay of environment and genetic diversity similarly results in increasing heterogeneity in physiologic responses. Whether creatinine clearance, cardiac output, or drug metabolism is measured, the heterogeneity of aging is manifested by the substantial increase in differ-

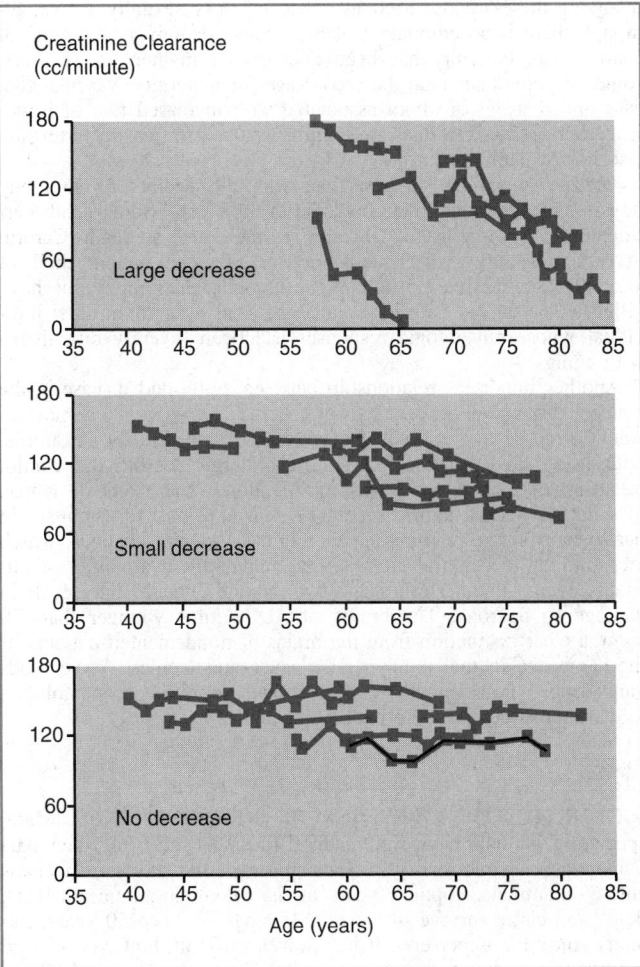

FIGURE 5–2. Individuality of aging changes in kidney function. Creatinine clearance was used to assay glomerular filtration rates in the Baltimore Longitudinal Study of the National Institute of Aging. *Top,* Individuals with extensive declines; *middle,* those with modest declines; *bottom,* a subgroup with no change during many decades. (From Finch CE: Longevity, Senescence, and the Genome. Chicago, University of Chicago Press, 1990. Redrawn from Lindemen, et al: J Am Geriatr Soc 33:278, 1985. Reproduced with the kind permission of the University of Chicago Press.)

ences between individuals. Thus, whereas pharmacologic response to specific drugs may be relatively similar among 20 year olds, predicting the response in 80 year olds is considerably more difficult. The normal heterogeneity of aging is further compounded in a clinical setting by the diseases acquired during a lifetime and the increased number of medications taken by older patients.

THE INTERPLAY OF DISEASE AND AGING

With aging, a number of important physiologic variables decline substantially and compromise the individual's ability to respond to pathologic insults. Some of these age-dependent factors include a decrease in vital capacity, renal clearance, immune function, and bronchiolar ciliary movement, as well as an increase in arterial wall stiffness. The changes decrease the ability of an older body to respond to specific insults such as infections or heart attacks. Thus, the risk of dying of pneumonia increases remarkably with aging and is probably related to both the decreased ability of the aged immune system to combat the pathogens and the impaired ability of the aged lungs to respond to this injury.

The decline of sexual activities after midlife also illustrates interactions between aging and disease. In women, menopause causes a loss of estrogen and progesterone. As a consequence, the reproductive tract mucosa tends to atrophy and become more subject to low-grade infections, either of which can make coitus painful (dyspareunia). Postmenopausal replacement of female sex steroids reverses many of these trends. Men also become less sexually active, although there is no equivalent of menopause or universal decline of testosterone. Paternity has been documented in men of 94 years, some 34 years later than the record age for maternity. Vascular disease and diabetes are both associated with increased risk of impotence, and β-blockers that are commonly used to treat hypertension also impair penile erections.

These associations suggest that, with the decline of so many physiologic functions, one could die of "old age." Some death certificates have even listed "old age" as the cause of death. Careful investigation, however, usually reveals that the patient died of a recognizable disease, such as pneumonia, that might not have killed a 20 year old but did produce the final blow to an older individual whose physiologic responses had been severely diminished with aging.

Another important relationship between aging and disease is the concept that age-dependent loss of specific cell populations may result in specific age-dependent diseases and disorders. For example, with aging, there is loss of cerebral cholinergic neurons that cannot be attributed to vascular disease or AD alone. The extent of neuron loss during normal aging is controversial and hard to establish, in part because large neurons tend to shrink. Vascular changes, which are common in cerebral arteries, may impair the availability of nutrients even without strokes and over a long enough time result in damage to neurons. The brains of AD victims younger than 70 show a clear distinction from the brains of nondemented patients of the same age in the numbers of plaques and tangles. At very advanced ages, however, it becomes difficult for the neuropathologist to distinguish between "normal" aging and AD.

LIFESPANS AND AGING IN OTHER SPECIES

GENETICS OF LIFESPANS OF OTHER SPECIES. Many species of animals have short natural lifespans reflecting their particular genes. Laboratory rodents possess the shortest lifespans among mammals, about 5 years at the maximum; domestic cats, dogs, and cattle survive in the middle range to 20 to 30 years; humans enjoy the upper end. It has proven difficult, however, to find specific genes that give superlongevity. The best-recognized effects of genes on the lifespan are the mutations that cause early-onset diseases. Just as in humans, mice have specific genes that cause early-onset malignant and vascular diseases. For example, the genetically inbred senescence-accelerated mice (SAM strains) show osteoporosis, cataracts, learning deficits, and tissue amyloid deposits at a comparatively young age.

In contrast to mammals, research on invertebrates has identified specific genes that can increase the lifespan as well as others that decrease it. The fruitfly *Drosophila* lives for about 2 months. Recent work shows that lifespans can be changed by genetic selection. The artificial evolution of short- and long-lived lines of flies was forced by choosing individuals that reproduce at younger versus later ages. The resulting selection for lifespan depended on existing genetic variation in the wild-caught flies rather than on new mutations. The conclusion was proved by switching the selection for the age of reproduction in the short- and long-lived lines. The particular survival-influencing genes are being sought, as are the causes of death.

The nematode *Caenorhabditis* also possesses "survival" genes that increase the organism's lifespan, which normally takes only 3 weeks from egg to senescence. Mutants have been found which double the lifespans because of slower accelerations of mortality (Gompertz rate). Other mutants have increased adult lifespans after slowed development; some molecule generated during the prolonged development may enhance lifespan. These studies on flies and nematodes give clues in the search for genes that favor longer lifespans in mammals.

ENVIRONMENTAL INFLUENCES ON THE LIFESPANS. Rodents also show plasticity in aging. By reducing their dietary intake to about half *ad lib* normal and avoiding vitamin or mineral deficiencies, the animals live up to 50% longer, with correspondingly slower accelerations of the mortality rate. Diet restriction also reduces age-related diseases, e.g., the lymphomas and kidney lesions that usually kill aging rodents. Moreover, diet restriction can delay infertility during aging by slowing the loss of ovarian oocytes. Contrary to what one might expect, the metabolic rate per gram of lean body mass does *not* decrease with diet restriction. Metabolic changes, however, do include a lower blood glucose and increased insulin efficiency, opposite to the usual trend during aging. Although the effect of diet restriction on human aging is unknown, diet restriction can have the same impact on lowering blood glucose and increasing insulin efficiency. These examples from other species demonstrate a wide range of environmental interventions that can modify the outcomes of aging. By implication, the recent increase of human life expectancy (see Fig. 5-1) could be due largely to environmental rather than genetic changes.

DO SOME SPECIES ESCAPE AGING? Extremely slow patterns of aging are found in many species. Plants give the best documentation through their annual growth rings. Bristlecone pines live at least 5000 years, and 1000 years is not unusual in other conifers. Some animals also can be dated by growth rings. Bivalve mollusks hold the record, with geoducks and quahogs living at least 200 years. In the northern Pacific, several species of rockfish can live at least 100 years and show no loss of fertility. Turtles may also exceed 100 years. Although no general signs of age-related dysfunctions are known in these long-lived examples, detailed studies remain to be done.

To experience a complete absence of aging, an organism would be required to repair all types of injuries and to rid itself of abnormal growths. Theoretically, the retention of a complete set of genes by cells throughout the body ('somatic cell genomic totipotency') could replace any damaged tissue. Achieving this goal through the control of gene activity, however, would not confer immortality because death still overtakes individuals, even in the absence of age-related disorders.

In humans, the safest of all ages occurs at about the time of puberty, when the mortality risk through accidents and disease equals about 1:2000 per year. If this risk were maintained indefinitely without the usual acceleration, then the life expectancy at birth would be about 1200 years, and the last survivor in a population of 4 billion would be 25,000 years old. Although fantastic improvements over the present human lifespans may be accomplished through disease reduction, the lesson is clear: We would still be subject to unavoidable dangers that statistically limit our ultimate lifespans.

THEORIES OF AGING

EVOLUTIONARY THEORY. Although true immortality seems unattainable, prospects are excellent for reducing many age-related dysfunctions that range from merely annoying changes, such as the common mild lapses of memory, to serious causes of morbidity, such as malignancies and osteoporotic fractures. A basis for optimism comes from the theories of aging that recognize multiple causes in the aging process. Evolutionary theory predicts a multiplicity of causes in aging.

The evolutionary view recognizes that young adults produce the most offspring. This would be so even if there were no menopause or reproductive declines, because mere living produces so many natural hazards. Natural annual mortality risks of 10% are not uncommon for mammals and birds. This statistic means that a small fraction survive to be grandparents. This demographic profile has great consequences, *because natural selection acts mostly on young adults,* who are the most responsible for the propagation of the species. Correspondingly, the force of natural selection against harmful or disadvantageous genes becomes progressively weaker with advancing age. As a consequence, theory predicts that mutations in the population gene pool are tolerated *if any adverse effects are delayed to older ages.* Among examples of genes with delayed adverse effects are hereditary AD and hereditary risks of breast cancer. Many different genes may cause particular diseases of aging.

MECHANISMS IN AGING. Numerous theories address specific aging changes in processes ranging from the molecular to organ system levels of function. One of the oldest is the *somatic mutation theory,* which originally focused on chromosomal genes. There is little doubt that somatic cells accumulate oncogenic mutations on a sporadic and scattered basis during the individual lifespan and that these are of great importance to the age-related increases in cancer. However, relatively few nuclear genes in any cell show evidence of damage through mutations. The somatic mutation theory has been expanded to include mitochondrial DNA mutations. In certain brain regions with high concentrations of the neurotransmitter dopamine, 1 to 5% of the mitochondria may have DNA deletions that impair ATP production.

Free-radical theories postulate that endogenously generated and highly reactive free radicals cause the somatic mutations described above. Free radicals can also damage proteins. Slowly replaced proteins such as collagen and elastin tend to show the accumulation of oxidized amino acids and the addition of glucose derivatives (glycation), both of which arise through free radicals. These modifications can change the molecular organization. Some features of diabetes such as diabetic lens opacity are associated with glycated proteins. Antioxidants and free radical trapping compounds may slow or reverse the oxidation of proteins during aging.

Oxidative damage from free radicals is being increasingly implicated in degenerative diseases of aging. Epidemiologic studies indicate that specific antioxidants protect individuals who are at risk for coronary artery disease and certain cancers. The gene for a familial type of amyotrophic lateral sclerosis has been mapped to the chromosomal locus for superoxide dismutase (SOD). The enzyme SOD converts the free radical of oxygen to hydrogen peroxide, which, in turn, is converted to harmless water and oxygen. Free radical damage also has been implicated in Parkinson's disease and AD. These findings have led policy organizations such as the Alliance for Aging to recommend that all adults consider supplementing their diets with vitamins C and E and β-carotene. In reality, it is impossible to totally abolish damage from free radicals; these chemical forms are ubiquitous and have key roles in our metabolism as well as causing slowly emerging damage.

Cell aging theories are based on the finite number of possible divisions made in culture *(in vitro)* by skin fibroblasts and by most other cells obtained from humans (the Hayflick phenomenon). The causes of clonal aging appear to involve the activities of genes that control cell proliferation, some of which are also crucial to malignancy, such as the p53 gene, which commonly mutates in human cancers and is thought to serve as a tumor suppressor. Most investigators agree that the nondividing status that follows repetitive proliferation does not lead to cell death. If kept carefully, nondividing cells can live for many months in culture dishes. The observation is consistent with the fact that our hearts and brains are full of cells that ceased dividing decades ago.

Cell senescence may also involve loss of DNA at the ends of chromosomes (telomers); immortal cancer cells, as well as the germ-like cells in the gonads, are protected against telomere shortening by an enzyme called *telomerase.*

Programmed cell death also relates to aging. During development excess numbers of neurons, lymphocytes, and other cells die through a genetically programmed sequence of changes called *apoptosis.* Cell death, however, can arise from other causes, such as ischemia or toxins, a process referred to as *necrotic cell death.* The cause of neuron death during AD and Parkinson's disease is being studied to resolve the relative contributions of apoptosis or necrotic cell death. In the aging prostate, apoptosis can be observed among benignly proliferating cells. Such natural mechanisms of cell death may protect against the progression of abnormal growths during aging.

Immune theories of aging are concerned with several changes. On the one hand, the primary immune response weakens, reflected in the increasing vulnerability to influenza and other infections found in the elderly. One factor is an increase in memory T cells at the expense of virgin T cells, with a net effect of reducing the response to novel antigens. On the other hand, there is a general increase of low-grade autoimmune and inflammatory processes, such as arthritis. The senile plaques of AD contain many inflammatory molecules, although T cells are not present. The net result indicates that hyperactivity in some immune functions coexists with hypoactivity in others. Ultimately, this complex situation may be understood in terms of the regulation of genes that control the proliferation of immune cell populations.

Endocrine theories account for a wide range of physiologic changes. Certain postmenopausal dysfunctions, as noted earlier, are clearly related to the exhaustion of ovarian follicles that produce estrogen and progesterone. The loss of estrogens accelerates osteoporosis. Moreover, the beneficial effects of estrogen, which also reduce the risk of heart attacks, strokes, and osteoarthritis, are lost at menopause. The event of menopause itself is clearly the consequence of the finite store of ovarian follicles and oocytes that are generated during development and not replaced.

Neuroendocrine theories address subtle changes in the output of the pituitary that accompany aging. The decreased secretion of growth hormone (GH), for example, is modest in most older adults. Some individuals may suffer GH deficits that cause skeletal muscle atrophy (myopenia), which can be corrected by GH replacement therapy. Nothing, however, suggests the presence of general deficits of GH that would warrant therapeutic replacement on the scale practiced for estrogen replacement after menopause. Many other age changes could be linked to altered functions of brain centers that influence the autonomic nervous system and metabolism. Such associations are largely speculative in humans. Hypothalamic age changes in female rodents importantly influence the irregularities of fertility (estrous) cycles that precede the exhaustion of the ovary. Glucocorticoids have been implicated in rodents as a cause of aging in some brain regions. No evidence, however, suggests a "death hormone" in humans or other mammals.

Wear and tear theories include mechanical and biochemical features of aging. Insects can wear out their irreplaceable wings. Tooth and joint erosion are common during human aging. At the molecular level, endogenously produced free radicals may damage certain irreplaceable molecules. Medical science has now come full circle in recognizing that molecules, like major body parts, are at risk for accumulating irreversible damage during aging.

SUMMARY

Aging changes appear to be very diverse and subject to numerous environmental and genetic influences. Aging processes thus show a great deal of plasticity and potential for modification. With the exception of the ovary, no other organ appears to have a programmed senescence that leads to predictable complete loss of function during aging in all human populations. Although some individuals carry genes that predispose them to early onset of specific degenerative diseases, there is much reason to anticipate that interventions will be possible. The slowed rates of death due to heart attacks in recent decades show the importance of lifestyle in the outcomes of aging. Many biologists and geriatricians are convinced that the potential for successful aging by maintaining health and independence at advanced ages is far greater than recognized by the general public.

General

Finch CE: Longevity, Senescence, and the Genome. Chicago, University of Chicago Press, 1990. *Comprehensive monograph on the comparative biology of aging, with references to many of the subjects treated in this chapter.*

Hazzard WR, et al.: Principles of Geriatric Medicine and Gerontology. 3rd ed. Healthcare Management Group, 1993. *Broad coverage and many special topics.*

Masoro EJ: Handbook of Physiology: Aging. Oxford, Oxford University Press, 1994. *Excellent chapters on aging of different organs and processes.*

Pliny the younger: Letters, Book V, Letter 6. New York, Penguin Press, 1961. E. Radice, translator.

Schneider EL, Rowe JW: Handbook on the Biology of Aging. 4th ed. San Diego, Academic Press, 1995. *A regularly updated and authoritative source of reviews by mainstream researchers.*

vom Saal FS, Finch CE, Nelson JF: The natural history of reproductive aging in humans, laboratory rodents and selected other vertebrates. *In* Knobil E (ed): Physiology of Reproduction. 2nd ed. New York, Raven Press, 1991, p 1213. *Detailed review on reproductive aging.*

Genetics of Aging

Brooks A, Lithgow GJ, Johnson TE: Mortality rates in a genetically heterogeneous population of *Caenorhabditis elegans.* Science 263:668, 1994.

Rose MR, Finch CE (eds): The Genetics of Aging. Genetica 91, Special Issue, 1994. *Current approaches to the genetics of aging in a wide range of species and select human conditions, including Alzheimer's disease.*

Theories of Aging

Dilman VM, Dean W: The Neuroendocrine Theory of Aging and Degenerative Disease. Pensacola, Fla, The Center for Bio-Gerontology, 1992. *Overview from a major theorist.*

Rose MR: The Evolutionary Biology of Aging. Oxford, Oxford University Press, 1991. *A lucid presentation of the evolutionary theory of aging.*

Sapolsky RM: Stress, the Aging Brain and Mechanisms of Neuron Death. Cambridge, MIT Press, 1993. *Definitive discussion of the stress hypothesis of aging.*

6 NEUROLOGIC PROBLEMS ASSOCIATED WITH AGING

Fred Plum

As the century approaches its end, the old get older, with those over 70 years being especially predisposed to several specific neurologic diseases listed in Table 6–1. Aging-related changes in the peripheral and central nervous systems produce worrisome symptoms in a far larger number. The process of aging importantly affects neurologic structures governing mood, intellectual processing, skilled movement, and the perceptions mediated by the special senses (Table 6–2). Symptoms of mild autonomic insufficiency, including constipation, nocturia, relative insomnia, sexual inadequacy, mild orthostatic hypotension, and increased susceptibility to hypothermia, affect many, if not most, persons more than 70 years of age. Almost half who survive beyond age 85 develop signs and symptoms of clinically diagnosable Alzheimer's disease, stroke, or both. Not surprisingly, many of the remainder become apprehensive about developing these conditions. Furthermore, many drugs used to ameliorate symptoms in various body systems also can cause brain dysfunction in the elderly. These considerations can make it difficult to distinguish benign neurologic symptoms from those related to disease (Table 6–3).

Most persons living beyond age 70 experience at least some recent memory loss, most have lost their life-long regular occupations, and few have developed active social, recreational, or athletic diversions to fill their time. Despite even television's lulling immanence, many become anxious and some depressed. Severe depression affects more than 15% of those older than 65 years, striking men more than women. Antidepressant medication often is effective but may be tolerated only at doses substantially lower than those indicated for younger persons. Chapter 7 discusses this problem at greater length.

No effective treatment for organic memory loss has appeared, but that due to anxiety or inattention may be helped by counseling or referral to appropriately concerned lay or religious support systems. The merely anxious do best with reassurance. Benzodiazepines or other tranquilizers seldom provide enduring benefit and sometimes make matters worse. Physiologic sleep in the elderly becomes less satisfying; deep, stage 4 sleep disappears and the remainder becomes more fitful and less lengthy. Furthermore, natural circadian rhythms intensify their effects, increasing the urge to postprandial drowsiness. A postlunch siesta can minimize or prevent the latter, heading off embarrassment and the appearance of senility among those who uncontrollably doze at meetings or social gatherings. Otherwise, strong reassurance is needed to alleviate overconcern about reduced ability to sleep. Sedative use for sleep problems in the elderly is almost never helpful and sometimes harmful. For the

already addicted, it may be impossible to discontinue such drugs. Otherwise their use should be confined briefly to emergencies or travel that extends beyond more than four to six time zones. In such instances, one-half the smallest available (0.125 mg) triazolam tablet, i.e., a dose of approximately 0.060 mg, usually brings at least brief sleep with minimal toxic side effects.

Delirium (see Ch. 394) is a common problem among elderly patients hospitalized acutely for systemic illness that independently lengthens institutional stay and worsens prognosis. Age over 80 years, pre-existing cognitive difficulties, and severity of illness provide the greatest vulnerability (Table 6–4). Definitive diagnostic features include acute onset, fluctuating course, inattention, disorganized thinking, and decreased arousal. Many drugs can impair cognition in the elderly; neuroleptics and narcotic pain relievers stand at the top of the list.

Effective treatment of elderly delirium can be difficult. Staff understanding and patience are crucial to management. More specifically, bedroom lights should be left on at night, restraints should be minimized (but not so much that falls occur), neuroleptics should be kept to minimal levels, and whenever possible attention by caregivers should be both gentle and maximized. Delirious patients should be kept out of bed as much as possible during waking hours, and incidental infections should be treated promptly. The presence of reassuring family members or other loved ones can help considerably in management.

Postural and musculoskeletal problems abound in the elderly. Joint and muscle-tendon pain sometimes can be difficult to separate from nerve root pain. Except for hip and knee replacements, however, few patients benefit from surgical treatment. Most of the symptoms derive from longstanding musculoskeletal wear and tear on joints and tendons, but changes in basal ganglia, postural reflexes, and perceptual functions contribute. Even in the absence of true parkinsonism, standing and walking become more stooped; the restless, normal, spontaneous muscular activity that characterizes more youthful life disappears; and physiologic tremor intensifies. Inadvertent falls become an increasing risk. The skeletal muscles lose their tone, reflex speeds slow down, and strength declines. All these changes reduce the sense of well-being but can be ameliorated somewhat by postural education and exercise. Even walking with briskly swinging arms can reduce discomfort and improve the sense of vigor. More extensive muscular activity must be appropriately individualized.

TABLE 6-1. NEUROLOGIC DISORDERS ESPECIALLY RELATED TO AGING

Alzheimer's disease and related dementias
Delirium
Cerebrovascular disease
"Idiopathic" degenerative disorders
  Parkinson's disease
  Senile tremor and allied movement disorders
  Motor neuron diseases
  Late-life ataxias
Spinal arthropathies with nerve root or spinal cord entrapment
Cranial arteritis
Herpes zoster
"Idiopathic" peripheral neuropathy
"Drop attacks" and falls
Hypothermia

TABLE 6-2. AGING CHANGES IN THE NERVOUS SYSTEM (65 TO 80 YEARS)

Brain shrinks and neuron counts decrease
  Frontal lobe (35%)
  Temporal lobe (45%)
  Basal ganglia (30%)
Cerebral blood flow and metabolism gradually decline
Speed of central and peripheral neural processing slows
Autonomic and muscle stretch reflexes lose sensitivity
Central and peripheral cholinergic systems decay
Olfactory, visual, and auditory-vestibular systems deteriorate
Susceptibility increases to degenerative, vascular, and immune-mediated disorders

TABLE 6-3. COMMON NONSPECIFIC SYMPTOMS OF NEUROLOGIC AGING

1. Recent memory loss
2. Depression or hopelessness
3. Insomnia-fatigue
4. Postural unsteadiness, giddiness, "spaciness," vertigo
5. Hearing difficulty—tinnitus, high-tone deafness, nerve deafness
6. Dimmed vision—cataracts, glaucoma, macular degeneration, presbyopia
7. Nocturia and/or incontinence
8. Male impotence, constipation
9. Vulnerability to therapeutic drugs

Pre-existing cognitive impairment
Age over 80 years
Severe illness or fractures
Acute infections
Male gender
Neuroleptics

Chronic feelings of dizziness, "spaciness," or giddiness plague the elderly. True vertigo is uncommon, but slowed or reduced baroceptor reflexes frequently induce brief orthostatic dysequilibrium. Similarly, contradictions among deteriorating visual, labyrinthine-vestibular, and proprioceptive perceptions develop and often generate a sense of giddiness or unsteadiness during standing or walking. Extending the head and looking skyward while walking or standing accentuate the contradictions between the senses, making matters worse. Among the very old, extremes of head extension (e.g., women leaning backward to the hairdresser's sink, men painting the ceiling) can induce true vertigo due to vertebral artery compression. All but the last of the above symptoms can be minimized by careful explanation because anxiety plays a role in every case. No drugs help the symptoms and many worsen them. Maneuvers that induce true vertigo should be specifically advised against.

Population surveys indicate that symptom-producing high-pitched, ringing tinnitus affects about 25% of all persons older than 60, probably reflecting gradual high-tone hearing loss. Only rarely is this distressing, and there is no effective treatment. The finding of progressive nerve deafness deserves referral to an otologist or neurologist. Most serious visual impairment in the elderly stems from cataracts, glaucoma, or macular degeneration (Part XXV). Once these conditions are excluded by ophthalmologic evaluation or treated, the physician can deal with nonspecific symptoms of visual fatigue or intermittent impairment of acuity by reassurance and common sense.

A variety of medications cause unwanted neurotoxic side effects in the elderly, including depression of mood, delirium, dyssomnia, and incoordination. Many produce side effects even at dosages and measured drug levels that lie within the "therapeutic ranges." Table 6-5 lists major pharmacal offenders, which should be prescribed cautiously.

The neurologic examination in healthy elderly patients reflects the inevitable decay that sooner or later affects nearly all neurologic systems. In addition, three fourths of those who live beyond 70 years have a major disorder of at least one other bodily system which reduces their sense of well-being. Nearly all have at least some difficulty with recent memory compared with their younger years. Nevertheless, many old persons retain sufficient cognitive and verbal activity to perform bedside mental status examinations at a normal level. Old-age changes in station, gait, mood, and neuromuscular functions have been mentioned above. As many as half of the very old have difficulty converging the eyes, and a substantial fraction show functionally unimportant limitations of conjugate upgaze. Pupillary miosis is common. As the skeletal muscles weaken, interosseous atrophy gradually, unavoidably affects the muscles of the hands and feet. The capacity to perform rapid skilled movements slows, and many persons develop a mild, non-parkinsonian tremor of the head or hands. Deep-tendon reflexes decline in amplitude and Achilles tendon jerks often disappear. Extensor plantar responses are *not* a normal finding. In asymptomatic patients, however, they sometimes can reflect osteoarthritic spinal cord encroachment rather than serious brain or spinal cord dysfunction. Perception of pain and touch and proprioceptive sensation remain essentially intact in normal elderly persons, but most have reduced vibratory perception in the distal lower extremities. A few develop peripheral neuropathy demonstrable more in the lower than the upper extremities and characterized chiefly by annoying paresthesias and a degree of proprioceptive impairment. Such patients should be evaluated for metabolic disorders or possible nerve root compression, but for most the cause remains unknown and the treatment symptomatic.

Hazzard WR, Andres R, Bierman EL, Blass JP (eds.): Principles of Geriatric Medicine and Gerontology, 2nd ed. New York, McGraw-Hill, 1990, p 1005. *Part 3, Section 1 provides a good background to the neurobiology of the aging brain and the specific diseases that affect the central and peripheral nervous systems.*
Inouye SK, Viscoli CM, Horwitz RI, et al.: A predictive model for delirium in hospitalized elderly medical patients based on admission characteristics. Ann Intern Med 119:474–481, 1993. *Among a large cohort of patients older than 70, visual factors, severe illness, pre-existing cognitive impairment, and dehydration were the greatest risk factors.*

TABLE 6-5. POTENTIAL NEUROTOXIC DRUG REACTIONS IN THE ELDERLY, MOSTLY DOSE-RELATED

Analgesics	
Aspirin (large doses)	Tinnitus, confusion
Nonsteroidal anti-inflammatory drugs	Confusion, aseptic meningitis
Opiates	Increased vulnerability to known effects
Anticholinergics	
Includes many agents employed for gastric difficulties (e.g., metoclopramide, atropine), urinary frequency, or parkinsonism; also tricyclic antidepressants and several tranquilizers	Confusion, hallucinations, glaucoma, urinary retention, constipation, hypothermia
Antihypertensives	Postural hypotension, erect giddiness, falls
Anticonvulsants	
Carbamazepine; phenytoin	Lethargic confusion; ataxia, mild confusion
Benzodiazepines	Depression, amnesia, confusion, drowsiness, falls
Cimetidine and other histamine H_2 blockers	Confusion
Corticosteroids	Delirium
Digitalis	Confusion, hallucinations
Dopaminergic agents	
Levodopa Bromocriptine	Dyskinesias, postural hypotension, confusion

7 NEUROPSYCHIATRIC ASPECTS OF AGING

Gene D. Cohen

Worldwide studies of older adults during the past 40 years have documented a 15% to 25% prevalence of serious mental disorders in later life. Organic mental disorders such as Alzheimer's disease (AD) and related dementias affect approximately 10% of persons older than age 65 and as many as 40% of those older than age 85. By no means, however, are Alzheimer-related illnesses the exclusive neuropsychiatric disorder of the elderly. Alcohol and substance abuse affect at least 2% to 5% of these persons, and as many as 15% experience worrisome depressive symptoms, with about 5% suffering severe depressions. Anxiety, like depression, is a variety of symptom states estimated to affect approximately 10% of older women and about 5% of older men. The frequency of dysfunctional personality disorders has been reported to be between 2% and 11%. Schizophrenia has about a 1% prevalence. Many if not most of these problems represent inextricable manifestations of both neurologic and psychiatric deterioration.

EVALUATION OF NEUROPSYCHIATRIC SYMPTOMS AND SIGNS IN LATER LIFE

MEMORY AND COGNITIVE CHANGES. At present, although increasing numbers of physicians are becoming aware of manifestations of AD, far fewer appreciate how much potentially treatable psychopathology affects the old and the very old.

With normal brain aging, cognitive functions remain relatively stable. Some mental skills actually improve in response to ongoing challenges, vocabulary especially. The implication is that cognitive impairment should be considered and investigated as a brain disease, not merely as evidence of the wastebasket diagnosis of benign cerebral senescence.

Mental Status Screening Tests. When a question of mental impairment arises, a useful quick approach to assess cognitive function is for the physician to apply a brief mental status screening instrument. An excellent example is the 19 item/30 point Mini-Mental State Examination (MMSE) (see Table 400–3); a score of 25 or greater is generally considered within normal range, with a score of 20 or less in older adults (including those of low education) suggesting the presence of dementia.

Clinically, dementia is characterized by the following:

Demonstrable evidence of significant impairment of short-term (as indicated by inability to learn new information) and long-term memory.

Impairment in abstract thinking, as indicated by difficulty in defining words and concepts previously known.

Impaired judgment, as indicated by inability to make reasonable plans to deal with interpersonal, social, and work-related problems.

Other disturbances of higher cortical function such as language problems (aphasia); motor skill problems despite physical capacity (apraxia); failure to recognize and identify familiar objects despite intact sensory function (agnosia).

Personality change, such as alteration or accentuation of premorbid traits (*note:* among healthy persons, personality remains stable with aging).

Normal or nearly normal results on mental status tests by patients complaining of memory loss suggest that mental illness rather than organic cognitive loss underlies their complaints. Many older adults complain of memory loss that is not apparent to others; often such complaints reflect not cognitive impairment, but depression—analogous to somatoform complaints in younger patients.

Excess Disability. When dementia or even severe depression from physical limitation is the correct diagnosis, it is important not to be misled by the commonly expressed nihilism that no treatment can help. Apart from the development of new drugs aimed at alleviating cognitive impairment, an extensive body of knowledge exists about how to treat excess disability in patients with early dementia, stroke, or other partial invalidisms. Just as depression, anxiety, and psychosis can interfere with concentration in the noncognitively impaired, when these symptoms accompany dementia they compound the cognitive or other age-related dysfunctions, causing the phenomenon known as "excess disability." By treating the overlay of depression, agitation, or delusions, physicians can reduce patient suffering, help patients to cope with their disorder, and lessen the burden on the family. A range of psychosocial interventions and judiciously used psychotropic medications can make a significant contribution to alleviating excess disability in patients with AD and related disorders.

Sleep Disturbances. Although older persons often complain of difficulty in sleeping, mere aging often is not the cause. Some sleep study reports describe a reduction in total sleep time; others do not. Undoubtedly, sleep stage changes occur normally, as do the number of nighttime awakenings, but this is a general principle not necessarily applying to each individual case. More relevant clinical considerations include whether any complaint is of recent onset and how much it departs from the patient's past sleep pattern. If an older person reports a noticeable reduction in sleep not attributed to daytime napping, an evaluation is indicated.

Apart from the role of arthritic, urologic, and cardiac problems, mental disorders are major inducers of sleep difficulty. Hallmarks include early morning awakening associated with depression and difficulty falling asleep or restless sleep with frequent awakenings associated with feelings of anxiety.

Change in Sexual Interest or Capacity. Sex life changes in later life, like sleep changes, often trigger patients to feel that "the ravages of aging are at work." Once again, group characteristics should be separated from the individual case. But even as a group, many or most healthy men and women with a past history of normal sexual activity demonstrate continuing interest in and capacity for some form of sexual relations. Reports of the prevalence of impotence in later life vary, with some studies reporting around 25% after age 65 and 50% after age 75, although as many as half of these are believed to be psychogenic in origin. As with sleep, clinically significant changes, particularly recent ones, should be evaluated. Factors that may induce marked changes include social situation (i.e., the opportunity for sexual relations), depression (interfering with motivation, arousal, satisfaction), drug and alcohol side effects (especially affecting erectile and ejaculatory capacity in men), as well as a range of general medical, neurologic (e.g., diabetic neuropathy), metabolic (e.g., thyroid dysfunction), urologic (e.g., recurrent cystitis and urethritis), and surgical disorders (e.g., rectal cancer surgery). Unfortunately, many doctors omit discussing sexual matters with older persons. Many patients with angina, for example, fear that an active sex life will place them at risk for a heart attack. Given the opportunity, physicians should offer both clarifying information and helpful interventions about elderly sexual activity.

Fear or Rumination about Death. That older people worry about death, and "wouldn't you, too, if you were elderly?" is a widely held view. But it does not accurately reflect the phenomenology of later life. Thinking about dying does not equal fearing it or dreading it. Not surprisingly, conversations about death are more common with elderly individuals because they have more peers and older relatives who have died or are dying. Dread of death is another matter—more common in midlife (as with the midlife crisis), when one takes a phenomenologic turn in contemplating for the first time how much time is left as opposed to how much has gone by. Once such individuals begin to think about time remaining, they confront an existential awareness of their own mortality, increasing the frequency of angst.

As time passes, older persons more than middle-aged ones come to terms with their mortality. Dread of death in later life arises more commonly in association with a terminal illness, personal losses, or major events that magnify one's sense of vulnerability. It is either the initial awareness that one is dying or the effect of depression—not the awareness of aging—that predisposes older individuals to death anxiety. Even with terminal illness, people eventually adjust. Dread of death should be viewed as a signal of distress, often of treatable depression.

MOOD CHANGES. Contrary to popular belief, most older adults are not depressed. Apart from normal grieving and bereavement, the prevalence of diagnosable clinical depression is reported at less than 5% in persons aged 65 years and older. Depressive symptoms, however, have been identified in as many as 15% in this age group, and studies of medical outcomes have shown that such symptoms can have adverse effects similar to those of a depressive disorder itself. Findings reveal that depressive symptoms have a greater influence on inability to carry out tasks and on days in bed than the following eight major general medical problems: hypertension, diabetes, advanced coronary artery disease, angina, arthritis, back problems, lung problems, and gastrointestinal disorders. Moreover, research indicates that over a 12-month period depressed persons in nursing homes have a 60% greater mortality than the nondepressed. Although completed suicide rates reported by countries throughout the world vary (World Health Organization, 1985/6), a generally consistent finding is that the elderly have the highest rates. Elderly men have the highest rates of all. (In the United States, male rates per 100,000 are 43.4 for those over age 60; 23.6 for those aged 30 to 59; 22.6 for those aged 15 to 29). These features highlight the importance of proper diagnosis and treatment of depression in older adults.

Diagnosis of Depression. As in the arena of cognitive impairment, brief depression scales are available for assessing whether or not the patient is depressed, such as the 15-question Geriatric Depression Scale (GDS).

Clinically, key features of major depressive disorder in later life are contained in Table 7–1. Apart from the emotional toll on the individual afflicted with depression and anguish for the family in trying to deal with the depression of an older loved one, the physical health of the depressed older person is also a concern. Weight loss, for example, can tilt the balance away from physical health by increasing vulnerability to other illness. The ability to treat depression in older adults through a combination of pharmacologic, be-

TABLE 7-1. GERIATRIC DEPRESSION SCALE—SHORT FORM

1.	Are you basically satisfied with your life?	yes/NO
2.	Have you dropped many of your activities and interests?	YES/no
3.	Do you feel that you life is empty?	YES/no
4.	Do you often get bored?	YES/no
5.	Are you in good spirits most of the time?	yes/NO
6.	Are you afraid that something bad is going to happen to you?	YES/no
7.	Do you feel happy most of the time?	yes/NO
8.	Do you feel helpless?	YES/no
9.	Do you prefer to stay home, rather than going out and doing new things?	YES/no
10.	Do you feel you have more problems with memory than most?	YES/no
11.	Do you think it is wonderful to be alive now?	yes/NO
12.	Do you feel pretty worthless the way you are now?	YES/no
13.	Do you feel full of energy?	yes/NO
14.	Do you feel that your situation is hopeless?	YES/no
15.	Do you think that most people are better off than you are?	YES/no

SCORING: Answers indicating depression are HIGHLIGHTED. Each answer counts one point; scores greater than 5 indicate probable depression.

Adapted from Yesavage J, Brink T, Rowe T, et al: Development and validation of a geriatric depression screening scale: A preliminary report. J Psychiatr Res 17:37, 1983.

havioral, and psychosocial interventions continues to improve and is discussed later in the treatment section.

Depression as excess disability in AD and related disorders aggravates problems with concentration, weight loss, sleep disturbances, and activities of daily living (ADL's) such as dressing and toileting. The aggravated sleep and ADL problems of the AD patient add measurably to a family's burden. Hence, treating excess disability in dementia patients not only helps them to cope better from day to day but also reduces the burden on the family, over 25% of whom, themselves, develop clinically significant symptoms of depression as a result of the stress associated with prolonged caregiving. Treatment also helps families wanting to keep their loved one home longer, postponing the need for nursing home placement. Studies show that ADL difficulties and sleep and appetite problems caused by depression in AD improve in as many as 85% of cases when the depression is treated through behavioral or combined behavioral and pharmacologic interventions.

PSEUDODEMENTIA. Pseudodementia (e.g., depression presenting like dementia) represents a clinical state in which mental disorders other than dementing diseases compromise cognitive functioning in older individuals. As many as 15% to 20% of depressed older adults exhibit signs of transient cognitive impairment in response to their mood disorder. Table 7-2 offers some general guidelines for differentiating depression from dementia when the two do not co-exist. Apart from the questions and criteria in Tables 7-1 and 7-2, and the clinical features of depression in Table

TABLE 7-2. DIAGNOSIS OF PSEUDODEMENTIA (CLINICAL FEATURES DIFFERENTIATING DEPRESSION FROM DEMENTIA)

Depression	Dementia
Cognitive impairment, when present, is usually more rapid in onset and brief in duration.	Cognitive impairment in Alzheimer's disease is gradual in onset, worsening over time.
Depressed mood typically prominent with complaints about cognitive impairment emphasized rather than concealed or denied.	Cognitive impairment typically more prominent than depressed mood, with complaints of the former often understated or denied.
Cognitive symptoms worsen or mitigate as depression becomes more or less severe.	Cognitive impairment less influenced by fluctuations in mood, remaining in the dementia range.
Mentation more likely to improve in response to treatment for depression.	Mentation less responsive to treatment for depression, remaining in the dementia range.
Past and family history of depression more likely.	Past and family history of depression less prevalent.

401-6, it may be necessary to test the effects of antidepressant medication as part of the diagnostic evaluation between depression and dementia.

INTERACTIONS BETWEEN MENTAL AND PHYSICAL HEALTH PHENOMENA WITH AGING

Studies during the past decade have increasingly disclosed that mental health problems can importantly influence the course of major medical and surgical diseases. Among patients with fractured femurs, for example, Levitan and Kornfeld showed that those who received psychiatric consultation not only had their hospital stay reduced 30%, but also had twice the likelihood of immediately returning home rather than entering a nursing home facility. The length of hospital stay and risk of nursing home placement were significantly greater in fracture patients not receiving psychiatric consultation. Mumford et al. reviewed and reported on more than 30 studies showing similar reductions in length of stay and improved hospital course among other older surgical and cardiac patients receiving mental health interventions along with their medical or surgical care.

The role of covert neuropsychiatric symptoms points to explanations of these outcomes. Consider that approximately 25% of older patients presenting to primary care physicians with nonpsychiatric problems reveal clinically significant symptoms of depression when also evaluated for co-existing mental disorder. Older patients with significant physical illness are at greater risk for depression than counterparts in the population who are in generally good physical health. Both biologic and psychological mechanisms—the two interacting—contribute to the adverse effect of depression on overall health outcomes. Psychoimmunologic studies of depression demonstrate the compromising effect of depressive disorder on immune function in both hospitalized and community-dwelling older adults; these studies suggest potential interference with healing processes in injuries and infections.

One study of older depressed caregivers of AD patients found the following immune system changes:

Lower percentages of total T lymphocytes, helper T lymphocytes, and helper/suppressor cell ratios than in comparison subjects (T cells are important in stimulating a number of other immunologic activities).

Lower levels of natural killer cells, thought to be an important defense against certain kinds of viruses and possibly cancer as well.

Significantly higher antibody titers to Epstein-Barr virus, the causative agent for infectious mononucleosis (presumably reflecting poor cellular immune system control over the expression of this latent herpesvirus).

From a psychodynamic vantage point, the depressed patient is less motivated to participate in aggressive rehabilitation and less confident of being able to function at home following hospitalization. The interaction and synergism of biologic and psychological factors increase the risk of a longer hospital stay and of further post-hospitalization convalescence at a skilled nursing facility.

Masked Depression. Just as infectious disease may be masked or present atypically in older patients, so too with mental illness. What on the surface may seem to be an exacerbation of a chronic physical disorder may underneath be the adverse influence of depression. For example, an older patient with congestive heart failure may be getting worse, making the family think that the deterioration is due to the progression of both the patient's age and cardiac disease. But underneath, what might be operating is a covert depression, causing the patient to give up, resulting in indirect suicidal behavior via poor medication compliance.

Similarly, with some labile diabetics, periods of depressive symptoms may explain episodic major fluctuations in glucose control. One may be witnessing not the natural clinical course of diabetes with aging but the effect of depressive episodes during which the patient is unmotivated or distracted from applying adequate diligence to insulin management. Anxiety or thought disorder (e.g., late-onset schizophrenia) may also compromise the ability of the physically ill patient to stick to treatment plans requiring a high level of attentiveness and consistency.

TABLE 7–3. GENERAL PRINCIPLES OF TREATMENT AND MANAGEMENT

Treatment planning
Identification of specific clinical problems: targeting signs and symptoms reflecting disturbances in mood, thought content, cognition
Identification of specific strengths: identifying remaining capacities and coping skills that can maximize functioning in the face of new deficits
Identification of individual satisfactions: identifying pleasant or satisfying experiences that enhance well-being or mitigate illness
Comprehensive approach to intervention
Behavioral and psychotherapeutic interventions
Psychopharmacologic treatment in combination with psychosocial support
Coordination of person/environment fit with attention to residential and care options within the expanding geriatric landscape

---

Contrary to popular view, psychodynamic studies reveal that older adults are less psychologically resistant than younger persons to unpleasant insights. Moreover, evidence indicates that today's cohort of older adults is highly receptive to behavioral and psychotherapeutic interventions.

BEHAVIORAL AND PSYCHOTHERAPEUTIC INTERVENTIONS. Clinical trials of behavioral and psychotherapeutic interventions have proven effective in treating nonpsychotic disorders in older adults (Table 7–3). A comparative study of three brief (16 to 20 individual sessions) psychotherapies (cognitive, behavioral, and psychodynamic) for major depression demonstrated comparable efficacy for each. Overall improvement was 70%, with 52% achieving remission and 18% significantly improving.

Pharmacotherapy. Two basic guidelines influence psychotropic drug use in later life: (1) "Start low and go slow" with dosage adjustments; (2) select medications as much from the perspective of side effects to avoid as desired effects to achieve.

Pharmacokinetics and Pharmacodynamics. Rational psychotropic drug choice and administration are influenced by *pharmacokinetics* (how the body acts on a drug) and *pharmacodynamics* (how a drug acts on the body). Pharmacokinetics includes *absorption, distribution, metabolism,* and *excretion.* Aging *per se* does not alter *absorption,* but the concomitant intake of other drugs, such as antacids, may delay absorption and hence the time it takes to reach peak plasma levels. Most psychoactive drugs (e.g., long-acting benzodiazepines) are lipid-soluble (lithium is water-soluble); an increase in body fat with aging influences *distribution,* resulting

in increased risk of accumulation, illustrating why a lower dose may be indicated. Most psychoactive drugs (exceptions include lithium) are *metabolized* in the liver; slower hepatic enzyme activity with aging also increases the risk of drug accumulation and the need for a lower dose. Renal excretion is the primary pathway for the removal of water-soluble lithium from the body; reduced renal function with aging increases the risk of accumulation. Pharmacodynamic considerations address central nervous system receptor sensitivity; increased sensitivity explains why a lower dosage of psychoactive drugs in older adults may achieve the same effect as a higher dosage in young adults.

Antidepressants. Table 7–4 reviews dosage and side-effect profiles of selected antidepressant drugs for treating elderly patients. Because of efficacy comparable to the tricyclic antidepressants and a different side-effect profile (less sedation, hypotension, anticholinergic and cardiac side effects) the selective serotonin reuptake inhibitors (SSRI's) are emerging as preferred antidepressants for older adults. Even so, the SSRI's are not without side effects (including nausea, anxiety, insomnia, drowsiness, and headache). Also, because they may be activating rather than sedating, SSRI's are typically given in the morning.

Not all antidepressants are included in Table 7–4. Monamine oxidase inhibitors represent a major category of antidepressants but because of their potentially serious side effects they are not first- or second-choice drugs in treatment of the elderly.

Finally, some points must be made about electroconvulsive therapy (ECT). Clinical experience and many controlled studies indicate that ECT is a safe and effective treatment for depression. It is typically reserved, however, for treating severely depressed patients who fail to respond to antidepressant medications or who are unable to tolerate their side effects.

Antianxiety Medications. Table 7–5 reviews dosage and half-life considerations of various anxiolytic drugs. Because drug accumulation in the body is a major concern, many physicians who treat older patients for anxiety prefer to use drugs with short half-lives. Oxazepam and lorazepam not only are short acting, but their half lives in older persons are essentially the same as in young ones. Note that oxazepam and lorazepam are often used in treating sleep problems in the elderly. Their effects often are better tolerated and they are less habit forming and less associated with rebound insomnia than are a number of hypnotics.

Neuroleptics. Antipsychotic medications are often considered in the treatment of schizophrenia, various delusional and severe mood disorders, and dementia. Like antidepressants, neuroleptics of choice are typically selected by side-effect profile because most are comparable in efficacy at equivalent dosages. High-dose/low-

TABLE 7–4. DOSAGE AND RELATIVE SIDE EFFECTS OF SELECTED ANTIDEPRESSANTS IN ELDERLY PATIENTS

Drug	Daily Dosage (mg)	Sedation	Hypotension	Anticholinergic Side Effects	Altered Cardiac Rate, Rhythm
Tertiary amines					
Imipramine	10–75	+	++	++/+++	++
Doxepin	10–75	++/+++	++	+++	++
Amitryptyline	10–75	+++	++	++++	+++
Trimipramine	10–75	+++	++	+++	+++
Clomipramine	10–250	+++	+++	+++	+++
Secondary amines					
Desipramine	10–75	+	+/++	+	+
Nortriptyline	10–50	+	+	++	+
Amoxapine	10–300	+	++	++	++
Protriptyline	5–20	+	++	+++	++
Maprotiline	10–75	++/+++	++	++	+
Selective serotonin reuptake inhibitors					
Fluoxetine	10–40	—	—	—	—
Paroxetine	10–40	—	—	—	—
Sertraline	25–150	—	—	—	—
Other					
Trazadone	25–200	++	++	+	+/++
Buproprion	75–300	—	–/+	—	—

Key: — indicates unusual or minimal or none; + indicates mild; ++ indicates moderate; +++ indicates strong; ++++ indicates very strong; / indicates in between (hence, +/++ indicates mild to moderate).
Adapted from Alexopoulos GS: Treatment of depression. *In* Salzman C (ed): Clinical Geriatric Psychopharmacology. Baltimore, Williams & Wilkins, 1992, 137.

TABLE 7–5. SELECTED ANTIANXIETY DRUGS: DOSAGES AND HALF-LIFE CHARACTERISTICS

Drug	Usual Geriatric Dose Range (mg/day)	Half-Life (hrs) Young Adults	Half-Life (hrs) Older Adults
Long-acting			
Diazepam	2–20	24	75
Chlordiazepoxide	10–40	10	30
Intermediate-acting			
Alprazolam	0.25–2	10	17
Short-acting			
Lorazepam	0.5–2	12	12
Oxazepam	10–45	10	10

Adapted from Salzman C: Treatment of anxiety. *In* Salzman C (ed): Clinical Geriatric Psychopharmacology. Baltimore, Williams & Wilkins, 1992, 189.

potency neuroleptics like thioridazine and chlorpromazine induce higher incidences of orthostatic hypotension, anticholinergic reactions, and sedation. Low-dose/high-potency neuroleptics like haloperidol and trifluoperazine are associated with higher incidences of extrapyramidal reactions and neuroleptic-induced parkinsonism. The low-dose/high-potency or intermediate range (e.g., trilafon) neuroleptics tend to be preferred by geriatric specialists when antipsychotic drugs are indicated.

Social/Environmental Considerations—The Geriatric Landscape.
The growth and diversification of "the geriatric landscape"—a term that describes the increasing number of sites where older persons both reside and receive treatment—have created new options for tailoring a disability–social environment fit for individual patients. In addition to home and nursing home, the new geriatric landscape includes settings such as congregate housing, assisted living facilities, life or continuing care communities, senior hotels, foster care, group homes, day care (where people reside during the day), and respite care as well as a growing diversity of retirement homes and communities. Clinicians who care for older patients with mental status impairments requiring increased supervision should familiarize themselves with community-based examples of the new geriatric landscape.

The Social Portfolio. Persons in the modern work force are advised to plan for economic security for their future—to strive for a balanced financial portfolio. At the same time, they pay too little attention to developing a balanced "social portfolio" based on sound activities and interpersonal relationships that they can carry into old age. The diagram (Table 7–6) of a social portfolio for the aging years reflects efforts to plan for the future balancing *individual* with *group* activities and balancing *active* endeavors (activities that require significant effort) with *passive* ones (those that require little physical exertion). Some activities that require low levels of physical effort can be drawn upon should illness reduce physical capacity. Others can buffer loneliness during a transition marked by the loss of a loved one.

The poet-physician William Carlos Williams suffered a stroke in his 60's that resulted in reduced physical capacity and a severe post-stroke depression. Although unable to return to the practice of medicine, he continued his poetry to which he turned full time; his writings in his 70's led to a Pulitzer Prize. Neuropsychiatrically, his history illustrates the importance of discerning physical changes from mental status changes and with mental status changes the importance of distinguishing changes in mood from changes in cognition. In the poetry he created in his later years, Williams wrote about "an old age that adds as it takes away."

TABLE 7–6. THE SOCIAL PORTFOLIO

	Group Efforts	Individual Efforts
Active Interests	Elder hostel	Gardening
	Dance lessons	Nature walks
	Tennis	Photography
Passive Interests	Movie club	Cooking
	Volunteerism	Reading/writing
	Art class	Telephone work

Birren JE, Sloane RB, Cohen GD (eds): Handbook of Mental Health and Aging. 2nd ed. San Diego, Academic Press, 1992. *An authoritative, comprehensive overview of both mental health and mental illness (including detailed attention to diagnosis and treatment) in later life, with concise chapters on both neuropsychiatric and neuropsychological assessment.*

Cohen GD: The geriatric landscape: Toward a health and humanities research agenda in aging. Am J Geriatr Psychiatry 3:185, 1994. *A discussion of the historic increase in settings where older persons reside and receive treatment, with attention to new practice, policy, and research options.*

Kiecolt-Glaser JK, Glaser R: Caregiving, mental health, and immune function. *In* Light E, Lebowitz BD (eds): Alzheimer's Disease Treatment and Family Stress: Directions for Research. U.S. Department of Health and Human Services Publication No (ADM)89–1569, 1989, p 245. *This reference summarizes major recent findings of the effect of chronic stress and depression on the immune system in older adults, in a book that looks at caregiver stress in general in AD.*

Mumford E, Schlesinger HJ, Glass GV: The effects of psychological intervention on recovery from surgery and heart attacks: An analysis of the literature. Am J Publ Health 72:141, 1982. *A comprehensive review of the literature identifying 34 studies involving a high percentage of older patients, showing similar results to an earlier Levitan and Kornfeld study (Am J Psychiat 138:790, 1981).*

Schneider LS, Reynolds CF, Lebowitz BD, et al. (eds): Diagnosis and Treatment of Depression in Late Life—Results of the NIH Consensus Development Conference. Washington, DC, American Psychiatric Press, 1994. *A state-of-the art collection of papers covering the nature, diagnosis, and treatment (psychotherapy, pharmacotherapy, and electroconvulsive therapy) of late-life depression.*

8 SPECIAL PROBLEMS IN THE GERIATRIC PATIENT
Judith C. Ahronheim

Biologic and chronologic ages are not well matched. However, certain physiologic changes and a higher prevalence of overt and subclinical disease in late life create specific vulnerabilities. The following discussion highlights special problems that confront this age group.

DRUGS AND RISKS

CLINICAL PHARMACOLOGY. The elderly experience more adverse drug events than any other age group. This is due to their exposure to larger numbers of medications, medication errors, drug-drug interactions, altered pharmacokinetics, and enhanced sensitivity to many agents.

Pharmacokinetic Changes. Certain physiologic changes that occur in late life lead to reduced drug elimination, prolonged half-life, and risk of toxicity. The most consistent age-related change is renal. Glomerular filtration rate (GFR) declines, on the average, by approximately 50% between the third and ninth decades of life. However, many individuals maintain normal or nearly normal GFR in late life, and it is difficult to predict individual renal function because serum creatinine does not reflect the age-related decline in GFR. This is because muscle mass, the source of serum creatinine, also declines with age.

In general, ordinary loading doses of renally eliminated drugs can be given safely and should be given when necessary. However, if a drug has a narrow therapeutic index (ratio of dose producing the desired effect to that producing a toxic effect), toxicity may occur after repeated doses unless the dose is adjusted according to actual renal function. This is the case for drugs such as digoxin and the aminoglycoside antibiotics. A 24-hour urine collection is difficult to obtain in elderly patients if they have functional impairments. Formulas for rapid estimation of GFR have been validated in subgroups of elderly patients and should be used when dosing decisions are rapidly needed. However, these estimates may be inaccurate in debilitated patients with muscle wasting and in the dynamic setting of acute illness. Serum drug levels should be obtained to guide dosing whenever there is uncertainty.

Controversy exists over the extent to which age-related hepatic changes affect drug metabolism. Hepatic blood flow may decrease with advancing age, reducing the efficiency with which the liver can handle drugs that present themselves for metabolic breakdown. Some but not all studies have demonstrated a decline in hepatic oxidative processes ("phase I" metabolism) with advancing age.

Likewise, unanimity is lacking over whether the inducibility or inhibition of the cytochrome P-450 system, responsible for most oxidative drug metabolism, changes with age. In contrast, there is general agreement that hepatic conjugation ("phase II" metabolism) is unaltered with age. Unlike oxidized metabolites, which are often active, metabolites produced by conjugation are usually inactive. It should not be assumed that these or any other hepatically metabolized drugs are necessarily "safe," however, because many have enhanced effects in the elderly regardless of metabolic pathway (see below).

With advancing age lean body mass declines and body fat increases. Thus, the volume of distribution tends to be lower for water-soluble drugs and higher for fat-soluble drugs among elderly patients. The onset of action of a water-soluble drug may be earlier than expected, and the steady-state concentrations of lipid-soluble drugs may not be reached until later than expected. In the latter situation, toxicity may occur in a delayed and unexpected fashion.

Serum protein levels may be altered in late life, and although these changes may have little impact on drug disposition, they may affect interpretation of serum drug levels. Serum albumin remains normal in healthy elderly but may decline swiftly during illness, owing to impaired protein synthesis and diminished reserves in late life. When serum albumin is low, standard clinical laboratory assays of drugs highly bound to albumin (such as phenytoin) may be misleading because they reflect total (bound plus free) drug. This might prompt the clinician to raise the dose, leading to toxicity. The reverse would be true for drugs that bind to α_1-acid glycoprotein, which is an acute phase reactant that tends to increase with advancing age.

Pharmacodynamics. The specific action of the drug at the tissue level may also be altered in late life. Although the effects of some agents may decrease, most alterations involve enhanced effects on the target or nontarget organ. These effects may be related to physiologic changes as well as the presence of overt or silent disease. Although enhanced effects are often due to reduced elimination (altered pharmacokinetics) rather than to any alteration in the receptor or tissue itself (pharmacodynamics), it is important to anticipate specific side effects that may occur regardless of the precise mechanism.

All of these problems are compounded by the important practical issues that arise, such as the risk of medication errors when the regimen is complex or the patient is cognitively impaired; the risk of drug interactions that is proportional to the number of drugs taken; the presence of multisystem disease leading the patient to seek the services of many doctors, who may dispense conflicting prescriptions.

BOWEL AND BLADDER PROBLEMS

CONSTIPATION AND FECAL IMPACTION. Contrary to popular belief, little evidence indicates an increased prevalence of constipation among community-dwelling elderly, although there is an increased use of laxatives, perhaps because of traditional beliefs about what constitutes normal bowel function. Constipation may be increased among institutionalized elderly, however. This has been attributed to immobility, decreased intake of fluid and fiber, prolonged intestinal transit time, impaired anorectal sensation, neurologic disease, bowel lesions, and use of constipating medicines. Constipating medications include tricyclic antidepressants, anticholinergics, some antihypertensive agents, calcium channel antagonists, opioid analgesics, aluminum-containing antacids, bile-acid resins, and others.

An important consequence of constipation is fecal impaction. Fecal impaction may present with fever, altered mental status, agitation, urinary retention, or paradoxical diarrhea. Because of these presentations, fecal impaction can be mistaken for other problems, leading to inappropriate treatment. In extreme cases, mechanical bowel obstruction may occur, necessitating surgical intervention, but fecal impaction can usually be treated with suppositories, enemas, or manual disimpaction. Prevention consists of strict attention to the patient's bowel habits, adequate hydration and adequate but not excessive dietary fiber, avoidance of constipating medications when possible, and judicious use of laxatives.

PROBLEMS WITH MICTURITION. Urinary Incontinence. Urinary incontinence affects 10 to 30% of community-

residing elderly and at least 60 to 70% of elderly residing in nursing homes. The prevalence of urinary incontinence is highest among the oldest old. Overactivity of the bladder detrusor is the most common cause of urinary incontinence in elderly men and women. In this condition (also called "detrusor hyperreflexia" or "detrusor instability"), the detrusor muscle contracts in response to inappropriately small volumes of urine, often preceded by a sense of urgency. Incontinence results if the patient is unable to get to the toilet on time or when other problems, such as urethral incompetence or bladder inflammation, co-exist.

Detrusor overactivity is believed to be caused by lack of inhibition of the brain stem detrusor reflex by higher cerebrocortical centers. However, most affected elderly have no clinically apparent neurologic disease. Detrusor instability has been linked epidemiologically to late adolescent enuresis, suggesting a lifelong predilection to bladder overactivity in many cases.

The symptoms of detrusor overactivity—frequency and urge incontinence—may be ameliorated by "bladder training," consisting of prolonging the interval between voidings using behavioral techniques. Patients who are physically disabled or cognitively impaired should be toileted frequently or on a schedule, and incontinence garments (adult diapers) may be used. Antispasmodic agents such as oxybutinin may be useful; this type of medication relaxes the bladder wall and promotes storage of urine, presumably by inhibiting cholinergically mediated detrusor contractions. Urodynamic subtypes of overactive bladder are the subject of active research and are likely to lead to targeted treatment approaches in the future. Currently, urodynamic studies are not required in all patients prior to selection of a treatment regimen. However, at a minimum, it is important to rule out "overflow incontinence" due to urinary retention prior to embarking on a treatment regimen (see below).

In elderly women, postmenopausal changes in pelvic musculature contribute to urinary incontinence by leading to loss of extrinsic support of pelvic organs and the bladder neck. Pelvic and distal urethral tissue contain estrogen and progesterone receptors, and the urethra may become patulous after the menopause. In this setting, intra-abdominal pressure may easily surpass intraurethral pressure, leading to leakage of urine. This "true stress incontinence" (i.e., occurring in the absence of a detrusor contraction) typically occurs after a cough or sneeze or, in severe cases, merely upon arising from a sitting position.

Stress incontinence may respond to treatment with exogenous estrogens, although controversy exists over the precise mode or site of action of these hormones. Clinical treatment trials have included few patients 75 years of age or older, and the efficacy of hormones at that age may be limited. Other treatment approaches include pelvic muscle exercises, and α-adrenergic agents, such as phenylpropanolamine, which act on urethral α-adrenergic receptors to increase urethral tone.

Chronic indwelling catheters should not be used in the management of incontinence. The prevalence of urinary tract infection is virtually 100% in chronically catheterized patients. A variety of maneuvers, including a closed drainage system, suprapubic catheterization, and systemic antibiotics may reduce the incidence of bacteriuria in the short term, but *no* maneuver has been shown to reduce the prevalence in the long term. Chronic antibiotic suppression merely leads to the production of resistant strains of organisms. Nor are indwelling catheters required for incontinent patients with sacral decubitus ulcers, which can generally be managed with meticulous nursing care. When indwelling catheters are the only alternative (as in urinary retention that cannot be managed with intermittent catheterization), antibiotic treatment should be reserved for symptomatic illness such as fever, lower abdominal discomfort, bacteremia with urine pathogens, or unexplained lethargy.

Urinary Retention. Urinary retention in men is most often related to prostatic outlet obstruction due to benign prostatic hyperplasia. Acute urinary retention may occur in elderly men and less often in women as the result of fecal impaction, the bedridden state, immobility, or anticholinergic drugs, such as tricyclic antidepressants, diisopyramide, first-generation antihistamines, and drugs used to treat urinary incontinence. Diuretics can also lead to urinary retention when they produce a volume of urine that overwhelms the compromised bladder. Urinary retention may develop following surgery; this is at least partly due to prolonged effects of anesthetic agents and opioid analgesics. Urinary retention that first begins in the hospital can become stubborn, but when there is no antecedent history of retention, the prognosis is good.

Diabetes mellitus may be associated with chronic urinary retention. In diabetic "cystopathy," disease of the peripheral nerves comprising the afferent limb of the spinal detrusor reflex leads to detrusor areflexia. Despite the high prevalence of diabetes in late life, most elderly diabetics do not have bladder dysfunction due to this problem, perhaps because of shorter disease duration or unknown factors related to the pathogenesis of late-onset diabetes.

Persistent urinary retention is relatively uncommon in elderly women. Anatomic problems such as cystocele may increase residual urine, and some patients may have incomplete bladder emptying because of modest detrusor hyporeflexia. In both sexes, it is important to distinguish frank urinary retention (the inability to void) from increased residual urine, defined as a postvoid residual urine volume greater than *approximately* 50 ml. Frank urinary retention requires immediate attention; it may present as "overflow incontinence," whereas increased postvoid residual urine may be asymptomatic and in and of itself does not require treatment.

FALLS AND FRACTURES

The incidence of fractures increases with age. Approximately 17% of men and >30% of all women sustain a hip fracture by age 90. This is due to two independent problems—bone loss and the tendency to fall.

Bone loss occurs at a rate of approximately 1% per year after the fourth decade of life in both sexes. At the time of menopause, the rate of bone loss in women accelerates to about 3% per year for approximately 7 years, and then the slower rate resumes. The accelerated phase is manifested first in trabecular bone of the vertebrae and the extreme ends of long bones. The rate of spinal compression fractures is about eight times higher, and the rate of wrist and hip fracture about twice as high in women as in men. Age-related bone loss is due largely although not entirely to osteoporosis. In osteoporosis, there is a proportional loss of the mineralized and nonmineralized phases of bone. However, many geriatric patients also have osteomalacia, a mineralization defect. Osteomalacia in the elderly is most often due to vitamin D deficiency, usually co-exists with osteoporosis, and resembles the latter clinically. Vitamin D deficiency in the housebound or institutionalized elderly is due to inadequate sunlight exposure. Contributing factors may include age-related impairments in intestinal vitamin D absorption and a reduced capacity to manufacture vitamin D in the skin. A seasonal variation in the rate of hip fractures parallels a seasonal variation in serum vitamin D levels. The peak fracture incidence in the late winter or early spring cannot be attributed solely to such factors as slipping on the ice, because most fractures among the elderly occur indoors.

Osteomalacia is preventable and treatable. It is believed that only 15 minutes of sunlight exposure twice a week is needed to optimize vitamin D status in light-skinned adults, but the elderly may require somewhat more; still more time is required in dark-skinned adults, in whom ultraviolet light does not penetrate the melanin layer as quickly. Elderly people regardless of race should ingest a minimum of 800 IU per day of vitamin D and higher doses if vitamin D deficiency is documented. Much higher doses should be continued only until the deficiency is corrected because of the danger of toxicity. Excessive sunlight exposure, on the other hand, does not produce hypervitaminosis D but is well known to produce skin damage.

There is no known effective treatment of established osteoporosis in the elderly. Antiresorptive agents such as estrogen and calcitonin may retard bone loss but do not replace bone that has already been lost. Estrogen instituted more than 10 years after the menopause probably plays a limited role. The effects of calcitonin are probably time-limited owing to antibody-mediated resistance or receptor downregulation. Bisphosphonates inhibit bone resorption, but etidronate, the only bisphosphonate currently approved for osteoporosis, also impairs mineralization when given long term. The overall effect of etidronate may be to reduce fracture risk when it is given cyclically with calcium. Calcium supplementation and physiologic doses of vitamin D may reduce fracture risk in elderly patients, calcium by retarding resorption and vitamin D by enhancing intestinal calcium absorption as well as preventing osteomalacia.

Standard methods of osteoporosis prevention, such as weight-bearing exercise and postmenopausal estrogen replacement, are of limited benefit when instituted in the geriatric patient with established osteoporosis. However, it is always important to identify and address preventable causes of bone loss, such as primary hyperparathyroidism, vitamin D deficiency, phosphate depletion, use of corticosteroids or heparin, cigarette smoking, excessive alcohol intake, and marginal calcium intake. Correction of negative calcium balance in elderly men and women generally requires a daily total intake of 1500 mg elemental calcium from dietary sources and supplements.

A key aspect of management in elderly patients is the prevention of falls. Vertebral wedging and fractures may occur without obvious trauma, but wrist and hip fractures are almost always related to a fall. The incidence of wrist (Colles') fracture increases in midlife among women but reaches a plateau by age 60. In contrast, the incidence of hip fracture rises steadily after age 60. These fracture patterns may be partly related to the mechanism of falling, in that an older person may lack the coordination to break a fall by quickly throwing out the arm. In addition, reduced muscle mass and subcutaneous fat may contribute to diminished absorption of energy on impact. Some hip fractures probably occur before or in the absence of a fall, perhaps because of torsion or other increased loading on a severely osteopenic femoral neck.

Hip fractures in the elderly are a surgical emergency. Initial radiographs sometimes fail to reveal a fracture. When an elderly patient has fallen and cannot bear weight or has severe pain on weight bearing, the hip must be deemed fractured until proven otherwise. If repeat radiography fails to reveal a fracture on frontal and lateral views, a bone scan or magnetic resonance imaging should be done. Surgery should be performed as soon as the patient is medically stabilized because morbidity and mortality rise exponentially if surgery is delayed beyond 24 to 48 hours. Assiduous medical management of these frail patients is essential and should be directed at prevention or treatment of pneumonia, deep vein thrombosis, pulmonary embolus, pressure sores, urinary tract infection, and fecal impaction. Postoperative delirium is common and may be due to one or more medical problems, to medications, or to prolonged effects of anesthesia.

Approximately one third of people 75 and older fall at least once annually. When fall-related injury occurs, it is just as important to assess the reason for the fall as to address the injury. Falls among the elderly are most commonly caused by acute or chronic neurologic disease, arthritis, musculoskeletal impairments, poor balance, postural instability, cardiac arrhythmias, generalized weakness due to acute or chronic medical illness (including acute myocardial infarction), orthostatic hypotension, or impaired coordination hampering the ability to fall "well." Additional factors are visual impairments, dementia, medications with sedating properties, and antihypertensive medications when they lead to overcorrection of hypertension.

Falls assessment should be performed by a careful history and physical examination, with appropriate laboratory tests directed by this initial evaluation.

FLUID BALANCE AND ELECTROLYTE DISORDERS

Geriatric patients may become easily dehydrated after a variety of insults, such as excessive environmental heat, diarrhea, or febrile illness. Underlying factors are an impaired renal concentrating ability and impaired urinary sodium conservation in response to salt deprivation. Responsible for these alterations are progressive nephron loss greater in the cortex, increase in basal and stimulated levels of atrial natiuretic hormone, and a decrease in the renin-angiotensin-aldosterone system. In addition, thirst response to dehydration is diminished even among healthy elderly. This problem is accentuated in neurologically impaired patients, who are even less likely to seek water when dehydrated. A variety of medical illnesses may therefore present with hypernatremia, hyperosmolarity, and obtundation.

Even more common is the occurrence of hyponatremia. Underlying this predilection is an exaggerated release of arginine vasopressin (AVP) after an osmotic stimulus, and a decreased ability to excrete a water load, which might be partly related to reduced GFR. Elderly patients also have a higher rate of disorders that predispose to hyponatremia, such as congestive heart failure (CHF) and central neurologic impairments, and to the syndrome of inappropriate antidiuretic hormone secretion (SIADH). The disproportionate occurrence of SIADH among the elderly is likely related to enhanced physiologic release of AVP as well as exposure to the many pharmacologic agents known to produce this syndrome.

Enteral tube feeding has frequently been associated with hyponatremia. Although hypotonic feeds may be partly to blame, hyponatremia in tube-fed patients may also be a marker for underlying central nervous system disease, which has been associated with SIADH. Serum sodium must be monitored in neurologically impaired tube-fed patients and attention paid to the amount of free water added to the feed or used to flush the feeding tube.

When saline solutions are given to correct dehydration, salt deficits, or fluid-electrolyte imbalance, they must be infused cautiously and with careful monitoring, as heart failure is a more likely consequence in the elderly. The risk of CHF may be related to underlying cardiac disease, decreased left ventricular compliance, or another age-related defect in sodium metabolism—the decreased ability of the kidney to excrete a sodium load.

PRESSURE SORES

Most pressure sores (decubitus ulcers) develop in elderly patients and occur within the first 2 weeks of hospitalization. The prevalence among nursing home patients is approximately 11%, but as many as 20% of these patients have hospital-acquired pressure sores when they are admitted to the nursing home.

Pressure sores develop when extrinsic pressure on the skin exceeds mean capillary pressure (32 mm Hg), thereby reducing blood flow and tissue oxygenation. In recumbent patients, pressures over the sacrum or greater trochanter reach as high as 100 to 150 mm Hg. Moisture, friction, and shear contribute to skin breakdown under these circumstances. Advanced age may increase the risk because of changes in the skin, including decreased thickness and vascularity of the dermal layer, delayed ability for wound healing, and redistribution of fat from subcutaneous to deeper layers. Conditions that increase risk include immobility, neurologic impairment, poor nutrition, and zinc, iron, or vitamin C deficiencies. Neurologic impairments as a cause of immobility have particular importance because the disease reduces the spontaneous movements that normally occur during sleep. Associated urinary and fecal incontinence exacerbate the problem by creating moisture and irritation.

Pressure sores can occur anywhere on the body. Typical sites include dependent areas possessing minimal subcutaneous fat, and bony prominences such as the sacrum, greater trochanter, scapula, lateral malleolus, thoracic spine, and heels. The last mentioned can be particularly stubborn when accompanied by arterial insufficiency.

Prevention offers the most important aspect of pressure sore management, and its hallmark is avoidance of pressure (Table 8–1).

Shallow ulcer craters should be kept clean and covered with a dressing if indicated; uncomplicated blisters should be managed without debridement or dressing, because blister fluid may enhance wound healing. Ulcers involving subcutaneous tissue may generate substantial necrotic tissue, which should be debrided promptly. Such cleansings often can be accomplished with dressings, enzymes, or debriding agents. Ulcers extending through fascia or involving bone, muscle, or supporting tissue require surgical debridement and often skin grafting.

Little evidence indicates that specific appliances, dressings, or debriding agents are superior to traditional meticulous nursing care, although they may ultimately reduce nursing time. Foam "egg crate" pads and mattresses redistribute pressure, and sheepskin padding absorbs moisture. Air-fluidized beds (warm air flowing through silicon beads) and alternating air pressure mattresses redistribute and reduce extrinsic pressure; although the air-fluidized bed may help to speed ulcer healing, it is expensive and difficult to clean. Specialized dressings help; for example, wet-to-dry dressings enhance debridement of necrotic tissue, but if the dressing is not exposed to air, it macerates healthy skin and enlarges the ulcer,

TABLE 8–1. PREVENTION OF PRESSURE SORES

Identify vulnerable patients early.
Lift, don't slide, bedridden patients.
Keep the skin dry without resorting to indwelling catheters.
Restore nutritional deficiencies.

From Ahronheim JC: Handbook of Prescribing Medications For Geriatric Patients. Boston, Little, Brown, 1991.

conversely, inappropriate use desiccates the tissue. Occlusive hydrocolloid dressings may enhance healing, avoid the problem of desiccation, and protect a pressure sore from external soilage; a covered wound cannot be inspected, however, and this sophisticated dressing, designed for leg ulcers rather than pressure sores, may create a false sense of security and reduce nursing vigilance when the key to treatment lies in removal of pressure.

Ulcer craters should not be treated with topical antibiotics: they promote antimicrobial resistance without enhancing wound healing. Systemic antibiotics should be used only when there is significant cellulitis or evidence of systemic infection related to the skin lesion.

MEDICAL DECISION MAKING FOR COGNITIVELY IMPAIRED ELDERLY

Patients have the constitutional right to refuse unwanted medical treatment, including life-sustaining treatment. The physician must inform a patient of the risks, benefits, and alternatives of proposed treatments and determine if he/she has the capacity to decide. A large proportion of geriatric patients lack decisional capacity because of significant dementia or other neurologic impairments. Nevertheless, they have the right to refuse treatment either through an advance directive (written or oral) or through an authorized surrogate decision maker, as discussed in Ch. 2.

Despite the general consensus that patients may refuse any form of medical treatment, controversy surrounds the refusal of long-term enteral tube feeding, a step that largely involves very old patients with advanced neurologic impairments. For many persons, tube feeding symbolizes the compassionate provision of food. From a medical perspective, however, tube feeding is an active treatment. Tube feeding requires technical skill, lacks a sensory component, does not heed feelings of satiety, may require mechanical restraints to prevent tube dislodgement, and can produce mechanical and medical complications. No evidence demonstrates that terminal dehydration from the withholding or withdrawal of tube feeding or even water leads to a painful death. Contrary evidence includes the diminished thirst response to dehydration and age-related physiologic changes leading to the early development of hyperosmolarity; the endogenous production of substances producing analgesia, such as endorphins; the rapid development of coma in neurologically impaired individuals; the frequent rejection of food or water by competent hospice patients; and observations by health professionals in the field. No evidence indicates that tube feeding prevents aspiration pneumonia or that gastrostomy or jejunostomy feeding lowers the risk of aspiration. Neurologically impaired patients with dysphagia may aspirate not only gastric contents but oropharyngeal secretions, independent of the presence or type of enteral tube. In patients with advanced neurologic impairments, tube feeding cannot be considered a palliative procedure.

Although the 1990 US Supreme Court *Cruzan* decision affirmed the right of patients with decisional capacity to refuse tube feeding and other medical treatments, the Court left it up to individual states to set specific legal standards for refusal by patients *lacking* decisional capacity. Some states require a high level of evidence of a patient's previously expressed wishes to refuse life-sustaining treatment, whereas other states possess separate legal standards for refusal of tube feeding. Physicians would be wise to familiarize themselves with such rules.

When conflict exists, health professionals who morally object to the withdrawal of life-sustaining treatments have the right to transfer care of the patient to another physician or facility that will uphold the patient's decision. They do not, however, have the right to decide unilaterally what patients should have.

Physicians are not required to provide futile treatment, but controversy surrounds what constitutes medical futility. A physiologic definition views futile treatment as one that cannot fulfill its intent. Narrowly interpreted, this implies that cardiopulmonary resuscitation (CPR) in terminal illness (such as advanced cancer) is not futile if it temporarily restores heart beat. An expanded definition, however, views CPR in this circumstance as futile because it does nothing for the underlying disease that will inevitably cause death. The first, narrow definition has been criticized because it goes beyond the goals of medicine, which are to heal or comfort. The second has been criticized because it makes value judgments that only the patient can make. Nonetheless, concerns about patient suffering as well as the consumption of limited and expensive resources to treat painfully terminal conditions may support the expanded definition over the organ-specific view.

As of this writing, lower courts have twice upheld family requests for treatment deemed medically futile by physicians. The arguments supporting such "futile" treatment have hinged on the need to maintain patient autonomy and affirm the family as the rightful decision makers for incompetent patients; they have not addressed the authority of physicians to make futility determinations. Fortunately, demands for treatment in such extreme cases are rare and in the courts have been vastly outnumbered by "right-to-die" disputes, in which patients or their surrogates have refused life-prolonging treatments imposed by physicians or institutions.

Ahronheim JC, Mulvihill M: Refusal of tube feeding as seen from a patient advocacy organization: A comparison with landmark court cases. J Am Geriatr Soc 39:1124, 1991. *This study suggests that case law does not adequately represent the types of clinical situations that most often occur.*

Allman RM: Pressure ulcers among the elderly. N Engl J Med 13:850, 1989. *Reviews pathophysiology and current treatment of pressure sores.*

Burke LB, Jolson HM, Goetsch RA, et al.: Geriatric drug use and adverse drug event reporting in 1990: A descriptive analysis of two national data bases. Annu Rev Gerontol Geriatr 12:1, 1992. *Recent data illustrating therapeutic drug use and incidence patterns of adverse drug events by age, sex, and drug class, in a large population.*

Mimran A, Ribstein J, Jover B: Aging and sodium homeostasis. Kidney Int 41(Suppl 37):S107, 1992. *Review of renal and endocrinologic changes affecting fluid and sodium balance. Extensive references.*

Riggs BL, Melton LJ: The prevention and treatment of osteoporosis. N Engl J Med 327:620, 1992. *Comprehensive, up-to-date review of pathophysiology, epidemiology, clinical syndromes, and treatment.*

Schneiderman LJ, Faber-Langendoen K, Jecker NS: Beyond futility to an ethic of care. Am J Med 96:110, 1994. *Critique of the debate over medical futility with an alternative view.*

Urinary Incontinence Guideline Panel: Urinary incontinence in adults: Clinical practice guidelines. AHCPR Pub. No. 92-0038. Rockville, MD, 1992. *Consensus panel guidelines with extensive references.*

Vestal RE, Cusack BJ: Pharmacology and aging. *In* Schneider EL, Rowe JW (eds.): Handbook of the Biology of Aging. 3rd ed. San Diego, Academic Press, 1990, p 349. *Thorough review of age-related factors in drug handling, highlighting controversies in a critical manner.*

9 PRINCIPLES OF PREVENTIVE HEALTH CARE
Albert Oberman

Concepts of preventive medicine have evolved rapidly over the past decade. A growing body of evidence links personal health behavior and preventive services to the reductions in mortality from the leading causes of death and disability in the United States. Total mortality has continued to decline, primarily from a nearly 3% annual reduction in cardiovascular disease (CVD) (Fig. 9–1). During the past decade, mortality from CVD has declined less in women than in men and less in the black population than in the white population. Nevertheless, life expectancy for the middle-aged adult has now increased, but chronic diseases are still the major cause of death and disability at all ages (Table 9–1). At the same time, other causes of preventable morbidity and mortality such as cancer, chronic obstructive pulmonary disease, HIV infection, and homicide (especially for young black men) have escalated.

PREVENTION STRATEGIES

There are two complementary strategies for prevention: a population approach and a clinical, high-risk approach. Both strategies rely on principles of changing behavior to reduce risk. A strong rationale exists for the population approach, in which interventions are offered on a broad scale to all segments of the population. This approach shifts the entire population distribution of risk to a lower level. Chronic diseases arise from the interaction of multiple risk factors at low to moderate levels rather than from a single aberrant risk factor. The current burden of ill health comes from the large numbers of those not apparently at risk rather than from the few who demonstrate obvious abnormalities. For example, most hypertensive complications and preventable deaths come from the larger numbers of those with "stage 1" hypertension (see Ch. 37) rather than from the much smaller numbers with severe hypertension. Although decision points must be made for clinical management, risk for chronic diseases is continuous, often curvilinear, so that even small shifts in the distribution of a risk factor have great impact. It has been estimated that a 3 mm Hg downward shift in the average systolic blood pressure in the United States might reduce the annual mortality from all causes by 4%, from coronary heart disease (CHD) by 5%, and from stroke by 8%.

The high-risk strategy targets those individuals judged more likely to develop disease and also more likely to benefit from intervention. This avoids the inefficiency of the mass approach with its need to interfere with many who neither desire such help nor are likely to benefit from population measures. This model is also more compatible with usual medical practice. Preventive policies that focus on high-risk individuals offer substantial benefits for them, but the potential impact on the total burden of disease is often disappointing.

CLINICAL PREVENTIVE SERVICES

Clinical preventive services include preventing disease, promoting health, immunization, screening, and counseling for individuals in the health care setting. Systematic review of preventive health services has revealed little scientific basis for performing many procedures routinely. Indiscriminate screening without adequate advice and follow-up serves no useful purpose. The periodic health examination (see Ch. 9.1) has evolved from a broad-based approach to targeting the prevention, detection, and treatment of specific diseases or risk factors for different age, gender, and race groups. Preventive services are often classified as primary, secondary, or tertiary. Primary prevention is directed toward preventing disease or injury before it develops (see Ch. 9.5); secondary prevention deals with early detection and treatment of preclinical disease to impede the progress of the condition. In contrast, tertiary prevention refers to rehabilitative activities after the onset of disease to minimize complications. Distinguishing between these phases of prevention may be confusing because detecting and treating hypertension could be considered secondary prevention of hypertensive disease but primary prevention for congestive heart failure and stroke. In any event, prevention can be perceived along a continuum of health from absence of predisposing factors or evidence of pathologic processes to premature death. The sooner the prevention, the more likely unnecessary illness, disability, and premature death can be avoided. Therefore, increasing emphasis has been placed on preventing risk factors themselves.

Likely changes in the health care system will draw greater attention to promoting health and prevention and to more community-based care. Physicians should consider each disorder in terms of the potential for preventing and the possibility of adverse events from intervening. Ample evidence and measures for primary prevention of morbidity and mortality for health problems are currently available (Table 9–2). Furthermore, many of these lifestyle changes benefit multiple systems and disorders. For example, cigarette smoking has been estimated to contribute to one of every six deaths in the United States (see Ch. 9.4); a low-fat diet (see Ch. 9.2) may lower the occurrence of both CHD and cancer; physical activity (see Ch. 9.3) improves glucose tolerance and blood lipids and most likely lowers the risk of CHD. Other procedures allow prevention at a later stage: e.g., the Papanicolaou test for cervical cancer, removing polyps for colon cancer, aspirin for strokes and recurrent CHD events, and treating hypertension for stroke and congestive heart failure.

Common misconceptions impede preventive health care. Many believe that diseases with a strong heritability component cannot be altered, but genetic traits for disease often result from the influence of multiple genes and require environmental factors for expression (see Part VI). In addition, chronic diseases are multifactorial, so that other factors can be changed to compensate for an elevated genetic risk. The notion that prevention is less useful in older persons excludes many who would benefit most from prevention. The elderly have a greater absolute risk of disease and have been shown to adhere and respond favorably to preventive measures. Also, life expectancy is frequently underestimated in the elderly—those who reach 65 years can now expect to live into their 80's.

Advances in understanding the determinants of risk, the demand for preventive measures in health reform, and the remarkable downward mortality trends provide the momentum for further primary preventive efforts. The United States still falls far short of the life expectancy achieved in many other countries and has a total death rate 50% greater than that of Japan. Furthermore, there is a broad spectrum of health care within the country; many segments of the US population, notably those of lower socioeconomic status, have not benefited equally from the decline in mortality.

With a larger aging population, decreased fatality rates, and im-

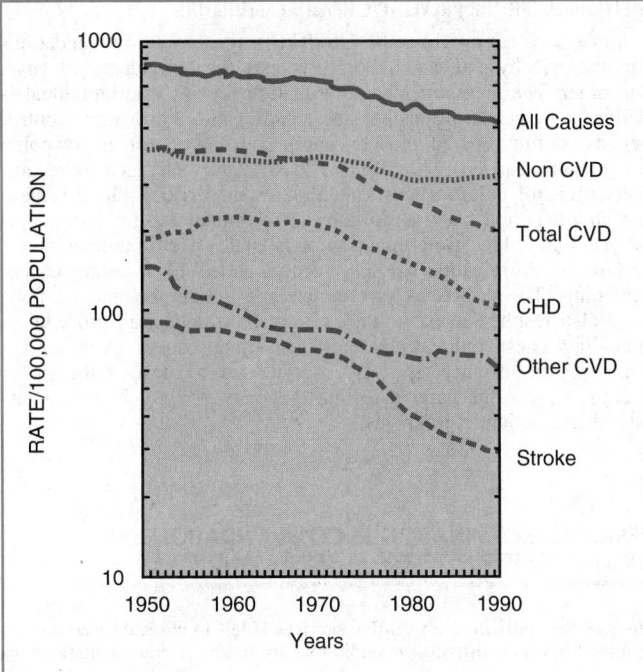

FIGURE 9-1. Age-adjusted death rates for selected causes of death in the United States, 1950 to 1990. All causes of mortality have steadily declined since 1950. Although there has been a modest reduction in mortality for noncardiovascular disease (non CVD), the most striking recent decline occurred in mortality for cardiovascular disease (total CVD), notably stroke and coronary heart disease (CHD). (From Kannel WB, Thom TJ: Incidence, prevalence, and mortality of cardiovascular diseases in the heart. *In* Schlant RC, Alexander RW [eds.]: The Heart: Arteries and Veins. 8th ed. New York, McGraw-Hill, 1994.)

TABLE 9-1. RANK OF THE TEN LEADING CAUSES OF DEATH FOR ADULTS BY AGE GROUP, UNITED STATES, 1992*

Cause of Death	Age Group			
	25–44	45–64	65–74	85+
Heart disease	4	2	1	1
Cancer	3	1	2	2
Cerebrovascular disease	8	3	3	3
Accidents	1	4	7	6
Chronic obstructive pulmonary disease	—	5	4	5
Pneumonia/influenza	10	10	5	4
Diabetes mellitus	9	6	6	8
Suicide	6	8	—	—
Cirrhosis	7	7	10	—
Atherosclerosis	—	—	—	7
Nephritis	—	—	8	9
Homicide	5	—	—	—
Septicemia	—	—	9	10
HIV infection	2	9	—	—

* Provisional estimate.
From the National Heart, Lung, and Blood Institute. US Department of Health and Human Services. Public Health Service. National Institutes of Health. Fact Book, Fiscal Year 1993. February 1994.

Report of the US Preventive Services Task Force: Guide to Clinical Preventive Services: An Assessment of the Effectiveness of 169 Interventions. Baltimore, Williams & Wilkins, 1989. *The most recent authoritative recommendation for clinical preventive services.*

Rose G: The strategy of preventive medicine. Oxford, Oxford University Press, 1993. *A concise discussion of the strengths and limitations of the various strategies of prevention.*

proved treatment of many disorders, it is essential that the focus be on primary prevention. Otherwise, the prevalence and associated morbidity of major diseases will increase and further consume available medical resources. It should be clearly understood that the purpose of prevention is not to postpone illness to a later age but rather to prevent the diseases themselves and the resultant disability. On the average, US citizens spend only 85% of their 75 + years of life expectancy in a healthy state unimpaired by disabilities, disease, or injuries. All US citizens should be able to reach the objective for Healthy People 2000—to attain at least 65 years of healthy life. Geoffrey Rose makes the best case for prevention: "It is better to be healthy than ill or dead. That is the beginning and the end of the only real argument for preventive medicine. It is sufficient."

Goldbloom RB, Lawrence RS (eds.): Preventing Disease Beyond the Rhetoric. New York, Springer-Verlag, 1990. *A careful documentation of the evidence for preventing disease, oriented toward primary care.*

Leaf A: Preventive medicine for our ailing health care system. JAMA 269:616, 1993. *A positive review of the role of preventive medicine in the health care system.*

National Center for Health Statistics: Health, United States, 1992. Hyattsville, MD, Public Health Service, 1993. *A report on the health status and trends of the nation supplemented with a Healthy People 2000 review of progress and objectives.*

9.1 The Preventive Health Examination
Richard K. Riegelman

Integrating prevention into the practice of adult medicine is an intellectual and administrative challenge. The annual physical examination has been replaced by the periodic health examination with intervals adjusted by age group. The complete physical and multiphasic screening laboratory workup has been replaced by the focused screening history and physical designed to detect risk factors for disease. Laboratory testing is now guided by principles designed to select tests that are likely to produce substantial benefit to groups of individuals at affordable cost. In addition, the preventive health examination should include active therapeutic interventions including counseling, vaccination, and chemoprophylaxis.

To help accomplish these multiple goals, a number of groups

TABLE 9-2. PRIMARY PREVENTION OF SELECTED HEALTH PROBLEMS

Health Problem	Potentially Modifiable Factors						
	Avoidable Exposure	Immunization	Tobacco	Alcohol	Adverse Dietary Pattern	Inappropriate Physical Activity	Occupational Hazards
Alcoholism	X			X			
Cancer	X		X	X	X		X
Cerebrovascular disease			X	X	X	X	
Dental disease			X		X		
Diabetes mellitus					X		
Gastrointestinal disease			X		X		
Infectious disease	X	X		X			X
Injury	X			X		X	X
Respiratory disease	X	X	X				X
Violence/homicide	X			X			

have developed guidelines for the preventive health examination. These include the American College of Physicians, the Canadian Task Force, and the United States Preventive Services Task Force (USPSTF). The widely used USPSTF recommendations have been intentionally limited to procedures for which there is adequate supportive evidence. A recommendation to screen for a disease, for instance, generally requires evidence that the disease causes substantial morbidity or mortality, that detection at the asymptomatic stage is feasible, and that early detection can alter outcome.

Thus it is important to view the USPSTF recommendations as a minimum set which are likely to increase in number over time as further evidence accumulates and new approaches are introduced. Other organizations, especially those with a specific disease or professional focus, generally recommend more intensive or aggressive examinations.

Table 9–3 summarizes the USPSTF screening recommendations for history, physical, and laboratory tests for individuals 19 years and older. The recommended examination for any one individual is derived by considering his/her age, gender, and risk factors. Controversies continue including over whom and how to screen for colon and prostate cancers. The USPSTF has recently changed its recommendation for colon cancer screening. Annual occult blood screening and/or periodic sigmoidoscopy is recommended for individuals 50 years and older. Determination of prostate-specific antigen levels and rectal examination are not recommended for prostate cancer screening. The efforts to systematize preventive recommendations have also resulted in excluding previously widely used procedures. Including chest radiography to detect lung cancer even among smokers, for instance, is not recommended by any of the major groups because the early detection that may occur does not generally alter a patient's prognosis.

TABLE 9–3. US PREVENTIVE SERVICES TASK FORCE PERIODIC EXAMINATION RECOMMENDATIONS: SCREENING HISTORY, PHYSICAL EXAMINATION, AND LABORATORY WORK—AGES 19 AND OVER

Schedule every 1 to 3 years age 19–64 and every year ≥65.
The recommended schedule applies only to the periodic visit itself. The frequency of the individual preventive services is left to clinical discretion except as indicated. The table indicates recommended ages and high-risk (HR) groups for whom the recommendations are made. Recommendations are applicable to age groups indicated in parentheses.

History

Dietary intake (≥19)
Physical activity (≥19)
Tobacco/alcohol/drug use (≥19)
Sexual practices (19–64)
Functional status (≥65)

Physical Examination

Height and weight (≥19)   Blood pressure (≥19)   Visual acuity (≥65)   Hearing (≥65)
Clinical breast exam (≥40 for 19–39 HR only)—Annually over 40, women aged 35 and older with a family history of premenopausally diagnosed breast cancer in a first-degree relative.
Testicular exam (HR 19–39)—Men with a history of cryptorchidism, orchiopexy, or testicular atrophy.
Symptoms of TIA (≥65)
Complete skin exam (HR ≥19)—Persons with family or personal history of skin cancer, increased occupational or recreational exposure to sunlight, or clinical evidence of precursor lesions (e.g., dysplastic nevi, certain congenital nevi).
Thyroid for nodules (HR ≥19)—Persons with a history of upper-body irradiation.
Auscultation for carotid bruits (HR ≥40)—Persons with risk factors for cerebrovascular or cardiovascular disease (e.g., hypertension, smoking, coronary disease, atrial fibrillation, diabetes) or those with neurologic symptoms (e.g., transient ischemic attacks or a history of cerebrovascular disease).
Complete oral cavity exam (HR ≥19)—Persons with exposure to tobacco or excessive amounts of alcohol, or those with suspicious symptoms or lesions detected through self-examination.

Laboratory Work

Nonfasting total cholesterol (≥19)
Papanicolaou smear (19–64, HR ≥65)—Pap smear every 1–3 years. At 65 and over only women who have not had previous documented screening in which smears have been consistently negative.
Fasting glucose (HR ≥19)—The markedly obese, persons with family history of diabetes, or women with a history of gestational diabetes.
Rubella antibodies (HR 19–39)—Women lacking evidence of immunity.
VDRL (HR 19–64)—Prostitutes, persons who engage in sex with multiple partners in areas in which syphilis is prevalent, or contacts of persons with active syphilis.
Urinalysis for bacteremia (HR 19–64)—Persons with diabetes.
Dipstick urinalysis (≥65)
Mammography (HR 35–49, and ≥50)—Women aged 35 and older with a family history of premenopausally diagnosed breast cancer in a first-degree relative; otherwise every 1–2 years beginning at age 50.
Chlamydial testing (HR 19–64)—Persons who attend clinics for sexually transmitted diseases, attend other high-risk health care facilities (e.g., adolescent and family planning clinics), or have other risk factors for chlamydial infection (e.g., multiple sexual contacts or a sexual partner with multiple sexual contacts, age less than 20).
Gonorrhea culture (HR 19–64)—Prostitutes, persons with multiple sexual partners or a sexual partner with multiple contacts, sexual contacts of persons with culture-proven gonorrhea, or persons with a history of repeated episodes of gonorrhea.
Counseling and testing for HIV infection (HR 19–64)—Persons seeking treatment for sexually transmitted disease; homosexual and bisexual men; past or present intravenous (IV) drug users; persons with a history of prostitution or multiple sexual partners; women whose past or present sexual partners were HIV infected, bisexual, or IV drug users; persons with long-term residence or birth in an area with high prevalence of HIV infection; or persons with a history of tranfusion between 1978 and 1985.
Hearing (HR 19–64)—Persons exposed regularly to excessive noise.
PPD (HR ≥19)—Household members of persons with tuberculosis or others at risk for close contact with the disease (e.g., staff of tuberculosis clinics, shelters for the homeless, nursing homes, substance abuse treatment facilities, dialysis units, correctional institutions); recent immigrants or refugees from countries in which tuberculosis is common, migrant workers; residents of nursing homes, correctional institutions, or homeless shelters; or persons with certain underlying medical disorders (e.g., HIV infection).
Fecal occult blood/sigmoidoscopy (HR)—Persons age 50 and older who have first-degree relatives with colorectal cancer; a personal history of endometrial, ovarian, or breast cancer; or a previous diagnosis of inflammatory bowel disease, adenomatous polyps, or colorectal cancer.
Colonoscopy (HR 19–39)—Persons with a family history of familial polyposis coli or cancer family syndrome.
Fecal occult blood/colonoscopy (HR ≥40)—Persons with a family history of familial polyposis coli or cancer family syndrome.
Fecal occult blood/sigmoidoscopy (≥50)—Annual fecal occult blood and/or periodic flexible sigmoidoscopy.
Bone mineral content (HR 40–64)—Premenopausal women at increased risk for osteoporosis (e.g., Caucasian race, bilateral oophorectomy before menopause, slender build) and for whom estrogen replacement therapy would otherwise not be recommended.
Electrocardiogram (≥19)—Men who would endanger public safety were they to experience sudden cardiac events, e.g., commercial airline pilots. (Men >40 with two or more cardiac risk factors (high blood cholesterol, hypertension, cigarette smoking, diabetes mellitus, family history of coronary artery disease) orsedentary or high-risk men planning to begin a vigorous exercise program.
Thyroid function tests (women ≥65)
Glaucoma testing by eye specialist (≥65)

It is increasingly viewed as the physician's responsibility to have in place a system to implement these recommendations. Successful implementation requires that physicians endorse, participate in, and take responsibility for the process. Success does not require, however, that physicians take sole responsibility for implementation. The preventive health examination should not be viewed as a one-shot effort. For some patients it may be best integrated into visits for specific problems. Patients, for instance, may be most receptive to smoking cessation recommendations when they are recovering from bronchitis.

Basic recommendations for implementation include using a tracking system such as flowsheets or checklists which organizes the preventive recommendations and serves as a reminder. Interventions that can be performed by other staff should be encouraged and formalized as a routine part of the practice. Active involvement by patients is essential to successful prevention. The recent introduction of Personal Health Guides allows patients to share in the responsibility for putting prevention into practice.

Hayward RSA, Steinberg SP, Ford DE, et al.: Preventive care guidelines. Ann Intern Med 114:758, 1991. *A comprehensive comparison of the recommendations of the ACP, CTF, and USPSTF.*

US Preventive Services Task Force: Guide to Clinical Preventive Services. 2nd ed. Baltimore, Williams & Wilkins, 1995. *A review of the methods, evidence, and recommendations of the USPSTF.*

US Public Health Service: Clinician's Handbook of Preventive Services. Washington, DC, US Government Printing Office 1994. *A guide to accompany the Office of Disease Prevention Health Promotion's Put Prevention into Practice program, which also include Personal Health Guides and patient educational materials.*

9.2 Diet
Roland L. Weinsier

HEALTH CARE REFORM

The two major components of medicine are prevention and cure. In recent times, the latter has received considerably more attention and funding. However, health care reform is rapidly under way to contain costs by improving the efficiency as well as the effectiveness of health care delivery. This is in response to the escalation of expenditures on health care in the United States, which in 1993 were almost three fourths of a trillion dollars and over 11% of our gross national product. Only a tiny fraction is invested in preventing disease and promoting health, despite the fact that nine preventable chronic diseases account for more than half of all deaths among Americans each year. According to recent reports, a large percentage of the health care dollar is spent on high-technology medicine, some of which might not even be needed if more were invested in preventive care. It is estimated that better control of fewer than 10 risk factors, including increasing exercise, decreasing smoking, wearing seat belts, and improving diet, could prevent 40 to 70% of all premature deaths, one third of all cases of acute disability, and two thirds of all cases of chronic disability.

Four factors contribute most significantly to our nation's public health—personal lifestyles, environment, heredity, and the medical care system. It has been suggested that our medical care system contributes in only a very small way to our overall health. By contrast, our personal lifestyles contribute most significantly, with diet being a major aspect. Although current health care reform legislation is intended to encourage and support preventive medical measures that enhance health, physicians and other health care providers cannot be expected—and should not spend most of their effort trying—to rectify a patient's lifetime of self-abusive habits. Individuals must accept greater responsibility for their own health. In support of this notion is the fact that during the decade of 1978 to 1988, there was a 29.2% reduction in the age-adjusted death rate from heart attacks in the United States. This reduction resulted largely from the public's assuming more healthful living habits rather than from medical treatments.

The themes of recent national studies and reports on our health care system are redundant. The emerging picture is one of focusing on health with emphasis on disease prevention and individual responsibility for health-related behaviors. Patients will become more fully informed participants in decisions regarding their own health. Accordingly, health professionals will be expected to incorporate prevention strategies into their practice—among them the provision of sound nutritional practices. As foreseen by Thomas Edison, "The doctor of the future will give no medicine, but will interest his patient in the care of the human frame, in diet and in the cause and prevention of disease."

NUTRITION IN PREVENTING DISEASE

It has been argued that it is more reasonable to identify individuals at risk who need intervention strategies than to modify the health behaviors of the general public. However, dietary recommendations aimed at reducing the risk for disease of the general population can have a major benefit for the nation's health. This is because even a relatively small reduction in risk for a disease that occurs in a large number of people at moderate risk could lead to a larger reduction in risk for the total population than a large reduction in risk for a smaller number of people at higher risk. For example, modifying diets to reduce coronary artery disease in the general population is thought to be worthwhile because most deaths occur not among those at high risk due to high serum cholesterol levels but in people who have only moderate elevations in serum cholesterol (i.e., < 240 mg/dl). Similarly, decreasing salt and fat intake may substantially reduce the risk of hypertension and certain cancers, although the effects on many individuals may be small or absent. Although genetic factors can affect individual susceptibility, they appear to account for only a small part of the observed variation in disease incidence among populations, as exemplified by the tendency of immigrants to acquire the disease rates of their adoptive countries. With future advances in understanding genetic variability and its interaction with the environment, we will be increasingly able to supplement recommendations for the general population with more sophisticated, individually based dietary intervention.

DIET-DISEASE PATTERNS/TRENDS

At the turn of the century, the leading causes of death were infectious diseases (i.e., environmental factors), and curing illness was the clinician's primary role. Today, most of the leading causes of death are largely attributable to how Americans live, and medical care is focused on treating diseases associated with specific lifestyles. These changes have demanded a shift in the health care practices of physicians to the acute manifestations of chronic disorders and to disease prevention. Heart disease, cancer, and stroke account for two thirds of all deaths in the United States; one third of us will die of coronary artery disease before age 65. Many others will be disabled by these illnesses and their complications.

Changes in eating patterns parallel these disease trends. In lieu of the high-fiber, low-fat foods once used, refined starches, sweets, saturated fats, and salt make up a major portion of today's typical diet in the United States. As shown in Table 9–4, of the 10 current leading causes of death, 5 can be attributed to an unhealthy diet. In addition, diet contributes greatly to hypertension, hypercholesterolemia, and obesity, which are associated with significant morbidity.

Traditionally, the goal, as well as measure of success, of our health care system has been increased life expectancy, regardless of well-being or quality of life. However, reducing morbidity—that is, improving the quality of life and maximizing the period of good health—may be the more important outcome. This is what preventive measures should accomplish and, if accepted, should be the effect of the following guidelines.

DIETARY GUIDELINES

CURRENT PRACTICES. Surveys suggest that people in higher education and income brackets have been more responsive to public health recommendations. Yet most North Americans do not follow published dietary guidelines. Intake of total fat has fallen from about 41 to 36% of calories, and Americans are now more likely to choose low-fat than whole milk; but use of high-fat cheeses has more than doubled during the same period, and cream intake is rising. Fruits and vegetables, specifically cruciferous vegetables (e.g., broccoli, cauliflower) and carotenoid vegetables (most green and

TABLE 9-4. RISK FACTORS ASSOCIATED WITH THE LEADING CAUSES OF DEATH IN THE UNITED STATES

Cause of Death	Percent of Total Deaths	High-fat, Low-fiber Diet	Obesity	Hypertension	Hypercholesterolemia	Diabetes	Alcohol Abuse	Sedentary Lifestyle	Smoking
Heart disease	35.7	*	*	*	*	*		*	*
Cancer	22.4	*	*					*	*
Stroke	7.0	*	*	*	*				
Accidents	4.4						*		*
Chronic obstructive pulmonary disease	3.7								*
Pneumonia, influenza	3.2								*
Diabetes	1.7	*	*					*	
Suicide	1.4						*		
Chronic liver disease	1.2						*		
Atherosclerosis	1.1	*			*	*			*

From Surgeon General's Report on Nutrition and Health, 1988 and National Center for Health Statistics Monthly Vital Statistics Rep 37:1, 1988.

yellow), thought to play a role in reducing cancer risk, are still consumed in relatively small amounts. According to the second National Health and Nutrition Examination Survey (1976 to 1980) of almost 12,000 Americans, the proportion who reported consuming any food considered protective against cancer was small: only 18% eat any cruciferous vegetables, and 21% eat fruits and vegetables high in carotene. By contrast, the proportion consuming foods that potentially increase cancer risk was high: 55% eat red meat, and 43% eat bacon and luncheon meats. White bread remains more popular than the unrefined, whole-grain breads; only 16% report eating high-fiber breads and cereals.

GOALS/GUIDELINES. At least five reports of dietary guidelines for Americans have been published in recent years. As well, there have been at least 19 reports of national dietary guidelines from outside the United States. It is noteworthy that there is almost complete agreement on the general recommendations made in these reports from different U.S. organizations and from the 20 different countries, lending great credence to the guidelines. These are listed below. Under each general category, specific recommendations are made based on current published guidelines for Americans. Table 9-5 outlines these specific dietary goals and compares them with current dietary practices.

1. EAT LESS FAT, PARTICULARLY SATURATED FAT

Aim: < 25% of calories as total fat; < 7% of calories as saturated fat; < 300 mg per day of dietary cholesterol. (Because there is no risk and great potential benefit, some experts suggest reducing total fat intake to as low as 10% of calories.) Eat less than three 3-oz servings of red meat a week (a 3-oz serving of meat is roughly the size of a deck of playing cards).

Comment: Fats, whether as oils, margarines, or butter, provide more than twice the calories (9 kcal per gram) of carbohydrates and protein (4 kcal per gram); hence, reducing all fats is the most important way to reduce energy intake and therefore to reduce risk of

TABLE 9-5. CURRENT DIETARY PRACTICES AND GOALS FOR AMERICANS

Dietary Factors	Current Practices	Goals*
Fat: Total (% of calories)	36	< 30 (< 25)
Saturated (% of calories)	13	< 10 (< 7)
Cholesterol (mg/day)	435 (men) 300 (women)	< 300 (< 200)
Carbohydrates (% of calories)	45	≥ 50 (≥ 55)
Vegetables and fruits (½-cup servings/day)	2½	5 (7) or more
Whole grain products/legumes (servings/day)	3	6 or more
Fiber (grams/day)	12 (men) 18 (women)	20–30
Red meat (3-oz servings/week)	6	< 3
Alcohol (as ethanol, oz/day)	†	< 1
Salt (grams/day)	10–12	< 6

* The listed dietary goals are considered minimal. In parentheses are those that many nutrition experts consider preferable.

† 30% of US population report drinking < 0.2 oz of ethanol/day; 21% drink 0.2 to 0.9 oz/day, and 10% drink ≥ 1 oz/day.

obesity and diabetes. Decreasing total fat intake may reduce risk of cancers such as colon, prostate, and breast; reducing saturated fat specifically lowers risk of coronary heart disease.

Saturated fats are solid at room temperature and are found primarily in meat and dairy products (butter, creams, cheeses, red meats) and some vegetable products (coconut, palm oil, cocoa butter, and vegetable oils that have been hydrogenated to make solid margarines). Dietary cholesterol comes solely from animal products. As a substitute for saturated fats, complex carbohydrates (i.e., fruits, vegetables, whole grain products) are preferred to polyunsaturated fats (i.e., oils and margarines) because the former are lower in energy content and higher in many essential nutrients and fiber. Saturated fat and cholesterol can be reduced by substituting fish, poultry without skin, lean meats, and low- or non-fat dairy products for fatty meats and whole-milk dairy products.

2. ADJUST ENERGY INTAKE FOR WEIGHT CONTROL

Aim: Ideal body weight.

Comment: Shakespeare admonished, "Leave gourmandizing. Know the grave doth gape for thee thrice wider than for other men." Found printed on Egyptian papyrus is an earlier warning about the adverse effects of excess energy intake: "Most of what we eat is superfluous. Hence, we only live off a quarter of all we swallow; doctors live off the other three quarters." Enough said.

3. EAT MORE FOODS CONTAINING COMPLEX CARBOHYDRATES AND FIBER

Aim: > 55% of calories as carbohydrate. Eat at least 7 servings of a combination of vegetables and fruits and at least 6 servings of a combination of unrefined starches and legumes.

Comment: Preferred carbohydrates include whole fresh fruit, green and yellow vegetables, whole-grain breads and cereals, beans, baked potatoes, and other unrefined starches. Eating these foods displaces food with higher energy density such as fats and simple sugars, which are conducive to obesity. They are good sources of carotenes, vitamin C, and fiber, all of which may protect against certain cancers. When these foods are eaten, fiber supplements are not necessary or recommended.

4. REDUCE SALT INTAKE

Aim: < 6 grams per day.

Comment: Taste for salt is acquired and can be modified. On average, Americans consume about 10 to 12 grams of salt per day, about 20 times their requirement of < 0.5 gram per day (equivalent to < 200 mg of sodium). Because susceptibility to salt-induced hypertension (i.e., salt-sensitive individuals) cannot be identified easily and because reducing salt intake has no detrimental effect, this recommendation is reasonable for the entire population and of specific benefit for the hypertension-prone. It entails avoiding table salt and infrequently using sodium-rich items such as soy sauce, steak sauce, chips, crackers, regular salad dressings, and many "convenience" foods.

5. DRINK ALCOHOL IN MODERATION, IF AT ALL

Aim: < 1 ounce of pure alcohol a day (equivalent to two cans of beer, two small glasses of wine, or two average cocktails). Pregnant women should avoid alcoholic beverages.

Comment: Although some studies suggest that moderate alcohol intake is associated with lower risk of coronary artery disease, it is not recommended that nondrinkers start because drinking poses other risks that may offset any potential advantages. Because alcohol is high in energy density (7 kcal per gram or 200 kcal per ounce of ethanol), alcoholic beverages may contribute significantly to total calorie intake.

DIETARY SUPPLEMENTS

Approximately one half of adults in the United States report using nutritional supplements. In many cases they are self-prescribed. Although a single daily dose of a multiple vitamin-mineral supplement containing 100% of the Recommended Dietary Allowances is not likely to be harmful, no data indicate that they are beneficial except when indicated for specific disorders or deficiencies. The desirable approach for the general public is to obtain the recommended levels of nutrients by eating a variety of whole foods as described in the foregoing section. When the diet is adequate, routine use of nutritional supplements is of little or no benefit, and unprescribed daily use of supplements in amounts exceeding the recommended allowances should be avoided.

SUMMARY

According to a recent blue-ribbon federal task force, researchers will confront the limit of technology's ability to continue the medical breakthroughs of the past century, making health increasingly a question of lifestyle. Current medical care is focusing more on treating diseases associated with specific lifestyles, which demands a shift in the health care practices of physicians to the acute manifestations of chronic disorders and to disease prevention. One of the public health goals for the year 2000 is to increase to at least 50% the proportion of primary care physicians who provide nutrition counseling and/or referral to qualified nutritionists. However, promoting health and preventing disease cannot be a national priority only for those whom we counsel. To be effective, it must also be a personal goal for all of us in the health care field.

As stated by a former U.S. government health official, "Two-thirds of all disease and premature death is preventable, but only if we as individuals recognize our responsibility to take care of ourselves. The priorities are obvious: quit smoking, stick to proper diet, control drinking, exercise, learn to handle stress and take preventive measures such as regular checkups." Wiser living is inexpensive and readily available; the alternative is inexcusable.

Consumer Reports: Are you eating right? October, 1992. *A nicely presented, easily understandable overview of the views of nutrition professionals on how to improve our dietary habits.*

Leaf A: Preventive medicine for our ailing health care system. JAMA 269:616, 1993. *Excellent commentary on the current overemphasis on curative medicine and mortality figures. Stresses the need to refocus on disease prevention and its impact on extending the period of health, not just extending life.*

National Research Council: Recommendations on diet, chronic diseases, and health. *In* Diet and Health: Implications for Reducing Chronic Disease Risk. Washington, DC, National Academy Press, 1989, p 665. *Extensive review of the criteria used for formulating dietary recommendations, their implications, potential adverse consequences, and positive public health impact.*

O'Neil EH: Health Professions Education for the Future: Schools in Service to the Nation. San Francisco, Pew Health Professions Commission, 1993. *A timely and thought-provoking report on the emerging challenges for health professions schools. Discusses the current health care crisis and proposes strategies for future health care practitioners.*

US Department of Health and Human Services, Public Health Service. Promoting Health/Preventing Disease: Year 2000 Objectives for the Nation. Washington, DC: Department of Health and Human Services, 1989. *Health promotion priorities and goals for the nation in areas such as nutrition, fitness, drugs, and sexual behavior. Preventive services for all age groups are proposed and outlined.*

9.3 Exercise
Michael Pratt

Regular physical activity is an important component of a healthy lifestyle. Over the past two decades a large body of epidemiologic and clinical evidence has accumulated which links physical inactivity with adverse health outcomes and regular physical activity with a variety of health benefits. Although the strength of the data supporting these associations varies greatly from condition to condition, physical inactivity clearly is a major contributor to premature

mortality and morbidity from chronic disease. To reduce the burden of disease resulting from physical inactivity, physicians should routinely assess the activity levels of their patients and provide appropriate counseling.

DEFINITIONS

Physical activity has been defined by Caspersen as "any bodily movement produced by skeletal muscles that results in energy expenditure." Activity performed at moderate or vigorous intensity has health benefits (Table 9–6). For most healthy adults brisk walking at 3 to 4 miles per hour is a moderate activity. Jogging, singles tennis, and moving heavy furniture are examples of vigorous activity. Exercise refers to physical activity that is planned or structured and may be done to improve or maintain one or more components of physical fitness. Both physical activity and exercise are behaviors, as opposed to physical fitness, which is "a set of attributes that people have or achieve that relate to the ability to perform physical activity," as defined by Caspersen. Physical fitness is generally considered to consist of five components: aerobic or endurance capacity, muscular strength, muscular endurance, flexibility, and body composition.

EPIDEMIOLOGY

National and state-based surveys indicate that approximately 30% of American adults are completely sedentary during their leisure time, and another 30% are minimally active. Only 40% of adults report being physically active on a regular basis (20 minutes or more at least three times per week). Among regularly active adults, only a few more than half are active at levels thought to ensure significant health benefits. Participation in leisure time physical activity appears to have increased from the 1960's through the 1980's but has reached a plateau over the past few years. Participation in physical activity declines with age and tends to be slightly higher among men than women and among whites than among members of other racial or ethnic groups. Higher levels of education and income are associated with greater participation in physical activity and account for most of the racial and ethnic differences observed for leisure time physical activity.

HEALTH BENEFITS OF PHYSICAL ACTIVITY

The physiologic and metabolic responses to exercise are at the root of the multiple health benefits associated with physical activity. Physical activity requires increased energy expenditure and imposes demands and stresses on multiple organ and enzyme systems. These demands lead to acute responses and to long-term adaptations of the circulatory, respiratory, nervous, endocrine, and skeletal systems. The most direct benefits of physical activity are cardiovascular and musculoskeletal adaptations, which increase functional capacity in these areas. Increased aerobic capacity and muscular strength and endurance have been well-documented following training programs in individuals of all ages. Maintenance of functional capacity and strength may be especially important for preventing disability and maintaining independence among older adults. Many disease- and risk factor–specific benefits of physical activity have also been postulated. Convincing data exist linking regular physical activity to health benefits in some areas such as coronary heart disease (CHD), mental health, glucose metabolism, and bone density, but much research remains to be done to better delineate other health consequences of physical activity and the underlying mechanisms.

CORONARY HEART DISEASE. The role of physical activity in preventing CHD has been studied extensively. Classic epidemio-

TABLE 9–6. DEFINING THE INTENSITY OF PHYSICAL ACTIVITY

Activity Type	METS*	Heart Rate†	Aerobic Capacity‡
Moderate	3–6	50–70%	40–60%
Vigorous	>6	>70%	>60%

* Ratio of metabolic rate during activity to resting metabolic rate. One MET is defined as the energy expended while sitting quietly.
† Percentage of maximum heart rate.
‡ Percentage of maximum aerobic capacity.

logic studies of three decades ago demonstrated that conductors on double-decker buses in London were less likely to develop heart disease than were less active drivers, and that among longshoremen the most active men had the least risk of CHD. Longitudinal studies of college alumni have shown a reduced incidence of CHD and lower CHD and all-cause mortality among regularly active men compared with their sedentary counterparts. Previously sedentary men who initiated regular physical activity in middle age also reduced their risk of death from CHD and all causes compared with men who remained sedentary. Increased physical fitness has been linked with lower all-cause and CHD mortality for both men and women (Fig. 9–2). A critical review of 43 studies of habitual physical activity and CHD indicates that the risk of CHD among sedentary men is about twice that of men who are habitually active. To date no randomized clinical trial of physical activity and CHD has been conducted. Methodologic and cost issues make such a study unlikely. However, the evidence linking regular physical activity with reductions in CHD mortality meets strict epidemiologic criteria for causality. The association is strong, consistent, graded, temporally appropriate, and biologically plausible (Table 9–7).

The evidence for a causal role for regular physical activity in the secondary prevention of CHD is at least as strong as that for primary prevention. Patients with CHD who engage in regular physical activity as part of a cardiac rehabilitation program have lower all-cause and CHD mortality than do nonparticipants 1 to 3 years after initial hospitalization. Exercise-based cardiac rehabilitation programs have also been shown to increase functional capacity and reduce CHD symptoms among patients and may improve quality of life. Appropriate physical activity should be a part of the management and rehabilitation of most patients with CHD.

WEIGHT CONTROL. Individuals who are regularly active tend to weigh less and have a lower percentage of body fat than do sedentary individuals. This occurs despite the fact that physically active persons are consistently observed to consume more calories than sedentary individuals. Regular physical activity increases caloric expenditure directly, and indirectly by raising the resting metabolic rate following activity, and perhaps by raising basal metabolic rate as well owing to metabolic changes and altered body composition. A combined program of diet and regular physical activity appears to be the most effective means of maintaining ideal body weight. Preliminary studies indicate that regular physical activity may also beneficially alter body fat distribution.

DIABETES. Physical activity increases muscle glucose uptake directly and also increases insulin sensitivity. Physical activity is commonly prescribed for managing non–insulin-dependent diabetes mellitus (NIDDM). Physical activity may also prevent NIDDM through its effects on insulin and glucose metabolism and maintenance of body weight. The incidence of NIDDM has been observed to be lower among regularly active male college alumni and physicians than among their sedentary counterparts in two well-conducted longitudinal studies.

OSTEOPOROSIS. Physical activity may play an important role in maintaining bone mineral density, preventing osteoporosis, and reducing fractures. Bone density is reduced by bed rest and can be increased by weight-bearing activity. Regular physical activity has been demonstrated to increase bone mass in young women, reduce the decline in bone mass seen in postmenopausal women, and may increase bone density in patients with osteoporosis. Postmenopausal women who walk approximately 1 mile per day have been observed to have higher bone mineral density and slower rates of bone loss than sedentary women. Regular physical activity also increases muscle mass and strength, perhaps reducing the risk of falls and protecting against fractures when falls do occur. It is not yet clear what combination of physical activity, estrogen replacement therapy, and calcium supplementation is optimal to promote bone health among women.

CANCER. Both regular physical activity and physical fitness have been associated with lower mortality from cancer in longitudinal studies. Although data for most specific cancers are limited, several studies of occupational and leisure-time activity do indicate that physical activity may protect against colon and breast cancer. The protective effects may be mediated by reduced intestinal transit time (colon cancer) and altered endocrine function.

MENTAL HEALTH. Regular physical activity and physical fitness are positively associated with mental health and well-being. Persons who are regularly active report less anxiety and depression and lower levels of stress than do sedentary persons. Exercise programs may be useful as an adjunctive therapy for treating mild to moderate depression. The mechanisms underlying the associations between physical activity and mental health remain unclear.

HEALTH RISKS

Risks as well as benefits are associated with physical activity. Musculoskeletal overuse injuries of the lower extremity are the most common negative consequence of physical activity. Three factors are strongly associated with the risk of musculoskeletal injury. First, previous injury is the strongest predictor of future injury. Second, increased duration of activity or mileage is associated with an increased risk of injury, and third, exercise intensity is associated with injury risk. The risk of injury is considerably higher with vigorous activity than with moderate activity. The clinician can reduce patients' risk of injury by making them aware of these associations and by advocating moderate physical activity and gradual increases in duration of activity or mileage.

Major cardiac events, although rare, have been associated with vigorous physical activity. The risk of cardiac arrest is transiently elevated during exercise for both those who are regularly active and to a greater extent for individuals who are irregularly active. However, the overall risk of cardiac arrest is reduced among men who are regularly active. The incidence of sudden death associated with jogging has been estimated at 1 per 360,000 hours of jogging. The majority of these deaths are due to underlying CHD. Physical activity may also exacerbate medical conditions such as asthma and diabetes. Most individuals with underlying disease or disability

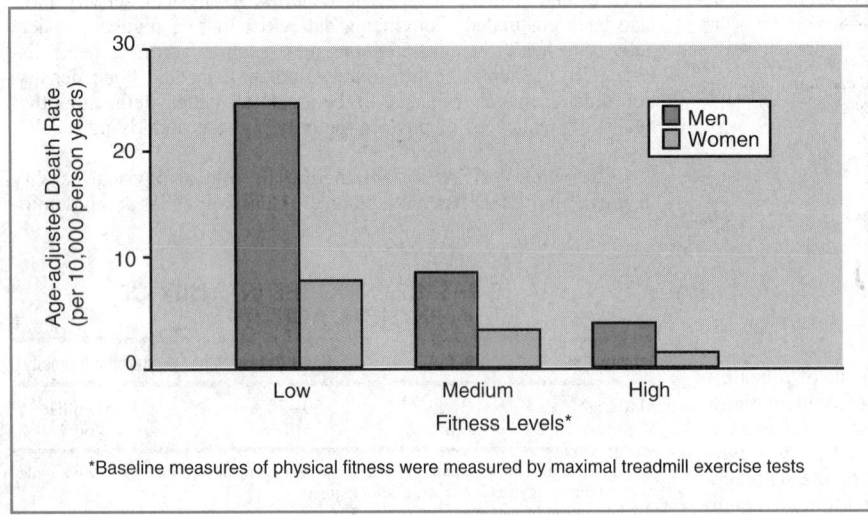

FIGURE 9–2. The relationship between level of physical fitness as measured by maximal treadmill exercise testing and cardiovascular mortality for men and women followed for an average of 8 years. (From Blair SN, Kohl HW, Paffenbarger RS, et al.: Physical fitness and all-cause mortality: A prospective study of healthy men and women. JAMA 262:2395, 1989.)

*Baseline measures of physical fitness were measured by maximal treadmill exercise tests

TABLE 9-7. MECHANISMS BY WHICH PHYSICAL ACTIVITY PREVENTS CHD

Reduces elevated systolic blood pressure
Reduces elevated diastolic blood pressure
Raises HDL cholesterol
Reduces triglycerides
Reduces weight gain and enhances weight maintenance
Increases glucose uptake and insulin sensitivity
Reduces platelet adhesion
Enhances fibrinolysis
May reduce thrombosis
Decreases sympathetic and increases parasympathetic drive, which reduces myocardial oxygen demand
May reduce ventricular arrhythmias
May increase myocardial oxygen supply

TABLE 9-8. THE EXERCISE PRESCRIPTION

Type of physical activity
   Continuous or intermittent
   Primarily aerobic
   Stretching for flexibility
   Resistance exercise for strength
Intensity
   Moderate (40–70% relative to capacity, "brisk walk")
   OR
   Vigorous (>70% relative to capacity)
Duration
   20–60 minutes per day
   200–300 kilocalories per day
Frequency
   Daily for intermittent moderate activity
   Three or more times per week for continuous, vigorous activity
Session
   For planned exercise: warm-up, 3–5 minutes
                        conditioning, 15–40 minutes
                        cool-down, 2–5 minutes
   For lifestyle activity: Incorporate activity into the daily routine. "Pulses" of activity should be at least 7–10 minutes long and at an intensity equal to brisk walking.
Progression
   Increase duration, intensity, and frequency gradually.
   Evaluate progress each visit.
Warning signs
   Severe musculoskeletal pain
   Claudication
   Chest pressure, pain, or discomfort
   Unusual shortness of breath
   Dizziness, nausea, vomiting

---

may still safely exercise if appropriate precautions are taken. The risks of cardiac, musculoskeletal, and medical injury may be reduced by decreasing the intensity of physical activity from vigorous to moderate.

MEDICAL EVALUATION

Appropriate medical evaluation depends upon the age and health status of an individual and the type of activity which he/she undertakes. Individuals free of disease who are initiating moderate-intensity physical activity, such as regular walking, do not require medical evaluation. Men over age 40 and women over age 50 who wish to become vigorously active should undergo a medical examination. Persons of any age with symptomatic cardiovascular disease or multiple risk factors for cardiovascular disease require medical evaluation. The evaluation of patients with cardiovascular disease should include a physician-supervised, symptom-limited exercise test with blood pressure and electrocardiographic monitoring.

ASSESSMENT AND COUNSELING

Health professionals should routinely counsel most of their patients to adopt and maintain an active lifestyle. The exercise prescription should take into account an individual's age, health, current activity level, and readiness to initiate behavior change. Research on both quitting smoking and initiating physical activity has shown that patients move along a behavioral continuum from precontemplation to contemplating change to making a change and finally to maintaining the new behavior. Physicians have greater success in changing their patient's physical activity practices if they can target their counseling to the patient's current activity level and behavioral stage. Brief, specific physical activity counseling reinforced by other providers, follow-up appointments, or educational materials can increase patient participation in physical activity.

How much and what type of physical activity should be prescribed? The traditional exercise prescription calls for 20 or more minutes of continuous aerobic activity three to five times per week at moderate to vigorous intensity (≥60% of maximum heart rate or 50% of aerobic capacity). This is an appropriate prescription for increasing fitness and improving health status. Reassessment of epidemiologic and clinical data on the health aspects of physical activity reveals that many of the health benefits attributable to physical activity are associated with the total quantity of activity performed even if the activity is discontinuous and of only moderate intensity. Moderate activities such as brisk walking, gardening, and stair climbing done on a daily basis can have major health impacts. The Centers for Disease Control and Prevention and the American College of Sports Medicine recommend that "every American adult should accumulate 30 minutes or more of moderate intensity physical activity on most, preferably all, days of the week."

The health professional may choose to prescribe physical activity using either the traditional exercise prescription or the new recommendation (Table 9–8). Both provide significant health benefits. Tailoring recommendations for physical activity to the patient's individual goals, interests, skills, available time, and barriers to activity increases the chances for success.

Most persons are aware that they should be more active. The health professional can encourage patients to become regularly active by reinforcing the importance of physical activity to health,

working with the patient to help build the skills and self-confidence needed to be active, and designing a program of physical activity that fits into the individual's lifestyle.

Bouchard C, Shepard RJ, Stephens T (eds.): Physical Activity, Fitness, and Health. Champaign, IL, Human Kinetics Publishers, 1994. *A compendium of detailed reviews of the health benefits and risks of physical activity and the underlying physiologic mechanisms.*
McGinnis JM, Foege WH: Actual causes of death in the United States. JAMA 270:2207, 1993. *A discussion and quantification of the major factors that contributed to mortality in the United States in 1990. Tobacco, diet, and activity patterns were identified as the most prominent contributors to mortality.*
Paffenbarger RS, Hyde RT, Wing AL, et al.: The association of changes in physical activity level and other lifestyle characteristics with mortality among men. N Engl J Med 328:538, 1993. *The most recent in a landmark series of publications documenting reductions in cardiovascular disease mortality among habitually active male college alumni compared with their sedentary counterparts.*
Powell KE, Thompson PD, Caspersen CJ, et al.: Physical activity and the incidence of coronary heart disease. Annu Rev Public Health 8:253, 1987. *A critical review of 43 epidemiologic studies of the association between habitual physical activity and the incidence of coronary heart disease.*

9.4 Tobacco
Neal L. Benowitz

EPIDEMIOLOGY. There are currently about 45 million cigarette smokers, including 28% of men and 23% of women, in the United States. People who are less well-educated and/or have unskilled occupations are more likely to smoke. Smoking is responsible for about 430,000 preventable US deaths annually. A lifelong smoker has about a one in four chance of dying prematurely from a complication of smoking. Smoking is the major preventable cause of death in developed countries.

Other forms of tobacco use include pipes and cigars (used by 8.7% of men and 0.3% of women) and smokeless tobacco (5.5% of men and 1% of women). Smokeless tobacco use in the United States is primarily oral snuff and chewing tobacco, whereas nasal snuff is used to a greater extent in the United Kingdom.

HARMFUL CONSTITUENTS OF TOBACCO.
Tobacco smoke is an aerosol of droplets (particulates) containing water, nicotine and other alkaloids, and tar. Tobacco smoke contains several thousand different chemicals, many of which may contribute to human disease. Major toxic chemicals in the particulate phase of tobacco include nicotine, benzo(a)pyrene and other polycyclic hydrocarbons, N'-nitrosonornicotine, β-naphylamine, polonium-210, nickel, cadmium, arsenic, and lead. The gaseous phase contains carbon monoxide, acetaldehyde, acetone, methanol, nitrogen oxides, hydrogen cyanide, acrolein, ammonia, benzene, formaldehyde, nitrosoamines, and vinyl chloride. Tobacco smoke may produce illness via systemic absorption of toxins and/or by local pulmonary injury by oxidant gases.

TOBACCO ADDICTION.
Tobacco use is motivated primarily by the desire for nicotine. Drug addiction is defined as compulsive use of a psychoactive substance, the consequences of which are detrimental to the individual or society. Understanding addiction is useful in providing effective smoking-cessation therapy. Nicotine is absorbed rapidly from tobacco smoke into the pulmonary circulation; it then moves quickly to the brain, where it acts on nicotinic cholinergic receptors to produce its gratifying effects, occurring within 10 to 15 seconds after a puff. Smokeless tobacco is absorbed more slowly and results in less intense pharmacologic effects. With long-term use of tobacco, physical dependence develops, associated with an increased number of nicotinic cholinergic receptors in the brain. When tobacco is unavailable, even for only a few hours, withdrawal symptoms often occur, including anxiety, irritability, difficulty concentrating, restlessness, hunger, craving for tobacco, disturbed sleep, and, in some people, depression.

Addiction to tobacco is multifactorial, including a desire for the direct pharmacologic actions of nicotine, relief of withdrawal symptoms, and learned associations. Smokers report a variety of reasons for smoking, including pleasure, arousal, enhanced vigilance, improved performance, relief of anxiety or depression, reduced hunger, and control of body weight. Environmental cues—such as a meal, a cup of coffee, talking on the phone, an alcoholic beverage, or friends who smoke—often trigger an urge to smoke.

Most tobacco use begins in childhood or adolescence. Risk factors for youth smoking include peer and parental influences, behavioral problems (e.g., poor school performance), and personality characteristics such as rebelliousness or risk-taking, depression, and/or anxiety, as well as genetic influences. Adolescent desire to appear older and more sophisticated, following more mature role models, is another strong motivator. Environmental influences such as advertising are also thought to contribute. Whereas smoking rates among adults have been declining over the past 30 years, initiation rates for youth have remained constant for the past 15 years. Approaches to preventing tobacco addiction in youth include educational activities in schools or in the media, reducing accessibility of tobacco to youth (such as taxation, enforcing restrictions against youth purchasing tobacco), changing the social and environmental norms, and deglamourizing smoking (restricting indoor smoking, educating parents not to smoke around children).

TOBACCO-RELATED DISEASES.
Tobacco use is a major cause of death from cancer, cardiovascular disease, and pulmonary disease. Smoking is also a major risk factor for peptic disease, osteoporosis, reproductive disorders, and fire-related injuries. Complications of cigarette smoking are summarized in Table 9–9.

Cancer. Smoking is the single largest preventable cause of cancer. It is responsible for about 30% of cancer deaths. A number of chemicals in tobacco smoke may contribute to carcinogenesis as tumor initiators, co-carcinogens, tumor promoters, or complete carcinogens. The cancers caused by smoking, with relative risks and attributable mortality, are shown in Table 9–10. Lung cancer is the leading cause of cancer deaths in the United States and is predominantly attributable to cigarette smoking. The risk of lung and other cancers is proportional to how many cigarettes are smoked per day and the duration of smoking. Workplace exposure to asbestos or alpha-radiation (see Ch. 13.1) (the latter in uranium miners) synergistically increases the risk of lung cancer in cigarette smokers. Alcohol use (see Ch. 11) interacts synergistically with tobacco in causing oral, laryngeal, and esophageal cancer. The mechanism of interaction may involve alcohol-solubilizing tobacco carcinogens, and/or alcohol-related induction of liver or gastrointestinal enzymes

TABLE 9-9. HEALTH HAZARDS OF TOBACCO USE (RISKS INCREASED BY SMOKING)

Cancer
See Table 9–10

Cardiovascular disease
Sudden death
Acute myocardial infarction
Unstable angina
Stroke
Peripheral arterial occlusive
 disease
Aortic aneurysm

Pulmonary disease
Lung cancer
Chronic bronchitis
Emphysema
Asthma
Increased susceptibility to
 pneumonia
Increased morbidity from viral
 respiratory infection

Gastrointestinal disease
Peptic ulcer
Esophageal reflux

Reproductive disturbances
Reduced fertility
Premature birth
Lower birthweight
Spontaneous abortion
Abruptio placentae
Premature rupture of membranes
Increased perinatal mortality

Oral disease (smokeless tobacco)
Oral cancer
Leukoplakia
Gingivitis
Gingival recession
Tooth staining

Other
Earlier menopause
Osteoporosis
Cataract
Premature skin wrinkling
Altered drug metabolism or effects

---

that metabolize and activate tobacco carcinogens. The tobacco-related risks of bladder and kidney cancer are enhanced by occupational exposure to aromatic amines, such as in the dye industry. Cervical cancer is more common in women who smoke, presumably the result of exposure to carcinogens in cervical secretions. Smoking appears to be involved in 20 to 30% of leukemia cases in adults, including both lymphoid and myeloid leukemia.

Cardiovascular Disease. Cigarette smoking accounts for about 20% of cardiovascular deaths in the United States. Risks are increased for coronary heart disease, including sudden death, cerebrovascular disease, and peripheral vascular disease, including aortic aneurysm. Cigarette smoking accelerates atherosclerosis and promotes acute ischemic events. The mechanisms of effects of smoking are not fully elucidated but are believed to include (1) hemodynamic stress: nicotine increases heart rate and transiently increases blood pressure; (2) endothelial injury; (3) development of an atherogenic lipid profile: smokers have on average higher LDL, more oxidized LDL, and lower HDL cholesterol than nonsmokers; (4) enhanced coagulability; (5) arrhythmogenesis; and (6) relative hypoxemia due to effects of carbon monoxide. Carbon monoxide reduces the capacity of hemoglobin to carry oxygen and impairs the release of oxygen from hemoglobin to body tissues, resulting in a state of relative hypoxemia. To compensate for this hypoxemic state, smokers develop polycythemia, with hematocrits often 50% or more. The polycythemia also increases blood viscosity, which adds to the risk of thrombotic events.

Cigarette smoking acts synergistically with other cardiac risk factors to increase the risk of ischemic heart disease. Although the risk of cardiovascular disease is roughly proportional to cigarette consumption, the risk persists even at low levels of smoking, that is, one to two cigarettes per day. Cigarette smoking reduces exercise tolerance in patients with angina pectoris and intermittent claudication. Vasospastic angina is more common and the response to vasodilator medication is impaired in patients who smoke. The number of episodes and total duration of ischemic episodes as assessed by ambulatory electrocardiographic monitoring in patients with coronary heart disease are substantially increased by cigarette smoking. The increase in relative risk of coronary heart disease due to cigarette smoking is greatest in young adults who, in the absence of cigarette smoking, would have a relatively low risk. Women who use oral contraceptives and smoke have a synergistically increased risk of both myocardial infarction and stroke.

Following acute myocardial infarction, the risk of recurrent myocardial infarction is higher and survival is half over the next 12 years, comparing smokers who continue to smoke with those who quit. Smoking interferes with revascularization therapy for acute myocardial infarction. After thrombolysis the reocclusion rate is fourfold higher in smokers who continue than in those who quit.

The risk of reocclusion of a coronary artery after angioplasty or the occlusion of a bypass graft is increased in smokers. Cigarette smoking is not a risk factor for hypertension per se but does increase the risk of complications, including the development of nephrosclerosis and progression to malignant hypertension.

Pulmonary Disease. More than 80% of chronic obstructive lung disease in the United States is attributable to cigarette smoking. Cigarette smoking also increases the risk of respiratory infection, including pneumonia, and results in greater disability from viral respiratory tract infections. Pulmonary disease from smoking includes the overlapping syndromes of chronic bronchitis (cough and mucus hypersecretion), emphysema, and airway obstruction. The lung pathology produced by cigarette smoking includes loss of cilia, mucous gland hyperplasia, increased number of goblet cells in central airways, inflammation, goblet cell metaplasia, squamous metaplasia, mucus plugging of small airways and destruction of alveoli, and a reduced number of small arteries. The mechanism of injury is complex and appears to include direct injury by oxidant gases, increased elastase activity (a protein that breaks down elastin and other connective tissue), and decreased antiprotease activity. A genetic deficiency of α_1-antiprotease activity produces a similar imbalance between pulmonary protease and antiprotease activity and is a risk factor for early and severe smoking-induced pulmonary disease.

Other Complications. Cigarette smoking increases the risk of duodenal and gastric ulcer, delays the rate of ulcer healing, and increases the risk of relapse after ulcer treatment. Smoking is also associated with esophageal reflux symptoms. Smoking produces ulcer disease by increasing acid secretion, reducing pancreatic bicarbonate secretion, impairing gastric mucosal barrier (related to decreased gastric mucosal blood flow and/or inhibition of prostaglandin synthesis), and/or reducing pyloric sphincter tone.

Cigarette smoking is a risk factor for osteoporosis, reducing the peak bone mass attained in early adulthood and increasing the rate of bone loss in later adulthood. Smoking antagonizes the protective effect of estrogen replacement therapy on the risk of osteoporosis in postmenopausal women.

Cigarette smoking is a major cause of reproductive problems, resulting in approximately 4600 U.S. infant deaths annually. Smoking during pregnancy increases the risks of adverse effects listed in Table 9–9. Growth retardation due to cigarette smoking has been termed the "fetal tobacco syndrome." Cigarette smoking causes reproductive complications by causing placental ischemia, mediated by the vasoconstricting effects of nicotine, hypoxic effects of chronic carbon monoxide exposure, and/or the general increase in coagulability produced by smoking.

Other adverse effects of cigarette smoking include premature facial wrinkling, an increased risk of cataracts, olfactory dysfunction, and fire-related injuries, the latter of which contribute significantly to the economic costs of tobacco use.

CIGARETTE SMOKING EFFECTS ON DRUG ACTION. Cigarette smoking potentially interacts with a variety of drugs. Two general mechanisms are involved: (1) cigarette smoking accelerates drug metabolism, and (2) nicotine and/or other constituents of tobacco have additive or antagonistic pharmacologic actions with other drugs. Significant drug interactions are summarized in Table 9–11.

HEALTH HAZARDS OF SMOKELESS TOBACCO. Smokeless tobacco refers to snuff and chewing tobacco. Oral snuff is placed (as a "pinch") between the lip and gum or under the tongue; chewing tobacco is actively chewed, which generates saliva that is spit out (hence the term "spit tobacco"). Smokeless tobacco products are usually flavored, many with licorice, and also contain sodium bicarbonate to keep the local pH alkaline so as to facilitate the buccal absorption of nicotine. Nicotine absorption from smokeless tobacco is similar in magnitude to that absorbed from cigarette smoking. In addition, other chemicals, including sodium, glycyrrhizinic acid (from licorice), and potentially carcinogenic chemicals such as nitrosoamines are absorbed systemically.

Smokeless tobacco is addictive and is associated with an increased risk of oral cancer at the site where the tobacco is usually placed (inside the lip, under the cheek or tongue) or nasal cancer in nasal snuff users. Other oral diseases including leukoplakia, gingivitis, gingival recession, and staining of the teeth are also associated with smokeless tobacco. Cardiovascular effects of smokeless tobacco include acute aggravation of hypertension or angina pectoris due to the sympathomimetic effects of nicotine, hypokalemia and hypertension due to effects of glycyrrhizinic acid (a potent mineralocorticoid), and excessive sodium absorption resulting in aggravated hypertension or sodium-retaining disorders.

ENVIRONMENTAL TOBACCO SMOKE. Considerable evidence indicates that exposure to environmental tobacco smoke (ETS) (i.e., passive smoking) is harmful to the health of nonsmokers. Recently, the U.S. Environmental Protection Agency (EPA) classified ETS as a class A carcinogen, meaning that it has been shown to cause cancer in humans. Health hazards of environmental smoke in nonsmokers are summarized in Table 9–12.

ETS consists of smoke that is generated while the cigarette is smoldering, as well as mainstream smoke that has been exhaled by the smoker. Seventy-five percent or more of the total combustion product from a cigarette enters the air. The constituents of ETS are qualitatively similar to those of mainstream smoke. However, some toxins, such as ammonia, formaldehyde, and nitrosoamines, are present in much higher concentrations in ETS than in mainstream smoke. The EPA has estimated that ETS is responsible for approximately 3000 lung cancer deaths annually in nonsmokers in the United States, is causally associated with 150,000 to 300,000 cases of lower respiratory tract infection in infants and young children up to 18 months of age and is causally associated with the aggravation of asthma in 200,000 to 1 million children. An appreciation of the hazards of ETS is important to the physician, as it provides a basis for advising parents not to smoke when children are in the home; for insisting that childcare facilities be smokefree; and for recommending smoking restrictions in work sites and other public places.

BENEFITS OF QUITTING. The benefits of quitting smoking are substantial for smokers of any age. A person who quits smoking before age 50 has half the risk of dying in the next 15 years that a continuing smoker has. Smoking cessation reduces the risks of developing lung cancer, with the risk falling to one-half that of a continuing smoker by 10 years, and one sixth that of a smoker after 15 years' cessation. The risk of acute myocardial infarction falls rapidly after quitting smoking and approaches nonsmoker levels within a year of abstinence. Cigarette smoking produces a progressive loss of airway function over time, characterized by an accelerated loss of FEV_1 with increasing age. FEV_1 loss to cigarette smoking cannot be regained by cessation, but the rate of decline slows after smoking cessation and returns to that of nonsmokers. Women who stop smoking during the first 3 to 4 months of pregnancy reduce the risk of a low birthweight baby to that of a woman who has never smoked.

After quitting, smokers gain an average of 5 to 7 pounds, which is perceived as undesirable and a reason not to quit by some smok-

TABLE 9–10. SMOKING AND CANCER MORTALITY

Type of Cancer		Relative Risk Among Smokers		Mortality Attributable To Smoking	
		Current	Former	Percentage	Number
Lung	Male	22.4	9.4	90	82,800
	Female	11.9	4.7	79	40,300
Larynx	Male	10.5	5.2	81	2,400
	Female	17.8	11.9	87	700
Oral cavity	Male	27.5	8.8	92	4,900
	Female	5.6	2.9	61	1,800
Esophagus	Male	7.6	5.8	78	5,700
	Female	10.3	3.2	75	1,900
Pancreas	Male	2.1	1.1	29	3,500
	Female	2.3	1.8	34	4,500
Bladder	Male	2.9	1.9	47	3,000
	Female	2.6	1.9	37	1,200
Kidney	Male	3.0	2.0	48	3,000
	Female	1.4	1.2	12	500
Stomach	Male	1.5	?	17	1,400
	Female	1.5	?	25	1,300
Leukemia	Male	2.0	?	20	2,000
	Female	2.0	?	20	1,600
Cervix	Female	2.1	1.9	31	1,400

Adapted from Newcomb PA, Carbone PP: The health consequences of smoking: Cancer. Med Clin North Am 76:305, 1992.

TABLE 9-11. INTERACTION BETWEEN CIGARETTE SMOKING AND DRUGS

Drug(s)		Interaction (Effects Compared with Nonsmokers)	Significance
Antipyrine	Lidocaine	Accelerated metabolism	May require high doses in smokers; reduced doses after quitting
Caffeine	Oxazepam		
Desmethyldiazepam	Pentazocine		
Estradiol	Phenacetin		
Estrone	Phenylbutazone		
Flecainide	Propranolol		
Heparin	Theophylline		
Imipramine			
Oral contraceptives		Enhanced thrombosis; increased risk of stroke and myocardial infarction	Do not prescribe to smokers, especially if over age 35
Cimetidine and other H$_2$ blockers		Lower rate of ulcer healing; higher ulcer recurrence rates	Consider using mucosal protective agents
Propranolol		Less antihypertensive effect, less antianginal efficacy. More effective in reducing mortality following myocardial infarction.	Consider use of cardioselective β-blockers
Nifedipine (and probably other calcium blockers)		Less antianginal effect	May require higher doses and/or multiple drug antianginal therapy
Diazepam, chlordiazepoxide (and possibly other sedative-hypnotics)		Less sedation	Smokers may need higher doses
Chlorpromazine (and possibly other neuroleptics)		Less sedation; possibly reduced efficacy	Smokers may need higher doses
Propoxyphene		Reduced analgesia	Smokers may need higher doses

ers. Smokers tend to be thinner because of the effects of nicotine—increasing energy expenditure and reducing compensatory increases in food consumption. After they quit smoking, ex-smokers tend to reach the weight expected had they never smoked. On balance, the benefits of quitting far outweigh the risks associated with weight gain, and patients should be counseled accordingly.

TREATMENT OF NICOTINE ADDICTION. Seventy percent of cigarette smokers would like to quit. Spontaneous quit rates are about 1% per year. Simple physician advice to quit increases the quit rate to 3%. Minimal intervention programs increase quit rates to 5 to 10%, whereas more intensive treatments, including smoking cessation clinics, can yield quit rates of 25 to 30%. A practical office smoking cessation program has been developed by the National Cancer Institute, consisting of "4 A's": (1) *Ask* about smoking at every opportunity; (2) *advise* all smokers to stop; (3) *assist* the patient in stopping and maintaining abstinence; and (4) *arrange* follow-up to reinforce nonsmoking. Assistance in quitting should include providing self-help material or quit kits, which are widely available from governmental health agencies, professional societies, and local organizations such as cancer, heart, and lung associations. The physician may offer additional education and counseling through the office (most efficiently provided by office staff and through teaching aids, such as videotapes) or through referral to community smoking-cessation programs. Smokers who are interested may be offered nicotine replacement therapy.

Currently, nicotine replacement medications include 2- and 4-mg nicotine polacrilex gum and transdermal nicotine patches. In all cases, a smoker should be instructed to quit smoking entirely before beginning nicotine replacement therapies. Both types of nicotine medication, if used properly, double smoking cessation rates compared with placebo treatments. Optimal use of nicotine gum includes instructions not to chew too rapidly, chewing 8 to 10 pieces per day for 20 to 30 minutes each, and using it for an adequate period of time for the smoker to learn a lifestyle without cigarettes,

usually 3 months or longer. Side effects of nicotine gum are primarily local, including jaw fatigue, sore mouth and throat, upset stomach, and hiccups.

Several different transdermal nicotine preparations are marketed—three deliver 21 or 22 mg over 24 hours, one delivers 15 mg over 16 hours. All have lower dose patches for tapering. Patches are applied in the morning and removed either the next morning or at bedtime, depending on the patch. Full-dose patches are recommended for most smokers for the first 1 to 3 months, followed by 1 to 2 tapering doses for 2 to 4 weeks each. Follow-up office visits and/or telephone calls during and after active treatment increase long-term smoking cessation rates. Even in the best treatment circumstances, 70% or more of smokers relapse. Most smokers go through a quitting process three or four times before they finally succeed. When a quit attempt fails, the health care provider should encourage the patient to try again as soon as he/she is ready.

Benowitz NL: Cigarette smoking and nicotine addiction. Med Clin North Am 76:415, 1992. *A review of the human pharmacology of nicotine, its role in producing tobacco addiction, and the basis for pharmacotherapy of addiction.*

Byrd JC: Environmental tobacco smoke—medical and legal issues. Med Clin North Am 76:377, 1992. *A review of health hazards of ETS, legislation on restricting smoking in public places, and relevant judicial activities.*

Manley MW, Epps RP, Glynn TJ: The clinician's role in promoting smoking cessation among clinic patients. Med Clin North Am 76:477, 1992. *A practical review of smoking cessation strategies that work in physicians' offices.*

Samet JM: The health benefits of smoking cessation. Med Clin North Am 76:399, 1992. *A review of the benefits of quitting smoking—useful data for patient education.*

Tang JL, Law M, Wald N: How effective is nicotine replacement therapy in helping people to stop smoking? Br Med J 308:21, 1994. *A recent review and analysis of trials of nicotine polacrilex gum and transdermal nicotine treatment to help people stop smoking; includes guidelines for using these treatments.*

TABLE 9-12. HEALTH HAZARDS OF ENVIRONMENTAL TOBACCO SMOKE IN NONSMOKERS

Children	Adults
Hospitalization for respiratory tract infection in first year of life	Lung cancer
Wheezing	Myocardial infarction
Middle ear effusion	Reduced pulmonary function
Asthma	Irritation of eyes, nasal congestion, headache
Sudden infant death syndrome	Cough

9.5 Violence and Injury
Elizabeth McLoughlin

DEFINITIONS. Violence in the United States is a public health emergency, manifested in institutional and personal behavior. The root causes of violence include inequitable social and economic conditions. *Personal violence* is the intentional use of physical or psychological force against another person or against oneself, which may result in injury or death. An **injury** is damage to tissue usually caused by excessive energy transfer. That energy can be kinetic (causing fractures, lacerations, and contusions), thermal (burns and scalds), electrical (electrocutions), or chemical (poisonings). The mechanism is somewhat different for drowning and suffocation, which result when tissue is deprived of oxygen. Injuries may be classified in many ways, primarily by type, by cause, and by intent. **Type** of injury includes, for example, a fracture, laceration, or burn. **Cause** groupings distinguish among, for example, injuries due to a car crash, a bullet, poisons, or a fall. **Intent** categories address whether the injury was unintentional, intentionally self-inflicted (the most severe outcome being suicide), or intentionally inflicted by another (the most severe outcome being homicide). Intentional or violent injuries are positioned at the intersection of violence in general and all injuries (Fig. 9–3).

EPIDEMIOLOGY. Injuries are the leading cause of death for all Americans aged 1 to 44. In 1990, injury caused death for 150,211 Americans. Table 9–13 presents injury mortality rates per 100,000 in the U.S. population for 1990, categorized by intent of injury. Within some subgroups, the death rate was far higher. For example, the unintentional injury death rate for Americans over age 85 was 257; the homicide death rate for black males aged 20 to 24 was 162; the suicide rate for white males over age 75 was 62.

The six leading external causes of injury death are motor vehicle crashes, firearms, falls, poisons, drownings, and fire/burns (Fig. 9–4). The two major consumer products most associated with injury death are the motor vehicle and the firearm; the rates for men far exceed those for women. The pattern for male motor vehicle and firearm deaths is remarkably alike across the age range (Fig. 9–5). Firearm deaths exceed motor vehicle deaths for men from age 25 through 84. Among firearm deaths, the peak among young men is primarily homicide, the peak among older men is primarily suicide. Motor vehicle deaths exceed firearm deaths among the young and the very elderly, age groups that are vulnerable to pedestrian as well as vehicle occupant deaths.

Less is known about nonfatal injuries, because until recently hospitals have not routinely included "external cause of injury" codes in medical records of injured patients. Estimates of nonfatal injuries, based on state samples and special studies, present causal patterns quite different from fatal injuries. Whereas motor vehicles and firearms together accounted for 54% of injury deaths in 1985, they accounted for only 25% of injuries requiring hospitalization and fewer than 10% of the less severe injuries. Falls accounted for one third of all injury-related hospital admissions (1985 data are cited because they are the most recent data for comparing three levels of severity by cause). The aggregate lifetime cost for the 57 million persons injured in 1985 was estimated at $158 billion—$45 million in direct medical and nonmedical care of injured persons, $65 billion for lost productivity due to temporary or permanent disability, and $48 billion in lost productivity due to premature death. Alcohol consumption is a major risk factor for all types of injury, both intentional (assault and suicide) and unintentional (particularly motor vehicle crashes).

Violence against girls and women by intimates, other relatives, and acquaintances far exceeds violence inflicted by strangers (Fig. 9–6). When asked in a context other than that of criminal behavior, 14% of American women acknowledged having been violently abused by a husband or boyfriend. Women victimized by strangers are almost six times more likely to report the violence to police than women victimized by intimates who fear reprisal from the offender.

PREVENTION. Injuries are preventable. Data on injury deaths from 1910 to 1990 show a significant decrease in other (i.e., non-motor vehicle) unintentional injury deaths (Fig. 9–7). This decrease was due in part to improved safety design of occupational machinery and other worker protections, labeling and packaging of drugs and toxic products, and improved medical care. The death rate from motor vehicle crashes increased 10-fold from 1910 to 1930 as cars became the primary form of transportation. However, there has been a 30% decrease in this death rate in the last two decades, owing in part to improved safety features in vehicles and roads, a temporary lowering of speed limits, the increased legal drinking age, and a public intolerance of drinking and driving. The homicide rate increased from 6 per 100,000 population in 1910 to 9 in 1930, decreased during World War II and the postwar period (1940's to 1960's) to approximately 5, then increased to 10 in the 1980's and 1990's. Recent increases are attributed to the enormous number of guns in circulation, currently estimated to be from 150 to 200 million, one third of which are handguns. The suicide rate has shown less variability but has been consistently higher than the homicide rate throughout this century. Firearm homicides and suicides now exceed deaths from motor vehicle crashes in seven states, and if trend lines (from 1968 to 1991) continue, deaths caused by firearms will exceed those from motor vehicles nationally by the year 2002.

The public health model for preventing both disease and injury indicates three sets of factors—host, agent, and environment—which can be modified to reduce the number or severity of injury.

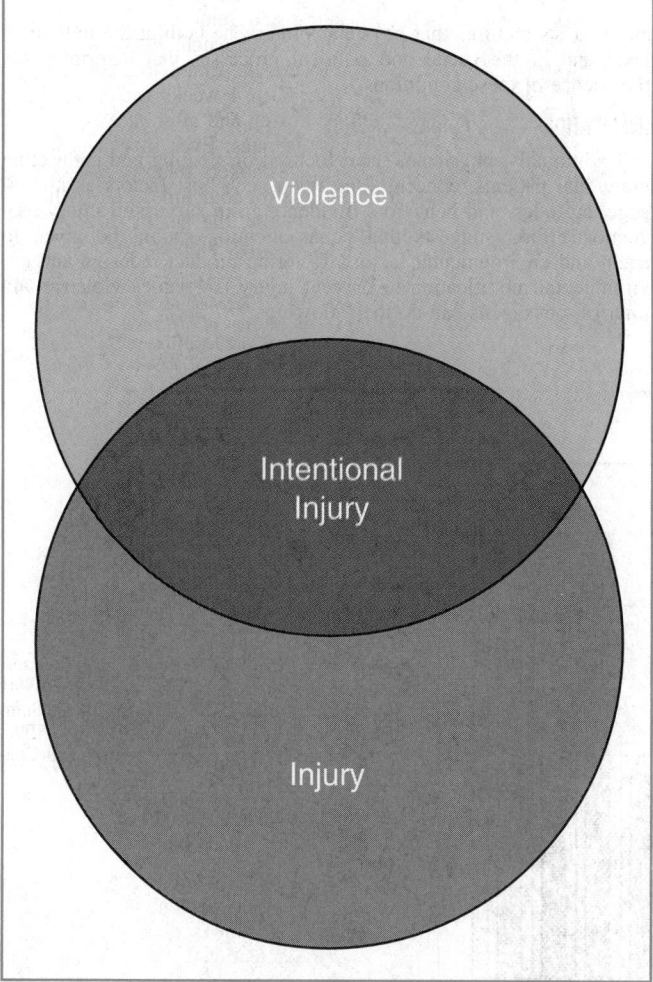

FIGURE 9–3. Intentional or violent injuries are positioned at the intersection of violence in general and all injuries.

TABLE 9–13. INJURY MORTALITY RATES FOR 1990*

Category by Intent	Total Number of Injury Deaths†	Rates		
		Male	*Female*	*Total*
Unintentional	91,983	48	18	32
Homicide	24,932	16	4	10
Suicide	30,906	19	4	11
TOTAL	150,211	84	27	55

* Numbers and age-adjusted injury rates per 100,000 population, by intent of injury, USA, 1990.

† Intent was not determined in 1.6% of the deaths.

Data from Injury Mortality, National Summary of Injury Mortality Data, 1984–1990; National Center for Injury Prevention and Control, (CDC.)

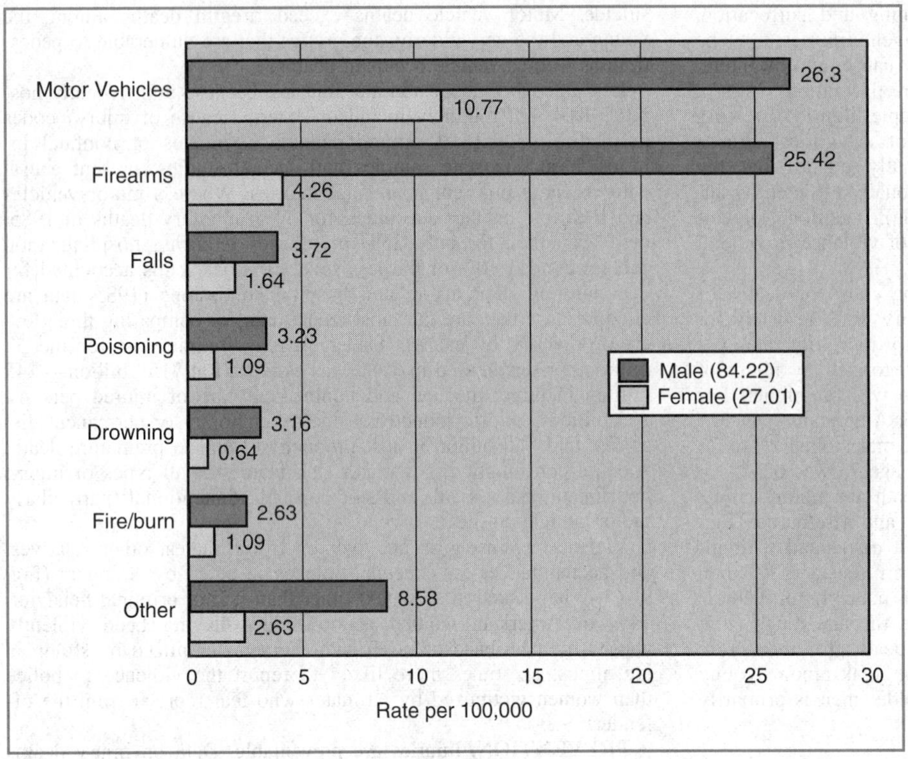

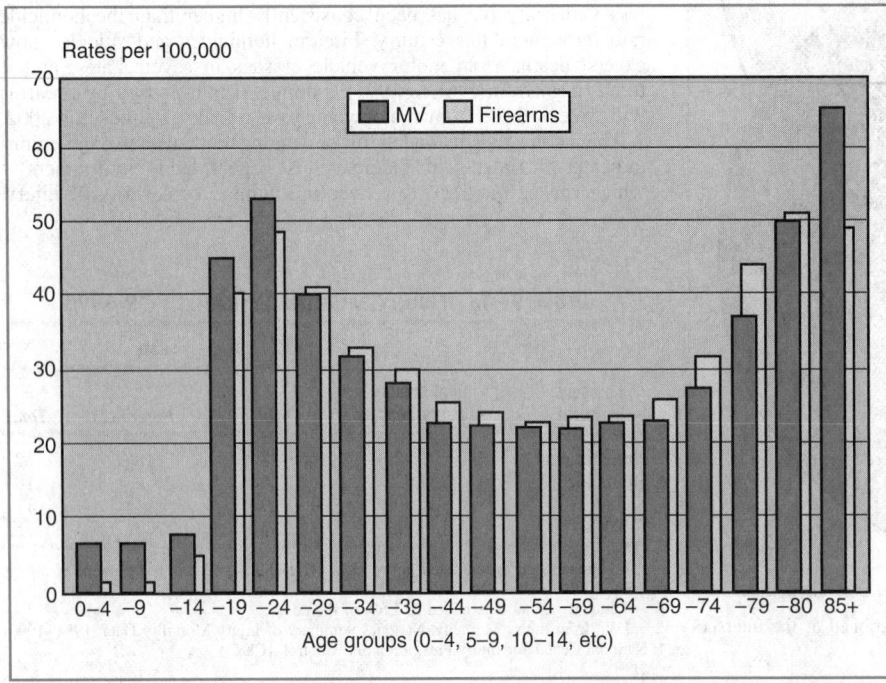

FIGURE 9-4. External cause of injury death: age-adjusted rates per 100,000, USA, 1990. (Data from Injury Mortality, National Summary of Injury Mortality Data, 1984–1990; National Center for Injury Prevention and Control, CDC.)

Host-related interventions modify the knowledge, attitudes, skills, and behaviors of individuals at risk. **Agent**-related interventions modify the objects (such as motor vehicles, guns, and bullets) that are directly involved in causing the injury. **Environment**-related interventions modify the physical environment (such as energy-absorbing or protective barriers and surfaces) and the social environment (such as norms and customs, laws and regulations), which influence the likelihood of an injury-causing event.

Violence and associated intentional injuries are complex, pervasive problems that must be reduced through comprehensive, multidisciplinary interventions. As is the case with preventing diseases such as smoking-associated cancers and AIDS, preventing violence and injuries requires that physicians intervene both at the individual level and in the social and political processes that determine the prevalence of these conditions.

IMPLICATIONS FOR MEDICAL PRACTICE

Traditionally, physicians have focused on treating and counseling individual patients, concentrating upon such host factors as knowledge, attitudes, and behaviors. Evidence from successful injury prevention efforts suggests that equal attention should be given to agent and environmental factors, fostering product redesign and environmental modification to prevent injury. To reduce violence and injuries, physicians can do the following:

FIGURE 9-5. Motor vehicles and firearms: male death rates by age groups, USA, 1990. (Data from Injury Mortality, National Summary of Injury Mortality Data, 1984–1990; National Center for Injury Prevention and Control, CDC.)

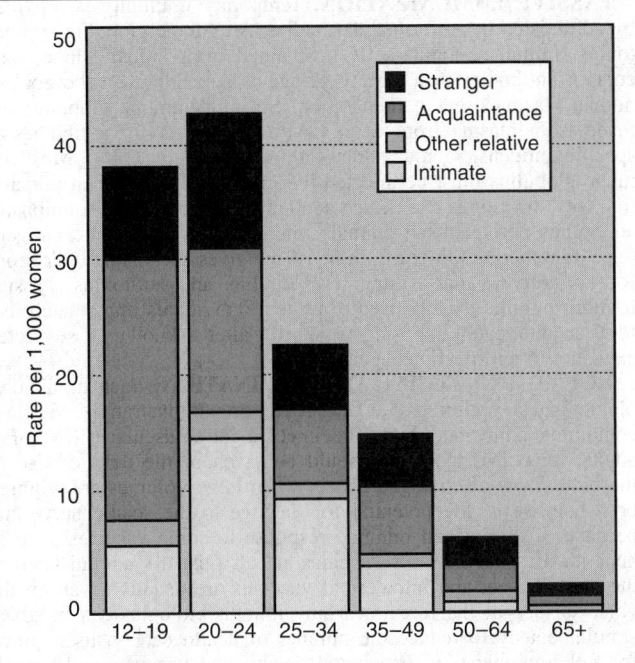

FIGURE 9–6. Violence against women: average annual rate of single-offender violent victimization per 1000 women, by victim-offender relationships and age group, 1987–1991, as determined by the National Crime Victimization Survey. (From Violence Against Women: A National Crime Victimization Survey Report, US Department of Justice, 1994.)

1. **Counsel patients about injury risk and prevention.** All physicians, regardless of specialty, have the opportunity to intervene with the "host." It is standard practice during history taking for physicians to inquire about tobacco and alcohol use, sexual practices, and exercise habits of adult patients, and to counsel parents about specific risks at different stages of child development. There are known risks for injury and protective strategies that patients can use to lower the risk of injury for themselves and their families. Risks for homicide in the home include a gun kept loaded in the home and a history of family violence; protective strategies include removing guns from the home (or at least unloading and locking them away), and identifying and referring battered women to protective services. Protective strategies regarding motor vehicle crashes include airbags in cars and the routine use of seatbelts, child car seats, and motorcycle and bicycle helmets. To prevent scald injuries, reduce the temperature settings in residential hot water heaters to 125°F. To prevent residential fire fatalities, install and maintain smoke detectors. To prevent young children drowning in home pools, install four-sided isolation fences with self-latching gates. To prevent fatal falls for children, install guards on balconies and windows in high-rise buildings, and for elders, improve lighting and install hand-grip devices in the home. Because alcohol consumption is a risk factor for all injuries, questions about drinking habits should be included in injury-prevention counseling. Although physician-patient counseling may not always result in behavior change, it can be a powerful educational message delivered by a trusted authority.

2. **Identify and refer abused patients.** Family violence is a serious and underdiagnosed problem in American society. Abused patients include children, battered spouses and/or partners, elders, and those raped and sexually abused by those with whom they have a personal or intimate relationship. Hospitals, clinics, and doctors' offices may provide the first opportunity for abused patients, particularly adult women, to acknowledge the abuse, receive support, find protection, and break the cycle of violence. Physicians treating women who are injured or who repeatedly seek medical care for complaints of pain should ask directly and empathetically if the injury was caused by a partner or spouse. Medical facilities and physicians should draw on available resources to prepare practice guidelines for the diagnosis and treatment of abused patients (e.g., AMA Guidelines). Policies and procedures should address state reg-

ulations about reporting the abuse to authorities. In any case, battered women should be given information about and referral to social and legal services and battered women's shelters.

3. **Emphasize rehabilitation and community follow-up.** Tertiary prevention involves minimizing functional disability, a consequence of serious injury. Physicians can help their patients return to productive lives by ensuring that patients receive appropriate physical and occupational therapy and that they have access to community services after discharge. The independent living movement and local centers for independent living, as well as state departments of rehabilitation, can provide role models and resources for people with disabilities. Because community social and mental health services are essential for prevention and rehabilitation, physicians can well serve their patients by publicly speaking out in support of these services.

4. **Improve the injury database for research and prevention.** Prevention must be grounded in good epidemiology that identifies high-risk products, situations, and populations. Injury epidemiologists depend upon the accuracy and reliability of coroner and hospital discharge data. Physicians who care for injured patients in a hospital or emergency department should describe the external cause and circumstances of the injury event in the medical record. This is then coded in the discharge record using the World Health Organization's International Classification of Disease External Cause of Injury "e-codes." Analyzing such data provides national, state, and local profiles of injury which can guide prevention program planning, evaluation, and allocation of resources.

5. **Advocate for solutions to the violence and injury problem, with focus on agent and environmental factors.** Physicians have played a leadership role in injury control in such diverse areas as traffic safety, burns from tap water and clothing ignition, and firearms policy. Today's injury problems call for leadership in the policy areas of firearms, alcohol, and other drugs. A rational firearms policy that reduces the availability of handguns and assault weapons will not stop violence, but it will reduce the lethality of violence. Alcohol policy that increases price, decreases underage drinking, and permits neighborhoods to control the density of alcohol outlets and advertising within their boundaries will reduce consumption and therefore injuries. The association of other drugs with injury is less through consumption than it is through trafficking. The debate about how to remove the profit from the illegal drug

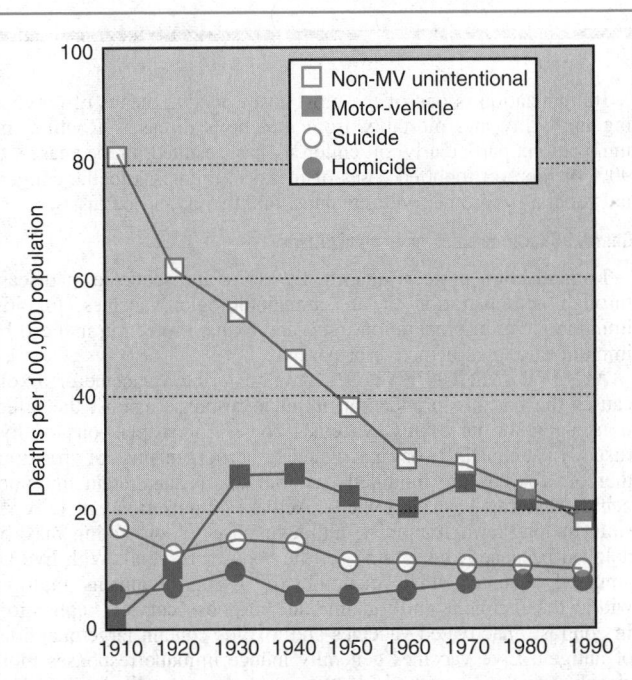

FIGURE 9–7. Trends in injury death rates, US, 1910 to 1990. (Adapted from Baker SP, O'Neill B, Ginsburg MJ, et al.: The Injury Fact Book. 2nd ed. New York, Oxford University Press, 1992.)

trade is heated, and proposed solutions are very controversial. These are issues that physicians concerned about injuries need to examine and form opinions about, and they should be willing to engage in the public debate. Legislators and journalists turn to physicians for information about disease and injury because physicians have daily contact with sick and injured people and thus can speak from personal experience about the problem. Informed physicians can advocate for solutions by testifying at legislative hearings, by granting media interviews, by presenting at professional meetings, and by teaching medical students and residents about injury prevention principles and strategies.

Baker SP, O'Neill B, Ginsburg MJ, et al: The Injury Fact Book. 2nd ed. New York, Oxford University Press, 1992. *Presents injury mortality data for 1980 to 1986. Chapters include 15 major causes of fatal injury and contain graphs, tables, findings from research on both fatal and nonfatal injuries, and a discussion of preventive strategies.*

Centers for Disease Control and Prevention, Public Health Service, USDHHS: (a) Injury Mortality: National Summary of Injury Mortality Data, 1984–1990 (June, 1993); (b) Injury Control. Position Papers from the Third National Injury Control Conference, April, 1991; (c) Injury Control for the 1990s: A National Plan for Action, Report to the Second World Conference on Injury Control, 1993. *CDC presents a national plan for injury control. It provides the plan's background papers developed by panels of experts in injury prevention and in treatment and rehabilitation of injured people and also contains tables of injury mortality data.*

Rice, MacKenzie, and Associates: Cost of Injury in the United States, A Report to Congress, 1989. San Francisco, University of California San Francisco, Johns Hopkins University, 1989. *Health economists and injury control specialists identify the magnitude of the economic effect of injury using 1985 injury data and the human capital approach to estimate the lifetime cost of injury. Included in these costs are direct medical costs, plus lost productivity resulting from disability or premature death.*

Robertson L: Injuries: Causes, Control Strategies, and Public Policy. Lexington, MA, Lexington Books, 1983. *Injury control options are examined as they relate to host, agent, and environment of injury. Control strategies, such as education, regulation, and legislation, are analyzed in light of research findings of effectiveness. The economics of injury, as well as the politics and future policy directions for injury control, are discussed.*

Rosenberg ML, Fenley MA (eds.): Violence in America: A Public Health Approach. New York, Oxford University Press, 1991. *This overview includes chapters on assaultive violence, child abuse and child sexual abuse, rape and sexual assault, spouse abuse, violence against the elderly, and suicide. These issues are examined using a framework of public health practice.*

10 VACCINATION/IMMUNIZATION
Walter A. Orenstein

Immunization is one of the most cost-effective means of preventing morbidity and mortality from infectious diseases. Routine immunization, particularly of children, has resulted in decreases of 90% or more in reported cases of measles, mumps, rubella, congenital rubella syndrome, polio, tetanus, diphtheria, and pertussis.

General Characteristics of Immunizations

Immunization protects against disease or the sequelae of disease through administration of an immunobiologic: vaccines, toxoids, immune globulin preparations, and antitoxins. Protection induced by immunization can be active or passive.

ACTIVE IMMUNIZATION. Administering a vaccine or toxoid causes the body to produce an immune response against the infectious agent or its toxins. Vaccines consist of suspensions of live (usually attenuated) or inactivated microorganisms or fractions thereof. Toxoids are modified bacterial toxins that retain immunogenic properties but lack toxicity. Active immunization generally results in long-term immunity, although onset of protection may be delayed because it takes time for the body to respond. With live attenuated vaccines small quantities of living organisms multiply within the recipient until an immune response cuts off replication. In contrast, inactivated vaccines and toxoids contain large quantities of antigen. Live vaccines generally induce immune responses more closely paralleling natural infection and are more likely to induce long-term immunity. Most induce active immunity in the majority of recipients after a single dose; killed vaccines, in contrast, often require multiple doses.

PASSIVE IMMUNIZATION. Temporary immunity is provided by administering preformed antibodies as immune globulins or antitoxins. Immune globulins (IG), obtained from human blood, may contain antibodies to a variety of agents depending on the pool of human plasma used in preparation. Specific immune globulins are made from plasma from donors with high levels of antibodies to specific antigens, such as tetanus immune globulin (TIG). Most immune globulins must be injected intramuscularly. A special preparation for intravenous use is also available. Antitoxins are solutions of antibodies derived from animals immunized with specific antigens (e.g., diphtheria antitoxin). Table 10–1 gives the major indications for currently available immune globulins and antitoxins. Passive immunization is usually used to protect individuals immediately before an anticipated exposure or shortly after a known or suspected exposure to an infectious agent.

ROUTE AND TIMING OF VACCINATION. Each immunobiologic has a preferred site and route of administration. Vaccines containing adjuvants should be injected intramuscularly (IM). For adults, most IM injections should be given in the deltoid. Use of the buttocks is discouraged except when large volumes are required both because of the potential for damage to the sciatic nerve and because of diminished immune response to some vaccines such as hepatitis B. Subcutaneous vaccines are also usually administered in the deltoid area, and intradermal vaccines are usually given on the volar surface of the forearm. Many immunobiologics can be given simultaneously to reduce the number of health care visits required for full immunization. In general, inactivated vaccines and toxoids can be given simultaneously at different sites. With vaccines that frequently cause side effects, such as cholera and parenterally administered typhoid vaccines, it may be best to separate administration by at least a week. With the exception of cholera and yellow fever vaccines, which should ideally be administered at least 3 weeks apart, live and inactivated vaccines can be administered at the same time. Measles, mumps, and rubella (MMR) vaccine can be administered with oral polio vaccine (OPV); OPV can be administered with yellow fever vaccine. For theoretical reasons, live vaccines not delivered on the same day should be separated by at least 1 month. Immune globulin may interfere with the take of live vaccines such as measles. Ideally, such vaccines should be administered at least 2 weeks prior to IG or depending upon the dose and type of IG, from 3 to 11 months after IG. IG does not appear to interfere with the response to OPV.

ADVERSE REACTIONS. Hypersensitivity to vaccine components can lead to local and systemic reactions ranging from mild to severe. Responsible components may include animal proteins, antibiotics, preservatives, and stabilizers. Egg proteins, contained in vaccines grown in chicken egg or chick embryo tissue culture, are a common allergen in measles, mumps, influenza, and yellow fever vaccines. In general, persons without anaphylactic type allergies to eggs can be given these vaccines safely. Persons with anaphylactic reactions to eggs, however, should receive these vaccines only with extreme caution under established protocols (see Greenberg and Birx, 1988).

No vaccine is completely safe or completely effective. Recommendations for use are based on an evaluation of the risks and benefits. Two major bodies make recommendations regarding immunization of adults: (1) the Task Force on Adult Immunization of The Infectious Diseases Society of America and the American College of Physicians (ACP), which publishes the Guide for Adult Immunization, and (2) the Advisory Committee on Immunization Practices (ACIP) of the US Public Health Service. The latter group publishes its information in the *Morbidity and Mortality Weekly Report*. The reader is referred to these sources for comprehensive information on vaccines, including indications, contraindications, precautions, and side effects.

ADVERSE EVENTS. Prior to licensure, vaccines are evaluated in prospective, randomized double-blind, placebo-controlled trials that can detect common adverse reactions attributable to vaccine. Uncommon and rare adverse events must usually be evaluated in postmarketing studies. Physician reporting of serious events temporally related to vaccination forms the basis for assessing whether such events are actually caused by the vaccine. Such events are usually called "adverse events" as opposed to "adverse reactions," which imply in advance that the vaccine produced the illness. It must be determined whether the clinical syndrome is distinctive from events not caused by vaccine and, if not, whether the frequency of the illness following vaccination is significantly greater than that expected from chance alone. Suspected adverse events should be reported to the Vaccine Adverse Events Reporting System (1–800-822-7967).

GENERAL CONSIDERATIONS. Immunizations for adults depend on age, lifestyle, occupation, and medical conditions. All adults should have a primary series of tetanus and diphtheria toxoids with boosters of combined toxoids (Td) every 10 years. Persons born in or after 1957 should have evidence of immunity to measles and mumps. Rubella vaccine is especially indicated for susceptible females of childbearing age. Pneumococcal vaccine and annual vaccination against influenza are indicated for all adults aged 65 years and older. Health care workers exposed to blood or blood products should receive hepatitis B vaccine (Hep B). Those caring for patients at high risk of complications from influenza should receive annual vaccination. Health care workers likely to come in contact with persons transmitting measles, mumps, or rubella should be immune to those diseases.

IMMUNOCOMPROMISE. Patients with conditions that compromise their immune systems should not receive live attenuated vaccines. Such patients include those with immunodeficiency diseases, leukemia, lymphoma, and generalized malignancy and those who are immunosuppressed from therapy with corticosteroids, alkylating agents, antimetabolites, and radiation. An exception is infection with human immunodeficiency virus (HIV). Asymptomatic patients should receive MMR vaccine. MMR should be considered for symptomatic patients with HIV. Because of the availability of enhanced potency inactivated polio vaccine (eIPV), all patients known to be infected with HIV should receive eIPV instead of OPV. Patients with leukemia in remission who are off all chemotherapy for at least 3 months may receive live-virus vaccines. Short-course therapy (<2 weeks) with corticosteroids, alternate-day regimens with low to moderate doses of short-acting corticosteroids, and topical applications or tendon injections do not ordinarily contraindicate live vaccines.

Immunocompromised patients can receive inactivated vaccines and toxoids, although the efficacy of such preparations may be diminished. Patients with known HIV infection should receive pneumococcal vaccine and annual influenza vaccination.

PREGNANCY. In general, live vaccines should not be given to pregnant women because of the theoretical concern that such vaccines could adversely affect the fetus. No significant adverse events attributable to vaccination with MMR of pregnant women have been documented, but pregnant women should not receive MMR, and women who do receive MMR should wait 3 months before becoming pregnant. Polio and yellow fever vaccines should not usually be given to pregnant women unless there is substantial risk of disease. Td is especially indicated for pregnant females who are not appropriately vaccinated to prevent neonatal tetanus in their infants. Vaccination is best performed after the first trimester. All pregnant women should be screened for hepatitis B surface antigen (HBsAg). Offspring of carrier mothers should receive Hep B and hepatitis B immune globulin (HBIG).

INDIVIDUAL IMMUNOBIOLOGIES (Table 10–2)

Tetanus and Diphtheria (Ch. 289 and 285)

Tetanus toxoid is one of the most effective immunizations, with over 95% protection following a primary series. The adsorbed is preferred over the fluid preparation because it induces protective levels of antitoxin that persist longer after fewer doses. In persons aged 7 years or older, it should always be used in combination with Td, which is more than 85% effective in preventing disease. A primary series consists of three doses (Table 10–2). There is no need to repeat doses if the schedule is interrupted. Boosters are recommended every 10 years. An easy way to remember is to schedule immunization at the middle of each decade (e.g., 25 years, 35 years, etc.). The ACP Task Force on Adult Immunization has recently suggested that a single Td booster at age 50 may be sufficient to maintain protective antibody levels in older adults who have received a primary series.

Following a wound, persons of unknown immunization status or

TABLE 10–1. PASSIVE IMMUNIZATIONS FOR ADULTS

Disease	Name of Material	Comments and Use
Tetanus	Tetanus immune globulin human (TIG)	Management of tetanus-prone wounds and treatment of tetanus
Cytomegalovirus	Cytomegalovirus immune globulin, intravenous (CMV-IGIV)	Prophylaxis for bone marrow and kidney transplant recipients
Diphtheria	Diphtheria antitoxin equine	Treatment of established disease, high frequency of reactions to serum of nonhuman origin
Rabies	Rabies immunoglobulin human (HRIG)	Postexposure prophylaxis of animal bites
Measles	Immune globulin, human (IG)	Prevention or modification of disease in contacts of cases; not for control of epidemics
Hepatitis A	Immune globulin, human (IG)	Protection of household contacts; control of epidemics; pre-exposure prophylaxis for travelers
Hepatitis B	Hepatitis B immune globulin, human	Prophylaxis for needle stick or mucous membrane contact with HBsAG-positive persons; for sexual partners with acute hepatitis B or hepatitis B carriers; for infants born to mothers who are carriers of HBsAg; for infants whose mother or primary caregiver has acute hepatitis B
Varicella	Varicella-zoster immune globulin (VZIG)	Persons under 15 years of age with underlying disease who have not had varicella and who are exposed to varicella; may be given to known susceptible adults, particularly if antibody-negative
Vaccinia	Vaccinia immune globulin (VIG)	Treatment of eczema vaccinatum, vaccinia necrosum, and ocular vaccinia following vaccinia (smallpox) vaccination
Erythroblastosis fetalis	Rh immune globulin (RIG)	Rh-negative women who give birth to Rh-positive infants or who abort
Hypogammaglobulinemia	Immune globulin, intravenous	Maintenance therapy
Idiopathic thrombocytopenic purpura	Immune globulin, intravenous	Therapy of acute episodes
Botulism	Trivalent A, B, and E antitoxin, equine	Treatment of botulism
Snakebite	Antivenin, equine (North American coral snake antivenin)	Specific for North American coral snake, *Micrurus fulvius*
	Antivenin, equine Crotalidae, polyvalent	Effective for viper and pit viper, including rattlesnakes, copperheads, moccasins
Spider bite	Antivenin, equine	Specific for black widow spider, *Latrodectus mactans,* and other members of the genus

TABLE 10–2. SELECTED IMMUNIZING AGENTS INDICATED FOR ADULTS*

Disease	Immunizing Agent	Indications	Schedule	Major Contraindications	Comments
Cholera	Inactivated vaccine	Meeting international travel requirements	Two 0.5-ml doses SC or IM or two 0.2-ml doses ID 1 week to 1 month apart; booster doses every 6 mo		Of limited effectiveness; cholera and yellow fever vaccine should be administered at least 3 weeks apart
Diphtheria	Tetanus and diphtheria toxoids combined (Td)	All adults	Two doses 4 wk apart; 3rd doses 6–12 mo after 2nd doses; booster every 10 yr; no need to repeat if schedule is interrupted	History of neurologic or severe hypersensitivity reaction following a previous dose	
Hepatitis B	Inactivated virus vaccine	Health care and public safety workers potentially exposed to blood; clients and staff of institutions for the developmentally disabled; hemodialysis patients; sexually active homosexual men; users of illicit injectable drugs; recipients of clotting factors; household and sexual contacts of HBV carriers; inmates of long-term correctional facilities; heterosexuals treated for sexually transmitted diseases or with multiple sexual partners; and travelers with close contact for ≥6 mo with populations with high prevalence of hepatitis B carriage	IM; three doses at 0, 1, and 6 mo		Pregnancy should not be considered a contraindication if the woman is otherwise eligible. All pregnant women should be screened for hepatitis B surface antigen (HBsAg), and infants of carrier mothers should be vaccinated at time of delivery with hepatitis B immune globulin and vaccine. Do not administer vaccine subcutaneously
Influenza	Inactivated influenza virus vaccine	All adults ≥65 yr, other adults with high-risk conditions; adults caring for persons with high-risk conditions, including medical personnel (see text)	Annual vaccination; see annual ACIP recommendation	Anaphylactic hypersensitivity to eggs	
Japanese encephalitis	Inactivated virus vaccine	Travelers to Asia spending at least 1 mo in endemic areas during transmission season	Three 1-ml doses SC on days 0, 7, 30; shortened schedule of 0, 7, 14 days may be used when necessary. Booster doses may be given after 2 yr	Persons with histories of urticaria at greater risk of adverse reactions to vaccine; pregnancy	No data exist on concurrent administration with vaccines other than DTP, drugs (e.g., chloroquine, mefloquine), or other biologics
Measles	Live-virus vaccine	All adults born after 1956 without history of live vaccine on or after 1st birthday, physician-diagnosed measles, or detectable measles antibody; persons born before 1957 can generally be considered immune	One dose sufficient for most adults; two doses at least 1 month apart indicated for persons entering college or medical facility employment, traveling abroad, or at risk of measles during outbreaks	Altered immunity (e.g., leukemia, lymphoma, generalized malignancy, congenital immunodeficiency, immunosuppressive therapy): immune globulin within prior 3–11 mo; untreated tuberculosis; anaphylactic hypersensitivity to neomycin; pregnancy	May be administered combined with mumps and rubella vaccines for persons who might be susceptible to these other diseases. Persons with anaphylactic allergies to eggs may be vaccinated with extreme caution using established protocols (see text). Vaccine should be administered to persons with asymptomatic HIV infection and should be considered for symptomatic HIV patients
Meningococcal disease	Polysaccharide vaccine containing tetravalent A, C, W135, and Y	Terminal complement component deficiencies; anatomic or functional asplenia; and travelers who will live in areas with hyperendemic or epidemic disease. May be useful during localized outbreaks	One dose		

TABLE 10–2. SELECTED IMMUNIZING AGENTS INDICATED FOR ADULTS* *Continued*

Disease	Immunizing Agent	Indications	Schedule	Major Contraindications	Comments
Mumps	Live-virus vaccine	All adults born after 1956 without history of live vaccine on or after 1st birthday, physician-diagnosed mumps, or detectable mumps antibody; persons born before 1957 can generally be considered immune	One dose	Altered immunity (e.g., leukemia, lymphoma, generalized malignancy, congenital immunodeficiency, immunosuppressive therapy); immune globulin within prior 3–11 mo; anaphylactic hypersensitivity to neomycin; pregnancy	Although persons born before 1957 are generally immune, vaccine can be given to adults of all ages and may be particularly indicated for postpubertal males who are thought to be susceptible. Persons with anaphylactic allergies to eggs may be vaccinated with extreme caution using defined established protocol (see text)
Pneumococcal disease	23-valent polysaccharide vaccine	Adults with cardiovascular disease, pulmonary disease, diabetes mellitus, alcoholism, cirrhosis, cerebrospinal fluid leaks, splenic dysfunction or anatomic asplenia, Hodgkin's disease, lymphoma, multiple myeloma, chronic renal failure, nephrotic syndrome, immunosuppression, HIV infection; high-risk populations such as certain native Americans and *all* adults ≥ 65 yr	One dose IM or SC. A 2nd dose should be considered 6 or more years later for adults at high risk of disease (e.g., asplenic patients) as well as those who lose antibody rapidly (e.g., nephrotic syndrome, renal failure, transplant recipients)		
Poliomyelitis	eIPV (inactivated), OPV (live attenuated)	Certain adults who are at greater risk of exposure to wild poliovirus than the general population, including travelers to countries where polio is epidemic or endemic; members of community or specific population groups with disease caused by wild polioviruses; laboratory workers handling specimens that may contain polioviruses; health care workers in close contact with patients who may be excreting wild polioviruses	For unvaccinated adults, eIPV is preferred: two doses, SC 4 wk apart; a 3rd dose 6–12 mo after the 2nd; if less than 4 wk available before protection is needed, a single dose of OPV or eIPV. For incompletely immunized adults, complete primary series with either vaccine; primary series consists of three doses of eIPV or OPV; no need to restart interrupted series. A single dose of OPV or eIPV can be given to adults who previously completed a primary series	OPV-immune deficiency diseases; patients with altered immune status (e.g., leukemia); household contacts of immunodeficient patients; household contacts in whom there is a family history of immunodeficiency until the immune status of individuals is established. On theoretical grounds, pregnant women should not receive eIPV or OPV. However, if immediate protection is needed, OPV can be used	Adults who have not been adequately immunized against polio are at a very small risk of polio when their children are vaccinated with OPV. The child can be vaccinated with OPV regardless of the immune status of the parents. An acceptable alternative provided that the full immunization of the child is not compromised is to vaccinate the parents first with eIPV
Rabies	Inactivated vaccine; human diploid cell rabies vaccine (HDCV); or rabies vaccine adsorbed (RVA)	High-risk persons including animal handlers, selected laboratory and field workers, and persons traveling for ≥ 1 mo to areas at high risk of rabies	Pre-exposure *prophylaxis:* three doses of 1.0 ml IM for HDCV or RVA on days 0, 7, and 28. For HDCV only, three doses of 0.1 ml ID on days 0, 7, and 21 or 28	History of severe hypersensitivity reaction	Further doses needed following exposure. If to be given concurrently with chloroquine, only an IM route should be used
Rubella	Live-virus vaccine	Adults, particularly women of childbearing age, who lack history of rubella vaccine and detectable rubella-specific antibodies in serum; both males and females in institutions where rubella outbreaks may occur, such as hospitals, the military, and colleges	1 dose SC	Pregnancy, altered immunity (e.g., leukemia, lymphoma, generalized malignancy, congenital immunodeficiency, immunosuppressive therapy), immune globulin within the 3–11 mo prior to vaccination, anaphylactic hypersensitivity to neomycin. Administration of blood products should not contraindicate postpartum vaccination. However, in this instance, serologic testing 6–8 wk after vaccination should be performed	Women should be counseled to avoid pregnancy for 3 mo following vaccination. Available data on previous and current rubella vaccines indicate the risk, if any, of causing defects compatible with congenital rubella syndrome is small. The ACIP believes that, although a final decision rests with the patient and her physician, vaccination of a pregnant woman should not ordinarily indicate that an abortion is necessary

Table continued on following page

TABLE 10–2. SELECTED IMMUNIZING AGENTS INDICATED FOR ADULTS* *Continued*

Disease	Immunizing Agent	Indications	Schedule	Major Contraindications	Comments
Tetanus	Tetanus and diphtheria toxoids combined (Td)	All adults	Three doses needed for primary series: two doses 4 wk apart; 3rd dose 6–12 mo after the 2nd dose; booster every 10 yr; no need to repeat if schedule is interrupted	History of neurologic or severe hypersensitivity reaction following a previous dose	Special recommendations for wound treatment (see text)
Typhoid fever	Heat-phenol–inactivated vaccine; live attenuated Ty2IA oral vaccine	Travelers to areas where the risk of prolonged exposure to contaminated food and water is high; may be considered for family and intimate contacts for carriers and laboratory workers who work with *S. typhi*	*Inactivated vaccine:* two 0.5 ml doses SC 4 or more wk apart. Boosters of 0.5 ml SC or 0.1 ml ID every 3 years. *Oral vaccine:* four doses on alternate days. Boosters every 5 years	Severe local or systemic reaction to a prior dose	Efficacy only 50%–77%. Food and water precautions essential
Yellow fever	Live attenuated virus (17 D strain)	Persons living or traveling in areas where yellow fever exists	One dose; booster every 10 years	Immunocompromised persons; history of anaphylactic allergies to eggs; pregnancy on theoretical grounds, although may be given if risk is high	

* See text and package inserts for further details, particularly regarding indications, dosage, mode of administration, side effects, and adverse reactions and contraindications. ACIP indicates Advisory Committee on Immunization Practices; eIPV, enhanced potency inactivated polio vaccine; OPV, live-virus trivalent oral polio vaccine.

those who have received fewer than three doses of tetanus toxoid should receive a dose of Td regardless of the severity of the wound. Td is also indicated for those who previously received three or more doses if more than 10 years have elapsed, in the case of clean, minor wounds, and if more than 5 years have elapsed for all other wounds. TIG should be administered simultaneously at a separate site to persons who have not received at least three doses of toxoid and who have wounds that are not clean and minor. Most reactions consist of local inflammation and low-grade fever. However, Guillain-Barré syndrome (GBS) has very rarely been associated with tetanus toxoid.

Measles (see Ch. 334)

Measles immunization is recommended for all persons born in or after 1957 who lack evidence of immunity to measles: prior physician-diagnosed measles, laboratory evidence of immunity, or appropriate vaccination. Prior to 1989, appropriate vaccination consisted of a single dose of live vaccine administered on or after the first birthday. Now, a routine two-dose schedule is recommended: the first dose, which is 93 to 98% effective, at 12 to 15 months of age and the second dose at entry to primary or middle school. Most adults are considered to have been appropriately vaccinated if they received one dose of vaccine administered on or after their first birthday. Some adults, however, who are at increased risk of measles (health care workers with direct patient contact, students in colleges, international travelers) should receive a second dose of vaccine unless they have documentation of prior physician-diagnosed measles or serologic evidence of immunity. Persons embarking on foreign travel should ideally have received two doses or have other evidence of measles immunity. Persons born before 1957 are usually immune as a result of natural infection and do not require vaccination, although there is no contraindication if they are believed to be susceptible.

During outbreaks of measles in institutions, all persons at risk who have not received two doses or who lack other evidence of measles immunity should be vaccinated. Measles vaccine is usually administered as combined measles, mumps, and rubella vaccine (MMR) to ensure immunity against all three diseases. There is no harm if individuals are already immune to one or more of the components.

Measles vaccine is contraindicated for pregnant women on theoretical grounds, for persons with moderate to severe acute febrile illnesses, and for persons with altered immunocompetence except those with HIV infection (Table 10–2). Patients with anaphylactic reactions to eggs should be vaccinated only with caution under established protocols.

Approximately 5 to 15% of susceptible recipients of measles vaccine develop fever of 39.4° C or higher with onset between 5 and 12 days after vaccination and lasting 1 to 2 days. About 5% develop transient rashes. Thrombocytopenic purpura following MMR has been reported rarely. The overall rate of reactions following the second dose of a measles-containing vaccine is substantially lower than after the first dose. Encephalopathy or encephalitis following measles vaccines has been reported at a rate lower than the background or expected rate.

Rubella (see Ch. 335)

Rubella vaccine is indicated for adults, particularly women of childbearing age, without a prior history of vaccination on or after the first birthday or laboratory evidence of immunity. A single dose of vaccine is 95% or more effective. Many persons receive two doses of rubella vaccine via the two-dose schedule of MMR.

Follow-up of 305 susceptible women who received rubella vaccines within 3 months of the estimated date of conception has failed to reveal any evidence of defects compatible with congenital rubella syndrome in their offspring. Nevertheless, vaccine is contraindicated in pregnant women on theoretical grounds.

Reactions occur only in susceptible persons. Up to 40% of susceptible adults develop arthralgia, usually of the small peripheral joints, and 10 to 20% develop frank arthritis. Joint symptoms usually begin 1 to 3 weeks following vaccination and persist for 1 day to 3 weeks. Very rarely patients have developed chronic recurrent or persistent joint symptoms following vaccination. In fact, such symptoms are considerably more common after the disease than after the vaccine. Other rare adverse events include transient peripheral neuritis and pain in the arms and legs. Thrombocytopenic purpura has been reported rarely when administered as MMR. Rubella vaccine is contraindicated for persons with moderate to severe acute febrile illnesses and for persons with reduced immunocompetence. When given with measles vaccine, it may be administered to those with asymptomatic HIV infection and considered for those with symptomatic infection. Rubella vaccine is grown in human diploid cells and can be administered without problems to persons with allergy to eggs.

Mumps (see Ch. 338)

Mumps vaccine is indicated for all persons, especially susceptible males, without a prior history of vaccination on or after the first birthday, physician-diagnosed mumps, or laboratory evidence of immunity. Most persons born prior to 1957 can be considered immune as a result of natural infection, although there is no contraindication if such persons are thought to be susceptible. In clinical trials, a single dose of vaccine has induced seroconversion in >90% of recipients.

Adverse events following mumps vaccine are uncommon—fever, parotitis, and allergic manifestations. Thrombocytopenic purpura has been reported rarely when administered as MMR. Mumps vaccine is contraindicated for pregnant women on theoretical grounds, for persons with moderate to severe acute febrile illnesses, and for persons with altered immunocompetence. Combined with measles vaccine, it may be given to those with asymptomatic HIV infection and considered for those with symptomatic infection. Patients with anaphylactic reactions to eggs should be vaccinated only with caution under established protocols.

Hepatitis B (see Ch. 117)

Hepatitis B vaccine is the first vaccine that can prevent cancer (an estimated 800 persons die annually in the United States from hepatitis B–related liver cancer; many times more do in the Third World). It can also prevent acute and chronic complications of hepatitis B, including an estimated 4000 deaths annually from cirrhosis and 250 deaths annually from fulminant hepatic disease in the United States. The original hepatitis vaccine in the United States consisted of purified, inactivated, alum-adsorbed, 22-nm hepatitis B surface antigen (HBsAg) particles obtained from human plasma. Currently produced vaccines are derived from inserting the gene for HBsAg into *Saccharomyces cerevisiae*. Hepatitis B vaccine, the first licensed vaccine made using recombinant techniques, produces adequate antibody responses in >90% of normal adults and >95% of normal infants, children, and adolescents when administered in a three-dose series. Dosage depends on the product, the age group, and the underlying clinical condition and can be determined by consulting the package insert. The duration of vaccine-conferred immunity is not known, although follow-up of vaccinees within 11 years indicates persistence of protection against clinically significant infections (i.e., detectable viremia and clinical disease). Booster doses are not currently recommended. Vaccine must be injected intramuscularly, preferably in the deltoid.

Because strategies targeting Hep B vaccine use only to high-risk populations has not had a significant impact on hepatitis B incidence, universal vaccination is now recommended (Table 10–2). Universal infant vaccination is now recommended for all populations and is under consideration for pre-adolescents and adolescents. Universal screening for HBsAg is recommended for all pregnant women, with administration of three doses of vaccine and one dose of HBIG recommended for infants of carrier mothers.

The major side effect is soreness at the injection site. GBS among adults following receipt of the plasma-derived vaccine shows borderline statistically significant increased risk after the first dose; however, the overall risk, if real, is very small and is outweighed by the substantial benefits of vaccination. Available data from reporting systems for adverse events do not indicate an association between receipt of recombinant vaccine and GBS. There is no risk of acquiring HIV infection from either vaccine.

Influenza (see Ch. 332)

Annual influenza vaccination is indicated for adults at high risk of complications from the disease: (1) persons with chronic cardiopulmonary disorders; (2) residents of nursing homes or other chronic care facilities; (3) persons aged 65 or older; (4) patients with other chronic diseases such as metabolic disorders (e.g., diabetes mellitus), kidney dysfunction, hemoglobin opathies, and immunosuppression; and (5) children on long-term aspirin therapy. In addition, transmission of influenza to high-risk patients can be reduced by annually vaccinating health care workers in institutions, offices, and homes who have contact with high-risk patients and immunization of household contacts of such patients.

The efficacy of influenza vaccine varies with host condition and the degree to which antigens in the vaccine match viruses in circulation the following season. Current vaccines contain whole or split inactivated viruses of three major antigenic types—A (H3N2), A (H1N1), and B. Provided that there is a good match, vaccine efficacy is usually 70 to 90% among normal healthy young adults. Ef-

ficacy is substantially lower, however, among the institutionalized elderly, often between 20 and 40%. Nevertheless, despite low efficacy at preventing illness, the vaccine appears to protect against pneumonia and death on the order of 60 to 80%. Ideally, vaccines should be administered between mid-October and mid-November of each year, although earlier in the fall suffices if circumstances require.

Persons with anaphylactic allergies to eggs should not be vaccinated without careful evaluation. The most common side effect is soreness at the injection site. Fever, malaise, and myalgia may begin 6 to 12 hours after vaccination and persist for 1 to 2 days, although such reactions are most common in children exposed to vaccine for the first time. Severe allergic reactions are rare. GBS may have been very rarely associated with influenza vaccine during the 1991 season among adults younger than age 65, suggesting that this illness may occasionally follow influenza vaccines besides those of New Jersey 76 (swine flu). Studies of influenza vaccines in years other than 1976 and 1991 have not supported a relationship to GBS.

Pneumococcal Vaccine (see Ch. 271)

Pneumococcal vaccine consists of the purified polysaccharide capsular antigens from the 23 types of *Streptococcus pneumoniae* that are responsible for 88% of the bacteremic disease in the United States. Most healthy adults, including the elderly and patients with alcoholic cirrhosis and diabetes mellitus, develop a twofold or greater rise in type-specific antibodies within 2 to 3 weeks of vaccination. Although serologic response is generally acceptable, estimates of vaccine efficacy in preventing disease vary widely. Efficacy may be lower in some patients, such as those with alcoholic cirrhosis or Hodgkin's disease. There is good evidence that vaccine is effective against bacteremic pneumococcal disease. However, evidence regarding efficacy against pneumonia among high-risk populations is not clear. Regardless, the preponderance of information supports use of pneumococcal vaccine in high-risk populations. Indications for vaccine are shown in Table 10–2.

Immunity may decrease 6 or more years after initial vaccination; boosters should therefore be considered at that time for adults at highest risk of disease (e.g., asplenic patients) as well as for those who lose antibody rapidly such as patients with nephrotic syndrome or renal failure.

Local reactions are frequent and may increase with revaccination. Fewer than 1% of vaccines experience severe local reactions or systemic illness such as fever and malaise. Severe events such as anaphylaxis are rare.

Special efforts should target hospitalized patients. Approximately two thirds of patients later admitted with pneumococcal disease had been hospitalized for other reasons within the preceding 5 years.

Poliomyelitis (see Ch. 425)

The last documented cases of indigenously acquired poliomyelitis caused by wild polio viruses in the United States were reported in 1979. All indigenous cases since 1981, approximately eight per year, have been linked epidemiologically and/or via laboratory tests to OPV exposure. Between 1980 and 1989, the overall risk of vaccine-associated polio was one case for every 2.5 million doses distributed. The risk is higher for immunodeficient persons; an estimated 0.5% of these recipients develop polio. Vaccine polioviruses may spread from recipients to contacts, and cases among the latter account for over half of the total vaccine-associated cases.

Adults are at increased risk of paralytic disease from receiving OPV; their routine vaccination is not warranted, therefore, given the small risk of exposure to wild virus in the United States. The major indication for adult vaccination is travel to areas where wild polio viruses are endemic or epidemic. For children, OPV is the vaccine of choice; for previously unvaccinated adults, however, eIPV is indicated. Travelers who have histories of partial vaccination should complete a primary series (three doses) of either eIPV or OPV. Persons who formerly completed a primary series should receive a booster of OPV or eIPV. Health care personnel who come in contact with wild viruses should be immune to polio. EIPV is the vaccine of choice in such persons to protect both the recipient and any immunocompromised persons with whom the health care worker has contact from exposure to OPV. Parents of children to be vaccinated with OPV may elect to receive eIPV before vaccinating their child. Most providers administer OPV to the child regardless of the parents' immune status.

A primary series of both OPV and eIPV consists of three doses (Table 10–2). There are no known serious side effects of eIPV. OPV should never be given to immunocompromised individuals or to a child living in a household with immunocompromised persons.

Meningococcal Polysaccharide Vaccine (see Ch. 281)

A quadrivalent meningococcal polysaccharide vaccine containing serogroups A, C, Y, and W135 is now available. These groups account for approximately 40 to 50% of meningococcal disease in the United States. Serogroups A and C vaccines have had 85 to 95% efficacy in epidemic settings, whereas vaccines for the other groups have documented good immunogenicity in adults. The duration of immunity is unknown, although protection in older children and adults probably persists at least 3 years. Protection in preschool children may be shorter. Routine vaccination is not recommended in the United States because of the low risk of infection. A single dose is indicated for high-risk persons (Table 10–2). Vaccination may also be useful during localized epidemics of serogroups in the vaccine. Meningococcal vaccine may be offered to travelers and persons who will live in areas with hyperendemic or epidemic disease, e.g., the "meningitis belt" of sub-Saharan Africa stretching from Mauritania to Ethiopia.

Booster doses are not currently recommended for adults. The major side effects are local reactions lasting 1 to 2 days.

Rabies (see Ch. 427)

Rabies vaccine is indicated for pre-exposure prophylaxis of high-risk persons, including animal handlers, selected laboratory and field workers, and persons traveling for more than 1 month to areas where rabies is a constant threat. The pre-exposure regimen consists of either three 1.0-ml intramuscular injections on days 0, 7, and 28 for all rabies vaccines or, for the human diploid cell vaccine (HDCV) only, three 0.1-ml intradermal injections on days 0, 7, and 21 or 28. Testing for serum antibody or a booster every 2 years is indicated for persons with continuing risk. Postexposure treatment depends on prior exposure to vaccine and is discussed in detail in Ch. 427.

Vaccines Intended Primarily for International Travelers (see Ch. 268)

YELLOW FEVER (see Ch. 345). Yellow fever now occurs only in areas of South America and Africa. Vaccination with a single dose of the live attenuated 17D strain of virus confers protection to almost all recipients for at least 10 years. Boosters are recommended every 10 years for those at risk. Side effects are uncommon. Yellow fever vaccine should not be given to immunocompromised persons or those with anaphylactic allergies to eggs. The vaccine is contraindicated in pregnant women on theoretical grounds, although if such women must travel to a high-risk area, they may be vaccinated.

TYPHOID VACCINE (see Ch. 292). Two types of vaccines, a live attenuated Ty21a oral vaccine and a parenteral heat-phenol–inactivated vaccine, appear to be of comparable efficacy (50 to 77%). Typhoid vaccine is indicated primarily for travelers to areas where the risk of prolonged exposure to contaminated food and water is high. The vaccine is not optimally effective; food and water precautions are still essential. The vaccine may also be considered for family or other intimate contacts of typhoid carriers and laboratory workers who work with *Salmonella typhi*. For adults and children age 6 and older, either vaccine may be used. For Ty21a, one enteric-coated capsule is taken every other day for four doses. Alternatively, two doses of inactivated vaccine separated by 4 or more weeks may be given. The duration of protection with Ty21a is not known; the manufacturer recommends a repeat primary series every 5 years for persons at risk. Boosters every 3 years are recommended for recipients of the inactivated vaccine if they continue to be at risk.

The parenteral vaccine is often associated with local reactions and fever. Reactions to the oral vaccine appear to be rare.

CHOLERA (see Ch. 296). Cholera vaccines offer only about 50% protection after completion of a primary series of two doses 1 week to 1 month apart. Peak protection appears about 2 months after the last dose, and protection wanes by 3 to 6 months. Vaccination often results in significant local reactions accompanied by fever. Neurologic reactions are rare. The major indication is to meet requirements imposed by some countries for entry.

JAPANESE ENCEPHALITIS VACCINE (see Ch. 424). Japanese encephalitis (JE) vaccine was licensed in 1992 and is primarily indicated for travelers to Asia who will spend a month or longer in endemic areas during the transmission season, especially if travel will include rural areas. In all instances, travelers should be advised to take personal precautions to reduce exposure to mosquito bites. The vaccine appears to be 80 to 91% effective in preventing clinical disease. The primary series consists of three subcutaneous 1-ml doses given on days 0, 7, and 30 (Table 10–2). A shortened schedule given on days 0, 7, and 14 may be used when necessary. Booster doses may be given after 2 years. Local reactions are common, occurring in about 20% of vaccinated persons, and systemic symptoms of fever, headache, chills, nausea, and abdominal pain have been noted in about 10%. A delayed urticaria-angioedema syndrome has been described following JE vaccination, occurring a median of 12 hours after the first dose of vaccine and up to 2 weeks after the second dose. Vaccinees should be observed for at least 30 minutes after inoculation and during the subsequent 10 days should remain in areas with ready access to medical care. The vaccine is contraindicated for pregnant women on theoretical grounds, although if such women travel to an area where the risk of JE is high, they may be vaccinated.

Other Vaccines

A number of other vaccines, used in selected circumstances, include (1) smallpox vaccine, which is used by the military and laboratory workers who handle orthopox viruses; (2) BCG vaccine, a vaccine used to prevent tuberculosis, which has very limited use in the United States; (3) oral adenovirus vaccines types 4 and 7 for use in the military; (4) anthrax vaccine, which is indicated in selected high-risk worker populations; and (5) plague vaccine, which may be considered for workers at risk and for some travelers. In addition, trivalent botulism antitoxin (ABE) is available from the CDC for treatment of suspected cases of botulism.

Although not available today, a number of vaccines are under development and may be licensed in the future. Extensive field trials have occurred with hepatitis A and varicella vaccines, which are probably the closest to completing development. Because of the biotechnology revolution, it is likely that many more vaccines will become available in the future.

ACP Task Force on Adult Immunization. Infectious Diseases Society of America. Guide for Adult Immunization, 3rd ed. Philadelphia, American College of Physicians, 1994, pp 1–218. *An excellent comprehensive guide covering all aspects of adult immunization. A must for the physician who cares for adults, whether in primary, secondary, or tertiary care.*

Centers for Disease Control: Health Information for International Travel. Washington, D.C., US Government Printing Office, 1993. *A complete guide for the international traveler, including required and recommended vaccinations. Revised annually.*

Centers for Disease Control: Update on Adult Immunization. Recommendations of The Advisory Committee on Immunization Practices (ACIP). MMWR (no. RR-12) 1991. *A compendium of ACIP statements on immunizations for adults as well as valuable information on other aspects of immunization. ACIP statements on individual vaccines are published as available in the Morbidity and Mortality Weekly Report.*

Centers for Disease Control and Prevention: General recommendations on immunization: Recommendations of The Advisory Committee on Immunization Practices (ACIP). MMWR 43 (No. RR-1) 1-38, 1994. *A comprehensive review of vaccination schedules, precautions, contraindications and adverse events, as well as information about federal laws on injury compensation and record keeping.*

Committee on Infectious Diseases, American Academy of Pediatrics: Report of the Committee on Infectious Diseases. 23rd ed. Elk Grove Village, Ill., American Academy of Pediatrics. 1994, pp 1–687. *The "Red Book" is published every 2 to 3 years and addresses in a comprehensive manner vaccination of children and adolescents as well as other issues relating to prevention, control, and treatment of infectious diseases.*

Greenberg MA, Birx DL: Safe administration of mumps-measles-rubella vaccine in egg-allergic children. J Pediatr 113:504, 1988. *A protocol for vaccinating persons with anaphylactic allergies to eggs. Also reviews other protocols.*

Howson CP, Howe CJ, Fineberg HV: Adverse effects of pertussis and rubella vaccines. A report of the committee to review the adverse consequences of pertussis and rubella vaccines. Institute of Medicine. Washington, DC, National Academy Press, 1991, pp 1–367. *An exhaustive review and evaluation of the adverse consequences of pertussis and rubella vaccines.*

Stratton KR, Howe CJ: Adverse events associated with childhood vaccines. Evidence bearing on causality. Institute of Medicine. Washington, DC, National Academy Press, 1994, pp 1–464. *A comprehensive review and evaluation of the adverse consequences of measles, mumps, polio, diphtheria, tetanus, Haemophilus, and hepatitis B vaccines.*

11 ALCOHOLISM AND ALCOHOL ABUSE

Ivan Diamond

EPIDEMIOLOGY

Nearly two thirds of Americans over age 14 drink alcoholic beverages. Their per capita consumption is the equivalent of 9.7 gallons of whiskey, 89 gallons of beer, or 31 gallons of wine per year. Heavy drinkers, who constitute 10% of the drinking population in the United States (7% of all adults), account for half of the alcohol consumed and nearly all of the socioeconomic and medical complications of alcoholism and alcohol abuse. The annual cost of these problems to American society is about $100 billion. Alcoholism and alcohol abuse occur in all socioeconomic classes and cultural groups; the prevalence of alcohol-related problems among hospitalized patients is 20 to 60%.

DEFINITIONS

Alcoholism is characterized by addiction to ethanol. Although there are behavioral and socioeconomic definitions of alcoholism, in a medical setting alcoholism refers to a chronic disease in which the alcoholic craves and consumes ethanol without satiation, becomes increasingly *tolerant* to the intoxicating effects of the drug, and, when drinking is discontinued, exhibits the symptoms and signs of withdrawal as evidence of *physical dependence* on ethanol. Individuals who drink prodigiously without evidence of physical dependence are considered to have *alcohol abuse*. They often continue excessive drinking, sometimes episodically *(binge drinking)*, despite significant socioeconomic and medical complications.

GENETIC FACTORS

Although environmental conditions influence drinking, many individuals are at risk to develop alcoholism because of genetic factors. Alcoholism tends to run in families, and studies of identical twins, alcoholic parents and children, and offspring from alcoholic parents adopted into nondrinking families suggest a genetically transmitted susceptibility for alcoholism. This is particularly evident for "male-limited" alcoholism in fathers and sons with antisocial, impulsive, novelty-seeking behavior, who become alcoholics in teenage years; they usually cannot abstain from drinking throughout life. Adoption studies indicate that this type of alcoholism in the biologic father is a much greater predictor for alcoholism in the son than is the environment in which the boy is raised. This is in contrast to other types of familial and nonfamilial alcoholism, in which individuals may begin drinking as teenagers but become alcoholic later in life without an apparent genetic predisposition. Such patients appear to be able to stop drinking with less difficulty.

PHARMACOLOGY OF ETHANOL

ETHANOL ABSORPTION, DISTRIBUTION, AND ELIMINATION. Ethanol is absorbed completely from the gastrointestinal tract and is detected in the blood within minutes of ingestion. Alcohol vapor can also be absorbed through the lungs. About 25% of ethanol enters the bloodstream from the stomach and 75% from the intestine, but many factors modify gastrointestinal absorption. These include food; the rate of drinking; the concentration, amount, and type of alcoholic beverage; and variations in gastrointestinal motility. Most foods in the stomach delay gastric absorption, and high concentrations of alcohol in the stomach can cause pylorospasm that slows gastric emptying and retards intestinal absorption. Rapid gastric emptying or gastrectomy increases rates of alcohol absorption from the small intestine.

Ethanol readily crosses biologic membranes and equilibrates rapidly into total body water. Ninety to 98% is metabolized in the liver, and the remainder is excreted by the kidneys, lungs, and skin. Elimination follows zero-order kinetics and is independent of concentration; a 70-kg man can metabolize 5 to 10 grams of ethanol per hour. Since the average drink contains 12 to 15 grams of ethanol, blood alcohol levels continue to rise when an individual drinks at a rate greater than metabolism, but when drinking is discontinued, blood levels fall about 10 to 25 mg per deciliter per hour.

ETHANOL METABOLISM. Ethanol oxidation to acetaldehyde by alcohol dehydrogenase in the liver is the rate-limiting step, accounting for more than 90% of ethanol metabolism *in vivo*. When blood alcohol concentrations are high, however, a microsomal ethanol-oxidizing system can also generate acetaldehyde. Moreover, this second enzyme system mediates ethanol effects on drug metabolism in the liver (see Ch. 118). Acetaldehyde is converted to acetate by aldehyde dehydrogenase, a metabolic event with important clinical ramifications. For example, 50% of Japanese and other Asians have a mutation in an aldehyde dehydrogenase isoenzyme that results in reduced enzyme activity *in vivo*. Shortly after drinking alcohol, blood acetaldehyde levels rise in affected individuals and they experience an *alcohol-flush* reaction, characterized by vasodilatation with facial flushing, hot sensations, tachycardia, and hypotension. These unpleasant experiences can deter drinking, and in Japan people with this mutation have a lower rate of alcoholism. Pharmacologically inhibiting aldehyde dehydrogenase causes even more severe aversive symptoms after drinking alcohol and is the reason disulfiram (Antabuse) has been used to help discourage drinking. Disulfiram inhibits aldehyde dehydrogenase (and other sulfhydryl-containing enzymes), but it is not ordinarily toxic when taken therapeutically without ethanol. After drinking alcohol, however, patients on prophylactic disulfiram therapy have significant increases in blood acetaldehyde levels and develop a more severe *acetaldehyde syndrome*. They can experience dysphoria, intense palpitations, sweating, thirst, throbbing headache, dyspnea, nausea and vomiting, weakness, vertigo, and syncope. Disulfiram does not cure alcoholism and is not widely used.

In peripheral tissues, acetate derived from acetaldehyde is converted to acetyl coenzyme A and subsequently to CO_2 and water. Complete oxidation of ethanol yields 7.1 kcal/gram, and some estimate that ethanol accounts for 10% of the total caloric intake in the United States. Alcoholics often obtain 50% of their calories from ethanol, and some develop serious nutritional deficiencies, particularly for protein, thiamine, folate, and pyridoxine (Table 11–1) (see Ch. 192.2). Moreover, as a consequence of ethanol metabolism, alcoholics can develop hypoglycemia, lactic acidosis, hyperuricemia, hypertriglyceridemia, and ketoacidosis.

ACUTE AND CHRONIC TOLERANCE TO ETHANOL. Tolerance is characterized by a reduced response to ethanol. Several hours after a drinking episode, when blood alcohol levels are no longer rising, normal subjects can appear to be sober at alcohol concentrations that are even higher than the levels that caused intoxication earlier. This is *acute tolerance*. Chronic alcoholics have greater resistance to the intoxicating effects of ethanol and may appear to be sober at levels of 400 to 500 mg per deciliter, concentrations known to produce stupor, coma, or death in naive individuals. This is *chronic tolerance*. The highest recorded level is 1510 mg per deciliter in an ambulatory chronic alcoholic who had stopped drinking 3 days earlier.

ACUTE ALCOHOL INTOXICATION

There is virtually no blood-brain barrier to ethanol, and shortly after drinking the concentration of alcohol in the brain is nearly the same as in the blood. In nonalcoholics, intoxication occurs at blood alcohol levels of 50 to 150 mg per deciliter (Table 11–2). Symptoms vary directly with the rate of drinking and are more severe when blood alcohol concentrations are rising than falling. Most individuals feel euphoric, lose social inhibitions, and manifest expansive, sometimes garrulous behavior; others may become gloomy, belligerent, or even explosively combative. Some people do not experience euphoria but become sleepy after moderate drinking; they rarely abuse alcohol. Neurologic signs of intoxication include impaired cognition, slurred speech, incoordination, mild truncal ataxia, and slow or irregular eye movements. Signs of increased sympathetic activity include mydriasis, tachycardia, and skin flushing. Cerebellar and vestibular function deteriorates at higher blood alcohol concentrations, and drunkenness is characterized by dysarthria, more severe ataxia, nystagmus, and diplopia. Patients may become lethargic with bradycardia, reduced blood pressure, and diminished respirations, sometimes complicated by vomiting and pulmonary aspiration. In nonalcoholics, stupor and coma may supervene at 400

TABLE 11-1. ALCOHOL-RELATED MEDICAL DISORDERS

Affected Organ or System	Disorder
Nutrition	Deficiencies of: Folate, thiamine, pyridoxine, niacin, and riboflavin Magnesium, zinc, calcium Protein
Metabolites and electrolytes	Hypoglycemia Hyperlipidemia Hyperuricemia Ketoacidosis Hypomagnesemia Hypophosphatemia
Brain	Hepatic encephalopathy Wernicke-Korsakoff syndrome Cerebral atrophy Amblyopia Central pontine myelinolysis Marchiafava-Bignami disease
Nerve	Neuropathy
Muscle	Myopathy
Liver	Fatty liver Hepatitis Cirrhosis Hepatoma
Heart	Hypertension Cardiomyopathy Arrhythmia
Blood	Anemia Leukopenia Thrombocytopenia Macrocytosis
Gut	Esophagitis and gastritis Pancreatitis
Endocrine	Pseudo–Cushing's syndrome Testicular atrophy Amenorrhea
Bone	Osteopenia

mg per deciliter and fatalities ensue at 500 mg per deciliter, usually because of respiratory depression with ventilatory acidosis and hypotension. The median lethal dose for ethanol is approximately 450 mg per deciliter.

Alcoholic blackouts sometimes complicate acute alcohol intoxication when large amounts of ethanol are consumed. These episodes, which can occur in alcoholics or sporadic drinkers, are characterized by amnesia for several hours without impaired consciousness. The patient reports an inability to remember new events but has no difficulty with long-term memory or immediate recall. These symptoms resemble the syndrome of transient global amnesia (see Ch. 419 and 399).

TABLE 11-2. BLOOD ETHANOL LEVELS AND SYMPTOMS

Blood Ethanol Levels (mg/dl)	Symptoms	
	Sporadic Drinkers	*Chronic Drinkers*
50–100	Euphoria, gregariousness incoordination	Minimal or no effect
100–200	Slurred speech, ataxia, labile mood, drowsiness, nausea	Sobriety or incoordination Euphoria
200–300	Lethargy, combativeness Stupor, incoherent speech Vomiting	Mild emotional and motor changes
300–400	Coma	Drowsiness
> 500	Respiratory depression, death	Lethargy, stupor, coma

EVALUATION AND MANAGEMENT. Severe acute alcohol intoxication can be fatal and is a medical emergency. The immediate history should include information about the quantity of alcohol consumed, the rate of drinking, use of other drugs including methanol, complicating medical and psychiatric disorders, and prior alcohol abuse or alcoholism. If the patient is stuporous and unable to walk, the airway must be evaluated immediately. Indications for endotracheal intubation and assisted ventilation include marked hypoventilation, accumulating secretions, or coma. In such patients, complications such as hypoglycemia, meningitis, and subdural hematoma must be considered. Evidence of head trauma or focal or lateralizing neurologic signs suggest urgent intracranial pathology and a CT scan should be performed immediately. Otherwise, routine CT scans for alcohol intoxication are not indicated. Gastric lavage may be performed if obtundation is due to recent and massive alcohol consumption, but only after endotracheal intubation. Hemodialysis should be considered if the blood ethanol level exceeds 600 mg per deciliter.

After a history and physical examination, patients with adequate vital signs and acceptable mental status and without evidence of other disorders can be kept calm under observation until sobriety returns. However, medical information is usually incomplete, and it is often necessary to anticipate complications commonly associated with severe alcohol intoxication or alcoholism (see Table 11–1). Routine blood counts and chemistries will uncover anemia (see Ch. 122), hypokalemia, hypophosphatemia, and hypomagnesemia. Alcoholic hypoglycemia (see Ch. 206.1) can be evaluated rapidly by determining a bedside blood glucose. If laboratory results are delayed, 12.5 to 25 grams of glucose should be given intravenously. Alcoholic ketoacidosis (see Ch. 75) is improved by infusion of 5% dextrose in 0.5 normal saline. Elevated serum ammonia levels support the diagnosis of hepatic encephalopathy (see Ch. 123). If the blood alcohol level is too low to account for the patient's obtundation, or if improvement does not occur as expected, it is necessary to search for other causes of stupor and coma (see Ch. 393), including other sedating agents.

ALCOHOL WITHDRAWAL SYNDROME

Ethanol is a central nervous system (CNS) depressant. In alcoholics, the nervous system appears to adapt to chronic exposure to ethanol by increasing the activity of neural mechanisms that counteract alcohol's depressant effects. When drinking is abruptly reduced or discontinued, these adaptive neural mechanisms are left unrestrained by ethanol, and a hyperexcitable *alcohol withdrawal syndrome* develops. This is evidence of *physical dependence* on ethanol. The alcohol withdrawal syndrome consists of several characteristic abnormalities that vary in severity. These include tremulousness, disordered perceptions, seizures, and delirium tremens (Table 11–3).

The general medical evaluation and management are as described for acute ethanol intoxication. Thiamine (100 mg) should be given parenterally to all patients undergoing ethanol withdrawal to prevent or treat Wernicke's encephalopathy (see Ch. 406), followed by daily multivitamins. It is important to search for evidence of alcohol-related medical disorders (see Table 11–1) and the associated complications of alcohol abuse, as described earlier. The alarming symptoms of ethanol withdrawal are best managed by substituting another CNS depressant. However, alcoholics undergoing withdrawal are very resistant to sedatives *(cross-tolerance)*, and large doses are often required to calm their agitation (see below).

TREMULOUSNESS. Tremor, the earliest, most common, and most apparent symptom, begins about 6 to 8 hours after the last drink, usually the morning after an overnight abstinence ("morning shakes"). Tremor is generalized, coarse, and rapid and often accompanied by irritability, nausea, and vomiting. The patient usually senses an inner tremulousness even when tremor is not severe. Self-treatment is usually a morning drink to "quiet the nerves," followed

TABLE 11-3. ETHANOL WITHDRAWAL SYNDROME

8 hours	Tremulousness, anxiety, irritability, nausea and vomiting
24 hours	Hyperexcitability, insomnia, disordered perceptions, convulsions
2–5 days	Delirium tremens

by drinking for the rest of the day. If the alcoholic does not resume drinking, tremor intensifies by 24 to 36 hours and is exacerbated by motor activity or stress. It can be so severe as to interfere with walking, eating, or talking. Accompanying symptoms and signs of sympathetic hyperactivity are also apparent. The patient is increasingly anxious and easily startled by minor stimuli and complains of insomnia and anorexia. There is increased sweating, facial flushing, mydriasis, tachycardia, and mild hypertension. Most abnormalities subside in a few days, but increased arousal and anxiety may persist for 2 weeks.

DISORDERED PERCEPTIONS. Disordered perceptions accompany tremor and sympathetic hyperactivity in approximately 25% of patients, become most pronounced at 24 to 36 hours, and clear in a few days. Vivid nightmares often interfere with sleep; while the patient is awake, ordinary visual, auditory, and tactile experiences become distorted and misinterpreted.

Alcoholics undergoing withdrawal may develop isolated and prolonged auditory hallucinations (*alcoholic hallucinosis*), despite being alert, oriented, and without memory loss. Hallucinations may persist for weeks even though other signs of ethanol withdrawal have improved and the patient is less agitated and tremulous. In the absence of sympathetic hyperactivity, persistent auditory hallucinations may be confused with acute schizophrenia. However, alcoholic hallucinosis is closely associated with ethanol withdrawal and usually subsides in weeks to months.

Benzodiazepines are widely used to manage tremulousness and disordered perceptions during ethanol withdrawal. The goal is to suppress symptoms and produce mild sedation, and drug dosage is adjusted to the severity of the withdrawal reaction. Patients with mild tremulousness and few associated symptoms usually respond to oral diazepam, 5 to 10 mg every 4 to 6 hours. Dosage is then reduced by 20 to 25% on successive days, or increased if symptoms of ethanol withdrawal return. Diazepam is used intravenously if symptoms are severe; some patients require much higher doses to achieve mild sedation. Once the symptoms of ethanol withdrawal are suppressed, it is necessary to avoid oversedation and the danger of respiratory depression by carefully titrating the dose of diazepam to just keep the patient calm.

ALCOHOL WITHDRAWAL CONVULSIONS. About one third of alcoholics develop generalized tonic-clonic seizures, most often within 12 to 24 hours after reducing or stopping drinking. Some propose that the first seizure in alcoholics may be a consequence of ethanol toxicity. However, ethanol dependence is followed by withdrawal seizures in animals, particularly in mice bred to develop convulsions during withdrawal, suggesting a role for genetic vulnerability in humans. Ethanol withdrawal seizures usually follow chronic daily drinking but can also occur after 5 to 7 days of binge drinking. Alcoholics who have seizures during one episode of withdrawal are likely to have convulsions again when alcohol withdrawal is repeated. There may be one isolated convulsion or several seizures, usually within a 6-hour period. Focal seizures are less common and should always suggest a focal lesion and an additional diagnosis. Status epilepticus occurs in about 3% of cases, and ethanol withdrawal accounts for about 15% of all patients who present with status epilepticus. Status epilepticus is a medical emergency and requires immediate treatment with anticonvulsants, as described in Ch. 433.

Most alcohol withdrawal convulsions are brief and self-limited and do not require specific anticonvulsant therapy. Phenytoin does not prevent recurrent seizures, but sedating doses of benzodiazepines are helpful. Complete evaluation for a convulsive disorder is indicated (see Ch. 433) if there is a suspicion of other CNS disorders, if the patient has focal seizures, if there are more than six convulsions, if the seizures persist beyond 6 hours, or if the postictal state is prolonged.

DELIRIUM TREMENS. Delirium tremens, the most alarming manifestation of the ethanol withdrawal syndrome, occurs in about 5% of alcoholics. It consists of agitated arousal, global confusion and disorientation, insomnia, and vivid and often threatening hallucinations and delusions. Signs of sympathetic hyperactivity include tremor, mydriasis, tachycardia, fever, and intense diaphoresis. In contrast to tremulousness, disordered perceptions, and seizures— which appear earlier after withdrawal—delirium tremens begins abruptly within 2 to 4 days of abstinence, often as a surprising development in an unrecognized alcoholic admitted to the hospital for other reasons. Patients are terrified by their hallucinations and can

be combative, destructive, and very dangerous. Episodes of delirium tremens last from 1 to 3 days and end as abruptly as they begin. However, relapses occur and the disorder may continue for days to weeks with intervening periods of lucidity.

Delirium tremens requires hospitalization and vigorous emergency treatment. When there are no signs of sympathetic hyperactivity, it may be difficult to distinguish delirium tremens from an acute psychosis. However, the diagnosis is usually suggested when symptoms evolve in a chronic alcoholic undergoing withdrawal. The differential diagnosis includes alcoholic hypoglycemia, overdose with anticholinergic agents, intoxication with amphetamines, cocaine, and phencyclidine, encephalitis, meningitis, thyrotoxicosis, and withdrawal from other sedating drugs. Seizures are unusual in delirium tremens and should be evaluated promptly because of the possibility of meningitis or other diagnoses. Mortality can reach 15%, primarily because of injuries or associated medical disorders complicated by hyperthermia and dehydration. Volume depletion accompanying delirium tremens may cause circulatory collapse, and fluid losses can require replacing 4 to 10 liters in the first day. The goal of treatment is to control behavior and suppress symptoms without endangering the patient. Five to 10 mg or more of diazepam is given intravenously every 5 to 15 minutes until the patient is calm, and maintenance therapy is continued every 1 to 4 hours, as needed. Initially, as much as 200 mg of diazepam may be required before agitation subsides, and some patients may need up to 1200 mg in the first 3 to 4 days of treatment to keep calm.

REHABILITATING ALCOHOLICS

Most alcoholics rarely admit to problem drinking and are often not recognized by their primary care physicians. Instead, alcoholics are usually identified because of the adverse socioeconomic consequences of heavy drinking or by developing medical complications and the alcohol-related disorders (see Table 11–1) that bring them to medical attention. After several days of detoxification under medical supervision, the patient should be referred to a rehabilitation program because alcoholism and alcohol abuse can rarely be treated by the physician alone. The patient needs encouragement to develop a high level of motivation to stop drinking and to readjust to a life without alcohol. The most successful treatment usually requires active participation of family members, friends, and peers, and the prognosis is best for alcoholics who enter treatment programs before the onset of associated medical disorders. Many patients and families find local support groups such as Alcoholics Anonymous and Al-Anon to be very helpful, and about 50 to 70% of socially stable, middle-class alcoholics can achieve abstinence. However, this success rate is not attributable to a specific kind of rehabilitation scheme.

Adinoff B, Bone GHA, Linnoila M: Acute ethanol poisoning and the ethanol withdrawal syndrome. Med Toxicol 3:172, 1988. *An extensive discussion of the presentation and management of ethanol intoxication and withdrawal.*
Begleiter H, Kissin B (eds.): Alcohol and Alcoholism, Vol. I—Genetics. New York, Oxford University Press, 1993. *A comprehensive review of the epidemiology and genetics of alcoholism.*
Goldstein DB: Pharmacology of Alcohol. New York, Oxford University Press, 1983. *An excellent introduction to the principles of ethanol pharmacology.*
Porter R, Mattson R, Kramer J, et al. (eds): Alcohol and Seizures: Basic Mechanisms and Clinical Concepts. Philadelphia, FA Davis, 1990. *Focuses on the pathogenesis and management of ethanol withdrawal seizures.*
US Department of Health and Human Services: Eighth Special Report to the US Congress on Alcohol and Health. Rockville, MD, National Institute on Alcohol Abuse and Alcoholism, 1993. *An excellent comprehensive discussion of the major biomedical and socioeconomic problems of alcoholism and alcohol abuse.*

12 DRUG ABUSE AND DEPENDENCE
Charles P. O'Brien

In the 1990's, substance abuse remains a significant problem in all strata of American society. The average physician is likely to encounter many patients exhibiting behavioral or medical complications of licit or illicit drug use, but the relationship of the symptoms to drugs often goes unrecognized. Early diagnosis—which is crucial for effective treatment—is difficult because, at an early stage, patients rarely fit the addict stereotype.

Clinicians tend to think of addicts as daily drug users who are unable to function in society. In reality, this image is a late stage of the syndrome. Drug use may be episodic rather than regular for several years as the condition progresses. *Tolerance* and *physical dependence* may not be apparent. Tolerance is an homeostatic process in which the body adapts to the presence of a drug and the user must increase the dosage in order to achieve the desired effect. *Withdrawal* symptoms occur in regular users who abruptly stop using the drug. *Physical dependence* is diagnosed by the presence of withdrawal symptoms. While these phenomena are present in late stages of drug dependence, physicians should be alert to the early behavioral signs of dependence—preoccupation with acquiring the drug, neglect of constructive activities, and impaired social functioning.

RECOGNITION. Because early diagnosis is so important, the physician should have a low threshold for including drug abuse in the differential diagnosis of any patient. The abuse pattern that presents the most difficulty is that of a successful middle-class adult whose substance abuse is detected incidental to a routine physical examination or during treatment of an unrelated disorder. Invariably the patient denies that drugs or alcohol is a problem. Physicians must be aware that denying problems and minimizing the drug or alcohol use are fundamental aspects of the syndrome. These patients usually do not admit to a problem until it becomes so severe that there is no alternative, and, of course, by that time, treatment is much more difficult.

The diagnosis of drug abuse or dependence is basically a clinical diagnosis. The physician should use all of the available information, including the patient's history, information from relatives or employer, physical examination, and laboratory tests. Blood or urine tests showing the presence of drugs or their metabolites can be useful but also can be misleading. The toxicologic tests, when properly done and confirmed, indicate use within a varying period of time depending on the drug and its dose. Such tests do not disclose pattern of use or the presence of dependence. Metabolites of some drugs, such as marijuana, remain in the urine for at least several days following a single dose. Thus the tests require interpretation and integration with other clinical information.

Clues on the physical examination include the presence of scars from numerous intravenous injections ("tracks"), edema of the arms, and difficulty finding veins. Chronic sinusitis or a scarred and perhaps perforated nasal septum suggests "snorting" of cocaine, a powerful vasoconstrictor. Frequent injuries due to falls or auto accidents are seen in sedative abusers as well as alcoholics. Infections such as abscesses, hepatitis, respiratory infections, and endocarditis are well known risks of drug abuse. The most devastating disease associated with drug abuse is acquired immunodeficiency syndrome (AIDS), and intravenous drug users now represent more than 30% of cases of HIV infection (see Part XXII).

Physicians must also be alert to the signs of drug abuse in order to avoid unwittingly prescribing medication that perpetuates the dependence. Patients taking sleeping medications, pain medications, or antianxiety agents on a chronic basis may visit several physicians in order to obtain a larger drug supply. Other patients deliberately feign illness, particularly pain syndromes. Some have read textbooks and recite classic descriptions of acute renal calculus, migraine headache, or pancreatitis. Physicians should be particularly wary of patients who ask for a specific medication or who claim to have an "allergy" to non-narcotic pain medication.

SEDATIVES

Sedatives are central nervous system depressants and they may produce abuse, tolerance, and physical dependence. Commonly used sedatives are barbiturates, alprazolam (Xanax), flurazepam (Dalmane), diazepam (Valium), lorazepam (Ativan), and zolpidem (Ambien). Their withdrawal syndromes are generally similar, although the sedatives come from different chemical categories (e.g., alcohol, barbiturate, benzodiazepine). Their effects are additive and they are often used in combination. This aspect is particularly im-

portant in considering interactions with the nonprescription sedative alcohol (see Ch. 11) and in treating patients who are dependent on multiple sedatives with different durations of action.

PATTERNS OF ABUSE. There are two basic patterns of sedative drug abuse other than that with alcohol: one is produced inadvertently by taking prescription sedatives without proper concern for their potential to produce dependence, and the second involves deliberately using sedatives to obtain a "high."

Prescription Sedatives. The problem of improper use of prescription sedatives is a concern to all physicians because these drugs are among the most widely prescribed of all drugs throughout the world. They have legitimate medical uses for seizure disorders and in the short-term treatment of insomnia and anxiety. The chronic use of medication for insomnia, however, often leads to problems because insomnia is merely a symptom. It may signal the presence of an underlying illness or it may simply require a change in activity patterns, but continuing sedatives simply adds a new problem. After daily use for several weeks, tolerance develops and sleep difficulties may return, often in a modified form. However, the patient becomes dependent on ingesting the sedative daily. If the drug is stopped, a rebound occurs with the appearance of symptoms worse than those experienced prior to treatment. Sedatives are not equal in their tendency to produce this iatrogenic insomnia. Long-acting benzodiazepines, for example, are unlikely to produce rebound effects at usual doses. However, other liabilities are associated with their use, such as "hangover" effects, which produce subtle neuropsychological deficits and may mimic dementia in older persons. On balance, insomnia should not be treated with drugs except for brief periods.

Another pattern associated with prescribing sedatives is that found when treating anxiety. Benzodiazepines (e.g., diazepam, alprazolam) are the most effective medications available to treat anxiety, and they produce relatively less sedation than older medications used for this purpose, such as meprobamate or phenobarbital. Anxiety symptoms are widespread, and one survey found that about 15% of all Americans received a prescription for one of these drugs in a single year. Although some argue that this suggests overprescribing, it is not out of line with other Western countries. Approximately 6% of the population take benzodiazepines chronically and this leads to *tolerance* and *physical dependence*. This does not imply a similar prevalence of *abuse* because the patient may be taking the benzodiazepine for a legitimate anxiety disorder. It does mean, however, that because the patient perceives less sedation, he/she may increase the dose. It also implies that the patient should be warned about withdrawal symptoms if the drug is terminated abruptly.

Deliberate Sedative Abuse. Sedatives are used at parties by groups of abusers, usually adolescents and young adults, to obtain a "high." The high appears to be a form of disinhibition or release and depends partially on the setting in which the drug is taken. As with alcohol, increasing the dose produces depression and eventual loss of consciousness. A dangerous aspect of sedative abuse is that tolerance to the sought-after subjective effects rapidly develops, but tolerance to the brain stem depressant effects remains low. As the experienced user increases the dose to obtain a high, he/she may unexpectedly reach the dose that depresses vital functions and threatens survival.

Abstinence Syndrome. The withdrawal syndrome following sedative dependence is similar to alcohol withdrawal (see Ch. 11). Among the sedatives, the syndrome varies in onset, duration, and severity depending on each drug's dose and duration of action and the duration of daily use. The long-acting benzodiazepines such as diazepam may have a withdrawal syndrome whose onset is delayed for several days after stopping the drug. At doses within the therapeutic range, withdrawal symptoms may consist of only mild irritability, complaints of peculiar sensations, diaphoresis, and sleep disturbance accompanied by rebound increases in rapid eye movement sleep. The symptoms may be similar to the anxiety symptoms for which the drug was initially prescribed. At higher doses, the sedative withdrawal syndrome is more severe and can be life-threatening. After the acute phase, irritability, anxiety, depressive symptoms, and neuropsychological deficits may persist for weeks or months.

Treatment. The acute withdrawal syndrome should be considered a serious medical illness usually requiring inpatient treatment. Close monitoring for cardiac arrhythmias or seizures is necessary.

Several detoxification techniques are available, each requiring the substitution of a prescribed sedative with cross-tolerance for the drug on which the patient is dependent. The physician should not simply accept the history but rather determine the level of dependence by giving a test dose of a known sedative such as diazepam or pentobarbital. If the patient shows no evidence of slurred speech or sedation after a test dose of 20 to 40 mg diazepam, a higher level of dependence is indicated and the daily dose should be adjusted accordingly. Gradual detoxification using diazepam can be accomplished over 1 to 3 weeks, although in some treatment centers where diazepam is the object of much drug-seeking behavior and manipulation by patients, phenobarbital is preferred. Patients dependent on both a short-acting sedative such as alcohol and a long-acting drug such as diazepam should be watched for a biphasic withdrawal. After detoxification, the patient must be put in a treatment program to prevent recurrence, as described at the end of this chapter.

STIMULANTS

Examples of stimulants include cocaine, dextroamphetamine, methylphenidate (Ritalin), and phenmetrazine (Preludin).

PATTERNS OF ABUSE. Although the rate of new cocaine users declined in the late 1980's, surveys in 1993 showed an increase in cocaine use among young people. Cocaine continues to be widely available at low prices. It can be administered in a powdered form, cocaine hydrochloride, through the nasal mucosa ("snorting") or taken intravenously, or the alkaloidal form (free base or "crack") can be inhaled after heating.

The sought-after effect of cocaine is an intense high or euphoria, which is often described in sexual terms but is claimed to be "better than sex." The euphoria may last only a few minutes depending on the dose and mode of administration. The aftereffect is one of depression and craving for more cocaine. During a period of regular cocaine use, the person becomes irritable and suspicious. High doses may result in persecutory delusions or hallucinations, but these are more common with longer-acting stimulants such as amphetamines. Families and friends of chronic cocaine users often note personality changes not noticed by the users themselves. Alcohol, sedatives, opioids, and marijuana are often taken concurrently to combat anxiety and irritability experienced with regular cocaine use. When regular users are deprived of cocaine, they experience intense craving, depression, apathy, fatigue, and sleepiness.

Dextroamphetamine has been prescribed by physicians for a variety of conditions including weight reduction, narcolepsy, and attention deficit disorder. Amphetamines have not been shown to be valuable in weight reduction programs, and their use for all purposes has been curtailed by legal restrictions. Because they produce effects that are pleasant to most people, patients have a tendency to increase the dose of all stimulants and to take them longer than the prescribing physician intended.

PHARMACOLOGY. Cocaine has several effects, but the crucial action for abuse potential is that it blocks reuptake of dopamine at central synapses, thus increasing dopaminergic synaptic activity. Systemic effects of cocaine and amphetamine include increased cardiac contraction, increased blood pressure and heart rate, dilated pupils, constriction of peripheral blood vessels, rise in body temperature, relaxation of the bronchial musculature, and increases in central venous pressure, pulmonary arterial pressure, and renal blood flow. Cocaine is an effective topical local anesthetic and vasoconstrictor of mucous membranes. Low doses of stimulants increase alertness and physical and cognitive ability. Stimulants do reduce appetite, but significant tolerance develops to this effect. When stimulants are discontinued, a rebound increase in weight often leaves the person heavier than before the drug was taken.

ADVERSE EFFECTS. The most common adverse effect of cocaine use is loss of control so that a severe dependence syndrome occurs and all constructive activities are neglected. *Acute cocaine toxicity* is dose related and is characterized by sympathomimetic effects including tachycardia, hypertension, hyperthermia, and arrhythmias, followed by seizures, brain stem depression, and cardiorespiratory collapse. Stroke, coma, intracranial vasculitis, myocardial infarction, and sudden death have each been occasionally observed by clinicians treating complications of cocaine binges. At lower doses the acute toxic effects may be marked by a brief period of paranoid behavior with hallucinations. *Acute amphetamine toxicity* is also characterized by excessive sympathomimetic stimulation. Grossly paranoid behavior mimicking acute paranoid schizophrenia is more commonly produced by amphetamine toxicity. There may be stereotyped compulsive behavior, tactile hallucinations consisting of "bugs" crawling under the skin, and visual or auditory hallucinations.

Chronic use of intranasal cocaine commonly causes ulceration or perforation of the nasal septum. Chronic users are typically debilitated and subject to infections as a result of neglect of hygiene, lack of sleep, and poor nutrition. Evidence of vascular damage and neuronal changes is found in the brains of animals treated chronically with high-dose stimulants. Schizophrenic disorders have been reported to be increased in chronic stimulant users. Chronic cocaine use among pregnant women is associated with a high incidence of premature, low birth weight, and behaviorally abnormal infants, but because of poor prenatal care and neglect, the role of pharmacologic factors is not clear.

TREATMENT. The anxiety reactions and irritability produced by cocaine or amphetamines can be treated with benzodiazepines. Acute psychotic reactions may require haloperidol if amphetamines are involved, but reactions produced by cocaine are usually self-limiting. Withdrawal from stimulant dependence requires a supportive environment and protection from the supply of cocaine. Intense craving for cocaine is the most prominent of the withdrawal symptoms, and these have been attributed to a state of dopamine depletion in the brain. The most difficult aspect of treatment is preventing relapse when the patient returns to his/her normal environment and is confronted with opportunities to re-establish the habit. This aspect of treatment is discussed at the end of this chapter.

OPIOIDS

Opioids may be divided into three categories: *Agonists* include morphine, methadone, hydromorphone (Dilaudid), oxycodone (Percodan), meperidine (Demerol), heroin, LAAM (alpha acetyl methadol), fentanyl (Sublimaze), codeine, and propoxyphene (Darvon). *Partial agonist-antagonists* include buprenorphine (Buprenex), nalbuphine (Nubain), pentazocine (Talwin), and butorphanol (Stadol). *Antagonists* include naloxone (Narcan), and naltrexone (Trexan).

Opiates are derivatives of the opium poppy plant, which contains >20 alkaloids. Heroin, morphine, and codeine are examples of commonly used *opiates*. Synthetic drugs that act via opiate receptors in the body are called *opioids*. The body also produces peptides that act at these receptors as neurohormones or neurotransmitters and are called *endogenous opioids* (see Ch. 200.1).

PATTERNS OF ABUSE. Opioid abuse has been a problem in the United States for well over 100 years. The patterns have changed considerably since the turn of the century, when most of the opium-dependent persons were either Civil War veterans or users of patent medicines. At the current time there are two abuse patterns in this country. The smaller group by far involves patients initially treated by a physician with opioid drugs for a legitimate pain problem. The pain may become chronic and the dose is increased, usually at the patient's demand. The treatment may have begun with a relatively weak medication such as propoxyphene or pentazocine, but it tends to progress through to the more potent opioids such as oxycodone or hydromorphone. Prescriptions may be refilled excessively, and patients may visit more than one physician for medication or may frequent emergency rooms. Such individuals vehemently deny being addicts; they are just seeking relief of pain. On closer examination, however, they are usually found to have symptoms of anxiety or depression that are temporarily relieved by opioids.

The second pattern is that of intentional misuse of opioids for their euphoria-producing properties. Intermittent heroin use, primarily among males in the inner city, typically begins during adolescence and dependence develops within a year or two of first use. Development in all areas—educational, social, occupational, and even psychosexual—is curtailed by use of heroin. It is not known how many people begin experimenting with heroin and stop using it. Those who continue to use heroin develop tolerance to its euphorigenic effects, continue to increase the dose, and soon find that they must use the drug daily to avoid withdrawal symptoms even while chasing that elusive first high.

Older users tend to introduce younger ones to injecting heroin and to techniques of crime required to support the "habit." Street heroin available in the United States has been of low potency, averaging 4% purity, until the 1990's, when increased availability produced dramatic increases in potency. The range of heroin potency in the 1990's has been 40 to 80%. This change means that users get more drug per bag of heroin and thus overdoses increase. Also, high-potency heroin can be administered by smoking rather than exclusively by intravenous injection, although some potency is lost and the effective dose then decreases.

Some heroin users discover that prescription medications are more reliable than street drugs because street drugs have no quality control. Hydromorphone, a very potent opioid, cannot be distinguished from heroin even by experienced users under double-blind conditions. Addicts may visit physicians or emergency rooms and feign pain syndromes to obtain opioids. Some unscrupulous physicians may simply sell prescriptions for whatever the addict requests. Another mechanism is used by addicts who have prescription pads printed with their own name and a fake DEA number in an effort to trick pharmacists. Some of the prescription drugs prized on the street are not even the more potent ones.

During the cocaine epidemic of the 1980's, heroin use spread from the inner city to the middle-class suburbs. The same supply system that distributes cocaine and marijuana also makes heroin available. Some educated and employed persons seeking a "thrill" prefer the effects of heroin. Others learn to use heroin to combat some of the unpleasant anxiety and irritability produced by chronic cocaine use.

PHARMACOLOGY. Opioids act at specific receptors that are widely distributed throughout the body in virtually all major organ systems. Because these receptors are well represented in the endocrine, cardiovascular, gastrointestinal, and nervous systems, the effects of opioids are many and varied. The potency of individual drugs appears to depend on receptor affinity as well as metabolism. Heroin, for example, is di-acetyl morphine, which has high lipid solubility and thus enters the brain rapidly. It is hydrolyzed to morphine, which is the metabolite active at opiate receptors. Other opiates and opioids have similar effects but reach brain receptors less rapidly. The partial agonist-antagonist drugs such as buprenorphine, pentazocine, butorphanol, and nalbuphine appear to act as agonists at kappa opiate receptors, but they also act as antagonists at mu (morphine) receptors. Thus, pentazocine can relieve pain on its own, but if given to someone already receiving morphine, displaces the morphine and precipitates withdrawal symptoms. Pure antagonists such as naloxone and naltrexone have no opiate-like effects, but they can reverse overdose and precipitate withdrawal if given *after* an opioid and prevent opiate effects if given *before* the opioid.

After heroin injection, traces of morphine can be found in the urine for about 12 to 48 hours, depending on the dose and the laboratory detection technique. Quinine, a common adulterant of street heroin, persists longer, but it is also found in legal substances such as tonic water. Parenteral injections of morphine or methadone have equal analgesic effects and persist for 4 to 6 hours, while heroin is three times as potent and meperidine and codeine are one tenth as potent as morphine. Codeine, meperidine, and methadone remain active when taken orally, and the duration of action of methadone is extended significantly by the oral route. For prevention of withdrawal in dependent persons, methadone is active for 24 to 30 hours, far longer than its analgesic effect.

Opioids appear to produce a state in which the patient can still feel pain but is less bothered by it. This state is produced, at least in part, by activation of an endogenous pain control system mediated via opiate receptors. Pain sensation is inhibited at the spinal level as well as within the brain. Opioids are much more effective against clinical pain with anxiety than on experimental pain in research subjects. Opioids produce a reduction in anxiety, some sedation, and a feeling of well-being or euphoria. This effect seems important to both their clinical usefulness and their abuse potential. This euphoria is sought after by street addicts and probably leads some medical patients to abuse prescribed opioids. Researchers have long sought a compound that relieves pain as effectively as opiates without the concomitant euphoria. It is not yet clear whether the effects are neurologically separable.

Tolerance to the euphoric effects of opioids develops rapidly, resulting in a tendency for users to increase their dose if possible. Only partial tolerance develops to other effects such as pupillary constriction, inhibited gastrointestinal contractions, and suppressed anterior pituitary function.

ADVERSE EFFECTS. *Acute opioid overdose* occurs when a user inadvertently injects a much higher dose than expected. This also can be seen when a previously tolerant person starts using opioids again after a long interval so that most of his/her tolerance has been lost. Also, in recent years heroin users may be surprised by the high potency of heroin purchased on the street. Street heroin may occasionally contain high-potency opioids such as fentanyl.

Many of the "overdoses" found with street heroin in the past are thought to have been due to a reaction to some of the adulterants rather than to the opiate. Acute reactions to adulterants including quinine, allergic reactions, and synergistic interactions among several drugs used simultaneously may produce the *acute heroin reaction*. The syndrome is marked clinically by the rapid development of cyanosis, pulmonary edema, respiratory distress, and varying levels of consciousness progressing to coma. Increased intracranial pressure and occasionally seizures are seen. Fever to 40° C may occur initially and may persist for 48 hours in association with leukocytosis. The pupils are usually pinpoint, although dilated nonreactive pupils may occur with hypoxia or multiple drug use. The pathologic picture includes pulmonary congestion and edema and frequently cerebral edema.

Opioids themselves are surprisingly nontoxic even when used in substantial daily doses for many years. Partial tolerance develops to their pharmacologic effects on the endocrine system. Thus females on methadone initially are amenorrheic, but the cycle usually returns in 6 to 12 months. Cortisol, luteinizing hormone, and testosterone are depressed while the patient is on methadone. Sexual response may be delayed; sperm count and ejaculate volume are reduced. Because street heroin users tend to have frequent periods of partial withdrawal, their endocrine systems are in turmoil. In contrast, a level dose of methadone induces some order and the effects are reversible when the opioid is terminated. Chronic constipation may persist throughout opioid use.

The major adverse effects of opioid use come from the adulterants found in street drugs and the nonsterile practices typically followed by users. Skin abscesses, cellulitis, and thrombophlebitis are the most frequent complications. Pentazocine injection causes chronic ulcers and sclerosis of muscle in the area of injection. Septicemia and bacterial endocarditis with involvement of either or both sides of the heart are seen. *Staphylococcus aureus* is frequently the causative agent in right-sided endocarditis. Peripheral and pulmonary embolic phenomena occur.

Viral hepatitis has long been common among intravenous drug abusers from sharing needles during an injection session. In recent years this has been overshadowed by the appearance of the AIDS virus. During the 1990's, up to 60% of patients applying to methadone programs in some large cities tested positive for HIV antibodies, and it has been suggested that this group is particularly susceptible because the drugs suppress host resistance. Studies of HIV seropositivity show relatively low levels for heroin addicts who remain in methadone treatment but high rates of infection for addicts out of treatment. IV drug abusers now represent more than 30% of all cases of HIV infection in the United States.

Among applicants for treatment, 75 to 80% of heroin users have significantly abnormal liver function tests. These findings may be related to persistent chronic hepatitis, but alcohol, malnutrition, allergic phenomena, and the toxic effects of adulterants may contribute. Pulmonary complications include pneumonia, abscess, infarct, and tuberculosis. Disseminated extrapulmonary tuberculosis has been reported. Angiothrombotic pulmonary hypertension and granulomatosis result from intravenously injecting foreign bodies, including talc and cotton. Other complications include nephropathy, local arterial occlusion, phlebitis, mycotic aneurysms, and necrotizing angiitis.

Neurologic complications of using street heroin include transverse myelitis, acute inflammatory polyneuropathy, peripheral nerve lesions, toxic amblyopia secondary to quinine, and muscle disorders including acute rhabdomyolysis with myoglobinuria and a fibrosing chronic myopathy. Septic states may lead to bacterial meningitis and brain, subdural, and epidural abscesses. Tetanus may result from dirty needles.

Pregnant addicts have a high incidence of toxemia and premature deliveries. About 50% of their newborns require treatment of withdrawal symptoms.

TREATMENT. More distinctly different kinds of treatment are available for dependence on opioid drugs than for any other type of drug dependence. As with other drugs, preventing relapse to drug-seeking behavior is the most difficult aspect (see below). The treatment of *acute overdose* is effective and straightforward. In any emergency situation in which opioid overdose is suspected, naloxone should be administered, preferably intravenously. The patient has constricted pupils, and a dose of 0.4 mg naloxone should cause an increase in pupil size, respiratory rate, and alertness within several minutes. Repeated doses may be necessary if the patient does not respond within several minutes to the first dose. Absence of a response to repeated naloxone injections excludes the diagnosis of opioid overdose.

Virtually no risk is associated with giving naloxone, but the potential benefits mean that it should be tried even in doubtful cases. Two pitfalls should be mentioned, however. One is that naloxone may not only reverse the overdose, but it may go beyond mere reversal and actually precipitate *withdrawal* symptoms in opioid-dependent persons. To avoid this, the dose of naloxone should be titrated according to the level of consciousness and respiratory rate. The second risk is that the rapid metabolism of naloxone may allow the overdose to recur if the overdose was caused by a long-acting drug such as methadone or LAAM. In cases of overdose, naloxone should be titrated via an intravenous drip or repeated every 2 to 3 hours with careful monitoring of vital signs for at least 24 hours.

The opioid withdrawal syndrome varies in severity and duration depending on the specific drug, dose, and duration of use. The typical heroin-dependent person notes the onset of withdrawal 6 to 10 hours after the last injection. Feelings of drug craving, anxiety, restlessness, irritability, sweating, rhinorrhea, and yawning develop early. These are followed by dilated pupils, sneezing, piloerection, anorexia, nausea, vomiting, diarrhea, abdominal cramps, bone pain, myalgias, tremors, sleep disturbance, and very rarely, convulsions or cardiovascular collapse. Untreated, these symptoms peak at 36 to 48 hours and gradually subside over 5 to 10 days. Withdrawal is generally not life-threatening and it has been compared with a severe case of the "flu." There is also a protracted abstinence syndrome consisting of mild symptoms of anxiety, sleep disturbance, and autonomic nervous system instability which may persist for 6 months after acute withdrawal. Longer-acting opioids such as methadone and LAAM produce an abstinence syndrome that develops more slowly and with less intensity but persists much longer.

Medically assisted withdrawal is usually accomplished using methadone, beginning with a test dose of 20 mg. If 20 mg has no appreciable effect on the signs and symptoms within 1 hour, an additional 20 mg can be given. The methadone can be gradually reduced over 7 to 10 days. An alternative is clonidine, an α_2-adrenergic agonist/partial agonist, which produces complex central effects that result in reduced central adrenergic outflow. Developed to treat hypertension, clonidine has also been found to reduce many of the signs of autonomic hyperactivity during opioid withdrawal. Thus clonidine can be useful in situations in which methadone is not available. Beginning with low doses of 0.1 to 0.2 mg to minimize the possibility of postural hypotension, clonidine can be increased to 1 to 1.5 mg daily in divided doses over 4 to 10 days and then tapered over the next 5 days.

Relapse after detoxification is very common so after several detoxification failures, many patients are treated with methadone maintenance. Methadone and LAAM, the recently approved new opioid maintenance medication, are described below.

CANNABIS (Marijuana and Hashish)

Cannabis is not a single drug but a complex preparation containing many biologically active chemicals. Δ-9-Tetrahydrocannabinol (Δ-9-THC) accounts for most of the pharmacologic effects of the complex.

PATTERNS OF ABUSE. Cannabis has been used in many societies as a form of folk medicine and for relaxation. Throughout the 1970's, its use increased explosively in the United States. Surveys indicate that use peaked in 1979, when more than 50 million Americans reported using the drug at least once and 9% of high school seniors reported daily use. In the 1980's, the popularity of this drug declined, but in the early 1990's use began to increase, particularly among junior high students. Domestic sources of marijuana have increased, and average potency is higher than in the past. The vast majority of users smoke marijuana cigarettes or hashish pipes in groups where the ritual of preparation and sharing is part of the social interaction. Few progress to a pattern of compulsive daily use with lives dominated by acquiring and using cannabis.

PHARMACOLOGY. Cannabis preparations are three to four times more potent when smoked than when taken orally. After inhalation, effects begin within 3 minutes and peak within 1 hour, and the subject reports feeling "normal" within 3 hours. Psychomotor effects, however, such as impairment on eye-tracking and vigilance tasks, may be evident for up to 11 hours after a single dose.

The acute physiologic effects of cannabis are dose related and include an increase in heart rate, conjunctival vascular congestion, decreased intraocular pressure, bronchodilation, increased airway conductance, and peripheral vasodilation. Dryness of mouth, fine tremors, ataxia, nystagmus, nausea, and vomiting have been noted. Sleep patterns are altered and orthostatic hypotension occurs infrequently.

Δ-9-THC is the main psychoactive factor in marijuana. A specific *cannabinoid receptor* has been identified and cloned. This receptor is widely represented in the brain, and an endogenous ligand named *anandamide* has recently been isolated. A derivative of arachidonic acid, anandamide may not be the only endogenous substance active at cannabinoid receptors, and the function of this system is still unknown. Psychoactive effects of marijuana depend on the dose, route of administration, personality and experience of the user, and environment in which the drug is used. Enhanced perceptions of colors, sounds, and tastes have been reported. Time seems to pass slowly, and ability to learn new facts is impaired. There is often some drowsiness and inattentiveness, which may account for some of the poor performance on driving simulators. *Motor vehicular driving performance is definitely impaired by cannabis,* and this impairment may persist for several hours after the period of obvious intoxication. Tolerance and physical dependence have been experimentally demonstrated with regular cannabis use. This is not relevant to the occasional user, but daily heavy users show clinical evidence of withdrawal when deprived of access to cannabis.

Cannabis contains chemicals with unusually high lipid solubility and thus a high affinity for brain tissue. Metabolites may persist for several weeks, although their biologic significance is unknown. Urine tests for marijuana can remain positive for more than 1 week after a dose and even longer in chronic users. Positive urine tests have also been experimentally demonstrated in subjects who simply sat in a room for several hours where marijuana was being smoked.

Cannabis derivatives have been investigated for their therapeutic potential in several illnesses. The antiemetic effect has been useful to some patients in reducing the nausea produced by cancer chemotherapy. The accompanying psychological effects have so far limited its usefulness. Glaucoma, convulsive seizures, asthma, and muscle spasticity are other conditions in which cannabis or a synthetic analogue may eventually prove useful.

ADVERSE EFFECTS. Most clinicians believe that regular cannabis use by adolescents impairs maturation and often results in poor social and scholastic adjustment. Although there is no way to experimentally demonstrate causality, cannabis use is associated with poor academic performance. Occasional users have fewer problems, but acute panic, paranoid reactions, and frightening distortions of body image are sometimes experienced. Rarely, these reactions are severe enough to require emergency room treatment. Such reactions seem to be more common with higher doses and with oral administration rather than smoking, which is easier to titrate. Patients with a history of schizophrenia may be particularly sensitive to adverse consequences of cannabis and should be warned to avoid it.

The cardiac stimulatory effects of cannabis may pose a threat to patients with cardiovascular disease. Chronically smoking cannabis inflames the bronchi and sinuses. Experimentally, cannabis is carcinogenic, but clinical studies are confounded by the concurrent use of tobacco by virtually all regular cannabis smokers.

TREATMENT. The acute anxiety reactions produced by cannabis are seldom severe enough to warrant medical attention. Treatment should be supportive and reassuring with frequent reminders of the drug-induced nature of the symptoms. Benzodiazepines may be indicated in more severely agitated states. For the chronic heavy user, treatment is much more difficult. Such patients typically insist that treatment is not necessary, and they feel no need to stop using cannabis on a daily basis. Meanwhile, they are failing in school or employment. Psychotherapy is unlikely to be of value unless cannabis use can be interrupted. Hospitalization or entering into a therapeutic community may be indicated if the patient can be so persuaded. Medication is usually not required to treat withdrawal, and the drug-free patient clears mentally over several weeks. Psychotherapy is usually necessary in addition to removing the cannabis.

HALLUCINOGENS

Hallucinogens include lysergic acid diethylamide (LSD), dimethyltryptamine (DMT), phencyclidine (PCP), mescaline, psilocybin, and 5-methoxy-3-4-methylene dioxyamphetamine (MDMA, "ecstasy").

Many drugs at some dose produce hallucinations, but the drugs classified here reliably produce distortions in perception or thinking as a primary effect, even at low dose. This category represents several chemical classes and different mechanisms of action. PCP, in particular, is quite different from the others in that it produces, in addition to hallucinations, analgesia and amphetamine-like stimulation.

PATTERNS OF ABUSE. Hallucinogenic drugs are among the oldest known psychoactive drugs, having long been used as an adjunct to religious practices in some societies. During the 1960's they became well known on college campuses, where they were used in an effort to "gain insight" or experiment in expanding the potential of the mind. Physicians in emergency rooms were frequently called upon to treat young people suffering from "bad trips" or adverse reactions to these substances. One of the problems with the use of illicit supplies of these drugs is their gross mislabeling. Chemical analysis of samples obtained from street purchases shows that PCP ("angel dust") and its by-products are often the active ingredient in LSD or psilocybin purchases. Thus, users often experience unexpected and severe effects. PCP as a veterinary anesthetic has been discontinued and now it is available only from clandestine laboratories where purity is quite variable. The toxic by-products produced during PCP synthesis may produce severe toxic symptoms.

The use of hallucinogenic drugs declined in the late 1970's and early 1980's, but PCP continues to be a problem in certain cities. There has also been increased interest in MDMA by college students. The typical pattern of hallucinogenic drug use involves intermittent rather than daily use. MDMA has been reported to facilitate insight and maturation and thus enhance the effects of psychotherapy. A few therapists have supported this notion and encourage their patients to use MDMA. The drug has never been studied rigorously for this use, however, and thus there is no evidence to support these claims. Similar claims were made for LSD in the past, but efforts to demonstrate a beneficial effect in controlled trials failed. Both MDMA and the closely related MDA produce long-term changes in serotoninergic nerve cells.

PHARMACOLOGY. LSD is the most potent hallucinogenic drug known. It has marked effects on serotoninergic systems in the central nervous system, but it affects other systems as well; the mechanism for its psychoactive effects is unknown. The usual illicit street dose is around 200 μg, but doses as low as 20 μg produce psychological effects in susceptible individuals. Central sympathomimetic stimulation occurs within 20 minutes of oral ingestion, and this is characterized by mydriasis, hyperthermia, tachycardia, elevated blood pressure, piloerection, increased alertness, and facilitation of monosynaptic reflexes. Nausea and vomiting occasionally occur.

Psychoactive effects of LSD, developing within 1 to 2 hours, vary with the subject, dose, setting, and expectation and mood of the subject. Perceptions are heightened and may become overwhelming. Afterimages are prolonged and may overlap with ongoing perceptions. There may be a sense of unusual clarity, and one's thoughts may assume extraordinary importance. Time seems to pass slowly and body distortions are commonly perceived. True hallucinations, usually visual, may occur in susceptible individuals. Mood

is highly variable and labile and may range from expansive reactions characterized by euphoria and self-confidence to a constricted reaction marked by depression and panic.

The syndrome begins to clear after 10 to 12 hours, but fatigue and tension may persist for an additional 24 hours. The duration of action of mescaline is about 12 hours and that of psilocybin 4 to 6 hours. Tolerance develops to repeated daily doses of LSD within 3 to 4 days, but recovery is rapid and weekly use of the same dose is possible.

PCP comes in various forms (powder, liquid, capsule, tablet) and often is taken inadvertently when the user is expecting something else. It produces a prompt stimulant effect similar to amphetamine and usually a feeling of euphoria. Ataxia, slurred speech, nystagmus, and numbness are commonly observed. At higher doses, frightening and bizarre visual hallucinations can arise. There may be hostile or aggressive behavior and amnesia for the episode. With still higher doses, catatonia and coma occur, with the patient's eyes open and the pupils partially dilated. Heart rate and blood pressure are elevated. Tolerance to the stimulant effects occurs, and some mild withdrawal symptoms have been observed in daily users.

ADVERSE EFFECTS. The acute reactions such as panic or psychosis ("bad trip") are the most common complications of psychedelic use. With LSD, these reactions vary in intensity and occasionally have led to suicide or self-injury. PCP is more likely to produce a severe reaction that results in suicide, often by drowning. Assaults and murders have been attributed to PCP, and certainly aggressive behavior can occur during the psychotic episode.

Prolonged psychotic episodes sometimes occur after psychedelic use. It is not known whether these can occur only in individuals who have pre-existing tendencies toward psychosis. Many clinicians believe that chronic or high-dose psychedelics, especially PCP, can produce prolonged psychosis even in healthy individuals. Overdose resulting in death can occur with PCP. The syndrome can progress rapidly from aggressive psychotic behavior to coma with elevated blood pressure, dilated pupils, muscular rigidity, arrhythmias, and seizures.

Another adverse effect of psychedelic use is known as "flashbacks." These are a brief reappearance of the hallucinations or distortions experienced during the acute ingestion but occur days or weeks after the last hallucinogenic dose. "Flashbacks" appear to be more common with heavy use, and they eventually disappear without treatment.

TREATMENT. Using medication in an emergency situation with a patient suffering from an unknown drug reaction can be dangerous owing to progression of the street drug effect with further absorption from the gut and to possible drug interactions with any prescribed medications. Thus treatment of acute panic reactions is best accomplished, when possible, by a supportive environment, observation, and reassurance. In severely agitated patients, intramuscular lorazepam or haloperidol can be used. Prolonged psychosis requires hospitalization and treatment with neuroleptics.

Treatment of PCP overdose may require support of vital signs. Gastric lavage with activated charcoal may prevent further absorption of the drug. To enhance the excretion of PCP, acidification of the urine may be accomplished acutely by intravenous ammonium chloride, 75 mg per kilogram per day in four divided doses, or ascorbic acid, 500 mg every 4 hours with repeated monitoring of blood pH, blood gases, blood urea nitrogen, blood ammonia, and electrolytes. If symptoms are mild, cranberry juice and 1 or 2 grams of ascorbic acid given orally four times per day may be sufficient.

Anticholinergic Compounds

Effects in some ways similar to hallucinogenic drugs may be produced by ingestion of the alkaloids *atropine, hyoscyamine,* and *scopolamine* in their natural plant forms. These are found in "herbal teas" and a variety of proprietary medications, and several deaths have occurred. Excessive use of *antihistaminic* compounds with anticholinergic effects also occurs. Psychoactive effects are those of an acute toxic delirium with confusion, visual or tactile hallucinations, and amnesia for the episode. Symptoms of the potent peripheral effects of the intoxication include dilated pupils, tachycardia, dry mouth, flushing, and hyperthermia. Treatment is symptomatic and consists of protecting the patient from self-injury, providing fluids, and reducing the fever. Administering cholinesterase inhibitors and lorazepam intramuscularly may be indicated in severe cases. Phenothiazines are contraindicated because of their anticholinergic effects. Anticholinergic drugs are sometimes sold as hallucinogenics, thus creating a potentially dangerous additive interaction if a phenothiazine is administered in the emergency room to treat a "bad trip."

INHALANTS

Chemicals that are volatile at room temperatures and that produce perceptible changes in brain function when inhaled have been popular among certain groups as a means of producing altered states of consciousness. Toluene (airplane glue), gasoline, amyl nitrite, kerosene, carbon tetrachloride, and nitrous oxide are commonly abused inhalants. There are characteristic patterns for each chemical.

Organic solvents such as toluene are typically used by children beginning at age 12. The material is usually placed in a plastic bag and the vapors inhaled. Dizziness and intoxication are described after several minutes of inhalation. Inhalant abuse also involves the use of aerosol sprays containing fluorocarbon propellents. Prolonged exposure or daily use may result in toxic effects on several organ systems including cardiac arrhythmias, bone marrow depression, cerebral degeneration, and damage to liver, kidney, and peripheral nerves. Death has occasionally been attributed to inhalant abuse, probably via the mechanism of cardiac arrhythmias especially accompanying exercise or upper airway obstruction.

Amyl nitrite is a yellowish, volatile, inflammable liquid with a fruity odor. It produces dilation of smooth muscle and has been used in the past to treat angina. In recent years, amyl nitrite has been used to enhance orgasm, particularly by male homosexuals. It is sold in the form of room deodorizers and can produce a feeling of "rush," flushing, and dizziness. Adverse effects include palpitations, postural hypotension, and headache progressing to loss of consciousness.

Nitrous oxide alone or in combination with oxygen and *halothane* is sometimes used as an intoxicant by medical personnel. Compulsive use and chronic toxicity have not been reported, but unauthorized use of such potent agents creates obvious acute dangers.

TREATMENT. Because the effects of solvents are brief, specific acute treatments are generally not indicated. When inhalant use is chronic or associated with other psychiatric diagnoses, specific psychiatric treatment and measures to prevent relapse are indicated.

NICOTINE (see Ch. 9.4)

The medical consequences of smoking tobacco products are covered in many chapters of this book because the effects are so widespread. As the dangers of smoking have become well known, it has become apparent that smoking cigarettes can produce a very powerful dependence on nicotine. Quitting smoking may be very difficult even in patients who strongly desire to remain abstinent.

PATTERNS OF ABUSE. Smoking has declined in almost all segments of the American population so that in various polls, 60 to 65% of Americans are nonsmokers. The proportion of those abstaining from tobacco increases with educational level and socioeconomic class. Those who begin smoking during adolescence have the most difficulty quitting.

PHARMACOLOGY. Nicotine in cigarette smoke is readily absorbed from the lungs and reaches the brain within 8 seconds after inhalation. Nicotine has very complicated effects that depend on the dose and experience of the user. Both alerting and relaxing effects can be produced. For example, EEG activation consistent with arousal is seen, hand tremor is increased, and heart rate and blood pressure are increased, but spinal reflexes are diminished. Memory is facilitated, but irritability and appetite are reduced. The overall effect of nicotine is considered pleasant, and each puff theoretically can produce a small reinforcement of smoking behavior. At 10 puffs per cigarette, a pack-per-day smoker could receive 200 reinforcements of the behavior each day.

Tolerance develops to some but not all of the effects of nicotine. The cardiovascular and subjective effects are greater with the first cigarette of the day than with later ones. If the supply of nicotine is terminated abruptly, heavy smokers frequently show a withdrawal syndrome beginning within the first 24 hours. It consists of irritability, headaches, drowsiness, sleep disturbance, and increased appetite. This syndrome is variable, but significant weight gain is common.

TREATMENT. Some smokers are able to stop smoking with no medical help and never return to the behavior. Those who are unable to stop on their own seek treatment from a variety of sources. About two thirds of these smokers are able to stop for a while, but at 12-month follow-up, 60 to 80% of these have relapsed to smoking. Thus, from a treatment perspective, nicotine dependence compares with alcoholism and opioid dependence in the difficulty of maintaining abstinence. Treatment is sometimes successful after multiple attempts. A nicotine patch or chewing gum as part of a formal treatment program increased the proportion of former smokers who were still abstinent 1 year after treatment.

ILLICIT SYNTHETIC DRUGS (Designer Drugs)

The so-called designer drugs are produced in clandestine laboratories, and they vary in their composition and purity. Fentanyl analogues have been produced which have extremely potent opioid actions and have resulted in overdose deaths. Other attempts at synthesis of opioids have resulted in toxic compounds. An example is MPTP, a toxic by-product of botched attempts to synthesize a meperidine (Demerol) analogue. MPTP produces an irreversible Parkinson's syndrome in people who have taken it intravenously. Other chemicals found in street samples are phenethylamines, which are analogues of amphetamine and various analogues of PCP. In evaluating the drug history of any patient, the physician must remember that the patient has no way of knowing what drugs he/she actually took if they were purchased on the street.

TREATMENT OF DRUG DEPENDENCE

The treatment of drug dependence involves four stages (Table 12–1).

ACKNOWLEDGING THE PROBLEM. Rarely does a patient in the early and most treatable phase of drug dependence spontaneously volunteer for treatment. Friends, relatives, or family members who observe the signs of a drug problem must confront the patient. Often the family physician is in a good position to notice the problem early and convince the patient to enter treatment. Confrontation is best accomplished when several concerned people approach the patient together in a firm but supportive way. Even when confronted with evidence of a substance abuse problem, the patient usually continues to deny its existence, making persistence necessary.

DETOXIFICATION. The pharmacologic aspects of detoxification were covered in the discussions of specific drug categories. In some cases hospitalization is mandatory, particularly when the degree of physical dependence is great. If, however, the drug taking can be interrupted while the individual remains an outpatient, detoxification can be far less expensive and just as effective. "Treatment programs" which advertise a 28-day inpatient treatment of drug dependence are misleading, because the heart of effective treatment is continued therapy usually lasting months or years, designed to prevent relapse after the patient returns to work or school. Frequently the patient has so much cognitive impairment during the detoxification period that he/she retains little of therapy or education provided during this first phase of treatment.

PHARMACOTHERAPY. This mode of therapy has been discussed under specific drug categories. For the most part, pharmacotherapy involves treating specific psychiatric disorders, such as affective disorders or psychosis commonly associated with a particular form of drug dependence. It must be remembered that patients who have abused one drug have a strong likelihood of abusing a prescribed psychoactive drug. For this reason, antianxiety agents or sedatives should rarely if ever be prescribed in the rehabilitation of drug-dependent persons.

Certain pharmacotherapies are directed at the drug-seeking behavior rather than an associated psychiatric disorder. Using disulfiram (Antabuse) to treat alcoholics is discussed in Ch. 11. Recent studies report lower relapse rates in alcoholics given the opiate antagonist naltrexone while in outpatient rehabilitation. The benefits are believed to be based on the effects of alcohol on the endogenous opioid system. Blocking opiate receptors thus reduces the reward from alcohol and reduces the likelihood of relapse.

Opioid-dependent patients who have repeatedly relapsed after detoxification can be transferred from illicit drugs to methadone maintenance. The patient can then be maintained on a steady

TABLE 12–1. TREATMENT OF DRUG DEPENDENCE

	Confrontation	Detoxification	Pharmacotherapy	Rehabilitation/ Psychotherapy
Sedatives	S	Diazepam or phenobarbital	Antidepressants as needed	S
Stimulants	I	Not usually needed	Antidepressants Neuroleptics	I
Opioids	M	Methadone Clonidine	Methadone Naltrexone	M
	I		Antidepressants	I
Cannabis		None	Antidepressants as needed	
	L			L
Psychedelics		None	Neuroleptics as needed	
	A			A
Inhalants		None	None	
	R			R
Nicotine		Nicotine gum or patch	None	

dosage of methadone as a substitute for his/her opioid drug of choice. The advantage is that the patient is stabilized owing to methadone's long duration of action and, properly managed, experiences no "highs" or "lows." Patients are able to function well on methadone and perform complex tasks competently. Methadone enables the patient to participate in a rehabilitation program including psychotherapy. Methadone may involve several years of maintenance and must be used only in authorized programs in which staff have received specialized training. In 1993 the FDA approved a new medication for maintenance called levo alpha acetyl methadol (LAAM). LAAM has a long duration of action and active metabolites so that maintenance can be accomplished on only three doses per week.

Naltrexone (Trexan) is a long-acting opioid antagonist. Before receiving this medication, the patient must first be thoroughly detoxified or the naltrexone will precipitate withdrawal. Because naltrexone blocks opiate receptors, the effects of impulsive opioid use are prevented while naltrexone is in the body. This treatment has been successful in conjunction with a comprehensive rehabilitation program including a wide range of psychotherapies. Naltrexone must be taken at least two or three times per week to protect against relapse, so it requires strong motivation on the part of the patient to remain opioid free.

PSYCHOTHERAPY. Psychotherapy is generally similar across all classes of drugs. It should be started as early as possible in the treatment program, but it is of little value when the patient is still intoxicated or confused. This treatment is, however, completely compatible with pharmacotherapy such as psychoactive medication, methadone, naltrexone, disulfiram, or nicotine patch. Such psychotherapy is broadly defined, and it involves counseling regarding job-finding or legal problems, family therapy, group therapy, individual therapy, all types of behavioral treatments, and self-help programs such as Narcotics Anonymous. The purpose of these treatments is to teach the patient alternate behaviors to ingesting drugs and to enable the patient to deal more effectively with problems of living. The general physician often can convince patients to join a specialized treatment program, and the physician can collaborate in the medical aspects of the treatment. Severe forms of drug dependence, however, are best managed by a treatment team specially trained in this area of medicine.

Mackler S, O'Brien CP: Cocaine abuse. In Stollerman G (ed.): Advances in Internal Medicine. St. Louis, Mosby-Year Book, 1992, p 21. *A comprehensive review of the medical complications of cocaine abuse.*

Metzger DS, Woody GE, et al.: Human immunodeficiency virus seroconversion among in- and out-of-treatment intravenous drug users: An 18-month, prospective follow-up. J AIDS 6:1049, 1993. *This study documents the spread of HIV among untreated opiate addicts and the protective value of methadone treatment.*

O'Brien CP: Opioid addiction. In Herz A (ed.): Handbook of Experimental Pharmacology, Vol. 104/II Opioids. Berlin, Springer-Verlag, 1992. *This chapter reviews the endogenous opioid system in relation to opioid tolerance and dependence.*

O'Brien CP, Jaffe J (eds.): Advances in Understanding the Addictive States. New York, Raven Press, 1991, p 291. *This volume summarizes the current state of knowledge on the biologic processes underlying addiction.*

13 PRINCIPLES OF OCCUPATIONAL AND ENVIRONMENTAL MEDICINE

Philip J. Landrigan

Work is a major part of life. Virtually every patient seen in a clinic, office, or hospital has spent 8 or more hours of every day and many months and years of life working. In their jobs, people can be exposed to dangerous chemicals, hazardous physical agents, and emotional stress, and they can suffer trauma. Any of these occupational exposures can cause disease—sometimes immediately and sometimes after an interval of years or decades.

The environment is another constant factor in human life that also can cause disease. Air pollution, lead, radon, and pesticides are examples of environmental agents that can cause illness and death. Tens of millions of people are exposed regularly to environmental toxins. Some are exposed to high levels in well-publicized disasters such as radiation at Chernobyl; lead near smelters; mercury in Minamata Bay, Japan; or the pesticide chlordecone (kepone) at Hopewell, Virginia. Many more are chronically exposed to lower levels.

Occupational and environmental toxins cause a broad range of illnesses, and these diseases can involve virtually every organ system. They include classic, well-described diseases such as lung cancer and malignant mesothelioma in workers exposed to asbestos; cancer of the bladder in dye workers; pneumoconiosis in coal miners; leukemia and lymphoma in people exposed to benzene; skin cancer in farmers and sailors chronically exposed to the sun; and chronic bronchitis in workers exposed to dusts. They also include newer entities recognized only in recent years such as dementia in persons exposed to solvents; sterility in men and women exposed to certain pesticides; and asthma and bronchitis in children and adults chronically exposed to particulate air pollution. Some of these diseases are acute; others are chronic. Some are manifest through obvious symptoms, whereas others involve more subtle degrees of dysfunction.

In the United States occupational exposures account each year for an estimated 50,000 to 70,000 deaths and for 350,000 new cases of illness. An additional 10 million people suffer traumatic injuries on the job each year and 10,000 die of occupational trauma. In the environment, the Centers for Disease Control and Prevention estimate that at least 3 million children suffer from lead poisoning and that tens of thousands have asthma induced by air pollution.

Occupational and environmental exposures always need to be considered in formulating a differential diagnosis. Because of the enormous numbers exposed and the wide range of illnesses, occupational and environmental exposures need to be sought when clinically evaluating every patient.

CLINICAL DIAGNOSIS OF OCCUPATIONAL AND ENVIRONMENTAL DISEASE

Occupational and environmental diseases are underdiagnosed. Many are incorrectly attributed to other causes, because frequently these diseases are not distinct in their clinical presentations and can closely resemble chronic diseases caused by other factors. Examples include (1) lung cancer caused by asbestos, radon, or beryllium incorrectly attributed to cigarette smoking; (2) severe abdominal pain caused by lead poisoning erroneously diagnosed as acute appendicitis; some such cases have resulted in unnecessary laparotomy; (3) dementia caused by organic solvents attributed to "old age" or to ethanol ingestion; and (4) renal failure caused by chronic exposure to cadmium ascribed to "idiopathic factors."

Only if a careful history of toxic occupational and environmental exposures is taken in these cases can a correct diagnosis be made. A barrier to accurate diagnosis is the long latency between occupational or environmental exposure and the appearance of disease. For some occupational and environmental cancers (e.g., mesothelioma caused by asbestos or lymphoma caused by benzene), this latency may span decades. Another impediment to diagnosis is that many people have had multiple toxic exposures at work or in the environment. At least until recently, workers were often not given the names of the materials with which they worked nor provided adequate information about the hazards of these materials.

The keys to properly diagnosing occupational and environmental disease are (1) obtaining an adequate history of occupational and environmental exposure for every patient; (2) possessing basic knowledge about the pathogenesis and clinical presentation of the major types of occupational and environmental disease; and (3) knowing how to report suspected cases of occupational and environmental illness to public health authorities so that additional cases caused by the same exposures can either be recognized or prevented.

Physicians should be especially knowledgeable about the occupational and environmental diseases that occur commonly in their practice areas, such as asbestosis and malignant mesothelioma in port cities with shipyards, pesticide intoxication in agricultural areas, and poisonings from solvents and exotic metals in regions that produce microelectronics.

OCCUPATIONAL AND ENVIRONMENTAL HISTORY

The history is the single most important instrument for obtaining information on the role of occupational and environmental factors in causing disease. Information about current and past exposures should routinely be sought at several logical points in taking a history on every patient. At each juncture, a few brief screening questions need systematically to be asked. Then if suspicious information is elicited, more detailed follow-up questions are needed. A routine screen for occupational and environmental disease consists of the following items:

1. In *the history of the present illness,* pay attention to any temporal relationship between onset of illness and toxic exposures in the workplace or the environment. For example, did symptoms begin shortly after the patient started a new job? Did they abate during vacation and then recrudesce after the patient resumed work? Were they related to the introduction of a new chemical or process? Did they correlate with episodes of pollution? Were there similar illnesses among co-workers or neighbors? Were the individuals who were more heavily exposed the more severely affected?

A possible occupational cause should be sought in every case of acute trauma (in children and adolescents as well as adults) and in every case of repetitive trauma, e.g., carpal tunnel syndrome.

2. In *the past medical history,* obtain a list of current and principal past occupations and of industries of employment. Each patient should be asked whether he/she ever developed illness as a consequence of his/her work.

3. In *the review of systems,* routinely ask every patient: "Do you now or have you previously had occupational or environmental exposure to asbestos, lead, fumes, chemicals, dusts, loud noise, radiation, or other toxic factors?" Also ask every patient whether he/she

believes that any of these factors may have caused or contributed to his/her illness. Even if a postulated connection between exposure and disease initially, appears tenuous, such suspicions always need to be carefully considered.

DETAILED EXPOSURE HISTORY. If information from the routine interview suggests an occupational or environmental cause, the physician should obtain a more detailed history of toxic exposures. Data on duration and intensity of exposures are particularly important. It is necessary to learn how the patient worked with the suspected toxin and to consider how he/she may have absorbed the material. Information should be obtained on all jobs ever held, places of employment, products manufactured, and materials with which the patient worked.

If toxic exposures are identified or strongly suspected and an occupational or environmental cause seems likely, further follow-up inquiries may need to be made through the patient's labor union, companies where he/she has been employed, company physicians, or state or local health departments. Information on toxic substances used in a workplace may be legally available to patients under the Records Access Standard and Hazard Communication Standard of the Occupational Safety and Health Administration and under state and local "right-to-know" laws.

REPORTING AND REFERRAL. If the diagnostic interview indicates or raises strongly the suspicion that disease is due to toxic occupational or environmental exposures, it is imperative that the physician report the case to state or local public health authorities. Many episodes of these diseases are in essence common-source outbreaks of highly preventable illness. Prompt reporting can lead to identifying additional cases earlier and to prevention by abating a common exposure source.

The physician may require access to specialized referral sources in occupational and environmental medicine. Two national organizations that maintain listings of occupational and environmental specialist physicians are the American College of Occupational and Environmental Medicine (Arlington Heights, Ill.) and the Association of Occupational and Environmental Clinics (Washington, DC). Another valuable resource is the US Public Health Service's National Institute for Occupational Safety and Health (Cincinnati, Ohio).

ESTABLISHING THE DIAGNOSIS OF OCCUPATIONAL OR ENVIRONMENTAL ILLNESS

If a history suggests an occupational or environmental cause, the following fundamental principles help make a diagnosis of occupational or environmental disease:

1. *Biologic Plausibility.* The likelihood that a disease is of occupational or environmental origin increases if the disease has previously been seen in other patients with the same or similar exposures, if a biologic mechanism is known, or if the disease has been seen in laboratory animals exposed experimentally to the chemical (or to a similar chemical). Bear in mind, however, that many thousands of chemicals to which workers are exposed regularly in industry and that have been dispersed into the environment have never been laboratory tested for their toxicity. Therefore, the possibility always exists of diagnosing a disease entity that has never previously been recognized, e.g., malignant mesothelioma in workers exposed to asbestos, hepatic angiosarcoma in workers exposed to vinyl chloride, and cancer of the bladder in aniline dye workers.

2. *Dose-Response.* The likelihood of occupational or environmental causation increases if the disease occurs more commonly and more seriously in the more heavily exposed members of a population. Bear in mind, however, that in the case of occupational and environmental carcinogens, there are no threshold levels of exposure below which safety is assured; any exposure to these agents is potentially carcinogenic, although heavier exposures carry greater risks. Also, agents that are allergens or chemical sensitizers can cause symptoms at very low exposure levels.

SENTINEL HEALTH EVENTS. To help physicians establish linkages between occupational exposures and disease, Rutstein and colleagues developed the concept of the sentinel health event. This is defined as "an unnecessary disease, disability, or untimely death whose occurrence signals a failure of prevention." Examples in-

TABLE 13-1. SELECTED LIST OF SENTINEL HEALTH EVENTS (OCCUPATIONAL)-OCCUPATIONALLY RELATED UNNECESSARY DISEASE, DISABILITY, AND UNTIMELY DEATH*

Condition	Industry/Occupation	Agent
Pulmonary tuberculosis	Physicians, medical personnel	*Mycobacterium tuberculosis*
Plague, tularemia, anthrax, rabies, and other infections	Farmers, ranchers, hunters, veterinarians, laboratory workers	Various infectious agents
Rubella	Medical personnel, intensive care personnel	Rubella virus
Hepatitis	Day-care center staff, orphanage staff, medical personnel	Hepatitis A, B, and C viruses
Ornithosis	Bird breeders, pet shop staff, poultry producers, veterinarians, zoo staff	*Chlamydia psittacy*
Malignant neoplasm of nasal cavities	Woodworkers, cabinet and furniture makers	Hardwood dust
		Formaldehyde
	Radium chemists and processors	Radium
	Nickel smelting and refining workers	Nickel
Malignant neoplasm of larynx	Asbestos industries and utilizers	Asbestos
Malignant neoplasm of trachea, bronchus, and lung	Asbestos industries and utilizers	Asbestos
	Topside coke oven workers	Coke oven emissions
	Uranium and fluorspar miners	Radon daughters
	Smelters, processors, users	Chromates, nickel, arsenic
	Mustard gas formulators	Mustard gas
	Ion exchange resin makers, chemists	Bis(chloromethyl) ether
Mesothelioma	Asbestos industries and utilizers	Asbestos
Malignant neoplasm of bone	Radium chemists and processors	Radium
Malignant neoplasm of scrotum	Automatic lathe operators, metalworkers	Mineral/cutting oils
	Coke oven workers, petroleum refiners	Soots and tars
Malignant neoplasm of bladder	Rubber and dye workers	Benzidine, naphthylamine, auramine, 4-nitrophenyl
Malignant neoplasm of kidney	Coke oven workers	Coke oven emissions
Lymphoid leukemia	Radiologists	Ionizing radiation
	Rubber industry; chemical industry	Benzene
Myeloid leukemia	Rubber industry; chemical industry	Benzene
	Radiologists	Ionizing radiation
Erythroleukemia	Rubber industry; chemical industry	Benzene
Nonautoimmune hemolytic anemia	Whitewashing and leather industry	Copper sulfate
	Electrolytic processes, smelting	Arsine
	Plastics industry	Trimellitic anhydride
Aplastic anemia	Chemical manufacture	TNT, benzene
	Radiologists, radium chemists	Ionizing radiation
Agranulocytosis or neutropenia	Explosives and pesticide industries	Phosphorus
	Pesticides, pigments, pharmaceuticals	Inorganic arsenic
		Benzene
Toxic encephalitis	Battery, smelter, and foundry workers	Lead
Parkinson's disease (secondary)	Manganese processing, battery makers, welders	Manganese
Inflammatory and toxic neuropathy	Pesticides, pigments, pharmaceuticals	Arsenic and arsenic compounds
	Furniture refinishers, degreasing operations	Hexane
	Plastics, rayon industries	Methyl butyl ketone, copper disulfide, other solvents
	Explosives industry	TNT
	Battery, smelter, and foundry workers	Lead
	Dentists, chloralkali plants, battery makers	Mercury
	Plastics industry, paper manufacturing	Acrylamide
	Microwave and radar technicians	Microwaves
	Radiologists	Ionizing radiation
	Blacksmiths, glass blowers, bakers	Infrared radiation
	Moth repellent formulators, fumigators	Naphthalene
Hearing loss	Many industries	Excessive noise
Raynaud's phenomenon (secondary)	Lumberjacks, chain sawyers, grinders	Vibration
	Vinyl chloride polymerization industry	Vinyl chloride monomer
Extrinsic asthma	Jewelry alloy and catalyst makers	Platinum
	Polyurethane, adhesive, paint workers	Isocyanates
	Plastics, dye, insecticide makers	Phthalic anhydride
	Foam workers, latex makers, biologists	Formaldehyde
	Bakers	Flour
	Woodworkers, furniture makers	Red cedar and other wood dust
Pneumoconiosis of coal workers	Coal miners	Coal dust
	Power plant workers	
Asbestosis	Asbestos industries	Asbestos
	Construction workers	
	Demolition workers	
	Building maintenance workers	
	Firefighters	
Silicosis	Quarrymen, sandblasters, miners, silica processors, mining, ceramic industries and foundries	Silica
Talcosis	Talc processors	Talc

TABLE 13–1. SELECTED LIST OF SENTINEL HEALTH EVENTS (OCCUPATIONAL)–OCCUPATIONALLY RELATED UNNECESSARY DISEASE, DISABILITY, AND UNTIMELY DEATH* *Continued*

Condition	Industry/Occupation	Agent
Chronic beryllium disease of the lung	Beryllium alloy workers, ceramic and cathode ray tube makers, nuclear reactor workers	Beryllium
Byssinosis	Cotton industry workers	Cotton, flax, hemp, and cotton-synthetic dusts
Acute bronchitis, pneumonitis, and pulmonary edema due to fumes and vapors	Alkali and bleach industries	Chlorine
	Silo fillers, arc welders	Nitrogen oxides
	Paper, refrigeration, oil industries	Sulfer dioxide
	Plastics industry	Trimellitic anhydride
Toxic hepatitis	Solvent utilizers, dry cleaners, plastics industry	Carbon tetrachloride chloroform, trichloroethylene
	Explosives and dye industries	Phosphorus, TNT
	Fumigators, fire extinguisher formulators	Ethylene dibromide
Acute or chronic renal failure	Battery makers, plumbers, solderers	Inorganic lead
	Electrolytic processes, smelting	Arsine
	Battery makers, jewelers, dentists	Inorganic mercury
	Fire extinguisher makers	Carbon tetrachloride
	Antifreeze manufacturers	Ethylene glycol
Male infertility	Pesticide formulators and applicators	Dibromochloropropane
Contact and allergic dermatitis	Leather tanning, poultry dressing plants, packing, adhesives and sealant industry, boat building and repair	Irritants (e.g., cutting fish oils, solvents, acids, alkalis, allergens)

* From Rutstein DD, Mullan RJ, Frazier TM, et al.: Sentinel health events (occupational): A basis for physician recognition and public health surveillance. Am J Public Health 73:1054, 1983.

clude unnecessary maternal deaths, an outbreak of cholera, or a single case of poliomyelitis. Extending the concept to occupational and environmental exposure, Rutstein and colleagues defined a sentinel health event (occupational) as "an unnecessary disease, disability or untimely death which is occupationally related." A selected list of these events is presented in Table 13–1. By scanning this list, physicians can identify work-related illnesses or exposures that may occur in their patients. Also, they can identify occupations and industries that may be pertinent to their local practice areas. This list represents an accessible starting point for developing competence in the differential diagnosis of occupational and environmental disease.

Goldman RH, Peters JM: The occupational and environmental health history. JAMA 246:2831, 1991. *A concise systematic approach to history taking.*

Rom WN: Environmental and Occupational Medicine. 2nd ed. Boston, Little, Brown, 1992. *The classic reference in the field.*

Rosenstock L, Cullen M: Clinical Occupational Medicine. 2nd ed. Philadelphia, WB Saunders, 1994. *A useful guide to common occupational and environmental health problems.*

Rutstein DD, Mullan RJ, Frazier TM, et al.: Sentinel health events (occupational): A basis for physician recognition and public health surveillance. Am J Public Health 73:1054, 1983. *A logical, accessible approach for linking occupational and environmental exposures to specific diagnoses.*

Terkel S: Working. New York, Ballantine Books, 1985. *A gifted writer records working people's first-hand stories of the hazards they face on the job.*

13.1 Radiation Injury

Arthur C. Upton

The term *radiation injury* denotes any abnormality of form or function caused by electromagnetic waves or accelerated atomic particles. The term is often applied also to the harmful effects of high-intensity ultrasound and electromagnetic fields. Because the different types of radiation differ markedly in their biologic effects, each must be dealt with separately in considering the injuries it can cause.

IONIZING RADIATION

Ionizing radiation occurs as electromagnetic waves of extremely short wavelength (Fig. 13–1) and also as accelerated atomic particles (e.g., electrons, protons, neutrons, alpha particles). The injuries

caused by ionizing radiation include mutagenic, carcinogenic, and teratogenic effects, as well as various acute and chronic tissue reactions (e.g., erythema, cataract of the lens, sterility, and depression of hematopoiesis).

ETIOLOGY. The biologic effects of ionizing radiation result from damage to DNA and other vital molecules by locally deposited energy. Doses of ionizing radiation are, therefore, measured in terms of energy deposition (Table 13–2).

All humans are exposed continuously to natural background ionizing radiation from (1) cosmic rays; (2) radium and other radioactive elements in the earth's crust; (3) potassium-40, carbon-14, and other radionuclides present normally in human tissues; and (4) inhaled radon and its daughter elements (Table 13–3). In people re-

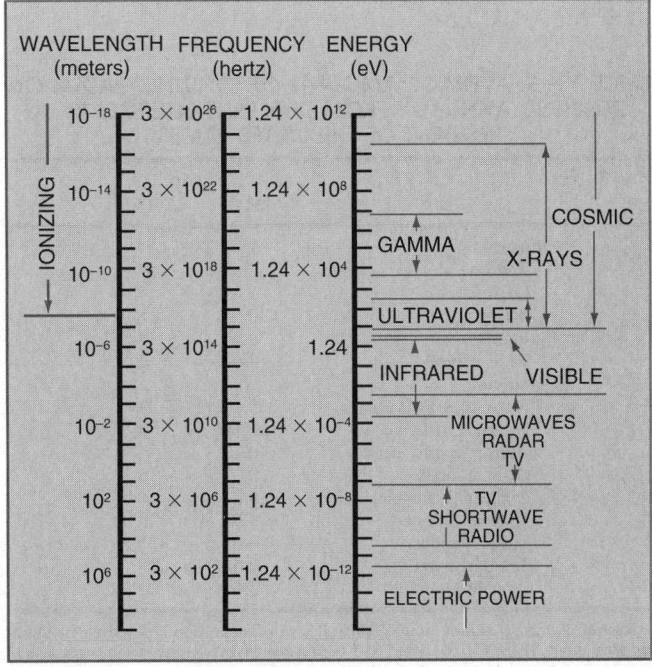

FIGURE 13–1. The electromagnetic spectrum. (From Mettler FA, Upton AC: Medical Effects of Ionizing Radiation. 2nd ed. Philadelphia, WB Saunders, 1994.)

TABLE 13–2. RADIATION QUANTITIES AND DOSE UNITS

Quantity	Dose Unit	Definition
Radioactivity	Becquerel (Bq)	One disintegration per second
Absorbed dose	Gray (Gy)	Energy deposited in tissue (1 joule/kg)
Equivalent dose	Sievert (Sv)	Absorbed dose weighted for the quality (potency) of the radiation
Effective dose	Sievert (Sv)	Equivalent dose weighted for the sensitivity of the exposed organs
Collective effective dose	Person-Sv	Effective dose applied to a population
Committed effective dose	Sievert (Sv)	Effective dose from a given intake of radioactivity, to be received over a period extending into the future

Modified from Phillips TL: Radiation injury. *In* Wyngaarden JB, Smith LH Jr, Bennett JC (eds): Cecil Textbook of Medicine. 19th ed. Philadelphia, WB Saunders, 1992, p 2351.

siding at mile-high elevations (as in Denver), the contribution from cosmic rays may be increased twofold, and at jet aircraft altitudes it may exceed 0.005 mSv (1 Sv = 100 rem) per hour. Likewise, in regions where the earth's crust is rich in radium, the contribution from this radionuclide may be similarly increased. Far larger in any case, however, is the contribution to the bronchial epithelium by inhaled radon and its daughters (Table 13–3).

In addition to the radiation they receive from natural sources, humans receive radiation from various man-made sources as well, the largest being x-rays used in medical diagnosis (see Table 13–2). Smaller amounts of radiation also are received from radioactive minerals in building materials, phosphate fertilizers, and crushed rock; radiation-emitting components of TV sets, smoke detectors, and other consumer products; radioactive fallout from atomic weapons; and nuclear power (Table 13–3).

Workers in various occupations are exposed to additional doses of ionizing radiation, depending on their job assignments and working conditions. The average annual effective dose received by monitored radiation workers in the United States is < 1 mSv, and < 1% approach the maximum permissible dose limit (50 mSv) in any given year.

INCIDENCE AND PREVALENCE. Precise data on the frequency of injuries caused by ionizing radiation are not available; however, most radiation therapy patients experience some injury of normal tissues within or adjoining the treatment field. Injuries attributable to excessive occupational exposure, although prevalent among radiation workers in the era preceding modern safety standards, are seldom encountered today. Nevertheless, some 285 nuclear reactor accidents were reported in various countries between 1945 and 1987 (excluding the Chernobyl accident in 1986), exposing more than 1350 persons and injuring 33 fatally. In most such accidents, the public was not directly affected; however, tens of thousands of inhabitants had to be evacuated from the surrounding area as a result of the Chernobyl accident, which caused radiation sickness in more than 200 emergency workers (injuring 31 fatally) and released enough radioactivity to result in a collective dose equivalent commitment of 600,000 person-Sv for the population of the Northern Hemisphere. Less catastrophic than reactor accidents, but even more numerous, have been accidents with medical and industrial gamma ray sources; a recent example, resulting from the improper disposal of a cesium-137 source in Goiania, Brazil, in 1987, injured dozens of unsuspecting victims, four of them fatally.

Another public health concern is the risk of cancer from exposure to ionizing radiation because carcinogenic effects of radiation have been well documented in pioneer radiologists, radium dial painters, Japanese atomic bomb survivors, radiation therapy patients, and uranium miners. To date, however, no definite evidence of such effects has been observed in contemporary radiation workers or populations residing in areas of high natural background radiation, and no more than 3% of all cancers in the general population are thought to be attributable to natural background ionizing irradiation, although a larger percentage of lung cancers may be attributable to indoor radon. Also of concern are heritable abnormalities resulting from the mutagenic and clastogenic effects of radiation, which have yet to be observed in humans although they are well documented in other organisms. From the available evidence, it is inferred that such effects probably account for < 1% of all genetically determined diseases in the human population.

Because prenatal irradiation has been observed in the past to cause death, malformations, cataracts, mental retardation, impairment of growth, and behavioral disorders, depending on the dose and the developmental stage of the embryo at the time of its exposure, special precautions are now taken to avoid exposing the embryo. As a result, such effects are largely prevented today.

EPIDEMIOLOGY. After its discovery by Roentgen in 1895, the x-ray was introduced so rapidly into medical practice that radiation injuries began to be encountered almost immediately. The first such injuries were predominantly acute skin reactions on the hands of those working with the early equipment, but in less than a decade other types of injury also were observed, including the first cancers attributed to radiation. Although clinical observations sufficed to identify the early reactions to radiation, epidemiologic studies have been necessary to identify and characterize most forms of radiation-induced cancer and other late effects.

PATHOGENESIS. Ionizing radiation, colliding randomly with atoms and molecules in its path, gives rise to ions and free radicals that break chemical bonds and cause other molecular alterations, ultimately injuring the affected cells. Any molecule may be thus altered, but DNA is the critical biologic target because of the limited redundancy of the genetic information it contains. A dose of radiation large enough to kill the average dividing cell (2 Sv) causes hundreds of lesions in its DNA molecules. The lesions produced by a densely ionizing radiation (e.g., proton or alpha particle) are generally less reparable than those produced by a sparsely ionizing radiation (e.g., x-ray or gamma ray).

TABLE 13–3. AVERAGE AMOUNTS OF IONIZING RADIATION RECEIVED ANNUALLY FROM DIFFERENT SOURCES BY A RESIDENT OF THE UNITED STATES

Source	Dose* (mSv)	Dose* (%)
Natural		
Radon†	2.0	55
Cosmic	0.27	8
Terrestrial	0.28	8
Internal	0.39	11
Total natural	3.0	82
Artificial		
X-ray diagnosis	0.39	11
Nuclear medicine	0.14	4
Consumer products	0.10	3
Occupational	< 0.01	< 0.3
Nuclear fuel cycle	< 0.01	< 0.03
Nuclear fallout	< 0.01	< 0.03
Miscellaneous‡	< 0.01	< 0.03
Total artificial	0.63	18
Total natural and artificial	3.6	100

Reprinted with permission from Health Effects of Exposure to Low Levels of Ionizing Radiation: BEIR V. Copyright 1990 by the National Academy of Sciences. Courtesy of the National Academy Press, Washington, DC.
* Average effective dose.
† Average effective dose to bronchial epithelium.
‡ Department of Energy facilities, smelters, transportation, etc.

Unrepaired or misrepaired damage to DNA may be expressed in the form of mutations, the frequency of which approximates 10^{-5} to 10^{-6} per locus per Sv. Because the mutation rate tends to increase in proportion with the dose, it is inferred that a single ionizing particle traversing a genetic target may suffice to cause a mutation. Radiation damage can also cause changes in chromosome number and structure, the yields of which are well enough characterized that their frequency in lymphocytes serves as a biologic dosimeter.

Radiation damage to genes, chromosomes, and other vital organelles may kill cells, especially dividing cells, which are radiosensitive as a class. Measured in terms of proliferative capacity, the survival of dividing cells tends to decrease exponentially with increasing dose, rapid exposure to 1 to 2 Sv generally sufficing to reduce the surviving population of such cells by about 50%. Except for lymphocytes and oocytes, which tend to die in interphase, most cells killed by irradiation die in mitosis.

Although the killing of cells is a stochastic process, too few cells are killed by a dose below 0.5 Sv to cause clinically detectable injury in most organs other than the testis and those of the embryo. The killing of dividing progenitor cells, if sufficiently extensive, can interfere with the orderly replacement of senescent cells, especially in tissues such as the epidermis, bone marrow, and intestinal epithelium, which are characterized by a normally high rate of cell turnover. The timing of the resulting atrophy varies, depending on the cell population dynamics within the tissue in question; in organs such as the liver and vascular endothelium, which are characterized by slow cell turnover, the expression of the injury is delayed. If the volume of tissue exposed is small or if the dose is accumulated slowly, the effects of irradiation may be counteracted in part by compensatory regenerative hyperplasia of surviving cells.

CLINICAL MANIFESTATIONS. Ionizing radiation injuries encompass a diversity of tissue reactions which vary markedly in dose-response relationships, manifestations, timing, and prognosis (Table 13–4). Except for mutagenic and carcinogenic effects, the reactions generally result from the killing of sizable numbers of cells in the exposed tissues and are not detectable unless the dose of radiation exceeds a substantial threshold. For this reason, the reactions are called *nonstochastic* (or *deterministic*) effects, in contrast to mutagenic and carcinogenic effects, which are presumed to have no thresholds and are considered to be *stochastic* in nature.

Tissues in which cells proliferate rapidly are generally the first to exhibit radiation injury. In such tissues, mitotic inhibition and cytologic abnormalities may be detectable immediately after irradiation, whereas ulceration, fibrosis, and other degenerative changes may not appear until months or years later.

Skin. After rapid exposure to a dose of 6 Sv or more, erythema typically appears within a day, lasts a few hours, and is followed 2 to 4 weeks later by one or more waves of deeper and more prolonged erythema, as well as epilation. Brief exposure to a dose in excess of 10 to 20 Sv may cause transepithelial injury, with moist desquamation, necrosis, and ulceration within 2 to 4 weeks. The ensuing fibrosis of the underlying dermis and vasculature may lead to atrophy and a second wave of ulceration months or years later.

Bone Marrow and Lymphoid Tissue. A dose of 2 to 3 Sv delivered rapidly to the whole body sufficiently destroys lymphocytes to depress the lymphocyte count and immune response within hours. Such a dose can also damage enough hematopoietic cells to cause profound leukopenia and thrombocytopenia within 3 to 5 weeks. If the dose exceeds 5 Sv, fatally severe infection and/or hemorrhage is likely to result (Table 13–5).

Intestine. The killing of epithelial stem cells is sufficiently extensive after an acute dose of 10 Sv to cause rapid denudation of the overlying intestinal villi. If the area affected is large, death from a fatal dysentery-like syndrome may ensue within days (see Table 13–5).

Respiratory Tract. Rapid exposure of the lung to a dose of 6 to 10 Sv damages alveolar cells and pulmonary vasculature sufficiently to result in acute pneumonitis within 1 to 3 months. If extensive, the process may lead to fatal respiratory failure within 6 months or pulmonary fibrosis and cor pulmonale months or years later.

Gonads. Spermatozoa are relatively radioresistant, but spermatogonia are highly radiosensitive; i.e., a dose of 0.15 Sv delivered rapidly to both testes causes oligospermia after a latent period of about 6 weeks, and a dose of 2 to 4 Sv may cause permanent sterility. Oocytes also are radiosensitive; a dose of 1.5 to 2.0 Sv de-

TABLE 13–4. ESTIMATED APPROXIMATE THRESHOLD DOSES OF CONVENTIONALLY FRACTIONATED X-RADIATION FOR CLINICALLY DETRIMENTAL NONSTOCHASTIC EFFECTS IN VARIOUS TISSUES

Organ	Injury at 5 Years	Threshold Dose (Gy)*	Irradiation Field (Area)
Skin	Ulcer, severe fibrosis	55	100 cm^2
Oral mucosa	Ulcer, severe fibrosis	60	50 cm^2
Esophagus	Ulcer, stricture	60	75 cm^2
Stomach	Ulcer, perforation	45	100 cm^2
Small intestine	Ulcer, stricture	45	100 cm^2
Colon	Ulcer, stricture	45	100 cm^2
Rectum	Ulcer, stricture	55	100 cm^2
Salivary glands	Xerostomia	50	50 cm^2
Liver	Liver failure, ascites	35	whole
Kidney	Nephrosclerosis	23	whole
Urinary bladder	Ulcer, contracture	60	whole
Testis	Permanent sterility	5–15	whole
Ovary	Permanent sterility	2–3	whole
Uterus	Necrosis, perforation	>100	whole
Vagina	Ulcer, fistula	90	5 cm
Breast, child	Hypoplasia	10	5 cm^2
Breast, adult	Atrophy, necrosis	>50	whole
Lung	Pneumonitis, fibrosis	40	lobe
Capillaries	Telangiectasis, fibrosis	50–60	—
Heart	Pericarditis, pancarditis	40	whole
Bone, child	Arrested growth	20	10 cm^2
Bone, adult	Necrosis, fracture	60	10 cm^2
Cartilage, child	Arrested growth	10	whole
Cartilage, adult	Necrosis	60	whole
CNS (brain)	Necrosis	50	whole
Spinal cord	Necrosis, transection	50	5 cm^2
Eye	Panophthalmitis, hemorrhage	55	whole
Cornea	Keratitis	50	whole
Lens	Cataract	5	whole
Ear (inner)	Deafness	>60	whole
Thyroid	Hypothyroidism	45	whole
Adrenal	Hypoadrenalism	>60	whole
Pituitary	Hypopituitarism	45	whole
Muscle, child	Hypoplasia	20–30	whole
Muscle, adult	Atrophy	>100	whole
Bone marrow	Hypoplasia	2	whole
Bone marrow	Hypoplasia, fibrosis	20	localized
Lymph nodes	Atrophy	33–45	—
Lymphatics	Sclerosis	50	—
Fetus	Death	2	whole

From Rubin P, Casarett GW: A direction for clinical radiation pathology: The tolerance dose. *In* Vaeth JM (ed.): Frontiers of Radiation Therapy and Oncology. Basel, Karger, 1972; and Nonstochastic effects of ionizing radiation. ICRP Publication 41. Ann ICRP 14:1, 1984, with kind permission from Elsevier Science Ltd, The Boulevard, Langford Land, Kidlington OX5 1GB, UK.

* Dose causing effect in 1% to 5% of exposed persons.

livered to both ovaries causes temporary sterility and a larger dose permanent sterility, depending on the woman's age at the time of exposure.

Lens of the Eye. Acute exposure of the lens to more than 1 Sv may lead within months to a microscopic posterior polar opacity, and 2 to 3 Sv received in a single brief exposure (or 5.5 to 14 Sv accumulated over a period of months) may result in a vision-impairing cataract.

Other Tissues and Organs. Other tissues and organs (see Table 13–4) are relatively less radiosensitive than the aforementioned, except for those of the embryo, as discussed below. All tissues, however, are more radiosensitive when rapidly growing.

Whole-Body Radiation Injury. Brief exposure of a major part of the body to more than 1 Sv may cause the *acute radiation syndrome.* This syndrome is characterized by (1) an initial prodromal stage in which there are malaise, anorexia, nausea, and vomiting; (2) an ensuing latent period; (3) a second (main) phase of illness; and (4) either recovery or death (see Table 13–5). The main phase of the illness usually takes one of four main forms: (1) hematologic, (2) gastrointestinal, (3) neurovascular, or (4) pulmonary, depending on the size and anatomic distribution of the dose (see Table 13–5).

TABLE 13-5. SYMPTOMS, THERAPY, AND PROGNOSIS OF WHOLE-BODY IONIZING RADIATION INJURY

	0–1 Sv	1–2 Sv	2–6 Sv	6–10 Sv	10–20 Sv	>50 Sv
Therapeutic needs	None	Observation	Specific treatment	Possible treatment	Palliative	Palliative
Vomiting	None	5–50%	>3 Gy, 100%	100%	100%	100%
Time to nausea, vomiting	—	3 hours	2 hours	1 hour	30 minutes	<30 minutes
Main locus of injury	None	Lymphocytes	Bone marrow	Bone marrow	Small bowel	Brain
Symptoms and signs	—	Moderate leukopenia	Leukopenia, hemorrhage, epilation	Leukopenia, hemorrhage, epilation	Diarrhea, fever, electrolyte imbalance	Ataxia, coma, convulsions
Critical period	—	—	4–6 weeks	4–6 weeks	5–14 days	1–4 hours
Therapy	Reassurance	Observation	Transfusion of granulocytes, platelets; antibiotics	Transfusion; antibiotics; bone marrow transplant	Fluids and salts; possible bone marrow transplant	Palliative
Prognosis	Excellent	Excellent	Guarded	Guarded	Poor	Hopeless
Lethality	None	None	0–80%	80–100%	100%	100%
Time of death	—	—	2 months	1–2 months	2 weeks	1–2 days
Cause of death	—	—	Infection, hemorrhage	Hemorrhage, infection	Enteritis, infection	Cerebral edema

Modified from Phillips TL: Radiation injury. *In* Wyngaarden JB, Smith LH Jr, Bennett JC (eds.): Cecil Textbook of Medicine. 19th ed. Philadelphia, WB Saunders, 1992, p 2354.

Localized or Regional Radiation Injury. In contrast to the acute radiation syndrome, manifestations of which are dramatic and relatively prompt, reactions to localized irradiation in most tissues tend to evolve more slowly and not to produce symptoms or signs unless the volume of tissue irradiated and the dose are large (see Table 13–4). When the injury is produced by a radionuclide, it follows the anatomic distribution of the radionuclide and the resulting radiation, which may be influenced by the physicochemical state in which the radionuclide(s) is encountered, as well as its portal of entry into the body.

Heritable (Genetic) Effects of Radiation. Radiation-induced heritable mutations and chromosomal abnormalities, although well documented in other organisms, have yet to be observed in humans, in spite of intensive study of more than 76,000 children of Japanese atomic bomb survivors, carried out over four decades, in whom no definite evidence of heritable radiation effects have been detectable, as measured by untoward pregnancy outcomes, neonatal deaths, malignancies, balanced chromosomal rearrangements, sex-chromosome aneuploids, alterations of serum or erythrocyte protein phenotypes, changes in gender ratio, or disturbances in growth and development. On the basis of the existing evidence, it is inferred that a dose of at least 1.0 Sv is required to double the rate of heritable mutations in human germ cells, and that, consequently, <1% of all genetically determined disease is attributable to natural background irradiation.

Carcinogenic Effects of Radiation. Many, but not all, types of benign and malignant growths have been observed as inducible by irradiation. The induced growths characteristically take years or decades to appear and possess no features distinguishable from those arising through other causes. With few exceptions, moreover, they have been detectable only after relatively large doses (>0.5 Sv) and have varied with the type of neoplasm as well as the age and gender of the exposed population. Because the existing data do not suffice to describe the dose-incidence relationship precisely or to define how long after irradiation the risk of cancer may remain elevated in an exposed population, assessment of the risks of low-level irradiation must be based on assumptions about these parameters. Such assessments (Table 13–6) have depended heavily on findings in the atomic bomb survivors, whose overall incidence of cancer appears to have increased as a linear nonthreshold function of their radiation dose. Such estimates cannot be assumed to predict the risk of cancer attributable to a dose accumulated over a period of weeks, months, or years, however, because experiments with laboratory animals have shown the carcinogenic potency of x-rays or gamma rays to decrease by a factor of 2 to 10 if the exposure is sufficiently prolonged.

Effects of Prenatal Irradiation. The embryo is especially vulnerable to killing if exposed before implantation, and it is susceptible to malformations and other developmental disturbances if exposed during subsequent stages in organogenesis. Evidence also suggests that the embryo and fetus are sensitive to the carcinogenic effects of radiation. Among various disturbances in growth and development, the dose-dependent increase in frequency of severe mental retardation and the dose-dependent decrease in IQ test scores in atomic bomb survivors who were irradiated between the 8th and the 15th week (and, to a lesser extent, the 16th and the 25th week) after conception are particularly noteworthy.

DIAGNOSIS. Any facility likely to deal with radiation injuries should be able to cope with such injuries and should have personnel on call who are appropriately trained and equipped for the purpose. At the outset, to evaluate the dose and to determine whether the patient has been contaminated with radionuclides, the nature of the exposure and any measurements by film badges or other detectors should be reviewed in detail. If exposure to radionuclides is known or suspected, radioactivity measurements of the whole body, skin, other tissue, blood, urine, and/or body fluid may be indicated to identify the isotope(s) and evaluate the dose. Malaise, anorexia, nausea, and vomiting suggest a total-body dose larger than 1 Sv, as do signs of erythema, hemorrhage, or infection in the skin, conjunctivae, or mucous membranes. The depth of lymphopenia within the first 24 hours also varies with the size of the total-body dose, and although the granulocyte count may be temporarily elevated during the first 24 to 48 hours, the rapidity with which it and the platelet count fall in the ensuing 2 to 4 weeks also varies with the total-body dose. Cytogenetic analysis of cultured lymphocytes for chromosomal aberrations can provide another useful index of exposure.

TREATMENT. In managing radiation injury, good medical judgment and first aid come first. Hence, even if the patient has been heavily irradiated, he/she should be evaluated for other forms

TABLE 13-6. ESTIMATED LIFETIME RISKS OF CANCER ATTRIBUTABLE TO 0.1 Sv RAPID IRRADIATION OF SPECIFIC TISSUES

Type or Site of Cancer	Excess Cancer Deaths per 100,000 (No.)	(%)*
Stomach	110	18
Lung	85	3
Colon	85	5
Leukemia (excluding CLL)	50	10
Urinary bladder	30	5
Esophagus	30	10
Breast	20	1
Liver	15	8
Gonads	10	2
Thyroid	8	8
Bone	5	5
Skin	2	2
Remainder	50	1
TOTAL	500	2

Modified from 1990 Recommendations of the International Commission on Radiological Protection. ICRP Publication 60. Ann ICRP 21:3, 1991, with kind permission from Elsevier Science Ltd, The Boulevard, Langford Lane, Kidlington OX5 1GB, UK.

* Percentage increase in the "spontaneous" risk of cancer of the same tissue expected for a nonirradiated population.

of injury (e.g., burns, mechanical trauma, smoke inhalation). If radioactive contamination is known or suspected, those handling the patient should wear gloves and other protective clothing and should take precautions to isolate all contaminated objects.

Apart from symptomatic treatment, management of the hematologic form of acute radiation syndrome is similar to that used for pancytopenic leukemia, including reverse isolation, antibiotics to combat infection, granulocyte and platelet transfusions as needed, and intravenous fluids as required to combat dehydration and electrolyte loss. Colony-stimulating factors and interleukin may be beneficial in patients exposed to 6 to 10 Sv. Bone marrow transplantation (see Ch. 130) may be life-saving after a dose of 7 to 10 Sv if a suitably matched donor is available (specimens of marrow and peripheral blood for tissue typing should be obtained as early as possible).

For localized injuries, the treatment depends on their anatomic location and severity. Dry and moist desquamation of the skin, most common injuries requiring treatment, are usually managed adequately by simple cleansing. Large or ulcerated lesions, on the other hand, should be covered with lanolin and closed dressings that are changed regularly; severe injuries may require resection of necrotic tissue and skin grafting.

In the event of radioactive contamination, steps to minimize the uptake and retention of isotope should be taken; e.g., contaminated areas should be rinsed; the mouth, nose, and bronchial tree lavaged; and the gastrointestinal tract purged, if necessary. Additional measures to inhibit the uptake and retention of specific radionuclides also may be indicated.

PROGNOSIS. After a total-body dose of 2 Sv or less, survival is probable with little or no treatment (see Table 13–5); in the 2 to 10 Sv range, appropriate treatment can afford a high rate of survival. If the injury is localized, the prognosis depends on the nature and severity of the reaction. While recovery is the rule after minor, acute reactions, delayed reactions (see Tables 13–4 and 13–5) tend to be irreversible and progressive.

PREVENTION. Because the mutagenic and carcinogenic effects of ionizing radiation have no thresholds, unnecessary exposures should be avoided, and any doses to radiation workers and patients should be kept as low as reasonably achievable, with particular care that they not exceed the relevant maximum permissible doses (e.g., 50 mSv per year occupational whole-body radiation). To this end, facilities using radiation or radiation sources should be appropriately designed and equipped and should provide specialized training and supervision for all workers who may be occupationally exposed. Inasmuch as indoor radon accounts for the bulk of the public's exposure to ionizing radiation, measures to limit excessive doses from this source also are warranted.

NONIONIZING RADIATION

ULTRAVIOLET RADIATION. The ultraviolet radiation (UVR) spectrum (see Fig. 13–1) is subdivided, for convenience, into three bands: UVA, or "black light," 400 to 320 nm; UVB, 320 to 280 nm; and UVC, which is germicidal, 280 to 100 nm. UVR does not penetrate deeply into human tissues, with the result that the injuries it causes are confined chiefly to the skin and eyes.

Etiology. The largest source of UVR for the public is sunlight, which varies in intensity with latitude, elevation, and season. Important man-made sources include sun and tanning lamps, welding arcs, plasma torches, germicidal and black-light lamps, electric arc furnaces, hot-metal operations, mercury-vapor lamps, and some lasers. Low-intensity sources include fluorescent lamps and certain laboratory equipment.

Incidence and Prevalence. Reactions of the skin to UVR, common among fair-skinned people, include sunburn, skin cancers (basal cell and squamous cell carcinomas and to a lesser extent melanomas), aging of the skin, solar elastosis, and solar keratosis. Injuries of the eye include photokeratitis, which may result from brief exposure to a high-intensity UVR source ("welder's flash") or more prolonged exposure to intense sunlight ("snow blindness"); cortical cataract; and pterygium.

Pathogenesis. The effects of UVR are attributable primarily to its absorption in DNA; pyrimidine dimers are produced, which cause mutational changes in exposed cells. Sensitivity to UVR may be increased by DNA repair defects (as in xeroderma pigmentosum), by agents (e.g., caffeine) that inhibit the repair enzymes, and

by photosensitizing agents (e.g., psoralens, sulfonamides, tetracyclines, nalidixic acid, sulfonylureas, thiazides, phenothiazines, furocoumarins, and coal tar) which produce UVR-absorbing DNA photoproducts. The carcinogenic action of UVR, in addition to being mediated through direct effects on the exposed cells, depresses local immunity as well. UVB in sunlight, although far less intense than UVA, plays a more important role in sunburn and skin carcinogenesis. UVA, however, also contributes to the latter, as well as to tanning, some photosensitivity reactions, and aging of the skin.

Clinical Aspects. See Parts XXVI (Skin Diseases) and XXV (Eye Diseases).

Prevention. Excessive exposure to sunlight or other sources of UVR should be avoided, especially in fair-skinned individuals. Protective clothing, UVR-screening lotions or creams, and UVR-blocking sunglasses should be used. To protect occupationally exposed workers, the National Institute of Occupational Safety and Health has recommended a limit of 1.0 mW per cm^2 (mW = milliWatts) for periods longer than 1000 seconds and 1000 mW per cm^2 (1.0 J per cm^2) for periods of 1000 seconds or less. Globally, the protective layer of ozone in the stratosphere is being depleted by chlorfluorocarbons and other air pollutants, and every 1% decrease in ozone is expected to increase the UVR reaching the earth by 1 to 2%, thereby increasing the rates of nonmelanotic skin cancer by 2 to 6%.

VISIBLE LIGHT. Visible light consists of electromagnetic waves varying in wavelength from 380 nm (violet) to 760 nm (red) (see Fig. 13–1). Too little illumination can cause eyestrain or seasonal affective disorder (SAD), whereas too bright a light can injure the retina.

Etiology. Bright, continuously visible light normally elicits an aversion response to protect the eye against injury, so few sources of light other than the sun in a solar eclipse are large and bright enough to cause a retinal burn under normal viewing conditions.

Pathogenesis. Photochemical reactions in the retina from sustained exposure to intensities exceeding 0.1 mW per cm^2, such as can result from fixing on a bright source of light, may suffice to produce photochemical blue-light injury, and brief exposure of the retina to intensities exceeding 10 W per cm^2, depending on image size, may cause a retinal burn.

Clinical Aspects. See Part XXV (Eye Diseases).

Prevention. Common sense usually suffices to prevent excessive exposure of the retina to light; however, in situations involving potential exposure to high-intensity sources such as carbon arcs or lasers, appropriate training, proper design of equipment, and protective eye shields are important.

INFRARED RADIATION. Infrared radiation (IR) consists of electromagnetic waves ranging in wavelength from 7×10^{-5} m to 3×10^{-2} m (see Fig. 13–1). The injuries caused by IR are chiefly burns of the skin and cataracts of the lens of the eye.

Etiology. Potentially hazardous sources include furnaces, ovens, welding arcs, molten glass, molten metal, and heating lamps.

Incidence and Prevalence. The warning sensation of heat usually prompts aversion in time to prevent burning of the skin by IR; however, the lens of the eye is vulnerable in lacking heat-sensing and heat-dissipating ability. As a result, glass blowers, blacksmiths, oven operators, and those working around heating and drying lamps are at increased risk of IR-induced cataracts.

Clinical Aspects. See Parts XXVI and XXV.

Prevention. Controlling IR hazards requires appropriately shielding sources, training potentially exposed persons, and using protective clothing and goggles.

MICROWAVE RADIATION. Microwave and radiofrequency radiation (MW/RFR) consists of electromagnetic waves ranging in frequency from about 3 kHz to 300 GHz (see Fig. 13–1). The injuries caused by MW/RFR consist primarily of burns of the skin and other tissues. MW/RFR can also interfere, however, with cardiac pacemakers and other medical devices.

Etiology. Sources of MW/RFR are used widely in radar, television, radio, other telecommunications systems, various industrial operations (e.g., heating, welding, and melting of metals; processing of wood and plastic; high-temperature plasma), household appliances (e.g., microwave ovens), and medical applications (e.g., diathermy and hyperthermia).

Incidence and Prevalence. Isolated cases of skin burns, thermal injury of deeper tissues, and even death from hyperthermia have been encountered in industrial MW/RFR sources. Burns have also resulted from faulty or improperly used household microwave ovens and from the overexposure of patients with impaired cutaneous pain and temperature senses that usually warn of impending injury. Other effects reported in the literature but as yet inconclusively documented include cataract of the lens, impairment of fertility, developmental disturbances, neurobehavioral abnormalities, depression of immunity, and increased risk of cancer.

Pathogenesis. The biologic effects of MW/RFR are primarily thermal in nature. Because of the deep penetration of MW/RFR, the cutaneous burns it causes tend to involve dermal and subcutaneous tissues and to heal slowly.

Clinical Aspects. See Part XXVI (Skin Diseases).

Prevention. Proper design and shielding of MW/RFR sources, along with appropriately training and supervising potentially exposed persons (especially those wearing cardiac pacemakers or other sensitive devices) are indicated. In general, because detectable heating of tissue requires MW/RFR power densities > 10 W per cm^2, avoiding such exposure, as prescribed by existing federal standards, suffices to prevent injury.

EXTREMELY LOW-FREQUENCY ELECTROMAGNETIC FIELDS. Extremely low-frequency electromagnetic fields (EMF's) are those ranging in frequency from 1 to 3000 Hz, including the 50 to 60 Hz fields associated with alternating currents in electric power distribution systems and appliances. Exposure to such fields is not known to be hazardous, but data suggesting that it may cause reproductive abnormalities and carcinogenic effects have aroused public health concern.

Etiology. The earth is surrounded by a naturally occurring EMF ranging in frequency from the low end of the extremely low-frequency region to radiofrequencies that exist briefly as a result of lightning discharges. Localized EMF's also are generated by electric power lines, transformers, motors, household appliances, video-display tubes (VDT's), and various medical devices, notably nuclear magnetic resonance (NMR) imaging systems. These localized fields are generally stronger than naturally existing ones; e.g., EMF flux densities near common household appliances may range up to 270 mG, compared with the average value of 0.6 mG for the earth's magnetic field.

Incidence and Prevalence. Exceptionally strong fields may affect electrically active tissues (nerves, neuromusculature, heart) and cardiac pacemakers and may raise body temperature. In addition, epidemiologic data have suggested that (1) residential exposure of children to weaker EMF's may increase their risks of leukemia, (2) occupational exposure of male utility workers may increase their risks of brain cancer and leukemia, and (3) chronic exposure of pregnant women through VDT's may increase their risks of miscarriages and of bearing children with birth defects. Although yet to be established, the possibility of such effects has led some public health authorities to urge caution.

Pathogenesis. Evaluation the epidemiologic data is complicated by the lack of any known biologic basis for their cause, especially because the 60-Hz currents emanating from normal nerve and muscle activity are far stronger than those attributable to 1 to 10 mG external 60-Hz fields. Such fields have, nevertheless, been reported to influence ion transport, melatonin secretion, and tumor promotion in some model systems.

Prevention. Persons wearing pacemakers should avoid EMF's stronger than 0.5 mT, such as exist around transformers, accelerators, NMR systems, and other electric devices; and areas containing such fields should be posted with warning signs. Exposure of workers should also be limited, in accordance with the guidelines recommended by the FDA and other authorities.

ULTRASOUND. Although frequently classified with nonionizing radiation, ultrasound actually consists of mechanical vibrations at inaudibly high frequencies (i.e., > 16 KHz) and is not a component of the electromagnetic spectrum. Deleterious effects from prolonged exposure to high-power ultrasound include headache, malaise, tinnitus, vertigo, hypersensitivity to light and sound, and peripheral neuritis. Low-level exposure to ultrasound has not been shown conclusively to cause injury, but the possibility of adverse effects on the embryo has been suggested.

Etiology. High-power, low-frequency ultrasound is used widely in science and industry for cleaning, degreasing, plastic welding, liquid extracting, atomizing, homogenizing, and emulsifying operations, as well as in medicine for such applications as lithotripsy. Low-power, high-frequency ultrasound is used widely in analytic work and in medical diagnosis (e.g., ultrasonography).

Incidence and Prevalence. Low-frequency ultrasound, transmitted through the air or through bodily contact with the generating source, has been observed to cause a variety of problems in occupationally exposed workers, including headache, earache, tinnitus, vertigo, malaise, photophobia, hyperacusis, peripheral neuritis, and autonomic polyneuritis. Similar complaints may result from excessive exposure to high-frequency ultrasound through bodily contact with the source; however, adverse effects have not been demonstrated to result from exposure to high-frequency ultrasound at the low power levels used in medical ultrasonography.

Pathogenesis. The biologic effects of ultrasound are similar in mechanism to those of mechanical vibration.

Prevention. Protection against ultrasound injury requires appropriately isolating and insulating generating sources, as well as proper training and ear protective devices for those working around such sources. Yearly audiometric and neurologic examinations of such workers also are advisable.

AMA Council on Scientific Affairs: Harmful effects of ultraviolet radiation. JAMA 262:380, 1989. *A good review of the biomedical hazards of ultraviolet radiation.*

Hall EJ: Radiobiology for the Radiologist. 3rd ed. Philadelphia, JB Lippincott, 1988. *Excellent introductory text on the biologic effects of ionizing radiation.*

Mettler FA, Kelsey CA, Ricks RC: Medical Management of Radiation Accidents. Boca Raton, Fl, CRC Press, 1990. *An excellent and comprehensive review of the management of people accidentally exposed to ionizing radiation.*

Mettler FA, Upton AC: Medical Effects of Ionizing Radiation. 2nd ed. Philadelphia, WB Saunders, 1994. *A comprehensive review of the effects of ionizing radiation on human beings.*

National Academy of Sciences-National Research Council: Health Effects of Exposure to Low Levels of Ionizing Radiation. BEIR V. Washington, DC, National Academy Press, 1990. *An authoritative review of the health hazards of low-level ionizing radiation.*

Office of Technology Assessment, US Congress: Biological Effects of Power Frequency Electric and Magnetic Fields—Background Paper. Washington, DC, US Government Printing Office, OTA-BP-E-53, 1989. *A detailed review of the biologic and medical effects of electric magnetic fields.*

Shapiro J: Radiation Protection: A Guide for Scientists and Physicians. 3rd ed. Cambridge, Harvard University Press, 1990. *Standard introductory text for radiation workers.*

Shore RE: Nonionizing Radiation. *In* Rom WN (ed): Environmental and Occupational Medicine. Boston, Little, Brown and Co, 1992, p 1093. *An excellent review of the medical effects of nonionizing radiation.*

1990 Recommendations of the International Commission on Radiological Protection. ICRP Publication 60. Ann ICRP 21:3, 1991. *An authoritative statement of principles and procedures for protection against ionizing radiation.*

13.2 Electrical Injury
Cleon W. Goodwin

DEFINITION AND PREVALENCE. Electrical injury manifests in a variety of forms, ranging from cardiopulmonary arrest and minimal tissue damage to devastating electrocution and vaporization of major body parts. Tissue damage is a direct consequence of the flow of electrical current, causing both thermal tissue damage and electrical breakdown of cell membranes. The extent of injury is proportional to current, voltage, duration of exposure, cellular architecture, and whether the electricity is alternating current (AC) or direct current (DC). AC, the more common cause of electrical injury, is more dangerous than DC because it can produce tonic muscle contractions, and the victim may be unable to release the source of electricity. Further, cardiac arrest and coma frequently accompany electrocution with AC, and these events are most likely to occur at current frequencies of 50 to 60 cycles per second. As frequency increases above 60 cycles per second, tissue damage and risk of cardiac arrest decrease. Tissue damage caused by line voltages <1000 volts arbitrarily is designated low-voltage injury. High-tension electrical injury is caused by line voltages >1000 volts.

Electricity causes injury by four mechanisms: direct contact, conduction, arc, and secondary ignition. Low-voltage electrical sources produce direct injury at the point of contact. Skin and subcutaneous tissue are involved most commonly, although occasionally muscle and bone beneath the cutaneous burn may be damaged. High-voltage current not only causes direct injury at the point of contact but also damages tissues that conduct the electricity through the body. Arc burns occur without the source of electricity actually contacting the body surface. Very high voltages are required to produce charge transfer, and when arcing occurs, extremely high temperatures (3000° C) are produced. The duration of the arc is brief, and the "flash" injury produced is usually limited to the body surface. A variant of arc injury occurs when electrical current being conducted along a body part surfaces and flashes over in the axilla and other flexion creases. Finally, burns occur when the electrical source ignites clothing and other flammable materials. Very deep flame burns may occur, especially if the patient is unconscious. The victim may not be able to verify actual circumstances, and patient evaluation and management must assume that diverse multisystem effects of electrical injury may be present.

In an adult, electrical burns are occupational hazards. However, in recent years, the increasing number of electrical injuries reflects the technologic sophistication of society. Sport parachuting and hot air ballooning and installation of home radio and television antennas have become common causes of electrical injuries. In urban environments, electric-powered mass transit conduits are one of the most common sources of such injuries. Household appliances cause most electrical injuries in children. Lightning injury affects all age groups, especially in rural areas. Electrical injuries comprise 1 to 5% of burn center admissions and up to 15% of deaths.

PATHOGENESIS. Meticulous laboratory investigations have verified that tissue damage associated with electrical injury occurs when electrical energy is converted to thermal energy and causes joule heating of tissue. The resulting injury is a thermal burn that produces physiologic responses similar to those caused by other mechanisms of thermal injury. Skin represents the initial barrier to current flow and is an effective insulator to deeper tissues. After electrical contact and the onset of current flow, the skin undergoes coagulation necrosis and desiccates. With low-voltage injuries, the charred skin at the point of contact terminates current flow and limits the extent of injury. The skin surrounding the contact point may sustain an arc burn as the increase in skin resistance terminates current flow (Fig. 13–2). At high voltages (>1000 volts), skin resistance initially is overcome, and current flow through deep tissue in the body is relatively unimpeded. Except for bone, these internal tissues act as a volume conductor, offering little resistance to flow. Current flow is terminated when the tissue at the point of electrical contact desiccates and resistance increases markedly. At this point, electrical arcing frequently occurs. The charred tissue then acts as an electrical insulator. Deep tissue damage is related to the density of current flow through these tissues. Heat production and hence thermal injury depend on the density of current flow. In body parts with small cross-sectional areas, such as an extremity, current density is high, and tissue destruction is severe. In large cross-sectional areas, such as the trunk, current density is reduced and deep injuries are unusual. Superficial tissues cool faster than deep tissues. Because bone has high resistance to current flow, it heats to higher temperatures than does surrounding soft tissue. As a result, the most severely damaged soft tissues are usually muscle and nerves directly adjacent to the bone, a position almost impervious to clinical detection. The most severe cutaneous and deep injuries are adjacent to contact sites, and damage decreases with increasing distance from contact points.

Recent investigations strongly suggest that in addition to joule heating of tissue, direct effects of electricity on the electrical and architectural properties of cell membranes are responsible for much of the resulting tissue damage, especially during the early phase of current flow. Experimental studies have shown that rhabdomyolysis and neurolysis may occur following electrical contact associated with only small increases in tissue temperature.

The extent of tissue injury appears to be determined at the time of electrical contact. Progressive soft tissue injury probably does not occur despite the clinical observation that muscle that appears to be viable immediately after electrical injury appears necrotic several days later. In addition, electrical energy may cause lesser degrees of damage without producing coagulation necrosis. This phenomenon may explain the transient abnormalities of visceral organ function that follow electrical injury. In the heart, this minor damage may have disastrous consequences. In electrically injured patients who experience fatal cardiac arrest, focal necrosis of the myocardium and the specialized tissue of the sinus and atrioventricular nodes and contraction band necrosis of smooth muscle cells of the coronary arteries are widespread.

CLINICAL MANIFESTATIONS. High-voltage electrical injuries commonly involve multiple organ systems and dictate treatment in specialized burn centers with broad multidisciplinary capabilities. Many of the abnormalities produced by electrocution may not be reflected by the surface appearance of the electrical burn and may manifest clinically at any time during hospitalization. Consequently, meticulous serial examinations and documentation of electrically injured patients are necessary for both medical and legal assessment and for planning.

Cardiopulmonary Arrest. Cardiopulmonary arrest is common in patients with high-voltage electrical injuries, particularly lightning injury. Arrhythmias, conduction disturbances, and infarct patterns may be present on the admission electrocardiogram. Most arrhythmias are transitory, whereas conduction delays and infarct patterns are likely to be permanent. In those few patients who have undergone long-term cardiac function studies and angiography, these permanent electrocardiographic findings appear to represent no physiologic abnormalities.

Burn Wound. In patients who survive to be admitted to the hospital, the electrical burn itself becomes a major focus of treatment. Most high-voltage electrical injuries present with contact burns at the locations where the electrical current has entered or left the body. These contact burns typically are charred and excavated, and deeper anatomic structures may be visible in the depths of the wound (Fig. 13–3). Contrary to popular notions, these contact wounds have no unique characteristics that identify them as so-called entrance or exit sites. These contact areas are usually surrounded by less severe burns of variable depth. If ignition of clothing has occurred, the patient may have extensive cutaneous burns unrelated to the site of electrical contact.

Underlying injury to major muscle compartments is accompanied by edema formation, which may be accentuated by concomitant fluid resuscitation. When the tissue pressure beneath this muscle fascia increases, signs of vessel and nerve compression appear. Loss of sensation, pain, and decreased pulses indicate the presence of a compartment syndrome. Palpation often demonstrates tense muscle compartments, especially when the affected extremity is compared with an opposite unburned extremity. Even with good blood flow, the burned extremity may be cool to the touch and have no palpable pulse. Therefore, circulatory integrity is best judged by Doppler ultrasonography of distal pulses. Compartment pressure can be

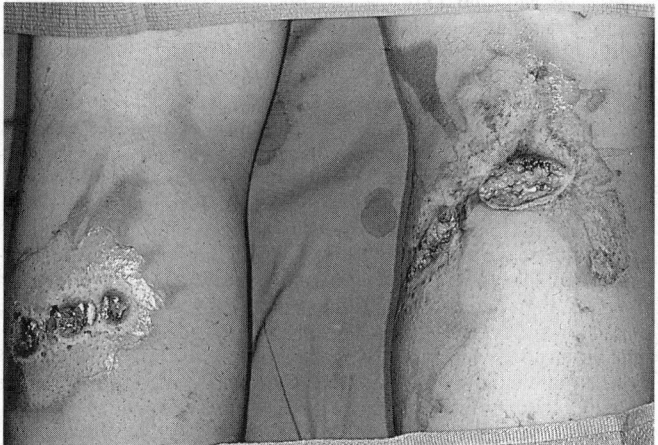

FIGURE 13–2. Charring of the skin of both calves indicates points of contact with a high-voltage electrical current. These contact points are surrounded by full-thickness cutaneous burns caused by arcing of current. The extent of deep tissue destruction is often not related to the size of the cutaneous presentation of the injury.

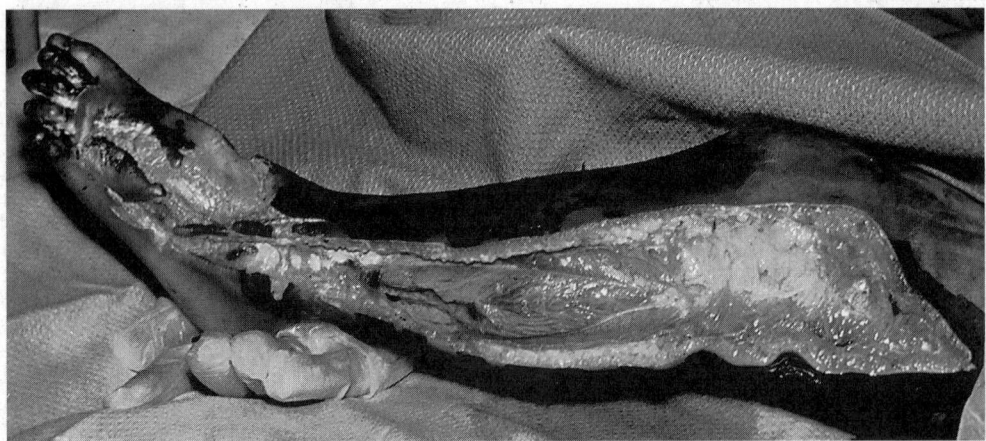

FIGURE 13-3. This severely burned lower extremity presented with no evidence of arterial circulation. Fasciotomy incisions were placed along the mid-medial and mid-lateral planes to decompress all muscle compartments. The incisional margins have separated because of massive edema in the proximal region of the incision. Necrotic muscle with overlying vessel thrombosis is seen distally. After the patient was stabilized, exploration and debridement were carried out in the operating room.

measured directly, and pressures >30 to 40 torr are associated with tissue damage.

Acute Renal Failure. Acute renal failure presenting as early oliguria or anuria is not uncommon after electrical injury and is caused by two mechanisms. Gross underestimation of the extent of injury and of fluid resuscitation requirements rapidly leads to hypovolemia and oliguria. In many patients, the majority of severely damaged tissue is muscle that is hidden from view, and the need for fluid replacement may not be appreciated immediately. Necrotic muscle releases myoglobin, which is directly toxic to renal tubular cells, Hypovolemia potentiates the toxicity of myoglobin in the tubules unless high urine flow is maintained (see Ch. 76). Myoglobin causes the urine to appear reddish brown in the absence of red blood cells. Deeply pigmented, concentrated urine typical of oliguric states may be mistaken for myoglobinuria. If uncertainty exists about the cause of urine pigments, a dipstick analysis can identify the heme nature of myoglobin. Visible myoglobinuria indicates massive acute muscle necrosis and impending renal failure. Life-threatening electrolyte abnormalities often accompany massive muscle injury and myoglobinuria.

Nervous System. The electrical injury may involve both the central and the peripheral nervous systems. A thorough neurologic examination on admission is essential, and because of the delayed presentation of many neurologic complications, serial examination should continue throughout hospitalization. Both normal and abnormal function should be documented. Because extremities sustain the majority of direct electrical injuries, associated peripheral nerves are most often damaged at the time of contact. Such injuries are usually permanent and may determine the ultimate salvageability of the extremity. Some patients may also present with signs of peripheral neuropathy in locations anatomically distant from the sites of electrical injury. The mechanism responsible is not known, but fortunately these deficits usually are reversible. Motor involvement is more common than are sensory abnormalities. Several days to weeks following electrical injury, a syndrome of polyneuritis affecting nerves away from the sites of surface injury may occur. Associated deficits may only partially resolve. Immediate signs of spinal cord symptoms tend to be temporary and readily reversible. Spinal cord injuries of delayed onset are more often permanent or only partially reversible and manifest as transverse myelitis, ascending paralysis, hemiplegia, or related syndromes.

Fractures. Early evaluation should include assessment for skeletal trauma. Long-bone fractures frequently accompany falls, and fractures of the vertebral column may be produced by the tetanic contraction of the paraspinous muscle at the time of electrocution. Both types of fractures can be identified on appropriate roentgenograms.

Internal Organs. Electrical injuries to the major viscera most commonly occur when the body wall overlying an organ is in direct contact with the electrical current. Otherwise, the volume of the torso is large by comparison with the extremities and allows the electrical current to be distributed over a large cross-sectional area at relatively low resistance. As a result, direct injury to internal organs rarely occurs. Dysfunction of the liver, pancreas, and gut may occur during hospitalization but usually reflects the patient's underlying condition rather than the unique effects of electrical injury.

TREATMENT. Cardiopulmonary Resuscitation (see Ch. 68 and 69). Cardiopulmonary arrest is common following electrical injury, and resuscitative effort should be instituted immediately. Patients in whom cardiac arrest has occurred frequently respond to cardiopulmonary resuscitation, particularly after lightning injury. All patients should be placed on cardiac monitors or telemetry for 48 hours, and continued monitoring is needed only if arrhythmias persist. The choice of antiarrhythmic agents is dictated by the nature of the rhythm disturbance. All persistent electrocardiographic alterations should receive thorough cardiologic investigation once the acute electrical injury has healed.

Fluid Therapy. As with any other tissue injuries, fluid loss into damaged tissue is one of the major physiologic derangements after electrical burns. Intravascular volume is replenished with lactated Ringer's solution sufficient to maintain a urinary output of 50 to 75 ml per hour. If the patient has grossly visible myoglobinuria, urinary output should be increased to 100 to 150 ml per hour by raising the fluid infusion rate. The increased urine production facilitates dilution of myoglobin and its washout from renal tubules. If myoglobinuria is severe or urinary output remains low in spite of an increased rate of fluid administration, mannitol (12.5 grams) is added to each liter of lactated Ringer's solution. In such cases, adding sodium bicarbonate to the resuscitation solution alkalinizes the urine and increases the solubility of myoglobin.

Wound Management. Wound care involves treating both cutaneous and deep soft tissue injuries. Immediately after electrical injury, second- and third-degree cutaneous wounds are debrided, cleansed, and placed in topical antimicrobial burn creams. Sulfamylon (mafenide acetate) is preferred for electrical injuries because of its superior ability to penetrate deeply injured tissue and its anticlostridial properties. Tetanus prophylaxis is brought up to date. Prophylactic antibiotics have not been shown to decrease episodes of infection and usually are not used. Extremity muscle compartment pressures are monitored by physical palpation and by Doppler ultrasonography of major arterial pulses. Tissue manometry using needle-tipped transducers appears to reflect compartmental pressures, and measurements >30 to 40 mm Hg are indications for surgical decompression. If the extremity has been injured by a circumferential third-degree burn, escharotomy is carried out. If the compartment symptoms persist, fasciotomy involving all major compartments is performed. Because blood loss may be difficult to control, fasciotomy usually should be carried out in an operating room. Although fasciotomy may allow preservation of nutrient blood flow to potentially viable tissue, it is likely that the ultimate extent of tissue damage is determined at the time of electrical injury and that progressive tissue loss seldom occurs.

Dead tissue promotes infection, which may be life-threatening, and definitive therapy of the electrical burns is directed toward the timely removal of necrotic tissue. At present, amputation of electrically injured extremities is not automatic. The availability of several diagnostic tools may allow definition of viable and nonviable tissue in wounds whose surface appearance may not reflect deeper injuries. Technetium-99m pyrophosphate scintigraphy is the most common diagnostic technique used to evaluate injured extremities and provides useful results within the first 24 hours (see Ch. 22). Normal isotopic uptake reflects normal perfusion, whereas totally nonviable tissue exhibits no uptake. Areas of potentially reversible injury demonstrate increased isotope uptake, and serial scanning may be useful in determining the need for debridement. In extremities with intact flow of the major arteries, arteriography may be helpful. Truncation of flow to nutrient muscle branches indicates irreversible injury. Finally, the viability of deep tissue is determined most accurately by serial surgical exploration of the injured extremity.

The timing of surgical intervention and the extent of debridement are determined by the stability of the patient and the nature of the burn wound. Generally, initial exploration and debridement may commence at the end of the resuscitation phase, within 24 to 48 hours of injury. Distal portions of electrocuted extremities that are desiccated and mummified should be amputated. More proximally, it may be impossible to determine grossly the extent of deep tissue injury. These areas should be explored thoroughly, using fasciotomy incisions if previously placed. All muscle groups should be inspected, especially those against bone. Only obviously necrotic tissue is removed, and every attempt should be made to salvage viable tissue. This approach requires daily wound examination and sequential operative debridements until all necrotic tissue is removed. Intervening complications, such as intractable hyperkalemia, severe myoglobinuria, or infection, may force abandonment of this sequential approach and require urgent amputation at a relatively high level. It is rarely advisable to proceed to early closure following amputation, and definitive closure of the debrided wound is carried out only when all necrotic tissue has been removed. Similarly, excising or grafting full-thickness cutaneous burns may be delayed until this time. Long-term care requires multidisciplinary rehabilitation and prosthetic services.

LATE COMPLICATIONS. Patients sustaining electrical injuries may develop a number of apparently related late complications that develop a few months to several years after injury. As with cutaneous burns, more than half of electrically injured patients develop post-traumatic stress disorders, especially if a body part has been lost. Associated psychiatric symptoms respond well to psychotherapy and medication. Contractures require extensive rehabilitation care and reconstructive surgery. Cholelithiasis occurs with increased frequency in patients who have sustained electrical burns. Cataracts are particularly troublesome and occur in up to 6% of electrically injured patients. The physical examination done on the admission of such patients should include a careful ophthalmologic evaluation to identify pre-existing cataracts. Although vision loss may be extensive, surgical correction is highly effective.

Amy BW, McManus WF, Goodwin CW Jr, et al.: Lightning injury with survival in five patients. JAMA 253:243, 1985. *Presentation and treatment of lightning injury are described, with emphasis on first responder care.*

Baker MD, Chiaviello C: Household electric injuries in children. Am J Dis Child 143:59, 1989. *As with other forms of thermal injury, electrical injuries to children commonly occur at home. Most can be prevented by using inexpensive safety devices.*

Hunt JL, Sato RM, Baxter CR: Acute electric burns: Current diagnostic and therapeutic approaches to management. Arch Surg 115:434, 1980. *An excellent description of electrical injury in a large series. The use of technetium-99m pyrophosphate scanning was introduced by these authors, and its efficacy in defining injured and nonviable tissue is confirmed.*

James TN, Riddick LR, Embry JH: Cardiac abnormalities demonstrated postmortem in four cases of accidental electrocution and their potential significance relative to non-fatal electrical injuries of the heart. Am Heart J 120:143, 1990. *Provides an exhaustive review of the effects of postmortem damage in young men presenting with fatal cardiac arrest.*

Lee RC, Gottlieb LJ, Krizek TJ: Pathophysiology and clinical manifestations of tissue injury and electrical trauma. Adv Plast Reconstr Surg 8:1, 1992. *The potential direct nonthermal electrical effects on cellular integrity are concisely summarized. Electroporation and cell membrane destruction appear to explain tissue defects when high tissue temperatures are unlikely to have occurred.*

Saffle JR, Crandall A, Warden GD: Cataracts: A long-term complication of electrical injury. J Trauma 25:17, 1985. *Cataracts occur in 5 to 10% of patients with electrical injury. Emphasizes the importance of early ophthalmologic examination, documentation, and long-term follow-up in determining disability.*

13.3 Chronic Poisoning: Trace Metals and Others

William O. Robertson

DEFINITION. Our chemical environment was recognized as a threat to health early in history. Well-documented outbreaks of occupational mercury and lead "poisonings" had been recorded and preventive measures implemented by 200 B.C. The Middle Ages saw arsenic poisoning used as a political weapon. More recent times have seen increasing recognition of industrial toxins, "accidental poisoning" in childhood, purposeful overdoses in adults, adverse reactions to drugs, medication mixups in hospitals, and environmental hazards for us all. The common theme is its metabolism. The term "poison" has undergone quantitative redefinition so that now such ubiquitous substances as table salt and drinking water are firmly established as being "poisonous." Recall that more than 400 years ago, Paracelsus cautioned "All substances are poisons: There is none that is not a poison. The right dose differentiates a poison and a remedy." Finally, the host-organism itself has contributed to a better comprehension of the word "poison," as genetic variability has been recognized to determine the impact of a given molecule in such hereditary disorders as phenylketonuria, glucose-6-phosphate dehydrogenase deficiency, and others. As our understanding of life has expanded, the connotation of poisoning has undergone substantial evolution.

ETIOLOGY. Approximately 1.2 million chemical entities had been identified and coded by 1950; the number had risen to more than 4.3 million by 1976. In 1995, the number exceeds 13 million. Although not all of these compounds have been marketed, many new organic compounds have appeared in the home and the workplace. For example, available formulations of pesticides have increased 50-fold over the past 35 years. Moreover, manufacturing processes have released additional compounds into the workplace or the environment that serve as poisons. Currently employed methods to determine carcinogenicity, mutagenicity, and teratogenicity indict chemicals as dangerous when simultaneous epidemiologic data from humans fail to support such contentions—e.g., formaldehyde, fluorides, dioxins. Because proving a negative remains so ephemeral, it appears likely that "scare incidents" that eventually prove groundless—e.g., cranberries in the 1960's, sturgeon (Hg) in the 1970's, and Agent Orange (dioxins) in the 1980's—will be even more commonplace.

New analytical techniques can promptly and completely identify poisonings and have uncovered the causes of such diverse entities as Minamata disease (teratogenesis consequent to methyl mercury), an outbreak of ascending paralysis affecting more than 4000 with more than 400 deaths in Iraq (also caused by methyl mercury), the "gray syndrome" in premature infants (caused by chloramphenicol), mesotheliomas induced by asbestos, and an epidemic of angiosarcoma of the liver among industrial workers (caused by vinyl chloride). Nevertheless, many unknowns remain and justify careful prospective monitoring of industry, of the home, and of the environment. Unfortunately, the combination of more "synthetic chemicals," vastly more precise testing techniques, a press far more devoted to Rachel Carson's *Silent Spring* than to Dupont's "better living through chemistry," and an increasingly litigious society has created an era of "toxic torts" and its consequences, plus a very anxious and concerned public and profession. As a consequence, primary care physicians are bound to be involved in disputes stemming from industrial, occupational, and environmental origins. This chapter emphasizes trace metal poisoning, which tends to have a chronic nature. Acute toxins are covered in Ch. 72.

Many metals and nonmetals in trace amounts are capable of causing human disease especially after chronic or repetitive exposure. In some cases poisoning is a consequence of workplace exposure. In others the disease results from using prescription or nonprescription medicines or as an adverse effect of medical procedures such as hemodialysis. Occasionally such poisoning results from attempts at suicide or homicide.

Over the past few decades, increased awareness of the health consequences of industrial substances, more stringent federal and state regulations, and fear of lawsuits have resulted in a healthier workplace. However, the majority of the potentially exposed work force is employed by small industries that may not have implemented protective measures.

We know a great deal about overwhelming exposure that results in acute illness, but our knowledge of the subtle consequences of chronic, low-level trace element exposure is still grossly inadequate. This is well illustrated by lead exposure. Acute lead poisoning in children or adults is readily diagnosed, but we are only beginning to understand the consequences of increased body lead burdens in the absence of the anemia, colic, or clinically apparent encephalopathy and its clinical significance—if any.

The interrelationships between trace elements are also poorly understood. For example, copper smelter workers are exposed not only to copper but also to lead, zinc, arsenic, gold, silver, cadmium, and mercury; in these workers pneumonitis or other acute illnesses may result from two or more metals acting in concert. In other instances excesses or deficits of a trace element may act indirectly by inducing deficiency or toxicity of another trace element.

LEAD

ETIOLOGY. In the past lead poisoning was ascribed to pica (abnormal ingestion) among children living in dilapidated houses with peeling layers of lead-based paints. In the past two decades lead intoxication has occurred with decreasing frequency. This may in part be related to less use of lead in paint and leaded gasoline; several studies relate environmental lead contamination to traffic density patterns.

In the United States, hundreds of occupations entail potentially significant exposure. It is estimated that more than 800,000 American workers have potentially significant lead exposure. Lead and other metal smelter workers or miners, welders, storage battery workers, and pottery makers are particularly heavily exposed. Workers in auto manufacturing, ship building, paint manufacture, and printing industries are also at substantial risk, as are house painters and those who repair old houses.

Lead-soldered kettles and cans and lead-glazed pottery can release lead when acidic fluids are stored or cooked in them. Demolition workers and those employed in firing ranges have become poisoned from intensive aerosol exposure. In the southern United States, moonshine whiskey is an important cause of poisoning. The stills are connected with lead solder, and old radiators containing lead are used as condensers; 20 to 90% of moonshine samples contain lead in the potentially toxic range.

In past centuries lead was added to wine to sweeten it, a deception that was eventually made punishable by death. Recently, adding lead to various herbal and folk medicines has resulted in poisoning. Retained bullets can result in lead poisoning, especially if a joint is involved, because synovial fluid appears to be a good solvent for lead. The interval between lodging of the bullet and clinical evidence of lead poisoning has ranged from 2 days to 40 years. Lead poisoning has also occurred in adults who have eaten fowl and inadvertently ingested lead pellets. Children have been poisoned by swallowing lead household objects, such as lead curtain weights, that are then retained in the gastrointestinal tract for a prolonged time.

Gasoline sniffing can produce lead poisoning; the organic tetraethyl lead appears to have a proclivity for the nervous system.

In a sense we are all lead poisoned; prior to the Industrial Revolution the total body burden of lead was about 2 mg, whereas currently in industrialized societies the whole body content is about 200 mg. One hundred fifty to 250 μg per day is ingested, 5 to 10% of which is absorbed. In children the percentage is even higher.

CLINICAL MANIFESTATIONS. The major toxic effects of lead are referable to the abdomen, the blood, and the nervous system.

Gastrointestinal Tract. The exact pathogenesis of lead colic remains uncertain. The crampy, diffuse, often intractable abdominal pain may be accompanied by nausea, vomiting, anorexia, constipation, or occasionally diarrhea. The pain may be confined to the epigastric, periumbilical, or other areas of the abdomen and may simulate a variety of surgical and nonsurgical diseases.

Blood. Lead interferes with a variety of red cell enzyme systems, including delta-aminolevulinic acid dehydratase and ferrochelatase. The former is needed to conjugate levulinic acid to form porphobilinogen; the latter facilitates the incorporation of iron into protoporphyrin IX. The red cell abnormalities include punctate basophilic stippling. Anemia is frequent in severe acute lead poisoning and may be normocytic normochromic but usually is microcytic hypochromic. Moreover, an inherited deficiency in delta-aminolevulinic acid dehydratase can lead to lead intoxication at modest blood lead levels.

Nervous System. Both the brain and the peripheral nerves may be involved. The central nervous system (CNS) symptoms at first are vague and are often mistakenly disregarded. These manifestations include irritability, incoordination, memory lapses, labile affect, sleep disturbances, restlessness, listlessness, paranoia, headache, lethargy, and dizziness. In more serious cases manifestations include syncope-like attacks, disorientation, flaccidity, severe mental impairment, ataxia, vomiting, cranial nerve palsies, localized neurologic signs, psychosis, somnolence, seizures, blindness, and coma. Severe lead encephalopathy is not restricted to children. Occasionally the brain manifestations mimic a space-occupying lesion. The cerebrospinal fluid may be under increased pressure and may show an increased protein content. Papilledema has been reported, as have grayish deposits surrounding the optic disc and optic atrophy. Frank encephalopathy is an ominous prognostic sign for both mortality and persistent brain damage. Most children who experience two or more bouts of clinically evident encephalopathy have neurologic residua.

Peripheral nerve involvement is seen more often in adults than in children. Wrist drop and foot drop are seen most often; the former, depending on type of occupation, may be asymmetric, and there may be paresthesias.

The spinal cord may also be involved, with manifestations having some similarity to those of amyotrophic lateral sclerosis.

Tetraethyl lead (organic lead) poisoning causes euphoria, nervousness, insomnia, hallucinations, convulsions, and frank psychosis.

Over the past generation increasing evidence has arisen of subtle brain damage in the absence of clinical evidence of encephalopathy. Inordinate body burdens of lead may result in mentation difficulties, emotional lability, deficits in intelligence and memory, impaired psychomotor and visual motor function, slowed nerve conduction, and behavioral aberrations in both children and adults, even in the absence of overt evidence of poisoning. These changes are postulated to occur at blood levels of 10 to 40 μg per deciliter (or even less in young children). However, the scientific community is sharply divided about the clinical significance of these observations.

Other Clinical Manifestations. In adults the kidneys are often involved (see Ch. 80), the characteristic lesion being interstitial nephritis; as the disease progresses, glomerular filtration rate falls. In children, Fanconi's syndrome, characterized by glycosuria, aminoaciduria, and phosphaturia, may occur transiently; and occasionally renal failure supervenes.

Polyarthralgias, mild hepatic dysfunction, and dysuria may also occur. Occasionally arrhythmias and cardiomegaly have been reported, as have abnormalities of liver function.

Lead readily crosses the placenta and is thought to be responsible for an increased incidence of spontaneous abortion and miscarriage and possibly for impairing the fetal CNS.

DIAGNOSIS. In the adult a high index of suspicion and a careful examination of the peripheral blood for basophilic stippling are mandatory; for occupational workers lead screening is warranted. Urinary coproporphyrin levels are increased because lead interferes with incorporation of iron into heme. Erythrocyte protoporphyrin (EP) can be measured rapidly fluorometrically; both EP and zinc protoporphyrin (ZPP) are reliable indicators of lead poisoning but are also elevated in iron deficiency anemia. Table 13–7 lists some indications of undue lead absorption.

Today blood lead levels are readily determined by atomic absorption spectrophotometry or anodic stripping voltometry. Specimens can be obtained by either venipuncture or finger stick; the latter technique is often difficult to interpret because of skin contamination.

Additional industrial exposure should not be permitted if blood

TABLE 13–7. POSITIVE SCREENING TESTS INDICATING UNDUE LEAD ABSORPTION

Whole-blood lead	Children	>25 μg/dl
	Adults	>40 μg/dl
Whole-blood erythrocyte protoporphyrin or zinc protoporphyrin	Children	>35 μg/dl*
	Adults	>50 μg/dl

* This value is unsettled.

levels exceed 25 to 40 μg per deciliter. Currently 26 states have lead registries to continuously monitor all lead analytic determinations in the state in an attempt to curtail problems.

TREATMENT. Three agents have been used to form tight complexes with lead and thus promote its biologic inactivation and elimination from tissues (Table 13–8). Dimercaprol (British antilewisite, BAL) is given in oil intramuscularly; calcium disodium edetate (calcium versenate) can be given either intramuscularly or intravenously; and D-penicillamine is administered by mouth. Chelation should be undertaken only after careful consideration for those with milder evidence of poisoning, because each of the agents may be associated with significant adverse effects. Because most of the body lead is stored in the bones, clinical improvement and reduction in blood lead levels (or reduction in EP or ZPP) may be temporary, to be followed by increases in blood lead concentrations and clinical evidence of repoisoning owing to mobilization of lead from bone. In such cases chelating agents may need to be readministered. Newer, less toxic oral dimercaprol analogues dimercaptosuccinic acid and dimercaptopropanesulfonate have recently been introduced with the hope of enhancing efficacy and reducing complications.

Treatment is ordinarily successful in extra-CNS disease but may not be so in patients with encephalopathy. Various degrees of mentation deficits may remain in both children and adults.

Although the Centers for Disease Control and Prevention (CDC) (1991) sees currently acceptable blood concentrations of lead for children to be 10 μg per deciliter, debate rages about that specific number. Blood lead levels have fallen dramatically in the United States (and some other countries) in the past 25 years, but no measurable increase in IQ has followed; if anything, hyperactivity, aggressiveness, and antisocial behavior have all increased.

More than 20 years ago, the extraordinary scientist and philosopher Rene Dubos observed: "The [lead] problem is so well-defined,

TABLE 13–8. CHELATION REGIMENS

	Children*	Adults*	Duration
CaNa$_2$ EDTA	50 mg/kg/day IM† or IV, or 1500 mg/m^2/24 hr (severe disease); 1000 mg/m^2/day (mild-moderate intoxication)	1.0 gram IV in 5% dextrose twice daily, or 2.0 grams/day IM in divided doses; longer term, 1 gram IM 3 × per week† until lead burden reduced to satisfactory levels	3 to 5 days
BAL	3 mg/kg/dose IM, or 300–450 mg/m^2/24 hr IM	2.5 mg/kg/dose IM	3 to 5 days
	(Given in divided doses every 4 hr)		
Penicillamine	30 mg/kg/day PO	1.0–1.5 grams/day PO	Until blood lead and FEP‡ levels approach normal§
**2,3-Dimercaptosuccinic acid (DMSA)	10 mg/kg tid for 5 days 10 mg/kg then bid for 14 days	—	

* CaNa$_2$ EDTA and BAL are ordinarily used together for symptomatic illness.
† Procaine must be used for IM injections of CaNa$_2$ EDTA.
‡ FEP = free erythrocyte protoporphyrin.
§ Must be monitored carefully because toxicity occurs in up to 20% of cases.
** Orphan drug approved only for children.

so neatly packaged with both causes and cures known, that if we don't eliminate this social crime, our society deserves all the disasters that have been forecast for it." Amen. On balance, however, the task has been accomplished.

MERCURY

ETIOLOGY. Mercury has been used for at least 2000 years. At present more than 60 occupations involve mercury exposure. These include chloralkali work; manufacture of pesticides, insecticides, and fungicides; manufacture of mercury-containing instruments, lamps, neon lights, batteries, paper, paint, dye, electrical equipment, and jewelry; and dentistry. However, exposure in dental offices has diminished substantially in recent years.

In addition to occupational or industrial exposure, poisoning has resulted from inadvertent contamination of grains by mercury-containing pesticides as well as from accidental or intentional ingestion or injection of elemental mercury or mercury-containing compounds. In the past, mercury was administered medicinally as a component of cathartics, teething powders, and anthelmintics. Today mercury compounds have no bonafide place in therapeutic medicine.

CLINICAL MANIFESTATIONS AND TREATMENT. The biologic effects, tissue distribution, and toxicity of mercury depend on the form in which it is introduced into the body.

Metallic Mercury. Elemental mercury is a liquid at environmental temperatures but vaporizes with agitation as well as gentle heating. Bulk mercury is used in dental amalgams; up to 10% of dental offices have been found to have excessive mercury vapor levels; and accidental spillage has occurred occasionally in homes or offices, and where carpeting has been involved mercury poisoning has followed. The greatest exposure to metallic mercury is in industry. Heavy aerosol exposure to mercury produces chills, fever, cough, chest pain, and hemoptysis; roentgenograms show diffuse pulmonary infiltrates. Oxidized elemental mercury is readily absorbed from the alveoli; subsequently it can enter the brain. With mild exposure the manifestations are likely to be subtle and diagnosis is difficult. Insomnia, nervousness, mild tremor, impaired judgment and coordination, decreased mental efficiency, emotional lability, headache, fatigue, loss of sexual drive, and depression are early manifestations and are often mistakenly ascribed to psychogenic causes. Abdominal cramps, dermatitis, and diarrhea may also occur, and the victim may complain of a metallic taste. As the poisoning becomes more severe, persistent involuntary tremors of the extremities are noted. Thereafter, other signs of mercury poisoning may appear, including amblyopia, polyneuropathy, erythroderma, acrodynia, joint pains, swollen gums with a blue line around the teeth, sialorrhea, and paresthesias. The major manifestation of chronic mercury vapor exposure may be renal damage, including the nephrotic syndrome.

Because of the body's metabolism of mercury, blood and urine levels may be unreliable, and clear evidence of poisoning may be documented only after administering drugs that augment mercury excretion in the urine.

In most cases improvement occurs after removal from exposure or treatment with appropriate chelating agents.

In contrast, ingesting even large amounts of metallic mercury usually produces no clinical disturbance. Aspiration of liquid mercury into the lungs is also usually benign, although roentgenologic visualization of mercury globules may be evident for many years. Even after intravenous injection of mercury, there may be no abnormalities other than roentgenologic densities or mild respiratory distress.

The wide range of clinical findings after elemental mercury exposure appears to relate in part to the rate of oxidation of mercury to its salts and the rapidity of their subsequent excretion through the kidneys, saliva, and urine.

Inorganic Mercury. Exposure to the salts of mercury, i.e., $HgCl_2$ and Hg_2Cl_2, occurs primarily in industry and results from ingestion. $HgCl_2$ is far more toxic than Hg_2Cl_2. The major manifestations are gastrointestinal and renal, with proteinuria, granular casts in the urinary sediment, the nephrotic syndrome, and pyuria from tubular damage. In some cases severe oliguria, and even anuria, may occur. Additionally, diarrhea, abdominal pain, hepatic dysfunction, and lesser evidence of CNS disease may be found. Rhabdomyolysis with striking muscle enzyme elevation and acrodynia have also been reported.

Organomercurials. Included are phenyl and methoxyethyl mercury salts found in fungicides and methyl mercury used in industry.

Methyl mercury—a devastating teratogen—is well absorbed from the intestinal tract, is widely distributed in the body, and readily passes through the placenta into the fetus and also into breast milk. About 10% localizes in the brain, and the ensuing damage is largely irreversible. Major epidemics have resulted from industrial contamination of water, with subsequent biotransformation of elemental and inorganic mercury into methyl mercury that was ingested by fish who were subsequently consumed by humans. Other epidemics have resulted from using grains contaminated by organic mercurial pesticides or animal ingestion of seeds treated with mercury. The epidemics in the Minamata and Niigata regions of Japan and in Iraq, Guatemala, Pakistan, and the United States have resulted in a high death rate and an appalling amount of permanent brain damage. In addition to the milder symptoms listed under elemental mercury poisoning, CNS manifestations include severe paresthesias, dysarthria, ataxia, visual field constriction, hearing loss, blindness, microcephaly, spasticity, paralysis, and coma.

ARSENIC

ETIOLOGY. Arsenic is ubiquitous in nature; it is present in the earth's crust in concentrations of 2 to 5 parts per billion. It is found in inordinately high concentrations in some well water. It is used in the glass, pigment, textile, tanning, and bronze-plating industries; in wood preservation; in a variety of metal alloys; in veterinary medicines; in some herbicides, insecticides, and rodenticides; in fire salts to produce multicolored flames; and by farmers and vintners. American industry uses about one half of the world's production of arsenic trioxide. Arsenic poisoning has also resulted from using certain herbal preparations, from ingesting illegal (moonshine) whiskey, from burning arsenate-treated wood, and from administering arsenic-containing folk and prescription medicines.

Elemental arsenic is not toxic even if ingested in substantial amounts. There are three toxic forms of arsenic: pentavalent salts, trivalent salts, and arsine gas. The arsenic in the earth's crust and in most foods is in the pentavalent form, the least toxic form. Trivalent arsenic, which is more toxic, accumulates in the body more readily than the pentavalent form. Arsenic gas (arsine) is extraordinarily toxic; it is formed by the hydrolysis of metallic arsenide or by the action of acids or nascent hydrogen on arsenical compounds, especially in the refining of certain metals. Arsine is used in the electronics industry and can be liberated in sewage plants.

CLINICAL MANIFESTATIONS. *Arsine gas* poisoning is usually overwhelming and frequently fatal. The onset of symptoms after exposure is usually between 1 and 6 hours. Fever, headache, muscle pains, nausea, vomiting, epigastric pain, dysuria, and explosive diarrhea characterize the acute episode. Because arsenic preferentially binds to red blood cells, hemolytic anemia and hemoglobinuria occur early, and red cell ghosts may be seen in the peripheral blood. There may also be profound hypoxia and cyanosis. Renal failure due to acute tubular necrosis (occasionally due to cortical necrosis) occurs in the first few days after onset of symptoms. This may be accompanied by shock and encephalopathy, characterized by agitation and disorientation. Both bone marrow depression and myocardial damage may occur. Those who do not die of intractable vascular collapse often develop subacute manifestations of arsenic poisoning, described below. Those who recover may develop chronic renal failure.

Arsenic Ingestion. Depending on dose and form, arsenic ingestion can be insidious or overwhelming with cramping abdominal pain and diarrhea. Other acute manifestations include nausea, vomiting, dysphagia, cyanosis, headache, hematuria, and weakness. Hyperesthesia, muscle cramps, conjunctivitis, syncope, excessive thirst, periorbital swelling, epistaxis, and tinnitus may also occur. The patient may complain of a metallic taste, and there may be a garlic odor to the breath which can also occur with selenium, tellurium, and phosphorus and dimethyl sulfoxide (DMSO) poisoning.

Skin, nails, and hair do not usually contain arsenic until 2 to 4 weeks after exposure, but occasionally hair accumulation can occur more rapidly.

Other manifestations that may occur in the first week include jaundice, hematuria, hepatomegaly with hepatic enzyme abnormalities; electrocardiographic abnormalities; a cardiomyopathy that can be lethal; pericarditis; rhabdomyolysis; pulmonary edema; evidence of encephalopathy; seizures; renal dysfunction; kidney failure with acute tubular necrosis; and respiratory muscle paralysis.

The most prominent manifestation after the first week of illness is symmetric polyneuropathy. At first, sensory manifestations predominate, the patient complaining of a burning sensation in a stocking-glove distribution. Motor involvement follows almost immediately with diminished or absent reflexes and severe weakness. Occasionally the neuropathy is unilateral. Prolonged encephalopathy and/or psychosis has been reported in a few instances.

In cases of subacute poisoning, Aldrich-Mees lines (transverse white bands) may be seen in the nails; like the garlic odor, these may be seen in other trace element intoxications.

Chronic exposure is associated with several other abnormalities. The most characteristic of these are the cutaneous lesions, particularly hyperpigmentation (arsenic melanosis) and hyperkeratoses located primarily on the palms and soles. Alopecia and so-called raindrop depigmentation may also occur. In about 5 to 10% of those chronically exposed, skin cancers appear after latent periods of 5 to more than 25 years; these tend to be multiple and are situated mainly on the trunk and upper extremities. In the United States the most frequent cause of such skin lesions in past years was the medicinal use of Fowler's solution, an inorganic trivalent arsenical. Currently most cases arise after occupational exposure, but a small number have been ascribed to chronic exposure to well water with high arsenic content.

Epidemiologic studies on gold ore and tin miners, vineyard workers, laborers in sheep-dip factories, and smelter workers show a clear increase in the incidence of squamous cell carcinoma of the lung, the risk of bronchogenic cancer correlating with the intensity and duration of arsenic trioxide exposure, and all are potentiated by smoking.

DIAGNOSIS. If the diagnosis is suspected, arsenic concentrations can be measured in blood, urine, hair, or nails by atomic absorption spectrophotometry or neutron activation techniques, but, as with mercury, interpretation can be difficult.

TREATMENT. The treatment of choice is dimercaprol (BAL), but it should be given within the first 24 hours after exposure. If the BAL is given later, it is less likely that improvement will be observed, and in many cases the peripheral neuropathy is refractory to treatment. Exchange transfusion or dialysis shortly after the onset of acute illness has also been reported to be beneficial. Penicillamine may also be useful, as may orally administered 2,3-dimercaptosuccinic acid (DMSA).

TRACE ELEMENTS WHOSE TOXICITY IS IN LARGE PART ASSOCIATED WITH HEMODIALYSIS

ZINC. The normal adult body zinc content is 1.5 to 3.0 grams. Usually daily intake ranges from 5 to 35 mg. Zinc is bound to metallothioneins synthesized in the liver and is excreted by both the urine and the gastrointestinal tract. It has a strong affinity for red cells and plasma proteins. Consequently, there is no loss across dialysis membranes; instead, depending on the dialysate, blood zinc concentrations may increase markedly during hemodialysis. There appear to be two well-documented zinc sources: adhesive plaster (containing zinc oxide) used to prevent dialysis coils from unwinding and the water of the dialysis fluid. Even if water has an initially low zinc content, galvanized iron pipes or tanks may release substantial amounts. This can be prevented by using deionized or distilled water.

The manifestations of zinc toxicity do not necessarily correlate well with plasma or whole-blood zinc levels. Nausea, vomiting, anorexia, lethargy, irritability, weakness, abdominal pain, and anemia are the most frequent manifestations. Other manifestations may include diarrhea, muscle pain, lymphadenopathy, hyperamylasemia with or without pancreatitis, intestinal bleeding, thrombocytopenia, oliguria, hypotension, and renal failure with tubular necrosis. Injecting large amounts of zinc has resulted in death. Intestinal manifestations may supervene after either orally or parenterally induced zinc intoxication.

Welders, smelter workers, and solderers are exposed to aerosolized zinc and may experience zinc fume fever, characterized by chills, fever, myalgias, a metallic taste, cough, nausea, lethargy, and occasionally hemoptysis. There may be diffuse roentgenologic infiltrates and pulmonary dysfunction. Ordinarily all manifestations disappear rapidly after cessation of exposure. If more prolonged pulmonary dysfunction occurs, it is thought to result from the effects of other metals to which the workers are simultaneously exposed.

ALUMINUM. Aluminum-induced dialysis dementia can be a fatal disease. The tap water used during dialysis is often to blame. Some waters naturally contain high concentrations of aluminum. In other cases aluminum sulfate had been added to the community water supply to remove organic materials. In still other cases the dialysis fluid appeared to be less responsible than aluminum-containing gels administered by mouth to reduce phosphate levels. If oral aluminum hydroxide is administered to nondialyzed patients suffering from renal failure, the encephalopathy syndrome rarely occurs in adults; young children appear to be particularly at risk. Dialysis encephalopathy occurs only after repeated dialyses, usually spanning months or years. Peritoneal dialysis can also be complicated by encephalopathy.

Early manifestations include malaise, memory loss, and a characteristic speech disturbance. As the disease progresses, dysarthria, asterixis, myoclonic twitches, dementia, somnolence, and seizures occur. The electroencephalogram shows slowing, together with bursts of delta activity and high-voltage, symmetric spikes. Using reverse osmosis or deionization treatment has markedly reduced the incidence of severe dialysis dementia, but there is increasing evidence of a mild form of encephalopathy in chronic dialysis patients, characterized by psychomotor dysfunction, memory defects, weakness, and mild myoclonus.

Unusual manifestations of aluminum intoxication include myalgias, proximal myopathy, and severe skeletal pain caused by profound osteodystrophy that is unresponsive to vitamin D and is followed by fractures. Aluminum is deposited at the calcified bone-osteoid junction, and bone formation is impaired (see Ch. 213 and 216). Aluminum also interferes with parathyroid function, and it may be associated with cardiomyopathy.

Aluminum toxicity is also characterized by a poorly understood microcytic anemia that may be related in part to aluminum binding to transferrin and interfering with iron incorporation into heme.

Although frequently lethal, in some cases the encephalopathy has regressed after intake of oral aluminum is curtailed. Treatment with deferoxamine (DFO), which complexes with aluminum, may be beneficial. Those with uremia should also be wary of community water supplies with inordinately high concentrations of aluminum.

Serum aluminum levels often do not reflect body loads; intoxication may be documented by a DFO mobilization test, but it can temporarily exacerbate the encephalopathy.

Those involved in aluminum processing or manufacturing, pottery or explosive making, or welding may be exposed to aluminum aerosols. Pulmonary granulomas, fibrosis, and in some cases postfibrosis emphysema may supervene. In bauxite smelters this is known as Shaver's disease. Those involved in aluminum smelting may develop wheezing, chest tightness, and evidence of airway obstruction (potroom asthma).

COPPER. Since the late 1960's, copper tubing in dialysis equipment has been known to release copper when exposed to acid water. For that reason it is no longer used. Copper levels may also be inordinately high in the dialysis water if the water is supplied through copper plumbing. Copper is a potent red cell toxin, damaging cell membranes and inhibiting a variety of red cell enzymes. Major manifestations of toxicity include hemolysis and gastrointestinal disturbances. Nausea, vomiting, diarrhea, abdominal pain, fever, chills, hemolytic anemia, jaundice, hemoglobinuria, and severe myalgias all occur frequently. Myoglobinemia, necrotizing pancreatitis, hepatic necrosis, and profound leukocytosis may also occur.

Copper poisoning may also occur after intentional or accidental ingestion; hematemesis, melena, hepatic necrosis, and shock may supervene.

Those exposed to metallic copper industrially may develop transient pulmonary manifestations (metal fume fever) and, rarely, green hair. These disappear rapidly when exposure is stopped.

COBALT. Patients with renal failure may have elevated tissue cobalt levels, often as a result of oral intake to combat anemia. Toxicity includes nausea, vomiting, anorexia, tinnitus, peripheral neuropathy, goiter resulting from blockage of iodine uptake, neuro-

genic deafness, hyperlipidemia, optic atrophy, and renal tubular damage.

Cobalt was added to beer in the 1960's as a foam stabilizer. This resulted in cardiomyopathy, often accompanied by pericardial effusion. Mortality from heart failure or arrhythmias ranged from 5 to 47% (see Ch. 43).

Persons exposed to cobalt industrially may also occasionally develop cardiomyopathy. Workers exposed to finely powdered cobalt may develop pulmonary interstitial fibrosis and cor pulmonale. Cobalt is often a component of alloys that are used in joint prostheses. Cases have been reported of joint pains, spontaneous dislocation of the prosthesis, and bone necrosis starting 9 months to 4 years postoperatively, apparently caused by a reaction to the cobalt in the alloy.

OTHER METALS. In one group of dialysis patients, *nickel* toxicity occurred when nickel leached from a stainless steel water heater tank into the dialysis fluid. Manifestations include nausea, vomiting, weakness, and headache. Symptoms developed within a few hours after dialysis and disappeared within 48 hours.

Tissue *tin* concentrations, especially in the liver, are also increased in patients undergoing hemodialysis. However, tin levels are even higher in uremic patients who have not been dialyzed. No definite clinical disease has been associated with these increased body tin burdens.

Patients undergoing maintenance hemodialysis are often treated with *iron* for anemia. In such patients parenteral and occasionally oral iron administration may be followed by hemosiderosis and occasionally hemochromatosis. Serum ferritin concentrations may exceed 500 ng per milliliter. A proximal myopathy has also been described. Treatment with deferoxamine may reduce the body iron burden.

CADMIUM

ETIOLOGY. Over 10 million pounds of cadmium are used industrially every year in the United States. The metal is a component of alloys; it is used to manufacture electrical conductors and in electroplating; and it is present in ceramics, pigments, dental prosthetics, plastic stabilizers, and storage batteries. It is also a by-product of zinc smelting and is used in the photographic, rubber, motor, and aircraft industries. Smelters, metal-processing furnaces, and the burning of coal and oil are responsible for much of the cadmium in air.

CLINICAL MANIFESTATIONS. *Acute intoxication* by cadmium fumes produces a characteristic clinical picture. Four to 10 hours after exposure, dyspnea, cough, and substernal discomfort supervene, often accompanied by prominent myalgias, fatigue, headache, and vomiting. In more severe cases, wheezing, hemoptysis, and progressive dyspnea caused by pulmonary edema may occur and may be accompanied by hypotension and renal failure.

In most cases, the pulmonary manifestations resolve rapidly, but pulmonary function abnormalities may not disappear for months; in these cases vital capacity is reduced, and there is a restrictive defect. Occasionally pulmonary edema is lethal.

Ingesting large amounts of cadmium results in nausea, vomiting, and abdominal pain, often accompanied by weakness, prostration, and myalgias. The onset of the gastroenteritis occurs shortly after ingestion and usually lasts for less than 24 hours.

Chronic cadmium exposure by aerosol for at least 10 years has resulted in emphysema in a small number of cases. The emphysema is not accompanied by bronchitis and may appear many years after industrial exposure has stopped. Workers exposed for at least 10 years also may suffer olfactory nerve damage; in some cases this progresses to total anosmia. The most frequent long-term consequence of aerosol or oral exposure is proteinuria. After prolonged and heavy contact, cadmium urinary excretion continues for years and is associated with damage to the proximal tubule.

On occasion the proteinuria may be accompanied by glycosuria and aminoaciduria. Only infrequently are the proteinuria and tubular damage followed by progressive renal failure. An exception to the relatively benign course of the renal damage is the disease in Japan known as itai-itai (ouch-ouch), which affected almost exclusively multiparous women of ages 40 to 70 who lived in an area contaminated by industrial cadmium waste. Manifestations included striking back and joint pains, a waddly gait, osteomalacia, bone deformities, and fractures, all presumably secondary to cadmium-induced renal tubular damage.

Some studies on workers exposed to cadmium have suggested an increased risk of lung or prostatic carcinoma, but the data are not convincing.

NICKEL

ETIOLOGY. Nickel is used widely industrially in various alloys, iron shell casings, ball bearings, and heart and joint prostheses. It is also used in nickel plating; as a catalyst; in magnetic tapes, dyes, and paints; and in acrylic plastics. It is found in petroleum and coal, in diesel fuels, and in soil and air. Municipal incinerators may contribute to the ambient air nickel concentrations.

Nickel is a potent contact allergen; the most frequent adverse effect for humans is nickel dermatitis, which may be both persistent and severe. Serious systemic reactions have occurred in allergic persons from nickel-containing dental prostheses, jewelry, pacemakers, or even fluids given intravenously through a nickel-containing needle. Prosthetic joints and heart valves have failed because of a reaction to the nickel in the prosthesis. In cases of recalcitrant nickel dermatitis, restriction in dietary nickel may be helpful.

CLINICAL MANIFESTATIONS AND TREATMENT. By far, the most toxic of the nickel compounds is nickel carbonyl, created by a reaction between nickel and carbon monoxide. Industrial aerosol exposure is followed immediately by headache, drowsiness, substernal pain, nausea, and vomiting. This is followed by a latent period of 1 to 5 days, after which the victim experiences fever, chills, dyspnea, a feeling of chest tightness, cough that is sometimes productive of blood-tinged sputum, muscle pains, weakness, and fatigue. Hepatic enzyme concentrations may be considerably elevated. In severe cases cyanosis, progressive respiratory difficulties, and convulsions ensue, and death may follow. The treatment of choice is diethyl dithiocarbamate (Dithiocarb); dimercaprol (BAL) is an alternative but less effective therapeutic agent. Although overwhelming pneumonitis caused by nickel carbonyl is now rare, milder pulmonary toxicity in occupations such as welding probably goes unrecognized under the general rubric of metal fume fever.

CARCINOGENESIS. Nickel is considered a potent respiratory tract carcinogen. Studies of nickel refinery workers have shown a fivefold increase in risk of lung cancer, a 150-fold increase in the risk of nasal cancer, and a substantially increased risk of laryngeal cancer. Those occupations most at risk among nickel workers are roasting, smelting, and electrolysis. Workers developing lung, laryngeal, and nasal cancers have usually been exposed for at least 10 years. Biopsies of nasal mucosa show potentially precancerous epithelial dysplasia in a substantial percentage of nickel workers. The cancer risk is so great that workers heavily exposed for over 10 years should probably have annual nasal mucosa biopsies as well as sputum cytologic studies and roentgenologic examinations every 4 to 6 months in an attempt at secondary prevention. The incidence of respiratory tract cancer in nickel workers depends on both the extent of nickel exposure and the effects of cocarcinogens, in particular, cigarette tobacco. Except for nickel miners and refinery workers, industrial nickel exposure has not been convincingly associated with increased risk of cancer.

OTHER TOXIC METALS

Thallium

ETIOLOGY AND PATHOGENESIS. Thallium is used in optical lenses, jewelry, low-temperature thermometers, semiconductors, luminescent tubes, dyes and pigments, scintillation counters, and fireworks. It forms a stainless alloy with silver and a corrosion-resistant alloy with lead and may be a by-product of lead and zinc production. In some areas it is still a component of rodenticides, pesticides, and insecticides. Thallium can enter the body through the respiratory tract, gastrointestinal tract, or skin. Like many other trace metals, thallium has a strong affinity for sulfhydryl groups and thus interferes with many enzyme systems. Additionally, it enters the cell, exchanging for intracellular potassium.

CLINICAL MANIFESTATIONS. Poisoning can be acute and overwhelming after suicidal ingestion, or it can be chronic and subtle. In acute poisoning, manifestations include nausea, vomiting, hematemesis, headache, lethargy, abdominal pain, diarrhea that may be bloody, insomnia, myalgias, muscle weakness, fever, hyperhidrosis, excessive thirst, confusion, delirium, seizures, coma, and respiratory failure. At least 10% of acutely poisoned persons die.

Among those who survive at least a week or who are exposed to smaller amounts of thallium, the most predictable manifestations are a combined sensory and motor, often painful, peripheral neuropathy and alopecia. Although the head alopecia is total, the facial, axillary, and pubic hair is spared, as is the inner one third of the eyebrows. Motor manifestations may predominate, and the ascending, predominantly motor paralysis may mimic Guillain-Barré syndrome. Abdominal colic, nausea, and vomiting occur frequently in both the acute and the subacute forms of thallium toxicity and may so dominate the clinical picture that a diagnosis of acute appendicitis is made. Other manifestations of subacute intoxication include dementia, headache, fatigue, sleep disorders, intractable thirst, hallucinations, blindness caused by optic neuritis, impotence, amenorrhea, a blue discoloration of the gingivae, centrilobular hepatic necrosis, renal tubular necrosis, orthostatic hypotension, paralytic ileus, and myoclonic twitches. Multiple cranial nerves may be involved, but the eighth nerve is almost always spared. The electrocardiogram may show arrhythmias and changes similar to those associated with hypokalemia.

DIAGNOSIS. Thallium can be measured in blood and urine, but blood levels are often deceptively low even during clinically apparent poisoning. Because thallium is excreted in the urine, thallium determinations on 24-hour specimens are more reliable.

In some cases there is no history of occupational, environmental, or intentional exposure. Unexplained abdominal pain, neurologic abnormalities, and alopecia suggest the diagnosis.

TREATMENT. Treatment consists of hemodialysis, which can remove up to half the thallium body burden, and administration of Prussian blue. Prussian blue, or activated charcoal given by mouth, absorbs thallium, so that fecal thallium concentrations increase. The half-life of thallium in the body is about 1 month, and repeated dialyses are usually needed.

PROGNOSIS. As many as 30% of those poisoned suffer some residual effects. The neuropathy may persist for many months before resolving, and some are left with variable amounts of dementia, neuropathy, ataxia, visual impairment, alopecia, and myoclonus.

Selenium

ETIOLOGY. Selenium is well absorbed from both the gastrointestinal tract and the lungs. The amount normally ingested varies markedly, depending on the local soil selenium content and on the geographic origins of foods consumed. The element is widely used in pigment, glass, electronics, ceramics, and steel industries.

CLINICAL MANIFESTATIONS. Both deficiency and toxicity syndromes are well described in animals. Deficiency, resulting from foraging on grains grown in soil deficient of selenium, produces white muscle disease, a diffuse, often severe myopathy. Excess caused by chronic ingestion of grains containing more than 10 parts per million of selenium results in two syndromes, alkali disease and the staggers. The former is milder and is characterized by anemia, emaciation, alopecia, and hoof deformity. The staggers is manifested by visual difficulties, anemia, liver cell degeneration, paralysis, and respiratory failure.

In humans a *selenium deficiency syndrome* has not been clearly defined. However, in the Republic of China, diffuse cardiomyopathy (Keshan disease) has been associated with low soil and blood selenium levels, and the incidence of the disease apparently has been strikingly reduced by selenium supplementation.

Selenium toxicity syndromes in humans can be divided into acute and chronic poisoning. Subjects with inordinate exposure to selenium fumes experience one or more of the following: intestinal disturbances, giddiness, apathy, lassitude, pallor, nervousness, depression, hair and nail loss, a garlic odor to the breath, and a metallic taste. Sore throat, dyspnea, and cough may also be noted. Symptoms usually disappear after removal from the occupational exposure. Among those ingesting excessive selenium, the following symptoms and signs have been reported: nausea, vomiting, abdominal pain, diarrhea, anorexia, fatigue, sore throat, arthralgias, emotional lability, a metallic taste, a garlic odor to the breath, brittle nails, brittle hair, hair loss, a bronze color to the skin, hepatic dysfunction, and diffuse dermatitis. Increased selenium burdens may be associated with an increased prevalence of dental caries.

EPIDEMIOLOGY. A most impressive epidemic of chronic selenium intoxication was observed in China in the 1960's. Subacute and chronic selenium toxicity may be seen with an increasing frequency because selenium is being promoted as a nonprescription supplement.

Manganese

Manganese toxicity occurs primarily in miners who have been exposed to manganese dioxide aerosols for prolonged periods. The manifestations, known as manganic madness, are limited to the CNS. The manganese is concentrated primarily in the basal ganglia and cerebellum, accounting for the extrapyramidal Parkinson-like facies, the rigidity, and the difficulty in walking. Other manifestations include compulsive behavior (including singing, dancing, fighting, and running), explosive and involuntary laughter, headache, muscular weakness, tremors, somnolence, dystonia, hypotonia, retropulsion and propulsion, dementia, speech disturbances, irritability, sialorrhea, impotence, hypersomnia, and memory defects. In some cases psychosis may be the dominant feature. There is no effective therapy. Manganese contamination of dialysates or ingestion has been associated with abdominal pain, liver dysfunction, and evidence of pancreatitis.

Barium

Barium compounds are used in printing; in the production of paints, glass, paper, leather, soap, and rubber; in ceramics, plastic, steel, oil, textile, and dye industries; as fuel additives; and in insecticides, rodenticides, and depilatories. There are two major adverse effects. After accidental or intentional ingestion of large amounts, abdominal pain, vomiting, and increased peristalsis occur. If enough is absorbed, potassium is displaced intracellularly, resulting in profound hypokalemia, which in turn may produce flaccid paralysis, potentially dangerous cardiac arrhythmias, renal failure, and respiratory paralysis. Poisoning has also been described after barium chloride skin burn. Treatment consists of administering potassium and efforts to promote barium excretion. Severe allergic reaction has followed barium enema; whether this is due to the barium or preservatives is not clear.

The other adverse effect from contact with barium is a benign pneumoconiosis that may supervene after 1 or more years of aerosol exposure. Chest roentgenograms show extensive, very dense bilateral nodules up to 4 to 5 mm in diameter. There is no prominent fibrosis and no clinically significant disease; the nodules often regress after occupational exposure is stopped.

Boron

There are few reports of boron toxicity. Ingesting boric acid can result in nausea; vomiting; diarrhea; anemia; seizures; a variety of skin eruptions characterized by intense erythema, desquamation, and exfoliation; and striking alopecia. Additionally, occupational aerosol exposure to diborane (B_2H_6) in high-energy fuels can produce acute pulmonary edema that resolves after the exposure is discontinued. Exposure to liquid boron hydride (B_5H_9) can produce dementia, cortical blindness, deafness, seizures, acidosis, and cardiac arrest. A subacute mild organic brain syndrome has also been observed.

Antimony

Industrial antimony toxicity is very rare, as is intentional ingestion or inadvertent poisoning from antimony released from inexpensive enamelware. Manifestations of acute poisoning include nausea, abdominal pain, weakness, headache, vomiting, diarrhea, hematemesis, myalgias, liver function abnormalities, acute renal tubular dysfunction, electrolyte abnormalities, and circulatory collapse. Gaseous SbH_3 (stibine) is as toxic as arsine, producing CNS toxicity and hemolysis. After antimonial injection for medicinal purposes, adverse effects include nausea, vomiting, cough, and muscle and joint pain. Hepatic dysfunction can occur, as can cardiac arrhythmias, including Adams-Stokes syndrome. Antimony is also considered one of the metals capable of causing metal fume fever. Treatment of oral ingestion consists of lavage, administration of ac-

tivated charcoal, and administration of dimercaprol or the less toxic analogues dimercaptosuccinic acid or dimercaptopropanesulfonic acid.

Chromium

Chromium is used extensively in metal and galvanizing industries and in the manufacture of dyes, enamel, and paints. Chromate exposure is associated with an increased incidence of lung and certain upper respiratory tract cancers. Additionally, chromium-exposed workers may show evidence of proximal renal tubule dysfunction and may suffer nasal septum perforations.

Molybdenum

In animals, molybdenum produces diarrhea, anemia, alopecia, diminished growth, and bone and joint abnormalities. No clearly defined molybdenum toxicity syndrome has been reported in humans.

Platinum

The major adverse effects observed in platinum workers are allergic pulmonary reactions, including bronchial asthma.

Plutonium

In experimental models, plutonium, because of its radioactivity, is a potent carcinogen. Workers have been generally well protected, but recent data suggest that occupational exposure may be a significant problem. Some still controversial epidemiologic studies have suggested that accidental community exposure has resulted in an increase in frequency of certain cancers and fetal malformations.

Tellurium

Used particularly in rubber, metallurgic, and electronics industries, tellurium can cause giddiness, headache, nausea, a metallic taste, and a garlic smell to the breath. In animals tellurium causes neuropathy, but this has not been convincingly demonstrated in humans.

Tin

Tin can be released into beverages or foods from tin cans; ingestion can produce nausea, vomiting, abdominal pain, and diarrhea. Such toxicity occurs infrequently. Additionally, there have been occasional reports of neurologic abnormalities following exposure to organic tin, including the triethyl, trimethyl, and triphenyl tins. These are used primarily in agriculture for their bactericidal, fungicidal, antiparasitic, and molluscacidal properties. Manifestations include ataxic dysmetria, disorientation, seizures, nystagmus, impaired vision, hearing loss, headache, vertigo, paresthesias, intracranial hypertension, paresis, and polyneuropathy. Aerosol exposure to tin may result in stannosis, a mild pneumoconiosis in which there may be dense bilateral infiltrates but usually no pulmonary dysfunction.

Vanadium

Vanadium is used in alloys and in the steel and chemical industries. Its inhalation can result in neurasthenia, anorexia, vertigo, throat pain, nasal irritation (even nasal hemorrhage), and acute bronchitis characterized by a cough that is sometimes accompanied by a whoop. The nasal mucosa of vanadium-exposed workers shows vascular hyperemia and round cell infiltration.

Agocs MM, et al.: Mercury exposure from indoor latex paint. N Engl J Med 323:1096, 1990. *A unique report of what ought be a nonexistent contamination problem.*
Brody DJ, Pirkle JL, Kramer RA, et al.: Blood lead levels in the US population. Phase 1 of the Third National Health and Nutrition Examination Survey (NHANES III, 1988 to 1991), JAMA 272:277, 1994.
Clarkson TW: Mercury. J Am Coll Toxicol 8:1291, 1989. *A thoughtful historical perspective that sets the stage for action.*
Clarkson TW (ed.): Mercury toxicity: ATSDR's case studies in environmental medicine #17. US Department HHS PHS, March 1992. *A readily available up-to-date clinical review.*
Dart RC: Chelation of heavy metals: The future. J Toxicol Clin Toxicol 30:491, 1992. *Provides insight into the pros and cons of chelation—with realistic parameters.*
Pirkle JL, Brody DJ, Gunter EW, et al.: The decline in blood lead levels in the United States. The National Health and Nutrition Examination Surveys (NHANES). JAMA 272:284, 1994.

14 CLINICAL DECISION MAKING

14.1 Approach to the Patient
Suzanne W. Fletcher

When a patient sees a doctor, the patient is seeking help—to regain or retain health. The physician's task is to work for the patient's health. The doctor does so by trying to attenuate disease, by relieving discomfort, by assisting the patient with any disability, by preventing premature death, and by maximizing contentment. (Some have summarized these activities as tackling "the five D's" of health—disease, discomfort, disability, death, and dissatisfaction.) Sometimes there is success in all these areas. In the best of circumstances, the doctor is able to prevent disease and help the patient remain healthy. In other cases, disease and death defeat us. In some cases none of the goals is achieved, but even that outcome must not stop us from trying. By focusing on the health of the patient, the doctor tests the myriad activities of clinical medicine against the health outcome of the patient.

In most clinical encounters the patient presents basic questions to the doctor: Am I sick? What is causing my illness? Will it go away? Will it kill me? Can you make me well? Better? Can you help me stay well?

These questions set the stage for making a diagnosis, determining prognosis, carrying out treatment, promoting health, and preventing disease. This is the bulk of daily clinical work. Although young physicians learn these skills one at a time, the master clinician blends them so skillfully that often it is difficult to discern which is occurring at any given moment. For example, when obtaining a history of performing a physical examination to arrive at a diagnosis, the master clinician all the while is considering prognosis and is treating the patient with appropriate attention, empathy, consolation, and therapeutic information, thus ensuring that the patient feels better just for having been with the doctor.

DIAGNOSIS

Diagnosis is accomplished with history, physical examination, and laboratory testing. Although modern medicine has shifted attention toward the laboratory, even today most of the diagnosis is accomplished through history taking and physical examination, which narrow the diagnostic possibilities before laboratory testing is used. And it is through history taking and physical examination that the doctor humanizes the medical encounter for the patient and sets the stage for successful treatment.

MEDICAL HISTORY. There are standard sections to a complete medical history (Table 14–1). It is usual, but not necessary, to obtain the complete history when a physician and patient meet for the first time. During follow-up visits active medical problems are the focus. If the patient's presenting complaint is urgent, it may not be feasible to obtain a complete medical history—for example, when a patient is admitted to the intensive care unit or seen in the emergency room, the presenting problem prevails. In every case, the doctor should start with what is most important in the history and, according to circumstances, adjust the rest of the history taking. The patient's medical history will unfold over time and should be augmented at each subsequent doctor-patient encounter.

History of the Present Illness. The present illness is like a newspaper story. For each major symptom, the doctor must determine *what* (e.g., pain, nausea, weakness), *where* (part of body), *when* (e.g., continuous, intermittent, time of day), *how much* (severity), *chronologic course* (beginning of symptom, end, improvement, worsening), and what makes the symptom *better* or *worse*. It is important to determine what medical care the patient has already received for the problem, including laboratory tests previously done, their results, the diagnosis reached, the treatment given, whether the patient adhered to the treatment, and results of the treatment. Finally, the physician must seek answers to questions that narrow the

TABLE 14–1. THE PATIENT'S MEDICAL HISTORY

Description of patient
  Age, gender, race, occupation, and, for women, parity
Chief complaint
  Four or five words, preferably quoting the patient, stating the purpose of the visit and the duration of the complaint. Occasionally the patient states a request (e.g., "I need a flu shot") instead of a complaint.
Other physicians involved in the patient's care
  Name, address, telephone number, and relationship to the patient
History of the present illness
  For each major symptom, what, where, when, how much, chronologic course, what makes the symptom better or worse, past medical care, questions to narrow diagnostic possibilities
Past medical history
  Previous illnesses and hospitalizations, immunizations, medications the patient takes, allergies, and alcohol, tobacco, and drug habits
Social and occupational history
  Description of a typical day in the patient's life and how the present illness affects it, social supports (family, friends, and colleagues) available to the patient, and occupational history
Family history
  History of genetically related diseases in the patient's family and longevity and cause of death of family members
Review of systems
  Systematic review of major organ systems: skin, hematopoietic system (including lymph nodes), head, eyes, ears, nose, mouth, throat, neck, breasts, and respiratory, cardiovascular, gastrointestinal, genitourinary, musculoskeletal, nervous, endocrine, and psychiatric systems

diagnostic possibilities. This step, the most difficult part of obtaining an understanding of the present illness, requires a great deal of diagnostic skill and knowledge. Skilled clinicians form diagnostic hypotheses early in the patient's story and are able to ask specific questions, the answers to which confirm or exclude a given diagnostic possibility. Parts of the history of the present illness (description of symptoms and treatment compliance) are best obtained from the patient, whereas others (details about previously performed laboratory tests and treatment) are best acquired from medical sources.

Clinical Interview Technique.
The interaction of a doctor and patient during the medical interview is a marvelous mixture of art and science. The art is the interaction of two unique human beings; the science, the biologic and behavioral bases of medicine.

Each physician must develop an interviewing technique that is comfortable and true to his/her own personality. Interview style also necessarily varies according to the particular patient. Some patients are loquacious to a fault, others right to the point, and still others mute. Some patients want to control the encounter, some are passive, a few are hostile. The doctor needs to adjust the interview accordingly. But at every encounter, the patient must be treated with both courtesy and dignity.

It is the physician's task to manage the pace and direction of the interview. At the outset, the doctor should introduce himself/herself and address the patient by name. It is helpful to indicate how long the encounter is likely to last. The physician should focus total attention upon the patient. A few minutes of complete attention are better than 30 minutes of distracted interaction.

In relating a history, most patients do not follow the precise order outlined above. The patient may include bits and pieces of social and family history while describing the current complaint. It is the physician's job to fashion order out of the story while still allowing the patient a chance to tell the story in his/her own way. Giving the patient this chance increases the likelihood of patient satisfaction with the clinical encounter as well as the patient's willingness to follow the doctor's advice about treatment. In addition, many doctors enjoy listening to their patients. Over a lifetime, a physician meets patients from almost every class, race, educational level, profession, moral persuasion, and personality type. Listening to patients' stories told in their own way reveals the rich variety of humanity open to the practicing physician.

After introductions, the physician asks why the patient has come. Then the doctor should listen. If questions are needed to help the patient along, they should be open-ended and nonspecific. After a few minutes, the doctor should begin to direct the interview more actively, by facilitating the patient's story with more directed questions. Often, it helps to summarize the history during the interview. Finally, the doctor must narrow the diagnostic possibilities with appropriate questions.

If time is short, the doctor must take charge of the interview more quickly, but in almost all circumstances, the patient should be given a chance to tell his/her story. If the physician takes charge too quickly, not only do patient satisfaction and cooperation decrease, but the chances for a missed diagnosis increase. This is especially true when the patient is uncomfortable or afraid to speak openly, as with teenage pregnancies or cases of sexual abuse.

Past Medical History, Social History, Family History, and Review of Systems.
These sections (see Table 14–1) are far more routine than the history of the present illness, and the questions in each section are best memorized. The doctor should explain briefly each new section so that the patient understands the shift in topic. ("Now I would like to ask you about other illnesses you may have had in the past.") Start with general questions. ("Have you ever been sick before?")

Usually, the social history seems least relevant for diagnosis and therefore physicians most frequently shorten or omit it. However, learning about a patient's daily life, how the current illness is affecting it, and what social supports the patient can call on for assistance are particularly important when trying to fashion an effective treatment for the patient.

Because most questions in the latter sections of the medical history are standard, answers can be obtained by giving the patient a printed questionnaire or by using a computerized questionnaire. Both are organized in a branching manner, so that affirmative answers can be explored further.

PHYSICAL EXAMINATION. The physical examination is done with the five senses, and probably a sixth as well. Physicians in training should practice the complete examination on as many patients as possible to master all parts thoroughly. A complete examination, with a thorough neurologic and pelvic examination, takes even skillful examiners a good deal of time. Sometimes, because of time, the doctor may have to conduct a complete examination over several visits.

Several principles are important every time a physician performs a physical examination. The physician must demonstrate respect for the patient, making sure to expose private parts of the body only for as long as necessary for a careful examination. The physical examination should follow a standard order and be carried out in a systematic manner. It should be as comfortable as possible for the patient and require a minimum amount of shifting and changing of position. The more uncomfortable parts of the examination, such as the rectal and pelvic examinations, generally should be performed last.

The physical examination begins with inspection, which starts when you enter the room. Next come the vital signs. The physician always should examine carefully those parts of the body related to the reason for the patient's visit. Whenever necessary, objective measurements—such as number and size of the nodes, breadth of the liver, circumference of the calf—should be taken, not only for accurate assessment of the clinical course but also for more precise communication with other clinicians who may next see the patient.

Physicians should strive to improve their physical examination skills throughout their careers. In this way, one begins to trust one's skills. One way to do this is to pick out one part of the examination and practice it on every patient seen during a given period. For example, a few weeks of extra attention to the thyroid improve those examination skills even if none of the patients so examined has thyroid disease.

Questioning and examining the patient are types of diagnostic tests and should be evaluated scientifically just as laboratory tests are. Some questions and examination techniques produce more accurate results than others. For example, the many different ways of examining the breast are not equally good for detecting lumps. Clinicians should master examination techniques that research has shown to be most accurate.

LABORATORY TESTS. Laboratory tests have become a standard part of the doctor-patient encounter; their correct use is complex and subject to a number of scientific principles (see Ch. 14.2). The physician must also explain clearly to the patient the purpose and use of tests. Although generally used for diagnosis or screening, occasionally a laboratory test is ordered as a therapeutic maneuver. For example, a patient with chest pain may be reassured by a normal chest radiograph.

PROGNOSIS

It is important to tell the patient the diagnosis (writing it down often helps) and discuss what to expect from the clinical course of the condition. For many patients, the prognosis of the illness is their greatest concern. If the illness is likely to resolve without sequelae, reassurance is often all that is needed.

The most difficult prognoses to discuss are those for fatal illnesses, especially many cancers. Most patients want to know even bad prognoses, but how much a physician tells a given patient should be determined primarily by the patient, not the physician. The physician has the duty to make the patient aware of his/her willingness to discuss the prognosis. Often detailed discussions are best conducted at follow-up visits, after the two have had a chance to get to know each other. The best physicians blend honest fact and hope together, helping the patient through the complicated steps of shock, denial, depression, and acceptance of a fatal illness. Most importantly, they make it clear that they will not abandon the patient.

Doctors should educate themselves about the clinical course of the medical illnesses they encounter. No matter the import of the disease, they should learn how long, on average, the pain of herpes zoster continues, the headache of sinusitis persists, and the patient with class IV congestive heart failure lives.

TREATMENT AND PREVENTION

Increasingly, patients visit doctors not for diagnosis but for treatment of ongoing medical problems. Even when a doctor must make the diagnosis, it is important to remember that making a diagnosis alone cannot improve the health of a patient. Only treatment and prevention can.

Two general principles should be kept in mind about treatment. First, the physician should treat the patient as well as the disease. With every clinical encounter, the physician should strive to ensure that the patient feels better just for having been with the doctor. When prescribing specific treatment, alleviation of symptoms, especially pain and nausea, is often as important to the patient as, say, antibiotics for an infection. Second, successful treatment of an illness, especially outside the hospital, usually requires the patient's active participation.

THERAPEUTIC PROCEDURES. Therapeutic procedures such as surgery, radiation, angioplasty, and chemotherapy (as well as invasive diagnostic tests) must be explained thoroughly to the patient; in most cases, signed consent must be obtained. The physician must help the patient understand what will happen during the procedure, the hoped-for outcome and its probability, and adverse effects of the procedure and their probabilities. Informed consent is a medical-legal requirement, but, just as important, it is a cornerstone of excellent clinical care. Technologic advances in medicine are complex, often costly, and rarely without the potential for adverse complications. True informed consent requires a great deal of clinical skill on the doctor's part. The physician should act as the patient's advocate. The patient should be given the necessary facts but not overwhelmed with incomprehensible technical details or a long list of terrifying and improbable adverse effects of a procedure. The physician should freely give professional advice but clearly communicate that the final decision is the patient's. If the patient remains undecided about a procedure after a thorough discussion, in most cases it is best to delay the decision. A patient who feels pressured by the doctor to undergo a risky procedure may be particularly upset if complications arise.

MEDICATIONS. Compliance with physicians' medication orders is a given in-hospital, but this is certainly not true in the ambulatory setting. With ambulatory patients it is especially important to explain the medication to the patient, its purpose in simple terms, its dosage schedule, and how long the patient should continue the medication.

It is useful to ask the patient to bring all medicines to each follow-up visit. Many patients do not know the names of their medicines; discussing pills in bottles is easier than abstract medication names. Often the doctor can make a rough estimate of medication compliance by the level of pills in the bottle (although for ongoing prescriptions patients may combine bottles or refill prescriptions before beginning to take the medication in a particular bottle, thus making accurate compliance measurement impossible). Sometimes the physician discovers that the patient does not have one of the prescribed medicines. The doctor may discover that the patient is taking medication prescribed by another physician. For each medicine discussed, the doctor should ask how often the patient is taking it and if there are any problems. If the patient is taking the medicine incorrectly, the physician can determine whether the problem is misunderstanding of the dosage schedule, forgetfulness, an adverse side effect, the cost of the drug, or some other reason.

To help the patient take prescribed medication, the physician should follow a few common-sense rules. The most important determinant of medication compliance is the number of medicines prescribed. Parsimony is key. In general, and especially for a patient on multiple medications, the doctor should strive for simple (once or twice daily) dosage schedules of the least expensive effective medication. At follow-up visits, the fewer the medication changes the better. For patients who have trouble remembering to take their medicines, written instructions or pill containers with alarms can help. Sometimes the physician can refer the patient to special pharmacy or nursing programs for help with medicine compliance.

PREVENTION AND HEALTH MAINTENANCE. Preventive and health maintenance activities (e.g., routine mammograms, smoking cessation, influenza vaccine) are indicated periodically according to an algorithm based on age, gender, and clinical status. Prompting systems, such as a prevention checklist, help incorporate appropriate prevention activities into the doctor-patient encounter. If there is no checklist or other system in place, the doctor should briefly consider what preventive activities are indicated in a patient of the given age and gender (see Ch. 9.1) and perform them.

Doctors perform three types of preventive and health maintenance activities: screening examinations to identify asymptomatic disease or risk factors, immunizations to prevent subsequent disease, and lifestyle counseling to stop harmful habits and promote healthful ones. It is much more difficult to get a patient to change daily habits than to agree to screening tests. Physicians who counsel patients to make lifestyle changes should expect many failures. Before beginning counseling, the patient's motivation for change should be determined. If the patient is motivated, and most are, counseling should concentrate on the actual steps the patient should take. Follow-up is especially important. Most patients fail the first few times they attempt to make a lifestyle change. If that happens, the doctor should encourage the patient to keep trying and avoid being judgmental. Success with even a small percentage of patients can lead to substantial health benefits. If doctors succeed in helping only 10% of their patients who smoke to break the habit, it has been estimated that more than 1 million American lives would be saved.

WRAP-UP

After taking the medical history, performing the physical examination, reviewing what laboratory tests are being ordered and why, and discussing recommended treatment and preventive activities, the doctor and patient should discuss follow-up plans and what to do if a problem occurs before the scheduled follow-up visit. The patient should be given the physician's name, *in writing,* and should know how to contact the doctor if the need arises. These steps are particularly important in the practice of internal medicine, in which most patient care involves chronic medical problems rather than episodic illness. The patient should be given a chance to ask any questions he/she may have. Arrangements should be made for the doctor to contact the patient with appropriate laboratory test results. At the end of the visit, the doctor should indicate that it was good to see the patient.

SUMMARY

A successful doctor-patient encounter requires a great deal of synthesis and judgment on the doctor's part. The physician must be thinking of many different elements at once, not only the diagnostic possibilities but also the prognostic implications, how and what to communicate to the patient, how to help the patient feel as comfortable as possible, which laboratory tests and therapy to choose, and how to explain them clearly to the patient. These elements must be addressed and updated constantly throughout the interview, often simultaneously. The doctor must translate all thought processes into effective interactions with the patient and must work to develop a partnership with the patient so that medically indicated diagnostic tests and treatments that are acceptable to the patient are identified and used. Overriding all of these activities, the doctor must keep asking how to improve and enhance the health of the patient, how to change those five D's.

Paradoxically, modern medicine, with its powerful technologies for diagnosis and treatment, requires more than ever that the physician emphasize one of medicine's most ancient activities, that of being a teacher. Fittingly, society requires that the doctor work with—not on—the patient. Although physicians may come to have a good deal of influence with some of their patients, the best carefully avoid trying to have power over their patients. Like great physicians of old, they know the truth of the classic maxim that the secret of the care of the patient is caring for the patient.

Fletcher RH, Fletcher SW, Wagner EH: Clinical Epidemiology—The Essentials. Baltimore, Williams & Wilkins, 1988. *Outlines the clinical-epidemiologic principles that underlie all doctor-patient encounters.*

Lipkin M, Putnam SA, Lazare A (eds.): The Medical Interview, New York, Springer-Verlag, 1994. *A textbook on the medical interview and related skills.*

Sackett DL, Rennie D: The science of the art of the clinical examination. JAMA 267:2650, 1992. *This editorial introduces a series of review articles on the accuracy and precision of different parts of the clinical examination.*

Schneiderman H: Bedside Diagnosis: An Annotated Bibliography of Recent Literature on Interviewing and Physical Examination. Philadelphia, American College of Physicians, 1992. *Lists references on the medical history and physical diagnosis, collected from a computerized search of the medical literature from 1974 through 1991 and other materials collected by the author.*

14.2 Clinical Decision Making: Handling and Analyzing Clinical Data

Stephen G. Pauker

The primary role of the physician is to make decisions—about what tests to order, about what test results mean, about what drugs to administer, about whether or not to perform surgery. Virtually all medical decisions are made beneath a cloak of uncertainty—about diagnosis, about the effectiveness of therapeutic alternatives, about prognosis. The benefits of formal approaches to decision making rest on their explicit nature, on their unyielding requirements for information, and on the ability to ask "What if?" What if this disease is more likely? What if surgery is more effective but also engenders a higher risk? What if the patient is an octogenarian? What if the optimal time for diagnostic testing has passed and the test's sensitivity is therefore diminished? Of course, these approaches also carry significant cost: They sometimes require extra effort and always require decision makers to confront uncertainty and to be explicit about their assumptions and the underlying data.

Clinical decision analyses must be distinguished from clinical algorithms or flow charts, which are used as media for representing and communicating management strategies and guidelines. Algorithms are compact schemata for summarizing a set of rules or "if-then" statements that can guide the clinician down an established management pathway. It would be possible, for example, to translate many of the management strategies in this book into algorithms. Of course, one needs a rational process for creating such rules. Although they are sometimes annotated to describe the rationale that underlies them, algorithms and guidelines are most often the implicit product of singular or communal experience. Indeed, one can use the formal techniques described in this chapter to help formulate algorithms.

THE NATURE OF CLINICAL INFORMATION

Be it the patient's history, the physical examination, imaging result, or laboratory data, clinical information virtually always reflects the variation in the underlying biology, the stage of the patient's disease, the coexistence of other diseases, the administration of treatments or drugs taken for other purposes, or imperfect observation and measurement. In any case, most clinical observations show a distribution of values: e.g., the duration of symptoms, the severity or nature of pain, the degree of organomegaly, the size of an abnormality on a radiologic or ultrasound image, the level of a metabolite or enzyme detected in blood or urine, the histologic appearance of a biopsy, and even the specific defect found on DNA analysis. Although such distributions are sometimes gaussian or "normal," more often than not they are skewed and asymmetric; occasionally they can even be multimodal. In such circumstances, it makes little sense to describe a normal range reaching from two standard deviations below the mean to two standard deviations above the mean. Rather, the trend has been to describe *reference intervals* which include 95% of normal individuals. But even this approach has limited clinical utility because the clinician must consider the distribution of results among both healthy individuals and patients with each potential diagnosis. The clinician must also consider the effects of comorbidities and variations in physiology on those distributions. For example, when interpreting the serum level of creatine kinase (CK) in a patient who may have had a myocardial infarction, the astute clinician must realize that CK levels in healthy men are far higher than CK levels in healthy women.

THE INTERPRETATION OF DATA

In making a diagnosis, the physician moves continually between two tasks: data gathering and data interpretation. The former task involves identifying potential data elements and deciding which elements to acquire. The latter task involves modifying a set of hypotheses based on new data elements; those new elements might be drawn from the patient's history, from the physical examination, from laboratory tests, or from the patient's response to diagnostic or therapeutic maneuvers. In each case, however, the new data might suggest new hypotheses to be added to the list of differential diagnoses and almost always will modify the clinician's strength of belief in existing hypotheses. Those beliefs can be most conveniently represented as *probabilities,* the likelihood of each diagnosis on a scale from 0 to 1, which can be manipulated by several basic rules:

1. The probability of a diagnosis being false ($P_{no\ dis}$) equals ($1 - P_{dis}$), where P_{dis} is the probability of the diagnosis.
2. The list of alternative diagnoses must be exhaustive, and the probabilities must sum to 1.0 (thus, one often includes the category "other" in the list of diagnoses).
3. The various hypotheses must be mutually exclusive (thus, if one hypothesis is that diseases a and b coexist, then the explicit hypothesis "both disease a and disease b" must be included).
4. Among mutually exclusive diagnoses, the probability that the patient has at least one of several diagnoses equals the sum of their probabilities [thus, $P_{dis-a\ or\ dis-b}$ equals ($P_{dis-a} + P_{dis-b}$)].
5. If events or findings are independent, their joint probability equals the product of their probabilities [thus, $P_{finding-a\ and\ finding-b}$ equals ($P_{finding-a} \times P_{finding-b}$)].
6. If events or findings are dependent, their joint probability equals the product of the probability of the first ($P_{finding-a}$) and the conditional probability of the second, given the first ($P_{finding-b|finding-a}$).

MULTIPLE TESTS (PANELS)

In clinical practice the clinician often must interpret a set of test results, be it a routine chemical panel, a stress test (which reflects physical performance, clinical symptoms, electrocardiographic ischemia, and myocardial perfusion) or perhaps even several genetic screening tests on a single blood sample. Some of these multiple results provide independent information, whereas other results may be correlated with one another. Suppose that several tests are performed, each having a modest false-positive rate; the chance that a healthy patient has at least one false-positive result can be quite substantial. For a panel of 12 independent tests, with the reference range of each test encompassing 95% of normal individuals, the chance that all 12 tests will be normal (based on rule 5) is 0.95^{12}, or 0.54, implying that 46% of healthy patients have at least one abnormal result. With a panel of 20 independent tests, the chance of at least one abnormal result is 64%; with 40 tests, the chance is 87%. As the Human Genome Project proceeds, we might expect as many as 1000 screening tests for genetic disease to be available; if each had a false-positive rate of 0.001 and if all these tests were done, 63% of patients screened would have at least one false-positive result. Thus, if not a part of a carefully designed strategy, routine screening panels can lead to substantial additional testing, with each test carrying its own risks, costs, anxiety, and inconvenience to the patient.

BAYES' RULE

In this context, data can be interpreted explicitly using a relation among probabilities that allows clinicians to modify their level of belief in each hypothesis based on incremental data. The technique begins with the probability of each disease before knowledge of the incremental finding is available (the *prior probability*), which in the absence of other clinical information can be estimated by the prevalence of disease but which can also be estimated by clinical prediction rules, by logistic regressions, or most commonly by the clinician's subjective impression. Next, for each disease the *conditional probability* of the incremental finding ($P_{finding|dis\ i}$) is specified. Although these probabilities can be combined using the equation for Bayes' rule,

$$P_{dis\ i|finding} = \frac{P_{dis\ i} \times P_{finding|dis\ i}}{\sum_{i=1}^{n} P_{dis\ i} \times P_{finding|dis\ i}}$$

it is almost always easier to use the tabular form of the technique (Table 14–2) or the cohort flow form (Fig. 14–1).

In the simplest case, the physician considers a single disease and interprets a diagnostic test, which is either positive or negative. In that situation, the probability of a positive test in a patient who has

TABLE 14–2. USING BAYES' RULE TO INTERPRET A SPUTUM CYTOLOGIC STUDY DEMONSTRATING ATYPICAL CELLS IN A NONSMOKER WITH A PULMONARY NODULE

A Diagnosis	B Prior Probability	C Conditional Probability of Observed Test Result	D Product (Col B × Col C)	E Revised or Posterior Probability (Col D/Sum)
Cancer	0.01	0.40	0.004	0.04 (a)
No cancer	0.99	0.10	0.099	0.96 (b)
			Sum = 0.103	

Step 1: List diagnoses in Column A.
Step 2: List prior probabilities in Column B.
Step 3: List conditional probabilities of finding in Column C.
Step 4: Multiply Columns B and C and place products in Column D.
Step 5: Divide each entry in Column D by sum of Column D and place quotients in Column E.
(a): for positive test results, this is sometimes called the *positive predictive value*
(b): for negative test results, this is sometimes called the *negative predictive value*

the disease, $P_{pos|dis}$, is called the *sensitivity* of the test, and the probability of a negative test in a patient who does not have the disease, $P_{neg|no\ dis}$, is called *specificity* of the test. Whenever one attempts to describe the diagnostic performance of a clinical finding, one needs a separate *gold standard* to define the presence or absence of each disease. When the test result is naturally a continuous variable (such as the serum level of an enzyme, the degree of ST segment depression on the ECG during exercise, or the size of the left atrium), the clinician (or the laboratorian) often selects a *criterion* to define a positive result (Fig. 14–2). The stricter that criterion, the more specific but the less sensitive is the test. For any given test, sensitivity and specificity are inversely related: the higher the clinician makes one, the lower the other becomes, a relation reflected by the test's *receiver-operator characteristic (ROC) curve* (Fig. 14–2). The only way to improve both measures of test performance simultaneously is to improve the test, that is, to further separate the two

overlapping distributions of results. Changing either the gold standard or the criterion of positivity changes the performance of the test (i.e., conditional probabilities of the findings). For example, using the data in Figure 14–1, if a positive exercise tolerance test is defined as one with ≥1 mm ST depression, then the sensitivity for the diagnosis of coronary disease would be (11,250 + 12,500 + 35,750 + 5,500)/(25,000 + 55,000) or 81% and the specificity would be 85%. On the other hand, if a positive result were defined as >2 mm ST depression, then the sensitivity would be only 23% but the specificity would be 99%. If "significant coronary artery disease" were defined as either three-vessel or left main coronary artery obstruction, then the test would likely be more sensitive and less specific than if it were defined simply as involvement of one or more coronary arteries.

Implicit test interpretation is fraught with error in several settings: (1) the setting of a low prior probability of disease and a positive result (here, the revised probability of disease is often not very high unless the test is extremely specific); (2) the setting of a high prior probability of disease and a negative finding (here, the revised probability of disease may not be very low unless the test is extremely sensitive); and (3) when several tests have produced conflicting results (the revised probability of disease depends on both the prior probability and the relative strength of information carried by each test as reflected in the finding's *likelihood ratio*, $P_{finding|dis}/P_{finding|no\ dis}$). Especially in those situations, it is important to interpret the finding in an explicit and formal manner. When interpreting a positive result of a screening test for low-prevalence disease, the test's specificity is of paramount importance and the revised probability of disease is approximately $P_{dis}/(P_{dis} + P_{pos|no\ dis})$. When screening for diseases having a low prevalence, false-positive test results can be far more common than true positive test results and the revised probability can be surprisingly low.

When interpreting a series of findings, the calculated posterior or revised probabilities based on the first finding become the prior probabilities for interpreting the next finding in a sequential application of Bayes' rule. If the several findings are not conditionally independent of one another, then appropriate conditional probabilities should be used. For example, in diagnostically eval-

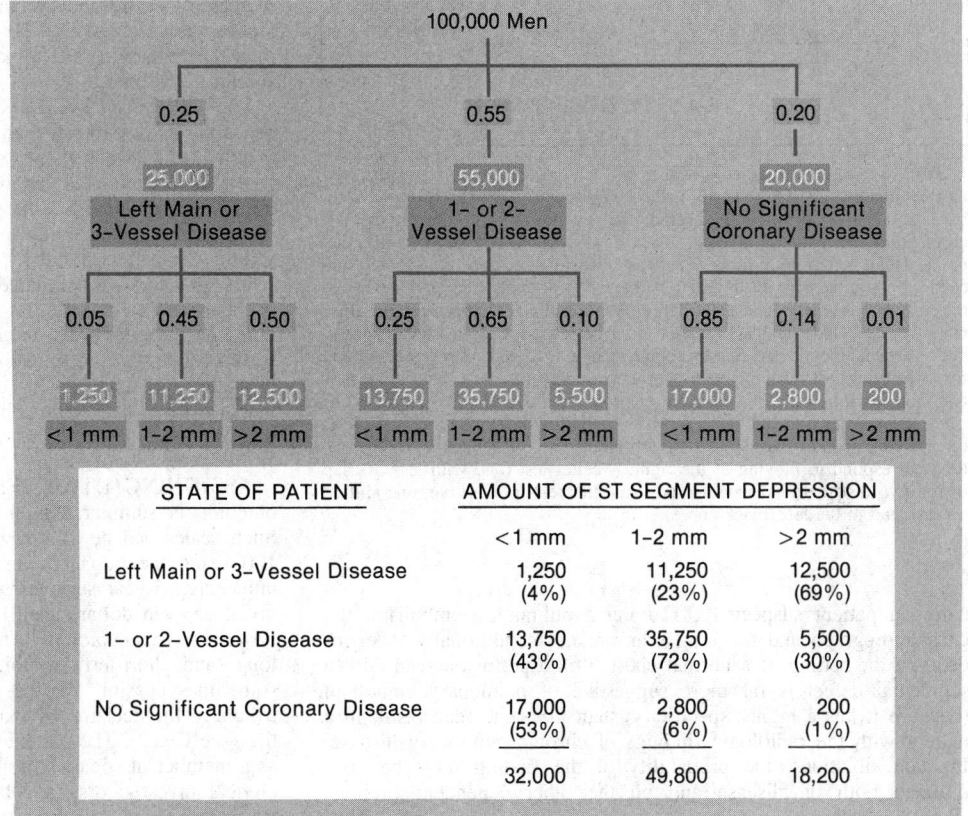

FIGURE 14–1. Cohort flow model of Bayes' rule used to interpret an exercise tolerance test in a 50-year-old man with typical angina. Consider a cohort of 100,000 such men: 25% have left main or 3-vessel disease, 55% have 1- or 2-vessel disease, and 20% are free of significant coronary disease. If the conditional probabilities of <1 mm, 1 to 2 mm, and >2 mm of ST depression are as shown and determine how many men from each diagnostic subgroup will have each finding, then of the 1,250 + 13,750 + 17,000 (or 32,000) men with <1 mm of ST depression, 17,000, or 53%, will have no significant coronary disease, 43% will have 1- or 2-vessel disease, and 4% will have left main or 3-vessel disease. (Based on data in Diamond GA, Forrester JS: Analysis of probability as an aid in the clinical diagnosis of coronary-artery disease. N Engl J Med 300:1350, 1979. Copyright 1979, the Massachusetts Medical Society.)

STATE OF PATIENT	AMOUNT OF ST SEGMENT DEPRESSION		
	<1 mm	1–2 mm	>2 mm
Left Main or 3–Vessel Disease	1,250 (4%)	11,250 (23%)	12,500 (69%)
1- or 2-Vessel Disease	13,750 (43%)	35,750 (72%)	5,500 (30%)
No Significant Coronary Disease	17,000 (53%)	2,800 (6%)	200 (1%)
	32,000	49,800	18,200

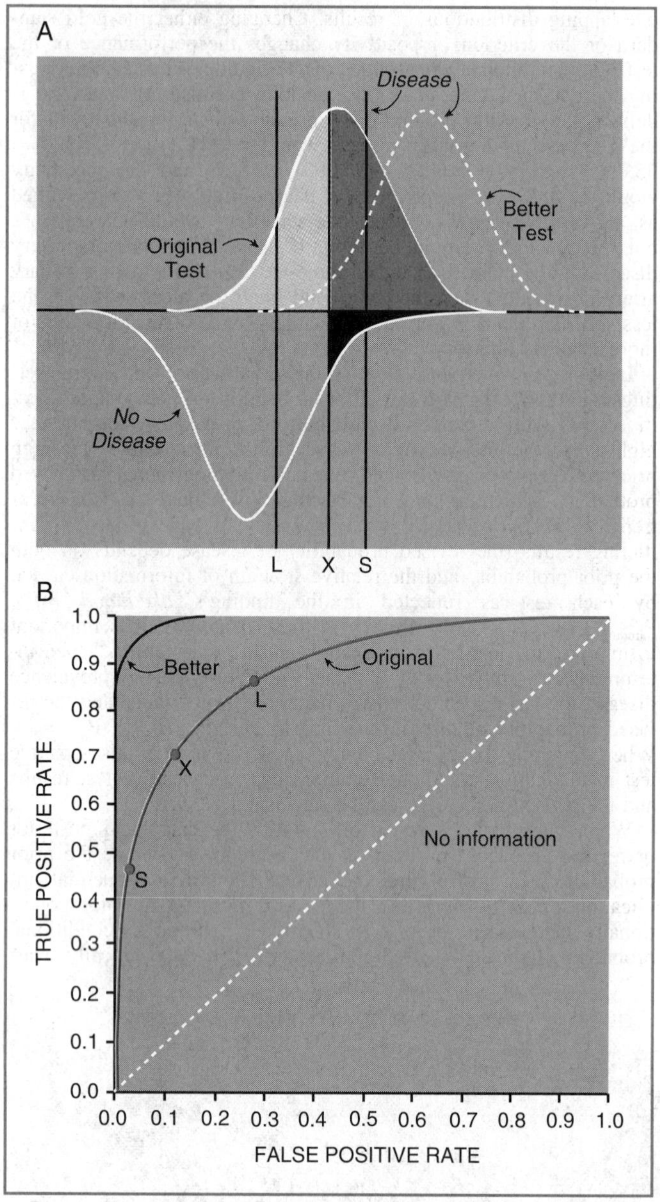

FIGURE 14-2. Distributions of test results and corresponding receiver-operator characteristic (ROC) curve. *A,* the upright solid distribution on the right corresponds to patients with disease; the inverted distribution on the left corresponds to patients without disease. If test results (horizontal axis) greater than criterion X are defined as positive, then the red shaded area corresponds to sensitivity or true-positive rate, the pink area corresponds to the false-negative rate, the unshaded area corresponds to specificity or true-negative rate, and the black shaded area corresponds to the false-positive rate. Vertical lines L and S correspond to more lax and more strict criteria for classifying test results. The broken curve depicts the results of a "better" test, one for which the two distributions have less overlap. *B,* The red ROC curve relates the true- and false-positive rates for different criteria. Stricter criteria correspond to moving to the left along the ROC curve; more lax criteria correspond to moving to the right. A better test (one with less overlap of the two distributions) would produce a different ROC curve, one shifted upward and to the left (black curve).

uating a patient suspected of having a pulmonary embolism, the chest radiograph and the lung scan are not conditionally independent: In the setting of a normal chest film, a perfusion scan with a segmental defect is far more suggestive of pulmonary embolism (because it has a higher specificity) than the same scan result in a patient with the radiologic findings of chronic pulmonary disease. In such situations, the probability of the finding must be conditioned both on disease and on the other dependent findings ($P_{finding\,|\,\text{"dis and other findings"}}$).

The physician managing a patient must choose among alternative plans. Such decisions often involve balancing risks and benefits. These choices often can be made more explicit and consistent by using formal *decision analysis.* The technique involves seven basic steps: (1) frame the question; (2) structure the problem; (3) determine the probability of the possible outcomes; (4) assign a value or utility to each possible outcome; (5) calculate the best strategy; (6) vary the assumptions and data over reasonable ranges to see whether the apparently optimal strategy changes; and (7) interpret the analysis.

For example, consider a 54-year-old man with acute myelogenous leukemia complicating longstanding lymphoma. The patient is immunosuppressed by chemotherapy and develops persistent fever, pulmonary infiltrates, and respiratory distress without a clear cause and despite empiric treatment with antibiotics and antituberculous drugs. The potential strategies of empiric therapy with amphotericin and open lung biopsy are raised.

FRAMING THE QUESTION. Formal decision analysis is designed to answer specific questions by evaluating well-specified alternatives and choosing the best. Rather than asking "How should this patient be managed?" the clinician should ask which of three alternatives is best: (1) empiric therapy with amphotericin, (2) conservative therapy, or (3) open lung biopsy with the amphotericin decision being based on the biopsy results.

STRUCTURING THE PROBLEM. The typical decision tree contains three basic elements: (1) decision nodes depicting choices, (2) chance nodes depicting events or diagnostic alternatives not under the control of the decision maker, and (3) outcome or terminal nodes summarizing events not explicitly occurring within the time horizon of the decision tree. This problem can be represented by the decision tree shown in Figure 14–3. The three choices are depicted by the decision node at the left. In both the "no amphotericin" and "amphotericin" strategies, prognosis is determined by whether a fungal infection is present and by the probability of short-term survival, conditioned on the presence or absence of fungal infection and on whether specific antifungal therapy is given. In the "lung biopsy" strategy, initially there is a chance of dying during the procedure. The biopsy may be either positive or negative, with the likelihood being determined by the prior probability of fungal infection and the sensitivity and specificity of the biopsy. If the biopsy result is positive, then the probability of fungal infection increases (the revised probability being calculated by Bayes' rule), and amphotericin should be administered. If the biopsy is negative, then the probability of fungal infection decreases and amphotericin should be withheld.

DETERMINING THE PROBABILITIES. In a decision tree, probabilities describe the present state of the patient (e.g., whether or not fungal disease is present) and the patient's prognosis. In both cases, these estimates can be based on the literature or on expert opinion. In either case, the physician uses descriptions of the past experience of other similar patients to predict the current and future state of the patient at hand.

In this case, we estimated the probability of fungal infection to be 30%; we estimated the chance of dying from untreated fungal infection to be 95% and the chance of dying from treated fungal infection to be 45%. If fungal disease is not present, we estimated the probability of death during this hospitalization to be 20%. We estimated that, in this setting, lung biopsy would be associated with a 5% mortality, a sensitivity of 80% in diagnosing fungal infection, and a specificity of 98%.

ASSIGNING UTILITIES. The relative value of each possible outcome is summarized on a single consistent scale by a utility. Such scales can be arbitrary (e.g., 0 being the worst outcome and 100 being the best) or can describe the outcomes in identifiable units (e.g., 5-year survival, years of life, years of disease-free survival, or even dollars spent). One useful metric can be *quality-adjusted life expectancy,* in which average survival is depreciated by long- and short-term morbidities. If such a metric is used, it is sometimes possible for the patient or the patient's family to contribute to the decision by expressing their attitudes about quality of life (see Ch. 2). The patient's quality of life and ability to function as a member of society can be important in many clinical decisions; clinical investigators have begun to measure explicitly the health status produced by different treatments. These studies examine

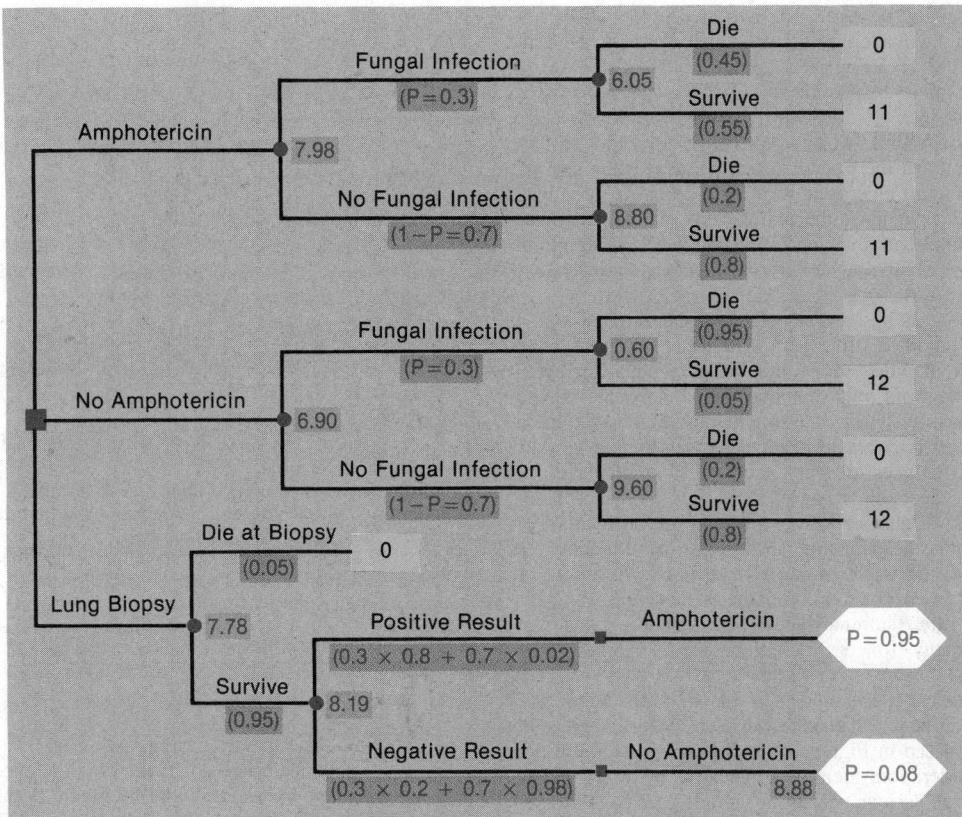

FIGURE 14–3. Decision tree depicting management choices in an immunosuppressed man with fever and pulmonary infiltrates. Decision nodes appear as squares. Chance nodes appear as circles. Outcome or terminal nodes appear as rectangles that contain the assigned utilities (in this case as quality-adjusted months of survival). Probabilities are shown (shaded red) within parentheses on each branch of each chance node. The hexagons at the end of the "lung biopsy" strategy represent the use of the "no amphotericin" and "amphotericin" subtrees (which are depicted in the first two branches of the main decision node), with the probability of fungal infection being modified to 0.95 and 0.08 after a positive and negative biopsy, respectively, by the application Bayes' rule. Calculated expected utilities are shown solid red to the right of each chance node. The sensitivity of the biopsy is taken as 0.8; the specificity is taken as 0.98. P = Probability of fungal infection. (Based on detailed analysis in Gottlieb JE, Pauker SG: Whether or not to administer amphotericin B to an immunosuppressed patient with hematologic malignancy and undiagnosed fever. Med Decision Making 1:75, 1981.)

more than just so-called "hard" outcomes, such as survival. New instruments allow "soft" outcomes to be measured reliably. Some health care systems have even begun to equate the quality of medical care with improved performance on such measures.

In this case, we shall use average survival modified by the short-term morbidity of amphotericin therapy. We estimated that survival would be 18 months if the patient achieves a remission of his leukemia but only 3 months if he does not. Because we assumed the chance of remission to be 60%, the average survival for this man, if he survived the acute event, would be 60% × 18 months plus 40% × 3 months, or 12 months. Although many physicians are very conservative in using amphotericin, the literature suggests that death and permanent renal failure are extremely rare complications of that drug; most side effects involve short-term toxicity. We assumed that the average duration of amphotericin therapy would be 2 months and that short-term morbidity would, on average, diminish quality of life during that period to half of what it otherwise would have been. Thus, we subtracted 1 month from the life expectancy to account for this morbidity, yielding a quality-adjusted survival of 11 months if amphotericin is administered. We assigned a utility of 0 to death during this acute illness.

CALCULATING THE EXPECTED UTILITY. In evaluating a tree (Fig. 14–3), the decision maker follows two basic rules: (1) When facing a choice, select the option with the highest utility or expected utility; (2) when evaluating a chance event, the expected utility is the weighted average of the utilities of its outcomes, with the weights being the respective probability of each outcome. In applying these rules, the decision maker begins at the distal outcome

nodes of the tree and sequentially calculates the average or expected utility of each node, moving toward the proximal decision node.

In this case, consider first the top branch of the decision node, the "amphotericin" strategy. The highest distal chance node describes the short-term consequences of a fungal infection treated with specific antifungal therapy. There is a 0.45 probability of dying (utility 0) and 0.55 probability of surviving (utility 11 quality-adjusted months). Thus, the average or expected utility of this chance node is 0.45 × 0 plus 0.55 × 11, or 6.05 quality-adjusted months. Similarly, the expected utility of amphotericin in the absence of a fungal infection (the second distal chance node) is 0.2 × 0 plus 0.8 × 11, or 8.8 quality-adjusted months. The expected utility of the "amphotericin" strategy is the weighted average of these two expected utilities: 0.3 × 6.05 plus 0.7 × 8.8, or 7.98 quality-adjusted months. In a similar fashion, we calculated the expected utility of "no amphotericin" to be 6.9 quality-adjusted months.

Next we consider the lowest branch of the main decision node—the "lung biopsy" strategy. As depicted at the end of the "positive" result branch, the expected utility is calculated using the "amphotericin" subtree, with the probability of fungal infection being increased to 0.95. In that case, the expected utility is 0.95 × 6.05 plus 0.05 × 8.8, or 6.18 quality-adjusted months. Similarly, the expected utility of the "negative" result branch is calculated with the "no amphotericin" subtree, with the probability of fungal infection being decreased to 0.08, yielding 0.08 × 0.6 plus 0.92 × 9.6, or 8.88 quality-adjusted months. The weighted average of these expected utilities depends on the probability of a positive result

(0.3 × 0.8 plus 0.7 × 0.02, or 0.25). The expected utility of the entire strategy is a weighted average of this result (8.19 quality-adjusted months) and the 5% chance of a procedure-related death (utility 0), providing an expected utility of 7.78 quality-adjusted months.

PERFORMING SENSITIVITY ANALYSES. Having calculated the expected utility in the baseline case, we next examine various central assumptions to determine whether reasonable variations in those assumed values change the conclusions. Such sensitivity analyses initially examine variables one at a time, usually beginning with the "softest" data. Such analyses are often called *one-way sensitivity analyses* (Fig. 14–4).

Typically, one strategy is best for all values of the variable below a certain cutoff, and another strategy is best for all values above that cutoff. The value at which the strategies have equal expected utility is called the *threshold* value for that variable. In addition to finding relevant threshold values, it is often important to examine the magnitude of the differences in expected values of the various strategies. If those differences are very small and potentially clinically insignificant, the decision may well be a *close call,* and there may be relatively little to gain or lose in selecting one management plan over another. With sufficient time and energy or with adequate computational support, the clinician can also examine the effect of simultaneous changes in two or more variables. Such multiway sensitivity analyses are often summarized by decision diagrams that specify the best strategy for each combination of values (Fig. 14–5).

In this case, the softest piece of data is the likelihood that this patient had a fungal infection. The one-way sensitivity analysis of this variable is summarized in Figure 14–4. If lung biopsy were not a strategy under consideration, then the probability of fungal infection above which amphotericin should be administered would depend only on the relative risks and benefits of treatment. In such circumstances the *therapeutic threshold* (the chance of disease above which treatment should be given) is simply $1/(1 + B/R)$, where B is the benefit of treatment in patients with disease (6.05 − 0.60, or 5.45 in Fig. 14–3) and R is the risk of treatment in patients without disease (9.60 − 8.80, or 0.80). In this example, the threshold is $1/(1 + 5.45/0.80)$, or 0.13. Another central variable is the effectiveness of amphotericin in enhancing survival in an immunosuppressed patient known to have fungal disease. We define the *efficacy* of therapy as $1 − (P_{die|Ampho}/P_{die|NoAmpho})$. Thus, the probability of dying despite appropriate therapy equals the probability of dying without therapy times $(1 − \text{efficacy})$. If efficacy were 0, then $P_{die|Ampho}$ would equal $P_{die|No\,Ampho}$; if efficacy were 100%, then

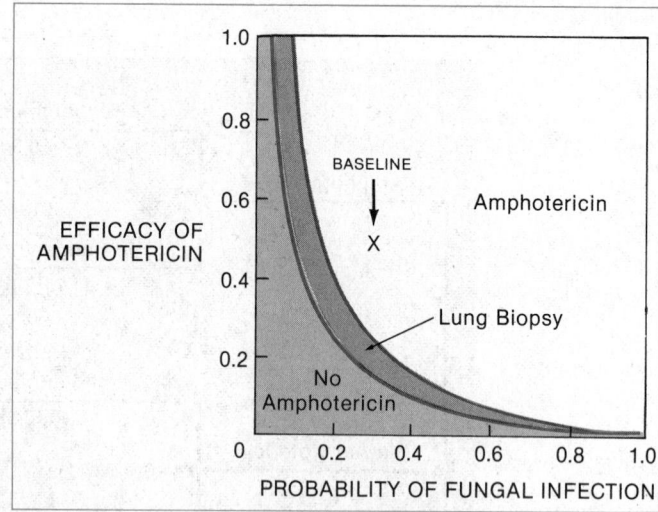

FIGURE 14–5. Two-way sensitivity analysis of the relation between the probability of fungal infection (horizontal axis) and the efficacy of amphotericin (vertical axis). Each combination of values corresponds to a unique point on the graph. All combinations falling in the lighter shaded area correspond to settings in which "no amphotericin" is the best strategy. All combinations falling in the darker shaded area correspond to settings in which "lung biopsy" is best. The baseline values correspond to the bold X, which lies within the settings in which "amphotericin" is best.

$P_{die|Ampho}$ would be 0. The baseline value is 0.53, and the threshold value for this variable is 0.28. If the efficacy exceeds that threshold, then empiric amphotericin should be given. If the efficacy is below 0.15, amphotericin therapy should be withheld. If the efficacy falls between these thresholds, lung biopsy is the best strategy. Clearly, if the efficacy of therapy is changed, then the threshold probability of fungal disease also changes, and vice versa. This two-way sensitivity analysis is summarized in Figure 14–5.

INTERPRETING THE ANALYSIS. Although there may well be a temptation to perform clinical decision analyses just to determine the best management strategy, the analyst would do the patient a disservice by stopping at that point. Every analytic model is merely an approximation of the underlying medical dilemma. The careful analyst must explore the model to discover its limitations. Only then can the clinician have reasonable confidence in its conclusions. One of the central benefits of a clinical decision analysis should be a better understanding of the clinical problem and a delineation of the settings in which the planned strategy is proper.

In this analysis, we see that empiric therapy with amphotericin is appropriate for any patient who has at least a moderate likelihood (>19%) of fungal infection. Therapy based on the results of lung biopsy is best only for the narrow wedge of patients falling in the darker shaded region of Figure 14–5. This region would be broadened if lung biopsy had a lower complication rate but would still be limited by the imperfect sensitivity of the test: Some patients with potentially treatable fungal infections would be denied therapy if their biopsy yielded falsely negative results. The major driving force is the surprisingly benign characteristics of amphotericin. Although patients receiving the drug have significant short-term morbidity, very few develop permanent renal insufficiency and even fewer die.

COST-BENEFIT AND COST-EFFECTIVENESS ANALYSIS

The practice of medicine in a world of limited resources sometimes leads the physician to consider not only what is "best" for the patient but also the resources that such medical care will use. In such contexts, cost-benefit and cost-effectiveness analyses can be used to guide policies. Because those policies may affect the way they practice medicine, physicians should understand some of the underlying principles. Although many physicians believe that there are ethical reasons to exclude any consideration of cost from the bedside, the economic realities that increasingly affect medical care often force the clinician to consider the cost of alternative care plans (see Ch. 4). The basic logic of such analyses is quite similar to that described above; the difference lies in the utility scales that

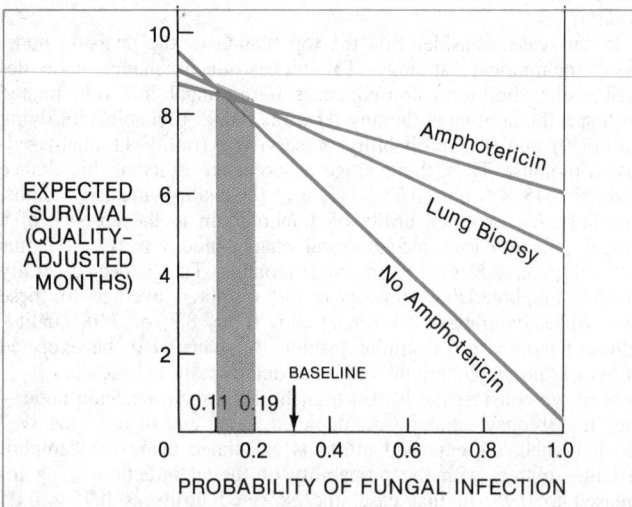

FIGURE 14–4. One-way sensitivity analysis in the decision tree shown in Figure 14–3. If the probability of fungal infection is zero, then the "no amphotericin" strategy is best. If the probability of fungal infection is 100%, the empiric amphotericin therapy is best. Lung biopsy is the optimal strategy in the narrow region between the two thresholds (vertical red bar) at 0.11 and 0.19. The baseline value of 0.3 is shown by the arrow.

measure the relative worth of the potential outcomes. When resources and societal issues are considered, outcomes are often measured by their economic impact. Economists argue that the magnitude of a cost depends on, among other things, *when* that cost is incurred. Money saved or spent immediately is worth more than money saved or spent in the future. This principle is called the *discounting* of future benefits and costs: Future costs and benefits are diminished by a fixed proportion for each year into the future when such costs and benefits occur. Although some analysts argue that discounting should be restricted to monetary factors, the balance of opinion favors the argument that all utility scales (e.g., survival and economic costs) should be discounted at the same rate.

When considering the economics of medical care, we should be careful to distinguish actual *costs* from *charges,* which may be quite distorted by particular billing practices or insurance plans. We also should consider *indirect costs* (e.g., heating and cleaning in the hospital and even malpractice insurance) and *induced costs* (e.g., the diagnostic evaluation of patients with falsely positive screening test results and even the medical care for treating cancer that develops years later in a patient who is "saved" from tuberculous pneumonia). Even among true direct costs, we must distinguish between average costs and variable costs (e.g., if a new policy eliminates the need for 30 CK tests each day, the hospital may not be able to decrease its laboratory personnel and thus may save only part of the cost of the tests). Finally, we must consider the *perspective* of the analysis—whose money is spent and whose survival or quality of life is improved.

In a *cost-benefit analysis,* economic impact is the only utility scale used: All benefits are measured in those terms. Thus, if a strategy increases survival, that benefit is translated into its monetary equivalent: Each year of life saved would be associated with a societal worth, perhaps based on economic productivity. If the benefits minus the costs of a given strategy are positive, the program contributes in the net to society. Presumably, the bigger the difference, the larger the contribution. But if the costs of a strategy exceed its benefits, the program should not necessarily be rejected. Society might well wish to underwrite such a program. For example, extending the life of a disabled, elderly nursing home resident might not provide net economic benefit to society, but our ethical values argue strongly against withdrawing care from such individuals, save perhaps at the very end of their lives.

Because the economic value of life and improved quality of life are difficult to quantify, we often turn to *cost-effectiveness* or *cost-utility analyses,* in which two separate utility measures are analyzed simultaneously, e.g., monetary costs and years of life saved. The results are expressed as the *ratio* of cost to benefits. That ratio does not measure the overall worth of a single strategy; rather, it is used to compare strategies. Often the strategy that engenders greater resource costs is also the strategy that provides the greater effectiveness. Thus, one usually examines the ratio of the difference in costs to the difference in effectiveness (the *marginal cost-effectiveness ratio*), which might be expressed as additional dollars spent per additional year of life saved or even as additional dollars spent per additional cancer detected (see Table 14–3). Such analyses rarely tell the decision maker which strategy is best in an absolute sense: They only provide a measure of cost per unit of gain.

Some external standard, perhaps established by society, must be applied to decide how much money is too much to spend to gain a year of life. Such analyses can also help when we must choose among alternate uses for a fixed amount of resource, i.e., when we have a budget. When we have only another $100,000 to spend, should we "buy" one heart transplant, five coronary bypass operations, or a year of therapy for 1000 hypertensive men? These are difficult decisions, but physicians must now contribute to the discussion, hopefully in a logical, explicit, and useful way.

Detsky AS, Naglie IG: A clinician's guide to cost-effectiveness analysis. Ann Intern Med 113:147, 1990. *Good introduction to performing and understanding the clinical relevance of cost-effectiveness analyses.*

Griner PF, Mayesski RJ, Mushlin AI, et al.: Selection and interpretation of diagnostic tests and procedures. Ann Intern Med 94:553, 1981. *Primer on Bayes' rule with many examples.*

Kassirer JP, Kopelman RI: Learning Clinical Reasoning. Baltimore, Williams & Wilkins, 1991. *A wonderful analysis of how doctors think, peppered with suggestions about how they might do it better.*

Pauker SG, Kassirer JP: Medical progress: Decision analysis. N Engl J Med 316:250, 1987. *A tutorial about new techniques, including the tabular approach to Bayes' rule.*

Stewart AL, Ware JE: Measuring Functioning and Well-Being: The Medical Outcomes Study Approach. Durham, Duke University Press, 1992. *Introduction to the reliable measurement of health status.*

14.3 Fundamental Statistics
Catarina I. Kiefe

The knowledge on which clinicians base medical decisions is growing explosively. Physicians must rely increasingly on the ability to quickly retrieve and integrate newly published data. Statistics allows a scientific approach to making inferences based on available data. Investigators use descriptive statistical tools to summarize data and inferential tools to test hypotheses.

DESCRIPTIVE STATISTICS

Many clinical variables, such as systolic blood pressure, are measured on a continuous numeric scale. For these continuous variables, appropriate measures of "central location" include a *mean* (average), *median* (50th percentile or middle value), and *mode* (most common value). Depending upon the data set, one of these measures most accurately summarizes the sample. Measures of dispersion quantify the amount of variability exhibited by variables. For those continuous variables distributed in a bell-shaped fashion (*gaussian* or *normal distribution*), the mean ± two *standard deviations* (SD) defines an interval containing 96% of the observed values. The *standard error of the mean* (SEM) measures the precision of the estimate of the mean itself. The SEM is always smaller than the SD, and it is not appropriate to use the SEM directly as a measure of dispersion. When a variable has a bell-shaped distribution, the sample mean ± 1.96 × SEM represents the 95% confidence interval for the mean. The length of this *confidence interval* describes the precision of the mean estimate. In general, when a certain parameter of interest, such as a mortality rate or a mean systolic blood pressure, is estimated from a given population sample, a 95% confidence interval for the parameter may be constructed from the same sample. Asserting that the parameter of interest is within its 95% confidence interval is true 95% of the time.

TABLE 14–3. CALCULATING THE MARGINAL COST-EFFECTIVENESS OF CORONARY BYPASS SURGERY AND PERCUTANEOUS TRANSLUMINAL ANGIOPLASTY*

A Strategy	B Cost ($)	C Effectiveness (Quality-Adjusted Life Years [QALY])	D Marginal Cost ($)	E Marginal Effectiveness (QALY)	F Marginal C/E Ratio ($/QALY)
Conservative therapy	44,000	5.8			
Angioplasty	50,000	6.7	6,000	0.9	6,667
Bypass surgery	60,000	7.2	10,000	0.5	20,000

Step 1: List strategies in Column A, in order of increasing cost.
Step 2: List discounted costs in Column B.
Step 3: List discounted effectivenesses in Column C.
Step 4: Calculate marginal (additional) cost of each strategy compared with next least expensive alternative (a strategy pair) and record in Column E.
Step 5: For each strategy pair, calculate marginal (additional) effectiveness achieved for that marginal cost and record in Column E.
Step 6: If entry in Column E is negative, then that next least expensive strategy has higher effectiveness and this strategy is dominated and eliminated from consideration.
Step 7: Divide each value in Column D by corresponding value in Column E and record marginal cost-effectiveness ratio in Column F.

* For a 55-year-old man with chronic stable angina in terms of additional cost per quality-adjusted life year gained (three-vessel disease and depressed ejection fraction).
Data from Wong JB, Sonnenberg FA, Salem DM, et al.: Myocardial revascularization for chronic stable angina. Ann Intern Med 113:852, 1990.

Many variables of clinical interest are not continuous. Vital status after a myocardial infarction is a *dichotomous* (nominal) variable taking on only the two values "alive" or "dead." Major blood group (A, B, AB, or O) is also a *nominal* variable with individuals classified into one of four categories, without intrinsic order to the categories. On the other hand, New York Heart Association functional status for congestive heart failure or stage of breast cancer are examples of *ordinal* variables, those that assume one of several possible values. The values are "ordered" in a meaningful manner, e.g., stage IV breast cancer is more advanced than stage II. Summarizing nominal or ordinal variables usually entails computing proportions of individuals in each category. Although it is common to code dichotomous variables by assigning values of 0 and 1 to the two categories, thus creating arbitrary values, it is usually inappropriate to use concepts such as SD to summarize nominal or ordinal variables.

HYPOTHESIS TESTING

Much clinical research is concerned with detecting associations between an exposure (tobacco smoking) and a disease (lung cancer) or between an intervention and a clinical response or outcome. For a typical study, investigators first develop a hypothesis: e.g., that the mean systolic blood pressure (SBP) in a group given an antihypertensive agent is lower than the mean SBP in a group given a placebo. Next, the investigators sample the populations of interest (treatment and control groups) and measure the variable of interest (SBP). To apply the standard statistical methodology, one formulates a *null hypothesis* of no effect, or no difference between groups. In our case, the null hypothesis would be that the two groups (treatment and control) were drawn from the same underlying population. Therefore, if the null hypothesis is true and the study is well designed, any observed difference in mean SBP's between the two groups is due to random sampling. Rejecting the null hypothesis thus becomes the goal. With a well-designed study, inferences based on population samples apply to the entire population. The underlying assumption is that the samples (treatment and control groups) are selected at random from the entire population. Any systematic violation of this assumption, such as preferentially including individuals on a low-salt diet in the treatment group, would introduce *bias* and jeopardize the validity of inferences to be drawn from the study. If a difference between two population samples is observed (e.g., SBP lower in treatment than control group), then the key statistical question is whether this difference could have been due to random sampling, i.e., chance.

The likelihood that an observed difference or an even more extreme difference is due to chance alone is called the *p-value*. In our study, if a certain difference between mean SBP's in treatment and control groups was observed, $p < 0.05$ would mean: given that the null hypothesis is true, there is a $< 5\%$ likelihood that this difference or a larger difference is due to random sampling. Thus, if the p-value is small, it is unlikely that an observed difference is due to random sampling, the null hypothesis is rejected, and it is inferred that real population differences or a real association exists between treatment and response.

An association may be demonstrated with statistical tools, but association does not necessarily establish causality. The decision of whether an association is due to cause and effect involves much more than statistics. Factors contributing to this decision include biologic plausibility, strength of association, consistency of association across well-designed studies performed in different settings, and dose-response effect.

A small p-value (the conventional level for "small" has been traditionally accepted as 0.05) safeguards against chance leading us to reject a null hypothesis which is true. A very low p-value strongly suggests that the observed data are inconsistent with the null hypothesis. The error of rejecting a true null hypothesis is called *type I error*. This occurs when chance leads to inferring differences or associations that do not exist. The probability of a type I error is usually called α or *significance level* and is traditionally chosen to be ≤ 0.05. In contrast, *type II error* occurs when a large p-value leads to the incorrect conclusion that a difference does not exist (incorrectly *not* rejecting a null hypothesis). The probability of a type II error is usually called β. Type II error occurs when the study lacks the statistical *power* to demonstrate a true association or dif-

ference. The power of the study, i.e., the probability of detecting a difference or an association that really exists, is $1 - \beta$. The power of the study increases with sample size and the magnitude of the difference that is considered clinically significant. On the other hand, a large amount of variability in the data (for continuous variables) decreases a study's power. A mistake commonly found in the medical literature is the conclusion that a certain effect does not exist because a study with low power failed to demonstrate it.

Conversely, impressive (very small) p-values may correspond to effects of small magnitude in studies with large sample sizes. For example, if a study documents an association between drug A and a drop in SBP at $p < 0.05$ and a further association between drug B and drop in SBP at $p < 0.001$, this should not be interpreted as meaning that drug B has a stronger effect than drug A. If, for example, the mean drop in SBP with drug B were only 1 mm Hg, this result would possess high statistical significance but no clinical significance. Thus, large sample sizes may lead to detecting statistically significant but clinically irrelevant differences.

Testing of statistical significance safeguards against chance threatening a study's validity. Other threats such as bias, confounding variables, or collecting faulty data are not addressed by statistical significance testing. Frequently, investigators overestimate their study's *external validity;* i.e., they generalize the results demonstrated by their data to a population inadequately represented in their study sample. For example, if results of a study performed on young men were to be applied to the population at large or to older women, it might lack external validity. Furthermore, if the study's data collection were questionable, the study would lack *internal validity* as well.

TESTS OF STATISTICAL SIGNIFICANCE

Once a hypothesis is clearly formulated and data have been collected in order to test that hypothesis, standard statistical procedures are used to interpret the data and assign p-values. These procedures are called tests of statistical significance. The choice of statistical tests depends on the nature of the data. Usually, when only one variable is measured, descriptive statistics are used. Most often tests of statistical significance come into play when data on at least two variables are collected. For example, in the aforementioned study comparing an active antihypertensive agent with a placebo, the two variables of major interest are the continuous variable SBP and the dichotomous variable describing the treatment group: active medication versus placebo. The null hypothesis of no effect is that the two groups have the same SBP distribution. Assuming that the SBP distributions are bell-shaped, the appropriate test of statistical significance for this situation is the *unpaired Student's t test*. The t test allows interpretation of the difference in mean SBP's between the two groups by assigning a p-value to this difference. Expanding our antihypertensive trial to include three (or more) randomization groups, such as diet, drugs, and placebo, means that analysis of variance, or *ANOVA*, is the most appropriate test of statistical significance. Both the Student's t test and ANOVA assign p-values to the differences between randomization groups. Sometimes, transformations such as applying logarithms are performed on nongaussian continuous variables to create new distributions approximating the gaussian curve. These transformed variables are easier to analyze with tools such as the t test or ANOVA.

ANOVA and t test are *parametric tests* in that they assume that data follow certain distributions described by parameters, such as the traditional bell-shaped curves. Unlike these parametric tests, *nonparametric* tests do not assume that data follow specified distributions. Table 14–4 names nonparametric analogues of parametric tests and statistics frequently found in the medical literature.

The study assessing effectiveness of an antihypertensive medication could have been designed somewhat differently, using each subject as his/her own control rather than a placebo. Here, investigators compare SBP before and after administering the antihypertensive agent, asking whether there was a difference between the initial mean SBP and the final one. Observations in the two groups of SBP are now paired and not independent. This situation calls for the use of the *paired Student's t test*.

A different situation arises when a dichotomous variable is the outcome of interest. For example, investigators studying the effect of administering a β-blocker on mortality after myocardial infarction might randomize subjects into two groups: one receiving a β-

TABLE 14-4. NONPARAMETRIC ANALOGUES OF FREQUENTLY USED PARAMETRIC STATISTICAL TOOLS

Normal Distribution(s)	Nonparametric
t test, unpaired	Mann-Whitney (Wilcoxon Rank Sum)
t test, paired	Wilcoxon Signed Rank
ANOVA	Kruskal-Wallis
Pearson correlation coefficient	Spearman rank correlation coefficient

blocker and the other receiving a placebo. The null hypothesis would be that the proportion of deaths is the same in both groups. The appropriate test of statistical significance in this case is the *chi-square*. Data that can be classified by two different nominal variables (β-blockers versus placebo and alive versus dead) are appropriate for display in a contingency table. The contingency table display suggests chi-square for statistical significance testing.

Certain situations call for evaluating the association between two continuous variables. For example, one might hypothesize that SBP increases linearly with age. Mathematically, this may be represented by the model

$$SBP = a + b \times age$$

with SBP and age varying with the individual, and fixed values a (regression constant) and b (regression slope or *regression coefficient*) to be determined. *Linear regression* provides a p-value for the null hypothesis that $b = 0$ and supplies values for the coefficients a and b. Furthermore, linear regression determines whether this model fits a given data set reasonably well. Assuming normally distributed data, the *Pearson correlation coefficient,* usually denoted by r, is a measure of the strength of linear association between age and SBP; r is always between -1 and 1, and r^2 (always between 0 and 1) measures how much of the variability in SBP is explained by age. Thus, a Pearson correlation coefficient of 0.6 would mean that approximately 36% (0.6 squared) of the variability in SBP is explained by age.

MULTIVARIABLE METHODS

Frequently, the complexity of clinical phenomena defies reduction to a simple equation with only one independent variable (age). For the above study, other factors, such as weight, may affect blood pressure while also being associated with age. The linear regression model described above neglects this *confounding variable* (weight) and may distort the association between SBP and age. We need a more sophisticated method to adjust for confounding variables, thus modeling the relationship more precisely (Table 14-5). Here, SBP is the dependent (outcome) variable and both age and weight are independent variables:

$$SBP = a + b \times age + c \times weight$$

Multiple linear regression allows us to determine the coefficients a, b, and c. We also assess goodness of fit of the model with the data and a p-value for each coefficient. This could, of course, be done with more than two independent variables.

When the dependent variable is dichotomous rather than continuous, and several continuous and/or nominal independent variables are being considered, *multiple logistic regression* has become a very popular tool to model clinical data. Recently, multiple logistic regression has been developed for polytomous (nominal with more than two categories) dependent variables as well. *Discriminant analysis* accomplishes a similar purpose of modeling a polytomous outcome variable being determined by several independent variables.

TABLE 14-5. COMMONLY USED MULTIVARIABLE METHODS AND THEIR DEPENDENT (OUTCOME) VARIABLES

Multivariable Methods	Dependent Variable
Multiple linear regression	Continuous
Multiple logistic regression	Dichotomous (polytomous)
Cox proportional hazards	Time to outcome event
Discriminant analysis	Nominal

Another multivariable analytic tool frequently found in the medical literature is *Cox proportional hazards regression,* in which the outcome variable is time to occurrence of a certain event. For example, a randomized controlled trial evaluating two different treatments for lung cancer might take survival time as its outcome variable. Cox regression allows one to model the effect of the treatment on survival time while adjusting for variables such as age, gender, and stage at diagnosis. The difference between Cox regression and multiple logistic regression is that the outcome variable in Cox regression is continuous (such as survival time) and the outcome in multiple logistic regression is dichotomous (such as survival at 5 years).

Multivariable modeling has become deceptively easy to perform because powerful statistical software is available. It is frequently misused in the medical literature. For example, suppose that multiple logistic regression is used to study the effect of β-blockers on mortality after myocardial infarction, and 20 deaths in a group of 200 subjects are observed. The outcome variable is vital status (alive or dead) at the end of the study. Investigators may be tempted to include in the model as independent variables—in addition to the use of β-blockers versus placebo—age, gender, co-morbidity, left ventricular ejection fraction, and a few other clinically relevant variables. Although no exact method is available to calculate the required number of outcome events (deaths), this modeling situation may well lead to *overfitting.* This means that the number of outcome events (deaths) is so low that the model is unreliable. In general, fewer than 5 to 10 outcome events per independent variable may result in a model that is inaccurate. Other issues such as violating the assumptions of normality and linearity also plague multivariable models in the clinical literature. These models are very powerful tools that are easily misused; hence they need to be handled with care.

In summary, statistics plays a very important role in interpreting and applying clinical data. One needs to be aware, however, that statistics only safeguards against random sampling error that causes erroneous inferences. Statistics cannot compensate for other threats to the validity of clinical research such as bias or collecting faulty data.

Bailar JC III, Mosteller F (eds.): Medical Uses of Statistics. 2nd ed. Boston, NEJM Books, 1992. *Essays on using statistics in medicine geared toward statistical ideas and their current use, not computational details. Addresses "why" rather than "how" questions.*

Concato J, Feinstein AR, Holford TR: The risk of determining risk with multivariable models. Ann Intern Med 118:201, 1993. *Useful review article that reports on how multivariable models are being used in medical journals and establishes a framework to critique their use.*

Rosner B: Fundamentals of Biostatistics. 3rd ed. Boston, PWS-KENT Publishing Co., 1990. *A concise and rigorous introductory biostatistics textbook with many clinical examples. Requires no background in statistics but provides useful information on most statistical tools used in clinical research, including multivariable analysis.*

Sackett DL, Haynes RB, Guyatt GH, et al.: Clinical Epidemiology: A Basic Science for Clinical Medicine. 2nd ed. Boston, Little, Brown, 1991. *Practical, insightful, and entertaining, this expanded, updated version of a classic series on how to read the medical literature clarifies statistical concepts, emphasizing their use in clinical practice and clinical research.*

15 THE DOMAIN OF THE GENERALIST PHYSICIAN

Susan C. Day

The purpose of this chapter is to define what the generalist physician needs to know in order to practice. Establishing the generalist's domain is the first step in creating a curriculum for training. It also provides a basis for assessing the performance of practitioners and setting a standard for competence in practice. Because identifying and caring for the problems of patients are the daily tasks that con-

TABLE 15-1. COMMON PATIENT PRESENTATIONS

A. Allergy/Immunology
1. The wheezing patient
2. The patient with allergies
3. The immunosuppressed patient

B. Cardiovascular
1. The patient with chest pain
2. The hypertensive patient
3. The patient with edema
4. The patient with a murmur
5. The patient with mitral valve prolapse
6. The patient with palpitations
7. The patient with new-onset congestive heart failure
8. The patient with chronic congestive heart failure
9. The patient with acute ischemia
10. The patient with chronic, stable angina
11. The patient with an abnormal stress test
12. The patient with atrial arrhythmias
13. The patient with asymptomatic ventricular arrhythmias
14. The patient with congenital heart disease
15. The patient with aortic valve disease
16. The patient with syncope
17. The patient with claudication
18. The patient with an abdominal aortic aneurysm
19. The patient with hyperlipidemia

C. Critical Care
1. The patient with acute pulmonary embolus
2. The patient with severe airway obstruction
3. The patient with massive gastrointestinal bleeding
4. The patient with chest pain
5. The decision to admit a patient to the ICU
6. The comatose or obtunded patient
7. The hyperthermic patient
8. The hypothermic patient
9. The patient who is pulseless and apneic
10. The patient with acute respiratory failure
11. The patient in shock
12. The patient with sepsis syndrome
13. The patient with anuria/oliguria
14. The agitated patient
15. The dying patient

D. Dermatology
1. The patient with a rash
2. The patient with skin cancer
3. The patient with a mole
4. The patient with sun-damaged skin
5. The patient with pruritus
6. The patient with hair loss
7. The patient with increased pigmentation
8. The patient with vitiligo
9. The patient with a decubitus ulcer
10. The patient with leg ulcers
11. The patient with acne
12. The patient with hives/urticaria
13. The patient with seborrhea
14. The patient with contact dermatitis

E. Disease Prevention/Health Promotion/Occupational
1. The periodic exam
2. The at-risk patient
   a. The geriatric patient
   b. The homosexual patient
   c. The asplenic patient
   d. The health care worker
   e. The parenteral drug user
   f. The patient with coronary risk factors
   g. The adolescent
3. The asymptomatic patient with a positive PPD
4. Management of contacts of the patient with tuberculosis
5. Asymptomatic patient with positive serologic test for syphilis
6. The asymptomatic patient with a positive HIV test
7. Management of contacts of STD patient
8. Recommendations for immunization
9. Recommendations for cancer screening
10. The worker
    a. with hearing impairment
    b. with low back strain
    c. with wheezing
    d. with contact dermatitis
    e. with stress
    f. with exposure to infections
    g. with exposure to carcinogens

11. The patient asking advice prior to travel
12. The patient undergoing surgery

F. Endocrinology, Diabetes, and Metabolism
1. The patient with diabetes mellitus
2. The patient with hyperthyroidism
3. The patient with hypothyroidism
4. The patient with a thyroid nodule
5. The patient with an enlarged thyroid
6. The patient on glucocorticoid therapy
7. The hypoglycemic patient
8. The adolescent patient with abnormal growth and development
9. The patient with an eating disorder
10. The patient with asymptomatic hypercalcemia
11. The hirsute patient

G. Gastroenterology
1. The patient with difficulty swallowing
2. The patient with heartburn
3. The patient with gastrointestinal bleeding
4. The patient with gallstones
5. The patient with acute pancreatitis
6. The patient with abnormal liver function tests
7. The patient with liver failure
8. The patient with jaundice
9. The patient with chronic abdominal pain
10. The patient with an acute abdomen
11. The patient with acute diarrhea
12. The patient with chronic diarrhea
13. The patient with functional bowel syndrome
14. The patient with nausea and vomiting
15. The constipated patient
16. The patient with excessive gas
17. The patient with ascites
18. The patient with rectal pain/itching
19. The patient with hemorrhoids
20. The patient with colonic polyps
21. The patient with peptic ulcer disease

H. Hematology
1. The patient with anemia
2. The patient with an abnormal bleeding time
3. The patient with an enlarged spleen
4. The patient without a spleen
5. The patient with purpura
6. The patient with sickle cell disease
7. The patient with easy bruising
8. The patient with a hypercoagulable state
9. The patient with a low platelet count
10. The patient with asymptomatic chronic lymphocytic leukemia
11. The patient with an abnormal serum protein

I. Infectious Disease
1. The patient with an upper respiratory infection
2. The patient with a sore throat
3. The patient with active tuberculosis
4. The patient with pneumonia/bronchitis
5. The patient with prostatitis
6. The patient with sexually transmitted disease
7. The patient with a penile discharge
8. The patient with a urinary tract infection
9. The patient with viral hepatitis
10. The patient with HIV infection
11. The febrile patient
    a. Fever of undetermined origin
    b. Fever in the hospitalized patient
    c. Fever in the compromised host
    d. Fever in the postoperative patient
12. The patient with a skin infection
13. The septic patient
14. The patient with herpes zoster
15. The patient with herpes simplex

J. Medical Ethics
1. The patient who refuses medical therapy
2. The patient with impaired decision-making capacity
3. The impaired health care professional
4. Withholding and withdrawing medical therapy
5. Duty to warn versus patient confidentiality
6. The patient who requests an abortion
7. Conflicts in advocacy

K. Nephrology/Urology
1. The patient with an abnormal urinalysis
   a. hematuria
   b. proteinuria

TABLE 15–1. COMMON PATIENT PRESENTATIONS *Continued*

    c. cellular casts
    d. pyuria
  2. The patient with dysuria
  3. The incontinent patient
  4. The patient with prostate cancer
  5. The patient with bladder outlet obstruction
  6. The patient with a scrotal mass/pain
  7. Evaluation (ECG recognition) and emergency treatment of hyperkalemia
  8. The patient with nocturia
  9. The patient with a renal mass
 10. The patient with renal colic/kidney stones
 11. The patient with hyperuricemia
 12. The patient with acute renal failure
 13. The patient with chronic renal insufficiency
 14. The patient with an acid-base disorder

L. Neurology
  1. The patient with an asymptomatic bruit
  2. The patient with transient neurologic symptoms
  3. The patient with a stroke
  4. The patient with seizures
  5. The patient with headaches
  6. The patient with dementia
  7. The dizzy patient
  8. The patient with progressive neurologic deficit
  9. The patient with an acute change in mental status
 10. The patient with paresthesia
 11. The patient with weakness
 12. The patient with tremor
 13. The patient with facial pain
 14. The patient with head trauma
 15. The patient with multiple sclerosis

M. Nutrition: Dietary recommendations in
  1. diabetes mellitus
  2. hyperlipidemia
  3. pregnancy/lactation
  4. hypertension
  5. osteoporosis
  6. renal calculi
  7. vegetarianism
  8. food fads, health food trends
  9. hepatic encephalopathy
 10. chronic renal failure
 11. lactase deficiency
 12. the elderly
 13. the obese patient

N. Obstetrics/Gynecology
  1. The patient with vaginitis
  2. The patient who requests contraceptive advice
  3. The patient with sexual dysfunction
  4. The patient with a menstrual disorder
  5. The menopausal woman
  6. The patient with galactorrhea
  7. The infertile patient (male and female)
  8. The patient with pelvic pain
  9. The pregnant patient
    a. with hypertension
    b. with diabetes
    c. with thyroid disease
    d. with valvular heart disease
    e. with thrombophlebitis/pulmonary embolism
    f. who needs immunization
 10. The postpartum patient
    a. with congestive heart failure
    b. with thyroid disease
 11. The patient with an abnormal pap smear
 12. The patient with a pelvic mass

O. Oncology
  1. The patient with a breast mass
  2. The patient who has been treated for breast cancer
  3. The patient with a positive fecal occult blood test
  4. The patient who has been treated for colon cancer
  5. The patient who has been treated for lung cancer
  6. The patient with involuntary weight loss
  7. The patient with a pathologic fracture
  8. The patient with bowel obstruction
  9. The patient with lymphadenopathy
 10. The patient with carcinoma of unknown origin
 11. The patient with superior vena cava syndrome

 12. The patient with cancer pain
 13. The cancer patient with hypercalcemia

P. Ophthalmology
  1. The patient with an abnormal fundoscopic examination
    a. papilledema
    b. glaucoma
    c. diabetic retinopathy
    d. optic atrophy
  2. The patient with red eye
  3. The patient with eye pain
  4. The patient with acute loss of vision
  5. The patient with elevated intraocular pressure
  6. The patient with exophthalmos
  7. The patient with cataracts

Q. Otolaryngology/Dental
  1. The patient with acute sinusitis
  2. The patient with chronic nasal congestion
  3. The patient with vertigo
  4. The patient with otitis
  5. The patient with impaired hearing
  6. The patient with epistaxis
  7. The patient with tinnitus
  8. The patient with hiccups
  9. The hoarse patient
 10. Screening for oral cancer
 11. The patient with a parotid mass

R. Pulmonary
  1. The patient with cough
  2. The patient with dyspnea
  3. The patient with a pulmonary infiltrate
  4. The patient with hemoptysis
  5. The patient with asthma
  6. The patient with chronic obstructive pulmonary disease
  7. The patient with a solitary pulmonary nodule
  8. The patient with pulmonary embolism/deep vein thrombosis/phlebitis
  9. The patient with pleural effusion
 10. The patient with a broken rib
 11. The patient with a pneumothorax

S. Psychiatry
  1. The patient with anxiety/panic attacks
  2. The depressed patient
  3. The patient with chronic fatigue
  4. The patient with insomnia
  5. The patient with neuroses
  6. The somatizing patient
  7. The patient with delirium
  8. The patient with altered mental status during hospitalization
  9. The patient who is under stress
 10. The patient with a conversion reaction
 11. The patient with factitious illness
 12. The patient with chronic schizophrenia

T. Rheumatology/Orthopedics
  1. The patient with back pain
  2. The patient with joint pain
    a. shoulder
    b. knee
    c. elbow/wrist/finger
    d. ankle/foot/toe
    e. hip
  3. The patient with neck pain
  4. The patient with osteoarthritis
  5. The patient with acute inflammatory arthritis (including gout)
  6. The patient with temporal arteritis/polymyalgia rheumatica
  7. The patient who falls
  8. The patient with polyarticular arthritis
  9. The patient with rash and arthritis
 10. The patient with muscle pain and weakness
 11. The patient with fibrositis
 12. The patient with sports-related injury
 13. The patient with osteoporosis

U. Substance Abuse
  1. The patient with excessive alcohol use
  2. The patient with alcohol withdrawal
  3. The patient who smokes cigarettes
  4. The patient with suspected drug overdose
  5. The drug-seeking patient
  6. The patient who uses cocaine

front the practitioner, the domain of the generalist is defined in terms of the problems that a practitioner encounters in the course of providing comprehensive medical care to an undifferentiated population of patients over time.

RATIONALE FOR USE OF A PROBLEM-BASED DEFINITION OF THE GENERALIST'S DOMAIN

Use of a problem-based definition of the generalist's domain is compelling for a number of reasons. First, it is consistent with the cognitive capabilities of the practitioner. A physician's ability to reason begins with a factual knowledge base, which appears to be acquired and retained in memory according to problems or cases. Further, studies of clinical problem-solving indicate little transfer of concepts or principles takes place from one case to another. A practitioner's performance varies from case to case, and how well an individual performs depends more on knowledge of specific, relevant content than general problem-solving skills. Thus, competence may be best described and evaluated in terms of the physician's ability to deal effectively with a defined series of problems.

Another advantage of a problem-based definition of the generalist's domain is that the list of patient presentations can be used by medical educators to assess whether a trainee has received adequate exposure to clinical problems and to generate cases for use in classroom or small group teaching sessions. Knowledge is more easily recalled and applied when it is acquired in the context in which it will subsequently be used. The problem-based approach ensures relevance and may increase the efficiency of learning.

BACKGROUND

A useful starting place for identifying the problems presenting to the generalist physician was provided by the American Board of Internal Medicine (ABIM). In the 1980's, the ABIM initiated a project to identify "core" conditions. Core conditions were defined as frequently encountered symptoms or diseases which are important in terms of patient health outcome and for which there is good evidence that medical intervention will have an effect.

To help define the frequency of conditions seen in practice, the ABIM began by turning to a study carried out by Mendenhall. This study surveyed a large sample of medical practices of specialists in all parts of the country and collected information regarding the reasons patients seek care. Having identified high-frequency conditions, the ABIM expanded this list to include treatable conditions that have a large impact on an individual's health status. This task was done by reviewing the work of medical educators who had developed curricula for primary care internal medicine programs, as well as available primary care textbooks.

Over the years since the ABIM first defined core conditions, the pattern of care delivery in the United States has changed, with fewer, shorter hospital stays and increased emphasis on the cost-effective, ambulatory care of patients. However, the reasons patients seek care have remained largely the same, as demonstrated through ongoing databases such as the National Ambulatory Medical Care Survey. Some gradual changes in disease frequency are to be anticipated with the aging of the population and the expanding impact of HIV and related infections on the patients being seen by the generalist.

The list generated by the ABIM was reframed in terms of patient presentations and updated and expanded to include a broader range of problems. These patient presentations are summarized in Table 15–1.

DESCRIPTION OF COMMON PATIENT PRESENTATIONS

To help interpret Table 15–1, a few points of clarification are in order. The list includes both common conditions and symptoms because patients present with pre-existing diagnoses as well as undifferentiated concerns. Problems posed by the healthy patient who asks to be screened and by the asymptomatic patient with abnormal findings are also listed. Diseases are not included on the list if they are rare or if most patients with active disease would likely be cared for by a specialist.

CLASSIFICATION OF PRESENTATIONS. Problems are listed by organ system for ease of reference, but many, if not all, of the undifferentiated symptoms and physical findings can be caused by problems in several organ systems (e.g., dyspnea or edema). Nonmedical specialties are included as well as traditional medical subspecialties because generalists must be able to identify and treat many of these problems. Three categories (disease prevention, critical care, and medical ethics) cover presentations that cut across organ systems.

PATIENT CHARACTERISTICS. The focus is on the adult patient. Problems are not clustered by patient age or gender. Although the emerging disciplines of geriatrics, adolescent medicine, and women's health have highlighted how the differential diagnosis of symptoms and the approach to care are often influenced by age and gender, most of the problems and symptoms on this list occur across the spectrum of adult patients.

SETTING. No setting is specified because patients may be seen with these problems in all practice settings. Because most patient visits occur in the outpatient environment, this might be assumed to be the predominant setting.

ROLE OF THE GENERALIST

For most conditions on the list, the generalist should be able to fully manage 80% of undifferentiated patients. This would be a daunting and unrealistic task if interpreted as the ability to manage 80% of patients with every disease that can cause a particular symptom. On the other hand, it is reasonable to expect a generalist to know how to manage the common diseases and cardinal symptoms very well and to be able to distinguish between benign or self-limited conditions and significant or systemic disease.

Referral is obviously indicated when a problem requires surgical intervention or advanced or invasive diagnostic testing, when seeking advice in managing complex patients, and when the physician is either not trained to deliver a service or cannot perform it because of time or logistic constraints. Defining the border between the generalist and other care providers requires recognizing the skills and limitations of each member of the health care team, as well as knowing the principles of cost-effective care.

SUMMARY

This list of common presentations is provided as a starting point in defining the domain of the generalist physician. Knowing the clinical features and natural history of each condition appropriately focuses the process of data collection, diagnostic testing, therapeutic recommendation, and long-term management. Each of these conditions and symptoms is discussed in depth in this textbook, as are the general clinical skills required to provide care.

For any given presentation, there are as many variations as there are patients. For any given practitioner, the profile of patients presenting with a given symptom varies with the practice setting and community. However, generalists practicing across all settings must know how to address a broad range of problems. To the extent that this list captures the range of patient problems that a generalist should be prepared to encounter in routine practice, it may be useful in directing the education and evaluation of the generalist physician.

Kassirer JP, Kopelman RI: Learning Clinical Reasoning. Baltimore, William & Wilkins, 1991. *Provides an overview of the processes of diagnostic and management decision making, then uses a series of clinical cases to demonstrate the principal aspects of clinical reasoning.*

Langdon LO, Grosso LJ, Day SC, et al.: A core component of the certification examination in internal medicine. J Gen Intern Med 8:497, 1993. *A summary of the development and evaluation of a core component for the certifying examination in internal medicine.*

Mendenhall RC: Medical Practice in the United States: A Special Report of the Robert Wood Johnson Foundation. Princeton, The Robert Wood Johnson Foundation, 1981. *Valuable reference document reporting on a 5-year study of the medical practices of 10,372 physicians of all specialties, including data from 450,210 actual patient encounters. Information was collected on practice characteristics, analysis of physicians' work day, and the type, site, and reason for patient visits.*

Norman GR, Schmidt HG: The psychological basis of problem-based learning: A review of the evidence. Acad Med 67:557, 1992. *Presents the theoretical benefits of problem-based learning (PBL), then reviews the related literature on the psychology of learning and the evidence for and against the argument that the PBL format enhances learning.*

Schappert SM: National Ambulatory Medical Care Survey: 1990 summary advance data from vital and health statistics. Hyattsville, MD, National Center for Health Statistics, 1992, No 213. *An example of the ongoing databases surveying physician practices. Data are collected periodically by the National Center for Health Statistics, Centers for Disease Control and Prevention, based on a national sample of physicians reporting details of their patients' office visits.*

16 PRINCIPLES OF DRUG THERAPY

Robert B. Diasio

It is generally appreciated that under different conditions a drug may produce diverse effects ranging from none to a desirable effect, or in other cases an undesirable, toxic effect. The physician caring for the patient must learn how to individualize the drug dosage under different conditions to ensure effective and safe therapy. This requires knowing both pharmacokinetics—examining the movement of a drug over time through the body—and pharmacodynamics—relating drug concentration to drug effect (Fig. 16–1). In this chapter, a review of the basic concepts of pharmacokinetics and pharmacodynamics is presented, followed by guidelines on how to use this information to optimize therapeutic applications. Finally, drug interactions and adverse drug responses are discussed with advice on how both can be recognized and minimized in clinical practice.

PHARMACOKINETIC PRINCIPLES

ADMINISTERING DRUGS. The most straightforward means of administering a drug into the systemic circulation is by intravenously injecting it as a bolus. With this route, the full amount of a drug is delivered to the systemic circulation almost immediately. The same dose may also be administered as an intravenous infusion over a longer time, resulting in a decrease in the peak plasma concentration as well as increasing the time the drug is present in the circulation. Many other routes of administration can be used, including sublingual, oral, transdermal, rectal, inhalation, subcutaneous, and intramuscular. Each of these carries not only a potential delay in the time it takes the drug to enter the circulation but also the possibility that a large fraction of it will never reach the circulation.

ABSORPTION. Absorption refers to the transfer of a drug from the site where it was administered to the systemic circulation. Most drugs use passive diffusion to cross a membrane barrier and enter the systemic circulation. Because passive diffusion in this setting depends on the concentration of the solute at the membrane surface, the rate of drug absorption is affected by the concentration of free drug at the absorbing surface. Factors that influence the availability of free drug affect drug absorption from the administration site. Understanding this effect can be exploited to design medications that provide a slow release of drug into the circulation by prolonging drug absorption. With certain sustained-released oral preparations, the rate of dissolution of the drug in the gastrointestinal tract determines the rate at which the drug is absorbed (e.g., time-released antihistamines). Similarly, one can obtain a prolonged drug effect by using transdermal medications (e.g., nitroglycerin) or intramuscular depot preparations (e.g., benzathine penicillin G).

First-Pass Effect. Some drugs that are administered orally are absorbed relatively well into the portal circulation but are metabolized by the liver prior to reaching the systemic circulation. This is known as a "first-pass" or "presystemic" effect. The oral route may therefore be less suitable than other routes of administration. A good example is nitroglycerin, which is well absorbed but efficiently metabolized during the first pass through the liver. The same drug can achieve adequate systemic levels when given sublingually or transdermally.

Bioavailability. The extent of absorption of drug into the systemic circulation may be incomplete. The bioavailability of a particular drug is the fraction (F) of the total drug dose that ultimately reaches the systemic circulation from the site of administration. This is calculated by dividing the amount of the drug dose that reaches the circulation from the administration site by the amount of the drug dose that would enter the systemic circulation following direct intravenous injection into the circulation (essentially the total dose). Bioavailability, or F, can therefore range from 0, in which no drug reaches the systemic circulation, to 1.0, in which essentially all of the drug is absorbed. The bioavailability of a drug in different formulations may change because the overall absorption may differ. This has become a recent concern with the increasing use of generic preparations.

DISTRIBUTION. Following delivery of drug into the systemic circulation either directly by intravenous injection or after absorption, the drug is transported throughout the body, initially to the well-perfused tissues and later to areas that are less perfused. The

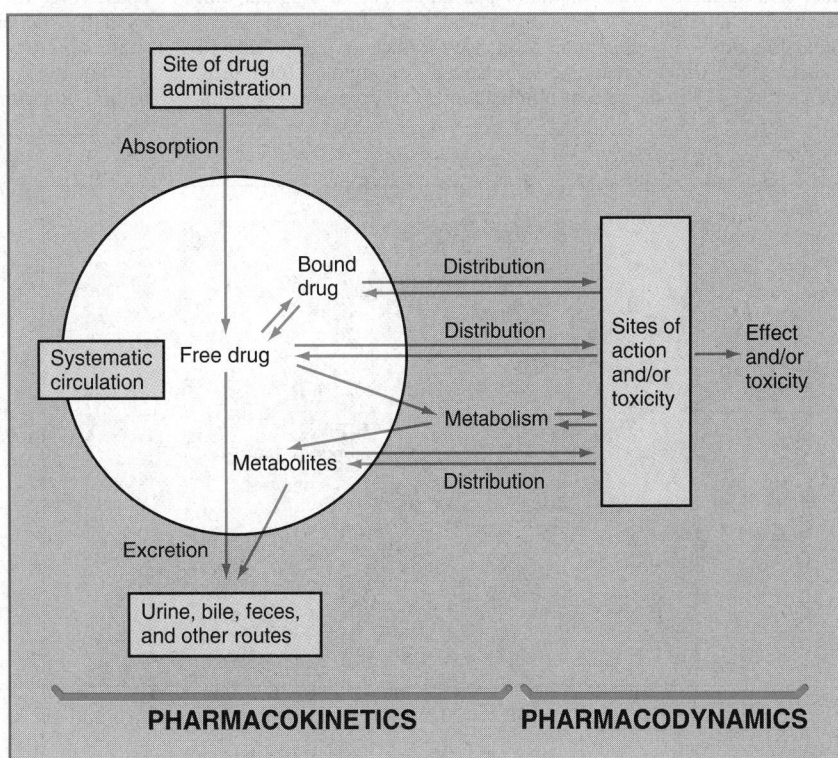

FIGURE 16–1. Schematic of drug movement through the body, from site of administration to production of drug effect. The relationship between pharmacokinetics and pharmacodynamics is shown.

PHARMACOKINETICS   PHARMACODYNAMICS

distribution phase can best be assessed by plotting the drug's plasma concentration on a log scale versus time on a linear scale, as is shown in Figure 16–2. The initial phase, from immediately after administration through the rapid fall in concentration, represents the distribution phase, during which a drug rapidly disappears from the circulation and enters the tissues. This is followed by the elimination phase (see below), when drug in the plasma is in equilibrium with drug in the tissues. It is during this latter phase that the drug's plasma concentration is thought to be related to drug effect.

Volume of Distribution. The volume of distribution (V_D) is a term used to relate the amount of drug in the body to the concentration of drug in the plasma. It is calculated by dividing the dose (that ultimately gets into the systemic circulation) by the plasma concentration at time zero (C_{p0}).

$$V_D = \frac{dose}{C_{p0}} \qquad (1)$$

The C_{p0} can be calculated by extrapolating the elimination phase back to time zero, as shown in Figure 16–2. The volume of distribution as defined above is best considered the "apparent V_D" because it represents the apparent volume needed to contain the entire amount of the drug, assuming that the drug is distributed throughout the body at the same concentration as in the plasma. Table 16–1 lists pharmacokinetic data for 20 commonly used drugs from several drug classes, demonstrating the wide variation in V_D. Thus, digoxin can be seen to have a large V_D (>5 liters), whereas valproic acid has a relatively small V_D (0.15 liter). As discussed below, the V_D is a useful pharmacokinetic term for calculating the loading dose and in appreciating how various changes can affect a drug's half-life.

ELIMINATION. Drugs are removed from the body by two major mechanisms; hepatic elimination, in which drugs are metabolized in the liver and excreted through the biliary tract, and renal elimination, in which drugs are removed from the circulation by either glomerular filtration or tubular secretion. For the vast majority of drugs, the rates of hepatic and renal elimination are proportional to the plasma concentration of the drug. This relationship is often described as a "first-order" process. Two measurements are used to evaluate elimination—clearance and half-life.

Clearance. The efficiency of elimination can be described by assessing how the drug clears from the circulation. Drug clearance is a measure of the volume of plasma cleared of drug per unit of time. It is similar to the measurement used clinically to assess renal function—the creatinine clearance—which is the volume of plasma from which creatinine is removed per minute. Total drug clearance (Cl_{tot}) is the rate of elimination by all processes (El_{tot}) divided by the plasma concentration of the drug (C_p):

$$Cl_{tot} = \frac{El_{tot}}{C_p} \qquad (2)$$

It is important to remember that drugs may be cleared by several organs, with renal and hepatic clearance being the two major mechanisms. Total drug clearance (Cl_{tot}) can therefore be best described as the sum of clearances by each organ. For must drugs this is essentially the sum of the renal and hepatic clearance:

$$Cl_{tot} = Cl_{Ren} + Cl_{Hep} \qquad (3)$$

Table 16–1 demonstrates the wide variation in clearance values among commonly used medications, with some drugs (e.g., ethosuximide and phenobarbital) having relatively low clearances (<5 ml per minute) whereas other drugs (e.g., aspirin and mexiletine) having relatively high clearances (>500 ml per minute). The contribution of renal clearance to overall clearance is also shown in Table 16–1. It can be seen that the antibiotics amikacin, gentamicin, and tobramycin are almost entirely cleared by the kidneys, whereas drugs such as aspirin, carbamazepine, and phenytoin are cleared <5% by the kidneys.

Drug clearance is affected by several factors, including (1) blood flow through the organ of clearance; (2) protein binding to the drug; and (3) the activity of the clearance processes in the organs of elimination (e.g., glomerular filtration rate (GFR) and tubular secretion in the kidney or enzyme activity in the liver). Drug clearance is not affected by distribution of drug throughout the body (V_D) because clearance mechanisms act only on drug in the circulation.

Half-Life. The amount of time needed to eliminate a drug from the body depends on both the clearance and the volume of distribution. The first-order elimination constant (k_e) represents the proportion of the apparent volume of distribution that is cleared of drug per unit of time during the exponential disappearance of drug from the plasma over time (elimination phase).

$$k_e = \frac{Cl}{V_D} \qquad (4)$$

The value of this constant for a particular drug can be determined by plotting drug concentration versus time on a log-linear plot (see Fig. 16–2) and measuring the slope of the straight line obtained during the exponential (elimination) phase.

The time needed to eliminate the drug is best described by the drug half-life, which is the time required during the elimination phase (Fig. 16–2) to decrease the plasma concentration of the drug by half. Mathematically, the half-life is equal to the natural logarithm of 2 (representing a reduction of drug concentration to half) divided by k_e. Substituting for k_e from Eq. 4 and calculating the natural logarithm of 2, the half-life can therefore be represented

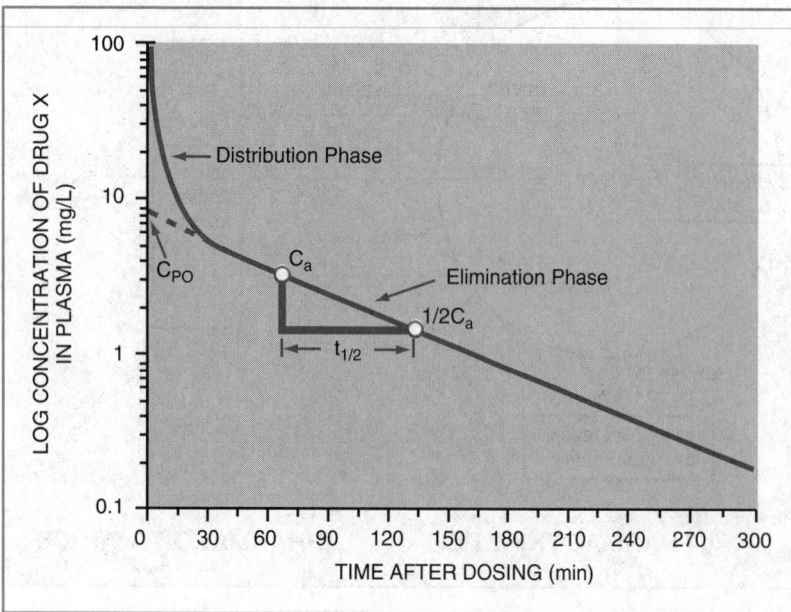

FIGURE 16–2. Representative "concentration versus time" plot used in pharmacokinetic studies where concentration of drug is plotted with a logarithmic scale on the ordinate and time is plotted with a linear scale on the abscissa. The resultant curve is seen to have two phases: the distribution phase, the initial portion of the plotted line when the concentrations of drug decrease rapidly; and the elimination phase, the later phase when there is exponential disappearance of drug from the plasma with time. The dotted line extrapolated from the elimination phase back to time zero is used to calculate C_{p0}. During the elimination phase, the $t_{1/2}$ can be calculated as the time it takes to decrease the concentration by half (shown here as the time needed to decrease from concentration C_a to $\frac{1}{2} C_a$).

TABLE 16-1. PHARMACOKINETIC PARAMETERS FOR SOME COMMONLY USED DRUGS

	V_D (liters/kg)	Protein Binding (%)	Total Cl (ml/min)	% of Cl_{Tot} as Renal Cl	$t_{1/2}$ (hr)	Therapeutic Range (mg/liters)
Amikacin	0.25	< 10	100	94–98	2–3	5–20 (TR) 20–30 (PK)
Aspirin (acetylsalicylic acid)	0.14–0.18	80–90	575–725	< 2	0.2–0.3	20–250
Carbamazepine	1.2	75–90	50–125	1–3	12–17	4–12
Digoxin	5–7.3	20–30	75	50–70	34–44	0.5–2.0
Disopyramide	0.6–1.4	50–65	1.3–1.4	40–60	4–10	2–4
Ethosuximide	0.7	< 10	3	20	60	40–100
Gentamicin sulfate	0.22–0.3	< 10	60	> 95	1.5–4 4–8 (PK)	0.5–2.0 (TR)
Lidocaine	3	60–80	700	< 10	1.5–2.0	1–5
Lithium carbonate	0.7–1	0	20–40	95–99	20–270	4–1.4*
Mexiletine	5.4	75	500–850	15	8–10	0.7–2.0
Penicillin G	0.5–0.7	45–68	—	20	0.4–0.9	Variable
Phenobarbital	0.6–0.7	20–45	4	25	2–6 Days	< 10–40*
Phenytoin	0.4–0.8	88–93	—	< 5	7–26	10–20
Primidone	0.6	< 20	45–100	15–25	10–12	5–12
Procainamide	2.2	14–23	470–600	40–70	2.5–4.7	4–8
Quinidine sulfate	2	80	180–300	10–20	6–8	0.3–6.0
Theophylline	0.3–0.7	60	36–50	< 10	4–16	5–20
Tobramycin	0.25–0.30	< 10	70	> 95	2–4 4–8 (PK)	0.5–2.0 (TR)
Valproic acid	0.15	80–95	7	< 10	5–20	50–100
Vancomycin	0.4–1.0	52–60	65	85	4–6	5–10 (TR) 25–35 (PK)

TR = Trough value; PK = peak value

* Therapeutic range varies depending on indication for drugs (e.g., *lithium carbonate*–range 0.4–1.3 mg/liter, appropriate for affective, schizophrenia disorder; whole range 1.0–1.4 mg/liter appropriate for mania; *phenobarbital*—concentration < 10 mg/liter appropriate for anticonvulsant, 40 mg/liter appropriate as hypnotic.

by the following equation:

$$t_{1/2} = \frac{0.693\ V_D}{Cl} \qquad (5)$$

From this equation one can therefore predict that, at a given clearance, as the volume of distribution increases, the half-life increases. Similarly, at a given V_D, as the clearance increases, the half-life decreases. Clinically, many disease states (see below) can affect both V_D and clearance. Because disease affects the V_D and clearance differently, the half-life may increase, decrease, or not change much. Thus, by itself, the half-life is not a good indicator of the extent of abnormality in elimination.

The half-life is useful to predict how long it takes for a drug to be eliminated from the body. Thus for any drug that has a first-order elimination, one would expect, as shown in Figure 16–2, that by the end of the first half-life the drug would be reduced to 50%, by the end of the second half-life to 25%, by the end of the third half-life to 12.5%, by the end of the fourth half-life to 6.25%, by the end of the fifth half-life to 3.125%, and so on. In general, a drug can be considered to be essentially eliminated after three to five half-lives when less than 10% of the effective concentration remains. Table 16–1 demonstrates the wide variation in $t_{1/2}$ for several commonly used drugs.

APPLYING PHARMACOKINETIC PRINCIPLES

USING A LOADING DOSE. In order to rapidly attain a desired therapeutic concentration, a loading dose is often used. In determining the amount of drug to be given, one needs to consider the "volume" within the body into which the drug may distribute. This is best described by the apparent V_D. The loading dose can be calculated by multiplying the desired concentration by the V_D.

$$\text{Loading dose} = \text{desired concentration} \times V_D \qquad (6)$$

Administering the entire loading dose rapidly may produce an initially high peak concentration that results in toxicity. This can be avoided either by administering the loading dose as a divided dose or by varying the rate of access to the circulation—for example, by administering the drug as an infusion (with intravenous drug) or by taking advantage of the slower access to the circulation from various other routes (e.g., oral dose). This approach is illustrated by phenytoin (Table 16–1), which may need to be administered with a loading dose to rapidly achieve a therapeutic level (10 to 20 mg per liter). Because the V_D for phenytoin is approximately 0.6 liter per kilogram, the loading dose calculated from Eq. 6 would be 420 mg in order to attain a minimally therapeutic level of 10 mg per liter in a 70-kg adult. Administering 420 mg of phenytoin by intravenous bolus carries the risk of cardiac arrest and death. By taking advantage of the reduced bioavailability (F = 0.8) and slow absorption of oral phenytoin, the loading dose can be safely administered as an oral dose of 500 mg.

The equation (Eq. 6) for the loading dose can also be used to calculate the dose needed to "boost" an inadequate blood level of drug to a desired therapeutic range. Thus, if the phenytoin level is observed on therapeutic monitoring to be 5 mg per liter and the desired level is 15 mg per liter, it is necessary to multiply the difference needed to achieve the desired concentration (10 mg per liter) by the V_D (0.6 liter per kilogram) to determine the dose (in milligrams per kilogram) necessary to achieve this drug level after distribution. Thus, in a 70-kg individual, one would multiply this latter amount by 70 kg to obtain the calculated loading dose (420 mg) that could be administered safely. A 500-mg oral dose with a bioavailability < 1 (e.g., F = 0.8) would deliver to the systemic circulation the approximate amount needed and avoid the risks associated with rapid intravenous administration, as discussed above.

DETERMINING DRUG ACCUMULATION. Continuing to administer a drug, either as a prolonged infusion or as repeated doses, results in accumulation until a "steady state" occurs. Steady state is the point when the amount of drug being administered equals the amount being eliminated so that the plasma and tissue levels remain constant. The elimination half-life determines not only the time of drug elimination but also the time course of drug accumulation. This "mirror image" pattern of drug accumulation and elimination is shown graphically in Figure 16–3. As with drug elimination, three to five half-lives determine the time it takes to reach steady state during drug accumulation. Whereas drugs with short half-lives accumulate rapidly, drugs with long half-lives require a longer time to accumulate, with a potential delay in achieving therapeutic drug levels. For drugs with long half-lives, a loading dose may be needed to rapidly achieve drug accumulation and in turn a more rapid therapeutic effect.

With each change in drug dose or rate of infusion, a change in steady state occurs. Although not obvious for drugs with short half-

$$D/t = Cl_{tot} \times C_p \qquad (8)$$

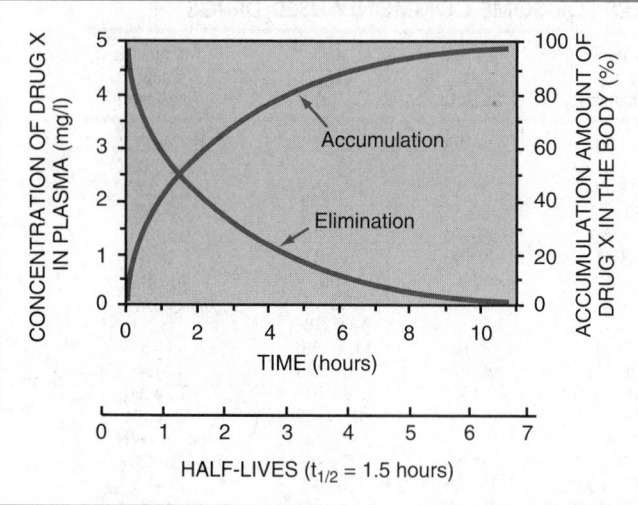

FIGURE 16-3. Representative plot of the "mirror image" relationship between elimination of drug (after drug is discontinued) and accumulation of drug (during infusion). The plot shows the concentration on the left y-axis and time on the upper x-axis. The lower x-axis shows the time in half-lives and the y-axis on the right shows the percentage of drug in the body. After three to five half-lives, elimination is essentially complete and accumulation is essentially at a steady state.

lives, the effects of dose adjustments for drugs with longer half-lives are delayed, with the time varying directly with the drug's half-life.

USING A MAINTENANCE DOSE. After steady state is reached in three to five half-lives with either a continuous infusion or intermittent doses, the rate of drug administered equals the rate of drug eliminated. For an intravenous drug, the administration rate is the infusion rate (I), whereas for a drug administered by another route (e.g., oral dose) the administration rate is the dose per unit time (D/t). From Eq. 3 the rate of elimination (total) can be seen to equal the $Cl_{tot} \times C_p$. Therefore, it follows with an intravenously administered drug, because the infusion rate equals the elimination rate at steady state, that:

$$I \times Cl_{tot} \times C_p \qquad (7)$$

Similarly, with an orally administered drug, the dose administered per unit time equals the elimination rate at steady state, with the result that:

These equations demonstrate the direct relationship between the dose and the resultant plasma concentration at steady state. This relationship is independent of the distribution of the drug. Using these equations, it is possible to determine the infusion rate or the interval and dose needed to achieve and maintain a specified drug concentration in the plasma.

When administered intermittently, a drug approaches steady-state concentration over time with a pattern similar to that observed with continuous infusion (Fig. 16–4). With intermittent drug administration, such as with an oral dose, the drug concentration fluctuates; the magnitude of fluctuation between the "peak" and "trough" concentrations depends on the interval of administration, drug half-life, absorption characteristics, and site of administration. The effect of a change in the interval of administration for an oral drug is shown in Figure 16–4. As the intervals decrease below the half-life, the fluctuation decreases and approaches the curve produced by an intravenous infusion. Orally administered drugs may reach the bloodstream more rapidly, attaining a higher peak concentration with one formulation, whereas the same drug administered as a time-released formulation is absorbed more slowly, with a lower peak concentration but lasting longer in the plasma. Finally, the same drug administered via different routes may have very different plasma profiles not only because of differing absorption characteristics but also because of other effects such as first-pass metabolism.

DECREASING THE DRUG LEVEL. At times it may be necessary to decrease the plasma drug level while maintaining therapy, e.g., when signs of toxicity become apparent or a potentially dangerously high concentration of drug is noted when monitoring drug levels (see below). The most effective and rapid response is to discontinue the drug, with the length of time off the drug determined by the estimated drug half-life in the specific patient. After discontinuing the drug for a time based on the drug's half-life, one can use the value for total clearance (Cl_{tot}) of the drug to determine what infusion rate (I) (Eq. 7) or dose and interval (D/t) (Eq. 8) must be used to achieve the new desired concentration (C_p).

DOSE-DEPENDENT PHARMACOKINETICS

Although one can use the above pharmacokinetic principles to help choose the dose of most drugs, not all drugs behave the same when the dose is increased. Most drugs are eliminated following first-order or linear kinetics, with the amount of drug eliminated directly proportional to the concentration of drug in the plasma (Fig. 16–5A). A few drugs have a different pattern when eliminated. Three of the most commonly used drugs that exhibit this different pharmacokinetic pattern are ethanol, phenytoin, and salicylate. These drugs have dose-dependent, nonlinear, saturation kinetics. As

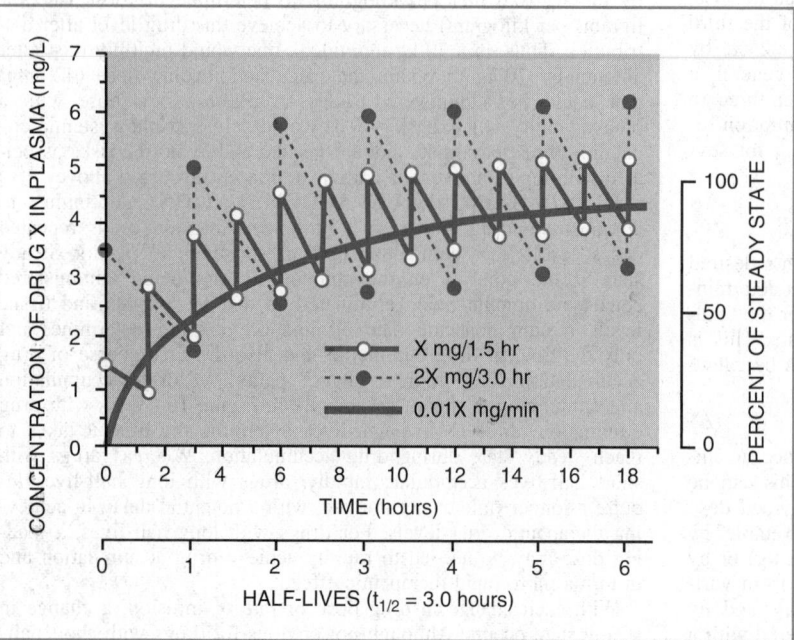

FIGURE 16-4. The accumulation of drug over time approaching a steady state is shown. Time is depicted in both hours (upper x-axis) and half-lives (lower x-axis), demonstrating that in three to five half-lives steady state is reached. The solid line depicts the pattern produced by an infusion of a hypothetical drug at a dose of 0.01X. The solid circles with the hatched line show the pattern resulting from orally administering a 2X dose every 3 hours, and the open circles with the solid line represent the pattern produced by orally administering a dose X every 1.5 hours.

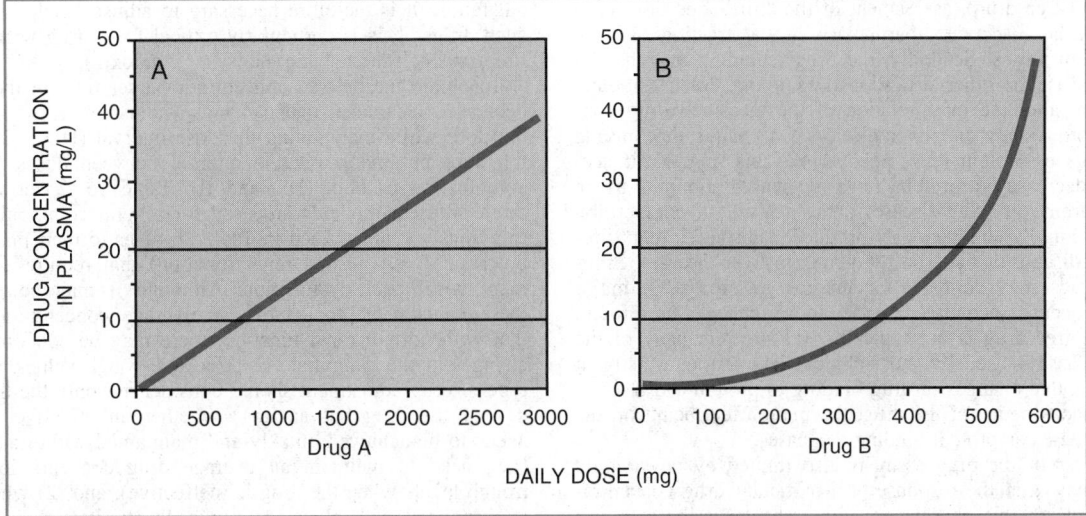

FIGURE 16–5. The effect of increasing dose on serum concentration for Drug A, which follows first-order of linear kinetics, and Drug B, which follows zero-order or nonlinear (or saturable) kinetics.

the dose of drug increases and the concentration of drug in the plasma in turn rises, the relative amount of drug being eliminated falls (i.e., the clearance decreases) until the rate of drug metabolism is at its maximum. At this point drug elimination is said to be "zero-order," and the drug concentration in plasma starts to increase much more (no longer a linear relationship) with each subsequent increase in dose (Fig. 16–5*B*).

MONITORING DRUG CONCENTRATION AS A GUIDE TO THERAPY

Although published pharmacokinetic data (usually population averages) such as are listed in Table 16–1 are useful to determine initial drug dosing, dose modification may still be needed in the individual patient. For some drugs (e.g., antihypertensives or anticoagulants), the therapeutic effects (e.g., blood pressure or coagulation) can be easily quantified over a range of concentrations, permitting adequate drug adjustment. For many other drugs (e.g., antiarrhythmics or antiseizure medications), therapeutic effects over a range of concentrations are not readily detectable. With these drugs, the plasma concentration of the drug may be used to provide further guidance in optimizing therapy. This is true only if the plasma drug concentration is a reflection of the concentration at the site of action and the drug effects are reversible. A third, much smaller group of drugs produces irreversible effects (e.g., aspirin inhibition of platelet aggregation). With these drugs, plasma drug concentration does not correlate with drug effect, and drug monitoring is therefore not useful.

To use drug concentrations as a guide to therapy, it is necessary to establish a range of concentrations from minimally to maximally efficacious with tolerable toxicity. This range of concentrations, or "therapeutic window," is usually determined from a dose-response curve generated from a population of patients who have been closely examined for therapeutic and toxic effects (Fig. 16–6). This graph may also be used to determine the "therapeutic index." This useful measure of drug toxicity is calculated by dividing the 50% value from the toxicity curve by the 50% value of the efficacy curve. Because these curves are generated from population data, the values may not be applicable for all individuals.

Table 16–1, in addition to providing useful pharmacokinetic data, also lists therapeutic ranges for several commonly used drugs for which measuring the drug concentration and knowing the therapeutic range may be useful in clinical management. Many of these drugs are typically used to treat serious or life-threatening diseases. It is essential to avoid inadequate doses because therapeutic effect is needed. At the same time, excessive doses must be avoided because of the risk of toxicity with many of these drugs that have a small therapeutic index. It is not necessary to assay drug levels for drugs used in noncritical diseases (no problem if inadequately treated) or for which the therapeutic index is large (therefore overtreatment not likely to produce toxicity).

PROBLEMS WITH INTERPRETING DRUG CONCENTRATION. The time of blood collection, perhaps more than any other factor, contributes to misinterpreting drug levels. As can be seen from Figure 16–2, if sampling is performed too early, while the drug is still in the distribution phase, the drug level may be high and not reflect drug concentration at the site of action. Therefore, it is important to sample after the distribution phase.

For many drugs administered intermittently, a trough level, obtained immediately before administering the next dose, is most useful for making decisions regarding dose adjustments. See Table 16–1 for examples of drugs that often are monitored using trough levels. For drugs that are administered by infusion or intermittently at short intervals (see Fig. 16–4), the best time to draw blood is during steady state.

Protein binding is another major factor that contributes to misinterpreting drug levels. Free drug (not bound to protein and thus able to equilibrate with tissues and interact with the site of action) is the critically important drug concentration when making therapeutic decisions. However, many drugs are tightly bound to plasma protein. Table 16–1 shows that many commonly used drugs, such as aspirin, carbamazepine, phenytoin, and valproic acid, have protein binding >75%. Because many of the commonly used drug assays determine total drug concentration (which includes both protein-

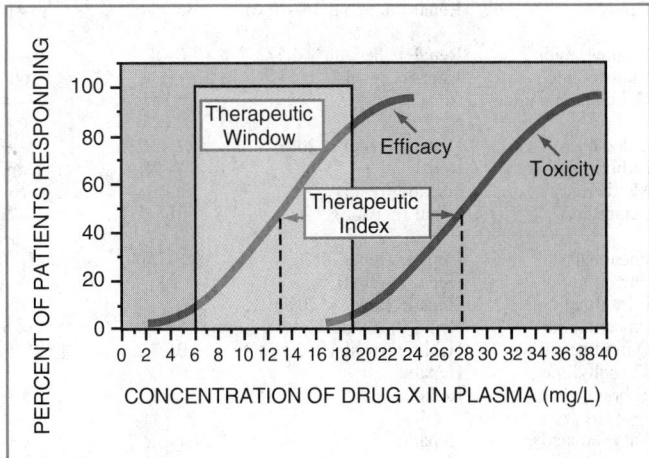

FIGURE 16–6. The pattern produced in a dose-response population study in which both effect and toxicity are measured. The therapeutic window is shown as the range of therapeutically effective concentrations, which includes most of the efficacy curve and less than 10% of the toxicity curve. The therapeutic index is calculated by dividing the 50% value on the toxicity curve by the 50% value on the efficacy curve.

bound drug and free drug), assessment of the "true" free drug concentration may be inaccurate, particularly if the fraction of drug bound to protein varies. Secondly, the drug's binding may be decreased by disease or other drugs, leading to increased unbound drug levels that alter the interpretation of the measured drug concentrations. Both kidney and liver disease can change the binding of certain drugs to protein (e.g., phenytoin). This may occur secondary to a decrease in protein (e.g., decreased albumin as in nephrotic syndrome or liver disease) or as a result of competition for protein binding by endogenously produced substances (e.g., uremia in kidney disease or hyperbilirubinemia in liver disease). Similarly, other drugs may compete for binding to protein. A major problem that occurs secondary to the above changes in protein binding is that free drug is not typically measured in many of the common drug assays used by most clinical laboratories. Lastly, it should be noted that changes in drug binding to protein can also affect the pharmacokinetics of the drug, the main affect being on the V_D, which increases as protein binding decreases.

The usefulness of the drug assay is also limited by physiologic changes that may alter the response at a particular drug concentration. An example of this pharmacodynamic change is the response produced at a certain digoxin level in the presence of altered electrolyte concentration (e.g., potassium, calcium, or magnesium). Tolerance, a reduced response to a given concentration of drug with continued use, is another pharmacodynamic change that may alter how a drug concentration is interpreted. This is commonly observed with the continued use of narcotics (e.g., in terminal cancer patients); initially adequate pain control is noted at a given drug concentration, but after chronic administration the same drug concentration is no longer associated with pain relief.

ADJUSTING DRUG DOSE WITH DISEASE

KIDNEY DISEASE. The major questions to be answered in determining whether drug dosage needs to be adjusted in the setting of kidney disease include (1) Is the drug primarily excreted through the kidneys? and (2) Are increased drug levels likely to be associated with toxicity? If both are true, it is likely that with decreased renal clearance a drug will accumulate and become toxic. With renal failure it is therefore necessary to adjust the dosing regimen of such drugs. This is particularly critical for a drug with a long half-life and small therapeutic index (e.g., digoxin).

To obtain the desired concentration over time in the presence of decreased clearance, one can make adjustments by (1) decreasing the dose while maintaining the dose interval (DD); (2) maintaining the dose but increasing the interval between doses (II); or (3) a combination of both (DD and II). Table 16−2 shows how these three different methods are used for several commonly used drugs (previously characterized in Table 16−1 as to their pharmacokinetic properties with normal renal function) that require dosage adjustment with renal dysfunction. Although it may be possible with these adjustments to achieve an average concentration similar to that with normal renal function, there may be concomitant marked changes in the magnitude of peak and trough values. Choosing the type of drug adjustment should consider not only the therapeutic index of the drug but also (1) whether an effective concentration needs to be achieved quickly and maintained within a narrow range (i.e., need to maintain an average drug concentration and avoid trough levels when the drug is ineffective); and (2) whether toxicity is associated with elevated drug concentrations (i.e., toxicity with peak drug concentration).

Renal drug clearance has been shown to correlate with creatinine clearance (whether the drug uses glomerular filtration or tubular secretion); therefore, any adjustment of drug dose in kidney disease can use the creatinine clearance to calculate the dose needed because the renal drug clearance is proportional to the creatinine clearance. The creatinine clearance, which is used as an estimate of GFR, may be directly calculated from the serum creatinine using the following equation:

$$Cl_{Cr} = \frac{(140 - age) \times weight\ (kg)}{72 \times serum\ creatinine\ (mg/dl)} \quad (9)$$

(The value should be multiplied by 0.85 for females) (*Note:* This calculation applies only when $C_{Cr} < 5$ mg/ml and the renal function is not rapidly changing.)

TABLE 16−2. ADJUSTMENT OF DRUG DOSAGE IN RENAL FAILURE

Drug	Type of Elimination	Half Life (hrs)		Method*	Adjustment for Renal Failure GFR (ml/min)			Removed by Dialysis†
		Normal	*End-Stage Renal*		*>50*	*10−50*	*<10*	
Amikacin	Renal	2−3	30	DD	60−90%	30−70%	20−30%	Yes
				II	12 hr	12−18 hr	24 hr	
Aspirin	Hepatic (renal)	2−19	Unchanged	II	4 hr	4−6 hr	Avoid	Yes
Carbamazepine	Hepatic (renal)	35	?	DD	Unchanged	Unchanged	75%	No
Digoxin	Renal (nonrenal 15−40%)	36−44	80−120	DD	Unchanged	25−75%	10−25%	No
				II	24 hr	36 hr	48 hr	
Disopyramide	Renal + hepatic	5−8	10−18	II	Unchanged	12−24 hr	24−40 hr	No
Ethosuximide	Hepatic, renal	55	60	DD	Unchanged	Unchanged	75%	Yes
Gentamicin sulfate	Renal	2	24−48	DD	60−90%	30−70%	20−30%	Yes
				II	8−12 hr	12 hr	24 hr	
Lidocaine	Hepatic (renal < 20%)	1.2−2.2	1.3−3.0	DD	Unchanged	Unchanged	Unchanged	No
Lithium carbonate	Renal	14−28	Prolonged	DD	Unchanged	50−75%	25−50%	Yes
Mexiletine	Hepatic (renal)	8−13	16	DD	Unchanged	Unchanged	50−75%	Yes
Penicillin G	Renal (hepatic)	0.5	6−20	DD	Unchanged	75%	25−50%	Yes
				II	6−8 hr	8−12 hr	12−16 hr	
Phenobarbital	Hepatic (renal 30%)	60−150	117−160	II	Unchanged	Unchanged	12−16 hr	Yes
Phenytoin	Hepatic (renal)	24	8	DD	Unchanged	Unchanged	Unchanged	No
Primidone	Hepatic (renal < 20%)	8	12	II	8 hr	8−12 hr	12−24 hr	Yes
Procainamide	Renal (hepatic 7−24%)	2.5−4.9	5.3−5.9	II	4 hr	6−12 hr	8−24 hr	Yes
Quinidine sulfate	Hepatic (renal 10−50%)	5.0−7.2	4−14	II	Unchanged	Unchanged	Unchanged	Yes
Theophylline	Hepatic	3−12	?	DD	Unchanged	Unchanged	Unchanged	Yes
Tobramycin	Renal	2.5	56	DD	60−90%	30−70%	20−30%	Yes
				II	8−12 hr	12 hr	24 hr	
Valproic acid	Hepatic	Biphasic 1 and 12	10	DD	Unchanged	Unchanged	Unchanged	No
Vancomycin	Renal	6−8	200−250	II	24−72 hr	72−240 hr	240 hr	No

* Method: DD (alone)—decrease dose (maintain same interval).
   II (alone)—increase interval between doses (maintain dose)
   DD and II (together)—combination of both approaches
† Dialysis refers to hemodialysis.
   GFR = Glomerular filtration rate.

Using Clearance for Dose Adjustment. The dose of a drug used in renal insufficiency ($Dose_{D-RI}$) can be shown to be proportional to the dose used with normal renal function ($Dose_D$) in the same ratio as the clearance of the drug in renal insufficiency (Cl_{D-RI}) to the clearance with normal renal function (Cl_D). Thus, by rearranging, the $Dose_{D-RI}$ is defined as:

$$Dose_{D-RI} = Dose_D \times \frac{Cl_{D-RI}}{Cl_D} \qquad (10)$$

One can estimate the Cl_{D-RI} by multiplying the Cl_D by the ratio of the creatinine clearance in renal insufficiency (Cl_{Cr-RI}) over the Cl_{Cr} with normal renal function.

$$Cl_{D-RI} = Cl_D \times \frac{Cl_{Cr-RI}}{Cl_{Cr}} \qquad (11)$$

It must be remembered, as shown in Eq. 3, that total clearance is the sum of clearance by renal and nonrenal (typically hepatic) mechanisms. Thus, if nonrenal clearance also occurs, this is assumed to remain normal, and only the renal clearance is adjusted, with total clearance being reduced only to the extent that renal clearance is reduced. The dose may then be calculated from the total (adjusted) clearance and the desired plasma concentration using either Eq. 7 or 8. However, the calculated dose is only an initial guide to the dose needed. By monitoring the drug response and/or the plasma drug concentration at various times after initial dosing, one can make further dose adjustments as necessary.

From a practical perspective, most clinical decisions today requiring dose adjustment of drugs in the presence of renal dysfunction use published tables that recommend reductions based on changes in GFR (Table 16–2); also provided is guidance on whether drugs are likely to be removed by dialysis.

Loading Dose in Renal Insufficiency. For those drugs that are typically administered with a loading dose with normal renal function, the same regimen may be used with renal insufficiency to ensure that the desired concentration is rapidly achieved. For other drugs that typically are administered without a loading dose with normal renal function, it should be recognized that the presence of a prolonged $t_{1/2}$ with renal insufficiency may delay drug accumulation to steady state. In this setting, a loading dose (equal to the amount needed to reach steady state with normal renal function) would be required.

Additional Considerations in Renal Insufficiency. Because of individual differences among patients, the approaches outlined above should be considered only initial approximations to prevent ineffective (too low) or toxic (too high) doses. In planning further maintenance therapy, it is desirable to monitor blood levels to guide further dosing.

If a metabolite of the drug is responsible for effect or toxicity and accumulates in renal failure, the drug level alone may not provide sufficient guidance for planning therapy in the setting of renal insufficiency. Thus, the major metabolite of procainamide is N-acetylprocainamide, which has similar toxicity to the parent drug but only modest antiarrhythmic activity. In the setting of renal failure, N-acetylprocainamide may accumulate dramatically because it is more dependent on renal elimination. Thus, measuring procainamide levels alone does not accurately assess either the levels needed for antiarrhythmic effect or the risk of toxicity.

LIVER DISEASE. Although many drugs are biotransformed in the liver, it is not possible to make any general recommendations for drug dose adjustments in liver disease. Unlike renal disease, no useful laboratory test is available on which to base dose adjustments. It has been suggested that if the liver's capacity to produce protein (reflected by albumin concentration and the prothrombin time) is significantly reduced, the clearance of drugs metabolized by the P-450 enzymes is probably also reduced.

One special situation that can develop with chronic liver disease and may require dose adjustment is the presence of portacaval shunts. This condition produces not only a potential hemodynamic alteration, leading to decreased hepatic blood flow with accompanying decreased clearance, but also possible bypassing of a first-pass effect, resulting in higher concentrations of drug reaching the systemic circulation. Drugs with a large hepatic extraction that are typically administered orally (e.g., propranolol) may then appear in the systemic circulation with higher, potentially toxic concentrations.

HEMODYNAMIC DISEASES. Decreased cardiac output or hypotensive conditions lead to decreased perfusion of the organs, including those responsible for eliminating drugs. As noted earlier with primary kidney disease, one can adjust doses for decreased renal perfusion by using the creatinine clearance. The effect of decreased hepatic blood flow on pharmacokinetics is more difficult to assess. For drugs that have a high hepatic extraction (e.g., lidocaine), decreased hepatic blood flow suggests a need to reduce doses.

Altered hemodynamics may also affect the distribution of selected drugs. Drugs that have a relatively large V_D (e.g., lidocaine, procainamide, and quinidine) may be affected by conditions leading to hypotension, such as shock resulting in a decrease in the apparent V_D. With a reduced V_D the loading dose of a drug should be reduced to avoid potentially toxic drug levels.

In general, in the setting of severely compromised hemodynamics, it is advisable to be conservative, avoiding potentially toxic loading and maintenance doses of drugs. One needs to monitor drug levels closely along with the clinical status and adjust doses as necessary.

APPROACH TO DRUG OVERDOSE

The pharmacokinetic principles discussed above can be useful to determine the best approach to drug removal in the setting of a drug overdose, particularly if hemodialysis or hemoperfusion is contemplated. The major goal is to increase the overall clearance of drug, removing a substantial fraction of the total body load of drug. Examining the V_D and Cl values can provide some guidance. For drugs with a very large V_D (e.g., digoxin in Table 16–1), only a small amount of drug can be removed because clearance affects only the amount of drug present in the plasma, and a large portion of the drug in the body is outside the plasma compartment. Similarly, for drugs with very high clearance values, hemoperfusion may only minimally increase the overall clearance and therefore is not indicated. Table 16–2 provides data for determining whether hemodialysis is likely to be useful to remove several commonly used drugs.

USING DRUGS IN THE ELDERLY

Administering drugs to the elderly is perhaps the most challenging area in adult therapeutics (see Part III). This is a consequence of several factors, including (1) the increasing likelihood of multiple illnesses often with multisystem involvement; (2) the need for these patients to be on multiple drugs (often prescribed by different physicians); and (3) the increasing probability of altered pharmacokinetics and pharmacodynamics. These factors together contribute to significantly increased frequency of drug interactions and adverse drug responses in this group of patients.

PHARMACOKINETIC CHANGES WITH AGE. These can be secondary to the effects of general physiologic changes of aging, such as the change in body composition or specific changes in pharmacokinetically important organs (e.g., kidneys or liver).

The distribution of drugs tends to change dramatically with age, mainly because of changes in body composition. Most typical is the increase in total body fat with the accompanying decrease in lean body mass and total body water. Changes may also occur in the concentration of plasma proteins, particularly albumin, which decreases as the liver ages. The changes in distribution are manifest as a change in the apparent volume of distribution. For water-soluble drugs that are not bound to plasma proteins, the apparent V_D is reduced, in contrast to lipid-soluble drugs, for which the V_D is increased. Minimal changes in metabolism accompany aging, but these alone cannot typically account for altered pharmacokinetics.

Excretion can be altered in the elderly. The clearance of a number of drugs is decreased. Both cardiac output and blood flow to the kidneys and liver may also be decreased. GFR may be reduced by as much as 50%. Hepatic elimination of drugs is less affected except for drugs with a high hepatic clearance (e.g., lidocaine). The elimination half-life of many drugs is increased with aging as a consequence of a larger apparent V_D and a decreased hepatic or renal clearance (see Eq. 5).

PHARMACODYNAMIC CHANGES WITH AGE. These are a result of changes in the responsiveness of the target organ. These pharmacodynamic changes require using smaller drug doses in the elderly, even if the pharmacokinetics are unchanged. Many examples exist of such changes with drugs commonly used in the elderly; e.g., antianxiety drugs and drugs from the sedative-hypnotic class may produce increased central nervous system depression in the elderly at concentrations that are well tolerated in younger adults. Similarly, anticoagulants (e.g., warfarin) may produce hemorrhage in the elderly at concentrations that are well tolerated in younger individuals.

GENERAL RECOMMENDATIONS. Several general principles apply to drug use in the elderly: (1) The clearance of drugs eliminated via the kidneys may be reduced by 50%; (2) drugs that are eliminated primarily by the liver typically do not require adjustment for age except for those with high hepatic clearances, which may be affected by age-related decrease in hepatic blood flow; (3) because of potential for increased target-organ sensitivity in the elderly, use only the lowest effective dose; and (4) conduct frequent reviews of the patient's drug history, including not only prescription but also over-the-counter medications, keeping in mind the increased potential risk for drug interactions and adverse drug responses.

INTERACTIONS BETWEEN DRUGS

Because patients are typically treated today with multiple agents even for a single disease, the possibilities for drug interactions are great. In general, most clinically important drug interactions typically involve a drug with a low therapeutic index (e.g., warfarin) and an easily detectable pharmacologic effect (e.g., bleeding), such that a small increase in the amount of drug produces a significant effect (toxicity).

EPIDEMIOLOGY. It is difficult to accurately assess the prevalence of drug interactions in either the inpatient or ambulatory settings, particularly because no formal surveillance mechanism is currently available. The risk for drug interactions appears to be increasing, particularly for critically ill, hospitalized patients who frequently are taking > 10 medications.

ETIOLOGY. There are basically two types of drug interaction: (1) pharmacokinetic drug interactions, caused by a change in the amount of drug or active metabolite at the site of action, and (2) pharmacodynamic drug interactions (without a change in pharmacokinetics), due to a change in drug effect.

Pharmacokinetic Drug Interactions

LESS DRUG AT THE SITE OF ACTION

DECREASED ABSORPTION. The gastrointestinal lumen is perhaps the best example of an area where two or more drugs have the opportunity to interact, resulting in decreased drug absorption. Several examples, including commonly used drugs, illustrate this type of interaction. For many of these drugs, a physicochemical interaction prevents the drug(s) from being absorbed. Drugs such as colestipol and cholestyramine (resins used to lower cholesterol and bind bile acids) can also bind other drugs simultaneously present in the gastrointestinal lumen. Among the drugs that can be bound are digoxin and warfarin. Because many other drugs can also be bound, it is generally recommended that other drugs not be administered within 2 hours of colestipol or cholestyramine. Metal ions (e.g., aluminum, calcium, and magnesium that are present in antacids and iron in supplements to treat iron deficiency) may form insoluble complexes with tetracyclines, which can act as chelating agents. Other commonly used medications that decrease absorption include kaolin-pectin suspensions used to treat diarrhea. These medications can significantly inhibit the absorption of co-administered drugs (e.g., digoxin).

Drugs that are particularly susceptible to pH changes may have decreased absorption when co-administered with drugs that either affect gastric acidity or alter the extent of exposure to low pH. Thus, histamine H_2-receptor antagonists such as cimetidine, ranitidine, and famotidine may elevate gastric pH, which can in turn inhibit the dissolution and subsequent absorption of drugs that are weak bases (e.g., ketoconazole). Medications that delay gastric emptying (e.g., belladonna alkaloids) can increase the degradation of a co-administered acid-labile drug (e.g., levodopa), resulting in decreased absorption.

ALTERED DISTRIBUTION. Drugs that use the same active transport process to reach their site of action can compete at the level of transport, resulting in lower levels of drug reaching the site of action. The classic example of this type of interaction is guani-

dinium-type antihypertensives co-administered with tricyclic antidepressants, phenothiazines, and certain sympathomimetic amines (e.g., ephedrine), which block the antihypertensive effects of the former.

INCREASED METABOLISM. A number of drugs (e.g., barbiturates such as phenobarbital, phenytoin, ethanol, glutethimide, griseofulvin, rifampin, and toxic compounds such as cigarette smoke and certain chlorinated hydrocarbons) can increase hepatic metabolism of other drugs (e.g., corticosteroids, cyclophosphamide, cyclosporine, certain β-adrenergic blockers, theophylline, and warfarin) by inducing the activity of the mixed-function oxidase (P-450) system.

MORE DRUG AT THE SITE OF ACTION

INCREASED ABSORPTION. Any drug that increases the rate of gastric emptying (e.g., metoclopramide) can potentially increase the absorption of acid unstable drugs. Also drugs that decrease intestinal motility (e.g., anticholinergics) may increase the absorption of drugs that are relatively poorly absorbed (e.g., digoxin tablets) by increasing the contact time of the drug with the absorbing surface.

ALTERED DISTRIBUTION. Drugs bound to protein are limited in their distribution (particularly to the site of action) and are not available for metabolism or excretion. Drugs can compete with each other for binding to plasma proteins, resulting in drug interactions. For example, sulfonamides can displace barbiturates bound to serum albumin, leading to increased levels of free barbituates with possible toxicity.

DECREASED METABOLISM. One of the most impressive drug interactions is produced when one drug inhibits the metabolism of another drug, leading to the second drug accumulating and thus significantly risking toxicity. For example, this type of interaction results from using 6-mercaptopurine, an antileukemic drug with a low therapeutic index, with allopurinol, often used in this setting to control hyperuricemia. The interaction may result in potentially life-threatening toxicity.

Some drugs can inhibit the metabolism of many other drugs. For example, cimetidine can inhibit the metabolism of diazepam, imipramine, lidocaine, propranolol, quinidine, theophylline, and warfarin. Amiodarone inhibits the metabolism of calcium-channel blockers, flecainide, phenytoin, quinidine, and warfarin. Of particular importance with amiodarone is its half-life of 1 to 2 months, so that it continues to inhibit drug metabolism for several months after being discontinued.

Other drugs are notable in that their metabolism is inhibited by a variety of different drugs. The metabolism of the commonly used anticoagulant warfarin is inhibited not only by cimetidine and amiodarone but also by many other drugs, including alcohol, allopurinol, disopyramide, disulfiram, metronidazole, phenylbutazone, sulfinpyrazone, and trimethoprim-sulfamethoxazole. Similarly, the metabolism of phenytoin is also inhibited by additional drugs, including chloramphenicol, clofibrate, dicumarol, disulfiram, isoniazid (slow acetylators), phenylbutazone, and valproic acid.

Although most of the examples above involved enzymes metabolizing the drug in the liver, it should be noted that drug-metabolizing enzymes located outside the liver may also be affected by certain drugs. The best known example is monoamine oxidase, which can be affected by nonspecific monoamine oxidase inhibitors, resulting in catecholamines accumulating at multiple sites which can be released after eating tyramine-containing foods.

DECREASED EXCRETION. Drugs can compete for the active transporters present in the kidney. Most of these interactions involve the acid transporters. The best-known interaction is the probenecid inhibiting penicillin transport, leading to decreased penicillin clearance with resultant increased plasma levels—an interaction that was used in the past to maximize penicillin therapy. A similar inhibitory effect on renal excretion of methotrexate can be produced by salicylates, phenylbutazone, and probenicid. The active transport of basic drugs (e.g., procainamide) can also be inhibited by other drugs (e.g., cimetidine or amiodarone).

Pharmacodynamic Drug Interactions

With pharmacodynamic interactions, drugs interact at the level of the receptor or may produce additive effects by acting at separate sites on cells. An example of the first is the interaction of propranolol and epinephrine, which blocks β-adrenergic receptors with the

TABLE 16–3. DRUGS WITH LOW THERAPEUTIC INDICES AT HIGH RISK FOR ADVERSE DRUG RESPONSE AND DRUG INTERACTIONS

Anticoagulants
Antiarrhythmics
Anticonvulsants
Digoxin
Lithium carbonate
Oral Hypoglycemics
Theophylline

result that the α-adrenergic effects of epinephrine are unopposed. This undesirable interaction can result in severe hypertension.

Many examples exist of additive effects between drugs. Aspirin, which can produce increased bleeding time by acting on platelets, can interact with warfarin, which affects clotting. The result is an increased risk of hemorrhage. Similarly, cardiac drugs such as β-adrenergic blockers and calcium channel blockers, when co-administered, have additive negative inotropic effects, resulting in an increased risk of cardiac failure.

DIAGNOSING AND PREVENTING DRUG INTERACTIONS. To recognize the presence of a drug interaction, the health professional must first consider the possibility that this may be occurring whenever multiple drugs are used together. Because of the ever-increasing list of known and suspected drug interactions, it is impossible for a clinician to remember all or even a significant number.

Several clinical settings should raise concern about the possibility of drug interactions: (1) The use of any drug with a low therapeutic index (Table 16–3). (2) As the number of drugs being used concurrently increases, there is a disproportionately greater risk of drug interactions, particularly with >10 drugs. (3) Critically ill patients who have multisystemic disease with compromised renal, hepatic, cardiac, or pulmonary function have an increased risk of drug interactions. This may be even more of a problem for patients with AIDS, who have an immunocompromised state as well as being on a great number of drugs. (4) Patients with various behavioral and psychiatric disorders (e.g., drug abusers taking a large number of prescription drugs, illicit drugs, and alcohol) are at risk to develop drug interactions.

Several steps can be taken to prevent drug interactions: (1) In taking the medical history, it is important to document all the drugs the patient is taking, including prescription, over-the-counter, and other addictive drugs. (2) It is desirable to minimize the number of drugs the patient is taking. This requires frequently reviewing the patient's drug list to ensure that each drug continues to be needed. (3) There should be a high degree of suspicion when medications with a low therapeutic index known to have a high risk of drug interactions (Table 16–3) are used. (4) High-risk clinical settings, such as occur with critically ill patients, should raise suspicion of adverse drug interactions. (5) Adverse drug interactions should be

considered in the differential diagnosis whenever any change occurs in a patient's course.

ADVERSE REACTIONS TO DRUGS

An adverse drug response is an undesired effect produced by a drug at standard doses which typically necessitates reducing or stopping the suspected agent and may require treatment for the noxious effect produced. Implied is the risk of further harm to the patient with continued or future therapy with the drug.

EPIDEMIOLOGY. The actual incidence of adverse drug responses is somewhat difficult to quantify, as many cases are not recognized. Several large studies have demonstrated that the incidence may be as high as 20% for inpatients (even higher for patients on >15 drugs) and 5 to 20% for outpatients. It is clear from recent surveys that a relatively small group of drugs (Table 16–3) continue to be implicated in most of the reported adverse drug responses. Current trends suggest that the incidence of adverse drug responses is likely to increase as a result of an increase in the number of both prescribed and over-the-counter medications.

ETIOLOGY. Most adverse drug responses are caused by either (1) exaggerated (but predictable) pharmacologic effect of the drug or (2) toxic or immunologic effect of drug or metabolite (not typically expected).

Exaggerated (Predictable) Response to a Drug. Exaggerated drug responses that cause adverse drug effects may be due to any condition that causes either altered pharmacokinetics or pharmacodynamics (discussed above).

Recently there has been interest in the role of genetic factors as a cause of increased susceptibility to adverse drug responses, primarily through an effect on drug metabolism. Genetic polymorphism of drug metabolizing enzymes can account for variability in pharmacokinetics and drug effect observed in population studies. Three of the best studied polymorphisms are the debrisoquine/sparteine, N-acetylation, and mephenytoin polymorphisms. These are each associated with an autosomal recessive inheritance and together are responsible for the metabolism of approximately 40 drugs (Table 16–4). Individuals with autosomal recessive genes are "poor metabolizers" with potentially altered pharmacokinetics that result in elevated plasma drug concentrations and can lead to toxicity. These defects are not noted until the patient is given the drug. They are often described as being "pharmacogenetic" syndromes.

Other genetic defects do not specifically affect metabolism and hence do not produce a range of quantitative changes. These defects can produce "qualitative" defects and are often associated with structural defects. The classic example is glucose-6-phosphate dehydrogenase (G6PD). Individuals who are deficient in this enzyme cannot tolerate oxidative stress that is produced by some drugs, leading to hemolysis (see Ch. 128). Drugs that can produce this clinical picture include aspirin, nitrofurantoin, primaquine, probenecid, quinidine, quinine, sulfonamides, sulfones, and vitamin K. Another similar defect is deficiency of methemoglobin reductase,

TABLE 16–4. GENETIC POLYMORPHISMS OF DRUG-METABOLIZING ENZYMES

Type	Primary Drug Examples	Other Drugs That Are Substrates	Incidence of "Poor Metabolizers" In Caucasians (%)	Enzyme Involved
Debrisoquine-sparteine polymorphism	Debrisoquine, sparteine, bufuralol	Antidepressants, antiarrhythmics, β-adrenergic–receptor blocking drugs, codeine, dextromethorphan, neuroleptics	5–10	Cytochrome P-450 IID6
Mephenytoin polymorphism	Mephenytoin	Mephobarbital, hexobarbital, diazepam, omeprazol	4 (Japanese, Chinese, 15–20)	Cytochrome P-450 IIC
Acetylation polymorphism	Isoniazid, sulfadiazine	Isoniazid, hydralazine, phenelzine, procainamide, dapsone, sulfamethazine, sulfapyridine aminoglutethimide, aminosalicylic acid, sulfadiazine, sulfasalazine	40–70 (Japanese, 10–20)	N-Acetyltransferase (NAT$_2$)
Methyl-conjugation (COMT) polymorphism	Catecholamines	L-Dopa, methyldopa	25–30	Catechol O-methyltransferase

which results in an inability to maintain iron in hemoglobin in the ferrous state, causing methemoglobinemia following exposure to oxidizing drugs such as nitrites, sulfonamide, or sulfones.

Toxic or Immunologic (Unpredictable) Response to Drug. This type of adverse drug response is not predictable and is not obviously due to either an increase in drug concentration (pharmacokinetic) or drug effect (pharmacodynamic). Toxic responses include direct reactions between drug and a specific organ (e.g., platinum-containing drugs such as cisplatin can produce direct toxicity in the kidney and the eighth cranial nerve). With other drugs, me-

tabolism of the drug to an active intermediate must first occur. With a standard dose of acetaminophen, no untoward effects occur because the relatively small amount of reactive metabolite formed by oxidative metabolism is rapidly detoxified by reduced glutathione. In the presence of an overdose, the glutathione is depleted and the remaining reactive metabolite can then damage the liver. Understanding the mechanism of this toxicity has provided a rationale for treating acetaminophen overdose. Thus, sulfhydryl-containing compounds (e.g., N-acetylcysteine), which can complex with the reactive metabolite, can be administered to reduce the amount of "free" toxic metabolite present, thereby protecting the liver.

Immunologic reactions to drugs (Table 16–5) in general are not

TABLE 16–5. ADVERSE DRUG REACTIONS

I. Multisystemic manifestations
- A. Anaphylaxis
  - 1. Macromolecules
    - Allergenic extracts
    - Dextrans (including iron dextran)
    - Enzymes
      - Asparaginase
      - Chymopapain
      - Trypsin
    - Heparin
    - Hormones (ACTH, insulin, etc.)
    - Human gamma globulin
    - Monoclonal antibodies
    - Protamine
    - Vaccines
    - Antisera
  - 2. Diagnostic agents
    - Fluorescein
    - Iodinated contrast media
  - 3. Antimicrobials
    - Aminosalicylic acid
    - Amphotericin B
    - Cephalosporins
    - Cinoxacin
    - Clindamycin
    - Demeclocycline
    - Ethambutol
    - Kanamycin
    - Lincomycin
    - Nalidixic acid
    - Penicillins
    - Streptomycin
    - Sulfonamides
    - Tetracyclines
    - Vancomycin
  - 4. Other drugs and other nonsteroidal anti-inflammatory drugs (NSAID's)
    - Aspirin
    - Benzyl alcohol
    - Bleomycin
    - Cisplatin
    - Colchicine
    - Cromolyn
    - Cytarabine
    - Dantrolene
    - Ethylenediamine
    - Etoposide
    - Flucytosine
    - Glucocorticoids
    - Indomethacin
    - Lidocaine
    - Local anesthetics
    - Mephyton
    - Meprobamate
    - Niacin
    - Opiates
    - Pentamidine
    - Probenecid
    - Procainamide
    - Sulfite
    - Thiopental
    - Tolmetin
    - Triamterene
    - Tubocurarine and other muscle-relaxing agents
    - Vitamin B_{12}
- B. Serum sickness
  - 1. Macromolecules
    - Dextrans
    - Heparin
    - Hormones (insulin, ACTH, etc.)
    - Vaccines
    - Antisera
  - 2. Antimicrobials
    - Cephalosporins
    - Griseofulvin
    - Lincomycin
    - Minocycline
    - Penicillins
    - Streptomycin
    - Sulfonamides
  - 3. Other drugs
    - Barbiturates
    - Hydralazine
    - Phenylbutazone
    - Phenytoin
    - Procarbazine
    - Propylthiouracil
- C. Drug fever
  - 1. Antimicrobials
    - 5-Aminosalicylic acid
    - Amphotericin B
    - Cephalosporins
    - Erythromycin
    - Isoniazid
    - Kanamycin
    - Nitrofurantoin
    - Norfloxacin
    - Penicillins
    - Pyrazinamide
    - Quinine
    - Streptomycin
    - Sulfonamides
    - Tetracyclines
  - 2. Other drugs
    - Allopurinol
    - Captopril
    - Heparin
    - Hydantoins
    - Hydralazine
    - Hydrochlorothiazide
    - Methyldopa
    - Penicillamine
    - Phenobarbital
    - Pneumococcal vaccine
    - Procainamide
    - Propylthiouracil
    - Quinine
- D. Vasculitis
  - Allopurinol
  - Atenolol
  - Busulfan
  - Carbamazepine
  - Colchicine
  - Diphenhydramine
  - Ethionamide
  - Furosemide
  - Hydantoins
  - Hydroxyurea
  - Ibuprofen
  - Indomethacin
  - Isoniazid
  - Meprobamate
  - Methamphetamine
  - Naproxen
  - Penicillins
  - Phenothiazines
  - Phenylbutazone
  - Propranolol
  - Propylthiouracil
  - Streptokinase
  - Sulfonamides
  - Tetracyclines
  - Thiazide diuretics
  - Vaccines
- E. Systemic lupus erythematosus syndrome
  - 5-Aminosalicylic acid
  - Chloroquine
  - Chlorpromazine
  - Ethosuximide
  - Griseofulvin
  - Hydralazine
  - Isoniazid
  - Methyldopa
  - Nitrofurantoin
  - Penicillamine
  - Penicillins
  - Phenytoin
  - Procainamide
  - Propylthiouracil
  - Quinidine
  - Tetracycline
  - Tocainide
  - Trimethadione

II. Skin
- A. Urticaria and angioedema
  - 1. Antimicrobials
    - 5-Aminosalicylic acid
    - Aminoglycosides
    - Cephalosporins
    - Isoniazid
    - Metronidazole
    - Miconazole
    - Nalidixic acid
    - Penicillins
    - Quinine
    - Rifampin
    - Spectinomycin
    - Sulfonamides
  - 2. Other drugs
    - Asparaginase
    - Aspirin and other NSAID's
    - Calcitonin
    - Chloral hydrate
    - Chorambucil
    - Cimetidine
    - Cyclophosphamide
    - Daunorubicin
    - Doxorubicin
    - Ergotamine
    - Ethchlorvynol
    - Ethosuximide
    - Ethylenediamine
    - Glucocorticoids
    - Melphalan
    - Penicillamine
    - Phenothiazines
    - Procainamide
    - Procarbazine
    - Quinidine
    - Tartrazine
    - Thiazide diuretics
    - Thiotepa
- B. Morbilliform-maculopapular rash
  - 1. Antimicrobials
    - 5-Aminosalicylic acid
    - Cephalosporins
    - Erythromycin
    - Gentamicin
    - Penicillins
    - Streptomycin
    - Sulfonamides
  - 2. Other drugs
    - Allopurinol
    - Barbiturates
    - Captopril
    - Coumarin
    - Gold salts
    - Hydantoins
    - Thiazide diuretics
- C. Toxic epidermal necrolysis, erythroderma, and exfoliative dermatitis
  - Allopurinol
  - Amikacin
  - Captopril
  - Carbamazepine
  - Chloral hydrate
  - Chlorambucil
  - Chloroquine
  - Chlorpromazine
  - Cyclosporine
  - Diltiazem
  - Ethambutol
  - Ethylenediamine
  - Glutethimide
  - Gold salts
  - Griseofulvin
  - Hydantoins
  - Hydroxychloroquine
  - Minoxidil
  - Nifedipine
  - NSAID's
  - Penicillin
  - Phenobarbital
  - Rifampin

TABLE 16-5. ADVERSE DRUG REACTIONS *Continued*

Spironolactone
Streptomycin
Sulfonamides
Trimethadione
Trimethoprim
Tocainide
Vancomycin
Verapamil
D. Erythema multiforme
Acetaminophen
Barbiturates
Carbamazepine
Chloroquine
Chlorpropamide
Clindamycin
Ethambutol
Ethosuximide
Gold salts
Hydantoins
Hydralazine
Hydroxyurea
Mechlorethamine
Meclofenamate
Penicillins
Phenolphthalein
Phenylbutazone
Rifampin
Streptomycin
Sulfonylureas
Sulindac
Vaccines
E. Photosensitive
1. Topical
Fluorouracil
Hexachlorophene
Para-aminobenzoic
acid esters
Promethazine
Sulfanilamide
2. Systemic
Carbamazepine
Chlorpromazine
Griseofulvin
Imipramine
Lincomycin
Nalidixic acid
Naproxen
Norfloxacin
Phenothiazines
Piroxicam
Quinethazone
Sulfonamides
Sulfonylureas
Thiazide diuretics
Triamterene
F. Fixed drug eruptions
Acetaminophen
5-Aminosalicylic acid
Aspirin
Barbiturates
Benzodiazepines
Cloroquine
Dapsone
Dimenhydrinate
Diphenhydramine
Gold salts
Hydralazine
Hyoscine
Ibuprofen
Iodides
Meprobamate
Methenamine
Metronidazole
Penicillins
Phenobarbital
Phenolphthalein
Phenothiazines
Phenylbutazone
Procarbazine
Pseudoephedrine
Quinine

Saccharin
Streptomycin
Sulfonamides
Tetracyclines
G. Erythema nodosum
Bromides
Oral contraceptives
Penicillin
Sulfonamides
H. Contact dermatitis
Ambroxol
Amikacin
Antihistamines
Bacitracin
Benzalkonium
chloride
Benzocaine
Benzyl alcohol
Cetyl alcohol
Chloramphenicol
Chlorpromazine
Clioquinol
Colophony
Ethylenediamine
Fluorouracil
Formaldehyde
Gentamicin
Glucocorticoids
Glutaraldehyde
Heparin
Hexachlorophene
Iodochlorhydroxyquin
Lanolin
Local anesthetics
Minoxidil
Naftin
Neomycin
Nitrofurazone
Opiates
Para-aminobenzoic
acid
Parabens
Penicillins
Phenothiazines
Proflavine
Propylene glycol
Streptomycin
Sulfonamides
Thimerosal
Timolol

III. Lungs
A. Asthma
Aspirin and other
NSAID's
Cromolyn
Sulfite
Tartrazine
Occupational exposures
to:
Cephalosporins
Glutaraldehyde
Pancreatic enzymes
Papain
Penicillins
Psyllium
Thimerosal
B. Eosinophilic pneumonitis
5-Aminosalycylic acid
Azathioprine
Captopril
Carbamazepine
Chlorpropamide
Cromolyn
Desipramine
Gold salts
Imipramine
Nitrofurantoin
Penicillins
Phenytoin
Sulfonamides
L-Tryptophan

C. Fibrotic and pleural
reactions
Bleomycin
Busulfan
Cyclophosphamide
Gold salts
Hydralazine
Hydrochlorothiazide
Melphalan
Methotrexae
Methysergide
Mitomycin
Nitrofurantoin
Procarbazine
IV. Liver
A. Cholestatic
Chlorzoxazone
Erythromycin estolate
Ethchlorvynol
Imipramine
Nalidixic acid
Nitrofurantoin
Phenothiazines
Sulfamethoxazole
Sulfonylureas
Troleandomycin
B. Hepatocellular
5-Aminosalicylic acid
Amphotericin B
Azapropazone
Ethacrynic acid
Furosemide
Gold salts
Griseofulvin
Halothane
Hydantoins
Isoniazid
Methyldopa
Monoamine oxidase
inhibitors
Nitrofurantoin
Propylthiouracil
Pyrazinamide
Quinidine
Rifampin
Sulfonamides
Trimethadione
C. Chronic active hepatitis
Methyldopa
Nitrofurantoin
V. Kidney
A. Glomerulitis
Allopurinol
Captopril
Gold salts
NSAID's
Penicillamine
Penicillins
Phenytoin
Probenecid
Sulfonamides
Thiazide diuretics
B. Interstitial nephritis
Allopurinol
Aztreonam
Captopril
Carbamazepine
Cephalosporins
Chloramphenicol
Cimetidine
Ciprofloxacin
Colistin
Furosemide
Minocycline
NSAID's
Penicillins, especially
methicillin
Phenytoin
Polymyxin B
Rifampin
Sulfonamides

Tetracycline
Thiazide diuretics
VI. Bone marrow and blood cells
A. Bone marrow aplasia
Chloramphenicol
Gold salts
Mephenytoin
Penicillamine
Phenylbutazone
Trimethadione
B. Anemia
Acetaminophen
5-Aminosalicylic acid
Captopril
Cephalosporins
Chlorpromazine
Cisplatin
Hydantoins
Ibuprofen
Insulin
Isoniazid
Levodopa
Mefenamic acid
Melphalan
Methyldopa
Methylsergide
Penicillins
Quinidine
Quinine
Rifampin
Sulfonamides
Sulfonylureas
C. Thrombocytopenia
Acetaminophen
Acetazolamide
Acetylsalicylic acid
5-Aminosalicylic acid
Carbamazepine
Chloramphenicol
Chlorpheniramine
Cimetidine
Digitoxin
Diltiazem
Ethchlorvynol
Gold salts
Heparin
Hydantoins
Isoniazid
Levodopa
Meprobamate
Methyldopa
Penicillamine
Phenylbutazone
Procainamide
Quinidine
Quinine
Ranitidine
Rauwolfia alkaloids
Rifampin
Sulfonamides
Sulfonylureas
Thiazide diuretics
D. Granulocytopenia
Captopril
Cephalosporins
Chloral hydrate
Chlorpropamide
Penicillins (semisyn-
thetic)
Phenothiazines
Phenylbutazone
Phenytoin
Procainamide
Propranolol
Tolbutamide
E. Lymphoid hyperplasia
Phenytoin
Mephenytoin

Adapted from Reed CE: Drug allergy. *In* Wyngaarden JB, Smith LH Jr, Bennett JC (eds.): Cecil Textbook of Medicine. 19th ed. Philadelphia, WB Saunders, 1992, pp 1480–1481.

produced by the drug alone. Like other small (< 1000) molecular weight compounds, they are typically not antigenic themselves. When a drug or reactive metabolite combines with a protein to form a drug-protein complex, it can become antigenic, capable of eliciting an immune response.

Perhaps the most impressive form of drug allergy is anaphylaxis, which is due to an IgE-mediated hypersensitivity. Many drugs from different classes have been shown to produce this type of drug allergy, as shown in Table 16–5. The best-known example is the anaphylactic response produced by penicillin. This can occur after administering penicillin by any route. Skin testing with penicillin G, penicilloic acid, or penicilloyl-polylysine can identify patients at risk and should be used in patients with suspected penicillin allergy who need to be treated with penicillin. If the skin test is positive, the patient must undergo desensitization prior to receiving penicillin. If the skin test is negative, penicillin can be administered but with caution.

DIAGNOSIS. Although it should be clear from the above discussion that many of the well-known adverse drug effects are due to a relatively small group of drugs, it should be emphasized that every drug can potentially cause an adverse drug response. Therefore, the physician should always consider the possibility of an adverse drug response in the differential diagnosis even if none has been reported previously for the particular drug. Table 16–5 lists a number of diverse clinical presentations associated with adverse drug responses. In many instances it is readily apparent that a specific drug has produced an adverse drug response, such as the appearance of a skin rash in an otherwise healthy patient who recently has been started on a single drug (e.g., penicillin). In other cases, the effect produced by the drug may be difficult to discern from other disease states. In still other cases the adverse effect may mimic the illness being treated (e.g., an arrhythmia developing in a patient being treated with an antiarrhythmic drug).

From a public health perspective, it is highly desirable to have a mechanism available for detecting, cataloging, and tracking the incidence and severity of adverse drug responses not only for drugs at various stages of development but also for drugs that were approved earlier. The Food and Drug Administration (FDA) tries to track adverse drug events through a voluntary reporting program, MedWatch. Health professionals are encouraged to report any adverse events or product problems on a one-page form that can then be sent by mail, FAX, or modem to the FDA. Although various methods for surveying adverse drug responses have been proposed, it is ultimately the cooperation of alert clinicians and health professionals that must be encouraged.

Bennett WM, Aronoff GR, Golper TA, et al.: Drug Prescribing in Renal Failure: Dosing Guidelines for Adults. 2nd ed. Philadelphia, American College of Physicians, 1991. *This recently updated manual provides useful data for adjusting doses in patients with renal dysfunction, including those on dialysis.*

Bloom HG, Shlom EA: Drug Prescribing for the Elderly. New York, Raven Press, 1993. *This manual provides not only recommendations on dose adjustments for many commonly used drugs in the elderly but also highlights potential drug interactions and adverse drug responses that occur with these drugs in this population.*

Evans WE, Schentag JJ, Jusko WJ: Applied Pharmacokinetics: Principles of Therapeutic Drug Monitoring. Vancouver, Applied Therapeutics, 1992. *Provides an excellent review of pharmacokinetic and pharmacodynamic principles that determine how best to optimize therapy. In addition, useful data are provided on many commonly used drugs.*

Meyer UA: Drugs in special patient groups: Clinical importance of genetics in drug effects. In Clinical Pharmacology: Basic Principles in Therapeutics. New York, McGraw-Hill, 1992, p 875. *The role of genetic factors as a source of interindividual variation in drug response is reviewed. This is the source for some of the data in Table 16–4.*

Montamat SC, Cusack BJ, Vestal RE: Management of drug therapy in the elderly. N Engl J Med 321:310, 1989. *An excellent review of the use of drugs in the elderly.*

Rizack MA, Hillman CDM: The Medical Letter Handbook of Adverse Drug Interactions. New Rochelle, The Medical Letter, 1993. *This paperback handbook provides a relatively comprehensive listing of drugs thought to produce interactions, with a description of adverse effects, their probable mechanism, clinical recommendations, and original references.*

Schrier RW, Gambertoglio JG (eds.): Handbook of Drug Therapy in Liver and Kidney Disease. Boston, Little, Brown, & Co, 1991. *This is an excellent guide to adjustments in drug dosing for renal and liver dysfunction.*

Scott G, Nierenberg D: Pharmacokinetic data for commonly used drugs. In Clinical Pharmacology: Basic Principles in Therapeutics. New York, McGraw-Hill, 1992, p 1029. *Excellent comprehensive summary of pharmacokinetic data from recent medical literature on >200 commonly used drugs. This is the source for some of the data in Tables 16–1 and 16–2.*

Wright JM: Drug interactions. In Clinical Pharmacology: Basic Principles in Therapeutics. New York, McGraw-Hill, 1992, p 1012. *Useful overview of how to recognize and prevent drug interactions.*

Problems of Overarching Importance Which Transcend Organ Systems

17 PAIN
Kathleen M. Foley

Pain is the most common symptom for which patients seek medical evaluation. Several national patient surveys have emphasized the magnitude of pain as a public health issue, citing its negative impact on patients' functional status and quality of life.

Improved medical and diagnostic methods, coupled with recent advances in our understanding of central nervous system (CNS) pain modulatory systems and their neuroanatomic and neuropharmacologic correlates, have led to specialized and innovative applications of pain management strategies. The consensus in pain therapy is that pain patients are managed most effectively by a multidisciplinary approach, using the expertise of a wide range of health care professionals. To facilitate clinical research and patient care, the International Association for the Study of Pain has proposed a taxonomy of pain syndromes to serve as a universal classification, with a working definition of pain as "an unpleasant sensory and emotional experience associated with either actual or potential tissue damage, or described in terms of such damage."

The physician's therapeutic task is twofold: to discover and treat the cause of the pain or to treat the pain itself, whether or not the underlying cause is treatable. In the majority of clinical pain syndromes, pain therapy serves to palliate the symptom. For such patients, the goal of pain treatment should be to improve the patient's quality of life by facilitating his/her functional status and social interactions.

TYPES OF PAIN

Clinically, pain can be classified *temporally* as acute or chronic; *quantitatively* as mild, moderate, or severe; *physiologically* as somatic, visceral, or neuropathic; and *etiologically* as medical or psychogenic.

TEMPORAL CHARACTERISTICS. Patients with *acute pain* usually give a clear description of its location, character, and timing, leading to an etiologic diagnosis. Objective signs and associated autonomic nervous system hyperactivity with tachycardia, hypertension, and diaphoresis are present. The setting of the pain, its meaning, and its duration influence the patient's ability to tolerate it. Acute pain (e.g., postoperative pain, acute traumatic pain) is usually self-limited. Subacute pain develops over several days, and episodic pain occurs for set periods of time on a recurring basis. *Chronic pain* is the persistence of pain for 3 months or longer. The acute signs of autonomic nervous system hyperactivity disappear with its adaption. Chronic pain leads to significant changes in personality, lifestyle, and functional ability, compromising the patient's quality of life. Multidisciplinary approaches to treatment play a critical role in addressing the multidimensional aspects of the pain. Other commonly used terms to describe pain include *baseline pain,* which refers to the average pain intensity expressed for 12 or more hours in a 24-hour period, and *breakthrough pain,* which is a transient increase in pain resulting from volitional (e.g., incident pain on movement) and nonvolitional factors (flatulence).

QUANTITATIVE CHARACTERISTICS. The intensity of pain is used to describe its severity. Pain intensity is the major factor in choosing drug therapy, and the use of a reliable pain intensity scale can enormously affect appropriate patient treatment. Numerous studies have shown that health care professionals underestimate patients' pain intensity, particularly if patients report pain as moderate or severe. This observation is one of the common causes of the undertreatment of pain. The repeated use of validated pain intensity scales, such as categorical scales, visual analogue scales, and numerical scales can facilitate appropriate pain assessment and treatment. Categorical scales use verbal reports and ask patients to describe their pain as mild, moderate, severe, or excruciating. Visual analogue scales consist of a 10-cm line anchored on either end by the two points, "no pain" and "worst possible pain," and the patient is asked to mark on the line the intensity of his/her pain. Numerical scales are often commonly used, asking patients to rate their pain as a number from 0 to 10 with 0 as "no pain" and 10 being the "worst possible pain."

PHYSIOLOGIC CHARACTERISTICS. Somatic pain results from activation of peripheral receptors and somatic sensory efferent nerves without injury to the peripheral nerve or CNS. The pain can be either sharp or dull but it is typically well-localized and describable. Visceral pain results from visceral nociceptive receptors and visceral efferent nerves being activated and is characterized by a deep, aching, cramping sensation often referred to cutaneous sites. Neuropathic pain results from direct injury to peripheral receptors, nerves, or the CNS. It is typically described as burning or dysesthetic and often occurs in an area of sensory loss (e.g., postherpetic neuralgia). The autonomic nervous system plays a significant modulatory role in all three types of pain but is most prominent in visceral and neuropathic pain. Somatic and visceral pain are readily managed with a variety of nonopioid and opioid analgesics as well as anesthetic and neurosurgical approaches. In contrast, neuropathic pain has a variable response to opioid analgesics. Various adjuvant analgesics have demonstrated their efficacy in neuropathic pain, and certain anesthetic and neurosurgical approaches provide relief in specific neuropathic pain syndromes.

ETIOLOGIC CHARACTERISTICS. Patients with chronic pain can generally be classified into one of three major etiologic groups, allowing for some overlap. The first group includes patients with chronic pain associated with structural disease. Such pain (e.g., metastatic cancer, sickle cell disease, rheumatoid arthritis) is usually characterized by prolonged episodes of pain alternating with pain-free intervals or by unremitting pain waxing and waning in severity. Successful treatment of the pain is closely allied with disease treatment, but in certain instances, treating the pain is the only therapeutic goal, e.g., the dying patient with pain. Psychological factors may play an important role in exacerbating or relieving the pain, but analgesic drugs are often the mainstay of therapy.

The second group comprises patients who suffer from *psychophysiologic disorders* causing pain. In these patients, structural disease, such as a herniated disc or torn ligament, may once have been present, but psychological factors have caused chronic physiologic alterations, such as muscle spasms, which produced pain long after the underlying defect has healed. Typically, such patients are physically inactive and spend much of their time thinking and talking about their pain, often leading to social and emotional isolation. Patients are more impaired by the "chronic illness behavior" than by a defined pathologic condition. They usually respond poorly to analgesic drugs and often suffer from iatrogenic complications such as adverse drug reactions and ineffective surgical procedures. Successful treatment can be expected only through a structured rehabilitation program designed to modify pain behaviors and not through medical intervention that corrects pathologic conditions. Multidisci-

plinary pain clinics that diagnose and treat these intractable chronic pain syndromes exist in many centers and should be used to evaluate and treat such patients.

Patients in the third group complain of pain that appears to have neither a structural nor a physiologic basis. These patients probably suffer from somatic delusions. Such patients usually have serious psychiatric disorders and the history of their pain is so vague and bizarre and its distribution so unanatomic as to suggest the diagnosis. These patients are rare and respond poorly to pain treatment strategies alone, requiring psychiatric treatment with a variable response rate.

ASSESSMENT OF PAIN

Table 17–1 outlines an approach to assessing the patient with pain. It begins with the premise that to manage pain, the physician must understand its multidimensional nature and must establish a relationship of mutual trust with the patient. The diagnosis of the specific pain syndrome and a complete understanding of the psychological state of the patient are not often achieved at the initial evaluation. A comprehensive assessment involves taking a careful history, performing a detailed medical, neurologic, and psychological evaluation, developing a series of diagnosis-related hypotheses, and ordering the appropriate diagnostic studies. The history of the pain complaint should include the patient's description of the site of the pain, its quality, its exacerbating and relieving factors, its temporal pattern, its associated symptoms and signs, its interference with activities of daily living, and its response to previous and current analgesic therapies.

Multiple pain complaints are common in patients with advanced disease and need to be prioritized and classified. In evaluating the patient with pain, it is imperative to clarify his/her current level of anxiety and depression and to obtain a history of previous psychiatric illness to define the psychological risk. Does the patient have a past history or family history of acute or chronic pain? Information on how the patient has handled previous painful events may provide insight into whether the patient has demonstrated chronic illness behavior. A personal or family history of alcohol or drug dependence may explain why the patient may be fearful or refuse to take opioid drugs. Has the patient seen someone die a painful death? Patients who have had such an experience are particularly fearful of their own death. Because each patient has his/her own understanding of the meaning of pain, it is useful to have the patient elaborate this meaning. Does he/she think it represents recurrent tumor, in the case of a patient with cancer? Or is he/she convinced that it is simply arthritis? The more serious the nature of the pain diagnosis, the more likely the patient's understanding of its meaning may produce psychological distress. Data suggest that psychological factors play a significant role in accounting for the differences in pain experiences among patients with the same pain diagnosis or illness. Awareness of the common psychiatric syndromes—anxiety and depression—that occur in patients with pain can facilitate the diagnosis during pain complaint assessment.

TABLE 17–1. CLINICAL ASSESSMENT OF PAIN

1. Believe the patient's complaint of pain.
2. Take a careful history of the pain complaint to place it temporally in the patient's history.
3. Assess the characteristics of each pain, including site, referral pattern, and aggravating and relieving factors.
4. Clarify the temporal aspects of the pain: acute, subacute, chronic, episodic, intermittent, breakthrough, or incident.
5. List and prioritize each pain complaint.
6. Evaluate the response to previous and current analgesic therapies.
7. Evaluate the psychological state of the patient.
8. Ask if the patient has a past history of alcohol or drug dependence.
9. Perform a careful medical and neurologic examination.
10. Develop a series of diagnosis-related hypotheses.
11. Order and personally review the appropriate diagnostic procedures.
12. Design the diagnostic and therapeutic approach to suit the individual.
13. Provide continuity of care from evaluation to treatment to ensure patient compliance and to reduce patient anxiety.
14. Reassess the patient's response to pain therapy.
15. Discuss advance directives for managing pain of dying patients.

Although it is crucial to know as much as possible about the individual patient with pain, such information may not be readily available in the first interview and, in some instances, may never be available because the patient lacks the intellectual competence to define clearly those various components. It is also necessary to verify the history from a family member who may provide information that the patient is unable or unwilling to provide; the family member may be more objective in assessing the disability of the patient who underreports his/her symptoms. Similarly, if a patient is a poor historian, a family member may provide essential information that may alter the diagnostic approach. In short, all attempts should be made to compile a careful history and to define the medical, neurologic, and psychological profile of the pain complaint.

In patients with advanced disease, it is crucial to request that they define what they would do if their pain is intractable or intolerable. Do they have suicidal thoughts or a pact with a family member because of the pain? Do they have a family history of suicide? Do they have drugs in reserve for such an event or a gun in the house that might be used if they feel desperate? Such questions may allow the patient to openly discuss his/her fears of pain. Such open discussions can allow the treating physician to better define for the patient the options for care and reassure the patient of his/her commitment to appropriate and adequate pain control. Patients rarely offer this information unless requested. Therefore, it is crucial that a repertoire of specific questions be developed that can be integrated into the initial history taking.

No patient should be evaluated inadequately because of a significant pain problem. Early management of the pain while investigating the source markedly improves the patient's ability to participate in the necessary diagnostic procedures. During the initial evaluation of the pain complaint, alternative methods of pain control including anesthetic and neurosurgical approaches should be considered, e.g., the temporary use of local anesthetics via an epidural catheter to manage pain from a vertebral body collapse or intravenous opioids to control acute severe abdominal pain. These approaches should not be considered only when all else fails but should be an integral part of the assessment. Continual reassessment of the response provides the best method to validate the initial diagnosis. However, in those patients in whom the effect of therapy is less than predicted or in whom the pain is exacerbated, reassessment of the treatment approach or a search for a new cause of the pain should be considered. In developing the diagnostic and therapeutic approach to suit the individual, careful judgment should be used in choosing diagnostic approaches that directly affect the choice of the therapeutic strategy or answer a specific question. The random use of diagnostic procedures in patients with pain is inappropriate and may have an adverse effect on their quality of life. This applies most commonly to patients with advanced cancer, in whom painful diagnostic procedures are inappropriate because they simply confirm the existence of disease for which treatment is unavailable or inappropriate. Lastly, in developing a strategy for managing pain in patients with advanced cancer or other untreatable medical diseases, it is important for the physician to know the patient's decisions about resuscitation, living wills, and symptom management if he/she becomes incompetent. These discussions improve the physician's ability to care for the pain patient with advanced disease appropriately and humanely.

MANAGEMENT OF PAIN

Recent advances in pain research provide the scientific rationale for using new, improved methods of treatment, including better and more effective use of standard drug therapy (nonopioid, opioid, and adjuvant analgesic drugs), the development of new drugs, the use of novel methods and routes of drug administration, and the use of selective anesthetic and neurosurgical approaches to control pain. The Agency for Health Care Policy and Research has published guidelines for management of acute traumatic and postoperative pain and cancer pain. These documents establish standards of care for using analgesic, anesthetic, and neurosurgical approaches for these populations of patients and have accompanying patient information booklets.

DRUG THERAPY. Analgesic drugs can be divided into three groups: group I: the nonopioid analgesics, such as aspirin and acetaminophen and the nonsteroidal anti-inflammatory drugs (NSAID's), act both peripherally and in some instances centrally, through inhibition of various enzyme systems, e.g., cyclo-oxygenase; group II: the opioid agonist and antagonist drugs, which activate opioid receptors in the central and peripheral nervous system; and group III: the adjuvant analgesic drugs that produce analgesia in certain pain states, (e.g., amitriptyline in neuropathic pain) or potentiate the opioid analgesics.

These three groups represent the mainstay of drug therapy for patients with acute and chronic pain. Their effective use requires an understanding of their pharmacologic characteristics and appropriate selection of a particular drug individualized to the needs of the patient and the specific pain syndrome.

Nonopioid Analgesics. Aspirin, acetaminophen, and the NSAID's are the first-line agents for management of mild to moderate pain, and in patients with severe pain, these drugs potentiate the effects of opioid analgesics. Nonopioid analgesics have a ceiling effect and their long-term use is compromised by gastrointestinal and hematologic side effects. The choice and use of these drugs must be individualized, with the patient receiving maximal levels of one drug before another is tried. If pain control is ineffective or the nonopioid agents are poorly tolerated, opioid analgesics are indicated.

Opioid Analgesics. Drugs in this class vary in potency, efficacy, and adverse effects. They are classified as agonist or antagonist drugs depending upon their ability to bind to the opiate receptor and produce analgesia. The opioid agonist drugs, such as morphine, bind to specific opiate receptors, resulting in analgesia. These agents are commonly used for moderate to severe pain. The opioid antagonist drugs block the effect of morphine at its receptor. Included in this category is a group of drugs with analgesic properties referred to as the mixed agonist-antagonist drugs. These drugs are often used in acute postoperative pain but are of limited use in chronic pain management for several reasons: They produce psychotomimetic effects with increasing doses. Only pentazocine is available in oral form and only in combination with naloxone, aspirin, and acetaminophen; they precipitate withdrawal in opioid-dependent patients.

Effective use of opioid analgesics requires balancing the desirable effects of pain relief with the undesirable side effects of nausea, vomiting, mental clouding, sedation, tolerance, and physical dependence. These undesirable effects may impose a practical limit on the dose one can give a particular patient. Recent studies suggest that aggressive treatment of opioid-induced side effects can facilitate dose titration, maximize analgesia, and minimize these effects. Much of the difficulty encountered with the clinical use of opioids arises from individual variation, consisting of differences in response of specific patients to the same drug or dose.

Table 17-2 lists a series of guidelines for the rational use of analgesics in patients with acute and chronic pain. Individualization of drug treatment is the cardinal rule of management. Both the type of pain and its intensity should dictate the drug selection, allowing the physician to start with a specific drug for a specific type of pain. To ensure adequate dosing schedules, one must know the clinical pharmacology of the opioid analgesics, including the relative potency of the drug, the duration of analgesic effect, its half-life, and the equianalgesic dose for both oral and parenteral routes of administration (Tables 17-3 and 17-4). For example, the plasma half-lives of the opioids vary widely and do not correlate with their analgesic time course. Both methadone with a half-life of 15 to 30 hours and levorphanol with a half-life of 12 to 16 hours produce analgesia for 4 to 6 hours. With repeated doses, these drugs accumulate in plasma and can result in excessive sedation and respiratory depression. It is often necessary to adjust the dosing schedule considering both the patient's degree of pain relief and the plasma half-life of the drug. Knowledge of the equianalgesic doses when a switch is made from one route of administration to another prevents undermedication. Medication should be administered on a regular basis with the interval between doses based on the duration of analgesic effect. The pharmacologic objective is to maintain the plasma level of the drug above the "minimal effective concentration" for pain relief. The time required to reach steady-state after repeated administration depends upon the half-life of the drug; full assessment of the analgesic efficacy of a drug regimen may take 24 hours for a drug such as morphine, or up to 5 to 7 days for methadone.

Combining drugs enables the physician to improve pain relief without escalating the opioid dose. Several combinations have

TABLE 17-2. GUIDELINES FOR THE USE OF ANALGESICS IN THE MANAGEMENT OF PAIN

1. Start with a specific drug for a specific type of pain.
2. Individualize the choice of drug, dose, timing, and route of administration.
3. Know the pharmacology of the drug prescribed.
   a. Relative potency of the drug
   b. Duration of the analgesic effect
   c. Pharmacokinetics of the drug
   d. Equianalgesic doses of the drug and its route of administration
4. Administer analgesics on a regular basis.
5. Use a combination of drugs to provide additive analgesia.
   a. Opioid plus nonopioid (e.g., aspirin, acetaminophen, and NSAID's)
   b. Opioids plus adjuvants (e.g., hydroxyzine and dextroamphetamine)
6. Gear the route of administration to the patient's needs:

Oral	Transdermal
Buccal	Subcutaneous
Sublingual	Intravenous
Transmucosal	Intrathecal
Intranasal	Intraventricular
Rectal	

7. Anticipate and treat side effects:

Sedation	Constipation
Respiratory depression	Multifocal myoclonus
Nausea and vomiting	Seizures

8. Know the difference between tolerance, physical dependence, and psychological dependence.
9. Prevent and treat acute withdrawal.
10. Know how to manage the tolerant patient:
    Use combinations of nonopioid and opioid drugs.
    Use combinations of drug therapy, anesthetic, and neurosurgical procedures.
    Switch to an alternative opioid analgesic starting with one fourth to one half the equianalgesic dose and titrate to analgesia.
    Use epidural local anesthetics alone or in combination with opioids.
11. Reassess the nature of the pain.
12. Do not use placebos to assess pain.

proven effective, including an opioid plus a nonopioid (aspirin, acetaminophen, or ibuprofen), an opioid plus an amphetamine (dextroamphetamine, 10 mg), and an opioid plus an antihistamine (100 mg of IM hydroxyzine). Drugs such as diazepam and chlorpromazine do not provide additive analgesia and may produce additive sedation. Oral administration of drugs is the most practical route, but the choice must be made according to the patient. Several routes or methods of drug administration have been developed to maximize analgesic effects and minimize the undesirable side effects associated with the standard methods. The approaches that are the most commonly used for managing acute or chronic pain with chronic medical illness include slow-release morphine preparations effective for 8 to 12 hours; rectal, intranasal, sublingual, and transdermal and continuous subcutaneous and intravenous infusions for patients who are unable to tolerate oral analgesics because of gastrointestinal obstruction or malabsorption and in whom repeated

parenteral dosing is difficult because of limited muscle mass or a bleeding diathesis; and epidural and intrathecal opioid administration via temporary catheters or implanted pumps. This last approach minimizes the distribution of drug to receptors in the brain stem and cerebral hemispheres, reduces the side effects of systemic administration, and is effective in selected patients with chronic cancer and nonmalignant pain who are unable to tolerate the excessive sedation or mental clouding associated with an oral or parenteral route.

Patient-controlled analgesia (PCA) is a useful approach to treat both acute pain associated with medical illness (postoperative pain, sickle cell pain) and chronic cancer-related pain. Parenteral infusions (intravenous or subcutaneous) of opioids can be self-administered by the patient using specially designed computerized pumps that can be set to deliver specific amounts of drug on demand or by continuous infusion. These devices allow patients to control their own pain management. Studies demonstrate that patients using PCA use less medication than patients who receive PRN medications for postoperative or chronic pain.

Side effects of the opioid analgesics should be anticipated and treated. Sedation and drowsiness vary with the drug, the dosage, and the route of administration. Reducing the individual dose and prescribing it more frequently; using dextroamphetamine (2.5 to 10 mg) or methylphenidate (5 to 15 mg) in combination with the morning opioid dose; switching to a different opioid—from morphine to hydromorphone or methadone; and discontinuing all other sedative drugs are useful approaches to counteract the sedative effects.

Respiratory depression is the most serious adverse effect, but tolerance develops rapidly, allowing for prolonged use and dose escalation for chronic pain. If respiratory depression occurs, it can be reversed by administering the specific opioid antagonist, naloxone, in a dose of 0.4 mg per milliliter. In patients receiving chronic opioids for pain who develop respiratory depression, diluted doses of naloxone (0.4 mg in 10 ml of saline) should be infused slowly to reverse the respiratory depression and to prevent severe withdrawal symptoms and recurrence of pain.

Opioids have emetic properties. The occurrence of nausea and vomiting with one drug does not mean that all produce similar symptoms. Changing to a different opioid or using an antiemetic in combination can obviate this effect. Tolerance rapidly develops to the emetic effects of opioids so that after several days antiemetics can often be discontinued. Constipation should be prevented by providing a regular bowel regimen including cathartics, stool softeners, and careful attention to diet. Opioids can produce multifocal myoclonus. The most common offender is meperidine because its active metabolite, normeperidine, accumulates, which can cause seizures. Because the half-life of the normeperidine is 16 hours, it may take several days for toxic side effects to clear. Multifocal myoclonus occurs more commonly in patients with renal dysfunction receiving the meperidine. Such patients should be switched to alter-

TABLE 17-3. ORAL NONOPIOID ANALGESIC DRUGS

Drug	Indications	Equianalgesic Dose	Starting Dose (mg/24 hr)	Comments
Aspirin	Often used in combination with opioids	650	650	Contraindicated in hepatic and renal dysfunction; avoid during pregnancy, in hemolytic disorders, and in combination with steroids
Choline magnesium trisalicylate	Like aspirin	ND	750–1500	Minimal impact on platelet function
Acetaminophen	Like aspirin	650	650	
Ibuprofen	Higher analgesic potential than aspirin	ND	200–400	Like aspirin
Fenoprofen	Like ibuprofen	ND	200–400	Like aspirin
Diflunisal	Longer duration of action than ibuprofen; higher analgesic potential than aspirin	ND	500–1000	Like aspirin
Naproxen	Like diflunisal	ND	250–1500	Like aspirin

ND = Analgesic relative potency studies are not available to determine equianalgesic dose to aspirin.

TABLE 17-4. OPIOID ANALGESIC DRUGS

Class	Drug	Indications	Equianalgesic Dose* for Mild to Moderate Pain (ORAL)	Starting Dose (mg/24 hr)	Comments
Morphine-like agonist, mild to moderate pain	Codeine	Often used in combination with nonopioid analgesics	32–65	32–65	Commonly used as first drug
	Oxycodone	Shorter acting; combination with nonopioid analgesics limits dose escalation	5	5–10	Fewer side effects than codeine, available alone or in combination with aspirin and acetaminophen
	Meperidine	Shorter acting; biotransformed to normeperidine, a toxic metabolite	50	50–100	Normeperidine accumulates with repetitive dosing, causing CNS excitation; not for use in patients with renal dysfunction or receiving monoamine oxidase inhibitors
	Propoxyphene hydrochloride (Darvon)	Used in combination with nonopioid analgesics; long half-life; biotransformed to potentially toxic metabolite (norpropoxyphene)	65–130	65–130	Propoxyphene and metabolite accumulate with repetitive dosing; overdose complicated by convulsions
Mixed agonist/antagonist	Pentazocine	Used in combination with nonopioids	50	50–100	May cause psychotomimetic effects; may precipitate withdrawal in opioid-dependent patients. Oral combination with naloxone to discourage parenteral abuse
	Butorphanol; (Stadol)	Used in combination with nonopioids	2	2–4	May cause psychotomimetic effects; may precipitate withdrawal in opioid-dependent patients; only available in intranasal and intramuscular preparations

Class	Drug	Indications	Equianalgesic Dose IM/PO†	Starting Dose (mg/24 hr) (ORAL)	Comments
Morphine-like agonists, moderate to severe pain	Morphine MSIR MS Contin Roxanol	Used for chronic pain, available in oral liquid, tablets, slow-release preparations, and rectal and parenteral routes	10–60	30–60	Standard of comparison for opioid-type analgesics; morphine-6-glucuronide, active metabolite, accumulates in renal failure
	Hydromorphone (Dilaudid)	Like morphine	1.5–8.0	4–8	Slightly shorter acting, high-potency IM dosage form available for tolerant patients
	Methadone (Dolphine)	Like morphine; may accumulate with repetitive dosing, causing excessive sedation	10–20	10–20	Good oral potency; long plasma half-life (15–30 hrs)
	Levorphanol (Levo-Dromoran)	Like methadone	2–4	2–4	Long plasma half-life (12–16 hrs)
	Fentanyl (Duragesic)	Like morphine, but available in a transdermal preparation applied every 3 days	NA	25–100 µg TD	Useful in patients who are unable to take drugs orally and require continuous opioid dosing
	Oxycodone	Like morphine	15/30	5–10	Available in immediate-release and slow-release tablets
	Oxymorphone	Like morphine, less histamine effect	1/10 PR	10 PR	Rectal and parenteral preparations only

* Equianalgesic doses for mild to moderate pain compared to 650 mg aspirin.
† Equianalgesic doses by IM/oral routes for severe pain compared to 10 mg IM morphine standard.
IM = Intramuscular; CNS = central nervous system; PR = per rectum; TD = transdermal.

native drugs such as fentanyl or methadone, which are not predominantly cleared by the kidney. Morphine has an active metabolite that accumulates in renal dysfunction and has been reported to play a role in its side effects. To prevent withdrawal, patients should be slowly tapered off their opioids. However, 25% of the total daily opioid dose prevents the development of abstinence symptoms. Tolerance is common in patients receiving opioid analgesics chronically for pain. The earliest sign is the decrease in the duration of effective analgesia. For reasons not well understood, the rate of tolerance development varies greatly among patients with pain. In-

creased opioid requirements are most commonly associated with disease progression rather than tolerance alone. With the development of tolerance, increases in the frequency or the dose of the opioid are required to provide continued pain relief. Because the analgesic effect is a logarithmic function of the dose of the opioid, doubling of the dose may be needed to restore full analgesia. There appears to be no limit to the development of tolerance and with appropriate dose adjustments, patients can continue to obtain pain relief. Cross-tolerance among the opioid analgesics is not complete; therefore, changing to an alternative opioid at a starting dose of one fourth to one half of the predicted equianalgesic dose may be advantageous. Tolerance is distinct from physical dependence, which is characterized by the appearance of withdrawal signs after drugs are abruptly withdrawn, and from psychological dependence, which is characterized by a concomitant behavioral pattern of drug abuse characterized by craving a drug for other than pain relief and overwhelming involvement in its procurement and use. The profound fear of causing psychological dependence plays a major role in physician's reluctance to prescribe opioid analgesics, particularly in patients with nonmalignant pain and in patients with cancer in the early phases of their disease. From the available data based on studies on the chronic use of opioids in patients with cancer, few patients develop psychological dependence on the drug. This issue is controversial in management of patients with chronic nonmalignant pain, but data indicate that such patients can be treated effectively with chronic opioid therapy. Guidelines for the use of chronic opioid therapy in nonmalignant pain have been developed (Table 17–5).

Adjuvant Analgesics. This group increases the analgesic effects of the opioids, counteract their side effects, or act as analgesics themselves. Clear evidence suggests the analgesic efficacy of

TABLE 17–5. GUIDELINES FOR MANAGING CHRONIC OPIOID THERAPY FOR NONMALIGNANT PAIN

1. Opioid therapy should be considered only after all other reasonable attempts at analgesia have failed.
2. A history of substance abuse, severe character pathology, and chaotic home environment should be viewed as relative contraindications.
3. A single practitioner should take primary responsibility for treatment.
4. Patients should give informed consent before the start of therapy; points to be covered include recognition of the low risk of true addiction as an outcome, potential for cognitive impairment with the drug alone and in combination with sedative/hypnotics, likelihood that physical dependence will occur (abstinence syndrome possible with acute discontinuation), and understanding by female patients that children born when the mother is on opioid maintenance therapy will likely be physically dependent at birth.
5. After drug selection, doses should be given around the clock; several weeks should be agreed upon as the period of initial dose titration; and although improvement in function should be continually stressed, all should agree to at least partial analgesia as the appropriate goal of therapy.
6. Failure to achieve at least partial analgesia at relatively low initial doses in the nontolerant patient raises questions about the potential treatability of the pain syndrome with opioids.
7. Emphasis should be given to attempts to capitalize on improved analgesia by gains in physical and social function; opioid therapy should be considered complementary to other analgesic and rehabilitative approaches.
8. In addition to the daily dose determined initially, patients should be permitted to escalate dose transiently on days of increased pain; two methods are acceptable: (a) prescription of an additional 4 to 6 "rescue doses" to be taken as needed during the month; (b) instruction that one or two extra doses may be taken on any day but must be followed by an equal reduction of dose on subsequent days.
9. Initially, patients must be seen and drugs prescribed at least monthly. When stable, less frequent visits may be acceptable.
10. Exacerbations of pain not effectively treated by transient, small increases in dose are best managed in the hospital, where dose escalation, if appropriate, can be observed closely and return to baseline doses can be accomplished in a controlled environment.
11. Evidence of drug hoarding, acquisition of drugs from other physicians, uncontrolled dose escalation, or other aberrant behaviors must be carefully assessed. In some cases, tapering and discontinuing opioid therapy are necessary. Other patients may appropriately continue therapy within rigid guidelines. Consideration should be given to consulting with an addiction specialist.
12. At each visit, assessment should specifically address:
    a. Comfort (degree of analgesia)
    b. Opioid-related side effects
    c. Functional status (physical and psychosocial)
    d. Existence of aberrant drug-related behaviors
13. Use of self-report instruments may be helpful but should not be required.
14. Documentation is essential and the medical record should specifically address comfort, function, side effects, and the occurrence of aberrant behaviors repeatedly during the course of therapy.

From Portenoy RK: Opioid therapy for chronic nonmalignant pain: Current status. In Fields HL, Liebeskind JC (eds.): Progress in Pain Research and Management, Vol 1. Seattle, IASP Press, 1994, p 247.

carbamazepine, baclofen, and pimozide in trigeminal neuralgia and of the tricyclic antidepressants in neuropathic pain. Similarly, several psychostimulants are effective in counteracting opioid-induced sedation (dextroamphetamine and methylphenidate) and in improving analgesia (dextroamphetamine and caffeine). For the other drugs in this group anecdotal or survey data suggest their usefulness in various types of neuropathic pain (Table 17–6), and the physician must consider the risks and benefits of polypharmacy when trying to provide analgesia for patients with difficult and complex pain syndromes. Certain phenothiazines also have potent analgesic effects. Methotrimeprazine (levoprome) has an analgesic potential close to that of morphine (15 mg IM is equivalent to 10 mg IM morphine). This drug is useful for severe pain in patients tolerant to opioid analgesics. It also has sedative and antiemetic properties. In treating neuropathic pain, the tricyclic antidepressants are efficacious. For lancinating neuropathic pains, not only carbamazepine and phenytoin but valproate and clonazepam have been reported to be effective. Mexiletine, an oral local anesthetic, demonstrates analgesic properties in patients with painful diabetic neuropathy. Corticosteroids have been reported to be useful as general purpose adjuvant analgesics. They ameliorate pain in patients with bone metastases and produce beneficial effects on appetite, nausea, mood, and fatigue. They have most commonly been used in patients with breast or prostate cancer to improve quality of life.

Specific adjuvants used in managing cancer pain have specialized effects, e.g., diphosphonates in malignant bone pain. The physician should become familiar with this class of compounds and consider their use in sequential trials to improve patients' quality of life and functional status.

ALTERNATE METHODS OF PAIN CONTROL. A variety of nonpharmacologic therapeutic approaches can be used alone or in combination with analgesic drugs. These include physical therapy, trigger point injections, transcutaneous nerve stimulation, and a variety of behavioral approaches—all of which should be familiar to general physicians. Pain experts should be consulted before using anesthetic and neurosurgical approaches.

Physical Therapy. Chronic pain is commonly associated with reduced physical activity and splinting or immobilization of the injured body part. A graded exercise program with appropriate use of splints and braces and reactivation of the injured part plays a pivotal role in re-establishing the functional status of the patient. Local rubbing and transcutaneous electrical stimulation for "counterirritation" may help to mobilize the patient with localized pain. Trigger point injections with either saline or a local anesthetic provide dramatic relief of painful muscle spasm.

Cognitive Behavioral Therapy. Cognitive behavioral interventions can help reduce the perception of distress caused by the pain through coping skills and modification of thoughts, feelings, and behaviors. Some patients may be able to use relaxation techniques to reduce muscular tension and emotional arousal or enhance pain tolerance. Other approaches, including meditation, imagery, music therapy, and biofeedback can reduce participatory anxiety that may lead to avoidance behaviors. Successful use of these therapies requires a cognitively intact patient and a health care professional skilled in their application.

Anesthetic and Neurosurgical Approaches. These approaches are most effective in treating patients with well-defined pain. Several factors are important in selecting an appropriate procedure for each patient. The role of these approaches is limited because diffuse pain problems rather than focal ones are the most common. Their use is limited by the number of professionals who have expertise in the performance of these procedures. Many of these procedures are most useful in patients with a limited lifespan, yet such patients often consider their pain to be an important marker for their disease and are frightened by the potential, although unlikely complications of these procedures. As a result, these procedures are often performed late in the course of the illness, and full evaluation of their effectiveness and duration of action is limited by the patient's overriding medical problems. These procedures are often not very effective in managing neuropathic pain, except for the use of local anesthetics. They are most helpful in managing somatic and visceral pain. These approaches include using nitrous oxide for patients with far-advanced disease to provide additive analgesia. Nitrous oxide is administered with oxygen through a nonrebreathing facemask in concentrations from 25 to

TABLE 17–6. ADJUVANT ANALGESIC DRUGS

Class	Drug	Indications	Starting Dose (mg) Range/24 hr	Comments
Anticonvulsants	Phenytoin	Neuropathic pain, acute lancinating type	100, 100–300	Use in paroxysmal nerve pain
	Carbamazepine	Acute lancinating type	100, 200–300	Use in paroxysmal nerve pain Start with low doses; titrate slowly
	Valproate	Neuropathic pain Acute lancinating type	125, 1000–3000	Anecdotal reports of efficacy in neuropathic pain
	Felbamate	Neuropathic pain Acute lancinating pain	300, 300–1200	Anecdotal reports of efficacy in neuropathic pain
Antidepressants	Amitriptyline, nortriptyline, desipramine, paroxetine*	Neuropathic pain, e.g., postherpetic neuralgia	10, 25–>150 10–>40*	Start at low dose and titrate slowly; have analgesic properties
Stimulants	Dextroamphetamine Methylphenidate Caffeine	Somatic and visceral postoperative pain and chronic pain Counteracts opioid-induced sedation	2.5 (5–10) 5 (5–15) 200 (200–400)	Additive analgesia in combination with opioids; reduces sedative effects
Antihistamines	Hydroxyzine	Somatic and visceral pain	25, 25–100	Additive analgesia in combination with opioids; antiemetic, antianxiety properties
Phenothiazine	Methotrimeprazine	Somatic and visceral pain; useful in opioid-tolerant patients with GI obstruction and pain	5 IM 5–20 IM	Has antianxiety and antiemetic effects; available only in IM preparation
Steroids	Prednisone	Somatic and neuropathic pain, e.g., inflammatory pain, reflex sympathetic dystrophy	5, 5–60	Anti-inflammatory, antiemetic, analgesic effects
	Dexamethasone	Somatic and neuropathic pain, e.g., inflammatory pain, reflex sympathetic dystrophy	0.5, 0.5–16	
Miscellaneous	Baclofen	Paroxysmal pain of trigeminal neuralgia and central pain states	10, 10–80	May be used with carbamazepine in trigeminal neuralgia
	Pimozide	Refractory trigeminal neuralgia	2, 4–12	Adverse effects include acute dystonia and akathesias
	Mexiletine	Neuropathic pain; useful in diabetic neuropathy	150, 150–600	Dose-response studies have not been done

*Refers to dose range for paroxetine.

75%. It has been demonstrated to be useful when combined with systemic opioid analgesics to control pain and anxiety in patients with advanced disease and pain. Similarly, intravenous barbiturates to manage dying patients who have inadequate analgesia or uncontrollable symptoms and who request that they be maintained in a sedated state represents another type of anesthetic approach.

A series of anecdotal reports and controlled studies support the use of intravenous, subcutaneous, transdermal, intrapleural, and epidural local anesthetics in managing patients with somatic, visceral, and neuropathic pain. Intravenous lidocaine represents both a diagnostic and a therapeutic treatment in patients with neuropathic pain. If such patients obtain an analgesic response, a trial of oral mexiletine or the use of continuous subcutaneous lidocaine may be considered. Transdermal lidocaine in a 2%, 5%, and 10% ointment has been reported to be useful in patients with superficial hyperesthesia, dysesthesias, and significant allodynia. Spreading the ointment on the painful site can often provide transient pain relief. This effect has been best demonstrated in patients with postherpetic neuralgia. Intrapleural local anesthetics are useful for acute pain in the chest wall and have been adapted for managing chronic cancer pain. Epidural local anesthetics are used to manage patients with localized pain syndromes, usually below the waist. Intermittent and continuous epidural infusions of local anesthetics are useful to manage difficult chronic pain associated with metastatic disease below the waist, often involving the sacrum and lumbosacral plexus. The use of continuous low-dose infusions of local anesthetics is associated with minimal systemic side effects.

Peripheral nerve blocks are used both diagnostically to localize the nerve distribution and therapeutically to interrupt pain transmission within a determined nerve distribution. This technique is limited to areas of the body in which interruption of both motor and sensory function does not interfere with the patient's functional status. This approach, therefore, is most commonly used in patients who have pain in the head, chest, or abdomen. These techniques are most useful in patients with somatic pain; neuropathic pain is rarely controlled by peripheral nerve blocks alone. Examples of successful blocks include gasserian ganglion blocks for craniofacial pain, intercostal blocks for chest wall pain, and paravertebral blocks for radicular pain. In patients with somatic pain who respond to a local anesthetic block, neurolytic blockade with either alcohol or phenol may provide more prolonged relief. A block produced by phenol tends to be less profound and of shorter duration than that produced by alcohol. Epidural and intrathecal neurolytic blocks are used primarily to manage patients with far-advanced disease whose pain is either unilateral in the chest or abdomen or midline in the perineum. These blocks are less useful in managing upper and lower limb pain associated with brachial and lumbosacral plexopathy because of the high risk of motor weakness associated with effective neurolytic blockade by this route. Patients should be selected for management with epidural or intrathecal agents on the basis of the following criteria: exhaustion of appropriate antitumor approaches; clear clinical and radiologic definition of the pain; poor candidacy for percutaneous cordotomy; failure of opioid, nonopioid, and adjuvants to produce adequate analgesia without significant side effects; and a favorable response to diagnostic epidural or intrathecal blocks, producing at least 75% pain relief.

The neurosurgical approaches include neuroablative, neurostimulatory, and neuropharmacologic approaches. Neuroablative procedures involve producing a surgical or radiofrequency lesion along the nociceptive neural pathway. Sectioning the posterior roots (rhizotomy), producing a lesion in the lateral dorsal horn (dorsal root entry zone lesion), and interrupting the ascending spinothalamic pathway (cordotomy) are examples of neuroablative procedures performed for pain relief. Cordotomy, either percutaneous or open, is the most common neuroablative procedure used to manage chronic pain, most commonly associated with cancer. It is the procedure of choice for patients with unilateral pain below the waist who have a relatively short life expectancy. Cordotomy is usually effective for 1 to 3 years with dysesthesias substituting for analgesia in patients living longer than 3 years. Pain in the chest wall or upper extremity may be successfully treated initially with cordotomy, but extensive data demonstrate that with time, the level of analgesia drops, limiting the effectiveness of this approach. Somatic pain appears to be most responsive to cordotomy; visceral and neuropathic pain are less responsive for reasons that are not fully understood. Percutaneous cordotomy can be performed in a supine, awake patient through a lateral C1-C2 approach. Such a lesion interrupts pain and temperature on the contralateral side of the lesioned site. Patients typically report spontaneously relief of pain in this lesioned area. Pain relief can be obtained in 60 to 80% of patients immediately after cordotomy; results at 6 to 12 months are 40 to 50%. Dorsal rhizotomy is the next most common neuroablative procedure used and is performed by sectioning the posterior sensory rootlets, and a specific localized dermatomal pain level can be identified. It can be performed by an operative section of the nerve or by a neurolytic block. This procedure is commonly used in patients with chest wall pain from tumor invasion and results in improved analgesia in 50 to 80% of patients treated.

Other neuroablative procedures are rarely used to manage patients with chronic pain, such as dorsal root entry zone lesions, myelotomy, and cingulotomy. Neurostimulatory procedures involving the peripheral nerve and spinal cord are generally based on the gate therapy of pain. Various percutaneous electrical nerve stimulators are available to treat chronic neuropathic pain. These devices deliver various patterns of electrical stimulation and take the form of either transcutaneous electrical nerve stimulation (TENS) or implanted devices producing nerve stimulation. Controversy exists about the usefulness of these techniques. The dorsal column—stimulating technique involves introducing an electrode into the epidural or intrathecal space and advancing it to the appropriate level overlying the dorsal columns. Once in place, the electrode is implanted subcutaneously, and an external transmitting electrode is placed over the receiving electrode and connected to a transmitter. The main indications for placing a dorsal column stimulator are intractable dysesthetic or deafferentation pain of the limbs or trunk. This procedure is effective in 43 to 75% of patients and carries a low morbidity rate. Its most common complication is failure of the device itself, which occurs in up to 10% of patients. Placing stimulating electrodes in the medial thalamus has also been reported to be useful for managing neuropathic pain from injury to the central and peripheral nervous systems. These anesthetic and neurosurgical approaches are most commonly performed by a pain expert in referral centers. They should be reserved for patients who have failed other pain management approaches and to whom the risks and benefits have been carefully explained.

MANAGEMENT OF CANCER PAIN

Figure 17–1 provides an algorithm for the management of cancer pain. It attempts to integrate assessment techniques, drug therapy, and anesthetic, neurosurgical, and behavioral approaches and stresses continuity of care. Treatment of cancer pain must begin with a careful diagnostic assessment that addresses not only the medical nature of pain, but also its psychological and social compo-

nents. At the time of assessment, a plan is developed to treat both the cancer, if possible, and the pain itself. If the anticancer treatment is effective, pain relief usually occurs, and the drugs used for analgesia can be discontinued without difficulty. Pain relief begins with analgesic drugs. Incorporated in Figure 17–1 is the World Health Organization's Cancer Pain Relief Program's three-step ladder. It proposes an analgesic drug ladder moving from nonopioid drugs alone or in combination with adjuvant drugs, through weak opioids to strong opioids. If pain relief is achieved with this program, no further therapy is necessary. In patients with severe, persistent pain unresponsive to analgesic drugs or in whom the side effects of the drugs are not tolerated, physicians should first try switching to an alternate analgesic. If the pain is unresponsive to analgesic drugs and is localized (e.g., intercostal pain from tumor infiltration of the chest wall), neurolytic blocks are indicated. If the pain is unilateral and below the waist, cordotomy should be considered. For more diffuse pain unresponsive to analgesics, neuropharmacologic procedures, including nitrous oxide inhalation, may be considered. Behavioral approaches, which include relaxation techniques, breathing exercises, and cognitive control of pain, serve as adjuvants and should be integrated into the management of patients with chronic pain.

As the algorithm indicates, whatever the techniques of pain management used in patients with cancer, the physician is responsible for delivering continuing care, constantly reassessing both the diagnosis and the treatment to achieve optimal relief of pain and suffering for both the patient and the family.

Acute Pain Management Guideline Panel: Acute Pain Management: Operative or Medical Procedures and Trauma. Clinical Practice Guideline. AHCPR Pub. No. 92-0032. Rockville, MD, Agency for Health Care Policy and Research, Public Health Service, US Department of Health and Human Services, February, 1992. *This monograph is a practical summary with recommendations for state-of-the-art acute pain treatment.*

Bonica JJ (ed.): The Management of Pain. 2nd ed. Philadelphia, Lea & Febiger, 1989. *An excellent compendium of pain pathophysiology for physicians.*

Foley KM: Supportive care and the quality of life of the cancer patient. *In* DeVita VT, Hellman S, Rosenberg SA (eds.): Cancer: Principles and Practice of Oncology. 4th ed. Philadelphia, JB Lippincott, 1993, p 2417. *This chapter provides a comprehensive review of the treatment of cancer pain.*

Jacox A, Carr DB, Payne R, et al.: Management of Cancer Pain. Clinical Practice Guideline No. 9. AHCPR Publication No. 94-0592. Rockville, MD, Agency for Health Care Policy and Research, US Department of Health and Human Services, Public Health Service, March, 1994. *This monograph provides a concise summary of the appropriate treatment of cancer pain.*

Portenoy RK: Opioid therapy for chronic nonmalignant pain: Current status. *In* Fields HL, Liebeskind JC (eds.): Progress in Pain Research and Management, Vol 1. Seattle, IASP Press, 1994, p 247. *An up-to-date review of the controversies and facts of drug therapy in patients with chronic pain.*

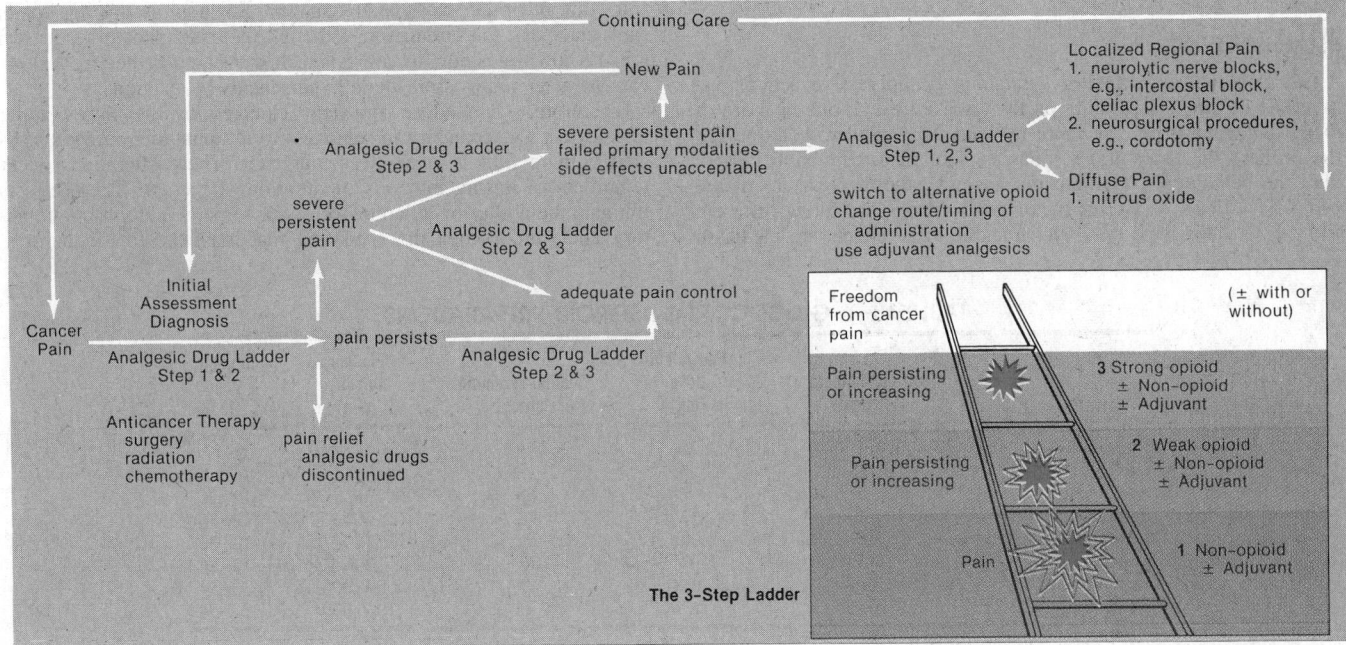

FIGURE 17–1. Algorithm for the management of cancer pain.

18 GLUCOCORTICOSTEROIDS IN RELATION TO INFLAMMATORY DISEASE

Paul Katz

For more than 50 years, glucocorticosteroids (GC) have been extremely important agents in treating diseases characterized by inflammation and exaggerated immune responses. The pioneering work of Hench and colleagues in rheumatoid arthritis demonstrated the possible potency of these agents in such pathologic states. Although substantial advances have been made in our understanding of the mechanisms by which GC exert beneficial effects, considerable gaps in our knowledge remain. Despite extensive data regarding the *in vitro* and *in vivo* activities of these drugs, it is probable that GC have different beneficial activities in different diseases. Furthermore, early studies did not recognize that the high concentrations of GC used *in vitro* were unattainable *in vivo* and that animal species differed from humans in responses to these drugs.

The potent anti-inflammatory and immunosuppressive actions of GC must be viewed in the context of the often substantial complications that accompany their use. The challenge of GC therapy continues to be the counterbalancing of desirable versus undesirable pharmacologic activities. Regrettably, our more precise understanding of the mechanisms of action of GC has not resulted in the development of regimens with minimal toxicity.

PHARMACOLOGY

A variety of GC preparations are available for systemic use (Table 18–1). These preparations differ in their relative anti-inflammatory potency, potential for sodium retention, and plasma and biologic half-lives. The biologic half-life of a compound is particularly important in selecting a GC. In general, shorter-acting preparations such as prednisone and prednisolone are preferable to longer-acting GC such as dexamethasone because tapering to an alternate-day schedule cannot be accomplished with drugs with prolonged (i.e., > 24 hour) biologic half-lives. Additionally, hydrocortisone and cortisone are rarely used to treat inflammatory and immunologically mediated diseases because of the considerable mineralocorticoid activity that accompanies their use.

MECHANISMS OF ACTION

GC exert anti-inflammatory and immunosuppressive actions via several pathways. Depending on the disease treated, one or more of these mechanisms may be more relevant than another. Additionally, the primary mechanism(s) responsible for efficacy probably differs with the pathologic condition. For example, the mechanisms of the beneficial effects of GC in rheumatoid arthritis are likely different from the actions in asthma. Nonetheless, these effects are mediated by (1) changes in leukocyte circulatory kinetics, (2) alterations in the function of inflammatory cells, and (3) modification of soluble mediators (summarized in Table 18–2).

Regardless of which of the above mechanisms is examined, the initial subcellular events appear to be similar. These actions are initiated by GC binding to cytoplasmic receptors. GC receptors are comparable among different leukocytes. The 800-amino acid receptor consists of three domains that differ in function: a hormone or ligand-binding carboxyl terminal region, a DNA-binding domain, and an amino terminal immunogenic area. GC receptors have been found in all leukocytes, with some heterogeneity within functional and phenotypic subsets of a given cell type. Following GC-receptor interaction, the complex traverses nuclear pores and binds to DNA at specific sites, which leads to changes in the transcription rates of GC-sensitive genes. This results in regulation of the synthesis of those proteins participating in the inflammatory response.

EFFECTS ON LEUKOCYTE CIRCULATORY KINETICS. GC have profound but transient effects on leukocyte trafficking, which differ depending on cell type. Irrespective of white cell type and regardless of duration of therapy or dosing interval, these effects are maximal at 4 to 6 hours after administering GC. In part, these effects derive from GC acting on vascular endothelial cells, which include alterations in adhesion molecule expression, changes in cytokine secretion, and decreased expression of major histocompatibility complex (MHC) class II antigens (see Ch. 229).

A significant neutrophilia is observed 4 to 6 hours after GC secondary to an increase in intravascular half-life, increased bone marrow release, and decreased egress from the circulation to extravascular sites of inflammation. By 24 hours after drug dosing, the neutrophilia has resolved. Therefore, although GC induce a transient increase in circulating neutrophils, these cells have a decreased ability to migrate to extravascular sites. In inflammatory diseases characterized by neutrophil-induced damage, this impairment is beneficial; however, poor migration to microbial foci is similarly reduced, increasing the likelihood of infection (see Complications, below).

Neutrophilia (see Ch. 140.2) is accompanied by lymphopenia secondary to the temporary migration of selected lymphocytes to bone marrow and spleen. Heterogeneity of lymphocyte trafficking is noted, depending on cell type. In this regard, a significant T lymphocytopenia occurs with a selective egress from the circulation of CD4+ "helper/inducer" T cells, whereas CD8+ "cytotoxic/suppressor" T cells are relatively resistant to these effects (see Ch. 221).

B lymphocytes are less susceptible to GC-induced effects than T cells, with little alteration in intravascular number or composition. Natural killer cells, identified by CD16 expression, are similarly resistant to GC. Monocytes, however, migrate to extravascular locales, assumed to be the same as lymphocytes, within the time frame of other GC-associated changes. Eosinophils and basophils transiently exit the circulation, although the exact sites of migration are unknown; eosinophils are noted, however, to be reduced at areas characterized by immediate hypersensitivity reactions.

Therefore, GC induce transient changes in the intravascular leukocyte pool secondary to relative and absolute alterations associated with migration to extravascular sites. These alterations occur regardless of dosing intervals or duration of therapy. These effects mitigate the ability of inflammatory cells to participate in inflammatory and immunologically mediated reactions, thereby inducing a

TABLE 18–1. GLUCOCORTICOSTEROID PREPARATIONS

	Anti-inflammatory Potency	Equivalent Dose (mg)	Sodium-retaining Potency	Plasma Half-life (min)	Biologic Half-life (hr)
Hydrocortisone	1	20	2 +	90	8–12
Cortisone	0.8	25	2 +	30	8–12
Prednisone	4	5	1 +	60	12–36
Prednisolone	4	5	1 +	200	12–36
Methylprednisolone	5	4	0	180	12–36
Triamcinolone	5	4	0	300	12–36
Betamethasone	20–30	0.6	0	100–300	36–54
Dexamethasone	20–30	0.75	0	100–300	36–54

From Garber EK, Targoff C, Paulus HE: *In* Paulus HE, Furst DE, Droomgoole SH (eds.): Drugs for Rheumatic Diseases. New York, Churchill Livingstone, 1987, p 446.

TABLE 18–2. EFFECT OF GLUCOCORTICOSTEROIDS ON INFLAMMATORY AND IMMUNE RESPONSES

Effects on leukocyte circulatory kinetics (transient and maximal 4 to 6 hours after administration)
1. Neutrophilia
2. Monocytopenia
3. Lymphocytopenia—selective depletion of CD4+ T cells
4. Eosinopenia
5. Basophilopenia

Effects on leukocyte function

1. Neutrophils	Little effect on chemotaxis, phagocytosis, and killing
2. Monocytes	Suppression of chemotaxis, cidal activity, and surface receptor expression
3. Eosinophils	Decreased chemotaxis and killing
4. T lymphocytes	Cutaneous anergy
	Suppression of activation, proliferation, and differentiation
	Reduced cytotoxic (CD8) responses
5. B lymphocytes	Reduction in serum immunoglobulins
	No effect on response to injected antigens
	Decreased activation and proliferation
6. Natural killer cells	No effect on cytotoxic activity

Effects on soluble mediators
1. Decreased production of prostaglandins, histamine, and leukotrienes
2. Decreased production of IL-1, IL-2, interferon-γ, and tumor necrosis factor-α
3. Little effect on complement
4. Decreased clearance of antigen-antibody complexes from circulation

favorable effect but also diminishing leukocyte participation in eliminating microbial invaders.

CHANGES IN LEUKOCYTE FUNCTION. Just as leukocytes vary in responsiveness to GC-induced circulatory changes, similar variability is observed in white cell intrinsic functional capabilities. Although neutrophils are quite sensitive to changes in trafficking after GC administration, these cells are relatively refractory to GC-associated changes in function. Thus, chemotaxis, lysosomal enzyme release, and killing are either resistant to GC effects or affected only with high doses. Conversely, cells of the monocyte/macrophage series are functionally sensitive to GC effects with reduced chemotaxis, cidal activity, and surface receptor expression such as class II antigens, Fc receptors, and the third component of complement (C3) receptors observed. Eosinophil chemotactic and cidal functions are reduced by GC.

A variety of lymphocyte functions, including activation, proliferation, and differentiation, are sensitive to GC. Although GC do not affect T-cell activation, downregulation of RNA synthesis decreases proliferation, which can be reversed *in vitro* with exogenous interleukin (IL)-2. Mitogen- and antigen-induced proliferative responses are reduced *in vitro;* the *in vivo* counterpart of these responses, cutaneous delayed-type hypersensitivity, is similarly impaired within 2 weeks of starting drug therapy. Similar effects on the mixed lymphocyte reaction are noted, which may in part explain the utility of GC in reversing allograft rejection. Cytotoxic T-cell (CD8+) responses are depressed by *in vivo* GC.

Unlike T cells, B-lymphocyte function is only modestly affected by GC. Within 1 month of GC therapy, reduction in serum immunoglobulins is noted secondary to increased catabolism. Antibody responses to injected antigens are not impaired. *In vitro,* GC suppress B-cell activation with abrogation of cell enlargement, expression of activation antigens, and responses to B-cell activators. Once *in vitro* activation and proliferation have occurred, immunoglobulin and antibody production are unaffected by GC. The cytotoxic activities of natural killer cells are resistant to *in vitro* and *in vivo* GC.

EFFECTS ON SOLUBLE MEDIATORS. GC may mediate some of the aforementioned activities by affecting soluble mediators. Prostaglandins (PG) arise from arachadonic acid after the action of phospholipase A_2 (PLA_2) on phospholipids. GC block PG production through effects on the inhibitors of PLA_2, called lipocortins, or directly on enzyme production. Additionally, transcription of the enzyme cyclo-oxygenase, which catalyzes the metabolism of arachidonic acid to PG, may also be blocked by GC.

Monocyte/macrophage–derived mediators are quite sensitive to

the effects of GC. IL-1, interferon-γ, IL-6, and tumor necrosis factor-α production and/or release are suppressed by GC. However, other monocyte-derived cytokines, such as migration inhibitory factor, are unaffected by GC. Substantial effects on the T cell–derived cytokine IL-2 are observed with GC. GC inhibit IL-2 synthesis, likely through effects on gene expression by suppressing RNA transcription, translation, and degradation, resulting in decreased production of this cytokine. Additionally, GC block IL-2–directed protein phosphorylation as well as the release of other T cell–derived mediators.

Basophil-derived histamine and leukotriene secretion are abrogated by GC. In general, complement metabolism is clinically unaffected by GC, although these drugs may have some effects on release of C3 and factor B. Profound effects on fibroblast activities are noted. GC inhibit the production of a variety of fibroblast-derived mediators including PG, glycosoaminoglycans, and IL-1. These effects may be clinically relevant in the inflammatory arthritides. The clearance of antigen-antibody (i.e., immune) complexes from the circulation is decreased by GC; this effect, which may be important in the therapy of autoimmune diseases, appears to be mediated by downregulation of reticuloendothelial Fc receptor activity.

CLINICAL USE OF GLUCOCORTICOSTEROIDS

GENERAL PRINCIPLES OF THERAPY. The decision to implement therapy with GC must be derived from a precise understanding of the use of these agents and the often formidable adverse reactions that accompany their use. This discussion focuses on the use of GC to treat inflammatory and immunologically mediated diseases. It is obvious, however, that these drugs have important roles in treating unrelated entities such as hypoadrenalism (see Ch. 207) and malignancy (see Ch. 162).

Prior to implementing GC therapy, it is incumbent upon the treating physician to determine that GC are the appropriate form of treatment and that other non-GC approaches are unlikely to be equally beneficial. Regrettably, the option for other forms of treatment may not exist and GC treatment becomes desirable if not mandatory. Under these circumstances, efforts at minimizing GC side effects while maintaining therapeutic efficacy must be maintained. Generally, these goals can be at least partially attained by using short-acting GC medications at the lowest possible dose and the greatest dosing interval for the shortest period of time.

SYSTEMIC GLUCOCORTICOSTEROID THERAPY. *Initiating and Tapering Therapy.* For most inflammatory and immunologically mediated diseases, short-acting GC preparations are desirable (see Table 18–1). In general, plasma half-life correlates with biologic half-life; use of longer biologic half-life preparations such as dexamethasone is associated with a greater chance of adverse effects. Therefore, shorter-acting GC such as prednisone or prednisolone are preferable to longer-acting preparations. These agents are less likely to result in toxicity, and their use facilitates tapering protocols to alternate-day regimens.

Therapy is usually initiated as a single oral morning dose of prednisone (0.5 to 1.0 mg per kilogram of body weight). A morning dose is preferable to dosing later in the day because morning administration mimics the natural diurnal variation in cortisol levels. When more potent anti-inflammatory and immunosuppressive effects are desired, the total daily dose can be divided into three to four doses, given the short half-life of this drug. Unfortunately, this regimen is associated with a greater likelihood of adverse effects and hypothalamic-pituitary-adrenal (HPA) axis suppression; therefore, as quickly as possible, efforts should be undertaken to consolidate the split-dose schedule to a single morning dose. For example, 15 mg of prednisone given four times per day is reduced to 20 mg three times daily, then to 30 mg twice daily and, finally, to a single dose of 60 mg. The duration of each of these steps is dictated by patient tolerance and by control of the underlying disease; in general, this should be accomplished within 3 weeks.

The once-daily regimen is maintained until the disease is stable and clinical improvement is recognized; obviously, this depends in large measure upon the process under therapy. An attempt at further tapering should not be undertaken until it is apparent that the process is clinically quiescent. At this point, reduction to an alternate-day regimen should be initiated with the goal of administering enough prednisone on the high-dose, or "on," day to suppress disease activity on the low-dose, or "off," day. This permits a return to normal HPA axis function while reducing the risk of GC side effects, notably opportunistic infection.

Several protocols for tapering to an alternate-day regimen have been used. For example, the single daily dose may be reduced in 5 to 10 mg decrements to one-half the initial dose. The dose on the "on" day can be doubled while the dose on the "off" day is gradually decreased. Therefore, once a daily dose of 30 mg of prednisone is achieved, the patient is changed to a regimen of 60 mg daily alternated with 30 mg per day, with subsequent 5-mg reductions on the low-dose day weekly until a 15-mg daily level is reached. This dose is then reduced in 2.5-mg amounts until discontinuation, at which point a 60-mg alternate-day regimen has been attained. Once alternate-day therapy has been realized, gradual reductions in GC should be attempted. An alternate approach is to reach a total daily dose of 30 mg daily and then reduce the drug on the low-dose day. This tapering scheme is feasible only when relatively short-acting GC are used; longer-acting drugs have biologic half-lives >24 hours, thereby negating the beneficial effects of an alternate-day regimen.

Clearly, this protocol is not uniformly effective. Failures may occur owing to attempts to begin tapering while the disease is still active, reducing the drug too rapidly, using decrements that are too large, failing to administer enough prednisone on the "on" day, and confusing GC "withdrawal" symptoms (e.g., myalgias, arthralgias, fever) with a recrudescence of the disease. In some instances, tapering can be facilitated by using GC-sparing drugs that help control the primary disease as GC are reduced. Thus, nonsteroidal anti-inflammatory agents, cytotoxic drugs such as methotrexate, azathioprine, and cyclophosphamide, and other agents may permit tapering to alternate-day GC regimens. Clearly, however, these agents may also have associated toxicities that limit utility.

Alternatives to Daily Therapy. Given the considerable toxicities that frequently accompany long-term therapy, alternate approaches to using systemic GC daily are desirable. That is, in many circumstances it may be appropriate to administer GC locally or to use systemic regimens that may reduce the likelihood of adverse effects.

Topical and ophthalmic GC preparations can often control cutaneous and ocular disease, respectively, without appreciable systemic absorption of the preparation. Similarly, GC administered nasally for allergic rhinitis, by inhalation for asthma or lower airway disease, and intra-articularly or by soft tissue injection for musculoskeletal inflammatory conditions may control the underlying disease without the adverse effects of systemic therapy. Certainly, however, these methods of delivering drugs are not without the potential for local toxicity, and caution should therefore be exercised. Deflazacort, an oral GC preparation not currently available in the United States, has been reported to have fewer adverse reactions, particularly osteoporosis, than conventional GC.

There are, obviously, instances when local GC therapy and even systemic daily oral treatment may be inadequate to control the underlying disease. In the 1960's, intermittent, short-term, high-dose intravenous methylprednisolone was used to treat renal allograft rejection, even in the setting of chronic daily immunosuppressive and GC therapy. Recently, similar protocols have been used in inflammatory and immunologically mediated diseases using 3- to 5-day regimens of methylprednisolone (20 mg per kilogram of body weight per day or 1 gram per square meter of body surface per day). The precise mechanism(s) of the beneficial actions of "pulse" therapy is unclear, particularly because these protocols are often efficacious despite daily GC usage. Pulse regimens have been successfully used in systemic lupus erythematosus with renal disease, some forms of vasculitis, rheumatoid arthritis, ankylosing spondylitis, and Goodpasture's syndrome.

This approach is not without the potential for side effects. Cardiac arrhythmias and sudden death have occurred, probably secondary to shifts in electrolytes in patients with electrolyte abnormalities, diuretic therapy, or underlying conduction disturbances. In these settings, ECG monitoring is advisable while slowly administering the drug over 1 to several hours. Other adverse reactions reported with pulse therapy have included seizures and systemic in-

TABLE 18–3. SIDE EFFECTS OF GLUCOCORTICOSTEROID THERAPY

Characteristic early in therapy: essentially unavoidable
  Insomnia
  Emotional lability
  Enhanced appetite or weight gain or both
Common in patients with underlying risk factors or other drug toxicities
  Hypertension
  Diabetes mellitus
  Peptic ulcer disease
  Acne vulgaris
Anticipated with use of sustained and intense treatment: minimize risk by conservative dosing regimens and steroid-sparing agents when possible
  Cushingoid habitus
  Hypothalamic-pituitary-adrenal suppression
  Infection diaathesis
  Osteonecrosis
  Myopathy
  Impaired wound healing
Insidious and delayed: likely dependent on cumulative dose
  Osteoporosis
  Skin atrophy
  Cataracts
  Atherosclerosis
  Growth retardation
  Fatty liver
Rare and unpredictable
  Psychosis
  Pseudotumor cerebri
  Glaucoma
  Epidural lipomatosis
  Pancreatitis

From Boumpas DT, Chrousos GP, Wilder RL, et al.: Ann Intern Med 119:1198, 1993.

fections; because many of these patients were critically ill, the precise relationship to pulse GC is unclear.

Indications for pulse regimens have included (1) recrudescence of disease despite chronic GC therapy; (2) a flare of disease activity in the setting of GC side effects; (3) the need to control disease until another modality (e.g., cytotoxic drug) becomes effective; and (4) the onset of a rapidly progressive GC-responsive syndrome.

COMPLICATIONS OF GLUCOCORTICOSTEROID THERAPY

Prolonged systemic GC therapy is invariably associated with toxicity. The major adverse effects of GC treatment are listed in Table 18–3. In general, side effects depend upon daily dose, dosing frequency, and duration of treatment, emphasizing the need to treat with alternate-day regimens or the lowest daily dose possible for as briefly as feasible. HPA axis suppression may occur with less than 2 weeks of systemic therapy and may be persistent despite cessation of the drug. The integrity of the HPA axis in the setting of GC therapy can be determined by measuring the change in serum cortisol level after cosyntropin infusion.

In general, the most effective way of preventing or minimizing GC adverse effects is to reduce GC dosage; unfortunately, this may not always be feasible. It is particularly important to closely monitor patients for the development of infection; typical signs of infection may be masked by GC treatment. GC-induced osteoporosis is especially problematic in older individuals, particularly those who are estrogen deficient. The precise prevention of this complication remains controversial, although there is enthusiasm for estrogen repletion, concomitant calcium supplementation, and, possibly, the addition of calcitonin and calcitriol.

Boumpas DT, Chrousos GP, Wilder RL, et al.: Glucocorticoid therapy for immune-mediated diseases: Basic and clinical correlates. Ann Intern Med 119:1198, 1993. *Clinically relevant information about how GC work. Update on usage and side effects.*

Boumpas DT, Paliogianni F, Anastassiou ED, et al.: Glucocorticosteroid action on the immune system: Molecular and cellular aspects. Clin Exp Rheumatol 9:413, 1991. *Excellent review of the mechanisms of action of GC.*

Neustadt DH: Systemic corticosteroids. In Katz WA (ed.): The Diagnosis and Management of Rheumatic Diseases. Philadelphia, JB Lippincott, 1988, p 805. *Information on the use of "pulse" GC.*

19 NSAID'S: ASPIRIN AND ASPIRIN-LIKE DRUGS

Gerald Weissmann

HISTORY

Salicylates as Antipyretics and Analgesics

On June 2, 1763, the Royal Society received a communication from Reverend Edmund Stone of Chipping Norton in Oxfordshire. Its opening lines are probably unmatched in clinical pharmacology:

> Among the many useful discoveries which this age has made, there are very few which better deserve the attention of the public than what I am going to lay before your Lordship. There is a bark of an English tree, which I have found by experience to be a powerful astringent and very efficacious in curing aguish and intermittent disorders.

The tree was the willow *(Salix alba)*, the astringent bark of which contains salicin, the glycoside of salicylic acid. Stone had discovered that salicylates reduced the fever and aches produced by a variety of acute, shiver-provoking illnesses, or agues.

In the 1990's the salicylate most commonly used is acetylsalicylic acid, aspirin. At over-the-counter doses (1 to 3 grams per day) aspirin is *analgesic* and *antipyretic.* In addition, at lower doses (80 to 325 mg per day) aspirin is used to prevent coronary and cerebral thrombosis by virtue of its *antiplatelet* effect. For 100 years very high doses (4 to 8 grams per day) have been used to reduce the redness and swelling of joints in rheumatic fever, gout, and rheumatoid arthritis.

Salicylates also have a variety of other biologic effects, only some of which are related to their current use in clinical medicine. Salicylates can dissolve corns on the toes—a *keratolytic* effect; provoke loss of uric acid from the kidneys—their *uricosuric* property; and kill bacteria *in vitro*—their *antiseptic* action. Aspirin inhibits the formation of prostaglandins and thereby inhibits the clotting of blood, induces peptic ulcers, and promotes fluid retention by the kidney. Cell biologists use aspirin and salicylates to inhibit anion transport across cell membranes, to interfere with the activation of white cells, and to uncouple oxidative phosphorylation by isolated mitochondria. Botanists use salicylates to induce flowering of *Impatiens;* indeed, the function of salicylates in plants such as the voodoo lily or skunk cabbage is to induce temperature rises of 12 to 16°C in the course of efflorescence. Salicylates therefore not only reduce fever but also produce it! Finally, molecular biologists use salicylates to activate genes that code for heat-shock proteins in the lampbrush chromosomes of *Drosophila.*

"About six years ago," wrote Stone in his letter to the Royal Society, "I accidentally tasted [the willow bark], and was surprised at its extraordinary bitterness; which immediately raised in me a suspicion of its having the properties of the Peruvian bark." Peruvian bark *(cinchona)* was a venerable remedy for the ague. Stone proceeded to offer a skillful rationale for using willow bark in febrile disorders: the traditional doctrine of signatures—i.e., that "many natural maladies carry their cures along with them, or their remedies lie not far from their cause." Because moist shires, like those drained by the Avon or Isis, abounded in both fevers and willows, Rev. Stone set out to test whether the former might be cured by the latter. Six years of careful clinical observation and the treatment of 50 patients with willow extracts prepared in water, tea, or beer culminated in his letter to the Royal Society. The eighteenth century had found a predictable remedy for fever.

Hippocrates (fourth century B.C.) had advocated the chewing of willow leaves to relieve the pains of childbirth, and there are references by Pliny (first century) and Galen (second century) to the *analgesic* property of willow, but it was Stone who put extract of willow bark into our pharmacopoeia as an effective *antipyretic* agent.

By 1828, at the Pharmacologic Institute of Munich, Buchner isolated a tiny amount of the active glycoside, salicin, in the form of bitter-tasting yellow, needle-like crystals. Two years later, Leroux in Paris improved on the extraction procedure and obtained 1 ounce of salicin from 3 pounds of the bark. By 1838, Raffaele Pira of Pisa, writing in the *Comtes Rendu de l'Academie de Science,* described how he obtained a pure substance from salicin by hydrolyzing the glycoside in a CrO_3-mediated oxidation via an aldehyde intermediate. He gave it the name by which we know it today: *"l'acide salicylique,"* or salicylic acid. Willow bark was not alone in providing a rich natural source of salicylates. Meadowsweet *(Spiraea ulmaria)* yielded ample quantities of an ether-soluble oil from which a *Spirsaure* was crystallized in 1835 by the Swiss chemist Karl Jakob Lowig. In 1839 Dumas demonstrated that the *Spirsaure* of Lowig was nothing else than the *acide salicylique* of Pira. Another Gallic pharmacologist, Auguste Andre Thomas Cahours (1843), showed that oil of wintergreen—a traditional remedy for aguish disorders—contained the methyl ester of salicylic acid and prepared *acide salicylique* from it.

As was to be the case in much of nineteenth century chemistry, French and British scientists were slightly ahead of the Germans in the study of natural products, whereas Germans held the edge in synthetic know-how. Forced to compete with the French and British dye industries which supplied their textile mills with pigments imported from overseas colonies, the Germans responded by inventing cheap aniline dyes, creating in their train such giant enterprises as I. G. Farben. By 1833, the pharmacist E. Merck of Darmstadt had obtained a clean preparation of salicin which was cheaper by half than the impure willow extracts used as antipyretics, but a cheap, pure, acceptable remedy was not available until 1860, when Kolbe and his students at Marburg succeeded in the first synthesis of salicylic acid and its sodium salt from phenol, CO_2, and sodium. Using industrial variations of the Kolbe synthesis, one of his students, Friedrich von Heyden, established in 1874 the first large factory in Dresden devoted to producing synthetic salicylates. The availability of cheap salicylic acid spread its clinical use far and wide.

SALICYLATES AS ANTI-INFLAMMATORY DRUGS. The first successful treatment of acute rheumatism was reported in 1876 by Stricker and Ries in the *Berliner Medizinische Wochenschrifft* and by Maclagan writing in *The Lancet.* Stricker and Ries reported the complete cure of acute "polyarthritis rheumatica" by sodium salicylate at doses of 5 to 6 grams per day. Almost simultaneously, Maclagan reported his results with salicylic acid and salicin at similar dosage levels; he paid tribute to the still prevalent doctrine of signatures, pointing out that cases of acute rheumatism were most abundant in moist areas where the willow grows.

Stricker and Ries and Maclagan had demonstrated a clinical property of high-dose salicylates which was not tested in the laboratory until the 1930's: They found that salicylates reduce not only fever and pain but also redness and swelling. That anti-inflammatory property was next used to advantage by the Parisian Germain See, who in 1877 introduced salicylates (both *acid salicylique* and salicin) as effective treatments for gout and "chronic poly-arthritis." See had great success among his well-off clientele with using salicylates in acute and chronic gout, so great indeed that the *British Medical Journal,* in an editorial note, called him to task for charging up to £80 sterling to treat a patient with gout by means of 6 to 8 grams of sodium salicylate per day, when the price of 1 gram of the drug was but 5 pence! There the matter rested, with high doses of sodium salicylate more or less accepted as a new treatment in many rheumatic diseases, whereas lower doses (1.5 to 2.0 grams per day) seemed to relieve aches and pains.

ASPIRIN. In 1898 a new chapter was written: Felix Hofmann was an aniline dye chemist at the Friedrich Bayer-Eberfeld division of the I. G. Farben cartel when his father complained to him of gastric irritation from the sodium salicylate he was taking for "rheumatism." Hofmann searched the chemical literature for less acidic derivatives and hit upon acetyl derivatives of sodium salicylate first described by G. Von Gilm in 1859 and 10 years later by a certain H. Kraut (sic). Although von Gilm and Kraut had outlined synthesis of the compound, they had no notion of what its biologic effects might be. Hofmann repeated the synthesis (via acetic anhydride) and tried acetylsalicylic acid first on himself and then on his father: It proved more palatable, less irritating to the stomach, and—he claimed—more effective. Hofmann took the material to his supervisor, Heinrich Dreser, head of Bayer's laboratory of pharmacology, who reported that it performed better in both laboratory and clinic and called the new drug *aspirin,* the *a* from *acetyl* and the *spirin* from the German *Spirsaure.*

THE ANILINE DERIVATIVES AS ANALGESICS AND ANTIPYRETICS. Competitors entered the field as the markets expanded for other drugs that could reduce fever and pain. Based on anecdotal accounts from the Alsace that a product formed from aniline treated with vinegar made a useful febrifuge, Karl Morner in 1889 synthesized the material—acetanilide—and isolated its metabolites. Acetanilide itself, unfortunately, caused bone marrow depression and anemias in a distinct number of patients, so other derivatives were sought. Acetanilide and the widely used phenacetin are metabolized to *N*-acetyl-*p*-aminophenol, which by various anagramatic combinations yields the generic names *acetaminophen* in the United States and *paracetamol* in the United Kingdom. In 1955 acetaminophen acquired a tradename in the United States that was to make it famous: *Tylenol*—also from acetyl-*p*-aminophenol.

NSAID's VERSUS CORTISONE. Neither acetanilide nor phenacetin proved as useful as aspirin for treating rheumatic fever or rheumatoid arthritis: They were not anti-inflammatory. For half a century (1900 to 1950) clinicians appreciated that there was something unique about high-dose salicylates. At levels over 4 grams per day, only salicylates—of all the analgesics—were anti-inflammatory. They also brought under control the erythrocyte sedimentation rate and levels of C-reactive protein in serum. Indeed, when James Reid in 1948 demonstrated an inverse relationship between plasma salicylate levels and signs of rheumatic inflammation, he asked, "Does sodium salicylate cure rheumatic fever?" The answer came from well-controlled and definitive studies in the 1950's that were prompted by the discovery of ACTH and cortisone, the most potent anti-inflammatory compounds ever described.

Each of more than two dozen studies concluded that neither steroids (cortisone and its derivatives) nor salicylates (aspirin or sodium salicylate) actually cured rheumatic fever or rheumatoid arthritis and that in the short run both types of agents are about equally effective at suppressing acute inflammation. Because the course of acute rheumatic fever is easier to document than that of rheumatoid arthritis, it is worth paying attention today to the back-to-back trials of steroids versus aspirin and sodium salicylate. These were performed by the Medical Research Council of Britain and the American Heart Association (reported in 1955) and the Combined Rheumatic Fever Study Group of the United States (reported in 1961) and showed that salicylates at doses high enough to yield plasma levels of 25 to 35 mg per deciliter (6 to 9 grams per day) were as effective anti-inflammatory agents as cortisone or prednisone in rheumatic fever.

NSAID's MODE OF ACTION: INHIBITION OF PROSTAGLANDIN SYNTHESIS

Unfortunately, until 1971 no useful hypothesis had emerged as to how salicylates exert their various effects. Pharmacologists had shown that salicylate analgesia was due to a peripheral effect—as opposed to morphine's central action. In contrast, physiologists maintained that salicylates did not reduce fever by peripheral action but worked directly on the fever centers of the hypothalamus. Renal physiologists found that low doses of salicylates raised uric acid in the blood by blocking tubular secretion by the kidney, whereas paradoxically, high doses of salicylates lowered uric acid by blocking its tubular absorption. Clinicians found that the latter property explained the utility of salicylates in both acute and chronic gout. It was more difficult to explain how aspirin inhibited platelet function, caused salt and water retention, and provoked severe dyspepsia. And why did some patients develop nasal polyps, with sniffles and wheezes: aspirin "hypersensitivity"?

The most important recent contribution to the story of aspirin-like drugs was made by John Vane (now Sir John), then at the Royal College of Surgeons in London, in 1971. Vane had been impressed that many forms of tissue injury are followed by release of prostaglandins (PG's), the oxidation products of arachidonic acid. PGE_1 and PGF_2 had been shown to be associated with acute vasodilation and fever. Vane and his colleagues found that aspirin-like drugs inhibited the biosynthesis of PGE_2 and $PGF_{2\alpha}$ from radiolabeled arachidonic acid in studies *in vitro*. Moreover, they found that platelets taken from volunteers given aspirin and indomethacin 1 hour before venipuncture failed to make prostaglandins in re-

sponse to thrombin and that catecholamine-induced release of prostaglandins from canine spleens could be inhibited by indomethacin, albeit less consistently than by aspirin or sodium salicylate.

All that remained was to show how and when prostaglandins caused redness and swelling with heat and pain and to study the exact means whereby aspirin-like drugs inhibited the enzyme that transformed arachidonic acid to the stable PGE_1 and PGE_2. The constitutive enzyme COX-1 (see below) has been found to be a 70-kDa homodimer localized to microsomal membranes; it has been cloned and sequenced and was first called "prostaglandin synthase" and then "cyclo-oxygenase," and today is known as "prostaglandin H synthase," or COX-1 (Fig. 19–1). This enzyme catalyzes two reactions: the bis-deoxygenation of arachidonic acid to form PGH_2 (cyclo-oxygenase activity) and the reduction of hydroperoxides to the corresponding alcohols. This enzyme—and COX-2, as well—produces stable prostaglandins of the E and F series via the unstable *endoperoxide* intermediates, PGG_2 and PGH_2. The endoperoxides, critical for platelet function, are transformed by platelets to a most potent vasoconstricting and platelet-aggregating substance, thromboxane B_2 (TxB_2). Meanwhile, Vane had isolated a potent vasodilator, prostacyclin (PGI_2), which was also made from arachidonate by the cyclo-oxygenase of endothelial cells. Because platelets make TxB_2—which constricts the smooth muscle of blood vessels—and because blood vessel walls make prostacyclin I_2, which powerfully relaxes blood vessels and inhibits platelet aggregation, the hunt was on for ways to inhibit the synthesis of thromboxane but not prostacyclin.

Vane and his associates in the 1970's had amassed convincing evidence that the prostaglandin hypothesis of aspirin action was largely correct. They pointed out that almost all aspirin-like drugs (by then generally called "nonsteroidal anti-inflammatory drugs," or NSAID's) inhibited prostaglandin synthetase and that the potency of these drugs (ID_{50}) in this regard pretty much paralleled their clinical potency or their effect in experimental animals; e.g., aspirin was anywhere from one fortieth to one two-hundredth as active as indomethacin and from one fifth to one fiftieth as active as ibuprofen. Indeed by 1990, more than 40 NSAID's had reached the clinic and each of them at one dose or another inhibits the synthetase. It should also be noted, however, that since 1971, inhibition of PG synthetase has been a *sine qua non* for their introduction! Only NSAID's, but not central analgesics such as morphine or codeine, inhibit PG synthetase, nor do antihistamines, antiserotonin drugs, or cortisone and its analogues. Moreover, concentrations of NSAID's that could be achieved in the circulation (allowing for protein binding) were in excess of those required to inhibit the enzyme in disrupted cell preparations.

Vane and his colleagues argued that stable prostaglandins not only were produced at sites of inflammation but, alone or in concert with other mediators, could provoke all the cardinal signs of inflammation. Indeed, PGE_1 and PGE_2 *do* induce vasodilation; they promote edema when dilated blood vessels have been made leaky by histamine; they produce fever when injected either into the cerebral ventricles or directly into the anterior hypothalamus, and they sensitize pain receptors of the skin to such other pain-provoking humors as bradykinin or histamine. Sound explanations were offered for a few troubling discrepancies. Acetaminophen ineffectively inhibited prostaglandin synthesis by enzyme preparations from a variety of tissues but was effective against the synthetase from brain. And although nonacetylated salicylates were roughly one tenth as potent as aspirin, *in vitro*, studies of urinary prostaglandin metabolites showed that sodium salicylate effectively diminished excretion of these metabolites in humans. Sodium salicylate also effectively reduced prostaglandin release in models of experimental inflammation in animals.

Cyclo-oxygenase products (COX-1, COX-2) and leukotrienes are associated with inflammation *in vivo*. Recent studies have documented that there are actually two PGH_2 synthase isozymes (COX-1 and COX-2), which share 62% homology at the message and protein level. Despite the close relationship of the cDNA's for COX-1 and COX-2, the mRNA for these two isozymes differs greatly with respect to size—2.8:3.0 Kb and 4.1 Kb for COX-1 and 2, respectively. The major difference between these two isozymes is that COX-1 is present in many cells constitutively, but COX-2 is expressed only after it is induced by tumor necrosis factor-α, interleukin 1 (IL-1)$_\alpha$ or lipopolysaccharide. Recent x-ray studies have

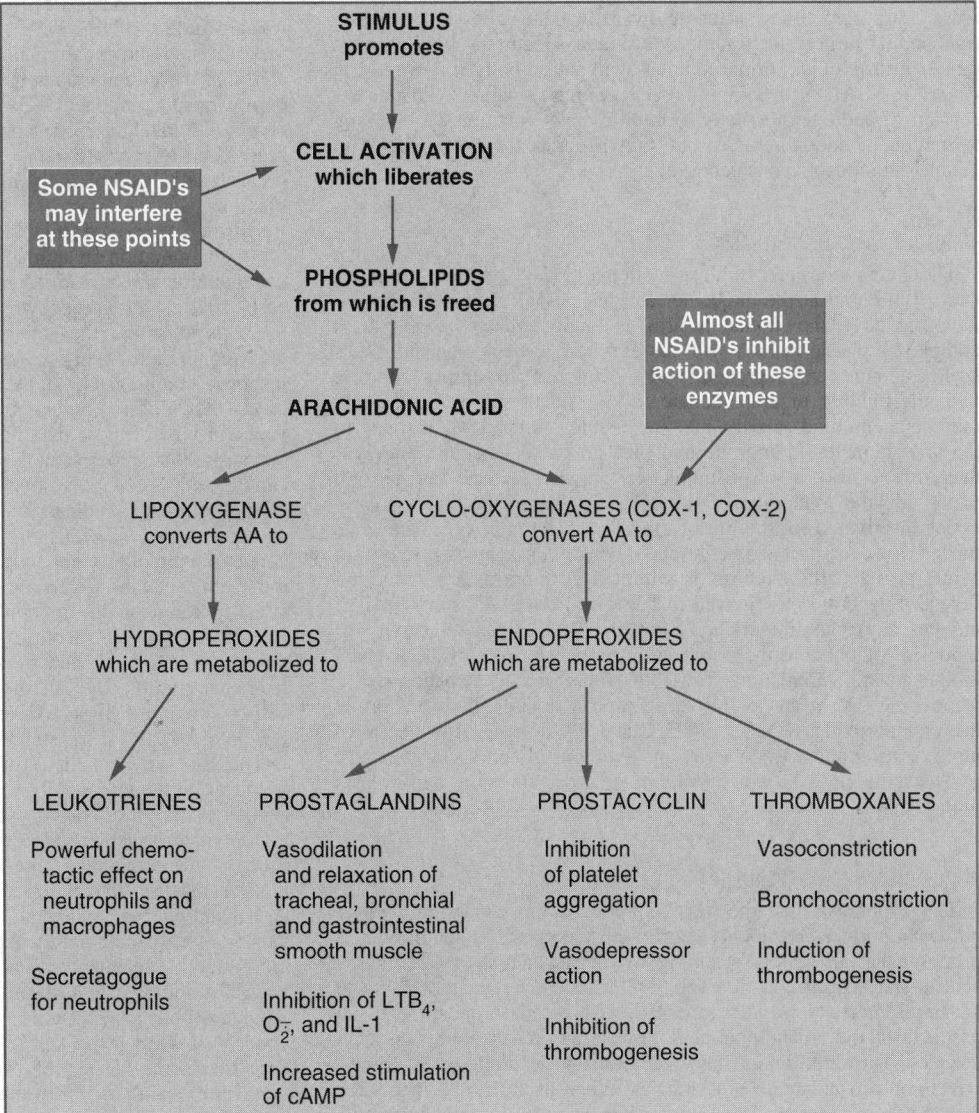

FIGURE 19-1. The inflammatory cascade. LTB_4 = leukotriene B_4; O_2^- = superoxide anion; IL-1 = interleukin 1; cAMP = cyclic adenosine monophosphate.

STIMULUS
promotes

CELL ACTIVATION
which liberates

Some NSAID's may interfere at these points

PHOSPHOLIPIDS
from which is freed

Almost all NSAID's inhibit action of these enzymes

ARACHIDONIC ACID

LIPOXYGENASE
converts AA to

CYCLO-OXYGENASES (COX-1, COX-2)
convert AA to

HYDROPEROXIDES
which are metabolized to

ENDOPEROXIDES
which are metabolized to

LEUKOTRIENES

Powerful chemotactic effect on neutrophils and macrophages

Secretagogue for neutrophils

PROSTAGLANDINS

Vasodilation and relaxation of tracheal, bronchial and gastrointestinal smooth muscle

Inhibition of LTB_4, O_2^-, and IL-1

Increased stimulation of cAMP

PROSTACYCLIN

Inhibition of platelet aggregation

Vasodepressor action

Inhibition of thrombogenesis

THROMBOXANES

Vasoconstriction

Bronchoconstriction

Induction of thrombogenesis

demonstrated that aspirin (ASA) irreversibly acetylates Ser 530 of COX-1, thereby blocking access of 20:4 to the active site. Other NSAID's sterically hinder access of 20:4 to the active site. By unknown means, ASA inhibition of COX-2 leads to the generation of 15-HETE. Its potential metabolite, 14,15-diHETE, is a potent inhibitor of neutrophil O_2^- generation. Engagement of two lipoxygenases (5- and 15-) leads to the synthesis of lipoxins A_4 and B_4, which inhibit several leukocyte functions. In contrast, linolenic acid is converted by endothelium to 13-hydroxyoctadecadienoic acid (13-HODE) via the 15-lipoxygenase pathway. 13-HODE is a potent chemorepellent, and studies have shown that when endothelial cells are activated by IL-1 to upregulate their vitronectin receptor, 13-HODE synthesis was decreased: The ratios of 15-HETE to 13-HODE determined the adherence of tumor cells to endothelium via that receptor. Many NSAID's selectively inhibit COX-1 or COX-2 (e.g., piroxicam, indomethacin, and sulindac sulfide are 10- to 40-fold selective for COX-1; 6-methoxy-2-naphthyl acetic acid, the active metabolite of nabumetone, is 15-fold selective for COX-2), whereas other agents inhibit COX-1 and COX-2 equally (flurbiprofen, S-ibuprofen, meclofenamic acid); ASA and sodium salicylate are equipotent with respect to COX-1 and COX-2 but differ in their effects on platelet and gastric mucosa. Another paradox!

NSAID SIDE EFFECTS

Perhaps the most persuasive aspect of the prostaglandin hypothesis (and especially the discovery of COX-2) was its explanation of

the clinical *side effects* of NSAID's. A major problem with NSAID's at anti-inflammatory doses is that they provoke stomach irritation and sometimes ulceration. Aspirin is the worst offender in this regard. The irritation derives from the need for endogenous prostaglandins by the gastric mucosa to regulate its overproduction of acid and to synthesize the mucous barrier that prevents its self-digestion. But now an *exogenous* PGE_1 analogue (misoprostol) has been approved for preventing and treating NSAID-induced ulcers.

Moreover, most NSAID's prevent the body from excreting salt and water properly, especially when heart or liver disease compromises renal blood flow. NSAID's block the formation of the vasodilator PGI_2 by kidney cells, and renal blood supply is reduced even further. It is no surprise, therefore, to learn that whereas kidney and stomach are rich in COX-1, COX-2 is induced in cells of inflammation such as macrophages.

Another side effect of NSAID's—but not sodium salicylate—is aspirin-sensitivity syndrome in those genetically susceptible: wheezing, sneezing, and polyp formation. Nowadays, thanks to the elucidation of arachidonic acid metabolism, we attribute these consequences to the diversion of arachidonate from blocked PGH synthase to the 5-lipoxygenase pathway, which is not inhibited by NSAID's. It is by means of the lipoxygenase pathways that leukotrienes (LT) C, D, and E are formed, and these have been implicated in aspirin hypersensitivity.

Finally, the most common side effect of NSAID's, and especially of aspirin, is their interference with platelet function. Patients on these drugs sometimes suffer untoward bleeding after tooth extraction, minor surgery, or trauma. Weiss and Aledort in 1967 showed that aspirin inhibits normal platelet aggregation both *in vitro* and *in vivo*. All NSAID's that inhibit PGH synthase—again with the exception of sodium salicylate—inhibit platelet function by blocking formation of endoperoxides and TxA_2, which are intermediates in platelet stimulus-response coupling.

INHIBITION OF PGH$_2$ SYNTHASE

The interaction of NSAID's with the PGH synthase has been studied in detail at the molecular and physiologic levels. Lands and Kulmacz have shown that aspirin and indomethacin interact in a complex, biphasic fashion with the enzyme, whereas other NSAID's such as ibuprofen, naproxen, and meclofenamate simply interfere with the binding of arachidonate to its oxidation site. Aspirin and indomethacin bind rapidly in a reversible, competitive manner to the arachidonate-binding site and then go on to inactivate the synthase irreversibly. Aspirin, moreover, acetylates serine residue 506 of the enzyme. When the PGH synthase is that of the platelet, it remains inactivated for the life of the cell and thromboxane cannot be made. However, in endothelial cells, which can synthesize new enzyme, prostacyclin synthesis is inhibited no more than a few days. Indeed, Fitzgerald has showed that low oral doses of aspirin (< 325 mg per day) can irreversibly block the PGH synthase activity of a pool of platelets in the portal circulation *before* salicylate appears in the general circulation. These two observations explain why it is possible, by means of low-dose aspirin, to inhibit formation of the endoperoxides (PGG_2, PGH_2), and TxA_2—all of which promote clotting and vasoconstriction—without inhibiting synthesis of prostacyclin (PGI_2), which inhibits platelet function and dilates blood vessels.

NSAID ACTIONS NOT DEPENDENT ON PROSTAGLANDINS

The hypothesis that the locally produced prostaglandins lead to *inflammation* has been only partly substantiated. Although Vane's proposal that all NSAID's inhibit the transformation of arachidonic acid to stable prostaglandins (i.e., PGE_2 and PGI_2) has turned out to be largely correct, we still cannot generalize this proposition to all products of the arachidonic acid cascade and to all NSAID's at all dosages. The three major antipyretic, analgesic drugs exert diverse effects on prostaglandin biosynthesis. When used to treat rheumatic diseases in dosages of 4 to 8 grams per day, aspirin has antipyretic, anti-inflammatory, and analgesic effects and can inhibit the synthesis of prostaglandins in disrupted cell preparations. At the intermediate dosage indicated for analgesia (650 mg every 3 to 4 hours), aspirin has antipyretic and analgesic but not anti-inflammatory activity. And at its lowest clinical dosage (80 to 325 mg per day), aspirin exerts only its antiplatelet effect. Plasma levels of salicylate in individuals given intermediate, analgesic doses of aspirin can inhibit prostaglandin biosynthesis *in vivo* by kidneys, platelets, and vascular endothelium, whereas the low levels of aspirin, to prevent thrombosis affect only prostaglandin synthesis by platelets. In contrast, higher plasma concentrations (18 to 30 mg per deciliter) are required to achieve an anti-inflammatory effect. Those observations suggest two possibilities: Either the PGH synthase of cells that provoke inflammation is relatively insensitive to aspirin or aspirin has a mode of action beyond its capacity to inhibit prostaglandin biosynthesis to which it owes its anti-inflammatory property.

Further evidence that aspirin-like drugs exert clinical effects that do not depend on inhibiting prostaglandin biosynthesis can be drawn from the properties of sodium salicylate and acetaminophen. Although sodium salicylate shares many of the properties of aspirin, it fails to inhibit prostaglandin biosynthesis is disrupted cell preparations at concentrations that may be achieved in plasma (approximately 5 mM). Moreover, clinical studies show that because nonacetylated salicylates do not inhibit platelet function *in vitro* or *ex vivo*, they do not cause bleeding. Indeed, acetaminophen, which also fails to inhibit prostaglandin biosynthesis, does not affect platelet aggregation, nor is it by any means anti-inflammatory. We must therefore conclude that pain and fever can effectively be reduced without inhibiting the synthesis of prostaglandins at all (Table 19–1).

PRO- and ANTI-INFLAMMATORY PROPERTIES OF PROSTAGLANDINS

The Vane hypothesis is further weakened by findings that stable prostaglandins (PGE_1, PGE_2, PGI_2) possess not only pro-inflammatory but also anti-inflammatory properties. It has been well appreciated that these compounds produce vasodilation, act in synergy with complement component C5a or LTB4 to produce edema, mediate fever and myalgia in response to IL-1, and act in synergy with bradykinin to provoke pain. They also inhibit the function of T suppressor cells. All of these are *pro-inflammatory* effects of prostaglandins.

On the other hand, high doses of these stable prostaglandins inhibit inflammation in animal models of arthritis, and much lower doses inhibit inflammation induced by local skin irritants. Since the early 1970's we have known that PGI_2 and stable prostaglandins of the E type inhibit the activation in vitro of neutrophils, platelets, and mononuclear phagocytes by interfering with their stimulus-response coupling. NSAID's increase cellular cAMP in these cells, levels of which are regulated via prostaglandin receptors. The relevance *in vivo* of these data obtained *in vitro* is supported by the observation that experimental arthritis or glomerulonephritis in rats can be reduced with systemic PGE_1. These are *anti-inflammatory* effects of prostaglandins.

As a class, NSAID's are planar organic anions that partition across the lipid bilayers of plasma membranes in accordance with the Nernst equation. The more acidic the pH (as at inflammatory sites), the greater the lipophilicity of NSAID's, which subsequently interfere with cell function, including assembly of a superoxide anion–generating system by a cell-free, membrane-rich preparation from neutrophils, the activity of phospholipase C in mononuclear cells, the 12-hydroperoxyeicosatetraenoic acid peroxidase in platelets, and signal transduction in neutrophils and lymphocytes.

The first effect of aspirin-like drugs on cell metabolism was found to be the uncoupling of oxidative phosphorylation by isolated mitochondria; until Vane's work in 1971 this was held to be their major mode of action! More recent studies have shown that aspirin (but not acetaminophen) alters the uptake of precursor arachidonate and its insertion into the membranes of cultured human monocytes and macrophages. Salicylates also inhibit anion transport across a variety of cell membranes. Again, the capacity of salicylates to inhibit anion movements is not shared by acetaminophen. Finally, NSAID's inhibit synthesis of cartilage proteoglycan and bone metabolism (both *in vitro* and *in vivo*), by mechanisms that do not depend on inhibiting the PGH synthase. It is a matter of clinical concern that some classes of NSAID's (e.g., salicylates), but not all (e.g., piroxicam), inhibit proteoglycan synthesis, thereby promoting loss of cartilage matrix.

NSAID's INTERFERE WITH NEUTROPHIL FUNCTIONS

Recent work has shown that aspirin-like drugs affect stimulus-response coupling in the most abundant cells of acute inflammation: neutrophils. Neutrophils injure tissues by releasing proteases, inflammatory peptides, reactive oxygen species such as O_2^- and H_2O_2, and lipid irritants such as platelet-activating factor and LTB_4. Activation of the neutrophil in response to soluble stimuli (chemoattractants) or to immune complexes follows general pathways of stimulus-response coupling secretory cells and is inhibited by all NSAID's studied so far.

NSAID's—indomethacin, piroxicam, diclofenac, and ibuprofen (at micromolar concentrations) and salicylates (at millimolar concen-trations)—inhibit the cell-cell aggregation of human neutrophils induced by chemoattractants and mediated by the cell surface adhesion molecule CD11b/CD18. Although *all* NSAID's inhibit aggregation, only some inhibit enzyme release and/or O_2^- generation. Millimolar concentrations of sodium salicylate and aspirin alike (levels achieved in treating rheumatoid arthritis or rheumatic fever) are required to inhibit the aggregation of neutrophils. However, at these concentrations sodium salicylate *does not* interfere with the activation of platelets or synthesis of TxA_2. In contrast, aspirin at one tenth to one hundredth of these concentrations inhibits platelet aggregation and completely inhibits thromboxane biosynthesis via its effect on PGH synthase. It is therefore likely that the shared anti-inflammatory effects of aspirin and sodium salicylate are related to their common inhibition of neutrophil activation rather than to their divergent actions on prostaglandin biosynthesis. In contrast to aspirin and sodium salicylate, acetaminophen does not affect neutrophil aggregation.

TABLE 19-1. EFFECTS OF COMMONLY USED ANALGESIC AND ANTIPYRETIC AGENTS

| | Acetylsalicylic Acid | | | | | |
	Low Dose*	Intermediate Dose*	High Dose*	Sodium Salicylate	Newer NSAID's†	Acetaminophen
Antipyretic	0	+	+	+	+	+
Analgesic	0	+	+	+	+	+
Anti-inflammatory	0	0	+	+	+	+
Inhibit PG synthesis of platelets	+	+	+	0	+	0
Inhibit PG synthesis systemically	0	+	+	±	+	0

*Low dose, 80 to 325 mg per day; intermediate dose, 650 mg to 3 grams per day; high dose, >3 grams per day.
†Includes indomethacin, ibuprofen, naproxen, diclofenac, piroxicam.

Inhibitory effects of NSAID's on neutrophil activation *in vitro* can also be demonstrated in the clinic. Indeed, neutrophils derived from the synovial fluid of patients with rheumatoid arthritis produced less superoxide anion following 10 days of therapy with piroxicam, whereas cells from normal volunteers given ibuprofen or piroxicam for 3 days failed to aggregate normally in response to chemoattractants. Sodium salicylate, an ineffective inhibitor of PGH synthase *in vitro,* is as effective as aspirin at inhibiting neutrophil activation.

It is somewhat paradoxical that both NSAID's and prostaglandins of the E series have similar *inhibitory* effects on the activation of such inflammatory cells as the neutrophil or platelet. Adding PGE_1 or PGE_2 to human neutrophils at nanomolar to micromolar concentrations fails to override piroxicam's inhibition of superoxide generation that is induced by chemoattractants. In the presence of piroxicam, superoxide anion generation was diminished by a fourfold factor of ~40 to 10 nmoles per liter of cytochrome c reduced per 10^6 cells. Recent studies with the clinically useful PGE_1 derivative misoprostol also show additive or synergistic rather than antagonistic effects between NSAID's and prostaglandins.

At anti-inflammatory concentrations, NSAID's appear to uncouple receptors with their effector molecules in the plasmalemma, including those regulated by at least one guanine nucleotide-binding (G) protein. Pertussis toxin, via its capacity for ADP-ribosylate, the alpha subunit of some plasma membrane G proteins, interferes with signal transduction in a variety of cells, including the neutrophil. Compared with pertussis toxin, sodium salicylate alone only modestly inhibits the production of superoxide induced by chemoattractants while inhibiting aggregation to a far greater extent. However, sodium salicylate blocks the inhibitory effect of pertussis toxin on neutrophils: Cells co-incubated with both pertussis toxin and sodium salicylate could still generate superoxide anion by inhibiting pertussis toxin. This paradoxical effect of salicylate suggests that salicylates interfere with the action of pertussis toxin near the site of its interaction with the alpha subunit of the G protein. NSAID's (salicylate, piroxicam, and indomethacin) block the pertussis toxin–dependent ADP-ribosylation of the G protein in purified neutrophil membranes, and salicylates and piroxicam inhibit, in part, the pertussis toxin–sensitive formation of diacylglycerol which follows cell activation.

THE PHYLOGENY OF NSAID STUDIES

A final blow to the generality of the prostaglandin hypothesis comes from the sea. The cell biology of marine sponges, such as *Microciona prolifera,* was first examined by Robert Hooke, who in 1685 suggested in *Microcosmographica* that all living creatures contain a commonality of substructure that under the microscope resembles the "cells of monks." We may recall that the name "cell" derives from Hooke's studies of onion root tips and sponges. *M. prolifera,* which is both the most primitive and most ancient of animal creatures (10^9 years in ancestry), offers a unique model for investigating the anti-inflammatory effects of NSAID's. The activation of sponge cells in the course of cell-cell aggregation is not influenced by stable prostaglandins, nor do sponge cells contain cyclo-oxygenase activity. Nevertheless, aggregation of marine sponge cells is inhibited by NSAID's—either by aspirin or sodium salicylate and by 12 other NSAID's tested but not by acetaminophen. After dispersing cells by treatment with EDTA and removing the chelator with calcium, cell-cell aggregation of the *M. prolifera* cells

is rapidly induced by phorbol esters or by adding an ionophore that raises cytosolic calcium. They are also aggregated by a species-specific aggregation factor called MAF, a 20×10^6 MW proteoglycan, and by arachidonic acid. Both aspirin and sodium salicylate (at millimolar concentrations) inhibit aggregation of these cells in response to MAF. Ibuprofen, piroxicam, and diclofenac (at micromolar concentrations) but not acetaminophen, also inhibit aggregation of these primitive cells. Because the concentrations of NSAID's that inhibit aggregation of marine sponges are the same as those that inhibit neutrophil aggregation and because marine sponges *cannot* make prostaglandins, we may conclude that these effects, like those of NSAID's on insects (*Drosophila* chromosomes), plants (voodoo lilies), or human cells (neutrophils), are unlikely to result from their inhibition of prostaglandin synthesis.

Abramson S, Weissmann G: The mechanisms of action of nonsteroidal antiinflammatory drugs. Arthritis Rheum 32:1, 1989. *The physicochemical properties of NSAID's may alter the fluidity of the plasma membrane and thereby disrupt molecular interactions required for normal signal transduction across the lipid bilayer. The alternative hypothesis to J. R. Vane's.*
Graham GG: Pharmacokinetics and metabolism of nonsteroidal antiinflammatory drugs. Med J Aust 147:597, 1987. *Review of the few controlled studies showing that plasma levels of NSAID's, when in the therapeutic range, correlate with response.*
Hennekens CH and the Steering Committee of the Physician's Health Study Research Group: Final report on the aspirin component of the ongoing Physicians' Health Study. N Engl J Med 321:129, 1989. *Aspirin at low doses prevents myocardial infarction.*
Kulmacz RJ: Topography of prostaglandin H synthase. Antiinflammatory agents and the protease-sensitive arginine 253 region. J Biol Chem 264:14136, 1989. *The best recent review of how NSAID's work on inhibition of the enzyme.*
Meade EA, Smith WL, DeWitt DL: Differential inhibitors of prostaglandin endoperoxide synthase (cyclo-oxygenase) isozymes by aspirin and other non-steroidal antiinflammatory drugs. J Biol Chem 268:6610, 1993. *How COX-1 and COX-2 differ in their response to aspirin-like drugs.*
Ritossa F: A new puffing pattern induced by temperature shock and DNP in Drosophila. Experentia 12:571, 1962. *Sodium salicylate induces heat shock protein in* Drosophila.
Vane JR: Towards a better aspirin. Nature 367:215, 1994. *A fine discussion of how COX-1 and COX-2 explain the toxicities of aspirin-like drugs.*

20 Antithrombotic Therapy
Laurence A. Harker

Antithrombotic therapy involves thrombolytic agents, antiplatelet drugs, and anticoagulants. In formulation of the appropriate antithrombotic strategy, thrombolytic therapy is the first consideration because it provides the means for removing already established thrombus. Subsequent antithrombotic therapy varies depending on whether the venous or arterial circulatory system is involved, the size and location of the involved vessel(s), the risks of extension, embolization, or recurrence, and the relative antithrombotic benefits and hemorrhagic risks. Suspected arterial or venous thrombosis or thromboembolism requires objective confirmation. Although angiography is the diagnostic reference standard, ultrasonography performed by skilled personnel is a suitable alternative for superficially accessible vessels and for cardiac assessment. Additional mechanical measures for restoring vascular patency include balloon catheter or surgical embolectomy. Occasionally, intravascular filters may be needed to prevent pulmonary thromboembolism. The agents, indications, regimens, and complications related to antithrombotic therapies are summarized in the following discussion.

THROMBOLYTIC THERAPY

Fibrinolytic therapy is useful for treating patients with acute arterial and venous thrombo-occlusive events. Early intravenous (IV) thrombolytic therapy is highly beneficial in patients with acute myocardial infarction (AMI), acute arterial thromboembolic occlusion, severe deep venous thrombosis (DVT), and threatening pulmonary embolism (PE). Overall, the clinical benefits, as well as the bleeding risks, are equivalent for the four approved thrombolytic agents: streptokinase (SK), recombinant tissue plasminogen activator (t-PA), anisoylated plasminogen-streptokinase activator complex (APSAC), and urokinase plasminogen activator (u-PA).

ACUTE ARTERIAL THROMBO-OCCLUSIVE EVENTS.
Acute Coronary Thrombosis (see also Ch. 41.2). Although it has been known for many years that coronary thrombosis is generally the cause of AMI, only in recent years has therapy been directed toward salvaging ischemic myocardium by re-establishing flow in the occluded artery within the first few hours after symptoms develop. Extensive clinical investigation has clearly established that IV thrombolytic therapy recanalizes 75% of occluded coronary arteries in the setting of AMI. Although t-PA appears to recanalize arteries more quickly than does SK or APSAC, this early advantage is lost within the first 24 hours, presumably because reocclusion occurs more frequently with t-PA.

Controlled trials convincingly show that thrombolytic reperfusion successfully salvages left ventricular function, especially in patients with anterior AMI who receive early therapy. Preservation of left ventricular function is equivalent for each of the three thrombolytic agents evaluated—t-PA, SK, and APSAC.

Recent clinical trials with more than 100,000 AMI patients unequivocally establish both early and late mortality benefits for IV thrombolytic therapy (Table 20–1). Moreover, the improvements in mortality are equivalent for SK, t-PA, and APSAC, as shown in several very large trials comparing the relative efficacy of two or more thrombolytic agents, e.g., GISSI-2 (Gruppo Italiano per lo Studio della Streptochinasia nell'Infarto Miocardio), ISIS-3 (Third International Study of Infarct Survival), and GUSTO (Global Utilization of Streptokinase and t-PA for Totally Occluded Coronary Arteries). See also Ch. 41.2 for further discussion and comparison.

These agents all efficiently convert plasminogen to plasmin (Table 20–2). Although systemic fibrinogenolysis is decreased by t-PA's fibrin-dependent generation of plasmin, t-PA is neither more effective nor safer. The explanation is related, at least in part, to the rapid clearance of t-PA and corresponding quickly diminishing of thrombolysis, with consequent enhanced early reocclusion. By contrast, SK and APSAC produce systemic fibrinogenolysis and high levels of fibrin degradation products that inhibit both platelet function and fibrin formation, thereby reducing rethrombosis.

Other medications should be included with thrombolytic agents in managing AMI, e.g., antiarrhythmics, narcotics, calcium channel antagonists, and β-adrenergic agonists and antagonists. Adjuvant aspirin (160 to 325 mg) adds significant antithrombotic benefit to AMI patients. Concurrent use of IV heparin is supported by GUSTO.

Systemic Thromboembolic Occlusive Events. Fibrinolytic therapy is an alternative to mechanical/surgical intervention for treating arterial thrombo-occlusive disease, but opinion varies regarding the relative importance and timing of each therapeutic strategy. Initial fibrinolytic therapy is the recommended approach, surgical intervention being reserved for resistant occlusive thrombi. In general, the local delivery of thrombolytic agents recanalizes occluded arteries effectively.

Bleeding complications occur with both local and systemic forms of therapy. Most episodes are at sites of arteriotomy produced during prior angiography and catheterization procedures. No controlled trials have directly compared outcomes using different thrombolytic agents.

VENOUS THROMBOSIS AND PULMONARY EMBOLISM.
Deep Venous Thrombosis (DVT) (see also Ch. 46). Fibrinolytic agents are indicated in the treatment of massive DVT. The theoretical advantages of managing proximal vein thrombosis with thrombolytic agents include (1) preserving native structures in the deep veins; (2) preventing postphlebitic syndrome; and (3) lysing thrombi more rapidly and completely. The accepted indications for fibrinolytic therapy in DVT include massive thrombus, symptomatic thrombus present for < 1 week, and absence of contraindications.

Acute Pulmonary Embolism (PE) (see also Ch. 40). Thrombolytic therapy is more effective than heparin in lysing acute PE, as measured by angiography, perfusion lung scans, and hemodynamic assessments. However, these lytic flow benefits disappear within 1 week, and there is no difference in mortality or short-term morbidity. However, bleeding is substantially more frequent in patients treated with thrombolytic agents. SK, u-PA, and t-PA produce approximately equivalent outcomes.

PHARMACOLOGIC AGENTS. Four thrombolytic agents are approved for IV administration in patients: SK, APSAC, u-PA, and t-PA. In general, thrombolysis is equivalent using SK, APSAC, u-PA, or t-PA in patients with AMI, DVT, and PE. The properties of these agents are compared in Table 20–2.

COMPLICATIONS OF THROMBOLYTIC THERAPY. Because severe bleeding is the primary limiting complication of thrombolytic therapy, medical thrombolysis is contraindicated in patients with recent surgery or trauma, malignant disease, recent stroke, active peptic ulcer disease, recent liver or renal biopsy, and recent arterial puncture. Invasive vascular procedures and their frequency and severity are influenced by the concomitant use of other antithrombotic therapies. The most dreaded bleeding complication is intracranial bleeding, which occurs in 0.3 to 1.0% of patients treated with intravenous SK, t-PA, or APSAC for AMI. Despite t-PA's fibrin specificity, clinical bleeding is equivalent for all of the thrombolytic drugs. Whereas adding aspirin has no effect on major bleeding, the addition of heparin to thrombolytic therapy significantly increases major bleeding. Invasive procedures should be avoided if at all possible.

ANTIPLATELET THERAPY

Coronary and cerebral atherosclerotic vascular diseases give rise to heart attacks and strokes by inducing thrombo-occlusive events at sites of plaque stenosis and rupture (see Ch. 40). These thrombotic processes are platelet-dependent and thrombin-mediated but largely unresponsive to conventional anticoagulation. The most useful overall validation of benefits resulting from antiplatelet therapy in patients with symptomatic vascular disease comes from the Antiplatelet Trialists' Collaboration. This meta-analysis includes more

TABLE 20–1. INTRAVENOUS THROMBOLYTIC THERAPY: COMPARISON OF AGENTS AND MORTALITY

Trial	n	Drugs	Follow-up	Mortality (5)			P
GISSI-2	12,490	SK, rt-PA	Hospital	SK 8.5	rt-PA 9		Not significant
International	20,891	SK, rt-PA	Hospital	SK 8.5	rt-PA 8.9		Not significant
ISIS-3	46,091	SK, APSAC, rt-PA	35 days	SK 10.5	APSAC 10.6	rt-PA 10.3	Not significant
GUSTO	41,021	SK, t-PA	30 days	rt-PA and heparin 6.3	SK and heparin 7.4	t-PA, SK, and heparin 7.0	0.001 for t-PA with heparin vs SK groups with heparin

TABLE 20–2. THROMBOLYTIC AGENTS

	Streptokinase (SK)	Anisoylated Plasmin-SK Activator Complex (APSAC)	Urokinase Plasminogen Activator (u-PA)	Tissue Plasminogen Activator (t-PA)
Structure	47-kD bacterial nonenzymatic trypsin-like protein	SK complexed with p-anisoylated plasminogen	54-kD human 2-chain serine protease	68-kD human single chain fibrin-dependent serine protease
Mode of action	SK forms complex with plasminogen, which converts plasminogen to plasmin	APSAC forms complex with plasminogen and generates plasmin gradually as active center panisoylated groups hydrolyze	u-PA directly cleaves plasminogen to form plasmin	t-PA forms complex with fibrin, which converts plasminogen to plasmin
Removal from plasma (T_{50})	30 min	100 min	15 min	5 min
Advantages/disadvantages	Relatively inexpensive; produces systemic fibrinogenolysis; immunogenic	Prolonged disappearance from plasma permits easy bolus administration; produces systemic fibrinogenolysis; immunogenic	Produces systemic fibrinogenolysis; not immunogenic	More rapid lysis; less systemic fibrinogenolysis; not immunogenic; expensive
Dose regimen: AMI (within 6 to 12 hrs)	1.5 million units IV over 60 min	30 units IV bolus	Not adequately validated	100 mg IV infusion over 90 min with heparin
DVT/PE	250,000 units IV bolus and 100,000 units/hr for 24 hours with heparin	Not adequately validated	4400 units/kg IV bolus and 4400 units/kg/hr for 24 hours with heparin	1–2 mg/kg per 24 hours for 2–4 days
Complications	Abnormal bleeding; allergic reactions	Abnormal bleeding; allergic reactions	Abnormal bleeding	Abnormal bleeding

than 200 randomized trials involving more than 100,000 patients. It confirms that aspirin and ticlopidine are beneficial in patients with atherosclerotic disease who are at high risk of vascular events, including males and females, diabetics and nondiabetics, old and young. Ticlopidine is at least as beneficial as aspirin and may be more effective. However, both aspirin and ticlopidine have adverse effects.

ATHEROSCLEROTIC VASCULAR DISORDERS. Aspirin and ticlopidine decrease the risk of thrombo-occlusion and thromboembolism for all major vascular distributions, irrespective of the anatomic site producing symptoms (Tables 20–3 and 20–4).

Cerebrovascular Disease (see also Ch. 418 and 419). Aspirin therapy in patients with either transient ischemic attacks (TIA's) or mild strokes reduces the risk of developing stroke, myocardial infarction, or vascular death by 22% (see Table 20–3), and the reduction in all strokes far outweighs the small increase in hemorrhagic stroke associated with aspirin. Although some of the trials used dipyridamole and aspirin, the benefits are not attributable to dipyridamole because aspirin alone showed equivalent outcomes, and a trial comparing placebo with dipyridamole alone failed to demonstrate any protection.

Compared with aspirin, ticlopidine reduces the risk of stroke and death from any cause by 12% and the relative risk of stroke by 21% (Ticlopidine-Aspirin Stroke Study). In patients with prior thromboembolic stroke, ticlopidine reduces the risk of the combined outcome of stroke, MI, and vascular death by 30% (Canadian-American Ticlopidine Study).

Coronary Artery Disease (see also Ch. 41.1 and 41.2). In patients with prior MI, aspirin reduces the risk of stroke, myocardial infarction, and vascular death by about 25% (see Table 20–3). Aspirin is also beneficial in AMI, reducing the risk of subsequent vascular events by 29% (see Table 20–3). Several large independent studies establish that aspirin decreases the risk of MI or cardiac death by about 50% in patients with unstable angina. Ticlopidine is also beneficial in coronary artery disease, although the experience is limited.

Coronary Artery Bypass Grafts (see also Ch. 41.3). Aspirin (160 to 325 mg) improves the patency of aortocoronary saphenous vein and internal mammary artery bypass grafts by approximately 40% (see Table 20–3). To maintain graft patency without increasing surgical bleeding, patients undergoing saphenous vein or internal

TABLE 20–3. EFFECTS OF ASPIRIN ON VASCULAR EVENTS

Category	Number of Trials	Percent Odds Reductions (SD) in MI, Stroke, and Vascular Deaths
Atherosclerotic disease		
Prior MI	11	25 (4)
Acute MI	9	29 (4)
Prior stroke/TIA	18	22 (4)
Other high risk	109	32 (4)
Primary prevention	3	10 (6)
All trials	150	25 (2)
Vascular procedures		
Coronary artery grafts	20	41 (6)
Peripheral vascular procedures	11	38 (9)
Angioaccess vascular grafts	9	70 (14)
All trials	40	44 (4)

MI = Myocardial infarction; TIA = transient ischemic attack.

TABLE 20–4. COMPARISON OF ANTIPLATELET AGENTS

	Aspirin	Ticlopidine
Mode of action	Irreversible acetylation of platelet cyclo-oxygenase within minutes of oral dose	Lasting inhibition of platelet recruitment initiated by all agonists after several days of oral dosing
Oral dose	160–325 mg daily	250 mg twice daily
Clinical indications	Symptomatic atherosclerotic vascular disease	Systemic atherosclerotic vascular disease (particularly aspirin failures)
	Vascular angioplasty and grafting angioplasty	Vascular angioplasty and grafting
Usefulness	Risk reduced by 25% for symptomatic disease and 44% for vascular procedures	Probably more effective by about 10%, but with greater complications and costs
Complications	Gastrointestinal bleeding increased with surgery; allergic reactions	Neutropenia in 1%; diarrhea in 10–20%; increased bleeding with surgery

mammary artery aortocoronary grafting should receive aspirin (325 mg per day) within hours after completing the procedure and continue aspirin therapy for 1 year.

Peripheral Vascular Disease (see also Ch. 46). Aspirin improves the patency after vascular angioplasty and grafting (see Table 20–3; $P < 0.0001$), although subsequent lesion formation is not decreased. Ticlopidine reduces fatal and nonfatal cardiovascular events in patients with peripheral vascular disease. For example, ticlopidine decreases the risk of stroke, myocardial infarction, or vascular death by 20% in patients with atherosclerotic peripheral arterial disease (Swedish Ticlopidine Multicentre Study).

Primary Prevention. Aspirin decreases vascular outcomes by 10% in primary prevention trials (see Table 20–3) but increases hemorrhagic stroke, with no net reduction in vascular deaths. Thus, it is generally concluded that administering aspirin to large numbers of asymptomatic individuals for prolonged periods is not justified.

CARDIOVASCULAR DEVICES. Prosthetic Heart Valves. Low-dose aspirin (100 mg daily) and anticoagulants are more effective than anticoagulants alone in reducing thromboembolic complications of prosthetic heart valves. However, adding aspirin to anticoagulation increases the incidence of serious gastrointestinal bleeding if the dose of aspirin exceeds 100 mg per day. When aspirin fails or is contraindicated, dipyridamole (100 mg four times daily) is combined with oral anticoagulant therapy in patients with prosthetic heart valves in the aortic and mitral position.

Prosthetic Vascular Grafts. Aspirin or ticlopidine reduces vascular occlusive events in patients with peripheral vascular disease undergoing grafting procedures and in hemodialysis patients receiving arteriovenous vascular angioaccess grafts (see Table 20–3). However, these therapies fail to decrease the formation of stenotic anastomotic lesions.

Although aspirin and anticoagulation have been used with endovascular stenting procedures to reduce the high frequency of thrombo-occlusion, no randomized controlled clinical studies have shown such therapies to be beneficial.

High-Risk Angioplasty. Thrombo-occlusive events complicate coronary angioplasty in high-risk patients despite treatment with aspirin and heparin. Aspirin resistance is explained by thrombin's mediation of the thrombotic process, an aspirin-independent pathway. Resistance to heparin is attributable to bound thrombin's inaccessibility to heparin and the local heparin-inhibiting effects of proteins secreted from activated platelets. A compelling strategy for interrupting resistant vascular thrombosis is the inhibition of glycoprotein (GP) IIb/IIIa–dependent platelet recruitment. Activated platelets express functional GP IIb/IIIa receptors (also referred to as integrin $\alpha_{IIb}\beta_3$) that mediate interplatelet bridging by circulating adhesive molecules, especially fibrinogen, containing the recognition peptide sequence ARG-GLY-ASP (RGD). Humanized monoclonal antibodies are capable of inhibiting platelet recruitment by blocking this common pathway of platelet cohesion. The administration of these antibodies for 12 hours to patients undergoing high-risk angioplasty inhibits vascular thrombosis and the corresponding acute coronary events, albeit in association with significant abnormal bleeding.

PHARMACOLOGIC AGENTS. Aspirin (see Table 20–4 and Ch. 19). Oral aspirin potently and irreversibly inactivates cyclooxygenase in circulating platelets, thereby interrupting the endoperoxide/thromboxane A_2 pathway of platelet recruitment and minimally impairing hemostasis. Although aspirin at 1 mg per kilogram is as effective as higher doses in the majority of patients at risk, some patients require 325 mg aspirin because of limited bioavailability. Because only 10% of non–aspirin-treated platelets are sufficient to generate full thromboxane A_2–dependent platelet aggregation in aspirin-treated platelets and 10% of the circulating platelets are produced daily, aspirin should be given every day to guarantee full benefit.

Ticlopidine (see Table 20–4). Ticlopidine (250 mg twice daily) is probably more effective than aspirin in patients at risk of vascular events and may be preferred in patients with TIA's, prior stroke, unstable angina, recent MI, and peripheral arterial disease. Ticlopidine produces dose-dependent global inhibition of platelet recruitment mediated by GP IIb/IIIa fibrinogen receptor. Ticlopidine requires several days of oral administration to manifest its maximum effect on platelet function; it has no direct inhibitory effect on platelets *in vitro*.

Intravenous anticoagulation with dose-adjusted heparin in hospital is indicated for managing acute DVT and PE, performing vascular procedures, and placing cardiovascular prosthetic devices. Subcutaneous dose-adjusted heparin is also indicated for the transient or chronic out-of-hospital prophylaxis of venous thrombosis during periods of increased risk, pregnancy, or resistance to oral anticoagulation. Monitored oral anticoagulation using coumadin drugs, usually warfarin, is indicated for long-term out-of-hospital prophylaxis of DVT, PE, and systemic thromboembolism.

ANTICOAGULANT THERAPY FOR VENOUS THROMBOSIS AND THROMBOEMBOLISM. Acute DVT and PE. Immediate treatment with heparin benefits patients presenting with DVT or PE by markedly reducing mortality from recurrent PE and preventing extension or embolization of DVT (Table 20–5). Immediate anticoagulation is obtained in hospital by bolus IV heparin.

Warfarin (0.1 mg per kilogram per day but not exceeding 10 mg) is begun after initiating the heparin infusion, while monitoring the response with the prothrombin time (PT) (Table 20–5). Because the risk of recurrence remains elevated for many weeks, uncomplicated DVT requires 3 months of warfarin therapy, and 6 months of treatment are generally recommended for major or complicated DVT. Patients with recurrent DVT or a continuing risk factor such as deficiencies in antithrombin III (AT-III), protein C, protein S, resistance to activated protein C, or malignancy should be treated indefinitely with oral anticoagulants. In patients developing new emboli despite adequate treatment with heparin or with absolute contraindications to antithrombotic therapy, vena caval umbrella may transiently protect the patient from pulmonary emboli.

Prophylaxis of Surgical DVT and PE. No specific prophylaxis is required for low-risk general surgery patients younger than 40 or those undergoing minor operations with no clinical risk factors other than early ambulation postoperatively.

Moderate-risk general surgery patients who are over age 40 and undergoing major surgery without additional risk factors should be treated prophylactically with low-dose heparin (5000 units subcutaneously every 12 hours). Low-dose subcutaneous heparin begun before surgery and continuing until a patient is ambulatory reduces the incidence of venous thrombosis by two thirds and pulmonary embolism by half. Patients older than 40 undergoing major surgery with additional risk factors should receive low-dose subcutaneous heparin (5000 U every 8 hours) or low-molecular-weight heparin every 12 hours.

Patients undergoing hip surgery should receive prophylaxis using low-molecular-weight heparin, adjusted-dose heparin (to prolong the activated partial thromboplastin time [aPTT] in the upper half of the normal range), or moderate-dose warfarin (to maintain the international normalized ratio [INR] at 2.0 to 3.0).

TABLE 20–5. ANTICOAGULANT THERAPY OF DEEP VEIN THROMBOSIS AND PULMONARY EMBOLISM

Initiate therapy with heparin
1. Administer heparin 5000 units IV and start an infusion of 1200 units/hour.
2. Check aPTT after 4–6 hours and adjust infusion to prolong aPTT to 1.5–2.5 times control.

Alternative: Administer heparin subcutaneously every 12 hours beginning with an initial dose of 18,000 units. Check aPTT after 4 hours and adjust subsequent doses to prolong aPTT to 1.5–2.5 times control; monitor and maintain range for 5–7 days.

Maintenance anticoagulation
  Oral anticoagulants
1. Give warfarin 5–10 mg during first hospital day.
2. Check PT daily.
3. Adjust dose to prolong PT to INR of 2–3 (1.3–1.5 times control with most rabbit brain thromboplastins).
4. Discontinue heparin after minimum of 5 days when PT reaches desired range.
5. Continue warfarin as outpatient for 3–6 months.
  Heparin
  Heparin subcutaneously every 12 hours in a dose to prolong the mid-interval aPTT to 1.5 times control.

aPTT = activated partial thromboplastin time; INR = international normalized ratio; PT = prothrombin time.

Patients undergoing intracranial neurosurgical procedures, major knee surgery, or urologic surgery should not receive anticoagulants but should be treated with intermittent pneumatic compression only.

Prophylaxis of Medical DVT and PE. Low-dose heparin is recommended for the prophylaxis of DVT and PE in medical patients at prolonged bed rest, such as patients with AMI or congestive heart failure. Full-dose anticoagulation is also effective. Similarly, prophylaxis should be provided for patients with ischemic stroke and lower-extremity paralysis using low-dose heparin or low-molecular-weight heparin.

DVT and PE During Pregnancy. Pregnant patients with a history of previous venous thromboembolic disease are at increased risk of developing DVT and PE; these patients should be given low-dose subcutaneous heparin (5000 units twice daily) throughout their pregnancy. Women who present with DVT during pregnancy should receive full-dose IV heparin by continuous infusion for 5 to 7 days, followed by twice-daily adjusted-dose subcutaneous heparin until term. If pregnancy is planned while the patient is receiving long-term anticoagulant prophylaxis, subcutaneous heparin anticoagulation should be substituted for the warfarin before pregnancy begins. Although no validating randomized studies have been carried out, pregnant patients with prosthetic heart valves or atrial fibrillation and documented systemic embolization should be treated with twice-daily adjusted-dose subcutaneous heparin from the time pregnancy is diagnosed until delivery.

PREVENTION OF SYSTEMIC THROMBOEMBOLISM.

Atrial Fibrillation and Valvular Heart Disease. Long-term warfarin therapy sufficient to maintain the INR at 2.0 to 3.0 should be given to patients with atrial fibrillation and valvular heart disease, except patients younger than age 60 who have no associated cardiovascular disease (Table 20–6). Long-term warfarin therapy (INR of 2.0 to 3.0) is also recommended for patients with rheumatic mitral valvular disease and normal sinus rhythm if the left atrial diameter is >5.5 cm. If systemic embolization recurs despite warfarin therapy, daily aspirin (100 mg) should be added to increase INR to 2.5 to 3.5.

Long-term antithrombotic therapy is not indicated in patients with aortic valve disease in the absence of associated mitral valve disease or atrial fibrillation. Additionally, antithrombotic therapy is not indicated in patients with mitral valve prolapse who have not experienced systemic embolism, unexplained TIA's, or atrial fibrillation. Warfarin therapy (INR of 2.0 to 3.0) should be given for 3 weeks before elective cardioversion of patients who have had atrial fibrillation for longer than 2 days and continued until normal sinus rhythm has been maintained for 4 weeks. However, antithrombotic therapy is not recommended for cardioversion of atrial flutter or supraventricular tachycardia or of patients who have been in atrial fibrillation for no more than 2 days unless other risk factors for systemic embolism are present.

Prosthetic Heart Valves. All patients with mechanical prosthetic heart valves should be treated with long-term warfarin at a dose sufficient to maintain the INR at 2.5 to 3.5. Aspirin (100 mg per day) in addition to warfarin (INR of 3.0 to 4.5) offers additional protection without increasing the risk of bleeding. Dipyridamole (400 mg per day) with warfarin may also produce a similar benefit.

Patients with mechanical prosthetic heart valves who suffer systemic embolism despite adequate therapy with warfarin should receive aspirin (100 mg per day) with warfarin. Dipyridamole (400 mg per day) with warfarin is an alternative therapy when aspirin cannot be used. Antiplatelet agents alone, without warfarin, do not offer sufficient protection against systemic embolism.

Patients with bioprosthetic mitral valves should be treated for the first 3 months after valve insertion with warfarin to maintain an INR of 2.0 to 3.0. Patients with bioprosthetic valves who have atrial fibrillation, exhibit left atrial thrombus at the time of surgery, have a history of systemic embolism, or show evidence of a left atrial thrombus at surgery should also be treated with long-term warfarin therapy (INR of 2.0 to 3.0).

Patients with bioprosthetic valves and sinus rhythm or valves in the aortic position may benefit from aspirin therapy (325 mg per day) without anticoagulants.

Acute Myocardial Infarction. Patients with anterior transmural AMI are at increased risk of systemic embolism and should receive full-dose heparin therapy by continuous infusion followed by warfarin therapy to maintain an INR of 2.0 to 3.0 for 1 to 3 months. Patients with AMI at increased risk of systemic embolism because of atrial fibrillation, history of previous systemic or pulmonary embolism, or congestive heart failure should also receive heparin therapy followed by warfarin therapy to prolong PT to an INR of 2.0 to 3.0 for at least 3 months. Although long-term anticoagulation therapy is not generally recommended in patients with AMI, long-term warfarin therapy is recommended in those with any risk factors for systemic or pulmonary embolism, i.e., atrial fibrillation, previous systemic embolism, venous thromboembolism, or severe heart failure.

PHARMACOLOGIC AGENTS. Standard Heparin (see also Ch. 153). Heparin is the anticoagulant of choice when rapid anticoagulant effects are required. Because heparin must be given parenterally, monitored regularly for its anticoagulant effects, and dosage adjusted frequently, its use is largely limited to in-hospital settings. Heparin is indicated for preventing DVT and PE, early treatment of unstable angina, chronic prevention of DVT and PE during pregnancy, treatment of resistant thrombotic processes, and transient anticoagulation when using cardiovascular devices and procedures. Tests of intrinsic clotting, such as the aPTT, have intermediate sensitivity to heparin, i.e., clotting times doubled by therapeutic heparin levels (0.2 to 0.3 IU per milliliter). Because the PT is only slightly prolonged by relatively high levels of heparin, it is a reliable means of assessing the status of oral anticoagulation during therapeutic heparin infusions.

Heparin may be administered intravenously by bolus injection, continuous infusion, or subcutaneous injection. Continuous infusion is associated with fewer bleeding complications than intermittent bolus injection and provides excellent protection against recurrent venous disease. The half-life of therapeutic heparin following bolus IV administration averages about 60 to 90 minutes, depending on the dose and the patient; response to heparin varies considerably among different individuals and even in the same individual at different times during the course of therapy.

After infusion into blood, heparin binds with a number of other basic proteins in plasma that compete with AT-III, including fibronectin, vitronectin, von Willebrand factor (vWF), histidine-rich glycoprotein, and platelet Factor 4. Variable binding of heparin to these proteins contributes to heparin's reduced bioavailability at low concentrations, variability in anticoagulant response after fixed dosing, and resistance to therapy. Additionally, heparin bound to vWF impairs vWF-dependent platelet hemostatic function. Heparin binding to endothelial cells and macrophages is thought to be responsible for the initial rapid saturable phase of heparin's clearance from blood after bolus injection. Consequently, the anticoagulant response to heparin is not linear but increases disproportionately in intensity and duration with increasing doses.

When given by continuous infusion, heparin requires an accurate administration and should be given a separate IV line. The initial loading dose is 75 IU per kilogram body weight by IV bolus injection, followed by infusion at 10 to 25 IU per kilogram per hour, depending on patient and clinical situation. The aPPT should be maintained at about 1.5 to 2 times baseline (heparin levels 0.2 to

TABLE 20–6. EFFECTS OF WARFARIN IN ATRIAL FIBRILLATION

	AFASAK	SPAF	BAATAF	CAFA
Control stroke events*	4.6	7.0	3.0	3.6
Warfarin stroke events*	1.9	2.3	0.4	2.1
Risk reduction	58	67	86	42
(95% CI) %	(7–81)	(21–86)	(51–96)	(68–80)
P values	.03	.01	.002	>.2
Intracerebral hemorrhage				
Control*	0.0	0.4	0.0	0.0
Warfarin*	0.4	0.4	0.2	0.4
Major bleeding				
Control*	0.0	1.2	1.6	0.8
Warfarin*	0.4	1.2	1.0	1.7

* Per 100 person-years.
AFASAK = Stroke Incidence and Risk Factors for Stroke in Copenhagen, Denmark; SPAF = Stroke Prevention in Atrial Fibrillation; BAATAF = Boston Area Anticoagulation Trial for Atrial Fibrillation; CAFA = Canadian Atrial Fibrillation Anticoagulation Study.

4 IU per milliliter). Appropriate therapeutic aPPT's are 50 to 80 seconds. The aPPT should be adjusted by changing the infusion rate. After each adjustment, the aPPT should be checked after 4 hours to assess effects of the dose change; monitor daily.

Plasma heparin levels are unexpectedly low after subcutaneous administration because entry of heparin into the intravascular space from the subcutaneous depots is delayed, thereby enhancing rapid saturable clearance due to binding to endothelium and macrophages. This effect seriously complicates initial therapy using subcutaneous heparin for DVT management by delaying the time required to attain full antithrombotic heparin levels.

Less intense anticoagulation is required to prevent venous thrombosis than to treat established thrombosis. Low-dose subcutaneous heparin (5000 IU two or three times daily) is used for prophylaxis during surgery or for medical patients at bed rest. Because individual variations are found in heparin levels when administered as a low-dose regimen, adjusted low-dose heparin (aPTT maintained just detectably prolonged) improves protection in patients at increased risk, e.g., patients undergoing hip surgery.

Low-Molecular-Weight Heparin.
Low-molecular-weight heparins (LMWH's) are effective and safe for preventing and treating venous thrombosis, and are now approved for this purpose. LMWH's are fragments of commercial-grade standard heparin produced by either chemical or enzymatic depolymerization and are approximately one third the size of standard heparin. Like standard heparin, they are heterogeneous in size, averaging 4000 to 5000 daltons. Depolymerization of standard heparin changes its anticoagulant profile, bioavailability, pharmacokinetics, and effects on platelet function and experimental bleeding. LMWH's produce their principal anticoagulant effect via pentasaccharide-dependent binding to AT-III. Whereas approximately one third of unfractionated heparin fragments exhibit these binding domains, a lower proportion of LMWH molecules bind AT-III. Although a minimum chain length of 18 saccharides (including the pentasaccharide sequence) is required for ternary complex formation with thrombin, inactivation of Factor Xa by AT-III depends only on the pentasaccharide. The various commercial LMWH's have anti–Factor Xa to antithrombin ratios varying between 4:1 and 2:1, compared with the 1:1 ratio for standard heparin.

Because LMWH's bind much less avidly to heparin-binding plasma proteins and endothelium than standard heparin, LMWH's exhibit superior bioavailability, longer rates of elimination, and more predictable anticoagulant responses in experimental animals. Compared with a gravimetric basis in experimental models of venous thrombosis, LMWH's are less effective than heparin as antithrombotic agents but produce much less bleeding than standard heparin in models measuring blood loss from a standardized injury, perhaps related to attenuated effects on platelet function and vascular permeability.

In patients, LMWH's also exhibit greater bioavailability, longer plasma half-life, and a more predictable anticoagulant response than standard heparin, allowing LMWH's to be administered once daily and without laboratory monitoring. LMWH's also produce less bleeding than standard heparin for an equivalent antithrombotic effect, thereby permitting patients to be treated with higher anticoagulant doses of LMWH's without compromising patient safety. This latter potential advantage of LMWH's has been demonstrated in patients undergoing hip surgery who are at high risk of thrombosis.

Coumarin-Type Anticoagulation.
Oral coumarin-type anticoagulation is indicated for preventing chronic out-of-hospital venous thrombosis, pulmonary embolism, and systemic embolism in patients at increased risk.

The PT is the most common laboratory test for monitoring oral anticoagulant therapy because it is sensitive to alterations in prothrombin and Factors X and VII, three of the vitamin K–dependent coagulation factors. The pharmacologic response of warfarin depends on the net effect on the activity levels of these factors because they have different half-lives; e.g., reduction in Factor VII, which has a 6-hour half-life, prolongs the PT within 24 hours following large doses of warfarin before significant changes occur in the other factors. It is therefore common practice to begin warfarin therapy with 10 mg for each of the first 2 days and then adjust the dose, usually downward, based upon the results of the daily PT until it equilibrates in the therapeutic range. PT's vary considerably in their dose-response curves, however, so they need to be carefully standardized. The range of response among different individuals is particularly wide; from 1 to 20 mg per day may be required to maintain a patient in the therapeutic range once equilibration has been achieved. During therapy the PT reflects the dose given 36 to 48 hours previously.

A properly standardized PT should be used for monitoring warfarin therapy. The variability among commercial thromboplastins renders the prolongation in absolute time unsatisfactory for this purpose. Moreover, because of relatively greater sensitivity to lower levels of Factor VII, the PT may not properly reflect the overall degree of anticoagulation during periods of instability.

The optimal therapeutic range for controlling anticoagulant therapy is a subject of confusion, primarily because different thromboplastin reagents respond variably to decreases in vitamin K–dependent clotting factors. Thromboplastins are prepared from brain, lung, or placental tissues and vary markedly in their responsiveness to the anticoagulant effects of warfarin. For example, to double the PT over baseline requires a lower dose of warfarin when using the more responsive thromboplastins employed in Europe than when using the less responsive thromboplastins currently used in North America. Differences in thromboplastins appear to be responsible for differing recommendations regarding warfarin dosage. Consequently, an international reference preparation of thromboplastin and a calibration system have been developed based on the assumption that a linear relationship exists between the logarithm of the PT ratios of the reference and test thromboplastins. Thus, to standardize the reporting of the PT, the observed PT ratio obtained with the local thromboplastin is converted into an INR, which is calculated as follows: $INR = observed\ ratio^c$, where C is the constant that represents the international sensitivity index (ISI). The INR, therefore, is the PT ratio that reflects the result that would have been obtained if the reference thromboplastin had been used to perform the test. For practical purposes, it is sufficient to know that the primary human brain reference thromboplastin, which is very responsive to the anticoagulant effects of warfarin, has an ISI of 1.0 and that the ISI value increases as the thromboplastin exhibits less responsiveness.

There is good evidence from clinical trials that a targeted INR range of 2.0 to 3.0 is effective in treating venous thrombosis after an initial course of heparin and in preventing venous thrombosis and systemic embolism.

Drug interactions significantly affect the dose of warfarin needed to maintain optimal therapy (Table 20–7).

COMPLICATIONS OF ANTICOAGULANT THERAPY. The major risk of anticoagulant therapy is bleeding secondary to excessive anticoagulation, the patient's underlying clinical disorder, or the concurrent use of high-dose aspirin. Patients treated with standard doses of either heparin or warfarin have a 2 to 4% per year frequency of major bleeding episodes, i.e., those requiring transfusion. The risk of a fatal hemorrhage is about 0.2% per year for patients on oral anticoagulants. The frequency of bleeding with heparin therapy is reduced when it is administered by continuous infusion and dose adjusted, as opposed to intermittent bolus injections. The risk of major bleeding is reported to be increased in patients over age 65, in patients with a history of stroke, gastrointestinal bleeding, atrial fibrillation, and co-morbid conditions such as uremia and anemia, and with infrequent monitoring. The most common minor episodes involve urinary, gastrointestinal, and vaginal bleeding. In general, any new or painful symptom in an anticoagulated patient should be considered a manifestation of a potential bleeding complication until proven otherwise.

The risk of clinically important bleeding is reduced by decreasing the therapeutic range of INR from 3.0 to 4.5 to 2.0 to 3.0. Bleeding episodes in patients on warfarin occurring while the anticoagulant effect is within this therapeutic range are frequently due to focal pathologic lesions, such as an occult neoplasm unmasked by the therapy, especially in the gastrointestinal or genitourinary tract.

Reversal of heparin is achieved by protamine sulfate, a basic nuclear histone containing one third of its residues as arginine. Protamine binds heparin more tightly than any plasma protein, including AT-III. It is routinely given after heparinization during cardiopul-

TABLE 20-7. FACTORS ALTERING THE PHARMACOKINETICS AND PHARMACODYNAMICS OF WARFARIN

Altered Absorption	Altered Hepatic Metabolism	
	Enhanced Anticoagulant Effects	*Impaired Anticoagulant Effects*
Enhanced anticoagulant effect	Drugs	Drugs
Low vitamin K intake	Phenylbutazone	Barbiturates
Reduced vitamin K absorption in	Metronidazole	Rifampin
fat malabsorption	Sulfinpyrazone	Griseofulvin
	Trimethoprim-sulfamethoxazole	Carbamazepine
	Disulfiram	Penicillin
	Amiodarone	
	Erythromycin	
	Anabolic steroids	
	Clofibrate	
	Cimetidine	
	Omeprazole	
	Thyroxine	
	Ketoconazole	
	Fluconazole	
	Isoniazid	
	Piroxicam	
	Tamoxifen	
	Quinidine	
	Vitamin E (megadoses)	
Impaired anticoagulant effect	Liver disease	Alcohol
Increased vitamin K intake	Hypermetabolic states	
Reduced absorption of warfarin	Pyrexia	
by cholestyramine	Thyrotoxicosis	

monary bypass surgery in approximately equal weight amounts to total administered heparin. The protamine may dissociate or metabolize more rapidly than heparin, thereby accounting for the occasional open-heart surgical patient who exhibits "rebound" heparinization observed after surgery.

Heparin-associated thrombocytopenia occurs in about 1 to 3% of treated patients. Thus, it is prudent to check a platelet count before heparin is given on the fifth day or with any bleeding episode. Thrombocytopenia may be induced by heparin derived from bovine or porcine sources, administered either intravenously or subcutaneously, or as LMWH derivatives. There are two main clinical types: the more common modest thrombocytopenia of early onset, possibly due to the platelet proaggregating effect of some contaminating fraction of heparin itself, and the less common severe delayed-onset thrombocytopenia caused by heparin-dependent immune destruction. Occasionally, patients with severe thrombocytopenia also develop threatening thromboembolic events attributable to platelet activation mediated by heparin-induced antibodies. The laboratory diagnosis of heparin-induced thrombocytopenia may be confirmed by demonstrating platelet activation by heparin-induced antibodies in the patient's plasma. In patients with severe thrombocytopenia, heparin should be stopped and warfarin commenced.

Alopecia and osteoporosis also complicate heparin therapy after prolonged use of full-dose heparin over several months. Rarely, "paradoxical" thrombosis occurs.

Management of bleeding in patients on warfarin depends on the seriousness of the bleeding episode. If the INR is outside the therapeutic range but < 6.0, the patient is not bleeding, and no invasive procedures are planned, several doses of warfarin are omitted and the drug is recommended at a lower dose. If the INR is between 6.0 and 10.0 and the patient is not bleeding, or more rapid reversal is needed to prepare for some invasive procedure, the IV injection of 1 mg vitamin K_1 often restores the INR to the therapeutic range within 24 hours. If the INR is between 10.0 and 20.0, an IV dose of 5 mg vitamin K_1 is recommended, with repeat dosing indicated if the INR remains prolonged at 12 to 24 hours. For more rapid reversal in patients with serious bleeding or an INR > 20.0, 10 mg IV vitamin K_1 should be given and the INR checked every 6 hours. Vitamin K_1 may need to be repeated every 12 hours and supplemented with plasma transfusion or factor concentrate, depending on the urgency of the situation. In the event that bleeding is life-threatening, replacement with factor concentrates is indicated in addition to supplemental intravenous vitamin K_1 (10 mg repeated every 12

hours until the INR is corrected). If the patient requires anticoagulant coverage after administered high-dose vitamin K, heparin should be used until the patient again becomes responsive to warfarin.

During the first trimester of pregnancy, warfarin therapy is associated with a fetal bony embryopathy. Women receiving warfarin should be advised against pregnancy because of this risk. If pregnancy develops, full-dose subcutaneous heparin should be substituted for warfarin. Poisoning with warfarin has occurred in children ingesting coumarin-type rat poisons and occasionally with factitious ingestion. Rarely, areas of skin necrosis are seen, particularly after large loading doses of warfarin. These lesions are associated with thrombi in the microcirculation. In a proportion of these patients, early depletion of protein C and protein S by warfarin in the absence of heparin coverage may explain this thrombotic complication.

Colman RW, Hirsh J, Marder VJ, et al. (eds.): Hemostasis and Thrombosis: Basic Principles and Clinical Practice. 3rd ed. Philadelphia, JB Lippincott Company, 1994. *Authoritative multiauthored textbook provides a comprehensive review of hemostasis, thrombosis, and antithrombotic therapy; useful source for conceptual formulations and reference citations.*

Dalen JE, Hirsh J: ACCP Conference on Antithrombotic Therapy. Chest 102 (Suppl):303S, 1992. *A comprehensive critical review summarizing the status of antithrombotic therapies and corresponding therapeutic recommendations based on objective analysis of published evidence. A very useful critical formulation of antithrombotic strategies.*

Thrombolytic Therapy

GISSI-2: A factorial randomised trial of alteplase versus streptokinase and heparin versus no heparin among 12,490 patients with acute myocardial infarction. Lancet 336:65, 1990. *This factorial randomized trial compared the effects of t-PA versus SK and heparin versus no heparin in the treatment of Italian AMI patients.*

The GUSTO Investigators: An international randomized trial comparing four thrombolytic strategies for acute myocardial infarction. N Engl J Med 329:673, 1993. *This study of 41,021 patients compared the relative efficacy of different thrombolytic agents with intravenous heparin as adjunctive therapy. The results suggest that t-PA plus IV heparin is of greater benefit than SK plus heparin or SK and t-PA with heparin.*

International Study Group: In-hospital mortality and clinical course of 20,891 patients with suspected AMI randomized between alteplase and SK with or without heparin. Lancet 336:71, 1990. *This study combined 8401 patients; there were no differences in mortality between the patients treated with SK and t-PA.*

ISIS-2 (Second International Study of Infarct Survival) Collaborative Group: Randomised trial of intravenous streptokinase, oral aspirin, both, or neither among 17,187 cases of suspected acute myocardial infarction: ISIS-2. Lancet 2:349, 1988. *This cooperative multicenter trial compared the effects of intravenous SK (1.5 million units over 1 hour) and low-dose oral aspirin (160 mg per day) using a four-way factorial design in 17,187 patients.*

ISIS-3 Collaborative Group: ISIS-3: A randomised comparison of streptokinase vs tissue plasminogen activator vs antistreplase and of aspirin plus heparin vs aspirin alone among 41,299 cases of suspected acute myocardial infarction. Lancet 339:753, 1992. *This study randomizing patients with AMI demonstrated that 35-day mortality was equivalent for patients receiving initial therapy with three different thrombolytic agents.*

Antiplatelet Therapy

Antiplatelet Trialists' Collaboration: Collaborative overview of randomised trials of antiplatelet therapy. I. Prevention of death, myocardial infarction, and stroke by prolonged antiplatelet therapy in various categories of patients. Br Med J 308:81, 1994.

Antiplatelet Trialists' Collaboration: Collaborative overview of randomised trials of antiplatelet therapy. II. Maintenance of vascular graft or arterial patency by antiplatelet therapy. Br Med J 308:159, 1994. *Large-scale meta-analyses showed that aspirin reduces vascular occlusive events in about one fourth of patients with symptomatic vascular disease and in patients undergoing vascular procedures.*

Harker LA, Gent M: Antiplatelet agents in the management of thrombotic disorders. *In* Colman RW, Hirsh J, Marder VJ, et al. (eds.): Hemostasis and Thrombosis: Basic Principles and Clinical Practice. 3rd ed. Philadelphia, JP Lippincott, 1994, p 1506. *Summarizes the evidence underlying the recommendation that all patients with symptomatic vascular disease be protected from nonfatal heart attacks, nonfatal strokes, and death by daily aspirin or ticlopidine therapy.*

Janzon L, Bergqvist D, Boberg J, et al.: Prevention of myocardial infarction and stroke in patients with intermittent claudication: Effects of ticlopidine. Results from STIMS, the Swedish Ticlopidine Multicentre Study. Scand J Intern Med 227:301, 1990. *Ticlopidine reduced the risk of stroke, myocardial infarction, or vascular death by about 20% in peripheral vascular disease.*

Anticoagulant Therapy

Furie B, Furie BC: Molecular and cellular biology of blood coagulation. N Engl J Med 326:800, 1992. *Summarizes the current understanding of the production, activation, and regulation of the coagulation serine proteases.*

Hirsh J: Heparin. N Engl J Med 324:1565, 1991. *Reviews heparin's mechanism of action and current therapeutic use.*

Turpie AG, Gent M, Laupacis A, et al.: A comparison of aspirin with placebo in patients treated with warfarin after heart-valve replacement. N Engl J Med 329:524, 1993. *Combining aspirin with warfarin reduces thromboembolic events more effectively than warfarin alone, without significantly increasing bleeding complications in patients with mechanical valves.*

21 PRINCIPLES OF OUTCOME ASSESSMENT

Albert W. Wu

Physicians treat patients to improve or maintain their health. How do we know when medical treatment has had a beneficial effect? For some complaints it is evident when the patient's health has improved. In other cases, the effects of treatment may not be immediately apparent. For a given patient, it may be difficult to know what treatment or course of action is likely to lead to the best outcome. Furthermore, several kinds of outcomes may be important to consider when evaluating a treatment.

Traditionally, data obtained from a medical history, physical examination, and laboratory tests form the basis of treatment evaluation. These include parameters such as clinical events, physical findings, laboratory abnormalities, symptoms, and mortality. However, as the emphasis in medicine has shifted from acute care to treating chronic diseases, conventional measures have not adequately addressed effects of treatment on the patient's overall health. Recently, new approaches for assessing patient outcome have been developed that use different data sources and evaluate a wider spectrum of outcomes than traditional clinical research. Some of these approaches use questionnaires to assess the quality of life and patient satisfaction, whereas others use insurance claims data to examine costs. As issues of cost-effectiveness and quality improvement are debated, outcome assessment is becoming increasingly important.

DEFINITIONS

Outcomes research is a comprehensive approach to determining the effects of medical care using a variety of data sources and measurement methods. Outcomes research includes the rigorous deter-

mination of what works in medical care and what does not and how different providers compare with regard to their effects on patient outcomes.

In outcomes research, a distinction is made between efficacy and effectiveness. *Efficacy* refers to how a treatment works in ideal circumstances, when delivered to selected patients by providers most skilled at providing it. *Effectiveness* refers to how a treatment works under ordinary conditions by the average practitioner for the typical patient.

Outcome assessment plays an important role in studies of the quality of care. *Quality of care* can be defined as the difference between efficacy and effectiveness that can be attributed to care providers. According to Donabedian's widely accepted model of quality of care, it is necessary to assess the "structure, process, and outcomes" of care. *Structure* refers to stable elements that form the basis of the health system, such as the type of facility, administrative organization, and provider qualifications. *Process* refers to what happens in the medical interaction and includes the technical and interpersonal skills of the physician and other providers. Process measures compare care delivered to relevant standards. In this framework, *outcomes* are the measurable events and observations that are presumed to occur in part due to the structure and process of medical care.

THE IMPORTANCE OF OUTCOME ASSESSMENT

Several factors have led to the current interest in patient outcomes. These include the rising cost of health care, changes in the organization of financing of care, findings of unexplained variation in physicians' practice patterns, recognition of the limitations of available information about the effects of many treatments, and increased adoption of a model of shared patient and physician decision making.

The cost of medical care in the United States has grown from $250.1 billion and 9.2% of gross domestic product (GDP) in 1980 to $903.3 billion and 14.4% of GDP in 1992. Rising costs, coupled with evidence that performance of some medical procedures may be inappropriate, have led to the desire to assess the relative effectiveness of different treatments. Treatments deemed less effective could be eliminated, resulting in reduced expenditures or allocation of those resources to treatments that produce greater benefits.

The growth of pre-paid care and prospective payment for hospital care has promoted increased competition among health care providers. Managed care organizations and insurers now compete for corporate buyers, and individual physicians compete for inclusion on preferred provider lists. Most of the competition is currently on the basis of price and services offered. However, "report cards" detailing performance of health plans, institutions, and individual physicians on a variety of outcomes are under development as mechanisms to improve consumer choice.

Researchers have documented substantial geographic differences in the use of medical procedures on apparently similar patients. For example, little variation exists in the incidence of inguinal herniorrhaphy, but large variations occur in rates of tonsillectomy (Fig. 21–1). Related studies have shown that the per capita costs of hospitalization for the residents of Boston are about twice those for the residents of New Haven. Whether these differences reflect overuse in high-use areas or underuse in low-use areas requires additional information.

A good deal is known about the efficacy and safety of drugs introduced since the 1960's. Less is known about the efficacy of many common diagnostic tests and procedures, such as endoscopy versus upper gastrointestinal series for patients with dyspepsia. Still less is known about using these tests in combination or repeatedly, e.g., the efficacy of repeated magnetic resonance scans for patients with persistent headache. Nearly nothing is known about the efficacy of cognitive and interpersonal services such as listening to or reassuring patients (see Ch. 14.1). Because less is known about effectiveness than efficacy, it is not surprising that practicing physicians face considerable uncertainty.

The traditional model of clinical decision making, in which patients delegate choice to the physician, is giving way to a model of shared decision making, in which patients actively participate in the choice of treatment. This model requires increased emphasis on patient preferences for risks and outcomes in the choices among treatment options, and increased patient understanding (see Ch. 2).

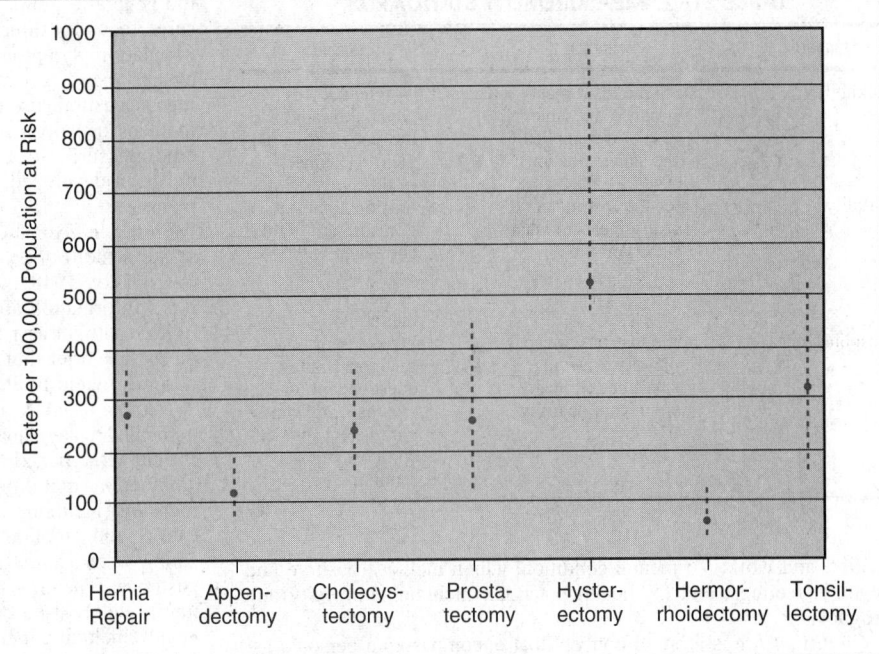

FIGURE 21–1. Mean and range of age- and sex-standardized rates for common surgical procedures in New England. (From McPherson K, Wennberg JE, Hovind OB, et al.: Small-area variations in the use of common surgical procedures: An international comparison of New England, England, and Norway. N Engl J Med 307:1310, 1982. Copyright 1982, the Massachusetts Medical Society.)

For all of the reasons stated above, activity directed at outcome assessment has grown rapidly. In 1986, the Health Care Financing Administration (HCFA) began to report hospital mortality rates for specific conditions. In 1987, the Joint Commission on Accreditation of Hospitals announced a shift from traditional structural measures of quality assurance to quality assessment based on outcomes adjusted for the severity of patients' disease. In 1989, Congress established the Agency for Health Care Policy and Research to promote research on medical outcomes and develop guidelines for clinical practice. The Health Security Act proposed in 1994 contained provisions for the ongoing collection of outcome data. It is hoped that outcomes research will make it possible to sort out what works best in medicine and how treatments should be used for a given patient. Better information should lead to improved clinical decision making, rational health policy at the local and national level, and appropriate payment rules.

TYPES OF HEALTH OUTCOMES

Outcomes research considers a broad range of indicators, including conventional clinical measures such as mortality, disease or treatment complications, persistence of pathology, physiologic or laboratory abnormalities, deformity, signs and symptoms, and adverse clinical events. In addition, outcomes research considers patient perspectives such as quality of life and satisfaction with care. Still other types of outcomes are important from a societal perspective. These include the use of health care resources and their associated costs and economic losses due to disability or death (Table 21–1). The principal outcomes of interest can be summarized as the six "D's" of death, disease, disability, discomfort, dissatisfaction, and dollars.

MEASUREMENT STANDARDS (Table 21–2)

To be useful, a test must meet standards for reliability, validity, and responsiveness. *Reliability* concerns the extent to which a measuring procedure yields consistent results on repeated trials. Although the measurement of any phenomenon always contains a certain amount of chance error, systematic error can lead to invalid results. For example, an intelligence test that focuses on knowledge specific to certain cultural groups can produce a spurious association between race and intelligence. *Validity* is the degree to which a test measures what it is intended to measure, e.g., if a pain questionnaire actually measures pain rather than the patient's mood. *Responsiveness* is the ability of a test to detect clinically meaningful changes. For example, if a treatment results in an important im-

provement in health-related quality of life, a measure should be able to detect that difference.

PATIENT-ASSESSED OUTCOMES

QUALITY OF LIFE. Several terms are used almost interchangeably to refer to the concept of "health," including quality of life, health status, functional status, and health-related quality of life. In 1948 the World Health Organization defined *health* as "a state of complete physical, mental, and social well-being, and not merely the absence of disease and infirmity." This definition reflects the positive and negative dimensions of health and its multidimensional nature.

Bergner identified five dimensions of *health status:* (1) genetic and inherited characteristics; (2) biochemical, physiologic, and anatomic condition, including impairment of these systems, disease, signs, and symptoms; (3) *functional status,* which includes performance of the usual activities of life, such as self-care, physical ac-

TABLE 21–1. HEALTH OUTCOMES

Outcome	Example for a Patient with Myocardial Infarction
Clinical	
Mortality	Death in hospital
Pathology	Coronary artery narrowing
Nonfatal clinical event	Stroke
Hospital re-admission	Re-admission within 30 days of hospital discharge
Complication of disease or treatment	Sternal wound infection after coronary artery bypass grafting
Physiologic test	Ejection fraction
Laboratory test	CPK-MB isoenzyme
Symptom	Angina pectoris
Patient-reported	
Health-related quality of life	Ability to perform usual physical activities
Satisfaction with care	Patient ratings of overall quality of care
Cost	
Utilization of health services	Number of physician visits
Direct cost	Cost of physician visits and prescription medications
Indirect cost	Loss of income due to missed days of work

TABLE 21-2. MEASUREMENT STANDARDS

Standard	Definition	Example
Reliability	Does the instrument produce the same results if reapplied to the same situation?	CD4 lymphocyte counts repeated for the same individual yield the same results.
Validity	Does the instrument really measure what it purports to?	Scores on a pain questionnaire are highly correlated with scores on established pain measures.
Responsiveness	Is the instrument capable of identifying small but clinically significant changes?	The mean score on a functional status questionnaire increases significantly with use of inhaled corticosteroids for asthma.

tivities, and work; (4) mental condition, which includes positive and negative feelings; and (5) health potential, including longevity and prognosis.

Quality of life is a broad concept that encompasses a person's assessment of all aspects of his/her experience. Because it includes important dimensions of life that are distant from medical concern (e.g., achievement and spiritual fulfillment), it is useful to focus on aspects of quality of life that may be affected by therapeutic measures. *Health-related quality of life* encompasses several dimensions of health status that are directly experienced by the person, including physical functioning, mental health, cognitive functioning, social and role functioning, energy, general health perceptions, symptoms, sexual functioning, and sleep (Table 21-3).

STRUCTURE OF MEASURES AND MODES OF ADMINISTRATION. Measuring health-related quality of life relies on assembling indicators of different dimensions. Some measures consist of a single global health item such as the question, "Would you say your health is excellent, very good, good, fair, or poor?" However, most instruments consist of a series of questions or "items" that are summed to yield a score for each specific dimension.

Questionnaires can be self-administered or given by trained interviewers. Interviews are labor intensive but ensure compliance and minimize misinterpretations. Interviews may be conducted in person or by phone. Sometimes a surrogate respondent is used to estimate results desired from the patient, such as a parent who reports on the child's health.

TYPES OF QUALITY-OF-LIFE MEASURES. There are two basic approaches to quality-of-life assessment: generic and disease-specific. The format of measures may be single indexes, health profiles, or utility measures.

Generic instruments are designed for use across different diseases, treatments, settings, and patient groups. The major advantage is that they can be used in any population and allow comparisons

TABLE 21-3. DIMENSIONS OF HEALTH-RELATED QUALITY OF LIFE

Dimension	Description
Physical functioning	Activities of daily living, strenuous activities
Mental health	Anxiety, depression, well-being, behavioral and emotional control
Social functioning	Quantity and quality of social contacts
Role functioning	Ability to perform work or usual activities
Cognitive functioning	Attention, memory, concentration
Energy	Energy and fatigue
General health perceptions	Global self-assessment of health
Pain	Severity and frequency of pain
Symptoms	Nausea, headache, dizziness, etc.
Sexual functioning	Performance and satisfaction
Sleep	Quantity and quality of sleep

of the relative impact of various health interventions. However, they may be unresponsive to changes in specific conditions and may be too general to guide clinical decision making. *Disease-specific* measures focus on dimensions of health related to a particular disease, population, symptom, or problem and may be more responsive to a change than a generic instrument. For example, the Health Assessment Questionnaire (Fries, 1982), widely used in studies of arthritis, includes questions about hand grip strength and pain. Disease-specific measures are easily understood by clinicians but to date have not been developed and tested to the same extent as generic instruments.

Single indices attempt to reduce several concepts to a unidimensional scale. For example, the Karnofsky Performance Status score (Karnofsky, 1948), which is commonly used in cancer trials, combines information about the ability to work, to carry out normal activities without assistance, and to care for personal needs. Single indices are brief but are less reliable than multi-item scales and generally yield limited information.

Health profiles attempt to measure all important dimensions of health-related quality of life. For example, the *Sickness Impact Profile* (Bergner, 1981) assesses a physical dimension (including ambulation, mobility, body care, and movement), a psychosocial dimension (including social interaction, alertness behavior, communication, and emotional behavior), and additional domains including eating, work, home management, sleep and rest, and recreation and pastimes. The *SF-36 health survey* (Ware, 1992) is a brief (36-item), widely used questionnaire that assesses several dimensions of health including general health perceptions, physical functioning, role functioning, social functioning, pain, mental health, and energy (Fig. 21-2).

Utility measures are derived from economic and decision theory. The term *utility* refers to the desirability or preference that the individual has for a particular condition. Utility is summarized as a score ranging from 0.0 representing death to 1.0 representing perfect health. This score reflects both the patient's health status and the value he/she places on that state. In economic analyses, utilities are used to justify devoting resources to a treatment. They can also be used to generate quality-adjusted life-years. However, because they are expressed as a single score, they are lacking in detail and do not describe the domains in which changes occur. The *Quality of Well-being scale* (Kaplan, 1988) is a widely used instrument that combines questions about various dimensions of functional status with community-derived preferences for these states to generate a score.

PATIENT SATISFACTION. *Patient satisfaction* refers to patients' subjective evaluations of their health care. Patient ratings of care reflect what they think is important about the quality of care, including the doctor-patient relationship and what they can judge about the adequacy of diagnosis and therapy. They also predict patients' subsequent behavior, including how they comply with medications prescribed, whether they return or go elsewhere, and whether they recommend a physician to others. The method used to elicit a patient's opinions of care can affect results dramatically. For example, when the response choices use the word *satisfied*, most patients choose the best possible answer. Rating scales (e.g., excellent to poor) result in a better distribution of responses. The Patient Satisfaction Questionnaire (PSQ) (Ware, 1988) and the Medical Outcomes Study 9-item Visit Rating Form (Rubin, 1993) are examples of carefully constructed instruments to assess general medical care and specific physician visits.

COST STUDIES

The basic formula of a cost study is a cost-benefit ratio. Studies most often examine direct costs (the costs of treatment itself) but may also include estimates of indirect costs (the costs of disability or loss of livelihood). Several types of cost analyses are possible (Table 21-4). *Cost-identification* studies enumerate the cost of applying a treatment to a specified population under a particular set of conditions. These studies describe the natural history of costs without comparing the benefits of one intervention with those of alternatives. *Cost-benefit* studies compare the costs of a treatment and cost savings due to benefits of the treatment in monetary units. A limitation is that all benefits, including decreased mortality, must be expressed in dollar terms. Techniques for assigning value to a human life are controversial. *Cost-effectiveness* analysis compares the costs and benefits of a treatment in terms of reduced mortality or

(circle one number on each line)

ACTIVITIES	Yes, Limited A Lot	Yes, Limited A Little	No, Not Limited At All
a. **Vigorous activities,** such as running, lifting heavy objects, participating in strenuous sports	1	2	3
b. **Moderate activities,** such as moving a table, pushing a vacuum cleaner, bowling, or playing golf	1	2	3
c. Lifting or carrying groceries	1	2	3
d. Climbing **several** flights of stairs	1	2	3
e. Climbing **one** flight of stairs	1	2	3
f. Bending, kneeling, or stooping	1	2	3
g. Walking **more than a mile**	1	2	3
h. Walking **several blocks**	1	2	3
i. Walking **one block**	1	2	3
j. Bathing or dressing yourself	1	2	3

FIGURE 21–2. Sample questions assessing physical functioning from the SF-36 health survey. (From Ware JE, Snow KK, Kosinski M, et al.: SF-36 Health Survey: Manual and Interpretation Guide. Boston, The Health Institute, 1993.)

morbidity, such as years of life saved or quality-adjusted life-years saved. *Cost-utility* analysis expresses the costs and benefits of treatment in terms of utility scores.

STUDY DESIGNS (see Ch. 14.3)

Outcome assessments employ a variety of research designs, including experiments (e.g., randomized controlled trials) and observational studies (e.g., cross-sectional, cohort, and case control studies). Meta-analysis is used to pool data from many studies. Appropriateness studies examine if treatments are used so that they produce more health than harm. Each of these study designs has strengths and limitations (Table 21–5).

RANDOMIZED CONTROLLED TRIALS. The randomized controlled trial (RCT) involves selecting representative subjects, randomly assigning them to treatment and control groups, and fol-

TABLE 21–4. TYPES OF COST STUDIES

Kind of Cost Studies	Description
Cost-identification	Enumerates cost of applying a treatment to a specified population under a particular set of conditions
Cost-benefit	Compares the costs of treatment and cost savings due to benefits of the treatment in dollar terms
Cost-effectiveness	Compares the costs and benefits of a treatment in terms of reduced mortality or morbidity such as years of life saved or quality-adjusted life-years saved
Cost-utility	Compares the costs and benefits of a treatment in terms of utility scores

TABLE 21–5. STUDY DESIGNS

	Strengths	Weaknesses
Experiment	Strongest evidence for cause and effect	Expensive Long duration Unsuitable for many questions Not useful for rare outcomes Limited generalizability
Cross-sectional	Short duration May study several outcomes Controls subject selection Controls measurements Yields prevalence	Does not establish causal relationships Unmeasured differences between groups
Cohort	Establishes sequence of events Avoids bias in measuring predictors Yields incidence, relative risk, excess risk	Relatively expensive Long duration Requires large sample size Not useful for rare outcomes
Case control	Useful for rare conditions Relatively inexpensive Short duration Yields odds ratio	Potential sampling bias Limited to one outcome variable Does not yield prevalence, incidence, or relative risk
Meta-analysis	Increases statistical power for outcomes Helpful when studies disagree	Quality of secondary data varies Requires combining data from different studies

lowing them for the outcomes of interest. The randomized double-blind placebo-controlled trial is considered the gold standard for evaluating treatment efficacy. The experimental design allows the greatest control of the influence of confounding variables and permits causal inferences. However, RCT's also have shortcomings. Data collection is time consuming and costly. Many research questions are not suitable for experimental designs, such as when ethical concerns rule out placebo controls or when outcomes are rare. Although blinding study subjects and physicians to treatment assignment is possible in studies of medications, it is more difficult when studying medical and surgical procedures. Inclusion and exclusion criteria often limit generalizability of the results.

OBSERVATIONAL STUDIES. Rather than assigning patients to a treatment of interest, observational studies examine the outcomes of medicine as it is practiced. In *cross-sectional studies,* all variables are measured at a single point in time. Although cross-sectional studies are relatively inexpensive and can provide useful descriptions of the prevalence of diseases, treatments, and outcomes, they provide weak evidence for causal associations because they do not account for temporal relationships.

In *cohort studies,* patients are followed over a period of time. Prospective cohort studies can provide evidence for cause-and-effect relationships between predictors and outcomes because the predictors are measured before the outcomes occur. If some patients receive a treatment and some do not, evidence for effectiveness can also be derived. In some cases, observational studies may use a *quasi-experimental design* to take advantage of "natural experiments" such as introducing a new treatment or changing insurance coverage. As in clinical trials, prospective data collection is expensive and time consuming, and cohort studies are not useful when outcomes are rare.

In *case-control studies,* the prevalence of risk factors in a sample of subjects who have a disease or outcome (the cases) is compared with that in a sample who do not (the controls). Case-control studies are inexpensive and uniquely efficient for studying rare conditions. However, a case-control study can examine only one outcome because cases are selected on this basis. In addition, because cases and controls are selected separately and data on predictors are collected retrospectively, these studies are susceptible to bias.

All observational studies are subject to significant confounding because groups may differ with regard to measured or unmeasured characteristics. Risk-adjustment methods are used to control for factors, such as patient demographics and severity of illness, that are unequally distributed between groups and that may be related to patient outcomes. However, inferences must be made cautiously because unmeasured variations in patients, practitioners, and processes may be the real explanation for differences in outcomes.

META-ANALYSIS/LITERATURE SYNTHESIS. Literature synthesis can be used to characterize the extent and quality of medical evidence and to summarize findings of existing studies. *Meta-analysis* is a systematic synthesis of literature that uses statistical methods (see Ch. 14.3) to obtain a quantitative estimate of the effect of a particular intervention from the effects reported in many studies. Its main purposes are to identify gaps in knowledge, increase statistical power for primary outcomes, and resolve controversy when studies disagree. Its primary disadvantage is that it relies on secondary data. If those data are inadequate, little additional information can be generated. In addition, it may be difficult to combine data from studies conducted at different times using different methods on different patient populations.

APPROPRIATENESS STUDIES. Appropriateness studies establish standard indications against which the use of a particular medical intervention is judged. Methods to produce indications involve careful analysis of what is known and the use of expert physicians to fill in gaps in knowledge and come to consensus about indications. Appropriateness studies can inform guidelines to help the practicing physician decide under what circumstances a procedure should or should not be done.

DATA SOURCES

Outcomes research uses a variety of sources of data, including patient questionnaires, medical records, and claims and administrative data files (Table 21–6).

PATIENT QUESTIONNAIRES. Outcomes research frequently uses a questionnaire-based approach to assess patient outcomes. Patients are commonly asked about their ability to function, how they feel, and their satisfaction with care received. Sometimes subjective data from patients can provide valuable information that may not be evident from physiologic measurements. Surprisingly, studies have shown that these data are at least as reliable as conventional biochemical or physiologic indices. However, although patient reports provide a unique perspective, measures must be chosen with care. Data collection requires cooperation of patients and providers, and selective nonparticipation can threaten generalizability. Study designs must recognize the limitations of patient recall and the fact that patients' evaluations of outcome may be affected by their expectations.

MEDICAL RECORD REVIEW. Detailed clinical information can be collected unobtrusively by retrospective review of medical records. To maximize reliability, abstraction must be performed by trained reviewers with a clinical background.

CLAIMS AND ADMINISTRATIVE DATA. Claims data analysis uses data files, such as those maintained by the Medicare program, to explore patterns of care and clinical outcomes. The HCFA maintains a database on all Medicare beneficiaries and providers.

Data elements include demographics, characteristics of hospitals and other providers, expenditures, diagnoses, procedures, dates of service, and complications. A large amount of data is available, including a longitudinal record of all utilization and costs for a 5% national sample of beneficiaries since 1967 and all submitted claims since 1991.

Medicare data have revealed striking variations in clinical practice, particularly in the performance of diagnostic and therapeutic procedures. They also provide population-based descriptions of frequency of death and complications and are used to monitor trends over time. However, several problems limit the value of claims data for assessing medical effectiveness or evaluating the quality of care. Claims data may not contain enough detail about clinical features thought to affect prognosis, such as the stage of colon cancer. Thus, it may be difficult to identify clinically relevant patient groups and to control for clinical factors likely to affect outcome.

CHALLENGES

Many challenges remain before outcome assessment can be applied to full advantage. In particular, there are large gaps in our understanding of how the structure and process of care influence patient outcomes.

Clinical trials are needed to examine the effectiveness as well as the efficacy of existing and newly developed treatments and procedures. Studies that measure the effectiveness of treatments need to examine short- and long-term outcomes. This requires data systems that can characterize variation in the use of treatments and patient outcomes to examine the effectiveness of services, to disseminate information, and to evaluate the quality of medical care. Better research tools and measurement techniques are needed, including more reliable, valid, and understandable measures of patient-reported outcomes tested in more diverse populations. Better risk-adjustment models are needed to facilitate valid reports and comparisons of patient outcomes.

Brook RH: Quality of care: Do we care? Ann Intern Med 115:486, 1991. *Forceful argument for improving the quality of US health care by creating national databases to increase knowledge about effectiveness and developing standards of medical practice.*

Guyatt GH, Feeny DH, Patrick DL: Measuring health-related quality of life. Ann Intern Med 118:622, 1993. *Outline of what makes a useful measure of health-related quality of life, and basic approaches to assessment.*

Hulley SB, Cummings SR: Designing Clinical Research. An Epidemiologic Approach. Baltimore, Williams & Wilkins, 1988. *Highly accessible primer that walks the reader step by step from conceiving a research question, through designing a study, to writing a grant proposal.*

Kaplan RM, Anderson JP: The quality of well-being scale: Rationale for a single quality of life index. *In* Walker SR, Rosser RM (eds.): Quality of life assessment and application. Lancaster, England, MTP Press, 1988, p 51. *Description of a widely used health status instrument that takes into account both morbidity and mortality.*

McDowell I, Newell C: Measuring Health: A Guide to Rating Scales and Questionnaires. New York, Oxford University Press, 1987. *A review of some 50 leading health measurement methods with critical comparisons between methods and summary tables comparing the scope of each instrument.*

Ware JE, Snow KK, Kosinski M, et al.: SF-36 Health Survey: Manual and Interpretation Guide. Boston, The Health Institute, 1993. *A user-friendly how-to manual that covers the conceptual basis, development, testing, and application of an extensively used brief self-administered health status questionnaire.*

TABLE 21–6. DATA SOURCES FOR OUTCOME ASSESSMENTS

Data Source	Advantages	Disadvantages
Patient surveys	Provides patient's perspective	Labor intensive
	Provides reliable data	Requires cooperation of patient ± providers
		Selective nonparticipation
		Patient may have trouble with recall
		Evaluations of outcome affected by expectation
Chart abstraction	Unobtrusive	Costly
	Detailed clinical information	Labor intensive
		May be unreliable
	Can be performed retrospectively	Variables may not be recorded consistently
Claims data	Unobtrusive	Data lack clinical detail for identifying patient groups or risk-adjustment
	Low cost	
	Large number	
	Broad cross-section of patients	May be inaccurate

22 OVERVIEW OF IMAGING TECHNIQUES FOR THE FUTURE

James M. Mountz and Hoby Hetherington

MANAGEMENT OF FUTURE CLINICAL IMAGING

Over the past decade, imaging technology has significantly advanced the accuracy of diagnosis owing to increased sensitivity and specificity of imaging modalities alone or combined with injectable contrast agents or radiopharmaceuticals. The clinical applications and expansion of the imaging techniques for the future depend on recognizing their clinical value, as demonstrated by patient outcome benefit.

Computers have become vital tools for radiologic clinical practice and have advanced the cost-effectiveness of imaging. Picture archiving and communications systems (PACS) have emerged as an important part of digital imaging technology. They enable image and multimedia data distribution, archiving, and transmission and represent the future of image management. The workstation will become the point of contact between a PACS and the radiologist or referring physician. These workstations must be able to handle efficiently the large volume of images and provide enough flexibility to allow the electronic systems to grow as medical imaging technology evolves.

ADVANCES IN CONVENTIONAL IMAGING MODALITIES

ULTRASONIC TECHNIQUES. Endoluminal ultrasonography has allowed the imaging of anatomy by inserting small ultrasonic probes into the major vessels or other body lumina to visualize nearly all organ systems of the body. Ultrasound probes are designed to pass through the instrument channel of ordinary fiberoptic or video endoscopes.

Intravascular ultrasonography (IVUS) is a new imaging system composed fundamentally of a miniature ultrasound (US) transducer mounted at the end of a catheter. The system may use either a single motor-driven rotating US element or a static ring of phased-array transducers. Ultrasound imaging frequencies range from 20 to 30 MHz in most clinical IVUS systems and up to 40 MHz in systems used for *in vitro* investigations. Catheter sizes range from 4.3 to 8.0 Fr. This catheter-based system, when introduced into an adequately sized blood vessel, produces real-time, two-dimensional (2D), cross-sectional images of the vascular structure. High-resolution images of vascular lumen, vessel wall, and vascular plaque are achievable (Fig. 22–1).

Applications for IVUS include guiding and evaluating endovascular interventional procedures, correlating IVUS results with histology in diseased vessels, early detection and sonographic tissue characterization of atherosclerosis, and three-dimensional (3D) voxel modeling of vascular structures by computerized reformation of 2D cross-sectional images. IVUS systems combined with other catheter-based therapeutic endovascular devices (e.g., angioplasty, atherectomy) are also under development.

With new techniques in transvaginal US, higher resolution allows earlier diagnosis of fetal developmental anomalies. Transvaginal echography is used to examine asymptomatic patients at risk for repeated abortion in the first trimester of pregnancy. It has been established that a reliable echographic finding—the normal sequential appearance of the yolk sac of the embryo and the presence of normal fetal heart activity—can be used prognostically for the future course of pregnancy. Transvaginal US is playing an increasing important role in detecting congenital heart defects among patients with high risk for fetal anomalies (see Ch. 27); they are usually performed at 12 to 16 weeks' gestation. A normal echocardiogram provides immeasurable reassurance to the family at risk. When a prenatal diagnosis of a structural abnormality is made, the health care team can outline a management strategy to optimize the care and support given to the fetus, mother, and family. Transvaginal US in the early second trimester is a useful tool both for detecting fetal cardiac structural defects and for providing anatomic evaluation of multiple organ systems in fetal development (Fig. 22–2).

US examination of the fetal heart has become increasingly sophisticated. Fetal echocardiography is now critical in making an early and accurate assessment of cardiovascular structure. A complete fetal echocardiographic study should include the structural and rhythm analysis using a combination of 2D imaging, M-mode scanning, pulsed- and continuous-wave Doppler measurements, and color-flow mapping.

Other endoluminal US modalities (e.g., transrectal or transesophageal US) may also be used to assess extraluminal anatomy and pathology, within the limits of the depth of penetration of the transducer. For example, a 20-MHz mechanical linear probe can be used within the upper gastrointestinal tract, pancreatic duct, biliary tree, and colon. Rotational mechanical sector scanning probes as well as phased array probes are also useful. US probes are best used for high-resolution imaging of focal endoscopically visible lesions. Endoscopic visualization enables direction of the probe to the lesion of interest.

ANGIOGRAPHIC TECHNIQUES. Digital subtraction angiography (DSA) is a valuable and frequently used diagnostic technique that allows the physician to evaluate vascular anatomy and pathology. More recently 3D time-of-flight magnetic resonance angiography (MRA) and intra-arterial DSA have been used to compare pre- and postoperative evaluation of the carotid bifurcation. Although MRA is emerging as an accurate modality for imaging carotid bifurcations, significant limitations still exist in its ability to adequately demonstrate the intracranial circulation.

Color-flow duplex surveillance of graft patency is a valuable tool to evaluate peripheral bypass procedures. For example, color-aided duplex Doppler sonography is valuable to rule out transplant renal artery stenosis and to determine the feasibility and safety of intra-arterial DSA in hypertensive renal allograft recipients on an outpatient basis. This imaging modality allows renal angiography to be reserved to those patients with an inconclusive US study.

Contrast-enhanced electron-beam computed tomography (CT) (100-msec scan time) is an ultrafast CT method which, among other applications, can effectively and noninvasively assess the clinical diagnosis of pulmonary embolism.

Spiral CT is a new technology that couples continuous tube rotation with continuous scan table movement. This allows a data set to be compiled that has continuous anatomic information without establishing arbitrary boundaries at section interfaces as in conventional CT. The unique method of data collection of the spiral CT scanner has been combined with dynamic intravenous (IV) contrast material bolus protocols to image the abdominal vasculature, including the aorta, renal arteries, and splanchnic circulation. Through various techniques of image processing, including surface renderings and maximum intensity projection (MIP) image display, it is possible to obtain excellent anatomic detail of the aorta and its major branches. Vessel contrast on spiral CT scans is excellent and can be used in evaluating renal artery stenosis, the degree of carotid artery stenosis (Fig. 22–3), and other pathologic conditions including celiac bypass graft occlusion, abdominal aortic dissection, and abdominal aortic aneurysm (Fig. 22–4).

FIGURE 22–1. Ultrasonic cross-sectional image *(left)* obtained *in vitro* (at 40 MHz) with the corresponding photomicrograph of the histologic cross-section *(right)* obtained from a mesenteric superior artery. Bright echoes of the internal elastic lamina and adventitia circumscribe the hypoechoic media. A distinct media was observed echographically in the absence of a lesion (at 10 o'clock). In the presence of an extensive lesion *(asterisk)* the media becomes invisible echographically. The corresponding histologic section reveals absence of the media in this region. (Verhoeff van Glieson stain [calibration 1 mm], magnification ×6.) (From Gussenhoven EJ, Frietman PAV, The SHK, et al.: Assessment of medial thinning in atherosclerosis by intravascular ultrasound. Am J Cardiol 68:1625, 1991.)

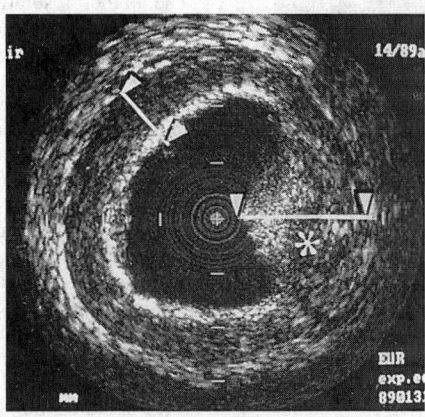
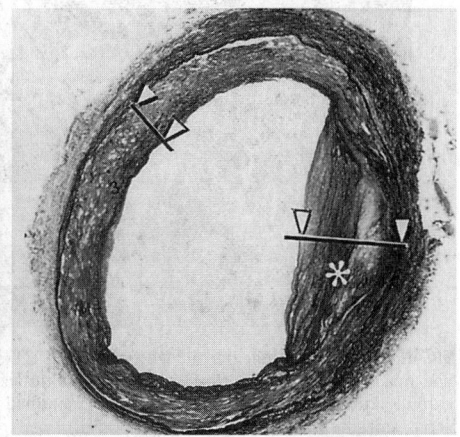

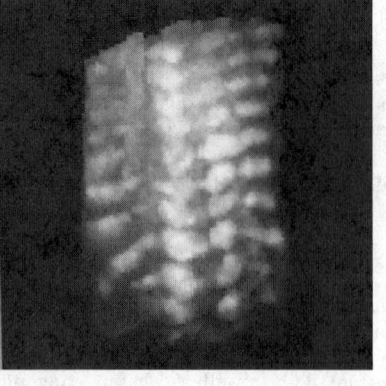

FIGURE 22-2. 3D ultrasound image of a 22-week gestational age fetus showing the posterior ribs and spine *(left)*. A magnified view of the lower thoracic spine and ribs *(right)* is obtained using the same acquisition volume data. 3D imaging provides improved visualization of the spine curvature and bony thorax. (Courtesy of TR Nelson, PhD, and DH Pretorius, MD, San Diego, CA.)

MAGNETIC RESONANCE IMAGING (MRI) (see Ch. 33.5)

Over the past 10 years remarkable progress has been made in the methods and equipment used to acquire MR images. With improvements in image quality and methods for achieving tissue contrast between healthy and abnormal tissue and decreases in the amount of time to acquire such images, MRI has become a powerful tool for clinical diagnosis. Four areas that should experience rapid growth during the next several years are (1) cardiac imaging of function and coronary angiography (see Ch. 33.6), (2) brain functional imaging, (3) spectroscopic imaging of metabolite content in human brain, and (4) high field high-resolution imaging. Just as much of the progress over the last 10 years was made possible by the availability of higher field superconducting magnets (0.5T to 1.5T) as opposed to their lower field resistive counterparts, similar improvements should be expected from the increasing use of the next generation of high field magnets, 3T and above. These improvements will be manifested as signal-to-noise ratio improves and spatial resolution increases.

BRAIN FUNCTIONAL IMAGING. Recently it has been demonstrated that images collected using a gradient echo sequence are sensitive to the oxygenation state of the cerebral venous system. Specifically, regions that increase their oxyhemoglobin: deoxyhemoglobin ratio show increases in image signal intensity. When performing a mental or physical task, blood flow to the affected area of the brain increases, typically outstripping the requirement for oxygen utilization. This in turn causes the venous system to have a higher oxyhemoglobin: deoxyhemoglobin content, thereby enhancing its signal intensity. By subtracting images acquired before and during the activating task, the region of the brain associated with the task is highlighted. This method has been used to localize the effects of visual stimulation, various motor functions, and word association. Figure 22–5 shows an activation image acquired during finger tapping. The activation (those regions of the brain that show

a significant increase in signal) is thresholded and then overlaid on a high-resolution anatomic image for reference. These images can be acquired with submillimeter resolution or with subsecond time resolution using rapid imaging methods. Although these studies can be performed at clinical field strengths of 1.5T, the effect of deoxyhemoglobin is quadratic with field strength such that much larger enhancements in signal intensity can be seen at higher field strengths. The increased sensitivity can then be used to generate higher resolution maps or acquire maps with more rapid temporal resolution. To date these methods have been used primarily as a tool for mapping cortical function in healthy subjects; however, their application in patients with neurologic disorders and the localization of the affected regions and their relative function is virtually limitless.

SPECTROSCOPIC IMAGING. Over the past 5 years there has been a dramatic expansion in the number of MRI systems that can perform spectroscopic measurements that permit the measurement of low concentration of cerebral metabolites. In epilepsy, measurements of *N*-acetyl aspartate (NAA), a specific marker for neurons, has allowed a noninvasive determination of neuronal loss, permitting lateralization of the affected areas. Similar measurements in Alzheimer's disease may also prove useful in localizing affected brain regions. In multiple sclerosis, measurements of choline—a compound that becomes elevated during membrane breakdown—permits an assessment of the degree of active demyelination. Although to date most of these measurements have been performed using methods that acquire a single region at a time, typically 8 cc or more, metabolic imaging methods (the creation of images representing the content of a metabolite) offer much for the future. Recent methods have permitted the planar and multislice imaging of these compounds. Seizure foci can be determined by using spectroscopic imaging (Fig. 22–6). By acquiring spectroscopic data in an image format, regions of the brain showing selective neuronal loss or membrane breakdown can be visualized. These spectroscopic images, when combined with high-resolution MRI, provide a correlation between anatomic and metabolic alterations.

HIGH-RESOLUTION IMAGING. The improved signal-to-noise ratio at 4.1T permits images of the human brain with 250 to 500 μM in plane resolution (a factor of 2 to 4 higher than that commonly obtained at 1.5T) from tomographic slices 3 mm thick. The higher resolution improves visualization of the basal ganglia and thalamus, frequently the site of small strokes (Fig. 22–7A). The images display excellent definition of a number of anatomic features of the brain (caudate head, globus pallidus, and putamen). The greater spatial resolution and gray/white matter contrast combine to improve the definition of the hippocampus, critical to diagnose temporal lobe epilepsy (Fig. 22–7B). Specifically, the parahippocampal gyrus, Ammon's horn with the alveus extending into the fornix, the subiculum, and the overlying superficial medullary stratum are well defined. The enhanced T_2^* contrast improves visualization of iron-rich structures such as the red nuclei and substantia nigra, which may aid in the diagnosis of idiopathic Parkinson's disease (Fig. 22–7C). Finally, the T_2^* contrast and high spatial resolution enable visualization of small cerebral vessels, which are not detectable in conventional clinical imaging studies (Fig. 22–7D). Although the number of high field systems at this time is limited, their potential for expanding our knowledge of disease states through imaging is

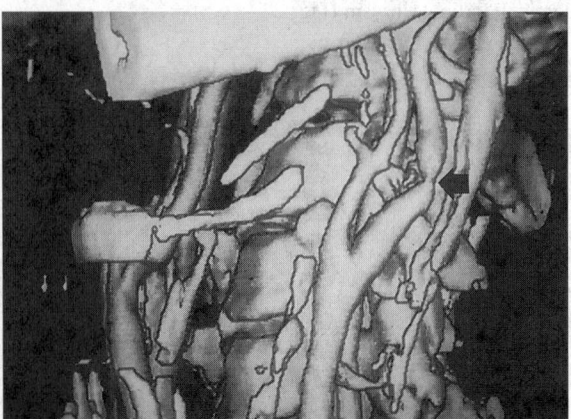

FIGURE 22-3. 3D rendered image from spiral CT of the neck. The bones and opacified vessels are clearly seen. A stenotic lesion of the left internal carotid artery distal to the bifurcation is identified *(arrow)*. (Courtesy of Jerry Arenson, Elscint, Inc., Hackensack, NJ.)

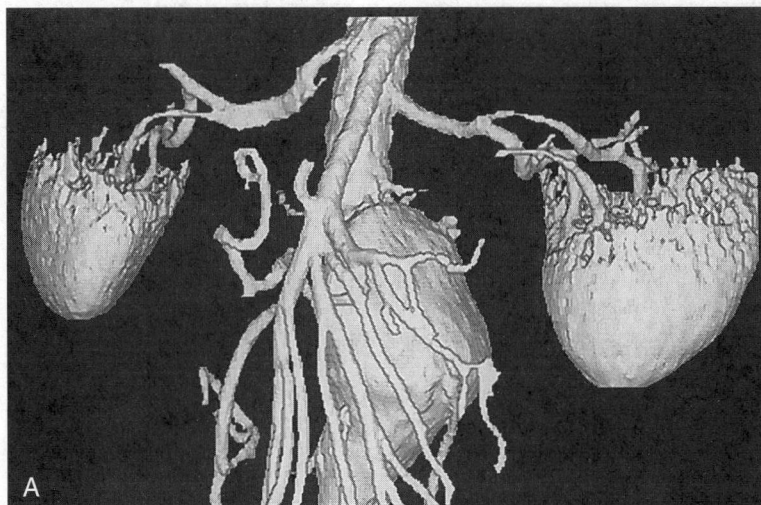

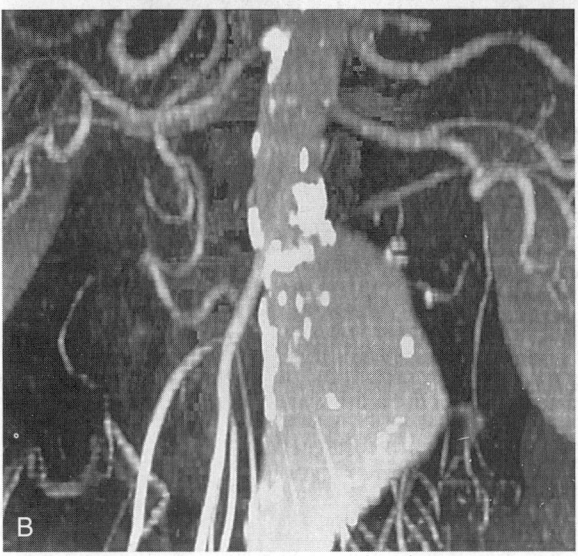

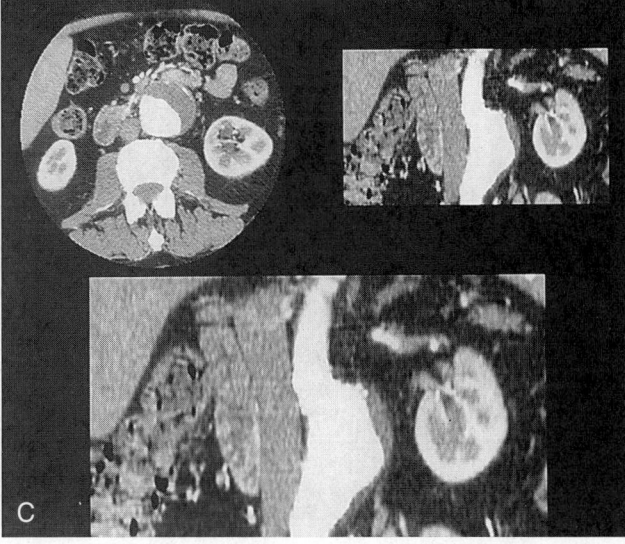

FIGURE 22–4. Abdominal aortic aneurysm. 3D image *(A)*, maximum intensity projection (MIP) image *(B)*, and cross-sectional images *(C)* of a 5-cm aneurysm. Mural thrombus within the aneurysm is best seen on the transverse slice. The relationship to the renal arteries is seen on the 3D and MIP images. The upper portions of the kidneys are not visualized on the 3D image because scanning begins before the contrast material reaches the capillary beds. The lower portions of the kidneys are visualized because the capillaries fill during the 30 seconds required for scanning from top to bottom. (From Mogavero GT, Wass JL, Kopecky KK: Angiography among top applications for spiral CT. Diagnostic Imaging [Spiral CT supplement], November:10–14, 1993.)

significant and will undoubtedly expand as their numbers increase and the costs associated with high field systems decline.

ADVANCES IN NUCLEAR MEDICINE IMAGING

BRAIN SPECT APPLICATIONS. Nuclear medicine imaging promises to evolve owing to the development of better imaging equipment and innovative tracers for diagnosing disease. The most

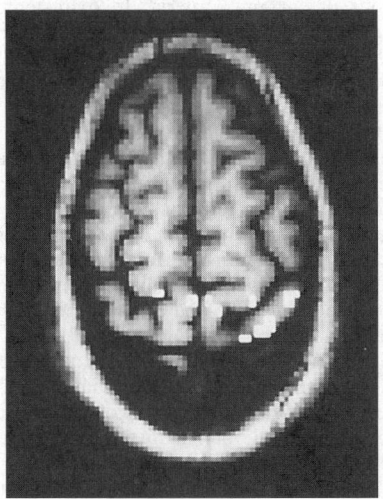

FIGURE 22–5. Functional brain activation image. The regions of the brain showing activation during finger tapping are highlighted and overlaid on an MRI of the same section. (Courtesy of Donald Twieg, PhD, and Graeme Mason, PhD, University of Alabama at Birmingham.)

rapid evolution of equipment has occurred in the area of single photon emission computed tomography (SPECT) and the associated radionuclides suitable for SPECT imaging. SPECT imaging can be performed by using a standard Anger camera acquiring multiple views of the radiotracer distribution over 360 degrees and reconstructing the radioactivity distribution of 3D space. The data are stored in a pixel matrix that can be displayed in the transverse, coronal, and sagittal planes.

Radionuclide tracers have also advanced, significantly enhancing disease diagnosis. The radionuclide technetium-99m hexamethylpropyleneamine oxime (Tc-99m HMPAO) is a brain blood flow tracer which is extracted by the brain in proportion to regional cerebral blood flow (rCBF). Brain rCBF evaluation is extremely useful clinically to evaluate the diagnosis of many central nervous system diseases including dementia, cerebrovascular disease, epilepsy, and psychiatric disorders.

Activation paradigm brain SPECT is possible because of rapid uptake of the tracer Tc-99m HMPAO (essentially within the time that the blood containing the tracer makes a first pass through the brain, approximately 30 to 45 seconds after IV injection), during which time there is tracer uptake, incorporation, and irreversible trapping. The brain radioisotopic tracer distribution retains this fixed cerebral distribution in essence permanently, dissipating only as dictated by the physical half-life of the tracer ($t_{1/2}$ = 6 hours). Owing to the irreversible binding and nonredistribution, this isotopic distribution is the end result of the actual brain SPECT image, which may commence many minutes after tracer injection and requires approximately 30 minutes acquisition time.

The rCBF uptake pattern over a short time interval (e.g., days) within the same subject is highly reproducible because the anatomy, location of brain functional regions, and brain metabolic activity do not appear to change significantly. This makes the tracer Tc-99m

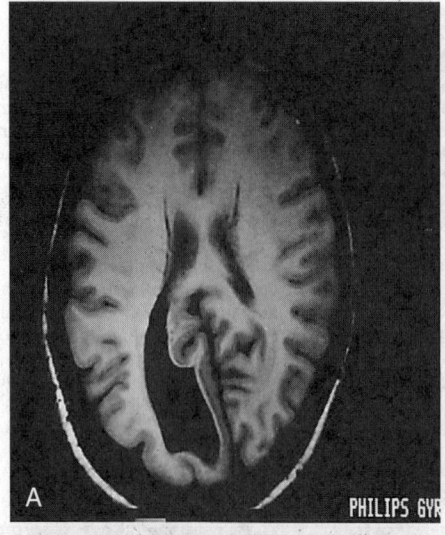

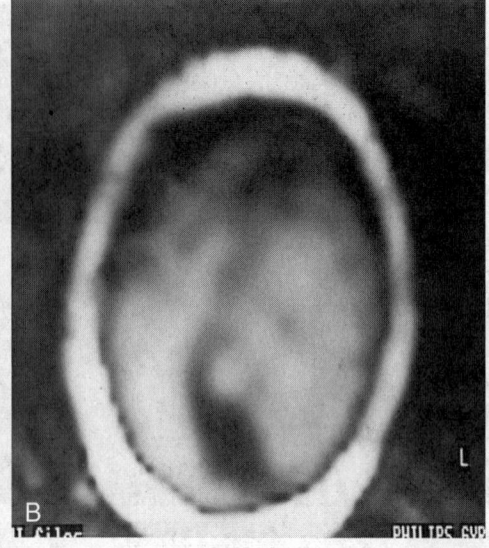

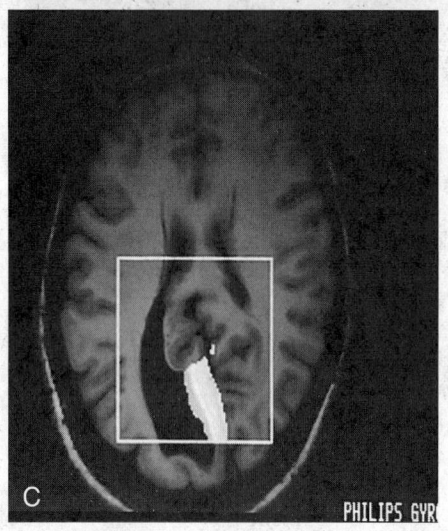

FIGURE 22-6. *A*, Axial MR image of a patient with a ventricular malformation and a history of seizures. Note the thickened gray matter adjacent to the malformation. *B*, Spectroscopic image of *N*-acetyl aspartate from the same section. *C*, The highlighted region corresponds to the brain regions having a creatine:*N*-acetyl aspartate ratio more than four standard deviations higher than that of normal gray matter. The highlighted region was overlaid on the image shown in *A*. The highlighted region corresponds to the thickened gray matter and was identified as epileptogenic by EEG. The data were acquired at 4.1T.

HMPAO especially well suited for brain activation studies because the change in distribution between mental states can yield information regarding which brain regions are responsible for the specific functional state under study. Clinically, mental stress activation has been useful to help diagnose psychiatric disease because tasks directed toward activating functionally abnormal brain regions show characteristic abnormal activation patterns.

Regional CBF brain SPECT can identify patients at risk for stroke who may benefit from neurosurgical revascularization procedures. Pharmacologic manipulation to detect cerebrovascular insufficiency is also possible using the cerebral vasodilator acetazolamide (Diamox). Diamox stress tests use a protocol employing two sequential brain SPECT scans. The first SPECT scan (rest scan) is obtained after injecting Tc-99m HMPAO (5 mCi) at rest. Then, Diamox (1 gram) is administered intravenously and, after a 20 minute waiting period for vasoreactive change, a second higher dose of Tc-99m HMPAO (20 mCi) is injected and the patient undergoes a second brain SPECT scan (stress scan) (Fig. 22-8). During the stress scan the vascularly comprised territories of brain blood flow show a relative decrease in tracer uptake compared with the rest scan.

Functional metabolic abnormalities and rCBF changes have been known to occur in partial seizures for many years. The rationale for injecting Tc-99m HMPAO during the ictal phase of a seizure is based on the observation that rCBF is temporally and focally increased during the ictal phase of seizure in patients with extra-temporal lobe epilepsy. The precise region of this neuronal hyperexcitability can be localized because Tc-99m HMPAO has rapid uptake without redistribution. Therefore, the patient can be stabilized after the seizure, and the subsequent brain SPECT scan several hours later reflects the dramatic increase in rCBF which occurred during the first few seconds of the seizure (not the actual rCBF at the time of the scan).

This injection and scan procedure is most revealing in extra-temporal lobe epilepsy patients without clear localization by any other laboratory or imaging criteria. In extra-temporal lobe epilepsy (particularly frontal lobe epilepsy), ictal rCBF brain SPECT studies have been shown to be extremely useful and highly localizing of the seizure focus. In patients undergoing limited brain resection guided by the abnormal rCBF brain SPECT scan, the ictal SPECT findings accurately localize the brain region responsible for seizures, as confirmed by the pathology of the resected tissue as well as the seizure-free postsurgery course.

Cerebral necrosis following brain tumor therapy is a significant problem because distinction between necrosis and residual or recurrent viable tumor cannot be accurately evaluated by either CT or MRI. This is because conventional anatomic neuroimaging modalities depend on alterations in blood-brain barrier permeability in order to evaluate tumor size.

Functional imaging of metabolic activity allows clear distinction between new, recurrent, or residual, viable, high-grade glioblastoma from brain necrosis. Therefore a variety of metabolic imag-ing protocols now play a central role in distinguishing cerebral necrosis from viable brain tumor. Functional imaging can not only determine tumor grade and viability status but can also measure tumor size. SPECT imaging using the radioisotopes thallium-201 (Tl-201) and Tc-99m 2-methoxy-isobutyl-isoni-trile (Tc-99m MIBI) have been shown to be both sensitive and specific for detecting viable portions of high-grade brain tumor. Tl-201 acts as a potassium analogue and

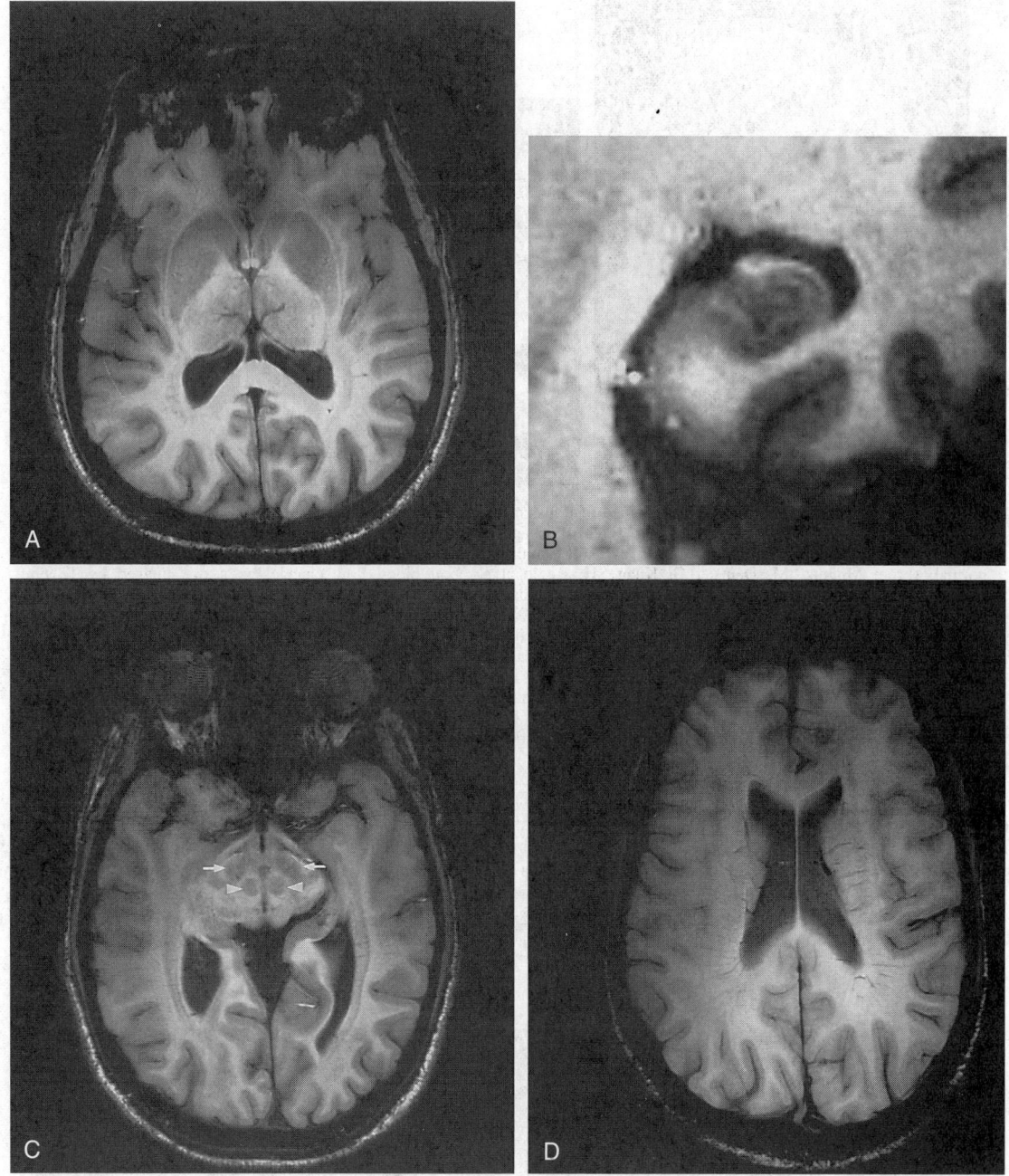

FIGURE 22–7. *A*, High-resolution MRI (460 μm in plane resolution from a 3-mm section) of a healthy human brain acquired at 4.1T at the level of the thalamus. *B*, Magnified portion of a coronal MRI of a healthy human brain displaying the internal structure of the hippocampus. *C*, Axial image at the level of the red nuclei *(arrowheads)* and substantia nigra *(arrows)*. *D*, Axial image displaying the multitude of small venous vessels.

is taken up into the metabolically active tumor cell based on the increased Na⁺K⁺-ATPase enzyme activity. Brain tumor evaluation with Tl-201 SPECT has now been well established for detecting viable tumor and for patient follow-up during therapy.

Brain SPECT has also made significant advances in using neuronal receptor–binding tracers to evaluate brain disease. The iodine-123–labeled tracer ((S)-(−)-3-iodo-2-hydroxy-6-methoxy-*N*-[(1-ethyl-2-pyrrolidinyl)-methyl]benzamide [iodine-123 IBZM]) is an example of a tracer that can map the dopamine D-2 receptor and has been used to investigate dopamine receptor distributions in movement disorders and schizophrenia. Muscarinic acetylcholine receptor distribution in Alzheimer's disease has been evaluated using the iodine-123–labeled tracer ((R)-3-quinuclidinyl-4-iodobenzilate [iodine-123 QNB]). The central benzodiazepine receptor distribution in epilepsy patients has been evaluated with iodine-123–labeled iomazenil. These tracer studies have elucidated the role of neurochemical receptors in the pathogenesis of neurologic and psychiatric disorders; this understanding is important for devel-

opment of pharmacologic therapies specifically targeted for these receptors.

MOLECULAR NUCLEAR MEDICINE IMAGING. Nuclear molecular imaging is an expanding new area of nuclear medicine that holds significant promise for noninvasively evaluating molecular events in the human body. Monoclonal antibodies have played an important role in the development of this target-specific imaging method. Recently a radiolabeled monoclonal antibody, indium-III CYT-103 (Onco Scint CR/OV), has been approved for clinical imaging of colorectal and ovarian carcinoma (Fig. 22–9).

POSITRON EMISSION TOMOGRAPHY (PET). Methods for whole-body PET imaging have been developed to provide a clinical tool for detecting and evaluating primary and metastatic cancers. A new generation of PET scanners that have introduced whole-body PET to the clinical setting has increased interest in developing protocols for the evaluation of both intracranial and somatic cancers. The value of PET in clinical oncology has been demonstrated with studies in a variety of cancers, including colorectal carcinoma, lung

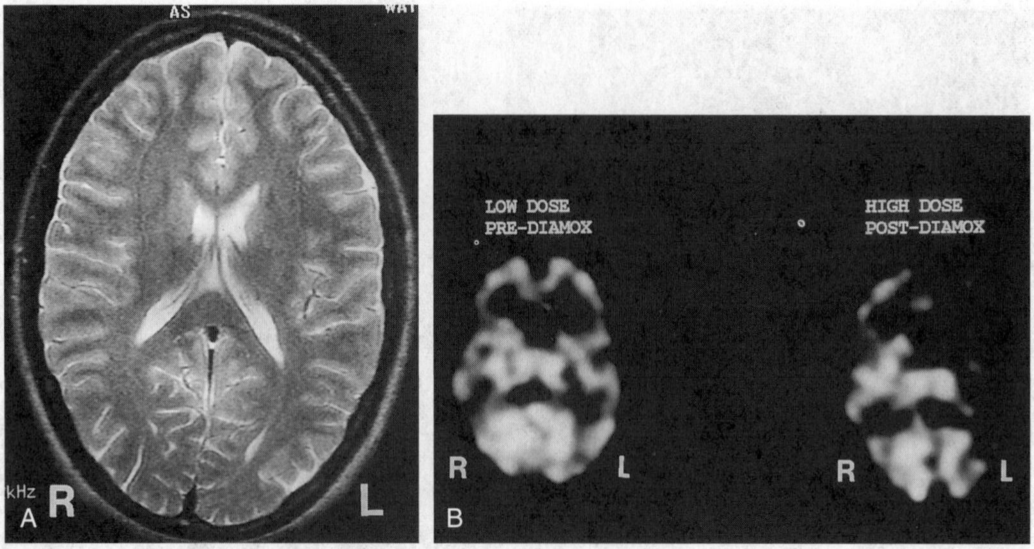

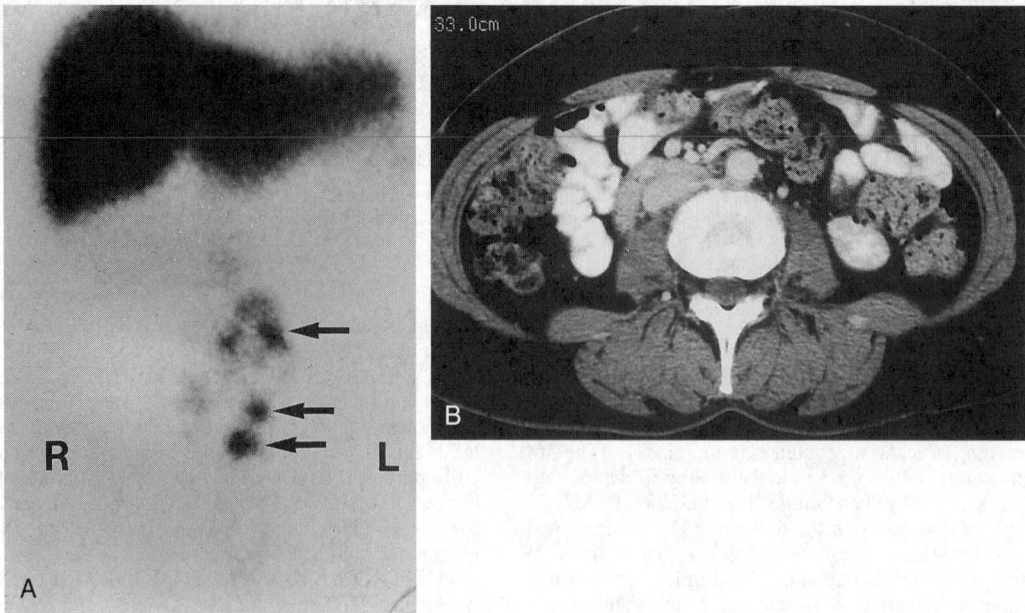

FIGURE 22-8. *A,* A 58-year-old man complained of transient neurologic deficits of motor function involving the right upper and lower extremities. Angiography showed 100% blockage of the left internal carotid artery. Owing to compromised cerebral blood flow, evaluation for a surgical revascularization procedure was performed. The illustrated MRI scan section is normal. (From Mountz JM, Deutsch G, Khan SH: Regional cerebral blood flow changes in stroke imaged by Tc-99m HMPAO SPECT with corresponding anatomic image comparison. Clin Nucl Med 18:1067, 1993.) *B,* A Diamox vascular stress test was performed to determine if the left internal carotid vascular territory was in viability jeopardy. The pre-Diamox SPECT scan demonstrates normal regional cerebral blood flow *(left),* but the post-Diamox scan showed a large region of decreased rCBF to the left frontal, temporal, and parietal lobes, representing severe rCBF compromise to the entire distribution of the left internal carotid artery *(right).* This case exemplifies the ability of the brain to provide effective vascular collateral supplies to the territory of a major arterial blockage. The cerebrovascular stress test clearly revealed the limitations of this collateral circulation. (From Mountz JM, Deutsch G, Kuzniecky R, et al.: Brain SPECT: 1994 update. *In* Freeman LM [ed.]: Nuclear Medicine Annual 1994. New York, Raven Press, 1994.)

cancer, head and neck cancer, primary and metastatic brain tumor, breast carcinoma, lymphoma, melanoma, bone cancer, and other soft tissue cancers (Fig. 22–10). A variety of radiopharmaceuticals are currently included in clinical tumor-imaging protocols, including metabolic substrates such as fluorine-18 fluorodeoxyglucose (fluorine-18 FDG).

Other investigations that will continue to demonstrate promise are those using true chemical composition of the tracer molecule to maintain biologic specificity of uptake. Incorporating carbon-11, oxygen-15, and nitrogen-13 into radiopharmaceuticals, for example, will allow production of numerous specific ligands to evaluate protein-specific receptors or metabolic pathways.

FIGURE 22-9. *A,* A 47-year-old woman was evaluated for metastatic ovarian carcinoma. After the injection of 6 mCi indium-111 CYT-103, numerous regions of increased tracer uptake representing metastatic carcinoma were found. Even in retrospect, the metastatic disease could not be identified on contrast-enhanced CT. *B,* A CT scan section through the level of the lower abdomen of the same patient shows no definite abnormalities. This illustrates the high sensitivity for detecting metastases which can be obtained using indium-111 labeled monoclonal antibody tracers.

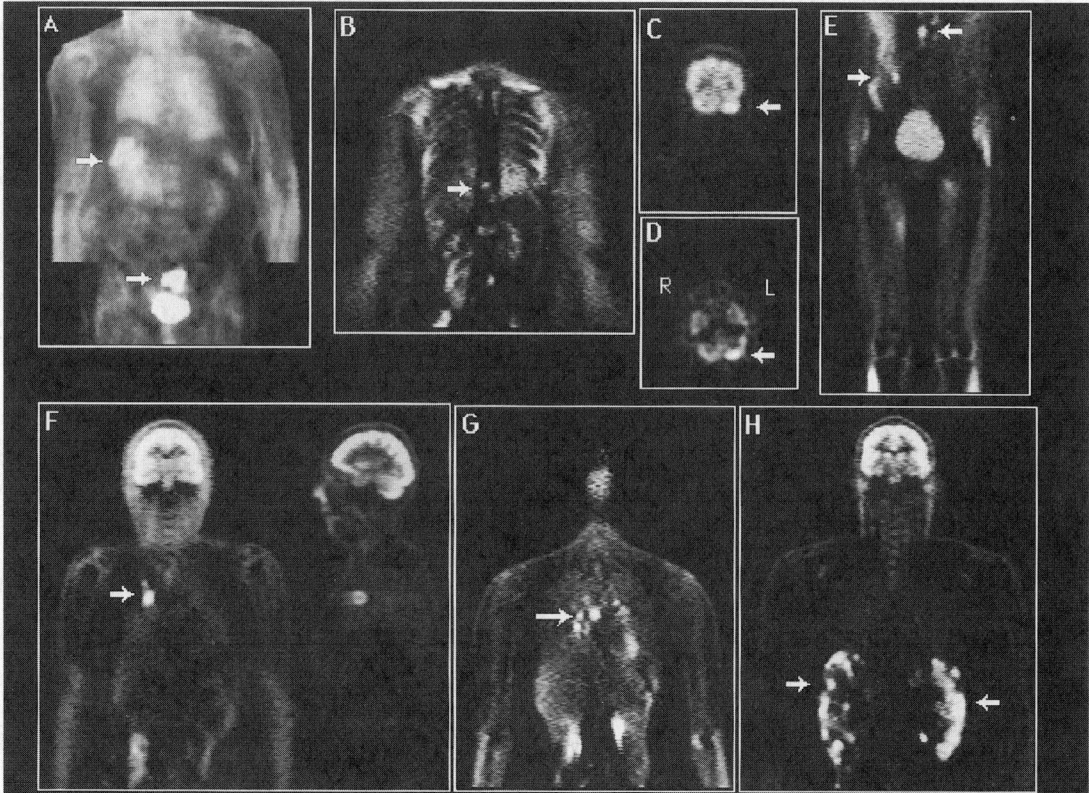

FIGURE 22–10. Whole-body fluorine-18 FDG PET scan images. All images were obtained on the Siemens 931 tomograph following injection of 10 mCi of fluorine-18 FDG (after a 40-minute uptake period) using the whole-body acquisition and processing technique. The images were not corrected for attenuation. *A,* Projection image (2D) of the torso of a patient with primary colorectal carcinoma *(lower arrow)* with metastases to the liver *(upper arrow).* The patient was fasting; therefore very little myocardial uptake is evident. Selected coronal tomographic sections *(B* and *C)* and transaxial *(D)* images from a breast cancer patient with metastases to the spine *(B,* multiple lesions at level of arrow and below), and the cerebellum *(C* and *D).* *E,* Coronal tomographic image illustrating abdominal metastases *(arrow)* in a patient with ovarian carcinoma. *F,* Coronal and sagittal tomographic image through the torso and head of a patient with a primary bronchogenic carcinoma *(arrow).* *G,* Coronal tomographic image of a patient with Hodgkin's disease with multiple thoracic nodal involvement *(arrow).* *H,* Coronal tomographic image of a patient with metastatic melanoma to the liver and spleen *(arrows).* (From Hawkins RA, Hoh C, Dahlbom M, et al.: PET cancer evaluation with FDG. J Nucl Med 32:1555, 1991.)

Arnold DL, Mathews PA, Francis GS, et al.: Proton magnetic resonance spectroscopic imaging for metabolic characterization of demyelinating plaques. Ann Neurol 37:235, 1992. *A description of the metabolic alterations in multiple sclerosis as visualized by NMR spectroscopy.*

Belliveau JW, Kennedy DN, McKinstry RC, et al.: Functional mapping of the human visual cortex using magnetic resonance imaging. Science 254:716, 1991. *An application of functional imaging to map visual activation.*

Dahlbom M, Hoffman EJ, Hoh CK, et al.: Whole-body positron emission tomography: Part I. Methods and performance characteristics. J Nucl Med 33:1191, 1992. *Describes methods and clinical examples of whole-body PET.*

Duyn JH, Moonen CT: Fast proton spectroscopic imaging of the human brain using multiple spin echoes. Magn Reson Med 30:409, 1993. *A rapid multiple-slice method for acquiring spectroscopic images.*

Friedman AH, Copel JA, Kleinman CS: Fetal echocardiography and fetal cardiology: Indications, diagnosis and management. Semin Perinatol 17:76, 1993. *A description of transvaginal ultrasonic evaluation of the fetal heart.*

Galanski M, Prokop M, Chavan A, et al.: Renal arterial stenoses: spiral CT angiography. Radiology 189:185, 1993. *Images from spiral CT angiographic analysis of renal artery stenosis.*

Gallup DG: Multicenter trial of 111-CYT-103 in patients with ovarian cancer. *In* Maguire RT, Van Nostrand D (eds.): Diagnosis of colorectal and ovarian carcinoma: Applications of immunoscintigraphy technology. New York, Marcel Dekker, 1992. *Description of the development and utility of indium-111 oncoscint.*

Kent DL, Haynor DR, Longstreth WT Jr, et al.: The clinical efficacy of magnetic resonance imaging in neuroimaging. Ann Intern Med 120:856, 1994. *Literature review of the efficacy of MRI.*

Kent DL, Haynor DR, Longstreth WT Jr, et al.: Magnetic resonance imaging of the brain and spine: A revised statement. Position paper of the American College of Physicians. Ann Intern Med 120:872, 1994. *Statement of clinical efficacy of MRI by the American College of Physicians.*

Kim SG, Ashe J, Georgopoulos AP, et al.: Functional imaging of human motor cortex at high magnetic field. J Neurophysiol 69:297, 1993. *Application of functional imaging to map the human motor cortex.*

Luyten PR, Marien AJH, Heindel W, et al.: Metabolic imaging of patients with intracranial tumors, ¹H MR spectroscopic imaging and PET. Radiology 176:791, 1990. *A description and application of ¹H spectroscopic imaging.*

Matthews PM, Andermann F, Arnold DL: A proton magnetic resonance spectroscopy study of focal epilepsy in humans. Neurology 40:985, 1990. *Application of magnetic resonance spectroscopy to the metabolic characterization of epileptic foci.*

Mountz JM, Deutsch G, Kuzniecky R, et al.: Brain SPECT: 1994 update. *In* Freeman LM (ed.): Nuclear Medicine Annual 1994. New York, Raven Press, 1994, pp 1–54. *A review of the clinical applications of brain SPECT.*

Ogawa S, Menon RS, Tank DW, et al.: Functional brain mapping by blood oxygenation level–dependent contrast magnetic resonance imaging. Biophysical J 64:803, 1993. *Study describing the blood oxygenation effect and presenting a model of its workings.*

Rubin GD, Dake MD, Napel SA, et al.: Three-dimensional spiral CT angiography of the abdomen: Initial clinical experience. Radiology 186:147, 1993. *Methods and results of spiral CT.*

Shulman RG, Blamire AM, Rothman DL, et al.: Nuclear magnetic resonance imaging and spectroscopy of human brain function. Proc Natl Acad Sci 90:3127, 1993. *An overview of the physical principles and applications of functional imaging.*

Whalen E: The impact of new imaging technology on worldwide health care, research, and teaching: Fifth international symposium, August 1992. Am J Roentgenol 160:195, 1993. *An overview of some economic considerations in imaging technology.*

Wilson MW, Webb RC, Marx MV, et al.: Intravascular ultrasound imaging of vascular responsiveness in isolated perfused canine arteries. Invest Radiol 26:248, 1991. *IVUS evaluation of arterial wall vasoconstriction using pharmacologic intervention.*

PART VI

PRINCIPLES OF HUMAN GENETICS

23 HUMAN HEREDITY
Harry W. Schroeder, Jr.

HISTORY OF GENETICS

Genetics as an experimental science owes its origins to Gregor Mendel and his cross-breeding of garden peas in 1865. He identified specific physical characteristics *(phenotypes),* such as seed color and plant height, that could be transmitted from one generation to the next. Each phenotype was ascribed to hereditary factors, later designated *genes,* that were inherited in pairs, one each from the male and female parent. True-breeding plants *(homozygotes)* inherited identical factors from the parental plants, whereas non–true-breeding plants *(hybrids* or *heterozygotes)* inherited alternative factors *(alleles)* from each parent. Some alleles were shown to have a greater effect on the phenotype of hybrids than others. In the case of a *dominant* allele, a single copy of the gene was sufficient to produce the same phenotype seen in homozygous organisms. Latent or *recessive* genes could not be detected by studying the phenotype of the hybrid parent. Detecting these genes in the hybrid required breeding the plants and demonstrating the presence of offspring that bore the recessive phenotype. Mendel's experiments led to the formulation of the laws of *unit inheritance* (that factors retain their identity from generation to generation and do not blend in the hybrid), of *segregation* (that two members [alleles] of a single pair of factors [genes] are never found in the same gamete but always segregate), and of *independent assortment* (that members of different pairs of genes [nonalleles] assort to gametes independently of one another). These laws were first applied to human disease by Sir Archibald Garrod in his studies of "inborn errors of metabolism" in 1908 (see Ch. 24).

MOLECULAR BASIS OF THE GENE AND THE TRANSMISSION OF GENETIC INFORMATION

Genetic information is encoded in the sequence of a linear polymer of purine and pyrimidine bases termed deoxyribonucleic acid (DNA). Each purine or pyrimidine pairs with a complementary base [A : T and G : C] (Table 23–1) to form two antiparallel polynucleotide strands that are twisted into a double helix. Each strand is thus complementary to the other. DNA strands are covered with histone and nonhistone proteins that allow them to be supercoiled and twisted into compact structures termed *chromosomes.* There are 23 pairs of chromosomes per somatic nucleus, 22 pairs of autosomes numbered by descending size, and one pair of sex chromosomes (X + X, female; X + Y, male). These chromosomes are located in the nucleus of the cell. During *mitosis,* the chromosomes are unwound and the DNA is split apart and copied. Each replicated strand creates a complete copy of the original DNA double helix, allowing the transmission of a complete set of genetic information into each daughter cell. In *meiosis* a reduction division of genetic information occurs. Allelic chromosomes are paired, duplicated, and separated. Only one of the allelic pair of chromosomes is allowed to segregate into the gamete. Thus, a *diploid* germ cell gives rise to

a *haploid* sperm or egg that contains an assortment of one of each of the 23 pairs of allelic chromosomes in the parental cell. During fertilization, sperm and egg unite to create a zygote with a complete set of 46 chromosomes. These fundamental properties of DNA and cell division are the basis of Mendel's laws of unit inheritance, segregation, and independent assortment.

The central dogma of molecular genetics holds that each gene encodes one polypeptide (Fig. 23–1). Each human cell contains approximately 3.9×10^9 base pairs of DNA per haploid genome, or enough to encode about 1 million polypeptides of average length. Estimates of the number of structural genes in humans ranges from 50,000 to 100,000; thus more than 90% of DNA does not encode peptide sequences. Noncoding DNA can play an important role in the function of the cell, forming regions important for the structural stability of the chromosome (e.g., *matrix-associated regions*) as well as specialized sequences that define the ends of the chromosome *(telomeres)* and the site of attachment at the time of meiosis and mitosis *(centromeres).* However, approximately 10% of cellular DNA consists of a repetitive sequence that has been randomly inserted throughout the genome. Although the function of this repetitive DNA is unknown, its presence has proven useful for gene mapping studies.

TABLE 23–1. THE GENETIC CODE

1st	2nd								3rd
	U		C		A		G		
U	UUU	Phe	UCU	Ser	UAU	Tyr	UGU	Cys	U
	UUC	Phe	UCC	Ser	UAC	Tyr	UGC	Cys	C
	UUA	Leu	UCA	Ser	UAA	Stop	UGA	Stop	A
	UUG	Leu	UCG	Ser	UAG	Stop	UGG	Trp	G
C	CUU	Leu	CCU	Pro	CAU	His	CGU	Arg	U
	CUC	Leu	CCC	Pro	CAC	His	CGC	Arg	C
	CUA	Leu	CCA	Pro	CAA	Gln	CGA	Arg	A
	CUG	Leu	CCG	Pro	CAG	Gln	CGG	Arg	G
A	AUU	Ile	ACU	Thr	AAU	Asn	AGU	Ser	U
	AUC	Ile	ACC	Thr	AAC	Asn	AGC	Ser	C
	AUA	Ile	ACA	Thr	AAA	Lys	AGA	Arg	A
	AUG	Met	ACG	Thr	AAG	Lys	AGG	Arg	G
G	GUU	Val	GCU	Ala	GAU	Asp	GGU	Gly	U
	GUC	Val	GCC	Ala	GAC	Asp	GGC	Gly	C
	GUA	Val	GCA	Ala	GAA	Glu	GGA	Gly	A
	GUG	Val	GCG	Ala	GAG	Glu	GGG	Gly	G

Three adjacent bases of RNA form a codon that specifies 1 of 20 different amino acids or 1 of 3 termination codons. A = adenine, C = cytosine, G = guanine, U = uridine. (In DNA, thymine (T) replaces uridine). The first base in the codon is identified on the right, the second base is identified at the top of the chart, and the third base is identified on the right. Each codon is followed by the amino acid it encodes. The amino acids are identified by their standard three-letter code. Ala = alanine, Arg = arginine, Asn = asparagine, Asp = aspartic acid, Cys = cysteine, Gln = glutamine, Glu = glutamic acid, Gly = glycine, His = histidine, Ile = isoleucine, Leu = leucine, Lys = lysine, Met = methionine, Phe = phenylalanine, Pro = proline, Ser = serine, Thr = threonine, Trp = tryptophan, Tyr = tyrosine, and Val = valine. Stop = termination codon.

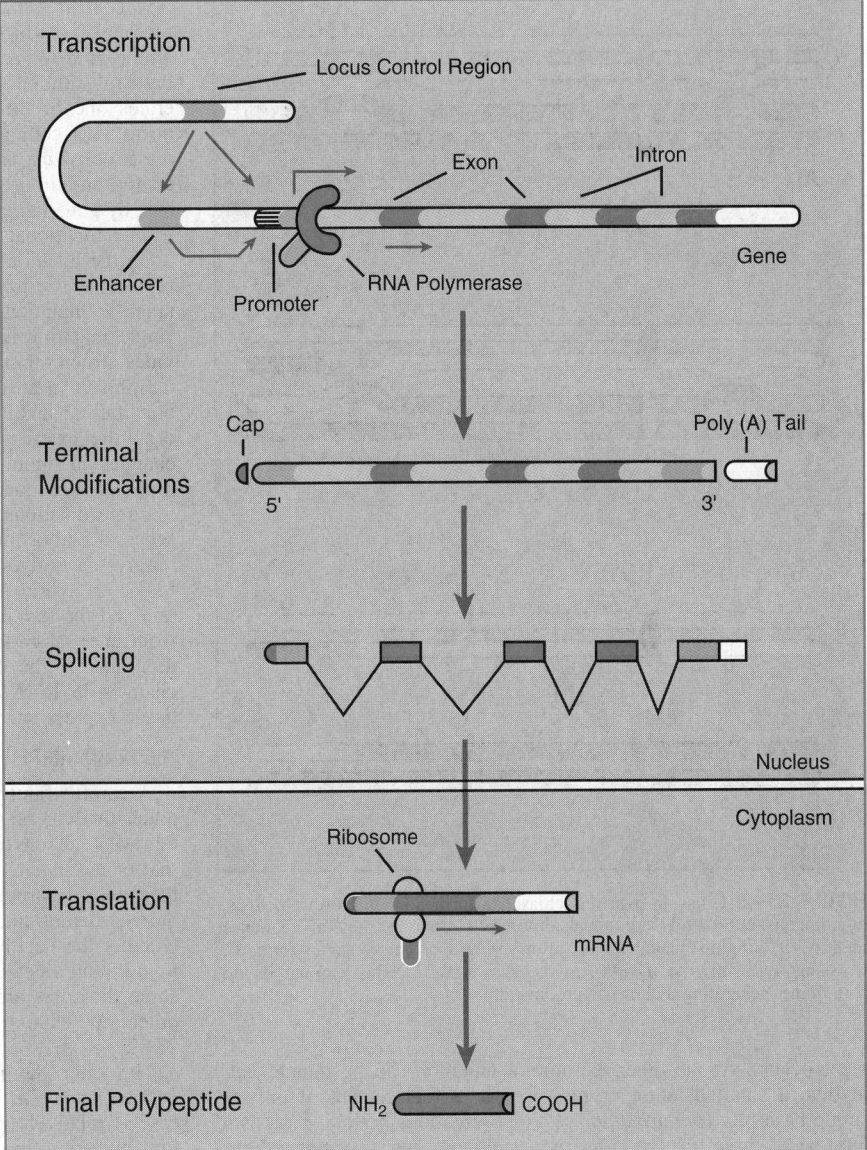

FIGURE 23-1. The flow of genetic information from gene to polypeptide proceeds in a stepwise fashion. Located near the gene are DNA control regions that specify the transcription start site *(promoters)*, define the tissue specificity of the gene *(enhancers)*, and control the use of linked genes during ontogeny *(locus control regions)*. The regions of DNA that specify the sequence of a polypeptide chain, or structural genes, are organized into discrete units *(exons)* that are separated by noncoding sequences *(introns)*. The sequence of the DNA is *transcribed* in the nucleus into RNA, a less stable nucleic acid that can be turned over rapidly. The termini of the RNA is modified to partially stabilize the final product, and the intervening introns are spliced out, generating messenger ribonucleic acid *(mRNA)*. The mRNA is transported from the nucleus to the cytoplasm, where it is *translated* by ribosomes into polypeptide strands.

RECOMBINATION

Genes linked and transmitted by chromosomes seem to violate Mendel's laws of independent assortment and segregation because effectively there would be only 23 sets of genes. During the process of meiosis, allelic chromosomes are brought into close juxtaposition (Fig. 23-2). Single-strand breaks occur in the chromosomes and allow bridges, or *chiasmata,* to form between homologous portions of the chromosomes. This *crossing over* of DNA strands allows allelic chromosomes to *recombine,* forming patchwork or *chimeric* chromosomes that contain portions of each of the parental chromosomes. Although recombination can occur anywhere in the chromosome, only a limited number of chiasmata form during each meiosis. Two genes that are on opposite ends of the chromosome may thus behave as if they were on different chromosomes, whereas recombination is less likely between genes that are very close linearly to each other. The increased frequency of the joint inheritance of two genes that are closely linked on a chromosome is termed *linkage disequilibrium.*

Distances between genes on a chromosome can be quantified by their physical distance from each other in millions of base pairs *(megabases)* or by their genetic distance, as measured by the frequency of recombination between the two genes per generation. One percent of genetic recombination is known as a *centimorgan.* On average, 1 centimorgan covers approximately 1 megabase of DNA. However, the relationship between linear and genetic distance is not absolute. The frequency of recombination and thus the genetic distance between genes in specific regions of the genome may differ depending on the sequence or the ancillary proteins that cover the DNA. Recombination frequencies in selected regions of the genome differ in male and female gametes, implying that DNA may be handled differently by testicular and ovarian cells. This disparity can lead to differences in the function of alleles, depending on whether they have been inherited from the mother or the father, a process termed *imprinting.*

MUTATION

Broadly defined, a mutation is a stable, heritable alteration in the DNA sequence which can be passed from a cell to its progeny. From the standpoint of evolution, mutations are essential to generate sufficient genetic diversity to permit species to adapt to their environment through the mechanism of "natural selection." The normal rate of mutation is approximately 10^{-7} base pair changes per generation; thus, on average, individuals pass on 390 base pair changes to their offspring. Alterations of DNA sequence in cells of the body that do not give rise to germ cells are termed *somatic mutations.* Although by definition these alterations are not transmitted to the gametes, the mutations are passed on to the progeny of the mutated cells. Somatic mutations in *oncogenes,* for example, underlie the development of many cancers (see Ch. 156).

Mutations may involve millions of base pairs in the structure of a chromosome, as in duplications, deletions, and translocations of a portion of one chromosome to another (see Ch. 26). Mutations can involve an entire human genome of 3.9 billion base pairs, as in triploidy, in which a third copy of the entire chromosomal comple-

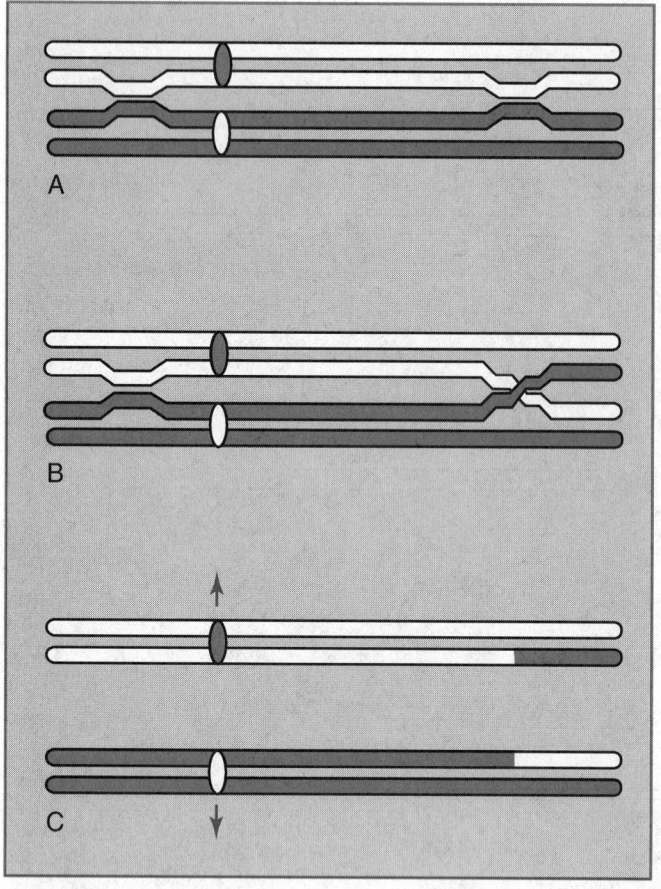

FIGURE 23-2. Crossing over and chiasmata formation. *A*, During meiosis, homologous chromatids are attached to each other at sites of sequence identity. *B*, Single-stranded breaks allow bridges or chiasmata to form. *C*, Crossing over of the DNA strands allows the allelic chromatids to recombine, generating a chimeric chromatid.

ment occurs. At the other extreme, a mutation can be minute and involve a small deletion or insertion, or a replacement of only a single base pair *(point mutation)*. Point mutations in coding regions may be of three types: (1) a *synonymous* or *silent* mutation (about 23% of random base substitutions in coding regions), in which the base replacement does not lead to a change in the amino acid but only to a different codon for the same amino acid; (2) a *missense* or *replacement* mutation (about 73% of base substitutions in coding regions), in which the base change results in substitution of one amino acid for another; and (3) a *nonsense* mutation (about 4% of base substitutions in coding regions), in which the base change generates one of the termination codons. Deletions or insertions that occur in a coding region can alter the reading frame distal to the mutation *(frameshift* mutations). Frameshift mutations frequently alter the protein sequence and can lead to premature peptide termination by generating a stop codon.

The functional consequences of mutations may vary depending upon the location of the mutation and the nature of the amino acid replacement. Enzymes, for example, exhibit a hierarchy of resistance to mutation. The catalytic site is exquisitely sensitive, and a single mutation may abrogate function. The hydrophobic core provides structural stability for the molecule, and amino acid changes may result in an unstable protein product that is temperature sensitive, falling apart at high temperature. Finally, portions of the hydrophilic exterior may serve primarily to promote solubility, and changes in amino acid sequence that preserve polarity may have minimal consequences.

Large deletions may interrupt a coding region and cause an absence of one or more closely linked protein products. If the deletion removes a bridge between two coding regions, the result may be a fusion or hybrid protein containing the initial sequence of one protein and the terminal portion of the other. Such deletions may result from unequal crossing over between homologous genes. Finally, alterations of the DNA in the surrounding regions may lead to changes in RNA splicing, transcriptional efficiency, or control of tissue expression.

THE FAMILY HISTORY

A careful family history is indispensable in the assessment and understanding of hereditary disease. The interviewer should ascertain whether anyone in the family has had a condition similar to that of the patient, and whether this condition or any other "runs in the family." Particularly in the case of rare disorders, one should inquire whether the parents are related and, if this is not known, whether they or their families came from the same village or community and whether their forebears may have intermarried. Because some disorders are more common in certain ethnic groups than in others, the ethnic origin of the parents should also be elicited (Table 23-2).

The rarer the recessive disorder in a specific population, the greater is the likelihood of parental consanguinity. Tay-Sachs disease is relatively rare in non-Jews, in whom the gene frequency is low, but a high proportion of non-Jewish parents of Tay-Sachs children are consanguineous. By contrast, Tay-Sachs disease is rela-

TABLE 23-2. EXAMPLES OF MENDELIAN DISORDERS THAT ARE PRESENT IN INCREASED FREQUENCY IN SOME ETHNIC GROUPS

Population	Disorder	Estimated Prevalence
African blacks	G6PD deficiency	1 in 10 (male), 1 in 5 (female)
(West Africa)	Sickle cell anemia	1 in 500
Ashkenazi Jews	21-Hydroxylase deficiency	1 in 30
	Facor XI deficiency (hemophilia C)	1 in 200
	Gaucher's disease	1 in 600
	Tay-Sachs disease	1 in 2,000
	Familial dysautonomia	1 in 3,600
Chinese (Hong Kong)	G6PD deficiency	1 in 28
East Asians	Acatalasia	1 in 250
Eskimos	21-Hydroxylase deficiency	1 in 282
French Canadians (Lac St. Jean)	Tyrosinemia	1 in 685
Hopi	Albinism	1 in 227
Mediterranean peoples	G6PD deficiency	~ 1 in 30
Native Americans	Adult lactase deficiency	1 in 1
Northern Europeans	Cystic fibrosis	1 in 2,000
Puerto Ricans	Albinism	1 in 2,000
Sephardic Jews	Familial Mediterranean fever	1 in 250
	Glycogen storage disease (type III)	1 in 5,400
Swedes	α_1-Antitrypsin deficiency	1 in 1,500
South Africans (whites)	Heterozygous familial hypercholesterolemia	1 in 85
	Porphyria variegata	1 in 330
Thais	Hemoglobin E	1 in 200

tively common in Jews of eastern European origin (Ashkenazis), in whom the gene frequency is relatively high. In parents of Jewish children with Tay-Sachs disease in the United States, the frequency of consanguinity is only slightly higher than in the general population.

Certain ethnic backgrounds increase the likelihood of certain diagnostic possibilities while decreasing that of others. Thalassemia (see Ch. 136.4) is chiefly a disorder of people of the Mediterranean region and of Southeast Asia, familial Mediterranean fever (see Ch. 139.2) is a disorder of Armenians and Sephardic Jews, acatalasia is a disease of Japanese and Koreans, and gout (see Ch. 251) is very common among the Maori. By contrast, cystic fibrosis (see Ch. 58) is rare in African blacks, phenylketonuria (see Ch. 176) is uncommon in Jews, and sickle cell anemia (see Ch. 137) does not occur in Northern Europeans.

PEDIGREE ANALYSIS

The chief method to study an inherited disease in humans is observing its pattern of distribution in families or *kindreds,* i.e., of its pattern in a *pedigree* (Fig. 23–3). The construction of a pedigree begins with the individual first detected, who is referred to as the proband or index case. The pedigree pattern allows one to judge whether the distribution conforms to mendelian principles of segregation and assortment and thus represents single-factor inheritance. Patterns that do not conform to mendelian principles may represent polygenic traits in which a number of genes each contributes a minor effect. Valid pedigrees depend on accurate and extensive information about the kindred. This information is likely to be more reliable when based on detection by the physician than when based on memory.

MAPPING THE HUMAN GENOME

Variation in the human genome can be detected by a number of different molecular techniques. One very useful technique takes advantage of repetitive sequences found in the genome, such as runs of dinucleotide repeats (e.g., CA_n). The repeat regions are subject to considerable evolutionary slippage, resulting in duplications and deletion. By means of the polymerase chain reaction *(PCR),* DNA oligonucleotide probes that bind uniquely to either side of a repeat region can be used to rapidly amplify and visualize the size of the repeat. These size variations create a number of different alleles, or PCR *markers,* for each repeat region. A series of markers on each chromosome can be used to create a genetic linkage map of the genome. The more closely a marker is linked to the gene or trait of interest, the more likely that the marker will be transmitted to the offspring along with that gene. By analyzing the inheritance of a series of markers in families with genetic disease, it becomes possible to find the rough location of the disease gene. A second type of genome map, the physical map, is an actual assemblage of DNA clones lined up in the same order as they appear on the chromosome. The ultimate goal is to use these maps to isolate and study the gene. A number of disease genes, most notably the genes for

cystic fibrosis, neurofibromatosis (see Ch. 417), Huntington's disease (see Ch. 411) and others, have already been isolated. It is likely that in the near future, the majority of genes that cause the major monogenic disorders will be identified.

MONOGENIC DISORDERS

Disorders caused by single mutant genes show one of four simple (mendelian) patterns of inheritance: (1) autosomal dominant, (2) autosomal recessive, (3) X-linked dominant, or (4) X-linked recessive. Dominant traits are those expressed in the heterozygote (as well as in the homozygote or hemizygote). Recessive traits are those expressed in the homozygotes (or hemizygotes) but silent in the heterozygote. The terms *dominant* and *recessive* refer to the phenotypic expression of the trait, not to the expression of the gene. Thus it is incorrect to speak of a dominant or recessive gene. A gene is either expressed or not expressed. Whether the trait is considered dominant or recessive often depends upon the level of observation. Sickle cell anemia is a recessive trait; i.e., it requires a double dose of the abnormal gene for expression at the clinical level. Nevertheless, the sickle gene is expressed in single dose as well, giving rise to carriers with SA hemoglobin. In a state of reduced oxygen tension, red cells in SA carriers may sickle. Recessive traits may thus be *codominant* when viewed biochemically at the level of the gene product or dominant in an altered environment.

With few exceptions, each of the more than 3000 mendelian diseases is rare. The overall population frequency of monogenic disorders is about 10 per 1000 live births, comprising about 7 per 1000 dominants, about 2.5 per 1000 recessives, and about 0.4 per 1000 X-linked conditions (Table 23–3).

If a particular disease shows a mendelian pattern of inheritance, its pathogenesis, no matter how complex, is likely due to a single abnormal gene. For example, in homozygous patients with sickle cell disease (SS), such seemingly unrelated disturbances as hemolytic anemia, painful crises, nephropathy, vascular occlusions, and *Salmonella* osteomyelitis are all physiologic consequences of a single missense mutation, resulting in a single amino acid substitution in both β-globin chains of hemoglobin ($\alpha_2\beta^s_2$). When two or more phenotypic characters are controlled by a single gene, that gene is said to have *pleiotropic* effects.

AUTOSOMAL DOMINANT TRAITS. Autosomal genes are those genes situated on chromosomes other than the X or Y. When there are two alleles—A and a—at a locus, three possible genotypes exist: AA, Aa, and aa. Genotypes AA and aa are *homozygotes;* Aa is a *heterozygote.*

Dominant traits are fully manifest in the presence of a gene in the heterozygous state, i.e., when only one abnormal gene *(mutant allele)* is present and the corresponding partner allele on the homologous chromosome is normal. Figure 23–4 shows a typical pedigree of transmission of an autosomal dominant trait. The following

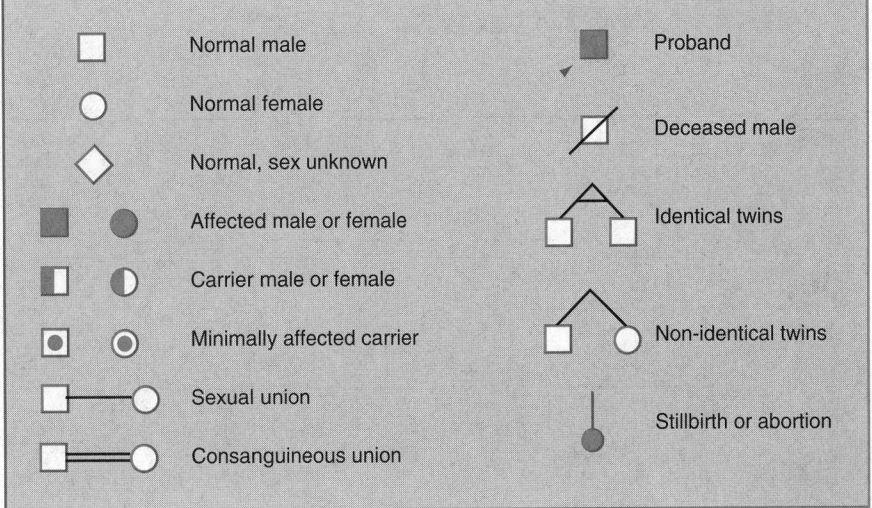

FIGURE 23–3. Standard pedigree symbols.

Normal male

Normal female

Normal, sex unknown

Affected male or female

Carrier male or female

Minimally affected carrier

Sexual union

Consanguineous union

Proband

Deceased male

Identical twins

Non-identical twins

Stillbirth or abortion

TABLE 23–3. ESTIMATED PREVALENCE OF SELECTED MONOGENIC DISORDERS IN THE UNITED STATES

Disorder	Estimated Prevalence
Autosomal dominant	
von Willebrand's disease	1 in 125
Familial hypercholesterolemia	1 in 500
Acute intermittent porphyria	1 in 500 (psychiatric admissions)
Polycystic kidney disease	1 in 1,250
Hypertrophic obstructive cardiomyopathy	1 in 1,500
Huntington's disease	1 in 2,500
Hereditary spherocytosis	1 in 5,000
Acute intermittent porphyria	1 in 10,000
Osteogenesis imperfecta tarda	1 in 15,000
Marfan's syndrome	1 in 20,000
Autosomal recessive	
Hemochromatosis	1 in 400
Sickle cell anemia	1 in 625 (US blacks)
Cystic fibrosis	1 in 2,500 (US Caucasians)
α_1-Antitrypsin deficiency	1 in 4,000
Tay-Sachs disease	1 in 3,000 (US Jews)
Cystinuria	1 in 7,000
Phenylketonuria	1 in 10,000
Albinism	1 in 10,000 (US blacks)
21-Hydroxylase deficiency	1 in 14,000
Albinism	1 in 18,000 (US Caucasians)
Mucopolysaccharidoses (all types)	1 in 25,000
Glycogen storage disease (all types)	1 in 50,000
Galactosemia	1 in 57,000
Wilson's disease	1 in 100,000
Homocystinuria	1 in 200,000
X-linked	
G6PD deficiency	1 in 10 (US blacks)
Fragile X syndrome	1 in 1,500 (males)
Duchenne muscular dystrophy	1 in 7,000 (males)
Hemophilia (A + B)	1 in 10,000 (males)

features are characteristic: (1) each affected individual has an affected parent (unless the condition arose by a new mutation in a germ cell that formed the individual); (2) an affected individual usually bears an equal number of affected and unaffected offspring; (3) males and females are affected in equal numbers; (4) each gender can transmit the trait to male and female; (5) normal children of an affected individual have only normal offspring; and (6) when the trait does not impair viability or reproductive capacity, *vertical* transmission of the trait occurs through successive generations. Three or more generations of male-to-male transmission argues against X-linkage of a rare gene.

Most autosomal dominant disorders show two additional characteristics that are not seen in recessive disorders: (1) marked variability in severity, or *expressivity,* and (2) delayed age of onset. Dominant traits in humans often exert only mild effects and are thus not completely dominant in a mendelian sense. Occasionally the expression of the abnormal gene is so weak that a generation appears to be skipped because the carrier of the abnormal gene is clinically normal. When this is the case, the trait is said to be *nonpenetrant.* When a gene of a dominant trait exists in the homozygous state, the effect may be very severe, perhaps lethal. Examples are common in animals in which experimental matings can be constructed, but rare in humans, because matings of two affected heterozygotes are exceptional. One example is homozygous familial hypercholesterolemia. Others possibly include achondroplasia and Osler-Weber-Rendu syndrome. Delayed age of onset is seen in Huntington's disease and adult polycystic kidney disease. These disorders do not become manifest clinically until adult life, even though the mutant gene has been present since conception.

In every autosomal dominant disease some affected persons owe their disorder to a new mutation rather than to an inherited allele. Because a reasonable estimate of the frequency of mutation is on the order of 5×10^{-6} mutation per allele per generation (or $\sim 1 \times 10^{-8}$ mutation per codon) and because a dominant trait requires a mutation in only one of the parental gametes, one would expect that about 1 in 100,000 newborns would possess a new mutation in any given gene. Many mutations are silent or recessive and are not manifest in a single gene dose. However, others cause a defective gene product that gives rise to a dominant trait.

Regions of trinucleotide repeats, such as $(CAG)_n$, appear to be at increased risk for slippage during DNA replication. The longer the repeat, the higher the risk of slippage. In genes that contain such repeats, this process appears to be the basis of *anticipation,* wherein the manifestations of a mutation are apparent at a younger age in each succeeding generation. Examples include myotonic dystrophy and the children of fathers with Huntington's disease.

The percentage of patients with dominant disorders that represent new mutations is inversely proportional to the effect of the disease upon *biologic fitness,* i.e., survival to adult life, and reproductive capacity. If a dominant mutation produces early death or absolute infertility, genetic transmission is impossible, and all cases represent new mutations. In tuberous sclerosis, the severe mental retardation reduces biologic fitness to about 20% of normal, and the proportion of cases due to new mutations is about 80%. In dominant conditions such as familial hypercholesterolemia, in which there is no reduction in biologic fitness, virtually all cases have a family pedigree showing classic vertical transmission.

For some genes, new mutations appear to be more frequent in the germ cells of fathers of relatively advanced age. Both Marfan's syndrome (see Ch. 183) and achondroplastic dwarfism display a "paternal age effect." Fathers of sporadic cases of both conditions are an average of 5 to 7 years older than the general population of fathers

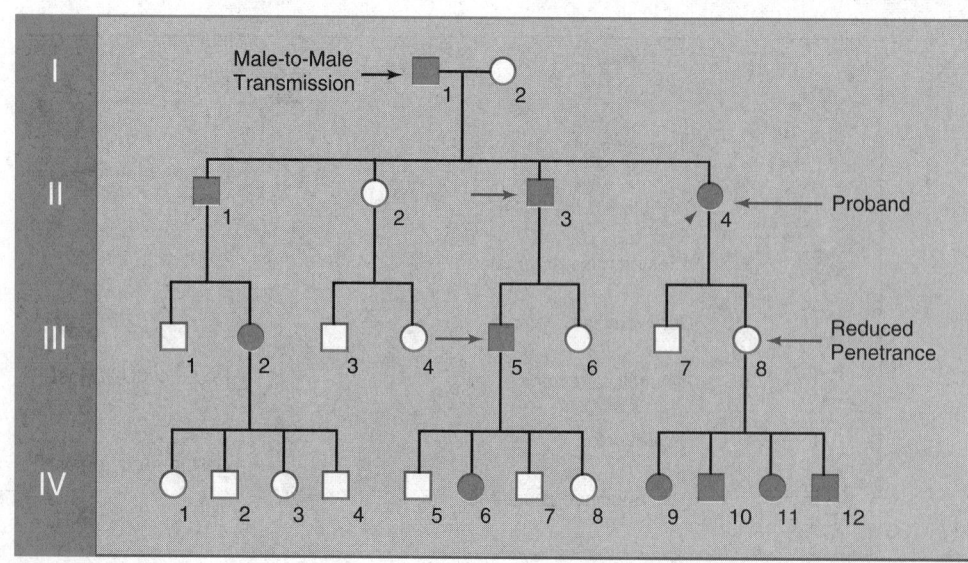

FIGURE 23–4. Pedigree of an autosomal dominant trait. Solid symbols indicate those affected. The generation is indicated by roman numerals, and individuals in each generation are sequentially assigned roman numerals. Three generations of male-to-male transmission provide strong evidence of the autosomal dominant transmission of the trait. Although the likelihood of inheriting the disease gene is 50% for each offspring, by chance alone all or none of the children in individual families may be affected. By phenotype, individual III.8 does not express the trait. (See text for further details.)

or than fathers who transmit these syndromes because of an inherited mutation. Diagnosis of a new mutation must exclude low expressivity of the trait in the carrier parent and also mistaken paternity.

Study of the molecular basis of autosomal dominant disorders has yielded a number of novel insights. Because in a dominant disorder the mutation expressed in only 50% of the gene product may be sufficient to cause disease, mutations can involve proteins that regulate complex metabolic pathways (such as membrane receptors as in familial hypercholesterolemia), and structural or nonenzymic proteins (such as hemoglobin or collagen) or a membrane protein (such as in hereditary spherocytosis). However, in hereditary retinoblastoma, the autosomal dominant trait reflects an absence of the *rb* gene on one allele and is nonpenetrant until a somatic mutation occurs on the second allele, creating a homozygous state. In this case, the autosomal dominant trait reflects increased susceptibility to the consequences of a second mutation. Conditions such as these emphasize that the distinction between recessive and dominant inheritance is one of perception and detection.

AUTOSOMAL RECESSIVE DISORDERS. Autosomal recessive conditions are clinically apparent only in the homozygous state, i.e., when both alleles at a particular genetic locus are mutant alleles. In most autosomal recessive disorders the clinical presentation tends to be more uniform than in dominant diseases, and the onset is often early in life. Figure 23–5 shows a typical pedigree of an autosomal recessive trait. The following features are characteristic: (1) The parents are clinically normal; (2) only siblings are affected; (3) males and females are affected in equal proportions; (4) if an affected individual marries a homozygous normal person, none of the children is affected but all are heterozygous carriers; (5) if an affected individual marries a heterozygous carrier, one half of the

children are affected, and the pedigree pattern superficially suggests a dominant trait; (6) if two individuals who are homozygous for the same mutant gene marry, all of their children are affected; (7) if both parents are heterozygous at the same genetic locus, one fourth of their children are homozygous affected, on average one fourth are homozygous normal, and one half are heterozygous carriers of the same mutant gene; and (8) the less frequent the mutant gene is in the population, the greater the likelihood that the affected individual is the product of consanguineous parents.

In actual practice, unless the kinship is very large, the ratio of affected to unaffected sibs is frequently greater than one in four. Including probands in the enumeration loads the results in favor of the trait. In a sibship of 10 or more children, the loading factor is not pronounced. However, in all ascertainable one-child sibships the involvement is 100%, in two-child sibships it is 67% (when the fundamental probability is 50%), in three-child sibships it is 57%, and so on. In small sibships a correction must be made for *bias of ascertainment.* The simplest method is to exclude the proband from the calculation and to determine the proportion of affected children among the remaining sibs.

A *completely* recessive disease is one in which the heterozygote is clinically normal. When some features of the disease are detectable in the heterozygote, the disease is sometimes said to show *intermediate inheritance,* or to be *incompletely recessive* or *incompletely dominant.* The ambiguity of these terms from classic genetic studies of phenotypes is further emphasized by results of different methods of detecting gene effects. In many instances of completely recessive inheritance, refined biochemical observations enable the recognition of the trait in the clinically normal heterozygote. An example is Tay-Sachs disease, in which clinically normal parents and some sibs can be shown to be heterozygotes by assay of hexosaminidase A in leukocytes. Because of its importance in genetic counseling, detecting healthy heterozygous carriers of genes that, in the homozygous state, cause overt disease is one of the most significant aspects of medical genetics. Because by definition a dominant trait is one that is detectable in the heterozygous state, Tay-Sachs disease (and many others) is recessive when the clinical phenotype is considered and dominant when the biochemical phenotype is determined.

In pure form a recessive disease requires the inheritance of identical mutant genes from both parents. When the mutant genes are rare, the likelihood that any two unrelated parents are carriers for the same defect is small. Inheriting two different mutant genes derived from the same locus gives rise to *heterollelic compounds.* The classic example is Hb SC disease, in which different abnormal β-globin genes have been inherited from each parent. As we identify and sequence a broad array of disease genes, many more such examples are being found. Alternative mutations contribute to varied manifestations of disorders of the same gene. Within a family, affected individuals are likely to have the same mutations. Therefore, ascertaining the effects of a mutation in a proband can have predictive value for other members of the family.

If the parents of a child with a recessive disorder have a common ancestor who carried a mutant gene, the likelihood that two of the descendants would each have inherited the gene increases. The less frequent the gene, the stronger is the likelihood that an affected individual has resulted from a consanguineous mating. First cousins share, on the average, one eighth of their genes. When two first cousins marry, an offspring has, on the average, one sixteenth of the loci homozygous for a gene derived from a common ancestor. In general, offspring of first-cousin mating are slightly more likely to have congenital malformations, as well as mental defects and metabolic diseases, than are children born to unrelated parents.

Increased frequency of consanguinity is not observed if the recessive disease is common. Sickle cell anemia, phenylketonuria, cystic fibrosis, and Tay-Sachs disease are examples in which the carrier (heterozygote) state is frequent in certain populations and in which consanguinity is usually not present in the parents. Consanguinity would also not be expected in dominant or X-linked traits or genetic compounds. When the disease allele is identical, it is likely that the gene was in fact inherited from a distant common ancestor, or *founder.*

A high percentage of recessive disorders involves abnormalities of enzyme proteins. In most reactions the normal maximal enzyme

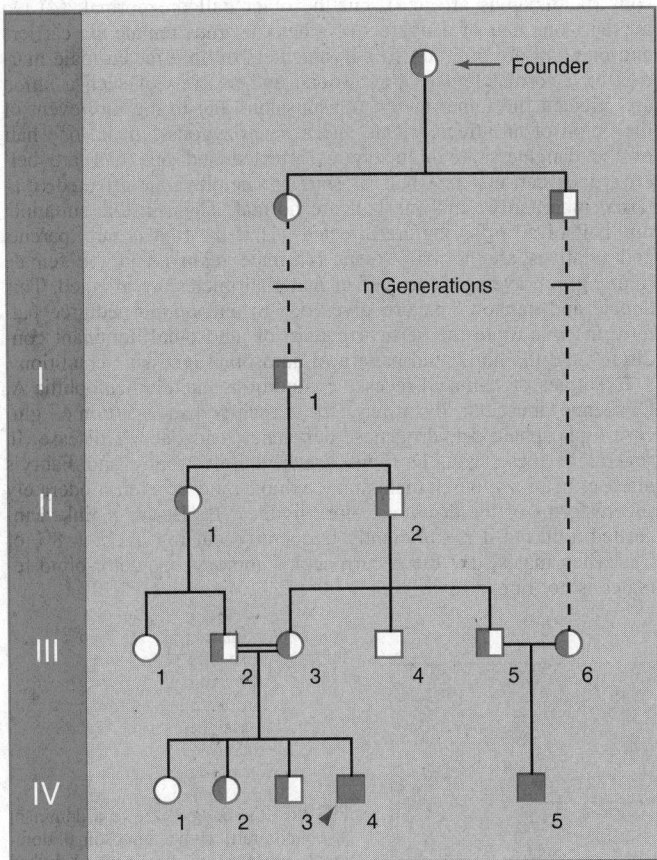

FIGURE 23–5. Pedigree of an autosomal recessive trait. Note that both parents (III.2 and III.3) of the affected proband (IV.4) are heterozygous for the trait. Two sibs of the proband are carriers, and one is normal (IV.1). The double line (====) indicates that the parents of the proband are related by descent (first cousins). In isolated populations, individuals are more likely to share a common ancestor (the *founder*). Although technically not consanguineous, marriage in an inbred society often leads to a higher risk for having affected offspring. (See text for further details.)

activity is greatly in excess of catalytic requirements; i.e., the concentration of a substrate is usually maintained at a point well below saturation for the enzyme that metabolizes it. Hence a reduction to 50% of normal activity in a heterozygote does not impair the health of the carrier, whereas a total or nearly total deficiency may result in a serious inborn error of metabolism (see Ch. 24).

X-LINKED INHERITANCE. Diseases or traits that result from genes located on the X chromosome are termed X-linked. Because the female has two X chromosomes, she may be either heterozygous or homozygous for the mutant gene, and the trait may exhibit recessive or dominant expression. The terms *X-linked dominant* and *X-linked recessive* refer only to expression of the trait in females. The male has only one X chromosome and therefore is *hemizygous* for X-linked traits. Males can be expected to express X-linked traits regardless of their recessive or dominant behavior in the female. This accounts for the large numbers of X-linked diseases. Males transmit their X chromosome to all of their daughters, making them all obligate carriers of an X-linked disease trait. Affected males do not transmit an X chromosome to their sons; thus, an important feature of X-linked inheritance is the absence of male-to-male transmission.

Because the female carries two X chromosomes in each cell, it might be expected that the concentrations of proteins determined by genes on the X chromosome would be twice that of males. This is not the case, and the explanation is provided by the process of X-inactivation first proposed by Mary Lyon, termed *lyonization* in her honor. Although both X chromosomes are active early in ontogeny, with differentiation one of the X chromosomes becomes inactive, condensing to form a *Barr body*. Inactivation is random so each cell has an equal probability that the paternally or maternally derived X chromosome will be inactivated. Once one of the two X chromosomes is inactivated, the same X chromosome remains inactive throughout all subsequent cell divisions. Thus, on the average one half of the cells of a female express the X chromosome of her father and one half of her mother. The single exception to this rule is a 2.5-megabase region at the tip of the X chromosome that shares homology with the tip of the Y chromosome, allowing recombination and pairing of the X and Y chromosomes during meiosis. Genes in this pseudoautosomal region escape X-inactivation.

For the vast majority of genes on the X chromosome, the normal female is a mosaic. If one of the X chromosomes carries a mutant gene, the probability is that the mutant phenotype is expressed in one half of her cells. However, this statistical probability may be disturbed in at least two ways: (1) Because inactivation of one of the X chromosomes occurs early in development and is random, some females may by chance have many more cells that carry an active X chromosome derived from one parent than from the other; and (2) if one of the X chromosomes carries a mutant gene that confers a metabolic disadvantage upon cells with that mutation, these cells may survive less frequently during development, and the female offspring may have cells that carry predominantly or exclusively the active X chromosome without the mutation.

Hemizygosity in males, patterns of X-inactivation, and the large numbers of X-linked diseases have driven mapping studies of the X chromosome. As a result, the X chromosome was the first to have a genetic map based upon restriction fragment length polymorphisms

(*RFLP's*), and a complete physical map is near completion. At present, more than 50 inherited disease genes of the X chromosome have been isolated by mapping approaches.

X-Linked Dominant Traits. This mode of inheritance (Fig. 23–6) is uncommon. Its characteristic features are as follows: (1) females are affected about twice as often as males; (2) heterozygous females transmit the trait to both genders with a frequency of 50%; (3) hemizygous affected males transmit the trait to all of their daughters and none of their sons; and (4) the expression is more variable and generally less severe in heterozygous females than in hemizygous affected males. Examples of X-linked dominant inheritance include the Xg(a+) blood group, vitamin D–resistant (hypophosphatemic) rickets (see Ch. 213) and pseudohypoparathyroidism (see Ch. 214).

Some rare X-linked dominant disorders occur only in the heterozygous female, because the condition is lethal in the hemizygous affected male. Additional characteristics of this form of inheritance are as follows: (1) an affected mother transmits the trait to one half of her daughters (heterozygotes), and (2) an increased frequency of abortions occurs in affected women, the abortions representing affected male fetuses. Examples of disorders that appear to fit this mode of inheritance include incontinentia pigmenti, focal dermal hypoplasia, orofaciodigital syndrome, and hyperammonemia caused by ornithine transcarbamylase deficiency.

X-Linked Recessive Traits. This mode of inheritance (Fig. 23–7) is relatively common. Its characteristic features are as follows: (1) The disorder is fully expressed only in the hemizygous affected male. (2) Heterozygous females are usually normal; occasionally they may exhibit mild features of the disorder; rarely they may be almost as severely affected as the hemizygous affected male (this variability is attributed to the probability that a disproportionate percentage of *normal* X chromosomes of the heterozygous female may have been inactivated early in development). (3) On average, a heterozygous female transmits the trait to one half of her sons (hemizygous affected), but the other half are normal. (4) On average, one half of daughters of a heterozygous female are carriers and one half are normal. (5) All daughters of an affected male married to a normal female are carriers, and no sons of such a union are affected (no father-to-son transmission). (6) In the rare event of the union of an affected male and a heterozygous female, one half of the daughters are homozygous affected and one half are heterozygous carriers; one half of sons are hemizygous affected (maternal inheritance) and one half are normal. Thus, in this situation, one half of all offspring are affected. (7) If the trait is rare, parents and relatives are normal except for male relatives in the female line; e.g., on average, one half of maternal uncles are affected. This "uncle and nephew" pattern gives rise to an *oblique* pedigree pattern, in contrast to the vertical pattern of autosomal dominant conditions and the horizontal pattern of autosomal recessive conditions.

Examples of X-linked recessive conditions include hemophilia A, Duchenne muscular dystrophy, the Lesch-Nyhan syndrome, glucose-6-phosphate dehydrogenase deficiency, and Fabry's disease. In several of these, e.g., Duchenne muscular dystrophy and Fabry's disease, heterozygous females may exhibit mild or even moderately severe forms of the disease. Color blindness is also an X-linked inherited trait, but it is sufficiently frequent (occurring in about 8% of Caucasian males) that the occurrence of homozygous color-blind females is not rare.

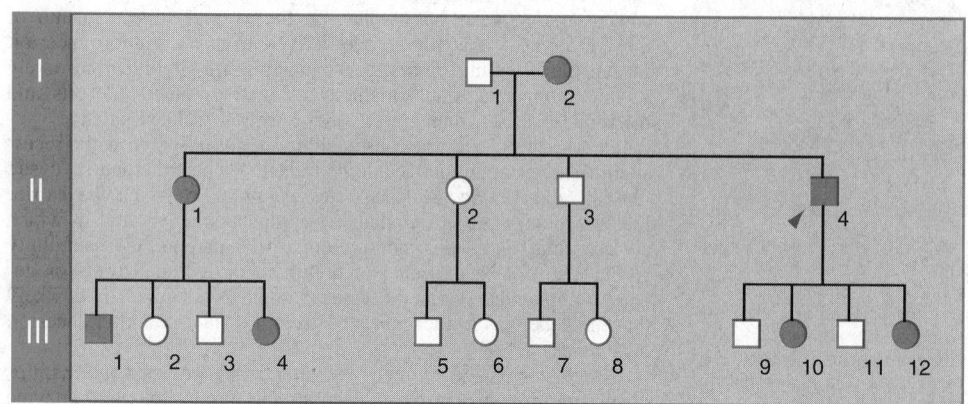

FIGURE 23–6. Pedigree of a dominant X-linked trait. Unlike autosomal dominant inheritance, dominant X-linked traits cannot be passed from a father to a son. (See text for further details.)

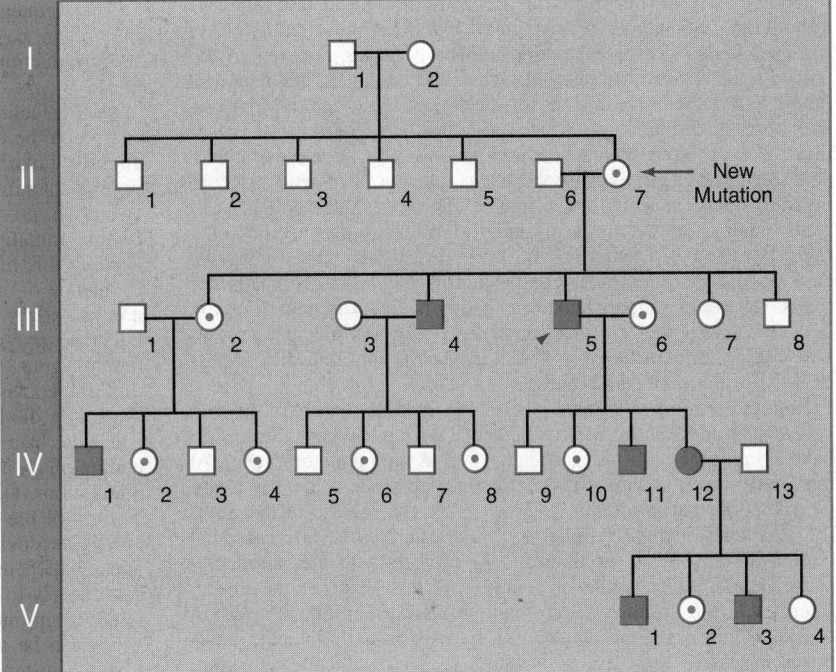

FIGURE 23-7. Pedigree on an X-linked recessive trait. Individual II.7 is the youngest daughter of a family of six siblings. She has two affected sons and five normal brothers. Most likely, the mutation took place in the aged father during spermatogenesis. (I.1). The proband (III.5) unfortunately married a female carrier and thus had an affected daughter (IV.12). All of her sons will be affected (e.g., V.1 and V.3). (See text for further details.)

It is important to distinguish between X-linked inheritance and *sex-influenced autosomal dominant inheritance*. Baldness and hemochromatosis are examples of autosomal dominant and recessive traits that are sex influenced. Heterozygous females express the gene for baldness only when a source of testosterone becomes available (e.g., a masculinizing tumor of the ovary). Homozygous females rarely develop clinical hemochromatosis because menstruation and pregnancy mitigate the accumulation of iron.

Y-LINKED INHERITANCE. A gene on the Y chromosome is transmitted through the father to all of his sons and none of his daughters. Only a small number of genes are located on the Y chromosome. Among them is the dominant gene for maleness, SRY.

POLYGENIC INHERITANCE

Most phenotypic traits are determined by many genes collaborating at different loci rather than by single gene effects. Polygenic inheritance is suggested for traits that show continuous variation in the form of a normal distribution curve. Height and intelligence are examples of polygenic traits in which the extremes of the distribution are not necessarily considered abnormal. Parents and offspring, and usually siblings also, have 50% of their genes in common. Second-degree relatives share on average one fourth of all genes [$(\frac{1}{2})^2$],

and third-degree relatives (cousins) share one eighth [$(\frac{1}{2})^3$]. As the degree of relation becomes more distant, the probability of inheriting the same combination of genes is reduced, and the degree of resemblance is likely to be less.

Many of the common chronic diseases of adults (e.g., essential hypertension, diabetes mellitus, hyperuricemia, hypercholesterolemia, coronary artery disease, and schizophrenia) and the common birth defects of children (e.g., cleft palate and lip and congenital heart disease) that tend to run in families fit best into the category of *multifactorial genetic disease*. This category should be suspected when the pedigree of a disease does not support inheritance in a simple dominant or recessive manner. Multifactorial genetic diseases have both a polygenic component and an environmental component of causative factors. In the population at large *risk* genes are present in low frequency. If any one individual has a particularly large number of risk genes, the latent disorder becomes overt. When an individual inherits just the right combination of risk genes, he/she passes beyond a "risk threshold" at which environmental factors may determine the expression and severity of disease (Fig. 23-8). In order for another family member to develop the same disease, that individual would have to inherit the same or a very similar combination of genes. The likelihood of such an occur-

FIGURE 23-8. The darkly shaded area represents the proportion of the population at risk for expression of a disease that conforms to a polygenic multifactorial model of inheritance. The shared inheritance of genes leads to an increased prevalence of disease among the relatives of affected individuals. This increased prevalence is most evident among first-degree relatives (hatched area).

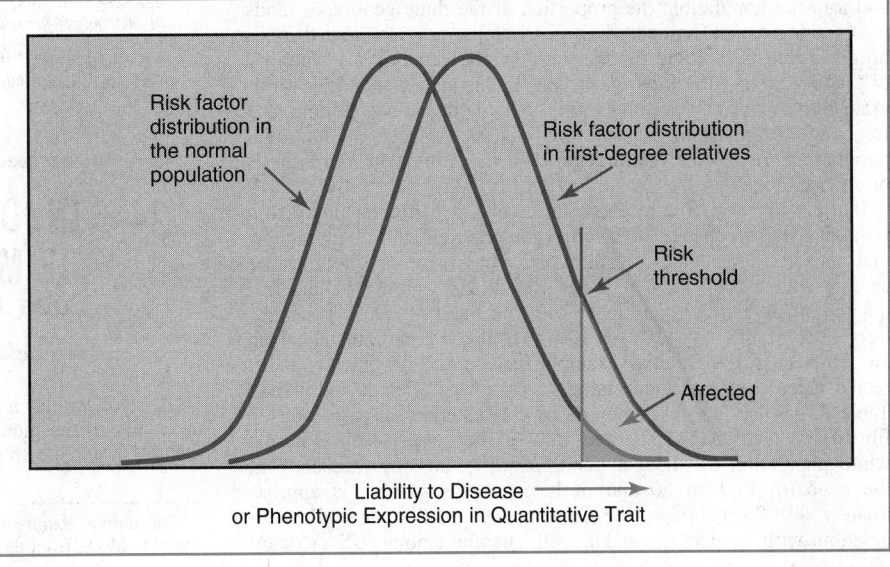

Risk factor distribution in the normal population

Risk factor distribution in first-degree relatives

Risk threshold

Affected

Liability to Disease ⟶ or Phenotypic Expression in Quantitative Trait

rence is clearly greater in first-degree than in more distant relatives. The chances of another relative inheriting the right combination of risk genes also decreases as the number of genes required to express a given trait increases. Elegant and complex mathematical models have been advanced for polygenic-multifactorial disease, but these should not obscure the fact that each of the risk genes must express itself, like any other gene, by way of a specific biochemical product. Eventually the vague concept of genetic susceptibility of polygenic inheritance must yield to the basic premise that genes control the synthesis of specific proteins with specific functions. To date the genetic loci most prominently associated with disease susceptibility are those composing the major histocompatibility (MHC) locus or human leukocyte antigen (HLA) system (see Ch. 229). We may anticipate that genetic mapping and linkage analyses will allow the identification of risk genes for common diseases, as well as for the monogenic ones.

Multifactorial or polygenic inheritance must not be confused with genetic heterogeneity. Hypercholesterolemia and hyperuricemia behave as multifactorial traits when viewed at the population level. At the family level, however, it is sometimes possible to identify a single mutation that is mainly responsible for the disease in that family. Examples include familial hypercholesterolemia, an autosomal dominant trait present in about 5% of subjects with premature myocardial infarctions, which in single-gene dosage produces atherosclerosis in the absence of any extraordinary environmental factor; or hypoxanthineguanine phosphoribosyltransferase deficiency, an X-linked recessive trait present in about 0.5% of subjects with gout, which in the hemizygous state produces marked purine overproduction without any relationship to obesity or alcohol consumption.

MITOCHONDRIAL INHERITANCE

Each mitochondrion contains several circular chromosomes that code for certain ribosomal and transfer ribonucleic acids (RNA's) and for 13 polypeptides involved in oxidative phosphorylation, the chief function of the mitochondrion. The mitochondrial code differs from that of nuclear DNA and that of any contemporary prokaryote; it is similar to that of bacteria. Mitochondrial inheritance is exclusively matrilineal. Diseases that are thought to involve mitochondrial mutations include Leber hereditary optic atrophy, infantile bilateral striatal necrosis, and myoclonic epilepsy with "ragged red fibers."

GENE FREQUENCY

The distribution of a mutant gene in the general population may be calculated on the basis of the Hardy-Weinberg equation. If the frequency of a particular gene A is p, then that of its alternative allele is $(1 - p) = q$. Three genotypes are found in the population: those who are homozygous AA, those who are heterozygous Aa, and those who are homozygous aa. In a randomly mating population, the frequencies of these genotypes are in the proportion p^2 (AA), 2 pq (Aa), and q^2 (aa). An important consequence of this distribution is that irrespective of the initial frequency of the genes A and a in the population, the proportion of the three genotypes tends to remain constant in succeeding generations, provided that there is no difference in biologic fitness of any of the genotypes. If viability or fertility among the three genotypes is unequal, if individuals migrate into or out of the population, or if mating is not random, the frequency calculations require considerable correction. In small populations major changes in gene frequency can occur on the basis of chance alone.

If the frequency of a recessive disease in a particular population is known, the frequency of heterozygous carriers and of the abnormal gene can be calculated. Thus for a recessively inherited disease aa (q^2) with a frequency of 1 per 10,000 (e.g., albinism), the frequency of the gene a (q) is 1 per 100, and that of heterozygous carriers is $2 \times p \times q = 2 \times 99/100 \times 1/100$ = approximately 1 in 50. Thus, in this particular example there are 200 clinically unaffected carriers of the abnormal gene for every affected individual. Table 23–3 lists the frequency of several inherited diseases. Cystic fibrosis, a recessively inherited disease, has a prevalence in the white population of about 1 per 2500 (q^2); thus the frequency of the gene (q) is 1 in 50 and of heterozygous carriers is approximately 1 in 25, or 4% of the Caucasian population. A similar calculation with respect to sickle cell anemia among US African-

Americans ($q^2 = 1/625$) yields a frequency of heterozygous carriers of 1 in 12.5, or 8% of this population.

The frequency of most genes in the population is relatively stable. When a gene is rare and severely disadvantageous, the rate of its introduction into a population by spontaneous mutation is balanced by the rate of elimination of the disadvantageous gene by natural selection. The frequency of the disadvantageous gene, however, can be stabilized at a high level if the heterozygotes are slightly favored (increased biologic fitness) and leave a greater number of progeny than either homozygote. When a rare form of a species is present at a frequency that cannot be maintained by recurrent mutation alone, a balanced polymorphism is said to exist. Usually this means that the rarer of two allelic forms occurs with a frequency of at least 1% of the population. When this is found, heterozygote advantage should be suspected. An example of such a balanced polymorphism is the increased resistance of individuals heterozygous for the sickle cell trait to falciparum malaria. Although persons with sickle cell disease (homozygotes, SS hemoglobin) often die before they can reproduce and thus remove the sickle cell gene from the population, the prevalence of heterozygotes (SA hemoglobin) may nevertheless reach 40% in certain West African populations. Death from falciparum malaria is much less frequent in carriers of the sickle cell trait than in noncarriers, and thus the heterozygote does have an advantage. Whether the extraordinary frequency of heterozygotes for the sickle cell gene in West Africa is due entirely to differential mortality or in part to differential fertility is uncertain, but this example suffices to illustrate that the effects of genes can be assessed only in relation to a particular environment. In most instances, however, a distinct advantage for the heterozygote of a polymorphic trait (of which there are many; see Ch. 24) cannot be demonstrated, and it is likely that certain polymorphic traits are genetically neutral.

The term genetic load has been used to describe the total genetic disability of a population. It comprises both a mutational load, based on recurrent mutation of a normal gene to a lethal or sublethal gene, and a segregational load, resulting from segregation of the harmful gene from advantaged heterozygotes, as in the example of sickle cell heterozygotes discussed above. Each individual has been estimated to have three to eight genes, which, if homozygous instead of heterozygous, would be lethal. The relative contribution of the segregational and mutational loads to the total genetic load is uncertain.

Beaudet AL, Scriver CR, Sly WS, et al.: Introduction to Human Biochemical and Molecular Genetics. New York, McGraw-Hill, 1990. A historical perspective and summation of what we know about basic principles of human genetics, which emphasizes causes (mutations), pathogenesis, and therapy.

Emery AEH, Rimoin DL, Sofaer JA: Principles and Practices of Medical Genetics. 2nd ed. Edinburgh, Churchill Livingstone, 1990. An authoritative textbook of medical genetics.

King RA, Rotter JI, Motulsky AG: The Genetic Basis of Common Diseases. New York, Oxford University Press, 1992. A review of the hereditary basis of diseases with a prevalence of 1% or greater in the population.

McKusick VA: Mendelian Inheritance in Man. 10th ed. Baltimore, Johns Hopkins University Press, 1993. A catalogue of autosomal dominant, autosomal recessive, and X-linked phenotypes, with brief descriptions and literature references for each.

Scriver CR, Beaudet AL, Sly WS, et al.: The Metabolic Basis of Inherited Disease. 7th ed. New York, McGraw-Hill, 1994. Authoritative discussions of all inborn errors of metabolism for which there is a substantial body of metabolic or biochemical information.

Vogel F, Motulsky AG: Human Genetics: Problems and Approaches. 2nd ed. Berlin, Springer-Verlag, 1986. A superb treatment of the principles of human genetics.

24 INBORN ERRORS OF METABOLISM

Louis J. Elsas II

Metabolism is a collective term for integrated biochemical processes of the intact organism, differentiated organ, cell, and subcellular organelle. Normal metabolism enables economical homeo-

The author acknowledges the chapter on this subject by James B. Wyngaarten, M.D., from the previous edition.

stasis for the organism by maintaining anabolic and catabolic flow of substrates to products. In the early twentieth century, Sir Archibald Garrod recognized heritable blocks in normal metabolic flow which conformed to mendelian mechanisms of inheritance. He first coined the term *inborn error of metabolism* in his Croonian Lectures of 1908, in which he described four diseases—alkaptonuria, albinism, cystinuria, and pentosuria—and their recessive patterns of inheritance. Garrod presumed that the patient expressing the full abnormality was homozygous for an abnormal gene affecting a specific metabolic flow while the parents were heterozygous for this same inherited block but were clinically normal. When he gave patients with alkaptonuria proteins or other precursors of homogentisic acid, excretion of alkaptones increased as evidenced by a darkening of the urine on standing. He theorized that this "block-in-reaction sequence" was controlled genetically because pedigree analyses were consistent with an *autosomal recessive* mode of inheritance. The enzyme defect in alkaptonuria was not discovered until 50 years later, when homogentisic acid oxidase was found to be missing from the liver and kidneys of patients with this disease.

First proof that an impaired protein function led to disease came from Gibson's observation in 1948 that erythrocyte methemoglobin reductase was impaired in patients with *methemoglobinemia.* By 1952, Pauling and Ingram had identified an abnormal hemoglobin structure in *sickle cell anemia.* During this same period, Cori and Cori identified a deficiency of hepatic glucose 6-phosphatase in *Von Gierke's disease* or *type I glycogen storage disease* and thus confirmed Garrod's theory by defining a block in the flow of hepatic glucose production from its stored glycogen.

It is important to understand that variations in human proteins do not usually produce disease. Heritable diversity in hemoglobins, phosphoglucomutase, lactate dehydrogenase, red blood cell acid phosphatase, haptoglobins, immunoglobins, and so forth were discovered and defined for normal populations. In some cases diversity is required for optimal health, as with the immunoglobulin proteins and the switch from fetal to adult hemoglobins. Several mechanisms produce a normal diversity of proteins. For example, the β-globin gene has many nucleotide sequence variations that produce different amino acid changes in the primary protein structure without producing a functional change. When no functional change occurs, the alteration is considered a *polymorphism.* Two different globin proteins coded for by different gene loci (alleles) form the functional tetramer, hemoglobin. Hemoglobin exemplifies how a protein may contain separate subunits, each encoded by different alleles ($\alpha2\beta2$, $\alpha2\delta2$, $\alpha2\gamma2$). There are many examples of proteins in which multiple alleles for subunits result in a wide array of multimeric functional proteins.

Another example of normal protein variation is the formation of immunoglobulins giving rise to required variations in these important molecules in response to foreign antigens (see Ch. 228). Examples of normal variation in proteins caused by alternative splicing of RNA are the insulin receptor, elastin, thyroid peroxidase, and tyrosine hydroxylase. Much of species and organ specificity for evolutionarily conserved genes occurs through post-translational modification of their encoded proteins. One example (of many) is the organ-specific isozyme of lactate dehydrogenase (LDH), a phenomenon used clinically to differentiate cellular damage in heart, liver, or lung.

The relatively rare circumstance in which a change in a protein impairs function is called a *mutation* and may produce an inborn error of metabolism. This circumstance provides insight into the functional role of the normal protein in human metabolism. Inborn

TABLE 24-1. CLASSIFICATION OF PROTEIN FUNCTION BY LOCATION IN THE ORGANISM

Proteins act as follows:
1. Catalyze plasma membrane functions
   a. Substrate transport
   b. Cellular signaling (receptors)
2. Catalyze major cellular metabolic pathways in the cytosol, lysosome, peroxisome, mitochondria, and nucleus.
3. Circulate in blood and provide and maintain various functions (clotting; metal, lipid, or vitamin transport; immunity; oxygen transport; regulate proteases, hormones, adhesion proteins)
4. Maintain structural integrity of organs and organelles (collagen, elastin, actin, dystrophin, fibrillins)

TABLE 24-2. CLASSIC PATHOLOGIC MECHANISMS FOR INBORN ERRORS OF METABOLISM

1. Accumulation to toxic concentrations of substrates in a blocked catabolic reaction. Examples: maple syrup urine disease, glucose-galactose malabsorption, galactosemia
2. Production of toxic by-products through a normally minor pathway. Examples: tyrosinemia type I and adenosine deaminase deficiency
3. Deficiency of an end-product in an anabolic pathway. Examples: albinism, orotic aciduria, and Zellweger syndrome
4. Loss of regulation resulting in overproduced intermediates to toxic levels. Examples: congenital adrenal hyperplasia, intermittent porphyria, familial hypercholesterolemia

errors of metabolism are classified here in accordance with the organ, cell, and subcellular location of normal protein function (Table 24–1) and the abnormal mechanisms that interfere with the normal metabolic flow resulting from impaired proteins (Table 24–2). Analysis of these inborn errors of metabolism defined the importance of normal proteins by their cellular location and catalyzed reactions. As we progress in protein and gene replacement therapy, this approach to disease classification provides a practical working model.

The most important clinical aspect in defining a metabolic disease as heritable rather than environmental is that one can predict, intervene, and prevent the disease. In general, the severity of an inborn error of metabolism depends on the degree of protein impairment rendered by the genetic mutation. Thus a "leaky" mutation may not be expressed until adulthood, whereas a complete block in the same metabolic pathway is lethal in infancy. A combination of the pathophysiologic mechanisms outlined in Table 24–2 and the effects of the environment produces loss of homeostasis and determines the extent of disease in the complex human organism. Outcome depends on the ability to engineer the environment, the degree of impaired protein function, and the timeliness of intervening to prevent irreversible organ damage.

Familial glucose-galactose malabsorption syndrome exemplifies defective transporter protein resulting in specific accumulation of its substrate to toxic levels (Tables 24–1 and 24–2).

Direct evidence for the genetic control of intestinal glucose transport in humans was obtained by *in vitro* studies of jejunal biopsy material from patients expressing refractory diarrhea on ingesting D-galactose or D-glucose. Biopsy material from asymptomatic first-degree relatives demonstrated partial impairment of this transport function and defined autosomal recessive inheritance. These physiologic data suggested that a single mutant gene affects sodium-dependent, active glucose transport by human jejunal (and proximal renal tubular) microvilli. Expression cloning of active transport has now confirmed the presence of an Na^+-glucose co-transporter gene, its deduced amino acid sequence, and specific codon changes producing the syndrome of familial glucose-galactose malabsorption. In fact, a whole family of glucose transporter genes is now known to be differentially expressed by specific organs.

The importance of membrane transporter proteins is supported by a large number of inherited defects involving the plasma membrane transport process (Table 24–3). Glucose transporters represent a family of proteins whose definitions of function have evolved through molecular genetic analysis (Table 24–4). Comparing the data from renal glycosuria and glucose-galactose malabsorption, it became evident that different Na^+-dependent active glucose transporters were present in kidney and gut epithelium. Other Na^+-independent, facilitative glucose transporters were cloned. An insulin-responsive, facilitative glucose transporter (GLUT4) is not Na^+-dependent and is expressed primarily in insulin-responsive tissues (fat cells, skeletal muscle). More than one glucose transporter is expressed by most cells. For example, the jejunal epithelial cell uses SGLT-1 to concentrate glucose from its luminal surface into the cytosol, then effluxes glucose at its basal-lateral surfaces through GLUT2. GLUT2 is also involved in regulating the amount of glucose transported into β cells of the pancreas, a process that regulates glucose stimulation of insulin release. Indirect evidence indicates that mutations in the GLUT2 gene are "sensitivity genes" involved in polygenic *insulin-dependent (type I, IDDM)* and *independent (type II, NIDDM) diabetes mellitus.*

TABLE 24–3. DISEASES CAUSED BY PLASMA MEMBRANE TRANSPORTER PROTEIN MUTATIONS

Disease	Tissues Affected	Substrate	Mode of Inheritance	Clinical Expression
B_{12} malabsorption	Ileum	Vitamin B_{12}	Autosomal recessive	Juvenile pernicious anemia
Blue diaper syndrome	Gut	Tryptophan	Autosomal recessive	Hypercalcemia
Congenital chloridorrhea	Gut	Chloride	Autosomal recessive	Diarrhea, alkalosis
Cystic fibrosis	Apical epithelia	Chloride	Autosomal recessive	Lung, intestinal obstruction
Cystinuria	Kidney + gut	Cystine + lysine, arginine, ornithine	Autosomal recessive	Renal lithiasis (cystine)
Familial hypophosphatemic rickets	Kidney + gut	Phosphate	X-linked dominant	Rickets
Folate deficiency	Lymphocyte, erythrocyte	Methyl tetrahydrofolate	Autosomal recessive	Aplastic anemia
Glucose-galactose malabsorption	Gut + kidney	Glucose and galactose	Autosomal recessive	Refractory diarrhea
Hartnup syndrome	Gut + kidney	Neutral amino acids	Autosomal recessive	Nicotinic acid deficiency (pellagra)
Hereditary hypophosphatemic rickets	Kidney	Phosphate	Autosomal dominant	Growth restriction, rickets, hypercalciuria
Hereditary renal hypouricemia	Kidney	Uric acid	Autosomal recessive	Urolithiasis (uric acid)
Hereditary spherocytosis	Erythrocyte	Sodium	Autosomal recessive	Hemolytic anemia
Hyperdibasic aminoaciduria (type I)	Kidney	Lysine Arginine Ornithine	Autosomal dominant	? Symptoms
Iminoglycinuria	Kidney + gut	Glycine Proline Hydroxyproline	Autosomal recessive	Benign ?
Isolated lysinuria	Kidney + gut	Lysine	Autosomal recessive	Growth failure, seizures
Lysinuric protein intolerance (type II)	Kidney, fibroblasts, hepatocytes, gut	Lysine	Autosomal recessive	Growth restriction, hyperammonemia, mental retardation
Methionine malabsorption (oasthouse disease)	Gut	Methionine	Autosomal recessive ?	Mental retardation, white hair, failure to thrive
Renal glycosuria	Kidney	Glucose	Autosomal recessive	Benign glycosuria
Renal tubular acidosis (type I)	Distal renal tubule	H+ secretion, citrate, calcium	Autosomal dominant	Hypokalemia, growth restriction, nephrocalcinosis
Renal tubular acidosis (type II)	Proximal renal tubule	Bicarbonate	"Familial"	Hyperchloremic metabolic acidosis

TABLE 24–4. HUMAN GLUCOSE TRANSPORTERS

	Protein kd (AA)	mRNA Size (kb)	Chromosomal Localization	Expression in Tissue and Cells	Function	Disorder
GLUT1	55 (492)	2.8	1p35 → p31.3	Fetal cells, blood-brain barrier, erythrocyte, fibroblast	Basal glucose transport across most cells, including blood brain barrier	Seizures with low CSF and normal blood glucose
GLUT2	58 (524)	2.8 3.4 5.4	3q26.1 → q26.3	Liver, kidney, intestine, B cell of the pancreas	Low affinity glucose transport	NIDDM and IDDM
GLUT3	54 (496)	2.7 4.1	12p13.3	Neurons, fibroblast, placenta, testes	Basal glucose transport	?
GLUT4	55 (509)	2.8 3.5	17p13	Fat, skeletal muscle, heart	Insulin-stimulated glucose transport	NIDDM
GLUT5	50 (501)	2.0	1p32 → p22	Small intestine	Fructose transport	?
GLUT7	60 (528)	?	?	Liver microsome	Glucose release from endoplasmic reticulum	Type IB glycogen storage disease
Concentrative glucose transporters						
SLGT1	75 (664)	2.2 2.6 4.8	22q11 → qter	Intestine, kidney	Intestinal absorption, renal reabsorption	Hypoglycemia, glucosegalactose malabsorption, renal glycosuria

IDDM, insulin-dependent diabetes mellitus; NIDDM, non–insulin-dependent diabetes mellitus.

Many diseases characterized by "hormone resistance" are caused by another family of proteins which function in the plasma membrane. The concept of failure to respond to hormone stimulation originated in the early 1940's with a description of *pseudohypoparathyroidism* (see Ch. 214). Heritability of resistance to parathormone was suggested before the existence of parathormone receptors or hormone-sensitive adenylate cyclases or guanine nucleotide–binding proteins was known.

Diseases caused by defective transmembrane signaling include *Laron dwarfism,* which results from growth hormone (GH) receptor defects. Deletions in the GH receptor gene of Asian Jews has been found. Phenotypic characteristics are *proportionate dwarfism,* hypoglycemia, craniofacial disproportion with a doll-like face, balding, frontal bossing, truncal obesity, and wrinkled skin. In this disorder, GH concentration is elevated in blood, peripheral tissue responses to GH are decreased, and insulin-like growth factor-1 concentrations in blood are low. An autosomal recessive mode of inheritance is defined. Other common causes for dominant or polygenic growth restriction may result from other mutations in the GH receptor. The GH receptor gene is found on chromosome 17q22-24. *Familial hypercholesterolemia* defines a phenotype of hypercholesterolemia, early onset heart disease, and decreased LDL-cholesterol binding to plasma membrane. This disorder affects a significant number of individuals in the general population, an estimated 1 in 500. An autosomal dominant mode is described for early-onset adult heart disease. Many different mutations are known in the LDL-cholesterol receptor gene which lead to decreased number or function of LDL-cholesterol receptors and to a loss in the cell's ability to downregulate endogenous cholesterol synthesis. Consequently there is increased intracellular and intravascular accumulation of LDL-cholesterol with resultant atherosclerosis and heart disease in the third and fourth decades of life (see Table 24–2). The gene is found on chromosome 19p13.1–13.2. The rare disorder, *leprechaunism,* has become a prototypic inborn error of severe insulin resistance and loss of cellular signal transduction through the insulin receptor. Affected infants have low birth weight, acanthosis nigricans, cystic changes in organs, and loss of glucose homeostasis. They also have remarkably elevated plasma insulin concentrations above 500 mIU per milliliter. Specific impairment in ^{125}I-labeled insulin binding is evident in cells cultured from patients and a spectrum of mutations produces a spectrum of diseases including adult-onset *type I diabetes.* Obligate heterozygotes (parents) of patients with leprechaunism have partially impaired insulin binding, which led to the discovery that leprechaunism was caused by a single gene (i.e., insulin-receptor gene) and that a mutation(s) affects specific domains of the receptor with a range of disease expression.

Sequencing of the cDNA for the insulin receptor whose gene is located on chromosome 19p indicated that both its α and β subunits are encoded by a single cDNA of 5 kb length. In families with leprechaunism and other variations of severe insulin resistance, several different mutations were found (Table 24–5). These mutations impair synthesis, receptor transfer to the plasma membrane, binding of insulin, autophosphorylation, and receptor signaling (Table 24–5). Thus mutations in the insulin receptor gene exemplify clinical *heterogeneity* in inborn errors of metabolism. This term signifies that different mutations produce different severity and variation of diseases even though they result from mutations in the same gene. Membrane receptors transduce signals to proteins bound on the inner cytoplasmic surface (second messengers). Thus, the insulin receptor transfers its signal by phosphotransfer to the insulin receptor signal protein 1 (IRS-1) protein, a protein of 180 kd. The IRS-1 gene is located on chromosome 2q, is rich in tyrosine residues, and acts as the phosphotransfer second messenger. Although no mutations in humans are as yet defined in IRS-1, some membrane receptors that signal through cyclic nucleotides have mutations in their signaling (G) proteins. An example is *Albright's hereditary osteodystrophy* or *pseudohypoparathyroidism* (see Ch. 214). A heterogeneous group of mutations has now been found in the gene for the parathyroid hormone receptor's guanine nucleotide–binding protein ($G_s a$) which links the receptor to adenylate cyclase and stimulates cAMP when the receptor is occupied by parathormone. This gene for $G_s a$ is located on chromosome 20q13, and both deletions and missense mutations are defined which produce Albright's hereditary osteodystrophy. Interestingly, somatic mutations in arginine 201 of the same gene turn the $G_s a$ protein constitutively "on" and produce another disease, the *Albright-McCune-Sternberg syndrome,* which includes nonossifying bone tumors and premature puberty.

Inborn errors affecting proteins of the cytosolic compartment within a cell are the more "traditional" inborn errors of metabolism (Table 24–6). They impair the catalytic reactions of anabolic or catabolic pathways and are usually classified by the type of micromolecules altered. Thus we consider disorders of sugar, amino acid, purine, and organic acid metabolism.

Galactose metabolism is important in infancy because the primary carbohydrate source of human milk is lactose, a disaccharide composed of glucose and galactose. Classic *galactosemia* results from mutations in the gene for galactose 1-phosphate uridyl transferase [GALT]. The gene is found on chromosome 9p13, and its cDNA codes for a protein of 379 amino acids. A common mutation is a substitution of arginine for glutamine at codon 188 (Q188R). This mutation eliminates GALT activity and produces classic neonatal disease. Untreated, the infant suffers liver, central nervous system, and renal damage and may succumb to bacterial sepsis. Variant forms of galactosemia with other mutations in the GALT gene are known to produce GALT activity ranging from 3 to 25% of normal. If excess lactose is ingested, cataracts, premature ovarian

TABLE 24–5. MUTATIONS IN THE INSULIN RECEPTOR (IR) GENE CAUSING INHERITED INSULIN RESISTANCE

Syndrome	Disease Mechanism
Recessive inheritance	
Leprechaunism	
1597 A → G Lys460 → Glu	Defective insulin binding
2233 C → T Gln672 → STOP	Reduced number of IR
476 G → C Arg86 → Pro	Defective binding
Homozygous	Activation of glucose transport and phosphotransfer
917T → C Leu233 → Pro	Defective processing by IR
Homozygous	
310 G → A Gly31 → Arg	Defective processing by IR
Not determined	
2908 C → T Arg897 → STOP	Reduced mRNA
Noncoding region IR gene	Reduced mRNA
1333 C → T Arg372STOP	Reduced mRNA
Noncoding region IR gene	Reduced mRNA
Del 1159-1161 Del Asn281	Defective binding (?)
Not determined	
302 T → C Val28 → Ala	(?)
1315 G → C Gly366 → Arg	
850 A → G His209 → Arg	Defective processing by IR
Homozygous	
Rabson-Mendenhall Syndrome	
264 C → A Asn15 → Lsy	Defective processing by IR
3217 → C → T Arg1000 → STOP	Reduced mRNA
Splice error intron 4	Reduced mRNA
Not determined	
Type I Insulin Resistance	
1363 T → G Phe362 → Val	Defective processing by IR
Homozygous	
1604 A → G Asn462 → Ser	Defective insulin binding
617 G → A Trp133 → STOP	Reduced mRNA
2424 G → T Arg735 → Ser	Defective cleavage IR
Homozygous	
3197 G → A Arg993 → Gln	Defective kinase
3217 G → T Arg1000 → STOP	Decreased mRNA
Delta exon 14	Receptor truncation
Not determined	
Lipodystrophy	
He485 → Thr	(?)
Dominant inheritance	
Type I insulin resistance	
3176 C → T Pro986 → Leu	Defective phosphorylation
3242 G → T Gly1008 → Val	Defective phosphorylation
Del 3300 → Ter Del 1013	Defective phosphorylation Truncated receptor
3619 G → A Ala1134 → Thr	Defective phosphorylation
3623 C → A Ala1135 → Glu	Defective phosphorylation
3678 G → A Met1153 → Ile	Defective phosphorylation
3818 G → C Trp1200 → Ser	Defective phosphorylation
Type II (non–insulin-dependent) diabetes mellitus	
3421 A → G Lys1068 → Glu	Defective phosphorylation
3710 G → A Arg1164 → Gln	Defective kinase

TABLE 24–6. DISEASES CAUSED BY IMPAIRED CYTOSOLIC ENZYMES

Disorder	Enzyme Defect	Phenotype	Inheritance
Carbohydrates			
Fructosuria	Fructokinase	Benign	Autosomal recessive
Hereditary fructose intolerance	Fructose 1-phosphate aldolase	Liver dysfunction, early death	Autosomal recessive
Galactosemia	Galactose-1-P-uridyl transferase	Liver dysfunction, cataracts, sepsis, death, mental retardation	Autosomal recessive
Hereditary fructose 1,6-bis-phosphate deficiency	Fructose 1,6-bisphosphatase	Apnea, ketosis, lactic acidosis	Autosomal recessive
Amino acids			
Phenylketonuria	p-Hydroxyphenylalanine hydroxylase	Mental retardation (teratogenic)	Autosomal recessive
Tyrosinemia			
Type II	Tyrosine aminotransferase	Palmar bullae, corneal lesions	Autosomal recessive
Type I	Fumarylacetoacetate hydrolase	Succinylacetone accumulation with acute porphyria	Autosomal recessive
Homocystinuria	Cystathionine B synthase	Marfanoid habitus, arterial thrombosis, lens dislocation, mental retardation	Autosomal recessive
Hyperornithinemia	Ornithine aminotransferase	Gyrate atrophy of the retina	Autosomal recessive
Lesch-Nyhan syndrome	Hypoxanthine phosphoribosyl-transferase	Hyperuricemia Neurologic dysfunction with self-destructive tendency	X-linked

failure, and growth and mental restriction may occur in the adult population. When individuals with these disorders are detected early, as with newborn screening programs (see Ch. 168), disease is prevented by replacing lactose with sucrose in infant's formula and by eating a diet restricted in galactose throughout life.

Phenylalanine is an essential amino acid for growth whose anabolic products include tyrosine, thyroid hormone, adenergic neurotransmitters, and melanin. *Phenylketonuria (PKU)* (see Ch. 176) is caused by mutations in the gene encoding the phenylalanine hydroxylase protein, the first enzyme in this anabolic flow which catalyzes tyrosine production.

Albinism is an example of an inborn error in an anabolic pathway in which the pathophysiologic mechanism is directly related to the lack of an end product (Mechanism 3, Table 24–2). Tyrosine is converted by the action of a cytosolic tyrosinase first to dopa and then dopamine. Dopamine can then be converted either to the red-yellow pigment phenomelanin or to the black-brown pigment eumelanin. These reactions occur in the melanosomes produced in the melanocytes and exported to the keratinocytes. Color of skin is an inherited factor that depends on several genes and is a function of the intensity of the pigment in the skin and not the number of melanocytes, which is constant for all humans. Although skin color is a polygenic trait, single genes can have a profound effect on this color, as evidenced by the albino phenotype. In humans, *oculocutaneous albinism* (OCA) is inherited as an autosomal recessive trait. An X-linked and autosomal recessive form of *ocular albinism* also exists. Individuals with OCA are classified as either tyrosinase-negative or positive for tyrosine activity in hair bulbs. Tyrosinase-neg-

ative individuals form no pigment, and prenatal monitoring for tyrosinase activity in cultured amniocytes is possible. A tyrosinase-positive OCA has been associated with an autosomal recessive gene located on chromosome 15q11-13 (the P gene). A wide variation in phenotypic expression of OCA is reported from very severe neurologic deficiency with ocular and sarcomatous skin cancers to mild cosmetic problems.

Inborn errors of the urea cycle (see Ch. 178) represent defects in the integration of both anabolic and catabolic pathways and the distribution of catalytic proteins between mitochondria and cytosol. The role of the urea cycle is to convert ammonia, a by-product of protein breakdown, to urea and to synthesize arginine (anabolic). Reactions of the complete cycle use two mitochondrial enzymes, three cytosolic enzymes, and two mitochondrial transporter proteins. Inherited disorders affecting the function of each of five enzymes are known. Individuals with defects in any of the enzymes present with varying degrees of hyperammonemia caused by protein ingestion. With the exception of the gene for ornithine transcarbamylase found on the short arm of chromosome X, the other four proteins are encoded on autosomes and defects are inherited as autosomal recessive traits. Many principles involved in the pathophysiology of inborn errors of metabolism are exemplified by disorders of the urea cycle.

A group of inborn errors of metabolism is caused by mutations in nuclear genes that encode mitochondrial proteins. Collectively they are considered disorders of organic acid metabolism (Table 24–7). For example, branched-chain α-ketoacid dehydrogenase is a multienzyme complex located on the matrix side of the mitochondrial

TABLE 24–7. ORGANIC ACIDEMIAS: DISORDERS OF METABOLISM BY MITOCHONDRIAL PROTEINS

Disorder	Enzyme Defect	Inheritance
Isovaleric acidemia	Isovaleryl CoA dehydrogenase	Autosomal recessive
Methylcrotonic aciduria	3-Methylcrotonyl CoA carboxylase	
Glutaconic aciduria	3-Methylglutaconyl CoA hydralatase	
Glutaric aciduria (I)	3-hydroxy-3-methylglutaryl CoA lyase	
Mevalonic aciduria	Mevalonate kinase	
Thiolase deficiency	2-methylacetoacetyl CoA thiolase	
Isobutyric aciduria	3-hydroxyisobutyryl CoA deacylase	
Propionic aciduria	Propionyl CoA carboxylase	Autosomal recessive
Methylmalonic aciduria	Methylmalonyl CoA mutase	Autosomal recessive
Lactic acidosis	Pyruvate dehydrogenase Pyruvate decarboxylase	Autosomal recessive
Acyl-CoA dehydrogenase deficiencies	Short-; medium-, and long-chain fatty acyl CoA dehydrogenases	Autosomal recessive
Branched-chain α-ketoacidemia	Branched-chain α-ketoacid dehydrogenase	Autosomal recessive
Respiratory chain defects	Electron transfer factor (ETF) deficiency	Autosomal recessive
Glutaric acidemia type II	Multiple acyl CoA dehydrogenases	Autosomal recessive

inner membrane in all tissues. When any one of these proteins is impaired, the autosomal recessive disorder *maple syrup urine disease* may result (see Ch. 179).

Another group of inborn errors of metabolism is collectively categorized as lysosomal disorders (see Ch. 174) to indicate the subcellular localization of these catalytic proteins.

I-cell disease is an inborn error that led to the discovery of how enzymes are imprinted to reside in lysosomes. Patients with I-cell disease have inherited defects in the recognition markers required to direct enzymes to the endocytic receptor of plasma membrane and to its capture in the acidic milieu of the lysosome. Patients lack all cellular lysosomal enzymes. Instead cells are filled with inclusion bodies (hence "I-cell"). The misdirected lysosomal enzymes are secreted and are present in excess in plasma but are missing from cells. These extracellular enzymes were found to lack mannose 6-phosphate residues, and this observation led to an understanding of the post-translational mechanisms by which enzymes are directed to the lysosome by adding phosphorylated mannose. Individuals with I-cell disease lack this phosphotransferase activity.

Inborn errors affecting single enzymes in the degradative pathway for mucopolysaccharides and gangliosides helped define the steps required for the breakdown of these complex macromolecules. Disorders of mucopolysaccharidose metabolism (Ch. 182) include Hurler syndrome; Scheie syndrome; Hunter syndrome; Sanfilippo syndrome types A, B, C, and D; Morquio syndrome types A and B; and Sly syndrome. Disorders of ganglioside metabolism include Fabry's disease, Gaucher's disease, Niemann-Pick disease, 11 mucopolysaccharidoses, Tay-Sachs disease, I-cell disease, fucosidosis, mannosidosis, sialidosis, and aspartylglycosaminuria.

Another group of inborn errors of metabolism in a subcellular organelle are *peroxisomal diseases* (Table 24–8). Peroxisomes are radiodense subcellular organelles of about 0.5 to 1 nm diameter bounded by a single trilaminar membrane. Both anabolic and catabolic reactions occur in this organelle. Primary pathways synthesize plasmalogens (unique fatty acids containing vinyl ethers), cholesterol, and bile acids. Other biosynthetic reactions include gluconeogenesis from amino acids and the formation of oxalic acid by the action of alanine:glyoxylate aminotransferase (see Ch. 172). Catabolic reactions include breakdown of hydrogen peroxide by catalase, the major protein of the peroxisome; polyamine oxidation; purine breakdown; ethanol oxidation; phytanic acid hydroxylation; and pipecolic acid degradation. A major function of the peroxisome is β-oxidation of very long chain fatty acids, those longer than 24 carbons.

An understanding of the importance of a number of reactions that occur in the peroxisome has come from identifying patients with either defects in individual biochemical pathways or lack of peroxisomes. The targeting signal for peroxisomal proteins may lie in their carboxyl terminal end, and mutations in the alanine:glyoxylate aminotransferase have resulted in mistargeting of this enzyme to mitochondria with consequent *familial hyperoxaluria* (see Ch. 172).

Disorders affecting the peroxisome are of two types: type 1, the absence of the peroxisome itself, and type 2, the absence of specific enzymes from the peroxisomal milieu. These disorders are listed in Table 24–8.

Several inborn errors are caused by abnormalities in proteins that function in the nucleus and are involved in DNA repair (category 2, Table 24–1). Patients expressing these inherited disorders carry a high risk for developing cancers. Among these inborn errors of DNA metabolism are xeroderma pigmentosum, Bloom's syndrome,

TABLE 24–9. SOME INBORN ERRORS OF PROTEINS THAT CIRCULATE IN BLOOD

Functional Class	Protein	Phenotype
Transport	Ceruloplasmin	Wilson's Disease
	Albumin	Analbuminemia
	Hemoglobin	Hemoglobinopathies
	α-Lipoprotein	Analphalipoproteinemia
	β-Lipoprotein	Abetalipoproteinemia
	Transcobalamin II	Megaloblastic anemia
Hormones	Growth hormone	Pituitary dwarfism
	Insulin	Diabetes mellitus (insulin-dependent)
	Somatomedin	Pituitary dwarfism
Coagulation	Factors I–XIII	Coagulopathies
	Kininogen	Kininogen deficiency
	Prekallikrein	Prekallikrein deficiency
Immune system	Complement components	Hypocomplementemias
	Immunoglobulins	Hypogammaglobulinemias
Inhibitors	α$_1$-Antitrypsin	Pulmonary emphysema and/or cirrhosis
	C'1 esterase inhibitor	Angioneurotic edema

ataxia-telangiectasia, Fanconi's anemia, and diseases associated with early aging such as progeria and Werner syndrome. Collectively the disorders show an increased sensitivity and delayed repair of damaged DNA due to ultraviolet, x-ray, or alkylating crosslinks.

A large number of inborn errors involve proteins that circulate in blood (class 3 of Table 24–1). Stable circulating proteins in blood perform a variety of functions, including immunologic, hemostatic, regulatory, hormonal, and interorgan transport of trace metals, lipids, and other nutrients. Some inherited disorders affecting circulating proteins are tabulated in Table 24–9. Proteins involved in oxygen transport, coagulation, and immunity are detailed in other chapters, but the pathophysiologic mechanisms and genetic approaches of screening, diagnosis, and intervention to prevent an expected outcome make them appropriate to consider here as inborn errors of metabolism.

Abnormal structural proteins produce inborn errors such as Marfan syndrome (fibrillin), osteogenesis imperfecta (collagen type I), spondyloepiphyseal dysplasia (collagen type II), and Sack syndrome (collagen type III) (see Ch. 182 to 186). These disorders exemplify category 4 of inborn errors of metabolism (Table 24–1). The enzymes involved in post-transitional processing of these proteins also cause these syndromes.

Inborn errors of matrix proteins are exemplified by collagen diseases. More than 20 different genes dispersed on 9 chromosomes are currently known to code for more than 11 different types of collagen. These disorders are detailed in Ch. 183, 184, and 185.

Elsas L, Priest J: Medical genetics. *In* Sodeman W, Sodeman T (eds.): Pathologic Physiology Mechanisms of Disease, 7th ed. Philadelphia, WB Saunders, 1985. *A traditional compilation of pathophysiologic mechanisms producing inheritance diseases.*

McKusick's Mendelian Inheritance in Man, 10th ed. Baltimore, Johns Hopkins Press, 1992. *The bible of human diseases caused by single genes of large effect. A resource of references to each.*

Scriver CR, Beaudet AL, Sly WS, et al.: The Metabolic Basis of Inherited Disease, 6th ed. New York, McGraw-Hill, 1989. *A two-volume resource for inherited metabolic diseases with complete biochemistry, pathophysiology, molecular genetics, and treatment and exhaustive referencing.*

TABLE 24–8. INBORN ERRORS OF PEROXISOMES

Disorders of peroxisomal biogenesis
  Zellweger syndrome (cerebro-hepato-renal syndrome)
  Neonatal adrenoleukodystrophy
  Infantile Refsum's disease
  Hyperpipecolic acidemia
  Leber amaurosis
  Rhizomelic chondrodysplasia punctata (Conradi syndrome)
Peroxisomal 3-oxoacyl CoA thiolase deficiency
Peroxisomal acyl CoA oxidase deficiency
X-linked adrenoleukodystrophy (impaired lignoceroyl CoA and hexacosanoyl CoA ligase)
Adult Refsum's disease (phytanic acid α hydroxylase deficiency)
Acatalasemia (H_2O_2 oxidoreductase deficiency)

25 GENE THERAPY
David T. Curiel

Gene therapy is a relatively new method of therapeutic intervention (Figs. 25–1 and 25–2) targeted at the level of cellular gene expression. In this approach, altering a pathophysiologic state is achieved by delivering nucleic acids into a cell. These nucleic acids may be genes, portions of genes, oligonucleotides, or RNA. In con-

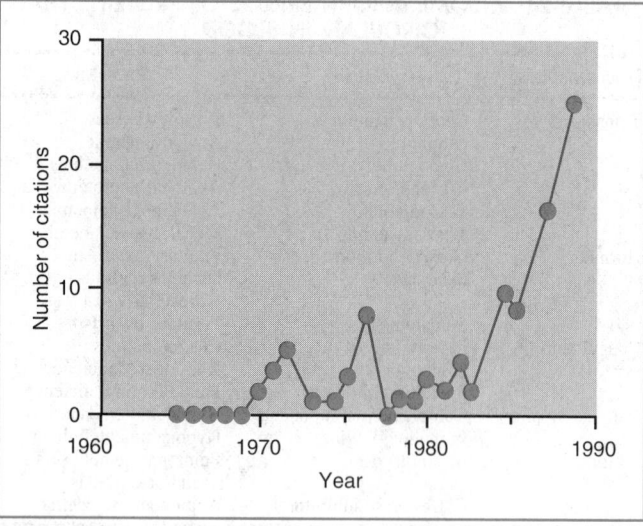

FIGURE 25-1. Growth in number of scientific publications on the subject of gene therapy.

ventional therapeutics, as in pharmacotherapy, altering a cell or tissue phenotype is accomplished by altering cell physiology or metabolism at the level of protein expression. For gene therapy, this is accomplished by changing the pattern of expression of the genes whose products may thus achieve the desired effect on the cellular phenotype. From a conceptual standpoint, gene therapy strategies may offer the potential to achieve a much higher level of specificity of action by virtue of the highly specific control and regulatory mechanisms of gene expression that may be targeted in this technique. Additionally, interceding at an earlier stage in disease pathogenesis may offer greater potential to achieve fundamental changes in phenotypic parameters of disease with a more favorable outcome.

Gene therapy was initially conceptualized as a method to treat acquired genetic diseases. In this regard, > 5000 monogenetic disorders exist in which the entirety of the disease state may be attributed to a single lesion at a specific genetic locus. Replacing or augmenting a defective gene by delivering its wild-type counterpart thus offers a potential means to rectify definitively the pathogenic basis of the disease state. Inherited genetic diseases, however, are not the only logical targets for gene therapy. The underlying basis for a variety of acquired disorders may be shown to be accumulated lesions in specific genetic loci, as in malignancies associated with mutations in dominant and recessive oncogenes. In these instances also, if the pathogenic basis is established to be lesions in cellular genes, a logical strategy is replacing or adding the mutated

genes with the wild-type counterpart to perform the deficient function.

The indications for this form of therapy must be established. The first and foremost criterion for any gene therapy is that the aberrant gene being targeted must be well characterized. In addition, it must be shown that the defined genetic abnormalities are the basis of the observed pathogenesis of the disease state. If the logic of genetic intervention thus exists, clearly defined endpoints of the therapy intervention must exist and an alternate, effective therapy for the targeted disease must not exist. This reflects the fact that at this juncture, gene therapy is still a radical, experimental therapy that may be justified only in this context.

Certain minimum criteria of potential efficacy also must be met. As a first step, it must be possible to deliver the therapeutic gene to the target cells of interest. After delivery, the introduced gene must be expressed at an appropriate level for the desired effect and for sufficient time for this effect to be achieved. Additionally, the delivery and expression of the therapeutic gene must be safe for the target cell and, by extension, for the individual being treated. From a conceptual standpoint, it must be recognized that these goals are all interrelated. Further, that all of them must be addressed to rationally implement any gene therapy strategy.

In practice, gene therapy implementation in human clinical trials has used two distinct strategies to meet the aforementioned criteria. In selected instances, target cells may be removed from the body, genetically modified extracorporally, and then reintroduced into the patient. This *ex vivo* strategy has been applied in those contexts in which the technical capacity exists to readily harvest and manipulate the relevant target cell. As an alternative strategy, the *in vivo* approach involves directly delivering the therapeutic gene to the relevant target cells *in situ* in an intact individual. Whereas both approaches have been used in human clinical trials, the preponderance of strategies to date have employed the *ex vivo* approach. Although this method may offer certain advantages in selected contexts, it must be recognized that using this route presents the technical difficulty associated with accomplishing direct *in vivo* delivery.

The advantages of the *ex vivo* approach are that it allows gene transfer to the target cells in a defined, *in vitro* setting, in which delivery efficiencies may be optimized. This approach also allows the modified cells to be characterized from the standpoint of safety prior to their being reintroduced to the patient. Despite these advantages, this method may be limited to very selected settings in which target cells can be propagated *ex vivo;* at present, this is viable for a very limited set of tissue types. The *in vivo* approach in theory overcomes this limitation of target tissue accessibility. Delivery *in vivo,* however, is at present fraught with considerably greater complexities than the *ex vivo* approach. Thus, the gene transfer vector in the direct-delivery approach must achieve delivery in the context of significant host barriers, including humoral, reticuloendothelial, and immunologic factors. This dichotomy highlights the fact that the ability to accomplish *in vivo* gene delivery currently represents the greatest challenge to implementing gene therapy strategies. Protocols to date have principally been of the *ex vivo* type and have relied on recombinant retroviruses as gene transfer vehicles.

The technology to derive recombinant retroviruses that can very efficiently transfer genes has been sufficiently developed that these vectors have been used for the overwhelming majority of human protocols (Fig. 25-3). They can accomplish effective gene transfer to a variety of target cells despite being rendered replication-incompetent by genomic deletions. In addition, because these viruses are integrative, they can produce permanent genetic modifications of target cells with the consequence of long-term heterologous gene expression. Whereas the vectors are suited for *ex vivo* modification of target cells, a variety of limitations has restricted their use in strategies to accomplish direct, *in vivo* gene transfer. The retrovirus requires proliferative target cells to mediate effective gene transfer. In addition, the virus particle is highly susceptible to humoral factors that ablate its gene-transfer capacity. Thus, the basic biology of recombinant retroviruses has been an additional factor restricting implemented gene therapy protocols to strategies using *ex vivo* methodologies.

To circumvent the limitations associated with recombinant retroviruses, alternative vector systems have been developed. These systems include both viral and nonviral approaches to accomplish gene transfer. In both of these approaches, the goal is to develop a system that can deliver genes *in vivo* after systemic administration.

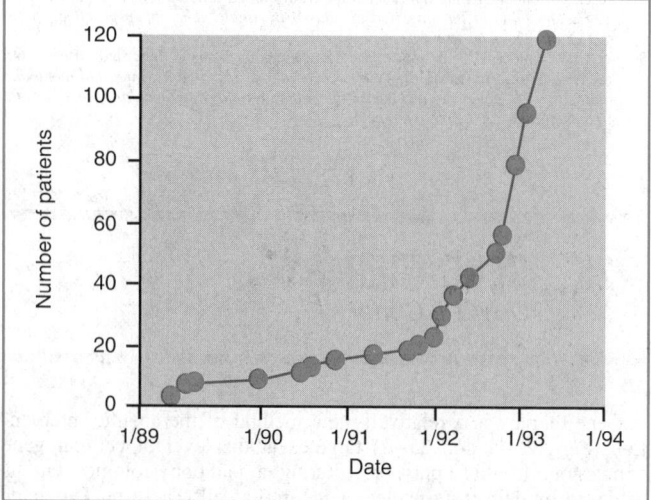

FIGURE 25-2. Growth in number of human recipients of experimental gene transfer as part of marking or therapy protocol.

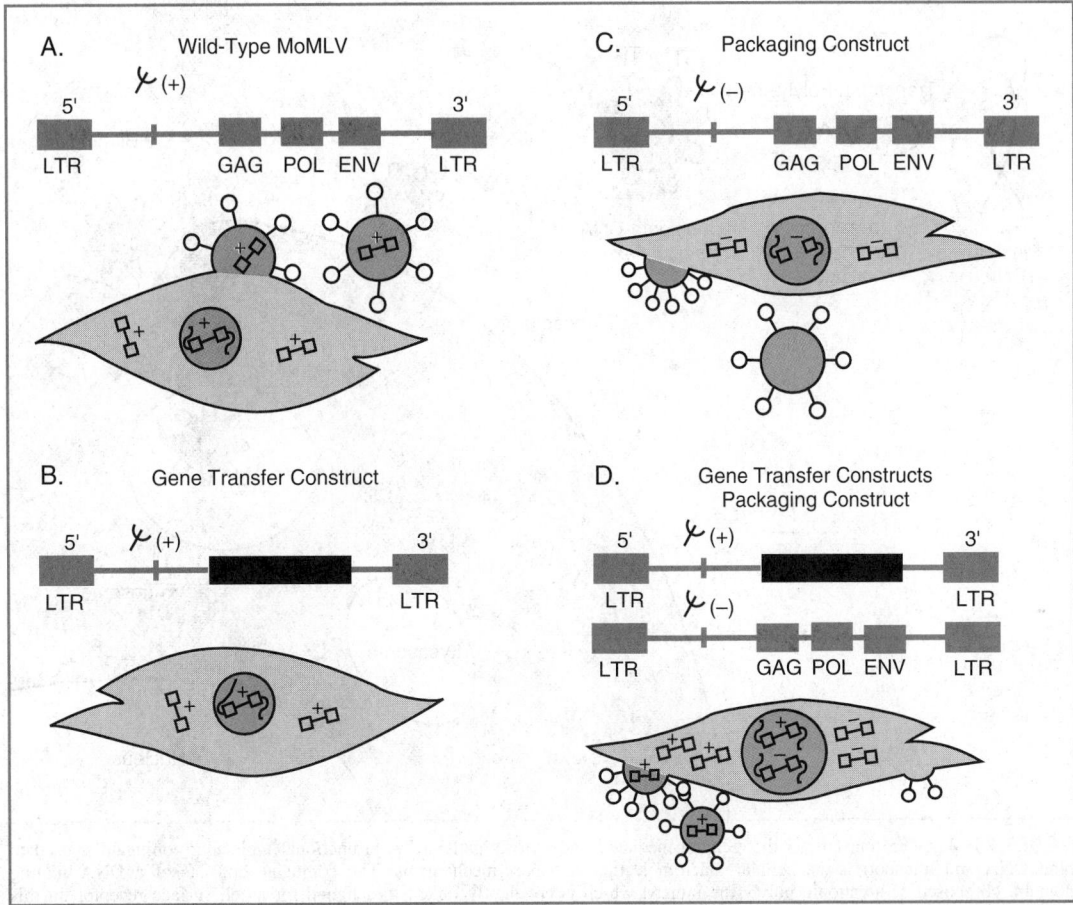

FIGURE 25–3. Strategy to derive recombinant retrovirus gene transfer vector. *A,* Retroviral genome produces RNA transcripts that are translated packaging functions as well as signals (+) allow the transcripts to pack into virions, which may be secreted by the infected cell. *B,* Gene transfer construct contains heterologous gene replacing packaging functions. *C,* Packaging construct contains viral packaging functions encoded in transcript which cannot be packaged due to deleted packaging function (−). *D,* Producer cell line contains both gene transfer construct and packaging construct. The packaging functions deriving from the packaging construct allow packaging of the gene transfer construct, as it possesses a packaging signal (+). The result is a recombinant virion capable of transferring the heterologous gene but not of achieving a replication cycles.

This development is a step toward deriving a "targetable-injectable" vector—a vector that can deliver therapeutic genes selectively to target cells after direct, *in vivo* administration. The development of such a vector system would have two very important consequences for potential gene therapy strategies: (1) it would allow the implementation of a variety of gene therapy strategies targeted to cell or tissue types that cannot currently be modified *ex vivo,* and (2) it would allow gene therapy to be carried out in a context other than its present restriction to highly specialized tertiary care medical centers possessing the support facilities involved in *ex vivo* approaches.

Nonretroviral viral vectors being actively developed include recombinant adenoviruses and the parvovirus adeno-associated virus (AAV). Adenoviruses have been evaluated for their ability to be directly delivered *in vivo* to a variety of organ systems, including the lung, liver, brain, and vasculature. Despite the desirable capacity, the present state of development of the system has a number of drawbacks, which predict very restricted use of these agents for human clinical trials. Principal among these is that the vector system is nonintegrative: Heterologous gene expression in any target cell is only transient. This phenomenon mandates that gene delivery must be carried out on a repetitive, perhaps chronic basis. Given the fact that these agents are extremely potent immunogens, it is not clear that repetitive delivery protocols will be possible. The AAV vector is much less highly developed but has also been associated with practical problems, including a very limited heterologous DNA-carrying capacity as well as extremely low viral titers.

A variety of nonviral systems have been developed and used in strategies to directly deliver genes *in vivo.* Liposomes are artificial lipid bilayer vesicles containing the foreign DNA. Their design overcomes the potential safety hazards associated with viral gene sequences contained in the viral vectors. Whereas initial formulations were associated with significant target cell toxicity, newer agents appear more promising in this regard. These vectors, delivered to selected target organs after direct *in vivo* delivery, have been used in human clinical trials targeting pulmonary disorders and cutaneous malignancies. Despite this systemic stability, delivery is at present nonspecific, as the liposomes lack any mechanism to achieve targeting. This goal is the principal logic behind the design of molecular conjugate vectors. These synthetic molecules exploit the endogenous cellular receptor-mediated pathway to transfer gene (Fig. 25–4). Their design characteristics allow a degree of targeting not available in other systems. The rapid appearance of alternative systems predicts that additional strategies can achieve the central goal of targeted gene delivery after the targeted vector is administered directly *in vivo.*

Initial strategies to accomplish gene therapy were designed for inherited genetic disorders. Since the first human clinical trial of gene therapy in 1990, a variety of genetic diseases—ADA deficiency, hyperlipidemia, and cystic fibrosis—have been treated using gene therapy. Specific strategies to treat a variety of other disorders are being developed, but the central problem of delivering genes to target cells has limited more general use of these methods for inherited genetic disorders.

Gene therapy is also rational in the context of acquired genetic disorders and thus has been used to target cancer; the overwhelming number of human gene therapy protocols in trial have been for cancer therapy. A variety of approaches have been developed based on the molecular pathogenesis of cancer. Specific strategies include the following: (1) a wild-type tumor suppressor gene for recessive oncogene mutations, (2) inhibitory gene constructs for overexpressed or dysregulated dominant oncogenes, (3) toxin genes selec-

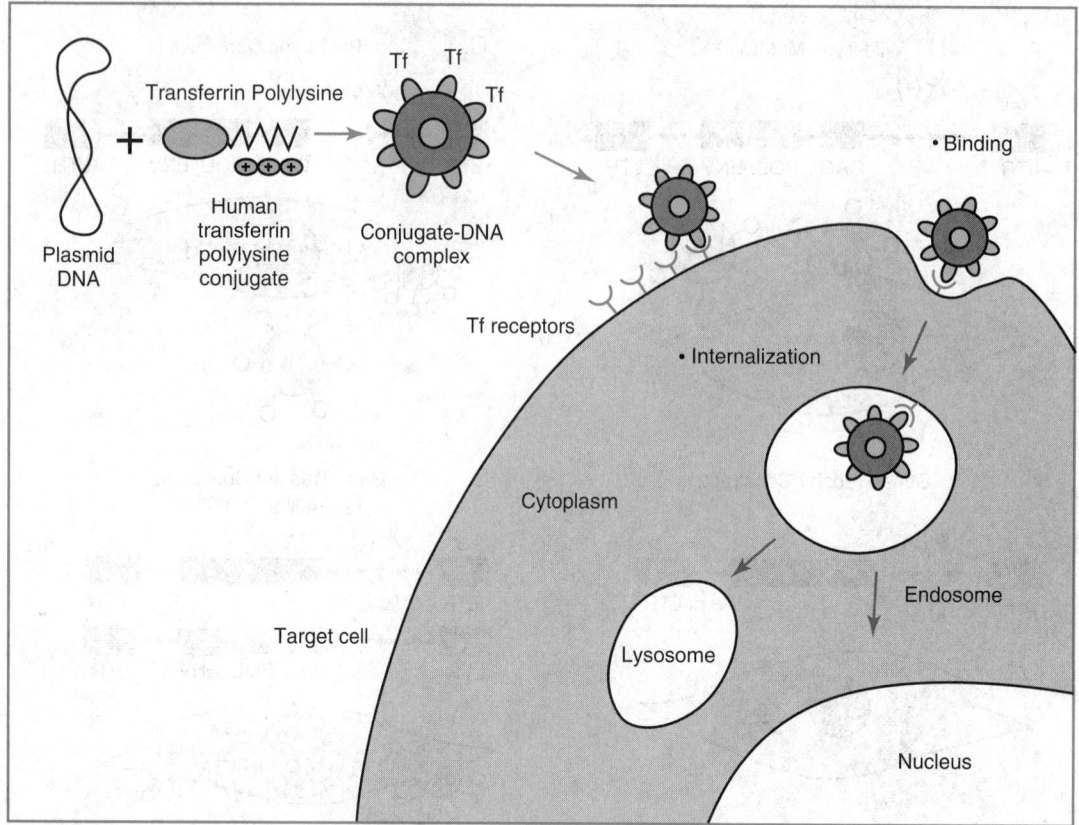

FIGURE 25–4. Gene transfer via the receptor-mediated endocytosis pathway. A bifunctional molecular conjugate is used to bind DNA and transport it via cellular macromolecular transport mechanisms. The conjugate consists of a DNA-binding domain, composed of a cationic polylysine moiety, which is covalently linked to a ligand for a cell surface receptor, in this case transferrin. Plasmid DNA bound to the polylysine moiety of the conjugate undergoes marked condensation to yield an 80- to 100-nm toroid with surface-localized transferrin molecules. When the transferrin ligand domain is bound by its corresponding cell surface receptor, the conjugate is internalized by the receptor-mediated endocytosis pathway, co-transporting bound DNA. Escape from the cell vesicle system is achieved by a fraction of the internalized conjugate-DNA complex to achieve nuclear localization where heterologous gene expression is affected.

tively delivered to cancer cells to eradicate them, and (4) immunomodulatory genes to increase the immunogenicity of tumors. Each of these specific strategies has a counterpart in human protocols that have been approved for clinical trials (Table 25–1).

Gene transfer may represent a therapeutic strategy applicable to contexts outside of genetic diseases. The ability to modulate specific patterns of gene expression may represent a viable option in certain inflammatory disorders. In this regard, specific genetic methods of abrogating selected patterns of gene expression have been shown to alter disease pathogenesis in models of inflammatory and fibrotic lung disease, postischemic hepatic injury, and postcatheterization arterial stenosis. Gene therapy thus offers a means for highly selected ablation of specific gene expression patterns. Using techniques of "anti-sense" inhibition, the "sense" informa-

tional flow from genes through the level of protein is interrupted by "anti-sense" nucleic acid molecules based upon sequence-specific hybridization. This strategy offers the potential to intervene at multiple sites in the gene expression pathway and with a level of specificity not achievable using strategies directed toward the level of aberrant proteins. Thus, gene therapy may ultimately represent another form of pharmacotherapy, albeit a form with mostly improved potentials based on exploitation of the exquisite specificity offered by the cellular apparatus of gene expression.

Anderson WF: Human gene therapy. Science 256:808, 1992. *State-of-the-art summary of clinical gene therapy.*
Blaese RM, Mullen CA, Ramsey WJ: Strategies for gene therapy. Pathol Biol 41:672, 1993. *Definitive summary of vector technologies for human application.*
Wivel NA, Walters L: Germ-line modification and disease prevention: Some medical and ethical perspectives. Science 262:533, 1993. *Discussion of ethical issues relevant to contemporary gene therapy.*

TABLE 25–1. GENE THERAPY APPROACHES FOR TREATMENT OF CANCER

Strategy	Molecular Mechanism of Anticancer Effect
Mutation compensation	Inhibition of expression of dominant oncogene
	Augmentation of deficient tumor-suppressor gene
	Abrogation of autocrine growth factor loops
Molecular chemotherapy	Selective delivery of toxin or toxin gene to cancer cells
Genetic immunopotentiation	Passive immunotherapy—augmentation by genetic enhancement of cell targeting or cell killing capacity of tumor-infiltrating lymphocytes
	Active immunotherapy—augmentation of immune recognition of cancer cells

26 CHROMOSOMES AND THEIR DISORDERS
R. Ellen Magenis

Cytogenetics is the study of chromosomes and their behavior as it relates to transmission of the genetic material from parent to offspring. Errors in chromosome behavior and structure are the cause of a wide range of clinical syndromes.

Every nucleated somatic cell in the human has a complete genome of about 6×10^9 base pairs of DNA, with an uncoiled total length of approximately 2 meters. The genome is packaged by supercoiling into 46 chromosomes, consisting of 22 pairs of homologous chromosomes (identical in regard to morphology and constituent gene loci) and one pair of sex chromosomes (X and Y), one partner of each pair being derived from the mother and one from the father. The 46 chromosomes in metaphase vary in length from 2 to 12 μm. The genes are arranged along the chromosomes in linear order, each gene having a precise position or locus. Genes that have their loci on the same chromosome are said to be *syntenic;* genes that are close together on the same chromosome and tend to travel together during meiosis (little crossing over) are said to be *linked.* Alternate forms of a gene that occupy the same locus are called *alleles.* Any one chromosome bears only a single allele at a given locus, although in the population as a whole there may be multiple alleles, any one of which can occupy that specific locus.

CELL DIVISION. The number of chromosomes found in somatic cells is constant and is termed the *diploid* (2n) number. Each gamete, however, has only half the diploid number and is said to be *haploid* (n). In order to maintain this regularity, two types of cell division occur: mitosis, which is the cell division occurring in somatic tissues during growth and repair, and meiosis, which is the specialized form of cell division occurring when gametes form.

Mitosis. The function of mitosis is to distribute and maintain the continuity of the genetic material in every cell of the body. This process consists of a number of different phases, which results in an equal distribution of the chromosomes to the two daughter cells. The cell cycle has four stages: mitosis (M), gap$_1$ (G$_1$), synthesis (S), and gap$_2$ (G$_2$). The G$_1$ phase follows mitosis, during which RNA and protein synthesis occurs. S is the period during which DNA replication takes place and the DNA content of the cell doubles, and G$_2$ is the period during which energy requirements for cell division are built up and any repair of errors in DNA synthesis takes place.

Meiosis. This process occurs only during the formation of the gametes and results in four daughter cells, each with the haploid number of chromosomes. In males each primary spermatocyte forms four functional spermatids that develop into sperm, while in females each oocyte forms only one ovum, the remaining products of meiosis being nonfunctional polar bodies.

Processes fundamental to meiosis include chromosome pairing, chromosome crossing over, and chromosome segregation. These processes result in halving the chromosome number, regular distribution of chromosomes to daughter cells, and independent assortment of the genetic material from both the cross-over events and maternal/paternal homologue distribution in meiosis I. The ultimate result ensures genetic variability.

METHODS FOR THE PREPARATION OF CHROMOSOMES. Because nondividing chromosomes cannot be analyzed, live dividing cells are required for chromosome analysis. The cell type most commonly used is the mitogenically stimulated peripheral blood lymphocyte. Skin fibroblasts, bone marrow cells, amniotic fluid cells, chorionic villus cells, and tumor cells are also used for special tests. Dividing cells are accumulated at metaphase. In order to accomplish this, a drug (Colcemide) that destroys the mitotic spindle is added to the culture medium toward the end of the culture period. The cells are subjected to hypotonic treatment followed by fixation and spreading on microscope slides. The slides are then stained.

Staining techniques may result in either a nonbanded or a banded appearance of the chromosomes. Laboratories today use at least one of several banding techniques; this results in a great deal of additional information. These methods provide a means to precisely identify each chromosome and extra or missing chromosomes as well as the precise localization of breakpoints in chromosome rearrangements.

High-Resolution Chromosomes. Cells are synchronized with the use of a methotrexate (or other) block; the block is released and the cells harvested at the times predicted to "catch" the chromosomes in late prophase or early metaphase, revealing more bands. With this approach, a band level of over 800 haploid cells can be achieved, which allows detection of a number of microdeletion syndromes (Fig. 26–1).

MOLECULAR CYTOGENETICS. Fluorescence *in situ* hybridization (FISH) is a recent advance in clinical cytogenetic technology that bridges the gap between molecular genetics and cytogenetics. Selected DNA sequences at least 2 to 3 kilobases long are used as probes. Probes are labeled by nick translation, usually with biotin or digoxigenin and then denatured by heat. Chromosomes are prepared by routine methods and are denatured using formamide and heat. The probe(s) is applied to these metaphase preparations and allowed to reanneal. The hybridization site(s) is detected by using fluorochrome conjugated reagents and fluorescence microscopy.

FISH allows the detection of submicroscopic deletions, subtle rearrangements, and small duplications, and it can identify marker chromosomes and the content of multiple rearranged chromosomes. FISH is also useful for detecting aneuploidy (extra or missing chromosomes) in interphase cells in cancers.

HUMAN CHROMOSOME NOMENCLATURE. The 46 human chromosomes consist of three types, designated by the position of the centromere or primary constriction. These are metacentric, submetacentric, and acrocentric, depending on whether the position of the centromere is median, submedian, or near terminal. Each individual chromosome pair can be recognized when banding techniques are used, and the chromosomes are numbered from 1 to 22 in descending order of length. In the female, the two sex chromosomes—designated X chromosomes—are identical, whereas in the male the two sex chromosomes—designated X and Y—are morphologically different.

The nomenclature used to describe the chromosomes and their bands, variants, and rearrangements is described in detail by the International System of Human Cytogenetic Nomenclature (ISCN). A shorthand notation is used to describe the chromosome complement of an individual. In this notation the number of chromosomes is specified first, followed by the listing of the sex chromosomes. Thus a normal female karyotype is designated 46,XX and a normal male karyotype 46,XY. Any deviations of the autosomes are written after the sex chromosomes. An individual autosome is referred to by its number, its short arm by the letter p, and its long arm by the letter q. A + or − sign written before a designated chromosome indicates that the chromosome is extra (+) or missing (−); e.g., 47,XX,+ 21 describes a female with 47 chromosomes, including an extra chromosome 21 in addition to the 46 chromosomes of the normal karyotype.

To describe a translocation between two autosomes the small letter t is used outside parentheses and the chromosome numbers are inside, as: 46,XY,t(9;21)(q34;p11). This indicates a male with a normal number of chromosomes and a reciprocal translocation between the long arm of chromosome 9 and short arm of chromosome 21 with designated breakpoints.

CHROMOSOME ABNORMALITIES

Chromosome abnormalities can be divided into two classes: abnormalities of number and structure.

ABNORMALITIES OF CHROMOSOME NUMBER. These arise from nondisjunction, that is, from *the failure of two homologous chromosomes in the first division of meiosis or of two sister chromatids in either mitosis or the second division of meiosis to pass to opposite poles of the cell.* Nondisjunction results in cells with abnormal chromosome numbers. If these cells are gametes, fertilization results in a zygote with an abnormal chromosome number. If nondisjunction occurs during an early cleavage division of a zygote, then chromosomal mosaicism (two or more cell lines differing in chromosome complement) may result.

ABNORMALITIES OF CHROMOSOME STRUCTURE. These result from chromosome breakage and reunion. When a chromosome breaks it can rejoin in its old form (restitution) or it can rejoin with another broken chromosome (reunion). Reunion leads to a structural rearrangement that can be balanced or unbalanced. If it is balanced, the amount of genetic material is presumed to be identical to that found in a normal cell, and there is a simple rearrangement of the distribution of this material. Types of balanced rearrangements include the balanced reciprocal translocation, Robertsonian translocations, and inversions. Balanced chromosome rearrangements do not usually lead to any clinical change. If the rearrangement is unbalanced, this indicates loss or gain of chromosome material. Such unbalanced rearrangements usually result in changes in the clinical phenotype.

Chromosome Deletion (Fig. 26–2A). Deletion is the loss of a chromosome segment following chromosome breakage. Dele-

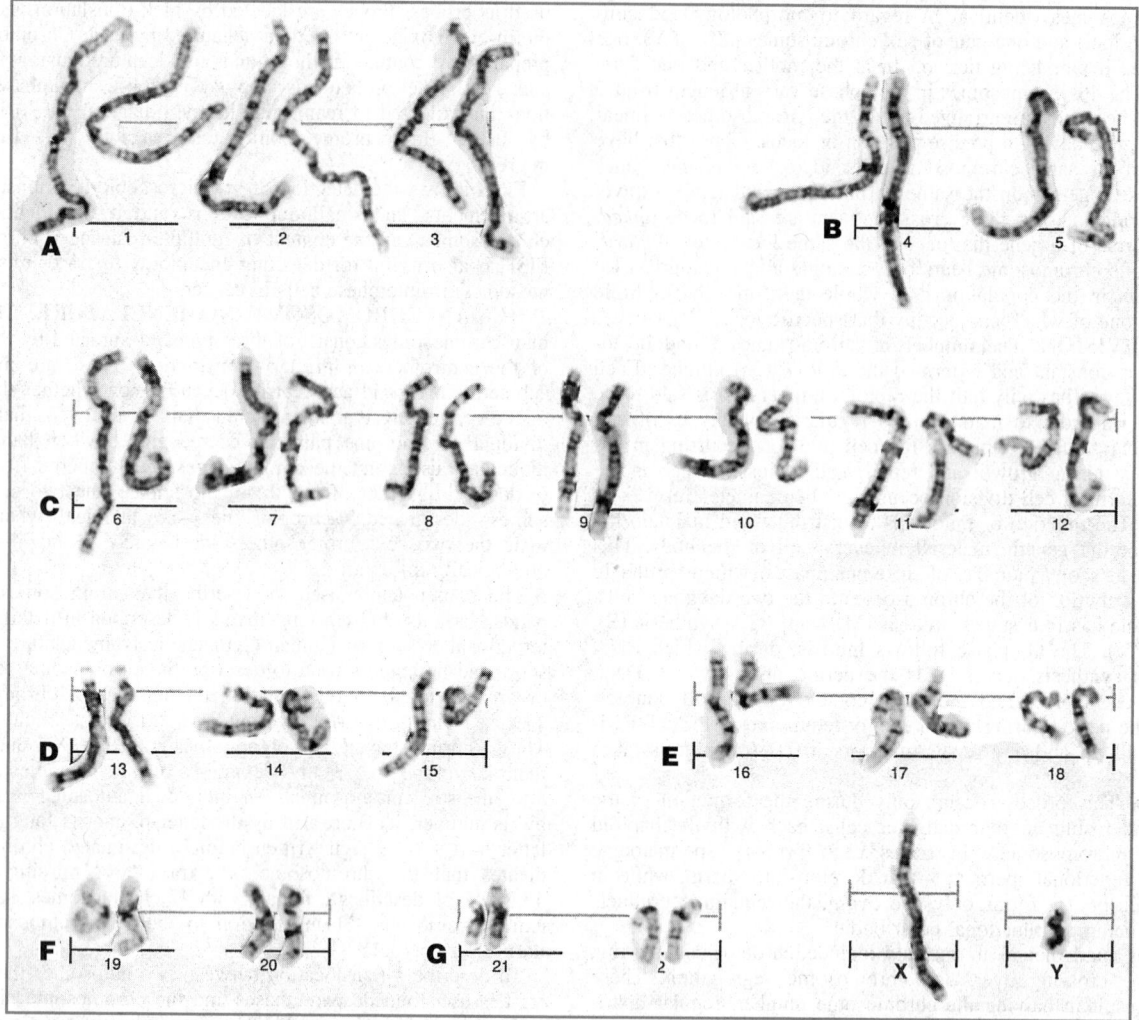

FIGURE 26–1. Normal Giesma-banded (G-band) male karyotype at the 850-band stage. This band level is the best to look for microdeletions, although the long chromosomes tend to curve, and overlapping of chromosomes is frequent.

tions may be terminal or interstitial or result in ring chromosomes.

CHROMOSOME DUPLICATION (Fig. 26–2B). Duplication is the addition of a chromosome segment and may be the result of breakage/reunion or of replication error.

INVERSIONS (Fig. 26–2C). These result from two chromosome breaks with inversion of the intervening segment and can be detected only by altered position of the centromere or by chromosome banding studies that show a changed banding sequence. Inversions result in disturbances in chromosome pairing and in the formation of unbalanced as well as balanced gametes.

BALANCED RECIPROCAL TRANSLOCATION (Fig. 26–2D). This results from exchange of chromosome segments between nonhomologous chromosomes. An individual carrying such a rearrangement has a higher frequency of abnormal gametes as the result of a disturbance in chromosome pairing at meiosis. Such individuals themselves have a balanced chromosome complement and are clinically normal, but they may have a high risk of having congenitally malformed children and/or spontaneous abortions. Normal children may also be born, and such persons require careful genetic counseling (see Ch. 29).

ROBERTSONIAN TRANSLOCATION (Fig. 26–2E). This is a specific type of unequal reciprocal translocation that occurs between acrocentric chromosomes, resulting in a new metacentric chromosome formed from two acrocentric chromosomes. Such rearrangements may be important in the transmission of Down syndrome when one of the chromosomes involved is chromosome 21. If the structural change occurs in the early embryo, mosaicism with some cells normal and some with the structural abnormality may result.

CONSEQUENCES OF CHROMOSOME IMBALANCE

FETAL LOSS. Through the processes of meiosis and mitosis, regular distribution of the chromosomes to daughter cells generally occurs. However, errors in these processes are frequent and account for a large portion of fetal loss. It is estimated that at least 50% of all conceptuses are lost in the first 2 to 3 weeks after conception, most due to major chromosome abnormalities. Chromosome studies of spontaneously aborted first trimester fetuses show a chromosome abnormality rate of close to 50%. The most common abnormalities each occurring in about 25% of the chromosomally abnormal cases are 45,X, missing a sex chromosome, and triploidy with three sets of chromosomes (3n). The remainder include trisomy for any of the autosomes with the exception of chromosome 1, which has been seen only in studies of the early zygote. Among the trisomies, trisomy 16 is the most frequent. No autosomal monosomies have been detected; it is postulated that they do occur at the same rate as the trisomies, as would be predicted from segregation events, but are so severely impaired that implantation does not occur.

Triploidy. Triploidy is characterized by cystic degeneration of the placenta, sometimes appearing as a hydatidiform mole, with an accompanying fetus. The fetus is small for gestational age and has low-set ears and syndactyly. There is a markedly increased incidence of toxemia of pregnancy, and eclampsia may ensue. Using chromosome heteromorphisms as a tool and confirmed using molecular techniques, it has been shown that most triploidy is due to double fertilization of a single egg.

The true mole may be confused with triploidy because it also has cystic degeneration of the placenta, the cysts appearing in grapelike clusters. However, there is no accompanying fetus and the chromo-

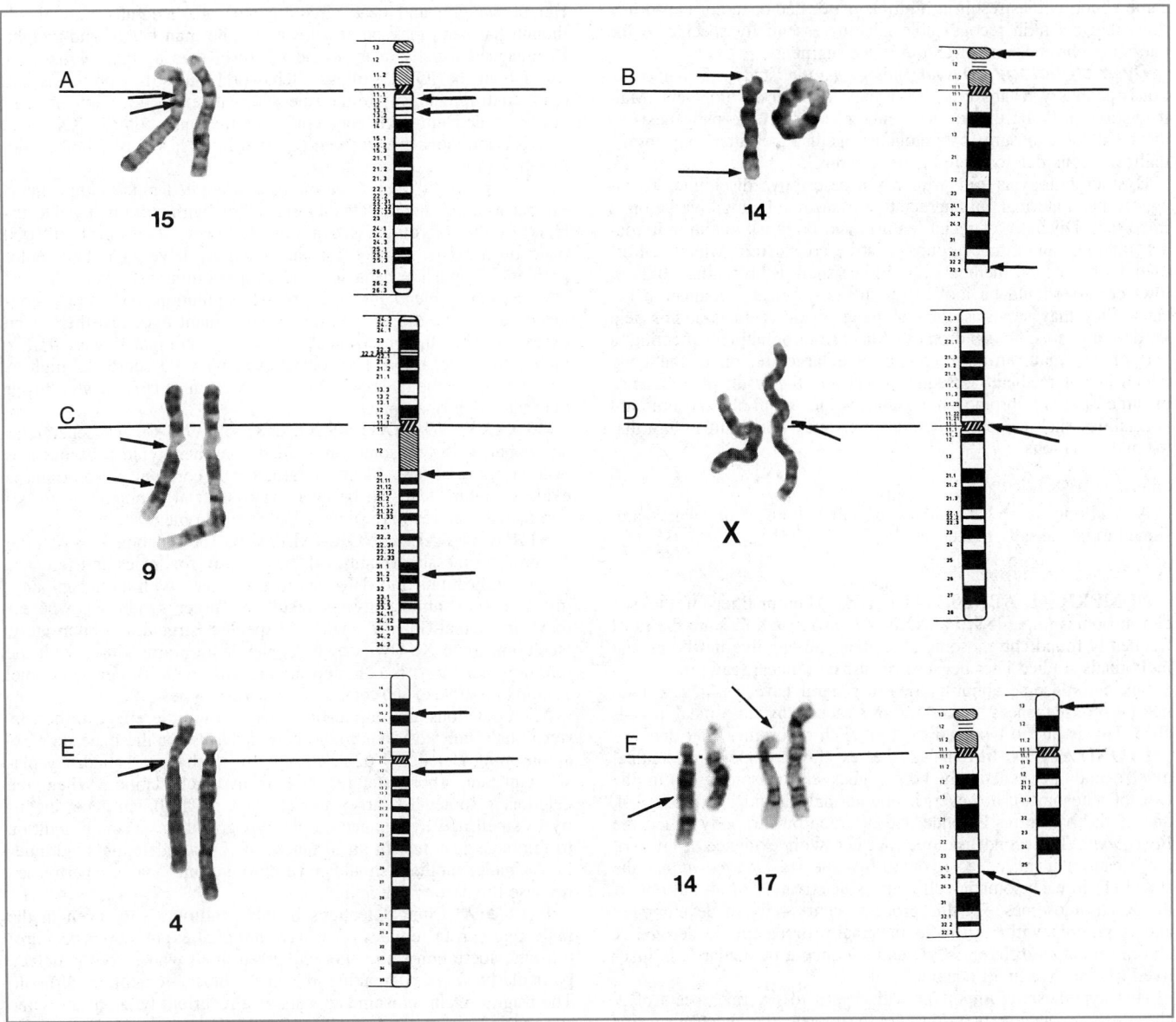

FIGURE 26-2. Partial karyotypes illustrating several types of structural chromosome aberrations. The abnormal chromosomes are placed on the right of each pair. *A,* Interstitial deletion: Chromosomes 15 from a patient with Angelman's syndrome. Ideogram and chromosomes are at the 850-band stage. Arrows on the ideogram and normal 15 indicate the small segment deleted. This same deletion is seen in 75 to 80% of *Prader-Willi* patients. *B,* Ring chromosome: Chromosomes 14 from a patient with nonspecific mental retardation. Both ends of the abnormal chromosome have very small deletions; the broken ends are joined in the form of a ring. Chromosomes are at the 550 band stage. *C,* Duplication: Chromosomes 9 at about the 850-band level. In the right-hand chromosome 9 there is an interstitial duplication of a large segment on the long arm, delineated by the arrows on the normal chromosome. The patient had multiple minor anomalies and mental retardation. *D,* Isochromosomes with duplication-deficiency: X-chromosomes from a patient with Turner's syndrome. Chromosomes at the 550-band stage show a deletion/duplication, in this case due to isochromosome formation. Both arms of the abnormal chromosome are long arms; the short arm is missing. One explanation for this recurring characteristic abnormality is centromere misdivision. The arrow points to the centromere of the abnormal chromosome. *E,* Inversion: Balanced chromosome 4 pericentric inversion delineated by arrows, from a normal woman. This inversion chromosome segregated throughout her family. Chromosomes are at the 550-band stage. *F,* Translocation: Balanced reciprocal translocation between chromosomes 14 and 17 from a normal individual. Arrows indicate breakpoints. Ideogram is at the 550-band level as are the chromosomes 14; the 17's are between the 550- and 850-band length. This likely is due to position in the metaphase spread; chromosomes at the periphery are often longer than those at the center.

somes are always apparently normal 46,XX. Both sets of chromosomes are paternal in origin, with no maternal contribution, likely the result of fertilization of an empty egg. The malignant potential of the true mole is high, while triploidy is rarely associated with malignancy.

45,X Fetuses. The 45,X fetuses are markedly edematous and have large cystic masses encircling the neck. They are small for gestational age and generally have characteristic facial features.

Autosomal Trisomy. Only three autosomal trisomies survive to term: trisomies of chromosomes 13, 18, and 21. Most trisomies 13

and 18 are lost before term, and those that survive to term usually live no more than 1 year. About 70% of trisomy 21 conceptions die before term; with modern treatment, many of those individuals doing well after birth may survive to old age. Mosaicism for autosomal trisomy along with a normal cell population may modify the phenotype and allow survival.

Birth Defects/Patterns of Malformation. About 7 to 10% of stillbirths and neonatal deaths are due to chromosome imbalance; trisomy 18 and trisomy 13 are frequent in this group. At least 0.5 to 1% of all liveborns have chromosome abnormalities. These chromosome abnormalities result in multiple major and/or minor malformations that occur in recognizable patterns essentially specific to the particular chromosome or chromosome segment.

Dysmorphology. *Dysmorphology* is the study of malformations secondary to abnormal embryonic or fetal development. Malformations may be the result of inborn errors in morphogenesis or the result of exposure to teratogenic agents; the latter may mimic malformations due to altered genetic control.

Dysmorphology is still primarily a descriptive discipline. To diagnose the abnormal, an appreciation of normal biologic variation is important. Diversity of facial features and body habitus in individuals, families, and ethnic groups must be considered. Minor malformations having no medical significance such as epicanthal folds or low-set ears should be looked for in the physical examination because they may serve as clues to more serious defects and/or help in defining specific syndromes. Major malformations affecting a part of an organ, an entire organ, or a larger region of the body which are of medical consequence may be the result of imbalance of large or small chromosome segments, but small chromosome abnormalities such as some microdeletions may not result in any major malformations.

CHROMOSOMAL SYNDROMES

A syndrome is a characteristic overall pattern of anomalies presumed to be causally related.

Sex Chromosome Syndromes

NUMERICAL ABNORMALITIES. Abnormalities of the sex chromosomes (e.g., 45,X; 47,XXX; 47,XXY; 47,XYY) are the most frequently found chromosome aberrations among live newborns and individuals studied later because of suspect clinical features.

Sex chromosome abnormalities in general have less severe phenotypic consequences than do those caused by autosomal imbalance. This is due to lyonization of all X chromosomes over one.

LYONIZATION. In females, the sex chromosomes are identical in size and are genetically homologous chromosomes (as in the case of autosomes); however, in the normal diploid interphase cell, one of the X's forms a condensed heterochromatic body called the *Barr body*. This condensation, together with evidence from coat color pattern in mice, led Lyon to hypothesize *X inactivation*. She stated (1) In each somatic cell there is inactivation of all but one of the X chromosomes; (2) this process occurs early in development and is random with respect to maternally or paternally derived X chromosomes in different cells; and (3) once a particular X is inactive, it is inactive in all daughter cells.

This hypothesis is important with regard to several aspects of X chromosome gene expression: (1) It reveals the mechanism for dosage compensation, a process which equalizes the amount of X chromosome gene expression between females with two X's and males having only one X chromosome; (2) it explains some of the phenotypic effects associated with additional or missing sex chromosomes, or the occasional manifesting XX carrier of an X-linked recessive disorder; and (3) this hypothesis indicates the complexity of testing for carrier status of X-linked diseases.

Evidence that dosage compensation has taken place in males with XXY or females with XXX is the fact that interphase cells in these cases have two condensed heterochromatic (Barr) bodies.

The 45,X Liveborn (Turner Syndrome). The most consistent features found in girls with a missing sex chromosome are short stature, usually beginning prior to birth, and gonadal dysgenesis. Although eggs may be present in the newborn gonad, early attrition takes place and eggs have disappeared by puberty. There is puffiness of the hands and feet usually disappearing in childhood, low posterior hairline and short and/or webbed neck, excessive pigmented nevi, deep-set nails, short fourth metacarpal, narrow maxilla, prominent ears, horseshoe kidney, and heart defect, usually coarctation of the aorta. Pubertal development usually does not occur in the absence of hormonal treatment.

47,XXY (Klinefelter Syndrome). This condition occurs in about one in 500 males and is the most common cause of male infertility. These males are tall with long limbs, have testes that remain small after puberty, have gynecomastia, are dull mentally (about 20% with IQ < 80), and are immature in behavior.

47,XXX. There are no characteristic major or minor malformations found in 47,XXX females; almost all appear normal at birth. Height, weight, and head circumference are generally normal, although the head may be at a lower centile than height and weight. Language is usually delayed and IQ lower than normal, particularly lower than the IQ of siblings. Behavioral and social problems and emotional immaturity are the rule. Normal sexual development generally occurs; although apparently not frequent, both 47,XXX and 47,XXY individuals have been reported in offspring of females with this condition.

47,XYY. The 47,XYY karyotype has elicited much public interest because of the reports of association with criminality. Occurrence of the karyotype is common, occurring in about 1 in 1000 male births. These males are tall and may have mild fine motor problems, impulsive behavior, and temper outbursts. Although most affected males blend into the general population, it is now recognized, after correction for earlier ascertainment bias, that there is an excess of aberrant or criminal behavior as compared with 46,XY males. Such behaviors may occur even with IQ scores as high as 146. However, the average IQ of 47,XYY males is somewhat lower than that of normal males.

48,XXXX; 48,XXXY; 49,XXXXX; 49,XXXXY. In general, as additional X chromosomes are added, the phenotypic consequences become more severe. Mental retardation is constant, dysmorphia is evident, stature tends to be small, and skeletal anomalies may occur. Facial features may suggest Down syndrome.

STRUCTURAL ABNORMALITIES. The outcome of structural X chromosome abnormalities differs greatly for males and females. Large duplications and deletions in the female with an accompanying normal X almost always result in Turner syndrome, whereas they are lethal in the male. A specific structural abnormality, isochromosome Xq (two copies of the X long arm joined with the missing short arm) is common among girls with Turner syndrome, comprising 20% of the total abnormal karyotypes.

Microdeletions and duplications may show little effect in the carrier female but have syndromic consequences for the male. For example, microdeletion Xp22.32 results in ichthyosis, chondrodysplasia punctata, short stature, and mental retardation. When the deletion is somewhat larger and includes the Kallman gene, inability to smell and hypogonadotropic hypogonadism occur in addition to the other features. In all instances of X microdeletion syndromes in the male, mothers should have chromosome analysis performed because the carrier rate is high.

Fragile X. Clinical features in this syndrome vary even in the male, and carrier females often have minimal expression. This chromosome aberration also is not expressed in all who carry the defect, particularly females, making diagnosis of the condition difficult. The fragile X chromosome appears as a recurrent break at the same site in Xq27 in about 4 to 50% of cells. The syndrome is frequent, occurring in 2 to 6% of retarded males. Birth weight is usually high and the head relatively large. The face is long and narrow with prominent chin and ears. There is usually macroorchidism. Mental retardation is moderately severe. About 15% exhibit autistic features.

With the recent finding of CGG trinucleotide repeat sequences in excess in the fragile X mental retardation 1 gene (FMR-1) in affected males, a molecular test has become available that can reliably diagnose carriers.

X/Y Translocations. The XX male with short stature, infantile testes, and mild intellectual difficulties is almost always the result of a cryptic translocation between the distal X short arm and distal Y short arm with transfer of the SRY gene (sex reversal Y) from the Y to the X.

Y-Chromosome Syndromes. Mosaicism for loss of the Y chromosome (45,X/46,XY) has varying results, probably depending on the percentage of cells missing a Y chromosome in the developing gonad. Peripheral blood cell mosaicism is compatible with normal male phenotype, with genital ambiguity, and with mixed gonadal dysgenesis or full Turner syndrome. In the latter case surgical extirpation and pathologic examination of the dysgenetic gonads is recommended because of the danger of gonadoblastoma.

Deletion of the distal short arm of the Y when it includes the SRY gene results in a female with gonadal dysgenesis and usually also lymphedema, as in Turner syndrome. However, these individuals are usually *not* short and may have excellent muscle strength.

Autosomal Aneuploidy

Of the three autosomal trisomies that may survive to a term birth, only one allows long-term survival—trisomy 21, Down syndrome. Trisomy 21 syndrome is both common and well-known, the features described by Down almost 130 years ago. It was the first syndrome known to have a chromosomal cause, the extra chromosome discovered by Lejeune in 1959. Increased incidence of the condition with increased maternal age was suspected by Mitchell in 1876 and shown statistically by Penrose in 1933. This increased incidence has led to the use of amniocentesis for prenatal diagnosis of Down syndrome in older mothers.

About 95% of individuals with Down syndrome have trisomy 21; the other 5% have translocation, predominantly Robertsonian translocation 14/21.

Clinical features do not differ between trisomy and translocation cases unless the translocation involves more distal breakpoints on chromosome 21. Clinical features in the newborn include hypotonia, hyperextensible joints, excess skin on back of neck, flat facial profile, slanted palpebral fissures, overfolded helices, protruding tongue, short fifth fingers with single creases, single palmar creases, plantar furrow. In the older individual, Brushfield spots may be more evident, strabismus and nystagmus may occur, fissured lips and furrowed tongue are common, pectus carinatum or excavatum may appear, and small genitalia may be noted. Moderate mental retardation is a constant feature. Congenital heart defects are present in about 50% of cases. There is an increased susceptibility to infection and an immunoglobulin imbalance. Antithyroid antibodies are found frequently and an increased rate of hypothyroidism.

Autosomal Structural Abnormalities

There is an almost unlimited number of different ways in which the 22 pairs of autosomes can be broken with pieces lost (deletions) or reattached (translocations/duplications). Therefore numerous described syndromes occur due to imbalance of such chromosome segments. Four such syndromes are summarized in order to illustrate certain points; all are microdeletion syndromes recognized by their recurring patterns of anomalies before recognition of their chromosomal origin. Other well-known syndromes that have recently been shown to be due to microdeletions are Williams syndrome (del 7q), Rubenstein-Taybi (del 16p), Miller-Dieker lissencephaly syndrome (del 17p), and Werdnig-Hoffmann syndrome (de 5q).

DEL(22) (q11q11) VCF (SPRINTZEN) AND DiGEORGE'S MICRODELETION SYNDROME. Velocardiofacial (VCF or Sprintzen) syndrome and DiGeorge's syndrome are now recognized

TABLE 26–1. MICRODELETION SYNDROMES— PHYSICAL FEATURES

VCF/(Sprintzen) DiGeorge Microdeletion syndrome

Common: cleft palate; conotruncal heart defects (interrupted aortic arch, tetralogy of Fallot, right side aortic arch, ventriculoseptal defect). *Also present:* pharyngeal hypotonia, retrognathia, malar flatness, small anomalous ears, tortuous retinal vessels, slender tapered digits, scoliosis, short stature. *Face:* mildly unusual: long with narrow palpebral fissures, thickening of helical rims; nose is prominent with squared nasal root, philtrum is long, mouth is often held open; velopharyngeal incompetence with or without cleft palate.

Prader-Willi syndrome

Face: narrow bifrontal diameter, almond-shaped eyes, thin upper lip, downturned mouth. *Genitalia:* particularly male, are hypoplastic; hypogonadism; delayed puberty. *Other:* Truncal obesity after age 1 to 4 years.

Angelman syndrome

Small head noted; occiput is flat, often a pronounced occipital groove. Eyes may be mildly wide spaced and deep set, nose is mildly prominent, mouth is large, teeth wide spaced. Ataxic gait. Happy demeanor.

to be the result of deletion of a small portion of the long arm of chromosome 22 near the centromere. The syndromes appear to be extremes along a clinical continuum not specifically related to the size of the deletion. The condition in some individuals is so mild that they blend into the normal population. The true incidence is unknown, but it may be as common as Down syndrome.

Although the deletion of chromosome 22(q11) may be so small that it cannot be detected at the microscope without FISH, major malformations may be present (Table 26–1 and Fig. 26–3A). Mild to moderate mental retardation may be present; speech is hypernasal even without clefting. Absent thymus, tonsils and adenoids and hypocalcemia in infancy have been noted. Affect is often very bland, including facial expression; phobias and psychosis may appear in adolescents and adults.

PRADER-WILLI/ANGELMAN SYNDROMES. Prader-Willi syndrome (PWS) was first described in 1956; that it is a chromosomal microdeletion syndrome was not known until 1981, when a small deletion of the proximal long arm of chromosome 15 was recognized. Clinical findings uniquely change with age. In the new-

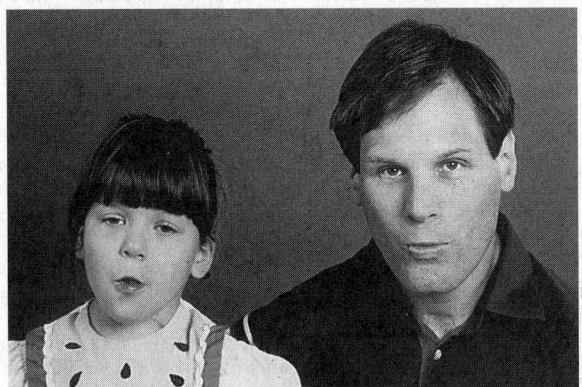

A

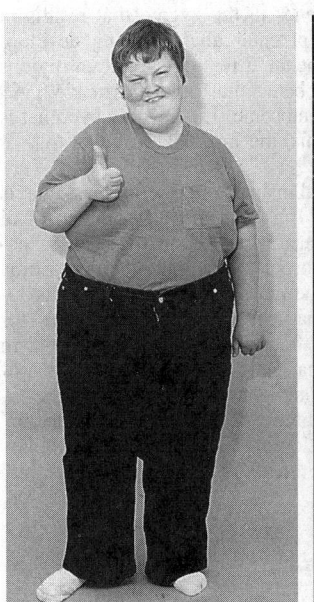

B

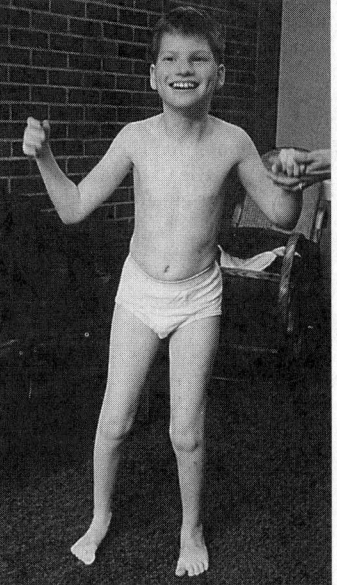

C

FIGURE 26–3. *A,* Father and daughter with velocardiofacial syndrome. Note masklike facial features and lack of ability to purse the lips for whistling. The father had had repair of a congenital heart defect (tetralogy of Fallot); the child had a normal heart. A small deletion of chromosome 22 long arm is found in most cases, sometimes detected only with molecular-cytogenetic techniques. *B,* Twenty-year-old male with Prader-Willi syndrome. He has a *de novo* deletion of the proximal long arm of chromosome 15, which occurred on the chromosome 15 homolog inherited from his father. *C,* Twelve-year-old male with Angelman's syndrome. He is ataxic and unable to walk without help, is happy and alert but severely mentally retarded, and has no speech. He had the same *de novo* deletion as the patient in Figure 26–3B, but the deletion occurred on the chromosome 15 inherited from his mother.

born period and infancy the infant may be so hypotonic that a primary muscle disorder is suspected; however, muscle biopsy and other neuromuscular studies show no abnormality. The infant is difficult to feed and weight gain is slow, as is motor development. The infant improves over time, and sometime after age 12 months and before 6 years, rapid increase in weight occurs and the child becomes progressively morbidly obese in the absence of intervention. Physical features are described in Table 26–1 and Figure 26–3B. Behavior problems are frequent in older children; stubbornness and obsessive-compulsive behavior are common, and temper tantrums may be sudden and severe.

In 1987 it was first reported that individuals with *Angelman syndrome,* a condition that clinically is very different from PWS, have a chromosome 15 proximal long arm deletion indistinguishable from that seen in PWS. Angelman syndrome is characterized by normal size at birth and normal appearance, incoordinated suck and swallow resulting in feeding difficulties, developmental delay noted at about age 6 months, limited babbling, absent speech, ataxic gait, happy disposition with frequent smiles and laughter, excessive drooling, and seizures. Table 26–1 and Figure 26–1 list physical features. After these individuals learn to walk around age 3 to 5, activity becomes almost ceaseless.

Parental Origin. As early as 1983, chromosome heteromorphism studies of individuals with PWS and their parents showed that in all cases the deletion of chromosome 15 had occurred on a paternally derived chromosome. Similar parental origin studies, using molecular techniques in addition to chromosome heteromorphisms of individuals with Angelman syndrome, have shown that the chromosome 15 deletion in all instances occurred on the maternally transmitted chromosome. These data forced the recognition that there must be gender-specific differences in the expression of certain genes in some regions of the human genome.

Uniparental Disomy. Some cases of Angelman syndrome and of PWS do not involve a cytogenetically visible deletion. In almost all the nondeletion PWS cases parental origin studies have identified characteristics that heretofore were thought *not* to occur in the human—findings of uniparental disomy, a situation in which both chromosomes 15 are maternal in origin and no paternal chromosome 15 is present. About 5% of the cases of nondeletion Angelman syndrome have shown uniparental disomy with two copies of chromosome 15 of paternal origin and no maternal copy. These findings further suggest that a gene or genes in the region 15q11 have differential expression, depending on the gender of the parent, now termed *imprinting.*

Imprinting. Imprinting is the differential epigenetic modification of certain maternal and paternal genes in the zygote that results in the differential expression of the parental alleles during development and in the adult. This phenomenon affects only certain regions of the human genome, one region being that involved in PWS/AS on the proximal long arm of chromosome 15. Several hypotheses have been formulated to explain this, the most likely being that of methylation differences.

RETINOBLASTOMA. The malignant tumor retinoblastoma is hereditary, originating in the eye. It is inherited as an autosomal dominant disorder with reduced penetrance. About 5% of these patients have a constitutional chromosomal deletion of chromosome 13, band q14. This suggests that the gene for retinoblastoma is located in the segment deleted and that it must be a tumor-suppressor gene. Studies using restriction fraction length polymorphism (RFLP) linked to the retinoblastoma locus have shown that loss of the homologous normal retinoblastoma gene is necessary for the tumor to develop. This would constitute the second event, the primary being the constitutional mutation or deletion of the retinoblastoma gene. These events would then fit Knudsen's "two-hit" hypothesis in tumor pathogenesis.

ACQUIRED CHROMOSOMAL ABNORMALITIES

Cancer Cytogenetics

Current thinking regarding the role of chromosome abnormalities in the pathogenesis of cancer is that the chromosomal change affects cancer-promoting or -suppressor genes, altering the stable normal behavioral characteristics of the cell to the unstable behavior

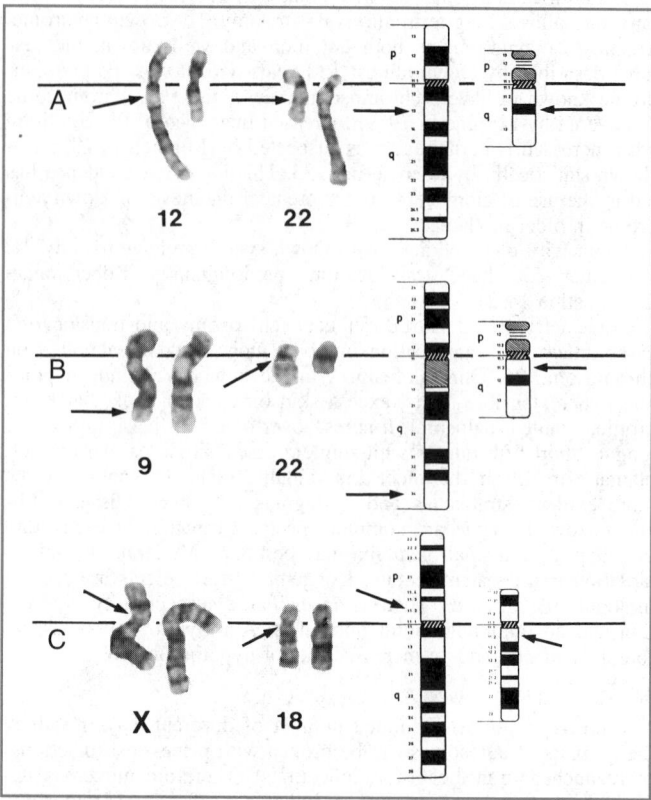

FIGURE 26–4. Partial karyotypes from three specific cancers illustrating recurring rearrangements in specific cancer types. The ideograms on the right are at the 400-band stage. *A,* Chromosomes 12 and 22 from a clear cell sarcoma. There is a breakpoint near the centromere of chromosome 12 long arm; arrow indicates the break site on the far left normal chromosome 12 and on the ideogram. The material distal to the break site is translocated to chromosome 22 as part of an apparently balanced exchange. Arrow points to breakpoint site on the normal chromosome 22 and ideogram. *B,* Chromosomes 9 *(far left)* and 22 from a patient with chronic myelogenous leukemia. Arrows point to break sites on the normal chromosomes beyond which the material on the abnormal chromosomes has been exchanged. This rearrangement results in a new fusion gene (BCR on chromosome 22 and ABL oncogene on 9) that alters the balance of certain hematopoietic cells. *C,* Translocation between the proximal short arm of the X chromosome and the proximal long arm of chromosome 18 is the hallmark of synovial sarcoma. Arrows point to the breakpoint region on the normal chromosomes (left chromosome of each pair) while the rearranged chromosomes are on the right. The fusion product has not yet been characterized.

typical of malignancy. These changes may occur through either loss or gain of a chromosome or chromosomal segment or rearrangement of chromosomal material which might alter function by virtue of an altered gene or infusion genes.

With loss of material due to terminal deletion it is suspected that there is concurrent loss of suppressor gene(s), but, if interstitial, the rejoined new segments may alter function of the splice point genes so that control is altered or a combined gene is formed. Gain of a chromosome or segment conceivably results in a dose effect of contained genes resulting in altered dynamics. Translocations recombine genes; gene function may be eliminated, new fusion genes created, and regulation damaged such that inactivation, activation, or up-regulation may occur (Fig. 26–4).

Over time, further chromosomal changes (evolution) usually occur in cancers as they progress, causing complex numerical and structural alterations. Although typical evolution is known for some malignancies as in chronic myelogenous leukemia, it is not known for most types of cancer (Fig. 26–5).

Cancer Categories

Cancers are classified in three major categories: (1) The hematologic malignancies, (2) lymphomas, and (3) solid tumors. Although

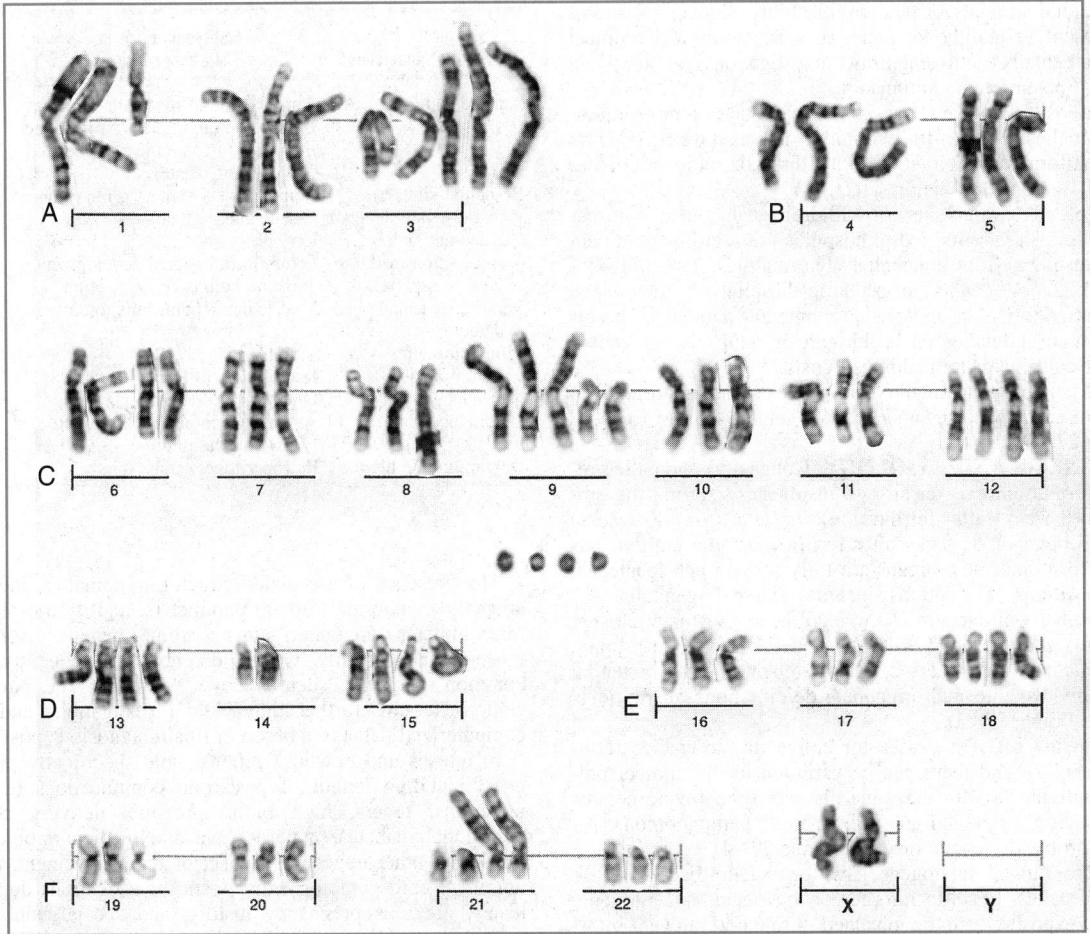

FIGURE 26–5. Karyotype from a metastatic malignant melanoma illustrating the complex numerical and structural abnormalities usually seen. The structural abnormalities involve chromosomes 1, 3, 4, 6, 8, 9, 14, and 21, and there are four small unidentifiable ring chromosomes. Note that all five chromosomes 9 are abnormal, with missing short arms, replaced in three with material from another chromosome.

tremendous advances have been made in the study of solid tumors, much more information is known in diagnosis, prognosis, and treatment of the leukemias (see Ch. 142 and 143). This is so despite the far greater numbers of solid tumors, because of difficulties in obtaining the appropriate solid tumor tissue, and culturing and obtaining good-quality chromosomes. Nevertheless, because there have been many improvements, a number of laboratories can perform solid tumor cytogenetics.

The number of recognized recurrent chromosome abnormalities in all categories is now large. For many cancers, malignancy behavior, prognosis, and treatment modalities may be determined by the specific chromosomal change(s).

Emery AEH, Rimoin DL: Principles and Practice of Medical Genetics. New York, Churchill-Livingstone, 1990. *An excellent practical text of medical genetics containing several outstanding chapters on basic and clinical cytogenetics.*

Gorlin RJ, Cohen MM, Levin LS: Syndromes of the Head and Neck. New York, Oxford University Press, 1990. *Almost encyclopedic in scope; the one you take to clinic with you.*

Heim S, Mitelman F: Cancer Cytogenetics. New York, Alan R Liss, Inc., 1987. *The overall most useful cancer cytogenetics text.*

ISCN: Harnden DG, Klinger HP (eds.): An International System for Human Cytogenetic Nomenclature. Published in collaboration with Cytgenet Cell Genet, Basel, S. Karger, 1985. Original Article Series, Vol 21, No 1, New York 1985. ISCN: F. Mitelman (ed.): Guidelines for Cancer Cytogenetics, Supplement to An International System for Human Cytogenetic Nomenclature, Basel, S. Karger, 1991. *The International Standing Committee on Human Cytogenetic Nomenclature met in Memphis, Tennessee, Fall 1994, to prepare new guidelines combining both constitutional and cancer cytogenetics in one volume; to be published in 1995. These volumes present internationally accepted official guidelines for naming and numbering human chromosomes, normal and abnormal.*

Schinzel A: Catalog of Unbalanced Chromosome Aberrations in Man. Berlin, Germany, Walter de Gruyter & Co., 1984. *A more comprehensive book of chromosome abnormalities; mildly difficult to use.*

27 CONGENITAL ANOMALIES
*Margot I. Van Allen
and Judith G. Hall*

DEFINITION. Structural abnormalities that result from errors in embryogenesis or the fetal period are called congenital anomalies (also called congenital malformations, birth defects, or structural anomalies). Structural anomalies can occur in any major organ system or part of the body, either in isolation or in association with other congenital anomalies. Major anomalies are defined as structural anomalies that require medical and/or surgical treatment and/or are cosmetically significant. Minor anomalies are structural alterations that pose no significant health or social burdens. When multiple congenital anomalies occur together and are etiologically related, they are called syndromes. When two or more congenital anomalies occur in nonrandom statistical association but are not known to be etiologically related, they are called associations. A sequence refers to a pattern of congenital anomalies which results from a single primary anomaly or from a single mechanical factor or disruptive event.

PREVALENCE. Major congenital anomalies are identified in 2 to 3% of all newborn infants, independent of ethnic group or country of origin. This rate doubles in the first year of life as congenital anomalies that are not diagnosed in the neonate become clinically apparent. By age 5, 7 to 10% of children have been diagnosed with a major congenital anomaly or learning disability. Congenital anomalies also present in adulthood, either in association with clinical disease, coincidentally with diagnostic investigations for unrelated disorders, or at postmortem examination.

Approximately 15% of newborn infants have one or more minor structural anomalies. Those with two minor defects have a 10% risk of a major malformation, and those with three or more minor defects have a 20% risk for a major defect.

Over half of all North American children evaluated in subspecialty medical clinics or admitted to hospitals are seen for treatment of disorders resulting from congenital abnormalities. Two thirds of infant and childhood deaths in pediatric hospitals in developed countries are caused by an underlying congenital anomaly. The effect of congenital anomalies on health care in adults is not known but is a major contributor to health care costs.

The rate of congenital anomalies and chromosomal abnormalities is higher in miscarried fetuses and stillborn infants than in liveborn infants (Table 27–1).

PATHOGENESIS AND ETIOLOGY. Congenital anomalies result from abnormal embryogenesis and histogenesis during the embryonic (up to 8 weeks after fertilization) and fetal (9 to 40 weeks) periods. By the end of 8 weeks after fertilization, the embryo has taken human form and most organs are fully formed and located in their final positions. Exceptions include external genitalia (12 weeks), abdominal wall closure (10 weeks), heart (postnatal closure of patent ductus arteriosus and atrial septal defect secundum), brain, and dental structures (Table 27–2). The pathogenesis of congenital anomalies is divided into malformations, deformations, disruptions, and dysplasias (Table 27–3).

There are many different causes for congenital anomalies (etiologic heterogeneity), and there can be variation in the clinical presentation of individuals with the same disorder (phenotypic heterogeneity). A specific congenital anomaly is rarely pathognomonic for a specific syndrome or genetic disorder (Table 27–4).

A number of human teratogens have been identified to cause congenital anomalies. Specific information on potential teratogenic effects of an exposure can be obtained through teratogen information services, computerized databases, and reference books. The most common teratogen used during pregnancy is alcohol. Other known teratogens frequently used in practice are antiepileptic drugs, metabolic teratogens from diabetes, ACE inhibitors, antimetabolite agents, isotretinoin, and others. Common *in utero* infections that affect the embryo and fetus include rubella, syphilis, HIV, toxoplasmosis, herpes, cytomegalovirus, parvovirus, and coxsackievirus.

CLINICAL MANIFESTATIONS. Congenital anomalies most commonly present in infants under age 2 months or are detected prenatally with sonograms.

Pertinent historical information includes age of presentation, appearance at the time of presentation and change with time, previous treatment and investigations, functional expectations, and current and future plans for treatment. Conduct a review of systems, with emphasis on identifying symptoms related to associated structural anomalies that commonly occur in association with the presenting anomaly. Examples of common associations are VACTERL (vertebral, anal, cardiac, tracheoesophageal, renal, and limb anomalies) and CHARGE (coloboma, heart defect, atresia choanae, retarded growth, genital anomalies, and ear anomalies). Assess the patient for sensory deficits, in particular hearing and vision.

TABLE 27–1. RATE OF CONGENITAL ANOMALIES AND CHROMOSOMAL ANOMALIES

Patient Group	Congenital Anomalies	Chromosomally Abnormal
Miscarried embryos	30%	60%
Miscarried fetuses (<20 weeks' gestation)	12.2%	29.2%
Stillborn fetuses (>20 weeks' gestation)	7.2%	6.0%
Liveborns	2–3% at birth 7–10% at age 5	0.57%

TABLE 27–2. EMBRYONIC TIMING OF COMMON CONGENITAL ANOMALIES

Structural Anomalies	Embryonic Error in Morphogenesis	Latest Time Post-conception
Anencephaly	Anterior neural tube fails to close	26 days
Cleft lip	Embryonic component parts of the lip fail to close (42% associated with cleft palate)	36 days
Branchial sinus and/or cyst	Remnant of fusion of primary or secondary palate	10 weeks
Cardiac anomalies	Variable	Variable
Transposition of the great vessels	Errors in directional development of the bulbus cordis septum	34 days
Ventricular septal defect	Ventricular septum fails to close	6 weeks
Limb anomalies	Variable	Variable
Radial aplasia	Radius fails to form	38 days
Syndactyly	Digits fail to separate	6 weeks
Omphalocele	Anterior abdominal wall fails to close in the midline	10 weeks
Diaphragmatic hernia	Retroperitoneal canal fails to close	6 weeks

The presence of associated structural anomalies, increased minor anomalies, abnormal growth parameters, and dysmorphic facial features indicates an underlying syndrome, genetic disorder, or chromosomal abnormality. Gestalt diagnosis is frequently possible for common syndromes such as Down syndrome. The majority of associations require further diagnostic investigations and searches in computerized databases before a final diagnosis is possible.

In fetuses and newborn infants, note specifically pregnancy history, including length of gestation, complications (e.g., bleeding, infections, fevers, high blood pressure, delivery complications, gestational diabetes, maternal age and medical problems, medications, and other exposures), onset of fetal movement, placental and umbilical cord pathology, diagnostic investigations during the pregnancy, previous pregnancy history, and special concerns that the pregnant mother had which she believes may have caused the problem.

In infants and children, as well as in individuals with intellectual disabilities, a history of developmental milestones should be determined. Informal developmental screening and/or formal developmental or intelligence testing is important for overall management and, at times, diagnosis. In general, individuals with congenital

TABLE 27–3. SCHEMATIC REPRESENTATION OF THE DIFFERENT TYPES OF ERRORS OF MORPHOGENESIS RESULTING IN CONGENITAL ANOMALIES AND THEIR DEFINITION

Error of Morphogenesis	Definition
Normal development	Normal development
Malformation	Morphologic defect of an organ, part of an organ, or a larger part of the body resulting from an intrinsically abnormal developmental process
Disruption	Morphologic defect of an organ, part of an organ, or a larger region of the body resulting from the extrinsic breakdown of, or an interference with, an originally normal developmental process
Deformation	Morphologic defect resulting in an abnormal form, shape, or position of a part of the body caused by mechanical forces
Dysplasia	Morphologic defect resulting from the abnormal organization of cells into tissues

TABLE 27–4. ETIOLOGY OF CONGENITAL ANOMALIES

Etiology	Percentage
Monogenic	7.5
Chromosomal	6
Multifactorial	20
Congenital infection	2–3
Maternal diabetes	1.5
Other maternal illnesses	<1.5
Maternal medication	1–2
Unknown	>50

TABLE 27–6. RECURRENCE RISKS FOR COMMON CONGENITAL ANOMALIES

Congenital Anomaly	One Affected Parent: Risk for First Child (%)	Normal Parents with One Affected Child: Risk for Subsequent Child (%)
Cleft lip and palate	3.2	4—unilateral lip 5.6—bilateral lip
Cleft palate	6	2
Clubfoot	3	3
Ventricular septal defect	3–4	4–5
Atrial septal defect	3.5	3
Neural tube defect	3	5
Congenital dislocation of the hip	3.5	3.5
Pyloric stenosis	25.4 (if mother affected)	3.2 (if brother affected) 6.5 (if sister affected)
Renal abnormalities	Variable	9

anomalies are more likely to be underestimated rather than overestimated in their abilities. In particular, certain minor facial anomalies can give an appearance that is interpreted by educators and others as indicative of "retardation" (e.g., blepharophimosis).

Many adults with congenital anomalies have received treatment as infants or young children and have no or poor recollection of their prior medical condition. Medical records may be the only source of information about the anomaly. Alternatively, history from parents or older siblings can sometimes be helpful. Many individuals with congenital anomalies of one organ system have associated structural anomalies that may present after childhood with clinical signs and symptoms specific for the involved organ system. Other signs of undiagnosed congenital anomalies include the presence of increased minor structural anomalies, certain skin lesions, abnormal growth, developmental delay, and mental retardation.

Family history is as important in assisting in the diagnosis of a disorder as other investigations.

Diagnosing the cause of a congenital anomaly is important because it helps predict an overall prognosis and natural history of the disorder. A differential diagnosis is helpful in directing investigations for potential complications and the presence of anomalies as well as excluding disorders that may have a more severe outcome. Preventive health care by early detection and treatment of potential complications of a specific disorder improves the patient's quality of life.

DIAGNOSTIC INVESTIGATIONS. Diagnostic investigations should determine whether the congenital anomaly is isolated or there are associated anomalies of the same or other organ systems. Indications for chromosome studies are summarized in Table 27–5.

RECURRENCE RISKS. Recurrence risks for common isolated structural anomalies are given in Table 27–6. These tables are applicable only after excluding monogenic, syndromic, chromosomal, and other possible causes for the congenital anomaly. A specific family may have an unrecognized monogenic disorder, and the recurrence risk may actually be higher (i.e., 25 to 50%) (see Ch. 26).

TREATMENT. Some structural anomalies are surgically correctable. More commonly, the congenital anomaly is not amenable to surgical treatment or requires multiple staged surgeries or operative palliation. Individuals with disabling or multiple congenital anomalies usually require the expertise of many medical and surgical specialists knowledgeable in the natural history of the disorder and are best managed by multidisciplinary teams.

TABLE 27–5. INDICATIONS FOR CHROMOSOME STUDIES

Stillbirths or neonatal details (7%)
Multiple congenital anomalies (23%)
Small for gestational age (10%)
Facial dysmorphia with a single major congenital anomaly
Significant mental retardation (12%)
Postnatal growth retardation
Microcephaly
Couple with more than two miscarriages

PROGNOSIS. The prognosis for a disorder depends on the specific structural anomaly. Review of that specific anomaly in the appropriate section of this text is recommended (e.g., atrial septal defect). When the diagnosis of a syndrome or a chromosomal or genetic disorder is made, reviewing previous medical history can provide information on long-term prognosis and the natural history of the disorder.

PREVENTION AND PRENATAL DIAGNOSIS. Using folic acid supplementation preconceptually and during the first 3 months of pregnancy reduces the risk of both occurrence and recurrence of neural tube defects (NTD's). Current recommendations are that all women of reproductive age receive at least 0.4 mg of folic acid supplementation per day. For couples at increased risk for recurrence of NTD's, women should take 4.0 mg of folic acid supplementation per day while planning pregnancy and for the first 3 months of pregnancy. Folic acid supplementation of 0.8 mg per day for women of reproductive age may also decrease the incidence of other congenital anomalies due to multifactorial inheritance.

COUNSELING ABOUT A CONGENITAL ANOMALY (see Ch. 29). Talking to a family once a congenital anomaly has been identified is rarely easy, in particular when the affected individual is a fetus or a newborn. It is the responsibility of the health professional to provide affected adults or parents and guardians of affected fetuses and children with sufficient and accurate information about the disorder so that they can make an informed decision regarding the medical and surgical management, obtain resource information in the community, and establish an appropriate social support network.

ACKNOWLEDGEMENT: We acknowledge the research assistance provided by Elena Lopez-Rangel, M.D., in the completion of this chapter.

Czeizel AE, Dudas I: Prevention of the first occurrence of neural tube defects by periconceptional vitamin supplementation. N Engl J Med 327:1832, 1992. *Prevention of the first occurrence of neural tube defects by periconceptional vitamin supplementation.*

Emery AE, Rimoin DL: Principles and Practice of Medical Genetics. New York, Churchill Livingstone, 1995. *A detailed text that provides specific clinical information and up-to-date research knowledge on genetic disorders.*

Gorlin RJ, Cohen MM, Levin LS: Syndromes of the Head and Neck. New York, Oxford University Press, 1990. *The most comprehensive text available on summaries of syndromes of the head and neck.*

Harper PS: Practical Genetic Counselling. 3rd ed. London, Wright, 1988. *A practical manual for information on congenital anomalies and genetic disorders for the practicing physician. It is particularly good for information on recurrence risks for isolated structural anomalies and a brief summary of the differential diagnosis of the most common causes of common structural anomalies.*

McKusick VA: Mendelian Inheritance in Man. Catalogs of Autosomal Dominant, Autosomal Recessive, and X-Linked Phenotypes. Baltimore, The Johns Hopkins University Press. Updated every two years. *A complete catalog of inherited disorders with up-to-date references.*

Stevenson RE, Hall JG, Goodman RM: Human Malformations and Related Anomalies. New York, Oxford University Press, 1993. *The most definitive book available on congenital anomalies.*

28 HEREDITARY SYNDROMES INVOLVING MULTIPLE ORGAN SYSTEMS

Kenneth Lyons Jones

The emergence of dysmorphology/clinical genetics as a specialty has led, over the last 20 years, to the recognition of a large number of multiple malformation syndromes. Although many of these disorders are due to the effect of a single altered gene, others are the result of a chromosome abnormality or of a teratogen such as alcohol. Although the majority of these conditions become apparent in early infancy or childhood, adolescent and adult patients with such conditions may initially present to internists and primary care physicians. The reader is referred to the textbooks listed below for general background information and diagnostic approaches to these disorders. The purpose of this chapter is to present information regarding the natural history of some of the more commonly recognized patterns of human malformation in order to provide a framework for managing adults with these disorders. In addition, data regarding etiology emanating from some of the newer molecular techniques are presented when available. Characteristics of these disorders are summarized in Table 28–1 and are further discussed below.

Briggs GC, Freeman RK, Yaffe SJ: Drugs in Pregnancy and Lactation. 3rd ed. Baltimore, Williams & Wilkins, 1990. *A reference guide to fetal and neonatal risk. Provides practical information regarding the effects of a large number of drugs on the unborn baby.*

Buyse ML (ed.): Birth Defects Encyclopedia. New York, Mosby, 1990. *A massive multiauthored reference book listing all known birth defects regardless of cause, with descriptions, illustrations, and references. For on-line search and retrieval, contact Maxwell Online, Inc., 8000 Westpark Drive, McLean, VA 22102 (telephone, 800-055-0906).*

de Grouchy J, Turlean J: Clinical Atlas of Human Chromosomes. 2nd ed. New York, John Wiley & Sons, 1984. *A good general reference volume for standard syndromes associated with cytogenetic abnormalities.*

Jones KL: Smith's Recognizable Patterns of Human Malformation. 4th ed. Philadelphia, WB Saunders, 1988. *The short "bible" for description of malformation syndromes. Many photographs and accounts of many different types of defects. Practically useful.*

McKusick V: Mendelian Inheritance in Man. 10th ed. Baltimore, Johns Hopkins University Press, 1992. *Standard reference source listing definite and possible monogenic diseases, traits, and syndromes with short descriptions and literature citations. Continuously updated and also available with computer access. Contact OMIM User Support, Welch Medical Library, 1830 E. Monument Street, Baltimore, MD 21205 (telephone, 301-955-7058).*

Schinzel A: Catalogue of Unbalanced Chromosome Aberrations in Man. New York, W. de Gruyter, 1984. *The definitive detailed reference for unbalanced chromosomal aberrations.*

Shepard TH: Catalog of Teratogen Agents. 7th ed. Baltimore, Johns Hopkins University Press, 1992. *The most comprehensive reference for teratogens in humans and animals.*

WILLIAMS SYNDROME. Ocular problems involve both estropia and hyperopia. Mean IQ of adults is in the mid-50's (range 17 to 87). The vast majority of individuals live with their parents, in group homes, or in supervised apartments. Although the most common cardiovascular defect is supravalvular aortic stenosis (occurring in about 70% of patients), pulmonary artery stenosis, aortic hypoplasia, and other vascular stenoses have been documented. Progression of the vascular stenosis including hypoplasia of the aorta and renal artery stenosis has been documented. The extent to which peripheral vascular lesions contribute to the hypertension is unknown. The presence of ectopic calcium deposits and hypercalcinuria indicates that the error in calcium metabolism assumed to be limited to early childhood does not disappear with age in all cases. Hyperparathyroidism secondary to the hypercalcinuria is often present. Gastrointestinal problems include obesity with subsequent diabetes mellitus, chronic constipation, peptic ulcer disease, cholelithiasis, and diverticulitis, and genitourinary problems include ureteral reflux and bladder diverticuli associated with recurrent infection. Nephrocalcinosis and renal insufficiency have been documented. Musculoskeletal defects including lordosis and limitation of joint movements are progressive.

Although most individuals with this disorder represent sporadic cases within otherwise normal families, parent-to-child transmission has been documented, implicating autosomal dominant inheritance. Recent studies using fluorescent *in situ* hybridization and quantitative southern analysis indicate that both inherited and sporadic cases of Williams syndrome are caused by a deletion of one elastin allele located within chromosome subunit 7q11.23.

Ewart AK, Morris CA, Atkinson D, et al.: Hemizygosity at the elastin locus in a developmental disorder, Williams syndrome. Nature Genet 5:11, 1993. *Hemizygosity at the elastin locus is identified in four familial and five sporadic cases of Williams syndrome.*

Morris CA, Leonard CO, Dilts C, et al.: Adults with Williams syndrome. Am J Med Genet (Suppl) 6:102, 1990. *A detailed clinical summary of 29 adults with Williams syndrome.*

NOONAN SYNDROME. Although rarely severe, mental deficiency occurs in approximately 25% of cases. Congenital heart defects occur frequently and include pulmonary valve stenosis due to a dysplastic or thickened valve, atrial septal defect, asymmetric septal hypertrophy, cardiomyopathy, and ventricular septal defect. Other problems that might affect long-term follow-up are uncommon. Rare cases of autoimmune thyroiditis have been documented. A small penis and cryptorchidism associated with delayed sexual development and infertility have been noted in some males. Most

TABLE 28–1. COMMON ABNORMAL SIGNS AND SYMPTOMS OF HEREDITARY SYNDROMES BY SYSTEM

Syndrome	Principal Features	Ocular	IQ	Neuro	Cardiovascular		Endo	GI	GU	MS	Tumor	Other
					Hypertension	*Anomaly*						
Williams	Prominent lips, hoarse voice, cardiovascular defect	+	+	+	+	+	+	+	+	−		−
Noonan	Neck webbing, pectus excavatum, pulmonic stenosis	−	+	−	−	+	+	−	+	+	−	Hematologic
Beckwith-Wiedemann	Overgrowth, macrocrania, poor coordination	−	−	−	−	+	+	−	+	+		−
Sotos	Overgrowth, macrocrania, poor coordination	−	+	−	−	+	+	−	−	+		−
Prader-Willi	Obesity, hypogenitalism, behavioral abnormalities	+	+	−	+	−	+	−	+	+	−	−
Stickler	Flat facies, myopia, spondyloepiphyseal dysplasia	+	−	−	−	−	−	−	−	+	−	Cleft palate Hearing loss
Saethre-Chotzen	Craniosynostosis, syndactyly, deviated nasal septum	−	+	−	−	−	−	−	−	+		−
Velo-cardio-facial	Cleft palate, cardiac defect, characteristic facies	−	+	−	−	+	+	−	−	−	−	Psychosis Immune deficiency
Bardet-Biedl	Pigmentary retinopathy, obesity, renal abnormalities	+	+	−	+	−	+	−	+	+		−
Werner	Cataract, gray sparse hair, skin changes	+	−	+	+	+	+	−	+	+	+	Short stature Metastatic calcifications

females are fertile. Malignant hyperthermia has been documented frequently. Hematologic abnormalities including Factor XI deficiency, von Willebrand disease, and thrombocytopenia occur.

Although most cases of this disorder are sporadic, parent-to-child transmission has been documented, implicating autosomal dominant inheritance as the cause. Because of the marked variability in expression of this disorder, in many cases a mildly affected parent is initially diagnosed following the birth of his/her severely affected child. Relative to the diagnosis of this disorder in adults, it is important to realize that a marked change of phenotype occurs with advancing age. In the teenager and young adult, the face becomes more triangular and facial features are sharper. In the older adult, the nasolabial folds become prominent, the anterior hairline becomes higher, and the skin becomes wrinkled and transparent.

Allanson JE, Hall JG, Hughes HE, et al.: Noonan syndrome: The changing phenotype. Am J Med Genet 21:507, 1985. *A review documenting the changing phenotype from the newborn period to adulthood.*
Mendez HMM, Opitz JM: Noonan syndrome: A review. Am J Med Genet 21:493, 1985. *An excellent review of the complete spectrum of defects.*

BECKWITH-WIEDEMANN SYNDROME (BWS). This disorder is the best known and most frequently recognized overgrowth syndrome. With increasing age, the typical facial features become less obvious. In the newborn period, the face is round to oval. Prominent cheeks give the impression of a narrow forehead. The tongue is extremely prominent through midchildhood. By adolescence the tongue no longer protrudes and the glabellar nevus, so prominent in early infancy, has faded. Creases on the ear lobes and indentations or pits on the posterior rim of the helix are typical at all ages. Regarding the overgrowth, height remains at or above the 95th percentile throughout adolescence while weight remains between the 75th and 95th percentile. Spontaneous pubertal development occurs at an appropriate time for chronologic age. Cardiovascular anomalies including both structural defects and cardiomegaly occur in approximately one third of patients. Malignant tumors, the majority of which include Wilms' tumor, adrenal carcinoma, and hepatoblastoma, occur in approximately 7% of cases. Although no consensus has been forthcoming regarding screening, most recommend abdominal and renal ultrasound scans at least every 6 months up to elementary school and then at yearly intervals until adolescence.

The gene for BWS is located at 11p15.5. In a normal situation, the maternal copy of BWS is inactivated such that a normal individual has only one active copy of the gene functioning at any one time, i.e., the paternal copy. BWS is one of a number of genetic disorders in which the presence of the phenotype depends on whether the gene has been inherited from the father or the mother, a mechanism known as genomic imprinting (see Ch. 23). In the case of BWS, the phenotype occurs as a result of a variety of different situations which produce a dosage imbalance or two rather than one active copy of the gene. For example, chromosomal abnormalities that cause duplication of the BWS locus at 11p15.5 result in the BWS phenotype if they are paternally derived and thus associated with two active copies of the gene. Chromosomal inversions and translocations involving the BWS locus produce the phenotype if they are inherited from the mother. Presumably, disrupting the locus activates a gene that is normally inactive. Also, the BWS phenotype has been seen in conjunction with paternal disomy, a situation in which both BWS loci are inherited from the father, giving two copies of the gene.

Hall JG: Nontraditional Inheritance. Growth Genetics Hormones 6:1, 1990. *An overview of genetic phenomena, including imprinting, which are not explained by traditional mendelian concepts.*
Normal AM, Read AP, Clayton-Smith J, et al.: Recurrent Wiedemann-Beckwith syndrome with inversion of chromosome 11p11.2p15.5. Am J Med Genet 42:638, 1992. *Possible mechanisms giving rise to this disorder are discussed.*

SOTOS SYNDROME. Although marked overgrowth is a consistent feature during infancy and childhood, adult height is usually within the normal range. The head, which is large at birth, remains so throughout life. In adulthood, mandibular growth is striking, and the chin becomes long and narrow. Mild mental deficiency with an average IQ of 72 has been reported in 85% of cases. Abnormal glucose tolerance testing has been observed in 14% of cases and tumors including Wilms' tumor, hepatocellular carcinoma, mixed parotid tumor, vaginal epidermoid carcinoma, osteochondroma, cavernous hemangioma, hairy pigmented nevus, and intestinal polyposis occur in 5%. Regarding cause, the majority of cases represent sporadic events in otherwise normal families. However, at least five

families have been reported in which both parent and offspring are affected, suggesting autosomal dominant inheritance.

Wit JM, Beemer FA, Barth PG, et al.: Cerebral gigantism (Sotos syndrome), compiled data of 22 cases. Eur J Pediatr 144:131, 1985. *An in-depth study of the clinical features, growth, bone age, cranial CT scans, and plasma somatomedin activity of 22 children with Sotos syndrome.*

PRADER-WILLI SYNDROME (PWS). Although severe hypotonia, failure to thrive, and hypogenitalism characterize this disorder in early life, hyperphagia, obesity, and the appearance of bizarre behavior that intensifies with advancing age usually become manifest by age 6. The insatiable appetite—leading in many cases to morbid obesity, limited sexual function, and severe behavioral abnormalities—results in significant problems that can have a devastating effect on the ability of adults with this disorder to successfully adapt to their families and society. Mental retardation, which occurs in the vast majority of affected individuals, is mild in 63%, moderate in 31%, and severe in the remainder. Almost three quarters of affected individuals receive special education and function at a sixth grade level or below in reading and third grade or below in mathematics. Secondary sexual characteristics are delayed and remain immature in the vast majority of cases. Sixty percent of females have amenorrhea, and the remaining 40% begin to menstruate between 10 and 28 years, with an average of 17 years. Obesity (see Ch. 196), sometimes severe enough to require gastric bypass surgery, contributes significantly to the health problems associated with this disorder, including elevated blood pressure, stroke, respiratory difficulties, and diabetes mellitus. Although sleep apnea has not been documented, REM-related oxygen desaturation is common and the severity is significantly correlated with severity of the obesity.

Typical maladaptive behaviors include temper tantrums, arguing, irritability, stubbornness, lying, skin picking, obsessions, and defiance. Aging may be associated with confusion, withdrawal, and fatigue.

More than 50% of affected individuals have a chromosome deletion involving band q11-12 of the long arm of chromosome 15. In all individuals with PWS, the origin of the deletion is the paternal parent. Individuals in whom the parental origin of the same deletion (15q11-12) is maternal have the Angelman syndrome—a disorder associated with severe mental retardation, a "puppet-like" gait, and paroxysms of laughter. Evidence that the expression of the clinical phenotype in these two conditions depends on the genetic material from the parent of origin gives further credence to the concept of genomic imprinting. Additional support for the concept of imprinting in these disorders comes from the observation that some individuals with PWS, who have no evidence of a chromosome deletion, have inherited both chromosome 15's from their mother, whereas some individuals with Angelman syndrome who have no evidence of a chromosome deletion have inherited both chromosome 15's from their father. The inheritance of both members of a chromosome pair from one parent is referred to as uniparental disomy. Recognizing that uniparental disomy occurs in some cases of PWS and Angelman syndrome indicates that these parents have genetic information in 15q11-12 that derives from only their mothers or their fathers, respectively. From a practical standpoint, recurrence risk for Prader-Willi syndrome is most likely less than 1 in 1000, and it is unlikely to occur in individuals with deletion of 15q.

Butler MG: Prader-Willi syndrome: Current understanding of cause and diagnosis. Am J Med Genet 35:319, 1990. *Review of all aspects (including detailed cytogenetics) of the syndrome.*
Dykens EM, Hodapp RM, Walsh K, et al.: Adaptive and maladaptive behavior in Prader-Willi syndrome. J Am Acad Child Adoles Psychiatry 31:1131, 1992. *Examination of the development and profiles of adaptive and maladaptive behavior of 21 adults and adolescents.*
Greenswag LR: Adults with Prader-Willi syndrome, a survey of 232 cases. Dev Med Child Neurol 29:145, 1987. *Review with special attention to adults.*

STICKLER SYNDROME. Marked variability of expression exists for this autosomal dominant disorder. Ophthalmologic abnormalities require the greatest follow-up. Although 75% of patients develop myopia by age 20, it does not occur in some patients until after age 50. Retinal detachment, leading to blindness, usually does not occur until after age 20. Mitral valve prolapse occurs in 50% of cases. Progressive degenerative arthropathy predominantly involving weight-bearing joints most commonly becomes a problem after age 30, leading in some cases to total hip replacement. Hearing loss, both sensorineural and conductive, frequently occurs.

Lieberfarb RM, Hirose T, Holmes LB: The Wagner-Stickler syndrome, a study of 22 families. J Pediatr 99:394, 1981. *Review of spectrum of defects documenting the variable expression.*

SAETHRE-CHOTZEN SYNDROME.

This is the most common heritable disorder in which coronal craniosynostosis is one feature. Although most affected individuals are of normal intelligence, mild to moderate mental deficiency has been documented occasionally. The degree of syndactyly is seldom of either cosmetic or functional significance. Deviated nasal septum is common. Facial appearance tends to become more normal with advancing age. Few, if any, medical complications should raise concern as one follows individuals with this autosomal dominant condition.

Cohen MM: Craniosynostosis: Diagnosis, Evaluation and Management. New York, Raven Press, 1986. *An excellent reference for all known syndromes associated with craniosynostosis.*

VELO-CARDIO-FACIAL SYNDROME (VCF).

One of the most common multiple malformation syndromes associated with oral clefting, this disorder is usually associated with submucous cleft palate or, even more likely, velopharyngeal incompetence with hypernasal speech. Ventricular septal defect with or without a right aortic arch is the most common cardiac defect. The characteristic facies includes vertical maxillary excess with a long face, a prominent nose with a squared nasal root and narrow alar base, a retruded mandible, and minor ear anomalies. Learning disabilities and mild intellectual impairment occur frequently with IQ ranging from 70 to 90. Hypocalcemia secondary to hypoparathyroidism (see Ch. 214) occurs infrequently in infancy but is virtually never a management problem following childhood. An excessive number of infections have been reported in a number of individuals with this condition. The extent to which this may relate to an immunologic deficiency is unclear. However, abnormal T-cell function and absent thymic tissue have been documented in a few instances, and adenoid hypoplasia has been noted frequently. Of perhaps greatest concern relative to natural history, a number of affected individuals have developed psychiatric disorders, primarily chronic schizophrenia with paranoid delusions with onset varying between ages 10 and 21. Regarding etiology, VCF is an autosomal dominant condition. Affected patients have been shown to have an interstitial deletion of chromosome 22q11. Of significance, this is the same region that is deleted in some cases of the DiGeorge sequence, a disorder that involves developmental defects of the third and fourth pharyngeal pouches, leading to thymic and parathyroid hypoplasia and cardiac defects. Based on a number of clinical studies in which a child with the DiGeorge sequence was born to a parent with VCF, it is now believed that the two disorders represent different manifestations of the same genetic defect.

Driscoll DA, Spinner NB, Budarf ML, et al.: Deletions and microdeletions of 22q11.2 in VCFS. Am J Med Genet 44:261, 1992. *A review of the karyotypic abnormalities in VCFS.*
Scrambler PJ, Kelly D, Williamson R, et al.: The velo-cardio-facial syndrome is associated with chromosome deletions which encompasses the DiGeorge syndrome locus. Lancet 339:1138, 1992. *Deletions of the DiGeorge syndrome critical region are described in a group of patients with VCFS.*

BARDET-BIEDL SYNDROME.

Visual acuity deteriorates rapidly with age such that by age 30 more than 90% of patients are legally blind, the result of severe retinal dystrophy. Markedly constricted visual fields, severe abnormalities of color vision, raised dark-adaptive thresholds, and extinguished or minimal rod-and-cone responses on electroretinography occur in the majority of cases. Mental deficiency is usually mild to moderate. Although structural and/or functional abnormalities of the kidneys associated in 50% of cases with hypertension occur in the vast majority of adults with this disorder, symptomatic renal impairment occurs in only a small minority. Genital hypoplasia manifest by small testes and a very small penis occurs in most males. Although no male with this disorder has reproduced, a few women have given birth. The hypogonadism has been described as primary germinal hypoplasia and also as hypogonadotrophic. Postaxial polydactyly, syndactyly, and brachydactyly are common. This is an autosomal recessive genetically determined condition with marked variability of expression even between affected siblings.

Green JS, Parfrey PS, Harnett JD, et al.: The cardinal manifestations of Bardet-Biedl syndrome, a form of Laurence-Moon-Biedl syndrome. N Engl J Med 321:1002, 1989. *Spectrum of clinical features in 32 patients ascertained through the Canadian National Institute of the Blind.*
Harnett JD, Green JS, Cramer BC, et al.: The spectrum of renal disease in Laurence-Moon-Biedl syndrome. N Engl J Med 319:615, 1988. *Review of abnormalities of renal structure and function.*

WERNER SYNDROME.

Usually not diagnosed until young adulthood, graying of the hair is the earliest sign, occurring at an average age of 20. This is followed by skin changes, primarily atrophy involving the face and distal extremities; loss of hair; development of an abnormally thin, high-pitched, or hoarse voice; visual symptoms or detection of cataracts; skin ulcers; and lastly, diabetes at a mean age of 34. Vascular calcifications, most commonly involving vessels of the legs, have been noted in all major vessels including the aorta. Hypertension occurs in about 50% of cases. Coronary artery disease is common. Hypogonadism, reduced fertility, and diabetes mellitus occur frequently. Testicular atrophy is the most striking pathologic feature of this disorder. Approximately 10% of patients develop malignant tumors, especially sarcomas and meningiomas. The mean stature of affected males is 61 inches and of affected females is 57.5 inches. Death occurs at an average age of 47, with a range from ages 31 to 63. The two most common causes of death are malignancies and vascular accidents. Werner syndrome is caused by a recessive mutation that has been mapped to chromosome 8p. Fibroblasts from skin biopsies grow more slowly, assume a senescent morphology more rapidly, and assume a markedly reduced lifespan *in vitro*. DNA repair is normal. Karyotype preparations show a normal number of chromosomes but multiple stable chromosome rearrangements, including deletion of a portion of a single chromosome and translocations involving several chromosomes, as well as an increase in chromosome breakage.

Epstein CJ, Martin GM, Schultz AL, et al.: Werner's syndrome: A review of its symptomatology, natural history, pathologic features, genetics. and relationship to the natural aging process. Medicine 45:177, 1966. *A detailed summary of clinical and laboratory characteristics of 125 cases of Werner syndrome.*
Thomas W, Rubenstein M, Goto M, et al.: A genetic analysis of the Werner syndrome region on human chromosome 8p. Genomics 16:685, 1993.

29 GENETIC COUNSELING
Margretta R. Seashore

Genetic counseling can be defined as a process in which an individual or family obtains information about a genetic condition that may affect them. The purpose of genetic counseling is to enable individuals and families to make important decisions about marriage, reproduction, and health management based on the facts of the genetic situation for which a risk is perceived. This process is part of a thorough genetic evaluation in which the diagnosis is made or confirmed, the genetic model is developed, the information is communicated, the options are discussed, and psychosocial support is offered. Any breakdown in this progression may lead to information being misunderstood, misinterpreted, or misused.

DIAGNOSIS

The first step in genetic counseling is to confirm the diagnosis. The worst error that can be made is to provide an elegant and sophisticated analysis for the wrong disorder. The importance of this step cannot be overemphasized. Many persons have been given general diagnosis, such as mental retardation, for which there can be a multitude of genetic as well as nongenetic explanations. The increasing definition of the molecular pathology of many disorders has heightened the importance of recognizing genetic heterogeneity. For example, at least 20 different forms of muscular dystrophy have been identified which are clinically similar. Both X-linked and autosomal recessive forms are known. At least two, Becker and Duchenne dystrophy, are X-linked conditions that are allelic but clinically quite distinct. Differentiations of this kind must be made with as much accuracy as possible if the patient and family are to be given the most precise answers.

The confirmation of the diagnosis uses five medical tools, four of which are very familiar to all clinicians. There are medical records, medical history, physical examination, conventional laboratory tests, and molecular genetic analysis. The importance of reviewing medical records seems obvious, yet it can be a difficult task to accomplish completely. Validation of the rate of progression of symptoms and signs, the development of the present physical findings, and the results of prior laboratory tests is best done from the medical records. In addition, the status of family members can sometimes be assessed from examination of their medical records. Often the medical geneticist has been told of a relative who "had the same problem" only to learn from that individual's medical records that the relative's problem was entirely different.

The medical history provides clues to the beginnings and progression of symptoms and signs which may provide valuable hints to diagnosis. The pattern of progression in the degenerative neurologic disorders provides important diagnostic information. A history of more than two spontaneous miscarriages may suggest a chromosomal translocation in one parent. Early death of infants in the pedigree may suggest an inborn error of intermediary metabolism.

The physical examination again provides the opportunity to consider genetic heterogeneity. For example, there are many genetic causes of short stature. The details of the physical examination may provide the information to determine the correct genetic diagnosis. Precise measurement of anthropometric features can be compared with values in the literature and the diagnostic considerations narrowed.

Conventional laboratory tests often provide helpful diagnostic information to complete the genetic diagnosis. Radiographic appearance of bones is often the critical information in diagnosing the chondrodystrophies, for example. Measurement of proteins, such as α_1-antitrypsin, can demonstrate the most important feature of a condition.

The development of molecular diagnostic tools that can provide precise definition of the mutation or utilize linkage to a specific genetic marker has revolutionized genetic counseling. In the past, the chromosomal location of specific genes was inferred from pedigree information for the X chromosome and linkage to specific protein markers for autosomes. Now the chromosomal location of many more genes is known, linkage to specific DNA markers has been established, and many genes of clinical importance have been cloned and sequenced. It is likely that within the next two decades, the entire human genome will be mapped and entirely sequenced. More than 2000 genes have now been mapped to specific locations in the human genome. Many of these comprise specific genes or linkage markers for some of the 6000 single gene conditions that appear in the McKusick catalog of mendelian phenotypes. The number of conditions that show linkage to known genetic markers or to anonymous DNA probes grows daily. These new tools can be used to enhance the precision of genetic diagnosis and counseling (see Ch. 25 for molecular methods). Table 29–1 lists examples of many of the genetic conditions that can be diagnosed using these molecular tools. This list is being expanded at a rapid rate and should not be considered complete. At least one disease has been mapped to each chromosome (Table 29–2). Any condition mapped to a specific chromosomal location can theoretically be diagnosed using molecular methods, given the appropriate molecular probes and informative family members.

THE GENETIC MODEL

The next essential step—development of the genetic model—should be taken before the genetic counseling visit with the patient and family takes place. The patient has come with the question "what is it and is it inherited?" Arrival at a diagnosis leads to the answer to the first part of the question. The second part is crucial to the process of genetic counseling. Development of the genetic

TABLE 29–1. SINGLE GENE CONDITIONS FOR WHICH DNA-BASED DIAGNOSIS HAS BEEN ACCOMPLISHED

Adult polycystic kidney disease	Neurofibromatosis type 1
Alport syndrome	Neurofibromatosis type 2
Duchenne muscular dystrophy	Ornithine transcarbamylase deficiency
Cystic fibrosis	Phenylketonuria
Fragile-X syndrome	Sickle cell anemia
Gaucher disease	Spinocerebellar ataxia type 1
Hemophilia A	Tay-Sachs disease
Huntington's disease	Thalassemias
Multiple endocrine neoplasia	Wiskott-Aldrich syndrome
Myotonic dystrophy	

TABLE 29–2. EXAMPLES OF ONE CONDITION MAPPED TO EACH CHROMOSOME

Genetic Condition	Map Location
Charcot-Marie-Tooth neuropathy 1	1q
von Hippel–Lindau syndrome	3p
Huntington's disease	4pter–p16
Familial polyposis of the colon	5q21–p22
Congenital adrenal hyperplasia	6p21.3
Cystic fibrosis	7q31–q32
Langer-Gideon syndrome	8124
Friedreich ataxia	9q13–q21
Multiple endocrine neoplasia IIB	10pter–q11
Wilms' tumor-aniridia syndrome	11p13
Stickler syndrome	12q14
Wilson's disease	13q14–q21
Variegate porphyria	14q
Xeroderma pigmentosum (comp group F)	15
Adult type polycystic kidney disease	16p13
Neurofibromatosis	17q11.2
Kidd blood group	18q11–q12
Myotonic dystrophy	19q13.3–q13.3
Alagille syndrome	20p12–p11
Alzheimer disease 1	21pter–q21
NF2 (bilateral acoustic neuroma)	22q11–q13.1
Duchenne muscular dystrophy	Xp21.3–p21.1

model requires the family history, the precise diagnosis, and knowledge of the possible genetic mechanisms. The diagraming of the pedigree from the family history may fit such an obvious genetic model that further analysis is simple. When the physical examination and laboratory studies are typical of a recognized genetic condition such as Duchenne muscular dystrophy and the pedigree demonstrates a clear pattern of X-linked inheritance, developing the genetic model is straightforward. More often, however, the pedigree is less clear. Where there is familial aggregation without an obvious mendelian pattern or the individual is the only affected member of the family at present, all possible genetic mechanisms must be considered and excluded or confirmed. The genetic model must then be used to identify those at risk for the condition.

Three general genetic mechanisms must be considered: chromosomal, mendelian, and multifactorial. The chromosomal disorders should be considered as a possible explanation for multiple anomalies, mental retardation, recurrent miscarriages, and unexplained stillbirths (see Ch. 26). Empiric figures must be used to predict the recurrence of chromosomal abnormalities in a family. These range between 1 and 10%, and the literature must be consulted with reference to the specific situation.

When a clear mendelian pattern is seen and the disorder is a recognized mendelian condition, counseling is based on that pattern. When the family history fails to demonstrate a mendelian pattern, the diagnosis is reviewed and the medical literature consulted to determine the inheritance pattern for the specific disorder. With autosomal recessive conditions the birth of an affected child may be the first signal that a set of parents is heterozygous for a rare recessive condition. Here the genetic model depends on the correct diagnosis and the known inheritance pattern for that disorder. For X-linked conditions, the decision must be made whether the affected individual represents a new mutation or inheritance from a heterozygous mother who by chance has no affected relatives. In the past, Bayesian calculations based on the pedigree have been the mainstay of this kind of analysis. Today, however, molecular diagnostic tools have refined the ability to determine heterozygosity in this situation. For dominantly inherited conditions, the literature must be consulted to determine the proportion of patients who represent new mutations, a figure that can approach 50%. When a new mutation is the explanation, others in the family are not at risk, but each offspring of the affected individual has a 50% risk of inheriting the gene. Variability expression can confound the analysis of a family demonstrating an autosomal dominant condition. The possibility of gonadal mosaicism, although rare, can never be eliminated. In general, however, the absence of the condition in any other family member makes the likelihood high that the patient represents a new mutation. Frequently no mendelian hypothesis can be sustained, yet

TABLE 29-3. SOME CONDITIONS THAT HAVE BEEN DIAGNOSED PRENATALLY

Disorder	Diagnostic Method
All defined chromosomal disorders	Cytogenetic analysis
Adrenoleukodystrophy	DNA and long chain fatty acid
Cystinosis	Cystine uptake
Cystic fibrosis	DNA analysis
Duchenne muscular dystrophy	DNA analysis
Ectodermal dysplasia	Fetoscopy, skin biopsy
Fabry's disease	α-Galactosidase A
Fragile-X syndrome	DNA analysis
Gaucher's disease	β-glucosidase; DNA analysis
GM$_2$-gangliosidosis I (Tay-Sachs)	Hexosaminidase A
Hemoglobinopathies	DNA analysis
Hemophilia A	DNA analysis
Metachromatic leukodystrophy	Aryl sulfatase A
Mucopolysaccharidosis I (Hurler)	α-L-iduronidase
Neural tube defects: spina bifida, anencephaly	α-Fetoprotein, ultrasound, amniotic fluid acetylcholinesterase
Omphalocele	α-Fetoprotein, ultrasound
Congenital malformations: hydrocephalus, limb, cardiac, renal anomalies	Ultrasound
Skeletal dysplasias	Ultrasound
Phenylketonuria	DNA analysis

See Milunsky for more information.

there is familial aggregation of the disorder. Many conditions, such as neural tube defects and cleft lip and palate, appear to be multifactorial in origin with both genetic and environmental components. Genetic counseling for these conditions must rely on empiric figures for the specific condition.

THE COUNSELING PROCESS

Once the genetic model has been established, this information can be communicated to the patient and family. The process of genetic counseling itself has the following components: transferring information about the genetic risks, putting the risks in perspective, providing a summary of the disorder, and discussing the options. It must begin with the individual who brought the original question. An explanation of the genetic risks requires imparting factual information using scientific concepts that are not familiar to everyone. It is important that the facts upon which the genetic model is based be clearly explained. However, it is neither possible nor desirable to present an entire course in medical genetics to the anxious patient and family. Therefore, the relevant facts must be carefully culled from the counselor's knowledge store and communicated clearly. It is important to remember that persons may be very anxious and find it difficult to absorb complex material, especially if they are fearful about the implications of the information. The strategy of first presenting a brief summary of the conclusions and their implications, stating that the evidence for this conclusion will presently be discussed, can allay some fears and relieve some of the distraction that prevents families from hearing this kind of information.

TABLE 29-4. INDICATIONS FOR GENETIC COUNSELING

Advanced parental age
  Maternal age over 35
  Paternal age over 50
Family history of inherited disease
Risk of chromosome disorder
  Previous child with chromosomal abnormality
  Parent with known chromosomal translocation
Heterozygote screening based on ethnicity
  Tay-Sachs (Ashkenazi-Jewish; French Canadian)
  Thalassemias (Mediterranean, Arab, Indo-Pakastani)
  Sickle cell anemia (West African, Mediterranean, Arab, Indo-Pakastani, Turkish, Southeast Asian)
Pregnancy screening abnormality
  Maternal serum α-fetoprotein
  Maternal serum triple screen

If the condition is a chromosome disorder, the structure and ways of identifying chromosomes must be mentioned and the specific disorder illustrated. Using teaching aids such as diagrams and photographs of chromosomes is helpful, the normal situation providing a frame of reference. When the condition is a mendelian disorder, the basic concepts of single gene inheritance must be discussed briefly, but the discussion should center on the mode of inheritance involved in the particular family and not be clouded with a great deal of extraneous material about other modes of inheritance. Families without a prior family history of the disorder may have difficulty with the fact that the disorder has never been seen in their family. An explanation of heterozygosity may help clarify autosomal recessive inheritance. Autosomal dominant inheritance is easy to understand when there are other affected individuals and the pedigree demonstrates a clear vertical pattern. Of more difficulty to the family is the new mutation. Careful examination of other family members must be performed before the presence of the condition can be excluded. As with the chromosome disorders, the use of such teaching aids as gene diagrams, sample pedigrees, and other models may be extremely valuable.

A second important component of genetic counseling is putting the risk in perspective. Many workers in the field (see Hsia) have noted that perception of risk may be of more importance in family decision making than the actual numerical value of the risk. This perception depends on at least two factors: risk compared to background risk, and overall burden, a combination of risk and severity. A risk of 1 in 4 of recurrence in a second child, in the case of PKU for example, is very much greater than a risk of 1 in 10,000 in the general population. Conversely, a risk of 1 in 10,000 may sound high to a couple who believe that the chances of something being wrong with an unborn child is 1 in a million. The presentation of such risk figures can change the perception of that risk. For example, a 1 in 4 chance of recurrence of PKU is also a 3 to 1 chance against recurrence. The judgment of burden, first put forth by C. O. Carter, is a very personal one. Physical handicap may be a severe burden for one family, whereas another may find that tolerable but

TABLE 29-5. REPRODUCTIVE OPTIONS FOR FAMILIES WITH GENETIC RISKS

Adoption
Reproductive assistance
  In vitro fertilization with a donor egg
  Artificial insemination by donor
Prenatal diagnosis

TABLE 29-6. PRENATAL DIAGNOSIS METHODS

Method	Use	Risk
Ultrasonography	Estimated fetal age Assess growth Evaluate anatomy and organ function	None recognized
Amniocentesis or chorionic villus sampling (CVS)	Fetal cells: analyze DNA, chromosomes proteins Amniotic fluid: analyze proteins, measure analytes of fetal origin	Amniocentesis (15–20 weeks) $\leq 0.5\%$ risk miscarriage CVS (9–11 weeks) $\leq 2\%$ risk miscarriage
Periumbilical blood sampling	Fetal blood: analyze cells, measure serum analytes	$\leq 2\%$ risk miscarriage

mental handicap unacceptable. Helping families to think about risks in these ways is an important component of genetic counseling.

Modern molecular tools have allowed some families to take advantage of presymptomatic diagnosis for inherited disorders such as α_1-antitrypsin deficiency, Huntington's disease, and breast cancer. The issues these families face depend on how they will be able to use that information. If treatment or prevention of disease is possible, the information may be welcomed. If, as in Huntington's disease, the affected person faces catastrophic outcome without any possible intervention, the choice to take the test may be a very difficult one. The physician must help the patient weigh the risks and benefits and discuss the impact of the results before the patient chooses testing.

Genetic counseling also includes a description of the disorder. Many persons go to their local library in an attempt to find literature about the disorder or ask medical friends to do so. Often this results in misinformation or information that is out of date. Providing written material about the disorder is often helpful. Many genetic counseling clinics have pamphlets, booklets, and other literature to provide. The family should also be furnished with a written report of the counseling summarizing the important points.

REPRODUCTIVE OPTIONS AND PRENATAL DIAGNOSIS

If risk to future unborn children is at issue, the family at risk for a genetic disorder must be told about the reproductive options available. Prenatal diagnosis is an important reproductive option that must be discussed. Appropriate referral to experts in areas of alternative reproductive options must be made. Aside from refraining from having children at all, the options can enhance the chances of having healthy children for the family at risk.

The methods in prenatal diagnosis depend on imaging the fetus, examining DNA in cells of fetal origin, analyzing chromosomes in fetal cells, and examining analytes and cells of fetal origin. The major autosomal and sex chromosomal aneuploidies can be diagnosed in this way, along with chromosomal rearrangements, deletions, insertions, and the like. Any DNA-based diagnosis that can be performed on cells can be performed on fetal cells.

Measurement of α-fetoprotein, human chorionic gonadotropin, and unconjugated estrogen in maternal serum (triple screen) allows detection of an estimated 60 to 70% of fetuses with Down syndrome or trisomy 18 regardless of maternal age, and is recommended regardless of prior risk. Indications, diagnostic uses, and risks of midtrimester amniocentesis, chorionic villus sampling (CVS), and periumbilical blood sampling are shown in the Tables 29–1 to 29–6. Recent studies of CVS suggest a slightly increased risk of limb hypoplasia in babies born following that procedure. Fetoscopy is done only when other diagnostic avenues have failed and is used to visualize fetal anatomy and to perform biopsy of fetal tissues such as liver or skin.

It is crucial that the pregnant woman undergoing prenatal diagnosis be given extremely clear counseling. Spelling out clearly the expectations and limitations of the testing prior to any procedures is critical. The diagnoses that are being sought must be explained. It is very easy for the woman to conclude that a normal test result shows that the baby will be "normal," when in fact a short list of pathologic conditions for which her risk was increased has been excluded. Normalcy is never completely assured. After these conditions have been excluded, the pregnancy stands at the same risk for other potential problems as others in the general population.

Much more difficult is the situation in which the result of the test is not normal. Although this possibility is best discussed beforehand and the options considered, it is no longer considered necessary that the woman make a decision before she learns the test results. The implications of the diagnosis must be reviewed with care, sensitivity, and accuracy. The options for the woman are to terminate the pregnancy or to carry it to term. The decision to terminate must be taken in collaboration with the obstetrician who will perform the procedure so that the process can be described and possible complications reviewed. The choice of procedure depends on the stage of pregnancy; the complications are specific to the particular procedure. Psychosocial support after the procedure is crucial. Most families who elect to terminate a pregnancy go through a period of grieving for the loss of the hoped-for normal child. Many such pregnancies were planned and wanted. The family should be offered the chance to visit with the genetic counselor to discuss their normal feelings of sadness and loss and to join a support group if one is available. There is no evidence for long-term psychological sequelae of genetic pregnancy termination.

Thoughtful genetic counseling challenges the skills of the physician in diagnosis, analysis, communication, and support. Rarely is it the province of only one person, but rather it requires the collaborative efforts of an experienced team. From the initial evaluation, through development of the genetic model and identification of those at risk to completion of the transfer of information, the use of these skills enables patients and their families to make intelligent, informed, and reasoned decisions for their futures.

Emery A, Pullen I: Psychological Aspects of Genetic Counseling. London, Academic Press, 1984. *Informative about the psychological aspects of genetic counseling, the impact of genetic information, and the challenge of information transfer.*

Frets P, Duivenvoorden H, et al.: Factors influencing the reproductive decision after genetic counseling. Am J Med Genet 35:496–502, 503–509, 1990. *Others in the series of articles on the psychodynamics of genetic counseling.*

Kevles D, Hood L: The Code of Codes: Scientific and Social Issue in the Human Genome Project. Cambridge, Mass., Harvard University Press, 1992. *Scholarly treatment of the social impact of the new molecular genetics.*

Lippman-Hand A, Fraser F-C: Genetic counseling—the post counseling period. II. Making reproductive choices. Am J Med Genet 4:73, 1979. *The third in a series of articles on the psychodynamics of genetic counseling.*

McKusick V: Mendelian inheritance in Man. 10th ed. Baltimore, Johns Hopkins University Press, 1992. *Exhaustive catalog of mendelian phenotypes.*

Milunsky A: Genetic Disorders and the Fetus, Diagnosis, Prevention and Treatment. 2nd ed., New York, Plenum Press, 1986. *Extensive textbook on prenatal diagnosis.*

Thompson M, McInnes R, Willard H: Genetics in Medicine. Philadelphia, WB Saunders, 1991. *Recent text of classic and molecular clinical genetics; short and accessible.*

Weatherall DG: The New Genetics and Clinical Practice. 3rd ed., Oxford, Oxford University Press, 1991. *Detail about modern methods of molecular diagnosis of genetic disorders.*

PART VII

CARDIOVASCULAR DISEASES

30 APPROACH TO THE PATIENT WITH CARDIOVASCULAR DISEASE

Thomas Woodward Smith

Common to the care of all patients with cardiovascular disease is a database on which sound diagnostic and therapeutic decisions can be made. This chapter outlines an approach to cardiovascular data collection that emphasizes general principles and strategies and is intended to complement the more specific consideration of disease entities in the chapters that follow. One of the endlessly fascinating aspects of medicine is that each patient presents to the physician a unique story of his/her past history and present illness. Textbook descriptions of disease therefore convey at best a set of findings that the author regards as typical but that never quite fit in detail the findings present in any one individual patient. Hence, an open mind is essential when evaluating each patient so that diagnostic possibilities are not overlooked or prematurely discarded.

A dazzling array of diagnostic tests is now available for evaluation of patients with evident or suspected cardiovascular disease. Sensitivity and specificity are known, or can be estimated, for each method under a given set of clinical circumstances. Redundancy must be avoided to achieve a favorable cost:benefit ratio (e.g., radionuclide ventriculography often yields information regarding ventricular function that can be obtained from a two-dimensional echocardiogram, and both methods may be superfluous if the patient undergoes left ventriculography as part of a cardiac catheterization procedure). The emerging discipline of decision analysis (see Ch. 14.2), with emphasis on the proper application of Bayes' theorem, should help in formulating strategies for developing an adequate cardiovascular database.

Although accurate diagnosis is a key element in patient care, prognosis is also vitally important to the patient and often to the physician, who must formulate a program of treatment. Information over and above that needed to establish a diagnosis is typically required to allow an accurate prediction of outcome. This exercise in probability statistics is challenging and deserves careful attention as an essential component of comprehensive patient care.

COMPONENTS OF THE CARDIOVASCULAR WORKUP

The three essential components of the clinical database are the history, physical examination, and laboratory studies. Although this sequence of data acquisition is typically followed, the value of returning to the bedside (often repeatedly) to refine the assessment of historical information and physical findings as the workup progresses cannot be overstated.

History

The cardinal symptoms of cardiovascular disease are listed in Table 30–1. *Dyspnea* (an abnormally uncomfortable awareness of breathing) and the related items in the first line are discussed in de-

tail in Ch. 34. Historical information is particularly important in distinguishing among heart failure, pulmonary disease (including pulmonary emboli), metabolic disturbances producing acidosis, and anxiety as factors causing dyspnea. The nature of onset and duration of symptoms, relation to position, and precipitating and alleviating factors all provide important clues to the underlying pathophysiologic process.

Fatigue and *weakness* are common to many physical and emotional disease states and are nonspecific; nevertheless, it is important to record quantitative information in the history (e.g., flights of stairs or distance on level ground that the patient can manage) for current and future reference. *Cough,* initially dry and irritative, is a common early manifestation of elevated left-heart filling (and hence pulmonary venous) pressures. *Hemoptysis* should be characterized in regard to color and nature of admixture of blood and sputum to help distinguish between pulmonary (e.g., bronchitis, pulmonary infarction) and cardiac causes (e.g., pulmonary edema, hemorrhage from loss of bronchial vein integrity, as in mitral stenosis). *Cyanosis* is discussed in Ch. 34.

Chest pain or discomfort should be characterized in terms of location, quality, course of onset and offset, duration, and precipitating and alleviating factors. Pain due to ischemic heart disease is considered in Ch. 41.1, but one should remember that the original meaning of the term angina is *choking* rather than pain, and it is often described by the patient with words such as "pressure" or "squeezing" discomfort. Pericardial pain is more likely to be left sided, sharp in character, and related to breathing and position. Pleuritic pain also tends to be localized and sharp and is related to breathing or coughing. Chest wall pain is often long lasting and associated with tenderness to pressure applied at the trigger area.

Palpitation refers to an awareness of the heart beat, usually occurring in response to a change in cardiac rhythm or rate or by increased contractile force. It is a common anxiety-related symptom in patients without heart disease. Awareness of irregularity of the heart beat is more closely correlated with cardiac rhythm disturbances. *Dizziness* and *syncope* are frequent manifestations of cardiac arrhythmias and demand careful evaluation, often with 24-hour electrocardiographic (ECG) monitoring. These symptoms also occur as a consequence of orthostatic hypotension due to reduced blood volume, vasodilator drugs, or autonomic dysfunction. Obstruction to venous return from any cause also predisposes to these symptoms. *Bradycardia* typically accompanies hypotension in neurocardiogenic (vasodepressor) syncope, which is usually evaluated by tilt table testing. *Claudication* refers to pain or an uncomfortable sensation of tiredness, usually in calf and/or thigh muscles, that occurs in re-

TABLE 30–1. CARDINAL SYMPTOMS OF CARDIOVASCULAR DISEASE

Dyspnea, orthopnea, paroxysmal nocturnal dyspnea, wheezing
Fatigue, weakness
Cough, hemoptysis
Cyanosis
Chest pain or discomfort
Palpitations, dizziness, syncope
Edema
Pain in extremities with exertion (claudication)

sponse to exertion and is relieved by rest. This common symptom of peripheral arterial insufficiency is further discussed in Ch. 46.

Edema refers to swelling, usually of a dependent part of the body, due to retention of excess fluid. It is typically maximal in the feet at the end of the day and resolves, at least partially, by morning. Local factors such as deep venous disease predispose to unilateral edema. Patients confined to bed usually accumulate fluid in the sacral area.

A careful family history must always be obtained because familial clustering is common in several forms of heart disease, including coronary atherosclerosis, hypertension, hypertrophic cardiomyopathy, Marfan's syndrome, and prolonged QT syndrome, among others.

The Physical Examination

Five elements constitute the cardiovascular physical examination. These are

1. Physical appearance
2. Venous pressure and pulse contours
3. Arterial pressure and pulse contours
4. Movement of the heart
5. Auscultation

PHYSICAL APPEARANCE. This is important in assessing the nature and severity of heart disease and also in providing clues to systemic diseases that affect the heart. Important cardiac problems are frequently encountered in patients with Marfan's syndrome, Turner's syndrome, Down syndrome, the pickwickian syndrome, scleroderma, and thyroid disease, all of which are often recognizable on the basis of careful inspection of the patient's appearance. The funduscopic examination yields important information with regard to hypertension, diabetes mellitus, and sometimes infective endocarditis (Roth's spots). Cheyne-Stokes respirations are often seen in patients with advanced heart failure. Sometimes a highly specific cardiac diagnosis can be made on the basis of the physical appearance, such as the association of atrial or ventricular septal defect with the bony abnormalities of the upper extremity that constitute the Holt-Oram syndrome. Central cyanosis and clubbing of the fingertips indicate right-to-left shunting in patients with congenital heart disease.

VENOUS PRESSURE AND PULSE. Both external and internal jugular veins require careful inspection: external for estimation of mean right atrial pressure and internal for wave form as well as pressure. Figure 30–1 illustrates the typical features of the normal jugular venous pulse and indicates the terminology applied to the various aspects of this wave form. The A wave reflects right atrial contraction and occurs immediately prior to the carotid arterial pulse and first heart sound. The X descent occurs with right atrial relaxation and continues with early right ventricular contraction. The C wave, often superimposed on the beginning of the A wave, coincides with the carotid pulse itself. The V wave in the normal jugular venous pulse represents passive right atrial filling behind a closed and competent tricuspid valve. The Y descent reflects sudden termination of the V wave with right ventricular relaxation and opening of the tricuspid valve. The X descent is normally the more evident of the two declining phases of the jugular venous pulse. These phenomena are best noted with the patient so positioned that the top of the venous column can be observed throughout the cardiac cycle. Estimation of the central venous pressure is accomplished by estimating its height in centimeters above the sternal angle of Louis, adding 5 cm to allow for the normal relation of the right atrium to the external chest wall. Normal venous pressure varies from 5 to 10 cm of H_2O. The A wave tends to be accentuated in disease states characterized by reduced right ventricular compliance, tricuspid stenosis, or rhythm disturbances in which the atrium contracts against a closed tricuspid valve ("cannon" A waves). Tricuspid insufficiency produces systolic or regurgitant waves that obliterate the normal jugular venous V waves. Abnormalities associated with pericardial disease are discussed in Ch. 44.

ARTERIAL PRESSURE AND PULSE. Examination of the arterial pulse yields crucial information regarding the cardiovascular system. Arterial pressure should always be measured in both arms because of the unexpected discrepancies that are encountered in disease states or that are occasionally due to congenital anomalies. Use

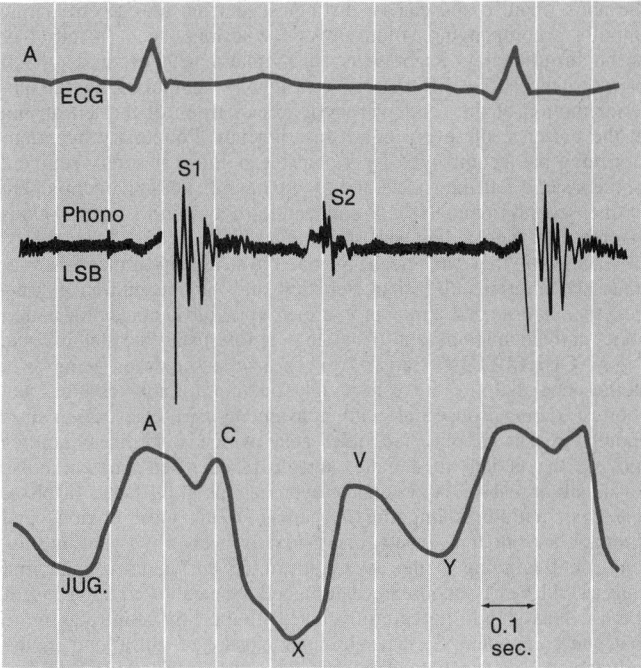

FIGURE 30–1. Normal jugular venous pulse.

of a cuff of appropriate size is essential, and the arterial blood pressure should be recorded in both supine and standing position to assess volume status and the adequacy of reflex vasoconstrictor responses. Pulsus paradoxus refers to a decrease in systolic blood pressure of > 10 mm Hg on inspiration and is a typical feature of pericardial tamponade.

The carotid arteries provide the most direct reflection of cardiac activity because of their central location in proximity to the left ventricle and aorta. The amplitude of the carotid pulse is typically increased under circumstances associated with higher cardiac output, including fever, anemia, hyperthyroidism, and arteriovenous fistulas. The regularity (or lack thereof) indicates disturbances of rhythm or hemodynamics as in pulsus alternans. The wave form of the arterial pulse yields clues regarding runoff from the aorta, as in aortic insufficiency or arteriovenous fistula; a bisferiens quality is often present in aortic insufficiency and should be distinguished from the spike-and-dome contour encountered in patients with hypertrophic cardiomyopathy with obstruction (i.e., hypertrophic subaortic stenosis). The volume of the carotid pulse is typically reduced in heart failure and in mitral or aortic stenosis. Peripheral arterial pulses other than the carotid pulses should be felt and compared, with particular attention to a pulse delay at the femoral artery as a manifestation of coarctation of the aorta. Patients with claudication should have their lower extremity pulses examined both at rest and with exercise because the latter often accentuates asymmetries.

MOVEMENT OF THE HEART. Observation, palpation, and percussion are the traditional means for physical examination of cardiac movements. Inspection of the precordium reveals asymmetries that serve as clues to chronic cardiac hypertrophy, particularly in congenital disease. The partial left lateral decubitus position is optimal for observation as well as palpation of the left ventricle in most patients. Diffuse left parasternal cardiac movement is often best appreciated with the heel of the palm, whereas higher frequency events (S_1, ejection clicks, S_2, opening snap, and thrills) are best felt with firm pressure and the tactile use of the fingertips. Precordial movements should be described at the apex, left parasternal area, and the right and left second intercostal spaces. The normal tapping impulse of the left ventricular apex is replaced by a more diffuse and sometimes dyskinetic impulse in patients with cardiac enlargement from a variety of causes. Displacement of the left ventricle is typically downward and to the left with cardiomegaly. Systolic overload with concentric hypertrophy increases the duration of the apex impulse and can be distinguished from the hyperdynamic impulse accompanying volume overload lesions, such as mitral or aortic insufficiency. Right ventricular enlargement produces a left parasternal systolic lift that is occasionally mimicked by the anterior motion of the heart with systolic expansion of the left atrium in the presence of severe mitral insufficiency. Pulmonary hypertension may be accompanied by a palpable pulmonary artery segment in the second left interspace and by a palpable pulmonic component of the second sound (P_2). Prominent third or fourth heart sounds can often be palpated as well as heard.

Thus, with the data gleaned from physical appearance, the venous and arterial pulse characteristics, and cardiac motion properties, the experienced clinician is armed with substantial information about cardiac anatomy and physiology before using the stethoscope.

AUSCULTATION. Satisfactory cardiac auscultation requires a stethoscope that fits the ears snugly but comfortably and has the shortest tubing consistent with convenient use. The examination should be carried out in a quiet area, which sometimes requires moving the patient to a more suitable place when ambient noise levels are excessive. A systematic approach, as in all facets of physical examination, is important. Apart from the most obvious and dramatic auscultatory events, one generally hears only what one listens for. Beginning at the apex, the timing and nature of the first and second heart sounds are determined. Separable components of these events should be carefully noted. If the first sound has more that one component, S_4, asynchronous closure of mitral and tricuspid valves, and ejection clicks must be distinguished. Higher frequency transient systolic and diastolic sounds are listed in Table 30–2 and should be listened for explicitly. Murmurs should be identified and characterized, using the diaphragm to distinguish high-frequency events and the bell for lower frequency sounds. The examination should include listening with the patient sitting and leaning forward, supine, and in the left lateral decubitus position. Variations during the respiratory cycle are often important. Position may have a particularly marked effect on the character and loudness of pericardial friction rubs. Standing, exercising, isometric handgrip, and the Valsalva maneuver are important in specific circumstances, as outlined in the chapters that follow.

The plethora of sophisticated laboratory examinations now available should refine, rather than render obsolete, physical diagnostic skills. Every opportunity should be taken to review physical findings with the additional insights provided by noninvasive and invasive laboratory studies.

Laboratory Studies

Laboratory studies of patients with cardiovascular disease run the gamut from routine examinations (chest radiograph, ECG) that should be performed on virtually every patient being evaluated to highly sophisticated techniques that would be appropriate for specific individual subsets of patients. Remarkable progress in noninvasive techniques now permits adequate evaluation of many patients without need for cardiac catheterization. Nevertheless, catheterization and angiography are essential components of the cardiovascular workup in most patients with advanced valvular or coronary artery disease.

ELECTROCARDIOGRAM. The standard 12-lead ECG remains a cornerstone of the clinical cardiologic evaluation. Although vectorcardiography and other more sophisticated approaches have their proponents, the standard 12-lead ECG remains a highly cost-effective screening test. It is reviewed in detail in Ch. 33.2. Detailed clinicopathologic correlations provide a wealth of background information. Important applications are in assessment of cardiac arrhythmias, in which analysis of the P wave and the QRS complex, and their temporal relation to each other, forms the basis for the definition and clinical diagnosis of rhythm disturbances. Existence and location of myocardial ischemia and infarction represent other important components of the information inherent in the ECG. Right and left ventricular hypertrophy patterns, as well as right and left atrial abnormalities, are well described. Characteristic electrocardiographic findings are frequently important in the assessment of congenital heart disease.

The 12-lead electrocardiogram augmented with a standard exercise protocol is important in the assessment of ischemic heart disease (see Ch. 41). Both establishment of coronary artery obstructive disease and useful prognostic information are available from this study. Risk stratification in patients who have had myocardial infarctions depends heavily on the exercise ECG. The predictive accuracy of the exercise ECG examination for coronary artery disease in specific patient subsets is well defined. It is important not only to classify ST-segment depression but also to assess duration of exercise, maximum heart rate achieved, blood pressure response, time of onset of ST-segment depression, and time of resolution. A decrease in blood pressure during exercise correlates closely with advanced three-vessel or left main coronary artery obstructive disease. As in all such examinations, the diagnostic and predictive accuracy depends on the population of patients studied, and false-positive exercise ECG results are relatively commonly encountered in women, especially from populations with a low predicted incidence of obstructive coronary artery disease.

Assessing symptoms of palpitations, dizziness, and syncope now rests heavily on the 24-hour (Holter) ECG. This approach is essential for evaluating cardiac arrhythmias and response to antiarrhythmic drug regimens. Recent technical advances permit the assessment of transient ST-segment and T-wave changes reflecting myocardial ischemia, findings of particular value in patients with variable threshold or "silent" ischemia.

CHEST RADIOGRAPHY. Posteroanterior and lateral views are a component of virtually every cardiovascular evaluation. Important findings are reviewed in Ch. 33.1. Chest radiography always supplements, rather than replaces, physical examination because the two approaches yield complementary information. Echocardiography yields more accurate and specific information regarding individual chamber sizes. Evidence of calcification of cardiac structures should be sought on the chest radiograph, although fluoroscopic examination and echocardiography both tend to be more sensitive for this purpose.

ECHOCARDIOGRAPHY. This noninvasive technique uses high-frequency sound waves that reflect from cardiac structures, permitting the imaging of cardiac anatomy and motion. The technique is considered in detail in Ch. 33.3. Two-dimensional echocardiography has largely replaced the M-mode display, although the latter provides superior quantitative details regarding wall thickness and chamber dimensions. This examination is now standard in the assessment of ventricular function (including regional wall motion) and valvular abnormalities.

The Doppler method is the standard technique for assessing intracardiac blood flow, shunts, and valvular stenosis and regurgitation. In selected patients, echocardiographic information, together with full clinical assessment, permits valvular surgery without prior cardiac catheterization. Echocardiography is diagnostic in cases of left atrial myxoma, mitral valve prolapse, and hypertrophic cardiomyopathy. It is frequently useful for visualization of vegetations on heart valves in patients with infective endocarditis. Pericardial fluid and tamponade are routinely assessed by echocardiography, which is also useful in guiding pericardiocentesis.

Transesophageal echocardiography gives high-resolution images of the heart and proximal great vessels and is particularly useful for evaluating suspected aortic dissection.

TABLE 30–2. SYSTOLIC AND DIASTOLIC SOUNDS

Systolic
 Early
  Ejection sounds (aortic, pulmonary)
  Systolic ejection clicks (mitral apparatus)
  Opening click of aortic valve mechanical prosthesis
 Mid to late
  Mitral valve clicks (prolapse)
Diastolic
 Early
  Opening snaps
  Early third sound of pericardial constriction or mitral regurgitation
  Opening click of mitral valve mechanical prosthesis
  "Tumor plop" of atrial myxoma
 Mid
  Third heart sound or gallop (S_3)
  Summation gallop ($S_3 + S_4$)
  Pericardial knock
 Late (presystolic)
  Fourth heart sound (S_4)

High-resolution B-mode ultrasonography with color Doppler imaging is of substantial value in the noninvasive diagnosis of both peripheral arterial (including carotid) and venous disease.

RADIONUCLIDE STUDIES. These tests involve injection of radioisotopes into the circulation with detection by special instrumentation. One of the most useful of these techniques is radionuclide ventriculography, also referred to as gated blood pool scanning. Technetium 99m (^{99m}Tc) bound to red blood cells stays in the blood pool and permits imaging of the size and contractile function of cardiac chambers. Special applications include detection of intracardiac shunts by "first pass" methods. Most commonly, the technique is used to assess left and right ventricular function by measuring end-systolic and end-diastolic dimensions, permitting evaluation of regional wall motion and the derivation of values for right and left ventricular ejection fractions.

Scanning with radioactive thallium (^{201}Tl) or ^{99m}Tc sestamibi permits assessment of myocardial perfusion. The radioisotope is injected at maximum exercise or pharmacologically induced stress and localizes in cardiac muscle as a function of coronary flow; areas of diminished myocardial perfusion are visualized as "cold" spots on the myocardial image. Viable but ischemic myocardium subsequently fills in with more homogeneous radionuclide distribution, whereas previous infarction produces a persistent cold spot. Viability of chronically ischemic hypocontractile myocardium is usefully assessed by ^{201}Tl reinjection protocols.

Scanning with ^{99m}Tc pyrophosphate or radiolabeled antimyosin antibody can be used to visualize areas of myocardial necrosis and is occasionally useful in evaluating patients with suspected myocardial infarction, transplant rejection, or myocarditis when other studies are equivocal.

CLINICAL APPLICATION. The safety of noninvasive techniques tempts the clinician to overutilize them, because no physical harm is likely to result and some incremental information is often obtained. Cost-effectiveness considerations must be kept in mind, however, and the use of these tests must be orchestrated so that the essential clinical decisions can be made without unnecessary cost and inconvenience to the patient. Some elements of noninvasive test information are superfluous if the patient is destined to undergo complete evaluation by cardiac catheterization and angiography. Newer noninvasive techniques including fast computed tomographic (CT) scanning and magnetic resonance imaging (MRI) need to be incorporated into cost-effective diagnostic strategies.

CARDIAC CATHETERIZATION. This invasive approach provides information on intracardiac and vascular pressures and flows. Gradients across stenotic valves and great vessels can be measured and systemic and pulmonary blood flows quantified. Contrast agents can be injected selectively to define the anatomy of cardiac chambers, coronary vessels, and pulmonary and peripheral vessels. The technique of cardiac catheterization and angiography is considered in detail in Ch. 33.6. This diagnostic approach is usually employed when a cardiac surgical or catheter-based interventional procedure is under consideration.

Other applications of cardiac catheterization include electrophysiologic studies with pacing and mapping procedures to evoke and localize the source of cardiac rhythm disturbances. Endomyocardial biopsy is a standard technique for assessing transplant rejection, unexplained cardiomyopathy, suspected myocarditis, suspected infiltrative diseases such as cardiac amyloidosis, or doxorubicin cardiotoxicity.

Cardiac catheterization procedures form the basis for therapeutic interventions, including percutaneous transluminal coronary angioplasty, or ablative procedures, such as those for managing selected patients with Wolff-Parkinson-White syndrome or other tachyarrhythmias (see Ch. 35).

Although cardiac catheterization involves substantial expense and a small but finite risk of morbidity and mortality, this approach remains indispensable for assessing a wide array of cardiac problems that remain unsolved after complete noninvasive assessment. A frequent problem is the adult patient with a chest pain syndrome consistent with angina pectoris but with a negative or equivocal exercise ECG. Such patients may be severely disabled by these symptoms and attendant anxiety. Even though coronary artery surgery may not loom as a likely therapeutic approach, coronary arteriography can be of substantial value, especially when normal coronary anatomy is found, directing the diagnostic evaluation in more productive directions and restoring a previously incapacitated patient to full activity.

TABLE 30-3. A COMPARISON OF THREE METHODS OF ASSESSING CARDIOVASCULAR DISABILITY

Class	New York Heart Association Functional Classification	Canadian Cardiovascular Society Functional Classification	Specific Activity Scale
I	Patients with cardiac disease but without resulting limitations of physical activity. Ordinary physical activity does not cause undue fatigue, palpitation, dyspnea, or anginal pain.	Ordinary physical activity, such as walking and climbing stairs, does not cause angina. Angina with strenuous or rapid or prolonged exertion at work or recreation.	Patients can perform to completion any activity requiring ≥ 7 metabolic equivalents, e.g., can carry 24 lb up eight steps; carry objects that weigh 80 lb; do outdoor work (shovel snow, spade soil); do recreational activities (skiing, basketball, squash, handball, jog/walk 5 mph).
II	Patients with cardiac disease resulting in slight limitation of physical activity. They are comfortable at rest. Ordinary physical activity results in fatigue, palpitation, dyspnea, or anginal pain.	Slight limitation of ordinary activity. Walking or climbing stairs rapidly, walking uphill, walking or stair climbing after meals, in cold, in wind, or when under emotional stress, or only during the few hours after awakening. Walking more than two blocks on the level and climbing more than one flight of ordinary stairs at a normal pace and in normal conditions.	Patient can perform to completion any activity requiring ≥ 5 metabolic equivalents but cannot and does not perform to completion activities requiring ≥ 7 metabolic equivalents, e.g., have sexual intercourse without stopping, garden, rake, weed, roller skate, dance fox trot, walk at 4 mph on level ground.
III	Patients with cardiac disease resulting in marked limitation of physical activity. They are comfortable at rest. Less than ordinary physical activity causes fatigue, palpitation, dyspnea, or anginal pain.	Marked limitation of ordinary physical activity. Walking one to two blocks on the level and climbing more than one flight in normal conditions.	Patient can perform to completion any activity requiring ≥ 2 metabolic equivalents but cannot and does not perform to completion any activities requiring ≥ 5 metabolic equivalents, e.g., shower without stopping, strip and make bed, clean windows, walk 2.5 mph, bowl, play golf, dress without stopping.
IV	Patient with cardiac disease resulting in inability to carry on any physical activity without discomfort. Symptoms of cardiac insufficiency or of the anginal syndrome may be present even at rest. If any physical activity is undertaken, discomfort is increased.	Inability to carry on any physical activity without discomfort—anginal syndrome *may be* present at rest.	Patient cannot or does not perform to completion activities requiring ≥ 2 metabolic equivalents. *Cannot* carry out activities listed above (Specific Activity Scale, Class III).

From Goldman, L., et al.: Comparative reproducibility and validity of systems for assessing cardiovascular functional class: Advantages of a new specific activity scale. Circulation 64:1227, 1981. Reproduced by permission of the American Heart Association, Inc.

ELEMENTS OF A COMPLETE CARDIOVASCULAR DIAGNOSIS

Coordinated use of the history, physical examination, and laboratory studies permits a full diagnosis to be established in nearly all patients, including the following five elements:

1. Etiology of the cardiovascular problem
2. Anatomic abnormalities, including quantification to the extent possible
3. Physiologic status, including pressures, flows, and relevant gradients
4. Functional capacity (Table 30–3)
5. Prognosis

Diagnostic Strategies

The most appropriate approach to a patient with suspected cardiovascular disease depends on the age and clinical presentation of the patient. A systolic ejection murmur at the base in a healthy teenager with an otherwise normal clinical evaluation, including ECG and chest radiograph, should ordinarily constitute adequate grounds for reassurance and avoidance of more elaborate studies. In an elderly patient with a systolic ejection murmur at the base, slow-rising carotid arterial pulses, and symptoms suggesting possible aortic stenosis, however, the chest radiograph, ECG, and echocardiogram with Doppler study are necessary, at a minimum, to determine whether further and more aggressive evaluation is warranted.

Because prevention is a highly desirable goal in cardiovascular medicine, certain diagnostic tests may be warranted in individual patients even in the absence of specific symptoms. In addition to careful history and physical examination, serum cholesterol measurements are appropriate in most patients, especially those with a family history of coronary artery disease, to assess risk and to guide therapeutic intervention. Exercise electrocardiography in sedentary, middle-aged individuals who are contemplating an exercise program remains controversial; many physicians would advocate this procedure, especially if the patient has risk factors for coronary artery disease.

There is no simple formula for defining the database that is adequate for clearing patients for noncardiac surgery. A simple, informal stress test of walking up one or more flights of stairs to observe the presence or absence of dyspnea or chest discomfort often obviates the need for more expensive and elaborate formal exercise testing. When extensive procedures such as peripheral vascular surgery or abdominal aortic aneurysm resection are contemplated in older patients with known or suspected coronary artery disease, aggressive diagnostic workup, sometimes including cardiac catheterization and coronary arteriography, may be necessary because of limitations imposed by vascular disease on exercise electrocardiography or other approaches to assessment of cardiac reserve requiring exercise stress.

Perloff JK: Physical Examination of the Heart and Circulation. 2nd ed. Philadelphia, WB Saunders, 1990. *A pocket-sized compendium of up-to-date information, well illustrated and referenced.*

31 EPIDEMIOLOGY OF CARDIOVASCULAR DISEASES
William T. Friedewald

COMPONENTS OF CARDIOVASCULAR DISEASE

Cardiovascular disease is a general diagnostic category consisting of several separate diseases. Coronary heart disease and cerebrovascular disease continue to be the major components of cardiovascular disease, with 478,530 dying of coronary heart disease and 144,070 dying of cerebrovascular disease in 1991. Another component, rheumatic heart disease, has had a dramatic 92% decline over the last 40 years in the age-adjusted death rate (Table 31–1). Al-

though 1.5 million people still have this disease, with slightly more than 6000 deaths in 1990, it has become a minor contributor to the overall cardiovascular disease problem.

CARDIOVASCULAR DISEASE MORTALITY

These diseases have not always been the major health problem of the United States. In 1900 the five leading causes of death were (1) pneumonia and influenza combined, (2) tuberculosis, (3) diarrhea, enteritis, and ulceration of the intestines, (4) diseases of the heart, and (5) intracranial lesions of vascular origin. These categories all had rates greater than 100 per 100,000 population. By 1940, only two disease categories still had rates >100 per 100,000: diseases of the heart and cancer and other malignant tumors. The infectious diseases had, to a large extent, been controlled, and their mortality rates have continued to fall. The "epidemic" of cardiovascular disease, especially coronary heart disease, had begun. By 1963, the mortality rate from coronary heart disease reached a peak; there has been a progressive and steady decline since then (Fig. 31–1). Despite the continued magnitude of the coronary heart disease problem, the focus recently has been on this dramatic reversal. Not only is the percentage of decline large (48% from 1950 to 1991), but also the impact on the total number of deaths in the United States is large and has led to an increase in life expectancy. To illustrate, if the rate of coronary heart disease mortality had not changed from its peak in 1963, in the year 1991 alone, an additional 518,000 Americans would have died from this cause.

Data from other countries during the same period offer a perspective on understanding the U.S. rates. The multinational data in Figure 31–2 are for coronary heart disease death rates age adjusted over the four 10-year age groups for men aged 35 to 74. During the period 1970 to 1988, among the 31 countries compared, the United States had the largest decrease in its coronary heart disease mortality rate and moved from third to sixteenth in rank. During this period, four other countries (Australia, Canada, Japan, and Israel) also had significant decreases, whereas several others, primarily the Eastern European countries, had significant increases. The largest absolute change was an increase of 85% for Romania. Although data for China and the USSR are not available for 1970, the data for 1988 rank China as having the second lowest rate and the USSR as having the third highest rate among the 33 countries reporting in 1988. The changes in coronary heart disease death rates for women from the same 33 countries are remarkably similar to those reported for men. The major difference is that the women uniformly have much lower rates than do the men in the same country. Although the large absolute difference in rates—especially for men by country in any given year—suggests that genetic differences among the populations account for this range, the large changes within a country over time demonstrate that regardless of genetic factors, the disease process can be significantly modified. Identifying the factors specifically responsible for these changes has proved to be difficult. Although the relative contributions of prevention efforts versus improved treatment modalities or improved general health measures have not been distinguishable, most likely all have contributed, with prevention efforts being the most significant.

ATHEROSCLEROSIS AND CARDIOVASCULAR DISEASE

The major pathologic process leading to disease of the heart and blood vessels is atherosclerosis, with hypertension either a contributing or a primary problem. Atherosclerosis in its most malignant and rare form begins in early childhood and becomes rapidly manifest as clinical coronary heart disease or sudden death in adolescence. The more common and highly prevalent form begins to develop in adolescence and slowly progresses over several decades, gradually occluding the arterial lumen and eventually manifesting clinically as a stroke, angina pectoris, claudication, myocardial infarction (MI), or, most devastatingly, sudden death. Although many factors may lead to an acute clinical event, such as arterial spasm, acute thrombosis, embolism, or plaque hemorrhage, the underlying problem is predominantly atherosclerosis.

Laboratory and clinical research efforts continue to search for the underlying causes of atherosclerosis, examining factors that may initiate the process as well as those that may cause the milder, highly prevalent forms of the disease (i.e., fatty streaks on the arterial surface) to progress in many individuals to the more serious, complicated, and obstructing form of the disease. Other research efforts concentrate on the later, preclinical stages of the process,

TABLE 31-1. AGE-ADJUSTED DEATH RATES* FOR MAJOR CARDIOVASCULAR DISEASES AND ALL OTHER CAUSES OF DEATH COMBINED IN THE UNITED STATES, 1905 TO 1991

			Cardiovascular Diseases			
Year	All Causes	All Causes Except Cardiovascular Diseases	*Total*	*Coronary Heart Disease*	*Cerebrovascular Disease*	*Rheumatic Heart Disease*
1905	1673.5	1315.9	357.6	NA	134.4	NA
1915	1443.4	1072.6	370.8	NA	123.3	NA
1925	1299.9	920.5	379.4	NA	114.2	NA
1935	1165.8	777.9	387.9	NA	94.4	NA
1945	947.4	556.9	390.5	NA	85.4	18.4
1955	764.6	368.5	396.1	200.0	83.0	11.2
1960	760.9	367.4	393.5	214.6	79.7	9.6
1965	739.0	364.8	374.2	215.8	72.7	7.4
1970	714.3	368.0	346.3	200.4†	66.3	6.3
1975	630.4	337.0	293.4	170.1†	53.7	4.8
1980	585.8	328.3	257.5	149.8	40.8	2.6
1985	546.1	320.8	225.3	125.5	32.3	1.9
1990	520.2	331.5	188.7	102.6	27.7	1.5
1991	507.9	324.4	183.5	97.0	26.5	1.4

* Rate per 100,000 population age adjusted to the United States population, 1940.
† Comparability ratio applied to convert rate to level comparable to rates for 1980 and onward.
NA = Not available.

searching for more quantitative diagnostic techniques. Meanwhile, epidemiologic research efforts continue to make major contributions to both prevention and treatment approaches.

RESEARCH IN CARDIOVASCULAR DISEASE

The research approach used in several large observational studies of cardiovascular disease is exemplified by the Framingham Heart Study, begun in 1948. A sample (5209 men and women aged 30 to 62) of the total population agreed to be part of this study, undergoing thorough examinations every 2 years, with intense follow-up for the development of disease. This population has remained under close scrutiny continuously since originally recruited. Similar studies have been performed in other groups in the United States, as well as around the world—in Tecumseh, Michigan; in Evans County, Georgia; in Albany, New York; and in Chicago, Illinois. The crucial elements of these studies have been (1) the inclusion of relatively large numbers of people to allow for sufficiently powerful subsample analyses; (2) enrollment of participants by methods that would make them reasonably representative of the total population from which they were recruited; (3) careful determination of all the variables (such as height, blood pressure, smoking and dietary histories, and blood chemical determinations) in a standardized, reproducible manner; and (4) meticulous follow-up of all the participants for the development of fatal and nonfatal events recorded and defined in a predetermined and standardized manner.

RISK FACTORS IN CARDIOVASCULAR DISEASE

From these U.S. studies and others worldwide, a consistent list of so-called risk factors for subsequent cardiovascular disease has been identified. These risk factors can be grouped into two broad categories: *unmodifiable* (such as age, male gender, and family history of premature heart disease) and potentially *modifiable* (such as cigarette smoking, high blood pressure, high blood cholesterol level, physical inactivity, diabetes, and the less prognostic factors of overweight and psychological conditions). These factors can be used to identify clearly those who are at especially high risk of developing cardiovascular disease.

CIGARETTE SMOKING. Cigarette smoking is established as a risk factor not only for lung cancer, emphysema, and bronchitis but also for coronary, cerebral, and peripheral vascular disease. This association has been seen in many countries, among widely diverse ethnic groups, in both genders, and across various adult age groups. In addition, the risk increases with increasing pack-years. This increased risk falls rapidly over time when people quit smoking. For coronary heart disease, approximately 40% of the increased risk is removed within 5 years of quitting, although it takes several more years of nonsmoking to achieve the level associated with the nonsmoker.

HIGH BLOOD PRESSURE. High blood pressure is a powerful risk factor for cerebrovascular disease as well as for coronary heart disease and the atherosclerotic process directly. An estimated 50

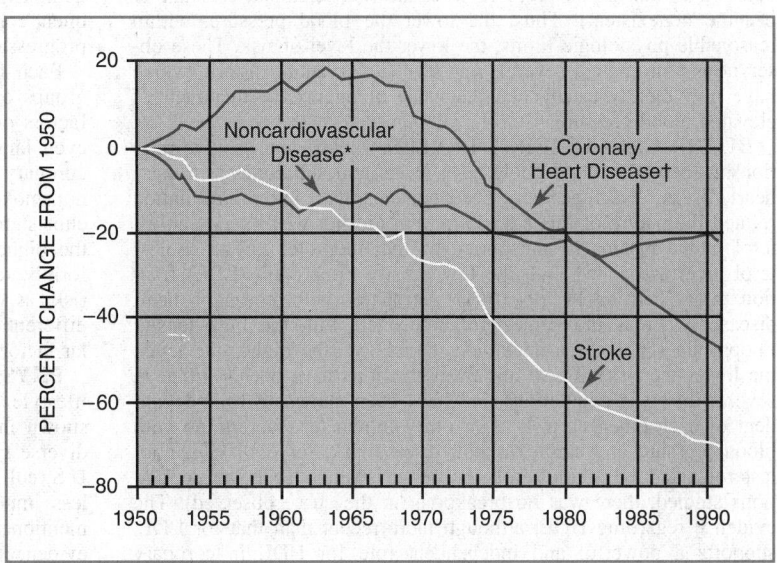

FIGURE 31-1. Percentage of change in age-adjusted death rates since 1950 (United States, 1950 to 1991). *Total mortality minus CVD (excluding congenital). †Comparability ratio applied to rates for years 1968 to 1970. (From Vital Statistics of the United States, National Center for Health Statistics.)

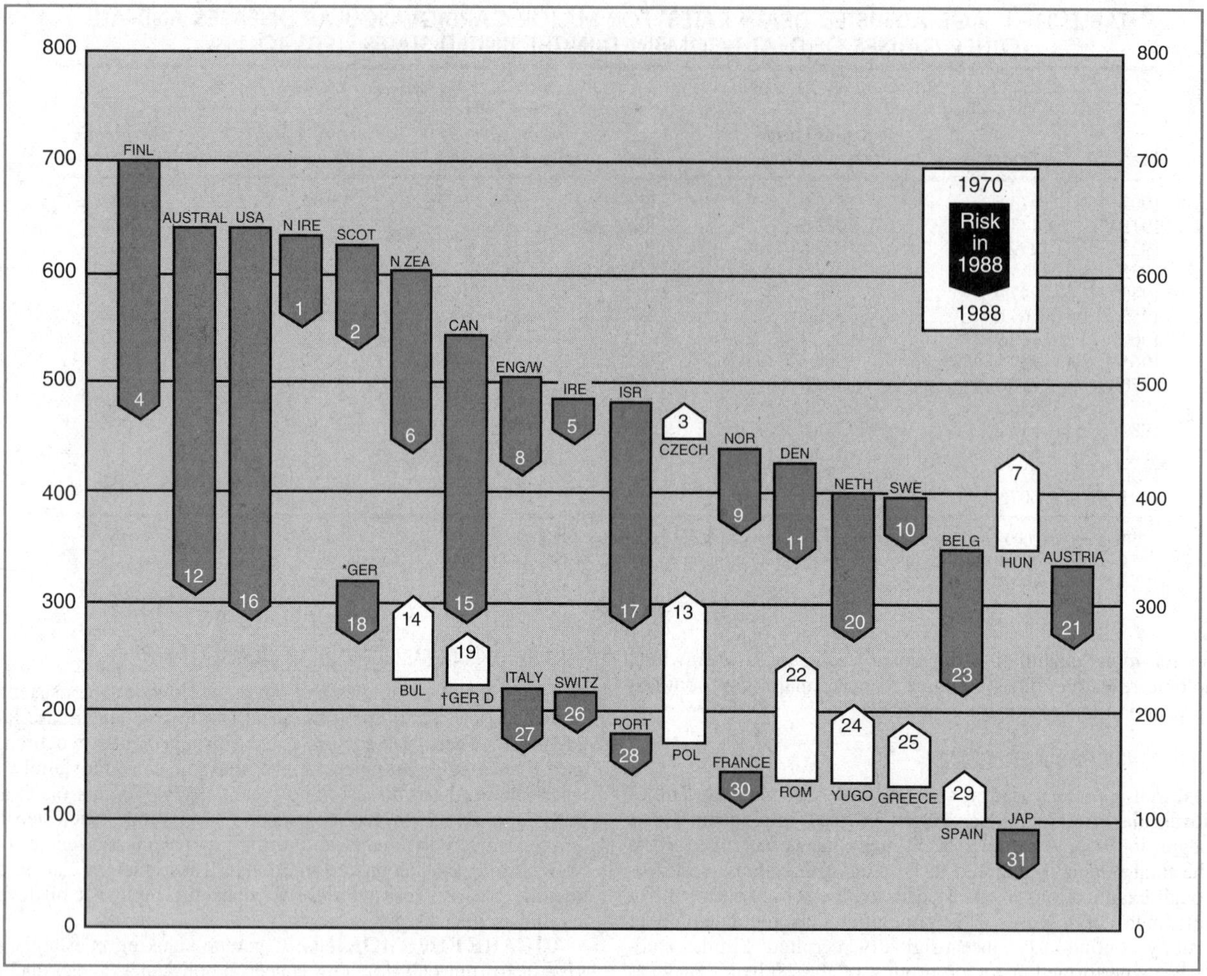

* Formerly West Germany
† Formerly East Germany

FIGURE 31–2. Age-adjusted coronary heart disease mortality rates per 100,000 population for men aged 35 to 74 by country, 1970 to 1988. (From World Health Organization, World Health Statistics Annual.)

million people have high blood pressure, defined as a level ≥ 140 mm Hg systolic or 90 mm Hg diastolic, or as being on a regimen of antihypertensive medication. An important result of the epidemiologic studies was the observation that the relationship between blood pressure and cardiovascular risk was not only a positive one (higher blood pressure results in higher disease rates) but also a smooth one (there was no sharp breakpoint in the curve such that below a certain blood pressure level the risk remained constant or became nonexistent). Thus, the lower the blood pressure, within reasonable physiologic limits, the lower the level of risk. These observations prompted several important intervention trials, which have now clearly established the value of aggressive treatment of elevated blood pressure.

BLOOD CHOLESTEROL LEVELS. A clear and positive relationship between blood cholesterol levels and subsequent coronary heart disease has repeatedly been demonstrated. Later information refined the nature of this association but did not weaken it. Cholesterol in the plasma is transported by the lipoproteins. The cholesterol level associated with the low density lipoprotein (LDL) fraction was seen to be positively correlated with coronary heart disease, whereas the cholesterol associated with the high-density lipoprotein (HDL) was negatively correlated (the higher the level, the lower the risk). These initial observations have been verified in several different populations and have been shown to be independent of each other, as well as of other known risk factors. As with blood pressure and cardiovascular disease risk, for both LDL cholesterol and HDL cholesterol, the curve is smooth (in the populations studied, there was no breakpoint in the curve observed). The evidence regarding HDL, although more recent than that for LDL, supports a powerful and independent role for HDL in coronary

heart disease risk and probably explains a significant portion of the difference in risk between men and women because women have higher average levels of HDL. Information from > 350,000 American men screened for eligibility in the Multiple Risk Factor Intervention Trial (MRFIT) demonstrated that even below levels of total blood cholesterol of 182 mg per deciliter, the risk continues to fall off. Recent intervention studies in hypercholesterolemic men have demonstrated that lowering blood cholesterol levels lowers subsequent coronary heart disease morbidity and mortality and the rate of progression of coronary atherosclerosis.

Each of these three risk factors can be used alone to separate groups of people into those at high or low risk. But as these risk factors occur simultaneously in individuals, the risk range becomes even larger (Fig. 31–3). Based on the MRFIT screenee data, the coronary heart disease mortality rate (1.6 per 1000 screenees) for nonsmokers in the lowest tertile of diastolic blood pressure and cholesterol is nine times lower than the rate (14.6 per 1000) for the highest risk group, using only these three variables. Age uniformly remains one of the most powerful factors at all levels of risk, as does being male, with women realizing a 10- to 20-year differential before attaining the same level of risk as men with similar factors.

PHYSICAL INACTIVITY. An association between a less active lifestyle and increased risk of coronary heart disease has been shown in multiple longitudinal and cross-sectional studies in such diverse groups as London transit workers, U.S. longshoremen, and U.S. college graduates. Traditionally this risk factor was considered less important and certainly less powerful than the three already mentioned. However, recent reviews of the total body of scientific evidence has led to the classification of this risk factor now as one

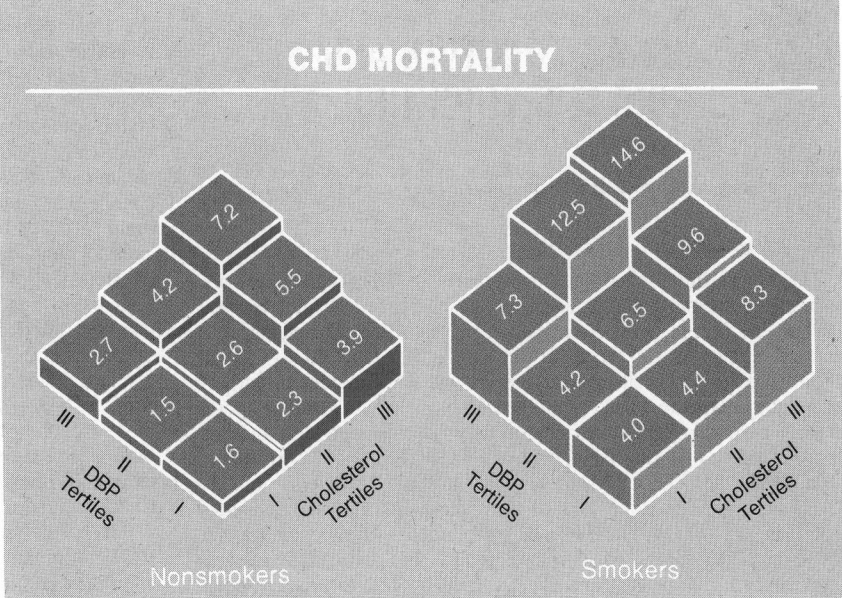

FIGURE 31-3. Age-adjusted CHD mortality rates per 1000 screenees for the Multiple Risk Factor Intervention Trial among smokers and nonsmokers for cholesterol tertiles (I = ≤ 196, II = 197–228, III = ≥ 229) and diastolic blood pressure (DBP) tertiles (I = ≤ 79, II = 80–87, III = ≥ 88).

of the four major modifiable risk factors for coronary heart disease. Consequently there are more consistent recommendations for an active lifestyle and recognition of its importance not only to health but also to disease prevention.

OBESITY. Initial epidemiologic data identified obesity as an important risk factor for coronary heart disease. Subsequent analyses, however, suggested that obesity was not a primary risk factor but rather acted indirectly through elevation of blood pressure and blood cholesterol levels. More recent analyses of the data from the Framingham Heart Study, with longer follow-up of people in the cohort, have once again suggested that obesity is indeed a primary risk factor acting independently of other factors. Clinically, the resolution of this issue of primary versus secondary causation is somewhat irrelevant. Weight reduction should lower the risk of coronary heart disease, whether it acts through a lowered blood pressure and/or cholesterol level or as a lowered risk factor itself.

DIABETES. Diabetes is a powerful and independent risk factor for cardiovascular disease, which remains the major cause of death in diabetic persons. An important remaining issue is whether an elevated blood glucose level is responsible for the observed higher rate of cardiovascular disease and, if it is, whether lowering or, preferably, normalizing the glucose level lowers the risk. Regardless of the answers, for the present the important observation is that diabetic individuals are at higher risk of cardiovascular disease, and thus careful attention should be paid not just to the blood glucose level and its control but also to the other risk factors that may coexist in a given patient and additionally elevate the risk.

RISK FACTORS AFTER MYOCARDIAL INFARCTION. For a patient who survives a MI, the primary risk factors become those related to the infarct itself and the damage to myocardial tissue (see Ch. 41.2). As part of the Coronary Drug Project clinical trial, 2789 post-MI patients were given usual medical care and observed over a period of 5 years. The most powerful factors increasing risk in this group were persistent resting electrocardiographic abnormalities (namely ST segment depression and ventricular conduction defects), use of diuretics, a higher (and therefore more activity restrictive) New York Heart Association functional classification (Table 30–3), and a higher heart rate. Although the traditional risk factors, such as cigarette smoking and elevated blood cholesterol levels and blood pressure, remained prognostic, they were weaker factors overshadowed now by primary damage to the myocardium. In addition, with sudden death as the initial clinical presentation of cardiovascular disease in approximately one quarter of patients, prevention is obviously important. Recent MI research clearly demonstrates the therapeutic value of using thrombolytic agents to minimize the extent of myocardial damage or even to pre-

vent the infarct entirely. Nonetheless, the greatest potential for the continuing decline in cardiovascular disease rates rests with preventing or treating the factors that lead to clinical presentation of disease and the atherosclerotic process.

CHANGE IN RISK FACTORS. Significant changes have occurred nationally in the major modifiable risk factors. In 1965, 51% of white men and 59% of black men aged 18 or older were cigarette smokers. In 1991 those figures had dropped to 27% for white men and 35% for black men. For women the change has been modest, falling from 34% for white women and 32% for black women to 24% for both groups in 1991. In the early 1970's, 36% of people with high blood pressure (defined as 160 mm Hg systolic or 95 mm Hg diastolic or as being on a regimen of antihypertensive medication) were being treated, and only 16% were effectively controlled. By the late 1980's, these figures had increased, with 73% treated and 55% controlled. During this same period, visits to a physician for high blood pressure increased by 89%. Average blood cholesterol levels fell from 220 mg per deciliter (217 in men and 222 in women) in the period between 1960 and 1966 to 205 (in both men and women) from 1988 to 1991. These impressive changes demonstrate that the American public can and will modify risk factors and suggest that additional gains in the prevention of the cardiovascular diseases can be made.

Goldman L, Cook EF: The decline in ischemic heart disease mortality rates: An analysis of the comparative effects of medical interventions and changes in lifestyle. Ann Intern Med 101:825, 1984. *An interesting attempt at quantifying the relative contribution of lifestyle and treatment factors to the decline in coronary heart disease mortality.*

Gordon T, Garcia-Palmieri MR, Kagan A, et al.: Differences in coronary heart disease in Framingham, Honolulu, and Puerto Rico. J Chronic Dis 27:329, 1974. *A valuable comparison of the relationship between risk factors and subsequent coronary heart disease in three geographically and ethnically diverse populations.*

Health, United States, 1992. National Center for Health Statistics, Public Health Service. DHHS Publication No. (PHS) 93-1232. August, 1993. *A frequently updated report presenting national data on morbidity and mortality, health delivery costs, and prevention programs, with detailed tables.*

Joint National Committee on Detection, Evaluation, and Treatment of High Blood Pressure: The Fifth Report of the Joint National Committee on Detection, Evaluation, and Treatment of High Blood Pressure. Arch Intern Med 153:154, 1993. *A succinct and authoritative review of the major clinical issues involving high blood pressure, with a list of key references.*

Second Report of the National Cholesterol Education Program Expert Panel on Detection, Evaluation, and Treatment of High Blood Cholesterol in Adults. Circulation 89:1329, 1994. *A concise review of the major issues involving blood cholesterol and health risks, with a list of key references.*

Surgeon General's Report on Nutrition and Health, 1988. US Department of Health and Human Services, Public Health Service. DHHS (PHS) Publication No. 88-50210, 1988. *A remarkably complete and reasonably concise summary of the relationship between major nutrients and disease.*

World Health Statistics Annual, 1992. Geneva, World Health Organization, 1993. *International vital statistics and population data in tabular form by country.*

32 CARDIAC FUNCTION AND CIRCULATORY CONTROL

John Ross, Jr.

FUNCTIONAL ANATOMY OF THE HEART

The myocardium is composed primarily of a branching network of muscle fibers (cells), connected by specialized boundaries between cells (intercalated discs) which serve to transmit tension and include regions of low electrical impedance (nexus junctions) which permit rapid cell-to-cell transmission of the action potential. An extracellular matrix (primarily collagen fibers) surrounds and supports the myocardial cells, and a rich coronary vascular network supplies approximately one capillary per muscle cell (Fig. 32–1). From the myocardial cell surface (sarcolemma) multiple transverse tubules (T-tubules) provide extensions of the sarcolemma into the cell interior (Fig. 32–1). Within the cell, surrounded by mitochondria, lie the sarcomeres composed of interdigitating thin actin filaments and thick myosin filaments (Fig. 32–1), which interact to produce muscle contraction following electrical activation. Within the cell, serially aligned sarcomeres from bundles, and surrounding each bundle is an intracellular tubular network, the sarcoplasmic reticulum (SR) (Fig. 32–1). The SR contains a high concentration of the protein calsequestrin, which avidly and reversibly binds Ca^{++}. The SR Ca^{++}-ATPase pumps located on the surface of the SR rapidly remove free Ca^{++} from the cell cytoplasm following activation, and a regulatory protein phospholamban lies adjacent to this Ca^{++}-ATPase (see below). Ca^{++} release channels (the ryanodine receptor) are situated on the SR beneath the sarcolemma, particularly along the T-tubules, and as Ca^{++} enters the cell via the sarcolemmal L-type Ca^{++} channels, the release channels signal the SR to release a much larger amount of Ca^{++}, which activates the myofilaments (so called Ca^{++}-generated Ca^{++} release).

The electrical subsystem of the heart includes the sinoatrial (SA) node, comprising special pacemaker cells with continuous phase 4 depolarization, and the atrioventricular (AV) node, which exhibits delayed or decremental conduction, allowing atrial depolarization to precede ventricular depolarization by approximately 140 msec and atrial contraction thereby to serve as a "booster pump" to fill the ventricles. From the AV junction (or node) the electrical impulse rapidly spreads through the specialized His-Purkinje conduction system in approximately 40 msec to reach the ventricles, which contract slightly out of phase (left before right), left ventricular contraction beginning about 50 msec after the onset of the QRS complex.

The nervous subsystem supplying the heart consists of sympathetic and parasympathetic divisions. There is a rich network of sympathetic nerve terminals containing norepinephrine distributed throughout the atria and ventricles, which allows reflex regulation of the contractility of the myocardium via β-adrenergic receptors on the myocardial cells, which also are accessible to circulating catecholamines. Sympathetic nerves also innervate the coronary arteries. The sympathetic nerves also heavily innervate the SA node and AV junction, where increases in sympathetic tone increase the heart rate (enhanced rate of phase 4 depolarization), improve conduction velocity through the AV junction, and enhance synchronicity of the ventricular muscle. Enhanced strength of muscle contraction and increased velocity of both muscle contraction and relaxation accompany the increased heart rate during sympathetic stimulation, as with excitement or exercise. Parasympathetic fibers from the vagus nerves containing acetylcholine provide heavy innervation to the right and left atria, the SA node, and the AV junction, but there are few parasympathetic nerve terminals in the ventricles or the conduction system below the AV junction. Activation of the parasympathetic system has a slowing effect on the SA node (reduced rate of phase 4 polarization) and slows conduction through the AV junction, providing reciprocal neural control with the sympathetic nervous system. The contractility of atrial muscle is depressed by parasympathetic stimulation, but there is minimal effect on the ventricles because of their sparse innervation by vagal fibers.

Unlike skeletal muscle, cardiac muscle can regulate its contractility, or inotropic state. The force of cardiac muscle contraction, as well as its velocity, is normally regulated to a large degree by the amount of free calcium (Ca^{++}) released within the cell when it is electrically activated. Ca^{++} enters the cell when the calcium "gate" is open during phase 2 of the action potential (Fig. 32–2). This provides some of the activating Ca^{++}, but the action potential (and the increasing Ca^{++} itself) trigger much more Ca^{++} release from the SR (Fig. 32–2). Ca^{++} then binds to a subunit of troponin on the actin filament, causing a conformational change that uncovers the active site and allows a tension-generating bond to occur between actin and myosin. More Ca^{++} allows more sites to bind. *Between* contractions, the SR rapidly and actively sequesters Ca^{++} (Fig. 32–2) so that the level at the myofilaments falls below that required for the actin-myosin interaction. Ca^{++} is also extruded more slowly against an electrical and chemical gradient. One important mechanism is a 3:1 sodium for calcium exchange across the sarcolemma by the Na^+/Ca^{++} exchanger (Fig. 32–2), which is driven mainly by the sodium gradient generated by the NaK-ATPase membrane pump. A Ca^{++}-ATPase pump on the sarcolemma (Fig. 32–2) also contributes to Ca^{++} extrusion but is relatively slow and unimportant in beat-to-beat Ca^{++} regulation.

Myocardial contractility is normally increased by catecholamines, which stimulate the β receptors and augment intracellular cyclic adenosine monophosphate (cAMP), which leads to phosphorylation of the calcium channel by cAMP-dependent protein kinase and increased Ca^{++} influx during the action potential. Phospholamban is also phosphorylated by cAMP-dependent protein kinase during β-adrenergic stimulation, as with excitement or exercise, and this phosphorylation results in enhanced SR-Ca^{++} uptake by causing disinhibition of the adjacent SR Ca^{++}-ATPase pump. This effect enhances the rate of ventricular relaxation and also increases Ca^{++} storage in the SR which, in turn, increases Ca^{++} release and enhances contractility during the next activation.

A variety of other mechanisms can stimulate myocardial contractility. Digitalis, by inhibiting membrane NaK-ATPase, increases intracellular sodium, which decreases the sodium gradient, thereby leading to increased intracellular Ca^{++} and enhanced contractility (Fig. 32–2). β-Adrenergic agonist drugs such as dobutamine are sometimes used to treat the acutely failing heart. Some positive inotropic agents (e.g., amrinone and milrinone) act largely by inhibiting phosphodiesterase, leading to increased intracellular cAMP, and new drugs are under study that may increase the sensitivity of the myofilaments to Ca^{++}.

DIASTOLIC PROPERTIES OF THE HEART. A major feature of relaxed cardiac muscle is its intrinsic stiffness while at rest. Skeletal muscle, when isolated from its bony supports, can be overstretched easily, but cardiac muscle at first stretches readily but then, when stretched further, reaches an elastic limit, giving a steep relation between length and resting tension at long muscle lengths. Thus, within the walls of the ventricles, particularly the left ventricle (LV), the extracellular matrix prevents overdistention with sudden changes in the venous return to the heart.

This property of heart muscle results in a nearly exponential relation between cardiac volume and pressure wherein small changes in volume produce large pressure changes as the ventricle is further filled beyond the upper limit of normal for left ventricular end-diastolic pressure (Fig. 32–3). Thus, the slope of this relation or chamber stiffness ($\Delta P/\Delta V$) increases as the ventricle is filled, and compliance ($\Delta V/\Delta P$) falls. The increased thickness and stiffness of the LV compared with the right ventricle (RV) result in a greater filling pressure and a higher upper limit of normal for the LV end-diastolic pressure (12 mm Hg versus 6 mm Hg for the RV) (Table 32–1).

When an abnormal chamber, such as a hypertrophied LV, is compared with a normal chamber at the same cardiac volume, the entire diastolic pressure-volume relationship is shifted upward and steepened (Fig. 32–3), and the abnormal chamber is said to be stiffer or less compliant than normal. Even in chronically dilated hearts (as in the normal heart), it does not appear possible to stretch sarcomere lengths much beyond 2.2 μm, so that the heart never appears to operate on a descending limb of the relation between resting sarcomere length and the active tension developed after muscle stimulation.

A thick, hypertrophied ventricle with decreased compliance in-

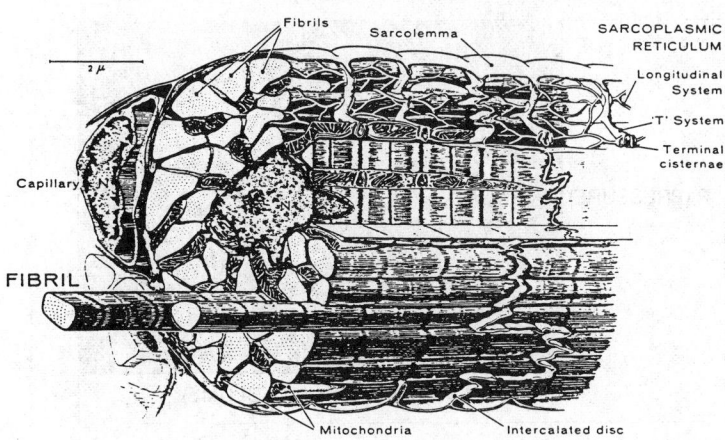

FIGURE 32–1. Portions of two myocardial cells (as reconstructed from electron micrographs) separated by a specialized cell boundary, the intercalated disc. N indicates nuclei of myocardial cell and a capillary. The transverse tubules invaginate from the sarcolemma, and the terminal cisternae of the sarcoplasmic reticulum abut the transverse tubules. (Adapted from Braunwald E, Ross J Jr, Sonnenblick EH: Mechanisms of Contraction of the Normal and Failing Heart. 2nd ed. Boston, Little, Brown & Co, 1976.)

creases resistance to filling and can lead to diastolic cardiac dysfunction even when systolic function is maintained. In this setting atrial dilation and hypertrophy occur in order to maintain the atrial contribution to ventricular filling. The importance of this contribution is apparent in patients with severe hypertrophy caused, for example, by aortic stenosis or hypertrophic obstructive cardiomyopathy. Loss of an appropriately timed atrial contraction often results in marked exacerbation of dyspnea and left heart failure. In these patients, during sinus rhythm the LV end-diastolic pressure is markedly elevated owing to a large A wave, whereas mean diastolic pressure, which is reflected back through the pulmonary veins into the lungs, is maintained at a lower level. When atrial contraction and the A wave "kick" are lost, as in atrial fibrillation, there is an increase in mean left atrial pressure to maintain the same level of end-diastolic pressure and cardiac output.

CARDIAC CONTRACTION AND ITS REGULATION

DETERMINANTS OF CARDIAC PERFORMANCE. There are four major determinants of the performance of both ventricles. These factors are interrelated but considered separately for convenience: (1) preload, (2) afterload, (3) contractility, and (4) heart rate.

The Preload. This refers to the loading condition on the heart at the end of diastole, which is primarily set by the venous return to the heart. In isolated heart muscle, it is defined as the force stretching the resting muscle to a given length prior to contraction. In the intact heart, it is less easily defined. Estimates of preload include measurements of the ventricular end-diastolic volume or the end-diastolic pressure (although the two are not linearly related, Fig. 32–3), and in acutely ill patients, it may be convenient to measure the ventricular "filling pressure" (the mean right or left atrial pressure, or the pulmonary artery wedge pressure) as an index of the preload. Within limits, as the preload increases, there is an increase in cardiac performance manifested by increased systolic pressure or increased volume of blood ejected. This represents the ascending limb of the familiar Frank-Starling relationship.

This overall relationship is often referred to as a ventricular function curve (Fig. 32–4). Some measure of cardiac performance, such as the stroke volume or stroke work (stroke volume × arterial pressure), is plotted as a function of some measure of the preload, such as the filling pressure or the end-diastolic pressure. The concept of the ventricular function curve is important because it allows an objective assessment of the contractility of the ventricles. For example, the normal ventricle has a steep function curve, relatively small changes in end-diastolic pressure producing large changes in performance, whereas the failing ventricle has a downwardly displaced and flattened curve (Fig. 32–4). Such curves can permit a comparison between subjective signs or symptoms and objective measurements. Because the failing LV operates near the peak of its ventricular function curve, the combination of a high filling pressure and low cardiac output (Fig. 32–4, point D) explains the clinical picture of dyspnea and fatigue (see Ch. 34).

An important distinction must be made between the right atrial

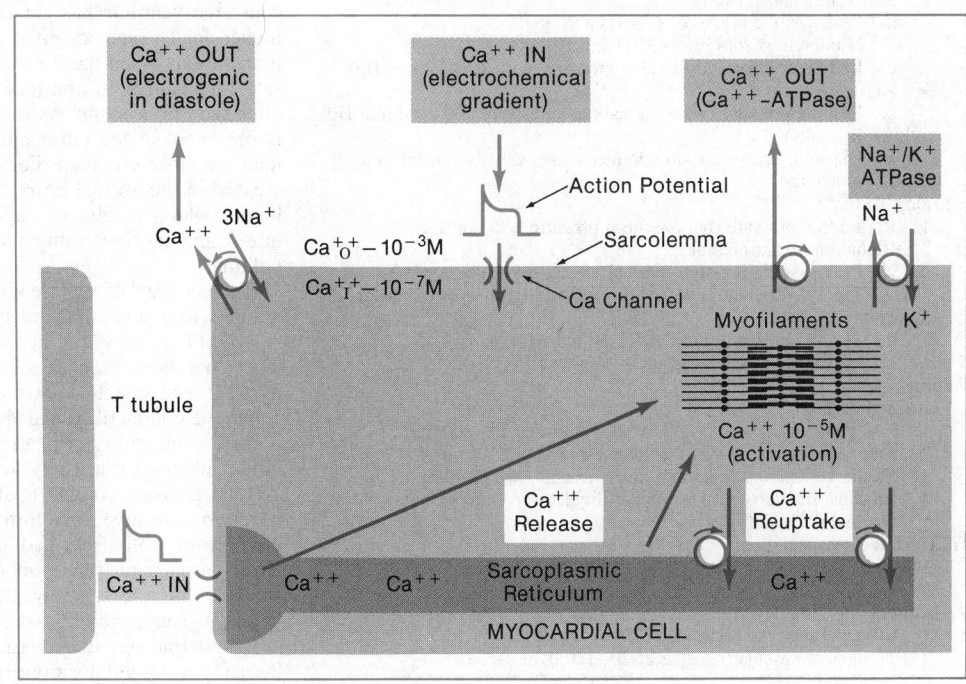

FIGURE 32–2. Movements of Ca^{++} during the cardiac cycle in a myocardial cell. Inward movement occurs across the sarcolemma during the action potential and also triggers Ca^{++} release from the sarcoplasmic reticulum. Free Ca^{++} is rapidly removed from the cytoplasm by the sarcoplasmic reticulum and extrusion across the sarcolemma also occurs by Na^{+}-Ca^{++} exchange and by a slower Ca^{++} pump (Ca^{++}-ATPase). (Adapted from West JB [ed.]: Best and Taylor's Physiological Basis of Medical Practice. 12th ed. Baltimore, Williams & Wilkins, 1991, p 204.)

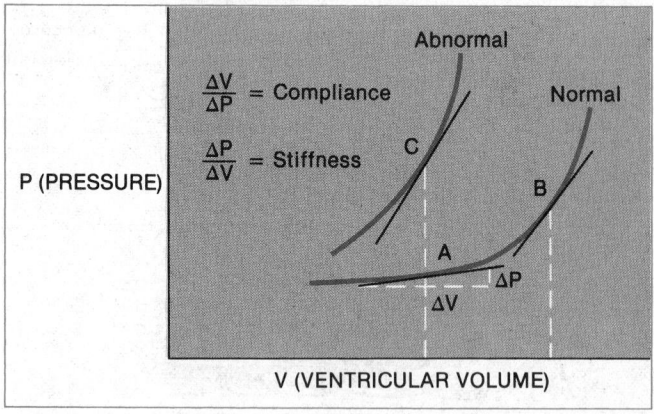

FIGURE 32–3. Diastolic pressure-volume curves of left ventricle under normal conditions and in the presence of severe ventricular hypertrophy (abnormal). Note the nearly exponential shape of the curves. The stiffness at any point on the normal curve ($\Delta P/\Delta V$) is shown by a tangent. Notice that ventricular stiffness increases (tangent A to tangent B) with ventricular filling to a larger ventricular volume. The stiffness of two ventricular chambers can be compared at a common volume, and comparison of the stiffness of the normal with that of the abnormal (hypertrophied) ventricle shows that the latter is markedly increased (tangent A versus tangent C). Compliance is the inverse slope ($\Delta V/\Delta P$) of the curve, and therefore the abnormal ventricle has a markedly reduced compliance. (Adapted from West JB [ed.]: Best and Taylor's Physiological Basis of Medical Practice. 12th ed. Baltimore, Williams & Wilkins, 1992, p 225.)

pressure, which represents the filling pressure of the RV and can be estimated from the jugular veins, and the left atrial pressure, which is the filling pressure of the LV. The mean left atrial pressure can be assessed from the mean pulmonary artery (or "capillary") wedge pressure, often measured by a flow-directed balloon catheter. In manipulating the volume status of the acutely ill patient, except in cases of isolated RV failure, it is preferable to measure the LV

TABLE 32–1. PRESSURES AND VOLUMES IN THE NORMAL HEART

Pressures
Left sided
 1. Left atrial pressure (normal mean pressure ≤ 12 mm Hg)
 2. Left ventricular pressure
  a. Peak systolic pressure (same as aorta)
  b. Maximum dP/dt (1200–3500 mm Hg/sec)
  c. Left ventricular end-diastolic pressure (normal ≤ 12 mm Hg)
 3. Aorta
  a. Systolic pressure (wide normal range, usually 100–150 mm Hg in adults)
  b. Diastolic pressure (wide normal range, usually 60–90 mm Hg in adults)
Right sided
 1. Right atrial pressure (normal mean pressure ≤ 6 mm Hg)
 2. Right ventricular pressure
  a. Peak systolic pressure (normal 15–30 mm Hg)
  b. Right ventricular end-diastolic pressure (normal ≤ 6 mm Hg)
 3. Pulmonary artery
  a. Systolic pressure (normal 15–30 mm Hg)
  b. Diastolic pressure (normal 4–12 mm Hg)
Volumes
Left sided (at rest)
 1. Left ventricular end-diastolic volume (normal 70–100 ml/m²)
 2. Left ventricular end-systolic volume (normal 25–35 ml/m²)
 3. Stroke volume (wide normal range, usually 40–70 ml/m²)
 4. Ejection fraction (stroke volume divided by end-diastolic volume [normal 0.55–0.80])
Time-related measurements
 1. Heart rate (wide normal range, usually 60–100 beats/minute)
 2. Cardiac index (2.5–4.2 liters/min/m²)
Resistances
 1. Systemic vascular resistance (770–1500 dynes sec cm⁻⁵)
 2. Pulmonary vascular resistance (20–120 dynes sec cm⁻⁵)

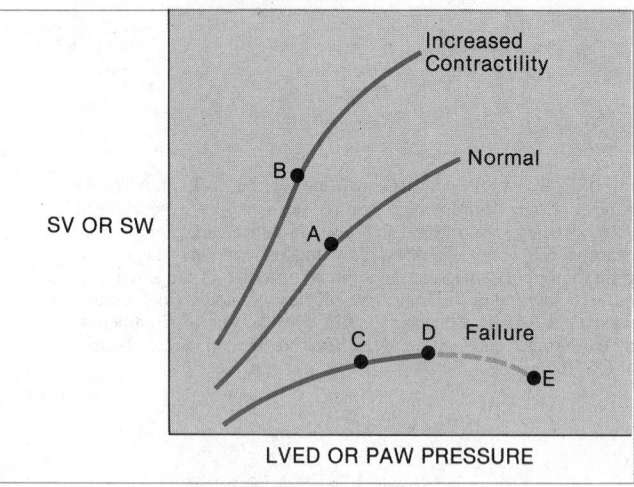

FIGURE 32–4. Left ventricular function curves relating the left ventricular filling pressure to ventricular performance expressed as stroke volume (SV) or stroke work (SW). The filling pressure can be expressed as either the left ventricular end-diastolic (LVED) pressure or the pulmonary artery wedge (PAW) pressure. Curves indicate normal, increased, and depressed ventricular contractility. Points A and B show the effects of a positive inotropic drug, which increases ventricular performance while reducing the filling pressure. See text for further discussion.

filling pressure, because the failing LV usually has a more important role in determining arterial pressure and the forward cardiac output.

The Afterload. Afterload refers to the load against which the ventricle must contract when it ejects blood. In isolated heart muscle, it can be accurately defined as the load (or force) resisting shortening after the muscle is stimulated to contract and lift a load. In the intact heart, afterload is often estimated as the systolic arterial pressure. A better measure of the afterload is the systolic wall stress, which can be related to the systolic pressure, heart size, and wall thickness through the simplified Laplace relation:

$$\sigma = \frac{PR}{2h}$$

in which σ = wall stress or force/cross-sectional area, P = intraventricular pressure, R = radius of chamber (radius of curvature of the wall), and h = wall thickness.

How afterload affects performance is relatively straightforward. As arterial pressure is increased, the stroke volume tends to fall because the ventricle has greater difficulty in ejecting blood against a higher load. Such an effect is seen most clearly in experimental preparations when the preload is held constant (and cannot compensate for changes in afterload), and an inverse relation between the afterload (or systolic ventricular pressure) and the stroke volume is observed. In the intact circulation, changes in preload and afterload are closely related. For example, as the arterial pressure is increased in the normal heart, the LF has greater difficulty in ejecting blood, which results in larger end-systolic and end-diastolic volumes, and the increasing preload then tends to restore the stroke volume.

Another way of representing ventricular function is the pressure-volume loop and the end-systolic pressure-volume relation (Fig. 32–5). (The slope of the latter relation, E_{max} or maximum elastance, has been used as a load-independent measure of contractility.) The end-systolic pressure-volume relation is shifted upward by enhanced contractility and downward with decreased slope by depressed contractility or heart failure (Fig. 32–5). The failing LV exhibits enhanced sensitivity to afterload (decreased slope of the end-systolic pressure-volume relation), and when it reaches the limit of its preload reserve, any further increase in afterload (expressed as pressure or wall stress in Figure 32–5), such as by increased systemic vascular resistance and/or progressive heart failure, causes the stroke volume to fall (Fig. 32–5, beat 2 to beat 3, and Fig. 32–4, point E). This condition has been termed "afterload mismatch."

If systemic vascular resistance and arterial pressure are reduced by using a vasodilator drug in a patient with heart failure, this mis-

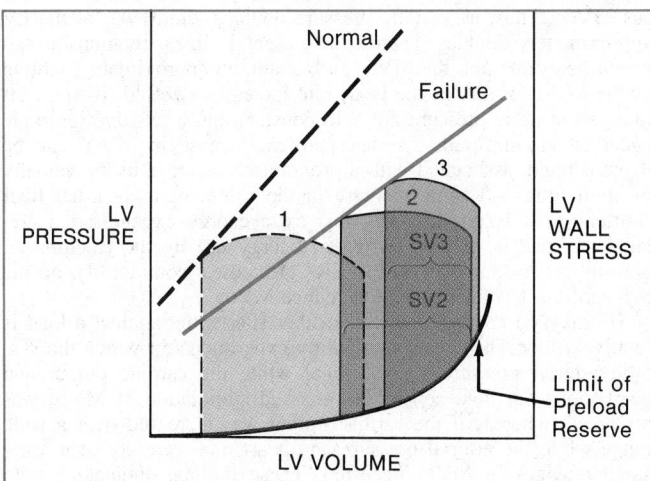

FIGURE 32–5. Left ventricular (LV) diastolic and end-systolic pressure-volume relations together with pressure-volume loops under normal conditions *(dashed lines)* and during heart failure when the linear end-systolic pressure-volume relation is shifted downward and to the right (failure). Beat 2 to beat 3 shows the effect of acutely increasing the LV systolic pressure with a vasoconstrictor when there is little or no preload reserve; the stroke volume drops (SV2 to SV3). In chronic heart failure, the LV may be operating under basal conditions similar to beat 3, and LV wall stress (right-hand ordinate) may be elevated despite a normal LV systolic pressure. Under these circumstances use of a vasodilator drug may relieve this "afterload mismatch" and allow the ventricle to improve the stroke volume by lowering the wall stress (beat 3 to beat 2). (Adapted from West JB [ed.]: Best and Taylor's Physiological Basis of Medical Practice. 12th ed. Baltimore, Williams & Wilkins, 1991, p 310.)

match is improved and the stroke volume and cardiac output increase (Fig. 32–5, beats 3 to 2, and Fig. 32–4, points E to D). Severe hypotension must be avoided because it compromises coronary blood flow and therefore reduces cardiac performance. The principle of afterload reduction has become one of the most important concepts in the therapy of both acute and chronic heart failure.

Contractility. The inotropic state, or contractility, refers to the vigor of contraction of heart muscle and is best defined in isolated heart muscle as an increased velocity and extent of shortening when the loading conditions (preload and afterload) do not change (or in the peak tension of isometric contractions). Contractility is altered under normal conditions primarily by reflex release of norepinephrine from adrenergic nerve terminals in the myocardium as well as by adrenal release of catecholamines during various forms of stress. One measure of increased contractility is a shift upward of the end-systolic pressure-volume relation with increased slope (increased E_{max}) compared with the normal resting relation (Fig. 32–5). Drugs such as digitalis increase contractility, whereas hypoxia, ischemia, acidosis, and certain antiarrhythmic agents and heart muscle damage reduce contractility. In terms of ventricular function curves, drugs that increase contractility shift the curve upward and to the left, increasing stroke volume or stroke work at a given end-diastolic pressure (Fig. 32–4). With depression of contractility, the ventricular function curve shifts down and to the right, with a reduction in stroke volume at a given LV end-diastolic pressure (Fig. 32–4).

Heart Rate. The frequency of contraction is an important determinant of cardiac performance and one of the most important mechanisms available to increase the cardiac output (cardiac output = stroke volume × heart rate), provided that the venous return is increased (see below). During the response to moderate exercise, when the venous return increases, a higher heart rate is mainly responsible for the change in cardiac output because the increase in stroke volume is relatively small.

The inotropic response to increased heart rate is also important. This increase of myocardial contractility to augmented cardiac frequency, called the force-frequency relation, reflects changes in Ca^{++} availability within the myocardial cell. It greatly augments the stimulation of contractility due to activation of β-adrenergic receptors alone consequent to sympathetic stimulation during exercise. Thus, myocardial contraction and relaxation are further en-

hanced by the higher exercise heart rate. This adaptation can be lost in heart failure.

The level of the resting heart rate may be an important indicator of the cardiovascular status of an individual patient. For example, in a patient with acute severe heart failure who has a sinus tachycardia of 140 beats per minute, the marked reduction in stroke volume is compensated for by the tachycardia in order to maintain an acceptable cardiac output. Other factors that can raise the resting heart rate must also be considered, including fever, anemia, thyrotoxicosis, and anxiety.

ASSESSMENT OF CARDIAC PERFORMANCE. Quantitative indices of cardiac performance can be measured in the cardiac catheterization laboratory or in critical care units. For reference, normal pressures, cardiac volumes, cardiac output, and vascular resistance are listed in Table 32–1. Volume measurements are normalized to allow interpatient comparison by dividing by the body surface area (square meters), obtained from a standard table based on height and weight. The maximum value of the first derivative of LV pressure during isovolumetric systole (dP/dt) is sometimes used as a measure of contractility. One very useful index of ventricular function is the *ejection fraction*, which is the stroke volume divided by the end-diastolic volume. A normal ejection fraction averages 0.65 (0.55 or greater), and in severe heart failure the ejection fraction may be reduced to less than 0.20.

As discussed above, shifts in *ventricular function curves* (Fig. 32–4) are often used to demonstrate changes in inotropic state, whereas changes in preload move the ventricle up and down on a *single* curve. Experimentally, they are produced by progressive infusions of fluid, whereas in the clinical setting often only two points on a curve are available, before and after an intervention.

Two ventricular function curves are generally compared at the same level of mean arterial pressure because the stroke volume of the ventricle is changed by altered afterload. Hence, decreased afterload shifts the relation between stroke volume and filling pressure upward, and increased afterload shifts the relation downward. In heart failure, such an effect is sometimes represented as an apparent "descending limb" of function. As discussed earlier, in such a setting, the preload reserve is exhausted and lowering the afterload improves the stroke volume and cardiac performance (Figs. 32–4 and 32–5).

Venous return and *cardiac output curves* can be used to represent cardiocirculatory responses under experimental conditions, and although venous return curves cannot be performed in humans, they allow insight into the highly important role of the venous return. The heart behaves as a demand pump, ejecting whatever blood is returned to it under normal conditions, and only in heart failure or when filling is impaired (as in constrictive pericarditis) does the heart itself become the limiting factor for cardiac output. Therefore, the return of blood to the heart (the venous return), which is regulated by a number of mechanical, neural, and humoral factors, through its influence on preload is a key determinant of cardiac performance under normal conditions.

In A. C. Guyton's analysis, cardiac function is represented by a cardiac output curve that intersects a venous return curve at any given steady-state condition (Fig. 32–6). Noncardiac factors that influence the venous return include the volume of blood in the vascular bed (transfusion shifts the venous return curve upward, whereas bleeding shifts it downward). The position of the venous return curve is also affected by neurohumoral factors, increased sympathetic tone shifting the venous return curve upward and to the right and vice versa; venoconstriction produced by increased sympathetic tone also displaces blood from the peripheral circulation toward the central (cardiopulmonary) circulation, whereas decreased tone to the veins causes pooling of blood in the peripheral circulation. With this framework, changes in *both* cardiac performance and peripheral circulatory regulation (venous return) can be represented as they influence the cardiac output. Positive inotropic interventions, decreased afterload, and other factors shift the cardiac output curve upward, and opposite effects, including heart failure, shift is downward (Fig. 32–6).

The importance of venous return can be illustrated by the response to electrical cardiac pacing to increase the heart rate. Myocardial contractility is increased, but since no significant effects on the peripheral circulation occur, no change in the cardiac output is

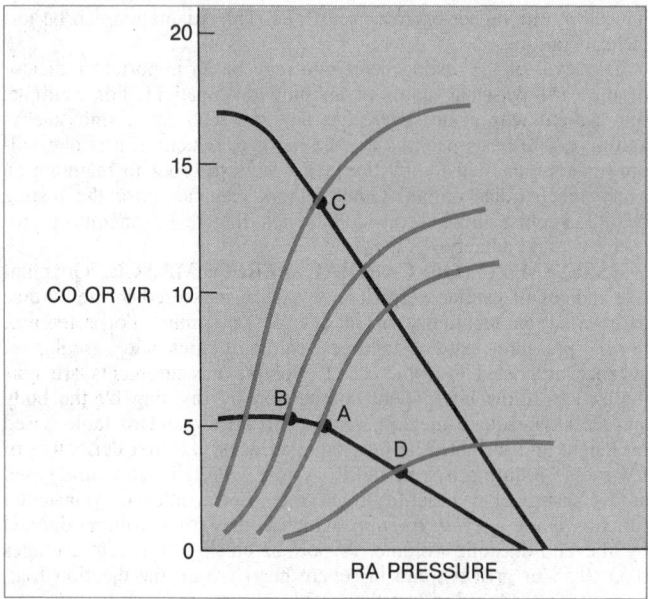

FIGURE 32–6. Relationship between the filling pressure of the heart, expressed as the right atrial (RA) pressure, and either cardiac output (CO) or venous return (VR). Venous return curves are represented as an inverse relation between the CO or VR and the RA pressure; the lower curve represents normal conditions and the upper curve shows the effect of marked sympathetic stimulation during exercise. The series of CO curves shows a positive relation between RA pressure and cardiac function. Any steady-state condition is represented by the intersection of these two curves. Shown are normal conditions (A), electrical pacing of the heart (B), severe exercise (C), and heart failure (D). See text for further discussion.

observed. This response occurs because the normal heart operates near the flat portion of the normal venous return curve (near the point of venous collapse), and therefore even though the cardiac output curve is shifted upward, the venous return curve is unchanged, and there can be no alteration of the cardiac output (Fig. 32–6, point A to B). The response to exercise using this diagram is discussed subsequently under integrated responses.

REGULATION OF MYOCARDIAL OXYGEN CONSUMPTION

The heart is almost entirely supplied with energy from ATP and creatine phosphate produced by aerobic metabolism, and for practical purposes, the total energy expenditure of the normal heart can be equated with its oxygen consumption. The myocardial oxygen consumption (MV_{O_2}) of the left ventricle can be determined using the Fick principle as the product of its coronary blood flow and the arteriovenous oxygen difference, calculated using blood samples from an artery and from the coronary sinus. Because the heart is a continuously active organ, its oxygen consumption is high relative to other organs, and the MV_{O_2} of the normal human LV at rest is approximately 6 to 8 ml per minute per 100 grams.

The determinants of the MV_{O_2} of the heart (most of which is used by the LV) consist of the basal oxygen consumption, which supplies energy for cell maintenance processes including the calcium and sodium pumps, protein synthesis, and so on. The remainder of the oxygen expenditure is controlled by the type of activity that the heart is called upon to perform. The determinants of MV_{O_2} are

1. Basal oxygen requirements
2. Systolic pressure (or wall stress)
3. Heart rate
4. Myocardial contractility (inotropic state)
5. Wall shortening against a load (related to cardiac work)

Systolic pressure, heart rate, and *contractility* are the major determinants of MV_{O_2}, whereas shortening of the wall uses relatively less oxygen. There is a nearly linear relation between systolic pressure developed by the LV and MV_{O_2}, and with the Laplace equation, this relation can also be expressed as systolic wall stress ver-

sus MV_{O_2}. Thus, as systolic pressure doubles, the MV_{O_2} of the LV approximately doubles. There is also a nearly linear relationship between heart rate and the MV_{O_2} and, again, an approximate doubling of the MV_{O_2} occurs as the heart rate increases twofold. If the heart rate and systolic pressure are held constant and a positive inotropic agent is administered, a rather marked increase in MV_{O_2} can be demonstrated, associated with a pronounced increase in the velocity of shortening and some increase in the extent of myocardial fiber shortening. It is possible that this extra energy expenditure is related, at least in part, to increased energy use by the calcium sequestration mechanism of the SR. Decreased contractility of the myocardium has been shown to reduce MV_{O_2}.

The oxygen cost of myocardial fiber shortening against a load is relatively low. This is exemplified by experiments in which the systolic arterial pressure was elevated while the cardiac output and heart rate were held constant. A marked stimulation of MV_{O_2} was produced, whereas if the cardiac output was increased over a wide range while the arterial pressure and heart rate were constant, only small changes in MV_{O_2} occurred. These findings indicate a high oxygen cost of "pressure work" and a relatively low oxygen cost of "volume work." The importance of heart rate and systolic pressure has resulted in the use of simplified indices of MV_{O_2}, such as the heart rate × blood pressure (the "double product"). In clinical studies, this provides a means of estimating the effect of an antianginal drug (such as β-blocker) on cardiac oxygen requirements during exercise.

The fact that myocardial energy expenditure, expressed as MV_{O_2}, is closely linked to mechanical cardiac performance carries important implications in various disease states. For example, in valvular heart disease, chronic mitral regurgitation places a large volume overload on the heart owing to the low impedance backward leak into the left atrium. In this condition, the systolic LV pressure is not elevated, and since the LV is performing extra "volume work," the MV_{O_2} of the LV is not significantly increased. Therefore, in the absence of coronary artery disease, oxygen supply-demand imbalance and angina pectoris are rarely seen in chronic mitral regurgitation. In contrast, in patients with aortic stenosis, the high LV systolic pressures with elevated MV_{O_2} of the entire chamber can lead to reduced coronary vasodilator reserve. Therefore, subendocardial ischemia with angina pectoris is quite common in aortic stenosis, particularly during exercise or when LV failure is beginning to occur, even in the absence of coronary artery disease. Of course, in chronic coronary artery disease, during exercise virtually all of the major determinants of MV_{O_2} are augmented, and in the presence of a stenosed coronary artery with impaired vasodilator reserve, coronary blood flow cannot keep pace with enhanced oxygen demands, and regional myocardial ischemia with angina pectoris occurs (see Ch. 41.1).

REGULATION OF CORONARY BLOOD FLOW

In keeping with the high energy requirements of the normal myocardium, coronary blood flow is relatively high, averaging 60 to 90 ml per minute per 100 grams in the normal human LV when an individual is at rest. Extraction of oxygen by the heart is the highest of any organ, so that little additional oxygen extraction can occur during stress. This means that changes in oxygen demand of the heart are met chiefly by alterations in oxygen supply through changes in coronary blood flow, reflected by a nearly linear positive relation between the MV_{O_2} and the coronary blood flow. Although cardiac metabolism (MV_{O_2}) is the main determinant of coronary blood flow, several additional factors can be of importance.

1. MV_{O_2}
2. Coronary perfusion pressure
3. Systolic compression
4. Endothelial-dependent relaxing factor
5. α-Adrenergic tone to the coronary arteries (or exogenous vasoconstrictors)
6. Exogenous vasodilators.

Because the MV_{O_2} is influenced by each of the major determinants of cardiac performance, coronary blood flow is altered in the appropriate direction. There is evidence that release of the ATP metabolite adenosine, a potent coronary vasodilator, is involved in some of the responses of the coronary blood flow to altered cardiac performance and metabolism, although a number of other stimuli to vasodilation (such as decreased P_{O_2}, decreased pH, and increased K^+ during enhanced metabolic activity) may also be important.

Under normal conditions, the mean coronary perfusion pressure is not a major determinant of coronary blood flow except as it affects the systolic arterial pressure and therefore the MV_{O_2}. On a moment-to-moment basis, the phasic pattern of coronary blood flow to the LV shows a slow fall during distole as the aortic pressure falls, as well as a sharp drop during systole as the squeezing action of the LV wall compresses the intramural vessels and shuts down coronary blood flow, particularly to the subendocardial layers. However, the mean flow has been shown to be independent of the mean coronary perfusion pressure within certain limits, a phenomenon termed "autoregulation." Studies in which the coronary arteries are perfused *separately* from the aorta show that between mean coronary perfusion pressures of about 60 and 150 mm Hg coronary blood flow is maintained constant, provided that the MV_{O_2} of the heart does not change (Fig. 32–7). When the coronary perfusion pressure drops below 60 mm Hg, the coronary bed reaches the limit of autoregulation and tends to become fully dilated; at that point, perfusion pressure becomes the major determinant of coronary blood flow, and flow drops as pressure falls below that value with a relation between pressure and flow typical of a passive blood vessel (Fig. 32–7). Obviously, in coronary artery disease the coronary perfusion pressure can become extremely important because the perfusion pressure beyond an area of stenosis may be relatively low.

Systolic compression of coronary vessels in the inner (subendocardial) LV wall almost entirely shuts off coronary blood flow during systole, but this does not occur in the outer wall (subepicardium). During diastole, flow to the subendocardium becomes slightly higher than in the outer wall, in order to compensate for the loss of flow during systole, a phenomenon that makes the vasodilator reserve in the subendocardium somewhat *less* than in the subepicardium. When the coronary bed becomes maximally dilated, this effect also makes subendocardial coronary blood flow highly dependent upon the time available for diastolic perfusion. For example, if heart rate increases under such circumstances, systolic time per minute is increased at the expense of diastolic time, and coronary flow falls. This can occur in coronary artery disease, when, during exercise, the heart rate increases and coronary blood flow consequentially falls beyond an area of coronary stenosis (decreased oxygen supply), in the face of increased oxygen demands. β-Adrenergic blockade is often used to treat angina pectoris in this setting (Ch. 41.1).

Endothelium-derived relaxing factor (EDRF), which appears to be nitric oxide or a closely related compound, has been established as an important endogenous regulator of coronary circulation (other substances produced by the endothelium, such as endothelin, may operate as endogenous vasoconstrictors). EDRF release is augmented by sheer stress on the endothelium, causing dilation of the coronary arteries whenever coronary blood flow increases, such as with augmented myocardial O_2 demands and vice versa. This flow-mediated dilation is often impaired or lost in atherosclerotic coronary vessels in which the endothelium is absent or damaged. EDRF release is also responsible for the coronary vasodilator properties of several substances, including acetylcholine and bradykinin.

α-Adrenergic constrictor influences on the coronary vascular bed have been demonstrated. Although such an effect is of relatively minor significance under normal conditions, under certain circumstances of reflex activation it can be greatly significant. There is recent evidence that under conditions of exercise-induced ischemia, α-adrenergic coronary vasoconstrictor tone exists and can be reduced by vasodilators or by α-adrenergic blockade.

A variety of substances can relax the smooth muscle of coronary arteries, including nitroglycerin and calcium channel blockers, and these are used to treat angina due to coronary artery spasm, as well as exercise-induced angina pectoris. Certain prostaglandins and agents such as vasopressin and ergonovine are coronary vasoconstrictors, and ergonovine is used as a diagnostic test to evoke coronary spasm in patients with variant angina.

REGULATION OF THE PERIPHERAL CIRCULATION

The heart pumps blood sequentially through the pulmonary and systemic circulations. Throughout the circulation, the small arterioles provide the main site for vascular resistance regulation. There is a wide variability in cardiac output distribution and in oxygen extraction by various organs; for example, the kidneys have a high blood flow (20% of the cardiac output) and a low oxygen extraction, whereas the coronary circulation has a lower flow but a much higher oxygen extraction. The large conduit arteries have a high velocity of blood flow (aorta = 31 cm per second), whereas in the capillaries, the enormous total cross-sectional area results in marked slowing of blood flow (0.05 cm per second), allowing exchange of metabolites. The veins contain 75 to 80% of the total blood volume in the circulation and serve a capacitance function, i.e., as a blood volume reservoir.

Systemic circulation is organized such that the arterial bed serves as a pressure reservoir from which the circulations to the various organs operate in parallel. Thus, each organ takes the blood supply that it requires by regulating its *local* vascular resistance primarily on the basis of metabolic needs (autoregulation, as discussed earlier for the coronary circulation), whereas the *total* peripheral vascular resistance (TPVR) is primarily controlled by cardiovascular reflexes and maintains the pressure in the arteries. Thus, blood pressure = cardiac output $\times$ TPVR and it is protected by the reflexes. For example, during tilting or standing abruptly, venous return and cardiac output fall (venous pooling), but a reflex increase in TPVR prevents a marked drop in the blood pressure.

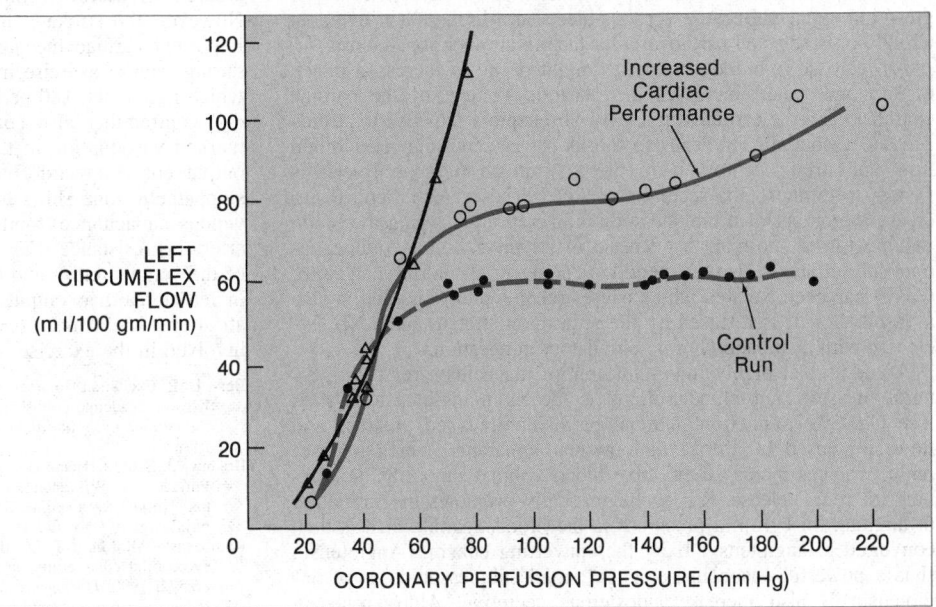

FIGURE 32–7. Autoregulation in the coronary circulation. When the left ventricular work is held constant and the coronary perfusion pressure is altered (coronary artery separately perfused from a controlled pressure source), coronary blood flow remains relatively constant over a wide range (*closed circles*, control run). At a coronary perfusion pressure below approximately 60 mm Hg, the limit of vasodilator reserve is reached, autoregulation is lost, and coronary flow is directly determined by the coronary perfusion pressure. The pressure-flow relation then falls on a curve of maximum vasodilation (passive pressure-flow curve of a distensible blood vessel, *open triangles*). Coronary blood flow is regulated at a higher level when cardiac performance and hence MV_{O_2} are increased (*open circles*, increased cardiac performance). (Adapted from West JB [ed.]; Best and Taylor's Physiological Basis of Medical Practice. 12th ed. Baltimore, Williams & Wilkins, 1991, p 163.)

REFLEX NEURAL CONTROL. The autonomic nervous system and certain neurohumoral factors maintain circulatory homeostasis by regulating heart rate, myocardial contractility, vascular tone in the arterioles and small veins, and the blood volume.

The high-pressure baroreceptors, which sense stretch in the walls of arteries, are located in the carotid sinuses and aortic arch. They increase their afferent impulse traffic when the blood pressure rises, and vice versa, and these nerve impulses affect the cardiovascular regulatory centers in the medulla. For example, as arterial pressure is increased, the enhanced impulse traffic stimulates the vagus to slow the heart rate and simultaneously inhibits the cardioaccelerator center. Simultaneously, the vasoconstrictor center is also inhibited, reducing sympathetic tone to the peripheral arterioles and also lowering venous tone. Thus, the reduced peripheral vascular resistance and venous return, together with the slowed heart rate, lower the increased blood pressure toward its previous level. With a decrease in blood pressure, as with moderate bleeding, opposite effects occur, tending to restore the lowered blood pressure. With a significant drop in blood pressure, reflex release of catecholamines from the adrenal glands also occurs.

Reflex control of the heart and circulation is also under the influence of higher brain centers, as when marked emotional stress activates the sympathetic nervous system. Such central stimulation, as well as reflex activation of the sympathetic nervous system via receptors in the exercising skeletal muscle, produce the marked sympathetic stimulation of exercise. At rest, there appears to be little sympathetic tone affecting heart rate or myocardial contractility, and the heart rate is primarily under the control of parasympathetic influences.

Low-pressure baroreceptors (stretch receptors) are also located in the heart, particularly in the atria and the pulmonary veins, with fewer in the ventricles (see also blood volume regulation). Increased stretch of the atrial receptors can induce tachycardia (the Bainbridge reflex). More marked stretch of these low-pressure receptors produces a depressor reflex — with withdrawal of sympathetic tone and a fall in peripheral vascular resistance — which contributes to high-pressure baroreceptor regulation of the blood pressure. Syncope in some patients with aortic stenosis and high intracardiac pressure may be due to sudden activation of these intracardiac receptors.

REGULATION OF BLOOD VOLUME. The magnitude of blood volume is an important factor affecting cardiovascular function, and it is important in long-term regulation of the blood pressure. Loss of fluid volume occurs primarily through the kidneys, whereas sweating, respiratory, and gastrointestinal losses are less important (except during extreme conditions). Because approximately 20% of the resting cardiac output passes through the kidneys, they provide an ideal location for regulating sodium and water balance. In addition, the hypothalamic osmoreceptors that regulate thirst and antidiuretic hormone (ADH) secretion are of great importance. Because these subjects are discussed in detail in Ch. 75, only selected cardiovascular factors are mentioned here.

An increase in blood volume, as might occur by increased intake of salt and water, increases the diastolic volume of the cardiac chambers and the cardiac output. Atrial receptors sensitive to stretch activate vasodilating reflexes to the kidneys, increasing renal blood flow, and atrial receptors also reflexly stimulate the central nervous system to diminish the secretion of ADH. These factors tend to increase the output of urine and sodium excretion, restoring the blood volume toward normal. A decrease in effective blood volume has opposite effects. Also, a peptide called atrial natriuretic factor (ANF) has been isolated which causes renal sodium loss and is also a vasodilator. It is released by the atria upon stretch, and ANF levels rise with acute and chronic circulatory congestion.

An additional highly important control mechanism regulating arterial pressure and blood volume is the renin-angiotensin system (see Ch. 37). Reduction in renal perfusion (reduced pressure and flow) is sensed by the juxtaglomerular apparatus, which releases renin, whereas increased effective blood volume shuts off the stimulus for renin release. Renin enzymatically promotes the formation of angiotensin I from a precursor in the bloodstream, which is then converted to angiotensin II by the converting enzyme. Angiotensin II is a powerful vasoconstrictor, but small subpressor doses of angiotensin II also increase aldosterone secretion. Aldosterone, in turn, acts on the kidney to promote retention of salt and water, thereby counteracting the original stimulus of decreased effective blood volume.

With congestive heart failure, there is increased retention of salt and water, which leads to edema formation and increased blood volume. There may be increased aldosterone levels in severe heart failure secondary to reduced renal perfusion and activation of the renin-angiotensin system. Diuretics are used in this setting, and in severe heart failure with hyponatremia that is unresponsive to diuretics, using an angiotensin-converting enzyme inhibitor may reverse this process by lowering angiotensin II and aldosterone levels as well as by lowering vascular resistance and afterload on the LV.

INTEGRATED CARDIOVASCULAR RESPONSES

It is important to emphasize the significance of interactions between the peripheral circulation and the heart in considering integrated responses. Certain peripheral circulatory factors, including the TPVR and the venous capacitance, affect two important mechanical determinants of cardiac performance — the preload and the afterload. Venous return primarily determines the cardiac output. In addition, feedback control by neurohumoral reflex mechanisms simultaneously regulates both the heart and the peripheral circulation.

CHANGES IN VENOUS RETURN. Venous return to the right heart varies with normal respiration. It increases during inspiration as intrathoracic pressure falls (thereby increasing the pressure gradient for right heart filling), and moment-to-moment operation of the Frank-Starling mechanism, in both ventricles to vary the stroke volume keeps the output per minute of the two sides of the heart in equilibrium.

Vasodilator drugs that have a considerable venodilating effect, such as nitroglycerin, nitroprusside and captopril, can differently affect the cardiac output in the normal circulation and in congestive heart failure. Thus, in the normal circulation the cardiac output falls with nitroprusside because the venous return curve is shifted downward as blood volume is displaced from the central circulation and pooled in the peripheral veins (decreased effective blood volume). However, during cardiac failure, the associated unloading of the LV by the arteriole-dilating action of this drug releases blood from the central circulation, which counterbalances the drug's venodilator effect. Therefore, the venous return curve is not shifted downward, and the marked shift upward of the cardiac output curve owing to reduced afterload results in an increased cardiac output (Fig. 32–6, D to A).

EXERCISE. Many mechanisms can come into play to cause the increased cardiac output that accompanies normal exercise. In nonsedentary individuals during low levels of exercise, increased stroke volume, combined with a mild increase in heart rate, augments the cardiac output. With marked exercise, as sympathetic stimulation and circulating catecholamine levels increase, the increased venous return causes further utilization of the Frank-Starling mechanism, and the stroke volume is further enhanced as increased myocardial contractility augments the ejection fraction. However, the stroke volume reserve is relatively small. The most important cardiac mechanism allowing a very high cardiac output during intense exercise in such individuals is augmented heart rate, which may reach 180 beats per minute or higher. Increased myocardial contractility also combines with decreased TPVR (caused by marked vasodilation in the exercising muscles) to shift the cardiac output curve upward (Fig. 32–6, A to C). In addition, increased sympathetic tone shifts the venous return curve upward (decreased venous capacitance), and it is steepened by decreased venous and arteriolar resistance (Fig. 32–6, A to C). Therefore, the intersection of the venous return and cardiac output curves occurs at a markedly increased cardiac output, with only a mild elevation of the right atrial pressure. Thus, *both* peripheral and circulatory adaptations are involved in the exercise response.

Bers DM: Excitation-Contraction Coupling and Cardiac Contractile Force. Boston, Kluwer Academic Publisher, 1991. *Detailed examination of Ca² movements during the cardiac cycle and their role in activating and controlling myocardial contractility.*

Braunwald E (ed.): Heart Disease: A Textbook of Cardiovascular Medicine. 4th ed. Philadelphia, WB Saunders, 1992, p 351. *Up-to-date review of cardiac performance from the cellular level to the intact heart. Also includes the pathophysiology of heart failure.*

Kambayashi M, Miura T, Oh BH, et al.: Enhancement of force-frequency effect on myocardial contractility by adrenergic stimulation in conscious dogs. Circulation 86:572, 1992. *Documents the augmentation of the force-frequency response effect on myocardial contractility produced by sympathetic stimulation or by exercise.*

Ross J Jr: Assessment of cardiac function and myocardial contractility. *In* Hurst JW (ed.): The Heart. New York, McGraw-Hill, 1993. *Current concepts concerning left ventricular function under normal and abnormal loading conditions, including heart failure and valvular heart disease.*

West JB (ed.): Best and Taylor's Physiological Basis of Medical Practice. 12th ed. Baltimore, Williams & Wilkins, 1991, p 110. *Basic physiology text that assumes little advanced knowledge. Pathophysiologic examples are concerned with cardiac function, circulatory control, myocardial oxygen consumption, coronary circulation, and heart failure.*

33 SPECIALIZED DIAGNOSTIC PROCEDURES

33.1 Radiology of the Heart

Murray G. Baron

The heart casts a homogeneous shadow on the chest film. No internal detail can be seen within its contours because the radiodensities of blood, myocardium, and other cardiac tissues are so similar that one cannot be distinguished from the others. Only two borders of the heart, where it contacts the radiolucent, air-containing lung, can be discerned in any one projection. Changes in the size and/or shape of the chambers of the heart and the great vessels usually alter the shape of the cardiac silhouette. However, because the heart is a three-dimensional structure and all of the cardiac chambers are not border-forming in any projection, multiple views are required for complete evaluation. With the advent of echocardiography, the need for this "cardiac series" has disappeared. However, a remarkable amount of information regarding the heart is presented on standard frontal and lateral films of the chest. As these are a part of most routine medical examinations, they are a useful tool for detecting disease as well as for evaluating the severity of known disease, documenting the progress of the disease, and assessing the efficacy of treatment.

ROENTGEN ANATOMY (Fig. 33–1)

On a frontal chest film, the right cardiac border has two components: a straight vertical upper half formed by the superior vena cava and a gently convex lower half representing the lateral wall of the right atrium. The break in the contour of this border of the heart indicates the cavo-atrial junction. Some patients are able to lower their diaphragms sufficiently during inspiration to uncover a small, straight segment of the inferior vena cava between the diaphragm and the right atrium.

The left cardiac border is composed of four distinct segments. The uppermost bulge represents the aortic knob, the most distal portion of the aortic arch, where it turns downward to become the descending aorta. The prominence below the knob is formed by the main pulmonary artery and the subvalvular portion of the outflow tract of the right ventricle. The lowermost third of this border represents the anterolateral wall of the left ventricle. Between this bulge and that of the pulmonary artery is a short, flat, or slightly concave segment where the left atrial appendage reaches the border of the heart.

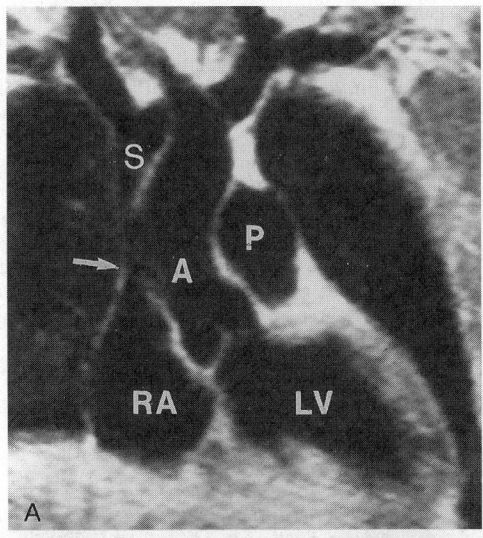
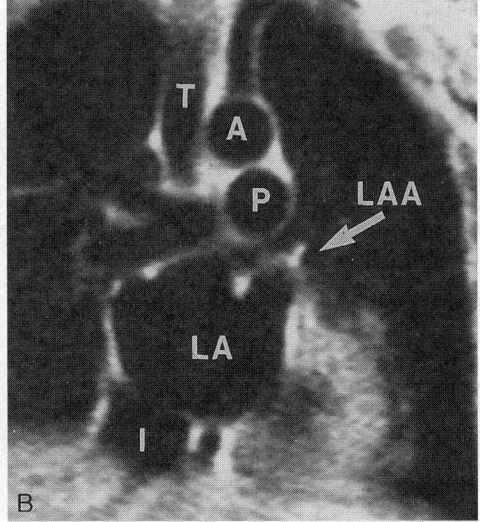
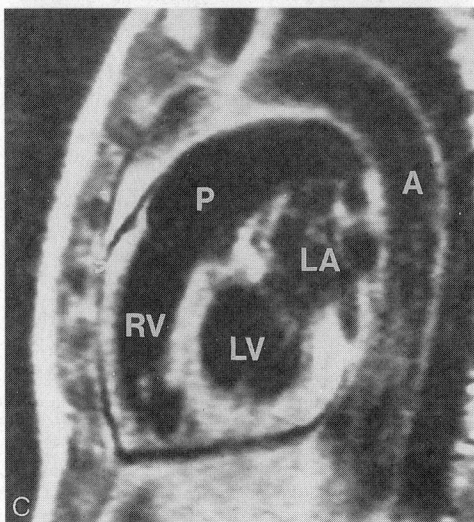

FIGURE 33–1. Normal roentgen anatomy. Magnetic resonance images. *A,* Coronal section at level of aortic valve. The right border of the cardiac silhouette is formed by the superior vena cava (S) and the right atrium (RA). The arrow indicates the cavalatrial junction. The lower portion of the left cardiac border is formed by the left ventricle (LV). A = Ascending aorta; P = main pulmonary artery. *B,* Coronal section at level of left atrium. The upper portion of the left cardiac border is formed by the aorta (A), main pulmonary artery (P), and left atrial appendage (LAA). LA = Left atrium; I = inferior vena cava; T = trachea. *C,* Sagittal section near midline. The right ventricle (RV) forms the anterior surface of the heart, abutting the sternum. The pulmonary artery (P) extends upward and posteriorly from the ventricle. The posterior border of the heart is formed by the left atrium (LA) and left ventricle (LV).

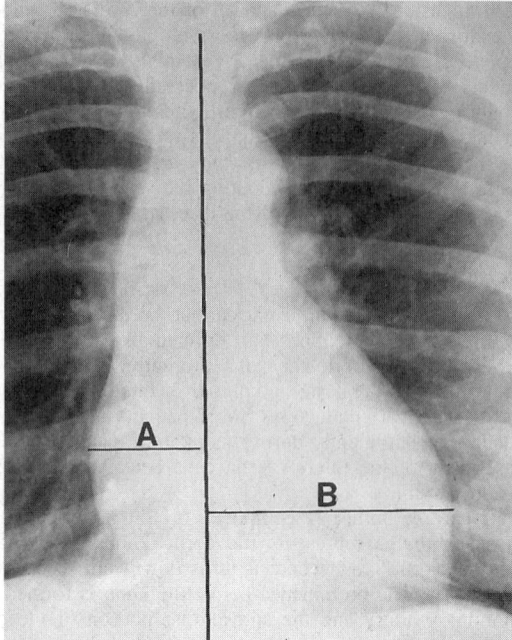

FIGURE 33-2. Measurement of the transverse cardiac diameter. Severe aortic stenosis with a 95-mm systolic gradient across the valve. The heart, although considerably hypertrophied, is normal in size and configuration. A vertical line is drawn through the heart. The greatest distances to the right cardiac border (A) and to the left cardiac border (B) are then measured. Transverse cardiac diameter = A + B.

In the lateral view (Fig. 33-1C), the anterior border of the cardiac silhouette is formed by the body and the outflow tract of the right ventricle. The heart lies in the anterior portion of the chest, and the right ventricle abuts the lower third of the sternum. Both the outflow tract and pulmonary artery slope posteriorly. Air-containing lung is interposed between this portion of the heart and the anterior chest wall, forming the "retrosternal clear space." The upper half of the posterior border of the cardiac silhouette, from the carina to the diaphragm, is formed by the posterior wall of the left atrium and the lower half by the posterior wall of the left ventricle. The shadow of the inferior vena cava can usually be seen extending

obliquely upward and anteriorly from the diaphragm. The posterior contour of the normal left ventricle crosses the shadow of the cava about 2 cm above the diaphragm.

Alterations in the contour of the heart usually reflect dilation and/or hypertrophy of the chambers. Many times the pattern of these changes, together with the appearance of the pulmonary vasculature, points to a specific underlying cardiac abnormality. Chest films are most sensitive for detecting chamber dilation. Cardiac hypertrophy is more difficult to recognize, as the thickened myocardium often encroaches on the lumen rather than extending outward and enlarging the heart (Fig. 33-2). With severe hypertrophy, as in hypertropic cardiomyopathy, the heart enlarges to the left and the apex becomes blunted and rounder than usual. This is not a pathognomonic appearance.

HEART SIZE

A normal cardiac silhouette is no guarantee that no cardiac disease is present. Angina, for example, no matter how severe, does not affect heart size until the left ventricle decompensates. Similarly, the patient with restrictive cardiomyopathy may be in severe congestive failure with a normal-appearing heart. On the other hand, an enlarged heart always indicates the presence of cardiac or pericardial disease. Therefore, accurate evaluation of heart size is important.

Over the years, various objective methods have been proposed for evaluating heart size. The simplest of these, the transverse cardiac diameter, is of little value because the normal range is so great and varies with the age, gender, and body habitus of the patient. However, when the transverse cardiac diameter is correlated with the patient's body surface area, a satisfactory distinction can be made between normal and abnormal. This is not a practical solution, because the data needed to calculate surface area are usually not available when reviewing chest films. In place of this value, the transverse diameter of the patient's chest can be used to provide a reasonable approximation of body size and habitus. The cardiothoracic ratio is measured by dropping a vertical line through the heart and measuring the greatest distance to the right and left cardiac borders (Fig. 33-2). The sum of the two is the transverse cardiac diameter. The transverse thoracic diameter is the greatest width of the chest, measured from the inner surfaces of the ribs. Dividing the cardiac diameter by the chest diameter gives the cardiothoracic ratio. A value of less than 0.6 can be considered within the limits of normal. Setting this value at 0.5, as is often done, produces too many false-positive results.

In most cases, exact measurement of the cardiac silhouette is not necessary, and a reasonably experienced observer can achieve an acceptable degree of accuracy by visual estimation. Regardless of

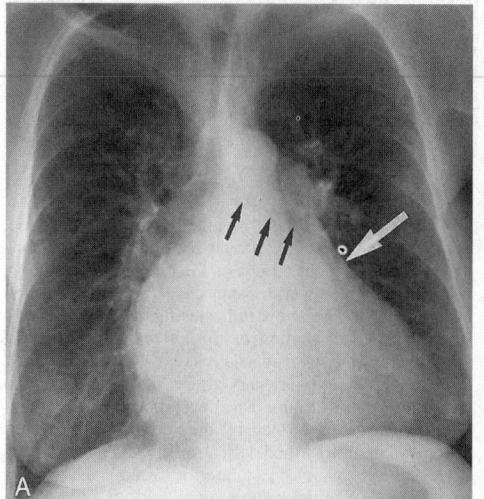 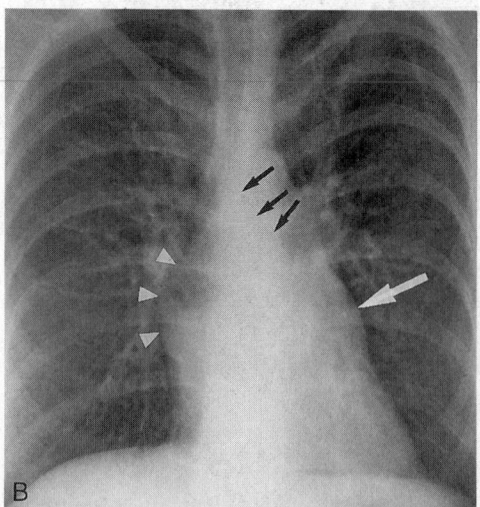

FIGURE 33-3. Left atrial enlargement in mitral valve disease. *A,* Patient 1: The enlarged left atrium causes the central portion of the cardiac silhouette to be abnormally dense. The right border of the atrium is seen within the right side of the cardiac silhouette. The left main bronchus *(small arrows)* is elevated. The region of the left atrial appendage *(white arrow)* is slightly concave because this structure was resected at the time of previous mitral commissurotomy. *B,* Patient 2: The enlarged left atrial appendage bulges from the left side of the heart *(white arrow)* while the body of the atrium *(arrowheads)* extends beyond the right atrium to form a part of the right heart border. There is no double density seen within the heart, and the left main bronchus *(small arrows)* is not elevated.

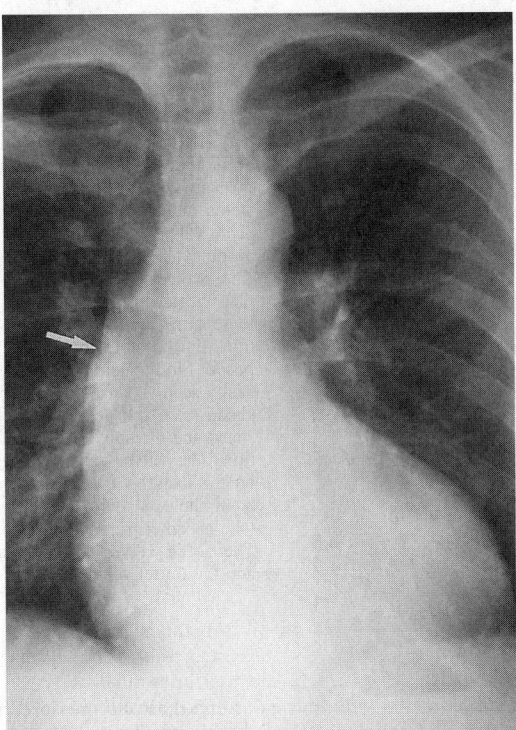

FIGURE 33–4. Left ventricular dilatation, aortic insufficiency. The apex of the heart is displaced downward and to the left. The ascending aorta *(arrow)* is diffusely dilated. The pulmonary vasculature is normal.

the method used, several cautions must be observed to avoid over-reading of abnormality. The single greatest effect on the apparent cardiac size is the degree of inspiration. The volume of the heart is essentially constant throughout the cardiac cycle. With expiration, as the diaphragm moves up, the vertical diameter of the heart is shortened and its transverse diameter increases. Because we gauge heart size primarily from its width, the heart appears larger on expiratory films. The degree of inspiration can be determined from the relationship of the diaphragm to the ribs. On a properly positioned frontal chest film, a reasonable degree of inspiration is indicated if the diaphragm is lowered to at least the level of the posterior portion of the ninth rib.

When the anteroposterior diameter of the chest is small, the heart may be compressed between the sternum and the spine so that it splays to one or both sides. For this reason, the heart often appears enlarged in patients with a straight back syndrome or with a pectus excavatum deformity of the sternum. An epicardial fat pad (actually it is truly extrapleural fat, outside of the pericardium) can occur in one or both cardiophrenic angles and makes the heart appear larger than it actually is. The cardiophrenic angle often appears obtuse or the cardiac apex is indistinct. In addition, the slightly more radiolucent image of the fat can usually be distinguished from the greater density of the heart.

A change in the size of the cardiac silhouette can also occur between systole and diastole. This is important because chest films are exposed at random with reference to the cardiac cycle, and the apparent size of the heart may be different on two films of the same patient made at different times. In the majority of cases, the difference in the transverse cardiac diameter between systole and diastole is small, measuring no more than several millimeters. However, in younger patients, especially the more athletic with a slow heart rate and a large stroke volume, phasic change in the cardiac diameter can be as much as 2 cm.

CHAMBER ENLARGEMENT

LEFT ATRIUM. Dilation of the left atrium alone, in the absence of a left-to-right shunt, is most often due to disease of the mitral valve, although it can also result simply from atrial fibrillation. The two "popular" roentgen signs of left atrial enlargement—a double contour within the right cardiac border and elevation of the left main bronchus—are both accurate when present, but are insensitive. They are not seen in about half the cases of mitral valve disease. In order to produce a discernible margin within the cardiac silhouette in the frontal projection, the thickness of the heart must increase sharply at some point. This occurs in mitral disease when the left atrium enlarges and protrudes posteriorly from the back of the heart. The right border of the left atrium is then silhouetted where it abuts the right lung and its contour is seen within the cardiac silhouette (Fig. 33–3A). This is not apparent with lesser degrees of left atrial enlargement. Conversely, when the right atrium also enlarges, as is common in longstanding mitral disease, it forms a continuous curve on the posterior cardiac border with the enlarged left atrium. Thus, the double contour is not seen with mild left atrial enlargement or in severe cases of mitral disease. Furthermore,

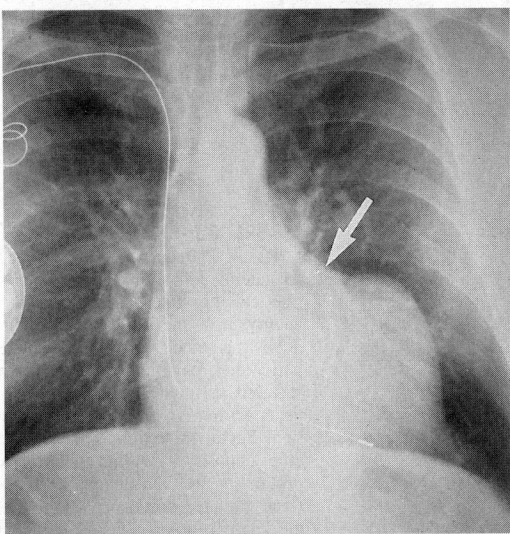

FIGURE 33–5. Left ventricular aneurysm. A bulge on the lower portion of the left cardiac border, formed by the anterolateral wall of the left ventricle, represents a ventricular aneurysm. The patient had suffered a myocardial infarct 1 year previously. The left atrial appendage segment *(arrow)* is normal. A transvenous pacemaker has been inserted through the right subclavian vein. The electrode tip is situated in the apex of the right ventricle.

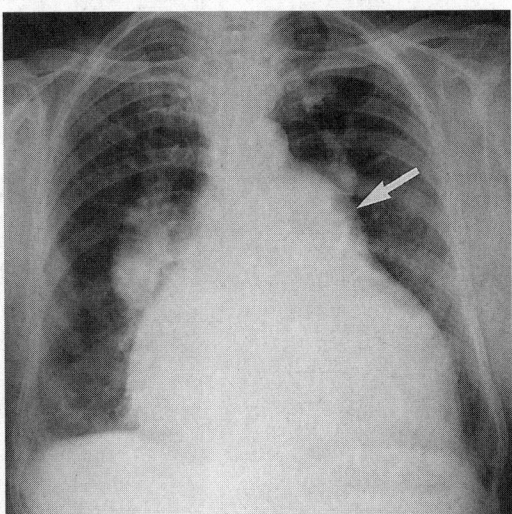

FIGURE 33–6. Right ventricular enlargement. Resistive pulmonary hypertension, secondary to atrial septal defect. The main pulmonary artery *(arrow)* and the right pulmonary artery are markedly dilated. The left pulmonary artery was also dilated but is hidden by the heart in this view. There is a sudden "cutoff" of the vascular shadows just beyond the hila. This is characteristic of resistive pulmonary hypertension. The right ventricle is enlarged, elevating the cardiac apex and displacing it to the left. The accentuation of the curvature of the lower right cardiac border and enlargement of the cardiac silhouette to the right are caused by dilatation of the right atrium.

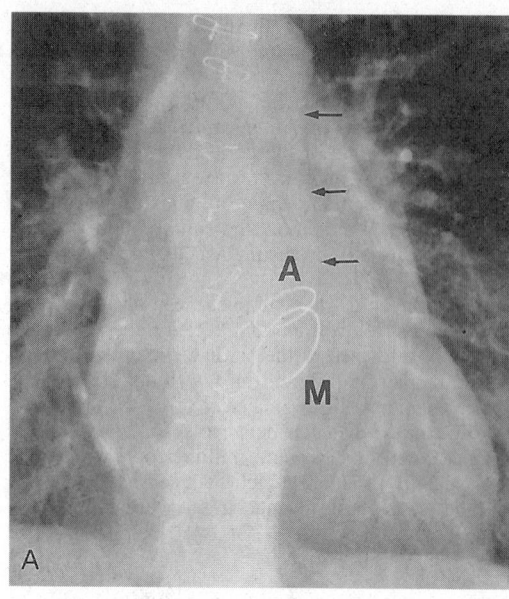
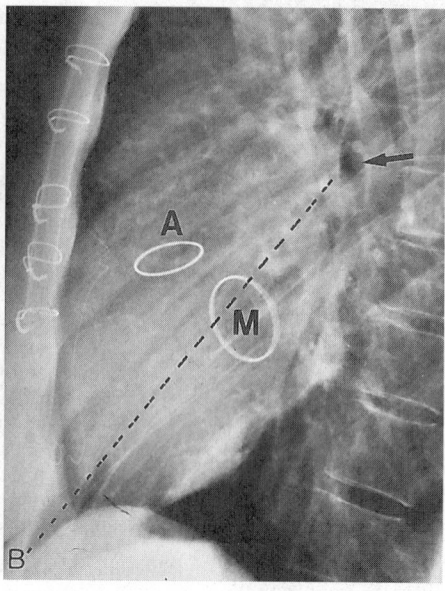

FIGURE 33-7. Location of the mitral and aortic valves. Both mitral and aortic valves have been replaced by porcine heterografts. The circular stents indicate the location and tilt of each valve. M = Mitral valve; A = aortic valve. A, Frontal projection. The two valves are normally in contact with each other, and it is difficult to separate them in the frontal projection. Furthermore, on a routinely exposed film, calcific deposits are not easily seen because of the overlapping shadows of the descending aorta *(arrows)* and the spine. B, Lateral projection. The valves can be differentiated on the lateral view by drawing a line from the left main bronchus *(arrow)* to the anterior costophrenic sulcus. The aortic valve lies above this line and the mitral valve below it.

the radiologic technique used for chest films is chosen to provide optimal images of the lungs. The heart, when enlarged, is underexposed, and the double contour may not be seen within its opaque silhouette. For the same reason, the position of the left main bronchus often cannot be clearly visualized through the mediastinal shadow.

LEFT VENTRICLE. The shape of the dilated left ventricle depends to a large extent on the underlying cause. When it is due to insufficiency of the aortic or mitral valve, the ventricle elongates and its apex is displaced downward, to the left, and posteriorly (Fig. 33-4). When the dilatation is due to coronary artery disease or primary myocardial disease, the ventricle tends to assume a more globular shape. In the lateral view, the downward extension of the enlarged left ventricle covers more of the vena caval shadow than normally, the crossing point of their posterior borders occurring nearer to the diaphragm than normal. Unfortunately, the usefulness of this sign is limited because even slight rotation of the patient from the true lateral position distorts the apparent relationship between the two structures.

Enlargement of the left ventricle produces a smoothly curved dilatation of the lower portion of the cardiac silhouette. A localized bulge in this contour most often represents a ventricular aneurysm (Fig. 33-5). Dilatation of the left ventricle is usually associated

with elevation of the left ventricular end-diastolic pressure. The latter increases the resistance to left atrial emptying and can result in dilation of the atrium. Therefore, left atrial enlargement in the presence of a large left ventricle does not necessarily indicate the presence of mitral valve disease.

RIGHT ATRIUM. Enlargement of only the right chambers of the heart is uncommon in adults. When seen, it is usually due to subacute bacterial endocarditis of the tricuspid and/or pulmonic valve, most often in drug addicts. Cardiac lesions involving the right side of the heart also occur with the carcinoid syndrome. Dilatation of the right atrium causes an accentuation and outward bowing of the curvature on the lower half of the right cardiac contour. With greater degrees of dilatation, the cardiac silhouette enlarges to the right (Fig. 33-6).

RIGHT VENTRICLE. The right ventricle is the most difficult of the four cardiac chambers to evaluate on chest films. Except for a small area in the subpulmonic region, the chamber is not border-forming in the frontal projection. Even moderate right ventricular enlargement may produce no abnormality in this view other than some elevation of the main pulmonary artery. As right ventricular size increases, the transverse diameter of the heart enlarges to the left, and the cardiac apex may be elevated (Fig. 33-6). Enlargement of either or both ventricles displaces the apex of the heart to

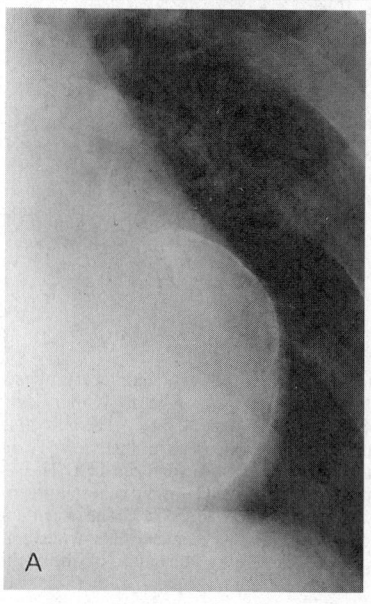
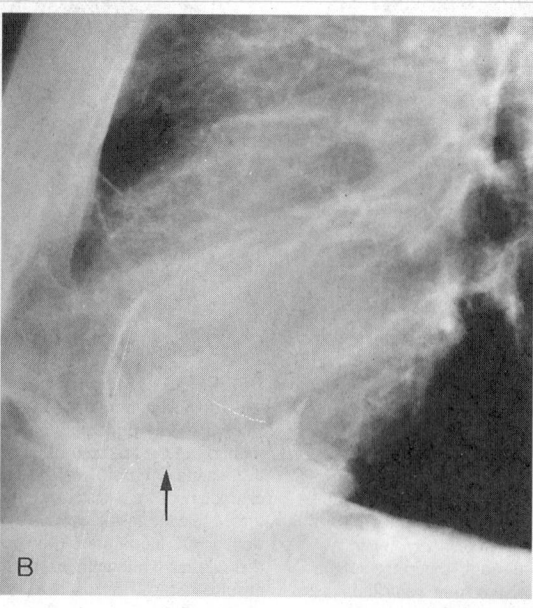

FIGURE 33-8. Calcified myocardial infarcts. A, Patient 1: Frontal projection. Anterolateral left ventricular aneurysm. The fine calcific line outlines an anterolateral aneurysm of the left ventricle. The calcific deposit is much finer than that seen with pericardial calcification. The patient had suffered a myocardial infarction several years earlier. B, Patient 2: Lateral projection. Septal infarction. The curvilinear calcific deposit is within the scarred lower portion of the ventricular septum. The infarct extended posteriorly along the base of the heart to involve the diaphragmatic wall of the left ventricle *(arrow).*

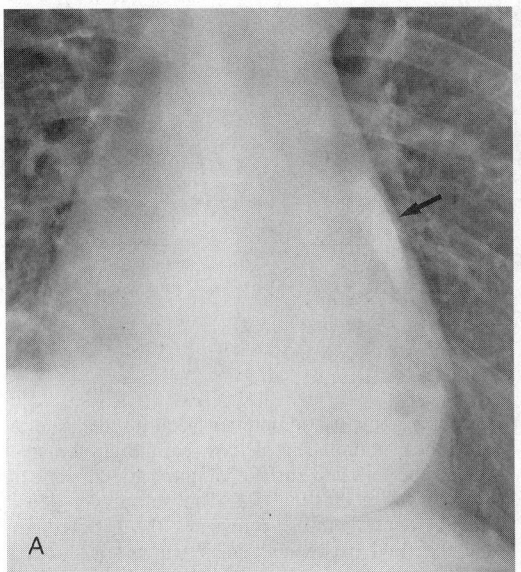

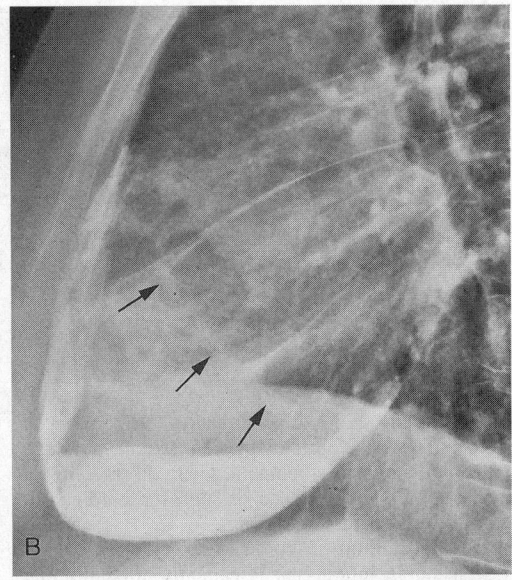

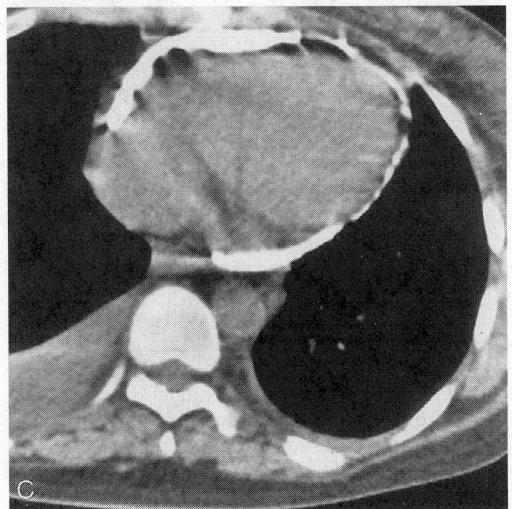

FIGURE 33–9. Calcific pericarditis. *A,* Frontal projection. There is a large, thick, calcific plaque *(arrow)* just below the level of the left upper lobe bronchus. More caudad, the calcific deposits become confluent and cover the diaphragmatic surface of the heart. *B,* The dense calcific peel around the cardiac apex and the diaphragmatic aspect of the heart is better seen. Linear calcific deposits *(arrows)* lie within the atrioventricular sulcus. *C,* A nonenhanced CT scan shows the irregular, thick, calcific peel almost encircling the heart.

the left. It is often not possible to distinguish between biventricular enlargement or dilatation of one or the other of the ventricles.

As the right ventricle enlarges, its area of contact with the sternum increases and tends to obliterate the retrosternal clear space in the lateral view. This is a nonspecific sign, as it also depends on the shape of the chest and the size of the left ventricle as well as the size of the right ventricle.

CALCIFICATION

Calcific deposits, because they have a greater radiodensity than the cardiac soft tissues, can be seen within the cardiac silhouette. Valvular calcification most often involves the mitral and aortic valves and usually indicates significant stenosis. This is particularly true of the mitral valve. The calcium is deposited in irregular clumps, near the valve commissures. Because the two valves are in contact—inserting on a common fibrous tendon—determining which valve is calcified may be difficult. They lie within the midportion of the cardiac silhouette in the frontal projection, just to the left of the spine (Fig. 33–7A). They can be separated by fluoroscopy as the axis of motion of the aortic valve approaches the vertical, whereas the orbit of motion of the mitral valve is oriented nearer to the horizontal. The distinction can also be made on lateral chest films. If a line is drawn from the left main bronchus (seen as a dark, circular shadow superimposed on the lowermost part of the trachea) to the anterior costophrenic angle, the mitral valve lies below the line and the aortic valve above it (Fig. 33–7B).

Calcification of the mitral annulus, most common in elderly women, can be distinguished from valvular calcification because it

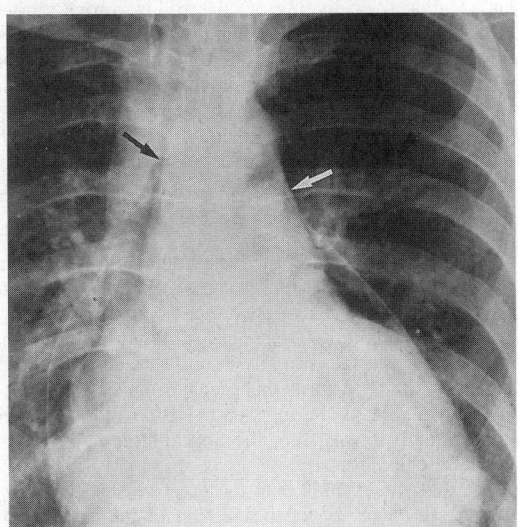

FIGURE 33–10. The superior pericardial reflection. Pericardial effusion following tap. During pericardiocentesis, some of the withdrawn fluid was replaced with air. The normal pericardium is now outlined between the intrapericardial air and the air in the lungs and is seen as a thin linear shadow along the outer border of the cardiac silhouette. The film is made in the erect position and the air has risen to the highest point of the pericardial cavity *(arrows),* above the level of the pulmonary hila and almost reaching the aortic arch.

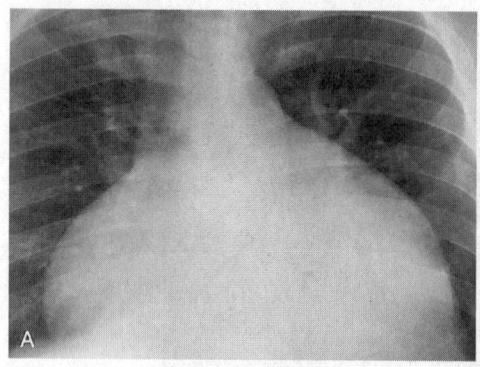
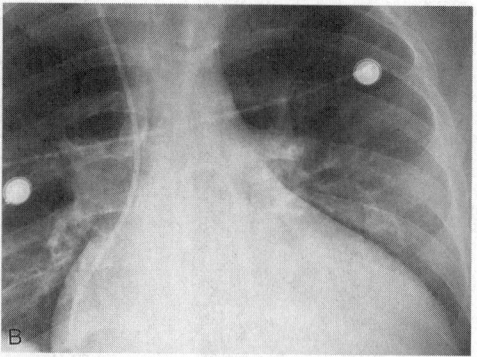

FIGURE 33–11. Hilum overlay sign. *A,* Pericardial effusion. The heart is diffusely enlarged. Its silhouette extends outward and obscures the hilar shadows in each lung. *B,* Dilated cardiomyopathy. The heart is diffusely enlarged. The failing left ventricle has caused congestion of the hilar vessels and they are more prominent than normal.

forms a heavy, relatively smooth curvilinear shadow in the form of an O or a C. Calcification of the wall of the left atrium, although rare, is virtually pathognomonic of rheumatic heart disease. It appears as fine, linear calcific shadows seen through the cardiac silhouette outlining the contour of the left atrium.

Calcification of the myocardium in coronary artery disease indicates a previous transmural infarct and frequently a ventricular aneurysm. The calcified scar is visualized as a fine, curvilinear density, most commonly on the anterolateral aspect of the heart, seen best in the frontal view (Fig. 33–8*A*), or in the lower portion of the interventricular septum, seen best in the lateral projection (Fig. 33–8*B*). Calcification of the pericardium is usually coarser and tends to occur in clumps. Often pericardial calcium is distributed primarily over the interventricular sulcus and the atrioventricular grooves, but when extensive, the deposits may coalesce and completely surround the heart (Fig. 33–9).

Calcification of the coronary arteries is a specific sign of atherosclerotic disease. Medial sclerosis and calcification do not occur in the coronary arteries, and calcium is deposited only in complicated atheromatous plaques, plaques in which previous hemorrhage has occurred. Not uncommonly, this type of plaque, which may not produce significant narrowing of the vessel, is the site of thrombosis and vascular occlusion leading to myocardial infarction. Although the calcium is often not deposited in the areas of high-grade stenosis, a very strong correlation exists between the extent of coronary artery calcification and the extent of coronary arterial sclerosis.

Calcification of the coronary arteries is difficult to visualize on chest films because the deposits are thin and their shadows are blurred by the motion of the heart. Fluoroscopy is more sensitive but not as accurate for detecting or quantifying coronary artery calcification as fast computed tomographic (CT) scanning. The stress ECG and thallium examinations, current screening methods for coronary artery disease, test only for secondary manifestations of coronary artery disease resulting from decreased perfusion of the myocardium beyond a stenosis. Radiologically detecting coronary artery calcification is the only noninvasive method for directly visualizing the atheromatous disease in the coronary arterial walls.

PERICARDIAL EFFUSION

The pericardium is a serosa-lined sac containing a small amount of fluid. It completely invests the heart, except for a small area on its posterior surface between the entrances of the pulmonary veins and the superior and inferior venae cavae. When fluid accumulates in the pericardium, the sac distends smoothly, enlarging the cardiac silhouette and giving it a flask-shaped appearance. A similar shape can occur with a dilated, failing heart. Differentiation of the two conditions is readily made from the appearance of the pulmonary hila on a frontal chest film.

The pericardial sac extends onto the great vessels reaching to, or slightly above, the level of the bifurcation of the main pulmonary artery (Fig. 33–10). As the sac distends with fluid, it tends to overlap and obscure the hilar vessels. On the other hand, when the heart fails, the vessels become congested and appear more prominent than normal (Fig. 33–11).

Posterior displacement of the epicardial fat line is a second reliable sign of pericardial effusion. In adults, fat is often insinuated between the myocardium and the visceral pericardium (the epi-

cardium). This is sometimes seen in the lateral projection as a curvilinear, radiolucent shadow paralleling the anterior aspect of the heart. The anterior surface of the parietal pericardium borders the retrosternal mediastinal fat. The soft tissue density between these two fat lines therefore represents the pericardium, the epicardium, and the fluid between them. When normal, this stripe is no more than 1 to 2 mm thick. As fluid accumulates in the pericardial sac, the epicardial fat line is displaced posteriorly and the pericardial stripe widens (Fig. 33–12).

PULMONARY VASCULATURE

Almost all of the linear shadows in the lung represent large and medium-sized pulmonary arteries and veins. The terminal branches of the vessels are too small to be visualized as individual structures. The same is true of the interstitial tissues that support the alveoli and form the primary and secondary interlobular septae. However, the summation of the minimal densities cast by these structures gives the pulmonary fields an overall grayish cast. The large vessels are seen because their soft tissue density is set off against the surrounding air-containing alveoli.

INTRACARDIAC SHUNTS. The caliber of the pulmonary vessels reflects the volume of blood flow through the lungs. When this volume is diminished owing to a right-to-left shunt, because venous blood is bypassing the lungs, the pulmonary fields appear abnormally radiolucent. Even with severe pulmonic valvular stenosis, so long as no intracardiac shunt occurs, the pulmonary vascularity is within normal limits. Increased size and prominence of the pul-

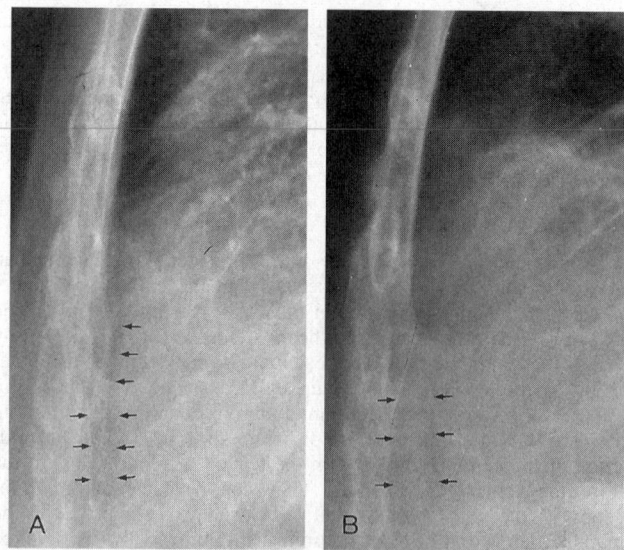

FIGURE 33–12. Pericardial effusion. Posterior displacement of epicardial fat line. The two lines of arrows point to the substernal fat and the subepicardial fat layers. *A,* Normal. The fine line of soft tissue density between the fat layers represents the epicardium, the pericardium, and the fluid between them. *B,* Same patient with a pericardial effusion. The epicardial fat line is displaced posteriorly, and the pericardial stripe is abnormally wide.

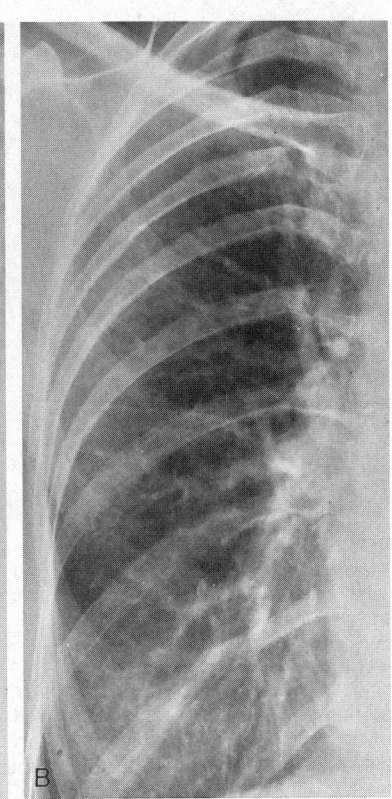

FIGURE 33-13. Pulmonary vasculature. *A,* Atrial septal defect, left-to-right shunt. All pulmonary vessels, to the lower lobes as well as the upper lobes, are dilated, indicating increased blood flow. *B,* Mitral stenosis, pulmonary venous hypertension with redistribution of the pulmonary vasculature. The lower lobe vessels are constricted and the upper vessels, which now carry more blood, are of greater caliber.

monary vessels, both central and peripheral, usually indicate an increase in pulmonary blood flow secondary to a left-to-right shunt (Fig. 33–13A). The vessels in the lower as well as the upper lung fields are dilated. Although pulmonary arteries and veins also become abnormally prominent in congestive failure, the vessels are usually not sharply outlined, and there are additional signs of pulmonary venous hypertension or interstitial edema.

The vessels to the lower lobes carry about 60 to 70% of the pulmonary blood flow and normally are of greater caliber than the vessels to the upper lobes. As pulmonary venous pressure increases, the lower lobe vessels become constricted. This increases local resistance to blood flow, so that more blood is distributed to the upper lobes, making their vessels more prominent. This redistribution of pulmonary vasculature is a reliable sign of pulmonary venous hypertension (Fig. 33–13B). With sufficient further increase in the venous pressure, pulmonary edema develops.

PULMONARY EDEMA. Normally, there is a constant, extravascular circulation of fluid in the lungs, from the capillaries through the interstitium and back to the bloodstream by way of the lymphatics. When pulmonary venous pressure increases, more and more fluid leaks from the capillary bed, the capacity of the lymphatics to remove the fluid is exceeded, and the interstitium be-

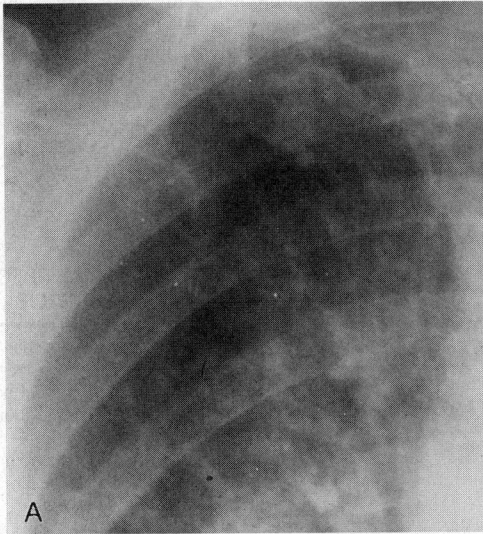
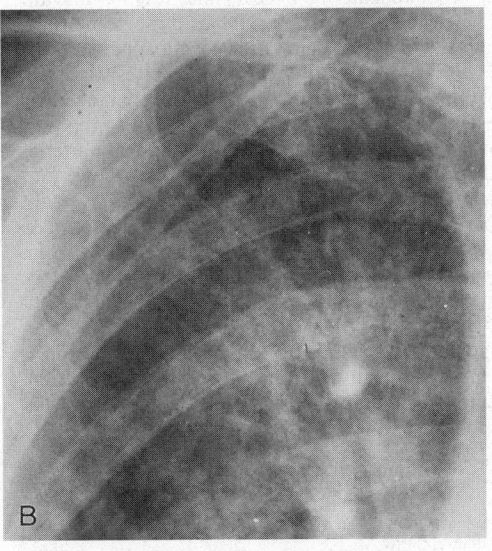

FIGURE 33-14. Interstitial pulmonary edema. *A,* Close-up of the right upper lobe. Portable film of a patient with acute myocardial infarct. The pulmonary vessels are well outlined. *B,* Two days later, the patient became tachypneic. There were no abnormal auscultatory findings in the lungs. Radiographically, the lung fields are noisy, with numerous random shadows obscuring the outline of the pulmonary vessels. The appearance and the time sequence of the changes are characteristic of interstitial pulmonary edema.

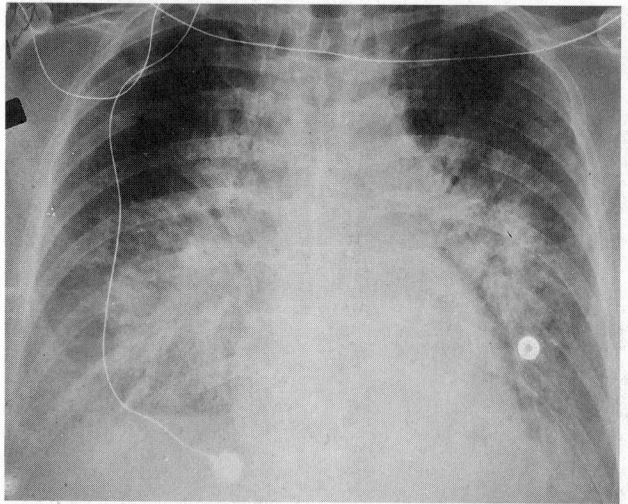

FIGURE 33-15. Alveolar pulmonary edema, acute myocardial infarction. There are patchy areas of consolidation in the perihilar regions of both lungs. Dilatation of the heart after a massive myocardial infarction may not be seen for the first 24 to 48 hours.

comes waterlogged. Because the interlobular septae in the outer portions of the lung bases are oriented parallel to the x-ray beam on an erect film, when thickened, they are seen as parallel, short horizontal lines extending to the pleural surfaces (Kerley B lines). Kerley A lines also represent thickened interlobular septae, but are longer and are seen in the upper lung fields. They are within the depth of the lung and usually do not reach the pleural surface. Most of the other septae, even when thickened, are too fine to be identified as individual structures. However, the summation pattern creates random "noise" on the film that obscures the shadows of the pulmonary vessels (Fig. 33-14). A "ground glass" appearance of the lung fields without identifiable vascular markings within them is characteristic of interstitial pulmonary edema. The patient is usually severely tachypneic at this stage, but rales are not present. Interstitial edema also causes thickening of the bronchial walls and peribronchial connective tissues, causing an increase in the thickness and indistinctness of the bronchial walls, seen where they are projected on end. This "peribronchial cuffing" is best visualized in the superior portion of the pulmonary hila, where the anterior segmental bronchus of the upper lobes is viewed on end. When the interstitium can no longer accommodate the excess fluid, it spills into the alveoli (Fig. 33-15). At this point, as air bubbles through the fluid, the typical auscultatory findings of pulmonary edema appear.

PULMONARY ARTERIAL HYPERTENSION. Resistive pulmonary hypertension can result from a left-to-right intracardiac shunt, mitral valve disease, or extracardiac disease such as repeated episodes of pulmonary embolization. The central pulmonary arteries become grossly dilated. Instead of gradually tapering as they bifurcate, there is a sudden, sharp change in the caliber of the vessels. The size and number of the smaller arterial branches decrease, making them look like a "pruned tree" (see Fig. 33-6). With severe pulmonary hypertension, the right heart chambers may dilate. Once this picture of resistive pulmonary hypertension develops, it is difficult to determine whether the original cause was cardiac or extracardiac. The radiographic appearance of pulmonary hypertension is relatively specific but not sensitive. Clinically significant hypertension can be present with a normal-appearing pulmonary vascular bed.

Baron MG: Radiology and Angiocardiography. *In* Onkman FFY (ed.): The Ciba Collection of Medical Illustrations. Vol 5: The Heart. Summit, NJ, CIBA Publications Department, 1969.

Chen JT: The plain radiograph in the diagnosis of cardiovascular disease. Radiol Clin North Am 21:609, 1983.

Felson B: The mediastinum. Semin Roentgenol 4:41, 1969.

Little WC: Angiographic assessment of the culprit coronary artery lesion before acute myocardial infarction. Am J Cardiol 66:44G, 1990.

Milne ENC: The radiologic distinction of cardiogenic and non-cardiogenic edema. Am J Roentgenol 144:879, 1985.

Stanford W, Thompson BH, Weiss RM: Coronary artery calcification: Clinical significance and current methods of detection. AJR 161:1139, 1993.

33.2 Electrocardiography

Nora Goldschlager

The electrocardiogram (ECG) is a recording of the electrical potentials produced by cardiac tissue. Formation of electrical impulses occurs within the conduction system of the heart; when excited, atrial and ventricular myocardial muscle fibers contract. The electrical currents produced by these electrical impulses spread through the body and are recorded from the body surface by applying electrodes at various body surface points and connecting them to a recording apparatus.

The ECG is valuable diagnostically to evaluate conduction delay of atrial and ventricular electrical impulses, origin of arrhythmias, myocardial ischemia and infarction, the effect of cardiac drugs (especially digitalis and certain antiarrhythmic agents), disturbances in electrolyte balance (especially potassium), evaluation of the function of electronic cardiac pacemakers, atrial and ventricular hypertrophy, pericarditis, and systemic diseases that affect the heart. Although the ECG is one of the most frequently performed examinations in clinical medicine, it is only a laboratory test whose interpretation must always be made in a specific clinical context. A patient with heart disease may have a normal ECG, and a normal individual may have an abnormal ECG.

LEAD SYSTEMS

12-LEAD ECG (I, II, III, aVR, aVL, aVF, V1-6). *Bipolar* standard leads (I, II, and III) record electrical potentials in the frontal plane. Electrodes are applied to the arms and legs; the right leg electrode serves as the ground. Lead I reflects the potential difference between the left and right arms, lead II the potential difference between the left leg and right arm, and lead III the potential difference between the left leg and left arm. The electrical potential recorded from any one extremity is the same regardless of where the electrode is placed on the extremity. Electrodes are usually applied just above the wrists and ankles. If an extremity has been amputated, the electrode can be applied to the stump. In a patient with tremor, an ECG relatively free of muscle "noise" can be obtained by applying the electrodes to the upper portions of the limbs. In exercise and in ambulatory ECG, the electrodes are applied near or on the torso.

A *unipolar* lead records electrical potentials from the small area of tissue underlying the lead, as well as all the electrical events of the cardiac cycle as viewed from that recording site. The unipolar leads most commonly used clinically are the augmented extremity leads, precordial leads, esophageal leads, and intracardiac leads. The frontal plane unipolar leads (aVR, aVL, and aVF) are related to the standard bipolar leads (I, II, and III). The precordial (V) leads record potentials in the horizontal plane without being influenced by potentials from an "indifferent" electrode (Table 33-1). Esophageal leads record atrial and ventricular potentials as seen from the esophagus, and intracardiac leads record potentials from the chamber or site in which they are positioned.

TABLE 33-1. POSITION OF UNIPOLAR PRECORDIAL LEADS ON THE BODY SURFACE

Lead	Precordial Position
V1	Fourth intercostal space, right sternal border
V2	Fourth intercostal space, left sternal border
V3	Equidistant between V2 and V4
V4	Fifth intercostal space, left midclavicular line. All subsequent leads (V5-9) are taken in the same horizontal plane as V4.
V5	Anterior axillary line
V6	Midaxillary line
V7	Posterior axillary line
V8	Posterior scapular line
V9	Left border of the spine
V3R-9R	Right side of the chest in the same location as the left-sided leads V3-9. V2R is therefore the same as V1.

THE CARDIAC VECTOR. The frontal plane vector, or axis, is the sum of the electrical potentials of the cardiac cycle as reflected in the frontal plane of the body. By combining frontal plane bipolar leads I, II, and III with frontal plane unipolar leads aVR, aVL, and aVF, a hexaxial reference system that illustrates all six leads of the frontal plane can be constructed (Fig. 33–16); and the mean QRS, P, and T wave vectors in the frontal plane can be approximated by determining their net magnitudes and direction in any two of the three standard leads. The normal QRS axis lies between 0 and + 110 degrees; superior axis deviation (between − 45 and − 90 degrees) and right axis deviation (between + 110 and ± 180 degrees) are considered abnormal. Leftward deviation of the mean frontal plane QRS axis can occur with advancing age in the absence of clinically overt heart disease. Both the normal frontal plane P wave and T wave axes usually correspond to the normal QRS axis and point in the same general direction. The unipolar precordial leads approximate the electrical potentials (vectors) in the horizontal plane (Fig. 33–17). Combining the electrical signals of frontal and horizontal planes produces a view of the electrical activity of the heart as a three-dimensional structure.

MONITOR LEADS. Although any lead or leads can be used in a specialized clinical area such as a coronary care unit, a modified bipolar chest lead (MCL) is most common. The positive electrode is placed in the V1; position and the negative electrode near the left shoulder; a third electrode is placed at a remote area of the chest and serves as the ground. This "MCL₁" lead is useful to evaluate cardiac rhythm. To monitor the patient for ST and T wave abnormalities due to ischemia, the positive electrode can be placed in any position that has been previously noted to show the abnormality.

THE ELECTROCARDIOGRAPHIC GRID. Electrocardiographic paper is graph paper with horizontal and vertical lines at 1-mm intervals (Fig. 33–18) with a heavier line every 5 mm. Time is measured along the horizontal lines with 1 mm = 0.04 second. Voltage is measured along the vertical lines and is expressed as millimeters (10 mm = 1 mV). In routine practice, the recording speed is 25 mm per second. The usual calibration is a 1-mV signal that

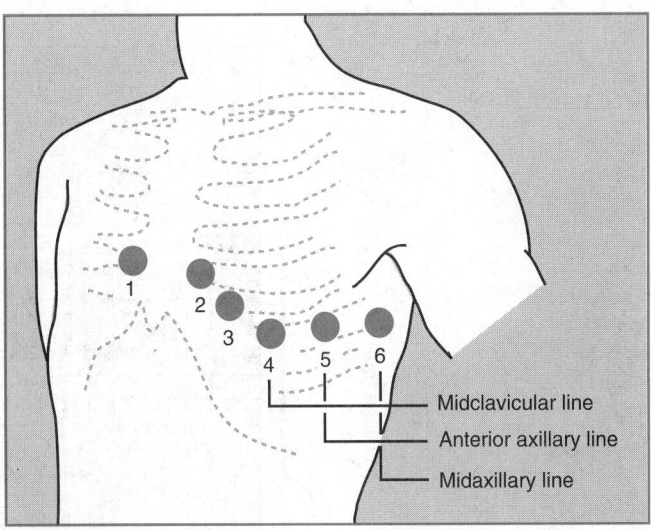

FIGURE 33–17. In a manner similar to determining mean frontal plane axes, to determine horizontal axis draw a perpendicular through the center of any unipolar precordial lead axis. An electrical force oriented in the positive half of the electrical field records a positive (upright) deflection in that lead; a force oriented in the negative half of the electrical field records a negative (downward) deflection in that lead. (Adapted from Goldschlager N, Goldman MJ: Principles of Clinical Electrocardiography. 13th ed. Norwalk, CT, Appleton & Lange, 1989.)

produces a 10-mm deflection. "Double standard," sometimes useful for identifying the atrial rhythm in patients with tachycardia, produces a 20-mm deflection; "half standard," useful when a markedly increased voltage precludes optimal visualization of QRS morphology, produces a 5-mm deflection; and "quarter standard," useful when recording intracardiac electrograms, produces a 2.5-mm deflection. Every ECG should be accompanied by a standard in order to properly interpret the tracing; currently available page-writing ECG machines, which can record multiple leads simultaneously, automatically inscribe the selected standard.

CELLULAR ELECTROPHYSIOLOGY OF THE HEART

CELL DEPOLARIZATION AND REPOLARIZATION. Much of clinical electrocardiography is based upon the behavior of cellular action potentials. Characteristics of transmembrane action potential vary with their site of origin and with different cell types and locations in the heart. Normal cardiac rhythm depends on normal generation of cellular action potential. Abnormally generated cellular action potentials can result in arrhythmias. Delays in conduction of the electrical impulses generated by transmembrane action potentials can result in both rhythm disorders and delayed depolarization of a cardiac chamber.

Four electrophysiologic events are involved in generating the ECG: (1) impulse formation in the primary pacemaker of the heart (usually the sinoatrial [SA] node); (2) impulse transmission through specialized conduction fibers; (3) activation (depolarization) of myocardial tissue; and (4) repolarization (recovery) of the myocardium. The potential difference between the inside and outside of the cell is known as the resting membrane potential, which is determined mainly by the 30:1 intracellular to extracellular potassium gradient across the membrane. The resting potential in most cardiac cells, with the exception of those of the SA and atrioventricular (AV) nodal areas, is − 80 to − 90 mV.

When cell depolarization begins, an abrupt change occurs in membrane permeability to sodium. Sodium and, to a lesser extent, calcium ions enter the cell through their respective channels, resulting in a sharp rise of intracellular potential to about ± 20 mV. This phase of depolarization is designated *phase 0* and reflects the sodium-dependent fast inward current typical of working myocardial cells and Purkinje fibers. The maximum rate of depolarization of ventricular cells is 200 volts per second, and that of atrial cells is 100 to 200 volts per second. Pacemaker cells in the SA and AV nodes are depolarized by a calcium-dependent slow inward current.

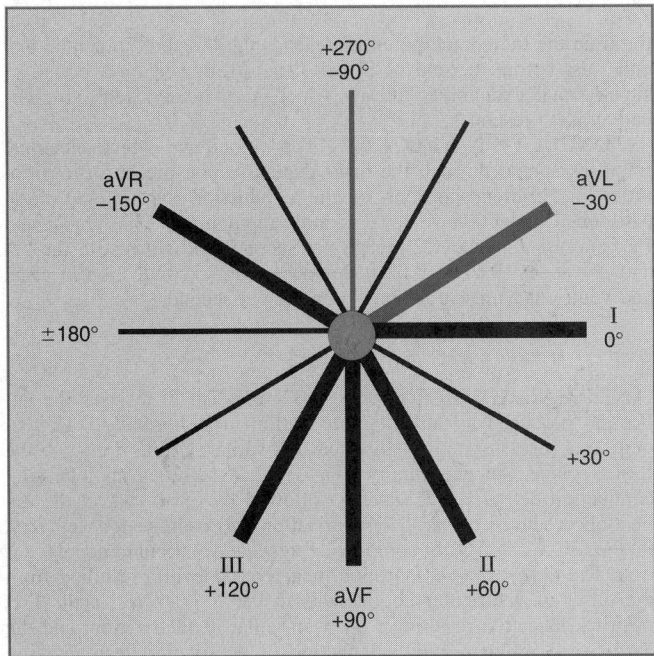

FIGURE 33–16. Hexaxial reference system depicting frontal plane ECG leads. By convention, the positive pole of lead I is designated as O° and the negative pole as ± 180°; the positive pole of aVF as + 90° and the negative pole as + 270° or − 90°; the positive pole of lead II as + 60°; the positive pole of lead III as + 120°; the positive pole of aVR as + 210° or − 150°; and the positive pole of aVL as + 330° or − 30°. If a perpendicular is drawn through the center of a given lead axis, any electrical force (vector) oriented in the positive half of the electrical field records an upright deflection in that lead; any force oriented in the negative half of the electrical field records a downward deflection. (Adapted from Goldschlager N, Goldman MJ: Principles of Clinical Electrocardiography. 13th ed. Norwalk, CT, Appleton & Lange, 1989.)

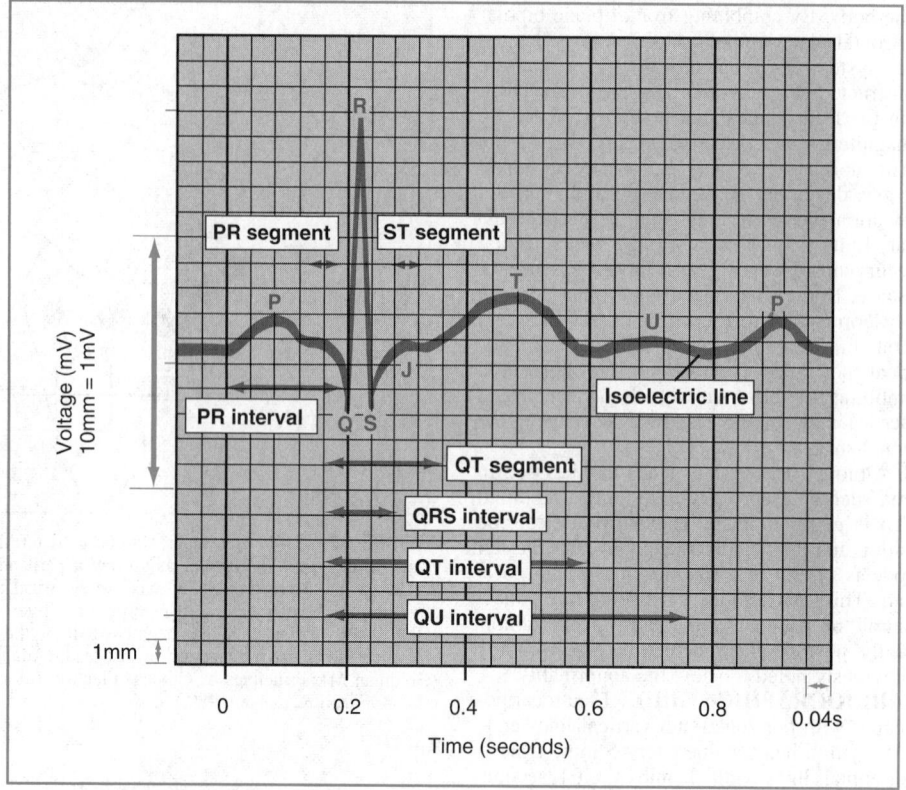

FIGURE 33–18. Schematic illustration of the electrocardiographic grid and normal complexes, intervals, and segments. (Adapted from Goldschlager N, Goldman MJ: Principles of Clinical Electrocardiography. 13th ed. Norwalk, CT, Appleton & Lange, 1989.)

Under some abnormal conditions, such as ischemia, cells whose fast inward sodium current is inhibited are depolarized by slow inward calcium currents.

Following cell depolarization, the potential gradually returns to resting potential. This repolarization process is characterized by *phase 1*—an initial rapid return of intracell potential to 0 mV, largely the result of sodium channels closing; *phase 2*—a plateau resulting from calcium entering slowly into the cell; and *phase 3*—return of the intracell potential to resting level, resulting from potassium extruding out of the cell. At the end of phase 3, the normal resting potential is re-established, and the excess of sodium and a deficit of potassium ions are rectified by a sodium pump. In calcium-dependent cells (SA and AV nodal cells) the phases of repolarization are less well demarcated.

The summation of all phase 0 potentials of atrial myocardial cells results in the P wave inscribed in the surface ECG. Phase 2 corresponds to the PR segment, which follows the P wave, and phase 3 corresponds to the T_a wave of atrial repolarization. The summation of phase 0 potentials of ventricular myocardial cells results in the QRS complex in the surface ECG. Phase 2 corresponds to the ST segment and phase 3 to the T wave.

EXCITATION AND THRESHOLD POTENTIAL. Excitation of a cardiac cell occurs when a stimulus reduces the transmembrane potential to threshold potential (about − 60 mV in atrial and ventricular muscle cells and about − 40 mV in SA and AV nodal cells). If the resting membrane potential is raised toward the level of the threshold potential, a relatively weak stimulus can evoke a response. Conversely, if the resting potential is lowered away from the threshold potential, a relatively stronger stimulus is required to produce a response.

REFRACTORINESS. The refractory period of myocardial cells and tissue consists of the absolute refractory period, during which no stimulus of any intensity can evoke a response, and a relative (effective) refractory period, during which only a strong stimulus can evoke a response. The relative refractory period begins at about the time the membrane potential reaches the threshold potential and ends just before the end of phase 3; it is followed by a period of supernormal excitability, during which a relatively weak stimulus can evoke a response.

CONDUCTION VELOCITY. The velocity at which electrical impulses spread through the heart depends upon the intrinsic properties of different portions of the conduction system and myocardium. Conduction velocity is most rapid in the His bundle and Purkinje system (about 2 meters per second) and slowest in the SA and AV nodes (0.01 to 0.02 meter per second); conduction in atrial and ventricular muscle is about 1 meter per second.

THE NORMAL ELECTROCARDIOGRAM

NORMAL COMPLEXES (Fig. 33–18). The *P wave* is the deflection produced by atrial depolarization; it is normally 0.12 second long or less and is directed leftward and inferiorly in the frontal plane. An abnormally long P wave signifies an interatrial conduction delay. The P wave is followed by the T_a wave, the deflection produced by atrial repolarization and usually not well seen in the ECG. The QRS complex represents ventricular depolarization. The *Q (q) wave* is the initial negative deflection resulting from the onset of ventricular depolarization; the *R (r) wave* is the first positive deflection resulting from ventricular depolarization; and the *S (s) wave* is the negative deflection of ventricular depolarization that follows the first positive (R) wave. A *QS wave* signifies a negative deflection that does not rise above the baseline. An *R' (r')* wave is a second positive deflection and follows an S wave; a negative deflection that follows the r' is termed the s' wave; if an s wave does not follow the initial R wave, the second positive deflection is still termed an R' (r') wave, and the QRS complex is described as an Rr' (rR') complex. Capital letters (Q, R, S) refer to waves over 5 mm; lower case letters (q, r, s) refer to waves under 5 mm. The morphology (and axis) of the QRS complex provides information regarding ventricular hypertrophy, myocardial infarction, and conduction delays in the bundle branches and myocardium. The *T wave* is the deflection produced by ventricular repolarization. The *U wave* is the (usually positive) deflection following the T wave and preceding the subsequent P wave; it is thought to be due to repolarization of the intraventricular (Purkinje) conduction system and is often accentuated in left ventricular hypertrophy and in hypokalemia and hypomagnesemia.

NORMAL INTERVALS. The *RR interval* is the interval between two consecutive R waves. If the ventricular rhythm is regular, this interval in seconds (or fractions of a second) divided into 60 (seconds) equals the heart rate per minute. If the ventricular rhythm is irregular, the number of R waves in a specific number of seconds is counted and converted into number per minute. The *PP interval* is the interval between two consecutive P waves. In regular sinus rhythm, the PP interval is the same as the RR interval. When the ventricular rhythm is irregular or when atrial and ventricular rhythms are regular but their rates are different from each other, the PP interval, measured from the same point on two successive P waves, is computed in the same manner as the ventricular rate. The *PR interval* measures the AV conduction time and includes the time required for atrial depolarization, normal conduction delay in the AV node (approximately 0.07 second), and impulse propagation through the His bundle and bundle branches, to the onset of ventricular depolarization (Fig. 33–19). The normal PR interval is 0.12 to 0.20 second and is related both to heart rate and to prevailing autonomic tone (Table 33–2).

The *QRS interval* represents ventricular depolarization time. The upper limit of normal is 0.11 second. Conduction delay in the bundle branches (Fig. 33–19) or in myocardial tissue results in a prolonged QRS interval. If the conduction delay is in one of the bundle branches, a specific ECG pattern of right or left bundle branch "block" is recorded (Table 33–3; Fig. 33–20).

The *QT interval* represents the duration of electrical systole and varies with heart rate and autonomic nervous system input (see Fig. 33–18). It includes the *QT segment*, which reflects calcium balance: A prolonged QT segment suggests hypocalcemia, whereas a short QT segment indicates hypercalcemia. The *QU interval* represents total ventricular repolarization time, including that of the Purkinje fibers. When the end of the T wave is not distinguished owing to superimposition of a U wave, the *QU interval* is measured in place of the QT interval. An abnormally prolonged QU interval is potentially clinically significant in patients with ischemia, syncope, or ventricular arrhythmias and potassium and magnesium imbalance (Fig. 33–21).

NORMAL SEGMENTS AND JUNCTIONS (Fig. 33–18). The *PR segment* is measured from the end of the P wave to the onset of the QRS complex; it is normally isoelectric but is often depressed in patients with ventricular hypertrophy or chronic pulmonary disease. The *J junction* defines the point at which the QRS complex ends and the ST segment begins.

The *ST segment* begins at the J point and ends at the onset of the T wave. This segment is usually isoelectric but may vary from −0.5 to +2 mm in the precordial leads; it is considered elevated or depressed compared with that portion of the baseline between the end of the T wave and the beginning of the P wave (TP segment). ST segment abnormalities are very important diagnostically in acute myocardial ischemia and infarction and in pericarditis. The *TP segment* defines the portion of the tracing between the end of the T wave and the beginning of the next P wave; at normal heart rates, it is usually isoelectric. At rapid

TABLE 33–2. COMMON CAUSES OF AV CONDUCTION DELAYS

Hypervagotonia (often associated with sinus bradycardia or sinus arrhythmia)
Digitalis
β-Blocking drugs
Some calcium channel–blocking drugs (verapamil, diltiazem)
Coronary artery disease
Lenegre's disease (diffuse fibrosis of the conduction system)
Infiltrative heart disease
Aortic root disease (syphilis, spondylitis)
Calcification of the mitral and/or aortic anulus
Acute infectious disease
Myocarditis

TABLE 33–3. SOME CAUSES OF BUNDLE BRANCH BLOCK PATTERN

Clinically normal individual
Lenegre's disease (idiopathic fibrosis of the conduction tissue)
Lev's disease (calcification of the cardiac skeleton)
Cardiomyopathy
  Dilated
  Hypertrophic (concentric or asymmetric)
  Infiltrative
    Tumor
    Chagas' disease
    Myxedema
    Amyloidosis
Ischemic heart disease
  Acute myocardial infarction
  Remote myocardial infarction
  Coronary artery disease without myocardial infarction
Aortic stenosis
Infective endocarditis with abscesses in the conduction system
Cardiac trauma
Hyperkalemia
Ventricular hypertrophy
Rapid heart rates
Massive pulmonary embolism

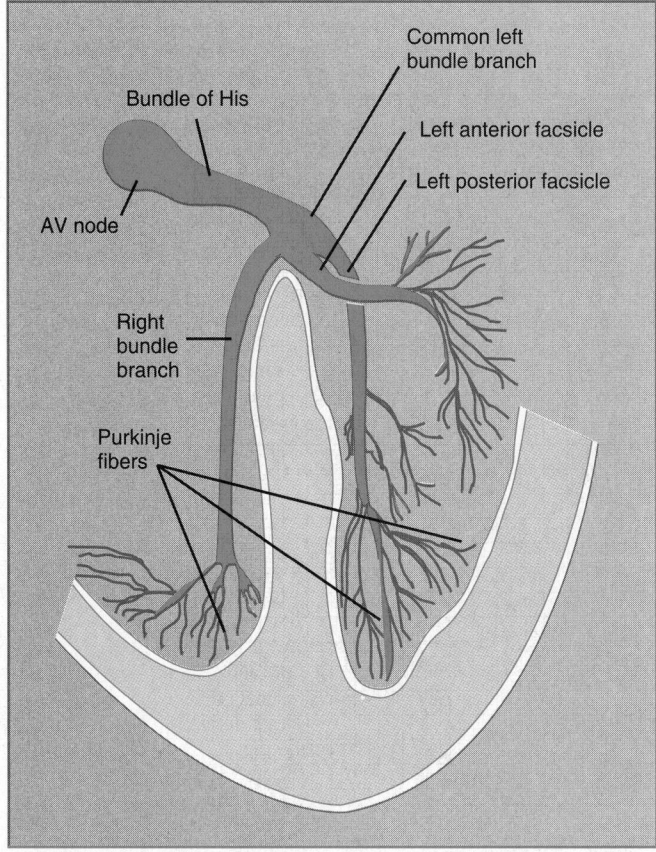

FIGURE 33–19. Schematic illustration of the AV node His-Purkinje conduction system. Sinus impulses are conducted along specialized interatrial conduction pathways (anterior, middle, and posterior internodal tracts) to the AV node, and from there through the His and bundle branches. The anterior and inferior fascicles of the left bundle branch are radiations rather than bundles of conduction tissue. Delay in conduction in the bundle branches does not affect the mean frontal plane QRS axis, whereas delays in the fascicles do. (Adapted from Goldschlager N, Goldman MJ: Principles of Clinical Electrocardiography. 13th ed. Norwalk, CT, Appleton & Lange, 1989.)

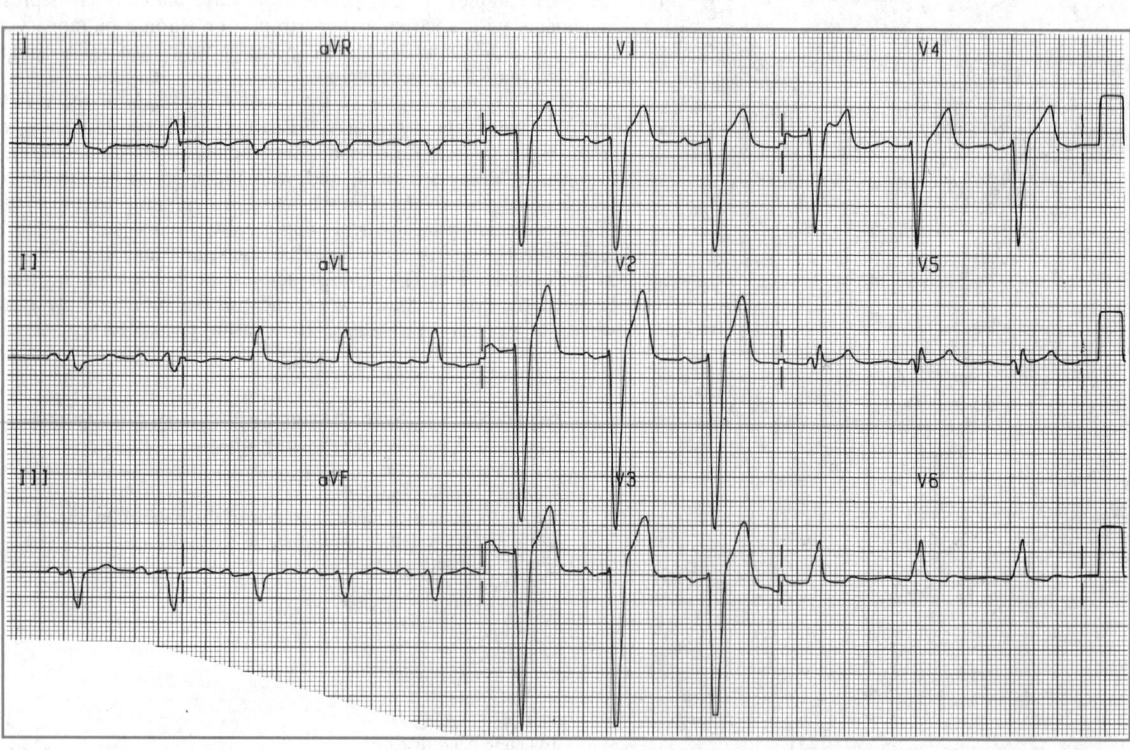

FIGURE 33-20. *A,* 12-lead ECG illustrating a markedly superior mean frontal plane QRS axis and right bundle branch block (deep, wide S wave in leads I, aVL, and V5–6 and rsR′ in V1). The ST segments are downsloping and depressed in leads overlying the region of conduction delay and thus may represent secondary abnormalities. The QU interval is also abnormally prolonged. *B,* 12-lead ECG illustrating left bundle branch block, indicated by the notched broad QRS complex in leads overlying the left ventricle (I, aVL, V5–6).

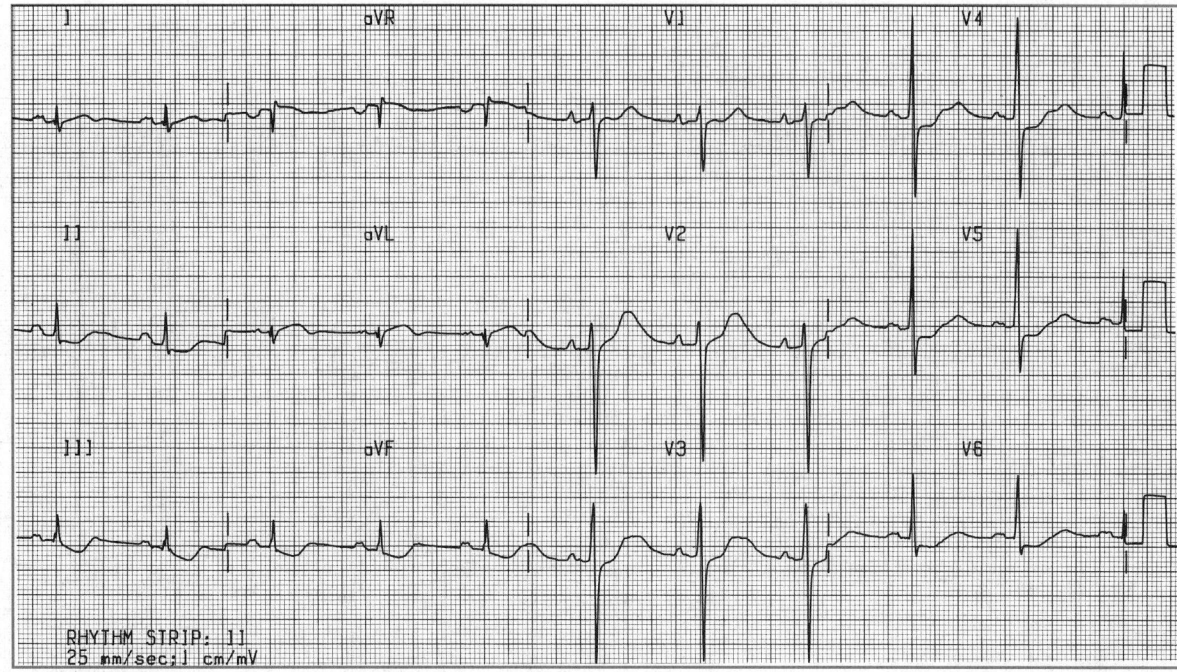

FIGURE 33–21. Sinus rhythm with a P wave duration of 0.13 second, diffusely depressed ST segments, and marked QU prolongation. The U wave is actually taller than the T wave in leads V4–5 and thus is termed a "giant" U wave. The patient had a serum potassium of 1.9 mEq per liter.

heart rates the P wave encroaches on the T wave, eliminating the TP segment.

In addition to the standard 12-lead ECG, recordings are used during exercise or pharmacologic stress testing to document myocardial ischemia, for ambulatory monitoring to detect arrhythmias or ischemic ST segment abnormalities, and for transtelephonic monitoring in patients with cardiac pacemakers or frequent rhythm disturbances. Newer ECG techniques such as body surface mapping (in which instantaneous depolarization and repolarization are plotted) and signal-averaged electrocardiography (in which the QRS complex is filtered to assess the presence of abnormal low-ampli-

tude terminal potentials to predict the risk of an arrhythmic event) are now clinically useful.

The availability of computerized ECG interpretation allows for rapid initial screening, which may be useful in some clinical circumstances; however, physician overread is mandatory to accurately interpret this clinical test.

STEPS IN ANALYZING AN ECG

Identify the atrial rhythm and measure its rate. Establishing the rate allows the atrial rhythm to be characterized as bradycardia (rate < 60 per minute), normal (rate between 60 and 100 per minute), and tachycardia (rate > 100 per minute). If atrial and ventricular rates are different from each other, their rates must be determined separately. Determine the regularity or irregularity of the rate. Irregular rhythms should be further described as totally irregular ("irregularly" irregular as, for example, in atrial fibrillation) or regular with periods of irregularity ("regularly" irregular as, for example, in atrial bigeminy).

Determine the P wave axis, duration, and morphology to provide information about the focus or origin of the atrial rhythm and whether the atria are being depolarized antegradely or retrogradely. If the atrial rhythm is sinus, the P wave morphology and duration can suggest the presence of atrial enlargement or hypertrophy.

Identify the ventricular rate and whether it is regular or irregular. Ascertain whether it is associated with the atrial rhythm and what their relationships are: Is there one P wave for each QRS complex? Do the P waves precede or follow the QRS complexes? What is the PR interval? Is it constant or does it change?

Determine the QRS axis and duration, and describe the QRS morphology. The duration, morphology, and axis of the QRS complexes can help define the origin of the ventricular rhythm. Rhythms originating above the ventricles usually use the normal His-Purkinje system to active ventricular muscle, and the QRS complexes are narrow and normal-appearing unless bundle branch block is present. QRS complexes originating from ventricular tissue, on the other hand, are broad and bizarre. If the ventricles are depolarized using the normal His-Purkinje pathways, the QRS morphology (including voltage), duration, and axis can suggest the presence of left and/or right ventricular hypertrophy (Table 33–4; Fig. 33–22).

Finally, compare the present ECG with previous records.

TABLE 33–4. SENSITIVITY AND SPECIFICITY OF ECG CRITERIA FOR VENTRICULAR HYPERTROPHY

ECG Criterion	Sensitivity (%)	Specificity (%)
Left ventricular hypertrophy		
RaVL + SV3 > 28 mm (men) or		
RaVL + SV3 > 20 mm (women)	42	95
Total QRS voltage > 175 mm	39	94
Romhilt-Estes point score system ≥ 5	37	95
SV1 + RV5 or RV6 > 35 mm	29	93
RV5 or RV6 ≥ 25 mm	19	97
RaVL > 11 mm	18	97
RI + SIII > 25 mm	16	98
Right ventricular hypertrophy		
Limb lead criteria		
R in I ≤ 0.2 mV	40	98
$S_1 S_2 S_3$	44	75
$S_1 Q_3$ pattern	—	92
Precordial lead criteria		
R/S ratio in V1 > 1	28	99
R wave height in V1 > 0.7 mV	30	97
S wave depth in V1 < 0.2 mV	22	100
S wave depth in V5–6 > 0.7 mV	14	98
R/S ratio in V5 or V6 < 1.0	10	100
QR in V1	—	100
Miscellaneous criteria		
QRS axis > + 90 degrees	16	100
P wave amplitude > 0.25 mV in II, III, aVF, V1, or V2	22	99

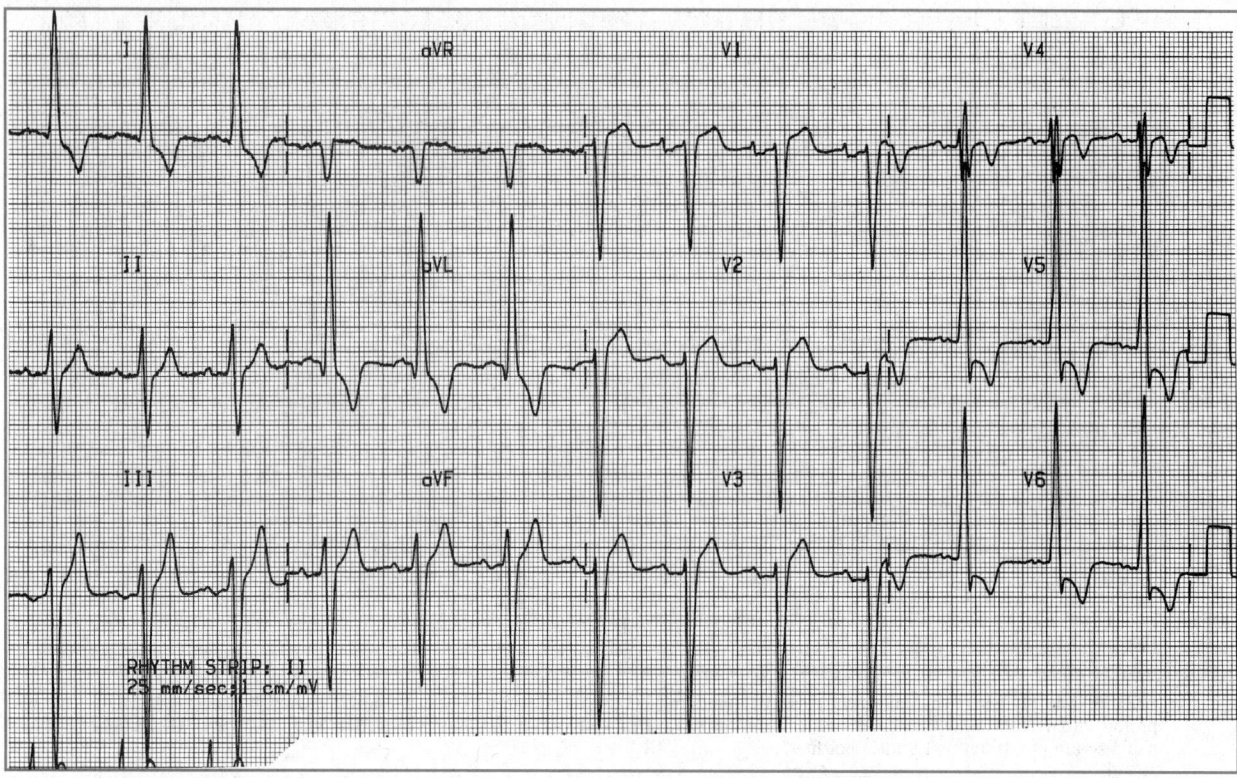

FIGURE 33–22. 12-lead ECG showing left ventricular hypertrophy with accompanying leftward deviation of the mean frontal plane QRS axis to about $-40°$ and depressed downsloping ST-T waves in leads overlying the left ventricle. The P waves are broad and notched, consistent with left atrial enlargement, a common accompaniment of left ventricular hypertrophy.

Chou T-C: Electrocardiography in Clinical Practice. 3rd ed. Philadelphia, WB Saunders, 1991. *A detailed, complete, clinically oriented, well-illustrated, and clearly written textbook.*

Fisch C: Electrocardiography of Arrhythmias. Philadelphia, Lea & Febiger, 1990. *An excellent exposition of cardiac arrhythmias with detailed and clear explanations and ladder diagrams.*

Goldschlager N, Goldman MJ: Principles of Clinical Electrocardiography. 13th ed. Norwalk, CT, Appleton & Lange, 1989. *A good introductory book, well-illustrated and including test tracings.*

33.3 Echocardiography

Richard L. Popp

PULSED REFLECTED ULTRASOUND

Echocardiography includes diagnostic procedures that use ultra-high-frequency sound waves to record the structure of the heart, and the blood flow velocities within the heart, throughout the cardiac cycle. Sound frequencies in the range of 1 to 10 million cycles per second, or megaHertz (MHz), are transmitted from a piezoelectric crystal along a carefully defined path within the thorax. A transducer is placed on the chest wall, and a short burst of ultrasound is transmitted through the chest and into the underlying cardiac structures. The transducer then acts as a sound receiver until the next pulse. At each interface of materials with differing acoustic impedance, part of the sound is reflected or refracted and the remaining sound energy is further transmitted for subsequent acoustic reflection. The acoustic reflecting interfaces oriented perpendicular to the path of sound travel produce reflected sound that is received by the transducer on the chest wall as an "echo" of the transmitted sound. The location of each reflecting surface relative to the transducer can be calculated from the known velocity of sound in tissue and the elapsed time between sending the sound wave and receiving the echo. This series of depth readings is displayed on an oscilloscope for each pulse of sound, as shown in Figure 33–23. The strength of each echo is indicated by the brightness of the signal on the display device. Blood within the heart chambers usually gives signals of low amplitude that are not displayed. This "brightness-modulated" (B-mode) record of the reflecting interfaces is the building block for both two-dimensional (2D) and time-motion (M-mode) echocardiography.

One thousand pulses per second are created with typical instruments used clinically. A high sampling rate facilitates tracking motion of cardiac structures, yet there is usually enough time for the sound to return from even the most distant reflectors before the next pulse. Sequentially directing the sound beam along a given path, usually a pie-shaped sector of a circular plane, for each successive pulse produces a 2D map of the structures underlying the transducer, called a 2D echocardiogram (Fig. 33–23). Clinical instruments sweep the sound beam through an arc of 60 to 90 degrees, by electronic or mechanical means, to create an imaging plane for visualizing a cross-section of the heart. Thus each 2D ultrasonic image is made up of multiple individual lines of sound reflection information. Depending on the basic pulse repetition rate, the time required for a single sound pulse to travel round trip through the thorax, and the number of such pulses per 2D image, 15 to 60 individual 2D image frames per second are available for interpretation. The images usually are presented on a digital scan converter that interpolates data between the scan lines and gives the impression of watching the heart in motion. The standardized examination provides multiple 2D cross-sectional planes through all parts of the heart using specific transducer locations, as shown in Figure 33–24. The dynamic three-dimensional structure of the heart can be understood by assembling these multiple slices mentally or by computer assistance. An electrocardiogram (ECG) is included as a reference signal in these studies.

A single direction of the sound beam, within the 2D image, may be selected for special attention and very high sampling rate. In this case, a given sound beam direction is repeatedly sampled, and the motion along the path of the sound beam is displayed with respect

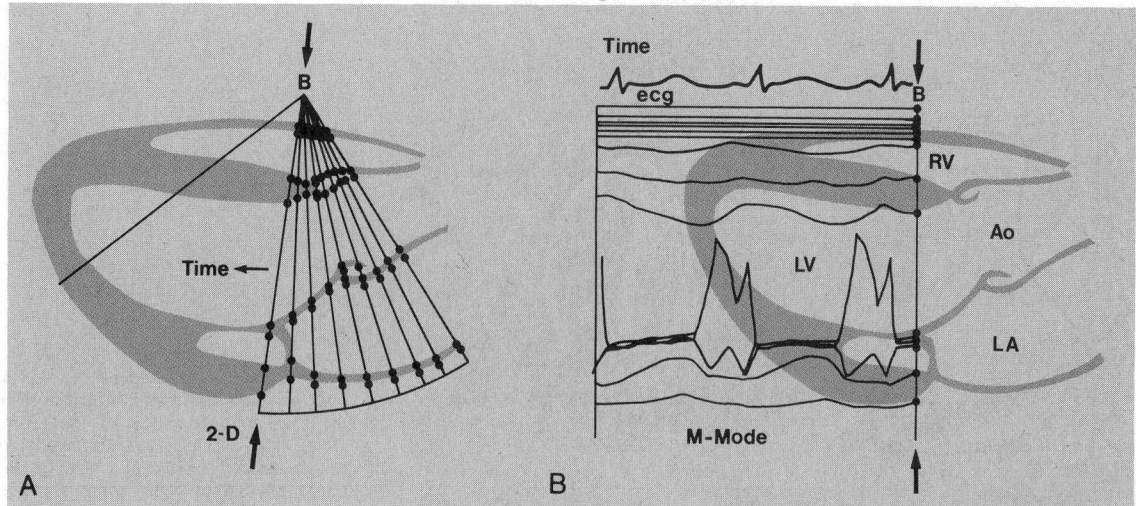

FIGURE 33–23. *A*, A schematic two-dimensional (2D) image of a cross-section of the heart oriented as displayed by echocardiography. The sound transducer is located on the anterior chest wall to the left of the sternum, at B. Sequential sound pulses and the returning echoes from reflecting interfaces are displayed as individual lines *(large arrows)*, with dots of light defining the loci of reflectors. B = Brightness-modulated display. Many such lines, accumulated over 1/60 to 1/15 second, make up a single 2D image. *B*, A schematic time-motion (M-mode) echocardiogram produced by tracing out the location of structures moving during the cardiac cycle under a stationary sound transducer. As in *A*, the transducer on the chest wall creates a B-mode (B, *arrows*) display of sequential pulses and traces the motion pattern of each echo-producing interface. The M- and W-shaped patterns represent the anterior and posterior mitral valve leaflets, respectively. Ao = Aorta; ecg = electrocardiogram; LA = left atrium; LV = left ventricle; RV = right ventricle. (Modified from Popp RL, Rubenson DS, Tucker CR, et al.: Echocardiography: M-mode and two-dimensional methods. Ann Intern Med 93:844, 1980.)

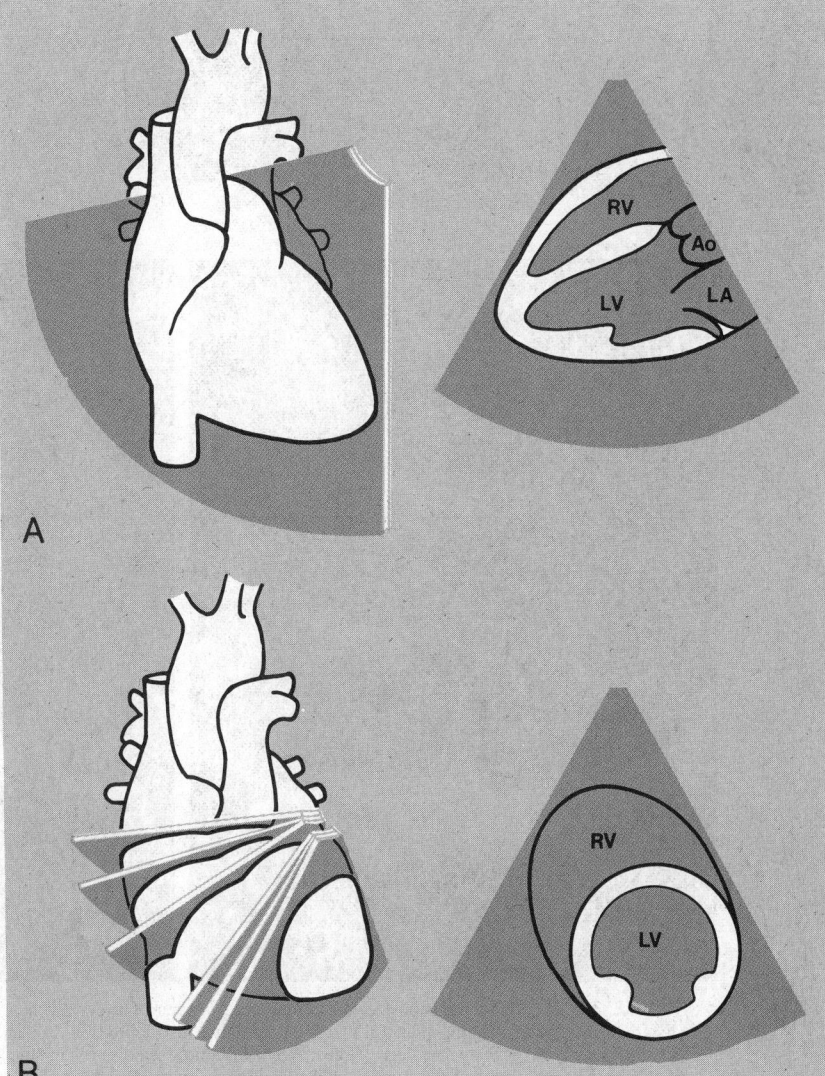

FIGURE 33–24. Schematic illustration of some standard 2D imaging planes used for clinical cardiac studies. *A*, Parasternal transducer position, with the imaging plane oriented parallel to the long axis of the left ventricle (LV) and intersecting a portion of the right ventricular outflow tract (RV), aortic root (Ao), and left atrium (LA). *B*, Transducer position as in *A*, but the imaging planes (six illustrated) are oriented parallel to the left ventricular short axis.

Illustration continued on following page

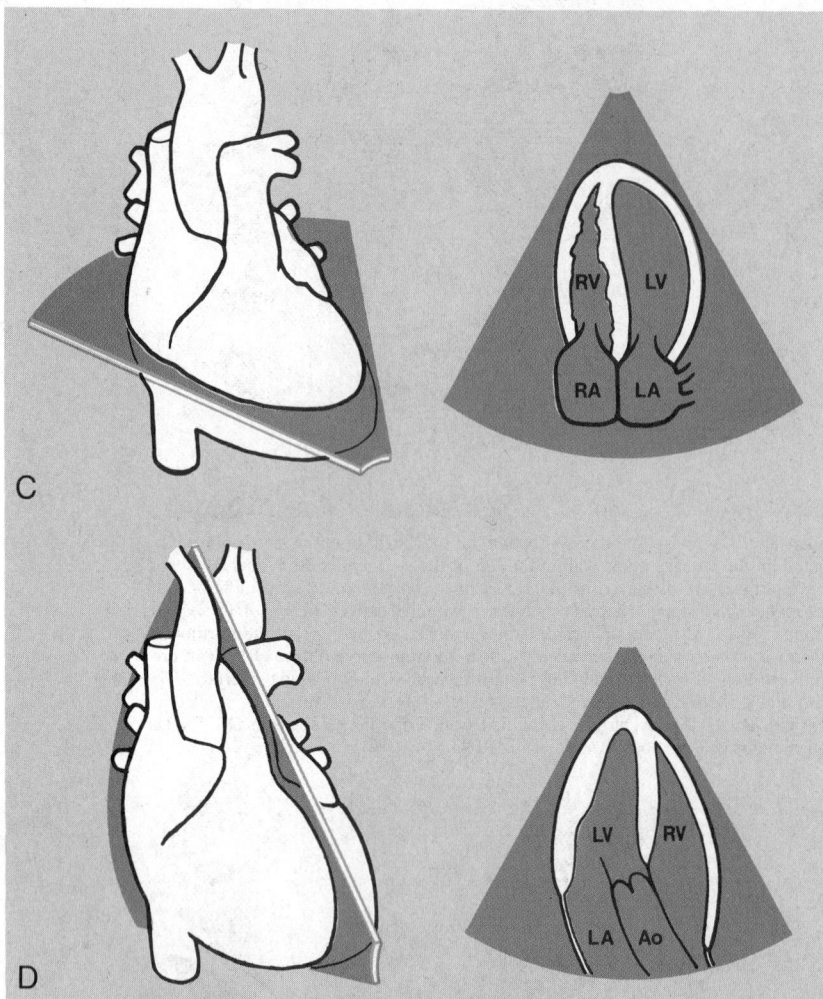

FIGURE 33–24. *Continued. C,* Apical transducer position, with the imaging plane oriented to show the four main chambers of the heart (4-chamber view). The 2D image is displayed relative to the transducer so that the cardiac apex is shown near the transducer. RA = Right atrium, *D,* Transducer position as in *C,* but the imaging plane is oriented parallel to the left ventricular long axis, as in panel *A.* (Redrawn from Popp RL, Fowles RE, Coltart DJ, et al.: Cardiac anatomy viewed systematically with two-dimensional echocardiography. Chest 75:579, 1979.)

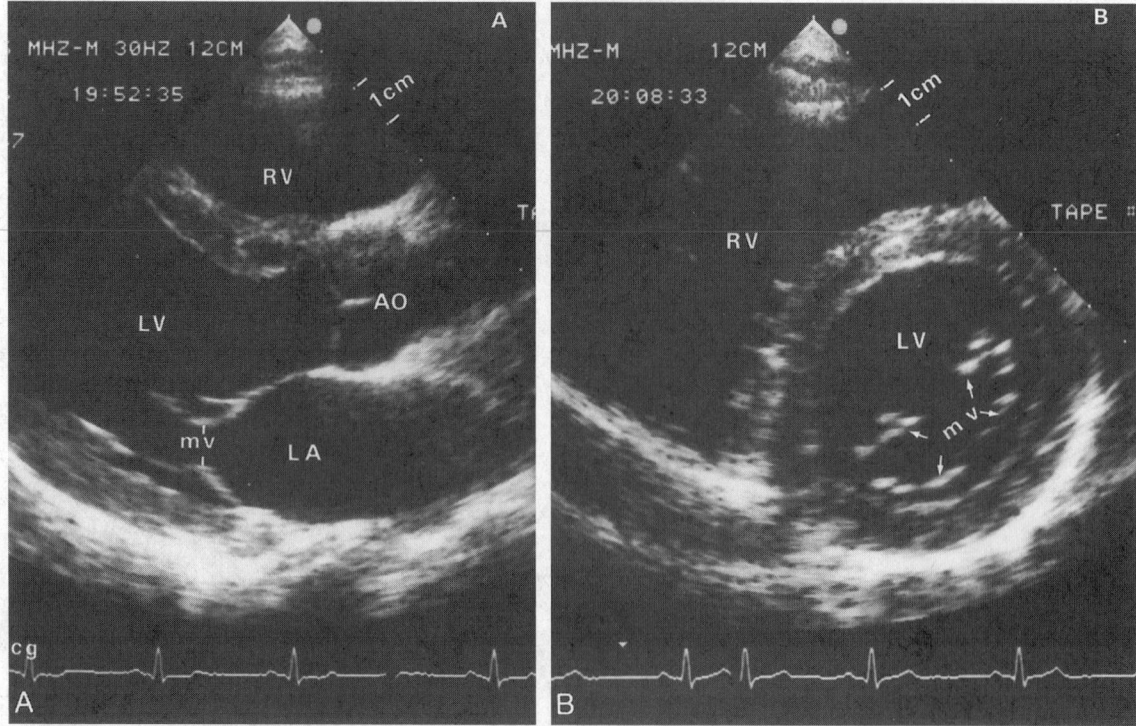

FIGURE 33–25. Two-dimensional echocardiographic images of a normal heart. Panels *A* and *B* were obtained with transducer positions and imaging plane orientations as shown in Figure 33–24*A* and *B,* respectively. Abbreviations as in Figure 33–24. mv = Mitral valve leaflets. (Note depth calibration scale at 1-cm intervals along right margin of each image.) The electrocardiograms (ecg) at the bottom of the panels are interrupted to indicate the timing of each image frame (late diastole in *A,* early diastole in *B*).

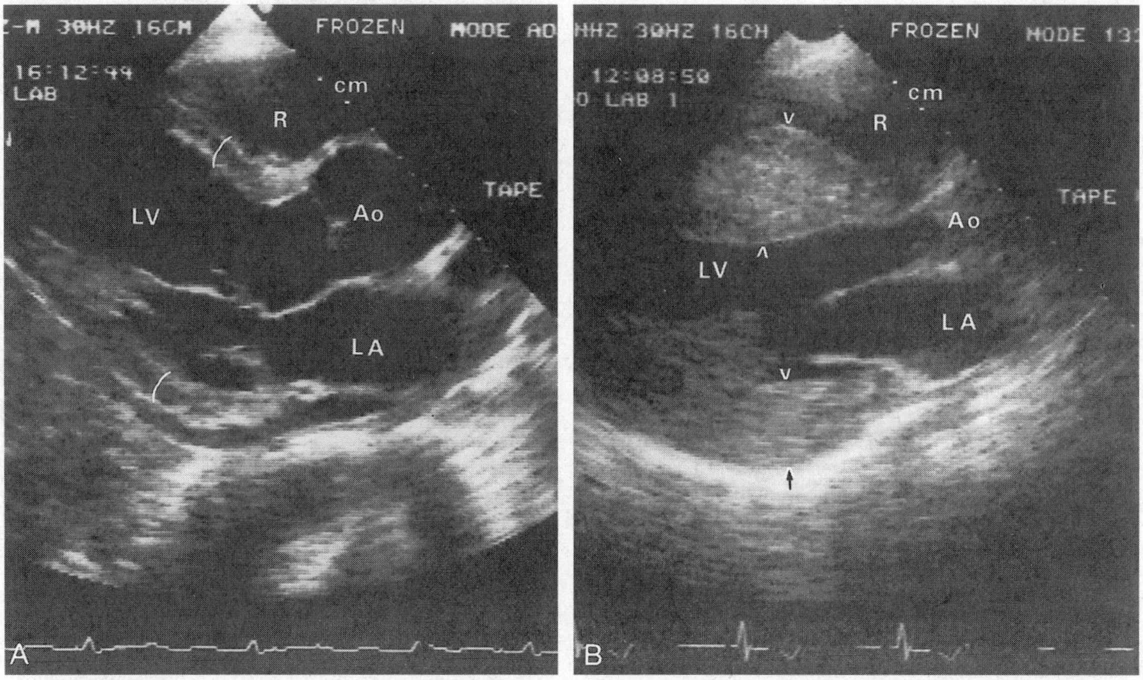

FIGURE 33–26. Two-dimensional echocardiographic images obtained with transducer position and image plane orientation as shown in Figure 33–24A. *A,* The left ventricle (LV) has normal wall thickness (white brackets). A relatively echo-free space posterior to the lower bracket, and extending toward the left atrium (LA), represents a small pericardial effusion. *B,* The LV cavity is small and the walls *(arrowheads)* are massively thickened in a patient with concentric hypertrophic cardiomyopathy. Ao = Aorta; cm = centimeter scale; R = right ventricle.

to time. The usual display is on an oscilloscope or strip chart recorder and is called a time-motion, T-M, or M-mode echocardiogram (right panel, Fig. 33–23). This recording method is especially useful for identifying precise timing of motion of cardiac structures, such as valves, with respect to the ECG, phonocardiogram, or Doppler echocardiogram (to be described below). Historically, the M-mode echocardiogram was the first to be used.

Normal or abnormal patterns of cardiac chamber size and connection, wall thickness, wall motion, valve structure, and valve motion all are well assessed by echocardiographic study (Figs. 33–25 and 33–26). It is the method of choice for visualizing many abnormal structures, such as vegetations of infective endocarditis, intracardiac tumors, mural thrombi, and pericardial fluid.

During acute and chronic ventricular ischemia and acute infarction, the echocardiographic images accurately show the extent of myocardial thinning and segmental akinesis or dyskinesis. Exercise-induced segmental abnormalities may also be observed. The acute complications of myocardial infarction detectable by imaging and Doppler echocardiography include pericardial effusion with or without cardiac tamponade, flail mitral leaflet (ruptured papillary muscle), acute mitral regurgitation of papillary muscle dysfunction, acute ventricular septal defect, myocardial rupture with pseudoaneurysm formation, infarct expansion producing true aneurysm, and right ventricular infarction.

Echocardiographic imaging also may be performed "invasively," as when transesophageal transducers are used or during thoracotomy by directly applying the transducer to the epicardium. These approaches produce superb images owing both to lack of sound scattering in the thorax and to the feasibility of using very high-frequency (5 to 10 MHz) ultrasound, which has high physical resolution but poor soft tissue penetration. Intravenous injections of many fluids, such as physiologic saline solution, contain myriad microbubbles of gas, which may be visualized by echocardiography as they travel through the right side of the heart. The gas does not pass through the pulmonary capillary bed, so if microbubble echoes are seen immediately in the left side of the heart, one may assume

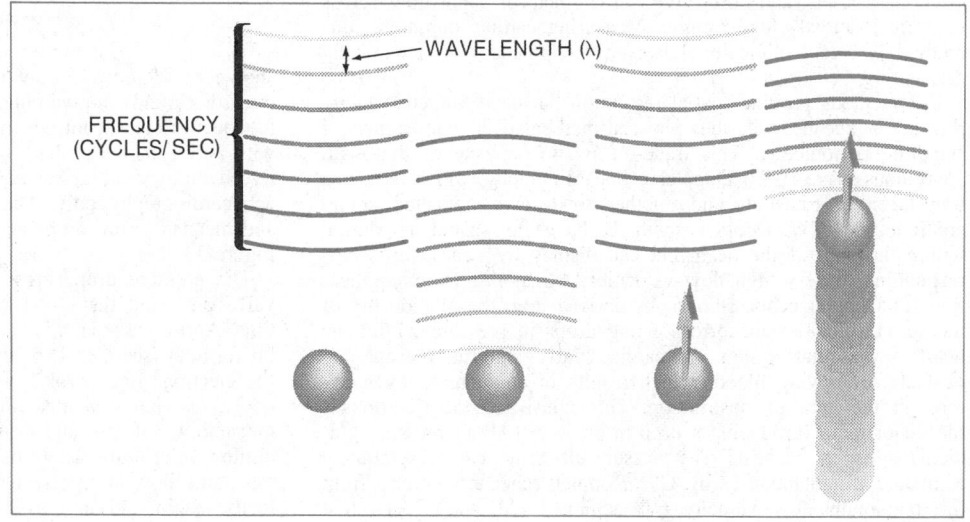

FIGURE 33–27. Schematic diagram of the Doppler principle as applied in echocardiography. From left to right: Sound waves of a given frequency (cycles/sec) and wave length (λ) are transmitted into the chest. Sound reflected from a stationary target has the same frequency as that transmitted. Sound directed toward a moving target interacts with the reflector and alters the frequency of the returning sound by a factor related to the speed of the moving target, the original sound frequency, and the angle of interception of the two.

an intracardiac shunt is present, and a delayed appearance implies an intrapulmonary shunt. Direct intra-aortic or intracoronary injection of various contrast agents has been used in attempts to visualize coronary perfusion areas of the left ventricle and experimentally to assess washout rates with altered coronary flow.

DOPPLER ULTRASOUND

Sound energy is transmitted as a series of compression-rarefaction waves with a given periodicity or wave frequency. Sound reflected from stationary surfaces has the same basic frequency as the transmitted sound, as shown in Figure 33–27. However, if the reflector or reflectors are moving relative to the direction of sound transmissions, the sequential interaction of the compression-rarefaction waves with the reflector results in a change in the frequency of the sound, as shown in Figure 33–27. This frequency shift is the Doppler effect, and it enables one to calculate the velocity of the reflector if one knows the originally transmitted frequency, the received frequency, the speed of sound in the medium (soft tissues), and the angle between the sound beam and the direction of the moving reflectors. The moving column of blood, with its cells and fluctuations in spatial distribution of cells, is the source of the Doppler frequency shift measured by echocardiography. An indicator of the beam direction undergoing Doppler frequency analysis is superimposed on the 2D image to help orientation and facilitate placing the beam in the general direction of flow. Fortunately, the change in frequency obtained with clinical instruments is in the audible range, so one may optimally match the direction of the sound beam with the direction of the blood flow by adjusting the transducer while listening to the signal. A beam-to-flow angle of zero degrees is desirable, since the calculated velocity is a function of the cosine of this angle (cos $0° = 1$), but an angle of up to 20 degrees produces underestimation of velocities of up to only 6%.

Blood flow toward or away from the transducer increases or decreases sound frequency, respectively, so both the velocity and the direction of the blood are measurable. These signals are usually displayed with velocities calculated from received Doppler shifted frequencies plotted versus time. The velocity spectrum is arranged above or below a baseline to convey information on flow direction, as shown in Figures 33–28 and 33–29.

Pulsed wave (PW) Doppler echocardiography is performed with pulses of ultrasound as described above, and frequency analysis is possible for sound returning from any given distance from the transducer. Thus, a signal received during systole from the left atrium and indicating high-velocity flow directed into the atrium from the ventricle signifies mitral regurgitation. This technique has proved especially valuable in locating intracardiac shunts, such as atrial or ventricular septal defects (Fig. 33–28) and patent ductus arteriosus. Since the product of the mean flow velocity (centimeters per second) and cross-sectional flow area (square centimeters) is volumetric flow (cubic centimeters per second), flow within the pulmonary artery or left ventricular outflow tract, or across the tricuspid or mitral valves, can be estimated. Comparing flows across the pulmonary artery and aorta gives an estimate of shunt flow across the septal defects, for example. Measuring cardiac output by this method is useful clinically; however, the procedure is technically demanding.

PW methods provide spatial resolution but have limited velocity resolution because of the physical-mathematical constraints of sampling periodically. This trade-off is the opposite of that with continuous wave (CW) Doppler echocardiography, which uses one transducer to transmit, and another to receive, reflected sound continuously. CW Doppler methods have no spatial resolution within the path of the beam but can display frequency shifts corresponding to very high flow velocities. A major series of applications of Doppler echocardiography derives from the relationship of measured velocities to corresponding drops in pressure within the heart or vascular system. A cardiac valve stenosis presents an obstacle to flowing blood, which results in an increased velocity through the area of obstruction. This convective acceleration is the major factor producing a drop in pressure (ΔP, or pressure gradient) across the stenosis. The pressure difference can be accurately estimated instantaneously by CW Doppler echocardiography from the maximum flow velocity (V) achieved ($\Delta P = 4V^2$), as first

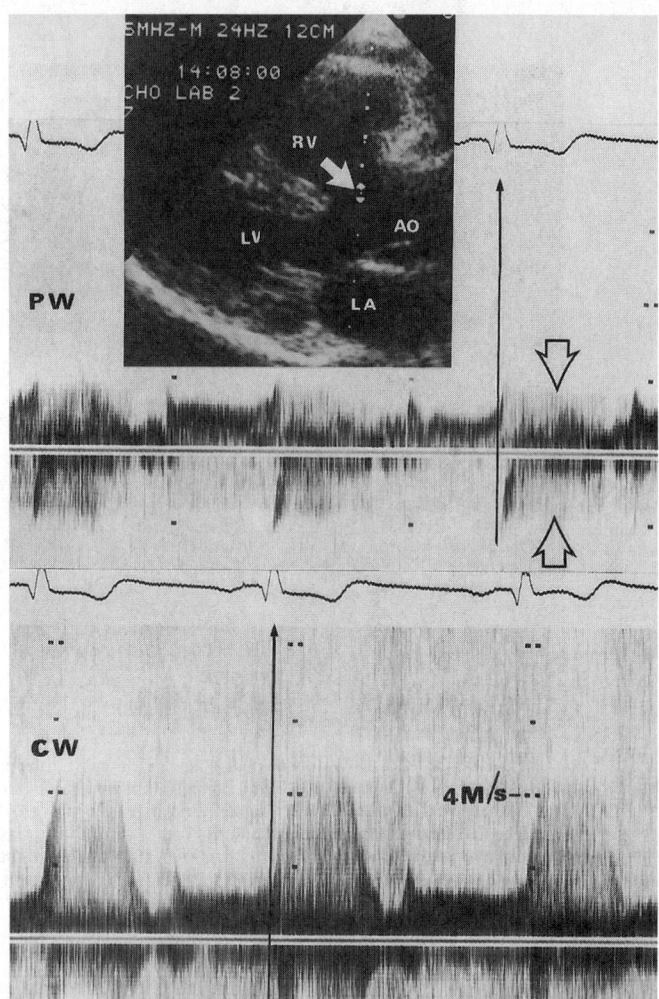

FIGURE 33–28. Methods of displaying a Doppler echocardiographic study in a patient with ventricular septal defect. The black panel above is a 2D image taken with transducer position and image plane orientation as in Figure 33–24A. The white arrow points to the sample volume indicator for pulsed-wave (PW) Doppler ultrasound analysis. This illustration is from a patient with a large defect of the septum between the right ventricle (RV) and left ventricle (LV). The white panels below are spectral displays of the Doppler ultrasound signals in a patient with a small ventricular septal defect. The PW record indicates a frequency shift *(open arrows)* from the area of the sample volume (above), which occurs in systole after the onset of the electrocardiographic QRS *(long arrow)*. The continuous-wave (CW) record indicates high-velocity (>4 M/s) flow somewhere along the dotted line shown above. The systolic pressure difference between the right and left ventricles can be calculated from the CW signal as shown in Figure 33–29. The location of the signal origin is defined by PW, while the CW signal defines high-flow velocity quantitatively but is ambiguous regarding signal locus. Other abbreviations as in Figure 33–23.

shown by Holen and co-workers (1976). The ability to obtain intracardiac and intravascular pressure information noninvasively has been a significant advance in echocardiography. Many patients with aortic or mitral stenosis or both now have adequate preoperative hemodynamic assessment on the basis of clinical features and echocardiography only. The method for calculating instantaneous and mean pressure drops across a stenotic aortic valve is shown in Figure 33–29.

The pressure drop across a stenotic valve depends on both the valve area and the blood volume crossing the valve per unit of time. Aortic valve area is accurately estimated by applying the Gorlin formula (see Ch. 33.6) using Doppler ultrasound-derived values for ejection time, stroke volume, and pressure gradient. Alternatively, one may calculate the flow per beat (see above) from the mean flow velocity and cross-sectional area of the left ventricular outflow tract immediately below the stenotic valve and assume that this same flow is represented by the product of the mean flow velocity within, and the cross-sectional area of, the stenotic valve. The

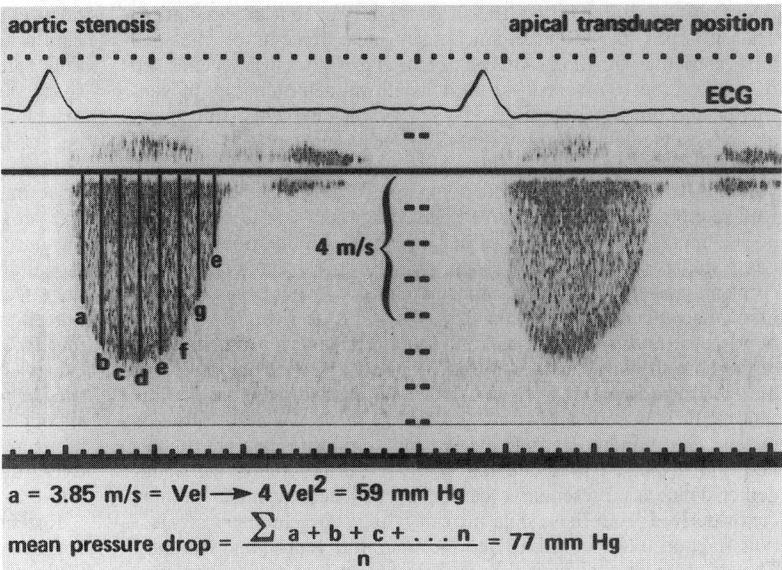

FIGURE 33-29. Continuous-wave Doppler ultrasound recording of aortic outflow velocities from a patient with aortic stenosis. The transducer is at the apex, so flow toward the aorta is registered below the baseline in this spectral display of velocity (M/S) versus time. The systolic signal occurs after each QRS of the electrocardiogram (ECG). Instantaneous (vertical lines a through e) maximum velocities (Vel) are assumed to occur in the narrowest part of the stenosis and to correspond to instantaneous pressure drops across the stenosis. The formulae for calculating the instantaneous and mean pressure drops in mm Hg are given below. n = Number of samples.

$$a = 3.85 \text{ m/s} = \text{Vel} \longrightarrow 4 \text{ Vel}^2 = 59 \text{ mm Hg}$$

$$\text{mean pressure drop} = \frac{\sum a + b + c + \ldots n}{n} = 77 \text{ mm Hg}$$

outflow tract flow velocity, outflow tract area, and aortic valve flow velocity are obtainable, permitting calculation of the aortic valve area. This method is reliable even when aortic regurgitation is present. It is fortuitous that the time required for the pressure drop across the mitral valve to reach one half of the maximum level is directly related to the valve area at virtually all clinically relevant flows. Thus mitral valve area may be accurately calculated from data developed by Holen and colleagues (1977) without needing to measure stroke volume.

Recording the velocity of blood flowing across a narrow orifice between any two chambers or cardiovascular loci permits calculation of the absolute pressure level in one chamber if the pressure in the other chamber is known. For example, the systolic pressure difference between the right ventricle and right atrium can be calculated from the velocities recorded from tricuspid regurgitant flow. The sum of jugular venous or right atrial pressure and the atrioventricular pressure difference is the right ventricular systolic pressure. The prevalence of tricuspid regurgitation detectable by Doppler echocardiography sufficient to perform this calculation ranges from 90% (in normal subjects) to 80% (in patients with cardiomyopathy and pulmonary hypertension). This concept is useful in assessing ventricular pressures in ventricular septal defect and is under investigation for several conditions. Quantitating the pressure gradient across prosthetic valves and assessing the central or perivalvular origin of regurgitant prosthesis leaks noninvasively are major advances because the alternative of catheter placement to get similar information may require trans-septal catheterization of the left side of the heart or direct left ventricluar puncture.

Advancing microprocessor technology for high-speed processing of ultrasonic echoes permits superposition of flow direction and velocity information, obtained from Doppler frequency shift analysis throughout the imaging field, upon the 2D image itself. The velocity data are coded in color and shade for direction and velocity, respectively, and are presented as a color velocity map within the cardiac chambers of the 2D image at frame rates of 12 to 30 per second. This flow velocity tomographic image is similar to angiographic projectional images in that it gives the appearance of blood moving normally or abnormally across the valves and within the chambers (see Color Plates 3A and 3B). Clinical instruments generally provide standard 2D, M-mode, PW, and CW Doppler audio and spectral displays as well as the color-flow velocity images.

Echocardiography has some advantages over competing imaging technologies. These include no risk from ionizing radiation, portability of equipment, noninvasive imaging, high imaging rate, no requirement for contrast injection, and generally low cost for the study. Its disadvantages include poor-quality images in 5 to 20% of various patient groups and lack of complete quantitative data from most clinical laboratories.

Feigenbaum H: Echocardiography. 3rd ed. Philadelphia, Lea & Febiger, 1986. *This encyclopedic text is useful for the neophyte as well as the advanced student. Its strength in discussion of M-Mode and 2D methods is not quite matched in areas discussing Doppler ultrasonography.*

Hatle L, Angelsen B: Doppler Ultrasound in Cardiology. 2nd ed. Philadelphia, Lea & Febiger, 1985. *The most authoritative text on this subject. The chapters on the physics of blood flow and Doppler analysis are excellent. The comprehensive illustrations of pathologic and normal flow velocity patterns are superb. Much of the information included is not published elsewhere.*

Holen J, Aaslid R, Landmark K, et al.: Determination of pressure gradient in mitral stenosis with a non-invasive ultrasound Doppler technique. Acta Med Scand 199:455, 1976. *The classic work describing the clinical use of the relationship between maximum blood velocity detected by Doppler ultrasonography and pressure gradient calculated from the velocity.*

Holen J, Aaslid R, Landmark K, et al.: Determination of effective orifice area in mitral stenosis from non-invasive ultrasound Doppler data and mitral flow rate. Acta Med Scand 201:83, 1977. *Original description of the pressure half-time method for estimation of mitral orifice area using Doppler ultrasonography.*

Popp RL: Echocardiography (Part 1). N Engl J Med 323:101, 1990. Echocardiography (Part 2). N Engl J Med 323:165, 1990. *A recent review of the clinically accepted uses of echocardiography.*

Popp RL, Macovski A: Ultrasonic diagnostic instruments. Science 210:268, 1980. *A more detailed discussion of the instrumentation for producing ultrasonic images than given in this chapter.*

33.4 Nuclear Cardiology
Barry L. Zaret

Nuclear cardiology is based upon the ability of externally placed instruments to detect, define, and quantify radiation emanating from cardiac structures after being injected with a radioisotope. The utility of nuclear procedures for defining pathophysiologic, prognostic, and diagnostic phenomena in cardiac patients has been established. The procedures can be safely repeated and are suitable for both imaging and biodistribution studies. Changes in cardiac function, ventricular volume, myocardial perfusion, viability, and metabolism can be evaluated in appropriate clinical circumstances.

CARDIAC PERFORMANCE

Assessment of global and regional cardiac performance is achieved with radionuclides that remain within the intravascular space during the period of study. Computer technology is critical. Cardiac performance can be assessed in two general ways: during the first pass of the isotope through the central circulation or following its equilibration in the cardiac blood pool. First-pass radionuclide angiocardiography is completed within 30 seconds following intravenous injection of a technetium-99m (^{99m}Tc) compound. There is temporal and anatomic segregation of the radioactive bolus during its first transit through the central circulation. Thus it is possible to make concomitant measurements of right and left ventricular function. Analysis of time-activity curves generated from the respective ventricular regions allows determination of ventricular ejection fraction (Fig. 33–30). Count rates emanating from a cardiac chamber are proportional to the volume of the chamber. In addition, rates of ventricular filling and emptying, ventricular volumes, and quantitative and qualitative assessments of regional wall motion can be made from the same data.

The more widely used approach involves equilibration radionuclide studies. Physiologic signals are introduced that convert the conventional static imaging procedure into a dynamic assessment of cardiac function. To obtain this goal, ^{99m}Tc is bound to the patient's own erythrocytes. The ^{99m}Tc label remains evenly distributed throughout the intravascular blood volume for several hours. Using the electrocardiogram, nuclear data are segregated according to the time of their occurrence within the cardiac cycle. Data are summed over several hundred cardiac cycles, and composite data are quantified and displayed as sequential 10- to 50-msec points, which together define a representative cardiac cycle. The ventricular volume curve derived from these data provides direct measurement of ejection fraction, rates of filling and ejection, and ventricular volumes. The data are also displayed as a series of images that, when projected in cinematic format, provide visual assessment of regional contraction patterns. Computer techniques for regional ejection fraction provide quantification of regional function. With the regional ejection fraction technique, the left ventricular blood pool in the left anterior oblique position is divided into five discrete areas corresponding to septal, apical, and lateral regions. Individual time-activity curves are obtained from each of these regions, thereby providing quantitative regional analysis.

Both first-pass and equilibrium techniques can be used to study cardiac performance under conditions of rest and exercise. Data may be accumulated during supine, semisupine, or upright bicycle exercise. Often critical data emerge only when the patient is evaluated during stress. The normal response to exercise involves an augmentation in the pump function of both ventricles, generally defined as an increase in ejection fraction of at least 5% (in absolute ejection fraction units) and the presence of normal regional wall motion. Abnormal exercise ventricular reserve may be encountered in a variety of conditions involving coronary, myocardial, valvular, and congenital heart disease.

The study of cardiac performance has been particularly useful in coronary artery disease. The ejection fraction is the single best clinical indicator of global ventricular pump performance. The index is of major prognostic importance in patients with coronary artery disease, either immediately following myocardial infarction (MI) or in the chronic or subacute phases of disease. Analysis is based upon radioactivity counts. It does not depend upon geometric assumptions concerning ventricular shape or ventricular volume. In coronary artery disease, particularly following MI, asymmetric contraction patterns are common. In these ischemic ventricles, cavitary shapes frequently cannot be approximated by idealized geometric models. Consequently, in coronary artery disease, ejection fraction is measured most accurately and reproducibly by the nuclear approach. Using portable equipment, it is possible to study cardiac performance at the bedside of the acutely ill. The important negative prognostic impact of functional left ventricular aneurysm forming during acute anterior infarction has been defined. Assessing regional and global function also is an important means of evaluating the effect of thrombolytic therapy for acute infarction.

Abnormalities of ventricular performance are found in approximately 85% of patients with coronary artery disease studied during exercise stress. Myocardial ischemia is reflected in abnormal ventricular reserve. Abnormal responses of the ejection fraction may be encountered in a variety of conditions, but the development of new regional abnormalities of wall motion is quite specific for coronary artery disease. Abnormal exercise performance has important prognostic implications, particularly following infarction.

Recent technical advances now also make it possible to monitor ventricular function in ambulatory patients using a miniaturized detector system employing the principles of equilibrium radionuclide angiocardiography. With this approach, abnormalities of ventricular performance have been noted during routine activities and during mental stress in patients with coronary disease. This new technique, still under active investigation, offers promise for studying silent myocardial ischemia.

Radionuclide assessment of ventricular performance may also be used to evaluate patients with valvular disease at rest or exercise. Resting measurement of cardiac function provides important preoperative prognostic data and may also be of value in defining the physiologic significance of valvular lesions. Assessing performance under hemodynamic stress may help define the advent of irreversible damage in valvular heart disease. This is particularly important in aortic regurgitation, in which irremediable change in left ventricular function is frequently present by the time valve surgery is considered.

Assessing ventricular performance and ventricular volumes is critical to understanding and treating congestive heart failure. Ejection fraction is a key prognostic indicator in this patient group. In addition, an important group of patients with primary diastolic dysfunction (normal systolic function and impaired measures of diastolic filling) has been defined well with nuclear techniques. This group may involve as much as 20 to 40% of patients presenting for evaluation of clinical congestive heart failure. It is highly important to define such patients because routine heart failure therapy is not

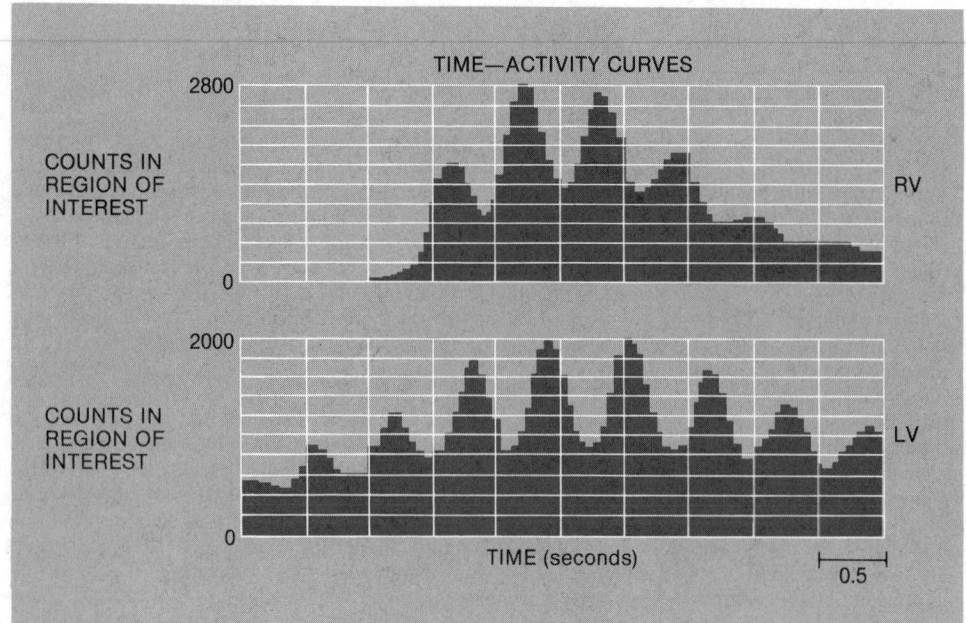

FIGURE 33–30. Right ventricular (RV) and left ventricular (LV) time-activity curves obtained at 20 frames per second with the computerized multicrystal scintillation camera. Analysis of these time-activity curves allows determination of ventricular ejection fraction. (Redrawn from Berger HJ, et al.: Semin Nucl Med 9:275, 1979.)

effective. These patients appear to respond to calcium channel blocking agents.

Radionuclide studies also have been used to evaluate myocardial function in patients with lung disease in which the major hemodynamic burden falls on the right ventricle. Right ventricular performance can probably be evaluated best with the first-pass technique. Abnormalities in right ventricular performance have been noted at rest and during exercise in patients with chronic obstructive pulmonary disease. Pharmacologic interventions may modify abnormal right ventricular performance.

These techniques also have been used for long-term studies assessing cardiac therapy. A prototype example has been the serial assessment of ventricular function in patients receiving the antineoplastic agent doxorubicin. Use of this agent has been limited by the frequent development of a drug-induced cardiomyopathy. Serial measurement of cardiac ejection fraction during the course of therapy has led to a set of dosage guidelines that help avert cardiotoxicity.

MYOCARDIAL PERFUSION IMAGING

Myocardial perfusion imaging uses radionuclides that traverse the myocardial capillary system and enter the myocardial cell. This is the most common nuclear cardiology procedure. The radionuclide currently employed most frequently for these studies is thallium-201 (^{201}Tl). This tracer is considered a potassium analogue, because its distribution generally mirrors that of intracellular potassium. Thallium-201 is produced in the cyclotron and has a physical half-life of approximately 72 hours. After intravenous injection it is rapidly extracted and distributed within the myocardium according to regional myocardial blood flow and regional cellular viability. Recently, ^{99m}Tc-sestamibi has become available as an alternative perfusion agent. This offers several advantages over ^{201}Tl. These include better imaging characteristics, ability to administer a higher dose, better suitability for tomographic studies, and biologic properties that involve lack of major washout following administration. This latter property allows for delayed imaging following administration, particularly in the acute situation, thereby allowing definition of risk zones in acute ischemic syndromes. The ability to administer a ^{99m}Tc bolus intravenously also allows for measurement of ejection fraction prior to perfusion imaging. The isonitrile images may also be electrocardiogram (ECG) gated, allowing for better image resolution as well as potential quantification of regional function. Thus, function and perfusion can be evaluated from the same study.

At rest, the normal myocardial perfusion image demonstrates homogeneous uptake in the left ventricular wall with a central area of decreased activity corresponding to the left ventricular cavity. In approximately 20% of normal persons, a region of decreased uptake at the cardiac apex corresponds to a normal relative apical thinning. Abnormal image patterns of decreased myocardial perfusion demonstrate a region of relatively decreased radionuclide uptake. Images are obtained in multiple positions. The normal right ventricle is not visualized at rest because it has a smaller mass than the left ventricle.

In the resting state, abnormalities usually represent either acute or remote MI. However, perfusion defects at rest may also be seen in some patients with severe obstructive coronary disease in the absence of clinical evidence of acute ischemia. Defects are noted with high sensitivity during the early hours of acute MI. Within the first 6 hours, virtually all infarcts may be identified. After 24 hours, sensitivity falls to 80 to 90%.

In most patients with coronary artery disease without previous infarction, myocardial perfusion patterns appear normal at rest. This is to be expected because coronary blood flow is relatively uniform at rest, even in the presence of relatively severe coronary obstruction. The major physiologic abnormality in coronary disease is diminished coronary vascular reserve. Therefore, to detect perfusion abnormalities in coronary disease it is necessary to study patients under conditions of increased myocardial blood flow. Exercise is employed frequently as an appropriate stress. Either ^{201}Tl or ^{99m}Tc-sestamibi is injected at peak exercise, and imaging is begun shortly after injection. The radioisotopes can be injected during the period of maximal heterogeneity of regional myocardial blood flow, and their distribution reflects this heterogeneity. Comparing images obtained immediately following exercise with those obtained following a redistribution phase 2 to 4 hours after exercise for ^{201}Tl or a

separate rest study for ^{99m}Tc-sestamibi allows definition of transiently ischemic zones. Defects present on exercise but not later are most consistent with transient ischemia; defects that are unchanged are most consistent with previous infarction and scar; and defects that are present at redistribution but are markedly increased during exercise are most consistent with transient ischemia superimposed upon the scar. Recently, it has been recognized that for ^{201}Tl delayed imaging may be important for detecting viable yet ischemic myocardium that appears as a fixed defect on the initial stress and redistribution images. For this purpose a second injection of radioisotope at rest has been used. In this manner, up to 40% of fixed ^{201}Tl defects have been demonstrated to have some reversibility. The overall sensitivity of this technique for detecting significant ischemic disease is approximately 80%. The specificity of the technique is excellent. This technique is of greatest value diagnostically in patients with equivocal exercise ECG's, abnormal baseline ECG's, or suspected false-positive or false-negative conventional exercise tests. Both imaging with the patient at rest and exercise/redistribution studies have been valuable in evaluating thrombolysis and reperfusion. Exercise studies also are of major value in assessing prognosis following infarction in stable coronary disease and in evaluating patients after coronary angioplasty. In addition to the magnitude of the perfusion defect, increased lung uptake has been demonstrated to be a potent prognostic index in coronary disease patients (Fig. 33–31). Generally, ^{201}Tl and ^{99m}Tc-sestamibi have comparable diagnostic sensitivity and specificity. ^{201}Tl is the preferred agent for assessing myocardial viability.

An alternative means of stress perfusion imaging involves using pharmacologic stress employing either dipyridimole, adenosine, or dobutamine. Thallium myocardial distributions following dipyridamole provide data comparable to those noted with exercise. How-

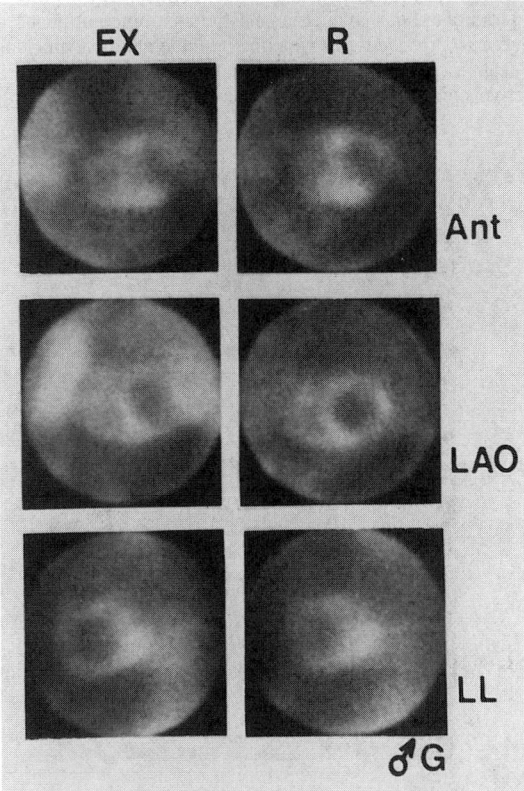

FIGURE 33–31. Planar thallium perfusion images obtained during exercise (EX, left column) and redistribution (R, right column) in a patient with a previous myocardial infarction. Anterior images (Ant) are shown in the upper panel, left anterior oblique (LAO) in the middle column, and left lateral position images (LL) in the lower column. A large, relatively fixed perfusion defect involves the anterior and lateral walls in both the exercise and redistribution studies. A partially reversible defect involves the inferolateral wall seen in the LAO view, with some redistribution noted. The marked lung uptake of thallium indicates a poor prognosis.

ever, with pharmacologic stress, evaluation is based upon differences in flow without necessarily implying ischemia; whereas with exercise, evaluation is based upon heterogeneity of flow, generally associated with ischemia. These studies are particularly valuable in patients unable to exercise. This type of study has been of value in identifying myocardial ischemia in peripheral vascular disease patients undergoing preoperative cardiac evaluation.

Planar imaging is now increasingly quantitative. Computer techniques provide objective definition of the presence and extent of defects as well as quantification of regional tracer washout kinetics. Contemporary evaluation of thallium imaging data should include quantitative interpretation of visual data.

Single photon emission computed tomography (SPECT) studies are currently employed widely (Fig. 33–32). In comparative studies with planar imaging, SPECT has been shown to have similar diagnostic accuracy. A major current use involves definition of multiple vascular bed involvement in coronary disease. SPECT is the preferred modality for defining specific vascular bed involvement.

INFARCT-AVID IMAGING

An additional radionuclide approach defines acute MI and regions of acute myocardial necrosis. This is performed with "infarct-avid" radiotracers, which bind selectively to regions of acute infarction. The current agents for this procedure are ^{99m}Tc stannous pyrophosphate clinically and indium-III antimyosin antibody imaging, which is still considered experimental. This general imaging approach is the least used nuclear cardiology procedure because competing clinical and nuclear techniques provide more timely and logistically feasible data. Acute infarcts are visualized as regions of increased radionuclide uptake.

POSITRON EMISSION TOMOGRAPHY (PET)

This technique involves imaging and quantifying the intracardiac distribution of positron-emitting radionuclides. By virtue of the types of radionuclides available and the instrumentation used, this technique has provided new insight into metabolism and coronary flow. Because carbon-11 is a positron emitter, a variety of biologically active compounds can be radiolabeled and used for imaging.

These include fatty acids, metabolites, receptor ligands, and neurotransmitters.

There has been great interest recently in PET studies of myocardial metabolism and perfusion. Of most immediate clinical impact has been the demonstration that increased regional glucose accumulation in areas that are hypoperfused represent viable tissue with a substantial likelihood of improved function with revascularization. This has been demonstrated using fluorodeoxygluocse as the radiopharmaceutical. This "glucose-perfusion mismatch" offers major opportunities for evaluating stunned and hibernating myocardium in ischemic heart disease as well as ischemic cardiomyopathy. PET studies of this type represent the current gold standard for assessing myocardial viability. Recent additional comparative studies have also involved radiolabeled acetate, palmitate, and glucose. Finally, tomographic perfusion imaging involving positron-emitting rubidium, water, and nitrogen-labeled ammonia has also shown promise. Because PET studies can be precisely quantified and corrected for attenuation, PET can be used to absolutely quantify regional myocardial blood flow and perfusion.

Zaret BL, Beller GA (eds.): Nuclear Cardiology: State of the Art and Future Directions. St. Louis, CV Mosby, 1993. *An up-to-date multiauthored book covering the state of the art of nuclear cardiology with respect to individual techniques, clinical applicability, current research, and future directions. The book contains 31 individual chapters.*

Zaret BL, Wackers FJT: Nuclear cardiology: Medical progress. N Engl J Med 329:775–783; 855–863, 1993. *An up-to-date review of clinical nuclear cardiology containing 179 references.*

Zaret BL, Wackers FJT, Soufer R: Nuclear cardiology. *In* Braunwald E (ed): Heart Disease: A Textbook of Cardiovascular Medicine. 4th ed. Philadelphia, WB Saunders, 1992, p 276. *A comprehensive review of nuclear cardiology, including both clinical and experimental aspects with 290 references.*

33.5 Cardiovascular Magnetic Resonance Imaging
Gerald G. Blackwell

Magnetic resonance imaging (MRI) methods are being increasingly applied in the care of patients with cardiovascular diseases. Using this technology, clinically useful information can be obtained regarding morphology and function of the cardiac chambers as well as the integrity of arterial and venous conduits throughout the body. Several primary indications for cardiovascular MRI have been established (Table 33–5). Cardiovascular MRI can also be used as an alternative technique to provide diagnostic information when other imaging modalities are typically attempted first (Table 33–6). This section of the chapter introduces some fundamental magnetic resonance (MR) principles and highlights the use of MRI for cardiovascular applications, a rapidly advancing, powerful, noninvasive diagnostic procedure that is expected to be widely used.

BASIC PRINCIPLES OF MRI

Medical MR images are tomographic representations of the distribution of hydrogen nuclei within the body. The production of these high-resolution images results from an elegant adaptation of the basic physical principle of nuclear magnetic resonance (NMR). Magnetism arises as a result of the motion of a charged particle. The hydrogen nucleus, which is ubiquitous in the human body primarily in the form of water (H_2O), both spins and has an electrical

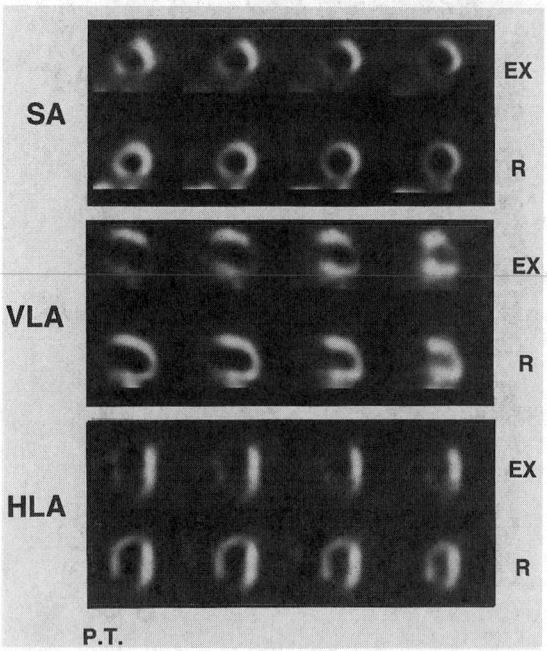

FIGURE 33–32. Technetium-99m-sestamibi SPECT study in a patient with myocardial ischemia. The short axis (SA) images are shown in the upper panels, the vertical long axis (VLA) in the middle panels, and the horizontal long axis (HLA) in the lower panels. For each orientation the exercise (EX) is shown above and the comparable rest (R) is shown immediately below. The study demonstrates a large reversible defect involving the entire septum in the SA views, the anterior apical wall in the VLA views, and the septum and apex in the HLA views. This defect is totally reversible, indicating the presence of ischemia alone.

TABLE 33–5. ESTABLISHED INDICATIONS FOR CARDIOVASCULAR MRI

Diagnosis and follow-up of stable patients with thoracic aortic disease (aneurysm, dissection, coarctation)
Diagnosis of abnormal pericardial thickening (constrictive pericardial disease)
Assessment of complex congenital heart disease
Assessment of known or suspected paracardiac masses
Assessment of angiographically occult runoff vessels in patients with lower extremity peripheral vascular disease

TABLE 33-6. APPLICATIONS OF CARDIOVASCULAR MRI AS AN ALTERNATIVE DIAGNOSTIC MODALITY

Assessment of global and regional biventricular function
Diagnosis and quantitation of valvular regurgitation and stenosis
Assessment of complicated pericardial effusion
Assessment of abdominal aortic aneurysm
Noninvasive cerebral and peripheral vascular angiography

charge associated with its isolated proton. Accordingly, it creates a microscopic magnetic field and can be thought of as resembling a tiny bar magnet (Fig. 33-33). In the absence of an external magnetic field, the body has no net magnetic moment because billions of atoms are randomly aligned in space and the charges cancel each other out. However, in the presence of a strong external magnetic field, the nuclei are constrained to lie in a preferred orientation and a detectable net magnetic moment is produced (Fig. 33-34). It is important to note that other atomic nuclei (those with an odd number of protons, neutrons, or both) are NMR "visible." However, hydrogen is both the most abundant and most NMR-sensitive nuclear species and therefore best suited for medical imaging.

Most commercial MRI instruments are composed of a large superconducting electromagnet that produces a homogeneous main magnetic field, a smaller set of magnets·(gradient coils) that produce local changes in the main magnetic field, a source for supplying and detecting radiofrequency energy (body and surface coils), and a powerful computer that integrates data collection and display. The challenge of MRI is to localize the hydrogen nuclei in three-dimensional (3D) space. All hydrogen nuclei spin at a specific frequency, which is given by the Larmor equation:

Larmor frequency = magnetic field strength × gyromagnetic ratio

where the gyromagnetic ratio is a physical constant for a given nuclear species. From this equation it can be appreciated that all hydrogen nuclei exposed to a certain external magnetic field spin at precisely the same frequency. Similarly, hydrogen nuclei exposed to a different external magnetic field spin at a different frequency. To identify the unique location of these atoms, it is necessary to create minor changes in the main external magnetic field (Fig. 33-35). These magnetic field "gradients" are accomplished in 3D by applying brief bursts of electromagnetic energy through the specialized gradient coils. In addition to applying these gradients, the selected imaging plane is bombarded with radiofrequency energy at the unique Larmor frequency for hydrogen atoms. Only hydrogen atoms that lie within the selected imaging plane can absorb the radiofrequency energy. The radiofrequency pulse is applied for a brief duration, after which the excited nuclei within the imaging plane relax back to an equilibrium state. In the process of relaxation, excited nuclei return absorbed radiofrequency energy to the environment. These emissions are detected by specialized coils and are faithfully recorded in an imaging matrix. Complex mathematical manipulations are performed on the acquired matrix and high-resolution MR images are produced. It is important to note that the radiofrequency energy used in MRI is nonionizing and devoid of known adverse biologic effects.

IMAGE APPEARANCE IN MRI

Image appearance in conventional radiographic imaging techniques is almost exclusively determined by tissue density. In MRI, hydrogen density is an important determinant of signal intensity, but image appearance is influenced by additional factors (Table 33-7). Blood flow within and through the imaging plane is a major source of MR image contrast. Tissues of varying composition (e.g., muscle, fat, blood) have different intrinsic magnetization properties (T1 and T2) and produce signal of varying intensity. Acquisition parameters such as how the magnetic field gradients are applied and the power and timing of the radiofrequency pulses (pulse sequences) also make a major impact on image contrast and can be selected by the operator.

Two basic acquisition sequences have been used in cardiovascular MRI—the spin-echo sequence and the gradient-echo sequence. The spin-echo sequence is often used to produce images with high spatial resolution which highlight morphology. With spin-echo imaging the blood pool typically appears black. The gradient-echo pulse sequence is used to produce multiphase images with excellent temporal resolution. With gradient-echo imaging the blood pool appears white and, when displayed in an endless loop cine format, closely resembles invasive contrast angiograms. Accordingly, this technique is often referred to as cine MRI. New and innovative

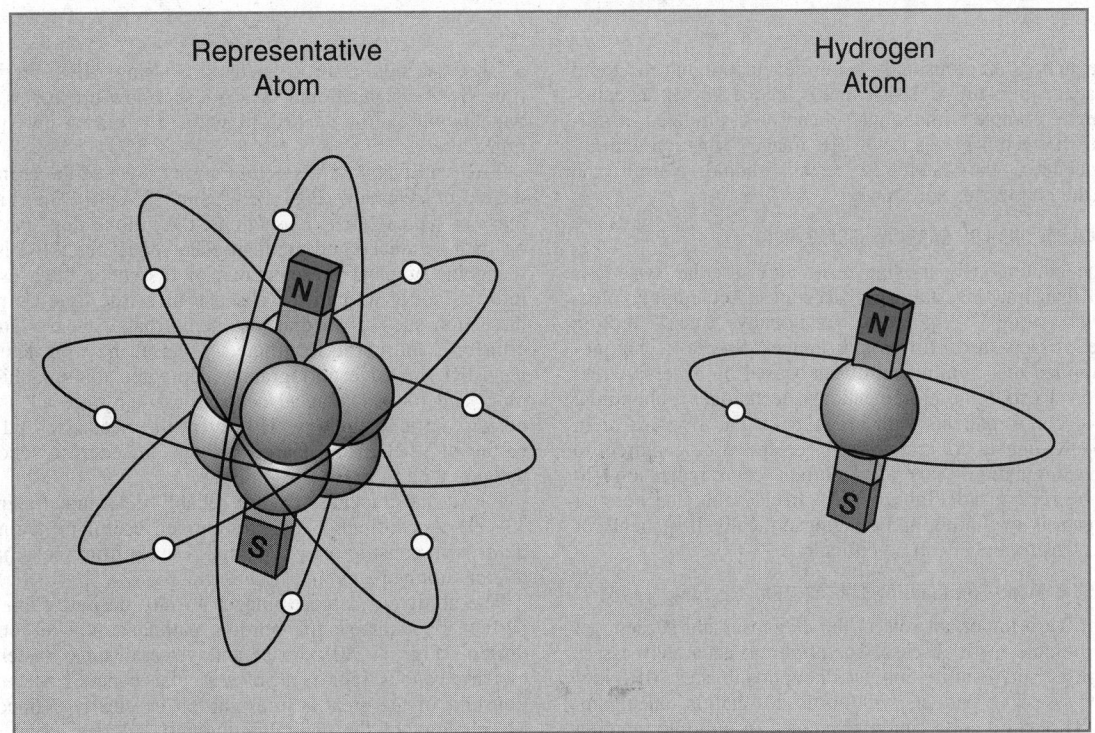

FIGURE 33-33. Spinning atomic nuclei which possess a net charge create microscopic magnetic fields and can be thought of as resembling tiny bar magnets having a north (N) and south (S) pole. Medical MRI exploits the magnetic properties of the abundant hydrogen nucleus. (From Blackwell G, Cranney GB, Pohost G: MRI: Cardiovascular System. New York, Gower Medical Publishing, 1992.)

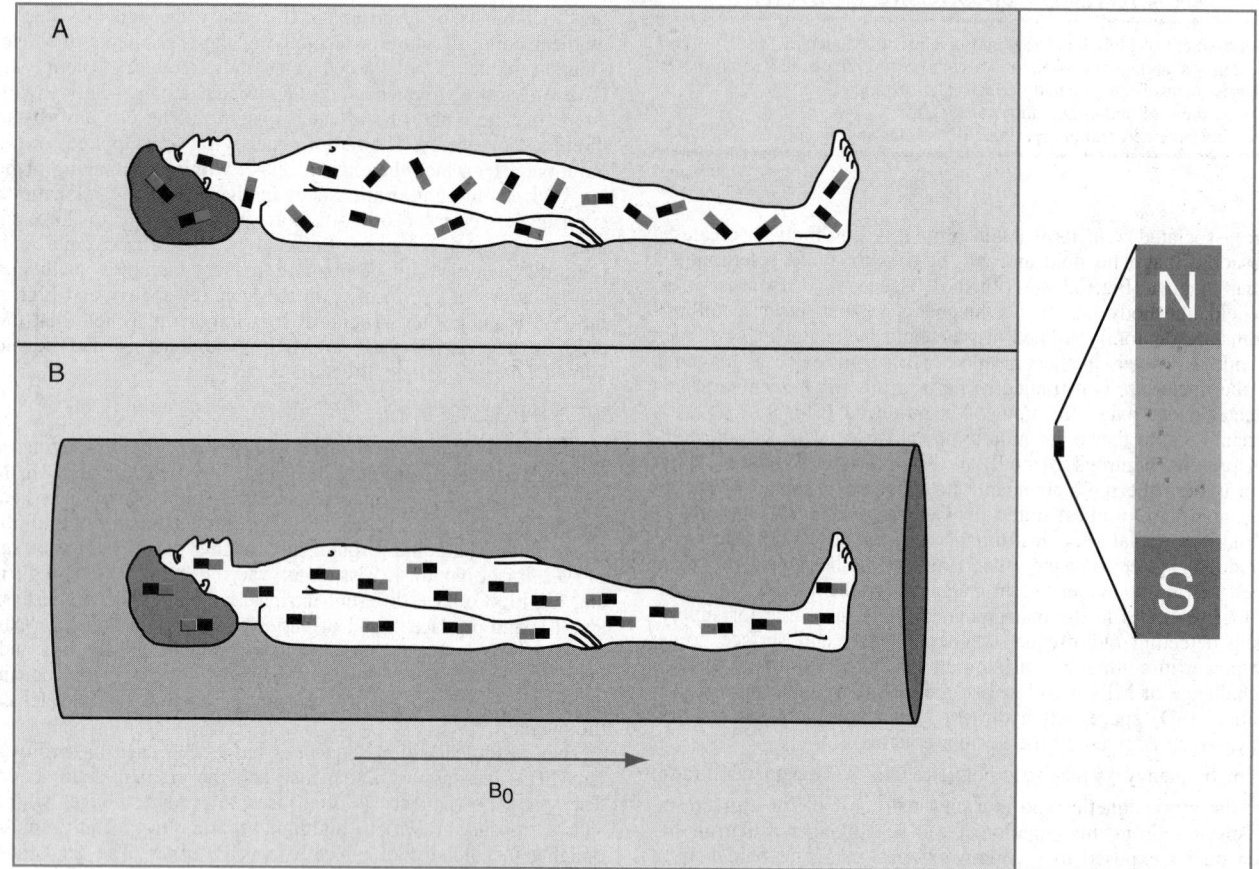

FIGURE 33–34. *A,* In the absence of an external magnetic field, hydrogen nuclei within the body, here depicted as tiny bar magnets, are randomly aligned and produce no net charge. *B,* In the presence of the external magnetic field of an MRI instrument, here depicted as a shaded cylinder, the nuclei are constrained to orient in a specific manner. Accordingly, a detectable magnetic moment (B_0) is produced. A typical external magnetic field strength for a commercial MRI instrument is 1.5 Tesla, or approximately 30,000 times the strength of the earth's magnetic field. (From Blackwell G, Cranney GB, Pohost G: MRI: Cardiovascular System. New York, Gower Medical Publishing, 1992.)

MRI pulse sequences are constantly being developed, and the trend is for faster acquisition times. Using the technique known as echoplanar imaging, a complete image matrix can be assimilated in milliseconds. For the technical details of MR image formation and acquisition sequences, the interested reader should consult the references at the end of this subchapter.

SPECIAL CONSIDERATIONS FOR CARDIOVASCULAR MRI

Imaging the continuously moving heart and vascular system is more difficult than imaging stationary structures. Accordingly, electrocardiographic gating is required to functionally "freeze" motion and minimize artifacts in cardiovascular images. Special techniques can also be applied that minimize artifacts caused by excessive respiratory motion. Despite the aforementioned techniques, suboptimal images often occur in patients with irregular cardiac rhythms or in patients who are unable to remain still for the time required to complete an examination. Several important contraindications to MRI should be recognized (Table 33–8). In addition, the bore of MRI instruments is confining, and imaging critically ill patients or patients with claustrophobia can be difficult.

ESTABLISHED INDICATIONS FOR CARDIOVASCULAR MRI (see Table 33–5)

MRI plays a very important role in the diagnosis and subsequent follow-up of thoracic aortic disease. The ability to accurately assess aortic dimensions and identify intimal disruption makes MRI ideally suited for assessing patients with aortic coarctation, aneurysm, or dissection. The entire aorta can be examined in multiple imaging planes using sequences that highlight morphology, complemented by sequences that assess flow within the aortic lumen. Figure 33–36 is a 3D reconstruction of an MR image from a patient with a large ascending aortic aneurysm. Using MRI, surgical interventions can be planned and subsequent follow-up studies performed in patients with aortic aneurysms without requiring invasive diagnostic procedures.

MRI can diagnose dissection at any level of the aorta with a high degree of accuracy (Figs. 33–37 and 33–38). The diagnostic hallmark of typical aortic dissections, the intimal flap, can be well seen on both spin-echo and gradient-echo sequences. MRI is also able to recognize atypical presentations of dissection such as hemorrhage into the aortic wall in the absence of a true flap. Complications of dissection such as mediastinal hemorrhage, pleural and pericardial effusions, and aortic insufficiency can all be well demonstrated using MRI. Invasive aortography, computed tomographic (CT) scanning, and transesophageal echocardiography are all useful in diagnosing aortic pathology. However, the accuracy and noninvasive nature of MRI make it arguably the procedure of choice in stable patients with thoracic aortic disease.

Pericardial thickness can be reliably determined using MRI (Fig. 33–39). Accordingly, MRI has proven useful in distinguishing patients with constrictive pericardial disease from those having restrictive cardiomyopathy.

The ability to acquire images in any desired plane makes MRI particularly valuable for defining pathoanatomy in congenital heart disease (Fig. 33–40). Atrial and visceral situs, systemic and pulmonary venous return, atrioventricular concordance, and the relationships of the great arteries can all be clearly defined using MRI. Morphology of the central pulmonary arteries, often an important issue in surgical management of these patients, can also be assessed. Cine MRI can also be useful for identifying shunt lesions and disturbed flow patterns in this patient population.

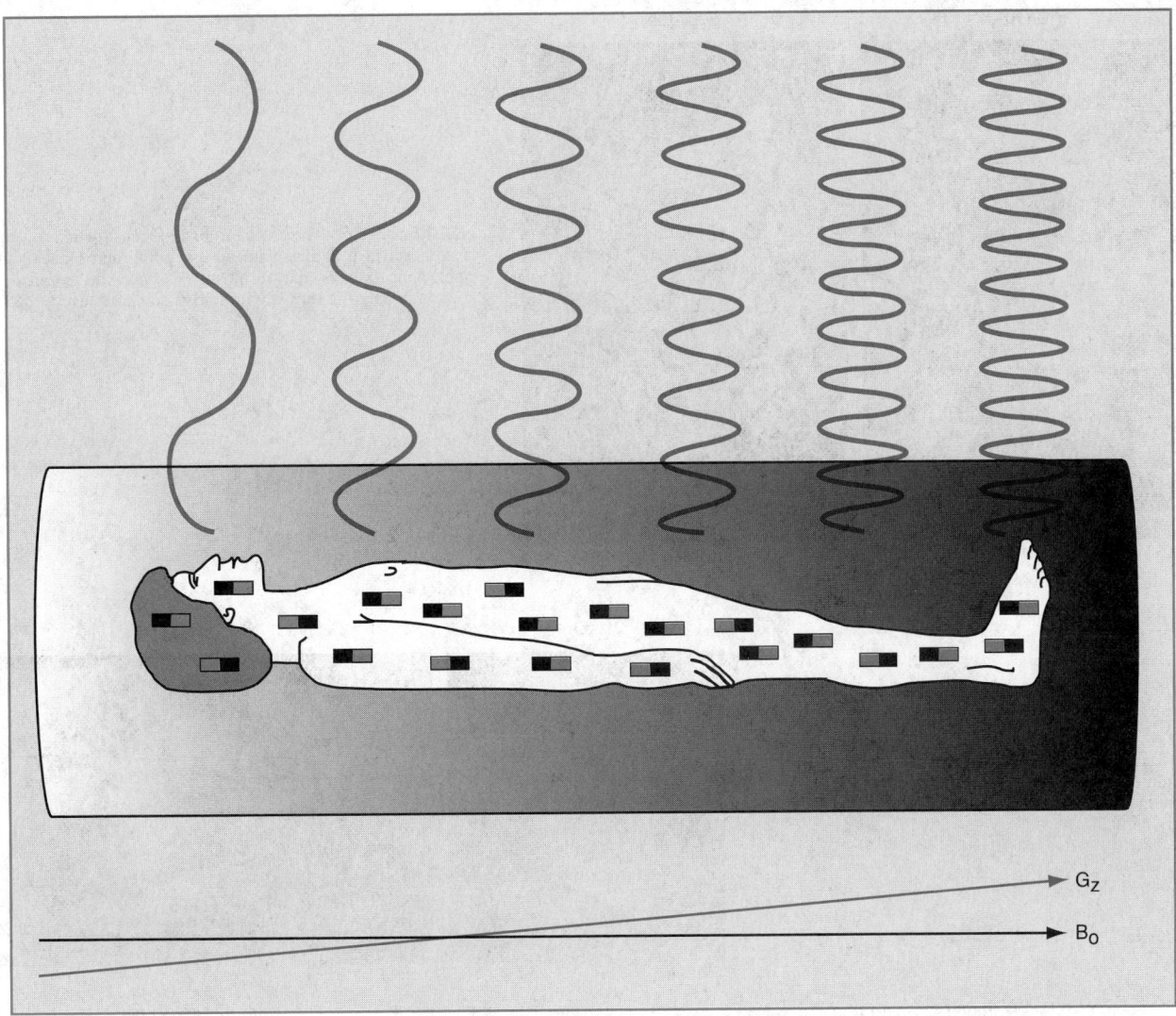

FIGURE 33–35. All hydrogen nuclei exposed to a uniform magnetic field strength spin at the same Larmor frequency, and spatial discrimination is not possible. In this figure the shaded cylinder represents a "gradient" (G_z) of progressively increasing magnetic field strength from head to toe. Hydrogen nuclei exposed to a higher magnetic field strength spin at a higher frequency and, therefore, can be distinguished from nuclei that spin at a lower frequency. Using magnetic gradients in three dimensions, precise spatial localization is possible with MRI. (From Blackwell G, Cranney GB, Pohost G: MRI: Cardiovascular System. New York, Gower Medical Publishing, 1992.)

The wide field of view of MRI makes it ideally suited for known or suspected paracardiac masses. Both the intracardiac and extracardiac extent of these lesions can be recognized. In addition, information regarding tissue characterization can occasionally be obtained. Lipomatous material in particular has a characteristic MRI signal intensity (Fig. 33–41).

A new indication for MRI is in assessing angiographically occult runoff vessels in patients with lower extremity peripheral vascular disease. Invasive x-ray angiography can be limited in these patients because an adequate concentration of contrast material cannot be delivered to the runoff vessels via collateral channels. The intrinsic vascular contrast and 3D nature of MRI are very useful in establishing the adequacy of runoff vessels, important information for surgically managing these patients.

APPLICATIONS OF CARDIOVASCULAR MRI AS AN ALTERNATIVE DIAGNOSTIC MODALITY (see Table 33–6)

Cardiovascular MRI provides diagnostic information in many circumstances; however, the availability of more cost-effective imaging modalities makes MRI applicable only when other modalities fail to provide sufficient information.

Global and regional left ventricular systolic function can be accurately assessed using MRI (Fig. 33–42). Stacked sets of tomograms allow left ventricular mass and volume to be determined without the need for major geometric assumptions. MRI is also valuable for evaluating morphology and function of the irregularly shaped right ventricle.

Cine MRI sequences are sensitive to disturbances of normal laminar flow. Accordingly, turbulent blood flow caused by either valvular regurgitation or stenosis can be readily appreciated. The sensi-

TABLE 33–7. DETERMINANTS OF SIGNAL INTENSITY IN MAGNETIC RESONANCE IMAGING

Density of hydrogen nuclei within the imaging plane
Blood flow within and through the imaging plane
Intrinsic magnetization properties of the tissues being imaged (T1 and T2)
Operator-determined acquisition parameters (pulse sequences)

TABLE 33–8. CONTRAINDICATIONS TO MAGNETIC RESONANCE IMAGING

Cardiac pacemakers and defibrillators
Cerebral aneurysm clips
Magnetically activated implants or foreign bodies

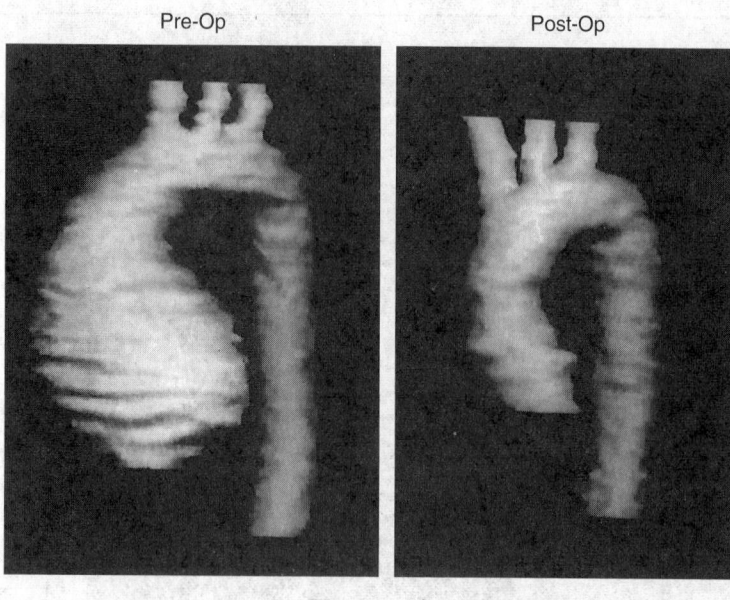

Pre-Op   Post-Op

FIGURE 33–36. Three-dimensional reconstruction of the thoracic aorta in a patient with an ascending aortic aneurysm. The right panel shows the result of a successful surgical repair. Anatomic detail is shown with unrivaled clarity using MRI.

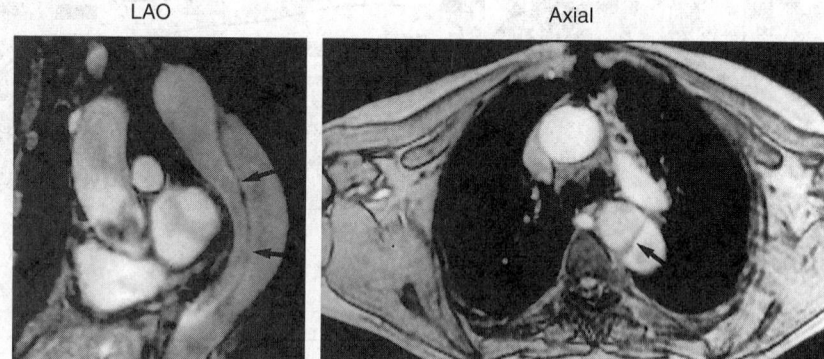

FIGURE 33–37. Type III (descending) aortic dissection. *Left,* Left anterior oblique (LAO) equivalent cine MRI frame. *Right,* Axial cine MRI frame. Arrows highlight the intimal flap separating the true and false lumina in the descending aorta. The ascending aorta appears normal.

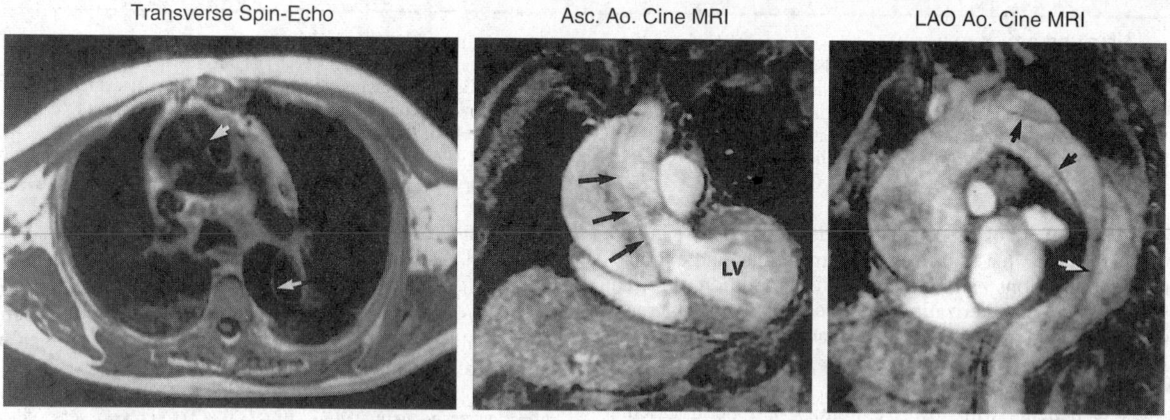

FIGURE 33–38. Type I (ascending) aortic dissection. *Left,* An intimal flap can be seen in both the ascending and descending thoracic aorta *(arrows)* on this spin-echo image. *Center,* Arrows highlight the flap in this ascending aortic cine MRI tomogram (LV = left ventricle). *Right,* Left anterior oblique (LAO) equivalent cine MRI frame displaying the spiral nature of the dissection in the descending thoracic aorta (arrows = intimal flap).

tivity and specificity of cine MRI for detecting valvular regurgitation are comparable to those of Doppler echocardiography.

Small loculated accumulations of pericardial fluid can often be identified by MRI in patients with nondiagnostic echocardiographic studies. The site and extent of abdominal aortic aneurysms can also be assessed via MRI. Although invasive angiography remains the gold standard, clinically useful 3D MR angiograms can be produced throughout the cerebral and peripheral vascular tree. In combination with flow data, reliable noninvasive screening for disease involving these vascular territories may be accomplished using MRI.

FUTURE DIRECTIONS

New frontiers will be opened for the field of cardiovascular MRI as ultrafast acquisition sequences are developed and refined. Preliminary information has demonstrated the feasibility of noninvasive MR coronary angiography. High-resolution, multislice MR perfusion imaging techniques are being investigated. MR quantitative flow packages are being developed that will facilitate calculation of stenotic gradients and vascular flow. Development of specific MR contrast agents for use in cardiovascular applications can also be expected.

Normal | Constrictive Pericardial Disease

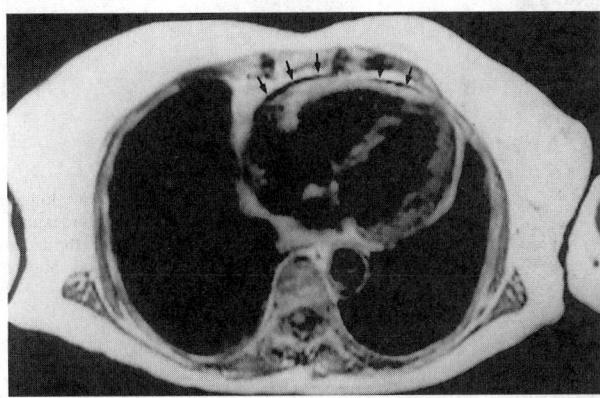 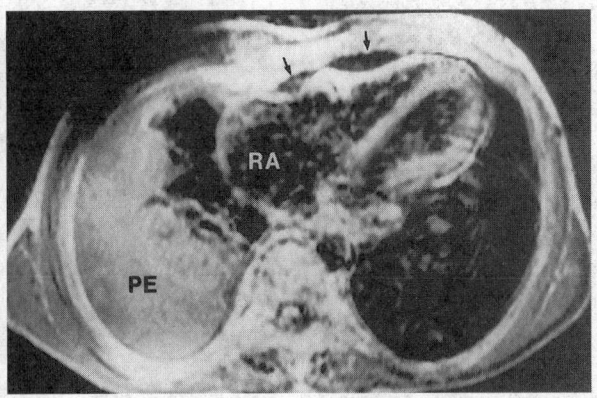

FIGURE 33–39. *Left,* MRI of the normal pericardium *(arrows). Right,* Marked pericardial thickening is seen *(arrows)* in this patient with constrictive pericardial disease. Associated findings include an enlarged right atrium (RA), pleural effusion (PE), and a distorted, tubular-shaped right ventricle.

FIGURE 33–40. Complex congenital heart disease. *Left,* Axial spin-echo image demonstrating dextrocardia, a common atrioventricular valve *(arrow),* and absence of the atrioventricular septum. *Right,* Coronal spin-echo image showing the enlarged ascending aorta (Ao) exiting the ventricular chamber.

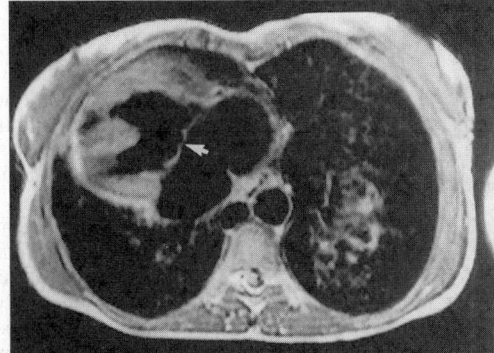 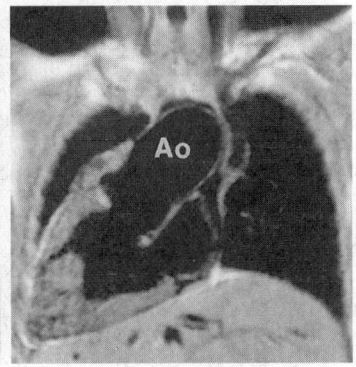

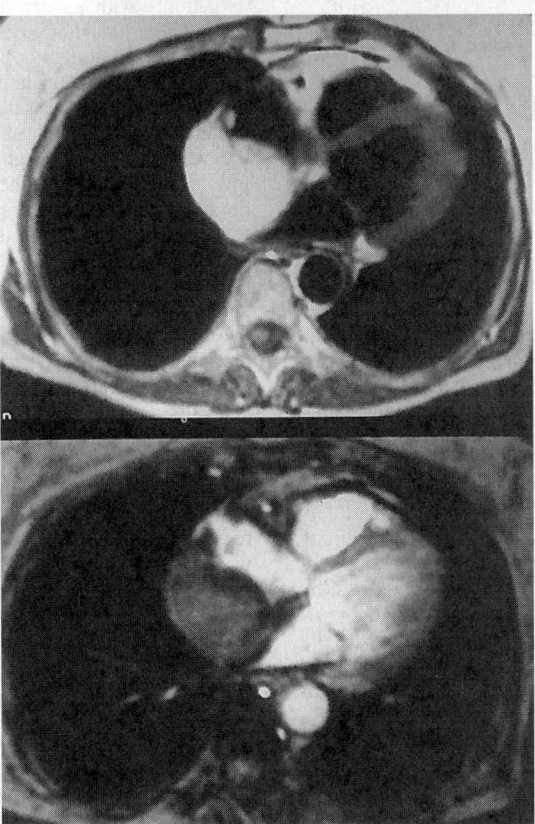

FIGURE 33–41. Right atrial lipoma. *Top,* A large, high MR signal intensity mass is seen occupying the right atrium on this axial spin-echo image. *Bottom,* Companion gradient-echo image. Bright MR signal intensity on spin-echo images is characteristic of lipomatous material. (From Blackwell G, Cranney GB, Pohost G: MRI: Cardiovascular System. New York, Gower Medical Publishing, 1992.)

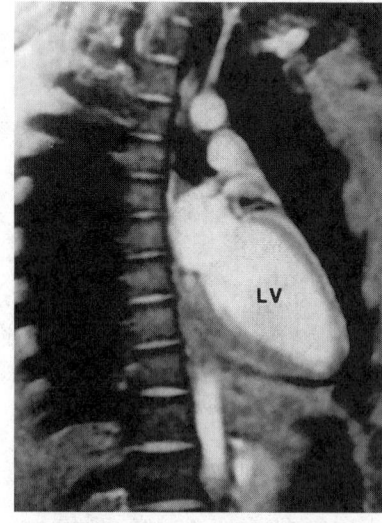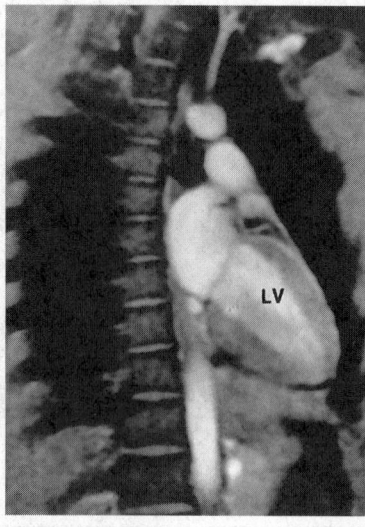

FIGURE 33–42. End-diastolic and end-systolic long-axis cine MRI frames. Accurate left ventricular (LV) volumes and ejection fraction can be obtained using cine MRI. Note the excellent discrimination between the left ventricular blood pool and myocardium.

Blackwell GG, Cranney GB, Pohost GM: MRI: Cardiovascular System. New York, Gower Medical Publishing, 1992. *A practical text and atlas designed to introduce cardiovascular specialists to the field of MRI.*

Blackwell GG, Pohost GM: The usefulness of cardiovascular magnetic resonance imaging. Curr Probl Cardiol 19:117, 1994. *Extensively referenced monograph highlighting the current clinical state of the art of cardiovascular MRI.*

Manning WJ, Li W, Edelman RR: A preliminary report comparing magnetic resonance coronary angiography with conventional angiography. N Engl J Med 328:823, 1993. *Report demonstrating the clinical feasibility of noninvasive MR coronary angiography.*

Nienaber CA, von Kodolitsch Y, Nicolas V, et al.: The diagnosis of thoracic aortic dissection by noninvasive imaging procedures. N Engl J Med 328:1, 1993. *Highlights accuracy of MRI in stable patients with aortic dissection.*

Pohost GM, O'Rourke R: Principles and Practice of Cardiac Imaging. Boston, Little, Brown, 1990. *Comprehensive section on basic principles of cardiovascular MRI.*

33.6 Cardiac Catheterization and Angiography
William H. Barry

Cardiac catheterization provides a unique, comprehensive, and quantitative assessment of cardiac structure and function and is frequently used to diagnose and manage patients with heart disease. With use of this procedure for bedside hemodynamic monitoring, intracardiac electrophysiologic testing, endomyocardial biopsy, percutaneous transluminal coronary angioplasty, and percutaneous balloon valvotomy, the internist must understand the indications, capabilities, and risks of cardiac catheterization.

INDICATIONS FOR CARDIAC CATHETERIZATION AND ANGIOGRAPHY

The accuracy of noninvasive evaluation has increased remarkably recently, because of the greatly improved sensitivity and specificity of two-dimensional Doppler echocardiography, radionuclide ventriculography, myocardial perfusion scintigraphy at rest and during therapy, and fast computed tomographic (CT) and magnetic resonance imaging (MRI). Therefore, cardiac catheterization is usually performed after noninvasive evaluation to quantify further the severity of disease present and to establish if a patient is a candidate for surgical intervention. Table 33–9 shows the diagnoses of a typical series of patients referred for cardiac catheterization. The vast majority of patients undergoing this procedure have coronary artery disease, with valvular disease a distant second. Table 33–10 lists the usual indications for cardiac catheterization and coronary angiography in patients with coronary artery disease or valvular heart disease.

TECHNIQUES AND THEIR HAZARDS

ARTERIAL AND VENOUS ACCESS. Vascular access can be achieved by skin incision and direct isolation and incision of the brachial artery and/or antecubital vein. However, the vast majority of catheterizations are currently carried out by the percutaneous approach. With this technique, an artery or vein is punctured percutaneously with a needle; a thin, flexible guidewire is inserted through the needle; and the needle is removed. Over the guidewire an arterial or venous sheath or a catheter is then introduced into the vessel. The percutaneous technique can be used to access the femoral artery and vein, the brachial artery, or the subclavian or internal jugular vein. Controlling postcatheterization bleeding may be difficult after the femoral approach, and patients must be relatively immobile for at least 4 to 6 hours. At present, the percutaneous femoral approach in which the femoral artery and femoral vein are punctured is most commonly used for cardiac catheterization and coronary angiography. However, the brachial approach is preferred in patients with severe atherosclerotic disease of the aorta or iliofemoral arteries or in those requiring early ambulation (i.e., for outpatient catheterization).

Catheterization and angiography can cause stroke or myocardial infarction due to vessel occlusion by clot from the tip of the catheter, dislodgement of atherosclerotic material, or dissection of the vessel wall, although the incidence of these complications is low (Table 33–11). Catheterization and angiography performed on the left side of the heart generally carry a much higher risk than on the right because the lung vascular bed can filter out thrombi. To decrease the risk of thrombosis and embolization, heparin is usually administered before catheterization of the left side of the heart. The anticoagulant effect of heparin is usually reversed with protamine at the end of the procedure, before the final withdrawal of the sheath or catheter. The risk is increased in patients over age 60, in patients with severe heart failure, and in patients with significant valvular heart disease.

PRESSURE MEASUREMENTS. Measuring intracardiac pressures, by attaching the end of the fluid-filled catheter to an external pressure transducer, is an essential part of the cardiac catheterization procedure. Phasic pressure waveforms up to 12 Hz may be recorded with this technique (Fig. 33–43), and all the pressures within the cardiac chambers are routinely measured, with the exception of the left atrial pressure. The pulmonary capillary "wedge" pressure, in which a segment of the pulmonary arterial tree is occluded either with the catheter tip or with a small balloon attached to the end of a catheter (a flow-directed Swan-Ganz type of catheter), is recorded to approximate the true left atrial pressure (Fig. 33–43). The normal values for intracardiac pressures are given in Ch. 32.

The shape as well as the magnitude of the intracardiac pressure waveforms contains diagnostic information. For example, in mitral regurgitation there is a large v wave in the left atrial or pulmonary artery wedge pressure (Fig. 33–44). A large v wave in the right atrial pressure tracing indicates tricuspid insufficiency. Simultaneous pressures measured in the pulmonary wedge position and left ventricle can quantitate the pressure gradient in diastole in mitral stenosis (Fig. 33–45). Left ventricular and aortic pressures are measured simultaneously to assess aortic valve function. Comparing pressures in different chambers can also be very useful. For exam-

TABLE 33-9. DIAGNOSES OF 562 PATIENTS CONSECUTIVELY STUDIED

Coronary Artery Disease (CAD)	Valvular Disease	CAD and Valvular Disease	Cardiomyopathy	Normal Persons	Congenital Heart Disease	Miscellaneous
62.6%	16.7%	6.0%	5.9%	6.4%	1.4%	0.9%

Adapted from Barry WH, et al.: Cathet Cardiovasc Diagn 8:401, 1979.

ple, in patients with pericardial constriction there is equalization of the right and left ventricular diastolic and the right atrial and pulmonary artery wedge mean pressures, and the mean right atrial pressure is usually greater than one third of the right ventricular systolic pressure. Measuring intracardiac pressures during exercise may provide useful information as well. For example, patients with mitral stenosis or mitral insufficiency may have relatively normal resting pressures but abnormally high pulmonary artery and wedge pressures with exercise.

MEASUREMENT OF CARDIAC OUTPUT. The most accurate way to measure cardiac output is by the Fick method, in which oxygen consumption is measured by determining the oxygen content in expired air collected over a 3-minute period. This allows determination of oxygen consumption in milliliters per minute. Collection of blood samples from the pulmonary artery (mixed venous sample) and a systemic artery allows determination of the arteriovenous (AV) oxygen difference. If the value for hemoglobin concentration in the blood is known, this allows calculation of the milliliters of blood that had to flow through the lungs to acquire the amount of oxygen consumed.

Cardiac output (liters/min)

$$= \frac{\text{oxygen consumption (ml } O_2/\text{min)}}{\text{A-V } O_2 \text{ difference (ml } O_2/\text{liter blood)}}$$

A-V O_2 difference (ml O_2/liter blood) = 13.9
$\times$ hemoglobin (gm/dl) $\times$ (% sat A $-$ % sat V)

TABLE 33-10. POSSIBLE INDICATIONS FOR CARDIAC CATHETERIZATION AND ANGIOGRAPHY

Suspected Coronary Artery Disease	Suspected Valvular Disease
1. Angina, especially if: unstable refractory to treatment strongly positive stress test young person with positive family history	1. Aortic stenosis angina syncope CHF
2. After acute myocardial infarction (including patients who have received thrombolytic therapy) if: angina positive stress test	2. Aortic regurgitation CHF angina progressive cardiac enlargement
3. In selected patients suspected to have "silent" ischemia by stress testing: occupational hazards strong family history of infarction/sudden death	3. Mitral stenosis* CHF refractory to digitalis and diuretics recurrent emboli with atrial fibrillation
4. Patients with ischemic cardiomyopathy and congestive heart failure (CHF)	4. Mitral regurgitation CHF progressive cardiac enlargement

5. In patients with high risk (age, diabetes, lipid disorder) prior to major noncardiac surgery; in patients at risk for coronary artery disease in whom cardiac surgery is planned

Additional Miscellaneous Indicators
  Congenital heart disease
  Pericardial disease
Other
  Percutaneous transluminal coronary angioplasty
  Electrophysiologic study
  Biopsy
  Hemodynamic monitoring
  Balloon valvotomy

* Operation may be performed without catheterization if diagnosis is certain.

Cardiac output may be normalized by dividing by body surface area (m^2) and expressed as cardiac index. In patients with intracardiac shunts, correction for the shunt must be made. This occurs most commonly in adult patients with atrial septal defects or ventricular septal defects with a left-to-right shunt. The pulmonary artery saturation in these conditions is elevated relative to the true mixed venous saturation, which is most closely approximated by the superior vena cava saturation. Standard methods exist to quantify left-to-right and right-to-left intracardiac shunts.

Another method commonly used to measure cardiac output is dye dilution, in which indocyanine green dye is injected into a peripheral vein, with continuous sampling of the dye concentration in blood drawn from a peripheral artery.

The cardiac output is calculated as $\frac{i}{c \times t}$ where i is the quantity of indicator injected, c is the average arterial concentration of the indicator during its first pass, and t is the total duration of the dye concentration curve. Cardiac output determined by dye dilution may be inaccurate in patients with extremely low outputs or with mitral or aortic regurgitation. The dye curve is also distorted by intracardiac shunts and in fact may be used in certain circumstances to diagnose the presence and direction of an intracardiac shunt.

With the "thermodilution" method the indicator is not dye, but cold saline injected into the right atrium. Temperature changes are detected with a thermistor in the pulmonary artery. The advantages of the thermodilution method are that it is relatively unaffected by mitral and aortic regurgitation and it may be repeated frequently to measure serial outputs. It is influenced by respiration, by shunts that increase pulmonary flow, and by tricuspid regurgitation. At the present time, the Fick method is most commonly used in the cardiac catheterization laboratory, and the thermodilution method is most commonly used in intensive care unit settings where patients are being monitored with catheters in the right side of the heart.

From measurements of cardiac output and pressure gradients across vascular beds, the systemic and pulmonary vascular resistances may be calculated. Elevations in systemic vascular resistance are important in patients with chronic congestive heart failure and may identify those patients who will respond favorably to vasodilator therapy. Pulmonary vascular resistance is frequently elevated in patients with severe left ventricular failure and elevated pulmonary venous pressures, in patients with mitral valve disease, in patients with left-to-right shunts, and always in patients with primary pulmonary hypertension. Measuring changes in pulmonary and systemic vascular resistances and in cardiac outputs and pressures before and after administering vasodilator drugs may be helpful in

TABLE 33-11. COMPLICATIONS OF CARDIAC CATHETERIZATION AND ANGIOGRAPHY*

	Percent Incidence In	
Complication	Patients with CAD†	Patients with Valvular‡ Heart Disease
Death	0.10	0.1
Myocardial infarction	0.06	0.2
Cerebrovascular accident	0.07	0.4
Arrhythmia	0.47	2.0
Vascular complications	0.46	1.7
Other	0.58	2.4
TOTAL	1.74	6.8

* Adapted from The Registry of Society for Cardiac Angiography and Interventions. Cathet Cardiovasc Diagn 17:5, 1989.
† Data on 222,553 patients.
‡ Data on 1,483 patients.

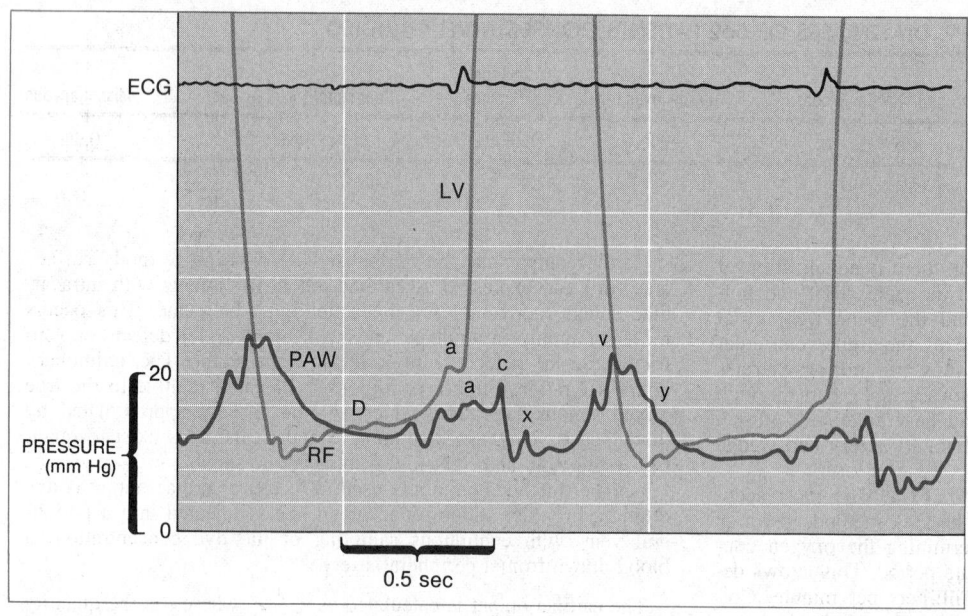

FIGURE 33-43. Simultaneous pulmonary artery wedge (PAW) pressure and left ventricular pressure (LV) in a normal patient. RF = Rapid LV filling; D = diastasis of LV filling; a = atrial contraction pressure wave. Note the delay of the PAW pressure relative to LV pressure.

guiding treatment of patients with specific disorders and is frequently used in the catheterization laboratory setting.

Determining cardiac output simultaneous with measurement of pressure gradients across the aortic, mitral, tricuspid, or pulmonic valve allows estimation of valve area by use of the Gorlin formula (see Fig. 33-45). The calculated valve area may differ significantly from the true valve area, particularly in the presence of very low cardiac output or valvular insufficiency. Nevertheless, this measurement is often useful in guiding surgical interventions.

ANGIOGRAPHY. During routine cardiac catheterization, angiography is commonly performed. For left ventriculography, contrast material is injected into the left ventricular chamber and cineangiographic filming is performed at 30 to 60 frames per second. Ejection fraction is determined as the fraction of end-diastolic ventricular volume ejected each systole. In patients with mitral regurgitation, the degree of regurgitation is usually graded on a simple 1+ to 4+ scale. In coronary artery disease, segmental contraction abnormalities are frequently present, and these may be quantified by a variety of regional indices of left ventricular performance.

Aortic root angiography allows assessment of the degree of aortic insufficiency, and right ventricular contrast injection allows assessment of the tricuspid valve. Pulmonary angiography may also be performed to detect pulmonary emboli.

Adverse effects of cardiac angiography include a negative inotropic effect due to calcium binding by the contrast agent and an intravascular volume-expanding effect due to hyperosmolality of the contrast material. The myocardial depressant effects of contrast agents are usually not a problem unless ventricular function is severely compromised. In these patients, the risks of left ventriculography may be reduced by using nonionic, non–calcium-binding contrast agents.

Coronary cineangiography is performed by injecting a contrast agent selectively into the right or left main coronary ostia. The degree of coronary artery obstruction in multiple views is assessed by measuring the percentage of narrowing of the artery at the site or sites of obstruction or by determining the percentage of area of stenosis by video-densitometric measurements. The presence and location of collateral vessels in relation to partially or totally occluded coronary artery narrowings are also determined. In patients with no or only minor coronary artery narrowings, but with a suggestive history of chest pain, ergonovine may be infused intravenously to precipitate coronary artery spasm, which then can be documented angiographically.

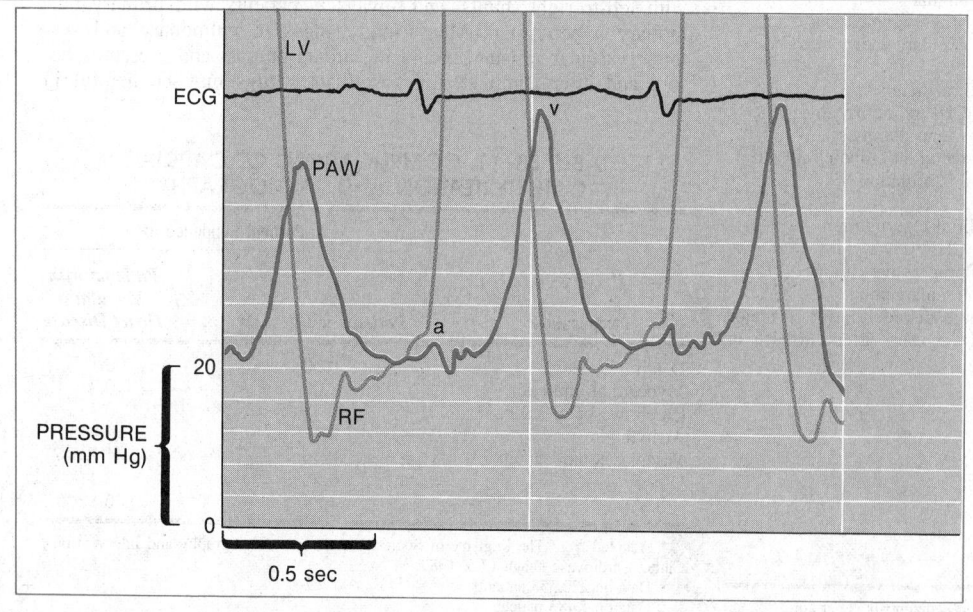

FIGURE 33-44. Simultaneous PAW and LV pressures in a patient with severe mitral regurgitation. Note large v wave with rapid y descent.

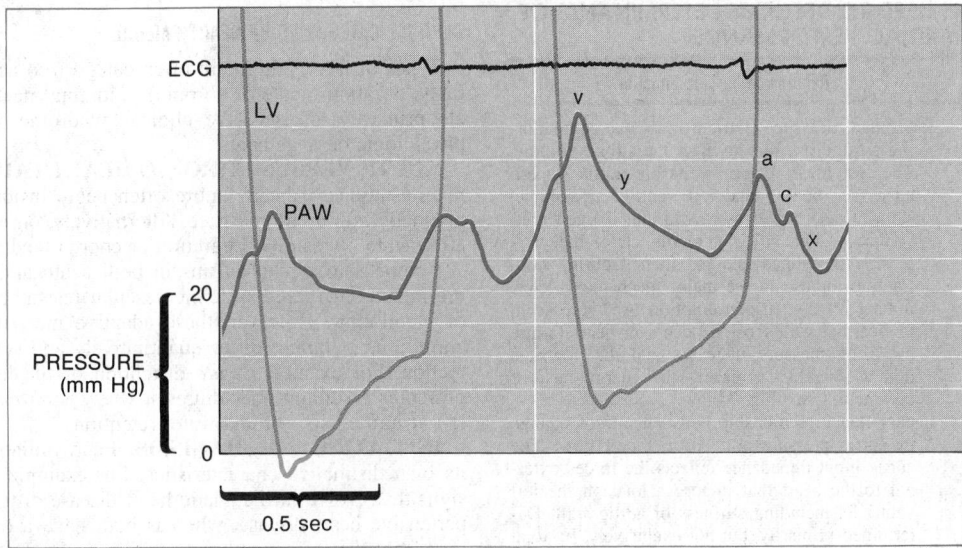

FIGURE 33–45. Simultaneous PAW and LV pressures in a patient with mitral stenosis. Note the slow y descent and the large gradient throughout diastole between PAW and LV diastolic pressures. The actual mitral valve area (M.V.A.) may be estimated as:

$$\text{M.V.A.} = \frac{\text{diastolic mitral flow (ml/sec)}}{38 \sqrt{\text{diastolic pressure gradient}}}$$

Thus, for a given M.V.A., the pressure gradient across the valve goes up as the *square* of mitral valve flow. This explains why the PAW pressure rises so markedly with increased cardiac output and hence increased mitral valve flow. Increased heart rate shortens diastolic time and hence increases the mitral valve flow rate per unit of diastolic time at any given cardiac output.

Descriptions of the indications, techniques, and risks of newer procedures that also involve cardiac catheterization and angiography, such as coronary angioplasty, endomyocardial biopsy, balloon valvotomy, and electrophysiologic study, are beyond the scope of this brief summary but may be found in the selected references included.

Grossman W, Baim DS: Cardiac Catheterization, Angiography and Interventions. 4th ed. Lea & Febiger, Philadelphia, 1991. *Excellent comprehensive text.*

Guidelines for Coronary Angiography: A report of the American College of Cardiology/American Heart Association Task Force on Assessment of Diagnostic and Theraputic Cardiovascular Procedures. Circulation 76:963A, 1987. *Summary of indications for coronary angiography.*

Guidelines for Percutaneous Transluminal Coronary Angioplasty: A report of the American Heart Association/American College of Cardiology Task Force on Assessment of Diagnostic and Theraputic Cardiovascular Procedures. Circulation 88:2982, 1993. *Summary of indications for PTCA.*

Latac B, Cribier A, Koning R, Lefelsure E: Aortic stenosis in elderly patients aged 80 or older: Treatment by percutaneous balloon valvuloplasty in a series of 92 cases. Circulation 80:1514, 1989. *Summary of results of percutaneous balloon aortic valvotomy.*

Palacios I, Block PC, Wilkins GT, Weyman AE: Follow-up of patients undergoing percutaneous mitrial balloon valvotomy. Circulation 79:573, 1989. *Summary of current results of percutaneous balloon mitral valvotomy.*

Registry Committee of the Society for Cardiac Angiography and Interventions: Complications of cardiac catheterization. Cath Cardiovasc Diagn 17:5, 1989. *Excellent current description of type and incidence of complications associated with cardiac catheterization and coronary angiography.*

34 HEART FAILURE
Thomas Woodward Smith

The heart generates the motive force to satisfy the metabolic needs of tissues by delivering blood containing oxygen and nutrients. The minute-to-minute adjustments in the distribution of the cardiac output according to physiologic priorities (e.g., muscular exercise, heat loss, and digestion) require a complex regulatory system that must also serve to protect vital organs such as the heart and brain when cardiac output is compromised.

The normal or failing heart, in terms of its structure and function, may be examined as a muscle, as a pump, or as a component of the circulatory system. This chapter addresses aspects of heart failure common to the various disease entities discussed in subsequent chapters.

GENERAL ASPECTS

Textbooks commonly define heart failure as a condition in which the heart cannot pump an adequate supply of blood at normal filling pressures to meet the metabolic needs of the body. Clinicians and clinical investigators, however, define heart failure operationally as a syndrome in which ventricular dysfunction is accompanied by reduced exercise capacity. Table 34–1 provides explanations of terms commonly used to describe determinants of cardiac performance.

Heart failure is encountered with increasing frequency. Most of this increase is attributable to an aging population with a high incidence of cardiovascular disease; heart failure in now the most common DRG throughout the United States for patients aged 65 and above.

Despite advances in the medical and surgical management of cardiovascular disease, the prognosis for patients with overt heart failure remains quite limited. About half of patients die within 4 to 5 years after this diagnosis; among the group with advanced heart failure, 50% or more die within 1 year. Several factors have been shown to be independent predictors of survival in patients with heart failure. The extent of impairment of ventricular function, usually judged by left or right ventricular ejection fraction, is correlated with prognosis, as are reduced cardiac index and elevated ventricular filling pressures. Exercise capacity, as well as peak O_2 consumption and New York Heart Association functional class, are valid predictors of survival. Neurohumoral activation as evidenced by elevated plasma norepinephrine levels, basal plasma renin activity, or plasma atrial natriuretic factor has adverse prognostic significance, as does hyponatremia. The occurrence of either ventricular or supraventricular arrhythmias is predictive of shorter survival. About 40 to 50% of deaths among heart failure patients occur suddenly and are due in large part to ventricular arrhythmias, and also to bradyarrhythmias and electromechanical dissociation, occurring at times when patients are relatively compensated and out of hospital. Antiarrhythmic drug therapy has not yet been shown to alter

TABLE 34-1. TERMS USED TO DESCRIBE DETERMINANTS OF CARDIAC PERFORMANCE

Term	Relation to Cardiac Function
Afterload	Resistance that the ventricle must overcome during systole in order to eject the stroke volume. The two major determinants are aortic impedance (see below) and left ventricular volume.
Energetics	Generally determined as myocardial oxygen consumption. For any contractile state, the wall tension developed and maintained during contraction represents the major mechanical determinant of oxygen consumption. An increase in myocardial wall tension occurs in heart failure as filling pressure increases and the ventricle dilates, thereby increasing the energy cost of contraction (see Fig. 34–3).
Impedance (during ejection)	Instantaneous relationship between rate of change in aortic pressure and aortic blood flow. The aortic input impedance reflects the forces external to the heart that impose a load on the left ventricle, including stiffness of aortic wall. Determined primarily, but not exclusively, by total peripheral vascular resistance to runoff from the arterial tree. Normal peripheral resistance is approximately 1500 dynes·sec/cm^{-5} or 15 peripheral resistance units (also known as Wood's units).
Inotropic state	A measure of contractility.
Preload	Rigorously, stretch of myocardial fibers at end-diastole; commonly used as a synonym for venous return to the heart or end-diastolic volume.

this troublesome situation, but the automatic implantable cardioverter/defibrillator shows promise.

Given the limited outlook despite application of all available treatment modalities for patients with heart failure, the clinician must do everything possible to *prevent* progression of heart disease to the point where cardiac reserve and compensatory mechanisms are exhausted and the syndrome of overt congestive heart failure supervenes.

The term *heart failure* is often used as a synonym for myocardial failure, emphasizing the impaired performance of the heart as a muscle and as a pump. It also provides a rationale for medical treatment. Subsequent chapters deal with syndromes in which the cause of circulatory compromise lies elsewhere, such as in abnormalities of the heart valves or pericardium or inappropriate heart rates.

Imbalance between circulatory demands and cardiac response sets the stage for the syndrome of heart failure. Volume overload is generally tolerated better than pressure overload. Aortic or mitral insufficiency produces *volume* overload that may be tolerated for years without overt heart failure; *pressure* overload from aortic stenosis, in contrast, usually results in earlier onset and more rapid progression of heart failure. Gradually developing overloads are accommodated better than acute overloads. Thus, gradually developing chronic mitral regurgitation is often present for years without signs of failure, whereas acute mitral regurgitation from a ruptured chorda tendineae can precipitate life-threatening pulmonary edema.

The myocardium adapts quite differently to volume and pressure loads. Volume overloads typically produce dilation followed by hypertrophy; pressure overloads characteristically elicit concentric hypertrophy until late in the natural history when dilation supervenes. Primary myocardial disease usually results in both dilation and hypertrophy.

Precipitating stresses (see Table 34–2) often tip the balance of the compromised heart toward decompensation and constitute important items for therapeutic attention.

Although the discussion in this chapter deals primarily with the abnormalities of the heart itself that underlie the syndrome of congestive heart failure, abnormalities of the peripheral circulation and neurohormonal milieu are also important factors in determining the

degree of functional limitation experienced by patients with heart failure.

CLINICAL CATEGORIES OF HEART FAILURE

Types of heart failure are often categorized according to five features: duration (acute or chronic), initiating mechanisms, the ventricle primarily affected, the clinical syndrome, and the underlying physiologic derangements.

ACUTE VERSUS CHRONIC HEART FAILURE. The clinical manifestations of heart failure often begin insidiously and progress gradually into a chronic state. Alternatively, onset may be abrupt, as after acute myocardial infarction or chorda tendineae rupture.

Compensatory mechanisms in both acute and chronic heart failure include increased systemic vascular resistance and redistribution of blood flow. However, these adaptive mechanisms in acute and chronic heart failure differ quantitatively and sometimes also in direction. For example, *acute* distention of the left atrium generally promotes a sodium-poor diuresis, whereas *chronic* distention of the left atrium elicits salt and water retention.

INITIATING MECHANISMS. Each initiating mechanism has its own distinctive characteristics. For example, the symptoms and signs that evolve in rheumatic heart disease differ from those of hypertensive heart disease, whereas both have a different natural history from that of cor pulmonale. Even a single cause, arteriosclerosis, may have distinctly different consequences, depending on the size and location of affected vessels. Progressive narrowing and gradual occlusion of distal branches of the coronary arteries may be so covert that shortness of breath and fatigue may be misinterpreted as the general physical decline of advancing age. In contrast, abrupt closure of a major coronary artery may result in myocardial necrosis followed by an acute low output state or by progressive chronic heart failure.

LEFT VERSUS RIGHT HEART FAILURE. One ventricle bears the brunt of many disease processes and fails before the other. Because of the prevalence of cardiac disorders that overload or damage the left ventricle, heart failure most often begins with that ventricle. Breathlessness is the most common presenting symptom and is a direct consequence of elevated left ventricular filling pressure and pulmonary congestion. When the right ventricle fails, systemic venous congestion and peripheral edema predominate. Left ventricular failure is the most common cause of right ventricular failure, and breathlessness may improve as right ventricular output falls and pulmonary congestion diminishes.

The mechanism by which left ventricular failure causes the right ventricle to fail is not clear. Pulmonary hypertension secondary to left ventricular failure may contribute, but the degree of pulmonary

TABLE 34-2. PRECIPITATING OR EXACERBATING FACTORS IN CONGESTIVE HEART FAILURE

Increased demand:
  Anemia
  Fever
  Infection
  Fluid overload
  Increased dietary salt intake
  High environmental temperature
  Renal failure
  Hepatic failure
  Thyrotoxicosis
  Arteriovenous (AV) shunt (Paget's disease of bone)
  Respiratory insufficiency
  Emotional stress
  Pregnancy
  Obesity
Arrhythmias
Pulmonary embolism
Ethanol ingestion
Thiamine deficiency
Uncontrolled hypertension
Poor compliance with therapeutic regimen
Drugs
  β-Adrenergic blockers
  Antiarrhythmic drugs (e.g., disopyramide)
  Salt-retaining drugs
    Steroids
    Nonsteroidal anti-inflammatory agents

hypertension is often insufficient to constitute a formidable burden on the right ventricle. Interdependence of the two ventricles, with failure of shared muscle in the ventricular septum, may also contribute. Right ventricular failure is an uncommon cause of left ventricular failure, but there is a relatively high frequency of independent left ventricular disease in elderly patients with right ventricular failure.

The combination of left and right ventricular (biventricular) failure, with elevated filling pressures of both ventricles causing pulmonary and systemic venous hypertension, results in the syndrome known as "congestive heart failure." This term implies reduced effort tolerance, breathlessness, distended neck veins, hepatic engorgement, and peripheral edema.

BACKWARD VERSUS FORWARD HEART FAILURE. "Backward failure" refers to elevated cardiac filling pressures and attributes to the consequent venous congestion a critical role in the evolution of the syndrome of heart failure. "Forward failure" refers to decreased cardiac output and inadequate perfusion of organs. This distinction has limited clinical usefulness and has largely been replaced by more specific consideration of ventricular filling pressures and cardiac output.

HIGH VERSUS LOW OUTPUT FAILURE. The separation into "high" and "low" output failure distinguishes certain clinical manifestations, rather than causes, of myocardial failure. It serves (1) to distinguish a type of myocardial failure ("high output failure") in which the circulation remains brisk and the extremities tend to remain warm despite elevated venous pressures and a lower cardiac output than existed prior to the onset of heart failure; (2) to emphasize that the cardiac output and the circulatory adjustments during heart failure are conditioned by the state that existed prior to heart failure; and (3) to relate cause to typical clinical features of heart failure. In regard to this last point, the more common causes—arteriosclerosis, myocardial disease, valvular disease, hypertension, and pericardial disease—tend to produce low output states; other, less common causes, including hyperthyroidism, Paget's disease of bone, anemia, beriberi, and arteriovenous fistula, tend to be associated with high output states. The essence of cardiac failure, however, remains the inability of the heart to increase its output appropriately in relation to demand.

CONGESTIVE FAILURE VERSUS CONGESTED STATE. Elevated volume of the circulation, with preserved ventricular function, characterizes the "congested state." It is commonly encountered in intensive care facilities, where vigorous volume infusions are often used to combat systemic hypotension. It is encountered on a chronic basis in severe anemia and chronic renal insufficiency and less often in Paget's disease or beriberi. In these situations, venous hypertension results from expanded intravascular volume, rather than from impaired myocardial contractile state.

In time, myocardial failure may supervene, with an inadequate increase in cardiac output for the increment in oxygen uptake during exercise. Correcting inciting factors and administering diuretics are effective in both the "congested state" and in "congestive heart failure."

SYSTOLIC VERSUS DIASTOLIC DYSFUNCTION. Recent studies indicate that up to one third of patients evaluated for symptoms and signs of heart failure have normal or nearly normal left ventricular ejection fractions, but because of the low compliance of the chamber they require substantially elevated filling pressures to maintain an adequate forward stroke output. These patients with diastolic dysfunction usually suffer from one (or more) of three underlying problems: (1) left ventricular hypertrophy (e.g., due to hypertension, aortic stenosis, or hypertrophic cardiomyopathy); (2) myocardial ischemia, which impairs ventricular relaxation; and (3) infiltrative disease (most commonly amyloidosis). Much of the discussion that follows focuses on the "classic" syndrome of congestive heart failure that accompanies a dilated heart with impaired systolic function. It is essential to distinguish these patients from those with predominant diastolic dysfunction, who require a distinctly different therapeutic approach (see below). Echo-Doppler study usually provides definitive information distinguishing these patient subsets, as does radionuclide ventriculography.

SUBCELLULAR BASIS FOR CONTRACTION

Cardiac contraction is initiated by depolarization of the sarcolemmal membrane, which activates slow calcium channels that undergo a transient increase in calcium permeability. The resulting calcium influx triggers the release of a much larger amount of calcium from the sarcoplasmic reticulum with consequent sarcomere shortening; the sarcoplasmic reticulum then resequesters calcium to turn off myofilament interaction, permitting myocardial relaxation.

Contractile force in heart muscle is generated by interactions among contractile proteins in repeating units (sarcomeres) that compose the individual muscle fibers (myofibrils). Within each sarcomere, the contractile proteins are arranged in thick filaments consisting of myosin and thin filaments consisting of actin and the modulator proteins troponin and tropomyosin. Interaction of calcium with one of three proteins composing troponin initiates the contractile process by removing a troponin-tropomyosin-induced inhibition of thick and thin filament interaction.

Changes in the length of heart muscle during contraction and relaxation are explained by the sliding filament hypothesis. During contraction, the thin actin filaments are propelled past the myosin thick filaments by force generated by ATP-dependent movement of cross-bridges consisting of the head portion of the myosin molecule. As the muscle shortens, the cross-bridges disengage and then engage other sites with a ratchet-like action. Depending on the number of cross-bridges that interact at a given time, different tensions are developed. Energy-dependent uptake of cytosolic calcium by the sarcoplasmic reticulum allows cross-bridge disengagement and relaxation to occur. Abundant mitochondria generate energy for the contractile machinery by oxidative phosphorylation fueled by free fatty acids and, to a lesser extent, glucose.

For the sarcomere, as for the whole heart (see Preload, below and Table 34–1), the tension developed during contraction is directly related to its end-diastolic length. Stretching to permit optimal thick and thin filament overlap increases the ability of individual contractile elements to develop force, and also enhances myocardial contractility by altering calcium homeostasis and excitation-contraction coupling. There are still many uncertainties regarding molecular details of the contractile process, and much is still to be learned about cardiac "success" as an essential background against which to examine basic mechanisms in cardiac "failure."

PATHOPHYSIOLOGIC INTERPLAY

Because of their location, structure, and function, the heart and lungs operate as a functional unit. The continuity of the muscle that surrounds the ventricular chambers, the shared ventricular septum, and the encasing pericardium ensure coordinate function, yet each ventricle functions as a separate muscular pump with its own atrial booster pump. In the normal heart, at least 50% of the ventricular end-diastolic volume is ejected with each beat. Although many properties of ejection are inherent in the architecture and physiology of cardiac muscle, adaptability to changing metabolic needs is provided by a superimposed set of neurohumoral adjustments that modulate cardiac rate, loading, and contractility.

Each ventricle has its own capacity to withstand and repair the stresses imposed by normal and abnormal function. The two ventricles also have different designs in keeping with their different physiologic functions. Before birth, both ventricles bear similar pressure loads. After birth, the right ventricular workload decreases as pulmonary arterial pressure falls. The greater workload of the mature left ventricle, together with the greater prevalence of diseases that compromise the left side of the heart and its blood supply, result in the preponderance of left over right ventricular dysfunction in groups of patients in whom ischemic disease and hypertension are common.

ASSESSMENT OF CARDIAC PERFORMANCE

In terms of its performance, the heart may be assessed as a pump, as a muscle, or as a component of the circulatory system. Hemodynamic pressure and flow measurements characterize its behavior as a pump. Principles of muscle mechanics are used to describe its behavior as a muscle. Its adequacy as a component of the circulatory system is reflected in the consequences of reduced cardiac output, redistribution of blood flow, organ hypoperfusion, and pulmonary or systemic venous congestion.

Heart as a Pump: Hemodynamics

By the time overt heart failure is apparent, the large functional reserve of the normal heart is compromised and a variety of mechanisms operate to compensate for its diminished performance. Despite an inappropriately low cardiac output, the blood pressure at rest tends to remain normal or even increases, albeit with frequent reduction in pulse pressure.

CARDIAC OUTPUT. In response to peripheral demands, a complex set of control mechanisms modulates heart rate and the extent of stretch and shortening of myocardial fibers and, hence, the stroke volume and the cardiac output (stroke volume times heart rate). Three principal variables determine the stroke volume (Table 34–1): preload, afterload (resistance to ventricular emptying during systole), and the contractile state of the heart. For practical purposes, three of the principal determinants of cardiac output—preload, afterload, and heart rate—are readily measured. Contractile (inotropic) state remains difficult to assess in formal quantitative terms, but noninvasive (echo-Doppler) and minimally invasive (radionuclide ventriculography) methods yield the requisite data for most clinical decision making. Ejection fraction is commonly used as a clinically useful index (albeit impure) of contractile state, and the maximum rate of pressure rise during the isovolumic phase of systole (dP/dt) is a useful measure in invasive hemodynamic investigations.

Relationships among these determinants vary with the state of the heart and circulation. Thus, when contractility is impaired, stroke output and cardiac output tend to be maintained by ventricular dilation (Frank-Starling mechanism), limiting the value of cardiac output as a measure of inotropic state to experimental circumstances in which preload, afterload, and heart rate can be held constant.

Indicator-dilution techniques can be used in the ICU or cardiac catheterization laboratory for determining cardiac output. In resting adults, the normal range is between 2.5 and 3.6 liters per minute per square meter of body surface area. Decreased cardiac output at rest occurs only in advanced stages of cardiac impairment. A blunted cardiac output response to exercise occurs much earlier. Supine exercise in normal subjects should increase the cardiac output by at least 600 ml per minute for each 100-ml increment in oxygen consumption; lower values indicate reduced cardiac performance. In heart failure the arteriovenous oxygen difference is abnormally wide, resulting chiefly from the low oxygen content of venous blood returning to the heart. Oxygenation of blood in the lungs remains nearly normal until pulmonary vascular congestion becomes sufficiently severe to create ventilation-perfusion mismatch with shunting, or abnormal diffusion barriers to oxygen transport.

During exercise, cardiac output normally increases as a linear function of oxygen consumption, although for any level of exercise the cardiac output tends to be lower in the upright position. Increases in cardiac output in the upright posture are accomplished principally by increases in heart rate rather than in stroke volume. In heart failure, cardiac output is particularly dependent on heart rate, both at rest and during exercise.

VENTRICULAR END-DIASTOLIC PRESSURE AND VOLUME. Impaired systolic ventricular emptying leads to an increase in the end-systolic residual volume of blood in the ventricle, predisposing to an increase in end-diastolic volume. Because this is inconvenient to measure or monitor, ventricular end-diastolic pressure is customarily followed for clinical purposes on the premise that a change in pressure is effected by a change in ventricular volume. Exceptions occur, however, including structural changes in the myocardium (fibrosis, edema, and hypertrophy) and pericardial constriction that cause disproportionate rises in end-diastolic pressure relative to volume. Acute ischemia also produces transient reduction in left ventricular compliance. Conversely, in some states of chronic volume overload, compliance increases so that increased volumes are accommodated at end-diastole with relatively modest pressure increases.

A left ventricular end-diastolic pressure greater than 12 to 15 mm Hg is abnormal. The corresponding upper limit for the right ventricle is 6 to 10 mm Hg. It is straightforward to estimate the right ventricular end-diastolic pressure by measuring the central venous pressure. In the absence of mitral obstruction or increased pulmonary vascular resistance, pulmonary arterial diastolic pressure approximates left ventricular end-diastolic pressure. Pulmonary capillary wedge pressure or diastolic pressure measured with a Swan-Ganz catheter is widely used in ICU settings to monitor left ventricular filling pressures.

To summarize, the performance of heart muscle depends on two essential components: fiber length (Frank-Starling mechanism) and inherent contractility (inotropic state). The normal heart autoregulates to maintain cardiac output. The variables involved are preload, afterload, contractility, and heart rate. With chronic overloading, the heart undergoes dilation, hypertrophy, or both.

PRELOAD. According to the Frank-Starling mechanism, an increase in end-diastolic volume (preload) results in more forceful contraction with enhancement of ventricular emptying and stroke volume. A unique ventricular function curve exists for each state of contractility (Fig. 34–1). The curve for a failing ventricle is shifted downward and flattened such that stroke volumes are reduced despite abnormally high end-diastolic volumes or pressures. The elevated filling pressures are responsible for congestion and edema in the venous beds leading to the failing ventricle.

In the normal heart, the Frank-Starling mechanism serves to match the stroke outputs of the two ventricles. In heart failure, this mechanism plays the additional role of helping to support the cardiac output.

AFTERLOAD. Afterload refers to the resistance that the ventricle must overcome during systole in order to eject the stroke volume. It incorporates all factors that oppose shortening of the ventricular fibers. In practice, it is estimated for the left heart either from the arterial blood pressure or from calculation of systemic vascular resistance (ratio of blood pressure to flow, expressed in units of $dynes \cdot sec/cm^{-5}$ or in peripheral resistance units). Right ventricular afterload (pulmonary artery pressure) can be estimated satisfactorily in most patients by echo-Doppler measurements.

In assessing patients, the relationship of blood pressure to cardiac output and peripheral resistance (P/Flow = R) is quite useful. Interventions that cause an increase in cardiac output without changing systemic blood pressure must cause vasodilation, thereby decreasing peripheral vascular resistance or afterload. Improved emptying of

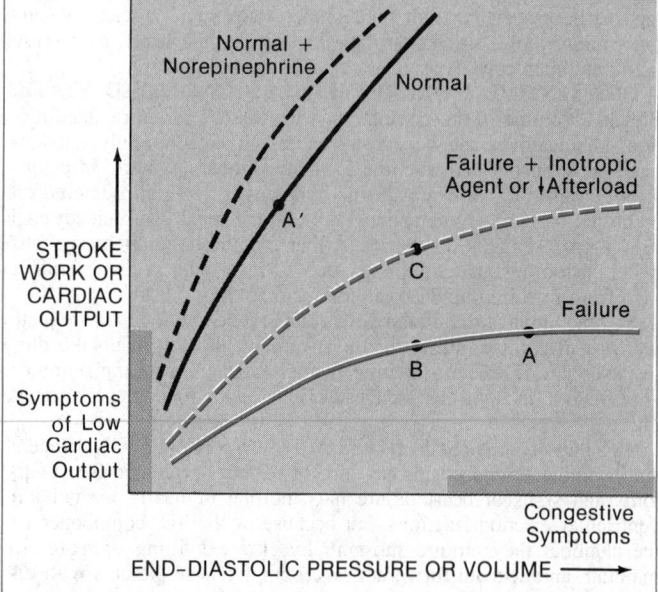

FIGURE 34–1. Schematic diagram demonstrating the relationship between ventricular end-diastolic pressure or volume and cardiac index in a normal and a failing heart. The normal left ventricle increases its stroke output as preload (often measured clinically as pulmonary capillary wedge pressure) increases, moving up the ascending limb of the curve until reserve is exhausted. In heart failure, the ventricular function curve is displaced downward and to the right. An increase in contractility, as after administration of norepinephrine or digitalis, displaces the curve to the left; i.e., a larger stroke output is accomplished at any given filling pressure. A and A′ represent the operating points at rest of a hypothetical patient with heart failure and of a normal person, respectively. Reduction of physical activity allows the failing heart to meet the demands of the metabolizing tissues. Treatment of heart failure by a reduction in preload (e.g., with a diuretic or a vasodilator acting predominantly on the venous bed) causes a shift from point A to B on the same ventricular function curve. Administration of a positive inotropic agent or a vasodilator producing afterload reduction shifts the curve as shown, resulting in improvement of the circulatory state in the direction shown by a shift from point A to C.

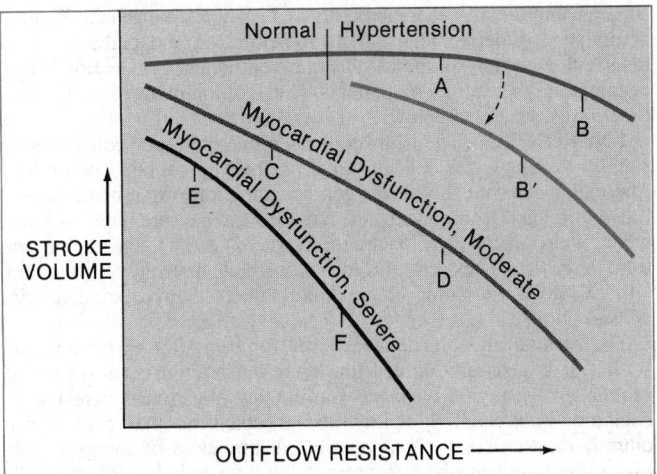

FIGURE 34–2. Relation of left ventricular stroke volume to systemic outflow resistance in normal and diseased hearts. A family of curves may be described, depending on the severity of the myocardial disease. If cardiac function is normal, a rise in resistance results in hypertension, because cardiac output remains fairly constant. Heart failure in a hypertensive patient could be shown by a move to either point B, a high resistance with normal function, or point B′, which represents a shift to a slightly depressed ventricular function curve. When myocardial dysfunction is more severe, as shown by the lower two curves, blood pressure is no longer directly determined by resistance because stroke volume and resistance are inversely related. Consequently, arterial pressure may be similar at points E and F despite marked differences in cardiac output and resistance. It is also apparent that a reduction in outflow resistance does not affect significantly the stroke volume of the normal ventricle. However, it can produce a marked increase in the stroke volume of the failing ventricle (F → E). (Adapted from Cohn JN, Franciosa JA: Vasodilator therapy of cardiac failure. N Engl J Med 297:27, 1977. Copyright 1977, the Massachusetts Medical Society.)

the left ventricle is usually accompanied by a decrease in its filling pressure (pulmonary capillary wedge or pulmonary artery diastolic pressure).

If preload and contractility remain constant, increasing afterload in the normal heart tends to decrease both the extent and the speed of contraction to a minor extent. Reduction in afterload has the opposite effects. Within broad physiologic limits, the normal ventricle maintains a relatively constant stroke volume as afterload is increased (Fig. 34–2). The impaired ventricle responds quite differently, with progressive diminution in its ability to eject blood against a given afterload as the severity of myocardial dysfunction advances. Figure 34–2 illustrates the rationale for afterload reduction in managing heart failure.

CONTRACTILITY (INOTROPIC STATE). Modulation of sympathetic nervous activity provides the major component of short-term adjustment of contractile state in the normal heart and also mediates increases in heart rate and venous tone. Unlike the Frank-Starling mechanism, the increase in force and velocity of contraction is accomplished without any increase in fiber length (end-diastolic volume). Contractility does not limit the output of the normal heart. By contrast, the failing heart is limited in its myocardial performance, indicated by displacement of the ventricular function curve as shown in Figure 34–1.

An objective index of myocardial contractility that could be measured independent of myocardial fiber length would be useful (1) to assess the effects on the myocardium of interventions such as administering digitalis or other inotropic agents; (2) to determine serial changes in inotropic state in an individual during the evolution of heart failure and in response to treatment; and (3) to compare the inotropic state in different individuals. However, distinction between the effects of loading conditions and intrinsic contractility is difficult because of the strong influence of loading on hemodynamic measurements. Changes in preload or afterload can modify ventricular performance greatly without affecting intrinsic inotropic state. Because conventional hemodynamic measurements do not take heart size into account, comparisons of contractility in hearts of different size are difficult to interpret.

Ejection Fraction. This term denotes the fraction of the right or left ventricular end-diastolic volume ejected per beat. It is useful

as an integrative measure of contractility and is determined by contrast ventriculography, by gated blood pool radionuclide imaging, or by echocardiography. The normal left ventricular ejection fraction ranges from 0.56 to 0.78. A reduced ejection fraction in a patient with normal valves and a dilated ventricle strongly suggests decreased contractility, particularly in the absence of increased afterload. Abnormalities of regional myocardial function are often evident in the pattern of ventricular contraction demonstrated by these techniques and suggest focal ischemic disease, but may also be observed in primary cardiomyopathic disorders.

Other Techniques. Simultaneous graphic recording of the electrocardiogram, phonocardiogram, and carotid arterial pulse contour provides another noninvasive means of assessing cardiac function but has been almost entirely supplanted by the more clinically useful echo-Doppler assessment. Accurate measurement of ventricular dP/dt can be accomplished at cardiac catheterization and provides a measure of contractile state less subject to the influence of loading conditions than most other approaches; its use is largely confined to research applications.

CHRONIC COMPENSATORY MECHANISMS. In chronic heart failure compensatory mechanisms include tachycardia, increased contractility due to sympathetic nervous activity, chamber dilation, and hypertrophy. The increase in sympathetic activity is a mixed blessing because it tends to increase systemic vascular resistance in addition to its salutary effects on cardiac output by increasing the heart rate and inotropic state. Peripheral vascular resistance is further augmented by activation of the renin-angiotensin system (see Ch. 37).

Heart Rate. Sustained tachycardia characterizes decompensated heart failure. The increase in rate stems in part from cardiac reflexes stimulated by distention of structures at the venoatrial junctions (Bainbridge reflex). Tachycardia is, in terms of energy, an expensive way to support the cardiac output, and induction of sustained tachycardia is a standard means to produce heart failure in experimental animal models. Clinical counterparts are recognized in sustained ectopic tachyarrhythmias, and sinus tachycardia may exert an independent deleterious influence in chronic heart failure.

Dilation. Progressive ventricular dilation typically occurs with the transition from compensation to overt failure. Dilation may serve as a useful compensatory mechanism for a time via the Frank-Starling relationship, but with progressive disease it ultimately becomes inadequate to maintain stroke output or does so only at the cost of markedly elevated filling pressures.

Mechanisms contributing to the ultimate inability of the dilated heart to maintain adequate function include (1) ultrastructural changes with slippage of sarcomeres during progressive dilation; as a result, they are not stretched to generate optimal contractility; and (2) increased wall tension (law of Laplace, Fig. 34–3) resulting in increased myocardial oxygen consumption; a corollary is that in contrast to the normal heart, in which the wall tension decreases in the course of systole, wall tension tends to remain high throughout contraction in the dilated heart. Thus chronic dilation has important limitations as a compensatory mechanism in cardiac failure.

Hypertrophy. Sustained abnormal pressure or volume loads lead to an increase in ventricular mass. This involves changes in gene expression and increased protein synthesis. Decreased protein degradation rates may occur as well in response to mechanical overload or dilation. The stimulus for hypertrophy appears to involve an increase in wall stress and possibly in the energy requirements of a chronically dilated heart with elevated filling pressures.

The hypertrophy pattern depends on the nature of the load. Chronic volume overloading leads to increased total mass as the chamber size enlarges, but wall thickness changes little ("eccentric" hypertrophy). By contrast, chronic exposure to increased pressure (e.g., systemic hypertension or aortic stenosis) leads to a "concentric" hypertrophy pattern in which end-diastolic volume remains unchanged but wall thickness increases.

Abnormal electrical conduction patterns can interfere with the normal, smoothly coordinated contraction pattern of the normal heart, as can myocyte loss with focal or diffuse fibrosis. Ischemic myocardial damage tends to cause hypertrophy and remodeling of residual muscle because the geometry of the abnormal ventricle causes it to operate at a mechanical disadvantage and also because

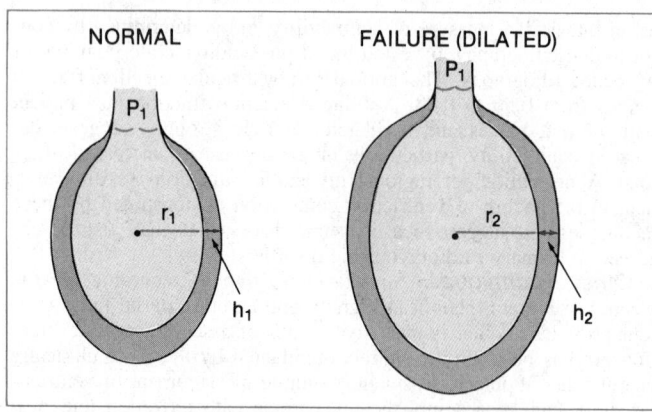

FIGURE 34-3. Laplace relationship applied to the dilated heart. The tension developed in the wall of the heart during systole (T) is a directional force that is proportional to the product of the mean pressure that the wall is supporting (P) and the mean radius (r). To a first approximation, $T = \dfrac{Pr}{2}$. Dilation of the heart ($r_2 > r_1$) at the same pressure ($P_1 = P_2$) increases wall tension ($T_2 > T_1$). Should the wall become thinner during dilatation, the wall stress would increase as the cross-sectional area of myocardium (h) decreased.

normal muscle must work, and expend energy, in moving and stretching adjacent damaged muscle or scar.

In early or mild hypertrophy, muscle mass and capillary vessels increase proportionately, preserving the nutritive and contractile properties of the myocardium. With progressive hypertrophy (in the absence of ventricular dilation), additional sarcomeres are laid down, wall thickness increases, and ventricular wall stress tends to be maintained at a normal level despite increased cavity pressure, as indicated in Figure 34–3. This process ultimately exacts a price, however, because increased wall thickness often leads to increased wall stiffness (reduced compliance), thus necessitating a disproportionate rise in filling pressure to maintain adequate end-diastolic ventricular volume. The increasingly recognized syndrome of diastolic ventricular dysfunction, which occurs relatively commonly in the presence of a preserved ventricular ejection fraction, leads to elevated pulmonary or systemic venous pressures, which contribute to symptoms of dyspnea or peripheral edema. In addition, beyond a certain point, coronary flow reserve diminishes and contractile function declines. Thus, once unremitting hypertrophy begins, the myocardium has embarked on the road to overt failure.

Despite the depressed contractile state associated with later stages of hypertrophy, circulatory function is maintained for a time by the combination of increased muscle mass, dilation, and augmented sympathetic drive. With continuing loss of myocardial contractility, or loss of muscle cells (e.g., from ischemic or inflammatory processes), circulatory compensation can no longer be maintained. The typical clinical and hemodynamic manifestations of congestive heart failure then emerge as cardiac output fails to meet demands and filling pressures increase.

Heart as a Muscle

Consideration of the ventricular performance of the failing heart usually centers on the contraction phase. Events during diastole, however, influence ventricular compliance and hence filling pressures, as well as the subsequent contraction and the energy supply for contraction and relaxation.

RELAXATION AND DISTENSIBILITY. Diastolic filling of the ventricle depends on the time available (a function of heart rate), the timing and properties of atrial systole, and the diastolic properties of the ventricle. Relaxation of cardiac muscle is an energy-requiring process (see above) that is quite vulnerable to adenosine triphosphate (ATP) depletion caused by ischemia. Although heart failure *per se* does not necessarily impair ventricular relaxation, associated processes of hypertrophy, fibrosis, and ischemia often reduce chamber distensibility and further increase filling pressures to levels producing pulmonary edema. This problem can be particularly severe in hypertrophic cardiomyopathy and in diseases

such as amyloidosis that markedly reduce left ventricular diastolic compliance. Elderly patients with hypertension and diabetes mellitus seem especially prone to diastolic ventricular dysfunction. Management of the subset of patients with predominant diastolic dysfunction is discussed below.

ENERGETICS. The heart depends on aerobic metabolism for its supply of energy, the bulk of which is spent to support contraction. The major determinants of oxygen consumption of the heart include the interrelated components of rate, ventricular pressure, volume, work, wall tension, and contractile state. The time integral of systolic tension relates closely to myocardial oxygen consumption, whereas fiber shortening has a minor effect on myocardial oxygen consumption.

The cellular and biochemical basis for heart failure remains unsettled. It is generally agreed that there are no consistent defects in protein synthesis and turnover. Current investigation is centered on excitation-contraction coupling and mechanisms that control calcium homeostasis as well as possible disturbances of energy metabolism that may contribute to progressive myocardial dysfunction.

Compensatory mechanisms in advanced heart failure tend to increase myocardial oxygen requirements by several mechanisms, including increased preload due to salt and water retention and enhanced sympathetic drive with consequently increased afterload, contractility, and heart rate. Increased preload and afterload are also the result of activation of the renin-angiotensin-aldosterone system.

Heart as Component of the Circulatory System

With loss of cardiac reserve and onset of overt heart failure, peripheral mechanisms are called upon to sustain blood pressure and to distribute the limited cardiac output to vital beds.

VENOUS HYPERTENSION. As the ejection fraction falls and the ventricle fails to empty properly during systole, the volume of unexpelled blood increases with an accompanying increase in diastolic pressure in the ventricles and in the atrium and proximal veins. Other elements that contribute to the venous hypertension include (1) increased tone in venous capacitance vessels; (2) blood volume expansion as a consequence of renal sodium and water retention; and, on occasion, (3) incompetence of mitral or tricuspid valves with regurgitation of blood from ventricle to atrium as the valve becomes incompetent from intrinsic valvular disease, papillary muscle dysfunction, ventricular dilation, or inadequate closure during an arrhythmia.

PERIPHERAL MECHANISMS TO SUSTAIN BLOOD PRESSURE AND CARDIAC OUTPUT. To sustain and distribute the cardiac output, and to maintain systemic arterial pressure, important peripheral mechanisms are activated.

In the normal circulation, the cardiac output doubles in response to a four- or fivefold increase in total body oxygen consumption. When functional impairment is such that the cardiac output cannot keep pace with peripheral demands, blood flow is redistributed to defend vital areas such as the brain and heart. The autonomic nervous system participates in this modulation of the circulation and contributes also to activation of mechanisms that mediate the retention of sodium and water.

Peripheral vasoconstriction and tachycardia characterize the common forms of heart failure. However, despite a generalized increase in sympathetic nervous activity, norepinephrine stores in the heart muscle are depleted because of its enhanced turnover rate. Pharmacologic agents such as reserpine or guanethidine further deplete cardiac catecholamine stores and can aggravate heart failure, as can β-adrenergic antagonists such as propranolol and the many other drugs of this class. At the same time, sustained activation of sympathetic nervous system activity has deleterious consequences and careful use of β-adrenergic blocking agents is undergoing intensive investigative scrutiny in patients with chronic heart failure.

The contribution of the parasympathetic nervous system to the control of heart rate and baroreceptor activity is impaired in heart failure, but therapeutic implications of these phenomena are not yet clear.

Peripheral Vasoconstriction. Peripheral arteriolar and venous constriction, mediated in large part by increased sympathetic nervous and renin-angiotensin system activity, is an important compensatory mechanism in heart failure that has both positive and negative consequences, as noted earlier.

Venoconstriction augments venous return by facilitating the return of blood to the central veins, increasing central venous pressure and hence preload. The principal determinant of elevated filling pressures, however, is the inability of the failing ventricle to eject the venous return.

Redistribution. Maintenance of oxygen and substrate delivery to brain and myocardium during states of limited cardiac output requires diversion of flow from skin, kidneys, splanchnic viscera, and skeletal muscle. This redistribution of blood flow initially occurs during activity or stress as cardiac output fails to increase sufficiently to meet the increment in metabolism; in severe heart failure, redistribution operates also at rest. The redistribution of blood flow to essential beds depends on the balance among sympathetic and renin-angiotensin system activities and local metabolism. The vasculature of skin, kidney, splanchnic beds, and skeletal muscle is richly innervated. Furthermore, these tissues have relatively low metabolic rates at rest, permitting sympathetic nervous and angiotensin II–mediated vasoconstriction to override local vasodilator effects of metabolites. By contrast, the circulations to brain and myocardium are less subject to α-adrenergically mediated vasoconstrictor influences because these organs, with their high oxygen consumption, produce metabolic dilator substances that offset increased sympathetic tone.

Under normal physiologic circumstances, exercise with the attendant need for heat dissipation induces an increase in cutaneous blood flow. Patients in heart failure, by contrast, fail to increase cutaneous flow despite this increased need for heat loss. Thus the patient in heart failure preserves systemic arterial pressure and flow to vital organs by suffering the consequences of impaired heat loss as well as limitation of blood flow to exercising muscle groups.

THE VALSALVA MANEUVER. An abnormal response to the Valsalva maneuver, in which intrathoracic pressure is maintained at approximately 40 mm Hg for 10 to 12 seconds, is characteristic of left ventricular failure. In normal subjects there is a characteristic decrease in blood pressure and pulse pressure and increase in heart rate; at cessation of straining, the blood pressure, pulse pressure, and bradycardia tend to overshoot. By contrast, in the presence of left ventricular failure there is a "square wave" response in which normal reflex responses are blunted. Hence blood pressure increases at the onset of straining, stays elevated throughout the maneuver, and decreases abruptly to baseline after the maneuver with no overshoot; tachycardia is absent.

SALT AND WATER RETENTION. As overt heart failure develops, there is typically a decrease in renal blood flow and glomerular filtration rate (GFR), with an associated redistribution of renal blood flow. These changes contribute to the sodium and water retention that characterizes heart failure, but the nature and extent of the response differ according to the severity of heart failure, as discussed subsequently under diuretics. Hemodynamic abnormalities are undoubtedly involved in activating the renin-angiotensin-aldosterone system both via direct effects on the kidney and via indirect effects stemming from activation of mechanoreceptors in the distended left atrium. Recognizing the role of hyperaldosteronism in the genesis of sodium and water retention has resulted in the development of aldosterone antagonists as useful adjuncts in the therapy of heart failure.

Sweat and saliva are sodium poor in patients with decompensated heart failure. Antidiuretic hormone (arginine vasopressin) levels tend to be elevated in heart failure and may contribute to elevated systemic vascular resistance, but probably are not important in salt or water retention.

An increase of about 10 to 20% in circulating blood volume contributes to maintenance of cardiac output and perfusion of vital organs in moderate-to-severe heart failure, augmenting ventricular end-diastolic volume and thereby tending to improve pump performance. The resulting elevation of filling pressure, however, promotes edema formation by raising venous and capillary pressures proximal to the failing ventricle. By the time the circulating blood volume has increased by 20%, the extravascular fluid volume may well have increased by a factor of two.

Exercise Testing

Graded treadmill or bicycle exercise testing has been used investigatively to determine maximum total body oxygen uptake (aerobic capacity). The endpoint of fatigue generally coincides with the point at which aerobic metabolism can no longer meet tissue demands and lactate production begins (anaerobic threshold). This ap-

proach has also been used to assess quantitatively the effects of therapeutic interventions for treating heart failure.

CLINICAL MANIFESTATIONS OF HEART FAILURE

The signs and symptoms of heart failure depend on which ventricle has failed and the severity and duration of failure. The clinical picture in left ventricular failure is dominated by *symptoms* of pulmonary congestion and edema. By contrast, right ventricular failure is dominated by *signs* of systemic venous congestion and peripheral edema. Weakness, fatigue, and effort intolerance are common to right or left ventricular failure as well as biventricular failure.

Left Ventricular Failure

The symptom of breathlessness predominates in patients with left ventricular failure and varies with position and activity. Noteworthy physical signs are most evident in the heart, lungs, or respiratory control mechanisms.

DYSPNEA. Dyspnea (breathlessness) during limited exertion is typically the earliest symptom of left heart failure and is usually associated with an increased rate of breathing (tachypnea). Although many details of the physiologic basis for the sensation of dyspnea remain unclear, some aspects of the origin of respiratory symptoms from pulmonary congestion deserve consideration. Because the bronchial capillaries drain for the most part via the pulmonary veins, congestion tends to develop in alveolar and bronchial vascular networks simultaneously. Interstitial edema surrounding pulmonary capillaries appears to stimulate juxtacapillary receptors known as J-receptors, which in turn elicits a reflexly mediated pattern of rapid and shallow breathing. At the same time, bronchial congestion stimulates mucus production, and the distended bronchial capillaries may rupture, with resulting cough and hemoptysis. Bronchial mucosal edema causes increased resistance in small airways, producing wheezing and respiratory distress known as cardiac asthma. The increased work of moving fluid-laden, noncompliant lungs must be accomplished in the face of decreased blood flow to respiratory muscles and also increased diffusion barriers to oxygen exchange across the alveolar-capillary interface, contributing to respiratory muscle fatigue and the sensation of dyspnea.

Thus, the symptom of dyspnea in left heart failure clearly relates to the increase in blood volume and interstitial fluid content of the lungs at the expense of air. Ventilation increases, and the awareness of dyspnea becomes more severe as minute ventilation approaches the maximal ventilatory capacity.

ORTHOPNEA. Dyspnea that occurs soon after lying flat (and is relieved by sitting up) is known as orthopnea. The pathophysiologic basis for orthopnea is the increase in venous return from the lower extremities and splanchnic bed to the lungs in the recumbent position, together with the reabsorption of peripheral edema that accumulates during the day. Orthopnea is a relatively reliable marker for left ventricular failure, whereas the dyspnea associated with chronic lung disease or musculoskeletal disorders is typically less aggravated by lying flat. Patients usually learn to avoid dyspnea of this sort by sleeping with the head and thorax on two or more pillows. In advanced heart failure, orthopnea may be so severe as to cause the patient to sleep upright in a chair. An orthopneic cough has the same significance as orthopnea and is presumably the consequence of venous congestion and edema. Patients with left heart failure may also complain of precordial distress in the supine position that is difficult to distinguish from symptoms caused by myocardial ischemia.

NOCTURIA. In early heart failure, limitation of renal blood flow with upright activity during the day gives way to more normal renal perfusion and diuresis while supine at night. This causes nocturia, a common early symptom of incipient heart failure.

PAROXYSMAL NOCTURNAL DYSPNEA. Severe respiratory distress may arouse the patient from sleep. Relief is urgently sought by sitting up and often by finding an open window. In addition to exacerbation of pulmonary vascular congestion and edema during supine sleep, blunting of the respiratory center response to sensory input from the lungs during sleep, together with increased venous return, allows pulmonary venous congestion and edema to accumulate and trigger the alarming episode of breathlessness.

ACUTE PULMONARY EDEMA. In an episode of acute left ventricular failure, pulmonary venous and capillary pressure can increase abruptly to levels exceeding plasma oncotic pressure, with consequent rapid accumulation of edema fluid in the interstitial spaces and alveoli. Interstitial pulmonary edema leads to an increase in respiratory rate (see foregoing discussion) and tends to produce alveolar hyperventilation and respiratory alkalosis. However, when free fluid enters the alveoli and bronchioles, respiratory acidosis may occur owing to an intolerable increase in the work of breathing. Hypoxemia also occurs commonly because of imbalances between alveolar ventilation and alveolar blood flow (ventilation-perfusion mismatch or "shunting").

Symptoms of pulmonary edema may begin with a nonproductive cough, with wheezing, or with frank dyspnea. Apart from tachypnea and possibly evidence of underlying heart disease on physical examination, few physical signs may be present initially. Later, as free fluid accumulates in distal airways, rales become audible at the lung bases and extend upward accompanied by rhonchi as the episode progresses. In severe acute pulmonary edema, the patient is typically pale, sweating, cyanotic, gasping for breath, and sometimes producing pink or blood-tinged frothy sputum.

HEMOPTYSIS. Rust-colored sputum containing heart failure cells (alveolar macrophages containing hemosiderin) sometimes occurs in severe chronic left heart failure and is seen with particular frequency in patients with advanced mitral stenosis. Frankly bloody sputum should suggest the possibility of pulmonary infarction, but expectoration of substantial quantities of blood can also occur as a consequence of rupture of engorged bronchial capillaries in patients with chronic left heart failure, including that caused by uncorrected mitral stenosis.

CHEYNE-STOKES RESPIRATION. Advanced heart failure may be accompanied by periodic breathing with alternate periods of apnea and hyperventilation. Because of slowing of the circulation time from lungs to brain, the arterial Po_2 reaches its peak and the arterial Pco_2 its nadir during apnea. At this time alveolar gas tensions are exactly opposite. During hyperpnea the alveolar Po_2 reaches its peak and the alveolar Pco_2 its nadir. Thus, changes in arterial blood gases are responsible for the cyclic ventilation, which in turn causes the changes in alveolar gas tensions. As would be expected from this delay of the normal negative feedback loop, the longer the circulation time, the longer are the cycles of hyperventilation and apnea. The neurologic changes of advanced age predispose to Cheyne-Stokes breathing, as does cerebrovascular disease.

Physical and Laboratory Signs of Left Heart Failure

The patient with decompensated left heart failure is generally tachypneic, pale, dusky, and sweaty. The handshake is cold because of peripheral vasoconstriction, and tachycardia is present. The pulse pressure is usually narrow, often with a modest increase in diastolic pressure. The neck veins are not distended if the left ventricle alone has failed.

THE HEART. Cardiac enlargement is often evident upon inspection, percussion, and palpation of the apical impulse and is confirmed by radiographic and echocardiographic examination, although this finding is more typical of valvular or primary myocardial disease than of ischemic heart disease. With increased left heart filling pressure, pulmonary venous pressure increases and the pulmonary arterial pressure must also increase. The pulmonic component of the second heart sound (P_2) therefore tends to increase in intensity. In the presence of left ventricular dilation, papillary muscle dysfunction, or both, the mitral valve leaflets may fail to appose properly, resulting in mitral incompetence.

Gallop Rhythm. The presence of a protodiastolic third heart sound (S_3 gallop) in an adult with heart disease usually signifies the presence of ventricular failure. The timing of the normal first and second sounds and the abnormal third sound, in conjunction with an increased heart rate, results in the characteristic cadence of the gallop rhythm. The third heart sound occurs in early diastole coincident with rapid ventricular filling. The S_3 gallop appears to be produced by vibrations of the ventricular walls as the rapidly inflowing blood is abruptly arrested. A third heart sound is a normal finding in children and in young adults.

Presystolic gallop rhythms result from the atrial contribution to ventricular filling. The atrial or S_4 gallop is characteristic of decreased ventricular compliance and typically results from left ventricular hypertrophy or ischemia rather than from myocardial dysfunction or failure, although an S_4 gallop is typically present in patients with symptoms and signs of heart failure due predominantly to diastolic dysfunction. When a patient with an audible fourth heart sound develops overt heart failure, a third sound may appear, causing a quadruple rhythm. If the heart rate is sufficiently rapid or the PR interval is prolonged, S_3 and S_4 may merge, producing a summation gallop. The presence of a summation gallop has the same clinical implication as other protodiastolic (S_3) gallop rhythms.

Pulsus Alternans. The presence of alternating strong and weak beats (the fundamental rhythm remaining regular) usually signifies advanced heart failure. Pulsus alternans can be detected by palpation or by sphygmomanometry and often follows an atrial or ventricular premature beat for several cycles. Mechanical alternans of this sort is only rarely associated with electrical alternans. Pulsus alternans has been attributed to a severe disturbance of excitation-contraction coupling, the detailed pathophysiology of which is unclear.

THE LUNGS. The sequence of pulmonary findings with advancing left heart failure has been described in the foregoing section on acute pulmonary edema.

THE ELECTROCARDIOGRAM. Electrocardiographic abnormalities result from underlying cardiac disease, therapeutic agents (e.g., digitalis), or both and yield little information regarding the functional status of the heart.

RADIOLOGIC ASPECTS. The chest radiograph is usually quite helpful in diagnosing and assessing left ventricular failure (see Ch. 33). The cardiac silhouette is typically, but not invariably, enlarged and may assume telltale configurations that are determined by the underlying disease process. In contrast to normal, the pulmonary vasculature is prominent in the upper lung zones, reflecting pulmonary venous hypertension and redistribution of blood flow because of encroachment upon the lower lung vessels by edema and possibly fibrosis. Enlarged hilar shadows and prominent septal lines, particularly near the costophrenic angles (Kerley's B lines), are typical findings. Alveolar edema results in a generalized clouding of the lung fields but can occur in focal or patchy distributions that are difficult to distinguish from pneumonia. Pleural effusions sometimes occur in predominantly left-sided heart failure but are more characteristic of biventricular failure. Interstitial and alveolar edema may lessen or disappear with onset of right ventricular failure. A widened superior vena cava shadow suggests right ventricular failure and systemic venous congestion.

NONINVASIVE ASSESSMENT. Echocardiographic study is a cost-effective approach to evaluating patients with heart failure, and together with Doppler study in most instances is advisable at an early stage in the workup of this group of patients (see Ch. 33.3). Valuable information can be obtained in every etiologic class of patients, including those with ischemic disease, cardiomyopathy, valvular disease, hypertensive disease, congenital disease, and cor pulmonale. Echo study is of particular value in making the important distinction between prominent systolic and diastolic ventricular dysfunction.

CARDIAC CATHETERIZATION. Invasive evaluation is usually appropriate in patients who are candidates for cardiac surgery or catheter-based interventional procedures such as coronary angioplasty or valvuloplasty, as discussed in Ch. 33.6. Right ventricular endomyocardial biopsy is valuable in patients suspected of having inflammatory or infiltrative disease and for assessment of myopathic effects of certain antineoplastic drugs (e.g., doxorubicin). Endomyocardial biopsy is routinely done using a percutaneous jugular approach at intervals following cardiac transplantation for assessing the adequacy of immunosuppressive therapy.

PULMONARY FUNCTION TESTS. With interstitial pulmonary edema, expiratory flow rates at low lung volumes are reduced and distal airways tend to close prematurely during expiration, trapping gas within the lungs and disturbing the normal relation of ventilation to perfusion. This produces a widening of the alveolar-arterial Po_2 difference and a decrease in arterial Po_2 due to venous admixture. Arterial oxygen saturation is typically nearly normal, however, unless intrinsic lung disease is present. The arteriovenous oxygen content difference increases with decreasing cardiac outputs as tissue extraction of oxygen becomes more complete. Systemic arterial Pco_2 remains normal or low unless ventilation is compromised in the course of pulmonary edema. Endotracheal intubation and assisted ventilation may be indicated if progressive carbon dioxide retention is documented by serial blood gas measurements.

Right Ventricular and Biventricular Failure

CLINICAL MANIFESTATIONS. Isolated right ventricular failure is uncommon in adults and is usually a consequence of cor pulmonale secondary to intrinsic lung disease or, on occasion, chronic volume overload from a congenital intracardiac left-to-right shunt (e.g., atrial septal defect). Right ventricular failure is encountered most often as a complication of left ventricular failure. In the presence of elevated right heart filling pressures, neck veins are distended and fill from below. Hepatic enlargement and tenderness to gentle palpation result from passive congestion, and manual compression over the liver causes further distention of the neck veins (hepatojugular reflux). In the presence of biventricular failure, signs of right ventricular failure may dominate, but the presence of dyspnea and rales should suggest additional left ventricular failure. Accompanying low cardiac output results in signs of increased sympathetic nervous activity and of organ hypoperfusion. It should be remembered that a critically lowered cardiac output from any cause sufficient to produce metabolic acidosis occasions hyperventilation in defense of acid-base balance, and this must be distinguished from the tachypnea of left heart failure. Advanced right-sided or biventricular failure may be associated with anorexia, weight loss, and malnutrition ("cardiac cachexia").

Cyanosis. Cyanosis is caused by 5 or more grams per 100 ml of unoxygenated hemoglobin in the subpapillary venous plexus of the skin. This occurs in right heart failure because the congested venules contain blood from which considerable oxygen has been extracted because of the slow flow. This is typically accompanied by relatively normal arterial Po_2 values unless intrinsic lung disease or intracardiac shunting is present. Cyanosis is usually absent in left heart failure unless caused by a complication (e.g., pneumonia) or by pulmonary edema.

Abnormal Heart and Lungs. Although dyspnea accompanying left ventricular failure may be partially relieved by onset of right ventricular failure, some dyspnea usually persists, together with tachypnea and basal rales. Tricuspid valvular insufficiency commonly accompanies severe right ventricular dilation and failure and contributes to systemic venous engorgement. The murmur of tricuspid insufficiency is distinguished from that of mitral insufficiency by its location (lower left border of sternum), by its tendency to increase during inspiration, and by associated physical signs, such as hepatic pulsation and systolic waves in the jugular venous pulse. Doppler echocardiography greatly assists in the assessment of this problem. Pleural effusion, often unilateral, is more common in right-sided or biventricular than in isolated left ventricular failure.

Systemic Venous Congestion. Elevated systemic venous pressure is a *sine qua non* of right heart failure. Responsible mechanisms include (1) the inability of the failing ventricle to eject the venous return without abnormally high filling pressures, causing (2) an increase in the volume of blood in the large systemic veins, and (3) increased venomotor tone resulting from increased sympathetic nervous system activity. Increased systemic venous pressure is responsible for the hepatomegaly, occasional splenomegaly, and peripheral edema that characterize decompensated right ventricular failure. Usually less apparent are the associated congestion and edema of the gastrointestinal tract.

Pressure in the jugular venous system, a useful index of right atrial pressure, may be estimated from the height of the column of blood distending the cervical veins. The cervical veins are normally flat in the upright posture in the absence of raised intrathoracic pressure, whereas in right heart failure they are prominent and distended. The wave form of venous pulsation is usually best appreciated when inspecting the right internal jugular vein, adjusting the angle of the patient's upper body to bring out the top of the venous pressure column. Tricuspid insufficiency distorts the normal venous pulse by producing a systolic or C-V wave that has no counterpart in the normal jugular venous pulse. Occasionally, compression over the liver is necessary to display the increased blood volume in the venous system, but the examiner must avoid being misled by venous distention from involuntary expiration against a closed glottis (Valsalva's maneuver).

Liver. The liver is typically enlarged and tender in right heart failure. If the onset is acute, right upper quadrant pain may result

from constraint of the swollen liver by its tight capsule. Splenomegaly is uncommon except in prolonged passive congestion of the liver, and pain or tenderness of the spleen should raise the question of superimposed systemic embolization and splenic infarction.

Early congestion of the liver may cause modest increases in the concentrations of hepatic enzymes such as alkaline phosphatase in serum, and increases in serum bilirubin may occur. Hyperbilirubinemia from this cause usually consists of a combination of conjugated and unconjugated bilirubin. Frank jaundice is uncommon unless hepatic congestion is associated with longstanding pulmonary congestion or pulmonary infarction.

Hypoglycemia may occur if cardiac output is severely compromised and hepatic congestion is marked and protracted. This is attributed to depletion of liver glycogen stores and increased formation of lactic acid from glucose induced by hypoxia.

Repeated and prolonged episodes of right heart failure with reduced hepatic blood flow and elevated venous pressures can cause atrophy and centrilobular necrosis of liver cells and can lead to extensive fibrosis ("cardiac cirrhosis") that is difficult to distinguish from posthepatitic cirrhosis. Hepatic failure with precoma or coma is a rare, preterminal complication of this sequence of events.

Extracellular Fluid Compartments. The fluid compartments of the body are normally maintained constant by neurohormonally mediated interplay among intake (governed by thirst and appetite), exchanges of fluid and electrolytes (governed by passive and active transport mechanisms), and excretion (regulated primarily by the kidneys). In heart failure, excessive retention of sodium and water by the kidneys results in an isosmotic expansion of extracellular fluid, including the circulating blood volume. In mild heart failure, retention of sodium and water may serve to expand the blood volume to sustain venous return and the forward output of the failing heart through the Frank-Starling mechanism. However, retention of salt and water only exacerbates pulmonary and systemic congestion and edema when the myocardium can no longer respond positively to increased filling pressure and volumes.

The distribution of excess extracellular ("third space") fluid varies among patients. Under the influence of gravity, edema accumulates in the feet and ankles of ambulatory patients but shifts to the sacral region in the bedridden patient. Localization occurs in areas of low tissue pressure, such as the back of the ankle. Colloid osmotic pressure and the integrity of the lymphatic system also influence extracellular fluid distribution.

Peripheral Edema. Dependent edema developing over the course of the day and subsiding by morning is a characteristic feature of right heart failure. It is a direct consequence of elevated systemic venous pressure and is typically preceded by a gain in weight. Persistent edema is accompanied relatively frequently by complications such as low-grade cellulitis, and the combination of edema and sluggish venous flow predisposes to deep venous thrombosis and pulmonary embolism.

Pleural Effusion. The infrequency of hydrothorax in isolated right ventricular failure dictates that the association of pleural effusion and cor pulmonale should lead one to search for another cause, such as pulmonary infarction. It is, however, common in biventricular failure. Hydrothorax results from impaired removal of isotonic fluid from the pleural space because of elevated venous pressures in both the pulmonary and the systemic circulations, compromising transcapillary exchange of water at the pleural surface and also impeding lymphatic drainage. Hydrothorax contributes to dyspnea reflexly, probably by stimuli from lungs and chest wall, as well as by displacing ventilated lung tissue from the relatively fixed volume of the thoracic space. Pulmonary embolism and infarction may contribute to pleural effusion in two ways: by transit of fluid from the infarcted area of the lung to the pleural space or by aggravation of heart failure.

Ascites. The presence of free fluid in the abdominal cavity is a late manifestation of right heart failure, usually associated with systemic venous hypertension, peripheral edema, and hydrothorax. It is commonly encountered in the setting of tricuspid valve disease or chronic constrictive pericarditis. Elevated pressures in portal and hepatic veins and in the systemic veins draining the peritoneum contribute to the formation of ascites, but renal retention of sodium and water is a prerequisite. It may contribute to anorexia and can cause abdominal discomfort or pain in patients with severe right ventricular failure.

Pericardial Effusion. Patients with chronic heart failure commonly have increased amounts of fluid in the pericardial sac that can be demonstrated echocardiographically. Only rarely, however, does it accumulate to an extent that produces further hemodynamic compromise (tamponade).

Anasarca. Advanced and protracted right ventricular failure without adequate treatment can cause edema fluid to accumulate throughout the body, most conspicuously in subcutaneous tissues as well as abdominal and thoracic cavities. Face and arms are typically spared until the preterminal stages of failure. This clinical picture occurs rarely in the present era of potent diuretics.

Gastrointestinal Tract. Systemic venous hypertension leads to edema of the bowel wall. These changes interfere with absorption of drugs or foods only when heart failure is severe, but reduced bioavailability of furosemide and perhaps other drugs can occur under these circumstances. In severe congestive heart failure, anorexia, nausea, and vomiting may occur from reflex, central, local, or drug-induced causes. Protein-losing enteropathy can occur in the setting of severe right heart failure.

Brain. Nonspecific complaints, including headache and insomnia, are common in heart failure and are usually attributable to some diminution of cerebral blood flow and triggering mechanisms such as dyspnea that contribute to insomnia. Neurologic or behavioral aberrations are more frequent when the burdens of a limited cardiac output are superimposed on antecedent neurologic disease (e.g., cerebrovascular disease or prior stroke) or on personality disorder. Irritability, restlessness, and limited attention span are associated with severe congestive heart failure. Stupor and coma supervene when cardiac output is critically reduced.

Kidney. Oliguria occurs with decompensation in isolated right or left heart failure but is more prominent in the latter or in biventricular failure. The urine is sodium poor but has a relatively high specific gravity (1.020 to 1.030). Prerenal azotemia is common, particularly in the presence of intrinsic renal disease or after vigorous diuresis. Azotemia with high urine specific gravity is characteristic of heart failure (and dehydration) and stands in contrast to the low specific gravity expected with renal insufficiency due to intrinsic renal disease. Blood urea nitrogen (BUN) is typically elevated out of proportion to serum creatinine. Proteinuria is common but does not usually exceed 1 gram per day.

Other Manifestations. In chronic severe congestive heart failure, weakness and gradual loss of tissue mass are frequent concomitants and may progress to cachexia. At this late stage, the patient is usually suffering from anorexia and often gastrointestinal symptoms and electrolyte disturbances as well. Although organ hypoperfusion and congestion play an important part in this syndrome, the physician must maintain vigilance to avoid additional contributions from overvigorous use of digitalis and diuretics.

Anxiety. This is a common feature of cardiac disease by the time the heart fails. Manifestations of anxiety may be difficult to distinguish from symptoms of the underlying cardiac disorder because of the nonspecific nature of complaints such as breathlessness. Symptoms related to hyperventilation as well as palpitations may contribute to the patient's anxiety by reinforcing the impression that organic heart disease is present. The physician must proceed with the separate assessment of organic and psychosomatic aspects of the disease process, recognizing that a careful history and physical examination, together with judicious use of noninvasive diagnostic methods, helps to establish the extent to which organic heart disease is responsible for the patient's symptoms.

CLINICAL MANAGEMENT OF HEART FAILURE
General Approaches

The management of congestive heart failure includes three general types of approaches. The first is removing the underlying cause. This deserves top priority in all cases and includes measures such as surgically correcting valvular lesions or congenital malformation. It also includes medical treatment of hypertension or infective endocarditis when present.

The second approach consists of removal of precipitating causes of heart failure. Frequently the initial development or exacerbation of heart failure is related not to worsening of the underlying cardiac condition but rather to a superimposed stress. Typical factors that can precipitate overt congestive heart failure, apart from changes in the status of the heart itself, are listed in Table 34–2.

The third set of measures, treatment of clinical manifestations of heart failure, occupies the remainder of this chapter. This approach may in turn be divided into three categories, as summarized in Table 34–3:

1. Measures to improve the contractile performance of the heart.
2. Measures to reduce cardiac work.
3. Measures to control excessive retention of salt and water.

As listed in Table 34–3, several therapeutic entities are available in each category. Cardiac glycosides and sympathomimetic agents constitute the principal drugs that enhance the pumping performance of the failing heart. In addition, placement of a pacemaker may improve pumping performance either by supporting a more appropriate heart rate or by restoring atrial augmentation of ventricular filling if synchronous atrioventricular contraction can be achieved (see Ch. 35).

Reducing the workload of the failing heart can be accomplished by physical and emotional rest, by appropriate treatment of obesity, and by vasodilator therapy. Under specific circumstances, assisted circulation with the intra-aortic balloon pump can usefully contribute to this goal.

Finally, controlling the excessive retention of salt and water is approached by instituting a low-sodium diet and using diuretic drugs. Under some circumstances, mechanically removing fluid is of value.

These measures are customarily applied in a stepwise fashion, as outlined in detail in Table 34–4.

Strategy of Heart Failure Management

The many causes and degrees of severity of heart failure demand an individualized approach to each patient. Nevertheless, certain general principles apply to the management of various subsets of patients. The comments that follow are relevant to patients with *systolic* ventricular dysfunction (i.e., reduced ejection fraction). In the past, it has not been considered appropriate to institute specific therapeutic measures until symptoms of overt heart failure occur—that is, until the patient makes the transition from functional class I to class II. The results of the SOLVD prevention and SAVE trials, however, support the earlier use of angiotensin-converting enzyme (ACE) inhibitors in patients with marked ventricular systolic dysfunction, even if signs and symptoms of overt heart failure have not become evident. The first approach (see Table 34–4) in all instances includes judicious limitation of activity, advising the patient to avoid physical exertion that produces undue dyspnea or exhaustion. The degree of restriction should be tailored to the severity of heart failure. It is important not to limit activity so severely that skeletal muscle deconditioning, rather than the underlying cardiac problem, becomes the limiting factor in the patient's activity. Physical activity should, however, be markedly restricted in the setting of

---

TABLE 34–3. MEASURES IN THE MANAGEMENT OF CONGESTIVE HEART FAILURE

A. Improve pump performance of the failing ventricle
  1. Cardiac glycosides (digoxin)
  2. Sympathomimetic drugs (dopamine, dobutamine)
  3. Other positive inotropic drugs (amrinone,* milrinone*)
  4. Pacemaker for bradycardia or loss of atrioventricular synchrony
B. Reduction of cardiac workload
  1. Rest (physical and emotional)
  2. Correction of obesity
  3. Vasodilator drugs
  4. Assisted circulation (e.g., intra-aortic balloon counterpulsation)
C. Control salt and water retention
  1. Limit dietary sodium intake
  2. Diuretics
  3. Mechanical removal of fluid
    a. Thoracentesis
    b. Paracentesis
    c. Dialysis
    d. Phlebotomy

* Available for short-term use in the ICU setting only.

TABLE 34-4. STEPS IN THE MANAGEMENT OF CHRONIC CONGESTIVE HEART FAILURE

Steps	Functional Class		
	II	*III*	*IV*
A	*Restrict physical activity:* Limit competitive sports and heavy labor	Reduce work schedule; rest periods during day	Limit to house and finally to bed and chair
B	*Dietary sodium restriction:* Eliminate salt shaker and heavily salted foods	Eliminate salt in cooking and at table (Na intake ~ 1.2 to 1.8 grams)	As in III, plus low-sodium foods (Na intake < 1 gram)
C	*Diuretics:* Thiazide or low-dose loop diuretic	Loop diuretic (progressive doses); consider adding distally acting (K-sparing) diuretic	Loop diuretic with distally acting (K-sparing) and/or thiazide diuretic
D	*Vasodilators:* ACE inhibitor (captopril, enalapril, or lisinopril)	Hydralazine and isosorbide dinitrate can be cautiously added or substituted for an ACE inhibitor (see text)	Intravenous nitroprusside
E	*Digitalis glycosides:* Conventional maintenance doses ————————————————→		Dose to maintain serum level in 1.5 ng/ml range
F			*Other inotropic drugs (intravenous):* Dopamine, dobutamine, amrinone, milrinone
G			*Consider cardiac transplantation* *Thoracentesis, paracentesis* *Dialysis* *Assisted circulation (e.g., intra-aortic balloon pump)*

acute decompensation of chronic heart failure, a situation in which hospitalization is generally advisable.

A comprehensive set of clinical practice guidelines for the management of patients with heart failure due to left ventricular systolic dysfunction formulated by an expert panel has recently been published (Konstam et al.).

PHARMACOTHERAPY. A diuretic, a vasodilator (usually an ACE inhibitor), or a cardiac glycoside may be added in early class II, with the choice of one or more based on the balance between risk and expected benefit. In many cases, modest doses of a mild diuretic such as a thiazide restore the patient to an essentially asymptomatic state. A vasodilator such as captopril or enalapril should be used if there is evidence of elevated peripheral vascular resistance (systemic hypertension) and no contraindications exist (e.g., postural hypotension or renal impairment with bilateral renal artery stenosis). These agents have also proved beneficial in large-scale clinical trials in delaying the progression of ventricular remodeling and emergence of overt heart failure in patients with left ventricular dysfunction. Dietary sodium restriction may be limited to avoiding heavily salted foods and the use of the salt shaker at the table. Special low-sodium foods are expensive and can be so unpalatable as to impair nutrition.

When symptoms persist or evolve on the simple regimen outlined above, combination therapy with diuretics, vasodilators, and cardiac glycosides is usually indicated. Intensifying the diuretic regimen is often necessary. Problems such as mitral regurgitation are particularly amenable to treatment with vasodilators, as discussed below.

As the severity of heart failure advances, increased restriction of physical activity is usually necessary, and patients often require rest periods during the day as class III symptoms evolve. When patients remain symptomatic during ordinary activity on a program that includes loop diuretics, digitalis, and vasodilators, detailed evaluation is advisable to search for precipitating causes and to consider the possibility of more aggressive approaches. In patients who have progressed to functional class IV, hospitalization is often advisable and the use of intravenous sympathomimetic agents can be considered, in addition to optimization of the vasodilator, diuretic, and cardiac glycoside regimens. In patients who meet appropriate criteria, cardiac transplantation should also be considered at this time if not earlier (see Ch. 48).

During episodes of decompensation, the hazards of deep venous thrombosis and pulmonary embolism must be guarded against, and the use of minidose heparin (see Ch. 46) is a relatively safe and effective approach during hospitalization. At these times, emotional as well as physical rest is important, and anxiety-provoking situations should be carefully avoided. Marked anxiety or insomnia may be treated with benzodiazepines such as diazepam or the shorter-acting agent triazolam.

DIET. Rigid salt restriction can usually be avoided until diuretics can no longer control the accumulation of salt and water. Water intake does not, in general, require specific restriction unless dilutional hyponatremia supervenes.

OXYGEN. Patients with hypoxia, and certainly those with pulmonary edema, benefit from oxygen inhalation, conveniently given by nasal prongs at 4 to 6 liters per minute. In general, supplemental oxygen is worthwhile whenever the arterial oxygen saturation falls below 90%. This is a particularly effective way of reducing right ventricular afterload because oxygen is a potent pulmonary arteriolar vasodilator.

PHYSICAL REMOVAL OF FLUID. The availability of potent diuretics limits the need for thoracentesis or paracentesis, but these procedures may be important diagnostically when the accumulation of fluid in serous cavities is not readily explained on the basis of heart failure alone. Pulmonary embolism, for example, is a relatively common cause of pleural effusion, and a diagnostic thoracentesis often provides critically important information leading to this diagnosis. Drainage of pleural or ascitic fluid should be carried out slowly, at a rate of not more than about 1500 ml per hour, and the total quantity of fluid removed on any single occasion should not exceed about 1500 ml because of the risk of fluid shifts from the vascular to the extravascular compartment, with consequently inadequate ventricular filling pressures. Particular caution is required in patients (such as those with aortic stenosis or hypertrophic cardiomyopathy) who have reduced ventricular compliance and require high ventricular filling pressures to maintain adequate stroke volume.

Acute Pulmonary Edema

Acute pulmonary edema is a medical emergency in which the immediate therapeutic goals are to (1) improve oxygenation; (2) reduce venous return (preload); (3) reduce anxiety; and (4) treat causal and precipitating factors. Placing flow-directed pulmonary artery (Swan-Ganz) and arterial lines to monitor pressures and arterial blood gases is often advisable. The patient is placed in a trunk-up, legs-down posture and given humidified 100% oxygen, by positive pressure mask if possible. Vital signs are monitored frequently, and an intravenous cannula is inserted for secure intravenous access. Arterial blood gas, BUN or creatinine, electrolyte, and complete blood count measurements are obtained at once. An electrocardiogram and chest radiograph (taken with a portable machine if necessary) should also be obtained, and electrical conversion of supraventricular or ventricular tachyarrhythmias should be considered if present and if not due to digitalis excess. Ultrasound (echocardiographic) study is indicated at the earliest opportunity if the nature and extent of underlying cardiac disease are not entirely clear.

Morphine given intravenously (2 to 10 mg, repeated every 10 to 15 minutes) reduces venous return and allays anxiety; naloxone should be available in case of respiratory depression. Nitroglycerin given sublingually or intravenously further reduces venous return; nitroprusside given intravenously may be used if the blood pressure is adequately maintained and afterload reduction is desirable. Furosemide should be given intravenously in a 20- to 40-mg dose and repeated in increasing doses as necessary to achieve a diuresis. Aminophylline, 250 to 500 mg given slowly intravenously (5.6 mg per kilogram), may be useful to relieve bronchospasm and promote diuresis but can exacerbate sinus or ectopic tachycardias.

If severe respiratory distress persists, tourniquets applied to three of four extremities and rotated every 15 to 20 minutes may be of value but are rarely needed in the current era, given the availability of potent diuretics and vasodilators. If respiratory acidosis (pH ≤ 7.10) or severe hypoxemia ($P_{O_2} < 50$ mm Hg) persists, endotracheal intubation and controlled positive-pressure ventilation should usually be instituted. Phlebotomy and hemodialysis deserve consideration in refractory cases. Digitalis has a secondary role in this clinical setting, except occasionally in the management of supraventricular tachyarrhythmias. Superimposed hypotension and low cardiac output states are considered in Ch. 69. Concurrently, vigorous attention should be directed to the identification and management of precipitating factors (see Table 34–2).

Diuretics

Salt and water retention with consequent expansion of the intravascular and interstitial compartments is a *sine qua non* of chronic congestive heart failure and accounts for many of the common signs and symptoms. Elimination of excess salt and water is an essential goal in management of heart failure.

Two stages characterize diuretic use: first, eliminating accumulated excess fluid; and second, maintaining optimal "dry" weight. Care of patients in the hospital typically focuses on eliminating excess fluid, which is facilitated by controlling salt intake and limiting activity of hospitalized patients. Maintaining optimal fluid balance out of hospital requires adjustments in the context of the individual patient's diet and activity. A sound approach is to use the mildest diuretic program that is consistent with maintaining appropriate fluid balance and a salt intake that promotes a nutritious diet. Severe sodium restriction is usually unnecessary except in very severe congestive heart failure. Overly rigorous restriction of sodium intake, together with use of potent diuretics, is a well-known formula for impaired renal function, oliguria, and prerenal azotemia, particularly in the elderly.

CONTROL OF SODIUM BALANCE. The key role of diuretics in managing heart failure relates to the central role of the kidney as a target of many of the neurohumoral and hemodynamic changes that occur in heart failure. Reduced cardiac output causes activation of the renin-angiotensin system in the kidney, with consequent reduction in renal blood flow and increased glomerular filtration fraction, leading to increased resorption of salt and water by the proximal tubule. Elevated plasma angiotensin II levels contribute to increased systemic vascular resistance and increase aldosterone release from the adrenal. Increased renal sympathetic nerve activity also tends to reduce renal blood flow and to release renin from the macula densa, as well as directly augmenting sodium resorption along other segments of the nephron. Intrarenal blood flow redistribution contributes to the formation of relatively concentrated urine (Fig. 34–4). Plasma vasopressin levels are frequently elevated in

patients with heart failure, further limiting free water clearance. Together with the increase in thirst of patients with advanced heart failure, this leads to a hyponatremic state that is a particularly ominous prognostic sign in heart failure.

Diuretics intervene in the pathophysiology of heart failure by reducing the reabsorption of sodium and its accompanying anions, as well as water, by the renal tubule. The four major classes of diuretics in current clinical use are summarized in Table 34–5. Each of these agents affects renal tubular function in a distinct way, and each tends to produce a characteristic set of abnormalities in electrolyte patterns, fluid balance, and acid-base homeostasis. The more potent the diuretic, the greater the potential risk for severe and sometimes life-threatening disturbances of electrolyte and acid-base balance.

THIAZIDES. Because of their effectiveness when administered orally, their predictable effects, and their relative freedom from toxicity, thiazide diuretics are very commonly used in managing heart failure. The thiazide diuretics include several agents with chemical and pharmacologic similarities. The prototype is chlorothiazide. Chlorthalidone and metolazone are heterocyclic compounds that share the basic benzothiadiazine nucleus. All of these drugs inhibit the Na^+-Cl^- cotransporter in the distal tubule. This effect does not depend upon the weak carbonic anhydrase inhibitory activities common to most of these drugs. By inhibiting sodium chloride transport in the distal tubule, dilution of tubular fluid is prevented and delivery of solute and water to the hydrogen- and potassium-secreting sites in the collecting duct is enhanced. Calcium reabsorption is also promoted by the thiazides, probably by enhancement of calcium entry into epithelial cells of the distal tubule and perhaps by mild volume depletion as well.

The thiazides are useful when initially managing mild to moderate congestive heart failure. Their utility is limited, however, by avid solute reabsorption in the more proximal nephron segments. Thiazides are largely ineffective when GFR < 30 ml per minute. They are often useful in the treatment of refractory edema in combination with loop diuretics, as discussed subsequently.

Potentially troublesome side effects include potassium depletion, hyperuricemia, glucose intolerance, and plasma lipid elevations, as discussed below. Care must be taken to avoid gastric and small bowel irritation from the potassium chloride supplements that are often required in conjunction with thiazide diuretics.

CARBONIC ANHYDRASE INHIBITORS. Related to the thiazides are the carbonic anhydrase inhibitors, of which acetazolamide is the only agent currently available. This drug results in urinary sodium and bicarbonate losses until the plasma bicarbonate level falls to the point at which renal tubular bicarbonate reabsorption (both proximal and distal) exceeds the filtered load of bicarbonate. Thus, these agents tend to have a transient effect. The sodium and potassium loss accompanying bicarbonate excretion is moderate, but acetazolamide may be of value in patients with high serum bicarbonate levels, as may occur in cor pulmonale or metabolic alkalosis. The presence of metabolic acidosis, e.g., from renal failure or hepatic failure, constitutes a contraindication to its use.

LOOP DIURETICS. These agents are the most potent diuretics in common clinical use and can induce a natriuresis of up to 20% of the filtered load of sodium for limited periods. They are of particular value in three situations: in acute pulmonary edema, used intravenously; in severe or refractory heart failure; or when renal function is impaired. Ethacrynic acid is chemically different from furosemide and its analogues but appears to share a similar set of pharmacologic properties. These diuretics act to inhibit the Na/K/2 Cl transport system that is responsible for solute reabsorption in the thick ascending limb of the loop of Henle. Each of these drugs is secreted into the tubular lumen by the organic acid secretory pathway, and their effects may therefore be delayed or decreased by exogenous (e.g., probenecid) or endogenous (organic anion accumulation in uremia) competitive inhibitors of the transporter.

Gastrointestinal absorption of furosemide, the most commonly used of the loop diuretics, is variable, with an average bioavailability of 60%. This is substantially diminished when the drug is given with meals. Congestive heart failure can decrease absorption rates of both furosemide and bumetanide. The nonsteroidal anti-inflammatory drugs, including aspirin, tend to blunt the natriuretic response to all of the loop diuretics.

The loop diuretics in general produce systemic hemodynamic changes that precede and are presumably unrelated to the degree

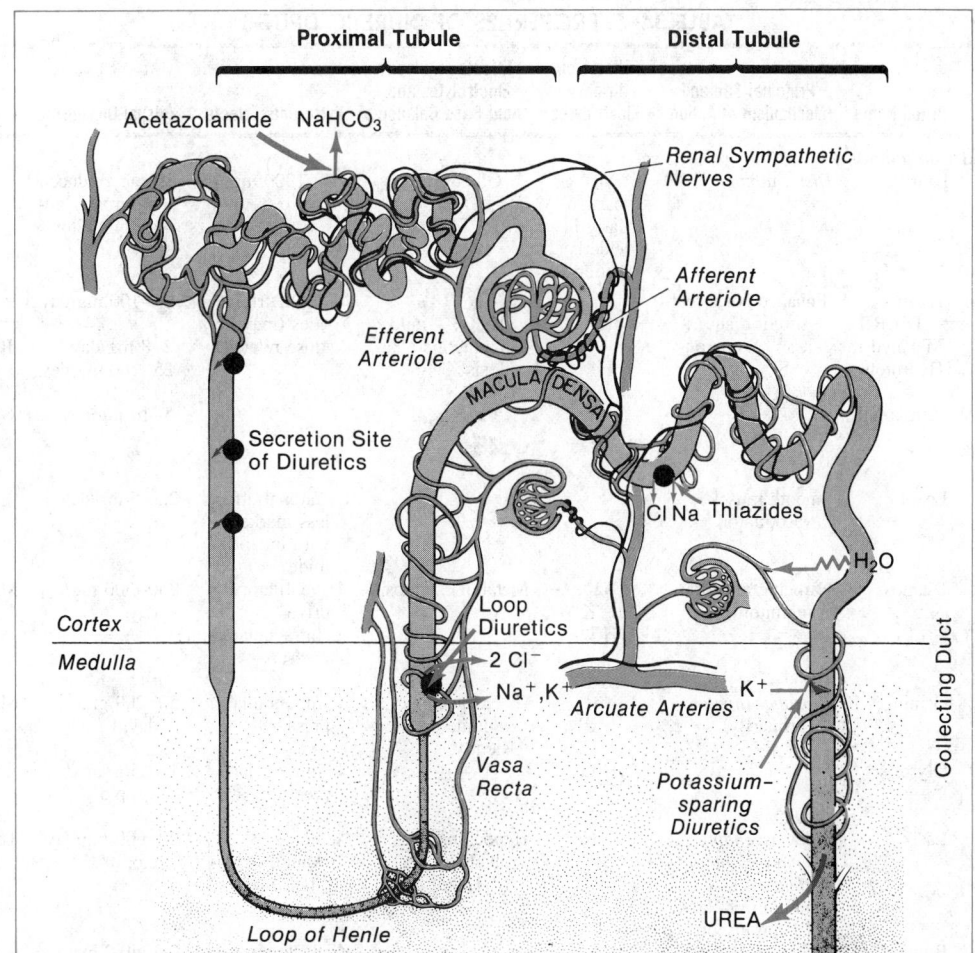

FIGURE 34–4. Sites of diuretic action in the mammalian nephron (see Ch. 74). Agents that alter the rate of formation of glomerular filtrate, such as ACE inhibitors, may enhance the delivery of solute and water to more distal segments of the nephron that are sensitive to diuretics. Nonsteroidal anti-inflammatory drugs may diminish the glomerular filtration rate, thus reducing the flow of urine to distal diuretic-sensitive portions of the nephron. A reduction in systemic blood pressure, or in renal artery pressure distal to the stenotic arterial lesion, below that necessary for formation of glomerular filtrate renders the kidney refractory to any diuretic. Most diuretics reach their site of action along the nephron after being secreted into the tubular lumen by the organic anion secretory transport system of the straight proximal tubule (pars recta).

The descending limb of Henle's loop is highly permeable to water, which leaves the nephron for the increasingly hyperosmotic medullary interstitium. Most of the solute transport responsible for maintaining the hypertonicity of the medullary interstitium occurs in the water-impermeable thick ascending limb of Henle's loop. Here, an NaK cotransport system in the luminal membrane is coupled to the uptake of two chloride ions. This Na/K/2 Cl cotransport system on the luminal membrane of the tubular cells is the site of action for the loop diuretics (furosemide, bumetanide, and ethacrynic acid). Inhibition of cation transport by loop diuretics prevents the normal generation of the hypertonic medullary interstitium, thus reducing the osmotic gradient for free water clearance of ADH-sensitive tubular cells in the collecting duct, and also delivers large amounts of solute and water to the distal nephron, thus overwhelming distal Na^+ and Cl^- resorption sites.

Loop diuretics may directly stimulate the release of renin by the juxtaglomerular apparatus (JGA), an action that may contribute to the extrarenal vascular effects of these drugs. The distal convoluted tubule begins beyond the macula densa. Na^+ and Cl^-, as well as other ions (e.g., Ca^{2+}), are resorbed in this segment. The thiazide diuretics and related drugs inhibit NaCl resorption in this segment. Thiazide-induced inhibition of NaCl resorption in this segment may lead to hyponatremia, particularly when accompanied by elevated ADH levels and increased thirst.

The cortical collecting duct actively resorbs NaCl via an aldosterone-sensitive mechanism. Antialdosterone drugs, such as spironolactone, competitively inhibit aldosterone's binding to its receptor, thereby limiting Na^+ permeability by the apical membrane and reducing K^+ secretion.

The blood supply to each nephron is derived from several sources. The afferent arteriole that enters the glomerulus is richly innervated with sympathetic nerve endings. Increased sympathetic discharge to the kidney results in increased net NaCl resorption. Elevated efferent sympathetic activity, as is often seen in decompensated congestive heart failure, would be expected to result in avid retention of solute due to reduced renal perfusion, increased renin release, and enhanced tubular resorption of solute. Dopamine is a potent renal vasodilator and may directly affect tubular epithelia to reduce NaCl resorption, thus acting as a natriuretic agent. Exogenously administered dopamine, particularly when infused at rates of 2 to 3 μg per minute, may be a useful adjunct to diuretic therapy in selected with advanced congestive heart failure.

and extent of diuresis they induce. Acute administration of furosemide causes a rapid increase in venous capacitance, with a consequent decline in cardiac filling pressures. This effect is accompanied by an increase in plasma renin activity that can produce an appreciable rise in systemic vascular resistance. These effects on the peripheral vasculature tend to plateau in the lower dose range at about a 20-mg intravenous dose of furosemide. Although the loop diuretics are potent inhibitors of Na/K/2 Cl cotransport, this process is not clinically important outside the kidney, except in the cochlea, where it is thought to account for the eighth nerve toxicity that is seen with loop diuretics, particularly ethacrynic acid. The ototoxic-

ity of loop diuretics is synergistic with that of aminoglycoside antibiotics.

Bumetanide tends to have higher bioavailability and greater potency than furosemide and may be slightly less ototoxic. Other differences among these closely related compounds appear to be small and probably clinically unimportant.

An important advantage of the loop diuretics is their rapid onset of action, with a diuretic response typically appearing within a few minutes of intravenous administration.

POTASSIUM-SPARING DIURETICS. Two groups of drugs fall into this class: (1) the aldosterone antagonists, and (2) the direct

TABLE 34–5. PROPERTIES OF DIURETIC DRUGS

Diuretic	Brand Name	Principal Site and Mechanism of Action	Effects on Urinary Electrolytes	Effects on Blood Electrolytes and Acid-Base Balance	Extrarenal Effects	Usual Dosage*	Drug Interactions
Thiazides and Related Compounds							
Chlorothiazide	Diuril	*Distal tubule:*	↓ Na⁺, particularly in elderly patients	↑ Glucose	500–1000 mg, IV or p.o.	Efficacy reduced by prostaglandin inhibitors	
Hydrochlorothiazide	Hydro-DIURIL	Enhance NaCl reabsorption and ↓ Ca²⁺ excretion	↑ Cl⁻, ↑ K⁺	↓ Cl, ↑ HCO₃⁻—mild metabolic alkalosis ↑ Uric acid	↑ LDL/triglycerides (may be dose related)	25–100 mg/day	
Trichlormethiazide	Metahydrin		↑ H⁺			2–8 mg/day	Reduces renal clearance of lithium
Chlorthalidone	Hygroton					25–100 mg/day	
Metolazone	Zaroxolyn		↑ Mg²⁺ ↓ Ca²⁺	↑ Ca²⁺		5–10 mg/day	Synergistic effects on NaCl and K⁺ excretion with loop diuretics
Indapamide	Lozol	Smooth muscle vasodilator			Extrarenal effects less marked with indapamide	2.5–5 mg/day	
Acetazolamide	Diamox	Carbonic anhydrase inhibitor	↑ Na⁺, ↑ K⁺ ↑ HCO₃⁻	Metabolic acidosis	↑ Ventilatory drive ↓ Intraocular pressure	250–500 mg/day	May be useful in alkalemia due to other diuretics
Osmotic Diuretics							
Mannitol	Osmitrol	*Proximal tubule* (primarily)	↑ Na⁺, ↑ Cl⁻	↑ Extracellular volume transiently	↓ Intracranial pressure	50–200 grams/day, IV	May enhance loop diuretic effectiveness by maintaining GFR
Glycerol	Glyrol		↑ H₂O		↓ Intraocular pressure	1–1.5 grams/kg, p.o.	
Loop Diuretics							
Furosemide	Lasix	*Thick ascending limb of loop of Henle:* Inhibition of Na/K/Cl cotransport	↑↑ Na⁺	Hypochloremic alkalosis (↑ HCO₃⁻)	Acute ↑ Venous capacitance	20–600 mg/day, p.o. or IV	Tubular secretion delayed by competing organic acids (renal failure) and some drugs
Bumetanide	Bumex		↑↑ Cl⁻		↑ Systemic vascular resistance	0.5–40.0 mg/day	
Torasemide			↑ K⁻ ↑ H⁺ ↑ Mg²⁺, Ca²⁺	↓ K⁺, ↓ Na⁺, ↓ Cl⁻ ↑ Uric acid (less than thiazide)	Chronic: ↓ Cardiac preload		Effectiveness reduced by prostaglandin inhibitors
Ethacrynic acid	Edecrin	↑ Renin, AII; ↑ PG's			Ototoxicity	50–150 mg/day	
Indacrinone				Uricosuric potency depends upon ratio of ± enantiomers in final drug			Additive ototoxicity with aminoglycosides Excessive hypotension may occur in patients treated chronically with diuretics and begun on ACE inhibitors
Potassium-Sparing Diuretics							
Spironolactone	Aldactone	*Aldosterone antagonist*	↑ K⁺ ↑ Na⁺ ↑ Cl⁻ ↑ HCO₃⁻	↑ K⁺, particularly in patients with ↓ GFR; metabolic acidosis	Gynecomastia Antiandrogen effects	25–200 mg/day	Useful adjunct to therapy with K⁺-wasting diuretics
Triamterene	Dyrenium	Inhibit Na⁺ conductance in collecting duct				100–300 mg/day	Triamterene with indomethacin may cause abrupt ↓ GFR
Amiloride	Midamor					5–10 mg/day	Triamterene may cause renal calculi

* Route of administration is p.o. except as noted.
AII = Angiotensin II; PG = prostaglandin; GFR = glomerular filtration rate; LDL = low density lipoproteins; ACE = angiotensin-converting enzyme inhibitor.

inhibitors of sodium permeability in the collecting duct. The aldosterone antagonist most frequently used is spironolactone, although canrenoate and canrenone have essentially identical effects. The aldosterone antagonists compete with the native hormone for cytoplasmic receptors in responsive cells, ultimately reducing sodium reabsorption. Therapeutic efficacy of these agents is limited when used alone, but they are often useful in combination with other potent diuretics.

Amiloride and triamterene are structurally related compounds that inhibit sodium uptake in collecting duct epithelial cells by inhibiting sodium conductance. A principal effect of these drugs is to reduce renal potassium secretion, which may be useful in concert with the action of potassium-wasting compounds such as the thiazides and loop diuretics but which may lead to clinically important hyperkalemia, particularly in patients with renal failure. The potassium-sparing diuretics tend to cause a mild metabolic acidosis. In patients with chronic obstructive pulmonary disease, these agents may be preferred to diuretics that enhance renal hydrogen losses and secondarily reduce ventilatory drive. Apart from causing hyperkalemia, these drugs are relatively benign. Spironolactone can cause troublesome gynecomastia.

OSMOTIC DIURETICS. These agents are rarely useful for managing heart failure, but it should be remembered that radiographic contrast dyes are filtered by the glomerulus and act as osmotic diuretics, increasing urinary loss of salt and water. This volume-contracting effect can be important in fragile patients, such as those with severe aortic stenosis. An important characteristic of osmotic diuresis is its ability to maintain urine flow even at very low GFR, as occurs in hypotension or dehydration.

COMBINED DIURETIC REGIMENS. Combined use of diuretics in patients with heart failure is usually considered for two main reasons: to avoid electrolyte disturbances that occur with the isolated use of a powerful agent such as a loop diuretic, especially in chronic therapy, and to augment salt and water excretion in the face of refractory edema. A third possible indication is the avoidance of ototoxicity from large doses of loop diuretics.

Combined use of potassium-sparing diuretics with a more proximally acting agent such as a thiazide or a loop diuretic constitutes a common practice. The potassium-sparing diuretics limit potassium and hydrogen ion loss induced by diuretics that act more proximally.

The combination of a loop diuretic with a thiazide or metolazone often results in a synergistic augmentation of salt and water excretion. This combination of agents can produce marked intravascular volume depletion and electrolyte disturbances. Potassium wasting can be severe, and serum potassium levels require close monitoring. In general, this combination of diuretics should be initiated in a hospital setting, carefully regulating the regimen on an outpatient basis, taking daily weight measurements, and frequently checking serum electrolyte and creatinine levels.

COMPLICATIONS OF DIURETIC THERAPY. Problems complicating diuretic therapy include intravascular volume depletion and hypotension from overly vigorous diuresis; hyponatremia, often due to prolonged diuretic therapy with inadequate sodium intake and often with excessive water intake; hypokalemia from the use of thiazides or loop diuretics, or both, with inadequate potassium supplementation, predisposing to cardiac arrhythmias with or without concomitant digitalis excess; hyperkalemia from administering potassium-sparing diuretic and potassium supplements, potentially augmented by the use of ACE inhibitors or β-adrenergic blockers; metabolic alkalosis with or without potassium depletion; hyperuricemia secondary to thiazide or loop diuretic administration; magnesium depletion, often occurring in parallel with potassium losses; and increased serum low density lipoprotein and triglyceride levels in patients receiving thiazides.

As a final comment, many patients treated for congestive heart failure spend a period of weeks developing the excessive fluid accumulation that characterizes this disease state; there is little virtue and much potential harm in attempting to correct this problem in an unduly short period of time. In general, in the absence of acute pulmonary edema, a reasonable goal (even in the era of DRG's) is about 1 kg of fluid loss per day.

Digitalis Glycosides

Cardiac glycosides have been used to manage heart failure for more than 200 years and remain the only drugs currently available for long-term ambulatory use that have a positive inotropic effect. The relatively narrow therapeutic-toxic ratio of cardiac glycosides renders them particularly difficult to use, and the clinician should have a detailed understanding of the actions and pharmacokinetics of one drug of this class, such as digoxin. Because digoxin has supplanted almost entirely the use of other cardiac glycosides in the United States, the discussion focuses on this agent.

BASIC MECHANISM OF CARDIAC GLYCOSIDE ACTION. A consensus exists that the sequence of events leading to the positive inotropic effect of digitalis on both normal and failing cardiac muscle is as summarized in Figure 34–5. The digitalis glycosides bind to a site on the extracellular facing aspect of Na^+-K^+-ATPase, the enzyme constituting the "sodium pump" that moves sodium and potassium across cell membranes against their respective concentration gradients. The complete amino acid sequences of the alpha and beta subunits of the enzyme are known. When a cardiac glycoside binds to the alpha subunit, that individual sodium pump unit is completely inhibited. When a fraction of Na^+-K^+-ATPase sites on a cardiac myocyte are occupied, intracellular sodium concentration tends to rise. Through the mechanism of sodium-calcium exchange, this leads in turn to augmentation of the intracellular calcium content. Because calcium constitutes the trigger that leads to the contractile event, the increase of intracellular calcium stores (up to a point) enhances the contractile state of both normal and failing myocardium.

The electrophysiologic toxicity commonly observed with excessive doses of digitalis is probably due to the same fundamental mechanism of sodium pump inhibition. At higher doses and myocardial concentrations of the drug, impaired sodium and potassium transport leads to characteristic disturbances of impulse formation and conduction, as discussed below. It is likely that intracellular calcium overload contributes to the cardiotoxicity of the digitalis glycosides, at least under circumstances that have been studied experimentally.

ELECTROPHYSIOLOGIC EFFECTS. Most of the antiarrhythmic effects of digitalis are the results of its actions at the level of the atria and atrioventricular junction. Conduction velocity is increased by cardiac glycosides in atrial and ventricular myocardium, but it is decreased in the conduction system and His-Purkinje system. Similarly, the effective refractory period is shortened in atrial and ventricular myocardium but tends to be lengthened in specialized conduction tissues. These effects are largely mediated by increased vagal tone, rather than by direct effects of cardiac glycosides, although the latter can be documented at the upper end of the dose range. Of particular importance in managing supraventricular tachyarrhythmias is the tendency of digitalis to lengthen the refractory period and to slow conduction in the atrioventricular node. At toxic doses and blood levels, digitalis enhances sympathetic nerve traffic to the heart, thus increasing the propensity to ectopic impulse formation at atrial, atrioventricular junctional, and ventricular levels.

HEMODYNAMIC EFFECTS. The positive inotropic action is a direct effect of digitalis on cardiac myocytes. Endogenous norepinephrine stores are not necessary to permit expression of this effect. A useful way to appreciate the effect of digitalis on the intact circulation is to consider the ventricular function curves shown in Figure 34–1. In contrast to diuretics, which reduce preload and shift the circulatory state to the left along a given ventricular function curve, a positive inotropic agent shifts the entire curve upward and to the left toward the normal curve. Because contractility does not limit cardiac output in the normal circulation, digitalis would not be expected to change output in normal subjects. This is the case. As soon as the contractile state becomes limiting, however, digitalis increases cardiac output and lowers filling pressures of both the right and the left ventricles. Thus, cardiac glycosides are of clinical value in patients with congestive heart failure in the presence or absence of supraventricular tachyarrhythmias such as atrial fibrillation or atrial flutter. Recent trials have demonstrated that patients with stable, mild to moderate heart failure and systolic ventricular dysfunction (left ventricular ejection fraction ≤0.35) who are in sinus rhythm benefit from standard maintenance doses of digoxin in terms of heart failure signs and symptoms and effort tolerance compared with randomized control patients withdrawn from digoxin. This benefit was superior to that in patients maintained on diuretics alone (PROVED trial) or diuretics plus an ACE inhibitor (RADIANCE trial). These patients must be carefully distinguished from those with predominant diastolic dysfunction (noncompliant ventricles and elevated filling pressures but normal ejection fractions) who are unlikely to benefit. Thus, patients who are most likely to

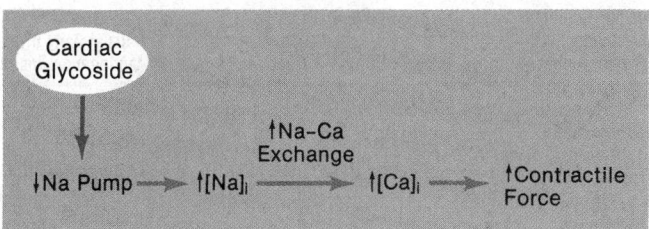

FIGURE 34–5. Schematic representation of the mechanism of inotropic action of cardiac glycosides. Binding of digitalis to Na^+-K^+-ATPase inhibits this enzyme and hence the active outward transport of Na^+ across the myocardial cell membrane. Na^+ pump inhibition leads to increased intracellular Na^+ ($[Na]_i$) content and activity, which in turn alters Na-Ca exchange with consequent increase in Ca influx, decrease of Ca efflux, or both. The resulting increase in intracellular Ca ($[Ca]_i$) is presumed to mediate the observed increase in myocardial contractile force.

benefit are those having cardiomegaly with impaired systolic contraction, often accompanied by S_3 gallops. There is no convincing evidence of desensitization or tolerance to the cardiac effects of digitalis, and the positive inotropic effects are sustained over periods of months and years in patients with congestive heart failure.

To summarize, as pathologic processes such as ischemia, volume or pressure loads, or primary myocardial disease lead to reduced contractility, compensatory mechanisms emerge. Elevated end-diastolic pressure and volume augment ventricular performance through the Frank-Starling mechanism. Sympathetic tone tends to increase, thus enhancing contractile state, and the process of ventricular hypertrophy generates additional contractile elements. Each of these mechanisms, however, exacts a price. Excessive elevation of filling pressures results in pulmonary or peripheral edema. Excessive sympathetic tone results in tachycardia and, together with elevated renin-angiotensin system activity, in increased peripheral vascular resistance as well as increased myocardial oxygen consumption. With the progression of underlying cardiac disease, the compensatory mechanisms ultimately fail, or the consequences of these mechanisms become limiting (for example, with emergence of pulmonary edema). Cardiac glycosides administered under these circumstances enhance myocardial contractility, decreasing the dependence of the circulation on compensatory mechanisms and providing improved cardiac reserve. Improved ventricular function yields a higher cardiac output at any given ventricular filling pressure. With the alternative therapeutic modalities now available, there is little virtue in giving cardiac glycosides to the brink of toxicity. Rather, conventional doses (see below) resulting in serum digoxin concentrations not exceeding 1.5 ng per milliliter appear to yield the best risk-benefit ratio.

PHARMACOKINETICS, BIOAVAILABILITY, AND DOSAGE CONSIDERATIONS. Summarized in Table 34–6 are the important pharmacokinetic variables and dosage ranges for cardiac glycosides in current clinical use. The values cited are averages, and individual variation is to be expected.

Digoxin. This is the most widely used preparation, particularly in hospitalized patients. Its virtues include flexibility of route of administration and intermediate duration of action. Digoxin is excreted exponentially (i.e., first-order kinetics) with a half-life of about 36 hours in young, healthy, normal subjects. In older patients with cardiac disease but without elevated BUN or serum creatinine levels, a half-life of 48 hours represents a more appropriate first approximation. Such patients excrete approximately one third of body stores daily, for the most part in unchanged form, although about 10% of patients excrete substantial quantities of the inactive metabolite dihydrodigoxin, which arises through bacterial biotransformation in the gut lumen. The excretion of digoxin by the kidney is directly proportional to GFR (and hence creatinine clearance) and is relatively independent of the rate of urine flow in patients with intact renal function. Clearance may decrease somewhat in patients with prerenal azotemia. There is also evidence for some secretion of the drug at the renal tubular level.

Therapy can be instituted in patients without urgent indications by starting the daily maintenance dose without a loading dose. This results in stable plateau concentrations of the drug in four to five excretory half-lives, or about 1 week. In patients with severe renal impairment, the half-life of the drug is prolonged to as much as 4 to 5 days, and steady-state levels are reached on a daily maintenance regimen only after 3 to 4 weeks.

Digoxin is extensively bound to tissues (large volume of distribution), and the drug is consequently not effectively removed from the body by hemodialysis. Lean body mass should be used for purposes of dosage calculation. Infants and children absorb and excrete digoxin much as do adults, although secretion at the renal tubular level may be somewhat more important in prepubertal patients.

An important interaction between digoxin and quinidine has been described, leading to a substantial increase in steady-state serum digoxin levels (averaging about twofold) when conventional quinidine doses are added to a maintenance digoxin regimen. Increases in the serum digoxin level are also observed when verapamil or amiodarone is given concurrently.

Bioavailability of digoxin in the standard tablet formulation is 55 to 75%. The higher estimate is usually used in converting oral to intravenous doses. A preparation in which digoxin is dissolved in an encapsulated gel gives higher bioavailability, requiring a slight adjustment in the standard maintenance doses, as noted in Table 34–6. Previously marketed preparations with poor bioavailability properties are no longer available in the United States.

The maintenance digoxin dose required to replace daily losses varies from about 37% of the body content in patients with normal renal function to 14% in patients with essentially no renal function. The latter figure is an average, however, and some patients require substantially more or less than the maintenance dose that would be predicted by the 14% figure. A useful approximation of daily percent of loss of digoxin from the body is given by the following expression:

$$\text{Percent daily loss} = 14 + \frac{C_{Cr} \text{ in ml/min}}{5}$$

Useful nomograms have been developed for loading and maintenance doses of digoxin, but it is important that these be used only as first approximations and that the patient be followed closely until a stable steady state is reached. Adjustments subsequently are required with changes in renal function, related either to intrinsic renal disease or to altered renal perfusion due to cardiac disease.

Digitoxin. This cardiac glycoside is the least polar and the most slowly excreted of the cardiac glycosides in current use. It is the principal constituent of the whole leaf of the digitalis plant. Gastrointestinal absorption of digitoxin is virtually complete. The drug binds avidly to serum albumin, and only about 3% of the drug circulates in the free, pharmacologically active state at conventional doses and serum levels. It thus differs substantially from digoxin, which is only about 23% bound to plasma proteins at usual doses. Because of the high degree of serum protein binding, renal clearance of digitoxin is minimal and the drug is metabolized to a variety of poorly defined derivatives, presumably in the liver. Some enterohepatic cycling occurs in the case of digitoxin but is not important for digoxin. The half-time for digitoxin excretion aver-

TABLE 34–6. PHARMACOLOGY OF CARDIAC GLYCOSIDES

Agent	Gastrointestinal Absorption	Onset of Action* (minutes)	Peak Effect (hours)	Average Half-Life†	Principal Metabolic Route (Excretory Pathway)	Average Digitalizing Dose Oral ‡	Average Digitalizing Dose Intravenous §	Usual Daily Oral Maintenance Dose ‖
Digoxin	55–75%¶ (Lanoxicaps 90–100%)	15–30	1½–5	36–48 hours	Renal; some gastrointestinal excretion	1.25–1.50 mg	0.75–1.00 mg	0.25–0.50 mg**
Digitoxin	90–100%	25–120	4–12	4–6 days	Hepatic#; renal excretion of metabolites	0.70–1.20 mg	1.00 mg	0.10 mg

Modified from Smith TW: Drug therapy: Digitalis glycosides. N Engl J Med 288:719, 1973. Copyright 1973, the Massachusetts Medical Society.
* For intravenous dose.
† For normal subjects (prolonged by renal impairment with digoxin and probably by severe hepatic disease with digitoxin).
‡ Divided doses over 12 to 24 hours at intervals of 6 to 8 hours.
§ Given in increments for initial subcomplete digitalization, to be supplemented by further small increments as necessary.
‖ Average for adult patients without renal or hepatic impairment; varies widely among individual patients and requires dose medical supervision.
¶ For tablet form of administration (may be less in malabsorption syndromes and in formulations with poor bioavailability).
# Enterohepatic cycle exists.
** Approximately 20% lower maintenance doses are required if gel solution in capsules (Lanoxicaps) is used.

ages about 5 to 6 days and is not appreciably affected by altered renal function.

Standard pharmacology texts give details of pharmacokinetics of other glycosides such as deslanoside and ouabain, which are rarely if ever used clinically at present in the United States.

DIGITALIS USE IN CONGESTIVE HEART FAILURE. The therapeutic use of digitalis in patients with normal sinus rhythm is complicated by the lack of any easily measurable therapeutic endpoint, such as that provided by the ventricular rate in patients with atrial fibrillation. Digitalis is of value in patients with symptoms and signs of heart failure due to ischemic cardiomyopathy, valvular disease, hypertensive heart disease, many types of congenital heart disease, and dilated cardiomyopathies and in some patients with cor pulmonale and overt right ventricular failure. The drug is of no demonstrated benefit in isolated mitral stenosis with normal sinus rhythm unless right ventricular failure is present. Similarly, little benefit can be expected in patients with pericardial tamponade or constrictive pericarditis. The latter disease states are all characterized by mechanical limitations to cardiac function, rather than by impairment of myocardial contractility. In hypertrophic cardiomyopathy with an obstructive element, digitalis may in fact be deleterious if left ventricular contractility increases and produces greater outflow obstruction. As noted previously, patients with symptoms of dyspnea on exertion due to high diastolic filling pressure from decreased ventricular compliance, but with well-preserved ejection fractions, are unlikely to benefit from digitalis if sinus rhythm is present.

The prophylactic use of digitalis in patients with diminished cardiac reserve who are expected to undergo a major stress such as surgery remains controversial. Many clinicians prefer to withhold digitalis until a specific indication arises.

The use of digitalis in the management of supraventricular rhythm disturbances is considered in Ch. 35. The drug is potentially dangerous in patients with Wolff-Parkinson-White syndrome.

INDIVIDUAL SENSITIVITY TO DIGITALIS. Table 34–7 lists factors that influence the sensitivity of individual patients to digitalis. These are factors intrinsic to the patient, rather than factors that influence *apparent* sensitivity, such as alterations in drug bioavailability or in the excretion pattern of the drug.

Electrolyte and Acid-Base Disturbances. Potassium depletion increases the likelihood that patients will develop digitalis toxicity. Hypokalemia has a primary arrhythmogenic effect of its own and also tends to increase cellular binding of digitalis glycosides. Potassium depletion must be guarded against carefully in patients on potassium-wasting diuretics. Magnesium depletion also predisposes to digitalis toxicity and is a common concomitant of diuretic therapy. Elevated serum calcium levels may enhance ventricular automaticity and may also predispose to digitalis toxicity.

Acid-base disturbances appear to exert their effects largely through shifts in serum potassium concentration, and the acid-base disturbances *per se* usually have little effect within the range commonly encountered clinically.

Drug Interactions. Several drugs, including cholestyramine, colestipol, and neomycin, decrease absorption of orally administered digoxin, as do nonabsorbable antacids and Kaopectate. Quinidine, verapamil, and amiodarone all increase steady-state serum digoxin levels.

Type and Severity of Underlying Heart Disease. The most important factor influencing individual digitalis sensitivity is the type and severity of underlying heart disease. Otherwise healthy subjects are remarkably tolerant of large doses of digitalis, and toxicity typically manifests itself as disturbances of atrioventricular conduction rather than life-threatening tachyarrhythmias. In patients with advanced heart failure or severe focal ischemia, however, the therapeutic ratio of digitalis is remarkably low, and these patients may experience potentially life-threatening toxicity at doses and serum levels no more than twice the optimal amount.

Digitalis and Ischemic Heart Disease. The effects of digitalis on myocardial oxygen consumption, and therefore its use in patients with ischemic heart disease, depend primarily on the prior state of the ventricle. In the normal-size ventricle, the enhanced contractile state may modestly increase oxygen consumption. If failure and ventricular dilation are present, however, digitalis administration tends to reduce cardiac dimensions and thereby reduces wall tension (Laplace's relation) such that myocardial oxygen consumption may not increase or may even be reduced. It is important,

TABLE 34–7. FACTORS INFLUENCING INDIVIDUAL SENSITIVITY TO DIGITALIS

Type and severity of underlying cardiac disease
Serum electrolyte derangement
   Hypokalemia or hyperkalemia
   Hypomagnesemia
   Hypercalcemia
   Hyponatremia
Acid-base imbalance
Concomitant drug administration
   Anesthetics
   Catecholamines and sympathomimetics
   Antiarrhythmic agents
Thyroid status
Renal function
Autonomic nervous system tone
Respiratory disease

therefore, to assess carefully the state of ventricular function prior to instituting digitalis therapy in patients with ischemic disease.

The role of digitalis therapy in acute myocardial infarction is limited. Other measures are generally preferable in the management of mild congestive heart failure in this setting. When symptoms and signs of overt left ventricular failure persist despite optimal use of diuretics and vasodilators, digitalis may be added at about 75% of the usual loading dose. The loading dose should be given over a period of 18 to 24 hours with cardiac rhythm closely monitored. It is customary to use digoxin in the presence of atrial fibrillation, which is typically a manifestation of heart failure in patients with acute myocardial infarction.

Some evidence suggests that patients may experience excess mortality when maintained on digitalis long-term following acute myocardial infarction, but most studies indicate that the mortality trends are accounted for by baseline variables such as greater severity of heart failure, rather than a deleterious effect of conventional doses of digoxin.

Advanced Age. It is unlikely that advanced age *per se* has an independent adverse effect on digitalis tolerance, but the reduced renal and pulmonary functions that attend advanced age require appropriate consideration.

Renal Failure. Factors influencing digitalis absorption and elimination, as well as rapid shifts in electrolytes with hemodialysis, predispose to digitalis toxicity. It is wise to leave an extra margin of safety in digitalis doses in managing these patients.

Thyroid Disease. Hyperthyroidism tends to reduce the response of patients to digitalis, whereas hypothyroidism increases the likelihood of digitalis toxicity. The failure of a patient with atrial fibrillation to respond to standard doses of digoxin with appropriate slowing of the heart rate should raise the question of occult thyrotoxicosis.

Pulmonary Disease. It is generally agreed that patients with chronic pulmonary disease, and especially with acute respiratory insufficiency, experience an increased frequency of digitalis intoxication. This may be related both to the underlying lung disease and hypoxia and to the sympathomimetic drugs that these patients often receive. It should be assumed that patients with a variety of pulmonary diseases may be sensitive to the arrhythmogenic effects of conventional doses and serum levels of cardiac glycosides.

SERUM DIGITALIS CONCENTRATIONS. Assay of serum digoxin concentration is routinely performed in most clinical laboratories, usually with the radioimmunoassay technique or one of its variants. There is a relatively constant ratio of serum or plasma to myocardial digoxin concentration, and thus the clinical effect of digoxin is directly related to the serum level. Nevertheless, there is considerable overlap in serum levels between patients with and without evidence of toxicity. Thus, serum concentration data must always be interpreted in the overall clinical context. Mean serum digoxin concentrations in groups of patients without evidence of toxicity, and with an expected therapeutic effect, average 1.4 ng per milliliter. Doubling the digoxin dose in a patient on a steady-state regimen can be expected to double the serum concentration when a new steady state is reached.

Serum digitoxin concentrations average about 10-fold higher than those of digoxin because of the binding of digitoxin to serum proteins.

The upper limit of the "therapeutic" range for digoxin is usually taken as about 2.0 ng per milliliter, but patients with supraventricular tachyarrhythmias, including atrial fibrillation and atrial flutter, may require appreciably higher levels to gain adequate control of the ventricular response. This is particularly true of patients with elevated sympathetic and decreased vagal tone—for example, in decompensated heart failure or during exercise. Such circumstances may be best dealt with by the judicious use of a β-blocker or verapamil added to conventional digoxin doses, bearing in mind the propensity of β-blockers and verapamil to reduce contractility of the impaired ventricle. Conversely, unusually sensitive patients may experience toxicity at serum levels as low as 1.0 ng per milliliter. It is not necessary to monitor serum digoxin levels routinely in patients who are doing well on standard maintenance doses of the drug. Serum levels may be of use, however, in assessing unexpected responses to therapy, including lack of the expected therapeutic response (Is the patient taking the drug?) or in situations in which digitalis toxicity is suspected (for example, multifocal ventricular premature beats in a patient with overt congestive heart failure who is taking digoxin).

DIGITALIS TOXICITY. At the cellular level, exposure to excessive levels of cardiac glycosides causes increased automaticity and decreased conduction. These abnormalities are reflected in a broad array of rhythm disturbances that are often difficult to distinguish from those caused by underlying heart disease. Commonly encountered rhythm disturbances, in decreasing order of incidence, include ventricular ectopic rhythms, AV block, atrial arrhythmias, sinoatrial arrhythmias, AV dissociation, and accelerated AV junctional rhythms.

Sinus Node and Atrium. Slowing of the sinus rate in patients with congestive heart failure is largely mediated by improved cardiac function and withdrawal of elevated sympathetic tone. Sinus rate is not a very useful indicator of digitalis effect because it tends to remain rapid in the presence of fever, infection, anemia, thyrotoxicosis, or a variety of other conditions that predispose to sinus tachycardia. At high toxic doses, digitalis can cause direct depression of sinus node automaticity, or more likely sinoatrial exit block, which produces bradyarrhythmias.

Atrioventricular Node. The effective refractory period of the atrioventricular (AV) node is prolonged by digitalis, chiefly through increased vagal activity. In addition, the conduction velocity through the AV junction is reduced. As digoxin doses are increased, first-degree block (PR interval >0.20 second) may appear, followed by second-degree AV block of the Mobitz type I or Wenckebach variety (see Ch. 35). With still higher doses, complete AV dissociation and third-degree block can occur. A typical manifestation of digitalis toxicity in the presence of atrial fibrillation is AV dissociation, often accompanied by increased automaticity of pacemakers in the AV junction. This causes regularization of a previously irregular ventricular rate.

His-Purkinje System. Digitalis-induced increase in the automaticity of cells in the His-Purkinje system is a relatively common manifestation of digitalis excess and is responsible for rhythm disturbances, including ventricular premature beats, ventricular bigeminy, and ventricular tachycardia.

Clinical Manifestations of Digitalis Toxicity. **Gastrointestinal Symptoms.** Anorexia, nausea, and vomiting are common consequences of digitalis toxicity. Unfortunately, these are present prior to the onset of rhythm disturbances in only about 50% of cases.

Neurologic Symptoms. Headache, fatigue, malaise, disorientation, confusion, delirium, and seizures can occur, and visual symptoms, including disturbances of color vision, are well known. In fact, the gastrointestinal symptoms actually arise from the effects of digitalis on the chemoreceptor trigger zone in the medulla rather than as a result of direct irritation of the gastrointestinal system.

Massive Cardiac Glycoside Overdose. Suicidal or accidental digitalis overdose can produce the entire array of typical cardiac arrhythmias, including refractory ventricular fibrillation. In addition, hyperkalemia is sometimes encountered owing to interference with sodium and potassium transport across cell membranes throughout the body. This must be taken into account when considering potassium supplements in cases in which massive toxicity may occur.

Treatment of Digitalis Intoxication. The most important element of successful treatment is early recognition that a cardiac rhythm disturbance is due to digitalis toxicity. For many of the most common manifestations, such as occasional ventricular premature beats, first-degree AV block, or atrial fibrillation with a slow ventricular response, temporary withdrawal of the drug with electrocardiographic monitoring (if indicated) until the arrhythmia has disappeared constitutes adequate management. The maintenance dose should then be adjusted to prevent recurrence. Arrhythmias that impair cardiac function because of rates that are too rapid or too slow, or those that suggest the possibility of progression to more malignant arrhythmias, require more aggressive management. Ventricular tachycardia due to digitalis toxicity requires immediate vigorous treatment. Bradyarrhythmias, including sinus bradycardia, sinoatrial arrest or exit block, and atrioventricular block of second or third degree can sometimes be treated effectively with atropine, 0.5 to 1.0 mg IV. Pervenous electrical pacing should be instituted if atropine is not rapidly effective.

Potassium. Potassium repletion is useful in treating ectopic tachyarrhythmias when hypokalemia is present or when the serum potassium level is in the low normal range. Potassium must be given with caution in other circumstances because of the risks of hyperkalemia, particularly in the presence of renal impairment or of conduction disturbances.

Lidocaine and Phenytoin. These are the most useful drugs in the treatment of ectopic rhythm disturbances caused by digitalis. They tend to have minimal adverse effect on sinoatrial or AV conduction. Lidocaine is given intravenously in 100-mg bolus doses every 3 to 5 minutes, followed by a maintenance intravenous infusion of 15 to 20 μg per kilogram of body weight per minute, as required to maintain control of the rhythm disturbance and to avoid neurologic signs and symptoms. Phenytoin* is given in a dose of 100 mg by slow intravenous infusion, repeated every 5 minutes until onset of toxicity or control of the arrhythmia.

Beta-Adrenergic Blocking Drugs. Beta blockade has been useful in the treatment of some arrhythmias caused by digitalis excess but tends to decrease conduction as well as myocardial contractility and therefore is not widely used in this setting.

Quinidine and Procainamide. These drugs carry a risk of depression of sinoatrial and atrioventricular node function and can also depress myocardial contractility. Other agents are usually preferable for use in digitalis toxicity.

Direct Current (DC) Countershock (also see Ch. 35). This is generally inadvisable in the presence of digitalis intoxication because it may evoke severe arrhythmias in this setting. However, it must occasionally be used when other methods have been ineffective in the presence of a life-threatening arrhythmia. Risk is decreased when lower energy levels are employed, and careful titration is essential. In general, ventricular tachycardia converts easily at an energy level of 25 watt-seconds or less. Cardioversion is generally a benign procedure in patients without digitalis-induced rhythm disturbances.

Steroid-Binding Resins, Hemodialysis, and Hemoperfusion. These techniques have not been demonstrated to be effective in managing advanced digitalis intoxication and are not recommended. Hemodialysis may be of value in controlling the serum potassium level in patients with refractory hyperkalemia.

Digoxin-Specific Antibodies. Purified Fab fragments of digoxin-specific antibodies are available for treatment of advanced digitalis toxicity of sufficient severity to be potentially life threatening. More than 20,000 patients have now been treated, with a high degree of efficacy and with adverse side effects largely limited to those expected from withdrawal of digitalis effects. This approach is recommended for patients in whom conventional measures are not rapidly effective.

Vasodilators

Cardiac loading has a strong dependence on the resistance and capacitance properties of the peripheral vascular bed. Thus, vasodilator therapy in heart failure is designed to reduce the preload or afterload, or both, of a failing ventricle by relaxing vascular smooth muscle in the periphery. Vasodilators have been shown to improve survival in patients with continuing symptoms of heart failure who are taking digitalis and diuretics.

---

* This use is not listed in the manufacturer's directive.

PRINCIPLES OF VASODILATOR THERAPY. As summarized in Figure 34–2, the normal ventricle is able to respond to increased afterload with an increase in the force of contraction such that there is little, if any, change in stroke volume until extreme elevations in afterload are encountered. As the ventricle fails, the relationship between afterload and stroke volume shifts downward and to the left so that a relatively modest change in outflow resistance causes a substantial alteration in stroke volume. This constitutes both a pathophysiologic problem and a therapeutic opportunity. The opportunity follows from the uniform increase in peripheral vascular resistance observed in untreated patients with decompensated congestive heart failure. Activation of the sympathetic nervous system and of the renin-angiotensin system accounts for most of the increase in peripheral resistance. These responses of the peripheral vascular system to a perceived decrease in cardiac output have survival value under conditions of hemorrhage or dehydration by redirecting the cardiac output to essential beds, including the brain and coronary circulation. Because congestive heart failure was presumably not an evolutionary pressure, it is not surprising that these primitive mechanisms for the defense of blood flow to vital organs prove maladaptive in the patient with chronic congestive heart failure.

As illustrated in Figure 34–1, the failing heart responds to a reduction in afterload by shifting its ventricular function curve toward normal, although the inotropic state remains unchanged. An attractive feature of afterload reduction is the ability to increase cardiac output without increasing preload or myocardial oxygen consumption.

VASODILATOR AGENTS. In the following discussion, primary consideration is given to vasodilator therapy for left ventricular failure, although the failing right ventricle also benefits from reduced pulmonary vascular resistance. The most potent afterload-reducing effect in the pulmonary circulation is oxygen; there is, as yet, no drug that reliably exerts a preferential afterload-reducing effect in the pulmonary circulation. Inhaled nitric oxide is under investigation for this purpose.

The action of vasodilator drugs is described in terms of effects on the venous bed (preload) or the arteriolar bed (afterload). Table 34–8 summarizes data on the vasodilators in current clinical use for managing heart failure.

Venous Dilators. These reduce the vascular smooth muscle tone in the systemic venous bed, increasing its capacitance and shifting blood volume from the arterial to the venous side of the circulation. Thus, patients with pulmonary vascular congestion and edema due to high left heart filling pressures obtain symptomatic relief, limited only by the necessity to maintain a level of preload that results in an adequate forward cardiac output. The most selective agents for this purpose are the nitrates, including nitroglycerin and the longer-acting orally administered compounds such as isosorbide dinitrate. Many investigators believe that much or most of the clinical benefit of vasodilator use derives from the venous dilator component. In chronic congestive heart failure, administering agents that preferentially dilate the arteriolar bed without a preload-reducing component, such as minoxidil and hydralazine, fail to show sustained benefit in placebo-controlled trials but may occasionally be of benefit when added to ACE inhibitors or nitrates in selected patients.

Arteriolar Dilators. These reduce left ventricular afterload and tend to redistribute blood flow among organ beds in ways that are, unfortunately, not always predictable. The improvement in blood flow to exercising skeletal muscle is relatively limited. Nevertheless, the forward stroke output of the left ventricle is delivered with a lower wall tension, such that myocardial oxygen consumption is favorably affected. The most selective agent routinely used in obtaining an afterload-reducing effect is hydralazine.

Balanced Vasodilators. The balanced vasodilators exert an effect on both preload and afterload through a generalized relaxing effect on vascular smooth muscle. The prototype short-acting agent of this kind is nitroprusside. This agent has found widespread application in managing acute heart failure states, including acute pulmonary edema. Used with care, it can also improve the circulatory state of patients with combined hypotension and low forward output, provided that adequate arterial pressure can be maintained by using volume loading or inotropic drugs or both. The tendency of nitroprusside to reduce systemic arterial pressure is offset to a considerable extent by the increased stroke output. The unloading effect of nitroprusside is most helpful when the left ventricular filling pressures are maintained in the vicinity of 15 mm Hg, which may require administering intravenous fluids. An important advantage of nitroprusside in ICU settings is its short duration of action, permitting minute-to-minute titration of the circulatory state.

A regimen yielding a balanced vasodilator effect is hydralazine and nitrates, the latter often given as the long-acting oral preparation isosorbide dinitrate. In an important multicenter study (V-HeFT I), the protocol randomly assigned patients who were symptomatic while taking digitalis and diuretics to hydralazine with isosorbide dinitrate, to prazosin, or to placebo. The group treated with hydralazine and nitrates showed a 38% mean reduction in mortality

TABLE 34–8. MAJOR VASODILATOR DRUGS*

Drug	Mechanism of Action	Venous Dilating Effect (Preload Reduction)	Arteriolar Dilating Effect (Afterload Reduction)	Usual Dosage	Comments
Nitroglycerin	Direct	+ + +	+	10–100 μg/min, IV 5–20 mg, transdermal 0.4 mg, s.l.	Tolerance may be a problem with sustained continuous use. May be used sublingually to control acute increases in left atrial pressure.
Isosorbide dinitrate	Direct	+ + +	+	5–20 mg q2 hr, s.l. 10–60 mg q4 hr, p.o.	Improved survival shows in chronic CHF when used with hydralazine.
Nitroprusside	Direct	+ + +	+ + +	5–150 μg/kg/min IV; usual dose, 50–75 μg/kg/min	Used IV only. Drug is light sensitive. Hazard of thiocyanate or cyanide toxicity with prolonged high doses.
Hydralazine	Direct	0	+ + +	10–75 mg q6 hr p.o.	Sustained benefit in heart failure not shown when used as sole vasodilator.
Prazosin†	α-Adrenergic blockade (alpha, selective)	+ + +	+ +	1–5 mg q6 hr p.o.	Extra caution required with initial doses. Tolerance requires dosage adjustments and complicates use in heart failure.
Captopril	Angiotensin converting enzyme (ACE) inhibitor	+ + +	+ +	6.25–25.0 mg q6–8 hr, p.o.	Approved by FDA for use in chronic CHF. Acute renal failure can occur with initial doses; initiate use with extra caution. Avoid potassium-sparing diuretics.
Enalapril	ACE inhibitor	+ + +	+ +	2.5–10 mg q12 hr p.o.	
Lisinopril	ACE inhibitor	+ + +	+ +	5–20 mg qd	

* All of these agents may cause severe hypotension, and special caution is required with initial use, particularly in patients with severe congestive heart failure. Heart rate changes with all agents listed are usually minor unless a hypotensive response elicits reflex tachycardia; prazosin can cause bradycardia with initial use. Calcium channel blocking drugs (verapamil, diltiazem, and dihydropyridines including nifedipine) are effective vasodilators but are not recommended for management of heart failure with systolic dysfunction because of their potential negative inotropic effects on the heart.

† Prazosin was not found to improve survival compared to placebo when added to diuretics and digoxin in patients with class II and III chronic heart failure.

CHF = congestive heart failure; FDA = Food and Drug Administration.

during the initial year of treatment, and the improved survival was sustained to the 3-year point. The prazosin-treated group showed no significant difference from the placebo group.

The ACE inhibitors captopril, enalapril, and lisinopril are available as balanced vasodilators for managing patients with heart failure. Multicenter trials have demonstrated sustained improvement in symptoms and exercise tolerance, and large-scale trials have shown that ACE inhibitors improve survival in patients with overt heart failure due to systolic ventricular dysfunction regardless of the cause or severity of symptoms. The CONSENSUS-I study demonstrated a 40% reduction in mortality at 6 months in patients with severe heart failure already treated with digoxin, diuretics, and other vasodilators who were randomized to enalapril rather than placebo. The arm of the SOLVD trial (1991) that randomized patients with symptomatic mild to moderate heart failure with left ventricular ejection fractions ≤35% to receive either enalapril or placebo reported a significant 16% reduction in overall mortality in the enalapril-treated group. A second arm of this trial that examined asymptomatic patients with similar left ventricular dysfunction did not demonstrate a statistically significant reduction in mortality among enalapril-treated patients (SOLVD, 1992), but there was a significant (29%) reduction in the combined endpoints of development of symptomatic heart failure and death due to any cause. The V-HeFT II trial (Cohn et al., 1991) showed a small but clear survival benefit in patients with mild to moderate heart failure randomized to receive enalapril versus the combination of hydralazine and isosorbide dinitrate. The SAVE trial (Pfeffer et al., 1992), which studied patients with recent acute anterior myocardial infarction and ejection fractions of 40% or less, showed a 20% reduction in mortality and a 36% reduction in the rate of progression to severe heart failure in the captopril-treated group after 12 months of follow-up. Both the SOLVD trials and the SAVE trial also demonstrated that enalapril and captopril, respectively, markedly reduced or prevented the increases in left ventricular end-diastolic and end-systolic volumes and decline in ejection fraction observed in patients randomized to receive placebo. Additional large-scale randomized trials of ACE inhibitors (AIRE, GISSI-III) have confirmed these general conclusions. Most clinicians find that captopril and enalapril provide a relatively simple and controllable approach to vasodilator therapy, and hence constitute vasodilators of choice. Special caution should be taken to use initial doses small enough to prevent hypotension and renal failure. An irritating, persistent dry cough is a class effect of ACE inhibitor drugs that occurs in up to 10% of patients.

Not all patients who appear to be reasonable candidates for vasodilator use in advanced heart failure can tolerate the drugs initially, and not all of the group that initially tolerates the regimen still show demonstrable benefit at the end of 3 months. Although results can be optimized by carefully selecting patients and judiciously using available agents, the fact remains that some patients with advanced heart failure are unable to tolerate vasodilators, chiefly because of postural hypotension or impaired renal function.

Combined Drug Therapy

Although patients with mild heart failure (early class II symptoms) can often be managed with a single class of drugs, accumulating evidence indicates that combination therapy with all three major classes of drugs tends to keep heart size and wall stress as well as symptoms at a minimum while allowing the patient maximal effort tolerance within the limits imposed by the underlying cardiac problem. Implicit in the scheme outlined in Table 34–4 is the working hypothesis that in patients with compromised contractile function, combination therapy with a diuretic, vasodilator, and digitalis yields optimal benefit while allowing each drug to be used at a dose level as far as possible from its toxicity threshold. There is substantial evidence documenting the additive beneficial hemodynamic effects of a vasodilator and a positively inotropic drug such as digoxin, as well as additive effects of combined use of digoxin and an ACE inhibitor on exercise tolerance. The experienced clinician usually elects to add these classes of agents to the regimen one at a time to permit assessment of the incremental response at each step, but in most cases evaluates the response to combined treatment with all three classes in patients who remain symptomatic at levels of activity they wish to maintain.

Treatment of Diastolic Ventricular Dysfunction

The elements of therapy in patients with predominant diastolic dysfunction differ in certain important ways from those in patients with "classic" congestive heart failure accompanying a dilated ventricle with impaired systolic function. Pulmonary congestion is appropriately treated in both subsets of patients with diuretics and other means of preload reduction, including venodilators. Nitroglycerin taken sublingually can be used effectively by patients to forestall or slow the progression of episodes of elevated left ventricular filling pressures that might otherwise progress to frank pulmonary edema. It is important to avoid excessive preload reduction in the predominant diastolic dysfunction patient, however, in order to avoid symptoms and signs of low cardiac output. Anti-ischemic and antihypertensive treatment should be pursued aggressively when these disorders and their attendant pathophysiology underlie diastolic ventricular dysfunction, with removal of ischemia and regression of hypertrophy as the goals of therapy. Atrial augmentation of ventricular systole is particularly important in these patients, and every effort should be made to maintain or restore normal sinus rhythm or pacemaker-induced AV synchrony. Tachycardia tends to be poorly tolerated in patients with diastolic dysfunction and should be managed as necessary with antiarrhythmic drugs and in some cases with β-adrenergic blocking agents, verapamil, or diltiazem. Calcium channel blocking drugs may be of benefit in some patients with predominant diastolic dysfunction but are generally to be avoided in the presence of severe systolic dysfunction because of their potential negative inotropic effects. Finally, positively inotropic agents such as digoxin have no established role in the management of patients with predominant diastolic dysfunction and are contraindicated in patients with hypertrophic cardiomyopathy and dynamic outflow tract obstruction.

Refractory Heart Failure

Therapeutic advances have left in their wake a subset of patients with marked impairment of ventricular function (often with left ventricular ejection fractions in the 10 to 20% range) who survive but are severely symptomatic on maximal tolerated doses of diuretics, digitalis, and vasodilators. Those who meet additional relevant criteria (including preserved function of other organ systems, no elevation of pulmonary vascular resistance, no active infection) may be referred for consideration of heart transplantation after detailed explanation of the potential risks and benefits of this procedure. This procedure now has relatively widespread application since the advent of cyclosporine for immunosuppression, and more than 150 centers in the United States now have active programs. Survival exceeds 65% in transplanted patients at 5 years in larger series, compared with an expected mortality well in excess of 50% at 12 months in patients treated by conventional means, and functional recovery is often gratifying. Expectations must be tempered by the very limited availability of donor hearts, however, which has recently plateaued in the 2000 per year range in the United States.

Treatment of acute decompensation using intravenous β-adrenergic or dopaminergic agonists, or the phosphodiesterase inhibitors amrinone or milrinone, is covered in Ch. 69. Longer-term use of orally active β-adrenergic agonist drugs has proved disappointing, in part because of rapid development of tolerance, and cannot be recommended. Phosphodiesterase inhibitor drugs have also shown a relatively high incidence of adverse outcomes (including excess mortality in longer-term ambulatory use at the milrinone dose studied) and these agents are not available for treatment of chronic heart failure. The artificial heart has been developed sufficiently for placement in several patients, but results to date have been disappointing because of unsolved thromboembolic problems, and mechanical assist devices are in current investigational use mainly to provide a bridge to heart transplantation in potentially suitable candidates (see Ch. 48).

ACKNOWLEDGMENT: Ralph A. Kelly, MD, has made major contributions to the coverage of diuretics, including Figure 34–4.

Berger BE, Warnock DG: Clinical uses and mechanisms of action of diuretic agents. *In* Brenner BM, Rector FC (eds.): The Kidney. Philadelphia, WB Saunders, 1986, p 433. *A compact summary of clinically relevant information as stated in the title.*

Cohn JN, et al.: A comparison of enalapril with hydralazine-isosorbide dinitrate in the treatment of chronic congestive heart failure. N Engl J Med 325:303, 1991. *The second Veterans Administration Cooperative Vasodilator-Heart Failure Trial (V-HeFT II).*

Kelly RA, Smith TW: Digoxin in heart failure: Implications of recent trials. J Am Coll

Cardiol 22:107A, 1993. *This brief review summarizes the available data from randomized clinical trials bearing on the efficacy of digoxin in patients with heart failure.*

Konstam M, et al.: Heart Failure: Evaluation and Care of Patients with Left-Ventricular Systolic Dysfunction. Clinical Practice Guideline No. 11. AHCPR Publication No. 94-0612. Rockville, MD, Agency for Health Care Policy and Research, Public Health Service, US Department of Health and Human Services, June 1994. *This comprehensive set of clinical practice guidelines includes decision algorithms and a detailed review and interpretation of available clinical data bearing on the management of patients with heart failure.*

Packer M (ed.): Physiologic determinants of survival in congestive heart failure. Circulation 75:IV-1, 1987. *This supplement to* Circulation *contains 14 papers reviewing the various factors influencing prognosis in heart failure and current aspects of vasodilator, inotropic, and antiarrhythmic therapy and their potential impact on survival.*

Packer M, et al.: Withdrawal of digoxin from patients with chronic heart failure treated with angiotensin-converting enzyme inhibitors. N Engl J Med 329:1, 1993. *The RADIANCE Trial randomized 178 patients with Class II or III heart failure and systolic dysfunction (left ventricular ejection fraction ≤ 0.35) to continuation or withdrawal of digoxin after a stable interval on digoxin, diuretics, and an ACE inhibitor.*

Pfeffer MA, et al. on behalf of the SAVE Investigators: Effect of captopril on mortality and morbidity in patients with left ventricular dysfunction after myocardial infarction. N Engl J Med 327:669, 1992. *The SAVE trial randomized 2231 patients within 3 to 16 days after myocardial infarction with ejection fractions ≤ 0.40 but without overt heart failure to placebo or captopril.*

Pouleur H (ed.): Diastolic function in heart failure: Clinical approaches to its understanding and treatment. Circulation 81:III-1, 1990. *This supplement to* Circulation *contains 21 papers covering virtually all clinically relevant aspects of diastolic dysfunction, including pathophysiology, role in heart failure, and therapeutic implications.*

Smith TW, Braunwald E, Kelly RA: The management of heart failure. *In* Braunwald E (ed.): Heart Diseases. 4th ed. Philadelphia, WB Saunders, 1992. *A detailed consideration of general and specific aspects of congestive heart failure management with more than 500 references.*

SOLVD Investigators: Effect of enalapril on survival in patients with reduced left ventricular ejection fractions and congestive heart failure. N Engl J Med 325:293, 1991. *The SOLVD treatment trial randomized 2569 patients with chronic heart failure and ejection fractions ≤ 0.35 receiving conventional treatment with diuretics and digoxin to enalapril (target dose 10 mg b.i.d.) or placebo.*

SOLVD Investigators: Effect of enalapril on mortality and the development of heart failure in asymptomatic patients with reduced left ventricular ejection fractions. N Engl J Med 327:685, 1992. *The SOLVD prevention trial randomized 4228 patients with asymptomatic left ventricular dysfunction (ejection fraction ≤ 0.35) to enalapril (target dose 10 mg b.i.d.) or placebo.*

35 CARDIAC ARRHYTHMIAS
J. Thomas Bigger, Jr.

Optimal management of cardiac arrhythmias requires knowing their (1) mechanism, etiology, and natural history and (2) effect on the hemodynamic state. Before selecting therapy, the physician should thoroughly assess the patient's physical, psychological, and biochemical state. The chosen treatment—whether drugs, devices, or surgery—must be monitored closely for its initial and continued effectiveness and for adverse effects. This chapter discusses mechanisms, electrocardiographic (ECG) recognition, and management of cardiac arrhythmias.

ANATOMIC CONSIDERATIONS

Normal Specialized Impulse-Generating and Conducting System

SINUS NODE. The sinus node is situated at the junction between the superior vena cava and the right atrium. The node surrounds a large central artery arising from the right (55%) or left circumflex coronary artery (45%). Two types of special muscle fibers are found in the node: P (pacemaker) and T (transitional) cells. P cells are small (diameter of 5 to 10 μg) ovoid or stellate cells that have a low density of mitochondria, sarcoplasmic reticulum, and myofibrils, suggesting a lack of contractile function. P cells occur in tight clusters and attach only to other P cells or T cells; intercellular attachments are sparse, correlating with the slow conduction in the sinus node.

T cells are intermediate in size, structure, and cellular organization between P cells and ordinary atrial myocardium. T cells may attach either to P cells or to working myocardial cells. T cells surround the sinus node and presumably serve both to organize impulses leaving the node and to hinder access of ectopic atrial impulses.

INTERNODAL TRACTS. Three internodal tracts connecting the sinus node to the atrioventricular (AV) node have been described: anterior, middle, and posterior. The *anterior internodal tract* also connects to the left atrium via the interatrial bundle of Bachmann. The three internodal tracts are widely separated in the interatrial septum but converge above and behind the AV node.

Internodal tracts contain working atrial cells interspersed with large cells that resemble ventricular Purkinje cells. Because internodal pathways are difficult to trace by serial microscopic sections, some doubt their presence or functional significance. Internodal tracts continue to function in high extracellular K^+ concentrations, a property that has been used to demonstrate their functional continuity and preferential internodal conductivity.

ATRIOVENTRICULAR NODE. The AV node lies beneath the endocardium of the right atrium near the septal leaflet of the tricuspid valve and immediately anterior to the ostium of the coronary sinus. The AV nodal artery usually arises from the right coronary artery. In the central portion of the AV node, the myocytes form tangled swirls with ample interconnections. Ultrastructurally, cells in the mid-AV node resemble sinus node T cells. Toward the distal end of the AV node, myocytes pallisade into linear arrays as they form the bundle of His.

The region between the ostium of the coronary sinus and the posterior margin of the AV node is richly supplied by cholinergic ganglia. Retronodal chemoreceptors may trigger vagal reflexes during ischemia of the posterior wall of the heart. These reflexes can produce marked bradycardia, peripheral vasodilatation, nausea, sweating, and salivation.

HIS-PURKINJE SYSTEM. The AV bundle (bundle of His) is a thick, cablelike structure about 15 mm in length that emerges from the anterior, inferior border of the AV node (Fig. 35–1). The bundle of His penetrates the central fibrous body and courses to the crest of the muscular interventricular septum where it divides into left and right bundle branches. The His bundle is the only normal route for AV conduction. Damage to the AV bundle can delay or block AV conduction. The His bundle is generously supplied with arterial blood from the anterior and posterior descending coronary arteries; therefore, extensive coronary disease is required to produce ischemic damage.

The left bundle branch is a broad sheet of fibers that cascade under the noncoronary cusp of the aortic valve and down the left side of the interventricular septum. The left bundle branch connects first with myocardium in the septum and near the papillary muscles, causing early activation of these regions.

The right bundle branch emerges from the bundle of His and courses down the right side of the interventricular septum to make its first connections with ventricular myocardium near the base of the anterior papillary muscle. From here, peripheral branches spread up the interventricular septum and the free wall of the right ventricle.

The terminal Purkinje fibers form extensive interconnected lacy networks on the endocardium of both ventricles. In human hearts, no Purkinje fibers are found in the outer two thirds of the ventricular walls. Purkinje cells are large—15 to 30 mm in diameter and 20 to 100 mm in length with a round, centrally located nucleus in the cell. Purkinje fibers contain fewer myofibrils and mitochondria than working ventricular muscle. External to the sarcolemmal basement membrane is a thick surface coat of negatively charged glycoproteins that function in Ca^{2+} binding and exchange. Intercalated discs are well developed in Purkinje fibers and provide low-resistance pathways for current flow and for diffusion of ions and small molecules.

Function of the Specialized Impulse-Generating and Conducting System

The normal heartbeat begins in the sinus node and spreads slowly through perinodal fibers to reach specialized atrial tracts and ordinary atrial muscle (Fig. 35–1). Specialized atrial tracts transmit the cardiac impulse rapidly from the sinus node to the AV node and to the left atrium. The cardiac impulse slows dramatically in the AV node, accounting for most of the PR interval in the ECG. Conduction accelerates tremendously in the His bundle, and excitation of the bundle branches and peripheral Purkinje fibers occurs with blazing speed. The great mass of ordinary ventricular muscle is activated almost simultaneously over much of its endocardial surface.

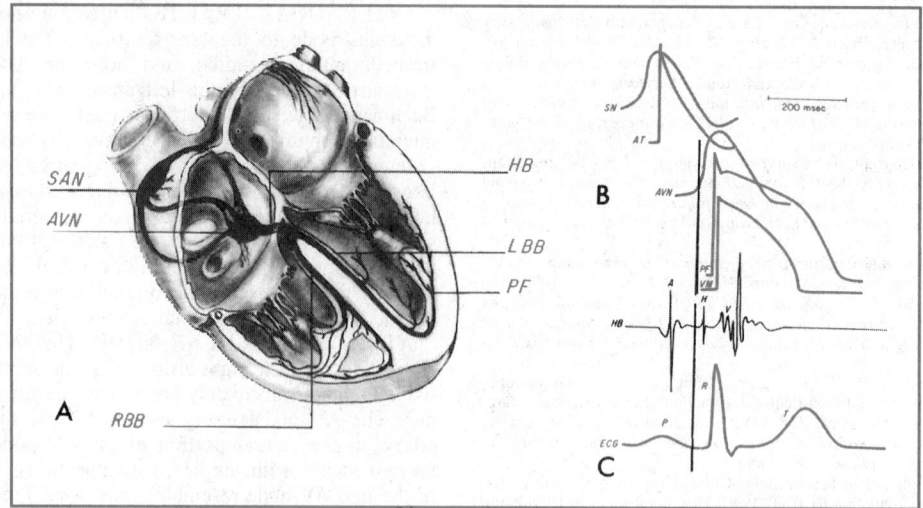

FIGURE 35–1. The anatomy and characteristic action potentials of the specialized impulse-generating and conducting system of the heart. *A*, A diagram of the conduction system of the heart. SAN = Sinoatrial node; AVN = atrioventricular node; HB = bundle of His; RBB = right bundle branch; LBB = left bundle branch; PF = Purkinje fiber. *B*, Typical action potentials from the sinus node (SN), atrium (AT), atrioventricular node (AVN), Purkinje fiber (PF), and ventricular muscle (VM). *C*, Relationship of deflections in the His bundle (HB) electrogram to depolarization of the sites shown in *B* and to the electrocardiographic deflections. Depolarization of the lower atrial septum (A), bundle of His (H), and ventricular septum (V) is recorded in the bipolar His bundle electrogram. The H deflection partitions the PR interval into two subintervals: the AH interval, representing atrioventricular nodal conduction, and the HV interval, which measures conduction to the His-Purkinje system. (From Braunwald E: Heart Disease: A Textbook of Cardiovascular Medicine. Philadelphia, WB Saunders, 1980.)

Then activation spreads to the epicardium to complete cardiac excitation.

BRIEF REVIEW OF CARDIAC CELLULAR ELECTROPHYSIOLOGY

RESTING POTENTIAL. The sarcolemma of cardiac cells is a hydrophobic phospholipid bilayer. Protein molecules that cross the entire width of the membrane provide hydrophilic channels and permit hydrated cations or anions to cross the sarcolemma. Ion-selective channels and energy-dependent ion pumping establish transmembrane gradients of Na^+ and K^+ that determine the resting voltage difference of about -80 to -90 mV across the sarcolemma, the *resting transmembrane voltage* (Vm).

ACTION POTENTIALS. When cardiac cells activate, a complex sequence of voltage changes occurs as a function of time and membrane ionic currents. Figure 35–2 diagrams the four phases of a Purkinje fiber *action potential.* Sinus and AV nodal cells have a slowly rising phase 0 and lack distinct phases 1, 2, and 3 (see Fig. 35–1). During phase 4, many cells have a steady transmembrane voltage, but automatic fibers in the sinus node and His-Purkinje system spontaneously depolarize and can initiate impulses that propagate to the rest of the heart.

OVERDRIVE SUPPRESSION. In the normal heart, P cells in the sinus node depolarize and overdrive subsidiary pacemaker cells in the atrial specialized tracts, coronary sinus region, or His-Purkinje system. The faster subsidiary pacemakers are overdriven, the more Na^+ enters the cell per unit of time. As the $[Na]_i$ increases, the activity of the Na^+/K^+ exchange pump becomes more electrogenic; i.e., the ratio of Na^+ out to K^+ increases, hyperpolarizing the cell and counteracting pacemaker activity. If the dominant pacemaker stops, there is a pause in rhythm. However, as the $[Na]_i$ is pumped out, outward pump current declines until spontaneous depolarization resumes. As the pump current declines, the firing rate in the subsidiary pacemaker increases gradually—the "warm-up" phenomenon.

FAST AND SLOW RESPONSES. Cardiac action potentials are classified as *fast* or *slow* responses (Table 35–1). The *fast response* (Fig. 35–3) is generated by intense inward i_{Na}, has a large, fast-rising phase 0, propagates rapidly, and has a large safety factor for conduction. Working myocardial cells in the atria, ventricles, and Purkinje fibers have fast responses. The *slow response* has a slowly rising phase 0, propagates slowly, and has a low safety factor for conduction (Fig. 35–3). Cells in the sinus node, pectinate muscles, AV node, and AV rings have slow responses. Depolarization in slow response fibers is due to slow inward current (i_s) carried by Ca^{2+} and, to a lesser extent, Na^+.

REFRACTORINESS. Refractoriness is involved in the pathogenesis of many arrhythmias and in the action of antiarrhythmic drugs. The effective refractory period (ERP), the minimum interval between two propagating responses, is closely linked to action potential duration (APD) in fast-response fibers because recovery from inactivation in the Na^+ channel closely parallels repolarization. However, in sinus and AV nodal cells (slow responses), refractoriness can outlast full repolarization so that the ERP is much longer than the APD.

RESPONSIVENESS AND CONDUCTION. The term *membrane responsiveness* applies to the response of a cardiac fiber to a stimulus. Changes in the maximum rate of depolarization during phase 0 ($\dot{V}_{max}$) provide an index of changes in availability of the Na^+ current. In cardiac Purkinje fibers and other fast-response

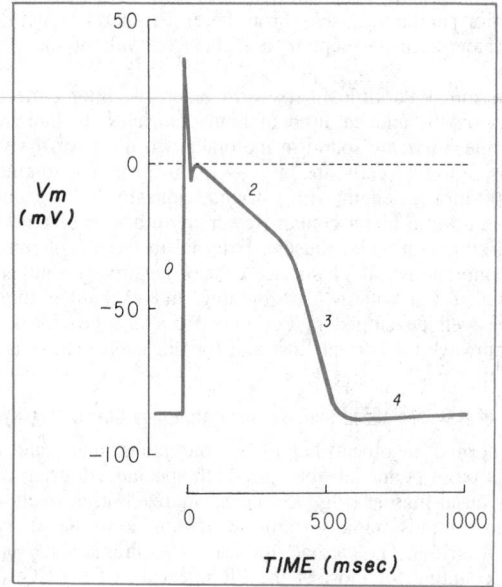

FIGURE 35–2. The cardiac action potential of a Purkinje fiber has five distinct phases: rapid depolarization (0), early repolarization (1), plateau (2), rapid repolarization (3), and diastole (4). (From Braunwald E: Heart Disease: A Textbook of Cardiovascular Medicine. Philadelphia, WB Saunders, 1980.)

TABLE 35–1. COMPARISON OF SLOW AND FAST ACTION POTENTIALS

Electrophysiologic Characteristics	Slow Potential	Fast Potential
Resting potential	Low (−40 to −70 mV)	High (−75 to −90 mV)
Action potential amplitude	40 to 80 mV	90 to 120 mV
Phase 0 V_{max}	1 to 10 V/sec	200 to 800 V/sec
Overshoot	0 to 15 mV	10 to 30 mV
Conduction velocity	0.01 to 0.1 m/sec	0.5 to 3.0 m/sec
Stimulus-dependent action potential amplitude	Yes	No
Threshold voltage	−50 to −30 mV	−75 to −65 mV
Depolarizing current carried by	Ca^{2+} (Na^+)	Na^+
Ionic current activates	Slow (10 to 20 msec)	Fast (0.5 msec)
Ionic current inactivates	Slow (50 to 100 msec)	Fast (0.5 msec)
Channel blocked by	Mn^{2+}, La^{3+}, verapamil, diltiazem, nifedipine	Tetrodotoxin, class 1 antiarrhythmics

TABLE 35–2. MECHANISMS RESPONSIBLE FOR CARDIAC ARRHYTHMIAS

I. **Abnormalities of impulse generation**
  A. Alterations of normal automaticity
  B. Abnormal automaticity
  C. Triggered activity
    1. Early afterdepolarizations
    2. Late afterdepolarizations

II. **Abnormalities of impulse conduction**
  A. Slowing of conduction and block
  B. Unidirectional block and reentry
    1. Ordered reentry
    2. Random reentry
    3. Summation and inhibition
  C. Conduction block, electrotonus, and reflection

III. **Combined abnormalities of impulse generation and conduction**
  A. Conduction showed by phase 4 depolarization
  B. Parasystole

fibers, $\dot{V}_{max}$ is strongly dependent on Vm at the instant of excitation; as soon as the fiber is fully repolarized, it is fully responsive. In slow-response fibers, responsiveness does not return until well after repolarization is complete. There is a considerable safety factor for conduction in fast-response fibers; $\dot{V}_{max}$ must be reduced to less than half normal before conduction velocity decreases. The safety factor is much lower in slow-response fibers so that premature impulses are likely to experience substantial conduction delay or block.

MECHANISMS OF CARDIAC ARRHYTHMIAS

An arrhythmia is an abnormality of rate, regularity, or site of origin of the cardiac impulse or a disturbance in conduction that causes an abnormal sequence of activation. Arrhythmias may arise because of alterations in impulse generation, impulse conduction, or both (Table 35–2).

Arrhythmias Due to Abnormalities of Impulse Generation

Many arrhythmias arise because of either depressed or enhanced normal automaticity. Abnormal automaticity and triggered activity also are important mechanisms for arrhythmogenesis.

ALTERED NORMAL AUTOMATICITY. Only a few cardiac cell types develop normal automaticity: sinus node, internodal tracts, fibers near the ostium of the coronary sinus, distal AV node, and the His-Purkinje system.

Sinus Node. The rate of firing in the sinus node can be altered by autonomic activity or intrinsic disease. Increased vagal activity can slow or stop sinus node pacemakers by increasing membrane K^+ conductance of P cells. Increased sympathetic nerve traffic to the sinus node causes sinus tachycardia.

Purkinje Fibers. Augmented automaticity due to increased sympathetic nerve activity in the His-Purkinje system commonly causes human arrhythmias. AV junctional pacemakers can fire faster than a normal sinus node because of selective traffic on sympathetic nerves, local release of catecholamines, or enhanced responsiveness of β-adrenergic receptors. Also, vagal and sympathetic activity can increase together; the vagus slows the sinus rate and AV conduction while sympathetic activity increases the firing rate in the His-Purkinje system.

In diseased hearts, automaticity in the His-Purkinje system may become reduced. In the sick sinus syndrome, it is typical for the ventricular escape pacemakers to be depressed, producing long pauses when the sinus node pacemaker fails. In AV block due to bundle branch disease, ventricular pacemakers also may be abnormally slow.

Abnormal Impulse Generation

Abnormal automaticity or triggered activity can generate impulses even in fibers that are incapable of normal automaticity, e.g., ordinary atrial or ventricular muscle cells.

ABNORMAL AUTOMATICITY. Abnormal automaticity refers to spontaneous diastolic depolarization in depolarized cells. Purkinje fibers, atrial cells, and ventricular cells can show spontaneous diastolic depolarization and repetitive automatic firing when their resting Vm is reduced to −60 mV or below. Abnormal automaticity is seen in Purkinje fibers depolarized by acute myocardial infarction. Abnormal automaticity and repetitive firing can be evoked in normal atrial or ventricular cells by applying depolarizing current. Abnormal automaticity is not readily suppressed by overdrive pacing.

TRIGGERED ACTIVITY. Repetitive firing in heart muscle can be caused by triggered activity. Triggered activity is *not* a form of automaticity but is capable of producing a sustained tachyarrhyth-

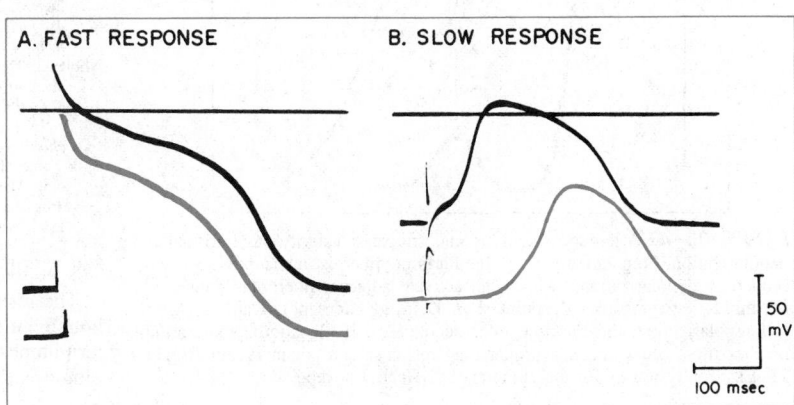

FIGURE 35–3. Two types of cardiac action potentials: (*A*) fast response potential, (*B*) slow response potential. (From Wit AL, Rosen MR, Hoffman BF: Electrophysiology and pharmacology of cardiac arrhythmias. II. Relationship of normal and abnormal electrical activity of cardiac fibers to the genesis of arrhythmias. Am Heart J 88:515, 1974.)

A. FAST RESPONSE   B. SLOW RESPONSE

50 mV

100 msec

mia. Two primary mechanisms can initiate triggered activity: early afterdepolarizations and delayed afterdepolarizations (Fig. 35–4).

Early Afterdepolarizations. Early afterdepolarizations are secondary depolarizations that occur before repolarization is complete, often from the action potential plateau (Fig. 35–4). Experimentally, early afterdepolarizations have been produced in cardiac Purkinje fibers by stretching or crushing, hypoxia, cooling, low $[K]_o$, high $[Ca]_o$, catecholamines, and chemicals and drugs (such as veratrine, aconitine, quinidine, sotalol, or N-acetyl procainamide). Torsades de pointes in humans is thought to be the counterpart of triggered activity due to early afterdepolarizations.

Delayed Afterdepolarizations. A delayed afterdepolarization is a secondary depolarization occurring just after full repolarization has been achieved. This event depends on the previous action potential (Fig. 35–4). Delayed afterdepolarizations can reach a threshold and cause a single premature depolarization or trigger a series of impulses. Delayed afterdepolarizations can be induced by digitalis, easily in the His-Purkinje system and with more difficulty in specialized atrial or ordinary ventricular cells. Some of the digitalis-induced ventricular tachycardias in humans behave like triggered activity. In the atria, coronary sinus, and mitral valve, delayed afterdepolarizations and triggered activity can be caused by catecholamines.

Arrhythmias Caused by Abnormalities of Impulse Conduction

Reentry seems to be a common cause of cardiac arrhythmias in humans, e.g., paroxysmal supraventricular tachycardia and constantly coupled ventricular premature complexes. Reentrant arrhythmias usually are started by an initiating premature complex; i.e., they are self-sustained but are not self-initiated. To start reentry, one-way conduction block must occur and there must be an anatomic or functional "barrier" that forms a circuit (Fig. 35–5). Also, the path length of the reentrant circuit must be greater than the wavelength of the cardiac impulse (wavelength = conduction

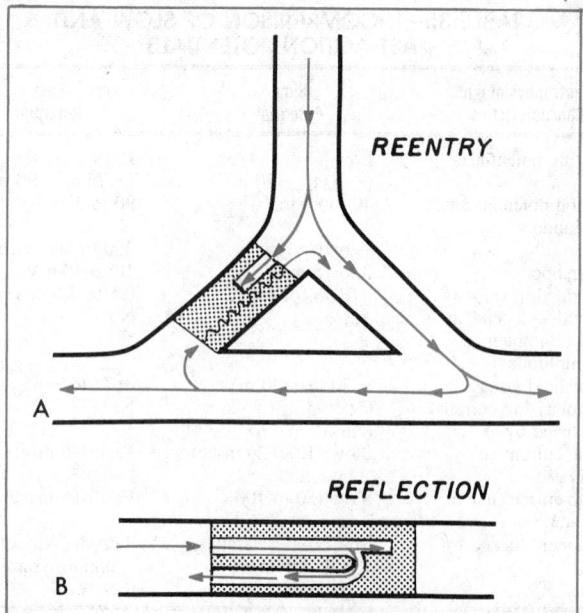

FIGURE 35–5. Two models of reentry according to Schmitt and Erlanger. *A*, Diagram showing a loop of cardiac fibers that could represent either a terminal branch of a Purkinje fiber ending on ventricular muscle or a loop of the Purkinje syncytium. In this case, one-way block and slow conduction permit reentry. *B*, A linear strand of cardiac muscle showing a depolarized zone in a portion of its cross-section. One-way block occurs in the depolarized zone, permitting the propagating impulse to reflect back in the direction from which it came. (From Braunwald E: Heart Disease: A Textbook of Cardiovascular Medicine. Philadelphia, WB Saunders, 1980.)

velocity × refractory period). For reentry to occur, conduction must be very slow, refractoriness very short, or both. Reentry has been demonstrated in anatomic loops (e.g., rings of Purkinje fibers) or anatomic obstacles (e.g., scars). Reentry occurring in unbranched bundles or sheets of cardiac muscle has been given specialized names, e.g., reflection or leading-edge reentry.

Reentry can be subdivided into random and ordered forms. In random reentry, the cardiac impulse conducts over circuits that change their location and size as a function of time, e.g., atrial and ventricular fibrillation. In ordered reentry, the circuit for reentrant activity is relatively constant.

LEADING-EDGE REENTRY. Reentrant excitation can be initiated *in vitro* by premature stimulation in small, thin pieces of normal atrium that contain no anatomic obstacles or loops of tissue. Conduction is slowed because activation occurs when the tissue is partially refractory. Block occurs in some regions because of local differences in refractory periods. The pathway for reentrant activity can stabilize and be sustained.

Fozzard HA, Haber E, Jennings RB, et al. (eds.): The Heart and Cardiovascular System, Scientific Foundations. 2nd ed. New York, Raven Press, 1991. *The section of cardiac electrophysiology and arrhythmias contains detailed reviews of current knowledge and thought on the electrophysiology of the heart, the genesis of cardiac arrhythmias, and the epidemiology of human arrhythmias. Other sections contain excellent reviews of the embryology, anatomy, and pathology of the heart. Profusely illustrated and exhaustively referenced.*

Hackel DB: Anatomy and pathology of the cardiac conducting system. *In* Edwards JE, Lev M, Abell MA (eds.): The Heart. Baltimore, Williams & Wilkins, 1974, p 232. *A concise description of the normal anatomy and pathology of the conduction system.*

Noble D: The Initiation of the Heartbeat. London, Oxford University Press, 1979. *An account of cardiac electrophysiology for medical students and clinicians who are unfamiliar with electronics and mathematics. Even the most difficult concepts of cardiac excitation are explained clearly and concisely. Selective references to the classic papers in electrophysiology.*

Task Force of the Working Group on Arrhythmias of the European Society of Cardiology: The Sicilian gambit. A new approach to the classification of antiarrhythmic drugs based on their actions on arrhythmogenic mechanisms. Circulation 84:1831, 1991.

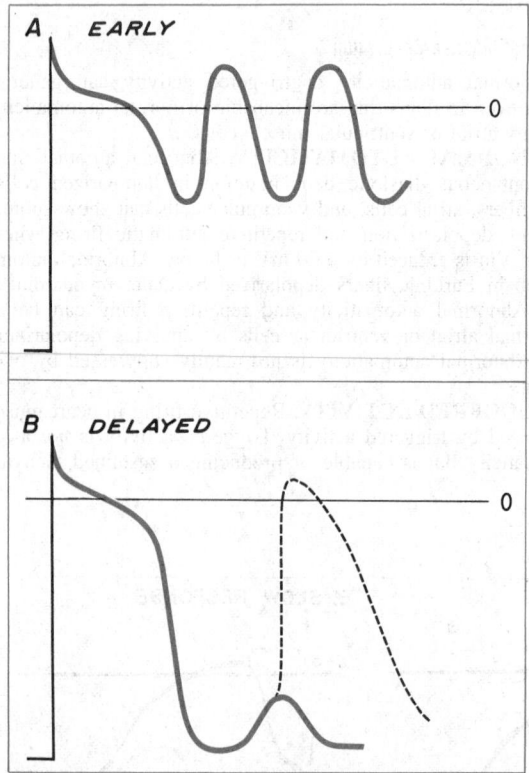

FIGURE 35–4. Afterdepolarizations and triggered activity. *A*, Early afterdepolarization. Repolarization of the Purkinje fiber is interrupted by two secondary depolarizations, which can activate adjacent fibers and cause arrhythmias, e.g., torsades de pointes. *B*, Delayed afterdepolarizations. After full repolarization, the Purkinje fiber depolarizes. If the afterdepolarization reaches threshold voltage, a propagating response can occur. (From Bigger JT: Electrophysiology for the clinician. Eur Heart J 5(Suppl B):1, 1984.)

DIAGNOSTIC APPROACHES TO CARDIAC ARRHYTHMIAS

The history, physical examination, 12-lead electrocardiogram, 24-hour continuous electrocardiographic recordings, exercise tests, intermittent electrocardiographic recordings, and clinical electrophysiologic studies are the primary tools used to diagnose cardiac arrhythmias. Decisions about treatment may require other laboratory studies to define better the cause of heart disease, other aspects of the functional status of the heart, e.g., left ventricular function or perfusion, or function of other organ systems (see Ch. 33).

History and Physical Examination

The primary purposes of the history are (1) to formulate a hypothesis about the presence and type of arrhythmia, (2) to detect factors that trigger the onset of the arrhythmia or intensify arrhythmic symptoms, (3) to establish the frequency and pattern of occurrence of the arrhythmia, and (4) to establish the functional consequences of the arrhythmia.

The physical examination provides information about the presence and type of heart disease and the degree of cardiac impairment. The physical examination in conjunction with the ECG can aid in the differential diagnosis of arrhythmias. A regular tachycardia, 150 beats per minute, with a wide QRS complex is compatible with many arrhythmias, and the physical examination can provide the key to the diagnosis.

Electrocardiography

The ECG is the most important test to obtain for arrhythmia diagnosis. A long continuous recording of a lead with clear-cut P waves should be made. Usually, a systematic analysis of the rhythm strip with the aid of calipers permits a definitive diagnosis. The rate and the regularity of P-P and R-R intervals, the constancy of the PR interval, and the ratio of atrial to ventricular complexes should be noted. Even when every P and QRS is identified, the ECG pattern may be compatible with more than one diagnosis. Ladder diagrams help display the possibilities in an unequivocal manner (Fig. 35–6).

Carotid Sinus Pressure

Taking ECG rhythm strips during carotid sinus pressure is a valuable bedside maneuver for diagnosis of cardiac arrhythmias.

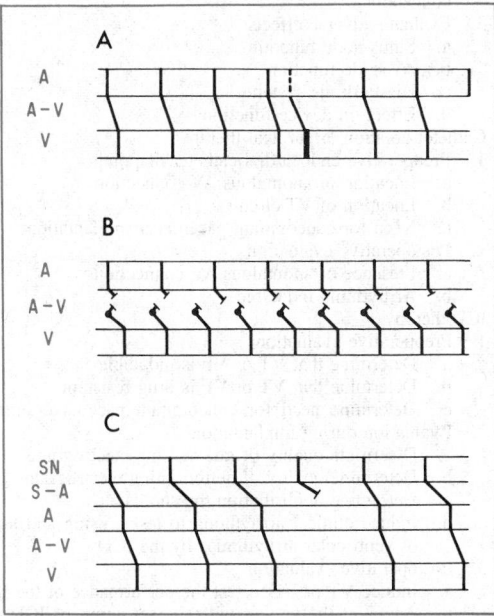

FIGURE 35–6. Ladder diagrams of cardiac rhythm. A = Atrium; A-V = atrioventricular junction (the A-V node and His-Purkinje system); V = ventricle; SN = sinus node; S-A = sinoatrial junction. *A,* Sinus rhythm with atrial premature complex (APC). Atrioventricular conduction of the APC is slower than for sinus impulses because the atrioventricular node is partially refractory. The broad line in the ventricular tier indicates aberrant ventricular conduction of the APC, which occurs because the premature impulse arrives during the relative refractory period of the His-Purkinje system. *B,* Atrioventricular junctional rhythm. The A-V junctional automatic rhythm captures the ventricles but shows retrograde block. The sinus node controls the atria, but the sinus impulse finds the A-V node refractory and is blocked; i.e., there is interference between the sinus and junctional rhythm. *C,* Type I (Wenckebach) sinoatrial block. The sinus impulse travels through the perinodal junctional tissues with increasing delay until block finally occurs. (From Braunwald E: Heart Disease: A Textbook of Cardiovascular Medicine. Philadelphia, WB Saunders, 1980.)

TABLE 35–3. EFFECT OF CAROTID SINUS PRESSURE ON TACHYARRHYTHMIAS

Arrhythmia	Response to Carotid Sinus Pressure
Sinus tachycardia	1. Gradual slowing during massage, gradual speeding after massage
Paroxysmal supraventricular tachycardia (AV nodal)	1. No effect, or 2. Abrupt conversion to sinus rhythm, or 3. Slight slowing
Paroxysmal supraventricular tachycardia (anomalous AV connection)	1. No effect, or 2. Abrupt conversion to sinus rhythm, or 3. Slight slowing
Nonparoxysmal supraventricular tachycardia	1. No effect, or 2. AV block, slowed ventricular rate, or 3. Gradual slowing of ventricular rate
Atrial flutter	1. AV block, slowed ventricular rate, or 2. No effect, or 3. Atrial fibrillation
Atrial fibrillation	1. AV block, slowed ventricular rate, or 2. No effect
Ventricular tachycardia	1. No effect, or 2. AV dissociation

Carotid massage activates a reflex arc that increases the vagal traffic to the heart. The most important use of carotid sinus pressure is to aid in the analysis of rapid, regular tachycardia when P waves are not clearly apparent. The responses of various arrhythmias to carotid sinus massage are listed in Table 35–3.

Carotid sinus pressure poses risks, particularly in older patients, i.e., syncope, convulsions, stroke, prolonged asystole, or ventricular tachyarrhythmias. In patients with digitalis toxicity, carotid sinus pressure may provoke malignant ventricular arrhythmias.

Special Procedures to Detect Atrial Activation

All of the P waves must be identified to make rhythm analysis reliable. P waves can be detected using special lead placement, e.g., the Lewis lead, esophageal electrograms, or intracavitary right atrial ECG.

Ambulatory ECG Recording

In 1961, Holter described the technique of ambulatory ECG recording. A light, portable tape recorder continuously records the ECG for 24 hours while the patient performs his or her usual daily activities and records the activities and symptoms in a diary. The primary indications for ambulatory ECG recordings are listed in Table 35–4.

INTERMITTENT RECORDERS. When symptoms occur only occasionally, intermittent recorders permit monitoring lasting from a few days to many weeks even though the ECG recordings are brief (seconds to minutes). These recorders may be attached to patients continuously or intermittently.

Hard-Wired Recorders. Intermittent recorders of the hard-wired type are continuously attached to the patient by electrodes and cables. Patients activate these recorders by pressing a button. Some units have 40 to 100 seconds of electronic memory and sample the ECG continuously, replacing old data with new. When activated, 30 to 60 seconds of ECG are recorded before the patient pressed the button. Data are retrieved from hard-wired systems either by direct playback or by telephonic transmission.

Intermittently Attached Recorders, Telephonic Transmission. These devices are typically about the size and shape of a radiopaging unit. The patient applies ECG leads when symptoms occur. Units with memory can store one to three ECG samples for subsequent telephone transmission. Commercial services provide immediate evaluation of the ECG. Transmissions are acted on according to the instructions of the patient's physician.

Intracardiac Recording and Stimulation (*Endocardial Electrical Stimulation*)

Over the past 30 years, intracardiac recording and stimulation have developed as a diagnostic and therapeutic tool for managing

TABLE 35-4. INDICATIONS FOR LONG-TERM CONTINUOUS ECG RECORDINGS

I. **Detect and quantify arrhythmias or conduction defects in patients with symptoms** (e.g., syncope or other central nervous system symptoms, palpitations, or angina pectoris)

II. **Quantify arrhythmias, conduction defects, or ischemia in patients with predisposing conditions**
 A. Sick sinus syndrome
 B. Pre-excitation syndromes
 C. AV conduction defects
 D. Pacemaker or ICD malfunction
 E. Mitral valve prolapse
 F. Long QT syndrome
 G. After myocardial infarction
 H. Angina pectoris
 I. Hypertrophic or dilated cardiomyopathy
 J. Heart failure

III. **Evaluate activity**
 A. To detect exercise-related arrhythmias or conduction defects
 B. To detect ischemia during activity

IV. **Evaluate therapy**
 A. Antiarrhythmic drug treatment
 B. Fad diets
 C. Drugs with cardiac adverse effects
 D. Pacemakers
 E. Implantable cardioverter/defibrillators
 F. Catheter ablation
 G. Surgery
  1. Ischemia or arrhythmias after coronary artery bypass graft surgery
  2. Pre-excitation after division of anomalous AV connection
  3. AV conduction after surgical division or catheter ablation of the His bundle

human cardiac arrhythmias. Local electrical activity can be recorded from the portions of the heart that are electrically silent on the body surface ECG, e.g., sinus node, His bundle, right bundle branch, left bundle branch, and Kent bundle. The sequence and time of activation of atria and ventricles can be mapped, and AV conduction can be partitioned into AV nodal and His-Purkinje components (Fig. 35-7). Recordings from selected sites are used with

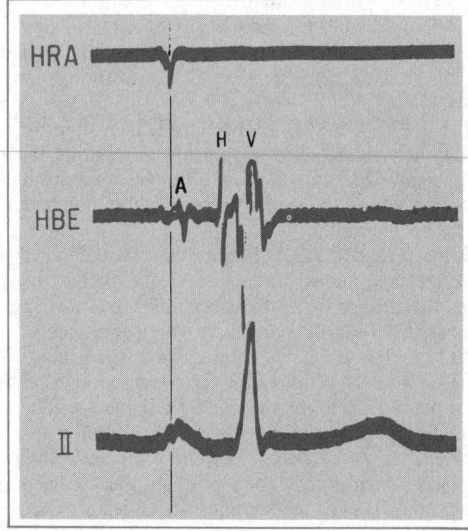

FIGURE 35-7. Intracardiac recordings. A high right atrial bipolar electrogram (HRA), His bundle bipolar electrogram (HBE), and tracing from lead II of the electrocardiogram. A = Atrial depolarization; H = depolarization of the His bundle; V = depolarization of the upper ventricular septum. The PA interval represents intra-atrial conduction time (upper to lower atrium); AH represents atrioventricular nodal conduction; and HV represents the His-Purkinje conduction time. The thin vertical line correlates the onset of atrial activation in the three recordings. (From Braunwald E: Heart Disease: A Textbook of Cardiovascular Medicine. Philadelphia, WB Saunders, 1980.)

pacing and programmed stimulation sequences to evaluate automaticity, conduction, refractoriness, and the causes of arrhythmias in intact humans. These techniques have not only enhanced our understanding of arrhythmias and conduction defects but also have improved our ability to select and evaluate therapy. Some of the major clinical uses of electrophysiologic studies are listed in Table 35-5.

Bigger JT Jr, Reiffel JA, Coromilas J: Ambulatory electrocardiography. *In* Platia EV (ed.): Nonpharmacologic Management of Cardiac Arrhythmias. Philadelphia, J.B.

TABLE 35-5. INDICATIONS FOR CLINICAL ELECTROPHYSIOLOGIC STUDIES—ENDOCARDIAL ELECTRICAL STIMULATION

I. **To evaluate mechanism, site, and extent of arrhythmia and/or conduction defect**
 A. Sick sinus syndrome
 B. Pre-excitation syndrome
 C. Supraventricular tachycardia
 D. Distinguish between supraventricular arrhythmias with aberration and ventricular arrhythmias
 E. Type I AV block with bundle branch block
 F. Type II AV block with normal QRS
 G. Bifascicular block occurring in acute myocardial infarction

II. **To search for a cause for syncope**
 A. Evaluate sinus node function
 B. Evaluate AV node function
 C. Evaluate function of His-Purkinje system
 D. Evaluate functional characteristics of anomalous AV connections
 E. Provoke arrhythmias
  1. Supraventricular tachycardia
  2. Atrial flutter or fibrillation
  3. Ventricular tachycardia

III. **To evaluate therapy**
 A. Drug therapy
  1. Prevent inducible arrhythmias
  2. Measure conduction and refractoriness in anomalous AV connections
  3. Evaluate adverse effects
   a. Sinus node function
   b. AV node function
   c. His-Purkinje system
   d. Effect on device function
 B. Catheter ablation or surgical therapy
  1. Preoperative endocardial catheter mapping
   a. Location of anomalous AV connections
   b. Location of VT circuit
   c. Need for concomitant pacemaker implantation
  2. Postoperative evaluation
   a. Presence of anomalous AV connections
   b. Arrhythmia inducible
 C. ICD therapy
  1. Preoperative evaluation
   a. Determine that VT or VF is inducible
   b. Determine that VT or VF is drug resistant
   c. Determine need for concomitant pacemaker implantation
  2. Evaluation during implantation
   a. Determine quality of rate-sensing electrograms
   b. Determine quality of defibrillating electrograms
   c. Determine defibrillation thresholds
   d. Induce clinical arrhythmia to test sensing and termination of ventricular arrhythmias by the ICD
  3. Postoperative evaluation
   a. Induce VT or VF to test the performance of the ICD
   b. Acquaint the patient with the sensation of ICD discharge
 D. Pacemaker therapy
  1. Evaluate condition for suitability for pacemaker therapy
   a. Supraventricular tachycardia due to reciprocation in the AV node
   b. Supraventricular tachycardia due to reciprocation in anomalous AV connections
   c. Reentrant ventricular tachycardia
  2. Determine the information needed to select pacemaker type and values for programmed features

IV. **To apply ablation therapy**
 A. Anomalous AV connections
 B. AV node or bundle of His
 C. Ventricular tachycardia (experimental)

ICD = Implantable cardioverter defibrillator; VT = ventricular tachycardia; VF = ventricular fibrillation.

Lippincott, 1986, p 36. *A comprehensive review of the technology, indications, and clinical used of ambulatory electrocardiography. Liberally illustrated and referenced.*

Josephson ME: Clinical Cardiac Electrophysiology: Techniques and Interpretations. Philadelphia, Lea & Febiger, 1993. *A detailed description of the techniques of clinical electrophysiology and the interpretation of the findings. Intended for the internist and clinical cardiologist without an extensive background in cardiac electrophysiology.*

Morganroth J: Ambulatory Holter electrocardiography: Choice of technologies and clinical uses. Ann Intern Med 102:73, 1985. *A concise review of the current status of ambulatory electrocardiography.*

Ward DE, Camm AJ: Clinical Electrophysiology of the Heart. London, Edward Arnold, 1987. *A comprehensive textbook with sections on (1) techniques and measurements, (2) diagnosis and assessment of bradycardias, (3) diagnosis and assessment of tachycardias, and (4) the strategy of using electrophysiologic technique for managing cardiac arrhythmias. Communicates clearly the role and uses of clinical electrophysiology.*

Wenger NK, Mock MB, Ringqvist I (eds.): Ambulatory Electrocardiographic Recording. Chicago, Year Book Medical Publishers, 1981. *Manuscripts from a workshop held at the National Heart, Lung, and Blood Institute. The topics of methodology, recording and analysis systems, quality control, and clinical, epidemiologic, and research applications are discussed thoroughly.*

SPECIFIC CARDIAC ARRHYTHMIAS

Clinically, cardiac arrhythmias are classified by their presumed site of origin, i.e., atrial, AV junctional, or ventricular, and as premature complexes, bradycardia, or tachycardia. It would be desirable to use the precise mechanism to classify clinical arrhythmias, but we do not know the precise mechanism of many cardiac arrhythmias. For some arrhythmias, e.g., the ventricular arrhythmias, prognostic significance can be assigned with reasonable precision. When this is the case, a prognostic classification is useful for guiding decisions about management. In this section, we use a classification based on the site of origin and rate as the framework within which to discuss the definition, pathophysiology, ECG diagnosis, significance, and management of each arrhythmia. The emergency and chronic treatments of cardiac arrhythmias are outlined in Tables 35–6 and 35–7.

Atrial Arrhythmias

SINUS RHYTHM

ECG DIAGNOSIS. Sinus rhythm is recognized in the ECG by a normal atrial rate and P wave vector, i.e., an upright P wave in leads III and a V_f and a normal PR interval. In adults, sinus rates below 60 or 50 per minute are called sinus bradycardia and those above 100, sinus tachycardia. Heart rate changes synchronized with breathing are called sinus arrhythmia and are caused by changing parasympathetic nervous activity. Sinus arrhythmia is more pronounced in children and young adults than in the elderly. Marked sinus arrhythmia can be difficult to distinguish from sinoatrial block or ectopic atrial rhythms.

CLINICAL FEATURES. Resting heart rate in sinus rhythm varies with age: from 130 to 160 per minute in infants to 50 to 100 per minute in adults. Gender, temperature, emotion, effort, and neurohumoral factors also influence sinus rate. The maximum heart rate during exercise varies from almost 200 per minute in healthy young persons to less than 140 per minute in the elderly. Many drugs increase or decrease the sinus rate, usually by interacting with autonomic mechanisms.

MANAGEMENT. Sinus bradycardia is treated only when symptomatic. When acute and symptomatic sinus bradycardia is due to increased vagus nerve activity, heart rate can be increased by intravenous (IV) atropine injection. Rarely, IV isoproterenol infusion may be needed. Chronic symptomatic sinus bradycardia is an indication for an electronic pacemaker. Treatment of sinus tachycardia is based on the cause, usually extracardiac.

ATRIAL PREMATURE COMPLEXES

Atrial premature complexes (APC's) arise in the atria outside the sinus node. APC's occur in normal and diseased hearts. In heart disease, APC's herald sustained atrial arrhythmias such as flutter fibrillation, or paroxysmal supraventricular tachycardia.

ECG DIAGNOSIS. APC's typically have premature P waves, abnormal P wave morphology, and a prolonged PR interval. Early APC's can be difficult to see because the P wave is superimposed on the T wave. Also, APC's can block in the AV node to produce pauses that can be misinterpreted as a sinus pause or sinoatrial block. Usually, APC's reset the sinus node so that the sum of the pre- and postextrasystolic PP intervals is less than two sinus cycles (Fig. 35–8). If sinus reset does not occur because the APC occurs late or the perinodal tissue is refractory, a compensatory pause occurs. An APC can conduct aberrantly, causing the QRS to be wide and bizarre like a ventricular premature complex (VPC) (Fig. 35–9). Aberrant conduction occurs when APC's activate one of the bundle branches, usually the right, during its relative refractory pe-

TABLE 35–6. EMERGENCY TREATMENT OF CARDIAC ARRHYTHMIAS

Arrhythmia	Usual First Treatment	Other Effective Treatments	Comments
Atrial fibrillation	Digitalis	Cardioversion; propranolol; acebutalol; verapamil; diltiazem	If hypotensive due to rapid ventricular rate, cardiovert. Avoid propranolol or verapamil in patients with heart failure or hypotension. Avoid digitalis or verapamil in Wolff-Parkinson-White syndrome.
Atrial flutter	Cardioversion	Digitalis; verapamil; diltiazem; propranolol; acebutalol; rapid atrial pacing	Very large doses of digitalis, e.g., 4–6 mg, often required to achieve AV block in atrial flutter.
Paroxysmal supraventricular tachycardia (AV nodal)	Vagal maneuvers; adenosine; verapamil; diltiazem	Digitalis; propranolol; acebutalol; procainamide	Do not treat wide QRS complex tachycardia with verapamil unless the diagnosis of PSVT is certain. Use cardioversion for PSVT with hypotension.
Paroxysmal supraventricular tachycardia (anomalous AV connection)	Vagal maneuvers; adenosine; verapamil	Cardioversion; procainamide	If the PR interval suggests anomalous AV connection, an electrophysiologic study should be considered.
Sick sinus syndrome	Pacemaker	Digitalis; pacemaker plus drug with class I antiarrhythmic action	Digitalis usually improves atrial tachyarrhythmias without aggravating sinus bradycardia or AV block.
Nonparoxysmal AV junctional tachycardia	Stop digitalis	Potassium; observation	If the arrhythmia is caused by digitalis toxicity and serum K^+ is low, digitalis should be stopped and potassium should be given.
Sustained ventricular tachycardia	Cardioversion	Lidocaine; procainamide	If VT is well tolerated, intravenous lidocaine or procainamide can be tried.
Ventricular fibrillation	Defibrillation	—	Lidocaine, bretylium tosylate, or propranolol may be helpful when ventricular fibrillation recurs several times immediately after cardioversion.
Digitalis-toxic atrial tachycardia with block or ventricular tachycardia	Lidocaine; phenytoin	Potassium	Avoid cardioversion or bretylium tosylate, which may precipitate ventricular fibrillation.
Digitalis-toxic asystole or AV block	Pacemaker	Fab fragments of digoxin-specific antibodies; dialysis	If associated with malignant hyperkalemia, these rhythms are always fatal unless treated promptly with Fab fragments of digoxin-specific antibodies.

TABLE 35-7. CHRONIC TREATMENT OF CARDIAC ARRHYTHMIAS

Arrhythmia	Usual First Treatment	Other Effective Treatments	Comments
Atrial fibrillation	Digitalis	Drug with class I antiarrhythmic action and digitalis; digitalis and propranolol; digitalis and verapamil	Drugs with class I antiarrhythmic action are used to maintain sinus rhythm; propranolol, acebutalol, or verapamil is used as adjunct to control ventricular rate in atrial fibrillation.
Atrial flutter	Drug with class I antiarrhythmic action	Digitalis; propranolol; verapamil	
Paroxysmal supraventricular tachycardia (AV nodal)	Digitalis	Flecainide or propafenone; propranolol	
Paroxysmal supraventricular tachycardia (anomalous AV connection)	Flecainide or propafenone	Drug with class IA antiarrhythmic action	Catheter ablation is preferable if patient also has atrial fibrillation with rapid ventricular response, if the anomalous AV connection has a short refractory period, or if the patient is noncompliant or has adverse effects from drugs.
Sick sinus syndrome	Pacemaker	Pacemaker and digitalis; pacemaker and drug with class I antiarrhythmic action	With the arrhythmias effectively treated, prognosis is determined by the severity of associated heart disease.
High-grade AV block	Pacemaker		No drugs are needed.
Symptomatic ventricular premature complexes or unsustained VT	β blocker	Drug with class I antiarrhythmic action	For benign and potentially malignant ventricular arrhythmias, β blockers are safest and often control symptoms. When heart failure is present, disopyramide and flecainide are relatively contraindicated.
Sustained VT	Drug with class III antiarrhythmic action	Drug with class I antiarrhythmic action	Treatment must be guided by a method with high predictive accuracy, e.g., endocardial electrical stimulation. Sotalol is tried first. If drugs fail or are not evaluable, an implantable cardioverter/defibrillator usually is the best treatment. In selected cases, surgical excision of the arrhythmogenic tissue is the best choice.

riod. Left bundle branch block aberrancy implies an abnormality in the left bundle branch (Fig. 35–9).

MANAGEMENT. The objective of treating APC's is to control symptoms or prevent sustained symptomatic arrhythmias. In patients with normal hearts, treatment should be focused on general hygienic measures; rest and reducing the use of tobacco, alcohol, or caffeine often reduces the frequency of APC's. In some patients with intermittent, sustained atrial arrhythmias, APC's should be treated with digitalis or class I, II, or IV antiarrhythmic drugs to prevent sustained arrhythmias.

PAROXYSMAL SUPRAVENTRICULAR TACHYCARDIA

ECG DIAGNOSIS. Typically paroxysmal supraventricular tachycardia (PSVT), also known as paroxysmal atrial or nodal tachycardia and reciprocating AV nodal tachycardia, has the following electrocardiographic features: a regular, rapid rate of 150 to 230 per minute; QRS duration less than 100 msec; and an abnormal P wave in a fixed relationship to each QRS. The P wave often is superimposed on the T wave or the QRS complex. PSVT starts abruptly, usually initiated by an APC or VPC. Often, the atrial rate in PSVT is about 185 per minute. The rate of PSVT often is faster in infants and children, in the Wolff-Parkinson-White (WPW) syndrome, and in thyrotoxicosis. The rate of PSVT is likely to be slower when AV node disease or certain drugs are present. The R-R intervals in typical PSVT are extremely regular except for the first or last few cycles of an episode. Carotid sinus massage either has no effect on PSVT or terminates it. In the presence of AV nodal disease or drugs that depress nodal conduction, e.g., digitalis or verapamil, fixed 2:1 AV block or AV Wenckebach can occur during PSVT.

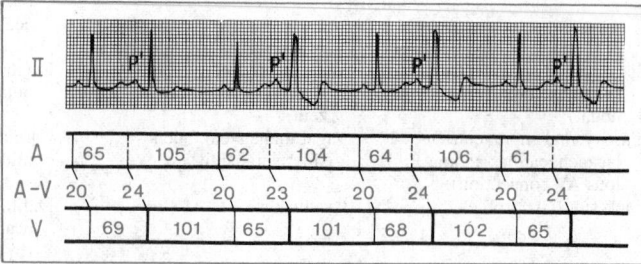

FIGURE 35–9. Atrial premature complexes (APC's) with aberrant conduction. The ladder diagram depicts the events in the lead II electrocardiographic strip above. A = Atrium; A-V = atrioventricular node and His-Purkinje system; V = ventricle. Time intervals are in msec × 10^{-1} (65 represents 650 msec). APC's are represented by dashed lines in the atrial tier; the wide QRS complexes are represented by a wide bar in the ventricular tier. APC's occur in a bigeminal pattern. The even (ectopic) P waves (P') are premature and have configurations slightly different from the odd P waves. Although the P-P' interval is relatively long (>600 msec), the P'-R interval is also prolonged, and the QRS complex following each P' is aberrant (left bundle branch block configuration)—a pattern of aberration suggesting bundle branch disease. Note that the QRS complex after the longest P-P' interval (second QRS) is least aberrant. (From Braunwald E: Heart Disease: A Textbook of Cardiovascular Medicine. Philadelphia, WB Saunders, 1980.)

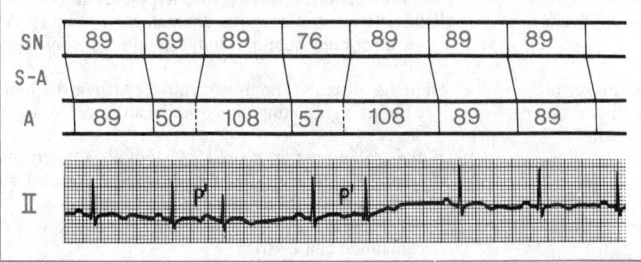

FIGURE 35–8. Atrial premature complex (APC). The ladder diagram correlates with the events in the lead II electrocardiographic strip below. SN = Sinus node; S-A = junctional tissues between sinus node and atrium; A = atrium. The time intervals in the ladder diagram are given in msec × 10^{-1} (e.g., 89 represents 890 msec). The third and fifth P waves are APC's (P'). These P' waves are premature and inverted. The P'R interval is prolonged, and QRS duration is normal. The APC's capture the sinus node and reset it; therefore, the pause following APC's is less than compensatory. (From Braunwald E: Heart Disease: A Textbook of Cardiovascular Medicine. Philadelphia, WB Saunders, 1980.)

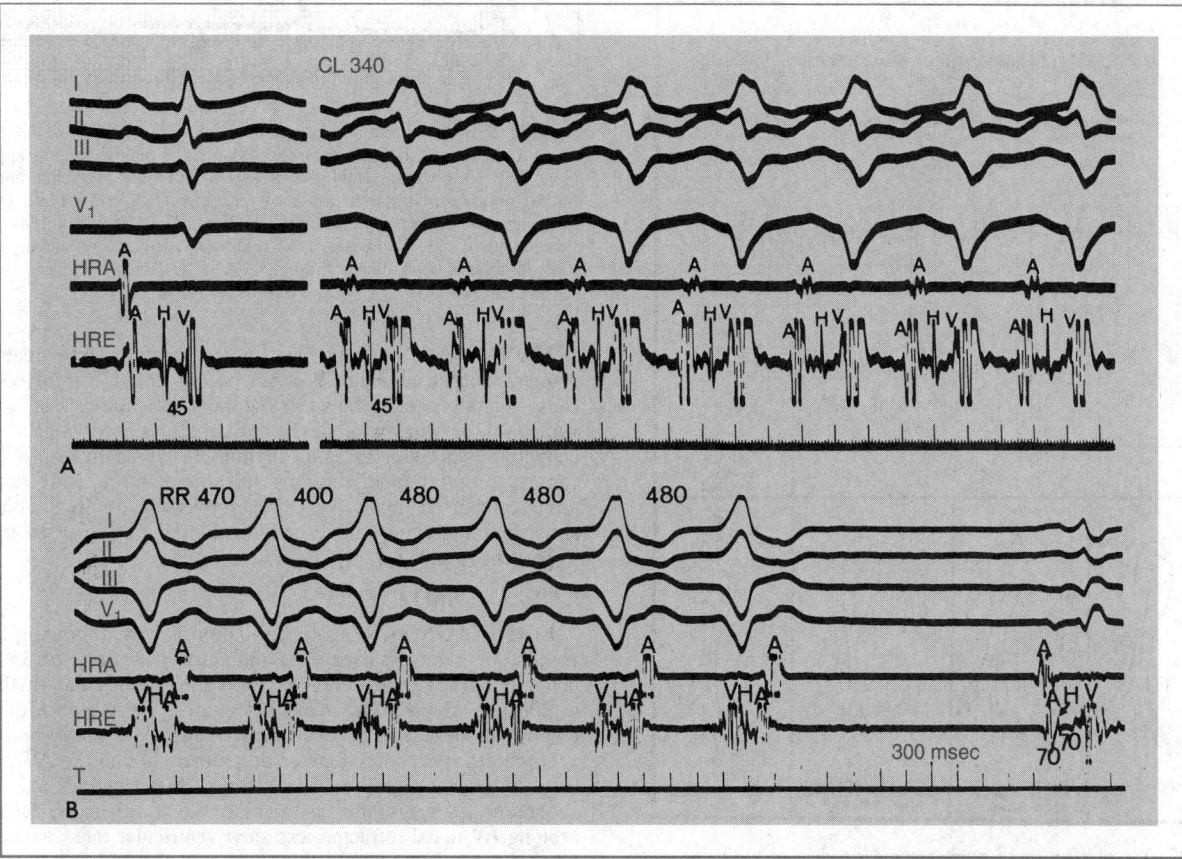

FIGURE 35–10. His bundle recording in regular tachycardia with a wide QRS complex. *A,* Supraventricular tachycardia. The left panel is a record taken during sinus rhythm; the QRS is normal. The right panel is a record taken during tachycardia; a left bundle branch block pattern is present. The normal HV interval in the His bundle electrogram (HBE) indicates that the rhythm is supraventricular tachycardia with aberrant conduction. *B,* Ventricular tachycardia. The last six depolarizations of a tachycardia and the first of sinus rhythm are shown. A left bundle branch block pattern is present during the tachycardia. In the His bundle electrogram, the ventricles depolarize (V) before the bundle of His (H), indicating that the rhythm is ventricular tachycardia. Ventriculoatrial conduction shows a stable 1:1 pattern. (From Caracta AR, Damato AN: Significance of His bundle electrocardiography. *In* Fowler NO (ed): Cardiac Diagnosis and Treatment. 3rd ed. New York, Harper and Row, 1980.)

The QRS complexes may be wide, resembling ventricular tachycardia, due either to a pre-existing wide QRS or to aberrant conduction of the rapid atrial rhythm. If AV dissociation can be documented, the rhythm originates in a subatrial location and is not PSVT. His bundle recording can differentiate between PSVT and ventricular tachycardia (Fig. 35–10).

The mechanism of PSVT is often AV nodal reentry initiated by an APC. The PSVT in the WPW syndrome is reentrant using the anomalous AV connection in the retrograde direction and the AV node in the antegrade direction (Fig. 35–11).

Nonparoxysmal atrial tachycardia probably is due to ectopic automaticity or triggered activity in the atrium. Atrial tachycardia with AV block suggests digitalis toxicity, particularly if the atrial rate is slow, e.g., 140 beats per minute.

CLINICAL FEATURES. PSVT occurs in normal as well as diseased hearts. Attacks of PSVT begin abruptly, cause palpitations, and may also end abruptly. The patient may learn maneuvers that are likely to stop the tachycardia, e.g., cough, Valsalva maneuver, or facial immersion. The hemodynamic effects of PSVT vary tremendously and depend on rate and the severity of heart disease. When PSVT is rapid, e.g., 180 to 220 beats per minute, systemic arterial pressure often falls and diastolic pressure rise in both ventricles, even in persons without heart disease. Prolonged and rapid supraventricular tachycardia can cause marked salt and water retention.

MANAGEMENT. Vagal maneuvers (e.g., Valsalva maneuver or carotid sinus massage), adenosine, or verapamil is effective in about 90% of the episodes. When PSVT causes hypotension or heart failure, DC cardioversion should be used. To prevent recurrences of PSVT due to AV nodal reentry, digitalis usually is tried first. If digitalis fails, potent drugs with class I antiarrhythmic action are quite effective. Catheter ablation usually is preferred to drugs

in the WPW syndrome with recurrent symptomatic tachyarrhythmias.

ATRIAL FLUTTER

ECG DIAGNOSIS. Typically, atrial flutter has the following ECG features: rapid atrial rate, 250 to 350 beats per minute, narrow QRS, and ventricular rate of 125 to 175 per minute, i.e., 2:1 AV conduction ratio (Fig. 35–12). In atrial flutter, the baseline of the ECG has a characteristic saw-toothed or undulating appearance best seen in leads II, III, and aV$_F$. Quinidine and other drugs with class I action can slow atrial flutter rate dramatically. In persons with a normal AV node, the AV conduction ratio usually is 2:1. Higher ratios suggest AV node disease or drug effect. Rarely, atrial flutter conducts to the ventricles with a 1:1 ratio, resulting in a ventricular rate of about 300 and hemodynamic collapse. The QRS complex usually is normal during atrial flutter but may be wide due to pre-existing bundle branch block.

CLINICAL FEATURES. Atrial flutter usually signifies either intrinsic heart disease or adverse extrinsic influences on the heart. Atrial flutter is associated with scarred atria due to rheumatic heart disease, coronary heart disease, or primary myocardial disease. Also, atrial flutter is associated with atrial enlargement, e.g., interatrial septal defect, mitral or tricuspid stenosis/regurgitation, or chronic ventricular failure. Atrial flutter occurs in toxic or metabolic conditions that affect the heart, e.g., thyrotoxicosis, alcoholism, or beri-beri, or when the pericardium is inflamed or infiltrated, e.g., with pneumonia or bronchogenic carcinoma. In all these conditions, atrial flutter is much less common than atrial fibrillation. Atrial flutter tends to be unstable, either reverting to sinus rhythm or converting to atrial fibrillation. Probably because the atria contract vigorously in atrial flutter, systemic emboli are less common during atrial flutter than during atrial fibrillation.

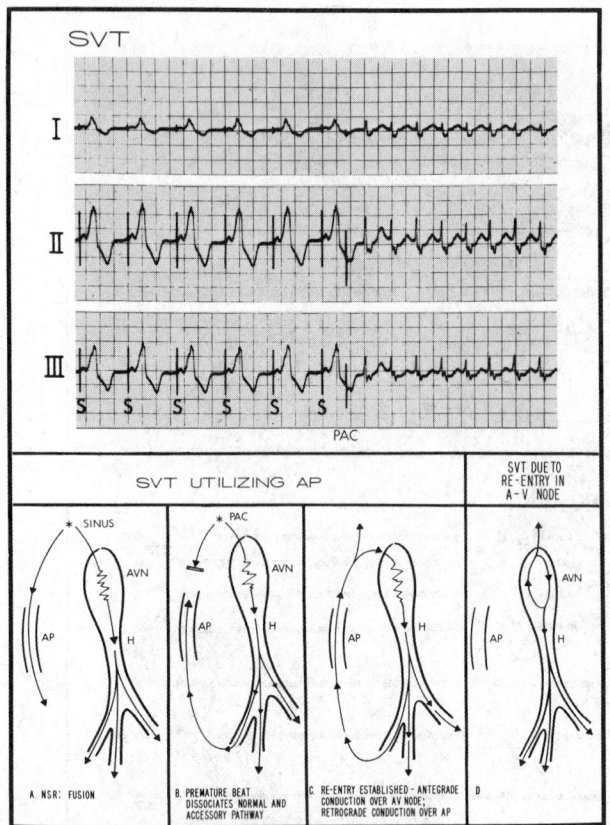

FIGURE 35–11. Mechanism of supraventricular tachycardia utilizing an accessory pathway. The upper panel demonstrates an electrocardiogram recorded in a patient with Wolff-Parkinson-White syndrome during straight atrial pacing and the introduction of a premature atrial complex. The first five beats are preceded by a stimulus artifact (S); a short PR interval and a wide QRS complex indicate the presence of pre-excitation. After a premature beat is introduced, a narrow QRS tachycardia is initiated. The events underlying this supraventricular tachycardia are diagrammatically shown in the lower panels. During sinus rhythm (A), fusion is present owing to conduction over the AV node (AVN) and the accessory pathway (AP). In B, an atrial premature complex blocks the accessory pathway and conducts with delay over the AV node, thus dissociating the activity of the normal and accessory pathways. In C, the impulse conducting through the ventricle travels retrograde over the accessory pathway and reenters the atrium, establishing a tachycardia. D demonstrates schematically the reentry circuit underlying supraventricular tachycardia resulting from reentry confined to the AV node.

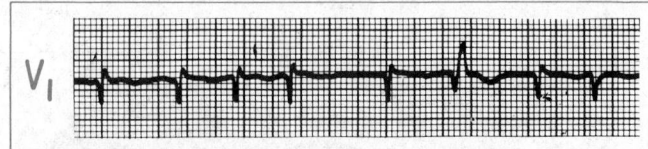

FIGURE 35–13. Aberrant conduction in atrial fibrillation (the Ashman phenomenon). The sixth QRS complex has a right bundle branch appearance. Note that this complex ends a long R-R—short R-R sequence and that its initial forces are similar to those of the other QRS complexes. These features suggest aberrant conduction of a supraventricular impulse. (From Braunwald E: Heart Disease: A Textbook of Cardiovascular Medicine. Philadelphia, WB Saunders, 1980.)

MANAGEMENT. The best choice for the acute treatment of symptomatic atrial flutter is atrial pacing or DC cardioversion because digitalis usually fails to slow the ventricular rate and digitalis, verapamil, or drugs with class I antiarrhythmic action usually fail to convert atrial flutter to sinus rhythm. IV verapamil or β blockers can be useful temporizing measures to control heart rate while arrangements are made for DC cardioversion. A drug with class I antiarrhythmic action alone or with digitalis is the usual treatment to prevent recurrence of atrial flutter.

ATRIAL FIBRILLATION

ECG DIAGNOSIS. Atrial fibrillation has the following features: absence of P waves; irregular atrial activity at a rate of 350 to 600 per minute; and rapid, irregularly irregular ventricular rhythm (150 to 200 per minute). The cardinal feature is the presence of fibrillatory waves best seen in ECG leads II, III, aV_F, or V_1 and at slow ventricular rates. Conditions or drugs that shorten the AV nodal refractory period, e.g., exercise, fever, hyperthyroidism, or catecholamines, increase the ventricular rate. Conversely, factors that prolong AV nodal refractoriness slow ventricular rate. Because atrial fibrillation is so common, this diagnosis should be entertained for any rapid rhythm that has irregularly irregular R-R intervals. Patients with the WPW syndrome may develop extremely rapid ventricular rates during atrial fibrillation.

Atrial fibrillation coexists with many other arrhythmias and conduction defects; two occur frequently and are critically important to diagnose correctly. The first is AV junctional arrhythmia caused by digitalis toxicity. As digitalis slows the ventricular rate, AV junctional automaticity increases. First, junctional escape complexes terminate long R-R intervals or the ventricular rate becomes regular at a slow rate. Then the junctional focus accelerates to produce nonparoxysmal AV junctional tachycardia. The second is aberrant conduction of supraventricular impulses that must be distinguished from VPC's. The duration of refractoriness in the His-Purkinje system is directly proportional to the preceding R-R interval. In atrial

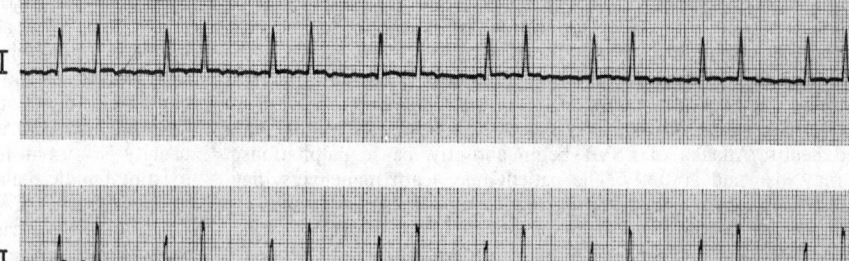

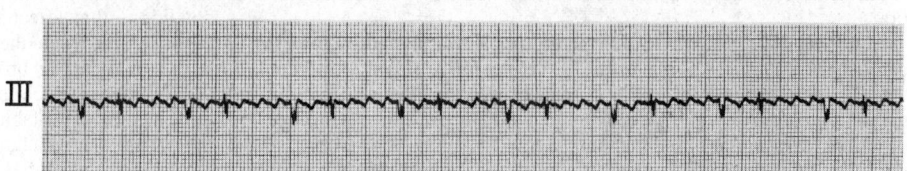

FIGURE 35–12. Atrial flutter with varying AV block. This ECG, recorded during a period of varying AV block induced by a vagal maneuver, demonstrates the characteristic "sawtoothed" appearance of P waves during atrial flutter.

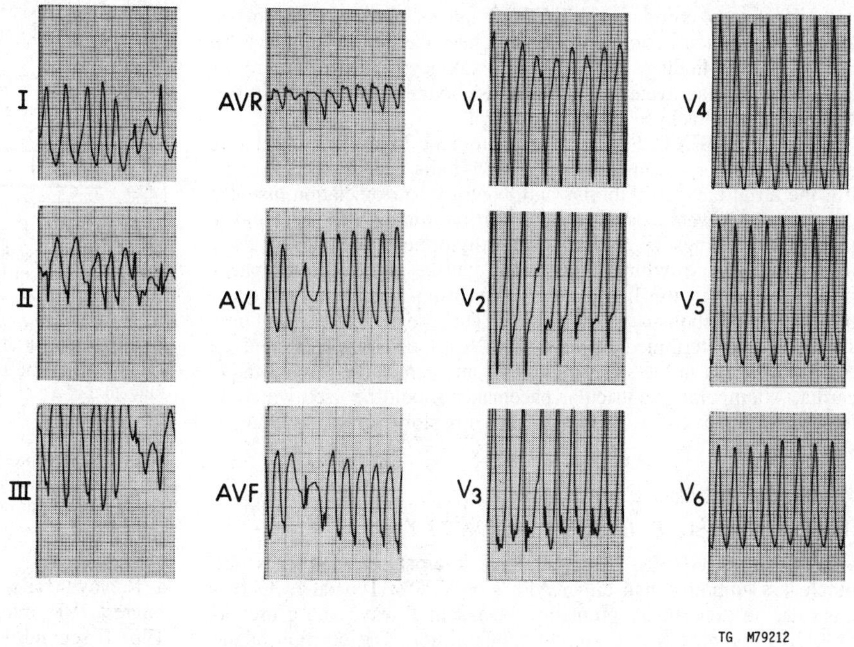

I

AVR

V₁

V₄

II

AVL

V₂

V₅

III

AVF

V₃

V₆

FIGURE 35-14. Atrial fibrillation in the Wolff-Parkinson-White syndrome. The ECG demonstrates the irregularly irregular response associated with anomalous-appearing QRS complexes resulting from atrial fibrillation with rapid conduction over the accessory pathway to the ventricle.

TG M79212

fibrillation, aberrant conduction is likely when a short R-R interval follows a long one—the Ashman phenomenon (Fig. 35-13). Aberrant conduction usually produces a triphasic (RSR') right bundle branch block configuration in lead V₁ and normal initial QRS forces. VPC's usually have a mono- or biphasic QRS pattern in lead V₁ and abnormal initial QRS forces and are followed by a longer pause. Another cause of repetitive aberrant QRS's in atrial fibrillation is the WPW syndrome (Fig. 35-14).

CLINICAL FEATURES. Like atrial flutter, atrial fibrillation implies myocardial or pericardial disease or adverse extrinsic influences. Atrial fibrillation is about 20 times as common as atrial flutter. Although atrial fibrillation may be paroxysmal, it is usually a chronic, stable rhythm. When atrial fibrillation occurs abruptly in patients with serious heart disease, the consequences may be dramatic, e.g., disconcerting palpitations, pulmonary edema, or angina pectoris. If the ventricular rate is well controlled with digitalis, atrial fibrillation may cause little hemodynamic impairment and is compatible with decades of uneventful survival. As with atrial flutter, atrial fibrillation occurs in many etiologic forms of heart disease. Chronic atrial inflammation and lack of effective atrial contraction promote left atrial thrombi and increased risk for systemic emboli. Atrial fibrillation may occur as an isolated arrhythmia in patients without heart disease or any other systemic illness. This condition has been called "lone atrial fibrillation."

MANAGEMENT. The objective of treating acute atrial fibrillation is to slow the rate. For symptomatic hypotension, immediate cardioversion in indicated. Usually, rate is controlled with IV digoxin (see Table 35-11). Verapamil or β-blocking drugs are useful adjuncts for achieving rate control but can aggravate heart failure or cause hypotension. Digitalis and verapamil are best avoided in patients with WPW because they can increase the ventricular rate and trigger ventricular fibrillation. The objectives of chronic treatment of atrial fibrillation are to (1) control ventricular rate, (2) prevent thromboemboli, and (3) maintain sinus rhythm.

MULTIFOCAL ATRIAL TACHYCARDIA

ECG DIAGNOSIS. The ECG features of multifocal atrial tachycardia are frequent APC's, often occurring in runs that have dramatically different P wave morphology and marked variability in P-P interval.

CLINICAL FEATURES. This rhythm occurs in patients with decompensated or overtreated chronic obstructive pulmonary disease. These patients often have severe derangement of arterial blood gases and electrolytes and are being treated aggressively with theophylline and/or catecholamines.

MANAGEMENT. Multifocal atrial tachycardia is resistant to digitalis therapy. Therapy is directed at improving ventilation and eradicating bronchial infection to improve arterial blood gases. The

dose of bronchodilators may need to be reduced as well. Verapamil can be used to control the arrhythmia while adjusting the other medications.

SINOATRIAL BLOCK

ECG DIAGNOSIS. Impulses generated in the sinus node may conduct slowly or block in the junction between the sinus node and atrium. First-degree SA block, i.e., a delay in conduction from sinus node to the atrium, cannot be recognized in the standard ECG but can be identified by electrophysiologic studies. Second-degree SA block can be diagnosed electrocardiographically. Type I second-degree SA block is recognized by Wenckebach periodicity of the P-P intervals (Fig. 35-15). In type II second-degree SA block, the P-P interval suddenly lengthens to a value almost precisely twice the usual P-P interval. Third-degree SA block causes atrial arrest.

CLINICAL FEATURES. SA block indicates intrinsic sinus node disease, electrolyte disturbance, or an adverse drug effect, most often digitalis. Drugs with class I antiarrhythmic action can cause SA block in patients with pre-existing sinus node dysfunction.

Sick Sinus Syndrome. The sick sinus syndrome is characterized by intrinsic inadequacy of sinus node pacemaking and/or conduction failure between the sinus node and the rest of the atrium. In the bradycardia-tachycardia syndrome, recurrent supraventricular tachyarrhythmias alternate with sinus bradycardia and/or subatrial bradyarrhythmias. Conduction disturbances are common in the atria, AV node, bundle branches, and ventricles, but ventricular ectopic activity is rare.

Symptoms in sick sinus syndrome may be intermittent, varied,

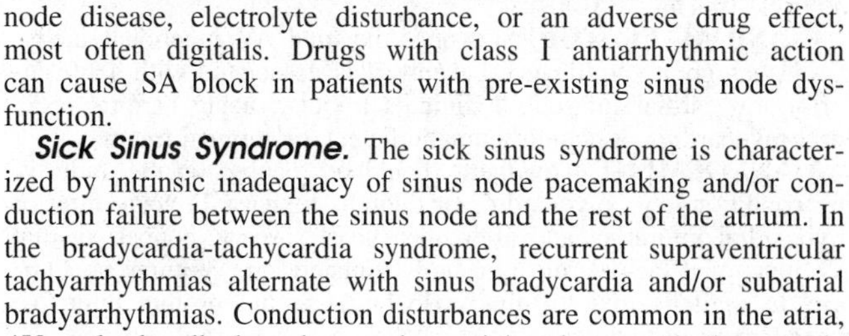

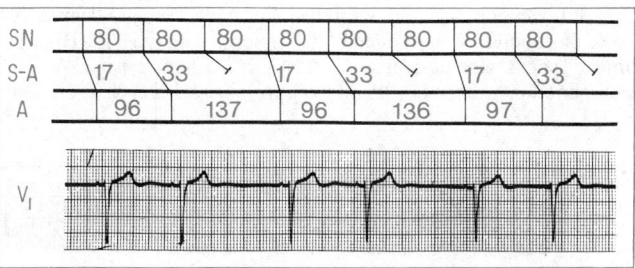

FIGURE 35-15. Second-degree sinoatrial block, type I (Wenckebach). The ECG shows periodicity of the P waves and QRS complex. The PR is constant. This pattern is consistent with a constant sinus node rate of 75 per minute (sinus cycle length = 800 msec) with 3:2 sinoatrial shock. The sinoatrial conduction times are assumed. (From Braunwald E: Heart Disease: A Textbook of Cardiovascular Medicine. Philadelphia, WB Saunders, 1980.)

and difficult to correlate with ECG changes. Syncope, dizziness, and palpitations are common, probably because these symptoms are used for case finding and diagnosis. Congestive heart failure or angina can be aggravated. Cerebral thromboembolism is common in the bradycardia-tachycardia syndrome.

MANAGEMENT. Persistent, symptomatic sinus bradycardia is an indication for pacemaker therapy. Digitalis can be used to control the atrial tachyarrhythmias and, contrary to expectation, usually does not aggravate coexistent bradyarrhythmias. After pacemaker implantation, drugs with class I antiarrhythmic action can be used to control tachyarrhythmias. Symptoms can be improved with pacemaker therapy in the bradycardia-tachycardia syndrome, but cerebral thromboembolism is still a risk. The prognosis of sick sinus syndrome is determined by associated heart disease. Treatment of atrial fibrillation in the sick sinus syndrome can cause severe bradycardia. A temporary ventricular pacemaker should be used when attempting to convert atrial fibrillation with slow ventricular rate to sinus rhythm.

AV Junctional Arrhythmias

AV JUNCTIONAL PREMATURE COMPLEXES

ECG DIAGNOSIS. AV junctional premature complexes are much less common than either APC's or VPC's. Typical ECG features are an abnormally premature or absent P wave and a premature QRS complex with a normal configuration. The position of the premature P wave (P') is critical to the diagnosis. The P' may occur 0.10 second or less before, during, or 0.20 second or less after the premature QRS. P' is inverted in leads II, III, and aV_F. The clinical significance of AV junctional premature complexes is similar to that of nonparoxysmal AV junctional tachycardia (see below).

NONPAROXYSMAL AV JUNCTIONAL TACHYCARDIA

ECG DIAGNOSIS. Nonparoxysmal AV junctional tachycardia is caused by enhanced automaticity in the AV junction. The junctional focus fires 70 to 130 per minute (Fig. 35–16). The QRS complex usually is normal or slightly aberrant. If the AV junctional focus captures the atria, the retrograde P may be positioned 0.10 second or less in front of the QRS, simultaneous with the QRS, or 0.20 second or less after the QRS. This arrhythmia often is associated with AV nodal conduction impairment and AV dissociation. The atrial rhythm may intermittently capture the junctional focus and ventricle (see Fig. 35–19).

CLINICAL FEATURES. Nonparoxysmal AV junctional tachycardia has great significance because it is associated with acute inferior myocardial infarction, digitalis toxicity, acute carditis (e.g., viral myocarditis or acute rheumatic fever), or surgical trauma.

MANAGEMENT. Treatment should be focused on the underlying condition, e.g., myocarditis or digitalis toxicity. In acute inferior myocardial infarction and after open heart surgery, nonparoxysmal AV junctional tachycardia is usually transient and requires no therapy. In digitalis toxicity, this arrhythmia should prompt intensive management of toxicity.

AV BLOCK

ECG DIAGNOSIS. AV block is classified as first, second, and third degree. First-degree AV block, i.e., a prolonged PR interval, is caused by conduction delay in the AV node. Second-degree AV block is subdivided into type I (AV nodal) and type II (His-Purkinje). Type I second-degree AV block has characteristic Wenckebach periodicity; i.e., the PR interval prolongs with each cycle until

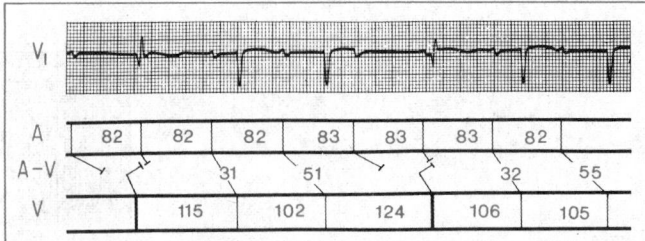

FIGURE 35–17. Sinus rhythm with type I second-degree atrioventricular block (Wenckebach) and junctional escape complexes. Sinus rhythm is regular at a rate of 73 beats per minute. The third P wave from the left begins a 3:2 Wenckebach cycle. The first PR interval of the cycle is quite long (0.31 sec), and the PR increment in the second cycle is large (an additional 0.20 sec). The third P wave of the cycle is blocked in the AV node. The PR interval following the pause is short (0.10 sec), and the QRS complex is aberrant; this is a junctional escape complex. The tracing demonstrates both impaired conduction and enhanced automaticity in the A-V junction. Type I A-V block nearly always occurs in the AV node, and A-V junctional escape complexes are presumed to arise in the bundle of His or the most proximal portions of the bundle branches. (From Braunwald E: Heart Disease: A Textbook of Cardiovascular Medicine. Philadelphia, WB Saunders, 1980.)

a P wave fails to conduct to the ventricles (Fig. 35–17). The longest R-R interval is less than twice the shortest R-R interval. Type II second-degree AV block is recognized by the sudden failure of a P wave to conduct to the ventricles without previous lengthening of the PR interval. Type II AV block nearly always occurs in patients with bundle branch disease, and the site of block is distal to the AV node.

In third-degree AV block, sinus or some other atrial rhythm controls the atria while the ventricles are controlled by an independent AV junctional or ventricular pacemaker. The QRS usually is prolonged, and the ventricular rate is between 35 and 50.

CLINICAL FEATURES. First-degree AV block causes no symptoms but may cause the first heart sound to be soft because the AV valves almost close before ventricular contraction. Second-degree AV block usually causes no symptoms unless the ventricular rate becomes very slow. It may be possible to discern second-degree AV block by characteristic pulse intervals, intermittent prominent A waves, and changing intensity of the first heart sound. In complete heart block with sinus rhythm, the pulse is slow, full, and regular; intermittent cannon A waves occur in the jugular venous pulse; and the first heart sound varies markedly in intensity.

MANAGEMENT. First-degree AV block requires no treatment. Type I second-degree AV block usually resolves without the need for a temporary pacemaker. When type I block is caused by a chronic AV junctional disease, block can progress slowly to complete AV block. Type II second-degree AV block usually results from chronic bundle branch disease and often progresses to complete heart block. Chronic, symptomatic second- or third-degree AV block should be treated with an implanted pacemaker.

Ventricular Arrhythmias

VENTRICULAR PREMATURE COMPLEXES

ECG DIAGNOSIS. The QRS is premature, wide, and often bizarre in appearance; the ST segment and T wave are opposite in direction to the QRS complex; and no premature P wave precedes the premature QRS complex (Fig. 35–18). As the impulse leaves its ectopic site of origin, it activates the ventricle in an abnormal sequence accounting for the striking QRS-T abnormalities. Typi-

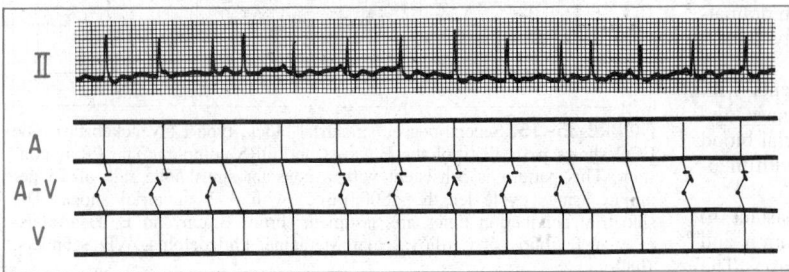

FIGURE 35–16. Nonparoxysmal atrioventricular junctional tachycardia with atrial capture of the ventricles. Two independent rhythms coexist: sinus tachycardia at 107 beats per minute and atrioventricular junctional tachycardia at 115 beats per minute. Sinus rhythm always controls the atria. The ventricles are usually controlled by the AV junctional focus, because its rate is faster. When time relationships are appropriate, atrial depolarizations propagate through the AV junction and capture the ventricles. (From Braunwald E: Heart Disease: A Textbook of Cardiovascular Medicine. Philadelphia, WB Saunders, 1980.)

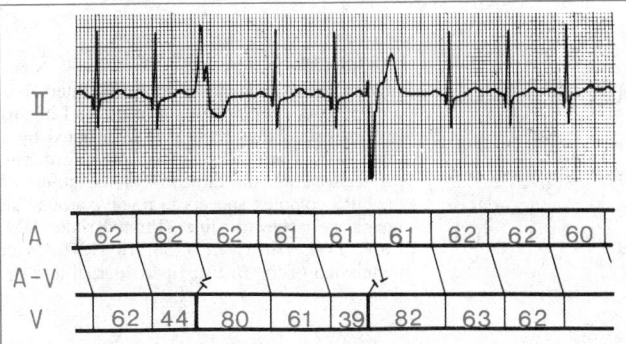

FIGURE 35–18. Multiformed ventricular premature complexes (VPC's). The third and sixth QRS complexes are VPC's with strikingly different configurations. Also, the coupling interval of the two VPC's differs by 50 msec. Such a difference in configuration may be due either to a different site of origin or to a difference in the sequence of ventricular activation from the same site of origin. (From Braunwald E: Heart Disease: A Textbook of Cardiovascular Medicine. Philadelphia, WB Saunders, 1980.)

cally, a VPC is followed by a fully compensatory pause; i.e., the RV interval plus the VR interval is equal to two R-R intervals in sinus rhythm (Fig. 35–18). VPC's may be *interpolated* between two successive sinus complexes. "Concealed" retrograde conduction of the interpolated VPC into the AV node causes the PR interval of the subsequent sinus complex to prolong. Certain patterns of VPC's have special names. When every other QRS is a VPC, the pattern is termed *bigeminy;* a VPC every third QRS is termed *trigeminy;* and two successive VPC's are termed a *pair* or a *couplet.*

CLINICAL FEATURES. Infrequent VPC's are commonly found even in young persons, and VPC frequency increases with age. While sporadic VPC's in persons with normal hearts do not seem to affect outcome adversely, VPC's confer significant risk of subsequent cardiac death in heart disease. When VPC's are caused by drug toxicity, e.g., digitalis, quinidine, or tricyclic antidepressants, lethal rhythm disturbances may ensue unless the drug is discontinued. A strong association exists between myocardial infarct size and the frequency of VPC's in acute myocardial infarction and a weak association between poor left ventricular function and frequency of VPC's during recovery.

MANAGEMENT. The most important issue in treating VPC is the selection of patients for treatment. In general, only very symptomatic VPC's need treatment, and drugs with class II antiarrhythmic action (β-adrenergic blockade) are the first choices for treatment of benign and prognostically important ventricular arrhythmias. IV lidocaine or procainamide is usually used to treat symptomatic VPC's occurring immediately after myocardial infarction or cardiac surgery.

VENTRICULAR TACHYCARDIA (VT)

ECG DIAGNOSIS. The most prevalent definition of VT is three or more VPC's in succession at a rate of 100 per minute or greater. VT may be unsustained, i.e., last less than 15 to 30 seconds, or sustained (Fig. 35–19). In a tachycardia with wide QRS complexes, two findings strongly suggest VT: *ventricular captures* and *fusion complexes.* Sinus impulses may capture the ventricle during VT, producing either a normal QRS (ventricular capture) or a QRS intermediate in contour between normal and VT (fusion complex). Sustained VT can be difficult to distinguish from supraventricular arrhythmias with a wide QRS complex. A His bundle recording can easily distinguish between these two possibilities (see Fig. 35–10).

CLINICAL FEATURES. Unsustained VT nearly always occurs in patients with heart disease, most often in those with coronary heart disease. Two weeks after myocardial infarction, about 10% of patients have VT detected by a single 24-hour continuous ECG recording. Patients with class III or IV heart failure have a 40 to 50% prevalence of VT in a 24-hour ECG. Most episodes of VT in either setting are brief, i.e., three to five consecutive VPC's, and asymptomatic, yet increase the risk of dying two- to fourfold. Sustained VT is rare and has a poor prognosis. As with other tachyarrhythmias, the severity of symptoms in sustained VT is related primarily to the rate of the tachycardia and left ventricular function. Blood pressure and mental status are not useful for distinguishing

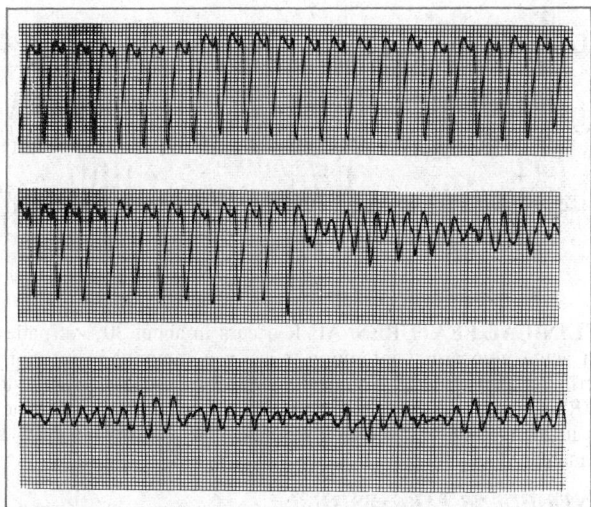

FIGURE 35–19. Ventricular tachycardia and ventricular fibrillation. Three continuous strips from lead V_4 of a Holter electrocardiograph. The top strip shows ventricular tachycardia at 214 cycles per minute. Ventricular fibrillation begins in the middle strip and continues on the bottom strip. Note the irregularity in amplitude and period of deflections recorded during ventricular fibrillation. (From Braunwald E: Heart Disease: A Textbook of Cardiovascular Medicine. Philadelphia, WB Saunders, 1980.)

between VT and PSVT with aberrant conduction. Sustained VT is prone to deteriorate into ventricular fibrillation (Fig. 35–19).

MANAGEMENT. The management of symptomatic, unsustained VT is the same as that described above for VPC's. Sustained VT in chronic heart disease is treated acutely with IV lidocaine or procainamide, if the patient is hemodynamically stable, or by DC cardioversion if unstable (Fig. 35–19). Baseline studies should include 48 hours of continuous ECG recording, exercise testing, endocardial electrical stimulation, and cardiac catheterization with coronary angiography. The drug/dose finding and long-term management of these patients should be guided by rigorous methods with high predictive accuracy. The standard method is endocardial electrical stimulation. A programmatic noninvasive approach using 24-hour continuous ECG recordings and exercise tests also can be used. The noninvasive approach predicts success in more patients and has predictive accuracy similar to endocardial electrical stimulation. dl-Sotalol is the drug of first choice. If an effective drug is not found, an implantable defibrillator is usually the best treatment. In selected cases, surgery is the best choice.

ACCELERATED IDIOVENTRICULAR RHYTHM (AIVR)

ECG DIAGNOSIS. AIVR is defined as three or more consecutive QRS complexes of ventricular origin with a rate between 50 and 100 (Fig. 35–20). Fusion QRS complexes often begin or end an episode of AIVR.

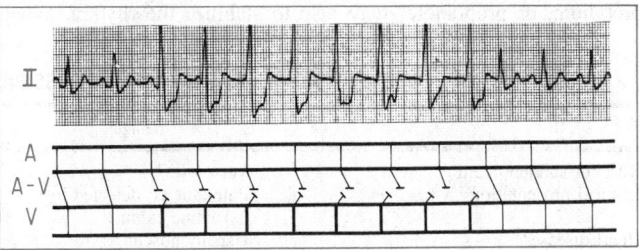

FIGURE 35–20. Accelerated idioventricular rhythm. Sinus rhythm at 88 cycles per minute is interrupted by a rhythm with wide QRS complexes at 95 cycles per minute. Note that the PR interval progressively shortens at the onset of the ventricular rhythm and that sinus rhythm continues unperturbed by the ventricular rhythm (atrioventricular dissociation). After eight QRS complexes of ventricular rhythm, sinus rhythm resumes. (From Braunwald E: Heart Disease: A Textbook of Cardiovascular Medicine. Philadelphia, WB Saunders, 1980.)

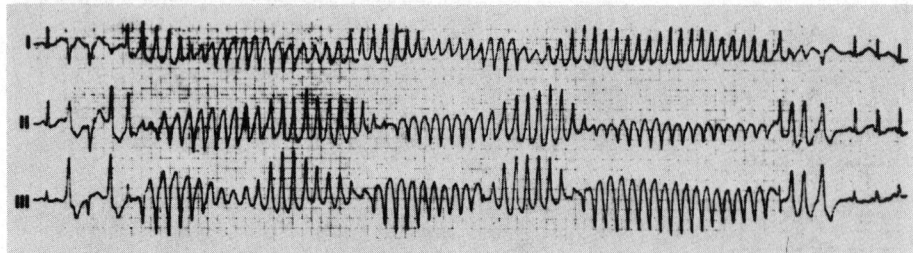

FIGURE 35–21. Torsades de pointes. Sinus rhythm associated with a long QT interval is present at the beginning and at the end of this rhythm strip. Sinus rhythm is interrupted by a rapid, wide QRS tachycardia. Note that during the tachycardia, the direction of the points of the QRS complex appears to revolve around an imaginary isoelectric line. (From Krikler DM, Curry DVL: Br Heart J 38:118, 1976. With permission of the British Heart Journal and authors.)

CLINICAL FEATURES. AIVR occurs in about 30% of patients with acute myocardial infarction, equally commonly in inferior or anterior infarcts. AIVR frequently follows coronary reperfusion. AIVR is usually asymptomatic and therefore needs no treatment. The incidences of ventricular fibrillation and hospital mortality are not increased in patients who have AIVR.

VENTRICULAR PARASYSTOLE

ECG DIAGNOSIS. Ventricular parasystole is an automatic rhythm in the His-Purkinje system that competes with sinus rhythm. Parasystole has two cardinal features: variable coupling of VPC's and a common denominator for interectopic intervals. Entrance block removes the parasystolic focus from the suppressant influence of the sinus impulses, permitting a stable automatic rhythm to emerge; the ectopic focus activates the ventricle every time it fires unless the ventricle is refractory (Fig. 35–20).

CLINICAL FEATURES. Parasystole often is resistant to antiarrhythmic drug therapy, and untreated patients seem to have a good prognosis.

VENTRICULAR FLUTTER AND FIBRILLATION

ECG DIAGNOSIS. The diagnosis of ventricular flutter is made when the ventricular tachyarrhythmia has large sinusoidal or zigzag QRS's and the rate is between 240 and 280 per minute. Multiform VT or torsades de pointes is recognized by the periodic twisting of the points of the QRS complexes (Fig. 35–21). Ventricular fibrillation is recognized in the ECG by the absence of QRS complexes and T waves and the presence of low-amplitude baseline undulations that are variable in both amplitude and periodicity (see Fig. 35–19).

CLINICAL FEATURES. Ventricular flutter is rarely recorded because it is unstable and tends to convert to sinus rhythm or, more often, to ventricular fibrillation. Ventricular flutter of fibrillation is catastrophic. Cardiac pumping ceases instantly, the patient loses consciousness, and, if cardiopulmonary resuscitation is not started within a few minutes, the patient dies. Identifiable causes are acute myocardial ischemia or infarction; marked electrolyte disturbances, e.g., hypokalemia; marked hypothermia; electrocution; and drug toxicity. Most victims of ventricular fibrillation who are resuscitated do *not* have one of these conditions but do have advanced coronary atherosclerosis and poor ventricular function.

MANAGEMENT. The only effective treatment for ventricular fibrillation is prompt defibrillation. In most cases, ventricular fibrillation does not recur after defibrillation. When it does, lidocaine, bretylium, or propranolol may help to stabilize the rhythm. When no transient or reversible cause for ventricular fibrillation is found (e.g., myocardial infarction, electrolyte abnormality, or drug toxicity), the process for evaluating long-term treatment is much the same as described above for sustained VT. Unfortunately, a smaller fraction of patients, about 60 to 70%, have VT induced by programmed ventricular stimulation. Nevertheless, the uninducible patients have a high recurrence rate for ventricular fibrillation.

The management of multiform VT (torsades de pointes) is based on its pathophysiology: toxic drug effects, hypokalemia and/or hypomagnesemia, and slow heart rates. Treatment may include avoiding drugs with class I antiarrhythmic action, ventricular pacing, reducing the level of the culprit drug, repleting electrolytes, treating with IV Mg^{2+}, or catecholamine infusion.

PROGNOSTIC CLASSIFICATION OF VENTRICULAR ARRHYTHMIAS. Table 35–8 outlines the classification of ventricular arrhythmias as determined by the presence of heart disease, left ventricular function, and arrhythmia characteristics. Prognosis is an important basis for deciding who to treat and how to sequence the treatment choices.

Bigger JT Jr, Reiffel JA: Sick sinus syndrome. Ann Rev Med 30:91, 1979. *A comprehensive review of the human sinus node dysfunction. Liberally referenced.*

Kastor JA: Arrhythmias. Philadelphia, WB Saunders, 1994. *This 430-page book has a short chapter for each arrhythmia, giving modern diagnostic and therapeutic approach for each. Intended to provide information for clinicians who are not clinical electrophysiologists. Contains the most pertinent recent references.*

Wagner G: Marriott's Practical Electrocardiography. Baltimore, Williams & Wilkins, 1994. *Designed to emphasize the simplicities of the ECG, provide only those concepts that make everyday ECG interpretation more intelligible, and provide illustrations and discussion of all important ECG patterns. Excellent for learning or reviewing the ECG patterns of arrhythmias.*

Mason JW for the Electrophysiologic Study versus Electrocardiographic Monitoring Investigators: A comparison of electrophysiologic testing with Holter monitoring to predict antiarrhythmic-drug efficacy for ventricular tachyarrhythmias. N Engl J Med 329:445, 1993. *A large randomized study showed that the predictive accuracy of noninvasive assessment was not significantly different from electrophysiologic testing for long-term antiarrhythmic drug efficacy in patients with malignant ventricular arrhythmias.*

Zipes DP: Specific arrhythmias: Diagnosis and treatment. *In* Braunwald E (ed.): Heart Disease. A Textbook of Cardiovascular Medicine. 4th ed. Philadelphia, WB Saunders, 1992, p 667. *Detailed description of the clinical features, electrocardiographic recognition, and treatment of cardiac arrhythmias. Contains 52 figures and 409 references.*

ANTIARRHYTHMIC DRUGS

Classification

Antiarrhythmic drugs have been classified according to their mechanisms of action into four classes (Table 35–9). One could think of digitalis as having class V drug action, i.e., a strong cholinergic action that can repolarize stretched or damaged atrial cells and

TABLE 35–8. PROGNOSTIC CLASSIFICATION OF VENTRICULAR ARRHYTHMIAS*

	Benign	Prognostically Important	Malignant
Risk for sudden death	Very low	Low to moderate	High
Clinical presentation	Palpitations; detected by routine exam	Palpitations; detected by routine exam or screening	Palpitations; syncope; cardiac arrest
Heart disease	Usually absent	Present	Present
Cardiac scarring and/or hypertrophy	Absent	Present	Present
VPC frequency	Low to moderate	Moderate to high	Moderate to high
Paired VPC and/or unsustained VT	Absent	Common	Common
Sustained VT	Absent	Absent	Present
Hemodynamic effects of arrhythmia	Absent	Absent to mild	Moderate to severe

VPC = Ventricular premature complex(s); VT = ventricular tachycardia

* The characteristics listed in this table are typical but do not represent the full range of observations. For example, benign ventricular arrhythmias can be frequent and occasionally repetitive. For prognostically important or malignant ventricular arrhythmias, the risk within a class depends strongly on left ventricular ejection fraction.

TABLE 35–9. CLASSIFICATION OF ANTIARRHYTHMIC DRUGS ACCORDING TO THEIR MECHANISM OF ACTION

Class	Action	Drugs
I	Sodium channel blockade	
B	Minimal phase 0 depression	Lidocaine, mexiletine, tocainide
	Slow conduction 0 to 1+ Shorten repolarization	
A	Moderate phase 0 depression Slow conduction 2+ Prolong repolarization*	Disopyramide, moricizine, procainamide, quinidine
C	Marked phase 0 depression Slow conduction 4+ Little effect on repolarization	Encainide, flecainide, indecainide, propafenone
II	β-Adrenergic blockade	Acebutalol, propranolol
III	Prolong repolarization	Amiodarone, bretylium, sotalol
IV	Calcium channel blockade	Diltiazem, verapamil

* Moricizine does not prolong repolarization.

thereby speed conduction. Digitalis glycosides slow conduction in the AV node, tending to slow or abolish reentrant rhythms that use the AV node. In 1991, an international task force published a critique of this classification and made recommendations for improvements—the Sicilian gambit.

Use-Dependent Block of Ionic Channels

Many antiarrhythmic drugs act on ionic channels in the sarcolemma. Drugs with class I antiarrhythmic action block the Na⁺ channel so that ionic conductance falls to zero until the drug dissociates from the channel (Fig. 35–22). Most drugs with class I antiarrhythmic action bind to open or inactivated channels; drug-associated channels have slow or incomplete reactivation. Drug binding and Na⁺ channel blockade increase with rate, producing *use-dependent block*. If the association and dissociation of drug from the Na⁺ channel both are rapid, use-dependent block attains a steady state after a few action potentials and, if the interval between action potentials is reasonably long, little block persists at the time of the next action potential upstroke. If dissociation is slow, use-dependent block requires many action potentials to develop fully as the degree of block increases with each depolarization. A spreadsheet of antiarrhythmic drug actions on ion channels, receptors, and membrane pumps is shown in Figure 35–23.

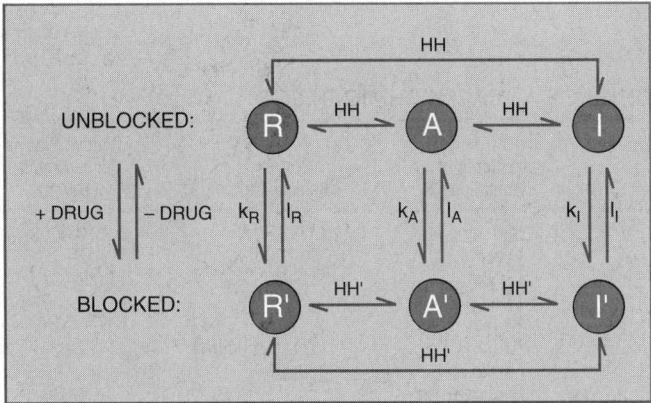

FIGURE 35–22. The modulated receptor model of the cardiac Na⁺ channel. The drug-free Na⁺ channel can exist in three states: (1) resting (R), (2) active or open (A), and (3) inactive (I). Drug-associated channels are indicated as R′, A′, and I′. Rate constants for drug binding to the channel are represented by k's and for drug unbinding by l's. Recovery of Na⁺ channels from I to R or from I′ to R′ is governed by the Hodgkin-Huxley (HH) voltage-dependent rate constant, h. (From Hondeghem LM, Katzung BG: Test of a model of antiarrhythmic drug action: Effects of quinidine and lidocaine on myocardial conduction. Circulation 61:1217, 1980.)

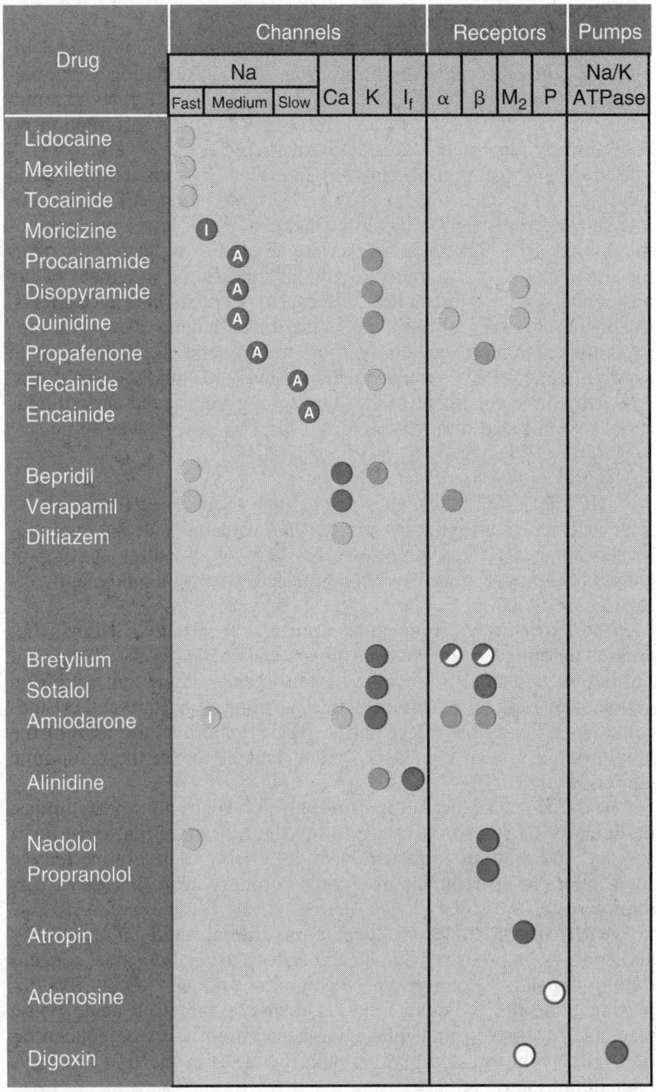

FIGURE 35–23. Summary of important actions of antiarrhythmic drugs on cardiac membrane channels, receptors, and ionic pumps. Some of the drugs shown are not yet approved for antiarrhythmic therapy. The drugs (rows) are ordered so that, in general, the entries for their predominant action(s) form a diagonal. However, drugs with multiple actions, e.g., amiodarone, depart strikingly from the diagonal trend. The actions of drugs on the sodium (Na⁺), calcium (Ca²⁺), potassium (K⁺), and i_f channels are indicated. Drugs that block Na⁺ channels are subdivided into three groups based on time constants for recovery from block (τ): fast (τ < 300 ms), medium (τ = 200–1500 ms), and slow (τ > 1500 ms). τ is a measure of use dependence and predicts the likelihood that a drug will slow conduction in Na⁺-dependent tissues in the heart and the chance that a drug will disturb conduction or aggravate arrhythmias. Where known, blockade of the Na channel in the inactivated (I) or activated (A) state is indicated. Information is incomplete on the state dependency of Na channel block for moricizine, propafenone, encainide, and flecainide. Drug interaction with receptors (alpha [α], beta [β], muscarinic subtype 2 [M₂], and A1 purinergic [P]), and drug effects on the Na⁺/K⁺ pump [Na⁺,K⁺-ATPase] also are indicated. Filled circles indicate antagonist or inhibitory actions; unfilled circles indicate direct or indirect acting agonists or stimulators. The intensity of the action is indicated by the various shadings, as described below. Half-filled circles for bretylium indicate its biphasic action, initially to increase the release of norepinephrine from cardiac sympathetic nerves and increase the occupancy of myocardial α and β receptors, followed by block of norepinephrine release and decreased occupancy of these receptors. Relative blocking potency: ◔ = low, ◑ = moderate, ● = high; ○ = agonist; ◐ agonist, antagonist; A = activated state blockers; I = inactivated state blockers. (From Schlant RC, Alexander RW [eds.]: The Heart, Arteries, and Veins. New York, McGraw-Hill, 1994, p 777.)

Specific Antiarrhythmic Drugs

This section gives a brief summary of the pharmacology and indications for each antiarrhythmic drug. This information is supplemented by information given in tables; Table 35–10 gives pharmacokinetic data for the drugs and Table 35–11 gives information on contraindications, precautions, and adverse effects.

Because of the findings in the Cardiac Arrhythmia Suppression Trial (CAST), the Food and Drug Administration (FDA) recommended more restrictive labeling of drugs with class I antiarrhythmic action. In 1991, these drugs were labeled as indicated for treating documented ventricular arrhythmias that, in the judgment of the physician, are life-threatening. Because of proarrhythmic effects, treatment of lesser arrhythmias with drugs having class I antiarrhythmic action is generally not recommended. Patients with asymptomatic VPC's should not be treated with this class of drugs. Antiarrhythmic treatment of life-threatening ventricular arrhythmias should be initiated in hospital.

DRUGS WITH CLASS IB ANTIARRHYTHMIC ACTION

LIDOCAINE. Lidocaine is a local anesthetic used frequently to treat ventricular arrhythmias in intensive care units. It has two major advantages: It reaches a steady state rapidly after starting or changing the dose, and it lacks significant adverse hemodynamic effects.

Pharmacology. Lidocaine prevents reentrant rhythms, decreases automaticity in Purkinje fibers, and increases the ventricular fibrillation threshold. Lidocaine has an intense depressant action on depolarized tissues but almost none on normal cardiac cells. Lidocaine has a negligible effect on the ECG. It shortens the ERP of the His-Purkinje system but has no significant effect on the autonomic nervous system.

Indications. Lidocaine is used only for ventricular arrhythmias, particularly those caused by acute myocardial infarction, open heart surgery, and digitalis intoxication. Lidocaine is relatively ineffective for ventricular arrhythmias in chronic coronary heart disease or cardiomyopathy.

Pharmacokinetics. Lidocaine is administered intravenously and, rarely, intramuscularly. Steady-state plasma lidocaine concentration depends strongly on hepatic blood flow. About 70% of plasma lidocaine is bound to α_1 acid glycoprotein, an acute phase reactant. At a given total plasma concentration, the free concentration falls as the α_1 acid glycoprotein increases in the first few days after infarction or surgery.

MEXILETINE. Mexiletine is an orally active local anesthetic, available in the United States since 1986, that is chemically and electrophysiologically similar to lidocaine.

Pharmacology. Mexiletine has an antiautomatic effect on Purkinje fibers and depresses phase 0 of fast-action potentials more than lidocaine. It shortens the action potential duration and ERP of

Purkinje fibers and ventricular muscle. Mexiletine has little effect on the ECG.

Indications. Like lidocaine, this drug is not indicated for atrial arrhythmias. In chronic coronary heart disease or cardiomyopathy, the drug is about 60% effective in controlling symptomatic, unsustained ventricular arrhythmias, less than drugs with class IA or IC antiarrhythmic action.

PHENYTOIN. Phenytoin is an anticonvulsant that has been used as an antiarrhythmic since the 1960's. Phenytoin is electrophysiologically similar to lidocaine and has no significant effect on the ECG. Phenytoin has complex central autonomic actions that decrease efferent traffic on cardiac sympathetic nerves during digitalis toxicity. Phenytoin has no peripheral cholinergic or β-adrenergic blocking activity.

Indications. Phenytoin is used to treat paroxysmal atrial flutter or fibrillation, supraventricular arrhythmias, and ventricular arrhythmias caused by digitalis but is ineffective for the common atrial arrhythmias, e.g., atrial flutter, atrial fibrillation, and PSVT. Phenytoin is effective against ventricular arrhythmias after acute myocardial infarction or open heart surgery, but lidocaine is easier to use. Plasma concentrations > 10 μg per milliliter are effective for reducing ventricular arrhythmias in the year after myocardial infarction. Phenytoin, like other drugs with class I antiarrhythmic action, is relatively ineffective against recurrent, sustained VT in patients with chronic coronary heart disease.

Pharmacokinetics. The enzymes that metabolize phenytoin can saturate at antiarrhythmic plasma concentrations, causing plasma concentration to rise sharply to toxic levels. Phenytoin should not be infused because its alkaline pH causes severe phlebitis.

TOCAINIDE. Tocainide is an orally effective analogue of lidocaine that was approved in 1984 for use in the United States. Tocainide has cardiac electrophysiologic effects almost identical to those of lidocaine and has almost no effect on the ECG. Also, it is well tolerated hemodynamically.

Indications. Tocainide is indicated for oral treatment of sustained or symptomatic unsustained ventricular arrhythmias. The drug is similar to mexiletine in its efficacy; i.e., it controls about 60% of the chronic unsustained ventricular arrhythmias. There is good concordance between the effect of IV lidocaine and oral tocainide on ventricular arrhythmias.

DRUGS WITH CLASS IA ANTIARRHYTHMIC ACTION

DISOPYRAMIDE. Oral disopyramide has been available in the United States for treatment of ventricular arrhythmias since 1978. Disopyramide suppresses normal automaticity in Purkinje fibers and depresses phase 0 of fast-action potentials and slows conduction. Disopyramide appears more potent than quinidine in increasing atrial or ventricular refractoriness but seems less potent in the His-Purkinje system. Therapeutic concentrations cause little change in heart rate or PR or QT intervals and increases the QRS duration by

TABLE 35–10. PHARMACOKINETIC PROPERTIES OF ANTIARRHYTHMIC DRUGS

Drug	Volume of Distribution (L/kg)	Half-time of Elimination (Hours)	Bioavailability	Major Route of Elimination	Protein Binding (%)	Effective Plasma Concentration (μg/ml)
Digoxin	10.0	24–72	50–80	Kidney	25	>0.0008
Lidocaine	1.0	1–3	—	Liver	70	1–5
Mexiletine	9.5	8–14	80–90	Liver	60	0.7–2.0
Phenytoin	0.7	18–30	60–80	Liver	90	8–20
Tocainide	3.0	10–14	80–90	Kidney, liver	10	6–15
Disopyramide	0.8	7–9	75–90	Kidney	Dose-dependent	2–5
Moricizine	4.5	3–5	35–45	Liver	>90	
Procainamide	2.0	3–6	75–85	Kidney, liver	15	4–20
Quinidine	2.5	5–9	70–80	Liver	90	2–6
Flecainide	10.0	13–30	>90	Kidney, liver	40	0.2–1.0
Propafenone	3.5	3–10	3–40	Liver	95	—
Acebutalol	1.2	2–4	35–45	Kidney, liver	25	
Propranolol	4.0	3–6	20–50	Liver	>90	0.04–0.9
Amiodarone	60.0	500–1000	30–40	Liver	>95	0.5–2.5
Bretylium	6.0	8–12	20–30	Kidney	5	—
dl-Sotalol	2.0	7–15	>90	Kidney	0	1.0–4.0
Diltiazem	5.5	2–6	40–50	Liver	75	0.5–2.0
Verapamil	4.0	4–10	10–35	Liver	90	0.1–0.2

TABLE 35–11. ADVERSE EFFECTS OF ANTIARRHYTHMIC DRUGS

	Contraindications	Precautions	Adverse Effects
Digoxin	Hypersensitivity to the drug	Reduce dose in renal insufficiency; hypokalemia, hypomagnesemia, and hypercalcemia predispose to digitalis toxicity; may accelerate the ventricular response to atrial flutter or fibrillation in Wolff-Parkinson-White syndrome; may worsen outflow obstruction in hypertrophic obstructive cardiomyopathy; serum digoxin concentration increased by quinidine and verapamil; absorption may be increased by some antibiotics; use cautiously with β blockers or calcium channel antagonists in atrial fibrillation	Ventricular arrhythmias, including ventricular tachycardia; accelerated junctional rhythms; atrial tachycardia with AV block; AV dissociation; progression of AV block Anorexia; nausea, vomiting; visual disturbances; weakness
Lidocaine	Known hypersensitivity to local anesthetics of the amide type; patients with Stokes-Adams syndrome, or with severe degrees of SA, AV, or intraventricular block in the absence of a pacemaker	Accumulation in heart failure or hepatic insufficiency or after prolonged infusions; reduce dosage in children and elderly patients; safety in malignant hyperthermia not established; cimetidine and propranolol increase plasma lidocaine concentration	Bradycardia, hypotension, and cardiovascular collapse Drowsiness, confusion, dizziness, respiratory depression, and arrest; vomiting; visual disturbances; convulsions; twitching; unconsciousness; allergic reactions secondary to lidocaine sensitivity
Mexiletine	Cardiogenic shock; pre-existing second- or third-degree AV block in the absence of a pacemaker	Patients with first-degree AV block, sinus node dysfunction, intraventricular conduction abnormalities; may worsen arrhythmias; mexiletine levels increased by cimetidine; use cautiously in patients with a history of seizures, hypotension, heart failure, or liver disease	GI distress, lightheadedness, tremor, coordination difficulties, diplopia, paresthesia, confusion
Phenytoin	History of hypersensitivity to hydantoin products; sinus bradycardia, SA block, second- or third-degree AV block; Stokes-Adams syndrome	Use cautiously in presence of hypotension and myocardial depression; may worsen arrhythmias; discontinue if skin rash develops; may cause hypoglycemia; multiple drug interactions; may be associated with congenital malformations	Hypotension and bradycardia with rapid IV injection Nystagmus, ataxia, slurred speech; Stevens-Johnson syndrome; sensory neuropathy; lymphadenopathy, pancytopenia; megaloblastic anemia, gingival hyperplasia, hyperglycemia, hypocalcemia
Tocainide	Hypersensitivity to this drug or to local anesthetics of the amide type; second- or third-degree AV block in the absence of a pacemaker	May cause blood dyscrasias, pulmonary fibrosis, pneumonitis; may aggravate heart failure or worsen ventricular arrhythmias; may accelerate the ventricular response in atrial fibrillation; accumulates in severe renal or hepatic insufficiency	Nausea, vomiting, lightheadedness, dizziness, tremor, diplopia, paresthesia, confusion, *agranulocytosis,* thrombocytopenia, hypoplastic anemia
Disopyramide	Cardiogenic shock; pre-existing second- or third-degree AV block in the absence of a pacemaker; congenital QT prolongation; known hypersensitivity to the drug	*Use cautiously with left ventricular dysfunction,* sick sinus syndrome, bundle branch block, or AV block; prior digitalization suggested for atrial flutter or fibrillation to prevent increase in ventricular rate. May precipitate myasthenic crisis, glaucoma, or urinary retention; may cause hypoglycemia; serum level may be lowered by phenytoin	*Heart failure;* worsening of arrhythmias; AV block; hypotension; may cause significant prolongation of QRS and QT intervals *Urinary retention;* dry mouth; constipation; blurred vision; impotence; cholestatic jaundice; fever; thrombocytopenia; granulocytopenia; gynecomastia
Moricizine	Second- or third-degree AV block unless a pacemaker is in place; cardiogenic shock; uncontrolled congestive failure; and hypersensitivity to moricizine	Monitor carefully when giving to patients with pre-existing sinus node dysfunction or intraventricular conduction abnormalities; reduce dose in patients with hepatic or renal impairment; cimetidine slows the clearance of moricizine; moricizine accelerates theophylline clearance	Can aggravate ventricular arrhythmias; dizziness; nausea
Procainamide HCl	Second- or third-degree AV block unless a pacemaker is present; torsades de pointes; lupus-like syndrome; hypersensitivity to the drug	Reduce dosage in renal insufficiency; may accelerate the ventricular response in atrial fibrillation or atrial flutter; may exacerbate myasthenia gravis	Hypotension; worsening of ventricular arrhythmias; myocardial depression; AV block *Lupus-like syndrome;* GI distress; *agranulocytosis;* hemolytic anemia; fever; thrombocytopenia; rash; myalgia; hallucinations; psychosis
Quinidine sulfate	Hypersensitivity to quinidine; complete AV block; complete bundle branch block or other severe intraventricular conduction defects exhibiting marked QRS widening; myasthenia gravis; arrhythmias due to digitalis toxicity	May accelerate the ventricular response to atrial flutter or atrial fibrillation; *concurrent use with digoxin increases plasma digoxin levels;* drugs that increase hepatic drug-metabolizing enzymes decrease the plasma concentration of quinidine; may worsen heart failure; test dose recommended because of idiosyncratic response; may require change in oral anticoagulant dose	Hypotension; worsening of ventricular arrhythmias; asystole; may increase AV or bundle branch block; may cause significant prolongation of QRS and QT intervals; *syncope; torsades de pointes* *Diarrhea;* nausea; *thrombocytopenia;* hemolytic anemia; granulocytopenia; fever; visual disturbances; hypersensitivity reaction; cinchonism; rash

Table continued on following page

TABLE 35-11. ADVERSE EFFECTS OF ANTIARRHYTHMIC DRUGS (Continued)

	Contraindications	Precautions	Adverse Effects
Flecainide	Second- or third-degree AV block or right bundle branch block with associated hemiblock unless a pacemaker is in place; cardiogenic shock; known hypersensitivity to the drug; asymptomatic ventricular arrhythmias after myocardial infarction	May worsen sinus node dysfunction; increases pacing thresholds; may suppress ventricular escape rhythms; avoid concurrent administration of disopyramide or verapamil	*New or worsened ventricular tachycarcia or ventricular fibrillation* in patients with sustained ventricular arrhythmias; *heart failure,* second- or third-degree AV block Dizziness; *visual disturbances;* dyspnea; hepatic dysfunction; blood dyscrasias
Propafenone	Uncontrolled congestive heart failure or cardiogenic shock; sinoatrial or AV block in the absence of an electronic pacemaker; bradycardia; bronchospastic disorders; manifest electrolyte disorders; and known hypersensitivity to the drug	Reduce dose in hepatic or renal dysfunction; may worsen arrhythmias; increases plasma digoxin or warfarin concentrations; decreases the clearance of some β blockers; quinidine or cimetidine increases plasma concentrations; use cautiously with β blockers or calcium entry blockers	New or worsened ventricular arrhythmias in patients with sustained ventricular arrhythmias; may increase mortality when used to treat prognostically important ventricular arrhythmias after myocardial infarction; aggravates asthma or chronic bronchitis; aggravates congestive heart failure; dizziness, taste disturbances, blurred vision; anorexia, nausea, and vomiting; agranulocytosis
Acebutolol	Severe sinus bradycardia; second- and third-degree AV block; overt cardiac failure; cardiogenic shock	Myocardial infarction or exacerbation of angina may occur following abrupt withdrawal; may mask symptoms of hypoglycemia or hyperthyroidism; cautious use in renal insufficiency or with concurrent α-adrenergic or catecholamine-depleting drugs	Congestive heart failure; bradycardia; hypotension; increase in AV block Fatigue; headache; dizziness; arterial insufficiency; bronchospasm; impotence
Propranolol	Cardiogenic shock; sinus bradycardia; second- or third-degree AV block; asthma; congestive heart failure	Exacerbation of angina or myocardial infarction may occur following abrupt withdrawal; may mask symptoms of hypoglycemia or hyperthyroidism; may cause severe sinus bradycardia following termination of tachycardia; may worsen hypertension in pheochromocytoma unless used with an α-adrenergic blocking drug	Congestive heart failure; bradycardia; increase in degree of AV block; hypotension Bronchospasm; arterial insufficiency; Raynaud's phenomenon; mental depression; sleep disturbances; weakness; impotence; disorientation; memory loss; blood dyscrasias
Amiodarone	Severe sinus node dysfunction; marked sinus bradycardia; second- or third-degree AV block; history of syncope due to bradycardia unless a pacemaker is in place	Raises serum digoxin concentration; potentiates the effect of oral anticoagulants; increases levels of quinidine, procainamide, phenytoin; may potentiate bradycardia or AV block when used with β blockers or calcium entry blockers; may worsen arrhythmias	Sinus bradycardia *Pulmonary fibrosis;* interstitial pneumonitis; corneal microdeposits; photosensitivity; blue-gray pigmentation; hypo- or hyperthyroidism; *hepatic injury;* nausea; vomiting, anorexia, constipation; tremor; malaise; gait disturbance; *peripheral myopathy or neuropathy*
Bretylium tosylate	*Severe hypotension may occur in patients with fixed cardiac output;* may aggravate digitalis toxicity; reduce dosage in renal insufficiency	*Hypotension, especially postural hypotension;* transient hypertension and increased frequency of ventricular arrhythmias Nausea and vomiting, usually with rapid IV infusion; increases sensitivity to catecholamines	
dl-Sotalol	Bronchial asthma; second- or third-degree AV block unless a pacemaker is in place; long QT syndromes; cardiogenic shock; uncontrolled congestive failure; and hypersensitivity to sotalol	Reduce dose in renal insufficiency; torsades de pointes and worsened ventricular tachycardia; especially in patients with sustained ventricular tachycardia or hypokalemia or hypomagnesemia; aggravation of heart failure; increase of sudden death in first 2 weeks after myocardial infarction; myocardial infarction or exacerbation of angina may occur following withdrawal	Torsades de pointes or aggravation of other ventricular arrhythmias; elevated liver enzymes (cause and effect not established); fatigue, dizziness; asthenia
Diltiazem	Sick sinus syndrome; second- or third-degree AV block in absence of a ventricular pacemaker; systolic BP <90 mm Hg	Cautious use in renal or hepatic insufficiency; additive effects on AV conduction when used with digitalis or β blockers	Bradycardia; hypotension; AV block Edema; headache; nausea; dizziness; rash; abnormal hepatic enzymes
Verapamil	*Severe left ventricular dysfunction; hypotension or cardiogenic shock;* sick sinus syndrome (except with a pacemaker); second- or third-degree AV block; concurrent intravenous β blockers and intravenous verapamil; known hypersensitivity to verapamil	Reduce oral dose with hepatic dysfunction; avoid use with disopyramide; use cautiously with renal insufficiency; β-blockers, quinidine, or severe hypertrophic obstructive cardiomyopathy; raises serum digoxin level; *may accelerate ventricular response in atrial flutter or fibrillation in the presence of the Wolff-Parkinson-White syndrome;* may potentiate activity of neuromuscular blocking agents	Hypotension; AV block; heart failure; bradycardia; asystole (with IV use); *severe hypotension or ventricular fibrillation when given IV to patients with ventricular tachycardia* Peripheral edema; headache; elevation of liver function tests; constipation

about 25%. It increases the ERP of the atrium and ventricle but not the AV node or His-Purkinje system. Disopyramide has a prominent anticholinergic action that counteracts its direct effects on the sinus and AV nodes.

Indications. Disopyramide is indicated for treating symptomatic, unsustained ventricular arrhythmias. It also terminates attacks of PSVT and decreases the frequency of recurrences. It is about as effective as quinidine for preventing recurrence of atrial fibrillation after cardioversion. Disopyramide prolongs the ERP of anomalous AV connections and can control arrhythmias in the WPW syndrome.

MORICIZINE. Moricizine is a phenothiazine derivative that was approved in 1990 for oral treatment of ventricular arrhythmias.

Pharmacology. Moricizine binds to Na^+ channels when they are open and inactivated. It slows phase 0 depolarization in atrial, His-Purkinje, and ventricular muscle cells but does not slow repolarization of these cardiac cell types. In humans, moricizine increases the PR and QRS interval of the ECG.

Pharmacokinetics. Clearance may be impaired in hepatic dysfunction and during concomitant cimetidine treatment. Moricizine increases theophylline clearance.

Indications. Like other drugs with class I antiarrhythmic action, moricizine is indicated for documented ventricular arrhythmias, e.g., sustained VT, that are judged to be life-threatening. Treatment should be initiated in hospital.

PROCAINAMIDE. Procainamide has been used since the 1950's to treat atrial and ventricular arrhythmias. The cardiac electrophysiologic effects of procainamide are similar to those of disopyramide and quinidine. It suppresses automaticity in cardiac Purkinje fibers, slows the phase 0 depolarization in fibers with fast action potentials, and delays repolarization and increases refractoriness in the atrium, His-Purkinje system, and ventricle. Procainamide produces a small increase in the PR and QT intervals in the ECG and lengthens the QRS duration by 20 to 30% at therapeutic plasma concentrations. Also, procainamide increases slightly the ERP of the atrium, has little effect on the refractoriness of the AV node, and prolongs the conduction time and ERP of the His-Purkinje system slightly in humans. Procainamide has no significant anticholinergic or α-adrenergic blocking properties.

Indications. Procainamide is indicated for treating atrial fibrillation, atrial flutter, PSVT, symptomatic, unsustained ventricular arrhythmias that do not respond to β-blockers, and sustained VT. It can suppress digitalis-toxic ventricular arrhythmias, but lidocaine or phenytoin is a better choice.

Pharmacokinetics. Procainamide is biotransformed in the liver to N-acetyl procainamide (NAPA), and steady-state plasma concentrations can equal or exceed those of procainamide. NAPA is qualitatively different electrophysiologically from procainamide; it has little class I action but a pronounced class III antiarrhythmic action. NAPA is eliminated by the kidney and can accumulate to toxic levels when renal or congestive heart failure is present. Procainamide's adverse effects often preclude chronic therapy.

QUINIDINE. Quinidine, an alkaloid derived from the bark of the cinchona tree, has been used to treat atrial and ventricular arrhythmias since the 1920's.

Pharmacology. Quinidine has powerful direct effects on most types of cardiac cells and has significant anticholinergic and α-adrenergic blocking activity. Quinidine has little effect on normal sinus nodes, but can markedly depress abnormal ones. Quinidine substantially decreases normal automaticity in cardiac Purkinje fibers but has little effect on abnormal automaticity. Quinidine increases atrial and ventricular pacing and fibrillation thresholds. Quinidine depresses phase 0 of atrial, ventricular, and Purkinje cells. Quinidine delays repolarization and increases the effective refractory period of atrial, ventricular, and Purkinje cells. In humans, quinidine causes a small increase in heart rate and in the PR, QRS, and QT intervals in the ECG, and usually prolongs the HV interval slightly.

Indications. Quinidine is indicated for the chronic treatment of atrial flutter or fibrillation, PSVT, and symptomatic ventricular arrhythmias. For symptomatic benign or potentially malignant ventricular arrhythmias that do not respond to β-blockers, quinidine can be used if the benefits outweigh the risks. Quinidine is selected for malignant arrhythmias if it renders them uninducible by programmed ventricular stimulation or if it abolishes unsustained VT from Holter recordings.

DRUGS WITH CLASS IC ANTIARRHYTHMIC ACTION

Two drugs with IC antiarrhythmic action are marketed in the United States: flecainide and propafenone. These drugs have little effect on the normal sinus node but can depress abnormal sinus nodes. They decrease spontaneous phase 4 depolarization in Purkinje fibers and markedly depress phase 0 in fast-response cardiac cells. They slow conduction substantially and shorten the ERP in atrium, ventricle, and His-Purkinje system. In humans, chronic oral doses prolong the refractory periods of the atrium, ventricle, and anomalous AV connections. They increase the AH and HV intervals and the PR, QRS, and QT intervals in the ECG much more than drugs with class IA or IB action. Propafenone has important active metabolites and significant β-blocking action.

Indications. At the present time, drugs with class IC antiarrhythmic action are indicated only for treating life-threatening ventricular arrhythmias when other drugs have failed. Treatment should be initiated in hospital. Flecainide and propafenone are effective against PSVT in the WPW syndrome, AV nodal PSVT, and paroxysmal atrial fibrillation and are approved for treatment of these arrhythmias in patients without structural heart disease. Encainide and flecainide increased the mortality rate in the CAST, a controlled study that enrolled patients with left ventricular dysfunction and asymptomatic or minimally symptomatic ventricular arrhythmias after myocardial infarction. It is prudent to assume that other drugs with class IC action and perhaps drugs with class IA or IB antiarrhythmic action have the same effect.

DRUGS WITH CLASS II ANTIARRHYTHMIC ACTION

Propranolol, the first β-blocker in the United States, was approved more than 25 years ago. Of the many β-adrenergic blocking drugs now available, only acebutolol and propranolol are approved for treating chronic atrial or ventricular arrhythmias; atenolol and metroprolol are indicated to reduce mortality in acute myocardial infarction (when started within hours of symptom onset); and propranolol and timolol are indicated to reduce cardiovascular mortality in patients who have survived the acute phase of infarction. Timolol also reduces nonfatal reinfarction. When there are no contraindications, drugs with class II antiarrhythmic action are the preferred treatment for prognostically important ventricular arrhythmias. There are many significant differences among the β-adrenergic blocking agents that govern the choice for an individual patient, e.g., cardioselectivity, intrinsic sympathomimetic action, electrophysiologic effects, and pharmacokinetics.

Pharmacology. β-Blockers decrease automaticity in the sinus node and His-Purkinje system when it is enhanced by sympathetic influences but have little effect when catecholamines are absent. Propranolol has little effect on phase 0 depolarization of cardiac fibers at low concentrations. At high concentrations, i.e., 1000 to 3000 ng per milliliter, phase 0 depolarization is depressed. Propranolol shortens while other β-blockers can prolong action potential duration in atrial, ventricular, and particularly His-Purkinje cells; these effects are unrelated to β-blocking activity. In humans, propranolol and other β-blockers increase the ERP of the AV node, a major antiarrhythmic effect, but have little effect on atrial or ventricular refractoriness.

Indications. Propranolol is indicated for supraventricular arrhythmias, particularly those induced by catecholamines and those associated with the WPW syndrome or thyrotoxicosis, for symptomatic APC's, and to control the ventricular rate in atrial flutter or fibrillation. It is also indicated for ventricular arrhythmias caused by catecholamines. Propranolol, acebutalol, or another β-blocker is the first choice for the treatment of symptomatic but benign or prognostically important VPC's.

DRUGS WITH CLASS III ANTIARRHYTHMIC ACTION

AMIODARONE. Amiodarone is a benzofuran derivative, 37% iodine by weight, originally developed as a smooth muscle relaxant and coronary vasodilator to treat angina pectoris. In 1986, amiodarone was approved by the FDA as a last-resort treatment for malignant ventricular arrhythmias. There have been no controlled studies of its efficacy.

Pharmacology. Amiodarone substantially prolongs action potential duration and ERP in atrium, ventricle, and Purkinje fibers (a class III action). Amiodarone slows sinus rate by a direct effect.

Under laboratory conditions, amiodarone can have a substantial class I antiarrhythmic effect. In humans, amiodarone slows the sinus rate and increases the PR and QT intervals in the ECG with less effect on the QRS. Also, it increases the atrial, AV nodal, and ventricular refractory periods and prolongs the HV interval (a class I action).

Indications. Amiodarone is indicated only for treating recurrent ventricular fibrillation or recurrent, hemodynamically unstable sustained VT that has not responded to other antiarrhythmic drugs or when other drugs cannot be tolerated. Treatment must be assessed by a method with high predictive accuracy. Endocardial electrical stimulation is the method of choice. About 20% of patients with inducible VT can be rendered uninducible, and these patients do well. In another 40 to 50%, the VT rate slows enough to control symptoms during sustained VT. In this group, recurrences of VT are not reduced much but usually are not fatal. Patients who have inducible symptomatic, sustained VT after being loaded with amiodarone should be considered for some alternate treatment. Because of the serious nature of the arrhythmias for which amiodarone is indicated and the unpredictable time course of effect, amiodarone should be started in a hospital setting.

BRETYLIUM TOSYLATE. Bretylium is a postganglionic adrenergic neuron blocker that was approved in the United States in 1978 for intramuscular or intravenous use as an antiarrhythmic drug.

Pharmacology. Bretylium causes marked lengthening of the action potential duration and ERP of ventricular muscle and Purkinje fibers (class III action). It is selectively taken up in peripheral adrenergic nerves and causes the acute release of norepinephrine; later, it produces chemical sympathectomy, preventing norepinephrine release when the nerve depolarizes. Bretylium has no significant effect on phase 0 depolarization or conduction (i.e., it has no class I action), but it does increase the ventricular fibrillation threshold. Bretylium does not depress myocardial performance but can cause severe postural hypotension by interfering with the efferent limb of the baroreceptor reflex.

Indications. Bretylium is indicated for the therapy and prophylaxis of ventricular fibrillation and for treating life-threatening ventricular arrhythmias, e.g., sustained VT, that have failed to respond to first-line antiarrhythmic drugs, e.g., lidocaine. Use of bretylium should be restricted to intensive care units. It is interesting that ventricular fibrillation usually responds within minutes while the full effect on unsustained VT and VPC's takes hours.

dl-SOTALOL. Sotalol is a β-adrenergic blocking drug that has been used in Europe for hypertension and angina pectoris for 20 years. In 1993 is was approved in the United States to treat life-threatening ventricular arrhythmias.

Pharmacology. dl-Sotalol has substantial class II and dose-dependent class III action. It decreases automaticity in the sinus node and increases the effective refractory period of atrial, AV nodal, His-Purkinje, and ventricular muscle cells and slows conduction in the AV node. It increases fibrillation threshold and decreases defibrillation threshold.

Indications. dl-Sotalol is indicated for treating ventricular arrhythmias, such as sustained VT, that are considered life-threatening. In the Electrophysiologic Studies Versus Electrocardiographic Monitoring (ESVEM) trial, dl-sotalol rendered 30% of sustained ventricular tachyarrhythmias uninducible, compared with 15% for six drugs with class I antiarrhythmic action; dl-sotalol also was more effective in preventing death and arrhythmia recurrences.

DRUGS WITH CLASS IV ANTIARRHYTHMIC ACTION

VERAPAMIL. Verapamil is a papavarine derivative that has been used since 1962 as a coronary vasodilator. Later, its calcium channel blocking properties were discovered and, in 1981, it was approved for use in the United States to treat angina pectoris and supraventricular arrhythmias.

Pharmacology. Verapamil slows spontaneous firing in isolated sinus node preparations; the effect is less marked *in vivo* because of reflex sympathetic nervous activity caused by peripheral vasodilation. Verapamil decreases normal automaticity in Purkinje fibers and abolishes delayed afterdepolarizations and triggered activity in experimental digitalis toxicity. Verapamil prolongs refractoriness and conduction in the AV node by blocking Ca^{2+} channels. This action

accounts for the ability of verapamil to terminate and prevent PSVT. Verapamil can abolish experimental VT due to slow potentials. Also, verapamil can delay ischemic injury and prevent arrhythmogenic electrophysiologic effects caused by transient ischemia. Verapamil also has α-adrenergic blocking properties. In humans, verapamil slows heart rate and increases the PR interval without any change in the QRS and QTc.

Indications. Intravenous verapamil is about 80% effective for a rapid conversion (45 to 60 seconds) of PSVT to sinus rhythm (see Table 35–11). Verapamil should not be given IV to patients with heart failure or those with wide QRS tachycardias until the rhythm is *proven* to be PSVT.

Verapamil can provide temporary control of rapid ventricular rate in atrial fibrillation. A 5- to 10-mg IV dose of verapamil slows the ventricular rate about 20% for 15 to 30 minutes while a more permanent treatment is being established. Verapamil can be used orally to prevent PSVT or to help control the ventricular rate in atrial flutter or fibrillation.

IV diltiazem is indicated for temporary control of rapid ventricular rate in atrial fibrillation or flutter and for rapid conversion of PSVT; a 20-mg IV injection can be used for either indication. IV infusion of 10 mg per hour can be used for up to 24 hours for rate control in atrial fibrillation.

DRUGS WITH MISCELLANEOUS ANTIARRHYTHMIC ACTION

ADENOSINE. Adenosine became available for use in the United States in 1990. It depresses automaticity in sinus node and conduction in the AV node; these are direct effects not blocked by atropine. A 10- to 20-mg IV dose of this drug terminates PSVT within 20 seconds in >90% of cases by blocking conduction in the AV node in AV reciprocating tachycardia or in the slow antegrade AV nodal pathway in AV nodal tachycardia. It is not effective for terminating intra-atrial reentry and therefore is ineffective for atrial tachycardia, flutter, or fibrillation. It has less adverse hemodynamic effect than verapamil but frequently causes transient, minor adverse effects.

Bigger JT Jr, Hoffman BF: Antiarrhythmic drugs. *In* Gilman AG, Goodman LS, Rall TW, Murad F (eds.): The Pharamcological Basis of Therapeutics, 8th ed. New York, MacMillan Publishing Company, 1990, p 840. *A concise summary of the pharmacology and clinical use of antiarrhythmic drugs. Selectively referenced.*

The Physicians Desk Reference, Montvale, NJ, Medical Economics. *A yearly publication that gives accurate full prescribing information for all drugs.*

ELECTRICAL MODALITIES IN THE MANAGEMENT OF CARDIAC ARRHYTHMIAS

Temporary or permanent cardiac pacemakers and DC cardioversion or external defibrillation are well-established forms of electrical therapy. In 1985, an implantable cardioverter/defibrillator was approved by the FDA and this mode of therapy continues to develop.

Cardiac Pacemakers

Permanent pacemakers were first implanted in the 1960's, and over the ensuing 30 years the pacemaker industry has matured, pro-

---

TABLE 35–12. DEFINITE INDICATIONS FOR IMPLANTED PACEMAKER

A. Complete heart block, permanent or intermittent with any one of the following complications:
   1. Symptomatic bradycardia
   2. Congestive heart failure
   3. Conditions that require treatment with drugs that suppress ventricular escape rhythms
   4. Asystole ≥ 3 seconds or ventricular rate < 40 per minute
   5. Mental confusion that clears with temporary pacing
B. Complete heart block or advanced second-degree AV block that occurs during myocardial infarction and persists
C. Chronic bi- or trifascicular block with one of the following
   1. Intermittent complete heart block
   2. Type II second-degree AV block associated with symptomatic bradycardia
D. Sinus node dysfunction with documented symptomatic bradycardia
E. Hypersensitive carotid sinus syndrome with recurrent syncope and asystole > 3 seconds provoked by minimal carotid sinus pressure
F. Symptomatic supraventricular tachycardia that does not respond to medical treatment

TABLE 35-13. CODE FOR PACEMAKER MODES

Chamber Paced	Chamber Sensed	Response to Sensing
V = Ventricle	V = Ventricle	I = Inhibited
A = Atrium	A = Atrium	T = Triggered
D = Double (atrium and ventricle	D = Double (atrium and ventricle)	D = Double (atrium and ventricle)
	O = None	O = None

viding highly sophisticated and diverse products for managing brad-yarrhythmias, and, to a lesser extent, tachyarrhythmias. About 100,000 pulse generators are implanted each year in the United States, about half of the world's pacemaker implants. There are approximately 500,000 patients with pacemakers living in the United States.

INDICATIONS FOR CARDIAC PACING. The joint report of the American College of Cardiology and American Heart Association divided indications into three classes: I, definitely indicated; II, possibly indicated; and III, not indicated (Table 35-12). Pacing is indicated for bradycardia with complete heart block or advanced second-degree AV block with symptoms such as transient dizziness, lightheadedness, near syncope or syncope, marked exercise intolerance, and congestive heart failure. Asymptomatic conditions that are definite indications are permanent high-grade AV block after myocardial infarction or surgical repair of congenital heart disease, or complete heart block with a ventricular rate less than 40 per minute.

LEAD PLACEMENT. More than 90% of permanent pacing leads are placed via cephalic, subclavian, or external jugular veins. Most transvenous leads are stainless steel, multifilament helical coil wires insulated with polyurethane or silicone rubber. These leads are small, steerable, and fracture resistant. Leads are anchored by tines or a screw-in arrangement at their tips. Both unipolar and bipolar electrodes are commonly used. For simple ventricular pacing, one lead is placed in the right ventricular apex. For dual-chamber pacing, a second lead is placed in the right atrium.

PULSE GENERATORS. Modern pacemaker generators weigh 40 to 50 grams, are powered by lithium batteries that last 7 to 10 years, and have circuitry for sensing intracardiac electrograms. Pacemakers can be interrogated to evaluate the pulse generator or reprogrammed to meet changing requirements. Multiprogrammability provides flexibility in obtaining diagnostic information and individualizing the pacemaker prescription.

MODES OF CARDIAC PACING. Pacemaker modes are expressed in the three- or five-letter notation proposed by the Inter-

Society Commission for Heart Disease Resources. Table 35-13 shows the first three letter codes. The three letters indicate the chamber paced, the chamber sensed, and the response to sensing. The fourth and fifth positions describe programmable and antitachycardia features and are used less frequently.

SELECTION OF THE PACEMAKER MODE. Selecting the appropriate pacemaker has become more complex as options have become more diverse. Table 35-14 summarizes common selections, considering the atrial rhythm and status of AV and VA conduction.

COMPLICATIONS. Transvenous implants are associated with cardiac perforation, arrhythmias, infection, thrombosis, emboli, and lead fracture or displacement. Thoracotomy carries the risk of general anesthesia, bleeding, infection, postoperative respiratory compromise, and late threshold increases. With either route of implantation, the pulse generator may erode through the skin. Pacemakers can be inhibited by intense magnetic fields such as large telephone transformers, microwave devices, diathermy, cautery, antitheft devices, and certain types of motors, e.g., electric razors. Unipolar pacemakers may be inhibited by local myopotentials. The "pacemaker syndrome" was first defined as lightheadedness or syncope related to long cycles of AV asynchrony that occurred during VOO or VVI pacing. The definition also includes (1) episodic weakness or syncope associated with alternating AV synchrony and asynchrony, (2) inadequate cardiac output associated with continued absence of AV synchrony or with fixed asynchrony (persistent VA conduction), and (3) patient awareness of beat-to-beat variation in vascular pulsation.

PACEMAKER FOLLOW-UP. Implanted pacing devices require careful follow-up. Regular transtelephonic monitoring permits early detection of battery depletion. At the present time, the principal problem in pacemaker follow-up is the diversity of pacemaker models and methods for interrogating pacemaker function.

DC Cardioversion

DC cardioversion was introduced in 1962 and has become a mainstay in managing cardiac arrhythmias. Cardioversion depolarizes all or most of the heart, interrupts reentrant circuits, and terminates arrhythmias. It is effective for atrial fibrillation, atrial flutter, PSVT, VT, or ventricular fibrillation. Drug-resistant arrhythmias, e.g., atrial flutter, may respond readily to DC cardioversion. Because of its speed, cardioversion is preferable to drug therapy for arrhythmias that adversely affect hemodynamics, such as rapid atrial arrhythmias, sustained VT, or ventricular fibrillation. Elective cardioversion is indicated for atrial fibrillation of recent onset (months) to control symptoms and hemodynamic abnormalities and lower the risk of systemic thromboembolism.

TABLE 35-14. INDICATIONS FOR PACING MODES

AV Conduction	Atrial Rhythm		
	Normal	*Bradycardia*	*Bradycardia-Tachycardia*
Normal	None indicated	AAI	AAI
AV block; normal VA conduction time	VDD, DDD	DDD, DVI	DVI, VVI
AV block; prolonged VA conduction time	DVI	DVI	DVI

AAI: Fixed-rate atrial pacing occurs unless inhibited by sensed atrial complexes. This mode can be used for patients with symptomatic sinus node dysfunction and normal AV conduction.

VDD: Ventricular pulses are delivered when atrial complex is sensed and inhibited when ventricular complex is sensed. The VDD mode is used when adequate atrial rates and sensing are present, along with high-grade AV block and normal VA conduction. VDD pacing provides atrial augmentation of ventricular filling and avoids the pacemaker syndrome but is contraindicated for patients with supraventricular tachyarrhythmias.

DVI: Both chambers are paced at a preselected rate and AV interval. Pacing is inhibited by ventricular but not atrial activity. The DVI mode is used when synchronous AV contraction is needed in patients with symptomatic atrial bradycardia. The pacing rate does not increase during exercise. DVI pacing is contraindicated in patients who have supraventricular tachyarrhythmias.

DDD: Both atria and ventricles are paced and sensed. The atrial or ventricular pacemaker pulses are inhibited when either atrial or ventricular premature activity is detected. When atrial activity is sensed, a ventricular pulse is provided. This mode of pacing provides synchronous AV contraction over a wide range of heart rates. DDD pacemakers are adaptive: totally inhibited in sinus rhythm with normal AV conduction; AAI pacing during sinus bradycardia with normal AV conduction; VDD pacing during sinus rhythm with impaired AV conduction; DVI pacing during sinus bradycardia with impaired AV conduction. DDD pacemakers are contraindicated in patients with persistent or frequently occurring atrial tachyarrhythmias and those with long VA conduction times who can develop pacemaker-mediated reciprocating tachycardia.

VVI: This mode can be used for any symptomatic bradyarrhythmia. The VVI mode is contraindicated in patients who have had the pacemaker syndrome, those with congestive heart failure, and those who need rate-responsive pacing.

Rate-Responsive Pacing (VVIR): Many patients who need increased heart rate during exercise have relative contraindications for DDD pacing, e.g., inadequate sinus node function or atrial fibrillation. Rate-responsive pacing is provided by sensing the activity level and increasing the pacing rate. Heart rate can be increased by as much as 90 per minute, i.e., from 60 at rest to 150 during exercise, providing an increase in cardiac output and exercise capability.

LIMITATIONS AND CONTRAINDICATIONS. Chronic atrial fibrillation, i.e., greater than 6 to 12 months long, is so likely to recur after cardioversion that digitalis therapy may be preferred. Contributing causes (e.g., hyperthyroidism, pericardial inflammation, pulmonary thromboembolism, chronic obstructive pulmonary disease, or alcohol abuse) should be controlled before cardioversion to avoid recurrence. Sinus rhythm is difficult to maintain after cardioversion of atrial fibrillation in patients with heart failure or large left atria (>45 mm in diameter by echocardiography). In the bradycardia-tachycardia syndrome, cardioversion often produces inadequate rhythms, and atrial fibrillation often resumes within a few hours. Cardioversion is contraindicated for arrhythmias caused by digitalis intoxication because it can precipitate ventricular fibrillation.

ANTICOAGULATION. Despite the lack of a controlled evaluation, a standard anticoagulation practice has evolved for patients with atrial fibrillation. Most patients who have been fibrillating for >3 weeks are anticoagulated, particularly those with (1) a history of embolization, (2) a prosthetic mitral valve, (3) an enlarged left atrium, or (4) congestive heart failure. The prothrombin time is kept at 1.3 to 1.8 (INR [international normalized ratio] of 2.0 to 3.0) times the normal value with warfarin for ≥3 weeks before and 1 week after cardioversion.

RESULTS. The immediate results of cardioversion are excellent (Table 35–15). The main long-term problem following cardioversion is reversion to atrial fibrillation. Class I antiarrhythmic drugs decrease the chance of recurrence of atrial fibrillation 1 year after cardioversion from about 75 to 50%.

COMPLICATIONS. Few complications attend technically excellent cardioversion. Occasionally, transient SA or AV block or ventricular arrhythmias occur immediately after DC shock, especially with excessive digitalis. In the sick sinus syndrome, the sinus may fail to resume control of cardiac rhythm after cardioversion. Atropine, isoproterenol, and/or external pacing usually maintains the patient until a temporary transvenous pacemaker can be inserted. Occasionally, worsening heart failure or frank pulmonary edema occurs within a few hours after cardioversion. The cause of this syndrome is unknown. Elevation of myocardial creatine kinase after DC cardioversion is rare.

Implantable Cardioverter/Defibrillators

The first automatic implantable defibrillator, a device that responded only to ventricular fibrillation, was implanted in 1980. The first implantable cardioverter/defibrillator (ICD) that provided cardioversion as well as defibrillation was implanted in 1982. The 1990's saw the advent of tiered therapy devices, backup bradycardia pacing, stored electrograms, and transvenous lead systems.

INDICATIONS. The ICD is indicated for patients who are at high risk of sudden cardiac death, usually patients who have survived cardiac arrest not associated with acute myocardial infarction.

IMPLANTATION. Until 1993, electrode systems were implanted via a thoracotomy. In 1993, transvenous lead systems were approved and most ICD systems now use them. During implantation, defibrillation thresholds and detection of ventricular tachycardia/fibrillation are tested to ensure proper ICD function.

FOLLOW-UP. An ICD pulse generator lasts 3 to 5 years, monitoring the ECG continuously. When ventricular tachycardia or fibrillation is detected and verified, it delivers therapy: antitachycardia pacing, low-energy cardioversion (0.3 to 5 joules), or high-energy defibrillation (20 to 30 joules). Some ICD's provide bradycardia pacing and store electrograms of detected arrhythmias. The ICD is a complex device that requires careful follow-up to detect (1) battery depletion, (2) lead breakage or migration, (3) inappropriate discharges, (4) infection, and (5) skin erosion. After implantation, the ICD should be evaluated every 2 to 3 months. The detection and therapy features are programmable to meet changing needs during follow-up.

Between 1980 and the end of 1993, >30,000 ICD's were implanted. At 1-year follow-up, a 10% cardiovascular death rate and a 2% sudden death rate are found for patients treated with ICD's. ICD therapy is highly effective for converting malignant ventricular arrhythmias, but it has not been shown to reduce all-cause mortality.

Estes NAM, Manolis A, Wang P (eds.): Implantable Cardioverter Defibrillator: A Comprehensive Text. New York, Marcel Dekker, 1994. *Has chapters on mechanisms of defibrillation, on indications for use of ICD's, on technical details of implantation and testing, on dealing with technical, medical, and emotional problems during follow-up, and on cost-effectiveness. Each of the ICD's currently available is described in detail.*

Frye RL, Collins JJ, DeSanctis RW, et al.: Guidelines for permanent cardiac pacemaker implantation, May 1984. J Am Coll Cardiol 4:434, 1984. *A report of a task force to review cardiac pacing. The report defines indications for cardiac pacing and makes recommendations about selecting devices for treatment of specific clinical problems. This report is used as a standard by the medical profession, regulatory agencies, and reimbursement sources.*

Mirowski M: The automatic implantable cardioverter-defibrillator: An overview. J Am Coll Cardiol 6:461, 1985. *A review of the concepts, evolution, clinical use, and follow-up of implantable cardioverter defibrillators by the originator of the devices.*

Winkle RA, Mead RH, Ruder MA, et al.: Long-term outcome with the automatic implantable cardioverter-defibrillator. J Am Coll Cardiol 13:1353, 1989. *The clinical events and outcome in 270 patients with ICD implants. Provides an excellent perspective on the current use of the device.*

ABLATION THERAPY FOR CARDIAC ARRHYTHMIAS

The objective of catheter ablation or surgical ablation of cardiac arrhythmias may be (1) to destroy or remove the arrhythmic focus, (2) to interrupt a reentrant pathway, or (3) to prevent the ventricles from responding to supraventricular tachyarrhythmias (Table 35–16). Recently, catheter ablation has proven >90% effective for

TABLE 35–15. ENERGY FOR CARDIOVERSION/DEFIBRILLATION

Arrhythmia	Recommended Initial Energy* (joules)	Comments
Atrial flutter	50	100% conversion; most convert with about 25 joules.
Atrial fibrillation	200	85–95% conversion; a few patients may require 300- to 400-joule DC shocks to cardiovert.
Paroxysmal supraventricular tachycardia	100	100% conversion
Ventricular tachycardia	50	90–95% conversion; 80% convert with <10 joules; a few need 100 joules or more.
Ventricular fibrillation	300–400	90–95% defibrillation; many convert at 200 joules or below but time is of the essence in successful defibrillation.

* An energy level with a high probability of converting the arrhythmia.

TABLE 35–16. ABLATION OF CARDIAC ARRHYTHMIAS

Arrhythmia	Operative Approach
Atrial fibrillation	Catheter ablation of AV node and implantation of a pacemaker The maze operation (experimental)
Ectopic atrial focus	Catheter ablation of the focus
PSVT (pre-excitation)	Catheter ablation of anomalous AV connection
PSVT (AV nodal)	Catheter ablation of AV slow pathway Retronodal surgical resection, division of His bundle, implantation of pacemaker
Ventricular tachycardia (coronary heart disease)	Endocardial resection guided by mapping
Ventricular tachycardia (arrhythmogenic right ventricular dysplasia)	Simple ventriculotomy; isolation of arrhythmic site
Ventricular tachycardia (after repair of tetralogy of Fallot)	Resection of infundibulectomy scar
Multiform ventricular tachycardia (long QT syndrome)	Left stellate ganglionectomy

AV reciprocating tachycardia and AV nodal reentrant tachycardia and has supplanted open-chest surgical ablation of these arrhythmias.

Supraventricular Arrhythmias

ATRIAL FLUTTER AND FIBRILLATION. Drug-resistant atrial flutter and fibrillation can be palliated by interrupting the His bundle and implanting a ventricular pacemaker. Catheter ablation with radiofrequency energy is the technique of choice. Rapid ventricular response is controlled by His bundle ablation, but loss of atrial transport function and vulnerability to thromboembolism are not. The maze procedure is a new operation that restores sinus rhythm. Experience with the operation is limited, but early reports suggest that atrial transport function is restored and risk of thromboembolism is reduced.

ABLATION OR EXCISION OF ECTOPIC ATRIAL FOCI. Rhythms originating in atrial automatic or tiny reentrant ectopic foci can be removed or ablated by catheter with radiofrequency energy or cryoablated during thoracotomy. The key to isolation, removal, or ablation is accurate localization by epicardial and/or endocardial activation mapping.

INTERRUPTING REENTRANT PATHWAYS. Surgery is effective and safe treatment for PSVT that depends on an anomalous AV connection or for atrial fibrillation with rapid ventricular response in the WPW syndrome. In the past few years, it has become possible to interrupt >90% of anomalous AV connections using catheter ablation, thus avoiding the need for thoracotomy. Also, >90% episodes of symptomatic PSVT due to reentrant AV nodal tachycardia can be cured with catheter ablation.

Sustained Ventricular Tachycardia

VT IN CORONARY HEART DISEASE. A large surgical experience is available for patients with recurrent, sustained VT and coronary heart disease; many of these patients have left ventricular aneurysms and severely impaired left ventricular function. Usually, VT is easily induced and relatively slow, which facilitates mapping during electrophysiologic studies. Accurate preoperative endocardial maps are critical because adequate endocardial maps are often impossible to obtain at surgery. During surgery, the arrhythmogenic tissue is removed or ablated with a cryoprobe. Map-guided excision, isolation, or cryoablation is about 80% effective in controlling sustained VT during 1 to 5 years of follow-up. The perioperative mortality is about 15% in patients with severe left ventricular dysfunction. Selection of ideal candidates lowers the mortality rate to about 5%. Ideal patients have (1) anterior aneurysms, (2) easily induced, easily mapped VT, (3) no concomitant valve replacement, (4) good function in the remaining left ventricle, and (5) amenability to excellent revascularization. Ideal patients have a 5 to 10% mortality rate. Those with prohibitive surgical risk are better managed with ICD's, catheter ablation, and/or drugs.

ARRHYTHMOGENIC RIGHT VENTRICULAR DYSPLASIA. Patients who have VT due to right ventricular arrhythmogenic dysplasia usually can be cured by an incision across the dysplastic area that shows the latest activation in sinus rhythm and earliest activation during VT. Small areas of dysplasia can be excised and large areas can be isolated if simple incision is not successful.

TETRALOGY OF FALLOT. VT occurs rarely in patients who have had total repair of tetralogy of Fallot. Epicardial excitation mapping at surgery shows that VT arises in the right ventricular infundibular scar, and scar resection effects a cure.

LONG QT SYNDROME. Patients with the congenital form of the long QT syndrome can have recurrent attacks of malignant, multiform VT of the torsades de pointes type. These rhythms are associated with cardiac arrest and sudden cardiac death. Unequal sympathetic nerve traffic to the heart contributes to the heterogeneous electrophysiologic condition of the ventricles. Excision of the left stellate ganglion and the first three or four left thoracic sympathetic ganglia markedly reduces the mortality rate in high-risk patients with the congenital long QT syndrome. Late failures have led some physicians to use ICD therapy in conjunction with sympathectomy.

Cox JL: The status of surgery for cardiac arrhythmias. Circulation 71:413, 1985. *A perspective on surgery for both supraventricular and ventricular arrhythmias.*

Cox JL: Patient selection criteria and results of surgery for refractory ischemic ventricular tachycardia. Circulation 79:163, 1989. *An update on selection of patients in the era of the automatic implantable cardioverter defibrillator.*

Cox JL, Boineau JP, Schuessler RB, et al.: Successful surgical treatment of atrial fibrillation. JAMA 266:976, 1991. *Atrial fibrillation is the most common of all sustained cardiac arrhythmias, yet it has no effective medical or surgical therapy. This article describes the development and early clinical experience with the maze procedure, a curative operation for atrial fibrillation.*

Cox JL, Gallagher JJ, Cain MM: Experience with 118 consecutive patients undergoing operation for the Wolff-Parkinson-White syndrome. J Thorac Cardiovasc Surg 90:490, 1985. *A review of a large, successful experience with surgery for anomalous AV connections.*

Guiraudon GM, Klein GJ, Sharma AD, Yee R: Surgical alternatives for supraventricular tachycardias. Am J Cardiol 64:92J, 1989. *A review of the operative treatment of a wide range of supraventricular tachycardias.*

Jackman WM, Beckman KJ, McClelland JH, et al.: Treatment of supraventricular tachycardia due to atrioventricular nodal reentry, by radiofrequency catheter ablation of slow-pathway conduction. N Engl J Med 327:313, 1992. *Technique, results, and follow-up in 80 patients.*

Jackman WM, Wang XZ, Friday KJ, et al.: Catheter ablation of accessory atrioventricular pathways (Wolff-Parkinson-White syndrome) by radiofrequency current. N Engl J Med 324:1605, 1991. *Technique, results, and follow-up in 166 patients.*

Klein GJ, Guiraudon GM: Surgical therapy of cardiac arrhythmias. Cardiol Clin 1:323, 1983. *A summary of concepts that form the basis for surgical treatment of cardiac arrhythmias.*

36 SUDDEN CARDIAC DEATH
Douglas P. Zipes

DEFINITION AND INCIDENCE

Sudden cardiac death is unexpected natural death from cardiac causes. The cardiac cause disturbs cardiac function, producing an abrupt loss of cerebral blood flow. Death occurs within 1 hour of the onset of acute symptoms. In 25% of patients who die of coronary heart disease, sudden cardiac death may be the first sign of trouble. Although some patients at risk for sudden cardiac death may be symptomatic prior to the event, their complaints are often too nonspecific to be helpful. An estimated 350,000 sudden cardiac deaths occur annually in the United States, or about one every 90 seconds. This represents almost half of all cardiovascular deaths and almost one fourth of all deaths. The incidence of sudden cardiac death due to coronary heart disease is declining, along with the overall decrease in coronary heart disease mortality. These decreases may relate to more frequent and effective treatment of hypertension, angina, and myocardial infarction and attention to additional risk factors.

The incidence of sudden cardiac death peaks between ages 0 and 6 months and between 45 and 75 years. Risk factors for sudden cardiac death parallel those for coronary heart disease and include being male, cardiac enlargement, obesity, cigarette smoking, glucose intolerance, hypertension, social isolation, stress, and excess alcohol consumption. The presence of coronary heart disease and past myocardial infarction (see Ch. 41.2) add additional risks. Following myocardial infarction, more than five to ten premature ventricular complexes (PVC's) per hour, three or more repetitive PVC's, late potentials recorded on signal-averaged electrocardiograms, and left ventricular dysfunction are variables identifying patients at increased risk of sudden cardiac death. Angiographic or hemodynamic characteristics are not significantly different between patients who have coronary artery disease and suffer sudden cardiac death and those who do not die suddenly.

Sudden cardiac death, stroke, and myocardial infarction all occur more frequently in the morning hours upon rising, from 6:00 A.M. to 12:00 noon, at a time when a hypercoagulable state with increased platelet aggregability or coronary vasoconstriction exists. Autonomic mechanisms may also be important in modulating this hypercoagulable state and in triggering sudden cardiac death. There appears to be an additional risk for sudden cardiac death during physical exertion.

This study was supported in part by the Herman C. Krannert Fund, Indianapolis; Grants HL-42370 and HL-07182 from the National Heart, Lung and Blood Institute, National Institutes of Health, Bethesda, Md; and the American Heart Association, Indiana Affiliate, Indianapolis.

TABLE 36-1. CAUSES AND CONTRIBUTING FACTORS IN SUDDEN CARDIAC DEATH

I. **Coronary artery abnormalities**
   A. Coronary atherosclerosis
      1. Chronic ischemic heart disease with transient supply/demand imbalance—thrombosis, spasm, physical stress
      2. Acute myocardial infarction
      3. Chronic atherosclerosis with change in myocardial substrate
   B. Congenital abnormalities of coronary arteries
      1. Anomalous origin from pulmonary artery
      2. Other coronary AV fistula
      3. Origin of left coronary artery from right sinus of Valsalva
      4. Origin of right coronary artery from left sinus of Valsalva
      5. Hypoplastic or aplastic coronary arteries
      6. Coronary-intracardiac shunt
   C. Coronary artery embolism
      1. Aortic or mitral endocarditis
      2. Prosthetic aortic or mitral valves
      3. Abnormal native valves or LV mural thrombus
      4. Platelet embolism
   D. Coronary arteritis
      1. Polyarteritis nodosa, progressive systemic sclerosis, giant cell arteritis
      2. Mucocutaneous lymph node syndrome (Kawasaki's disease)
      3. Syphilitic coronary ostial stenosis
   E. Miscellaneous mechanical obstruction of coronary arteries
      1. Coronary artery dissection in Marfan syndrome
      2. Coronary artery dissection in pregnancy
      3. Prolapse of aortic valve myxomatous polyps into coronary ostia
      4. Dissection or rupture of sinus of Valsalva
   F. Functional obstruction of coronary arteries
      1. Coronary artery spasm with or without atherosclerosis
      2. Myocardial bridges

II. **Hypertrophy of ventricular myocardium**
   A. Left ventricular hypertrophy associated with coronary atherosclerosis
   B. Hypertensive heart disease without significant coronary atherosclerosis
   C. Hypertrophic myocardium secondary to valvular heart disease
   D. Hypertrophic cardiomyopathy
      1. Obstructive
      2. Nonobstructive
   E. Primary or secondary pulmonary hypertension
      1. Advanced chronic right ventricular overload
      2. Pulmonary hypertension in pregnancy

III. **Myocardial diseases and heart failure**
   A. Chronic congestive heart failure
      1. Ischemic cardiomyopathy
      2. Idiopathic congestive cardiomyopathy
      3. Alcoholic cardiomyopathy
      4. Hypertensive cardiomyopathy
      5. Post-myocarditis cardiomyopathy
      6. Postpartum cardiomyopathy
   B. Acute cardiac failure
      1. Massive acute myocardial infarction
      2. Acute myocarditis
      3. Acute alcoholic cardiac dysfunction
      4. Ball-valve embolism in aortic stenosis or prosthesis
      5. Mechanical disruptions of cardiac structures
         (a) Rupture of ventricular free wall
         (b) Disruption of mitral apparatus
            (1) Papillary muscle
            (2) Chordae tendineae
            (3) Leaflet
         (c) Rupture of interventricular septum
      6. Acute pulmonary edema in noncompliant ventricles

IV. **Inflammatory, infiltrative, neoplastic, and degenerative processes**
   A. Acute viral myocarditis with or without ventricular dysfunction
   B. Myocarditis associated with the vasculitides
   C. Sarcoidosis
   D. Progressive systemic sclerosis
   E. Amyloidosis
   F. Hemochromatosis
   G. Idiopathic giant cell myocarditis
   H. Chagas' disease
   I. Cardiac ganglionitis
   J. Arrhythmogenic right ventricular dysplasia
   K. Neuromuscular diseases (e.g., muscular dystrophy, Friedreich's ataxia, myotonic dystrophy)
   L. Intramural tumors
      1. Primary
      2. Metastatic

M. Obstructive intracavitary tumors
      1. Neoplastic
      2. Thrombotic

V. **Diseases of the cardiac valves**
   A. Valvular aortic stenosis/insufficiency
   B. Mitral valve disruption
   C. Mitral valve prolapse
   D. Endocarditis
   E. Prosthetic valve dysfunction

VI. **Congenital heart disease**
   A. Congenital aortic or pulmonic valve stenosis
   B. Right-to-left shunts with Eisenmenger's physiology
      1. Advanced disease
      2. During labor and delivery
   C. After surgical repair of congenital lesions, e.g., tetralogy of Fallot

VII. **Electrophysiologic abnormalities**
   A. Abnormalities of the conducting system
      1. Fibrosis of the His-Purkinje system
         (a) Primary degeneration (Lenègre's disease)
         (b) Secondary to fibrosis and calcification of the "cardiac skeleton" (Lev's disease)
         (c) Post-viral conducting system fibrosis
         (d) Hereditary conducting system disease
      2. Anomalous pathways of conduction
   B. Prolonged QT interval syndrome
      1. Congenital
         (a) With deafness
         (b) Without deafness
      2. Acquired
         (a) Drug effect
         (b) Electrolyte abnormality
         (c) Toxic substances
         (d) Hypothermia
         (e) CNS injury
   C. Idiopathic ventricular fibrillation
      1. Absence of identifiable structural or functional causes
      2. Sleep-death in Southeast Asians
         (a) Bangungut
         (b) Pokkuri
         (c) Nonlaitai

VIII. **Electrical instability related to neurohumoral and central nervous system influences**
   A. Catecholamine-dependent lethal arrhythmias
   B. CNS-related
      1. Psychic stress, emotional extremes
      2. Auditory-related
      3. "Voodoo" death in primitive cultures
      4. Diseases of the cardiac nerves
      5. Congenital QT interval prolongation

IX. **Sudden infant death syndrome and sudden death in children**
   A. Sudden infant death syndrome
      1. Immature respiratory control functions
      2. Susceptibility to lethal arrhythmias
      3. Congenital heart disease
      4. Myocarditis
   B. Sudden death in children
      1. Eisenmenger's syndrome, aortic stenosis, hypertrophic cardiomyopathy, pulmonary atresia
      2. After corrective surgery for congenital heart disease
      3. Myocarditis
      4. Unexplained

X. **Miscellaneous**
   A. Sudden death during extreme physical activity
   B. Mechanical interference with venous return
      1. Acute cardiac tamponade
      2. Massive pulmonary embolism
      3. Acute intracardiac thrombosis
   C. Dissecting aneurysm of the aorta
   D. Toxic/metabolic disturbances
      1. Electrolyte disturbances
      2. Metabolic disturbances
      3. Proarrhythmic effects of antiarrhythmic drugs
      4. Proarrhythmic effects of noncardiac drugs
   E. Mimics of sudden cardiac death
      1. "Cafe coronary"
      2. Acute alcoholic states ("holiday heart")
      3. Acute asthmatic attacks
      4. Air or amniotic fluid embolism

From Meyerburg RJ, Castellanos A: Cardiac arrest and sudden cardiac death. *In* Braunwald E (ed.): Heart Disease: A Textbook of Cardiovascular Medicine. 4th ed. Philadelphia, WB Saunders, 1992, pp 761–762.

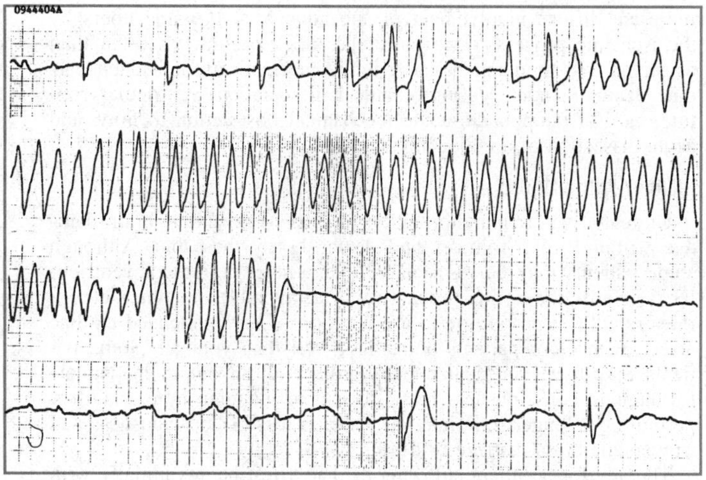

FIGURE 36-1. Continuous ECG recordings in a dying patient. The top tracing demonstrates the presence of complete AV block with a junctional escape rhythm that evolves into ventricular tachycardia. The latter spontaneously terminates *(third tracing)* and is replaced by complete AV block and ventricular asystole interrupted by two ventricular escape complexes *(bottom tracing).*

CAUSES

SUBSTRATE AND TRIGGERS. Ventricular myocardial abnormalities such as hypertrophy, dilated cardiomyopathy, inflammatory changes, diseases of the heart valves, and primary electrophysiologic abnormalities (Table 36-1) are responsible for about 25% of sudden cardiac deaths, with the remaining 75% due to coronary artery disease. Drugs such as cocaine (see Ch. 12) are assuming greater importance as causes of sudden cardiac death. Occasionally, patients without structural heart disease suffer ventricular fibrillation. The long QT syndrome is one of several electrophysiologic abnormalities that can predispose to sudden cardiac death (Table 36-1). It may be acquired by exposure to several antiarrhythmic drugs such as quinidine, phenothiazines, and tricyclic antidepressants or may result from electrolyte disturbances such as hypokalemia or hypomagnesemia. Less commonly, drugs such as terfenadine (Seldane) or erythromycin can be responsible. It may also be congenital, with (Jervell-Lange-Nielsen syndrome) and without (Romano-Ward syndrome) neural deafness. Preliminary information suggests that a specific electrophysiologic mechanism is responsible, called early afterdepolarizations.

At autopsy, $\geq 90\%$ narrowing of at least one coronary artery is noted in three quarters of patients dying of sudden cardiac death, and almost two thirds have three vessels with $\geq 75\%$ stenosis. Old myocardial infarction is found in about two thirds of autopsies. Significant narrowing of the proximal left anterior descending coronary artery has been associated with an increased risk of sudden cardiac death. Acute thrombotic occlusion is noted in 60 to 75%, usually at the site of a fissured plaque, providing clues about mechanisms of sudden cardiac death. For example, in sudden cardiac death, as in unstable angina, plaque rupture with thrombus formation may result in myocardial ischemia and precipitate fatal ventricular arrhythmias. Also, platelet microthrombi from ulcerated arterial plaques can produce multiple areas of myocardial necrosis that can cause electrical instability and ventricular fibrillation. It is likely that a non-flow-limiting intimal plaque serves as a nidus for acute formation of a lumen-occluding thrombus in a significant number of patients with sudden cardiac death. Coronary artery spasm or other factors that reduce myocardial blood flow without an increase in demand, as well as an increase in myocardial oxygen demand with a fixed supply, may be critical. Blacks may be at higher risk for cardiac arrest and subsequent death than whites.

Only 20% of patients who are successfully resuscitated from ventricular fibrillation progress to an acute myocardial infarction. This means that if thrombosis of a coronary artery causes the ischemia responsible for the ventricular fibrillation, it is transient because flow must be restored to prevent infarction. Ventricular fibrillation recurs in 30% within 1 year and 45% by 2 years in those survivors who do not, versus only about 2% in those who do suffer a transmural myocardial infarction after resuscitation. Therefore, patients without infarction are at increased risk for sudden cardiac death.

Ischemia is conducive to developing arrhythmias. Myocardial ischemia results in loss of membrane integrity with cellular efflux of potassium and influx of calcium, development of acidosis, reduction of transmembrane resting potentials, and enhanced automaticity in some tissues. Reperfusion causes continued influx of calcium, which may result in arrhythmias. The electrophysiologic changes following myocardial ischemia can create areas of slow conduction and unidirectional block, changes necessary for reentry to occur, as well as areas of abnormal automaticity and triggered activity. These factors can lead to ventricular tachycardia/fibrillation. Tissue healed after previous injury and hypertrophied myocardium appear more susceptible to the electrical destabilizing effects of acute ischemia. The combination of a triggering event such as a PVC's and a susceptible myocardium may be the fundamental combination for developing a lethal arrhythmia. Triggering events and a susceptible myocardium may be dissociated from each other so that in the absence of a susceptible myocardium, triggering events such as autonomic factors may occur innocuously. Similarly, the presence of a susceptible myocardium without a triggering event may not give rise to arrhythmias.

ARRHYTHMIAS. More than 90% of sudden cardiac deaths are due to a lethal cardiac rhythm disturbance, approximately 80% to ventricular tachycardia/fibrillation (Fig. 36-1), and 20% to a severe bradyarrhythmia or ventricular asystole (Fig. 36-2). Loss of sinus rate variability, decreased baroreceptor sensitivity, and ST-T wave alternans occur in the electrically unstable ventricle. Ventricular tachycardia leading to ventricular fibrillation is often preceded by increases in sinus rate, advancing grades of ventricular ectopy, and loss of sinus arrhythmia (suggesting a decrease in vagal tone and/or an increase in sympathetic activity). Only a small percentage of patients have ischemic ST changes. Bradycardia and ventricular asystole occur more commonly in a severely diseased heart and may

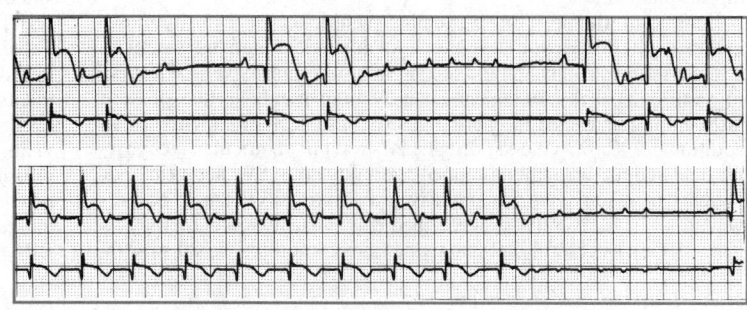

FIGURE 36-2. AV block during chest pain. The patient has atypical angina characterized by episodes of chest pain with ST segment elevation. Sinus rhythm conducts with first-degree AV block. Short episodes of atrial flutter block entirely, causing long periods of ventricular asystole.

represent diffuse involvement of subendocardial Purkinje fibers by the ischemic process. Atrioventricular block occurs less often than asystole. Less frequent nonarrhythmic mechanisms of sudden cardiac death include electromechanical dissociation, ventricular rupture, cardiac tamponade, acute mechanical obstruction to flow, and acute dissection of a major blood vessel.

THERAPY AND OUTCOME

Untreated ventricular fibrillation produces irreversible brain damage within 3 to 5 minutes and death shortly thereafter. Although some patients may be resuscitated after longer periods of ventricular tachyarrhythmia, the probability of a favorable outcome deteriorates rapidly in proportion to the duration of the unattended cardiac arrest, with older patients doing less well than younger. Some patients may have ventricular tachycardia with an output inadequate to maintain consciousness but sufficient to maintain brain viability, permitting a longer time interval between loss of consciousness and irreversible brain damage or death.

Therapy for a patient suffering cardiac arrest begins initially with establishing the diagnosis of the cardiac arrest, delivering a blow to the chest to attempt "thumpversion" of ventricular tachycardia, and clearing the airway. Basic life-support activities including mouth-to-mouth ventilation and chest compression should be started and continued until advanced life-support activities begin, which initially include electrical cardioversion/defibrillation to treat ventricular tachycardia/fibrillation, pacing for bradyarrhythmia/asystole, and drug administration. After successful resuscitation, the patient is admitted to a monitoring unit, where treatment goals are to provide hemodynamic support, prevent a second cardiac arrest, and evaluate causes of the first.

Early ventricular defibrillation is the most important factor influencing survival. In hospital, no time should be wasted in instituting electrical cardioversion or defibrillation. Out of hospital, prompt cardiopulmonary resuscitation (CPR) (see Ch. 67) by bystander laypersons awaiting the arrival of emergency rescue personnel significantly improves the percentage of patients subsequently discharged alive from the hospital. Presumably this difference is due to CPR-related protection of the central nervous system.

Elements required to achieve the highest survival rates from out-of-hospital cardiac arrest include witnessed arrest, rapid telephone notification of the emergency medical service, early initiation of cardiopulmonary resuscitation, rapid arrival of emergency personnel equipped with a defibrillator, early advanced airway management, and prompt intravenous drug therapy. Significant risk factors for death after cardiopulmonary resuscitation include hypotension and pneumonia prior to arrest, time for restoration of normal rhythm exceeding 15 minutes, need to intubate, the presence of hypotension, and, after resuscitation, a need for vasopressors.

The rhythm disturbance responsible for the cardiac arrest influences outcome dramatically. Patients who have ventricular tachycardia have the best prognosis but comprise the smallest group, only about 10% of all cardiac arrests. It is possible that many more cardiac arrests begin as sustained ventricular tachycardia and progress to ventricular fibrillation and that patients found with ventricular tachycardia do better because their arrest is treated earlier. Of patients who have ventricular fibrillation, 40 to 60% are successfully resuscitated and admitted to the hospital alive, and about half of those are ultimately discharged. Patients who have bradyarrhythmia or asystole as the initiating event or at initial contact have the worst prognosis, with only about 10% admitted to hospital alive and few if any subsequently surviving. Similarly, patients whose rhythm following defibrillation is a bradyarrhythmia of less than 60 beats per minute also have a poor prognosis, with 95% dying prior to or during hospitalization.

Long-term therapy for preventing ventricular tachyarrhythmias includes pharmacologic, electrical, and surgical options (see Ch. 35). Serial electrophysiologic testing and/or noninvasive assessment of ventricular arrhythmias can identify drug regimens that prevent arrhythmia recurrence in approximately 20 to 40% of patients. In an additional 20% of patients, drugs can slow the ventricular tachycardia and reduce arrhythmia-related mortality to <3% per year. For patients in whom ventricular tachycardia/fibrillation cannot be prevented or significantly slowed, medical antiarrhythmic therapy is generally unsuccessful and the sudden death mortality is 20 to 40%

per year. In these patients, surgically resecting the arrhythmogenic substrate or implanting a pacemaker/cardioverter/defibrillator may be indicated; both methods are highly effective in preventing sudden cardiac death. The choice of procedure depends on the arrhythmia diagnosis and the nature of the cardiac disease. Because operative mortality is 5 to 15% for surgical resection versus <1% for nonthoracotomy device implantation, with left ventricular function being the most important predictor of risk, defibrillator implantation appears to be replacing endocardial resection. Arrhythmic mortality following device implantation is <2% per year.

Bardy GH, Hofer B, Johnson G, et al.: Implantable transvenous cardioverter defibrillators. Circulation 87:1152, 1993. *An original article reporting the outcome in 84 patients with ventricular tachycardia, fibrillation, or both who received an implantable cardioverter-defibrillator, with 98% patient survival over 11 months follow-up.*
Cohen TJ, Goldner BG, Maccaro PC, et al.: A comparison of active compression-decompression cardiopulmonary resuscitation with standard cardiopulmonary resuscitation for cardiac arrests occurring in the hospital. N Engl J Med 329:1918, 1993. *A prospective randomized trial between standard CPR versus using a suction device providing active compression-decompression, showing the latter to be superior.*
Mason JW: A comparison of electrophysiologic testing with Holter monitoring to predict antiarrhythmic-drug efficacy for ventricular tachyarrhythmias. N Engl J Med 329:445, 1993. *A prospective randomized comparison of noninvasive versus invasive testing to determine antiarrhythmic drug efficacy, showing no significant difference in the success of drug therapy as selected by the two methods.*
Myerburg RJ, Kessler KM, Castellanos A: Sudden cardiac death: Epidemiology, transient risk and intervention assessment. Ann Intern Med 119:1187, 1993. *A review of the causes of sudden cardiac death.*
Vlay SC, Burger L, Vlay LC, et al.: Prediction of sudden cardiac arrest: Risk stratification by anatomic substrate. Am Heart J 126:807, 1993. *An original study showing that significant narrowing of the maximal left anterior descending coronary artery was associated with an increased risk of sudden cardiac death.*

37 ARTERIAL HYPERTENSION
Suzanne Oparil

Systemic hypertension is the most prevalent cardiovascular disorder in the United States, affecting >50 million Americans. Almost 40% of all black adults and more than half of the entire population over age 60 have hypertension. In spite of increasing public awareness and a rapidly expanding array of antihypertensive medications, hypertension remains one of the most common risk factors for cardiovascular morbidity and mortality. Efforts to prevent, diagnose, and treat hypertension remain an important concern of national health care. Advances in diagnosing and treating hypertension have played a major role in the decline in coronary heart disease and stroke mortality that has occurred in the last 20 years (Fig. 37–1). Recent data from the National Health and Nutrition Examination Surveys (NHANES) indicate that major progress has been made in public awareness of the importance of hypertension, introducing antihypertensive therapies, and in controlling hypertension in the population (Fig. 37–2). However, the adverse metabolic effects of some classes of antihypertensive drugs and the disappointing results of antihypertensive treatment in preventing coronary disease have raised questions that challenge traditional approaches to managing the hypertensive patient. Antihypertensive treatment should be undertaken in the context of overall management of cardiovascular disease risk factors, and its ultimate goal should be to reduce overall cardiovascular risk.

DEFINITION

Hypertension in individuals aged ≥18 years is defined and classified by the Joint National Committee on Detection, Evaluation, and Treatment of High Blood Pressure (JNC V report), as shown in Table 37–1. The diagnosis of hypertension in adults is made when the average of two or more diastolic blood pressure (BP) measurements on at least two subsequent visits is ≥90 mm Hg or when the average of multiple systolic BP readings on two or more subsequent visits is consistently >140 mm Hg. The patient should be clearly informed that a single elevated reading does not constitute a diagnosis of hypertension but is a sign that further observation is required. *Isolated systolic hypertension (ISH)* is defined as systolic BP ≥140 mm Hg and diastolic BP <90 mm Hg. *Essential, pri-*

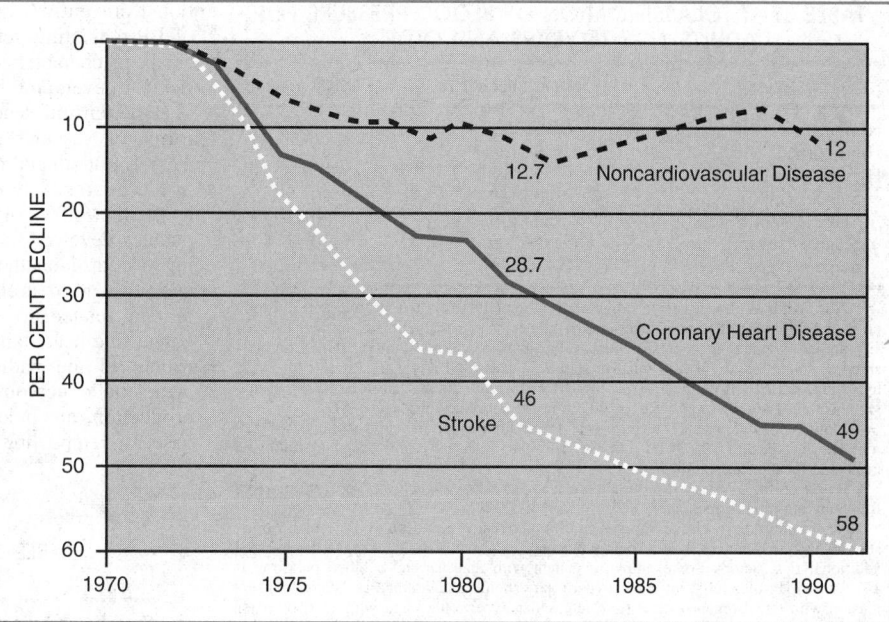

FIGURE 37-1. Temporal trends in death rates, adjusted for age, from noncardiovascular disease, coronary heart disease, and stroke in the US population from 1972 to the present. The numbers refer to percent decline from 1972 figures to 1982 and 1992. (Modified from Joint National Committee on Detection, Evaluation, and Treatment of High Blood Pressure: The Fifth Report of the Joint National Committee on Detection, Evaluation, and Treatment of High Blood Pressure (JNC V). Arch Intern Med 153:154, 1993.)

mary, or *idiopathic hypertension* is systemic hypertension of unknown cause. More than 95% of all cases of hypertension are in this category. *Secondary hypertension* is systemic hypertension of known cause. Fewer than 5% of all cases of systemic hypertension are in this category. The importance of identifying patients with secondary hypertension is that they sometimes can be cured by surgery or can be easily controlled by specific medical treatment. Thus the morbidity and mortality of potentially ineffective empiric medical therapy can be avoided and the cumulative cost of medical treatment reduced. The most common causes of secondary hypertension are summarized in Table 37-2.

Malignant hypertension is the syndrome of markedly elevated BP (diastolic BP usually >140 mm Hg) associated with papilledema. *Accelerated hypertension* is the syndrome of markedly elevated BP associated with hemorrhages and exudates (grade 3 Kimmelstiel-Wilson [K-W] retinopathy). If untreated, accelerated hypertension presumably progresses to a malignant phase. Both accelerated and

malignant hypertension are associated with widespread degenerative changes in the walls of resistance vessels. These syndromes are characterized by extreme BP elevations, sudden onset, fulminant course, and evidence of severe, generalized vascular damage, including grade 3 or 4 K-W retinopathy, hypertensive encephalopathy, hematuria, and renal dysfunction. Malignant hypertension is usually fatal unless treated promptly and vigorously. If BP can be controlled, prognosis depends on the state of renal function.

Complicated hypertension is the descriptive term for arterial hypertension of any cause in which there is evidence of cardiovascular damage related to the BP elevation. Hypertensive complications commonly include stroke, congestive heart failure, renal failure, myocardial infarction, and arterial aneurysm.

People with *high normal BP* tend to maintain pressures that are above average for the general population and are at greater risk of developing definite hypertension and of experiencing nonfatal and fatal cardiovascular events than the general population. As a group,

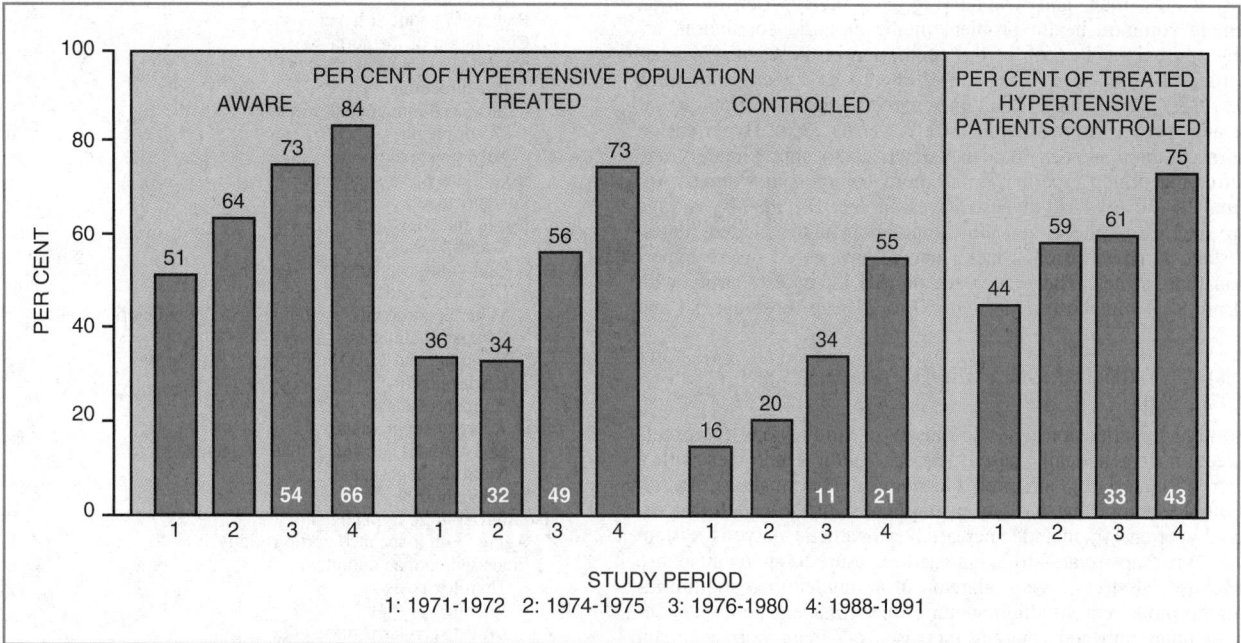

FIGURE 37-2. Hypertension awareness, treatment, and control rates reported in the National Health and Nutrition Examination Surveys (NHANES). Numbers outside bars are based on a hypertensive threshold of ≥160/95; numbers inside bars are based on a hypertensive threshold of ≥140/90. (From Thom TJ, et al.: Trends in blood pressure control and mortality. *In* Izzo JL, Black HR (eds.): Hypertension Primer. Dallas, American Heart Association, 1993, p 207.)

TABLE 37–1. CLASSIFICATION OF BLOOD PRESSURE FOR ADULTS AGE 18 YEARS AND OLDER*

Category	Systolic (mm Hg)	Diastolic (mm Hg)
Normal†	<130	<85
High normal	130–139	85–89
Hypertension‡		
Stage 1 (mild)	140–159	90–99
Stage 2 (moderate)	160–179	100–109
Stage 3 (severe)	180–209	110–119
Stage 4 (very severe)	≥210	≥120

* Not taking antihypertensive drugs and not acutely ill. When systolic and diastolic pressures fall into different categories, the higher category should be selected to classify the individual's blood pressure status. For instance, 160/92 mm Hg should be classified as stage 2, and 180/120 mm Hg should be classified as stage 4. Isolated systolic hypertension (ISH) is defined as systolic BP ≥ 140 mm Hg and diastolic BP <90 mm Hg and staged appropriately (e.g., 170/85 mm Hg is defined as stage 2 ISH).

† Optimal blood pressure with respect to cardiovascular risk is systolic BP <120 mm Hg and diastolic BP <80 mm Hg. However, unusually low readings should be evaluated for clinical significance.

‡ Based on the average of two or more readings taken at each of two or more visits following an initial screening.

Note: In addition to classifying stages of hypertension based on average blood pressure levels, the clinician should specify presence or absence of target-organ disease and additional risk factors. For example, a patient with diabetes and a blood pressure of 142/94 mm Hg plus left ventricular hypertrophy should be classified as "stage 1 hypertension with target-organ disease (left ventricular hypertrophy) and with another major risk factor (diabetes)." This specificity is important for risk classification and management.

From Joint National Committee on Detection, Evaluation, and Treatment of High Blood Pressure: The Fifth Report of the Joint National Committee on Detection, Evaluation, and Treatment of High Blood Pressure (JNC V). Arch Intern Med 153:154, 1993.

these people manifest increased cardiac output, more rapid heart rate, and higher left ventricular ejection rate than either the normotensive population or the population of patients with stable hypertension.

White coat hypertension refers to the situation in which a patient's BP is elevated when measured by a physician or other health care personnel but normal when measured outside of the health care setting. The syndrome is best diagnosed by 24-hour ambulatory BP monitoring or home BP monitoring but may be suspected based on any reliable BP measurements outside of the health care setting.

INCIDENCE AND PREVALENCE

The prevalence of hypertension increases with age in all groups: blacks, whites, men, and women (Fig. 37–3). Hypertension is an extremely common health problem in the geriatric population, afflicting approximately 65% of the population in the 65- to 74-year-old group. Blacks have a higher prevalence of hypertension than whites (38% versus 29%), and men have a higher overall prevalence of hypertension than women (33% versus 27%). Hypertension is more common in men than in women up to approximately age 50; after that time, hypertension is more common in women. Approximately 70% of all hypertensives in the 18- to 74-year age group, or 15% of the entire adult population of the United States, have stage 1 hypertension. Blacks tend to have more severe hypertension than whites. The prevalence of ISH increases sharply with age from <5% in those under age 50 to 22% in those age 80 and older.

ETIOLOGY AND PATHOGENESIS OF ESSENTIAL HYPERTENSION AND ITS CARDIOVASCULAR COMPLICATIONS

Essential hypertension tends to cluster in families and represents a collection of genetically based diseases and/or syndromes with a number of underlying inherited biochemical abnormalities. Pathophysiologic factors that have been implicated in the genesis of essential hypertension include increased sympathetic nervous system activity—perhaps related to heightened exposure to and/or response to psychosocial stress, overproduction of an unidentified sodium-retaining hormone, chronic high sodium intake, inadequate dietary intakes of potassium and calcium, increased or "inappropriate" renin secretion, deficiencies of vasodilators such as prostaglandins and nitric oxide, congenital abnormalities of the resistance vessels, diabetes mellitus, insulin resistance, obesity, increased activity of vascular growth factors, and altered cellular ion transport. The tools of

molecular biology provide for the first time the means of defining the genetic basis of the hypertensive diseases and for designing rational preventive and therapeutic strategies. To date, no specific set of BP-regulating genes has been identified, nor have genetic markers been characterized that permit early detection of individuals at risk for developing hypertension.

Hypertension leads to atherosclerosis (see Ch. 40) and other forms of vascular pathology by damaging the endothelium (Fig. 37–4). Endothelial damage results in the cascade of events depicted in the figure. If hypertension is accompanied by hyperlipidemia, as it is in >40% of the US population, lipid-rich atherosclerotic plaques develop. In the absence of hyperlipidemia, intimal thickening occurs. Nonatherosclerotic hypertension-induced vascular damage can lead to stroke and end-stage renal disease, and increased afterload related to systemic hypertension is a leading cause of congestive heart failure. Further, the neurohumoral factors that contribute to the pathogenesis of hypertension, including increased sympathetic nervous system activity and enhanced angiotensin II production, are independent causes of myocardial hypertrophy and vascular remodeling.

TABLE 37–2. CAUSES OF SECONDARY HYPERTENSION

Systolic and diastolic hypertension
  Renal
    Renal parenchymal disease
      Chronic nephritis
      Polycystic disease
      Collagen vascular disease
      Diabetic nephropathy
      Hydronephrosis
      Acute glomerulonephritis
    Renal vascular disease
    Renal transplantation
    Renin-secreting tumors
  Endocrine
    Adrenal
      Primary aldosteronism
      Overproduction of 11-deoxycorticosterone (DOC), 18-OH-DOC, and other mineralocorticoids
      Congenital adrenal hyperplasia
      Cushing's syndrome
      Pheochromocytoma
    Extra-adrenal chromaffin tumors
    Hyperparathyroidism
    Acromegaly
  Pregnancy-induced hypertension
  Coarctation of the aorta
  Neurologic disorders
    Dysautonomia
    Increased intracranial pressure
    Quadriplegia
    Lead poisoning
    Guillain-Barré syndrome
  Postoperative
  Drugs and chemicals
    Cyclosporine
    Oral contraceptives
    Glucocorticoids
    Mineralocorticoids, including licorice and carbenoxolone
    Sympathomimetics
    Tyramine and MAO inhibitors
    Erythropoietin
    Antidepressants
    Appetite suppressants
    Nonsteroidal anti-inflammatory agents
    Nasal decongestants
    Phenothiazines
Isolated systolic hypertension
  Aging, with associated aortic rigidity
  Increased cardiac output
    Thyrotoxicosis
    Anemia
    Aortic valvular insufficiency
  Decreased peripheral vascular resistance
    Arteriovenous shunts
    Paget's disease of bone
    Beriberi

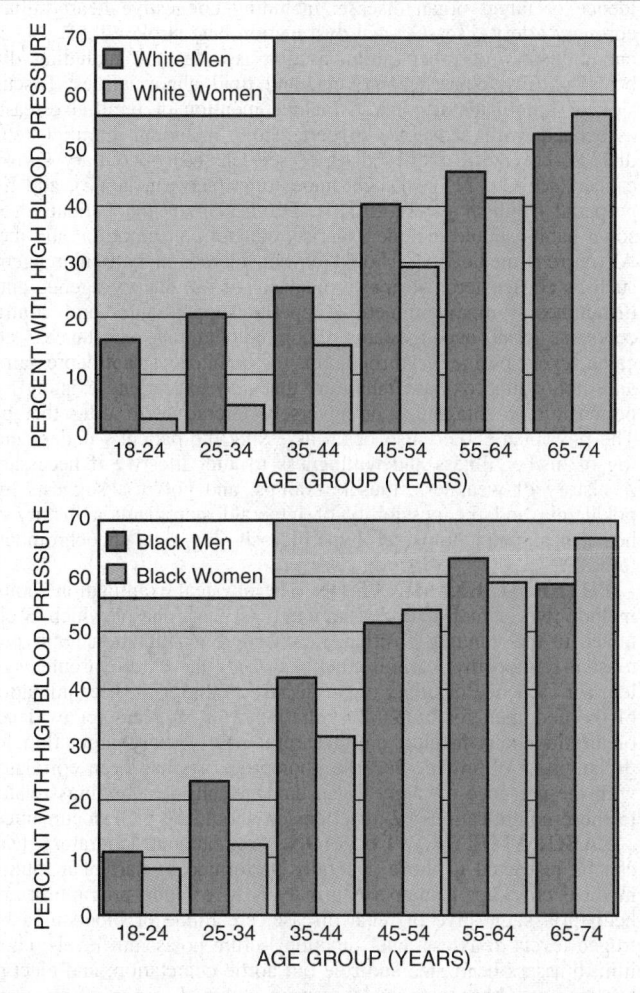

FIGURE 37–3. Prevalence rates of high blood pressure by race, gender, and age. Second National Health and Nutrition Examination Survey, 1976–1980. Based on the average of three blood pressure measurements with systolic blood pressure ≥ 140 mm Hg and/or diastolic blood pressure ≥ 90 mm Hg. (From Drizd T, et al.: Blood pressure levels in persons 18–74 years of age in 1976–80, and trends in blood pressure from 1960 to 1980 in the United States. Vital Health Stat 234:1, 1986.)

DIAGNOSIS

INITIAL EVALUATION. The initial evaluation of the hypertensive patient should determine baseline arterial BP, assess the degree of target organ disease, screen for secondary causes of hypertension, identify other cardiovascular risk factors, and characterize the patient (gender, race, age, lifestyle, concomitant illnesses) to facilitate the choice of therapy, in particular drug selection.

BP MEASUREMENT. The accurate and reproducible measurement of BP by the cuff technique is the most crucial part of the diagnostic evaluation. On the initial visit, the BP should be taken after the patient has been seated comfortably for at least 5 minutes with his or her arm bared. The upper arm should not be constricted by a rolled sleeve, as it distorts the BP measurement. Two or three measurements should be taken at each visit, and at least 2 minutes should be allowed between readings. Proper cuff size is critical to accurately measuring BP. The width should be about two thirds the width of the arm (15 cm in most adults), and, more important, the bladder cuff should be long enough to circle the arm. Falsely elevated readings can be obtained when the bladder is too short, and the error is magnified if the cuff is also too narrow. Mercury manometers are more accurate, but aneroid manometers can be used if they are standardized frequently against a mercury manometer.

To obtain an accurate systolic BP, the cuff should be inflated rapidly to at least 30 mm Hg above the systolic BP, as determined by palpating the radial artery. This inflation is necessary to avoid underestimating the BP because of the auscultatory gap, an unexplained disappearance of Korotkoff's sounds for some interval between systole and diastole. The systolic reading is taken as the level of BP at which clear Korotkoff's sounds are heard with each heart beat. The diastolic reading is taken at the level both when sounds become muffled (Korotkoff phase IV) and when sounds disappear (phase V). Both readings should be recorded. It is not known whether the level of muffling or of disappearance more accurately reflects the intra-arterial diastolic BP, so selecting one over the other as the clinical measurement of diastolic BP is a matter of convenience and reproducibility. Baseline BP should be calculated from the average of two separate measurements determined at least 2 weeks apart. However, patients with diastolic BP's >115 mm Hg or elevated BP with evidence of ongoing target organ damage should be started on therapy immediately.

Measurement of BP by patients or family members and/or automated ambulatory BP monitoring often helps verify the diagnosis and assess the severity of hypertension. BP values obtained outside of the clinic setting have consistently been shown to be lower and to better correlate with target organ damage than BP measurements

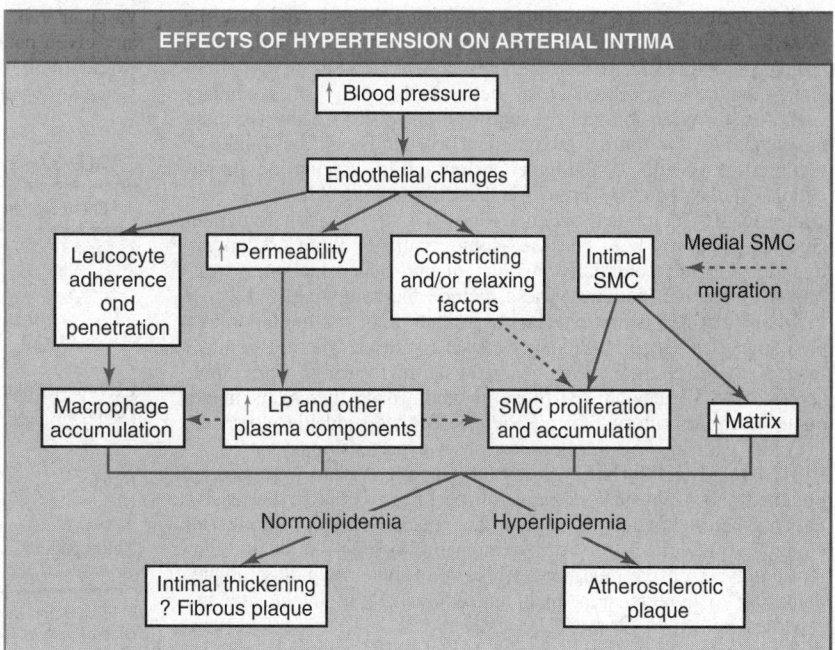

FIGURE 37–4. Mechanism by which hypertension produces accelerated atherosclerosis and vascular remodeling. SMC = smooth muscle cell; LP = lipoprotein. (Modified from Chobanian AV: 1989 Corcoran Lecture: Adaptive and maladaptive responses of the arterial wall to hypertension. Hypertension 15:666, 1990.)

by health care personnel. Therefore, assessment of the need to treat and the efficacy of treatment is augmented by considering both clinic and outside-of-clinic BP measurements. The superiority of home or workplace BP measurements depends on use of accurate and calibrated BP monitors and careful and repeated instruction in how to measure BP.

In patients with stage 1 and early stage 2 untreated hypertension (diastolic BP 90 to 104 mm Hg), the prevalence of white coat hypertension is approximately 20%. In patients receiving antihypertensive therapy, the white coat phenomenon is just as common, occurring in 30% of patients. In patients with more severe hypertension (diastolic BP $\geq$ 105 mm Hg), this syndrome is seen in only 5% of patients. The cause of white coat hypertension is unknown but is likely an anxiety response to having one's health assessed or perhaps a conditioned response, i.e., an initial anxiety response that has been reinforced and perhaps amplified through patient/physician interactions (see Ch. 14.1).

The long-term significance of white coat hypertension is unknown, so treatment recommendations are not well defined. White coat hypertension, like primary hypertension, has an increased association with other coronary risk factors, such as obesity, insulin resistance, and elevated LDL levels. However, evidence of increased target organ damage has not been found consistently in patients with white coat hypertension. Until long-term prospective studies can clarify this issue, a conservative therapeutic approach is recommended. BP's obtained outside of the clinic setting should be monitored. Nonpharmacologic antihypertensive therapy should be prescribed for all patients. In subjects who have white coat hypertension without evidence of target organ damage, pharmacologic therapy is likely unnecessary; however, if target organ damage is present—particularly if it is progressive—pharmacologic therapy may be beneficial but should be administered cautiously to avoid overtreatment. Repeat ambulatory BP measurements may be useful in avoiding overmedication.

Determining BP accurately can be particularly difficult in elderly patients owing to stiffening of arterial walls. The loss of arterial wall compliance can result in falsely elevated BP measurements by using a standard sphygmomanometer, so-called *pseudohypertension*. Such an occurrence should be suspected in elderly patients diagnosed as having hypertension but lacking evidence of target organ damage. The *Osler maneuver* can sometimes identify this phenomenon. During the Osler maneuver, the BP cuff is inflated above the level of systolic BP. If the pulseless radial or brachial artery remains palpable, stiffening of the artery may be sufficient to falsely elevate the BP measurement. Intra-arterial BP determinations may be necessary to accurately diagnose hypertension in this setting.

Selection of Patients for Evaluation for Secondary Hypertension

Once a diagnosis of stable hypertension has been established, the need for antihypertensive treatment should be assessed, and, where indicated, diagnostic evaluation for secondary causes of hypertension should be undertaken. In view of the rarity of secondary causes of hypertension and the high cost and risk of elaborate diagnostic studies, the routine pretreatment workup should be limited to defining the severity of the hypertension and identifying its complications and associated cardiovascular risk factors. All of the secondary causes combined account for < 5% of the adult hypertensive population, but because some patients with secondary hypertension are potentially curable, diagnostic evaluation is warranted in selected patients. These include the following: (1) Those in whom routine history, physical examination, or routine laboratory data suggest a specific secondary cause; (2) those who are younger than 30 because they have the greatest prevalence of correctable secondary hypertension; (3) those in whom drug therapy is inadequate or unsatisfactory; (4) those whose BP has suddenly worsened; (5) older patients who develop new-onset hypertension.

MEDICAL HISTORY. A careful, complete history should be obtained and a physical examination performed in all hypertensive patients before therapy is started. The medical history should include any previous history of hypertension, including prior and current antihypertensive treatment; a history of factors regarded as predisposing to hypertension, including excessive salt intake, the use of drugs known to elevate BP (see Table 37–2), stressful occupation, and a family history of hypertension and its complications; ev-

idence of target organ disease, including congestive heart failure, coronary artery disease, renal dysfunction, and stroke (Table 37–3); and a history of other cardiovascular risk factors, including diabetes, obesity, cigarette smoking, and lipid abnormalities. Discussion of family history should include mention of familial diseases associated with secondary hypertension, including familial renal disease, polycystic kidney disease (see Ch. 89), medullary thyroid cancer (see Ch. 215), pheochromocytoma (see Ch. 204.2), and hyperparathyroidism (see Ch. 214). Discussion of the patient's personal habits should include exercise, ethanol consumption, and diet. All current medications should be considered, in particular agents such as corticosteroids, nonsteroidal anti-inflammatory agents, antihistamines, sympathomimetics, appetite suppressants, oral contraceptives, nasal decongestants, licorice-containing substances, cocaine, cyclosporine, erythropoietin, phenothiazines, antidepressants, and monoamine oxidase inhibitors that may exacerbate existing hypertension or antagonize or adversely interact with drug therapy. The physician should also begin assessing the patient's understanding of his/her illness and willingness to alter lifestyle if necessary. A history of weakness, muscle cramps, and polyuria suggests hypokalemia and the possibility of hyperaldosteronism; a history of headaches, palpitations, or hyperhidrosis suggests pheochromocytoma.

PHYSICAL EXAMINATION. The physical examination should include two or more BP measurements, at least one of which is obtained in the standing position; funduscopic examination for hypertensive retinopathy; careful examination of the cardiovascular system for evidence of target organ disease (Table 37–3); examination of the abdomen for bruits; auscultation over all scars for evidence of arteriovenous fistulas; and a careful neurologic examination for the stigmata of stroke. Because poor prognosis has been correlated with the presence of target organ damage, physical findings related to these complications of hypertension should be well documented.

LABORATORY EVALUATION. Pretreatment laboratory tests can be restricted to those generally performed as part of a routine medical checkup: hematocrit; urinalysis to exclude proteinuria and hematuria suggestive of renal disease; creatinine or blood urea nitrogen levels to assess renal function; serum potassium levels; chest film to assess heart size and rule out aortic coarctation; and electrocardiogram. Other tests, which can be obtained as part of most automated blood chemistry batteries, such as the blood glucose and serum cholesterol, triglyceride, and uric acid levels, help assess other cardiovascular risk factors and can be used as a baseline for monitoring the effects of antihypertensive treatment. Serial electrocardiograms (ECG) and echocardiograms (see Ch. 33.2 and 33.3) may help assess the effects of hypertension and antihypertensive treatment on the heart.

TREATMENT

The goal of antihypertensive therapy is to reduce overall cardiovascular risk and thus cardiovascular morbidity and mortality. In any given patient, the decision to initiate therapy is governed by the extent of the BP elevation and the presence or absence of cardiovascular complications, additional cardiovascular risk factors, or

TABLE 37–3. MANIFESTATIONS OF TARGET ORGAN DISEASE

Organ System	Manifestations
Cardiac	Clinical, electrocardiographic, or radiologic evidence of coronary artery disease
	Left ventricular hypertrophy or "strain" by electrocardiography or left ventricular hypertrophy by echocardiography
	Left ventricular dysfunction or cardiac failure
Cerebrovascular	Transient ischemic attack or stroke
Peripheral vascular	Absence of one or more major pulses in the extremities (except for dorsalis pedis) with or without intermittent claudication; aneurysm
Renal	Serum creatinine $\geq$ 130 μmol/L (1.5 mg/dl)
	Proteinuria (1+ or greater)
	Microalbuminuria
Retinopathy	Hemorrhages or exudates, with or without papilledema

From Joint National Committee on Detection, Evaluation, and Treatment of High Blood Pressure: The Fifth Report of the Joint National Committee on Detection, Evaluation, and Treatment of High Blood Pressure (JNC V). Arch Intern Med 153:154, 1993.

both. Antihypertensive treatment is indicated in patients with diastolic BP measurements of ≥ 95 mm Hg and in those with lesser elevations (90 to 94 mm Hg) who are at high risk of developing cardiovascular morbidity or mortality. The high-risk group includes patients with target organ damage, diabetes mellitus, and/or other major risk factors for coronary artery disease. The initial goal of therapy is to lower diastolic BP to levels < 90 mm Hg and systolic BP in ISH to the 140 to 160 mm Hg range with minimal adverse effects. The ultimate theoretical goal is to achieve optimal BP levels with respect to cardiovascular risk, i.e., < 120/80 mm Hg. However, such aggressive BP lowering is poorly tolerated by many patients and therefore impractical for the general population of hypertensives. Further, concerns have been raised that excessively reducing diastolic BP (to levels < 85 mm Hg) may increase the risk of ischemic heart disease, presumably secondary to coronary hypoperfusion, the so-called J curve hypothesis. This concern appears to be most relevant to hypertensive patients with pre-existing coronary artery disease, as no data support a similar relationship of BP reduction to adverse effects on cerebral or renal function. Data currently available that deal with this issue are predominantly retrospective and contradictory. Large prospective studies are needed to clarify this issue. In the meantime, it seems prudent to lower BP cautiously in patients with known coronary artery disease. An effort should be made to correct other cardiovascular risk factors in all hypertensive patients.

In patients with stages 2 to 4 hypertension, even partial BP reduction has been shown to decrease cardiovascular morbidity. Therefore, in these patients, a more limited therapeutic goal may be accepted if side effects of antihypertensive therapy are intolerable at doses necessary to achieve normal BP. For patients with diastolic BP in the range of 90 to 94 mm Hg who are otherwise at low risk, an initial trial of nonpharmacologic therapy with careful BP monitoring should be carried out. If the diastolic BP remains > 90 mm Hg despite nonpharmacologic therapy for a 3- to 6-month period, antihypertensive drugs should be added. Nonpharmacologic therapy should be encouraged in all patients with hypertension, as it may reduce the dosage of medication required to adequately control BP.

Antihypertensive treatment is indicated in ISH because pharmacologic therapy has recently been shown to be well tolerated and effective in both lowering BP and reducing cardiovascular morbidity and mortality, particularly through reductions in stroke and myocardial infarction, in this group. Patients with systolic BP > 160 mm Hg are generally considered to deserve treatment.

Pharmacologic treatment is not indicated in high normal BP in the absence of other risk factors for cardiovascular disease or target organ damage. Careful monitoring and nonpharmacologic therapy are indicated for these patients.

Lifestyle Modification

Because the nonpharmacologic interventions (lifestyle modifications) useful in hypertensives are not costly and are generally beneficial in promoting good health, their gradual introduction should be attempted in all hypertensive patients. Although permanent modifications in diet and lifestyle are difficult to achieve, in motivated patients, they may obviate the need for drug treatment or reduce the dosage requirements of antihypertensive drugs to adequately control BP. The recent Treatment of Mild Hypertension Study (TOMHS) demonstrated that well-motivated patients with stage 1 and 2 hypertension were able to adhere to lifestyle-modification regimens that resulted in significant weight loss, reduced sodium and alcohol intake, and increased physical activity. Lifestyle modification alone was associated with a significant reduction in BP that was maintained over an average of 4.4 years of follow-up. Adding drug therapy produced a further reduction in BP that did not differ among the five therapeutic classes of antihypertensive agents tested. These findings suggest that in well-motivated patients with stage 1 and 2 hypertension, modifying lifestyle effectively lowers BP and may be more important than the initial choice of antihypertensive drug. Further, the same lifestyle-modification strategies that are effective in treating hypertensive patients may be useful in the primary prevention of essential hypertension.

WEIGHT REDUCTION. There is a clear, direct relationship between body weight and resting BP. Epidemiologic studies have consistently shown that overweight individuals have an increased risk of hypertension and increased cardiovascular risk. Weight loss is closely correlated with reduction in BP and is potentially the most efficacious of all nonpharmacologic measures to treat hypertension. This effect is independent of dietary sodium restriction and is seen in both obese and nonobese hypertensive individuals (see Ch. 196). In addition to reducing BP, weight loss independently reduces cardiovascular risk and tends to improve the patient's self-image and sense of well-being. Patients should avoid appetite suppressants, which contain sympathomimetics such as phenylpropanolamine that can elevate BP.

ALCOHOL RESTRICTION. Alcohol consumption elevates BP, both acutely and chronically, and cross-sectional studies have demonstrated an association between increased BP and increased levels of alcohol consumption (see Ch. 11). Regularly ingesting 30 ml of alcohol per day (two drinks) is estimated to raise systolic BP by 2 to 6 mm Hg. However, moderate alcohol consumption has recently been shown to reduce overall cardiovascular risk in the general population. The issue of whether this risk reduction also occurs in the hypertensive population needs further study.

EXERCISE. Both cross-sectional and longitudinal studies have demonstrated a lower prevalence of hypertension in physically active people. Regular isotonic exercise, such as jogging, bicycling, or swimming, produces modest reduction in BP in persons with mild to moderate hypertension. Exercise also reduces cardiovascular risk independent of weight loss while promoting a sense of well-being. Current recommendations for reducing BP and overall cardiovascular risk include aerobic exercise maintaining 70 to 80% of maximal heart rate (maximal heart rate calculated by subtracting age from 220) for 20 to 30 minutes three times a week. Patients should work gradually toward this goal.

RESTRICTING DIETARY SODIUM. Although restricting dietary sodium is commonly recommended by physicians to hypertensive patients, studies evaluating the antihypertensive efficacy in unselected patients with essential hypertension have not demonstrated a clear benefit. A recent meta-analysis of published studies found little evidence that lower sodium intake has a beneficial effect on BP control. Further, BP increases have been observed in some hypertensive patients when dietary sodium intake is reduced. The observed heterogeneity in BP response to restricted dietary sodium has given rise to attempts to classify hypertensive patients as "salt sensitive" or "salt resistant" and to develop biochemical indices of salt sensitivity. Patients with low renin activity, such as elderly and black patients, are more likely to respond to sodium restriction with a decrease in BP. Sodium restriction can minimize diuretic-induced hypokalemia and may enhance the ease of BP control with diuretic therapy, and so should be encouraged in patients who are receiving diuretics. Moderate sodium restriction (4 to 6 grams of salt per day) can be generally recommended to hypertensive patients, realizing that only a subset of patients will benefit. This can be effected by the simple and tolerable measures of not adding salt to food during preparation or at the table and avoiding processed foods containing salt as the preservative. Salt substitutes in which sodium is replaced with potassium are useful in hypertensive patients who do not have renal dysfunction. Patients should be instructed to avoid concomitant decreases in calcium and potassium intake.

SUPPLEMENTING DIETARY CALCIUM. Epidemiologic studies have suggested an inverse relationship between dietary calcium intake and BP: Hypertensive persons, according to their dietary recalls, ingest less calcium than normotensive persons. Clinical studies of the BP-lowering effects of calcium supplementation have produced mixed results: Only a fraction of the hypertensive patients given oral calcium supplementation (1 gram of elemental calcium per day) show significant reductions in BP. Patients with salt-sensitive essential hypertension who ingest a high salt diet appear to be sensitive to the BP-lowering effects of dietary calcium, whereas patients with salt-resistant hypertension are not. This issue requires more study, but early data suggest that patients with salt-sensitive essential hypertension may benefit from supplementing oral calcium. Maintaining oral calcium intake at levels ≥ 1 gram per day may also be beneficial for other reasons, such as preventing osteoporosis and gastrointestinal malignancy.

SUPPLEMENTING DIETARY POTASSIUM. Epidemiologic studies have demonstrated an inverse relationship between dietary potassium intake and BP, and several recent controlled studies have demonstrated a small but significant reduction in BP with dietary potassium supplementation. The antihypertensive effect of supplementing potassium appears to be related to concomitant sodium intake, in that the higher the sodium intake, the more effectively potassium supplementation reduces BP. Hypertensive patients should maintain adequate potassium intake ($\sim$ 100 mEq per day) by eating enough fresh fruits and vegetables and, if necessary, by using potassium supplements. Potassium supplementation should be avoided or used only with extreme caution in patients with renal insufficiency, in diabetics, and in patients receiving potassium-sparing diuretics. Hypokalemia (see Ch. 75), whether due to diuretic use or poor dietary intake, should be treated. Hypokalemia should particularly be avoided in patients receiving digoxin and in patients with known coronary artery disease, as it predisposes to arrhythmia. Using potassium-sparing diuretics should be considered in patients who are hypokalemic prior to initiation of diuretic therapy or who develop hypokalemia while receiving a non–potassium-sparing diuretic (see Ch. 75).

SUPPLEMENTING DIETARY MAGNESIUM. There appears to be an inverse relationship between dietary magnesium intake and BP in the general population. However, no convincing data justify recommending increased magnesium intake as an antihypertensive measure.

SPECIAL DIETS. Dietary manipulations, such as changing to a vegetarian diet, increasing total fiber intake, decreasing total fat intake while increasing polyunsaturated fats relative to saturated fats, or increasing ingestion of fish oils, have been shown in preliminary studies to lower BP. They may, in addition, reduce other cardiovascular risk factors. Further studies are necessary to evaluate the role of these special diets in lowering BP, and it is premature to recommend them to patients with essential hypertension who lack other cardiovascular risk factors.

SMOKING CESSATION AND CAFFEINE RESTRICTION. Caffeine and nicotine raise BP acutely, but neither cigarette smokers nor coffee drinkers have an increased incidence of sustained hypertension, and there is no evidence that quitting smoking or caffeine products benefits BP control. Accordingly, patients should be advised to avoid cigarettes and coffee or tea immediately prior to having their BP checked. Because of the high incidence of associated malignancy and accelerated cardiovascular disease, all patients should be strongly urged to quit smoking.

RELAXATION/REDUCING STRESS. Relaxation and stress management lower BP only a bit, even in highly motivated patients. Therefore, although these techniques have beneficial side effects, including decreasing anxiety and an improved sense of well being, they have limited clinical application in treating hypertension.

OVERALL RECOMMENDATIONS FOR MODIFYING LIFESTYLE AS PRIMARY OR ADJUNCTIVE THERAPY IN ESSENTIAL HYPERTENSION. Lifestyle modifications should be used in all hypertensive patients, either as definitive treatment or as an adjunct to drug therapy (Fig. 37–5). Therapy should be tailored to the individual characteristics of each patient, for example, weight reduction and exercise for the overweight patient and moderation in alcohol consumption for the heavy drinker. A reasonable generalized approach for all patients includes (1) reduced dietary sodium and increased dietary calcium and potassium; (2) weight loss for the overweight patient; (3) regular exercise; (4) moderation of alcohol consumption; and (5) smoking cessation. Such an approach has been shown to produce significant sustained reductions in BP while reducing overall cardiovascular risk.

Pharmacologic Therapy

THERAPEUTIC BENEFIT. Epidemiologic studies have clearly demonstrated that elevated BP is correlated with an increased incidence of cardiovascular disease, including stroke, renal failure, congestive heart failure, and myocardial infarction. The risk of cardiovascular complications is proportional to the degree of BP elevation, and the benefit of antihypertensive treatment is greatest in patients with the highest pretreatment BP. Clinical trials have shown that the pharmacologic treatment of stage 2 to 4 hypertension reduces overall cardiovascular morbidity and mortality, producing significant reductions in stroke, congestive heart failure, and end-stage renal disease; the benefits of treating stage 1 hypertension are less clear. A meta-analysis of 14 randomized trials of antihypertensive therapy averaging 5 years and involving $\sim$ 37,000 subjects showed a 21% reduction in mortality from all vascular causes, a 42% reduction in incidence of stroke, and a 14% reduction in incidence of myocardial infarction in subjects assigned to drug (diuretic or β-blocker) therapy (Fig. 37–6). Diastolic BP was reduced by a mean of 5 to 6 mm Hg in the drug-treated groups compared with controls. Three more recent trials in older patients have shown a

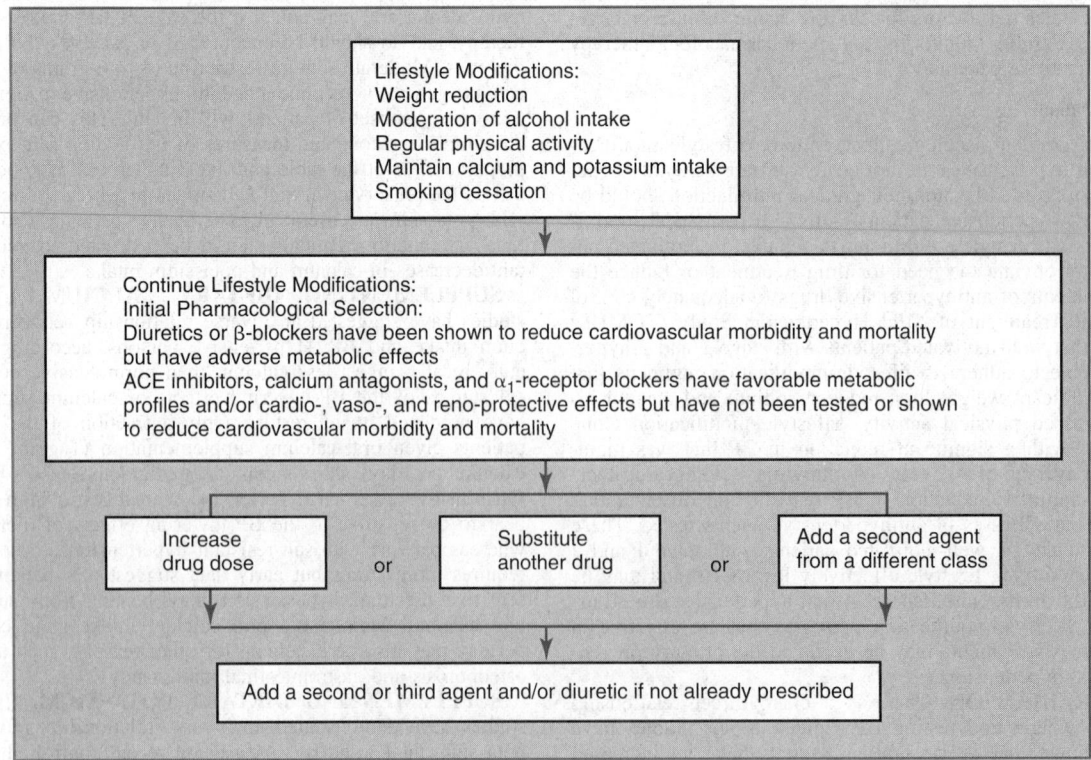

FIGURE 37–5. Treatment algorithm for patients with essential hypertension. If goal blood pressure is not achieved in response to a given intervention, the additional interventions indicated in the lower boxes are added.

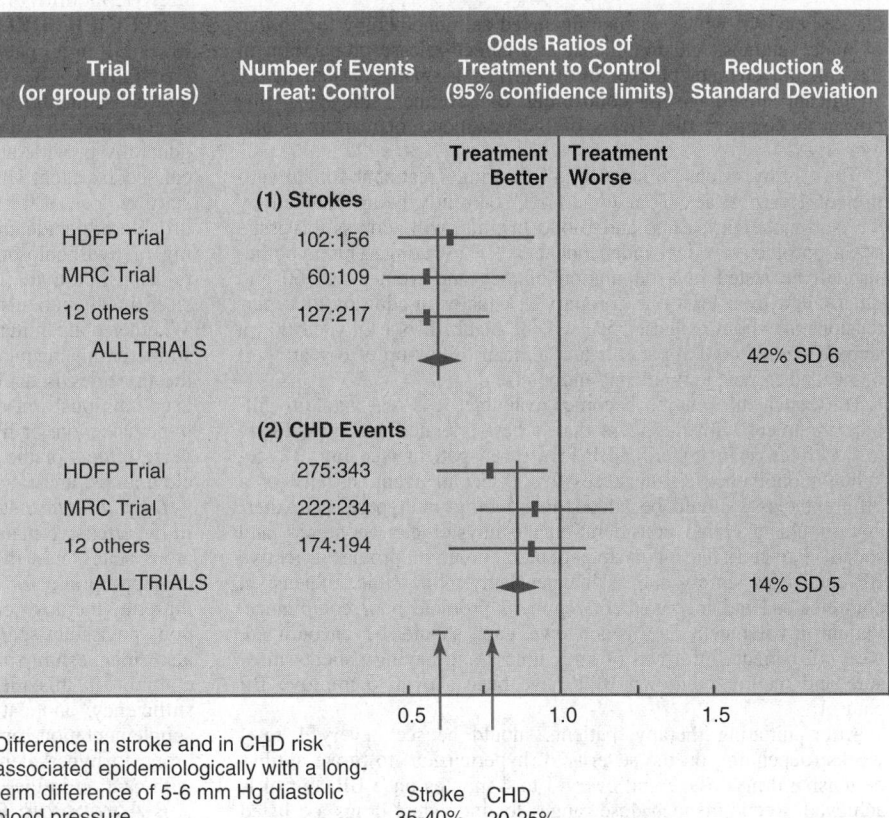

FIGURE 37-6. Reduction in the odds of developing stroke and coronary heart disease (CHD) in the treatment versus placebo groups of the Hypertensive Detection and Followup trial (HDFP), the Medical Research Council trial (MRC), and 12 other smaller unconfounded randomized trials of antihypertensive therapy in which mean differences in diastolic blood pressure between treatment and control groups were 5 to 6 mm Hg over a 5-year follow-up period. (Modified from Collins R, Peto R, MacMahon S, et al.: Blood pressure, stroke, and coronary heart disease. Part 2: Short-term reductions in blood pressure: Overview of randomised trials in their epidemiological context. Lancet 335:827, 1990.)

greater (17%) reduction in incidence of fatal and nonfatal myocardial infarction. Although the reduced incidence of stroke in these randomized trials approximated that expected on the basis of epidemiologic studies, the reduced incidence of myocardial infarction was about half that expected. The disappointing lack of efficacy of antihypertensive treatment in preventing myocardial infarction has been explained in several ways. Some experts have postulated that the adverse metabolic effects of antihypertensive agents may increase coronary risk and offset the benefit of BP reduction. Others have noted that the expected results were calculated from 30 years of observational data in populations, and the results of clinical trials reflect the outcome of only 5 years or fewer of intervention. When clinical trial populations are observed beyond 5 years, the efficacy of antihypertensive treatment in preventing myocradial infarction becomes more evident.

GENERAL CONSIDERATIONS. The increasing number and variety of drugs available for use in hypertension, coupled with our rapidly expanding knowledge of the pathophysiology of hypertension and of the adverse effects of these drugs in individual patient groups, make it increasingly possible to individualize antihypertensive treatment. When used as monotherapy, most agents effectively control BP in >50% of patients with stage 1 or 2 disease. Thus, it is possible to use a single agent to effectively control BP with minimal side effects in many patients. However, the ultimate test of antihypertensive therapy is its ability to reduce morbidity and mortality owing to cardiovascular disease. The recent report of the JNC V stresses that diuretics and β-blockers are the only classes of antihypertensive drugs that reduce morbidity and mortality from cardiovascular causes in long-term controlled clinical trials. Therefore, they were recommended as first-choice agents unless they are contraindicated or poorly tolerated or there are special indications for other agents in any given patient. This recommendation has aroused much debate and controversy because the diuretics and β-blockers have adverse biochemical effects and the newer classes of antihypertensive drugs—including the calcium channel-blocking agents, the angiotensin-converting enzyme (ACE) inhibitors, and the α-adrenergic blocking agents—have favorable metabolic profiles and salutary effects on the cardiovascular system that are, at least in part, independent of BP lowering. Further, the newer classes of drugs have not yet been tested in long-term controlled clinical trials with cardiovascular events as endpoints. The adverse metabolic ef-

fects of some classes of antihypertensive drugs may increase coronary risk and offset the benefit of BP reduction (see Table 37-7).

The ACE inhibitors have cardio-, vaso-, and reno-protective effects in animal models and humans. ACE inhibitors reduce left ventricular hypertrophy, decrease mortality from congestive heart failure, and reduce cardiovascular morbidity and mortality in patients with asymptomatic left ventricular dysfunction. ACE-inhibitor therapy started after acute myocardial infarction and continued long term increases survival and reduces morbidity and mortality due to major cardiovascular events in patients with asymptomatic left ventricular dysfunction. The ACE inhibitors, like the calcium channel blockers, do not alter circulating lipid/lipoprotein levels and appear to reduce insulin resistance. A large multicenter trial has recently demonstrated that the ACE inhibitor, captopril, preserves renal function, reduces the need for dialysis and transplantation, and reduces mortality rate in patients with insulin-dependent diabetic nephropathy. The protective effect was independent of the ACE inhibitor's antihypertensive properties because BP control was comparable in the inhibitor group and the control group that received conventional antihypertensive therapy. Whether the renoprotective effects of the ACE inhibitors are generalizable to nondiabetic patients, to patients with type II diabetes, and to diabetic patients with normal renal function and without proteinuria is uncertain.

The α-adrenergic blocking agents have a beneficial effect on the serum lipid profile, decreasing total and/or LDL cholesterol and increasing HDL cholesterol. These agents are also useful in benign prostatic hypertrophy, appear to decrease insulin resistance, and may reduce left ventricular hypertrophy and platelet aggregability and stimulate synthesis of tissue plasminogen activators.

Although the evidence cited above seems to favor using one particular class of antihypertensive agents over others to treat at least certain subsets of hypertensive patients, only two randomized trials have compared the effects of representatives of all major classes in large numbers of patients with uncomplicated stage 1 and 2 essential hypertension. The TOMHS is a randomized, double-blind, placebo-controlled clinical trial that compared the effects of five antihypertensive agents. BP control and the other outcome measures did not differ significantly among the five drug treatment groups; all were significantly better than placebo. The Department of Veterans Affairs Cooperative Study Group on Antihypertensive Agents compared the effects of six antihypertensive drugs from different classes, each of which was administered as monotherapy to a group of male veterans, and found that a sustained-release preparation of the calcium channel blocker diltiazem had a small but statistically significant advantage in controlling BP. Neither study had the power to compare the effects of the treatments on cardiovascular outcomes.

The Antihypertensive and Lipid-Lowering Treatment for Prevention of Heart Attack Trial (ALLHAT) currently being planned by the National Heart, Lung and Blood Institute will address this issue of vasoprotective effect independent of BP lowering. This hypothesis will be tested in a population of men and women age 60 and older, all with at least one coronary risk factor in addition to hypertension, of whom at least 55% will be black. It is estimated that a sample size of 40,000 patients and a mean follow-up of 6 years will be needed to reach significant endpoints.

Until such information becomes available, it is reasonable to initiate treatment with the agent that is best tolerated and most likely to be effective in lowering BP in a given patient (see Fig. 37–5). When monotherapy is unsuccessful, a second agent, usually of a different class, should be added. Prescribing antihypertensive therapy should take into consideration the physiologic, economic, and social characteristics of each patient in order to provide effective BP control as simply and as inexpensively as possible. Expensive, complicated, and inconvenient regimens promote poor compliance. Patient involvement in his/her own care should be encouraged. Keeping patients informed of their illness and having patients measure and record their own BP's have been shown to improve BP control.

After initiating therapy, patients should be seen every 1 to 4 weeks (depending on the severity of hypertension) to titrate antihypertensive drug dosage and every 3 to 4 months once BP control is achieved. Recommended dose ranges for individual drugs are listed Tables 37–4 and 37–5 and for combination agents in Table 37–6. Common adverse effects are summarized in Table 37–7.

Step-down therapy, or withdrawing antihypertensive medication under close monitoring, should be attempted in patients with stage 1 or 2 hypertension whose BP has been adequately controlled for 1 year or more. Dosages should be titrated slowly downward and medications discontinued one at a time, if possible. Step-down therapy is generally most effective in patients who are also making lifestyle modifications for their hypertension.

SPECIFIC DRUGS. *Diuretics.* *Thiazide diuretics* effectively lower BP in all patient groups, particularly in blacks and the elderly (see Table 37–4). They are inexpensive and generally well tolerated and consequently are widely used. Diuretics have been used safely in combination with all other classes of antihypertensive agents and generally provide additional BP reduction and, therefore, are a logical second agent when combination therapy is needed. A reasonable starting dose of thiazide diuretic is the equivalent of 12.5 mg of hydrochlorothiazide in the general hypertensive population and 6.25 mg of hydrochlorothiazide in the elderly hypertensive patient. The thiazides, particularly when given in high doses, lower serum potassium in all patients and produce significant hypokalemia in some. Whether concomitant potassium supplementation or use of a potassium-sparing agent can neutralize the arrhythmogenic potential of the thiazides is unclear at present. The thiazide diuretics should be used cautiously in diabetics and in patients with a history of gout, hypercalcemia, or hyperlipidemia. The most common subjective adverse effects of the thiazides are impotence, decreased libido, muscle cramps, and fatigue.

Loop diuretics, such as furosemide and bumetanide, are indicated in hypertensive patients with congestive heart failure or other edematous states or with renal insufficiency. *Potassium-sparing diuretics* are appropriate for patients who are hypokalemic prior to starting diuretic therapy or who develop hypokalemia from using a non–potassium-sparing diuretic. Potassium-sparing diuretics are also magnesium-sparing and may prevent the hypomagnesemia common in thiazide diuretic use. Diabetics, patients with renal insufficiency, and patients receiving ACE inhibitors, oral potassium supplementation, or salt substitutes high in potassium chloride are prone to hyperkalemia. Potassium-sparing diuretics should be used with caution in these patients.

β-Adrenergic Receptor Blocking Agents. β-Blockers have been used effectively and safely in combination with all other classes of antihypertensive agents. They must be used cautiously in combination with calcium channel blockers that have significant negative inotropic and chronotropic activity, as these effects of the two classes of agents may be additive. β-Blockers are routinely used in combination with vasodilators to blunt reflex tachycardia. β-Blockers are more effective in lowering BP in younger patients

TABLE 37–4. DIURETICS FOR AMBULATORY TREATMENT OF HYPERTENSION

Generic Name	Trade Name (Manufacturer)	Adult Dosage (mg/day)	Duration (hr)	Dispensing Unit (mg)
Benzothiadiazine diuretics				
Thiazides				
Chlorothiazide	Diuril (Merck)	250–1000	6–12	250, 500
Hydrochlorothiazide	Esidrix (CIBA)	12.5–100	12–18	25, 50, 100
	HydroDIURIL (Merck)			
	Oretic (Abbott)			
Bendroflumethiazide	Naturetin (Squibb)	5.0–20	18–36	5.0, 10.0
Benzthiazide	Exna (Robins)	25–100	12–18	50
Hydroflumethiazide	Saluron (Apotecon)	25–100	18–24	50
	Diucardin (Wyeth-Ayerst)			
Methyclothiazide	Aquatensen (Wallace)	2.5–5.0	24–48	2.5, 5.0
	Enduron (Abbott)			
Polythiazide	Renese (Pfizer)	2–4	24–48	1, 2, 4
Trichlormethiazide	Naqua (Schering)	2–4	24–48	2, 4
Indapamide	Lozol (Rhone-Poulenc Rorer)	1.25–5.0	18–24	1.25, 2.5
Phthalimidines				
Chlorthalidone	Thalitone (Horus)	15–50	24–72	15, 25
	Hygroton (Rhone-Poulenc Rorer)	12.5–100	24–72	25, 50, 100
Metolazone	Mykrox (Fisons)	0.5–1.0	12	0.5
	Zaroxolyn (Fisons)	2.5–5.0	12–24	2.5, 5.0, 10.0
Quinazolines				
Quinethazone	Hydromox (Lederle)	50–100	18–24	50
Loop diuretics				
Furosemide	Lasix (Hoechst-Roussel)	20–1000	3–6	20, 40, 80
Ethacrynic acid	Edecrin (Merck)	50–400	3–6	25, 50
Bumetanide	Bumex (Roche)	0.5–2.0	1–4	0.5, 1.0, 2.0
Potassium-sparing diuretics				
Spironolactone	Aldactone (Searle)	50–100	3–6	25, 50, 100
Triamterene	Dyrenium (SKB)*	50–100	3–6	50, 10.0
Amiloride	Midamor (Merck)	5–10	24	5.0

*SKB = SmithKline Beecham

TABLE 37-5. ANTIHYPERTENSIVE DRUGS IN AMBULATORY TREATMENT OF HYPERTENSION

Generic Name	Trade Name (Manufacturer)	Adult Maintenance Dose (mg/day)	Frequency of Administration (Times/day)	Duration of Action (hr)
Sympatholytic agents				
Centrally acting agents				
Methyldopa	Aldomet (Merck)	500–2000	2–3	6–12
Clonidine	Catapres (Boehringer-Ingelheim)	0.2–0.8	2	6–12
Clonidine patch	Catapres-TTS (Boehringer-Ingelheim)	1 patch (0.1, 0.2, 0.3 mg)	Weekly	7 days
Guanfacine	Tenex (Robins)	1–3	1	12–24
Guanabenz	Wytensin (Wyeth-Ayerst)	8–64	2	8–12
Reserpine and rauwolfia alkaloids		0.1–0.25	1	24
β-Adrenergic blocking agents				
Propranolol	Inderal (Wyeth-Ayerst)	40–640	2	6–12
Propranolol sustained release	Inderal LA (Wyeth-Ayerst)	80–640	1	24
Carteolol	Cartrol (Abbott)	2.5–10	1	24
Betaxolol	Kerlone (Searle)	10–20	1	24
Metoprolol	Lopressor (CIBA)	100–450	2	12
Metoprolol sustained release	Toprol XL (Astra)	50–400	1	24
Bisoprolol	Zebeta (Lederle)	2.5–40	1	24
Atenolol	Tenormin (Zeneca)	50–100	1	24
Nadolol	Corgard (Bristol)	40–320	1	24
Timolol	Blocadren (Merck)	20–60	2	6–12
Pindolol	Visken (Sandoz)	10–60	2	6–12
Acebutolol	Sectral (Wyeth-Ayerst)	400–1200	1 or 2	12–24
Penbutolol	Levatol (Reed & Carnrick)	20	1	24
α-Adrenergic blocking agents				
Prazosin	Minipress (Pfizer)	2.5–20	2 or 3	3–6
Terazosin	Hytrin (Abbott)	1–20	1	24
Doxazosin	Cardura (Roerig)	2–16	1	24
Mixed α- and β-adrenergic blocking agent				
Labetalol	Normodyne (Schering) Trandate (Allen & Hanbury's)	200–1200	2	3–6
Ganglion blocking agent				
Mecamylamine	Inversine (Merck)	2.5–25	1–3	12–24
Peripherally acting sympatholytic agent				
Guanethidine	Ismelin (CIBA)	10–50	1	24
Angiotensin-converting enzyme inhibitors				
Captopril	Capoten (Squibb)	75–450	2–3	4–8
Enalapril	Vasotec (Merck)	5–40	1 or 2	12–24
Lisinopril	Prinivil (Merck) Zestril (Stuart)	10–40	1	24
Quinapril	Accupril (Parke-Davis)	5–80	1 or 2	12–24
Ramipril	Altace (Hoechst-Roussel)	2.5–20	1 or 2	12–24
Benazepril	Lotensin (CIBA)	10–80	1 or 2	12–24
Fosinopril	Monopril (Mead-Johnson)	10–80	1 or 2	12–24
Spiropril*	(Schering)	12.5–50	1 or 2	12–24
Perindopril	Aceon (Ortho-McNeil)	2–16	1 or 2	12–24
Moexipril*	(Schwarz-Pharma)	7.5–30	1 or 2	12–24
Calcium channel blocking agents				
Nifedipine	Procardia (Pratt) Adalat (Miles)	30–180	3 or 4	6–8
Nifedipine sustained release	Procardia XL (Pratt) Adalat CC (Miles)	30–90	1	24
Diltiazem	Cardizem (Marion)	90–360	3 or 4	6–8
Diltiazem sustained release	Cardizem SR (Marion)	120–360	2	12
	Cardizem CD (Marion) Dilacor XR (Rhone-Poulenc Rorer)	120–360	1	24
Verapamil	Isoptin (Knoll) Calan (Searle)	240–480	3	6–8
Verapamil sustained release	Isoptin SE (Knoll) Calan SR (Searle)	120–480	1 or 2	12–24
Nicardipine	Cardene (Syntex)	30–120	3	6–8
Nicardipine sustained release	Cardene SR (Syntex)	60–120	2	12
Isradipine	DynaCirc (Sandoz)	2.5–20	2	12
Amlodipine	Norvasc (Pfizer)	5–10	1	24
Felodipine sustained release	Plendil (Merck)	5–20	1	24
Direct vasodilators				
Hydralazine	Apresoline (CIBA)	20–300	2–4	6
Minoxidil	Loniten (Upjohn)	5–100	1 or 2	Up to 72

* These agents have not been approved by the FDA for the treatment of hypertension.

than in the elderly and in whites than in blacks. Because β-blockers are effective in treating angina and in the secondary prevention of myocardial infarction, they are the initial drugs of choice in hypertensive patients with known coronary artery disease. β-Blockers are the drugs of choice in hypertensive patients with sympathetic hyperactivity, as indicated by a rapid resting heart rate and a wide pulse pressure.

The most common adverse effects of β-blockers are bradycardia, atrioventricular block, and congestive heart failure in susceptible patients. β-Blockers should be used with caution in patients with chronic obstructive pulmonary disease (COPD) or peripheral vascular disease because β₂ blockade may exacerbate bronchospasm, peripheral vascular constriction, and Raynaud's phenomenon. Central nervous system (CNS) side effects such as fatigue, impotence, and decreased mental acuity can occur with β-blockers, particularly in the elderly. These can be minimized by using lipophilic agents, such as atenolol, acetobutolol, nadalol, labetalol, and timolol, which are less likely to enter the brain. β-Blockers should be used with caution in insulin-dependent diabetics, as they mask symptoms and delay recovery from hypoglycemia. β-Blockers adversely affect the serum lipid profile by reducing HDL cholesterol and increasing triglycerides.

Labetalol has both α- and β-adrenergic antagonist properties; its most prominent pharmacologic effect is α₁-adrenergic receptor antagonist activity, similar to prazosin. Labetalol is particularly effective in lowering BP in individuals with labile hypertension with a marked neurogenic component. It has no significant effect on serum lipid levels and has been used safely in patients with COPD and peripheral vascular disease.

Calcium Channel Blockers.
Calcium channel blockers are effective in reducing BP in most hypertensive patients; like the diuretics, they are particularly efficacious in blacks and the elderly.

The calcium channel blockers have been used safely and successfully in combination with all the other classes of antihypertensive agents, but they (particularly verapamil) should be used cautiously in combination with β-blockers because of common negative inotropic and chronotropic properties.

The availability of sustained-release formulations of the calcium channel blockers has made these agents well tolerated and convenient for general use. Verapamil should be avoided in patients with left ventricular dysfunction and should be used cautiously in patients with conduction abnormalities because of its negative chronotropic effects. Adverse effects are less common with sustained-release preparations. Calcium channel blockers generally are free of CNS side effects, including sexual dysfunction. They are metabolized by the liver and may require dosage adjustment in patients with hepatic disease but can be used safely in patients with renal disease. All of the calcium channel blockers can increase serum digoxin levels, but this is a particular problem with verapamil.

Angiotensin-Converting Enzyme Inhibitors.
ACE inhibitors effectively lower BP in all of the major subgroups of hypertensive patients, including the elderly. Blacks are generally less sensitive to their antihypertensive effects than are whites, but increasing the dose of ACE inhibitor or adding a diuretic abolishes the racial difference. ACE inhibitors reduce afterload and are the drugs of choice in patients with hypertension and congestive heart failure. ACE inhibitors are particularly useful in hypertensive patients with diabetes because they decrease proteinuria and stabilize renal function in patients with diabetic nephropathy. They are also particularly effective in controlling hypertension secondary to renovascular disease. However, in patients with renal artery stenosis in a solitary kidney, bilateral renal artery stenosis, or transplant renal artery stenosis, ACE inhibition may precipitate acute renal failure. Renal function should be monitored closely if ACE inhibitors are used in this setting. ACE inhibitors are well tolerated and generally free of adverse effects on

TABLE 37-6. COMBINATION AGENTS FOR TREATMENT OF HYPERTENSION

Generic Name	Trade Name (Manufacturer)	Daily Dose (pills/day)	Pill Content (mg/mg)
Centrally acting agents and diuretics			
Methyldopa/chlorothiazide	Aldoclor (Merck)	2–4	250/150, 250/250
Methyldopa/HCTZ	Aldoril (Merck)	2–4	250/15, 250/25, 500/30, 500/50
Clonidine/chlorthalidone	Combipres (Boehringer-Ingelheim)	1–2	0.1/15, 0.2/15, 0.3/15
Reserpine/chlorothiazide	Diupres (Merck)	1–2	0.125/250, 0.125/500
Reserpine/methychlothiazide	Diutensen-R (Wallace)	1–4	0.1/2.5
Reserpine/HCTZ	Hydropres (Merck)	1–2	0.125/25, 0.125/50
Reserpine/polythiazide	Renese-R (Pfizer)	0.5–2	0.25/2
Reserpine/hydroflumethiazide	Salutensin-Demi (Apothecon)	1–2	0.125/25
	Salutensin (Apothecon)	1	0.125/50
Reserpine/chlorthalidone	Demi-Regroton (Rhone-Poulenc Rorer)	1	0.125/25
	Regroton (Rhone-Poulenc Rorer)	1	0.25/50
Deserpidine/methychlothiazide	Enduronyl (Abbott)	0.5–1	0.25/5
	Enduronyl-Forte (Abbott)		0.5/5
Guanethidine/HCTZ	Esimil (CIBA)	1–2	10/25
Rauwolfia/bendroflumethiazide	Rauzide (Princeton)	1–4	50/4
Other combinations			
Reserpine/hydralazone/HCTZ	Ser-Ap-Es (CIBA)	1–2	0.1/25/15
Combination diuretics			
HCTZ/spironolactone	Aldactazide (Searle)	1–2	25/25, 50/50
HCTZ/triamterene	Maxzide (Lederle)	1–2	25/37.5, 50/75
HCTZ/triamterene	Dyazide (SKB)	1–4	25/50
HCTZ/amiloride	Moduretic (Merck)	1–2	50/5
ACE inhibitors and diuretics			
Captopril/HCTZ	Capozide (Squibb)	2–3	25/15, 25/25, 50/15, 50/25
Enalapril/HCTZ	Vaseretic (Merck)	1–2	10/25
Lisinopril/HCTZ	Zestoretic (Stuart)	1–2	20/12.5, 20/25
β-Blocking agents and diuretics			
Propranolol/HCTZ	Inderide (Wyeth-Ayerst)	1–2	40/25, 80/25
Propranolol LA/HCTZ	Inderide LA (Wyeth-Ayerst)	1	80/50, 120/50, 160/50
Atenolol/chlorthalidone	Tenoretic (Zeneca)	1	50/25, 100/25
Timolol/HCTZ	Timolide (Merck)	1–2	10/25
Nadolol/bendroflumethiazide	Corzide (Bristol)	1	40/5, 80/5
Bisoprolol/HCTZ	Ziac (Lederle)	1–2	2.5/6.25, 5/6.25, 10/6.25
Vasodilators and diuretics			
Hydralazine/HCTZ	Apresazide (CIBA)	2	25/25, 50/25, 50/50
	Hydra-Zide (Par)	1	25/25, 50/50, 100/50
Prazosin/polythiazide	Minizide (Pfizer)	2–4	1/0.5, 2/0.5, 3/0.5

HCTZ = Hydrochlorothiazide

TABLE 37–7. COMMON ADVERSE EFFECTS OF ANTIHYPERTENSIVE DRUGS

Drugs	Side Effects	Precautions and Special Considerations
Diuretics		
Thiazides and related sulfonamides	Hypokalemia, hyperuricemia, glucose intolerance, hypercholesterolemia, hypertriglyceridemia, sexual dysfunction	May be ineffective in renal failure; hypokalemia increases digitalis toxicity; and hyperuricemia may precipitate acute gout.
Loop diuretics	Same as for thiazides	Effective in chronic renal failure; cautions regarding hypokalemia and hyperuricemia same as above; hyponatremia may occur, especially in the elderly.
Potassium-sparing agents	Hyperkalemia	Danger of hyperkalemia in patients with renal failure or diabetes or those receiving ACE inhibitors.
Amiloride hydrochloride	Sexual dysfunction	—
Spironolactone	Gynecomastia, mastodynia, sexual dysfunction	—
Adrenergic antagonists		
β-Adrenergic blockers	Bradycardia, fatigue, insomnia, bizarre dreams, sexual dysfunction, hypertriglyceridemia, decreased HDL cholesterol	Should not be used in patients with asthma, chronic obstructive pulmonary disease, congestive heart failure, heart block (> first degree), and sick sinus syndrome. Use with caution in patients with diabetes and peripheral vascular disease. Sudden withdrawal of these drugs may be hazardous.
Centrally acting agents	Drowsiness, dry mouth, fatigue	Rebound hypertension may occur with abrupt discontinuance.
Methyldopa	—	May cause liver damage and positive direct Coombs' test (rare hemolytic anemia).
Reserpine	Sexual dysfunction, nasal congestion, lethargy	Contraindicated in patients with a history of depression; use with caution in patients with a history of peptic ulcer.
α₁-Adrenergic blockers	"First-dose" syncope, orthostatic hypotension, weakness, palpitations, dizziness, headache, fluid retention	Use cautiously in elderly patients.
Combined α- and β-adrenergic blockers	Nausea, fatigue, dizziness, headache, orthostatic hypotension	Use with caution in patients with cardiac failure, chronic obstructive pulmonary disease, sick sinus syndrome, heart block (> first degree), diabetes.
Vasodilators		
Vasodilators	Headache, tachycardia, fluid retention	May precipitate angina in patients with coronary heart disease.
Hydralazine hydrochloride	Positive antinuclear antibody (without other changes)	Lupus syndrome may occur (rare at recommended doses).
Minoxidil	Hypertrichosis, ascites (rare)	May cause or aggravate pleural and pericardial effusions.
Angiotensin-converting enzyme inhibitors		
Angiotensin-converting enzyme inhibitors	Cough	Can cause reversible acute renal failure in patients with bilateral renal artery stenosis; neutropenia may occur in patients with autoimmune collagen disorders; proteinuria may occur (rare at recommended doses).
Calcium channel blocking agents		
Calcium channel blocking agents	Headache, hypotension, dizziness	Use with caution in patients with congestive heart failure or heart block.
Verapamil hydrochloride	Constipation, bradycardia	

the CNS, sexual function, and metabolism. Specifically, they do not adversely affect lipid levels, glucose tolerance, or uric acid levels and have positive effects on quality of life.

Class-specific adverse effects of ACE inhibitors include hyperkalemia, acute renal failure, angioedema, and cough, which tends to be nonproductive and worse at night. Cough is the most common adverse effect of the ACE inhibitors, with an incidence that approaches 25%.

Centrally Acting Agents. The traditional centrally acting antihypertensive agents—clonidine, methyldopa, and guanabenz—have been a mainstay of antihypertensive therapy for several decades. However, until recent years their use has been limited by a high incidence of side effects and the need for frequent dosing. The availability of transdermal clonidine and long-acting guanfacine, both of which allow for more convenient dosing with fewer side effects, expands the role of centrally acting agents in treating hypertension.

The centrally acting agents are predominantly α₂-adrenoceptor agonists, stimulating adrenoceptors in the brain stem and hypothalamus, thereby inhibiting sympathetic outflow from the CNS and decreasing BP, heart rate, and peripheral vascular resistance. These agents have no significant effects on glucose regulation, serum lipid levels, or renal function. The most common side effects of the centrally acting agents—dry mouth, drowsiness, and fatigue—occur

initially in as many as 30% of patients but tend to diminish with continued therapy. Less frequent side effects include orthostatic hypotension, sexual dysfunction, and decreased mental acuity. Abruptly discontinuing the traditional agents, particularly clonidine, has been associated with a withdrawal syndrome characterized by headache, nausea, anxiety, vomiting, and rebound hypertension that may require emergency therapy. In this setting BP can be reduced and symptoms alleviated by reinitiating previous therapy. The withdrawal syndrome has not been associated with transdermal clonidine or guanfacine. Approximately 10 to 20% of patients receiving methyldopa develop a positive direct Coombs reaction, but only a very small percentage (<1%) develop hemolytic anemia. Drug-induced hepatitis and/or fever is rarely associated with using methyldopa. Transdermal clonidine is associated with a local rash in 10 to 15% of patients. The rash is generally a mild, localized erythema, but vesicular eruptions have been reported. It disappears when therapy is discontinued or the patch is moved.

The centrally acting agents should be used cautiously in the elderly because of their adverse effects on baroreflex and CNS function. Transdermal clonidine with its once-weekly dosing is well suited for patients who are forgetful, who do not like to be reminded daily of their illness, or who have their medicines administered to them by family or friends. The centrally acting agents have been used safely and successfully in combination with all of the major classes of antihypertensive agents, including diuretics.

α-Adrenergic Receptor Blockers. The α-adrenergic antagonists are effective in all major subgroups of hypertensive patients and have been used safely in combination with all of the major classes of antihypertensive agents, including diuretics and β-blockers. The major adverse effects of the α-antagonists include headache, dizziness, weakness, and mild fluid retention. Orthostatic hypotension is most prominent with the initial dose and can be minimized by initiating therapy with a small dose at bedtime. The α-antagonists are generally free of CNS-mediated side effects, such as dry mouth, fatigue, and sexual dysfunction. The development of longer-acting α-antagonists with minimal side effects and positive effects on serum lipid levels expands the role of these agents as an initial antihypertensive therapy, particularly in patients with underlying diseases such as COPD, peripheral vascular disease, diabetes, and hyperlipidemia.

Vasodilators. Common side effects of the direct vasodilators include tachycardia, fluid retention, palpitations, headache, nasal congestion, and, in patients with underlying coronary artery disease, myocardial ischemia (Table 37–7). The lupus reaction with hydralazine generally resolves after stopping therapy but occasionally may require several years for complete resolution. Side effects of minoxodil include hirsutism (which makes it unacceptable to female patients), nausea, fatigue, and skin rash. Minoxodil use has been associated with unexplained pericardial effusion, occasionally with tamponade.

The combination of a vasodilator and diuretic with a β-blocker (triple therapy) is effective in treating patients with severe, refractory, essential, or renal hypertension.

New Classes. Several new classes of antihypertensive agents are under investigation and/or are available outside of the United States. Many of these agents potentially provide unique therapeutic benefits and likely will become available for clinical use in the near future. *Trimazosin* is a selective α₁-adrenergic receptor antagonist structurally related to prazosin that may also have some direct vasodilator properties. *Ketanserin* is a selective antagonist of serotonin S_2 (5-HT$_2$) receptors and a weak selective α₁-adrenergic receptor antagonist. *Indoramin* is a competitive antagonist of α₁-adrenergic, serotoninergic, and histaminergic H₁ receptors that is structurally similar to procainamide. BP reduction is accomplished in large part through indoramin blocking α₁-adrenergic receptors, but it may also decrease sympathetic nerve activity through a CNS mechanism. *Urapidil* acts as an α₁-adrenergic blocker that also has some CNS effects, possibly secondary to antagonism of central adrenergic receptors, stimulation of serotonin receptors, or both. *Rilmenidine* appears to reduce BP by stimulating CNS imidazoline receptors and shows promise of having a favorable adverse effect profile.

Renin inhibitors are an experimental class of antihypertensive agents that selectively inhibit the renin-substrate reaction and consequent generation of angiotensin I. Because angiotensinogen is the only known substrate for renin in humans, the renin inhibitors are selective for the renin-angiotensin system and are free from adverse effects unrelated to those—such as cough and angioneurotic edema—that are found with the ACE inhibitors and are thought to be secondary to inhibiting the degradation of bradykinin and substance P. Clinical use of the orally active renin inhibitors has been precluded by limited bioavailability and brief duration of action. Recent reports suggest some progress in overcoming these limitations. *Angiotensin II antagonists,* like the renin inhibitors, show promise in effectively reducing BP by interrupting the renin-angiotensin system without the adverse effects common to the ACE inhibitors. The angiotensin II antagonists are available as orally active compounds and are undergoing clinical trials.

SPECIAL PATIENT GROUPS. The Elderly. The drugs used to treat diastolic hypertension or ISH in the elderly are the same as those used in younger patients. Because older persons are particularly sensitive to pharmacologic intervention, antihypertensive medications should be prescribed cautiously at lower than the recommended starting dose for the general population of hypertensives and adjustments made slowly (6- to 8-week intervals). Elderly persons are more prone to orthostatic hypotension because of decreased sensitivity of their baroreceptors. Accordingly, supine and standing BP's should be checked regularly to avoid orthostasis. Agents particularly prone to cause severe orthostatic hypotension (guanethidine, prazosin, and guanadrel) should be avoided. All of the major classes of antihypertensive drugs have been shown to be effective in elderly patients, although the β-blockers may be slightly less effective in this group.

Diabetics. Hypertension is twice as common in diabetics as in the general population. Diabetics with hypertension have a greatly increased risk of developing cerebrovascular disease, coronary artery disease, and renal disease compared with normotensive diabetics. Nonpharmacologic approaches, including weight loss, exercise, and decreased alcohol consumption, benefit both glucose and BP control. Because of their proven effectiveness and lack of significant adverse effects, recommended first-line agents for BP control in diabetics include calcium channel blockers, ACE inhibitors, and α-adrenergic blockers. The ACE inhibitors are gaining favor for treating hypertension in diabetic patients, particularly type 1 diabetics, because they reduce proteinuria and slow the rate of deterioration in renal function due to diabetic nephropathy. α-Blockers are favored as antihypertensive treatment in diabetics because of their positive effects on the serum lipid profile. Diuretics are effective in lowering BP in hypertensive diabetics, but their effects are particularly worrisome in this group. Similarly, β-blockers are effective but they tend to mask the symptoms of hypoglycemia and inhibit recovery of glucose levels. Potassium supplements and potassium-sparing diuretics should be used with caution in diabetics because of the frequent occurrence of hyporeninemic hypoaldosteronism in patients with diabetic nephropathy.

Blacks. Hypertension is more common, earlier in onset, and more severe in blacks than in whites. Organ damage secondary to hypertension also occurs more frequently in blacks than in whites. However, hypertension can be treated as successfully in blacks as in whites.

Secondary Hypertension. Renovascular Hypertension. Renovascular disease is the most common (1 to 2%) cause of curable hypertension. Any lesion that obstructs either large or small renal arteries can cause renovascular hypertension. The most common and clinically important of these are intrinsic lesions of the large vessels, because they can be physically removed and the hypertension either cured or ameliorated. Atherosclerotic disease is found in two thirds of patients with renovascular hypertension; fibrous or fibromuscular disease in one third. Patients with atherosclerotic renal artery lesions tend to be older and to have higher systolic BP's and more frequent extrarenal arterial disease than patients with essential hypertension and are more likely to develop target-organ damage. Patients with fibromuscular disease tend to be younger and predominantly female and are less likely to develop cardiovascular complications.

Patients most likely to have renovascular hypertension include those with hypertension of abrupt onset, especially in the young or in late middle age or old age; with malignant hypertension or sudden acceleration of benign hypertension; and who fail to respond to medical therapy. These patients generally have moderately severe to severe fixed diastolic hypertension. The presence of an upper abdominal bruit, particularly one that is systolic-diastolic or continuous in timing, high pitched, and radiates laterally from the midepigastrium, strongly suggests functionally significant renal artery stenosis. Such bruits have been described in one half to two thirds of patients with surgically proven renovascular hypertension.

Screening tests for renovascular hypertension include abdominal ultrasonography and the captopril renogram. *Abdominal ultrasonography* provides an inexpensive, noninvasive means of assessing renal size and ureteral anatomy that does not require administering radioactive isotopes. It is useful in evaluating patients in whom renal parenchymal disease and obstructive uropathy are part of the differential diagnosis. The *captopril renogram*—a renal scan performed after administering the ACE inhibitor captopril—has replaced the rapid-sequence or hypertensive intravenous pyelogram as the most commonly used screening test for renovascular hypertension. A positive captopril renogram indicates that a stenotic lesion is both hemodynamically and functionally significant and predicts a good result from renal revascularization. Definitive diagnosis of functionally significant renal artery stenosis has traditionally been made by combining *selective renal angiography* and *differential renal vein renin measurement.* Renal angiography defines the anatomy of the stenotic renal artery, information needed to plan the approach to revascularization. With the advent of safe and highly effective percutaneous techniques for renal revascularization, many angiographers now elect not to perform renal vein renin determinations in patients with typical lesions, but to proceed immediately to angioplasty and use the BP response as a test of the functional significance of the lesion. In some centers, the captopril renogram has replaced renal vein renin determinations as a functional test in patients with documented renal artery stenosis.

In general, the therapeutic approach to patients with renovascular hypertension is to attempt revascularization with percutaneous transluminal angioplasty at the time of diagnosis in patients with anatomically favorable lesions. If angioplasty is unsuccessful or if restenosis occurs after successful dilatation, the procedure can be repeated. If repeat angioplasty is unsuccessful, surgical revascularization should be attempted in patients with favorable lesions who can tolerate the procedure, particularly if BP is uncontrolled on medical treatment or renal function is deteriorating. Only patient with anatomically unfavorable lesions and those who are not surgical candidates should receive medical treatment without a prior attempt at revascularization.

ACE inhibitors, given alone or in combination with a diuretic, are generally effective in controlling BP while sparing renal function and maintaining negative sodium balance in patients with hypertension due to unilateral renal artery stenosis. These simple regimens are well tolerated and represent the medical treatment of choice in most patients with renovascular hypertension. The ACE inhibitors induce acute, reversible renal failure in a subset of patients with renovascular hypertension: those with bilateral renal artery stenosis or renal artery stenosis in a solitary kidney, whether native or allograft, or with unilateral renal artery stenosis and severe parenchymal disease in the contralateral kidney. This form of reversible renal insufficiency results from impaired autoregulation of glomerular filtration secondary to blockade of the intrarenal renin-angiotensin system when renal artery perfusion pressure is reduced. Normal autoregulation of glomerular filtration rate, which depends on an intact intrarenal renin-angiotensin system, is lost when an ACE inhibitor is administered.

Renal size and function must be carefully monitored in patients being treated medically for renovascular hypertension, even if BP is satisfactorily controlled. Renal function can deteriorate and renal mass can be lost very rapidly in patients with atherosclerotic disease who are treated medically. Significant reduction in renal length is the most sensitive index of loss of renal mass. Serial (every 3 to 6 months) estimates of renal size are important to follow patients who are receiving medical treatment for renovascular hypertension.

Adrenal. Primary aldosteronism and pheochromocytoma are relatively rare causes of hypertension that are clinically important because the associated hypertension can usually be cured with appropriate surgical or targeted drug therapy. These syndromes are discussed in detail in Ch. 204.

Oral Contraceptive–Induced Hypertension. A small percentage of women who use oral contraceptives experience the onset of hypertension, which resolves by stopping oral contraceptive therapy. The diagnosis of oral contraceptive–induced hypertension can be made by documenting the onset of hypertension *de novo* during contraceptive therapy and the resolution of the hypertension upon drug withdrawal. This form of hypertension usually begins during the first year of taking oral contraceptives.

Hypertensive Crisis. Hypertensive crises are subclassified as *hypertensive urgencies* or *emergencies,* depending on evidence of ongoing target-organ damage. In the absence of neurologic, cardiovascular, or renal deterioration and funduscopic abnormalities, patients with severely elevated BP's ($> 200/120$ mm Hg) do not require immediate BP reduction. However, with evidence of ongoing target-organ damage, patients with severely elevated BP's should immediately be treated with parenteral medications in an intensive care unit. A BP of 190/130 mm Hg may be well tolerated in a patient with chronic hypertension, whereas that BP reading in another patient may precipitate acute renal insufficiency, left ventricular failure, cerebral edema, or other vascular crisis, thereby creating a medical emergency. The triggering mechanism for the arteriolar lesion responsible for the development of accelerated or malignant hypertension is unknown but has been related to the absolute level or rate of rise of arterial pressure, the presence of disseminated intravascular clotting, or activation of the renin-angiotensin system. The syndrome is perpetuated by the deposition of fibrin in arteriolar walls which leads to retinopathy, renal damage, and increased renin release. Usually the cause of any particular hypertensive crisis is not known, and therapy must be generalized. However, when the cause is known, specific treatment should be instituted whenever possible (Table 37–8).

Symptoms of hypertensive crisis include headache, malaise, dizziness, blurred vision, chest pain, palpitations, and shortness of breath. Clinical and laboratory signs of hypertensive crisis include funduscopic changes (arteriolar narrowing, arteriovenous nicking, hemorrhages, exudates, papilledema); changes related to renal insufficiency; microangiopathic hemolytic anemia; signs of left ventricular dysfunction (gallops, jugular venous distention, cardiomegaly, tachycardia, pulmonary edema); and evidence of increased intracranial pressure (confusion, somnolence, stupor, neurologic deficits, seizures). Patients with hypertensive emergencies may present with stroke, subarachnoid hemorrhage, intracranial hemorrhage, aortic dissection, left ventricular failure, or myocardial ischemia. Importantly, however, severely elevated BP is often discovered coincidentally without any related signs or symptoms.

Evaluation of a patient with hypertensive crisis includes a pertinent history, with a special attempt to elicit symptoms relating to the cause or consequences of the severely elevated BP. Physical examination includes determining supine, sitting, and standing BP's, neurologic evaluation, funduscopic examination, cardiac auscultation with evaluation of left ventricular size and function, and palpation of distal pulses. Chest radiography, ECG, complete blood cell

TABLE 37–8. HYPERTENSIVE EMERGENCIES AND TREATMENT RECOMMENDATIONS

Emergency	Recommended Treatment	Drugs to Avoid
Hypertensive encephalopathy	Nitroprusside, labetalol, diazoxide	β-Antagonists, clonidine, methyldopa
Subarachnoid hemorrhage	Nimodipine, nitroprusside, labetalol	β-Antagonists, clonidine, methyldopa, diazoxide
Ischemic stroke	Nitroprusside, labetalol	β-Antagonists, clonidine, methyldopa, diazoxide
Intracerebral hemorrhage	No treatment, nitroprusside, labetalol	β-Antagonists, clonidine, methyldopa, diazoxide
Myocardial ischemia or infarction	IV nitroglycerin, labetalol, calcium antagonists, nitroprusside	Hydralazine, diazoxide
Left ventricular failure	Nitroprusside, IV nitroglycerin	β-Antagonists, labetalol
Aortic dissection	β-Antagonist with nitroprusside or trimethaphan, labetalol	Hydralazine, diazoxide
Hyperadrenergic states (cocaine overdose, clonidine withdrawal, pheochromocytoma, diet pills, amphetamines)	Phentolamine, labetalol, nitroprusside, clonidine (for clonidine withdrawal only)	β-Antagonists without α antagonism
Acute renal insufficiency	Nitroprusside, nicardipine, labetalol	β-Antagonists, trimethaphan
Eclampsia	Magnesium sulfate, hydralazine, labetalol, calcium antagonists	ACE inhibitors, diuretics, trimethaphan
Postoperative crisis	Labetalol, nitroglycerin, nicardipine, nitroprusside	Trimethaphan

From Calhoun D, Oparil S: Topics in acute care/handling hypertensive emergencies. Hosp Med 29:39, 1993.

TABLE 37-9. ANTIHYPERTENSIVE DRUGS FOR MANAGEMENT OF HYPERTENSIVE EMERGENCY

Drugs	Intramuscular (mg*)	Single Dose (mg*)	Continuous Infusion (µg/kg/min)	Onset of Action	Adverse Effects
Parenteral agents					
Direct vasodilators					
Sodium nitroprusside (Nipride)	—	—	0.5–10	Instantaneous	Nausea, vomiting, muscle twitching, apprehension, sweating, thiocyanate intoxication
Diazoxide (Hyperstat)	—	50–100 at 5–10–min intervals until satisfactory BP response is achieved	Rarely used	3–5 min	Tachycardia, palpitations, flushing, headache, nausea, vomiting, aggravation of angina or congestive heart failure or both, hyperglycemia, hyperuricemia, hypotension
Hydralazine (Apresoline)	10–40 min at 30-min intervals until satisfactory BP response is achieved	10–20 at 30-min intervals until satisfactory BP response is achieved	Rarely used	Intramuscularly 30 min; 5–10 min intravenously	Tachycardia, palpitations, flushing, headache, vomiting, aggravation of angina or congestive heart failure or both
Sympathetic blocking drugs					
Ganglion-blocking agents					
Trimethaphan camsylate (Arfonad)	—	—	4–90	5–10 min	Urinary retention, paralytic ileus, paralysis of pupillary reflex and accommodation of eye, dry mouth, orthostatic hypotension
CNS-active agents					
Methyldopate hydrochloride (Aldomet ester)		250–500; may be repeated at 6-hr intervals		2–3 hr	Drowsiness
α-Adrenergic-receptor-blocking agents					
Phentolamine (Regitine)	5-15	5–15 (rapid injection essential)	—	Instantaneous	Tachycardia, flushing
Labetalol	—	20 mg initially over 2 min, then 40–80 mg at 10-min intervals as needed up to 300 mg total	2 mg/min to a total dose of 300 mg	Instantaneous	Postural dizziness with or without postural hypotension; paradoxical pressor responses have been reported; nausea, vomiting, scalp tingling, burning in throat and groin
Nicardipine (Cardene)	—	5/hr initially, titrated upward by 1–2.5/hr every 15 min as needed up to 15/hr	—	1–5 min	Hypotension, flushing, headache, diaphoresis, dizziness, nausea, tachycardia

* Start with the lowest dose shown. Subsequent doses and intervals of administration should be adjusted according to the BP response. Constant surveillance is mandatory.

count with blood smear, and renal chemistries and urinalysis should be performed. If by history, physical examination, or laboratory data the patient has evidence of ongoing (new or worsening) end-organ damage, the patient should be considered to be having a medical emergency.

The goal in treating *hypertensive emergencies* is a prompt but gradual reduction in BP to just above normotensive levels. Precipitous or excessive reductions in BP may impair the body's ability to autoregulate blood flow, causing target organ hypoperfusion. Ideally, BP should be reduced to 150 to 160/100 to 110 mm Hg and maintained at that level for a few days. Then, with initiation or reinitiation of long-term therapy, BP can slowly be returned to the normotensive range.

Patients presenting with *hypertensive emergencies* require parenteral antihypertensive therapy administered in an intensive care setting. The antihypertensive drugs most commonly used to manage hypertensive emergencies, with recommended doses and common adverse effects, are summarized in Table 37–9.

Hypertensive urgencies do not require immediate BP reduction. Recent studies have demonstrated that patients experiencing hypertensive urgency require only initiation of maintenance therapy without acute oral loading for effective and sustained BP reduction. The prior practice of immediately reducing BP with oral loading of clonidine, nifedipine, or other antihypertensive agents exposes the patient to the unnecessary risk of acute end-organ hypoperfusion secondary to abrupt, uncontrolled decreases in BP. However, after initiating maintenance therapy or adjusting existing therapeutic regimens, early follow-up is essential to ensure efficacy of and compliance with the prescribed therapy.

Collins R, Peto R, MacMahon S, et al.: Blood pressure, stroke, and coronary heart disease. Part 2: Short-term reductions in blood pressure: Overview of randomised drug trials in their epidemiologic context. Lancet 335:827, 1990. *A meta-analysis of 14 randomized trials of antihypertensive drugs including 37,000 individuals treated for a mean of 5 years shows significant treatment-related reduction in stroke and coronary artery disease.*

Izzo JL, Black HR: Hypertension Primer. Dallas, American Heart Association, 1993. *An up-to-date introduction to the basic biology, pathophysiology, and clinical and epidemiologic aspects of hypertension prepared by the Council for High Blood Pressure Research of the American Heart Association.*

Joint National Committee on Detection, Evaluation, and Treatment of High Blood Pressure: The Fifth Report of the Joint National Committee on Detection, Evaluation, and Treatment of High Blood Pressure (JNC V). Arch Intern Med 153:154, 1993. *Detailed recommendations for diagnosis and pharmacologic and nonpharmacologic treatment of systemic hypertension.*

Neaton JD, Grimm RH Jr, Prineas RJ, et al.: Treatment of Mild Hypertension Study: Final results. JAMA 270:713, 1993. *Demonstration that both lifestyle modification and pharmacologic treatment are effective in lowering blood pressure in patients with stage 1 essential hypertension and that agents from each of the five major classes of antihypertensive drugs appear to be equally potent in controlling blood pressure in this patient group.*

Prisant LM, Carr AA, Hawkins DW: Treating hypertensive emergencies. Controlled reduction of blood pressure and protection of target organs. Postgrad Med 93:92, 1993. *An up-to-date discussion of the epidemiology, pathophysiology, and treatment of hypertensive urgencies and emergencies—emphasizes the hazards of precipitous blood pressure lowering in patients with ongoing target organ damage.*

SHEP Cooperative Research Group: Prevention of stroke by antihypertensive drug treatment in older persons with isolated systolic hypertension: Final Results of the Systolic Hypertension in the Elderly Program (SHEP). JAMA 265:3255, 1991. *Demonstration that treating isolated systolic hypertension in the elderly is successful in both lowering blood pressure and preventing cardiovascular morbidity and mortality, particularly stroke.*

38 PULMONARY HYPERTENSION

Joseph S. Alpert

Pulmonary hypertension is defined as pressure within the pulmonary arterial system elevated above the normal range. Pulmonary hypertension may be acute or chronic; right ventricular failure may develop in either setting as a result of the increase in right ventricular pressure work. Severe pulmonary hypertension even affects left ventricular function: Right ventricular dilatation secondary to severe pulmonary hypertension causes the interventricular septum to shift to the left, thereby decreasing left ventricular volume and compliance.

A variety of pathologic disorders can cause pulmonary hypertension. These entities lead to changes in pulmonary circulatory function that elevate pulmonary pressure. Certain normal physiologic events can also elevate pulmonary pressures. For example, exercise-induced increases in cardiac output result in moderate elevations in pulmonary arterial pressure. Increased blood viscosity secondary to increased red cell mass, e.g., polycythemia vera, can also cause pulmonary hypertension. Moreover, increased resistance in any of the various zones of the pulmonary circulation can lead to pulmonary hypertension. For example, increased pulmonary arteriolar resistance in a patient with congenital heart disease causes severe, chronic pulmonary hypertension. Finally, elevated pulmonary venous pressure in the setting of left ventricular failure or mitral stenosis is associated with an immediate increase in pulmonary arterial pressure which maintains forward blood flow through the lungs despite the increase in pulmonary venous pressure.

Chronic pulmonary hypertension is an important cause of right ventricular failure in the United States. Many of the 30,000 individuals who die each year of chronic obstructive pulmonary disease (COPD) succumb secondarily to right ventricular failure resulting from pulmonary hypertension. In addition, it has been estimated that approximately 200,000 deaths occur yearly from acute pulmonary embolism, a common cause of sudden-onset pulmonary hypertension and acute right ventricular failure.

HEMODYNAMICS OF THE PULMONARY CIRCULATION

In normal individuals at sea level, pulmonary arterial blood pressure is quite low because pulmonary arteriolar resistance is low—one-twelfth of the value found in the systemic circulation. Therefore, normal mean pulmonary arterial pressure is only 12 to 15 mm Hg (Table 38–1). Normal left atrial pressure is also low at 6 to 10 mm Hg. Consequently, the driving pressure or *pressure gradient* across the pulmonary vascular bed is only 6 to 12 mm Hg; i.e., a normal cardiac output of 5 to 6 liters per minute flows across the pulmonary vascular bed to the left atrium with a pressure drop of 6 to 12 mm Hg. This compares with a pressure drop of approximately 90 mm Hg across the systemic circulation.

The distensibility and low vascular resistance of the pulmonary circulation are the result of the thin muscular medial layer of the pulmonary arterioles. Systemic arterioles have a medial muscle layer that is considerably thicker. The lower resistance and hence pressure within the pulmonary circuit, compared with its systemic counterpart, are reflected in the right ventricle, which is less than half as thick as the left ventricle.

TABLE 38–1. NORMAL VALUES AT SEA LEVEL AND AT ALTITUDE FOR RESTING PULMONARY PRESSURES

Variable	Sea Level	14,900 feet
Pulmonary arterial pressure (mm Hg, systolic/diastolic, mean)	20/12, 15	38/14, 25
Left atrial pressure (mm Hg)	5	5
Gradient (difference) between pulmonary arterial mean pressure and left atrial pressure (mm Hg)	10	20
Pulmonary vascular resistance (dynes·sec·cm^{-5})	120	266

Modified from Fishman AP: Pulmonary hypertension, *In* Wyngaarden JB, Smith LH Jr, Bennett JC (eds.): Cecil Textbook of Medicine. 19th ed. Philadelphia, WB Saunders, 1992, p 270.

Pressure within the pulmonary arteries (P_{pa}) is directly proportional to three factors: the pressure within the pulmonary veins (P_{pv}), the cardiac output (CO), and the pulmonary vascular resistance (PVR). This relationship is expressed in the following formula:

$$P_{pa} = CO \times PVR + P_{pv}$$

Pulmonary hypertension develops when flow or resistance to flow across the pulmonary vascular bed increases. As already noted, a variety of physiologic and pathophysiologic mechanisms can lead to such increases in pulmonary pressures, e.g., exercise. In normal individuals, marked increases in right ventricular cardiac output during severe exertion are associated with small increments in pulmonary arterial pressure: Pulmonary pressure increases minimally during exercise in normals because pulmonary vascular resistance falls with increasing cardiac output. This fall in vascular resistance is due in part to arteriolar vasodilation and in part to opening or recruitment of previously closed microvessels.

Another "physiologic" cause of pulmonary hypertension is hypoxia, which is associated with ascent from sea level (Table 38–1). The pulmonary hypertension of altitude results from hypoxic arteriolar vasoconstriction.

Other factors that may affect pulmonary pressures are blood viscosity and intrathoracic pressure. Poiseuille's law predicts that pressure change along a tube containing a moving fluid is directly proportional to the viscosity of the contained fluid. Therefore, marked increases in the number of red blood cells per cubic milliliter of blood produce elevations in blood viscosity that can cause pulmonary hypertension. Another factor that can increase pulmonary arterial pressure is elevation in intrathoracic pressure, which is directly transmitted to the pulmonary vasculature. Increased intrathoracic pressure is a causative factor in the pulmonary hypertension observed in patients who are being mechanically ventilated, especially if positive end-expiratory pressure (PEEP) ventilation is used.

PATHOPHYSIOLOGY OF PULMONARY HYPERTENSION

As already mentioned, a number of different pathophysiologic scenarios can produce pulmonary hypertension: increases in pulmonary flow, vascular resistance, blood viscosity, and intrathoracic pressure. "Hyperkinetic" pulmonary hypertension can be seen in patients with congenital heart disease who have extensive left-to-right cardiac shunts that produce a large pulmonary blood flow (Table 38–2). Other disease entities associated with pulmonary hypertension result from increased pulmonary vascular resistance of the arterial, arteriolar, or venous segments of the pulmonary vascular bed.

Increased resistance to blood flow through the pulmonary arterial circulation can be the result of large pulmonary emboli or loss of pulmonary arterial cross-sectional area from various disease entities, e.g., pulmonary fibrosis, extensive pulmonary resection, vasculitis, or infiltration of the lung with tumor (see Table 38–1).

Increased pulmonary arteriolar resistance is commonly the result of hypoxia and/or acidosis, which cause pulmonary arteriolar vasoconstriction. Certain specific vasoactive chemical compounds, e.g., pyrrolizidine alkaloids, can also increase pulmonary arteriolar tone. Patients with congenital heart disease with left-to-right shunts can

TABLE 38-2. PATHOPHYSIOLOGY OF PULMONARY HYPERTENSION

Mechanism	Disease Entities
Increased pulmonary blood flow	Congenital heart disease with left-to-right shunts; marked increase in cardiac output, e.g., severe anemia; severe bronchiectasis with systemic-to-pulmonary artery shunts
Abnormalities in the pulmonary arteries: Increased resistance to flow or loss of cross-sectional area	Pulmonary embolism; pulmonary fibrosis; sarcoidosis; scleroderma; extensive pulmonary resection; severe COPD; thoracic deformities, e.g., kyphoscoliosis, severe pectus excavatum; schistosomiasis; extensive neoplastic or inflammatory infiltration
Abnormalities in the pulmonary arterioles: vasoconstriction and/or obliteration	Hypoxia, e.g., altitude; COPD, hypoventilation syndromes, e.g., sleep apnea; acidosis; toxic substances; primary pulmonary hypertension
Abnormalities in pulmonary veins or venules: elevated pulmonary venous pressure and vascular resistance	Left atrial hypertension, e.g., mitral stenosis, left ventricular failure; pulmonary venous thrombosis; pulmonary veno-occlusive disease; mediastinitis, e.g., methysergide-induced sclerosing mediastinitis
Increased blood viscosity	Polycythemia vera; leukemia with very high leukocyte counts
Increased intrathoracic pressure	COPD; mechanical ventilation, especially with positive end-expiratory pressure

COPD = Chronic obstructive pulmonary disease

develop markedly increased pulmonary arteriolar vascular resistance through a pathophysiologic process that begins as vasoconstriction and ends with obliteration and loss of pulmonary microvessels. Finally, primary pulmonary hypertension is the result of abnormal increases in pulmonary arteriolar tone. The resultant pulmonary hypertension in these patients leads to thickening of the intimal and medial layers of the pulmonary arterioles, which, in turn, further exacerbates the degree of pulmonary hypertension. A vicious spiral is thereby engendered in which ever-increasing levels of pulmonary arterial hypertension lead to further arteriolar thickening, which leads to worsening pulmonary hypertension. This pathophysiologic sequence is also seen in patients with congenital heart disease who develop pulmonary vascular disease and pulmonary hypertension.

Increased pulmonary venous pressure and vascular resistance are other causes of pulmonary hypertension: Increased pulmonary venous pressure leads to augmented pulmonary capillary and pulmonary arterial diastolic pressure. Pulmonary arterial pressure must increase in this setting to maintain forward cardiac output. Disease entities that increase pulmonary venous pressure and resistance to blood flow include pulmonary venous thombosis, e.g., sickle cell anemia, pulmonary venous occlusive disease, mitral stenosis, and left ventricular failure.

Pulmonary hypertension can be divided into three classes based on the location of the abnormal increase in pulmonary vascular resistance: precapillary, passive, and reactive. Patients with increased pulmonary arteriolar and/or arterial resistance are classified as having precapillary pulmonary hypertension. The pathologic changes involve the pulmonary circulation proximal to the pulmonary capillaries, i.e., in the pulmonary arterioles and/or arteries. Pulmonary arterial pressure is increased, but pulmonary capillary wedge and pulmonary venous pressures are normal. The gradient between the mean pulmonary arterial pressure and the pulmonary capillary or pulmonary venous pressures is >12 mm Hg. Examples include hypoxic pulmonary hypertension (increased arteriolar resistance) and pulmonary embolism (increased arterial resistance).

Individuals with increased pulmonary venous pressure secondarily causing pulmonary arterial hypertension are said to exhibit passive pulmonary hypertension because the increase in pulmonary arterial pressure occurs passively—without active pulmonary arterial

vasoconstriction. Pulmonary arterial, capillary, and venous pressures are all elevated. The gradient between the mean pulmonary arterial pressure and the pulmonary capillary or pulmonary venous pressures is ≤12 mm Hg. Examples of passive pulmonary arterial hypertension include mitral stenosis and left ventricular failure.

The third form of pulmonary arterial hypertension is termed reactive and contains elements of both precapillary *and* passive pulmonary hypertension. Reactive pulmonary hypertensive patients have elevated pulmonary venous pressure as well as pulmonary arteriolar vasoconstriction. The gradient between the mean pulmonary arterial pressure and the pulmonary capillary or pulmonary venous pressures is >12 mm Hg. Patients with reactive pulmonary arterial hypertension usually have longstanding mitral stenosis.

DIAGNOSIS OF PULMONARY HYPERTENSION

Unfortunately, no simple, inexpensive technique, such as the blood pressure cuff, exists for measuring pulmonary arterial blood pressure. Accurate noninvasive measurement of pulmonary arterial blood pressure can be obtained with the Doppler echocardiogram, but this technique is costly, time consuming, and not as portable as the indirect method employed to measure arterial blood pressure (cuff and stethoscope). Consequently, the physician must rely on clinical information obtained from the history and physical examination to select individuals for Doppler echocardiographic examination.

HISTORY AND PHYSICAL EXAMINATION. Patients with mild to moderate pulmonary hypertension are often asymptomatic. Individuals with more severe pulmonary hypertension usually complain of dyspnea on exertion secondary to exercise-induced decreases in cardiac output and increases in pulmonary arterial pressure. Other symptoms can include easy fatigability, exertional chest discomfort and/or syncope, cough, hemoptysis, and rarely, hoarseness secondary to compression of the left recurrent laryngeal nerve by a dilated pulmonary artery.

Physical examination (Table 38-3) in the patient with pulmonary arterial hypertension may disclose increased intensity of the pulmonic component of the second heart sound, a diastolic murmur of pulmonic regurgitation in patients with severe pulmonary hypertension, evidence of right ventricular dilatation (left parasternal lift or heave), or signs of right ventricular failure: jugular venous distension, right ventricular S_3 (increased loudness of the S_3 on inspiration), hepatomegaly, ascites, and/or peripheral edema. Patients with severe emphysema and increased thoracic anteroposterior diameter may not display the findings usually associated with advanced pulmonary hypertension because chest expansion make palpation and auscultation more difficult.

THE ELECTROCARDIOGRAM. Electrocardiographic (ECG) diagnosis of right ventricular hypertrophy (RVH) is often the first suggestion that pulmonary hypertension is present (Table 38-4). However, the finding of RVH by ECG is often a late finding in patients with pulmonary hypertension. Acute right ventricular strain (an S wave in lead I, and a Q wave and inverted T wave in lead III) develops in patients with major pulmonary embolism. Chronic right ventricular pressure overload leads to right axis deviation and an R/S ratio greater than 1.0 in lead V_1 (Fig. 38-1). Incomplete or complete right bundle branch block may also be observed.

ECHOCARDIOGRAPHY AND DOPPLER ECHOCARDIOGRAPHY. Echocardiographic findings that may be present in patients with pulmonary hypertension include right ventricular dilata-

TABLE 38-3. COMMONLY USED CLINICAL CLUES SUGGESTING THE DIAGNOSIS OF PULMONARY HYPERTENSION

Increased loudness of the pulmonic component of the second heart sound
Right ventricular enlargement on physical examination: left parasternal impulse or lift
Signs of right ventricular failure present on physical examination: jugular venous distention, right ventricular S_3, hepatomegaly, ascites, hepatojugular reflux, peripheral edema
Right ventricular hypertrophy on the ECG
Enlargement of the right ventricle and/or pulmonary arteries on the chest radiograph, echocardiogram, radionuclear ventriculogram, or CT/MRI
Pulmonary arterial systolic blood pressure > 30 mm Hg by Doppler echocardiography or catheterization

TABLE 38-4. LABORATORY FINDINGS IN PATIENTS WITH PULMONARY HYPERTENSION

Disease Entity	ECG	Chest X-ray	Other Useful Tests	Catheterization
Precapillary Pulmonary Hypertension				
PPHT	RVH	↑↑ PA, ↑ RV, clear lungs with tapered periph. arteries	PFT's nl; lung scan nl or min. abn	PAP ↑↑, nl PCW, ↑ RAP, PAgram nl
Pulmonary embolism	nl or acute cor pulmonale (S₁Q₃T₃ or new IRBBB or RBBB)	nl or infiltrate, unilateral pulm. effusion	abnl ABG's: ↓ Po₂, ↑ pH, ↓ Pco₂; lung scan: seg. perf. defects, nl ventil. scan	PAP ↑, nl PCW, RAP nl or ↑; + PAgram
Disorders of ventilation	nl or RVH	Specific abnl in various entities	ABG's, PFT's: abnl	PAP ↑, PCW nl, RAP nl or ↑
Congenital heart disease	RVH	Clear lungs, ↑↑ PA, ↑ RV, tapered distal arteries, specific abnl in various entities	Cardiac echo: specific abnl in various entities	↑↑ PAP, nl PCW, RA ↑ or nl, ↑↑ Po₂
Passive Pulmonary Hypertension				
Mitral stenosis	AF or NSR, LAE, RVH or no VH	Pulm. congestion, ↑ LA, ↑ RV	Echo: LAE, abnl MV, nl LV	Gradient across MV, PAP ↑ PCW ↑, RAP nl or ↑
Left ventricular failure	Abnl depends on specific entity: LVH, MI, BBB	↑↑ or ↑ LV, ↑ LA or nl RV, pulm. congestion	Echo: abnl LV function, LAE	Abnl LV function, ↑ LVEDP, ↑ PCW, ↑ PAP
Reactive Pulmonary Hypertension				
Longstanding mitral stenosis	AF, RVH	↑↑ PA, ↑↑ RV, ↑↑ LA, pulm. congestion	Echo: very abnl MV, ↑↑ RV, ↑↑ LA	MV gradient, PCW ↑↑, ↑↑ PAP, ↑ RAP
Pulmonary veno-occlusive disease	RVH	↑↑ PA, ↑↑ RV	Lung scan: nl or minor defects	Absent MV gradient, PCW ↑ or nl, LAP nl, LVP nl

Abbreviations: PPHT = primary pulmonary hypertension; PA = pulmonary artery; RV = right ventricle; RA = right atrium; LV = left ventricle; LA = left atrium; PAP = pulmonary artery pressure; RAP = right atrial pressure; LVP = left ventricular pressure; PCW = pulmonary capillary pressure; LAP = left atrial pressure; nl = normal; abnl = abnormal or abnormality; pulm. = pulmonary; ABG's = arterial blood gases; PFT's = pulmonary function tests; seg. = segmental; PAgram = pulmonary angiogram; RVH = right ventricular hypertrophy; LVH = left ventricular hypertrophy; NSR = normal sinus rhythm; VH = ventricular hypertrophy; LAE = left atrial enlargement; AF = atrial fibrillation; MI = myocardial infarction; BBB = bundle branch block; LVEDP = left ventricular end-diastolic pressure; min. = minimal; MV = mitral valve; periph. = peripheral; perf. = perfusion; ventil. = ventilation; + = positive; ↑↑ = markedly increased; ↑ = increased; ↓ = decreased.

tion and/or hypertrophy, right atrial dilatation, and the parodoxical septal wall motion associated with right ventricular overload (Table 38-4). Doppler studies predict with considerable accuracy the level of pulmonary arterial systolic and mean pressures. Associated pathologic entities, e.g., mitral stenosis, can also be identified and their severity quantitated.

RADIONUCLEAR DIAGNOSTIC TECHNIQUES. A number of radionuclide diagnostic studies are useful in patients with known or suspected pulmonary hypertension. Pulmonary scintigraphy is the most sensitive noninvasive diagnostic test for pulmonary embolism, but it is not very specific (Table 38-4). Ventricular size and func-

tion can be measured using radionuclear ventriculography in patients in whom adequate echocardiographic studies are unobtainable. Certain pulmonary conditions that may cause pulmonary hypertension, e.g., sarcoidoisis, are associated with abnormal gallium lung scans.

COMPUTED TOMOGRAPHY (CT) SCANNING/MAGNETIC RESONANCE IMAGING (MRI). Tomographic studies of the chest with CT or MRI (see Ch. 33.5) often yield important information about cardiac and/or pulmonary pathologic changes in patients with pulmonary hypertension. Right and left ventricular size and shape are clearly visualized, as are the major pulmonary

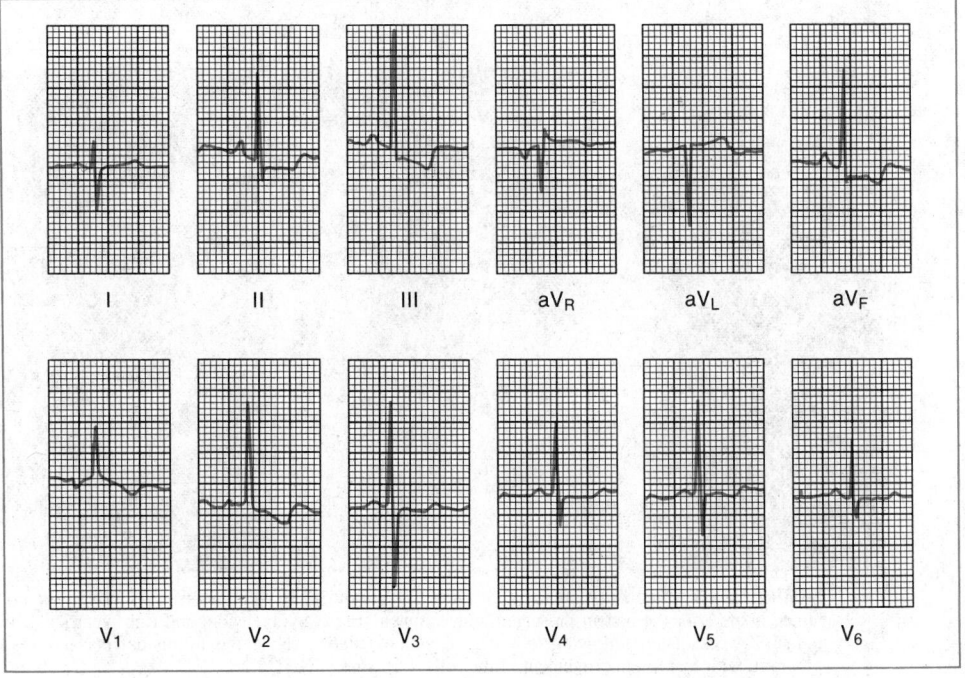

FIGURE 38-1. Unsuspected primary pulmonary hypertension: A routine ECG in an symptomatic 32-year-old man demonstrates right ventricular hypertrophy, the first clue to the presence of primary pulmonary hypertension.

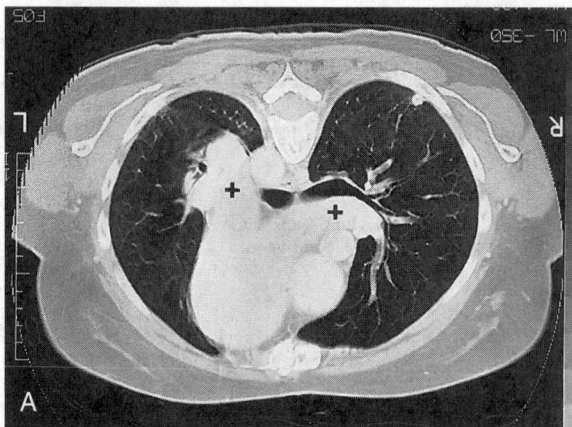

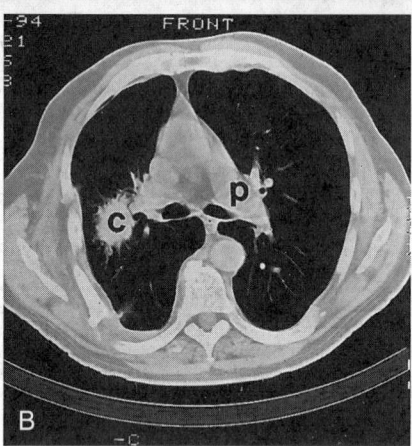

FIGURE 38–2. *A*, MRI from a 47-year-old woman with an atrial septal defect and pulmonary vascular disease producing severe pulmonary hypertension. Note the marked enlargement of the main pulmonary arteries (+) and the dearth of peripheral pulmonary arteries ("pruning"). (Courtesy of Dr. Howard I. Molitch, Radiology Department, University of Arizona Health Science Center.) *B*, MRI from a 62-year-old man with severe, chronic asthmatic bronchitis leading to pulmonary hypertension. Note the markedly enlarged left main pulmonary artery (p). There is a bronchogenic carcinoma in the right lung (c). (Courtesy of Dr. Theron W. Ovitt, Radiology Department, University of Arizona Health Science Center.)

arteries. Pulmonary parenchymal alterations are also disclosed (Fig. 38–2).

CARDIAC CATHETERIZATION AND ANGIOGRAPHY. Precise measurement of pulmonary arterial, capillary, and venous pressures are obtained by right, and at times left, heart catheterization. Pressures may be unexpectedly low if the patient has undergone vigorous diuresis prior to the hemodynamic study. Precapillary pulmonary hypertension can be distinguished from venous (also termed passive) pulmonary hypertension by hemodynamic observations (Table 38–4). Cardiac catheterization also identifies patients with congenital or acquired intracardiac shunts and pulmonary hypertension. The severity of right ventricular failure can be quantitated.

Pulmonary angiography is the most accurate technique for identifying pulmonary embolism (Fig. 38–3). Angiographic studies are usually combined with hemodynamic measurements of right heart function.

SPECIFIC ENTITIES ASSOCIATED WITH PULMONARY HYPERTENSION

Myriad disease entities are associated with pulmonary hypertension (see Table 38–2). For many of these conditions, pulmonary hypertension is an epiphenomenon, i.e., the major pathophysiologic abnormality is not the increased pressure in the pulmonary vascular bed. On the other hand, there are diseases for which pulmonary hypertension is the central theme. A number of these latter conditions are discussed in this section.

PRECAPILLARY PULMONARY HYPERTENSION. *Primary Pulmonary Hypertension.* Although primary pulmonary hypertension (PPHT) is an uncommon disease, it represents the purest form of pulmonary hypertension without other disease entities present. PPHT is a disease of unknown cause, although abnormal pulmonary vascular reactivity seems to underlie this condition in many individuals. Some authorities argue that recurrent episodes of asymptomatic pulmonary embolism lead to PPHT. In support of this theory is the common autopsy finding of clinically silent organizing or recanalized pulmonary thrombi in the pulmonary arterial bed. It is possible, however, that these thrombi are the result of *in situ* thromboses. Abnormalities of coagulation such as increased platelet reactivity and defective fibrinolysis have been described in patients with PPHT.

Increased pulmonary vascular reactivity and vasoconstriction have been documented in many patients with PPHT; this appears to be the underlying pathophysiologic abnormality in the majority of patients with this condition. However, it remains unclear why patients with PPHT demonstrate this abnormality. Because the increase in vascular resistance is present in the pulmonary arterioles, PPHT is one of the forms of precapillary pulmonary hypertension.

A number of pathologic findings are common to all patients with PPHT: intimal thickening and fibrosis in small pulmonary arteries

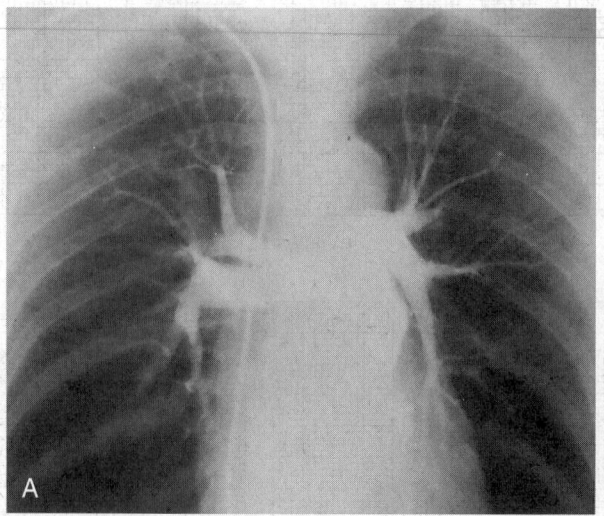

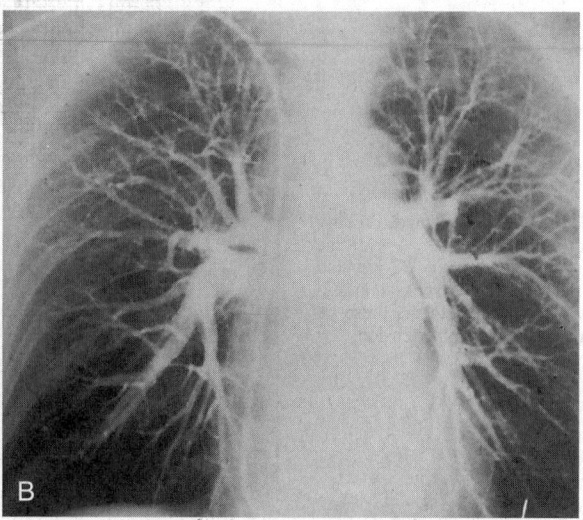

FIGURE 38–3. Pulmonary angiography in a 67-year-old man with massive pulmonary embolism. *A*, Angiogram was obtained hours after the patient presented with dyspnea at rest, hypotension, and right ventricular failure. *B*, Angiogram was obtained 2 weeks later, following 2 weeks of anticoagulation. Note the filling defects and vessel cut-offs in the initial angiogram, with marked improvement in the follow-up study.

and arterioles; increased medial thickening of small muscular pulmonary arteries and arterioles; necrotizing arteritis and fibrinoid necrosis in small muscular pulmonary arteries; dilated, thin-walled side branches to muscular pulmonary arteries called plexiform lesions.

The majority of patients with PPHT come to medical attention late in the course of the illness. Women outnumber men 3 to 4:1. Familial or autosomal dominant inheritance is occasionally observed. Patients usually complain of exertional dyspnea without orthopnea and fatigue. Other complaints include exertional syncope, angina-like chest discomfort, palpitations, cough, and hemoptysis. Physical examination discloses findings consistent with pulmonary hypertension with or without right ventricular failure (see Table 38–3). Routine laboratory tests are usually unremarkable. The aforementioned abnormalities in platelet function and fibrinolysis may be observed. The ECG reveals signs of RVH and, at times, right atrial enlargement. Chest roentgenograms disclose clear lung fields, enlarged central pulmonary arteries, and marked tapering of peripheral pulmonary arteries. Pulmonary function tests are usually normal except for arterial blood gases, which disclose evidence of hyperventilation: low $Paco_2$ and normal or modestly reduced Po_2.

Pulmonary scintigraphy is usually normal or demonstrates minor subsegmental defects. Patients with advanced PPHT may develop hypotension during pulmonary scintigraphy secondary to obstruction of many of the remaining pulmonary microvessels. Pulmonary angiography is a diagnostically important but clinically dangerous procedure in patients with PPHT. Angiography demonstrates small tapering pulmonary arteries in a "pruned tree" pattern and *absence* of pulmonary emboli. Hypotension or frank shock may develop during angiography in patients with PPHT. Consequently, small selective injections of angiographic dye are usually used.

The differential diagnosis of PPHT includes mitral stenosis, recurrent pulmonary embolism, congenital cardiac defects with severe pulmonary vascular disease, sickle cell anemia, collagen vascular disease, and rare entities such as cor triatriatum.

Pulmonary Embolism. Acute pulmonary embolism is probably the most common cause of pulmonary hypertension in the United States. The cause of the increase in pulmonary arterial pressure is obstruction of the pulmonary arterial bed by embolized thrombus. Therefore, pulmonary embolism represents another example of precapillary pulmonary hypertension.

Massive embolism, defined as thrombus obstructing 50% or more of the pulmonary arterial circulation, is associated with pulmonary arterial systolic pressures in the range of 50 to 60 mm Hg in individuals without prior heart or lung disease. Patients with heart and/or lung disease and pre-existing pulmonary hypertension may demonstrate pulmonary arterial systolic pressures that are considerably higher. Pulmonary hypertension is relieved in patients with acute pulmonary embolism as the degree of embolic obstruction declines. Chronic pulmonary hypertension secondary to unresolved embolism is rare. It is usually the result of multiple episodes of symptomatic but unrecognized pulmonary embolism.

Patients may present with dyspnea and tachypnea at rest, pleuritic chest discomfort, or hypotension. Physical examination discloses clear lungs or localized rales and/or wheezes. Signs of right ventricular dilatation and/or failure are usually restricted to patients with massive embolism. Abnormal arterial blood gases (decreased Po_2 and Pco_2 and increased pH) are the rule in acute pulmonary embolism. The ECG is abnormal only in patients with massive embolism, disclosing the pattern of acute right ventricular strain (S_1, Q_3, T_3) (see Fig. 38–1). The chest radiograph is often normal or it may reveal unilateral platelike atelectasis and/or a small pleural effusion. Pulmonary ventilation/perfusion scintigraphy is the most useful noninvasive test in patients with acute pulmonary embolism, demonstrating subsegmental perfusion defects that fail to ventilate. Pulmonary angiography represents the diagnostic gold standard for the diagnosis of pulmonary embolism: Intraluminal filling defects are identified in patients with acute embolism (Fig. 38–3). The differential diagnosis includes congestive heart failure and a variety of pulmonary or pleural infectious processes, e.g., bacterial pneumonia or viral pleuritis.

Disorders of Ventilation. A number of ventilatory disorders cause pulmonary hypertension by three different pathophysiologic sequences: hypoxic vasoconstriction, anatomic restriction of the pulmonary vascular bed, and a combination of both vasoconstriction and restriction of the vasculature. Patients with high-altitude

pulmonary hypertension and COPD develop pulmonary vasoconstriction and hypertension secondary to alveolar hypoxia. Patients with COPD exacerbate existing hypoxic pulmonary vasoconstriction by means of acidemia secondary to CO_2 retention.

Anatomic restriction of the pulmonary vascular bed as a cause of pulmonary hypertension is seen in patients with sarcoidosis and idiopathic pulmonary fibrosis. The combination of vasoconstriction and anatomic restriction of the vascular bed is observed in patients with kyphoscoliotic pulmonary disease.

In patients with ventilatory disorders and pulmonary hypertension, the symptoms and signs of pulmonary hypertension (see Table 38–3) are mixed with the clinical manifestations of the underlying pulmonary disorder. Similarly, laboratory abnormalities depend on the underlying pulmonary disease. For example, ECG evidence of RVH may be obscured in patients with COPD and marked hyperinflation. In general, the ECG is a reasonable reliable marker for RVH in patients with pulmonary hypertension secondary to restriction of the pulmonary vascular bed. However, the ECG is much less reliable in patients with vasoconstrictive pulmonary hypertension. The differential diagnosis of pulmonary hypertension is extensive in patients with ventilatory disorders (see Table 38–2).

Congenital Heart Disease with Severe Pulmonary Vascular Disease. Patients with congenital cardiac lesions and left-to-right shunts may develop progressive pulmonary vascular disease with associated pulmonary hypertension. As pulmonary vascular disease progresses, pulmonary hypertension worsens and the magnitude of the left-to-right shunt declines. Eventually, there is minimal shunting of blood or even a net right-to-left shunt that results in arterial desaturation, so-called Eisenmenger's reaction. The pathologic changes associated with severe pulmonary vascular disease resemble those observed in patients with PPHT. A number of different underlying congenital cardiac defects can be associated with Eisenmenger's reaction, including atrial septal defect, ventricular septal defect, patent ductus arteriosus, and more complex lesions such as transposition of the great arteries (see Fig. 38–2A). As with PPHT, the long-term prognosis is guarded for these patients although better than once thought.

Patients with Eisenmenger's reaction usually complain of dyspnea on exertion. They may also experience angina-like chest discomfort, hemoptysis, and exertional syncope. The ECG discloses RVH, and the chest radiograph demonstrates clear lung fields, central pulmonary arterial enlargement, and marked tapering of distal pulmonary arteries. Echocardiography and/or catheterization with angiography usually reveals the correct diagnosis. The differential diagnosis includes PPHT, severe mitral stenosis, and a variety of end-stage pulmonary diseases.

PASSIVE PULMONARY HYPERTENSION. *Mitral Stenosis.* Increased left atrial pressure in patients with mitral stenosis is accompanied by pulmonary arterial hypertension, as noted earlier. Pulmonary hypertension is largely reversible in these patients following successful valvuloplasty or valve replacement. Rarely, pulmonary hypertension fails to regress in patients with severe and longstanding mitral stenosis.

Patients complain of dyspnea on exertion, fatigue, and occasionally hemoptysis. Physical examination discloses the typical murmur of mitral stenosis and evidence of right ventricular enlargement. The patient is often in atrial fibrillation. The ECG may reveal RVH; left atrial enlargement is commonly present. The chest radiograph demonstrates pulmonary congestion and right ventricular and left atrial enlargement. Echocardiography and/or cardiac catheterization with angiography confirms the diagnosis. The differential diagnosis includes PPHT, a variety of entities leading to left ventricular failure and the rare condition cor triatriatum.

Left Ventricular Failure. Any disease that causes left ventricular failure with resultant left atrial hypertension is accompanied by pulmonary hypertension. The most common causes of left ventricular failure include coronary artery disease, systemic hypertension, and cardiomyopathy. Patient complaints are similar to those expressed by individuals with mitral stenosis. The physical examination often reveals the underlying cause of left ventricular failure, e.g., the murmur of aortic stenosis combined with abnormal carotid upstroke and left ventricular enlargement. A left ventricular S_3 is commonly present in patients with overt left ventricular failure regardless of cause. The ECG findings depend on the nature of the underlying cause of left ventricular failure, e.g., myocardial infarction in a patient with coronary artery disease or left ventricular hypertrophy in a patient with aortic stenosis. The chest radiograph usually reveals pulmonary congestion as well as left ventricular enlargement. The differential diagnosis of left ventricular failure includes mitral stenosis, aortic stenosis, coronary artery disease and myocardial infarction, hypertensive heart disease, cardiomyopathy, and other less common entities affecting the left ventricle, e.g., myocarditis.

REACTIVE PULMONARY HYPERTENSION. A small number of patients with chronic passive pulmonary hypertension develop pulmonary arteriolar vasoconstriction, i.e., precapillary pulmonary hypertension, on top of pre-existing passively elevated pulmonary arterial pressure. In these individuals, pulmonary arterial pressure is elevated disproportionately to the level of pulmonary venous pressure. The gradient between mean pulmonary arterial pressure and pulmonary capillary or venous pressure is >12 mm Hg. Medial hypertrophy and possibly intimal hyperplasia are found in pulmonary arterioles of patients with reactive pulmonary hypertension. The most common disease entity resulting in reactive pulmonary hypertension is mitral stenosis with longstanding passive pulmonary hypertension. Other pathologic conditions that cause pulmonary venous hypertension, e.g., aortic stenosis or left ventricular failure secondary to myocardial infarction, usually result in the patient's death before reactive pulmonary hypertension can develop.

Patients with reactive pulmonary hypertension are usually very symptomatic. Dyspnea and fatigue are the dominant complaints. The physical examination usually reveals right ventricular enlargement and other findings associated with severe pulmonary hypertension (see Table 38–3). The ECG demonstrates RVH; the chest roentgenogram shows right ventricular enlargement and very large central pulmonary arteries. Marked cardiomegaly secondary to right ventricular dilation is often present. Successful mitral valvuloplasty or valve replacement often results in marked amelioration of reactive pulmonary hypertension. However, some elevation in pulmonary arterial pressure may persist secondary to permanent loss of pulmonary microvessels.

Pulmonary veno-occlusive disease is a poorly understood condition characterized by diffuse involvement of pulmonary veins and venules. Affected veins demonstrate fibrous narrowing or obliteration of the lumen. The result is severe, chronic pulmonary venous and capillary hypertension that eventually results in irreversible reactive pulmonary arterial hypertension. Patients complain of dyspnea and fatigue; the clinical picture may resemble advanced mitral stenosis or PPHT.

TREATMENT OF PULMONARY HYPERTENSION

Because a variety of disease entities with varying pathophysiologic abnormalities lead to pulmonary hypertension, it is impossible to recommend one specific remedy for all forms of increased pulmonary vascular pressure. In general, however, effective therapy should reduce pulmonary vascular resistance directly. If pulmonary pressures are reduced in proportion to a decrease in cardiac output, little therapeutic gain is achieved. General therapeutic measures include supplementing inspiratory oxygen, correcting acid-base abnormalities, and ensuring that inspired air is cool, dry, and free of inhaled irritants.

Specific measures are discussed at greater length, including interventions such as vasodilators, bronchodilators, antibiotics for pulmonary and/or bronchial infection, return to sea level for patients with high-altitude pulmonary hypertension, anticoagulants for pulmonary embolism, relief of mitral stenosis, and measures to improve left ventricular function in patients with left ventricular failure.

Specific Measures for Treating Pulmonary Hypertension

Patients with PPHT represent a difficult therapeutic challenge because increased pulmonary vascular abnormalities may be so far advanced that they cannot be ameliorated when these individuals come to medical attention. Therefore, survival statistics are often poor for these patients (Fig. 38–4). When first seen, most patients with PPHT have lost microvasculature, rendering pulmonary hypertension irreversible; cardiopulmonary or pulmonary transplantation are the only effective means of therapy. Earlier in the course of the illness, however, pulmonary vasoconstriction may still be present.

Calcium channel blockers given in high dose, e.g., diltiazem, 120 mg three times a day, can lower pulmonary vascular resistance by dilating pulmonary resistance vessels if vasoconstriction is still present. In patients with PPHT and residual pulmonary vasoconstriction, therapy with calcium channel blockers has been shown to reduce pulmonary arterial pressure and vascular resistance, leading to regression of RVH (Fig. 38–5). Unfortunately, only a minority of patients with PPHT still exhibit pulmonary vasoconstriction when they first seek medical attention. Lifelong anticoagulation is advised by some authorities for these individuals, who are at high risk for pulmonary embolism.

Patients with acute pulmonary embolism can usually be successfully managed with intravenous heparin followed by oral warfarin therapy. Patients continue to receive oral anticoagulation for 3 to 6 months or until the factor that predisposed them to pulmonary embolism has resolved. Use venous interruption in patients who have strong contraindications to anticoagulation, e.g., active gastrointestinal hemorrhage. Thrombolytic therapy or surgical embolectomy is usually reserved for patients with massive, life-threatening embolism.

Therapy for patients with disorders of ventilation varies, depending on the particular pulmonary disorder. Thus, patients with COPD may experience a lowering of pulmonary arterial pressure when given supplemental inspiratory oxygen, bronchodilators, and appropriate antibiotics for bronchial or pulmonary infection. Patients with high-altitude pulmonary hypertension improve with supplemental inspiratory oxygen or return to sea level. Kyphoscoliotic pulmonary disease may improve following appropriate corrective orthopedic surgery. Individuals with severe pulmonary sarcoidosis may experience amelioration when given corticosteroids.

Patients with congenital heart disease complicated by pulmonary vascular disease may require cardiopulmonary or pulmonary transplantation if pulmonary vascular changes are advanced. If there is a reversible component to the increased pulmonary vascular resistance in these individuals, it can often be identified by measuring pulmonary arterial resistance during inspiration of 100% oxygen. In patients with reversibly increased pulmonary vascular resistance, successful obliteration of the left-to-right shunt may result in subsequently lower vascular resistance. However, in some patients, pulmonary vascular resistance continues to increase despite closing the congenital cardiac defect.

In patients with passive pulmonary hypertension, pulmonary arterial pressure and resistance usually fall following successful therapy for the condition producing elevated pulmonary venous pressure. Thus, relieving mitral valvular obstruction in patients with mitral stenosis results in decreased pulmonary venous and arterial pressures and pulmonary vascular resistance. Similarly, successful therapy for left ventricular failure leads to lower pulmonary pressures and resistance. Even patients with longstanding mitral stenosis and reactive pulmonary hypertension usually demonstrate a marked im-

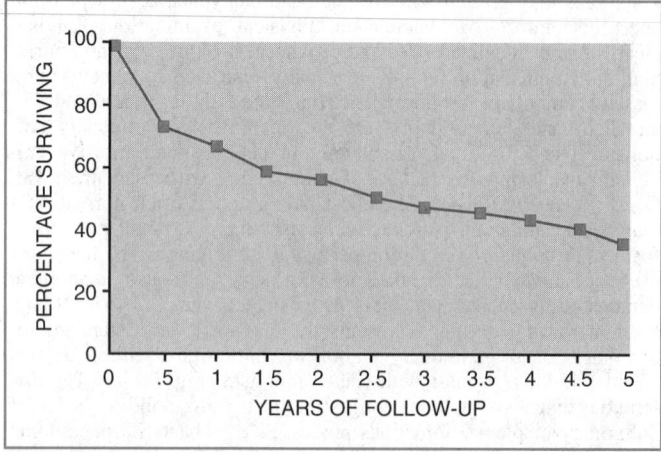

FIGURE 38–4. Approximate percentage of patients with primary pulmonary hypertension surviving during 5 years of follow-up after initial cardiac catheterization. (Data from the National Prospective Registry of Primary Pulmonary Hypertension. Reproduced with permission from D'Alonzo GE, Barst RJ, Ayres SM, et al.: Survival in patients with primary pulmonary hypertension—Results from a National Prospective Registry. Ann Intern Med 115:349, 1991.)

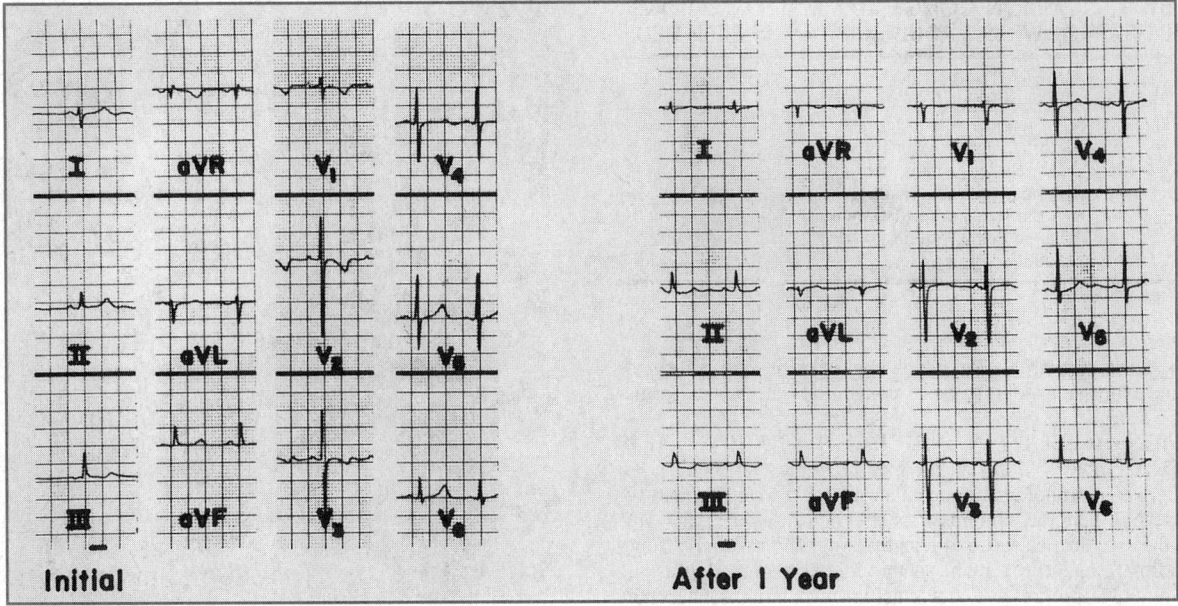

FIGURE 38–5. Regression of electrocardiographic right ventricular hypertrophy following 12 months of calcium channel blocker therapy in a patient with primary pulmonary hypertension. This patient had a marked decrease in pulmonary arterial pressure secondary to calcium channel blocker therapy. (From Rich S, Brundage BH: High-dose calcium blocking therapy for primary pulmonary hypertension: Evidence for long-term reduction in pulmonary arterial pressure and regression of right ventricular hypertrophy. Circulation 76:135, 1987. By permission of the American Heart Association, Inc.)

provement in pulmonary pressures and resistance after relieving mitral valvular obstruction. Patients with pulmonary veno-occlusive disease usually require cardiopulmonary or pulmonary transplantation because the diagnosis is usually made late in the course of the illness. In many instances, the diagnosis of pulmonary veno-occlusive disease is first made when the involved lungs are examined pathologically following removal for cardiopulmonary or pulmonary transplantation.

D'Alonzo GE, Barst RJ, Ayres SM, et al.: Survival in patients with primary pulmonary hypertension—Results from a National Prospective Registry. Ann Intern Med 115:343, 1991. *Results from a national registry of 194 patients with primary pulmonary hypertension followed at 32 clinical centers in the United States between 1981 and 1988.*

Dinh-Xuan AT, Higenbottam TW, Clelland CA, et al.: Impairment of endothelium-dependent pulmonary artery relaxation in chronic obstructive lung disease. N Engl J Med 324:1539, 1991. *Endothelial-dependent pulmonary arterial relaxation is impaired in arteries taken from patients with chronic obstructive pulmonary disease. Such impairment may play a role in development of pulmonary hypertension in these patients.*

Fuster V, Steele PM, Kaufmann L, et al.: Primary pulmonary hypertension: Natural history and the importance of thrombosis. Circulation 70:580, 1984. *Extensive retrospective review of the Mayo Clinic experience with primary pulmonary hypertension. Contains both pathologic and clinical data.*

Rich S, Brundage BH: High-dose calcium blocking therapy for primary pulmonary hypertension: Evidence for long-term reduction in pulmonary arterial pressure and regression of right ventricular hypertrophy. Circulation 76:135, 1987. *Selected patients with primary pulmonary hypertension exhibit a marked reduction in pulmonary arterial pressure during high-dose calcium channel blocker therapy.*

Rubin LJ: Primary pulmonary hypertension. Chest 104:236, 1993. *A concise but complete review of the cause, pathophysiology, diagnosis, and management of primary pulmonary hypertension.*

39 CONGENITAL HEART DISEASE IN ADULTS

Joseph K. Perloff

Congenital heart disease should be considered not only in terms of age of onset but also in terms of the age range that survival now permits. Because of advances in diagnostic techniques, surgical skills, and medical management, 90% of infants born annually in the United States with congenital heart disease can expect to survive to adulthood. The quality of care provided by pediatric cardiologists from birth to maturity must now be matched with care of

equal quality during adulthood. In response to this need, congenital heart disease in adults has become a new area of special cardiovascular interest and is the central concern of this chapter, which focuses on five general topics: facilities for caring for adults with congenital heart disease, survival patterns, medical considerations, surgical considerations, and postoperative residua and sequelae.

FACILITIES FOR THE CARE OF ADULTS WITH CONGENITAL HEART DISEASE

Special facilities devoted to congenital heart disease in adults reflect the collaboration of cardiologists and cardiac surgeons. The combined expertise of medical and pediatric cardiologists, at least currently, is superior to that of either of these specialists acting alone. The next generation is likely to include cardiologists trained in both disciplines.

Patients enter adult congenital heart disease facilities either during adolescence (recognizing adolescent medicine as a bridge between pediatric and adult medicine), at age 18, or when judged to have achieved appropriate psychological and physical maturity. It is not uncommon for patients in their late teens or 20's to be physically small, emotionally immature, and dependent upon a pediatric cardiology setting to provide them with a sense of security. Every effort should be made not to reinforce that dependency.

Pediatric cardiologists can continue to care for patients beyond adolescence provided that those cardiologists are well versed in acquired cardiac and medical diseases of adults. Cardiologists with a primary interest in adult medicine may interest themselves in congenital heart disease, provided they are well versed in the complexities of the discipline. In either case, adult care is best provided in an adult setting, whether outpatient or inpatient. Noninvasive, catheterization, and angiographic laboratories must meet the standards established by pediatric laboratories for infants and children.

Consultants in individual specialties are incorporated into adult congenital heart disease facilities so that experience is gained with problems peculiar to that patient population. Ad hoc consultations are less useful even when rendered by consultants of otherwise high quality. Specialties include hematology, nephrology, metabolism, pulmonary medicine, anesthesiology, obstetrics and gynecology, genetics and epidemiology, electrophysiology, psychiatry, pathology, and insurability and vocational counseling.

SURVIVAL PATTERNS IN PATIENTS WHO HAVE NOT UNDERGONE CARDIAC OR VASCULAR SURGERY

The term *natural survival* has come to be a misnomer because survival patterns are materially affected not only by surgical intervention but also by current medical expertise. The care of adults with congenital heart disease must take into account acquired disor-

TABLE 39–1. COMMON CONGENITAL MALFORMATIONS OF THE HEART IN WHICH ADULT SURVIVAL IS EXPECTED

Bicuspid aortic valve
  Functionally normal
  Stenotic/incompetent
Aortic cuspal inequality
Coarctation of the aorta
Pulmonary valve stenosis
Atrial septal defect (secundum)
Patent ductus arteriosus
Fallot's tetralogy

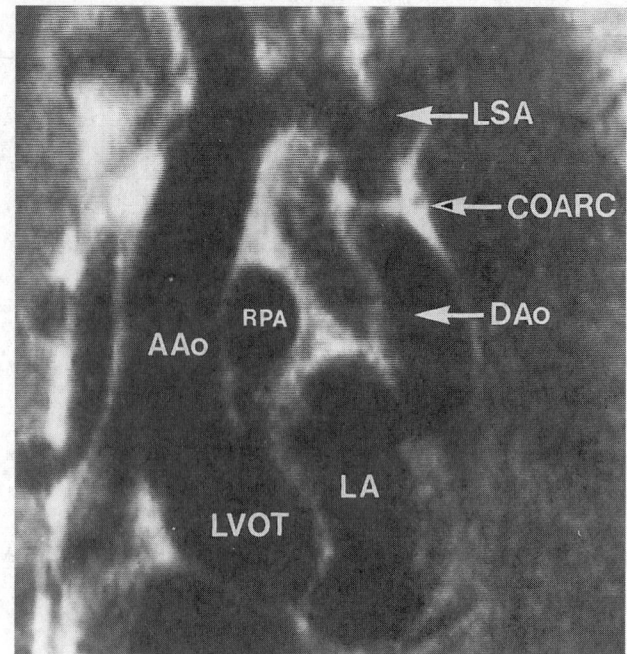

FIGURE 39–2. Magnetic resonance image (sagittal plane) from a 21-year-old man with coarctation (COARC) of the aorta just distal to the left subclavian artery (LSA). DAo = Descending aorta; AAo = ascending aorta; RPA = right pulmonary artery; LA = left atrium; LVOT = left ventricular outflow tract.

ders of the heart and circulation which coexist with and modify the physiologic expressions of the basic congenital cardiac malformation.

COMMON DEFECTS IN WHICH ADULT SURVIVAL IS EXPECTED (Table 39–1). A *bicuspid aortic valve* is the most common gross morphologic congenital anomaly of the heart or great vessels. When the commissures are not fused and the free edges of the two leaflets are sufficiently long, the valve is "functionally normal" and can remain so throughout a normal lifespan. More commonly, progressive fibrocalcific thickening renders the valve stenotic (Fig. 39–1A). Alternatively, the valve gradually becomes incompetent because of eversion of the redundant edge of either or both cusps. An important and less recognized feature of bicuspid aortic valves is the relationship to an intrinsic aortic root abnormality that can express itself as a dissecting aneurysm (Fig. 39–1B).

The importance of diagnosing a functionally normal bicuspid aortic valve is underscored by its susceptibility to infective endocarditis, which may convert a functionally normal valve into catastrophic acute severe aortic regurgitation. Clinical suspicion sets the stage for confirmation by two-dimensional echocardiography with color flow imaging.

Coarctation of the aorta (Fig. 39–2) produces significant symptoms either in early infancy or after the third or fourth decade. The majority of patients who remain unoperated survive infancy and reach adulthood. Diagnosis requires nothing more than palpating brachial and femoral pulses and recording cuff blood pressures in anticipation of repair. Longevity and morbidity are influenced by coexisting congenital cardiac and vascular malformations, the most common of which is the bicuspid aortic valve (see above). Dissecting aortic aneurysm just distal to the coarctation has a peak incidence in the third and fourth decades, and pregnancy increases the risk. Less common is a coexisting congenital aneurysm of the circle

of Willis (Fig. 39–3), which may announce itself as a fatal rupture, usually in the second or third decade.

Pulmonary valve stenosis is typically represented by a conical, dome-shaped, pliant valve with a narrow outlet at its apex (Fig. 39–4). Apart from pinpoint pulmonary stenosis in neonates, survival into adolescence and adulthood is the rule. Longevity depends upon the initial severity of obstruction, upon whether a given degree of obstruction remains constant or progresses, and upon the functional response of the pressure-overloaded right ventricle. The physical, electrocardiographic, and radiologic signs permit clinical recognition, with few exceptions. Echocardiography provides virtually all necessary diagnostic information. Relief of obstruction is usually by balloon dilatation.

Ostium secundum atrial septal defect may be overlooked in children because the soft, impure midsystolic murmur is mistaken for a normal or innocent pulmonary midsystolic murmur of childhood.

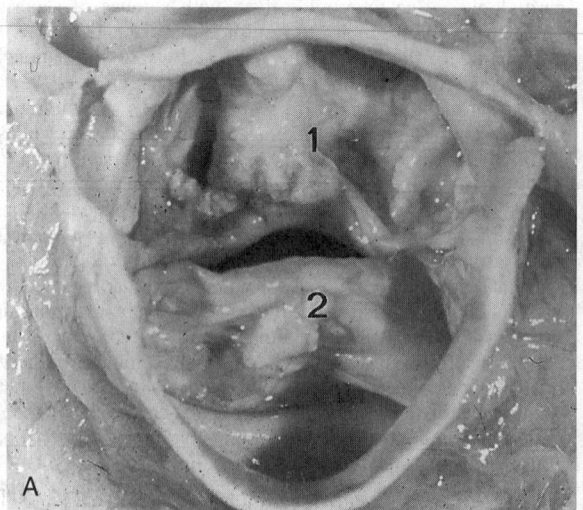

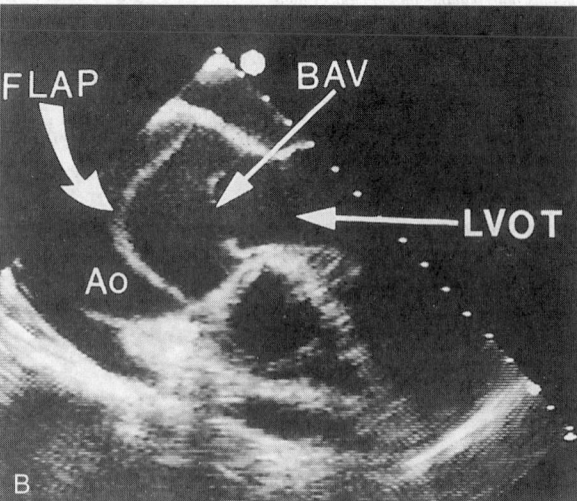

FIGURE 39–1. *A*, Gross morphology of a functionally normal bicuspid aortic valve (1,2 cusps) that became stenotic because of calcification. *B*, Transesophageal echocardiogram from a 37-year-old man with a bicuspid aortic valve (BAV) and an acute dissecting aneurysm of the ascending aorta (Ao). Curved arrow identifies the dissected, mobile intimal flap. LVOT = Left ventricular outflow tract.

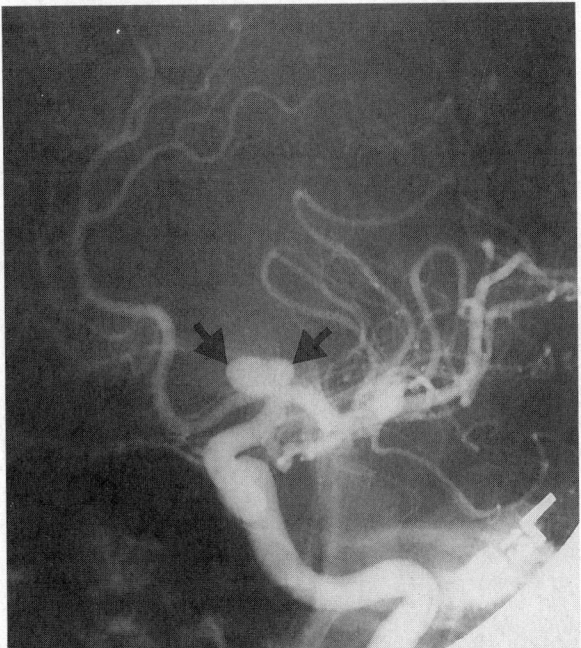

FIGURE 39-3. Carotid arteriogram from a 23-year-old woman with an 11-mm congenital aneurysm within the circle of Willis *(arrows)*. The patient had Fallot's tetralogy with pulmonary atresia rather than coarctation of the aorta.

However, the physical signs, electrocardiogram (ECG), and chest radiograph should prevent error. Echocardiography with color flow imaging and Doppler interrogation (echo/Doppler) identifies the defect and the left-to-right shunt. The stage is then set for operative closure.

The major reasons for symptomatic deterioration are the age-related decrease in left ventricular distensibility, the advent of atrial tachyarrhythmias that augment the left-to-right shunt and precipitate right ventricular failure (Fig. 39-5), and mild to moderate pulmonary hypertension in the presence of a persistent large left-to-right shunt. Almost all patients who survive beyond the sixth decade are symptomatic. The clinical signs may then be atypical.

Patent ductus arteriosus should not go unrecognized except perhaps for the small ductus with its soft, localized continuous murmur

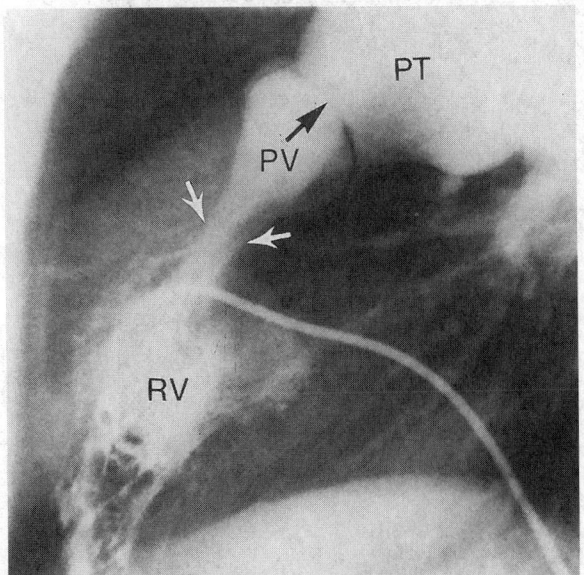

FIGURE 39-4. Right ventriculogram (RV) from a 35-year-old man with severe pulmonary valve stenosis (PV), poststenotic dilatation of the pulmonary trunk (PT), and secondary hypertrophic subpulmonary stenosis *(paired arrows)*.

that might be overlooked. More characteristic is the "machinery" murmur that begins in systole and continues through the second heart sound into all or part of diastole. A chest radiograph may disclose calcification of the ductus in older adults (Fig. 39-6A). Echo/Doppler interrogation establishes the diagnosis (Fig. 39-6B). There is an accrued risk of infective endocarditis, especially if the ductus is restrictive (high-velocity continuous flow). Patients with a nonrestrictive ductus seldom reach adulthood unless a rise in pulmonary vascular resistance curtails pulmonary arterial blood flow and relieves the left ventricle of excessive volume overload. The shunt is then reversed, and the continuous murmur vanishes and is replaced by auscultatory signs of pulmonary hypertension and distinctive differential cyanosis. Unoxygenated blood selectively reaches the feet, because the reversed flow is delivered into the aorta just distal to the left subclavian artery.

Ventricular septal defects are among the most common congenital cardiac malformations present at birth. Patients who survive into adulthood comprise two main groups: those with defects that have closed spontaneously or decreased in size so that they are clinically inapparent (Fig. 39-7A), and patients with nonrestrictive defects accompanied by a rise in pulmonary vascular resistance that relieves the left ventricle of volume overload while imposing no additional increase in afterload upon the systemic right ventricle (Eisenmenger's complex) (Fig. 39-7B).

Fallot's tetralogy accounts for the largest proportion of unoperated adults with cyanotic congenital heart disease, a point that speaks as much for the poor outlook of other types of cyanotic congenital heart disease as for virtues inherent in the tetralogy. Acyanotic or mildly cyanotic patients come to attention because of a prominent systolic murmur. When the murmur is soft, cyanosis is obvious. Echo/Doppler establishes the diagnosis.

UNCOMMON DEFECTS IN WHICH ADULT SURVIVAL IS EXPECTED

(Table 39-2). *Dextrocardia in situs inversus (mirror image)* usually occurs with a structurally normal heart. Patients therefore experience normal longevity and are susceptible to acquired cardiac and noncardiac diseases, the symptoms of which often result in discovery of the hitherto unsuspected cardiac malposition. The pain of angina pectoris or myocardial infarction radiates to the right anterior chest, right shoulder, and right arm. The pain of acute appendicitis is in the *left lower* quadrant, and the pain of biliary colic is in the *left upper* quadrant (Fig. 39-8) because of the mirror image locations of the appendix and gallbladder.

Congenital complete heart block would not escape diagnosis if infants and children with slow heart rates had nothing more than a routine scalar ECG. Most patients reach adulthood, although mortality in childhood is not negligible. Optimism is further dampened by the fate of adolescents and adults when congenital complete heart block goes unrecognized.

Congenitally corrected transposition of the great arteries is characterized by inversion (right-to-left interchange) of the ventricles and their atrioventricular valves, resulting in atrioventricular and ventriculo–great arterial discordance (Fig. 39-9). Blood from a given atrium reaches the relevant great artery—hence the term "congenitally corrected." Longevity in the uncomplicated malformation is good but not normal because of the vulnerability of a morphologic right ventricle in the systemic location (Fig. 39-9A) and

TABLE 39-2. UNCOMMON CONGENITAL MALFORMATIONS OF THE HEART IN WHICH ADULT SURVIVAL IS EXPECTED

Dextrocardia
    In situs inversus (mirror image)
    In situs solitus
Congenital complete heart block
Congenitally corrected transposition of the great arteries
Ebstein's anomaly
Primary pulmonary hypertension
Ruptured sinus of Valsalva aneurysm
Lutembacher's syndrome
Pulmonary arteriovenous fistula
Coronary arteriovenous fistula
Congenital pulmonary valve regurgitation
Idiopathic dilatation of the pulmonary trunk

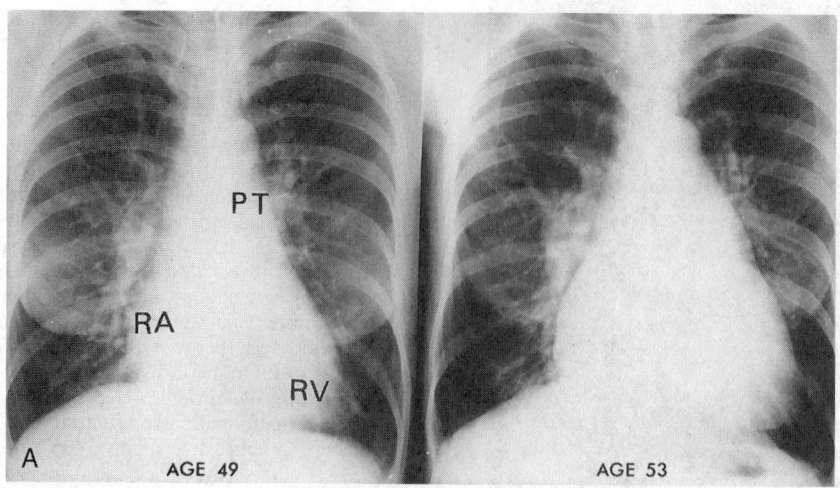

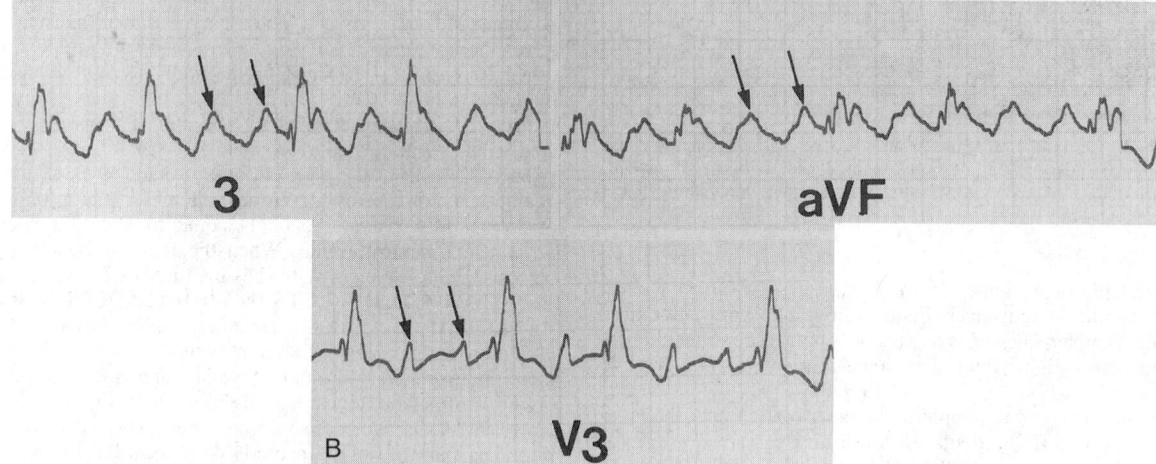

FIGURE 39–5. *A,* Chest radiograph in a 49-year-old woman with an ostium secundum atrial septal defect. Pulmonary arterial vascularity is increased and there is moderate enlargement of the pulmonary trunk (PT), right atrium (RA), and right ventricle (RV). The radiograph at age 53 was done 3 months after the onset of atrial fibrillation. There is a significant increase in size of the pulmonary trunk, right atrium, and right ventricle. *B,* Leads 3, aVF, and V₃ from a 60-year-old woman with a nonrestrictive ostium secundum atrial septal defect and atrial flutter *(arrows identify flutter waves).*

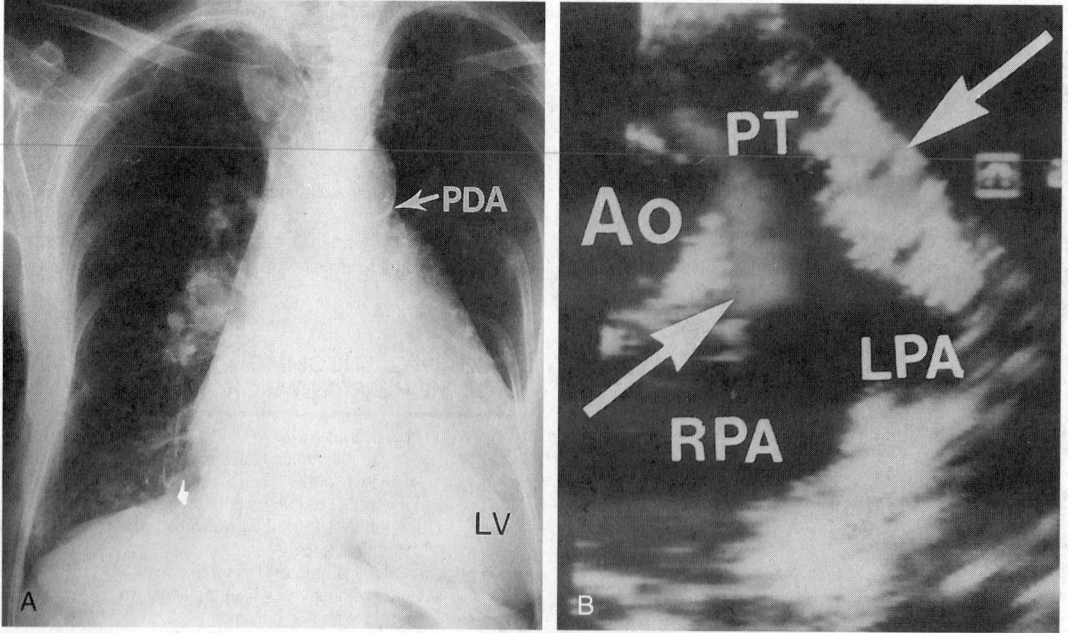

FIGURE 39–6. *A,* Chest radiograph from an 84-year-old man with a calcified, moderately restrictive patent ductus arteriosus (PDA). The pulmonary trunk, right pulmonary artery, and left ventricle (LV) are enlarged. *B,* Black and white print of color flow imaging (short axis) showing typical ductal flow tracking down the lateral wall *(upper right arrow)* and up the medial wall *(lower left arrow)* of the pulmonary trunk (PT). LPA, RPA = left and right pulmonary arteries, respectively. Ao = Aorta.

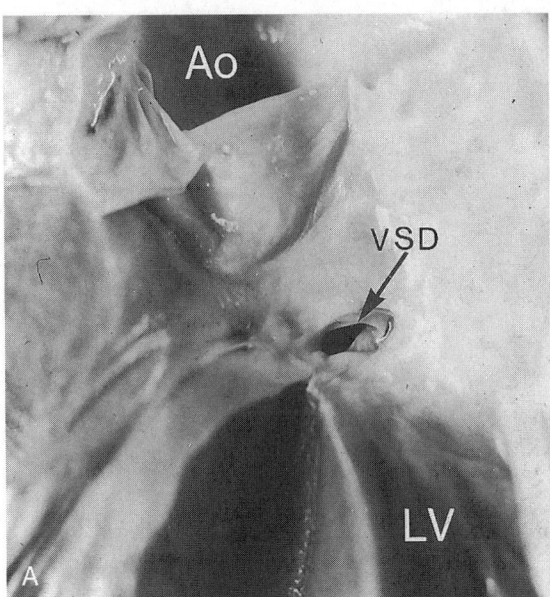
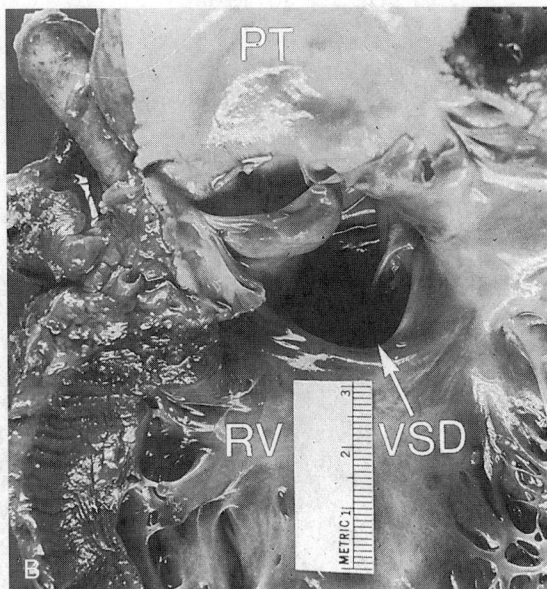

FIGURE 39–7. Two widely disparate types of ventricular septal defects. *A*, Tiny membranous ventricular septal defect (VSD) found incidentally at necropsy. LV = Left ventricle; Ao = aorta. *B*, Nonrestrictive perimembranous defect (VSD) with suprasystemic pulmonary vascular resistance (Eisenmenger's complex). Compare VSD size to centimeter rule. RV = Right ventricle; PT = pulmonary trunk.

because of the risk of complete atrioventricular block that accrues at a rate of about 2% per year.

In *Ebstein's anomaly of the tricuspid valve,* longevity depends on the physiologic consequences of the malformed tricuspid valve and atrialized right ventricle, on the presence of an interatrial communication (right-to-left shunt), and on atrial tachyarrhythmias, especially when accompanied by accelerated conduction through accessory pathways (Fig. 39–10). The ECG and chest radiograph are distinctive, and echocardiography with color flow imaging provides all necessary diagnostic details.

Primary pulmonary hypertension (Fig. 39–11) is an idiopathic obstructive disease that resides in pulmonary arterioles and typically presents in young women at a mean age of 21 to 30. Longevity is related to the degree and progression of the pulmonary vascular disease and the right ventricular afterload.

An *aneurysm of a sinus of Valsalva* (Fig. 39–12) typically ruptures in the late teens or 20's with a marked male predominance.

The acute development of a large perforation announces itself dramatically with chest pain and unremitting biventricular failure.

Lutembacher's syndrome is a congenital interatrial communication upon which *acquired* mitral stenosis is imposed. Mitral stenosis augments the left-to-right interatrial shunt, and the atrial septal defect decompresses the left atrium (Fig. 39–13).

Congenital pulmonary arteriovenous fistulas commonly occur in association with hereditary telangiectasia—the Rendu-Osler-Weber syndrome. A substantial majority of fistulas go unrecognized until adulthood when patients come to attention because of cyanosis or recurrent bleeding from telangiectasia. The chest radiograph shows one or more densities in the lower lobes or right middle lobe connected to the hilus by afferent and efferent vascular channels (Fig. 39–14).

Coronary arteriovenous fistulas represent the most common major congenital malformation of the coronary circulation which permits adult survival. Initial suspicion is generally prompted by an

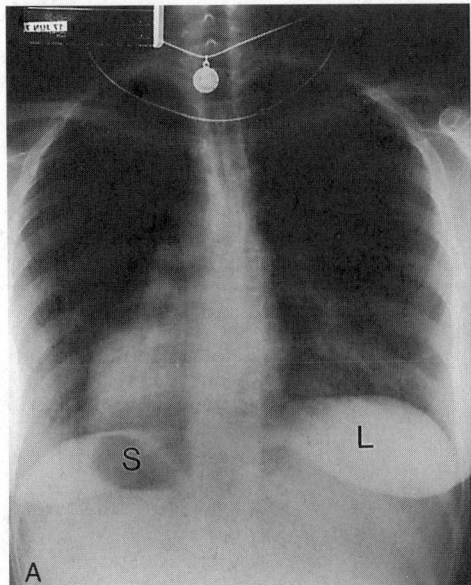
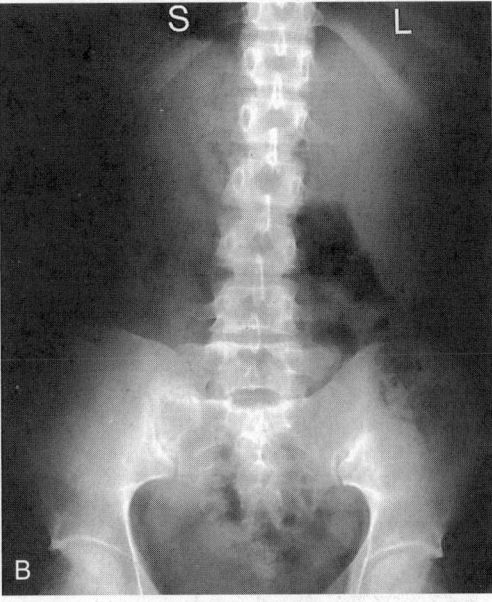

FIGURE 39–8. *A,* Chest radiograph from a 28-year-old woman with complete situs inversus. The heart was normal except for the malposition. The stomach (S) is in the *right* upper quadrant and the liver (L) is in the *left* upper quadrant. *B,* The patient presented with biliary colic in the *left* upper quadrant because of the mirror image location of the liver (L).

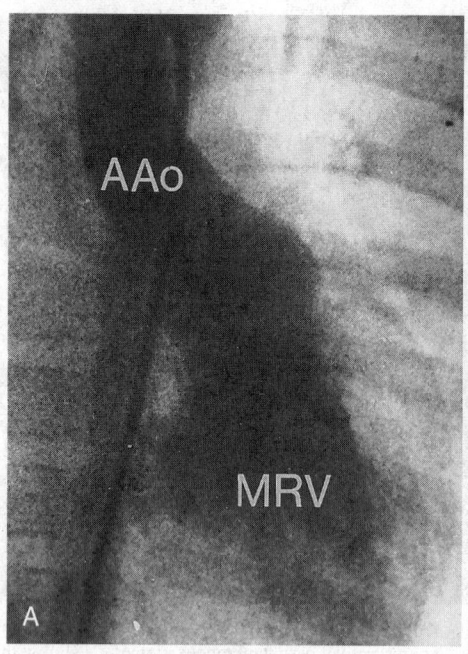
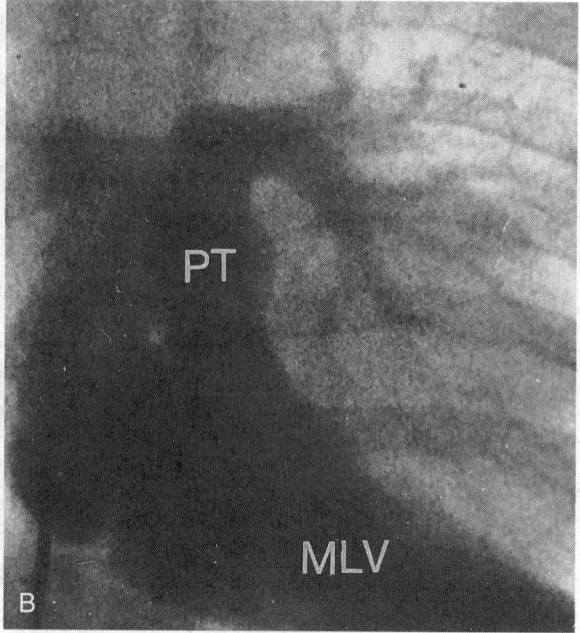

FIGURE 39–9. Angiocardiograms from a 23-year-old woman with isolated, uncomplicated congenitally corrected transposition of the great arteries (ventricular inversion). *A,* The morphologic right ventricle (MRV) is subaortic (AAo = ascending aorta). *B,* The morphologic left ventricle (MLV) is subpulmonary (PT = pulmonary trunk).

atypical continuous murmur. Selective coronary angiography confirms the origin and insertion of the fistula (Fig. 39–15).

Congenital pulmonary valve regurgitation is often overlooked because of the unfamiliar murmur of low-pressure pulmonary incompetence. The majority of patients tolerate the anomaly into adulthood because the degree of regurgitation is moderate and because

the right ventricle adapts well to low-pressure volume overload. Echocardiography with color flow imaging establishes the diagnosis (Fig. 39–16).

MEDICAL CONSIDERATIONS

Refinements in medical care of unoperated or inoperable adults with congenital heart disease have contributed appreciably to increased longevity and decreased morbidity. The major medical considerations are listed in Table 39–3.

Children with chronic illnesses, such as congenital heart disease, are prone to develop *psychosocial disorders* because of the stressful, frustrating effects of the illness, because of the detrimental effects of low self-esteem, and because of inappropriate parental attitudes. Maladaptive behavior expresses itself during adolescence and adulthood against the backdrop of experiences that differ significantly from those of normal, healthy children. The overprotected child becomes the overprotected adolescent or adult whose immaturity is often reinforced by long-term care in a pediatric setting. Cyanosis is believed to impair intellectual acuity. However, the degree of impairment is generally mild and is often overestimated because IQ tests depend on gross motor function at a young age. Early reparative surgery appears to improve intellectual and psychological development, although circulatory arrest with deep hypothermia may have subtle adverse effects on intellectual function.

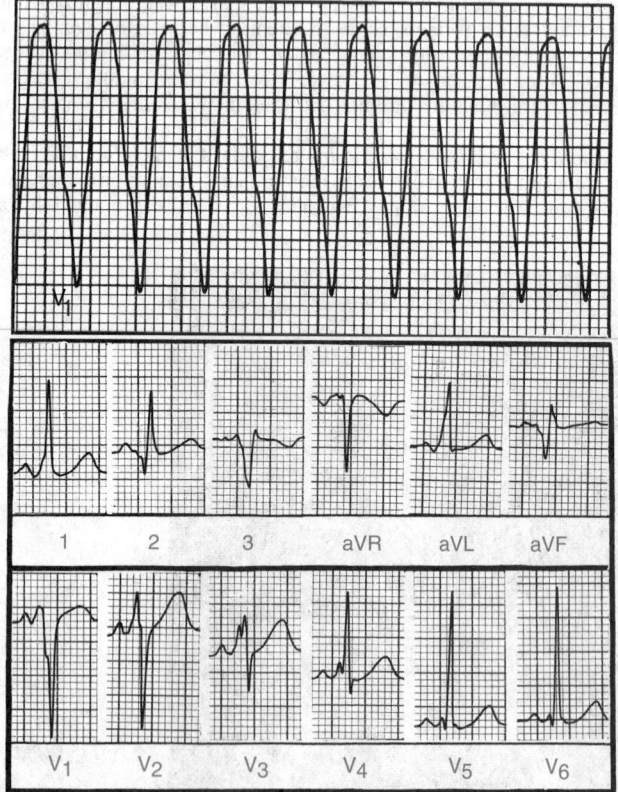

FIGURE 39–10. *Top,* Rapid wide QRS tachycardia in a 32-year-old man with Ebstein's anomaly of the tricuspid valve, atrial fibrillation, and antegrade conduction via an accessory pathway. *Bottom,* After electrical cardioversion, the 12-lead electrocardiogram shows delta waves directed superior and posterior, typical of a right atrioventricular bypass tract in Ebstein's anomaly.

TABLE 39–3. MEDICAL CONSIDERATIONS IN ADULTS WITH CONGENITAL HEART DISEASE

Psychosocial concerns
Electrophysiologic abnormalities
Ventricular function
Infective endocarditis
Cyanotic congenital heart disease
    Hematologic disorders
    Renal function
    Urate metabolism
    Gallstones and cholecystitis
    O_2 uptake and control of ventilation
Pregnancy
Genetics and epidemiology
Exercise and athletics
Neurologic complications
Acquired cardiac and vascular disease
Insurability and employability

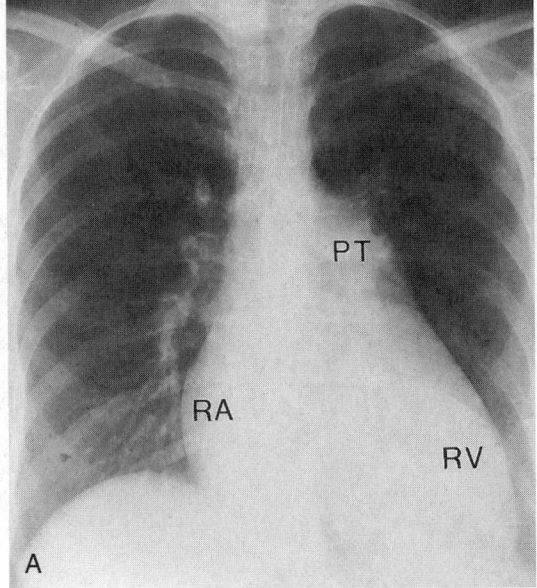
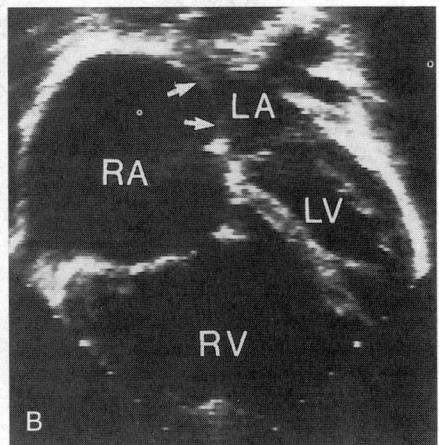

FIGURE 39–11. *A*, Chest radiograph from a 24-year-old woman with primary pulmonary hypertension. There is striking dilatation of the pulmonary trunk (PT), right atrium (RA), and right ventricle (RV). *B*, Two-dimensional echocardiogram (apical four-chamber view) from a 12-year-old girl with primary pulmonary hypertension. There is striking dilatation of the right atrium (RA) and right ventricle (RV). The left ventricular cavity (LV) is small. The atrial septum bows from right to left *(arrows)* because of the high right atrial pressure.

Electrophysiologic abnormalities are among the most prevalent medical concerns in adolescents and adults with congenital heart disease. There are three general categories: (1) rhythm and conduction disturbances that are inherent components of certain unoperated congenital malformations and that persist as obligatory residua after reparative surgery; (2) electrophysiologic disturbances that reflect the hemodynamic or hypoxic stress imposed upon the heart by the basic congenital malformation and that may or may not persist as postoperative residua; (3) electrophysiologic disturbances that are not present prior to reparative surgery but instead develop as sequelae of operation.

Rhythm disturbances that are inherent components of certain unoperated malformations are represented in ostium secundum atrial septal defects. The incidence of supraventricular arrhythmias—especially atrial fibrillation and atrial flutter (see Fig. 39–5)—increases with age, and approximately half of patients who survive to age 60 experience atrial tachyarrhythmias that respond poorly to pharmacologic suppression until after operative repair. In Ebstein's anomaly of the tricuspid valve, supraventricular tachyarrhythmias—atrial fibrillation, atrial flutter, re-entrant supraventricular tachycardia—occur in 25 to 30% of patients. Accessory atrioventricular pathways in such patients set the stage for accelerated conduction, which can have serious consequences (see Fig. 39–10).

Intra-atrial baffle operations (Mustard, Senning) for complete transposition of the great arteries require extensive reconstruction and are followed by electrophysiologic sequelae that include atrial arrhythmias and injury to sinus and atrioventricular nodes. Disturbances of atrial rhythm are matters of grave concern whether or not the ventricular rate is controlled.

A Fontan repair (right atrial to pulmonary arterial connection or total caval to pulmonary arterial connection) in patients with single ventricle or tricuspid atresia requires the coordinated atrial contraction inherent in sinus rhythm to support the subaortic ventricle. Atrial tachyarrhythmias adversely affect left ventricular function, provoking a rise in end-diastolic pressure that translates into impaired forward flow from the caval or right atrial connection to the pulmonary artery.

Electrical instability after an intracardiac repair through a right ventriculotomy is a major electrophysiologic concern. Fallot's tetralogy is a case in point (Fig. 39–17). The older the patient is at the time of intracardiac repair, the greater the degree of postoperative right ventricular hemodynamic overload (residual obstruction, postoperative pulmonary regurgitation); and the greater the depression of right ventricular function, the greater the probability of right ventricular ectopic rhythms, ventricular tachycardia, ventricular fibrillation—and sudden death.

Ventricular function is more complex in congenital than in acquired heart disease. Gross morphologic considerations must take into account whether there are two ventricles or one ventricle; whether the ventricles are noninverted or inverted; and whether a single ventricle is a morphologic left or a morphologic right ventricle.

The long-term durability of a morphologic right ventricle in the systemic location has a been a matter of lively interest (see Fig. 39–9A). Normal stroke volume of an inverted right ventricle is maintained at a comparatively lower ejection fraction than that of a systemic left ventricle without necessarily implying abnormal function of the right ventricle.

In patients with univentricular hearts, the single ventricle qualifies on morphologic grounds as either a finely trabeculated left ventricle, a coarsely trabeculated right ventricle, or a ventricle with an indeterminate trabecular pattern. A univentricular heart, irrespective of its morphology, exhibits abnormal systolic and diastolic function and a relatively low ejection fraction. Insufficient mass relative to ventricular volume reflects poor adaptation to overload, especially in univentricular hearts of the right ventricular type.

An *increase in ventricular mass* beyond normal growth is influenced not only by the type and duration of the inciting stimulus but

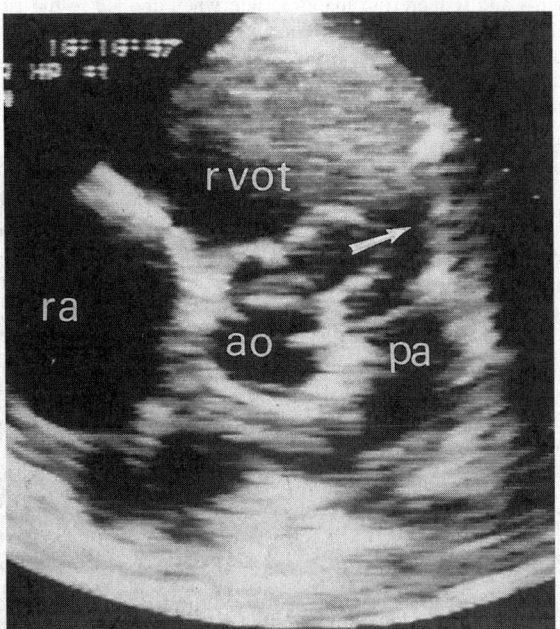

FIGURE 39–12. Two-dimensional echocardiogram (short axis) from a 22-year-old man with perforation of an aneurysm of a sinus of Valsalva into the right ventricular outflow tract (RVOT) *(arrow)*. Ao = Aorta; pa = pulmonary artery; ra = right atrium.

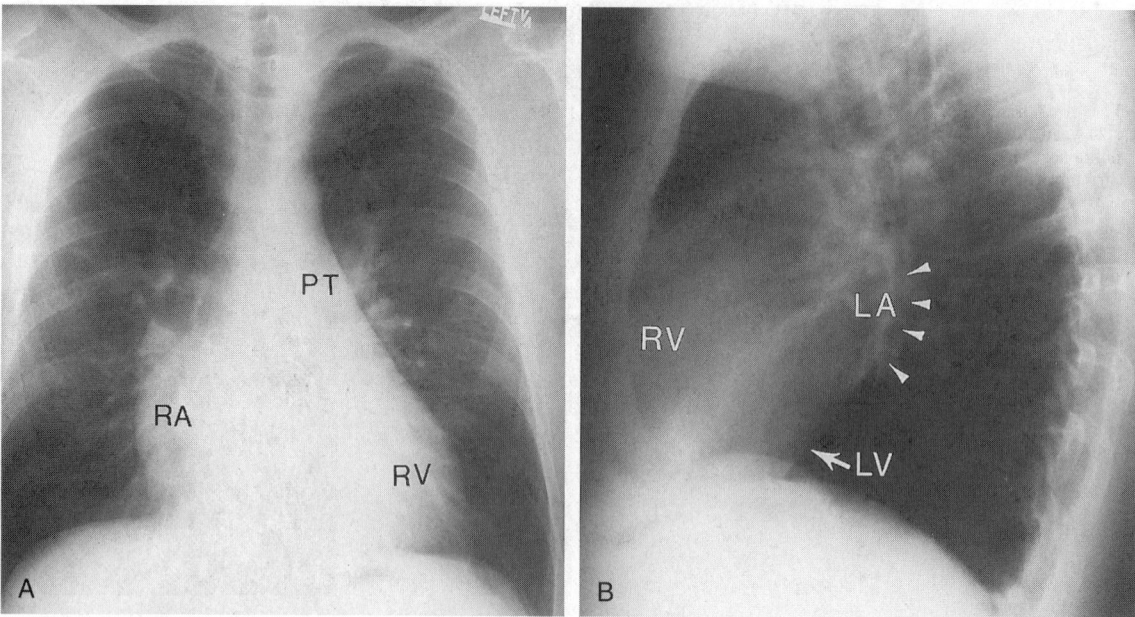

FIGURE 39–13. Chest radiograph from a 46-year-old man with Lutembacher's syndrome (ostium secundum atrial septal defect with rheumatic mitral stenosis). *A*, Posteroanterior view shows marked dilatation of the right atrium (RA) and right ventricle (RV), the latter of which occupies the apex. There is moderate dilatation of the pulmonary trunk (PT). *B*, Lateral view shows the dilated retrosternal right ventricle (RV), mild dilatation of the left atrium (LA), and a normal-sized left ventricle (LV).

also by myocardial maturity (or immaturity) at the time the inciting stimulus becomes operative. The immature heart retains its intrauterine capability of myocyte replication (hyperplasia) for 6 to 8 months after birth. When overload or hypoxia is imposed upon an immature heart, ventricular mass increases chiefly because of myocyte hyperplasia, which is an appreciably different response to analogous stimuli imposed upon a mature heart that is equipped with terminally differentiated myocytes.

Infective endocarditis is an important medical consideration because the number and age range of susceptible patients have increased owing to survival into adolescence and adulthood (see Ch. 278). Among unoperated congenital lesions, those at highest risk are adults with a bicuspid aortic valve, a restrictive ventricular septal defect, Fallot's tetralogy, or lesions associated with obstruction to ventricular outflow or high-pressure valvular regurgitation. In Fallot's tetralogy, infective endocarditis on an abnormal aortic valve can result in acute severe biventricular aortic regurgitation (Fig. 39–18). Surgical interventions have had a significant impact upon the risk of infective endocarditis. Certain operations (ligation of a patent ductus arteriosus) eliminate the risk, whereas other opera-

tions (prosthetic valves or conduits) materially increase the risk. Nonchemotherapeutic prophylaxis is important and includes day-to-day oral hygiene, skin care, nail care, and female contraception. The spongy, fragile gums of patients with cyanotic congenital heart disease are a special concern. Skin care is important, particularly in cyanotic patients who are prone to develop acne and pustules that are widely distributed beyond the face. Biting of nails or picking of fingers predisposes to paronychial infection with staphylococci.

There are a number of *medical considerations peculiar to cyanotic congenital heart disease* (Table 39–3). These include hematologic disorders, renal function, urate metabolism, gallstones and cholecystitis, and respiratory function.

The *adaptive increase in red cell mass* prompted by the hypoxemia of cyanotic malformations is properly designated erythrocytosis. *Polycythemia* (see Ch. 141.1) refers to an increase in all formed elements and is therefore inappropriate when applied to the isolated increase in red cell mass that characterizes the response in cyanotic congenital heart disease patients whose platelet counts are generally in the low range of normal and whose leukocyte counts and leukocyte alkaline phosphatase activity are normal.

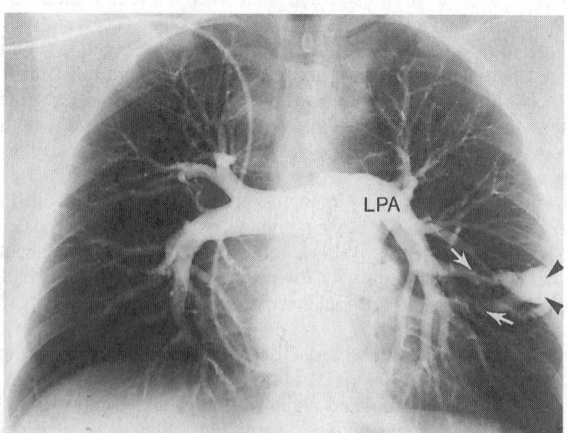

FIGURE 39–14. Pulmonary arteriogram from a cyanotic 35-year-old woman with a solitary congenital pulmonary arteriovenous fistula *(black arrows),* and Rendu-Osler-Weber telangiectasia. The white arrows point to the afferent and efferent vascular channels of the fistula. LPA = Left pulmonary artery.

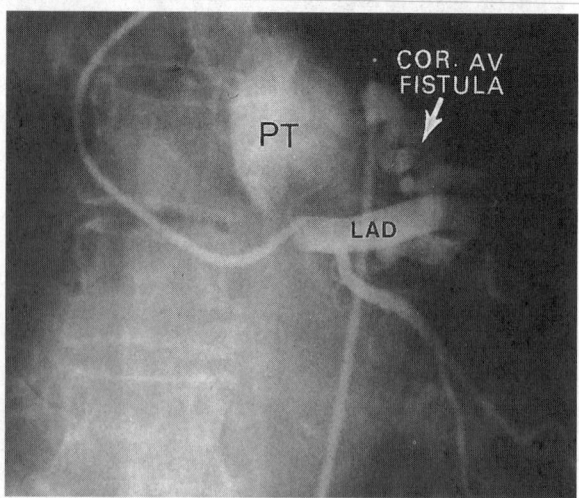

FIGURE 39–15. Coronary arteriogram from a 62-year-old woman with a congenital coronary arteriovenous fistula (COR. AV FISTULA) from left anterior descending artery (LAD) to pulmonary trunk (PT).

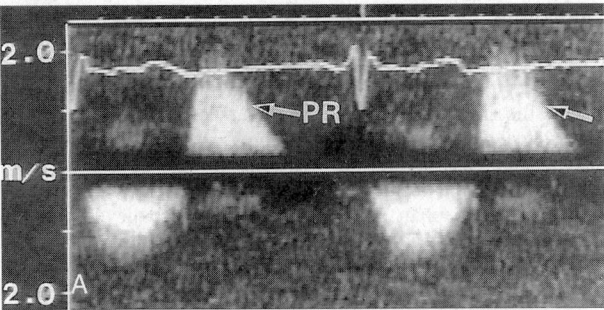

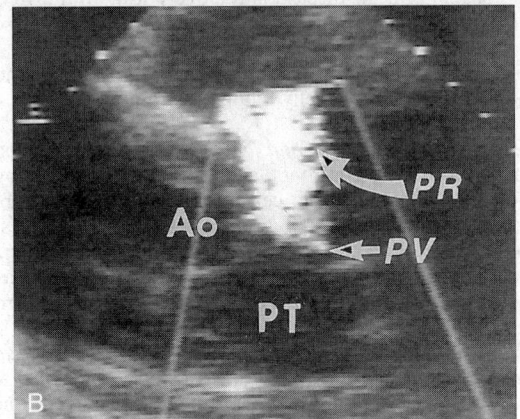

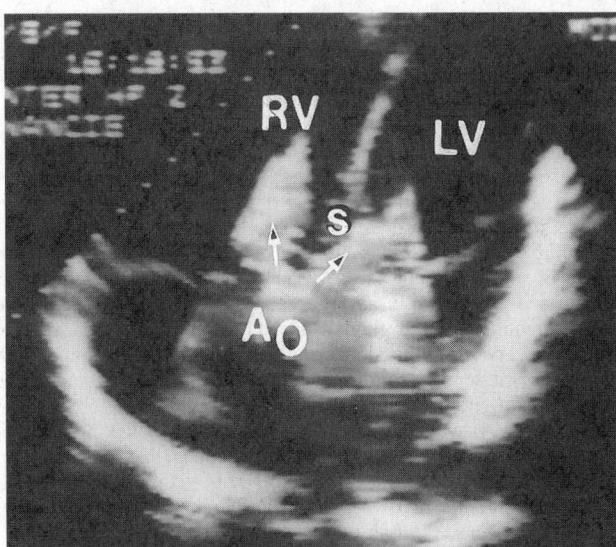

FIGURE 39-18. Black and white print of color flow imaging from a 28-year-old woman with Fallot's tetralogy and pulmonary atresia. Infective endocarditis on the biventricular aortic valve caused acute severe aortic regurgitation into both the right and left ventricles *(arrows)*. S = Ventricular septum; RV, LV = right and left ventricles, respectively; Ao = aortic valve.

FIGURE 39-16. *A*, Continuous-wave Doppler from an 18-year-old man with congenital pulmonary valve regurgitation (PR) *(arrows)*. The peak regurgitant velocity was low because the pulmonary arterial pressure was not elevated. *B*, Black and white print of color flow imaging in same patient (short axis) showing the low-pressure pulmonary regurgitation (PR). PV = Pulmonary valve; Ao = aorta; PT = pulmonary trunk.

Cyanotic patients are divided into two hematologic subgroups. Those with compensated erythrocytosis establish equilibrium hematocrit levels in iron-replete states and have absent, mild, or moderate hyperviscosity symptoms, even at high hematocrit levels. Decompensated erythrocytosis occurs in patients who fail to establish equilibrium conditions; who manifest unstable, rising hematocrit levels that are uncontrolled by negative feedback inhibition; and who experience marked to severe hyperviscosity symptoms. Hematocrit levels should be based upon automated determinations, because microhematocrit centrifugation results in plasma trapping and falsely elevated levels. Adults with cyanotic congenital heart disease and erythrocytosis are often phlebotomized and occasionally anticoagulated because of an assumed risk of cerebral arterial thrombotic stroke. However, the presumed risk of stroke due to cerebral arterial thrombosis has not withstood scrutiny. Furthermore, the circulatory effects of phlebotomy are transient, and phlebotomy-induced iron deficiency results in an increase in whole blood viscosity at an equivalent red cell mass (nondeformable microspherocytes). For patients with compensated erythrocytosis, phlebotomy is not advised irrespective of hematocrit level as long as symptoms attributed to hyperviscosity are absent, mild, or moderate. When the hematocrit

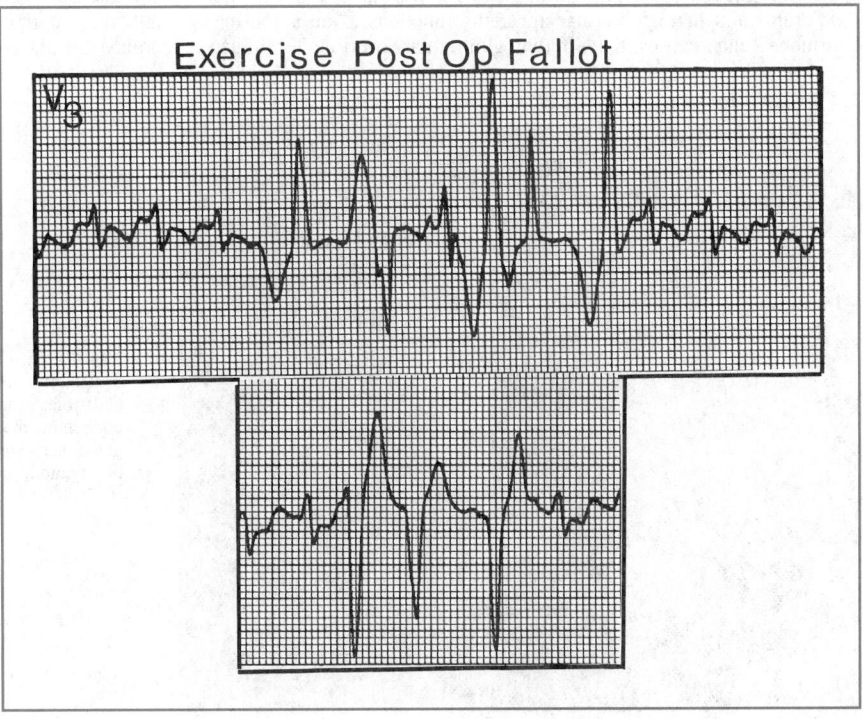

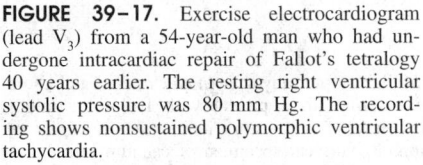

FIGURE 39-17. Exercise electrocardiogram (lead V_3) from a 54-year-old man who had undergone intracardiac repair of Fallot's tetralogy 40 years earlier. The resting right ventricular systolic pressure was 80 mm Hg. The recording shows nonsustained polymorphic ventricular tachycardia.

level is <65%, hyperviscosity symptoms are almost always due to iron deficiency. Phlebotomy further depletes iron stores and aggravates rather than alleviates the symptoms, which respond instead to careful iron repletion. The firmest indication for isovolumetric phlebotomy is marked to severe symptomatic hyperviscosity in patients with hematocrit levels >65%, provided that dehydration is not the cause. The volume of blood withdrawn should be the minimum required to achieve the short-term goal of temporary symptomatic relief. One unit usually suffices.

Abnormal hemostasis is a feature of cyanotic congenital heart disease. Bleeding tendencies are usually mild to moderate and are characterized by easy bruisability, petechial hemorrhages (skin and mucous membranes), and gingival bleeding. However, epistaxis and hemoptysis vary from occasional and moderate to copious and infuriatingly recurrent, and serious bleeding can occur with accidental trauma or with surgical procedures. Cyanosis, turbulent blood flow, and pulmonary vascular disease appear to be independently associated with reductions in or absence of large von Willebrand factor multimeric forms (see Ch. 153). Aspirin reinforces the intrinsic hemostatic defects, and nonsteroidal anti-inflammatory agents and anticoagulants increase the risk of bleeding.

Platelet counts are generally in the low range of normal in adults with cyanotic congenital heart disease, but moderate or marked reduction sometimes occurs. The platelet is unique among cells in higher-order vertebrates because it never possesses a nucleus. Megakaryocytes or large cytoplasmic fragments are released from bone marrow into the systemic venous circulation and are believed to undergo physical fragmentation in the pulmonary circulation, producing platelets. Right-to-left shunts permit large platelet precursors to bypass the lungs and enter the systemic circulation, where they are trapped in systemic arterioles and capillaries. The trapped, degranulated megakaryocytes or megakaryocyte fragments release platelet-derived growth factor, which is believed to initiate protein synthesis, connective tissue formation, and cell proliferation that result in clubbing of the fingers and toes and hypertrophic osteoarthropathy.

Renal histopathology in cyanotic congenital heart disease is characterized initially by dilated glomerular hilar arterioles, increased glomerular capillary diameter, enlarged glomeruli, red cell engorgement of glomerular capillaries, increased mesangial cells and matrix, and increased cellularity of the juxtaglomerular apparatus. Late-stage histopathology includes hyalinized glomeruli, focal subcapsular scars, interstitial fibrosis, and tubular atrophy. Intrinsically high resistance in the glomerular tuft, coupled with an increase in viscosity of erythrocytotic blood, results in high glomerular hydrostatic pressure. Nitric oxide synthesized in mesangial cells of the glomerulus and juxtaglomerular apparatus functions as an autocrine "hormone" that causes the afferent glomerular arteriole to dilate,

thus increasing glomerular blood flow and contributing to, if not causing, the increase in size and vascularity of the glomerular tuft. Platelet-derived growth factor released from megakaryocytes or from large cytoplasmic fragments trapped in glomerular tufts may contribute to the abnormalities of glomerular morphology.

Hyperuricemia commonly accompanies cyanotic congenital heart disease in adults. High plasma uric acid levels are not caused by urate overproduction from red blood cell nucleoprotein but instead are secondary to enhanced urate reabsorption believed to result from renal hypoperfusion reinforced by a high filtration fraction. Asymptomatic hyperuricemia does not require treatment. The incidence of acute gouty arthritis in patients with the hyperuricemia of cyanotic congenital heart disease is relatively low, with a frequency similar to that in other forms of secondary hyperuricemia (see Ch. 251). In treating acute gouty arthritis, intravenous colchicine results in a rapid clinical response and avoids undesirable hemoconcentration that accompanies the dehydrating gastrointestinal side effects of oral administration.

The risk of *cholelithiasis and cholecystitis* caused by calcium bilirubinate gallstones confronts adults with cyanotic congenital heart disease. An expanded red cell mass provides the substrate for an increase in unconjugated bilirubin and pigment stones (Fig. 39–19B) because the compound is largely insoluble in water. Gallstones may announce themselves years after the cyanosis has been eliminated by surgical repair of the congenital cardiac malformation (Fig. 39–19A).

Abnormalities of *oxygen uptake and the control of ventilation* in cyanotic congenital heart disease have adverse functional consequences. The diversion of systemic venous blood from the pulmonary circulation into the systemic arterial circulation is a fundamental pathophysiologic fault in cyanotic congenital heart disease. The fall in systemic vascular resistance induced by isotonic exercise serves to increase the degree of venoarterial mixing and materially influences the dynamics of oxygen uptake and ventilation (Fig. 39–20). These observations underscore the need to modify the New York Heart Association's functional classification that largely reflects the symptomatic response to heart failure. A functional classification more appropriate for congenital heart disease is shown in Table 39–4.

Pregnancy in congenital heart disease requires planning and careful monitoring. The common congenital malformations of the heart and circulation in which unoperated survival into childbearing age can be anticipated are listed in Table 39–5. Reparative surgery not only prolongs the lifespan of women with anomalies that have inherent tendencies for adult survival but also permits increasing numbers of women with disorders that were previously fatal in early life to reach reproductive age. Central to this topic is the intricate interplay between maternal circulatory and respiratory physiology and maternal congenital heart disease and the effects of that interplay on the fetus, which is exposed to immediate risks that

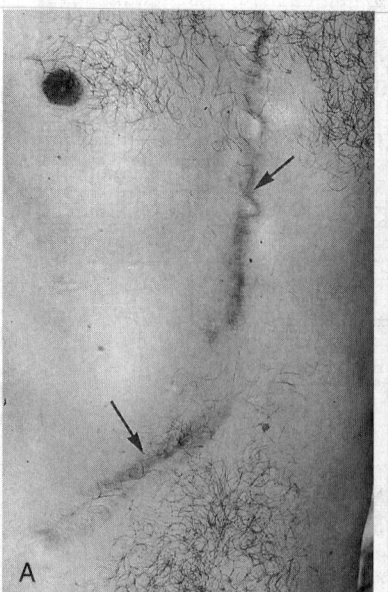
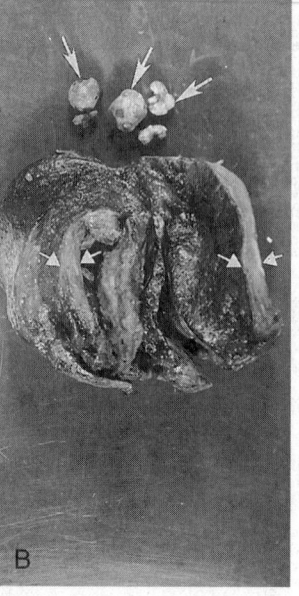

FIGURE 39–19. *A*, Midline sternotomy scar *(upper arrow)* and cholecystectomy scar *(lower arrow)* in a patient with Fallot's tetralogy. Gallstones announced themselves years after intracardiac repair of the congenital malformation. *B*, Surgical specimen of calcium bilirubinate gallstones *(upper arrows)* and thick-walled gallbladder from a 39-year-old cyanotic man with Eisenmenger's complex.

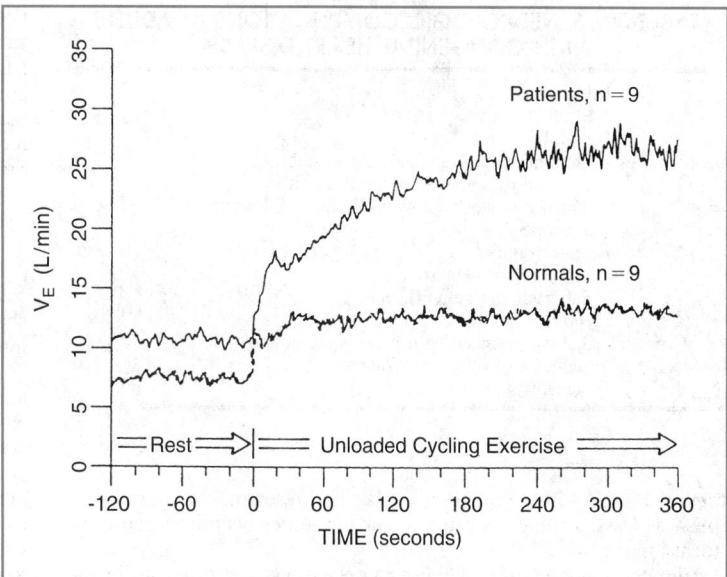

FIGURE 39-20. Recording of the increase in ventilatory response to unloaded cycle ergometric exercise in nine adult patients with right-to-left shunts and in nine normal subjects. Minute ventilation at rest and in response to exercise was higher in patients than in normal subjects. (From Sietsema KE, Cooper DM, Perloff JK, et al.: Control of ventilation during exercise in patients with central venous to systemic arterial shunts. J Appl Physiol 64:234, 1988.)

threaten its viability and to remote risks that express themselves as developmental defects or transmitted congenital anomalies. Certain congenital cardiac malformations impose such a formidable threat to maternal survival that pregnancy is proscribed or should be interrupted irrespective of functional class. The two major maternal cardiac risks are pulmonary vascular disease and pulmonary edema. Pulmonary vascular disease limits or precludes appropriate adaptive responses to the circulatory changes of pregnancy and to the volatile hemodynamic changes during labor, delivery, and the puerperium. Pulmonary edema is less common in congenital than in acquired heart disease, but the functional adequacy of the ventricle that serves the systemic circulation is much to this point.

In women with mild unoperated lesions or successful intracardiac repair, managing labor and delivery is essentially the same as for normal women except for the risk of infective endocarditis. High-risk patients should be attended by a high-risk obstetrician, a neonatologist, and a cardiologist knowledgeable in congenital heart disease. It is often wise to admit such patients prior to term for elective induction of labor so that delivery can be accomplished during daytime working hours. Labor in the lateral decubitus position attenuates the hemodynamic fluctuations associated with major uterine contractions in the supine position. A strong consensus favors spontaneous vaginal delivery with the fetus passing through the pelvis in response to the force of uterine contractions unassisted by straining in order to minimize the undesirable circulatory effects of the Valsalva maneuver. Injecting fentanyl into the epidural space provides analgesia during labor without unfavorably affecting muscle tone and without loss of sympathetic tone. Cesarean section is reserved for obstetric indications (cephalopelvic disproportion) or for preterm labor in a gravida on oral anticoagulants. A flotation catheter permits hemodynamic surveillance, but individual judgment is required. In Eisenmenger's complex, for example, the risks of a flotation catheter outweigh the benefits. It seems intuitive to administer oxygen during labor and delivery in cyanotic patients, although oxygen is without proven efficacy. Oxygen dries nasal mucous membranes and predisposes to epistaxes in cyanotic patients with intrinsic hemostatic defects.

The risk of thromboembolism increases during the postpartum period, and patients with lesions susceptible to paradoxical embolism are at particular risk. Meticulous leg care, use of elastic support hose, and early ambulation are important preventive measures.

Immediate risks to the fetus are determined chiefly by the functional class of the mother (Table 39-4), maternal cyanosis, and maternal oral anticoagulants. Cyanosis threatens the growth, development, and viability of the fetus and materially increases fetal wastage. Anticoagulants confront the fetus with risks that cannot be satisfactorily resolved. It is best to plan pregnancy carefully, replace warfarin with heparin prior to conception, and continue heparin through at least the first trimester. Whatever subsequent regimen is selected in using warfarin and heparin, the patient should be advised of her options before she conceives.

An important fetal risk is parental transmission of congenital heart disease. Fetal echocardiography is a major diagnostic step forward. The incidence of genetic transmission is believed to be higher if the mother rather than the father has congenital heart disease. Two hypotheses are relevant—cytoplasmic (mitochondrial) maternal transmission and the effects of parental imprinting (methylation) on inheritance of nuclear genes (see Ch. 23).

Exercise and athletics (recreational or competitive) are medical concerns in patients with congenital heart disease. Consideration must be given to the type, intensity, and duration of exercise, the training program required for a given sport, the emotional response (stress) that the athlete experiences in anticipation of or during a sporting event, and the risk of injury to the athlete or to the spectator if the athletic activity results in body collision or induces loss of consciousness. Moderate steady-state (isotonic) exercise is often permitted because the patient can safely desist in anticipation of or at the onset of symptoms. High-intensity isotonic exercise, especially of prolonged duration, requires individual physician judgment. Isometric exercise, even mild or moderate, should be minimized. Strenuous isometric exercise is seldom permissible.

Neurologic complications in adults with congenital heart disease are listed in Table 39-6. Brain abscess is suspected when cyanotic adults present with headaches, seizures, focal neurologic signs, and fever. A recent brain abscess can be diagnosed by computed tomog-

TABLE 39-4. CONGENITAL HEART DISEASE FUNCTIONAL CLASS (PRESENCE AND DEGREE OF SYMPTOMS)

Class 1	Asymptomatic
Class 2	Symptoms are present but do not interfere with normal activities
Class 3	Symptoms interfere with some but not most activities
Class 4	Symptoms interfere with most if not all activities

TABLE 39-5. COMMON ACYANOTIC AND CYANOTIC MALFORMATIONS WITH EXPECTED ADULT SURVIVAL*

Acyanotic
  Atrial septal defect (secundum)
  Patent ductus arteriosus
  Pulmonary valve stenosis
  Coarctation of the aorta
  Aortic valve disease
Cyanotic
  Fallot's tetralogy

*Malformations are listed in descending order of prevalence among women.

TABLE 39–6. NEUROLOGIC COMPLICATIONS IN ADULTS WITH CONGENITAL HEART DISEASE

Infectious
    Brain abscess
Ischemic
    Cerebral emboli (paradoxical, systemic)
    Cerebral thrombosis (venous, arterial)
    Subclavian steal following Blalock-Taussig shunt
    Syncope
Hemorrhagic
    Intracerebral hemorrhage
    Subarachnoid hemorrhage
Hypoxic
    Spells associated with Fallot's tetralogy
    Sequelae of open heart surgery
    Seizures

raphy (Fig. 39–21). Seizures may be the presenting symptom of a fresh abscess or may persist or recur long after healing because of focal injury.

Cerebral emboli can be bland or infected and can originate in either the systemic circulation or peripheral or pelvic veins—paradoxical embolization. Paradoxical emboli in adults with cyanotic congenital heart disease pose a therapeutic dilemma because anticoagulants reinforce intrinsic hemostatic defects and increase the risk of hemorrhage. Paradoxical emboli in hospitalized cyanotic patients can be avoided by inserting a particle/air filter into the intravenous line (Fig. 39–22). Paradoxical emboli in acyanotic patients sometimes occur because an interatrial communication—ostium secundum atrial septal defect or patent foramen ovale—permits inferior caval blood to cross the atrial septum, carrying the offending embolus. Provocation (the Valsalva maneuver or vigorous coughing) is often required to initiate the transient venoarterial mixing that provides the physiologic substrate for a paradoxical embolus through a foramen ovale. Systemic emboli may also originate from an atrial septal aneurysm in the absence of a right-to-left shunt.

Cerebral hemorrhage in adults with congenital heart disease occurs because of the injudicious use of anticoagulants or aspirin in cyanotic patients with intrinsic hemostatic defects and because of rupture of a congenital aneurysm of the circle of Willis (see Fig. 39–3), especially in patients with coarctation of the aorta.

Syncope in patients with congenital aortic stenosis is due principally to an exaggerated, prolonged, exercise-induced fall in systemic vascular resistance mediated by left ventricular baroreceptors.

Malignant ventricular arrhythmias *per se* seldom initiate syncope but are the chief cause of death *after* a faint. Syncope-induced hypotension is more likely to provoke ventricular arrhythmias and sudden death in older adults with calcific aortic stenosis and coexisting coronary artery disease than in young patients with congenital aortic stenosis and normal coronary arteries. Congenital complete heart block, either isolated or in the context of congenitally corrected transposition of the great arteries, may be accompanied by Stokes-Adams episodes that require a pacemaker to prevent recurrence.

The subclavian steal is an occasional neurologic complication of a Blalock-Taussig anastomosis. The anastomosis may create an anatomic and physiologic substrate identical to that of an atherosclerotic subclavian steal. Symptoms may appear decades after the shunt is created, depending upon the development of cervical and intrathoracic collateral arteries.

Acquired disorders of the heart and circulation, especially systemic hypertension, coronary artery disease, and valvular heart disease, may coexist with and modify the physiologic expressions of congenital heart disease in adults. In ostium secundum atrial septal defect, systemic hypertension or coronary artery disease impairs left ventricular diastolic function and augments the left-to-right shunt, and the incidence of mitral regurgitation increases with age. In Fallot's tetralogy, systemic hypertension imposes an increase in afterload upon both left *and* right ventricles (biventricular aorta). In Eisenmenger's complex, systemic hypertension reduces the right-to-left shunt but at the price of increased afterload imposed upon the right and left ventricles. Control of the systemic hypertension must be meticulous, because an inappropriate reduction in systemic vascular resistance increases the right-to-left shunt.

Insurability and employability in adults with congenital heart disease are closely coupled. An appreciable number of young adults who have undergone successful repair of their congenital heart lesion can anticipate normal or nearly normal lifespans and lifestyles, but exclusion from health insurance plans because of pre-existing disease imposes financial burdens. Job discrimination is an important factor affecting work opportunities. Employers are often reluctant to hire patients with a thoracotomy scar. Job applicants may feel compelled to withhold medical information in order to secure employment and often remain at work that they dislike because of fear that other employers will not hire them or that they will lose existing health benefits.

SURGICAL CONSIDERATIONS

Surgical considerations in adults with congenital heart disease apply to patients who have had palliative procedures, reparative surgery, or cardiac catheterization as a therapeutic intervention and to those who require noncardiac surgery. The cardiac surgeon often

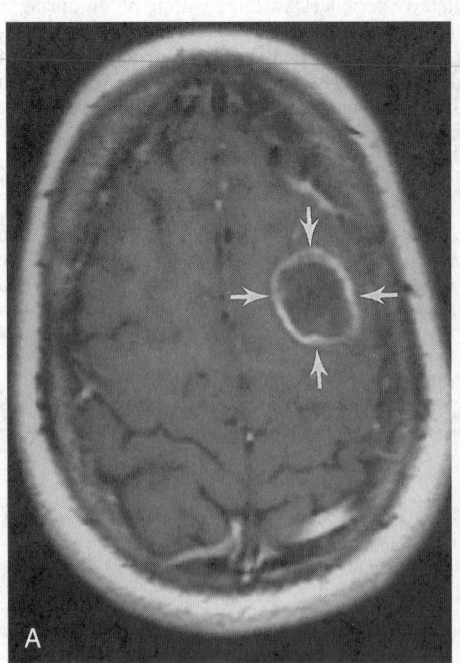
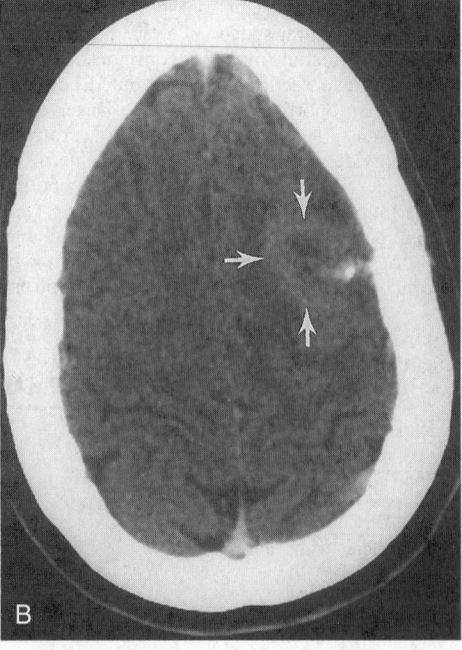

FIGURE 39–21. Computed tomography of fresh brain abscess *(arrows)* from a cyanotic 23-year-old woman with Fallot's tetralogy and pulmonary atresia. *A,* Typical ring enhancement of the fresh abscess. *B,* Abscess immediately after aspiration drainage.

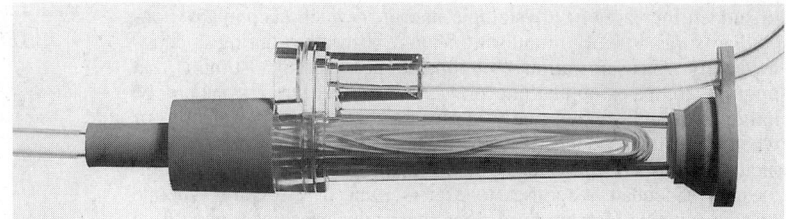

FIGURE 39–22. An air/particle filter for insertion into intravenous lines to prevent paradoxical air or particle emboli in patients with cyanotic congenital heart disease.

confronts an uncharted course at reoperation, including coexisting acquired coronary artery disease and valvular heart disease.

In adults with cyanotic congenital heart disease, hematocrit levels above 65% carry an increased risk of perioperative hemorrhage. Preoperative phlebotomy that reduces the hematocrit level to just below 65% is believed to decrease that risk. Phlebotomized units are stored for potential autologous transfusion. Hemostatic defects in cyanotic congenital heart disease reinforce the risk of bleeding inherent in excessive tissue vascularity in such patients. Two other issues are relevant in adults with cyanotic congenital heart disease confronting operation or reoperation—the effect of erythrocytosis on renal function (see above) and the risk of a recurrence of acute gouty arthritis during the stress of surgery, even if the gout has long been quiescent (see Ch. 251).

Prosthetic materials have materially influenced survival patterns after surgery for congenital heart disease. There are three categories of prosthesess—patches, valves, and conduits. Bioprosthetic valves and conduits often require replacement (reoperation) when the patient outgrows a device placed in childhood or when a bioprosthetic valve or conduit begins to malfunction.

Cardiac catheterization as a therapeutic intervention is currently the preferred primary treatment for certain types of congenital cardiac malformations and also serves as an adjunct to surgical management in increasing numbers of pediatric and adult patients. The intervention can be reparative or palliative. An example of a reparative if not corrective procedure is balloon dilatation of typical pulmonary valve stenosis (Fig. 39–23). Balloon dilatation of a mobile stenotic bicuspid aortic valve is an example of palliation. Preoperative occlusion of aortic to pulmonary collaterals in cyanotic congenital heart disease is a catheter procedure that is an adjunct to surgery.

Noncardiac surgery in adults with congenital heart disease includes patients who have *not* undergone cardiac surgery and those who have undergone reparative or palliative surgery. First, let us cite a few examples of patients with *acyanotic* congenital heart disease who have not been operated upon.

Situs inversus with dextrocardia may go unrecognized until an illness requiring noncardiac surgery brings the patient to clinical attention (see above). In otherwise asymptomatic congenital complete heart block, the heart and circulation may not respond appropriately

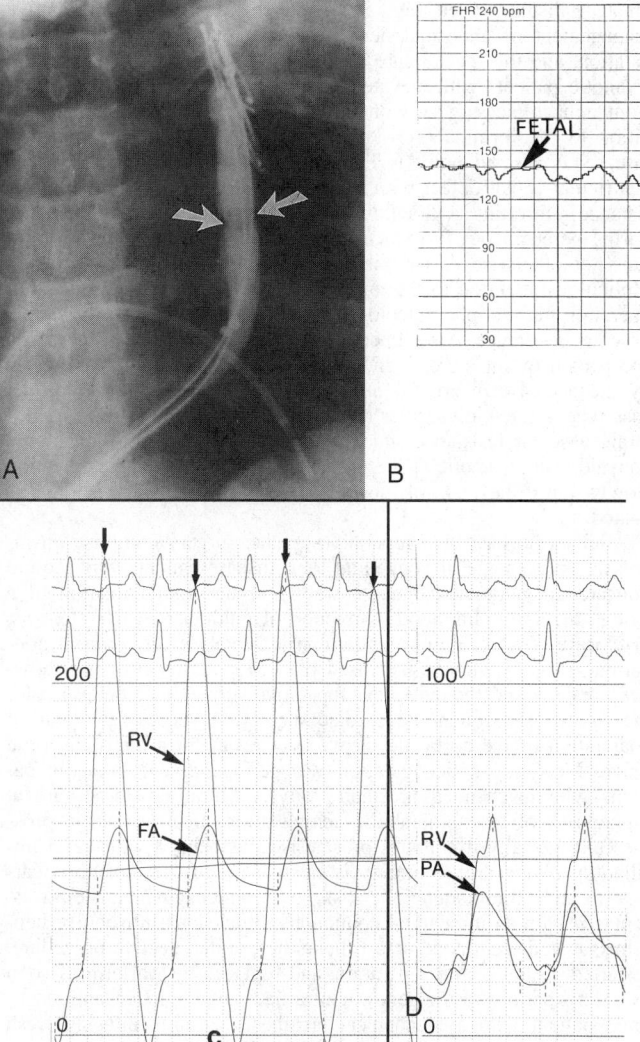

FIGURE 39–23. *A*, Cineangiogram frame from an 18-year-old woman with severe pulmonary valve stenosis. She was near term in her first pregnancy. The dilated single balloon is indented *(arrows)* by the stenotic pulmonary valve. *B*, Monitor of fetal heart rate. *C*, Right ventricular (RV) systolic pressure was more than twice the femoral arterial (FA) pressure. Note the right ventricular pulsus alternans *(arrows)*. *D*, After balloon dilatation, the gradient was about 20 mm Hg. Subsequent delivery of a normal infant was uneventful.

to sudden increases in physiologic demands which accompany noncardiac surgery. ECG monitoring should be routine during and immediately after operation. Intraoperative vagotonic stimuli that might accompany ophthalmic or gastrointestinal surgery should be minimized and treated with intravenous atropine expectantly or when there is a sudden decrease in heart rate. Higher risk patients includes those with relatively slow heart rates, wide QRS complexes, inadequate responses to exercise, and a history of syncope or near-syncope. A temporary right ventricular pacemaker should be inserted before surgery in high-risk patients.

In patients with primary pulmonary hypertension, noncardiac surgery incurs risks that are not to be ignored. Even the seemingly mild stress of a minor procedure can culminate in circulatory demands that are poorly tolerated. Preoperative sedation reduces anxiety, intraoperative or postoperative systemic hypotension is hazardous, and inserting a flotation catheter for hemodynamic monitoring is, in itself, not devoid of risk.

Unoperated young adults with an ostium secundum atrial septal defect confront cardiac surgery with comparatively little risk, but there are two caveats. Sudden blood loss results in a rise in systemic vascular resistance and a decrease in venous return, a combination that augments the left-to-right interatrial shunt, sometimes appreciably. Paradoxical emboli from leg or pelvic veins represent an additional postoperative risk. Thrombi carried by the inferior vena cava tend to stream through a secundum atrial septal defect into the systemic circulation. Meticulous leg care and early ambulation minimize venous stasis.

Infective endocarditis is a potential risk in patients undergoing noncardiac surgery. A case in point is the bicuspid aortic valve, whether functionally normal, stenotic, or incompetent (see above).

In adults with *cyanotic* congenital heart disease, attention should focus on certain concerns discussed earlier, namely, calcium bilirubinate gallstones (see Fig. 39–19) (see Ch. 126), perioperative management of abnormal hemostasis, the question of oxygen inhalation, and the special care of intravenous lines (see Fig. 39–22). Cyanotic patients with elevated pulmonary vascular resistance confront noncardiac surgery with risks inherent in the cyanosis, in addition to the formidable risks inherent in the pulmonary vascular disease. A case in point is Eisenmenger's complex (nonrestrictive ventricular septal defect with suprasystemic pulmonary vascular resistance). Inserting a flotation catheter poses the risk of bleeding during percutaneous introduction and provides little or no information not otherwise easily achieved by a fingertip pulse oximeter. Meticulous attention to the pulse oximeter before, during, and after operation permits pharmacologic control of fluctuations in systemic vascular resistance. A perioperative fall in systemic resistance is accompanied by an increase in right-to-left shunt identified promptly by the decrease in arterial oxygen saturation. The converse is the case when systemic vascular resistance rises. Because a drop in systemic vascular resistance suddenly augments the right-to-left shunt, convalescent cyanotic patients are advised to change position slowly until the risk of postoperative postural hypotension has abated.

Adults who have had reparative cardiac surgery comprise an increasing percentage of congenital heart disease patients who require noncardiac operations. Patients who have undergone ligation of a patent ductus in childhood, correction of pulmonary valve stenosis, or closure of an ostium secundum atrial septal defect confront noncardiac surgery without increased risk. More often than not, however, residua and sequelae after reparative surgery (see below) color the risk of subsequent noncardiac surgery. A successful repair of coarctation of the aorta may leave as a residuum a bicuspid aortic valve. Managing anticoagulation is a perioperative concern in patients with mechanical prosthetic valves. Mitral prostheses are at higher risk of thromboembolic complications than are aortic prostheses, especially if a mitral prosthesis is associated with atrial fibrillation. If noncardiac surgery is elective and if the prosthesis carries a high thromboembolic risk, oral anticoagulants should be replaced with an in-hospital continuous intravenous infusion of heparin that is discontinued 4 to 6 hours before the elective procedure, restarted 48 hours after operation, and replaced by warfarin as soon as safety permits. Emergency noncardiac surgery in an anticoagulated patient with a mechanical prosthesis requires infusing fresh frozen plasma, not administering vitamin K.

TABLE 39–7. RESIDUA AFTER REPARATIVE SURGERY FOR CONGENITAL HEART DISEASE

Electrophysiologic
Valvular
Ventricular
  Chamber morphology
  Chamber mass
  Chamber function
  Myocardial connective tissue
Vascular
  Anatomic (morphologic) vascular anomalies or defects
  Elevated resistance and/or pressure—systemic, pulmonary
Noncardiovascular
  Developmental abnormalities
  Somatic defects
  Medical disorders

Electrophysiologic sequelae may be present after reparative cardiac surgery for congenital heart disease and require attention during noncardiac surgery. Systemic hypertension can be a concern in managing adults during noncardiac surgery. Adequacy of ventricular function (left, right, or single ventricle) is a major determinant of perioperative risk. Excessive intravenous fluids should be avoided, and hemodynamic monitoring should be used when the morphologic substrate permits.

The medical management of adults with congenital heart disease undergoing noncardiac surgery must take into account not only the congenital malformation—unoperated or operated—but also age-related acquired diseases of the heart and circulation, especially coronary artery disease and systemic hypertension, as well as coexisting medical illnesses that prevail in adults.

RESIDUA AND SEQUELAE

Residua are represented by preoperative cardiac, vascular, or noncardiovascular disorders that are intentionally left behind at the time of reparative cardiac surgery (Table 39–7). *Sequelae* are alterations or disorders that are incurred—occasionally or invariably—at the time of reparative surgery and are looked upon as necessary and acceptable consequences of operation (Table 39–8). By contrast, *complications* are unintentional aftermaths of reparative surgery that range in severity from inconsequential to fatal. Cardiac surgery is considered to be *curative* if no residua, sequelae, or complications of the heart and circulation occur after operation. This ideal is seldom realized, and curative cardiac surgery does not preclude noncardiovascular residua (see Table 39–7). Electrophysiologic residua include axis deviation, especially left; conduction defects, especially atrioventricular; disorders of impulse formation, especially of the sinus node; and arrhythmias, especially atrial. Valvular residua include congenitally malformed cardiac valves that are functionally normal and therefore do not require attention during reparative surgery; intrinsically normal cardiac valves that are rendered incompetent because of the physiologic stress imposed by the congenital malformation that prompted the surgical repair; and residually incompetent or stenotic congenitally malformed valves that do not lend themselves to complete repair.

TABLE 39–8. SEQUELAE OF REPARATIVE SURGERY FOR CONGENITAL HEART DISEASE

Electrophysiologic
  Atriotomy
    Intra-atrial repair
    Intraventricular repair
  Ventriculotomy
  The incision site
    The intracardiac repair
Native valves
  Left ventricular or right ventricular *outflow* repair
  Left ventricular or right ventricular *inflow* repair
Prosthetic materials
  Patches
  Valves
  Conduits
Myocardial and endocardial sequelae

Residual ventricular abnormalities after reparative surgery are represented by disorders that are permanent, such as chamber morphology, or disorders that change with the passage of time, such as alterations in chamber mass, function, and myocardial connective tissue. Vascular residua after reparative surgery consist of anomalies or defects that involve the aorta and the cerebral and coronary arteries or that consist of elevated resistance and/or pressure in the systemic or pulmonary circulation. A residual bicuspid aortic valve may be accompanied by aortic root disease that suddenly announces itself as a dissecting aortic aneurysm (see Fig. 39–1*B*). A residual congenital aneurysm of the circle of Willis (see Fig. 39–3) may announce itself by sudden rupture. Residual coronary artery disease— intimal proliferation, medial thickening, premature atherosclerosis—may persist after otherwise successful repair of coarctation of the aorta or supravalvular aortic stenosis, and elevated systemic arterial pressure is a potential residuum after coarctation repair. The preoperative status of the pulmonary resistance vessels is a major determinant of the presence and degree of residual postoperative pulmonary vascular disease.

Noncardiovascular residua can be important long-term concerns after reparative surgery. Examples are Down syndrome, Turner's syndrome, and specific somatic defects that include facial dysmorphism and limb abnormalities (Fig. 39–24). Medical and psychosocial disorders may persist as important postoperative residua. A brain abscess (see Fig. 39–21) can serve as a focus of a residual seizure disorder, and cataracts or deafness persist as medical residua after division of a patent ductus in children with the rubella syndrome.

Sequelae of reparative surgery for congenital heart disease are listed in Table 39–8. Electrophysiologic sequelae result from the surgical incision per se or from intra-atrial or intraventricular repair, and are among the most important and prevalent concerns after reparative surgery for congenital heart disease. Valvular sequelae (affecting native valves) are, in part, represented by pulmonary regurgitation after direct repair or balloon dilatation of congenital pulmonary valve stenosis or outflow repair of Fallot's tetralogy.

Prosthetic materials represent a special category of sequelae after reparative surgery because biologic and nonbiologic materials are introduced as essential parts of the operative procedure. Patches can be devoid of sequelae, but that is not the case with prosthetic valves or conduits.

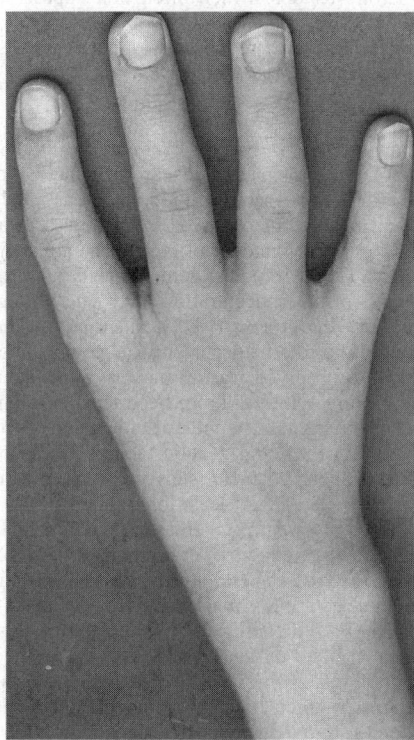

FIGURE 39–24. Hand of a 26-year-old woman with the Holt-Oram syndrome, here represented by absence of the thumb. The patient had a nonrestrictive ostium secundum atrial septal defect.

Myocardial sequelae after intracardiac repair usually originate at the site of the atrial or ventricular incision. The major sequelae are, as a rule, electrophysiologic. Morphologic or mechanical sequelae at these sites are generally of less concern, unless there is aneurysm formation, which is more properly considered a complication rather than a sequela.

Perloff JK: The Clinical Recognition of Congenital Heart Disease. 4th ed. Philadelphia, WB Saunders, 1994. *In each congenital malformation, clarification of the anatomic derangements and physiologic consequences leads to understanding of the natural history, physical signs, electrocardiogram, chest radiograph, and echo/Doppler from birth through adulthood.*

Perloff JK: Systemic complications of cyanosis in adults with congenital heart disease. Cardiol Clin 11:689, 1993. *Reviews the hematologic derangements (red cell mass, hemostatic defects), renal involvement, and urate metabolism in adults with cyanotic congenital heart disease, providing a rational basis for management.*

Perloff JK, Child JS: Congenital Heart Disease in Adults. Philadelphia, WB Saunders, 1991. *Deals with congenital heart disease in adults as a new area of specialized cardiovascular interest and includes sections on background and facilities, survival patterns (unoperated and postoperative), medical considerations, surgical considerations, and postoperative residua and sequelae.*

Perloff JK, Marelli AJ: Neurologic and psychosocial disorders in adults with congenital heart disease. Heart Dis Stroke 1:218, 1991. *A comprehensive review of the neurologic and psychosocial disorders in patients with congenital heart disease. Neurologic abnormalities include infectious, ischemic, hemorrhagic, hypoxic, and seizure disorders. Psychosocial issues include psychosocial adjustment and intellectual and cognitive development.*

Perloff JK, Marelli AJ, Miner PM: The risk of stroke in adults with cyanotic congenital heart disease. Circulation 87:1954, 1993. *Examines and calls into question the previously assumed relationship between an increase in red cell mass and stroke caused by cerebral arterial thrombosis. A rational basis for clinical management is recommended, and criteria for phlebotomy are redefined.*

40 ATHEROSCLEROSIS
Russell Ross

Atherosclerosis is responsible for the majority of cases of myocardial and cerebral infarction and thus represents the principal cause of death in the United States and western Europe. Atherosclerosis is the descriptive term for thickened and hardened lesions of the medium and large muscular and elastic arteries. It is a lipid-rich lesion, in contrast with arteriosclerosis, which is the generic term used for thickened and stiffened arteries of all sizes. Other forms of arteriosclerosis include focal calcific arteriosclerosis (Mönckeberg's arteriosclerosis) and arteriolosclerosis, a disease of small vessels.

The lesions of atherosclerosis occur within the innermost layer of the artery, the intima, and are largely confined to this region of the vessel. The lesions are generally eccentric and, if they become sufficiently large, can occlude the artery and thus the vascular supply to a tissue or organ, resulting in ischemia or necrosis. If this occurs, it often leads to the characteristic clinical sequelae of myocardial infarction, cerebral infarction, gangrene of the extremities, or sudden cardiac death.

THE NORMAL ARTERY

The normal artery consists essentially of a tube lined on its luminal aspect by a continuous layer of endothelium and on its outer aspect by loose connective tissue containing fibroblasts and smooth muscle cells; these package an intermediate layer of pure smooth muscle cells that are bound together in such a manner that, by working with the elastic laminae and the collagen and proteoglycans that surround the cells, the smooth muscle cells contract and maintain the tonus of the artery wall as the blood flows through with each systole and diastole.

The cells lining the artery, the endothelium, represent the interface with the cells of the blood. At this interface different blood cell types can interact with the endothelium and, under appropriate circumstances, develop into lesions of atherosclerosis. These cells are the platelet, the monocyte, and the lymphocyte. Their potential roles in atherogenesis are discussed below.

THE LESIONS OF ATHEROSCLEROSIS

The two principal forms of atherosclerosis are the early lesion, or fatty streak, and the advanced lesion, or fibrous plaque, which can become an advanced complicated lesion.

THE FATTY STREAK. The fatty streak is the most common and ubiquitous lesion of atherosclerosis. It occurs at all ages and in Western society is present at birth in some infants and is common in young children. The lesions of atherosclerosis are confined principally to the intima. Initially, the fatty streak appears to contain two cell types: foam cells that consist of macrophages filled with lipids (principally in the form of cholesteryl esters) and T lymphocytes (principally CD8+ with some CD4+ cells). The macrophages are derived from blood-borne monocytes that are chemotactically attracted into the artery wall, where they develop into foam cells. As the fatty streak enlarges, it does so with monocytes continuing to attach and migrate into the intima, and consequently to develop into macrophages. Subsequently, smooth muscle cells appear to migrate into the intima from the media and also begin to accumulate lipid and take on the appearance of foam cells. As the fatty streak becomes larger and more advanced, it contains varying numbers of smooth muscle cells mixed together with lymphocytes and the predominant lipid-filled macrophages. Fatty streaks can be found in young individuals at the same anatomic sites that are later occupied by advanced lesions, as well as at sites where they may either regress and disappear or remain as fatty streaks throughout life.

THE FIBROUS PLAQUE. The fibrous plaque is also located in the intima and characteristically leads to the eccentric thickening of the artery that often results in an occluded lumen. The fibrous plaque is typically covered at its luminal aspect by a thickened cap of dense connective tissue containing a special form of flattened, pancake-shaped smooth muscle cell that has formed the dense collagenous matrix in which it is embedded. Beneath this cap, the lesion is highly cellular and contains large numbers of smooth muscle cells, some of which may be full of lipid droplets. It also contains numerous macrophages, many of which take the form of foam cells, together with variable numbers of T lymphocytes. These collections of cells usually overlie a deeper area of necrotic foam cells and debris. This necrotic area sometimes becomes calcified and often may contain cholesterol crystals. (Figure 40–1 details the cellular composition of a fibrous plaque.)

THE COMPLICATED LESION. The complicated lesion is a fibrous plaque that has degenerated extensively and often calcifies. It may contain ulcerations, cracks, and fissures, which serve as sites for platelet adherence, aggregation and thrombosis, and subsequent organization. Many cases of sudden death have been reported to result from fibrous plaques with poorly developed fibrous caps which are thin at the shoulders. At these shoulders, or margins of the lesions which may be enriched in macrophages, breaks or tears may permit hemorrhage into the necrotic core, thrombosis, and sudden death.

MORBID ANATOMY OF THE LESIONS. Fatty streaks are flat lesions that often appear as yellow discolorations on the surface of the artery but seldom intrude into the lumen and thus cause no clinical sequelae. The fibrous plaques and complicated lesions are raised lesions that are often pearly gray in appearance but may be discolored when associated with erythrocytes and thrombi.

LOCALIZATION OF THE LESIONS. The arteries most commonly involved with atherosclerosis are the aorta; the femoral, popliteal, and tibial arteries; the coronary arteries; the internal and external carotid arteries; and the cerebral arteries.

In the aorta, the abdominal portion is commonly involved with lesions of atherosclerosis at an earlier age, and, as in the thoracic aorta, lesions most commonly form around orifices of branches and bifurcations of the artery. There is a greater incidence of atherosclerotic lesions in the leg arteries, whereas they are relatively rare in the upper limbs. Atherosclerosis of the smaller arteries, particularly those of the legs and the coronary arteries, is more common in cigarette smokers and in individuals who have glucose intolerance.

Coronary atherosclerosis is most prominent in the main stems of the coronary arteries, particularly in the segments closest to the ostia of the coronary vessel. The degree of luminal narrowing in the coronary arteries can be variable; however, atherosclerosis is generally present in the epicardial segment of the vessels, whereas the intramural coronary arteries are generally spared. Typically, after coronary bypass surgery, the perianastomotic site of the bypass is often (30% of the time) involved in new atherosclerotic lesions developing, which is probably related to mural thrombi that readily form at these sites.

The carotid and cerebral arteries generally have patchily distributed atherosclerotic lesions, which often first appear at the base of the brain in the carotid, basilar, and vertebral arteries.

The pulmonary arteries are generally spared of lesions, except when associated with pulmonary hypertension.

RISK FACTORS

The risk factor concept evolved from epidemiologic studies of the incidence of coronary artery disease conducted in the United States and in Europe. Prospective studies demonstrated a consistent association of characteristics observed in apparently healthy individuals with the subsequent incidence of coronary artery disease in the same individuals. These studies demonstrated an association between an increase in the concentration of plasma lipoproteins, principally low density lipoprotein (LDL) and thus plasma cholesterol (see Ch. 173) and the rate of occurrence of new events of coronary artery disease. Also observed was an increased incidence of the disease in relation to cigarette smoking, hypertension, clinical diabetes, age, being male, obesity, stress and particular personality characteristics (denoted as type A), and genetic factors. Because of these associations, each of these characteristics was termed a risk factor for atherosclerosis (see Ch. 31). At least three independent predictors of risk are valuable in anticipating increased incidence of atherosclerosis: hyperlipidemia, cigarette smoking, and hypertension.

HYPERLIPIDEMIA. There is a clear association between chronic hypercholesterolemia and increased incidence of ischemic heart disease. The Framingham Study demonstrated this association, particularly in men between ages 20 and 40. When the plasma cholesterol levels are >220 mg per deciliter, there is a marked increase in the relative incidence of myocardial infarction, which is most easily demonstrated in individuals with familial hypercholesterolemia. The range of normality is not entirely clear in defining cholesterol and triglyceride levels for a given population as they relate to increased risk of ischemic heart disease. However, in the United States, 200 mg per deciliter is considered to be the upper

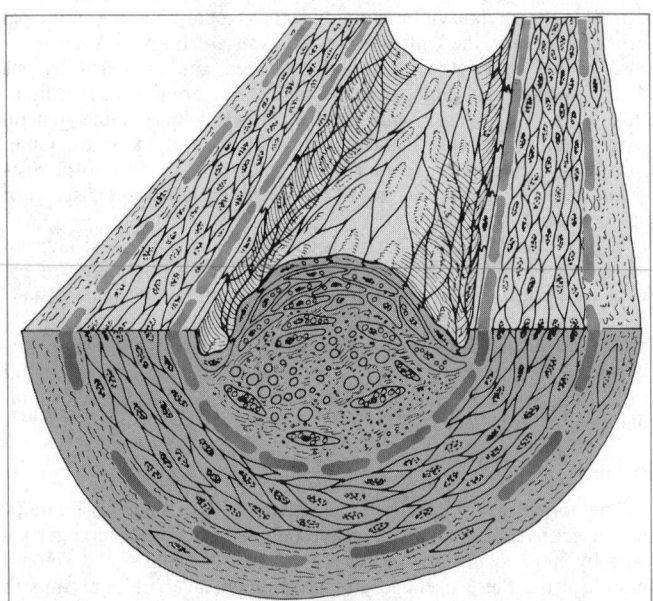

FIGURE 40–1. The *fibrous plaque,* which characteristically consists of numerous proliferated smooth muscle cells together with macrophages and variable numbers of lymphocytes. In this diagram, the fibrous plaque is covered by an intact endothelial monolayer and contains a fibrous cap of smooth muscle cells. These smooth muscle cells lie in a dense connective tissue matrix that covers a deeper collection of smooth muscle cells and macrophages, both of which may contain numerous lipid droplets and take the form of foam cells mixed together with variable numbers of lymphocytes. These collections of cells lie in a mixture of connective tissue matrix and free extracellular deposits of lipid. The fibrous plaque usually intrudes into the lumen owing to its proliferative nature. This diagram represents only in general terms the relative appearance of such a lesion.

limit of normal for the plasma cholesterol level, which increases from birth through young adulthood until approximately age 50 in men and to somewhat older ages in women. Similarly, there is an age-related increase in plasma triglyceride levels. Triglyceride is associated with increases in very low density lipoproteins (VLDL), whereas elevated plasma cholesterol level is generally associated with increase in LDL.

Lipoproteins can accumulate abnormally in the plasma from overproduction and/or deficient removal. There are numerous forms of genetically derived hyperlipoproteinemias that are either monogenic or polygenic. Perhaps more common are forms of hyperlipoproteinemia secondary to other disease, such as diabetes, renal disease, alcoholism, hypothyroidism, and the dysglobulinemias (see Ch. 173).

Homozygous Familial Hypercholesterolemia. Patients with homozygous familial hypercholesterolemia (FH disease) represent one of the best demonstrations of the capacity of hypercholesterolemia to induce the cellular changes that lead to atherogenesis. Although FH disease is much rarer than the secondary hyperlipoproteinemias or other forms of genetic hyperlipidemia, we know a great deal about its course in humans and in an animal model, the Watanabe heritable hyperlipidemic rabbit, as well as diet-induced hypercholesterolemia in the nonhuman primate. In the case of genetic hyperlipidemia, the plasma cholesterol and LDL levels are inordinately high owing to faulty or missing LDL receptors. When LDL is bound to its normal receptor, it suppresses the activity of the rate-limiting enzyme for cholesterol synthesis, HMG-CoA-reductase. In individuals with FH disease, the liver and peripheral cells continue to synthesize large amounts of cholesterol because absent or faulty receptors fail to generate a feedback inhibitory signal and cholesterol synthesis goes on unabated. Under these conditions, plasma cholesterol levels reach 500 to 1000 mg per deciliter or higher, and rampant atherosclerosis develops, with advanced occlusive lesions. This can occur at very young ages, and myocardial infarcts have been described in young children with this disease.

Treatment of Hypercholesterolemia. The Lipid Research Clinic Trials have demonstrated that it is beneficial to lower plasma levels in patients with chronically elevated VLDL. These studies showed that the decrease in plasma cholesterol levels can be correlated with a reduced incidence of myocardial infarction and thus atherosclerosis. Premature ischemic heart disease is usually associated with hypercholesterolemia, particularly when levels of plasma cholesterol are > 240 mg per deciliter. When this occurs, the incidence of atherosclerotic disease can be as high as fivefold greater than for individuals with plasma cholesterol levels < 200 mg per deciliter.

Hypertriglyceridemia is usually associated with increases in VLDL in the plasma, which may be complicated by increases in cholesterol as well. Patients with increased VLDL levels who come from families with familial combined hyperlipidemia are at increased risk for atherosclerosis, whereas those with elevated VLDL levels from families with monogenic familial hypertriglyceridemia are not at increased risk. Increased VLDL levels can increase the risk of atherosclerosis if it accompanies other risk factors, such as diabetes mellitus or cigarette smoking.

It is important to examine all patients over age 20 for hyperlipidemia, particularly if they have a family history of premature ischemic heart disease. This is best done by measuring the concentrations of cholesterol and triglyceride in plasma after an overnight fast. Cholesterol levels > 200 mg per deciliter or triglyceride levels > 250 mg per deciliter, or both, indicate hyperlipidemia, requiring attention and therapy, the first step being dietary intervention. Such patients should be brought to normal weight if this is excessive and maintained on a diet low in saturated fat and cholesterol. Those with hypertriglyceridemia should limit or eliminate alcohol intake. In general, reducing intake of calories, cholesterol, and saturated fat is the best approach to begin with in most patients. Severe hyperlipidemia with cholesterol levels > 350 mg per deciliter or triglyceride levels > 400 mg per deciliter, or both, usually represents a genetic disorder and often first manifests with xanthomas. Such patients' families, particularly first-degree relatives, should also be examined.

Recent studies suggest that increased LDL is harmful when it is modified as it is transported by the endothelial cells into the artery wall or during exposure to macrophages or smooth muscle. The principal form of modification is oxidation, which can lead to oxidized LDL (oxLDL). In diabetics, LDL may be modified by glyca-

tion. Both oxLDL and glycated LDL form free radicals. Treating hypercholesterolemic rabbits and nonhuman primates with antioxidants reduces lesion size and decreases macrophages.

If dietary approaches are unsuccessful, then regimens including bile acid-binding resins, nicotine acid, or HMG-CoA-reductase inhibitors (statins) should be considered (see Ch. 173). Use of such agents depends not only on their efficaciousness, but on their long-term effects as well. Their use before puberty and during pregnancy is currently not recommended. Although further investigation is necessary, the possible use of antioxidants to treat and prevent atherosclerosis may represent a component of future therapy.

HIGH DENSITY LIPOPROTEIN (HDL). In epidemiologic studies, elevations of HDL particles in the plasma are inversely related to the incidence of atherosclerosis and its sequelae. Elevated HDL cholesterol level is "protective" against ischemic heart disease; conversely, the individuals with abnormally low levels of HDL are at increased risk.

HDL has been postulated to participate in transferring cholesterol out of cells. Women generally have elevated HDL levels prior to menopause. If their HDL level is decreased in association with diabetes or obesity, they are at increased risk for ischemic heart disease. Regular strenuous exercise, decreased cigarette smoking, and diet rich in some fish oils (eicosapentaenoic acid) are associated with increased HDL levels, although the basis for the increase is poorly understood.

CIGARETTE SMOKING. Cigarette smoking is one of the most common risk factors associated with increased incidence of atherosclerosis, and when it is reduced or eliminated, the risk of developing the disease decreases. Stroke, myocardial infarction, and intermittent claudication are common in male cigarette smokers, who, together with female smokers, show an increased incidence of symptoms associated with atherosclerosis. In addition to atherosclerosis of the large coronary arteries, cigarette smokers characteristically have occlusive disease of the leg arteries. There is a mean increase of approximately 70% in the death rate and a three- to fivefold increase in the risk of ischemic heart disease in males who smoke more than one pack of cigarettes per day, compared with nonsmokers.

Sudden death is frequently associated with cigarette smoking, and it is particularly important to note that quitting smoking, within 1 year, reduces the risk of the sequelae of atherosclerosis to the levels of nonsmokers.

GLUCOSE INTOLERANCE AND DIABETES MELLITUS. Both insulin-dependent and non–insulin-dependent diabetics show at least a twofold increase in the incidence of myocardial infarction, compared with nondiabetics. Younger diabetics have a marked increase in the risk of atherosclerosis and thus of ischemic heart disease, and diabetic women appear to be even more prone than diabetic men. Gangrene of the lower extremities is one of the principal sequelae of atherosclerosis in diabetics. Diabetics form modified proteins termed *advanced glycosylation endproducts* (AGE's). LDL can be modified and AGE-LDL may play a role in atherogenesis similar to oxLDL.

HYPERTENSION. Elevated blood pressure is an important risk factor associated with increased incidence of atherosclerosis and is particularly important because this is a factor that is easily diagnosed and highly treatable. The risk of atherosclerosis and its sequelae increases progressively with increase in blood pressure, and when the blood pressure is > 160 mm Hg systolic and 95 mm Hg diastolic in middle-aged men the risk is five times greater than in normotensive men with blood pressure of 140 mm Hg systolic and 90 mm Hg diastolic or less. After age 50, hypertension may be more important as a risk factor in predicting increased incidence of atherosclerosis than hypercholesterolemia. Recent intervention studies of individuals with hypertension have demonstrated that reducing diastolic pressure levels below 105 mm Hg can significantly reduce the incidence of symptomatic cerebrovascular disease, ischemic heart disease, and congestive heart failure in men (see Ch. 37). When multiple risk factors are present, including hypertension, it is particularly important to treat the hypertension because it is the most easily accessible and treatable aspect of this disease process.

OBESITY. When body weight is > 20% above the norm, there is an increased risk of ischemic heart disease. Obesity may particularly accelerate atherosclerosis in individuals below age 50. Obesity is generally associated with hypertriglyceridemia, hypercholesterolemia, glucose intolerance, and hypertension.

PHYSICAL ACTIVITY (see Ch. 9.3). There are many studies related to the value of increased physical activity in reducing the incidence of ischemic heart disease. The Framingham Studies suggest that sedentary individuals are more susceptible to atherosclerosis and to sudden death than individuals who maintain an active lifestyle. It has been suggested that increased physical activity may elevate the level of HDL. Appropriately supervised physical training can improve exercise performance in patients with angina due to ischemic heart disease.

GENETIC FACTORS. Clearly, genetic factors are critical in atherosclerosis. The best example of this is the increased incidence of atherosclerosis in individuals with homozygous familial hypercholesterolemia and familial combined hyperlipidemia. Other risk factors, such as hypertension and diabetes mellitus, can also be inherited, and it is possible that protective factors, such as increased HDL, may also be inherited, although the latter is not well understood. As a consequence, family history must be included in assessing the risk for a given individual.

THE PATHOGENESIS OF THE LESIONS OF ATHEROSCLEROSIS

The lesions of atherosclerosis as they occur in the intima of the artery essentially consist of three biologic entities. First and foremost of these is an increase in the number of intimal smooth muscle cells, together with an accumulation of macrophages and variable numbers of lymphocytes. The increased number of smooth muscle cells is responsible for the second entity, the formation of large amounts of connective tissue matrix containing collagen, elastic fibers, and proteoglycans. The third entity, lipid, accumulates in hyperlipidemic individuals within the smooth muscle cells and the macrophages and in many instances causes them to develop into foam cells. Lipid also accumulates within the surrounding connective tissue matrix but may be absent from lesions of patients who are normocholesterolemic, subject to other risk factors. Thus the advanced lesions of atherosclerosis represent the culmination of a usually longstanding chronic inflammatory, proliferative disease process in which it becomes important to understand the basis for smooth muscle proliferation, macrophage accumulation, new connective tissue formation, and lipid accumulation.

THE RESPONSE TO INJURY HYPOTHESIS OF ATHEROSCLEROSIS. During the past 20 years, a hypothesis has been formulated, tested, and revised that takes into account most of what is known concerning risk factors, the biology of the artery wall, the cells involved, and the biologic processes that result in the lesions of atherosclerosis.

The response to injury hypothesis of atherosclerosis suggests that some form of "injury" affects the lining endothelial cells. The injury may alter the functional characteristics of the endothelium, leaving the endothelium morphologically intact. Thus endothelial injury could alter the permeability of the endothelium, its nonthrombogenic character, its ability to form vasoactive substances and growth factors, and its capacity to regenerate. At the other extreme, endothelial injury may lead to endothelial cell-cell disjunction and endothelial retraction, exposing the underlying connective tissue or accumulated foam cells, such as macrophages, that form the first and ubiquitous lesion of atherosclerosis, the fatty streak.

In hypercholesterolemic animals, including nonhuman primates, swine, rabbits, and rats, the first change that occurs in the artery wall is the formation of a series of adhesive cell surface glycoproteins of several classes including selectins, vascular cell adhesion molecules (VCAM's), and intercellular adhesion molecules (ICAM's). Consequently, circulating monocytes and lymphocytes increasingly adhere to the surface of the endothelial cells in clusters throughout the arterial tree. The adherent monocytes migrate on the surface of the endothelium, penetrate between endothelial junctions, localize subendothelially, accumulate lipid, and become intimal foam cells. The accumulation of these intimal lymphocytes and monocytes that become converted to lipid-laden macrophages represents the initial lesion of atherosclerosis, the fatty streak. These fatty streaks expand by continuing to attract and accumulate lymphocytes and monocytes in the artery. They also expand with some smooth muscle cells migrating from the underlying media into the intima, where they localize beneath the accumulated macrophages and also accumulate lipid.

With increasing time, level, and duration of hypercholesterolemia, endothelial cell-cell junctions separate and endothelial cells retract, permitting lipid-laden macrophages to enter the circulation and home to the spleen and lymph nodes. This occurs particularly at branches and bifurcations of the artery. Sometimes the exposed macrophages or connective tissue, or both, can be thrombogenic and induce platelets to adhere at these sites. Sites where mural thrombi have formed become loci of increased migration and proliferation of smooth muscle cells that accumulate and form large amounts of connective tissue matrix. Thus sites where platelets adhere and aggregate subsequently may become sites where intimal smooth muscle proliferates.

At other anatomic sites, the endothelium may remain intact, but the fatty streak expands by continuing to attract and accumulate monocytes. Many of the macrophages in the lesions also synthesize DNA and replicate, further aggravating the proliferative component of the lesions.

Numerous investigations have attempted to determine the factors responsible for the migration and proliferation of smooth muscle cells in the intima. Growth factors able to induce these actions can be formed and secreted by several cells. Particularly important is that platelets can release growth factors and activate macrophages to release the same as well as other types of growth factors. The growth factors that may play a critical role in atherogenesis include platelet-derived growth factor (PDGF), a potent growth factor for mesenchymal connective tissue cells such as fibroblasts and smooth muscle, and transforming growth factor beta (TGF-β), a factor that may act in an inhibitory fashion and can induce formation of large amounts of connective tissue.

PDGF is a potent mitogen that, at nanogram and picogram levels, can induce cells such as smooth muscle to multiply and TGF-β can induce them to form new connective tissue. PDGF and TGF-β can be derived from platelets, from activated macrophages which are probably the principal cellular source of PDGF, and from appropriately stimulated or "injured" endothelial cells. Thus, if endothelial injury occurs, appropriate opportunities may be present to release mitogens such as PDGF from all three cells. Such growth factor release may be related to increased incidence of atherogenesis in experimental animals. There is also evidence that smooth muscle cells, once they have been induced to proliferate in the artery wall, may themselves be able to express the gene for PDGF and secrete this growth factor so that they may, in effect, stimulate themselves in an autocrine fashion to continue proliferating.

The response to injury hypothesis of atherogenesis suggests that the "injury" to the endothelium results in cellular changes that lead to a modified form of inflammation in which monocytes and lymphocytes enter the artery wall and the monocytes become macrophages that can secrete growth factors, act as scavenger cells, and accumulate lipid and become foam cells. The fatty streak then becomes converted into a smooth muscle proliferative lesion, or fibrous plaque, and probably does so by locally releasing within the artery growth factors derived from activated macrophages, injured endothelium, and/or platelets that may interact with the artery wall at sites where the protective cover of the endothelium may be altered. These changes are diagrammatically shown in Figure 40–2, which suggests how the lesions of atherosclerosis may form.

The response to injury hypothesis also offers an opportunity to consider means of preventing lesions of atherosclerosis from forming. Clearly, altering lifestyle habits, including changing dietary habits and altering risk factors associated with increased incidence of atherosclerosis, could be potentially important in preventing these cellular changes from occurring and possibly in inducing lesion regression.

REGRESSION OF ATHEROSCLEROSIS. In experimental animals the fatty streak can clearly regress and disappear entirely if hypercholesterolemic animals are placed on a normocholesterolemic regimen for a sufficient time. Evidence suggests that fatty streaks can also regress in humans, based on examination of individuals who decreased their dietary intake of lipids and atherogenic foods. Fibrous plaques or complicated lesions in humans may also be partially reversible, based upon angiographic studies. It is not yet clear how far a lesion must progress before it becomes irreversible. Cessation of cigarette smoking is associated with decreased risk, and this in combination with treatment of hypertension, dietary intervention, treatment of diabetes mellitus, and removal, when possible, of other associated causes may be important in inducing regression

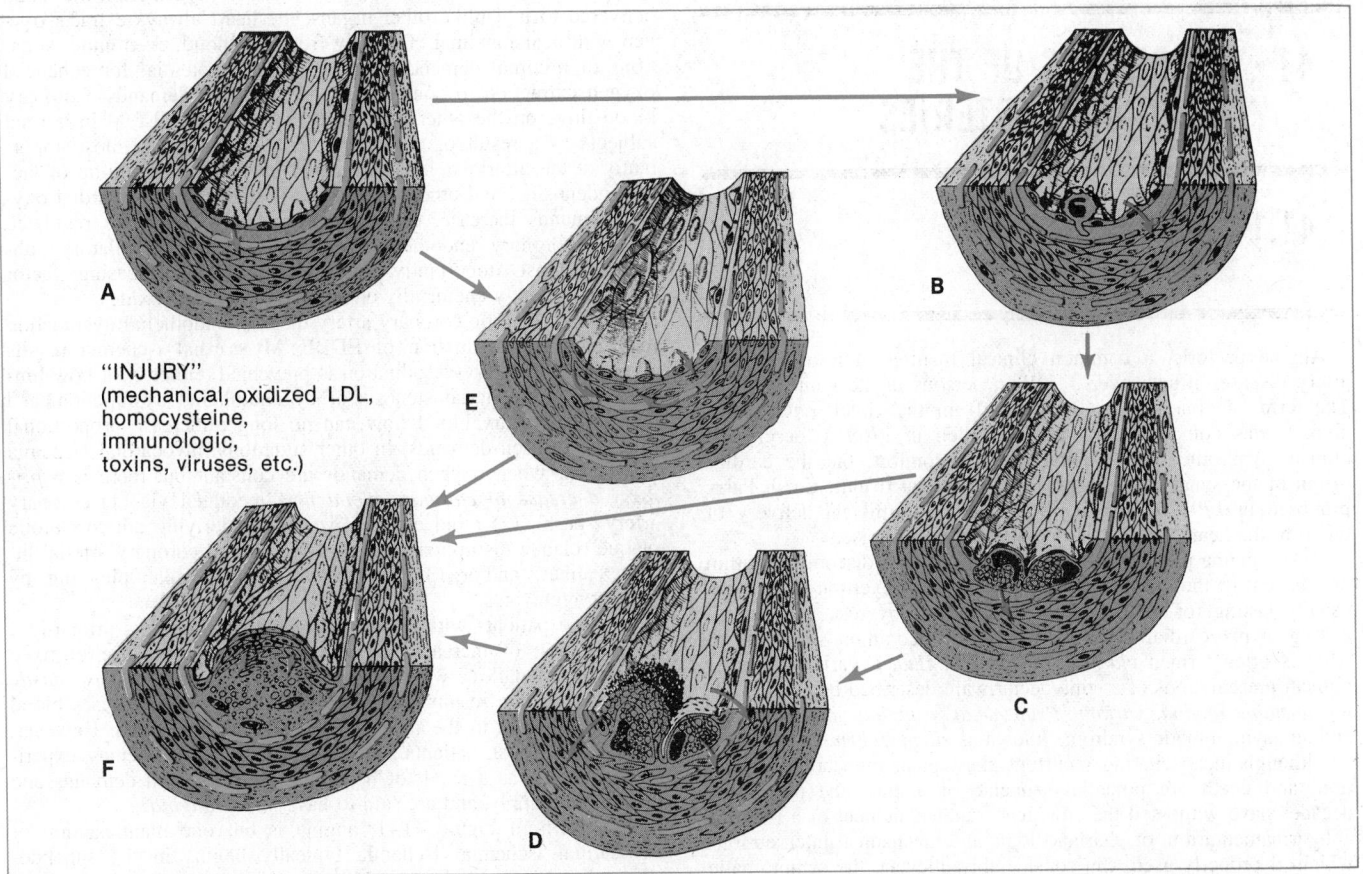

FIGURE 40-2. Endothelial injury: The response to injury hypothesis. Advanced intimal proliferative lesions of atherosclerosis may occur by at least two pathways. The pathway demonstrated by the clockwise *(long)* arrows to the right has been observed in experimentally induced hypercholesterolemia. Injury to the endothelium *(A)* may induce growth factor secretion *(short arrow)*. Monocytes attach to endothelium *(B)*, which may continue to secrete growth factors *(short arrow)*. Subendothelial migration of monocytes *(C)* may lead to fatty streak formation and release of growth factors such as platelet-derived growth factor (PDGF) *(short arrow)*. Fatty streaks may become directly converted to fibrous plaques *(long arrow from C to F)* by releasing growth factors from macrophages or endothelial cells or both. Macrophages may also stimulate and/or injure the overlying endothelium. In some cases, macrophages may lose their endothelial cover and platelet attachment may occur *(D)*, providing three possible sources of growth factors—platelets, macrophages, and endothelium *(short arrows)*. Some of the smooth muscle cells in the proliferative lesion itself *(F)* may form and secrete growth factors such as PDGF *(short arrows)*.

An alternative pathway for development of advanced lesions of atherosclerosis is shown by the arrows from *A* to *E* to *F*. In this case, the endothelium may be injured but remain intact. Increased endothelial turnover may result in growth factor formed by endothelial cells *(A)*. This may stimulate migration of smooth muscle cells from the media into the intima, accompanied by PDGF produced endogenously by smooth muscle as well as growth factor secreted from the "injured" endothelial cells *(E)*. These interactions could then lead to fibrous plaque formation and further lesion progression *(F)*. (From Ross R: The pathogenesis of atherosclerosis—an update. N Engl J Med 314:496, 1986. Copyright 1986, the Massachusetts Medical Society.)

of atherosclerotic lesions. More remains to be learned concerning this approach to reversing the disease process.

Prevention of atherosclerosis, rather than treatment, has to be the principal goal for all patients. Considering the association between hyperlipidemia and increased atherosclerosis, and recognizing the decline in the death rate in the United States from premature ischemic heart disease, it becomes increasingly important to understand that early detection of risk and approaches toward changing dietary habits and lifestyles are important for preventing atherosclerosis in individuals who may potentially be at increased risk. It is important to detect those who may be at increased risk on a familial basis, who may be hypertensive, who are cigarette smokers, or whose dietary habits could be altered to reduce their risk. Treating hypertension, as well as giving advice regarding diet, cigarette smoking, and exercise, can be valuable adjuncts to helping a patient deal with these problems. Pharmacologically treating hyperlipidemia should be limited to individuals whose plasma cholesterol is > 240 mg per deciliter or who do not respond adequately to dietary management. The long-term value of antiplatelet drugs and, potentially in the future, of drugs that may affect growth factor activity could be important for reducing the incidence of atherosclerosis and the long-term sequelae of this disease process.

Brown BG, Albers JJ, Fisher LD, et al.: Treatment study: A randomized trial demonstrating coronary disease regression and clinical benefit from lipid altering therapy among men with high apolipoprotein B. N Engl J Med 323:1289, 1990.

Fuster V, Badimon L, Badimon JJ, Chesebro JH: The pathogenesis of coronary artery disease and the acute coronary syndromes. N Engl J Med 326:242, 1992.

Gordon T, Castelli WP, Hjortland MC, et al.: Diabetes, blood lipids, and the role of obesity in coronary heart disease risk for women. The Framingham Study. Ann Intern Med 87:393, 1977.

Gordon T, Castelli WP, Hjortland MC, et al.: High density lipoprotein as a protective factor against coronary heart disease. The Framingham Study. Am J Med 62:707, 1977. *These two papers represent epidemiologic studies that relate the role of several of the principal risk factors to atherosclerosis and indicate the potential protective effect of HDL in atherosclerosis.*

Report of the Working Group of Arteriosclerosis of the National Heart, Lung, and Blood Institute. Vol. 2. Department of Health, Education and Welfare (National Institutes of Health) Publication No. 82–2035. Washington, DC, Government Printing Office, 1981. *An overview of a large number of individuals who have examined both the epidemiology and the nature of the lesions of atherosclerosis.*

Ross R: The pathogenesis of atherosclerosis: A perspective for the 1990s. Nature 362:801, 1993.

Ross R: The pathogenesis of atherosclerosis—an update. N Engl J Med 314:488, 1986.

Ross R, Glomset JA: The pathogenesis of atherosclerosis. N Engl J Med 295:369, 1976. *These two papers review the anatomic structure of the artery wall, lesions of atherosclerosis, and the potential roles of the cells in atherosclerosis. They provide a hypothesis for how atherogenesis may come about.*

Steinberg D: Metabolism of lipoproteins and their role in the pathogenesis of atherosclerosis. Atherosclerosis Rev 18:1, 1988.

41 DISORDERS OF THE CORONARY ARTERIES

41.1 Angina Pectoris
William J. Rogers

Angina pectoris, a common clinical manifestation of coronary artery disease, afflicts over 3 million persons in the United States. The term "angina pectoris," derived from the Greek *ankhein* (to choke), was coined by William Heberden in 1768 to describe a clinical syndrome of exertional chest discomfort, but the cardiac origin of the syndrome was not fully appreciated until Caleb Parry proposed in 1799 that angina was due to insufficient delivery of blood to the heart muscle, particularly during exercise.

Today angina pectoris is generally defined as a discomfort within or adjacent to the chest, typically provoked by exertion or anxiety, usually lasting for several minutes, alleviated by rest, and not resulting in myocardial necrosis. Besides this common syndrome of what is often termed *classic exertional angina,* a variety of other clinical presentations of angina pectoris are described below, including *unstable angina, variant (Printzmetal's) angina, mixed angina,* and an asymptomatic syndrome known as *silent ischemia.*

Although incapacitating recurrent chest pain, myocardial infarction, and death are potential sequelae of angina, the past three decades have witnessed the emergence and refinement of a remarkable armamentarium of pharmacologic and mechanical interventions which, if properly used, can considerably alleviate the symptomatic manifestations and extend the survival of most patients with this common condition.

PATHOPHYSIOLOGY AND CLASSIFICATION

Angina pectoris is a symptom of myocardial ischemia, occurring when the requirement for oxygen by either ventricle exceeds its supply (Fig. 41–1). The most common underlying disease is atherosclerotic coronary artery disease, although occasionally angina occurs secondary to other entities, such as hypertrophic cardiomyopathy, aortic stenosis, and coronary arteritis.

Myocardial oxygen demand is primarily determined by heart rate, contractility, and ventricular wall tension, a function of ventricular volume and intraventricular pressure. An increase in one or more of these determinants—as might occur with exercise, emotional stress, or other states of heightened adrenergic activity—triggers an increase in myocardial oxygen demand, and myocardial ischemia results unless myocardial oxygen supply rises proportionately.

Myocardial oxygen supply is governed by coronary blood flow and the ability of the myocardium to extract oxygen from the blood delivered to it. Unlike other organs, the heart always extracts oxygen with near maximal efficiency from the blood, even under situations of minimal demand, so there is little potential for enhanced oxygen extraction to counter increased oxygen demands. Coronary blood flow, on the other hand, can increase several-fold in normal subjects as a result of coronary arterial vasodilation, most importantly at the arteriolar level, triggered by the local build-up of lactate, adenosine, and other vasoactive substances as myocardial oxygen demands increase. Coronary arterial vasodilation is regulated by the coronary endothelium, which releases vasodilatory substances, most importantly endothelium-derived releasing factor (EDRF), recently chemically characterized as nitric oxide.

In atherosclerotic coronary artery disease, endothelial dysfunction may diminish production of EDRF. Myocardial ischemia results when autoregulatory vasodilation is prevented, either by a flow-limiting coronary arterial stenosis or by endothelial dysfunction, and therefore coronary blood flow can no longer increase proportional to rising oxygen demands. In other situations, myocardial ischemia may occur when oxygen demands are constant but there is a *primary decrease in coronary blood flow* mediated via (1) coronary artery spasm, (2) rapid evolution of the underlying atherosclerotic plaque (plaque disruption) leading to a reduced coronary arterial lumen caliber, and/or (3) intermittent microvascular plugging by platelet aggregates.

In some patients with *exertional angina,* ischemia is primarily a manifestation of increased oxygen demands in the face of fixed coronary blood flow, whereas in patients with primary *vasospastic angina,* ischemia results when coronary artery spasm causes blood flow to diminish in the face of stable oxygen demands. However, many, if not most, patients fall between these two extremes, experiencing angina as a result of both heightened oxygen demands and diminished supply, and are said to have *mixed angina.*

As shown in Figure 41–1, angina is but one manifestation of myocardial ischemia. Ischemia typically begins in the subendocardium, where wall tension is high and compressive forces limit coronary microvascular flow, and then spreads like a wavefront toward the epicardium. The electrocardiogram often depicts ST segment depression or T-wave inversion as manifestations of subendocardial ischemia but may show ST segment elevation (injury current) if ischemia is prolonged and extends transmurally. These electrocardiographic changes may occur without typical anginal symptoms, a condition termed *silent ischemia.*

Abnormalities in segmental left ventricular contraction occur in the region of the myocardium served by the coronary arterial branches distal to the stenosis responsible for the ischemia (the culprit lesion), and, if about 10% or more of the myocardium is rendered ischemic, reduced global function of the left ventricle may be detectable. In addition to abnormal systolic function during ischemia, increased diastolic stiffness of the left ventricle manifests by a rising left ventricular end-diastolic pressure and rising pulmonary venous pressure. Consequently, transient clinical evidence of left ventricular failure may occur during episodic ischemia and

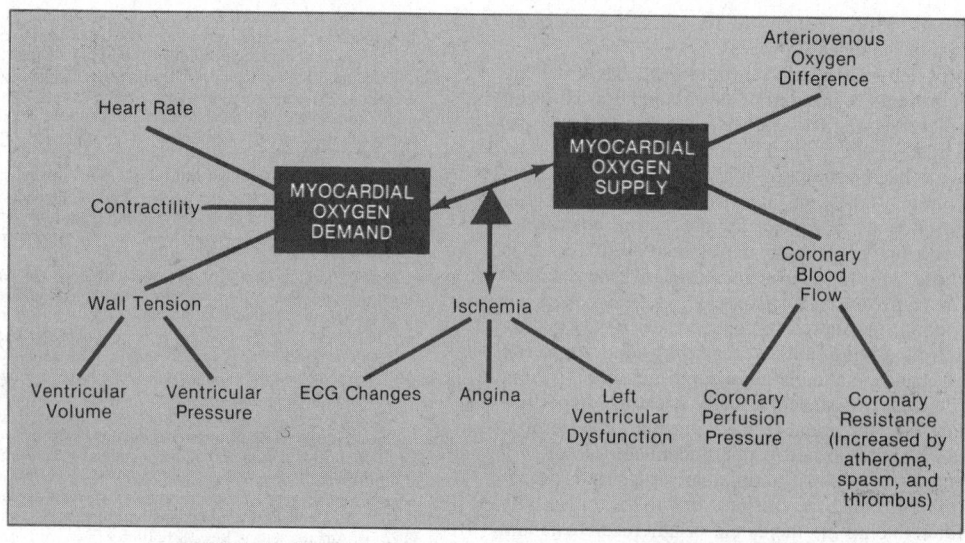

FIGURE 41–1. Ischemia occurs when oxygen demand exceeds supply.

may explain why many patients describe their angina not as pain but as a feeling of "breathlessness" or "chest tightness."

It is prognostically and clinically useful to classify anginal syndromes as stable or unstable. *Unstable angina* refers to angina of recent onset (within 2 months) or angina that has begun to intensify or to occur at rest or with a lower level of exertion within the previous 2 months. *Stable angina,* as the name implies, describes a relatively constant pattern of pain with regard to its severity and precipitating factors within the recent months. Some authorities classify angina of recent onset as "stable angina" if it is precipitated by moderate or severe levels of exertion and maintains a constant threshold over time, because "stable angina" has to begin at some point in time.

Of patients with unstable angina, up to 20% progress to acute myocardial infarction within the next 3 months. Coronary angiography and angioscopy reveal that >50% of patients with unstable angina have multivessel disease with eccentric, irregular, or ulcerated atherosclerotic lesions associated with endothelial disruption and adherent thrombus. Left main coronary artery disease occurs in about 10% of patients with unstable angina. It is likely that unstable angina represents a point on a continuum between stable exertional angina and acute myocardial infarction.

Variant angina, originally described by Printzmetal, is characterized by rest pain accompanied by transient ST segment changes (often ST elevation resembling acute myocardial infarction, although ST depression can also occur) and ventricular arrhythmias. Variant angina is a form of unstable angina caused by coronary arterial spasm, usually within a coronary artery narrowed by plaque, but occasionally within an angiographically normal appearing artery.

HISTORY AND PHYSICAL EXAMINATION

The diagnosis of angina pectoris often requires considerable clinical skill because there is no totally specific symptom, physical finding, or laboratory examination to confirm its presence. The history is probably the most powerful tool for diagnosing angina and provides the skilled interviewer an assessment of both the stability (or instability) of the syndrome as well as its severity (Table 41–1). The patient should be instructed to describe the chest discomfort according to its character, location, radiation, duration, precipitating and alleviating factors, accompanying symptoms, and change in pattern over the past few weeks or days.

As indicated above, the typical *history* is that of exertional chest discomfort of several minutes duration alleviated by rest. The discomfort typically involves the region of the sternum (substernal or, more properly, retrosternal location) but may instead manifest itself in any region between the jaw and epigastrium. Commonly the discomfort radiates to the shoulders or arms, especially the left, to the neck or jaw, and less commonly to the back or epigastrium. Most patients perceive angina as a deep or visceral (rather than superficial) sensation and describe it as a "tightness," "heaviness," or "choking sensation" rather than as a definite pain. The discomfort usually lasts several minutes; discomfort of <1 minute is rarely angina, and discomfort at full intensity >20 minutes should arouse

suspicion of myocardial infarction or discomfort unrelated to myocardial ischemia. The pain of unstable angina, however, may wax and wane repeatedly over several hours.

Typically angina is provoked by exertion, especially walking uphill, climbing stairs, vigorous arm work, coitus, or exercising in cold weather (when peripheral vascular resistance is greater). The discomfort may also be provoked by emotion (fear, anger, anxiety), may follow a meal, or may occur on lying down (angina decubitus) owing to increased ventricular filling pressure, or may occur during sleep (nocturnal angina), perhaps owing to increased adrenergic output related to dreams. Typically, exertional angina is relieved promptly (within 5 minutes) by rest; emotionally triggered angina may last longer; both usually are alleviated within 3 to 5 minutes with sublingual nitroglycerin. For patients with exertional angina, quantitation of the severity of the discomfort by a scale such as that of the Canadian Cardiovascular Society can be useful (Table 41–1).

During an episode of angina, *the physical examination* may be normal or may disclose one or more of the following: an increased heart rate and blood pressure; paradoxical splitting of the second heart sound; a precordial presystolic bulge or fourth heart sound (S_4), both due to enhanced atrial contraction into a ventricle rendered stiff by ischemia; a systolic bulge due to left ventricular dyskinesis; a diastolic bulge or S_3 gallop as evidence of significant left ventricular failure; a mid- to late systolic murmur of mitral regurgitation related to ischemia-induced mitral papillary muscle dysfunction; or transient rales or other evidence of pulmonary venous congestion.

Other conditions that should be considered in the *differential diagnosis* of angina include the following: gastrointestinal disease—especially disordered esophageal motility, gastroesophageal reflux, peptic ulcer disease, and cholecystitis; exertional bronchospasm related to asthmatic bronchitis; chest wall discomfort related to costochondritis, muscle spasm, herpes zoster, or anxiety states, the last often presenting as submammary sharp pain of a few seconds' duration; and other cardiac and vascular diseases such as pericarditis, myocardial infarction, aortic dissection, or pulmonary embolism. These should be readily distinguished from angina in most cases by a detailed history, physical examination, and appropriate laboratory tests.

LABORATORY EVALUATION

Certain laboratory studies may help establish a diagnosis of angina pectoris by confirming the presence and extent of underlying coronary artery disease.

ELECTROCARDIOGRAM (see Ch. 33.2). Although often normal at baseline, electrocardiogram (ECG) *during* an episode of spontaneous or provoked angina may demonstrate horizontal or downsloping depression of the ST segment, T-wave peaking or inversion, and, rarely, transient ST-segment elevation. Such ECG changes, when transitory and accompanied by typical anginal discomfort, make the diagnosis of myocardial ischemia with a high degree of confidence. However, taken alone, and occurring on the resting ECG, such ST and T wave changes are regarded as nonspecific because they accompany many other conditions including hyperventilation, electrolyte abnormalities, left ventricular hypertrophy, pericarditis, myocarditis, and the administration of digitalis and other drugs.

EXERCISE ECG. The exercise ECG or graded exercise test is a widely used clinical provocative test for myocardial ischemia in which the patient is required to exercise, usually on a treadmill or bicycle, at gradually increasing workloads until ischemic electrocardiographic changes, angina, or other limiting symptoms occur. With the increasing workload of progressive exercise, heart rate and systolic blood pressure should rise. The product of heart rate and systolic blood pressure (the double product) correlates with myocardial oxygen demand and defines an anginal threshold for a given subject. During exercise a clinically positive response is typical anginal chest discomfort, whereas an electrocardiographically positive response is a 0.1 mV horizontal or downsloping ST depression at 0.08 second after the J point of the ECG.

The sensitivity of the graded exercise test for diagnosing coronary artery disease ranges from 54 to 94% and is greatest in patients with the most extensive coronary artery disease. The speci-

TABLE 41–1. CANADIAN CARDIOVASCULAR CLASSIFICATION OF ANGINA SEVERITY

Class I	"Ordinary physical activity does not cause . . . angina, such as walking and climbing stairs. Angina with strenuous or rapid or prolonged exertion at work or recreation."
Class II	"Slight limitation of ordinary activity. Walking or climbing stairs rapidly, walking uphill, walking or stair climbing after meals, or in cold, or in wind, or under emotional stress, or only during the few hours after awakening. Walking more than two blocks on the level and climbing more than one flight of ordinary stairs at a normal pace and in normal conditions."
Class III	"Marked limitation of ordinary physical activity. Walking one to two blocks on the level and climbing one flight of stairs in normal conditions and at normal pace."
Class IV	"Inability to carry on any physical activity without discomfort—anginal syndrome *may be* present at rest."

From Campeau L: Grading of angina pectoris. Circulation 54:522, 1976. Reproduced by permission of the American Heart Association, Inc.

ficity (negative test when coronary disease is absent) ranges from 67 to 97%. False-positive tests are *more common* when the test is used in patients with a low probability of coronary disease (as for example, with the screening of asymptomatic subjects), and false-positive exercise tests are *least common* in patients with a history of typical exertional angina.

Exercise testing is useful not only for diagnosing the presence of obstructive coronary artery disease but also for following the natural course of the disease in patients with chronic stable angina, detecting high-risk coronary artery disease, and estimating prognosis. Left main or multivessel coronary artery disease is suggested by exercise-induced hypotension, by 3.0 mm or more ST-segment depression, by downsloping ST segments, and by ischemic ST depression occurring within the first 3 minutes of exercise and/or persisting 5 or more minutes after exercise. A good prognosis is suggested by a negative exercise test or one that becomes positive only after the patient has exercised for more than three stages (> 9 minutes), or to a heart rate exceeding 160 beats per minute.

Exercise testing is generally safe; experienced laboratories report a mortality of about 1 per 10,000 tests and a morbidity requiring hospitalization of 2.4 per 10,000. Exercise testing should not be performed in patients with significant aortic stenosis, hypertension, congestive heart failure, or unstable angina, and, when exercise testing is performed, resuscitative equipment should be immediately available.

RADIONUCLIDE STUDIES. To enhance the sensitivity and specificity of exercise testing for detection of myocardial ischemia, either myocardial perfusion imaging (with thallium-201 or technetium-99m sestamibi) or serial assessment of left ventricular function by the "first pass" or "multiple gated" ("MUGA") approach can be used (see Ch. 33.4). For patients unable to exercise, pharmacologic stress with intravenous dipyridamole, adenosine, or dobutamine may be combined with thallium imaging. The radionuclide tests may localize the ischemic myocardial zone and are generally not influenced by factors that alter interpretation of the baseline ECG such as ST-T wave changes. However, compared with the conventional exercise test, the radionuclide studies are expensive and are not routinely required. Perfusion scintigraphy or radionuclide assessment of left ventricular function during exercise can, however, be useful in interpreting the physiologic significance of angiographically proven coronary lesions, in assessing equivocal or suspected false-positive conventional exercise tests, in evaluating patients with chest pain following coronary revascularization surgery or angioplasty, and in screening for residual ischemia in patients following myocardial infarction.

STRESS ECHOCARDIOGRAPHY. Echocardiographic imaging may be used in conjunction with exercise stress to detect regional left ventricular wall motion abnormalities secondary to ischemia. Pharmacologic stress echocardiography, particularly with intravenous dobutamine, is currently advocated as an alternative to imaging with thallium-201.

CORONARY ARTERIOGRAPHY. Coronary arteriography, selectively visualizing the major epicardial coronary arteries by radiographic contrast material, is the most precise means currently available to document the presence and extent of obstructive coronary artery disease. The results of coronary arteriography coupled with assessment of left ventricular systolic function (ejection fraction) provides powerful prognostic information concerning the natural history of coronary artery disease and, along with the clinical evaluation, can suggest the need for coronary artery revascularization by angioplasty or bypass graft surgery.

Coronary arteriography is indicated in patients with angina whose symptoms are severe (class III to IV) or unstable, in patients with angina or other evidence of myocardial ischemia following myocardial infarction, and in many patients with recurrent chest pain of uncertain cause. Coronary arteriography is also often performed in certain categories of patients in whom angina may or may not be present, for example, those over age 40 about to undergo cardiac valve replacement or other noncoronary cardiac surgery, those with refractory ventricular arrhythmias, survivors of out-of-hospital cardiac arrest, those with heart failure thought secondary to coronary artery disease, and those with convincing electrocardiographic evidence of extensive ischemia, either during exercise testing or during electrocardiographic monitoring at rest or during normal daily activities.

Coronary artery stenoses of ≥ 70% diameter narrowing are generally considered flow limiting and thus clinically significant; however, coronary stenoses may be considerably underestimated on arteriography. If the coronary arteriograms are normal, the smooth muscle constrictor, ergonovine maleate, may be carefully administered intravenously in an attempt to evoke angiographic and electrocardiographic evidence of localized coronary arterial spasm in patients suspected of having coronary vasospasm.

The risks of coronary arteriography are low and are related to the skill and experience of the operator and to the severity of the patient's cardiac disease; complications are increased in patients with severe left main coronary artery disease and in those with severe left ventricular dysfunction. Experienced operators report procedural mortality in 0.2%, myocardial infarction in 0.25%, embolization in 0.1%, and severe vascular complication at the entry site in 0.7%.

GENERAL MANAGEMENT

Patients diagnosed with angina pectoris should be counseled concerning the potential serious and unpredictable nature of the condition but also advised that powerful new pharmacologic and mechanical interventions are available that may ameliorate symptoms and, in many cases, extend survival. Patients with unstable angina should be admitted to the hospital to rule out myocardial infarction, to receive intensive pharmacologic therapy, and, in most cases, to undergo coronary arteriography. All patients with angina should be thoroughly instructed in how to modify risk factors, particularly managing intake of dietary cholesterol and saturated fat, quitting smoking and controlling blood pressure. A search should be made for potentially correctable conditions such as aortic stenosis, severe anemia, thyrotoxicosis, and tachyarrhythmias that might be contributing to the myocardial oxygen supply/demand imbalance causing angina.

PHARMACOLOGIC THERAPY

The goals of pharmalogically treating angina pectoris are to rectify the imbalance between myocardial oxygen demand and supply by reducing oxygen demands, increasing coronary blood flow, or both. The most important categories of antianginal drugs are the nitrates, β-blockers, and calcium channel blockers. Additionally, patients with unstable angina benefit from heparin and aspirin.

NITRATES. When taken up by vascular smooth muscle, nitrates are thought to be converted to nitric oxide, the substance believed to be EDRF. Thus, administering nitrates may compensate for inadequate production of nitric oxide in patients with endothelial dysfunction due to coronary atherosclerosis or other causes.

Nitrates alleviate angina predominantly by reducing oxygen demands, but they also improve coronary blood flow and may oppose platelet aggregation and adhesion. Nitrates reduce oxygen demands by relaxing vascular smooth muscle, producing venodilation at low dosages but arterial and arteriolar dilation as well at higher dosages. Their major effect at usual dosages is peripheral venous pooling, which diminishes systemic venous return, thus reducing left ventricular end-diastolic pressure and volume, left ventricular wall tension, and myocardial oxygen demands. To a lesser extent, the diminished peripheral arteriolar resistance lessens myocardial oxygen demands by reducing systemic blood pressure and left ventricular wall tension. Unfortunately, the fall in systemic blood pressure may trigger a slight rise in heart rate which augments oxygen demands. Nitrates may also improve coronary blood flow by dilating coronary vessels, reversing or preventing coronary spasm, and enhancing collateral blood flow. Furthermore, the effect on lowering left ventricular end-diastolic pressure, noted above, may allow better perfusion of subendocardial tissue.

The most commonly used nitrate preparations are nitroglycerin and isosorbide dinitrate. Nitroglycerin is available in a variety of formulations (Table 41–2), each with different onset and duration of action. For an acute anginal attack, one of the rapidly acting preparations such as sublingual nitroglycerin is preferable, whereas for chronic prophylaxis of angina a longer-acting nitroglycerin formulation such as isosorbide dinitrate is helpful. Failure to respond to long-acting nitrates may occur if inadequate doses are used; however, to minimize adverse reactions, these preparations should

TABLE 41-2. AVAILABLE DOSAGE FORMS OF NITROGLYCERIN, ISOSORBIDE DINITRATE, AND ISOSORBIDE MONONITRATE

Medication	Dosage Form	Recommended Dosage	Onset of Action (min)	Antianginal Duration
Nitroglycerin	Intravenous	Start at 10–20 μg/min	Immediate	Transient
	Aerosol spray	0.4 mg prn	2	10–30 min
	Sublingual	0.3–0.8 mg prn	2–5	10–30 min
	Oral sustained release*	2.6–6.5 mg t.i.d.	15–45	2–6 h
	Topical ointment, 2%*	1.2–5.0 cm q6–8h	15–60	3–8 h
	Transdermal disc or patch*	10–30 mg/24 h	30–60	Up to 24 h
Isosorbide dinitrate	Sublingual	5–10 mg q3h	5–20	45–120 min
	Oral	10–40 mg q6h	15–45	2–6 h
	Oral sustained release*	40–80 mg b.i.d.	15–45	Up to 8 h
Isosorbide mononitrate	Oral sustained release*	20 mg b.i.d.	20–60	Up to 10 h

*A daily "nitrate-free" interval of 12 to 15 hours is recommended for sustained-release preparations to prevent nitrate tolerance.

be initiated at low doses and then titrated upward until the desired clinical response or limiting side effects occur. Intravenous nitroglycerin is useful to treat unstable angina in hospitalized patients. The drug is usually begun at doses of 10 to 20 μg per minute and titrated upward by dosage increments of 10 to 20 μg at intervals of 10 to 15 minutes until chest pain is controlled or limiting side effects, such as hypotension, occur. Once pain is stabilized with intravenous nitroglycerin, one can usually substitute one of the long-acting preparations.

Adverse reactions to administering nitrates include cutaneous flushing, headaches, postural dizziness, nausea, and vomiting. Attenuation or resolution of these side effects usually occurs with continued administration of the drug. Nitrate tolerance or hyporesponsiveness has been noted with preparations providing constant plasma levels over many hours. It is believed that nitrate tolerance can be prevented by using the smallest effective dose of nitrate, by using less frequent dosing, and by allowing a nitrate-free interval of 12 to 15 hours daily. For example, sustained-release isosorbide dinitrate produces less tolerance when administered at 8:00 A.M. and 2:00 P.M. than when given at 8:00 A.M. and 8:00 P.M.; furthermore, nitroglycerin patches are more apt to retain effectiveness if there is an overnight patch-free interval.

BETA-BLOCKERS. β-Adrenergic blockers alleviate angina predominantly by reducing oxygen demand. These drugs competitively inhibit the action of catecholamines on β receptors throughout the body. By blocking the β_1 or cardiac β receptor, these agents lower heart rate, blood pressure, and myocardial contractility, three major determinants of myocardial oxygen utilization, and thus attenuate the rise in oxygen consumption normally occurring during exercise. By slowing the heart rate, β-blockers also prolong diastole, allowing more time for diastolic coronary perfusion to occur, thus indirectly augmenting coronary flow.

Four β-blockers are currently available (Table 41-3) in the United States to treat angina. The available agents differ according to various pharmacologic properties, and these differences may favor the use of one agent over another in certain clinical situations.

For example, cardioselectivity, a feature of some β-blockers, permits selective blockade of the cardiac β_1 receptor and is potentially advantageous in patients with reactive airways disease who depend upon chronic β_2 stimulation. Selectivity is lost, however, as the dose of the cardioselective β-blockers is increased; furthermore, patients with true asthma rarely tolerate β-blockade, regardless of the agent used. β-blockers with predominantly renal clearance tend to

have longer half-lives, allowing once-daily dosing and, theoretically, better patient compliance. The ultrashort-acting intravenous β-blocker esmolol (currently approved only for treating supraventricular tachycardia) may be useful in patients with unstable angina when rapid onset of action is desired and rapid reversal would be advantageous should adverse hemodynamic effects occur.

β-blockers are generally administered orally in small doses and titrated upward at 1- to 2-day intervals until clinical benefit is observed, an adverse reaction occurs, or some physiologic marker of β-blockade is noted, such as a slowing of the resting heart rate to 50 to 60 beats per minute. Side effects include bradycardia, hypotension, atrioventricular (AV) block, heart failure, and central nervous system complaints (fatigue, depression, nightmares). β-blockers are, of course, contraindicated in patients already having any of those findings. β-blockers may contribute to lack of recognition of hypoglycemia and are thus relatively contraindicated in patients with brittle diabetes. Discontinuing β-blocker therapy should be done by gradual tapering because rebound unstable angina and myocardial infarction may occur with sudden cessation.

CALCIUM CHANNEL BLOCKERS. Calcium channel blockers alleviate angina by reducing myocardial oxygen demands as well as by increasing coronary blood flow. Calcium channel blockers limit the uptake of calcium by vascular smooth muscle and cardiac muscle required for excitation-contraction coupling and thereby produce systemic arteriolar dilation, systemic venodilation, and reduced inotropism, all of which reduce myocardial oxygen demands. Furthermore, coronary arteries are dilated and spasm is opposed, thus enhancing myocardial oxygen delivery.

The available calcium channel blockers are considerably dissimilar in chemical structure and adverse clinical actions (Table 41-4). Verapamil and diltiazem reduce sinus node automaticity, decrease atrioventricular conduction, and thus often slow the resting heart rate. Nicardipine and nifedipine, on the other hand, are potent arterial dilators, often causing mild hypotension and reflex sinus tachycardia. With the possible exception of amlodipine, calcium channel blockers should be used with caution in patients with significantly impaired systolic left ventricular dysfunction (ejection fraction < 30%) and discontinued if heart failure worsens. Mild peripheral edema is common with nicardipine and nifedipine, constipation is common with verapamil, and atrioventricular block may occur in response to verapamil or diltiazem, especially with concomitant β-blocker use and in patients with baseline conduction abnormalities. Serum digoxin levels may rise when introducing a calcium channel

TABLE 41-3. β BLOCKERS AVAILABLE IN THE UNITED STATES TO TREAT ANGINA

Medication	Cardio-selective	ISA*	Primary Clearance	Half-Life (hrs)	Usual Dosage
Atenolol	Yes	No	Renal	6–9	50–100 mg q.d.
Metoprolol sustained release	Yes	No	Hepatic	3–7	50–100 mg b.i.d. 100–200 mg q.d.
Nadolol	No	No	Renal	20–24	40–80 mg q.d.
Propranolol sustained release	No	No	Hepatic	4 10	40–80 mg b.i.d.–q.i.d. 80–320 mg q.d.

*ISA = Intrinsic sympathomimetic activity

TABLE 41-4. CALCIUM CHANNEL BLOCKERS AVAILABLE IN THE UNITED STATES TO TREAT ANGINA

Medication	Initial Dosage	Unique Adverse Reactions*			
		Resting Heart Rate	AV Block	Edema	Constipation
Amlodipine	5 mg q.d.	Unchanged	No	++	No
Bepridil†	200 mg q.d.	Unchanged	No	No	No
Diltiazem	30 mg q.i.d.	Decreased	++	+	No
sustained release	60 mg b.i.d.‡				
	180 mg q.d.‡				
Nicardipine	20 mg t.i.d.	Increased	No	+++	No
Nifedipine	10 mg t.i.d.	Increased	No	+++	No
sustained release	30 mg q.d.				
Verapamil	80 mg t.i.d.	Decreased	+++	+	Yes
sustained release	180 or 240 mg q.d.‡				

* All calcium channel blockers can cause hypotension, and all but amlodipine are known to exacerbate heart failure.
† Bepridil causes electrocardiographic QT and QTc prolongation, may rarely cause torsades and agranulocytosis, and is therefore recommended for use only as a last resort.
‡ Initial dosage recommended to treat hypertension.

blocker, especially verapamil. Bepridil prolongs the QTc interval, may in rare instances cause torsades or agranulocytosis, and is therefore reserved for patients inadequately controlled with conventional therapy.

Calcium channel blockers particularly benefit patients with vasospastic or mixed angina but are also effective in those having exertional angina. Therapy is generally begun with the doses shown in Table 41–4 and gradually advanced over 2- to 3-day intervals until symptoms or other evidence of ischemia improves or until a limiting adverse reaction occurs.

COMBINATION THERAPY AND CHOICE OF AGENT. The antianginal therapy preferred in a given clinical situation may be dictated by the type of anginal presentation and by concomitant medical conditions (Table 41–5). Therapy is usually begun with sublingual nitroglycerin to treat acute anginal attacks and a sustained release nitrate preparation for anginal prophylaxis, owing to the relatively low cost and reasonably few side effects with these agents. In most patients, angina is incompletely controlled with nitrates alone; a second drug is necessary. For patients having exertional angina, β-blockers may be combined with nitrates and often prove synergistic; i.e., β-blockers prevent the nitrate-induced reflex tachycardia while the vasodilating action of nitrates reduces the tendency of β-blockers to precipitate heart failure. For patients suspected of having vasospastic or mixed angina, a combination of nitrates and a calcium channel blocker is often effective. For patients having recurrent angina despite two-drug therapy, a third drug

TABLE 41-5. CHOICE OF ANTIANGINAL THERAPY

Situation	Choice of Therapy*
Type of anginal presentation	
Stable exertional angina	N, BB, CaB
Unstable angina†	N, BB, CaB
Vasospastic angina	N, CaB
Asymptomatic (silent) myocardial ischemia	BB, CaB, N
Concomitant conditions in patient with angina	
Hypertension	BB, CaB
Diabetes	N, CaB
Heart failure	N, BB,‡ CaB‡
AV block	N, CaB (other than diltiazem or verapamil)
COPD, peripheral vascular disease	N, CaB, cardioselective BB‡
Bradyarrhythmias	N, CaB (other than diltiazem or verapamil)
Tachyarrhythmias	BB, diltiazem or verapamil
Recent myocardial infarction	BB, ASA

* Drug of first choice for monotherapy is listed first. Combination therapy may also be used in most instances.
† Intravenous heparin and aspirin are also useful adjuncts in unstable angina.
‡ Use with caution in this situation.
Abbreviations: BB = β blocker; CaB = calcium channel blocker; N = nitrate; AV = atrioventricular; COPD = chronic obstructive pulmonary disease.

(triple therapy) is often added. For patients with persistent symptoms, attention should be directed toward maximizing the dose of each agent while considering the feasibility of mechanical revascularization.

ANTIPLATELET AND ANTITHROMBIN THERAPY. With the recognition that intracoronary thrombus is often present in patients with unstable angina has come the demonstration that both aspirin and heparin reduce the incidence of myocardial infarction and death in patients with unstable angina. Low doses of aspirin also reduce the frequency of myocardial infarction and death in patients with stable angina. Therefore, patients with stable angina should be maintained on 81 mg aspirin daily, and patients with unstable angina should be given 325 mg aspirin daily. Hospitalized unstable angina patients should be treated with intravenous heparin with or without concomitant aspirin. For patients with unstable angina intolerant to aspirin, ticlopidine (currently approved for stroke prophylaxis) may be substituted. Thrombolytic therapy has not been found to be effective in improving the outcome of patients with unstable angina.

CORONARY REVASCULARIZATION

Pharmacologic therapy, when used aggressively, can control the symptoms of angina in many patients and return them to a normal or nearly normal lifestyle. However, many physicians and patients elect to proceed with mechanical interventions for improving coronary blood flow—coronary artery bypass surgery or percutaneous transluminal coronary angioplasty. These procedures are each being performed in more than 250,000 patients annually in the United States.

Coronary artery bypass surgery, popularized as a treatment for ischemic heart disease approximately 25 years ago, consists of anastomosing a reversed segment of saphenous vein between the ascending aorta and one or more stenotic coronary arteries. The procedure carries an operative mortality of approximately 1 to 3%, higher in patients with disease of the left main coronary artery, with significant left ventricular dysfunction, older than 65, and with prior bypass surgery. Perioperative myocardial infarction occurs in 2.5 to 10% of the patients. About 10% of the grafts occlude within the first year postoperatively, 2% occlude per year during the next 6 years, and 5% occlude per year over the next 5 years. Owing to graft occlusion and progression of coronary artery disease in native vessels, angina recurs in 2 to 4% of patients each year postoperatively. Recently, following the demonstration of lower rates of graft occlusion (1% per year or less), internal mammary arteries rather than free saphenous vein grafts have been used as conduits, especially for left anterior descending artery revascularization.

Percutaneous transluminal coronary angioplasty was introduced by Gruentzig in 1979, primarily to treat isolated, discrete, noncalcified, proximal stenoses in patients with single-vessel disease. As equipment has improved and operator experience has grown, the range of coronary artery lesions approachable by balloon angioplasty has expanded to encompass almost the entire spectrum formerly managed by bypass surgery. Currently, the only categories of patients having coronary artery disease in whom angioplasty is contraindicated are those with minimal coronary narrowing (no lesion of 60% or greater diameter stenosis), left main stenoses, and severe diffuse multivessel disease. Angioplasty should not be performed unless in-hospital cardiovascular surgery backup is available.

Elective angioplasty is successful initially in approximately 90% of patients; failures are due primarily to inability to cross the lesion with the balloon catheter or to abrupt reclosure of the vessel by dissection or thrombus following dilation. Procedure-related complications of elective angioplasty are as follows: death, 1%; myocardial infarction, 4 to 5%; emergency bypass surgery, 4 to 5%. Complications are higher with emergency procedures, with multivessel disease, or when angioplasty is performed on complex (eccentric, angulated, or long) atherosclerotic lesions. A major limitation of coronary angioplasty is restenosis of the dilated artery in 25 to 30% of patients, usually occurring within the first 6 months following angioplasty and usually amenable to repeat angioplasty. Intracoronary stenting has been recently shown to reduce restenosis. Other interventional technology, including mechanical atherectomy and laser angioplasty, have not yet substantially reduced the frequency of restenosis but have proven to be useful adjuncts to conventional balloon angioplasty.

Patients undergoing balloon angioplasty have much shorter hospitalizations than those undergoing bypass surgery and are probably more likely to return to normal life. The long-term role of angioplasty compared with bypass surgery for patients with multivessel disease is the subject of several ongoing randomized clinical trials. Initial results of the trials suggest that, after 2 to 3 years follow-up, death and myocardial infarction occur at similar frequencies with either procedure, but recurrence of angina and repeat coronary arteriography and repeat revascularization are more common in patients initially managed with angioplasty.

Revascularization with either angioplasty or bypass surgery is unequivocally indicated under two circumstances: (1) to alleviate incapacitating angina when medications have failed, and (2) to improve survival in certain patient subsets. Bypass surgery has been shown to improve longevity compared with continued medical therapy in patients with > 50% stenosis of the left main coronary artery, in those with three-vessel coronary artery disease and abnormal ventricular function (ejection fraction between about 30 and 50%), in those with multivessel disease with proximal left anterior descending artery involvement, and in those with residual ischemia (spontaneous or exercise-provoked) following myocardial infarction. Continued medical therapy rather than mechanical revascularization is recommended for patients with minimally obstructive (< 60% diameter stenosis) coronary artery disease, especially if coronary artery spasm is suspected; for patients with chest pain atypical for angina and lacking confirmation of ischemia by objective testing; for patients without left main disease who have normal ejection fraction and good symptomatic response to antianginal therapy; for patients with left main coronary artery stenoses < 50%; for patients with prior bypass surgery and chest pain but without objective evidence of ischemia; for patients with severe left ventricular dysfunction (ejection fraction < 20%) whose primary limitation is heart failure rather than myocardial ischemia; and for elderly patients (> 75 years) who have coronary disease but lack disabling angina.

Haynes RB, Sandler RS, Larson EB, et al.: A critical appraisal of ticlopidine, a new antiplatelet agent. Arch Intern Med 152:1376, 1992. *Review of recent randomized trials of the new antiplatelet agent ticlopidine, shown to reduce vascular death and nonfatal myocardial infarction in patients with unstable angina.*

Julian DB (ed.): Angina Pectoris. New York, Churchill Livingstone, 1985. *An exhaustive discussion of the historical background, epidemiology, prognosis, hemodynamics, clinical classification, physical examination, laboratory findings, and medical and surgical management of angina pectoris.*

Juul-Moller S, Edvardsson N, Jahnmatz B, et al.: Double-blind trial of aspirin in primary prevention of myocardial infarction in patients with stable chronic angina pectoris. The Swedish Angina Pectoris Aspirin Trial (SAPAT) Group. Lancet 340:1421, 1992. *Randomized clinical trial demonstrating that routine, low-dose aspirin in patients with stable angina reduced the incidence of sudden death and myocardial infarction at 50 months follow-up by 34%.*

Lubsen J: Medical management of unstable angina. What have we learned from the randomized trials? Circulation 82 (Suppl II): 82, 1990. *Clinical trials suggest that β blockers should be used before considering calcium channel blockers in unstable angina.*

Parisi AE, Folland ED, Hartigan P, on behalf of the Veterans Affairs ACME Investigators: A comparison of angioplasty with medical therapy in the treatment of single-vessel coronary artery disease. N Engl J Med 326:10, 1992. *Patients with single-vessel coronary artery disease and exercise-induced myocardial ischemia randomized to coronary angioplasty rather than medical therapy had less angina and better exercise tolerance 6 months later.*

RITA Trial Participants: Coronary angioplasty versus coronary artery bypass surgery: The Randomised Intervention Treatment of Angina (RITA) trial. Lancet 341:573, 1993. *RITA, one of several clinical trials comparing coronary angioplasty with bypass surgery, demonstrated after 2 years follow-up no significant difference in risk of death or myocardial infarction with the two treatments, but less angina, less repeat coronary arteriography, and less repeat coronary revascularization procedures in the bypass surgery group.*

Theroux P, Waters D, Qiu S, et al.: Aspirin versus heparin to prevent myocardial infarction during the acute phase of unstable angina. Circulation 88:2045, 1993. *In patients with unstable angina, both aspirin and heparin prevent myocardial infarction, but heparin is more efficient in doing so.*

The TIMI IIIB Investigators: Effects of tissue plasminogen activator and a comparison of early invasive and conservative strategies in unstable angina and non–Q-wave myocardial infarction: Results of the TIMI III B Trial. Circulation 89:1545, 1994. *Randomized clinical trial showing no benefit from thrombolytic therapy in patients with unstable angina. The trial also assessed the need for routine coronary arteriography and revascularization in patients who stabilized during hospitalization and concluded that such invasive management was a feasible option but not mandatory.*

van Rugge FP, van der Wall EE, Bruschke AVG: New developments in pharmacologic stress imaging. Am Heart J 124:468, 1992. *A comprehensive discussion of the use of dipyridamole, adenosine, and dobutamine in conjunction with radionuclide imaging, echocardiography, and magnetic resonance imaging.*

Weiner DA, Frishman WH (eds.): Therapy of Angina Pectoris. A Comprehensive Guide for the Clinician. New York, Marcel Dekker, 1985. *An extensive description of the pathophysiology, clinical evaluation, and pharmacologic and mechanical therapy of angina pectoris.*

Willard JE, Lange RA, Hillis LD: The use of aspirin in ischemic heart disease. N Engl J Med 327:175, 1992. *Excellent review of the mechanism of action and benefits of aspirin in stable and unstable ischemic heart disease.*

41.2 Acute Myocardial Infarction
Burton E. Sobel

DEFINITIONS AND HISTORICAL CONSIDERATIONS.
Literally, acute myocardial infarction is a focus of necrosis resulting from inadequate perfusion of the tissue. What is generally implied by the term, however, is the clinical syndrome resulting from such ischemia and manifested by sudden cardiac death; "typical" signs and symptoms of infarction such as crushing chest pain and diaphoresis, malignant ventricular arrhythmia, and congestive heart failure or shock; or atypical presentations that can be clinically silent or subtle with new-onset or accelerated angina, atypical chest pain mimicking "indigestion," impaired cerebral perfusion with syncope or signs simulating those of a cerebrovascular accident or psychosis. Coronary thrombosis was recognized as a potential cause as early as 1910 in Obrastzow and Straschesko's report of coronary thrombosis with "status anginous" and respiratory embarrassment, and in 1912 by Herrick, who described clinical features typical of sudden coronary occlusion. Although the diminishing perfusion has not been questioned, the contribution of thrombotic occlusion with severe atherosclerosis as a primary phenomenon rather than an epiphenomenon was resolved only recently. Its pivotal role was established unequivocally by early angiographic study of afflicted patients. Early catastrophic complications of infarction include ventricular fibrillation, rupture of the ventricular free wall, ventricular septal rupture (with shock and left-to-right shunting), or papillary muscle rupture (with profound mitral or tricuspid regurgitation). Later complications include ventricular mural thrombus with peripheral embolization and cerebrovascular accident, congestive heart failure with or without ventricular true or pseudoaneurysm, ventricular dilatation and infarct expansion, and sudden cardiac death. Progression of underlying coronary artery disease in survivors or acute myocardial infarction may result in unstable angina pectoris, "silent ischemia" (with electrocardiographic [ECG] changes without symptoms), recurrent infarction, or sudden death.

INCIDENCE AND ETIOLOGY

INCIDENCE. Heart disease, the leading cause of death in the United States, accounts for 25% of all adult deaths, most of which are attributable to acute myocardial infarction. Age-adjusted death rates for infarction have declined dramatically, however, since 1950 (from > 300 per 100,000 population to slightly < 200). Nevertheless, because of population growth, the total number of infarct-related deaths in the United States has not declined, and heart disease remains responsible for more years of potential life lost before age 65, regardless of gender or race, than any other illness.

Infarction accounts for 750,000 hospital admissions in the United States annually. Diagnosed coronary disease is present in as many as 7 million Americans and kills > 500,000 annually. Sudden death, precluding hospitalization, occurs in more than 350,000. Even among those who die after the prehospital phase, death is most often sudden. The impressive decline in age-adjusted death rates attributable to acute myocardial infarction over the past 25 years, a decrease of as much as 47% according to some estimates, probably reflects a decreased incidence and severity of coronary atherosclerosis antedating the recent intense interest in diet, fitness, and smoking cessation. It may reflect in part early and aggressive treatment of predisposing conditions such as hypertension, widespread use of β-adrenergic blockers in patients with angina, the benefits of community-based CPR and defibrillation programs, the impact of coronary care units, and consequences of aggressive revascularization.

ETIOLOGY. Although most infarcts result from thrombotic occlusion superimposed on severe coronary atherosclerosis, severe atherosclerotic disease may exist for years with no change in severity of effort-induced angina. Angina that occurs with progressively less effort or at rest, protracted angina simulating the pain of infarction, and accelerated angina despite intense medical management and the absence of exacerbating factors such as anemia, arrhythmia, hypertension, congestive heart failure, thyrotoxicosis, or obesity often reflect dynamic changes in obstructing plaques with consequent intermittent thrombosis. *Q-wave infarcts* (previously called transmural) appear to result when occlusive thrombi persist, as documented angiographically in >90% of patients with infarction. *Non–Q-wave* infarcts (previously called subendocardial) result often from incomplete or spontaneously recanalized thrombotic occlusions after ischemia persistent enough to elicit necrosis. Reocclusion with early recurrent infarction is common. A common denominator of all acute coronary syndromes (sudden cardiac death, new-onset angina, unstable angina, acute myocardial infarction) appears to be instability of atherosclerotic plaques with intramural hemorrhage, fissuring, and plaque rupture, all of which may precipitate acute thrombotic occlusion.

Risk factors for infarction parallel those for atherosclerosis in general. Hypercholesterolemia, hypertriglyceridemia, diabetes mellitus, hypertension, truncal obesity, smoking, increased concentrations of low density lipoprotein (LDL) cholesterol and decreased concentrations of high density lipoprotein (HDL) cholesterol in plasma, increased concentrations of lipoprotein (a), elevated plasma homocysteine, and genetic predisposition to atherosclerosis manifested by a strong family history apply to both, as discussed in Ch. 40. Changes such as hyperglycemia, elevated triglycerides, and diminishing serum cholesterol early after infarction may be inappropriately interpreted as indicative of diabetes or hyperlipidemia when in fact they reflect transiently impaired insulin release because of reduced pancreatic blood flow, augmented glycogenolysis secondary to catecholamines, increased gluconeogenesis secondary to 17-OH corticosteroids, increased concentrations of plasma free fatty acids, and augmented hepatic synthesis of triglycerides. Conversely, the decreased cholesterol secondary to hepatic dysfunction may be misinterpreted as the absence of hypercholesterolemia that would otherwise have been evident. The fall in LDL cholesterol is greater than that of total cholesterol and may persist for 6 to 8 weeks.

Several causes of acute myocardial infarction (Table 41–6) other than atherosclerosis merit particular consideration. These include coronary arterial emboli secondary to infective or marantic endocarditis (associated with drug abuse or collagen vascular disease), calcium deposits or thrombi from prosthetic or calcified valves, ventricular mural thrombi, or atrial thrombi or myxomas. Coronary thrombosis caused by trauma or by oral contraceptives in women, perhaps attributable to diminished antithrombin III or increased plasminogen activator inhibitor type I (PAI-1) in plasma; vasculitis; vasospasm (idiopathic or associated with cocaine or amphetamine abuse); coronary vascular degeneration (including accelerated atherosclerosis) after cardiac transplantation; or inflammatory small vessel coronary disease (0.1- to 1.0-mm diameter vessels) associated with diabetes, collagen vascular diseases, or disorders affecting extracellular matrix may be implicated.

Occasionally, acute myocardial infarction may occur with syndrome X (angina with "normal" coronary arteries) or variant angina. Diminished elaboration of endothelial cell-derived relaxing factor or release of vasoconstrictors such as endothelin may contribute.

PATHOLOGY AND PATHOPHYSIOLOGY

PATHOLOGY. Coronary atherosclerosis is particularly prominent at branch points of vessels. Atherosclerotic lesions appear initially as "fatty streaks"—i.e., lipid-laden cells, presumably monocytes or macrophages, adhering to the endothelial surface and ultimately penetrating the intima. More advanced fibrous plaques comprise not only lipid-laden cells but also connective tissue and proliferating smooth muscle cells. The most advanced lesions, called complicated plaques, exhibit fibrocalcific degeneration with intra- and extracellular lipid, calcium, fibrous tissue, necrotic debris, extravasated blood, and a fibrous tissue cap. Platelet-rich mural thrombi are often associated with the surface. Atherogenesis may reflect endothelial injury; permeation of atherogenic lipoproteins

TABLE 41–6. CONDITIONS OTHER THAN CORONARY ATHEROSCLEROSIS THAT MAY CAUSE ACUTE MYOCARDIAL INFARCTION

Coronary emboli	Causes include aortic or mitral valve lesions, left atrial or ventricular thrombi, prosthetic valves, fat emboli, intracardiac neoplasms, infective endocarditis, and paradoxical emboli.
Thrombotic coronary artery disease	May occur with oral contraceptive use, sickle cell anemia and other hemoglobinopathies, polycythemia vera, thrombocytosis, thrombotic thrombocytopenic purpura, disseminated intravascular coagulation, antithrombin III deficiency and other hypercoagulable states, macroglobulinemia and other hyperviscosity states, multiple myeloma, leukemia, malaria, and fibrinolytic system shutdown secondary to impaired plasminogen activation or excessive inhibition.
Coronary vasculitis	Seen with Takayasu's disease, Kawasaki's disease, polyarteritis nodosa, lupus erythematosus, scleroderma, rheumatoid arthritis, and immune-mediated vascular degeneration in cardiac allografts.
Coronary vasospasm	May be associated with variant angina, nitrate withdrawal, cocaine or amphetamine abuse, and angina with "normal" coronary arteries.
Infiltrative and degenerative coronary vascular disease	May result from amyloidosis, connective tissue disorders such as pseudoxanthoma elasticum, lipid storage disorders and mucopolysaccharidoses, homocystinuria, diabetes mellitus, collagen vascular disease, muscular dystrophies, and Friedreich's ataxia.
Coronary ostial occlusion	Associated with aortic dissection, luetic aortitis, aortic stenosis, and ankylosing spondylitis syndromes.
Congenital coronary anomalies	Including Bland-White-Garland syndrome of anomalous origin of the left coronary artery from the pulmonary artery, left coronary artery origin from the anterior sinus of Valsalva, coronary arteriovenous fistula or aneurysms, and myocardial bridging with secondary vascular degeneration.
Trauma	Associated with and responsible for coronary dissection, laceration, or thrombosis (with endothelial cell injury secondary to trauma such as angioplasty); radiation; and cardiac contusion.
Augmented myocardial oxygen requirements exceeding oxygen delivery	Encountered with aortic stenosis, aortic insufficiency, hypertension with severe left ventricular hypertrophy, pheochromocytoma, thyrotoxicosis, methemoglobinemia, carbon monoxide poisoning, shock, and hyperviscosity syndromes.

such as oxidized LDL; platelet and monocyte mitogens; and impaired reverse cholesterol transport attributable to low HDL. It is undoubtedly linked intimately to thrombosis. For example, platelet-derived growth factors may contribute to atherogenesis, impaired endothelial cell function caused by early atherosclerosis may predispose to platelet adhesion and activation, diminished endothelial elaboration of activators of fibrinolysis or augmented release of inhibitors may predispose to thrombosis, and vasospasm in atherosclerotic vascular segments may potentiate platelet activation through augmentation of sheer forces.

The spectrum of injury manifest in myocardium depends not only on the intensity of impaired myocardial perfusion but also on its duration. Accordingly, no conventional microscopic or gross changes may be evident in hearts of patients who die suddenly as a result of an acute coronary event. Typical infarction is manifest by coagulation necrosis followed ultimately by fibrosis. Contraction-band necrosis occurs when ischemia is followed by reperfusion or accompanied by massive adrenergic stimulation, often with myocytolysis.

In patients who succumb with a history of preceding unstable angina, morphologic manifestations of frank infarction may be lacking. However, one can see platelet microemboli and vascular mural thrombosis of diverse ages, which is indicative of the underlying pathophysiology involving repetitive thrombotic phenomena initiated by dynamic changes in complicated atherosclerotic plaques. In victims of infarction reflected by evolutionary ECG changes, the classic differentiation of transmural from nontransmural infarction based on ECG criteria (the presence or absence of Q waves after complete evolution of the insult) serves only as a crude generalization in view of bidirectional overlap of morphologic lesions associated with each ECG pattern.

PATHOPHYSIOLOGY. The right and left coronary arteries arise independently from individual ostia associated with right and left aortic valve cusps. The left anterior descending (LAD) and circumflex coronary arteries arise as the left main coronary artery bifurcation and supply the anterior left ventricle, the bulk of the interventricular septum, and the lateral and posterior left ventricular walls. The apex, lateral wall, and posterior wall may be supplied by the right posterior descending coronary artery, diagonals from the LAD, and the posterior left ventricular branch of the right coronary artery, respectively. When the posterior descending coronary artery that supplies the posterior interventricular septum arises from the left circumflex, the circulation is called left dominant. More often, the posterior descending artery arises from the terminal portion of the right coronary artery (right dominant circulation). The posterior left ventricular branch of the right coronary artery supplies the atrioventricular (AV) node in 90% of subjects. Another right coronary artery branch (in 55% of subjects) supplies the sinus node. The right ventricle is supplied by the right coronary artery. Although the posterior division of the left bundle branch has a dual blood supply (from both the left and right coronary arteries), the anterior fascicles of the left bundle and the right bundle are each supplied primarily by branches of the LAD.

In view of anatomic considerations it is not surprising that right coronary artery occlusion is manifested frequently by sinus bradycardia, AV block, right ventricular infarction, or left ventricular infarction of modest extent. Conversely, markedly impaired left ventricular function with pulmonary congestion or edema indicative of extensive injury and intraventricular conduction defects such as hemiblock is more typical of left coronary artery occlusion.

Acute insults are generally attributable to thrombosis initiated by hemorrhage or rupture of complicated atheromatous plaques with deprivation of blood flow to myocardium as a final common denominator. Even if recanalization is induced relatively promptly (spontaneously, mechanically, surgically, or with fibrinolytic drugs), regional myocardial perfusion may not be sustained (the "no reflow" phenomenon) because of endothelial cell swelling, platelet and leukocyte plugs, or complement-mediated microvascular inflammation. In addition to hypoxia, decreased removal of noxious metabolites, including potassium, calcium, amphiphilic lipids, and oxygen-centered free radicals, impairs ventricular performance and may evoke lethal arrhythmias. Inflammation of endocardial surfaces and stasis associated with dyskinesis can lead to ventricular mural thrombi. Epicardial inflammation may initiate the pericardial involvement seen with as many as 20% of Q-wave infarcts.

Systolic Function. Even transitory oxygen deprivation and accumulation of metabolites are manifest promptly by diminished regional systolic contractile function and wall thickening detectable by echocardiography, abnormal wall motion detectable by radionuclide ventriculography, diminished cardiac cycle–dependent variation of backscattered ultrasound detectable by tissue characterization, and, if extensive, diminished stroke volume. Restoring perfusion may promptly restore function of depressed myocardium even after prolonged intervals ("hibernating" myocardium). Often, however, impaired function persists even if blood flow is restored early ("stunning")—when injury is not yet irreversible. In general, hypokinesis and dyskinesis reflect the locus and extent of myocardial injury. Expansion of infarction and ventricular dilatation begin as early as 24 hours after the onset of infarction with thinning of the infarct zone and realignment of layers of tissue within and adjacent to it. Rupture, seen in 20% of fatal infarcts, may result, particularly when cardiogenic shock, malignant arrhythmia, or antecedent ventricular hypertrophy is present. Rupture may occur also with small infarcts because the well-preserved ventricular function increases wall stress.

Ventricular aneurysms are seen with early cardiac imaging in as many as 20% of patients with Q-wave infarction. Clinically, they may be recognized only late, manifested by congestive heart failure, recurrent ventricular arrhythmia, or recurrent emboli. They may be accompanied by persistent ST-segment elevation in ECGs obtained ≥6 weeks after infarction.

Because coronary artery disease is usually generalized, ischemia "at a distance" may be evident. As left ventricular end-diastolic volume and pressure increase because of impaired regional pump function, intramural diastolic ventricular pressure increases and myocardial perfusion declines. Peripheral arterial vasoconstriction and systemic venous constriction can no longer compensate for diminished stroke volume, and blood pressure falls. With decreased cardiac output and accelerated heart rate, coronary flow declines further. Ischemia at a distance may be manifest simply as an ECG derangement or may result in a vicious circle in which stuttering infarction ultimately leads to profound left ventricular failure and cardiogenic shock.

Normally perfused zones may initially exhibit compensatory hyperfunction with excessive wall thickening in systole. However, as the heart dilates over 24 to 48 hours, hyperfunction regresses.

Diastolic Function. Early after the onset of infarction, distensibility of ischemic myocardium first increases and then decreases. Effective ventricular filling can be maintained only with an increase in left ventricular end-diastolic volume and pressure (LVEDP). The increased LVEDP results in elevated pulmonary venous pressure, decreased pulmonary compliance, interstitial and ultimately alveolar pulmonary edema, hypoxemia, and exacerbation of myocardial ischemic injury. As the infarct thins and shrinks and if infarct expansion does not predominate, ventricular dilatation may regress, and diastolic cardiac and pulmonary pressures may return toward normal.

Right Ventricular Function. Impaired right ventricular function was recognized initially in the extreme, when right coronary artery occlusion led to gross right ventricular infarction. However, similar manifestations can occur when inferior left ventricular infarction and right coronary or left circumflex occlusion exist in the presence of a left dominant circulation. Right ventricular dysfunction diminishes cardiac output disproportionally to left ventricular injury. High-grade bradyarrhythmias are common, including those resulting from third-degree heart block, occasional profound arterial oxygen desaturation because of augmented right atrial pressure and right-to-left shunting through a patent foramen ovale, and exacerbation or extension of left ventricular infarction because of hypotension and diminished cardiac output.

Compensatory Mechanisms. Reflexly augmented sympathoadrenal and vagal discharge may give rise to tachycardia, ventricular arrhythmia, and bradycardia (sinus node depression or heart block), as well as pallor, cutaneous vasoconstriction, and diaphoresis. Initially, compromised cardiac output is maintained by the combination of increased heart rate and ventricular dilatation with recruitment of the Frank-Starling mechanism. Right ventricular infarction impairs hemodynamics most dramatically early in its course. As healing progresses and the right ventricle becomes less compliant, its conduit function is restored, permitting maintenance of cardiac output at the expense of augmentation of right ventricular filling pressure.

Effects of Myocardial Infarction on Organs Other Than the Heart. Augmentation of pulmonary venous pressure may cause diminished pulmonary compliance, dyspnea, pulmonary vascular redistribution (detectable radiographically), interstitial and alveolar pulmonary edema, respiratory decompensation, and hypoxemia.

Cerebral hypoperfusion may result in restlessness or, rarely, psychosis. Coupled with dyspnea in the elderly, it may be manifest only as confusion and combativeness. Increased sympathoadrenal tone reflected by markedly elevated plasma catecholamines and adrenocortical stimulation may be prominent as well. Plasma concentrations of atrial natriuretic peptide decrease initially but then increase, perhaps because of heart failure and atrial stretch. Elevated plasma concentrations of vasopressin, angiotensin (with β-adrenergic stimulation of renin release), and aldosterone contribute to fluid retention and hyponatremia. Impaired pancreatic blood flow inhibits insulin secretion.

In addition to the typical increase in erythrocyte sedimentation rate and leukocytosis, modestly increased plasma fibrinogen and augmented circulating PAI-1 occur as part of the acute phase reaction to infarction. Impaired fibrinolysis and augmented platelet activation by circulating catecholamines may predispose to continuing coronary and ventricular mural thrombosis. Plasma viscosity increases because of increased fibrinogen, α_2 globulins, and hemoconcentration several days after the onset of infarction, most markedly when left ventricular failure or shock supervenes.

Determinants of Prognosis. Immediate survival depends primarily on whether ventricular fibrillation occurs, and if so, whether it can be treated instantly. Community-based emergency systems that have defibrillators and appropriately trained personnel, rapid hospitalization, and in some instances dedicated chest pain facilities for patients with suspected evolving infarction have improved early survival. Even among hospitalized patients, fatality is generally attributable to ventricular fibrillation, which can, of course, often be interrupted by immediate defibrillation.

Judging from ambulatory ECG's and recordings obtained in coronary care units, mortality associated with acute myocardial infarction is attributable to primary ventricular fibrillation in ≥85% of instances. Only rarely is electrical asystole responsible. The association between primary ventricular fibrillation and "warning arrhythmias" (high-grade ventricular ectopy and R-on-T phenomena) is not strong, although ectopy as well as fibrillation may reflect intermittent or severe ischemia with compromised ventricular performance exacerbating ischemia, thereby predisposing to fibrillation. Ventricular premature complexes activating the ventricle during its vulnerable period can, of course, trigger fibrillation. Nevertheless, pharmacologically suppressing ventricular ectopy per se does not necessarily protect the heart against fibrillation. In fact, suppression with type IA or IC agents, β blockers, calcium channel blockers, or type III agents may increase the incidence of asystole in patients being treated with lidocaine.

In some instances mortality may result from fibrillation secondary to cardiac decompensation accompanying profound congestive heart failure, hypotension, or shock (secondary ventricular fibrillation). Accordingly, determinants of late mortality include "infarct size" measured enzymatically or by other means at the time of the index infarct (Fig. 41-2). Diminished left ventricular ejection fraction is a powerful descriptor.

Late mortality is determined also by the likelihood of recurrent infarction and the frequency and severity of episodic ischemia. Both may reflect progression of underlying atherosclerotic coronary artery disease and thrombosis. Complex ventricular ectopy after hospital discharge predicts subsequent mortality as well. Most late cardiac death is sudden, arrhythmic death (Fig. 41-3).

The Status of the Infarct-Related Artery. Coronary thrombolysis and mechanical revascularization have revolutionized primary treatment of acute myocardial infarction largely because they salvage myocardium when implemented early after the onset of ischemia. In addition, however, the prognostic benefit of an open infarct-related artery is evident even when recanalization can be in-

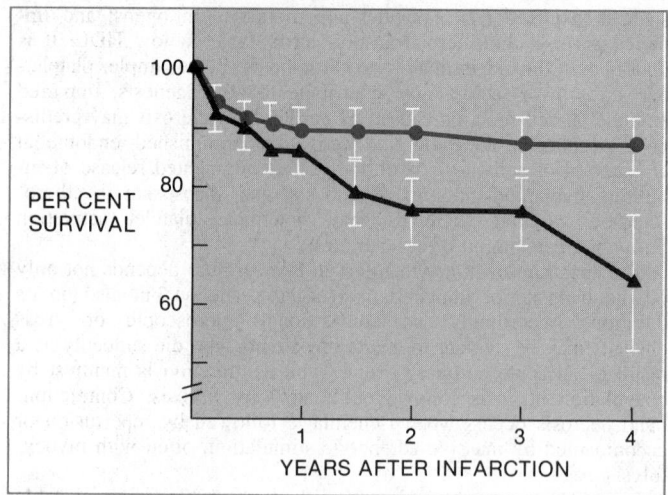

FIGURE 41-2. The influence of the extent of an initial infarct on survival. Infarct size index was estimated enzymatically and expressed as CK-g-equivalents per square meter of body surface area in 173 patients who survived for at least 24 hours. Survival was greater for those with small (< 15 CK-g-eq) *(circles)* than with large (≥ 15 CK-g-eq) *(triangles)* infarcts. (From Geltman EM, et al.: Circulation 60:805, 1979. Reproduced by permission of the American Heart Association, Inc.)

duced only 6 hours or more after onset of symptoms, when salvaging substantial amounts of jeopardized ischemic myocardium is no longer likely. An open infarct-related artery may potentiate improved ventricular function, improved collateral blood flow, decreased infarct expansion, decreased ventricular aneurysm formation, improved ventricular remodeling, diminished left ventricular dilatation, decreased late arrhythmia associated with ventricular aneurysms, decreased late potentials on the signal-averaged ECG, and decreased mortality.

SIGNS AND SYMPTOMS

"Typical" Q-wave infarction is manifested by prodromal symptoms of fatigue, chest discomfort, or malaise in the days preceding the event. Onset of infarction occurs often in the early morning hours, presumably in part because of the increased catecholamine-induced platelet aggregation and diminished plasma concentrations of PAI-1 after awakening. Onset is generally not directly associated with severe exertion.

Typical pain is intense, severe, unremitting for 30 to 60 minutes,

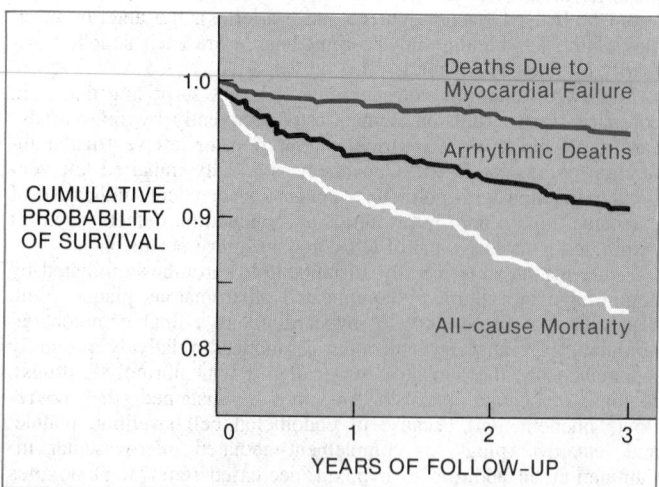

FIGURE 41-3. The large contribution of arrhythmia (sudden cardiac death) to overall mortality throughout the follow-up interval in victims of acute myocardial infarction. The ordinate shows survival from the time of hospital discharge after acute myocardial infarction. The number of patients alive and in follow-up were 0 years, 867; 1 year, 777; 2 years, 704; and 3 years, 314. (Adapted from Marcus F, et al.: Am J Cardiol 61:8, 1988; with permission.)

crushing or squeezing in nature, retrosternal, and often radiating down the ulnar aspect of the left arm and into the neck, teeth, or jaw. Occasionally the pain is epigastric. Diaphoresis, weakness, a sense of impending doom, profound restlessness, confusion, presyncope, hiccuping (presumably reflecting irritation of the diaphragm), nausea and vomiting, and palpitations are common. Decreased systolic ventricular performance accounts for impaired perfusion of vital organs and reflexly mediated compensatory responses to hypotension such as restlessness and impaired mentation, pallor, cutaneous vasoconstriction and sweating, tachycardia, and prerenal failure. Impaired left ventricular diastolic function leads to pulmonary vascular congestion with shortness of breath and tachypnea and pulmonary edema with orthopnea. Impaired right ventricular diastolic function leads to systemic venous hypertension, edema, hepatomegaly, and further compromise of left ventricular cardiac output.

Myocardial infarction may be clinically silent (in as many as 1% of patients), with the diagnosis established only retrospectively by electrocardiographic criteria. The patient may recall only an episode of "indigestion" or nothing. Stoicism, an unusually high pain threshold, disorders impairing function of the nervous system such as diabetes mellitus, or obtundation caused by medications or impaired cerebral perfusion may prevent recognition of typical chest pain.

PHYSICAL FINDINGS TYPICAL OF ACUTE MYOCARDIAL INFARCTION. Typical clinical findings can be summarized as follows:

General Appearance. Pallor, diaphoresis, restlessness.

Vital Signs. Heart rate is often increased secondary to sympathoadrenal discharge, ventricular ectopy, accelerated idioventricular rhythm, ventricular tachycardia, atrial fibrillation or flutter, or other supraventricular arrhythmias, especially when atrial infarction or heart failure is present. Bradyarrhythmias attributable to impaired sinus node function. AV nodal block, or infranodal block may be evident. The blood pressure is generally elevated initially with arterial vasoconstriction, in contrast to the case with acute pulmonary embolism, in which initial hypotension is frequent. However, with right ventricular infarction or severe left ventricular dysfunction, hypotension occurs. The respiratory rate is usually increased in response to pulmonary congestion. Coughing, wheezing, and production of frothy sputum may occur. Fever is usually present within 24 to 48 hours and may exceed 39° C.

Funduscopic Examination. Manifestations of atherosclerotic vascular disease including copper wiring of arterioles, hypertension with arterial narrowing and hemorrhages, or conditions predisposing to atherosclerosis such as diabetes with microaneurysms may be evident. Funduscopic examination is particularly important to detect hemorrhage, which is a relative contraindication to treatment with fibrinolytic agents.

Arterial and Venous Pulses. Pulsus alternans, although rare, may reflect impaired left ventricular function, as may brevity of the carotid pulse secondary to decreased stroke volume. Jugular venous distention may accompany right ventricular infarction or right ventricular failure secondary to profound left ventricular dysfunction and pulmonary hypertension.

Chest. Rales secondary to pulmonary venous hypertension are common with extensive left ventricular infarction; pleural effusions occur generally only with biventricular failure.

Heart. Lateral displacement of the apex impulse, dyskinesis, a palpable S_4, and a soft S_1 may indicate diminished contractility of the compromised left ventricle; paradoxical splitting of S_2 may reflect left bundle branch block or prolongation of the pre-ejection period with delayed aortic valve closure despite decreased stroke volume; accentuated S_4 and S_3 may reflect diminished left ventricular compliance; a mitral regurgitation murmur indicative of either papillary muscle dysfunction or rupture or annulus dilatation may be audible even if cardiac output is diminished markedly; a pericardial friction rub may be evident. Premature ventricular beats, brief runs of ventricular tachycardia, or accelerated idioventricular rhythm is common.

Abdomen. Hepatojugular reflux may be elicited even when hepatomegaly is not marked.

Extremities. Peripheral cyanosis, edema, and pallor may indicate vasoconstriction, and diminished cardiac output may reflect right ventricular dysfunction or failure.

Neurologic Findings. Patients with acute myocardial infarction are prone to frank cerebrovascular insults as a result of ventricular mural thrombi and consequent embolization (with an incidence of approximately 1%). Recrudescence of signs or symptoms of a prior cerebrovascular accident may occur secondary to diminished cerebral perfusion. Conversely, the incidence of myocardial infarction in patients with cerebrovascular accidents is substantial.

The incidence of myocardial infarction appears to be greater and its prognosis worse in patients with depression. Infarction may precipitate reactive depression whether or not β-adrenergic blocking agents or other central nervous system (CNS)-active agents are administered.

HEMODYNAMIC MANIFESTATIONS. Hemodynamic observations are of inestimable value in guiding therapy. A categorization of hemodynamic subsets of patients is shown in Table 41–7.

Patients Requiring Invasive Monitoring. Not all patients with infarction require hemodynamic monitoring with right heart catheterization and/or invasive arterial pressure monitoring. Those who are hemodynamically stable without apparent complications such as tachycardia, refractory arrhythmia, respiratory compromise, impaired cerebral, hepatic, or renal function, or persistent or recurrent pain indicative of recurrent or refractory ischemia, pericarditis, or incipient cardiac rupture can generally be managed without invasive hemodynamic monitoring. Effective management may be facilitated by balloon flotation right heart catheter hemodynamic monitoring in patients with pulmonary congestion indicative of pulmonary venous hypertension reflected by physical findings or chest roentgenographic abnormalities, but many patients with mild complications can be managed conservatively. Patients with peripheral hypoperfusion despite initial administration of fluids to replete or expand vascular volume and those with severe, refractory, or progressive congestive heart failure, potentially catastrophic complications of acute infarction, refractory

TABLE 41–7. HEMODYNAMIC SUBSETS AMONG PATIENTS WITH ACUTE MYOCARDIAL INFARCTION

Subset		Systemic Arterial Blood Pressure	Cardiac Index (L/m²/min)	Left Ventricular Filling Pressure (Pulmonary Artery Occlusive Pressure; mm Hg)
I	Normal hemodynamics	Normal	2.7 ± 0.5	≤ 12
II	Hyperdynamic state	Increased	>3.0	<12
III	Hypovolemia*	Decreased	≤ 2.7	≤ 9
IV	Left ventricular failure			
	A. Mild	Normal	≤ 2.5	$>18, \leq 22$
	B. Severe	Normal or decreased	≤ 1.8	≥ 22
V	Cardiogenic shock	Decreased	≤ 1.8	≥ 18
VI	Shock attributable to right ventricular infarction†	Decreased	≤ 1.8	≤ 18

Adapted from information appearing in The New England Journal of Medicine: Forrester JS, et al.: Medical therapy of acute myocardial infarction by application of hemodynamic subsets. N Engl J Med 295:1404, 1976.

*Relative hypovolemia may result in hypertension even if pulmonary artery pressure is moderately elevated (≤ 18) if left ventricular compliance is decreased associated with infarction or failure.

†Central venous (systemic venous) pressure is often markedly elevated (upper limit of normal = 6 mm Hg).

arrhythmias, persistent pain, or hemodynamic instability should be evaluated by balloon flotation right heart catheter hemodynamic monitoring.

Monitoring catheters should generally be introduced through compressible sites, particularly because of the high likelihood that thrombolytic agents will be used early in the treatment of infarction. They should remain in place for no more than 72 hours to avoid the risk of infection and can often be removed much more promptly. Sometimes ascertaining systemic and pulmonary venous pressure, cardiac output, and peripheral vascular resistance is sufficient for subsequent management without the need for continuous monitoring. In other instances the effects of vasodilators, diuretics, agents with positive inotropic effects, and therapeutic alterations of vascular volume should be monitored over the ensuing 48 to 72 hours.

Hemodynamic Subsets. Patients are categorized with respect to cardiac output (increased, normal, or diminished), systemic arterial blood pressure (increased, normal, or diminished with or without increased or decreased systemic vascular resistance), and the presence or absence of pulmonary venous hypertension (augmented pulmonary arterial wedge pressure) (Table 41–7).

Patients without diminished systemic arterial blood pressure or pulmonary venous hypertension may have normal or hyperdynamic hemodynamics (the latter reflected by a high cardiac output with or without hypertension caused by sympathoadrenal stimulation). Systemic arterial hypotension may be attributable to relative or absolute hypovolemia or to right ventricular infarction (generally reflected by augmented systemic venous pressure). Rarely, it reflects decreased peripheral vascular resistance caused by vagotonia or sepsis. The noncompliant left ventricle requires augmented filling pressure to sustain cardiac output. Accordingly, relative hypovolemia may exist despite moderately elevated left ventricular filling pressure. Central venous pressure cannot be relied upon for assessment of vascular volume.

Right ventricular failure with or without concomitant tricuspid regurgitation leads to increased central venous pressure without concomitantly increased pulmonary venous or pulmonary arterial occlusive (indicative of left atrial) pressure. Pulmonary venous hypertension without systemic arterial hypotension is often indicative of left ventricular failure (differentiated as mild or severe in terms of normal or depressed cardiac output). Profound hypotension and pulmonary venous hypertension are manifestations of cardiogenic shock. The vicious circle of cardiogenic shock—progressive infarction with declining cardiac output, further compromise of perfusion, and ultimately extensive necrosis with profound failure and shock—is generally irreversible without prompt mechanical support of the circulation and coronary revascularization with thrombolytic drugs, angioplasty, or surgery.

In general, hemodynamic status reflects the extent of left ventricular infarction. However, an infarct of modest extent superimposed on a previous infarct can profoundly compromise hemodynamics. Initial impairment of ventricular performance may exceed that attributable to irreversible injury because of myocardial stunning early after the onset of infarction. Right ventricular involvement may compromise cardiac output more than anticipated from the extent of left ventricular injury alone.

LABORATORY DETERMINATIONS

The objectives of acquiring laboratory data include determination of the presence or absence of infarction (diagnosis and differential diagnosis); characterization of the locus, nature (Q or non-Q), and extent of infarction (estimation of infarct size); detection of recurrent ischemia or infarction (extension of infarction); detection of early and late complications of infarction; and estimation of prognosis.

The complete blood count and platelet count (which may decrease after heparin) are useful not only diagnostically but in assessing suitability for treatment with thrombolytic drugs. The leukocyte count may be normal initially but generally increases within 2 hours and peaks in 2 to 4 days with predominance of polymorphonuclear leukocytes and a shift to the left. Elevations generally persist for 1 to 2 weeks. Other components of the acute phase reaction contribute to elevations of the erythrocyte sedimentation rate (ESR) within 48 hours with subsequent changes paralleling those in leukocyte count. Because of increased pulmonary and sometimes systemic venous pressure, contraction of plasma volume is common after acute myocardial infarction, manifested not only by hemoconcentration but also by prerenal failure with elevation of plasma creatinine and blood urea nitrogen. Arterial blood gases should be assayed if necessary to evaluate hypoxemia resulting from pulmonary congestion, atelectasis, or ventilatory impairment secondary to complications of infarction or excessive sedation or analgesia. Fingertip oximetry may be adequate and can obviate the need for arterial puncture and bleeding in patients treated with thrombolytic drugs. The chest radiograph is particularly useful in determining the presence or absence of cardiomegaly (often correlated with the presence or absence of increased LVEDP, left atrial pressure, and pulmonary venous hypertension), pulmonary edema, pleural effusions, Kerley B lines, and other criteria of congestive heart failure. A small cardiac silhouette and clear lung fields in a patient with systemic hypotension may indicate relative or absolute hypovolemia. A large cardiac silhouette with similar hemodynamics may reflect hemopericardium and tamponade or right ventricular infarction compromising cardiac output. Chest radiographic findings indicative of pulmonary venous hypertension may occur later and persist longer because of delay in fluid shifts between vascular, interstitial, and alveolar spaces.

Sequential ECG findings remain hallmarks of diagnosis despite the occasional occurrence of infarction without any acute changes and the nonspecific nature of some of the ECG changes that may be seen. The diagnosis can be established with certainty when typical ST elevation persists for hours and is followed by inversion of T waves within the first few days and development of Q waves subsequently. However, initial ST depression or T-wave inversion is difficult to differentiate from that seen with ischemia without infarction or in unrelated conditions (Table 41–8). ST-segment depression followed by T-wave inversion without evolution of Q waves can result from non–Q-wave infarction or subendocardial ischemia without infarction. Q-wave infarction cannot be differentiated from non–Q-wave infarction initially if ST elevation is lacking and Q waves have not yet developed. Infarction is often associated with nonspecific ECG changes including intraventricular conduction delays; ventricular and supraventricular arrhythmias; signs of atrial infarction, such as changes in P-wave morphology, elevation or depression of the PQ segment, atrial flutter or fibrillation, or a wandering atrial pacemaker; and signs of right ventricular infarction such as ST elevation or Q waves detectable in right-sided precordial leads. The appearance of abnormalities in a large number of ECG leads often indicates extensive injury or concomitant pericarditis. Anterior and anterolateral infarcts tend to involve more left ventricular myocardium than inferior or true posterior infarcts.

MACROMOLECULAR MARKERS OF INFARCTION. Detection of elevated concentrations in plasma of macromolecules released from irreversibly injured myocardium has become the definitive diagnostic criterion of infarction. Enzymes including creatine kinase (CK), aspartate serum transaminase (AST), and lactate dehy-

TABLE 41–8. CONDITIONS ASSOCIATED WITH ELECTROCARDIOGRAPHIC CHANGES THAT MAY OBSCURE OR SIMULATE THOSE INDICATIVE OF ACUTE MYOCARDIAL INFARCTION

Abnormality	Example
Intraventricular conduction abnormalities	Left bundle branch block, left anterior superior fascicular block, infranodal arborization block, right ventricular transvenous or epicardial pacing
Electrolyte disturbances	Hypo- or hyperkalemia, hypocalcemia
Pre-excitation	
Early repolarization	
Cerebrovascular accident	
Myocarditis	Inflammatory, infiltrative, viral, collagen vascular disorders, pheochromocytoma, cardiac allograft rejection, neuromuscular disorders such as muscular dystrophy and Friedreich's ataxia
Left ventricular hypertrophy	Hypertrophic cardiomyopathy, dilated cardiomyopathy, valvular heart disease, hypertension
Right ventricular hypertrophy	Cor pulmonale, acute pulmonary embolus, pneumothorax
Cardiac tumors	
Pericarditis	

drogenase (LDH); myoglobin; myosin light chains; and cardiac troponin I among numerous other constituents egress from irreversibly injured ischemic myocardium within several hours after the onset of the insult. Their elevated concentrations in plasma constitute sensitive diagnostic findings. Specificity is limited, however, because of their ubiquitous distribution in skeletal muscle and other tissues. Assay of activity in plasma of the MB isoenzyme of CK (MB CK) is the cornerstone of diagnosis because of the marked abundance of this isoenzyme in myocardium and virtual absence from most other tissues, and its consequent sensitivity (detection of necrosis of < 100 mg of myocardium). Characteristic sequential changes of plasma MB CK include elevations above normal within 4 hours, a 2- to 10-fold peak in 16 to 24 hours, and a return to baseline within 3 to 4 days. The magnitude and persistence of elevations are useful in estimating the extent of infarction.

Initially normal enzyme values are seen often when patients present very early after the onset of infarction. Thus, discharge from an emergency room of a patient with a history consistent with myocardial infarction should not occur without several hours of observation and repeat determinations. If infarction has occurred more than 24 hours before admission, is of very modest magnitude, or is stuttering in nature, enzyme elevations may be lacking because of the predominance of clearance over rates of release into the circulation. Assay of myosin light chains, troponin I, or the $LDH_1:LDH_2$ isoenzyme ratio, which remains elevated for several days after infarction because of the slow clearance of LDH, may be helpful. Late detection of infarction is sometimes facilitated by myocardial infarct scintigraphy with technetium-99m (^{99m}Tc)-pyrophosphate or radiolabeled antimyosin antibodies.

Generally, MB CK is assayed at admission and at 12- to 24-hour intervals until the diagnosis is established. Determination of total CK is less specific and is redundant. Recently, assays detecting post-translational conversion of individual isoenzymes of CK to isoforms have been shown to permit even earlier diagnosis (within 2 to 3 hours of infarction). Recanalization is reflected by sudden washout of the tissue isoform into plasma. Isoform analysis is likely to become useful for monitoring interventions such as coronary thrombolysis. Determining plasma concentrations of myoglobin, a protein with a short half-life in the circulation, offers similar promise, but results may be distorted by changes in renal function with prerenal failure.

IMAGING. Several noninvasive modalities permit detection of regional wall motion and hypo- or dyskinesis, as well as estimation of overall ventricular performance (Fig. 41–4). These include two-dimensional and color flow Doppler echocardiography, radionuclide ventriculography, ultrafast (cine) computed tomography, and gated magnetic resonance imaging. Because of cost considerations and convenience, only the first two are used widely. Both sensitivity and specificity of abnormal wall motion as criteria of acute myocardial infarction exceed 90%, particularly in patients without previous infarction. Assessing segmental function and overall left ventricular performance has prognostic implications and is essential when infarction is extensive (elevations of MB CK > 150 IU per liter) or complicated by shock or profound heart failure, in part to identify potentially surgically correctable complications and to detect ventricular true or false aneurysms and thrombi (Fig. 41–5) that can be treated with anticoagulants or fibrinolytic drugs. Imaging is useful also to detect pericardial effusion, concomitant valvular or congenital heart disease, and marked depression of ventricular function that may interdict treatment with calcium antagonists or β-adrenergic blockers. Doppler echocardiography is particularly useful to estimate the severity of mitral or tricuspid regurgitation, detect ventricular septal defects secondary to rupture, assess diastolic function, and monitor cardiac output calculated from flow velocity and aortic valve area. When right ventricular infarction is suspected or when infarction is superimposed on a previous insult or associated with electrocardiographic phenomena such as left bundle branch block which obscure diagnosis, assessment of right ventricular function and delineation of regional wall motion may be particularly helpful.

Infarct-avid agents such as ^{99m}Tc-pyrophosphate and radiolabeled antimyosin antibodies can sensitively detect infarction and define its locus. However, positive results with infarct scintigraphy cannot be obtained generally until ≥ 24 hours after the onset of infarction and may be simulated by accumulation of tracer in temporally remote infarcts. Perfusion scintigraphy with tracers such as thallium-201 or ^{99m}Tc-sestamibi (an isonitrile) is sometimes useful when the diagnosis is obscure.

Positron emission tomography with tracers of intermediary metabolism (Fig. 41–6), perfusion (Fig. 41–7), or oxidative metabolism (Fig. 41–7) permits quantitative assessment of the distribution and extent of impairment of myocardial oxidative metabolism and regional myocardial perfusion (Fig. 41–8). It has been particularly useful in defining the efficacy of therapeutic interventions designed to salvage myocardium and has been used diagnostically to differentiate reversible from irreversible injury in hypoperfused zones.

DIFFERENTIAL DIAGNOSIS

The diagnosis is straightforward when the history of acute myocardial infarction is typical, the initial ECG abnormal and followed by definitive sequential changes, and MB CK elevated in the initial or subsequent plasma samples with typical sequential changes. A

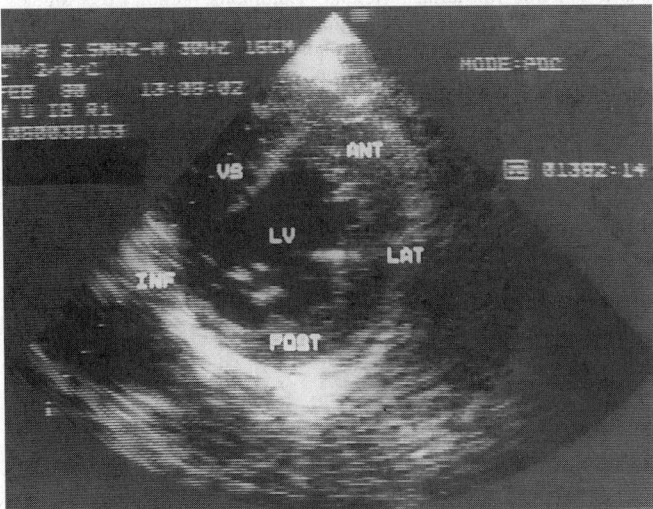

FIGURE 41–4. A still-frame short-access two-dimensional echocardiogram illustrating an inferoposterior left ventricular aneurysm after acute myocardial infarction evident as an outpocketing of the thinned left ventricular wall on the perimeter of the left ventricular cavity in the region corresponding to 6 to 9 o'clock, with the center of the clock face envisioned as central. The echo densities within the left ventricular cavity posteriorly and laterally are caused by papillary muscles. ANT = Anterior; LAT = lateral; POST = posterior; INF = inferior; VS = ventricular septum; LV = left ventricular cavity. (Courtesy of Dr. J. E. Perez, Washington University School of Medicine, St. Louis, MO.)

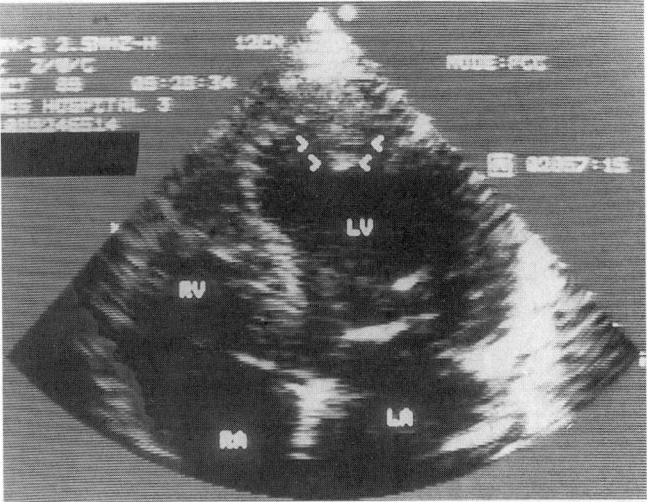

FIGURE 41–5. An apical four-chamber two-dimensional echocardiographic still frame demonstrating thrombus in the apex of the left ventricle (arrows) associated with acute myocardial infarction. LV = Left ventricle; RV = right ventricular; RA = right atrium; LA = left atrium. (Courtesy of Dr. J. E. Perez, Washington University School of Medicine, St. Louis, MO.)

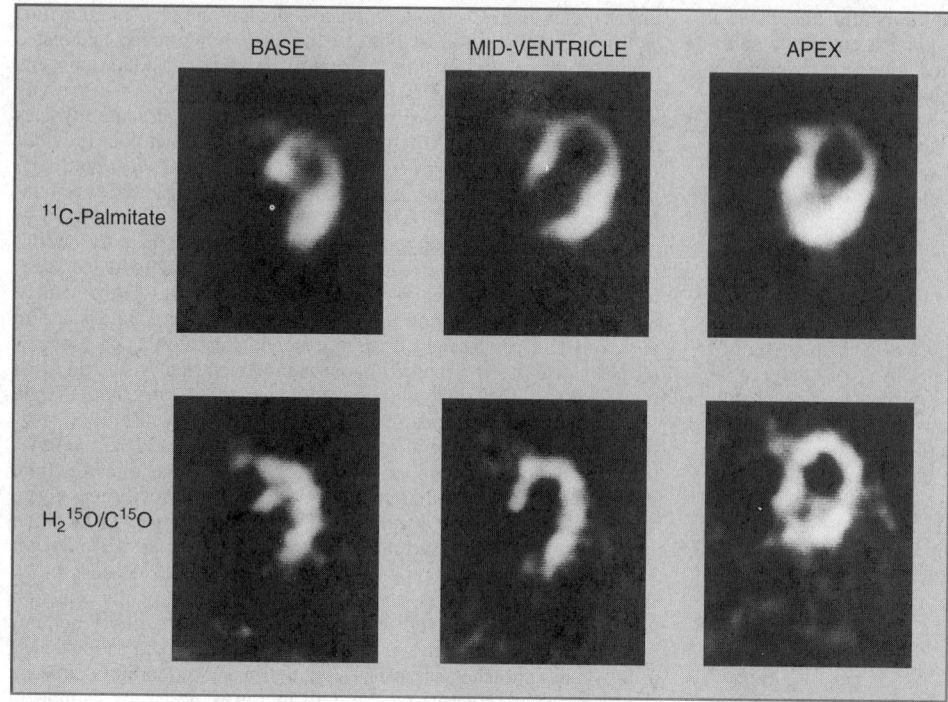

BASE   MID-VENTRICLE   APEX

^{11}C-Palmitate

H$_2$^{15}O/C^{15}O

FIGURE 41-6. Positron emission tomograms at three levels of the left ventricle obtained from a subject with myocardial infarction after late spontaneous coronary recanalization. Anterior myocardium is at the top right, the left ventricular free wall at the bottom right, and posterior myocardium at the bottom left. Reconstructions acquired after intravenous administration of ^{11}C-palmitate show the persistent anterior defect despite homogeneous myocardial perfusion imaged with H$_2$^{15}O and blood pool subtraction with C^{15}O. The discontinuity posteriorly in some tomographic sections is attributable to the mitral valve apparatus. (From Bergmann SR, et al.: Prog Cardiovasc Dis 28:165, 1985; with permission.)

presumptive diagnosis can be made when any two of these criteria are present. Unfortunately, however, the diagnosis may be obscure in patients seen very early after the onset of infarction and in those with ECG manifestations of prior ischemic or other types of heart disease, electrocardiographically silent infarcts, or atypical presentations. Differentiation from ischemia without infarction (unstable angina, aortic stenosis in the elderly, ischemia attributable to right ventricular overload, new-onset angina, or inadequate myocardial perfusion in markedly hypertrophied left ventricles or in association with marked aortic insufficiency) and from pericarditis with pain simulating that of infarction may be difficult without the aid of laboratory tests and cardiac imaging. A critical differential diagnostic consideration is aortic dissection. It should be suspected whenever pain is atypical or not associated with ECG changes typical of infarction.

Pleurodynia, pulmonary embolism or infarction, pneumothorax, pneumonitis, musculoskeletal pain associated with bursitis, the shoulder/hand syndrome, pectoral lymphadenopathy, herpes zoster before eruption of the typical vesicles, myalgia, and costochondritis may simulate infarction superficially but can usually be differenti-

ated easily on the basis of physical findings, results of laboratory tests, and chest radiography. Pain orginating in the abdomen that may masquerade as infarction includes that caused by cholecystitis or cholelithiasis, pancreatitis, duodenal or gastric ulcer, gastritis, esophagitis, esophageal spasm, or esophageal reflux associated with a hiatal hernia.

CARE OF THE PATIENT

The focus of treatment differs in the prehospital, hospital (coronary care unit and step-down unit), and convalescent phases despite considerable overlap of objectives in each. Most death caused by infarction occurs early and is attributable to primary ventricular fibrillation. Thus, initial objectives are immediate ECG monitoring and reversal of ventricular fibrillation should it occur.

TREATMENT IN THE PREHOSPITAL PHASE. Community-based systems in Belfast, Ireland; Columbus, Ohio; Los Angeles, California; and Seattle, Washington, have conclusively documented the effectiveness of rapidly responding rescuers such as police and firefighters trained in defibrillation. Approximately 65% of deaths caused by infarction occur in the first hour. More than 60% (39%

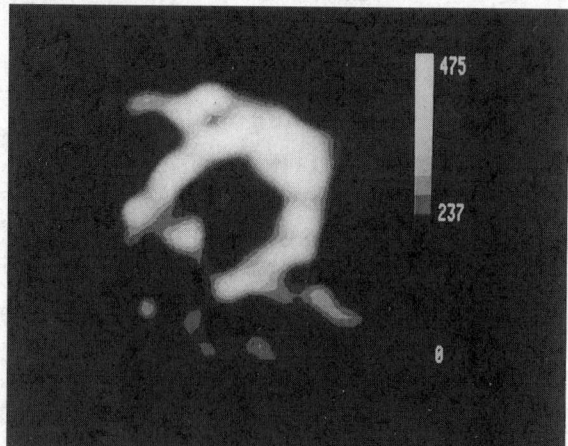

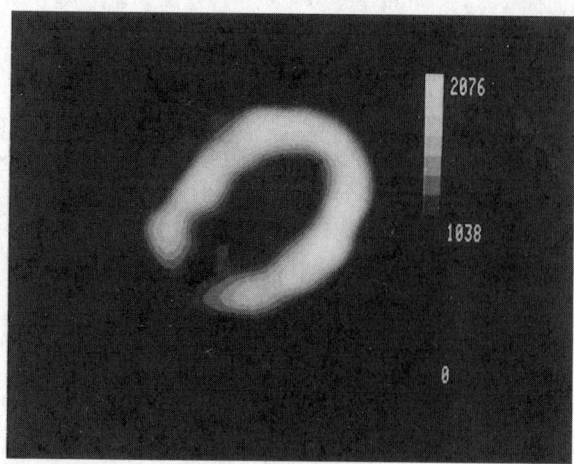

FIGURE 41-7. A single midventricular positron emission tomographic reconstruction obtained from a normal subject. Perfusion *(left)* assessed with H$_2$^{15}O and myocardial oxidative metabolism *(right)* assessed with ^{11}C-acetate are homogeneous. The scales indicate counts per pixel. Orientation is the same as in Figure 41-6. (Courtesy of Dr. S. R. Bergmann, Washington University School of Medicine, St. Louis, MO.)

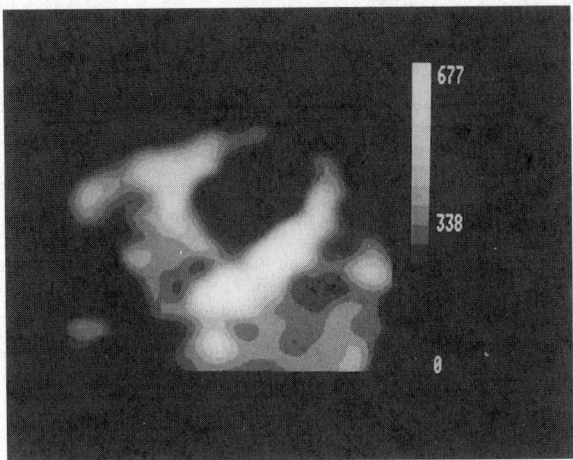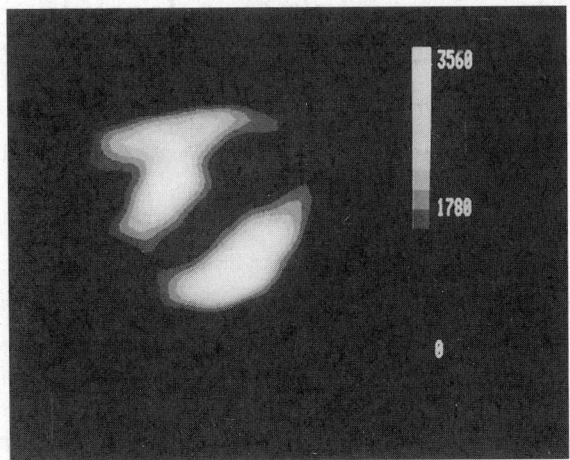

FIGURE 41–8. Midventricular tomographic reconstructions of perfusion *(left)* and oxidative metabolism *(right)* obtained after intravenous administration of $H_2^{15}O$ and ^{11}C-acetate after acute anterior myocardial infarction. A large perfusion deficit is evident anteriorly with a concordant decrease in myocardial oxygen consumption reflected by decreased ^{11}C-acetate uptake. (From Walsh MN, Geltman EM, Brown MA, et al.: Noninvasive estimation of regional myocardial oxygen consumption by positron emission tomography with carbon-11 acetate in patients with myocardial infarction. J Nucl Med 30:1798, 1989; with permission.)

of those who would succumb) can be saved by defibrillation initiated by a bystander or first-responding rescuer. Additional objectives of prehospital care by paramedical and emergency room personnel include adequate analgesia (generally with morphine), reduction of excessive sympathoadrenal and vagal stimulation pharmacologically, prophylaxis and treatment of malignant ventricular arrhythmias (generally with lidocaine), and support of cardiac output, systemic blood pressure, and respiration. Atropine (0.5 mg IV at 5-minute intervals to a maximum of 2 to 4 mg) is particularly useful to counteract excessive vagal tone that often underlies bradyarrhythmias and hypotension. It is indicated when heart rate is disproportionately diminished with respect to blood pressure, when hypotension (sometimes secondary to morphine) is refractory despite augmentation of left ventricular filling pressure, or when impaired AV nodal conduction with Wenckebach block is evident. If bradycardia persists, pacing may be required.

The advent of coronary thrombolysis as primary therapy for acute myocardial infarction has already revolutionized management of patients in the hospital. Prehospital phase coronary thrombolysis initiated by paramedical personnel under medical supervision appears likely to become important as well because of its promise for salvaging more myocardium because of earlier interruption of ischemia.

TREATMENT IN THE HOSPITAL PHASE. Cardiac care units (CCU's) have reduced early mortality attributable to acute myocardial infarction by approximately 50%, largely by immediately implementing defibrillation. They have proven to be optimal facilities for continuous ECG monitoring, invasive hemodynamic monitoring when indicated, implementation and titration of measures designed to limit the extent of infarction and salvage jeopardized ischemic myocardium, and induction of recanalization of infarct-related arteries pharmacologically.

Care in the CCU. In addition to continuous ECG monitoring, several general measures should be implemented. Diet should include liquid only during the first 24 hours because of the risk of aspiration with the frequent nausea and vomiting, and possible cardiac arrest. Stool softeners are helpful to avoid constipation, straining, and consequent circulatory derangements. Prophylaxis (oral sucralfate, 1 gram twice a day), or an H_2 antagonist (famotidine, ranitidine, or cimetidine orally or intravenously at 6- to 12-hour intervals) for stress ulcers is appropriate for patients at high risk, including those with sepsis, hypotension or shock, bleeding diathesis, a requirement for prolonged mechanical intervention, or elevated intracranial pressure. Patients with uncomplicated infarction need be confined to bed for only 1 day. Physical activity should be limited (bed-chair regimen) throughout the 2- to 3-day CCU stay, with gradual and carefully monitored resumption of ambulatory activity in the late hospital phase. Sedative, anxiolytic, and hypnotic

drugs at night may be helpful but cannot replace optimal communication by compassionate physicians and nurses and the reassurance it provides. Patients requiring mechanical ventilation need special consideration (Table 41–9). Oxygen should be given to avoid hypoxemia. High doses may be counterproductive because of vasoconstriction and lack of augmented myocardial oxygen delivery in normoxemic patients.

Refractory or severe pain should be treated with intravenous morphine, meperidine, or pentazocine. Repeated intravenous doses of 4 to 8 mg of morphine at intervals of 5 to 15 minutes can be given with relative impunity until the pain is relieved or toxicity is manifest by hypotension, vomiting, or depressed respiration. Prodigious quantities are sometimes required (2 to 3 mg per kilogram). Should toxicity occur, a morphine antagonist such as naloxone can reverse it. Morphine-induced hypotension in a patient without incipient or overt pulmonary edema can be minimized by maintaining the patient in a supine position, elevating the legs, administering fluids, and, if heart rate does not increase, atropine.

Continuing chest pain indicative of ischemia should be treated with agents diminishing myocardial oxygen requirements and potentiating myocardial perfusion. Intravenous nitroglycerin titrated (10 to 200 μg per minute) to avoid hypotension reduces peripheral arterial resistance and ventricular afterload. Higher doses diminish systemic venous tone, blood pressure, and ischemic zone perfusion. Favorable effects are probably mediated by diminished afterload and preload and decreased LVEDP facilitating myocardial perfusion. Although coronary vasodilation in intramural vessels is often already maximal when vasodilator metabolites accumulate locally, nitrates may dilate epicardial vessels and reduce vasospasm, thereby reducing shear forces that otherwise contribute to platelet activation and potentially propagate coronary thrombi. Tolerance to continuously administered intravenous nitrates occurs rapidly, often within hours.

Oral calcium channel blockers such as nifedipine and diltiazem are often useful because they reduce ventricular afterload (nifedipine) and modestly reduce heart rate and contractility as well (diltiazem). However, prognosis appears to be affected adversely in patients with congestive heart failure or impaired left ventricular function that persists after myocardial infarction by treatment with diltiazem and possibly other calcium channel blockers as well. Oral or intravenous conventional or ultra-short-acting β-adrenergic blockers such as esmolol may ameliorate ischemia and pain by lowering heart rate and hence myocardial oxygen requirements. Theoretically, cardioactive calcium antagonists, including verapancil and diltrazem, and β-adrenergic blockers may exert anti-injury effects as well by diminishing inward calcium flux in cardiac myocytes.

Despite the use of effective analgesia with nitrous oxide given by inhalation in concentrations of 20 to 50% combined with oxygen in

TABLE 41–9. AGENTS USED FOR SEDATION AND NEUROMUSCULAR BLOCKADE FOR PATIENTS REQUIRING MECHANICAL VENTILATION

Agent	Dosage	Remarks
Haloperidol	1. 2–5 mg parenterally initially* 2. Twofold increased amounts every 20 min until efficacy or side effects occur 3. 50% effective dose every 4 h subsequently	Particularly useful to treat agitation or episodes of psychosis
Midazolam	1. 1 mg IV repeated at 2–5 min intervals until desired effect is achieved 2. 1–10 mg/h infusion subsequently titrated to effectiveness	A short-acting benzodiazepine with antagonism to platelet-activating factor Doses near 10 mg/h can lead to escalation of effects because of accumulation of the agent.
Fentanyl	1. 25 μg IV, repeated at 2–5 min intervals until desired effect is achieved 2. 25–300 μg/h infusion subsequently titrated to efficacy	A short-acting opiate, often useful in combination with midazolam to avoid the need for high doses of the benzodiazepine in continuous infusions. Fentanyl is approximately 100 times more potent than morphine but is relatively devoid of vasodilator effects.
Pancuronium or Vecuronium or Atracurium	1. 0.04–0.1 mg/kg IV loading dose 2. Maintenance with 0.05–0.1 mg/kg IV every 1–2 h 1. 0.1 mg/kg IV loading dose 2. maintenance with 0.05–0.1 mg/kg every 1–2 h 1. 0.4 mg/kg IV loading dose 2. 0.4–1.2 mg/kg/h	Neuromuscular blocking agents; monitoring efficacy with the aid of a peripheral nerve stimulator is necessary at least every 8 h; continuous infusions should be avoided for pancuronium and vecuronium; durations of action are: pancuronium = 40–60 min; vecuronium = 30–45 min; atracurium = 20–40 min.

* Most sources indicate intramuscular administration is preferred. However, in an intensive care unit setting, intravenous administration is often used.

Europe and elsewhere, this agent is not used widely in the United States. Its effects on ventricular afterload are favorable, and it is generally well tolerated for intervals as long as 24 to 48 hours when used intermittently.

Limitation of Infarct Size. Because the evolution of infarction is dynamic and determined in part by the imbalance between myocardial oxygen requirements and oxygen supply, early treatment focuses not only on prompt recanalization of the infarct-related artery but also on diminution of myocardial oxygen requirements without compromise of perfusion of vital organs. Myocardial protection can be enhanced with β-adrenergic blockers to reduce heart rate; arterial vasodilators such as nifedipine, nitrates, or angiotensin-converting enzyme (ACE) inhibitors to reduce ventricular afterload; and diuretics with pulmonary venous dilating properties such as furosemide and ethacrynic acid to reduce left ventricular preload. β-Adrenergic blockers are likely to be useful in most patients without specific contraindications such as heart failure, bradycardia, or bronchial constriction. Other agents should be titrated to optimize left ventricular filling pressure (often to as high as 18 to 22 mm Hg because of decreased ventricular compliance) and cardiac output while maintaining adequate systemic arterial blood pressure (Table 41–10).

Coronary Thrombolysis. The potential value of coronary thrombolysis has been recognized for more than 30 years. Its emergence as primary therapy was delayed, however, until the pivotal role of thrombosis in causing Q-wave infarction was established unequivocally by coronary arteriography, the impact of extensive infarction on mortality had been established, and salvage of myocardium by decreasing oxygen requirements had been found to be limited. The "modern" era of coronary thrombolysis began in the late 1970's with the demonstration that intracoronary administration of plasminogen activators recanalized occluded arteries and immediately relieved pain. Recanalization was soon documented in 70 to 75% of patients given intracoronary streptokinase. However, intracoronary dosing entailed serious disadvantages including risk and delay associated with the obligatory cardiac catheterization. Intravenous administration was soon shown to be effective in recanalizing approximately 50% of infarct-related arteries when streptokinase was used and 75 to 80% (comparable to the optimal recanalization rates with any agent by any route of administration) when tissue-type plasminogen activator (t-PA) was used (Fig. 41–9). The superiority of intravenously administered second- compared with first-generation plasminogen activators in recanalizing coronary arteries may reflect (1) more modest plasminemia with its

TABLE 41–10. THERAPEUTIC INTERVENTIONS TAILORED TO SPECIFIC HEMODYNAMIC SUBSETS

	Hemodynamic Subset	Intervention	Remarks
I	Normal hemodynamics	None required	
II	Hyperdynamic state	β-Adrenergic blockade	Analgesics and anxiolytic drugs may be helpful.
III	Hypovolemia	Intravenous fluids to augment effective vascular volume	Marked increases in pulmonary artery occlusive pressure reflecting pulmonary venous hypertension and increased left ventricular filling pressure may occur if heart failure is unmasked or exacerbated; manifestations may include dyspnea, hypoxemia, bronchospasm and rales, and pulmonary congestion evident radiographically.
IV	Left ventricular failure A. Mild B. Severe	Systemic arterial vasodilators Systemic arterial vasodilators and diuretics	Diuretics may be useful if failure is refractory. Cardiotonic agents may be helpful if hypotension supervenes, but their use can exacerbate the imbalance between myocardial oxygen requirements and supply; sympathomimetic and dopaminergic agents may be helpful, but their benefit on hemodynamics is usually only transitory and may exacerbate ischemic injury.
V	Cardiogenic shock	Coronary recanalization and circulatory support	
VI	Shock attributable to right ventricular infarction	Augmentation of vascular volume and cardiotonic agents	

Adapted from information appearing in The New England Journal of Medicine: Forrester JS, et al.: Medical therapy of acute myocardial infarction by application of hemodynamic subsets. N Engl J Med 295:1404, 1976.

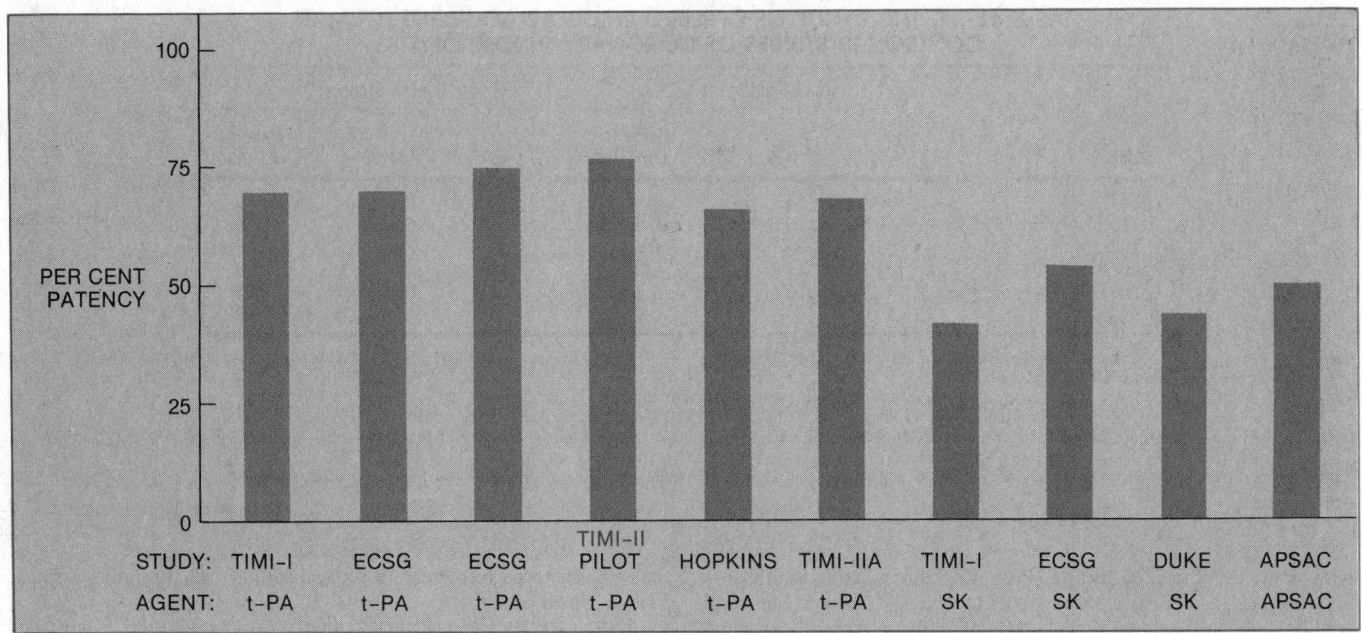

FIGURE 41–9. Angiographically defined patency of infarct-related arteries 90 minutes after treatment within 4 to 8 hours after onset of symptoms with streptokinase (SK), tissue-type plasminogen activator (t-PA), or acetylated plasminogen streptokinase activator complex (APSAC) reported in 10 large studies involving 1654 patients. TIMI = Thrombolysis in Myocardial Infarction; ECSG = European Cooperative Study Group. (From Tiefenbrunn AJ, Sobel BE: Fibrinolysis 3:1, 1988; with permission of Churchill Livingstone.)

consequent procoagulant and platelet-activating effects counteracting thrombolysis; (2) a lack of "plasminogen steal" with consequent maintenance of high concentrations of clot-associated plasminogen available for activation to plasmin induction of lysis; and (3) the feasibility of safe administration of high concentrations of activator with less degradation of hemostatic proteins.

Coronary thrombolysis with intravenously administered activators of plasminogen improves ventricular function and decreases mortality both early and late after infarction, particularly when initiated within a few hours after the onset of ischemia. Even when initiated only 6 hours or more after the onset of infarction, restoring patency of the infarct-related artery appears to confer benefits reflected by improved collateral blood flow, improved ventricular remodeling, decreased infarct expansion, decreased late potentials manifest in signal-averaged ECG's potentially indicative of arrhythmogenicity, improved late ventricular function, decreased ventricular aneurysm formation, decreased late arrhythmia associated with those aneurysms that do develop, and decreased mortality.

It is convenient and useful to consider two generations of fibrinolytic drugs. The first, typified by streptokinase, urokinase, and APSAC (acetylated plasminogen streptokinase activator complexes) induces activation of free plasminogen and clot-associated plasminogen indiscriminately. First-generation drugs invariably elicit a systemic lytic state characterized by depletion of circulating fibrinogen, plasminogen, and hemostatic proteins and by marked elevation of concentrations of fibrinogen degradation products in plasma. Their lack of clot selectivity is therefore associated with an increased risk of bleeding and possible protection against early reocclusion in inadequately anticoagulated patients.

Second-generation drugs, typified by t-PA and single-chain urokinase plasminogen activator, activate plasminogen in the fibrin domain preferentially compared with free plasminogen in the circulation. Thus they exhibit relative clot selectivity. In optimal dosage they induce clot lysis without inducing a systemic lytic state. They are less prone to predispose to hemorrhage that requires transfusion.

Recanalization is more frequent (occurring in 80 to 90% of infarct-related arteries) and more rapid (within 90 minutes) with second-than with first-generation agents, perhaps in part because of clot selectivity and lack of induction of plasminemia, which may induce procoagulant effects that attenuate fibrinolysis and plasminogen steal and diminish the intensity of fibrinolysis. Furthermore, clinical outcome is superior, as shown in the recently reported GUSTO trial in which 24-hour mortality; 30-day mortality; 1-year mortality; net clinical benefit (survival without a disabling stroke); the incidence of cardiac complications, including ventricular fibrillation, ventricular tachycardia, acute mitral regurgitation, asystole, and sustained hypotension; and preservation of ventricular function were all significantly better in patients treated with the fibrin-selective agent t-PA plus intravenous heparin than in those treated with streptokinase, with or without intravenous heparin.

The risks of coronary thrombolysis with plasminogen activators include bleeding, most of which is confined to sites of vascular access. Marked depletion of fibrinogen indicating a systemic lytic state may be a marker of pharmacologic effects that can lead also to bleeding. Marked prolongation of bleeding time may reflect bleeding risk somewhat more specifically. Although intracranial hemorrhage had been feared, the incidence of cerebrovascular accidents in patients treated with thrombolytic agents is no greater than that seen with conservative treatment without fibrinolytic drugs (Table 41–11). The incidence of hemorrhagic stroke is somewhat greater and that of thrombotic or embolic stroke somewhat less, but the disparity is not reflected by an increased incidence of fatal cerebrovascular accidents and is more than offset by the favorable impact of fibrinolytic agents on survival after infarction.

Plasminogen activators should not be given to patients with active internal bleeding or a bleeding diathesis, suspected aortic dissection, hemorrhagic retinopathy, recent trauma (including surgery or prolonged and traumatic cardiopulmonary resuscitation), intracranial neoplasm, or hypertensive crisis. Relative contraindications include peptic ulcer disease, remote cerebrovascular accident, and hepatic failure. Safety has not been established for pregnant women. In general, thrombolytic agents should be used in patients ≤75 years of age who present with suspected Q-wave infarction within 6 hours after the onset of symptoms in whom contraindications are not present. Treatment may be helpful in some patients first seen ≥6 hours after the onset of symptoms. Its impact on non–Q-wave infarction, infarction in patients of very advanced age, and unstable angina is not yet clear.

Adjunctive and Conjunctive Measures. Clinical efficacy of coronary thrombolysis depends on the frequency, rapidity, and persistence of recanalization, all of which depend not only on the intensity of fibrinolysis but also on the inhibition of coagulation and platelet-induced thrombosis that undoubtedly occur concomitantly. Intravenous heparin (Table 41–12) is the agent of choice, coupled

TABLE 41-11. INCIDENCE OF CEREBROVASCULAR ACCIDENT (CVA) IN CONTROLLED STUDIES OF CORONARY THROMBOLYSIS

Study	Thrombolytic Agent			Control Group		
	n	*Agent*	*Percent with CVA*	*n*	*Agent*	*Percent with CVA*
GISSI	5860	SK	1.1	5852	Placebo	0.9
AIMS	502	APSAC	0.4	502	Placebo	1.0
ISIS-2	8592	SK	0.7	8595	Placebo	0.8
ASSET	2516	t-PA	1.1	2495	Placebo	1.0
ECSG*	722	t-PA	1.1	366	Placebo	0.5
TOTAL	18,192		0.9	17,810		0.9

Adapted from Tiefenbrunn AJ, et al.: Coronary thrombolysis—It's worth the risk. JAMA 261:2107, 1989. Copyright 1989, American Medical Association.

* Two studies, one with placebo, one with t-PA with and without angioplasty.

GISSI = Gruppo Italiano per lo Studio della Streptochinasi nell'Infarto Miocardico; AIMS = APSAC Intervention Mortality Study; ISIS-2 = International Study of Infarct Survival; ASSET = Anglo-Scandinavian Study of Early Thrombolysis; ECSG = European Cooperative Study Group.

SK = Streptokinase; APSAC = anisoylated plasminogen streptokinase activator complex; t-PA = tissue-type plasminogen activator.

with orally administered aspirin. Promising direct-acting antithrombins such as hirudin (investigational) are likely to supersede conventional heparin, however. Even optimally effective coronary thrombolysis is compromised by early thrombotic reocclusion in 6 to 20% of patients with initial recanalization unless vigorous conjunctive anticoagulation is initiated immediately.

Calcium antagonists have potential value as anti-injury agents in the setting of reperfusion, as antiplatelet agents, and as coronary vasodilators, effects that may minimize activation of platelets in the vicinity of lysed thrombi by reducing sheer forces. Nitrates may diminish excessive coronary reactivity and hence ischemia. Reperfusion arrhythmias, if they compromise hemodynamics or threaten to degenerate into ventricular fibrillation, can often be suppressed with lidocaine. α-Adrenergic blocking agents are attractive theoretical alternatives. Accelerated idioventricular arrhythmia often does not require pharmacologic intervention. Perhaps of most importance are conjunctive anticoagulation with a powerful antithrombin such as heparin or hirudin (currently investigational) and conjunctive use of antiplatelet agents such as aspirin *or* antibodies and antagonists to the platelet glycoprotein IIb/IIIa receptor, prostacyclin and PGE_2 analogues, thromboxane receptor antagonists and synthetase inhibitors, and serotonin antagonists (all investigational at present).

Contrary to initial expectations, not all patients treated with thrombolytic drugs should be subjected to obligatory early cardiac catheterization and angioplasty. A strategy comprising arteriography and angioplasty in only those patients who exhibit recurrent or persistent symptoms and signs of ischemia appears to be safer (Table 41–13) and as effective as obligatory angiography for all patients in preserving ventricular function and reducing mortality. The value of rescue angioplasty, i.e., angioplasty performed when occlusion

has proven to be refractory to recanalization with fibrinolytic drugs, has not been established.

Mechanical Revascularization. Compared with pharmacologic thrombolysis, mechanical recanalization (angioplasty or surgery) may enhance flow more markedly or more rapidly in patients who sustain infarction while in a cardiac catheterization laboratory. However, except in such rare instances or in centers dedicated to immediate angioplasty as primary therapy, it has not yet proven to be superior. Immediate angioplasty or surgery cannot be provided universally because of contention for facilities, the need for large teams of highly trained personnel on a 24-hour per day basis, and other logistic constraints. Risks of primary angioplasty exceed those of elective angioplasty for coronary artery disease with angina. Surgical facilities and personnel should be readily available in view of the 10% incidence of life-threatening complications encountered. Restenosis rates after balloon angioplasty or other investigational approaches such as laser or mechanical atherectomy generally exceed 40% within 6 months despite vigorous use of anticoagulants, antiplatelet drugs, calcium antagonists, vasodilators, and intracoronary stents. Although restenosis rates after coronary surgery are much lower, morbidity is substantial, and the mortality risk for patients with evolving infarction is not trivial. In view of the remarkably low early mortality attainable with intravenous fibrinolytics (approximately 5% in appropriately selected patients in several large studies with second-generation agents), the sustained benefit of coronary thrombolysis, and the effectiveness of late mechanical intervention when indicated after initial coronary thrombolysis, mechanical revascularization is generally indicated as

TABLE 41-12. COMMONLY USED PROTOCOL FOR CONJUNCTIVE USE OF HEPARIN

aPTT Measured (sec)	Modification of Dose				Time at Which Repeat aPTT Should be Obtained
	Repeat Bolus Dose	*Stop Infusion for Designated Interval*	*Change Infusion Rate (U/h)*		
<50	5000 units	0	+100		6 h
50–59	0	0	+100		6 h
60–85	0	0	0		12 h
86–95	0	0	−100		12 h
96–120	0	30	−100		6 h
>120	0	60	−200		6 h

A loading dose of 5000 U is given as an intravenous bolus followed by an infusion of 1200 U/h.

The first aPTT is obtained 6 h after the initial bolus, with subsequent adjustments made as indicated.

The normal aPTT range is 25–36 sec.

The target range of 60–85 sec indicates a concentration of heparin of 0.2–0.4 U/ml.

Adapted from Cruickshank MK, et al.: Arch Intern Med 151:333, 1991. Copyright 1991, American Medical Association.

TABLE 41-13. OUTCOME AFTER INVASIVE VERSUS CONSERVATIVE MANAGEMENT*

Event	Management Strategy after Thrombolysis		
	Invasive	*Conservative*	*P Value*
Death	5.2%	4.7%	0.49
Death or reinfarction	10.9%	9.7%	0.25
Coronary artery bypass grafting	11.9%	10.5%	0.18
Intracranial hemorrhage	0.9%	0.7%	0.70
Any adverse endpoint†	13.0%	10.6%	0.04

Adapted from information appearing in The New England Journal of Medicine: The TIMI Group: Comparison of invasive and conservative strategies after treatment with intravenous tissue plasminogen activator in acute myocardial infarction: Results of the thrombolysis in myocardial infarction (TIMI) phase II trial. N Engl J Med 320:618, 1989. Inclusion and exclusion criteria are delineated in the referenced article.

* The percentages of adverse clinical events during the initial 42 days of follow-up are shown in these results from a study of 3262 patients with Q-wave infarction randomized to treatment with (invasive strategy) or without (conservative strategy) obligatory angiography and angioplasty early after acute myocardial infarction treated initially with tissue-type plasminogen activator (t-PA). The invasive strategy was not superior.

† Death, nonfatal reinfarction, intracranial hemorrhage, or coronary bypass grafting after angioplasty.

primary therapy only for patients with contraindications to pharmacologic thrombolysis, those with immediate life-threatening conditions such as cardiogenic shock refractory to coronary thrombolysis, and those with infarction resulting from occlusion of previously placed coronary artery bypass grafts amenable to angioplasty. The role of salvage angioplasty for occlusions refractory to fibrinolysis remains to be established, in part because candidates are likely to have already sustained extensive irreversible injury by the time failure of thrombolysis can first be established.

PROPHYLAXIS AND TREATMENT OF ARRHYTHMIA. Continuous ECG monitoring is essential for 72 hours after the onset of infarction and optimally throughout hospitalization by telemetry to immediately detect ventricular fibrillation and numerous arrhythmias that may occur. Some degenerate into ventricular fibrillation because of augmentation of myocardial oxygen requirements, impaired ventricular performance with consequent exacerbation of ischemia, or both.

Both primary and secondary (to hemodynamic decompensation, hypoxemia, electrolyte disturbances, or progressive cardiac or pulmonary failure) ventricular fibrillation should be treated by immediate electrical countershock. Fibrillation may be confused with electrical asystole when the vector of fibrillation is perpendicular to the axis of the recording lead used for monitoring. True asystole requires confirmation with multiple leads and differentiation from fine ventricular fibrillation. If the distinction between ventricular fibrillation and asystole cannot be made with certainty, fibrillation should be assumed to be present. Other established components of cardiopulmonary resuscitation and advanced cardiac life support are invaluable, but the primacy of immediately restoring effective cardiac rhythm cannot be overemphasized. Electrical countershock should be implemented immediately rather than deferred until after endotracheal intubation and other emergency measures. If true electrical asystole is documented, immediate external, transvenous, or transthoracic cardiac pacing is essential, although prognosis in this situation is grim.

When ventricular fibrillation accompanies acute myocardial infarction, lidocaine is the drug of choice to prevent immediate recurrence. Prophylactic administration is not necessary when the patient is in a setting in which defibrillation can be implemented immediately and pharmacologic treatment can be initiated promptly. Adverse effects of prophylactic lidocaine (central nervous system depression, seizures, proarrhythmic, asystolic, and cardiodepressant effects) may offset potential benefit. However, repeat bolus injections of 0.5 to 1.0 mg per kilogram body weight every 5 minutes to a total of 4 mg per kilogram, followed by maintenance infusions of 1 to 2 mg per minute are used for this purpose in younger patients without prior cardiac disease who can be treated within the first few hours after the onset of infarction when the risk of primary ventricular fibrillation is greatest. After successful resuscitation when ventricular fibrillation has occurred, lidocaine should be administered by continuous infusion (20 to 50 μg per kilogram of body weight per minute), particularly if frequent, closely coupled, multiform, or repetitive ventricular premature complexes or ventricular tachycardia occurs. Blood levels should be maintained in the range of 2 to 5 μg per milliliter. Recurrent ventricular fibrillation, refractory to lidocaine, may be suppressed after a considerable lag period by intravenous bretylium given in 5- to 10-mg per kilogram doses or by amiodarone (0.75 μg per kilogram loading dose followed by infusion of 5 to 10 μg per minute [still investigational in the United States]). Other promising antifibrillatory drugs are currently investigational in the United States.

High-grade ventricular ectopy or bursts of ventricular tachycardia should be treated with lidocaine. If they persist for more than a few hours after hospitalization, their management is similar to that applicable in other circumstances. Procainamide and quinidine are generally the drugs of choice. Torsades de pointes may respond to overdrive pacing or intravenous magnesium sulfate. Accelerated idioventricular rhythm should not be treated unless hemodynamic decompensation occurs, in which case sequential or atrial overdrive pacing or atropine may be effective. Administering magnesium sulfate (1 gram over 5 minutes intravenously followed by an 8-gram infusion over 24 hours) appears to reduce the incidence of primary lethal arrhythmias and to reduce mortality in patients treated with or without thrombolytic agents. Benefits have been ascribed to induction of more favorable myocardial energetics as well as to antiarrhythmic effects.

Supraventricular Arrhythmias. Treatment of these arrhythmias is the same as when they occur under other circumstances and is indicated when they impair hemodynamics or compromise myocardial viability by augmenting oxygen requirements. Sinus tachycardia is usually secondary to excessive sympathoadrenal tone associated with extensive infarction and impaired ventricular performance, pericardial inflammation and irritation of the sinus node, relative or absolute hypovolemia, hypoxemia secondary to pulmonary venous congestion and respiratory impairment, congestive heart failure, or other potentially remediable factors. Atrial fibrillation or atrial flutter may indicate failure or atrial infarction. In the absence of the Wolff-Parkinson-White syndrome, these conditions should be treated with calcium channel blockers such as verapamil, digitalis glycosides, or a short-acting β-adrenergic blocker such as esmolol to control ventricular rate. Procainamide (intravenous or oral) or quinidine (oral) is often effective in restoring and maintaining sinus rhythm. When decompensation is evident, rapid atrial pacing (to terminate atrial flutter) or electrical cardioversion (to terminate either atrial fibrillation or flutter) should be used. When hemodynamics are compromised or myocardial viability is threatened, paroxysmal supraventricular tachycardias should be managed initially by augmentation of vagal tone with carotid sinus compression or the Valsalva maneuver, calcium channel blockers, intravenous adenosine, or electrical cardioversion. The safety of adenosine in patients with infarction has not yet been established unequivocally.

Bradyarrhythmias. Sinus bradycardia occurs often, particularly in patients with inferior myocardial infarction. If refractory to atropine, it may require temporary transvenous pacing. A wandering atrial pacemaker or first-degree AV block rarely requires specific treatment. Higher degrees of AV block or AV block associated with hypotension refractory to atropine may require sequential pacing to sustain adequate hemodynamics.

Long-term pacing is needed only when heart block persists throughout the hospital phase, sinus node function is markedly impaired, Mobitz II second- or third-degree block occurs intermittently, or block is associated with newly acquired bundle branch block or other criteria of conduction system impairment. It is difficult to prove that long-term pacing improves survival after myocardial infarction because mortality is so high, with the extensive infarction frequently responsible. Nevertheless, temporary transvenous pacing may stabilize hemodynamics, and long-term pacing may be justified prophylactically in patients at high risk.

TREATMENT TAILORED TO HEMODYNAMICS. Invasive hemodynamic monitoring is of inestimable value in patients with clinically complicated acute myocardial infarction. It permits rapid delineation of left ventricular filling pressure, effective vascular volume, the presence or absence of mitral regurgitation and its severity, ventricular septal rupture (with oximetry), right ventricular systolic and diastolic pressure and function, and cardiac output and peripheral vascular resistance. Selection of therapy based on hemodynamics is delineated in Table 41–10 and is predicated on the following considerations:

1. Hypertensive patients with increased cardiac output and normal pulmonary artery wedge pressure may benefit from infusions of β-adrenergic blockers such as esmolol to reduce myocardial oxygen requirements.

2. Hypotension associated with relative or absolute hypovolemia reflected by lack of substantial elevation (>18 mm Hg) of left ventricular filling pressure generally responds to augmentation of vascular volume with intravenous fluids. Pulmonary artery wedge pressure should be monitored to preclude excesses leading to pulmonary edema. Hypotension with markedly elevated right ventricular diastolic, right atrial, and central venous pressures may implicate right ventricular infarction, which responds often to augmented vascular volume and stimulation of contractility with cardiotonic agents such as dobutamine, dopamine, or β-adrenergic agonists. Systemic arteriolar vasodilators secondarily decrease impedance of right ventricular outflow if they ameliorate left heart failure and can be used when systemic arterial diastolic pressure is adequate.

3. Sudden and profound hypotension may reflect a catastrophic insult such as pulmonary embolism (manifested by pulmonary arterial hypertension and hypoxemia) or rupture of the ventricular sep-

tum (detectable by augmented right ventricular and pulmonary artery pressure associated with an oxygen step-up in the right ventricle). Alternatively, it may reflect left ventricular papillary muscle rupture with mitral regurgitation manifested by large V waves in the pulmonary artery wedge pressure recording. When caused by free wall rupture with hemopericardium, hemodynamic manifestations of pericardial tamponade are apparent, with a diastolic pressure plateau in all four cardiac chambers, impaired right ventricular filling, and confirmatory echocardiographic findings of pericardial fluid and diastolic right atrial and right ventricular collapse. Mechanical insults should be treated by immediate surgery if hemodynamic stability can be maintained with only pharmacologic and circulatory support. Surgery can be delayed for 1 to 2 weeks if stability can be maintained without such measures and the patient can be monitored meticulously.

4. Hypotension associated with markedly elevated pulmonary artery wedge pressure generally indicates severely impaired left ventricular performance and cardiogenic shock. Supportive measures and cardiotonic agents are generally ineffective unless the ischemia responsible can be relieved by coronary thrombolysis, angioplasty, or surgery. Mechanical circulatory support may be necessary to obtain definitive diagnostic information pertinent to potentially remediable insults such as septal or free wall rupture, mitral regurgitation, or coronary reocclusion. Intra-aortic balloon counterpulsation or circulatory support with a left ventricular assist device may be particularly useful as a temporizing measure or as a bridge to cardiac transplantation.

5. Pulmonary venous hypertension with normal systemic arterial pressure indicates relative or absolute excess of vascular volume and left heart failure that should be treated with vasodilators to reduce both ventricular preload and afterload, diminish the commonly associated mitral regurgitation accompanying left ventricular failure, and diminish left atrial and pulmonary venous hypertension. Intravenous nitroprusside, nitroglycerin, or parenteral or oral ACE inhibitors may be effective. Caution must be exercised to avoid marked changes in concentrations of electrolytes in plasma. If pulmonary congestion is severe or pulmonary edema is present but cardiac output is reasonably well maintained and associated with an adequate systemic arterial blood pressure, contraction of vascular volume by removing fluid (phlebotomy with reinfusion of blood cell elements, slow continuous ultrafiltration, and rarely peritoneal dialysis) may be effective. If pulmonary congestion persists or if cardiac output and systemic arterial pressure are low, loop diuretics (having the advantage also of pulmonary venodilation) may be helpful. Hemodialysis is dangerous because of the risk of precipitous changes in filling pressures and cardiac performance. Cardiotonic agents (dobutamine or dopamine, digitalis, and phosphodiesterase inhibitors such as amrinone or milrinone [investigational]), previously a mainstay of therapy for congestive heart failure with diminished cardiac output and hypotension, may be necessary but entail the risk of exacerbating imbalance between myocardial oxygen supply and demand and are generally not dramatically effective alone.

6. Hypotension with or without pulmonary venous hypertension indicative of left heart failure is generally associated with increased peripheral vascular resistance in patients with infarction. In rare instances it may be decreased, in which case vasoconstrictors (such as dopamine in relatively high doses, epinephrine particularly if cardiac rate is not accelerated, and rarely, although usually fruitlessly, norepinephrine) may be indicated. The decrease of resistance is often caused by other factors, such as occult sepsis, which must of course be recognized. In patients with profound ventricular failure, circulatory support with intra-aortic balloon counterpulsation or left ventricular assist devices may permit performance of diagnostic catheterization and identification and treatment of surgically remediable lesions.

Care in the Step-Down Unit. Patients with uncomplicated myocardial infarction require CCU care generally for no more than 72 hours. Subsequent care is facilitated in a step-down unit equipped with telemetry for continuous ECG monitoring. Therapeutic objectives include immediate recognition and treatment of ventricular tachycardia, ventricular fibrillation, and bradycardia caused by sinus node dysfunction or AV block; daily clinical and appropri-

ate laboratory monitoring for prompt detection and treatment of complications, including deep venous thrombosis (sometimes manifest by fever and Homans' sign), pulmonary emboli, postmyocardial infarction pericarditis with a friction rub, tachycardia, and fever (generally managed with aspirin to avoid impaired infarct healing that may occur with nonsteroidal anti-inflammatory agents or corticosteroids), ventricular thrombi, ventricular true or false aneurysm, or catastrophic mechanical complications including cardiac rupture; treatment to minimize the risk of recurrent infarction; assessment of prognosis based on evaluation of left ventricular function, exercise tolerance, and the severity of spontaneous or inducible ischemia; and gradual and judicious progressive ambulation followed by a rehabilitation program after discharge.

In patients who have been treated with thrombolytic agents, heparin can be discontinued after 5 to 7 days, and secondary prevention of thrombosis can be continued with daily aspirin. For those with ventricular mural thrombus or extensive hypokinesis, congestive heart failure, or ventricular aneurysm predisposing to mural thrombus, anticoagulation with warfarin is appropriate for 6 months. Patients with non–Q-wave infarction without congestive heart failure should be treated with calcium channel blockers to prevent recurrence. Those with Q-wave infarction without failure or other contraindications should be treated for 6 months or more with β-adrenergic blockers devoid of intrinsic sympathomimetic activity to reduce the incidence of reinfarction and enhance survival.

Complications detected by telemetry (episodic ischemia with ST-segment deviation, arrhythmia, heart block, new-onset bundle branch block, tachycardia with minimal exertion), physical findings suggestive of congestive heart failure, markedly impaired ventricular performance documented echocardiographically or by radionuclide ventriculography, or manifestations of recurrent coronary occlusion such as recurrent pain, unexplained tachycardia, exacerbation or appearance of heart failure, hypotension, or impaired ventricular performance justify consideration of coronary arteriography before discharge from the hospital, with mechanical revascularization if indicated. In patients without such complications and particularly those treated initially with thrombolytic drugs, submaximal (7 to 10 days) or symptom-limited (predischarge) exercise testing should be performed to determine whether arteriography is indicated. Exercise-induced ischemia manifested by ST-segment depression of ≥ 1 mm, reversible thallium perfusion defects, a hypotensive response to modest workloads, ventricular arrhythmias, diminution of ejection fraction, or induction of wall motion abnormalities with or without angina pectoris is an indication for coronary arteriography. Marked impairment of ventricular performance (resting ejection fraction < 40%) or anticipated stringent physical occupational requirements are relative indications. Thallium scintigraphy or exercise echocardiography may be useful when baseline ECG abnormalities obscure interpretation. Dipyridamole thallium scintigraphy or dobutamine stress echocardiography may substitute for exercise testing in patients unable to exercise for noncardiac reasons. Risk for development of sustained ventricular tachycardia or ventricular fibrillation can be estimated by high-resolution ECG with frequency- or time-domain analysis of signal-averaged recordings, which provides criteria, independent of left ventricular dysfunction (Fig. 41–10). Ambulatory continuous ECG monitoring is often used, but the occurrence of the complex ventricular ectopy targeted for detection is generally concordant with severe left ventricular dysfunction after infarction.

CONVALESCENCE

Most patients can be discharged within 1 to 2 weeks. Any complications may require a longer hospital stay. Objectives of management during convalescence include (1) preventing recurrent infarction (continued use of β-adrenergic blockers after Q-wave infarction, calcium channel blockers after non–Q-wave infarction with preserved left ventricular function, and aspirin); (2) preventing late complications of infarction such as peripheral or cerebral embolus from ventricular mural thrombus with continued anticoagulation for 3 to 6 months in patients at high risk or harboring mural thrombi; (3) modifying risk factors including cessation of smoking, treatment of hypertension, diabetes, and hyperlipidemia (with a target of reducing LDL cholesterol to 100 mg per deciliter), and implementation of a carefully monitored exercise rehabilitation program under supervision or for appropriately motivated patients at home; (4) promptly detecting and evaluating potential progression

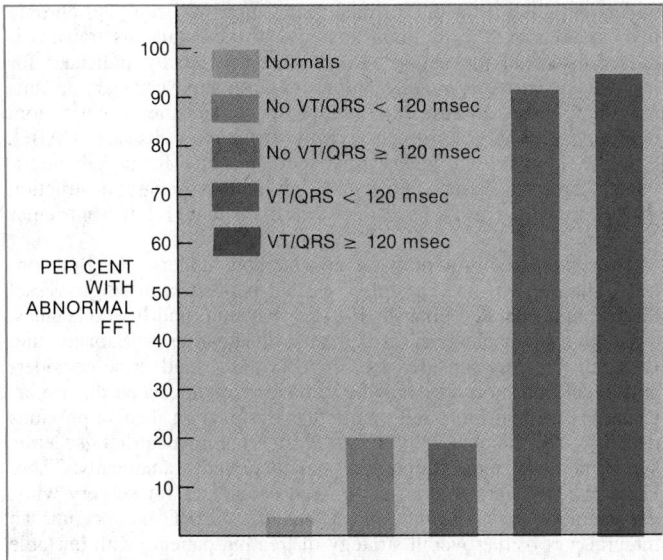

FIGURE 41–10. The predictive value for risk of sustained ventricular tachycardia (VT) of abnormalities detectable by high-resolution electrocardiography performed by fast-Fourier transform (FFT) frequency domain analysis in 169 subjects with and without coronary artery disease and myocardial infarction categorized with respect to the presence or absence of QRS complex prolongation indicative of left bundle branch block or other intraventricular conduction delays. High-resolution ECG abnormalities correlated closely with the likelihood of occurrence of sustained VT whether or not conduction disturbances were present. (From Lindsay BD, et al.: Circulation 77:122, 1988. Reproduced by permission of the American Heart Association, Inc.)

of underlying coronary artery disease manifested by signs or symptoms of ischemia including angina pectoris; and (5) preventing sudden cardiac death with β-adrenergic blockers in patients without specific contraindications. Indiscriminate use of antiarrhythmic agents, particularly type I_c drugs, to suppress asymptomatic ventricular ectopy should be avoided because of the risk of increasing mortality (Fig. 41–11).

Patients with non–Q-wave infarctions require special consideration. This syndrome appears often to be a manifestation of incomplete or nonsustained thrombotic coronary occlusion. Early prognosis is good compared with prognosis for patients with Q-wave infarction. However, mortality late after infarction may exceed that after Q-wave infarction because of reocclusion, reinfarction, or sudden cardiac death reflecting recurrent ischemia. Survivors of non-Q infarction in whom ventricular function is well maintained benefit from treatment with calcium channel blockers. Beta-blockers are

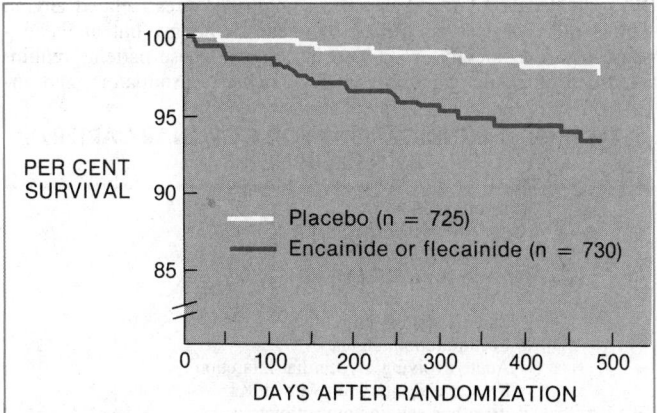

FIGURE 41–11. Survival among 1455 patients randomly assigned to treatment with encainide or flecainide compared with those assigned to placebo calculated with respect to death attributable to arrhythmia or cardiac arrest. (Reprinted by permission of The New England Journal of Medicine. Adapted from Cardiac Arrhythmia Suppression Trial Investigators: N Engl J Med 321:406, 1989.)

more likely to improve survival after Q-wave infarction; aspirin is indicated in both groups.

THE OUTLOOK

Early mortality associated with acute myocardial infarction has declined dramatically over the past three decades. Before the advent of CCU's, hospital mortality was approximately 30%. Aggressive defibrillation reduced it by half. Protection of jeopardized ischemic myocardium and early pharmacologic coronary recanalization followed by mechanical revascularization when indicated have lowered mortality even further, to $\leq 5\%$ among patients ≤ 75 years of age with no contraindications to thrombolysis in whom treatment can be initiated within several hours after the onset of symptoms. Consolidating these gains requires close observation and management of patients throughout convalescence to recognize and prevent recurrent ischemia; retard progression of coronary artery disease; promptly recognize its occurrence; and supply vigorous medical, mechanical, and surgical intervention when required.

Bergmann SR: Positron emission tomography. *In* Gerson M (ed.): Cardiac Nuclear Medicine. New York, McGraw-Hill, 1990. *A comprehensive and elegant review addressing technology, instrumentation, applications in research, and utility in diagnosis.*

Braunwald E: Thirty-five years of progress in cardiovascular research. Circulation (Suppl III) 70:III-8, 1984. *Lucid and thorough articulation of the major conceptual themes and paradigms underlying treatment of acute myocardial infarction and their evolution during the modern era.*

The Cardiac Arrhythmia Suppression Trial Investigators: Preliminary report: Effect of encainide and flecainide on mortality in a randomized trial of arrhythmia suppression after myocardial infarction. N Engl J Med 321:406, 1989. *A noteworthy report of the unexpected adverse influences of type I_c antiarrhythmic agents when used to treat ventricular ectopy in asymptomatic patients who have sustained acute myocardial infarction.*

Collen D, Topol EJ, Tiefenbrunn AJ, et al.: Coronary thrombolysis with recombinant human tissue-type plasminogen activator: A prospective, randomized, placebo-controlled trial. Circulation 70:1012, 1984. *The initial study demonstrating effective coronary thrombolysis with sparing of fibrinogen in patients with acute myocardial infarction treated with tissue-type plasminogen activator produced by recombinant DNA technology.*

DeWood MA, Spores J, Notske R, et al.: Prevalence of total coronary occlusion during the early hours of transmural myocardial infarction. N Engl J Med 303:897, 1980. *Demonstration of the high incidence of occlusive coronary thrombi in patients studied angiographically soon after the onset of chest pain who have sustained acute Q-wave infarctions.*

Ellis AK, Little T, Masud Z, et al.: Early noninvasive detection of successful reperfusion in patients with acute myocardinal infarction. Circulation 78:1352, 1988. *A recent report demonstrating the value of macromolecular markers such as myoglobin in the detection of recanalization.*

Forrester JS, Litvack F, Grundfest W, et al.: A perspective of coronary disease seen through the arteries of living man. Circulation 75:505, 1987. *Angioscopic illustrations supporting the hypothesis that acute coronary syndromes are attributable to dynamic changes in complex atherosclerotic plaques with characteristic durations of thrombosis accounting for differences between the syndromes.*

Fry ETA, Sobel BE: Coronary thrombolysis. *In* Zipes DP, Rowlands DJ (eds.): Progress in Cardiology. Philadelphia, Lea & Febiger, 1990, p 199. *A recent review of the impact of coronary thrombolysis on acute myocardial infarction with extensive reference to clinical trials performed with diverse plasminogen activators.*

Geltman EM, Ehsani AA, Campbell MK, et al.: The influence of location and extent of myocardial infarction on long-term ventricular dysrhythmia and mortality. Circulation 60:805, 1979. *An investigation establishing the association between the extent of myocardial injury sustained and long-term morbidity and mortality after acute myocardial infarction.*

Gruppo Italiano per lo Studio della Streptochi-nasi nell'Infarto Miocardico (GISSI): Long-term effects of intravenous thrombolysis in acute myocardial infarction: Final report of the GISSI study. Lancet 2:871, 1987. *The pivotal report demonstrating improved survival after coronary thrombolysis in patients with acute myocardial infarction.*

Gunnar RM, Bourdillon PDV, Dixon DW, et al.: ACC/AHA guidelines for the early management of patients with acute myocardial infarction. J Am Coll Cardiol 16:249, 1990. *This task force report summarizes the rationale and accepted approaches to treatment of all aspects of acute myocardial infarction based on full understanding of pertinent pathophysiologic principles.*

The GUSTO Investigators: An international randomized trial comparing 4 thrombolytic strategies for acute myocardial infarction. N Engl J Med 329:673, 1993. *A critical review of the major advances in coronary thrombolysis that addresses minimization of untoward effects and maximization of prompt and sustained induction of patency in thrombotically occluded coronary arteries. Authorities highlight areas of rapidly evolving fundamental and clinical investigation, clarify the importance of conjunctive and adjunctive measures needed for optimal coronary thrombolysis, and summarize historical, mechanistic, and clinical aspects of coronary thrombolysis in depth.*

Kanovsky MS, Falcone RA, Dresden CA, et al.: Identification of patients with ventricular tachycardia after myocardial infarction: Signal-averaged electrocardiogram, Holter monitoring, and cardiac catheterization. Circulation 70:264, 1984. *Delineates the relationship between changes evident by high-resolution electrocardiography and the risk of ventricular tachycardia after acute myocardial infarction.*

Kennedy JW, Martin GV, Davis KB, et al.: The Western Washington intravenous streptokinase in acute myocardial infarction randomized trial. Circulation 77:345, 1988. *Report of a major clinical trial supporting the hypothesis that an open infarct-re-*

lated coronary artery is beneficial even if recanalization cannot be induced very early after the onset of symptoms.

Lindsay BD, Markham J, Schechtman KB, et al.: Identification of patients with sustained ventricular tachycardia by frequency analysis of signal-averaged electrocardiograms despite the presence of bundle branch block. Circulation 77:122, 1988. *Observations indicating that frequency-domain analysis of signal-averaged electrocardiograms provides information to predict risk of sustained ventricular tachycardia even when intraventricular conduction abnormalities are present.*

Marcus FI, Cobb LA, Edwards JE, et al.: Mechanism of death and prevalence of myocardial ischemic symptoms in the terminal event after acute myocardial infarction. Am J Cardiol 61:8, 1988. *The prominence of arrhythmia as a cause of death late after acute myocardial infarction is underscored by these findings from a longitudinal study of survivors of acute myocardial infarction.*

Maroko PR, Kjekshus JK, Sobel BE, et al.: Factors influencing infarct size following experimental coronary artery occlusions. Circulation 43:67, 1971. *Laboratory observations demonstrating that myocardial infarction is a dynamic process favorably modified by reducing myocardial oxygen requirements.*

Puleo PR, Perryman B, Bresser MA, et al.: Creatine kinase isoform analysis in the detection and assessment of thrombolysis in man. Circulation 75:1162, 1987. *The value of assay of creatine kinase isoforms in plasma for early detection of recanalization induced by fibrinolytic agents is demonstrated.*

Roberts R, Croft C, Gold HK, et al.: Effect of propranolol on myocardial infarct size in a randomized blinded multicenter trial. N Engl J Med 311:218, 1984. *Despite favorable effects in experimental animals, reducing myocardial oxygen requirements in victims of acute myocardial infarction does not appear to reduce the extent of necrosis judging from results of this large-scale randomized multicenter study.*

Seacord LM, Abendschein DR, Nohara R, et al.: Detection of reperfusion within 1 hour after coronary recanalization by analysis of isoforms of the MM creatine kinase isoenzyme in plasma. Fibrinolysis 2:151, 1988. *A report demonstrating that serial assay of plasma creatine kinase isoforms permits very prompt detection of coronary recanalization.*

Sobel BE (ed.): Coronary thrombolysis. Review in depth. Coronary Artery Dis 1:1, 1990. *A review with components from Collen and Lijnen, Sheehan, Ohman and Califf, Guerci, and Muller and Topol addressing features of first- and second-generation fibrinolytic drugs, similarities and differences between the two, and mechanisms responsible for both.*

Sobel BE, Collen D (eds.). Coronary Thrombolysis in Perspective. Principles Underlying Conjuntive and Adjunctive Therapy. New York, Marcel Dekker, 1993. *This long-awaited prospective trial comparing fibrin-selective and nonselective thrombolytic agents (t-PA compared with streptokinase) demonstrated definitively that using a clot-selective agent with intravenous heparin and aspirin was associated with a lower mortality and higher net clinical benefit (survival without disabling stroke) compared with using a nonselective agent alone with subcutaneous or intravenous heparin and aspirin or in combination with t-PA.*

Tiefenbrunn AJ, Sobel BE: The impact of coronary thrombolysis on myocardial infarction. Fibrinolysis 3:1, 1989. *A review of pathophysiologic mechanisms, principles underlying treatment with plasminogen activators, and benefits resulting from early coronary thrombolysis.*

The TIMI Study Group: Comparison of invasive and conservative strategies after treatment with intravenous tissue plasminogen activator in acute myocardial infarction: Results of the thrombolysis in myocardial infarction (TIMI) phase II trial. N Engl J Med 320:618, 1989. *A definitive report from a large number of centers comparing survival after coronary thrombolysis with that following obligatory early angiography and demonstrating the advantages of a conservative strategy focusing on thrombolysis alone.*

Topol EJ, Califf RM, George BS, et al.: A randomized trial of immediate versus delayed elective angioplasty after intravenous tissue plasminogen activator in acute myocardial infarction. N Engl J Med 317:581, 1987. *Lack of benefit of immediate angioplasty after coronary thrombolysis was demonstrated initially in this important trial.*

Woods KL, Fletcher S, Roffe C, et al.: Intravenous magnesium sulphate in suspected acute myocardial infarction: Results of the second Leicester Intravenous Magnesium Intervention Trial (LIMIT-2). Lancet 339:1553, 1992. *Using magnesium to treat patients with heart disease has been advocated intermittently over many decades. Recently, objective information demonstrated benefit attributable not only to improved electrophysiologic stability of the heart but also to protection of myocardium. Results in this study provide strong support for treatment with magnesium in patients with acute myocardial infarction.*

41.3 Surgical Treatment of Coronary Artery Disease

Lawrence H. Cohn

Surgical treatment of coronary heart disease by coronary artery bypass grafting (CABG) is an important therapy for patients with acute and chronic syndromes of ischemic heart disease. Despite the enormous advances in interventional cardiology, thrombolytic therapy, and pharmacologic therapy of patients with coronary heart disease, surgical therapy continues to be the most comprehensive and totally flexible method of direct reperfusion of the ischemic human myocardium. In 1993 approximately 300,000 patients underwent CABG for one of many indications of acute and chronic myocardial ischemia. Balloon angioplasty (percutaneous transluminal coronary angioplasty [PTCA]) is now generally indicated for less severe anatomic manifestations of obstructed coronary lesions for single-vessel disease but is used in some patients with more than one coronary lesion, especially two-vessel disease. CABG, however, continues to be the treatment of choice for severe multivessel coronary disease, especially left main coronary obstruction and particularly in those patients with decreased left ventricular function.

The wide spectrum of patients who now undergo CABG contrasts sharply with the carefully selected patients with single-vessel disease first operated upon in 1967 by Favaloro and his colleagues, although a few isolated cases had been done earlier by Sabiston and Debakey. Patients considered for CABG today tend to be considerably older and more acutely ill and have more advanced diffuse arterial disease and more left ventricular dysfunction than in previous decades. The number of patients with acute myocardial ischemic syndromes who require operation has increased dramatically. These latter patients were seldom considered candidates for surgery when the operation was first introduced, but now CABG has become an integral part of the overall strategy of treating patients with unstable angina and acute evolving myocardial infarction either primarily or after failure. The increasingly wide spectrum of operative indications requires considerable ingenuity, better operative techniques including coronary bypass conduits, markedly improved myocardial protection, and more sophisticated techniques for life support during and after surgery.

INDICATIONS FOR CORONARY BYPASS SURGERY

In general, the patients selected for CABG should be those who have failed intensive medical therapy for treating chronic angina or acute myocardial ischemia and who, by demonstration on coronary arteriography, have one or more significant lesions >70% luminal diameter in the coronary arterial system. With exercise testing, radionuclear ventriculography, and coronary arteriography, the patient's diseased coronary arteries and the impact on his/her cardiac function can be completely evaluated. In addition, patients to undergo CABG should not have other life-threatening comorbidities. Table 41–14 lists clinical indications for CABG.

SILENT ISCHEMIA. Patients with "silent" ischemia are those with exercise electrocardiogram (ECG) evidence of ischemia with documented coronary arterial obstruction who have no anginal symptoms. These patients may present with an episode of "sudden death" after physical exertion. Considerable controversy has arisen about the logistics required to identify these patients and whether or not a positive exercise tolerance test alone should be indication for angiography and coronary bypass. Data now suggest that those with severe hemodynamic alterations during or after exercise testing and with multivessel disease are especially good candidates for CABG in this setting.

CHRONIC STABLE ANGINA. This is the largest group of patients considered for CABG. These patients, predominantly men in the sixth decade of life, have effort angina or stress-related angina that is more or less controlled by medical therapy but at the expense of a considerable reduction in activity. These patients require intense β blockade, calcium channel blockers, vasodilators, and an-

TABLE 41–14. INDICATIONS FOR CORONARY ARTERY BYPASS SURGERY

Chronic ischemia
  "Silent" ischemia
  Chronic stable angina
Acute myocardial ischemia
  Unstable angina
  Subendocardial infarction
  Postinfarction angina
  Acute evolving myocardial infarction
  Myocardial infarction with shock
With other cardiac operations
  Valve surgery
  Mechanical sequelae of myocardial infarction
    Ventricular septal defect
    Ruptured septal defect
    Left ventricular aneurysm

tiplatelet aggregation agents, which may produce a considerable number of untoward effects. Arteriography of patients in this category usually shows at least two- but most commonly three-vessel coronary artery disease. They may have normal left ventricular function but often have reduced function, especially as measured by the left ventricular ejection fraction, owing to prior myocardial infarction(s). Occasionally, CABG may be considered for a patient with single-vessel disease who is symptomatic despite medical treatment, who is not a candidate for or who has failed angioplasty, and whose single diseased coronary artery is unusually large and dominant.

UNSTABLE ANGINA. Unstable angina refers to a condition of accelerated anginal patterns not controllable by the usual medical therapy; this includes rest angina, nocturnal angina, or continuous anginal pain with ECG abnormalities indicating ischemia but not infarction, and requiring intensive therapy in a coronary care unit. Patients with unstable angina should be stabilized, if possible, by intravenous vasodilators such as nitroglycerin and adjunctive heparin. In the severest cases these patients may require intra-aortic balloon support pump for the stabilization of hemodynamics, relief of anginal symptoms, and amelioration of ECG abnormalities. A national prospective randomized study in the 1970's showed that stabilizing patients prior to bypass surgery is far preferable to operating on patients in a truly unstable condition. By decreasing left ventricular myocardial oxygen consumption with intensive β blockade and vasodilation, operative mortality is similar to that in the elective patient when patients are operated upon with this syndrome after stabilization.

SUBENDOCARDIAL INFARCTION. The patient with a subendocardial myocardial infarction has a small leak of myocardial enzymes not associated with a Q-wave infarction on ECG. Clinically, these patients are very similar in presentation to patients with unstable angina. The angiographic patterns of obstructive disease are the same as those of unstable angina, and patients are considered for operation with the same degree of aggressiveness as are patients with unstable angina, provided that they are otherwise good candidates for surgery.

EVOLVING MYOCARDIAL INFARCTION. Patients with evolving myocardial infarction present in the throes of a myocardial infarction, with pain and unstable ECG findings, usually from occlusion of the anterior descending artery, and are considered for operation when circumstances allow operation within 6 hours of the onset of chest pain. A number of cardiac centers with excellent logistic set-ups have performed large numbers of operations in these patients with excellent results and reduction or prevention of myocardial necrosis. These large studies evolved from earlier anecdotal experiences with patients who had sustained an acute coronary occlusion in the cardiac catheterization laboratory, who underwent a CABG, and were prevented from sustaining a major myocardial infarction. The patients currently candidates for CABG for an evolving myocardial infarction usually have triple-vessel coronary disease; those with single-vessel disease are excellent candidates for thrombolytic therapy and/or PTCA.

POSTINFARCTION ANGINA. Postinfarction angina is an important clinical syndrome that occurs in patients who have had a transmural myocardial infarction but in whom additional myocardium is threatened by extension in the area of the infarction or in a new area of ischemia. A major advance in the therapy of coronary heart disease has been the aggressive treatment by CABG of this syndrome, which may occur within hours to days of the completed myocardial infarction. Results of surgery for this syndrome are similar to those for unstable angina, provided that the patient is not in shock preoperatively.

MYOCARDIAL INFARCTION WITH CARDIOGENIC SHOCK. In this group of patients, CABG is performed after suffering an occlusion of a coronary artery which has produced a major infarct of the left ventricle, involving at least 40% of left ventricular volume. This syndrome often leads to sudden death, but in some instances, by support with appropriate pharmacologic (including thrombolytic agents) and mechanical devices, the patients are stabilized to be considered for emergency CABG. Carefully evaluating the residual left ventricular function in nonischemic areas and the anatomy of the distal coronary vessels is critical in these patients because patients with poor residual myocardial function or poor distal vessels do not do well after CABG preoperative shock. This

treatment has best results in patients previously in good health and generally in the younger age group. Operative mortality in the best of centers is about 25 to 30%.

CORONARY BYPASS WITH OTHER CARDIAC OPERATIONS. When a mechanical abnormality is associated with a myocardial infarction requiring operation, coronary bypass is often adjunctively done. These "conditions" include infarction ventricular septal defect, ruptured or dysfunctional papillary muscle that produces mitral regurgitation, left ventricular aneurysm, pseudoaneurysm, or left ventricular rupture. These sequelae of a transmural myocardial infarction may occur days to weeks following the original infarction and are often associated with multiple-vessel coronary disease requiring CABG.

In cardiac valve disease, a high percentage of patients in the adult population, especially the elderly with aortic valve disease, have coexistent coronary artery lesions. These patients require a concomitant coronary bypass operation because of the increased demand for coronary blood flow to the left ventricular myocardium imposed by the hemodynamic burden produced by the valve lesion. In some series of patients operated upon for aortic valve disease, 30 to 40% of the patients require concomitant CABG. The long-term outlook for patients with valve disease and coronary disease, despite the fact that the coronary disease may be grafted completely, is not as satisfactory as for those who have valve disease without concomitant coronary artery disease. In the workup of any adult patient for valvular heart surgery over age 40, coronary arteriography is indicated.

ANATOMIC INDICATIONS FOR CORONARY ARTERY BYPASS GRAFTING. There are anatomic indications for CABG regardless of symptoms or clinical syndrome. Severe occlusive lesion of the left main coronary artery of >70% diameter is an indication for immediate surgery, regardless of the severity of the patient's clinical symptoms. Similarly, acute failure of a coronary angioplasty of any vessel may require emergency CABG, either because of failure to improve the lesion over subsequent dilations or because a failed angioplasty may result in an acute myocardial infarction and cardiogenic shock.

BASIS OF SURGICAL TREATMENT OF CORONARY HEART DISEASE

The basis of the surgical treatment of coronary arterial disease is the "vascular bypass" principle, which has been used for many decades to treat ischemic problems in many arterial beds, including aortofemoral, renal artery, distal femoral-tibial, and cerebral circulations. In the coronary bypass operation, a conduit is sutured distal to the obstructing lesion in the artery and then connected proximally to either the aorta or naturally by *in situ* connection such as the internal thoracic artery to the subclavian artery. CABG uses only autogenous conduits because artificial grafts, at the present time, have not been developed to the point that they are satisfactory to maintain long-term patency in 1- to 2-mm coronary arteries. Cryopreserved homograft veins and glutaraldehyde heterograft vessels (cow, pig) are very rarely used in desperate situations. The reversed autogenous saphenous vein graft continues to be a reliable and flexible conduit for coronary bypass. The best readily available conduit is the internal thoracic (mammary) artery, which runs under the chest wall bilaterally, supplying blood to the chest wall and breast. These arteries may be dissected off the chest wall and used as a conduit to a coronary artery beyond the blockage, particularly the left anterior descending coronary artery. The advantages of this conduit are a better size relationship to the coronary artery into which it is anatamosed, its natural *in situ* connection to the subclavian artery obviating a proximal anastomosis, and the major clinical advantage of significantly improved long-term patency over that of any other conduit, thus reducing the need for reoperation postoperatively. It is the bypass graft of choice, particularly for the left anterior descending coronary artery. More recently, the right internal thoracic artery, the right gastroepiploic artery, and even the radial artery have been used for autogenous arterial conduits for coronary bypass surgery.

Operations are performed on cardiopulmonary bypass with moderate systemic hypothermia and using cardioplegic solutions administered both in the ascending aorta (antegrade) and in the coronary sinus (retrograde) to render the heart totally flaccid and motionless, markedly reducing myocardial energy requirements while performing these precise anastomoses. Hemodilution and other blood salvage techniques to minimize blood loss and avoid blood transfusions are extensively used.

Over the quarter century that CABG has been performed several facts have become clear. Complete revascularization—placing a graft beyond every major significant coronary arterial stenosis—yields significantly better long-term survival and freedom from cardiac events than incomplete revascularization. Thus, in the average patient with multivessel coronary artery disease who undergoes coronary bypass, at least three to four bypass grafts are common.

The surgical mortality after coronary bypass surgery varies with the acuity of the presenting clinical syndromes, the state of left ventricular function, size and diffuseness of the coronary artery disease, and patient comorbidities. The operative mortality of coronary bypass in a multivessel CABG in the younger age group, <60, with good left ventricular function is about 1%. In acute ischemic syndromes, operative mortality may vary from 2 to 25%, depending upon whether the indication is postinfarction angina with a normal ventricle or acute myocardial infarction with cardiogenic shock. Operative mortality in patients older than 70, particularly women, and those operated upon for acute ischemic events have an increased operative risk. The rates of ventilator dependency, stroke, and other organ system complication are higher in the older age group undergoing CABG. Although older patients tolerate elective CABG exceedingly well, if this age group presents with acute ischemic syndromes, there is a significant increase in operative mortality.

Postoperative care of the CABG patient consists of managing all organ subsystems including renal, pulmonary, cerebral, and general metabolic functions. Low cardiac output following cardiac surgery is monitored by cardiac output, pulmonary vascular resistance, and left and right ventricular filling pressures. Acute atrial fibrillation is common postoperatively despite prophylaxis, occurring in about 30% of patients. Perioperative myocardial infarction diagnosed either by new ECG Q waves or significant CK enzyme leak occurs between 2 and 5% of the time. Postoperative antiplatelet therapy is important and includes daily aspirin to prevent platelet "stickiness" in the grafts. One of the major morbid factors associated with patients undergoing CABG is stroke. Stroke rate in the previous decade has been about 7% in the over-70 group undergoing CABG, and it has now been attenuated by paying very close attention to atherosclerotic changes in the ascending aorta using Doppler echo (see Ch. 22) frequently to diagnose aortic pathology. The use of a single aortic cross-clamp during the anastomoses to prevent a showering of platelet emboli to the brain is now considered preferable. Using these techniques of aortic diagnosis and decreased handling, the stroke rate is now <2%.

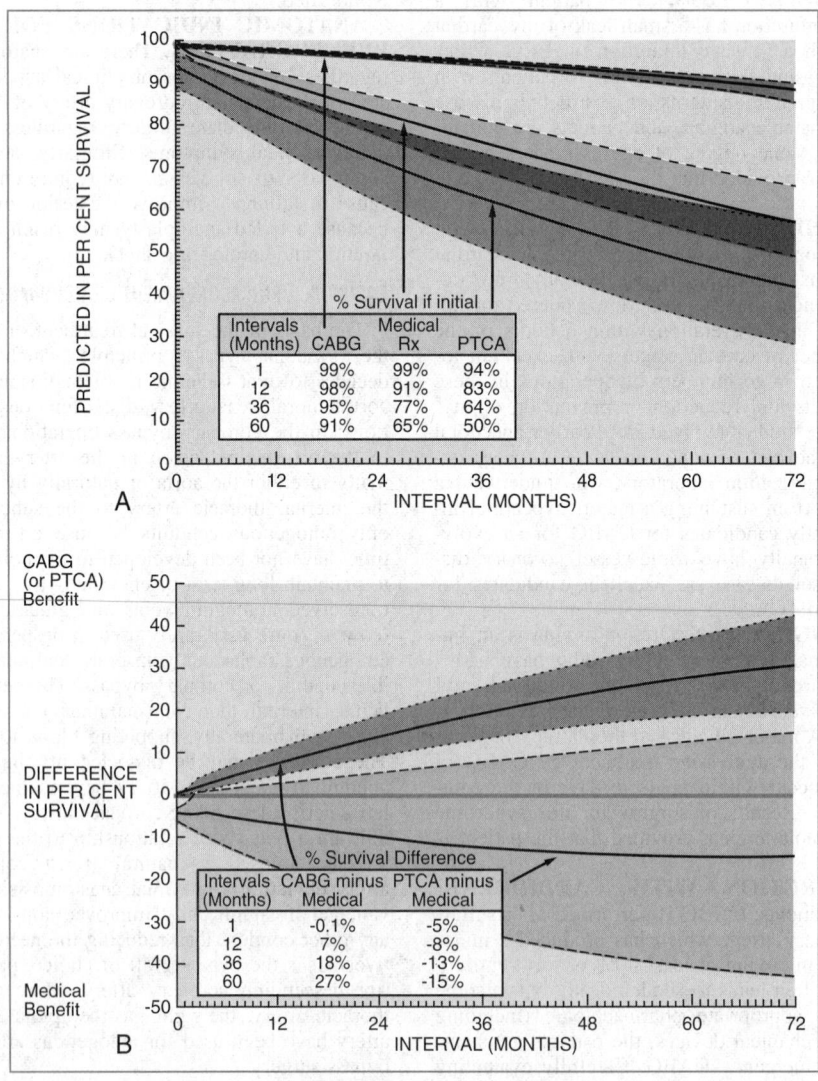

FIGURE 41-12. Nomogram depicting the predicted patient-specific comparative benefit of the coronary artery bypass (CABG) operation, using the internal thoracic (mammary) artery to left anterior descending coronary artery (and of coronary angioplasty [PTCA]) compared with initial medical treatment in a 65-year-old man with three-vessel coronary disease showing predicted percent survival in *A* and comparative benefit in *B*. (From Kirklin JW, et al.: ACC/AHA Task Force Report. J Am Coll Cardiol 17:543, 1991. Reprinted with permission from the American College of Cardiology.)

Coronary bypass surgery is palliative. Unless the atheromatous coronary disease is controlled biochemically, symptoms may recur as a result of progression of native disease and/or disease in the bypass grafts, and reoperation may be required. Increased use of the internal thoracic artery bypass graft to at least the left anterior descending artery delays reoperation significantly. Indications for reoperative CABG are similar to primary operative indications, but ischemia should be well documented prior to undertaking reoperations because the risk is somewhat higher, about 5 to 8%, and the benefits to be gained are somewhat less than with primary operation. Operative risk is higher owing to the possibility of myocardial ischemia from manipulating partially obstructed atheromatous grafts and the increased risk of bleeding from adhesions. Currently utilizing a "no touch" technique with early onset of femerofemoral cardiopulmonary bypass and improved retrograde cardioplegia myocardial protection, the risk of reoperative surgery has now decreased to that of almost primary operations.

LATE RESULTS OF CORONARY BYPASS SURGERY

The current operative mortality has stabilized at 2 to 5% despite the increased number of aged patients, complexity of disease, numbers of reoperations, left ventricular dysfunction, and extension of the operation to almost all forms of acute myocardial ischemia. The probability of long-term survival and prevention of late cardiac events is also related to the function of the left ventricle, complete revascularization, type of conduits used (internal thoracic arteries versus saphenous veins), and to some extent patient rehabilitation. In general, the 5-year late survival of patients with multivessel disease completely revascularized is 90 to 95% and the 10-year survival is 85 to 90% (Fig. 41–12). The long-term graft patency is clearly better with an internal thoracic artery than with a saphenous vein (95% versus 75 to 80% at 5 years). In the long term, it is now clear that patients with left main coronary stenosis or with severe triple-vessel disease and perhaps some form of two-vessel disease have improved survival and protection from cardiac events over similar medical patients analyzed in both prospective randomized studies and retrospective studies. Effects on ventricular function are less easy to document, but it is apparent that the ischemic or "stunned" myocardium may show significant improvements in left ventricular function after CABG, and moreover CABG may prevent further deterioration of function in the severely dysfunctional left ventricle.

American College of Cardiology/American Heart Association: Guidelines and Indications for Coronary Artery Bypass Graft Surgery. A report of the American College of Cardiology/American Heart Association Task Force on Assessment of Diagnostic and Therapeutic Cardiovascular Procedures (Subcommittee on Coronary Artery Bypass), J Am Coll Cardiol 17:543, 1991. *A multispecialty, multiorganizational compendium of the most current guidelines for performing coronary artery bypass graft surgery. Summarizes medical and surgical literature into 50 comprehensive and authoritative pages of indications for this important operation.*

Beyersdorf F, Mitrev Z, Sarai K, et al.: Changing patterns of patients undergoing emergency surgical revascularization for acute coronary occlusion. J Thorac Cardiovasc Surg 106:137, 1993. *Analyzes the changes over time of the patient undergoing emergency coronary bypass for acute coronary occlusion, documenting that these patients are older and have more extensive disease, more preoperative cardiogenic shock, and previous infarctions. Despite this increase in patient morbidity, the hospital mortality decreases owing to maximal protection of the ischemic and remote myocardium.*

Califf RM, Harrell FE, Lee KL, et al.: The evolution of medical and surgical therapy for coronary artery disease. JAMA 261:2077, 1989. *A 15-year perspective on evolution of medical and surgical treatment, indicating that surgical treatment, particularly in the last decade, has produced markedly improved early and late survival over that with medical therapy because of newer revascularization techniques and better myocardial protection.*

Cohn LH: Surgical treatment of acute myocardial infarction. Cardiology 76:167, 1989. *A review of the various acute ischemic syndromes related to coronary occlusion and the results of both pure bypass surgery and surgery associated with the mechanical sequelae of myocardial infarction.*

Frye RL, Kronmal R, Schaff HV, et al.: Stroke in coronary artery bypass surgery: An analysis of the CASS experience. Int J Cardiol 36:213, 1992. *Stroke is the most important complication following coronary bypass surgery, and this is a large analysis of stroke patients in the coronary artery surgery registry study analyzed in this multicenter study.*

Loop FD, Bruce WL, Cosgrove DM, et al.: Influence of the internal-mammary-artery graft on 10-year survival and other cardiac events. N Engl J Med 314:1, 1986. *A long-term follow-up of patients treated with internal thoracic arteries versus those treated with only saphenous vein grafts for anterior descending coronary bypass. This is a classic, documenting a large, well followed-up series (including angiography) showing conclusively that the internal thoracic artery is the preferable conduit for coronary bypass surgery.*

42 VALVULAR HEART DISEASE
Charles E. Rackley

Recognizing a heart murmur on physical examination is the usual means of initially diagnosing valvular heart disease. Thus, the clinical examination remains important for detecting valvular heart disease, recognizing cardiac deterioration, and assessing follow-up status. The noninvasive technologies of electrocardiography, chest radiography, echocardiography, radionuclide angiography, and stress testing play an important role in assessing the impact of valvular heart disease on cardiac function and determining the timing of operative intervention. In recent years advances in echocardiography have resulted in more accurate assessment of valvular orifice size, and catheterization is reserved to confirm impressions and identify underlying coronary artery disease.

GENERAL APPROACH TO THE PATIENT WITH VALVULAR HEART DISEASE

HISTORY. The patient with valvular heart disease often recalls a history of a heart murmur, and therefore the first recognition of the murmur may be helpful in establishing the etiology. A heart murmur detected in early adulthood often suggests a congenital or rheumatic basis, whereas a murmur developed in later years is often due to the degenerative changes in valvular structure. The physician should carefully assess the patient's physical activities and note the initial onset of dyspnea or fatigue. Symptoms dictate the appropriate timing of noninvasive and invasive cardiac studies as well as the decision for surgical correction.

AORTIC STENOSIS

ETIOLOGY AND PATHOLOGY. Aortic stenosis (Table 42–1) can result from a congenital abnormality, rheumatic fever, or degeneration with calcification in the aging patient. A bicuspid valve is the most common congenital abnormality, and invariably a raphe in one of the cusps indicates failure of the commissure to develop. Rarely, a unicuspid valve can be present at birth. Although the bicuspid valve may not be initially stenotic, fibrosis and thickening lead eventually to a reduced orifice size with calcification. Rheumatic fever scars the leaflet margins, and eventually the commissures fuse and calcify. More than 50% of adults with aortic stenosis are found to have a bicuspid valve, but fibrosis and calcification may make it difficult to determine whether the valve is bicuspid or tricuspid. In the aging patient with degenerative aortic stenosis, calcium deposits usually develop in the sinuses and annulus, whereas the margins of the leaflets remain free.

In any of the conditions producing hemodynamic stenosis of the aortic valve, systolic hypertension in the ventricular chamber is compensated by concentric hypertrophy of the myocardial wall. As myocardial failure develops from depression of the contractile state, dilatation of the ventricle occurs. Myocardial oxygen consumption remains high owing to elevation of systolic pressure within the left ventricle and increase in left ventricular mass. Thus, significant aortic stenosis creates conditions in which high myocardial oxygen demands are inadequately supported by reduced oxygen supply, which leads to subendocardial ischemia. Eventually, with a decline in the inotropic state of the myocardium, the ventricle dilates and the ejection fraction is decreased below the normal range. Further elevation of the left ventricular end-diastolic pressure results in pulmonary venous hypertension. The increased myocardial oxygen demands in aortic stenosis with the underperfused subendocardial myocardium can produce arrhythmias, chest pain, and even sudden death. Adults may have coexistent coronary artery disease, which further contributes to myocardial ischemia.

CLINICAL FEATURES. Chest pain, syncope, and heart failure are the characteristic symptoms of aortic stenosis, even though a gradient across the valve can exist for years before the patient develops symptoms. Children with a severe gradient can suddenly develop symptoms, whereas in adults the increase in mortality occurs later in the course of the disease.

TABLE 42–1. AORTIC STENOSIS

Etiology	Physiology	Symptoms	Physical Examination	Electro-cardiogram	Chest	Echocar-diogram	Catheterization	Medical Therapy	Surgical Therapy
Congenital Rheumatic Degenerative	LV* pressure overload LV hypertrophy Decreased LV compliance	Chest pain Syncope Heart failure	Delayed arterial pulse wave Aortic thrill Diamond-shaped aortic area, left sternal border and apex	LV hypertrophy	Normal cardiac size Poststenotic dilatation of ascending aorta	Anatomy of aortic valve/calcium Number of cusps LV wall thickness Echo Doppler estimate of valvular gradient Valvular area	Valvular gradient LV function Valvular area Coronary anatomy Mitral lesions	Endocarditis prophylaxis	Symptoms Gradient > 50 mm Hg Valvular area < 0.8 cm²

* LV = left ventricular.

Chest discomfort is exertional and indistinguishable from that of ischemic heart disease. Approximately 50% of patients older than 40 with aortic stenosis have underlying coronary artery disease whether exertional chest pain is present or not. Syncope can be an initial symptom of aortic stenosis and is probably related to the same mechanism as the chest pain, that is, critical reduction in myocardial oxygen supply with increased demands. Arrhythmias due to myocardial ischemia can also contribute to syncope and sudden death. When aortic stenosis is found at autopsy, approximately 15% of the patients have died suddenly without previous symptoms.

Heart failure in aortic stenosis generally reduces life expectancy to less than 2 years, whereas patients with syncope or angina may survive, on the average, 2 to 5 years. With calcification of the aortic valve, hemolytic anemia due to destruction of red cells can develop; furthermore, patients with aortic stenosis have an increased incidence of gastrointestinal bleeding resulting from angiodysplasia. Finally, patients with aortic stenosis are susceptible to infective endocarditis.

PHYSICAL EXAMINATION. In aortic stenosis, the typical physical findings include a delay in the upstroke of the peripheral pulse, a diamond-shaped crescendo-decrescendo systolic murmur, and hypertrophy of the left ventricle. The peripheral pulse is diminished in amplitude, delayed in upstroke, and prolonged owing to sustained ejection across the aortic valve (pulsus tardus et parvus). The harsh murmur is often transmitted to the carotid vessels, and a palpable thrill develops with a substantial gradient across the aortic valve.

Because the contour of the heart does not become enlarged with concentric hypertrophy, abnormalities may not be visible on chest examination. When the ventricle dilates owing to myocardial failure, the impulse is displaced laterally and becomes more diffuse. Palpable systolic vibrations over the primary aortic area, with the patient in the sitting position during full expiration, often correlate with a gradient across the aortic valve of >40 mm Hg. An atrial (S₄) gallop is usually audible, and an ejection click may be heard along the left sternal border. The aortic second sound becomes diminished, except in calcific stenosis of the elderly, in whom the margins of the leaflets usually maintain their mobility. Fibrosis and fusion of the aortic leaflets may result in a single S₂ at the base. Mechanically or electrically prolonged left ventricular systole can create reverse splitting of S₂. The diamond-shaped ejection murmur develops after the first sound, peaks in mid- and late systole, and disappears before the second heart sound. The murmur is most intense over the aortic area and along the left sternal border, but in the elderly patient the musical quality of the murmur can sometimes be loudest at the apex. The intensity in the apical area can be confusing and may cause difficulty in distinguishing this murmur from that of mitral regurgitation. A faint diastolic blow is often audible along the left sternal border because the severely stenotic valve may have a mild degree of incompetence.

LABORATORY STUDIES. Electrocardiogram. Left ventricular hypertrophy is the most common finding on the electrocardiogram, with an increase in QRS amplitude and ST-T changes of a strain pattern. Left-axis deviation can develop as well as conduction disturbances and left bundle branch block. As the left ventricle becomes noncompliant, the left atrium may be enlarged with a negative P wave in lead V₁. Because of myocardial fibrosis, Q waves can develop in the precordial leads, but these, as well as the ST-T wave abnormalities, can be indistinguishable from underlying coronary artery disease.

Chest Radiograph. Cardiac size remains unchanged in the early phase of aortic stenosis because hypertrophy does not increase the cardiothoracic ratio. Poststenotic dilatation and prominence of the ascending aorta may be present. Heart failure enlarges the left ventricle and causes pulmonary congestion.

Echocardiogram. The echocardiogram can demonstrate thickening of the aortic leaflets, determine the number of leaflets, detect calcification of the valves, and estimate left ventricular wall thickness and function. Echocardiography can estimate the size of the aortic orifice, and the Doppler technique can assess accurately the systolic pressure gradient across the valve. Thus, available echocardiographic techniques can accurately detect and assess aortic stenosis (Fig. 42–1).

Cardiac Catheterization. The pressure gradient across the aortic valve can be accurately measured with simultaneous measurements of left ventricular and aortic pressures. A decline in car-

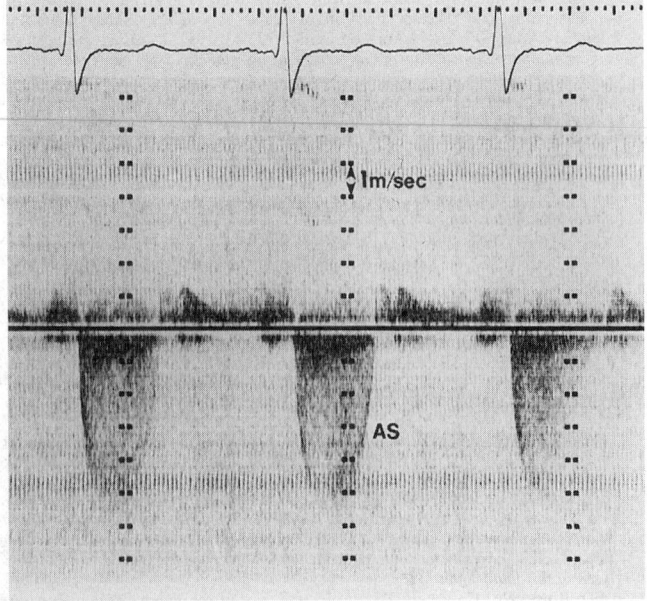

FIGURE 42–1. Continuous-wave Doppler recording from the ascending aorta in a patient with severe aortic stenosis. The peak velocity is approximately 5 meters per second. Using the modified Bernoulli equation, a peak instantaneous gradient across the aortic valve of 100 mm Hg can be calculated. Peak-to-peak gradient at catheterization was 80 mm Hg.

diac output is associated with a reduced pressure gradient across the valve, and the valvular area tends to be overestimated when the cardiac output is reduced and only the pressure gradient is analyzed.

The size of the normal aortic orifice is 2.5 to 3 sq cm, and mild stenosis develops when the orifice is reduced to 0.75 to 1.5 sq cm. Moderate stenosis is present when the valvular size is <0.75 sq cm and severe stenosis when the valvular area is <0.5 sq cm. Surgery is usually advised when the aortic valve gradient is >50 mm Hg or the valve area is <0.8 sq cm. Left ventricular angiography is helpful for determining the presence of mitral regurgitation. With the information available from echocardiography, cardiac catheterization may be primarily indicated for coronary arteriography because 50% of patients over age 40 have underlying coronary artery disease.

DIFFERENTIAL DIAGNOSIS. In children, valvular aortic stenosis has to be differentiated from congenital forms of both supravalvular and infravalvular lesions. In hypertrophic cardiomyopathy with obstruction, the systolic ejection murmur is similar to that of valvular aortic stenosis, but the peripheral pulse is hyperdynamic with a rapid upstroke and a double-notch or bisferious contour compared with the delayed upstroke observed in valvular stenosis. With rupture of the chordae or papillary muscle, acute mitral regurgitation may produce a harsh systolic murmur. This murmur can be transmitted to the left atrial wall and aorta, resulting in a palpable and audible "aortic" murmur. However, the murmur of acute mitral regurgitation transmitted into the aortic area is holosystolic rather than midsystolic. A systolic ejection murmur accompanies significant aortic regurgitation and is generally caused by turbulence of the large stroke volume across the aortic valve.

MEDICAL THERAPY. Prophylaxis with antibiotics is indicated for dental, genitourinary, and gastrointestinal procedures in the asymptomatic patient to reduce the likelihood of infective endocarditis. Prophylaxis should be routine throughout life in a patient with a stenotic or prosthetic valve (Table 42–2). If the patient with aortic stenosis develops a supraventricular tachycardia, digitalis and an antiarrhythmic drug may be necessary to slow the ventricular response. Chest pain warrants catheterization to evaluate underlying coronary artery disease, but the use of nitrates should be undertaken with great caution because arterial pressure may fall and further reduce coronary blood flow. Because life expectancy is reduced when aortic stenosis becomes symptomatic, chest pain, syncope, or heart failure warrants appropriate studies and consideration for surgery. Asymptomatic patients with hemodynamically significant aortic stenosis are at significant risk for cardiac events within 2 years and should be followed closely.

SURGICAL THERAPY. In children with aortic stenosis, surgery may be considered before symptoms develop. If the pressure gradient is high, valvuloplasty can sometimes be performed before calcification occurs. The operative mortality for aortic valve replacement is 2 to 3% and is <5% if coronary bypass surgery is also performed. A mechanical valve requires long-term coagulation, but the porcine valve can be used in older patients or in those in whom anticoagulation is contraindicated. Currently, the porcine valve usually lasts 10 years or longer in adults before it deteriorates, but it is not recommended in children or adolescents. If indicated, coronary bypass surgery should also be performed at the time of valve replacement. The 10-year survival of combined aortic valve replacement and coronary revascularization approaches 55%. Late cardiac events occur at a rate of approximately 6% per year

and include thromboembolic neurologic insults, myocardial infarction, congestive heart failure, endocarditis, bleeding, peripheral thromboembolism, and reoperation. Valvuloplasty is an option in severely ill or elderly patients, but the restenosis rate remains high.

AORTIC REGURGITATION

ETIOLOGY AND PATHOLOGY. Aortic regurgitation (Table 42–3) can be caused by disease conditions that render the aortic leaflets incompetent or affect the ascending aorta with dilatation of the annulus of the aortic valve. Rheumatic fever produces scarring and fibrosis of the valvular margins. Hypertension, as well as arteriosclerosis, can be associated with scarring of the aortic valve and mild incompetence. Congenital lesions, such as bicuspid aortic valve, are predominantly stenotic, but scarring and calcification can result in associated incompetence as well.

Conditions that affect the ascending aorta and produce valvular incompetence include syphilis, heritable disorders of connective tissue, arthritic diseases, and cystic medial necrosis of the aorta. Myxomatous degeneration of the aortic valve occurs in Marfan's syndrome. Ankylosing spondylitis, rheumatoid arthritis, and Reiter's syndrome are arthritic conditions that can cause aortic root dilatation and aortic cusp thickening. Cystic medial necrosis and aortic ectasia can produce extreme dilatation of the aorta with secondary aortic regurgitation. Acute aortic regurgitation can result from dissection of the aorta, valve perforation with infective endocarditis, sinus of Valsalva rupture, and mechanical complications of a prosthetic aortic valve.

PHYSIOLOGY. Although the end-diastolic pressure may be normal or slightly elevated in the early phases, progressive regurgitation dilates the chamber by myocardial fibers slippage and sarcomere replication with eventual hypertrophy and elevated left ventricle end-diastolic pressure. These compensatory mechanisms support a large left ventricular stroke volume, which is often achieved with an ejection fraction above 50%.

Systolic wall stress or afterload can be maintained within the normal range by hypertrophy of the myocardium, but myocardial oxygen demand is significantly increased. A progressive decline in aortic diastolic pressure due to regurgitation of blood into the left ventricle can reduce coronary blood flow in severe chronic aortic regurgitation and thus create conditions for subendocardial ischemia.

The gradual volume overload of chronic aortic regurgitation can be tolerated for years before the inotropic state of the myocardium deteriorates. Eventually, the declining ejection fraction and inotropic state, along with limits to the dilatation/hypertrophy mechanism, markedly elevate the left ventricular filling pressure with pulmonary venous capillary congestion.

Left ventricular hemodynamics in acute aortic regurgitation, compared with those in chronic aortic regurgitation, are immediately disturbed because the regurgitant volume may be imposed on a normal end-diastolic volume. Sudden incompetence of the aortic valve can severely elevate the left ventricular filling pressure because acute dilatation of the left ventricle is limited.

CLINICAL COURSE. Because the chronic volume overload of aortic regurgitation is well tolerated, patients may remain asymptomatic for long periods. The accelerated development of angina,

TABLE 42–2. ANTIBIOTIC PROPHYLAXIS IN AORTIC STENOSIS

Category	Drug	Dose and Route of Administration
Dental, oral, upper respiratory tract procedures		
Standard regimen in patients at risk (includes prosthetic valves and other high-risk patients)	Amoxicillin	3 grams amoxicillin 1 hour before and 1.5 grams 6 hours later
Allergic to amoxicillin/penicillin	Erythromycin or Clindamycin	Erythromycin ethylsuccinate 800 mg or erythromycin stearate 1 gram orally 2 hours before procedure and then 1/2 dose 6 hours later Clindamycin 300 mg orally 1 hour before procedure and 150 mg 6 hours later
Gastrointestinal and genitourinary tract procedures and instrumentation		
Most patients	Ampicillin and gentamicin	Ampicillin 2 grams IV plus gentamicin 1.5 mg/kg IV 30 minutes before procedure, followed by ampicillin 1.5 grams 6 hours later
Allergic to amoxicillin/ampicillin/penicillin	Vancomycin and gentamicin	Vancomycin 1 gram IV over 1 hour plus gentamicin 1.5 mg/kg IV 1 hour before procedure. May be repeated 8 hours later.

TABLE 42-3. AORTIC REGURGITATION

Etiology	Physiology	Symptoms	Physical Examination	Electro-cardiogram	Chest	Echocar-diogram	Catheterization	Medical Therapy	Surgical Therapy
Chronic									
Rheumatic fever Connective tissue disorders Hypertension, atherosclerosis Syphilis Cystic medial necrosis Aortic ectasia Cogenital heart disease	Chronic volume over-load LV* dilatation LV hypertrophy	Fatigue Dyspnea Edema	Wide arterial pulse pressure Enlarged LV Diastolic aortic murmur Systolic ejection murmur Third sound Apical diastolic rumble	LV hypertrophy and strain	Enlarged LV Dilated aorta	Valvular anatomy Aortic root size Enlarged LV Mitral valve fluttering LV function	Contrast from aorta to LV LV function	Preload and afterload reduction Diuretics Digitalis	LV systolic echo dimension > 55 mm Ejection fraction < 50%
Acute									
Endocarditis Aortic dissection Ruptured sinus of Valsalva Prosthetic valve	Acute LV diastolic pressure and volume overload	Pulmonary edema	Loud diastolic musical murmur Right and left sternal border radiation with thrill Soft S₁ and third sound Continuous murmur if rupture into right side of heart	LV strain	Pulmonary edema Normal heart size	Vavular anatomy Aortic size and intimal flap	Contrast from aorta to LV Aortic and intimal flap	Preload and afterload reduction	Urgent surgery

* LV = left ventricle or left ventricular.

heart failure, or sudden death within several years has been observed in patients with a pulse pressure > 140/40 mm Hg and left ventricular enlargement demonstrated on electrocardiography or chest radiograph. Dyspnea, orthopnea, and paroxysmal nocturnal dyspnea result from impaired left ventricular contractility and pulmonary venous hypertension. Chest pain is often associated with underlying coronary artery disease, and syncope is usually attended by arrhythmias.

With acute aortic regurgitation, pulmonary edema is often the presenting manifestation. Severe chest pain suggests aortic dissection when acute aortic incompetence develops.

PHYSICAL EXAMINATION. In aortic regurgitation, the physical findings reflect the large left ventricular stroke volume ejected into the systemic circulation and the rapid diastolic run-off into the left ventricle. The peripheral pulse is characteristically bounding, and additional manifestations of the wide pulse pressure include head bobbing, pulsing retinal arterioles, bounding carotid pulse, pistol shot sounds over the femoral arteries, a to-and-fro murmur elicited from the femoral artery with slight compression of the stethoscope, and capillary pulsations in the nail beds. Connective tissue and arthritic diseases that produce aortic regurgitation may create characteristic changes in habitus, such as the musculoskeletal type in Marfan's syndrome and kyphosis of the thoracic spine in ankylosing spondylitis.

The auscultatory hallmark is the high-pitched, blowing, decrescendo diastolic murmur heard best along the left sternal border during full expiration while the patient is in the sitting position. As the regurgitation becomes more severe, a diastolic rumble or Austin Flint murmur due to vibration of the anterior leaflet of the mitral valve in the regurgitant jet may be audible at the apex. If the ascending aorta is dilated, the diastolic murmur may be heard along the right sternal border as well.

With acute aortic regurgitation due to disruption of an aortic leaflet or dissection dilating the aortic annulus, the diastolic murmur may be harsh with palpable vibrations along the left sternal border. A perforated or prolapsed aortic leaflet, as well as the detached aortic intima from dissection, can generate prominent musical qualities in the diastolic murmur.

LABORATORY STUDIES. *Electrocardiogram.* The electrocardiogram typically reveals left ventricular hypertrophy with increased QRS voltage amplitude and ST-T wave changes of the strain pattern. With acute aortic regurgitation, the hypertrophy may be absent, and the ST-T wave changes can indicate myocardial ischemia.

Chest Radiography. Significant cardiomegaly usually attends chronic aortic regurgitation, with the increase in size due to dilatation of the left ventricle. The ascending aorta is often prominent. Left ventricular failure is accompanied by pulmonary congestion and venous prominence.

Echocardiogram. Echocardiography has become the most useful noninvasive tool to recognize anatomic abnormalities of the aortic valve and to assess dimensions of the annulus and ascending aorta. The intensity of the regurgitant flow can be appreciated by the vibrations of the anterior mitral leaflet, and the echo Doppler and color techniques can estimate the severity of the regurgitation. Left ventricular chamber dimensions and wall thickness permit calculation of end-diastolic volume and hypertrophy. Finally, an end-systolic dimension of 55 mm has been proposed by several investigators to represent the limit of surgically reversible dilatation of the left ventricle, so aortic valve replacement should be performed before this chamber size is exceeded.

Exercise Testing. Although exercise capacity can be measured and followed periodically in patients with aortic regurgitation, exercise testing is best clinically used in combination with radionuclide angiography. An exercise ejection reduced by ≥5% is considered by some an indication for surgery even in the absence of symptoms.

Cardiac Catheterization. The primary clinical indications for catheterization are recognition of coexisting lesions, such as mitral regurgitation, and detection of coronary artery disease.

DIFFERENTIAL DIAGNOSIS. In evaluating diastolic murmur along the left sternal border, aortic insufficiency is far more common than pulmonic insufficiency. The pulsatile characteristics of the peripheral circulation can be helpful in differentiating an aortic from a pulmonic origin of the diastolic murmur. In systemic hypertension, accentuated tambour qualities of the second heart sound can sometimes suggest mild aortic regurgitation, but the level of the diastolic blood pressure can be helpful in distinguishing incompetence from reverberations of the second sound. Any condition that causes aortic stenosis through immobility of the valve leaflets is often accompanied by some degree of aortic regurgitation.

MEDICAL THERAPY. Antibiotic prophylaxis is indicated to prevent endocarditis. When symptoms of heart failure develop, vasodilating agents such as hydralazine and angiotensin-converting enzyme (ACE) inhibitors may be beneficial, but benefits are rarely maintained. Thus, using digitalis, diuretics, and afterload-reducing agents is primarily of short-term benefit in aortic regurgitation.

SURGICAL THERAPY. The echocardiographic dimensions and evidence of reduced left ventricular function are now being used to advise valve replacement before symptoms of heart failure are manifested. Even after heart failure has developed, patients still improve clinically after aortic valve replacement. Valve replacement can be undertaken with a mortality of <3 to 5%. The type of prosthetic valve depends on the patient's age and the ability to be anticoagulated. In aortic dissection, there may also be replacement of the ascending aorta because acute regurgitation requires intervention.

MITRAL STENOSIS

ETIOLOGY AND PATHOLOGY. Rheumatic fever remains the predominant cause for mitral stenosis (Table 42–4). Calcification of the mitral valve annulus in the elderly patient can occasionally cause hemodynamic obstruction. Space-occupying lesions, such as left atrial myxoma, or thrombus formation can rarely obstruct the mitral valve. The characteristic pathologic change in rheumatic fever is fibrosis and scarring, particularly at the margins of the valve. Pulmonary venous hypertension causes thickening of the pulmonary veins and capillaries with eventual intimal and medial proliferation of the pulmonary arteries. With longstanding mitral stenosis and pulmonary hypertension, right ventricular hypertrophy and fibrosis develop.

PHYSIOLOGY. The hemodynamic abnormalities in mitral stenosis result from obstructed diastolic blood flow into the left ventricle. The normal cross-sectional area of the mitral valve ranges from 4 to 6 sq cm, and turbulence of diastolic blood flow occurs when the valvular orifice is reduced below 2 sq cm. Increased demands for cardiac output, such as exercise or fever, may be necessary to produce the diastolic murmur when the mitral valve orifice is as small as 1.5 to 2 sq cm. In the second stage of progressive reduction in the mitral orifice size, a diastolic gradient develops between the left atrium and left ventricle under resting conditions when the valvular area is 1 to 1.5 sq cm. In the advanced stage, mitral orifice size is <1 sq cm, and left atrial and pulmonary hypertension becomes significant. The pulmonary capillary pressure often exceeds 20 to 25 mm Hg, and this leads to significant pulmonary arterial hypertension, pressure overload on the right ventricle, and compensatory hypertrophy of the right ventricle. Another hemodynamic complication in chronic mitral stenosis is atrial fibrillation due to left atrial enlargement. A rapid ventricular rate can aggravate hemodynamic abnormalities by reducing the diastolic filling period and leading to further elevation of pressure in the lungs.

CLINICAL FEATURES. Rheumatic fever occurs on average at age 10 to 12, and generally there is a 10-year period before the murmur of mitral stenosis can be detected. Mitral stenosis affects women more than men, and symptoms usually develop between ages 25 and 30. Dyspnea is the most common symptom secondary

to pulmonary venous hypertension and can be precipitated by any circumstance that increases cardiac output, such as exercise or febrile conditions. Paroxysmal atrial fibrillation can precipitate symptoms by increasing the ventricular rate. As the stenosis progresses, patients experience symptoms with minimal effort or at rest.

Systemic embolization resulting from underlying atrial fibrillation and left atrial thrombus development can also be a manifestation of mitral stenosis. Women can become symptomatic in the second trimester of pregnancy, when the blood volume increases significantly and elevates pulmonary pressures. With severe enlargement of the left atrium and infringement on the mainstream bronchus, persistent cough may develop. Hemoptysis can result from rupture of small vessels in the bronchi due to longstanding venous hypertension.

PHYSICAL EXAMINATION. The classic physical findings of mitral stenosis are an accentuated first sound at the apex, an opening snap, and a diastolic rumble. Patients may display typical "mitral facies" with florid congestion of the cheeks. Distended neck veins indicate right ventricular failure with secondary tricuspid regurgitation. If tricuspid stenosis coexists with mitral stenosis, a prominent α wave may be observed in the jugular vein.

Inspecting the precordium may reveal activity along the left sternal border, indicating right ventricular enlargement and pulmonary hypertension. On palpation, the accentuated first sound, the opening snap, and the diastolic rumble can sometimes be felt at the apex. With significant right ventricular dilatation, the left ventricular apical impulse may be displaced laterally, and the right cardiac border may be percussed to the right of the sternum. The higher the left atrial pressure, the closer the opening snap to the second heart sound (S_2), and thus the S_2–opening snap interval indicates the severity of the mitral stenosis. The opening snap is a high-pitched sound and is heard best with the patient in the left lateral decubitus position. The diastolic rumble at the apex is a low-pitched murmur following the opening snap. If sinus rhythm is present, there is presystolic accentuation due to atrial contraction. Because the murmur of mitral stenosis may be faint in the early stages, to complete the physical examination, a complete examination should include mild exercise to increase heart rate and intensify the diastolic rumble.

The diastolic murmur of pulmonic insufficiency should be sought along the left sternal border, but this can be difficult to distinguish from aortic regurgitation. A widened systemic pulse pressure favors aortic over pulmonic insufficiency with mitral stenosis. Rarely, tricuspid stenosis can simultaneously occur with the mitral stenosis. The murmur of tricuspid stenosis is heard along the lower left sternal border and is greatly accentuated with inspiration. Finally, some degree of mitral incompetence often accompanies mitral stenosis and produces an apical systolic murmur of varying intensity.

LABORATORY STUDIES. *Electrocardiogram.* The electrocardiographic changes of mitral stenosis include left atrial enlargement and right ventricular hypertrophy due to pulmonary hypertension. Characteristic notching and a prolonged P wave are most prominent in leads II, III, and aV_F. The terminal portion of the P wave is usually negative in lead V_1. Right-axis deviation and an increased amplitude of the R wave in V_1 are evidence of right ventricular hypertrophy.

TABLE 42–4. MITRAL STENOSIS

Etiology	Physiology	Symptoms	Physical Examination	Electro-cardiogram	Chest	Echocardiogram	Catheterization	Medical Therapy	Surgical Therapy
Rheumatic Myxoma Calcification Congenital	Pressure overload LA* and pulmonary veins	Dyspnea Fatigue Palpitations Hemoptysis	Loud S₁ Opening snap Diastolic rumble Signs of pulmonary hypertension: RVH* ↑P₂ Diastolic blow	Broad, notched P wave in lead II	Enlarged LA Prominent pulmonary veins	Square wave of EF slope of mitral valve Estimation of gradient and orifice size	Elevated PA* wedge pressure and normal LV diastolic pressure	Dental prophylaxis Digitalis for atrial fibrillation Warfarin (Coumadin)	Symptoms Vavular area < 1.0 cm²

*LA = left atrium; RVH = right ventricular hypertrophy; PA = pulmonary arterial.

Chest Radiograph. Radiographic evidence of mitral stenosis includes left atrial enlargement, pulmonary venous hypertension, and right ventricular prominence. The enlarged left atrium produces a double contour along the right cardiac silhouette, as well as straightening of the left cardiac border due to the large left atrial appendage. This change elevates the left mainstem bronchus. The pulmonary venous hypertension redistributes the blood flow to the apices of the lungs, with a reduction in blood volume of the lower lung. Kerley's B lines due to fibrosis and lymphatic engorgement appear as transverse linear densities at the lung bases above the diaphragm.

Echocardiogram. The echocardiogram is the most accurate noninvasive technique for detecting mitral valve stenosis (Fig. 42–2) and is recognized by the characteristic square wave motion of the E-to-F slope of the valve during diastole. The concordant movement of anterior and posterior mitral valve leaflets is one of the cardinal echocardiographic findings in mitral stenosis. Calcification produces additional echoes from the stenotic valve. The two-dimensional echo can accurately measure the diastolic area of the mitral valve, and the echo Doppler technique can estimate the pressure gradient across the valve, as well as left atrial and left ventricular dimensions, and provide an assessment of left ventricular function. Transesophageal echo can identify thrombus or a myxoma in the left atrium.

Exercise Testing. Exercise testing can be useful in following the young patient with mitral stenosis during the early stages of the disease. The response of the heart rate to exertion and early symptoms of fatigue or dyspnea can be documented with an exercise test.

Cardiac Catheterization. Hemodynamic confirmation of mitral stenosis requires measuring the diastolic pressure gradient across the mitral valve. Left atrial pressure can be obtained directly through trans-septal puncture or as reflected in the pulmonary capillary wedge pressure and recorded simultaneously with the left ventricular pressure. The Gorlin formula (see Ch. 33.6) permits calculation of the mitral orifice size based on the diastolic flow derived from the forward cardiac output and the simultaneous pressure gradient across the valve. The mitral valve gradient can vary from 5 to 25 mm Hg. In an individual without symptoms, mitral valve area can range from 1.5 to 2.0 sq cm. In those exhibiting symptoms with usual activity, valvular size may be ≤ 1.5 sq cm, and patients with marked limitations usually have an orifice size < 1.0 sq cm. Sometimes, a minimal mitral valve gradient is obtained under resting circumstances, but exercise can markedly increase pulmonary pressures to the level of heart failure. At the time of catheterization,

associated valve lesions should be assessed, such as mitral regurgitation, aortic stenosis, and aortic regurgitation. If the patient is older than age 40, coronary arteriography should also be performed.

DIFFERENTIAL DIAGNOSIS. A left atrial myxoma can produce dyspnea or syncope with an opening snap and a diastolic rumble. Primary pulmonary hypertension in young women can be associated with dyspnea and an accentuated pulmonic second sound, but other auscultatory findings are lacking. An atrial septal defect can mimic mitral stenosis with an accentuated first sound, opening snap, and diastolic rumble. However, the accentuated first sound is due to tricuspid valve closure, the opening snap is a split pulmonic second sound, and the diastolic rumble is created by flow across the tricuspid valve.

MEDICAL THERAPY. Medical therapy is directed at reducing the recurrence of rheumatic fever, prophylaxis for infective endocarditis, control of atrial fibrillation with a rapid ventricular response, and anticoagulation for thromboembolic phenomena. The patient should continue on rheumatic fever prophylaxis until age 30.

Because atrial fibrillation can aggravate and precipitate symptoms of pulmonary congestion, digitalis, β blockers, or calcium blockers should be administered to control ventricular response. Anticoagulation on a chronic basis should be considered in all patients with mitral stenosis and atrial fibrillation. Pulmonary edema with atrial fibrillation is an indication for cardioversion. Ideally, the patient should be anticoagulated 2 weeks prior to elective cardioversion for atrial fibrillation. An antiarrhythmic agent should be started 2 days before the elective procedure, and if digitalis has been administered, this may be discontinued 1 day before the cardioversion. If cardioversion is successful, the patient should remain on long-term anticoagulation and an antiarrhythmic drug. For thromboembolic phenomena from the left atrium, anticoagulation is indicated. For acute embolism to the extremities or abdomen, surgical embolectomy may be beneficial.

Valvuloplasty via catheter is optional in selected patients with mitral stenosis, particularly in children, in young women desiring to become pregnant at a later date, and in the elderly at high surgical risk.

SURGICAL THERAPY. The decision to operate is based on symptoms of pulmonary congestion developing during activity or at rest. In addition to pulmonary congestion, recurrent atrial fibrillation with aggravation of pulmonary congestion, thromboembolic phenomena, and hemoptysis can be indications for surgery. Mitral commissurotomy remains the procedure of choice with a pliable mitral valve without calcification or mitral regurgitation and carries an operative mortality of < 1%. This procedure should be considered particularly for the young woman who wants to become pregnant. Sometimes commissurotomy can be performed before significant symptoms develop. Patients may benefit for 5 to 20 years after commissurotomy, but if symptoms occur at a later time, mitral valve replacement may be required. Mitral valve replacement carries an operative mortality rate of 2 to 3%. In a young woman, the type of mitral valve depends on her age as well as the circumstances for anticoagulation. The porcine valve can be inserted without the need for chronic anticoagulation but may require replacement after 10 years. If the valve is calcified or if the patient has had a previous commissurotomy, a prosthetic device is preferred. When there is a contraindication to anticoagulation, as in the aging patient, the porcine valve can be inserted.

Anticoagulation and antibiotic prophylaxis are required in patients with a prosthetic valve. If atrial fibrillation persists with a rapid ventricular response, an agent to slow atrioventricular (AV) conduction still must be administered. Long-term complications of prosthetic mitral valves, such as thrombus formation, infection, and mechanical dysfunction, are estimated to occur at a rate of 1 to 2% per year. Thromboembolism occurs at a rate of 3% per year with a mechanical mitral valve, whereas with the porcine valve, the incidence is 1 to 2% per year.

MITRAL REGURGITATION

ETIOLOGY AND PATHOLOGY. *Mitral valve prolapse* has now become the leading cause of mitral regurgitation (see next section). Coronary artery disease, annular calcification, connective tissue disorders, and any condition producing left ventricular dilatation can create incompetence of the mitral valve. Several congenital cardiac conditions, such as partial AV canal, corrected transposition of the great arteries, and isolated cleft of the mitral valve seen with

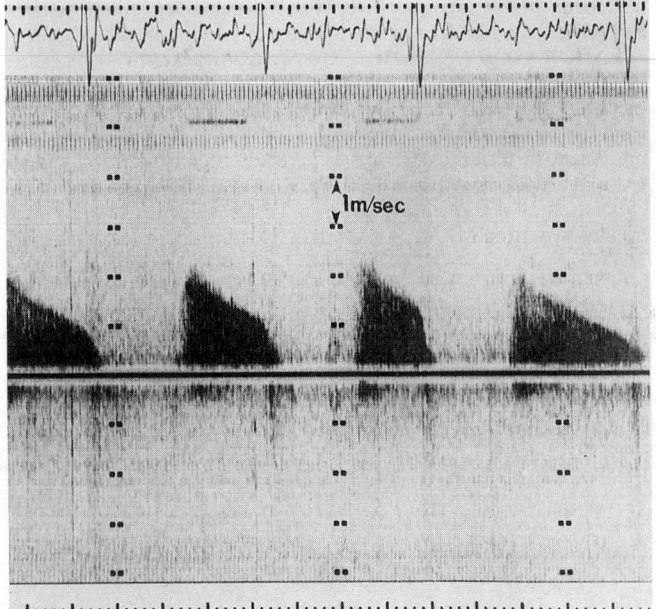

1m/sec

FIGURE 42–2. Continuous-wave Doppler echocardiogram of mitral valve flow in a patient with mitral stenosis and atrial fibrillation.

the ostium primum atrial septal defect, can be associated with mitral valve regurgitation.

Acute mitral regurgitation can result from sudden disruption of the normal function of the mitral valve apparatus. Ruptured mitral valve chordae from endocarditis, myxomatous degeneration of the valve, or trauma can produce sudden mitral regurgitation. Acute myocardial infarction can rupture the papillary muscle, and infective endocarditis can perforate the mitral valve leaflet or the chordae. Mechanical disturbances with a prosthetic mitral valve can lead to mitral incompetence.

PHYSIOLOGY. In chronic mitral regurgitation, a volume overload is imposed on the left ventricle, and the size of the regurgitant volume determines the increase in the end-diastolic volume. Systolic regurgitation into the left atrium produces a prominent v wave, which accentuates the normal filling of the left ventricle from the pulmonary venous inflow. With chronic mitral regurgitation, distensibility of the left atrium and pulmonary veins and increased compliant properties of the left ventricle permit rapid ventricular diastolic filling.

In *chronic mitral regurgitation,* the large total left ventricular stroke volume maintains the forward stroke volume despite the regurgitant volume into the left atrium. Eventually, the contractile properties of the left ventricular myocardium decline, and the end-systolic volume is abnormally increased. The ejection fraction declines, even though the value may remain near the normal range in the early stage of left ventricular decompensation. An increase in the end-systolic volume elevates the pressure and wall stress values beyond those that can be attributed solely to changes in wall thickness or hypertrophy. This situation has been designated a mismatch in afterload and preload.

In coronary artery disease, mitral regurgitation results from abnormalities of wall motion and papillary muscle function. Ischemia of the papillary muscle has been proposed as a mechanism, and disturbances in wall motion are usually present with mitral regurgitation. Severe dilatation of the left ventricle from either a primary volume overload or secondary myocardial decompensation eventually results in mitral regurgitation. Dilatation of the left ventricular chamber displaces the papillary muscles so that coaptation of the leaflets is impaired during systolic ejection.

In *acute mitral regurgitation,* a sudden pressure overload is imposed on the left atrium and pulmonary veins from the left ventricular regurgitant volume. This pressure overload is intensified by the inability of the left atrium and left ventricle to dilate suddenly and often produces pulmonary edema.

CLINICAL FEATURES. When mitral regurgitation results from primary defects in the mitral apparatus, significant enlargement of the left ventricle develops, but the patient may remain symptom-free with normal exercise tolerance. Because pulmonary venous hypertension and congestion are not early features of mitral regurgitation, fatigue due to reduced forward cardiac output is a more frequent symptom than dyspnea. Gradual impairment of the contractile state is attended by further enlargement of end-systolic and end-diastolic volumes and elevation of the left ventricular end-diastolic and left atrial pressures. Atrial fibrillation commonly develops when the left atrium enlarges and further aggravates heart failure.

In coronary artery disease, significant mitral regurgitation is usually accompanied by symptoms of impaired left ventricular function, such as dyspnea, fatigue, and orthopnea. This condition is sometimes designated the *ischemic cardiomyopathy syndrome.* In acute syndromes of mitral regurgitation, pulmonary edema is often the initial presentation because of the suddenly imposed pressure and volume overload on the left atrium and pulmonary venous system.

PHYSICAL EXAMINATION. The typical physical finding of mitral regurgitation is the apical holosystolic murmur, but the intensity, variation during the ejection phase, and radiation over the precordium are influenced by the underlying mechanism. The precordium may reveal a diffusely hyperdynamic impulse, and the first heart sound at the apex is diminished. The characteristic holosystolic murmur radiates into the axilla and often to the left sternal border. A protodiastolic or ventricular gallop sound is frequently audible and may be followed by an early diastolic rumble due to the large inflow of blood from the left atrium. When mitral regurgitation is caused by left ventricular dilatation and depression of the contractile state, the systolic murmur may be mid-, late, or holosystolic. Under these circumstances, the systolic murmur is usually

grade II/VI or less and is accompanied by a left ventricular (S_3) gallop sound.

In acute mitral regurgitation due to rupture of the mitral valve apparatus, the murmur is harsh, grade III or IV/VI, and accompanied by a palpable thrill at the apex.

LABORATORY STUDIES. *Electrocardiogram.* In chronic mitral regurgitation, the electrocardiogram shows evidence of left ventricular hypertrophy with increased QRS voltage and ST-T wave changes in the lateral precordial leads. Left atrial enlargement produces a negative P wave in lead V_1, but atrial fibrillation often develops in the late stages.

Chest Radiograph. Left ventricular enlargement due to the volume overload can be appreciated from the standard chest film. Left atrial enlargement causes a prominence along the right sternal border, but the pulmonary venous pattern may show no abnormalities until venous congestion and heart failure have developed.

Echocardiogram. The echocardiogram can define the anatomy of the mitral valve apparatus as well as left atrial and left ventricular chamber dimensions and function. Calcification of the valve leaflets and the annulus can be recognized. With acute mitral regurgitation, a flail leaflet, ruptured chordae, or nidus of infection with infective endocarditis can sometimes be identified by the echocardiogram. The echo Doppler and color techniques can assess the intensity of the regurgitant jet into the left atrium. Finally, left ventricular end-systolic dimension < 50 mm can identify the optimal time for mitral valve replacement before irreversible myocardial deterioration has taken place.

Exercise Testing. The standard exercise tests and radionuclide angiography can quantify functional capacity and document early deterioration in patients with mitral regurgitation.

Cardiac Catheterization. Left ventriculography confirms mitral regurgitation by demonstrating systolic regurgitation of contrast material into the left atrium. The difference between the angiographic left ventricular stroke volume and the forward stroke volume, calculated from the Fick or thermodilution method, yields the regurgitant stroke volume per beat across the mitral valve. Coronary artery disease and the wall motion abnormalities can also be confirmed at catheterization. Cardiac catheterization can also detect coexistent lesions in the aortic valve. Because the left ventricular ejection fraction may be maintained in the normal range despite a deteriorated contractile state, additional assessment of the contractile state is important in all causes of mitral regurgitation.

DIFFERENTIAL DIAGNOSIS. A holosystolic murmur identifies mitral regurgitation, even though the mechanism may not be apparent. Tricuspid regurgitation can cause a holosystolic murmur at the lower left sternal border, but inspiration accentuates the murmur more than in mitral regurgitation. If the murmur is not holosystolic, conditions such as aortic stenosis could be considered, along with papillary muscle dysfunction and mitral valve prolapse. In calcific aortic stenosis of the elderly patient, the murmur may sometimes be more prominent in the apex and may be confused with that of mitral regurgitation. A ventricular septal defect also causes a harsh holosystolic murmur at the lower left sternal border, but this generally radiates to the right of the sternum, compared with the axillary radiation of the murmur in mitral regurgitation.

MEDICAL THERAPY. In the early phase of mitral regurgitation without symptoms, only antibiotic prophylaxis is warranted. The same antibiotic program as described for mitral stenosis should be administered to these patients. When atrial fibrillation develops, digitalis is indicated to slow the ventricular response. Afterload-reducing agents, such as nitrates and antihypertensive drugs, have been found useful to maintain the forward stroke volume in mitral regurgitation. Once heart failure develops, surgery should be considered.

SURGICAL THERAPY. The operative mortality of mitral valve replacement in mitral regurgitation has remained higher than the 2 to 3% in mitral stenosis and for the symptomatic patient may range from 5 to 10%. In the past, surgery has been delayed until patients develop symptoms, but the advanced symptomatic stage and depressed left ventricular function contribute to high operative mortality rates. When the ejection fraction falls below 20%, operative mortality for mitral valve replacement may be as high as 25%. Therefore, surgery should be considered before the patient becomes extremely symptomatic. An echocardiographic systolic dimension

< 50 mm has been proposed as a predictor for mitral valve replacement. When technically feasible, valvular reconstruction is used to preserve the anatomy and ejection fraction. The mechanical prosthetic valve in the mitral position is more likely to develop thrombotic material than in other locations, so anticoagulation must be maintained. Any contraindication to anticoagulation warrants considering a porcine valve. Thromboembolism in patients with mechanical valves who are on anticoagulation occurs at a rate of 3% per year, and for preoperative functional classes I through III, there is a yearly mortality rate of 3% over a 10-year follow-up period. With a porcine valve, the rate of thromboembolism is lower but may reach 1.5% per year.

MITRAL VALVE PROLAPSE

ETIOLOGY AND PATHOLOGY. Echocardiography has identified prolapse of the mitral valve in as much as 5% of the adult population. A variety of synonyms include the midsystolic click–late systolic murmur, click murmur syndrome, and Barlow's syndrome. Pathologic findings include myxomatous degeneration of the valve and redundancy of the valve leaflets. These changes can also involve the chordae as well as the mitral valve. Changes in the mitral valve are seen with several connective tissue diseases, including Marfan's syndrome and osteogenesis imperfecta, and sometimes with coronary artery disease.

PHYSIOLOGY. The abnormalities of mitral valve prolapse can affect both anterior and posterior leaflets, but the posterior leaflet is more frequently involved. When the valve closes, redundancy of the leaflets results in further upward motion of the valve into the left atrium. Sudden cessation of the valvular motion is thought to generate the click, and the lack of proper positioning of the two leaflets results in the systolic regurgitant murmur in mid- and late systole.

CLINICAL FEATURES. Symptoms include palpitations, fatigue, chest pain, orthostatic changes, and psychological aberrations. Frequently, symptoms fail to correlate with the prominence of the physical findings and the extent of mitral regurgitation. Circulatory studies on changes in tilting, along with heart rate and blood pressure response, have led to the designation of dysautonomia in some of these patients. In 10 to 15% of affected individuals, palpitations may become frequent, and in a smaller number there may be progressive mitral regurgitation. Infective endocarditis occurs with a slightly higher incidence than in the normal population. Sudden death has been rarely associated with this syndrome.

Physical Findings. Patients are often women, with a thin habitus and a narrow anteroposterior chest diameter. The principal findings are the early to midsystolic click and a mid- or late systolic murmur. Often the murmur is crescendo and decrescendo, but it can be sustained in its frequency. The click or the murmur may be present alone, and not infrequently, both click and murmur are absent. Maneuvers that decrease ventricular filling, such as standing and the Valsalva maneuver, result in movement of the click closer to the first sound, followed by early onset of the murmur. Conditions that increase filling of the ventricle, such as the squatting maneuver, can delay the onset of the click and the murmur.

LABORATORY STUDIES. *Electrocardiogram.* Most commonly, the T wave is slightly inverted in the inferior and lateral precordial leads, and occasionally there is associated ST-segment depression. Rarely, QT prolongation with deep coving of the T wave is seen in the precordial leads. Runs of premature beats, both from the atrium and the ventricle, can be recorded by Holter monitoring.

Chest Radiograph. The habitus is asthenic; the chest has a narrow anteroposterior diameter, and the cardiac silhouette is elongated.

Echocardiography. The echocardiogram is the diagnostic technique of choice for mitral valve prolapse (Fig. 42–3). In one form, late systolic prolapse of the posterior leaflet resembles an inverted question mark. In the second form, there may be prolapse of the posterior leaflet throughout the systolic ejection phase with a hammock type of configuration. The diagnostic standard for mitral valve prolapse is the two-dimensional echo, which can define the plane of the mitral annulus and demonstrate whether the mitral valve leaflets extend beyond the annulus into the left atrium. Color Doppler imaging can display the amount of mitral regurgitation.

Exercise Testing. Stress testing can aggravate or precipitate cardiac irritability in these patients. Furthermore, the exercise test

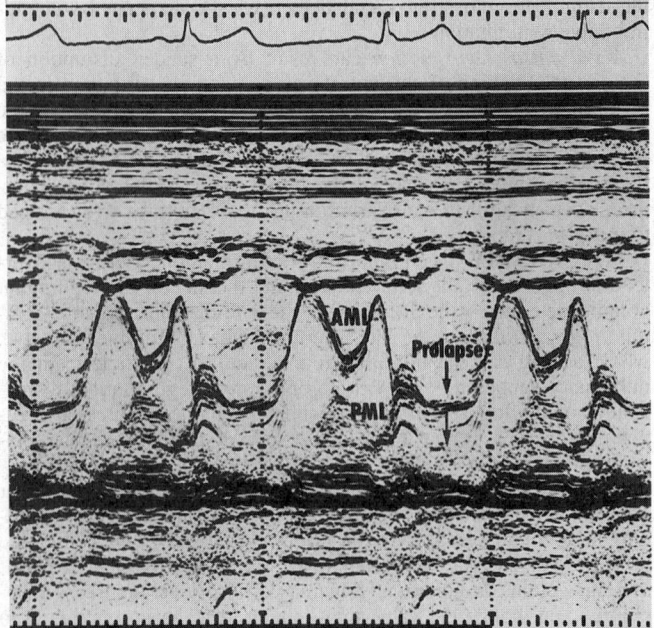

FIGURE 42–3. M-Mode echocardiogram of a patient with mitral valve prolapse. Note the systolic posterior motion of the anterior (AML) and posterior (PML) mitral valve leaflets.

can document the patient's fatigue and musculoskeletal symptoms, which often are at variance with the echocardiographic findings.

Cardiac Catheterization. The precision of echocardiography has obviated the necessity of catheterization in the majority of patients with prolapse. Atypical chest discomfort sometimes requires coronary arteriography to exclude coronary artery disease. Wall motion abnormalities have been recognized on the ventriculogram, but these do not correlate with coexisting abnormalities in the coronary arteries. Prolapse of the tricuspid valve can also occur. With mitral valve prolapse in connective tissue disorders, there may be associated aortic regurgitation.

DIFFERENTIAL DIAGNOSIS. The mid- and late systolic murmur, as well as the crescendo-decrescendo qualities of mitral valve prolapse, can be similar to the murmur of regurgitation in papillary muscle dysfunction. In coronary artery disease or hypertrophic cardiomyopathy with obstruction, the crescendo-decrescendo murmur may be similar to that of mitral valve prolapse. However, the harsh intensity of the murmur is much louder with the hyperdynamic contraction of hypertrophic cardiomyopathy. Maneuvers that increase the murmur of mitral valve prolapse intensify the murmur of cardiomyopathy with obstruction even more. However, in the latter condition, the murmur is often holosystolic. If ventricular irritability is present, the intensity of the murmur of hypertrophic cardiomyopathy with obstruction is much louder in the post-extrasystolic beat.

TREATMENT. Ventricular ectopy and symptoms of palpitations can be effectively managed with β-blocking drugs. However, fatigue in these patients can sometimes be aggravated with β blockade. With a prolonged QT interval or syncope, treatment with an antiarrhythmic is warranted. Infrequently, control of ectopy may be difficult despite using standard antiarrhythmic agents.

Infective endocarditis is a potential problem in these patients. Studies now suggest that only those patients with an audible click and murmur should be treated with antibiotic prophylaxis. Patients with prolapse demonstrated on echocardiography without a click or murmur may be at no greater risk than the normal population. When mitral regurgitation becomes progressive with chamber enlargement or with ruptured chordae, mitral valve replacement may be necessary. Mitral valve reconstruction or annuloplasty is preferred by some surgeons to total valve replacement. Fortunately, for the majority of patients, reassurance and conservative follow-up constitute the best treatment.

TRICUSPID STENOSIS

Rheumatic fever remains the most common cause of stenosis of the tricuspid valve, but this condition is invariably associated with involvement of left-sided valves by the same rheumatic process.

Rare conditions such as carcinoid tumor, endocardial fibroelastosis, and right atrial myxoma can create stenosis or obstruction of the tricuspid valve. Tricuspid stenosis causes right atrial hypertension and elevated systemic venous pressure. Stenosis of the tricuspid valve may serve as a protective mechanism for the pulmonary vascular bed in patients with mitral stenosis. Symptoms of tricuspid stenosis are dyspnea and fatigue, but the pulmonary manifestations of mitral stenosis can diminish with the development of significant stenosis of the tricuspid valve. Pulsations in the neck veins and peripheral edema develop.

Physical examination reveals a prominent, often giant, α wave in the neck veins caused by the vigorous atrial contraction against the stenotic valve. The diastolic murmur is heard best along the left lower sternal border and is presystolic if sinus rhythm is present or midsystolic with atrial fibrillation. The murmur increases prominently with inspiration, but an opening snap is rarely heard. Because mitral stenosis is usually concurrent, the auscultatory maneuvers must specifically locate the tricuspid stenosis murmur. If tricuspid stenosis is the dominant hemodynamic lesion, pulmonary hypertension and right ventricular hypertrophy are not detected on the physical examination.

The electrocardiographic finding is a tall, tented P wave in leads II, III, and aV_F, with absence of right ventricular hypertrophy. The chest radiograph should reveal a large right atrium without prominent pulmonary arteries. The echo Doppler technique may detect and assess the gradient across the tricuspid valve. Treatment consists of antibiotics. If surgery is performed for lesions in the left side of the heart, correcting the tricuspid lesion can also be undertaken.

TRICUSPID INSUFFICIENCY

Tricuspid insufficieny is, most commonly, secondary to right ventricular dilatation and hypertrophy. Tricuspid regurgitation can result from infective endocarditis, myocardial infarction, trauma, prolapse, or congenital heart disease such as atrial septal defect or Ebstein's anomaly. Symptoms of tricuspid regurgitation are those of hepatic congestion or peripheral edema.

On physical examination, atrial fibrillation is commonly present and large cv waves can be detected in the jugular veins. The murmur is holosystolic along the left sternal border and increases with inspiration. The electrocardiogram often reveals atrial fibrillation without other significant features. The chest film reveals a prominent right atrium and ventricle. The echocardiogram can document prolapse of the tricuspid leaflets as well as a nidus of infection or disruption of a chorda. Color and echo Doppler techniques can detect and assess the amount of tricuspid regurgitation. Therapy usually consists of treating conditions leading to right ventricular failure. Should surgery be performed for left-sided lesions, the tricuspid valve can be inspected. Often the leaflets are anatomically normal, and annuloplasty is indicated rather than valve replacement.

PULMONIC REGURGITATION

Regurgitation of the pulmonic valve is most commonly secondary to severe pulmonary hypertension, which can be caused by mitral stenosis, chronic lung disease, or pulmonary emboli. Inflammatory diseases and endocarditis can sometimes render the pulmonic valve incompetent; and previous surgery for congenital heart disease may create pulmonic regurgitation. The murmur (Graham Steell) is typically a high-pitched diastolic blow along the left sternal border similar to that in aortic regurgitation. No characteristic electrocardiographic changes are found, but the chest radiograph often demonstrates a prominent pulmonary artery. With echo the color Doppler technique easily detects regurgitation in the pulmonary outflow tract. Treatment consists of managing pulmonary hypertension with medical agents or occasionally with mitral valve surgery.

PULMONIC STENOSIS

Stenotic lesions of the pulmonic valve are almost always caused by congenital malformations (see Ch. 39). Rarely, hypertrophic cardiomyopathy can involve the right side of the heart with obstruction of the right ventricular outflow tract.

Aortic Valve Disease

Pellikka PA, Nishimure RA, Bailey KR, et al.: Natural history of adults with asymptomatic hemodynamically significant aortic stenosis. J Am Coll Cardiol 15:1012, 1990. *Clinical guidelines for the asymptomatic patient.*
Rappaport E, Rackley CE, Cohn LH: Aortic valve disease. *In* Schlant RC, Alexander RW (eds.): The Heart. 8th ed. New York, McGraw-Hill, 1994, p 1457. *A current review of aortic valve disease.*

Mitral Valve Disease

Duran DR, Recker AE, Dunning AJ: Long-term follow-up of idiopathic mitral valve prolapse in 300 patients: A prospective study. J Am Coll Cardiol 11:42, 1988. *Clinical events in the most common abnormality of the cardiac valves.*
Gaasch WH, O'Rourke RA, Cohn LH, et al.: Mitral valve disease. *In* Schlant RC, Alexander RW (eds.): The Heart. 8th ed. New York, McGraw-Hill, 1994, p 1483. *A thorough, contemporary review of mitral valve disease.*
Rappaport E: Natural history of aortic and mitral valve disease. Am J Cardiol 36:221, 1975. *A 10-year follow-up of stenotic and regurgitant lesions of the aortic and mitral valves; a classic study.*

Valve Surgery

Kirkland JW, Barratt-Boyes BG: Cardiac Surgery, 2nd ed. New York, Wiley, 1993. *An extensive review of techniques and results in cardiac valve surgery by pioneers in the field.*
Wisenbaugh T, Skudicky D, Careli P: A prediction of outcome after valve replacement for rheumatic mitral regurgitation in the era of chordal preservation. Circulation 89:191, 1994. *Guidelines for mitral valve replacement.*

43 DISEASES OF THE MYOCARDIUM
Lynne Warner Stevenson

The word *cardiomyopathy* means heart muscle disease. This term distinguishes those disorders originating in the myocardium from those in which myocardial dysfunction results from other cardiovascular disease. General usage, however, frequently also includes the diffuse dilation and hypocontractility that can result from severe coronary artery disease as "ischemic cardiomyopathy," which is discussed in Ch. 41.

GENERAL PRESENTATION OF CARDIOMYOPATHY

Patients presenting with cardiomyopathy usually describe progressive exertional intolerance. Patient perception often does not allow distinction between limitation due to inadequate cardiac output reserve and that due to excessive rise in ventricular filling pressures. Decreased ventricular compliance and fluid retention can cause left-sided congestive symptoms of dyspnea on minimal exertion, orthopnea, and paroxysmal nocturnal dyspnea; right-sided congestion causes discomfort during bending, hepatic distention, abdominal discomfort, and peripheral edema. As these congestive symptoms occur commonly in all types of cardiomyopathy, the term *congestive heart failure* does not clarify the type of cardiomyopathy, although it has commonly been used to denote systolic failure with a dilated ventricle and low ejection fraction.

In some patients, tachyarrhythmias or bradyarrhythmias may be the presenting symptom of cardiomyopathy. Chest pain occurs in almost one third of patients with cardiomyopathy despite normal epicardial coronary arteries and may result from pulmonary hypertension, pericardial involvement, microvascular ischemia, or unknown factors. Systemic emboli are occasionally the first sign of cardiomyopathy, arising from dilated ventricles or atria, frequently associated with atrial fibrillation.

Once a patient has been diagnosed as having abnormal cardiac function, the first question is whether this can be attributed to primary myocardial disease or to other cardiovascular conditions such as coronary artery disease, valvular disease, pericardial disease, or persistent tachycardias. Chronic severe hypertension was once the most common cause of dilated heart failure and continues to be a common cause of diastolic dysfunction, particularly in the elderly. If these other conditions are absent or inadequate to explain the degree of cardiac dysfunction, the next task is to distinguish between dilated, restrictive, and hypertrophic cardiomyopathy, which may be most efficiently accomplished using echocardiography (Fig. 43–1).

DILATED CARDIOMYOPATHY

Dilated cardiomyopathy is characterized by increased left ventricular or biventricular dimensions with decreased ventricular ejection fraction (Table 43–1). Myocardial contractility is severely impaired, labeled "systolic failure," with variable impairment detected in re-

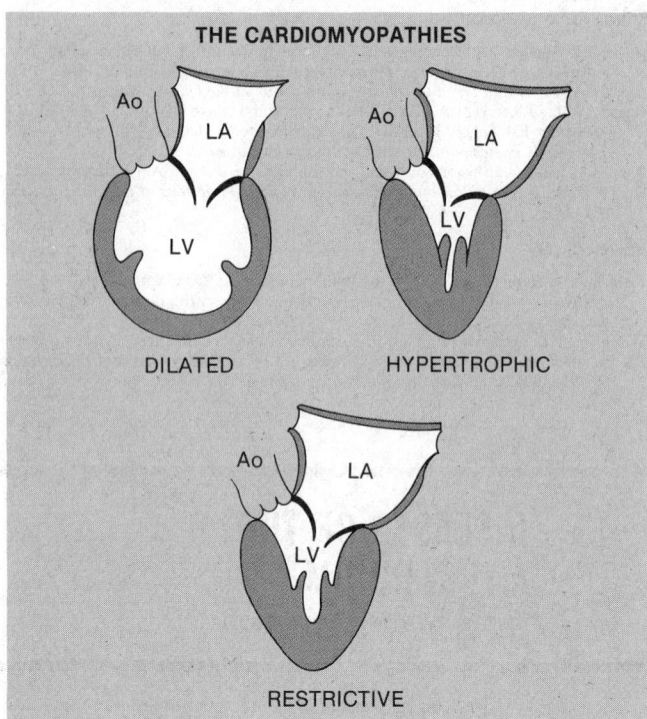

THE CARDIOMYOPATHIES

DILATED

HYPERTROPHIC

RESTRICTIVE

FIGURE 43-1. Diagram illustrating geometric differences between dilated, restrictive, and hypertrophic cardiomyopathies. (Modified from Roberts WC, Ferrans VJ: Pathologic anatomy of the cardiomyopathies. Human Pathol 6:287, 1975.)

laxation and compliance, labeled "diastolic failure." The diagnosed incidence of dilated cardiomyopathy has been increasing, estimated at 8 in 100,000 after 1980. The prevalence is estimated at 37 in 100,000, half of whom are under age 55, and one third have New York Heart Association Class III or IV symptoms at diagnosis. The frequency of unrecognized mild disease would render the true prevalence considerably higher.

ETIOLOGY. The major causes of dilated cardiomyopathy are listed in Table 43–2. Myocardial injury of many types and time courses can create the same final picture of dilated cardiomyopathy (see Color Plate 2J). A brief primary injury such as toxic exposure may be fatal to some myocytes, after which the remaining myocytes adapt to the increased burden with hypertrophy that initially preserves global function but can eventually limit contractility and relaxation. Some agents, such as ethanol, may reversibly impair

global contractility without directly causing cell injury but cause irreversible dysfunction if continued chronically. Inflammatory myocarditis may combine irreversible cell death with reversible depression from inflammatory mediators such as cytokines. Many injuries may also affect the collagen scaffolding of the myocardium, influencing stiffness and the potential for ventricular dilation. Most cardiomyopathies reflect the sum of irreversible myocyte loss plus secondary abnormalities, some of which may be reversible, in the remaining myocardium struggling to compensate.

Myocarditis. As causes of *viral myocarditis,* the cardiotropic enteroviruses, specifically coxsackie group B and the echoviruses, have been most extensively studied. In the susceptible mouse, the initial active viral replication of coxsackie B infection is exacerbated by exercise and immunosuppression. Subsequently, active replication ceases, although some viral DNA may still be detectable, and thymus-derived lymphocytes appear to cross-react with myocardial cells. Infected animals may die, recover, or develop dilated hearts with areas of fibrosis.

Viral myocarditis in humans may be suspected from the clinical picture of recent febrile illness often with prominent myalgias, followed by rapid onset of cardiac symptoms. Elevated creatine phosphokinase, with or without elevated MB fraction, supports the diagnosis as many cardiotropic infections also affect skeletal muscle. The diagnosis is supported by increasing viral titers, particularly to coxsackie and echoviruses. Myocarditis, according to the strict definition that requires extensive lymphocyte infiltration with adjacent myocyte necrosis on endomyocardial biopsy (see Color Plate 2I), is identified in fewer than 20% of patients biopsied within the first few weeks of typical symptoms, and less often later. Biopsies performed in patients without recent onset of symptoms frequently show scattered lymphocytes but meet criteria for myocarditis in fewer than 5% of cases. The diagnosis and role of antibody-mediated injury remain controversial.

It has been assumed that the majority of otherwise unexplained human cardiomyopathy represents sequelae of previous viral myocarditis, but the data are lacking. Even with a history of recent viral symptoms, primary causation is difficult to demonstrate because most systemic viral infections can depress myocardial function at least transiently owing to induction of cytokines. Many cases presumed to be acute myocarditis may represent chronic asymptomatic cardiomyopathy exacerbated by acute viral illness.

Prognosis and Therapy. The general prognosis of new-onset heart failure due to viral myocarditis is major improvement in left ventricular function in up to half of patients, one quarter stabilizing at low function, and one quarter deteriorating to need transplantation urgently (see Ch. 48). The presence or absence of histologic myocarditis does not change this prognosis. Treatment for biopsy-proven acute myocarditis, presumed to be postviral, has included azathioprine and prednisone, and more recently cyclosporine. The rationale for immunosuppressive therapy is based in part on the dramatic response of transplant rejection, which has equivalent histology. In addition, immunosuppressive therapy in animal trials has

TABLE 43-1. PROFILES OF SYMPTOMATIC CARDIOMYOPATHY

	Dilated	Restrictive	Hypertrophic
Ejection fraction (normal ≥ 55%)	< 30%	25–50%	> 60%
Left ventricular diastolic dimension (normal < 55 mm)	≥ 60 mm	< 60 mm	Often decreased
Left ventricular wall thickness	Decreased	Normal or increased	Markedly increased
Atrial size	Increased	Increased, may be massive	Increased
Valvular regurgitation	Mitral first during decompensation, tricuspid regurgitation in late stages	Frequent mitral and tricuspid regurgitation	Mitral regurgitation
Common first symptoms*	Exertional intolerance	Exertional intolerance	Exertional intolerance, may have chest pain
Congestive symptoms*	Left before right, except right prominent in young adults	Right often exceeds left	Primary exertional dyspnea
Risk for arrhythmia	Ventricular tachyarrhythmia. Conduction block in Chagas' disease; giant cell, and some families. Atrial fibrillation.	Ventricular uncommon except in sarcoidosis. Conduction block in sarcoidosis and amyloidosis. Atrial fibrillation.	Ventricular tachyarrhythmias Atrial fibrillation

* Left-sided symptoms of pulmonary congestion; dyspnea on exertion, orthopnea, paroxysmal nocturnal dyspnea. Right-sided symptoms of systemic venous congestion: discomfort on bending, hepatic and abdominal distention, peripheral edema.

TABLE 43-2. MAJOR CAUSES OF DILATED CARDIOMYOPATHY

I. Inflammatory myocarditis
    Infective
        Viral
        Rickettsial
        Bacterial
        Mycobacterial
        Spirochetal
        Parasitic
        Fungal
    Noninfective
        Collagen vascular disease
        Peripartum cardiomyopathy
        Hypersensitivity myocarditis
        Transplant rejection
        Giant-cell myocarditis: infectious or noninfectious?

II. Toxic
    Alcohol
    Chemotherapeutic agents: doxorubicin; cyclophosphamide, interferon-α
    Heavy metals: lead, mercury
    Occupational exposure: hydrocarbons, arsenicals
    Catecholamines: amphetamines, cocaine

III. Metabolic
    Nutritional deficiencies: thiamine, selenium, carnitine
    Electrolyte deficiencies: calcium, phosphate, magnesium
    Endocrinopathy: thyroid disease, diabetes, pheochromocytoma
    Obesity

IV. Familial
    Cardiac and skeletal myopathy
        Duchenne's dystrophy
        Becker's dystrophy
        Facioscapulohumeral dystrophy
        Erb's limb-girdle dystrophy
        Friedreich's ataxia
        Kearns-Sayre syndrome
    Isolated cardiomyopathy—dystrophin promoter defect
    Associated with other systemic diseases
    Susceptibility to immune-mediated myocarditis

V. Overlap with restrictive
    Hemochromatosis
    Amyloidosis
    Sarcoidosis

VI. Idiopathic
    Primary left ventricular or biventricular
    Arrhythmogenic right ventricular dysplasia

---

lated cytokine secretion. The role of secondary factors is supported by the frequent improvement observed in impaired ventricular function. Detecting viral particles in myocytes, however, supports a direct causation. Pericardial effusions as well as myocarditis may occur.

Chagas' disease (see Ch. 376), due to infection with *Trypanosoma cruzi,* carried by the reduviid bug, affects up to 15% of the rural population in South America and is also common in Central America. The acute tissue-invasive phase can present as myocarditis but is usually silent. Subsequent progression of myocardial disease occurs over years, with a predilection to develop apical aneurysms and right bundle branch block. Destruction of parasympathetic ganglia may contribute to cardiac dysfunction. Because organisms are no longer detected in tissue, the chronic process has been attributed to a triggered autoimmune reaction, perhaps similar to that induced by viral infection. However, frequent eruption of generalized trypanosomal infection during immunosuppression following transplantation for chronic Chagas' disease implies continued presence of viable organisms. The prognosis of seropositive patients with a normal electrocardiogram at presentation was for normal 10-year survival; an abnormal electrocardiogram and extensive wall motion abnormality without symptoms, 80% 5-year survival; and symptomatic heart failure, 20% 5-year survival, almost half of the deaths occurring suddenly. There is no specific therapy for the chronic stage of the disease, although pacemaker implanta-

TABLE 43-3. CARDIAC LESIONS IN AIDS

Myocardial involvement
  Infections (opportunistic)
    Bacterial
      Mycobacterium tuberculosis
      Mycobacterium avium—intracellulare
    Fungal
      Cryptococcus neoformans
      Aspergillus fumigatus
      Candida albicans
      Histoplasma capsulatum
      Coccidioides immitis
    Protozoan
      Toxoplasma gondii
    Viral
      Cytomegalovirus
      HIV
      Herpes simplex
  Noninflammatory myocardial necrosis
    Microvascular spasm?
    Catecholamine excess
    Vascular disease
    Infection
    Toxic drug reaction
  Right ventricular hypertrophy or dilation with pulmonary hypertension resulting from
    Pulmonary infections
    Pulmonary emboli
  Neoplastic
    Kaposi's sarcoma
    Lymphoma
Pericardial involvement*
  Infectious
    Bacterial—tuberculosis *(M. tuberculosis, M. avium—intracellulare),* nocardiosis
    Viral—herpes simplex
    Fungal—histoplasmosis, cryptococcosis
    Idiopathic (?) HIV organism
  Uremia
  Neoplastic
    Kaposi's sarcoma
    Lymphoma
Endocardial involvement
  Marantic endocarditis (nonbacterial thrombotic endocarditis)
  Infective endocarditis
    Bacterial
    Fungal

* As evidenced by effusion with or without tamponade, or pericarditis without effusion and with or without constriction. (From Kaul S, Fishbein MC, Siegel RJ: Cardiac manifestations of acquired immunodeficiency syndrome: A 1991 update. Am Heart J 122:535, 1991.)

---

been shown to decrease late mortality but to increase early mortality when given during active viral replication. Controlled trials in humans, however, have shown no benefit of immunosuppressive therapy on outcome and thus no convincing reason to biopsy for suspected myocarditis. The suspicion remains that some patients who show a progressive downhill course may benefit from immunosuppression. A common current approach is to defer biopsy and give no immunosuppressive treatment in the first few weeks after presentation. If the patient continues to deteriorate despite standard therapy, the prognosis for recovery is very poor and biopsy may then be considered, presuming that severe persistent inflammation, if present, may respond to a brief course of immunosuppression, which could prevent the need for transplantation and lifelong immunosuppression.

Occasionally, acute viral myocarditis may present over a few days with a "fulminant" picture, characterized by fevers and compromise of hepatic and renal function, as well as cardiac function. Such patients are assumed to be undergoing active viral infection during which immunosuppression would be deleterious. The equally likely outcomes of dramatic improvement or demise often declare themselves within the next week. Biopsy, which could be complicated by the coagulopathy that frequently occurs, may show dramatic lymphocyte infiltration but is generally deferred.

Cardiomyopathy defined by echocardiographic abnormalities occurs in 10 to 40% of patients clinically infected with the *human immunodeficiency virus* (HIV). Causes and presentations of cardiac involvement vary greatly (Table 43–3). Lymphocytic myocarditis has been found in up to 50% of autopsied hearts. The causative role of the HIV virus itself is difficult to isolate from the contribution of other co-infecting organisms such as cytomegalovirus and their re-tion may decrease deaths from heart block. Recent evidence suggests that cardiomyoplasty may improve prognosis, perhaps in part by harnessing the ventricle before dilation is advanced.

Toxoplasmosis (see Ch. 378) can cause myocarditis, with intermittent rupture of cysts in the myocardium leading to atypical chest pain, arrhythmias, pericarditis, and symptomatic heart failure. The endomyocardial biopsy may show focal lymphocytic infiltration and rarely a fortuitous cyst. Diagnosis is made from antibody titers. Therapy is with pyrimethamine and sulfadiazine, on which relapses are common.

Heart failure developing during the last month of pregnancy and first 3 months post partum is termed *peripartum cardiomyopathy.* The frequency is between 1 in 3000 and 1 in 15,000 deliveries, with increased risk for mothers with older age, increased parity, twins, malnutrition, toxemia, or hypertension. Lymphocytic myocarditis has been found in 30 to 50% of biopsies, suggesting an immune component postulated to be cross-reactivity between uterine and cardiac myocyte proteins. Presentation is usually with orthopnea and excessive dyspnea on minimal exertion, often with persistent or exacerbated fluid retention and edema. Many patients are already improving by the time the diagnosis is made, and the frequency may be higher than appreciated. Normal systolic ventricular function recovers during the next 6 months in approximately half of patients, with the best chance for recovery in those with preserved cardiac output at diagnosis. It has been recommended that breast feeding, which requires vigorous hydration, be discontinued after diagnosis and that diuretics be used as needed to facilitate postpartum diuresis. It is not known whether therapy with angiotensin-converting enzyme (ACE) inhibitors improves likelihood of recovery.

Myocardial inflammation may occur without preceding infection, often associated with *systemic immunologic disorders.* Lymphocytic myocarditis has been documented in systemic lupus erythematosus (SLE), although pericarditis and coronary artery vasculitis are more common. *Hypersensitivity* reactions, particularly to drugs, can cause myocarditis characterized by infiltration of eosinophils in addition to lymphocytes. Such hypersensitivity is frequently unsuspected and may complicate cardiomyopathy of other causes. Response to withdrawing the offending agent and to steroid therapy has been described.

Rejection after cardiac transplantation is the paradigm for lymphocyte-mediated myocarditis (see Ch. 48). The human leukocyte antigens (HLA) on the donor myocardium and endothelium represent a major target of T lymphocytes derived from the recipient. Lessons derived from this "model" include (1) the frequent reversibility of myocardial depression, which implicates cytokine release rather than widespread myocyte injury; (2) the rapid response to immunosuppression, which validates its use at least in this setting; (3) the potential importance of "humoral," antibody-mediated rejection even when lymphocytic infiltration is mild or absent; and (4) the association between chronic immune stimulation and coronary vascular disease. The average transplant recipient experiences one to two episodes of rejection requiring enhanced immunosuppression with increased cyclosporine, glucocorticoids, or antilymphocyte sera. Only 10% of rejection causes clinical compromise, and 95% of all episodes resolve.

An unusual form of myocarditis which may or may not be infectious is *giant-cell myocarditis,* accounting for 10 to 20% of biopsy-positive cases of myocarditis. The giant cells appear to arise from macrophages rather than myocytes, although this is controversial. Onset is usually rapid with chest pain, fever, and hemodynamic compromise. There is a higher incidence of ventricular tachycardia and atrioventricular block than in lymphocytic myocarditis. Giant-cell myocarditis has been associated with thymomas, thyroiditis, pernicious anemia, and SLE. The time course and histology of the disease suggest that it is distinct from sarcoidosis, although some believe that it may be related (see Ch. 61). Immunosuppression has not appeared to improve the unfortunate outcome, but it has been suggested that cyclosporin A might be more effective.

Many substances have been reported to cause acute cardiac injury or chronic cardiomyopathy. Ethanol is implicated in >10% of cases of heart failure. Although *alcoholic cardiomyopathy* was once attributed to associated nutritional abnormalities and at one time to cobalt additives in beer, alcohol and its direct metabolite acetaldehyde are direct cardiotoxins acutely and chronically. Atrial fibrilla-

tion may be particularly common. It is important to recognize that ethanol can contribute to heart failure with another primary cause, such as coronary artery disease. This myocardial depression is initially reversible but if sustained can lead to irreversible injury characterized histologically by vacuolization, mitochondrial abnormalities, and fibrosis. Even in chronic stages, however, the heart failure represents a sum of reversible and irreversible depression. The amount of alcohol necessary to produce symptomatic cardiomyopathy in susceptible individuals is not known but has been estimated to be six drinks (about 4 ounces of pure ethanol) a day for 5 to 10 years. Frequent binging without heavy daily consumption may also be sufficient. Alcoholic cardiomyopathy can develop in patients without social evidence of an alcohol problem. It is crucial to convince them of the value of abstention, which leads to improvement in at least half of patients with severe symptoms, some of whom normalize left ventricular ejection fraction (Fig. 43–2). Patients with other causes of heart failure should also avoid alcohol (see Ch. 11).

Adriamycin (doxorubicin) cardiotoxicity causes characteristic histologic changes on endomyocardial biopsy, with vacuolar degeneration and myofibrillar loss. Potential mechanisms of cardiotoxicity include free radical formation, release of histamines and catecholamines, and effects on mitochondrial function and nucleic acid synthesis. Between 5 and 10% of patients receiving at least 500 mg per square meter of body surface area develop overt heart failure, but more than half of patients receiving multiple courses have 10%

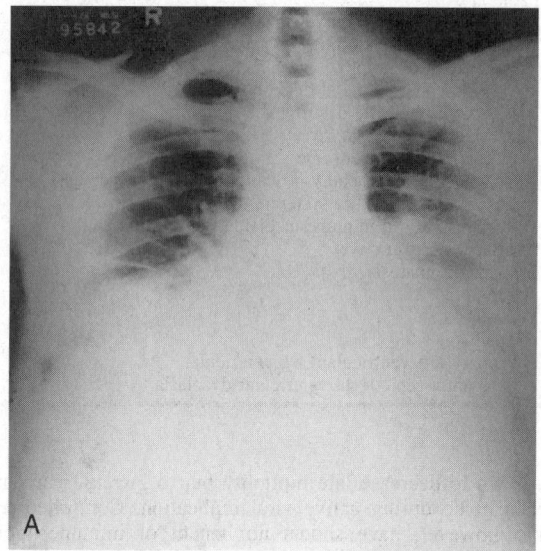

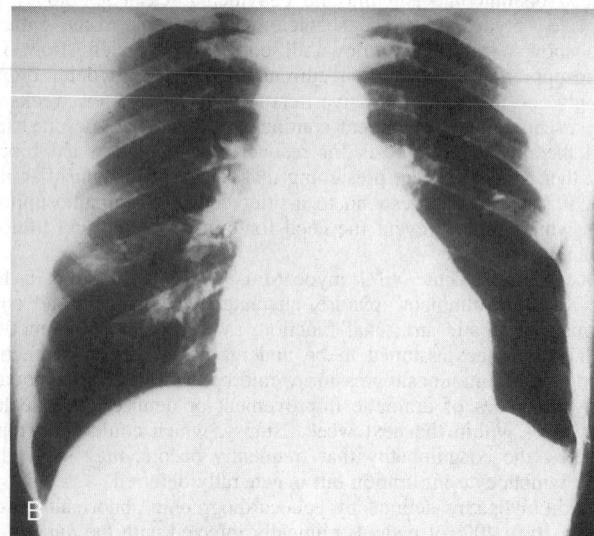

FIGURE 43–2. *A,* Chest radiograph from a 36-year-old man diagnosed with alcoholic cardiomyopathy, demonstrating the marked cardiomegaly and large right pleural effusion. *B,* Chest radiograph from the same patient after 6 weeks of abstinence from alcohol. (From Stevenson LW, Perloff JK: The dilated cardiomyopathies. Cardiol Clin 6:187, 1988.)

decline in resting ejection fraction. Patients with higher doses and lower baseline ejection fractions have higher risk for clinical heart failure. The dysfunction may continue to progress, with 63% of pediatric patients who have received at least 500 mg per square meter having some cardiac dysfunction detected after 10 years. Clinical status may improve with supportive hemodynamic therapy, but chronic cardiac function rarely improves. Use of slower, less frequent infusion appears to decrease toxicity, but may not be as effective against some tumors.

Cyclophosphamide has been associated with more acute cardiac dysfunction during therapy or the first few weeks, frequently with decreased electrocardiographic voltage. Pericarditis with effusion has been seen, and increased left ventricular mass has been attributed to hemorrhagic necrosis. Ifosfamide is a newer, similar compound that can cause acute severe heart failure and malignant ventricular arrhythmias. Death from cardiogenic shock and recovery of normal left ventricular function have both been reported.

Cardiomyopathy has been associated with *catecholamine excess,* which may injure the heart by compromising the coronary microcirculation but also through direct toxic effects on myocytes exposed to excessive stimulation and calcium loading. Pheochromocytoma can cause a reversible cardiomyopathy, as can heavy use of cocaine, which inhibits the re-uptake of catecholamines. Anecdotal evidence implicates heavy use of adrenergic bronchodilators, with an increased incidence of cardiomyopathy in patients with lung disease.

Nutritional deficiencies are not commonly implicated in cardiomyopathy in developed Western countries. Thiamine deficiency can lead to beri-beri heart disease, which is initially a vasodilated state with high cardiac output, later deteriorating to low output. This can result from poor nutrition in some Asian areas and to alcoholism but has also been reported in teenagers with diets dominated by processed foods. Abnormal regulation of carnitine can cause dilated or restrictive forms of cardiomyopathy, particularly in children. Calcium deficiency due to hypoparathyroidism, gastrointestinal abnormalities, or chelation directly compromises myocardial contractility, as does deficiency of phosphate, needed for high-energy compounds. Hypophosphatemia may occur in alcoholism, in diabetes, during recovery from malnutrition, and in hyperalimentation. Magnesium, a cofactor for thiamine-dependent reactions and for sodium-potassium adenosine triphosphatase, may be depleted by impaired absorption or increased renal excretion.

Endocrinopathies have multiple systemic effects that may affect the heart. Hyperthyroidism may impair cardiac reserve, in part due to tachycardia and to enhanced adrenergic sensitivity in addition to direct affects of triiodothyronine. Hypothyroidism depresses contractility and conduction and may cause pericardial effusions. Diabetes has been associated with cardiomyopathy independently of the epicardial coronary atherosclerosis for which it is a risk factor. Particularly in combination with hypertension, cardiomyopathy with diabetes may present a picture in which diastolic function is more impaired than systolic function. In addition to aggravating heart failure by increasing demand, massive obesity is implicated as a cause of cardiomyopathy with increased ventricular mass and decreased contractility, which improve following weight loss.

Inherited genetic factors have been implicated in *familial dilated cardiomyopathy,* although with much less frequency than in hypertrophic cardiomyopathy. Many of the early examples described varying degrees of cardiomyopathy associated with specific conduction system abnormalities. The most distinct examples of familial cardiomyopathies are the *neuromyopathic disorders* (see Ch. 454) such as Duchenne's muscular dystrophy and Becker's X-linked slowly progressive muscular dystrophy, both caused by mutations in the gene for dystrophin, a cytoskeletal protein. Recently a deletion in a cardiac promoter region associated with this gene was demonstrated in a family with X-linked cardiomyopathy without skeletal myopathy. Mitochondrial abnormalities have also been reported in familial cardiomyopathies, such as the Kearns-Sayre syndrome of cardiomyopathy, ophthalmoplegia, retinopathy, and cerebellar ataxia. In addition to abnormalities of muscle proteins and metabolism, heritable factors may influence susceptibility to external triggers for anticardiac immune responses. Kindreds have been described with heart failure presenting after viral infection or during pregnancy. Although previously thought to be very rare, familial involvement has recently been described in up to 20% of dilated cardiomyopathy.

Isolated *right ventricular cardiomyopathy* is characterized by focal fibrous-fatty replacement. The right ventricular free wall and the atria are primarily involved, giving rise to ventricular and supraventricular arrhythmias, which are often the presenting symptom. Proposed causes include congenital hypoplasia of myocardial tissue and focal injury with fibrous replacement.

Diseases causing primarily restrictive cardiomyopathies can occasionally cause a picture consistent with dilated cardiomyopathy, particularly when the ventricle is not severely dilated. Hemochromatosis and sarcoidosis should be considered when evaluating all cardiomyopathy.

EVALUATION OF DILATED CARDIOMYOPATHY

The usual history for a patient with dilated cardiomyopathy is gradual exertional intolerance and onset of congestive symptoms, occasionally including dysrhythmic or embolic events, as described above for cardiomyopathy in general. An acute presentation may reflect a new problem, such as hyperthyroidism, superimposed on an unrecognized chronic cardiomyopathy of other origin. Rapid development over days to weeks, however, suggests postviral or giant-cell myocarditis. Chest pain, typical of pericarditis or mimicking acute myocardial infarction, may result from acute myocarditis, as can ventricular arrhythmias in the absence of detectable left ventricular dysfunction. Regardless of cause, however, many patients describe an upper respiratory syndrome during the preceding 6 months, as do most people without cardiomyopathy. Adequate history regarding alcohol and cocaine use requires tactful diligence. Family history of possible cardiomyopathy may be helpful, with careful questioning about sudden deaths attributed to "massive heart attacks." Other specific clues such as toxic occupational exposure, residence in rural South America, or frequent exposure to raw meat products can suggest specific causes.

CLINICAL EVALUATION. The physical examination for all types of cardiomyopathy should address systemic circulatory compensation, evidence of intracardiac abnormalities, and any extracardiac clues for the specific cause of cardiomyopathy. Resting hemodynamic status is assessed for congestion, including history of orthopnea and detection of elevated jugular venous pressures, abnormal hepatojugular reflux, hepatic distention and ascites, peripheral edema, and the presence of rales, which is the least sensitive sign of congestion in chronic heart failure. Adequacy of perfusion is best assessed by blood pressure, specifically the difference between systolic and diastolic, which generally exceeds 25% of systolic if the cardiac index is over 2.2 liters per minute per square meter. Tachycardia, vague or obtunded mental status, and cool extremities may indicate severe hypoperfusion. Pulsus alternans and periodic breathing may be detected in some patients with marked decompensation. If resting hemodynamics appear to be normal, functional cardiac reserve may be assessed initially by a 6-minute walk around the corridor and more objectively by exercise testing analyzing oxygen uptake and anaerobic threshold.

The specific cardiac examination varies according to the type of cardiomyopathy. In dilated cardiomyopathy, the left ventricular impulse is often displaced far laterally, although considerable posterior dilation can occur without detectable lateral displacement. The impulse is generally diffuse but not sustained. A separate right ventricular impulse may be felt along the left sternal border, and beneath the xiphoid process during inspiration. Third and fourth heart sounds, "gallops," are often heard, with increasing prominence of the third heart sound for a given patient frequently reflecting more ventricular volume overload. Absence of gallops does not mean that heart failure is absent. Mitral regurgitation is usually significant once hemodynamic decompensation has developed but is not always audible. This murmur, heard best in the axilla, may overlap with a sternal area murmur of tricuspid regurgitation, which generally develops later during decompensation. A short medium-pitched murmur of pulmonic regurgitation may occur early in diastole in patients with marked pulmonary hypertension.

ROUTINE LABORATORY ASSESSMENT. The electrocardiogram usually shows left ventricular dilation, with poor R wave progression and higher voltage in V_6 than in V_5. Left atrial abnormality is generally present. Atrial fibrillation may be present. Left bundle branch block occurs in approximately 20%, and many other patients have nonspecific QRS prolongation. Right bundle branch block is uncommon except in Chagas' disease. Prolongation of the P-R interval is common and has been associated with worse survival in some series. More profound conduction block may suggest giant-cell myocarditis or sarcoidosis. Nonspecific T-wave abnormalities are usually present.

The chest radiograph usually shows cardiomegaly, although in some patients marked left ventricular dilation occurs posteriorly before the silhouette enlarges on the anteroposterior view. The degree of cardiomegaly on radiography often reflects more the degree of right than left ventricular dilation, which may explain its prognostic significance, as right ventricular failure carries a more ominous prognosis.

Creatine phosphokinase may be elevated in acute myocarditis, reflecting both cardiac and skeletal myositis. It may also be elevated in the chronic dystrophies. Serial viral titers may support a diagnosis of myocarditis, and titers for toxoplasmosis, Chagas' disease, or antistreptolysin may also be considered. Peripheral blood eosinophilia should stimulate search for a systemic allergic reaction that could be causing a hypersensitivity myocarditis. Serologic evidence of active collagen-vascular disease should raise the question of cardiac involvement. In the absence of active inflammation, the erythrocyte sedimentation rate is generally below normal in patients with decompensated heart failure. A sensitive assay for thyroid-stimulating hormone is usually an adequate screen for thyroid disease. Other endocrinologic diagnoses, particularly pheochromocytoma, should be entertained but do not all need to be excluded by extensive laboratory testing. Studies of iron and transferrin should exclude hemochromatosis (see Ch. 189). Low sodium and chemistries indicating compromise of renal and hepatic function usually reflect the degree of hemodynamic compromise rather than any specific cause.

Echocardiography is the initial cardiac laboratory examination in most patients, identifying left ventricular and often right ventricular dilation and hypocontractility, allowing distinction of dilated cardiomyopathy from other forms of cardiomyopathy (see Fig. 43–1; Table 43–1). In addition, primary valve disease and septal defects can be detected if present. Primary mitral regurgitation may be difficult to distinguish from mitral regurgitation secondary to dilated heart failure but is more likely if the leaflets or chordae tendineae are abnormal. In general, congestive symptoms with severe mitral regurgitation and ejection fraction >30% are due to primary valve disease, whereas secondary mitral regurgitation develops at lower ejection fractions. Focal wall motion abnormalities often result from coronary artery disease but are common in Chagas' disease and in sarcoidosis and may be seen in any cardiomyopathy. Disproportionate left ventricular hypertrophy may implicate previous hypertension or "burned out" hypertrophic cardiomyopathy as primary cardiac diagnoses.

Thallium imaging may occasionally be useful in the restrictive cardiomyopathies but has little role in dilated cardiomyopathy. Focal thallium defects make coronary disease more likely but are also found in nonischemic cardiomyopathy. Gallium scans have been used to screen for myocardial inflammation but do not correlate well with biopsy findings.

Coronary arteriography should be seriously considered in most patients presenting with dilated heart failure, in order to exclude coronary artery anomalies or atherosclerotic disease. Cardiac catheterization may be needed to confirm a diagnosis of primary valve disease suspected from echocardiography. Determining cardiac output and filling pressures with right heart catheterization may be useful to confirm information from the clinical assessment and to guide subsequent therapy when hemodynamic decompensation is present.

The only definite indications for endomyocardial biopsy are monitoring of cardiac transplant rejection and anthracycline cardiotoxicity. The two other major groups of dilated cardiomyopathy patients in whom biopsy is considered, however, are (1) those presenting with <3 to 6 months of symptoms and (2) patients with chronic cardiomyopathy without obvious cause. Lymphocytic myocarditis is detected in 5 to 20% of the first group, with uncertain implications as described above, and occasional unsuspected diagnoses are made. In the second group, lymphocytic myocarditis is detected in <10%, occasionally with other diagnoses. The majority of patients with chronic cardiomyopathy show abnormalities of varying myocyte size, nuclear hypertrophy ("box-car" nuclei), and fibrosis. Although these have frequently been considered "diagnostic," they do not have unique therapeutic implications. Diagnoses commonly made on endomyocardial biopsy that may affect therapy are transplant rejection, anthracycline cardiotoxicity, giant-cell myocarditis, amyloidosis, sarcoidosis, hypereosinophilic syndrome, hemochromatosis, and occasionally other metabolic storage diseases. Sampling error limits recognition of toxoplasmosis or Chagas' disease and can lead to false-negative biopsies for sarcoidosis as well. In the individual patient, decisions regarding biopsy must reflect the likelihood that a diagnosis will be made, with its therapeutic and prognostic implications. The utility of biopsy will expand as new biochemical analyses supersede the current techniques of staining and microscopy.

PROGNOSIS AND THERAPY

The more common causes of dilated cardiomyopathy with specific prognostic and therapeutic features have been discussed above. Even after a careful evaluation, however, most patients do not have a specific cause identified, although the newer genetic information promises to diminish this group. Patients with recent-onset cardiomyopathy have almost a 50% chance of significant recovery, lower in patients with the most severe compromise at presentation. For patients with chronic cardiomyopathy of unknown cause, the prognosis is determined by the stability or deterioration of their left ventricular function and hemodynamic compensation, as described in Ch. 34.

Patients considered to have a recent process with some potential for improvement, such as new-onset cardiomyopathy, peripartum cardiomyopathy, or alcoholism, are often advised to avoid vigorous exercise for the next 3 to 6 months. This proscription is derived weakly from data that swimming enhanced mortality in the murine model of acute viral myocarditis and from anecdotal human experience. Patients should be advised, however, to remain mobile and to avoid excessive bedrest, which leads to deconditioning and depression.

When no cause dictates specific therapy, it is important to rule out contributing factors such as thyroid disease or rapid atrial fibrillation which could be treated. If there are no such factors, the therapy for cardiomyopathy is as described in Ch. 34 for various stages of heart failure, with prescription of ACE inhibitors in almost all patients, digitalis glycosides in many, and diuretics and additional vasodilators as dictated by hemodynamic profile. Beta-blocking agents improve ventricular function in a subset of patients yet to be precisely defined. When symptoms of congestion or dyspnea on minimal exertion persist despite empiric therapy with vasodilators, diuretics, and digoxin, compensation can frequently be restored and maintained on a regimen tailored to hemodynamic goals, which include near-normal filling pressures and systemic vascular resistance. For patients who are truly refractory to medical therapy but have no other conditions that would compromise long-term survival, cardiac transplantation may be considered. The limited supply of donor hearts restricts transplantation, however, to approximately only 2000 to 2500 patients annually (see Ch. 48).

RESTRICTIVE CARDIOMYOPATHY

The restrictive cardiomyopathies are the least common of the three major categories of cardiomyopathy. Although characterized primarily by decreased distensibility ("diastolic dysfunction"), the restrictive cardiomyopathies are frequently accompanied by some degree of depressed contractility and ejection fraction ("systolic dysfunction"). Hemodynamically, end-diastolic pressures and consequently atrial pressures are elevated early, with relative preservation of cardiac output until disease is advanced. Although classically considered to be "nondilated," with normal ventricular dimensions, many restrictive cardiomyopathies are associated with some global or focal ventricular dilation, although less than for equivalent degrees of congestive symptoms in the primary dilated cardiomyopathies. The atria, however, frequently become very enlarged after chronic exposure to high filling pressures.

The initial challenge is to distinguish restrictive cardiomyopathy from dilated cardiomyopathy or pericardial disease. Echocardiography in restrictive disease usually shows left ventricular diastolic dimension <6 to 6.5 cm and ejection fraction >30% (see Table 43–1). Symptomatic congestion, the major clinical feature of restrictive cardiomyopathy, rarely occurs in primary dilated cardiomyopathy until the ejection fraction is <30%. Echocardiographic profiles of abnormal relaxation and diastolic filling are helpful in confirming physiologic impairment in patients with near-normal ejection fraction but are less helpful in distinguishing restrictive from other cardiomyopathy, in which the degree of volume overload determines filling pattern. The difficult distinction between primary restrictive disease and extrinsic pericardial disease often requires comparison of right and left ventricular filling during invasive hemodynamic measurement and pericardial imaging by computed tomography or magnetic resonance imaging, particularly in patients with a history of mediastinal radiation, which can cause both myocardial and pericardial disease.

Most restrictive cardiomyopathies result from deposition of abnormal substances in the myocardium (Table 43–4). These are commonly divided into "infiltrative" diseases, in which the abnormal substance is largely between the myocytes, and "storage" diseases, in which abnormal substances accumulate within myocytes.

INFILTRATIVE DISEASE. *Amyloidosis* (see Ch. 248) is the most common cause of infiltrative cardiomyopathy. Clinically evident cardiac amyloidosis usually results from primary amyloidosis or the amyloidosis associated with multiple myeloma, in which immunoglobulin light chains are the major amyloid protein. Instead of an immunoglobulin, however, amyloid deposits in familial amyloidosis contain an abnormal prealbumin (transthyretin) associated with different specific point mutations, many of which involve the kidney or liver without cardiac compromise. Secondary amyloidosis and senile amyloidosis rarely cause clinical cardiac involvement.

Amyloid infiltration of the interstitium stiffens the ventricles and also replaces some contractile elements (Fig. 43–3). Although it is also found in the atria, it is not extensive enough to prevent atrial dilation. Deposits frequently affect the conduction system, leading to bradyarrhythmias. Amyloid also surrounds the arterioles, which may compromise the microcirculation, further impairing systolic and diastolic function and leading to anginal chest pain in some patients.

Like other cardiomyopathies, the earliest symptom may be dyspnea with exertion. Congestion occurs earlier in the course than with dilated cardiomyopathy, frequently with disproportionate right-sided congestive symptoms of abdominal discomfort and peripheral edema. Syncope may reflect sinus or atrioventricular node involvement. Occasional angina may be due to small vessel ischemia. Some patients may present with orthostatic hypotension due to amyloid autonomic neuropathy. Evidence of involvement elsewhere such as carpal tunnel syndrome, skin friability, or nephrotic syndrome may also suggest the diagnosis of amyloidosis.

Electrocardiograms characteristically show markedly decreased voltage despite increased wall thickness on echocardiography. Specific diagnosis in some cases can be made from a characteristic

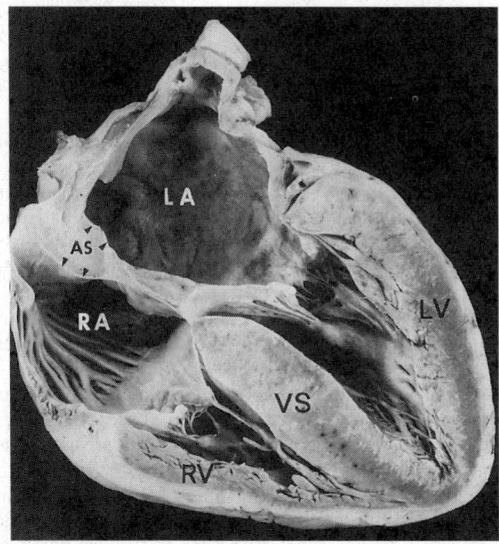

FIGURE 43–3. A necropsy specimen of an amyloid heart demonstrating the thickened ventricular septum (VS), atrial septum (AS), and free walls of the left ventricle (LV) and right ventricle (RV), and the dilated left atrium (RA). (Courtesy of Dr. William Edwards, Mayo Clinic, Rochester, Minnesota.)

sparkling refractile pattern on echocardiography. More than 80% of patients have a monoclonal protein identified from either serum or urine. Technetium pyrophosphate cardiac scans may be positive. Biopsy of subcutaneous fat or the rectum frequently reveals amyloidosis. Endomyocardial biopsy, which carries a higher risk of perforation in the amyloid-infiltrated heart, reveals infiltration in the interstitium and around the coronary vasculature with deposits that are pale pink on hematoxylin-eosin stain and are birefringent with the specific Congo red stain. Symptomatic patients generally have >25% of myocardial areas involved.

Once amyloidosis has been associated with heart failure, the median survival is <1 year, with <5% 5-year survival. Most deaths occur suddenly. Patients with familial amyloidosis may have a slower course than those with a monoclonal gammopathy. Making the diagnosis is important to exclude potential candidates for cardiac transplantation, after which amyloidosis can recur rapidly. Symptomatic therapy focuses on the congestive picture. Vasodilator therapy is less effective than in dilated cardiomyopathy, owing to less pronounced systolic dysfunction, greater reliance on high filling pressures, and the frequently accompanying autonomic neuropathy, which predisposes to postural hypotension. Digoxin has not been associated with clear benefit and may carry increased toxicity, particularly through aggravating conduction block. Therapy with colchicine or the combination of melphalan and prednisone for patients with associated monoclonal gammopathy has yielded response rates of only 20 to 30%.

Sarcoidosis (see Ch. 61) is a disease of unknown cause characterized by granulomatous involvement of multiple organs. In patients with extracardiac sarcoidosis, clinical cardiac involvement is present in <5%, but the noncaseating granulomas have been found in 25% of autopsied hearts, where they may be surrounded by lymphocytic infiltrates and patchy fibrosis. Granulomas can be replaced by connective tissue, leading to focal aneurysmal dilation. Predilection for the upper ventricular septum leads to a high incidence of heart block, which may present with syncope or sudden death, although these are frequently due to ventricular tachycardias in this disease. Echocardiography may show global or regional ventricular dysfunction, usually without marked dilation. Diagnosis of the focal lesions is often missed on endomyocardial biopsy. Technetium pyrophosphate, gallium, and thallium imaging have all been used. Most patients with cardiac sarcoidosis have evidence of involvement elsewhere, usually pulmonary. Steroid therapy decreases dysrhythmias and improves ventricular function in some patients and has been recommended for proven cardiac sarcoidosis. The prognosis is often determined more by the consequences of pulmonary parenchymal involvement and pulmonary hypertension.

TABLE 43–4. CAUSES OF RESTRICTIVE CARDIOMYOPATHIES

Infiltrative
  Amyloidosis
  Sarcoidosis
  Gaucher's disease—glucocerebroside-laden macrophages
  Hurler's disease—mucopolysaccharide-laden macrophages
Storage
  Hemochromatosis
  Fabry's disease
  Glycogen storage diseases
Fibrotic
  Radiation
  Scleroderma
Metabolic
  Carnitine deficiency
  Defects in fatty acid metabolism
Endocardial
  Possibly related diseases
    Tropical endomyocardial fibrosis
    Hypereosinophilic syndrome (Löffler's endocarditis)
  Carcinoid syndrome
  Radiation
  Doxorubicin
Dilated cardiomyopathy overlap
  Early stage ("minimally dilated cardiomyopathy")
  Partial recovery from dilated cardiomyopathy
  Myocardial metabolic defects
Idiopathic

STORAGE DISEASES. Although amyloidosis and sarcoidosis infiltrate around myocytes, compromise from the storage diseases results primarily from intracellular accumulation. *Hemochromatosis* is the most common example in adults, frequently arising from an autosomal recessive disorder in the gene that regulates iron absorption. The estimated frequency of homozygosity for the mutant allele is 5 per 1000. The gene is closely linked to HLA-A3 but has not been identified yet. In the absence of the genetic defect in iron regulation, hemochromatosis can result from iron overload due to hemolytic anemia and transfusions. Iron is deposited primarily in the perinuclear areas of myocytes. Disrupted cellular architecture and mitochondrial function lead to cell death and replacement fibrosis. The atrioventricular node may be involved. The degree of left ventricular dilation is variable, leading to both dilated and restrictive pictures, with the restrictive aspects dominating earlier in the course. Dilation is generally to left ventricular diastolic dimensions of ≤ 60 mm, but ejection fractions in severe cases are often $<30\%$, unlike the other restrictive diseases. The diagnosis is generally made from the clinical picture and the serum iron proteins but may be confirmed by endomyocardial biopsy tissue stained for iron. Early diagnosis is important, as phlebotomy and iron chelation therapy may improve cardiac function before cell injury has become irreversible. Deaths from hemochromatosis result more from cirrhosis and liver carcinoma than from cardiac disease.

Specific metabolic enzyme deficiencies can lead to abnormal metabolites accumulating in the myocardium, causing increased ventricular mass and restrictive cardiomyopathy. Fabry's disease (see Ch. 174.1) results in intracellular glycolipid accumulation in myocardium and valves, vessel walls, skin, cornea, kidneys, gastrointestinal tract, and central nervous system (CNS). Mortality from this X-linked disorder in men results from multiple organ involvement in the fourth or fifth decade. Some heterozygous women have also developed cardiomyopathy. Glycogen storage disease (see Ch. 170) results from enzyme deficiencies that lead to excessive deposition of normal glycogen in myocardium, skeletal muscle, and liver. The most common is type II, Pompe's disease, associated with dramatic thickening of ventricular septal and free walls, large QRS amplitude, short PR interval, and death usually within the first few years of life.

Gaucher's disease (see Ch. 174.2) of glucocerebroside metabolism and Hurler's disease of mucopolysaccharide metabolism result in infiltration of the myocardium by cells filled with abnormal metabolites and may more properly be considered with the infiltrative cardiomyopathies.

FIBROTIC RESTRICTIVE DISEASE. Restrictive myocardial disease can occur with diffuse fibrotic changes in the absence of abnormal substance accumulation. Radiation for thoracic malignancy can produce restrictive cardiomyopathy, usually presenting within several years, although occasionally up to 15 years later. Patients treated with both doxorubicin and radiation may be at higher risk. This consequence of radiation is less common, however, than pericardial disease, from which it must be distinguished.

Fibrosis in the scleroderma heart accumulates in the interstitium but may also result from small vessel ischemia with microinfarction. Left ventricular dilation is uncommon, and the congestive symptoms may be refractory to therapy.

ENDOCARDIAL RESTRICTIVE DISEASE. The picture of restrictive cardiomyopathy can be caused also by specific involvement of the endocardium with relative sparing of the remaining ventricular wall thickness. In equatorial Africa, endomyocardial fibrosis accounts for 15 to 25% of cardiac deaths. It can involve either ventricle, most commonly both, with dense thickening of the ventricular inflow tracts and atrioventricular valves while sparing the underlying myocardium and systolic function. Diuretics can decrease but rarely resolve the congestive symptoms. Extensive surgical resection has been performed for otherwise refractory disease, but with high perioperative morbidity and mortality.

Endomyocardial fibrosis may represent part of the spectrum of hypereosinophilic syndrome (Löffler's endocarditis), characterized by persistent eosinophilia of >1500 eosinophils per cubic millimeter without other cause leading to dysfunction of the heart, CNS, or other organs. The eosinophilic contents are thought to injure the endocardium, which is then the site of platelet thrombi and fibrosis. The apices may be obliterated, creating a characteristic echocardi-ographic picture. The mitral and tricuspid valves are affected, leading to prominent atrioventricular valve regurgitation. The thrombotic surface can be the origin of multiple systemic emboli. Geographic, infectious, and metabolic factors have been implicated but not verified. Immunosuppressive therapy can reduce the burden of eosinophils and the cardiac injury caused by the eosinophilic granules.

Endocardial injury can also result from the 5-hydroxyindoleacetic acid released by carcinoid tumors. The major sites affected are the tricuspid valve and right ventricular endocardium.

IDIOPATHIC RESTRICTIVE DISEASE. Restrictive cardiomyopathy may occasionally be diagnosed in the absence of any specific cause. Although isolated systolic function may be relatively spared, the ejection fraction is usually in the 30 to 45% range, in which cardiac output may become compromised from restricted filling and secondary valvular regurgitation. For a given patient with slightly reduced left ventricular ejection fraction and slightly elevated left ventricular volume, overt congestive symptoms and abnormal diastolic filling pattern suggest a restrictive cardiomyopathy, whereas a relative lack of symptoms is more consistent with a "minimally dilated cardiomyopathy." Some patients who demonstrate marked improvement of left ventricular function after an obvious dilated cardiomyopathy attributed to viral infection or alcohol may be left with an ejection fraction $>40\%$ but significant exertional dyspnea related to reduced compliance. Restrictive disease occasionally occurs in families, in whom a genetic defect affecting myofilament relaxation has been postulated but not identified.

Because systolic function is relatively preserved, some patients with restrictive disease may be misdiagnosed for many years as hypochondriacal or deconditioned. Prolonged exposure to elevated filling pressures can cause irreversible pulmonary hypertension, analogous to that with mitral stenosis, and occasionally true cardiac cirrhosis prior to diagnosis. When congestive symptoms develop, they may be dominated by refractory pleural effusions, ascites, and sometimes dramatic cachexia. Therapy with diuretics is helpful but not curative. The theoretical rationale for calcium channel blockers to improve diastolic relaxation has not been validated. Despite frequently preserved ejection fraction, these patients can sometimes be helped only with cardiac transplantation, which should be done before severe inanition develops.

HYPERTROPHIC CARDIOMYOPATHY

Hypertrophic cardiomyopathy has been diagnosed in approximately 2.5 in 100,000 per year in one population study. The prevalence is estimated at 20 per 100,000. Although probably less than half as common as dilated cardiomyopathy, the disease serves as an important example for studying genetic factors causing cardiomyopathy, stimuli for hypertrophy, abnormalities of myocardial relaxation and compliance, the substrate for malignant ventricular arrhythmias, and appropriate screening for competitive athletics. The cardinal features are marked left ventricular hypertrophy not due to other cardiac disease, frequently with asymmetric involvement of the septum, accompanied by supranormal contractility and decreased left ventricular systolic cavity dimension (see Table 43–1). The mitral valve moves anteriorly in systole (SAM). The descriptor —"obstructive" or "nonobstructive"—refers to whether a pressure gradient is generated which impedes left ventricular outflow at rest or with maneuvers that decrease left ventricular volume. Previous names for this syndrome included asymmetric septal hypertrophy (ASH), hypertrophic obstructive cardiomyopathy (HOCM), and idiopathic hypertrophic subaortic stenosis (IHSS) but have been largely replaced by hypertrophic cardiomyopathy (HCM) because hypertrophy can be concentric and the majority of patients do not demonstrate obstruction to outflow.

The hypertrophied ventricular walls can exceed three times normal thickness, resulting in marked encroachment on the ventricular cavity (Fig. 43–4). Classically the septum is most involved, but hypertrophy can be asymmetric elsewhere or global. Pathologically, the myocytes show marked disarray in a characteristic whorled pattern and disorganization of the larger muscle bundles as well. Intramural coronary arteries usually have thickened vessel walls and reduced lumina. Although the left ventricle is the usual site, some patients have associated right ventricular hypertrophy and, rarely, right ventricular gradients.

Genetic transmission occurs as an autosomal dominant trait. The disease can be caused by multiple single mutations; the best charac-

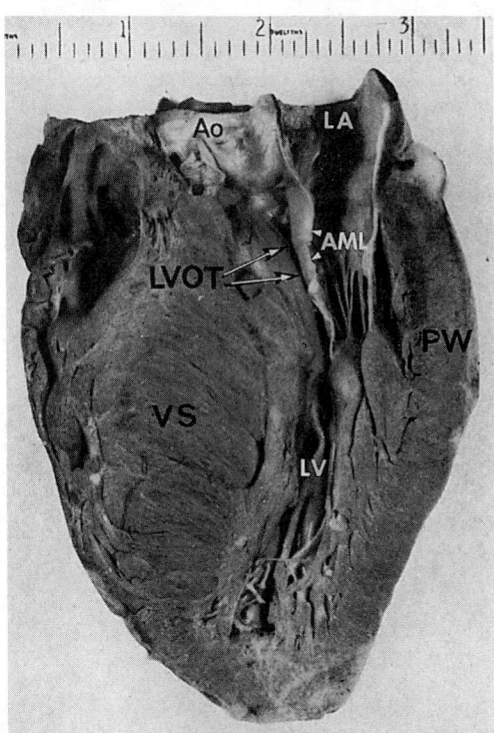

FIGURE 43–4. One of the original described cases of hypertrophic cardiomyopathy, demonstrating the marked hypertrophy of the ventricular septum (VS) in contact with the anterior mitral leaflet (AML), impinging on the left ventricular outflow tract (LVOT). The left ventricular (LV) cavity is severely reduced. Ao = Aorta; LA = left atrium. (From Teare D: Asymmetric hypertrophy of the heart in young adults. Br Heart J 20:1, 1958. Labels superimposed.)

terized are those of the myosin heavy chain gene on chromosome 14. Although producing similar hypertrophy, some mutations appear to be associated with more benign clinical courses. Similar mutations may occur spontaneously, causing sporadic disease that becomes familial without earlier family history.

Abnormal calcium channels and fluxes may play a role in the myocyte dysfunction. Evidence indicates that early catecholamine-related stimulation contributes to this condition, which may reflect failed regression of the septal hypertrophy normally seen in fetal and neonatal hearts. In many patients with the disease, the asymmetric hypertrophy may not develop fully until adolescence.

PHYSIOLOGY. The affected ventricle is hypercontractile with a supranormal ejection fraction, at times almost obliterating the left ventricular cavity. Diastolic distensibility is decreased, leading to elevated filling pressures that can cause shortness of breath, particularly with exertion. Impaired ventricular filling at rapid heart rates may limit cardiac reserve and exercise performance. Anginal-type chest pain occurs frequently and may reflect relative myocardial ischemia without focal epicardial coronary artery lesions.

Outflow obstruction, present in about 25% of patients, is usually due to the anterior mitral valve leaflet apposing the septum. When present, the midsystolic gradient can approach levels seen in severe aortic stenosis. The gradient may be elicited or enhanced by maneuvers that decrease left ventricular volume, such as vasodilation, the Valsalva maneuver, or standing after squatting. Enhanced contractility, such as in the beat following a premature ventricular contraction, also aggravates a gradient. Handgrip increases systemic resistance and decreases the gradient. Syncope can result from an increased gradient leading to decreased cardiac output, from elevated intraventricular pressures activating vagal tone, or from ventricular arrhythmias arising within the areas of abnormal myocyte organization.

CLINICAL DIAGNOSIS. Most patients present between ages 20 and 40, although occasional patients present after age 50. Presenting symptoms may be dyspnea on exertion, chest pain, palpitations, or syncope. When syncope occurs, it is generally during or shortly after heavy exertion. Cardiac examination in asymptomatic patients may be unrevealing except for slightly prominent

left ventricular impulse. Decreased compliance during atrial filling may lead to a palpable and audible presystolic sound (S_4). When present, the murmur is usually best heard at the left lower sternal border, and represents a sum of the outflow murmur and mitral regurgitation. It is typically harsh, and increases in intensity with the maneuvers described above, which decrease ventricular size. When a gradient impedes ejection, the carotid impulse may transmit both an early and late systolic pulse. Enhanced *a* wave in the jugular venous pulse usually reflects decreased right ventricular compliance due to the abnormal septum rather than right heart failure.

Electrocardiographic abnormalities most commonly include left ventricular hypertrophy and increased Q waves occasionally misdiagnosed as infarction. Left atrial abnormality may be detected in the P waves, and a short PR interval with slurred QRS upstroke may be misdiagnosed as pre-excitation. Echocardiography establishes the diagnosis, and frequently Doppler interrogation can identify resting gradients. Classic asymmetric septal hypertrophy is defined as a septal–posterior wall thickness ratio of at least 1.5, but asymmetry is not necessary to diagnose hypertrophic cardiomyopathy. Cardiac catheterization is often performed to quantify the gradient and in older patients to exclude coexistent coronary disease as a component of their chest pain.

Considerable debate exists over appropriate screening for hypertrophic cardiomyopathy, which is the most common cause identified in sudden deaths occurring in athletes. It is unclear whether the increased recognition in athletes results from the addition of their physiologic ventricular hypertrophy or their high public profile.

THERAPY. Therapy in asymptomatic patients focuses on preventing progression and sudden death (Fig. 43–5). The risk of sudden death appears increased in asymptomatic patients with nonsustained ventricular tachycardia and may be reduced by amiodarone, although amiodarone may increase mortality in patients with severe symptoms. β-Adrenergic blocking agents and calcium channel blockers could reduce hypertrophy and the chance of sudden death but have not been clearly beneficial in asymptomatic patients. Owing to the risk of sudden death during exertion, competitive sports are generally contraindicated.

Symptoms of exertional dyspnea or chest pain may improve with β-adrenergic blocking agents and calcium channel blockers. Verapamil improves left ventricular diastolic filling and may offer additional benefit. Disopyramide may be useful in hypertrophic cardiomyopathy owing to its negative inotropic effect. Amiodarone, another antiarrhythmic agent, may also improve clinical status. Symptoms from diastolic dysfunction are aggravated at high heart rates owing to reduced filling time, particularly when the atrial booster pump function is lost during atrial fibrillation, which should be aggressively suppressed. Digoxin, however, is not indicated in hypertrophic cardiomyopathy.

When symptoms become severe, high filling pressures may lead to fluid retention requiring diuretic therapy, which must be carefully modulated. When combination medical therapy fails to maintain adequate functional capacity, recent experience with dual-chamber pacing suggests improvement in symptoms and up to 50% reduction in gradients, when present. The benefits have been attributed to altering the sequence of ventricular activation and possibly to decreasing mitral regurgitation with short atrioventricular interval. Ventricular septal myotomy-myectomy, in which a small portion of the ventricular septum is surgically removed, may be considered in patients with gradients > 50 mm Hg and refractory symptoms. This procedure can usually eliminate the resting gradient and improves symptoms in about 70% of patients, most of whom continue to have some limitation due to the intrinsic diastolic dysfunction. Mitral valve replacement may be performed simultaneously or as an isolated procedure in patients with atypical distribution of hypertrophy.

PROGNOSIS. The natural history of hypertrophic cardiomyopathy reflects referred populations in whom disease is more severe, with annual mortality rates of 1 to 4%, higher in children. Sudden death is most common in people < 35 years, in those with a family history of sudden death, and in those with syncope. Despite the prominence of death during vigorous exertion, two thirds of sudden deaths occur during rest or mild activity, and most occur in patients with few or no symptoms.

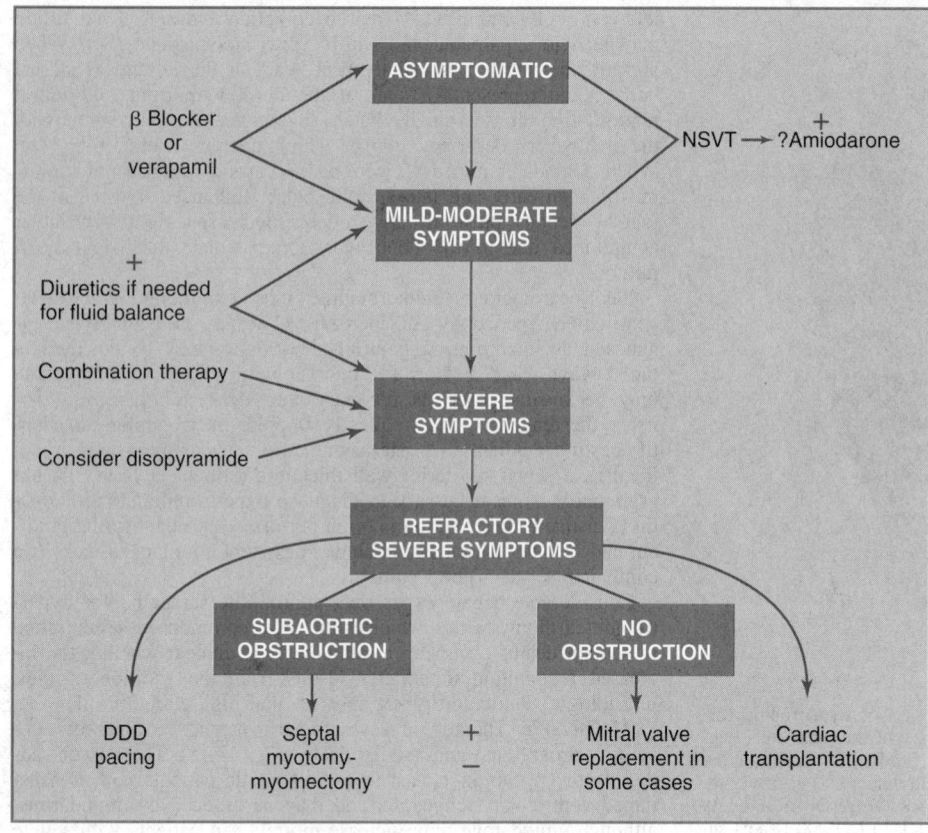

FIGURE 43–5. Approach to therapy of hypertrophic cardiomyopathy according to symptom severity. (Adapted from Maron BJ: Hypertrophic cardiomyopathy. Curr Prob Cardiol 18:637, 1993.)

Hypertrophic cardiomyopathy is observed to "burn out" into a dilated cardiomyopathy with low ejection fraction in approximately 10 to 15% of symptomatic patients. Therapy then is tailored to the hemodynamic compromise but may require close adjustment, as the residual diastolic dysfunction leads to severe congestive symptoms at higher ejection fractions than in primary dilated cardiomyopathy.

A separate entity of apical hypertrophic cardiomyopathy has recently been recognized, predominantly in Japan, where it accounts for one fourth of hypertrophic cardiomyopathy. It is characterized by systolic apical obliteration that creates a "spade-like" cavity on angiography, and frequently by giant negative T waves in the precordial electrocardiogram. There is no intraventricular gradient. Symptoms are usually mild. Malignant ventricular arrhythmias appear less commonly than in other forms of hypertrophic cardiomyopathy. Some patients, particularly elderly women, have marked symmetric hypertrophy, which is disproportionate to the degree of their hypertension. As with other hypertrophic or restrictive disease, these patients with congestive symptoms may describe a history of previous misdiagnosis and therapy for dilated cardiomyopathy.

Codd MB, Sugrue DD, Gersh BJ, et al.: Epidemiology of idiopathic dilated and hypertrophic cardiomyopathy. Circulation 80:564, 1989. *A meticulous study directed at defining the frequency of cardiomyopathy in a regional Minnesota population, which may not necessarily be representative of other regions.*

Davidoff R, Palacios I, Southern J, et al.: Giant cell versus lymphocytic myocarditis. A comparison of their clinical features and long-term outcomes. Circulation 83:953, 1991. *A comparison of clinical features between lymphocytic myocarditis and the less common but more devastating giant-cell myocarditis.*

Espinosa R, Carrasco HA, Belandria F, et al.: Life expectancy analysis in patients with Chagas' disease: Prognosis after one decade (1973–1983). Int J Cardiol 8:45, 1985. *A detailed analysis of the varying presentations and prognoses for patients with this common disease, which is not sufficiently understood outside of endemic areas.*

Kasper EK, Agema WRP, Hutchins GM, et al.: The causes of dilated cardiomyopathy: A clinicopathologic review of 673 consecutive patients. J Am Coll Cardiol 23:586, 1994. *Results of systematic endomyocardial biopsy in a large referral population. Results are representative of other series except for a slightly higher incidence of myocarditis, which included "borderline myocarditis."*

Kaul S, Fishbein MC, Siegel RJ: Cardiac manifestations of acquired immune deficiency syndrome: A 1991 update. Am Heart J 122:535, 1991. *An excellent summary of the multiple factors that may affect cardiac function in this disease.*

Kelly DP, Straus AW: Inherited cardiomyopathies. N Engl J Med 330:913, 1994. *A thoughtful summary of recent progress in the identification of specific genetic defects causing cardiomyopathy.*

Maron BJ: Hypertrophic cardiomyopathy. Curr Prob Cardiol 18:637, 1993. *An extensive review of current pathophysiologic concepts, therapy, and prognosis in hypertrophic cardiomyopathy.*

Mason JW, O'Connell JB: Clinical merit of endomyocardial biopsy. Circulation 79:971, 1989. *The most thorough clinical review available of the current rationale and limitations of endomyocardial biopsy to diagnose cardiomyopathy.*

O'Connell JB, Constanzo-Nordin MR, Subramanian R, et al.: Peripartum cardiomyopathy: Clinical, hemodynamic, histologic, and prognostic characteristics. J Am Coll Cardiol 8:52, 1986. *An excellent clinical series describing the spectrum of patients with peripartum cardiomyopathy.*

Olson LJ, Edwards WD, Holmes DR, et al.: Endomyocardial biopsy in hemochromatosis: Clinicopathologic correlates in six cases. J Am Coll Cardiol 13:116, 1989. *A careful description of clinical and histologic findings demonstrating the variable profile of hemochromatosis.*

Watkins H, Rosenzweig A, Hwang DS, et al.: Characteristics and prognostic implications of myosin missense mutations in familial hypertrophic cardiomyopathy. N Engl J Med 326:1108, 1992. *A fascinating demonstration of the impact of molecular biology on understanding the pathogenesis and prognosis of clinical cardiomyopathy.*

Webb JG, Sasson Z, Rakowski H, et al.: Apical hypertrophic cardiomyopathy: Clinical follow-up and diagnostic correlates. J Am Coll Cardiol 15:83, 1990. *A series describing the characteristics and relatively mild course of disease in this patient population. This description of North American patients extends previous experience, which focused on the Japanese population.*

Wynne J, Braunwald E: The cardiomyopathies and myocarditides: Toxic, chemical and physical damage to the heart. In Braunwald E (ed.): Heart Disease: A Textbook of Cardiovascular Medicine. Philadelphia, WB Saunders, 1992, p 1394. *A definitively detailed and referenced source of information on all of the clinical aspects of the cardiomyopathies.*

44 DISEASES OF THE PERICARDIUM

Ralph Shabetai

Diseases of the pericardium typically present in one or more of three clinical forms: acute pericarditis, pericardial effusion, and pericardial constriction. Pericardial involvement may progress from inflammation to effusion and then constriction, or it may present as effusion or constriction without clinical evidence of preceding inflammation.

The pericardium may be involved in a large number and variety of diseases. The most important are listed in Table 44–1. Pericardial disease may be asymptomatic but may alternatively cause dramatic symptoms and signs (Table 44–2).

INFECTIONS WITH LIVING AGENTS. *Virus Infection.* Many viruses may cause pericarditis; the common offenders are listed in Table 44–1. The number of cases of idiopathic pericarditis caused by preceding viral infection is unknown.

Bacterial Infection. Bacterial pericarditis is still important, although the spectrum has altered. Pneumococcal pericarditis, once a frequent complication of pneumonia, is now uncommon, whereas infection by staphylococci, fungi, and exotic organisms is more

TABLE 44–1. MAJOR CAUSES OF PERICARDIAL DISEASE

1. Inflammation
   Virus
       Coxsackie (usually B) — (E)
       Echo — (E)
       AIDS — (E)
       Other
   Bacterial
       Pneumococcus — (E)
       Staphylococcus — (E,C)
       Meningococcus — (E,C)
       Mycobacterium tuberculosis — (E,C)
       Haemophilus influenzae — (C)
       Other
   Fungus
       Histoplasma capsulatum — (E,C)
       Other
   Other living organisms
       Parasites — (E)
       Protozoa — (E)
   Nonliving agents
       Trauma — (E,C)
       Radiation — (E,C)
       Chemical
           Chemotherapeutic agents
2. Idiopathic
   (Many may be viral, but unproven) — (E,C)
3. Neoplastic
   Secondary to carcinoma of
       Lung — (E,C)
       Breast — (E,C)
       Other
   Lymphoma — (E)
   Primary
       Mesothelioma — (E)
       Other
4. Metabolic
   Chronic renal disease
       Associated with dialysis — (E)
       End-stage uremia — (E)
   Myxedema — (E)
   Chylopericardium — (E)
   Hypoalbuminemia — (E)
5. Myocardial injury
   Myocardial infarction
       Acute
       Dressler's syndrome — (E)
   Congestive heart failure — (E)
6. Trauma — (E,C)
   Postpericardiotomy syndrome — (E)
   Postoperative — (E,C)
7. Connective tissue disorders and hypersensitivity
   Acute rheumatoid fever
   Rheumatic arthritis — (C)
   Systemic sclerosis
   Lupus erythematosus
   Drugs
       Procainamide
       Others
8. Congenital
   Absence of left pericardium
       Partial
       Complete
   Cyst
   Other

(E) = effusion common; (C) = constrictive pericarditis common.

TABLE 44–2. CLINICAL SYNDROMES OF PERICARDIAL DISEASE

Dry, fibrinous pericarditis
    Usually acute (R)
Lax pericardial effusion
    Chronic effusive
Cardiac tamponade (R)
Constrictive pericarditis
    Subacute
    Chronic
    Transient
Effusive-constrictive pericarditis

(R) = Relapse or recurrence common.

common, especially in persons at either extreme of age and in the immunologically compromised host.

Tuberculosis. Although tuberculous pericarditis has become less common, it must be considered in immigrants and those at risk for tubercular infection. Pulmonary tuberculosis may be present, but often pericardial effusion is an isolated manifestation. *Mycobacterium tuberculosis* can be recovered from only one third of effusions. Even pericardial biopsy findings are not uniformly positive. Evidence based on molecular biologic methods such as polymerase chain reaction holds promise. Commonly, the diagnosis is presumptive and based on circumstantial evidence, such as a positive skin test result or a history of recent contact.

Haemophilus influenzae infection is an important cause of constrictive pericarditis in children.

Fungal Infection. In an otherwise normal population fungal pericarditis is uncommon, but infection with *Histoplasma capsulatum* should be considered in patients who reside in the Ohio Valley. Similarly, coccidioidomycosis should be considered in patients who have been in the San Joaquin Valley of California. Patients with AIDS are particularly susceptible to fungal infection.

PERICARDIAL INFLAMMATION CAUSED BY NONLIVING AGENTS. *Trauma.* Blunt or sharp trauma is an important cause of pericarditis and may lead to pericardial effusion with or without tamponade and ultimately to constrictive pericarditis. Common examples of acute trauma include gunshot and knife wounds. Impact against a steering wheel, explosions, and crushing are the major blunt injuries.

Radiation. The pericardium may be exposed to considerable injury when radiotherapy is used to treat neoplasia, for example, Hodgkin's disease and lung or breast cancer. The latent period between radiation and clinical pericardial disease may extend for many years.

PERICARDIAL DISEASE IN METABOLIC DISORDERS. *Renal Disease.* Pericardial disease continues to be an important major complication of chronic dialysis and may cause cardiac tamponade, but its incidence is declining. Fortunately, constrictive pericarditis is rare. The cause is not understood: It may be a manifestation of end-stage renal disease, but the process of dialysis itself may be responsible in whole or in part.

Myxedema. Pericardial effusion may occur and accounts in part for cardiomegaly; it may also contribute to the low voltage and T-wave inversion that, in addition to sinus bradycardia, characterize the electrocardiogram. Pericardial effusion may contain cholesterol crystals.

CHYLOPERICARDIUM. Chylopericardium, a pericardial collection of fluid bearing a large quantity of chyle, may be idiopathic but often follows surgical or other trauma of the thoracic duct.

MYOCARDIAL INFARCTION. Acute dry, fibrinous pericarditis can be detected by auscultation in about one third of patients with acute myocardial infarction and is not a contraindication to thrombolytic therapy. Autopsy evidence is more common. Acute pericarditis early in the course is often contiguous inflammation but may also represent reaction to myocardial injury. Rupture of an infarction, aneurysm, or pseudoaneurysm creates greater or lesser degrees of hemopericardium, the former usually ending fatally.

In some patients, pericarditis (often accompanied by effusion) occurs in the weeks or months following acute myocardial infarction. This syndrome (Dressler's) is thought to be a delayed autoimmune reaction and is often recurrent.

CONNECTIVE TISSUE DISORDERS. Pericardial reaction may occur in virtually all of these disorders. Acute pericarditis is a constituent of rheumatic pancarditis but does not progress to constriction. On the other hand, subacute constrictive pericarditis can occur in rheumatoid arthritis. Pericarditis is an important manifestation of lupus erythematosus, both spontaneous and induced by drugs such as procainamide, and can cause tamponade.

HEART FAILURE. In patients with fluid retention, small pericardial effusion may be seen by echocardiography.

CONGENITAL LESIONS AND CYSTS. Partial absence of the pericardium produces a striking abnormality on the chest radiograph. Cysts are more frequent. They are filled with clear fluid and most often occupy the right cardiophrenic angle. They are benign and produce no symptoms.

ACUTE (FIBRINOUS) VIRAL OR IDIOPATHIC PERICARDITIS

SYMPTOMS. Findings are often preceded by generalized malaise and fever. The chief symptom is chest pain, which may be either sharp or crushing. Frequently, the pain is precordial but may shift to the left side, simulating pleurisy. Characteristically, the pain is relieved by sitting up and exacerbated by deep inspiration. Thus, pericardial pain has features that may suggest either myocardial ischemia or pleural inflammation. Referral of pain to the right trapezius ridge is a specific but uncommon sign of its pericardial origin.

CLINICAL FINDINGS. *Pericardial Friction Rub: The Pathognomonic Sign of Pericardial Inflammation.* Classically, the rub has components accompanying atrial systole, ventricular systole, and ventricular diastole (see LMSB line, Fig. 44–1). Commonly, the rub is biphasic and must be distinguished from to-and-fro murmurs. When it is monophasic, it must be differentiated from systolic murmurs. It is typically superficial and scratchy, and although it may be widely distributed over the precordium, it is usually most apparent at the left sternal edge. Appreciation is enhanced by firm pressure with the diaphragm of the stethoscope. Changes in posture and the respiratory cycle may alter the intensity. Pericardial friction rubs are often transient and should be sought frequently when pericarditis is suspected. Pericardial effusion does not abolish the rub. It must be distinguished not only from cardiac murmurs but also from mediastinal crunch due to air in the mediastinum, crepitations from surgical emphysema, and artifacts produced by movement of the skin against the stethoscope.

LABORATORY FINDINGS. *Electrocardiogram.* The typical findings of pericarditis are shown in Figure 44–2. ST-segment elevation, although widespread, is not uniform, depression being usual in leads aV_R and V_1. Depression of the PR segment, although highly specific, is less common than ST-segment elevation.

On a single tracing and without clinical information, ST-segment elevation cannot always be distinguished from the early repolarization normal variant or from the early stage of acute myocardial infarction. In the latter, evolution of the pattern in serial tracings is helpful. In acute pericarditis, the ST segment returns to baseline without inversion of the T wave (which may occur later if pericarditis becomes chronic), whereas in acute myocardial infarction, T-wave inversion typically occurs before the ST segment becomes isoelectric.

Other Laboratory Findings. The erythrocyte sedimentation rate is elevated and there is variable leukocytosis. Viral titers may confirm the origin of the illness but are seldom performed in clinical practice. Gallium radioisotope scanning may display the inflamed epicardium, but this expensive test is required only in exceptional cases. Plasma levels of cardiac enzymes may be elevated, but this determination need not be made routinely.

DIAGNOSIS. The diagnosis can usually be made reliably from symptoms and signs. When any of the conditions listed in Table 44–1 is suspected, the symptoms and signs of pericarditis should be specifically sought and the diagnosis confirmed by electrocardiography. Effusion detected by echocardiogram is very helpful. Its absence, however, does not diminish the likelihood of the diagnosis. When the pain simulates that of pleurisy, pneumonia or pulmonary infarction must be considered. When it is retrosternal and crushing, myocardial infarction must be ruled out. On occasion, other major causes of chest discomfort, such as acute pulmonary embolism or dissection of the aorta, need to be considered.

CLINICAL COURSE, PROGNOSIS, AND MANAGEMENT. Commonly, this is a self-limiting disease. It usually responds rapidly to treatment with nonsteroidal anti-inflammatory agents such as indomethacin (25 to 50 mg three to four times a day) or ibuprofen. Even aspirin is often satisfactory. Resistant cases may require steroid treatment—for instance, prednisone, starting with 75 mg a day and rapidly tapering to the minimum dose that suppresses symptoms and signs.

Detectable pericardial effusion occurs in a small proportion of cases and may progress to cardiac tamponade. Similarly, acute pericarditis may rarely lead to chronic constrictive pericarditis.

Recurrent Pericarditis. Perhaps the most troublesome of all complications is frequent recurrence over a period of years. The patient is greatly disturbed by the frequent occurrence of disabling pain, and when steroidal agents must be used for resistant cases, their side effects may become significant.

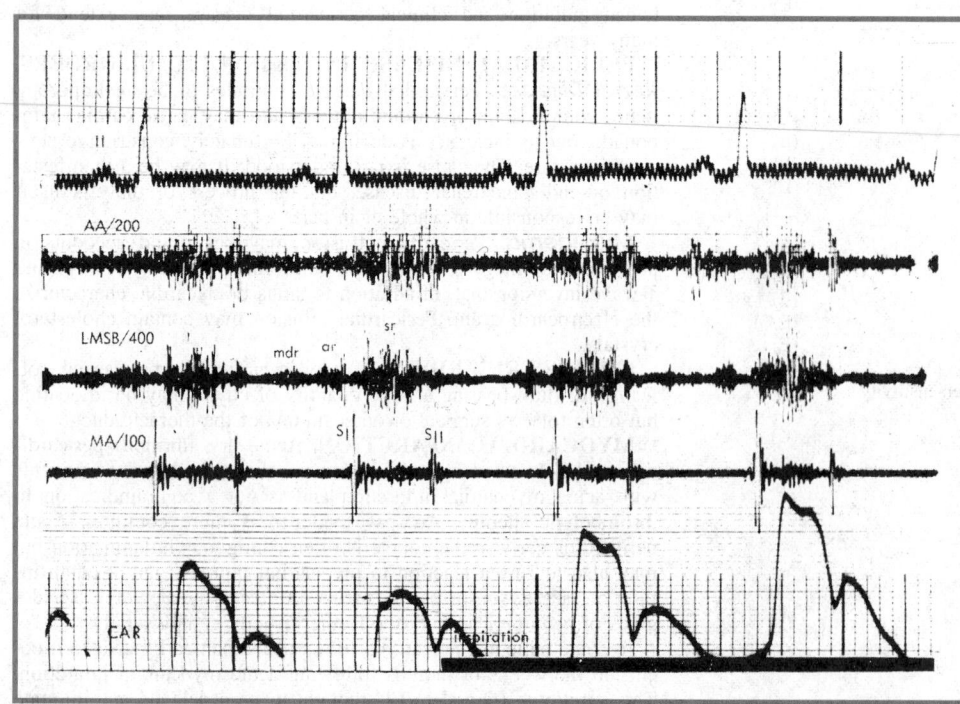

FIGURE 44–1. Phonocardiography of pericardial friction rub. AA = Aortic area; LMSB = left mid-sternal border; MA = mitral area. Note the three-component rub heard along the left mid-sternal border. Numbers refer to filter settings. (Reproduced by permission from Spodick DH: Am Heart J 81:114, 1971.)

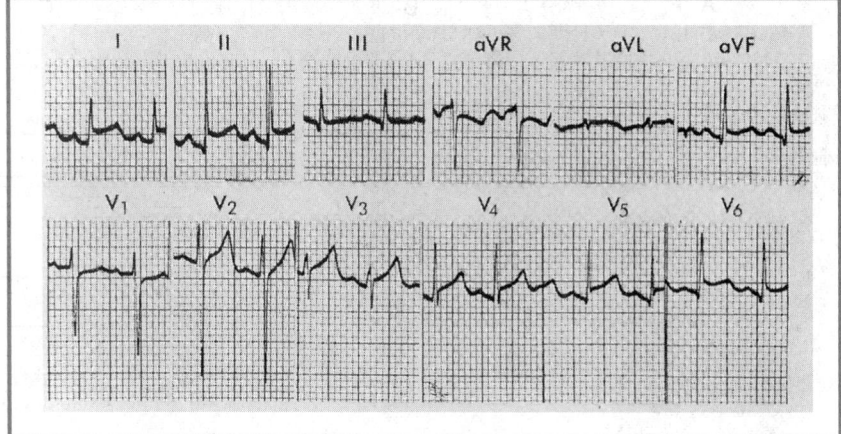

FIGURE 44–2. ECG from a case of acute pericarditis. Note the ST-segment elevation in leads I, II, aVF and V$_4$ to V$_6$ and ST segment depression in leads aV$_R$ and V$_1$. (From Shabetai R: The Pericardium. New York, Grune & Stratton, 1980.)

PERICARDIAL EFFUSION

LAX PERICARDIAL EFFUSION. Pericardial effusions that do not raise intrapericardial pressure more than 3 or 4 mm Hg do not cause symptoms. The physical findings are variable and frequently do not provide valuable clinical clues. Pericardial effusion should be strongly suspected in the setting of acute pericarditis if the cardiopericardial silhouette is enlarged on the chest radiograph. A previous radiograph showing a normal-sized silhouette is particularly helpful. The diagnosis can be made with certainty by echocardiography (Fig. 44–3).

PERICARDIAL EFFUSION COMPLICATING ACUTE PERICARDITIS. When echocardiograms are performed routinely in acute pericarditis, effusion is found in a considerable proportion of cases. However, in clinical practice, echocardiography is not required if the heart size remains normal, no evidence of cardiac tamponade or myocarditis is seen, and the findings subside within 48 to 72 hours after beginning treatment. Myocarditis should be suspected when depolarization changes, such as left or right bundle branch block, or conduction abnormalities develop and when a third heart sound is audible. In such cases, echocardiography is often useful in distinguishing cardiac chamber enlargement from pericardial effusion.

ETIOLOGY OF PERICARDIAL EFFUSION. The causes of pericardial effusion are indicated in Table 44–1. Pericardial effusion must always be considered in patients who have or are likely to have one of these disorders, but especially when there is or has been evidence of acute pericarditis or when there is circulatory compromise. When the patient has a possible cause of cardiac tamponade or constrictive pericarditis, pericardial disease must be ruled out before attributing circulatory abnormalities to heart disease.

PERICARDIOCENTESIS. When the venous pressure is normal, systemic arterial hypotension is absent, and the cause of pericardial effusion has been established with reasonable certainty, pericardiocentesis is seldom needed. On the other hand, if the clinician suspects or diagnoses purulent effusion, or cardiac tamponade that is not responding satisfactorily to medical treatment, removing pericardial fluid via a needle or open drainage becomes necessary. In a smaller fraction of cases, pericardiocentesis is required to establish a tissue or bacteriologic diagnosis. In such instances, the relative merits of the less traumatic and less expensive pericardiocentesis, versus surgical drainage, must be weighed against local experience and preference and the relative importance of pericardial biopsy in establishing the diagnosis.

Lax pericardial effusions have minimal hemodynamic effects, but when large and chronic, as, for example, in idiopathic chronic effusive pericarditis, a number of clinicians recommend surgical drainage.

CARDIAC TAMPONADE

ETIOLOGY AND PATHOPHYSIOLOGY. Pericarditis of virtually any cause may be associated with pericardial effusion, and virtually any pericardial effusion can progress to cardiac tamponade. The important causes are indicated in Table 44–1. The pathophysiology is illustrated in Figure 44–4, taken from cardiac catheterization data from a patient with severe cardiac tamponade.

Normal pericardial pressure is subatmospheric (Fig. 44–4F) and approximates pleural pressure. When pericardial effusion rapidly accumulates, pericardial pressure rises abruptly because the parietal pericardium can stretch acutely only to a limited extent (Fig. 44–4D). A few hundred milliliters accumulating rapidly can generate intrapericardial pressures in excess of 20 mm Hg, whereas a slowly developing effusion may assume gigantic proportions with only minimal elevation of intrapericardial pressure. In clinical practice, cases may be encountered anywhere between these two extremes.

To maintain effective circulation, systemic venous pressure must rise to equal intrapericardial pressure to maintain venous return. Figure 44–4E indicates equilibration of right atrial and pericardial pressure. Unless the pre-existing left ventricular diastolic pressure was higher than pericardial pressure during cardiac tamponade, this pressure also must rise to the same level to maintain filling of the left ventricle. Figure 44–4A to E shows equally elevated pulmonary wedge, right atrial, right ventricular diastolic, and intrapericardial pressures. During inspiration the normal inspiratory drop of systemic venous pressure is maintained (Fig. 44–4A), but the normal systemic arterial systolic and pulse pressure drop is exaggerated during inspiration (Fig. 44–4C). The latter finding is termed pulsus paradoxus (Fig. 44–5). Systemic arterial hypotension is absent (Fig. 44–4C) in mild-to-moderate cardiac tamponade. Surgical causes such as trauma or rupture of the heart or the aorta into the pericardium are usually associated with profound hypotension. In medical cases, cardiac output is often reduced to the range shown in Figure 44–4, but in surgical cases still lower cardiac outputs are often observed.

CLINICAL FINDINGS. The chief component in recognizing tamponade is thinking of it. Cardiac tamponade must be considered whenever evidence suggesting heart disease or heart failure devel-

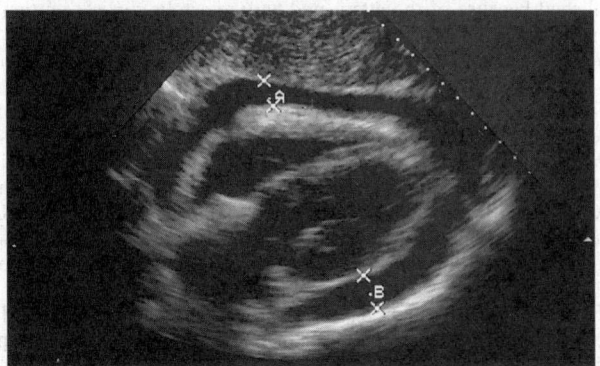

FIGURE 44–3. Echocardiogram showing large circumferential pericardial effusion. A is the anterior effusion in front of the right ventricle. B is the posterior effusion behind the left ventricle. x x marks the pericardial and epicardial boundaries of the effusion.

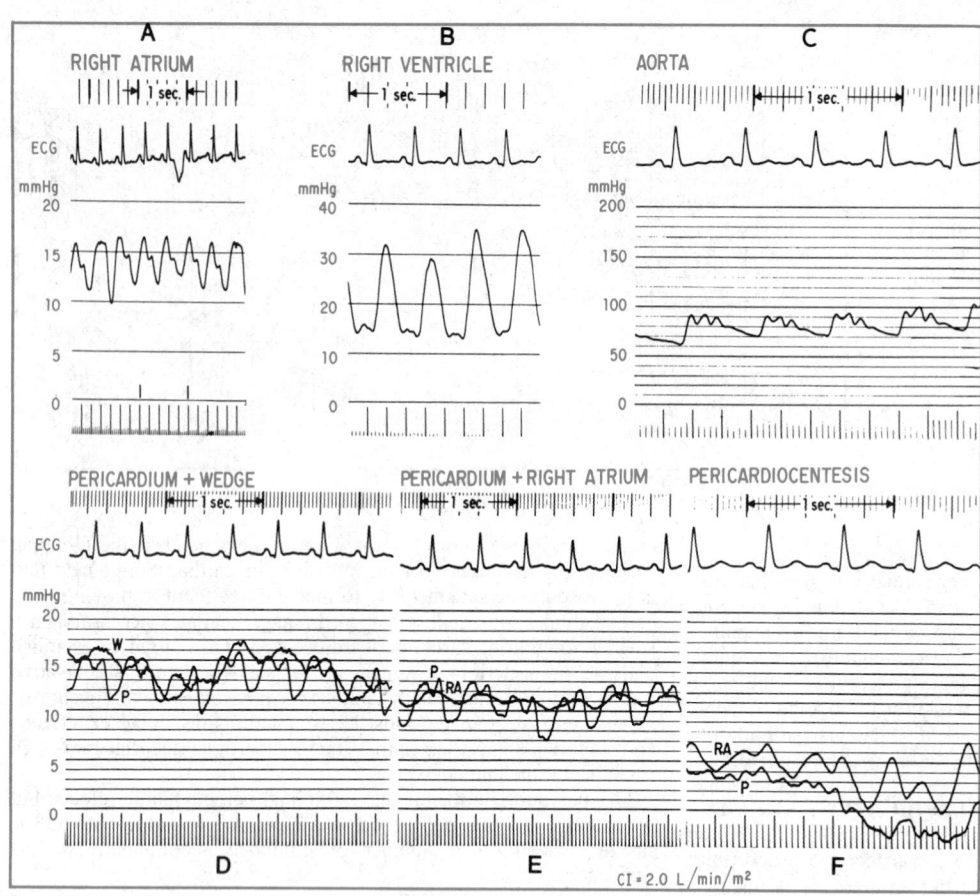

FIGURE 44-4. Hemodynamic data from a patient with cardiac tamponade. See text for discussion.

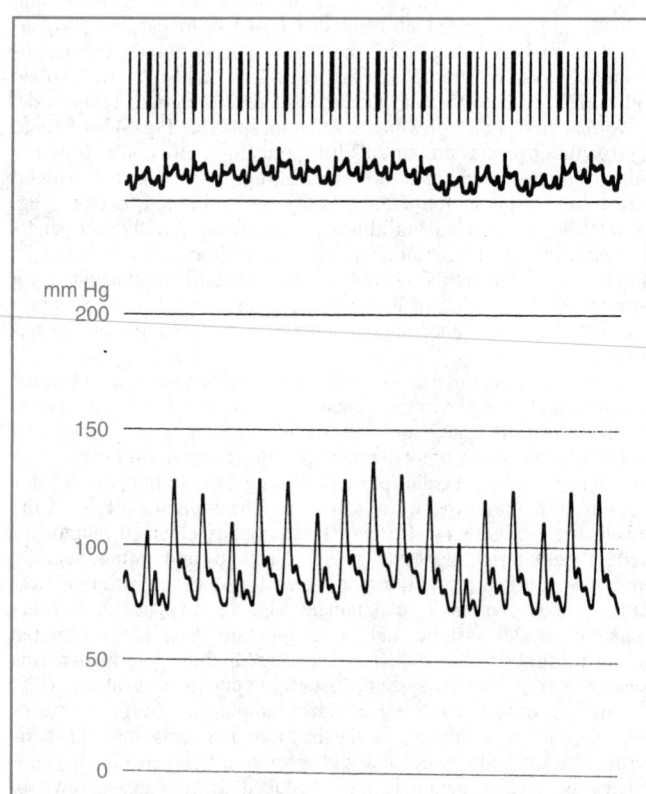

FIGURE 44-5. Radial arterial tracing showing pulsus paradoxus. During inspiration systolic and pulse pressures decline. Diastolic pressure is little affected.

ops in a patient who may reasonably be suspected of a disorder listed in Table 44-1. In extreme cases consciousness may be impaired, and arterial blood pressure may drop to shock levels. Frequently there is oliguria, because cardiac tamponade—with the resulting drop in cardiac output and blood pressure—is a powerful stimulus for the kidney to retain sodium. Pericardial pain may or may not be present; often there is a sensation of fullness of the chest and sometimes frank dyspnea.

Venous Pressure. Important evidence of cardiac tamponade includes abnormal jugular venous pulses. The venous pressure is elevated, usually considerably so, unless there is concomitant acute blood loss or severe dehydration. The right atrial (and therefore the jugular) pulse is monophasic, the normal inspiratory drop is maintained, and the predominant wave is the x descent, occurring when the ventricle ejects (Fig. 44-4A). The prominent x descent is detected as a sharp inward movement of the internal jugular pulse synchronous with the carotid pulse. The y descent is reduced or abolished because of the attenuated early diastolic dip of ventricular pressure (Fig. 44-4B).

Pulsus Paradoxus. Severe pulsus paradoxus (Fig. 44-5) may be detectable by palpating any arterial pulse. When extreme, the pulse disappears during inspiration; when less extreme, it diminishes but is palpable. In the presence of severe hypotension, pulsus paradoxus may be difficult to detect. Pulsus paradoxus is quantified with a sphygmomanometer. As the cuff is deflated, pulsus paradoxus is estimated as the difference between pressure occurring when the first blood pressure sound can be heard only during expiration and that when the sound is heard throughout the respiratory cycle.

Friction Rub. In some cases of cardiac tamponade, a pericardial friction rub is present; otherwise, precordial examination tends not to be helpful.

LABORATORY FINDINGS. The echocardiogram proves that effusion is present and may show compression of the right atrium and ventricle (Fig. 44-6). The chest radiograph usually shows car-

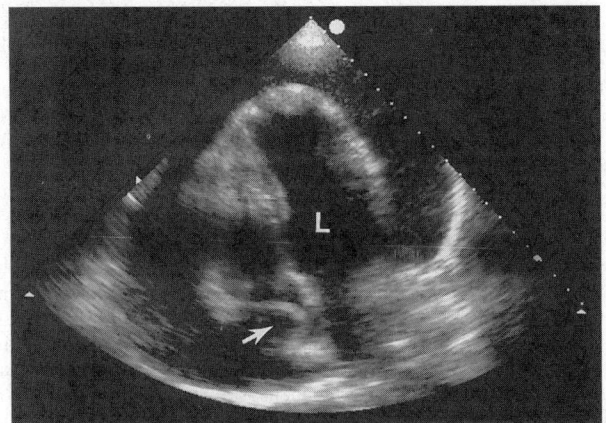

FIGURE 44-6. Echocardiogram of large pericardial effusion causing tamponade. The cardiac apex is at the top of the figure and the left ventricle (L) on the right. The right atrium at the lower right corner of the figure normally has a convex outer wall. Here it is severely compressed *(arrow)* and therefore appears sharply concave.

diac enlargement, but in acute cases the volume of pericardial effusion may be too small to increase the cardiothoracic ratio. The electrocardiogram is often not helpful, but when pericardial effusion is large, especially in cardiac tamponade secondary to neoplasm, electrical alternans may occur. Alternation is usually confined to the QRS complex; more specific for pericardial effusion, but less common, is alternation of P, QRS, and T waves.

TREATMENT. Unless tamponade is mild and rapidly improves following medical treatment, prompt removal of pericardial fluid is mandatory. In acute cases only a small portion of the fluid need be removed, because of the steep pressure-volume curve of the pericardium. In experienced hands, pericardiocentesis is safe. When experience is limited, tamponade is recurrent, or biopsy is needed, subxiphoid surgical drainage is preferred.

CONSTRICTIVE PERICARDITIS

DEFINITION AND ETIOLOGY. Constrictive pericarditis produces thickening, fibrosis, and sometimes calcification of the pericardium with restriction of a cardial filling. The most common causes are listed in Table 44-1. In the United States and western Europe, constrictive pericarditis most often is idiopathic, secondary to neoplasm or radiation, post-traumatic, or due to connective tissue disease. Tuberculosis and pyogenic infection are less common. More subacute and fewer chronic cases are seen, and heavy calcification of the pericardium is infrequent.

PATHOPHYSIOLOGY. The pathophysiology and hemodynamics are shown in Figure 44-7 from the study of a stock car driver with post-traumatic pericarditis. Panel A shows pressures recorded simultaneously from both ventricles. In early diastole there is a prominent dip of pressure, and in mid and late diastole the pressure forms a plateau. The two plateaus are elevated and of equal amplitude. During early diastole, ventricular filling is faster than normal, signified by the early diastolic dip, at the end of which cardiac volume reaches the limit set by the rigid pericardium. The ventricular diastolic pressures are then elevated but do not rise through the remainder of diastole, signifying absence of further ventricular filling. Elevated left ventricular diastolic pressure to approximately 20 mm Hg causes elevation of right ventricular systolic pressure.

Panel B shows simultaneous pressure records from the right ventricle and right atrium. In contradistinction to cardiac tamponade, right atrial pressure is biphasic, showing a prominent x descent with ventricular ejection and prominent y descent coincident with the early diastolic dip of ventricular pressure. The y descent can be recognized at the bedside as a sharp inward movement of the jugular pulsation out of phase with the carotid pulse. Respiratory variation is absent. Panel C shows simultaneous pulmonary wedge and superior vena cava pressures, confirming equilibration of filling pressures on the two sides of the heart. Panel D shows pressures simultaneously recorded from the pulmonary artery and the pulmonary

wedge position. In late diastole all cardiac pressures equilibrate around 20 mm Hg.

CLINICAL FINDINGS. Elevated filling pressure of the left side of the heart causes dyspnea and pulmonary congestion, which in severe cases is evident on the chest radiograph. Elevated filling pressure of the right side of the heart causes peripheral edema; hepatic enlargement, congestion, and dysfunction; and frequently ascites.

When ventricular filling is suddenly checked at the end of the early diastolic pressure dip, a loud third heart sound ("pericardial knock") is frequently audible. The apex beat may not be palpable, or there may be systolic retraction. Ascites is often prominent in relation to peripheral edema. The liver is usually enlarged and pulsatile. When present, palmar erythema, spider angiomas, and mild jaundice testify to severe, chronic hepatic congestion.

The abnormally small ventricular end-diastolic volume reduces stroke volume even when systolic function is well maintained, as it usually is.

LABORATORY FINDINGS. By chest radiography, the heart is normal in size to moderately enlarged. In chronic cases, particularly those associated with tuberculosis, pericardial calcification may be seen. The electrocardiogram usually shows T-wave inversions and frequently a wide, notched P wave due to chronic elevation of left atrial pressure. In longstanding cases, atrial fibrillation supervenes. Liver function test results are abnormal, and hypoalbuminemia may be compounded by protein-losing enteropathy.

Echocardiography. The echocardiogram is less helpful than in pericardial effusion. Sometimes increased thickness of the pericardium can be detected, especially if there is also a small effusion. The cardiac walls move abruptly in early diastole and are stationary throughout middle and late diastole, corresponding to the hemodynamic alterations. Motion of the interventricular septum is often abnormal.

Other Imaging Techniques. The thickened pericardium is well visualized by computed tomography. Magnetic resonance imaging, which, although more expensive, is slightly more accurate.

DIAGNOSIS. Systemic venous congestion not explained by heart failure or other causes should suggest the possibility of constrictive pericarditis, especially when one of the causes listed in Table 44-1 is present or suspected.

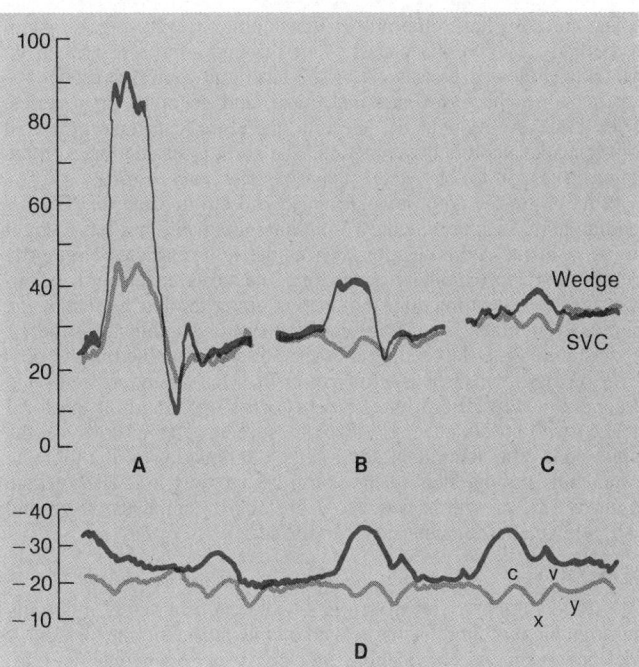

FIGURE 44-7. Hemodynamic data from a case of constrictive pericarditis. See text for details. (From Shabetai R: Profiles of constrictive pericarditis, restrictive cardiomyopathy and cardiac tamponade. *In* Grossman W [ed.]: Cardiac Catheterization and Angiography. 2nd ed. Philadelphia, Lea & Febiger, 1980.)

In patients with massive edema and liver dysfunction, the most common erroneous diagnosis is cirrhosis of the liver. This major error can be avoided by examining the venous pressure in the neck. When the venous pressure is elevated, anasarca is due to cardiac or pericardial, not hepatic, causes.

Imaging shows normal systolic function and cardiac valves. The ventricles are often small and fill rapidly in early diastole but not at all for the remainder of diastole.

Restrictive cardiomyopathy is a disease of heart muscle (see Ch. 43) that mimics constrictive pericarditis. In some cases, endomyocardial biopsy and occasionally exploratory thoracotomy are needed to establish the correct diagnosis.

TREATMENT. For the vast majority of patients, the treatment is pericardiectomy. The patient should be prepared by modest diuresis. With modern techniques of cardiopulmonary bypass, especially in cases that are not too far advanced, the operation yields gratifying clinical improvement, although full benefit may not be evident for about 3 months.

Engel PH: Echocardiographic findings in pericardial disease. *In* Fowler NO (ed.): The Pericardium in Health and Disease. Mt. Kisco, NY, Futura Publishing Company, 1985. *An up-to-date, well-written discussion.*

Klopfenstein HS, Schuchard G, Wann LS, et al.: The relative merits of pulsus paradoxus and right ventricular diastolic collapse in the early detection of cardiac tamponade. An experimental echocardiographic study. Circulation 71:829, 1985. *Describes the correlation between hemodynamics and echocardiographic abnormalities in cardiac tamponade.*

Oh JK, Hatle LK, Seward JB, et al.: Diagnostic role of Doppler echocardiography in constrictive pericarditis. J Am Coll Cardiol 23:154, 1994.

Shabetai R: The Pericardium. New York, Grune & Stratton, 1980. *A comprehensive monograph dealing with the normal pericardium and pericardial diseases.*

Shabetai R, Fowler NO, Fenton JC, et al.: Pulsus paradoxus. J Clin Invest 44:1882, 1965. *An experimental study of the mechanisms of pulsus paradoxus.*

Spodick DH: Pathogenesis and clinical correlations of the electrocardiographic abnormalities of pericardial disease. Cardiovasc Clin 8:201, 1977. *A well-illustrated and complete account of theory and clinical application.*

45 DISEASES OF THE AORTA
Lawrence S. Cohen

The aorta is vital to the proper functioning of every organ system in the body. The coronary arteries are the first arteries to arise from the aorta, followed by vessels of the head and central nervous system and then the gastrointestinal, renal, and genitourinary arteries. Disease in any segment of the aorta, therefore, can have profound consequences upon bodily function. The aorta is susceptible to three major disease processes: *aneurysm, dissection,* and *aortitis.*

At its origin the aorta is approximately 3 cm in diameter. The ascending aorta is approximately 5 cm long, coursing in a left-to-right direction in the same ejection axis as the left ventricle. The aortic arch is also approximately 5 cm long and takes an upward, posterior, and leftward direction, terminating along the left border of the thoracic vertebrae. The aortic arch lies entirely within the superior mediastinum. The descending thoracic aorta is contained in the posterior mediastinum. It is a bit narrower than the ascending aorta and is approximately 20 cm long. It runs to the diaphragm at the level of the twelfth thoracic vertebra and supplies the arteries to the spinal cord. The abdominal aorta is the continuation of the thoracic aorta, ending at the level of the fourth lumbar vertebra. The average length is 15 cm, with an average diameter of 2 cm at its origin and a slightly smaller diameter at its lower end.

ANEURYSM

DEFINITION. An aneurysm is a widening of a vessel involving the stretching of fibrous tissue within the media of the vessel. A true aneurysm is a widening of the vessel, whereas a false aneurysm represents a localized rupture of the artery with sealing over by clot or adjacent structures. The natural history of aneurysms is to enlarge. Not only does the process tend to continue and progress but also the law of Laplace is a factor. As described by Laplace, the tension in the wall of a spherical chamber enclosing a fluid under pressure is related to the pressure under which the

fluid is kept and the radius of curvature of the containing vessel. As the radius increases so does wall tension. Hence, enlargement of the vessel begets more enlargement.

It is convenient to classify aneurysms according to cause, morphology, and location. Arteriosclerosis is the most common cause of aneurysms. Other causes are cystic medial necrosis, trauma, and infection, including syphilis. Rarer causes are rheumatic aortitis, Takayasu's syndrome, temporal arteritis, and relapsing polychondritis. Marfan's syndrome is characterized by cystic medial necrosis (Ch. 183). In some forms of Ehlers-Danlos syndrome, rupture of blood vessels, including the aorta, may occur. Aneurysms can be classified into three morphologic types: (1) fusiform, in which the aneurysm encompasses the entire circumference of the aorta and assumes a spindle shape; (2) saccular, in which only a portion of the circumference is involved and in which there is a neck and an asymmetric outpouching of the aneurysm; and (3) dissecting, in which an intimal tear permits a column of blood to dissect along the media of the vessel. This is often called a dissecting hematoma. Aneurysms are also classified by location, involving (1) the ascending aorta, including the sinuses of Valsalva; (2) the aortic arch; (3) the descending thoracic aorta, originating just distal to the left subclavian artery; and (4) the abdomen, most commonly distal to the renal arteries.

The most proximal portion of the ascending aorta comprises the sinuses of Valsalva. Aneurysms in this location are usually congenital in origin. Most involve either the right sinus or the right portion of the noncoronary sinus. Aneurysms of the sinus of Valsalva are often silent until they rupture into the right side of the heart, usually the right ventricle or right atrium. This event may occur spontaneously or may be a consequence of infective endocarditis. Other causes of aortic sinus aneurysm are Marfan's syndrome, syphilis, and infective endocarditis. Aneurysms of the ascending aorta may be arteriosclerotic, but cystic medial necrosis with or without other features of Marfan's syndrome is more common. Syphilis was once a common cause of ascending aortic aneurysm but has all but disappeared as a cause. The more distal the aortic location of the aneurysm, the more likely it is to be arteriosclerotic.

CLINICAL MANIFESTATIONS. Clinical manifestations of aneurysms of the thoracic aorta (other than rupture) are due to compression, distortion, or erosion of surrounding structures. Pain is the most common symptom. Pain in a gradually enlarging aneurysm is insidious and may be described as boring and deep. Increasing intensity of pain is an ominous sign and may presage impending rupture.

Aortic valve regurgitation may be associated with aneurysms of the ascending aorta. Distortion of the aortic annulus and separation of the aortic valve cusps accounts for the regurgitation. If regurgitation occurs rapidly, the clinical consequences can be dramatic, with the patient developing acute pulmonary edema. Many patients develop a murmur of aortic regurgitation gradually and may be relatively asymptomatic. Aneurysms of the transverse aortic arch are less common than are aneurysms in other sites. The consequences of such aneurysms are often formidable because the innominate and carotid arteries arise from the transverse aortic arch. In addition, the arch is contiguous with other vital structures such as the superior vena cava, pulmonary artery, trachea, bronchi, lung, and left recurrent laryngeal nerve. Symptoms may include dyspnea, stridor, hoarseness, hemoptysis, cough, or chest pain.

The most common site of an aneurysm of the descending thoracic aorta is between the origin of the left subclavian artery and the diaphragm. Arteriosclerosis is the most common cause, with age, hypertension, and probably smoking contributing as risk factors. One factor in the pathogenesis of aneurysms of the descending aorta may be the immobility of the aorta at this site and the unique stresses imposed on the aorta immediately distal to the left subclavian artery. Distortion of the architecture in this area may result in sufficient turbulence to cause elastic tissue degeneration, accelerated arteriosclerosis, and localized dilatation.

Pain from descending thoracic aortic aneurysm is often intrascapular but can vary considerably. Hoarseness may occur from stretching of the left recurrent laryngeal nerve. Hemoptysis may occur owing to leakage into the left lung. Thoracic aortic aneurysms, like those of the abdominal aorta, threaten life by potential rupture. They are rarely complicated by thrombosis or embolism. Thoracoabdominal aneurysms involve the celiac, superior mesenteric, and renal arteries. Fortunately, they are not common, for they represent a great challenge to the vascular surgeon. Although some are caused by cystic medial necrosis, most are of arteriosclerotic origin and occur in older men.

The most common form of aneurysm is the abdominal aortic aneurysm. The prevalence of this aneurysm at autopsy is in the 1 to 3% range but is even more common in men over 60. Its frequency in men outnumbers that in women by 6:1. Almost all of these aneurysms are below the renal arteries. Most are of arteriosclerotic origin, but trauma, infection (including syphilis), and arteritis make up a small fraction. A fortunate feature of these aneurysms is their accessibility on physical examination. Rupture of an abdominal aneurysm is the greatest threat and may lead to a rapid demise because of shock and hypotension. Other less acute symptoms may also occur. Pain in the lower back is a sign of enlargement of the aneurysm and at times is a warning of impending rupture. Almost all abdominal aortic aneurysms are lined with clot or have ulcerated plaques. Embolization of atherothrombotic material may lead to a variety of symptoms, ranging from digital infarction to anuria from a shower of emboli to the kidneys.

The likelihood of rupture increases with increasing aortic aneurysm size. Sixty to 80% of patients with lesions ≥ 7 cm die of rupture, and 95% of patients with lesions > 10 cm die of aneurysm rupture. The risk of rupture in aneurysms ≤ 5 cm is considerably lower. Given these data, general guidelines about surgical repair have emerged. Aneurysms associated with aortic thrombosis or distal embolic events should be repaired promptly. Aneurysms suspected of rupture or acute expansion should be treated surgically immediately. Although there are differences of opinion concerning when elective repair of asymptomatic aneurysms should be undertaken, once the aneurysm exceeds 5 cm in diameter, the prognosis on continued medical management becomes increasingly guarded.

DIAGNOSIS. Palpation is usually the first step in diagnosing abdominal aneurysms. Ultrasound imaging is an excellent technique to confirm the diagnosis, as it is noninvasive, inexpensive, and accurate to within 2 to 3 mm of aneurysm size when compared with the findings at surgery. Computed tomographic (CT) scanning utilizing contrast material is as effective as ultrasonography for detecting and sizing abdominal aortic aneurysms. Often lumbar spine radiographs clearly outline the walls of an abdominal aortic aneurysm if there is calcium in the walls. Aortography, either arterial or venous with digital subtraction, may not reflect the true size of the aneurysm; an extensive laminated clot may reduce the lumen.

Joyce JW: Aneurysmal disease. *In* Spittell JA Jr (ed.): Clinical Vascular Disease. Philadelphia, FA Davis, 1983, p 89. *A concise summary of aneurysmal disease, including management guidelines for aneurysms in all aortic locations.*

Spittell JA Jr: Abdominal aortic aneurysms. Hosp Pract 21:105, 1986. *This is a short, well-illustrated practical management update. Modern diagnostic tools are discussed, and management strategies are reviewed.*

DISSECTING ANEURYSM OF THE AORTA

The incidence of aortic dissections is not known exactly, but it is estimated that approximately 2000 acute cases occur in the United States each year.

Classification of aortic dissection is based on duration and anatomic location of the dissection. Dissection is considered acute if it occurred within 2 weeks and chronic if it occurred more than 2 weeks before starting therapy.

Aortic dissection is more commonly classified by site of the intimal tear and extent of dissecting hematoma. In type I and type II dissections, the intimal tear is in the ascending aorta, usually within a few centimeters of the aortic valve. In type I aneurysms, the dissecting hematoma extends and involves at least the aortic arch and often the descending aorta as well. Type II aneurysms involve the ascending aorta only. Type III aneurysms are characterized by an intimal tear in the descending aorta, usually immediately distal to the left subclavian artery. The dissecting hematoma usually propagates distally but at times may extend in a retrograde manner to the aortic arch (Fig. 45–1).

ETIOLOGY. The most consistent causative factor in aortic dissection is hypertension. Other conditions are associated with dissection in the absence of hypertension. Marfan's syndrome is discussed below. There is a peculiar association between pregnancy and dissection. It is postulated that hormonal changes during pregnancy may alter the composition of the aorta and make it more susceptible to rupture. Stresses and strains of labor may also be a factor.

Valvular aortic stenosis, particularly that due to a bicuspid valve, is associated with dissection. Turbulence established beyond the

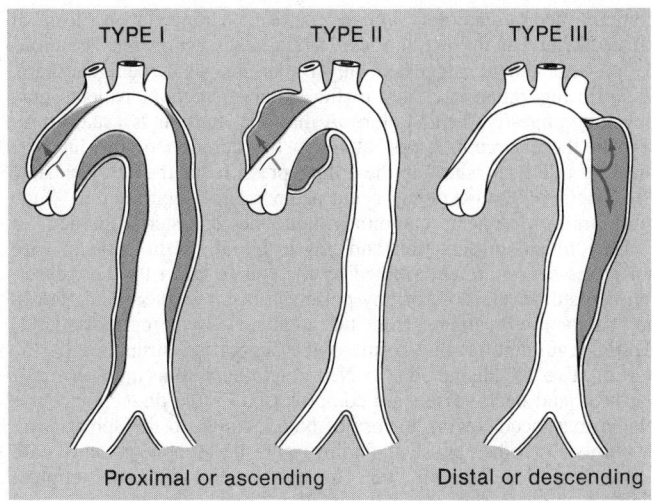

FIGURE 45–1. Classification of dissecting aneurysms of the aorta. (Modified from DeBakey.)

stenotic valve increases lateral forces, thereby enhancing the likelihood of an intimal tear and development of a dissection. The association between coarctation of the aorta and dissection is well known. The years of proximal aortic hypertension before repairing the coarctation may establish the conditions that ultimately lead to aortic dissection. In addition, a high incidence of bicuspid aortic valves is seen in patients with coarctation of the aorta. Before the advent of antimicrobial agents, syphilitic aortitis was the most common cause of aortic dissection; it is now unusual. Trauma may be a cause of dissecting aneurysm. Other unusual causes are the Ehlers-Danlos syndrome and relapsing polychondritis.

PATHOGENESIS. Aortic dissection begins most frequently in an intimal tear in the ascending aorta a short distance above the aortic valve. The primary tear is often referred to as the *entry intimal tear.* The *re-entry* or *secondary tear* occurs more distally. The basic pathologic condition resides in the underlying media, the chief supporting layer of the aorta. Most tears are transverse or circumferential, reflecting the direction of the muscular fibers of the media.

The two key ingredients of aortic dissection are arterial hypertension and medial degeneration. In any given patient, one or the other of these abnormalities may be the more important. Many patients with Marfan's syndrome or the Ehlers-Danlos syndrome develop dissecting aneurysms without ever developing hypertension. Alternatively, individuals with longstanding hypertension may develop dissection without any apparent specific weakness of the aortic medial wall. Additional factors in the pathogenesis of aortic dissections are the anatomy and motion of the heart and great vessels themselves. The heart beats an average of 70 times per minute, over 80,000 times per day, and over 35 million times per year. The heart is not absolutely fixed in place but is limited in its anterior-posterior movement by the sternum and vertebral column, respectively. Its motion is both side to side and twisting as it ejects blood into the ascending aorta. This produces a flexing stress in the ascending aorta and contributes to the frequency of ascending aortic dissections. The descending aorta becomes fixed distal to the left subclavian artery, accounting for the alternative predilection for dissection to occur at that site. Once an intimal tear occurs, the dissecting hematoma is propagated through the weakened medial wall. The forces that continue the propagation are the arterial pressure and the pulse wave properties (dp/dt) of left ventricular ejection. Some dissecting hematomas rupture back into the aortic lumen at a distal site. Rupture may also occur externally into the pericardial or pleural space.

CLINICAL MANIFESTATIONS. Pain is often excruciating and may occur primarily in the anterior chest. It may migrate to the back as the dissecting hematoma works it way down the aorta. Patients sometimes describe an accentuation of the pain with each heart beat, suggesting the driving force of the pulse wave. Pain may occur in the neck, jaw, or teeth if the aortic arch is involved. Less common symptoms are syncope, stroke, paraplegia, or loss of pulses in any of the extremities. Rarely, a dissection may be clinically silent and be suggested only by an abnormal roentgenogram. If aortic regurgitation occurs owing to the dissection, patients may develop congestive heart failure. A diastolic murmur is usually present in these circumstances, although the duration of the murmur may be relatively short if the filling pressure in the left ventricle rises rapidly because of the acute nature of the regurgitation. Such murmurs may be heard commonly along the right sternal border.

The clinical presentation and physical findings in patients with aortic dissection are determined by the course taken by the dissecting hematoma. (1) Loss of any pulse can occur as the circulation to any major artery arising from the aorta may be compromised. (2) Aortic regurgitation may result if the supporting structures of the aortic valve are disrupted. (3) Neurologic symptoms may occur if the head and neck vessels are compromised by the dissection. Paraplegia may occur owing to loss of blood supply to the spinal cord. A number of other physical findings may be seen in patients with aortic dissection. These include Horner's syndrome due to compression of the superior cervical ganglion, vocal cord paralysis and hoarseness due to pressure against the recurrent laryngeal nerve, superior vena cava syndrome, pulsating neck masses, dyspnea due to tracheal or bronchial compression, hemorrhagic pleural effusion, myocardial infarction if the hematoma dissects retrograde across a coronary ostium, and symptoms and signs of mesenteric infarction. Persistent fever has also been described.

DIAGNOSIS. Time is often of utmost importance in management. Once the patient is stabilized, aortography should not be delayed. Routine laboratory tests do not generally add much to the diagnosis. Leukocytosis is a common but nonspecific finding. A chest roentgenogram may be normal but often shows widening of the aortic shadow (Fig. 45–2). Aortic angiography was once the definitive procedure, yielding precise information necessary for proper management. The extent of the dissection, the entry and reentry sites, the competence or degree of regurgitation of the aortic valve, and aortic branch vessel involvement can all be ascertained (Fig. 45–3).

However, development of accurate noninvasive methods of making the diagnosis has altered the diagnostic approach to suspected aortic dissection. CT scanning, magnetic resonance imaging (MRI), and transesophageal echocardiography have each been used to diagnose dissection. When available, transesophageal echocardiography should be considered first owing to its safety, speed, accuracy, and

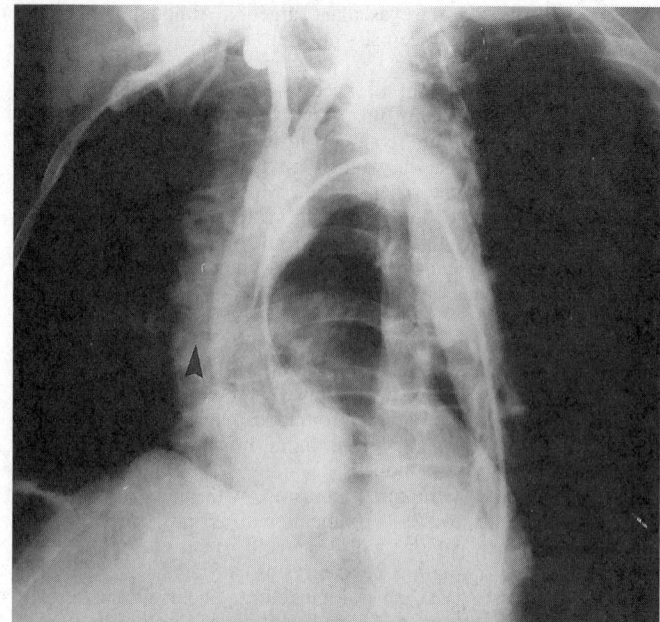

FIGURE 45–3. Aortic root angiogram in the left anterior oblique projection. The black arrowhead demonstrates the false lumen caused by the aortic dissection.

convenience (Fig. 45–4) MRI (see Ch. 33.5) is perhaps even a bit more accurate than esophageal echocardiography, but its use is sometimes not practical in an acute situation because the patient is often receiving intravenous antihypertensive agents and may be intubated. CT scanning is a reasonable alternative if transesophageal echocardiography or MRI scanning is not available. Two-dimensional transthoracic echocardiography does not require the use of contrast agents or ionizing radiation and is easily performed (Fig. 45–5). False-negative and false-positive diagnoses remain a problem with this procedure, but, at outlying hospitals, it may be the most available diagnostic procedure.

The differential diagnosis of a patient with chest or back pain, pulmonary edema with a new murmur of aortic regurgitation, any acute neurologic syndrome, or sudden loss of pulse in an extremity should include aortic dissection.

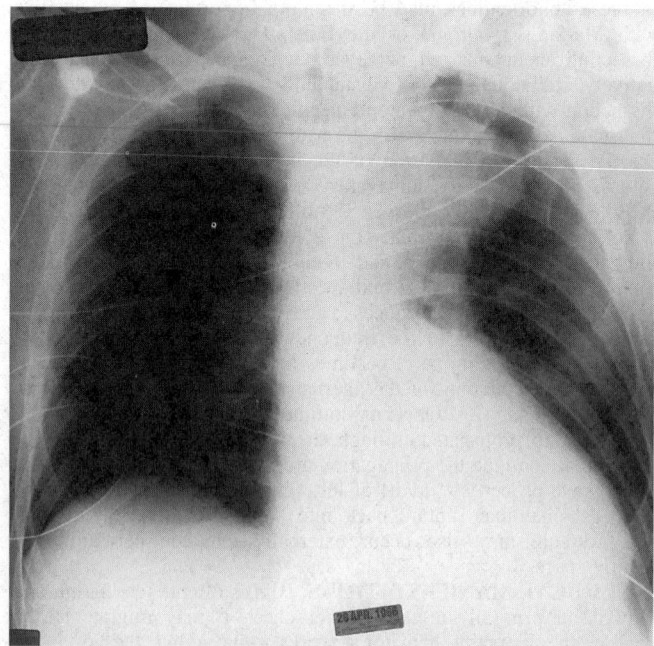

FIGURE 45–2. Chest roentgenogram of a patient with a dissecting aneurysm demonstrating marked enlargement of the aortic arch and descending aorta.

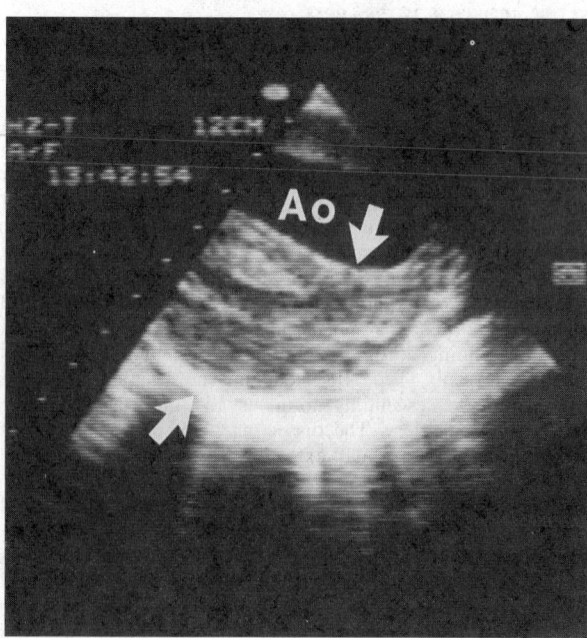

FIGURE 45–4. Transesophageal echocardiogram demonstrating an ascending aortic dissection. The top arrow points to an intraluminal clot. The bottom arrow points to the outer aortic wall.

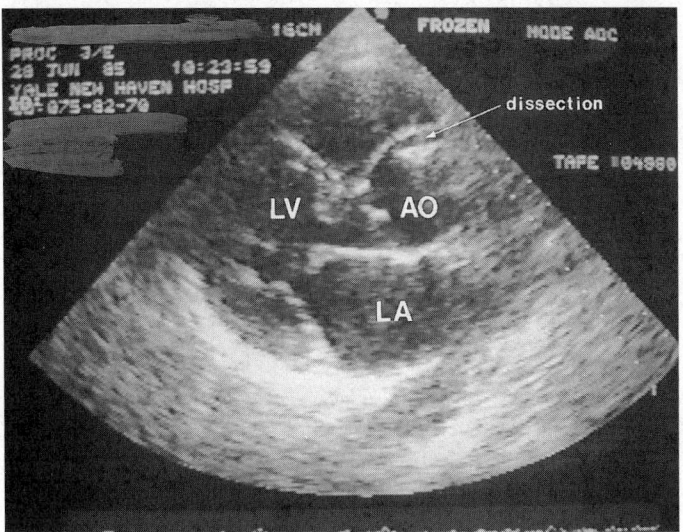

FIGURE 45-5. Echocardiogram, long-axis parasternal view of a patient with dissecting aneurysm. The dissection arises in the proximal aortic root. LV = Left ventricle; AO = aortic root; LA = left atrium.

PROGNOSIS. In untreated aortic dissection, the prognosis is poor. Approximately 20% of patients die in 24 hours, 60% in 2 weeks, and 90% in 3 months. The principal cause of death is not the initial intimal tear but is related to the effects of propagation of the dissecting hematoma. Progressive aortic regurgitation may occur if the hematoma dissects in a retrograde direction. Rupture into the pericardial or pleural space is often a fatal complication.

TREATMENT. Prompt diagnosis and institution of therapy are critical to the success of treatment. Because the most important known factors in the propagation of the dissecting hematoma are hypertension and the rate of rise of the aortic pressure pulse (dp/dt), efforts must be undertaken to alter both of these. An intravenous drip of sodium nitroprusside is started, and the infusion is titrated to reduce the systolic blood pressure to 100 to 120 mm Hg. The infusion rate can usually be started at 1 μg per kilogram per minute. Simultaneously, propranolol should be given in intermittent intravenous boluses of 0.5 to 1.0 mg until the heart rate is in the range of 60 beats per minute. When possible, an intra-arterial line to measure blood pressure accurately and a central venous line or Swan-Ganz catheter should be used. Once the patient's blood pressure and other hemodynamic and clinical features are stable, aortography should be performed. CT scanning or echocardiography may be of some diagnostic aid at this stage while awaiting aortography.

Operative intervention is usually indicated if the dissection involves the ascending aorta, as in types I and II aneurysms. These aneurysms are unstable and pose the threat of retrograde dissection, rupture, severe aortic regurgitation, or fatal pericardial tamponade. This type of acute dissection can be corrected surgically with a mortality rate in the range of 20%. Type III aneurysms that involve the distal or descending aorta can generally be treated medically. If the patient's condition stabilizes, drug therapy can be continued into the chronic phase. Surgical intervention for the patient with a type III aneurysm is indicated if there is evidence of increasing size of the dissecting hematoma, impending rupture, inability to control pain, or bleeding into the pleural space.

The operative approach must be flexible and individualized. For patients with ascending aortic dissection and involvement of the annulus or root, it is often necessary to replace the entire aortic root and aortic valve with a composite conduit, which is attached proximally to the aortic annulus and distally to the aorta after obliteration of the false lumen. The coronary ostia are then reimplanted into the tubular graft. If the ascending aorta is involved but the sinuses of Valsalva are spared, operative repair consists of resection of the aneurysmal portion with replacement by a synthetic tubular graft. This same technique applies for descending aortic dissections. In all cases, the false lumen is obliterated. Management and follow-up of patients initially treated either surgically or medically is the same. Continued meticulous control of blood pressure and administration of β-blockers to control dp/dt are warranted. The systolic blood pressure should be kept below 130 mm Hg at rest and the heart rate below 72 beats per minute at rest.

MARFAN'S SYNDROME

Patients with Marfan's syndrome (see Ch. 183) develop both aortic aneurysm and aortic dissection. Myxomatous degeneration of valve leaflets may also occur. The mitral valve cusps may be involved. The chordae tendineae may elongate or rupture, predisposing to mitral valve prolapse, or flail mitral valve with mitral regurgitation. Regurgitation at either the mitral or the tricuspid valve may be the most prominent finding in certain patients. However, the most commonly affected tissue is the aorta. The aorta enlarges, beginning with the sinuses of Valsalva. The enlargement most often extends to the innominate artery, although at times the entire aorta may be involved in what has been referred to as annuloaortic ectasia. Aortic dilation may begin as early as the fifth year of life or as late as the sixth decade.

Aortic regurgitation may occur secondary to participation of the aortic root in the development of an aortic aneurysm. Dissection of the aortic root may lead to acute aortic regurgitation. Dilation of the pulmonary artery is common.

DIAGNOSIS. Dilation of the aortic root is easily measured by echocardiography. Two-dimensional echocardiography shows the classic flask-shaped dilation of the aorta extending from the aortic valve to the innominate artery (Fig. 45-6). Echocardiography may also be used to demonstrate the major complications of aortic root dilation, dissection of the aorta, and aortic regurgitation. The echocardiogram has also helped in defining the optimal time for operative intervention. MRI can also give excellent definition to abnormalities of the aorta (Fig. 45-7).

THERAPY. It is now generally agreed that β blockade may inhibit the pace of aortic dilation. Therefore, it is appropriate to obtain serial echocardiograms in patients thought to have Marfan's syndrome. When incipient dilation of the aorta is recognized, institution of a β blocker is warranted. By diminishing the velocity with which the left ventricle ejects blood, the forces on the weakened aortic wall may be lessened.

Complications of aneurysms in the ascending aorta account for more than 90% of deaths from Marfan's syndrome. The likelihood of both aortic dissection and aortic regurgitation increases as the size of the aortic root increases. Operation in the face of an acute dissection is fraught with considerable hazard. Therefore, prophylactic operation is recommended if the aortic root enlarges to 6 cm on echocardiography. The operation most commonly utilized for patients with Marfan's syndrome is replacing the ascending aortic aneurysm with a composite tube graft that includes a prosthetic valve at its proximal end. The coronaries are anastomosed to the

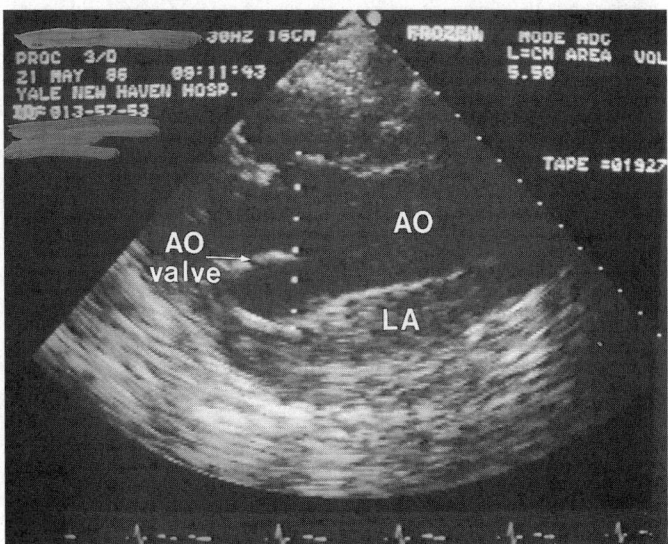

FIGURE 45-6. Echocardiogram, long-axis parasternal view of a patient with Marfan's syndrome. The sinuses of Valsalva are flared and the aortic root is dilated.

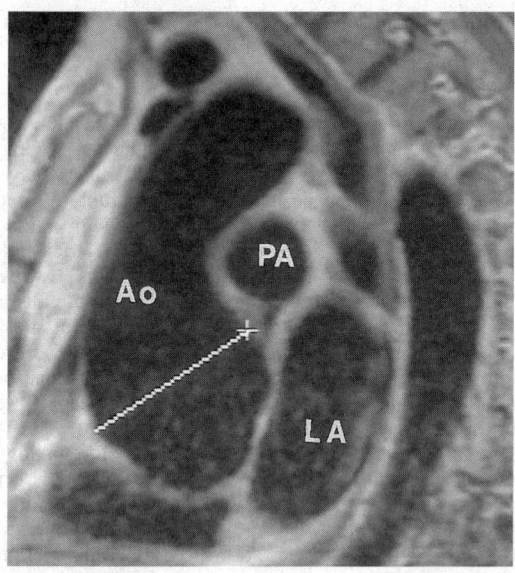

FIGURE 45-7. Magnetic resonance image, sagittal view, showing an aneurysm of the ascending aorta in a patient with Marfan's syndrome.

lower extremities round out the clinical picture. A chest roentgenogram may show mediastinal widening. Prompt surgical intervention may be life saving.

Cigarroa JE, Isselbacher EM, DeSanctis RW, et al.: Diagnostic imaging in the evaluation of suspected aortic dissection. N Engl J Med 328:35, 1993. *This excellent review assesses the sensitivity, specificity, indications, and contraindications of diagnostic modalities.*

Gott VL, Pyeritz RE, Magovern GJ Jr, et al.: Surgical treatment of aneurysms of the ascending aorta in the Marfan syndrome. N Engl J Med 314:1070, 1986. *Results of ascending aorta replacement with a composite graft in 50 consecutive Marfan's syndrome patients are reported. Because of the unfavorable natural history of Marfan's syndrome, prophylactic repair is recommended when the aneurysm reaches a diameter of 6 cm.*

Halpern BL, Char F, Murdoch JL, et al.: A prospectus on the prevention of aortic rupture in the Marfan syndrome with data on survivorship without treatment. Johns Hopkins Med J 129:123, 1971. *This is one of the first articles to advocate the prophylactic use of β blockers in Marfan's syndrome in order to prevent further dilation and dissecting aneurysm.*

Lupi-Herrera E, Sanchez-Torres G, Marcushamer J, et al.: Takayasu's arteritis: Clinical study of 107 cases. Am Heart J 93:94, 1977. *A review of 107 Takayasu's arteritis patients. This entity is not limited to Asians; it is a nonspecific inflammatory process affecting the aorta and its main branches.*

Shores J, Berger KR, Murphy EA: Progression of aortic dilatation and the benefit of long-term β-adrenergic blockade in Marfan's syndrome. N Engl J Med 330:1335, 1994.

sides of the tube graft. The aneurysm is wrapped around the tube graft to help establish hemostasis. The overall hospital mortality of the procedure is 2%. Although it may seem radical to recommend aortic replacement to a patient who may be asymptomatic, the adverse prognosis of the patient with Marfan's syndrome whose aorta dilates to >6 cm in diameter probably warrants this recommendation.

MISCELLANEOUS FORMS OF AORTITIS AND THE AORTIC ARCH SYNDROME

ARTERITIS. A number of inflammatory processes can involve the aortic arch and its major branches. Aortic arteritis, no matter what the cause, may narrow or occlude the major arch vessels. Blood supply to the areas supplied by the innominate artery, the left common carotid artery, and the left subclavian artery may be impaired. Symptoms may include transient ischemic attacks, syncope, disorders of vision or speech, claudication of the upper extremities or of the muscles of the jaw, decreased pulses in the neck and upper extremities, or symptoms of basilar artery insufficiency. As a group, these entities are called the aortic arch syndrome. They include aortitis due to syphilis, tuberculosis, giant cell arteritis, polyarteritis nodosa, Takayasu's syndrome, and dissecting aneurysm. Kawasaki's mucocutaneous lymph node syndrome may cause an aortitis, but the coronary arteries are the principal vessels involved. Giant cell arteritis may cause the aortic arch syndrome in addition to temporal and ophthalmic artery disease.

Takayasu's arteritis may be a more specific form of aortitis. Initially it was thought that the arteritic process was limited to the aortic arch and its branches. Subsequent studies have demonstrated that the arteritis is not confined to these areas. Three varieties are now recognized. In one type, the involvement is localized to the aortic arch and its branches. The second type involves the descending thoracic aorta and abdominal aorta without the arch. The third type contains features of both. There is a preponderance of females with "pulseless disease." Although early reports were more common in Japan, increasing numbers of patients are being recognized in the United States. The presence of hypertension with absent pulses in the upper extremities has caused this syndrome to be called *reversed coarctation.*

TRAUMATIC AORTIC DISEASE

The most common form of trauma to the aorta is due to deceleration injuries, often seen in automobile accidents. Because the descending aorta is relatively immobile, deceleration injuries characteristically affect the portion of the aorta immediately distal to the left subclavian artery. Nonpenetrating aortic injury may cause internal bleeding with no external evidence of chest injury. Hypotension or shock, left hemothorax, absence of femoral pulses, and pale

46 VASCULAR DISEASES OF THE LIMBS
Hermes A. Kontos

VASCULAR DISEASES OF THE LIMBS CAUSED BY ABNORMAL RESPONSES OF VASCULAR SMOOTH MUSCLE

Raynaud's Phenomenon and Disease

DEFINITION. Raynaud's phenomenon is a syndrome manifested by attacks of pallor and cyanosis of the digits in response to cold or to emotion. As the attack abates, these color changes are replaced by redness. When the disorder is primary, it is called Raynaud's disease; when it is secondary to another disease or cause, it is called Raynaud's phenomenon.

ETIOLOGY AND INCIDENCE. Raynaud's disease is the most common cause of Raynaud's phenomenon, accounting for 60% of patients with this disorder. Although Raynaud's disease can begin at any age, it commonly manifests clinically between ages 20 and 40. It is much more common in women than in men. There are two theories about its cause. Raynaud believed that it is caused by increased sympathetic nerve activity. However, measurements of the sympathetic nerve traffic in the median nerve failed to show differences between patients with Raynaud's disease and normal individuals. Lewis discovered that attacks of Raynaud's phenomenon could be induced after interrupting the sympathetic nerves. His conclusion: The cause of the disorder was a fault in the arterial wall that rendered the vessels hyperresponsive to the vasoconstrictive effects of cold. He ascribed the vasospastic attacks to spasm of the digital arteries as a result of this hypersensitivity. Little is known about the defect in the vessel wall, which renders the vessel hypersensitive to cold. The circulation of the digits of patients with Raynaud's disease is not hypersensitive to infused norepinephrine. Also, determining the arteriovenous concentration differences of norepinephrine and epinephrine across the hand showed no excessive release of catecholamines from the hands of patients with Raynaud's disease. More recently, accelerated destruction of platelets and release of agents such as serotonin or thromboxane A_2 have been proposed as causing vasoconstriction in some patients with Raynaud's phenomenon. It is not known whether platelet destruction is the cause of spasm in such patients or a consequence of it. The skin of the fingers of patients with Raynaud's disease and of those with Raynaud's phenomenon secondary to scleroderma were found to have lower density of calcitonin gene-related peptide-containing nerve fibers than those of normal controls. Based on these findings, it was hypothesized that abnormal synthesis and release of this powerful vasodilator peptide might be causally related to the pathogenesis of Raynaud's phenomena.

In a recent study, 26% of patients with the variant type of angina pectoris were found to have migraine, and 24% were found to have Raynaud's phenomenon. This suggested that some patients with Raynaud's phenomenon may have a generalized defect that predisposes arteries in many regions to vasospasm. An association of Raynaud's phenomenon with idiopathic pulmonary hypertension has also been reported. This association may reflect a very high level of peripheral vascular tone secondary to the severe reduction in cardiac output.

Secondary Raynaud's phenomenon is observed frequently as a manifestation of the diseases listed in Table 46–1.

When arterial obstruction is present, vasoconstrictive stimuli that normally do not cause clinical manifestations result in more severely reduced blood flow and may cause Raynaud's phenomenon.

Raynaud's phenomenon is very often associated with connective tissue diseases, particularly scleroderma. Almost all patients with scleroderma develop Raynaud's phenomenon at some time during the course of their illness. There is a distinctive syndrome consisting of calcinosis, Raynaud's phenomenon, abnormal esophageal motility, sclerodactyly, and telangiectasia (CREST syndrome). Raynaud's phenomenon may be the presenting manifestation in connective tissue diseases and may precede the appearance of other manifestations by several years. The presence of abnormal nail fold capillaries in patients with Raynaud's phenomenon may predict future development of scleroderma. Structural changes in the vessel wall that limit flow and increase the sensitivity to vasoconstrictive influences appear to account for the frequent occurrence of Raynaud's phenomenon in these diseases. Vascular injury may also result from repetitive minor occupational trauma or from a severe exposure to cold, as in frostbite. Consequent hypersensitivity to cold causes Raynaud's phenomenon. Occupationally induced Raynaud's phenomenon is frequently secondary to exposure to a source of vibration. It is referred to as vibration white finger. It usually develops after several years of using hand-held vibrating power tools.

Neurogenic lesions cause Raynaud's phenomenon because of irritation of sympathetic nerves and consequent vasoconstriction. Intense or sustained vasoconstriction caused by drugs may also result in Raynaud's phenomenon, as in 3 to 6% of patients taking β-adrenergic receptor–blocking drugs. Propranolol is the main offender. These drugs block a β-adrenergic vasodilative mechanism in the digits and may also enhance the vasoconstrictive effects of norepinephrine. A high incidence of Raynaud's phenomenon was described during administration of certain antimetabolite drugs, such as cisplatin, vinblastine, and bleomycin. Raynaud's phenomenon

TABLE 46–1. CAUSES OF SECONDARY RAYNAUD'S PHENOMENON

1. Occlusive arterial disease
   a. Arteriosclerosis obliterans
   b. Buerger's disease
   c. Arterial embolism
   d. Vasculitis
   e. Arterial thrombosis
2. Connective tissue diseases
   a. Scleroderma
   b. Rheumatoid arthritis
   c. Systemic lupus erythematosus
3. Vascular injury
   a. Repetitive minor occupational trauma, as in pneumatic hammer operators, pianists, typists, or users of hand-held vibrating tools
   b. Frostbite
4. Neurogenic causes
   a. Thoracic outlet compression by cervical rib, by scalenus anticus muscle, or in hyperabduction syndrome
   b. Carpal tunnel syndrome
   c. Sympathetic causalgia
   d. Spinal cord diseases
5. Drugs or exposure to chemicals
   a. Ergotamine
   b. Ergotism
   c. Methysergide
   d. Polyvinyl chloride
   e. β-Adrenergic receptor blockers
   f. Antimetabolite drugs (cisplatin, vinblastine, bleomycin)
6. Intravascular coagulation or aggregation
   a. Cryoglobulinemia
   b. Cold agglutinins

was associated with hypomagnesemia, which might have been responsible for vasoconstriction.

Intravascular aggregation of coagulation of blood elements may obstruct the vessels and cause ischemia and Raynaud's phenomenon.

PATHOPHYSIOLOGY. The pallor during the attack of Raynaud's phenomenon is explained by intense vasoconstriction or spasm of the digital arteries. This results in severely reduced blood flow. In a later stage of the attack, the vasoconstriction becomes less severe, and the capillaries and veins are partially filled with blood whose hemoglobin becomes markedly deoxygenated. This accounts for the cyanosis. Upon rewarming, cyanosis is replaced by an intense red color associated with reactive hyperemia. Between attacks, blood flow to the digits is usually reduced, especially in patients who have trophic changes, but may be normal in some patients. In patients without trophic changes, blood flow to the hand during maximum vasodilation is the same as in normal individuals, but it is severely reduced in those with trophic changes, a reflection of structural changes in the blood vessels.

PATHOLOGY. In the early stages of the disease, the digital blood vessels are histologically normal. In longstanding cases, the intima becomes thickened, and the media may be hypertrophied. In severe progressive cases, complete obstruction from thrombosis may occur, and gangrene of the tips of the digits may ensue.

CLINICAL MANIFESTATIONS. The onset of Raynaud's disease is usually gradual. The patient notices an occasional mild and short-lasting attack during winter. Over succeeding years, the severity and duration of the attacks may increase. A wide variation in severity is present. Most commonly, the attacks are provoked by exposure to cold. In some patients, attacks are also precipitated by emotion. The attacks may be terminated by rewarming, or they may abate spontaneously. Between attacks, in a warm environment, the patient is asymptomatic, and physical examination shows no abnormalities. Some patients, however, complain of chronically cold hands and feet, and they may have cyanotic, cold fingers on examination. In a typical attack of Raynaud's phenomenon, the digits become pale. Usually, all digits are affected symmetrically. The pallor is sharply demarcated at the level of the metacarpophalangeal joints, reflecting spasm of the digital arteries. At a later stage during the attack, pallor is replaced by cyanosis. The patient may have feelings of coldness, numbness, and occasionally pain. Upon rewarming, the cyanosis is replaced by intense redness, and the patient may feel tingling or throbbing. Most commonly, only the hands are affected. Frequently, both hands and feet are affected. Rarely, the nose, cheeks, ears, and chin are affected also.

Atypical attacks are not infrequent. In these, the involvement of the digits may be asymmetric with only one or two digits being affected. In some cases, only a portion of the digit is affected. In these instances, the most severely affected portion of the digit is the most distal one. Thus, one may see pallor of the fingertip or of the terminal phalanx of one digit. In other cases, more than one phalanx may be involved.

In severe, progressive cases, trophic changes may occur after a few years of involvement. The hair may disappear from the dorsal aspect of the digits. The nails grow more slowly and become brittle and deformed. The skin becomes atrophic, thin, and tight (sclerodactyly). Ulcerations may develop at the fingertips or around the nail bed. These heal slowly and may become infected. They are extremely painful, especially at night. When they heal, they leave characteristic small, pitted scars.

DIAGNOSIS. The diagnosis of Raynaud's phenomenon can usually be made on the basis of the history of vasospastic attacks in the digits, precipitated by cold and relieved by warming. In atypical cases or when the patient's description of the attack is not clear, provocation of an attack is done by immersing the hands in water at a temperature of 10 to 15°C. Whole-body exposure to cold is more successful in provoking attacks. A negative result does not exclude Raynaud's phenomenon.

In typical cases, Raynaud's phenomenon is easily distinguished from acrocyanosis, but when involvement is atypical, the differentiation may be more difficult. Distinguishing features include the following: The color changes in Raynaud's phenomenon are episodic, whereas in acrocyanosis they are sustained. Pallor is not a prominent feature of acrocyanosis. Cyanosis is the more typical color change, whereas in Raynaud's disease digital pallor is characteristic. In Raynaud's disease, only the digits are involved, whereas in acrocyanosis the color changes usually involve the whole hand or foot and sometimes even more proximal portions of the limbs. In Raynaud's disease the skin of the palms is usually dry, whereas in acrocyanosis it is wet and clammy with sweat. Finally, acrocyanosis rarely causes trophic changes and ulcerations.

Obstruction of major arteries from arteriosclerosis, angiitis, embolism, or thrombosis changes skin color in the digits that simulate Raynaud's phenomenon. The distinction is made by the demonstration of changes in arterial pulses and by the fact that the color changes in these disorders are likely to be confined to one limb rather than symmetric. Arteriography, which demonstrates the arterial lesion, is helpful. However, secondary Raynaud's phenomenon may be superimposed on any of these diseases. In Raynaud's phenomenon, Doppler velocity studies show patent arteries and sharply peaked blood flow velocity patterns in the digits. Arteriography shows normal major arteries and diffuse spasm of the digital arteries.

Raynaud's disease is distinguished from secondary Raynaud's phenomenon by excluding disorders known to cause the latter. Exclusion of obstructive arterial disease is discussed above. Connective tissue disorders, particularly scleroderma, are excluded by the absence of arthralgias or arthritis, alterations of esophageal motility, and the absence of a pulmonary oxygen diffusion defect. The presence of a normal sedimentation rate and the absence of circulating autoantibodies, such as antinuclear antibodies, provide additional reassurance. A careful occupational history is necessary to exclude Raynaud's phenomenon secondary to minor repetitive trauma. A history of drug ingestion or exposure to chemicals is helpful in identifying drug-induced Raynaud's phenomenon. Neurologic disorders can be recognized by their somatic neurologic manifestations. Thoracic outlet compression syndromes can be excluded by the appropriate maneuvers. The presence of intravascular agglutination or coagulation of the blood elements may be suspected if, in the presence of cyanosis, the blood cannot be expelled from vessels by pressure, and when there are isolated areas of redness as the attack abates during rewarming. Confirmation is obtained by demonstrating the cold agglutinins or cryoglobulins in the patient's blood.

PROGNOSIS. The prognosis of patients with Raynaud's disease is good. There is no mortality associated with the disease and morbidity is low; it is generally limited to loss of portions of digits as a result of ulcerations. In approximately 50% of patients with Raynaud's disease, the disorder improves and may disappear completely after several years. In only a fraction of 1% of patients is amputation necessary. Approximately 15% of patients with Raynaud's phenomenon eventually develop a connective tissue disorder, particularly scleroderma (see Ch. 241).

The prognosis in secondary Raynaud's phenomenon depends on the course of the primary disorder. In scleroderma, the prognosis is unsatisfactory, particularly when the disease has caused digital ulcerations.

TREATMENT. Managing patients with Raynaud's phenomenon must be tailored to the individual needs of the patient, taking into consideration the frequency and severity of the attacks (Table 46–2). All patients benefit from reassurance and protective measures against exposure to cold. The patients should limit their exposure to cold to the greatest extent possible. They should wear heavy clothing, protecting not only the hands and feet but also the face and trunk, especially when there is a cold wind; this is important because exposure to cold of other portions of the body may reflexly induce vasoconstriction in the digits and precipitate Raynaud's phenomenon. When prolonged exposure to cold is unavoidable, using electrically powered or solid fuel–powered hand and foot warmers is advisable. These patients should be taught to recognize and terminate attacks by returning promptly to a warm environment, placing their hands in warm water, or using a warm-air hairblower to warm their hands rapidly. Smoking causes cutaneous vasoconstriction; therefore, tobacco smoking is contraindicated in Raynaud's phenomenon. Using induced vasodilation by placing the hands in warm water ($43°C$) has been reported to raise skin temperature and minimize the severity of attacks of Raynaud's phenomenon. Biofeedback to teach patients to raise skin temperature voluntarily

TABLE 46–2. TREATMENT OF RAYNAUD'S PHENOMENON

Frequency and Severity of Vasospastic Attacks	Suggested Treatment
1. Rare or mild attacks	Protective measures, cessation of smoking, and no drug therapy
2. Frequent or severe attacks without trophic changes	Protective measures and calcium antagonists
3. Frequent attacks with trophic changes but no open ulcers	Protective measures plus calcium antagonists or oral reserpine plus liothyronine
4. Frequent attacks with active, painful ulcers	Intravenous PGE_1, intra-arterial reserpine followed by calcium antagonists; or reserpine plus liothyronine; or oral misoprostol

has been shown to limit the duration and frequency of vasospastic attacks, but its effect is nonspecific because it is also seen in control patients who received no such treatment and in those in whom biofeedback is used to teach relaxation. In patients with Raynaud's phenomenon secondary to vibration, the use of vibrating tools must cease. However, terminating exposure to vibration does not always eliminate Raynaud's phenomenon.

The simple measures outlined above usually suffice for patients with infrequent or mild attacks. When Raynaud's phenomenon is more frequent or more severe, and especially when it has resulted in trophic changes or ulcerations, these measures need to be supplemented by drugs. Drug therapy is aimed at inducing vascular smooth muscle relaxation, thereby relieving spasm, raising resting blood flow, and limiting the degree of ischemia during attacks. The drugs most frequently used in treating patients with Raynaud's phenomenon are shown in Table 46–3. For most patients, the drug of choice is a calcium antagonist. Nifedipine* has been found to be effective in several well-controlled, double-blind studies. The drug is administered at a dose of 10 to 20 mg three or four times daily. Diltiazem,* at a dose of 60 mg three or four times daily, may be substituted if nifedipine is not well tolerated or if it causes side effects. In one study of very severely affected patients, verapamil was found not to be effective. The angiotensin-coverting enzyme inhibitors enalapril and captopril also effectively reduce the frequency and decrease the severity of Raynaud's phenomenon. Although less extensively studied than calcium antagonists, they appear equally effective. Enalapril is administered by mouth in a dose of 10 to 20 mg once daily, and captopril in a dose of 25 to 50 mg two or three times daily.

Reserpine* is the best-studied drug among the group that interferes with the function of the adrenergic nervous system. It is administered by mouth in doses of 0.1 to 0.5 mg daily. In cases in which ulcerations have developed, it may be given intra-arterially in a dose of 0.5 to 1 mg, dissolved in saline and administered into the

TABLE 46–3. SOME DRUGS USEFUL IN TREATING RAYNAUD'S PHENOMENON

1. Calcium antagonists
   a. Nifedipine*
   b. Diltiazem*
2. α-Adrenergic receptor blockers
   a. Phenoxybenzamine*
   b. Tolazoline
   c. Prazosin*
3. Drugs that interfere with sympathetic nerve activity
   a. Reserpine*
   b. Guanethidine*
   c. Alpha-methyldopa*
4. Vasodilators
   a. PGE_1*
   b. PGE_2*
   c. PGI_2*
   d. Iloprost
   e. Misoprostol*
5. Miscellaneous
   a. Liothyronine*

* Investigational drug for this purpose.

brachial or radial artery by slow infusion over several minutes. The drugs in this group may also be administered by means of tourni-quet-controlled intravenous injection (Bier's block). Administration by the last two routes gives a much higher local concentration and largely avoids systemic side effects.

In controlled trials, nitroglycerin* ointment or topical prosta-glandin E$_2$* (PGE$_2$) has been found effective in Raynaud's phenom-enon. The topical application of these drugs is advantageous be-cause their local relaxant action is not counteracted by reflex vasoconstriction secondary to changes in blood pressure that may occur when they are given systemically.

Prostaglandin E$_1$* (PGE$_1$) or prostacyclin* (PGI$_2$) administered intravenously has a beneficial effect in patients with Raynaud's phenomenon. These drugs can be given by constant intravenous infusion in a dose of 6 to 10 ng per kilogram per minute for a few hours or up to 3 days. Iloprost is an experimental stable ana-logue of PGI$_2$. It is administered intravenously in a dose of 0.5 to 2 ng per kilogram per minute for several hours. Misoprostol* is an analogue of PGE$_1$. It is administered by mouth in a dose of 0.2 mg three or four times daily. It is reported that the beneficial effect outlasts this therapy by several weeks. All these drugs act by inducing vasodilation and also by inhibiting platelet aggrega-tion.

A novel but effective way of inducing vasodilation in the digits is via the iatrogenic induction of hyperthyroidism by administering sodium liothyronine* (triiodothyronine), 75 μg daily. The resultant hypermetabolism elicits thermoregulatory reflex cutaneous vasodila-tion. The combination of triiodothyronine and reserpine has been found to be most effective.

Preganglionic sympathectomy to eliminate vasoconstrictor tone may have a beneficial immediate result, but the long-term results are disappointing. The duration of benefit is limited by nerve regen-eration. If sympathectomy is contemplated, it is advisable to try sympathetic blockade with local anesthetics to verify a beneficial result. A recently devised technique that involves surgical stripping of the palmar and digital arteries to bring about a local sympa-thectomy may also be tried, but its results have not been fully eval-uated.

---

* Investigational drug for this purpose.

Bunker CB, Terenghi G, Springall DR, et al.: Deficiency of calcitonin gene-related peptide in Raynaud's phenomenon. Lancet 336:1530, 1990. *Demonstration of re-duced density of calcitonin gene-related peptide–containing nerve fibers in pa-tients with Raynaud's phenomenon, suggesting the involvement of deficiency in this vasodilator peptide in the pathogenesis of Raynaud's phenomenon.*
Coffman JD: Raynaud's phenomenon: An update. Hypertension 17:593, 1991. *A review of current views concerning the pathogenesis of Raynaud's phenomenon and a consideration of methods of treatment.*
Fagius J, Blumberg H: Sympathetic outflow to the hand in patients with Raynaud's phenomenon. Cardiovasc Res 19:249, 1985. *Demonstration that sympathetic nerve activity in patients with Raynaud's phenomenon under baseline conditions and during maneuvers that increase sympathetic nerve traffic does not differ from that in normal controls. The results do not support the theory that Raynaud's disease is caused by increased sympathetic nerve activity.*
LeRoy EC, Medsger TA Jr: Raynaud's phenomenon: A proposal for classification. Clin Exper Rheumatol 10:485, 1992. *An attempt to clarify the confusion regarding Raynaud's phenomenon, syndrome, and disease.*

Acrocyanosis

DEFINITION. Acrocyanosis is a rare disorder characterized by persistent cyanosis of the skin of the hands and, less commonly, of the feet associated with reduced skin temperature.

ETIOLOGY. Acrocyanosis is a primary disorder of unknown cause. It is much more common in women than in men. The onset of the disease is usually in young adults or middle-aged people. The high incidence of the disease among patients with psychiatric disorders is of unknown significance.

PATHOPHYSIOLOGY. The smaller precapillary vessels (arteri-oles) are abnormally constricted, reducing blood flow and account-ing for cyanosis and reduced skin temperature. The veins are secon-darily dilated. The arterioles constrict under normal environmental conditions and even more so when exposed to cold because these vessels are abnormally sensitive to cold. An important feature of acrocyanosis is the reduced venous tone. No venous obstruction is present. These features can be demonstrated by elevating the in-volved limb and eliminating the blue color or intensifying the blue color by placing the limb in a dependent position and overfilling the veins.

CLINICAL MANIFESTATIONS. Patients with acrocyanosis persistently have blue-colored hands and, less commonly, discolored feet. In some cases, the blue color extends to more proximal por-tions of the limbs. The skin is cold, and the palms are wet and clammy from sweat. No pallor is usually present. In some cases, there may be spots of pallor surrounded by confluent cyanosis. The blue color is intensified by exposure to cold, and it is converted into purplish or red color by exposure to heat. There are few ac-companying symptoms. The patient has feelings of coldness and, occasionally, numbness. Ulcerations and other trophic changes are distinctly unusual. Patients with acrocyanosis seek medical advice either because they are frightened or because the cyanosis is cos-metically unappealing.

DIAGNOSIS. The distinction between acrocyanosis and Ray-naud's phenomenon is discussed above in the section on Raynaud's phenomenon. Differentiation from cyanosis secondary to arterial ob-struction can be made on the basis of normal pulses, by the bilat-eral and symmetric occurrence of acrocyanosis, and, if necessary, by angiographically verifying the absence of obstruction. Cyanosis limited to the hands and feet that improves in a warm environment and no reduced arterial blood saturation distinguish acrocyanosis from generalized, systemic cyanosis.

TREATMENT. Since acrocyanosis is a benign disease, no drug therapy is usually required.

Livedo Reticularis

DEFINITION. Livedo reticularis is a reticular, bluish discol-oration of the skin of the extremities that produces a lacy, irregular appearance outlining central areas of normal-appearing skin. The cause is not known. The disorder usually begins in young individu-als before age 20 to 30 years. It is equally common in men and women but more often symptomatic in women. An association be-tween generalized livedo reticularis and ischemic cerebrovascular manifestations has been described (Sneddon's syndrome). About one fourth to one third of patients with Sneddon's syndrome have high concentrations of anticardiolipin antibodies, suggesting that the pathogenesis of the vascular lesions in this rare disorder may be similar to what is seen in the antiphospholipid syndrome described in some patients with systemic lupus erythematosus (see Ch. 240).

PATHOPHYSIOLOGY. The mechanism of livedo reticularis is presumed to be similar to that of acrocyanosis, namely, constriction of arterioles followed by stasis and dilation of capillaries and veins. The latter are filled with desaturated blood. The reticular appear-ance of livedo reticularis reflects the anatomic arrangement of the affected vessels. It is believed that the bluish areas represent the ar-borizations of peripheral capillaries from central penetrating arteri-oles. Blood flow is faster in the central regions closer to the pene-trating arteriole, whereas the more distant areas have lower flow, with consequent stasis and cyanosis.

TREATMENT. In most cases no treatment is required. Protec-tion from cold and abstinence from tobacco are useful. In severe cases, drugs useful in the treatment of Raynaud's phenomenon, such as nifedipine and reserpine, may be tried. Aspirin has helped some patients with Sneddon's syndrome.

Sneddon IB: Cerebral vascular lesions and livedo reticularis. Br J Dermatol 77:180, 1965. *Description of the association between livedo reticularis and ischemic cere-brovascular manifestations.*

VASCULAR DISEASES OF THE LIMBS CAUSED BY DAMAGE FROM COLD

Frostbite

DEFINITION AND ETIOLOGY. Frostbite results from freez-ing of the tissues and consequent vascular injury. In most cases, frostbite occurs during prolonged exposure to temperatures below 0°C. Other environmental factors include high wind and humidity. Predisposing factors include vascular disease, inadequate clothing, lack of acclimatization, and general debility.

PATHOPHYSIOLOGY. Tissue damage results from cold-influ-enced vasoconstriction. Freezing causes water crystal formation in cells and dehydration. Endothelial damage with increased perme-ability to protein ensues, causes edema, and further contributes to stasis and eventual thrombosis.

PATHOLOGY. The vessels show endothelial swelling and vac-uolization and proliferative changes. Subsequently, there are inflam-matory reactions and atrophic changes in the skin.

CLINICAL MANIFESTATIONS. Initially, the patient notices a prickling sensation followed by numbness. The skin becomes bloodless and appears white and cold. This is followed by redness, swelling, and increased temperature. Blisters may form 24 to 48 hours after thawing. They are filled with either serous yellow or hemorrhagic fluid. There may be hemorrhages under the nail beds. Necrosis and gangrene may supervene. The subsequent course may be similar to that of sudden arterial occlusion, including ischemia and gangrene. Spontaneous amputation may require several weeks or months. After an attack of frostbite, the affected extremities may remain sensitive to cold for a period of time or permanently, and secondary Raynaud's phenomenon may occur.

TREATMENT. Frostbite should be treated with immediate rewarming. If frostbite affects deep tissues, rewarming should be done with water at 40 to 44°C. Avoid exercise or massage of the involved limb because this tends to increase edema and pain. If pain is severe, it should be treated with analgesics or narcotics. After the tissues have thawed, the exposed parts should remain at room temperature. Vesicles should be left untouched, and the limb should be left exposed, without dressings. If infection is present, antibiotic therapy should be used. Sympathectomy has been reported to be beneficial in the initial stages as well as in preventing the delayed sequelae of frostbite.

Chilblain (Pernio)

DEFINITION. Chilblain is an inflammatory condition of the skin of the extremities induced by cold and characterized by erythema, itching, and ulceration. The cause is unknown. It is more common in cold, damp climates, as in England, than in the United States. Women are affected more commonly than men. In most patients, the disease begins before the age of 20 years.

PATHOLOGY. In chronic cases, the lesions consist of angiitis with intimal proliferation, thickening of the arterial wall, and perivascular infiltration with lymphocytes and polymorphonuclear leukocytes. There may be necrosis of the adipose tissue and chronic inflammatory infiltrates in the subcutaneous tissue.

CLINICAL MANIFESTATIONS. The disease has both acute and chronic forms. The typical patient is a young woman who, in the winter, notices bluish-red discoloration and edema of the skin of the lower limbs associated with burning and warmth. The lesions are persistent and are associated with itching. They generally last from 7 to 10 days and then clear up, sometimes leaving residual pigmentation of the skin. In severe cases, the lesions may become hemorrhagic, or blebs may appear. Infection may supervene.

With repeated exposure to cold, susceptible persons may develop chronic lesions. These are erythematous, ulcerative, and hemorrhagic lesions that begin as raised, red areas 0.5 to 1 cm in diameter. These lesions are then transformed into blebs and finally ulcerate. Healing occurs in the summer, leaving a permanently pigmented region.

DIAGNOSIS. Acute chilblain is distinguished from other forms of dermatitis by its characteristic distribution and by its relationship to cold. Chronic chilblain needs to be distinguished from erythema induratum and erythema nodosum. Erythema induratum of Bazin is caused by *Mycobacterium tuberculosis*. If the infection is active, the differential diagnosis may be made by finding it microscopically or culturing the bacteria. Erythema induratum affects the upper part of the legs more frequently than the lower part. The lesions are more nodular, deeper, and infiltrative. They are also more permanent, whereas those of chronic chilblain clear up in the summer. Erythema nodosum is a more acute process, and it is usually associated with a systemic reaction, consisting of fever, malaise, and arthralgias. There is no seasonal association.

TREATMENT. In mild cases, protecting the skin from cold, locally applying anti-inflammatory ointments, avoiding scratching, and cessation of smoking are usually sufficient. In more severe cases, drugs useful in treating Raynaud's phenomenon, such as reserpine or nifedipine, may be effective.

Rustin MHA, Newton JA, Smith NP, et al.: The treatment of chilblain with nifedipine: The results of a pilot study, a double-blind placebo-controlled randomized study and a long-term open trial. Br J Dermatol 120:267, 1989. *Report of a controlled trial showing that nifedipine accelerated the clearance of chilblain and prevented new lesions. It also caused symptomatic relief and resolution of edema and perivascular infiltration.*

VASCULAR DISEASES OF THE LIMBS CAUSED BY ORGANIC ARTERIAL OBSTRUCTION

Arteriosclerosis Obliterans

DEFINITION. Arteriosclerosis obliterans consists of segmental arteriosclerotic narrowing or obstruction of the lumen in the arteries supplying the limbs.

ETIOLOGY AND INCIDENCE. The cause of arteriosclerosis in general is discussed in another chapter (see Ch. 40).

Arteriosclerosis obliterans is the most common cause of arterial obstructive disease of the extremities. The disease usually manifests clinically between the ages of 50 and 70. It is unusual in individuals younger than 30. Men are affected more often than women. The lower limbs are involved much more frequently than the upper limbs. The most commonly affected vessel is the superficial femoral artery. The distal aorta and its bifurcation into the two iliac arteries and the popliteal artery are the next most frequent sites of involvement. The presence of diabetes mellitus influences arteriosclerosis obliterans in a number of important ways. In diabetics, arteriosclerosis obliterans is likely to be more progressive. This is reflected in a much higher incidence of intermittent claudication in diabetics. The disease affects arterial vessels of smaller caliber and more distally located vessels more frequently than in nondiabetics. The incidence of involvement of vessels below the knee with arteriosclerosis obliterans in diabetics is considerably higher than in nondiabetics.

PATHOLOGY. The lesions of arteriosclerosis obliterans are typical atheromatous plaques involving the intima of the arteries. As a rule, there is superimposed thrombus formation. The media of the vessels shows degenerative changes. Calcification of the media is frequent and may take the form of a ringlike arrangement, as in Mönckeberg's sclerosis. Medial calcification is twice as frequent in diabetics as in nondiabetics. These arteriosclerotic lesions are segmental, and they are typically multiple. Weakening of the media may give rise to aneurysmal dilation of the involved artery. Such arteriosclerotic aneurysms are most common in the popliteal fossa or in the femoral artery below the inguinal ligament. They may be filled with thrombi.

PATHOPHYSIOLOGY. Stenoses that decrease the cross-sectional area of the vessel by <75% do not usually affect resting blood flow. When the prevailing flow rates are high, as in exercise, decreases of 60% or more in cross-sectional area are required before a reduction in flow occurs.

CLINICAL MANIFESTATIONS. The symptoms of arteriosclerosis obliterans are intermittent claudication, pain at rest, and trophic changes in the involved limb. Intermittent claudication denotes pain that develops in a limb during exercise and disappears when the patient rests. The pain is usually described as a cramp or a tightness or as severe fatigue of the exercising muscles. The pain is usually bilateral. The amount of exercise it takes to induce the pain is usually constant for any given patient. In some patients, the pain disappears by slowing the pace of walking without completely stopping exercise. The location of the pain is distal to the arterial obstruction. The most frequently affected muscles are in the calf, because of the high frequency with which the femoral artery is involved. The muscles of the lower part of the back, the buttocks, the thigh, and the foot may also be affected.

Pain at rest occurs when a pronounced reduction in resting blood flow is present. It is a sign of severe disease. The pain—usually burning or gnawing—may be localized to one or more toes, or it may have a stocking-type distribution. It is generally worse at night. It is improved by placing the limb in a dependent position and by cooling. There may be associated coldness and numbness, together with cyanosis or pallor of the extremity.

Examination discloses reduced or absent arterial pulses distal to the obstruction. There may be bruits audible over the aorta or its branches. These may be systolic, or they may be continuous. In advanced cases, examination may reveal signs of ischemia. The skin temperature may be abnormally low, or there may be pallor or cyanosis. Ischemic damage may cause persistent reddish or reddish-blue discoloration. There may be trophic changes, including a dry, scaly, and shiny skin. The hair may disappear, and the toenails may become brittle, ridged, and deformed. There may be ulcerations or gangrene. The ischemic ulcers are usually at pressure points and may be inflamed and painful.

Leriche's syndrome refers to isolated aortoiliac disease, which produces a fairly characteristic clinical picture. There is intermittent claudication of the lower back, buttocks, and thigh or calf muscles. The limbs atrophy and the skin in the feet and legs is pale. Impotence may also be present. Arterial pulses in the legs are absent; they may be present but weak in the femoral arteries. Systolic bruits may be audible over the femoral arteries and lower abdomen.

Arteriosclerotic aneurysms may occur and present as pulsatile, expansible masses in the popliteal fossa or in the femoral artery below the inguinal ligament. These may cause symptoms by pressure on adjacent structures and, occasionally, by embolism of peripheral vessels or by hemorrhage into the tissues.

DIAGNOSIS. The diagnostic approach to the patient with arteriosclerosis obliterans should be directed at establishing the site of the arterial obstruction, its severity, the degree of ischemia, and the adequacy of the collateral circulation. Palpation of the arterial pulses and auscultation of bruits usually suffices to determine the presence and site of arterial obstruction. Several tests may be helpful. With the patient in a warm environment, so that vasoconstrictor tone is low, the leg is raised to a 45-degree angle while the patient is supine. The color of the plantar surface of the foot is observed. Pallor during this test indicates arterial insufficiency. The systolic blood pressure in the dorsalis pedis or posterior tibial arteries can be determined with the use of a Doppler velocitometer at rest as well as during exercise. As a rule, pressures <30 mm Hg indicate ischemia of sufficient severity to cause gangrene.

Arteriography confirms arterial obstruction, which is essential to establish the exact anatomy of the arterial vessels and to determine the advisability of surgery.

Arterial embolism is usually distinguishable from arteriosclerosis obliterans because of the sudden onset of the ischemic manifestations and the usually unilateral involvement. Intermittent claudication may occur in severe anemia, in venous disease, and in muscle phosphorylase deficiency (McArdle's syndrome). These conditions are distinguished from arteriosclerosis obliterans by the presence of normal pulses. Ergotamine or methysergide toxicity may cause severe vasospasm, which may affect the large arteries and diminish pulses. The history of drug ingestion may help distinguish these from arteriosclerosis obliterans. In difficult cases, angiography shows the generalized vasospasm and absence of segmental obstructions.

TREATMENT. Patients with arteriosclerosis obliterans without evidence of ischemia should be treated medically. Limiting physical activity, avoiding smoking tobacco (which causes vasoconstriction), and a regular exercise program are advisable. Treating hyperlipidemia, if present, may prevent new arteriosclerotic lesions from developing. Control of diabetes, if present, is required. Patients should maintain the skin of the affected limbs clean, dry, and soft and protect it from cold and trauma. Infections and trauma should be treated promptly. There is no evidence that vasodilative drugs effectively treat arteriosclerosis obliterans. In fact, they may be harmful under certain circumstances by lowering arterial blood pressure and reducing collateral blood flow or by diverting blood to proximal healthy areas, thereby reducing the perfusion pressure in the more distal portions of the limb. Pentoxifylline, 400 mg orally three times daily, has been shown in controlled trials to prolong the duration of exercise and the distance the patient is able to walk before claudication begins. The drug acts by increasing red cell membrane deformability, thereby reducing effective blood viscosity.

Surgical treatment is advisable when ischemia is present or if intermittent claudication seriously interferes with the patient's activities. Surgery involves either endarterectomy of the stenotic artery or a bypass operation. Axillofemoral or femorofemoral grafts for aortoiliac disease have been successful. The larger the size of the vessels grafted, the higher the rate of successful restoration of blood flow.

Nonsurgical revascularization techniques, such as balloon angioplasty, laser angioplasty, and rotational atherectomy, offer attractive alternatives to surgery in treating arteriosclerosis obliterans. These techniques are simple, have low morbidity, and are less costly than surgery. With balloon angioplasty, the segmental stenosis or obstruction is dilated by suddenly inflating—at the site of the lesion—a balloon introduced into the artery by percutaneous catheterization. High success rates and good long-term rates of patency of the dilated vessel have been reported. Angioplasty is more successful in larger vessels, when the stenotic segment is relatively short and when the vessel is not completely occluded. Restenosis of lesions dilated by angioplasty occurs in 20 to 30% of patients within

a year. It may be due to thrombosis or more commonly to intimal and medial proliferation. Laser angioplasty uses a cold excimer laser, which ablates by a photochemical process. The rotational atherectomy device is a debulking bur covered with diamond chips that rotates quickly. It selectively cuts the atherosclerotic lesion by pulverizing hard material into small particles without damaging soft tissue. Laser angioplasty and atherectomy are helpful in dealing with fibrotic or calcified lesions, particularly in smaller vessels. Frequently, after using these devices balloon dilatation is used to optimize the angiographic result. A new device—the intravascular stent—is a wire mesh collar crimped on a deflated balloon that is placed across the lesion. The stent is then expanded by inflating the balloon. Subsequently, the balloon is deflated and removed, leaving the stent, which acts as a scaffold to maintain a widely patent lumen. This approach is used to manage lesions of the iliac artery when the prevailing high flow rates make chronic anticoagulation unnecessary. Very high patency rates exceeding 90% after a year have been reported. Using stents in more distal vessels also gives excellent acute angiographic outcomes; it requires short-term anticoagulation to prevent thrombosis at the site of the stent prior to endothelialization.

If the anatomy of the disease makes surgery impossible and ischemic manifestations are present, bed rest is essential. The affected extremity should be kept in a slightly dependent position at 20 to 30 degrees below horizontal, and direct application of heat should be avoided. The limb is best kept warm by placing it under a cradle, under which the temperature is regulated below 38°C. Analgesics or narcotics may be required to control pain. Ulcers should be kept clean with warm saline soaks and debrided. Appropriate antibiotics should be used if infection is present. Administering PGE$_1$* intra-arterially may help in patients with gangrene or ulceration in whom surgery is not possible. To arrest advancing gangrene, amputation may be necessary; its level is chosen by the presence of warm, viable tissue having normal color.

Long-term anticoagulants are of questionable value, except when used with invasive revascularization procedures. Systemic fibrinolytic therapy with intravenous thrombolytic agents is helpful in some patients but is associated with risk of bleeding. For this reason, it is not extensively used. Intra-arterially administered thrombolytic agents are an important adjunct to interventional procedures. Acute and chronic thrombotic lesions can be recanalized using prolonged low-dose intravascular infusion of thrombolytic agents. Following recanalization, balloon angioplasty or other nonsurgical revascularization procedures can be used to treat the residual atherosclerotic obstruction.

Preganglionic lumbar sympathectomy may be performed as an acute intervention to treat ischemic manifestations of arteriosclerosis obliterans. Before surgery, it must be demonstrated that interrupting sympathetic nerves is likely to improve circulation of the limb. This is done by inducing temporary sympathetic blockade with local anesthetics. This is essential, especially in diabetics in whom peripheral neuropathy may have already produced spontaneous sympathectomy. Sympathectomy does not influence the long-term prognosis of intermittent claudication.

PROGNOSIS. Arteriosclerosis obliterans in the absence of diabetes is a slowly progressive disease. No significant deterioration may be detected for several years. When diabetes is present, the disease tends to progress more rapidly, and the prognosis is less satisfactory. The location of obstructing lesions also influences the prognosis. When the lesions are in larger arteries, the probability of successful surgical intervention or percutaneous angioplasty is higher, and the prognosis is better. Frequently arteriosclerosis obliterans is only one of the manifestations of a generalized arteriosclerotic process. Mortality results from arteriosclerotic involvement of other vascular beds, such as the coronary or the cerebral circulation, with death from myocardial infarction or stroke.

Thromboangiitis Obliterans (Buerger's Disease)

DEFINITION. Thromboangiitis obliterans is an obstructive arterial disease caused by segmental inflammatory and proliferative lesions of the medium and small arteries and veins of the limbs.

---

* Investigational drug for this purpose.

ETIOLOGY. The cause of thromboangiitis obliterans is unknown. Almost all patients with this disease are moderate or heavy smokers, particularly of cigarettes. Many show cutaneous hypersensitivity to intradermally injected tobacco products. There is a high prevalence of HLA-A9 and HLA-B5 antigens in affected persons. An autoimmune mechanism is suggested by a study of cellular and humoral immune responses of 39 patients with thromboangiitis obliterans. Lymphocytes from 77% of these patients exhibited cellular sensitivity to human type I and type III collagen, both of which are constituents of the vascular wall. In addition, approximately 50% had significant levels of anticollagen antibodies in their blood. By contrast, normal controls and patients with arteriosclerosis obliterans had considerably lower levels of cellular sensitivity to collagen and no circulating anticollagen antibodies.

INCIDENCE. Thromboangiitis obliterans is a disease mostly of young males. The disease begins most frequently between the ages of 20 and 40 years, and the ratio of men to women affected varies from 9:1 to as high as 75:1. There is a higher prevalence of the disorder in Israel, the Orient, and in India than in the United States and Western Europe.

PATHOLOGY. The disease affects small and medium-sized arteries and veins in segmental fashion. Acute lesions are manifested by proliferation of the intima and thrombosis. There is inflammatory infiltration with polymorphonuclear leukocytes, lymphocytes, and giant cells of all coats of the artery or vein, extending into the thrombus.

CLINICAL MANIFESTATIONS. The typical patient with thromboangiitis obliterans is a young man who smokes cigarettes heavily, has manifestations of ischemia of the extremities, and has a history or evidence of superficial thrombophlebitis. Common presenting complaints are Raynaud's phenomenon with digital ulcerations or pain from ischemia. Pain in thromboangiitis obliterans may be of several types. The most frequent is pain at rest in one or more digits. This pain may be accompanied by manifestations of ischemia, such as color or temperature changes of the skin. This type of pain may be a forerunner of ulceration or gangrene. When these trophic lesions are present, there may be localized, aching pain that is more severe at night. Another type of pain may occur along the course of the inflamed blood vessels. Ischemic neuropathy may result and cause a paroxysmal, shocklike pain, which may follow the distribution of sensory nerves. Paresthesias may accompany this type of pain. Typical intermittent claudication occurs commonly in the lower extremities. It most often occurs in the arch of the foot because of involvement of the vessels of the leg and sparing of the femoral and iliac arteries. Some patients have intermittent claudication of the forearm or hand. Sensitivity to cold with paresthesias and the development of secondary Raynaud's phenomenon are common. Migratory superficial thrombophlebitis is manifested by the development of inflamed, tender, red segments of the superficial veins, which subside over a period of several weeks.

Physical examination discloses impaired arterial pulsations in the more distal portions of the limbs, such as the radial, ulnar, dorsalis pedis, and posterior tibial arteries. The more proximal arteries are normal, a finding that contrasts with arteriosclerosis obliterans. There may be cyanosis or pallor or persistent redness in the digits, and associated changes in temperature may be noted. Postural changes in color are also common. Gangrene or ulcerations of the digits may be present in both upper and lower extremities. Edema of the foot is common. Occasional patients have involvement of visceral arteries with stenosis or occlusion of mesenteric, coronary, cerebral, or renal arteries and manifestations of ischemia of these organs.

DIAGNOSIS. Consider the diagnosis of thromboangiitis obliterans when there is evidence of ischemia of the extremities from arterial occlusive disease in association with migratory superficial thrombophlebitis. The age and sex of the individual and the involvement of the upper extremities are additional helpful characteristics. Arteriography may help disclose segmental multiple occlusions of the medium-sized and small arteries associated with collateral vessel visualization. The larger arteries are generally spared, a finding that also helps distinguish the disorder from arteriosclerosis obliterans. Final confirmation may be obtained only from biopsy material of an early lesion and histologic demonstra-

tion of the characteristic inflammatory and proliferative lesion of the disease.

PROGNOSIS. Thromboangiitis obliterans is not usually life-threatening except in rare individuals in whom the visceral arteries are involved. The disease, however, results in disability and amputation of the extremities in a high percentage of cases. It is generally more rapidly progressive than arteriosclerosis obliterans, especially in individuals who refuse to stop smoking.

TREATMENT. Cessation of tobacco smoking is essential, as continuation results in a progressive course. If the patient stops smoking, new lesions do not develop or they develop more rarely. Patients with thromboangiitis obliterans generally are treated as are patients with advanced arteriosclerosis obliterans. Treatment consists of conservative measures, including protection from cold, local care in the event of ulceration or gangrene, and eventually amputation, if these lesions occur. Sympathectomy is tried frequently and may be effective, at least temporarily, if vasospasm is a prominent feature. Vasodilative drug therapy can be tried in cases of Raynaud's phenomenon with ulcerations, but its effectiveness is questionable.

Sudden Arterial Occlusion

DEFINITION. Sudden arterial occlusion may result from obstruction of an artery of the extremity by embolism or by thrombosis *in situ*. The clinical manifestations are the result of the consequent ischemia.

ETIOLOGY. The major cause of sudden arterial occlusion is arterial embolism. The heart is the most frequent source of emboli in this syndrome. Emboli may arise from thrombi in the left atrium with atrial fibrillation or mitral valve disease, usually mitral stenosis. Emboli may also arise from mural thrombi from a myocardial infarction or in the presence of a cardiomyopathy. Septic emboli may arise from vegetations from the mitral or aortic valves in the presence of bacterial endocarditis. Less commonly, emboli originate from an arteriosclerotic plaque in more proximal parts of the arterial tree or from aneurysms. In rare cases, the embolus may arise from the venous side and enter the arterial tree via a patent foramen ovale (paradoxical embolism). More rarely, the embolus consists of calcium fragments from a calcified valve leaflet, cholesterol crystals from an arteriosclerotic plaque, or foreign materials such as a bullet.

Sudden arterial thrombosis occurs in about 10% of the cases of arteriosclerosis obliterans. The condition is rare in thromboangiitis obliterans or in polyarteritis nodosa. Acute arterial thrombosis may occur in conditions in which the coagulability of the blood is increased in normal vessels, such as in polycythemia vera (see Ch. 141.1) or in cryoglobulinemia (see Ch. 149). Rarely, arterial thrombosis may occur in the presence of normal vessels in infections such as septicemia, pneumonia, peritonitis, tuberculosis, ulcerative colitis, and other debilitating diseases. Trauma from penetrating wounds, as from arterial puncture or catheterization, may cause arterial occlusion.

PATHOPHYSIOLOGY. The sudden arterial occlusion causes reduced blood flow to the more distal portions of the limb and consequent ischemia. Vasoactive agents released from the emboli, such as serotonin from platelets, may contract vascular smooth muscle in more distal portions of the vascular tree and result in vasospasm that further aggravates ischemia. The severity and extent of ischemia depend on the size of the vessel occluded and on the extent of collateral circulation. The larger the occluded vessel, the more likely it is that severe ischemia will result.

CLINICAL MANIFESTATIONS. Sudden arterial occlusion abruptly causes severe pain accompanied by manifestations of ischemia in about half the patients. In the remainder, the onset is gradual with either mild pain or numbness and paresthesias. Pain is present in about 75% of the cases. There may be muscular weakness or outright paralysis. A saddle embolus of the aortic bifurcation causes abdominal pain, nausea, and vomiting and may result in a shocklike state.

Examining the patient discloses diminished or absent pulses distal to the occlusion. Evidence of ischemia is present with low skin temperature and pallor or cyanosis or a combination of the two. If the occluded artery is superficial, the site of lodgment of the embolus may be identified as a tender region. The subsequent course depends on the adequacy of the collateral circulation. If this is adequate, gradual improvement occurs. Otherwise, gangrene supervenes.

DIAGNOSIS. The diagnosis of sudden arterial occlusion is usually relatively easy in the patient who has the acute onset of pain and ischemia of an extremity. If the cause is an embolus, its source may be evident. Rarely, patients with acute thrombophlebitis of the iliac and femoral veins may have feeble or absent arterial pulses and show manifestations resembling those of ischemia from an arterial embolus. In these cases, the demonstration of the feeble pulse and the presence of distended veins and pronounced edema help make the differentiation possible.

PROGNOSIS. The outcome of acute arterial obstruction depends on the size of the vessel affected, the age of the patient, the extent of the collateral circulation, and the timing of therapeutic intervention. When a large artery is occluded, the prognosis is poor without surgical treatment. In older patients with pre-existing arterial occlusive disease, the prognosis is poor because of obstruction of multiple vessels, including collateral vessels.

TREATMENT. The goal of therapeutic intervention is to remove or dissolve the thrombus and re-establish patency of the occluded artery. This can be achieved by surgical embolectomy or by thrombolytic therapy. Urgent embolectomy is the preferred treatment method when a large artery is occluded, such as with a saddle embolus of the bifurcation of the aorta. When smaller vessels are occluded and the thrombus is not easily accessible or when the patient's general condition does not permit surgical intervention, intravenous or intra-arterial streptokinase or urokinase may be given, if there are no contraindications for their use. Streptokinase is given intravenously as a bolus of 250,000 IU, followed by an infusion of 100,000 IU per hour. The infusion is continued for 72 hours. Intra-arterial administration can be used instead, in a dose of about one tenth of the intravenous dose; it can be coupled with angioplasty. Thrombolytic therapy is followed by conventional anticoagulants. The success rate of thrombolytic therapy is critically dependent on how early it is administered after symptoms begin. It is more effective for thrombotic lesions than embolic ones. Streptokinase or urokinase cannot be safely followed by surgery because of the danger of bleeding from the arteriotomy. The choice of therapy, therefore, must be carefully considered.

If neither therapeutic approach can be used, the patient should be treated conservatively. The patient should rest. The limb is placed in a slightly dependent position under a cradle whose temperature is controlled at 30 to 35°C. Anticoagulation with heparin should begin as soon as possible to prevent extension of the thrombus and to prevent additional emboli. If vasospasm is prominent, lumbar sympathectomy may be tried to reduce vasomotor tone and improve blood flow to the limb.

When a patient is treated conservatively, he/she should be followed closely for evidence of deterioration. If this occurs, immediate surgical intervention and embolectomy are attempted. The results of embolectomy depend, to a large extent, on the timing of intervention. Therefore, surgery should not be delayed longer than a few hours. If therapy fails, gangrene may supervene, and amputation may become necessary.

VASCULAR DISEASES OF THE LIMBS CAUSED BY ABNORMAL COMMUNICATION BETWEEN ARTERIES AND VEINS

Arteriovenous Fistula

DEFINITION. Arteriovenous fistula is an abnormal direct communication between an artery and a vein.

ETIOLOGY. Arteriovenous fistulas in the limbs may be congenital or acquired. Congenital fistulas are usually multiple; acquired ones are usually single. The most common type is iatrogenic, created to carry out renal dialysis. Acquired arteriovenous fistulas may also result from trauma caused by penetrating wounds or surgical procedures.

PATHOPHYSIOLOGY. The low resistance of the direct communication between artery and vein results in a high arterial inflow into the vein, resulting in an increase in venous pressure. The elevated venous pressure engorges and distends the vein and may lead to varicose veins. In the region of the fistula, blood flow is high, whereas more distal portions are deprived of capillary blood flow and may show ischemia and trophic changes.

Large fistulas reduce systemic vascular resistance and impose a burden on the heart because of the associated increase in cardiac output. Total blood volume may be increased. Left ventricular failure may eventually result.

CLINICAL MANIFESTATIONS. The patient may be totally asymptomatic, and the discovery of the fistula may be accidental. In other cases, there may be pain near the fistula, edema, varicosities, and asymmetry in limb size. In some cases, the presenting symptoms may be those of cardiac decompensation with dyspnea on exertion, palpitations, and orthopnea. Examining the involved limb reveals tortuous, dilated superficial veins and venous pulsation at the fistula site. Skin temperature may be high, and distal portions of the limb may show ischemic changes. A bruit or a thrill may be heard over the fistula during systole. At other times, a continuous bruit may be present. The extremity may be swollen, or the girth of the limb may be increased because of hypertrophy of the soft tissues. Temporary compression of the artery proximal to the fistula immediately increases systemic vascular resistance and leads to reflex decrease in heart rate (Branham's sign), a change that may be helpful diagnostically.

DIAGNOSIS. When the fistula is superficial and large, the diagnosis can be made easily. If this is not possible from the physical examination, arteriography should be attempted for a definitive diagnosis. The oxygen saturation of the venous blood from the involved limb is higher than that of its contralateral part, and this comparison may help make the diagnosis.

TREATMENT. The treatment of choice is surgical intervention: closing the fistula and re-establishing the continuity of the involved artery and vein. If such restoration is not possible, ligation of the artery or vein or both may be necessary, but this may lead to arterial or venous insufficiency of the limb. In some cases, the fistula involves an anomalous artery. In this case, the ligation of the artery and the obstruction of the veins by injecting sclerosing solutions may give a satisfactory result. It may not be practical to surgically treat patients with multiple fistulas. In these cases, conservative measures consisting of local care, pain relief, and elastic bandages may be helpful. If the fistula is inoperable and cardiac decompensation is present or threatened, amputation may be necessary.

Glomus Tumor (Glomangioma)

DEFINITION. Glomangioma, or glomus tumor, is a benign tumor of the glomus body.

PATHOLOGY. The glomus tumor is an encapsulated structure consisting of a hypertrophied arteriovenous anastomosis. The tumor varies in size from 0.5 to 2.5 cm in diameter. It can be found in various parts of the upper and lower extremities but is most frequently located in the nail beds.

CLINICAL MANIFESTATIONS. The most common symptom is severe burning pain near the tumor. The pain may precede the appearance of the tumor. Pain may occur spontaneously, or it may be precipitated by exposure to heat or cold. Occasionally, the tumor is exquisitely sensitive to touch, and even the slightest pressure from contact with clothing may cause severe pain. Severe disability and atrophy of the limb from disuse may occur secondary to fear of pain. Examining the involved area shows a reddish, purplish, or bluish mass that is sharply demarcated. At times, the tumor may not be easily visible or palpable. In this case, pressure with the head of a pin may help identify the location of the tumor. When it is located under the nail bed, the nail and the phalanx may be visibly deformed, thereby giving a clue to the location of the tumor. Ultrasonography or magnetic resonance imaging is useful to diagnose small glomus tumors.

TREATMENT. The glomus tumor is a benign tumor. Surgical excision results in complete relief without recurrence.

Heys SD, Brittenden J, Atkinson P, et al.: Glomus tumour: An analysis of 43 patients and review of the literature. Br J Surg 79:345, 1992. *Consideration of the clinical and pathologic features and diagnosis of a large number of patients with glomus tumors.*

DISEASES OF THE VEINS OF THE LIMBS

Thrombophlebitis and Deep-Vein Thrombosis

DEFINITION. Thrombophlebitis refers to venous thrombosis with accompanying inflammation of the venous wall. For important practical reasons, superficial thrombophlebitis is distinguished from deep-vein thrombosis. Superficial thrombophlebitis does not cause embolic complications, but deep-vein thrombosis frequently causes pulmonary embolism.

PATHOLOGY. Thrombi in veins consist mostly of red cells with a few platelets held together with fibrin. They propagate in the direction of the bloodstream by extending the thrombotic process. They attach to the wall of the vein at one end, while the more proximal end floats freely into the lumen of the vessel. This is the portion that is commonly broken off and travels to the lungs. Varying degrees of inflammatory reaction of the venous wall may be present. Venous thrombosis may exist in the absence of inflammation, as is the case in some patients with malignancy. This is referred to as "phlebothrombosis." In most cases, however, inflammation and thrombosis coexist. The disorder may start as a pure thrombotic process, and inflammation usually occurs secondary to the presence of the thrombus.

INCIDENCE. Deep-vein thrombosis is a common disorder. It is more common in women than in men. The incidence of the disease increases with advancing age. Approximately one third of the patients over age 40 who have undergone major surgery or have had an acute myocardial infarction develop deep-vein thrombosis. The incidence is even higher after certain operations such as repair of hip fractures or prostatectomy. Patients with thrombotic strokes have an equally high incidence of deep-vein thrombosis. This occurs almost exclusively in the paralyzed limb.

Superficial thrombophlebitis occurs most commonly in patients with varicose veins, possibly as a result of minor trauma. It is also frequent after pregnancy. A migratory type of superficial thrombophlebitis also occurs in patients with thromboangiitis obliterans.

PATHOGENESIS. Venous stasis, injury to the venous wall, and a hypercoagulable state are the three main factors that lead to venous thrombosis. The combination of venous stasis and changes in the clotting mechanism of the blood accounts for the increased incidence of deep-vein thrombosis in pregnancy and during administration of oral contraceptives. Venous stasis is the major factor in the development of venous thrombosis in patients with heart disease, in paralyzed patients, in patients undergoing major surgery, in those who have varicose veins, and in healthy individuals after long trips. Increased viscosity, leading to stasis, and alterations in the clotting factors of the blood account for the high incidence of polycythemia vera. Patients with familial deficiencies of certain anticlotting factors are susceptible to recurrent thrombophlebitis. These include deficiencies of antithrombin III, protein S, protein C, and heparin cofactor II. Injury to the venous wall may result from use of certain vasoconstrictive or chemotherapeutic agents, or it may result from infectious agents. Patients with malignancies may have migrating thrombophlebitis, which has been attributed to low-grade activation of intravascular coagulation.

CLINICAL MANIFESTATIONS. The presence of superficial thrombophlebitis is usually easily ascertained by finding the inflamed vein. This may be apparent as a red, tender cord. By contrast, deep-vein thrombosis frequently causes few distinctive clinical features; about one half of patients with deep-vein thrombosis are asymptomatic. The first manifestation of deep-vein thrombosis may be the occurrence of pulmonary embolism. Pain in the region of the thrombosed veins at rest or only during exercise and edema distal to the obstructed veins are the usual symptoms of deep-vein thrombosis. Edema or pitting of the malleolar fossa may be present and may cause loss of the normal concavity of that portion of the leg. There may be a difference between the two legs in the calf circumference. A difference in maximal circumference >1.4 cm in men and 1.2 cm in women is highly suspicious. The temperature of the skin may be increased as a result of the inflammatory reaction, and palpation may disclose the thrombosed veins in the calf or in the popliteal fossa. There may be tenderness to palpation. Increased resistance or pain on voluntary dorsiflexion of the foot (Homans' sign) may be present.

Thrombosis of the iliac and femoral veins usually presents with a characteristic clinical picture consisting of rapidly advancing swelling of the entire limb. The thrombosed vein may be tender if it extends below the inguinal ligament. Collateral distended veins may be present in the upper thigh.

Thrombosis of the subclavian vein may result in swelling of the upper extremity, and collateral veins may be present. In axillary thrombosis, a similar clinical picture occurs; the thrombosed vein may be felt in the axilla. A history of walking on crutches or sleeping in a sitting position on a bench with the arms behind the backrest may encourage a positive diagnosis. Thrombosis of the superior vena cava increases venous pressure in the neck and face, distending the neck veins in the upper part of the chest.

In septic thrombophlebitis, there may also be systemic manifestations of infection, such as fever, chills, and leukocytosis. In cases in which septic phlebitis begins from infected needles or catheters, an inflamed, tender cord may appear at the site of the venipuncture.

DIAGNOSIS. Ileofemoral thrombophlebitis is usually easily recognized by the rapid swelling of the entire limb, engorged collateral veins in the thigh, and signs of inflammation, such as increased skin temperature.

By contrast, in the majority of cases of deep-vein thrombosis involving the calf, popliteal area, and thigh, the clinical picture is not sufficiently distinctive to allow diagnosis with a high degree of confidence. Confirmation of the diagnosis must be provided by resorting to one or more of a number of diagnostic tests. The most commonly used tests, their important features, and main usefulness are listed in Table 46–4.

DIFFERENTIAL DIAGNOSIS. A number of conditions that cause localized pain or edema in the lower extremities may be confused with deep-vein thrombosis. A ruptured popliteal synovial membrane or cyst (Baker's cyst) may simulate most of the manifestations of venous thrombosis. The diagnosis can be suspected if there is a history or physical findings of arthritis of the knee joint. The diagnosis may be confirmed by an arthrogram revealing the entry of dye from the joint into the calf muscles. Ruptured calf muscles may cause pain, tenderness, and edema and may simulate thrombophlebitis. The diagnosis can be made from the history of strenuous or unusual exercise, the presence of ecchymosis from extravasated blood, and the palpation of a hematoma. Sometimes the patient reports an audible snap during the activity when the pain first occurred. The differential diagnosis is important because anticoagulants are contraindicated in this condition. A severe muscle cramp may cause pain and swelling for a considerable period of time. Other manifestations of thrombophlebitis are, however, lacking in this situation. The pain of a lumbar disc may be localized in the calf. There are no other manifestations of venous thrombosis, however, and there may be neurologic findings to identify the cause of the pain. Lymphedema is recognized by its slower and gradual onset and the absence of signs of inflammation and of collateral veins. Finally, cellulitis may be confused with superficial thrombophlebitis.

COMPLICATIONS. Pulmonary embolism is a frequent and serious complication of deep-vein thrombosis. About 80 to 90% of pulmonary emboli arise in the deep veins of the lower limbs. Although deep-vein thrombosis may begin frequently in the veins of the calf, it is only when the thrombosis extends above the knee that serious pulmonary embolism occurs.

About 5% of patients with deep-vein thrombosis develop venous insufficiency with stasis dermatitis (postphlebitic syndrome). This is more likely to occur in those with more proximal venous obstruction. A rare complication of iliofemoral thrombophlebitis is venous claudication, in which the patient develops pain on exercise which is relieved by rest, as in arterial occlusive disease.

PROPHYLAXIS. Prophylactic therapy against deep-vein thrombosis should be attempted in high-risk patients (Table 46–5). The exact regimen used must take into consideration the risk of deep-vein thrombosis and consequent pulmonary embolism and the potential risk of hemorrhagic complications from the prophylactic therapy. Low-dose heparin is currently the most commonly used prophylactic technique. For surgical patients, this consists of 5000 IU of heparin administered subcutaneously 2 hours before surgery and then every 8 to 12 hours until the patient is ambulatory.

This method is effective in reducing the incidence of deep-vein thrombosis and pulmonary embolism in patients subjected to a variety of surgical procedures. It is also effective in reducing the incidence of deep-vein thrombosis in patients following acute myocardial infarction, but it is not known whether there is also a reduction in the incidence of pulmonary embolism. Low-dose heparin has been shown to be ineffective in patients undergoing surgery for hip fracture and hip replacement, and its effectiveness has not been established in urologic procedures. High-dose heparin adjusted to give an activated partial thromboplastin time (aPTT) in the upper limits of the therapeutic range has been reported to be more effective than low-dose heparin. In addition, the administration of dihydroergotamine mesylate, 0.5 mg subcutaneously, together with low-dose heparin, is more effective in preventing deep-vein thrombosis than heparin alone in surgical patients. Ergotamine acts by inducing venoconstriction and also by altering the coagulability of the blood.

TABLE 46–4. DIAGNOSTIC TESTS FOR CONFIRMATION OF DEEP-VEIN THROMBOSIS

Tests	Underlying Principle	Features	Main Use
X-ray venography	Injection of contrast medium in venous system to detect obstruction or filling defect	Most accurate test available. Occasionally complicated by local inflammation and thrombosis	Considered the "gold standard." Used when other test results are not conclusive
Radionuclide venography	Injecting radioisotope-labeled albumin in venous system coupled with external counting	Less sensitive and specific than x-ray venography	Used when x-ray or contrast is not advisable
Radioisotope-labeled fibrinogen	Intravenously injecting ^{125}I-labeled fibrinogen coupled with external counting	Requires 1–2 days to detect radioactivity. Not suitable for pelvic vein thrombosis because of high background radioactivity	Longitudinal screening of high-risk populations
Liquid crystal thermography	Detects small differences in skin temperature due to underlying venous inflammation	Very sensitive but not very specific	Monitors patients at risk
Ultrasonography	Detects venous obstruction by ultrasonography	High-degree stenosis needed for detection. Distinction of compression versus obstruction difficult	Most sensitive for thrombosis above the knee
Duplex ultrasonography	Ultrasound imaging coupled with Doppler evaluation of blood flow	Excellent specificity and sensitivity for thrombosis above knee	The best noninvasive substitute for venography
Impedance plethysmography	Detects volume changes by electrical impedance	High sensitivity and specificity	Good alternative to duplex ultrasonography

TREATMENT. Anticoagulation is not necessary to treat superficial thrombophlebitis. Local measures, sometimes coupled with anti-inflammatory drugs, such as indomethacin, sufficiently heal and relieve symptoms.

Full anticoagulation is the preferred treatment for deep-vein thrombosis. Heparin is preferred to initiate treatment because of its immediate action, whereas warfarin-type drugs may not become fully effective for a considerable period of time. Heparin inhibits coagulation by binding and activating antithrombin III, an inhibitor of activated Factor X. Heparin is best administered by constant infusion. Initially a bolus of 5000 IU is given intravenously, followed by constant infusion of 750 to 1000 IU per hour. The dose is adjusted by monitoring the aPTT so that a level about two times the normal control is achieved. aPTT is checked 4 to 6 hours after the initial bolus and once a day thereafter. An alternative method is intermittently administering 5000 to 10,000 IU intravenously every 4 to 6 hours. If no suitable veins are found, heparin may be administered subcutaneously in a dose of 15,000 to 30,000 IU every 12 hours. Low molecular weight heparin fragments have high bioavailability and a longer biologic half-life. They are administered subcutaneously and do not require monitoring; they may, therefore, eliminate the need for hospitalization of patients with deep-vein thrombosis.

One day after initiation of heparin therapy, oral warfarin at a dose of 10 to 15 mg daily is begun. The prothrombin time (PT) is monitored 48 hours after the onset of warfarin therapy and daily thereafter. Dosage is adjusted to achieve an international normalized ratio (INR) in the PT test between 2 and 3. Heparin therapy is discontinued in 5 to 7 days, provided that PT time is in the desired therapeutic range.

Warfarin brings about anticoagulation by decreasing the level of Factors II, VII, IX, and X. Many drugs interact with warfarin. Some of them potentiate its action and others inhibit it. If the patient requires other drug therapy while on warfarin, each drug should be carefully screened for potential interaction. If bleeding occurs in the course of heparin therapy, its effect can be counteracted by administering 1 mg of protamine per 100 IU of heparin. If bleeding develops in the course of warfarin treatment, the patient should receive vitamin K_1 intramuscularly to reduce PT to the therapeutic range (0.25 to 1.0 mg usually suffices). If bleeding is serious, blood or fresh frozen plasma may be necessary.

Thrombolysis with fibrinolytic agents, such as streptokinase or urokinase, administered intravenously in patients with deep-vein thrombosis has been shown to more completely dissolve the thrombus and preserve the venous architecture than conventional anticoagulants. These drugs activate plasminogen to plasmin, thereby dissolving the thrombus. Streptokinase is administered intravenously as an initial bolus of 250,000 to 500,000 IU, followed by an infusion of 100,000 IU per hour for 24 to 72 hours. The effectiveness of the drug diminishes after the first 24 hours. Urokinase is less likely to cause anaphylactic reactions, but it is more expensive. It is given in a dose of 4400 IU per kilogram as a bolus, followed by an infusion of 4400 IU per kilogram per hour for the same duration as streptokinase. Human recombinant tissue-type plasminogen activator can also dissolve venous thrombi and pulmonary emboli. Thrombolytic therapy is the preferred method to treat patients with iliofemoral or subclavian-axillary vein thrombosis. In patients with more distal deep-vein thrombosis, the high effectiveness of heparin and its lower rate of hemorrhagic complications make it the preferred method of treatment.

In patients in whom anticoagulation is contraindicated, simple measures—elevating the extremity and local heat—should be used. When the risk of pulmonary embolism is low, as is the case of deep-vein thrombosis limited to the calf, these measures suffice. In

TABLE 46–5. PREVENTION OF VENOUS THROMBOEMBOLISM

Representative patient groups	1. Medical patients without predisposing factors on short bed rest 2. Young patients without predisposing factors undergoing brief (<1 hr) general surgical procedure	1. Medical patients with predisposing factors or on prolonged bed rest 2. Middle-aged or old patients without predisposing factors undergoing general surgical procedure longer than 1 hr	1. Patients with hip fracture 2. Patients undergoing extensive orthopedic or pelvic surgery 3. Middle-aged or old patients with predisposing factors or with previous venous thrombosis undergoing general surgical procedure longer than 1 hr
Approximate incidence of venous thrombosis	5%	20–40%	50–70%
Approximate incidence of pulmonary embolism	Almost zero	5%	10%
Suggested prophylaxis	None	Low-dose heparin or intermittent pneumatic compression	Warfarin, low-dose heparin plus either intermittent pneumatic compression or dihydroergotamine, or higher dose heparin

patients with deep-vein thrombosis extending above the knee, in whom the risk of pulmonary embolism is high, implanting an inferior vena caval filter or ligating the inferior vena cava may also be considered. This form of therapy should also be used when anticoagulation needs to be terminated because of complications, when recurrent thromboembolism occurs in the presence of adequate anticoagulation, and when there is septic thromboembolic disease not controlled by antibiotics.

Bed rest should be continued until local signs of inflammation, including tenderness and edema, subside. After 7 to 15 days the patient is allowed to walk wearing elastic stockings. If no discomfort occurs, resumption of full activity is allowed 1 to 2 weeks later. Anticoagulation for 3 months is usually sufficient to prevent recurrence of deep-vein thrombosis.

Beisaw NE, Comerota AJ, Groth HE, et al.: Dihydroergotamine/heparin in the prevention of deep-vein thrombosis after total hip replacement. J Bone Joint Surg 70A:2, 1988. *Report of a controlled, randomized multicenter trial showing greater effectiveness of the combination of dihydroergotamine plus heparin than either drug alone in the prophylaxis of deep-vein thrombosis in patients undergoing total hip replacement.*

Bergqvist D: Review of clinical trials of low molecular weight heparins. Eur J Surg 158:67, 1992. *Review of clinical trials of low molecular weight heparins.*

Grassi CJ, Goldhaber SZ: Interruption of the inferior vena cava for prevention of pulmonary embolism: Transvenous filter devices. Herz 14:182, 1989. *A consideration of the uses of inferior vena cava filters to prevent pulmonary embolism.*

Hirsh J: Antithrombotic therapy in deep vein thrombosis and pulmonary embolism. Am Heart J 123:1115, 1992. *A comprehensive review of the clinical use of anticoagulants in deep vein thrombosis and pulmonary embolism.*

Hull RD, Raskob GE, Hirsh J: Prophylaxis of venous thromboembolism: An overview. Chest 89:374S, 1986. *A concise and thoughtful analysis of the methods for preventing deep-vein thrombosis.*

Peterson CE, Kwaan HC: Current concepts of warfarin therapy. Arch Intern Med 146:581, 1986. *A concise consideration of the pharmacology and use of warfarin in the treatment of thrombotic disease.*

Rogers LQ, Lutcher CL: Streptokinase therapy for deep vein thrombosis: A comprehensive review of the English literature. Am J Med 88:389, 1990. *A comprehensive review of the literature on using streptokinase for deep-vein thrombosis.*

White RH, McGahan JP, Daschbach MM, et al.: Diagnosis of deep-vein thrombosis using duplex ultrasound. Ann Intern Med 111:297, 1989. *A review of the use of duplex ultrasonography in the diagnosis of deep-vein thrombosis.*

Varicose Veins

DEFINITION. Varicose veins are prominent, abnormally distended, and tortuous veins.

INCIDENCE. Approximately 20% of adults develop varicose veins. A familial history is present in 15% of patients. They are more common in women than in men by a ratio of 5 to 1. Most women date the onset of varicose veins from the time of pregnancy. The veins of the lower extremities are most frequently affected because of the effects of gravity on venous pressure.

ETIOLOGY. Congenitally absent or defective valves are a recognized cause of varicose veins in early life. Varicose veins may develop secondary to sustained elevations of venous pressure from obstructed veins. The cause of the obstruction may be thrombosis secondary to thrombophlebitis or external pressure, as is the case in pregnancy, ascites, and tumors. However, in most affected individuals, no clearly identifiable cause or precipitating factor can be found. Individuals with lower-extremity varicose veins may have a variety of structural, functional, and biochemical abnormalities in unaffected veins. These include increased venous distensibility and reduced amounts of collagen and hexosamine, reduced responsiveness to vasoconstrictor agents, abnormally depressed endothelium-dependent relaxation responses, reduced protein content, and increased endothelin content. With such a generalized defect, a sustained elevation in venous pressure from the effects of gravity in the lower extremities or from other factors may lead to stretching of the walls and, finally, to incompetence of the valves and overdistention of the veins. Varicose veins associated with hemorrhoids and diverticulosis of the bowel suggest the possibility that increased intra-abdominal pressure during bowel movements may play a role in their pathogenesis.

CLINICAL MANIFESTATIONS. Most patients are asymptomatic, especially in the early stages of the disease. They may seek attention because the dilated, tortuous varicosities are cosmetically unappealing. In some cases, aching in the lower extremities and edema, especially after prolonged standing or exercise, may be present. The edema usually subsides overnight. When the communicating veins are incompetent, symptoms are more common. Prolonged venous insufficiency leads to the postphlebitic syndrome,

with sustained edema, induration, and fibrosis. Eventually, trophic changes with brownish discoloration of the skin and ulceration may result. Ulcers usually occur above the medial malleolus. An incompetent communicating vein may be identified near the ulcer. The arterial pulses are normal, and no evidence of ischemia is present.

DIAGNOSIS. Clinical inspection suffices to make the diagnosis. The Trendelenburg test can identify the presence of defective valves and incompetent communicating veins: With the patient recumbent, the leg is elevated to empty the veins, and a tourniquet is then applied to occlude the superficial veins. The patient is instructed to resume the erect position, and the tourniquet is released. If the venous valves are incompetent, the veins immediately become distended as a result of the backflow. If two tourniquets are applied, the distention of the veins in the intervening portion of the limb identifies the presence of incompetent communicating veins. The patency of the deep venous system can be examined by venography. It is prudent to exclude other causes of edema, such as congestive heart failure and renal disease.

PROGNOSIS. The prognosis of uncomplicated superficial varicose veins is excellent. The postphlebitic syndrome, once established, is usually progressive and resistant to treatment.

TREATMENT. Simple measures usually suffice to treat uncomplicated varicose veins. These consist of frequent periods of rest while elevating the limbs, external pressure with elastic stockings or bandages, and avoiding obstructing of the veins by garments such as girdles. In more severe or advanced cases, ligation and stripping of the saphenous veins or injecting sclerosing solutions may become necessary to prevent the postphlebitic syndrome. An injection/compression technique in which the sclerosing solution is injected into a vein emptied of blood, followed by compression by external pressure, is simple, cheap, and effective. It is widely used in Europe. When stasis ulcers are present, local care with warm, wet dressings is necessary. If infection is present, local and systemic antibiotics may be administered. If considerable fibrosis is present, it may be necessary to excise the entire area and carry out skin grafting to eliminate ulceration.

DISEASES OF THE LYMPHATIC VESSELS OF THE LIMBS

Lymphangitis

DEFINITION. Lymphangitis is an inflammation of the lymphatic vessels. It is usually of bacterial origin.

ETIOLOGY. In most cases the responsible infective agent is the hemolytic streptococcus or *Staphylococcus aureus,* both of which are coagulase-positive. The bacteria gain access to the lymphatics via local trauma or ulcerations. In many instances no identifiable portal of entry can be found. Infection spreads from the lymphatics to the regional lymph nodes.

PATHOLOGY. Various stages of inflammation are found in the subcutaneous tissue and regional lymph nodes.

CLINICAL MANIFESTATIONS. The local manifestation of lymphangitis consists of a red streak that appears where the infective organism initially entered and extends to the regional lymph nodes. The latter are swollen and tender. There may be a surrounding area of cellulitis. Systemic accompaniments of infection may constitute the presenting manifestations.

DIAGNOSIS. The local manifestations of lymphangitis and the accompanying systemic reaction are usually sufficient to make the diagnosis. Leukocytosis with predominance of polymorphonuclear leukocytes may be present. Confirmation is obtained by culturing the organism from the portal of entry or from the subcutaneous tissues. Acute lymphangitis may be difficult to distinguish from a generalized cellulitis or from thrombophlebitis.

PROGNOSIS. With treatment the prognosis is good when one is dealing with an initial attack in an otherwise normal limb. In the case of recurrent attacks, lymphedema may develop and residual increase in the girth of the limb may occur.

TREATMENT. This consists of systemically administering the appropriate antibiotics. In addition, surgically draining the focus of infection is important. Supportive measures, including rest and elevating the infected limb and local warm, wet dressings, also help. Elastic support hose may be necessary for several weeks to prevent lymphedema. In recurrent cases, the causes of secondary lymphedema should be sought.

Schinger A, Martin WJ, Spittell JA: Acute lymphangitis and cellulitis. Minn Med 48:191, 1965. *Concise consideration of the clinical features, diagnosis, and treatment of lymphangitis.*

DEFINITION. Lymphedema refers to edema from accumulated lymph secondary to obstruction to its flow.

ETIOLOGY AND INCIDENCE. Lymphedema can be primary or secondary. The most frequent type of primary lymphedema is simple congenital lymphedema, which is not familial and is present at birth. A congenital familial form (Milroy's disease) is inherited as an autosomal dominant trait. Another hereditary form is associated with Noonan's syndrome in about 15% of cases. Lymphedema praecox becomes manifest in puberty and is associated with congenital hypoplasia of the lymphatics. A late form may become manifest in middle age.

Primary lymphedema is more common in women. Most cases are manifest at birth or become apparent before age 40. A syndrome characterized by yellow nails, recurrent pleural effusion, and lymphedema is believed to be secondary to multiple lymphatic abnormalities in the areas involved. A familial syndrome consisting of recurrent intrahepatic cholestasis and lymphedema is probably due to defective hepatic lymphatic vessels as well as those in the extremities.

Secondary lymphedema results most commonly from trauma. It commonly results from surgically removing lymph nodes and from fibrosis secondary to radiation following surgery for cancer. Lymphoma or metastatic carcinoma involving the lymph nodes may also obstruct the flow of lymph and lymphedema. Filarial infection (see Ch. 388) in the tropics is a cause of secondary lymphedema.

CLINICAL MANIFESTATIONS. Typically, lymphedema begins gradually—the involved limb is enlarged without other manifestations. The swollen extremity is soft and pitting. The edema subsides at night. With time, the skin becomes thickened and cannot be raised into a fold, and the edema becomes more persistent. The lower extremities are involved most often. In about half the patients the edema is unilateral. Superimposed lymphangitis and cellulitis may occur, and in longstanding cases lymphangiosarcoma may develop.

DIAGNOSIS. The diagnosis of lymphedema may be confirmed with a radioisotope lymphogram. ^{99m}Tc-labeled rhenium sulfur colloid, ^{99m}Tc-labeled antimony trisulfide colloid, or ^{99m}Tc-labeled human serum albumin microcolloid is injected in the web spaces of the foot. The ilioinguinal region is scanned 30 and 60 minutes later. In lymphedema, the uptake of isotope by the lymph nodes is reduced, whereas in edema due to venous obstruction it is greater than normal owing to increased lymph flow. The precise diagnosis of the type of lymphedema is made by lymphangiography. Contrast medium is injected directly into a lymphatic vessel in the foot, or a water-soluble contrast agent is injected intracutaneously and taken up by the lymphatics. By this technique, a distinction can be made between absence or hypoplasia of the lymphatic vessels on one hand, which characterizes congenital lymphedema, and the hyperplasia and numerous small lymphatics, which characterize secondary lymphedema, on the other.

PROGNOSIS. Primary lymphedema is usually a slowly progressive disorder, not easily amenable to treatment. The prognosis of secondary lymphedema depends on the cause. In cases in which it results from infection, it can be effectively managed with antibiotics.

TREATMENT. In primary lymphedema treatment is aimed at keeping the limb as free of edema as possible to prevent fibrosis and secondary infection. Frequently elevating the limb, using elastic stockings, and diuretics may be useful. In cases not controlled by these simple measures, benzopyrones have been reported to be useful. These drugs break down protein by activating macrophages; hence, they reduce viscosity and facilitate the flow of lymph. Surgery may be tried in advanced cases to remove subcutaneous tissue and to induce new lymph vessel formation. Anastomosis of small lymphatic vessels with veins by microsurgery has been reported to give good results in some cases.

Browse NL, Stewart G: Lymphedema: Pathophysiology and classification. J Cardiovasc Surg 26:91, 1985. *An up-to-date description of the pathophysiology and classification of lymphedema.*

Casley-Smith JR, Morgan RG, Piller NB: Treatment of lymphedema of the arms and legs with 5,6-benzo-[α]-pyrone. N Engl J Med 329:1158, 1993. *Report of a clinical trial of benzopyrones in lymphedema demonstrating benefit manifested in slow and safe reduction in lymphedema.*

Gloviczki P, Calcagno D, Schirger A, et al.: Noninvasive evaluation of the swollen extremity experiences with 190 lymphoscintigraphic examinations. J Vasc Surg 9:683, 1989. *Report of the use of lymphoscintigraphy with ^{99m}Tc-labeled antimony trisulfide in the diagnosis of lymphedema.*

Weissleder H, Weissleder R: Lymphedema: Evaluation of qualitative and quantitative lymphoscintigraphy in 238 patients. Radiology 168:729, 1988. *Report of the application of lymphoscintigraphy using ^{99m}Tc-labeled human serum albumin microcolloid in the diagnosis of lymphedema.*

47 MISCELLANEOUS CONDITIONS OF THE HEART: TUMOR, TRAUMA, AND SYSTEMIC DISEASE

Joshua Wynne

CARDIAC TUMORS

Although the heart is resistant to the development of primary malignancies, it is a frequent site of secondary involvement by metastatic tumors. Primary tumors of the heart are noted in 1 per 2000 to 4000 unselected autopsies, whereas metastatic involvement may be found in up to 20% of cancer patients. Recognition of cardiac involvement by tumor often is delayed because of a low index of suspicion, yet it is almost always detectable by standard noninvasive techniques (echocardiography, computed tomography, and magnetic resonance imaging). The clinical presentation of a patient with a cardiac tumor is determined less by the histology of the tumor than by its location and size. Intracavity tumors typically involve a cardiac valve and may produce valve dysfunction (with obstruction and/or regurgitation). Intramyocardial tumors may be clinically silent or may lead to arrhythmia or heart block. Intrapericardial tumors generally become manifest when they compress the heart chambers, usually by tamponade due to an effusion but occasionally by constriction. Conversely, tumor type most directly determines management and prognosis. Most primary cardiac tumors are benign, whereas all secondary are malignant (Fig. 47–1).

The most common primary tumor by far is the myxoma; others include fibromas, lipomas, fibroelastomas, and rhabdomyomas. Only an occasional malignant primary tumor is encountered, usually a sarcoma. Secondary tumor involvement of the heart is much more common than a primary neoplasm and is dominated by cancers of the lung and breast, reflecting their relative frequency overall. Together they account for more than half of all cases of cardiac tumors. Cardiac involvement is common as well with lymphomas, esophageal cancer, leukemia, and melanoma, and may be seen on occasion with other malignancies.

INTRAPERICARDIAL TUMORS. Tumor involvement of the heart most commonly occurs by contiguous spread and direct extension of neoplasms involving the chest cavity, usually with invasion of the pericardium. Lung and breast cancers typically invade the heart in this manner and, because of their relative frequency, make pericardial involvement the most common mode of presentation of secondary tumors, often with attendant pericardial effusion and cardiac tamponade. Because tumor invasion often extends beyond the pericardial space to involve the myocardium as well, there often is little expectation of long-term therapeutic success. Nevertheless, pericardiocentesis (often guided by echocardiography), balloon pericardiotomy, or surgical drainage and limited pericardiectomy ("pericardial window") often are life-saving short- and intermediate-term palliative procedures. Even very debilitated patients may benefit from a subxiphoid pericardiectomy, a quick and low-morbidity procedure that may provide brief palliation.

INTRACAVITY TUMORS. The most common intracavity tumor is the *myxoma*, a benign globular neoplasm that usually is located within the left atrium attached to the interatrial septum. Sometimes, it also is seen in the right atrium and rarely in the ventricles. Myxomas are more common in women and usually are an

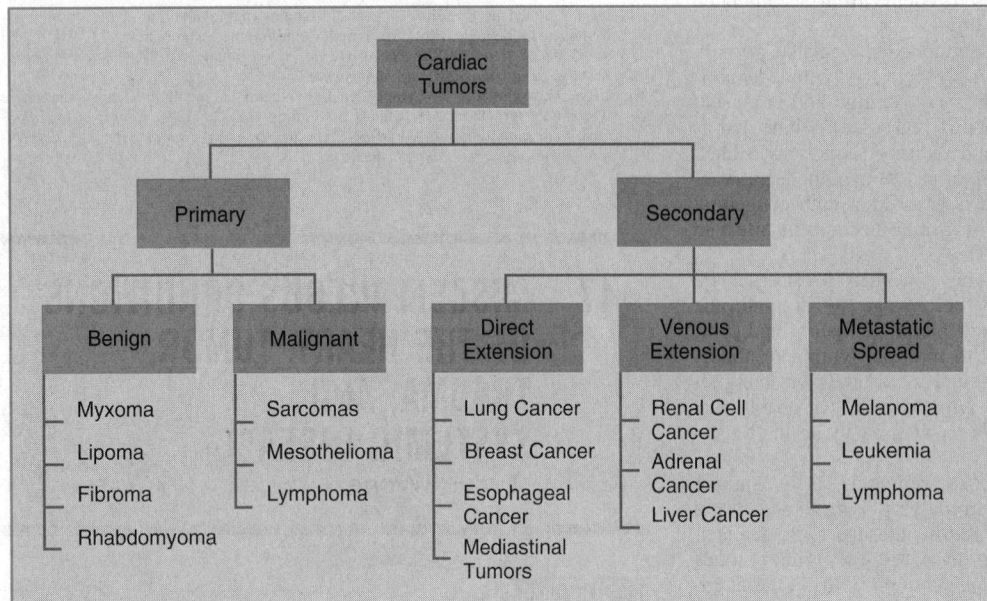

FIGURE 47–1. Classification of the most common primary and secondary tumors. (Adapted from Salcedo EE, Cohen GI, White RD, Davison MG: Cardiac tumors: Diagnosis and management. Curr Probl Cardiol 17:75, 1992.)

isolated finding, although they can be familial or are found in association with other systemic abnormalities (such as pigmented skin lesions and noncardiac tumors). Although they may not be clinically apparent when small, myxomas usually produce findings due to tumor embolization, mitral valve obstruction similar to mitral stenosis, and constitutional symptoms such as fever, malaise, and arthralgias. During diastole, a left atrial myxoma often is drawn into the mitral orifice and may produce obstruction to blood flow from the left atrium to the left ventricle, simulating rheumatic mitral stenosis. Even the physical examination may be misleading, with a tumor "plop" simulating an opening snap and a diastolic rumble similar to the murmur found with rheumatic involvement.

If the diagnosis is suspected, echocardiography provides the definitive diagnosis; most myxomas are discovered when embolization or valve dysfunction leads to an echocardiographic study. Once diagnosed, the tumor is removed surgically, which usually is a low-risk procedure that results in cure. Myxomas can be multiple or recurrent, so even after successful removal, continued surveillance is indicated.

Other intracavity tumors are uncommon. Papillary fibroelastomas are frondlike excrescences that typically arise from a cardiac valve and usually are detected incidentally during echocardiography. They may produce symptoms by virtue of systemic or coronary embolization. Angiosarcomas occur in men more frequently than women and have a predilection for the right atrium, where they may cause obstruction and attendant right-sided congestive heart failure. A unique type of cardiac involvement that occurs most commonly with renal cell carcinoma (and occasionally with adrenal and hepatic neoplasms) consists of venous extension of the tumor via the inferior vena cava, with resultant tumor involvement of the right atrial cavity.

INTRAMYOCARDIAL TUMORS. The least common location for cardiac tumors is within the myocardium, where the tumors may be clinically silent, produce arrhythmias, or protrude into a cardiac chamber with attendant obstructive features. Lipomas are encapsulated benign primary cardiac tumors that often are clinically silent. Sarcomas (angiosarcomas, rhabdomyosarcomas, fibrosarcomas) often demonstrate widespread cardiac involvement, with protrusion into the cardiac chambers and extension into the pericardial space. No good therapy is available for these tumors.

Secondary tumor involvement usually is the result of hematogenous or lymphatic spread and frequently is seen with melanoma, leukemia, and lymphoma.

CARDIAC INVOLVEMENT IN SYSTEMIC DISEASE

CARCINOID (see Ch. 125). More than half the patients with carcinoid syndrome metastatic to the liver have cardiac involvement, usually consisting of thickening and scarring of the endocardium and of the tricuspid and/or pulmonary valves and producing both stenosis and regurgitation. Left-sided valvular involvement as well as myocardial metastasis and pericardial effusions occur on occasion. It has been speculated that the endocardial changes are produced by serotonin and other vasoactive amines that are released by the tumor but usually are inactivated by the liver and lungs. It is thought that the hepatic metastases that are ubiquitous in carcinoid heart disease permit these vasoactive compounds to bypass the liver and thus escape inactivation. Dyspnea is a common finding, and right heart failure may contribute to the death of one third of the patients. Treatment usually is with a somatostatin analogue, and in selected patients valve replacement seems to have improved symptoms and perhaps retarded or prevented the development of advanced right heart failure. Nevertheless, the median survival in carcinoid heart disease is <2 years.

CARDIOTOXICITY OF CANCER THERAPY (see Ch. 162). Cardiotoxicity following chemotherapy is most common with doxorubicin (Adriamycin), with dose-related systolic (and diastolic) dysfunction appearing, and often clinical congestive heart failure (with or without ventricular arrhythmias) that may appear months to years after treatment. Although less common with current dosing schemes that use more frequent but lower doses, doxorubicin cardiotoxicity continues to be associated with a poor prognosis and significant mortality. It often is irreversible, although occasional improvement of ventricular function is seen; the best "treatment" is discontinuing the doxorubicin once preclinical evidence of cardiotoxicity is found. This is achieved with radionuclide ventriculography (manifested by a fall in left ventricular ejection fraction and/or failure of an appropriate increase with exercise), echocardiography, or right ventricular endomyocardial biopsy (with the demonstration of characteristic histologic abnormalities such as myofibrillar dropout and sarcotubular dilatation). Cardiotoxicity appears to be potentiated in the setting of mediastinal irradiation, preexisting cardiac disease, young or advanced age, and concomitant administration of other chemotherapeutic drugs. Once congestive heart failure appears, usual treatment strategies (e.g., digitalis, diuretics, vasodilators) may produce symptomatic improvement.

Cardiotoxicity may be seen with other chemotherapeutic agents. Cyclophosphamide occasionally produces often fatal hemorrhagic myocardial necrosis. Myocardial ischemia and infarction may be seen during 5-fluorouracil infusions, and some but not all patients appear to respond to nitrates. Taxol has been associated with a variety of often asymptomatic arrhythmias and abnormalities of the conducting system.

Cardiotoxicity as a consequence of radiation therapy has declined in frequency with better shielding of the heart, use of improved dosing schedules, and use of multiple radiation portals. Nevertheless, cardiac damage occurring months and years after radiation therapy continues to be seen, most commonly consisting of pericardial inflammation and effusion that may progress to chronic constrictive pericarditis. Other manifestations include accelerated coronary artery atherosclerosis (often involving the coronary ostia), myocardial fibrosis, and occasionally valvular dysfunction and abnormalities of the conducting system.

ENDOCRINE DISORDERS. The heart often is involved in diabetics, although there is continued debate as to whether there is a unique cardiomyopathy due only to the diabetes or the observed cardiac abnormalities simply are the consequence of the coronary artery disease and hypertension that so frequently accompany diabetes. The weight of evidence favors the existence of a distinctive diabetic cardiomyopathy that is marked by myocardial deposits of collagen, lipids, and glycoprotein along with abnormalities of the smaller intramyocardial coronary arteries. The clinical expression of these abnormalities is one of a restrictive cardiomyopathy, with impairment of ventricular filling.

Hyperthyroidism (see Ch. 203) commonly results in a hyperkinetic cardiovascular state, manifested by a fall in systemic vascular resistance, an increase in cardiac output, and enhanced left ventricular emptying. Other effects include atrial fibrillation, and, especially with pre-existing heart disease, congestive heart failure is seen on occasion. Those with coronary artery disease often experience an exacerbation of angina pectoris. Hypothyroidism may be associated with hypertension, bradycardia, and a pericardial effusion that rarely progresses to cardiac tamponade. Because myocardial ischemia often is exacerbated in myxedematous patients with pre-existing coronary artery disease as therapy is begun, thyroid hormone replacement should be started with very low doses that are increased slowly.

Pheochromocytomas (see Ch. 204.2) are associated with histologic evidence of catecholamine-induced myocardial damage in about half the patients, consisting of focal myocardial contraction band necrosis, inflammation, and fibrosis, but these abnormalities only occasionally culminate in clinical congestive heart failure. The effects of direct myocardial toxicity are exacerbated by the accompanying systemic hypertension. Treatment with adrenergic receptor blockers (initially α and then β) usually is effective in treating both the hypertension and the cardiotoxicity.

INFILTRATIVE DISEASES. Involvement of the cardiovascular system is the most frequent cause of death in cardiac amyloidosis and occurs in one (or more) of four clinical presentations: diastolic dysfunction (restrictive cardiomyopathy); systolic dysfunction; conduction disturbances and arrhythmias; and orthostatic hypotension. Focal cardiac amyloid (see Ch. 248) deposits occur commonly in elderly patients (often involving the atria) but usually are clinically silent. Hemochromatosis (see Ch. 189) usually presents with abnormalities of ventricular filling (restrictive cardiomyopathy) along with impaired systolic performance and should be suspected when cardiomyopathy occurs in association with diabetes mellitus, hepatic cirrhosis, and increased skin pigmentation. Iron overload is reduced with deferoxamine therapy, which appears to improve cardiac function as well. Myocardial sarcoidosis typically occurs in concert with obvious pulmonary sarcoidosis and produces both diastolic and systolic ventricular dysfunction. Arrhythmias and abnormalities of atrioventricular conduction often are distinctive features.

NEUROMUSCULAR DISEASES. Cardiac involvement is common in Friedreich's ataxia, with symmetric or asymmetric left ventricular hypertrophy, often grossly resembling hypertrophic cardiomyopathy. Associated ST-segment and T-wave abnormalities of the electrocardiogram are common. In Duchenne's muscular dystrophy (see Ch. 454), a peculiar form of myocardial necrosis occurs that principally involves the posterobasal portion of the left ventricle and the adjacent papillary muscle. The echocardiogram often is distinctive, as is the electrocardiogram, which demonstrates tall R waves in the right precordial leads and deep Q waves in the limb and lateral precordial leads. Myotonic dystrophy produces a variety of electrocardiographic abnormalities, especially abnormalities of atrioventricular conduction with the attendant risk of syncope and sudden death.

COLLAGEN VASCULAR DISEASES. Whereas demonstrable cardiac involvement is common in rheumatoid arthritis, clinical manifestations are rare. The endocardium, myocardium, or pericardium may be involved, but the most common manifestation is pericarditis, with variable amount of pericardial effusion. Pericardial involvement also is common in systemic lupus erythematosus (SLE) (see Ch. 240), and there may be inflammation and scarring of the myocardium, aortic and/or mitral valves, and coronary arteries, producing clinical myocarditis, valvular regurgitation (with so-called Libman-Saks endocarditis), or coronary arteritis. The existence of a distinct SLE cardiomyopathy is controversial, and in any event the prevalence of overt clinical manifestations is relatively low.

In progressive systemic sclerosis (see Ch. 241), there may be focal myocardial necrosis and fibrosis, culminating in a dilated cardiomyopathy. Ankylosing spondylitis and the associated seronegative arthropathies (Reiter's syndrome, psoriatic arthritis) may be associated with involvement of the proximal aortic root, with the production of often clinically important aortic regurgitation.

CARDIAC TRAUMA

Cardiac damage may result from trauma as a consequence of either penetrating or nonpenetrating injury. The usual cause of penetrating trauma is a bullet or stab wound, whereas deceleration injuries as a consequence of automobile accidents are the most common cause of nonpenetrating injury. Either often results in death before the patient comes to medical attention, usually due to hemopericardium and attendant tamponade, or massive hemorrhage.

NONPENETRATING INJURY. The most common manifestation of blunt trauma is myocardial contusion, often the result of the impact of the chest wall against the steering wheel. Although the diagnosis of contusion is straightforward when new electrocardiographic changes or arrhythmias are noted, the diagnosis is more difficult in the typical chest trauma patient. In such cases, the demonstration of new regional left ventricular wall motion abnormalities on echocardiography or radionuclide ventriculography or a positive radionuclide scan using infarct-avid agents such as pyrophosphate helps secure the diagnosis. Other less common manifestations include traumatic ventricular septal defect, myocardial rupture and/or pseudoaneurysm formation, coronary artery trauma with myocardial infarction, and valvular regurgitation.

The most feared complication of blunt trauma is traumatic transection of the descending aorta, which occurs just distal to the ligamentum arteriosum. It results from the shear forces that occur during deceleration injury as the more mobile aortic arch continues to move anteriorly while the descending aorta remains fixed because of its attachment to the posterior mediastinum. It usually is fatal if not rapidly repaired surgically. However, occasional patients may show long-term survival even without operative repair.

PENETRATING INJURY. Bullet and stab wounds, the most common form of penetrating trauma, usually result in hemopericardium and tamponade, or exsanguination, depending on the site of injury. Associated cardiac damage is not uncommon, including traumatic valvular regurgitation, intracardiac shunts, and, occasionally, coronary artery injuries. Immediate thoracotomy is indicated when life-threatening hemorrhage or tamponade is present; repair of any associated cardiac defects often can wait for definitive diagnosis and management at a later time.

Allen A: The cardiotoxicity of chemotherapeutic drugs. Semin Oncol 19:529, 1992. *Review of clinical manifestations, findings, and management of the cardiotoxicity associated with doxorubicin and other drugs less commonly associated with cardiac effects; 135 references, although many are dated.*

Pellikka PA, Tajik AJ, Khandheria BK, et al.: Carcinoid heart disease. Clinical and echocardiographic spectrum in 74 patients. Circulation 87:1188, 1993. *The most definitive recent description of the echocardiographic, Doppler, and clinical features of carcinoid heart disease.*

Rhoden W, Hasleton P, Brooks N: Anthracyclines and the heart. Br Heart J 70:499, 1993. *A short review article summarizing the pathogenesis, clinical manifestations, prevention, and treatment of anthracycline cardiotoxicity; extensive bibliography.*

Salcedo EE, Cohen GI, White RD, Davidson MB: Cardiac tumors: Diagnosis and management. Curr Probl Cardiol 17:75, 1992. *Reasonably up-to-date review of pathologic, clinical, and management issues of primary and secondary cardiac tumors.*

48 CARDIAC TRANSPLANTATION
Robert C. Bourge

Cardiac transplantation, once considered an experimental procedure, has emerged as the therapy of choice for many appropriately selected patients with life-threatening, irremediable heart disease. Congestive heart failure (CHF), the primary indication for cardiac transplantation, is the most commonly reported reason for hospital admission in the United States Medicare population. A knowledge of cardiac transplantation medicine is therefore important for all physicians, as transplantation should be considered a therapeutic option for many of these patients.

In the past, post–cardiac transplant care was largely performed by specialized transplant physicians, primarily cardiologists and cardiovascular surgeons. As survival after cardiac transplantation markedly improved over the last decade, the population of patients who are long-term survivors after heart transplantation has grown. Primary care physicians, as well as cardiologists not based at cardiac transplant centers, often assist in the care of these patients, most often in consultation with cardiac transplant physicians. In addition, a physician may be called on to assist in the management and evaluation of a potential cardiac donor.

THE CARDIAC TRANSPLANT RECIPIENT

INDICATIONS FOR CARDIAC TRANSPLANTATION. Cardiac transplantation should be limited to those patients who will most benefit from it, with a significant predicted improvement in both quality of life and life expectancy. This is based on the facts that (1) cardiac transplantation is not a surgical "cure" for advanced heart disease, as it commits a patient to both a lifelong complex medical regimen and the need for frequent medical follow-up; (2) the procedure and its postoperative medical regimen result in significant chance of morbidity and mortality; and (3) there is a relative shortage of cardiac donors throughout the world, making each cardiac allograft a precious resource to be used judiciously.

Patients with New York Heart Association (NYHA) class IV CHF or symptoms at rest despite optimal medication therapy have < 50% 1-year survival and therefore should be considered for transplantation. This includes patients who are dependent on intravenous inotropic support or mechanical cardiac support or have undergone mechanical cardiac replacement. Patients with NYHA class III heart failure have 1-year survival rates of 30 to 70% and therefore should also be evaluated for cardiac transplantation. Patients with NYHA class II symptoms may benefit from evaluation and subsequent transplantation if other concomitant cardiac conditions, such as malignant ventricular arrhythmias, adversely affect predicted survival.

The most common underlying disease leading to cardiac transplantation in the United States is ischemic heart disease (IHD). Owing to the often unstable and rapidly changing nature of this disease, an estimation of projected mortality may be difficult. Most large studies have shown that patients with CHF secondary to IHD have a higher mortality than those with nonischemic causes. Evidence of ischemic myocardium despite maximum tolerated medical therapy, either symptomatic (refractory angina) or detected by noninvasive studies (such as thallium scintigraphy), which is not amenable to revascularization is predictive of a poor prognosis. Patients with sustained ventricular tachycardia refractory to all forms of therapy, including the implantable cardioverter-defibrillator (ICD), should be referred for cardiac transplantation.

In the United States, the second most common disease leading to cardiac transplantation is idiopathic dilated cardiomyopathy. In most patients with severe left ventricular dysfunction, factors that correlate with a high mortality should be considered, especially if symptoms are "borderline" in severity. These factors include (1) a very low peak oxygen consumption on an exercise gas exchange study (< 11 to 14 ml per kilogram per minute); (2) a low plasma sodium, especially after intensive medical management; (3) high right ventricular and/or left ventricular filling pressures (a very high right atrial or jugular venous pressure and/or pulmonary capillary wedge pressure), especially after medical management; (4) a very low ejection fraction (< 15 to 20%, not predictive alone however); (5) complex ventricular arrhythmias; (6) a very large left ventricular cavity (end-diastolic maximal dimension > 70 to 75 mm); and (7) the need for recurrent hospitalizations to treat worsening symptoms despite maximum medical therapy. In addition to IHD and dilated cardiomyopathies, other cardiac diseases may be treated with cardiac transplantation. These include sarcoidosis (especially if limited to the heart), restrictive cardiomyopathy, hypertrophic cardiomyopathy, congenital heart disease (not amenable to surgical palliation or correction), and valvular heart disease (when the risk of cardiac surgery is prohibitively high).

EVALUATION FOR CARDIAC TRANSPLANTATION.
Evaluation of Underlying Disease and Estimation of Risk of Mortality. The evaluation for cardiac transplantation should, in general, be performed at an experienced cardiac transplantation center. This evaluation typically involves an attempt at identifying the underlying cardiac disease (if not already established), considering other acceptable (or preferable) treatment options, evaluating the patient for other comorbid conditions that may limit survival or increase morbidity after transplantation, and educating the patient (and family) regarding the rigors of the *post-transplant* medical regimen. Table 48–1 lists studies typically performed during a cardiac transplantation evaluation.

A comprehensive evaluation for the underlying cardiac condition leading to CHF is important both in terms of considering other treatment options and in terms of refining an estimation of mortality. This evaluation most importantly includes a complete history and physical examination, which may help to direct further tests (see Ch. 34).

The transplantation evaluation includes an assessment of the immunologic state of the potential recipient. Typically, a panel (or percentage) reactive antibody (PRA) study is performed to assess the presence or absence of pre-existing antibodies to other (non-"self") human leukocyte antigens (HLA) (Table 48–1). A high PRA (a higher percentage of the panel that is positive) predicts a higher likelihood of post-transplant rejection and death. Patients with a high PRA require a negative crossmatch between their sera and a potential donor's lymphocytes before transplantation. An appropriate donor may be impossible to locate depending on the specificity of the antibodies to more common HLA types. A very high PRA may preclude transplantation.

Evaluation for Comorbid Conditions. Many other coexisting medical conditions are relative contraindications to transplantation and should be considered in reference to predicted survival with and without transplantation. Table 48–2 lists conditions that could affect morbidity or mortality following transplantation.

An evaluation of social and financial resources is very important during the transplantation evaluation. The charges for the initial cardiac transplantation hospitalization in the United States averaged approximately $90,000 in 1987. The cost of follow-up procedures is formidable, even if no post-transplant complications occur (see Routine Post-transplant Life below). Charges for follow-up care for the first year (excluding medications) range from $5,000 to $30,000. Medications for the first year after transplantation cost from $6,000 to $20,000. Most insurance carriers and Medicare help defray some of the costs, but the patient's portion may be significant. Therefore, an assessment of an individual patient's need for financial support after transplantation should be performed before transplantation (see Patient and Family Education below and Ch. 4). Noncompliance due to inability to pay for medications is life-threatening.

Patient and Family Education. The decision by an institution to offer cardiac transplantation includes a responsibility to assist in the ongoing medical care of the patient. Although transplantation promises the severely ill cardiac patient a greater likelihood of a longer life and an improved lifestyle, it is not a "cure" for underlying cardiac disease, as it imparts a significant risk of postoperative complications, including death. It is important that the prospective organ recipient understand the individualized risks involved with the decision to proceed with transplantation, including the possible complications that may occur. Both the medical regimen and the potential cost of this regimen should be described in detail.

RECIPIENT MEDICAL CARE: "THE WAITING LIST." Occasionally, a patient is deemed "too well" to be listed for trans-

TABLE 48-1. EVALUATION FOR CARDIAC TRANSPLANTATION

General

Complete history and physical examination

Nutritional status evaluation*

Blood chemistries including liver and renal profiles [bilirubin, SGOT, alkaline phosphatase, BUN, creatinine, calcium, phosphorus, magnesium]

Hematology and coagulation profile [complete blood cell count, differential, platelet count, prothrombin time (or International Normalized Ratio), partial thromboplastin time, fibrinogen]

Urinalysis

    24 hour urine for creatinine clearance (and protein if diabetic or urinalysis positive for protein*)

Nuclear renal scan with measurement of effective renal plasma flow*

Pulmonary function testing with arterial blood gases

Stool for heme ($\times 3$)

Mammography

Prostate-specific antibody (PSA)*

Abdominal ultrasound study (liver, pancreas, gallbladder, kidney, and aorta evaluation)

Social evaluation

Psychiatric evaluation

Neuropsychiatric evaluation (neurocognitive evaluation)*

Dental evaluation

Cardiovascular

Electrocardiogram

Chest x-ray (PA and lateral)

2-dimensional echocardiogram with Doppler study

Exercise test with oxygen consumption (peak VO_2)*

Right heart catheterization with detailed hemodynamic evaluation

Shunt series*

Left heart catheterization with coronary angiography*

Myocardial biopsy*

Radionuclide angiogram (gated blood pool study)*

Nuclear imaging study for myocardial viability (thallium-201 or positron emission tomography)*

Immunology

ABO blood type and antibody screen

Panel reactive antibody (PRA) screen

Human leukocyte antigen (HLA) typing (if to be listed for transplantation)

Infectious disease screening

Serologies for hepatitis A, B, and C; herpes virus, human immunodeficiency virus, cytomegalovirus (CMV), toxoplasmosis, varicella, rubella, Epstein-Barr virus, capsid IgG and IgM antibodies, Lyme titers*, histoplasmosis and coccidioidomycosis complement fixing antibodies*

Venereal disease research laboratory testing and/or fluorescent treponemal antibody test

Urine for CMV and adenovirus cultures*

Throat swab for viral cultures (CMV, adenovirus, herpes simplex virus)*

Urine culture and sensitivity*

Stool for ova and parasites*

PPD (purified protein derivative) skin test with controls (i.e., mumps, dermatophytin, histoplasmosis, and coccidioidomycosis)*

---

* Performed only if appropriate or indicated.

Adapted from Mudge GH, et al.: Twenty-fourth Bethesda Conference: Cardiac transplantation: Recipient guidelines/prioritization. J Am Coll Cardiol 22:21, 1993; and O'Connell JB, et al.: Cardiac Transplantation: Recipient election, donor procurement, and medical follow-up. Circulation 86:1061, 1992.

---

plantation—when the estimated risk of transplantation is higher than the risk of continued medical care (or a surgical intervention). The transplant center and the referring physician(s) continue ongoing assessment of the patient. Most patients should be re-evaluated and risk stratified at intervals of 3 to 12 months until either (1) the underlying cardiac problem improves or resolves, which occasionally occurs; or (2) worsening symptoms or risk factors for death develop, which would prompt the decision to proceed with transplantation.

In the United States, the responsibility for cadaveric donor organ procurement and distribution is contracted to the United Network for Organ Sharing (UNOS). Regionalized organ procurement organizations (OPO's) exist throughout the United States which are members of UNOS. Patients are "listed" for transplantation by being placed on a national computerized list maintained by UNOS. Donor organs are distributed by location of the donor (within an OPO), ABO blood type, size, and occasionally the need for specialized immunologic testing (a crossmatch, see above). Furthermore, organ distribution is made based on (1) the time that a patient has

waited on the list, and (2) a status system, which varies slightly within different regions. Patients are typically listed as follows: *UNOS Status 1:* patients in a hospital intensive care unit receiving inotropic agents and/or mechanical ventricular assistance (these patients have highest priority); *UNOS Status 2:* all other patients active on the computerized list (there are some variations of status 2 in some areas according to clinical variables); or *UNOS Status 7:* temporarily inactive. In mid 1994, almost 3000 patients were awaiting cardiac transplantation. In 1993, approximately 2300 heart transplant operations were performed. Unfortunately 10 to 30% of patients listed die before an appropriate donor is located.

Once the decision is made to list the patient, the goals of ongoing medical care should be to (1) keep the listed patient alive, (2) improve and maintain the patient's functional class and quality of life, and (3) avoid medical complications that could delay or prevent transplantation. Prolonging the survival of patients awaiting transplantation involves risk-stratifying as to risk of dying while waiting for a donor heart. A patient may require adjustments in his/her medical regimen, the implantation of an ICD as a bridge to transplantation, hospitalization for continuous intravenous inotropic agents or electrocardiographic monitoring, intra-aortic balloon counterpulsation to improve or maintain adequate hemodynamic stability, or a ventricular assist device (VAD) to sustain life. Patients are usually followed at a cardiac transplantation center at 4- to 12-week intervals. Patients with left ventricular failure routinely undergo periodic right heart catheterization to re-assess pulmonary arterial resistance and pulmonary arterial pressures. Medication changes are tailored to the individual patient's hemodynamic parameters so that elevated pulmonary arterial pressures and an elevated pulmonary vascular resistance can be avoided. If not corrected, these elevated hemodynamic parameters could preclude transplantation or lead to death soon after transplantation (see Evaluation for Comorbid Conditions above).

THE CARDIAC DONOR

IDENTIFYING AND EVALUATING A CARDIAC DONOR. Vascularized organs such as the heart must be obtained for use while still functioning from donors declared brain dead. Criteria in the United States specify that brain death may be declared only when all brain functions, both cortical and brain stem, have ceased and are considered irreversible (Table 48–3). Even with the Uniform Anatomical Gift Act (Table 48–3), it is estimated that only 10 to 20% of potential cardiac donors are procured in the United States, in large part owing to the failure of medical professionals to pursue organ donation with a brain-dead patient's family. It is crucial to the success of cardiac transplantation that attending physicians understand the importance of organ donation and consider re-

---

TABLE 48-2. CONDITIONS THAT MAY AFFECT MORBIDITY AND MORTALITY AFTER CARDIAC TRANSPLANTATION

* Active severe infection
* Neoplasm (other than excisable carcinoma of the skin)
* Infection with HIV

Severe, irreversible pulmonary arterial hypertension

Coexistent systemic illness with a poor prognosis

Irreversible renal dysfunction

Irreversible hepatic dysfunction

Insulin-dependent diabetes with end-organ damage

Irreversible pulmonary parenchymal disease

Acute pulmonary thromboembolism

Severe peripheral vascular disease

Severe cerebrovascular disease

Active diverticulosis or diverticulitis

Active peptic ulcer disease, especially with recent or recurrent hemorrhage

Myocardial infiltrative and inflammatory diseases

Prior sternotomies

Severe obesity

Severe osteoporosis

Age

Psychosocial instability, substance abuse, or both

---

* Near-absolute contraindications to cardiac transplantation.

Adapted from Mudge GH, Goldstein S, Addonizio LJ, et al.: Twenty fourth Bethesda Conference: Cardiac Transplantation. Recipient guidelines/prioritization. J Am Coll Cardiol 22:21, 1993. (Reproduced by permission from the American College of Cardiology.)

TABLE 48-3. IDENTIFICATION/EVALUATION/MANAGEMENT OF POTENTIAL DONORS FOR CARDIAC TRANSPLANT

Identification
US criteria for irreversible brain death
1. Documentation of persistence over time (often 12 to 24 hours)
2. Documentation of an established cause of brain injury
3. No evidence of hypothermia, drug intoxication, or shock

Uniform Anatomical Gift Act of 1968
A. Persons over age 18 may choose to donate their organs in the event of brain death; often conveniently stated on the back of a driver's license.
B. The decision to donate organs, unless a person has declared to the negative before death, is made by the next of kin.

Evaluation
Past medical history, specifically cardiac
  Risk factors for early ischemic heart disease (diabetes, hypercholesterolemia)
  History or evidence of infection or malignancy
Physical examination
  Thorax examination for chest trauma, effusions, infection, pulmonary edema
  Cardiovascular examination for *any* abnormal findings
    Measure central venous pressure directly
    ECG—examine for pathologic Q waves.
      —may have ST and T wave changes secondary to any CNS event.
  Chest radiograph for evidence of infection, lung congestion, cardiac or vascular abnormalities
  Echocardiogram to assess global and segmental ventricular function and valve function and to exclude structural abnormalities.

Management
May need to place a pulmonary flotation catheter (Swan-Ganz catheter)
Anticipate early transient increase in sympathetic tone, which may result in severe hypertension and tachycardia; control with IV nitroprusside (vasodilator) and esmolol (short-acting β-adrenergic blocker)
If hypovolemia develops, treat by maintaining the central venous pressure at 8 to 12 mm Hg. If needed, administer dopamine to maintain a systolic blood pressure of 100 mg Hg. DO NOT USE prolonged high doses of catecholamines to prevent the possibility of negative effects on post-transplantation heart function thought due to subendocardial ischemia, and decreased blood flow to the donor kidneys and liver.
If present, treat diabetes insipidus by adequate fluid and electrolyte replacement and low-dose, continuous IV vasopressin (dose adjusted to maintain urine output at 100–300 ml/ hr).
  Avoid high-dose or bolus vasopressin to prevent the possibility of deleterious effects on the liver and renal vasculature.

---

ferral of a brain-dead or a recently expired patient to an OPO for consideration for solid organ (heart, kidney, lung, pancreas, intestine) or tissue (heart valve, bone, skin, cornea) donation. The organ procurement specialist from the OPO will assist in both the initial discussions with the family regarding brain death, if the attending desires, or will discuss the concept of organ donation after brain death is declared.

A physician may occasionally be asked to provide a cardiac consultation of a potential cardiac donor. The evaluation should cover elements listed in Table 48–3. In general, any brain-dead patient with adequate heart function is a potential cardiac donor. In practice, donors are usually considered cardiac donors if the age is less than 40 to 50. Older donors are considered under special circumstances, e.g., if a critically ill recipient is near death. In some cases, coronary angiography may be requested if the combination of age and risk factors indicates a relatively high possibility of IHD. Serologic tests are ordered and reviewed by the OPO coordinator to exclude infectious diseases, including human immunodeficiency virus (HIV), hepatis, and other blood- or tissue-borne pathogens. In addition, the OPO coordinator assists in all aspects of the cardiac consultation and handles all necessary consent forms and legalities associated with organ donation and subsequent organ procurement.

DONOR MANAGEMENT. The potential cardiac donor should preferably be managed in an intensive care unit setting by trained OPO personnel. After brain death is declared, the emphasis of medical care shifts to maintaining the function of the organ to be transplanted (Table 48–3). Brain death may be associated with multiple hemodynamic and hormonal problems that may lead to cardiac arrest and the loss of potentially transplantable organs. It is important

to consider the potential negative effects of any intervention on transplantable organs. An early transient increase in sympathetic tone may result in severe hypertension and tachycardia.

THE CARDIAC TRANSPLANTATION

PREOPERATIVE ASSESSMENT. Critically ill patients awaiting cardiac transplantation are usually located in an intensive care unit at the cardiac transplant center. Although such patients may be cared for by other physicians at another medical facility, it is logistically difficult and also dangerous to move a critically ill patient to the transplant center just prior to the transplant operation. A longer donor heart ischemic time (the time that the donor heart is not beating and is stored in cold cardioplegic preservative solution) is associated with a higher risk of death after transplantation. Therefore it is best to keep the ischemic time to a minimum—if possible, to less than 4 hours.

The transplant admission begins with a rapidly performed history and physical examination, chest radiography, and drawing blood for laboratory studies. This assessment is geared to detect occult infection and evaluate the patient's renal function. In patients with established or suspected problems with pulmonary arterial pressures, a pulmonary flotation catheter (Swan-Ganz catheter) may be placed to help control the patient's intraoperative volume status and help in the possible institution of vasodilators early during the procedure. Occasionally, a patient with unstable hemodynamics, especially one with IHD, decompensates when the stress of the upcoming operation is manifested. In these patients, careful sedation and reassurance and occasionally intravenous nitrates or inotropic agents are sometimes required before surgery.

MEDICAL CARE AFTER TRANSPLANTATION

ROUTINE POST-TRANSPLANT FOLLOW-UP. The maximum mortality from two of the most common causes of death following transplant—allograft rejection and infection—occurs during the first days to weeks after transplantation. Hence, the most intense medical scrutiny is in the first 6 to 8 weeks after the operation. During this period, most transplant centers require that the recipient reside within a reasonable distance. During this time patients are evaluated twice weekly as outpatients (Table 48–4). Although the optimal routine biopsy frequency is not known (see Rejection below), endomyocardial biopsies are typically performed once per week for the first 4 to 8 weeks and then at gradually longer intervals. Additionally, serum or whole blood cyclosporine levels are

---

TABLE 48-4. MEDICAL CARE AFTER TRANSPLANTATION

During the first 6 to 8 weeks after operation
Most centers require the recipient to reside within a reasonable distance from the center; many require a family member or friend to remain with the recipient
Patients are seen twice weekly (outpatient)
A directed history and physical is performed at each visit to assess for signs or symptoms of infection, rejection, or graft dysfunction

Weekly Studies	
Chest radiograph	Screens for early infection
ECG	Evaluates allograft conduction system
Echocardiogram	Assesses left ventricular function
Serologic studies	Assesses early liver or kidney dysfunction
Serum or whole blood Cyclosporine levels	To guide dosing
White blood cell counts	Assesses response; screens for overtreatment with azathioprine

Early postoperative period and first few weeks after transplant

Lifestyle changes	Directed exercise program
	Proper nutrition

After third to sixth month, every 3 months for 1 to 2 years
Repeat examination
Endomyocardial biopsy
ECG
Hematology profile
Renal function studies
Liver enzymes

After 2 years
Mid-year evaluation as in every 3-month evaluation above
Yearly examination at transplant center
  Examination and testing as in every 3-month evaluation above
  Screen for cardiac allograft vasculopathy with coronary angiography
  Possible coronary artery intravascular ultrasound study

drawn to guide dosing (see below). White blood cell counts are performed to assess response and screen for overtreatment with azathioprine (Imuran).

After the first 3 to 6 months, barring any significant complications, patients are usually followed every 3 months for the first 1 to 2 years. At these visits patients have a repeat examination, endomyocardial biopsy, electrocardiography, hematology profile, renal function studies, and liver enzymes. Follow-up after this is adjusted to an individual patient's rejection history and other concomitant medical problems.

Routine Immunosuppression. Immunosuppression for the cardiac transplant recipient begins with the preoperative administration of azathioprine and often cyclosporine. Intraoperative corticosteroids are often given and continued intravenously in the immediate postoperative period. Cyclosporine and azathioprine are started soon after surgery and may be given intravenously until oral medications are tolerated. Although controversial, the use of anti–T cell monoclonal antibodies (OKT3) or polyclonal antibodies (ATGAM, RATG) as *induction therapy* remains the practice at many transplant centers. Such cytolytic preparations are used for the first 5 to 14 days postoperatively to delay the onset of rejection and allow the use of lower doses of cyclosporine early after transplantation. Induction therapy is associated with a significant incidence of immediate side effects (such as vasodilation and hypotension, fever, and chills) and repeated use of such preparations may increase the risk of post-transplant lymphoproliferative disease (see below).

Routine chronic immunosuppression for most patients consists of *triple-drug therapy,* which includes prednisone, azathioprine, and cyclosporine. Because the risk of rejection is highest soon after transplantation, doses and target serum levels of cyclosporine are higher during this period. However, the use of higher dosages of cyclosporine, especially in the immediate postoperative period, may induce renal insufficiency, especially in patients with preoperative renal dysfunction, relative hypovolemia, or a marginal cardiac output. Doses of cyclosporine are subsequently tapered over 1 to 3 months to maintenance doses adequate to maintain target cyclosporine levels (the specific target level depends on the cyclosporine assay and the transplant center). Cyclosporine use is associated with many potential side effects and drug interactions (see Medication-Related Medical Problems below).

Corticosteroids affect nearly all immune responses by inhibiting gene transcription for the production of cytokines. *Prednisone* (initial dose of 1.0 mg per kilogram per day) is tapered over 4 to 8 weeks to maintenance doses of 0.1 to 0.2 mg per kilogram on alternating days. Prednisone dosing is kept as low as possible to minimize potential complications, although some patients require higher maintenance doses to remain free of rejection.

Azathioprine (Imuran) is metabolized in the liver to 6-mercaptopurine, an antimetabolite that inhibits purine synthesis and cell proliferation. Although it may affect all dividing cells, it does have some selective anti–T cell activity. Dosing is usually 1.5 to 5 mg per kilogram per day as a single dose, usually in the evening. Dosing is adjusted to changes in patient weight, degree of bone marrow suppression, and any underlying liver dysfunction. Rarely leukopenia, anemia, and thrombocytopenia may be severe. In general, the azathioprine dose is lowered if the white blood cell count falls consistently below 4,000 to 5000 cells per milliliter.

Prophylactic Drug Administration/Immunizations. In addition to routine immunosuppressive agents and drugs given to treat other common post-transplant medical conditions, such as hypertension and diabetes mellitus, a number of agents are administered prophylactically in an attempt to lower medical complication rates following transplantation (Table 48–5).

Immunosuppressed patients should not receive certain live viral vaccines (see Ch. 10), such as Sabin oral polio vaccine or MMR (mumps, measles, rubella). Sabin oral polio vaccine should not be given to close contacts of transplant patients, as viral shedding does occur. Contacts may receive MMR immunization, as transmission of these attenuated viruses does not occur. Diphtheria, pertussis, tetanus, Salk polio, pneumococcus, and *Haemophilus influenzae* vaccines can be given safely; however, the immune response generated by the transplant recipient may be suboptimal. Routine use of influenza vaccine, while controversial, is of little risk and may offer some protection against epidemic influenza outbreaks.

POST-TRANSPLANT MEDICAL PROBLEMS. *Allograft Rejection.* Incidence. Cardiac allograft rejection is the result of

TABLE 48–5. PROPHYLACTIC DRUG ADMINISTRATION/IMMUNIZATIONS

Prophylaxis Against	Drug
Oral *Candida* infections (thrush)	Oral daily clotrimazole or nystatin
Herpes zoster (shingles)	Oral acyclovir (Zovirax), 200 mg tid
Cytomegalovirus (CMV)	IV ganciclovir (Cytovene)*
Pneumocystis carinii	Oral trimethoprim-sulfamethoxazole (Bactrim, Septra) three times per week OR pentamidine (NebuPent), 300 mg inhaled once per month
Toxoplasma gondii	Pyrimethamine and sulfadiazine (or clindamycin in sulfa-allergic patients)

* Intravenous ganciclovir used primarily in recipients with negative CMV serologies who receive a heart from a CMV serology-positive donor.

the recipient's immune system attempting to rid the body of foreign alloantigenic tissue. Cardiac rejection may be cell mediated (cellular rejection), the most common form, or antibody mediated (humoral rejection), which is probably less common but may be potentially more dangerous. The International Society of Heart and Lung Transplantation (ISHLT) has established a standardized nomenclature for the pathologic grading of acute rejection. A mononuclear infiltrate is the hallmark of early cellular rejection. Higher grades of rejection are classified according to the presence and extent of myocyte infiltration, myocyte necrosis, hemorrhage, and/or vasculitis (Table 48–6). The incidence of cardiac rejection is highest early after transplantation and then subsequently decreases to a low but constant rate, as illustrated in Figure 48–1.

Detection. Symptoms associated with rejection are nonspecific and include malaise, lethargy, fatigue, low-grade fever, and mood changes. If the rejection is associated with diastolic or systolic cardiac dysfunction, then symptoms such as dyspnea may occur. In

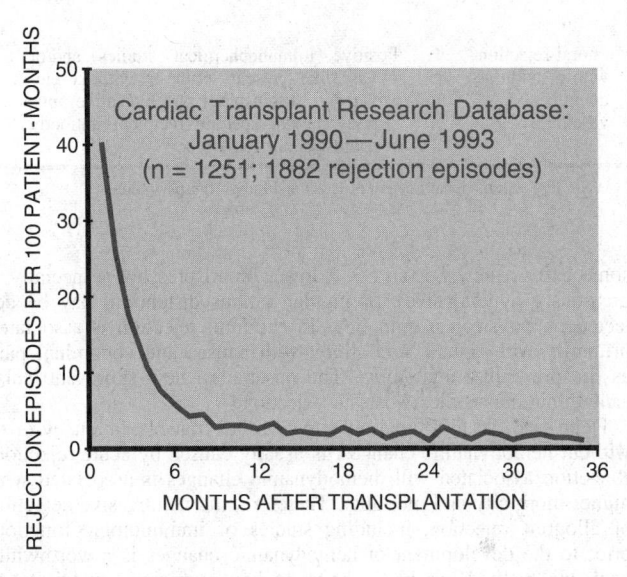

FIGURE 48–1. Rejection incidence over time following initial cardiac transplantation for 1251 patients with follow-up of at least 12 months. The incidence of rejection episodes, calculated as the number per 100 patients followed occurring each month after transplant, is highest in the first month following transplantation (41 rejections per 100 patient-months) and then rapidly declines over time. The average rejection rate after the first year following transplantation is 1.8 rejections per 100 patient-months. (Data from the Cardiac Transplant Research Database population as described in Kubo SH, Naftel DC, Mills RM, et al.: Risk factors for late recurrent rejection after cardiac transplantation: A multi-institutional, multivariable analysis. J Heart Lung Transplant, 14:409, 1995.) (The author would like to thank David C. Naftel, Ph.D., for his assistance with data analysis and preparation of the figures.)

TABLE 48–6. A GENERAL MANAGEMENT PROTOCOL FOR THERAPY OF ACUTE OR PERSISTENT CARDIAC ALLOGRAFT REJECTION

ISHLT* Biopsy Score	Biopsy Description; Other Studies	Therapy
0	No rejection	None
1A Acute cellular rejection	Focal (perivascular or interstitial) infiltrate without necrosis	None (treated as per 1B at some institutions)
1B	Diffuse but sparse infiltrate without necrosis	*< 3 months post transplant:* Oral prednisone bolus, 1.5 mg/kg/day for 3 days, then rapid taper to baseline; re-biopsy in 1 week *> 3 months post transplant:* No treatment unless persistent, re-biopsy in 2–4 weeks
2	One focus only with aggressive infiltration and/or focal myocyte damage	*< 3 months post transplant:* Intravenous methylprednisolone, 1.5 mg/kg/day for 3 days (maximum 1 gram), then return to baseline steroid dose, re-biopsy in 1 week *> 3 months post transplant:* Oral prednisone, 15 mg/kg/day for 3 days, then rapid taper to baseline prednisone dose; re-biopsy in 1–2 weeks
3A	Multifocal aggressive infiltrates and/or myocyte damage	*< 6 months post transplant:* Intravenous methylprednisolone, 1.5 mg/kg/day for 3 days (maximum 1 gram), then return to baseline steroid dose; re-biopsy in 1 week; if recurrent, augmentation of baseline prednisone dose; re-biopsy in 1 week *> 6 months post transplant:* Oral prednisone, 1.5 mg/kg/day for 3 days, then rapid taper to baseline prednisone dose; re-biopsy in 1 week
3B	Diffuse inflammatory process with necrosis	Intravenous methylprednisolone, 15 mg/kg/day for 3 days (maximum 1 gram); then return to baseline steroid dose; *plus* antilymphocyte therapy (OKT3 or ATGAM) for 5 to 10 days; re-biopsy in 1 week; consider augmentation of baseline immunosuppression (cyclosporine, azathioprine, steroids)
4	Diffuse aggressive polymorphous infiltrate, ± edema, ± hemorrhage, ± vasculitis, with necrosis	Plasmapheresis, once per day for 3 days; *plus* intravenous methylprednisolone, 15 mg/kg/day for 3 days; *plus* antilymphocyte therapy (OKT3 or ATGAM) for 5 to 10 days (dose after plasmapheresis); *plus* augmentation of baseline immunosuppression; re-biopsy in 1 week
Persistent rejection, grade 1B or 2	Biopsy description as in grade 1B or 2 above, present in follow-up biopsy	Intravenous methylprednisolone, 15 mg/kg/day for 3 days (maximum 1 gram), then return to baseline steroid dose; *plus* augmentation of baseline immunosuppression; re-biopsy in 1 week
Persistent rejection, grade 3A or 3B	Biopsy description as in grade 3A or 3B above, present in follow-up biopsy	Intravenous methylprednisolone, 15 mg/kg/day for 3 days (maximum 1 gram), then return to baseline steroid dose; *plus* consider antilymphocyte antibody therapy (OKT3 or ATGAM) for 5 to 10 days; re-biopsy in 1 week; consider augmentation of baseline immunosuppression; consider total lymphoid irradiation, methotrexate, or long-term intermittent photochemotherapy
Hemodynamic compromise, with or without biopsy	Biopsy performed if feasible, not performed if patient unstable	Intravenous methylprednisolone, 15 mg/kg/day for 3 days (maximum 1 gram), then return to baseline steroid dose; *plus* antilymphocyte antibody therapy (OKT3 or ATGAM) for 5 to 14 days; *plus* acute plasmapheresis if hemodynamic compromise is severe; re-biopsy in 3 to 7 days; consider augmentation of baseline immunosuppression; consider total lymphoid irradiation, methotrexate, or photochemotherapy
Humoral rejection with or without documented vasculitis	Positive immunochemical studies and/or vasculitis present; with or without elevated post-transplant panel reactive antibody, and/or specific recipient antibody against donor HLA type	Intravenous methylprednisolone, 15 mg/kg/day for 3 days; *plus* plasmapheresis (1 treatment/day for 3 days); *plus* long-term intermittent photochemotherapy; *plus* chronic cyclophosphamide (stop azathioprine); *plus* augmentation of baseline immunosuppression

* ISHLT = International Society of Heart and Lung Transplantation.

some cases a new S4, an S3, a lower blood pressure (especially if previously hypertensive), or jugular venous distention may be detected on physical examination. In children, rejection is associated primarily with right heart failure, with nausea and abdominal pain as the presenting symptoms. The onset of a new supraventricular arrhythmia may indicate cardiac rejection.

Depressed cardiac function after cardiac transplantation, with or without hemodynamic changes, is usually caused by acute rejection. Rejection associated with hemodynamic changes is associated with higher morbidity and mortality. Therefore, the noninvasive detection of allograft rejection, including studies of immunologic function, prior to the development of hemodynamic changes is a worthwhile goal. No method has been shown to have sufficient sensitivity or specificity to allow it to replace surveillance endomyocardial biopsies, especially within the first 6 months after transplantation.

Therapy. The therapy of acute allograft rejection varies among transplant centers but generally is related to the severity and type of rejection (cellular or humoral), the time from the transplantation operation, and the presence or absence of hemodynamic compromise. The therapy of ISHLT grade 1A (Table 48–6) *acute cellular rejection* at many centers involves augmentation of baseline immunosuppression, although other centers do not specifically treat grade 1A rejection in the absence of hemodynamic changes or changes in left ventricular function on echocardiography. The therapy of ISHLT Grade 1B or 2 rejection is individualized; however, there is general

agreement that ISHLT grade 3A or greater rejection warrants acute therapy. Table 48–6 outlines a reasonable approach to the therapy of acute cardiac allograft rejection. *Hyperacute rejection* is a form of humoral rejection in the immediate postoperative period, due to preformed antibodies to the HLA type of the donor heart present in the recipient. This condition results in sudden severe allograft dysfunction and often death. Plasmapheresis, cyclophosphamide, antilymphocyte therapy, and retransplantation have been used with variable but generally poor survival.

Infection. Infection is the most common cause of death in the first year after transplantation despite the development of more selective immunosuppressive drugs such as cyclosporine. Notwithstanding, only one third of post-transplant patients develop a serious infection (defined as requiring intravenous antibiotics or considered life-threatening and treated with oral antibiotics) during the first year after transplant. Lung and blood-borne infections are most common, accounting for 50% of serious infections. Within the first year after transplant, bacterial infections (see Ch. 269) account for 46%, viral 40% (most are cytomegalovirus) (see Ch. 340), fungal 7% (see Ch. 347), and protozoal (see Ch. 373) 6% of serious infection episodes. The risk of a bacterial infection is highest in the early postoperative period (at 1 week). The risk of a viral infection is highest at 1 to 1.5 months, fungal infection within the first month, and protozoal infection from 2 to 5 months following transplant (Fig. 48–2).

Malignancy. Immunosuppressed transplant recipients of any organ have an estimated risk of developing a malignancy of 1 to 2% per year. The overall risk is 6%, approximately 100 times that of the nontransplant age-controlled population. The risk of malignancy in cardiac transplant patients may be somewhat higher than this owing to the higher baseline immunosuppression than for renal transplant recipients. Solid organ transplant recipients appear to be at higher risk than the general population for squamous cell carcinoma of the skin, lymphoma, Kaposi's sarcoma, other sarcomas, carcinoma of the vulva and perineum and of the kidney, and hepatobiliary tumors.

Medication-Related Problems. **Cyclosporine-Related Problems.** The use of cyclosporine has both improved survival after transplantation and created a host of drug-related medical problems and complications. Cyclosporine-induced *hypertension* occurs in >90% of heart transplant recipients within the first year. Drug dosing should allow for diurnal blood pressure changes with dosing timed to have a peak effect in the morning. To control blood pressure, vasodilators (direct and calcium entry blocking drugs) and angiotensin-converting enzyme (ACE) inhibitors are equally effective. β-Adrenergic blocking drugs should be avoided because the denervated heart relies on circulating catecholamines to increase heart rate and systolic function with exercise.

Cyclosporine *renal toxicity* is a common phenomenon. Cyclosporine decreases glomerular filtration rate and raises the serum creatinine. Acute nephrotoxicity may occur with the first perioperative dose of cyclosporine (see Ch. 76 and 77). This is thought to be secondary to drug-induced renal afferent arteriolar vasoconstriction superimposed on chronic renal hypoperfusion present in patients with a low cardiac output prior to transplantation. In addition, there is evidence for some direct dose-dependent toxic effects of cyclosporine on the renal tubules. Cilastatin (present in intravenous imipenem) may ameliorate early cyclosporine toxicity, probably by affecting renal tubular function.

Renal tubular acidosis may occur secondary to cyclosporine use. If severe, treatment with oral bicarbonate preparations may avoid the long-term complications of chronic metabolic acidosis. Cyclosporine is also rarely associated with the *hemolytic-uremic syndrome.*

Hepatic dysfunction following transplantation may be due to many causes, including intraoperative or perioperative hepatic hypoperfusion, cyclosporine, azathioprine, or viral hepatitis. It occurs in up to 10% of patients. Cyclosporine-induced hepatotoxicity is dose-dependent and usually occurs when serum levels are extremely high. Cyclosporine decreases urate clearance by the kidney; *hyperuricemia and gout* commonly occur. Acute gouty arthritis may be difficult to treat owing to the additive nephrotoxicity of nonsteroidal anti-inflammatory drugs and the increased immunosuppression, diarrhea, and bone marrow toxicity associated with colchicine use (especially if there is underlying renal insufficiency). Single-dose intravenous colchicine may be very useful. Allopurinol use is associated with a decrease in azathioprine metabolism.

Table 48–7 illustrates cyclosporine *drug interactions* and *additive toxicities* associated with various drugs according to mechanisms of action. These interactions should always be considered carefully when prescribing these drugs in combination with cyclosporine.

Corticosteroid-Related Problems (see Ch. 12). Corticosteroid use after transplantation may result in or worsen *glucose intolerance.* Corticosteroids often increase appetite, making transplant recipients who were obese prior to transplantation more obese following transplantation. An ongoing program of dietary education and a structured exercise program may help to prevent this problem. *Hyperlipidemia* occurs or worsens in the majority of transplant recipients, largely due to corticosteroid use and obesity.

Corticosteroids, especially in high doses early after transplantation, may precipitate *osteoporosis* and its complications, increasing bone resorption and decreasing bone formation. Patients at most risk are older patients and postmenopausal women. Calcium supplementation, vitamin D, and, in postmenopausal women, estrogen therapy, are used as preventive measures with varied success.

Azathioprine-Related Problems. The most common adverse effects associated with azathioprine use are secondary to bone marrow toxicity—most commonly *leukopenia* and less commonly thrombocytopenia, megaloblastic anemia, red cell aplasia, and reticulocytopenia. Suppression of these myeloid elements usually appears 7 to 14 days after initial dosing or elevations in dosing.

Drug Effects on the Cardiac Allograft. In addition to the many drug interactions associated with the routine pharmacologic therapy of the cardiac transplant recipient, the denervated cardiac allograft results in certain differences in response to medications. Although postganglionic parasympathetic neurons remain in the donor heart, transplanted hearts are effectively *denervated* because conduction does not traverse the atrial anastomotic suture lines. Any drug that affects the heart via either a change in vagal tone or a direct increase in sympathetic nerve activity has little effect on the transplanted heart. However, systemic effects still occur. Thus, for example, atropine, which increases heart rate primarily by a vagolytic effect, does not increase the heart rate in cardiac allograft recipients. However, it still affects peripheral vasodilation, the eyes, and mucous membranes.

The denervated heart is, however, more sensitive to both β-adrenergic agonists such as isoproterenol and to β-adrenergic antagonists. Ocular β blockers can occasionally cause profound bradycardia. Isoproterenol, by virtue of its chronotropic effect, is used routinely to stimulate heart rate in cases of sinus node dysfunction early after transplantation. The denervated heart is especially *hypersensitive to adenosine;* therefore, extreme care should be used to avoid bradycardia or ventricular asystole if the drug is used during vasodilator diagnostic cardiovascular nuclear imaging studies or to convert or slow supraventricular arrhythmias. A starting dose of adenosine to attempt to convert supraventricular tachycardia is 25% of the usual administered dose.

Cardiac Allograft Vasculopathy. Cardiac allograft vasculopathy (CAV) is a vascular disease that affects all vessels in the transplanted heart (including veins) and leads to vessel lumen obliteration. It is the leading cause of death after the first year of transplantation. Depending on the means used to detect it, the incidence of the disease ranges from 10 to 50% at 1 year to 50 to 90% at 5 years after transplantation. Despite changes in immunosuppression, there appears to be no change in the incidence of the disease in the last two decades. Histologically, the disease manifests as hyperplasia of smooth muscle cells, intimal proliferation, mononuclear cell infiltration of the intima, and the presence of lipid-laden macrophages in all areas of the vessel wall. These pathologic changes are usually concentric. The process is thought to be multi-

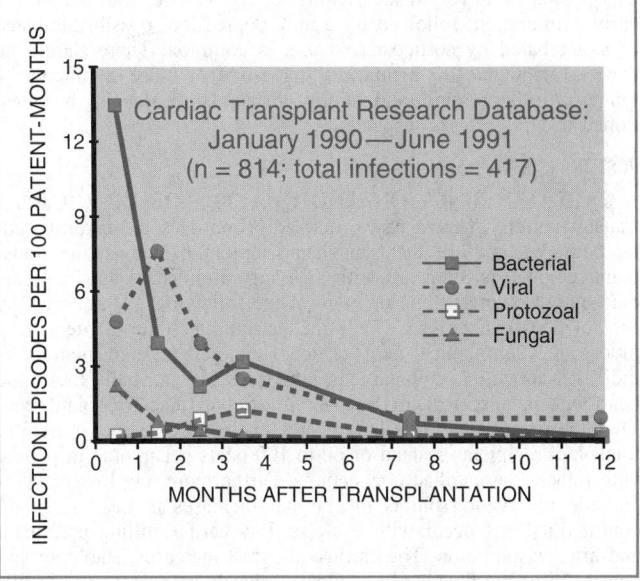

FIGURE 48–2. Incidence of the four major types of severe infections—bacterial, viral, protozoal, and fungal—during the first year after cardiac transplantation. A severe infection was defined as one requiring intravenous antibiotics or one considered life-threatening. Bacterial and fungal infections peak during the first month, viral infections during the second month, and protozoal infections during the fourth month. (Data from the Cardiac Transplant Research Database population described in Miller LW, Naftel DC, Bourge RC, et al.: Infection after heart transplantation: A multi-institutional study. J Heart Lung Transplant 13:381, 1994.)

TABLE 48-7. CYCLOSPORINE DRUG INTERACTIONS

Increase cyclosporine levels by inhibition of hepatic cytochrome P-450

cimetidine (*mild effect*)
diltiazem (*moderate effect*)
erythromycin (*marked effect*)
fluconazole (*moderate effect*)
ketoconazole (*marked effect*)
itraconazole (*moderate effect*)
metoclopramide (*mild effect*)
nicardipine (*mild to moderate effect*)
verapamil (*mild to moderate effect*)
oral contraceptive drugs (*mild effect*)

Increase cyclosporine levels by increased rate and extent of absorption

metoclopramide (*mild effect*)
erythromycin (*mild effect*)

Decrease cyclosporine levels by induction of hepatic cytochrome P-450 enzyme system

carbamazepine (*marked effect*)
ethambutol (*moderate to marked effect*)
ethanol (*varied dose dependent effect*)
glutethimide
isoniazid (*mild effect*)
nafcillin (*moderate effect*)
phenobarbital (*marked effect*)
phenytoin (*marked effect*)
primidone (*moderate effect*)
rifampin (*moderate to marked effect*)
sulfamethoxazole (*mild effect*)

Decrease cyclosporine levels by decreasing bioavailability

cholestyramine
octreotide (decrease pancreatic secretion)

Additive renal toxicity

acetazolamide
amphotericin B
aminoglycoside antibiotics
cephradine
cefotaxime
cefuroxime
ciprofloxacin
fluoroquinolone antibiotics
nonsteroidal anti-inflammatory drugs
melphalan
trimethoprim-sulfamethoxazole

Lessens cyclosporine renal toxicity

cilastatin (alters renal tubular cell function; limited data available)

Increased effect or level of other drug

prednisone, methylprednisolone (cyclosporine inhibits metabolism, results in greater effect)
probucol, lovastatin; (3-hydroxy-3-methylglutaryl coenzyme A reductase inhibitors) (cyclosporine increases drug levels; higher incidence of myositis and rhabdomyolysis with possible renal failure; drugs may be used with low initial dosing)

Drugs that interact with the alcohol carrier in oral cyclosporine with disulfiram-like reaction (flushing, tachycardia, nausea, dyspnea)

disulfiram
metronidazole
chlorpropamide
cefamandole

---

factorial in origin but probably stems from an initial and/or an ongoing immunologically mediated or possibly infection-induced (cytomegalovirus) injury to the vascular endothelium.

Social and Psychological Problems. Adapting to cardiac transplant life involves an interplay of many variables, including the patient's pretransplant condition including the duration of illness, the patient's personality, intelligence, social support, and financial support. It is common for end-stage cardiac patients to become depressed about their condition. Acknowledging the need for cardiac transplantation is very disheartening for some. After transplantation, early exhilaration, followed by a mild depression, possibly induced or exacerbated by corticosteroid use, is common. There should be constant vigilance for symptoms suggestive of more significant or longer-term depression, and family or friends should also be questioned if depression is suspected.

POST-TRANSPLANT LIFE

CARDIAC FUNCTION AND QUALITY OF LIFE. Cardiac transplantation, in most cases, markedly improves the cardiovascular hemodynamics of the transplant recipient. However, the transplant recipient is often left with a slightly diminished maximal cardiac output owing to one or more of the following: (1) denervation (neural decentralization), (2) limited atrial function, (3) decreased myocardial compliance, and (4) donor-recipient size mismatch. As indicated above, parasympathetic influences that normally lower the heart rate in normal hearts are absent after cardiac transplantation. Thus the resting heart rate is typically 95 to 115 beats per minute in transplant recipients instead of 60 to 100 beats per minute in people with intact neurocardiac connections. Furthermore, the loss of sympathetic innervation blunts the normal increases in heart rate and contractility that occur with exercise, low cardiac filling pressures, and after vasodilation. The cardiac allograft increases heart rate and contractility, and thus cardiac output primarily by an increase in filling pressure and secondarily by means of the effects of circulating catecholamines. As the transplanted heart is in some ways dependent on these effects, β-adrenergic receptor antagonists should be used with caution in this population (see above). In transplant recipients, the native and donor atria do not contract in unison, further decreasing the atrial component of ventricular filling.

Immediately after transplantation, the cardiac allograft exhibits compliance abnormalities as evidenced by a restrictive hemody-

namic pattern. This usually gradually improves over a few days to weeks. From 10 to 15% of transplant recipients develop a chronic restrictive hemodynamic pattern with marked volume dependence to maintain adequate cardiac output, despite a normal ejection fraction. Some patients may develop this as a response to acute cardiac rejection episodes, whereas in others the cause is not clear. An undersized heart may also create a situation of volume-dependent hemodynamics and a higher resting heart rate.

In a recent study, 80 to 85% of patients were found to be physically active after cardiac transplantation. Preoperative psychological problems and personality problems do influence quality of life and survival after transplantation. These problems may worsen with the stresses and uncertainties of post–cardiac transplant life and therefore negatively influence perceived quality of life. One important measure of quality of life is financial stability. In the National Transplantation Study, only 33 to 50% of patients were employed. Barriers to employment primarily involve employer fears regarding cardiac transplant recipient reliability and the costs of ongoing health care in these patients. These barriers, the need to maintain government-sponsored health coverage due to disability, and in some patients physical limitations preclude gainful employment in many cardiac transplant recipients.

SURVIVAL. Cardiac transplantation is associated with both an early risk of mortality and morbidity and then a subsequent ongoing risk of death. Data from the Cardiac Transplant Research Database reveals that in major North American cardiac transplant centers from 1990 to 1993, survival at 1 year for 1719 recipients of their first allograft was 85%, and 2-year survival was 83%. It is estimated that, in the current era of immunosuppression, 5-year survival for the average recipient will be approximately 75 to 80% at major US cardiac transplant centers.

HEART-LUNG TRANSPLANTATION (see Ch. 66)

Combined heart and lung transplantation (HLT) involves the transplantation of the heart and lung block from a donor to an appropriate recipient in a single operation. In a recipient with normal right atrium and aortic anatomy, HLT has been described as, in some ways, a technically easier procedure than heart transplantation because it involves only right atrial, aortic, and tracheal anastomoses. It is estimated that <20% of heart donors are potential heart-lung donors. The primary indications for HLT proposed by the

American College of Cardiology are (1) patients with congenital cardiac abnormalities and severe pulmonary hypertension (Eisenmenger's complex), (2) patients with irremediable primary lung disease and associated severe secondary right ventricular failure, and (3) patients with primary end-stage cardiac disease and secondary irreversible pulmonary arterial hypertension that would preclude isolated cardiac transplantation.

Baumgartner C, Reitz BA, Achuff SC: Heart and Heart-Lung Transplantation. Philadelphia, WB Saunders, 1990. *An excellent text with chapters on all areas of heart and heart-lung transplantation. Provides moderate to extensive detail on most areas, including surgical techniques.*

Billingham ME, Cary NR, Hammond ME, et al.: A working formulation for the standardization of nomenclature in the diagnosis of heart and lung rejection: Heart Rejection Study Group. J Heart Transplant 9:587, 1990. *The standardized nomenclature and pathologic description of the degree of allograft rejection from myocardial biopsy specimen.*

Bourge RC, Naftel DC, Costanzo-Nordin M, et al.: Pre-transplant risk factors for death after cardiac transplantation: A multi-institutional study. J Heart Lung Transplant 12:549, 1993. *The first large-scale multi-institutional risk factor analysis evaluating pretransplant variables and their relationship to post-transplantation survival, from the group now referred to as the Cardiac Transplant Research Database Group.*

Hunt SA (Conference Chairman), 24th Bethesda Conference: Cardiac transplantation. J Am Coll Cardiol 22:11, 1993. *A comprehensive and well-referenced state-of-the-art overview covering the current status of cardiac transplantation and containing recommendations for future directions in research and policy.*

Hosenpud JD, Shipley GD, Wagner CR: Cardiac allograft vasculopathy: Current concepts, recent developments, and future directions. J Heart Lung Transplant 11:9, 1992. *A well-written and well-referenced review describing different proposed causes, pathology, clinical course, and possible therapies.*

Loop FD (Guest ed.): Mechanical circulatory support. Semin Thorac Cardiovasc Surg 6:129, 1994. *A series of 12 papers reviewing the topic by various authors. Excellent illustrations of the various mechanical support devices used as a bridge to transplantation.*

O'Connell JB, Bourge RC, Costanzo-Nordin MR, et al.: Cardiac transplantation: Recipient selection, donor procurement, and medical follow-up. Circulation 86:1061, 1992. *An excellent overview of indications and contraindications for cardiac transplantation, donor-related matters, and post-transplant care.*

United States General Accounting Office Report: Heart Transplants, Concerns About Cost, Access, and Availability of Donor Organs, May 1989, GAO/HRD-89-61. *A general review of the topic with specific cost data from multiple transplant centers.*

Young JB, Naftel DC, Bourge RC, et al.: Matching the heart donor and cardiac transplant recipient: Clues for successful expansion of the donor pool, a multivariable, multi-institutional report. J Heart Lung Transplant 13:353, 1994. *Expands the risk factor analysis for death after transplantation from the CTRD group (Bourge et al., above) to include a larger number of patients with an emphasis on donor-related factors and their influence on survival.*

PART VIII

RESPIRATORY DISEASES

49 APPROACH TO THE PATIENT WITH RESPIRATORY DISEASE

Gerard M. Turino

The respiratory system is subject to a number of diseases which are primary to that organ system but also reflects disease in other organs. The process of respiration includes many structural and functional components (see Ch. 50) in addition to the lungs, such as the nose, pharynx, sinuses, chest cage and musculature, pleura, diaphragms, extrathoracic airways, cerebral regulatory respiratory centers, and cardiovascular system. Thus, in addressing the patient with pulmonary disease, the physician must maintain a circumspect approach to possible pathogenic factors. Pulmonary infiltrates on chest film may be manifesting a pulmonary infection or primary lung tumor but also may be the result of metastatic cancer from extrapulmonary sites. Pulmonary densities of various types on chest film may be manifesting more generalized systemic diseases such as lupus erythematosus (see Ch. 240), scleroderma (see Ch. 241), rheumatoid arthritis (see Ch. 237), or embolic disease (see Ch. 59). Abnormal blood gas composition may result from defective regulation of ventilation rather than intrinsic lung disease.

The function of the lungs contributes vital processes to all other organ systems of the body. Pulmonary O_2 and CO_2 exchange is necessary for body metabolism and contributes to acid-base homeostasis. The circulation of the lungs is interposed between the circulations of the right and left heart and therefore is subject to hemodynamic disturbances originating in the cardiac chambers but may also contribute to circulatory disease by pulmonary hypertension (see Ch. 38). The lungs are the gaseous and particulate interface between the external atmosphere and the body, so lung function must be considered in terms of the hazards of exposure to atmospheric toxins. Also the lungs contain a large variety of cells, about 40, which not only are necessary for the normal respiratory and circulatory functions of the lung but also contribute to extrapulmonary processes such as blood pressure control through the action of angiotensin-converting enzyme, which resides on pulmonary endothelium.

The essential starting point to determine the cause of the symptoms and signs of the patient with disease of the respiratory system is a complete history and physical examination, along with the chest roentgenogram.

HISTORY

A detailed account of the patient's primary symptoms is essential, but other information concerned with the respiratory system must also be elicited: the amount and exposure to tobacco smoke (including passive exposure), and exposure to possible atmospheric pollutants such as nitrogen dioxide, beryllium, asbestos, coal and silica dust (see Ch. 13.3), fumes from industrial processes, and animal danders. If the patient is exposed to a potentially toxic industrial process, precise historical details on the place and duration of occupational exposure are necessary. The family history of lung disease with respect to asthma, allergies, cystic fibrosis (CF), lung cancer,

and emphysema is also important. A family history of emphysema may be present in cases of serum α_1-antitrypsin deficiency. Living in certain regions of the country may predispose to histoplasmosis (see Ch. 348) or coccidioidomycosis (see Ch. 349), as occurs in those living in the southwestern United States.

Infections such as *Pneumocystis carinii* pneumonia, chronic sinusitis, pneumococcal pneumonia, and tuberculosis are recognized common complications of human immunodeficiency virus (HIV) infection (see Part XXII). The history should therefore explore the possibility of exposure to HIV infection such as homosexuality, intravenous substance abuse, promiscuous heterosexuality, and travel to areas of high HIV prevalence.

A history of the medications taken previously and currently is necessary to evaluate certain pulmonary infiltrative lesions such as interstitial pulmonary fibrosis as a complication of therapy with bleomycin, cyclophosphamide, methotrexate, and nitrofurantoin. Bronchospasm may be initiated or exacerbated by β-adrenergic blocking drugs. Cough and angioneurotic edema are complications of angiotensin-converting enzyme blocking drugs in a small percentage of patients.

PHYSICAL EXAMINATION

The common physical signs associated with various pulmonary abnormalities are outlined in Table 49–1. In the physical examination, the general body habitus should be noted such as obesity, which affects the mechanics of breathing and predisposes to sleep apnea. The configuration of the thorax should also be noted, such as increased anteroposterior diameter, which may be evidence of pulmonary hyperinflation, or shortening and deformation of the thorax, as occurs in kyphoscoliosis of the spine. Lagging of one side of the chest may be evidence of unilateral fibrothorax or atelectasis. Accessory muscles of ventilation are frequently used in severe airway obstruction.

If there is audible wheezing on ventilation it is essential to distinguish airway obstruction in the tracheobronchial tree from that in the larynx and pharynx. In this regard, extrathoracic airway obstruction in the upper airway is frequently more marked during the inspiratory phase, whereas lower airway obstruction is more marked in the expiratory phase. The presence of nasal voice and/or tenderness over sinus regions of the face can be a manifestation of acute or chronic sinus disease. Full inspection of the nose and pharynx is essential for lesions such as polyps or septal deviations to explain postnasal secretions.

Clubbing of the fingers may be a manifestation of carcinoma of the lung but is frequently present in cystic fibrosis with hypoxemia and severe bronchiectasis, as well as in hypoxemia associated with congenital lesions of the heart.

Physical examination of the heart and cardiovascular system is essential to evaluating the patient with pulmonary disease. Thus a loud pulmonary second sound and a right ventricular heave may be manifestations of pulmonary hypertension, whereas left ventricular enlargement and a gallop sound may be manifestations of poor left ventricular function. Systemic hypertension or arrhythmias may be considered as a basis for high filling pressures of the left ventricle.

CHEST ROENTGENOGRAM, COMPUTED TOMOGRAPHY, AND MAGNETIC RESONANCE IMAGING OF THE THORAX

The chest roentgenogram is essential to the workup. It can indicate diaphragmatic and rib cage abnormalities as well as the air-containing volumes of each lung. It also defines the presence of infiltrates, cavitary lesions, pneumothorax, pleural fluid or pleural

TABLE 49-1. PHYSICAL SIGNS OF PULMONARY DISEASE

Pathogenic Process	Chest Wall Motion and Configuration	Breath Sounds	Percussion	Fremitus
Asthmatic and bronchitic airway obstruction	Increased AP diameter, use of accessory muscles of ventilation	May be decreased; prolonged expiration; inspiratory and expiratory wheezes and rhonchi	Hyperresonant	Decreased
Airway obstruction of emphysema	Increased AP diameter, reduced chest wall musculature with general weight loss, use of accessory muscles of ventilation	Markedly diminished; prolonged expiratory phase; maybe rhonchi	Hyperresonant	Decreased
Atelectasis	Inspiratory lag on affected side	Absent over affected area	Dullness	Decreased
Consolidation of acute pneumonia	Splinting of chest wall on affected side	Bronchial breath sounds, whispered pectoriloquy, rales and/or rhonchi	Dullness	Increased
Pleural effusion	Lag on affected side	Absent or decreased	Flatness	Absent
Pneumothorax	Lag on affected side, tracheal deviation away from affected side	Absent	Hyperresonant	Absent
Diffuse alveolitis or fibrosis	Restricted inspiratory and expiratory excursion	May be increased with diffuse fine rales	Decreased resonance or normal	Increased or normal

thickening, cardiac size and chamber contours, along with pulmonary congestion, pulmonary edema, and enlargement of the pulmonary arteries.

Computed tomography (CT) and magnetic resonance imaging of the thorax have contributed substantially to the finer definition of pulmonary lesions and can yield information not seen on the posteroanterior chest film. These techniques can outline lesions with respect to contours, density, homogeneity, their relationship to bronchi and adjacent vascular structures, and the presence, location, and extent of lymphadenopathy.

EVALUATING BLOOD GAS COMPOSITION AND PULMONARY FUNCTION TESTING

Unless the patient is severely hypoxemic, giving rise to polycythemia and visible cyanosis, significant degrees of hypoxemia can go undetected clinically unless blood gas composition is measured. Similarly, significant degrees of hypercapnia may be present without symptoms of somnolence or headache, which is present when the P_{CO_2} levels are in the higher ranges above 70 mm Hg. Thus, as part of evaluating the patient with pulmonary disease, in many instances an arterial blood gas measurement is essential to rule in or out significant hypoxemia and/or hypercapnia and can be done as single measurements or as part of a complete evaluation of pulmonary function in the laboratory.

Pulmonary function testing, including blood gas measurements during rest and exercise, is essential to fully characterize and quantify pulmonary dysfunction. Simple spirometry can quantify airway obstruction as well as determine the response to bronchodilator therapy. Spirometry may also establish the presence or absence of airway obstruction that also may be essential to the clinical evaluation. Lung volume measurements can establish whether the air-containing volume of the lung is reduced and a restrictive pattern of lung disease is present, as occurs in interstitial alveolitis, sarcoidosis, or fibrosis. The pulmonary diffusing capacity is a sensitive measurement of interstitial reactions of the lung such as interstitial alveolitis and fibrosis (see Ch. 54), when the surface area of the pulmonary capillary membrane is reduced and the thickness of the alveolar capillary membrane is increased. In airway obstructive disease, diffusing capacity can be a method of determining the presence of pulmonary emphysema. A low diffusing capacity indicates alveolar destruction and the presence of emphysema as a primary process or in association with chronic bronchitis or asthma.

Detecting pulmonary hypertension and estimates of pulmonary artery pressure can now be provided by echocardiography. For more thorough evaluation of the hemodynamics of the pulmonary circulation, measurements of pulmonary artery pressure and pulmonary vascular resistance should be obtained by right heart catheterization, in which measurements of cardiac output can be obtained along with pulmonary artery pressure to accurately quantify pulmonary vascular resistance. Also, when indicated, a pulmonary angiogram can be obtained if pulmonary embolism is clinically suspected and the ventilation-perfusion scans are equivocal.

INVASIVE TECHNIQUES IN PULMONARY DIAGNOSIS

In certain conditions such as suspected pulmonary neoplasm or in investigating hemoptysis, fiberoptic bronchoscopy is essential with sampling of bronchial cells by brushing or bronchial biopsy or, where indicated, bronchoalveolar lavage, to determine the cell composition in alveoli. If pleural disease is detected, pleural biopsy, along with evaluating the cellular and protein composition of pleural fluid with respect to exudates or transudates, is necessary. CT-guided needle aspiration of intrapulmonary lesions is most useful. Within the past few years thoracoscopy has been introduced as a technique to evaluate lesions on the pleural surface of the lung by biopsy or local resection.

MAJOR MANIFESTATIONS OF PULMONARY DISEASE

Although a wide array of pathologic factors can produce respiratory symptoms and signs, the four most common manifestations of pulmonary disease which bring patients to the physician are cough, shortness of breath or dyspnea, chest pain, and hemoptysis.

COUGH WITH AND WITHOUT SPUTUM. Cough results from sensory stimuli in the tracheobronchial tree transmitting nervous impulses to the integrative cough centers in the brain. Cough may be a transient symptom or persistent. Usual causes of transient cough are inflammatory reactions of the surface of the trachea or bronchial branches, usually from bacterial or viral infections. Occasionally noxious vapors in the atmosphere can induce cough, e.g., tobacco smoke, volatile chemical compounds, and vehicular exhaust. For persistent cough, one of the most prominent causes is an allergic inflammatory reaction of the bronchi associated with asthma. In this disease, cough may be the earliest presenting manifestation, rather than shortness of breath or wheezing.

Another significant cause of tracheobronchial irritation leading to cough is regurgitation of acidic gastric contents into the tracheobronchial tree during sleep. Such regurgitation and aspiration result from failure of gastric emptying due to gastric outlet obstruction or an incompetent gastroesophageal junction (see Ch. 97). Many individuals regurgitate gastric and esophageal contents during sleep and are totally unaware of this phenomenon.

An important cause of persistent cough is a tumor in the tracheobronchial tree that leads to distortions of the bronchial wall and increases stimuli to the cough center. In any patient with persistent cough as a symptom, and particularly in smokers, the possibility of a bronchial carcinoma or adenoma must be considered. Extrabronchial lesions must also be considered, such as mediastinal or esophageal tumors or aortic aneurysms compressing bronchi, or cardiac chamber enlargement, particularly of the left atrium, compressing the left main bronchus. Sinusitis with persistent nasal secretions into the pharynx and upper airway is a frequent cause of therapy-resistant chronic cough and deserves consideration.

Diagnostic investigations of cough include chest radiography and, if necessary, sinus radiography and CT of the thorax. When indicated, bronchoscopy and laryngoscopy should be done. The presence of sputum—and its type and amount—can be useful in differential diagnosis. Acute onset of sputum with cough suggests acute pulmonary infection or sinusitis. Longstanding sputum production, usually in the morning, is characteristic of chronic bronchitis from smoking. Large volumes of sputum throughout the day are characteristic of bronchiectasis or lung abscess. Foul-smelling sputum is characteristic of anaerobic infection associated with lung abscess. In asthma, sputum production may vary in occurrence and amount throughout the day. Yellow or green sputum is usually a sign of infection. The latter results from the release of myeloperoxidase by leukocytes.

SHORTNESS OF BREATH. "Shortness of breath," "a feeling of not being able to get enough air," and "labored breathing" are all terms used by patients to describe the symptom of dyspnea. The cause of dyspnea may be pulmonary or circulatory disease or, in certain circumstances, both. It is the physician's responsibility to define the causative mechanisms of shortness of breath so that diagnostic techniques and therapies can be directed appropriately. The most consistent correlate of the symptom of dyspnea is increased mechanical work of breathing, usually brought on by increased airway resistance as occurs in asthma, chronic bronchitis, and emphysema, or decreased distensibility of the lungs as occurs in interstitial fibrotic reactions (Fig. 49–1). In the latter diseases increased effort is required to produce a higher negative pressure in the pleural space to inflate the lungs. The increased mechanical work done on the lungs to overcome obstruction to air flow or decreased distensibility is perceived as an effort to breath and produces the symptom of dyspnea.

An increased drive to ventilate may also be a cause of dyspnea. Such stimuli might come from hypoxia, usually when arterial oxygen tensions are <60 mm Hg. Stimuli coming from inflamed lung parenchyma, as occurs in bacterial pneumonia or alveolitis from immunologic reactions of lung parenchyma, also give rise to stimuli to the respiratory centers of the brain which constitute abnormal drives to ventilation. These stimuli often induce abnormally low levels of resting P_{CO_2}, below the normal of 40 mm Hg. Such abnormal drives in the presence of normal or abnormal lung mechanics can give rise to dyspnea, especially on mild exertion.

It is especially important to recognize that patients with pulmonary emboli may present only with shortness of breath. Their chest roentgenograms may be normal and there may be no discernible cause for dyspnea such as airway obstruction, decreased lung distensibility, or low arterial P_{O_2}. However, the inefficiency of the embolized lung for gas exchange requires abnormally high ventilatory rates to maintain a normal arterial P_{CO_2}. Unless this particular presentation of pulmonary embolism is appreciated, many patients with embolic disease go unrecognized until they suddenly die or become extremely compromised with pulmonary hypertension and right heart failure.

Because of the high prevalence of heart disease and congestive heart failure in the general population, most patients coming to physicians with dyspnea are found to be suffering from cardiac abnormalities. The basis of the dyspnea is usually a high filling pressure of the left ventricle, which then causes high left atrial pressures and high pulmonary capillary and pulmonary arterial pressures, which increase the pulmonary blood volume under increased pressure and reduce lung compliance. If the pulmonary capillary pressure is in the range of 25 mm Hg, there will be transudation of capillary fluid into the pulmonary matrix, which additionally reduces lung compliance, causing increased work of breathing and the symptom of dyspnea. The main causes of increased filling pressures of the left ventricle are myocardial ischemia from coronary atherosclerosis, afterload increases from arterial hypertension or stenosis, and regurgitation of the aortic or mitral valves. Echocardiography is diagnostic in detecting abnormal ventricular or valvular function and should be done in any patient in whom the cause of dyspnea is not readily apparent.

CHEST PAIN. Chest pain is also a common presenting symptom of lung disease. One common type of chest pain is pleuritic pain, which is sharp and severe, is magnified by breathing, and may be associated with a pleural friction rub. Pericarditis (see Ch. 44) causes chest pain that may not be related to breathing and often is relieved by leaning forward. Pericardial friction rubs may be audible in synchrony with the heart beat. However, pleuropericardial friction rubs may induce pain related to breathing as well as friction rubs related to cardiac contraction.

The chest pain of myocardial ischemia from coronary artery disease should be discernible on the basis of its relation to physical exertion and by the characteristic of a pressure-type anterior chest pain, often with radiation to the left shoulder or arm or occasionally to the right shoulder and arm, the neck, and the jaw.

The chest pain of pulmonary embolism may also be characterized by a feeling of anterior chest pressure, which may persist for hours and be related to pulmonary hypertension.

HEMOPTYSIS. The fourth symptom is hemoptysis. The most common cause of hemoptysis is pneumonia or pulmonary infection. Blood streaking of purulent sputum occurs during pneumonia or severe bronchitis and subsides as the infection is treated. The sudden appearance of hemoptysis without other cause must be considered a possible manifestation of lung tumor, either benign or malignant.

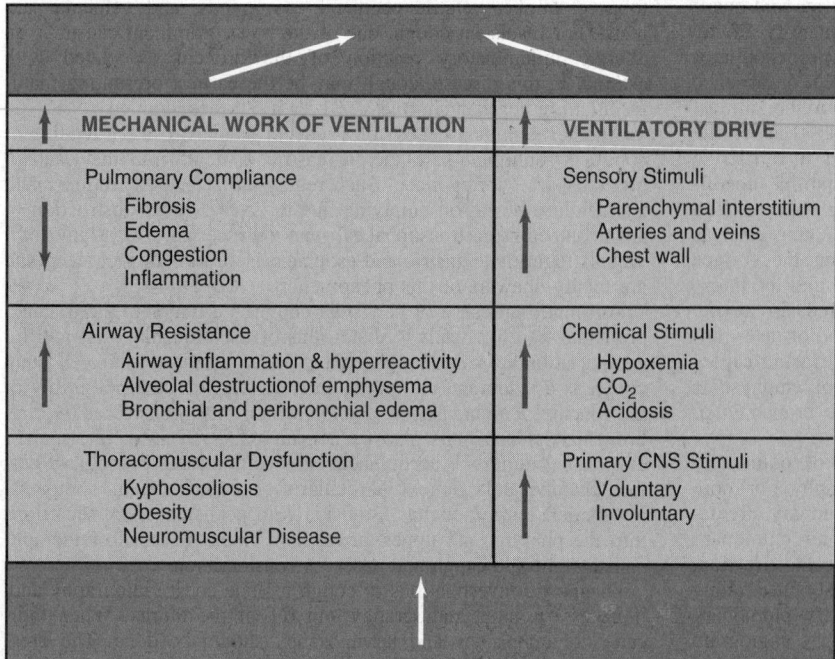

DYSPNEA

MECHANICAL WORK OF VENTILATION	VENTILATORY DRIVE

Pulmonary Compliance
  Fibrosis
  Edema
  Congestion
  Inflammation
	Sensory Stimuli
	  Parenchymal interstitium
	  Arteries and veins
	  Chest wall

Airway Resistance
  Airway inflammation & hyperreactivity
  Alveolal destructionof emphysema
  Bronchial and peribronchial edema
	Chemical Stimuli
	  Hypoxemia
	  CO_2
	  Acidosis

Thoracomuscular Dysfunction
  Kyphoscoliosis
  Obesity
  Neuromuscular Disease
	Primary CNS Stimuli
	  Voluntary
	  Involuntary

VENTILATORY MUSCLE FATIGUE

FIGURE 49–1. The symptom of dyspnea can best be related to increases in the mechanical work of breathing and/or increases in ventilatory drive as a result of the effect of different pathogenic factors on ventilatory mechanics and increased ventilatory stimuli, as shown. Ventilatory muscle fatigue is an added factor (see text).

Such hemoptysis necessitates full investigation diagnostically in terms of chest radiographs, CT scans of the thorax, and bronchoscopy. A pulmonary embolism that leads to pulmonary infarction almost always results in hemoptysis. It is usually associated with a pulmonary infiltration as a manifestation of infarction, which occasionally then excavates to leave a cavity in the lung parenchyma. Bronchiectasis commonly gives rise to hemoptysis. Hemoptysis is not uncommon in cystic fibrosis of the lung and can be severe and even life-threatening. A certain proportion of patients have sudden and usually mild hemoptysis for which no cause can be found. Such episodes of hemoptysis may result from a ruptured blood vessel or varix in the bronchial mucosa. In this regard, clotting parameters should be checked. Bronchopulmonary aspergillosis or an aspergilloma also causes persistent hemoptysis, and the diagnostic workup should investigate this possibility when accompanying manifestations are suggestive. Pulmonary tuberculosis, especially with cavity formation, is a prominent cause of hemoptysis and must constantly remain under diagnostic consideration, especially in patients with HIV infection.

Cooper A, White D, Matthay RA: Drug-induced pulmonary disease. Am Rev Respir Dis 133:321, 1986. *A thorough review of the pathologic responses of the lung to a variety of cytotoxic agents.*

Fishman AP (ed.): Pulmonary Diseases and Disorders. 2nd ed. New York, McGraw-Hill, 1988. *A well-indexed and well-referenced text that considers in depth clinical and pathologic concepts in lung disease.*

Irwin RS, Curley FJ, French CL: Chronic cough: The spectrum and frequency of causes, key components of the evaluation and outcome of specific therapy. Am Rev Respir Dis 141:640, 1990. *A thorough study of the major causes of chronic cough and the methods of evaluation and therapy in 108 patients.*

Loudon RG: The lung exam. Clin Chest Med 8:265, 1987. *A useful and practical guide to physical examination of the lungs.*

Murray JF, Nadel JA (eds.): Textbook of Respiratory Medicine. Philadelphia, WB Saunders, 1988. *A lucid and comprehensive text of respiratory function in relationship to pathophysiologic mechanisms.*

50 RESPIRATORY STRUCTURE AND FUNCTION

James D. Crapo

The primary function of the lung is to enable gas exchange, which facilitates movement of oxygen into the bloodstream and the removal of carbon dioxide (CO_2). In addition, the respiratory system carries out a large number of other ventilatory-related and nonventilatory functions. The complex effects of lung structure on its gas exchange and nonventilatory functions are critical to understanding how the lung responds to both intrapulmonary and systemic diseases.

LUNG STRUCTURE

UPPER AIRWAYS. The nasopharynx plays a critical role in humidifying inhaled gases and in clearing particles and reactive substances contained in those gases. In addition to contributing to the senses of smell and taste, the nasopharynx removes a large fraction of inhaled particles and reactive gases. Turbulent gas flow past the nasal turbinates and the right-angle turn at the posterior pharynx cause impaction of most large particles before inhaled gas enters the trachea. In addition, very highly soluble or reactive gases may be almost completely removed by the nasopharynx. Lymphoid tissue at the posterior pharynx plays a role in immune processing at this critical junction of the body with its external environment.

AIRWAYS. The primary airways consist of the trachea, the bronchi, and smaller bronchioles. The adult human trachea is approximately 25 cm in length and 2.5 cm in diameter and is given a somewhat rigid shape by 15 to 20 horseshoe-shaped cartilaginous rings. The posterior portion of the trachea, representing the membranous portion or open part of the cartilaginous rings, contains the trachealis muscle. The trachea divides into two main-stem bronchi, which then rapidly divide in an irregular dichotomous pattern into progressively smaller bronchi. Cartilaginous support surrounding or partly surrounding bronchi continues for a number of generations, at which point the airways are termed bronchioles. As the size of

the cartilage decreases in smaller bronchi, the relative mass of smooth muscle becomes more prominent and these medium-sized bronchi can be a significant site of bronchoconstriction. Smooth muscle becomes more scarce as it extends into the bronchioles and is virtually absent from terminal bronchioles. The shortest path from the trachea to a terminal bronchiole involves approximately seven divisions and has a total length of 7 to 8 cm. The longest pathway would encounter approximately 25 branch divisions and have a total length of >22 cm. The cross-sectional area of each daughter branch is decreased, but the increasing number of branches leads to an increase in the total cross-sectional area as one moves deeper into the lung. The increase in airway cross-sectional area is nearly exponential and leads to a fall in airway resistance distal to the conducting airways. This means that the primary site of air flow resistance is in the large, central airways. Gas flow rates also slow as the cross-sectional area increases and the flow pattern becomes less turbulent and more laminar. The final airway segments are termed terminal bronchioles, which then branch into two to four respiratory bronchioles (airway segments with alveolar or gas exchange outpockets) before entering alveolar ducts. The terminal bronchioles are approximately 250 μm in internal diameter, do not have smooth muscle, and are covered only with a thin, serous fluid coat. They are not normally a site of significant airway resistance but may become so during a number of disease processes.

The airways and large vessels in the lung make up about 10% of the substance of the lung and account for about 25% of the lung cells. More than 40 different cell types are found in the lungs, representing virtually every major class of tissue. The most common type of cell in the lung is the capillary endothelial cell, which represents almost 40% of the cells in the alveolar gas-exchange region. The epithelial cells lining the airways include ciliated cells, secretory cells, basal cells, and mucous cells, as well as mucus-secreting glands. Under normal conditions the airway epithelium has a low rate of cell turnover, but these cells can potentially be exposed to a variety of inhaled carcinogens and are the site of origin of the most common cancer in humans. The upper airways in the human lung are covered by a thick mucous coat, which can be more than 10 μ thick. The mucous covering of the airways thins as one moves more distally into the lung, becoming a thin serous coat over the terminal airways and leaving this region of the lung most vulnerable to inhaled reactive substances. The small airways, in conjunction with the most proximal portions of the alveolar gas-exchange region, are the primary sites where lung injury is caused by most inhaled substances.

The lungs are divided into three lobes on the right and two on the left and have a normal total of ten segments on the right and eight segments on the left side. A lung lobule is the smallest unit separated by fibrous septa. It is approximately 2 cm in size and contains about four to eight terminal bronchioles.

ALVEOLAR REGION. The alveolar region is a branching system of alveolar ducts whose walls are made up of alveoli. The number of alveolar duct branches ranges from 3 to 13, ending in alveolar sacs whose walls are composed of alveolar outpockets. The human lung contains about 500 million alveoli that are each roughly spherical and about 225 μm in diameter. The mouths of the alveoli, which form the walls of alveolar ducts and alveolar sacs, contain large collagen and elastin bundles, while adjacent alveoli are interconnected by collagen fibers laced through the alveolar walls. The connective tissue bundles lining alveolar duct walls are arranged in a spiral or helical fashion and are critical in determining the overall structure and compliance of the gas-exchange region (Fig. 50–1).

Gas exchange occurs across alveolar walls that have a high vascular content, with the surface area of subadjacent capillaries virtually matching that of the alveolar surface (Fig. 50–2). Capillary blood is separated from air by a fine tissue sheet whose thickness can be as little as 0.5 μm. An oxygen (O_2) molecule penetrating an alveolar wall to reach a red cell must traverse, at the least, a highly attenuated epithelial cell, basement membrane, and a highly attenuated endothelial cell that make up the tissue barrier and, after entering the capillary, cross the plasma, penetrate the red cell, and bind to hemoglobin. The efficient function of the lung as a gas-exchange surface depends upon a thin air-blood barrier, a small tissue resistance to diffusion of O_2 and CO_2 molecules, a large alveolar surface

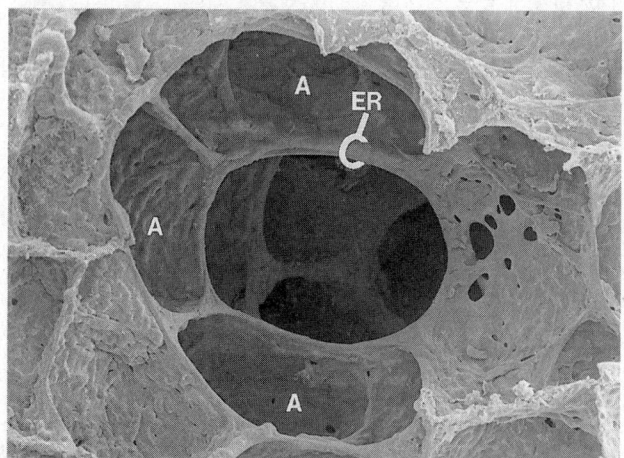

FIGURE 50–1. Scanning electron micrograph of human lung showing an alveolar duct with concentrically arranged alveoli (A). The free edge of an alveolar septum is reinforced with thick bundles of connective tissue that form the entrance rings (ER). X 380. (From Gehr P, Bachofen M, Weibel ER: The normal human lung: Ultrastructure and morphometric estimation of diffusing capacity. Respir Physiol 178:112, 1978.)

for gas exchange, and a relatively large capillary blood volume uniformly distributed below the alveolar surface. In a normal human the total surface area of the alveolar region of the lung is about 100 m^2, or approximately the size of a tennis court. The human lung contains approximately 200 ml of blood in the pulmonary capillaries, which have a microvascular surface area approximately equal to the alveolar surface.

The lung structural parameters that most influence its ability to efficiently carry out gas exchange are the thickness of the air-blood barrier, the alveolar and capillary surface areas, and the volume of blood distributed within the pulmonary capillaries. To maintain this highly efficient gas-exchange function while minimizing the work of breathing, a number of highly efficient supportive functions have developed within the lung. For example, the surface tension at the air-liquid interface over the alveolar surface is reduced dramatically by the presence of surfactant. Surfactant creates a phospholipid monolayer distributed uniformly over the aqueous subphase lining the alveolar surface and, by lowering the surface tension, both enables alveoli to be stable at low lung volumes and allows alveolar volume to change with a relatively small expenditure of energy. The alveolar epithelial surface is covered by two types of specialized epithelial cells. Ninety-eight percent of the alveolar surface is covered by type I alveolar epithelial cells, which are large cells each covering an enormous surface area (approximately 5000 μm^2 per cell) with a thin, highly attenuated cytoplasm that minimizes the thickness of the air-blood barrier. About 2% of the alveolar surface is covered by the highly metabolic, cuboidal-alveolar type II epithelial cells. These cells secrete surfactant and carry out a number of other biologic functions, including regeneration of the alveolar epithelium, transport of electrolytes and fluids across the epithelium to maintain "dry" alveolar air spaces, and secretion of substances that help regulate immune and inflammatory functions in the lung.

LYMPHATICS. The lung has an extensive system of lymphatics which clears fluid from both the pleural space and the lung. The pleural network lies in the visceral pleura lining the outer lung surface and connects to the deep or parenchymal plexus, which follows the bronchovascular bundles and the lobular septa. The two systems connect at the boundaries between lobes or lobules and the pleura, and both systems drain toward hilar lymph nodes through larger lymphatic channels equipped with valves. The parenchymal lymphatic channels begin at the level of respiratory bronchioles. Alveolar walls do not contain lymphatic channels. The pleural space is also lined by a parietal pleura, which is the pleural membrane on the chest wall side. The balance of oncotic and hydrostatic pressures in the capillaries lining the parietal and visceral pleuras is different owing to the fact that parietal pleura capillaries are supplied by the systemic vasculature. Mean capillary hydrostatic pressure in the parietal pleura is about 25 cm H_2O. The visceral pleura

capillaries, which derive primarily from the low-pressure pulmonary vascular circuit, have a mean capillary pressure of 5 to 10 cm H_2O. Under normal conditions, the oncotic pressure in blood is approximately 15 cm H_2O greater than that in the surrounding extravascular tissues; thus, the oncotic pressure gradient is the primary force moving fluid back into the capillaries. The oncotic pressure in the systemic and pulmonary capillary systems is similar. The effects of the normal hydrostatic and oncotic pressure differences in pleural capillaries lead to fluid movement from systemic capillaries in the parietal pleura into the pleural space. The pleural fluid can be absorbed either into low-pressure visceral or parietal pleural lymphatics or into pulmonary capillaries lying within the visceral pleura. The negative intrathoracic pressures during the respiratory cycle also contribute to the presence of a large fluid flux out of the parietal pleura. The low-pressure pulmonary vascular circuit creates an even larger positive gradient favoring resorption of fluid from the pleural spaces (and, in a similar fashion, from the alveolar air spaces). Unless disturbed by disease, fluid moves continuously into and out of the pleural spaces, but the pleural spaces are maintained free of excess fluid by the high absorptive capacity of the visceral pleura and of lymphatics. In a similar manner, any fluid in alveolar air spaces is rapidly absorbed by the pulmonary capillary bed, and the alveolar air spaces are kept "dry" and thereby available for gas exchange. Diseases which affect the permeability barrier created by pulmonary capillary walls, disturb pulmonary lymphatic drainage, or increase pulmonary hydrostatic pressure can alter these forces, leading to rapid accumulation of pleural effusions and/or intra-alveolar flooding.

CLEARANCE. The lung has a large surface area exposed to the external environment. More than 99% of the mass of particles inhaled under normal conditions are cleared by the nasopharynx and larger airways in the lung. Particles impacting the upper airways are primarily cleared by the epithelial mucociliary escalator. Airway epithelial cells are covered by a mucous coat that increases in thickness as it moves upward. This mucous coat is continually moved proximally by the ciliated cells lining all levels of the airways. Under normal conditions, once airway mucus reaches the posterior pharynx, it is swallowed; up to 1 liter of fluid moves by this pathway from the lungs to the gastrointestinal tract per day.

Small particles (< 10 μm aerodynamic diameter) have a finite probability of reaching alveolar gas exchange surfaces. Once particles deposit in the alveolar region, clearance is primarily via alveolar macrophages. In the normal lung, each alveolus contains about 12 macrophages, and this number may be 2 to 10 times greater in

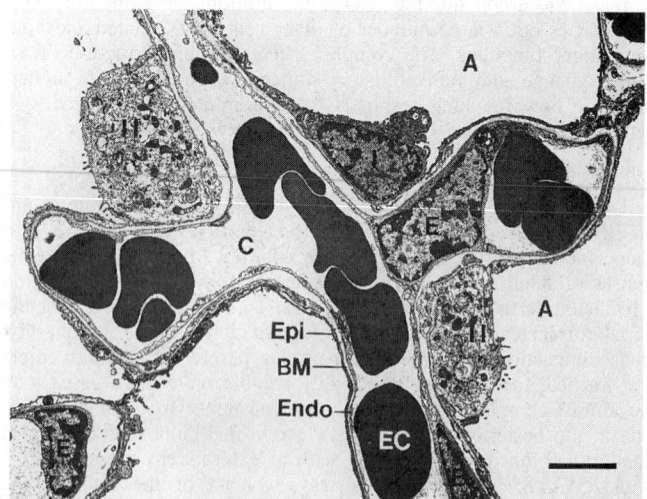

FIGURE 50–2. Transmission electron micrograph of a normal human lung illustrating relationships of the alveolar air spaces (A) to pulmonary capillaries (C). Alveolar septal tissues include epithelial type I cells (I), epithelial type II cells (II), and capillary endothelial cells (E). Note the thin alveolar septal tissue barrier over much of the surface. The barrier for O_2 diffusion across the thin portions of the septa into erythrocytes (EC) consists of the epithelium (Epi), a common basement membrane (BM), and the endothelium (Endo). (Bar = 4 μm.) (Modified from Crapo JD, Bevry BE, Gehr P, et al.: Cell number and cell characteristics of the normal human lung. Am Rev Respir Dis 125:740, 1982.)

the proximal alveoli of a smoker or an individual exposed to high levels of environmental air pollutants. These free-moving cells on the alveolar surface process inhaled particles, antigens, bacteria, and viruses by phagocytosis. A critical function of the lung is to clear and/or process inhaled antigens and infectious agents or other toxic material without stimulating an amplified immune response. The alveolar surface is constantly bombarded with inhaled materials. Despite this, the thin, delicate alveolar septa are generally maintained in a noninflamed state and gas exchange is undisturbed. A variety of chemical and structural elements contribute to regulation of immune processes in the lung, creating a milieu in which widely dispersed inhaled particulate material or infectious agents can be processed without creating an exaggerated or unnecessary immune response. Disorders in these immune regulatory pathways, which are at the present time poorly understood, are likely to be important elements of hyperimmune or inflammatory lung diseases.

METABOLISM. Although gas exchange is the obvious primary function of the lung, the lung also has several critical metabolic functions. The lung is the only organ in the body in which 100% of the blood passes through a capillary bed on each circulation. Thus, the lung is in a critical position to act as a mechanical filter of the blood and to regulate vascular levels or responses to a variety of small peptides. Angiotensin-converting enzyme on the lung endothelial surfaces plays a critical role in regulating systemic blood pressure, both by metabolizing bradykinin and by activating angiotensin I to angiotensin II (see Ch. 38). The lung has an active uptake pathway for a variety of vasoactive amines or peptides. The lung vascular bed is also a primary site where circulating polymorphonuclear leukocytes are sequestered. Under normal conditions, approximately half of the circulating polymorphonuclear leukocytes are sequestered in the pulmonary capillary bed. These neutrophils are available both for rapid response to invading inhaled pathogens in the lung and for distribution through the systemic circulation, although the regulation, function, and control of these lung-sequestered neutrophils is not yet well defined.

PHYSIOLOGIC FUNCTION

PULMONARY FUNCTION TESTS. Pulmonary function tests provide an objective measurement of lung function. They can be used to assess both heart and lung function, identify basic functional categories of lung disorders, assess responses to a variety of inhalation injuries, and assess lung injury occurring via the pulmonary circulation. Although an enormous array of pulmonary function parameters can be measured, the primary parameters of value to the practicing physician are summarized in Table 50–1. These include basic measurements of lung volumes. Spirometric examination is the most commonly used test and consists of measurement of the pattern of air movement into and out of the lungs during controlled ventilatory maneuvers. The primary spirometric parameters of interest are forced expiratory volume in 1 second (FEV_1), forced vital capacity (FVC), and the ratio of FEV_1 to vital capacity (VC). Carbon monoxide (CO) diffusing capacity and arterial blood gases are the other most commonly helpful pulmonary function parameters.

LUNG VOLUMES. The lungs and the chest wall are elastic structures, and both function in parallel to determine the gas volume in the lungs at rest and the work involved in various breathing maneuvers. Functional residual capacity (FRC) is defined as the volume of gas in the lung at rest when the elastic inward pull of the lung is exactly balanced by the outward pull of the chest wall and diaphragm (Fig. 50–3). This is the most reproducible of the pulmonary function tests because it is independent of patient effort. The gas remaining in the lung at the end of a maximal exhalation maneuver is termed residual volume. Total lung capacity (TLC) is the volume of gas contained in the lungs at the end of a maximal inspiration maneuver.

In healthy persons, lung volumes vary according to gender, age, height, and ethnic group. In determining predicted normals, it is essential to have standardized data that closely approximate the subject's characteristics. Using 95% confidence intervals for the predicted normals is recommended as the best index for determining whether a given subject is within or outside their predicted normal range. A simple and commonly used substitute for 95% confidence intervals is to define as abnormal a measured lung functional parameter that falls below 80% of its predicted normal. Thus, ± 20% of predicted normal is a crude estimator of the range of values of pulmonary function found in a normal population.

Total gas in the lungs is commonly measured by one of three methods: (1) washout of an inert gas (N_2), (2) equilibration with an inert test gas, or (3) whole-body plethysmography. Lung volume measurements initially determine FRC because that lung volume is most easily reproduced by the patient and is independent of patient compliance. Exhalation from FRC gives the expiratory reserve volume (ERV). Residual volume (RV) can then be calculated by subtracting ERV from FRC. TLC can be calculated by adding the VC to the residual volume. Accurate measurements of lung volume done by washing out nitrogen (N_2) or by equilibrating with an inert test gas (helium) require that the test gas communicate from or to all compartments of the lung. All gas-containing compartments must be freely washed out or exchanged. Poorly communicating blebs or bullae can cause lung volumes to be significantly underestimated when using N_2 washout or helium dilution techniques. Lung volumes can also be measured by body plethysmography, which involves placing the subject in a large air-tight box and having him/her breathe through a mouthpiece connected to the outside. A shutter occludes the mouthpiece and as the subject then pants against the closed shutter, the volume of gas in the chest is compressed and expanded, creating a similar change in gas volume in the box. By measuring either changes in pressure in the box or flow through a calibrated orifice in the box, the total volume of gas in the thorax can be calculated. This calculation uses Boyle's law, which states that the pressure times the volume of a gas is a constant at a constant temperature. Body plethysmography measures all gas contained in the thorax and does not require that bullae or blebs be communicating in order for their volume to be measured.

TABLE 50–1. PULMONARY FUNCTION TESTS

Lung volume	
TLC	Total lung capacity
FRC	Functional residual capacity
ERV	Expiratory reserve volume
RV	Residual volume
Expiratory flow	
FEV_1	Forced expiratory volume (in 1 second)
FVC	Forced vital capacity
FEV_1 %	FEV_1/VC ratio
Diffusing capacity	
DL_{CO}	Diffusing capacity for carbon monoxide
Arterial blood gases	
Pa_{O_2}	Arterial O_2 pressure
Pa_{CO_2}	Arterial CO_2 pressure
pH	

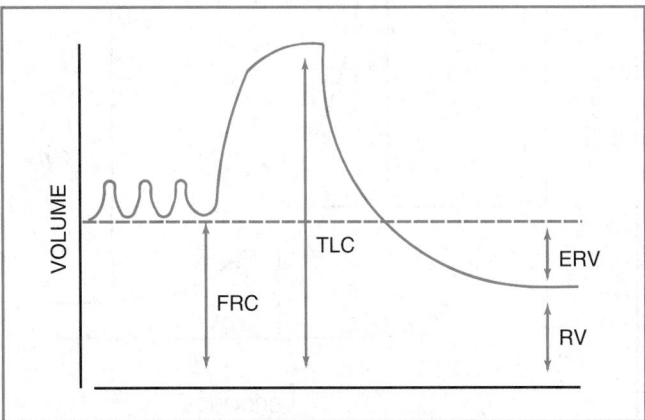

FIGURE 50–3. Ventilatory tracing showing normal resting ventilation followed by a forced inhalation to total lung capacity (TLC) and then a forced exhalation to residual volume (RV). Functional residual capacity (FRC) is the resting lung volume at the end of a normal exhalation. Expiratory reserve volume (ERV) is the volume of air that can be exhaled from FRC down to RV.

Finally, posteroanterior and lateral chest radiographs can be used to estimate lung volumes using planimetry and a nomogram that correlates thoracic gas volume with the projected area of the lungs on two perpendicular views of the chest.

SPIROMETRIC MEASUREMENTS OF EXPIRATORY FLOW. With common computerized equipment, >20 spirometric variables are often reported. The use of large numbers of variables can lead to false-positive findings, and it is recommended that only a few basic variables from the lung spirogram be used. The primary variables are FEV_1, FVC, and the ratio of FEV_1 to VC (Fig. 50–4). FVC is the maximal volume of air that can be exhaled during a forced exhalation beginning at TLC. FEV_1 is the volume of gas that can be exhaled during the first 1 second of a forced exhalation maneuver beginning at TLC. Spirometric measurements of lung function are most useful when the patient has physical findings, symptoms, or risk factors suggesting pulmonary disease. Lung functional studies can be used to define the basic class of a lung disorder, evaluate the severity of the abnormality being quantitated, or follow the progression of the disease process. It has been shown that physicians cannot consistently and reliably identify obstructive and restrictive ventilatory defects from history taking or physical examination. Age-related declines in lung function must be considered in evaluating test results. Nonsmokers lose FEV_1 at a rate of 20 to 30 ml per year. In some smokers this rate of decline can increase by two- to three-fold. In smokers under age 35, quitting smoking can result in an increase in lung function. In smokers over age 35 who quit smoking, the rate of decline of lung function generally slows to the normal rate associated with aging. Measurement of lung function can be a critical part of a preoperative evaluation because enhanced risk of postoperative pulmonary complications occurs when FVC or FEV_1 falls to <50% of predicted value or significant hypoxemia or hypercapnia is present.

The magnitude of functional impairment in obstructive lung disease can be assessed using pulmonary function testing. Table 50–2 gives a simple, but reliable approach for assessment of predicted exercise impairment in a middle-aged person of normal body size. When the predicted FEV_1 is close to 4 liters, the subject should not have a history of a significant exercise impairment until the FEV_1 falls below 3 liters per second. In that individual, an FEV_1 between 2 to 3 liters per second would be consistent with a history of mild exercise limitation. Mild exercise limitation means that the subject is able to walk significant distances but cannot do so at high rates of speed. An FEV_1 of between 1 to 2 liters per second is consistent with a moderate degree of exercise impairment,

TABLE 50–2. ASSESSMENT OF EXERCISE LIMITATION IN OBSTRUCTIVE LUNG DISEASE

FEV_1 (liters/second)	Impairment*
> 3	None
2–3	Mild
1–2	Moderate
< 1	Severe

* This assumes a middle-aged person of normal body size having a predicted FEV_1 of close to 4 liters/second. Applying this simple formula commonly requires some adjustment for age and body size.

meaning that intermittent rest periods are required to walk significant distances or to climb stairs. An FEV_1 < 1 liter per second predicts a severe exercise impairment, limiting the person to very short walking distances, perhaps restricting him/her to home. These guidelines for assessing severity of an exercise impairment in obstructive lung disease must be adjusted for age and body size in the same manner that predicted FEV_1 varies. It is important to correlate predicted functional capacity by pulmonary function testing with the history of exercise limitation described by the patient. A significant variation in the functional capacity predicted by pulmonary function testing with that described by the patient can be an important indicator of the presence of other nonpulmonary disease processes.

DIFFUSING CAPACITY. The diffusing capacity of the lung is defined as the lung's ability to take up an inhaled nonreactive test gas, such as CO, which binds to hemoglobin (Fig. 50–5). CO binds to hemoglobin with a high affinity so that virtually all the CO that reaches an alveolar space, crosses the alveolar air-blood barrier, and reaches a red cell binds to hemoglobin and thus is removed from the exhaled gas. Measurement of lung-diffusing capacity is critically influenced by three parameters: (1) the ability of the test gas to reach the alveolar gas-exchanging surfaces, (2) the ability of the test gas to cross the alveolar septa, and (3) the mass of red cells in the pulmonary capillary bed available to bind the test gas. A defect in any one of the above three components influences measured lung-diffusing capacity. Airways obstruction and ventilation-perfusion mismatching prevent the test gas from reaching the alveolar gas-exchange surfaces and lower the diffusing capacity in proportion to the maldistribution of ventilation. Thickening of the air-blood barrier can increase the resistance of gas movement across the tissue barrier, increasing diffusing capacity. Alveolar filling, as in pulmonary edema, reduces the alveolar surface area available for test gas exchange. Finally, the volume of red cells in the alveolar capillary bed is crucial in determining how much CO is retained in the capillary bed. Of the parameters that influence CO uptake in the lung during a diffusing capacity measurement, the uniformity of ventilation and the volume of red cells in the pulmonary capillary

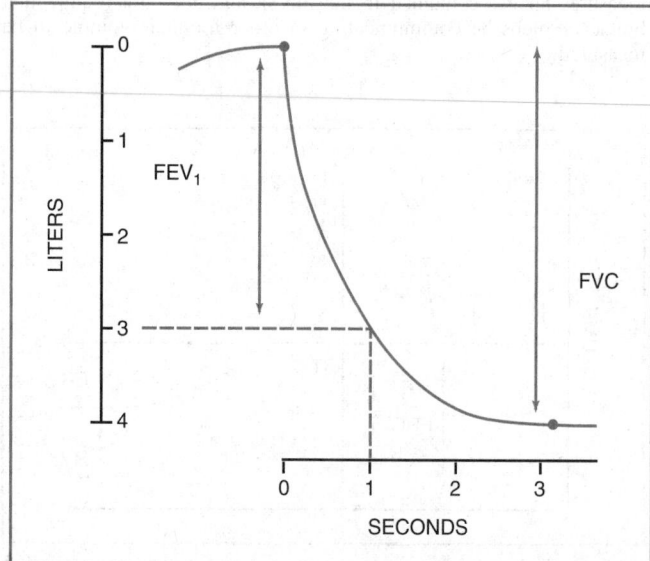

FIGURE 50–4. A portion of a normal spirogram showing the forced exhalation from total lung capacity. FEV_1 is the volume exhaled in 1 second, and forced vital capacity (FVC) is the total volume that can be forcibly exhaled from total lung capacity.

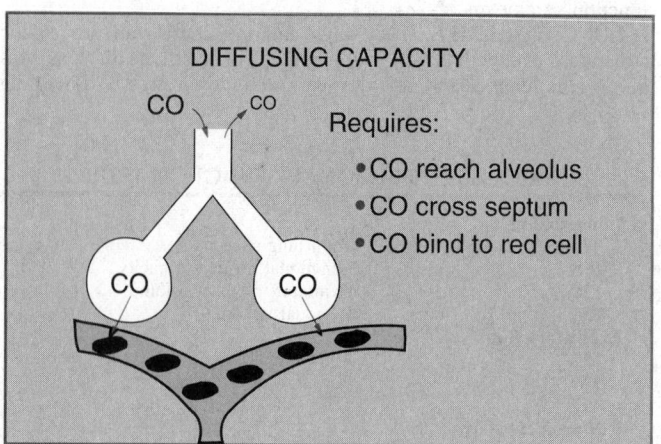

FIGURE 50–5. Measurement of pulmonary diffusing capacity for CO. The critical elements in measurement of DL_{CO} are illustrated. An altered DL_{CO} may be due to an alteration in any one of the fundamental elements required for the uptake of CO in the lung.

bed dominate the overall reaction kinetics. Diffusing capacity measurements are less sensitive to changes in thickness of the air-blood barrier because CO has a high capacity for diffusion across pulmonary tissues.

The normal values for CO diffusing capacity vary widely between laboratories, and both the absolute values and their reproducibility are strongly influenced by the measurement techniques. Diffusing-capacity measurements are most commonly useful in following changes in a patient's lung function when measured by consistent techniques applied by the same laboratory.

ABNORMALITIES OF CO-DIFFUSING CAPACITY. Based on the above discussion, it should be apparent that DL_{CO} can be altered in patients with a variety of cardiopulmonary disorders. Disorders of distribution of ventilation such as chronic obstructive pulmonary disease (COPD) and asthma are perhaps the most common causes of disordered diffusing capacity. Because of the high sensitivity of DL_{CO} to changes in pulmonary capillary blood volume, any disorder that alters pulmonary capillary blood volume significantly changes DL_{CO}. Thus, mitral stenosis or congestive heart failure, by increasing pulmonary vascular volumes, can increase DL_{CO}. When congestive heart failure is sufficiently severe to produce pulmonary edema, the alveolar filling decreases the surface area available for interaction with the test gas and may decrease measured DL_{CO}. Anemia or polycythemia can alter measured DL_{CO}, although the reported value is commonly corrected for changes in blood red cell content by measuring hemoglobin in venous blood near the time the test is carried out. Pulmonary vascular disorders such as pulmonary emboli and vasculitis can decrease the volume of blood in the pulmonary capillary bed and thereby decrease DL_{CO}. It is also decreased in patients with a loss of lung tissue, either by surgical resection or by destruction of the lung by a disease process such as emphysema. Finally, DL_{CO} may be decreased by interstitial lung diseases, which are characterized by interstitial fibrosis and thickening of the air-blood barrier. These processes were originally thought to be alveolar capillary block syndromes in which the block was thought to be an enhanced tissue thickness that the CO molecules had to cross to reach the pulmonary vascular bed. It is now recognized that these diseases also destroy the pulmonary capillary bed and that the primary cause for a low DL_{CO} in these conditions is a decrease in capillary blood volume rather than an alveolar capillary block associated with thickening of the blood-gas barrier.

GAS EXCHANGE. The expected product in pulmonary gas exchange is to maintain physiologically normal levels of P_{O_2} and P_{CO_2} in the arterial blood. Inhaled air is rapidly warmed to body temperature (37°C) and fully humidified. At sea level (barometric pressure 760 mm Hg), this gives a P_{H_2O} of 47 mm Hg. This water vapor dilutes the N_2 and O_2 in the inhaled gas to a total of 713 mm Hg, with O_2 contributing 150 mm Hg. In the alveoli O_2 is taken up and CO_2 is exchanged into the gas phase. Because under normal metabolic conditions more O_2 is taken up than CO_2 liberated, the respiratory exchange ratio is closer to 0.8. This may vary with diet and other factors influencing metabolic interrelations of O_2 and CO_2. The alveolar oxygen tension ($P_{A_{O_2}}$) can be calculated using the alveolar gas equation:

$$PA_{O_2} = PI_{O_2} - PA_{CO_2}\left[FI_{O_2} + \frac{1 - FI_{O_2}}{R}\right]$$

where PI_{O_2} equals the P_{O_2} of the expired gas, PA_{CO_2} equals alveolar P_{CO_2} (this is usually assumed to be equal to the arterial P_{CO_2}), FI_{O_2} equals the fractional concentration of O_2 in the inspired gas, and R

equals the respiratory exchange ratio. At sea level with an assumed R of 0.8, the alveolar gas equation simplifies to alveolar $P_{O_2} = 150 - Pa_{CO_2} \times 1.2$.

The estimated alveolar oxygen tension ($P_{A_{O_2}}$) should be compared with the measured arterial oxygen tension (Pa_{O_2}) to determine the A−a O_2 gradient. It is normal for there to be a small gradient (5 to 15 mm Hg) due to nonuniform distribution of ventilation and/or a small right-to-left shunt. A wide A−a O_2 gradient strongly suggests a disorder of gas exchange in the lung or an intracardiac right-to-left shunt. A normal A−a O_2 gradient indicates normal gas exchange in the lung. Hypoxemia in the setting of a normal A−a O_2 gradient suggests that hypoventilation (e.g., drug overdose, neuromuscular dysfunction) rather than lung dysfunction is the primary cause.

The partial pressures of gases (at sea level) in various compartments are shown in Table 50-3. Dry air is fully humidified as it enters the respiratory system, decreasing the partial pressures of both N_2 and O_2. The exchange of O_2 for CO_2 in alveolar spaces actually causes a small increase in the partial pressure of N_2 because the respiratory exchange ratio is normally <1.0. Note that the total pressure of soluble gases in both the arterial and venous systems is less than total atmospheric pressure. Tissues throughout the body are in equilibrium with venous blood and are thus also subatmospheric. When gas or a bubble forms in a tissue space (e.g., a pneumothorax), that gas equilibrates with venous blood except for N_2, which is elevated to a supra-atmospheric level as the total pressure in the pneumothorax becomes equal to atmospheric pressure. This creates a gradient for removing N_2 from the pneumothorax and, in combination with continuous re-equilibration of the other gases with venous blood, leads to resorption of all free gas in the pleural space. This mechanism keeps the lung expanded against the chest wall and removes any gas forming in or placed in any other body spaces.

DISORDERS OF VENTILATION

Lung diseases are commonly divided into two broad categories—obstructive lung disease and restrictive lung disease—based on fundamental differences in the pulmonary function assessment.

OBSTRUCTIVE VENTILATORY DISORDERS. This term is used for the constellation of diseases characterized by limitation of expiratory air flow. The primary criterion for air flow obstruction is a reduced $FEV_1/VC\%$. In the presence of a normal or elevated TLC, the absolute value of the FEV_1 can be used to estimate severity of the obstructive lung disease. The obstruction may be caused by a variety of airway diseases including chronic bronchitis, bronchiectasis, and mucous gland hyperplasia, leading to physical obstruction or plugging of airways. In emphysema extensive destruction of alveolar and/or airway walls occurs, leading to loss of elasticity and collapse of airway walls during exhalation, thus trapping gas in the distal lung. Emphysema is also associated with abnormalities of diffusing capacity due to extensive destruction of the alveolar capillary bed. Reversible forms of airway obstruction such as asthma are classified as obstructive lung diseases in which the abnormality is primarily due to restriction of size of the airway walls by inflammation, enhanced muscular tone, and/or enhanced mucus secretion. If underlying tissue destruction does not occur, this form of obstructive lung disease can be reversible.

RESTRICTIVE VENTILATORY DISORDERS. This class of lung dysfunction is characterized by fibrotic reactions of the alveo-

TABLE 50-3. PARTIAL PRESSURE (mm Hg) OF GASES IN VARIOUS BODY SPACES

	Dry Air	Humidified Air	Alveolar	Arterial	Venous	Tissue Bubble or Pleural Gas
N_2	600	563	571	571	571	633
O_2	160	150	102	95	40	40
H_2O	—	47	47	47	40	47
CO_2	—	—	40	40	40	40
TOTAL PRESSURE	760	760	760	706	651	760

TABLE 50-4. LUNG VOLUMES IN RESTRICTIVE LUNG DISEASES

	Pulmonary Fibrosis	Obesity (Chest Wall Restriction)	Neuromuscular Disorders
TLC	↓	↓	↓
FRC	↓	↓	Normal
ERV	↓	↓ ↓	↓
RV	↓	Normal	↑
Collapse point	Zero	RV	FRC

lar septa and commonly includes the walls of small airways. The increased fibrotic tissue increases the elastic recoil in parenchymal lung tissue, and because these walls are interconnected to airway walls, this can hold airways open. The hallmarks of restrictive lung diseases are a low TLC and a fall in VC. Where caused by a fibrotic process, it is associated with smaller alveoli having thickened walls, increased amounts of elastic and connective tissues, and destruction of portions of the pulmonary capillary bed. Airways are generally held open by enhanced elastic recoil. The enhanced elastic recoil increases the resistance against inspiration, making it difficult for the patient to inhale and lowering the FVC. The enhanced elastic recoil facilitates rapid exhalation; thus $FEV_1/VC\%$ is generally increased in patients with restrictive lung diseases. Other forms of restrictive ventilatory impairments can include (1) diseases of the chest wall with altered chest wall compliance (obesity, kyphoscoliosis), (2) neuromuscular diseases in which the patient has difficulty carrying out ventilatory maneuvers (Guillain-Barré syndrome, myasthenia gravis), (3) diseases of the pleura which may entrap the lung (extensive pleural thickening), (4) space-occupying lesions in the lung (tumors, cardiac enlargement, pleural effusions), and (5) removal of portions of the lungs via surgical resection.

Table 50-4 gives the common changes in lung volumes in various classes of restrictive lung diseases. Note that fibrotic lung diseases cause significant decreases in all lung volumes as the fibrosis creates a smaller, less compliant lung. In contrast, massive obesity tends to preserve the RV because the underlying lung is normal and the primary problem is inspiring against the excess weight of the chest wall. The ERV is often markedly reduced out of proportion to the other lung volumes in obesity and the FRC approaches RV as the heavy chest wall pushes the "zero energy point" downward. Neuromuscular diseases create a restrictive lung disorder in which all lung volumes move closer to FRC. These patients lack the respiratory strength to fully inhale or exhale from FRC and thus have a low TLC with an elevated RV. The simplified analysis shown in Figure 50-4 assumes that other processes such as atelectasis are not complicating the classic presentation of these forms of restrictive lung disease.

EXERCISE. Most pulmonary function measurements are taken while the subject is at rest. Defects in pulmonary function can be brought out by assessing pulmonary function under conditions of exercise. In addition, complaints of fatigue or exercise limitation can be more rigorously assessed by complete cardiopulmonary exercise testing in which cardiac and pulmonary function are simultaneously quantified under conditions of gradually increasing exercise. Measurements of heart rate, electrocardiogram, arterial blood gases, and exhaled gases can allow simultaneous assessment of cardiac and pulmonary function and can both separate disorders of heart and lung function and distinguish these from exercise limitation due to poor cooperation or deconditioning. These tests can also facilitate the diagnosis of pulmonary vascular and parenchymal infiltrative diseases.

Crapo RO: Pulmonary-function testing. N Engl J Med 331:25, 1994. *Excellent review of the use of spirometry in assessing patients with pulmonary disorders.*

Gehr P, Geiser M, Stone KC, Crapo JD: Morphometric analysis of the gas exchange region of the lung. *In* Toxicology of the Lung. 2nd ed. New York, Raven Press, 1993, p 111. *Review of the structural parameters that are critical determinants of gas exchange.*

Murray JF: The Normal Lung: The Basis for Diagnosis and Treatment of Pulmonary Disease. 2nd ed. Philadelphia, WB Saunders, 1986. *An excellent review of normal lung anatomy and pulmonary physiology.*

51 ASTHMA
Jeffrey M. Drazen

DEFINITION

Asthma is a clinical syndrome characterized by recurrent episodes of airway obstruction that resolve spontaneously or as a result of treatment; its cause remains unknown. Unlike patients with chronic obstructive lung diseases, those with asthma periodically have normal lung function. Asthma is also associated with an exaggerated bronchoconstrictor response to stimuli that have little or no effect in nonasthmatic subjects; this phenomenon is known as airway hyperresponsiveness. Current evidence suggests that the syndrome we now recognize as asthma is an inflammatory condition that comprises a number of distinct disease entities.

EPIDEMIOLOGY AND STATISTICS

Asthma is an extremely common disorder affecting men and women equally; approximately 5% of the US population has signs and symptoms consistent with a diagnosis of asthma. Although most cases begin before age 25, asthma may develop at any time throughout life. Asthma is also a common reason to seek medical treatment; in the United States in 1988 there were 15 million outpatient visits to physicians for asthma and nearly 2 million inpatient hospital days of treatment. Over $4 billion per year are spent on asthma care.

PATHOGENESIS AND PATHOLOGY

Despite the high prevalence of asthma, its cause remains unknown. The episodic airway narrowing and resulting reduced airflow that constitute an asthma attack result from obstruction of the airway lumen. Although it is now well established that infiltration of the airway with inflammatory cells (including TH_2 lymphocytes, eosinophils, and mast cells) is a common feature of asthma, the links between these cells and the pathobiologic processes that account for asthmatic airway obstruction have not been clearly delineated. Three possible links have been postulated: (1) constriction of airway smooth muscle, (2) thickening of the airway epithelium, and (3) the presence of liquids within the confines of the airway lumen. Among these mechanisms, the constriction of airway smooth muscle due to the local release of bioactive mediators or neurotransmitters is the most widely accepted explanation for the acute reversible airway obstruction in asthma attacks. Several bronchoactive mediators are thought to be of importance in asthma.

MEDIATORS OF THE ACUTE ASTHMATIC RESPONSE. *Acetylcholine.* Acetylcholine released from intrapulmonary motor nerves constricts airway smooth muscle by directly stimulating muscarinic receptors of the M_3 subtype. The effectiveness of atropine and its congeners in the treatment of asthma constitutes the major evidence for the importance of acetylcholine in the pathogenesis of this condition.

Adenosine. Adenosine is a purine nucleoside formed during the rapid extracellular metabolism of adenosine triphosphate. In the past, adenosine was considered a potentially important effector molecule because its activity was antagonized at the tissue-receptor level by therapeutic levels of theophylline. However, current evidence suggests that adenosine receptor stimulation in asthma is unlikely to be a major bronchoconstrictor pathway.

Histamine. Histamine, or β-imidazolylethylamine, was identified as a potent endogenous bronchoactive agent more than 80 years ago. Mast cells, which are prominent in the airway tissues of asthma patients, constitute the major pulmonary source of histamine. Recent studies with novel potent antihistamines indicate a minor role for histamine in the bronchospasm of asthma.

Kinins. Bradykinin and related molecules are cleaved from plasma precursors by enzymes known as kallikreins; at least one type of kallikrein is released from activated mast cells. Although no bradykinin synthesis inhibitors or receptor antagonists are under clinical study or in clinical use, bradykinin is potentially significant because of its potency and the release of kinin-forming enzymes from mast cells.

Leukotrienes. The cysteinyl leukotrienes LTC$_4$, LTD$_4$, and LTE$_4$, as well as LTB$_4$, are derived by the sequential lipoxygenation of arachidonic acid, which is released from cell membrane phospholipids during cellular activation. The enzyme 5-lipoxygenase, a membrane protein known as 5-lipoxygenase–activating protein, LTA$_4$ hydrolase, and LTC$_4$ synthase are required to produce the leukotrienes; only the first three enzymes are needed to produce LTB$_4$. Mast cells, eosinophils, and alveolar macrophages have the enzymatic capability needed to produce cysteinyl leuko-trienes from membrane phospholipids, whereas polymorphonuclear leukocytes produce largely LTB$_4$. LTB$_4$ is predominantly a chemoattractant molecule, whereas LTC$_4$ and LTD$_4$ are potent contractile agonists. Clinical trials with leukotriene receptor antagonists or synthesis inhibitors have documented efficacy in the treatment of exercise- and antigen-induced asthma; these agents are especially potent for treating aspirin-induced asthma. Agents active on this pathway may be available for asthma treatment in the near future.

Neuropeptides. Neuropeptides are small peptides found in pulmonary nerves. Two prophlogistic peptides, substance P and neurokinin A (substance K), are found in the terminal axon dendrites of certain sensory nerves. When these nerves are excited by appropriate sensory stimuli, peptides are released into the airway microenvironment, where they can induce constriction of airway smooth muscle and bronchovascular leak through action at NK$_1$ and NK$_2$ receptors, respectively. Vasoactive intestinal peptide is found in sensory and autonomic pulmonary nerves; this endogenous bronchodilator is believed to play a homeostatic role in the airways. Ordinarily, the peptides released from nerves are rapidly degraded by specific peptidases located at or near the site of their action or release; inhibition of the function of these peptidases enhances the biologic effects of released peptides. The recent identification of nonpeptide antagonists at neuropeptide receptors may elucidate the role of these peptides in the asthmatic response.

Nitric Oxide. NO· is produced enzymatically by airway epithelial cells and by inflammatory cells found in the lung in asthma. Free NO· has a half-life on the order of seconds in the airway and is stabilized by conjugation to thiols to form RS-NO. NO· and RS-NO can cause bronchodilation and may play a homeostatic role in the airway. Paradoxically, high levels of NO· may form toxic oxidation products, such as OONO$^-$, which could damage the airway epithelium.

Platelet Activating Factor (PAF). PAF—a phospholipid with an ether-linked fatty acid (C$_{16}$–C$_{20}$) in the *sn-1* position, an acetyl moiety in the *sn-2* position, and phosphatidylcholine in the *sn-3* position—is derived from lyso-PAF by the action of specific acetyltransferases and is produced by a variety of inflammatory cells, including mast cells and eosinophils. PAF had been thought to induce airway hyperresponsiveness and airway inflammation, but the failure of recent studies with PAF receptor antagonists to show efficacy in chronic stable asthma casts doubt on the role of PAF as a mediator of the asthmatic response.

PATHOLOGY OF THE ASTHMATIC RESPONSE. The pathology of mild asthma, as delineated by bronchoscopic and biopsy studies, is characterized by edema and hyperemia of the mucosa and by infiltration of the mucosa with mast cells, eosinophils, and lymphocytes bearing the TH$_2$ phenotype. Such cells produce interleukin (IL)-3, IL-4, IL-5, and granulocyte-macrophage colony-stimulating factor and thereby promote the synthesis of IgE, an important allergic effector molecule. Within the airway wall, there is thickening of the lamina propria, with deposition of type III and type V collagen (Fig. 51-1). In more severe asthma there is thickening of the airway wall due to hypertrophy and hyperplasia of airway glands and secretory cells, hyperplasia of airway smooth muscle, and further deposition of submucosal collagen. The shedding of airway epithelium may lead to a denuded airway. These changes occur in a patchy fashion in mild asthma and become more widespread as the disease becomes more severe. Morphometric studies of airways from asthmatic subjects have demonstrated airway wall thickening sufficient to increase airflow resistance and enhance airway responsiveness. In severe asthma the airway wall is markedly thickened; in addition, there is patchy airway occlusion by a mixture of hyperviscous mucus and shed airway epithelial cells.

PHYSIOLOGIC CHANGES IN ASTHMA. The consequence of the airway obstruction induced by smooth muscle constriction, thickening of the airway epithelium, or free liquid within the airway

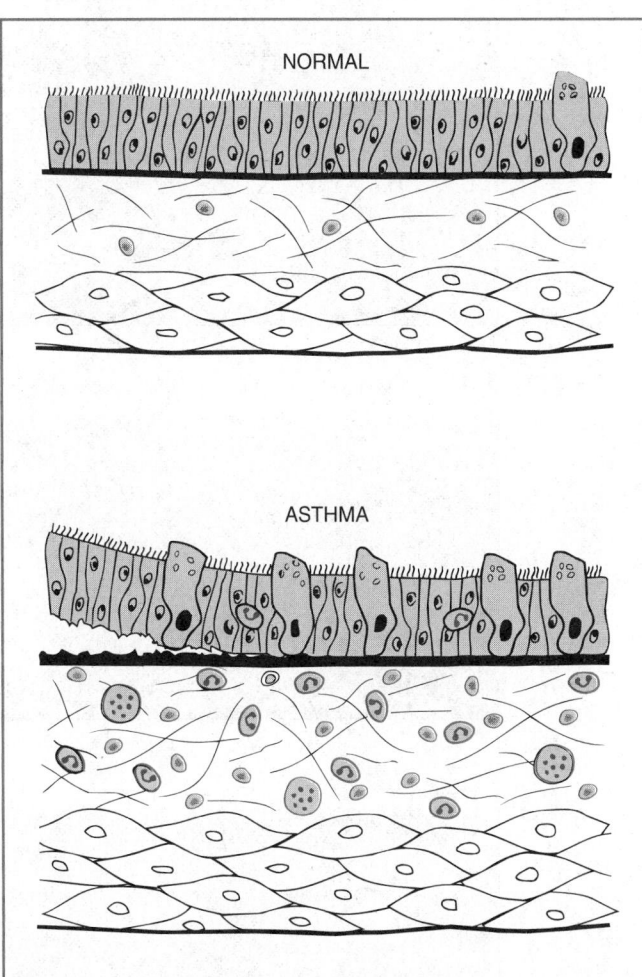

FIGURE 51-1. Schematic diagram of the airway epithelium in normals and asthmatics. The airway in asthma has more goblet cells, is loosely attached to a thickened basement membrane, and has a thickened lamina propria infiltrated with eosinophils and mast cells. Furthermore, there is both hypertrophy and hyperplasia of the airway smooth muscle layer.

lumen is an increased resistance to airflow, which is manifested by increased airway resistance (R$_{aw}$) and decreased flow rates throughout the vital capacity. At the onset of an asthma attack, obstruction occurs at all airway levels. As the attack resolves, these changes reverse—first in the large airways (i.e., mainstem, lobar, segmental, and subsegmental bronchi) and then in the more peripheral airways. This anatomic sequence of onset and reversal is reflected in the physiologic changes monitored during an asthmatic episode (Fig. 51-2). Specifically, as an asthma attack resolves, flow rates normalize first high in the vital capacity and only later low in the vital capacity. Because asthma is an airway disease, no primary changes occur in the static pressure-volume curve of the lungs. However, during an acute attack, airway narrowing may be so severe as to result in closure. Individual lung units tend to close at a volume that is near their maximal volume; this closure results in a change of the pressure-volume curve such that, for a given contained gas volume within the thorax, there will be decreased elastic recoil. The decreased elastic recoil, at a given overall lung volume, further depresses expiratory flow rates.

Additional factors influence the mechanical behavior of the lungs during an acute attack of asthma. During inspiration, the pleural pressure drops far below the 4 to 6 cm H$_2$O subatmospheric pressure usually required for tidal airflow. The expiratory phase of respiration also becomes active as the patient tries to force air from the lungs. As a consequence, peak pleural pressures during expiration, which normally are only a few centimeters of water above atmospheric, may be as high as 20 to 30 cm H$_2$O. The low pleural pressures during inspiration tend to dilate airways, whereas the high

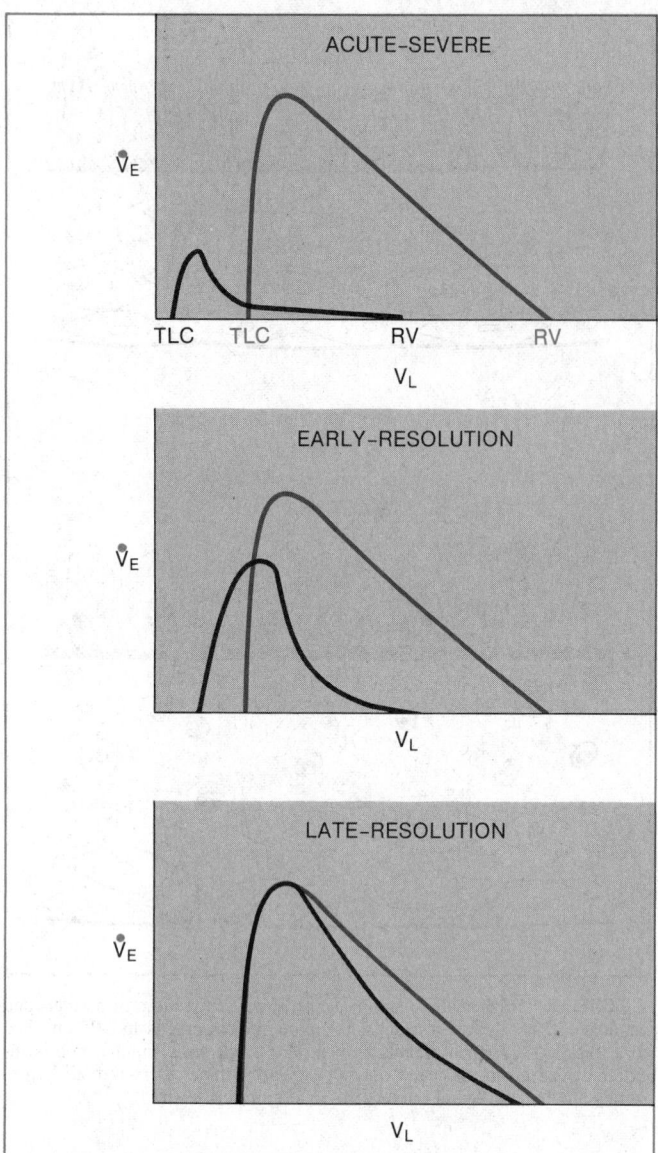

ACUTE-SEVERE

$\dot{V}_E$

TLC   TLC   RV   RV

V_L

EARLY-RESOLUTION

$\dot{V}_E$

V_L

LATE-RESOLUTION

$\dot{V}_E$

V_L

FIGURE 51–2. Schematic flow-volume curves in various stages of asthma; in each figure the dashed line depicts the normal flow-volume curve. Predicted and observed total lung capacity (TLC) and residual volume (RV) are shown in the top panel. V_E = Expiratory flow rate; V_L = lung volume.

pleural pressures during expiration tend to narrow them. During an asthma attack, the wide pressure swings coupled with alterations in the airway wall lead to an expiratory airflow resistance that is much higher than the inspiratory resistance.

The respiratory rate is usually rapid during an acute asthmatic attack. This tachypnea is driven not by abnormalities in arterial blood gas composition but rather by stimulation of intrapulmonary receptors with subsequent effects on central respiratory centers. One consequence of airway narrowing combined with these rapid airflow rates is a heightened mechanical load on the ventilatory pump. During a severe attack, the load can increase the work of breathing by a factor of 10 or more and can predispose the ventilatory muscles to fatigue.

The patchy nature of asthmatic airway narrowing results in a maldistribution of ventilation relative to pulmonary perfusion. There is a shift from the normal preponderance of $\dot{V}/Q$ units with a ratio near unity to a large number of alveolar-capillary units with a $\dot{V}/Q$ ratio of less than unity. The net effect is to induce arterial hypoxemia. In addition, the hyperpnea of asthma is reflected as hyperventilation with a low arterial PCO_2.

HISTORY. During an asthma attack, patients seek medical attention for shortness of breath accompanied by cough, wheezing, and anxiety. The patient's degree of breathlessness is not closely related to the degree of airflow obstruction but is often influenced by the acuteness of the attack. Dyspnea may occur only with exercise (exercise-induced asthma), after ingesting aspirin (aspirin-induced asthma), after exposure to a specific known allergen (extrinsic asthma), or for no identifiable reason (intrinsic asthma). There are variants of asthma in which cough, hoarseness, or an inability to sleep through the night is the only symptom. Identifying a provoking stimulus through careful questioning helps establish the diagnosis of asthma and may be therapeutically useful if the stimulus can be avoided. Most patients with asthma complain of shortness of breath when exposed to rapid changes in the temperature and humidity of inspired air. For example, in less temperate climates during the winter months, patients commonly become short of breath when leaving a heated house. Airway narrowing induced by breathing cold, dry air is one of the diagnostic tests for asthma.

An important factor to consider when taking a history from a patient with asthma is the potential for occupational exposures leading to the asthmatic diathesis. In such cases pre-existing asthma may be exacerbated or asthma may occur *de novo* after workplace exposure; this clue eventually leads to the diagnosis of *occupational asthma.* Rapid reversal of symptoms upon removal from the offending environment may not occur; indeed, it is now appreciated that once airway inflammation is established it may take years or longer for the clinical manifestations to resolve if they resolve at all. Information about a number of common specific syndromes is detailed in Table 51–1.

PHYSICAL EXAMINATION. *Vital Signs.* Common features of acute asthma attacks include a rapid respiratory rate (often 25 to 40 breaths per minute), tachycardia, and pulsus paradoxus (an exaggerated inspiratory fall in the systolic pressure); the magnitude of the pulsus is related to the severity of the attack.

Thoracic Examination. Inspection reveals that the patient experiencing an acute attack of asthma is using accessory muscles during inspiration; the skin over the thorax may be retracted into the intercostal spaces during inspiration. The chest is usually hyperinflated, and the expiratory phase is prolonged relative to the inspiratory phase. Percussion of the thorax demonstrates hyperresonance, with loss of the normal variation in dullness due to diaphragmatic movement. Auscultation reveals wheezing, which is the cardinal physical finding in asthma but does not establish the diagnosis (Table 51–2). Wheezing is commonly heard during both inspiration and expiration, although it is louder during the latter phase of respiration. The wheezing is characterized as polyphonic in that more than one pitch may be heard simultaneously. Accompanying adventitious sounds may include rhonchi, which are suggestive of free secretions in the airway lumen, or rales, which are indicative of localized infection or cardiac failure. Decreased intensity or the absence of breath sounds in a patient with asthma indicates severe airflow obstruction.

LABORATORY FINDINGS. *Pulmonary Function Findings.* Decreased airflow rate throughout the vital capacity is the cardinal pulmonary function abnormality in asthma. Although essential to diagnose asthma, this abnormality is not specific. The peak expiratory flow rate (PEFR), the forced expiratory volume in the first second (FEV_1), and the maximal midexpiratory flow rate (MMEFR) are all decreased in asthma. In very severe asthma the dyspnea may be so extreme as to prevent the patient from performing a complete spirogram. In this case, if 1 second of forced expiration can be recorded, useful values for PEFR and FEV_1 can be obtained. Gradation of attack severity *must* be assessed by objective measures of airflow; no other methods yield accurate and reproducible results. Table 51–3 relates the severity of the asthma attack to the relative depression of airflow rates. As the attack resolves, the PEFR and the FEV_1 increase in concert while the MMEFR remains substantially depressed. Further resolution of obstruction is indicated by a normalization of both the FEV_1 and the PEFR while the MMEFR remains depressed. Even when the attack has resolved clinically, residual depression of the MMEFR is not uncommon; this depression may resolve over a prolonged course of treatment. Representative schematic flow-volume curves during an asthma attack are shown in Figure 51–2. If the patient is able to cooperate fully, mea-

TABLE 51-1. COMMON OCCUPATIONAL CAUSES OF ASTHMA

High Molecular Weight Compounds[1]			Low Molecular Weight Compounds[2]		
Agent	*Occupation*	*Prevalence[3]*	*Agent*	*Occupation*	*Prevalence[3]*
Animals			**Metals**		
Laboratory animals (rats, mice, rabbits, guinea pigs)	Laboratory workers, veterinarians	Moderate	Platinum	Platinum refining	High
Chicken	Poultry workers		Vanadium	Hard metal industry	High
Crab	Crab processing	Moderate	**Other**		
Shrimp	Shrimp processing	High	Trimetallic anhydride	Epoxy resin, plastics	High
Hoya	Oyster farming	High	Toluene diisocyanate	Polyurethane industries, varnishing, plastics	Moderate
River fly	Contact with riverside power plants	Low	Western red cedar	Carpenter, cabinet makers, sawmill workers	Low-moderate
Screw worm fly	Flight crews	High	Azidocarbonamide	Plastic and rubber workers	Moderate
Bee moth	Fish bait breeders	Moderate	Formalin	Hospital workers	
			Urea formaldehyde	Insulation workers, affected homeowners	
Plants/Vegetables					
Grain dust	Grain handlers				
Wheat/rye flour	Bakers, millers				
Gum acacia	Printers	High			
Biologic Enzymes					
Bacillis subtilis	Detergent industry	High			
Trypsin	Plastics, pharmaceutical	High			
Papain	Packing	High			

Abbreviated and adapted from Chan-Yeung M: Occupational asthma. Chest 98:1485, 1990.
[1] High molecular weight compounds are usually considered to induce occupational asthma via an allergic mechanism.
[2] Asthma is induced by low molecular weight compounds by acting as haptens; other mechanisms which are not clearly elucidated also exist.
[3] Prevalence is indicated by low, i.e., ≤ 3% of exposed individuals; moderate, i.e., 3–20% of exposed individuals; high, i.e., > 20% of exposed individuals.

surements of lung volumes show an increase in total lung capacity (TLC) and residual volume during an acute attack which resolve with treatment.

Arterial Blood Gases. Blood gas analysis need not be undertaken in individuals with mild asthma. If the asthma is sufficiently severe to merit prolonged observation, however, blood gas analysis is indicated; in such cases hypoxemia and hypocarbia are the rule. With the subject breathing room air, the Pa_{O_2} is usually between 55 and 70 torr and the Pa_{CO_2} between 25 and 35 torr. At the onset of the attack, an appropriate pure respiratory alkalemia is evident; with attacks of prolonged duration, the pH normalizes as a result of compensatory metabolic acidemia. A normal Pa_{CO_2} in a patient with moderate to severe airflow obstruction is reason for concern, as it may indicate that the mechanical load on the respiratory system is greater than can be sustained by the ventilatory muscles and that respiratory failure is imminent. When the Pa_{CO_2} rises in such settings, the pH falls quickly because the bicarbonate stores have become depleted as a result of renal compensation for the prolonged preceding respiratory alkalemia. Because this chain of events can take place rapidly, close observation is indicated for asthmatics with "normal" Pa_{CO_2} levels and moderate to severe airflow obstruction.

Other Blood Findings. Asthmatic subjects are frequently atopic; thus blood eosinophilia is common. In addition, elevated serum levels of IgE are often documented; epidemiologic studies indicate that asthma is unusual in subjects with low IgE levels. If indicated by the patient's history, specific RAST assays for IgE directed against likely offending antigens can be conducted. In rare instances asthma alone can result in the elevated serum concentrations of aminotransferases, lactate dehydrogenases, muscle creatine phosphokinase, ornithine transcarbamylase, and antidiuretic hormone.

Radiographic Findings. The chest radiograph of subjects with asthma is often normal. Severe asthma is associated with hyperinflation, as indicated by depression of the diaphragm and abnormally lucent lung fields. Complications of severe asthma, including pneumomediastinum or pneumothorax, may be detected radiographically.

TABLE 51-2. DIFFERENTIAL DIAGNOSIS OF WHEEZING OTHER THAN ASTHMA

Common
Acute bronchiolitis (infectious, chemical)
Aspiration (foreign body)
Bronchial stenosis
Cardiac failure
Chronic bronchitis
Cystic fibrosis
Eosinophilic pneumonia
Uncommon
Airway obstruction due to masses
  External compression
    Central thoracic tumors, superior vena cava (SVC) syndrome, substernal thyroid
  Intrinsic airway
    Primary lung cancer, metastatic breast cancer
Carcinoid syndrome
Endobronchial sarcoid
Pulmonary emboli
Systemic mastocytosis
Systemic vasculitis (polyarteritis nodosa)

TABLE 51-3. RELATIVE SEVERITY OF AN ASTHMATIC ATTACK AS INDICATED BY PEFR, FEV₁, AND MMEFR

Test	Percent of Predicted Value	Asthma Severity
PEFR	80% or greater	
FEV_1	80% or greater	No spirometric abnormalities
MMEFR	80% or greater	
PEFR	80% or greater	
FEV_1	70% or greater	Mild asthma
MMEFR	55%–75%	
PEFR	60% or greater	
FEV_1	45%–70%	Moderate asthma
MMEFR	30%–50%	
PEFR	Less than 50%	
FEV_1	Less than 50%	Severe asthma
MMEFR	10%–30%	

PEFR = peak expiratory flow rate; MMEFR = maximal midexpiratory flow rate; FEV_1 = forced expiratory volume in the first second.

In mild to moderate asthma without adventitious sounds other than wheezing, a chest radiograph need not be obtained; if the asthma is severe enough to merit hospital admission, a chest radiograph is advised.

Electrocardiographic Findings. In acute asthma the electrocardiogram is usually normal, save for sinus tachycardia. However, right axis deviation, right bundle branch block, "P pulmonale," or even ST-T wave abnormalities may arise during severe asthma and resolve as the attack resolves.

Sputum Findings. The sputum of the asthmatic patient may either be clear or opaque with a green or yellow tinge. The presence of color does not invariably indicate infection, and examination of a Gram-stained and Wright-stained sputum smear is indicated. Often the sputum contains eosinophils, Charcot-Leyden crystals (crystallized eosinophil lysophospholipase), Curschmann's spirals (bronchiolar casts composed of mucus and cells), or Creola bodies (clusters of airway epithelial cells with identifiable cilia) which can impact color in the absence of infection.

DIFFERENTIAL DIAGNOSIS. Asthma is easy to recognize in a young patient without comorbid medical conditions who has exacerbating and remitting airway obstruction accompanied by blood eosinophilia. A rapid response to bronchodilator treatment is usually all that is needed to firmly establish the diagnosis. However, in the patient with cryptic episodic shortness of breath, airway challenge testing by a laboratory familiar with this procedure is indicated. Challenge testing performed when airway obstruction is minimal determines the presence and magnitude of airway hyperresponsiveness. In such tests, subjects are exposed to increasing amounts of inhaled bronchoconstrictor agonists or breathe graded levels of cold, dry air. Subjects with asthma usually require smaller amounts of a stimulus to reach a given endpoint in airway response than do nonasthmatic subjects. Airway hyperresponsiveness strongly suggests asthma, although its absence does not exclude asthma as a possibility. However, in the absence of airway hyperresponsiveness, other causes of wheezing, as detailed in Table 51–2, should be investigated.

TREATMENT

The treatment of asthma is directed at airway obstruction and inflammation; resolution of obstruction should be documented by objective measures of airflow obstruction, such as FEV_1 or PEFR. Inexpensive and easy-to-use peak flow meters make the latter measurement feasible in virtually all cases. Treatment of asthma consists of using bronchodilators, anti-inflammatory drugs, specific receptor antagonists, and other agents. The intensity of treatment depends on the severity of disease. It is now well established that asthma is a chronic disease that in all but its mildest forms should be treated chronically. The treatment outlined below for chronic stable asthma is based on the recommendations of both the National Asthma Education Program (US) and the World Health Organization.

BRONCHODILATORS. *Beta-Adrenergic Agents.* Inhaled β-adrenergic agents are the mainstay of bronchodilator treatment for asthma. Constricted airway smooth muscle relaxes when β_2-adrenergic receptors are stimulated. β-Adrenergic agents with varying degrees of β_2 selectivity are available for use in inhaled (by nebulizer or metered-dose inhaler), oral, or parenteral preparations. Patients with very mild asthma (i.e., fewer than three or four attacks of mild severity per year) or with asthma manifesting in known settings (for example, with exercise) may be given treatment on an as-needed basis. This treatment should consist of a moderate-duration β_2 selective inhaler. Two "puffs" from the inhaler separated by a 3- to 5-minute interval are recommended; this interval is thought to allow enough time for the first puff to dilate narrowed airways, thus giving the agent better access to affected areas of the lung. Patients should be instructed to exhale to near residual volume, to breathe in slowly, and to actuate the inhaler as they inspire. Inspiration to near TLC is followed by holding the breath for 5 seconds to allow the smaller aerosol particles to deposit in more peripheral airways. Patients should receive specific instructions in correct inhaler use; careful attention should be paid to female patients, who historically use their inhalers improperly. Aerosol "spacers" are available from many manufacturers for patients who have difficulty coordinating inspiration and inhaler actuation. Patients with mild to moderate disease should use their inhalers only on an as-needed basis. Patients consistently requiring four or more treatments per day with inhaled β agonists should be considered to have asthma of moderate severity and should receive treatment with an inhaled steroid.

Theophylline. Theophylline and aminophylline are bronchodilators of moderate potency that are useful in both inpatient and outpatient management of asthma. The mechanism by which they exert their effects has not been established with certainty but likely is related to the inhibition of certain forms of phosphodiesterase. The utility of theophylline is limited by its toxicity and by wide variations in the rate of its metabolism, both in a single individual over time and among individuals in a population. Because of this variability, monitoring plasma theophylline levels is indicated to ensure that patients are appropriately treated. Acceptable plasma levels for therapeutic effects are between 10 and 20 μg per milliliter; higher levels are associated with gastrointestinal, cardiac, and central nervous system (CNS) toxicity, including symptoms such as anxiety, headache, nausea, vomiting, diarrhea, cardiac arrhythmias, and seizures. The latter catastrophic complications may occur without antecedent mild side effects when plasma levels exceed 20 μg per milliliter. Because of these potentially life-threatening complications of treatment, plasma levels need to be measured very frequently in hospitalized patients receiving intravenous aminophylline and less frequently in stable outpatients receiving one of the long-acting theophylline preparations. Treatment with theophylline is recommended only for patients who are receiving inhaled steroids as a potential treatment to prevent the need for escalation to oral steroid treatment.

ANTI-INFLAMMATORY AGENTS. *Systemic Corticosteroids.* Corticosteroids are widely used and effective to treat moderate to severe asthma. Their mechanism of action in asthma has not been established with certainty but has been linked to the diminished phlogistic potential of the normal cells that reside within the airway and to a reduction in the number of inflammatory cells within the airway.

No consensus exists on the specific type, dose, or duration of corticosteroid to be used in the treatment of asthma. In nonhospitalized patients with asthma refractory to standard therapy, a steroid "pulse" with initial doses of prednisone on the order of 40 to 60 mg per day, tapered to 0 mg over 7 to 14 days, is recommended. For patients who cannot stop taking steroids without having recurrent uncontrolled bronchospasm, alternate-day administration of oral steroids is preferable to daily treatment. For patients whose asthma requires in-hospital treatment but is not considered life-threatening, an initial intravenous bolus of 2 mg per kilogram of hydrocortisone, followed by continuous infusion of 0.5 mg per kilogram per hour, has been shown to be beneficial within 12 hours. In attacks of asthma that are considered life-threatening, intravenous methylprednisolone (125 mg every 6 hours) has been advocated. In each case, as the patient improves, oral steroids are substituted for intravenous steroids and the oral dose is tapered over 1 to 3 weeks; adding inhaled steroids to the regimen when oral steroids are started is strongly recommended.

Inhaled Corticosteroids. Inhaled corticosteroids, which have less systemic impact for a given level of therapeutic effects, are effective therapeutic adjuncts to bronchodilators for moderate to severe asthma. A number of studies have shown that when administering recommended doses of inhaled steroids, it is possible to discontinue treatment with oral steroids in steroid-dependent asthmatic patients. Recent studies have suggested that two to six times the recommended dose of inhaled steroid (i.e., 6 to 20 inhalations twice a day) results in even greater improvement in indices of airflow obstruction and asthmatic symptoms. Adding inhaled steroids to the regimen of any asthmatic patient who has required a course of oral steroids is strongly recommended. The major adverse effect of inhaled steroids at recommended doses is oral thrush. The risk and severity of this complication can be reduced by means of aerosol spacers and good oropharyngeal hygiene. When high doses of inhaled steroids are used, adverse reactions similar to those observed among patients receiving oral steroids may occur; the precise dose at which such reactions begin to be elicited is not known.

Other Anti-Inflammatory Drugs. Disodium chromoglycate is a mast cell membrane–stabilizing agent that is valuable in the prophylaxis of asthma. It is most useful when an identifiable stimulus (such as exercise or allergen exposure) elicits an asthmatic response.

The use of systemic gold (as in rheumatoid arthritis), methotrexate, or cyclosporine has been suggested as adjunctive treatment for patients with severe chronic asthma who cannot otherwise discontinue high-dose corticosteroid treatment. However, these agents are experimental and their routine use is not advocated.

RECEPTOR ANTAGONISTS. *Antihistamines.* Potent H_1 receptor antagonists, such as terfenadine and astemizole, although not widely used for the treatment of asthma, have been shown to produce bronchodilation and to alleviate asthmatic symptoms. They are considered third-line agents for asthma and are used most frequently in patients with a concomitant allergic diathesis.

Anticholinergics. For more than a century, atropine has been known to be useful for treating asthma. It is thought to inhibit the effects of acetylcholine released from the intrapulmonary motor nerves that run in the vagus and innervate airway smooth muscle. The adverse CNS effects of atropine (which limited its utility in the past) have been overcome with the development of ipratropium bromide, now available for use in a metered-dose inhaler. Although ipratropium bromide has a salutary effect on cough in asthma and is useful as an adjunct to inhaled β_2 agonists in chronic stable asthma, it has not been shown to be effective for acute asthmatic bronchospasm.

Other Receptor Antagonists or Mediator Synthesis Inhibitors. Antagonists active at the putative receptor for LTD_4 or inhibitors of 5-lipoxygenase are valuable in chronic stable asthma. These agents are in the late stages of clinical study but are not yet available for clinical use.

SPECIFIC TREATMENT SCENARIOS. *Asthma in the Emergency Room.* When a patient with asthma presents for acute emergency care, objective measures of the severity of the attack, including quantification of pulsus paradoxus and measurement of airflow rates (PEFR or FEV_1), should be evaluated in addition to the usual vital signs. If the PEFR or FEV_1 is <40% of the predicted value but the attack does not appear clinically to be life-threatening, inhaled β_2 agents and intravenous aminophylline (at a dose determined by the patient's previous treatment status) should be given. If the attack is prolonged and fails to respond to treatment with bronchodilators, intravenous steroids (40 to 60 mg methylprednisolone) should be administered. Inhaled treatment should be repeated at 20- to 30-minute intervals until the PEFR or FEV_1 rises to >40% of the predicted values. If this point is not reached within 2 hours, admission to the hospital for further treatment is strongly advocated.

When patients have PEFR and FEV_1 values >60% of the predicted value on admission to the emergency room, treatment with inhaled β_2 agonists alone is likely to result in an objective improvement in airflow rates. If a significant improvement takes place in the emergency room, such patients can usually be treated as outpatients and given inhaled β_2 agonists plus inhaled corticosteroids; the dose of steroids depends on the severity of the attack and the rapidity of its response to treatment.

For patients whose PEFR and FEV_1 are between 40 and 60% of the values predicted at the time of initial evaluation in the emergency care setting, a plan of treatment varying in intensity between the two cited above is indicated. Failure to respond to treatment by objective criteria (PEFR or FEV_1) is an indication for more intense therapy.

Status Asthmaticus. The asthmatic subject whose PEFR or FEV_1 does not increase to >40% of the predicted value with treatment, whose Pa_{CO_2} increases without improvement of indices of airflow obstruction, or who develops major complications such as pneumothorax or pneumomediastinum should be admitted to the hospital for close monitoring. Frequent treatments with inhaled β agonists, intravenous aminophylline (at doses yielding maximal plasma levels), and high-dose intravenous steroids are indicated. Oxygen should be administered by face mask or nasal cannula to yield Sa_{O_2} values between 92 and 94%; a higher FI_{O_2} promotes absorption atelectasis. If there is objective evidence of an infection, give appropriate treatment for that infection. If no improvement occurs with treatment and respiratory failure appears imminent, bronchodilator treatment should be intensified to the maximum tolerated by the patient. If indicated, tracheal intubation and mechanical ventilation can be instituted; in this case the goal should be to provide a level of ventilation just adequate to sustain life but not sufficient to normalize arterial blood gases. For example, a Pa_{CO_2} of 50 to 60 Torr is acceptable for a patient in status asthmaticus.

The Pregnant Asthmatic. Asthma may be exacerbated, remain unchanged, or remit during pregnancy. There need not be substantial departures from the ordinary management of an asthmatic during pregnancy. However, no unnecessary medications should be administered; systemic steroids should be used sparingly to avert fetal complications, and certain drugs should be avoided, including tetracycline (as a treatment for intercurrent infection), atropine and atropine-like drugs (which may cause fetal tachycardia), terbutaline (which is contraindicated during active labor because of its tocolytic effects), and iodine-containing mucolytics such as SSKI. Moreover, use of prostaglandin $F_{2\alpha}$ as an abortifacient should be avoided in asthmatics.

Guidelines for the management of asthma—a summary. Br Med J 306:776, 1993. *Guidelines for asthma treatment formulated by an expert panel in the United Kingdom.*

Holgate S: Mediator and cytokine mechanisms in asthma. Thorax 48:103, 1993. *A comprehensive review of how inflammatory cells could lead to the asthmatic diathesis.*

McFadden ER, Gilbert IA: Medical progress—asthma. N Engl J Med 327:1928, 1992. *A review comparing inflammatory and mechanical changes in asthma.*

National Asthma Education Program: Guidelines for the Diagnosis and Management of Asthma. Bethesda, Md, US Department of Health and Human Services, 1991. *Guidelines for asthma treatment formulated by an expert panel in the United States.*

52 CHRONIC AIRWAYS DISEASES
*Richard A. Matthay and
Alejandro C. Arroliga*

CHRONIC BRONCHITIS AND EMPHYSEMA

This chapter covers chronic generalized airway disorders that are not the direct result of a "specific" bronchopulmonary disease. Common to most of these diseases is chronic airways obstruction, caused most frequently by a diffuse involvement of peripheral (small) airways or, more rarely, by localized obstruction of central (large) airways. The designation *chronic obstructive pulmonary disease* (COPD) is an imperfect, although widely used, term because it includes several specific disorders with different clinical manifestations, pathologic findings, therapy requirements, and prognoses.

Four *diffuse* airway disorders are examined in this chapter: simple chronic bronchitis, asthmatic bronchitis, chronic obstructive bronchitis, and emphysema. Some classifications include all of these entities in the broad term COPD. Moreover, various combinations of these disorders coexist; for instance, patients often have chronic obstructive bronchitis as well as emphysema. Localized airways obstruction, above and below the tracheal bifurcation, is discussed in a separate section of this chapter.

DEFINITIONS OF TERMS. Unfortunately, *chronic bronchitis* has been used variably to refer to a simple smoker's cough or, as in the British literature, to severe COPD. To reduce ambiguity, in this discussion, chronic bronchitis is considered "simple," "obstructive," or "asthmatic," and thus these three terms are applied. It is useful clinically to differentiate between the extremely common simple chronic bronchitis and the less common but often devastating form, chronic obstructive bronchitis. These two entities are therefore described in separate sections.

Simple chronic bronchitis, a syndrome characterized primarily by a chronic productive cough, is the result of low-grade exposure to bronchial irritants in an individual without hyperreactive airways. This syndrome is associated with enhanced mucus secretion, reduced ciliary activity, and impaired resistance to bronchial infection. Simple chronic bronchitis is defined in clinical terms: (1) excessive production of mucus; (2) presence of symptoms, largely cough, on most days for at least 3 months annually during 2 or more successive years; and (3) exclusion of bronchiectasis, tuberculosis, or other causes of these symptoms. The term does not describe the underlying process, which may vary widely. Chronic obstructive bronchitis, which develops in a relatively small proportion

TABLE 52–1. FEATURES OF THE EMPHYSEMATOUS AND BRONCHIAL TYPES OF COPD

	Emphysematous (Type A)	Bronchial (Type B)
Clinical features		
Dyspnea	Insidious onset, slowly progressive	Often noted first only during chest infections
Sputum	Usually scant and mucoid	Often copious and purulent
Weight loss	Often marked	Usually slight or absent
Chronic cor pulmonale with heart failure	Infrequent until terminal stages of the disease	Common
Chest examination	Quiet chest (except slight wheeze at end expiration), marked hyperinflation	Noisy chest, slight hyperinflation
Chest radiograph	Hyperlucent, overinflated lung; often regional attenuation of vessels	Often evidence of old inflammatory disease
Physiologic tests		
Total lung capacity	Increased	Normal or slightly decreased
Residual volume	Markedly increased	Moderately increased
Lung compliance, static	Increased	Near normal
Lung compliance, dynamic	Normal or slightly low	Very low
Lung recoil	Markedly reduced	Variable
Inspiratory airways resistance	Normal	Increased
Diffusing capacity	Markedly reduced	Variable
Arterial P_{O_2}	Slight reduction at rest; usually falls with exertion	Often very low at rest; variable change with exertion
Arterial P_{CO_2}	Usually normal or low	Often chronically elevated
Resting pulmonary artery pressure	Normal or slightly elevated at rest; increases with exertion	Often markedly elevated at rest
Cardiac output	Often low	Usually near normal

From Matthay RA: Chronic airways diseases. *In* Wyngaarden JB, Smith LH Jr, (eds.): Cecil Textbook of Medicine. 18th ed. Philadelphia, WB Saunders, 1988, p 411.

of individuals with simple chronic bronchitis, results in irreversible narrowing of airways. Because the obstruction is in bronchioles and bronchi ≤ 2 mm in diameter, the term *small airways disease* has been used.

Exposure to bronchial irritants in individuals with hyperreactive, or "twitchy," airways can lead to bronchospasm (i.e., bronchial smooth muscle constriction), frequently accompanied by excessive mucus production and edema of bronchial walls. Recurrent episodes of symptomatic bronchospasm are called *asthma* (see Ch. 51). The present discussion must consider bronchospasm because a degree of reversible airways obstruction often accompanies other reactions to inhaled noxious agents. In fact, episodic airways obstruction is common in individuals with chronic bronchitis. This combination, called *asthmatic bronchitis,* may closely resemble classic asthma. The term *chronic asthmatic bronchitis* is applied in patients with persistent airways obstruction, a chronic productive cough, and a major problem of episodic bronchospasm.

Emphysema, another lung response to noxious stimuli, is characterized by abnormal, permanent enlargement of air spaces distal to the terminal bronchioles, accompanied by destruction of their walls, and without obvious fibrosis. The alterations in emphysema reduce lung elastic recoil, which permits excessive airway collapse upon expiration and leads to irreversible airflow obstruction.

These definitions are not mutually exclusive; there is considerable crossover between the emphysematous (type A) and bronchial (type B) findings listed in Table 52–1. For example, most individuals with emphysema also have a chronic productive cough. It may be difficult to determine the relative importance of emphysema and chronic obstructive bronchitis, with obliteration of small airways. Accordingly, general terms such as *COPD* have been used to describe this clinical syndrome.

PATHOPHYSIOLOGY OF AIRWAYS OBSTRUCTION. Airways obstruction denotes slowing of forced expiration. As outlined in Ch. 50, the speed of forced expiration is determined primarily by three factors: intrinsic resistance of the airways, compressibility of the airways, and lung elastic recoil. Reduced maximal expiratory flow ($\dot{V}max$) results from high airways resistance, reduced lung recoil, and/or excessive airways collapsibility.

In general, a low FEV_1/FVC* ratio indicates airflow obstruction; the amount of reduction in FEV_1 itself establishes the severity of the obstruction (Fig. 52–1). Some prefer to use $FEF_{25-75\%}$, the average flow over the middle half of a forced expiration.

Actual $\dot{V}max$ values have been measured, commonly at 50% or

75% of the forced expired volume ($\dot{V}max_{50\%}$ or $\dot{V}max_{75\%}$, respectively*). $\dot{V}max_{75\%}$ has become popular in epidemiologic studies because it appears to be more sensitive than the FEV_1.

In clinical practice, FEV_1 is used more widely because it is easy to measure, is quite reproducible, has a relatively narrow normal range, and reflects the clinical severity of disease.

A variety of physiologic abnormalities are associated with obstructive airways disorders (also discussed in Ch. 50). Increased venous admixture and hypoxemia develop owing to ventilation-perfusion mismatching. Unless there is an increase in overall ventilation, this mismatching may also lead to increased physiologic dead space and hypercapnia. Carbon dioxide retention is likely when airways obstruction is severe, respiratory muscles become fatigued, and the drive to breathe is depressed. Air trapping and an increase in residual volume develop because obstructed airways tend to close prematurely during a maximal exhalation. In emphysema, total lung capacity may be enhanced as well. The pulmonary diffusing capacity measurement is usually reduced in emphysema owing to loss of functioning alveolar-capillary membrane surface area.

Because of the large total cross-sectional diameter of the small airways, marked alterations are required to produce discernible changes in the FEV_1 values. Several potentially more sensitive tests have been proposed to detect mild abnormalities of the small airways: closing volume, helium response of the maximal expiratory flow volume (MEFV) curve, and frequency dependence of compliance. Although these tests are not used routinely, they may prove useful in research studies for detecting subclinical disease.

---

* Because use of these symbols has caused confusion, it has been suggested that $\dot{V}max_{50\%}$ and $\dot{V}max_{75\%}$ be expressed as $FEF_{50\%}$ and $FEF_{75\%}$, respectively. Moreover, $\dot{V}max_{75\%}$ as defined herein has sometimes been reported as $\dot{V}max_{25\%}$, the 25% referring to the portion of the FVC remaining when the flow measurement is made.

Burrows B: Airways obstructive diseases: Pathogenetic mechanisms and natural histories of the disorders. An overview of obstructive lung disease. Med Clin North Am 74:547, 1990. *This is the lead article of an 18-chapter symposium on obstructive lung diseases. The entire symposium is recommended reading and an excellent source of original references.*

Fishman AP: The spectrum of chronic obstructive disease of the airways. *In* Fishman AP (ed.): Pulmonary Diseases and Disorders. 2nd ed. New York, McGraw-Hill, 1988, p 1159. *A concise, clearly written description of the different types of airways obstructive disorders and how they overlap.*

Snider GL, Kleinerman J, Thurlbeck WM, et al.: The definition of emphysema. Am Rev Respir Dis 132:182, 1985. *Succinct statement of the definition, anatomic subtypes, and clinical diagnosis of emphysema.*

Thurlbeck WM: Pathophysiology of chronic obstructive pulmonary disease. Clin Chest Med 11:389, 1990. *Overview of pathophysiology associated with airways obstruction.*

---

* FEV_1 = forced expiratory volume in 1 second; FVC = forced vital capacity; FEF = forced expiratory flow.

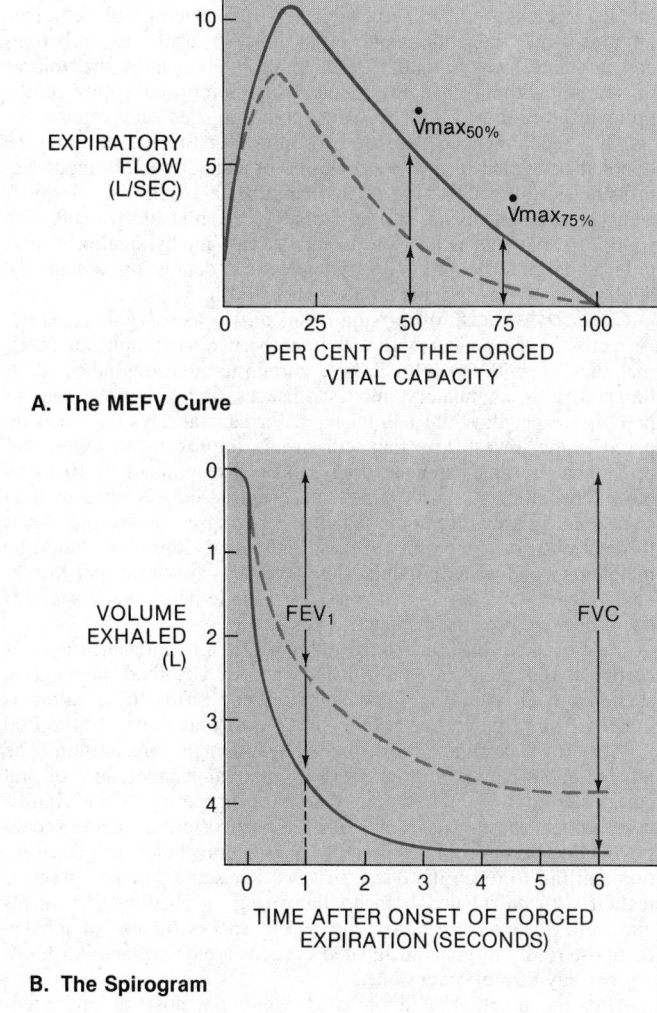

A. The MEFV Curve

EXPIRATORY FLOW (L/SEC)

Vmax$_{50\%}$
Vmax$_{75\%}$

PER CENT OF THE FORCED VITAL CAPACITY

B. The Spirogram

VOLUME EXHALED (L)

FEV$_1$ FVC

TIME AFTER ONSET OF FORCED EXPIRATION (SECONDS)

FIGURE 52–1. Solid lines are used to show a normal maximal expiratory flow-volume (MEFV) in *A* and a normal spirogram in *B*. Broken lines indicate typical curves for a patient with mild airways obstruction. Measurements of the forced vital capacity (FVC), the forced expiratory volume at 1 second (FEV$_1$), and forced flow rates at 50% and 75% of the FVC V̇max$_{50\%}$ and V̇max$_{75\%}$) are depicted as vertical lines. (Adapted from Burrows B: Chronic airways disease. *In* Wyngaarden JM, Smith LH Jr [eds.]: Cecil Textbook of Medicine. 17th ed. Philadelphia, WB Saunders, 1988, p. 412.)

Simple Chronic Bronchitis and Asthmatic Bronchitis

PREVALENCE AND PATHOGENESIS. "Simple chronic bronchitis" refers to a productive cough for at least 3 months of the year for 2 consecutive years. It affects 10 to 25% of the adult population. Cough with sputum production is more common in men than in women and more common in persons over the age of 40 than in younger individuals. All forms of chronic bronchitis are strongly linked to cigarette smoking. Thus, a large proportion of cigarette smokers, particularly those over age 45, fit the diagnostic criteria for simple chronic bronchitis. Some occupations (e.g., those involving dust, handling grain, and mining) are associated with an abnormally high incidence of chronic bronchitis, even after statistics are corrected for smoking habits. Few individuals with simple chronic bronchitis consult a physician, and then the visit is usually prompted by acute or recurrent respiratory tract infections or wheezing in addition to chronic cough. *Chronic asthmatic bronchitis* tends to develop in elderly individuals; most commonly, they are smokers.

Three direct effects of inhaling bronchial irritants cause chronic bronchitis: (1) stimulation of mucus secretion in the airways, (2) impaired mucus clearance due in part to interference with ciliary activity, and (3) lowered resistance to bronchopulmonary infection because of disturbed alveolar macrophage function. Cough de-

velops owing to accumulation of secretions. As a result of bacterial colonization by organisms usually found in the nasopharynx, normally sterile bronchi now harbor organisms.

Although cigarette smoking is the most important of the identifiable causes, not all smokers experience mucus hypersecretion, and no more than 15 to 20% develop airflow obstruction. Little is known about why susceptibility to hypersecretion and airflow obstruction varies in smokers or why reversible airways obstruction develops in many patients with chronic bronchitis. Retention of secretions may be a major factor in some instances. Immunologic factors and other mediators of bronchoconstriction may play a role because some patients have bronchospasm resembling classic asthma.

Occupational exposure to an irritant agent causes chronic bronchitis. Exposure to dust, gases, or fumes at the workplace may be associated with productive cough and inflammatory changes in the airways. Evidence of obstructive airways disease may be present with prolonged exposure (see Ch. 54.1).

PATHOLOGY. Enlarged mucous glands in the large airways, the most characteristic abnormality, is primarily due to increased numbers of their constituent cells (hyperplasia) rather than to enlargement of cells (hypertrophy). Retained bronchial secretions and variable degrees of inflammatory changes in the bronchial walls are also identified. Narrowing or obliteration of some small airways, increased mucus in these airways, and scattered centrilobular emphysema may be found, even though clinically significant obstruction is absent. Because asymptomatic smokers may have similar small airways and emphysematous changes, it is unclear whether these alterations are related to simple chronic bronchitis, except through a common association with cigarette smoking.

CLINICAL MANIFESTATIONS. When the disease is mild, *cough* occurs when the patient arises or usually after he/she smokes the first cigarette of the day. The cough produces a small amount of mucoid sputum and occurs most regularly in the winter months. As the severity increases, the patient coughs throughout the day, symptoms are present throughout the year, sputum volume increases, and episodes of severe coughing develop. Near the end of a severe paroxysm of coughing, wheezing may occur, probably owing to cough-induced bronchospasm. Lying down may induce wheezing, which is probably caused by retained secretions, for cough often provides relief.

Symptoms associated with purulent sputum, suggesting overgrowth of bacteria, may reappear after a viral respiratory infection. *Haemophilus influenzae* and *Streptococcus pneumoniae* may be present, but sputum cultures usually show normal nasopharyngeal flora.

Bacterial organisms probably represent secondary pathogens rather than the primary cause of these exacerbations of symptoms. During exacerbations, various degrees of bronchospasm may also develop, blurring the distinction between such episodes and asthma. Whereas *blood-streaked sputum* is noted occasionally, severe or repeated hemoptysis may indicate a more serious entity, such as a pulmonary neoplasm.

The sputum may become chronically purulent as the disorder progresses, and the term *mucopurulent bronchitis* may be applied at this stage of the disease. Rarely, drug-resistant organisms (e.g., *Pseudomonas aeruginosa*) are identified on sputum cultures, especially if the patient has received multiple antibiotics.

In mild disease, the physical examination may be normal. As the disease advances, variable coarse crackles, which may clear or change location with coughing, and scattered wheezes are heard. A forced expiratory maneuver often induces a wheeze or a paroxysm of coughing.

If reversible airways obstruction is present, the patient may resemble the typical asthmatic person, with wheezing and slowing of forced expiration as prominent features.

LABORATORY FINDINGS. The chest radiograph and the blood cell counts are all normal in the uncomplicated case. Leukocytes and a mixed flora of organisms are noted on sputum examination. Although spirometry often shows some slowing of forced expiration, flow rates may be normal in simple bronchitis. Individuals with *chronic asthmatic bronchitis* may have severe airways obstruction even between acute attacks. During episodes of bronchospasm in patients with asthmatic bronchitis, functional abnormalities are more severe, and both blood and sputum eosinophilia may be present.

COURSE AND PROGNOSIS. In patients with simple chronic bronchitis, symptoms may fluctuate widely. Increased cigarette use, inclement weather, and acute respiratory infections all tend to enhance cough and sputum production. Cessation of smoking in mild cases usually leads to disappearance of symptoms. A slight reduction in ventilatory function is common in simple chronic bronchitis, but progressive respiratory insufficiency does not necessarily develop.

The long-term outcome of patients with asthmatic bronchitis is variable. Some patients may become asymptomatic for years after an initial excellent response to therapy, whereas others require progressively more medication to control bronchospasm. Progress to irreversible airways obstruction occurs in at least a few patients despite good medical management.

DIFFERENTIAL DIAGNOSIS. A persistent, productive cough not attributable to an upper respiratory tract disorder, a specific endobronchial disease, or parenchymal lung disease justifies the diagnosis of chronic bronchitis. A chest radiograph is required to exclude a parenchymal lesion. Moreover, physicians should carefully examine the upper airway, and physical findings, such as a persistent, localized wheeze, must be sought to identify a localized airways disorder. Cystic fibrosis must be excluded in children and in young adults who have severe symptoms of chronic bronchitis (see Ch. 58). In addition, in individuals with one of the rare immotile cilia syndromes, symptoms of chronic bronchitis may be noted (see Ch. 58).

When there is no identifiable source of chronic bronchial irritation, the diagnosis of simple chronic bronchitis should be made with caution. Sputum and blood eosinophilia should be sought in a nonsmoking patient whose symptoms are associated with exposure to allergens or in a patient with episodes of combined wheezing and dyspnea. Asthmatic bronchitis, which may respond to bronchodilators or corticosteroids, is suggested by high eosinophil levels.

Bronchoscopy or a computed tomography (CT) scan of the chest may be indicated to rule out an endobronchial lesion or localized bronchiectasis in patients with severe or repeated hemoptysis or with physical findings suggesting localized disease. In the routine case, these procedures are not indicated.

Severe mucopurulent bronchitis may be difficult to distinguish from bronchiectasis. In fact, in persons with severe bronchitis, the bronchi may show mild, diffuse, cylindrical dilatation. Saccular bronchiectasis is suggested by (1) repeated pneumonias in the same lung zone, (2) honeycombed areas on the chest radiograph, and (3) recurrent hemoptysis. Bronchography provides an accurate diagnosis but is invasive and is indicated only if resection of the bronchiectatic area or areas is considered. High-resolution CT scan of the chest is a noninvasive technique with a high sensitivity and specificity to diagnose localized and diffuse bronchiectasis.

TREATMENT. Smoking cessation is mandatory, and physicians must offer counseling about currently available smoking cessation strategies. Other bronchial irritants should be removed because this step alone may relieve symptoms. If the symptoms persist after the maximal effort to avoid provoking factors, the following measures are applied.

Antibiotic Therapy. Infection is considered present when the patient is producing a noneosinophilic, purulent sputum. A 7- to 10-day course of tetracycline, double-strength sulfamethoxazole-trimethoprim, or erythromycin or amoxicillin-clavula irate should be administered. If this antibiotic therapy fails to clear the sputum, a sputum culture and sensitivity tests are warranted. Successive doses of different antibiotics should be avoided because this may lead to resistant flora.

The antibiotic may have to be changed on the basis of drug susceptibility studies when resistant organisms are cultured from the sputum. (For severe, purulent exacerbations, penicillin has proved to be inadequate therapy.)

Bronchodilators. The bronchodilator agents are the mainstays for managing bronchospasm associated with simple chronic bronchitis and for controlling any reversible component of COPD. They are also useful in conjunction with bronchial hygiene therapy, described below. Inhaled bronchodilators have a rapid onset of action and are very effective. Careful instruction about the proper technique for using inhalers is necessary. β-Adrenergic agonists have been the mainstay of treating COPD for years and are useful in re-

lieving bronchospasm. Oral β-adrenergic agonists have a high incidence of side effects and are used only if patients are unable to use inhaled agents. Anticholinergic agents—ipratropium and nebulized atropine—are bronchodilators efficacious in acute exacerbations and in stable patients with COPD. Ipratropium reduces the volume of sputum without changing its viscosity. Ipratropium may be the optimal, basic drug for COPD and should be used on a regular basis. The recommended dose of two puffs four times a day may be doubled or tripled to achieve maximal bronchodilation without significant side effects. Using methylxanthine in COPD is controversial, yet these agents are still commonly used in stable patients with COPD. In patients with acute exacerbations, methylxanthines offer only a marginal benefit. The principles and details for therapeutic application of these agents are described in Ch. 51.

Corticosteroids. When significant airways obstruction persists or recurs in the patient with asthmatic bronchitis in spite of maximal therapy with bronchodilators, corticosteroids are indicated. If the patient is ambulatory, modest dosages (e.g., 20 to 40 mg of prednisone per day) are administered for several days and then tapered to the lowest dose that will sustain improvement. Often, improvement is rapid, and the drug can be discontinued in 10 to 14 days. Thereafter, a short "burst" of corticosteroids is used to treat occasional relapses. In some patients, tapering corticosteroids leads to recurrence of symptoms. In these individuals, the dose should be maintained as low as possible to relieve bronchospasm and to prevent recurrent attacks. Alternate-day single-dose corticosteroids should be used for maintenance if possible.

Once bronchospasm has been relieved and a maintenance dose of corticosteroid achieved, an inhaled, poorly absorbed preparation such as beclomethasone should be added. This medication is inhaled from a pressurized container, two to four puffs (100 to 200 μg) two to four times daily, depending upon the preparation. The inhaled agent may permit reduction in the maintenance dose of oral corticosteroid without recurrence of bronchospasm. When significant bronchospasm is present, inhaled corticosteroid agents should be avoided because this medication may aggravate bronchoconstriction and fail to reach the distal airways. For some patients, premedication with an inhaled bronchodilator (e.g., a β-adrenergic agent) may relieve airway irritation and permit successful use of inhaled corticosteroids. In general, inhaled corticosteroids replace 7.5 to 10 mg per day of oral prednisone.

After the addition of an inhaled agent, the dose of oral prednisone should be reduced slowly (over several months) to avoid adrenal insufficiency in a corticosteroid-dependent patient who has received months or years of systemic medication. In up to 30% of patients, oropharyngeal candidiasis occurs because of inhaled corticosteroids. This condition responds, however, to specific therapy and rarely requires discontinuation of the inhaled preparation.

Bronchial Hygiene. These measures are designed to clear retained bronchial secretions. Deep breathing followed by deliberate coughing is the most important maneuver. Sputum production may be more effective if the most involved lung regions are in the superior position (postural drainage) and chest percussion and vibration are applied.

Bronchial hygiene measures may be better tolerated and more effective if the patient is premedicated with an inhaled bronchodilator and then inhales a bland mist to loosen secretions. Although some patients are convinced of its efficacy, objective benefits of bland mist therapy have been difficult to establish. Because patients' reactions to this therapy vary, and occasionally acute bronchospasm develops, only measures that prove effective should be continued because the full program is uncomfortable and time consuming.

Patients should be encouraged to keep well hydrated. Intravenous fluids may be required for acute exacerbations. Although the efficacy of expectorant medications has not been established, some authorities recommend 10 to 12 drops of a saturated solution of potassium iodide three times daily. This program is associated with a high rate of side effects, some of them severe. Cough syrups and lozenges have little effect on the viscosity of bronchial secretions, but they may relieve a "tickle" in the throat of many persons with bronchitis. Cough sedatives should be used only for acute episodes of a severe, nonproductive cough and are otherwise contraindicated.

Treatment of Severe Exacerbations. Severe exacerbations of asthmatic bronchitis can be life threatening, particularly when associated with severe airways obstruction. The approach to status asthmaticus outlined in Ch. 51 is appropriate, although the patient with asthmatic bronchitis may require more attention to bronchial hygiene measures to clear secretions than does the person with asthma.

Callahan CM, Dittus RS, Katz BP: Oral corticosteroid therapy for patients with stable chronic obstructive pulmonary disease: A meta-analysis. Ann Intern Med 114:216, 1991. *A review of the effectiveness of oral corticosteroids in patients with stable COPD.*

Ferguson GT, Cherniak RM: Management of chronic obstructive pulmonary disease. N Engl J Med 328:1017, 1993. *A complete review of the current management of patients with COPD.*

Fisher EB Jr, Lichtenstein E, Haire-Joshu D, et al.: Methods, successes, and failures of smoking cessation programs. Annu Rev Med 44:481, 1993. *Extensive, lucid review of the addictive and conditioning processes of cigarette smoking and the different types of intervention currently available for smoking cessation.*

Murphy TF, Sethi S: Bacterial infection in chronic obstructive pulmonary disease. Am Rev Respir Dis 146:1067, 1992. *Extensive review of the role of bacterial infection in COPD and current antibiotic therapy.*

Stoller JK, Aboussouan LS: Chronic obstructive lung diseases: emphysema, chronic bronchitis, bronchiectasis, and cystic fibrosis. *In* George RB, Light RW, Matthay MA, et al. (eds.): Chest Medicine. 3rd ed. Baltimore, Williams & Wilkins, 1995. *Comprehensive discussion of the various obstructive lung diseases and their management.*

Chronic Obstructive Bronchitis and Emphysema

PREVALENCE AND PATHOGENESIS. As a major cause of chronic disability in older individuals, chronic obstructive bronchitis and emphysema (COPD) rank behind only heart disease and schizophrenia in the United States. Trends over the past two decades suggest a 60% increase in the prevalence of COPD. This disease is the fourth leading cause of death in the United States, and there has been an increase in the death rate from this condition over the past 20 years. Approximately 75,000 individuals per year die of COPD in the United States, approximately one half the number of persons dying annually of lung cancer.

Emphysema is common, and its incidence increases with age. Death rates from emphysema peak in the 75 to 84 age group.

Chronic obstructive pulmonary disease is usually diagnosed in people between the ages of 55 and 65. The greater incidence in men than in women most likely reflects the lower incidence of smoking in women in earlier decades. Recent trends, however, show that more teenage girls than boys are starting to smoke. Thus, in several decades COPD may be as common, or more common, in women.

Smoking. Patients with COPD have some combination of chronic obstructive bronchitis and pulmonary emphysema, both of which are closely associated with cigarette smoking. Longitudinal studies confirm a dose-response relationship between cigarette smoking and the rate of pulmonary function decline in patients with COPD. The chronic, progressive destruction of the alveolar structures characteristic of emphysema is thought to occur because of an imbalance between the proteases (proteolytic enzymes) and antiproteases in the lower respiratory tract. According to this concept, proteases, particularly polymorphonuclear neutrophil (PMN) elastase and elastases in pulmonary alveolar macrophages (PAM's), work unimpeded to destroy alveolar structures and their elastin network. Cigarette smokers have increased numbers of PAM's, and PMN's are recruited into their lungs, so that increased numbers of both cell types are recoverable on bronchoalveolar lavage. Recruitment of PMN's into the lungs may occur as a result of the elaboration of chemotactic factors by PAM's stimulated by cigarette smoke. Moreover, smoke components can cause elastase to be released by PMN's by inducing cytotoxic reactions and by stimulating secretion from viable cells. Macrophages exposed to cigarette smoke *in vitro* or *in vivo* increase secretion of an elastase-like enzyme. This potential for a greatly increased protease (primarily elastase) burden must be counteracted by the antiprotease defense system of the lungs.

The protease-antiprotease theory of the pathogenesis of emphysema has received further support from the recognition that patients with severe (homozygous phenotype) α_1-antitrypsin deficiency have markedly reduced levels of serum α_1-antitrypsin and progressive panacinar emphysema. As might be expected, when studied by bronchoalveolar lavage, patients with severe α_1-antitrypsin deficiency have little or no α_1-antitrypsin in their lower respiratory tracts. Nor do they have alternate antiprotease protection against neutrophil elastase.

Severe genetic deficiency of serum α_1-antitrypsin occurs in 0.5 to 2% of patients with COPD. Typically, in such individuals, emphysema is likely to develop by age 40 in smokers and by age 60 in nonsmokers. Prolonged exposure to irritants, primarily cigarette smoke, induces recruitment of PMN's and PAM's that liberate elastases, causing destruction of the lung parenchyma.

Compared with nonsmokers, cigarette smokers without α_1-antitrypsin deficiency also show reduced elastase inhibitory capacity because of inactivation of α_1-proteinase inhibitor (alpha$_1$-PI). Chemical oxidation of alpha$_1$-PI by material in cigarette smoke is postulated as a major cause of the observed decrease in elastase inhibitory capacity. Smoking may interfere with elastin repair mechanisms, as documented by studies both *in vivo* and *in vitro*.

The protease-antiprotease hypothesis of the pathogenesis of emphysema does not readily explain all of the observations in experimental and human emphysema. For instance, experimental enzyme-induced emphysema is panacinar rather than centrilobular, the more common type in humans with chronic airflow obstruction. Further, it does not explain the predominant localization of centrilobular emphysema to the upper lung zones or of panacinar emphysema to the lung bases or of paraseptal emphysema to the regions beneath the pleura and adjacent to fibrous septa. A close relationship exists between slowing of forced exhalation and cigarette smoking. The average heavy smoker has a 38- to 59-ml per year decline in FEV$_1$, whereas the average nonsmoking adult shows a decline of only 29- to 37-ml per year. Nonsmokers with α_1-antitrypsin deficiency have approximately an 80-ml per year decline in FEV$_1$; cigarette smokers with this deficiency have approximately a 150-ml per year decline. When individuals with α_1-antitrypsin deficiency stop smoking, this excess rate of decline in FEV$_1$ ceases. Nevertheless, the average effect of cigarette smoking alone does not explain the more severe reduction in FEV$_1$ noted in patients with COPD. Moreover, why is it that only a minority of smokers develop clinically significant COPD? Some individuals may be particularly susceptible for various reasons: respiratory disorders in childhood, intercurrent respiratory infections, and genetic factors, for example.

Can COPD be detected early by screening lung function in young to middle-aged adults? Longitudinal studies are attempting to identify susceptible cigarette-smoking individuals with an excessive rate of decline in pulmonary function throughout adult life. The hypothesis is that the individual who will develop COPD later in life should be identifiable by age 40 because he/she will show at least a mild ventilatory abnormality by then. There is no direct evidence yet, however, that any physiologic test applied early in life detects the individual who will develop disabling COPD.

Alpha$_1$-Antitrypsin Deficiency. A deficiency in serum antiproteolytic activity associated with a susceptibility to COPD has been noted in several families. The protease inhibitor, or "Pi," phenotype of the subject determines the serum's trypsin inhibitory capacity. Two M genes (Pi MM phenotype) are present in normal individuals. When only Z genes are present (Pi ZZ phenotype), serum α_1-antitrypsin levels are severely reduced (< 15 mg per deciliter, 7 μM), and the α_1-antitrypsin that is present in plasma is less effective in inhibiting neutrophil elastase than the α_1-antitrypsin in individuals with the Pi MM phenotype. Patients with the Null variants, in which there is no measurable serum protein inhibitor, have 100% risk of developing emphysema by age 30. Deficiency of α_1-antitrypsin is transmitted as a codominantly autosomal recessive trait. This antiproteolytic deficiency, present in approximately 1 in 4000 of the population, is associated with neonatal hepatitis and the development of emphysema in the third, fourth, and fifth decades. Present in 3 to 5% of the population, the heterozygotic state (Pi MZ phenotype) is associated with a moderately reduced serum antiproteolytic activity, but no predilection for developing an excess of respiratory disorders. Several other Pi genes have been identified (of which S is the most common), but only the Z gene clearly leads to COPD. In Ch. 121 the hepatic manifestations of α_1-antitrypsin deficiency are discussed.

PATHOLOGY. Alveolar wall destruction with a nonuniform pattern of enlarged air spaces is the basic abnormality in emphysema. The orderly appearance of the acinus and its components is disturbed and may be lost, as air spaces are fewer in number but enlarged. In centrilobular emphysema, the process is most severe in the central portion of the lobule, whereas in panacinar emphysema, the defect occurs uniformly throughout the acinus. Both centrilobular and panacinar emphysema may be noted in the same lung. In severe centrilobular emphysema, the entire acinus may ultimately become involved. Centrilobular emphysema generally is the most common form of emphysema in patients with chronic airflow obstruction caused by smoking. Panacinar emphysema is generally associated with α_1-antitrypsin deficiency.

In large airways, inflammation is noted in and around air passages, with narrowing of the lumina, impaction of mucus, and obliterative changes. Abnormalities of the small airways are usually not obvious on cursory examination and require careful morphometric studies.

CLINICAL MANIFESTATIONS. Dyspnea is usually the predominant complaint, but some patients consult a physician initially because of cough, wheezing, recurrent respiratory infections, or, occasionally, weakness or weight loss. Patients may date the onset of chronic symptoms to an acute respiratory infection. In some, shortness of breath is present only during acute exacerbations.

A productive cough is usually present, associated with a thick or "sticky" sputum varying widely in quantity. Copious amounts of purulent sputum, coupled with a severe cough, are noted by some patients.

The physical examination may yield normal findings early in the illness. Auscultation of the chest may reveal rhonchi, or the chest may be quiet, particularly in patients with extensive emphysema. Wheezing, which may be absent on quiet breathing, can often be heard on forced exhalation. As the disease progresses, marked hyperinflation with low diaphragm and a reduced area of cardiac dullness are common. Labored breathing, at times through pursed lips, may be noted after minimal exertion or even at rest. Patients tend to lean forward on their elbows when sitting, assuming a stooped posture, while using accessory muscles of respiration. Cyanosis and dependent edema may be noted.

Occasionally, patients first seek medical attention when signs of right ventricular failure due to cor pulmonale appear. In such cases, the FEV_1 is likely to be below 1 liter and the arterial Po_2 below 45 mm Hg. The pulmonary hypertension in these patients with COPD and cor pulmonale is most closely related to the severity of hypoxemia.

Table 52–1 shows features of relatively distinctive COPD clinical syndromes and their associated underlying pathologic conditions. These two clinical types of COPD, emphysematous (type A) and bronchial (type B), represent extremes of presentation; most individuals, if followed chronically, develop a mixture of findings from the type A and type B groups. Type A patients, described as "pink puffers," often hyperventilate, maintaining a normal or nearly normal arterial O_2 tension. In contrast, type B patients, "blue bloaters," often have a low arterial O_2 tension, high CO_2 tension, cyanosis, and right-sided congestive heart failure. The "blue bloater" syndrome may also result from disordered breathing during sleep, a common problem in patients with COPD.

LABORATORY FINDINGS. The routine blood count and differential study are normal except for erythrocytosis in some COPD patients with hypoxemia. When eosinophilia is found, a reversible (asthmatic-bronchitic) component of the disease should be suspected.

Early in the disease, the chest radiograph may be normal; however, in severe emphysema, lung hyperinflation and an increased retrosternal air space, with flattening of the diaphragm and regional attenuation of blood vessels, are usually noted. Frank bullae outlined by hairline margins are present in some cases. The chest radiograph should not be the sole basis for the diagnosis of COPD, for individuals with perfectly normal lung function may have radiographic findings suggesting the disease. Chest CT has been used to determine with accuracy the presence of emphysema and to quantify its severity.

Persistent reduction in FEF rates is the most typical finding in COPD. The residual volume and the ratio of residual volume to total lung capacity, are elevated. When the diffusing capacity is very depressed and the total lung capacity is clearly increased, emphysema is likely to be extensive. Ventilation-perfusion mismatch and nonuniformity of ventilation are also typical findings, whereas arterial hypoxemia and physiologic shunting vary among patients.

Ventilation-perfusion lung scans should be interpreted cautiously when pulmonary emboli are suspected. These scans reveal the uneven ventilation and perfusion typical of COPD. Areas of diminished perfusion may be mistaken for pulmonary emboli. Accord-

ingly, when pulmonary embolism is suspected in a patient with COPD, a pulmonary angiogram is often required for definitive diagnosis.

The electrocardiogram tends to be normal, particularly early in the course of the disease. Later, the axis is shifted to the right, and there are early R waves in the precordial leads V_1 and V_2 and net negative electrical forces in leads V_5 and V_6. Especially during exacerbations, peaked P waves ("P pulmonale") are present. Unfortunately, these changes do not correlate well with pulmonary artery hypertension and cor pulmonale. The presence of R waves over the right precordium is the most reliable indication of cor pulmonale.

COURSE AND PROGNOSIS. Initially, the response to bronchodilator therapy is variable, depending on the degree of bronchospasm. Thereafter, the disease progresses slowly, with an annual average decrement in FEV_1 of 50 to 75 ml. Because the variability in FEV_1 may be greater than the true annual decline, a follow-up of several years is required to determine the rate of loss of lung function. If the patient stops smoking, cough and sputum production may cease. However, most other symptoms progress gradually.

In terms of absolute FEV_1, patients are dyspneic upon moderate exertion when the value is 1.2 to 1.5 liters; they are forced to be relatively sedentary at 1.0 liter; and they are often invalids when the FEV_1 is ≤ 500 ml. As the FEV_1 drops below 1 liter, severe arterial hypoxemia, hypercapnia, and cor pulmonale are often evident.

Median survival varies considerably. Despite initially very low FEV_1 values, some individuals live 12 to 15 years. Generally, however, when the FEV_1 is more than 1.2 liters, patients survive about 10 years; when the FEV_1 is 1.0 liter, survival is approximately 5 years; and when the FEV_1 is < 700 ml, survival is about 2 years. Signs of a poor prognosis include a low FEV_1, a resting tachycardia, severe arterial hypoxemia or hypercapnia or both, and evidence of cor pulmonale. If a patient resides at altitudes higher than 3500 feet, longevity is reduced.

Increased cough and dyspnea are hallmarks of periodic worsening of the disease. Symptoms characteristically occur after an acute respiratory infection and may be accompanied by bronchospasm. Such exacerbations in patients with severe COPD may be life threatening and may lead to acute respiratory failure as well as right ventricular failure. The latter occurs secondary to pronounced increases in pulmonary artery pressure and pulmonary vascular resistance, which, in turn, are due primarily to hypoxic pulmonary vasoconstriction.

DIFFERENTIAL DIAGNOSIS. Three criteria are required to diagnose COPD: (1) The FEV_1 must be reduced, and this reduction must be proportionately more than any lowering in the FVC (i.e., both the predicted percentage of FEV_1 and the FEV_1/FVC ratio must be depressed); (2) in spite of intensive, prolonged medical treatment, this slowing of forced expiration must persist; and (3) other bronchopulmonary disease that might explain the observed physiologic abnormalities must be excluded. Sufficient evidence for the last criterion generally includes absence of extensive parenchymal abnormalities on the chest radiograph and absence of any signs of upper airways obstruction, such as neck mass, stridor, or narrowing of the upper airway seen on the chest radiograph. Irreversibility of the obstructive ventilatory defect may be more difficult to establish. This factor is discussed further in the treatment section.

Assessing the relative contribution of emphysema and intrinsic airway changes can also be difficult. Emphysema is usually severe when the diffusing capacity is very depressed and the chest radiograph shows hyperlucent lungs with attenuated vascular markings. In contrast, if the diffusing capacity is normal or nearly normal, extensive emphysema is unlikely. Esophageal balloon measurements, which are required to assess lung elastic recoil (the best guide to the severity of emphysema), are seldom justified as part of the clinical evaluation.

If there is a family history of emphysema or emphysema-type COPD develops at an early age, a homozygous α_1-antitrypsin deficiency should be considered. Suspicion is heightened when the patient is a nonsmoker or a woman or when the chest radiograph shows a bibasilar distribution of emphysematous changes. Laboratory confirmation is provided by almost complete absence of α_1 globulin, by a markedly reduced serum trypsin inhibitory capacity, and, most specifically, by a ZZ phenotype on crossed immunoelectrophoresis of the serum.

TREATMENT. The following are therapeutic goals in patients with COPD: (1) to relieve the portion of airway obstruction that is reversible; (2) to control cough and sputum production; (3) to eliminate and prevent airway infections; (4) to increase exercise tolerance to the maximum allowable at the individual's level of physiologic deficit; (5) to control remedial disease complications, such as arterial hypoxemia and cardiovascular problems; (6) to avoid smoking and other airway irritants, narcotics and sedatives, and noncritical surgery, all of which aggravate the disease; and (7) to relieve the anxiety and depression of the COPD patient.

Despite treatment, most patients with severe COPD show progressive ventilatory deterioration; yet therapy should not be withheld. A comprehensive therapeutic program can reduce symptoms, decrease the frequency of hospital admissions, prevent premature death, and permit patients to lead a more active and satisfying life. A formal rehabilitation program using a team approach is effective. Nevertheless, good results can also be obtained by a dedicated physician, assisted, perhaps, by an office nurse who can help patients with physical therapy and bronchial hygiene measures.

Initial Treatment. During the initial visit, it is impossible to predict with certainty the degree of reversibility of airways obstruction in a patient with COPD. Therefore, all patients should be considered as having potentially reversible disease. Smoking should be discontinued and other bronchial irritants avoided. Bronchodilators should be administered according to tolerance, as outlined in the therapy for asthmatic bronchitis and asthma. As mentioned in the therapy for simple chronic bronchitis, bronchial hygiene measures and, when indicated by purulent mucus production, antibiotics should be used. In addition, the pneumococcal vaccine and yearly administration of the influenza vaccine are indicated.

The effects of this initial therapy both on symptoms and on pulmonary function test results should be determined and adjustments made in medication to minimize side effects. Apparently ineffective measures (e.g., postural drainage that leads to no symptom relief or sputum production) should be discontinued. Next, if further reversibility of the disease is considered possible, a 3- to 4-week trial of corticosteroids can be initiated. If the acute inhalation of bronchodilator produces a 20% improvement in FEV_1 or if there is a similar increase in FEV_1 several days or weeks after intensive bronchodilator therapy, corticosteroids are likely to be beneficial. Several other findings suggest that corticosteroids may help: (1) a noisy chest or wheeze upon auscultation, (2) sputum or blood eosinophilia, (3) evidence of atopy (e.g., history of hay fever, an elevated serum immunoglobulin E [IgE] level, positive results of allergy skin tests), or (4) associated nasal polyps or vasomotor rhinitis.

Generally, 20 to 40 mg of prednisone daily is given for 3 to 4 weeks, and spirometry tests are used to assess the efficacy of this medication. Other bronchodilators are continued at full doses. If improvement is noted, (e.g., increase in $FEV_1 > 20\%$), the corticosteroid dose should be tapered to the lowest maintenance dose possible, as outlined for asthmatic bronchitis. If there is no significant improvement in FEV_1, corticosteroids should be tapered slowly and discontinued.

Maintenance Therapy. Frequently, objective improvement (i.e., increase in FEV_1) cannot be demonstrated with bronchodilator therapy. Yet inhaled ipratropium and β-adrenergic agents, combined with oral theophylline are recommended to prevent superimposed bronchospasm. In COPD, theophylline can (1) enhance respiratory muscle function, in both the fatigued and the nonfatigued state; (2) augment right and left ventricular systolic pump function while decreasing pulmonary artery pressures and pulmonary vascular resistance (potentially helpful in patients with cor pulmonale); and (3) in some patients, reduce dyspnea. The β-adrenergic agents also improve biventricular systolic pump performance and decrease pulmonary vascular resistance. Whether any of these potentially salutary effects are additive or synergistic when oral theophylline is administered in conjunction with β-adrenergic agents has not been established.

Aerosolized adrenergic agents are also used (1) to relieve acute attacks of dyspnea; (2) prior to exposure to known bronchial irritants, such as cold air; or (3) as a regular part of a bronchial hygiene program.

Those patients with a productive cough, retained secretions, or repeated episodes of bronchopulmonary infection should be treated with the same measures as described for simple chronic bronchitis. In addition, some other forms of treatment are uniquely applicable to patients with COPD.

Physical Therapy. Exercise has not been shown to improve lung function, but it may enhance cardiovascular fitness and train skeletal muscles to function more efficiently, thus increasing exercise tolerance. Accordingly, unless contraindicated by an underlying cardiac abnormality, progressively increasing exercise (usually walking) should be prescribed. In most cases, the program can be recommended directly by the physician, but if the patient is severely disabled, a trained physical therapist can initiate an appropriate exercise program. Arterial blood gas levels should be obtained when the patient is at rest and after exercise, prior to instituting a vigorous exercise program. Supplemental oxygen should be used during exercise if the patient becomes severely hypoxemic. Some patients benefit from vocational rehabilitation and occupational therapy.

Although breathing exercises probably do not alter the usual breathing pattern of COPD, occasionally they are recommended to encourage diaphragmatic breathing. Perhaps it is more useful and more realistic to teach patients slow, deep breathing as a quicker, more effective method for relieving dyspnea than rapid, shallow "panic" breathing. Breath holding should be avoided during exertion. Some authorities recommend inspiratory muscle training by breathing against a graded resistor, although there is little clinical evidence of benefit from respiratory muscle training.

Oxygen Therapy. In some individuals with COPD, there are clear indications for home oxygen therapy. Supplemental oxygen therapy improves survival in patients with COPD and hypoxemia. Survival is best with continuous oxygen (19 to 24 hours) and intermediate with 12 to 15 hours of oxygen per day. Patients should be started on continuous supplemental oxygen if they have persistent hypoxemia at rest ($PaO_2 < 55$ mm Hg, < 88% oxygen saturation). Furthermore, patients with a $PaO_2 < 59$ mm Hg or oxygen saturation < 89% with cor pulmonale or polycythemia or congestive heart failure require continuous oxygen supplement as well. The goal of therapy is to achieve an oxygen saturation > 90%. The need for continuous oxygen supplement should be reevaluated with arterial blood gases after 1, 3, and 6 months of therapy. Oxygen may be administered by nasal cannula, although oxygen-saving devices are available. Transtracheal oxygen therapy is useful when high flows are needed. Supplemental oxygen improves exercise performance, neuropsychological function, and quality of life, and reduces pulmonary artery pressure. It may increase survival in patients who have low oxygen saturation only during sleep.

Environmental Control. All patients with severe COPD should be cautioned to avoid high altitudes, and supplemental oxygen may be required for those with severe hypoxemia when they travel by air. Moreover, COPD patients with severe hypoxemia should reside at altitudes below 4000 feet. A change in residence may be indicated in patients who live in areas with heavy air pollution.

Cold winter climates are avoided by some patients who find relief in either warm desert climates or warm, humid regions. No specific climate has been shown to alter the overall course of the disease. Accordingly, the economic and social hardships of a move should be weighed carefully against the potential symptomatic benefit provided by relocation to a more agreeable climate.

Treatment of Edema and Cor Pulmonale. Even in the absence of frank right-sided congestive heart failure, pedal edema is common, and control is usually obtained with small doses of diuretics. Ankle edema associated with cor pulmonale is more difficult to control, but oxygen combined with careful diuretic administration often suffices. Digitalis is useful for enhancing right ventricular function only if there is concomitant left ventricular failure. Phlebotomy is not required in most oxygen-treated patients but may transiently relieve central nervous system symptoms, especially when the hematocrit is > 60%.

Treatment of Hypercapnia. Chronic hypercapnia is common in late stages of COPD, but it requires no therapy. However, during exacerbations, blood gases must be monitored closely for severe respiratory acidosis, and all narcotics, sedatives, and tranquilizers should be avoided. In patients with stable chronic hypercapnia, mechanically assisted ventilation and respiratory stimulants are unnecessary.

Surgical Therapy. In the absence of significant emphysema (e.g., that manifested by a moderate to severe reduction in diffusing capacity), bullectomy may benefit patients with large bullae compressing normal or nearly normal lung. Careful, detailed preoperative evaluation is required to select suitable candidates for operation. Lung transplantation is increasingly becoming a therapeutic option for selected patients with end-stage emphysema, which is currently the most common indication for single lung transplant. The 3-year survival is 75%.

Supportive Measures. Careful, detailed education of the patient regarding the nature of the disease is essential. The significance of symptoms such as purulent sputum production, potential side effects of medication, and therapeutic goals should be explained. A prompt, prearranged treatment plan for intercurrent exacerbations should be discussed with the patient. Malnutrition is common in patients with COPD, and close attention to the nutritional status is needed.

Replacement Therapy In Severe Alpha₁-Antitrypsin Deficiency Emphysema. Chronic, weekly, biweekly, or monthly replacement therapy with intravenous α_1-antitrypsin concentrate of normal plasma is given to individuals with severe α_1-antitrypsin deficiency who are nonsmokers, older than age 18, and have fixed airflow obstruction. After therapy, serum and bronchoalveolar lavage α_1-antitrypsin levels are elevated to levels that probably have effective antielastase protection. The incidence of adverse reactions after transfusion is low. Fever is the most common side effect in <1% of the patients.

Recently, recombinant DNA methodology has been used to produce α_1-antitrypsin molecules. The future may bring widespread clinical application of this potentially less expensive material administered by intravenous infusion or by inhalation to patients with the PiZZ phenotype.

Treatment of Exacerbations. Antibiotics, increased bronchodilator medications, and even corticosteroids are often indicated for acute exacerbations. Immediate hospitalization is required for severe hypoxemia, increasing CO_2 tension, or congestive heart failure. Ch. 34 and 65 outline the management of decompensated cor pulmonale and acute respiratory failure, respectively. The same management used in patients with status asthmaticus is indicated in COPD patients with superimposed refractory bronchospasm.

Crystal RG, Brantly ML, Hubbard RC, et al.: The alpha ₁-antitrypsin gene and its mutations: Clinical consequences and strategies for therapy. Chest 95:196, 1990.
Patterson GA, Cooper JD: Lung transplantation. Chest Surg Clin North Am 3:1, 1993. *Comprehensive monograph on lung transplantation.*
Salvaterra CG, Rubin LJ: Investigation and management of pulmonary hypertension in chronic obstructive pulmonary disease. Am Rev Respir Dis 148:1414, 1993. *Current review of the management of cor pulmonale.*
Snider GL: Emphysema: The first two centuries and beyond. Part I and II. Am Rev Respir Dis 146:1334, 1615, 1992. *A comprehensive review of the pathogenesis of emphysema.*
Snider GL: Pulmonary disease in alpha₁-antitrypsin deficiency. Ann Intern Med 111:957, 1989. *Succinct, up-to-date statement on the pathogenesis and therapy of lung disease in patients with α₁-antitrypsin deficiency.*
Tiep BL: Long-term home oxygen therapy. Clin Chest Med 11:505, 1990. *Extensive discussion of the rationale of oxygen therapy for patients with COPD.*

LOCALIZED AIRWAYS OBSTRUCTION

Extrinsic compression of airways, intraluminal obstruction, and diseases of the airways themselves all can cause localized airways obstruction. Signs and symptoms depend upon the location of the obstruction and upon whether it is partial or complete, variable or fixed. The discussion of localized lesions is divided into obstructions above and below the bifurcation of the trachea.

Obstruction Above the Tracheal Bifurcation

PARTIAL OBSTRUCTION. Stridor, frequently accompanied by inspiratory retraction of the intercostal spaces, is the principal finding in partial obstruction above the main (tracheal) carina. On both forced inspiration and forced expiration, airflow rates are reduced, and there may be a characteristic appearance to the MEFV curve. As shown in Figure 52–2, the site and nature of the obstruction determine the findings on spirometry. When the obstruction is severe, hypoxemia and hypercapnia may result owing to reduced overall ventilation.

Among the intrinsic airways diseases that can cause partial airways obstruction are (1) tonsil and adenoid enlargement, especially in young children; (2) stenosing lesions secondary to trauma or prolonged or traumatic intubation; (3) neoplams or granulomatous processes (e.g., sarcoidosis, fungi) involving the hypopharynx, lar-

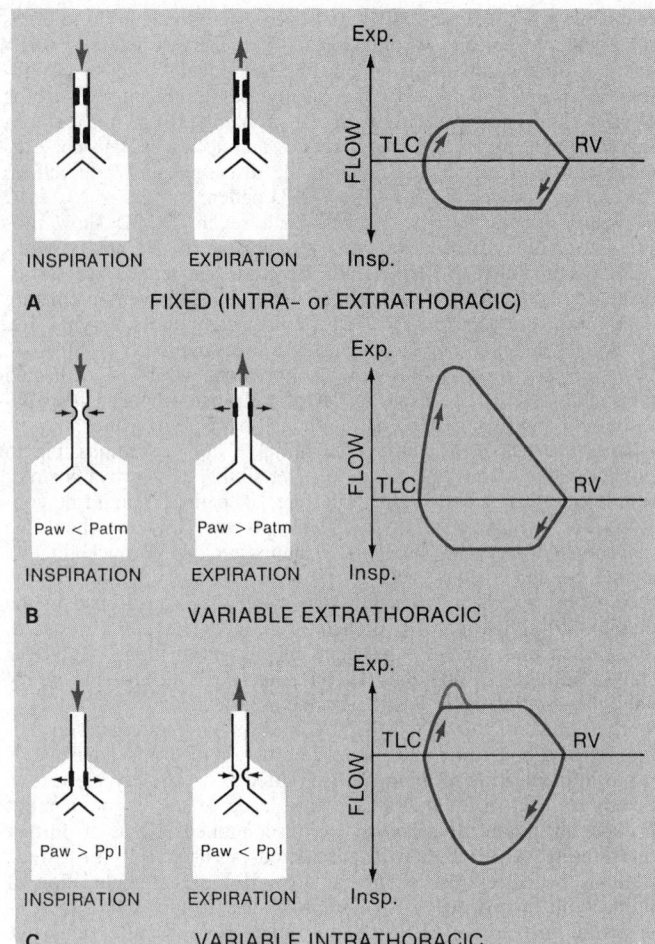

FIGURE 52–2. Airways obstruction above the carina may produce characteristic flow-volume abnormalities, depending on the type and site of obstruction. *A,* If the obstruction is fixed, both inspiratory and expiratory flows are decreased whether the obstruction is intrathoracic or extrathoracic (for purposes of illustration, obstruction is shown in both locations). Note that this pattern is usually seen when the obstruction is at the level of the thoracic inlet. *B,* When a variable obstruction is extrathoracic in location, the airway narrows during inspiration when airway pressure (P_{aw}) is less than atmospheric pressure (P_{atm}) and inspiratory flow is diminished. Expiratory flows are often limited, but to a lesser extent. *C,* When a variable obstruction is intrathoracic in location, airway pressure is less than pleural pressure (Ppl) during expiration and expiratory flow is diminished. Inspiratory flows are often limited, but to a much lesser extent. (Reproduced with permission from Burrows B, Knudson RJ, Quan SF, et al: Respiratory Disorders—A Pathophysiologic Approach. 2nd ed. Copyright © 1983 by Year Book Medical Publishers, Inc., Chicago.)

ynx, vocal cords, or trachea; (4) bilateral paralysis of the vocal cords; (5) spasm or edema of the larynx; (6) inflammation in several locations—the pharynx (e.g., peritonsillar abscess), the larynx (e.g., croup), or the trachea (e.g., diphtheria); or (7) vasculitis (Wegener's granulomatosis). An enlarged thyroid, a paratracheal neoplasm, or a mediastinal infection can extrinsically compress the airways. An artificial airway, tracheostomy, or surgical repair is indicated when the primary cause of the obstruction cannot be eliminated.

COMPLETE OBSTRUCTION. Rapid asphyxiation results unless complete obstruction above the main carina is relieved promptly. There is a pathognomonic presentation, with absent airflow at the mouth in spite of both inspiratory efforts and inspiratory retraction of the intercostal muscles. Aspiration of poorly chewed food (so-called "café coronary") is the most common cause of acute obstruction. If a sharp blow to the back fails to dislodge the obstructing material, forced pressure is applied to the epigastrium—the *Heimlich maneuver.*

When the glossopharyngeal structures fall back in some obese individuals, complete obstruction of the upper airway occurs. Local abnormalities in the hypopharynx may also cause complete upper airways obstruction, resulting in disordered breathing, especially during sleep. Frequent awakening, a troubled sleep, and somnolence are characteristic. This clinical picture, often confused with the pickwickian syndrome and other forms of sleep disorders, is discussed in Ch. 196.

Obstruction Below the Tracheal Bifurcation

PARTIAL OBSTRUCTION. A primary neoplasm, compressing or growing into an airway, is the most common cause of obstruction below the tracheal bifurcation. Other causes include aspiration of foreign bodies, acute or chronic inflammatory lesions of the bronchi, and compression of bronchi by enlarged hilar lymph nodes or mucous plugs. A localized expiratory wheeze over the site of obstruction and hyperinflation of the lung distally are characteristic. Spirometry may be normal or only mildly abnormal because airflow from the remaining lung is unimpaired; yet other tests show nonuniformity of ventilation. A ventilation lung scan may reveal an area of diminished airflow. Bronchoscopy usually provides a definitive diagnosis, and treatment is directed at the cause of obstruction.

Infection and perhaps an abscess may develop with partial bronchial obstruction due to impaired secretion clearance from the distal lung. Partial obstruction of the proximal bronchus should be suspected in patients with recurrent infections in the same lung zone, slow resolution of pneumonia, or a lung abscess.

COMPLETE OBSTRUCTION. "Obstructive atelectasis" is a condition caused by absorption of air into the bloodstream from the lung distal to a complete obstruction. This condition is discussed in Ch. 53. Complete occlusion of a bronchus and resultant obstructive atelectasis may develop with progression of any of the above-mentioned causes of partial obstruction.

McCaffery TV: Management of subglottic stenosis in the adult. Ann Otol Rhinol Laryngol 100:90, 1991. *Addresses the issue of surgical management of subglottic stenosis in adults.*

Mehta AC, Lee FYW, Cordasco EM, et al.: Concentric tracheal and subglottic stenosis. Chest 194:673, 1993. *A report of the current management of stenotic lesions using laser and rigid bronchoscopic dilatation.*

Zalzal GH: Stridor and airway compromise. Pediatr Clin North Am 36:1389, 1989. *Discusses the most common lesions of the upper airways in children, and the diagnosis and management of those lesions.*

53 LOCALIZED ABNORMALITIES OF LUNG AERATION

Richard A. Matthay and Alejandro C. Arroliga

LOCALIZED HYPOAERATION (ATELECTASIS)

Atelectasis, or reduced aeration of the lung, is present in many bronchopulmonary disorders and assumes a variety of forms. A total loss of ventilation to a lung region (i.e., with total airway collapse) leads to an "absolute" shunt wherein blood traversing this region fails to participate in gas exchange and behaves as if it were moving directly from the right to the left side of the heart. The absolute shunt is not fully corrected by inhaling 100% oxygen.

TYPES OF ATELECTASIS AND THEIR PATHOGENESIS. *Obstructive atelectasis* is a condition of alveolar collapse that develops when an airway is obstructed distal to the tracheal bifurcation. The collapse occurs because gas in the lung behind the obstruction is slowly absorbed into the bloodstream. If the lung is filled with oxygen-rich gas rather than ambient air, the alveoli collapse more rapidly. Nitrogen in ambient air is poorly soluble, whereas oxygen is rapidly absorbed into the bloodstream. As a result, high inspired oxygen tensions encourage the development of atelectasis behind obstructing mucous plugs.

Contraction atelectasis occurs when fibrotic changes in a local area of the lung increase its recoil. Contraction, or shrinkage, of the involved lung, rather than complete airlessness, results.

Patchy atelectasis develops throughout the lung owing to alveolar instability in adult and infant (newborn) respiratory distress syndromes.

A large pneumothorax, pleural effusion, or other space-occupying lesion in the thorax can increase intrapleural pressure, causing a portion of the lung to decrease in volume. This *compression atelectasis* is more appropriately called *relaxation atelectasis* because the atelectasis results from the tendency of the lung to recoil when the distending forces are relaxed. As small airways close in the affected region because of marked relaxation atelectasis, any air remaining distally is absorbed into the bloodstream.

Although its pathologic significance is unclear, *platelike atelectasis* may be visible on the chest radiograph. This condition is characterized by horizontal radiopaque streaks, usually in the lung bases. Commonly associated with poor lung aeration, these streaks are seen when the patient has been unable to breathe deeply for a sustained period or when the diaphragm is elevated, such as after intraabdominal surgery.

CLINICAL MANIFESTATIONS. The chronicity and extent of the process determine the physiologic and clinical consequences of atelectasis. When the obstruction evolves slowly, typical of bronchial neoplasms, usually few or no symptoms develop and hypoxemia is minimal. In contrast, profound dyspnea and severe hypoxemia often develop after the acute collapse of a large section of the lung. As blood flow through the nonventilated lung diminishes over several hours, symptoms and hypoxemia lessen. The acute situation typically involves obstructive atelectasis due to aspirating a foreign body or retaining secretions (which may develop in the postoperative period).

The type of atelectasis determines the physical findings. In obstructive or contraction atelectasis, these findings depend upon the amount of lung involved. In major atelectasis, the trachea and mediastinum shift to the affected side, the diaphragm is elevated, and the involved hemithorax is smaller and shows less respiratory motion than does the unaffected side. Patchy atelectasis is associated with findings like those of the respiratory distress syndrome reviewed in Ch. 65. The underlying condition (e.g., pleural effusion, pneumothorax, space-occupying lesion) determines the findings in relaxation atelectasis. Platelike atelectasis is primarily diagnosed on the basis of a chest radiograph and presents no distinctive abnormalities on physical examination.

DIAGNOSIS, TREATMENT, AND OUTCOME. The chest radiograph confirms the presence of atelectasis. When obstructive atelectasis is suspected, bronchoscopy is required to establish the cause; it may be possible to remove the occluding material through the bronchoscope. However, a bronchogenic neoplasm should always be considered when obstructive atelectasis is present and the patient is not severely ill.

Treatment is directed at the underlying disorder in nonobstructive forms of atelectasis.

When relaxation atelectasis is relieved (e.g., by inserting a chest tube for a large pneumothorax), the lung usually returns to normal. However, obstructive atelectasis often is accompanied by secondary complications, such as infection, which lead to abscess formation, localized bronchiectasis, and fibrosis. Moreover, after prolonged collapse, the affected lung may fail to reexpand after the obstruction is removed. The *middle lobe syndrome* exhibits a typical sequence of events. In this syndrome, the middle lobe bronchus in the right lung has usually been compressed by large hilar lymph nodes in tuberculosis or other granulomatous lung diseases. Even after the lymph nodes finally decrease in size, the affected lung fails to expand fully, there are often bronchiectatic changes, and the lobe may be a site of recurrent or chronic infection. Although less common, the same sequence of events may occur in other lung regions. The involved lung may have to be resected if recurrent pneumonia, chronic suppuration, or repeated episodes of hemoptysis develop.

LOCALIZED HYPERAERATION

BLEBS AND BULLAE. Blebs are the uncommon result of dissection of air from the lung interstitium into the lung septa and thence into and between the layers of visceral pleura. Blebs are not clinically important except on the rare occasions that they rupture and cause a spontaneous pneumothorax. Sometimes blebs are visible on the plain chest radiograph, particularly in the lung apex; they are more easily seen when there is a pneumothorax and partial collapse of normal surrounding lung.

Bullae are larger air spaces in the parenchyma of the lung that are associated with destruction. A bulla denotes severe, localized emphysema causing the formation of a large air space. Bullae may occur with several different types of emphysema and are common in patients with chronic obstructive bronchitis and emphysema. Individuals without diffuse emphysema may also develop bullae.

Bullae are commonly located in the apices of the lungs and are often multiple. They may range from 1 cu cm to a size that fills a hemithorax. A lack of an endothelial lining distinguishes bullae from cysts. Moreover, on the chest radiograph, bullae have "hairline" (thin) margins and, unlike cysts, are usually irregularly shaped, are frequently trabeculated, and rarely contain fluid.

When they become large enough to compromise the function of the remaining normal lung and cause shortness of breath, bullae are clinically important. However, like blebs, when small, they are of little significance, unless they rupture and lead to a pneumothorax.

A difficult clinical problem may be to ascertain whether dyspnea is secondary to diffuse emphysema of the lungs or to bullae. Surgery may be indicated in the latter case, and may also be contraindicated in the former. Ventilation-perfusion radionuclide lung scans, computed tomography (CT) scans, and pulmonary angiograms may be necessary to make this distinction and to evaluate the remaining lung. As a rule, unless associated generalized obstructive airways disease is present, bullae that occupy less than half a hemithorax do not cause severe dyspnea or impair function significantly. Moreover, when diffuse disease is present, severe slowing of expiratory airflow is unusual, even with very large bullae. An ideal surgical candidate has moderate to severe dyspnea, bullae that fill most of a hemithorax, only mild slowing of flow rates on forced expiration, good perfusion of normal remaining lung on lung scan and pulmonary angiogram, and no evidence of significant emphysema (e.g., the diffusing capacity measurement is normal or only moderately reduced, and lung compliance studies are normal).

The diagnosis is usually made on the basis of the chest radiograph; however, on physical examination, a tympanitic percussion sound and reduced breath sounds may be noted over very large bullae. The radiolucency of a very large bulla on the chest film may be mistaken for a pneumothorax.

BRONCHOGENIC CYSTS. Bronchogenic cysts may occur in the mediastinum or within the lung parenchyma. These congenital malformations can be differentiated from bullae by their epithelial lining. On the chest radiograph, mediastinal cysts are seen as masses in the hilar, the paraesophageal or paratracheal, and, most commonly, the subcarinal and paratracheal regions. In the parenchyma, these cysts are most often found in the lower lobes and are usually filled with a proteinaceous material, unless they become infected and communicate with the bronchial tree. They may have thin walls. During early development, acquired lung cysts often have relatively thick walls; later even those resulting from lung abscesses may have very thin walls simulating those of bullae.

Large cysts may cause respiratory symptoms in young children, but adults with these large lesions are usually asymptomatic, and the abnormality tends to be an incidental finding on the chest radiograph. In the differential diagnosis, mediastinal cysts must be distinguished from other mediastinal masses. Lung cysts must be differentiated from acute lung abscesses, cavitated carcinomas, previous pulmonary infarcts, thin-walled cavities secondary to granulomatous infections, and cystic bronchiectasis. Frequently, thoracotomy and resection of the lesion are required to obtain a specific diagnosis, although chest CT combined with needle aspiration has been useful for diagnosis and drainage.

Only when they have a bronchial connection (communication) do bronchogenic cysts manifest as abnormalities in lung aeration. Although often partially filled with fluid, they may appear as air spaces when there is a bronchial communication. Infection in fluid-filled cysts is unusual, but if it occurs and does not resolve after a course of antibiotics, the cysts may have to be removed surgically. Cysts containing air can often be distinguished from bullae by their regular outline, lack of trabeculation, and the presence of a fluid level.

BRONCHOPULMONARY SEQUESTRATION. In *bronchopulmonary sequestrations* of the intralobular type, cystic lesions may be identified. This sequestration is caused by abnormal budding in the tracheobronchial tree of the early embryo. The involved area is found most often in the bases of the lungs posteriorly, and

the affected lung region is nonfunctional. On the chest radiograph, involved areas are opaque.

Only when there is a bronchial communication do air-containing cysts develop, and in such situations secondary infection is the prime concern. These lesions are asymptomatic and are incidental findings on the chest radiograph unless infection develops. An aortogram that shows an abnormal vascular supply distinguishes a sequestration from a simple cyst. Magnetic resonance imaging may alleviate the need for angiography (see Ch. 33.6). The arterial supply to some sequestrations arises at least partially from below the diaphragm. Surgical excision is the only treatment.

THE UNILATERAL HYPERLUCENT LUNG. Swyer-James (also called Macleod's) syndrome, a rare disorder, is generally discovered on the chest radiograph. It results from repeated viral or mycoplasmal infections during childhood, causing localized bronchiolitis obliterans. This bronchiolitis causes a nonvalvular obstruction of the bronchi and bronchioles, resulting in emphysema affecting one or several areas of the lungs. The areas affected become hypoventilated and hypoperfused. Increased translucency of one hemithorax is noted because of diminished vascular markings in the lung on that side. On the inspiration chest radiograph, the affected lung is usually not hyperinflated. However, air trapping has been described, and an expiration chest radiograph may show hyperinflation of the affected lung relative to the other uninvolved lung and shift of the mediastinum to the unaffected side. Dyspnea, a productive cough, and occasionally hemoptysis may occur.

Patency of the pulmonary artery on the angiogram differentiates Swyer-James syndrome from pulmonary artery stenosis or atresia. On the affected side, the lung scan shows reduced ventilation and perfusion. Pulmonary function test findings are variable and usually include some evidence of airways obstruction and an increase in residual volume, suggesting air trapping. Severe expiratory obstruction of airflow is uncommon.

Resection is not indicated, and treatment is usually limited to managing infection.

Felker RE, Tonkin ILD: Imaging of pulmonary sequestration. AJR 154:241, 1990. *A comprehensive review of the embryology, different variants, and imaging techniques used for proper diagnosis of the sequestration spectrum.*

Klingmann RR, Angelillo VA, DeMeester TR: Cystic and bullous disease. Ann Thorac Surg 52:576, 1991. *Concise review of the controversies of the pathophysiology of bullous disease, selection of the operative candidate, and operative procedures for cystic and bullous lung diseases.*

Ohri SK, Rutty G, Fountain SW: Acquired segmental emphysema: The enlarging spectrum of Swyer-James/Macleod's syndrome. Ann Thorac Surg 56:120, 1993. *Good description of the histopathologic features of the Swyer-James/Macleod's syndrome.*

Suen HC, Mathisen DJ, Grillo HC, et al.: Surgical management and radiological characteristics of bronchogenic cysts. Ann Thorac Surg 55:476, 1993. *A recent series of patients with bronchogenic cysts. The authors recommend complete excision in most instances.*

54 INTERSTITIAL LUNG DISEASE
Galen B. Toews

GENERAL DESCRIPTION

The interstitial lung diseases (ILD) represent a large and heterogeneous group of lower respiratory tract disorders that are considered together because of several consistent themes among their clinical, radiographic, and physiologic presentations. They also share certain pathogenetic mechanisms and histopathologic features. The target structure in ILD is the alveolar interstitium, which encompasses the space between the alveolar epithelium and the capillary endothelium, including the connective tissues surrounding blood vessels, lymphatics, and airways. Although distinctive pathologic changes may be present, the common denominator among ILD is that they are all characterized by widespread disruption of alveolar walls with loss of functional alveolar capillary units and accumulation of collagenous scar tissue. In the majority of cases, disrupted alveolar architecture is the consequence of inflammatory injury, followed by a dysfunctional process of wound repair.

A working diagnostic classification is presented in Table 54–1. The array of conditions that lead to ILD is so broad and includes so

TABLE 54–1. CLINICAL CLASSIFICATION OF INTERSTITIAL LUNG DISEASE

Primary lung diseases
 Idiopathic pulmonary fibrosis*
 Sarcoidosis*
 Bronchiolitis obliterans with organizing pneumonia*
 Lymphocytic interstitial pneumonia
 Histiocytosis X
 Lymphangioleiomyomatosis
ILD Associated with Systemic Rheumatic Disorder
 Rheumatoid arthritis*
 Systemic lupus erythematosus*
 Scleroderma*
 Polymyositis-dermatomyositis*
 Sjögren's syndrome
 Mixed connective tissue disease*
 Ankylosing spondylitis
ILD Associated with Drugs or Treatments
 Antibiotics*
 Anti-inflammatory agents
 Cardiovascular drugs*
 Antineoplastic agents*
 Illicit drugs
 Dietary supplements
 Oxygen
 Radiation
 Paraquat
Environment/Occupation–Associated ILD
 Organic dusts/hypersensitivity pneumonitis (>40 known agents)
  Farmer's lung*
  Air conditioner-humidifier lung*
  Bird breeder's lung*
  Bagassosis
 Inorganic dusts
  Silicosis*
  Asbestosis*
  Coal workers' pneumoconiosis*
  Berylliosis
 Gases/fumes/vapors
  Oxides of nitrogen
  Sulfur dioxide
  Toluene diisocyanate
  Oxides of metals
  Hydrocarbons
  Thermosetting resins
Alveolar Filling Disorders
 Diffuse alveolar hemorrhage
 Goodpasture's syndrome
 Idiopathic pulmonary hemosiderosis
 Pulmonary alveolar proteinosis
 Chronic eosinophilic pneumonia*
ILD Associated with Pulmonary Vasculitis
 Wegener's granulomatosis
 Churg-Strauss syndrome
 Hypersensitivity vasculitis
 Necrotizing sarcoid granulomatosis
Inherited Disorders
 Familial idiopathic pulmonary fibrosis
 Neurofibromatosis
 Tuberous sclerosis
 Gaucher's disease
 Niemann-Pick disease
 Hermansky-Pudlak syndrome

Disorders marked with a dot are the most common causes of ILD or less common conditions in which ILD is a prominent manifestation of disease.

many diverse, rare disorders that a comprehensive consideration of all diagnostic possibilities is impossible. Faced with this daunting task, a clinician must appreciate the value and limitations inherent in each step of a diagnostic evaluation. Virtually all ILD may involve breathlessness, exercise intolerance, progressive respiratory insufficiency, and diffuse parenchymal abnormalities on chest roentgenograms. Therefore, the key element of the history is to carefully identify the exposures to exogenous agents and symptoms of associated systemic illnesses that point to specific conditions. The physical examination may suggest the presence of ILD, but occasionally, ancillary findings (such as evidence for a pleural effusion or a systemic rheumatic disease) also suggest or discount specific diagnoses. The radiographic features of ILD may be entirely nonspecific or may be tremendously valuable in narrowing the diag-

nostic possibilities. Pulmonary function testing is most useful for demonstrating physiologic abnormalities consistent with ILD and for managing patients and assessing responses to therapy. Only occasionally does physiologic testing help narrow the differential diagnosis. Having sifted through this initial evaluation, the clinician is often left with only a presumptive diagnosis. The accompanying dilemma is to decide when to obtain tissue for histopathologic examination, knowing that even lung biopsy findings may be nonspecific. As discussed in subsequent sections, this difficult and complex decision is highly individualized, based not only on the differential diagnosis at hand but also the realization that the implications for therapy and outcome may vary dramatically among individuals.

EPIDEMIOLOGY

The prevalence of ILD is estimated to be 20 to 40 per 100,000 of the population. ILD accounts for 100,000 hospital admissions yearly. The increased use of pneumotoxic drugs to treat malignant and cardiovascular disease and organ transplantation and the increased identification of occupationally induced ILD are likely to contribute to an increased incidence of ILD.

CLINICAL PRESENTATION

HISTORY. Breathlessness is the most prevalent complaint. Initially, dyspnea develops only on exertion. This symptom is often denied or attributed to other causes ("out of shape," "overweight," "viral infection"). As the disease progresses, dyspnea occurs even at rest. Nonproductive cough and fatigue are also prominent complaints. Cough is a frequent complaint in patients with bronchiolitis obliterans/organizing pneumonia (BOOP), eosinophilic pneumonia, and idiopathic pulmonary fibrosis (IPF). Pleuritic chest pain may occur with ILD associated with systemic rheumatic disease and some drug-induced disorders. Pleuritic chest pain and sudden worsening of dyspnea should suggest spontaneous pneumothorax, a characteristic finding in lymphangioleiomyomatosis (LAM), neurofibromatosis, tuberous sclerosis, and pulmonary histiocytosis X. Hemoptysis may be the presenting complaint of patients who have diffuse alveolar hemorrhage syndromes or in lymphangioleiomyomatosis but is infrequent in other ILD. Hemoptysis should prompt a search for complications such as pulmonary embolus, superimposed infection, or malignancy. Substernal chest discomfort may be noted late in the disease due to pulmonary hypertension.

The history must include an exhaustive search for a causative agent. If a specific diagnosis is made, it is most often because of information gathered during the history. A detailed, lifelong occupational history must be obtained. A record of the patient's present occupation is inadequate; ILD have long latency periods between occupational exposure and onset of symptoms and radiographic abnormalities. Specific work duties and known exposures to inhaled agents should be explored (see Ch. 54.1). Exposure to agents that cause ILD may also occur as a result of hobbies or recreational activities (bird breeder's lung, wood dust worker's lung, farmer's lung, sauna taker's disease). Accordingly, exposures outside the occupational setting should also be explored. Specific questions relating to medications that induce ILD must be asked. The agents to which the patient has been exposed and the circumstances, intensity, and duration of exposure must be determined. Fever and chills are common symptoms in hypersensitivity pneumonitis and are often temporally related to the workplace or to hobbies. Symptoms may diminish or disappear after a weekend, vacation, or an absence from the workplace for several days, only to reappear on return. Patients with IPF or BOOP may date the onset of their symptoms to a preceding upper respiratory tract infection. A smoking history should be obtained. Ninety per cent of patients with histiocytosis X are active smokers. The pulmonary component of Goodpasture's syndrome occurs in only 20% of affected individuals who are nonsmokers, but in 100% of smokers. Hypersensitivity pneumonitis is very infrequent in patients who are active smokers. Smoking adversely affects the course of IPF and asbestosis. A family history of ILD should be sought; genetic factors may play a role in these disorders. An autosomal dominant inheritance pattern has been described for familial IPF, tuberous sclerosis, and neurofibromatosis, and an autosomal recessive pattern of inheritance is found in Gaucher's disease, Niemann-Pick disease, and Hermansky-Pudlak syndrome (see Ch. 174).

PHYSICAL EXAMINATION. Bilateral, basilar, crepitant "Velcro-like" rales are found in most patients with ILD. Wheezing, rhonchi, and coarse rales are occasionally heard. The lung examination may be normal. With advanced disease, patients may have tachypnea and tachycardia, even at rest. Clubbing of the fingers and toes is a common but nonspecific finding in many fibrotic lung disorders; it is most often seen in patients with IPF and is unusual in sarcoidosis. The syndrome of hypertrophic pulmonary osteoarthropathy is rare. The appearance of digital clubbing in a patient with known ILD should prompt a search for a complicating lung malignancy. The heart examination is normal early in the course of the disease. Later, with the onset of pulmonary hypertension and cor pulmonale, an accentuated P_2, tricuspid insufficiency, a right ventricular heave, and peripheral edema may be noted. Physical findings characteristic of associated diseases (rash of systemic lupus erythematosus [SLE], skin changes of scleroderma) may be noted.

LABORATORY STUDIES. Laboratory tests can either confirm or suggest a diagnosis in ILD, but these studies are seldom diagnostic. Rheumatoid factor and antinuclear antibodies are occasionally present in patients with ILD; their presence does not necessarily indicate the presence of an underlying collagen vascular disorder. Plasma immunoglobulin may be elevated, but this finding is nonspecific. If hypersensitivity pneumonitis is suspected, serum-precipitating antibodies to a limited number of inhaled organic antigens may be measured. Tests for antineutrophil cytoplasmic antibodies (ANCA) should be obtained if Wegener's granulomatosis is suspected. Tests for anti–basement membrane antibodies should be obtained when Goodpasture's syndrome (see Ch. 79) is suspected. The electrocardiogram (ECG) is usually normal in ILD. With progressive loss of alveolar capillary units, the ECG may demonstrate a pattern of right atrial and ventricular strain.

CHEST RADIOGRAPHY. The chest radiograph plays a major role in establishing the presence of ILD and may suggest a specific diagnosis (Table 54–2). The majority of ILD cause infiltrates in the lower lung zones. A diffuse ground glass pattern is seen early in the disease. More typically, a chest radiograph demonstrates nodules, linear (reticular) infiltrates, or a combination of the two (reticulonodular infiltrates). Alveolar filling disorders produce a diffuse abnormality on chest radiography, characterized by ill-defined alveolar nodules (acinar rosettes). Air bronchograms may be noted in these patients. As the disease progresses, the infiltrates become coarser and lung volume is lost. Cystic areas (honeycomb pattern) appear late in the course of ILD. Five to 10% of patients with biopsy-proven disease have a normal chest radiograph.

HIGH-RESOLUTION COMPUTED TOMOGRAPHY. High-resolution computed tomography (HRCT) shows greater morphologic detail of the lung parenchyma than standard chest radiography. Although further studies are needed to define its clinical utility, HRCT appears to offer advantages over standard chest radiology in (1) detecting early ILD, (2) diagnosing specific ILD, and (3) quantifying extent of ILD. HRCT can detect ILD in subjects with normal chest radiograms in asbestosis, silicosis, sarcoidosis, and scleroderma. HRCT abnormalities may be present before pulmonary function tests are abnormal, but HRCT may be normal in biopsy-proven ILD. Normal findings on HRCT should not be used to exclude ILD. HRCT may be valuable for identifying a suitable site for transbronchial or open lung biopsy.

PULMONARY FUNCTION TESTS. Physiologic testing can document the physiologic abnormalities associated with ILD, determine the severity, and determine the course and response to treating ILD. The classic physiologic alterations in ILD include reduced lung volumes (vital capacity, total lung capacity [TLC]), reduced diffusing capacity ($D_{L_{CO}}$), and a normal or supernormal ratio of forced expiratory volume in 1 second (FEV_1) to forced vital capacity (FVC). Static lung compliance is decreased (decreased lung volume for any given transpulmonary pressure) and maximal transpulmonary pressure is increased (a very high negative pressure must be generated to open the fibrotic alveoli). There are exceptions to this classic presentation—histiocytosis X, lymphangioleiomyomatosis, neurofibromatosis, sarcoidosis, tuberous sclerosis—and in these diseases, primary airway disease results in an increase in TLC and airflow limitation. A mixed restrictive and obstructive pattern is also seen in BOOP.

Arterial blood gas analysis typically shows mild hypoxemia. Carbon dioxide retention is rare, even late in the course of the disease. Most patients with ILD have marked increases in minute ventilation both at rest and at exercise, resulting in a reduced P_{CO_2} and a compensated respiratory alkalosis. The increased minute ventilation is accomplished by increases in respiratory rate rather than in tidal volume. Hyperventilation is not due to abnormalities in acid-base status or to hypoxemia but rather to an increased stimulation of the respiratory center from neural signals arising from altered mechanoreceptors in the deranged lung parenchyma. The exercise tolerance of ILD patients is markedly limited. With exercise, arterial P_{O_2} falls and the P_{CO_2} remains constant. Hypoxemia in patients with ILD results from abnormal ventilation-perfusion relationships and from diffusion abnormalities. The abnormalities in diffusion were originally believed to be the result of thickened alveolar walls; it is now recognized to be due to loss of capillary cross-sectional area and the passage of red blood cells through functioning pulmonary capillaries at a rate that is too rapid to permit full saturation of hemoglobin. Arterial pH is usually normal in ILD but can fall with exercise as a result of anaerobic metabolism in oxygen-deprived muscles.

BRONCHOSCOPIC STUDIES. Patients with suspected ILD are often evaluated by fiberoptic bronchoscopy to make a definitive diagnosis and to rule out infectious or neoplastic diseases. Bronchoalveolar lavage (BAL) is often performed with this procedure to analyze the cellular constituents, cellular products, and proteins of the distal airspaces of the lung. BAL has clinical utility in diagnosing some ILD. A predominance of eosinophils in conjunction with an appropriate clinical/radiographic picture can diagnose eosinophilic pneumonia. A predominance of lymphocytes in BAL ($\geq 35\%$) narrows the diagnostic considerations to berylliosis, drug-induced ILD, hypersensitivity pneumonitis, lymphocytic interstitial pneumonia, sarcoidosis, or lymphoma. An asbestos body count of > 1 per milliliter of BAL fluid documents significant asbestos exposure. In histiocytosis X, ultrastructural studies of BAL mononuclear cells reveal the typical Birbeck granule of the Langerhans cell. Monoclonal antibodies can be used to specifically identify these cells. Cytoplasmic lipid vacuoles within alveolar macrophages are seen in patients with lipoid pneumonia. The utility of BAL for predicting the underlying pathology (fibrosis versus inflammation), staging of disease, and determining response to therapy is less clear.

TABLE 54–2. RADIOGRAPHIC FEATURES THAT SUGGEST SPECIFIC ILD

Hilar or Mediastinal Lymphadenopathy
  Sarcoidosis
  Silicosis (egg shell calcification)
  Lymphocytic interstitial pneumonia
  Amyloidosis
  Gaucher's disease
Pleural Disease
  Asbestosis (pleural effusion, thickening, plaques, mesothelioma)
  Systemic rheumatic disorders
  Lymphangioleiomyomatosis (chylous effusion)
  Nitrofurantoin
  Radiation pneumonitis
Pneumothorax
  Histiocytosis X
  Lymphangioleiomyomatosis
  Neurofibromatosis
  Tuberous sclerosis
Preserved Lung Volumes or Hyperinflation
  Bronchiolitis obliterans organizing pneumonia
  Chronic hypersensitivity pneumonitis
  Histiocytosis X
  Lymphangioleiomyomatosis
  Neurofibromatosis
  Sarcoidosis
  Tuberous sclerosis
Upper Lobe Distribution
  Ankylosing spondylitis
  Berylliosis
  Histiocytosis X
  Silicosis
  Chronic hypersensitivity pneumonitis
  Necrobiotic nodules of rheumatoid arthritis

TABLE 54–3. GUIDELINES FOR RECIPIENT SELECTION FOR LUNG TRANSPLANTATION IN PATIENTS WITH ILD

Recipient Selection Guidelines
  Untreatable, end-stage ILD
  Substantial limitation of daily activities
  Limited life expectancy (< 12 to 18 months)
  No other significant medical disease
  Ambulatory, good rehabilitation potential
  Acceptable nutritional status
  Acceptable psychosocial profile and support system
Relative Contraindications
  Presence of active systemic disease
  Significant disease of other organ systems
  Significant psychosocial problems, substance abuse, or history of non-
    compliance
  Poor nutritional status
  Poor rehabilitation potential

LUNG BIOPSY. The diagnosis of most ILD depends on histologic studies of lung parenchyma. Transbronchial biopsy can be performed at the time of bronchoalveolar lavage. Transbronchial biopsy should be performed if sarcoidosis or alveolar filling diseases are likely. An open-lung or thoracoscopic biopsy is required to secure a specific diagnosis and accurately stage most patients with ILD who do not have systemic rheumatic disease or drug-induced injury. Open or thoracoscopic biopsy is performed if the diagnosis remains questionable after reviewing the clinical, radiographic, bronchoalveolar lavage, and transbronchial biopsy data and if the patient is not at high risk for this procedure because of age or other serious medical disease. The mortality rate for open lung biopsy is < 1% and the morbidity is < 3%. A specific diagnosis is established in 92% of cases.

THERAPY. The principal aims of therapy are (1) to remove exposure to injurious agents, (2) to suppress inflammation to prevent further destruction of the pulmonary parenchyma, and (3) to palliate the manifestations of these diseases. Corticosteroids are the mainstay of therapy. The initial treatment of choice is prednisone, 1 mg per kilogram of ideal body weight per day (up to 80 mg per day) given in one dose for 3 months, with a gradual taper (5 mg weekly) over several months to a maintenance dose of 15 to 20 mg per day. The rate of taper should be individualized using clinical and physiologic parameters. Corticosteroids are continued until pulmonary functions are stable for 1 year. Relapses require returning to high-dose steroids, but their efficacy in this circumstance is usually limited. Cytotoxic agents or immunosuppressive agents may be used in patients who progress on steroid therapy or who cannot tolerate corticosteroids. Cyclophosphamide, 1 to 2 mg per kilogram ideal body weight, may be useful. Azathioprine has been suggested as an alternative agent.

Supplemental oxygen is recommended for patients who have an arterial oxygen tension of < 55 mm Hg at rest or with exercise. Patients with cor pulmonale and right ventricular failure or those with significant erythrocytosis should also receive oxygen therapy. Respiratory tract infections should be treated promptly. Influenza and pneumococcal vaccines should be given.

LUNG TRANSPLANTATION. Lung transplantation is now an accepted therapy for patients with end-stage ILD refractory to medical therapy (see Ch. 66). Guidelines for selecting patients for transplantation are outlined in Table 54–3. Single lung transplantation is the preferred therapy for most patients. Two-year survival ranges from 60 to 80%, with most deaths due to infections that complicate immunosuppressive therapy or to chronic allograft rejection.

PATHOGENESIS

ILD are the result of the superimposed processes of inflammation and tissue injury and attempted repair (Fig. 54–1). If the events associated with a self-limited inflammatory response are altered, the result may be a persistent inflammatory response with ongoing injury and structural derangement rather than normal repair.

The causes of most ILD are not known. Bacteria, viruses, fungi, toxic agents, and environmental agents have all been implicated. Causative agents may activate resident pulmonary inflammatory or immune cells, which, in turn, generate inflammatory or immune responses. Alternatively, the causative agents may directly injure ep-

ithelial or endothelial cells. In this instance, the inflammatory response might be initiated by the injured tissue.

INTRA-ALVEOLAR INFLAMMATION. The earliest detectable lesion in ILD is a lower respiratory tract inflammatory exudate. Macrophages, neutrophils, and lymphocytes are all present in increased numbers in the alveolar walls and the alveolar air spaces. Cellular recruitment can be divided into four steps: (1) sequestration of inflammatory cells in pulmonary vessels, (2) transmigration of the vascular wall, (3) migration through extracellular matrix, and (4) selective tissue retention. A number of cytokines are released and adhesion receptors are upregulated on endothelial cells at sites of inflammation (see Ch. 228). Selectins are critical for leukocytes to attach to endothelial cells. Leukocyte deformability also is important in the sequestration of cells in the lung. Directed migration of inflammatory cells in ILD depends on cytokines and chemokines. Chemoattractants involved include leukotriene B$_4$ (LTB$_4$), interleukin-8 (IL-8), and C5a for neutrophils; C5a, fibronectin fragments containing the RGD cell-binding domain and monocyte chemoattractant protein-1 (MCP-1) for monocytes; and IL-1 and RANTES in the case of lymphocytes. Alveolar macrophages, endothelial cells, fibroblasts, and epithelial cells are all important sources of these cytokines.

Specific immune responses are also generated. T lymphocytes are activated following the recognition of major histocompatability complex (MHC)–associated antigens on the surface of antigen-presenting cells such as dendritic cells and recruited monocytes. An immune response results in an increase in immunocompetent cells in involved pulmonary tissues.

INJURY. Epithelial cell injury is a hallmark of ILD. Oxidants, proteases, immune and inflammatory cells, and viral infections have all been proposed as mechanisms of injury. Loss of the epithelial barrier results in transudation of plasma and the formation of a fibrin-rich exudate. Epithelial cells are lost and the alveolar basal lamina may be destroyed. The persistence and activation states of inflammatory cells (macrophages, lymphocytes, polymorphonuclear leukocytes) likely determine the type and amount of alveolar wall injury.

INTRA-ALVEOLAR FIBROSIS/ALVEOLAR COLLAPSE. Whether the repair process results in fibrosis or in a return to normal lung anatomy depends, in part, on the success of clearing the intra-alveolar exudate and debris. The forming alveolar exudate contains a new group of cytokines and mediators, including growth factors (platelet-derived growth factor, transforming growth factor-β), fibronectin, thrombin, and fibrinopeptides. Alveolar epithelial cells and macrophages regulate both the formation and clearance of intra-alveolar fibrin. If the intra-alveolar exudate is not cleared, the exudate is invaded by fibroblasts and other cells. Under the influence of growth factors, these cells proliferate and produce new matrix proteins, converting the fibrin-rich exudate into scar. Proliferating type II epithelial cells eventually resurface the organized exudate. Alveolar surface area is lost as a result of intraluminal fibrosis and also as a result of alveolar collapse. Connective tissue deposition in these collapsed airspaces results in irreversible loss of gas exchange units.

PRIMARY LUNG DISEASE

IDIOPATHIC PULMONARY FIBROSIS (IPF). IPF is the "classic" fibrotic lung disease, but it also remains the most enigmatic ILD. The exact prevalence of IPF is unknown, but it is estimated to occur in 5 per 100,000 population. Typically, IPF is diagnosed in patients between ages 40 and 60. No geographic, gender, racial, or seasonal predilections have been noted. Most patients present with the insidious onset of breathlessness with exercise and a dry, nonproductive cough. Constitutional symptoms including fever, fatigue, weight loss, myalgias, and arthralgias are present in some patients. Chest examination reveals late inspiratory fine (Velcro) rales at the lung bases. A right-sided heave, an augmented P$_2$, and an S$_3$ gallop are present in late stages of disease. Chest radiographs typically show a reticular or reticulonodular infiltrate that is most prominent in the lower lung zones. Multiple cystic or honeycombed areas with translucencies measuring 0.5 to 1 cm in diameter are seen late in the course of the disease and indicate a poor prognosis. Spontaneous pneumothorax may occur secondary to rupture of honeycomb cysts. Early in the course of the disease HRCT findings in-

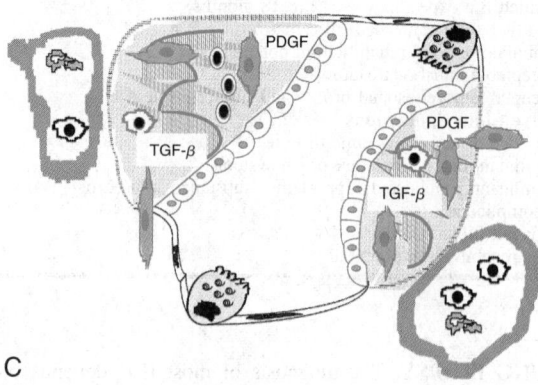

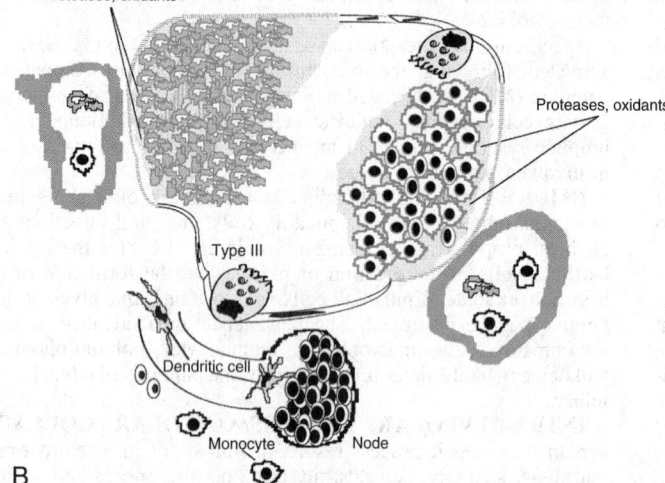

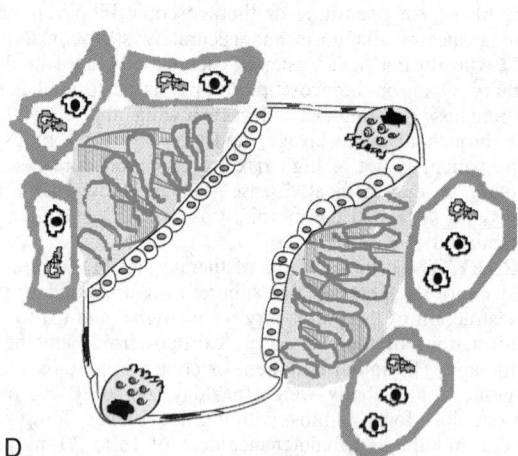

FIGURE 54-1. Pathogenesis of ILD. *A,* The development of an intra-alveolar exudate of polymorphonuclear leukocytes or mononuclear cells depends on inflammatory cell sequestration in pulmonary vessels. Chemokines cause leukocytes to emigrate into the parenchyma and alveolar spaces. Specific cellular immunity depends on migration of antigen-presenting cells to local nodes, clonal expansion of specific lymphocytes, and recirculation of these lymphocytes to the lung. *B,* Inflammatory cells cause epithelial cell injury, epithelial cell loss, and basal lamina destruction. A fibrin-rich exudate forms. *C,* Fibroblasts migrate through the injured basal lamina, multiply, and produce new matrix proteins. Epithelial cell migration and proliferation covers the scar, completing the process of intra-alveolar fibrosis. *D,* Alveolar collapse results from loss of basal lamina. Folded basal lamina is found in areas of new matrix formation. Multiple alveoli may collapse to form a conglomerate scar.

clude a patchy, predominantly peripheral airspace opacification or "ground glass" lung density that does not obscure the underlying lung parenchyma. The interlobular septa are thickened. These findings are thought to correlate with alveolar septal inflammation and the filling of airspaces by mononuclear cells. Later there is a predominantly lower lung zone reticular infiltrate which consists largely of thickened interlobular septa. Honeycombing and subpleural fibrosis are also present. Physiologic testing reveals a restrictive impairment with normal airflow parameters. The $D_{L_{CO}}$ frequently is reduced; this reduction may precede the restrictive abnormalities. Arterial blood gases may be normal or reveal hypoxemia (secondary to ventilation-perfusion mismatch) and respiratory alkalosis. The resting P_{O_2} usually falls with exercise equivalent to walking up a single flight of stairs.

Lung tissue obtained by thoracoscopic or open lung biopsy is required to establish the diagnosis of IPF. Alveolar walls are thickened by an inflammatory cell response. Alveolar epithelial cells and their basement membranes are abnormal. Alveolar cell hyperplasia and metaplasia are noted. Later in the course of the disease, capillaries are lost and increased numbers of mesenchymal cells and deranged collagen fibers are noted. The disease is patchy (nonhomogeneous) in its distribution until late in the course of disease. Assessing lung tissue provides not only diagnostic information but also the best estimate of the stage of the disease. Active inflammation and minimal fibrosis suggest early disease, whereas severe fi-

brosis with minimal inflammation is consistent with late or end-stage disease. BAL has also been used to stage this disease, although its role in planning therapy and predicting outcome remains controversial. BAL lymphocytosis correlates with a cellular biopsy and with therapeutic responsiveness to corticosteroids. Persistence of increased numbers of neutrophils and/or eosinophils indicates a poorly responsive, progressive disease.

The mean survival after diagnosis of IPF is 5 to 7 years. Few patients spontaneously regress or stabilize; accordingly, the great majority of patients require treatment. Corticosteroids are the mainstay of therapy, although favorable clinical response occurs in only 10 to 20% of patients (see earlier section for treatment). Lung transplantation is an accepted therapy for selected patients who are unresponsive to medical therapy and have end-stage disease.

SARCOIDOSIS. Sarcoidosis is a multisystem granulomatous disease characterized by noncaseating granulomas and derangement of normal tissue architecture. Sarcoidosis is described in detail in Ch. 61 and is not further discussed here.

BRONCHIOLITIS OBLITERANS ORGANIZING PNEUMONIA (BOOP). BOOP is a clinical entity that shares certain features of IPF and bronchiolitis obliterans. The distinct onset of a flulike illness with a nonproductive cough is the most common presentation. Fever, malaise, weight loss, and fatigue are usually present for 2 to 4 months prior to the onset of dyspnea. Patients have often been unsuccessfully treated with multiple courses of antibiotics. Rales are common but wheezing is rare. A restrictive defect with a reduction in DL_{CO} is present in a majority of patients. An obstructive defect is present in 20% of patients, most of whom are current or past smokers. Chest radiography reveals bilateral diffuse alveolar opacities with normal lung volumes. A peripheral distribution of infiltrates similar to that seen in chronic eosinophilic pneumonia or migratory infiltrates may be present. Reticulonodular infiltrates and honeycombing are rare. In selected instances the diagnosis can be made by transbronchial biopsy, but thoracoscopic or open lung biopsy is usually required to confirm this diagnosis. Honeycombing and diffuse alveolar wall fibrosis are not features of BOOP. Corticosteroid therapy is the most common treatment and results in recovery in two thirds of patients. Clinical improvement is rapid (days to a few weeks) in some individuals, but relapse may occur when steroids are withdrawn. Retreatment of these patients with steroids is often successful. Cyclophosphamide has been used to treat patients with progressive disease.

LYMPHOCYTIC INTERSTITIAL PNEUMONIA (LIP). LIP is an uncommon cause of ILD. LIP must be differentiated from other lymphocytic infiltrations of the lung, including primary lymphomas and lymphomatoid granulomatosis. An idiopathic form of this disease exists, but it is frequently associated with other conditions such as hypo- or hypergammaglobulinemic states, acquired immunodeficiency syndrome (AIDS), systemic rheumatic disorders, and bone marrow transplantation. Infectious complications occur in LIP associated with AIDS and hypogammaglobulinemia. Corticosteroid therapy is successful in approximately 50% of patients, although some patients progress to end-stage lung disease or lymphoma.

HISTIOCYTOSIS X (see Ch. 147). *Histiocytosis X* is a term that encompasses three systemic diseases (eosinophilic granuloma, Letterer-Siwe disease, and Hand-Shüller-Christian disease) that have in common an abnormal proliferation of a mononuclear cell, the Langerhans' cell. "Langerhans' cell granulomatosis" has been proposed as an alternate term to histiocytosis X because current evidence suggests that the histiocytes are Langerhans' cells. "Pulmonary Langerhans' cell granulomatosis" has been proposed as an alternative to eosinophilic granuloma of the lung. Most new patients are age 20 to 40, with an equal gender distribution. A history of cigarette smoking is obtained in >90%. Patients present with nonproductive cough and exertional dyspnea. Hemoptysis, fever, weight loss, and wheezing are occasionally noted. Pleuritic chest pain and acute dyspnea secondary to spontaneous pneumothorax occur in 25% of patients. Cystic bone lesions (skull, ribs, pelvis) accompany the pulmonary disease in 10% of cases. Diabetes insipidus complicates 10% of cases and indicates poor prognosis. Chest radiography reveals reticulonodular opacities and 5- to 10-mm cysts in the upper and mid-lung zones. Lung volumes are normal or increased. Pulmonary function studies demonstrate a mixed obstructive and restrictive pattern. DL_{CO} is reduced and hypoxemia at rest or with exercise is present.

Definitive diagnosis requires a thoracoscopic or open lung biopsy. Morphologically, a granulomatous reaction develops in a bronchocentric distribution but also involves the walls of blood vessels and the interstitium. Langerhans' cells, monocytes, eosinophils, and lymphocytes are present in these lesions. A granulomatous vasculitis may also be noted. Langerhans' cells may be detected by their characteristic X body or Birbeck granule and/or by monoclonal antibody staining for the CD1a (T6) surface antigen. The clinical course of histiocytosis X is variable; spontaneous remission, stabilization, and disease progression may all occur. Corticosteroids have been reported to be effective in some cases.

LYMPHANGIOLEIOMYOMATOSIS. LAM is a rare disorder occurring only in women of child-bearing age. It is characterized by smooth muscle cells proliferating in the lymphatic, peribronchial, perivascular, and interstitial tissues of the lung. Very little inflammation is present, but in most cases, the alveolar walls are eventually destroyed. Patients present with dyspnea, chylous pleural effusions (secondary to obstruction of the pleural lymphatics), and recurrent pneumothorax (due to rupture of emphysematous cysts). Coarse reticular infiltrates with areas of cystic dilatation are noted on chest radiography. Lung volumes are increased. Pleural effusions or recurrent pneumothoraces may be the sole radiographic manifestation. Septal (Kerley B) lines may be seen because of lymphatic obstruction. Thoracoscopic or open lung biopsy is required to make the diagnosis. Most patients die of respiratory failure within 10

years of onset of symptoms. Hormonal influences are thought to be important in the pathogenesis because LAM occurs predominantly in premenopausal women and is accelerated during pregnancy, the postpartum period, and exogenous estrogen therapy. Progesterone is the drug of choice for therapy. Lung transplantation has been successful in patients with LAM.

ILD ASSOCIATED WITH SYSTEMIC RHEUMATIC DISORDERS

The systemic rheumatic disorders are a heterogeneous group of immunologically mediated inflammatory diseases. The association between systemic rheumatic diseases and ILD is well established; all systemic rheumatic disorders are associated with ILD. The airways, alveoli, vascular system, and pleura are all variably affected in systemic rheumatic diseases. ILD associated with systemic rheumatic diseases accounts for 1600 deaths per year, which is 25% of all mortality associated with ILD and 2% of all respiratory deaths. Pulmonary manifestations of systemic rheumatic diseases are outlined in Table 54–4.

RHEUMATOID ARTHRITIS (see Ch. 237). Although rheumatoid arthritis (RA) is more common in women (2:1 to 4:1), RA associated with ILD is more common in men (3:1) and occurs in patients with late-onset RA. The majority of cases occur between ages 50 and 60. Symptoms are similar to those seen with IPF. Tachypnea and bibasilar rales are common. Associated pleural rubs may be

TABLE 54–4. PULMONARY MANIFESTATIONS OF SYSTEMIC RHEUMATIC DISORDERS

Rheumatoid Arthritis
ILD
Pleural disease (pleuritis with or without effusion, empyema, pyopneumothorax)
Bronchiolitis obliterans with or without organizing pneumonia
Caplan's syndrome
Pulmonary vascular disease
Apical fibrobullous disease
Central airway obstruction secondary to cricoarytenoid arthritis
Systemic Lupus Erythematosus
Pulmonary infection
ILD—acute, chronic
Pleuritis with or without effusion
Pulmonary hemorrhage
Pulmonary vascular disease, thromboembolic disease
Bronchiolitis obliterans
Diaphragmatic dysfunction
Central airway obstruction
Systemic Sclerosis (Scleroderma)
ILD
Pulmonary hypertension
Aspiration pneumonia (gastroesophageal reflux)
Bronchogenic carcinoma (scar carcinoma)
Polymyositis/Dermatomyositis
Aspiration pneumonia (pharyngeal/esophageal disorder)
ILD
BOOP
Respiratory muscle dysfunction (pneumonia, atelectasis, hypoventilation, respiratory failure)
Malignancy (primary, metastatic)
Sjögren's Syndrome
ILD
Lymphocytic interstitial pneumonitis
BOOP
Lymphoma
Chronic bronchitis
Recurrent pneumonia
Mixed Connective Tissue Disease
ILD
Pleuritis with or without effusion
Pulmonary hypertension
Aspiration pneumonia (esophageal disorder)
Ankylosing Spondylitis
Upper lobe fibrobullous disease
Pleural disease (pleural thickening, pneumothorax)
Mycobacterial infections (tuberculous and nontuberculous)
Aspergillomas
Abnormal chest wall mobility
Bronchogenic carcinoma (scar carcinoma)

heard, and clubbing occurs in as many as 75% of cases. Pulmonary symptoms most often follow the onset of arthritis, but simultaneous onset of ILD and arthritis may occur. In one fifth of the cases ILD precedes joint manifestations. Pleural disease accompanies ILD in 20% of patients. The physiologic abnormalities of rheumatoid ILD are identical to those of other fibrosing lung diseases. Bronchoalveolar lavage reveals an increase in macrophages and neutrophils. A subset of patients with RA but without clinical lung disease have a BAL lymphocytosis. Open lung biopsy early in the course of the disease reveals interstitial pneumonitis with perivascular, peribronchiolar, and interstitial infiltration by lymphocytes, plasma cells, and macrophages. This prominent lymphocytic infiltrate, which may contain germinal follicles adjacent to vessels and airways, is useful in differentiating rheumatoid ILD from IPF. The presence of rheumatoid nodules, pleural fibrosis, and adhesions is also helpful diagnostically. Rheumatoid ILD appears to be more indolent and less severe than IPF; prolonged periods of symptomatic and clinical stability may occur. Gold salts and methotrexate, common therapies for RA, can also induce ILD. It is difficult to distinguish between drug-induced and rheumatoid-induced ILD, except that the drug-induced disease may reverse when the drug is discontinued.

Progressive bronchiolitis obliterans is also associated with RA. Clinical manifestations include the abrupt onset of dyspnea and dry cough associated with rales and mid-inspiratory squeaks, occurring particularly in middle-aged women with seropositive RA. Pulmonary function studies reveal airflow obstruction, arterial hypoxemia, and respiratory alkalosis. A bronchiolitis with lymphoplasmacytic infiltration of the small airway walls and obliteration of the bronchiolar airspace with granulation tissue is the predominant lesion. The prognosis is poor because treatment is ineffective. BOOP has also been described in patients with RA. It has a more favorable prognosis than obliterative bronchiolitis alone.

SYSTEMIC LUPUS ERYTHEMATOSUS (SLE) (see Ch. 240).

Acute lupus pneumonitis is characterized by the acute or subacute onset of tachypnea, tachycardia, dyspnea, cough, and cyanosis. Fever is common, hemoptysis is infrequent, and clubbing is absent. In 50% of patients with acute lupus pneumonitis, the acute pneumonitis is the presenting manifestation of SLE. An evolution from acute to chronic ILD likely occurs in some individuals because persistent disease after an acute onset can occur. Clubbing is seen in some of these patients, but less frequently than in rheumatoid ILD. The overall impact of ILD on mortality in SLE appears small; acute and chronic ILD cause death in 2.5% of cases of SLE. Strong consideration should be given to the possibility of pulmonary infections in patients with acute infiltrates in SLE because infections outnumber SLE pneumonitis >30:1. High doses of corticosteroids are indicated in severely ill patients with acute pneumonitis; azathioprine can be added for refractory cases.

SYSTEMIC SCLEROSIS (see Ch. 241).

ILD is the most common pulmonary manifestation of scleroderma. Morphologic changes are found in 90% of patients at autopsy and radiographic evidence of ILD has been noted in 14 to 67% of cases. Clinical manifestations include dyspnea, initially with exertion and later at rest, but these symptoms may be denied because of marked limitation of physical activity. Cough is usually present. Primary pulmonary hypertension may occur in the absence of pulmonary fibrosis and is often the cause of cor pulmonale. In general there is poor correlation between the severity of pulmonary and cutaneous manifestations in scleroderma. Pulmonary symptoms may antedate either cutaneous changes or Raynaud's phenomenon by intervals as long as 14 years. Reticulonodular densities may be noted on chest radiographs in both CREST syndrome (calcinosis, Raynaud's phenomenon, esophageal involvement, sclerodactyly, and telangiectasia) and diffuse scleroderma, but ILD is much less common in the former. A strikingly high incidence of calcified pulmonary granuloma (65%) has been noted in the CREST syndrome. A restrictive ventilatory defect with impaired DL_{CO} is found on pulmonary function testing. Bronchoalveolar studies of scleroderma have demonstrated an alveolitis in a significant proportion of patients with or without ILD. Pulmonary function abnormalities have significant prognostic implications; those with normal function have a >90% 5-year survival, whereas those with restrictive spirometry have a 58% 5-year survival. Patients with a DL_{CO} of <40% predicted have a dismal 9% 5-year survival rate. No consistently effective treatment of sclero-

derma ILD exists. No data support a favorable long-term effect of corticosteroid therapy. D-Penicillamine may diminish the rate of visceral disease, but no data show improvement in lung function.

There is a significant association between the development of bronchogenic carcinoma and chronic pulmonary fibrosis in scleroderma. The majority of bronchogenic carcinomas are either bronchoalveolar cell or adenocarcinomas.

POLYMYOSITIS/DERMATOMYOSITIS (see Ch. 247).

The clinical presentation includes progressive dyspnea on exertion, nonproductive cough, and basilar rales, but a rapidly progressive syndrome (Hamman-Rich) may occur. Lung disease may precede muscle complaints by months to years or be superimposed on established muscular disease. No correlation exists between the severity or duration of the muscular disease and the ILD. Interstitial pneumonitis and BOOP are the most common histologic patterns identified in patients with polymyositis/dermatomyositis. Active inflammation on lung biopsy, especially BOOP, predicts a good therapeutic response. Corticosteroids have stabilized and improved symptoms and physiologic abnormalities in up to 40% of patients. Methotrexate and azathioprine have been used as therapies; both can cause ILD.

SJÖGREN'S SYNDROME (see Ch. 242).

Diffuse ILD is the most common lung abnormality identified in patients with primary Sjögren's syndrome. Malignant lymphomas may occur in primary Sjögren's and are usually fatal. Corticosteroids and immunosuppressive drugs are used in patients with extraglandular involvement. LIP or BOOP may be present and often responds well to corticosteroid or immunosuppressive therapy.

MIXED CONNECTIVE TISSUE DISEASE (see Ch. 241).

Evidence of pulmonary dysfunction has been reported in as many as 80% of patients with mixed connective tissue disease. A proliferative vasculopathy with intimal thickening and medial muscular hypertrophy that affects pulmonary arteries and arterioles is a prominent pathologic lesion. The vasculopathy is more prominent than the associated interstitial fibrosis. It has been suggested that evidence of early interstitial lung disease should be sought in these patients and corticosteroid therapy and/or immunosuppressive therapy instituted early. However, preventing progression to irreversible pulmonary fibrosis has not been documented.

ANKYLOSING SPONDYLITIS (see Ch. 238).

Upper lobe fibrobullous disease, the most common pulmonary manifestation of ankylosing spondylitis, is found in patients with advanced disease. The disease is usually bilateral; diffuse reticulonodular infiltrates in the upper lung zones and cyst formation as a result of parenchymal destruction are seen on chest radiographs. Patients with ankylosing spondylitis appear to be predisposed to typical and atypical tuberculosis. Additionally, aspergillomas are a late complication of colonization of the apical fibrobullous cavities. No therapy is available for the apical fibrobullous disease.

DRUG-INDUCED ILD

More than 100 drugs are known to alter the structure or function of the lower respiratory tract (Table 54–5). Most drug-induced ILD is reversible if recognized early and the responsible drug is discontinued. Drugs can cause acute, subacute, or chronic ILD. Acute and subacute forms of drug-induced ILD usually present with fever and cough and may be mistakenly treated as bacterial pneumonia. Rales, tachypnea, tachycardia, and occasionally cyanosis are noted. A diffuse reticulonodular infiltrate, perhaps accompanied by a pleural effusion, is noted on chest radiography. Blood eosinophilia is frequently noted. Pulmonary function studies reveal a restrictive defect, and arterial blood gas analysis reveals hypoxemia and hypocarbia. The chronic form of drug-induced ILD is more difficult to associate with a specific causative agent because of the insidious nature of this disease. Mild, nonproductive cough is the most common symptom. Fever and eosinophilia are less common. The pathogenesis of most drug-induced reactions is poorly understood.

ANTIBIOTICS. Nitrofurantoin-induced ILD is one of the most commonly reported drug-induced pulmonary diseases. Both acute and chronic ILD occur. The mechanisms of acute and chronic ILD secondary to nitrofurantoin appear to be different; chronic reactions can occur without previous acute ILD. The acute ILD begins 2 hours to 10 days after the onset of therapy and does not appear to be dose related. A reticulonodular or alveolar infiltrate, most prominent at the bases, is noted. The infiltrate may be asymmetric; a pleural effusion (usually unilateral) is present in one third of pa-

TABLE 54–5. DRUG-INDUCED ILD

Antibiotics
  Nitrofurantoin
  Cephalosporins
  Sulfonamides
  Penicillin
  Isoniazid
Anti-inflammatory Agents
  Methotrexate
  Gold
  Penicillamine
  Phenylbutazone
  Nonsteroidal anti-inflammatory agents
Cardiovascular Drugs
  Amiodarone
  Tocainide
  β blockers (propranolol, practolol, pindolol, acebutolol)
  Hydralazine
  Procainamide
  Hydrochlorothiazide
Anti-neoplastic Agents
  Bleomycin
  Busulfan
  Cyclophosphamide
  Methotrexate
  Nitrosoureas (BCNU, CCNU, methyl-CCNU, DCNU)
  Melphalan
  Chlorambucil
  6-Mercaptopurine
  Mitomycin-C
  Procarbazine
Central Nervous System Drugs
  Phenytoin
  Carbamazepine
  Chlorpromazine
  Imipramine
Oral Hypoglycemic Agents
  Tolbutamide
  Tolazamide
  Chlorpropamide
Illicit Drugs
  IV use of drugs formulated for oral use
Opiates
  Heroin
  Propoxyphene
  Methadone
Oxygen
Radiation

tients. Discontinuing the drug is the only treatment required. Chronic nitrofurantoin-induced ILD mimics the presentation of IPF. Dyspnea and nonproductive cough begin 6 months to several years after initiating therapy. In these cases, fever, eosinophilia, and pleural effusion are unusual. A diffuse interstitial process with lower zone predominance is noted on chest radiographs. A restrictive pattern is present on pulmonary function testing. Withdrawing the drug is an important part of treatment, but permanent loss of function can occur. Corticosteroid therapy can be used if no improvement occurs after 2 months, but data regarding its use are scanty. Chronic nitrofurantoin-induced ILD is fatal in approximately 8% of cases.

ANTI-INFLAMMATORY DRUGS. Methotrexate causes a granulomatous pneumonitis in 5% of patients on low-dose methotrexate for RA or other chronic inflammatory conditions. Most patients present with dyspnea, fever, rales, and hypoxemia. No eosinophilia is noted. Granulomatous pneumonitis is noted after administering approximately 10 mg of methotrexate per week for an average of 80 weeks. BAL reveals a marked lymphocytosis. Most patients respond favorably to discontinuing methotrexate, but deaths have been associated with this pneumonitis.

CARDIOVASCULAR DRUGS. Amiodarone, an antiarrhythmic drug used predominantly for treating refractory ventricular dysrhythmias, causes ILD in 5 to 10% of patients. Risk factors include maintenance dose (less frequent if dose < 400 mg per day) and previous pulmonary disease.

Two clinical patterns exist. The most common presentation includes the insidious development of dyspnea, cough, fever, and malaise accompanied by weight loss. Pleuritic chest pain occurs in

10 to 20% of patients. Diffuse reticulonodular infiltrates are present on chest roentgenograph. Other patients may present with a more abrupt onset of an acute illness characterized by fever and localized alveolar infiltrates. This clinical presentation may strongly mimic an infectious pneumonia or, in severe cases, the adult respiratory distress syndrome (ARDS). The combination of amiodarone and general anesthesia, cardiopulmonary bypass, or pulmonary angiography is synergistic for developing acute lung injury. Multiple, nodular pulmonary infiltrates with necrotizing pneumonia and cavities have also been reported. Amiodarone-induced ILD is unlikely in the absence of a 15% decline in DL_{CO}. Histologic findings include phospholipid-laden lamellar inclusions within lung parenchymal cells. These distinctive histologic findings may be seen in any patient receiving amiodarone and do not prove a drug-induced lung injury. If reasonable alternative antiarrhythmic therapy is available, amiodarone should be withdrawn if ILD is present. In patients with severe cardiac disease and refractory ventricular arrhythmias, the ultimate prognosis may be largely dependent upon the underlying heart disease. In spite of significant toxicity, withdrawal of the drug may adversely affect outcome. If the drug is to be continued, a trial of corticosteroid therapy is reasonable.

ANTINEOPLASTIC AGENTS. Chemotherapeutic drug-induced ILD is a major cause of morbidity and mortality in immunocompromised patients and patients with malignancies. Diffuse pulmonary infiltrates may be the result of drug toxicity in 20% of these patients. The diagnosis of chemotherapeutic drug-induced ILD is one of exclusion. Dyspnea occurs within the first few weeks of treatment, followed by cough and intermittent fever. Auscultation reveals dry rales; clubbing has not been reported. Symptoms frequently precede chest radiographic findings. An asymmetric infiltrate limited to a single lobe may be the initial radiographic presentation, but the infiltrate generally becomes diffuse and uniform in distribution. Pulmonary function studies invariably show a restrictive pattern with a reduction in DL_{CO}.

Bleomycin-induced lung disease is common. Ten per cent of patients develop parenchymal lung disease; the mortality rate approaches 50%. The incidence of pulmonary reactions to bleomycin increases in the presence of risk factors such as age (> 70), administering oxygen, radiation therapy, multidrug regimens, and a cumulative dose of > 450 units. *Busulfan*-induced ILD, the first reported chemotherapeutic drug-induced ILD, occurs in 2 to 3% of patients and frequently develops a year after onset of therapy. The ILD usually does not respond to withdrawing the drug or to corticosteroids. *Cyclophosphamide*-induced lung disease can begin a few weeks to 6 years after initiating therapy. The course of the ILD is variable; both steroid-responsive and nonresponsive disease has been reported. *Methotrexate*-induced ILD presents with cough, dyspnea, and fever within a few days to weeks after initiating the drug. Hilar lymphadenophathy is seen in 10 to 15% of patients and pleural effusion is present in 10%. Peripheral eosinophilia is seen in approximately half of patients; eosinophils are not found in the lung parenchyma. Methotrexate-induced ILD is usually reversible by discontinuing the drug, but adding corticosteroids is necessary to resolve some cases. *Nitrosourea* (BCNU and methyl-CCNU)–induced ILD has been reported in as many as 50% of patients who have received doses of > 1500 mg per square meter. These agents may have a synergistic effect with cyclophosphamide. *Procarbazine* causes an acute ILD with peripheral and pulmonary eosinophilia and pleural effusions.

ENVIRONMENTAL/OCCUPATION–ASSOCIATED ILD

ILD associated with inhalation of organic dusts (hypersensitivity pneumonitis) and inorganic dusts are discussed in Ch. 54.1.

ALVEOLAR FILLING DISORDERS

Alveolar filling diseases occur when airspaces distal to the terminal bronchiole are filled with blood, lipid, protein, water, or inflammatory cells. An acinar infiltrate characterized roentgenographically by small nodular densities with ill-defined margins is noted. Virtually all of the alveolar filling disorders can ultimately result in interstitial lung disease.

GOODPASTURE'S SYNDROME (see Ch. 79). Goodpasture's syndrome is characterized by diffuse pulmonary hemorrhage, progressive glomerulonephritis, circulating anti–glomerular basement membrane (anti-GBM) antibodies, anti–alveolar basement membrane (anti-ABM) antibodies, and ILD. Goodpasture's syndrome occurs primarily in young men between ages 18 and 35. The most common presenting symptoms are hemoptysis, dyspnea, cough, and fatigue. Hemoptysis may be modest but can be massive and life-threatening. Gross hematuria, nausea, and vomiting are present in 50% of patients. Fever and weight loss are noted in approximately one fourth of patients. Hypochromic, microcytic anemia is characteristic of Goodpasture's syndrome. Bilateral, symmetric alveolar or acinar infiltrates are present on chest radiographs. When active bleeding stops, the alveolar infiltrates fade within 48 hours, leaving residual reticulonodular infiltrates. The DL_{CO} increases during intrapulmonary bleeding due to CO uptake by the intra-alveolar erythrocytes. An increase in DL_{CO} ($\geq 30\%$) highly suggests diffuse hemorrhage. The differential diagnosis of Goodpasture's syndrome includes SLE, Wegener's granulomatosis, Henoch-Schönlein syndrome, polyarteritis nodosa, and cryoglobulinemia. Serologic assays for anti-GBM antibodies are positive in 95% of patients. The diagnosis is confirmed by immunofluorescent studies of renal tissue in some patients; lung biopsy is seldom necessary.

Spontaneous remissions of Goodpasture's syndrome can occur but are rare. Severity of renal involvement best predicts the outcome. Therapy consists of corticosteroids and cytotoxic drugs together with plasmapheresis until circulating anti-GBM antibodies have been removed.

IDIOPATHIC PULMONARY HEMOSIDEROSIS (IPH). IPH is a rare disorder characterized by intermittent, diffuse alveolar hemorrhage without evidence of vasculitis, inflammation, granulomas, necrosis, circulating anti-GBM antibodies, elevated pulmonary venous pressure, or systemic disease. Iron deficiency anemia and ILD frequently accompany this disorder. Although predominantly a disease of children, about 20% of patients with IPH are adults, usually younger than age 30. There is a 2:1 male predominance in adults. Respiratory symptoms include cough, fatigue, substernal chest pain, and malaise due to anemia. Tachycardia, tachypnea, fever, and hepatosplenomegaly (20%) may be found. Roentgenographic examination usually reveals diffuse, bilateral, acinar infiltrates. Following repeated episodes, a chronic interstitial infiltrate, infrequently associated with hilar and mediastinal adenopathy, remains. Systemic corticosteroids appear to be beneficial in improving the immediate outcome of acute exacerbations, but a long-term beneficial effect has not been demonstrated.

PULMONARY ALVEOLAR PROTEINOSIS. Pulmonary alveolar proteinosis is characterized by the accumulation of an acellular, periodic acid–Schiff positive, lipoproteinacious material within alveoli. Approximately one half of patients with alveolar proteinosis have been exposed to various dusts or solvents, including silica, asbestos, tin, cadmium, molybdenum, or cement dust. Pulmonary alveolar proteinosis has been associated with hematologic abnormalities (10% of cases), including myeloblastic leukemia, chronic myelocytic leukemia, paraproteinemia, and Fanconi's anemia. Melanoma metastatic to the lung, dermatomyositis, and busulfan-induced ILD have also been associated with alveolar proteinosis. Alveolar proteinosis may present with (1) an abnormal chest roentgenogram in an asymptomatic patient; (2) the abrupt onset of cough, fever, and chest discomfort due to a superimposed infection; or (3) the insidious onset of cough and dyspnea related to accumulation of large amounts of intra-alveolar lipoproteinaceous material. Roentgenographic findings include diffuse, bilateral, symmetric lower lobe alveolar infiltrates associated with air bronchograms. Opportunistic infections are associated with pulmonary alveolar proteinosis in 15% of patients; specific organisms include *Nocardia* (most common), *Cryptococcus, Aspergillus, Histoplasma, Mycobacterium, Pneumocystis,* and cytomegalovirus (CMV). The diagnosis of alveolar proteinosis can often be established by bronchoscopic transbronchial lung biopsy. Open lung biopsy may be required in some instances. The treatment of choice is therapeutic whole lung lavage using 40 to 60 liters of fluid via a double-lumen endotracheal tube while the patient is under general anesthesia. The clinical course in alveolar proteinosis is highly variable and may include (1) a progressive disease with superimposed pulmonary infection despite frequent, repeated lavages; (2) stable, recurrent disease requiring repeat lavages (every 6 to 24 months); (3) improvement without relapse; or (4) development of severe ILD.

CHRONIC EOSINOPHILIC PNEUMONIA. There is a wide spectrum of clinical illness at presentation ranging from no symptoms to respiratory failure. Cough, fever (as high as 40° C), dyspnea, weight loss, malaise, and night sweats are the most common symptoms. Wheezing is part of the syndrome in one third to one half of patients, but some patients never wheeze. Peripheral blood eosinophilia is present in 85% of patients during the course of chronic eosinophilic pneumonia but may be absent at initial presentation in as many as one third of patients. The proportion of eosinophils in peripheral blood may be as high as 65%, although it is more commonly 10 to 40%. BAL eosinophils may be greater than 40% during exacerbations. The abnormalities on chest roentgenograms are variable, but a classic, almost pathognomonic group of findings occurs in about 25% of cases. These classic findings include (1) peripheral, nonsegmental alveolar infiltrates, (2) rapid resolution within 2 to 4 days after treating with corticosteroids, and (3) recurrence of roentgenographic abnormalities in the same distribution with clinical relapses. The dense peripheral infiltrates have been characterized as the "photographic negative of pulmonary edema." Dense apical or axillary peripheral infiltrates, lobar consolidation, patchy perihilar infiltrates, nodules with cavities, and bilateral reticulonodular infiltrates also have been described. Although the diagnosis of chronic eosinophilic pneumonia often can be made with enough certainty to justify a therapeutic trial of corticosteroids, transbronchial biopsy and BAL should be performed unless contraindications exist. Open lung biopsy is rarely required.

Corticosteroids almost universally lead to rapid improvement in chronic eosinophilic pneumonia; failure to improve on corticosteroids should raise doubts about the accuracy of the diagnosis. Improvement often occurs within hours, and chest roentgenograms usually clear in 2 to 4 days. Prolonged therapy is often required (6 to 12 months); there is a high rate of relapse even after a year of corticosteroid therapy.

ILD ASSOCIATED WITH PULMONARY VASCULITIS

The pulmonary vasculitic syndromes are a diverse, rare group of diseases with overlapping clinical and pathologic manifestations. Although ILD is not a common presenting feature of the pulmonary vasculitides, most ultimately develop significant pulmonary fibrosis.

WEGENER'S GRANULOMATOSIS (see Ch. 245). Wegener's granulomatosis is a systemic disease in which a granulomatous, necrotizing vasculitis involves the upper and lower respiratory tracts and the kidneys. All patients have respiratory tract involvement, but certain patients with a limited form of the disease have no apparent renal disease. Chest radiographs usually reveal multiple nodular or cavitary infiltrates, but single nodules may be found. Patients in whom Wegener's granulomatosis is expected should be tested for ANCA. A negative ANCA does not rule out Wegener's granulomatosis. An open lung biopsy is the procedure of choice for establishing a diagnosis. Cyclophosphamide (1 to 2 mg per kilogram per day orally) in conjunction with oral corticosteroids (60 mg prednisone daily) is the standard initial therapy for Wegener's granulomatosis. After clinical manifestations have subsided, the prednisone dose can be decreased. Initial remission occurs in >90% of patients. Relapses occur in 25 to 30% of patients after a successful course of therapy or during the period of corticosteroid dose reduction. The serum C-ANCA is a useful monitor of disease activity.

CHURG-STRAUSS SYNDROME (ALLERGIC ANGIITIS AND GRANULOMATOSIS) (see Ch. 244). This systemic necrotizing vasculitis affects the upper and lower respiratory tracts and is almost invariably preceded by allergic manifestations such as asthma, allergic rhinitis, or a drug reaction. Chest radiographs reveal bilateral patchy, fleeting infiltrates, diffuse nodular infiltrates without cavitation, or diffuse reticulonodular disease. Open lung biopsy provides definitive histologic evidence for Churg-Strauss syndrome.

INHERITED DISORDERS

ILD may result from a group of rare inherited disorders. Both autosomal dominant and recessive disorders may be associated with ILD.

FAMILIAL IDIOPATHIC PULMONARY FIBROSIS. This is an autosomal dominant disease with clinical, roentgenographic, physiologic, and morphologic features that are indistinguishable from nonfamilial IPF. Symptoms begin between ages 20 and 40.

There is evidence of alveolar inflammation in clinically unaffected family members of patients with familial IPF.

NEUROFIBROMATOSES (see Ch. 417). ILD occurs in 20% of patients with neurofibromatosis. The onset of ILD is usually noted between ages 35 and 60, and dyspnea is the predominant symptom. The ILD has histologic features similar to those of IPF. There is no known therapy.

TUBEROUS SCLEROSIS (see Ch. 417). Hamartomas are the characteristic histologic lesion and may be found in the lungs, central nervous system, bones, eyes, kidneys, skin, and heart. Lesions of tuberous sclerosis are found in the lung in 1% of patients. The clinical, physiologic, radiographic, and pathologic picture strongly resembles that of lymphangioleiomyomatosis.

AUTOSOMAL RECESSIVE DISEASES. ILD has been described in several autosomal recessive diseases, including Gaucher's disease, Niemann-Pick disease (see Ch. 174), and Hermansky-Pudlak syndrome (partial oculocutaneous albinism, a hemorrhagic defect due to platelet dysfunction, and accumulation of ceroid in the reticuloendothelial system).

BAL Cooperative Group Steering Committee: Bronchoalveolar lavage constituents in healthy individuals, idiopathic pulmonary fibrosis, and selected comparison groups. Am Rev Respir Dis 141:S169, 1990. *A review of standardized techniques and normal values of BAL constituents in normal individuals and patients with ILD.*

Cooper JAD Jr (ed.): Drug-induced pulmonary disease. Clin Chest Med 2:1, 1990. *Reviews the clinical findings and pathogenesis of drug-induced interstitial lung disorders.*

Crouch E: Pathobiology of pulmonary fibrosis. Am J Physiol 259:L159, 1990. *Reviews the processes involved in both inflammation and repair of the alveolar walls.*

Katzenstein AA, et al. Bronchiolitis obliterans and usual interstitial pneumonia. Am J Surg Pathol 10:373, 1986. *A review of the pathology of the interstitial lung diseases.*

Kelley J (ed.): Cytokines in the Lung. New York, Marcel Dekker, 1992. *An exhaustive treatment of the role of cytokines in the biology and pathobiology of the lung.*

Muller NL, Ostrow DN: High resolution computed tomography of chronic interstitial lung diseases. Clin Chest Med 12:97, 1991. *Reviews the use of HRCT in chronic interstitial lung diseases.*

Schwarz MI, King TE Jr (eds.): Interstitial Lung Disease. St. Louis, Mosby-Yearbook, 1993. *An exhaustive review of all interstitial lung diseases.*

54.1 Occupational Pulmonary Disorders

Jonathan M. Samet

Interstitial lung diseases (ILD) damage the pulmonary interstitium by disrupting alveolar structures and the small airways. Occupational diseases affecting the pulmonary interstitium include primarily the pneumoconioses, or dust diseases of the lung (Table 54–6), and hypersensitivity pneumonitis. The principal pneumoconioses—asbestosis, coal workers' pneumoconiosis, and silicosis—typically occur after sustained exposures to dust concentrations that are no longer legally permissible in many developed countries, including the United States. Although these diseases are declining, cases still occur in locales where industries have been historically associated with high dust exposures and as "sentinel" cases, signaling unsuspected and uncontrolled occupational exposures. New agents introduced into the workplace may also cause unanticipated diseases. People with occupational ILD may present to health care providers through diverse paths. Physicians may evaluate previously undiagnosed patients with occupational ILD who present with dyspnea or unexplained radiographic infiltrates or previously diagnosed patients who present for assessment of the extent of associated physiologic impairment, often in the context of a legal proceeding or a claim for disability. Current or former workers exposed to agents causing lung disease may also present for screening for adverse effects.

The occupational ILD result from inhaling and retaining dusts with induction of inflammation and fibrosis. Dust particles in the respirable size range are generated in workplaces by diverse processes; power-driven equipment, such as drills and grinders, place their operators at risk for diseases caused by dust. The lung is defended against dust particles by a system that includes the physical barrier posed by the upper airway that filters out larger particles, the mucociliary escalator that removes inhaled particles, and the

TABLE 54–6. PRINCIPAL PNEUMOCONIOSES CAUSED BY MINERAL DUSTS

Agent	Disease	Radiograph Appearance
Asbestos	Asbestosis	Reticular, basilar predominance
Coal dust	Coal workers' pneumoconiosis	Nodular, upper lobe predominance
Cobalt	Hard metal disease	Reticular, basilar predominance
Silica	Silicosis	Nodular, upper lobe predominance
Talc	Talcosis	Rounded, irregular, or both

alveolar macrophages that scavenge inhaled and deposited particles in the small airways and alveoli. Particle size determines the likelihood and site of deposition. During quiet breathing, most particles larger than 10μ in aerodynamic diameter are deposited in the upper airways, although some particles in this size range may enter the lung during exertion. Particles between approximately 3 and 10μ tend to deposit in the larger airways of the lung, whereas smaller particles down to about 0.1μ are preferentially deposited in the small airways and alveoli.

Induction of inflammation and subsequent fibrosis are central in the pathogenesis of the occupational ILD, although the mechanisms underlying the distinctive pathologic responses found in the different pneumoconioses are currently not characterized. Present concepts of pathogenetic mechanisms for the pneumoconioses emphasize the roles of alveolar macrophages in the initial response to dust inhalation, of cytokine release, and of interactions among macrophages, lymphocytes, neutrophils, and fibroblasts. Hypersensitivity pneumonitis reflects cell-mediated immune responses to inhaled antigens.

Preventing these diseases rests largely on controlling exposures in the workplace through regulations that limit exposures to levels considered to be safe and that specify respiratory protection. Medical screening for early evidence of disease represents a complementary but secondary control approach. In the United States, the standard-setting agencies are the Occupational Safety and Health Administration (OSHA) and the Mine Safety and Health Administration (MSHA). Physicians who make a diagnosis indicating a failure of control measures should follow through by contacting relevant agencies, and with permission and possibly preservation of confidentiality, the employer or the union, as appropriate. The burden of respiratory morbidity and mortality in workers at risk for occupational lung disease can also be reduced by preventing and stopping smoking (see Ch. 9.4). For the nonmalignant occupational lung diseases, the adverse effects of cigarette smoking on lung function appear additive to those of the occupational agents, whereas for lung cancer, synergism with smoking has been found for most occupational carcinogens. New genetic approaches may eventually provide strategies for identifying workers with the greatest susceptibility; however, we still lack the scientific and ethical framework for implementing control programs based upon genetic screening, and prevention will continue to be based on workplace controls for the foreseeable future.

For patients with clinically significant impairment, supportive treatment, as for other chronic lung diseases, is warranted. Patients should receive pneumococcal and influenza vaccines and oxygen therapy, as needed. Physical activity should be encouraged, and a comprehensive pulmonary rehabilitation program may benefit some patients. As for other patients with advanced chronic lung diseases, lung transplantation may be a consideration (see Ch. 66).

EVALUATING THE PATIENT WITH SUSPECTED OCCUPATIONAL INTERSTITIAL LUNG DISEASE

GENERAL APPROACH. Diagnosis of an occupational ILD is based on an appropriate clinical picture and documentation of exposure, related in a temporally appropriate fashion to the occurrence of the disease. As indicated, workup may also be needed to exclude other disorders associated with a comparable clinical picture. For example, in an elderly man with a history of underground mining and of cigarette smoking, a lung nodule might represent complicated silicosis or a primary cancer of the lung. The clinical history should cover the cardinal respiratory symptoms—cough, phlegm, dyspnea, and wheezing; emphasis should be placed on quantifying the degree of dyspnea. Graded questions should be used for this purpose that inquire, for example, about having dyspnea while hurrying on the level ground or walking up a slight hill, about walking slower on level ground than same-age peers, about stopping for breath after walking about 100 yards, and about having dyspnea during such routine activities as dressing and bathing. On physical examination, the physician should look for finger clubbing or cyanosis, indicative of advanced disease. On examining the chest, the physician should note the quality of the breath sounds and the timing (early or late) and the type (fine or coarse) of any crackles (see Ch. 49).

HISTORY. A comprehensive occupational history should be taken from all patients with suspected occupational disease. The history needs to cover each job systematically, describing the industry in which the patient worked, the specific occupation and job duties, materials handled, required and actual use of respiratory protective equipment, and occurrence of disease in fellow workers. Seasonal, part-time, and temporary jobs should not be omitted, as such jobs may have a greater likelihood of hazardous exposure. The dates of specific jobs may also be relevant because exposures for many agents were higher during past decades. The history should inquire about specific materials, e.g., asbestos, and also about exposure through hobbies and the jobs of family members. A temporal association between entering the workplace and symptoms may indicate an exposure that triggers hypersensitivity pneumonitis.

The history should also cover cigarette smoking and other tobacco use (see Ch. 9.4). Chronic bronchitis and chronic airflow obstruction associated with smoking may explain cough and dyspnea or complicate the diagnosis of a distinct occupational lung disease.

IMAGING OF THE CHEST. In addition to a comprehensive occupational history, the diagnostic workup of patients with suspect occupational ILD also includes imaging of the lungs to establish the presence of disease and the characteristics of any infiltrates. All patients suspected to have an occupational ILD need to have standard posteroanterior (PA) and lateral radiographs. Most patients with a pneumoconiosis have an abnormal chest radiograph; but 10 to 20% do not. The type of infiltrates, nodular or reticular, and the distribution provide an indication of the underlying disease (Table 54–6). The International Labour Organization has developed a standardized system for classifying the abnormalities found on the PA radiograph in pneumoconioses. Although intended for use in epidemiologic research, the scheme is now widely applied clinically. In this system, small parenchymal opacities are classified by shape (irregular or rounded), size, distribution, and profusion or concentration. The profusion, scored on a 12-point scale, is indicative of the degree of histopathologic derangement. The pneumoconiosis is termed "simple" if all opacities are < 1 cm diameter and "complicated" if ≥ 1-cm opacities are present.

High-resolution computed tomography (HRCT) is increasingly used to evaluate patients with ILD, including occupational diseases. The narrow slice thickness of 1 to 2 mm provides visualization of fine parenchymal detail and detects interstitial changes and emphysema. Although the role of HRCT is still evolving, it should be considered for patients who have a normal chest radiograph but are suspected of having an occupational ILD. HRCT may also prove valuable for quantifying the degree of abnormality and the extent of coexisting emphysema, but it cannot be recommended for these purposes at present.

PULMONARY FUNCTION TESTING. Spirometry should be performed on all patients at risk for an occupational ILD and the results compared with predicted values based on gender, race, age, and height. If the results are within the limits of normal, further testing is not indicated except for patients complaining of dyspnea or having roentgenographic abnormalities indicative of pneumoconiosis. Those patients, as well as patients with abnormal spirometry, should have measurements of the single breath diffusing capacity for carbon monoxide and lung volumes (total lung capacity [TLC] and residual volume). Exercise testing with blood gases and gas exchange parameters measured may be needed to evaluate dyspnea and to quantitate exercise impairment.

INVASIVE DIAGNOSTIC MEASURES. Invasive procedures are rarely indicated to establish the diagnosis of an occupational ILD, although biopsy may be warranted on clinical grounds to ex-

clude alternative diagnoses. Bronchoalveolar lavage, the least invasive approach, provides fluid that can be analyzed for dusts and fibers and for cell populations; it is primarily a research tool at present. Transbronchial lung biopsy specimens obtained via the fiberoptic bronchoscope may yield a specific diagnosis, and the specimens can be analyzed for dusts and fibers, as can those obtained by open lung biopsy. Polarized light microscopy, which is routinely available, can detect crystals, and ferruginous bodies—ferritin-coated fibers—can be identified with routine optical microscopy. More sophisticated techniques can be used to quantify and identify particles in lung tissue, but these techniques are not routinely available. They should be considered for patients with an interstitial disease but uncertain exposure history and if needed for medical-legal purposes.

McLoud TC: Occupational lung disease. Radiol Clin North Am 30:1121, 1992. *This monograph provides an updated discussion of imaging approaches for occupational lung diseases, including conventional radiography and newer modalities such as HRCT.*

Rom WN: Environmental and Occupational Medicine. 2nd ed. Boston, Little, Brown & Co, 1992. *This comprehensive text reviews the full scope of occupational medicine, touching on workplace assessment, clinical evaluation, and specific agents and disease entities.*

PNEUMOCONIOSES

ASBESTOSIS. *Definition.* Asbestosis refers to fibrosis of the lung parenchyma and not to the pleural fibrosis and plaques that are frequently found in asbestos-exposed workers. Asbestos exposure is also associated with mesothelioma of the pleura and peritoneum, lung cancer, larynx cancer, and possibly gastrointestinal cancers.

Etiology. Asbestos refers to several fibrous silicate minerals having unique physical-chemical properties that make them effective for insulation, reinforcing materials, friction products, and other purposes. All types of asbestos fibers are associated with asbestosis, pleural disease, and lung cancer. Chrysotile, the type principally used in the United States, is a serpentine mineral that undergoes gradual physical and chemical dissolution in tissues. Crocidolite, anthophyllite, and amosite, the other principal asbestos types used, are in the amphibole mineral group and are more needle-like than the curly chrysotile fibers and not as prone to dissolution. Chrysotile asbestos appears to be a weaker cause of mesothelioma than the amphiboles.

Epidemiology. Asbestos fibers have been widely used during the twentieth century, and large numbers of workers directly handling asbestos have been exposed, along with indirectly exposed nearby workers and even family members exposed to fibers brought home on clothing. The exposed worker groups include asbestos miners and millers, workers manufacturing asbestos products such as textiles and brake linings, and workers using asbestos products such as insulators and other construction trades. With a large number of buildings now having asbestos-containing materials, custodial and maintenance workers may also be exposed, as may workers involved in removing asbestos and demolishing buildings. Exposures for general building occupants are quite low and in a range not associated with asbestosis. The risk of asbestosis increases with cumulative exposure to asbestos fibers; with the exception of extraordinarily high exposures, manifestations of disease are not usually present until 15 to 20 years have elapsed since first exposure. With the widespread recognition of the disease risks associated with asbestos, exposures have been lowered and substitutes introduced in many developed countries, including the United States. The cohort of workers at greatest risk for asbestosis comprises workers exposed through the early 1970's, and the incidence of asbestosis should diminish as these workers age.

Pathology. In experimental models of asbestosis, the earliest lesions are found in the alveolar ducts and peribronchiolar regions where deposited asbestos fibers attract alveolar macrophages. The lungs of asbestos-exposed workers show an inflammatory and fibrotic lesion of the small airways, termed "mineral dust–induced small airways disease." As disease progresses, the fibrotic process becomes more extensive and may ultimately involve the entire lung. In advanced cases, extensive fibrosis may destroy the normal architecture of the lung to cause honeycombing, cystic spaces bounded by fibrosis. In advanced disease, the lungs are small and stiff with macroscopically visible fibrosis and honeycombing. Asbestos bodies are typically visible with conventional microscopy.

Clinical Manifestations. Patients with asbestosis present with the same clinical picture found in other interstitial lung diseases:

cough and exertional dyspnea. Some cases of asbestosis may also be detected by screening exposed worker populations. Bibasilar fine crackles are heard on auscultation of the chest in most patients, and clubbing may be present in advanced cases. The chest radiograph shows irregular opacities that are typically most prominent in the lung bases; pleural disease, particularly in the form of localized and often calcified plaques, is often present as well. The degree of physiologic impairment on lung function testing varies with the severity of the asbestosis. The small airways lesions produce airflow obstruction, manifest by changes in the shape of the expiratory flow-volume curve, with corresponding reduction of flow rates at lower lung volumes. Airflow obstruction cannot be readily attributed to asbestos exposure in individual patients who have smoked cigarettes. In patients with clinically significant dyspnea, spirometry typically shows a reduced forced vital capacity (FVC) with preservation of the ratio of the forced expiratory volume in 1 second (FEV_1) to FVC, and reduced TLC and diffusing capacity; however, this typical physiologic profile is not invariably observed. Progressive exercise testing shows pulmonary limitation of exercise capacity and desaturation in many patients with asbestosis.

Diagnosis. Asbestosis can be diagnosed with confidence if there is a history of significant exposure to asbestos; radiographic, clinical, and physiologic evidence of ILD compatible with asbestosis; and no indication of another disease process associated with a comparable clinical picture of interstitial lung disease, e.g., scleroderma (see Ch. 241). The exposure should have started at least 15 years before the disease developed. Pleural plaques provide a strong indication of past asbestos exposure. In patients with biopsy-proven ILD without a firm history of exposure, the presence of asbestos bodies should increase suspicion for asbestosis. More formal counting of asbestos bodies or of fibers may be warranted.

Treatment. At present, there is no effective treatment for asbestosis, other than oxygen therapy as needed. Lung transplantation may be considered for selected patients. Because of the increased risk of asbestos-exposed individuals for lung cancer, perhaps particularly those with asbestosis, smoking cessation should be counseled for current smokers.

Prognosis. The course of radiographically identified asbestosis is variable, with some cases showing progression whereas others remain static. Factors influencing progression are not well established but appear to include the cumulative exposure to asbestos, the duration of exposure, and the type of asbestos exposure.

Becklake MR: Asbestos and other fiber-related diseases of the lungs and pleura. Chest 100:248, 1991. *A succinct introduction to the extensive literature on nonmalignant diseases associated with asbestos exposure.*

COAL WORKERS' PNEUMOCONIOSIS. *Definition.* Coal workers' pneumoconiosis is the parenchymal lung disease caused by inhaling coal mine dust. The disease is termed "simple" if all radiographic opacities are < 1 cm in diameter. Progressive massive fibrosis complicates simple coal workers' pneumoconiosis if any nodular opacities of ≥ 1 cm are present on the chest radiograph. Exposure to coal mine dust is also associated with industrial bronchitis and loss of lung function at a rate beyond that associated with aging; these consequences of such exposure are not considered coal workers' pneumoconiosis, although they do contribute to the respiratory morbidity experienced by coal miners. The group of lung diseases caused by coal mine dust are commonly referred to as "black lung."

Etiology. Coal refers to a group of carbonaceous materials characterized by the hardness or "rank," ranging from peat, the softest, to anthracite, the hardest. Inhaling coal dust causes coal workers' pneumoconiosis, but inhaling more pure carbon materials—lampblack and carbon black—has also been associated with a comparable lung disease. Silica in the coal dust may also contribute to the development of coal workers' pneumoconiosis. Determinants of progression from simple coal workers' pneumoconiosis to progressive massive fibrosis, other than coal rank and coal mine dust exposure, have not been identified.

Epidemiology. Extensive epidemiologic information shows that the risk of coal workers' pneumoconiosis increases with dust level in the mine and cumulative exposure to coal mine dust. Risk also increases with the rank of the coal, being greatest for the harder coals. In studies of the mortality of underground coal miners, progressive massive fibrosis increases risk of death, whereas simple

coal workers' pneumoconiosis has a lesser adverse effect. Reduced exposures for US miners since the passage of the Coal Mine Health and Safety Act of 1969 should reduce risks for those recently starting to mine.

Pathology. The characteristic lesion of coal workers' pneumoconiosis is the coal macule, an inflammatory lesion consisting of focal collections of coal mine dust–laden macrophages surrounding respiratory bronchioles. The coal macule may extend to the alveoli and be accompanied by fibrosis of the small airways and alveoli and by focal emphysema. Larger "coal nodules" may develop which are grossly firm and contain dust-filled macrophages in collagen and reticulin. Progressive massive fibrosis is diagnosed pathologically if nodules reach at least 2 cm, although the radiographic definition is based on opacities of at least 1 cm. These lesions are also collagen-containing and tend to disrupt the lung's architecture. In Caplan's syndrome, or rheumatoid pneumoconiosis, multiple lung nodules, ranging from 1 to 5 cm, are present, typically in the periphery.

Clinical Manifestations. Coal mine dust–exposed miners may present with cough and sputum production reflecting industrial bronchitis and dyspnea associated with pulmonary function impairment, whether secondary to progressive massive fibrosis involving the parenchyma or accelerated loss of ventilatory function related to dust-induced airways disease. Other than characteristic radiographic findings, there are no specific clinical manifestations of simple coal workers' pneumoconiosis; in spite of widespread radiographic abnormalities, many miners are asymptomatic or have only mild adverse changes in lung function, whereas some may have significant impairment with little or no radiographic abnormality. In simple disease, the chest radiograph typically shows small nodules that tend to predominate in the upper lung zones. Reticular opacities may also be present, more often in cigarette smokers.

Progressive massive fibrosis is associated with progressive dyspnea, pulmonary hypertension, and even respiratory failure. The chest radiograph shows the characteristic nodules of progressive massive fibrosis, often with contraction of the affected lung, typically upper lobes, and compensatory hyperinflation, typically lower lobes. The nodules may cavitate and produce melanoptysis. In progressive massive fibrosis, lung function is typically impaired, particularly if larger nodules are present. Both airflow obstruction (reduced FEV_1 and FEV_1/FVC ratio) and lung restriction (reduced TLC) can occur. The single-breath diffusing capacity for carbon monoxide is also reduced, and there may be resting hypoxemia or desaturation with exercise. Caplan's syndrome should be considered in miners with multiple peripheral nodules; this uncommon syndrome may develop in miners with rheumatoid arthritis or with circulating rheumatoid factor without arthritis (see Ch. 237).

Diagnosis. Coal workers' pneumoconiosis is diagnosed on the basis of an appropriate history of exposure and characteristic radiographic abnormalities. Miners with noncoal experience are at risk for both silicosis and coal workers' pneumoconiosis. In patients with probable progressive massive fibrosis, consideration should be given to alternative causes of lung masses, including lung cancer.

Treatment. No effective treatment is currently available for coal workers' pneumoconiosis. Appropriate supportive care and rehabilitation should be provided for those with impaired lung function.

Prognosis. Total coal mine dust exposure and increasing severity of simple pneumoconiosis predict the development of progressive massive fibrosis, which is associated with more severe morbidity and increased overall mortality. Simple pneumoconiosis alone does not increase mortality.

Attfield M, Wagner G: Respiratory disease in coal miners. *In* Rom WN (ed.): Environmental and Occupational Medicine. 2nd ed. Boston, Little, Brown & Co, 1992, p 325. *A recent review chapter covering epidemiology, clinical features, and control.*

SILICOSIS. *Definition.* Silicosis refers to the parenchymal lung diseases associated with crystalline silica exposure, including acute, accelerated, and chronic or classic silicosis. These entities are distinguished by their clinical pictures and time course in relation to silica exposure. In acute silicosis, an alveolar filling process follows heavy exposure within a few years. Accelerated silicosis occurs within 5 to 10 years of exposure and has a clinical picture comparable to that of chronic silicosis, which develops after a longer latent period.

Etiology. Crystalline silicon dioxide, the causal agent, is abundant and ubiquitous in the earth's crust and is used in a variety of industrial applications. Quartz is the most common form. Consequently, large numbers of workers, probably millions in the United States, are still exposed (Table 54–7).

Epidemiology. As for the other pneumoconioses, the risk of developing disease increases with the level and duration of exposure. Although the hazard posed by silica exposure has long been recognized and exposure standards have been promulgated, new cases continue to occur, even of acute silicosis, which has been recently reported in sandblasters, ground silica workers, and rock drillers.

Pathology. Like coal workers' pneumoconiosis, chronic silicosis occurs in a simple form and as progressive massive fibrosis. The earliest lesions are collections of dust-laden macrophages in the peribronchiolar and paraseptal or subpleural areas. The silicotic nodule has an acellular core composed of collagen surrounded by a cellular capsule with macrophages, lymphocytes, and fibroblasts. Silicotic nodules may also involve the hilar lymph nodes. Silicotic nodules coalesce to form the lesions of progressive massive fibrosis, masses of dense hyalinized connective tissue with little inflammation. Accelerated silicosis progresses rapidly to progressive massive fibrosis, whereas acute silicosis has a distinct pattern with few or no nodules and alveolar filling with proteinaceous material. Polarized light microscopy may show birefringent particles indicative of silica in the lungs of silica-exposed persons, including those with silicosis.

Clinical Manifestations. Chronic silicosis without progressive massive fibrosis is associated with little physiologic impairment. Cough and sputum production may reflect underlying bronchitis related to dust exposure or cigarette smoking. As in coal workers' pneumoconiosis, progressive massive fibrosis can be associated with significant impairment on lung function testing and clinically significant dyspnea. Both airflow obstruction and lung restriction may be present. Acute silicosis presents with rapidly progressive dyspnea. Persons with silicosis are at increased risk for mycobacterial infection (see Ch. 311), and they may present with manifestations of infection such as fever and weight loss.

In chronic silicosis, the chest radiograph shows small nodules that tend to predominate in the upper lobes. Calcification of the nodules is rare, as is so-called eggshell calcification of enlarged hilar nodes, which may be present. In progressive massive fibrosis, the mass lesions are typically in the upper lobes and often associated with compensatory hyperinflation of the lower lobes. Widespread consolidation is present on the chest radiograph in acute silicosis. Caplan's syndrome may also occur in silica-exposed workers, but it is rare.

Diagnosis. The diagnosis of chronic silicosis is made on the basis of characteristic radiographic findings and history of employment in a job associated with exposure to silica-containing dust. Before accepting a diagnosis of progressive massive fibrosis in a silica-exposed worker, other causes of lung masses should be considered, including specifically lung cancer and mycobacterial infection. Acute silicosis should be considered in heavily exposed individuals with a diffuse consolidating process. Unless the epidemiologic features of the case make the diagnosis of acute silicosis certain, lung biopsy may be indicated to establish the diagnosis and to exclude other diseases.

Treatment. As in any chronic lung disease, supportive therapy, oxygen, and rehabilitation may be indicated. One report suggested possible short-term benefits of corticosteroid therapy, but steroid therapy cannot be recommended at present. Because of the increased risk of mycobacterial diseases, particularly *Mycobacterium tuberculosis,* all persons with silicosis should receive yearly tuberculin skin tests and workup for active tuberculosis if the test is positive. Isoniazid prophylaxis is recommended if the test is positive and active disease is not present. Some studies indicate that prolonged antituberculous therapy may be indicated in patients with silicosis and active tuberculosis (see Ch. 311).

Prognosis. The prognosis of accelerated and acute silicosis is poor; both are associated with progressive loss of function and acute silicosis may be rapidly fatal. Progressive massive fibrosis has a more variable course, which may also lead to progressive impairment and respiratory failure. Factors determining progression from chronic silicosis to progressive massive fibrosis are uncertain.

Balaan MR, Banks DE: Silicosis. *In* Rom WN (ed.): Environmental and Occupational Medicine. 2nd ed. Boston, Little, Brown & Co, 1992, p 345. *A review chapter covering the full spectrum of silicosis.*
Valiante DJ, Rosenman KD: Does silicosis still occur? JAMA 262:3003, 1989. *Provides a recent perspective from one state on the occurrence of new cases of silicosis.*

OTHER PNEUMOCONIOSES. Inhaling other minerals and metals may also cause pneumoconioses (see Table 54–6). Silicates other than asbestos have been linked to interstitial lung disease, including talc, kaolinite, mica, and vermiculite. Benign pneumoconioses are associated with inhaling forms of barium (baritosis) and tin (stannosis). Hard-metal disease occurs in workers exposed to cobalt in applications involving its use in alloys and abrasives. This diffuse interstitial disease, which can be associated with clinically significant impairment, should be considered in workers in foundries and in industries involving grinding of metals, gems, and other materials. Some workers exposed to man-made fibers develop small opacities, but a distinct pneumoconiosis has not yet been identified from exposure to these newer fibers. Mixed-dust pneumoconiosis is a nonspecific label often used for the presence of both rounded and irregular opacities on the chest radiograph of a worker with exposure to several types of dust. Typically, there is exposure to silica and to an additional mineral.

Rom WN: Benign pneumoconioses. *In* Rom WN (ed.): Environmental and Occupational Medicine. 2nd ed. Boston, Little, Brown & Co, 1992, p 479. *A review chapter that covers a wide range of agents associated with pneumoconiosis.*

BERYLLIUM DISEASE. Beryllium disease is a granulomatous lung disease that results from inhaling beryllium, a rare metal now widely used in high-technology applications (Table 54–8). The typical cases currently observed present with gradual onset and are referred to as chronic beryllium disease; a more acute form was reported with past higher levels of exposure. When first recognized, the disease was found in workers who extracted and produced beryllium and in workers making fluorescent lamps containing a beryllium phosphor. Cases have been reported in bystanders not working directly with the metal and in persons residing in the vicinity of beryllium processing plants. More contemporary industries place a large number of workers at risk. In a recent study of nuclear weapons workers, about 5% of exposed workers were shown to be sensitized to beryllium.

Advances in understanding of the pathogenesis of beryllium disease have provided both a screening test for sensitization and a marker for individual susceptibility. The beryllium lymphocyte transformation test can be used to establish sensitization to the metal and as a workplace screening tool. In this *in vitro* assay, blood lymphocytes or lung lymphocytes obtained by bronchoalveolar lavage are exposed to beryllium salts; cells from sensitized individuals show proliferation. Recently, a genetic marker for susceptibility to beryllium disease has been identified. A strong association has been reported between a specific phenotype associated with the major histocompatibility complex (MHC) HLA-DPβ1 (see Ch. 229) and beryllium disease. This marker may eventually prove useful to identify workers at greatest risk and to better understand the pathogenesis of beryllium disease.

TABLE 54–7. PRINCIPAL OCCUPATIONS ASSOCIATED WITH SILICON EXPOSURE

Abrasives workers	Silica flour workers
Foundry workers	Silica millers
Glass makers	Stone workers
Pottery workers	Surface mine drillers
Quarriers	Underground miners
Sandblasters	

TABLE 54–8. CURRENT INDUSTRIES USING BERYLLIUM

Aerospace	Electronics	Plating
Beryllium extraction, fabrication, smelting	Foundries	Telecommunications
Ceramics	Nuclear reactors	Tool and die
Dental alloys and prostheses	Nuclear weapons	

Although interstitial fibrosis is classically considered to be a granulomatous disorder, some patients may have interstitial fibrosis without granulomas. If granulomas are present in lung or other tissue specimens, the differential diagnosis includes sarcoidosis and hypersensitivity pneumonitis. The lymphocyte transformation test can confirm beryllium exposure, but the metal can also be measured in tissue specimens and urine. Patients with beryllium disease may have both respiratory and systemic symptoms and chest radiograph findings extending from normal to diffuse interstitial infiltrates and hilar adenopathy. Corticosteroid therapy may be beneficial, but life-long treatment is needed.

Kreiss K, Mroz MM, Zhen B, et al.: Epidemiology of beryllium sensitization and disease in nuclear workers. Am Rev Respir Dis 148:985, 1993. *This recent article describes risk factors for beryllium sensitization applying the blood beryllium lymphocyte transformation assay.*

Richeldi L, Sorrentino R, Saltini C: HLA-DPβ1 Glutamate 69: A genetic marker of beryllium disease. Science 262:242, 1993. *This report describes a new genetic marker for beryllium disease with implications for screening and for research on pathogenesis.*

HYPERSENSITIVITY PNEUMONITIS. Hypersensitivity pneumonitis, typically a granulomatous ILD, results from inhaling diverse environmental antigens and chemicals. Hypersensitivity pneumonitis may present as an acute illness, but it may also present in a chronic form with pulmonary fibrosis. The workplace is often a site of exposure to antigens generated by microbial contaminants of heating, ventilating, and air conditioning systems or other moist devices or materials. Chemical agents associated with hypersensitivity pneumonitis include isocyanates and trimellitic anhydride. The diagnosis is made on the basis of the clinical picture, exposure history, and demonstration of precipitating antibodies to antigens.

54.2 Physical, Chemical, and Aspiration Injuries of the Lung

Claude A. Piantadosi

PHYSICAL AND CHEMICAL INJURIES OF THE LUNG

The lung's large and delicate surface area is protected from toxic substances in the environment by extensive defense mechanisms. Normally, inspired gas is fully humidified and warmed to body temperature, and all large particulate substances are cleared by the upper airways. These normal defenses are not adequate to handle exposure to many physical and chemical substances that cause lung injury. This section discusses lung disorders initiated by inhalation or aspiration of injurious chemicals or by exposure to potentially harmful physical environments.

Thermal Injuries and Smoke Inhalation

After major burns, about one third of patients have pulmonary complications; these complications account for the majority of burn-related deaths. Thermal injury to the lung is associated with three groups of complications: (1) *immediate reaction*—direct thermal injury to upper airways leading to upper airway obstruction, carbon monoxide poisoning, and smoke inhalation; (2) *adult respiratory distress syndrome* (ARDS) developing 24 to 48 hours after the thermal injury; and (3) *late-onset pulmonary complications,* which include pneumonia, atelectasis, thromboembolism, and chest wall restriction caused by circumferential thoracic burns.

The constituents of smoke are by-products of pyrolysis and incomplete combustion. Many of these products are potent mucosal irritants and bronchoconstrictors and contribute to both upper and lower lung injury. Certain constituents of smoke have been identified consistently as contributors to respiratory injury (Table 54–9). Smoke inhalation rarely causes thermal injury to the lung parenchyma; the large capacity of the upper airways to humidify and modify the temperatures of inhaled air protects the alveolar tissue from heat. Exceptions are steam burns and explosions in an enclosed space.

CLINICAL MANIFESTATIONS. The initial signs and symptoms of smoke inhalation are tachypnea, cough, dyspnea, wheezing,

TABLE 54–9. TOXIC BY-PRODUCTS OF SMOKE IMPLICATED IN RESPIRATORY INJURY

Source	By-products
Cotton, paper, wood	Acrolein, CO, acetaldehyde
Petroleum products	Acrolein, CO, benzene
Polyvinyl chloride (PVC)	Hydrocyanic acid, CO, chlorine, phosgene
Nylon, silk, wool	Hydrocyanic acid, ammonia
Nitrocellulose	Oxides of nitrogen
Sulfur compounds	Sulfur dioxide

cyanosis, hoarseness, and stridor (an ominous sign). Facial burns may provide a clue to smoke inhalation and thermal injury to the upper airway. During the 12 to 48 hours after the injury, the patient can manifest increasing hypoxemia, and lung compliance may decrease owing to noncardiogenic pulmonary edema. Roentgenograms of the chest may reveal a pattern of diffuse, patchy infiltrates. A major complication is infection, often caused by *Pseudomonas aeruginosa* or *Staphylococcus aureus.* The lung defenses against infection are compromised by thermal and chemical injury to the airway epithelium as well as by the presence of an endotracheal or tracheostomy tube. The pathway for infection is either by inhaling airborne organisms or by hematogenous spread from cutaneous burns.

The ARDS may develop 24 to 48 hours after the initial injury. The causes of ARDS are controversial in burn patients, but possibilities include a chemical pneumonitis from constituents in smoke, a circulating burn toxin, disseminated intravascular coagulation, microembolism, and neurogenic pulmonary edema. The extent of surface thermal injury does not correlate with the degree of respiratory distress that occurs subsequently.

TREATMENT. The most immediate life-threatening complications in the patient presenting with major burns or with a history of smoke inhalation are upper airway obstruction and carbon monoxide (CO) intoxication. The patient should be closely observed for evidence of these complications. Laryngeal and tracheobronchial inflammation may be detected by fiberoptic bronchoscopy. Arterial blood gases should be measured and prompt intubation or tracheostomy performed if there is evidence of significant airway obstruction. Corticosteroids may help treat edema of the upper airways but must be used with caution because infection is a major concern for managing both skin and pulmonary injury. Prophylactic antibiotics are of no value in preventing pneumonia and may predispose to infection with resistant organisms. Careful pulmonary toilet, humidification, and sterile suctioning should be used to reduce the risk of pneumonia. Serial bronchoscopy may be necessary to remove mucous plugs and thereby prevent segmental atelectasis and postobstructive infection.

Late-onset pulmonary burn complications—atelectasis, thromboembolism, and pneumonia—are discussed in Ch. 53, 59, and 271 to 274, respectively.

Carbon Monoxide Poisoning

Smoke inhalation is invariably accompanied by the body taking up CO. In some fires, CO exposure is complicated by cyanide poisoning from the combustion of plastic compounds. CO poisoning also is encountered frequently after exposure to automobile exhaust, and in the winter when victims are exposed to fumes from faulty furnaces. As a result, CO is the leading cause of accidental poisoning in the United States.

CO toxicity is a consequence of tissue hypoxia created by the displacement of oxygen from hemoglobin. CO competes with oxygen for binding at the iron-porphyrin centers of hemoglobin. These centers bind CO reversibly, but with an affinity more than 200 times greater than that for oxygen. The oxygen affinity of heme not occupied by CO is also increased in the presence of carboxyhemoglobin (HbCO). This HbCO-related increase in oxygen affinity shifts the oxyhemoglobin dissociation curve to the left and impairs the release of oxygen to the tissues. These two effects of CO on hemoglobin decrease the partial pressure of oxygen in the tissues. Tissue hypoxia has serious functional consequences for organ systems that require a continuous supply of oxygen, such as the brain and the heart. In addition, when tissue P_{O_2} is low, CO binds to intracellular hemoproteins such as myoglobin and cytochrome c oxidase, inhibiting their functions.

CLINICAL MANIFESTATIONS. The clinical features of acute CO poisoning are diverse but most often related to the central nervous system. In normal, nonsmoking individuals, symptoms may appear when HbCO levels reach 10%. Patients with chronic obstructive pulmonary disease (COPD) and coronary artery disease are more sensitive to the effects of HbCO. Smokers often maintain HbCO levels of 3 to 10%, and they may tolerate slightly higher levels without symptoms. Common symptoms of CO poisoning include headache, nausea, vomiting, confusion, and visual disturbances. More severe CO poisoning can produce seizures, transient unconsciousness, coma, and death. Metabolic acidosis, pulmonary edema, and rhabdomyolysis may also accompany serious CO poisoning. The "classic" clinical findings of cherry red lips and nail beds are rare. The differential diagnosis includes drug overdoses, other poisonings (e.g., cyanide), and cerebrovascular accidents. The clinical diagnosis is confirmed by an elevated blood HbCO level measured by CO-oximetry. The severity of the clinical illness, however, may not correlate well with the HbCO level but relates instead to the duration and extent of the exposure.

TREATMENT AND OUTCOME. Symptoms of mild CO poisoning generally subside within minutes to a few hours after removing the patient from the noxious environment. Patients with more severe CO intoxication benefit from inspiring high concentrations of oxygen to hasten the removal of CO from hemoglobin. In obtunded or comatose patients, 100% oxygen should be administered via an endotracheal tube until the HbCO level is < 5%. Pure oxygen reduces the halftime for eliminating HbCO from the body from approximately 240 minutes to 60 minutes. Patients with loss of consciousness or other neurologic impairment, cardiac symptoms or signs, or HbCO levels >25% should receive hyperbaric oxygen if it is readily available. Hyperbaric oxygen at 2.5 atmospheres absolute (ATA) reduces the HbCO halftime to approximately 20 minutes. Oxygen dissolved in plasma under hyperbaric pressure also bypasses the impairment of oxygen transport to tissues imposed by HbCO. As a result, potentially serious neurologic sequelae may be averted if the therapy can be instituted promptly. Adjunctive therapy, such as corticosteroids, hyperventilation, mannitol, and hypothermia, has been recommended for treating serious cases of CO intoxication, but benefit from these modalities is unproved.

Neurologic recovery in patients with mild to moderate CO poisoning is good. The prognosis after severe CO intoxication is variable and correlates with the extent and duration of the insult. Short-term memory impairment, depression, and syndromes related to lesions of the basal ganglia are well described. A syndrome of delayed neurologic deterioration occurs in 3 to 10% of victims of serious CO intoxication. Risk factors for the delayed syndrome include age over 40, prolonged exposure, and abnormalities of the brain on computed tomography (CT). Hyperbaric oxygen therapy has been reported to decrease the incidence of the delayed syndrome.

Other Toxic Inhaled Gases

A large number of gases and chemicals, to which exposures most frequently occur in an industrial setting, can acutely and sometimes chronically injure the respiratory system. A few agents cause an "asthma-like" reaction with cough, chest pain, and wheezing. Toluene di-isocyanate and other isocyanates (liberated as a gas in making polyurethane foams), aluminum soldering flux, and platinum salts are typical examples. Reaginic and precipitating antibodies against platinum salts and soldering flux have been found in symptomatic individuals, suggesting an immunologic basis for the reaction. An allergic basis has not been demonstrated for the reaction to toluene diisocyanate. The symptoms usually subside after removal from exposure; however, chronic lung injury may occur if the exposure is prolonged.

A number of highly irritating gases cause an *acute chemical pneumonitis.* Such gases include chlorine (used in the chemical and plastic industries and to disinfect water), ammonia (used in refrigeration), sulfur dioxide (used in making paper and smelting sulfide-containing ores), ozone (generated in welding and in photochemical smog), nitrogen dioxide (released from decomposed corn silage), and phosgene (used in producing aniline dyes).

An important injury of this type is *silo-filler's disease* (nitrogen dioxide). During the exposure, there may be no symptoms, there may be tracheobronchitis with cough and shortness of breath, or there may be immediate acute pulmonary edema. Signs of ocular and oropharyngeal mucous membrane irritation may be present. The symptoms can rapidly progress, but commonly the initial symptoms resolve and are followed by a period of minimal symptoms (cough) lasting up to 48 hours. Fever, myalgias, dyspnea, and progressive hypoxemia then occur, and the radiographic picture is that of pulmonary edema. These severe symptoms can resolve, only to recur 2 to 5 weeks later and lead to progressive bronchiolitis obliterans. Treatment with corticosteroids (prednisone, 1 mg per kilogram per day) can dramatically improve the acute illness. Bronchodilators, mechanical ventilation, and supplemental oxygen may be necessary. Because improvement after the initial exposure may be temporary, observation for a period of 48 hours is advisable.

The clinical response caused by each irritant gas varies but appears to be closely related to the degree of acute irritation it causes and to its water solubility. The less irritating gases, such as ozone and the oxides of nitrogen, phosgene, mercury, and nickel carbonyl, can be inhaled for prolonged periods and thereby cause injury throughout the respiratory system. Highly irritating and soluble gases, such as ammonia and hydrochloric acid, are less likely to be inhaled deeply and tend to result in immediate injury to the upper airways and have potential for obstruction secondary to mucosal edema. Less soluble substances, such as chlorine, cadmium, zinc chloride, osmium tetroxide, and vanadium, can cause injury to the entire tracheobronchial tree and generally do not produce upper airway obstruction as the initial presentation. Bronchiolitis and pulmonary edema are common, ultimately leading to bronchiolitis obliterans. Long-term consequences vary with the gas. Cadmium, for example, can cause diffuse emphysema and severe airway obstruction but only minimal fibrosis.

Different mechanisms are involved in the injury caused by irritant gases. Most of them cause injury by acting as a strong acid, a strong base, or an oxidant. Gases of chemicals that are strong acids or bases in water solution, such as hydrogen chloride, sulfuric acid, sulfur dioxide, and ammonia, tend to react more in the upper airways, where they change tissue pH and thereby cause cell damage.

Pulmonary Oxygen Toxicity

Oxygen is toxic to the lungs when used in high concentrations for prolonged periods. This toxicity occurs clinically in patients in intensive care units who are on mechanical ventilators. The toxic effects of hyperoxia are believed to result from excessive generation of superoxide, an unstable free radical produced by the single electron reduction of oxygen. Superoxide is produced as a normal by-product of oxidative metabolism and scavenged by the protective enzymes, the superoxide dismutases, that catalyze its dismutation to hydrogen peroxide (Fig. 54–2). If it is not scavenged enzymatically, superoxide anion can react with hydrogen peroxide in the presence of transition metals, e.g., iron, to form hydroxyl radical (OH·). Hydroxyl radical is highly reactive and can initiate lipid peroxidation and oxidize protein and nucleic acids.

In the adult, the major site of oxygen injury is the pulmonary capillary endothelium. Pathologically, the lungs are atelectatic, congested, and edematous. Hyaline membranes are often present. Oxidant injury attracts inflammatory cells to the lung, including neutrophils. Advanced injury destroys the capillary bed with resultant interstitial and alveolar edema, hypoxemia, and sometimes death. Alveolar epithelium is also injured, causing hyperplasia of type II cells. An acute tracheobronchitis also occurs, and histologic changes have been found in the ciliated epithelium and Clara cells in the small airways.

CLINICAL MANIFESTATIONS. Oxygen toxicity usually occurs in acutely ill patients who are receiving oxygen in high concentrations and mechanical ventilation for lung injuries that obscure the onset of pulmonary toxicity. Lung compliance progressively falls; the alveolar-arterial oxygen gradient gradually widens, and increasing concentrations of oxygen are needed to maintain adequate oxygenation of arterial blood. This cycle progresses to pulmonary edema, respiratory failure, and death.

The earliest symptoms of oxygen toxicity are those of acute tracheobronchitis. A dry, hacking cough and substernal pain may occur after 6 to 12 hours of breathing pure oxygen. Vital capacity decreases, and respiratory rate increases. The flow of tracheal mucus decreases after short exposures to excess oxygen, probably reflecting functional injury of airway epithelium. These patients are therefore more susceptible to mucus impaction and to infection caused by failure to clear inhaled pathogens adequately.

TREATMENT AND OUTCOME. The only proven therapy is to prevent the insult by judicious use of high oxygen concentrations. The physician often faces a dilemma in that increasing concentrations of oxygen are needed to save the patient immediately, but eventually can kill the patient. Alternative methods to enhance arterial oxygen content should be used whenever possible. These include positive end-expiratory pressure (PEEP) and transfusion of packed red cells to maintain the hematocrit near 30%. Maintaining cardiac output and measures to decrease the tissue oxygen demand by reducing fever or agitation are appropriate.

The safe maximal concentration of oxygen is not known. Many authors recommend 40 to 50% oxygen as a safe limit because little injury has been demonstrated in normal animals or human volunteers breathing such concentrations for prolonged periods. The diseased lung, however, may be more susceptible to oxygen injury. A rational therapy is to use only enough oxygen to provide adequate arterial blood saturation, e.g., an SaO_2 of 90%. Corticosteroids have no benefit and may actually worsen the lung injury caused by hyperoxia. If the patient survives oxygen toxicity, some residual damage to the lung parenchyma may remain, with septal fibrosis replacing areas where the pulmonary capillary bed was destroyed by the hyperoxia.

Radiation Lung Injury (See also Ch. 13.1)

Ionizing radiation produces oxidant lung injury related to the degree of the radiation exposure. The clinical occurrence of radiation pneumonitis is determined by the total radiation dose, the number of fractions, and the duration of time over which the radiation is given. Chemotherapeutic drugs that produce oxidant-based lung toxicity, such as bleomycin, may potentiate lung injury from radiation. A total lung dose of less than 2000 Gy generally is not associated with severe radiation pneumonitis, whereas a total dose in excess of 4000 Gy, even if distributed over as many as 30 fractions, has virtually a 100% risk of radiation pneumonitis.

The reaction of the lung to radiation injury can be divided into three phases. (1) An *acute phase,* occurring 1 to 2 months after radiation exposure, is characterized by vascular damage, congestion, edema, and mononuclear cell infiltration. Alveolar type II cells and alveolar macrophages are increased in number. (2) A *subacute phase* occurs 2 to 9 months later. The alveolar walls become infiltrated with mononuclear inflammatory cells and fibroblasts. (3) The *chronic* or *fibrotic phase* generally occurs more than 9 months after irradiation. Alveolar fibrosis and capillary sclerosis are its predominant histologic features.

CLINICAL MANIFESTATIONS. Signs of bronchial irritation, e.g., cough, may appear immediately after radiation therapy, followed shortly thereafter by esophagitis. Some patients may have no symptoms for 6 to 12 weeks. If large volumes of lung have been irradiated, or if high radiation doses have been given over short periods, the patient can develop dyspnea, tachypnea, and fever. These symptoms can be severe and either progress to severe dyspnea and death or gradually subside, leaving varying degrees of respiratory impairment due to lung fibrosis. Permanent fibrosis takes 6 to 24 months to evolve and then usually remains stable if no further exposure occurs. Auscultation of the chest is usually normal, although rales, signs of consolidation, and pleural rubs may be found. Clubbing does not develop after radiation injury. Laboratory findings include a mild leukocytosis and an increased erythrocyte sedimentation rate. If the irradiated area is extensive, arterial hypoxemia may develop. Radiographic changes generally appear 1 to 3 months after treatment. The affected areas are generally demarcated by a "straight edge" defining the margins of the radiation portal and have a "ground-glass appearance"—a hazy increase in density with indistinct pulmonary markings. In the later phases of the radiation injury, fibrosis and contraction of the irradiated region are the predominant radiographic findings. Pulmonary function tests do not change until clinical symptoms appear, and then pulmonary restriction may be noted. Capillary sclerosis is associated with a decrease in blood flow to the affected region and a decrease in CO diffusing capacity.

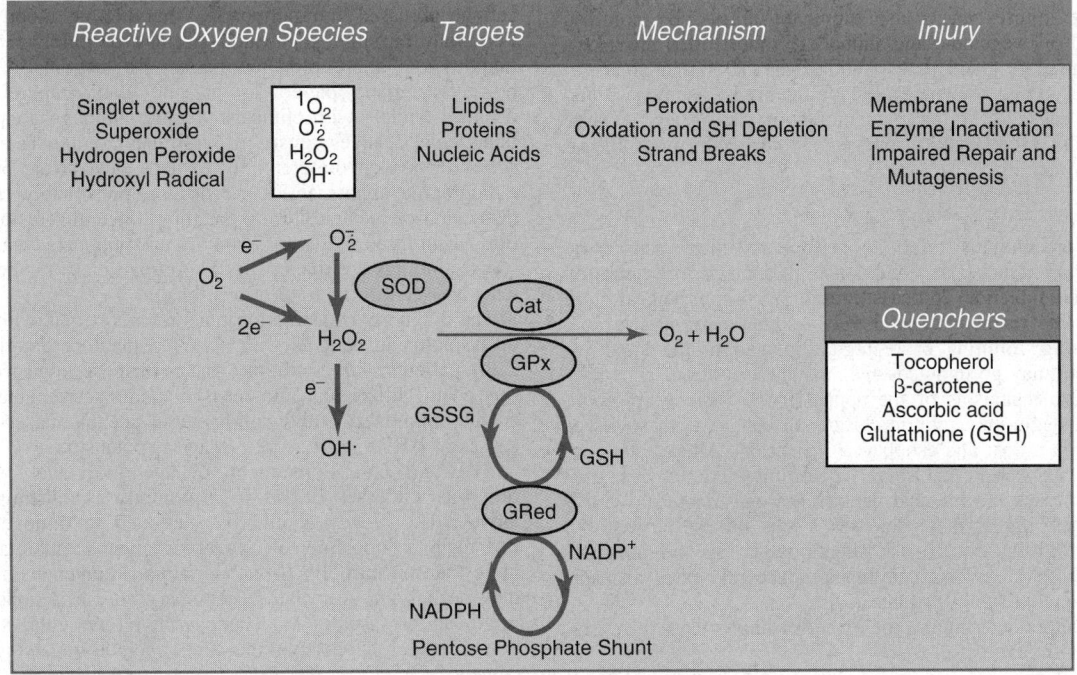

FIGURE 54–2. Reactive oxygen species and antioxidant defenses. When oxygen (O_2) is reduced incompletely, toxic oxygen species are formed such as singlet oxygen ($^1O_2$), superoxide anion, (O_2^-) and hydrogen peroxide (H_2O_2). H_2O_2 in the presence of iron (Fe^{2+}) or other reduced transition metals can generate highly reactive hydroxyl radical ($OH\cdot$). Reactive oxygen species can oxidize lipids (lipid peroxidation) proteins and nucleic acid (DNA strand breaks). Quenchers react with reactive oxygen species or with oxidized cellular molecules to prevent further oxidation. The enzymatic antioxidant defenses consist of the superoxide dismutases (SOD), catalase (Cat), and the glutathione peroxidase-reductase system (GPx and GRed). These enzymes detoxify (O_2^-) and H_2O_2 to prevent undesirable biologic oxidations. NADPH is required both for reduction of glutathione and for pathways for repair of oxidant damage. Glucose 6-phosphate dehydrogenase determines availability of NADPH because it is the rate-limiting step in the pentose phosphate shunt.

The diagnosis of acute radiation pneumonitis may be difficult to establish because of coincidental disease. The clinical picture is often complicated by the immunocompromised state of many of the patients, resulting in increased risk of bacterial or opportunistic pneumonias, e.g., those caused by *Pneumocystis carinii,* or by the signs and symptoms of the original neoplasm. Radiation pneumonitis in parts of the lung outside the radiation portal has been suspected in a few patients on the basis of typical clinical and radiographic features. Complications of radiation pneumonitis include small pleural effusions and, occasionally, spontaneous pneumothorax.

TREATMENT AND OUTCOME. The patient who develops radiation pneumonitis requires supportive care, including cough suppression, antipyretics, and supplemental oxygen for hypoxemia. Corticosteroids (prednisone, 1 mg per kilogram of body weight) have been advocated for treating severe cases of radiation pneumonitis, although there have been no controlled clinical trials. There is no evidence to support use of prophylactic corticosteroids, but using them at the very onset of pneumonitis appears to be more effective than later therapy. On occasion, the response may be dramatic, with complete resolution of symptoms within 24 hours. Corticosteroids should be tapered carefully after achieving maximal clinical benefit. Pneumonitis has been reported occasionally after withdrawing steroids. No other effective therapeutic strategies are known. Antibiotic therapy should be reserved for patients in whom the clinical findings suggest infection. Because the lesion involves occlusion and thrombosis of many small blood vessels, anticoagulation has been tried, but there is no evidence of its effectiveness.

Rosiello RA, Merrill WW: Radiation-induced lung injury. Clin Chest Med 11:65, 1990.
A summary of the clinical features of radiation-induced lung disease.

ASPIRATION-RELATED INJURIES

Injury to the respiratory system by aspiration can be categorized by the nature of the aspirate as (1) *infectious material,* (2) *chemical* or *inflammatory substances,* and (3) *inert material.* Contamination of the lungs by aspirating oropharyngeal bacterial flora is discussed in Ch. 56. Aspirating gastric acid is the most common example of chemical aspiration in adults; hydrocarbon aspiration occurs predominantly in children but is encountered occasionally in adults. Both of these injuries can cause fulminant illness. By contrast, lipids (mineral oil, vegetable and animal fats) most often provoke a chronic inflammatory reaction. Aspirating inert material such as water causes injury (e.g., drowning), predominantly by asphyxia. Food particles can cause a fibrotic, granulomatous lesion or, if large enough to occlude the larynx or trachea, sudden death by asphyxiation ("cafe coronary").

Aspiration Pneumonitis

Aspiration pneumonitis refers to pulmonary injury caused by acidic stomach contents. This condition is in contrast to "aspiration pneumonia," an infectious process caused by oropharyngeal flora contaminating the tracheobronchial tree. Aspiration of gastric acid can occur during vomiting or regurgitation, and in the latter instance the event may go unnoted—i.e., "silent aspiration." The normal protective mechanisms of the upper airway include epiglottic closure during deglutition, glottic closure on contact with solids or fluids, the cough reflex, and esophageal sphincters. Altered states of consciousness, anesthesia and surgery, neuromuscular disease, gastrointestinal disease, and medical devices (nasogastric tubes or tracheostomy tubes) impair these defenses. Protecting the airway is a major concern in these high-risk situations. Using low-pressure, high-volume cuffs on endotracheal tubes reduces the extent of aspiration of gastric contents in patients at risk.

The main factors determining the extent of illness caused by gastric acid aspiration are as follows:

1. *pH of the aspirate.* The acidity of the material is the single most important contributor to the lung injury. A pH of 2.5 or less has been proposed as a critical value for inducing severe pneumonitis from acid aspiration.

2. *The presence of food particles.* Aspiration of gastric food substance causes a severe pneumonitis and peribronchial inflammatory reaction in the absence of acid.

3. *Volume of the aspirate.* Aspirating >0.4 ml per kilogram of body weight of gastric acid is sufficient to cause pneumonitis.

4. *Distribution of the aspirate.* Many patients who aspirate immediately begin to cough, which may partially protect the lung from injury or may enhance dispersion of the acid over a greater area and create a diffuse injury.

After intratracheal instillation, acid is rapidly distributed in the lungs and can reach the pleura in 12 to 18 seconds. It is rapidly neutralized by bronchial secretions; in less than 30 minutes, the pH at the bronchial surface returns to normal. Acid causes chemical burns of the bronchi, bronchioles, and alveolar walls, with subsequent exudation of fluid into the lungs. Plasma volume may decrease by as much as 35% in severe injury without fluid replacement, and cardiac output and systemic arterial blood pressure may fall. Pulmonary artery wedge pressure is normal or low, indicating a nonhydrostatic cause of the pulmonary edema. The characteristics of phospholipids in the alveolar surface lining layer (surfactant) are altered, increasing surface forces and promoting early alveolar collapse. Lung compliance decreases secondary to the increase in interstitial fluids and altered surface forces. These disturbances of airways, alveoli, and vascular elements profoundly unbalance the normal ventilation-perfusion relationships. Increased intrapulmonary shunting is also common. As a result, hypoxemia is invariably present and usually severe.

CLINICAL MANIFESTATIONS. Some patients aspirate a large volume of gastric acid and almost immediately become apneic and hypotensive and die. More often, the patient survives the initial crisis but later develops a fulminant illness marked by dyspnea, cough, and frothy sputum. Alternatively, aspiration may not be accompanied by immediate coughing and agitation. After such silent aspiration, the patient may develop acute respiratory failure without an obvious reason for a precipitous deterioration in gas exchange. Within 1 to 5 hours after aspiration of gastric acid, tachypnea, rales, and rhonchi occur, and wheezing, cyanosis, cough, and hypotension may be present. Fever in the first 36 hours occurs in about 50% of patients.

Laboratory tests are nonspecific. A moderate leukocytosis with left shift develops early. Arterial blood gases show hypoxemia, and the arterial oxygen tension does not reach predicted levels after the patient has been breathing 100% oxygen for several minutes, indicating increased intrapulmonary shunting of blood. The arterial P_{CO_2} may be slightly elevated, normal, or mildly reduced. Abnormalities on chest roentgenograms are extremely variable, and no characteristic pattern is present. Radiographic abnormalities do not correlate with clinical outcome, although about 50% of patients have changes consistent with pneumonitis. The acid is sometimes distributed preferentially to dependent areas, but usually the radiographic abnormalities are diffuse, presumably from enhanced dispersion of the acid during coughing. Pleural effusions and cavitation of infiltrates are not seen in uncomplicated cases. Bronchoscopic findings are diagnostic if food particles or other gastric contents are seen in the trachea or bronchi.

The diagnosis of aspiration pneumonitis begins with a high index of suspicion in patients with abrupt respiratory deterioration, especially patients with conditions that predispose to gastric acid aspiration. The differential diagnosis includes cardiogenic pulmonary edema, pulmonary embolism, bacterial pneumonia, and many of the causes of ARDS, such as sepsis and hypotension.

TREATMENT. Treatment of the individual whose aspiration was witnessed begins with promptly establishing an adequate airway. The airway should be suctioned to remove any particulate matter. Supplemental oxygen is given to maintain a PaO_2 of more than 60 mm Hg. Bronchodilators (intravenous aminophylline) may be helpful. Associated pulmonary edema is noncardiogenic in origin and is usually associated with intravascular volume depletion. General supportive measures include replacing fluids judiciously.

The prophylactic use of antibiotics for acid aspiration is not indicated because they do not reduce morbidity or mortality and may increase the risk of subsequent infection with a resistant organism. The acid-damaged respiratory tract is more susceptible to bacterial infection, and up to one half of patients with significant aspiration develop bacterial pneumonia. Such patients undergo new deterioration after 2 or 3 days, with increasing fever, leukocytosis, production of purulent sputum, worsening hypoxemia, and new infiltrates on the chest radiograph.

Systemic corticosteroids in aspiration pneumonitis should not be used routinely. As for other forms of ARDS, administering corticosteroids does not decrease morbidity or mortality.

Positive-pressure ventilation is helpful after severe cases of aspiration to improve arterial oxygen tension. Mortality rates probably decrease with its use. Other measures useful to treat ARDS, such as maintaining a normal pulmonary capillary wedge pressure, are beneficial after aspiration injury of the lung. PEEP to improve oxygenation is commonly used in the management of gastric acid aspiration. Caution should be used in applying PEEP because it can produce a marked increase in extravascular water content in the acid-injured lung.

Aspiration pneumonitis carries a high mortality rate despite treatment, and because it largely occurs in a defined population at increased risk, efforts should be made at prevention. Elevating the head of the bed retards regurgitation. In intubated patients, placing a nasogastric tube should be considered to keep the stomach decompressed. Aspiration may occur even in the presence of a cuffed endotracheal tube. Elective general anesthesia should be given with the stomach empty, after at least a 12-hour fast. Preoperatively, the pH of gastric contents can be raised by a single dose of an H_2 receptor blocker or by a single 10-ml oral dose of antacid given 2 hours before surgery.

OUTCOME. Mortality from aspiration pneumonitis is high, reaching 28 to 62% of cases. Factors associated with highest mortality are age over 50 years, the early development of shock or apnea, severe and prolonged hypoxemia, very low pH of gastric contents at the time of aspiration, and the development of secondary bacterial pneumonia. Most patients survive the early moments but deteriorate over 12 to 24 hours. Some then show steady improvement, with radiographic resolution within a week. Others have a second episode of deterioration, an event that should suggest a new problem, such as bacterial infection, pulmonary embolism, heart failure, or another aspiration. Still others pursue a relentlessly worsening course to death. Few data exist regarding long-term clinical follow-up, but pulmonary fibrosis of varying degrees may occur in some of the survivors.

Bernard GR, Luce JM, Sprung CL, et al.: High dose corticosteroids in patients with the adult respiratory distress syndrome: A randomized double-blinded trial. N Engl J Med 317:1565, 1987. *Corticosteroid therapy does not improve morbidity or mortality after development of ARDS.*

Hydrocarbon Pneumonitis

Hydrocarbon pneumonitis results from the direct toxic effects of volatile hydrocarbons on the respiratory epithelium and vasculature. It occurs in individuals who, having ingested the hydrocarbons, aspirate them into the respiratory tract. The problem occurs most often in children, particularly those below age 5. It is an uncommon problem in adults, occurring most often in industrial accidents, in patients attempting suicide, in siphoning of gasoline, and in uninformed alcoholics seeking an ethanol substitute.

Different hydrocarbons cause respiratory injury of varying extent, depending on the viscosity and volume of the aspirate. The lower the viscosity or the larger the volume, the worse the lesion. As lipid solvents, these compounds are directly toxic to respiratory tissues. The lungs of children dying of hydrocarbon pneumonitis demonstrate hemorrhage, pulmonary edema, atelectasis, hyaline membrane formation, and necrosis of airway epithelium and alveolar septa. These compounds also have systemic toxicity, and in fatal cases, degenerative changes have been seen in the liver and kidneys.

CLINICAL MANIFESTATIONS. Aspiration usually occurs when hydrocarbons are ingested, and a history of vomiting after ingestion is obtained in fewer than half the patients. Dyspnea, tachypnea, tachycardia, and high fever quickly ensue. Sputum may be bloody. Lethargy is common, but more severe disturbances of consciousness also occur, such as confusion, coma, and seizures. Auscultation is frequently normal, but rales and rhonchi may be present.

Laboratory tests give nonspecific results. A moderate leukocytosis with left shift is common. Arterial hypoxemia of various degrees develops owing to shunting and to ventilation-perfusion mismatching. The chest radiograph is particularly helpful, as infiltrates may occur within 20 to 30 minutes after aspirating some types of hydro-

carbons. The multiple, fluffy, ill-defined infiltrates favor dependent areas of the lungs. Some patients present a picture of bilateral perihilar infiltrates, a pulmonary edema pattern. Pleural effusions, pneumothorax, and pneumomediastinum occur but are uncommon. Pneumatoceles can form later, especially in children.

The differential diagnosis is that of sudden respiratory distress. Frequently, the patient has an impaired sensorium at presentation. The adult patient is often an alcoholic. Gastric acid aspiration, cardiogenic pulmonary edema, pulmonary embolism, and acute bacterial pneumonia can all manifest similarly. The correct diagnosis requires the history of hydrocarbon ingestion or aspiration. The diagnosis is also suggested by the odor of the patient's breath and by extensive radiographic abnormalities in a patient with a clear chest on auscultation.

TREATMENT. Emesis to remove residual hydrocarbons is contraindicated. Gastric lavage by nasogastric tube may cause vomiting and should be performed only after placing a cuffed endotracheal tube in the patient who has recently ingested a large volume of hydrocarbons. Supplemental oxygen should be given to maintain a PaO_2 greater than 60 mm Hg. Mechanical ventilation and PEEP may be necessary. No data support the routine use of antibiotics. Systemic corticosteroids (prednisone, 1 mg per kilogram per day) during the acute illness have been suggested by anecdotal reports of improvement after their use in children and adults.

OUTCOME. Hydrocarbon pneumonitis in adults is rare, so that estimates of morbidity and mortality are not available. In children, death occurs in about 10% of cases, but most children have a prompt clinical recovery. Bronchiectasis, recurrent bronchitis, and/or pulmonary fibrosis ensues in an unknown portion of cases. After recovery, children frequently have normal chest examinations and radiographs, although pulmonary function abnormalities suggestive of small airway (<2-mm diameter) disease have been found in asymptomatic patients as late as 8 to 14 years after hydrocarbon pneumonitis.

Lipoid Pneumonia

Lipoid pneumonia is a chronic inflammatory reaction of the lungs to the presence of lipid substances. Exogenous lipoid pneumonia results from the aspiration of vegetable, animal, or (most commonly) mineral oils. This material differs greatly from the excessive accumulation of endogenous lipids in the lungs occurring in fat embolism, cholesterol pneumonia, pulmonary alveolar proteinosis, and the lipid storage diseases (endogenous lipoid pneumonia).

The most frequently implicated agent is mineral oil used as a laxative and to reduce dysphagia, either in clear liquid form or as petroleum jelly. Mineral oil is bland and, when introduced into the pharynx, can enter the bronchial tree without eliciting the cough reflex. It also mechanically impedes the ciliary action of the airway epithelium. The risk of mineral oil aspiration is increased in debilitated or senile patients, in those having neurologic disease that interferes with deglutition, and in patients with esophageal disease. Mineral oil taken as nose drops to relieve nasal dryness has caused lipoid pneumonia and years ago was a frequent cause of the illness. Inhalation of mineral oil mist by airplane and automobile mechanics has also been implicated as a cause of the problem.

Mineral oils cannot be hydrolyzed in the body and provoke a chronic inflammatory reaction that may not become clinically overt until years later. In the alveolar spaces, macrophages accumulate and phagocytize the emulsified oil. Some macrophages disintegrate, releasing their lysosomal enzymes and oil. The alveolar septa become thickened and edematous, containing lymphocytes and lipid-laden macrophages. Oil droplets are seen in the pulmonary lymphatics and hilar nodes. Later, fibrosis develops, and the normal lung architecture is effaced. It is usual in a single specimen to find both the early inflammatory and the later fibrotic picture, in keeping with repetitive aspirations over many months or years. If nodular, the lesion may grossly resemble tumor and is called a paraffinoma.

CLINICAL MANIFESTATIONS AND TREATMENT. Most patients are asymptomatic, coming to the physician's attention because of an abnormal chest radiograph. When patients are symptomatic, cough and exertional dyspnea are the most frequent complaints. Chest pain (sometimes pleuritic), hemoptysis, fever (usually low grade), chills, night sweats, and weight loss may occur. The physical examination may be completely normal, or fever, tachypnea, dullness on percussion of the chest, bronchial or bronchovesicular breath sounds, rales, and rhonchi may be found. Clubbing and cor pulmonale are rare.

In mild lipoid pneumonia, arterial blood gas values may be normal with the patient at rest but may show hypoxemia after exercise. In more severe disease, resting hypoxemia, hypocapnia, and mild respiratory alkalosis develop. Pulmonary function testing reveals a restrictive ventilatory defect; lung compliance is decreased. The only specific laboratory finding is the presence in sputum of macrophages with clusters of vacuoles 5 to 50 μm in diameter that stain deep orange with Sudan IV and extracellular droplets that stain similarly.

Radiographically, the earliest abnormalities are air space infiltrates, unilateral or bilateral, localized or diffuse, but most often in the dependent portions of the lung. Air bronchograms may be seen. Hilar adenopathy and pleural reaction are rare. As fibrosis develops, volume loss occurs and linear and nodular infiltrates appear. A solid lesion that closely resembles bronchogenic carcinoma may develop.

The differential diagnosis is extensive, particularly in the late phase, when multiple other causes of pulmonary fibrosis must be considered. The key to the correct diagnosis before biopsy is the history of chronic oral or intranasal use of an oil- or a lipid-based product, or an occupational exposure to oil mists. The presence of lipid-laden macrophages in the sputum confirms the diagnosis.

Once the diagnosis has been made and the aspiration stopped, the subsequent course is variable. Some patients have no change in symptoms. Others improve in some or all parameters, whereas a few patients deteriorate, with worsening pulmonary function and cor pulmonale. Because the only way the lung can dispose of mineral oil is by expectoration, the patient should be instructed in coughing exercises to be performed many times each day for months. Expectorants have not been shown to help. Systemic corticosteroids are recommended by some on the basis of improvement seen in a few uncontrolled reports. The rationale has been that the cellular reaction, rather than the oil itself, is the destructive factor. Because of the well-recognized side effects of systemic corticosteroids, their use for lipoid pneumonia should be limited to those patients who have significant symptoms and then for as brief a period as possible.

Wright BA, Jeffrey PA: Lipoid pneumonia. Sem Respir Infect 5:314, 1990. *A good review of the clinical and pathologic features of exogenous lipoid pneumonia; with 24 references.*

Near-Drowning

Drowning is one of the three leading causes of accidental death in children and young adults. In adults, alcohol consumption and shallow water blackout during breath-hold diving are common aggravating factors. Pathophysiologically, drowning can be of two types: (1) "wet" drowning—initial laryngospasm but early relaxation and subsequent aspiration of copious amounts of fluid; the majority of drownings are of this sort: (2) "dry" drowning—asphyxiation secondary to intense glottic spasm that persists beyond the point of apnea, so that when the muscles relax, little or no water is aspirated; this accounts for 10 to 20% of drownings. The immediate cause of death in many victims of drowning is cardiac arrhythmia. Victims who survive the initial episode frequently develop ARDS a few hours to a few days after the event (secondary drowning).

The most important consequences of near-drowning are attributed to asphyxia. Asphyxia results in severe hypoxemia, hypercarbia, and metabolic acidosis. The metabolic consequences of drowning in fresh water or salt water appear to differ little except for drowning in water with very high mineral content (e.g., the Dead Sea). In both cases, hypoxemia is caused by the occlusion of airways with water and particulate debris, by changes in surfactant activity, by direct injury to the alveolar septa, and by bronchospasm. Right-to-left shunting is markedly increased, and physiologic dead space is increased. Life-threatening electrolyte disturbances caused by water aspiration in humans are rare. Cardiac arrhythmias and central nervous system and renal insufficiency often occur after near-drowning. Brain anoxia is usually global anoxia, and if it is of sufficient duration and magnitude, it leads to diffuse cerebral edema.

Autopsies of drowned persons demonstrate wet, heavy lungs with varying amounts of hemorrhage and edema and some disruption of alveolar walls. In about 70% of victims, vomitus, sand, mud, and aquatic vegetation are aspirated. Specimens from victims dying of secondary drowning show desquamation of alveolar epithelial cells, hemorrhage, hyaline membrane formation, acute inflammatory infiltrates, and foreign body reactions to particulate matter. Cerebral edema and diffuse neuronal injury are seen. Changes of acute tubular necrosis are found in the kidneys.

CLINICAL MANIFESTATIONS. The initial appearance of the patient can vary widely, from coma to agitated alertness. Cyanosis, coughing, and the production of frothy pink sputum are common. Tachypnea, tachycardia, and a low-grade fever in the first few hours are seen if the patient did not become hypothermic during submersion. Rales, rhonchi and, less often, wheezes are heard. Neurologic signs vary and can fluctuate in any given patient but usually derive from diffuse cerebral dysfunction. Signs of associated trauma to the head and neck should be sought.

Laboratory studies reveal mild hypokalemia, hypernatremia, and hyperchloremia. A moderate leukocytosis may be present. Hematocrit and hemoglobin usually are normal at first measurement; in fresh water aspiration, the hematocrit may fall slightly in the first 24 hours owing to hemolysis. An isolated increase in serum-free hemoglobin without a change in hematocrit is more common. Occasionally, the clinical picture of disseminated intravascular coagulation occurs in near-drowning. Arterial blood gas values, usually obtained after preliminary resuscitation, show severe hypoxemia and metabolic acidosis. The most common electrocardiographic changes are sinus tachycardia and nonspecific ST segment and T wave changes, which revert to normal within hours; however, other, more ominous abnormalities may occur—ventricular arrhythmias, complete heart block, or myocardial infarction. The chest radiograph may be normal initially despite severe respiratory disturbances. It often shows patchy infiltrates, and sometimes a classic pattern of pulmonary edema is seen.

TREATMENT. Treatment of the near-drowning victim begins with establishing an adequate airway and, if necessary, emergency cardiopulmonary resuscitation. Oxygen in high concentrations is necessary because hypoxemia is present in essentially all victims. Even the patient who quickly becomes apparently normal should be hospitalized for 24 hours to watch for a subsequent clinical picture of ARDS. During transportation to a hospital, supplemental oxygen should be continued and precautions taken for potential head and neck injuries and other serious trauma.

In the hospital, therapy is dictated largely by the arterial blood gas values and the degree of respiratory failure. Continuous positive airway pressure or PEEP is particularly helpful for managing hypoxemia. Bronchospasm should be treated with nebulized β-agonists and intravenous theophylline. Patients with persistent localized atelectasis or localized wheezing should undergo bronchoscopy to exclude a foreign body as the cause. Prophylactic antibiotics have not been shown to be beneficial, although many victims of near-drowning develop pneumonia, sometimes caused by unusual microorganisms. Corticosteroids for the pulmonary lesions of near-drowning have no controlled prospective human studies to support their use. Animal models and retrospective studies in humans have failed to demonstrate any benefit.

The therapeutic approach to brain resuscitation after near-drowning is also controversial. If evidence of cerebral edema exists, intracranial pressure (ICP) monitoring may be useful to guide therapy. In the event of increased ICP, PEEP should be minimized because it may increase ICP. Hyperventilation to maintain a $PaCO_2$ of 25 to 30 mm Hg decreases ICP at the expense of cerebral blood flow. Mannitol may decrease cerebral edema. It should be used to maintain the serum osmolarity near 300 mOsm per liter. Corticosteroids are used widely (e.g., dexamethasone, 10 mg given intravenously initially and then 4 to 6 mg given intravenously every 4 hours) but are not of proven benefit for the brain injury. Seizures should be treated with anticonvulsants. Shivering or random, purposeless movements can increase ICP and should be controlled. If these maneuvers fail to lower ICP, then barbiturate coma for 24 to 48 hours has been recommended, although its benefit is questionable.

OUTCOME. Outcome in near-drowning is best judged by the neurologic status, i.e., the presence or absence of coma. The shorter the interval between recovery from the water to first spontaneous gasp, the better the prognosis for recovery. The absence of sponta-neous respiration after resuscitation from near-drowning is an omi-nous sign associated with severe neurologic sequelae. Permanent neurologic sequelae persist in about 20% of comatose victims. Common sequelae include minimal brain dysfunction, spastic quad-riplegia, extrapyramidal syndromes, optic and cerebral atrophy, and peripheral neuromuscular damage. Survival without neurologic damage is best in children who are hypothermic when recovered and may occur even after 40 minutes of submersion. Similar reports of survival after prolonged immersion in adults are very rare.

Modell JH: Near drowning. Circulation 74(Suppl IV):27, 1986. *An excellent summary of the pathophysiologic mechanisms involved in drowning.*

DISORDERS CAUSED BY ALTERED BAROMETRIC PRESSURE

Significant alterations in environmental pressure are encountered by humans during ascent to altitude and during underwater diving. As altitude increases, barometric pressure falls from approximately 760 mm Hg at sea level to 380 mm Hg (0.5 ATA) at 18,000 feet. In seawater, the pressure of the water column increases by an amount equal to the barometric pressure for every 33 feet of depth. Hence at 33 feet of seawater, the absolute pressure is doubled (2 ATA). As a result, participants in activities such as mountaineering and scuba diving are often exposed to extremes of environmental pressure. Rapid pressure changes produce notable physiologic effects related to the behavior of atmospheric gases in the lungs and body tissues.

Diseases of High Altitudes

At high altitudes, the low barometric pressure causes physiologic effects due primarily to the decrease in the partial pressure of in-spired oxygen. Physiologic changes, characterized primarily by hy-perventilation, appear at 8000 to 10,000 feet. At altitudes above 10,000 feet the physiologic responses become more pronounced owing to the shape of the oxygen-hemoglobin dissociation curve, which has a steep downslope below a Po_2 of approximately 60 mm Hg. A small drop in Po_2 below this level results in a relatively large decrease in arterial saturation. At 10,000 feet (3048 meters), the alveolar Po_2 is approximately 60 mm Hg, and some individuals manifest impairment of memory, judgment, and the ability to per-form complex calculations. At 18,000 feet (5486 meters), the alveo-lar Po_2 is 40 mm Hg, and unacclimatized individuals develop seri-ous neurologic signs and symptoms.

Exposure to high altitude occurs most commonly in commercial aviation. In general, aircraft cabins are maintained at a pressure equal to or greater than that encountered at 8000 feet, so that sup-plemental oxygen is not required. Some patients with reduced car-diac reserve or with COPD may have difficulty tolerating even a small drop in arterial oxygen saturation and may require oxygen during flights. Aircraft regulations require that the flight crew re-ceive supplemental oxygen when the cabin pressure drops below that at 10,000 feet and that passengers receive supplemental oxygen should the cabin pressure drop below that at 15,000 feet.

ACUTE MOUNTAIN SICKNESS (AMS). Ascent to high alti-tude produces a wide spectrum of illness that depends on factors such as the absolute altitude, the rate of ascent, the length of stay, and individual susceptibility. Altitude illness may be classified into several syndromes, as shown in Table 54–10. The acute syndromes probably reflect a common pathophysiology initiated by a relatively abrupt lack of oxygen, although the precise mechanisms remain uncertain. The ventilatory response to hypoxia and poor physical conditioning may play a role in susceptible individuals. The most common malady is AMS, and self-limited symptoms of headache, anorexia, malaise, and disturbed sleep may appear within a few hours of arriving at altitudes above 8000 feet. Symptoms may be-come worse with exercise owing in part to further oxygen desatura-tion of arterial blood. Mild AMS may affect half of unacclimatized visitors to 14,000 feet. At altitudes above 9500 feet, AMS may be severe and followed sometimes by the more serious conditions of high-altitude pulmonary edema (HAPE) and high-altitude cerebral edema (HACE) (Table 54–10), which frequently coexist. High-alti-tude retinal hemorrhages (HARH) are prevalent above 14,000 feet and probably share a similar pathophysiology with cerebral edema. Retinal hemorrhages are not significant unless they produce visual symptoms; the latter circumstance usually indicates involvement of the macula and mandates immediate descent. The more serious forms of AMS are discussed below.

TABLE 54–10. HIGH-ALTITUDE SYNDROMES

Syndrome	Clinical Description
Acute mountain sickness (AMS)	Common, self-limited; characterized by headache, anorexia, and malaise after ascent to altitudes > 8000 ft; "normal puna"
High-altitude pulmonary edema (HAPE)	Noncardiac pulmonary edema recognized by dyspnea and tachypnea at rest, cough, and bibasilar crackles; usually at altitudes > 9500 ft; "pulmonary puna"
High-altitude cerebral edema (HACE)	Uncommon, severe central nervous system dysfunction following AMS, character-ized by severe headache, memory loss, ataxia, hallucinations, and confusion; may progress to coma and death; "ner-vous puna"
High-altitude retinal he-morrhages (HARH)	Dilated retinal vessels and peripheral flame-shaped or dot hemorrhages; occa-sionally cause visual symptoms
Chronic mountain sickness (Monge's diseases)	Cor pulmonale with minimal lung disease in long-term residents of high altitude

HIGH-ALTITUDE PULMONARY EDEMA (HAPE). Acute pulmonary edema is a potentially fatal complication of rapid ascent to altitudes above 9500 feet. HAPE occurs by noncardiogenic mechanisms, although pulmonary hypertension appears to be in-volved in its pathogenesis. Symptoms begin after 6 to 36 hours at high altitude and may follow an episode of AMS. Dyspnea at rest, tachypnea, and crackles are characteristic features of HAPE. Cyanosis, orthopnea, and hemoptysis commonly develop in more advanced cases.

At autopsy, the lungs are typically heavy, congested, and edema-tous and have hyaline membranes in small airways and alveoli. Why hyaline membranes form is not known; this is not a character-istic finding in death caused by other forms of hypoxia. Hemody-namic studies have shown elevated pulmonary artery pressure with normal pulmonary venous pressure. The pulmonary edema may be due to an increase in pulmonary capillary pressure in small regions of the pulmonary capillary bed or to increased permeability in lung capillaries.

HIGH-ALTITUDE CEREBRAL EDEMA (HACE). HACE is relatively uncommon, occurring in perhaps 1.5% of individuals af-fected by AMS. Hypoxemia produces cerebral vasodilation and in-creased cerebral blood flow, which may lead to mild brain edema and produce the symptoms of AMS. Cerebral edema may also be aggravated by hypoxic inhibition of the adenosine triphosphate (ATP)-dependent sodium pump. By factors yet to be defined, the brain edema may progress and become life threatening. Signs and symptoms of HACE include severe, progressive headache, ataxia, confusion, anxiety, hallucinations, and coma. Papilledema and meningeal signs occur. Examining the cerebrospinal fluid reveals high opening pressures and perhaps hemorrhage or leukocytosis. Pathologically, the pattern of cerebral edema appears to be hetero-geneous, and focal areas of capillary damage, red cell sludging, and platelet aggregation are seen.

TREATMENT OF ACUTE HIGH-ALTITUDE DISEASE. The simplest approach to preventing and treating acute altitude ill-ness is to ascend to altitude gradually and to descend when trou-bling symptoms appear. Gradual ascent allows time for the body to adapt. If possible, the rate of ascent should be limited to approxi-mately 1000 feet per day between altitudes of 7000 and 10,000 feet. Slower ascent (500 feet per day) is recommended for altitudes above 10,000 feet. If slow ascent is impractical, prophylactic treat-ment with acetazolamide is effective in preventing AMS. Acetazol-amide increases renal bicarbonate excretion and lessens the degree of respiratory alkalosis. The recommended regimen is 250 mg every 8 hours the day before, during, and for 1 day after the ascent. Some physicians use one half to one third of this amount of acetazol-amide to avoid dehydration and potassium depletion. Other diuret-ics have not proved to be effective, and in practice, liberal water intake appears to hasten bicarbonate excretion and prevent hemoconcentration. Dexamethasone also reduces the incidence and early symptoms of AMS; however, it is not recommended because of potential side effects.

Management consists of rest, mild analgesics, alcohol avoidance, and adequate hydration. The symptoms usually abate within a few days. The definitive treatment for HAPE, HACE, and severe HARH is oxygen administration and descent to lower altitude. High-altitude pulmonary edema may improve dramatically with a descent of only a few thousand feet. If the descent is delayed, the combination of oxygen and PEEP or continuous positive airway pressure, or placing the victim in a pressurized bag or chamber, is effective. Nifedipine and dexamethasone also have been reported to be effective for treatment of serious AMS when descent is not feasible.

CHRONIC MOUNTAIN SICKNESS (MONGE'S DISEASE). Chronic mountain sickness occurs in people living at high altitudes, usually at over 14,000 feet, for many years. These "high-landers" have a blunted respiratory drive in response to hypoxia and have a lower minute ventilation at high altitudes than do those who normally reside at lower altitudes. Chronic mountain sickness is characterized by an exaggerated response to hypoxia resulting in cor pulmonale. Physiologic responses include erythrocytosis with hemoglobin levels as high as 25 grams per deciliter, a decreased minute ventilation with an elevated Pco_2, hypoxemia, and impaired sensitivity of the respiratory center to hypoxia. Clinical manifestations are similar to those of polycythemia rubra vera and include cyanosis, dyspnea, cough, palpitations, headache, giddiness, muscular weakness, pain in the extremities, sensory and motor changes, and episodic stupor. The only therapy is to move the patient to a lower altitude. Subacute forms of this illness, in which cyanosis and alveolar hypoventilation are absent, also occur. A similar syndrome, brisket disease, has been described in cattle.

Sutton JR: Mountain sickness. Neurol Clin 10:1015, 1992. *A nice summary of the pathophysiology and treatment of high-altitude disorders; with 43 references.*

Decompression Illness

Ambient pressure changes outside the body must be reflected across the lungs by proportional changes in the partial pressures of various gases dissolved in the tissues of the body. This condition is a consequence of the physical behavior of gases and their interactions with solutions. Because the quantity of gas dissolved in tissue varies directly with atmospheric pressure, changes in gas concentrations in the body are most pronounced during diving with compressed air, when, in order for divers to expand their lungs, the density of the breathing gas must be increased in proportion to the column of water around them. Nitrogen uptake is most important in this respect because it comprises 80% of the atmosphere and, unlike oxygen, it is inert (not metabolized). Inert gases like nitrogen must be eliminated from the body after a decrease in ambient pressure, e.g., return from a compressed air dive or rapid ascent to high altitude. The process of eliminating inert gas is called decompression.

During decompression, inert gas dissolved in the tissues may come out of physical solution if environmental pressure falls too rapidly. Bubbles of inert gas form within the tissues and venous blood and produce various clinical manifestations known as decompression illness (DCI), or Caisson's disease. DCI, however, is not entirely explained by gas bubbles in blood and tissue, and not all bubbles cause symptoms. Bubbles produce a number of secondary manifestations attributed to surface activity at the interface between the bubble and the blood or tissue. These secondary effects, such as activation of complement, platelet aggregation, and release of vasoactive mediators, may lead to ischemia and some of the manifestations of DCI.

CLINICAL MANIFESTATIONS. DCI can occur during decompression after diving to more than 25 feet of seawater (1.75 ATA) or during rapid ascent from sea level to 18,000 feet (0.5 ATA). DCI is most commonly encountered in compressed air (or gas) divers after prolonged or repetitive dives or after severe exercise and in divers with excessive body fat, poor physical conditioning, and increasing age. The signs and symptoms of DCI usually appear within a few minutes to a few hours after the end of the dive. Historically, DCI has been classified as either mild (type 1) or serious (type 2). This distinction is somewhat arbitrary because both mild and serious manifestations of DCI occur simultaneously in about one third of patients. Type 2 DCI usually involves the ner-

TABLE 54–11. CLASSIFICATION OF DECOMPRESSION ILLNESS (DCI)

Organ System	Signs and Symptoms
	Mild DCI (Type 1)
Skin	Pruritus, mottling, urticaria
Musculoskeletal	Pain (bends) usually in the joints, numbness, edema
	Serious DCI (Type 2)
Central nervous system	
Cerebral	Loss of consciousness, ataxia, vertigo, aphasia, hemiparesis
Audiovestibular	Vertigo, nystagmus, auditory symptoms
Spinal cord	Back pain, paraparesis, bladder and bowel dysfunction
Cardiopulmonary	Cough, substernal pain, tachypnea, asphyxia (chokes)
Systemic	Extreme fatigue, hypovolemic shock

vous system, although in its most serious form, gas exchange and hemodynamic compromise occur. The common clinical features of DCI are outlined in Table 54–11.

TREATMENT AND OUTCOME. The first step in treating DCI is administering high concentrations of oxygen by face mask. Prompt recompression in a hyperbaric chamber with 100% oxygen usually relieves symptoms in a matter of minutes. If recompression therapy is delayed for more than a few hours, the illness is more difficult to treat. The rationale for recompression is based on (1) enhancing the dissolution of gas bubbles by compression and (2) lowering the concentration of inert gas in venous blood with oxygen, thus increasing the rate of nitrogen removal from body tissues and bubbles. With prompt treatment, complete recovery is to be expected. If therapy is delayed for more than 24 hours, the outcome is less certain, although many patients, even those with serious neurologic disease, respond to recompression after delays of several days.

Pulmonary Barotrauma and Arterial Gas Embolism

Pulmonary barotrauma and arterial gas embolism (AGE) may occur in compressed air divers when they ascend to the surface, particularly with failure to exhale normally. They are also encountered during explosive decompression at high altitude and in blast injury of the thorax. Under these circumstances, ambient hydrostatic or barometric pressure decreases rapidly, and gas within the lungs expands reciprocally according to Boyle's law. Under water near the surface, small decreases in depth result in large increases in gas volume. If the expanding gas is not allowed to escape, it may create a pressure gradient exceeding the compliance of lung tissue. This positive-pressure gradient between alveolar gas and the pulmonary interstitium may lead to alveolar disruption and pulmonary interstitial emphysema and then to soft tissue or mediastinal emphysema, pneumothorax, or pneumopericardium. This condition is known as pulmonary barotrauma. Free gas may also enter pulmonary venous blood and travel through the left side of the heart to the systemic circulation. Air can be embolized throughout the arterial system, including the cerebral, coronary, and renal arteries.

CLINICAL MANIFESTATIONS. The clinical manifestations of AGE usually occur within minutes after the diver surfaces. Signs and symptoms that suggest distribution of gas to the carotid arteries frequently develop. This condition leads to acute cerebral dysfunction characterized by severe headache, blindness, loss of consciousness, seizures, or paralysis. Depending on the amount of pulmonary barotrauma, the quantity of embolized gas may be very large. This serious complication of ascent can occur in compressed air diving after very brief exposures or at very shallow depths, when DCI is not a diagnostic consideration.

TREATMENT AND OUTCOME. Severe central nervous system deficits from AGE are more likely to be permanently disabling or lethal in the absence of adequate treatment than is DCI. Recompression therapy should commence within minutes if good neurologic recovery is to be ensured. The management is similar to that of DCI, but the magnitude, length, and number of recompression treatments are generally greater. If treatment is delayed more than 24 hours, the likelihood of benefit from recompression therapy is low.

55 OVERVIEW OF PNEUMONIA

Waldemar G. Johanson, Jr.

Pneumonia is a term used to indicate inflammation of the distal lung—terminal airways, alveolar spaces, and interstitium. To improve the precision of communication, the term *pneumonia* is usually further qualified with words that imply a cause, mechanism, anatomic site, or clinical course. Thus, descriptors such as "viral bronchopneumonia," "aspiration pneumonia," "chronic interstitial pneumonia," and "acute bacterial pneumonia" serve to identify patients with clinical illnesses characterized by signs and symptoms of lung inflammation in a variety of clinical situations. This chapter also provides the background for the chapters that deal with specific forms of bacterial pneumonia (see Ch. 271, 273, and 274).

PATHOPHYSIOLOGY

Bacterial pneumonia results when host defense mechanisms are insufficient against a bacterial challenge presented to the lungs. Bacteria may be introduced into the lungs by any of four routes (Table 55–1). The most common routes are aspirating contaminated oropharyngeal secretions and inhaling airborne bacteria. The bloodstream may transport organisms to the lung that may produce pneumonia, but the originating site of infection and the severe systemic effects of sepsis usually outweigh the importance of the resulting pneumonia. Direct extension from a focus of infection adjacent to the lungs is uncommon, and the initial site of infection is always more important.

EXPOSURE TO PATHOGENIC BACTERIA. Aspiration of contaminated oropharyngeal secretions is by far the most common route of lung inoculation leading to pneumonia. The term *aspiration* is often mistakenly equated with inhaling large volumes of material into the tracheobronchial tree; it is less commonly appreciated that normal individuals aspirate small quantities of oropharyngeal secretions during sleep. The frequency and amount of aspiration are increased in patients with altered consciousness. The concentration of aerobic bacteria in upper respiratory tract secretions is about 10^8 organisms per milliliter, whereas that of anaerobic bacteria is about 10 times greater. Thus, aspirating even small quantities of oropharyngeal secretions causes inoculation of the lung with an enormous bacterial challenge.

Organisms that are to be aspirated into the lungs must first colonize the respiratory tract. This is facilitated by bacteria adhering to the regional epithelium. Mucosal cells of the upper respiratory tract contain cell-surface receptors for a variety of bacteria that are major determinants of the resident flora. The oropharyngeal flora of normal humans may include highly pathogenic organisms. In contrast, pathogenic viruses do not establish a chronic colonization state. The chemical nature of receptors for different species of bacteria is highly variable, and the site of the receptor may be either an integral part of the cell surface or contained in proteins attached to the cell. The availability of epithelial receptors and therefore susceptibility to colonization vary with the underlying disease, antimicrobial therapy, or concurrent viral infections.

Organisms present in ambient air are highly selected by environmental conditions, as they must have survived aerosolization, drying, temperature changes, and ultraviolet irradiation. Further, because few, if any, microorganisms are inhaled with each breath, only highly virulent organisms capable of causing infection with a very small inoculum can produce disease; this is not the case for most pathogenic bacteria. The infecting dose of *Mycobacterium tuberculosis* may be as low as a single organism, and many viruses are transmitted by the airborne route as well. However, the list of bacteria capable of being transmitted by this route is short and includes only organisms that are unusually invasive, such as the plague bacillus, and organisms particularly adapted to certain environments, such as *Legionella*, so that they are present in large numbers in the air in confined spaces, such as buildings served by contaminated air conditioning systems. Organisms capable of airborne transmission often produce outbreaks of infection when groups of susceptible people are exposed, a striking characteristic of *Legionella* infections or influenza, for example.

TABLE 55–1. ROUTES OF BACTERIAL INOCULATION OF THE LUNGS

Route	Examples
Aspiration of oropharyngeal secretions	Most bacterial pneumonias; anaerobic pleuropulmonary infections
Inhalation of airborne microorganisms	*Mycobacterium tuberculosis; Legionella;* many viruses including influenza
Bacteremia	*Staphylococcus aureus* sepsis
Direct extension into lungs	Amebic liver abscess

HOST DEFENSES. The anatomy of the upper air passages (see Ch. 50) is an important aspect of defense against inhaled particulates, including bacteria. Droplets that exceed 10 μm in diameter are deposited by inertial impaction in the upper airways, a process that is promoted by the angulation of these structures. About 90% of particles 5 to 10 μm in diameter are deposited along the tracheobronchial tree, whereas particles 0.5 to 3 μm in diameter are deposited in the alveoli. Smaller particles behave like gas molecules and are exhaled to a large extent. *Droplet nuclei* is the term applied to particles about 1 to 3 μm in diameter containing a single bacterium, the likely infecting unit for organisms transmitted by the airborne route.

The first line of defense against bacteria deposited in the lungs is the mucociliary escalator, an integrated multifaceted system consisting of the ciliated cells lining the airways, the secretory cells (goblet cells and submucosal glands), and the secretions. Cilia beating 10 to 20 times per second propulse the secretions toward the mouth. However, the effectiveness of this activity depends on maintaining the depth and viscosity of secretions and coordination of ciliary activity. Processes that impair ciliary movement, cause excessive secretion of respiratory mucus, or change the viscosity of secretions may each hinder the effectiveness of this transport system (Table 55–2).

Bacteria that penetrate to the distal airways or alveoli are killed *in situ* by phagocytic cells. Nonspecific opsonization, which aids phagocytosis, may be provided by lung surfactant or fibronectin. Alveolar macrophages that reside in the lungs can ingest and kill enormous numbers of nonpathogenic bacteria, such as most of the normal oropharyngeal flora, without eliciting an inflammatory response. For bacteria that are more pathogenic, the situation is more complicated; some species promptly recruit neutrophils and bacterial killing appears to depend much more upon the availability of neutrophils than on the presence of alveolar macrophages. Clearing these organisms from the lung is enhanced by the presence of specific antibody. IgG is the predominant immunoglobulin in the alveolus, comprising about 10 to 15% of the protein in alveolar fluid.

If bacteria on the alveolar surface are not promptly engulfed and killed, an inflammatory response swiftly develops that is characterized by interstitial and alveolar edema and an influx of neutrophils. The chemoattractants responsible for the latter include bacterial products, C5a, and neutrophil chemotactic factors including IL-8 secreted by alveolar macrophages and perhaps other cells (see also Ch. 140.2 and 222). As neutrophils and bacteria accumulate, the

TABLE 55–2. FACTORS THAT IMPAIR MUCOCILIARY FUNCTION

Factor	Mechanism	Examples
Genetic	Altered secretions Ciliary dysfunction	Cystic fibrosis Dysmotile cilia syndromes
Environmental	Mucus hypersecretion, epithelial cell injury	Cigarette smoke, irritant gases, dust
Bacterial infection	Decreased ciliary beating, cell injury	*Pseudomonas aeruginosa* *Bordetella pertussis* *Mycoplasma pneumoniae*
Viral infection	Epithelial cell injury	Influenza

milieu becomes acidic and hypoxic, and bacterial ingestion and killing are remarkably retarded. Spreading edema and inflammation at the periphery of the lesion continue until specific antibody appears (days 5 to 7) or effective antibiotic therapy is initiated.

Community-acquired pneumonias are usually due to a single organism, an observation that appears to contradict the aspiration mechanism that necessarily includes multiple species. The susceptibility of individual bacterial species to lung defenses varies widely. As a result, the lung's defenses select the organism (or organisms) that go on to cause pneumonia—the species most capable of evading phagocytosis and killing. The spectrum of causative organisms varies to some extent with certain clinical factors. The most common organisms in several settings are shown in Table 55–3. Conditions clinically associated with an increased risk of bacterial pneumonia are shown in Table 55–4.

Organisms gain access to the systemic circulation early in the development of pneumonia. In dogs, pneumococci introduced into the lungs were recovered from hilar lymph nodes within 15 minutes. Bacteremia and positive cultures of spleen and liver occur when the lung bacterial burden exceeds 10^4 per gram of lung tissue. Successful host defense against the systemic spread of infection requires a functioning reticuloendothelial system, opsonins, and adequate numbers of neutrophils. Patients who present with overwhelming sepsis due to pneumonia generally lack one or more of these

CLINICAL MANIFESTATIONS

SIGNS AND SYMPTOMS. The signs and symptoms associated with bacterial pneumonia vary widely, depending on several factors, most importantly the nature of the offending pathogen and the state of the host. Extremes in presentation can be easily described, although most patients fall somewhere in between. At one extreme is the previously healthy person with pneumococcal pneumonia. Such patients complain of a brief prodromal upper respiratory illness followed by fever, a single shaking chill, pleuritic chest pain, and a cough productive of purulent or "rusty" sputum. Physical examination reveals signs of consolidation, which are readily confirmed by chest radiography. Gram stain of the sputum reveals numerous neutrophils and abundant pneumococci. In such a patient there is no doubt that a lower respiratory tract infection is present, and the stain of the sputum strongly suggests the cause. At the other extreme might be an elderly, confused patient who presents with only deterioration in mental function. Physical examination reveals only rhonchi without signs of consolidation, and the chest radiograph shows only bilateral lower lobe interstitial infiltrates that might represent acute or chronic changes. Gram stain of the sputum (obtained with difficulty) shows many squamous epithelial cells, a few neutrophils, and a pleomorphic bacterial flora that includes both gram-positive and gram-negative organisms. In such patients it may not be clear whether or not the patient has pneumonia, and the information at hand offers few clues regarding cause.

The history-taker should explore the presence of risk factors, including chronic illnesses, recent acute illnesses, illness in family members, use of alcohol or other drugs, and possible exposures to infectious agents. A thorough physical examination, posteroanterior and lateral chest radiographs, and blood leukocyte count with differential should be performed. On the basis of the data available

TABLE 55–4. COMMON RADIOGRAPHIC PATTERNS OF PNEUMONIA AND ASSOCIATED PATHOGENS

Pattern	Pathogens
Lobar or segmental consolidation	S. pneumoniae, K. pneumoniae, H. influenzae, other gram-negative bacilli
Inhomogeneous infiltrates (patchy or streaky opacities)	M. pneumoniae, viruses, Legionella sp.
Diffuse interstitial infiltrates	Legionella sp., viruses, P. carinii
Cavitary infiltrates	M. tuberculosis, gram-negative bacilli, S. aureus (multiple nodules)
Pleural effusion plus infiltrate	S. pneumoniae, S. aureus, anaerobes, gram-negative bacilli, Streptococcus pyogenes

from these steps, it is usually possible to conclude that pneumonia is present. The remaining task is to determine its cause.

MICROBIOLOGIC DIAGNOSIS. Controversy exists over the proper microbiologic evaluation of the patient with pneumonia because of questions of sensitivity, specificity, cost, and benefit. These problems are created basically by the presence of abundant organisms in the upper tract and the resultant contamination of expectorated specimens. Further, because most patients with pneumonia respond satisfactorily to simple, relatively nontoxic antibiotic regimens, the need to document the cause of the process is uncertain. It is impossible to define rules that apply to all patients, and knowledgeable physicians differ in their approach to an individual patient.

Sputum should be examined microscopically. The portion chosen should be purulent and contain <10 squamous cells and >25 leukocytes per low-power field. A well-done Gram stain discloses whether one species of organism predominates. Often, such specimens contain a vast preponderance of a single species, and if these are encapsulated gram-positive cocci (pneumococci) or small pleomorphic gram-negative coccobacilli (Haemophilus), a presumptive diagnosis can be made. Problems arise when a predominant organism is less apparent, when enteric gram-negative bacilli are present, or when an adequate specimen cannot be obtained.

Aerobic culture of expectorated sputum suffers from a lack of sensitivity (organisms causing pneumonia are not detected) and specificity (organisms are present that did not cause pneumonia); both have been estimated to occur in up to 50% of cases. The results may be improved by microscopic screening of the specimen prior to culture. Quantitative culture techniques have not become routine in evaluating sputum specimens.

Contamination of sputum by oral secretions may be avoided by collecting the specimen proximal to the mouth. The most direct approach involves puncturing the trachea with a large-bore needle and inserting a plastic cannula into the trachea, a technique called transtracheal aspiration. If secretions cannot be harvested by suction, a small amount of sterile saline is injected through the cannula and suction is reapplied. Transtracheal aspiration is an excellent method of identifying anaerobic bacteria responsible for pleuropulmonary infections, if this diagnosis cannot be made by other means, but has few other indications.

TABLE 55–3. COMMON ETIOLOGIC AGENTS OF COMMUNITY-ACQUIRED PNEUMONIA IN APPROXIMATE ORDER OF FREQUENCY*

Outpatient Evaluation Age < 60 Years, No Underlying Disease	Hospitalized Patient	Severe Pneumonia, ICU Care
Streptococcus pneumoniae	S. pneumoniae	S. pneumoniae
Mycoplasma pneumoniae	Haemophilus influenzae	Legionella sp.
Respiratory viruses	Aerobic gram-negative bacilli	Aerobic gram-negative bacilli
Chlamydia pneumoniae	Legionella sp.	M. pneumoniae
Miscellaneous, including Legionella sp.	Miscellaneous including M. pneumoniae, viruses	Respiratory viruses

* Adapted from American Thoracic Society: Guidelines for the initial management of adults with community-acquired pneumonia: Diagnosis, assessment of severity, and initial antimicrobial therapy. Am Rev Respir Dis 148:1418, 1993.

Another method for bypassing the mouth to collect specimens is to aspirate directly from the area of lung consolidation, using either physical findings or fluoroscopy to guide the approach. This technique, called transthoracic lung aspiration, has proved to be a valuable technique in children with complicated pneumonias because sputum samples may be impossible to obtain. In adults, especially those with underlying lung disease, the rate of complications, particularly pneumothorax and bleeding, limits its usefulness. This direct approach is further compromised by the fact that the false-negative rate may be as high as 30%.

Fiberoptic bronchoscopy provides a relatively safe way to collect specimens from the periphery of the lung. Specially designed protected specimen brushes (PSB) are available that permit the operator to obtain endobronchial specimens that have not been contaminated by proximal airway secretions, even though the instrument has traversed the upper airways. Complications of the procedure are infrequent, and the major limiting factors are expense and time. In addition to the small specimens collected by brushing the peripheral airways, sterile fluid can be instilled and aspirated to obtain material from a larger area of the lung (bronchoalveolar lavage, BAL). PSB samples must be cultured quantitatively; organisms present in concentrations of $\geq 10^3$ bacteria per milliliter are causative agents. BAL samples can be quantitatively cultured or concentrated by centrifugation and used for a variety of special stains and/or cultures. The large sample size of BAL is a major advantage.

Immunologic techniques, such as immunofluorescence, enzyme-linked immunoassay, and DNA hybridization, hold great promise for determining the cause of pneumonia. However, compared with conventional cultures, these techniques are expensive and relatively insensitive. They detect the presence of only a narrow spectrum of related organisms. Because of this specificity, they have a limited role in evaluating patients with pneumonia and should be considered only when specific organisms are strongly suspected on clinical grounds. Because PSB or BAL samples avoid upper tract contamination, they provide better materials for immunodiagnosis than expectorated sputum.

Last, it must be remembered that cultures of the blood and pleural fluid, if positive, provide results that are highly specific. However, only about 30% of patients with bacterial pneumonia are bacteremic. About the same percentage of pleural fluid aspirates are positive in the absence of antibiotic therapy, but because only 10 to 15% of patients with pneumonia have a pleural effusion, the applicability of this approach is limited. Nevertheless, blood cultures should be obtained in patients with serious illness due to pneumonia, and a diagnostic thoracentesis should be performed in patients with effusions large enough to be aspirated safely.

Proper use of these techniques must be individually determined for each patient with pneumonia. In many patients, the history, physical examination, radiographic studies, and evaluation of the sputum by Gram stain provide all the data that might be reasonably required. Additional procedures should be reserved for those patients in whom a delay in making an accurate diagnosis has serious consequences or those in whom the diagnosis cannot be reasonably suspected on the basis of simpler approaches.

RADIOGRAPHIC PATTERNS. Carefully examining posteroanterior (PA) and lateral chest radiographs is an invaluable adjunct in the diagnosis of pneumonia and should be part of the evaluation of every patient with suspected pneumonia. Although a specific microbiologic diagnosis is seldom, if ever, possible on the basis of radiographic data alone, important clues to the cause of pneumonia and its distribution and severity may be gained by this technique. Pathogens frequently associated with particular radiographic patterns are summarized in Table 55–4.

Lobar or segmental consolidation suggests a bacterial cause for pneumonia, especially *Streptococcus pneumoniae* or *Klebsiella pneumoniae*. Consolidation may obscure the borders between the lung and adjacent structures (e.g., heart border or diaphragm). This obliteration is termed the "silhouette sign" and is very useful to localize infiltrates.

Less well-defined and inhomogeneous radiographic densities, often described as "patchy" or "streaky" infiltrates, may be observed in bronchopneumonia and in infections caused by a variety of organisms, including bacteria and viruses. Diffuse pulmonary infiltrates are most commonly caused by infection with viruses (such as cytomegalovirus or influenza), *Legionella pneumophila*, or opportunistic pathogens such as *Pneumocystis carinii*.

Cavitary shadows generally suggest the presence of a necrotizing infection with destruction of lung tissue. Organisms that frequently produce this radiographic picture include *Staphylococcus aureus* (see Ch. 279), gram-negative bacteria, anaerobes, and *M. tuberculosis* (see Ch. 311). Less commonly, non-necrotizing infection occurring in an area of the lung containing cysts or bullae may have a cavitary appearance on the radiograph in the absence of frank lung destruction.

The chest radiograph may also yield valuable information about infectious involvement of structures outside the parenchyma of the lung, including the pleural surface and thoracic lymph nodes. Pleural effusions occur in a variety of respiratory infections. Lateral decubitus radiographs help document the presence of free pleural fluid, and thoracentesis is necessary to distinguish transudative and uncomplicated parapneumonic effusions from complicated parapneumonic effusions or empyema, which may require drainage (see Ch. 56 and 63). Enlargement of mediastinal and hilar lymph nodes is rare in acute bacterial infection of the lung. When present in association with pneumonia, this finding should suggest infection by fungi or mycobacteria or the presence of an underlying lung cancer. Loss of volume of a pulmonary segment or lobe (partial or complete atelectasis) should raise suspicion of an obstructing endobronchial lesion with distal infection.

American Thoracic Society: Guidelines for the initial management of adults with community-acquired pneumonia: Diagnosis, assessment of severity, and initial antimicrobial therapy. Am Rev Respir Dis 148:1418, 1993. *A well-referenced guide to diagnosis and initial therapy of patients with community-acquired pneumonia. A patient-stratifying scheme is suggested that uses age, underlying disease, and severity to modify therapy.*

Cole P, Wilson R: Host-microbial interrelationships in respiratory infection. Chest 95(Suppl):217S, 1989. *A thoughtful review of host defenses, emphasizing the effects of bacteria and bacterial products on those defenses.*

Østergaard L, Anderson PL: Etiology of community-acquired pneumonia: Evaluation by transtracheal aspiration, blood culture, or serology. Chest 104:1400, 1993. *A recent large-scale effort to determine the cause of community-acquired pneumonia with results similar to many before—a causative agent definitively identified in only 34% of patients.*

Reynolds HY: Pulmonary host defenses: State of the art. Chest 95 (Suppl):223S, 1989. *A thorough review of defense mechanisms, emphasizing host factors.*

56 LUNG ABSCESS
John G. Bartlett

DEFINITION. Lung abscess literally means a collection of pus within a destroyed portion of the lung; thus there are numerous possible causes of such a lesion (Table 56–1). As used clinically, however, the term *lung abscess* refers to a pulmonary infection with parenchymal necrosis, generally caused by bacteria other than mycobacteria. Lung abscesses are usually solitary, but occasionally multiple discrete lesions are observed. Numerous small abscesses confined to a given region of the lung are sometimes referred to as "necrotizing pneumonia." Because they share a common pathogenesis, there is considerable overlap among aspiration pneumonia, lung abscess, and necrotizing pneumonia, and each of these may lead to and coexist with an empyema (a collection of pus within the pleural space).

ETIOLOGY. As indicated in Table 56–1, many different underlying processes can lead to the formation of a lung abscess. By far the most important are necrotizing pulmonary infections, and, of these, anaerobic bacteria are responsible for the majority. These organisms account for essentially all "putrid" lung abscesses and nearly all that have been classified as "nonspecific" or "primary." Most of these infections involve multiple bacterial species, which may include aerobic organisms. The dominant bacteria are *Fusobacterium nucleatum, Prevotella melaninogenicus, P. intermedia,* peptostreptococcus, aerobic streptococci, and microaerophilic streptococci.

Pneumonia, particularly cases caused by *Staphylococcus aureus* and *Klebsiella pneumoniae*, may also be complicated by abscess formation. Less frequent but well-documented agents of lung ab-

TABLE 56–1. DIFFERENTIAL DIAGNOSIS OF A CAVITARY LESION IN THE LUNG

Necrotizing infections
  Bacteria: Anaerobic bacteria, *Staphylococcus aureus,* enteric gram-negative bacteria, *Pseudomonas aeruginosa, Legionella, Streptococcus pyogenes, Haemophilus influenzae, Pseudomonas pseudomallei, Actinomyces, Nocardia, Rhodococcus equi, Streptococcus pneumoniae* (?)
  Mycobacteria: *Mycobacterium tuberculosis, M. kansasii, M. avium-intracellulare*
  Fungi: *Coccidioides immitis, Histoplasma capsulatum, Blastomyces hominis, Cryptococcus neoformans, Aspergillus, Phycomycetes (Mucor)*
  Parasites: *Entamoeba histolytica, Paragonimus westermani*
  Septic embolism: *S. aureus,* anaerobes, and so on
Cavitary infarction
  Bland infarction (with or without superimposed infection)
  Vasculitis: Wegener's granulomatosis, periarteritis
Neoplasms
  Bronchogenic carcinoma, metastatic carcinoma, lymphoma (with or without superimposed infection)
Miscellaneous lesions
  Cysts or bullae with fluid collections, sequestration

scess include *Streptococcus pyogenes* (group A beta-hemolytic streptococci), *Streptococcus pneumoniae* (especially type 3), *Streptococcus milleri, Haemophilus influenzae* (type B), *Pseudomonas aeruginosa, Pseudomonas pseudomallei* (melioidosis), *Actinomyces* (actinomycosis), *Legionella, Nocardia, Rhotococcus equi, Paragonimus westermani* (lung fluke), and *Entamoeba histolytica* (amebiasis). Enteric gram-negative bacilli other than *K. pneumoniae* may cause lung abscess, but this occurs almost exclusively in debilitated patients with severe associated medical-surgical conditions. Necrotizing alveolitis is a separate entity diagnosed by microscopic examination and usually caused by *P. aeruginosa;* sometimes these microabscesses coalesce to form radiographically detectable cavities.

INCIDENCE AND PREVALENCE. The incidence of primary lung abscess has decreased substantially since the prechemotherapeutic era. Nevertheless, most large academic centers encounter 10 to 30 cases annually.

EPIDEMIOLOGY. Most lung abscesses, and nearly all involving anaerobic bacteria, involve the normal flora of the oropharynx. Abscesses involving *S. aureus* or gram-negative bacilli are more likely to be nosocomial in origin. Amebic lung abscess results from an hepatic abscess directly extending through the diaphragm into the lung. *Nocardia* causes lung abscess almost exclusively in immunocompromised hosts, especially in those receiving corticosteroids. Septic pulmonary emboli commonly lead to multiple solitary abscesses in noncontiguous sites and are usually caused by *S. aureus,* most often found in intravenous drug abusers with tricuspid valve endocarditis. Lung abscesses due to *P. westermani* and melioidosis are usually acquired in the Far East or Indonesia.

PATHOGENESIS. The formation of an anaerobic lung abscess nearly always involves two coexisting abnormalities: (1) periodontal infection, such as gingivitis or pyorrhea, which provides the inoculum; and (2) aspiration, which provides access to the lung parenchyma. The usual causes for aspiration are those that compromise consciousness and the gag reflex, such as alcoholism, drug addiction, general anesthesia, seizure disorder, sedative use, or neurologic disorders. Other factors predisposing to aspiration include dysphagia resulting from esophageal disorders or neurologic deficits; disruption of the usual mechanical barriers, as with nasogastric intubation, tracheostomy, or nasogastric feeding tubes; or pharyngeal anesthesia, as seen with dental procedures or surgery involving the upper airway. Most healthy persons periodically aspirate small inocula from the upper airways, but these are readily cleared by the normal cough reflex and other pulmonary defense mechanisms without deleterious consequences. Patients who develop aspiration pneumonia and lung abscesses presumably do so because of the relatively large inocula of bacteria and failure of the usual protective mechanisms.

The initial lesion is pneumonitis, or "aspiration pneumonia," that typically involves dependent pulmonary segments, e.g., those favored by gravitational flow. The dependent pulmonary segments in patients who aspirate in the recumbent position are the superior

segments of the lower lobes or posterior segments of the upper lobes. Aspiration in the upright or semi-upright position favors involvement of the basilar segments of the lower lobes. Patients who have a defined period of known or probable aspiration demonstrate with sequential radiographs that 7 to 14 days are usually required for a typical air-fluid level to appear on chest radiograph.

CLINICAL MANIFESTATIONS. Patients with anaerobic abscesses tend to have indolent symptomatology with medical complaints for 2 or more weeks before presentation. The usual symptoms are fever, malaise, cough, sputum production, and pleuritic pain. The frequent observation of weight loss and anemia provides testimony to the chronicity of the infection. Frank rigors are rare, and their presence suggests organisms other than anaerobes. The cough often becomes more productive at the time of cavitation, and it is at this time that the patient is most likely to note the onset of putrid sputum, which is considered diagnostic of anaerobic infection. Putrid sputum is found in 60% of patients with a confirmed anaerobic origin. Many patients also note that the sputum has an unusually noxious taste. Most patients have a history of compromised consciousness or other risk factors for aspiration, and many have periodontal infection. Nevertheless, about 10% of patients with anaerobic lung abscesses have no identifiable predisposing condition. Occasional patients with anaerobic lung abscesses are edentulous; the incidence of underlying bronchogenic neoplasms seems particularly high in this group. Patients with lung abscesses due to *S. aureus,* gram-negative bacilli, and amebae usually have a more fulminant course, with the precipitous onset of symptoms. Other features that may be noted in this group include chills, the lack of putrid discharge, and the absence of the usual associated findings. The physical findings in the early phases of disease are those of pneumonia, with or without a pleural effusion. At a later stage there may be amphoric or cavernous breath sounds, pleural effusions are common, and approximately 25% of patients have an associated empyema.

DIAGNOSIS. The diagnosis of lung abscess is usually established on the basis of a chest radiograph showing a parenchymal infiltrate with a cavity containing an air-fluid level (Fig. 56–1). The differential diagnosis of this roentgenographic finding is included in Table 56–1. Certain roentgenographic features may provide clues to the presence of an infected cyst, bulla, or sequestration. Massive pulmonary fibrosis with necrosis from occupational exposure is usually distinctive. A loculated empyema with an air-fluid level may be differentiated from lung abscess with computed tomography.

Studies for an etiologic agent are often limited to expectorated sputum. These specimens are useful for detecting mycobacteria, pathogenic fungi, and parasites, and they may be used for cytologic studies. However, routine aerobic cultures often give erroneous results, and they are not valid for meaningful anaerobic culture owing to the universal presence in oral secretions of anaerobes. Blood cultures are useful, primarily for patients with infections involving *S. aureus* or gram-negative bacilli, but most patients with anaerobic abscesses do not have bacteremia. Pleural fluid is a valuable culture source for both aerobic and anaerobic bacteria in any patient with an empyema. For most patients with anaerobic pulmonary infections restricted to the pulmonary parenchyma, the preferred specimen source is from a transtracheal aspiration, from a transthoracic needle aspirate, or from a fiberoptic bronchoscopy using a double-lumen catheter with a distal occluding plug combined with quantitative cultures. Collecting specimens before instituting antibiotic therapy is preferred. In most cases of anaerobic abscesses, the etiologic agents are not defined, and the therapeutic regimen is selected empirically. Bronchoscopy, which used to be performed routinely in patients with lung abscesses, is now usually restricted to patients who fail to respond to antibiotic treatment or who have an atypical clinical presentation. Major concerns are a cavitating neoplasm, an obstructing tumor, or a foreign body.

TREATMENT. The most important facets of the treatment are administering appropriate antibiotics and adequately draining any associated empyema. Physiotherapy with postural drainage should be used when possible; however, this must be done with considerable caution in patients with large lung abscesses because of the possibility of spillage of purulent contents, with extensive involvement of other lobes.

The drugs of choice for treating abscesses caused by aerobic pyogenic microorganisms, *Mycobacterium tuberculosis,* fungi, and *Entamoeba histolytica* are reviewed in detail elsewhere in this vol-

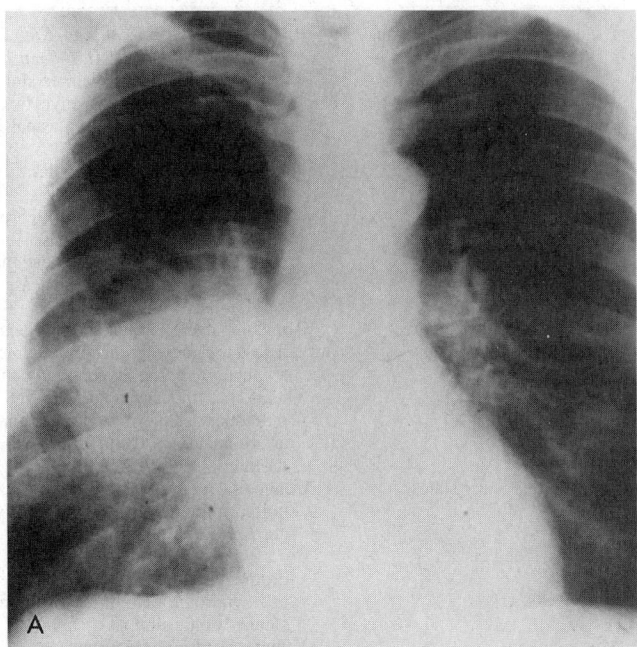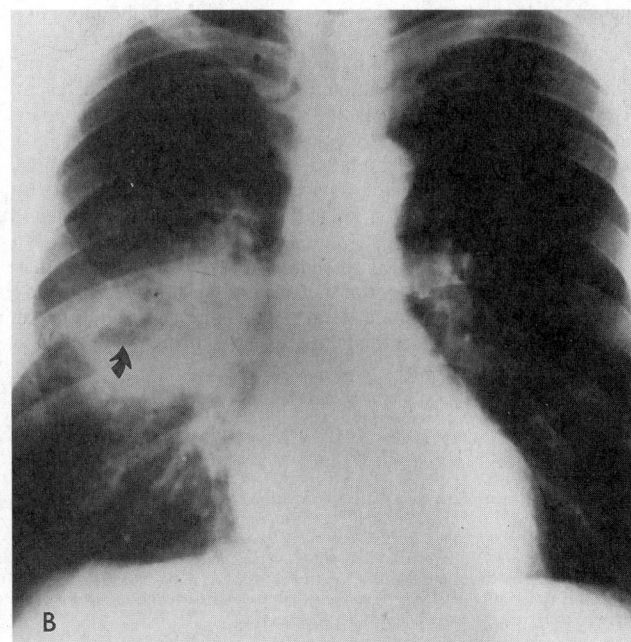

FIGURE 56–1. Chest radiographs of a 55-year-old alcoholic man. The first film *(A)* shows pneumonitis involving the superior segment of the right lower lobe, a common segment for aspiration pneumonia. The second radiograph *(B),* taken 1 week later, shows cavitation with an air-fluid level as indicated by the arrow. A transtracheal aspirate yielded *Fusobacterium nucleatum, P. melaninogenicus,* and anaerobic streptococci. The final diagnosis was aspiration pneumonia with progression to lung abscess due to anaerobic bacteria.

ume. (See index for discussion of specific organisms.) For aspiration-related lung abscess involving anaerobic bacteria, the three antimicrobial regimens recommended are penicillin, clindamycin, or penicillin plus metronidazole. Penicillin has traditionally been regarded as a favored drug using initial doses of 10 to 20 million units intravenously per day. When there is clinical improvement, treatment is often changed to intramuscular or oral penicillin using penicillin G, penicillin V, ampicillin, amoxicillin or amoxicillin-clavulanate, each in doses of 500 to 750 mg three or four times daily. Some authorities suggest an arbitrarily selected total duration of treatment of 3 to 6 weeks, whereas others continue treatment until the chest radiograph changes have cleared or there is only a small, stable residual lesion. The latter criterion commonly requires 2 to 4 months or longer but may be necessary to prevent relapses.

Clindamycin is active against most penicillin-resistant anaerobes that are found in 20 to 25% of cases, and many regard clindamycin as the preferred agent for all lung abscesses due to anaerobic bacteria. The usual regimen is 600 mg given intravenously every 6 to 8 hours until the patient is afebrile and clinically improved, followed by 300 mg orally four times daily. An alternative regimen is penicillin G (above doses) combined with metronidazole (2 gm orally per day in two to four divided doses). Metronidazole is active against nearly all clinically important anaerobes, but penicillin must be added owing to the probable importance of aerobic and microaerophilic streptococci.

The necessity to treat the aerobic components of mixed aerobic-anaerobic infections is controversial, but this is generally advocated for patients who are seriously ill or fail to respond to clindamycin. Most penicillins are considered equally effective against oral anaerobes, including penicillin G, penicillin V, ampicillin, amoxicillin, ticarcillin, mezlocillin, and piperacillin. However, antistaphylococcal penicillins, such as nafcillin or oxacillin, are considered inferior and unacceptable. Most cephalosporins other than ceftazidime are considered nearly equivalent to penicillins in terms of *in vitro* activity, although the clinical experience is limited. Imipenem and any combination of a β-lactam–β-lactamase inhibitor are considered almost universally active against clinically important anaerobes. The activity of tetracyclines and macrolides (erythromycin, clarithromycin, and azithromycin) is variable. Quinolones and trimethoprim-sulfamethoxazole are unacceptable for infections caused by anaerobic bacteria.

Patients with lung abscesses involving *S. aureus* should be treated with a penicillinase-resistant penicillin, a first-generation cephalosporin, vancomycin, or clindamycin based on *in vitro* sensitivity and penicillin tolerance. Penicillin G is the preferred agent for infections involving group A beta-hemolytic streptococcal infection. Antibiotic selection for infections involving gram-negative bacilli requires *in vitro* sensitivity data. This usually consists of an aminoglycoside combined with an expanded-spectrum penicillin, such as ticarcillin for *P. aeruginosa* or a cephalosporin for Enterobacteriaceae. Sulfonamides are preferred agents for *Nocardia* infections.

The expected response to antimicrobial agents is subjective improvement with decreased fever within 3 to 7 days and fever eliminated within 7 to 14 days. The putrid odor of the sputum, when initially present, usually resolves in 3 to 10 days. Delayed response may indicate large cavity size, poor host status, obstruction, erroneous antimicrobial selection, a wrong diagnosis, drug fever, a complicating empyema requiring drainage, or an abscess that requires drainage by physiotherapy, bronchoscopy, or surgery. Radiographic response is delayed; in fact, there is often extension of the infiltrate and increased cavity size or new cavity formation during the first week. Chest radiographs should be followed at 2- to 3-week intervals with the expectation that infiltrates will clear or there will be a small residual scar or a thin-walled cyst. Resolution often takes months.

Bronchoscopy is indicated in patients with an atypical presentation and in those who fail to respond to recommended antimicrobial regimens. The major purpose of the procedure is to differentiate cavitating neoplasms and to detect underlying lesions, such as bronchogenic neoplasms, bronchostenosis, or a foreign body. It may also be used to facilitate drainage.

The major indications for surgery are an uncontrollable or life-threatening hemorrhage, a bronchogenic neoplasm, a bronchial obstruction, or a lung abscess that proves refractory to medical treatment. Medical failures are rare but are most common in patients with an obstructed bronchus, those with extremely large abscesses, those with abscesses that have been present for an extended period before the institution of treatment, and those with infections involving certain bacteria such as gram-negative bacilli. The usual surgical procedure is lobectomy.

PROGNOSIS. The natural course of lung abscesses was best studied in the prechemotherapeutic era. The mortality rate was about 33%, and an additional third developed chronic debilitating disease with bronchiectasis, recurrent pneumonias, or chronic empyemas. Drainage with the Jackson bronchoscope had no important impact on this prognosis. With the availability of penicillin, the frequency of lung abscess decreased substantially and the mortality rate decreased to 5 to 10%. Findings that herald a relatively poor prognosis include (1) large cavity size, particularly cavities >6 cm in diameter; (2) prolonged symptoms prior to presentation, especially symptoms for >6 weeks; (3) necrotizing pneumonia characterized by multiple small abscesses in contiguous segments; (4) patients who are elderly, debilitated, or immunologically compromised; (5) abscesses associated with bronchial obstruction; and (6) abscess due to aerobic bacteria, including *S. aureus* and gram-negative bacilli.

PREVENTION. The major preventive measures are factors that reduce the incidence or magnitude of aspiration, provide appropriate care of periodontal disease, treat pneumonia early, and ensure adequate courses of antimicrobials to prevent relapses.

Bartlett JG: Anaerobic bacterial infections of the lung. Chest 91:6, 1987. *A review of anaerobic pleuropulmonary infections, including 83 cases of lung abscesses with bacteriology, clinical features, and management guidelines.*

Hagan JL, Hardy LD: Lung abscess revisited. A survey of 184 cases. Ann Surg 197:755, 1983. *Surgical point of view concerning lung abscess; 11% were operated on.*

Landay MJ, Christensen EE, Bynum LJ, et al.: Anaerobic pleural and pulmonary infections. AJR 134:233, 1980. *Review of the roentgenographic features of anaerobic pleuropulmonary infections, including response to antibiotic treatment.*

Levison ME, Mangura CT, Lorber B, et al.: Clindamycin compared to penicillin for the treatment of anaerobic lung abscess. Ann Intern Med 98:466, 1983. *The authors show the superiority of clindamycin versus intravenous penicillin in terms of response rates, relapse rates, and time to defervescence.*

57 BRONCHIECTASIS
Roger C. Bone

DEFINITION

The definition of bronchiectasis is primarily an anatomic one, characterized by *irreversible* dilation of one or more proximal and medium-sized bronchi due to destruction of the muscular and elastic supporting tissues of the bronchial walls. Bronchiectasis may be accompanied by massive collapse, in which all airways and alveoli distal to the site of bronchial collapse are also deflated, resulting in an airless lobe; the condition may thus be localized to a lobe or, alternatively, generalized throughout the bronchial tree. Destruction is generally the result of recurrent or chronic inflammation and intermittent healing with deposited fibers and fibrosis. Chronic cough and copious sputum production are nearly universal, although "dry" bronchiectasis with little or no sputum production has been described; dyspnea and orthopnea occur in severe cases.

HISTORICAL PERSPECTIVE AND CURRENT ETIOLOGIES

Before the advent of antibiotics and vaccines, bronchiectasis contributed much more significantly to patient morbidity and mortality than it does today. Measles, pertussis, tuberculosis, and a variety of childhood respiratory infections commonly set the stage for bronchiectasis to develop. Immunization and aggressive antibiotic therapies have reduced the significance of these diseases as precursors to bronchiectasis in the United States; in developing countries, however, these diseases remain common antecedents.

Immunization and antibiotics also reduce the absolute incidence of bronchiectasis. Although infection remains a major component in the disease, those cases that do occur are often in patients with one or more predisposing conditions (Table 57–1).

BRONCHIAL OBSTRUCTION. The aspiration of foreign bodies (most notably in children), tumors, and, occasionally, mucous impaction can lead to infection, dilated bronchi, and subsequent destructive changes. These processes are generally focal rather than diffuse. Bronchiectasis may develop years after aspirating foreign bodies or inhalational injury. Obstruction *per se* does not appear to cause bronchiectasis but facilitates the condition by interfering with bronchial clearance, which promotes infection. On the other hand, some have argued that peripheral obstruction may tend to promote bronchiectasis by increasing the intra-alveolar pressures around the

TABLE 57–1. PREDISPOSING FACTORS FOR BRONCHIECTASIS

Bronchopulmonary infections	Pertussis, measles; *S. aureus, Klebsiella, M. tuberculosis, H. influenzae;* adenovirus, influenza, herpes simplex; viral bronchiolitis; mycotic (histoplasmosis) or mycoplasmal infection
Bronchial obstruction	Foreign body aspiration; neoplasm; hilar adenopathy (tuberculosis, sarcoidosis); mucoid impaction; chronic obstructive pulmonary disease (COPD, chronic bronchitis, asthma); acquired tracheobronchial disease; amyloidosis
Congenital anatomic defects	Bronchomalacia, bronchial cysts, cartilage deficiency, tracheobronchomegaly, ectopic bronchus, endobronchial teratoma, tracheoesophageal fistula; pulmonary sequestration, pulmonary artery aneurysm; yellow-nail syndrome
Immunodeficiency states	Congenital agammaglobulinemia; acquired immune globulin deficiency; chronic granulomatous disease
Hereditary defects	Ciliary defects (immotile cilia syndrome, ciliary dyskinesia, Kartagener's syndrome); α_1-antitrypsin deficiency; cystic fibrosis
Miscellaneous	Young's syndrome; recurrent aspiration pneumonias (alcoholism, neurologic disorders, lipoid pneumonia); irritant inhalation (ammonia, nitrogen dioxide, smoke, talc, silicates, detergents); post–heart/lung transplantation (associated with obliterative bronchiolitis)

Adapted with permission from Swartz MN: Bronchiectasis. *In* Fishman AP (ed.): Pulmonary Diseases and Disorders. 2nd ed. New York, McGraw-Hill, 1988, p 1559.

affected airway. Although this "chicken or egg" question continues to attract attention, most physicians agree that bronchiectasis is associated with both obstruction and infection.

CONGENITAL OR HEREDITARY CONDITIONS. The cilia of individuals with immotile cilia syndrome exhibit ultrastructural alterations (dynein arms are absent or aberrant) that render them immotile or dyskinetic. The syndrome is probably transmitted as an autosomal recessive gene. This lack of ciliary motility is apparent in several body systems. For instance, males with the condition are infertile, owing to immotile sperm; females have decreased fertility as well. Such patients are prone to the recurrent infections characteristic of bronchiectasis because cilia of the respiratory tract are either dysfunctional or totally unable to beat. Mucociliary clearance of bacteria and phagocytic debris is inhibited; chronic sinusitis and bronchiectasis may result (see Ch. 64).

Patients with Kartagener's syndrome—a subset of immotile cilia syndrome—may exhibit situs inversus in addition to bronchiectasis and sinusitis. Situs inversus is presumed to be the chance result of embryonic migration of viscera rather than the normally cilia-dependent placement of internal organs.

In patients with cystic fibrosis, bronchiectasis is a reflection of defects in exocrine gland secretion. In the United States, nearly half of the cases of bronchiectasis in children or young adults are attributable to cystic fibrosis. Copious amounts of thickened secretions promote the development of infection (see Ch. 58).

Intralobar sequestration of the lung is a congenital malformation that can cause bronchiectasis. This condition involves a detached segment of pulmonary tissue, which has a systemic arterial blood supply and is attached to normal lung and covered by the same pleura. In adults, pneumonia may occur in this segment. In general, the detached segment is not attached bronchially to the rest of the lung and therefore is not filled with air. With infection, however, connections may become established, allowing progression to bronchiectasis.

Bronchiectasis is also associated with immunodeficiency states; defects in humoral immunity more frequently lead to the disorder than do defects in cellular immunity. Panhypogammaglobulinemia, especially, may lead to bronchiectasis. Such patients are much more susceptible to repeated bacterial infections and so are at increased risk.

OTHER CAUSES. Although no longer common in the United States, bronchiectasis can follow necrotizing pneumonias caused by the tubercle bacillus, staphylococci, or other infectious agents. Because of the resurgence of drug-resistant forms of the tubercule bacillus (see Ch. 311), this cause of bronchiectasis may be seen more often in the future and clinicians should be aware of its possible consequences. Previously, necrotizing pneumonia was not uncommon, secondary to measles, pertussis, and influenza. In addition, one third to two thirds of all patients with Young's syndrome, a combination of obstructive azoospermia and chronic sinopulmonary infections, develop bronchiectasis. Central bronchiectasis is a finding associated with allergic bronchopulmonary aspergillosis. There is also the very rare "yellow-nail syndrome"—a combination of lymphedema of the lower extremities, recurrent pneumonia, bronchiectasis, and yellowed nails. Unfortunately, in the majority of patients with bronchiectasis, no specific cause is ever determined, although most of these have lower lobe disease, indicating that some process similar to the above described causes (obstruction and infection) has taken place.

PATHOGENESIS AND PATHOLOGY

Infection and at least some degree of obstruction are likely necessary to develop bronchiectasis. Bronchiectatic changes may become irreversible if obstruction persists or if infection produces further bronchial inflammation, destruction, and dilation.

Current views on the pathogenesis of bronchiectasis describe the following scenario. An inhalational or parenteral injury occurs (e.g., corrosive chemical, infectious agent, particulate agent). If the precipitating event is a respiratory infection, it is not necessarily a serious one. Obstruction and stasis occur because secretions, epithelial injury, or a relatively minor obstruction inhibit drainage and clearance and allow infection to continue. The process may be exacerbated in a vulnerable host (one with immunodeficiency, ciliary dysfunction, or reactive airways). Often, the initial insult is unknown; it may be that in the susceptible host, repeated cycles of bacterial infection with increasing airway obstruction and destruction develop.

Bronchial dilation involves predominantly medium-sized bronchi but may extend to more distal regions. Bronchi may be dilated to greater than four times their normal size and are often filled with purulent secretions. Peripheral airways in involved regions are often obstructed, and viscous secretions often further slow mucociliary clearance. The proteolytic activity of polymorphonuclear leukocytes involved in the inflammatory process may directly destroy tissues. There is also evidence that the purulent secretions themselves are rich in proteases (elastase, collagenase, and cathepsin G) and may at least partially contribute to the enzyme-mediated breakdown of tissue protein. The mucosal surface is swollen, inflamed, frequently ulcerated, and sometimes necrotic. Granulation tissue formation may alter the bronchial epithelial lining. This is often described as a "polypoid" appearance in which the healthy ciliated columnar epithelium is replaced by cuboidal cells or fibrous tissue.

Bronchiectasis is most likely to develop in the lower lobes, the left much more often than the right, presumably because of anatomic differences in drainage. In bronchiectasis of the left lower lobe, the posterior basal segment is almost always involved and the apical segment is usually spared.

The radiologic appearance of bronchiectasis can be classified into three types of increasing severity. In *cylindrical* or *fusiform* bronchiectasis, the bronchi are relatively straight and not greatly increased in diameter. Bronchi in *varicose* bronchiectasis are typically dilated and irregular, exhibiting bulbous, distorted terminations. The bronchial lumen may be totally obliterated by fibrous tissue; distal portions may become epithelium-lined and fluid-filled. *Saccular* or *cystic* bronchiectatic segments are dilated, ballooning into pus-filled cavities called saccules as they approach the periphery. These saccules represent totally destroyed and fibrosed segments of the bronchial tree. Larger, more proximal segments may remain relatively unchanged except for marked inflammation in the bronchial walls and polyposis of the epithelium. The morphology of saccular bronchiectasis probably can be attributed to an extension of the inflammatory process from the bronchial wall to the supporting structures and surrounding lung parenchymal tissue, which are destroyed or fibrosed by this inflammation. Polyposis of the bronchial mucosa

proximal to these saccular regions partially obstructs the bronchi and prevents drainage. As a result, these more proximal regions become distended with pus. Squamous metaplasia is a common sequela in saccular bronchiectasis, although it is uncommon in the other types of bronchiectasis.

CLINICAL MANIFESTATIONS AND CLINICAL COURSE

Today, most clinically significant bronchiectasis originates in early childhood but may not become apparent until much later. Predisposing factors such as cystic fibrosis, immotile cilia syndrome, or immunodeficiency states are usually present.

Cough (sometimes paroxysmal) and sputum production (frequently purulent)—often more severe upon awakening—are observed in 90% of all bronchiectasis patients. In pre-antibiotic times, sputum volumes of as much as 600 ml per day were seen in those with advanced, untreated disease. Fetid sputum and foul breath were also common. Today, these extreme presentations are less likely because antibiotics and postural drainage techniques have greatly reduced the volume of sputum and have prevented the development of secondary anaerobic bacterial infection that contributes to such purulence.

Recurrent episodes of infection exacerbate established bronchiectasis. Intercurrent infections may be accompanied by fever, cough, sputum production, and dyspnea. Anorexia and weight loss are associated with multiple bronchiectatic episodes, as is wheezing. Hemoptysis was very common in the past but is not as common today because the infectious aspect of the disease can be treated. Sinusitis sometimes accompanies bronchiectasis, especially in patients with ciliary defects and immunodeficiency states.

Bronchiectatic patients usually show abnormalities during the physical examination. Persistent, medium to coarse "moist crackles" over the involved lobes are the most significant finding. The crackles begin early in inspiration, continue to mid-inspiration, then fade by the end. Diffuse rhonchi and prolonged expiratory phases may also be evident. In patients with extensive disease, dullness and decreased breath sounds may be heard over involved regions. Respiratory expansion may be either increased or decreased. Patients with advanced disease or disease complicated by emphysema may show hyperexpansion, although this sign is more common in children.

Before antibiotics, clubbing and cyanosis were common (40% of cases) as the disease progressed, and metastatic abscesses, especially in the brain, were well known. These days, such signs are rarely seen. The incidence of cor pulmonale has also declined dramatically among bronchiectasis patients, except for those with cystic fibrosis and considerable lung destruction. Secondary amyloidosis is rare (see Ch. 248).

DIAGNOSIS

Because the definition of bronchiectasis is an anatomic one, diagnosis of the disease is based on demonstrating morphologic alterations in the bronchial tree—usually through radiologic techniques. Patients should also be evaluated for the presence of one of the heritable causes of bronchiectasis (Table 57–2) unless there has been an obvious precipitating event. Bronchiectasis should be suspected in any patient presenting with chronic productive cough (especially if sputum is purulent or there is intermittent blood streaking).

CHEST RADIOGRAPHY. Chest radiographs are crucial to document regions of increased markings, cavities, and atelectasis. However, routine chest radiographs may appear normal, especially in the early phases of bronchiectasis (in 7 to 10% of bronchiectasis patients). Often, all that may be seen are nonspecific markings in localized segments of lung. Tubular shadows (tram tracks, tram lines), mucoid impactions, or gloved finger shadows are more significant. Tubular shadows reflect the thickening of bronchial walls, peribronchial fibrosis, and alveolar collapse. Mucoid impactions or gloved finger shadows appear when secretions and pus fill airways with radiodense material. Compensatory hyperinflation of uninvolved lung regions is common, especially in patients with cystic fibrosis.

BRONCHOGRAPHY. Previously, bronchography was considered to be the best method to confirm bronchiectasis and evaluate the extent of its progress. However, it is rarely used now because severely compromised patients or those with bronchospasm may react adversely to the technique; bronchographic studies should not

TABLE 57-2. DIAGNOSTIC FEATURES OF FAMILIAL BRONCHIECTASIS

Disorder	Clinical Findings	Laboratory Tests
Cystic fibrosis (see Ch. 58)	Pancreatic insufficiency Mucoid *Pseudomonas* strain Obstructive azoospermia Infertility	Sweat chloride
Immotile cilia syndrome	Infertility, sinusitis, otitis media, Kartagener's syndrome (with or without dextrocardia)	Electron microscopy of cilia Absent mucociliary clearance Immotility in living cells (nasal, sperm)
α_1-Antitrypsin deficiency	Emphysema, cirrhosis	Serum α_1-antitrypsin, Pi typing
IgG deficiency	Recurrent infections	Quantitative Ig, IgG subclass
IgA deficiency	Autoimmune phenomena Atopy	Quantitative Ig
Williams-Campbell syndrome	Disease restricted to chest	Bronchographic expiratory collapse of proximal bronchi
Neutrophil deficiencies	Recurrent infections (with or without thrombocytopenia, with or without pancreatic disease)	Blood smear Differential leukocyte count Nitroblue tetrazolium dye test
Complement deficiencies	Recurrent infections	C3 levels CH_{50} determination

be performed in patients with active disease. Bronchography is rarely indicated today and should not be performed unless the results will be important in deciding upon a treatment. For example, it could be used to document localized bronchiectasis that might be amenable to surgery. If needed, bronchograms should be obtained several months following the development of bronchiectasis, when reversible damage to airways has had time to resolve.

COMPUTED TOMOGRAPHY (CT). In almost all instances, CT replaces bronchography. Adequate visualization of bronchiectatic segments is usually possible, and the problems noted above do not occur with this technique.

BRONCHOSCOPY. Though not useful in diagnosing bronchiectasis, bronchoscopy is useful in identifying obstructions or sources of hemoptysis and in removing secretions. The technique may be used to obtain biopsy material of bronchial (or nasal) mucosa for electron microscopic evaluation to confirm ciliary dyskinesia.

SINUS RADIOGRAPHY. Radiographic evaluation may help to identify patients in whom sinusitis accompanies bronchiectasis (e.g., immotile cilia syndrome, Young's syndrome).

PULMONARY FUNCTION. Patients with extensive bronchiectasis show impairments similar to those seen in chronic bronchitis or emphysema. Cough may prematurely collapse the large bronchi in patients with saccular or varicose bronchiectasis, which can result in obstructed expiratory airflow and air trapping, probably due to the inflammatory destruction of proximal bronchial walls. Ineffective cough leads to the retention of secretions, predisposing patients to further infection.

Disturbances in respiratory function depend on the anatomic type of bronchiectasis and the degree of lung compromise. Pulmonary function tests in patients with diffuse involvement usually reveal airway obstruction, although with disease progression, both obstructive and restrictive defects may be noted. The forced vital capacity (FVC), forced expiratory volume in one second (FEV_1), FEV_1/FVC, and the forced expiratory flow ($FEF_{25-75\%}$) are all decreased, and the residual volume is increased. Decreased ventilation, perfusion, and ventilation/perfusion ratios are found in involved regions. Nitrogen washout studies may indicate that inspired air is maldistributed. Hypoxemia may occur in severe bronchiectasis; however, CO_2 retention tends to occur only in those patients with concomitant severe bronchitis or advanced emphysema. Persistent or pro-

gressive hypercapnia is an ominous finding, one that reflects advanced disease and cor pulmonale.

ADDITIONAL STUDIES. Sputum cultures may yield evidence of *Haemophilus influenzae, Streptococcus pneumoniae, Streptococcus pyogenes, Pseudomonas aeruginosa, Pseudomonas cepacia, Staphylococcus aureus,* or *Aspergillus,* as well as a number of other organisms. Accurately identifying infective organisms has obvious implications for antibiotic therapies.

White blood cell counts and differentials may help confirm active infection and distinguish bronchiectasis from lymphoproliferative disorders. Arterial blood gas levels may be used to help assess severe respiratory compromise. Sweat chloride tests in patients with bronchiectasis may detect previously undiscovered cystic fibrosis. Quantitative immunoglobulin determinations should be obtained if immunodeficiency is suspected. Nasal or bronchial biopsy is indicated when immotile cilia syndrome is suspected.

DIFFERENTIAL DIAGNOSIS. Bronchiectasis represents permanent lung destruction and needs to be distinguished from the reversible changes caused by such entities as pneumonia, bronchitis, and atelectasis, as well as from aspirating foreign bodies, tuberculosis, and lung abscess. Also, the presence of any of the numerous predisposing conditions needs to be determined.

COMPLICATIONS

Severe complications are relatively uncommon, although hemoptysis does occur. Early onset of the disease, especially in those with cystic fibrosis or immune deficiencies, is associated with a shorter life span. Such complications as lung abscesses, pneumonia, progression of infection through the pleura producing bronchopleural fistulas, or empyema are more common in this population than in those who acquire bronchiectasis later in adult life.

TREATMENT AND PROGNOSIS

Because the anatomic destruction seen in bronchiectasis is irreversible, most efforts are directed at medical therapies to prevent disease progression and control symptoms. The most important treatments consist of chest physiotherapy, including instructing the patient on postural drainage and antibiotics. The following techniques should be used, as appropriate: hydration, discontinuation of smoking, bronchodilators (in patients with either bronchospasm or other forms of airway obstruction), oxygen (for hypoxemic patients during acute exacerbations or for those with chronic respiratory insufficiency), and treatment for sinusitis. Patients should also receive annual influenza vaccines.

The choice of antibiotics should be guided by results of sputum culture. However, these cultures typically grow "normal flora," so ampicillin is often administered empirically. Trimethoprim-sulfamethoxazole or tetracycline is appropriate for patients for whom penicillins are contraindicated. Antibiotic therapy for 1 to 3 weeks may be required to achieve the desired therapeutic effects. Longterm, continuous antibiotic therapy may not be appropriate for patients with bronchiectasis because it may predispose them to gramnegative infection with such organisms as *P. aeruginosa.* On the other hand, regular courses of inhaled antibiotics may be effective, particularly if the patient has cystic fibrosis.

Progression within involved bronchial segments is common, but extension to normal regions is unusual. Underlying diseases such as cystic fibrosis, asthma, and immotile cilia syndrome may render the entire bronchial system vulnerable. Appropriate use of antibiotics effectively controls symptoms and minimizes dysfunction and disease progression.

Resection may cure the small subset of patients with severe localized disease and significant hemoptysis. On the other hand, patients with advanced, bilateral disease may do well with medical therapies alone. Rarely, surgery is indicated for a patient with massive hemoptysis resulting from vascular deformity within a bronchiectatic segment. If the patient cannot tolerate surgical resection, bronchial artery embolization may be warranted. Some patients with end-stage bronchiectasis may be candidates for lung transplantation.

Barker AF, Bardana EJ Jr: Bronchiectasis: Update of an orphan disease. Am Rev Respir Dis 137:969, 1988. *A concise review with 214 references, outlining pathology, cause, host-insult pathogenesis, prognosis, and suggested evaluation.*

Eppler GR: Bronchiolitis obliterans and other bronchiolar airflow disorders. *In* Bone RC (ed.) Pulmonary and Critical Care Medicine. St. Louis, Mosby-Year Book, 1993, p 1. *A concise review with 54 references of bronchiolitis obliterans and other bronchiolar airflow disorders.*

Le Roux BT, Mohlala ML, Odell JA, et al.: Suppurative diseases of the lung and pleural space. Part II: Bronchiectasis. Chicago, Year Book, 1986, p 95. *Review with exhaustive bibliography and excellent section on historical perspective; focuses primarily on surgical management of bronchiectasis.*

Slutzker AD, Kinn R, Said SI: Bronchiectasis and progressive respiratory failure following smoke inhalation. Chest 95:1349, 1989. *Case presentation of patient who developed bronchiectasis following inhalational injury.*

Swartz MN: Bronchiectasis. *In* Fishman AP (ed.): Pulmonary Diseases and Disorders. 2nd ed. New York, McGraw-Hill, 1988, p 1553. *Comprehensive, well-referenced, and well-illustrated examination of the subject.*

58 CYSTIC FIBROSIS

Roger C. Bone

DEFINITION

Cystic fibrosis (CF) is a heritable disease that follows an autosomal recessive pattern of transmission. It is the most common lethal genetic disease in the United States, with the approximate frequency among Caucasians being 1 in 2000. On the basis of this figure, it is estimated that 1 in 20 are carriers of the defective gene. Blacks and Asians are seldom affected. CF is characterized by abnormal eccrine and exocrine gland function; mucous glands produce viscous secretions, which lead to chronic pulmonary disease, insufficient pancreatic and digestive function, and abnormally concentrated sweat.

HISTORICAL PERSPECTIVE

Although there are numerous historical associations between salty skin and early death, CF was first described as a distinct clinical entity in the late 1930's. It was first referred to as CF of the pancreas, to describe the histologic appearance of that organ late in the course of the disease. Only later was it recognized that all exocrine glands were involved.

PATHOLOGY AND PATHOGENESIS

The gene for CF is located on the long arm of chromosome 7 and has only recently been isolated. The encoded protein contains 1480 amino acids, is very similar to other membrane proteins, and may, in fact, be an ion channel. It is believed that the defective CF protein may be at least partially responsible for altering cAMP-mediated chloride secretion, a defect that could modify all exocrine secretions.

The first CF-associated mutation described consists of a three-base-pair deletion in the genetic code, resulting in the loss of a phenylalanine residue at position 508; others have been described and many may exist. Mutations at position 508 account for 70% of all CF cases, although that percentage varies by race and location.

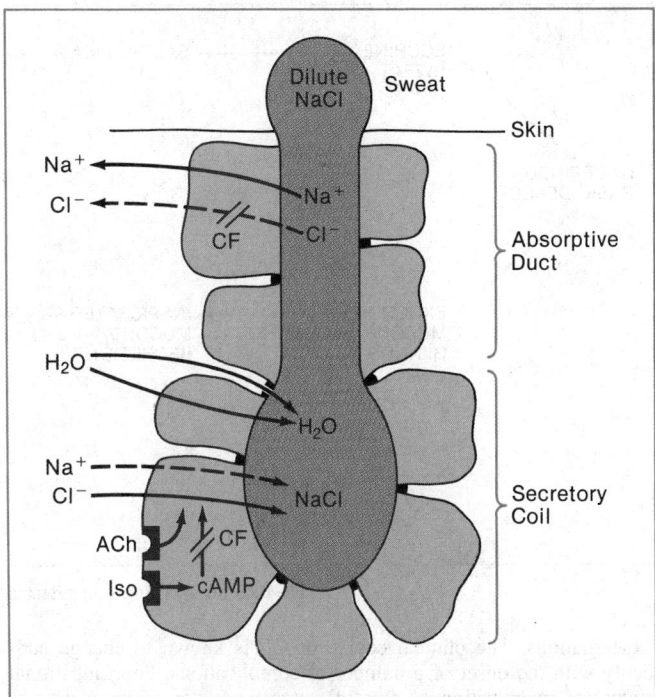

FIGURE 58-2. Electrolyte transport by sweat glands. (From Welsh MJ, Fick RB: Cystic Fibrosis. J Clin Invest 80:1524, 1987, by copyright permission of the American Society for Clinical Investigation.)

Amino acid 508 is found in nucleotide-binding fold 1 of the intramembrane channel (Fig. 58-1), a region that may bind to ATP. Thus, the molecule's inability to use the driving force of ATP hydrolysis may result in its becoming a nonfunctional ion pump. There has been some association between specific mutations and their effects. For instance, the above deletion at 508 may be more likely to result in pancreatic insufficiency than other mutations. Unfortunately, there has been no clear demonstration that a particular mutation can be associated with the detrimental effects that CF has on the lung.

Following the isolation in 1989 of a genetic defect that presumably leads to CF, a unifying hypothesis regarding the function of chloride channels in CF has begun to emerge. In normal individuals, chloride channels are located on the luminal membranes of epithelial cells. When these channels are open, chloride ions move into the airway lumen, producing an osmotic gradient that draws water into the lumen (Fig. 58-2). Abnormal electrolyte levels in the sweat of CF patients probably result from the impermeability of the sweat duct epithelium to chloride. Anomalous mucus found in the lungs and other organs of CF patients occurs when there is an inadequate amount of water on the luminal side of epithelial membranes. This results from excessive sodium reabsorption or failure to secrete chloride. Evidence suggests that several secretory products of CF patients contain inadequate amounts of water and that the physical properties of mucous secretions are highly dependent on water content.

CLINICAL MANIFESTATIONS AND CLINICAL COURSE

Patients with CF present with symptoms that can mimic other clinical entities (Fig. 58-3). Early gastrointestinal involvement (i.e., meconium ileus, failure to thrive) leads to a diagnosis of CF at birth or during infancy in more than 10% of all CF patients. More typical presentations, however, include the early onset of respiratory symptoms such as cough and recurrent respiratory infections later in life.

In many patients, intermittent episodes of acute respiratory infections persist longer than would be expected because mucociliary clearance of mucus is inhibited by its high viscosity. Coughing increases and becomes worse at night and upon awakening. Sputum is viscous and purulent. Disease progression is often marked by gradual decline in pulmonary function and is punctuated by acute

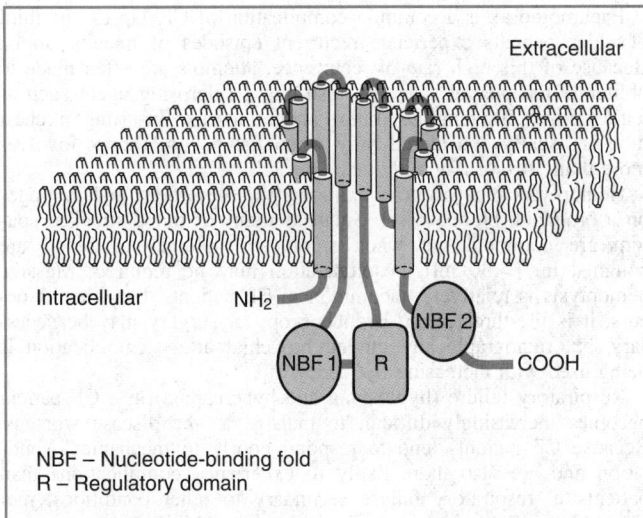

NBF – Nucleotide-binding fold
R – Regulatory domain

FIGURE 58-1. The cystic fibrosis transmembrane channel.

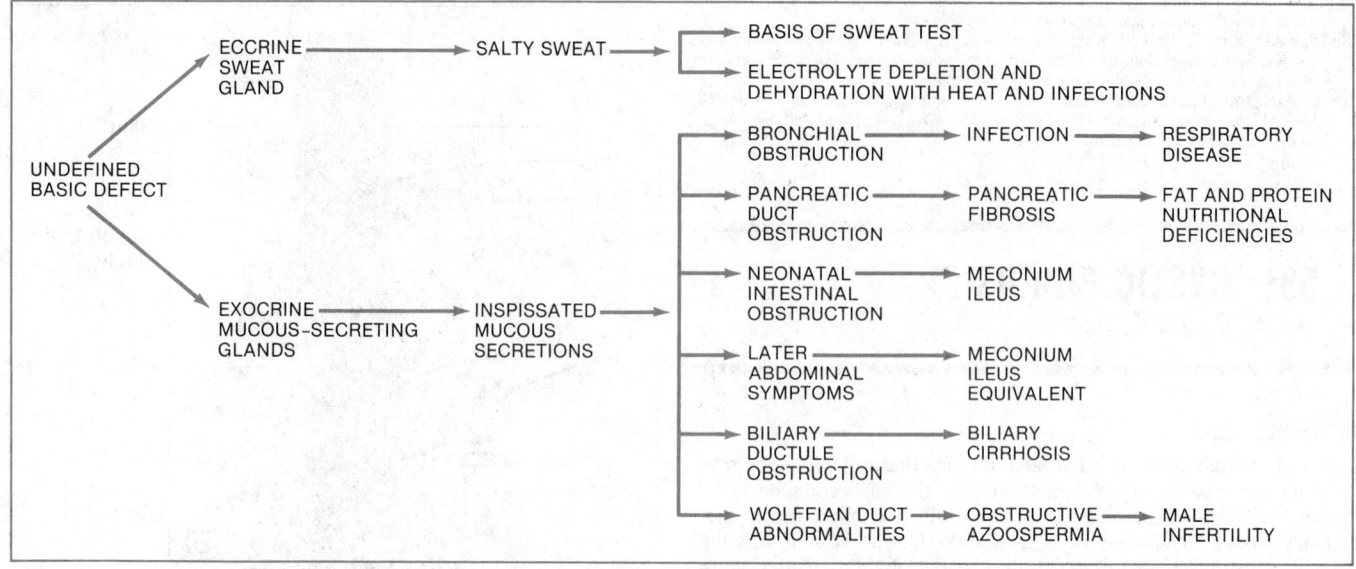

FIGURE 58–3. Clinical manifestations of cystic fibrosis.

exacerbations. The clinical course of CF is known to change suddenly with the onset of a number of complications. Poor nutritional status (or malnutrition, if present) often correlates with severity of the pulmonary disease.

DIAGNOSIS

RADIOLOGY. Hyperinflation is noted early in the course of CF. As the disease progresses, hyperinflation and evidence of bronchitis (see Ch. 329) increase and there may also be evidence of peripheral cuffing, mucus impaction, or bronchiectasis (see Ch. 57).

PULMONARY FUNCTION. It is thought that newborns with CF have normal lung function, but within a short time many children show evidence of decreasing function. There is usually demonstrable obstruction of small airways (e.g., decreased maximum mid-expiratory flow rates, reduced expiratory flow rates at low lung volumes, increased residual volume/total lung capacity ratios). Spirometry, lung volume measurements, and oxygenation levels are most frequently used to monitor pulmonary function and disease progression. Oxygenation gradually worsens throughout life; when arterial P_{O_2} values remain below 55 mm Hg, pulmonary hypertension is often present. Significant arterial P_{CO_2} elevations or forced expiratory volume in 1 second (FEV_1) values < 30% of predicted portend end-stage disease; survival then averages 29 months. Patients with CF often display airway hyperreactivity, which can be demonstrated by exercise testing, histamine challenge, or response to bronchodilators.

SPUTUM CULTURE. Although *Staphylococcus aureus, Pseudomonas aeruginosa,* and *Pseudomonas cepacia* are sometimes found in sputum cultures from patients with pulmonary diseases other than CF, their association with this disease is so consistent that attempts to obtain sputum cultures have become an integral part of evaluating any suspected CF patient. Sputum cultures may also be useful during exacerbations of the disease.

PANCREATIC FUNCTION (see Ch. 107). Ninety to 95% of CF patients exhibit some degree of exocrine pancreas dysfunction. Enzyme deficiency leads to maldigestion of protein and fat, which produces bulky, foul-smelling stools. If untreated, these patients fail to gain weight and growth is inhibited. Poor growth can also be the result of increased energy expenditures associated with the work of breathing in those with severe respiratory symptoms.

SWEAT. The discovery that excessive loss of salt occurs in the sweat of CF patients has been used as its most important diagnostic criterion. Although the sweat glands of CF patients are histologically normal, they function abnormally—producing secretions that are nearly isotonic, rather than the hypotonic solutions excreted by normal individuals.

Quantitative pilocarpine iontophoresis, performed in laboratories with established expertise, remains the standard criterion for diagnosing CF. To perform this test, a minimum of 100 mg of sweat needs to be collected, and results should be confirmed by a second

test. In children, sodium and chloride concentrations exceeding 60 mEq per liter are considered diagnostic of CF; in adults the level is 70 mEq per liter.

LABORATORY. Since the defective CF gene was discovered in 1989, the use of cDNA probes has permitted a fairly rapid and accurate assessment of the patient's genetic makeup with regard to CF. Four out of five babies born with CF come from parents with no family history of CF. Although some have called for widespread screening for the CF gene, this is not likely to occur for some time. The Office of Technology Assessment predicts that better DNA tests for CF will soon become widely available. However, the patient's choice is still the essential factor in determining whether a DNA test takes place.

COMPLICATIONS

RESPIRATORY. The major source of morbidity in CF patients is pulmonary disease associated with chronic and recurrent bacterial infections. The resultant high levels of antigens, antibodies, inflammatory cells, and inflammatory mediators have detrimental cumulative long-term effects on the pulmonary tissue. To date, trials of anti-inflammatory drugs have not shown that they prevent inflammation-related damage in CF. Atelectasis is not uncommon in CF, and it is usually associated with few symptoms. Evidence of bronchiectasis is common in CF patients by age 5 to 10. Chest physiotherapy and antibiotics are often successful in re-expanding atelectatic regions. Surgical resection is only rarely considered because the bronchiectasis is diffuse.

Pneumothorax is a common complication of CF. Up to one third of older patients experience recurrent episodes of pneumothorax. Because of this high rate of recurrence, attempts are often made to obliterate the pleural space by instilling a sclerosing agent such as tetracycline following an initial pneumothorax. Inserting a chest tube is usually considered only when the pneumothorax involves more than 10% of a hemithorax.

Hemoptysis may occur if pulmonary tissue erodes and impinges on a bronchial blood vessel. Small amounts of blood-streaked sputum are common, but when significant volumes of blood are coughed up (> 30 ml), hospitalization may be required. Massive hemoptysis is relatively uncommon in CF patients, but when it occurs, it is life-threatening. Bronchoscopy or surgery may be necessary, but radiographically guided bronchial artery embolization is being used with increasing frequency.

Respiratory failure (hypoxemia and hypercapnia) in a CF patient becomes increasingly difficult to manage as the disease worsens. Because CF patients tend to respond poorly to mechanical ventilation and are also more likely to experience complications than patients in respiratory failure secondary to other conditions, mechanical ventilation is generally instituted only if there are acute precipitating events such as infectious pneumonia or other reversible complications. With disease progression, hypoxemia increases and pulmonary hypertension and cor pulmonale develop in virtually all CF patients.

Although as many as 50% of CF patients exhibit antibodies to *Aspergillus fumigatus* in their serum, only a small number develop allergic aspergillosis (see Ch. 355). Expectoration of rusty brown plugs of sputum is suggestive of this condition.

Digital clubbing occurs in nearly every CF patient and is often present early in the course of pulmonary manifestations of this disease. Severity seems to correlate with the degree of pulmonary dysfunction. Hypertrophic pulmonary osteoarthropathy occurs in up to 15% of adolescent and adult CF patients and is often characterized by pain in the joints when walking. Symptoms tend to subside when pulmonary symptoms improve.

OTHER. Because the abnormal physiology seen in CF affects many body systems, it is not surprising that a variety of complications may be seen in the disease (Table 58–1). Intestinal obstruction (caused by meconium ileus or meconium ileus equivalent) can usually be treated medically; intussusception or rectal prolapse usually requires surgical intervention. Patients with CF are often prone to episodes of acute or chronic, crampy, lower-right quadrant abdominal pain, reflecting partial intestinal obstruction. These episodes can usually be treated with oral mineral oil and *N*-acetylcysteine used with hyperosmolar enemas that contain agents such as diaztrizoate methylglucamine.

Symptomatic biliary cirrhosis occurs in 2 to 5% of CF patients. Patients present with hyperbilirubinemia, ascites, and peripheral edema. Although bleeding esophageal varices are an infrequent complication of CF, they are seen in some patients secondary to hepatic cirrhosis and portal hypertension. Endoscopy is generally used to sclerose the affected vessels.

As fibrosis of the exocrine pancreas continues, hyperglycemia may be encountered in CF patients, especially in the second and third decades. Diabetes mellitus occurs in approximately 10% of adult CF patients. If diabetes occurs, insulin therapy should be initiated because oral agents are usually ineffective.

Metabolic alkalosis and volume depletion can be serious complications of CF. These occur most commonly during hot weather, when excessive chloride and sodium losses are not replaced.

Although spermatogenesis can be demonstrated by testicular biopsy, more than 97% of male CF patients are sterile (azoospermia) because of incompletely developed wolffian ducts. Many women with CF are anovulatory secondary to chronic lung disease, but fertility may be as high as 20%. Viscous cervical mucus may also prevent conception.

Pregnancy in a CF patient can complicate disease progression. If prepregnancy pulmonary function and nutritional status are good, return to pregravid levels can be anticipated. Women with severely compromised pulmonary and nutritional status before pregnancy often show accelerated deterioration after pregnancy. Infants of mothers with CF have a 2.5% risk of also having the disease.

TABLE 58–1. COMPLICATIONS IN CYSTIC FIBROSIS

Complication	Frequency
Genitourinary	
Azoospermia	97%
Anovulation	80%
Intestinal	
Meconium ileus	10% of all fetuses
Obstruction	17% of all adults
Liver	
Biliary cirrhosis	2–5%
Bile duct proliferation/portal fibrosis	30% at death
Cholelithiasis	<20%
Pancreas	
Diabetes mellitus	8–10%
Malabsorption	85%
Pulmonary	
Atelectasis of lobe or segment	5% overall; 50% in adults
Clubbing	~100%
Hemoptysis, massive (>500 ml blood)	8%
Hemoptysis, minor	50%
Pneumothorax	5–8% of all patients; <19% of all adults
Pulmonary hypertrophic osteopathy	5–15%
Right heart failure	~33% at death
Infection	~100%

The psychosocial aspects of CF are formidable. Many patients are in prolonged pain. Complications such as hypertrophic osteoarthropathy may cause continuous and intense pain. Problems associated with right heart failure may necessitate mechanical ventilation and long-term intensive care. When possible, patients should be cared for in special centers, so that the multifaceted problems of the disease can be dealt with by health care teams who are experienced in managing these patients.

TREATMENT

Because more than 98% of CF patients die of either respiratory failure or pulmonary complications, the therapeutic goals are to prevent and treat the complications of obstruction and infection in the airways, enhance mucus clearance, and improve nutrition. Antibiotics are the key element to increasing survival in this patient population. Frequent courses of antibiotic therapy are usually necessary; some patients may require them nearly continuously. Antibiotic selection should be guided by sputum culture.

Several species demonstrate great affinity for the respiratory tracts of CF patients—*S. aureus, P. aeruginosa,* and more recently, *P. cepacia.* Indeed, their presence suggests CF. Patients with demonstrable infection by *S. aureus* (see Ch. 279) are most often treated using dicloxacillin, cephalexin, the newer cephalosporins, or chloramphenicol. Ciprofloxacin is also being increasingly used but is recommended only for patients over age 10. Early in the course of disease, *Pseudomonas* organisms may be sensitive to tetracycline, trimethoprim-sulfamethoxazole, or chloramphenicol, but infection by these organisms is most often treated using a combination of an intravenously administered aminoglycoside and a semisynthetic penicillin (more popular combinations include gentamicin/carbenicillin and tobramycin/ticarcillin). Once found in the sputum, however, *P. aeruginosa* is rarely if ever eradicated. Therapeutic benefit therefore seems to be derived from reducing the microbial load rather than eliminating infecting organisms. However, studies indicate that it may be possible to delay this chronic form of *P. aeruginosa* infection for several years through early antimicrobial treatment, which may further extend the lives of CF patients.

Of late, *P. cepacia* is emerging as a serious problem for CF patients. This species tends to develop resistance to multiple anti-biotics and has been associated with severe, frequently fatal pneumonia. *Haemophilus influenzae* infection is most often treated with ampicillin, trimethoprim-sulfamethoxazole, or chloramphenicol.

CHEST PHYSIOTHERAPY. Percussion and postural drainage are mainstays in treating CF. Clearing pulmonary secretions to prevent the complications that result from plugging of the airways with viscous mucous secretions and the infections that may arise distal to obstruction constitutes a crucial component of therapy.

DNase. Although the water content of bronchial secretions is probably the critical determinant of their viscosity, DNA from lysed cells may also add to this index. A recent phase II clinical study has shown that aerosolized application of human recombinant DNase to the respiratory tree is safe and improves pulmonary function in CF patients. Phase III trials are underway to confirm these results.

BRONCHODILATORS. Although beneficial effects can be demonstrated in laboratory studies, the long-term benefit of using bronchodilators for CF patients has not been established.

NUTRITION. Most patients can be maintained on normal diets supplemented with pancreatic enzymes (usually enteric-coated capsules taken with meals). Because defective fat metabolism may lead to deficiencies in the fat-soluble vitamins (i.e., vitamins A, D, E, and K), it is often necessary to provide these vitamins as a supplement. Many CF patients also have higher than normal caloric needs, presumably resulting from the increased workload of breathing and maldigestion.

EXERCISE AND REHABILITATION. Exercise tolerance in CF patients correlates with severity of pulmonary obstruction. Although exercise does not improve pulmonary function, it does improve cardiorespiratory fitness, and a program of physical conditioning is recommended. Long-term oxygen therapy can be used for chronic hypoxemia.

GENE THERAPY (see Ch. 25). The most recent advances in genetic research are coming close to providing clinicians with a tool to essentially "cure" CF patients. In preliminary human testing, a normal CF gene has been transfected into the nasal epithelial cells of patients with CF, resulting in improved function of the transmembrane chloride channel, as assessed by an increase in the voltage across the nasal epithelium. The transfecting E1-deficient adenovirus did not appear to replicate or cause any other ill effects aside from the transient inflammation associated with infections of the nasal epithelial cells. These are preliminary results; however, the ability to induce normal chloride ion conductance in cells within the bronchial tree may soon be within our grasp. As new cells replace old cells in the epithelium, it would be necessary to infect them with renewed doses of the adenovirus. Also, recent advances in our ability to detect the defective gene may some day provide us with the next best treatment to totally eliminate the CF gene from the human genome.

PROGNOSIS

Over the past three decades there can be no question that comprehensive treatment programs have increased the overall survival of CF patients. In the 1950's patients lived only a few years; at present, median survival is to age 24, and significant numbers of patients survive well beyond that. Patients with CF who initially present with respiratory symptoms seem to have poorer prognoses. Once lung disease is established, colonization by *Pseudomonas* may be indicative of poor prognosis.

Until now, the use of marker techniques to screen for carriers of the genetic defect has been possible only within families of living CF patients. Recent advances in our ability to detect the defective gene promise to have profound effects on our ability to identify heterozygote carriers of CF. Carriers of the gene may then undergo effective counseling with regard to the heritability and likelihood that their children will suffer this devastating and fatal disease. It seems increasingly likely that in the relatively near future, various forms of gene therapy may be used to cure this disease or at least alleviate its symptoms.

Barker PE: Gene mapping and cystic fibrosis. Am J Med Sci 299:69, 1990. *Report describing the location of the genetic defect and purported relationships to the cellular alterations of CF.*

Fiel SB: Clinical management of pulmonary disease in cystic fibrosis. Lancet 341:1070, 1993. *An excellent assessment of approaches to the treatment of respiratory disease in CF patients.*

Fiel SB: Cystic fibrosis. *In* Bone RC (ed.): Pulmonary and Critical Care Medicine. St. Louis, Mosby-Year Book, 1993, p 1. *Outstanding review, with particularly clear description of diagnostics, genetic defects, and treatment; 77 references.*

Koch C, Hoiby N: Pathogenesis of cystic fibrosis. Lancet 341:1065, 1993. *A recent update on the pathogenesis of cystic fibrosis.*

Michel BC: Antibacterial therapy in cystic fibrosis: A review of the literature published between 1980 and February 1987. Chest 94(2 Suppl):129S, 1988. *Numerous comparative tables compiled over a 7-year period; 67 references.*

Ranasinha C, Assoufi B, Shak S, et al.: Efficacy and safety of short-term administration of aerosolized recombinant human DNase I in adults with stable stage cystic fibrosis. Lancet 342:199, 1993. *Most recent of the DNase studies—demonstrates the recombinant drug's safety and indicates that it has the potential to greatly improve pulmonary function in CF patients.*

Zabner J, Couture LA, Gregory RJ, et al.: Adenovirus-mediated gene transfer transiently corrects the chloride transport defect in nasal epithelia of patients with cystic fibrosis. Cell 74:207, 1993. *Original description of viral transfection of the gene into the cells of CF patients to bring about normal Cl⁻ transport.*

59 PULMONARY EMBOLISM
Robert M. Senior

DEFINITION

Pulmonary embolism is the impaction of material into branches of the pulmonary arterial bed. Although they may completely prevent blood flow, most pulmonary emboli do not produce necrosis of lung parenchyma ("pulmonary infarction") because (1) a dual circulation (bronchial and pulmonary) supports lung parenchymal tissue and (2) exchange of oxygen and carbon dioxide can occur directly between the tissue and alveolar gas. Most pulmonary emboli are blood clots ("thromboemboli"); more rarely, neoplastic cells, fat droplets (see Ch. 60), air bubbles, exogenous materials (such as talc and cornstarch particles in intravenous drug abusers), or pieces of

intravenous catheters and catheter introducers occlude pulmonary vessels. The ensuing discussion deals with pulmonary thromboembolism.

PATHOGENESIS

Pulmonary thromboembolism is a complication of venous thrombosis: that is, emboli come from thrombi in peripheral veins, principally the proximal deep veins of the lower extremities and pelvis, and "travel" through the circulation to the pulmonary artery. In approximately 70% of patients with pulmonary thromboembolism, coexisting thrombi can be found in the deep veins of the thighs or pelvis. In the remaining cases, it is presumed that the emboli come from other sites that escape detection or represent the entire thrombus that originated in the lower extremities or pelvis. Although thrombosis of superficial veins of the lower extremities does not lead to pulmonary thromboemboli, pulmonary emboli can result from thrombosis that is confined to deep veins of the calf. The renal veins can be a source of thromboemboli, particularly in patients with the nephrotic syndrome, but in nephrotic patients they do not necessarily arise only from the renal veins. Pulmonary thromboemboli seldom originate in veins of the upper extremities, head, or neck, but intravenous lines inserted into internal jugular or subclavian veins predispose to intracardiac thrombi that can embolize to the lungs. Mural thrombi in the right side of the heart, in the absence of intracardiac catheters, are another source of pulmonary thromboemboli. When venous thromboemboli reach the heart, they may be trapped in the right atrium or right ventricle, from which they embolize to the lungs intact, or they may fragment in the heart and shower the lungs with emboli at one time or intermittently.

Venous thrombosis can be attributed to one or more of the following: stasis of blood, increased tendency for blood to coagulate, and endothelial injury. Many clinical situations have been associated with risk of proximal deep venous thrombosis (Table 59–1).

Without prophylaxis against deep venous thrombosis, the risk of pulmonary embolism is approximately 1% in patients over age 40 following abdominal or thoracic surgery. The risk is 5 to 10% after surgery for hip fracture. In general, the risks associated with surgery are increased by advanced age, obesity, a lengthy operative period, underlying malignancy, pre-existing venous disease, prolonged bed rest after surgery, and postoperative infection. Venous stasis due to immobilization is probably a major reason for venous thrombosis associated with surgery, but other factors come into play: increased blood coagulability associated with release of tissue thromboplastin and exposure of subendothelium, decreased blood fibrinolytic activity postoperatively, and vessel damage, particularly in surgery of the lower extremities or pelvis.

Cancers of the lung, breast, and abdominal viscera are strongly associated with deep venous thrombosis and thromboembolism, and the thrombosis may antedate clinical recognition of the malignancy. Factors released from tumors may increase blood coagulability, decrease fibrinolytic activity, and alter endothelial surfaces. Malignan-

TABLE 59–1. RISK FACTORS FOR DEEP VENOUS THROMBOSIS AND PULMONARY THROMBOEMBOLISM

Common	Uncommon
Prior deep venous thrombosis	**Acquired**
Surgery with > 30 min general anesthesia	Antiphospholipid antibody syndrome (lupus anticoagulant, anticardiolipin antibodies)
Surgery or trauma of pelvis or lower extremities	Nephrotic syndrome
Congestive heart failure	Inflammatory bowel disease
Myocardial infarction	Thrombocytosis
Immobilization (bed rest, stroke, prolonged travel, and so forth)	Polycythemia vera
Malignancy	Paroxysmal nocturnal hemoglobinuria
Pregnancy, especially in the puerperium and after cesarean section	**Inherited**
	Antithrombin III deficiency
Estrogen therapy	Protein C deficiency
Obesity	Protein S deficiency
Advanced age (over 70 years)	Abnormal fibrinogens
	Abnormalities of plasma fibrinolytic system
	Homocystinuria

cies also predispose to deep venous thrombosis by leading to venous stasis through immobilization and surgical interventions. Prolonged bed rest from any cause and paralysis resulting from stroke or spinal cord injury are associated with a high incidence of venous thrombosis. Pulmonary embolism is common at autopsy in patients who die of congestive heart failure.

In pregnancy, multiple factors predispose to venous thrombosis: (1) venous stasis induced by compression on pelvic veins, increased intra-abdominal pressure, and hormonal relaxation of vascular smooth muscle; (2) altered blood rheologic properties; and (3) increased concentrations of factors in the coagulation cascade (fibrinogen and Factors VII, VIII, IX, and XII), with concomitant reductions in antithrombin III and fibrinolytic activity. There may be increased risk of thromboembolism during pregnancy, but there is clearly an increased risk after cesarean section. Estrogen therapy increases the incidence of venous thrombosis, and the risk appears related to the dose, but the precise degree of increased risk and the mechanisms involved are not certain. Multiple possibilities have been considered, including reduction in antithrombin III concentration, decreased plasminogen activator level, increased platelet aggregability, increased blood viscosity, and increased distensibility of peripheral veins predisposing to venous stasis.

When pulmonary embolism occurs without an obvious predisposing factor, the possibility of a hereditary hypercoagulable state most commonly due to deficiencies of antithrombin III, protein C, or protein S should be considered. Features that suggest a hereditable basis are age under 40, recurrent deep venous thrombosis, thrombosis at uncommon sites, and a family history of venous thrombosis.

INCIDENCE

Extrapolations from acute care hospital discharges suggest that 170,000 patients per year experience a first-time episode of pulmonary thromboembolism in the United States and an additional 90,000 other patients are hospitalized for recurrent thromboembolic disease. However, these figures almost certainly underestimate actual incidence because autopsy data indicate a much higher incidence of pulmonary embolism than is diagnosed during life, and noninvasive studies of lower extremity veins show that deep venous thrombosis is often clinically silent. Pulmonary thromboembolism is rare before the age of 20. The incidence rises gradually between ages 20 through 60 and then increases sharply, so that in people over age 70 the incidence is four to eight times greater than in younger individuals. Autopsy data indicate that pulmonary emboli are a major factor in 10 to 15% of in-hospital deaths, with massive pulmonary embolism present in approximately 6%.

PATHOPHYSIOLOGY

Pulmonary emboli produce respiratory and hemodynamic responses that reflect the extent of pulmonary vascular obstruction, the time elapsed since embolization, and the presence or absence of pre-existing heart or lung disease.

HYPERPNEA AND ALVEOLAR HYPERVENTILATION. Acute pulmonary embolism stimulates ventilation. The increase in minute ventilation, manifested clinically by increased respiratory rate, usually offsets the increased physiologic dead space produced by obstruction of the pulmonary vascular bed, so that the arterial carbon dioxide (Pa_{CO_2}) does not rise. On the contrary, the Pa_{CO_2} typically falls below 35 mm Hg, indicating that hyperpnea does not occur solely to preserve a normal Pa_{CO_2}. Similarly, alveolar hyperventilation is not due to hypoxemia, as it occurs even when arterial oxygenation is normal, and it cannot be abolished with supplemental inspired oxygen. The stimulus for alveolar hyperventilation is unknown but presumably involves reflexes initiated from the pulmonary parenchyma in the area of the obstructed vessel. A reduction of Pa_{CO_2} below baseline may occur even among those with chronic hypercapnia. Although a lower than normal Pa_{CO_2} is usual, the Pa_{CO_2} rises in individuals who cannot increase their minute ventilation adequately to compensate for the increased physiologic dead space—for example, in those with neuromuscular disease, those receiving controlled mechanical ventilation, or those with severe pleuritic pain. The Pa_{CO_2} may also rise when massive embolization confines pulmonary blood flow to a severely reduced portion of the pulmonary vascular bed.

HYPOXEMIA. A decrease in arterial oxygen tension (Pa_{O_2}) is common in acute pulmonary embolism. The mechanisms are complex. Ventilation-perfusion (V/Q) inequality seems to be the pre-dominant mechanism early in the course of pulmonary embolization, with intrapulmonary shunting as the dominant cause after 48 hours. Regional bronchoconstriction, atelectasis, and pulmonary edema are postulated as the anatomic basis for these physiologic defects. If cardiac output fails to keep up with metabolic demands, as is common with massive pulmonary embolism, mixed venous oxygen saturation falls and accentuates the effects of abnormal V/Q and intrapulmonary shunting. If pulmonary hypertension develops and a patent foramen ovale is present, blood may be shunted from right to left within the heart; this is another factor causing arterial hypoxemia.

PULMONARY HYPERTENSION AND ACUTE COR PULMONALE. Pulmonary thromboembolism is the most common cause of acute pulmonary hypertension (see Ch. 38). The rise in pulmonary arterial pressure results primarily from mechanical blockage of the pulmonary vascular bed. Vasoconstrictive reflexes and mediators may also contribute. The rise in mean pulmonary arterial pressure tends to match the extent of blockage of the pulmonary arterial tree, but in patients without pre-existing cardiac or pulmonary disease, mean pulmonary arterial pressure is usually < 20 mm Hg unless pulmonary vascular obstruction exceeds 50%. Pressures of 20 to 40 mm Hg occur only with 50 to 75% obstruction. The pressure seldom goes above 40 mm Hg because the normal right ventricle cannot generate higher pressures. A mean pulmonary arterial pressure > 40 mm Hg indicates chronic right ventricular hypertrophy secondary to recurrent pulmonary emboli or other diseases. When a sudden and marked increase in pulmonary vascular resistance pushes mean pulmonary arterial pressure toward 40 mm Hg, several events occur. Right ventricular diastolic pressure, right atrial pressure, and systemic venous pressure all increase. The cardiac index falls below 2.5 liters per minute per square meter, and systemic hypotension and other clinical signs of hemodynamic distress appear.

PATHOLOGY

Most episodes of acute pulmonary embolism involve multiple emboli. Both lungs are affected about two thirds of the time. Lower lobe vessels are involved more often than upper ones, and the right lung is affected more often than the left. Emboli in the main branches of the right or left pulmonary arteries are seen in only a small percentage of patients. A large embolus obstructing the main pulmonary artery or straddling the pulmonary artery bifurcation (so-called saddle embolus) is uncommon even in fatal acute pulmonary embolism. When a thromboembolus is poorly organized, it is likely to fragment when passing through the heart and is thus more likely to impact smaller vessels than are organized thromboemboli.

The likelihood that emboli will cause pulmonary infarction is determined by the size of the vessels involved, the extent of obstruction, the potential for delivery of bronchial arterial blood flow, and the adequacy of ventilation to the lung tissue supplied by the blocked pulmonary arteries. Occlusions of segmental arterial vessels or smaller branches are more likely to lead to infarction than are emboli lodged in larger vessels. Infarction is also more likely with elevated pulmonary capillary pressure from any cause—hence the frequency of infarction in patients with congestive heart failure—but otherwise healthy individuals can develop infarcts. Histologically, pulmonary infarction is characterized by intra-alveolar hemorrhage and necrosis of alveolar walls but little inflammation. Cavitation rarely develops without coexisting pulmonary infection or an infected thrombus.

CLINICAL MANIFESTATIONS

The most common symptoms of acute pulmonary embolism are dyspnea and pleuritic pain, each occurring in at least two thirds of the patients (Table 59–2). Hemoptysis, often considered typical of pulmonary embolism, is not common, so its absence is not evidence against pulmonary embolism. Similarly, leg pain or leg swelling occurs in only about one fourth of the patients. A respiratory rate of at least 20 breaths per minute is the most common sign and is found in most patients. Occasionally, unexplained arrhythmia or refractory congestive heart failure is the principal manifestation of pulmonary embolism.

TABLE 59–2. SYMPTOMS AND SIGNS IN 117 PATIENTS WITH ACUTE PULMONARY EMBOLISM WITHOUT PRE-EXISTING CARDIAC OR PULMONARY DISEASE

Symptoms	Percentage	Signs	Percentage
Dyspnea	73	Tachypnea (≥ 20/min)	70
Pleuritic pain	66	Rales (crackles)	51
Cough	37	Tachycardia (> 100/min)	30
Leg swelling	28	Fourth heart sound	24
Leg pain	26	Increased pulmonary component of second sound	23
Hemoptysis	13		
Palpitations	10	Deep venous thrombosis	11
Wheezing	9	Diaphoresis	11
Angina-like pain	4	Temperature $>38.5°C$	7
		Wheezes	5
		Homans' sign	4
		Right ventricular lift	4
		Pleural friction rub	3
		Third heart sound	3
		Cyanosis	1

Adapted from Stein PD, Terrin ML, Hales CA, et al.: Clinical, laboratory, roentgenographic and electrocardiographic findings in patients with acute pulmonary embolism and no pre-existing cardiac or pulmonary disease. Chest 100:598, 1991.

The symptoms and signs of acute pulmonary embolism depend upon the extent of pulmonary arterial tree blockage, whether there is pre-existing cardiopulmonary disease, and whether pulmonary infarction occurs. Marked disturbances in pulmonary and systemic hemodynamics seldom occur unless there is extensive vascular obstruction or pre-existing heart or lung disease. Pleuritic pain and signs of pulmonary consolidation and pleural effusion indicate that embolization involves one or more peripheral pulmonary arterial branches. Discrepancies may exist between the severity of embolization and symptoms; some patients with massive embolization may appear remarkably comfortable, whereas others with minimal embolization may show great distress. Asymptomatic high probability lung scans are common among patients with deep venous thrombosis, further indicating that pulmonary emboli may be clinically silent.

The picture of sudden apprehension, chest discomfort, and dyspnea, with physical findings of acute cor pulmonale (accentuated pulmonic closure sound in the second left interspace, right ventricular lift, and jugular venous distention), and systemic hypotension is uncommon, but it is this presentation that may culminate in death within a few minutes.

DIAGNOSIS

Although the history and physical examination may lead a clinician to suspect pulmonary embolism, a diagnosis based on clinical grounds alone is likely to be incorrect because many other conditions resemble acute pulmonary embolism. The differential diagnosis of acute pulmonary embolism is lengthy but principally includes conditions that produce acute shortness of breath or pleuritic pain (Table 59–3). Several features point away from the diagnosis of pulmonary thromboembolism: (1) the absence of risk factors for deep venous thrombosis, (2) recurrent chest pain in the same location, (3) pleuritic pain of more than 1 week's duration that is increasing in severity, (4) pleuritic pain with negative findings on the chest radiograph, (5) hemoptysis of >5 ml with negative findings on the chest radiograph, (6) purulent sputum, (7) pericardial friction rub, and (8) spiking fever $>39°$ C lasting more than 1 week.

DIAGNOSTIC STUDIES. When pulmonary embolism is suspected, confirming the diagnosis depends on establishing the presence of intravascular obstruction to pulmonary arterial blood flow. The definitive method of making the diagnosis is pulmonary angiography. Ventilation-perfusion lung scanning is also useful to visualize the pulmonary circulation, but its limitations must be appreciated (see below). Other imaging methods such as ultra-fast computed tomography and magnetic resonance imaging, as well as visualizing intrapulmonary thrombi using radiolabeled platelets or monoclonal antibodies to platelet antigens and fibrin, are under development.

Because most pulmonary emboli originate in lower extremity veins and because residual thrombi usually remain in these veins after thromboembolism has occurred, studying the veins of the lower extremities for thrombi has become a valuable addition to ventilation-perfusion lung scanning. Noninvasive methods for assessing lower extremity veins, such as venous duplex imaging, are proving to be quite reliable for detecting deep venous thrombosis above the knee, the site most often implicated as the source of pulmonary thromboemboli. The finding of normal lower extremity veins tends to point away from a diagnosis of pulmonary thromboembolism. On the other hand, detecting proximal deep venous thrombosis supports pulmonary embolism and from a practical standpoint settles the issue about whether to use anticoagulant therapy.

Arterial blood gas measurement, the electrocardiogram, the chest radiograph, and thoracentesis may help evaluate patients suspected of having pulmonary embolism, either by pointing toward or away from diagnoses with which pulmonary embolism can be confused, but these studies lack specificity and therefore cannot be used in place of imaging the pulmonary circulation. However, quantification of plasma D-dimer, a unique plasmin-mediated fragment of fibrin, appears promising as a sensitive and reliable screening test for pulmonary embolism.

ARTERIAL BLOOD GASES. Typically in pulmonary embolism the Pa_{O_2} and Pa_{CO_2} are reduced concomitantly. In patients with angiographically proven acute pulmonary embolism who do not have previous cardiopulmonary disease, Pa_{O_2} values are <50 mm Hg in 13%, 50 to 59 mm Hg in 19%, 60 to 80 mm Hg in 55%, and >80 mm Hg in 13%. Those with a normal Pa_{O_2} usually have an increased alveolar-arterial oxygen difference, reflecting reduced efficiency of alveolar gas exchange, but even a normal alveolar-arterial oxygen difference does not exclude the diagnosis. A $Pa_{O_2} < 50$ mm Hg is confined to those patients with $>50\%$ occlusion of major pulmonary arterial branches; however, in individuals with underlying cardiopulmonary disease, less severe degrees of pulmonary vascular obstruction can be associated with severe hypoxemia. Arterial blood gas abnormalities have no specificity for pulmonary embolism; similar abnormalities occur in conditions with which pulmonary embolism is confused.

ELECTROCARDIOGRAM. The main value of the electrocardiogram is to help exclude acute myocardial infarction and pericarditis. The most common finding in pulmonary embolism is sinus tachycardia. Emboli that substantially raise pulmonary arterial and right-sided cardiac pressures may induce patterns of S_1, Q_3, T_3, inverted T waves in leads V_1 to V_3, right ventricular strain, right-axis deviation, right bundle branch block, and atrial arrhythmias. These changes tend to be transient, lasting only a few hours or less and disappearing as the pulmonary arterial pressure returns toward normal.

CHEST RADIOGRAPHY. A normal chest radiograph is uncommon in acute pulmonary embolism, but the usual radiographic findings are nonspecific: Elevation of one of the hemidiaphragms, basilar atelectasis, parenchymal densities, and unilateral pleural effusion are the typical abnormalities. The parenchymal densities tend to be in the lower lung fields, pleural-based, and associated with pleural effusions. These densities usually represent extravascular blood rather than infarcted tissue. Cardiac dilatation, dilatation of the main branches of the pulmonary artery, and zones of oligemia in the lung fields may occur with massive embolization. The principal value of the chest radiograph is to help exclude other diagnoses.

TABLE 59–3. DIFFERENTIAL DIAGNOSIS OF ACUTE PULMONARY EMBOLISM

Myocardial infarction
Pericarditis
Congestive heart failure
Pneumonia
Asthma
Chronic obstructive pulmonary disease
Pneumothorax
Pleurodynia
Pleuritis from collagen vascular disease
Thoracic herpes zoster ("shingles")
Rib fracture
Musculoskeletal pain
Primary or metastatic intrathoracic cancer
Infradiaphragmatic processes (e.g., acute cholecystitis, splenic infarction)
Hyperventilation syndrome

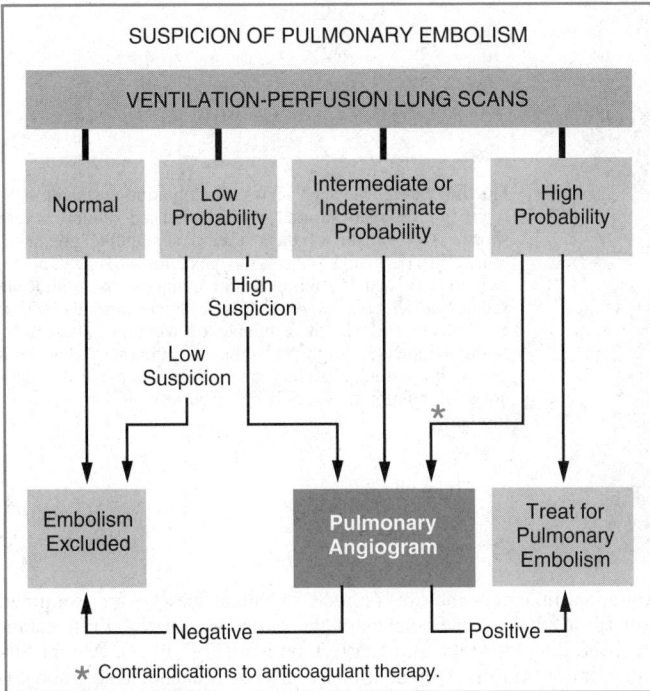

SUSPICION OF PULMONARY EMBOLISM

VENTILATION-PERFUSION LUNG SCANS

Normal | Low Probability | Intermediate or Indeterminate Probability | High Probability

High Suspicion

Low Suspicion

*

Embolism Excluded | Pulmonary Angiogram | Treat for Pulmonary Embolism

Negative | Positive

* Contraindications to anticoagulant therapy.

FIGURE 59–1. Ventilation-perfusion lung scanning in the evaluation of the patient suspected of having pulmonary embolism.

THORACENTESIS. Pleural effusion, usually unilateral, is common with pulmonary embolism. The pleural fluid is most often an exudate and is often hemorrhagic (but has a low hematocrit).

VENTILATION-PERFUSION LUNG SCANS. Isotopic scans of pulmonary perfusion ("Q scans") provide a sensitive, safe means of assessing regional pulmonary blood flow and therefore are valuable in evaluating patients suspected of having pulmonary embolism. Q scans can be performed alone or with isotopic scans of ventilation ("V scans"). The combination of scans ("V/Q scans") is more specific than the Q scan alone, and therefore every effort is made to include a V scan. V/Q scanning has become accepted as the initial means of assessing the pulmonary circulation in the patient suspected of pulmonary embolism (Fig. 59–1). The interpretation of V/Q scans is summarized in Table 59–4.

A Q scan requires intravenous administration of technetium-99m–labeled particles of macroaggregated albumin in a supine patient, followed by scanning the thorax with a gamma camera in a minimum of six views (anterior, posterior, right and left lateral, and right and left posterior oblique). The particles, which are slightly larger in diameter than the precapillary vessels of the pulmonary circulation, are injected into a peripheral vein; flow through the peripheral and central venous circulation, the right side of the heart, and the main pulmonary arteries; and finally lodge in precapillary vessels, where they remain for hours. The standard dose of particles blocks <0.2% of the pulmonary precapillary vessels in the normal

pulmonary vascular bed. For a ventilation scan, the patient usually inhales and then rebreathes air containing radioactive gas, most often xenon-133, or aerosolized radiolabeled particles. Images of the initial breath, equilibration, and washout of the tracer are obtained. Typically, the xenon ventilation scan is performed before the perfusion scan in the posterior projection with oblique views during washout. The patient is upright if possible. Besides ^{133}Xe, two other isotopes used for ventilation scanning are (1) krypton-81m and (2) ^{99m}Tc-labeled particles in aerosols, which have the advantage over ^{133}Xe of allowing scans to be obtained in the same views as the perfusion scan with minimal radiation exposure.

A normal Q scan reveals a homogeneous distribution of radioactivity with an image that conforms to the lungs. This finding almost always eliminates the diagnosis of pulmonary embolism. When a pulmonary embolus is present, the radiolabeled particles are prevented from reaching vessels distal to the embolus, and the scan shows one or more perfusion defects (Fig. 59–2). The sensitivity of the Q scan to pulmonary arterial obstruction is excellent, as obstruction of vessels 3 mm in diameter or more leads to defects. Perfusion defects generally show some resolution within 4 to 5 days, but substantial abnormalities can persist for several weeks and may be permanent.

The limitation of the Q scan is its nonspecificity. Besides emboli, perfusion defects can be caused by lesions that compress pulmonary vessels, by increased pulmonary vascular resistance, by regional alveolar hypoxia, and by regional loss of pulmonary parenchyma as in pulmonary emphysema. In practice, chronic obstructive lung disease (COPD) is the most common clinical condition causing perfusion defects not due to pulmonary embolism.

Ventilation ("V") scans increase the specificity of Q scans for diagnosing pulmonary emboli because pulmonary emboli do not usually disrupt regional ventilation as much as regional blood flow, unlike other causes of perfusion defects, especially COPD. V scans may reveal (1) the preservation of ventilation at sites of perfusion defects ("V/Q mismatches"), (2) the loss of ventilation where there are perfusion defects ("V/Q matches"), and (3) nonuniform delays of washin or washout of respiratory gas, indicative of obstructive lung disease. V/Q mismatches establish a higher probability of pulmonary emboli than Q defects alone. With some patterns of V/Q mismatch the diagnosis of pulmonary embolism can be made with virtual certainty, particularly when there is a strong suspicion on clinical grounds. Matched V/Q defects are less likely to represent pulmonary embolism, but pulmonary embolism is not excluded.

In addition to the V scans, Q scans may be interpreted in conjunction with the chest radiograph. Perfusion defects that do not have a corresponding abnormality on the chest radiograph are scored by number and size for the probability of pulmonary embolism. Single defects smaller than segments carry low probability of pulmonary embolism, whereas multiple defects that are segmental or larger carry a substantially higher probability of pulmonary embolism. Perfusion defects that have corresponding abnormalities on the chest radiograph are called indeterminate, although some evidence indicates that a perfusion defect can be assigned a probability of embolus based upon its size relative to the radiographic abnormality.

TABLE 59–4. INTERPRETATION OF VENTILATION-PERFUSION (V/Q) LUNG SCANS

Category	Pattern	Approximate Frequency of Pulmonary Embolism Detected by Pulmonary Angiogram (%)
Normal	No perfusion defects	0
Low probability	Small V/Q mismatches	15
	V/Q matches without corresponding roentgenographic changes	
	Perfusion defect substantially smaller than roentgenographic density	
Intermediate probability	Marked, diffuse obstructive pulmonary disease with perfusion defects	30
	Perfusion defect of same size as roentgenographic change	
	Single segmental mismatch*	
High probability	Two or more segmental mismatches*	90
	Perfusion defect substantially larger than roentgenographic density	

* Controversy exists regarding the important categorization of a single segmental mismatch. This has been considered either of high or intermediate probability. The more conservative interpretation, that is, intermediate probability, has been used in this table.

Adapted from Biello DR: Radiological (scintigraphic) evaluation of patients with suspected pulmonary thromboembolism. JAMA 257:3257, 1987; with permission. Copyright 1987, American Medical Association.

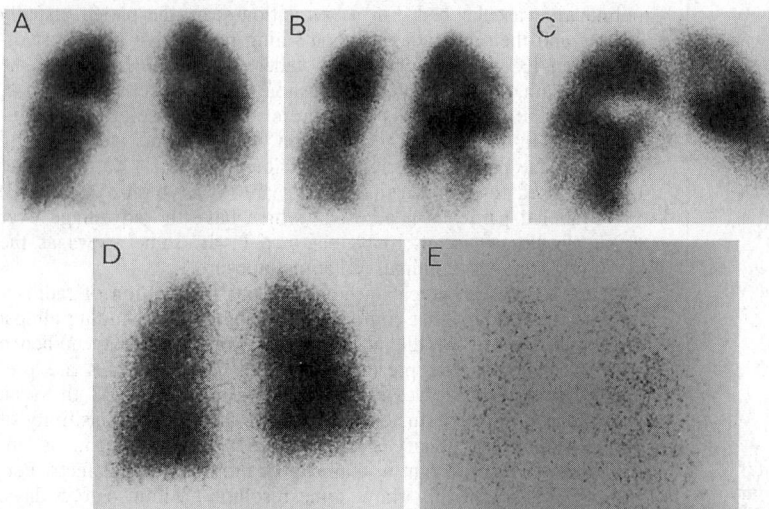

FIGURE 59–2. Selected views of ventilation-perfusion lung scans in a 60-year-old man who experienced sudden, severe shortness of breath 14 days after a suprapubic prostatectomy. The perfusion scans—*(A)* posterior, *(B)* right posterior oblique, and *(C)* left posterior oblique—show multiple segmental defects; the ventilation scans are normal—*(D)* at equilibrium and *(E)* at 1 minute of washout. These scan findings indicate a high probability of pulmonary embolism and with the clinical setting are sufficient to make the diagnosis of pulmonary embolism. (Courtesy of Dr. Keith C. Fischer.)

A multicenter study to evaluate the sensitivity and specificity of V/Q scanning to diagnose pulmonary embolism has recently been completed. This study, the Prospective Investigation of Pulmonary Embolism Diagnosis (referred to as the PIOPED), used V/Q scanning and pulmonary angiography in a large number of randomly selected individuals suspected of having acute pulmonary embolism. The results support the findings of earlier studies: (1) high-probability V/Q scans are usually confirmed by pulmonary angiography; (2) normal V/Q scans are rarely associated with findings of emboli by pulmonary angiography; and (3) intermediate-probability V/Q scans do not help predict the results of pulmonary angiography. It is essential to note that among the patients with positive pulmonary angiograms in the PIOPED study, only 41% had high-probability V/Q scans. To restate this important point, 59% of patients with acute pulmonary embolism do not have high-probability scans. Thus, one must not equate low- or intermediate-probability lung scans with exclusion of pulmonary embolism.

PULMONARY ANGIOGRAPHY. Pulmonary angiography is the definitive test to diagnose pulmonary embolism. It involves inserting a catheter into the pulmonary artery, usually percutaneously, through one of the femoral veins. After the catheter is advanced at least as far as the right or left main branch of the pulmonary artery, or more selectively into lobar or segmental branches, the contrast medium is injected and films are taken in rapid sequence. Radiographic images—anterior, oblique, or lateral views—are examined for filling defects in branches of the pulmonary artery; these establish the diagnosis of pulmonary embolism (Fig. 59–3). Abrupt terminations ("cutoffs") of pulmonary arterial branches also point toward that diagnosis, although less definitely. The filling defects or cutoffs should be present in vessels of at least 2 to 3 mm in diameter. Other types of abnormalities, including delayed filling and diminished number of small vessels, are not diagnostic. A negative study has rarely been proven wrong.

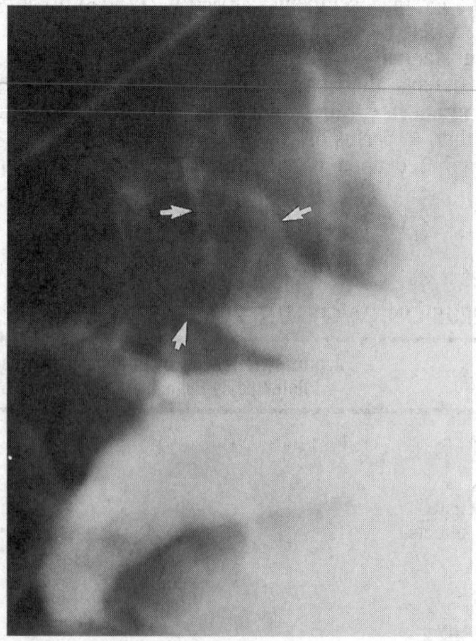

As shown in Figure 59–1, pulmonary angiography is indicated when V/Q scanning is of intermediate probability. It is also warranted (1) when V/Q scanning shows high probability but there are serious concerns about using anticoagulation therapy; (2) before using thrombolytic agents; (3) when there are contraindications to anticoagulation therapy so that other forms of treatment will be needed; and (4) when there is an apparent failure of anticoagulation therapy and interruption of the inferior vena cava or embolectomy is being contemplated. When V/Q scans are interpreted as low probability, it is reasonable to be guided by clinical suspicion as to the need for pulmonary angiography. Angiography should be done in those patients in whom there is either a strong or uncertain clinical suspicion of pulmonary embolism, as it may be positive in 40% of patients in whom the diagnosis is strongly suspected clinically, according to the PIOPED study. In contrast, when the clinical suspicion is low, the likelihood of a positive result by angiography is only 4%. Assessing the proximal deep veins of the lower extremities may be valuable in this setting. Negative results by this approach are reasonable reassurance that future pulmonary embolism is unlikely. In one large prospective series, the scenario of an abnormal V/Q scan, but not of high probability, combined with normal results on serial noninvasive tests for thrombosis of proximal veins, carried an excellent prognosis without anticoagulant therapy.

Many experts in this field believe that pulmonary angiography is underused because physicians have unwarranted concerns about the safety of the procedure. When performed by an experienced staff, pulmonary angiography has sufficiently low risk to justify its use for diagnosing pulmonary embolism. In large series, major nonfatal complications occur in about 1 to 3% and death happens in ≤0.5%.

THERAPY

Nearly all patients with acute pulmonary embolism who survive long enough to have the diagnosis confirmed survive the acute episode. Accordingly, the primary goal of therapy is to prevent a potentially fatal recurrence. Additional goals are to reduce the morbidity of the acute episode and to prevent chronic pulmonary hypertension.

The overall therapeutic approach is summarized in Figure 59–4. Because most patients with acute pulmonary embolism are hemodynamically stable and do not have a contraindication to anticoagulants, the cornerstone of therapy is anticoagulant drugs. Patients who are treated with therapeutic doses for an appropriate period seldom have a recurrence of pulmonary embolism, and fatal recurrences are rare. Thrombolytic therapy accelerates restoration of pul-

FIGURE 59–3. Pulmonary angiogram showing filling defects in branches of the pulmonary artery, indicative of pulmonary embolism. (Courtesy of Dr. Noah Susman.)

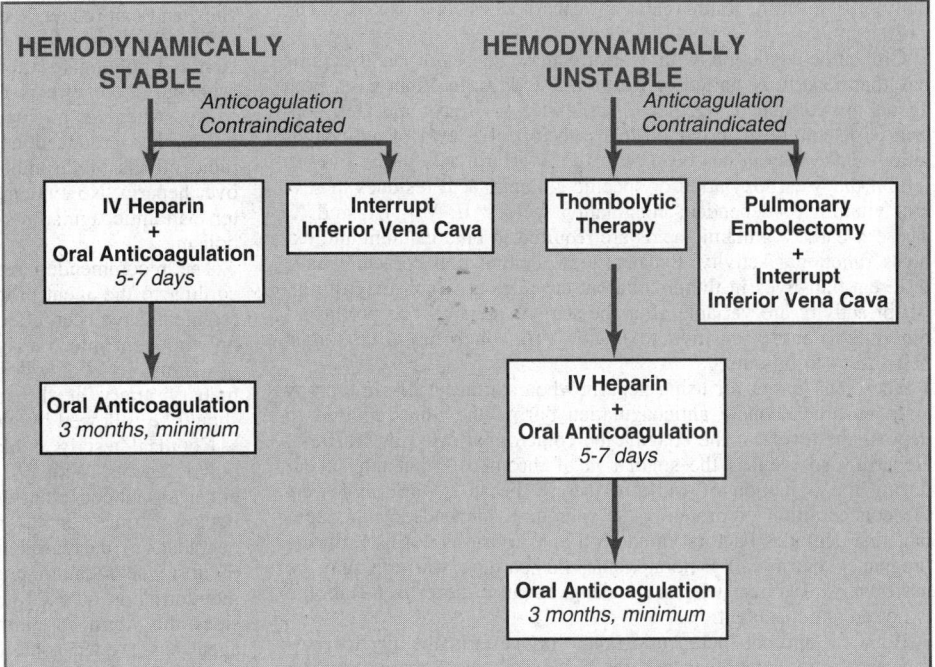

FIGURE 59-4. Therapy of acute pulmonary thromboembolism.

monary blood flow and normal pulmonary hemodynamics and therefore is the initial therapy for massive pulmonary embolism that has produced hemodynamic instability. When anticoagulants and thrombolytic agents are contraindicated or prove ineffective, therapy consists of interruption of the inferior vena cava, combined with pulmonary embolectomy for patients with hemodynamic instability.

Supportive measures can reduce the morbidity of the acute episode and on occasion are essential to help the patient through a period of hemodynamic crisis. These include supplemental oxygen to correct hypoxemia, analgesics for pleuritic pain, and hemodynamic and ventilatory support.

ANTICOAGULANT THERAPY. Anticoagulant therapy prevents future embolization by stopping the formation of new deep venous thrombi and the propagation of residual thrombi in the deep venous system. During anticoagulant therapy, pulmonary emboli and residual deep venous thrombi either organize or undergo dissolution or both. Anticoagulation does not, however, hasten resolution of the thromboemboli within the lungs.

Table 59-5 presents a regimen for using anticoagulants. Heparin is an acidic glycosaminoglycan obtained from pig intestinal mucosa or beef lung. It produces an anticoagulant effect by accelerating the inhibitory effect of antithrombin III upon the coagulation enzymes, thrombin, and Factors IXa, Xa, XIa, and XIIa. Heparin exerts its effect immediately and therefore is used to begin therapy in patients with suspected or proven pulmonary thromboembolism. If pulmonary embolism is suspected, an intravenous bolus of heparin (5,000 to 10,000 units) should be given while diagnostic studies are underway, unless there is active intracranial bleeding, intracranial lesions predisposed to bleed, or other active internal bleeding, all of which are contraindications to heparin.

Heparin is usually administered intravenously by continuous infusion. Intermittent intravenous injection and subcutaneous injection are alternatives, but bleeding occurs more often with intermittent injection, and it is difficult to establish the correct dose with the subcutaneous route. Insufficient dosage is probably the most common error in administering heparin for acute pulmonary thromboembolism. The recommended dose of heparin is that amount which maintains the activated partial thromboplastin time (aPTT) at 1.5 to 2.5 times control at all times. However, this aPPT range (which amounts to extending the aPTT about 15 to 60 seconds beyond the control) may be low because it is reached at plasma heparin levels below levels that correlate with clinical efficacy. Accordingly, an aPTT of 1.5 times control must be regarded as the minimum for effective heparin therapy. The effect of heparin therapy on the aPTT should be monitored particularly closely during the first few days after the thromboembolic event because the heparin requirements

are greatest then. On the average, at least 31,000 units daily (> 1300 units per hour) are required to maintain a therapeutic effect. Heparin therapy should be continued for 5 to 10 days. Low molecular weight heparins, which are approved by the Food and Drug Administration for prophylaxis of deep venous thrombosis after hip replacement surgery, are not approved for use in pulmonary thromboembolism.

The most common and most serious complication of heparin therapy is bleeding. The risk of bleeding does increase with dose and effect on the whole blood clotting time and the aPTT, but clear-cut correlations between bleeding and results of *in vitro* coagulation tests do not exist. The risk of bleeding has also been related to comorbid conditions such as renal failure and liver disease. Thrombocytopenia (platelet counts < 100,000 per cubic millimeter) complicates heparin therapy in about 1 to 5% of patients. It is an indication to stop heparin therapy because the falling platelet count may be due to antibody-mediated platelet and endothelial injury that can produce arterial thromboembolism and worsen existing venous thrombosis. Thrombocytopenia seldom occurs until after several days of therapy. Heparin therapy at high dose (> 15,000 units

TABLE 59-5. GUIDELINES FOR ANTICOAGULANT THERAPY WITH HEPARIN AND WARFARIN FOR PULMONARY EMBOLISM

Suspected embolism	Give a bolus of heparin, 5000 units IV, and order imaging study
Confirmed embolism	Rebolus with heparin 5,000–10,000 units IV and start maintenance infusion at 1300–1600 units/hour (heparin 20,000 units in 500 ml D₅W, infused at 33 ml/hour)
	Check aPTT at 6 hours and adjust the heparin infusion to keep the aPTT between 1.5–2.5 times control*
	Check platelet count daily
	Start warfarin therapy on day 1 at 10 mg daily for first 2 days, then administer warfarin daily at estimated daily maintenance dose
	Stop heparin therapy after 5 to 7 days of joint therapy when INR is 2.0–3.0 off heparin
	Anticoagulate with warfarin for 3 months at an INR of 2.0–3.0

aPTT = activated partial thromboplastin time; PT = one-stage prothrombin time; IV = intravenous; INR = International Normalized Ratio.

* For recommendations about adjustment of the heparin infusion, see Cruickshank MK, Levine MN, Hirsh J, et al.: A standard nomogram for the management of heparin therapy. Arch Intern Med 151:333, 1991.

Adapted from Hyers TM, Hull RD, Weg JG: Antithrombotic therapy for venous thromboembolic disease. Chest 102:408S, 1992.

daily) for several months can cause marked osteoporosis (see Ch. 217).

Oral anticoagulation with warfarin may be begun on the same day that heparin is started or within a few days. In either case, both agents are continued together for at least 5 to 7 days and then heparin is discontinued, provided that a therapeutic level of anticoagulation with warfarin has been achieved. Warfarin acts in the liver to inhibit the γ-carboxylation of specific glutamic acid residues in several vitamin K–dependent coagulation factors: II, VII, IX, and X. These γ-carboxyglutamic acids are required to bind calcium and express functional activity. Because these coagulation cofactors have different half-lives in the circulation, the rates at which they diminish in activity are variable after the start of therapy. The prothrombin time is most sensitive to Factor VII, which has the shortest half-life (4 to 6 hours).

The main reason for using heparin when starting warfarin therapy is to ensure adequate anticoagulation during the time required to depress the levels of the coagulation cofactors affected by warfarin. Heparin also reduces the small risk of thrombosis that may occur during the induction of warfarin therapy because warfarin lowers the concentration of protein C, a vitamin K–dependent anticoagulant that degrades Factors Va and VIIIa. Warfarin is not used during pregnancy because it is teratogenic. Postpartum, warfarin may be used even in women who are nursing, because the drug metabolite is not an anticoagulant.

Both the optimal therapeutic range for warfarin therapy for pulmonary thromboembolism and the proper means of monitoring the anticoagulant effect of warfarin have undergone a number of revisions over the years. The current recommendation is that warfarin dosage should be adjusted to achieve an International Normalized Ratio (INR) of 2.0 to 3.0, rather than a ratio of the patient's prothrombin time (PT) to the PT of the laboratory control, as has been the usual practice for many years. The INR corrects the ratio of the patient's PT to the PT of the laboratory control by a factor that adjusts for the activity of the laboratory's thromboplastin by comparing it to a World Health Organization (WHO) thromboplastin reference standard. Using the INR helps avoid problems of either under- or over-anticoagulation resulting from wide differences in activity among the thromboplastins in use in laboratories; however, use of the INR is not foolproof. It is influenced by the instruments used to measure the PT, and it does not give consistent results during the first week of warfarin therapy owing to variable depression of clotting factors when therapy is begun. Therefore, the INR is not recommended at the start of therapy. Although commercial suppliers of thromboplastin reagents provide the conversion factor of their product (called the International Sensitivity Index) so that clinical laboratories can convert the PT ratio to an INR, many laboratories in the United States do not use the INR.

The optimal duration of warfarin therapy following pulmonary thromboembolism is not known. It is generally advised to continue therapy for at least 3 months in all patients, to extend therapy as long as risk factors for deep venous thrombosis are resolving, and to give therapy indefinitely to patients who have permanently increased risk for deep venous thrombosis.

THROMBOLYTIC THERAPY. Thrombolytic agents lead to lysis of pulmonary thromboemboli and thrombi in the deep venous system by converting endogenous plasminogen, an inactive proenzyme, to plasmin, a potent fibrinolytic proteinase. Three thrombolytic agents are available—streptokinase (SK), urokinase (UK), and tissue-type plasminogen activator (t-PA). Variants of these agents are likely soon. SK is a product of β-hemolytic streptococci. UK is derived from human cells in culture, and t-PA is produced by mammalian cells into which the human t-PA cDNA has been inserted. SK and UK convert circulating plasminogen to plasmin— SK by forming a complex with plasminogen, allowing expression of plasminogen's normally hidden active site, which then cleaves other plasminogen molecules to plasmin; UK by cleaving plasminogen to plasmin directly. Unlike both SK and UK, t-PA appears to act preferentially upon plasminogen that is associated with fibrin. Although the plasmin formed by thrombolytic agents lyses the fibrin in pulmonary emboli and venous thrombi, it also cleaves other circulating molecules, including fibrinogen and Factors V and VIII, and it leads to consumption of circulating plasmin inhibitors, in particular α₂-antiplasmin. Thus, these agents can lead to the breakdown of hemostatic plugs where they are important, such as at incisional sites, and can reduce hemostatic competence generally.

Thrombolytic agents can restore pulmonary parenchymal perfusion and pulmonary arterial pressure toward normal faster than heparin, but these effects do not result in improved patient survival except when an angiographically proven massive pulmonary embolism has produced hemodynamic instability. In this setting, the rapid effects of thrombolytic therapy offer a life-saving advantage over heparin. No evidence indicates that thrombolytic drugs are better than anticoagulants in reducing the recurrence of pulmonary embolism.

The recommended regimens for thrombolytic therapy vary according to the agent (Table 59–6). In small series of patients, other regimens have been effective, such as a single large bolus of thrombolytic agent into the right atrium over a few minutes, or continuous infusions of low-dose thrombolytic agent directly into the pulmonary artery at the clot site. Any thrombolytic regimen used should be followed by anticoagulant therapy.

No ideal test is available for monitoring patients given thrombolytic agents. With SK or UK, the usual approach is to document either an anticoagulant effect (lengthening of the PT, partial thromboplastin time, or thrombin time), evidence of fibrinogen/fibrin degradation (decreased fibrinogen concentration or increased titers of fibrin degradation products), or both. With t-PA, no laboratory monitoring is advised. Because these agents digest substrates besides the fibrin in pulmonary emboli, proof that a thrombolytic agent has exerted some effect by these tests does not prove an effect upon pulmonary emboli, nor is it possible to use results from these tests to titrate the thrombolytic dose; however, clinical effectiveness is usually apparent from improvement in the patient's cardiopulmonary status.

Because thrombolytic agents may start or aggravate bleeding, they are contraindicated when there is active or recent internal bleeding, history of hemorrhagic stroke, recent cranial surgery, or head injury. They are relatively contraindicated within 10 days of major surgery or trauma, within 10 days of biopsies of internal organs, during pregnancy and the first 10 days postpartum, within 1 year of nonhemorrhagic stroke, and in the presence of uncontrolled severe hypertension. Some bleeding occurs at the site of catheter insertion for pulmonary angiography in approximately 20%. Despite the possible bleeding hazard, in the patient who is critically ill from pulmonary emboli, the potential benefits of thrombolytic therapy must be weighed against the risks and effectiveness of alternative forms of therapy.

INTERRUPTION OF THE INFERIOR VENA CAVA. As with anticoagulant therapy, the purpose of interrupting the inferior vena cava (IVC) is to prevent future pulmonary thromboemboli. The principal indications for IVC interruption are (1) contraindications to anticoagulant therapy because of active internal bleeding or complications of anticoagulation such as heparin-induced thrombocytopenia, (2) recurrent pulmonary emboli despite adequate anticoagulation, and (3) as prophylaxis in patients who are at high risk

---

TABLE 59–6. GUIDELINES FOR THROMBOLYTIC AGENTS FOR PULMONARY THROMBOEMBOLISM

Stop heparin infusion and start thrombolytic intravenous infusion when the aPTT or thrombin time (TT) is ≤ 1.5 times control.

Thrombolytic Agent	Dose*
Streptokinase	250,000 IU† loading dose
	100,000 IU/hour maintenance for 24 hours
Urokinase	4,400 IU/lb loading dose
	4,400 IU/lb/hour maintenance for 12 hours
Tissue plasminogen activator	100 mg (56 million IU) over 2 hours

After terminating thrombolytic infusion, restart heparin infusion without a loading dose or with a small loading dose when aPTT or TT is ≤ 1.5 times control.

* All medications given intravenously.
† IU = international units.
Adapted from Hyers TM, Hull RD, Weg JG: Antithrombotic therapy for venous thromboembolic disease. Chest 102:408S, 1992.

for fatal pulmonary embolism, such as patients with extensive deep venous thrombosis and chronic pulmonary hypertension. Because collateral veins bypassing the interruption can enlarge and provide routes for thromboemboli to reach the lungs and because thrombi may form above the site of interruption, IVC interruption may not provide permanent protection against pulmonary thromboembolism.

IVC interruption is usually done with filters inserted percutaneously through jugular or femoral veins under local anesthesia. The filters produce channels in the IVC small enough to limit the passage of large thrombi without blocking blood flow. Except when anticoagulation is contraindicated, anticoagulant therapy should be used in conjunction with IVC interruption.

It must be remembered that most bleeding during anticoagulant therapy is controllable and not life-threatening and that fatal pulmonary embolism is rare during therapeutic anticoagulation. Therefore, a conservative approach is advised regarding interruption of the IVC.

PULMONARY EMBOLECTOMY. Embolectomy for acute pulmonary embolism is performed rarely because few patients meet the criteria for this surgery and survive long enough to have it done. Embolectomy is restricted to patients with massive pulmonary emboli who have hypotension and end-organ (brain and kidney) dysfunction despite maximal medical support and who have absolute contraindications to thrombolytic therapy or in whom full-dose thrombolytic therapy has proved ineffective. The mortality for emergency pulmonary embolectomy is at least 25%. Removing emboli by suction via a transvenous catheter approach has been used with some success and is an alternative to surgical embolectomy. In contrast to emergency surgery for acute emboli, elective surgery for symptomatic, unresolved, chronic pulmonary emboli in large branches of the pulmonary artery has proved effective and reasonably safe. The procedure to remove chronic emboli—which amounts to an endarterectomy for removing organized thromboemboli—can improve functional status, reduce pulmonary arterial pressure, and normalize pulmonary arterial perfusion and arterial oxygenation.

PROGNOSIS

Most deaths due to pulmonary thromboembolism occur either too quickly for therapy to be given, because a therapeutic level of anticoagulant therapy was not maintained, or because the condition was not recognized. Among patients who do receive adequate anticoagulant therapy promptly, death due to pulmonary embolism occurs in about 2% and recurrent emboli are seen in about 8%. By contrast, if pulmonary embolism goes untreated, death occurs from recurrent thromboembolism within a few weeks of the first episode in about 30% of patients.

Although anticoagulant therapy provides a large therapeutic margin against a fatal outcome from pulmonary thromboembolism, an episode of acute pulmonary embolism carries serious implications. Despite anticoagulant therapy and a low incidence of fatal pulmonary embolism, approximately 25% of the patients in the PIOPED study died within 1 year of other causes, especially cancer, left-sided congestive heart failure, and chronic lung disease. Therefore, long-term survival after pulmonary embolism is strongly associated with comorbid conditions. Because other serious conditions are more likely with advancing age, long-term survival after pulmonary embolism correlates inversely with age.

In patients who die of pulmonary embolism, systemic hypotension is usually present at the onset of the fatal episode, and pulmonary vascular obstruction is usually >75%. Even the presence of hypotension and acute cor pulmonale at the onset of acute pulmonary embolism, however, does not necessarily mean a fatal outcome. Clinical signs of massive embolization can subside quickly, presumably because vascular obstruction decreases as a result of fragmentation or remodeling of the emboli or because pulmonary vasoconstrictive reflexes and mediators dissipate. The presence of pulmonary infarction has no effect on survival.

In <1% of those who survive acute pulmonary thromboembolization, the emboli do not lyse and instead become organized. Organized thromboemboli involving large branches of the pulmonary artery can result in a syndrome of progressive exertional dyspnea, pulmonary hypertension, and cor pulmonale. Importantly,

TABLE 59–7. RECOMMENDATIONS FOR PROPHYLAXIS FOR DEEP VENOUS THROMBOSIS

	Patients	Recommendation
Low risk	Hospitalized medical patients without risk factors (see Table 59–1)	Ambulation, leg exercises
	Surgical patients under age 40, surgery lasting < 30 min, no additional risk factors	Ambulation, leg exercises
Moderate risk	Hospitalized medical patients with ≥ 1 risk factors (see Table 59–1)	Low-dose heparin*
	Surgical patients over age 40 having abdominal or thoracic surgery lasting > 30 min	Low-dose heparin*
	Neurosurgery or other patients with high bleeding risk	Intermittent pneumatic compression of the legs
High risk	Hip fracture	Warfarin†
	Hip replacement	Warfarin† or low molecular weight heparin
	Knee replacement	Warfarin† and intermittent pneumatic compression of the legs
	Open prostatectomy	Intermittent pneumatic compression of the legs
	Gynecologic malignancy	Intermittent pneumatic compression of the legs

* 5000 units subcutaneously every 8–12 hours.
† Low-dose regimen.

not all of the individuals diagnosed with chronic thromboembolic pulmonary hypertension have a history of deep venous thrombosis or acute pulmonary embolism.

PREVENTION

Prophylaxis for deep venous thrombosis reduces the occurrence of pulmonary thromboembolism. A number of mechanical and pharmacologic approaches suitable for varying clinical situations lower, but do not eliminate, the occurrence of deep venous thrombosis (Table 59–7). Low-dose heparin is indicated for hospitalized medical patients who have risk factors for deep venous thrombosis and for surgical patients over age 40 undergoing abdominal or thoracic surgery. Therapy should be started preoperatively. Intermittent pneumatic compression of the calves and/or thighs is a satisfactory alternative for patients in whom bleeding could prove disastrous, such as those who are having eye or neurologic surgery. In patients at high risk for deep venous thrombosis because they are having hip or knee replacement or repair of a hip fracture, anticoagulant therapy with warfarin has a positive effect, but low molecular weight heparin is proving to be more effective. If physicians are to save lives from pulmonary thromboembolism, they must routinely evaluate their patients for the risk for deep venous thrombosis and administer therapy that will reduce the likelihood of this potentially lethal problem.

Carson JL, Kelley MA, Duff A, et al.: The clinical course of pulmonary embolism. N Engl J Med 326:1240, 1992. *A prospective study of mortality and recurrence of pulmonary embolism in 399 patients showed a low rate of recurrence or death from pulmonary embolism among those properly treated.*

Dalen JE, Hirsh J (eds.): Third ACCP Conference on Antithrombotic Therapy. Chest 102:303S, 1992. *Authoritative, practical reviews of anticoagulant therapy.*

Goldhaber SZ, Braunwald E: Pulmonary embolism. *In* Braunwald E (ed.): Heart Disease: A Textbook of Cardiovascular Medicine. 4th ed. Philadelphia, WB Saunders, 1992, p 1558. *A comprehensive, fully referenced review of pulmonary thromboembolism.*

Moser KM, Fedullo PF, LittleJohn JK, et al.: Frequent asymptomatic pulmonary embolism in patients with deep venous thrombosis. JAMA 271:223, 1994. *About one third of patients with deep venous thrombosis have high probability lung scans without pulmonary symptoms.*

Stein PD, Athanasoulis C, Alavi A, et al.: Complications and validity of pulmonary angiography in acute pulmonary embolism. Circulation 85:462, 1992. *This prospective analysis of the complications of pulmonary angiography for diagnosing suspected pulmonary embolism in 1111 patients concludes that the risks from the procedure are low enough to justify its use in the appropriate setting.*

60 FAT EMBOLISM SYNDROME
Robert M. Senior

DEFINITION. Fat embolism syndrome refers to the constellation of clinical manifestations that may develop when fat droplets become impacted in the pulmonary microvasculature and other microvascular beds, especially in the brain. The principal clinical features of fat embolism syndrome are respiratory failure, cerebral dysfunction, and petechiae.

CLINICAL SETTING. Fat embolism syndrome occurs almost exclusively as an early complication of traumatic fractures of the pelvis and of long bones, particularly the shaft of the femur. Delays in stabilization of fractures and periods of systemic hypoperfusion after trauma increase the risk of the syndrome. The syndrome develops in approximately 2 to 25% of people with fresh long bone fractures, depending on criteria for the diagnosis and selection of patients at risk. It seldom follows elective orthopedic surgery on long bones, even though fat droplets can be found routinely in the venous blood draining the operative sites, and recent studies with transesophageal echocardiography indicate that echogenic material commonly appears in the right side of the heart during surgical procedures involving long bones. Other forms of trauma that rarely result in the fat embolism syndrome include massive soft tissue injury, severe burns, and liposuction. Nontraumatic settings occasionally lead to the syndrome. These include conditions associated with fatty liver, prolonged corticosteroid therapy, acute pancreatitis, osteomyelitis, and conditions that cause bone infarcts such as sickle cell hemoglobinopathy.

DIAGNOSIS. The diagnosis of the fat embolism syndrome is made on clinical grounds and is based on the presence of at least one of the following features within the first 72 hours after traumatic fracture: (1) otherwise unexplained dyspnea, tachypnea, arterial hypoxemia, and diffuse alveolar infiltrates on the chest radiograph; (2) otherwise unexplained confusion or other signs of cerebral dysfunction; and (3) petechiae over the upper half of the body, including the axillae, conjunctivae, and oral mucosa. The diagnosis is definite if all three features are present and is further supported by fluffy retinal exudates and hemorrhages and unexplained fever. The diagnosis is unlikely if the signs and symptoms of pulmonary dysfunction begin more than 72 hours after the injury. In these situations, more probable causes of respiratory distress are pulmonary edema from massive fluid replacement, aspiration, sepsis, pneumonia, or venous thromboembolism. No laboratory tests are diagnostic of fat embolism syndrome; however, bronchoalveolar lavage and staining the lavage cells for neutral fat with oil red O may be helpful. Numerous, large intracellular fat droplets have been reported in typical cases of fat embolism syndrome, whereas fat droplets are rare in lavage cells from normal individuals or patients with other causes of respiratory distress.

Microscopic examination for fat globules in blood aspirated from a Swan-Ganz catheter in the pulmonary capillary wedge position is another method that has been used to support a diagnosis of fat embolism syndrome. Looking for fat droplets in peripheral blood and urine is not helpful in making the diagnosis, as droplets may not be present in patients who clearly have the syndrome but may be found after traumatic fractures in patients without evidence of the syndrome.

PATHOGENESIS. The mechanisms leading to the fat embolism syndrome are not fully understood, but it is clear that the syndrome is not simply a consequence of fat droplets mechanically obstructing small blood vessels. An important aspect of the pathogenesis appears to be endothelial injury caused by fatty acids released from impacted fat droplets by lipoprotein lipase, with ensuing increased microvascular permeability and fluid leakage into interstitial spaces.

The fat droplets found in small vessels are from the trauma site. As the first microvascular bed encountered by fat droplets in the venous circulation, the lungs bear the brunt of fat embolization. Presumably, fat emboli in other organs, especially the brain, reach those sites by passing through the pulmonary microvasculature or through right-to-left intracardiac shunts. Recent transesophageal echocardiographic studies during surgical treatment of long bone fractures have shown paradoxical embolization of echogenic material through a patent foramen ovale.

Although the effects of fatty acids upon endothelium appear to be important in the mechanism of lung injury, the pathogenesis of respiratory failure may be more complex in some cases. Other tissue components besides fat may be liberated from fracture sites, and these as well as the injured pulmonary endothelium may activate the clotting, complement, and contact systems. Thus, the pathogenesis of lung injury may be multifactorial, as in other forms of the adult respiratory distress syndrome, involving thrombi, mediators of inflammation, and products of inflammatory cells.

Hypoxemia explains brain dysfunction in some cases, but not all. Cerebral symptoms may reflect direct brain injury, with many fat emboli and associated hemorrhage and necrosis. Moreover, patients with comparable hypoxemia from causes other than fat embolism syndrome seldom have brain dysfunction, and occasional patients with fat embolism syndrome have neurologic features that precede hypoxemia or are disproportionately severe for the degree of hypoxemia.

The reason for petechiae is not known, although some patients may have thrombocytopenia and disseminated intravascular coagulation. There is also no explanation for the striking localization of the petechiae to the pectoral regions and conjunctivae.

THERAPY. Management of fat embolism syndrome is supportive and consists primarily of ensuring good arterial oxygenation. Supplemental oxygen is given to maintain the arterial oxygen tension in the normal range, 75 to 90 mm Hg. If endotracheal intubation and ventilatory support are necessary, positive end-expiratory pressure may reduce the need for high concentrations of inspired oxygen. Restricting fluid intake and even giving diuretics, if systemic perfusion can be maintained, may minimize fluid accumulation in the lungs. The role of corticosteroids is controversial; there is no clear-cut evidence that they are helpful.

In patients with acute long bone fractures, the risk of fat embolism syndrome is reduced by prompt surgical stabilization of the fractures and by correcting or preventing decreased systemic perfusion. Although corticosteroids have not proved to be of benefit once the syndrome is manifest, administering corticosteroids for a short period (for example, 1.5 mg per kilogram of methylprednisolone intravenously at 8 hour intervals for 2 days) seems to prevent development of the syndrome.

PROGNOSIS. The mortality from fat embolism syndrome is $\leq 10\%$ and thus is much lower than the 50% or greater mortality for most causes of the adult respiratory distress syndrome. Even severe respiratory failure is seldom fatal.

Castella X, Vallés J, Cabezuelo MA, et al.: Fat embolism syndrome and pulmonary microvascular cytology. Chest 101:1710, 1992. *Fat globules were found in blood aspirated from a Swan-Ganz catheter in the wedge position in a patient with typical clinical features of the fat embolism syndrome.*

Chastre J, Fagon J-Y, Soler P, et al.: Bronchoalveolar lavage for rapid diagnosis of the fat embolism syndrome in trauma patients. Ann Intern Med 113:583, 1990. *Looking for fat droplets in alveolar macrophages and neutrophils recovered by bronchoalveolar lavage may be helpful in diagnosing the fat embolism syndrome.*

Fabian TC: Unraveling the fat embolism syndrome. N Engl J Med 329:961, 1993. *Concisely reviews the mechanical and biochemical theories of the pathogenesis of the fat embolism syndrome and current methods of diagnosis.*

Kallenbach J, Lewis M, Zaltzman M, et al.: "Low-dose" corticosteroid prophylaxis against fat embolism. J Trauma 27:1173, 1987. *Persuasive evidence for the efficacy of corticosteroids to prevent fat embolism syndrome in young adults with fresh fractures of the long bones of the lower extremities.*

Pell ACH, Hughes D, Keating J, et al.: Brief report: Fulminating fat embolism syndrome caused by paradoxical embolism through a patent foramen ovale. N Engl J Med 329:926, 1993. *Transesophageal echocardiography during intramedullary nailing of a hip fracture demonstrated echogenic material filling the right atrium and right ventricle that was followed by pulmonary hypertension and passage of the intracardiac material through a patent foramen ovale into the left side of the heart.*

61 SARCOIDOSIS
Barry L. Fanburg

DEFINITION

Sarcoidosis, a multisystem granulomatous disease, begins most frequently in people between 20 and 40 years old. The cause is unknown, but alterations in the immune system are clearly involved in its pathogenesis. Organ involvement is usually asymptomatic, and the disease most frequently regresses spontaneously, but it may progress to a more chronic state of fibrosis with severe functional impairment of various organs. No natural animal models of sarcoidosis have been discovered.

EPIDEMIOLOGY AND GENETICS

Sarcoidosis occurs with similar manifestations worldwide, but its incidence differs strikingly, from 0.04 per 100,000 in Spain, for example, to 64 per 100,000 in Sweden. The reported numbers are susceptible to considerable error based upon procedures for evaluation, but large unexplained differences in prevalence clearly exist. The occurrence in blacks has been reported to be more frequent than that in whites. The majority of cases occur during adulthood, but sarcoidosis is also present in the pediatric population.

The disease has been reported to be transmissible in experimental animals, but this work still has not been rigorously tested for confirmation. Sarcoidosis is not contagious in humans.

Familial occurrences have been reported, but no specific patterns of parent-child or sibling relationships have emerged. Sarcoidosis has been reported in twins, with a preponderance of monozygotic over dizygotic twins. The disease seems not to be linked with specific human leukocyte antigen (HLA) types.

IMMUNOLOGY

A postulated schema for the immunopathology of sarcoidosis is presented in Figure 61–1. The macrophage most likely initiates the cellular response of sarcoidosis, possibly in response to some unknown presenting antigen. Recurrence of sarcoidosis in allograft lung transplants suggests an importance of circulating constituents. Various factors released by the macrophage, such as interleukin 1, cause accumulation and proliferation of helper T lymphocytes. Factors secreted by the lymphocytes attract and immobilize other inflammatory cells. In addition, B lymphocytes are stimulated to produce increased amounts of immunoglobulins, and fibroblasts are stimulated to proliferate. As the response becomes less active, the number of T lymphocytes decreases, and suppressor T lymphocytes predominate. Although elevated in bronchoalveolar lavage fluid, CD4+ cells may have limited importance in sarcoidosis because it is now known that sarcoidosis and HIV infection may coexist.

As a result of these various immunologic interactions, (1) inflammatory cells proliferate in the affected organ (forming the granuloma), (2) cutaneous delayed hypersensitivity responses to common antigens are depressed, and (3) immune globulins are synthesized and circulate in excess. In addition, circulating antibodies to common environmental antigens and immune complexes may be present.

Intradermally injected extracts of homogenized tissue of involved organs from patients with sarcoidosis can produce a delayed inflammatory reaction in patients with sarcoidosis. This antigen that causes the so-called *Kveim-Siltzbach reaction* has not been purified, and the basis for its response has not been defined. The reaction differs from a cutaneous delayed hypersensitivity reaction in that it takes 4 to 6 weeks to develop and then persists for several months.

CLINICAL PRESENTATION

Sarcoid lesions may develop in almost any organ system, so the clinical presentation is quite varied (Fig. 61–2). In fact, "silent" granulomas are frequently present in multiple organs. Most characteristically, the patient is asymptomatic, but the disease is detected by an abnormal chest radiograph, usually showing bilateral symmetric hilar adenopathy often associated with paratracheal adenopathy (Fig. 61–3) and/or reticulonodular parenchymal infiltrates. Pa-

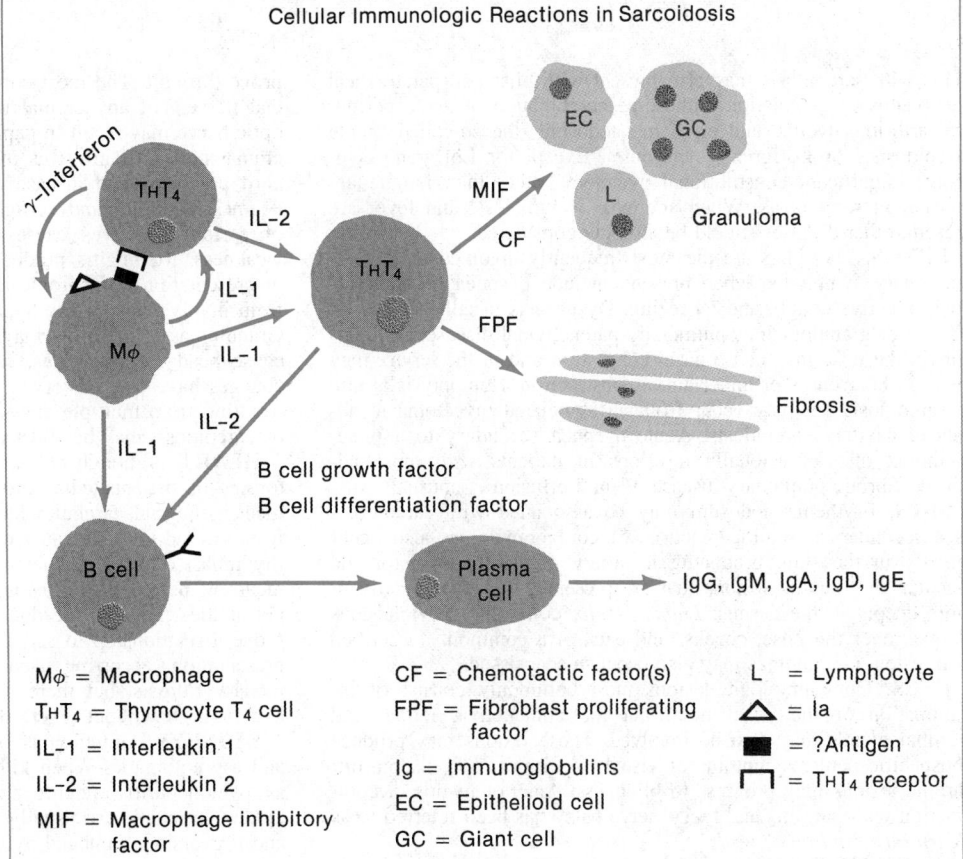

FIGURE 61–1. Immunologic abnormalities associated with sarcoidosis.

Cellular Immunologic Reactions in Sarcoidosis

Mφ = Macrophage
THT4 = Thymocyte T4 cell
IL-1 = Interleukin 1
IL-2 = Interleukin 2
MIF = Macrophage inhibitory factor

CF = Chemotactic factor(s)
FPF = Fibroblast proliferating factor
Ig = Immunoglobulins
EC = Epithelioid cell
GC = Giant cell

L = Lymphocyte
= Ia
= ?Antigen
= THT4 receptor

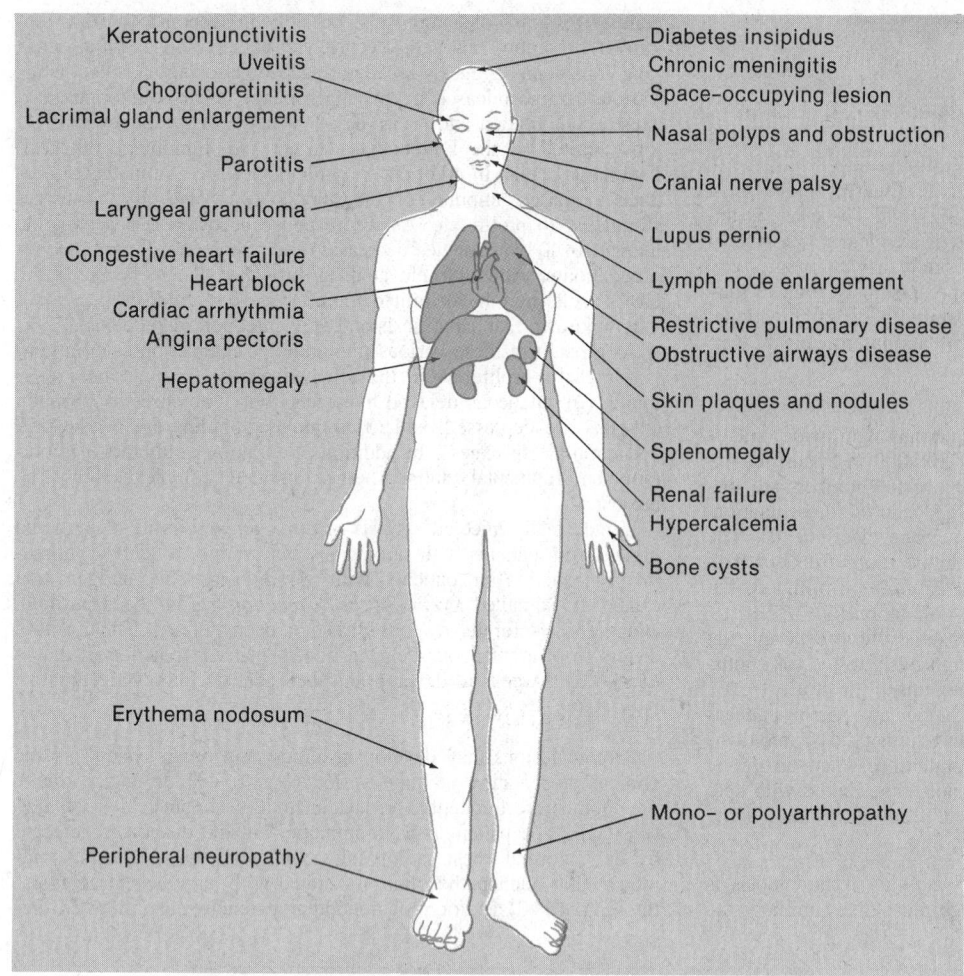

Keratoconjunctivitis
Uveitis
Choroidoretinitis
Lacrimal gland enlargement

Parotitis

Laryngeal granuloma

Congestive heart failure
Heart block
Cardiac arrhythmia
Angina pectoris

Hepatomegaly

Diabetes insipidus
Chronic meningitis
Space-occupying lesion

Nasal polyps and obstruction

Cranial nerve palsy

Lupus pernio

Lymph node enlargement

Restrictive pulmonary disease
Obstructive airways disease

Skin plaques and nodules

Splenomegaly

Renal failure
Hypercalcemia

Bone cysts

Erythema nodosum

Mono- or polyarthropathy

Peripheral neuropathy

FIGURE 61-2. Organ abnormalities associated with sarcoidosis.

tients with sarcoidosis may also present with hilar and paratracheal adenopathy in association with some combination of acute peripheral arthritis, uveitis, and erythema nodosum (the so-called "acute sarcoidosis," or Löffgren's syndrome). Except for Löffgren's syndrome, significant constitutional symptoms other than fatigue are unusual in sarcoidosis. When anorexia, weight loss, and fever are present, other diseases should be strongly considered.

LUNGS. The lungs are the most frequently involved organ, and pulmonary symptoms, when present, include dyspnea on exertion, nonproductive cough, and wheezing. Dyspnea is usually caused by fibrotic or granulomatous pulmonary parenchymal disease. Granulomas in the nose may cause nasal congestion and in the larynx may result in hoarseness or upper airway obstruction. Hemoptysis is rare in sarcoidosis but may occur from an associated mycetoma in advanced cavitary sarcoidosis. Acute dyspnea secondary to a pneumothorax also occasionally develops in patients with more advanced fibrotic pulmonary disease. Pleural effusion is unusual.

SKIN. Erythema nodosum may be associated with sarcoidosis as a secondary vasculitic reaction. Sarcoid granulomas also occur directly in the skin, producing a variety of small, asymptomatic macular and papular lesions that are present either superficially or more deeply in the dermis. *Lupus pernio,* consisting of violaceous plaques over the nose, cheeks, and ears, is a commonly described skin lesion. Granulomas may also occur in scar tissue.

EYES. Ophthalmologic lesions most commonly consist of inflammation of the uveal tract, but the conjunctiva, retina, and lacrimal glands may also be involved. These lesions may produce nonspecific ocular symptoms of visual impairment and discomfort; chronic lesions may progress to blindness. Anterior uveitis in combination with parotitis and facial nerve palsy has been referred to as *Heerfordt's syndrome.*

NERVOUS SYSTEM. Almost any portion of the neurologic system may be affected by sarcoidosis, and the diagnosis may prove difficult. The most common cranial nerve involved is the facial nerve, but any cranial nerve may be affected. Disease of the optic nerve may result in papilledema. Palsies of the ninth and tenth cranial nerves manifest as dysphagia, absent gag reflex, and vocal cord paralysis, and disease of the eighth cranial nerve occurs as deafness, tinnitus, and vertigo. Mononeuropathy or polyneuropathy of peripheral nerves causes sensory loss, paresthesias, or motor weakness. Meningitis produced by sarcoidosis is usually insidious in presentation and chronic in its course. Diabetes insipidus results from involvement of the hypothalamus or posterior pituitary gland. Granulomas of the brain may produce a space-occupying lesion and cause headaches, seizures, or focal symptoms. Rarely, personality changes have been observed, and the total constellation of findings resulting from multiple areas of involvement of the nervous system by sarcoidosis may bewilder the diagnostician.

HEART. Although cardiac granulomas are often present on autopsies of patients with sarcoidosis, symptomatic cardiac involvement is unusual. Granulomatous or fibrotic cardiac lesions resulting from sarcoidosis may cause congestive heart failure, heart block, arrhythmias (often ventricular), angina pectoris, ventricular aneurysm, recurrent pericardial effusion, or sudden death. Because these abnormalities may also be due to other causes, it may be difficult to prove a relationship to sarcoidosis. Cor pulmonale is an infrequent presentation, occurring usually in association with advanced pulmonary fibrosis, but there has been the rare report of pulmonary hypertension without severe restrictive lung disease.

KIDNEYS. Granulomas of the kidneys are usually infrequent and asymptomatic. When kidney failure occurs, other lesions such as pyelonephritis, nephrocalcinosis, and hyalinization of various kidney structures are usually present. The kidneys may be severely and irreversibly damaged by calcium nephropathy caused by altered calcium metabolism that produces hypercalcemia and hypercalciuria. Symptoms of kidney failure may be the predominant feature

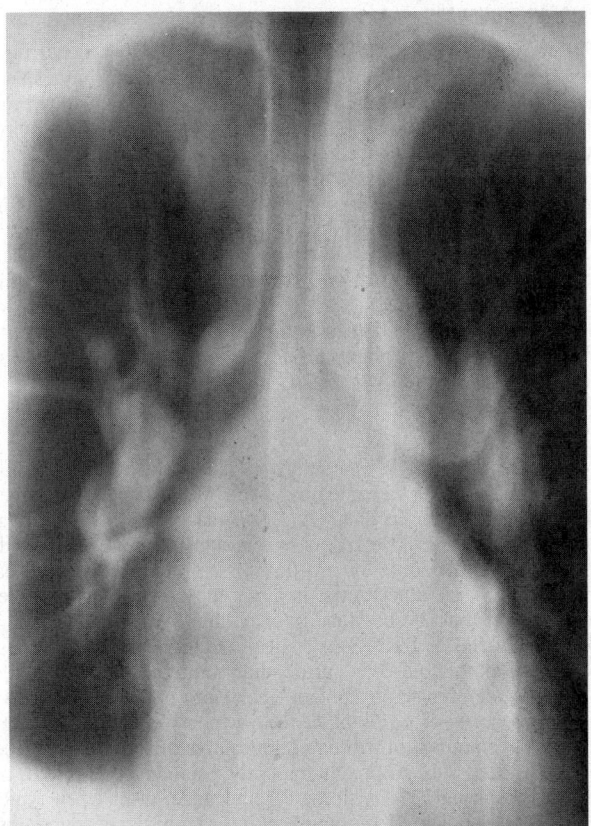

FIGURE 61–3. Tomogram of chest showing hilar and paratracheal adenopathy. (From Murray JF, Nadel J: Textbook of Respiratory Medicine. 2nd ed. Philadelphia, WB Saunders, 1994.)

of sarcoidosis in these cases. Sarcoid lesions can enzymatically activate vitamin D precursors to 1,25-dihydroxycholecalciferol, thereby increasing intestinal absorption of calcium. The result may be hypercalcemia and hypercalciuria, with renal damage from nephrocalcinosis and recurrent nephrolithiasis.

MUSCULOSKELETAL SYSTEM. Bones, joints, and muscles are frequently involved in sarcoidosis. Bone changes are found most often in chronic cases and are particularly common in blacks with chronic skin disease. The phalanges, metacarpals, and metatarsals are the bones most frequently involved. Osteoporosis, cystic or reticulated changes, and external manifestations of digital deformation and dystrophic nails may be present. Joints are usually spared destructive changes except in the vicinity of bone lesions.

Arthritic changes may also manifest acutely by monoarthralgias or polyarthralgias or arthritis of the larger joints, such as the ankles, knees, wrists, or elbows. The associated symptoms may be migratory and usually recede with no residual deformities. Although, like the liver, muscles frequently contain asymptomatic granulomas, acute myositis and chronic myopathy with associated muscular enzyme abnormalities are uncommon findings in sarcoidosis. Gout may complicate sarcoidosis, presumably owing to overproduction of purines in widespread granulomas.

MISCELLANEOUS. Although diffuse granulomas may be present, clinical manifestations of liver, gastrointestinal, or pancreatic disease are very unusual. Similarly, clinical evidence for involvement of the endocrine and reproductive systems is rare. As noted earlier, posterior pituitary and hypothalamic involvement may result in diabetes insipidus. Hypopituitarism from anterior pituitary disease occurs very rarely. Sarcoidosis of the genital tract is very uncommon. Alteration in fertility by sarcoidosis has not been described. Peripheral lymph nodes, in contrast to hilar nodes, are seldom more than moderately enlarged and usually go unnoticed by the patient; rarely, peripheral nodes may be grossly enlarged. Although the spleen is moderately enlarged in 5 to 10% of patients, gross enlargement that causes discomfort and predisposes to rupture occurs rarely. Thrombocytopenia is occasionally present and may be associated with hypersplenism. Hypercalcemia may produce nonspecific anorexia and vomiting.

PHYSICAL FINDINGS

Physical findings in the chest are usually normal despite radiographic abnormalities that may be extensive. Fever is absent, except with Löffgren's syndrome. Other physical findings usually relate to granulomatous or fibrotic involvement of a specific organ system. Skin lesions may be readily apparent or found only with careful examination. Subcutaneous or muscle nodules may be identified. Slit-lamp examination may be necessary to demonstrate ocular lesions. Lymph nodes are often palpable but usually only moderately enlarged. As noted above, hepatosplenomegaly may be present. Digits may be deformed by bone lesions, and the nails may be dystrophic in cases of chronic disease. Acute arthritic changes may be apparent, in particular in association with erythema nodosum, and must be differentiated from associated gout.

ROUTINE LABORATORY STUDIES

Routine laboratory evaluation may reveal lymphopenia, hyperglobulinemia, hypercalcemia, and/or hypercalciuria. The platelet count is rarely decreased. It is unusual for the sedimentation rate to be significantly elevated, except with Löffgren's syndrome. Liver function tests may be moderately abnormal, and, in particular, alkaline phosphatase levels may be elevated. With complications of the disease, the expected but nonspecific changes in arterial blood gases and serum chemistries accompany respiratory or renal failure, respectively. Cerebrospinal fluid examination may show nonspecific pleocytosis and increased protein in meningitis caused by sarcoidosis.

DIFFERENTIAL DIAGNOSIS

The differential diagnosis of sarcoidosis depends largely upon the clinical presentation of the patient. With hilar lymphadenopathy, lymphoma is most frequently considered; with pulmonary parenchymal disease, a wide variety of diffuse interstitial diseases must be considered (see Ch. 55). Tuberculosis and other granulomatous pulmonary infections must always be ruled out. Eosinophilic granuloma is another diagnostic possibility, particularly when diabetes insipidus is present. Exposure to beryllium may produce disease very similar to sarcoidosis. Pulmonary sarcoid nodules raise the possibility of primary or metastatic tumor. Similarly, sarcoid nodules in the breast or brain may be thought to be tumor. Conglomerate lesions with hilar retraction or eggshell calcification of lymph nodes may be confused with silicosis. Sarcoidosis presenting with airways obstruction may be confused with asthma. Hypercalcemia in sarcoidosis raises the question of a number of metabolic or malignant disorders, especially primary hyperparathyroidism (see Ch. 214). Arthritis or arthralgia associated with sarcoidosis may be confused with acute rheumatic fever or gout. The isolated finding of granulomas on biopsy of various tissues raises the possibilities of foreign body reactions, fungal or tubercular infections, and malignancy associated with granulomatous reactions. Granulomas occurring only in the liver may result in confusion between granulomatous hepatitis and sarcoidosis. Granulomas present in the intestinal wall may suggest Crohn's disease. Finally, renal and hepatic impairment or cardiac abnormalities occurring in sarcoidosis may be caused by more common coexisting diseases rather than by sarcoidosis itself.

RADIOLOGIC EVALUATION

Radiologic evaluation of the chest is particularly useful in sarcoidosis because the disease is so often asymptomatic and so often involves the thorax. Radiologic abnormalities that occur in sarcoidosis have been arbitrarily classified as follows: grade 0—absence of abnormal radiographic findings; grade 1—lymph node enlargement without pulmonary parenchymal abnormalities; grade 2A—combination of lymph node and diffuse pulmonary parenchymal disease; grade 2B—diffuse parenchymal disease without lymph node enlargement; and grade 3—radiographic changes indicating more chronic disease with pulmonary fibrosis ("honeycombing" or hilar retraction). The most frequent parenchymal abnormality is reticulonodularity, consisting of fine linear densities and small, irregular nodules measuring 3 to 5 mm in diameter (Fig. 61–4). Large, conglomerate lesions may be present in association with hilar retraction (Fig. 61–5). Parenchymal infiltrates are at times "fluffy" and have an alveolar pattern. Single or multiple large nod-

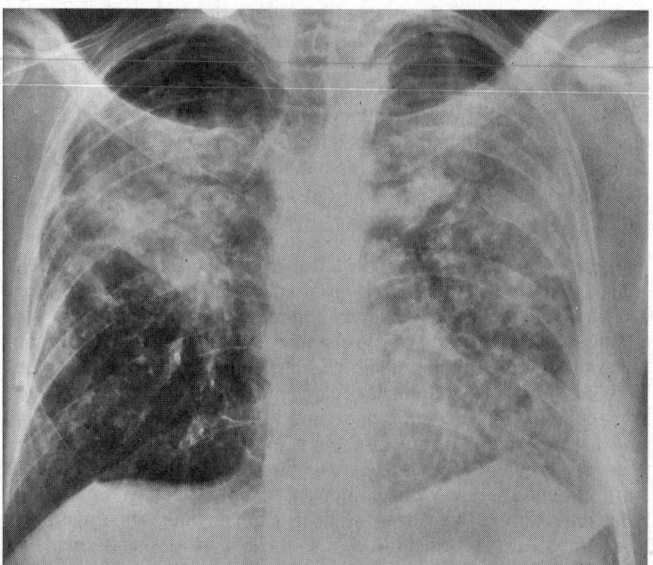

FIGURE 61-4. Chest radiograph showing typical reticulonodular appearance of parenchymal sarcoidosis. (From Murray JF, Nadel J: Textbook of Respiratory Medicine. 2nd ed. Philadelphia, WB Saunders, 1994.)

ules may occur and may be confused with tumor. Small nodules may cause a miliary pattern suggestive of tuberculosis.

A large variety of other changes may be present on the radiograph. Pleural effusion occurs rarely in sarcoidosis. Mediastinal or hilar lymph nodes may show eggshell calcification. In addition to bullous changes, true cavities may be present that, at times, contain mycetomas. Lobar atelectasis may be caused by intrabronchial granulomas, and postobstructive bronchiectasis may be present. In addition to the more common locations in the short tubular bones of the hands and feet, lytic or sclerotic bone lesions may occur in the ribs.

Computed tomographic (CT) scans can demonstrate lymphadenopathy more clearly and, in particular, can detect anterior mediastinal and subcarinal lymph nodes that have gone undetected on conventional films of the chest (Fig. 61–6). Intra-abdominal nodes may be noted serendipitously. CT examination, however, is needed in only a limited number of patients with sarcoidosis. Magnetic resonance imaging has been useful for detecting CNS sarcoidosis.

PHYSIOLOGIC CHANGES

The most common pulmonary physiologic changes occurring in sarcoidosis are decreases in vital capacity and diffusing capacity. Although useful in determining the extent of functional impairment at the onset and in following the course of the disease, physiologic changes do not correlate well with symptoms or radiologic abnormalities. At times pulmonary function studies are totally normal despite radiologic evidence of pulmonary disease. Conversely, functional abnormalities, especially of diffusing capacity, may be present when the lung parenchyma appears normal radiographically. Evidence of airway obstruction may also be present, and, at times, this is the predominant feature of sarcoidosis, confusing it with asthma. An elevation in arterial P_{CO_2} is unusual, but moderate arterial hypoxemia may be present. As with other interstitial diseases, arterial hypoxemia often worsens with exercise.

APPROACH TO DIAGNOSIS

With a very typical presentation (i.e., bilateral symmetric hilar and paratracheal lymphadenopathy in an asymptomatic patient 20 to 40 years of age or in one with erythema nodosum, uveitis, and arthralgias), the clinical diagnosis of sarcoidosis can be made with a high degree of certainty by physicians familiar with this disease (Table 61–1). In all other cases in which the diagnosis is less clear, further support must be obtained by examining biopsy material.

DIAGNOSIS BY BIOPSY. Typical sarcoid granulomas consist of whorls of epithelioid cells surrounding multinucleated giant cells, which may or may not contain inclusion bodies (Fig. 61–7). Mononuclear cells are present at the periphery of the granulomas, and various amounts of fibrosis and/or hyalinization are present throughout the tissue. Although some necrosis may be present, true caseation is unusual. The histologic appearance, even when typical, is always nonspecific. To strengthen the diagnosis of sarcoidosis, infectious agents and foreign bodies must be excluded by special stains, cultures, and examination under polarized light.

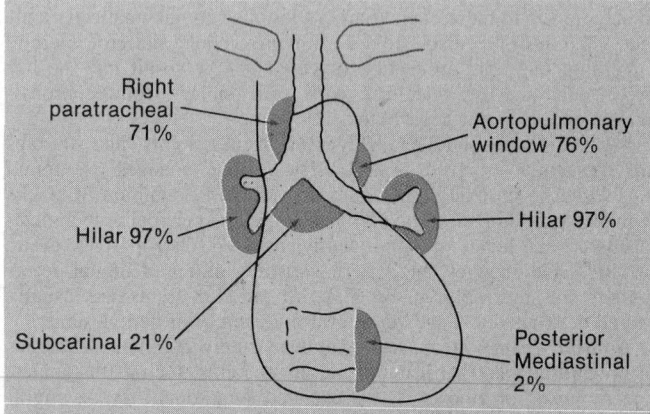

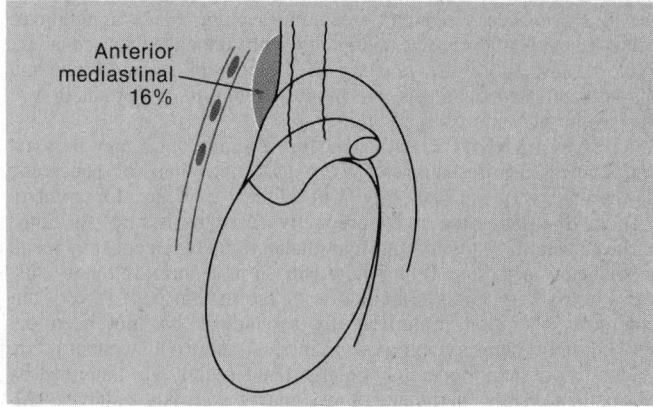

FIGURE 61-6. Schematic representation of CT detection of thoracic lymphadenopathy in sarcoidosis. (Reprinted from Rodan BA, Putman CE: Radiologic alterations in sarcoidosis. In Fanburg BL [ed.]: Sarcoidosis and Other Granulomatous Diseases of the Lung. New York, Marcel Dekker, 1983. By courtesy of Marcel Dekker, Inc.)

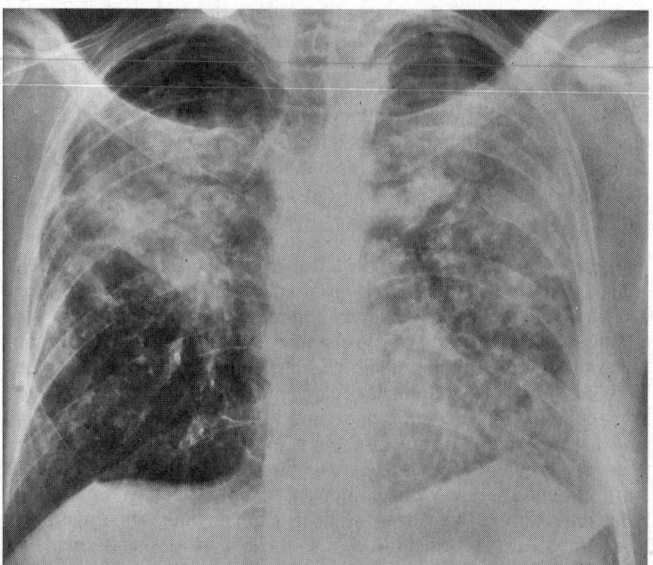

FIGURE 61-5. Chest radiograph showing large conglomerate lesions associated with hilar retraction. (From Murray JF, Nadel J: Textbook of Respiratory Medicine. 2nd ed. Philadelphia, WB Saunders, 1994.)

TABLE 61–1. FEATURES CONSIDERED IN THE DIAGNOSIS OF SARCOIDOSIS

Primary
1. Clinical and radiologic presentation
2. Biopsy material showing granuloma, but no mycobacteria, fungi, or refractile material

Secondary
1. Anergy to skin tests
2. Positive Kveim-Siltzbach reaction (infrequently performed)
3. Significant elevation of serum angiotensin I-12 converting enzyme with exclusion of other obvious diseases associated with elevation (e.g., Gaucher's disease, leprosy)

Current Research Modalities
1. Evaluation of cells obtained by bronchial lavage
2. Gallium–67 scanning

What tissue should be examined by biopsy? In the absence of specific skin lesions, transbronchial biopsy of the lung is usually most specific because rarely, if ever, are nonspecific granulomas found (in contrast to liver or lymph nodes). Approximately 60% of patients with sarcoidosis show granulomas on transbronchial lung biopsy even if their chest radiographs are normal; this number increases to 90 to 95% when there is a parenchymal abnormality on chest radiograph. If the transbronchial biopsy yields negative findings but a high suspicion of sarcoidosis exists and there is obvious parenchymal disease on the chest radiograph, a repeat transbronchial biopsy may be justified. Other reasonable approaches at this time include mediastinoscopy or, at times, open lung biopsy.

Blind conjunctival, lacrimal gland, or gingival biopsies are frequently not rewarding in the absence of overt disease at these locations. When these tissues are involved, however, the yield is high. Biopsies of skin lesions are particularly useful because they may show granuloma and, in association with other findings, may provide an easy diagnosis if foreign body granuloma can be excluded. Biopsy of identifiable subcutaneous or muscle lesions may also be diagnostic. Biopsy of lesions of erythema nodosum shows a nonspecific panniculitis or vasculitis and therefore is not diagnostic. Other localized lesions, such as those of the pharynx or larynx, re-

quire direct biopsy for diagnosis. Diagnosis by biopsy sometimes becomes problematic for neurologic disease caused by sarcoidosis when other tissues do not provide a positive diagnosis because the involved tissue is often not easily accessible.

OTHER AVAILABLE TESTS. The Kveim-Siltzbach test is not precise and the required antigen is not readily available. It is therefore rarely used. Anergy to delayed hypersensitivity skin test antigens is a frequent finding but is obviously not diagnostic of sarcoidosis. Similarly, characterization of cells obtained by bronchial lavage and the use of gallium–67 scanning of the lungs are not in themselves diagnostic of sarcoidosis, although abnormalities consistent with that diagnosis may be found. For this reason, and because of cost and radiation exposure, these last two tests are not routinely justified currently for diagnosis in clinical practice. However, gallium–67 scanning may be useful in detecting unsuspected organ involvement by sarcoidosis, such as that of parotid glands. This observation may support the diagnosis.

Serum angiotensin I–converting enzyme activity is often elevated in sarcoidosis, but a number of other diseases may be similarly associated with its increased activity (e.g., miliary tuberculosis, leprosy, Gaucher's disease). If these diseases can be readily excluded, measurement of this enzyme may be useful. This is the case when the primary diagnostic considerations are lymphoma and sarcoidosis because angiotensin I–converting enzyme activity is not increased in lymphoma. Elevations of other proteolytic enzymes in serum, such as lysozyme and thermolysin-like metalloendopeptidase, have been evaluated but are not yet commonly used for diagnostic purposes.

ACTIVITY OF DISEASE

Sarcoidosis may remit spontaneously; the concept of "activity of disease" is therefore useful when considering therapeutic strategies (Table 61–2). Activity of disease is very difficult to define because occult granulomatous lesions may exist throughout many tissues of the body. Clinical findings provide some indication of activity of disease, but often in a nonquantitative and imprecise way, especially when the patient is relatively asymptomatic. Changes in radiologic and pulmonary function study may also help assess activity of disease. Bronchoalveolar lavage to measure the percentage of lymphocytes as a reflection of parenchymal inflammation has been advocated. A high percentage of lymphocytes has been referred to as high-intensity alveolitis, denoting a poorer prognosis, but this approach has not gained wide acceptance. Gallium–67 scanning of the lung, which is also thought to reflect inflammation, has been proposed to indirectly monitor the intensity of alveolitis; the utility of this assessment of disease activity, similar to that of bronchoalveolar lavage, needs to be determined by more extensive prospective testing. Because elevated activity of serum angiotensin I–converting enzyme in sarcoidosis may be derived from epithelioid cells or granulomas, it has been suggested, without convincing evidence, that serum levels of this enzyme may reflect the granuloma "load" of the body. On the basis of this premise, its measurement is sometimes used to follow disease activity, but its validity for this purpose has not been fully verified.

THERAPY

Many patients with sarcoidosis show spontaneous total remission in a period up to 3 years. As many as 80 to 90% of those with hilar and mediastinal lymphadenopathy or Löffgren's syndrome alone may have remission; fewer patients with parenchymal involvement experience remission spontaneously. Other patients show arrest of the disease with moderate fibrosis, and a small percentage of patients develop progressive fibrosis and organ impairment. Once the

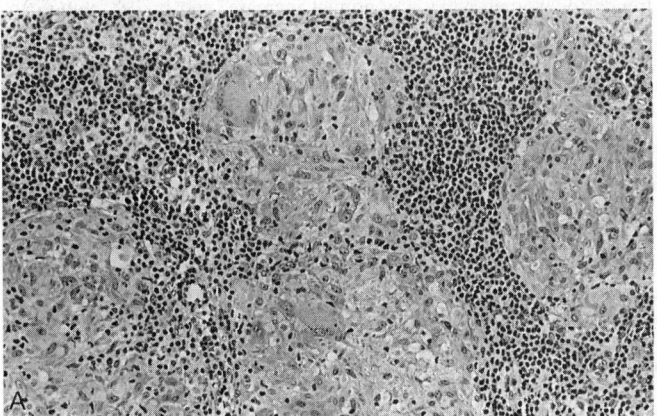

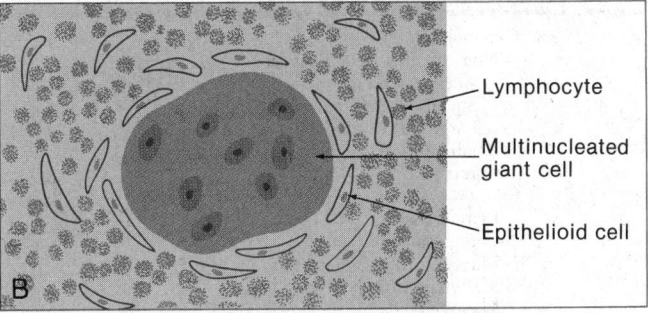

FIGURE 61–7. Typical histologic appearance of the granuloma of sarcoidosis with accompanying schematic representation.

TABLE 61–2. INDICATORS OF "ACTIVITY" OF SARCOIDOSIS

1. Clinical features present
2. Symptoms worse
3. Pulmonary function tests/chest radiograph worse
4. Elevated serum calcium level
5. Elevated serum angiotensin I–converting enzyme level
6. Positive gallium scan
7. Evidence of alveolitis on bronchial lavage

disease remits spontaneously, only rarely does it recur. Treatment with corticosteroids causes granulomas to regress but does not appear to affect the natural course of the disease because granulomas may recur if therapy is stopped. Because the disease may remit spontaneously and steroids may cause significant side effects, treatment is usually started only if the function of a vital organ (lungs, kidneys, eyes, heart, or CNS) seems to be interfered with or hypercalcemia is present. All patients with sarcoidosis should be followed carefully so that therapy can be started as soon as deterioration of organ function has been detected.

Prednisone is usually the drug of choice to treat sarcoidosis. The usual starting dosage is 30 to 40 mg per day, but at times a schedule of 50 to 60 mg every other day is used for initial therapy. A response in terms of symptoms or radiologic findings should be seen within 2 to 4 weeks. The steroid dose should be tapered after several weeks, and the eventual maintenance dose should be the lowest one that is effective in maintaining the response that is being followed (see below). Often 10 to 15 mg of prednisone every other day, a dosage that has a low risk of side effects, suffices. Attempts to stop therapy may be tried after several months, but evidence of disease activity (symptoms, chest radiographic abnormalities, or worsening of pulmonary function) may recur, and prednisone may have to be restarted.

What are the best parameters to follow as indicators of disease activity? Measurements of disease activity are imprecise. Certainly, clinical symptoms should be assessed carefully, and chest radiographic and pulmonary function changes often give indication of disease activity. However, both radiographic abnormalities and pulmonary function changes correlate poorly with clinical parameters. Serum angiotensin I–converting enzyme levels are easily obtained and may provide clues to activity, but tests such as bronchial lavage and gallium–67 scanning are still largely experimental. Failure of response may indicate irreversible fibrosis, in which case steroid therapy causes more potential risk than benefit. In advanced cases lung transplantation may be considered.

All of the usual side effects associated with steroid therapy may occur in patients treated for sarcoidosis (see Ch. 18). The dose can usually be reduced sufficiently, however, so that infection with opportunistic organisms occurs rarely. Cosmetic problems of weight gain and fluid accumulation are often the most bothersome side effects. However, these can be controlled for many patients by care with dietary intake. More difficult decisions about steroid therapy arise when there are associated disorders, such as diabetes mellitus, that may be exacerbated by these agents. Because tuberculin skin tests become positive in patients with sarcoidosis who contract tuberculosis, appropriate prophylaxis or treatment should be given when the tuberculin skin test is positive or converts to positivity.

Topical steroids have been used for dermatologic and ophthalmologic lesions, and chloroquine and methotrexate have been used for sarcoidosis of the skin. Anecdotal effectiveness of immunotherapy has been reported. Indomethacin and other nonsteroidal anti-inflammatory agents may be useful for arthritis occurring in Löffgren's syndrome. Aerosolized steroids approved for use in the United States have not been effective for pulmonary sarcoidosis, but other aerosolized preparations are being tried in Europe. Sarcoidosis that manifests with bronchoconstriction does not respond well to conventional bronchodilator therapy other than steroids. It remains to be determined whether avoidance of sunlight significantly influences calcium metabolism in sarcoidosis. Dietary calcium restriction may be considered when hypercalcemia is present.

Bascom R, Johns CJ: The natural history and management of sarcoidosis. Adv Intern Med 31:213, 1986. *This is an excellent general review of this controversial area, with 138 references.*

Fanburg BL: Sarcoidosis and Other Granulomatous Diseases of the Lung. New York, Marcel Dekker, 1983. *A comprehensive textbook covering both clinical and experimental aspects of sarcoidosis.*

James DG, Williams WJ: Sarcoidosis and Other Granulomatous Disorders. Philadelphia, WB Saunders, 1982. *Another good monograph with an extensive review of all phase of sarcoidosis. Excellent clinical descriptions and comprehensive references.*

Lowery WS, Whitlock WL, Dietrich RA, Fine JM: Sarcoidosis complicated by HIV infection: Three case reports and a review of the literature. Am Rev Respir Dis 142:887, 1990. *Addresses sarcoidosis in the AIDS patient.*

Rockoff SD, Ronatagi PK: Unusual manifestations of thoracic sarcoidosis. Am J Radiol 144:513, 1985. *A comprehensive coverage of radiologic features of sarcoidosis.*

Sharma OP, Maheshwari A, Tharer K: Myocardial sarcoidosis. Chest 103:253, 1993. *An update of sarcoidosis of the heart.*

Thomas PD, Hunninghake GW: Current concepts of the pathogenesis of sarcoidosis. Am Rev Respir Dis 135:747, 1987. *A review with emphasis on immunologic features in sarcoidosis.*

Venet A, Hance AJ, Saltini C, et al.: Enhanced alveolar macrophage-mediated antigen-induced T-lymphocyte proliferation in sarcoidosis. J Clin Invest 75:293, 1985. *Further information about immunologic abnormalities in sarcoidosis.*

62 PULMONARY NEOPLASMS
York E. Miller

DEFINITION

Lung cancer is the leading cause of cancer death in both men and women in the United States. More than 99% of malignant lung tumors arise from the respiratory epithelium and are termed bronchogenic carcinomas. For practical purposes, bronchogenic carcinomas can be divided into two subgroups: small cell lung cancer (SCLC) and non–small cell lung cancer (NSCLC), which includes the subtypes adenocarcinoma, squamous cell carcinoma, and large cell carcinoma (Table 62–1). A correct tissue diagnosis is crucial, because SCLC has a high response rate to chemotherapy and radiation and is appropriately treated by surgery only in rare situations. On the other hand, NSCLC can be cured by surgery in certain stages and is not highly responsive to chemotherapy. The overall 5-year survival rate for lung cancer is a disappointing 13%. Smoking is the major risk factor for developing lung cancer (see Ch. 9.4 and 157).

INCIDENCE AND PREVALENCE

In the first decade of the twentieth century lung cancer was a rare disorder. In 1993, there were approximately 170,000 new cases of lung cancer in the United States, with approximately 150,000 deaths. Lung cancer is now the most common cause of cancer death for both genders and accounts for 28% of the overall cancer death rate. In terms of both cancer deaths and years of life lost, the effect of lung cancer is greater than that of breast, prostate, colon, and rectal cancer combined. Lung cancer incidence for middle-aged white men recently peaked and is now declining slightly. However, trends for women show a continual increase, and in 1987 lung cancer surpassed breast cancer as the leading cause of cancer deaths in women. On a worldwide basis, lung cancer will continue to be a major problem into the twenty-first century, owing to introducing tobacco smoking and exporting tobacco products to underdeveloped countries.

EPIDEMIOLOGY

Modifiable Risk Factors

TOBACCO PRODUCTS. Tobacco smoke causes approximately 87% of cases in men and 85% in women. There is a dose-dependence relationship between both duration and intensity of smoking and mortality from lung cancer. SCLC has the strongest association

TABLE 62–1. MALIGNANT PULMONARY NEOPLASMS

	Incidence
Common (99%)	
Non–small cell lung cancer	~75%
Adenocarcinoma	~35%
Squamous cell carcinoma	~30%
Large call carcinoma	~10%
Small cell lung cancer	~20%
Carcinoids	~5%
Rare (<1%)	
Lymphoma	
Carcinosarcoma	
Mucoepidermoid carcinoma	
Malignant fibrous histiocytoma	
Melanoma	
Sarcoma	
Blastoma	

with smoking, with attributable fractions of 97% and 91% for men and women, respectively. Overall, one in nine smokers develops lung cancer. Smoking cessation causes a gradual drop in lung cancer over a number of years, with a decrease to a risk ratio of approximately 1.5 after 10 to 15 years of abstention. Excellent laboratory evidence ties cigarette smoking to lung cancer. Cigarette smoke contains a number of active carcinogens and procarcinogens. Furthermore, the pattern of mutations (transversions versus transitions) seen in oncogenes and tumor suppressor genes isolated from smokers with lung cancer is that expected from the mechanism of action of the major cigarette smoke carcinogens (see Ch. 156).

PASSIVE SMOKE EXPOSURE. The Environmental Protection Agency has classified passive smoke exposure as carcinogenic. In support of this association, increased levels of carcinogens are measurable in the blood of passive smokers. A number of studies have shown increased risk for lung cancer in the spouses of smokers. The tobacco smoke exposure of a smoker's child is greater than that of a spouse. Exposure to 25 smoker years in childhood approximately doubles the risk of lung cancer in a nonsmoker.

OCCUPATIONAL AND OTHER EXPOSURES (see Ch. 54.1). Asbestos is an important environmental carcinogen. In addition to its association with mesothelioma, asbestos exposure also increases the risk for all histologic subtypes of lung cancer. The relative risk of a nonsmoking asbestos worker is approximately five. The effect of smoking and asbestos exposure is synergistic, with a risk ratio of between 50 and 100. Common sources of asbestos exposure include the shipbuilding industry, nautical engine rooms, automotive (particularly brake lining) work, painting, and the construction industry. Exposures that may seem trivial can be significant; for example, cases of mesothelioma have been reported in the spouses and children of asbestos workers who brought their work clothes home to be washed. Exposure to asbestos fibers is now closely regulated. Because risk of asbestos exposure and smoking is synergistic, the most important intervention in an individual with both exposures is to stop smoking.

The association between ionizing radiation (see Ch. 13.1) and lung cancer was made in classic studies of uranium miners exposed to radon daughters. Other miners in areas of significant subterranean radioactivity can also be exposed. Recently, it has been appreciated that some home environments have significant levels of radon. Modern insulation practices lead to increased radon levels. It is estimated that between 5000 and 15,000 excess lung cancer deaths, mostly in smokers, are caused annually in the United States by radon. As with asbestos and smoking, the risks of ionizing radiation exposure and smoking are synergistic. A variety of other environmental or occupational lung carcinogens have been identified, including arsenic, chromium, chloromethyl ethers, mustard gas, nickel, polycyclic hydrocarbons, vinyl chloride, and certain manmade fibers (see Ch. 13.3).

AIR POLLUTION. Air pollution is associated with a variety of respiratory disorders and has long been suspected as a possible pulmonary carcinogen. A number of studies demonstrate an increased incidence of lung cancer in urban versus rural environments, but other factors could also explain these differences.

CHRONIC OBSTRUCTIVE PULMONARY DISEASE. The presence of chronic obstructive pulmonary disease (COPD), either airflow obstruction on pulmonary function testing or symptoms of chronic bronchitis, increases the risk of lung cancer several-fold. COPD is a risk factor by itself and is not just a reflection of the number of cigarettes smoked.

DIET (see Ch. 9.2). Epidemiologic studies demonstrate increased risk for lung cancer in individuals with a diet low in β-carotene and vitamin A. Vitamin A and its derivatives have potent effects on the differentiation of the respiratory epithelium. Animal studies demonstrate that rodents fed a diet deficient in vitamin A develop dysplastic changes in their airways. Finally, 13-*cis*-retinoic acid has recently been shown to be an effective chemopreventive agent in aerodigestive cancers. In addition to vitamin A, β-carotene, and related compounds, additional micronutrients, including selenium, and vitamins C and E may have protective effects.

Nonmodifiable Risk Factors

GENDER AND RACIAL DIFFERENCES. There is currently a male predominance in lung cancer incidence and mortality in the United States. The incidence rates for women are rising rapidly, however, while those for middle-aged men are reaching a plateau. The largest factor in gender differences in incidence of lung cancer is differences in cigarette smoking habits. There is no agreement as to whether a gender difference in susceptibility to lung cancer exists. Black men have the highest incidence of lung cancer. Racial differences in lung cancer incidence are confounded by differences in socioeconomic status and smoking behavior. One study has concluded that black men and black women appear to have higher rates of lung cancer than do whites, after adjustment for differences in these factors.

GENETIC SUSCEPTIBILITY. A recent study has demonstrated that segregation analysis within families is consistent with mendelian inheritance of a major autosomal gene governing susceptibility to lung cancer. Individuals with early age of onset are most likely to carry this gene (see Ch. 23). It is estimated that segregation at this locus accounts for 69%, 47%, and 22% of lung cancers diagnosed at ages 50, 60, and 70, respectively.

A number of genes potentially determine susceptibility to lung cancer (see Ch. 156). Three major categories of such genes include proto-oncogenes and tumor suppressor genes, genes encoding enzymes that metabolize procarcinogens to active carcinogens, and enzymes that detoxify carcinogens. Although kindreds with germ line abnormalities of either the p53 or the retinoblastoma tumor suppressor genes have higher incidences of lung cancer, this does not appear to be a common mechanism in the general population. The P-450 enzyme system, which metabolizes and in many cases activates carcinogens, has been investigated as a potential determinant of susceptibility to lung cancer. Multiple members of the P-450 gene family exist, making analysis complex. Two P-450 isozymes, CYP2D6 and CYP1A1, have been implicated in susceptibility to lung cancer.

PATHOGENESIS

The respiratory epithelium develops as an outpouching from the endoderm of the primitive foregut. All respiratory epithelial cells differentiate from the primitive respiratory epithelium. Animal studies demonstrate that in the airway epithelium, both the secretory and basal cells can dedifferentiate and subsequently redifferentiate into the various epithelial subtypes. In the alveolar epithelium, the Type II cell is the stem cell that can proliferate. All histologic subtypes of bronchogenic carcinoma are believed to be derived from the respiratory epithelium. The different histologic subtypes are a reflection of the differentiation pathway taken by a particular tumor. The plasticity of this differentiation is demonstrated by the occurrence of mixed tumors expressing differentiation markers for more than one histologic subtype. In addition, experimental expression of specific oncogenes in lung cancer cell lines can alter their differentiation characteristics.

Premalignant Biology

Currently, the favored model for the development of bronchogenic carcinoma is that of multistep carcinogenesis with the successive accumulation of mutations in a number of genes involved in regulating growth. Premalignant lesions have been accurately described only for squamous cell carcinoma. Microdissection of a limited number of bronchial epithelial dysplasias has allowed the identification of genetic lesions including chromosome 3p deletion, chromosome 17p deletion, and p53 gene mutations in premalignant dysplasias.

Increased cellular proliferation is also necessary for carcinogenesis. Pulmonary neuroendocrine cells contain a variety of bioactive peptides, several of which, including the bombesin-like peptides and calcitonin gene–related peptide, are growth factors for bronchial epithelial cells. Exposing animals to tobacco smoke causes a neuroendocrine cell hyperplasia, and increases in bombesin-like peptide levels have been reported in the lower respiratory tract of a subset of human tobacco smokers. It is likely that additional growth factors, derived not only from neuroendocrine cells but also from inflammatory and epithelial cells, may be elevated in tobacco smokers and play a role in pathogenesis of lung cancer.

Tumor Biology

GENETIC ALTERATIONS. Bronchogenic carcinomas (see Ch. 156) have highly abnormal tumor karyotypes, but certain consistent

TABLE 62–2. CHARACTERISTIC CHROMOSOMAL DELETIONS COMMON IN LUNG CANCER

Chromosomal Region Deleted	Tumor Suppressor Genes Inactivated
3p14–25	Unknown, probably multiple, ? VHL
5q	? APC, MCC
9q	Unknown, linked to interferon gene cluster
11p	? WT 1
13q14	Rb ($\sim$ 100% SCLC, $\sim$ 20% NSCLC)
17p13	p53 ($\sim$ 90% SCLC, $\sim$ 60% NSCLC)

Abbreviations: VHL = von Hippel-Lindau; APC = adenomatous polyposis coli; MCC = mutated in colon carcinoma; WT 1 = Wilms' tumor; Rb = retinoblastoma (see Ch. 156).

chromosomal abnormalities have been noted both in SCLC and NSCLC, including deletions involving chromosomes 3p, 5q, 9p, 11p, 13q, and 17p (Table 62–2). These abnormalities typically result in loss of heterozygosity but not homozygous deletion of a region. The deleted regions are likely the loci of tumor suppressor genes. Indeed, two tumor suppressor genes, Rb and p53, have been assigned to regions typically deleted in lung cancer and are frequently inactivated. For other regions, such as the short arm of chromosome 3, tumor suppressor genes have not been identified. Although Rb and p53 mutations are found in both SCLC and NSCLC, the incidence of both is significantly higher in SCLC. Overexpression of p53 is reported to be a poor prognostic marker.

Transforming oncogenes can be activated by a number of mechanisms, including point mutation, gene amplification, and overexpression (Table 62–3). Abnormalities of the Ki-*ras, her2/neu,* and *myc* family oncogenes have been described and noted to negatively affect prognosis. *Bcl*-2 oncogene overexpression has been reported to have a favorable effect. Because abnormalities in tumor suppressor and proto-oncogenes in lung cancer have prognostic significance, it is likely that in the future treatment plans will be altered on the basis of these abnormalities.

AUTOCRINE GROWTH FACTORS. Bronchogenic carcinomas produce a variety of autocrine growth factors. The bombesin-like peptides are a family of neuropeptides that include gastrin-releasing peptide and neuromedin B in humans. Both SCLC and, to a lesser extent, NSCLC produce bombesin-like peptides and express receptors for these ligands. Disrupting this autocrine growth factor loop, either with monoclonal antibodies or with peptide antagonists, can result in growth inhibition. Other autocrine growth factors expressed by bronchogenic carcinomas include insulin-like growth factor 1, transforming growth factor-α, the c-*kit* ligand (stem cell growth factor), and the *her2/neu* ligand. In addition, nicotine receptors have been demonstrated in lung cancer cell lines and modulate cell growth under certain conditions. Clinical trials are under way in humans using strategies to disrupt stimulation by autocrine growth factors.

Pathology

NON–SMALL CELL LUNG CANCER. *Adenocarcinoma* has increased in incidence and is now the most frequent histologic sub-

TABLE 62–3. ONCOGENE ABNORMALITIES

	Abnormality	
Oncogene	*SCLC*	*NSCLC*
Ki-*ras*	0	30% of adenocarcinomas (activating mutation)
H-*ras*	0	Rare mutation; overexpression occurs
N-*ras*	0	Rare mutation; overexpression occurs
myc (c,L,N)	Majority	Occurs (gene amplification, overexpression)
her2/neu	—	30% (overexpression)
c-*kit*	Overexpression	—
bcl-2	?	Overexpression

type. Adenocarcinomas may be derived from either the periphery of the lung or the central airways. Approximately one half of adenocarcinomas exhibit markers for Type II or Clara cells, such as mRNA for the surfactant proteins A, B, and C. The hallmark of adenocarcinomas is the tendency to form glands. Special stains demonstrate that the tumor cells contain mucins. *Bronchoalveolar carcinoma* is a subcategory of adenocarcinoma which arises in the periphery and tends to spread in a lepidic fashion along pre-existing alveolar septa. Peripheral adenocarcinomas are sometimes associated with pulmonary scars. It is likely that in a few cases the carcinoma arose from the scar and in most that the carcinoma caused the scar either by producing a localized infarct or by instituting a desmoplastic cellular reaction. Precursor lesions for adenocarcinomas have not been well described. *Squamous cell carcinoma* tends to originate in the central airways. Histologically, squamous cell carcinomas are characterized by keratinization with keratin "pearl" formation, i.e., flattened cells surrounding central cores of keratin. Squamous carcinomas are also characterized by predominant desmosomes that can be visualized on histologic sections as intercellular bridges. *Large cell carcinoma,* often referred to as large cell undifferentiated carcinoma, is a group of carcinomas undifferentiated at the light microscopic level. Large cell carcinomas may exhibit neuroendocrine or glandular differentiation markers when studied by immunohistochemistry or electronmicroscopy. Ten percent of large cell carcinomas may contain dense core granules and express neuroendocrine markers on more detailed study. Two rare subtypes of large cell carcinomas exist: the giant cell carcinomas, associated with peripheral leukocytosis, and clear cell carcinomas, which resemble renal cell carcinomas. *Bronchial carcinoids* are well-differentiated neuroendocrine tumors. Carcinoids often cause localized bronchial obstruction and present in young individuals. Although they tend not to metastasize widely, they can exhibit a spectrum of biologic behavior.

SMALL CELL LUNG CANCER. SCLC is characterized by small, dark-staining cells with little cytoplasm. The nuclear chromatin is finely distributed and nucleoli are inconspicuous. Biopsies frequently exhibit a "crush artifact," in which the tumor cells are compressed and distorted. The Pathology Committee of the International Association for the Study of Lung Cancer has promoted a nomenclature that includes the categories small cell carcinoma, mixed small cell/large cell carcinoma, and combined small cell carcinoma. The mixed small cell/large cell carcinoma may actually present with a predominant large cell component, and it is estimated that 10% of large cell carcinomas are actually mixed small cell/large cell tumors. Rarely, SCLC tumors comprise a combination of cells with SCLC and NSCLC features and are termed combined small cell carcinomas. When SCLC recurs after chemotherapy, NSCLC elements often increase. The diagnosis of SCLC is not usually a difficult one to make, but in certain situations, such as fine-needle aspirations of lymph nodes, applying immunohistochemical markers can be helpful.

CLINICAL MANIFESTATIONS

Lung cancer is clinically silent for the majority of its course. The presence of symptoms is usually accompanied by late disease, and prognosis is worse than with a carcinoma which presents as an asymptomatic radiographic abnormality. Symptoms can be divided into four categories: (1) those caused by tumor growing locally, (2) those caused by tumor invading adjacent structures, (3) those caused by metastatic disease, and (4) paraneoplastic syndromes.

LOCAL. Either a new cough or a change in the nature of a chronic cough is the most common presenting symptom of bronchogenic carcinoma. The presence of this symptom in a smoker should always cause concern. Cough productive of copious thin secretions, often with a salty flavor, has been described as classically occurring in bronchoalveolar carcinoma, but it occurs in only a minority of cases. Hemoptysis, either gross or minor, commonly occurs when mucosal lesions ulcerate. Although the most common cause of hemoptysis is bronchitis, this symptom in a high-risk individual should prompt investigation. Tumors that obstruct major airways can produce wheezing. In particular, wheezing that is localized to one side suggests a localized obstruction. Airway obstruction can result in atelectasis or postobstructive pneumonia. Bronchogenic carcinomas are often associated with cavitation and lung abscess formation, due either to airway obstruction with postobstructive pneumonia or to necrosis of a large tumor mass. Clinical signs particularly indicative of malignancy-associated lung abscess include chronicity of symptoms, lack of high fever, and lack of leukocytosis.

LOCAL INVASION. Local invasion can produce chest pain, dyspnea from pleural effusion, and symptoms referable to nerves, heart, and great vessels. Malignant pleural effusions occur in approximately 10 to 20% of patients at the time of diagnosis and are most frequently a sign of lack of surgical resectability. Invasion of the pericardium can lead to cardiac tamponade as well as arrhythmias. A number of syndromes have been described in locally invasive disease. The *superior vena cava syndrome* is characterized by facial suffusion and swelling due to blockage of the superior vena cava by either tumor or associated thrombosis. Although this is no longer considered a medical emergency, it should be treated promptly. *Horner's syndrome* results from disruption of the cervical sympathetics and is characterized by unilateral facial anhidrosis, ptosis, and miosis in its full-blown form. Hoarseness can occur from invasion of the recurrent laryngeal nerve, usually by either tumor directly extending into the mediastinum or adjacent malignant nodes. The symptom of hoarseness is important because vocal cord paralysis denotes lack of resectability. The *Pancoast syndrome* occurs in tumors involving the apex and superior sulcus of the lung and results from local invasion into the brachial plexus as well as the cervical sympathetics. Clinical manifestations are dominated by shoulder and arm pain and may include Horner's syndrome. The tumor may not be readily apparent on plain radiographs, and computed tomography (CT) scanning or magnetic resonance imaging (MRI) may be necessary for diagnosis.

METASTATIC DISEASE. Common sites of metastases of bronchogenic carcinomas include brain, bone, adrenal, and liver. In smokers who present with space-occupying lesions in these sites, the possibility of bronchogenic carcinoma should be immediately considered. In addition, metastatic carcinoma is a frequent cause of cervical and supraclavicular lymphadenopathy. Metastases to skin are relatively rare but important to recognize clinically because of the ease of making a diagnosis with a noninvasive biopsy.

PARANEOPLASTIC SYNDROMES. Paraneoplastic syndromes occur in approximately 10% of patients with bronchogenic carcinoma and occasionally are the presenting symptom. Paraneoplastic manifestations of bronchogenic carcinoma can be divided into the following categories: systemic, endocrine, neurologic, cutaneous, hemologic, and renal. Systemic manifestations are often nonspecific and can include weight loss, anorexia, and fever. The endocrine and neurologic manifestations of bronchogenic carcinoma are more specific (see Ch. 158.1).

Digital clubbing is seen in a variety of pulmonary conditions but occurs most commonly in association with bronchogenic carcinoma. Clubbing is caused by soft tissue subungual thickening that most commonly involves the fingernails, resulting in loss of the normal angle between the fingernail and nail bed. In addition, the fingernails are easily compressed against the nail bed, with a spongy feel. Hypertrophic pulmonary osteoarthropathy (see Ch. 158.1) is often associated with clubbing and commonly presents with exquisite tenderness over the long bones. Hypercoagulable states can result from bronchogenic carcinoma. Invasion of the bone marrow can produce leukocytosis with a leukoerythroblastic reaction, as well as anemia.

ASYMPTOMATIC RADIOGRAPHIC ABNORMALITY. High-risk individuals, i.e., smokers with COPD, receive frequent chest radiographs for a variety of indications. A significant number of patients with lung cancer are initially detected as an asymptomatic radiographic abnormality. Lack of symptoms should not delay workup, as these patients are the most likely to be cured by appropriate therapy. A large number of these patients present with a solitary pulmonary nodule, defined as a mass <6 cm in diameter, completely surrounded by aerated lung.

DIAGNOSIS AND STAGING

General Principles

In many cases the decision of whether or not to aggressively investigate a patient for lung cancer is an obvious one (Fig. 62–1). In other situations, such as when a relatively low-risk patient presents with an asymptomatic radiographic abnormality, the decision to initiate a workup may be difficult. A variety of factors must be considered, including patient age, smoking history, exposure to other environmental carcinogens, family history of lung cancer, exposure to

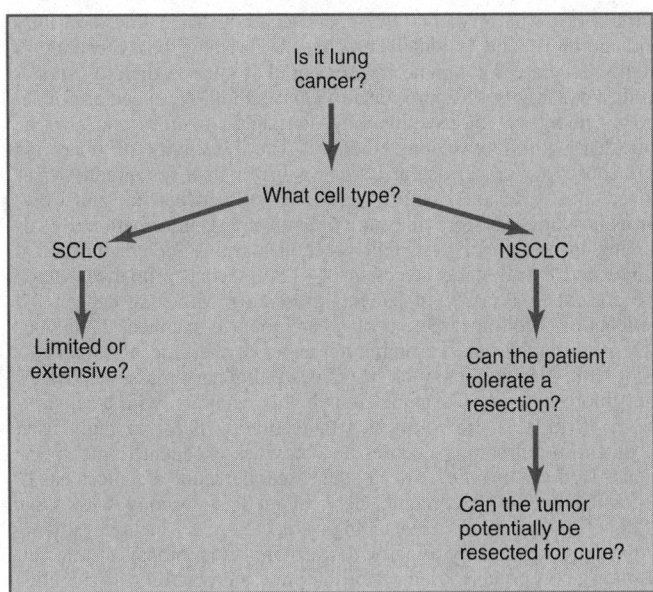

FIGURE 62–1. Questions to determine therapy for lung cancer.

fungal and other infectious diseases that might cause pulmonary nodules, general health and operative risk of the patient, and finally the patient's personality and tolerance for uncertainty regarding a diagnosis. Once a decision to investigate is made, a firm tissue diagnosis should be obtained. It is imperative that the clinicians directing the patient's workup consult closely with the pathologist who is interpreting tissue biopsy and cytologic results. When the cell type is in doubt, there should be no hesitation in obtaining additional tissue for pathologic study. Many clinicians are reluctant to base treatment plans on a cytologic diagnosis only.

IMAGING STUDIES. The chest radiograph is the most important radiologic study to diagnose lung cancer. When an abnormality is visualized on a chest radiograph, it is extremely helpful to obtain old chest radiographs if available. The stability of the lesion over time can be very helpful in suggesting either a benign or malignant diagnosis. Doubling times of <6 weeks or >18 months strongly suggest a benign diagnosis (doubling is calculated on the basis of volume, i.e., proportional to the cube of the radius of a lesion). Another reliable sign of benignity is the presence of heavy calcification within a lesion, particularly when present in a concentric, solid, or popcorn pattern. It must be kept in mind, however, that carcinomas can arise adjacent to calcified granulomas; therefore, if a lesion that contains a significant amount of calcium enlarges over time, it should be considered likely to be malignant. CT scanning of the thorax is now frequently undertaken in patients with suspicious nodules. In many cases, calcification can be detected, suggesting a benign diagnosis. CT scans also reliably detect enlarged lymph nodes, although biopsy is required to determine whether the lymphadenopathy is due to metastatic tumor. The CT scan can easily be extended to include the liver and adrenals, assessing common sites of metastatic disease. MRI studies are particularly useful to detect vertebral, spinal cord, and mediastinal structure invasion in selected patients.

PATHOLOGIC DIAGNOSIS. Sputum cytology is the least invasive means to establish a tissue diagnosis. Sputum cytology is approximately 60 to 70% sensitive for central lesions, but it is much less accurate for small peripheral lesions. In some instances, the diagnosis of cell type can be difficult on sputum cytology, and many clinicians believe that it is preferable to obtain biopsies of a tumor if at all possible. Other relatively noninvasive means of establishing a diagnosis include pleural fluid cytology, biopsy or aspiration cytology of enlarged cervical and supraclavicular lymph nodes, and biopsies of skin lesions. More invasive means of establishing a tissue diagnosis include either bronchoscopy, needle biopsy, video-assisted thoracoscopy, cervical mediastinoscopy, and thoracotomy. Flexible fiberoptic bronchoscopy allows visualization of all the central, lobar, segmental, and subsegmental airways. It can be performed on awake patients with local sedation, has a low morbidity and mortality, and is widely practiced. Fiberoptic bronchoscopy is highly accurate for diagnosing lesions that can be directly visualized; a sensitivity of approximately 95% should be expected for lesions undergoing biopsy this way. Peripheral nodules can also be biopsied with fluoroscopic guidance. The sensitivity of fiberoptic bronchoscopy for peripheral lesions is lower than for directly visualized airway lesions, with a sensitivity of between 60 and 70%. Bronchoscopy also provides important staging information by allowing inspection of potential resection margins for endobronchial tumor and by allowing detection of occult second primaries, which are present in 1 to 3% of patients presenting with lung cancer. All patients in whom a resection of a carcinoma is planned should undergo a bronchoscopic examination either at the time of surgery or prior to it. Needle biopsy of suspicious pulmonary masses under either fluoroscopic or CT guidance is highly accurate, with a sensitivity of 90 to 95%. Video-assisted thoracoscopy is increasingly used to diagnose pulmonary nodules and provides excellent tissue specimens. Lesions that lie close to the visceral pleura are most easily accessible by this technique. Cervical mediastinoscopy with sampling of lymph nodes is also highly accurate in selected patients with lymphadenopathy. Finally, thoracotomy with biopsy of a lesion is often appropriately used when the pretest probability of a malignancy is high, such as when a peripheral nodule has been demonstrated to increase in size on serial chest radiographs.

Staging

Accurate staging of lung cancer is necessary to predict prognosis and determine the appropriate therapy. The staging systems for NSCLC and SCLC are different: in NSCLC a TNM staging system is used, whereas in SCLC patients are divided into those with limited and extensive disease (Tables 62–4 to 62–6).

All patients with lung cancer should have a history and physical examination with attention to detecting lymphadenopathy and neurologic and bone abnormalities. Laboratory studies include a complete blood count, liver function tests, and serum calcium. Routine radiographic studies include a chest radiograph with posteroanterior and lateral views. In most patients chest CT with extension through the liver and to the adrenals is useful. There are subsets of patients, for instance those with obvious hilar and mediastinal adenopathy on plain chest radiograph and those with small peripheral T1 lesions, in whom the chest CT may not be necessary. Owing to the high incidence of metastasis in SCLC, CT of the brain and abdomen is frequently ordered in asymptomatic patients with this tissue diagnosis.

Intrathoracic lymph nodes that exceed 1 cm in size have a high likelihood of harboring metastatic disease. However, a variety of benign conditions including pneumonia, healed tuberculous and fungal infection, silicosis, and sarcoidosis can all cause significant lymphadenopathy. Therefore, enlarged intrathoracic lymph nodes should always undergo biopsy and metastatic disease should be proven before therapy plans are altered in patients with NSCLC. Cervical mediastinoscopy is most commonly used; needle biopsy (either transbronchial or transthoracic), video-assisted thoracoscopy, and mediastinal exploration at thoracotomy are also useful in certain patients.

The presence of metastatic disease outside the chest predicts a poor prognosis, and these patients are almost never referred for surgery. In the absence of any localizing clinical signs, symptoms, or laboratory abnormalities, routine brain, liver, and bone scans are not cost-effective for detecting occult metastasis. Bone scans are complicated by a high rate of false positives due to old fractures. CT of the upper abdomen may be useful in the asymptomatic patient for detecting occult metastasis, particularly silent metastasis involving the adrenal. Because of the high incidence of adrenal adenomas in the normal population, most adrenal lesions should be histologically confirmed as metastatic disease before altering treatment plans.

PHYSIOLOGIC ASSESSMENT FOR RESECTION. Before considering a patient for surgical resection of a bronchogenic carcinoma, it must be determined that adequate pulmonary reserve exists to permit this therapy. Simple spirometry and an arterial blood gas are the only tests routinely required. Patients predicted to have a postoperative forced expiratory volume in 1 second (FEV_1) < 800 to 1000 ml have an unacceptably high operative and postoperative mortality. Loss of FEV_1 is approximately proportional to loss of normal lung tissue. The right lung contains approximately 55 to 60% of pulmonary function in most individuals and the left lung contains 40 to 45% of function. When pulmonary function does not appear to be evenly distributed between right and left lungs, perfusion scanning, which correlates well with ventilation, may help estimate the contribution of each side. CO_2 retention on arterial blood gas analysis, unless solely on the basis of a low respiratory drive, is a predictor of bad postoperative outcome. Hypoxemia is not a strong indicator of poor outcome. The roles of exercise testing and pulmonary artery pressure measurement are unclear.

With the advent of lung-sparing operations, including sleeve and wedge resections, many patients who previously would not have been considered surgical candidates are now undergoing pulmonary resection. Close collaboration between internists and thoracic surgeons is necessary to determine whether marginal candidates are indeed appropriate for surgical therapy.

TREATMENT

NSCLC Therapy

SURGICAL. Surgery offers the best chance for curing appropriately staged patients with NSCLC: 5-year survival rates range from 60 to 80% for patients with stage I disease to 15% for selected patients with stage IIIA. Stages I–IIIA NSCLC are those routinely considered for surgery. Over the past 30 years significant advances have been made surgically in treating lung cancer. Operative mortality has dropped from 10 to 20% to approximately 3%. The inci-

TABLE 62–5. NSCLC STAGING DEFINITIONS

Tumor	
T0	No tumor
TX	Positive cytology, no apparent tumor
TIS	Carcinoma *in situ*
T1	Tumor < 3 cm diameter; no visceral pleural or lobar bronchial involvement
T2	Tumor < 3 cm diameter, visceral pleural or > 2 cm from carina
T3	Direct extension to pleura or chest wall, or < 2 cm from carina
T4	Invades heart, great vessels, esophagus, trachea, carina, vertebrae, or malignant pleural effusion
Nodes	
N0	No involvement
N1	Peribronchial or ipsilateral hilar
N2	Ipsilateral mediastinal or subcarinal nodes
N3	Contralateral mediastinal or hilar nodes; any supraclavicular or scalene nodes
Metastasis	
M0	None detected
M1	Any

TABLE 62–4. SCLC STAGING

Limited	Tumor confined to chest plus supraclavicular nodes, but excluding cervical, axillary nodes
Extensive	Tumor outside of above confines

TABLE 62–6. STAGE GROUPING AND SURVIVAL FOR NSCLC

Stage	Definition	5-Year Survival	
		Clinical Staging	Pathologic Staging
I	T1 or T2; N0; M0	45%	60–85%
II	T1 or T2; N1; M0	25–30%	~45%
IIIA	T1 or T2; N2; M0	~15%	~25%
	T3; N0, 1 or 2; M0		
IIIB	T1–4; N3; M0	<5%	
	T4; N0, 1 or 2; M0		
IV	Any T, any N, M1	~1%	

Refer to Table 62–5 for definitions.

dence of "fruitless thoracotomy," in which a lesion is discovered to be inoperable at the time of thoracotomy, has decreased from 25% to approximately 5%. The increased use of lung-sparing resections including sleeve lobectomy, segmentectomy, wedge resection, and thoracoscopic wedge resection has allowed surgical therapy to be applied to a group of patients with less pulmonary reserve than in the past. A prospective trial comparing conventional lobectomy with wedge resection has demonstrated that local recurrence rates are higher with the latter procedure. Nevertheless, wedge resection is still an acceptable alternative in patients with diminished pulmonary reserve.

Before a decision for surgical therapy is made in a given patient, three questions must be addressed (Fig. 62–1). (1) Is the cell type NSCLC? With the exception of peripheral solitary pulmonary nodules without hilar or mediastinal lymphadenopathy, a firm tissue diagnosis should almost always be obtained prior to surgical therapy. Owing to the rarity with which SCLC presents with stage I disease and the likelihood that surgical therapy does benefit patients in this subset, it may not be necessary to obtain tissue diagnosis for all patients in this group prior to surgical therapy. (2) Is the patient physiologically capable of tolerating resectional surgery? General medical criteria such as absence of a recent myocardial infarction should be applied. In addition, physiologically assess whether the planned resection will leave the patient with adequate pulmonary reserve. (3) Can the disease be completely resected? This requires adequate staging with detection of both distant metastases and local lymph node involvement. As surgical therapy provides the best hope for long-term survival in NSCLC, physiologic assessment and staging should be accurate and objective.

RADIATION THERAPY. Radiation therapy of NSCLC often effectively controls local disease. Significant physiologic impairment does result, however, so most patients who might be considered for curative radiation therapy are also candidates for curative surgical therapy. There have been few trials of radiation therapy in early-stage lung cancer. It is estimated that between 10 and 20% of localized lesions can be cured by radiation. Radiation therapy is most commonly used to palliate symptoms. Endobronchial symptoms, including hemoptysis and obstruction, respond frequently to radiation. Distant metastases also are frequently treated primarily with radiation. Radiation therapy as an adjuvant to surgical therapy in NSCLC is currently undergoing trial.

CHEMOTHERAPY. Using chemotherapy for NSCLC has been controversial. A number of drugs are frequently used: cisplatin, mitomycin, vinca alkaloids, ifosfamide, and etoposide. There is no group of patients with NSCLC in whom chemotherapy is unequivocally effective. Trials comparing chemotherapy with best supportive care for stage IV NSCLC have yielded conflicting results; meta-analyses suggest a small (several months increased survival) benefit from chemotherapy. Several trials treating stage III patients with chemotherapy plus radiation have demonstrated a longer survival than for patients treated with radiation alone. Further trials of this are now underway. In selecting patients with NSCLC for chemotherapy, several factors should be kept in mind: Survival is reduced and side effects of chemotherapy are increased in patients who are not fully ambulatory. Benefits to this group are likely to be minimal. Response to therapy needs to be evaluable. Patients must be fully informed of the limitations of chemotherapy in NSCLC. Many physicians discontinue treatment if there is no clinical response after two or three cycles of chemotherapy. Most patients with NSCLC are not cured by surgery; the controversy over chemotherapy for this subgroup emphasizes the major need for new agents and approaches to deal with this problem.

ADJUVANT THERAPY. In patients with resectable stage II or III NSCLC, there is a high risk for failure of surgical therapy secondary to local, mediastinal, or distant metastatic recurrence. A trial in this group of patients comparing mediastinal irradiation with no adjuvant therapy has been completed. Adding radiation therapy decreases the risk of mediastinal recurrence but does not improve overall survival. It has been attempted, therefore, to control occult metastatic disease by adding chemotherapy. Several trials have demonstrated increased disease-free survival in stage II and III resected NSCLC patients treated with either chemotherapy or radiation therapy plus chemotherapy. Unfortunately, although increased disease-free survival has been demonstrated, overall survival has not been increased. Additional trials are underway investigating the role of adjuvant therapy in resected NSCLC. Neoadjuvant therapy (administering chemotherapy and/or radiation therapy prior to resection) has not been fully studied yet and its clinical use remains unclear.

Therapy of SCLC

Before effective chemotherapy for SCLC, the median survival was approximately 6 to 12 weeks for extensive disease and approximately 6 months for limited-stage SCLC. Overall 5-year survival rate was <1%. With optimal therapy, current median survival for limited-stage SCLC exceeds 1 year and for extensive-stage disease is approximately 10 months. Five-year survival rate has increased to between 5 and 10%.

Chemotherapy is the cornerstone of treatment for both limited- and extensive-stage SCLC. A variety of agents have activity. Many experts believe that regimens containing etoposide and either carboplatin or cisplatin offer the best combination of efficacy and lack of toxicity. In patients with limited-stage SCLC, the most frequent site of recurrence is the primary lesion. Therefore, adding radiation therapy to thoracic disease has been studied. At the present time, either concurrent or alternating chest radiation therapy with chemotherapy is preferred in patients with limited-stage disease. No evidence indicates that prophylactic cranial irradiation improves survival, but it is associated with increased CNS morbidity. In patients with extensive-stage SCLC, radiation therapy is generally not used in the initial management because chemotherapy produces initial palliation in 80% or more of cases. The addition of radiation therapy does not seem to increase survival, but it does increase toxicity. Radiation therapy is used as palliation in patients who fail initial chemotherapy. A small proportion (<1%) of patients with SCLC present with stage I or II disease. This rare subset of patients has a 5-year survival of 50 to 70% if treated by surgery followed by chemotherapy with or without radiation therapy. Surgery for patients with SCLC with stage III or greater disease should be confined to experimental trials and not routinely performed. A number of trials have examined whether increased duration or intensity of chemotherapy for SCLC is beneficial. At the present time, no data support the efficacy of more than four to six cycles of chemotherapy. Increasing dose intensity above standard results in increased toxicity and is not currently supported.

PROGNOSIS

The overall prognosis for patients with lung cancer remains grim, with a 5-year survival rate of 13%. Owing to the high incidence of bronchogenic carcinoma, this 13% survival rate represents a large number of patient years that are potentially salvageable, however. Certain subgroups, including patients with stage I and stage II NSCLC treated by surgery, do have a 40 to 85% 5-year survival rate, making it critical for the physician to recognize and appropriately diagnose and treat these individuals. Long-term survivors of both NSCLC and SCLC are a high-risk group for second primary lung cancers, with an incidence of 3 to 5% per year.

PREVENTION

The most important preventive measure is deterring young individuals from starting to smoke (see Ch. 9.4). This public health issue is mainly a social, economic, and political problem. It has been shown that increasing the cost of tobacco products, through increased taxes, is an effective strategy for keeping people from starting this habit. Negative advertising and measures that make it less socially acceptable and glamorous to smoke are also effective.

Smoking cessation is also an important strategy and results in a gradual decrease in risk for lung cancer over 10 to 15 years. Approximately 30% of patients who enter a smoking cessation program are successful. Physician input is crucial in this process.

Large trials examining the value of early detection efforts carried out in the 1970's failed to show a benefit in terms of long-term survival. Women and high-risk smokers were not studied. It is possible that early detection may become a viable strategy, especially if improved screening tests are developed and high-risk groups targeted.

Chemoprevention of lung cancer may be possible. The use of 13-cis-retinoic acid in patients with laryngeal cancer has been shown to decrease the incidence of second primaries in the aerodigestive system. A number of clinical trials are currently underway investigating the efficacy of retinoic acid derivatives and carotenoids in high-risk groups. Additional compounds including vitamin E, vitamin C, selenium, and pharmacologic agents that interfere with growth factor signal transduction are being evaluated. Owing to the large reservoir of smokers and ex-smokers at risk, chemoprevention has considerable potential.

Carbone DP, Minna JD: The molecular genetics of lung cancer. Adv Intern Med 37:153, 1992. *An up-to-date review of this rapidly evolving field.*

Cook RM, Miller YE, Bunn PA: Small cell lung cancer: Etiology, biology, clinical features, staging, and treatment. Curr Probl Cancer 17:71, 1993. *A general review of SCLC.*

Ihde DC: Chemotherapy of lung cancer. N Engl J Med 327:1434, 1992. *Authoratative and concise review of the role of chemotherapy in SCLC and NSCLC. Adjuvant therapies are also discussed.*

Miller DL, Allan MS: Rare pulmonary neoplasms. Mayo Clin Proc 68:492, 1993. *A review of over 10,000 patients treated for primary lung cancer in the past decade yielded 80 patients with rare neoplasms. The experience in this series is recounted and references to the literature are provided.*

Mountain CF: Lung cancer staging classification. Clin Chest Med 14:43, 1993. *A guide for determining staging for possible surgery and prognosis of patients with lung cancer. Includes illustrations of tumor and nodal stages as well as a valuable section on staging indicators for specific unusual clinical situations.*

Samet JM: The epidemiology of lung cancer. Chest 103 (Suppl):20S, 1993. *A concise review that documents the evidence for classifying various exposures as carcinogenic. Extensively referenced.*

63 DISEASES OF THE DIAPHRAGM, CHEST WALL, PLEURA, AND MEDIASTINUM

Bartolome R. Celli

THE DIAPHRAGM

This, the most important muscle of respiration, is shaped like a thin dome and separates the thoracic and abdominal cavities. It has two components—the central noncontractile tendon and the muscle fibers that arise from it and radiate down and outward to insert distally in the circumferential caudal limits of the ribcage. There is a hiatus for each of the structures that passes from thorax to abdomen. The diaphragm is neurologically controlled by the phrenic nerve, the motoneurons of which arise in the cervical spinal cord at levels C3 to C5. The anatomic arrangement of the diaphragm and its coupling to the ribcage-abdomen explain its mechanical action. Diaphragmatic contraction displaces the abdominal contents downward and raise the ribs outward, resulting in the negative intrapleural inspiratory pressure. Like the heart, the diaphragm, and to a lesser degree the other respiratory muscles, must intermittently contract throughout a person's life. Unlike the heart, it has no intrinsic contractile mechanism, and the respiratory cycle is regulated by a complex set of centrally organized neurons and several peripheral feedback mechanisms that synchronize the diaphragm with many other muscles. This must be so because the diaphragm serves other nonrespiratory functions such as speech, defecation, and parturition. The blood supply to the diaphragm is rich and is arranged to minimize interruption during contraction. Nevertheless, the muscle itself is highly oxygen-dependent.

DYSFUNCTION AND FATIGUE. Diaphragmatic dysfunction is most frequently caused by lung hyperinflation—acute as in asthma or chronic as in chronic obstructive pulmonary disease (COPD). Hyperinflation shortens the diaphragmatic fibers and changes its shape to a flatter one in which the horizontal fibers do not generate the normally expanding action on the ribcage but rather an inward deforming change in the lower ribcage (Hoover's sign in COPD). These changes, coupled with the increased loads secondary to airways resistance and changes in lung and chest wall compliance, result in increased work by the diaphragm. If the increased energy demand outstrips the energy supply, the diaphragm fatigues and ventilation may fail.

Diaphragmatic fatigue can be determined by using pressure measurements across the diaphragm (transdiaphragmatic pressure, or Pdi) or by the more elaborate power spectrum analysis of elec-

tromyographic signals. Both correlate well with the simpler clinical signs of increased respiratory rate with progressively shallow breathing. As fatigue progresses, ventilation is maintained by intermittent expansions of ribcage and abdomen (respiratory alternans) and then paradoxical inward abdominal motion during inspiration (abdominal paradox). The strategies to improve diaphragmatic function in impending fatigue are listed in Table 63–1. If fatigue results in hypercapnia and acidosis, the respiratory muscles must be rested with mechanical ventilation. This should be maintained for at least 1 to several days because this kind of muscle fatigue may take that long to recover.

DISORDERS OF DIAPHRAGMATIC MOTION. Unilateral diaphragmatic paralysis is usually secondary to phrenic nerve involvement by a tumor (bronchogenic carcinoma being the most frequent). It may result from neurologic diseases such as myelitis, encephalitis, poliomyelitis, and herpes zoster, from trauma to the thorax or cervical spine, or from compression by benign processes such as substernal thyroid, aortic aneurysm, and infectious collections. With the advent of cardiac surgery, paralysis secondary to phrenic nerve cooling has increased. Occasionally, the paralysis may be idiopathic. In patients with normal lungs, unilateral paralysis is usually asymptomatic and rarely requires treatment. The diagnosis is suspected when, in the chest roentgenogram, the diaphragmatic leaflet is elevated and is confirmed fluoroscopically by observing paradoxical diaphragmatic motion on sniff and cough. Bilateral paralysis usually results from high cervical trauma (C3 to C5) or from myopathies. The myopathy may be generalized (muscular dystrophy, polymyositis, hypothyroidism) or limited, primarily affecting the diaphragm (acid maltase deficiency, collagen vascular disorders). In many cases the cause remains unknown. Patients become symptomatic early. The dyspnea is characteristically worsened by the supine position because abdominal contents displace the diaphragm into the thorax. This also results in a significant drop in the vital capacity (> 500 ml) and in oxygen saturation. Fluoroscopy is less reliable because the flaccid diaphragm may lag behind the ribcage expansion when accessory muscles contract, thus giving the impression of diaphragmatic contraction. The diagnosis is suspected by the presence of abdominal paradoxical retraction. It is confirmed by measuring transdiaphragmatic pressure with and without electromyographic recording. Phrenic nerve conduction establishes the diagnosis of neuropathy. Treatment of ventilatory failure secondary to bilateral paralysis consists of intermittent ventilation, which has been achieved with different methods (external negative ventilation, nasal positive pressure ventilation, and rocking beds). In some cases, such as cardiac surgery, the paralysis recovers and ventilation may be discontinued. When permanent but with intact muscle function (e.g., high quadriplegics), diaphragmatic pacing has been lifesaving.

Hiccup (singultus) is a common disorder produced by spasm of the diaphragm followed by sudden closure of the glottis during an inspiratory effort. Hiccups are usually self-limited but may persist for days or weeks. In most patients a cause is never found, but it

TABLE 63–1. THERAPEUTIC MODALITIES TO IMPROVE DIAPHRAGMATIC FUNCTION

Reduce mechanical load
1. Decrease airways resistance (bronchodilators, treat infection, decrease inflammation).
2. Reduce hyperinflation.
3. Decrease ventilatory requirement (administer oxygen, control fever, avoid caloric loads).

Improve respiratory muscle contractility and endurance
1. Administer oxygen therapy.
2. Improve nutrition.
3. Improve cardiovascular performance.
4. Correct electrolytes (sodium, potassium, calcium, phosphorus).
5. Administer drugs that improve contractility (theophylline, β_2-agonist, caffeine).
6. Check for hypothyroidism or drugs that impair contractility (aminoglycosides).
7. Give ventilatory muscle training.

Improve respiratory muscle coordination and energy conservation
Rehabilitation
Respiratory muscle resting

may occasionally be a sign of serious disease such as central nervous system (CNS) disorder (encephalitis, stroke, tumor), uremia, herpes zoster, and pleural or abdominal processes that irritate the diaphragm. Prolonged hiccups are sometimes psychogenic in origin. In general, hiccups subside spontaneously or when the initiating disease improves. When hiccups are chronic or debilitating, local anesthesia or phrenic nerve crushing may be required (permanent paralysis may occur with the latter). Diaphragmatic flutter is a rare disorder in which rhythmic contractions of the diaphragm occur at a rate of 1 to 8 per second. The cause and treatment are similar to those of hiccups.

Diaphragmatic hernias occur through congenitally weak or incompletely fused areas of the diaphragm, or they may result from traumatic rupture of the muscle or through the esophageal hiatus (>70% of all hernias). Anterior hernias occur through the foramina of Morgagni, are rare, and tend to occur in obese patients. They usually show as a rounded density in the right cardiophrenic angle. Posterior hernias through the foramina of Bochdalek are more common, especially in infants. They occur more frequently in the left. Diaphragmatic hernias usually contain omentum but may also contain stomach, bowel, or liver anteriorly or kidney and spleen posteriorly. The diagnosis is suspected on chest roentgenograms and in some cases when there is borborygmus over the chest. Computed tomographic (CT) scans, gastrointestinal contrast films, radioisotope scan of the liver, and induction of a pneumoperitoneum with a follow-up film help establish the diagnosis. In infants, large hernias may compromise ventilation, requiring immediate surgical correction. In the asymptomatic adult with previous evidence of a hernia, observation is indicated. Surgery may be needed for diagnosis or to relieve strangulation of sac contents. Traumatic diaphragmatic hernias may result from penetrating injuries or abdominal compression.

Symptom severity depends on the extension of abdominal contents into the thorax and the presence of strangulation. They may be asymptomatic for several years before respiratory and abdominal symptoms recur. Treatment in these cases is surgical. Eventration may resemble a hernia but consists of a localized elevation of the diaphragm resulting from impaired muscle development or weakness. It is more frequent in the right anteromedial portion and tends to occur in middle-aged obese persons. Once differentiated from neoplasm, it rarely requires surgical treatment.

Celli BR: Clinical and physiologic evaluation of respiratory muscle function. Clin Chest Med 10:199, 1989. *Comprehensive, up-to-date review covering the clinical aspects and practical application of respiratory muscle function.*
Rochester DF: The diaphragm: Contractile properties and fatigue. J Clin Invest 75:1397, 1985. *Excellent review of the anatomy and physiology of the diaphragm. It covers our understanding of dysfunction and fatigue.*

THE CHEST WALL

It is an integral part of the ventilatory pump. It consists of the bony thoracic cage (ribs, sternum, and vertebrae) and the various muscles of respiration. Besides the diaphragm, the intercostals and scaleni are active even during quiet breathing in normals. Other muscles such as the sternocleidomastoid, pectoralis minor and major, serratus anterior, latissimus dorsi, and trapezius partake in respiration during increased ventilatory demand. Even the abdominal muscles can participate in ventilation, by contracting during exhalation. The thoracic cage is a major determinant of ventilation and of static and dynamic lung volumes. Diseases that disrupt the system alter the ventilation and ventilation-perfusion relationship, thus causing hypoxemia or hypercapnia. Primary disorders of the chest wall may occur from impairments of the neuromuscular apparatus or the bony thoracic cage. Because alterations in the neuromuscular apparatus are dealt with in different parts of the text, this section discusses primary alterations of the bony thoracic cage.

Most diseases of the bony thoracic cage are listed in Table 63–2. They are all linked by a similar pathophysiologic process: (1) alveolar hypoventilation, (2) changes in chest wall compliance, (3) variable lung compression, (4) ventilation-perfusion imbalance, and (5) pulmonary hypertension and cor pulmonale. Clinical symptoms include dyspnea without significant cough, sputum, or pain. Physical examination usually establishes the diagnosis and helps determine the presence of cor pulmonale.

KYPHOSCOLIOSIS. Deformities of the dorsolumbar spine are the most common causes of symptomatic derangements of the chest wall. Scoliosis consists of lateral angulation and rotation of the spine and can be categorized as right (most frequent) or left according to the direction of the convexity of the curvature. Kyphosis is less important and consists of anteroposterior angulations of the spine. The severity of scoliosis is quantified by measuring the angle (Cobb's angle) between the upper and lower portions of the spinal curve on a roentgenogram. Only when this angle exceeds 70 degrees is any abnormality of respiratory function detectable. When the angle is >120 degrees, dyspnea and respiratory failure are expected. The ribs over the convex side are separated and rotated posteriorly, giving rise to the kyphoscoliotic hump. On the concave side, the ribs are crowded and displaced anteriorly. This, combined with decreased thoracic height, results in forward bulging of the anterior wall.

Kyphoscoliosis is usually idiopathic and begins in childhood. Ventilatory failure may result in death in the fourth to sixth decade. If the scoliosis is not severe and progressive, life expectancy may be normal. Static lung volumes, chest wall, and to a lesser degree, lung compliance are also decreased. Ventilation-perfusion imbalances result in hypoxemia. When the mechanical load, caused by progressive scoliosis or superimposed infection, is such that the muscles fail, the hypoxemia may be associated with hypercapnia. Hypoventilation and hypoxemia may worsen during sleep, which accounts for the frequent worsening of some patients with otherwise stable kyphoscoliosis.

Several therapeutic approaches are available. Surgical correction includes traction, plasters, and rods. The effects appear mostly cosmetic, and improvement in function is minimal. In hypoxemic patients, oxygen is beneficial. Kyphoscoliosis is one of the few diseases for which administering intermittent positive pressure ventilation increases tidal volume, temporarily improving compliance and lung volumes. In chronic ventilatory failure, night time ventilatory assistance is beneficial. Efforts must be made to induce the patient to stop smoking. Bronchospasms and respiratory infections must be treated aggressively. If obese, the patient should decrease weight.

ANKYLOSING SPONDYLITIS. This inflammatory disease results in fusion of costotransverse and vertebral joints but may also involve sternomanubrial and clavicular joints. With relative fixation of the ribcage in an inspiratory position, most of the ventilatory movement is performed by the diaphragm-abdomen, which is already placed in a mechanical disadvantage, as shown by a normal or greater than normal functional residual capacity. In contrast to kyphoscoliosis, cor pulmonale and ventilatory failure are rare. Some patients may develop upper lobe fibrosis with minimal alterations in gas exchange.

PECTUS EXCAVATUM. This is a congenital deformity of the lower portion of the sternum, with symmetric bowing of the anterior ribs. In infants it tends to occur with multiple abnormalities and is associated with high mortality. It may also be associated with mitral valve prolapse. With severe deformity, the heart and mediastinal structures are laterally displaced. Although some patients may fail to normally increase cardiac output during exercise, functional impairment is usually limited. Surgical correction is mainly cosmetic.

THORACOPLASTY. This is the term applied to surgical procedures employed from 1940 to 1950 to treat tuberculosis. They included resection of several ribs with collapse of the underlying lung. This results in paradoxical retraction of that portion of the chest wall. It was originally thought to have minimal physiologic consequences, but the incidence of cardiorespiratory failure is increased in those patients.

FIBROTHORAX. Resulting from pleural diseases such as hemothorax or asbestosis, it is also considered a primary disease of

TABLE 63–2. MOST IMPORTANT RIBCAGE DERANGEMENTS

Spine
    Scoliosis (idiopathic, cogenital, paralytic)
    Kyphosis
    Ankylosing spondylitis
Sternum, ribs, or pleura
    Pectus excavatum
    Thoracoplasty
    Fibrothorax

chest wall because the lung itself may not be affected. It may result in ventilatory and cardiac failure. The treatment is similar to that for kyphoscoliosis. Occasional pleurectomy may help patients with fibrothorax secondary to pleural fibrosis.

FLAIL CHEST. This is produced by double fractures of three or more adjacent ribs or by combined sternal and rib fractures. The flail segment paradoxically moves inward during inspiration. The inefficient ventilation increases the work of breathing, which may worsen ventilation owing to the frequent association with neuromuscular impairment. Flail chest occurs most frequently with accidental chest trauma and/or after cardiopulmonary resuscitation. Ventilation-perfusion and lung contusion cause hypoxemia. In most cases supportive care with attention to oxygenation, clear airways, and infection prevention is the preferred therapy. Artificial ventilation should be reserved for patients with ventilatory failure. When the flail segment is large, chest fixation may be considered.

Holppner VH, Cockcroft DW, Dosman JH, et al.: Nighttime ventilation improves respiratory failure in secondary kyphoscoliosis. Am Rev Respir Dis 129:240, 1984. *Reviews the use of nighttime ventilation and its effectiveness in reversing ventilatory failure in cases of "pump fatigue."*
Todd TR, Shamji F: Pathophysiology of chest trauma. *In* Roussos C, MacKlem PT (eds.): The Thorax, New York, Marcel Dekker, 1985, p 979. *Excellent review of the pathophysiologic changes in respiratory function secondary to chest trauma. Reviews the controversies in treatment.*

THE PLEURA

ANATOMY AND PHYSIOLOGY. The pleura consists of a layer of mesothelial cells with a smooth semitransparent appearance. It is supported by a network of connective and fibroelastic tissue, lymphatics, and vessels. The mesothelial cells are rich in microvilli, and their most important function is to deliver glycoproteins rich in hyaluronic acid, which decrease friction between lung and chest wall. The parietal pleura covers the surface of the chest wall diaphragm and mediastinum. It is supplied with blood from the systemic circulation, and contains sensory nerves. The visceral pleura covers the surface of the lungs, including the interlobar fissures. Its blood supply arises from the low-pressure pulmonary circulation and has no sensory nerves. Both layers are separated by a virtual cavity lubricated by 5 to 10 ml of fluid, which facilitates lung expansion. It also helps maintain lung inflation by coupling it with the chest wall. Both functions decrease the work of breathing.

The pleural fluid has a low protein concentration (< 2 grams per deciliter) with a pH and glucose similar to that of blood. Pleural fluid is formed primarily from the parietal pleura, and part of its turnover depends on the same Starling forces that govern vascular and interstitial fluid exchange. The parietal pleura has a hydrostatic pressure similar to that of the systemic circulation (30 cm H_2O), whereas that of the visceral pleura depends on the pulmonary circulation (10 cm H_2O). Oncotic pressure is similar in both (25 cm H_2O), but the pressure within the pleural cavity is affected by the gravity gradient. Thus the pleural space is heterogeneous with a nondependent portion where Starling forces favor outpouring of fluid to the cavity and into parenchymal capillaries. The stomas or "lacuna," present over the parietal surface of the low mediastinum, low chest wall, and diaphragm, seem to empty into lymphatics. These subpleural lymphatics represent the major pathway for liquid and solute drainage. Alterations of this formation-resorption mechanism frequently result in the accumulation of pleural fluid. Increases in hydrostatic forces or decreases in oncotic pressures result in low protein "transudates." Increased outpouring by capillaries or cells and/or blocking of lymphatics results in high protein "exudates" (Table 63–3).

DIAGNOSTIC PROCEDURES. *History and Physical Examination.* Although suggestive, a patient's history of pain, dyspnea, or cough is neither sensitive nor specific. These symptoms may be absent in some large effusions and in critically ill patients. When present, the pain is usually unilateral and sharp and worsens with inspiration or cough. It may radiate to shoulder, neck, or abdomen. Dyspnea may result from compression of lung tissue. It may also result from mechanical alterations in the respiratory muscles as the fluid changes their length-tension relationship. The degree of dyspnea relates to fluid volume and intrathoracic pressure and their effect on mechanics and gas exchange. Finally, pleural effusions in patients with minimal lung compromise are well tolerated, whereas similar effusions in patients with lung disease may cause ventilatory failure. The physical examination shows decreased breath sounds and excursions in the affected hemithorax (splinting). Percussion shows dullness with absent tactile fremitus over the area. Frequently there are E to A changes (egobronchophony) at the upper fluid border.

Radiologic Examination. An effusion is suspected when there is blunting and medial displacement of the sharp costophrenic angle. Fluid accumulation between the lung and the diaphragm (subpulmonic effusion) is suspected when there is apparent elevation of the hemidiaphragm or widening of the shadow between the gas-containing stomach and the lower left lung margin. Up to 300 ml of fluid may fail to be seen in a posteroanterior chest roentgenogram, whereas as little as 150 ml may be seen in a lateral decubitus view. A supine film (frequent in patients in intensive care units) may obscure the diagnosis as the fluid layers posteriorly. A pseudotumor occurs when fluid loculates in an interlobar fissure, most commonly in the minor fissure, and gives the radiologic appearance of a tumor. A clue to the diagnosis is the presence of pleural fluid elsewhere and a biconvex lenticular configuration of the mass. A collection of pleural air and fluid (hydropneumothorax) usually produces horizontal and not concave margins. A pneumothorax is identified by the contrast between the water density of the visceral pleura centrally and the gas lucency without vascular markings laterally. Small pneumothoraces may be harder to diagnose, but an expiratory film may help outline them. Pleural plaques may be seen when calcified or may be detected when viewed tangentially but not *en face.* Ultrasonography and CT scans may provide better definition of pleural and parenchymal abnormalities.

Thoracentesis and Pleural Fluid Analysis. Thoracentesis may be performed for diagnosis or therapy. A thoracentesis is diagnostic in approximately 75% of patients, and even when not diagnostic it helps exclude other important diagnoses such as empyema. Diagnostic thoracentesis requires a relatively small amount of material (30 to 50 ml). As a rule, newly discovered effusions should be tapped. Although there are no absolute contraindications to a diagnostic thoracentesis, relative contraindications include a bleeding diathesis, anticoagulation, a small volume, mechanical ventilation, and low benefit-to-risk ratio. Therapeutic thoracentesis involves removing larger amounts of fluid (no more than 1000 to 1500 ml at one time because edema may occur in the re-expanded underlying lung, especially in cases of tension effusions). Although the classification of "transudate" or "exudate" is not absolute, it is helpful in orienting the directions to follow and suggesting possible diagnosis. To differentiate transudates and exudates, it is cost effective to obtain total protein, lactate dehydrogenase (LDH), white blood cell count (WBC) with differential and either glucose or pH (Table 63–4). *Transudates* are due to imbalances in hydrostatic and oncotic pressures such as seen in congestive heart failure or hypoalbuminemia. They may result from movement of fluid from the peritoneum to the pleural space. *Exudates* (Table 63–5) are defined by the presence of at least one of the following criteria: (1) pleural

TABLE 63–3. MECHANISMS THAT LEAD TO ACCUMULATION OF PLEURAL FLUID

1. Increased hydrostatic pressure in microvascular circulation (congestive heart failure)
2. Decreased oncotic pressure in microvascular circulation (severe hypoalbuminemia)
3. Decreased pressure in the pleural space (complete lung collapse)
4. Increased permeability of the microvascular circulation (pneumonia)
5. Impaired lymphatic drainage from the pleural space (malignant effusion)
6. Movement of fluid from peritoneal space (ascites)

TABLE 63–4. CHARACTERISTICS OF PLEURAL FLUID TRANSUDATES

	Absolute Value	Pleural Fluid/ Serum Value
Protein	< 3 g/dl	< 0.5
Lactate dehydrogenase (LDH)	< 200 IU/L	< 0.6
Glucose	> 60 mg/dl	1.0
White blood cell count	< 1000	—

TABLE 63–5. CORRELATION OF PLEURAL FLUID EXUDATE FINDINGS AND CAUSATIVE DISEASE

Tests	Disease(s)
pH < 7.2	Empyema, malignancy, esophageal rupture; rheumatoid, lupus, and tuberculous pleuritis
Glucose (< 60 mg/dl)	Infection, rheumatoid pleurisy, tuberculous and lupus effusions, esophageal rupture
Amylase (> 200 μ/dl)	Pancreatic disease, esophageal rupture, malignancy, ruptured ectopic pregnancy
Rheumatoid factor, ANA, LE cells	Collagen vascular diseases
Complement (decreased)	Lupus erythematosus, rheumatoid arthritis
Red blood cells (> 5000/μl)	Trauma, malignancy, pulmonary embolus
Chylous effusion (triglycerides > 110 mg/dl)	Violation of thoracic duct (trauma, malignancy)
Biopsy (+)	Malignancy, tuberculosis

fluid/serum protein ratio > 0.5; (2) pleural fluid/serum LDH ratio of < 0.6, and (3) pleural fluid LDH greater than two thirds of serum LDH. The diagnoses that can be established by thoracentesis include malignancy, empyema (pus), tuberculosis (positive acid-fast bacillus for smear or cultures), fungal infection (positive KOH or culture), lupus pleuritis (LE cells), chylothorax (high triglycerides or presence of chylomicrons), urinothorax (pleural fluid/serum creatinine ratio > 1), and esophageal rupture (increased pleural fluid amylase and pH around 6.0). Because many diagnoses produce overlapping values, acid-fast and Gram stains, aerobic and anaerobic cultures, cell count and differential, and cytologic analysis should be included in the study of these effusions. A predominance of polymorphonuclear leukocytes is most compatible with bacterial infection, whereas lymphocytes (particularly with paucity of mesothelial cells) suggest tuberculosis. Lymphocytes are also seen in lymphoma and leukemic effusions. Eosinophils are nonspecific and suggest longstanding fluid. A bloody effusion when not due to trauma is most likely due to malignancy or pulmonary infarction. A white effusion suggests either chyle, cholesterol, or lymphoma. A black fluid suggests aspergillosis. A yellow-green color may be seen in rheumatoid pleurisy. A putrid odor is diagnostic of anaerobic empyema, whereas an ammonia odor suggests urinothorax. The value of other diagnostic markers such as adenosine deaminase (ADA), β_2-microglobulin, and lysozyme remain to be determined. The complications of thoracentesis include pain, bleeding (local, pleural, or abdominal), pneumothorax, infection, and spleen or liver puncture. With therapeutic thoracentesis, up to 50% of patients experience a temporary fall in Pa_{O_2} of as much as 20 mm Hg.

Percutaneous Pleural Biopsy. Biopsy is indicated to evaluate patients with undiagnosed exudative effusion (particularly those with lymphocytic predominance) because the most frequently diagnosed disease is malignancy or tuberculosis (TB). The procedure is performed under local anesthesia using a hook type needle (Cope or Abrams). The contraindications are a small or loculated pleural effusion, an uncooperative patient, and anticoagulation or bleeding diathesis including azotemia with abnormal bleeding time. Because pleural seeding may not be uniform, multiple samples are needed. The overall diagnostic yield is around 60% for malignancy and 75% for TB.

Exploration of the Pleura. In most of the 5 to 10% of patients with undiagnosed effusion, the effusion itself disappears spontaneously or the cause becomes evident. When it is considered necessary to make a diagnosis, a biopsy can be obtained through thoracoscopy (introducing a rigid scope with a cold light source). Thoracoscopy may be performed under local anesthesia and has a high yield (> 85%). In some other cases it is necessary to perform an open pleural biopsy under general anesthesia. The main advantage is the possibility of obtaining larger specimens and concomitant lung tissue.

TRANSUDATIVE EFFUSION. Congestive heart failure is the most common cause and results from biventricular failure with venous hypertension. Effusions are often bilateral, usually larger on the right, and on the chest roentgenogram are associated with vascular congestion and cardiomegaly. In chronic heart failure (months) the total protein may be > 3 grams per deciliter. Thoracentesis is indicated if the patient is febrile, the effusion is large and unilateral, or there is pain or unexplained hypoxemia. Transudates occur in 5 to 10% of patients with liver cirrhosis, secondary to movement of ascitic fluid through diaphragmatic defects or lymphatic channels. The effusion is more frequent on the right (70%). If in doubt, radioactive tracer injected in the ascitic fluid shows up in the chest. The effusion often improves with improvement of the ascites. Occasionally, chemical pleurodesis has effectively relieved symptomatic, recurrent effusions. The transudate seen in up to 20% of patients with nephrotic syndrome is due to decreased oncotic pressure (hypoalbuminemia) and increased hydrostatic forces. Frequently bilateral, it improves by correcting the protein-losing nephropathy. Peritoneal dialysis and atelectasis may also cause transudative effusions. The rarely seen urinothorax is an ipsilateral pleural transudate that occurs with urinary system obstruction. The effusion has the characteristic odor of urine. Relieving the obstruction promptly resolves the effusion.

EXUDATIVE EFFUSIONS. *Infections.* Parapneumonic effusion (pleural fluid associated with pneumonia or lung abscess) is the most common cause of exudates. They may be uncomplicated, which resolve spontaneously or with antibiotics, or complicated, which require drainage. Complicated effusions are rich in white cells (empyema) and/or have positive Gram stains or cultures. Uncomplicated effusions are usually small, contain moderate amounts of polymorphonuclear neutrophils (PMN's), a glucose similar to blood, a pH > 7.30, and an LDH < 500 units per liter. In contrast, complicated effusions have large numbers of PMN's, many times > 100,000 per cubic millimeter, pH < 7.20, glucose < 40 grams per deciliter, and LDH > 1000. If the effusion is also purulent and has bacteria, immediate drainage is necessary. The more of these criteria the effusion has, the more likely it is that drainage is needed. Drainage itself is best achieved with a chest tube. If the fever persists over 48 to 72 hours, either the drainage is inadequate (such as when fluid becomes loculated), the antibiotic is inappropriate, or the diagnosis is wrong. If drainage is not effective because of loculation, inserting an additional tube or instilling intrapleural streptokinase has been effective. Poorly treated empyemas may result in communications with the bronchial tree (bronchopleural fistula) or skin (bronchopleurocutaneous fistula). These require surgical therapy (open drainage with rib resection, decortication, and extensive reconstruction). In some patients with uncontrolled pleural sepsis, a thoracotomy with drainage and decortication may be life-saving. Pleural involvement by nonbacterial, nontuberculous infection is uncommon and when present is usually small. Fungal diseases rarely affect the pleura except for coccidioidomycosis, which may cause a hypersensitivity pleuritis.

Other Infective-Inflammatory Disorders. Exudative effusions may result from subdiaphragmatic processes such as upper abdominal abscess, of which a subphrenic site is the most common location. Frequently postoperative in origin, they may result from hepatic diseases and gastrointestinal perforations. The patients are usually febrile and dyspneic and manifest elevated hemidiaphragm with ipsilateral splinting. Abscesses may also arise in the liver or spleen. Antibiotics alone may not be sufficient; drainage may be necessary. Pancreatitis and pancreatic pseudocyst can cause pleural effusions, more often on the left or bilaterally. These exudates may be blood tinged. The amylase level is higher than that in the serum. They tend to resolve as the pancreatic problem improves. Esophageal rupture is an urgent cause of pleural effusion. Close to half of cases are secondary to endoscopy or esophageal dilatation. They may also be secondary to a foreign body or trauma or occur spontaneously (Boerhaave's syndrome). Patients complain of chest pain, dyspnea, and dysphagia. Fever is universal, and half have subcutaneous emphysema. The roentgenogram may confirm the emphysema and may show pneumothorax, more frequent on the left. Pleural effusion occurs in 75% of patients, with the findings depending on the time of thoracentesis. Early on the exudate has abundant PMN's, followed by high concentrations of salivary amylase. Later, anaerobic mouth organisms seed the space, and the pH approaches 6.0. The diagnosis is established by using barium sulfate or water-soluble compounds. Early diagnosis and prompt surgical correction result in >90% survival. If surgical closure is delayed, antibiotics for anaerobes, parenteral nutrition, and mediastinal and pleural drainage are necessary.

TUBERCULOSIS. Pleural effusion occurs in most cases of pulmonary TB but is frequently inapparent. The effusion may accompany the primary infection, in which case it is serous and results from a hypersensitivity phenomenon. These patients, usually febrile, may recover without treatment, but close to two thirds develop active TB within 5 years. A second form occurs when a subpleural focus of *Mycobacterium tuberculosis* ruptures into the pleural space. The fluid is usually rich in protein (>4 grams per deciliter), with a leukocyte count around 5000 cells (90 to 95% lymphocytes). A PMN predominance may occur the first few days after the bacillus reaches the pleural space. The glucose may be low, but rarely lower than 20 mg per deciliter. The pH ranges between 7.00 and 7.30, with pH >7.40 virtually excluding TB. The fluid is characteristically free of mesothelial cells. Recently, the presence of adenosine deaminase and lysozyme has been found to correlate with TB. Using an enzyme-linked immunosorbent assay (ELISA) or polymerase chain reaction (PCR) to demonstrate mycobacterial antigen is gaining acceptability. Acid-fast bacilli in a smear are seen in <10% of cases. Multiple samples from a closed pleural biopsy are positive in 50 to 80% of cases, whereas positive cultures range from 30 to 70%. With all methods combined, the yield is close to 95%. The clinical presentation simulates an acute pneumonia (60% of cases) with fever, nonproductive cough (80%), chest pain (75%), or a subacute or chronic fever. Chest roentgenogram shows small to moderate effusion (4% are large), with parenchymal disease seen in one third of cases. Intermediate-strength PPD is positive in 70% of patients, and if repeated after 6 to 8 weeks it may become positive in those with a prior negative test. Treatment results in resolution of the fever within 2 weeks but may persist for 6 or 8 weeks. The effusion resolves by 6 weeks but may persist for 3 to 4 months. Very ill patients may be helped by short-term corticosteroid treatment. Rarely surgical drainage of tuberculous empyema or decortication may be necessary.

OTHER INFECTIOUS EFFUSIONS. Actinomycosis (see Ch. 306) caused by the anaerobic organism *Actinomyces israelii* may cause purulent effusions. They may bulge the thoracic wall and drain through the chest. Sulfur granules (whitish yellow or brown interwoven filaments) can be identified in the fluid. Pleural effusions are also common in *Nocardia* infection (see Ch. 307). The effusion is usually purulent with abundant PMN's. Sulfonamides are the treatment of choice. Aspergillosis (see Ch. 355) of the pleura is uncommon, but an inflammatory, thickened pleura is frequently seen in progressive invasive aspergillosis. Pleural effusions due to parasitic diseases are still uncommon but are increasing among Third World immigrants. Paragonimiasis (see Ch. 386) causes pleural thickening or effusion in up to 48% of patients. This effusion has a triad of low glucose (<10 grams per deciliter), high LDH (>1000 units per liter) and low pH (<7.10). Complement-fixation antibodies >1:64 are diagnostic. Amebiasis and echinococcosis are rare.

HEMOTHORAX. Frank blood in the pleural space (hematocrit >20%) is usually the result of trauma, hemothorax, hematologic disorders, or pleural malignancies. Left-sided pneumothorax, particularly with a widened mediastinum, may indicate rupture of the aorta. Pleural blood often does not clot and can be readily removed by lymphatics if small. Larger effusions require tube drainage. Persistent bleeding requires surgical correction.

CHYLOTHORAX. Leakage of the lymph (chyle) from the thoracic duct most commonly results from mediastinal malignancy (50%), lymphoma being the most frequent. It may also result from thoracic surgery (20%) or trauma (5%). Because chyle collects within the posterior mediastinum, the chylothorax may not appear for days, until the mediastinal pleura ruptures. The usual milky appearance of the effusion may be confused with a cholesterol effusion or effusion with many leukocytes. The best diagnostic criterion is the presence of a triglyceride concentration >110 mg per deciliter, with rare instances of values between 50 and 110 mg per deciliter. The major complications are malnutrition and immunologic compromise, as fat, protein, and lymphocytes are depleted with repeated thoracentesis or chest tube drainage. Treatment

should include draining the pleural space, decreasing chyle formation by intravenous hyperalimentation, and decreasing oral intake, possibly adding medium-chain triglycerides, which are directly absorbed into the portal circulation. Thoracic duct ligation should be considered if the cause is traumatic. If secondary to tumor, the treatment should be that of the primary cause. The triad of slow-growing yellow nails, lymphedema, and pleural effusion (yellow-nail syndrome) is due to hypoplastic or dilated lymphatics.

IMMUNOLOGIC CAUSES OF PLEURAL EFFUSIONS. Clinical rheumatoid pleurisy occurs in close to 5% of patients with rheumatoid disease (see Ch. 241), even though autopsy studies suggest up to 50% involvement. It has a male predominance and appears within 5 years after onset of the disease; nevertheless, effusions have occurred up to 20 years before the onset of articular disease. The fluid is an exudate with low glucose (<30 mg per deciliter) and pH and a high LDH. The complement level is usually low, with high titers of rheumatoid factors. The patient may complain of pleuritic pain or dyspnea. Fever is not common, in contrast with lupus pleuritis. The effusion does not resolve quickly but rather over months and occasionally persists over years. The major complication is fibrosis with lung trapping so that anti-inflammatory agents and corticosteroids may be tried. Pleuritic pain or effusion can be the presenting manifestation in 5% of patients with systemic lupus erythematosus (SLE) and occurs at some point in the course in close to 50% of patients. Pain (86%), cough (64%), dyspnea (50%), pleural friction rub (71%), and fever (57%) are commonly seen. The effusions are exudates that in the majority of cases have normal pH and glucose. The hemolytic complement (especially C3 and C4 components) are low, and classic LE cells may be present. LE pleuritis is likely if ANA in the fluid is >1:160. Spontaneous resolution of LE pleuritis is uncommon but usually disappears within 2 weeks after beginning corticosteroids. Sarcoidosis, Wegener's granulomatosis, Sjögren's syndrome, and immunoblastic lymphadenopathy (see Ch. 54) are rare causes of pleural effusions.

OTHER CONDITIONS. *Asbestosis* (see Ch. 54.1). This is frequently associated with pleural disease. It is often unilateral, small, and serosanguineous. The cell count is <6000 cells per microliter, with either PMN's or mononuclear predominance. Eosinophilia of up to 50% of cells has been described. The diagnosis is suspected with known exposure. Exclusion of malignant mesothelioma in the presence of pleural plaques may be difficult and requires follow-up of 2 to 3 years. The effusion tends to resolve in 1 month to 1 year, leaving a blunted angle in >90% of patients, with 50% showing diffuse pleural thickening. Calcification of the plaques occurs late (20 to 40 years after exposure). Close to 5% of patients may have underlying pulmonary parenchymal asbestosis.

Meigs' Syndrome. This consists of the triad of benign fibroma or other ovarian tumors, ascites, and large effusions (usually on the right side). Most commonly seen after menopause, the symptoms are malaise, chest pain, and increased abdominal girth. Fluid moves from the abdomen through small diaphragmatic defects or lymphatics. The fluid is usually an exudate with a paucity of mononuclear cells. When suspected, besides the pelvic examination, an abdominal CT scan documents the ovarian tumor. Removing it resolves the effusion within 2 to 3 weeks.

Uremia. In contrast to the urinothorax and hydrothorax of the nephrotic syndrome, the effusion of uremia accompanies a polyserositis. It is usually a bloody exudate that resolves with treatment of the uremia. Repeated thoracentesis may be needed if the patient is symptomatic (dyspnea, cough, chest pain).

Other causes of inflammatory effusions include radiation therapy, esophageal sclerotherapy, enteral feeding misplacement, drug-induced pleural disease (nitrofurantoin, dantrolene, methysergide, methotrexate, procarbazine, amiodarone, practolol, mitomycin, bleomycin, and minoxidil). Pleuritis in a lupus-like syndrome has been associated with procainamide, hydralazine, isoniazid, and quinidine. It usually resolves after discontinuing the medicine and may occasionally require corticosteroids.

MALIGNANCY. Malignant effusions probably are the most common cause of exudate in patients over age 60. Invasion by lung cancer is the most frequent, whereas spread from liver metastasis or chest wall lymphatic invasion is the most frequent mechanism in breast cancer. Ovarian and gastric cancer represent close to 5%, whereas 7% may have an unknown primary at time of diagnosis. Patients may be asymptomatic or develop cough, pain, and dyspnea. The effusion is an exudate with abundant red cells (30,000 to 50,000 per milliliter and mononuclear cells (lymphocytes >50%). Occasionally (5 to 10%) they are transudative, and close to one third may have pH <7.3 or glucose <60 mg per deciliter. Cytology is positive in close to 60% of cases, but biopsy increases the yield only to 70%. Thoracentesis should be repeated if the diagnosis is still suspected. Malignant pleural effusion carries a very poor prognosis, with the exception of breast and small cell carcinoma of the lung, both of which may respond temporarily to therapy. The best method, short of pleurectomy or pleural abrasion, to control recurrent malignant effusion consists of instilling tetracycline intrapleurally after chest tube drainage.

Lymphomas may cause exudative effusions, frequently diagnostic in the case of non-Hodgkin's lymphoma. Mediastinal invasion with lymphatic blockage and effusion on this basis is suggestive of Hodgkin's lymphoma. Although the prognosis in these patients is poor, they frequently respond to chemotherapy.

MALIGNANT MESOTHELIOMA. This is related to asbestos exposure in 80 to 90% of cases. Patients may present with dyspnea, cough, weight loss, and pain. Smoking is not a factor. The tumors often encase the underlying lung. The effusion may be massive and often bloody and in 70% of cases have pH <7.30. Cytology is controversial because even when positive, it may be difficult to differentiate from metastatic carcinoma. Elevated levels of hyaluronic acid and special stains and electromicroscopy of biopsy tissue may help in the diagnosis. Median survival is 6 to 12 months after diagnosis. Malignant mesotheliomas may be confused with benign mesothelioma, which have the histology of a fibroma. Benign mesotheliomas may reach a large size and be pedunculated (migrating with position changes). They are often associated with hypertrophic pulmonary osteoarthropathy and clubbing. Treatment involves surgically removing the mass.

PNEUMOTHORAX. Pneumothorax is defined as an accumulation of gas in the pleural space. It may be caused by (1) perforation of the visceral pleura and entry of gas from the lung; (2) penetration of the chest wall, diaphragm, mediastinum, or esophagus; or (3) gas generated by microorganisms in an empyema. When gas originates in the lung, the rupture may occur in the absence of known disease (simple pneumothorax) or as a result of parenchymal disease (secondary pneumothorax).

Simple spontaneous pneumothorax occurs most commonly in previously healthy men aged 20 to 40 and is due to spontaneous rupture of subpleural blebs at the apex of the lungs. The right lung is more frequently involved, and recurrence is frequent (30% ipsilateral, 10% contralateral). Patients usually present with acute pain, dyspnea (related to size of pneumothorax), and cough. Physical examination shows decreased breath sounds and tactile fremitus with ipsilateral hyperresonance. The chest roentgenogram classically shows the visceral pleural line, but small pneumothoraces may become evident only with expiratory or lateral decubitus film. Small amounts of fluid (sometimes blood) are present in 25% of patients.

Tension pneumothorax (caused by increased positive pressure through a "ball-valve" air leak) can cause mediastinal shift and compromise circulation. With small pneumothorax (<20% of the hemithorax) in an asymptomatic patient, observation may suffice because it reabsorbs in 7 to 14 days. Larger pneumothoraces can be treated with air aspiration. Pneumothorax that occupies >50% of the hemithorax, symptomatic patients, or tension pneumothorax requires a chest tube, which can be connected to suction or placed under water seal. The tube should be left in for 2 to 4 days until the leak seals. Because of frequent recurrences, chemical pleurodesis or surgical correction may be necessary.

Secondary or complicated pneumothorax results from trauma or pulmonary diseases. Widespread emphysema is the most common cause, but it may result from rupture of an abscess with spillage of pus into the pleural space (pyopneumothorax). Less frequently but also seen are asthma, certain interstitial lung diseases (idiopathic fibrosis, eosinophilic granulomatosis, sarcoidosis, tuberous sclerosis), neoplasms (sarcoma, bronchogenic carcinoma), some rare diseases such as Marfan's and Ehlers-Danlos syndromes, and endometriosis (catamenial pneumothorax). Iatrogenic injuries (e.g., insertion of central lines) and barotrauma are frequently seen in the intensive care unit. The patient should be hospitalized and a chest tube inserted because spontaneous expansion is rare and the decreased reserve resulting from the pneumothorax may cause ventilatory com-

promise. Surgery must not be taken lightly because the rate of complications is high, but it may be life-saving in some patients. In patients on ventilatory support, a pneumothorax is always under tension and requires immediate insertion of a chest tube. If a bronchopleural fistula persists, a portion of the minute ventilation exits through it; hence, it is necessary to increase ventilation to compensate for this loss. For severe leak, high-frequency low-pressure ventilation or synchronized chest tube occlusion may be helpful. Frequent complications of chest tube insertion include re-expansion pulmonary edema, lung trauma or infarction, subcutaneous emphysema, bleeding, and infection.

Light RW: Management of spontaneous pneumothorax. Am Rev Respir Dis 148:245, 1993. *Reviews the pathogenesis and treatment of pneumothorax. Summarizes results of the VA study of 118 patients.*
Light RW, MacGregor MI, Luchsinger PC, et al.: Pleural effusions: The diagnostic separation of transudates and exudates. Ann Intern Med 77:507, 1977. *Classic paper that separates effusions into transudative or exudative on the basis of pleural fluid to serum ratios of LDH and protein.*
O'Rourke JP, Yee E: Civilian spontaneous pneumothorax: Treatment options and long-term results. Chest 96:1302, 1989. *Retrospective review of 130 patients with discussion of therapeutic options.*
Pistolesi M, Miniati M, Giuntini C: Pleural liquid and solute exchange. Am Rev Respir Dis 140:825, 1989. *It summarizes the new concepts that have increased the importance of lymphatic drainage for fluid and solute exchange.*
Sahn SA: The pleura: State of the art. Am Rev Respir Dis 138:184, 1988. *Extensive in-depth review of pleural effusions: cause, presentation, and differential diagnosis. With 594 references, the most complete review.*
Wied U, Halkier E, Holier-Madson K, et al.: Tetracycline versus silver nitrate pleurodesis in spontaneous pneumothorax. J Thorac Cardiovasc Surg 86:591, 1983. *Controlled trial that determined superiority of tetracycline over silver nitrate.*

MEDIASTINUM

The mediastinum is the anatomic space that lies in the midthorax and separates the two pleural cavities. It is limited by the diaphragm below and the suprasternal thoracic outlet above. The mediastinum contains several vital structures in a small space. Thus, regardless of the cause, mediastinal abnormalities can produce important symptoms. For clinical purposes it is convenient to divide the mediastinum into anterior, middle, and posterior (Fig. 63–1). The anterior compartment contains the thymus, substernal extensions of the thyroid and parathyroid glands, blood vessels, pericardium, and lymph nodes. The middle compartment contains the heart, great vessels, trachea, main bronchi, lymph nodes, and phrenic and vagus nerves. The posterior compartment contains the vertebrae, descending aorta, esophagus, thoracic duct, azygous and hemizygous veins, lower portion of the vagus, sympathetic chains, and posterior mediastinal nodes.

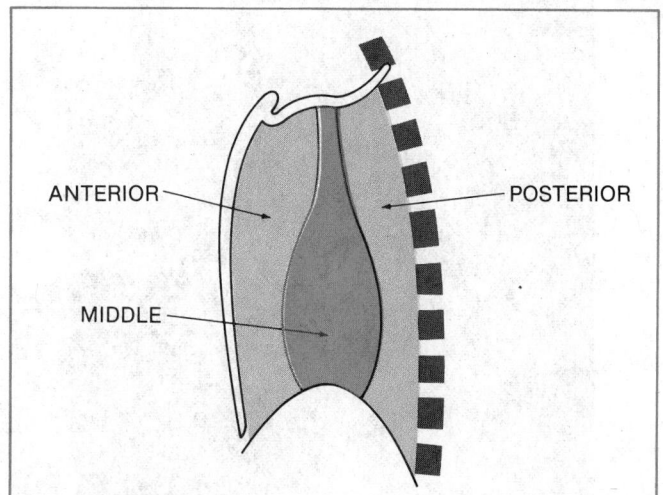

FIGURE 63–1. Anatomic compartments of the mediastinum. The anterior compartment is bound posteriorly by the pericardium, ascending aorta, and brachiocephalic vessels and anteriorly by the sternum. The middle compartment extends from the posterior limits of the anterior compartment to the posterior pericardial line. The posterior compartment extends from the pericardial line to the dorsal chest wall.

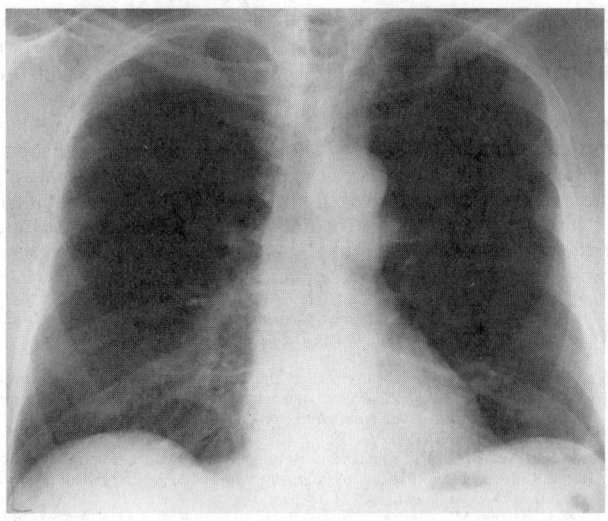

FIGURE 63–2. Posteroanterior roentgenogram of a patient with a mass in the superior portion of the anterior mediastinum.

SIGNS AND SYMPTOMS. Most patients with mediastinal masses are asymptomatic, and the finding is incidental on a chest roentgenogram obtained for another reason. The most common symptoms are chest pain, cough, hoarseness, and dyspnea, whereas stridor, dysphagia, and Horner's syndrome are less frequent. Occasionally some syndromes are associated with a primary mediastinal lesion. Myasthenia gravis is seen in nearly half of thymoma patients. Hypoglycemia has been seen in patients with mesotheliomas, fibrosarcomas, and teratomas. Parathyroid tumors may induce hypercalcemia, whereas neurogenic tumors may cause neurologic symptoms. The physical examination is usually nonspecific. The mass may produce superior vena caval obstruction with facial edema, dilated veins, and arm edema. The masses may erode trachea, esophagus, and great vessels with life-threatening consequences.

DIAGNOSIS. Most mediastinal masses are detected on a plain chest roentgenogram (Figs. 63–2 and 63–3). Chest CT is the initial

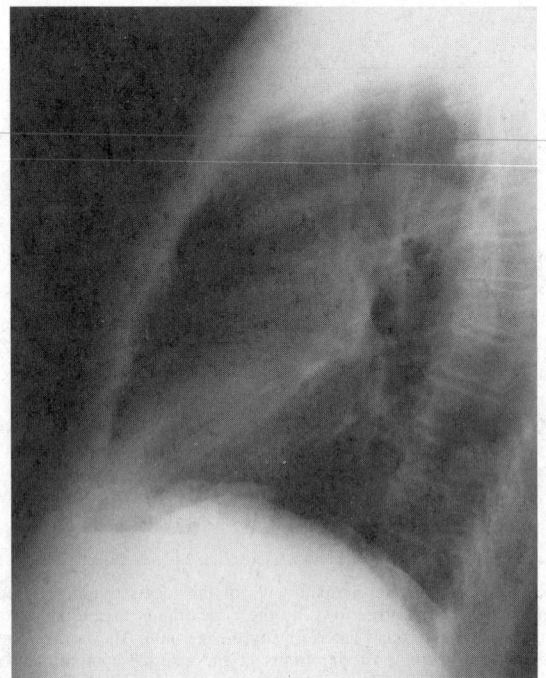

FIGURE 63–3. Lateral chest radiograph of same patient as in Figure 63–2.

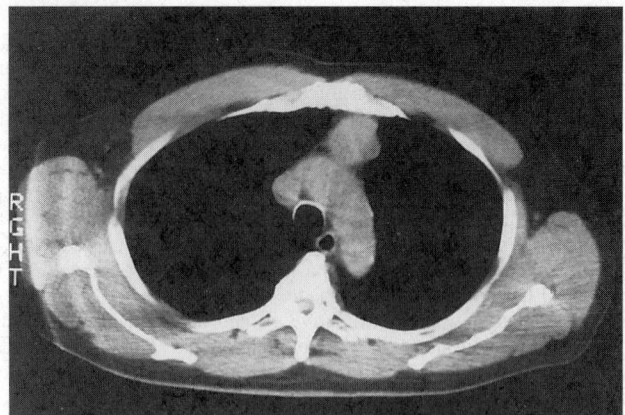

FIGURE 63–4. CT of same patient as in Figures 63–2 and 63–3. The mass proved to be a thymoma. (Courtesy of Elon Gale, M.D., Department of Radiology, Boston Veterans Affairs Medical Center.)

procedure of choice (Fig. 63–4) because it provides good definition of mediastinal structures. If the patient is asymptomatic and the noninvasive information obtained by CT—with and without contrast—suggests a benign process, careful follow-up is justified. The radiologic evaluation may include angiography and an esophagogram. The role of magnetic resonance imaging (MRI) is currently being investigated, specifically for evaluating vessels and blood flow without contrast solution. In some patients it may be necessary to obtain tissue for histologic diagnosis. Classically, anterior and middle compartment lesions are reached through mediastinoscopy or mediastinotomy. Thoracotomy may be needed for middle and posterior compartment lesions or when surgery is the treatment of choice for the suspected lesion. Direct sampling using fluoroscopy or CT-guided needle aspiration has proven useful in patients whose underlying conditions make thoracotomy or mediastinoscopy a risky procedure.

SPECIFIC DISEASES. Tumors. The most common cause of a mediastinal mass in older patients is a metastatic carcinoma (most commonly bronchogenic carcinoma). In young adults primary mediastinal pathology is more frequent. The common origin of tumors by location is shown in Table 63–6.

Neurogenic tumors located in the posterior mediastinum are the most common (20%). Nonspecific chest pain and nonproductive cough with occasional compression of intercostal nerves and trachea and bronchi are the most frequent symptoms. Most tumors are benign, originating in the nerve sheath (neurilemoma, neurofibroma) or sympathetic ganglion cells (ganglioneuroma). Neuroblastoma (malignant tumor of sympathetic ganglion cells) has a better prognosis than the same tumor occurring in the adrenals. Neurofibromas may occur in association with von Recklinghausen's disease. Ganglioneuromas and neuroblastomas may secrete hormones that cause flushing, diarrhea, and hypertension. Pheochromocytomas may occasionally arise in the mediastinum. Neurogenic tumors should be resected and postoperative radiation given to neuroblastomas.

Lymphoreticular. Thymomas account for 20% of mediastinal tumors and are located in the superior portion of the anterior mediastinum. Two thirds of them are malignant. Myasthenia gravis is seen in 40% of cases, and other paraneoplastic syndromes such as Cushing's, refractory anemia, and hypogammaglobulinemia have been reported. All thymomas should be regarded as malignant and

TABLE 63–6. MOST FREQUENT CAUSES OF MEDIASTINAL MASSES

Anterior	Middle	Posterior
Thymona	Lymphoma	Neurogenic tumors
Lymphoma	Cancer	Enteric cysts
Teratogenic tumors	Cysts	Esophageal lesions
Thyroid	Aneurysms	Aneurysms
Parathyroid aneurysms	Hernia (Morgagni)	Diaphragmatic hernias (Bochdalek)

surgical resection should be followed with radiation. Lymphatic tumors (17%) also arise in the anterior mediastinum. Hodgkin's lymphoma is the most frequent and carries the best prognosis. Non-Hodgkin's lymphoma, plasmacytomas, and angiomatous lymphoid hamartomas with similar clinical presentation carry a worse prognosis. Teratomatous tumors comprise 10% of mediastinal tumors, and one third of them are malignant. Also located in the anterior compartment, they are embryologically and histologically linked to the thymus. Cystic teratomas are more frequent and may contain squamous cells, hair follicles, sweat glands, cartilage, and linear calcifications. Intrathoracic goiter (10%) is usually a benign nodular or follicular enlargement of the thyroid gland. Three quarters of patients present with stridor, cough, and dyspnea. Most frequently located in the anterior mediastinum, they occasionally cause superior vena cava syndrome. Benign cysts are usually asymptomatic and occur as an incidental radiographic finding. Bronchogenic cysts develop around the paratracheal area or carina and are seen in the middle and posterior compartments. They are filled with liquid and are lined with respiratory epithelium and cartilage but do not communicate with the tracheobronchial tree. Pericardial cysts occur in the anterior compartment and cardiophrenic angle. They contain clear liquid and flattened endothelial or mesothelial lining with a bland fibrous wall. Enteric cysts are located in the posterior mediastinum and are lined by gastric or intestinal epithelium. All cysts may become infected, bleed, or rupture into the mediastinum or pleural cavity.

Vascular tumors may have a primary origin in the mediastinum. The vascular hamartomas, lymphangiomas, and hemangiomas are benign tumors, whereas hemangiopericytomas are malignant. Mesenchymal benign (lipoma) or malignant (liposarcoma, mesothelioma, rhabdomyosarcoma, and mesenchymoma) masses rarely cause mediastinal masses.

Hernias through the diaphragm may also show as mediastinal masses. They may be retrosternal through the foramen of Morgagni, posterolateral through the foramen of Bochdalek, or most commonly through the esophageal hiatus. When gas is contained in the herniated organ, the presumptive diagnosis is easily made.

Pneumomediastinum. This may occur secondary to a tear in the esophagus or tracheobronchial tree or from dissecting air from ruptured alveoli. Tears in esophagus and tracheobronchial tree commonly have a traumatic origin, whereas alveolar rupture may occur spontaneously or as a complication of artificial ventilation. Air may track to the neck and the body, producing subcutaneous emphysema, or may cause pneumothorax. The patient complains of retrosternal pain and dyspnea. There may be subcutaneous emphysema with the classic crepitus. Auscultation may reveal a crunching sound synchronous with the heart beat (Hamman's sign). Rarely, cardiac function is compromised. A lateral chest roentgenogram is usually diagnostic. Simple spontaneous pneumomediastinum usually resolves without treatment. When severe or resulting from organ rupture, surgical drainage and repair are required.

Superior Vena Cava Syndrome (SVC). This results from obstruction of blood flow through the superior vena cava. Besides dilatation of collateral veins of the upper thorax and neck and edema and congestion of face, patients may have headache, dyspnea, dysphagia, and wheezes. Malignancy is the most frequent cause of SVC, with bronchogenic carcinoma responsible for >70% of cases and lymphoma a distant second. Fibrosing mediastinitis after granulomatous diseases such as histoplasmosis or associated with methysergide ingestion can also be seen. Aortic aneurysm and retrosternal thyroid are relatively benign causes of SVC. Because of vessel dilatation, invasive procedures are contraindicated. An effort must be made to obtain tissue elsewhere, and irradiation or chemotherapy should be begun before attempts are made to obtain mediastinal tissue.

Benjamin SP, McCormack LJ, Effler DB, et al.: Primary tumors of the mediastinum. Chest 67:297, 1972. *Excellent experience on 215 patients with mediastinal tumors managed by two surgeons. It establishes the prevalence and localization of primary mediastinal masses.*

Putgatch RD, Faling LJ, Robbins AH, et al.: CT diagnosis of benign mediastinal abnormalities. Am J Roentgenol 135:685, 1980. *Examines the evidence supporting the concept that CT scan of the thorax should be the initial procedure used to evaluate mediastinal masses.*

Weisbrod GL: Percutaneous fine needle aspiration biopsy of the mediastinum. Clin Chest Med 8:27, 1987. *Reviews the experience with fluoroscopy and CT-guided needle aspiration. It reiterates that experience and good cytopathologic interpretation are important for a successful procedure.*

64 UPPER AIRWAY DISEASES
Kingman P. Strohl

The nose, ears, pharynx, and larynx are involved in such functions as conducting airflow to and from the lungs, taste, deglutition, speech, hearing, and smell. These chambered, highly specialized structures develop from the foregut and second through fourth branchial arches and are highly served by neural systems for motor control and sensation. Disease in any segment of the upper airway can have several functional consequences, and loss of any function can arise from both local processes and neural mechanisms. Because the larynx and pharynx act in series as the conducting airway to the trachea, bronchi, and the more distal gas-exchanging units of the lungs, dyspnea and air hunger result from swelling, encroachment, or neural dysfunction of these segments. Other presentations of upper airway disease include rhinorrhea and nasal obstruction, sneezing, postnasal and pharyngeal secretions, cough, dysphagia, changes in voice, swelling of the upper and lower jaw, hearing loss, tinnitus, snoring and apneas during sleep, epistaxis, and pain.

Anatomic and functional assessments often reveal the cause of symptoms. For example, muffled speech and drooling in the presence of neck or jaw swelling indicate encroachment of the pharyngeal airway and require assessment and monitoring of airway patency. Watching the patient with dysphagia while he/she drinks and eats may differentiate a neural from an anatomic process. Examining the upper airways requires an appreciation of the anatomic complexities of the area and a facility with the otoscope, tongue blade, tuning fork, and manual (gloved!) palpation of the mouth. Knowledge of salivary gland and lymph node locations, bimanual examination of the floor of the mouth, and percussion of the teeth are needed to distinguish among periodontal abscess, mandibular swelling, fracture, or tumor. Referral to the appropriate specialist (orthodontist, oral surgeon, or otolaryngologist) saves time, prevents progression and complications, and/or avoids unnecessary procedures.

Clues to a systemic illness may arise from examining the upper airways in the absence of symptoms. Nasal polyps are associated with both aspirin-sensitive asthma and cystic fibrosis. Nasal ulceration, nasal drip, and sinusitis may be seen in chronic cocaine use and withdrawal as well as in pulmonary vasculitis, especially that of Wegener's granulomatosis (see Ch. 245). Parotid gland enlargement is associated with sarcoidosis and with collagen vascular diseases. Hereditary hemorrhagic telangiectasia (Rendu-Osler-Weber syndrome) presents to the internist with gastrointestinal bleeding and is characterized by dilated thin-walled capillaries and draining veins seen in the nose, lips, and mouth.

The remainder of this chapter discusses presentations and common diseases found in the upper airway.

HEARING DEFICITS (see Ch. 403.3)

OTITIS (also see Ch. 403.3)

Otitis media may occur at any age; however, the most frequent presentation is under age 10. Presenting symptoms include pain and conductive hearing loss, more often unilateral. In acute presentations, most patients acknowledge a preceding upper respiratory tract infection; symptoms improve with antibiotics. When the presentation is subacute or chronic, treatment is also directed at mechanical factors, such as eustachian tube functional or anatomic obstruction and/or tympanic membrane rupture—as well as using antibiotics. This condition requires surgical collaboration. A list of the more common presentations of otitis media is provided in Table 64–1.

There are special concerns about otitis relevant to internal medicine. First, there may be serious complications from untreated or inadequately treated disease. Infection from the middle ear extending into the mastoid sinus and adjacent structures in the temporal bone may result in unilateral distal facial nerve palsy, osteomyelitis, infection of the basal structures of the skull, and/or intracranial

TABLE 64-1. OTITIS MEDIA

Type	Mechanisms	Treatment
Acute	*Streptococcus pneumoniae,* and *Haemophilus influenzae;* rarely *Staphylococcus aureus, Streptococcus pyogenes, Proteus, Pseudomonas*	Oral antibiotics
Serous	Failure to clear fluid (Starling effect)	Antihistamines and decongestants
Chronic	Persistent eustachian tube obstruction (rarely tuberculosis)	Drainage tubes ± all of the above

extensions, including dural abscess, brain abscess, and meningitis. Patients can present with sepsis and/or coma with increased intracranial pressure. Identifying the infecting organism is crucial. Problems in the inner ear may be addressed surgically, but only after definitive intravenous antibiotic therapy. Second, the spectrum of organisms in immunocompromised hosts is wider than that listed in Table 64-1. In particular, fungal infections (*Aspergillus* and *Candida*) occur and, if undetected, lead to complications. A third special circumstance is patients with longstanding endotracheal or nasogastric intubation. Nasal inflammation can block the eustachian tube and produce otitic and sinus infections with nosocomial organisms. Unexplained fever in the medical intensive care unit should involve examination of the upper airway and, occasionally, radiographic imaging and aspiration of the middle ear or sinuses for culture.

External otitis is characterized by severe pain and discharge from the auditory meatus. In contrast to otitis media, the ear and the tragus are painful to the touch, and otoscopic examination is painful. Often there is a history of water in or trauma to the ear canal. Culture could reveal *Pseudomonas* organisms but usually is not needed. Treatment with topical broad-spectrum antibiotics combined with topical corticosteroids, so-called otic drops, results in resolved symptoms and cure over 3 to 5 days. Oral antibiotics are indicated when regional lymphadenitis or erythema/cellulitis is present.

Infections of the external ear can present more severely in immunocompromised hosts and especially in diabetic patients, who have decreased host defenses and reduced sensation. This condition is sometimes called *"malignant" otitis* (see Ch. 421). Spread of infection from the ear inferiorly results in facial nerve paralysis (not to be dismissed as Bell's palsy); infection of the jugular foramen; involvement of the glossopharyngeal, vagus, and accessory nerves; and infection of the sheath of the jugular vein, with extension inferiorly and contralaterally into the neck and rostrally into the lateral sinus. Medial spread involves the middle ear and the mastoid, and anterior spread to the temporomandibular joint. Broad-spectrum intravenous antibiotics should be promptly instituted. Surgical intervention to identify organisms is indicated when nerve involvement or foreign body obstruction is suspected.

With recurrent external otitis, a history of repetitive trauma or exposure to water (so-called *swimmer's ear*) is likely. In the former, counseling may be needed on proper ear hygiene; in the latter, over-the-counter ear drops containing an alcohol/glycerine mixture can be recommended for use after bathing or swimming.

RHINITIS (also see Ch. 225)

Rhinitis comprises a group of disorders characterized by nasal itching, drip, and obstruction. These symptoms relate to irritation and inflammation of the mucosa and increased nasal secretions. Antigen challenge in susceptible hosts, histamine challenge, or activating nonmyelinated nerves with substance P can reproduce symptoms found in acute allergic reactions and acute rhinitis. Subacute and chronic symptoms and nasal obstruction result from the activation of mucosal prostanoids and cytokine networks to promote the nasal inflammatory response, recruit inflammatory cells, and promote healing. Acute insults take 3 to 5 days to resolve unless bacterial superinfection, concomitant eustachian tube or sinus obstruction, or repeated exposure to a causative noninfectious agent or allergen occurs. A persistent inflammatory state can develop in sus-

ceptible individuals and result in chronic symptoms, nasal polyps, and altered or decreased sense of smell (anosmia).

The most frequent cause of acute rhinitis is the common cold (see Ch. 328). An *upper respiratory tract infection* is usually self-limiting. The severity of viral infections can be attenuated by amantadine or similar agents if taken near the time of exposure. Antihistamines, decongestants, and cool mist relieve symptoms. Topical decongestants like oxymetrazoline, used as directed, relieve nasal obstruction; however, rebound congestion and the potential complications of chronic vascular constriction follow if therapy is prolonged beyond 1 week. Bacterial superinfection presenting as sinusitis or otitis should be suspected if recurrent fever, regional lymphadenopathy, persistent mucopurulent discharge, or persistent symptoms last longer than 5 days. In this instance, oral antibiotics are useful.

SINUSITIS

A mucopurulent discharge and a painful face suggest *sinusitis,* an inflammation of the lining of the paranasal sinuses. Most cases occur as a complication of the common cold or other upper respiratory tract infections, with occasional presentations due to extension of a periodontal infection under the maxillary sinus. Less than 1% of upper respiratory tract infections result in the clinical syndrome of acute sinusitis. Fewer meet the criteria for chronic sinusitis. Sinusitis is more common in adults, perhaps because the paranasal sinuses do not develop fully until the second and third decade of life. Bedside transillumination can suggest the presence of sinusitis. Normal light transmission to the frontal sinus from the supraorbital ridge or to the maxillary sinus through the hard palate excludes sinusitis; reduced or absent transmission is less helpful because considerable intraindividual anatomic variation exists. Radiographic evaluation is relatively sensitive. A coronal computed axial tomography image with bone window settings is the preferred test. Magnetic resonance imaging and ultrasonography have limited but specialized applications. Sinus aspiration and endoscopic sinuscopy may be necessary to recover organisms or to effect drainage. Surgical interventions are indicated for treatment failure, suppurative complications, diagnosis of nosocomial infection, and fever of unknown origin with sinus opacification.

Most causes of sinusitis are bacterial infections such as those that produce otitis (see above). The course of acute sinusitis is 3 to 4 weeks, secondary to the anatomic difficulties in drainage. Decongestants and antihistamines improve nasal obstruction and may improve sinus drainage. Oral antibiotics are often prescribed. Occasionally, surgical interventions are used when disease is chronic and resistant to empiric therapy. Fungal sinusitis is uncommon and presents with a chronic course. *Aspergillus* is most common, but *Candida, Mucor,* and *Penicillium* organisms may be recovered from infected sinus aspirates. Invasive disease with eye, mouth, and brain extension occurs in patients with acquired immunodeficiency disease or on chemotherapy. Finally, *maxillary antrum tumors* produce a unilateral bloody nasal discharge that can be confused with sinusitis. Clues to a malignant process are a chronicity of symptoms, refractoriness to conventional therapy, and the presence of bony destruction of the antrum on radiographic examination.

MASSES, SWELLING, AND PAIN OF THE JAW (also see Ch. 96)

Occasionally the internist sees patients with swelling of the face and jaw. The differential diagnosis is based on careful history and examination. Duration of symptoms, presence of a fever, history of local trauma, orthodontic difficulties, shortness of breath, or dysphagia may help localize lesions and identify potential complications (see above). The anatomic locations of the salivary glands and lymph nodes are distinct (Fig. 64-1). The site of swelling of the jaw is determined on physical examination by palpation, running the finger intraorally along the inner and outer borders of the mandible, and comparing the right and left sides. Inspection and tooth percussion with a metal rod localize periodontal processes.

Fracture of the lower jaw usually presents with a history of trauma, although sometimes minor in nature. Jaw fractures are treated like compound fractures because the teeth communicate with the oral cavity. Occasionally, soft tissue swelling from secondary infection obscures a fracture. *Aseptic necrosis* caused by a vascular disease or a mandibular hairline fracture can also present with swelling and pain. *Periodontal abscess* results from poor dental hygiene or tooth trauma, particularly in the elderly, the diabetic,

LYMPH NODES   SALIVARY GLANDS

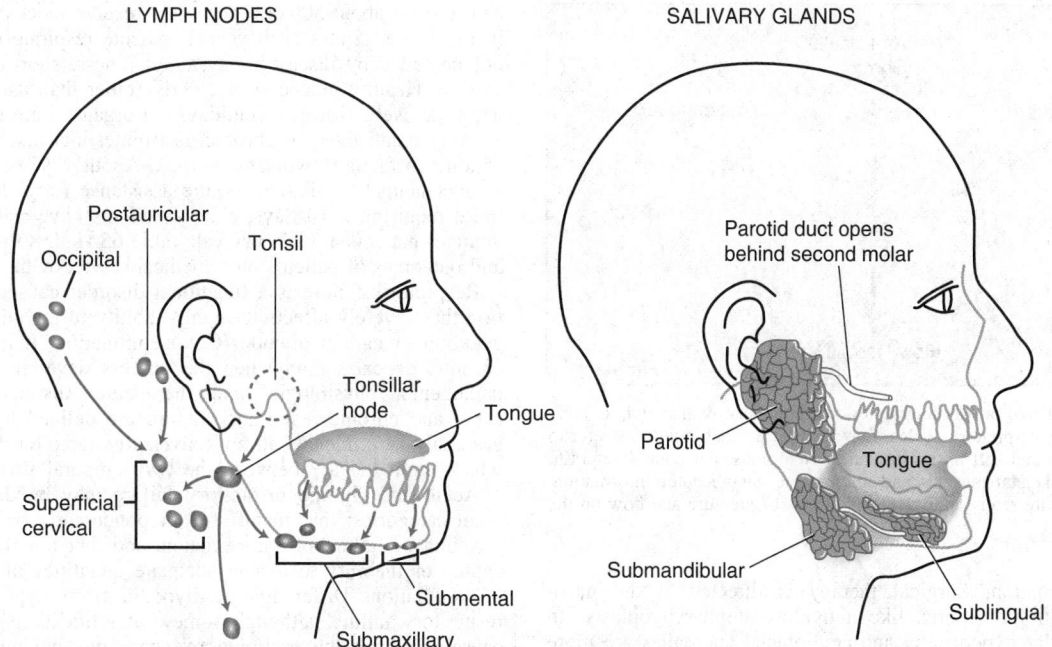

FIGURE 64-1. Approximate position of the lymph nodes *(left)* and the salivary glands *(right)*. Arrows indicate routes of lymphatic drainage.

or the immunocompromised host. Complications result from periodontal abscess because infection can track rapidly along tissue planes to the basal structures of the skull and to the neck and mediastinum. *Ludwig's angina* (see Ch. 290) is an infection presenting with a painful swelling of the anterior floor of the mouth, drooling, and dysphagia. Left unrecognized or untreated, it can progress rapidly to respiratory obstruction. Intravenous antibiotics and corticosteroids must frequently be accompanied by surgical exploration and drainage.

Nonpainful swelling of the lower jaw suggests tumor of the bone or soft tissues. The most common nonmalignant tumor is an *epulis* (meaning "on the gum"), a granulomatous and fibrous tissue growth. Other growths include *osteoma, cyst, ameloblastoma* (a tumor of the cells that make enamel), and *malignant epithelioma*. Bilateral enlargement of the mandible occurs in *acromegaly, Paget's disease, osteitis fibrosa* from hyperparathyroidism, and *leontiasis ossea*. The last is a rare condition with jaw changes resembling acromegaly but without enlargement of the hands or feet.

Pain in the lower jaw without swelling is commonly due to *dental caries, periodontal disease,* or *temporomandibular dysfunction* (otomandibular syndrome). *Trigeminal neuralgia* presents with a unilateral dull pain, a rigid anatomic distribution, and a trigger zone for intense pain; and neuralgia occurs in cranial nerve VII division II more than in III or I. In contrast, *herpes zoster* involves more commonly division I. Pain from cardiac angina also may be referred to the jaw and has been mistaken for periodontal disease.

DYSPHAGIA (see Ch. 97)

HOARSENESS

Simple hoarseness is the inability to pitch the voice and results from failure to use the larynx to produce tones. This change in voice occurs with voluntary acts, e.g., whispering, or with diseases affecting vocal cord motion and position. The most common cause of an acute onset of hoarseness is a bacterial or viral *infection*. Inhaled *irritants* (smoke or fumes) and *overuse* of the larynx present similarly. Inflammation and edema inhibit precise tension or closure of the cords. Treatment is rest and avoidance of irritants. Inhaled corticosteroids may produce cough and further irritation. Stridor suggests involvement of more than edema and inflammation of the vocal folds and warrants evaluation for extrinsic or intrinsic airway encroachment. Intermittent or recurrent hoarseness is usually associated with *smoking* and/or *allergy*.

Hoarseness persisting 2 weeks or more should be investigated by directly examining the laryngeal structures. Chronic hoarseness can result from benign and malignant processes, including *polyps,*

chronic sinusitis, gastroesophageal reflux, laryngeal carcinoma, hypothyroidism, goiter, and infections *(tuberculosis, syphilis,* and *histoplasmosis)*. Chronic hoarseness due to malignancy in the chest, with entrapment of the left recurrent laryngeal nerve, and to pharyngeal or esophageal carcinomas, with entrapment of nerves or extrinsic compression, usually occurs after the primary tumor has declared itself by other symptoms. Hoarseness due to recurrent laryngeal nerve paralysis may present years after thyroid or parathyroid surgery, trauma to the neck, or goiter and is attributed to fibrosis and/or aging. Hoarseness following endotracheal intubation is common but should resolve within 3 to 5 days after removing the tube. Idiopathic, isolated unilateral, and bilateral vocal cord paralysis is rare. Treatment of chronic hoarseness is directed at the underlying cause. Nerve-grafting procedures can restore function in a paralyzed cord and laser therapy can be used for vocal folds entrapped after prolonged intubation, tracheostomy, or granuloma formation.

SNORING AND OBSTRUCTIVE SLEEP APNEA (also see Ch. 397)

Snoring is produced by vibrations of the soft tissues of the nasopharynx initiated by turbulent flow through a narrowed airway. Airway caliber is determined by anatomic factors, neuromuscular tone to skeletal muscles, and the pressure differences across the airway wall (Fig. 64-2). Snoring occurs during sleep, a state in which postural tone to the skeletal muscles and reflex adjustments to respiratory loads are reduced. The airway closing at the level of the nasopharynx and/or oropharynx during sleep produces apnea (cessation of airflow) and is believed to represent an extension of the process that produces snoring. Heavy snoring and apneas are terminated by state changes or brief arousals from sleep. Repetitive apneas during sleep result in inadequate sleep, excessive daytime sleepiness, and asphyxia, with cardiorespiratory and central nervous system (CNS) effects.

So common is snoring (30 to 50% of the population at age 50 report snoring) that it is the theatrical signature for sleep and the subject of social comment. Loud snoring, enough to be heard in the next room, is present in 5 to 10% of the population. In adults, examination reveals a reddened soft palate with or without anatomic narrowing of the nasal and oropharyngeal passages, micrognathia, or hypothyroidism. Other predisposing factors may include family history, obesity, respiratory depressants (alcohol and drugs), sleep restriction, nasal obstruction, and aging. Treatment is symptomatic for the bed partner, and one must first exclude hypothyroidism and then address predisposing factors. Medical therapy is directed toward weight loss, nasal decongestants, and drugs to reduce upper

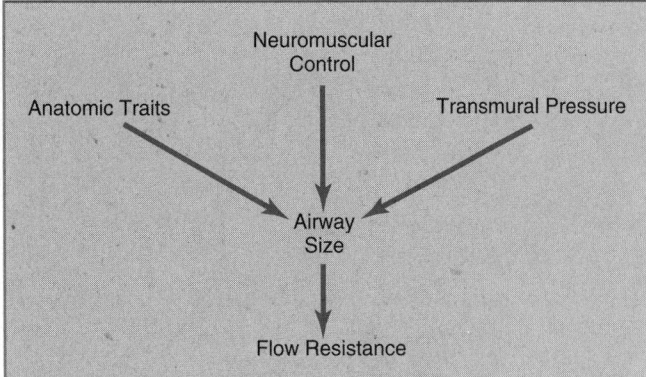

FIGURE 64–2. Three factors interact to determine airway size and, as pressure is applied by respiratory cycles, flow resistance. Anatomic traits refer to craniofacial bony and soft tissue structures. Neuromuscular control refers to motor drive to skeletal muscles and afferent mechanoreceptor information. Transmural pressure refer to the dynamic effects of pressure and flow on the airway wall.

airway inflammation. Surgical therapy is directed at the naso-oropharynx with procedures like a uvulopalatopharyngoplasty. In children, tonsillar hypertrophy and craniofacial anomalies are more common, and surgical intervention is more successful.

Recent epidemiologic studies have discovered an association between snoring and increased risk of hypertension, myocardial infarction, and stroke, even when adjusted for obesity, smoking, and age. The link may be through the 17-fold increase in risk for apnea in people who report snoring. A clue to the presence of apnea is the bed partner reporting observed apneas or respiratory pauses followed by a loud snort during sleep. Multiple apneas (> 10 per hour of sleep) during sleep may result in daytime symptoms, commonly excessive daytime sleepiness. Because snoring is very common, the trait by itself should not trigger a search for sleep apnea. Snoring, hypertension, or obesity alone is a poor indication for a sleep apnea workup. Snoring in combination with observed apneas, excessive daytime sleepiness, hypertension poorly controlled by medical therapy, and heart disease is a better indication for examining the patient during sleep to quantify the presence, type, number, and severity of respiratory disturbances during sleep.

Blomquist IK, Bayer AS: Life-threatening deep facial infections of the head and neck. Infect Dis Clin North Am 2:237, 1988. *An exhaustive review of the subject with references.*

Mathew OP, Sant'Ambrogio G (eds.): Respiratory Function of the Upper Airway. New York, Marcel Dekker, 1988. *Written by leading expert contributors, this book compiles much of what is known of the upper airway anatomy and physiology.*

Newman LJ, Platts-Mills TAE, Phillips CD, et al.: Chronic sinusitis. Relationship of computed tomographic findings to allergy, asthma, and eosinophilia. JAMA 271:363, 1994. *The presence of peripheral eosinophilia in patients with sinusitis indicates a high likelihood of extensive disease.*

Oppenheimer RW: Sinusitis. How to recognize and treat it. Postgrad Med 91:281, 1992. *A practical guide to a common problem, with references to the literature.*

Phillipson E: Sleep apnea—a major public health problem. N Engl J Med 328:1271, 1993. *This editorial discusses current epidemiologic studies and refers to the relevant literature on snoring and sleep apnea. An article in the same issue relates the first North American study of the prevalence of sleep apnea.*

65 RESPIRATORY FAILURE

Warren R. Summer

Respiratory failure, whether acute or chronic, is a frequently encountered medical problem and a major cause of death in the United States. Chronic obstructive lung disease (COPD), which ends in death from respiratory failure, is the only chronic disease that continues to show a yearly increase in mortality. More than 70% of the deaths in patients with pneumonia are attributed to respiratory failure. Authorities estimate that 34% of patients in critical care units—about 500,000 persons—receive mechanical ventilation in the United States each year. For acute respiratory failure (ARF) not preceded by disease or systemic illness, short-term survival is > 85%. Healthy independent elderly (older than age 80) people do nearly as well. However, multisystem organ failure (MSOF) or pre-existing renal, liver, or chronic gastrointestinal disease with malnutrition substantially worsens outlook. About 17% of patients placed on mechanical ventilation require assistance for > 14 days. Among those requiring > 14 days, elderly patients have a 9% survival and younger patients a 36% survival. Table 65–1 lists the characteristics and outcomes of patients on a medical service with ARF.

Respiratory failure is a functional disorder caused by any condition that severely affects the lungs' ability to maintain arterial oxygenation or carbon dioxide (CO_2) elimination. It may be acute or chronic, depending on when the process develops with important pathogenic, physiologic, and therapeutic distinctions. Although acute and chronic respiratory failure are defined by arterial blood gas analysis, clinicians do not universally agree on the exact values, which seem to vary between the two temporal varieties of failure.

Acute and chronic respiratory failure may be divided into two main categories: that manifested preponderantly or entirely by hypoxemia or failure of gas exchange and that manifested by hypercapnia or inability to exhale adequate quantities of CO_2, a failure of ventilation. Differentiating hypoxic from hypercapnic-hypoxic respiratory failure, although somewhat artificial, is convenient because it allows the grouping of conditions having related pathophysiology or common clinical presentations (Table 65–2). In addition, this grouping focuses on related therapeutic strategies.

ACUTE RESPIRATORY FAILURE

DEFINITION. *Hypoxic respiratory failure* (HRF) may be defined as any condition producing severe arterial hypoxemia (Pa_{O_2} < 50 mm Hg) that cannot be corrected by increasing the inspired oxygen concentration to > 50% (Fi_{O_2} > 0.5). Although both Pa_{O_2} < 50 mm Hg and Fi_{O_2} > 0.5 are arbitrary levels, they represent critical physiologic landmarks. At a Pa_{O_2} level of 50 mm Hg, hemoglobin is about 80% saturated, and further small reductions in the Pa_{O_2} produce significant reductions in arterial oxygen (O_2) content. Under those circumstances the O_2 reserve is minimal and patients become symptomatic. An Fi_{O_2} of 0.5 is probably the highest level that can be readily achieved in a patient's airway, without requiring a

TABLE 65–1. CHARACTERISTICS OF PATIENTS AND CIRCUMSTANCES ASSOCIATED WITH RESPIRATORY FAILURE

Mean Age	Male	Assisted Ventilation	Hospitalization
60 yrs	54%	3 days median, 10 days mean	14 days median, 26 days mean

Common Etiology*	Frequency (%)	Survival (%)
ARDS	7	60
Cardiogenic pulmonary edema	16	60
Cardiopulmonary arrest†	10	20
COPD	12	65
CNS: trauma, stroke, hemorrhage, seizures	11	60
Drug overdose	7	95
Metabolic coma	8	30
Neuromuscular disease‡	8	36
Pneumonia	10	38
Asthma	< 1	90
Other§	10	50

* A large portion of patients have more than one condition leading to respiratory failure.

† Overlaps with other causes—sepsis, pneumonia, renal failure. Includes cardiac patients and those undergoing various hospital procedures. Does not represent patients already critically ill in an ICU.

‡ Guillain-Barré syndrome, myasthenia gravis, tetanus, amyotrophic lateral sclerosis, etc.

§ Multiple cause of respiratory failure—hard to define single reason. MSOF and sepsis common.

TABLE 65–2. FEATURES OF HYPOXIC AND HYPERCAPNIC-HYPOXIC ACUTE RESPIRATORY FAILURE

Feature	Condition	
	Hypoxic	*Hypercapnic-Hypoxic*
Physiologic	Large right-to-left intrapulmonary shunt; hyperventilation usual	COPD: hypoventilation due to marked wasted (dead space) ventilation; minute ventilation normal to increase; V/P imbalance with increased A-a gradient. Neuromuscular and overdose: hypoventilation due to decreased minute ventilation, normal A-a gradient
Anatomic	Extensive edema; atelectasis or consolidation; hyaline membranes	Mucous gland hyperplasia (bronchitis); alveolar wall destruction (emphysema); hypertrophied bronchial muscle and mucus impaction (asthma); upper airway obstruction (fixed or variable); normal
Clinical presentation		
Age	Any	Any; bronchitis and emphysema >55 years
Medical history	Well; hypertension; heart disease	Chronic shortness of breath; history of depression; weakness and wheezing
Present illness	Acute shortness of breath temporally related to some serious event (e.g., car accident, sepsis, worsening blood pressure, chest pain)	Recent upper respiratory infection; gradual worsening of shortness of breath, increased cough, sputum, and wheezing; drug overdose; new or increased muscle weakness
Physical examination	Evidence of acute illness, tachypnea (>35); tachycardia; hypotension; diffuse crackles; signs of consolidation	Tachypnea (<30); tachycardia; prolonged expiration; decreased breath sounds; wheezing; pedal edema; reduced strength; altered consciousness
Laboratory examination		
Chest roentgenogram	Small, white lungs; multiple patchy, diffuse infiltrates; lobar atelectasis or consolidation	Hyperinflation; large black lungs, bullae; wide interspaces; prominent bronchovascular marking with COPD or asthma; Hypoinflation, small black lungs; with overdose or neuromuscular disease
Electrocardiogram	Sinus tachycardia; acute myocardial infarction; left ventricular hypertrophy	Right ventricular hypertrophy; "P" pulmonale; low voltage; clockwise rotation; normal
Laboratory	Nonspecific. Hemoglobin low to normal; respiratory alkalosis; metabolic acidosis; raised BUN	Hemoglobin normal to high; respiratory acidosis; mixed metabolic and respiratory acidosis; low potassium

closed system (intubation) or specialized nonrebreathing masks, necessitating management in an intensive care unit (ICU). In addition, an FI_{O_2} of 0.5 usually corrects the hypoxemia associated with hypercapnic-hypoxic respiratory failure and nearly all conditions in which right-to-left shunting is not the dominant clinical problem. If hypoxemia is corrected by an FI_{O_2} of 0.5, patient management is notably simplified. In HRF the low Pa_{O_2} is due to a large right-to-left shunt and therefore increases minimally with increasing FI_{O_2} so that the alveolar-arterial gradient increases markedly and the Pa_{O_2}/FI_{O_2} ratio remains low (usually < 200 mm Hg) at all levels of FI_{O_2}. The exact level of arterial oxygen tension (Pa_{O_2}) depends on the amount of blood that bypasses the gas-exchanging portion of the lung, the alveolar O_2 tension (FI_{O_2}), and the mixed venous oxygen tension (Pv_{O_2}). In the presence of a large right-to-left shunt, small changes in Pv_{O_2} caused by decreases in cardiac output or increases in metabolism can result in a major reduction in Pa_{O_2}. The calculated right-to-left shunt is usually between 25 and 50% in most patients.

Hypercapnic-hypoxic respiratory failure (HHRF) may be defined as a life-threatening condition with inadequate CO_2 excretion. CO_2 excretion, and thus Pa_{CO_2}, are inversely related to the alveolar ventilation (VA), i.e., $Pa_{CO_2} = kVco_2/VA$, where Vco_2 is the amount of steady-state CO_2 produced each minute as determined by the patient's metabolic rate. Thus, a rise in the Pa_{CO_2} level is by convention a reduced alveolar ventilation or hypoventilation. The mechanism for the failure in CO_2 excretion varies with the condition, preventing the elimination. It is usually associated with severe airflow obstruction seen in COPD or asthma. Nonetheless, hypercapnia may occur even when the lungs are normal, e.g., following alterations in the control of breathing (sedative drug overdose) or when the neuromuscular apparatus is inadequate.

HHRF is often defined by the level of Pa_{CO_2}. It is difficult to assign absolute values as representative of *failure,* however, because they depend on the precipitating condition and the previous state of the patient. A Pa_{CO_2} > 55 mm Hg is considered failure in patients with known COPD and previously normal Pa_{CO_2} values. By contrast, a Pa_{CO_2} > 45 mm Hg has greater importance in patients suffering from acute asthma, drug overdose, or neurologic weakness. No Pa_{CO_2} value indicates with certainty the extent of deterioration in

a patient with known chronic hypercapnia. Because of renal compensation and the development of base excess, the arterial pH does not always reflect the rate at which Pa_{CO_2} rose. About 25% of patients with ARF on admission have a compensated pH resulting from transient increases in VA. During hypoventilation the PCO_2 and PO_2 levels change in opposite directions by nearly the same amount, with no significant increase above normal in alveolar-arterial O_2 gradient. For example, normal Pa_{CO_2} (40 mm Hg) + Pa_{O_2} (90 mm Hg) = 130. If the change in Pa_{CO_2} does not account for the change in Pa_{O_2} (Pa_{CO_2} 60 + Pa_{O_2} 70 = 130 mm Hg), some additional cause of hypoxia other than pure hypoventilation must be present. The primary mechanism of hypoxemia in HHRF secondary to COPD and asthma is perfusion of poorly ventilated lung units or ventilation-perfusion (V/P) mismatch (Pa_{CO_2} 60 + Pa_{O_2} 40 = 100 mm Hg). Low V/P ratios can be recognized by giving a patient 100% O_2; this causes any alveolar-arterial difference present while the patient is breathing room air to decrease and arterial Pa_{O_2} to increase to normal values (550 mm Hg). Because the degree of V/P mismatch varies, the increase in Pa_{O_2} with low levels of supplemental O_2 cannot be predicted, and the targeted Pa_{O_2} must be reached by trial and error. By contrast, because arterial hypoxemia of pure hypoventilation is not associated with an increase in alveolar-arterial O_2 gradient, modest increases in FI_{O_2} easily displace the remaining alveolar nitrogen and substantially improve the Pa_{O_2} value.

CLINICAL MANIFESTATIONS. The clinical presentation is dictated primarily by the condition causing the functional impairment (Table 65–2). Manifestations are strongly influenced by the level of arterial Pa_{O_2} and in the most severe cases, tissue hypoxia. Arterial hypoxemia increases ventilation by stimulating carotid body chemoreceptors. The degree of ventilatory response depends on the ability to sense hypoxemia and the capacity of the respiratory system to respond. Activity of the sympathetic nervous system increases with secondary vasoconstriction and elevated cardiac output. Severe hypoxia impairs mental performance and may progress to myocardial ischemia and permanent brain damage. Manifestations of hypoxic respiratory failure are more pronounced in the presence of underlying hematologic or circulatory abnormalities.

Acute hypercapnia depresses central nervous system activity but does so primarily by lowering the cerebrospinal fluid pH. Thus, low pH, rather than absolute levels of CO_2, best correlates with altered mental status. Although hypercapnia stimulates ventilation in normal subjects, the mechanism leading to hypercapnia often impairs or depresses any effective increases in minute ventilation. Symptoms of hypercapnia may overlap those of hypoxemia. Precipitating neurologic disorders, overmedication with sedatives, myxedema, or head trauma may mask the physiologic effect of both hypercapnia and hypoxemia. Clinical manifestations of hypoxemia and hypercapnia are listed in Table 65–3.

ACUTE HYPOXIC RESPIRATORY FAILURE

Diseases or conditions most frequently associated with severe hypoxemia are listed in Table 65–4. Most of these processes are discussed elsewhere (see Table 65–4 for cross-references), and only a fraction of patients develop severe hypoxemia. All of these diseases are common, however, so even a small percentage of cases with ARF is a significant number of persons. It is important to include these processes in the differential diagnosis because they require specific therapies in addition to managing the severe hypoxemia.

ADULT RESPIRATORY DISTRESS SYNDROME (ARDS) (see also Ch. 68)

Because it is an important cause of hypoxic respiratory failure and is unique in its clinical presentation, pathogenesis, and management, ARDS is discussed here. ARDS is a form of acute lung injury often seen in previously healthy patients. It is characterized by rapid respiratory rates, a sensation of profound shortness of breath, severe hypoxemia not responsive to supplemental oxygen (Pa_{O_2}/FI_{O_2} < 200), and widespread pulmonary infiltrates (involvement of three of six lung regions) not explained by cardiovascular disease or volume overload. The functioning lung tends to be small, which is indicated by a diminished thoracic gas volume and a reduction in the amount of air that can enter the lung at usual pressures (low compliance of < 40 ml of air per centimeter of H_2O, where normal approximates 100 ml per centimeter). Each year in the United States there are 100,000 cases of ARDS. It tends to follow a diverse array of systemic and pulmonary insults (Table 65–5), although 80% of ARDS is associated with systemic or pulmonary infection, severe trauma, or aspirating gastric contents. The likelihood of developing ARDS is highest in patients with severe sepsis or septic shock (30%) (see Ch. 70) and increases in the presence of multiple risk factors. The generic term ARDS belies the nonuniformity of possible mechanisms and diverse precipitating events. Nonetheless, lumping seemingly unrelated lung injuries is practical because it is frequently difficult to isolate a particular cause and there is a common strategy of supportive care once this syndrome is fully manifest.

PATHOGENESIS. Despite the many risk factors and different initiating processes, the crucial stimulus seems to be an inflammatory response to distant or local tissue injury. ARDS is often only part of an inflammatory systemic disease that can evolve into

TABLE 65–4. CAUSES OF HYPOXIC RESPIRATORY FAILURE

Adult respiratory distress syndrome (see Ch. 68)
Pneumonia—lobar, multilobar* (see Ch. 55 and 365)
Pulmonary emboli (massive) (see Ch. 59)
Atelectasis (acute lobar) (see Ch. 53)
Cardiogenic pulmonary edema (see Ch. 34)
Lung contusion or hemorrhage—trauma, Goodpasture's disease, idiopathic pulmonary hemosiderosis, systemic lupus (see Ch. 54)

* AIDS patient with *Pneumocystis carinii* pneumonia, diffuse alveolar damage or extensive TB, coccidioidomycosis, and histoplasmosis may result in severe hypoxemia.

MSOF. The initial insult causes injury to the pulmonary endothelium and is followed by release of cytokines, mediators from cell membranes (arachidonic acid and platelet-activating factor), and activation of a number of cascades (complement, coagulation, and kinin). Neutrophils activating and adhering to endothelial cells with release of oxygen radicals (O_2^-) and proteases may contribute to endothelial cell damage, with a subsequent sequence of events (Fig. 65–1). Data from numerous experimental models suggest that many substances are involved in initiating injury and its progression, whereas few if any biologic substances are critical to the development of endothelial leak. These events take several hours to evolve, with continued injury extending to basement membranes, interstitial matrix, and alveolar epithelium. Although ARDS is usually defined by a level of hypoxemia (Pa_{O_2}/FI_{O_2} < 200), it is likely that a spectrum of *acute lung injury* (ALI) exists and less severe cases frequently can be identified (Pa_{O_2}/FI_{O_2} < 300), especially following severe sepsis. The extent of ALI depends on the magnitude of initial damage, repeated insults such as persistent septicemia or retained necrotic and inflamed tissue, and added insults from treatment including barotrauma, hyperoxia, and nosocomial infection. Experimental and clinical evidence shows that some cases of ARDS resolve rapidly (postictal, heroin overdose), whereas others progress relentlessly through several stages to severe fibrosis and lead to death from persistent respiratory failure. Surprisingly, there is a

TABLE 65–5. DISORDERS ASSOCIATED WITH ADULT RESPIRATORY DISTRESS SYNDROME

Aspiration
  Gastric contents
  Fresh and salt water
  Hydrocarbons
Central nervous system
  Trauma
  Anoxia
  Seizures
  Increased intracranial pressure
Drug overdose or reactions
  Acetylsalicylic acid
  Heroin
  Plaquenil
  Propoxyphene
  Paraquat
Hematologic alterations
  Disseminated intravascular coagulation
  Massive blood transfusion
  Leukoagglutination reactions
Infection
  Sepsis (gram-positive or -negative)
  Pneumonia–bacterial, viral, fungal
  Tuberculosis
Inhalation of toxins
  Oxygen
  Smoke
  Corrosive chemicals (NO_2, Cl_2, NH_3, phosgene)
Metabolic disorders
  Pancreatitis
  Uremia and diabetes mellitus seem to contribute to other risk factors
Shock (rare in caridogenic or embolic; uncommon in pure hemorrhagic)
Trauma
  Fat emboli (long bones usually)
  Lung contusion
  Nonthoracic (severe)
  Cardiopulmonary bypass

TABLE 65–3. CLINICAL MANIFESTATIONS OF HYPOXIA AND HYPERCAPNIA

Hypoxemia*	Hypercapnia*
Tachycardia	Somnolence
Tachypnea	Lethargy
Anxiety	Restlessness
Diaphoresis	Tremor
Altered mental status	Slurred speech
Confusion	Headache
Cyanosis	Asterixis
Hypertension	Papilledema
Hypotension	Coma
Bradycardia	
Seizures	
Lactic acidosis†	

* Listed in order of development with progressive alteration in Pa_{O_2} or Pa_{CO_2}.
† Usually requires additional reduction in oxygen delivery due to inadequate cardiac output, severe anemia, or redistribution of blood flow.

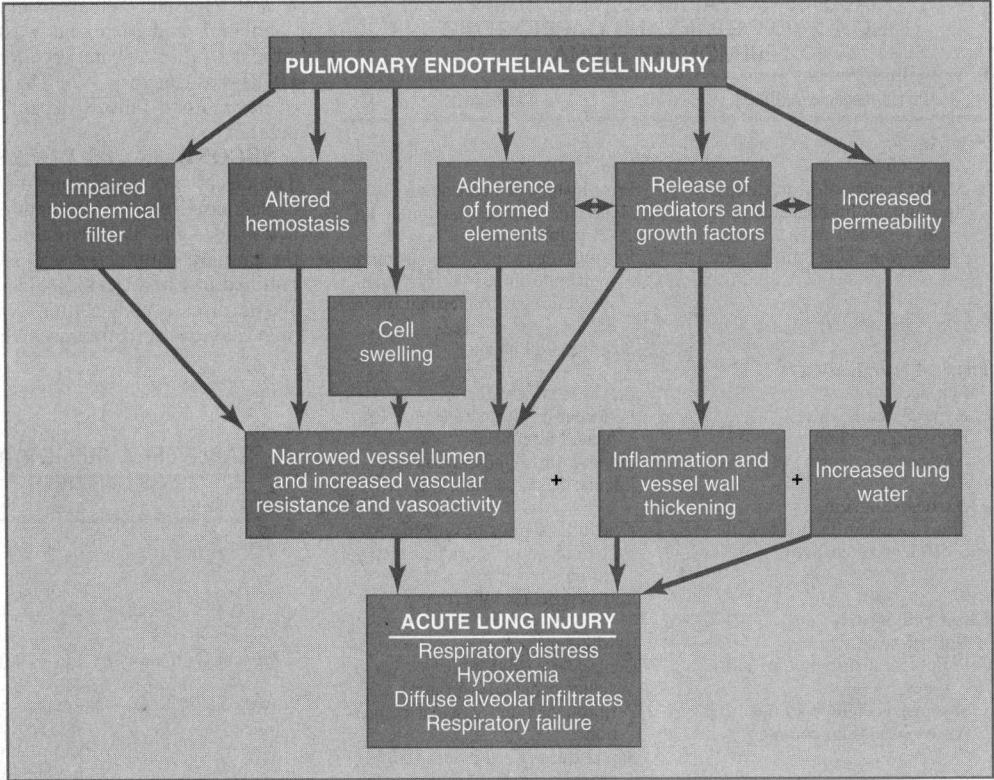

FIGURE 65–1. Possible pathogenesis of acute lung injury following damage to the pulmonary endothelial cell. The mechanism for endothelial cell injury is unknown, but various cytokines have been implicated. (From Block ER: Pulmonary endothelial cell pathobiology: Implications for acute lung injury. Am J Med Sci 304:136, 1992.)

poor correlation between Pa_{O_2} levels, measurements of extravascular lung water, and extent of chest radiographic densities.

DIFFERENTIAL DIAGNOSIS. Although several generalized and focal disease processes can result in severe hypoxemia, in most cases underlying risk factors and temporal relationships focus the differential diagnosis primarily between hydrostatic or cardiogenic pulmonary edema and permeability pulmonary edema (as in ARDS). Table 65–6 outlines the distinguishing characteristics between noncardiogenic and cardiogenic pulmonary edema. For many patients, historical information may be absent and physical and noninvasive laboratory findings may overlap so that even in expert hands clinical distinctions can be accurate in only 60 to 80% of cases. If accurate indices of volume status and cardiac function are unavailable, ascertain hemodynamics by right-sided heart catheterization. One must remember that high left-sided filling pressures may resolve rapidly after an acute episode of left ventricular ischemia or by introducing vasodilator and diuretic therapy. The intrapulmonary edema may take several days to clear roentgenographically. Transesophageal echocardiography may reveal left atrial volume and biventricular function as a useful guide to subsequent therapy.

TREATING ACUTE HYPOXIC RESPIRATORY FAILURE. The predisposing condition producing the diffuse lung injury and pulmonary capillary leak should be identified and treated because removing ongoing inflammatory stimuli limits further injury and allows gradual resolution. No therapies have been proved to directly repair endothelial and alveolar permeability or increase removal of alveolar and interstitial fluid.

Corticosteroids have been evaluated repeatedly in clinical trials and have shown no effect on lung mechanics, gas exchange, or outcome in early established ARDS. Corticosteroids apparently have no role in conditions that predispose to ARDS, such as sepsis syndrome, because when corticosteroid-treated patients were compared with placebo-treated controls, high doses (30 mg per kilogram every 6 hours for four doses) did not prevent ARDS or reduce mortality. *Nonsteroidal anti-inflammatory agents* such as ibuprofen have been shown to slightly modify the evolution of sepsis-induced lung injury and are under active clinical investigation. *Surfactant levels* or component ratios are reduced in patients with ARDS, and bronchoalveolar lavage fluid from patients has been shown to contain

diminished surface tension–reducing properties. Direct instillation in animal models and patients with neonatal respiratory distress syndrome has shown rapid and impressive improvements in gas exchange and radiographic clearing. Recent attempts to aerosolize surfactant into adults with ARDS, however, have not improved outcome. Current techniques may not deliver sufficient amounts of surfactant to the alveolae most in need of replacement. Alternatively, the outcome in many of these patients may be primarily influenced by MSOF and not the lung injury. Recently, preliminary data in patients with sepsis-induced ARDS have shown an encouraging reduction in the number of organs developing dysfunction and a trend toward improvement in survival after administering *free radical scavengers*. Prevention of acute lung injury by administering antibodies or receptor blockers to endotoxin, TNF-α, and interleukin-1 is also under active study, but initial results are not particularly encouraging.

SUPPORTIVE THERAPY. Major energy and attention should be directed to supportive therapy. The primary goals of treatment are to maintain adequate Pa_{O_2} levels and O_2 transport while preventing complications such as O_2 toxicity, volume overload, gastrointestinal bleeding, local or systemic infection, thromboembolism, malnutrition, and ventilator-associated problems (Table 65–7). See Ch. 68 for respiratory therapy and care in ARDS.

VENTILATORY MANAGEMENT. Because too few randomized clinical trials have been done, one cannot strongly advocate an optimal mode of ventilatory support for patients with acute hypoxic respiratory failure. Nonetheless, several principles should guide the use of mechanical ventilation in patients with ARDS: (1) Physiologic targets do not have to be in the normal range. Allowing Pa_{CO_2} to rise to 60 to 70 mm Hg (permissive hypercapnia) and Pa_{O_2} to fall below 55 mm Hg may be reasonable rather than risk lung overdistention, air trapping, circulatory compromise, or oxygen toxicity. (2) Alveolar overdistention with excess end-inspiratory volume can damage capillary and alveolar walls, resulting in increased fluid leakage with worsening pulmonary edema and/or air rupture, producing barotrauma such as pneumothorax and mediastinal emphysema. Direct measures of overdistention in the ICU are difficult and are guarded against by monitoring easily obtained end-inspiratory pressure. (3) A ventilator manipulation designed to improve one physiologic relationship may have an equally undesirable effect

TABLE 65-6. FEATURES DIFFERENTIATING NONCARDIOGENIC AND CARDIOGENIC PULMONARY EDEMA

Noncardiogenic (ARDS)	Cardiogenic
Prior history	
Age < 60	Age > 60
Absent history of heart disease	Prior history of heart disease
Appropriate fluid balance (difficult to access after resuscitation from shock, trauma, etc.)	Hypertension, chest pain, new onset palpitations
	Recent dietary indiscretion, minor metabolic stress—urinary tract infection, gastrointestinal bleed, etc.
	Positive fluid balance
Physical examination	
Flat neck veins	Elevated neck veins
Hyperdynamic pulses	Left ventricular enlargement, lift, heave, dyskinesis
Physiologic gallop	3rd and 4th sounds; murmurs
Absence of edema	Edema: flank, sacrum, legs
Electrocardiogram	
Sinus tachycardia, nonspecific ST-T wave changes	Evidence of prior or ongoing ischemia, supraventricular tachycardia
	Left ventricular hypertrophy
Chest radiograph	
Normal heart size	Cardiomegaly
Peripheral distribution of infiltrates	Central or basilar infiltrates
Vascular pedicle < 48 mm	Vascular pedicle (> 53 mm)
Air bronchogram common (80%)	Peribronchial and vascular congestion
	Septal lines (Kerley lines), air bronchograms (25%)
	Pleural effusion
Hemodynamic measurements	
Pulmonary artery wedge pressure < 15 mm Hg and cardiac index > 3.5 L/min/m²	Pulmonary artery wedge pressure > 18 mm Hg and cardiac index < 3.5 L/min/m²

on another relationship (e.g., increasing PEEP to improve Pa_{O_2} may decrease cardiac output, thereby reducing O_2 delivery to tissues). (4) In severe ARDS, only a small fraction of compliant lung is capable of gas exchange; therefore, tidal volume settings should be relatively small. (5) Peak inspiratory flow rates should match the patient's inspiratory demands with settings at 70 to 100 liters per minute. (6) The imposed resistive loads created by ventilator equipment and endotracheal intubation should be minimized by using very low ventilator-trigger sensitivities and some PEEP. (7) Mechanical ventilation is associated with a number of adverse consequences that require specialized knowledge and constant vigilance. Complications of ventilator management are discussed in Ch. 68. (8) The underlying pathophysiology varies over time, requiring repeated assessments of ventilator modes and setting. (9) Clinicians should always choose the ventilator mode with which they are familiar and not the most recent modification recommended by experts. The guidelines in Table 65-8 help ensure that these principles are satisfied and complications of ventilator assistance are minimized

OUTCOME. Survival in ARDS is 60% and is highest when it occurs as an isolated event (> 85%) and lowest when it is part of MSOF (30%). Nosocomial pneumonia significantly increases mortality. In the majority of patients who survive to extubation, lung damage completely resolves (60%), with only a small percentage left with significant functional impairment.

ACUTE HYPERCAPNIC-HYPOXIC RESPIRATORY FAILURE

Acute HHRF is a physiologic derangement that results from many pathologic events. It may occur in previously healthy people without specific lung injury or with underlying pulmonary disease. In the presence of severe COPD, a minor event may precipitate acute decompensation. The presentation and treatment of HHRF can be divided into conditions in which the hypercapnia results from decreased minute ventilation (Table 65-9, categories I–III and IVa)

and those in which the respiratory failure results from severe ventilation-perfusion mismatch (Table 65-9, category IVb). Categories V and VI usually result from varying degrees of decreased minute ventilation and increased wasted ventilation. Their presentation is similar to that of category IVb. About half of the clinical cases of HHRF are category IVb. The observed frequency of specific causes of respiratory failure depends on a particular hospital's referral base.

SECONDARY TO DECREASED MINUTE VENTILATION. The diseases or conditions that may present with HHRF secondary to decreased minute ventilation are numerous. Each entity has characteristic signs and symptoms that initially or ultimately point to the primary pathogenesis. Discussion of each of these conditions is outlined in Ch. 425, 432, 445–452, and 453–459.

The disease presentation varies from a sudden onset, as seen in high cervical cord trauma or botulism, to the subacute course seen

TABLE 65-7. SUPPORTIVE MANAGEMENT OF ARDS

Principle	Goal	Strategy
Improve Pa_{O_2}	Pa_{O_2} 60 mm Hg, Sat 90%	Initiate therapy with 100% O_2
	Accept Pa_{O_2} < 60 mm Hg, esp. in young	Usually requires intubation
Prevent O_2 toxicity	FI_{O_2} < 0.6	Monitor pulse oximetry
Provide adequate O_2 transport	Normalize blood pressure, pulse pressure, and organ perfusion; maintain cardiac index > 3.5 L/min/m² Hemoglobin > 10 g/dl	Recruit lung units by adding PEEP Fluid replacement for adequate venous return following increased PEEP Vasoactive drugs to maintain blood pressure and organ perfusion; measure cardiac index if uncertain
Optimize fluid status	Lowest tolerated filing pressures Keep dry	Limit extraneous IV fluids, follow intake and output; diurese empirically Measure pulmonary capillary wedge pressure if fluid status unclear
Meet ventilatory demands	Reduce work of breathing and O_2 consumption of respiratory muscles; eliminate CO_2	Assisted ventilation, sedation, rarely paralysis. Follow arterial blood gases. Permit hypercapnia 60–70 mm Hg
Avoid gastrointestinal bleeding	Gastric pH > 4; protect gastric lining	H_2 blockers, sulcrafate
Prevent thromboembolism	Reduce clotting and venous stasis	Pneumatic and elastic compression stocking, subcutaneous heparin
Supply adequate nutrition	Replace resting energy expenditure	25–30 kcal/kg, 1.5 gm protein/kg Enteral feed preferred, total parenteral nutrition if gut dysfunctional
Prevent respiratory and system infection	Maintain sterile techniques, promote gastric emptying, minimize lung congestion and atelectasis	Hand washing and good respiratory therapy technique, elevate bed 30°, jejunal enteral feeding, frequent or continuous mechanical turning
Weaning and extubation	Remove from ventilator and extubate ASAP	Take every opportunity to reduce PEEP and do not prolong weaning or extubation any longer than absolutely necessary
Minimize anxiety, pain, discomfort	Keep sedated but easily aroused	Regular intermittent sedation, anticipate analgesic needs as clinically dictated, try frequently to communicate with patient

TABLE 65-8. VENTILATOR GUIDELINES TO MAXIMIZE EFFICIENCY AND MINIMIZE COMPLICATIONS

Parameter	Target
FI_{O_2}	< 0.5. Balance against PEEP, relative risk problematic
PEEP	< 10 cm H_2O, can increase to ≥ 20 cm H_2O to maintain FI_{O_2} < 0.8
Tidal volume	6–8 ml/kg. May allow Pa_{CO_2} to rise
Plateau pressure*	< 35 cm H_2O end inspiration
Flow rate	> 70 L/min
Sensitivity	– 0.5 to – 1.5 cm H_2O
Respiratory rate†	Assist-control at 10–15/min

* Usually measured by inducing a brief inspiratory hold. Pressure falls from peak inspiratory pressure but often only 5 to 10 cm depending on inspiratory flow rate and degree of airway resistance secondary to endotracheal tube and small airways reactivity.

† In spontaneously breathing patients rate is determined by inspiratory drive and/or ventilatory demand. Select inspiratory flow and resulting inspiratory: expiratory ratio to prevent hemodynamic compromise and air trapping. Reductions in tidal volume or patient sedation may be necessary to achieve these goals.

in polyneuritis or myasthenia gravis. An even slower onset is observed in hypothyroidism and muscular dystrophy. Kyphoscoliotic cardiopulmonary disease and obesity-hypoventilation syndrome are generally present for decades before respiratory failure develops. In many chronic neuromuscular or musculoskeletal conditions, a minor acute respiratory insult may precipitate sudden respiratory failure by worsening the underlying neuromuscular condition (as in myasthenia gravis) or abruptly reducing the pulmonary function (as with aspiration pneumonia in parkinsonism).

In conditions that alter control of respiration, the degree of respiratory failure may not correlate with the level of consciousness. This is best illustrated by the effects of barbiturate and morphine overdoses, the former often resulting in coma without elevated Pa_{CO_2} and the latter showing profound hypercapnia with only moderate reductions in the level of consciousness. Respiratory failure should be suspected in all unconscious or obtunded patients and in all having neuromuscular insults. The diagnosis is established by evaluating arterial blood gases. All patients having a neuromuscular disease should be followed up with frequent measurements of their vital capacity and negative inspiratory force. When the vital capacity is < 1 liter, or the inspiratory force cannot exceed 15 cm H_2O, ARF should be anticipated and patients transferred to an ICU for close monitoring.

Early intubation for a potentially reversible disease with ARF is indicated. Assisted ventilation can be easily accomplished because the underlying lung produces little resistance to adequate ventilation or gas exchange. Methods of artificial ventilatory support without

TABLE 65-9. COMMON CAUSES OF HYPERCAPNIC-HYPOXIC RESPIRATORY FAILURE

I. **Altered control**
   Primary intracranial disease (tumor, hemorrhage)
   Trauma and raised intracranial pressure
   Drugs, poisons, and toxins
   Central hypoventilation
   Excess oxygen administration in hypercapnic patient
II. **Neuromuscular disease**
   Spinal cord lesions (trauma, tumor, vascular)
   Acute polyneuritis
   Myasthenia gravis
   Polymyositis, dermatomyositis
   Parkinson's disease
III. **Metabolic derangements**
   Severe acidosis
   Severe alkalosis
   Hypokalemia
   Hypophosphatemia
   Hypomagnesemia
IV. **Lungs and airway disease**
   a. Upper airway disease (fixed, variable, or sleep-dependent)
   b. Lower airway disease (COPD, asthma)
V. **Musculoskeletal alterations**
   Kyphoscoliosis
   Ankylosing spondylitis
VI. **Obesity-hypoventilation syndrome**

intubation, such as external negative pressure ventilation or nasal continuous or intermittent positive air pressure ventilation (CPAP and BIPAP), may suffice in some patients but are often unreliable (see Ch. 68). Hypoxemia should always be corrected. Inspiratory O_2 > 30% is necessary only in such superimposed conditions as atelectasis, pneumonia, or pulmonary embolism. Maintaining good airway toilet and postural drainage usually prevents significant respiratory complications. Minor episodes of aspiration pneumonia are frequent; however, transient low-grade fevers or minor leukocytosis without pulmonary infiltration should be treated by increased respiratory toilet alone and a careful search for any nonpulmonary site of infection. Left lower lobe infiltrates often elude detection in patients in intensive care units because routine chest roentgenograms are usually obtained by portable anteroposterior techniques. Right and left lateral decubitus films are helpful in ruling out suspected left lower lobe pneumonia.

Recovery from HHRF with decreased minute ventilation depends on the underlying condition and the supportive care. Some patients with neuromuscular disease may require prolonged or even permanent assisted ventilation. After extubation, long-term nocturnal ventilatory assistance with CPAP or BIPAP may support patients with moderate daytime hypoventilation. Electrophrenic pacing of both diaphragms may be helpful in some central hypoventilation syndromes. A long-term commitment to respiratory support with an artificial ventilator should be avoided in patients with progressive neuromuscular disease who are not suffering from an acute reversible cause of respiratory failure.

SECONDARY TO LOWER AIRWAY DISEASE. COPD and asthma represent the major causes of acute HHRF. The diagnosis and general treatment of these conditions are covered in Ch. 51 and 52. Many of these patients have the diagnosis and have experienced multiple exacerbations and past episodes of ARF (see Table 65–2). Examination usually reveals an anxious person in severe respiratory distress. Breathing is labored and the rate is moderately increased. Accessory muscles are active. If respiratory depressant drugs are given (often for agitation or insomnia), respiratory rate and depth may not seem abnormal and the patient may appear calm. This particular clinical presentation is characteristic of patients who have received high inspiratory O_2 en route to the hospital. Cyanosis may be obvious, but its absence does not rule out severe hypoxemia. Papilledema is occasionally seen, most often in comatose patients but occasionally as the only impressive finding of respiratory failure. Supraventricular arrhythmias and signs of right ventricular failure are common in patients with severe COPD.

A chest film may reveal the presence of obvious chronic lung disease or acute pulmonary infiltrates; however, in a number of patients with HHRF, the chest roentgenogram is not helpful. Leukocytosis suggests infection, but severe leukoerythroblastic responses may follow the stress of severe hypoxemia.

TREATMENT SECONDARY TO CHRONIC OBSTRUCTIVE LUNG DISEASE. Principles of patient care that apply to most cases include (1) applying immediate lifesaving measures; (2) determining the precipitating factors; (3) treating the airways dysfunction; and (4) monitoring. Appropriate lifesaving measures for acute respiratory failure center on the immediate correction of hypoxemia, need for emergency intubation or assisted ventilation, and adequate circulatory support. If, as in most cases, the patient is alert or only minimally confused and has a stable cardiovascular status, low-flow O_2 is the principal therapy. Adequate oxygenation is nearly always achieved; however, it may take serial elevations in inspiratory FI_{O_2} to as high as 0.5. The patient should be transferred to an ICU or other appropriate setting for monitoring immediately after administering supplemental O_2. COPD patients usually maintain their minute ventilation with O_2 therapy. The expected modest rise in Pa_{CO_2} is attributed largely to increased dead space ventilation secondary to O_2-induced changes in V/P mismatch and is generally of little concern unless Pa_{CO_2} continues to rise to extremely high levels (> 75 mm Hg) or obtundation develops. Reducing FI_{O_2} under these circumstances is dangerous. Closely follow blood gases, systemic arterial pressure, respiratory rate, vital capacity, and cardiac rhythm. Also, monitor hemoglobin, electrolyte, and urinary output levels.

Most patients with COPD who develop HHRF have a reversible precipitating factor that decreases alveolar ventilation. The most common precipitating event is increased bronchospasm associated with a change in weather, minor infection, or failure to take medication. Infection may also increase bronchial secretions, reduce functional pulmonary parenchyma, or increase CO_2 production, overwhelming an already limited respiratory system. Occasionally, inadvertently administering sedatives or more obvious factors such as pneumothorax, cardiac arrhythmias, left ventricular failure, or dehydration may have developed. If adequate oxygenation can be maintained without major worsening of respiratory acidosis, conservative measures can usually be applied to reverse all of these precipitating conditions (Table 65–10). Respiratory stimulants are rarely effective to reduce hypercapnia because minute ventilation is normal or increased and mechanical work is already excessive.

ASSISTED VENTILATION. Most patients hospitalized with HHRF improve after conservative therapy without needing artificial ventilatory support. Mortality has decreased significantly, as relying on more conservative therapy has replaced early use of artificial ventilation. If a patient continues to deteriorate despite controlled supplemental O_2, bronchodilators, antibiotics, and correction of fluid and electrolyte status, assisted ventilation is indicated. The need for ventilator assistance is best assessed by a physician at the bedside. Arterial blood gas values are of limited use in making this judgment. High respiratory rates (> 36 per minute), excessive use of accessory muscles, paradoxical thoracoabdominal movement, subjective sense of exhaustion, and even minor mental status changes should be considered probable indications. Nasal BIPAP has been effective in sustaining or augmenting alveolar ventilation and allowing time for specific therapy to improve airway dysfunction in some patients.

If hypoventilation is to be effectively reversed by a mechanical ventilator, an endotracheal tube must be inserted. Intubation results in laryngeal and tracheal irritation, loss of effective cough, and increased risk of infection. It is also a source of discomfort in the conscious and alert patient. With careful handling, endotracheal

TABLE 65–10. THERAPY FOR ACUTE HYPERCAPNIC-HYPOXIC RESPIRATORY FAILURE SECONDARY TO AIRWAY DISEASE

Condition	Therapy	Route	Dose	Expected Response or Target	Advantage/Comment
Hypoxia	O_2	Nasal prongs	2–3 L/min	$Pa_{O_2} > 55$ mm Hg	Reduce pulmonary hypertension and airway resistance, improve diuresis
		Venti mask	0.24–0.3 FI_{O_2}	Lower initial Pa_{O_2}, lower initial target	Low FI_{O_2} reduces Pa_{CO_2} increase
Airway obstruction	Albuterol	MDI and spacer	400–600 μg q1–4h	Improve FEV_1 or peak flow	Cost effective; use only when patient alert, cooperative, coordinated
		Aerosol solution	2.5–7.5 mg q1–4h	Same as above	More reliable than MDI when intubated Deep breath improves deposition; maximum dose determined by response and toxicity
	Ipratropium	MDI and spacer	80–120 μg q4–6h	Same as above	Little to no toxicity, slower onset than albuterol. Drug of choice with any cardiac arrhythmia
		Aerosol solution	500 μg q4–6h	Same as above	Limited experience in acute failure
	Theophylline	IV	5.6 mg/kg load 0.3–0.6 mg/kg/hr	Same as above May improve air trapping, shorten hospital stay	Not first line. Add if patient not improving, keep blood levels < 15 mg/L; clearance influenced by numerous other drugs, diseases, age
Anti-inflammatory	Methylprednisone	IV	40–80 mg q8–12h	Reduced inflammation Improved FEV_1	Recommend in all patients; takes hours to days for response Controversial in asthma; not well studied in COPD
Infection	2nd-generation cephalosporin	IV	Depends on preparation	Resolve pneumonia quicker, improve bronchitis, fewer relapses	Usually concerned about *Streptococcus pneumoniae* and *Haemophilus influenzae*
	Ampicillin/ clavulanate	p.o.	500 mg q8h		Use with productive sputum, elevated temperature, presumed acute bronchitis, suspected pneumonia
	SMX/TMP	p.o.	1 b.i.d.		
Prevention of deep venous thrombosis and pulmonary embolism	Heparin	sc	500 units	Reduce clotting, less morbidity	Graduated elastic stocking of some value, encourage leg movement
Gastrointestinal bleeding	H_2 blocker	IV or p.o. various compounds	q12h	Gastric pH > 4	Not all patients have low pH; standard dose achieves target in only 80%
	Sucralfate	p.o.	1 g q.i.d.	Protect mucosal lining	Must be placed in stomach if not eating
Agitation	Lorazepam	IV	1–3 mg q3–4h	Mild sedation and amnesia	Only when on ventilator
Arrhythmias	Improve respiratory failure, reduce theophylline or β_2 agonists, correct K, Mg, alkalosis			If symptomatic supraventricular tachycardia, treat with cardizem, adenosine, or digoxin	Usually more of a nuisance than a real problem; do not be distracted. Avoid β blockers, esp. in asthma
Dehydration	0.45 normal saline	IV	100 cc/hr	Volume expansion Better cardiac output	Better slightly wet, esp. on ventilator 1^+ edema safe
Volume overload	Diuretics	IV	40 mg furosemide	Improvement in gas exchange	Have impaired capacity to excrete water load. Assisted ventilation reduces atrial natriuretic factor, increase SIADH
Electrolytes	KCl, etc.	IV	40 mEq in 100 cc as needed	Normalize serum K^+, prevent alkalosis	Often hypokalemic, may be total body depleted even with normal values
Thick secretions	Correct dehydration, treat infection, postural drainage, vibration, percussion		q4–12h as tolerated	Improved expectoration Improved FEV_1	Encourage cough, nasotracheal suction Monitor O_2 saturation with drainage or suction Continue drainage procedures only if productive

tubes may be kept in place for at least 2 weeks. When artificial ventilation is required for >2 weeks, a tracheostomy usually is performed. The most important indication for early tracheostomy is the presence of copious, tenacious secretions that cannot be adequately removed through the endotracheal tube. Tracheostomy carries some risk of bleeding, pneumothorax, local infection, and an increased incidence of aspiration.

VENTILATION PRINCIPLES IN HYPERCAPNIC-HYPOXIC RESPIRATORY FAILURE. Principles of artificial ventilation are similar to those discussed under HRF. Additional principles are as follows: (1) Stabilize alveolar ventilation; once Pa_{CO_2} has stopped climbing, goals can be reassessed. (2) Correct severe respiratory acidosis by increasing Pa_{CO_2} removal. (3) Measure end-expiratory alveolar pressure or dynamic hyperinflation (auto-PEEP or intrinsic PEEP) and direct management toward limiting or reversing the adverse consequences of air trapping by using the lowest minute ventilation and the longest expiratory to inspiratory time that produces adequate alveolar ventilation. Maneuvers likely to accomplish this goal are reducing tidal volume, increasing inspiratory flow rate, and relieving respiratory drive. Acceptance of hypercapnia is often necessary. (4) In patients with known baseline elevated Pa_{CO_2}, do not reduce Pa_{CO_2} below that level. (5) Keep end inspiratory plateau pressures at <35 cm H_2O, although its relationship to barotrauma is less clear than in ARDS.

Short-term outcome following acute HRF is generally good (see Table 65–1). Long-term prognosis is dictated by underlying disease and functional impairment before acute failure. Only 25% of COPD patients survive 2 years after an episode of ARF.

CHRONIC RESPIRATORY FAILURE

Any process that affects the airways, lung parenchyma, chest wall, or neuromuscular system can evolve into chronic respiratory failure. Diagnosis is usually well established. If historical information is not available, however, specific diagnosis may be difficult because many end-stage primary lung diseases clinically overlap. Obstruction can be separated from restriction, although patients may not be able to perform the necessary rigorous pulmonary function tests. At times, superimposed infection, pleural disease, or previous surgery also blurs these distinctions. In the most severe cases of chronic HRF, progressive lung destruction also impairs ventilation and hypercapnia develops.

The majority of patients with chronic HRF have end-stage fibrosis (honeycomb lung). Diagnosing and treating conditions leading to this outcome are discussed in Ch. 54. At this time only supportive care with oxygen for severe hypoxia and diuretics for excessive edema is helpful. About two thirds of delivered O_2 per breath escapes into the environment. Various O_2-conserving devices are available and may allow for more cost-effective supplementation and longer periods away from home. If patients are under age 60 and have no other significant problems, lung transplantation should be considered.

Diagnoses and management of diseases leading to chronic HRF are discussed in Ch. 51 and 52. Progressive elevation in Pa_{CO_2} levels indicates a poor prognosis. Using periodic negative- and positive-pressure devices may relieve dyspnea and provide some modest long-term ventilatory support in patients with neuromuscular disease and kyphoscoliosis. The major contraindication is a swallowing dysfunction because aspiration may be more likely. Using these devices in COPD is controversial. Short-term hospitalization with volume or pressure adjustments that document improved alveolar ventilation is required before attempting home management. Transtracheal O_2 may decrease the work of breathing, improve dyspnea, and reduce costs of O_2 therapy. Younger patients with α_1-antitrypsin deficiency, cystic fibrosis, and other causes of bronchiectasis are good candidates for lung transplantation. Quality of life is always an issue for elderly patients, and relieving suffering may be the agreed major therapeutic goal of both patient and physician.

Block ER: Pulmonary endothelial cell pathobiology: Implications for acute lung injury. Am J Med Sci 304:136, 1992. *Excellent review of the chemical and cellular insults that may lead to ARDS.*

Hill NS: Noninvasive ventilation. Am Rev Respir Dis 147:1050, 1993. *A review of alternative methods to improve ventilation.*

Pingleton SK, Hall JB: Prevention and early detection of complications of critical care. Principles of Critical Care. 218:587, 1992. *Recent compendium of this perplexing problem.*

Slutsky AS: Mechanical ventilation. Chest 104:1833, 1993. *A consensus conference review of physiologic principles and guidelines necessary to apply mechanical ventilation at the bedside.*

66 LUNG TRANSPLANTATION
Norman W. Rizk

INTRODUCTION AND HISTORICAL PERSPECTIVE

Although the first unilateral human lung transplant was performed in 1963, lung transplantation did not emerge as a successful therapy until the last decade. Between 1963 and 1980, the approximately 40 recipients of lung transplants unfortunately succumbed to early postoperative respiratory failure, graft rejection, sepsis, and bronchial anastomotic leaks. Studies conducted largely in laboratory animals during that period developed partial solutions to these technical problems. In particular, lung preservation techniques improved so that graft ischemia and the resulting postperfusion acute lung injury diminished. Likewise, the introduction of the immunosuppressive agent cyclosporin A (CSA) in 1976 improved engraftment and lessened rejection without impairing bronchial healing.

These advances helped enable Reitz and colleagues in 1981 to achieve successful heart-lung transplantation (HLT) in humans. In 1983 the Toronto Lung Transplant Group reported extending the triumph to single lung transplantation (SLT) in patients with pulmonary fibrosis. In this they were aided by the development of omental pedicle wrapping of the bronchial anastomosis, which minimized the problem of anastomotic dehiscence. The same group shortly thereafter introduced double lung transplantation (DLT) therapy for patients with emphysema. Since 1989, sequential bilateral lung transplantation (BLT), rather than *en bloc* DLT, has become standard because of improved bronchial healing and the desirability of avoiding heart-lung bypass at surgery.

Currently the availability of HLT, SLT, and BLT provides physicians novel life-saving modalities that are increasingly commonly used to treat hitherto untreatable conditions in selected patients. With the immediate surgical technical issues largely resolved, attention has now turned to refinement of indications for surgery, the crisis of graft availability, therapy and prophylaxis of infections, and management of rejection, particularly chronic rejection, as the limiting factors in lung transplantation.

INDICATIONS FOR LUNG TRANSPLANTATION

The frequency of specific diseases commonly treated by transplantation is summarized in Figure 66–1 as a guide to current indications. Table 66–1 details general selection criteria for lung transplant recipients. In practice, the most difficult selection criterion is accurately estimating life expectancy for the diversity of specific diseases treatable by transplantation. For some disorders, accurate predictors of prognosis are available and transplant centers should incorporate them into the more general guidelines for these diseases. In cystic fibrosis (see Ch. 58), for example, a forced expiratory volume in 1 second (FEV_1) <30% predicted, Pa_{O_2} <55 mm Hg, and Pa_{CO_2} >50 mm Hg all carry a 2-year mortality >50%; females and younger patients with these markers of severity fare particularly poorly. In primary pulmonary hypertension, right atrial pressure >20 mm Hg, mean pulmonary arterial pressure >85 mm Hg, cardiac index <2 liters per minute, presence of Raynaud's phenomenon (see Ch. 46), and functional impairment at the New York Heart Association III or IV level predict a very short survival. This contrasts with a median survival from diagnosis of 2.8 years overall in primary pulmonary hypertension.

Prognosis in idiopathic pulmonary fibrosis is more difficult to pinpoint. The available but limited data suggest that total lung capacity <60% predicted, diffusion capacity <40% predicted, and severe functional impairment predict short survival, but the pace of progression of fibrosis and responsiveness to therapy must be factored in as well. Severity of disease as judged by computed tomography (CT) cross-sectional imaging and the presence of pulmonary hypertension on echo/Doppler examination probably also are important.

Estimating survival in chronic obstructive lung disease (COPD) is the most difficult of all. Markers of disease severity, i.e., FEV_1

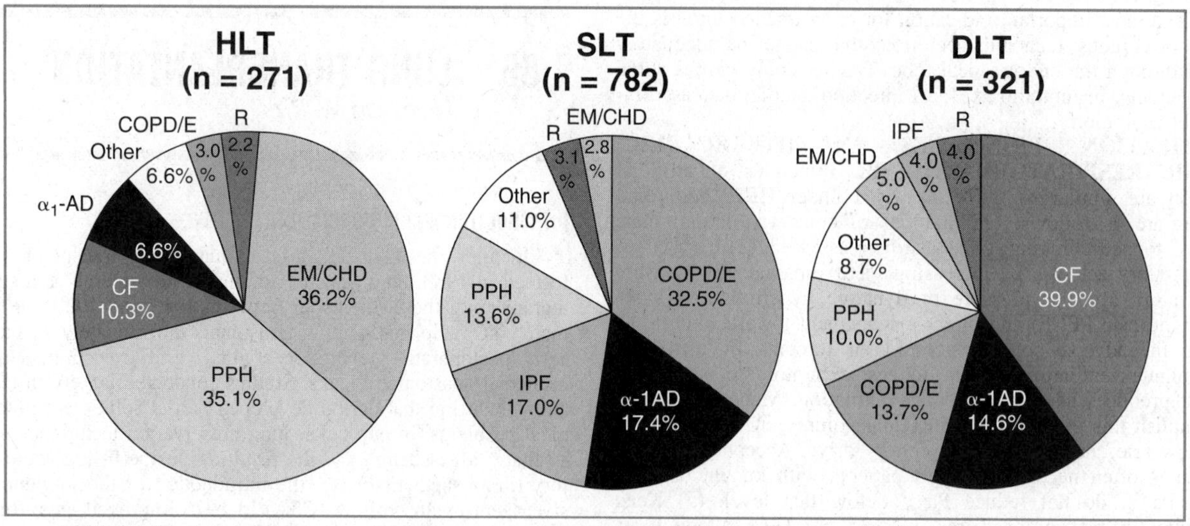

FIGURE 66–1. Indications for specific types of lung transplantation in the United States (October 1987 to December 1992). PPH = Primary pulmonary hypertension; IPF = idiopathic pulmonary fibrosis; CF = cystic fibrosis; COPD/E = chronic obstructive pulmonary disease/emphysema; α_1-AD = α_1-antitrypsin deficiency; EM/CHD = Eisenmenger's/congenital heart disease; R = retransplant. (Data from the United Network for Organ Sharing.)

< 30% predicted, DL_{CO} < 35% predicted, hypoxemia, and hypercapnia, may not be adequate predictors of survival. Quality, rather than quantity, of life is extremely important in these patients. Intolerable limitation of the activities of daily living, such as inability to complete dressing in less than 1 hour, or dismal functional status, e.g., a 6-minute walking distance < 300 meters with profound desaturation despite rehabilitative efforts, might be the best inclusion criteria for those patients with documented severe physiologic derangement.

For many disorders less frequently treated with transplantation—e.g., sarcoidosis, eosinophilic granuloma, lymphangiomyelomatosis—there are no clear guidelines, so clinical experience and use of the collected judgment of a panel of physicians are the best approach.

In addition to general and disease-specific selection criteria for recipients, certain contraindications have been established. Multisystem disease, e.g., systemic vasculitis or malignancy without a 5-year disease-free interval, is a clear contraindication. Abnormal hepatic and renal function, if substantial, contributes to perioperative mortality and complicates use of immunosuppressives, particularly CSA. Transplantation also should not be offered to patients with active or systemic infections, e.g., invasive aspergillosis, unless bilateral transplantation will remove the infected source, because immunosuppression will otherwise exacerbate the disease. Patients in overall good condition with isolated severe pulmonary disease are the best candidates.

CHOICE OF PROCEDURE

Determining the type of transplantation to perform rests upon the physiologic derangement present in particular patients. SLT is clearly appropriate for pulmonary fibrosis patients. More recently, acceptable post-transplant outcomes in selected patients with COPD treated by SLT have overcome initial theoretical concerns about using SLT in these patients. These concerns included the specter of

TABLE 66–1. SELECTION CRITERIA FOR LUNG TRANSPLANT RECIPIENTS

End-stage lung disease, with a life expectancy of 18 to 24 months, despite optimal management
No other major medical diseases
Substantial and progressive functional impairment
Ambulatory status, with rehabilitation potential postoperatively
Satisfactory psychosocial profile, free of alcohol and tobacco abuse
Adequate nutritional status

native lung hyperexpansion, with graft compression and atelectasis, and refractory ventilation-perfusion mismatches. Although these clearly occur occasionally, they have proved to be uncommon in patients without serious bullous disease, and COPD is now the most common indication for SLT. SLT may also adequately correct the physiology of primary pulmonary hypertension, although many groups prefer BLT to minimize the complications of postoperative reperfusion pulmonary edema seen in these patients. Some centers have used SLT to treat Eisenmenger's syndrome with correctable anomalies (e.g., atrial septal defect), but the latter patients, because of their associated cardiac disease and long intraoperative time, present special perioperative problems.

BLT is the preferable procedure for cystic fibrosis and generalized bronchiectasis because of the risk of cross-contamination of infected material when a native lung is left in place. BLT, compared with SLT, has significant perioperative disadvantages, including much greater anesthesia and graft ischemia time, and greater blood loss, resulting in an overall higher perioperative mortality rate. This disadvantage may be offset by the patient's acquiring more pulmonary reserve to deal with both acute and chronic rejection and intercurrent infection, so that long-term survival may prove to be superior. SLT does have the advantage of making more organs available for the large number of patients anxiously awaiting transplantation. At the present time SLT is performed twice as often as BLT.

HLT is best reserved for patients with severe combined pulmonary and cardiac disease because cardiac transplantations may be complicated by asynchronous cardiac rejection and the accelerated coronary artery disease that accompanies it. Separating the indications for heart and lung transplantation also frees up cardiac allografts for patients with cardiac disease alone. Severe combined pulmonary and cardiac disease occurs in Eisenmenger's syndrome with irreparable cardiac defects, in disabled pulmonary patients with cardiac ischemia, and in some patients with pulmonary hypertension (see Ch. 38), be it primary or secondary. Left ventricular (LV) dysfunction, as judged by an ejection fraction < 35%, is a clearer indication for HLT than impaired right ventricular (RV) dysfunction because RV function may quickly improve after the lowering of pulmonary vascular resistance that accompanies successful allografts. However, in patients with end-stage lung disease or pulmonary vascular disease, severe RV dysfunction, defined by an ejection fraction of < 20%, remains in some centers an indication for HLT. Adequate assessment of LV and RV function should include radionuclide MUGA or echo/Doppler examinations of the heart. Cardiac catheterization (see Ch. 33.6) is useful primarily for defining reparable cardiac defects and coronary artery disease in those patients at high risk for it.

In the United States, access to lungs for transplantation is controlled by local organ procurement organizations, which subscribe to regulations promulgated by the United Network for Organ Sharing (UNOS). Allograft selection criteria are provided in Table 66–2. Age criteria may vary from center to center. Under certain circumstances, lungs with remediable problems, like pulmonary edema, contusion, or atelectasis, may be suitable despite an abnormal chest radiograph. Using lungs subjected to < 10 days of mechanical ventilation minimizes the risk of unsuspected infection and lung injury and hence is desirable. Some standard of gas exchange, like a Pa_{O_2} > 300 on FI_{O_2} = 1.0, should also be applied. Acceptable graft ischemia time is currently up to 6 hours; hypothermic atelectasis and flushing the explanted lung with donor blood or Eurocollins solution maintains graft viability.

Under agreements regulated by UNOS, individual centers may offer donor lungs to potential recipients based on ABO status, lung volume compatibility, and length of time on the waiting list. There is no provision regarding urgency of need, unlike in cardiac transplantation. Death rates of recipients while awaiting transplantation are in the 5 to 25% range and relate to local availability of donor lungs, number of patients on the waiting list, and stability of the potential recipient's underlying disease. The latter consideration accounts for the approximately 5% death rate of COPD patients, compared with 15 to 20% for those with pulmonary fibrosis or cystic fibrosis. Median waiting time in the United States currently is 13 months, but there is considerable regional variability.

MANAGING THE LUNG TRANSPLANT RECIPIENT

As in routine cardiac or thoracic surgery, the immediate postoperative course is dominated by concern for hemodynamic stability and by the frequent development of low-grade pulmonary edema, attributable to interrupted lymphatic drainage, graft ischemia during preservation, the effects of reperfusion, and surgical manipulation of the lung. Early mobilization and extubation, fluid restriction, and clearance of retained secretions in the denervated lung are the main goals.

INFECTION. The transplanted lung is at special risk for infection owing to a variety of reasons, including lung denervation, interruption of lymphatic clearance and bronchial circulation, impaired mucociliary clearance, and immunologic paresis due to immunosuppressive drugs. In the immediate period after transplantation extending up to 30 days postoperatively, bacterial pathogens, particularly *Staphylococcus aureus* and organisms of the Enterobacteriaceae family, predominate. In particular, *Pseudomonas* species frequently colonize airways, eventuating later in a syndrome of chronic purulent bronchitis, particularly in patients with chronic rejection. After the first 30 days, organisms more commonly associated with drugs that impair CD4 lymphocyte function appear. Among these, *Pneumocystis carinii* was particularly common until the widespread adoption of prophylaxis with trimethoprim-sulfamethoxazole, usually given thrice weekly. Monthly aerosolized pentamidine may be an effective alternative in patients intolerant to sulfa drugs. Prior to prophylaxis, *P. carinii* typically appeared in the third to sixth month postoperatively and affected as many as two thirds of allograft recipients.

Cytomegalovirus (CMV) (see Ch. 340) is the most common nonbacterial cause for pneumonia in lung transplant patients, usually occurring 4 to 8 weeks postoperatively. The incidence of infection is directly related to donor and recipient CMV serologic status. Primary CMV infection usually causes more serious illness than reactivation disease; the lung is the primary site of organ involvement in half of cases, with the remainder having multiple organ involve-

ment of varying severity. Because of this, all CMV-seronegative recipients should receive only blood products that have been screened and found to be serologically negative. Serologic samples that show IgM antibodies or a fourfold rise in IgG antibodies are useful in diagnosing infection. CMV lung infection, but not disease, is easily demonstrated by bronchoalveolar lavage fluid analysis, which should include conventional culture and cytologic examination for nuclear inclusion bodies. These studies are best supplemented by the rapid shell vial assay for CMV that employs immunostaining of viral antigen to achieve rapid identification of the organism. To demonstrate CMV pneumonitis, which presents similarly to acute rejection with fever, cough, and radiographic infiltrates, a biopsy showing the characteristic histopathology is necessary. Although prompt treatment with ganciclovir offers an approximately 90% recovery rate, long-term chronic rejection and infection due to other organisms appear to be more common in survivors of CMV pneumonia. In addition, they probably have lower long-term survival rates. Because of this, many centers are instituting prophylaxis regimens with ganciclovir.

The other major viral pathogens following transplant are Epstein-Barr virus (EBV) (see Ch. 341) and herpes simplex (see Ch. 339). The former is associated with a mononucleosis-like syndrome and a lymphoproliferative lesion that possesses the genome of EBV. Herpes simplex virus causes disease in up to half of all patients, varying from simple herpes labialis or genitalis to esophagitis and disseminated disease.

In decreasing order of frequency, *Candida albicans, Aspergillus fumigatus,* and *Cryptococcus neoformans* are the most common fungal invaders. Preoperative screening for *Histoplasma capsulatum* and *Coccidioides immitis* helps identify patients at special risk for reactivation from these disorders, although they are much less frequently encountered. Identifying any of these organisms in clinical specimens from transplant recipients should initiate a thorough search for extent of disease and should prompt early aggressive therapy. In general, candidal infections are more easily treated and prevented than *Aspergillus* infections and require lower total doses of amphotericin B for control. Individual transplant centers are exploring low-dose amphotericin and triazole prophylaxis.

REJECTION

Allograft rejection is usually classified by histopathology and onset after transplantation. In general, hyperacute rejection in lung transplants is encountered extremely rarely, if at all, and is due to preformed alloantibodies directed against graft endothelium. Its rarity is due to preoperative screening of recipient serum against a panel of cells that represent possible donor antigens, because time constraints make crossmatching of cadaveric grafts against recipient serum impossible.

Acute rejection commonly occurs in the first 120 days but may be seen up to several years after transplant. Within the first 30 days it presents stereotypically as dyspnea, fever, and hypoxemia in a patient with chest radiograph infiltrates. After the first 30 days its presentation is highly variable, and typical histopathologic change may be present even in patients who are asymptomatic. Immunologically it is mediated primarily by CD4 and CD8 lymphocytes reacting against foreign human leukocyte antigen (HLA) complex–encoded cell surface molecules. Both class I molecules, ubiquitously expressed on most cell lines, and class II molecules, expressed primarily on B lymphocytes, macrophages, and monocytes but inducible on other cells, are involved. Cytotoxic T cells and delayed hypersensitivity mechanisms cause graft injury in a complex cascading process that histopathologically is characterized by perivascular mononuclear infiltrates, with or without lymphocytic bronchitis or bronchiolitis (Table 66–3).

Because it frequently presents as a nonspecific syndrome, the differential diagnosis of acute rejection is large and includes infection, particularly CMV, pulmonary edema, and postoperative acute lung injury. Transbronchial biopsy via bronchoscopy is the procedure of choice to establish the diagnosis and is particularly valuable when combined with bronchoalveolar lavage to exclude infection.

Chronic rejection is defined by the presence of bronchiolitis obliterans, with or without fibrointimal thickening of vessels. Bron-

TABLE 66–2. SELECTION CRITERIA FOR LUNG ALLOGRAFTS

Donor age < 65 for lung, < 50 for heart-lung
Clear chest radiograph
Negative HIV screen
Absence of infection, demonstrated bronchoscopically
ABO blood type compatibility
Appropriate total lung capacity for recipient

TABLE 66-3. HISTOLOGIC CLASSIFICATION SCHEME FOR PULMONARY REJECTION

Type of Rejection	Pathologic Features
Acute rejection	Perivascular mononuclear infiltrates with or without lymphocytic bronchitis or bronchiolitis
Active airway damage without fibrous scarring	Lymphocytic bronchitis or bronchiolitis without perivascular infiltrates or scarring
Chronic airway rejection	Bronchiolitis obliterans, involving membranous and respiratory bronchioles
Chronic vascular rejection	Fibrointimal thickening of arteries and veins
Vasculitis	Mononuclear mural infiltrate, sometimes with necrosis of vessels larger than arterioles and venules

Adapted from The Working Formulation of the Lung Rejection Study Group: J Heart Transplant 9:593, 1990.

chiolitis obliterans is the most common cause of late death after transplantation and affects one quarter to one third of patients. Prior infection with CMV and repetitive acute rejection are probably risk factors. The onset of bronchiolitis obliterans is variable but averages 6 to 12 months after transplant. Clinically it presents either as a cough with sputum production (but no rhinorrhea) or as subacute onset of dyspnea. Surveillance for it by periodic pulmonary function testing is mandatory in transplant recipients because bronchiolitis obliterans is often first discovered by recognizing airway obstruction on testing; a staging system based on FEV_1 level has been proposed. Many programs supplement formal testing with home spirometry as an early warning system. Decrements in FEV_1 of >10% should always raise the possibility of chronic rejection, but the alternative diagnosis of infection requires consideration. The sensitivity of transbronchial biopsy for chronic rejection, as opposed to acute rejection, is quite variable, and the diagnosis should not be excluded by negative transbronchial biopsies. In fact, if infection has been excluded and the clinical picture and pulmonary function tests are consistent with bronchiolitis obliterans, presumptive therapy is warranted. Unfortunately, augmenting immunosuppression is effective only in about two thirds of patients. Because more than half of the responders relapse, allograft function usually declines over time; changes similar to bronchiectasis and pulmonary fibrosis sometimes develop, and recurrent infection is problematic, leading frequently to graft failure and death.

A major challenge for transplant physicians is the successful management of immunosuppressive regimens. They are used for successfully inducing tolerance at the time of transplant, maintaining the graft, and treating superimposed rejection. Although there is some variability in use of the major agents, Table 66–4 details a representative treatment regimen. Managing these agents requires knowledge of their complex pharmacokinetics and interactions to minimize bone marrow suppression, nephrotoxicity, and infectious complications.

OUTCOME OF TRANSPLANTATION

As experience with transplantation has accrued, the prognosis of recipients has progressively improved. In the immediate perioperative period, technical surgical problems and acute graft failure are still the major causes of mortality but account for only 25% of all fatalities. After 15 days, infection is the leading cause of death, followed by chronic rejection in the form of bronchiolitis obliterans. Overall, survival appears to depend upon both the type of procedure and the underlying diagnosis. As shown in Figure 66–2, adult SLT worldwide has a 73.1% actuarial survival at 1 year, 66.5% at 2 years, and 62.7% at 3 years. BLT recipient survival, also depicted in Figure 66–2, is somewhat lower at every time point in international data, but US studies show approximately equal survival for SLT and BLT. As longer follow-up data emerge, BLT recipients may prove to have advantages related to the greater pulmonary re-

serve conferred by bilateral allografts. HLT recipients have a somewhat worse prognosis, with a 1-year survival of 59.9%, and a 3-year survival of 49%.

Part of the discrepancies in survival among different transplantation procedures is due to the specific diagnoses characteristically treated by them. Primary pulmonary hypertension patients, for example, have a slightly inferior prognosis, no matter how treated, but comprise a larger fraction of HLT recipients than SLT recipients and so contribute to the worse prognosis of HLT. Alternatively, emphysema patients do particularly well with transplantation and are most frequently treated by SLT, so that survivorship of the SLT group as a whole is enhanced. These interactions mean that outcome data must be evaluated both by specific diagnosis and by treatment procedure and that selecting procedure type for specific diagnoses must be individualized, with particular attention to local transplant center outcome.

Part of the rationale for transplantation is to improve recipients' functional status, and it is effective in this. Physiologic studies document marked improvement in both static pulmonary function and in exercise tolerance. SLT recipients regain most but not all of the lung function afforded by BLT and HLT. In particular, SLT recipients' FEV_1 and FVC average 60 to 65% of predicted lung function, compared with 75 to 85% of predicted lung function in BLT and HLT patients. For each group, lung function tends to continue to improve until 6 months postoperatively and then stabilizes. Maximal oxygen uptake 6 months following transplantation averages 40 to 60% of predicted lung function and is not limited by ventilatory capabilities. This is a level of function that permits moderate levels of work and exercise. SLT, BLT, and HLT recipients achieve similar levels of exercise despite their differences in spirometry. The chief determinant in maximal oxygen uptake appears to be level of conditioning achieved in postoperative rehabilitation, although peripheral muscle dysfunction in oxygen extraction may play a role as well.

Finally, quality of life studies following transplantation have shown that most patients would choose again to undergo it and would recommend transplantation to others, reinforcing the notion that this therapy has now come of age.

TABLE 66-4. IMMUNOSUPPRESSIVE DRUGS IN LUNG TRANSPLANTATION*

Induction and maintenance

Cyclosporine	Initial and maintenance dose of 1.0–4.0 mg/kg/d IV or p.o., beginning on day +1, adjusted to achieve gradually declining but therapeutic blood levels. Monitor Mg^{2+}, K^+, renal function
Azathioprine	Initial and maintenance dose 2 mg/kg/d IV or p.o., titrated to maintain WBC >5000/cu mm beginning on day 0
Corticosteroids	Intraoperatively at graft reperfusion, methylprednisolone in dose of 500 mg IV
	Postoperatively methylprednisolone 125 mg q8h IV × 3 doses at day +1
	Maintenance dose of 0.6 mg/kg/d at day +15, tapered to 0.2 mg/kg/d over 3–4 weeks
Antilymphocyte agents	For induction, give either (a) OKT3, 5 mg IV q.d., day +1 to +14, or (b) RATG, 2.5 mg/kg IV q.d., day +1 to +5

Rejection

Acute rejection	Methylprednisolone, 1 g IV q.d. × 3, then augment maintenance dose to 0.6 mg/kg/d × 3 weeks
Recurrent rejection (individualized)	Methylprednisolone, 0.5 gm to 1 gm IV q.d. × 3, then augment maintenance dose to 0.6 mg/kg/d × 3 weeks
	Consider antilymphocyte agents for steroid resistance
Chronic rejection	Methylprednisolone, 1 g IV q.d. × 3
	Consider antilymphocyte agents in induction doses

* Used at Stanford University Transplant Program in February 1994.

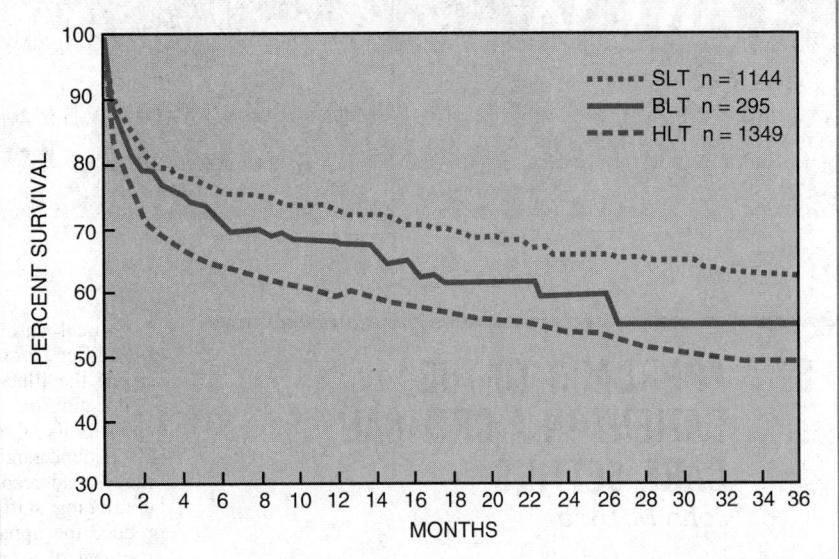

FIGURE 66-2. Actuarial survival by transplant procedure (international data). HLT data represent adult recipients only. (Data from Registry of the International Society for Heart and Lung Transplantation.)

American Thoracic Society: Lung Transplantation: Report of the ATS workshop on lung transplantation. Am Rev Resp Dis 147:772, 1993. *Consensus report by a panel of experts on the current state of lung transplantation.*

Marshall SE, Kramer MR, Lewiston NJ, et al.: Selection and evaluation of recipients of heart-lung and lung transplantation. Chest 98:1488, 1990. *Details specific methods of evaluation of potential recipients.*

Registry of the International Society for Heart and Lung Transplantation—1993. J Heart Lung Transplant 12:541, 1993. *Most recently published international database of outcomes in heart-lung and lung transplantation, stratified in a variety of ways.*

Trulock EP: Management of lung transplant rejection. Chest 103:1566, 1993. *Overview of both diagnostic methods and therapy of acute and chronic rejection in lung transplantation.*

PART IX

CRITICAL CARE MEDICINE

67 APPROACH TO THE PATIENT IN A CRITICAL CARE SETTING

John M. Luce

CHARACTERISTICS OF CRITICAL CARE MEDICINE

Critical care medicine is a body of knowledge that is applied to the management of severely ill patients in critical care units. Many kinds of patients require critical care, but most have dysfunction or failure of one or more organ systems. Circulatory and respiratory failures are the most common kinds of organ system failure dealt with in critical care units. Patients who manifest dysfunction or failure of two or more organ systems are said to have multiple organ system dysfunction or failure (MOSF).

Critical care medicine is practiced for the most part by internists, anesthesiologists, surgeons, and pediatricians. The parent boards of these disciplines recognize that critical care medicine may become a specialty and now provide certification of special competence in critical care medicine. The American Board of Internal Medicine gave its first critical care certifying examination in 1987. This and subsequent examinations have been taken primarily by pulmonologists, cardiologists, and general internists. These physicians are expected to be familiar with all areas of internal medicine that are relevant to severely ill patients, in addition to ethical issues in critical care.

Although physicians usually direct the care of critically ill patients, critical care medicine is a team approach that involves representatives of the other disciplines. Nurses are essential team members, as are respiratory care practitioners, nutritionists, biomedical technologists, and other health professionals. Also essential are mental health experts, clergy, social workers, and other persons who serve as counselors to patients and families and sources of support for the critical care team.

ATTRIBUTES OF CRITICAL CARE UNITS

Critical care units were first developed in the 1950's for patients who required mechanical ventilation because they had poliomyelitis or were recovering from anesthesia. Currently, various kinds of critical care units are found in almost all acute care hospitals in the United States with more than 200 beds. These units are defined by their ability to provide the environment, facilities, and personnel for the care of severely ill patients. The important features of critical care units are listed in Table 67–1.

Critical care units may have a general orientation, treating all kinds of severely ill patients, or be more specialized, accepting only specific categories of patients as defined by the kind of illness (e.g., burn units), organ system involved (coronary and acute neurologic units), specialty service designation (medical and surgical units), or the patient's age (neonatal and pediatric units). In addition to having the basic attributes listed in Table 67–1, specialized units provide medical personnel specifically skilled in the units' areas of care and have available particular forms of technology specific to treat the category of patients they receive.

Critical care units need administrative policies and procedures that differ from those of other hospital areas. Because of the severity of the illness of their patients, critical care units require clear delineation of administrative and medical lines of authority and responsibility. Critical care units also must have general guidelines for patient admission and discharge, specifically described roles for nurses and respiratory therapists, standing orders, and programs of continuing staff education and quality improvement. Such policies reduce the apparent ambiguity often inherent in the difficult environment of a critical care unit and enable prompt decision making by health professionals.

APPROACH TO THE CRITICALLY ILL PATIENT

Patients are admitted to critical care units from a variety of settings, including the emergency department, medical or surgical service, or operating room. Although a few patients may be admitted solely for monitoring purposes, such admissions have become less prevalent because of the relative scarcity of critical care beds in many hospitals and the introduction of prospective reimbursement practices that discourage the inappropriate use of critical care services. Thus most critical care patients are, by definition, acutely and severely ill. In addition, because they frequently manifest dysfunction or failure of more than one organ system, they are complicated patients as well.

Due to the nature of critical illness, the initial assessment of the critically ill patient generally should be rapid (Table 67–2). This assessment should focus on real or potentially life-threatening processes that require immediate diagnostic and therapeutic intervention. As a result, history taking, physical examination, and the gathering of laboratory information should be abbreviated. An example of this rapid approach is the resuscitation of a patient with cardiopulmonary arrest, which may take place elsewhere in the hospital but continues in the critical care unit. The pace of resuscitation is necessarily quick; physical examination may be restricted initially to the central nervous (CNS), cardiovascular, and respiratory systems; and interventions may be limited to the essential ABC's of airway, breathing, and circulation.

After initial resuscitation, or in lieu of this step if the patient has not experienced cardiopulmonary arrest or another major catastrophe, time should be available to form a broader and more comprehensive diagnostic and therapeutic plan. Now the history taking (often from family, friends, or onlookers) should be more detailed and the physical examination more complete. Laboratory tests, such as radiographic studies, should be called for and collected. Monitoring should be initiated, and treatment should be begun. For example, the cause of the cardiopulmonary arrest should be ascertained in the previously mentioned patient, if it is not known already. Continuous external electrocardiographic monitoring and measurement of blood pressure should be commenced, and diuretics, vasoactive drugs, and other appropriate agents should be administered if the cause is congestive heart failure.

TABLE 67–1. FEATURES OF CRITICAL CARE UNITS

High nurse–patient ratio
Ready accessibility of physicians
Ability to provide invasive cardiovascular and respiratory monitoring
Availability of respiratory support techniques
Ability to provide supervised continuous infusion of pharmacologic agents

Rapid initial assessment and intervention
Formulation of a broader and more comprehensive diagnostic and treatment
  plan
Management based on understanding of physiology and pathophysiology
Appreciation of organ system interdependence
Directed and dynamic management approach

Management of the critically ill patient should be based for the most part on an understanding of physiology and pathophysiology. This is not to slight the contributions of cell and molecular biology to critical care medicine, but for the moment, physiology and pathophysiology are the intellectual underpinnings of this discipline. Indeed, the critical care unit resembles somewhat the physiology laboratory, wherein variables such as heart rate and blood pressure are measured in an on-line manner and the effects of interventions such as the giving of vasoactive drugs can be observed directly. The critical care unit offers great therapeutic benefit because so many physiologic data are available. Yet practitioners must avoid the temptation to collect data for their own sake in such a setting, and they must exercise clinical judgment in caring for the critically ill.

Consistent with this pathophysiologic approach, the interdependence of organ systems must be kept in sharp focus in critical care practice. Limited attention to one component of an illness, even if it is predominant, frequently will yield a therapeutic approach that is detrimental to the patient as a whole. For example, treatment directed toward reducing intravascular volume in a patient with MOSF to improve respiratory function may affect renal and CNS function adversely. Conversely, increasing intravascular volume to raise cardiac output in a patient with left ventricular infarction may result in noncardiogenic pulmonary edema if parenchymal lung injury pre-exists. Physicians caring for severely ill patients must synthesize an overall management strategy that supports several organ systems and often incorporates the view of numerous consultants. This is one of the major challenges of critical care.

Finally, management should be directed and dynamic. Diagnostic studies should be performed for good reasons, not just because the results are intellectually interesting, and treatments should be initiated with specific endpoints in mind. Although many such treatments constitute therapeutic trials, both their potential benefits and their adverse effects should be appreciated. Practitioners also should appreciate that the status of critically ill patients frequently (and often swiftly) changes and that such change should be accounted for. Thus, although standing orders may be appropriate in many circumstances, other orders should be revised regularly. Similarly, while making rounds, critical care physicians should review not only the patient's overall course but also the functioning of all organ systems at least once a day.

PROGNOSIS OF CRITICALLY ILL PATIENTS

Critical care units have been used in more or less their present form for approximately 25 years, yet their contribution to health care has not been well quantified. Studies of patients suspected of having a myocardial infarction have suggested that if there are no early indications of complications (initial 2 hours in one study, at 24 hours in another), management in a coronary care unit does not offer any advantage over care in a hospital room or at home. Similarly, the outcome of patients with bacteremic pneumococcal pneumonia has not been found to be appreciably improved by critical care.

Other diseases commonly encountered in the critical care setting continue to have a poor outcome. The mortality rate of patients with cardiogenic shock remains approximately 75% despite pulmonary artery catheterization, a finding that has led to questions regarding the value of this monitoring technique. Cardiopulmonary resuscitation (CPR), when performed on hospitalized patients or persons older than age 70 out of the hospital, may be successful less than 10% of the time. The survival rate of patients with three or more organ failures after 5 days in a critical care unit approached zero in one large investigation.

Data such as these imply that critical care is of little or no value in several categories of illness. Yet patients in the postoperative pe-

riod and patients with cardiac arrhythmias, narcotic and sedative drug overdose, reversible neuromuscular disease, hypovolemic shock, and asthma and chronic obstructive pulmonary disease clearly benefit from critical care. Furthermore, the prognosis of certain diseases seems to be improving. For example, 90% of patients with a severe form of the adult respiratory distress syndrome died in a series from the 1970's compared with only 50% of comparable patients in a series from the last several years.

Establishing prognosis is difficult in critically ill patients because such patients are heterogeneous and because their prognosis changes over time. In recent years, a number of prognostic scoring systems based on the findings from large groups of patients have been developed to help quantify the severity of illness and determine whether individual patients will survive to hospital discharge. For example, the Acute Physiology and Chronic Health Evaluation (APACHE) III system uses major medical and surgical disease categories, acute physiologic abnormalities, age, pre-existing functional limitations, major comorbidities, and treatment location prior to critical care admission for these purposes. Mortality estimated by APACHE III is comparable with that estimated by physicians in most circumstances, and this and other systems are used increasingly as adjuncts to clinical judgment in critical care medicine.

ETHICAL ISSUES IN CRITICAL CARE MEDICINE

Despite their potential usefulness, prognostic scoring systems such as APACHE III are rarely used to restrict unit admission. This is so because most clinicians treating severely ill patients have hope that the patients will survive, and they thus request that critical care be provided, almost regardless of the likely prognosis. One reason for this is that prognostication is difficult in individual patients despite data derived from groups. Another is that patients and their families usually desire critical care if it will prolong life, assuming that self-awareness and social interaction are maintained. A third reason is that physicians may respond to what has been called the "technologic imperative": the desire to do everything possible despite the ratio of benefit to cost (see Ch. 4).

Critical care is extraordinarily expensive. The issue of who should be admitted to critical care units and how aggressively they should be treated is a social, as well as medical, concern. This concern is likely to increase under health care reform because funds may be shifted from tertiary care to support primary and preventive care services. Until this issue is resolved, physicians should base decisions regarding critical care primarily on the wishes of well-informed, mentally capable patients or their surrogates. Patients and surrogates who request critical care should receive it if they can benefit and if space permits. On the other hand, the wishes of mentally capable patients who choose against therapies such as endotracheal intubation and mechanical ventilation should be respected, as should the wishes of the surrogates who speak for them (see Ch. 2).

Orders not to initiate CPR, which are also called "do not resuscitate" or "DNR" orders, may be written at the request of patients or may be initiated by physicians when, to the best of their knowledge, CPR will not be successful in the broad sense of restoring meaningful life. In most instances, such decisions should be discussed with the patient and, when appropriate, with the family. The order should then be written in standard fashion on the order sheet, and a note describing the basis for the order and the decisions that took place should be included in the chart. Such orders clarify the ambiguity that surrounds the decisions concerning critical care for patients with irreversible illnesses and relieve nurses or uninvolved physicians from the responsibility of deciding not to initiate CPR.

Some patients with pre-existing DNR orders may still benefit from critical care. Treating airways obstruction, metabolic abnormalities, or arrhythmias may at least temporarily improve the patient's condition, making the existence of DNR orders a moot point. Nevertheless, a recent study has shown that, when written in a critical care unit, DNR orders usually represent the start of withholding or withdrawal of life support. Life-sustaining care was withheld or withdrawn from only 5% of the patients in a recent study, but it precipitated about half the deaths occurring in critical care units. The reason for limiting care was a poor prognosis, including brain death, the complete and irreversible loss of the functions of the cerebral hemisphere and brain stem. Most of the patients from whom life support was withheld or withdrawn were not mentally capable of participating in the decision-making process. Only a few had previously expressed their wishes regarding critical care in a "living will" or other format (see Ch. 3). As a result, family members or other surrogates usually had to make decisions limiting treatment on the basis of the physician's recommendations. Developing the prognostic knowledge to make such recommendations on a more rational basis and managing the death of severely ill patients are among the major responsibilities of those who participate in critical care medicine.

Jayes RL, Zimmerman JE, Wagner DP, et al.: Do-not-resuscitate orders in intensive care units: Current practices and recent changes. JAMA 270:2213, 1993. *Recent study demonstrating an increased use of do-not-resuscitate orders in critically ill patients.*

Kelly MA: Critical care medicine—A new specialty? N Engl J Med 313:24, 1988. *Traces the evolution of critical care medicine.*

Knaus WA, Wagner DP, Draper EA, et al.: The APACHE III prognostic system: Risk prediction of hospital mortality for critically ill hospitalized adults. Chest 100:1619, 1991. *A description of the most recent version of the Acute Physiology and Chronic Health Evaluation (APACHE) system.*

Luce JM: Ethical principles in critical care. JAMA 263:696, 1990. *A recent review of the application of ethical principles in the critical care unit.*

Schuster DP: Predicting outcome after ICU admission: The art and science of assessing risk. Chest 102:1861, 1992. *An explanation of how prognostic scoring systems work.*

Smedira NG, Evans BH, Grais LS, et al.: Withholding and withdrawal of life support from the critically ill. N Engl J Med 322:309, 1990. *This recent study documents why, how, and under what circumstances life support was withheld or withdrawn from patients in two large critical care units.*

68 RESPIRATORY ASPECTS OF CRITICAL CARE MEDICINE

John M. Luce

RESPIRATORY FAILURE

The word *respiration* describes the exchange of oxygen and carbon dioxide between humans (or other animals) and the environment. Human respiration may be divided into the following four processes: (1) *ventilation,* in which oxygen (O_2) is inhaled and carbon dioxide (CO_2) is excreted into the atmosphere, (2) *arterial oxygenation,* in which O_2 is transferred from the alveoli into mixed venous blood in the pulmonary capillaries in exchange for CO_2, (3) *oxygen transport,* in which O_2 is carried in systemic arterial blood to the tissues, and (4) *oxygen extraction and utilization,* in which the tissues take up O_2 from the blood and give up CO_2, which is transported in venous blood to the lungs.

Impairment in any or all of these processes could result in respiratory failure. Nevertheless, the term *respiratory failure* traditionally has been used to describe blood gas abnormalities of a high systemic arterial CO_2 tension (Pa_{CO_2}) and a low oxygen tension (Pa_{O_2}) or both. The traditional definition of respiratory failure is described at greater length in Ch. 65. In this chapter, care and treatment of conditions involving all four processes of respiration are discussed (Table 68–1).

RESPIRATORY MONITORING

Physical Examination

Physical examination may be very helpful in assessing respiratory function. For example, retracted intercostal muscles may reflect respiratory distress. Inward movement of the abdominal wall during inspiration, a sign called *abdominal paradox,* signifies that the diaphragms are not contracting normally and frequently presages ventilatory failure. In addition, hypoxemia may be suspected if there is cyanosis of the lips and palate. Nevertheless, cyanosis is an insensitive finding, and respiratory failure can only be diagnosed through systemic arterial blood gas analysis.

Assessment of Ventilation

Samples of systemic arterial blood for measurements of Pa_{CO_2} and Pa_{O_2}, pH, and bicarbonate concentration ($[HCO_3^-]$) may be obtained from either repeated percutaneous arterial punctures or indwelling arterial catheters. The Pa_{CO_2} is used to assess the adequacy of ventilation and diagnose hypercapnic respiratory failure, also called *ventilatory failure.* Similarly, the pH and $[HCO_3^-]$ measurements can be used to determine whether hypercapnia is acute or chronic. Table 68–2 lists normal values for these and other respiratory variables.

An approximation of Pa_{CO_2} may be made by measuring the end-tidal carbon dioxide tension (PET_{CO_2}) in expired gas. This is most conveniently measured in mechanically ventilated patients. If the PET_{CO_2} is to substitute for the Pa_{CO_2}, the two values should be correlated using several paired measurements. The PET_{CO_2} usually is slightly less than the Pa_{CO_2}.

Ventilatory variables such as respiratory rate (F) and tidal volume (V_T) and their product, minute ventilation ($\dot{V}E$), may be accurately measured by a technique called *respiratory inductance plethysmography,* which uses wire coils embedded in bands that fit around the chest and abdomen to detect movements of these areas. These variables also may be measured by a pneumotachograph or other types of spirometers in patients who are breathing through endotracheal tubes. The ratio of F to V_T (F/V_T) increases as patients breathe rapidly and shallowly. An F/V_T of 100 or more usually indicates the need to start or continue mechanical ventilation.

Neither alveolar ventilation ($\dot{V}A$) nor dead space ventilation ($\dot{V}D$) can be measured directly, although the value of $\dot{V}A$ may be inferred if $\dot{V}E$ and $\dot{V}D$ are known. The ratio of $\dot{V}D$ to V_T per breath can be calculated in patients whose Pa_{CO_2} and PET_{CO_2} are known using the modified Bohr equation:

$$V_D/V_T = \frac{Pa_{CO_2} - PET_{CO_2}}{Pa_{CO_2}} \tag{1}$$

The V_D/V_T is usually 0.30 to 0.35 in healthy persons breathing spontaneously. In patients with normal lungs being mechanically ventilated it is ~ 0.50.

CO_2 production ($\dot{V}CO_2$) may be measured by closed systems in patients breathing spontaneously or receiving mechanical ventilation. Once $\dot{V}CO_2$ is measured, V_D/V_T is calculated from Equation 1, and $\dot{V}A$ is inferred, one can determine which abnormality in the alveolar ventilation relationship is responsible for ventilatory failure. This relationship is captured in the equation

$$Pa_{CO_2} = \frac{K(\dot{V}CO_2)}{\dot{V}A} \tag{2}$$

where K is a constant and $(\dot{V}A) = (\dot{V}E) - (\dot{V}D)$. (See Ch. 65 for further explanation.)

Three other variables that reflect ventilatory capability are the maximum inspiratory pressure (MIP), the vital capacity (VC), and the ratio of the forced expiratory volume in 1 second (FEV_1) to the forced VC. In the MIP maneuver, a manometer is used to measure the negative pressure patients can generate when inspiring from a low lung volume. An MIP that is > -20 cm H_2O suggests the need for ventilatory support, whereas an MIP that is < -20 cm H_2O correlates with successful weaning from mechanical ventilation.

The VC, the greatest amount of gas that can be inhaled or exhaled in a single breath, can be measured with any of a variety of spirometers. The normal VC is ~ 50 ml per kilogram of body weight. A VC of < 10 ml per kilogram usually indicates the need for mechanical ventilation. The FEV_1 also can be measured by spirometry. Normally the FEV_1 is ~ 75 to 80% of the forced VC; reductions in this ratio may occur in patients with airways obstruction due to asthma or chronic obstructive pulmonary disease (COPD).

Assessment of Respiratory System Compliance

The amount of pressure required to increase the volume of the lungs and the thoracic cavity is termed the *compliance of the respiratory system* (C_{RS}). When determined in a patient who is being mechanically ventilated, effective respiratory system compliance (C_{EFF}) equals the maximum or peak airway pressure (Pmax) required to deliver a given V_T minus the amount of positive end-expiratory pressure (PEEP) the patient is receiving. Thus

TABLE 68-1. KINDS OF RESPIRATORY FAILURE

Failure	Definition	Abnormality	Examples
Ventilatory failure	Inadequate alveolar ventilation	High Pa_{CO_2}	Narcotic or sedative drug overdosage Pleural diseases Asthma Chronic obstructive pulmonary disease Neuromuscular diseases
Failure of arterial oxygenation	Inadequate oxygenation of systemic arterial blood	Low Pa_{O_2}	Pneumonia Asthma Chronic obstructive pulmonary disease
Failure of oxygen transport	Inadequate supply of oxygenated blood to tissues	Low Ca_{O_2} or $\dot{Q}T$ or both Low $P\bar{v}_{O_2}$, $S\bar{v}_{O_2}$, $C\bar{v}_{O_2}$ Increased $C(a - \bar{v})_{O_2}$ Lactic acidosis	Anemia Carbon monoxide poisoning Hypovolemic shock Cardiogenic shock Cardiorespiratory arrest
Failure of oxygen extraction	Inadequate tissue oxygen uptake	Low $\dot{V}_{O_2}$ High $P\bar{v}_{O_2}$, $S\bar{v}_{O_2}$, $C\bar{v}_{O_2}$ Decreased $C(a - \bar{v})_{O_2}$ Lactic acidosis	Cyanide poisoning Adult respiratory distress syndrome? Multiple organ system failure?

Note: Pa_{CO_2} = systemic arterial carbon dioxide tension; Pa_{O_2} = systemic arterial oxygen tension; Ca_{O_2} = systemic arterial oxygen content; $\dot{Q}T$ = cardiac output; $P\bar{v}_{O_2}$ = mixed venous oxygen tension; $S\bar{v}_{O_2}$ = mixed venous oxygen saturation; $C\bar{v}_{O_2}$ = mixed venous oxygen content; $C(a - \bar{v})_{O_2}$ = arterial–mixed venous content difference; $\dot{V}_{O_2}$ = oxygen consumption.

$$C_{EFF} = \frac{V_T}{(P_{max} - PEEP)} \quad (3)$$

Because it is a dynamic measurement made when gas is flowing, C_{EFF} includes the resistance to gas flow in the airways and ventilator tubing, as well as the volume and pressure characteristics of the lungs and chest wall. It will be influenced by airways obstruction, or secretions, and the diameter of the endotracheal tube.

Static respiratory system compliance (Cstat) is a measure of the airway pressure (Pstat) required to distend the lungs and maintain the increase in volume after a V_T has been delivered and gas is not flowing into or out of the lungs. The amount of PEEP should be subtracted to determine this pressure. Thus

$$Cstat = \frac{V_T}{(Pstat - PEEP)} \quad (4)$$

Because it is a static measurement, Cstat reflects only the compliance of the lungs and chest wall and is not affected by resistance to gas flow. It will be decreased (normal level is 50 to 60 ml per cen-

TABLE 68-2. NORMAL VALUES FOR SELECTED RESPIRATORY VARIABLES

Variables	Symbol	Value
Systemic arterial carbon dioxide tension	Pa_{CO_2}	40 mm Hg
Fraction of inspired oxygen	FI_{O_2}	0.21
Systemic arterial oxygen tension	Pa_{O_2}	95 mm Hg
Carbon dioxide production	$\dot{V}_{CO_2}$	200 ml/min
Oxygen consumption	$\dot{V}_{O_2}$	250 ml/min
Minute ventilation	$\dot{V}_E$	6 L/min
Dead space ventilation (per breath)	V_D	150 ml
Tidal volume	V_T	450 ml
Dead space to tidal volume ratio (per breath)	V_D/V_T	0.3–0.35
Respiratory rate	F	12–22/min
pH	pH	7.40
Bicarbonate concentration	$[HCO_3^-]$	24 mg/dl
Hemoglobin	Hb	15 grams/ml
Systemic arterial oxygen saturation	Sa_{O_2}	98%
Systemic arterial oxygen content	Ca_{O_2}	20 ml/dl
Mixed venous oxygen tension	$P\bar{v}_{O_2}$	40 mm Hg
Mixed venous oxygen saturation	$S\bar{v}_{O_2}$	75%
Mixed venous oxygen content	$C\bar{v}_{O_2}$	15 ml/dl
Arterial to mixed venous oxygen content difference	$C(a - \bar{v})_{O_2}$	5 ml/dl
Shunt fraction	$\dot{Q}S/\dot{Q}T$	<7%
Maximum inspiratory pressure	MIP	-40 cm H_2O
Vital capacity	VC	50 ml/kg
Forced expiratory volume in 1 second	FEV_1	75% of VC

timeter of water) by conditions such as the adult respiratory distress syndrome (ARDS) that decrease lung volume. Weaning from mechanical ventilation is difficult if Cstat is < 25 ml per centimeter of water.

Assessment of Intrinsic Positive End-Expiratory Pressure

Another measurement that may be made on mechanically ventilated patients is intrinsic or auto-PEEP. Auto-PEEP occurs in patients with airways obstruction and other disorders who fail to complete expiration either during spontaneous breathing or before they receive the next breath from a mechanical ventilator. This results in air trapping that produces positive pressure at end expiration. The auto-PEEP effect can reduce cardiac filling pressures and $\dot{Q}T$; it also can elevate readings of vascular pressures inside the chest unless it, like intentionally administered PEEP, is accounted for. Auto-PEEP can be measured in mechanically ventilated patients by stopping airflow at end expiration just before the next breath, allowing the pressure in the airways and the ventilator tubing to equilibrate, and reading the pressure from the ventilator manometer.

Assessment of Arterial Oxygenation

Just as measuring Pa_{CO_2} is used to diagnose ventilatory failure, failure of arterial oxygenation can be diagnosed only by determining the Pa_{O_2}. Introducing the values for Pa_{CO_2} and the inspired O_2 tension (PI_{O_2}) into the alveolar gas equation determines the alveolar O_2 tension (PA_{O_2}). Subtracting the Pa_{O_2} from the PA_{O_2} yields the alveolar-arterial O_2 tension difference [$P(A - a)_{O_2}$]. This information in turn provides insight into the probable cause of hypoxemia in a given patient. The alveolar gas equation is

$$PA_{O_2} = PI_{O_2} - \frac{Pa_{CO_2}}{RQ} \quad (5)$$

where RQ is the respiratory quotient, which is usually assumed to be 0.8.

Because systemic arterial blood sampling may be associated with complications, a less invasive approximation of the state of arterial oxygenation often is desirable. This may be accomplished through pulse oximetry, in which the differential absorption of certain wavelengths of light passed through a finger or other appendage is used to calculate the systemic arterial saturation (Sa_{O_2}). This technique accurately measures Sa_{O_2} > 80% in patients with adequate peripheral blood flow. It is particularly helpful as a continuous measurement in patients who are relatively stable and in whom a normal oxyhemoglobin saturation curve enables good correlation between Sa_{O_2} and Pa_{O_2}. The Sa_{O_2} measured by oximetry does not account for hemoglobin that is saturated by substances other than O_2, such as carbon monoxide (CO).

Assessment of Oxygen Transport and Extraction

The Sa_{O_2} also may be derived from the Pa_{O_2}. The Sa_{O_2}, the hemoglobin (Hb) concentration, and Pa_{O_2} are the determinants of the systemic O_2 content (Ca_{O_2}). Once Ca_{O_2} is known, it can be multiplied by the cardiac output ($\dot{Q}T$) obtained by pulmonary artery catheterization (see Ch. 33.6) to determine the systemic O_2 transport ($\dot{T}o_2$).

Thus systemic arterial blood gas analysis helps diagnose failure of $\dot{T}o_2$, determine the abnormalities responsible for such failure, and assess its severity.

Pulmonary arterial blood gas analysis provides information about the mixed venous oxygen tension, saturation, and content ($P\bar{v}_{O_2}$, $S\bar{v}_{O_2}$, $C\bar{v}_{O_2}$). In addition, $S\bar{v}_{O_2}$ may be measured continuously with oximetric pulmonary artery catheters. Combined with values for $\dot{Q}T$ and Ca_{O_2} obtained by systemic arterial blood gas analysis, the $C\bar{v}_{O_2}$ may be inserted into the Fick equation to calculate the O_2 consumption ($\dot{V}o_2$):

$$\dot{V}o_2 = \dot{Q}T[C(a - \bar{v})_{O_2}] \qquad (6)$$

where $C(a - \bar{v})_{O_2}$ is the arterial–mixed venous content difference.

Alternatively, $\dot{V}o_2$ may be determined directly by measuring concentrations of oxygen in inspired and expired gas and the inspired and expired volumes. Even if $\dot{V}o_2$ is not calculated or precisely known, the decrease in $P\bar{v}_{O_2}$, $S\bar{v}_{O_2}$, and $C\bar{v}_{O_2}$ and the increase in $C(a - \bar{v})_{O_2}$ that characterize inadequate $\dot{T}o_2$ can be assessed by analysis of systemic and pulmonary artery blood gas samples, as can the increase in $P\bar{v}_{O_2}$, $S\bar{v}_{O_2}$, and $C\bar{v}_{O_2}$ and the decrease in $C(a - \bar{v})_{O_2}$ that characterize inadequate O_2 extraction.

Assessment of Shunt Fraction

Finally, combined systemic and pulmonary artery blood gas analysis may be used to quantitate the contribution to hypoxemia of right-to-left intrapulmonary shunting of blood. This may be performed in patients receiving an inspired O_2 fraction (Fi_{O_2}) of 1.0 using the following shunt equation:

$$\frac{\dot{Q}s}{\dot{Q}T} = \frac{Cc'_{O_2} - Ca_{O_2}}{Cc'_{O_2} - C\bar{v}_{O_2}} \qquad (7)$$

where $\dot{Q}s$ is the volume of shunted blood and Cc'_{O_2} is an approximation of end-capillary blood oxygen content, assuming Pc'_{O_2} to be the same as PA_{O_2} and calculating Cc'_{O_2} on the basis of that assumption. The shunt equation is based on the Fick equation. A simpler but less precise way of estimating intrapulmonary shunt, which also is based on the Fick equation and assumes a normal $C(a - \bar{v})_{O_2}$ of 5 ml per deciliter of blood, is to divide the $P(A - a)_{O_2}$ by 20. The normal $\dot{Q}s$ is $\leq 7\%$ of $\dot{Q}T$.

Assessment of Tissue Oxygenation

As suggested by the preceding discussion, the data obtained from combined systemic and pulmonary arterial blood gas analysis may be very helpful in managing critically ill patients. Nevertheless, not all such patients require such sophisticated monitoring techniques, and the techniques still cannot provide an ideal assessment of oxygenation of a tissue level. The same can be said for serial measurement of serum lactate levels, which some physicians use as a monitoring tool.

Recently, measuring the gastric intramucosal pH through a tonometer tube situated in the stomach that measures intraluminal P_{CO_2} has been proposed as a way of estimating the adequacy of oxygenation of that organ and, by inference, the body as a whole. Measuring intramucosal pH has been shown to be more sensitive than lactate levels and other variables in predicting outcome from circulatory failure. However, despite this and other technologic advances in critical care monitoring, assessing tissue oxygenation probably is best performed by analyzing individual organ system function by simple biochemical tests, such as renal and hepatic indices, measuring urine output, and observing mental status.

GENERAL MANAGEMENT OF RESPIRATORY FAILURE

Abnormalities in ventilation, arterial oxygenation, $\dot{T}o_2$, and O_2 extraction may exist separately or coexist in critically ill patients. As a result, managing such patients may require therapy to improve these processes either independently or simultaneously. The following section provides a general approach to improving ventilation, arterial oxygenation, $\dot{T}o_2$, and O_2 extraction.

Therapy to Improve Ventilation

The Pa_{CO_2} may be improved by manipulating the variables that affect it: $\dot{V}co_2$ and $\dot{V}A$ ($\dot{V}A$ is equal to $\dot{V}E - \dot{V}D$). Manipulating $\dot{V}A$ may involve any or all components of the respiratory system. These include the respiratory control centers in the brain stem that regulate $\dot{V}A$, the nerves that transmit messages from the control centers to the respiratory muscles, the muscles themselves, the chest wall to which the muscles are attached, the pleura that lines the lungs, the lung parenchyma, and the upper and lower airways.

Ventilation may be improved in patients who have overdosed on narcotics by administering intravenous naloxone in 0.4-mg doses as required. Similarly, the sedating effects of benzodiazepines can be antagonized by intravenous flumazenil in 0.2-mg doses. The excretion of some other drugs that depress ventilation may be enhanced by hemodialysis or charcoal hemoperfusion. At the very least, narcotics and sedatives should be administered cautiously to patients at risk of ventilatory failure. Intravenous doxapram in a bolus of 140 mg and a continuous infusion of 2 mg per minute has been used to overcome drug-induced ventilatory depression and to forestall mechanical ventilation in a variety of patients whose ventilatory failure is thought to be reversible, such as those recovering from anesthesia or having exacerbated COPD. However, neither this agent nor other ventilatory stimulants can forestall mechanical ventilation indefinitely.

Disorders of the chest wall such as massive obesity and kyphoscoliosis usually are not amenable to specific treatment. However, this is not true of neuromuscular diseases that cause respiratory muscle weakness or paralysis, as will be discussed. Beyond therapies for neuromuscular diseases, there are few measures that improve respiratory muscle weakness. Theophylline has been shown to increase ventilatory capacity in some, but not all, patients with COPD. Nutrition also improves respiratory muscle function to a limited extent, but it also increases $\dot{V}co_2$, which may offset any increase in $\dot{V}E$.

Pleural and parenchymal diseases limit $\dot{V}A$ by restricting lung expansion and by increasing $\dot{V}D$. These disorders also increase the work of breathing, which increases $\dot{V}co_2$ and may fatigue the respiratory muscles. Using tube thoracostomy to evacuate the pleural space is called for in patients compromised by pneumothorax, hemothorax, or pleural empyema.

Anatomic obstruction of the upper airways should be removed or bypassed when it causes or could cause hypercapnia; this applies to excessive soft tissues as well as to aspirated material. Inspissated secretions frequently cause or contribute to ventilatory failure in a variety of patients, including those with neuromuscular diseases, asthma and COPD, and ARDS. Secretion removal may be facilitated by chest physiotherapy or gentle endotracheal suctioning. Iodinated glycerol has been shown to facilitate secretion clearance in outpatients with COPD, although the effects of this oral mucolytic agent on $\dot{V}A$ and Pa_{CO_2} have not been determined.

The $\dot{V}co_2$ may be reduced by lowering the metabolic rate and thereby the need for increased ventilation. For example, seizures may respond to phenytoin (50 mg per minute intravenously up to a loading dose of 1000 mg, followed by 300 mg per day). Shivering may be prevented by chlorpromazine (25 to 75 mg intramuscularly). Fever may be reduced with antipyretics such as aspirin or acetaminophen, which are more effective than cooling blankets or sponge baths in decreasing core temperature.

Unfortunately, the increase in $\dot{V}D$ caused by obliterated pulmonary vasculature due to disorders such as ARDS rarely is amenable to medical measures. Increases in the $\dot{V}D$ caused by pulmonary thromboembolism may be treated with thrombolytic agents such as streptokinase and prevented with heparin.

Therapy to Improve Arterial Oxygenation

The Pa_{O_2} may be improved by manipulating the variables that affect it: Pa_{CO_2}, Pi_{O_2}, and $P(A - a)_{O_2}$. Thus, if hypoventilation is the sole cause of hypoxemia, as might be the case in a narcotic overdosage, the Pa_{O_2} increases as the Pa_{CO_2} decreases in response to naloxone. Similarly, if the Pi_{O_2} is reduced by the combustion of O_2 in a fire or by living at high altitude, the Pa_{O_2} should improve if the patient breathes supplemental O_2. Patients whose $P(A - a)_{O_2}$ is increased require therapy for the underlying cause of their hypoxemia as well as supplemental O_2.

POSITIONING. Alveolar collapse, also called *atelectasis*, commonly occurs in dependent regions of the lung. Atelectasis is particularly problematic in supine patients whose lung expansion is limited by obesity, pain on deep breathing, or the presence of restricting bandages over the abdomen or chest. Positioning such patients upright from time to time and relieving their pain with narcotics may greatly improve the Pa_{O_2}.

Adults with unilateral parenchymal lung disorders such as infectious pneumonia may become more hypoxemic when their diseased lung is dependent. The Pa_{O_2} of these patients may improve when they lie on the side of the nondiseased lung. Pulmonary edema tends to collect in dependent lung regions because the intravascular hydrostatic pressure is greatest there. For this reason, the Pa_{O_2} of patients with pulmonary edema may improve, at least temporarily, if they are moved from the supine to the prone position. Unfortunately, such positioning may complicate nursing care.

OXYGEN DELIVERY SYSTEMS. Hypoxemia usually responds to increasing the $F_{I_{O_2}}$ and thereby the $P_{I_{O_2}}$. The hypoxemia associated with disorders such as asthma and COPD that are characterized by ventilation-perfusion mismatching but not by intrapulmonary shunt usually are relieved by supplementing O_2 at a low $F_{I_{O_2}}$. An $F_{I_{O_2}}$ of 0.24 to 0.35 usually can be achieved by delivering O_2 through nasal prongs at flow rates of 5 to 6 liters per minute; higher flow rates dry the nasal mucosa and do not further increase the $F_{I_{O_2}}$ because patients dilute the oxygen with ambient air. Open face masks provide a higher flow of humidified, premixed air and O_2 at an $F_{I_{O_2}}$ of up to 0.5. Such masks can be used with a Venturi device that allows precise setting of the $F_{I_{O_2}}$ to avoid ventilatory depression in patients who have chronic CO_2 retention.

Tightly fitting face masks with a nonrebreathing valve and reservoir bag can be used to provide even higher concentrations of O_2 to patients whose hypoxemia is caused by shunting associated with disorders such as severe infectious pneumonia and ARDS. However, these masks are uncomfortable and may cause nasal necrosis if left in place for several days.

Endotracheal Intubation

INDICATIONS FOR INTUBATION. Humidified O_2 at an $F_{I_{O_2}}$ higher than 0.50 is most reliably delivered through the closed system provided by an endotracheal tube. The other indications for endotracheal intubation are listed in Table 68–3. Although intubation often precedes mechanical ventilation, it should be stressed that the indications for these two therapies and their timing are not necessarily the same. For example, some patients who are intubated to prevent aspiration of gastric contents never require mechanical ventilation.

KINDS OF INTUBATION. Endotracheal intubation may be performed either via the translaryngeal route through the nose or mouth or via a tracheostomy. Tracheostomy tubes once were used routinely in patients requiring intubation for longer than 1 or 2 days. However, the development of low-pressure and high-compliance cuffs that limit tracheal damage from nasal or oral tubes, demonstration that such tubes can be left in place for weeks and even months without severe sequelae, and documentation of complications after tracheostomy have led to a preference for orotracheal or nasotracheal intubation over tracheostomy in all but a few patients. Such patients include those with laryngeal fractures and those who will require intubation for longer than a month or so. Tracheostomy tubes generally are more comfortable than translaryngeal tubes; they also are easier to suction through, and talking may be made possible by fitting the tubes with a device that directs a stream of air retrograde through the larynx above the cuff site.

Nasal intubation provides good support for the endotracheal tube and often allows patients to swallow their secretions better than when the tube passes orally. Oral intubation may allow passage of a tube with a larger diameter (≥ 8 mm) than the nostril will accommodate and usually is the preferred route during emergency intubations. Whichever route is chosen, the tube diameter should be sufficient to seal the trachea without cuff pressures > 20 to 25 mm Hg. These pressures should be monitored regularly. Tube position

should be determined by chest radiograph immediately following insertion and on a regular basis thereafter. Intubation of the right mainstem bronchus, which extends from the trachea at less of an angle than the left mainstem bronchus, should be looked for in particular.

COMPLICATIONS OF INTUBATION. Many patients receiving endotracheal intubation suffer adverse consequences. Excessive cuff pressure requirements (> 20 mm Hg), self-extubation, and inability to seal the airway are the most common complications with nasotracheal and orotracheal tubes. Problems associated with tracheostomy include stomal hemorrhage, excessive cuff pressure requirements, and subcutaneous emphysema. Follow-up studies of patients receiving intubation and mechanical ventilation reveal a higher incidence of tracheal stenosis after tracheostomy compared with translaryngeal intubation, although laryngeal complications are more common with nasal and oral tubes.

WEANING FROM INTUBATION. In general, endotracheal tubes may be removed when the original indications for their insertion are no longer present. For example, extubation frequently follows the return of consciousness and an adequate gag reflex in previously comatose patients or restored adequate ventilation and arterial oxygenation in patients with respiratory failure. If an endotracheal tube has been in place only briefly, it may be removed after secretions have been suctioned from above the cuff site and the patient has been seated upright. Depending on physical and mental status, a patient with a tracheostomy may be progressed from a cuffed to a noncuffed or fenestrated tube and then may be extubated.

Mechanical Ventilation

INDICATIONS FOR MECHANICAL VENTILATION. Mechanical ventilation may be necessary in patients who have inadequate ventilation, inadequate arterial oxygenation, or both. Furthermore, severe airway obstruction caused by asthma and COPD or parenchymal disease caused by disorders such as ARDS may increase the work of breathing to levels that cannot be maintained by spontaneous breathing. Finally, mechanical ventilation may be required in clinically unstable patients such as those in shock and in patients who require hyperventilation to decrease cerebral blood flow and intracranial pressure. These indications and severe physiologic abnormalities that may indicate the need for mechanical ventilation are listed in Table 68–4.

KINDS OF MECHANICAL VENTILATION. Mechanical ventilators include devices to assist ventilation, negative- or positive-pressure ventilation, and extracorporeal ventilation. The simplest kind of mechanical ventilation consists of devices that function like the diaphragm. One such device is the rocking bed, which swings the patient in a 45-degree arc, forcing the weak or paralyzed diaphragm into inspiratory and expiratory positions by gravity. Another is the pneumobelt, which is used by patients in the sitting position. The pneumobelt intermittently squeezes the abdomen and forces the diaphragm cephalad. It then falls due to gravity, creating a marginally effective inspiration in the process.

Negative-Pressure Ventilation. Ventilation also can be supported by devices that generate a negative pressure around the chest during inspiration to substitute for the negative pleural and airway pressures normally created by contracting the respiratory muscles. Negative-pressure ventilation can be achieved either by

TABLE 68–3. INDICATIONS FOR ENDOTRACHEAL INTUBATION

To provide a closed system for mechanical ventilation or oxygen delivery, especially at a high fraction of inspired oxygen
To prevent or reverse upper airway obstruction
To protect against aspiration of gastric contents
To facilitate tracheobronchial toilet

TABLE 68–4. INDICATIONS FOR MECHANICAL VENTILATION

Acute hypercapnia
Minute ventilation > 10 L/min
Ratio of respiratory rate to tidal volume ≥ 100
Vital capacity $< 10-15$ ml/kg body weight
Maximum inspiratory pressure more positive than -20 cm H_2O
Dead space to tidal volume fraction ≥ 0.60
Acute hypoxemia ($Pa_{O_2} < 50-60$ mm Hg, especially if inspired oxygen fraction ≥ 0.4 or $P(A - a)_{O_2} > 300$ mm Hg on inspired $F_{I_{O_2}}$ of 1.0)
Clinical instability
Need for hyperventilation therapy

Note: Pa_{CO_2} = systemic arterial carbon dioxide tension; Pa_{O_2} = systemic arterial oxygen tension; $P(A - a)_{O_2}$ = systemic alveolar to arterial oxygen pressure difference; $F_{I_{O_2}}$ = fraction of inspired oxygen.

including the entire body except the head and neck in an "iron lung," by encompassing the thorax in a garment wrap, or by fitting a cuirass to the anterior chest. As with machines that substitute for the diaphragm, negative-pressure ventilators are best suited for stable patients with neuromuscular diseases whose lungs are normal and who do not require endotracheal intubation to deliver O_2 at a high F_{IO_2}.

Positive-Pressure Ventilation. Due to the limitations of the aforementioned devices, positive-pressure ventilation (PPV) is the kind of mechanical ventilation most widely used today. With PPV, gas is delivered under positive pressure, usually through an endotracheal tube, into the airways and the lungs. In contrast to negative-pressure ventilation, PPV produces a positive airway pressure during inspiration. This inflates the alveoli, providing both ventilation and arterial oxygenation while reducing the work of breathing.

Most PPV's may be used to deliver gas up to either a preset pressure or volume. The first approach allows establishable limits on the Pmax and Pstat used for lung inflation but allows VT and hence $\dot{V}E$ to vary, depending on CRS. Alternatively, the ventilators may deliver a preset VT at whatever Pmax is required to inflate the lungs, which guarantees $\dot{V}E$ but may increase Pmax and Pstat. Standard ventilators are cycled whenever a certain pressure or volume is reached or at preset time intervals. Time-cycled ventilation is used primarily in infants or in adults who are ventilated at a high F that precludes pressure or volume cycling.

Modes of Positive-Pressure Ventilation. Perhaps the simplest mode of PPV is *controlled mechanical ventilation* (CMV), in which the ventilator delivers gas at a preset F and either a preset Pmax or VT (Table 68–5). Volume-cycled CMV is used most often in patients who are unconscious due to illness or drugs, who are being intentionally hyperventilated, or who are recovering from anesthesia. Patients whose ventilatory drives are intact often must be hyperventilated or given sedatives to diminish their tendency to breathe asynchronously with the ventilator while receiving CMV. As with most other modes of PPV, an inspiratory-to-expiratory (I:E) ratio of 1:3 or less generally is used with CMV to allow adequate time for expiration and thereby avoid auto-PEEP. Because patients receiving CMV cannot increase their $\dot{V}E$ voluntarily, their ventilatory status must be followed closely. Thus the advantage of CMV—complete control of ventilatory function—is also its major limitation.

Assisted mechanical ventilation (AMV) is a PPV mode in which the patient triggers the ventilator to deliver a preset VT. Triggering is accomplished by generating an airway pressure less than that in the ventilator and tubing; if the ventilator is sensitive to this pressure, it will increase F and $\dot{V}E$ in response to patient demands. The machine will not trigger if it is insensitive, however, and if it is unduly sensitive, it will trigger in response to small fluctuations in airway pressure in addition to attempts to breathe. The latter problem may be circumvented by establishing a proper sensitivity or, if this is not possible, by sedating the patient. Because sedation or neurologic changes may prevent patients from adjusting $\dot{V}E$, an obligatory backup (or CMV) rate that will provide the minimum allowable $\dot{V}E$ should be used with AMV. The combination of AMV and CMV, which is called the *assist/control mode,* offers the great advantage of responding to changes in patient status without the close monitoring needed with CMV. Traditionally, AMV and CMV have been referred to as *intermittent positive-pressure ventilation* (IPPV).

Intermittent mandatory ventilation (IMV) is a PPV mode in which the ventilator delivers a preset VT at specific intervals while also providing a flow of gas for spontaneous breathing. The form of IMV used most often today is *synchronized IMV* (SIMV), in which ventilator breaths are delivered only after the end of a spontaneous expiration so that patients are not hyperinflated by receiving spontaneous and machine-delivered inspirations simultaneously. With SIMV, the ventilator F may be set high enough to provide most, if not all, of the patient's $\dot{V}E$ initially; F then may be lowered as the patient improves. The potential benefits of SIMV include less asynchronous breathing and lower sedation requirements, reducing mean airway pressure by combining spontaneous and machine breaths and improving respiratory muscle function by allowing patients to breathe spontaneously. Disadvantages include the lack of a backup to guarantee $\dot{V}E$ in unstable patients and the possibility of causing respiratory muscle fatigue in patients who receive SIMV at a low ventilator F.

High-frequency ventilation (HFV) delivers gas to the lungs using either a conventional ventilator with very high internal compressibility, high-pressure jet sources, or an oscillator that entrains ambient air. The ventilator F with HFV is > 60 per minute, the I:E ratio is very small, and the VT is either greater than the patient's anatomic VD (convective flow HFV) or less than the VD (nonconvective flow HFV). Although adequate ventilation with a VD/VT > 1.0 would seem to be physiologically impossible, nonconvective flow HFV can adequately eliminate CO_2 in some patients probably by enhancing diffusion in the lung. Both convective and nonconvective flow HFV usually produce a Pmax that is less than that with other modes of PPV, although the small I:E ratio usually produces auto-PEEP. The lower Pmax supports using HFV to treat patients with bronchopleural fistulas and conditions such as ARDS. However, ventilation and arterial oxygenation may be inadequate with HFV.

Pressure-support ventilation (PSV) augments spontaneous ventilatory efforts with a level of positive airway pressure that is preset to achieve a desired VT. This mode of ventilation allows patients to set their own F and timing of breaths, which may be more comfortable than other modes of PPV. PSV also is useful in overcoming the work of breathing through an endotracheal tube. Inasmuch as patients must initiate breaths with PSV, it should not be used in unstable patients and is most applicable during weaning.

TABLE 68–5. MODES OF POSITIVE-PRESSURE VENTILATION

Mode	Description	Advantages/Disadvantages
Controlled mechanical ventilation (CMV)	Ventilator F, VT (and thus $\dot{V}E$) preset.	May be used with sedation or paralysis; ventilator cannot respond to ventilatory needs.
Assisted mechanical ventilation (AMV) or assist/control	Ventilator VT preset but patient can increase F (and thus $\dot{V}E$).	Ventilator may respond to ventilatory needs; ventilator may under- or overtrigger depending on sensitivity.
Intermittent mandatory ventilation (IMV)	Ventilator delivers preset VT and F, but patient also may breathe spontaneously.	May decrease asynchronous breathing and sedation requirements; ventilator cannot respond to ventilatory needs.
Synchronized intermittent mandatory ventilation (SIMV)	Same as IMV, but ventilator breaths only delivered after patient exhales.	Same as IMV, plus patient not overinflated by receiving spontaneous and ventilator breaths at same time.
High-frequency ventilation (HFV)	Ventilator F is increased, and VT may be smaller than VD.	May reduce peak airway pressure; may cause auto-PEEP.
Pressure-support ventilation (PSV)	Patient breathes at own F; VT determined by inspiratory pressure and respiratory system compliance.	Increased comfort and decreased work of breathing; ventilator cannot respond to ventilatory needs.
Pressure-control ventilation (PCV)	Ventilator peak pressure, F, and respiratory time preset.	Peak inspiratory pressures may be decreased; hypoventilation may occur.
Inverse-ratio ventilation (IRV)	Inspiratory time exceeds expiratory time to facilitate inspiration.	May improve gas exchange by increasing time spent in inspiration; may cause auto-PEEP.

F = rate; VT = tidal volume; VD = dead space; $\dot{V}E$ = minute ventilation; PEEP = positive end-expiratory pressure.

With *pressure-control ventilation* (PCV), gas is not delivered at a constant VT. Instead, it is delivered until a preset Pmax is reached, and the patient's V̇E is determined by the preset Pmax, ventilator F, and inspiratory time. In contrast to the squarewave gas flow pattern used with CMV and AMV, inspiratory flow with PCV decelerates when the Pmax is reached. Advocates of this mode state that complications are reduced with PCV because Pmax is limited. In addition, the decelerating waveform is thought to provide ventilation of more alveoli. This might be particularly helpful in patients with ARDS, although PCV may not provide a V̇E that is sufficient to prevent hypoventilation.

In *inverse-ratio ventilation* (IRV), the I:E ratio is increased above the normal level of 1:3 or less to 1:1 or more. The rationale for this approach is that the longer duration of inspiratory positive pressure will open stiff or fluid-filled alveoli, and the shorter expiratory time will not allow these alveoli to collapse. Peak airway pressure also may be lower than with other modes of PPV, although the increase in I:E time probably increases auto-PEEP. One drawback to IRV is that it is often uncomfortable and requires sedation or paralysis of the patient.

Complications of Positive-Pressure Ventilation. One possible result of PPV is that inflating lungs at high pressure may damage them. Such damage has been described traditionally as barotrauma, implying that it is the consequence of pressure changes. However, because alveolar distention occurs as a result of changes in pressure and probably is responsible for the damage, *volutrauma* may be a better term. Pneumothorax is a common kind of volutrauma, but subcutaneous and mediastinal emphysema, parenchymal lung cysts, and systemic air embolism also may occur. Some investigators believe that PPV at high pressures and volumes also causes bronchopulmonary dysplasia and diffuse alveolar damage that is identical to ARDS and may either cause or perpetuate the syndrome.

In addition to these respiratory effects, PPV also may compromise the cardiovascular system. This occurs because the positive airway pressure during inspiration reduces venous return to the chest and may depress Q̇T. This effect may be increased if auto-PEEP is produced by PPV. On the other hand, it may be decreased if adequate time is allowed for airway and alveolar pressure to return to ambient levels during exhalation.

Weaning from Positive-Pressure Ventilation. Mechanical ventilatory support generally can be withdrawn when the reasons for its initiation are no longer present. This generally means complete or near-complete resolution of the patient's disease process, whether or not it involves the lungs. Such resolution should be reflected in clinical stability, a return of V̇E to <10 liters per minute, spontaneous VT to between 10 and 15 ml per kilogram, F/VT to <100, MIP to < −20 cm H_2O, VD/VT to <0.6, Pa_{O_2} to >50 to 60 to 100 mm Hg on an FI_{O_2} of 0.4, and P(A − a)$_{O_2}$ to <300 mm Hg on an FI_{O_2} of 1.0.

Weaning from AMV and other modes of PPV may be accomplished by connecting the endotracheal tube to a piece of tubing, called a *T-piece,* which is connected to a source of O_2 that is diluted with air to create the desired FI_{O_2}. The patients then may breathe spontaneously through the T-piece at their own F and VT until they meet some or all of the weaning criteria just described. Otherwise healthy persons recovering from anesthesia or drug overdosages may be put on a T-piece when they wake up and may be extubated after a brief (15- to 30-minute) period. Chronically ventilated patients may be put on a T-piece for a few minutes each hour or a few hours each day. When their respiratory muscles are less fatigued and they can tolerate longer periods on a T-piece, discontinuing the ventilator may be appropriate.

To wean a patient from SIMV, progressively reduce the ventilator F until he/she can maintain an adequate V̇E by breathing spontaneously. Patients initially receiving AMV or other PPV modes can be weaned with SIMV without ever using a T-piece. Finally, SIMV and PSV may be combined to facilitate weaning. The PSV level is reduced as long as the patient's VT remains adequate; SIMV is begun at an intermediate rate and reduced to an F of 2 or so to periodically inflate the lungs and limit atelectasis.

Extracorporeal Ventilation. Mechanical ventilation also can be extracorporeal, in that gas exchange takes place entirely or in part outside the body. With extracorporeal membrane oxygenation (ECMO), venous blood is circulated through a CO_2 scrubber and membrane oxygenator and returned to the body as arterial blood with a normal Pa_{CO_2} and Pa_{O_2}. Extracorporeal CO_2 removal (EC$_{CO_2}$R) also uses an extracorporeal circuit to remove CO_2 from venous blood, but oxygenation is achieved by insufflating O_2 into the lungs at high flow rates while the lungs are inflated with PPV at a low rate and held open with small amounts of PEEP to recruit alveoli. Both ECMO and EC$_{CO_2}$R are used only occasionally, the first in neonates for the most part and the latter in patients with ARDS.

Positive End-Expiratory Pressure

INDICATIONS FOR POSITIVE END-EXPIRATORY PRESSURE (PEEP). PEEP improves arterial oxygenation by increasing lung volume. This prevents or reverses atelectasis and redistributes intra-alveolar edema either into a thinner meniscus within the alveoli or out into the lung interstitium. The end result is that alveoli are recruited for better O_2 exchange. It should be noted that PEEP does not improve ventilation; in fact, the Pa_{CO_2} may increase because PEEP increases VD/VT by distending the airways and alveoli.

One indication for PEEP is to prevent or reverse atelectasis (Table 68–6). For example, low levels such as 5 cm H_2O of PEEP commonly are given to intubated patients who are supine in bed. Some investigators believe that low levels of PEEP facilitate weaning from mechanical ventilation by maintaining higher lung volumes while patients breathe through an endotracheal tube. They therefore continue PEEP during T-piece trials and when patients are receiving SIMV at a low ventilator F, with or without PSV.

The other major indication for PEEP is to improve arterial oxygenation in patients with diffuse parenchymal lung disorders such as ARDS. Because their hypoxemia is primarily due to interpulmonary shunt, such patients often cannot be oxygenated adequately even at an FI_{O_2} of 1.0, as illustrated in Figure 68–1. Administered in levels >5 cm H_2O, PEEP usually improves the Pa_{O_2} of these patients. It also allows the FI_{O_2} to be reduced to levels of 0.6 or less, thereby minimizing the risk of O_2 toxicity.

MODES OF POSITIVE END-EXPIRATORY PRESSURE. PEEP may be administered to spontaneously breathing patients through either a tightly fitting face mask or an endotracheal tube, in which case it is called *continuous positive airway pressure* (CPAP). It also may be combined with IPPV to create what is called *continuous positive-pressure ventilation* (CPPV). The improvement in oxygenation that may be produced by these two modes of PEEP depends primarily on the increase in lung volume they achieve, which, in turn, depends on the increase in airway pressure. As illustrated in Figure 68–2, the increase in airway pressure generally is greater with CPPV than with CPAP. Because of this, patients who merely have atelectasis often may be managed solely with CPAP. However, because they also have edema and their ventilatory needs are greater, patients with diffuse parenchymal lung disease generally receive CPPV.

COMPLICATIONS OF POSITIVE END-EXPIRATORY PRESSURE. As with its benefits, the complications of PEEP are related to lung volume and airway pressure. Delivering gas at high pressure to achieve an increase in lung volume throughout the ventilatory cycle is more likely to cause volutrauma than is delivering pressurized gas solely during inspiration. It also is more likely to decrease venous return to the chest and thereby depress blood pressure and Q̇T. Although the incidence of complications due to PEEP has not been well studied, these complications appear to be significant if high levels are used.

WEANING FROM POSITIVE END-EXPIRATORY PRESSURE. Patients who are receiving low levels of PEEP for atelectasis usually can be weaned without difficulty. However, premature withdrawal or reduction of PEEP from patients with diffuse parenchymal lung disorders can worsen oxygenation and cause clinical deterioration that requires hours or days of therapy to reverse. For this reason, PEEP should be withdrawn slowly, in small (2 to 5

TABLE 68–6. INDICATIONS FOR POSITIVE END-EXPIRATORY PRESSURE

To prevent or reverse atelectasis
To facilitate weaning from mechanical ventilation
To improve arterial oxygenation at a low inspired oxygen fraction

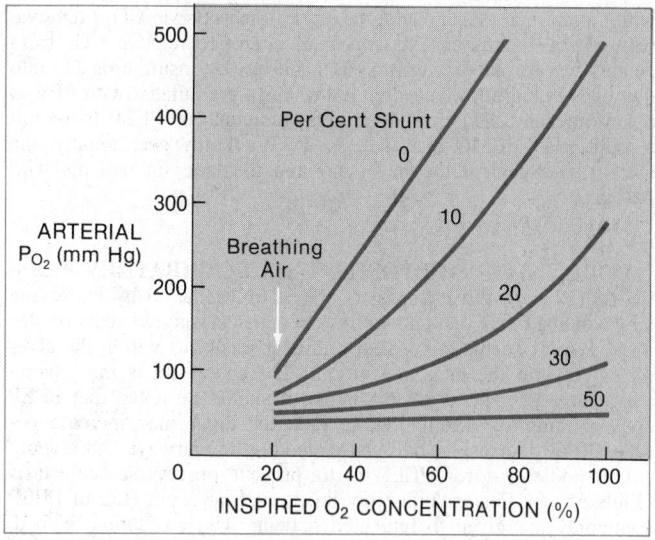

FIGURE 68–1. The relationship of the partial pressure of oxygen in systemic arterial blood (Pa_{O_2}) to the fraction of inspired oxygen (FI_{O_2}) with increasing amounts of shunt. Note that with 30% of the cardiac output being shunted, there is only a slight increase in Pa_{O_2}. (From West JR: Pulmonary Pathophysiology: The Essentials. Baltimore, Williams & Wilkins, 1977.)

cm H_2O) increments, with close monitoring of Pa_{O_2} or Sa_{O_2} in such patients. Prematurely reduced PEEP can be avoided if the disease process for which PEEP was initiated has resolved or is substantially improved, if the Pa_{O_2} is ≥ 80 mm Hg on an FI_{O_2} ≤ 0.4, and if these conditions have been present for several hours.

Therapy to Improve Oxygen Transport

To_2 may be improved by manipulating the variables that affect it: Ca_{O_2} and $\dot{Q}T$. The major determinants of Ca_{O_2} are the hemoglobin (Hb) concentration and Sa_{O_2}. Most physicians are familiar with the need to optimize Sa_{O_2} by the methods discussed earlier, but

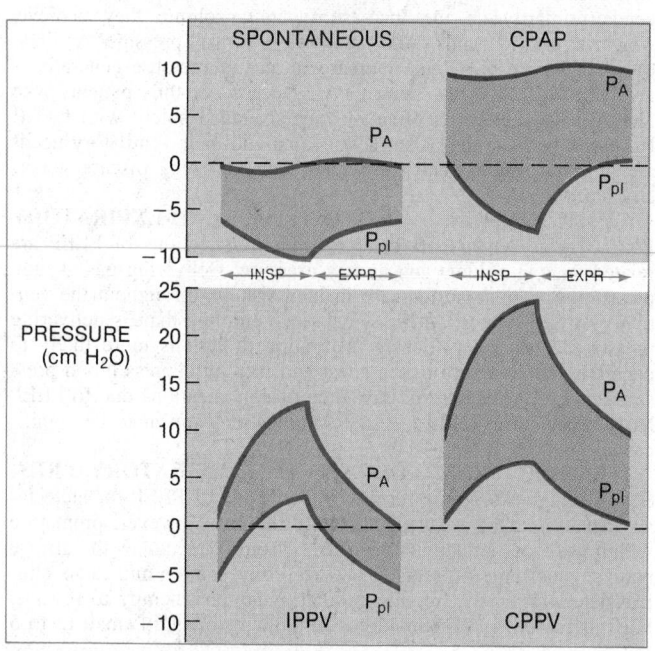

FIGURE 68–2. Schematic representations of airway (Pa) and pleural (Ppl) pressures with spontaneous respiration, spontaneous respiration with continuous positive airway pressure (CPAP), intermittent positive-pressure ventilation (IPPV), and continuous positive-pressure ventilation (CPPV). Note that with CPAP and CPPV, the pressure gradient between the airway and the pleural space is increased compared with spontaneous respiration and IPPV, respectively. (From Hinshaw HC, Murray JF [eds.]: Diseases of the Chest. Philadelphia, WB Saunders, 1980.)

many forget that To_2 often can be improved by restoring the Hb concentration to normal, as depicted in Figure 68–3.

CO poisoning causes a functional anemia that may impair To_2. The oxyhemoglobin dissociation curve also is shifted to the left in patients with CO poisoning, which results in less O_2 being available to the tissues. However, because the Pa_{O_2} is normal, the possibility of CO poisoning may be overlooked unless the Sa_{O_2} and the Ca_{O_2} are measured directly. CO poisoning is treated with supplemental O_2 at an FI_{O_2} of 1.0 and occasionally with hyperbaric oxygenation. Both these maneuvers improve To_2 by dissolving O_2 in plasma and displacing CO from Hb.

Manipulating $\dot{Q}T$ in patients with failure of To_2 often involves administering fluids and drugs. An adequate intravascular volume is necessary for stroke volume to be optimized. The drugs most commonly used to improve $\dot{Q}T$ in critically ill patients are dopamine and dobutamine. Dopamine may be given in low doses (usually 2.0 to 5.0 μg per kilogram per minute) to enhance renal and mesenteric perfusion through its dopaminergic effects. Intermediate-dose (5.0 to 10.0 μg per kilogram per minute) dopamine improves $\dot{Q}T$ through its β_1 effects, whereas high-dose (> 10.0 μg per kilogram per minute) dopamine increases PSA through its α_1 properties. The pharmacologic effects of dopamine are not always predictable in all patients, and the drug must be titrated carefully to achieve its desired effects.

Unlike dopamine, dobutamine does not selectively enhance renal and mesenteric perfusion because it lacks dopaminergic properties. It also does not generally increase blood pressure because its α_1 properties are balanced by its β_1 properties; in fact, dobutamine may reduce blood pressure in some labile patients when its β_2 properties predominate. However, dobutamine improves $\dot{Q}T$ through its β_1 properties. If blood pressure is reduced, dobutamine may be combined with high-dose dopamine or other α_1 agonists. The usual dose of dobutamine is 2.5 to 10 μg per kilogram per minute up to a maximum dose of 30 μg per kilogram per minute.

Therapy to Improve Oxygen Extraction

O_2 extraction may be improved by increasing $\dot{V}_{O_2}$. In patients with cyanide poisoning, this traditionally has involved administering amyl nitrate by inhalation and sodium nitrite intravenously; these drugs produce methemoglobin, which binds free cyanide ions. Intravenous sodium thiosulfate then is given to enhance conversion of cyanide to thiosulfate, which is less toxic and is readily excreted. Vitamin $B_{12}A$ is now available for treating cyanide poisoning in the United States.

Unfortunately, no simple antidote exists for the disturbances in O_2 extraction associated with ARDS and multiple organ system failure (MOSF). The general approach to these conditions is to improve To_2, as will be discussed.

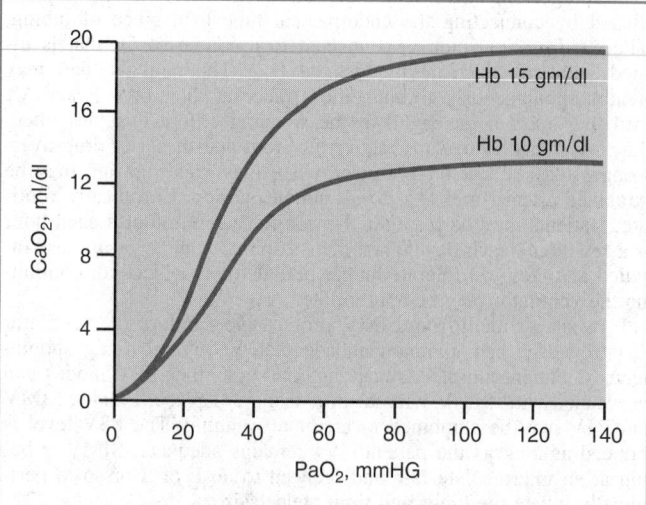

FIGURE 68–3. Importance of blood hemoglobin (Hb) concentration in oxygen transport. At a Pa_{O_2} of 80 mm Hg, arterial blood oxygen content (Ca_{O_2}) can be increased by 50% by raising Hb from 10 to 15 grams per 100 ml in an anemic patient. (From Luce JM, Pierson DJ, Tyler ML: Intensive Respiratory Care. 2nd ed. Philadelphia, WB Saunders, 1993.)

Neuromuscular Diseases Causing Respiratory Failure

Many neuromuscular diseases cause weakness or paralysis that may lead to hypercapnic respiratory failure. These disorders may involve the upper motor neurons (e.g., traumatic quadriplegia), lower motor neurons (e.g., amyotrophic lateral sclerosis), peripheral nerves (e.g., Guillain-Barré syndrome), myoneural junction (e.g., myasthenia gravis), or the muscles themselves (e.g., muscular dystrophies). The overall approach to patients with these conditions is to diagnose and treat the specific neuromuscular disease if possible, diagnose precipitating factors prompting admission to the critical care unit, evaluate the need for respiratory support, provide such support on an acute basis, and consider chronic support when required.

Once weakness or paralysis is appreciated, most neuromuscular diseases causing these symptoms can be differentiated by clinical characteristics (see Ch. 453), cerebrospinal fluid analysis, provocative tests such as administering cholinergic drugs, nerve conduction studies and electromyography, and occasionally muscle biopsy. In terms of specific therapy, plasmapheresis is used for patients with the Guillain-Barré syndrome (see Ch. 454). Myasthenia gravis is treated with relatively long-acting anticholinesterase agents such as pyridostigmine, as well as with plasmapheresis, corticosteroids, and thymectomy (see Ch. 459). Specific therapy for botulism involves eliminating malabsorbed neurotoxin from the gut with enemas and gastric lavage, administering trivalent antitoxin, administering high-dose penicillin, and accomplishing surgical debridement of contaminated wounds (see Ch. 286).

Although some patients with neuromuscular disease need critical care solely because of progressive muscle dysfunction, admission often is precipitated by other factors. For example, patients with bulbar involvement may aspirate or develop upper airway obstruction, whereas atelectasis and pneumonia are more common in patients with generalized weakness. Pulmonary hypertension (see Ch. 38) and right-sided heart failure should be anticipated in chronically hypoxemic patients, including those whose muscle weakness is compounded by kyphoscoliosis. Intercurrent illnesses, such as urinary tract infection and pulmonary thromboembolism, also may occur.

The need for respiratory support in patients with neuromuscular disease can be assessed by the MIP and VC maneuvers. As noted earlier, intubation and mechanical ventilation generally are required if the $F/V_T \geq 100$, MIP > -20 cmH$_2$O, and the VC $\simeq 10$ ml per kilogram. It should be noted that impaired secretion clearance may occur at a VC < 30 ml per kilogram and may require intubation but not mechanical ventilation.

Hypoxemic respiratory failure in patients with neuromuscular disease usually can be treated adequately with supplemental O$_2$ (nasal prongs or a face mask), coupled with frequent positioning and delivering CPAP via a tightly fitting face mask to treat atelectasis. However, intubation and mechanical ventilation usually are called for if muscle strength and lung volumes have declined to the level mentioned previously and always are necessary if hypercapnia is acute and severe. Patients with rapidly reversible muscle weakness or paralysis should be intubated by the translaryngeal route in most instances, but tracheostomy is indicated if patients require intubation for longer than a month or so.

No particular kind of ventilatory support has been demonstrated as superior in patients with neuromuscular disease, although PPV is preferred over negative-pressure ventilation in the critical care unit, especially if admission has been prompted by pneumonia or some other intermittent illness that requires supplemental O$_2$ at a high F$_{O_2}$. The value of various modes of PPV is also open to debate. Nevertheless, because SIMV can be used only in those patients who can generate substantial inspiratory pressures, patients with severe weakness or paralysis are ventilated at least initially with CMV or AMV. In patients who are improving, SIMV may be used if it does not cause fatigue. Weaning by SIMV, T-piece, or PSV should be attempted only when patients demonstrate improvement in the MIP and VC.

Ṫo$_2$ usually is adequate in patients with neuromuscular disease who are not hypoxemic or anemic and do not have concurrent cardiac disease. Nevertheless, autonomic dysfunction in patients with Guillain-Barré syndrome and other disorders may take the form of either over- or underactivity of the sympathetic nervous system. Hypertension, diaphoresis, and tachycardia may be treated with titratable agents such as esmolol to prevent overswings in heart rate and blood pressure. The hypotension that often accompanies spinal cord injury and other conditions may be treated with intravenous fluids or α_1 agonists such as phenylephrine or high-dose dopamine. Bradycardia is treated with atropine. Patients with profound vagal tone in whom bradycardia progresses to asystole may be candidates for cardiac pacing.

Asthma and Chronic Obstructive Pulmonary Disease

The primary pathophysiologic abnormalities in asthma and COPD are an increased resistance in airflow resulting from narrowing of the airways by bronchospasm, inflammation, and mucus or loss of airway tethering forces by parenchymal lung destruction. The airflow resistance causes air trapping and an abnormal increase in lung volume. Patients also have hypoxemia caused by mismatching of ventilation and perfusion and hypercapnia caused by the airways obstruction itself plus fatigue of the respiratory muscles.

In patients with asthma and COPD, Pa$_{CO_2}$ usually begins to increase when the FEV$_1$ is reduced to ~ 750 ml or 25% of the predicted value. This reduction may result from gradually progressive disease but more often occurs in the setting of acute exacerbations of obstruction due, for example, to acute bronchitis. An increase in Pa$_{CO_2}$ without a deterioration in FEV$_1$ may result from decreased ventilatory drive due to narcotic or sedative drugs or inhaling O$_2$ at a high F$_{O_2}$. Alternatively, it may result from increased Ṽco$_2$ in a patient with a limited ability to increase Ṽ$_A$. As described previously, the distinction between acute and chronic respiratory acidosis can be determined by analyzing the relationships among Pa$_{CO_2}$, pH, and [HCO$_3^-$]. Acute hypoventilation obviously dictates a more prompt response than chronic partially compensated respiratory acidosis, as is also true in patients with neuromuscular disease.

Metabolic acidosis is a more ominous finding than pure respiratory acidosis with airways obstruction. It implies a failure of Ṫo$_2$ to meet the demands imposed by the increased work of breathing. This failure may result from a decrease in Ca$_{O_2}$ due to processes such as hypoxemia or anemia or a decrease in Q̇$_T$ due to concurrent ischemic heart disease, inadequate intravascular volume, or auto-PEEP caused by air trapping. Unless patients with inadequate Ṫo$_2$ improve, their condition will deteriorate rapidly.

Patients with asthma (see Ch. 51) and COPD may be treated with β_2-adrenergic agonists, theophylline, anticholinergic agents, and corticosteroids. β_2-Agonists such as metaproterenol and albuterol relax bronchial smooth muscle though their action on β_2 receptors in the airways and have little effect on β_1 receptors in skeletal muscles, systemic vessels, and the heart. They therefore are preferred to agents such as epinephrine and isoproterenol that have mixed β_1 and β_2 properties. The usually mild tachycardia, tremulousness, and other cardiovascular side effects of β_2-agonists can be minimized if the drugs are taken in aerosol form. Average doses of aerosolized metaproterenol and albuterol are 15 and 2.5 mg, respectively, given every 2 to 4 hours. See Ch. 51 for additional therapeutic modalities.

Although hypoxemia invariably is present in patients with severe airways obstruction, the degree of reduction in Pa$_{O_2}$ is generally not sufficient to require respiratory support other than supplemental O$_2$ delivered with external devices. Hypoxemia usually should be corrected only to a Pa$_{O_2}$ of ~ 60 mm Hg using as low an F$_{O_2}$ as possible to avoid ventilatory depression. If a high F$_{O_2}$ must be used in patients with intercurrent illnesses such as pneumonia, endotracheal intubation and mechanical ventilation may be required.

One cannot definitely state criteria for intubating and ventilating patients with severe airways obstruction. Arterial blood gas and pH values at a single point in time showing marked acute respiratory acidosis with or without metabolic acidosis may be sufficient information to decide whether to mechanically ventilate. More commonly, however, it is necessary to evaluate the patient during the time drugs are being administered and to evaluate the response to therapy. If blood gas values are worsening or not improving despite maximal treatment, mechanical ventilation is the next logical step. In addition to the objective evaluation provided by arterial blood gas and pH measurements, subjective assessments are also of value. Patients who are confused, somnolent, or uncooperative may require ventilatory support because their mental status may indicate inadequate $\dot{T}_{O_2}$ and because they cannot cooperate with conservative management.

Severe airways obstruction presents a difficult situation in which to apply PPV. There is need to allow adequate expiratory time to avoid auto-PEEP, but slow inspiratory flows are also desirable to optimize the distribution of ventilation and to minimize the airway pressure required to deliver a preset V_T. To accomplish these goals, at least early in the course of mechanical ventilation, it often is necessary to sedate the patient receiving CMV or AMV in order to provide a slow ventilator F, which allows a small I:E ratio to be used. Some patients will benefit from SIMV in this situation. The V_T should be between 7 and 10 ml per kilogram, and the $F_{I_{O_2}}$ should be adjusted to provide an adequate Pa_{O_2}. The Pa_{CO_2} may rise due to the relatively low F and V_T, but severe drops in pH can be treated with HCO_3^- if necessary. If the Pa_{CO_2} remains elevated, or if the patient already has chronic hypoventilation, it is important not to reduce the Pa_{CO_2} rapidly because doing so will result in uncompensated metabolic alkalosis.

PEEP would appear to be contraindicated in patients with asthma and COPD whose lung volumes already are increased above normal. Certainly, high levels of PEEP are potentially dangerous; they also are unnecessary because these patients do not have failure of arterial oxygenation due to diffuse parenchymal lung disease. Nevertheless, PEEP in levels of ∼ 5 cm H_2O does not commonly cause hyperinflation in patients with airways obstruction. Indeed, low levels of PEEP may reduce the work of breathing of some obstructed patients by preventing airway collapse during expiration.

The adequacy of $\dot{T}_{O_2}$ in patients with asthma and COPD generally can be assessed by physical examination, measuring urine output, and monitoring blood pressure. Central venous and pulmonary artery catheterizations rarely are required but may help evaluate patients whose $\dot{Q}_T$ is known or suspected to be depressed and evaluate their response to fluids and agents such as dopamine or dobutamine. Intrathoracic vascular pressures evaluated by auto-PEEP should be taken into account when estimating intravascular volume. Serial measurements of C_{EFF} in ventilated patients may be useful to assess the severity of airways obstruction and the response to therapy.

In patients with airways obstruction, weaning from mechanical ventilation also may present difficulties. Patients with asthma usually may be weaned and extubated quickly after they have responded to treatment. However, patients with COPD may at best have marginal lung function with persistent retention of CO_2. In general, the arterial blood gas pattern that exists when the patient is "well" should be approximated while mechanical ventilation is still being used. Ideally, weaning with SIMV or a simple T-piece with or without PSV and small amounts of PEEP then can proceed using previously described criteria.

In some instances, patients with COPD never meet the objective criteria for weaning and extubation. When this occurs, the decisions regarding weaning and extubation are based on subjective criteria, such as level of alertness, patient cooperation, and prognosis. These factors obviously cannot be quantitated. Once the patient has demonstrated the ability to maintain a desired $\dot{V}_E$ spontaneously for 30 to 60 minutes, the endotracheal tube should be removed.

Infectious Pneumonia

Infectious pneumonias may be divided epidemiologically into the community-acquired type, implying that the pathogens were acquired in the patient's normal environment, and the nosocomial or hospital-acquired type (see Ch. 267). Another approach, which is based on the characteristics of the human host, is to describe infectious pneumonia as either routine, in that it occurs in an immunocompetent patient (see Ch. 266) or opportunistic, in that the patient is immunocompromised by, for example, cancer or infection with the human immunodeficiency virus (HIV).

Microorganisms reach the lungs either by direct inhalation from air or from respiratory therapy devices, aspiration of secretions from the mouth and nasopharynx, hematogenous spread from other body sites, or direct penetration of the chest wall (see Ch. 274). Usually the mouth and nasopharynx are populated predominantly by anaerobic bacteria that are kept out of the lungs by intact gag and cough reflexes and the mucociliary clearance mechanisms of the trachea and bronchi. However, these resident flora are rapidly replaced by aerobic bacilli, including those found in critical care

units and in the lower gastrointestinal tract, when illness supervenes. Approximately one fourth of patients who become colonized in this manner go on to develop either bacterial tracheobronchitis or pneumonia, in large part because their gag and cough reflexes and mucociliary clearance mechanisms are depressed by disease, medications, or the presence of an endotracheal tube.

Bacteria that proliferate in the alveoli generally elicit an inflammatory response characterized by complement activation and phagocytosis by alveolar macrophages and neutrophils that are attracted to the lung. This is accompanied by an increase in permeability of the endothelium of the pulmonary capillaries and the epithelium of the alveolar wall. The increased permeability allows water and proteins to leak from the vessels into the air spaces even though the hydrostatic pressure within the capillaries is normal. As the lung tissues become consolidated, local pulmonary compliance diminishes, and hypoxemia results from mismatching of ventilation and perfusion in the lung.

Spontaneously produced sputum or secretions that have been suctioned from the tracheobronchial tree should be Gram stained and examined for abundant neutrophils as a reflection of purulence and for potentially pathogenic bacteria. Several types of bacteria may be seen in critically ill patients, especially those who are intubated, if their pneumonia is due to more than one microorganism. Sputum and tracheobronchial secretions also should be cultured to determine which microorganisms are predominant. However, it should be noted that the presence of positive cultures does not confirm the diagnosis of either tracheobronchitis or pneumonia, in that critically ill patients without these disorders may have positive cultures due to airway colonization.

Some clinicians treat any respiratory infection in hospitalized patients, reasoning that if tracheobronchitis is present, pneumonia cannot be far behind. Most, however, prefer not to give antibiotics for mild to moderate cases and wait until tracheobronchitis is severe or, more often, until pneumonia is documented by chest radiograph. Antibiotic therapy may be empirical or based on the results of Gram stain, culture, or both. Therapeutic recommendations are included in Table 68-7.

Many kinds of mechanical ventilation can be used in patients with infectious pneumonia who require ventilatory support, although the CMV, AMV, and SIMV modes of PPV are most commonly used. Patients with diffuse, bilateral pneumonia usually require PEEP, as do patients with other forms of ARDS, as will be discussed. PEEP must be applied cautiously to patients with unilateral pneumonia, in whom this therapy may cause overdistention of nondiseased alveoli rather than expansion of diseased alveoli and thereby worsen arterial oxygenation.

Most bacterial pneumonias respond to antibiotic treatment, maneuvers to aid secretion clearance, and mechanical ventilation, if indicated, so radiographic infiltrates should begin to clear after several days. This may not be the case in critically ill patients, however; because their infiltrates are due to some other cause such as atelectasis, they cannot ward off an identified pathogen due to its virulence or their depressed host defenses, the pathogen is insensitive to the antibiotics being given, or the patients are infected with an undiagnosed and perhaps opportunistic, nonbacterial microorganism. Because of the last possibility, patients who do not improve with treatment may be subjected to diagnostic tests more invasive than sputum analysis, such as bronchoscopy with protected brush catheterization of the lower airways or bronchoalveolar lavage.

Adult Respiratory Distress Syndrome and Multiple Organ System Failure

A constellation of clinical, radiographic, and pathophysiologic findings that result from diffuse injury to the lung parenchyma defines ARDS. The characteristics of this syndrome are (1) severe hypoxemia due to intrapulmonary shunting of blood, (2) decreased C_{RS} due to decreased compliance of the lung, and (3) the presence of diffuse infiltration on the chest radiograph. The common abnormality that accounts for these features is an increase in the permeability of the endothelium of the pulmonary capillary and the epithelium of the alveolar wall. This allows fluid to leak from the capillary into the alveolus even though the hydrostatic pressure within the capillary is normal; hence noncardiogenic pulmonary edema results.

ARDS is associated with a variety of clinical conditions, the most common of which is sepsis syndrome. A partial list of these conditions is found in Table 68-8. The injury to the lung that oc-

TABLE 68-7. INFECTIOUS PNEUMONIAS

Kind of Patient	Likely Offending Microorganisms	Initial Antimicrobial Therapy (Pending Sensitivities)	Average Dose	Route	Interval
Normal young host with community-acquired pneumonia	*Mycoplasma*				
	Mycoplasma pneumoniae	Erythromycin or tetracycline	0.5 gram 0.5 gram	PO PO	qid qid
	Gram-positive aerobic bacteria				
	Streptococcus pneumoniae	Penicillin G or erythromycin	600,000 units 0.5 gram	PO, IM, IV PO, IM, IV	bid qid
	Viruses				
	Influenza A Adenovirus	No therapy or amantadine	0.2 gram	PO	qid
	Fungi (in endemic areas) *Coccidioides immitis* *Histoplasma capsulatum*	Usually untreated unless dissemination occurs or pulmonary infection becomes chronic. Then use amphotericin B as below.			
Elderly host, heavy smoker or alcoholic individual with nosocomial pneumonia	Gram-positive aerobic bacteria				
	Streptococcus pneumoniae	Penicillin G or erythromycin	600,000 units 0.5 gram	IM, IV IM, IV	bid qid
	Staphylococcus aureus	Nafcillin or vancomycin	1–2 grams 1 gram	IV IV	q4h q12h
	Gram-negative aerobic bacteria				
	Haemophilus influenzae	Ampicillin or cefuroxime	0.5–1 gram 1.0 gram	IV, PO IV	qid q8h
	Klebsiella pneumoniae	Cefazolin and gentamicin or tobramycin	1.5 mg/kg 1.5 mg/kg	IV IV	q8h q8h
	Legionella pneumophilia	Erythromycin	0.5–1 gram	IV	qid
	Anaerobic bacteria				
	Bacteroides fragilis	Metronidazole or clindamycin	500 mg 0.3 gram	IV IV, PO	q8h qid
Normal young or elderly host with nosocomial pneumonia	Gram-positive aerobic bacteria				
	Staphylococcus aureus	Nafcillin or vancomycin	1–2 grams 1 gram	IV IV	q4h qid
	Streptococcus fecalis (nonendocarditis)	Ampicillin and gentamicin or tobramycin	1 gram 1.5 mg/kg	IV IV	q8h q8h
	Gram-negative aerobic bacteria	?			
Normal young or elderly host with nosocomial pneumonia	*Escherichia coli*	Ampicillin alone or gentamicin or tobramycin and carbenicillin or ticarcillin	1 gram 1.5 mg/kg 3–6 grams	IV IV IV	qid qid q4h
	Pseudomonas aeruginosa	Piperacillin or ticarcillin and gentamicin or tobramycin	3–6 grams 1.5 mg/kg	IV IV	q4h q8h
	Proteus mirabilis	Ampicillin or ticarcillin	1 gram 3–6 grams	IV IV	qid q4h
	Klebsiella pneumoniae	Cefazolin and gentamicin or tobramycin	1–2 grams 1.5 mg/kg	IV IV	q8h q8h
	Enterobacter species	Piperacillin and gentamicin or tobramycin	3–6 grams 1.5 mg/kg	IV IV	q4h q8h
Immunocompromised host with community- or hospital-acquired pneumonia	Gram-negative aerobic bacteria, as above	As above; prefer combination			
	Viruses				
	Cytomegalovirus	Gancyclovir			
	Varicella-zoster	Acyclovir			
	Herpes simplex	Acyclovir			
	Fungi				
	Candida albicans	Amphotericin B	0.025–0.1 gram	IV	qd
	Aspergillus fumigatus	Amphotericin B	0.025–0.1 gram	IV	qd
	Cryptococcus neoformans	Amphotericin B	0.025–0.1 gram	IV	qd
	Protozoa				
	Pneumocystis carinii	Trimethoprim with sulfamethoxazole or pentamidine isethionate	20 mg/kg 4 mg/kg	IV, PO IV	qid qid

TABLE 68-8. CONDITIONS ASSOCIATED WITH ARDS AND MOSF

Sepsis syndrome
Severe trauma
Diffuse pneumonia
Burns and smoke inhalation
Multiple transfusions
Pancreatitis
Anaphylaxis
Drug overdosage
Cardiorespiratory arrest

curs in these conditions may be delivered either via the airways or via the circulation. In many instances (e.g., gastric aspiration or diffuse pneumonia), lung injury would appear to be direct. In others (e.g., sepsis syndrome or pancreatitis), the injury presumably is indirect and is mediated by circulating substances.

Regardless of the type or mechanism of injury, the damage to the lungs of patients with ARDS is diffuse compared with diseases such as unilateral pneumonia. However, the damage is nonhomogeneous, and some areas of lung parenchyma may be spared. In damaged areas, the lung is atelectatic, edematous, and hemorrhagic. Microscopic examination reveals intra-alveolar collections of proteinaceous fluid, red blood cells, and inflammatory cells. Microthrombi or white cell aggregates may be seen in small vessels. After 24 to 48 hours, hyaline membranes formed by fibrin that has escaped through the capillaries line the alveoli. Subsequently, as repair of the injury occurs, fibrosis may ensue.

Reduced lung volume is characteristic of ARDS and is caused by a combination of atelectasis, edema fluid, and inflammation and perhaps fibrosis replacing alveolar air. This decrease in lung volume contrasts with the increase in lung volume of patients with airways obstruction. It is largely responsible for the decrease in CRS associated with ARDS, which traditionally has been attributed primarily to lung stiffness. The work of breathing considerably increases because of the decreased CRS.

The major and most frequent gas exchange abnormality in ARDS is hypoxemia caused by the loss of functional alveoli. In severe forms of ARDS, as the process evolves from injury to repair, CO_2 exchange abnormalities also evolve. Lung fibrosis may result in obliterated capillaries and coalesced alveoli, producing an increased VD/VT. Unless $\dot{V}E$ can be increased, which may be difficult, hypercapnia will result.

Some, but not all, patients with ARDS develop dysfunction or failure of one or more organ systems sequentially or simultaneously. By contrast, other patients develop MOSF without having ARDS, although they may have less severe degrees of parenchymal lung injury. MOSF is associated with the same clinical conditions as ARDS. Furthermore, as with ARDS, it is associated most commonly with sepsis syndrome. This suggests that ARDS is a respiratory manifestation of MOSF, just as shock is a cardiovascular manifestation. Alternatively, ARDS and MOSF may be aspects of sepsis syndrome. Indeed, some investigators have broadened the use of the term *sepsis syndrome* to include any generalized inflammatory process that may cause or contribute to widespread organ dysfunction.

This generalized inflammatory process may be mediated by a variety of circulating substances with vasoactive, inflammatory, and tissue damaging properties. These substances, which may include endotoxin, histamine, arachidonic acid metabolites, complement, myocardial depressant factor, and tumor necrosis factor, may cause systemic vasodilatation, microvascular vasoconstriction, altered myocardial contractility, capillary microembolization, and endothelial cell disruption. The end result is increased capillary permeability with intravascular fluid loss, interstitial fluid accumulation, impaired microcirculatory blood flow, and inadequate tissue oxygenation in the lungs and other organs. Patients may die of refractory hypotension, hypoxemia attributable to ARDS, or other manifestations of MOSF such as disseminated intravascular coagulation.

The diagnoses of ARDS and MOSF are made clinically because there are no reliable markers for the disorders. The diagnoses are supported by documenting the presence of the associated conditions

just discussed. Pulmonary artery catheterization, which may aid in management, also suggests the diagnosis of ARDS and MOSF if the characteristic patterns of distributive shock and inadequate oxygen extraction are observed.

It is not clear whether the term *sepsis syndrome* should be applied to patients with ARDS and MOSF who are not truly infected. Nevertheless, such patients probably should be assumed to be infected unless there is another explanation for their condition. If bacterial infection is suspected or known to exist, broad-spectrum antibiotics such as ampicillin, metronidazole, and gentamycin should be given intravenously to cover gram-positive and gram-negative pathogens and then tailored to culture results. Suspected or documented infections with other organisms, including those causing infectious pneumonia, should be treated appropriately. In addition, abscesses should be searched for by computed tomography and other techniques when appropriate. If detected, they should be drained percutaneously or at surgery.

The unusual patient with MOSF who does not have severe parenchymal lung disease may benefit from endotracheal intubation and mechanical ventilation merely because he/she is hemodynamically unstable. Vital organ perfusion also may be enhanced if the work of breathing is reduced by mechanical ventilation. Patients with ARDS, however, invariably require both PPV and PEEP to improve arterial oxygenation. The need for such support may be evaluated by monitoring the Pa_{O_2} and $P(A - a)_{O_2}$. Respiratory or metabolic acidosis is ominous in this setting. Because patients with ARDS, MOSF, or both may deteriorate rapidly, it generally is better to provide intubation and mechanical ventilation earlier rather than later.

The use of PPV in patients with ARDS and MOSF varies. Many physicians probably administer CMV, AMV, or SIMV with a VT of 10 to 15 ml per kilogram, an I:E ratio of 1:3 or greater, and a Pmax as required to deliver a VT in the aforementioned range. PEEP is used at levels necessary to reduce the $F_{I_{O_2}}$ to ≤ 0.6. However, increasing concern over the possible effects of high alveolar pressures and volumes in causing volutrauma has led some investigators to advocate using HFV, PCV, and IRV even though these newer modes of PPV have not been shown to be superior to older ones. When older modes of PPV are used, it is argued, VT should be as low as 5 to 7 ml per kilogram, ventilators should be pressure cycled, and high levels of PEEP should be avoided if possible, even if the $F_{I_{O_2}}$ exceeds 0.6 in the process.

It is not clear that the current concepts of the pathogenesis of lung injury and therapies based on them will prove superior to concepts and therapies accepted earlier. Nevertheless, it does appear prudent to use all modes of PPV and PEEP carefully. Most patients with ARDS and MOSF probably can be ventilated and oxygenated adequately by CMV, AMV, and SIMV at a relatively low VT and a Pmax of < 35 cm H_2O. If Pmax exceeds this amount, PCV may be added with or without IRV. PEEP should be used at the lowest possible level to achieve an $F_{I_{O_2}}$ of ≤ 0.6.

Because volutrauma is such a concern, Pmax and Pstat should be monitored frequently in patients receiving PPV and PEEP. In addition, the amount of auto-PEEP should be measured by the method cited previously. Although the auto-PEEP often caused by PCV and IRV has been considered undesirable, investigators note that auto-PEEP is just as potentially useful as intentionally administered PEEP in recruiting alveoli. The important point is to include the amount of auto-PEEP in the overall measurement of PEEP so that its effects can be anticipated.

Appropriately using intravenous fluid is an essential component in managing ARDS and MOSF. Because pulmonary capillary permeability is increased, administering fluid, which increases the capillary hydrostatic pressure, tends to increase the amount of lung water. The relationship between capillary hydrostatic pressure and extravascular lung water is shown schematically in Figure 68-4. A recent study has demonstrated that patients with ARDS whose extravascular lung water is reduced by fluid restriction require fewer days of mechanical ventilation than patients with increased extravascular lung water.

On the other hand, adequate pulmonary perfusion may be important in preventing or ameliorating lung damage, and systemic perfusion clearly is essential in maintaining renal, cardiac, and CNS function. Thus the effects of administering crystalloid, colloid, or red blood cells should be monitored carefully with clear endpoints in mind. In addition to measuring blood pressure and other vari-

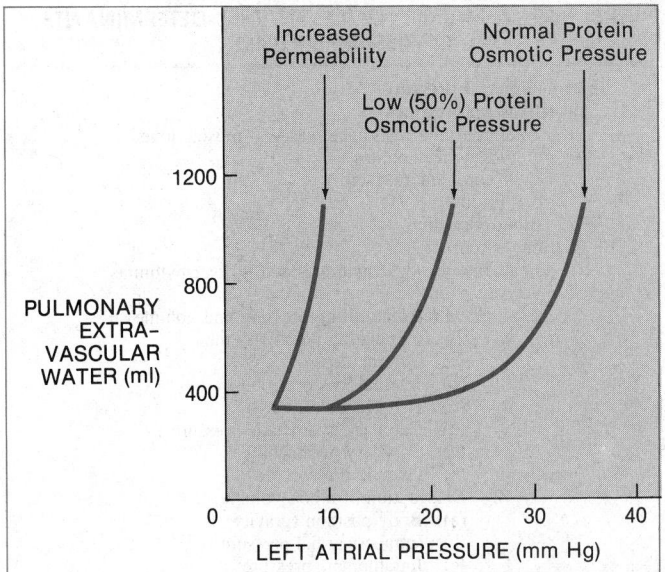

FIGURE 68–4. Schematic representation of the relationship of pulmonary extravascular water volume and left atrial or pulmonary artery occlusion pressure. Curve at right represents the relationships when both microvascular permeability and plasma protein osmotic pressures are normal; middle curve represents normal permeability but a reduction in plasma protein osmotic pressure of 50%; left curve shows relationship when permeability of the capillaries is increased. (From Hopewell PC, Murray JF: Adult respiratory distress syndrome. *In* Moser KM, Spragg RG [eds.]: Respiratory Emergencies. 2nd ed. St. Louis, C.V. Mosby, 1982.)

ables, indices of organ perfusion such as urine output and mental status should be followed.

Pulmonary artery catheterization may be extremely helpful in assessing hemodynamic status, at least early in the course of ARDS and MOSF. Although the correlation between the pulmonary artery occlusion pressure and the outcome of these disorders has not been determined, it appears reasonable to maintain the pressure at a normal or slightly below normal level as long as perfusion of vital organs is maintained. If perfusion is inadequate or if $\dot{Q}T$ is depressed by the patient's underlying disease or its treatment, the circulation can be supported with dopamine or dobutamine.

Ideally, the combination of specific therapy for associated conditions such as sepsis syndrome and appropriate cardiovascular and respiratory system support should improve $\dot{T}o_2$ in patients with ARDS and MOSF. It is important to keep this goal in mind for at least three reasons. First, $\dot{T}o_2$ and its components (Ca_{o_2} and $\dot{Q}T$) can be quantified, and therapies that increase one component at the expense of the other may be modified. Second, because there is no specific antidote for the inadequate oxygen extraction that so often characterizes ARDS and MOSF, therapies to improve $\dot{T}o_2$ are the only ones available.

A third reason to improve $\dot{T}o_2$ is that the apparent failure of O_2 extraction in patients with ARDS and MOSF may actually be a complicated form of $\dot{T}o_2$ failure. This is supported by the demonstration that $\dot{V}o_2$ appears to be dependent on $\dot{T}o_2$ at some critical level of $\dot{T}o_2$ in these conditions. It also is supported by the finding that some patients with ARDS and MOSF increase $\dot{V}o_2$ and resolve their lactic acidosis with increases in $\dot{T}o_2$. Given this finding, some investigators have advocated fluid loading, hypertransfusion with red blood cells, or administering dobutamine to patients with ARDS and MOSF to increase Ca_{o_2} and $\dot{Q}T$ to arbitrarily high levels. The benefit of this approach has not been demonstrated prospectively, however. Furthermore, recent studies in which $\dot{V}o_2$ is measured directly and not merely calculated have cast doubt on the earlier findings that $\dot{V}o_2$ is dependent on $\dot{T}o_2$ and that $\dot{V}o_2$ can be increased by increasing $\dot{T}o_2$. As a result, there is little reason at present to increase $\dot{T}o_2$ beyond normal levels in patients with ARDS and MOSF.

Kelly BJ, Luce JM: The diagnosis and management of neuromuscular diseases causing respiratory failure. Chest 99:1485, 1991. *Recent review describing management of patients with neuromuscular disease.*

Mitchell JP, Schuller D, Calandrino FS, et al.: Improved outcome based on fluid management in critically ill patients requiring pulmonary artery catheterization. Am Rev Respir Dis 145:990, 1992. *Lower positive fluid balance, especially in patients with pulmonary edema, regardless of cause, is associated with reduced extramuscular lung water and days in mechanical ventilation.*

Ronco JJ, Fenwick JC, Tweeddale MG, et al.: Identification of the critical oxygen delivery for anaerobic metabolism in critically ill septic and nonseptic humans. JAMA 270:1724, 1993. *Recent study demonstrating that sepsis does not alter the critical oxygen delivery level for anaerobic metabolism or tissue oxygen extraction ability.*

Ronco JJ, Fenwick JC, Wiggs BR, et al.: Oxygen consumption is independent of increases in oxygen delivery by dobutamine in septic patients who have normal or increased plasma lactate. Am Rev Respir Dis 147:25, 1993. *Oxygen consumption remained relatively constant despite large increases in oxygen transport in septic patients, and increased concentration of plasma lactate did not predict dependence of oxygen consumption on oxygen delivery.*

Russell JA, Ronco JJ, Lockhat D, et al.: Oxygen delivery and consumption and ventricular preload are greater in survivors than in nonsurvivors of the adult respiratory distress syndrome. Am Rev Respir Dis 141:659, 1990. *Despite recent studies suggesting that oxygen consumption is not pathologically dependent on oxygen transport in patients with ARDS, these patients whose oxygen transport is relatively high (generally ≥600 mg per minute per square meter) are less likely to develop MOSF and more likely to survive than patients whose oxygen transport is relatively low.*

Slutsky AS: Mechanical Ventilation. Chest 104:1833, 1993. *This comprehensive review covers the physiology and administration of all forms of mechanical ventilation.*

Stauffer JL, Olson DE, Petty TL: Complications and consequences of endotracheal intubation and tracheotomy. Am J Med 70:65, 1981. *The only large prospective study of the complications of endotracheal intubation by translaryngeal route or via tracheostomy.*

Tobin MJ: Respiratory monitoring in the intensive care unit. Am Rev Respir Dis 138:1625, 1988. *Comprehensive review of respiratory monitoring.*

Yang KL, Tobin MJ: A prospective study of indexes predicting the outcome of trials of weaning from mechanical ventilation. N Engl J Med 324:1445, 1991. *Demonstrates that rapid shallow breathing, as reflected by an increased ratio of ventilatory frequency to tidal volume (F/VT), is the most accurate predictor of failure of weaning from mechanical ventilation.*

69 CARDIOGENIC SHOCK

David W. Ferguson

Shock—a rude unhinging of the machinery of life.

SAMUEL GROSS, 1872

Rather than a specific disease, shock is a complex clinical syndrome, the successful treatment of which requires vigilant medical attention, precise hemodynamic monitoring, and a thorough understanding of the basic principles of circulatory physiology and the pharmacology of cardiac and vasoactive medications. Cardiogenic shock comprises one of four broad categories of shock, the others being hypovolemic shock, vascular obstructive shock, and distributive shock. This chapter reviews the basic principles of circulatory control as they relate to all these common shock syndromes, the systemic and cellular mechanisms involved in the pathogenesis of the shock state, and the clinical characteristics and management goals specific to patients with cardiogenic shock.

DEFINITION. The term *shock* (Fr. *choc*), first used by the French physician LeDran in 1773 to describe the clinical characteristics of patients after severe gunshot trauma, is a nonspecific term now used to describe complex pathophysiologic syndrome(s) arising from any of a multitude of causes. Common to all these syndromes is a failure of the circulatory system to maintain cellular perfusion and function. Shock usually results from a critical impairment of blood flow to vital organs and tissues and/or the inability of those tissues to utilize essential nutrients. The common denominator in all forms of shock is microcirculatory insufficiency. The end result of irreversible shock is cellular membrane dysfunction, abnormal cellular metabolism, and eventually cellular death. Shock is inferred from clinical evidence of major organ hypoperfusion in the setting of hemodynamic instability usually associated with relative or absolute hypotension.

Cardiogenic shock is a pathophysiologic state arising from various potential underlying etiologies, the common feature of which is a marked inadequacy of tissue perfusion due to a *primary* myocardial impairment. In common usage, *cardiogenic shock* refers to conditions in which cardiac output is inadequate to meet peripheral metabolic demands, usually as a result of inadequate forward stroke volume rather than an inadequacy of heart rate (e.g., a primary, hemodynamically significant tachyarrhythmia or bradyarrhythmia). A strict hemodynamic definition, requiring invasive hemodynamic monitoring, is essential to define cardiogenic shock and to exclude nonmyocardial etiologies (e.g., hypovolemia) as the cause of the shock state (Table 69–1).

An understanding of the pathophysiology operative in cardiogenic shock, which is a prerequisite for implementing effective therapy, requires a broader understanding of normal circulatory control mechanisms.

MECHANISMS OF CIRCULATORY CONTROL—NORMAL AND DURING SHOCK

The basic underlying abnormality in all forms of shock is a state of disordered cellular metabolism, manifested by reduced or insufficient cellular oxygen consumption. Since all cellular functions depend on adequate tissue perfusion, the pathophysiology of shock requires an understanding of the normal determinants of tissue perfusion.

Major Determinants of Tissue Perfusion (Table 69–2)

The basic functions of the circulation are the delivery of oxygen and essential nutrients to peripheral tissues and the removal of metabolic wastes from those tissues. In most cases of shock, there is either insufficient delivery or inappropriate distribution of oxygen and nutrients. The major determinants of normal tissue perfusion are listed in Table 69–2. Perfusion of any organ depends on systemic arterial pressure (the driving force for blood flow through the organs), the resistance offered by the vasculature of that organ, and the patency of nutritional capillaries within the organ.

Systemic arterial pressure is determined by cardiac output and the resistance of the total vascular tree:

Arterial pressure = cardiac output × Total vascular resistance

Vascular resistance is predominantly a function of the caliber of blood vessels, which is influenced by neurogenic, humoral, and myogenic factors that regulate the tone of vascular smooth muscle. Thus blood flow to any one organ depends on cardiac function, vascular muscle tone, and the caliber of resistance beds both in the systemic arterial tree and within the organ itself. The microcirculation determines the exchange of substrates and metabolites within the tissue. A patent nutritional capillary network is the critical interface between the circulation and the cell. The following discussion reviews the critical cardiac, vascular, and microcirculatory determinants of tissue perfusion which are important in understanding the pathophysiology and treatment of shock.

CARDIAC FACTORS. *Cardiac Output.* Cardiac output is the product of heart rate and stroke volume:

Cardiac output = heart rate × stroke volume

In normal resting adults, a heart rate of 70 beats per minute and a stroke volume of 70 to 75 ml per beat produce a cardiac output of approximately 5 liters per minute. A decrease in cardiac output to less than 2 liters per minute per square meter of body surface area (cardiac index) may result in severe shock, particularly if imposed over a short time interval.

Heart Rate. Normal individuals tolerate a wide range of heart rates, from approximately 30 to 180 beats per minute. An increase in heart rate is one of the earliest physiologic responses to a fall in arterial pressure and is modulated by the autonomic nervous system. Physiologic ranges of tachycardia usually increase cardiac output, but marked increases in heart rate may limit cardiac diastolic

TABLE 69–1. CARDIOGENIC SHOCK: HEMODYNAMIC AND CLINICAL DEFINITION

Primary myocardial insult
Arterial hypotension (intra-arterial measurement): Systolic pressure ≤ 90 mm Hg or > 60 mm Hg below baseline
Adequate preload (pulmonary artery catheter): Pulmonary capillary wedge pressure ≥ 15–18 mm Hg
Impaired cardiac output (pulmonary artery catheter)
  Cardiac index ≤ 2.2 L/min/m²
  Widened arterial–mixed venous oxygen content difference (pre-shunt)
Clinical evidence of hypoperfusion
  Diminished mental function
  Peripheral vasoconstriction/cyanosis
  Oliguria or anuria (urine output < 30 ml/hr)

TABLE 69–2. MAJOR HEMODYNAMIC DETERMINANTS OF TISSUE PERFUSION

I. **Systemic arterial pressure**
  A. Total vascular resistance
    1. Total arteriolar resistance, vascular muscle tone
      a. Tissue metabolites
      b. Neurohumoral factors
      c. Toxins
    2. Blood viscosity
  B. Cardiac output
    1. Heart rate: Bradyarrhythmias and tachyarrhythmias
    2. Stroke volume
      a. Preload (cardiac filling pressure and volume)
        (1) Total circulating blood volume
          (a) External loss
          (b) Internal loss or sequestration
          (c) Red blood cell mass
          (d) Capillary hydrostatic pressure
          (e) Capillary permeability
          (f) Oncotic pressure
        (2) Distribution of blood volume
          (a) Body position (gravity)
          (b) Intrapericardial pressure
          (c) Intrathoracic pressure
          (d) Venous tone
          (e) Skeletal muscle pump
        (3) Atrial contraction
          (a) Contractile state
          (b) Timing (AV synchrony)
        (4) Diastolic filling time (heart rate)
      b. Inotropic state
        (1) Total functioning ventricular muscle mass
        (2) Intrinsic (myocardial) control mechanisms
          (a) Adrenergic receptors
          (b) Excitation-contraction coupling
         (3) Extrinsic (noncardiac) neurocirculatory control mechanisms
          (a) Circulating catecholamines
          (b) Autonomic nervous system
          (c) Myocardial depression
        (4) Myocardial perfusion (oxygen supply)
          (a) Aortic diastolic pressure
          (b) Fixed and nonfixed coronary obstructions
          (c) Metabolic coronary vasodilation
          (d) Neurogenic control mechanisms
        (5) Myocardial oxygen demand
          (a) Heart rate
          (b) Cardiac size
          (c) Afterload
          (d) Contractility
          (e) Pharmacologic agents
        (6) Physiologic depressants
          (a) Acidosis
          (b) Hypoxemia
          (c) Alkalosis (severe)
        (7) Pharmacologic depressants
        (8) Humoral agents
          (a) Catecholamines
          (b) Myocardial depressant factors
      c. Afterload
        (1) Aortic diastolic pressure
          (a) Systemic vascular resistance
          (b) Arterial viscoelasticity
          (c) Aortic root blood volume
        (2) Ventricular size (law of Laplace)
          (a) Impedance
II. **Organ vascular resistance**
  A. Occlusive vascular disease
  B. Local arteriolar and venular resistance
    1. Neurogenic factors
    2. Humoral factors
    3. Local autoregulation
  C. Blood viscosity
III. **Nutritional microcirculatory patency**
  A. Precapillary sphincter tone
  B. Postcapillary venular tone
  C. Intracapillary aggregation of blood components
  D. Capillary endothelial integrity

filling time and thereby result in a low cardiac output and a fall in arterial blood pressure. The tolerable limits for heart rate decrease with underlying cardiovascular impairment. For example, the onset of a rapid tachyrhythmia in a patient with an acute myocardial infarction (associated with marked reduction in ventricular compliance) may result in significant shortening of ventricular diastolic filling time. This may produce an abrupt and profound fall in ventricular filling volume (preload) and thereby impair cardiac output, resulting in arterial hypotension. Prompt treatment of the tachyrhythmia (e.g., electrical cardioversion) is required to restore normal cardiac rate and rhythm.

Managing the patient in shock who is noted to be tachycardic requires an appreciation of the differential diagnosis of the tachycardia. A "compensatory sinus tachycardia" is often seen in patients with fever, anemia, sepsis, hemorrhage, heart failure, or severe hypovolemia. In these settings, sinus tachycardia is an appropriate reflex circulatory adjustment to maintain cardiac output. It would be deleterious to attempt to treat the tachycardia alone (e.g., with β-adrenergic or calcium channel blocking agents) without determining the underlying etiology of the tachycardia (e.g., hypovolemia) and correcting the primary defect rather than its physiologic compensatory response.

Marked bradycardia also may reduce cardiac output and result in hypotension. In many situations, bradycardia is vagally mediated and responds to anticholinergic maneuvers (e.g., atropine). Many commonly used medications (e.g., β-adrenergic and calcium channel blockers) may aggravate bradycardia in patients with acute circulatory insults or may attenuate normal sympathetically mediated tachycardic responses. Sinus bradycardia and atrioventricular (AV) block are often seen immediately following myocardial infarction and should be reversed if they contribute to hypotension or other hemodynamic instability (e.g., heart failure).

Stroke Volume. Stroke volume is the amount of blood ejected by the ventricle with each cardiac contraction and is determined by cardiac preload, inotropic state, and afterload. A decrease in stroke volume may be caused by (1) a decrease in cardiac filling (preload), (2) a decrease in myocardial contractility (inotropic state), or (3) an increase in cardiac afterload (Figs. 69–1 and 69–2).

Preload is defined as the stretch or tension on an individual sarcomere just prior to the onset of fiber shortening. Clinically, preload refers to the volume of blood filling the ventricle at the end of diastole (presystole). Ventricular preload regulates the subsequent force of cardiac contraction as described by Starling's law of the heart. Preload is often assessed clinically as ventricular filling pressure rather than volume. The clinician must remember that it is the *compliance* (distensibility) of the ventricle that determines the relationship between pressure and volume:

$$\text{Compliance} = \text{change in volume/change in pressure}$$

The compliance of the ventricle varies with the underlying ventricular structure and any acute physiologic insult. Compliance may change rapidly and managing the patient in shock requires an appreciation of the potential for minute-to-minute changes in the relationship between ventricular pressure and volume.

The most important determinant of cardiac preload is the total circulating blood volume. A reduction in blood volume may be either absolute or relative to the capacity of the vascular tree. Absolute reduction in blood volume is apparent when blood or fluids are lost, leading to hypovolemic shock.

Total blood volume must be not only adequate but also appropriately distributed for preload to be sufficient to maintain stroke volume. The chief determinants of the distribution of preload include body position (gravity), venous tone, intrathoracic and intrapericardial pressure, and the skeletal muscle pump.

Another important determinant of ventricular preload is atrial contraction and the rate of diastolic filling of the ventricle. Although atrial contraction in a normal heart may determine only 5 to 10% of the subsequent ventricular stroke volume, in a diseased heart the contribution of atrial contraction to the subsequent ventricular stroke volume may be as great as 40 to 50%. This is the primary reason that patients with hypertrophic cardiomyopathy, critical aortic stenosis, or acute myocardial infarction undergo rapid hemodynamic decompensation with the onset of atrial fibrillation and loss of an organized atrial component to ventricular preload.

Inotropic state is physiologically defined as the magnitude and rate of myocardial fiber contraction under a given set of loading conditions. From the clinical standpoint, inotropic state refers to the contractile strength of the heart and is determined by a number of factors. These include the total mass of functioning ventricular muscle, myocardial perfusion, intrinsic and extrinsic neurocirculatory control mechanisms, and the presence or absence of physiologic and pharmacologic stimulants or depressants. In addition, certain shock states (e.g., sepsis) may be associated with circulating "myocardial depressant factors" that impair cardiac performance.

Detailed autopsy studies in patients dying of cardiogenic shock following myocardial infarction have demonstrated that loss of > 30 to 35% of functioning left ventricular muscle mass results in marked impairment of cardiac inotropic performance to a degree that is usually incompatible with maintenance of an effective cardiac output.

An important determinant of cardiac contractile performance is the sympathetic nervous system via activation of β-adrenoreceptors in the heart that increase cardiac contractile vigor and heart rate. These effects are mediated both by efferent sympathetic nerves impinging on the myocardium and by catecholamines released from the adrenal medulla. The effectiveness of such cardiac stimulants depends on the number and sensitivity of cardiac β-adrenergic receptors. These receptors in turn are modified by various disease states, the most important of which is underlying chronic heart failure, in which receptor number and sensitivity are diminished.

Myocardial performance depends on the relationship between myocardial oxygen demand and supply. Myocardial oxygen supply depends primarily on myocardial perfusion, which is determined to a significant extent by the level of arterial diastolic pressure and the presence of fixed (e.g., atherosclerotic) or reactive (e.g., vasospastic) obstructions to coronary blood flow. A significant fall in arterial

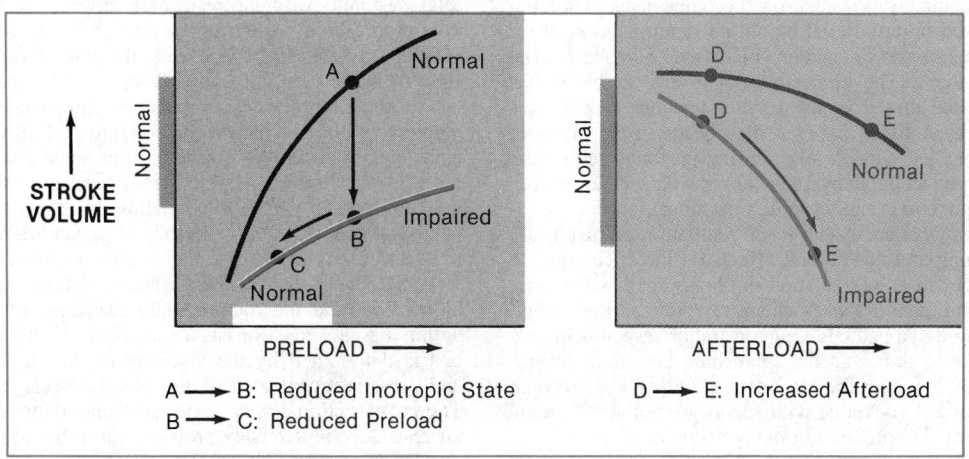

A — B: Reduced Inotropic State

B — C: Reduced Preload

D — E: Increased Afterload

FIGURE 69–1. Effects on stroke volume of alterations in preload, afterload, and contractility.

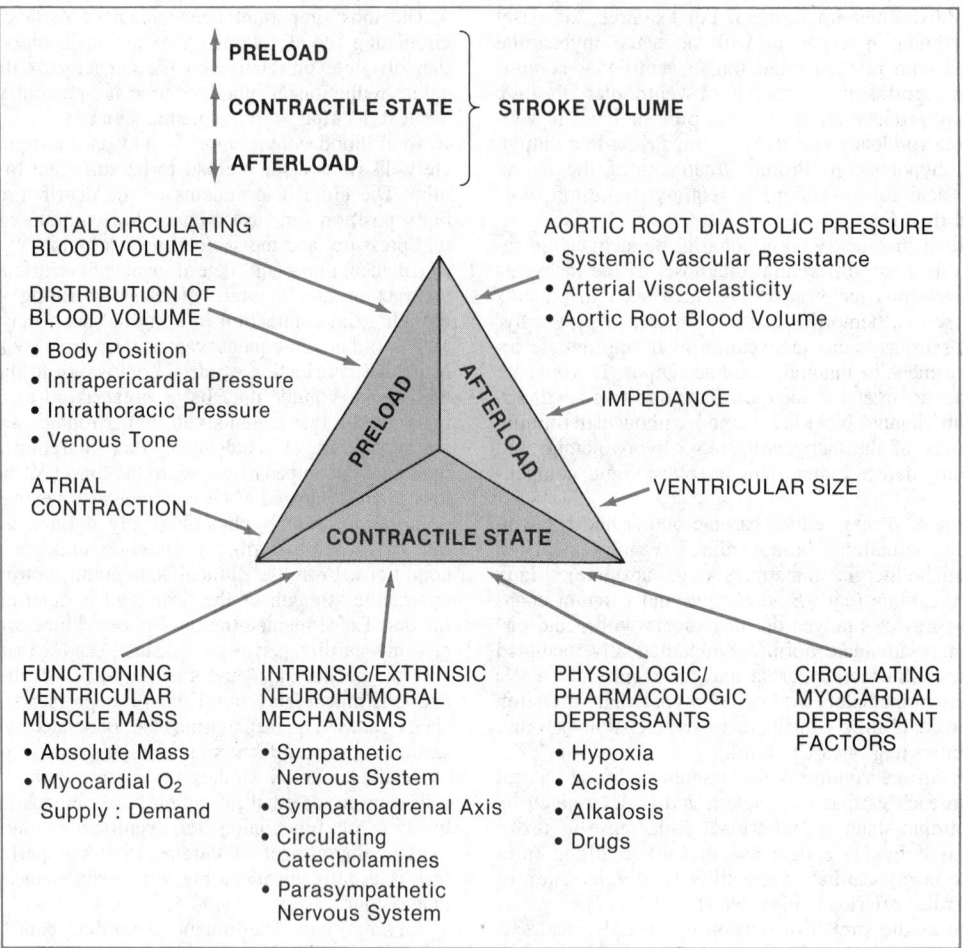

FIGURE 69-2. Determinants of stroke volume.

diastolic pressure (e.g., to < 60 mm Hg) may produce myocardial ischemia that further impairs overall hemodynamic performance by further reducing cardiac output. In the presence of coronary artery disease, resistance to flow is due largely to structural changes in the coronary vessel wall, and maximal vasodilation tends to occur distal to the site of coronary stenosis because excessive vasodilator metabolites accumulate. In this setting, arterial pressure determines perfusion to the ischemic segment through collateral vessels or across a coronary narrowing.

Among the pathophysiologic depressants common in shock are *hypoxia* and *acidosis.* Tissue hypoxia is a cellular diagnosis that is clinically inferred by evidence of organ dysfunction in the setting of cardiovascular abnormalities known to be associated with impairment of tissue perfusion. Hypoxemia, on the other hand, is a laboratory diagnosis based on an arterial blood gas determination of reduced oxygen tension (Po_2) and/or increased alveolar-arterial oxygen tension gradient. The clinician often relies on blood gas analyses of arterial and mixed venous oxygen tensions to infer cellular hypoxia. However, tissue hypoxia may occur in the presence of normal arterial oxygen tension (e.g., during profound reductions of cardiac output), and cellular hypoxia may be present in the absence of arterial hypoxemia (e.g., cyanide poisoning).

In shock, hypoxemia often results from ventilation-perfusion abnormalities in the lung and has several effects on the circulation. A direct vascular effect causes vasodilation in organs such as the heart and brain. Hypoxemia also activates chemoreceptors in the carotid sinus region, causing a sympathetic vasoconstrictor response in vessels of skeletal muscle, skin, and the splanchnic bed, thus permitting redistribution of blood to the vital organs with higher oxygen demand. Severe arterial hypoxemia with secondary cellular hypoxia is a cause of myocardial depression in many forms of shock.

Acidosis results from anaerobic metabolism that releases lactate, from decreased renal perfusion that accumulates organic acids, and from hypoventilation with secondary respiratory acidosis. Acidosis reduces myocardial contractility and the vasoconstrictor response to various endogenous and exogenous neurohumoral agents.

Finally, a number of pharmacologic agents used to treat critically ill patients directly or indirectly depress the myocardium and should be avoided if at all possible. These include sedative-hypnotic agents, anesthetic agents, antiarrhythmic agents, β-adrenergic blocking agents, and calcium channel antagonists.

Afterload is best understood as the sum of forces that the ventricle must overcome in order to eject blood. Afterload is determined primarily by the diastolic arterial pressure at the root of the aorta, ventricular size (law of Laplace), and vascular impedance. The diastolic pressure at the root of the aorta is determined primarily by total systemic vascular resistance, arterial viscoelasticity, and the volume of blood present in the root of the aorta at the onset of ventricular contraction. Impedance is the sum of factors opposing blood flow from the ventricle and is determined by inertial, viscous, resistance, and compliance components. Impedance relates to the dynamic relation of changes in pressure and flow. In general, clinicians cannot accurately measure impedance and therefore rely on a *calculated resistance,* derived from measuring the ratio of pressure gradient to flow across a circulation, to assess afterload (i.e., calculated systemic vascular resistance = [mean arterial pressure − mean right atrial pressure]/[systemic cardiac output]).

VASCULAR FACTORS. These determine the resistance to blood flow and the transcapillary exchange of gases and nutrients within tissue beds. Resistance to flow of blood through an organ bed is determined by the viscosity of the blood and by the length and cross-sectional area of the blood vessels perfusing that organ. The cross-sectional area is the most important component, as vascular resistance is inversely proportional to the fourth power of the radius of the vessel. The radius is in turn determined by the tone of vascular smooth muscle in the wall of the vessel. Vascular smooth muscle tone is modulated by neurogenic influences mediated primarily through the sympathoadrenal system and by circulating humoral and local metabolic factors.

Neurogenic Control. Sympathoadrenal discharge to the circulatory system is regulated by medullary neurons in the vasomotor centers of the brain stem. Neuron activity is modulated by afferent neural impulses originating in various peripheral sensory receptors located in strategic areas throughout the body. Important among these receptors are the arterial (sinoaortic) and cardiopulmonary baroreceptors, chemoreceptors, and somatic receptors in skeletal muscle. Activities originating in higher portions of the central nervous system also impinge on the brain stem vasomotor centers and thereby centrally modulate sympathetic and parasympathetic output.

The heart functions both as a muscle pump and as a peripheral sensory and endocrine organ. *Cardiopulmonary baroreceptors,* located primarily in the posterior wall of the left ventricle, are tonically active mechanoreceptors that are activated when the myocardium expands and stretches. When activated by an increase in cardiac preload, these "low-pressure" receptors exert an afferent inhibitory influence on brain stem cardiovascular centers and thereby decrease efferent sympathetic outflow from these centers. Conversely, reduction in the stretch of these ventricular receptors, as during hypovolemia or sitting upright, lessens their tonic afferent inhibition on brain stem centers and releases efferent sympathetic activity to cause reflex vasoconstriction, tachycardia, and the release of renin.

The *arterial baroreceptors,* located in the carotid sinus and aortic arch regions, are "high-pressure" mechanoreceptors that are activated by an increase in arterial pressure. When activated, these receptors exert an afferent inhibition on the brain stem vasomotor centers, thereby decreasing efferent sympathetic drive and resulting in vasodilation and bradycardia. Conversely, when deactivated by a fall in arterial pressure, the afferent inhibitory arterial baroreceptor input to the brain stem is decreased, resulting in an increase in sympathetic efferent tone with compensatory vasoconstriction and tachycardia.

In addition to inhibitory receptors such as the cardiac and arterial baroreceptors, peripheral excitatory afferent mechanisms also exist which contribute importantly to reflex control of the circulation. Severe hypoxia, often found associated with shock, activates excitatory *chemoreceptors* located in the carotid sinus region. This exerts an excitatory afferent influence on the brain stem centers, resulting in an increase in efferent sympathetic tone and vasoconstriction. *Somatic receptors* are metabolic receptors in exercising muscle that are activated by metabolic products of exercise and produce an afferent excitatory influence on the brain stem cardiovascular centers. This effect results in an increase in efferent sympathetic discharge to nonexercising muscles, with resultant vasoconstriction and increase in blood pressure to compensate for metabolic vasodilation occurring in exercising muscle beds.

During circulatory perturbations, synergistic and/or antagonistic activation of these multiple reflex pathways may occur. The net effect on cardiovascular homeostatic mechanisms depends on the relative influence of these various regulatory pathways and interaction with other neurohormonal responses.

HUMORAL FACTORS. A number of circulating humoral agents play important roles in cardiovascular homeostasis. The release of hormones such as renin, vasopressin, adrenal steroids, prostaglandins, kinins, atrial natriuretic factor, and catecholamines is partially mediated through the autonomic nervous system and partly through direct and indirect cellular effects of toxins, ischemia, and antigens in various organs. These hormones have direct cardiovascular and renal effects and indirect effects on central and/or peripheral adrenergic transmission.

Renin-Angiotensin. The release of renin, synthesized primarily in the juxtaglomerular apparatus of the kidney, is regulated by various stimuli, including renal afferent arteriolar pressure, sodium concentration within the macula densa, stimulation of renal sympathetic nerves, circulating angiotensin II, and electrolyte concentration in circulating plasma. A fall in arterial blood pressure or an increase in sympathoadrenal discharge to the kidney results in the release of renin. Renin functions as a proteolytic enzyme, converting inactive angiotensinogen to angiotensin I, which is converted to angiotensin II by angiotensin-converting enzyme, primarily in the lung. Angiotensin II is a very potent direct-acting vasoconstrictor that also facilitates the release of norepinephrine from sympathetic

nerve terminals. The net result is peripheral vasoconstriction in an attempt to maintain arterial pressure. In addition, the increase in angiotensin II increases the release of aldosterone, consequently retaining sodium and water.

Vasopressin. This important osmolality-regulating and vasoconstrictor hormone is released from the posterior pituitary primarily in response to increases in osmolality as well as in response to hypovolemia. Vasopressin appears to play a role in the circulatory control response to shock by being both an antidiuretic and a vasoconstrictor. In addition, vasopressin stimulates release of adrenocorticotropin (ACTH) and cortisol. Release of vasopressin is reduced by stretch of left atrial receptors during hypervolemia and by stretch of the arterial baroreceptors during hypertension; conversely, during hemorrhage and systemic hypotension, or when patients are on cardiopulmonary bypass, blood levels of vasopressin increase significantly. Vasopressin may be released by as little as a 10% reduction in blood volume. Thirst and the release of vasopressin may be induced by a central nervous system (CNS) action of angiotensin. From the standpoint of managing the shock patient, it is important to realize that vasopressin secretion is stimulated by nausea, morphine, and hypoxia and may be inhibited by catecholamines and alcohol.

Kinins. A variety of potent vasodilator polypeptides are formed by the action of certain proteolytic enzymes on plasma protein precursors. Bradykinin serves as the prototype for this class of endogenous peptides. Their major physiologic role may be locally regulating blood flow and function of such organs as the salivary glands, pancreas, and kidney. In pathophysiologic states, kinins are believed to play a part in the hyperemia associated with inflammation and as vasodilators in hypotension produced by anaphylactic reactions. Renal kinins may cause diuresis and natriuresis.

Serotonin and Histamine. Serotonin released from platelets and histamine released from mast cells during anaphylaxis or during complement activation in shock may play an important role in regulating local vascular tone and capillary permeability.

Prostacyclin and Thromboxane A$_2$. Prostaglandins may be released in various organs during ischemia and may contribute to reactive hyperemia and vasodilation. The prostaglandin endoperoxides formed in platelets and in blood vessels are pivotal in the synthesis of two potent substances with opposing effects on thrombus formation. Prostacyclin, a powerful vasodilator and inhibitor of platelet aggregation, is synthesized in the vascular wall, mostly in the endothelial layer, from endoperoxides. In the platelets, however, endoperoxides are converted to thromboxane A$_2$, which causes vasoconstriction and platelet aggregation. In shock, damage to endothelial cells may inhibit synthesis of prostacyclin; in addition, platelets may release thromboxane A$_2$, causing intravascular platelet aggregation, clumping, and vasoconstriction.

Neuropeptides. Recent experimental and clinical studies in shock have emphasized the potentially important role of certain neuropeptides in regulating cardiovascular adjustments to shock and trauma. Among these important mediators are endogenous opioids (e.g., β-endorphin), thyrotropin-releasing hormone (TRF), and ACTH. β-Endorphin and adrenocorticotropin are stored in the pituitary gland and secreted concomitantly under stress. These agents appear to modulate autonomic function through CNS action, and they may play a role in peripherally integrating autonomic nervous system activity. The β-endorphins, in particular, may play an important role in the pathophysiology of certain types of shock, most notably hemorrhagic, endotoxic (septic), and spinal shock. β-Endorphins may contribute directly or indirectly to myocardial depression during shock states. Experimental and limited clinical studies have suggested that blocking the action of such endogenous opiates pharmacologically with specific antagonists such as naloxone may improve cardiovascular stability in certain shock states. However, the precise role of these agents in such therapy remains to be defined (see Management).

TRF is a neuropeptide with potent central cardiovascular actions. Although frequently thought of primarily as a hypothalamic hormone with specific endocrinologic actions (e.g., stimulating release of thyroid-stimulating hormone from the pituitary), a major fraction of TRF is found outside of the hypothalamus in the brain and spinal cord. Experimental studies have suggested that exogenously administered TRF improves cardiorespiratory function in certain shock states, possibly through antagonism of adverse physiologic effects of endogenous opioids. The clinical importance of TRF in shock states in humans remains to be defined.

Atrial Natriuretic Factors. These biologically active peptides are released from specific granules in atrial myocytes and to a lesser extent from ventricular myocytes. These peptides bind to specific high-affinity receptors located in adrenal, renal, and vascular beds. These peptides produce direct vasorelaxant effects on vascular smooth muscle and natriuretic effects in the kidney. In addition, atrial natriuretic factor inhibits the action of renin and the production of aldosterone. Animal studies have suggested that these agents may alter the sensitivity of baroreceptors. While atrial natriuretic factor has been found to be elevated in pathophysiologic states such as severe heart failure, the exact role of these peptides in severe hemodynamic disorders such as shock remains unclear.

Catecholamines. The catecholamines norepinephrine and epinephrine are potent modulators of cardiovascular homeostasis. Released primarily from sympathetic nerve terminals, norepinephrine increases myocardial contractility and heart rate by activating β-adrenoceptors and therefore increases cardiac output. In addition, norepinephrine has potent α-adrenergic actions and produces vasoconstriction, although the magnitude of this effect varies from tissue to tissue. Norepinephrine is a potent vasoconstrictor in skin, muscle, and splanchnic beds, whereas it may produce vasodilation in coronary vascular beds through a β_2-adrenergic mechanism. Epinephrine is released primarily from the adrenal glands, where the ratio of its release to that of norepinephrine is $10:1$. Epinephrine has α, β_1, and β_2 effects and produces a modest increase in cardiac output through β effects. However, epinephrine redistributes cardiac output away from the kidney and splanchnic circulation toward skeletal muscle, where its β_2 effect predominates with vasodilation. In other beds, epinephrine has significant α-vasoconstricting effects. Epinephrine also may effect release of norepinephrine from adrenergic nerve terminals through a prejunctional action.

Local Autoregulatory Mechanisms. Blood vessels have an intrinsic ability to autoregulate vascular tone and thereby maintain blood flow over a wide range of perfusion pressures. This property is independent of systemic neurogenic influences or humoral factors. Different vascular beds vary with respect to their ability to maintain blood flow. The cerebral, coronary, and renal circulations have the most developed autoregulatory mechanisms. Thus, during a fall in arterial pressure, vasodilation in these vascular beds maintains blood flow and oxygen delivery to the brain and heart and helps to preserve sodium and water balance. Although a myogenic response intrinsic to the smooth muscle may partially explain the phenomenon, accumulation of tissue metabolites following a transient period of ischemia also may cause vasodilation and restore blood flow. The specific mediator of metabolic vasodilation is not known, but it is likely that a combination of changes in oxygen, carbon dioxide, hydrogen ions, and other cations, in osmolality, in the amount of adenosine compounds, and in Krebs cycle intermediates and other metabolites released in the immediate environment of blood vessels contributes to adjustments in vascular tone.

Finally, apart from neural and humoral influences, the presence of occlusive vascular disease may play an important role in determining resistance to flow through regional circulations. This effect depends on both fixed physical obstruction to the cross-sectional area of the perfusion bed and abnormalities in vascular reactivity induced by atherosclerotic changes in the vascular endothelium.

MICROCIRCULATION AND TRANSCAPILLARY EXCHANGE. The most critical aspect of the pathogenesis of shock takes place at the level of the microcirculation. In essence, all shock can be considered a form of microcirculatory failure. Delivery of a significant amount of blood to an organ does not guarantee that all the segments of that organ and all capillaries are perfused appropriate to the regional metabolic demand.

Intraorgan Blood Flow Distribution. Adequate tissue perfusion depends on blood flow through vascular channels in which diffusion between the blood and tissues can occur. These channels are referred to as *nutritional capillaries,* as contrasted to nonnutritional vessels, which do not permit capillary exchange. The latter are referred to as *arteriovenous shunts.* An example of the importance of the intraorgan redistribution of blood flow is observed in myocardial infarction, in which an increase in coronary blood flow may

not increase perfusion to the infarcted segment. Under some circumstances, a coronary vasodilator may redistribute flow away from ischemic into nonischemic regions (e.g., a potent intravenous vasodilator given to a patient with severe fixed coronary obstruction with consequent induction of a coronary steal phenomenon). Similarly, the pattern of intraorgan blood flow may be crucial in the kidney. Acute tubular necrosis associated with shock may reflect a reduction in glomerular filtration in the outer cortex because of a localized increase in vascular resistance in this region and a selective reduction in blood flow. Interventions that alter total renal blood flow can produce significant redistribution of flow within the kidney; for example, renal vasoconstriction following adrenergic discharge tends to shunt blood away from the outer cortex, whereas renal vasodilators (including the loop diuretic furosemide) shunt blood toward the outer cortical nephrons.

Pre- and Postcapillary Resistance. The precapillary sphincters regulate the patency of nutritional or "exchange" capillaries. The tone of these sphincters may be modulated by neurohumoral factors that contribute to the circulatory adjustments in shock. The metabolic products at the local tissue level are important determinants of the tone of these sphincters, which regulate the total functional capillary surface area and in turn determine the potential capillary area available for intravascular-to-extracellular fluid and solute exchange. The capillary hydrostatic force driving fluid out of the capillaries into the extracellular space depends on the ratio of post- to precapillary resistances. In hypovolemic or hemorrhagic shock, the fall in arterial pressure activates the sympathoadrenal system, constricts precapillary resistance vessels, and decreases capillary hydrostatic pressure, facilitating movement of fluids from the extracellular to the intravascular space. This partially restores intravascular volume. Hematocrit, viscosity of blood, and plasma oncotic pressure fall. With persistent hypotension and ischemia, the vasoconstrictor response of precapillary resistance vessels becomes less pronounced because of tissue acidosis, while resistance of postcapillary vessels (venules) increases. This creates a situation in which more fluid is lost from the vascular to the interstitial space. Thus venular resistance and the reactivity of venules to the various vasoactive agents involved in shock become important. Venules may even be relatively more reactive than precapillary resistance vessels to catecholamines, which activate α-vasoconstrictor receptors. This differential effect in favor of postcapillary vasoconstriction also further increases hydrostatic pressure and intravascular fluid loss.

Capillary Permeability and Oncotic Pressure. Colloid osmotic pressure is a major determinant of intravascular volume. Albumin is the main osmotically active protein in plasma. The balance between colloid osmotic pressure and capillary hydrostatic pressure determines the balance between intravascular and extracellular fluid spaces. A significant degree of hypovolemia and hemoconcentration may take place either because of excessive capillary hydrostatic pressure from an increase in the ratio of post- to precapillary resistance or because of a reduction in plasma protein and consequent reduction of plasma oncotic pressure. Fewer plasma proteins may circulate as a result of increased capillary permeability and loss of plasma proteins from the intravascular to the extracellular space. The balance between oncotic and hydrostatic pressures also determines the level of pulmonary edema and is critical in the management of the shock lung syndrome. An appreciation of the important interplay between hydrostatic and colloid pressures is crucial to selecting appropriate intravenous volume replacement in the therapy of many types of shock. Similarly, nutritional support of the critically ill patient is important to maintain adequate production of albumin.

Shock resulting from increased vascular permeability, as in anaphylactic shock or snake venom poisoning (see Ch. 390), is characterized by a dramatic reduction of plasma volume. Hematocrit rises sharply and oncotic pressure drops. This increase in capillary permeability may be partly related to release of histamine, metabolites, or humoral factors that alter endothelial permeability.

Intravascular Hemaglutination and "Blood Sludging." Erythrocytes, leukocytes, and platelets undergo agglutination to a variable degree in association with the shock syndromes in thermal burn, sepsis, trauma, and perhaps even hemorrhage. These aggregates may obstruct nutritional capillaries as well as arterioles. The precipitating events are numerous. They may include platelet aggregation by catecholamines, damage to endothelial lining of small blood vessels and capillaries with subsequent fibrin deposition and accumulation of microthrombi, hypoxia increasing the rigidity of red blood cells, oxygen free radicals generated by endothelial cells or neutrophils, and release of vasoactive peptides and anaphylatoxins as a result of complement activation. These also may damage endothelial cells and increase the tone of precapillary sphincters, leading to further reduction in tissue perfusion and cellular injury.

PATHOPHYSIOLOGY AND STAGES OF SHOCK

Conceptually, shock can be considered to progress through stages of lesser to greater severity and from reversible to irreversible derangements of metabolic processes. This conceptual framework involves stages of compensated, decompensated, and irreversible shock as summarized in Figure 69–3 and Table 69–3.

STAGE I—COMPENSATED SHOCK. In early shock, hypotension may arise from either a fall in cardiac output or peripheral vasodilation. The fall in cardiac output and arterial pressure triggers compensatory mechanisms, which attempt to restore arterial pressure and blood flow to vital organs such as the brain and heart. At this stage, symptoms and signs of hemodynamic impairment are often subtle, and a high degree of clinical suspicion is required to identify early signs of hemodynamic compromise. Arterial pressure is usually maintained or mildly reduced, there is an increase in heart rate and a narrowing of pulse pressure, and there may be mild anxiety and early peripheral vasoconstriction. If shock is identified and vigorously treated at this stage, the syndrome may be successfully reversed in many cases.

STAGE II—DECOMPENSATED SHOCK. At this stage in the progression of shock, the compensatory mechanisms invoked during stage I to maintain perfusion of vital organs are insufficient to compensate for the hemodynamic insult. Patients can demonstrate impaired major organ perfusion, as manifested by altered mental state (impaired cerebral perfusion), reduced urine output (renal hypoperfusion), and myocardial ischemia (coronary flow impairment). The patient in this stage demonstrates the classic clinical picture of shock with hypotension, tachycardia, tachypnea, and narrowed pulse pressure (rapid, weak, and thready pulse). The external appearance of the patient reflects excessive sympathetic drive with acrocyanosis, peripheral vasoconstriction, and diaphoresis (cold and clammy extremities). Rapid aggressive intervention is required to restore cardiac output and perfusion of the tissues in this stage, prior to the onset of irreversible shock.

STAGE III—IRREVERSIBLE SHOCK. Excessive and prolonged reduction of tissue perfusion leads to significant alterations in cellular membrane function, aggregation of blood cells in the microcirculation, and "sludging" in the capillaries. The vasoconstriction that has taken place in the less vital organs in order to maintain blood pressure is now excessive and has reduced perfusion to such a point that cellular damage occurs. In this stage of shock, arterial pressure continues to fall progressively to a critical level at which vital organ perfusion is reduced. A physiological vicious circle of hemodynamic insults occurs during this stage, with cascading impairment of tissue perfusion leading to further metabolic derangements, which, in turn, provoke further degradation of organ functions. The net result is the onset of multiple organ system failure (MOSF). Critical impairment of renal perfusion leads to acute tubular necrosis. Ischemia of the gastrointestinal tract leads to necrotic damage of the mucosa with a breakdown of this natural barrier and the subsequent absorption into the circulation of bacteria and their toxins with secondary detrimental effects on other organs. A generalized endothelial damage and disseminated intravascular coagulation may occur. Bacterial toxins may react with neutrophils and cause the release of vasodilator polypeptides that contribute to the fall in arterial pressure. Severe acidosis results from anaerobic metabolism as peripheral organs fail to receive nutrients sufficient to maintain aerobic metabolic pathways. Decreased perfusion of the coronary circulation, particularly in patients with coronary disease, results in further impairment of myocardial function with a further decline in cardiac output. Damage to capillary endothelium leads to loss of fluid and protein through the capillaries, with exacerbation of hypovolemia and hypotension. Ultimately, damage to cellular membranes from ischemia leads to leakage of lysosomal enzymes and other intracellular constituents, to progressive reduction in high-energy phosphate levels, and to cellular destruction. This terminal stage of shock is characterized by irreversible impairment of subcellular machinery, as discussed in the following section.

CELLULAR AND BIOCHEMICAL FACTORS IN SHOCK

MITOCHONDRIAL FUNCTION. Mitochondrial electron transport–linked mechanisms provide >95% of the body's energy needs under normal resting conditions. To do this, mitochondria utilize >90% of the available cellular oxygen. The delivery of this essential oxygen depends on maintaining adequate tissue perfusion and the integrity of the capillary-interstitial-cellular interface. Shock of many diverse etiologies has been shown to result in progressive defects in mitochondrial metabolism.

Possible mechanisms involved in mitochondrial abnormalities during shock include structural changes (e.g., swelling), altered enzyme systems secondary to loss of critical cofactors, decreases in mitochondrial magnesium levels, increase in mitochondrial calcium concentration, altered mitochondrial sodium and potassium content, inhibited mitochondrial function by agents such as free fatty acids, and free radical oxidation of phospholipids in the mitochondrial membranes.

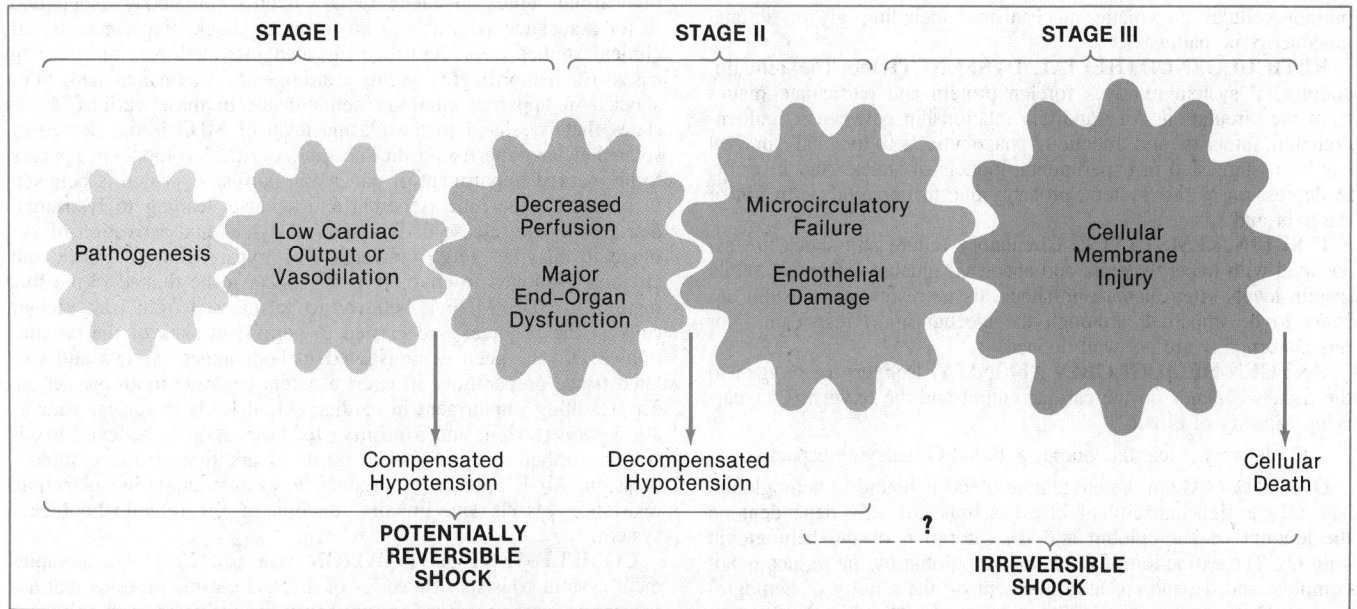

FIGURE 69–3. Pathophysiology of shock.

TABLE 69–3. PATHOPHYSIOLOGIC STAGES OF SHOCK—CLINICAL SIGNS

Clinical Parameters	Stage I (Compensated)	Stage II (Decompensated)	Stage III (Irreversible)
Arterial pressure	N or (−)	(− −)	(− − −)
Heart rate	(+)	(+ +)	(+ + +) to (− − −)
Pulse pressure	(−)	(− − −)	(− − −)
Respiratory rate	N	(+ +)	(+ + +) to (− − −)
Cardiac output	(−)*	(− −)	(− − −)
Mental status	Anxiety	Impaired/ Obtunded	Coma
Urinary output	N or (−)	(− −)	Anuric
Skin	Cool*	Mottled	Cold, cyanotic

N = no change; (−) = decreased; (+) = increased.
* A high cardiac output and warm skin may be present in early stages of septic shock.

It is unclear whether the degree of mitochondrial damage is a uniform feature in all tissues of the patient with shock or is manifested to a greater degree in some organs than in others. In experimental models, hepatic mitochondrial damage appears to dominate, whereas cerebral mitochondrial function appears to be preserved until very late in the experimental shock state. Experimental studies suggest that mitochondrial dysfunction may be reversed by intervening in the very early stages of shock, but the limits of this crucial period of reversibility are unknown at present.

METABOLIC ALTERATIONS. Survival of aerobic cells depends on the availability of substrates and oxygen to the mitochondria, which provide most of the high-energy phosphate needs of the cell and utilize most of the available oxygen in the process. During shock, a lack of oxygen in metabolically active organs such as the liver and kidney results in anaerobic metabolism. This is demonstrated by an early and marked impairment in ATP production. With advanced shock, this impairment is seen in other organs such as skeletal muscle. In these organs, anaerobic metabolism becomes the predominant mechanism of energy production and cellular levels of lactate and pyruvate increase owing to both anaerobic glycolysis and decreased use of these substrates.

CELLULAR TRANSPORT MECHANISMS. While water is freely diffusible across cellular membranes, the normal transport of important solutes requires diffusion, facilitated diffusion, or active transport. Experimental evidence suggests that important disturbances in cellular transport mechanisms occur during shock. Hemorrhagic and septic shock have been shown to produce marked decreases in electrical potentials across hepatic and skeletal muscle membranes. This impairment and the consequent derangements in cellular electrolytes and water result in further impairment of important cellular enzymatic mechanisms, including glycolytic and gluconeogenic pathways.

RETICULOENDOTHELIAL DYSFUNCTION. The reticuloendothelial system removes foreign protein and particulate matter from the circulation. An important relationship between reticuloendothelial integrity and function, phagocytic activity, and survival has been suggested in experimental models of shock. Shock results in depression of this system, probably due to impaired perfusion of the liver and spleen.

INSULIN RESISTANCE. Circulatory failure and shock are associated with hyperglycemia and abnormal glucose tolerance. While insulin levels often increase in shock, tissue response to insulin appears to be impaired, although the mechanism(s) responsible for this abnormality are not well defined.

OXYGEN-HEMOGLOBIN AFFINITY. Delivery of oxygen to the tissues depends on the cardiac output and the oxygen (O_2)-carrying capacity of blood:

$$O_2 \text{ delivery} = \text{cardiac output} \times \text{blood } O_2\text{-carrying capacity}$$

Over 98% of O_2 in the circulating blood is bound to hemoglobin. The O_2-carrying capacity of blood is thus critically dependent on the amount of hemoglobin and the saturation of the hemoglobin with O_2. The extraction of O_2 from hemoglobin by the tissues is not complete and depends to a large extent on the affinity of hemoglobin for O_2, i.e., the shape of the oxygen-hemoglobin dissociation curve.

Hydrogen ions (Bohr effect), carbon dioxide (CO_2), and 2,3-diphosphoglyceric acid (2,3-DPG) cause greater dissociation of O_2 from hemoglobin because of their preferential affinity for reduced hemoglobin. The concentration of 2,3-DPG in red cells results from a side reaction of glycolysis and increases during anemia, hypoxia, and acidosis. A drop in hemoglobin, hypoxemia, and acidosis may thus be partly compensated for by a shift of the O_2 dissociation curve to the right, favoring greater delivery of O_2 to the tissues at the same P_{O_2}. This compensatory mechanism, in addition to the increase in cardiac output, provides for better oxygenation as extraction of O_2 increases at the expense of the O_2 reserve in venous blood. In certain tissues, however, such as the myocardium, O_2 extraction at rest is already large, and any additional O_2 demand or a decrease in oxyhemoglobin dissociation such as in alkalosis requires greater delivery of O_2, i.e., higher coronary blood flow.

In shock, the pH, CO_2, and 2,3-DPG levels are changing, and one cannot calculate O_2 extraction from values of arterial P_{O_2} because the shape of the oxyhemoglobin dissociation curve cannot be predicted accurately. It is preferable to measure O_2 content or saturation of venous and arterial blood; if saturation is lower than predicted from values of P_{O_2}, one can deduce that there is a shift of the dissociation curve to the right, and vice versa. Overzealous correction of acidosis with bicarbonate may, through the Bohr effect on hemoglobin affinity for O_2, actually reduce O_2 delivery to the tissues. Hypophosphatemia (reported during hyperalimentation) may decrease 2,3-DPG and O_2 delivery.

LYSOSOMAL ABNORMALITIES. While present in most tissues, the higher concentrations of lysosomes in the body are found in the liver, kidney, and spleen. Lysosomes are cytoplasmic vesicles that contain a variety of potent hydrolytic enzymes bound in a latent form. These enzymes can hydrolyze a variety of intra- and extracellular macromolecules. When released from organelles as a consequence of certain forms of cellular injury, these enzymes may contribute to the pathogenesis or the propagation and perpetuation of shock. They are most active at an acid pH, which makes them potentially more destructive in the setting of hypoxia and shock.

Numerous morphologic and biochemical observations implicate the lysosomal enzymes in the perpetuation of shock. In organs such as the liver, spleen, and intestine, the lysosomes enlarge during the early phases of shock. This is associated with a decrease in the total activity of lysosomal hydrolases in tissues and a corresponding increase in activity in the soluble fraction of the tissue homogenate. This indicates a loss of lysosomal membrane integrity *in vivo*. The lysosomes obtained from animals in shock demonstrate an enhanced release of enzymes *in vitro*. A reduction in lysosomal membrane integrity also has been observed in animals after administration of endotoxin. In several animal studies, the levels of hydrolases found in blood, lymph, or serum seem to correlate with severity of shock.

MYOCARDIAL DEPRESSANT FACTOR(S). Initially described in 1966 in the plasma of cats following hemorrhagic shock, myocardial depressant factor (MDF) is an incompletely understood factor associated with almost all forms of shock. Experimental and clinical studies have described elevated plasma levels of MDF in cases of hemorrhagic, septic, cardiogenic, traumatic, and burn shock. An apparent common denominator in these various shock states that is related to the plasma level of MDF is the degree of splanchnic hypoperfusion that occurs. A critical component appears to be marked impairment of pancreatic perfusion, which is believed to result in pancreatic ischemia and acidosis leading to lysosomal disruption. The release of lysosomal enzymes and activation of zymogenic enzymes (e.g., conversion of trypsinogen to trypsin and chymotrypsinogen to chymotrypsin) appear to be related to the formation of MDF. MDF is believed to be released from leaky acinar cells in the pancreas and carried to peripheral sites of the circulation. MDF has been demonstrated in both intact animals and isolated tissue preparations to exert a potent negative inotropic action. The resulting impairment in cardiac output leads to further pancreatic hypoperfusion, and a positive feedback loop is believed to result in further release of this agent. In addition to the cardiodepression, MDF appears to produce vasoconstriction in splanchnic resistance vessels and impairs function of the reticuloendothelial system.

COMPLEMENT ACTIVATION (see Ch. 222). The complement system consists of a series of discrete plasma proteins that are present as inactive precursors until they are activated by highly specific biochemical reactions. Activating the complement system results in the cleavage of several low-molecular-weight vasoactive peptides from the complement molecules. These peptides in turn have a variety of significant biologic effects. For example, during activation of C2, a cleavage product occurs that has kinin-like activity, which then can significantly influence capillary permeability. Two other activation peptides, C3a and C5a, release histamine from mast cells, have chemotactic activity, and constrict vascular smooth muscle. Another fragment, C3B, acts as an opsonin and facilitates phagocytosis. Polymorphonuclear leukocytes may be attracted chemotactically through activation of esterases on their surface and may release their lysosomal enzymes if the concentration of the complement reaction product C5a is large enough. Platelets may increase their procoagulant activity. In addition to the direct and indirect effects of the fragments of activated complement on cells, their aggregation as complexes on the surface of cell membranes destroys cells. The expressions of all these effects are increased capillary permeability, increased leukocyte accumulation and infiltration, release of lysosomal enzymes, and activation of intravascular coagulation factors. Clinically, these result in such entities as glomerulitis, necrotizing vasculitis, the Schwartzmann reaction, thrombocytopenia, and other manifestations of microcirculatory collapse and intravascular plugging seen in prolonged shock and endotoxemia.

Although the side effects of complement activation in shock are detrimental, leading to cellular death, the fundamental biologic activities of the complement components are beneficial—in enhancing phagocytosis and mediating the inflammatory response to local infection or irritation, in neutralizing viruses, and finally, in modulating the immune response.

EICOSANOIDS. These lipid substances, derived from arachidonic acid (eicosatetraenoic acid), have recently been implicated as important mediators of ischemic and circulatory shock. During ischemic and shock states, a number of these substances are produced, the most important of which are the vasoconstrictor prostaglandins (PG), thromboxanes (TX), and leukotrienes (LT).

PGF_2-α has been found to be increased in animals with hemorrhagic, endotoxic, cardiogenic, and burn shock, has been identified as a potent vasoconstrictor of coronary, mesenteric, and renal vessels, and is believed to play some role in the pathogenesis of circulatory shock. TXA_2 is believed to play three important roles in shock: (1) inducing vasoconstriction, (2) aggregating circulating platelets, and (3) inducing leakage in lysosomal membranes. It is believed to play a role in myocardial ischemia, sudden death, and circulatory shock. Recent experimental evidence suggests that TX synthetase inhibitors may play a protective role in certain types of myocardial ischemia, trauma, and endotoxic shock.

LT's are the major biologically active products of the lipoxygenase pathway of arachidonic acid metabolism and are produced by pulmonary parenchymal cells, macrophages, mast cells, white blood cells, and connective tissue cells. These agents appear to be potent vasoconstrictors and bronchoconstrictors. The exact role, if any, that these agents play in the pathogenesis of shock remains to be defined experimentally.

OXYGEN FREE RADICALS. Oxygen free radicals may be generated in tissues during shock states. The unpaired electron in these radicals may react with any cellular component, but particularly with unsaturated fatty acids and sulfhydryl amino acids, and cause cellular damage. The clinical documentation of the relative importance of these factors and the effectiveness of their elimination awaits further experimentation in humans.

TUMOR NECROSIS FACTOR. Tumor necrosis factor (TNF, cachectin) was the first of a family of cytokines recognized to play a role as endogenous mediators of shock and inflammation. TNF is derived from mononuclear phagocytes being exposed to lipopolysaccharide endotoxin, and TNF appears to be responsible for many of the deleterious effects of endotoxin. TNF appears to be one of the primary mediators of experimental septic shock, with many of the lethal cytotoxic effects of endotoxin being due to host cell effects mediated by this agent. Biologic effects attributed experimentally to TNF include the suppression of lipoprotein lipase biosynthesis by adipocytes, induction of antigenic determinants on fibroblasts and endothelial cells, stimulation of products of PGE_2 and collagenase, and activation of neutrophils. This latter effect appears responsible for many of the inflammatory changes seen in sepsis which lead to tissue damage. TNF also exerts a catabolic effect on bone and cartilage and is an endogenous pyrogen. TNF appears to share many of the same bioactivities of other inflammatory cytokines such as interleukin-1 and IL-6. The precise role of TNF in clinical shock is under active investigation.

ETIOLOGY OF SHOCK—CLASSIFICATION

Understanding and recognizing cardiogenic shock require an appreciation for the other potential (e.g., noncardiac) etiologies of shock. The clinician caring for a patient who presents in a shock state must entertain a wide differential diagnosis in initially approaching the patient in order to avoid misdiagnosis and mismanagement. When initially encountering a patient in shock, the clinician should entertain four broad categories of etiologies in the differential diagnosis. A brief overview of the etiologic classification of shock is therefore presented.

While the end result of most shock syndromes involves irreversible deterioration of cellular and subcellular metabolic processes and structural integrity, it is clinically useful to consider the differential diagnosis of shock from a functional standpoint. This classification scheme emphasizes potential initiating pathogenic mechanisms. Most cases of shock can be considered to arise from one of four basic abnormalities: (1) hypovolemia, (2) cardiac functional impairment, (3) obstruction of major vascular conduits, and (4) inappropriate distribution of cardiac output secondary to abnormal vasodilation. Common clinical syndromes representative of the functional types of shock are discussed below.

HYPOVOLEMIC SHOCK. Perfusion of major organs and peripheral tissues depends on the integrity of a vascular pump (heart), a capacitance vascular tree, and an intravascular blood volume. Hypovolemic shock is the most common type of shock and is due to an absolute and often sudden reduction in circulating blood volume relative to the capacity of the vascular system. The classic hemodynamic features of this type of shock include tachycardia, hypotension, reduced cardiac filling pressures, and peripheral vasoconstriction (see Table 69–3). An important aspect of this type of shock is the *rapidity* with which hypovolemia occurs. A sudden reduction in circulating blood volume of 10% in previously healthy individuals mildly reduces arterial pressure and moderately reduces cardiac output. A sudden reduction in blood volume of 20% produces moderate hypotension and moderately severe reductions in cardiac output. The loss of 40% of circulating blood volume produces profound reductions in arterial pressure and cardiac output. These hemodynamic consequences are accentuated in patients with pre-existing cardiovascular, pulmonary, renal, or cerebrovascular disorders. In contrast, a similar degree of volume loss occurring over a longer period of time (days to weeks) may not be accompanied by the same magnitude of hemodynamic impairment.

Hypovolemia may occur as a result of loss of blood volume secondary to hemorrhage (internal or external) or may arise as a result of the loss of fluid and electrolytes. This latter form of hypovolemia may occur following severe loss of gastrointestinal fluids (e.g., diarrhea, vomiting), renal losses (e.g., polyuria), external losses of fluids secondary to impairment of surface tissue integrity (e.g., burns), or internal losses of fluids without a change in total body water (e.g., third-space sequestration of fluids).

As previously noted, hypovolemia usually results in the induction of neurohumoral compensatory mechanisms that produce the characteristic features of shock (e.g., tachycardia, tachypnea, and peripheral vasoconstriction). However, it has been known for some time, although poorly appreciated by clinicians, that profound exsanguinating hemorrhage may present as paradoxical bradycardia (or absence of tachycardia) due to activation of cardiac mechanoreceptors in the setting of vigorous contraction of a "volume-depleted" ventricle. Recent observations in normal humans have demonstrated that abrupt decreases in cardiac filling pressures can result in sympathetic inhibition with profound hypotension and bradycardia. This afferent inhibition from ventricular receptors may override the hypotension-induced deactivation of arterial baroreceptors. Thus the presentation of a patient with obvious hypovolemic hypotension in the absence of tachycardia should alert the clinician to the possibility of massive volume loss and the need for vigorous volume resuscitation.

DISTRIBUTIVE SHOCK. This functional classification involves shock syndromes manifested by decreased vascular resistance that is not adequately compensated for by alterations in cardiac output. The classic example of distributive shock is endotoxin sepsis (see Ch. 70).

The incidence of septic shock in the hospital setting appears to have increased over the past several decades, probably as a consequence of multiple medical advances in other areas. It is estimated that 1% of hospital admissions are complicated by gram-negative sepsis, and the mortality from septic shock ranges from 30 to 80%. Sepsis is now the thirteenth leading cause of death in the United States, affecting over 2.5 million patients per year. Rather than a primary community-acquired phenomenon, septic shock more commonly arises in hospitalized patients and is one of the most common causes of mortality in intensive care unit patients (see Ch. 267).

Septic shock is most commonly associated with gram-negative infections, and approximately 40% of gram-negative bacteremias are complicated by shock. Gram-negative septic shock is most often an example of an opportunistic infection. The most common gram-negative organisms associated with septic shock include *Escherichia coli, Klebsiella, Enterobacter,* and *Pseudomonas* species. The most common sources for these infectious agents are the genitourinary and gastrointestinal tracts, followed by respiratory tract, wounds, and sites of indwelling vascular access. Important non–gram-negative organs associated with septic shock include some gram-positive *Staphylococcus* and *Streptococcus* species and fungal organisms such as *Candida.*

Host factors important in the propensity for developing septic shock include advanced age, diabetes, debilitation and malnutrition, chronic alcohol or intravenous drug use, neoplastic diseases, immunocompromised state (especially granulocytopenia), and MOSF.

Septic shock often follows a trimodal pattern of hemodynamic presentation: "warm" shock, "cold" shock, and MOSF. Early sepsis is often associated with a decrease in systemic vascular resistance, due most likely to the release of vasodilatory mediators such as bradykinin and histamine and an increase in cardiac output ("warm" shock). The early stages of sepsis are characterized hemodynamically by low cardiac filling pressures, increased cardiac output, tachycardia, fever, and decreased whole-body oxygen consumption. This latter effect is likely due to impaired mitochondrial oxygen utilization and deficient oxygen delivery to cells despite an increase in overall cardiac output (maldistribution of cardiac output). Late in the sequence of septic shock, there is a decline in cardiac output and profound hypotension with severe acidosis, hypoxemia, and hypoxia ("cold" shock). Recent evidence suggests that the initial increase in cardiac output is often followed by a decrease in ventricular ejection fraction, possibly due to a myocardial depressant factor, myocardial edema, or altered responsiveness to adrenergic stimuli.

Lipopolysaccharide endotoxin appears to be a common etiologic factor in septic shock, as previously reviewed in this chapter (Cellular and Biochemical Factors in Shock). The end stages of septic shock are often associated with MOSF with profound derangements in cardiovascular, pulmonary, and renal systems. The adult respiratory distress syndrome is a common complication of septic shock and is discussed later.

VASCULAR OBSTRUCTIVE SHOCK. Although often included in the category of cardiogenic shock, vascular obstructive shock usually arises as the result of insults that are not intrinsically myocardial in nature. However, vascular obstructive etiologies, especially those involving the pericardial and valvular portions of the heart, must be considered in the differential diagnosis of cardiogenic shock. The most common example of shock secondary to acute obstruction of the vascular tree is acute cardiac tamponade that results in impaired diastolic ventricular filling. This may arise as a result of trauma, infection, neoplasm, or cardiac rupture. It is the rapidity of accumulation of pericardial volume, rather than the absolute volume, that is the critical determinant of the hemodynamic impairment in cardiac tamponade. Rapid accumulations of as little as 100 to 200 ml of blood in the pericardium may produce tamponade. Similarly, therapeutic removal of small amounts of fluid (e.g., 50 to 100 ml via percutaneous pericardiocentesis) may be all that is required to relieve tamponade and allow diastolic ventricular filling to resume and cardiac output to rise. Other examples of vascular obstructive shock include tension pneumothorax, left ventricular inflow obstruction by an atrial myxoma or large thrombus, massive pulmonary embolism with obstruction of the right ventricular

outflow or pulmonary artery, or abrupt occlusion of the aorta secondary to dissection or arterial embolism.

CARDIOGENIC SHOCK. Cardiogenic shock may arise from a number of underlying etiologies, the common denominator of which is a primary myocardial insult (Table 69–4). The usual common denominator in these conditions is inadequate ventricular stroke volume. As noted previously, a strict hemodynamic operational definition, based on invasive hemodynamic monitoring, is necessary to differentiate cardiogenic from hypovolemic shock (see Table 69–1).

Cardiogenic shock most commonly presents as an acute deterioration of cardiac function, although this may be superimposed on chronic impairment. The most common etiology of cardiogenic shock is *acute myocardial infarction.* Approximately 5 to 15% of myocardial infarctions are complicated by cardiogenic shock, a rate which has remained constant over the past two decades. Despite marked advances in the management of patients with myocardial infarction, cardiogenic shock in this setting is still associated with a high mortality (70 to 90%), which has not changed significantly since the mid-1970's. Cardiogenic shock complicating acute myocardial infarction may arise because of impairment of a critical mass of myocardium, as the result of a mechanical lesion producing acute regurgitant lesions (e.g., ventricular septal defect or mitral insufficiency), or secondary to rupture of the ventricular free wall with hemopericardium and tamponade.

Shock following myocardial infarction is more common in the setting of anterior infarctions than inferior infarctions. This reflects, to some extent, the greater mass of myocardium supplied by the left anterior descending coronary artery (the site of coronary occlusion in many anterior infarctions) than that supplied by either the circumflex or right coronary arteries. However, large inferoposterior infarctions also may be complicated by cardiogenic shock. Furthermore, inferior infarctions that are associated with significant right ventricular involvement also may produce cardiogenic shock. De-

TABLE 69–4. DIFFERENTIAL DIAGNOSIS OF CARDIOGENIC SHOCK

I. **Acute myocardial infarction**
   A. Involvement of critical muscle mass or location:
      1. Large anterior wall infarction
      2. Large inferoposterior wall infarction
      3. Massive right ventricular infarction
      4. Extensive subendocardial infarction
   B. Acute mechanical lesion:
      1. Ventricular septal rupture
      2. Acute mitral valve insufficiency (rupture or dysfunction)
      3. Left ventricular free wall rupture
      4. Left ventricular aneurysm (chronic)

II. **Critical valvular heart disease**
   A. Critical aortic stenosis
   B. Critical mitral stenosis
   C. Severe aortic insufficiency
   D. Severe mitral insufficiency

III. **Obstructive nonvalvular myocardial lesions**
   A. Cardiac tamponade
   B. Hypertrophic obstructive cardiomyopathy
   C. Constrictive pericardial disorders
   D. Atrial myxoma with ventricular inflow obstruction
   E. Ball-valve left atrial thrombus
   F. Severe restrictive cardiomyopathy

IV. **Inflammatory or infectious myocardial lesions**
   A. Fulminant myocarditis
   B. Acute endocarditis with severe myopathic or valvular involvement

V. **Physiologic myocardial depressants:**
   A. Severe hypoxia
   B. Severe acidosis or alkalosis

VI. **Pharmacologic myocardial depressants:**
   A. β-Adrenergic blocking agents
   B. Calcium channel blocking agents
   C. Antiarrhythmic agents
   D. Cardiotoxic chemotherapeutic agents
   E. Anesthetic agents

VII. **Miscellaneous etiologies:**
   A. End-stage idiopathic cardiomyopathy
   B. Postpartum cardiomyopathy
   C. Post-cardiopulmonary bypass myocardial depression
   D. Myocardial depressant factor (e.g., pancreatitis, sepsis)

tailed anatomic studies of patients succumbing to cardiogenic shock following acute infarction, in the absence of mechanical lesions, have demonstrated that impairment of 30 to 35% or more of functioning ventricular muscle accompanies this syndrome.

In addition to being the result of large losses of functioning ventricular muscle mass, cardiogenic shock complicating an acute myocardial infarction may arise from the acute development of intracardiac mechanical defects. These include acute ventricular septal rupture, acute mitral insufficiency (papillary muscle dysfunction or rupture), and left ventricular free wall rupture. The frequency of shock due to acute mitral insufficiency and ventricular septal rupture is evenly divided between anterior and inferior infarctions. Left ventricular free wall rupture develops in about 10% of patients with fatal myocardial infarctions. While previously considered to be an unpredictable event, recent evidence suggests that this mechanical complication is more common in women, hypertensive patients, patients aged >60 years sustaining a first infarction, and the setting of inferoposterolateral infarctions related to circumflex coronary artery occlusions. Rupture is often preceded by one or more episodes of abrupt, transient hypotension, bradycardia, and unexpected alterations in T waves, probably reflecting a stuttering process with progressive tears and bleeding into the infarcting myocardium. These mechanical complications may occur within days to weeks following the acute infarction.

Non–infarction-related etiologies of cardiogenic shock include critical valvular heart disease (e.g., critical aortic stenosis), disorders of pericardial restraint (e.g., constrictive pericarditis), obstructive myopathic cardiac disorders (e.g., hypertrophic obstructive cardiomyopathy), acute cardiomyopathies of diverse etiologies (e.g., acute fulminant viral myocarditis), and as the result of various physiologic or pharmacologic myocardial depressants (e.g., severe acidosis, overdose, marked disturbances of cardiac rate and rhythm). In addition, an element of myocardial depression may be a significant factor in the pathogenesis of shock from sepsis and severe hemorrhage.

COMMON COMPLICATIONS OF SHOCK

DISSEMINATED INTRAVASCULAR COAGULATION. Disseminated intravascular coagulation (DIC) is a syndrome often seen in shock, particularly that due to gram-negative septicemia, and is associated with a high mortality rate. The clinical hallmark of DIC is the simultaneous occurrence of intravascular clotting and fibrinolysis, although bleeding dominates the clinical picture in most cases. The syndrome causes renal cortical necrosis, generalized ischemic damage of multiple organs, consumption of coagulation factors, and bleeding and also may contribute to the pathogenesis of shock lung.

ADULT RESPIRATORY DISTRESS SYNDROME. The adult respiratory distress syndrome (ARDS), previously known as "shock lung," is a common complication of various shock syndromes and emphasizes the disastrous complications of microcirculatory failure. ARDS is defined physiologically as the presence of severe hypoxemia ($Pa_{O_2}/Fi_{O_2} < 150$ mm Hg), chest roentgenographic evidence of generalized pulmonary infiltrates, reduced lung compliance, absence of significant elevations of pulmonary venous pressures as confirmed by invasive hemodynamic monitoring (e.g., pulmonary capillary wedge pressure <18 mm Hg), and absence of alternative explanations for the clinical presentation.

ARDS is seen most commonly in association with sepsis but also may complicate major trauma, aspiration of gastric contents, cardiogenic shock, multiple blood transfusions, drug overdose, and primary pneumonic infections. The onset of ARDS may be extremely rapid (e.g., within 1 to 2 hours) but more often follows the initiating event by 24 to 48 hours. In most series, the mortality associated with ARDS is >50% and as great as 90% in patients with combined ARDS and sepsis. The presence of other shock-associated disorders, such as MOSF or severe infections, increases the mortality.

Three pathologic phases of ARDS have been described. An early exudative phase (24 to 96 hours) is characterized by death of alveolar type I cells, regional microatelectasis, and accumulation of protein-rich edema and fibrin with endothelial cell swelling. Complement-mediated neutrophil activation is a prominent early feature and likely contributes to endothelial damage. A second proliferative phase is characterized by the formation of hyaline membranes and rapid proliferation of type II alveolar cells. A chronic or late proliferative phase is characterized by widespread fibrosis. ARDS appears to produce inhomogeneous lesions in the lung, with the dependent portions being affected to a greater extent.

The physiologic consequences of ARDS include severe hypoxemia, reduced lung compliance, reduced functional residual lung capacity, increased dead space ventilation, pulmonary hypertension, and a nidus for superimposed pulmonary infection. The cause of death in patients who develop ARDS in the setting of shock is usually not respiratory failure. Early deaths are usually due to the underlying illness, and late deaths are related to complications of the treatment of this type of patient. Secondary lung infection is a common complication of ARDS. In those patients surviving ARDS, approximately one third have persistent pulmonary symptoms.

ACUTE RENAL FAILURE. Acute renal failure is a common complication of shock, regardless of primary etiology, and is responsible for considerable morbidity and mortality in this syndrome. Current mortality rates for acute renal failure developing in all hospitalized patients average 40 to 60%. The most common causes of acute renal failure in hospitalized patients include decreased renal perfusion (of particular concern in the shock patient), administration of radiographic contrast agents, and administration of nephrotoxic drugs, particularly the aminoglycoside antibiotics.

The most common mechanism of acute renal failure in the setting of shock is probably acute tubular necrosis, otherwise known as vasomotor nephropathy. The pathogenesis of this disorder usually involves severe reductions in renal cortical blood flow due to marked preglomerular vasoconstriction. Vasomotor nephropathy is usually manifested by oliguria but can occasionally present as total anuria, persists for 1 to 3 weeks, and can be followed by a recovery phase associated with marked diuresis. In most patients, the serum creatinine rises 1 to 4 mg per deciliter per day, and the mortality increases with total increases of 3 mg per deciliter or more.

In management of the shock patient, close attention needs to be paid to monitoring urine output and ensuring that cardiac preload and cardiac output are adequate to maintain renal perfusion. The onset of anuria requires that postrenal obstructive etiologies be excluded rapidly. In the case of trauma, consideration must be given to vascular insults (renal artery or renal vein occlusion) and to rhabdomyolysis as possible etiologies of renal failure.

CLINICAL PRESENTATION AND DIAGNOSIS OF CARDIOGENIC SHOCK

The classic presentation of any patient in shock is that of hypotension (systolic arterial pressure <90 mm Hg or >60 mm Hg below baseline), tachycardia with a weak and thready pulse, hyperventilation, cold clammy extremities, and a dulled sensorium ranging from agitation to stupor or coma. The patient is frequently oliguric (urine output < 30 ml per hour) or anuric.

Patients with cardiogenic shock may manifest some or all of the preceding characteristics depending on the nature of the cardiac insult. A high index of clinical suspicion is required for early diagnosis of the cardiogenic shock state. The prognosis of these patients varies both with the underlying cardiac insult and with how quickly shock is recognized clinically and the initiation of proper (and avoidance of improper) medical therapy. The clinical presentation also may be altered by pre-existing noncardiac disease or by chronic use of pharmacologic agents. If possible, a rapid assessment of medical history and medication regimens should be obtained during the initial assessment.

Cardiogenic shock following myocardial infarction may present in one of three general patterns: (1) rapid onset of fulminant cardiovascular collapse with pulmonary edema and profound hypotension, usually as the result of a massive myocardial infarction or rupture of the left ventricle; (2) abrupt onset of shock with pulmonary edema several days following an otherwise uncomplicated infarction, due to abrupt rupture of the interventricular septum or mitral valve dysfunction/rupture, accompanied by the appearance of a new systolic murmur; or (3) gradual progression into a low-output shock state over a period of many days following an initial cardiac insult, due to recurrent "piecemeal" necrosis of the myocardium in the setting of infarct extension.

The onset of other forms of cardiogenic shock depends on the underlying etiology. For example, shock secondary to critical valvular stenosis (aortic or mitral) may appear only in the presence of onset of a rapid tachyarrhythmia (e.g., atrial fibrillation). Cardiogenic shock due to fulminant viral myocarditis may present insidiously with progressive heart failure and low-output state weeks to months following a mild or asymptomatic viral-like illness. Rupture of a myxomatous mitral valve, producing massive mitral insufficiency with pulmonary edema and shock, may occur suddenly in a previously asymptomatic individual with an unrecognized myxomatous mitral valve.

Common to these varied presentations is evidence of severe impairment of forward cardiac output, often associated with severe pulmonary vascular congestion. Patients often complain of dyspnea, orthopnea, paroxysmal nocturnal dyspnea, severe fatigue, and exercise intolerance and may have syncope or presyncope.

Assessing the Cardiogenic Shock Patient

GENERAL PRINCIPLES. There are five major goals in managing the patient in cardiogenic shock: (1) rapidly recognizing the shock state, (2) correcting the initial insult, (3) correcting the secondary consequences of the shock state, (4) maintaining the function of vital organs, and (5) identifying and correcting aggravating factors. All five goals are approached simultaneously in an organized and methodical way so as to ensure optimal therapy (Fig. 69–4). The prognosis of a patient in shock is determined in part by the etiology of the shock state (e.g., hypovolemic traumatic shock in a young, healthy adult carries a mortality of < 20% in many centers, whereas cardiogenic shock due to massive anterior wall myocardial infarction carries a mortality of > 70% even in the most aggressive medical center). Prognosis is also affected by the duration of shock and consequent secondary organ dysfunction and by the speed of recognition and appropriateness of medical intervention. Finally, the prognosis of the patient in shock is also affected by the preshock status of the patient with respect to pre-existing medical conditions.

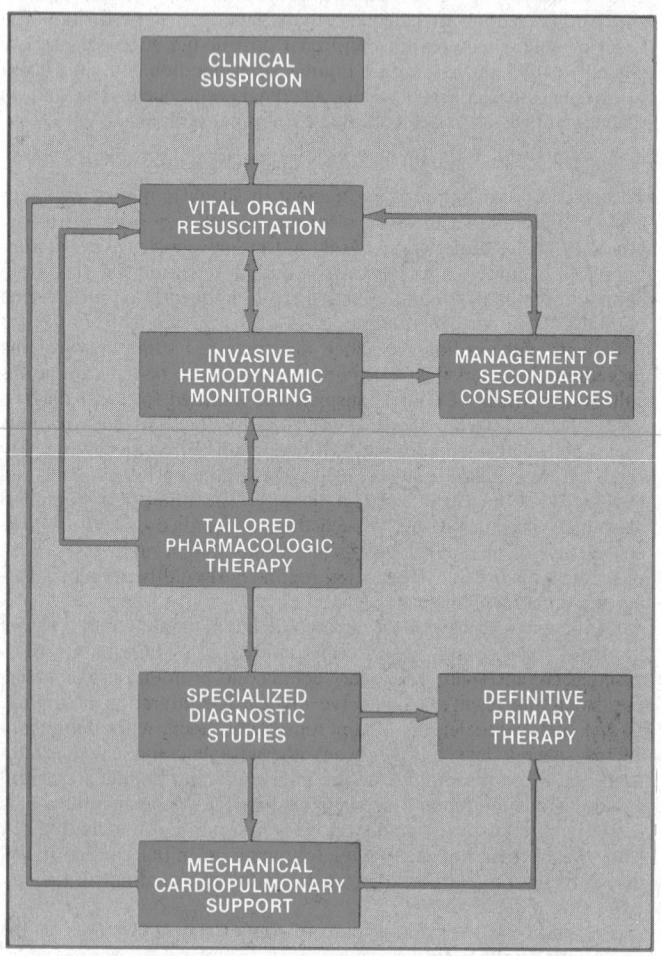

FIGURE 69–4. Strategy for management of the shock patient.

CRITICAL CARE TEAM. Successful and sophisticated management of a patient in shock requires an integrated team approach that begins to function on initial contact with the patient and extends through periods of resuscitation, early stabilization, diagnostic evaluation, definitive therapy, and recovery phases of treatment. In addition to a primary physician knowledgeable in critical care who is responsible for the overall coordination of patient care efforts, managing these patients requires a number of other highly motivated, well-trained, and objective but empathetic professionals. Such a team includes critical care nurses, respiratory therapists, hemodynamic monitoring technicians, special procedure and diagnostic technicians, nutrition/dietetic consultants, and physical therapists. Finally, the immediate availability of multiple surgical and medical subspeciality consultants is essential to care for these complexly and critically ill patients.

MEDICAL HISTORY AND PHYSICAL EXAMINATION. A rapid but thorough medical history and a complete but directed physical examination should be performed during the initial assessment and early management of the shock patient. Particular attention should be directed to the recent medical history and the details of the present illness in an effort to rapidly identify precipitating or causative factors of shock. Pertinent medical history should be obtained with emphasis placed on pre-existing cardiopulmonary, renal, hepatic, neurologic, and hematologic disorders. A complete listing of current medications and known allergies should be obtained from the patient, medical record, or closest relative.

Examination of the patient in presumed cardiogenic shock should be directed at determining the presence or absence of tachyarrhythmias or bradyarrhythmias, hypotension, narrowed pulse pressure, neck vein engorgement, Kussmaul's sign, pulmonary edema, ventricular and atrial gallop sounds, murmurs of valvular stenosis or insufficiency, peripheral signs of low cardiac output, and stigmata of other disease entities (e.g., splinter hemorrhages in the setting of infective endocarditis). The clinician must remember, however, that many of the murmurs of critical cardiac lesions may be diminished in the presence of a low-flow state or difficult to hear in the presence of severe pulmonary edema.

The most important initial assessment of the patient should be directed to the patency and adequacy of the airway. If the patient is unable to ventilate or cannot adequately protect the airway, endotracheal intubation is indicated. Initial assessment of circulatory reserve can be obtained by palpating central arteries (e.g., femoral) and by sphygmomanometrically measuring blood pressure. Particular attention should be focused on the pulse pressure, since a narrow pulse pressure suggests marked impairment of stroke volume.

Sinus tachycardia is one of the earliest compensatory mechanisms for a fall in arterial pressure or cardiac output, and the differential diagnosis of this increase in heart rate includes the seven H's of hypovolemia, hypotension, heart failure, hypoxemia, hyperthermia, hyperthyroidism, and reflex hyperadrenergic state (e.g., reflex tachycardia seen in some cases of anterior wall myocardial infarction). Other important possible causes of tachycardia include anxiety and pulmonary embolism. The clinician must remember that unexplained tachycardia may be one of the earliest indications of impending cardiovascular collapse, and it therefore must not be ignored or inappropriately treated until the differential diagnosis is appropriately addressed.

INTRAVENOUS ACCESS. At least two large-bore intravenous catheters (16 gauge or larger) should be inserted in peripheral extremities, and at least one central venous sheath (8 Fr or greater) should be inserted under optimal sterile conditions as rapidly as possible. During placement of these venous access catheters, blood can be obtained for essential hematologic and chemical studies and for blood typing and cross-matching. In most circumstances, isotonic fluids (e.g., normal saline or Ringer's lactate) should be infused through these catheters pending further assessment of the patient.

INITIAL HEMATOLOGIC/BIOCHEMICAL DETERMINATIONS. Essential initial laboratory determinations should include those which may alter immediate therapy. These include complete blood count, serum electrolytes (sodium, potassium, calcium, magnesium), and arterial blood gases. Additional laboratory parameters should be obtained as indicated by the patient's presentation and the most likely etiologies for the shock state (e.g., blood culture; toxicology screen; cardiac enzyme panels).

A key element in the therapy of a patient in cardiogenic shock is hemodynamic monitoring.

Patient Monitoring

Managing the patient in shock requires accurate and serial measurements of heart rate and rhythm, respiratory rate and adequacy of gas exchange, systemic arterial pressure and cardiac filling pressures, tissue perfusion, and end-organ function. A reference for normal hemodynamic parameters in adults is provided in Table 69–5.

ELECTROCARDIOGRAPHIC MONITORING. Continuous electrocardiographic monitoring permits assessment of cardiac rate and rhythm and allows prompt detection of serious cardiac arrhythmias such as ventricular tachyarrhythmias, atrial fibrillation, high-degree AV block, and marked sinus bradycardia. It is essential to use a monitoring lead, or preferably several leads, that provide adequate assessment of atrial as well as ventricular rhythms (e.g., MCL_1). Serial standard 12-lead electrocardiograms permit indirect assessment of myocardial ischemia and may be required to analyze complex rhythm disorders.

ARTERIAL PRESSURE MONITORING. An indwelling arterial catheter is essential for continuous on-line assessment of arterial pressure and also provides a convenient access for obtaining blood samples. Assessment of arterial pressure by sphygmomanometry is not adequate for most patients with shock, is often an unreliable indicator of true core blood pressure in the hypotensive patient, and fails to provide continuous on-line assessment of blood pressure in patients with rapidly changing cardiovascular states. The choice of insertion site for arterial line placement depends on the status of the patient being monitored, the presence and severity of peripheral vascular disease, and the expertise of the critical care team. In general, the more severe the shock state, the more central should the arterial catheter be placed in order to assess core blood pressure. In contrast, the more central the placement, the higher the complication rate with long-term use of these catheters. The clinician must therefore assess the risk-benefit ratio of arterial cannulation sites in each individual patient. In patients with intense endogenous adrenergically medicated vasoconstriction or under the influence of potent vasoconstricting drugs, monitoring pressure in small peripheral arteries such as the radial may be inadequate owing to vessel constriction. In the most severely ill patient, rapidly inserting a femoral arterial catheter under optimal sterile conditions provides the most accurate means of monitoring blood pressure. This catheter can always be removed and replaced with a more distal one as the patient's hemodynamic status improves. Alternative sites for arterial pressure monitoring include the radial, brachial, axillary, and dorsalis pedis arteries.

TABLE 69–5. NORMAL RESTING ADULT HEMODYNAMIC PARAMETERS

Parameter	Wave	Range (mm Hg)
Hydrostatic Pressures		
Systemic arterial pressure		
Systemic arterial	Systolic	100–140
	Diastolic	60–90
	Mean	70–105
Right heart pressures		
Right atrial	"a"	2–10
	"v"	2–10
	Mean	2–8
Right ventricular	Systolic	15–30
	Diastolic	2–8
Pulmonary arterial	Systolic	15–30
	Diastolic	4–12
	Mean	9–18
Pulmonary capillary wedge	"a"	3–15
	"v"	3–15
	Mean	2–10
Cardiac output determinations		
Cardiac index (L/min/m²)		2.6–4.2
Arterial–mixed venous oxygen content difference (ml/dl)		3.0–5.0

From Grossman W: Cardiac Catheterization and Angiography, 3rd ed. Philadelphia, Lea & Febiger, 1986.

Complications associated with arterial pressure monitoring include bleeding, arterial thrombosis, vasospasm, infection, aneurysm or pseudoaneurysm formation, embolization (distal and proximal), limb ischemia, and pain. Appropriate care must be taken to ensure adequate collateral circulation prior to inserting the arterial line, if possible, and to follow the patient closely for early signs of ischemia, infection, or embolization at or distal to the insertion site. These catheters should be changed to a new site, under sterile conditions, at least every 72 hours.

CARDIAC FILLING PRESSURE ASSESSMENT. Cardiac preload must be assessed invasively in patients with cardiogenic shock, since the physical examination is often not sensitive enough to determine accurately the state of cardiac filling, much less to monitor rapidly changing trends in this important determinant of cardiac output and blood pressure. The relative risk-benefit ratio of invasive hemodynamic monitoring must be assessed in each individual patient. In those patients requiring invasive monitoring, assessment of central venous pressure (e.g., superior vena caval pressure) alone is inadequate for patients in cardiogenic shock, since this pressure reflects only diastolic filling of the right ventricle. In the critically ill shock patient, use of a flow-directed pulmonary artery catheter with cardiac output capability is required for optimal management.

A flow-directed pulmonary artery balloon catheter (Swan-Ganz catheter) is an essential component for monitoring patients in cardiogenic shock. This catheter can be inserted either peripherally from a median antecubital vein or through more central venous access sites such as the percutaneous internal jugular, external jugular, subclavian, or femoral venous approach. Such a catheter can be inserted "blindly" by pressure waveform analysis or under fluoroscopic guidance. During initial catheter insertion, measurements should be obtained of right atrial, right ventricular, pulmonary arterial, and pulmonary capillary wedge pressures during held end expiration without a Valsalva maneuver. These measurements assess the preload of the right ventricle (right atrial and right ventricular end-diastolic pressures) and of the left ventricle (pulmonary arterial diastolic and pulmonary capillary wedge pressures). In the absence of significant vascular obstruction between the pulmonary artery and the left ventricle (e.g., severe fixed pulmonary arteriolar hypertension, pulmonary venous occlusive disease, mitral stenosis), the pulmonary capillary wedge pressure should reflect left ventricular end-diastolic pressure and thereby provide an index of left ventricular preload. In the presence of very rapid heart rates or acute severe aortic insufficiency, the pulmonary capillary wedge pressure may not reflect true left ventricular filling pressure. The clinician must remember, however, that the left ventricular volume is the critical determinant of preload, and the relation between this volume and the left heart filling pressure depends on the compliance (distensibility) of the ventricle.

At the bedside, the clinician can determine in vivo Starling curves in the individual patient by assessing cardiac output at various levels of cardiac filling pressure during incremental volume loading. This also allows an assessment of the compliance of the ventricle by relating the volume infused to the resulting filling pressure. By measuring heart rate, blood pressure, cardiac output, pulmonary capillary wedge pressure, and arterial O_2 tension, the optimal preload in an individual patient can be determined, which provides adequate perfusion without compromising ventilation.

A series of oximetry blood samples should be obtained when first inserting the pulmonary artery catheter. This is most important in the patient with presumed cardiogenic shock in the setting of a new systolic murmur in whom the differential diagnosis includes ventricular septal rupture (diagnosed by step-up in O_2 saturation from the right atrium to the pulmonary artery) versus mitral insufficiency. It is essential to obtain blood samples from the superior vena cava, right atrium, pulmonary artery, and systemic artery to perform an adequate oximetry series. As a rule of thumb, there should be no greater than a 7% step-up in O_2 saturation from the superior vena cava to the pulmonary artery in the absence of a left-to-right intracardiac shunt.

In general, only right-sided heart catheters that can also assess cardiac output should be used to monitor the shock patient. A proximal lumen for right atrial injection, coupled with an in-line thermistor for assessment of temperature at the tip of the catheter in the pulmonary artery, permits bedside assessment of cardiac output by the thermodilution technique. This indicator-dilution technique utilizes injection of cold saline into the right atrium and the time-dependent appearance of the "cold" indicator in the pulmonary artery to construct an indicator-dilution curve to assess cardiac output.

In addition, the Swan-Ganz catheter provides a distal monitoring port in the pulmonary artery which can be utilized for drawing pulmonary artery blood samples for chemical determinations. Important among these is the assessment of mixed venous O_2 saturation and content. Simultaneously obtaining arterial and mixed venous (pulmonary arterial blood in the absence of a left-to-right intracardiac shunt) blood samples permits assessment of arterial-mixed venous O_2 content difference (where O_2 content difference [ml/dl] = hemoglobin [grams $\times$ saturation difference] $\times$ 1.38 [ml O_2 per gram hemoglobin that is 100% saturated]). This provides an inverse assessment of cardiac output by the Fick principle and is complementary to the thermodilution technique for measuring cardiac output. As cardiac output increases, arterial–mixed venous O_2 content difference should narrow, and vice versa, assuming constant hemoglobin content and O_2 consumption. The normal arterial–mixed venous oxygen content difference is 3.0 to 5.0 ml per deciliter and is a clinically useful reflection of O_2 extraction as well as an indicator of the adequacy of cardiac output in relation to systemic metabolic demand.

Newer modifications of the pulmonary artery catheter with an in-line fiberoptic system permit continuous assessment of pulmonary artery saturation (mixed venous saturation), based on reflectance spectrophotometry. The mixed venous O_2 saturation is determined by the relationship between O_2 delivery and O_2 consumption in the systemic circulation and can be considered a reflection of "oxygen reserve." In general, mixed venous O_2 saturations >65% represent adequate reserves, whereas those <35% indicate severe impairment of tissue oxygenation (assuming an arterial F_{IO_2} = 0.21, room air).

Continuous monitoring of mixed venous O_2 saturation with fiberoptic catheters provides another complementary continuous assessment of a patient's hemodynamic status. A reduction in mixed venous O_2 saturation may be produced by a decrease in cardiac output, decrease in arterial O_2 saturation, decrease in hemoglobin, or increase in O_2 consumption (e.g., hyperthermia, pain, seizures). Conversely, an increase in mixed venous O_2 saturation may indicate an increase in cardiac output, an increase in inspired O_2 concentration, a decrease in O_2 consumption (e.g., hypothermia, pharmacologic paralysis, anesthesia), a decrease in peripheral tissue O_2 extraction (e.g., sepsis), a left-to-right shunt, or an artifactual increase in mixed venous saturation due to a wedged catheter.

A reduction of mixed venous O_2 saturation to <50% is frequently associated with the development of anaerobic metabolism. An important exception to this generalization is sepsis, in which a decrease in tissue oxygenation is associated with an increase in mixed venous O_2 saturation, probably due at least in part to peripheral AV shunting.

Finally, assessment of pulmonary arterial blood gases permits analysis of pH, P_{CO_2}, and P_{O_2} in the systemic venous return and may have important applications for monitoring the success of cardiopulmonary resuscitation in certain patients.

Further modifications of the Swan-Ganz catheter have permitted monitoring of intracardiac electrocardiograms, the passage of temporary pacing wires into the right ventricle for external electrical pacing of patients with hemodynamically significant bradyarrhythmias, and the incorporation of in-line Doppler echo crystals that permit beat-to-beat assessment of ventricular stroke volume and cardiac output.

The clinician must remember that the Swan-Ganz catheter is expensive to insert and monitor, and complications such as arrhythmias, infection, and pulmonary infarction may occur. Rigorous attention to detail and expertise in the use of this catheter are essential to ensure an optimal risk-benefit ratio during its use. These catheters should be inserted only by physicians adequately trained in using these devices who possess extensive knowledge pertaining to indications, potential complications, and analysis of the information they provide. The patient with indwelling Swan-Ganz and arterial catheters requires continuous monitoring of pressure waveforms to detect catheter migration or occlusion. Rigorous attention to ster-

ile technique should be employed in the care of the patient with such catheters.

URINARY CATHETER. An indwelling bladder catheter permits hourly assessment of urinary output, a reflection of effective renal perfusion. A decline in urinary output to < 20 ml per hour often indicates inadequate renal perfusion. The most frequent cause of oliguria in the setting of shock is hypovolemia. The diagnosis of anuria should be made only once it is confirmed that the bladder catheter is patent and there is no obstruction from the renal pelvis to the catheter.

SPECIALIZED DIAGNOSTIC STUDIES

In addition to the standard diagnostic studies (e.g., electrocardiogram, chest roentgenogram, hematologic and biochemical blood studies) used to manage a shock patient, certain auxiliary specialized studies also may be beneficial.

ECHOCARDIOGRAPHY. Two-dimensional echocardiography with Doppler capability provides a rapid, noninvasive, and sensitive bedside tool to evaluate the patient with unexplained shock. The echocardiogram is particularly useful for (1) rapid assessment of generalized and regional myocardial systolic function, (2) evaluation for intrapericardial fluid accumulation and echocardiographic suggestion of tamponade physiology (diastolic right ventricular and right atrial collapse), (3) assessment of cardiac valves for stenosis, regurgitation, and vegetations, (4) evaluation for intracardiac shunts (e.g., ventricular septal rupture) and left ventricular aneurysm, (5) assessment of prosthetic valve function, and (6) assessment for aortic dissection (transesophageal echocardiography).

NUCLEAR MEDICINE STUDIES. A variety of isotope imaging studies may be beneficial for managing the shock patient. Ventilation-perfusion lung scans may be useful to diagnose or exclude massive pulmonary emboli. First-pass radionuclide ventriculograms provide important information about systolic and diastolic function of the right and left ventricles. In occasional patients, use of myocardial perfusion imaging with thallium-201, technetium-99m sestamibi, or positron emission tomography may identify viable but jeopardized myocardium that may benefit from attempts at interventional (e.g., coronary angioplasty) or surgical revascularization.

COMPUTED TOMOGRAPHY AND NUCLEAR MAGNETIC RESONANCE IMAGING. These techniques provide noninvasive anatomic detail of most major regions of the body and can often be very useful to evaluate selected patients in shock (e.g., suspected aortic dissection).

INTERVENTIONAL CARDIOVASCULAR RADIOLOGY STUDIES. Cardiac catheterization is an essential component in the initial evaluation and management of the patient with cardiogenic shock. In addition to providing necessary anatomic diagnosis as a guide to definitive surgical therapy in some patients, cardiac catheterization may provide the route for definitive nonsurgical therapy in certain forms of cardiogenic shock. This includes use of percutaneous transluminal balloon coronary angioplasty for reperfusion therapy in cardiogenic shock following myocardial infarction and balloon valvuloplasty as therapy for cardiogenic shock in high surgical risk patients with critical aortic stenosis (see below). Other noncardiac vascular diagnostic procedures are often required to localize vascular trauma (e.g., aortic dissection), confirm suspected massive pulmonary embolism, and achieve definitive therapy in certain cases (e.g., percutaneous insertion of inferior vena cava filter in survivors of submassive pulmonary emboli despite adequate anticoagulation).

Techniques under development for further specialized monitoring of shock patients include transcutaneously monitoring arterial O_2 and CO_2 tensions, tissue electrodes to directly measure tissue oxygenation, measurement of respiratory muscle strength by assessing maximum airway pressures, assessment of respiratory muscle fatigue by measuring tension-time index of the diaphragm, continuous monitoring of end-tidal P_{CO_2} by capnography to assess arterial P_{CO_2}, thermal dye techniques to measure extravascular lung water, and double-indicator dilution techniques to evaluate pulmonary endothelial integrity.

THERAPEUTIC GUIDELINES FOR MANAGING CARDIOGENIC SHOCK

Management of the patient in cardiogenic shock consists of primary therapy directed at the underlying cardiovascular insult and secondary therapy directed at the consequences of the shock state. Primary therapy depends on identifying the cause of the shock state. An example of primary therapy is pericardiocentesis for cardiac tamponade. Major efforts in the initial management of patients with shock are simultaneously directed at identifying and reversing the primary etiology while at the same time managing the secondary consequences of the shock state (see Fig. 69–4). Selected aspects of this management are reviewed.

PAIN CONTROL. Patients in shock are often in pain and may be frightened or agitated. Care must be taken to avoid approaches to these problems that can worsen the underlying hemodynamic instability of the patient. Essentially all pharmacologic agents used for pain control or anxiolysis produce some degree of hemodynamic compromise and must therefore be carefully titrated with close observation of the patient's hemodynamic and ventilatory status. In the setting of shock, all medications must be administered intravenously, since absorption of intramuscular or subcutaneous medication is unpredictable and therefore unreliable.

In general, severe pain can be managed most easily by judicious use of a reversible narcotic such as morphine sulfate (2- to 4-mg IV increments). Potential side effects following morphine include vasodilation with hypotension (mediated by histamine release, direct vasodilation, and neurogenic mechanisms), vagally mediated bradyarrhythmias, respiratory depression, nausea and vomiting, and biliary spasm. The primary route of morphine metabolism is hepatic glucuronic acid conjugation. Patients with hepatic dysfunction, common in shock states, may be very sensitive to the effects of morphine, as may be the elderly. An advantage of morphine and similar opioid agonists is the capacity for rapid pharmacologic antagonism with agents such as naloxone should adverse effects follow their administration. Naloxone may have additional benefits in shock, as discussed below.

ADMINISTERING OXYGEN. Oxygen is a drug, and its use should be guided by considerations applicable to the use of other drugs in treating shock. In general, O_2 should be administered initially to most patients in shock, in view of the likelihood of impaired peripheral O_2 delivery. However, the administration should be performed via a high-flow system (one that delivers the entire inspired O_2 atmosphere) so that the fraction of inspired O_2 administered to the patient (Fi_{O_2}) is controlled. This permits bedside assessment of the degree of arterial hypoxemia (defined by the alveolar-arterial O_2 gradient), since the calculation of alveolar Po_2 depends on a known Fi_{O_2}. Clinically useful high-flow systems include Venturi masks in the nonintubated patient and ventilators in the intubated patient. An attempt should be made to provide sufficient O_2 to achieve an arterial O_2 saturation $\geq 90\%$. In the patient requiring positive-pressure ventilation, an attempt should be made to achieve this with an $Fi_{O_2} \leq 0.60$ in order to reduce the incidence of pulmonary O_2 toxicity. This may be facilitated by the judicious use of positive end-expiratory pressure (PEEP). A cutaneous pulse oximeter may be useful to continuously monitor peripheral tissue O_2 saturation. However, the reliability of these noninvasive measurements should be verified by analysis of arterial blood gases on a frequent basis. In addition, the clinician must be aware of potential physiologic abnormalities that alter the normal oxygen-hemoglobin affinity (saturation) relationships (as previously discussed). Furthermore, use of peripheral cutaneous monitoring in patients with intense peripheral vasoconstriction may not be a reliable indicator of true arterial oxygen-carrying capacity.

Endotracheal intubation of the patient in shock is indicated if the patient is unable to protect the airway or as a means to permit mechanical ventilation.

Mechanical ventilation is indicated for managing the shock patient for the following: (1) apnea or ventilatory failure (acute respiratory acidosis), (2) failure to adequately oxygenate with high-flow system, (3) mechanical splinting of the flail chest wall, (4) relief of the metabolic stress of the work of breathing in selected patients, and (5) adjunctive therapy for other interventions. During mechanical ventilation, careful attention must be paid to the hemodynamic effects of positive intrathoracic pressure. Positive-pressure mechanical ventilation results in increased intrathoracic pressures and therefore tends to partially impair venous return to the right side of the heart, resulting in a fall in cardiac preload. The magnitude of this effect varies with the underlying condition of the patient and the magnitude of the positive pressure used. In managing the shock patient who requires mechanical ventilatory support, adjuvant use of an indwelling pulmonary artery catheter is required to determine and compensate for the effects of this positive pressure on cardiac preload, cardiac output, and arterial pressure.

EXCLUSION OF HYPOVOLEMIA. Excluding hypovolemia as an etiology for low cardiac output in patients with presumed cardiogenic shock is an essential step in the management of these patients. Indeed, hypovolemia is one of the most common causes of hypotension in patients following acute myocardial infarction. This relates to the fact that many infarction patients present in a state of relative volume depletion due to diaphoresis, reduced intake of fluids secondary to nausea or vomiting, and venodilation brought about by administering nitroglycerin or morphine to manage chest pain. Hypotension in these patients, in the absence of evidence of acute pulmonary edema, should be managed initially by judicious administration of isotonic volume expanding agents (e.g., intravenous normal saline), carefully monitoring blood pressure and heart rate and auscultating lung fields. If the hypotension does not resolve with volume expansion, or if a shock state intervenes, then promptly initiating invasive hemodynamic monitoring is required for further management.

While the normal left ventricular filling pressure is 2 to 10 mm Hg (see Table 69–5), an acute myocardial ischemic process often results in a stiff and noncompliant ventricle that requires higher filling pressures to maintain an adequate end-diastolic volume (preload). Only when relative hypovolemia has been excluded by invasive monitoring may the diagnosis of cardiogenic shock be seriously entertained (see Table 69–1). In the setting of acute infarction with hypotension, invasive monitoring with a pulmonary artery catheter should be utilized to guide therapeutic interventions directed at achieving and maintaining a left ventricular filling pressure of 15 to 18 mm Hg in order to provide a reasonable level of cardiac preload. Further adjustment of cardiac filling pressure (achieved with use of volume administration or vasodilator medications) can be adjusted by determining the optimal filling pressure for the patient. This "optimal" level of preload is determined by defining that filling pressure that yields the optimal forward cardiac output without producing significant pulmonary vascular congestion and worsening hypoxemia, as determined by serial measurement of arterial blood gases.

CORRECTION OF ACIDOSIS. A significant secondary complication in shock of any etiology is the development of metabolic acidosis as a consequence of tissue ischemia. Severe acidosis impairs metabolic processes, impedes normal neurovascular interactions, and may prevent effective pharmacologic actions of various vasopressor and inotropic agents administered to the shock patient.

The differential diagnosis of metabolic acidosis is aided by calculation of the anion gap, where the anion gap = $[Na^+] - ([Cl^-] + [HCO_3^-])$ and should be approximately 12 to 16 mEq per liter. Increases in the anion gap are due to increased endogenous acid production (e.g., lactic acidosis, diabetic ketoacidosis, alcoholic ketoacidosis, starvation), increased exogenous acids (e.g., aspirin toxicity, methanol, ethylene glycol, paraldehyde), or decreased acid excretion (e.g., renal failure). A metabolic acidosis with normal anion gap is usually due to gastrointestinal or renal loss of bicarbonate or may be a complication of parenteral hyperalimentation.

If arterial pH < 7.00 and respiratory acidosis has been excluded as the etiology, intravenous sodium bicarbonate should be administered and titrated to maintain a pH ≥ 7.3. Care must be taken to avoid overcorrection and metabolic alkalosis, as this may also impair cardiac function and decrease O_2 delivery to the tissues by shifting the oxyhemoglobin dissociation curve to the left. In addition, inappropriately administering sodium bicarbonate may produce sodium and water overload, can induce hypokalemia, and may worsen CNS acidosis.

TREATING ARRHYTHMIAS. In general, the physician managing the patient in shock should treat disturbances of cardiac electrical activity only if these disturbances produce hemodynamic instability (e.g., hypotension, heart failure, myocardial ischemia) or if the specific rhythm is of clear prognostic significance (e.g., high-degree AV block in the setting of an anterior wall myocardial infarction). It must be remembered that all the currently available antiarrhythmic agents possess known adverse side effects, and many of them have negative inotropic properties to some degree. Thus an attempt to "abolish" the appearance of premature ventricular complexes on the monitor in an otherwise electrically stable patient is not appropriate. It is the patient and not the monitor which must be evaluated and treated.

Ventricular fibrillation is managed with nonsynchronized electrical countershock, delivered as rapidly as possible. Standard cardiopulmonary resuscitation may be required until a shock can be delivered or during intervening periods between defibrillation attempts.

Sustained ventricular tachycardia with profound hemodynamic instability should be treated with synchronized electrical countershock. An initial electrical dose of 100 to 200 joules should be applied, and repeated if necessary, prior to increasing energy dose. If the ventricular tachycardia is sustained and causes severe hemodynamic compromise, the patient may be treated with intravenous lidocaine, with an initial bolus of 1.0 to 1.5 mg per kilogram, followed by a continuous infusion at 2 mg per minute and a repeat bolus of 0.5 to 0.75 mg 10 to 15 minutes later. Patients who are prone to serious complications following lidocaine are those 65 years of age or older, those in severe heart failure, and those with compromised hepatic function. These are important factors to consider in management of the shock patient. In particular, care must be taken to follow plasma drug levels in those patients who require sustained infusions. Every effort should be made to discontinue these drugs as soon as possible once the patient has been stabilized in order to avoid drug-related toxicity. Alternative agents for management of sustained ventricular tachycardia include bretylium and procainamide.

Sinus tachycardia is often an initial autonomically mediated compensatory response to a fall in arterial pressure and cardiac output. Particularly in the young patient, rapid rates of sinus tachycardia must be distinguished from other forms of supraventricular tachycardia in order to avoid inappropriate attempts at converting this rhythm. Sinus tachycardia should be considered a diagnostic sign rather than a dysrhythmia.

Supraventricular tachyarrhythmias (atrial tachycardias, atrial flutter, atrial fibrillation) that are associated with marked hemodynamic compromise are best treated with synchronized electrical cardioversion. Atrial flutter may respond to energies as low as 10 to 20 joules, whereas atrial fibrillation may require 100 to 200 or more joules. Medical therapy of these arrhythmias includes use of digitalis glycosides, calcium channel blockers, and/or β-adrenergic blockers. However, these latter two classes of drugs are relatively contraindicated in the shock patient. Inappropriate administration of potent intravenous calcium channel blockers for treatment of supraventricular tachycardias in patients with underlying shock has been associated with adverse outcomes, including death.

Sinus bradycardia may be a manifestation of vagally mediated responses to local (e.g., cardiac receptor) or generalized (e.g., pain) noxious stimuli. Sinus bradycardia is commonly seen following inferior wall myocardial infarction, owing to activation of cardiac afferents and inhibitory cardiac reflexes. Sinus bradycardia usually responds to atropine (0.6 to 1.0 mg IV). Care must be taken to avoid too small a dose of atropine (e.g., ≤ 0.4 mg), as this may induce a centrally mediated vagal response that paradoxically worsens the bradycardia. An adult patient should not be considered "atropine-resistant" until he/she has received a total intravenous dose of 3.0 mg atropine.

Conduction disturbances such as AV block carry a variable prognosis, and the approach to therapy depends on the underlying mechanism and clinical state. In the setting of acute inferior wall myocardial infarction, AV block is usually neurogenically mediated by afferent inhibitory cardiac reflexes, responds to atropine, and has a good prognosis. In contrast, AV block in the setting of anterior wall infarction is usually due to ischemic impairment of the AV node or His bundle, frequently does not respond to atropine, and has a poor prognosis, because it reflects a large infarction. If atropine fails to counteract and reverse the hemodynamic compromise of AV block, external (transthoracic) or internal (transvenous) electrical pacing can be used. In general, it is preferred to re-establish organized AV synchrony, with associated atrial loading of ventricular preload, rather than rely on ventricular pacing alone. This may occasionally require using combined atrial and ventricular synchronized electrical pacing modalities.

SYMPATHOMIMETIC AMINES. These drugs are used to increase cardiac output through their inotropic action and to redistrib-

ute blood flow to vital organs by their selective vasoconstricting action. The net desired effect of these agents is therefore an increase in arterial pressure and/or cardiac output with improved perfusion of ischemic regions. Unfortunately, no single agent appears to produce the effects desired in all forms of shock. There are also two potential problems associated with use of these types of agents. If arterial pressure is elevated significantly, the hypertension can cause a detrimental increase in cardiac afterload and increase myocardial O_2 demand (see Fig. 69–1). Thus judicious elevation of arterial pressure to levels adequate for peripheral perfusion is the goal, while avoiding excessive hypertension. The blood pressure range needed to meet these criteria varies with each patient. Reasonable guidelines are to achieve a systolic arterial pressure of 110 to 130 mm Hg and to maintain diastolic arterial pressure in the 60- to 80-mm Hg range. The second and related potential problem associated with these agents is their vasoconstricting effect. While some degree of vasoconstriction is desired in nonessential organ beds, it should be avoided in critical organs. Thus proper use of sympathomimetic amines requires a thorough knowledge of their cardiovascular effects. These effects depend primarily on the affinity of the individual agent for various types of adrenergic receptors.

ADRENERGIC RECEPTORS. The adrenergic receptors are classified as α or β receptors with respect to their cardiac and vascular actions. Over the past 10 years, both prejunctional and postjunctional adrenergic receptors have been identified, and various subtypes of receptors have been characterized. Several have been cloned and their primary structure has been defined. However, from a practical clinical standpoint, the catecholamines used to treat shock can be understood by considering three specific types of postsynaptic adrenergic receptors. The α receptors are located primarily in blood vessels and mediate vasoconstriction. The β receptors are present in the blood vessels as well as the myocardium. Activation of β_1 receptors in the heart produces an increase in myocardial contractility and heart rate. Activation of β_2 receptors in blood vessels produces vasodilation. The same catecholamine may activate both α and β receptors, depending on the dose and the organ in which it is acting (Table 69–6). The net effect depends to a large extent on the relative distribution of the various receptor subtypes in the organ. The sympathomimetic amines that are commonly used clinically in management of the patient in shock include dopamine, dobutamine, epinephrine, norepinephrine, and isoproterenol. The relative actions and potencies of these agents are summarized in Table 69–6.

Each of these catecholamines carries the potential for adverse side effects. Common to all these agents are the potential complications of cardiac arrhythmias, nausea, vomiting, ischemia of major organs with prolonged infusions of potent vasoconstrictors, and localized skin necrosis with inadvertent extravasation of these agents.

INOTROPIC AND VASOPRESSOR AGENTS. *Norepinephrine.* Norepinephrine is the primary neurotransmitter of the sympathetic nervous system. It increases myocardial contractility by activating β_1 receptors and thus may increase cardiac output. In blood vessels, it activates primarily α receptors, thereby producing vasoconstriction. The magnitude of its effect on blood vessels varies from one organ to another. Norepinephrine is a very potent vasoconstrictor in skin, muscle, and splanchnic beds, whereas in the coronary vessels it activates the β_2 receptors as well as the α receptors. Because there is a paucity of α receptors in the coronary vessels (in contrast to other vascular beds), norepinephrine dilates the coronary arteries.

TABLE 69–6. INITIAL HEMODYNAMIC EFFECTS OF CATECHOLAMINES

Catecholamine	Heart Rate	Arterial Pressure	Cardiac Output	Systemic Resistance
Norepinephrine	(+)	(++)	(+)/NC	(++)
Epinephrine	(+)	(+)	(+)	(+)/NC
Dopamine	(+)	(+)	(+)	(+)/NC
Isoproterenol	(+)	(−)/NC	(++)	(−)
Dobutamine	NC/(+)	NC	(+)	NC/(−)

Note: There may be marked regional variations in reactions of different vascular beds to these agents. (+) = increase; (−) = decrease; NC = no change.

Norepinephrine offers several distinct advantages for treating some forms of shock, especially septic shock. It increases cardiac output and redistributes blood flow away from the extremities and toward the heart and brain and increases arterial pressure. This in turn increases coronary blood flow to ischemic myocardium. Because it is a potent peripheral vasoconstrictor, norepinephrine may be particularly useful in septic shock, a condition associated with significant peripheral vasodilation and resultant hypotension. However, because of its intense peripheral vasoconstricting action, with a resulting increase in afterload and impedance to ventricular emptying, norepinephrine is not a drug of first choice for managing patients with known cardiogenic shock. Only if more preferred agents (e.g., dobutamine or dopamine alone or in combination with vasodilators and mechanical circulatory support) fail to achieve desired hemodynamic stability should norepinephrine be considered in this setting.

Norepinephrine should be administered intravenously through a secure catheter, preferably a centrally placed one, in order to diminish the risk of extravasation, which can result in severe tissue necrosis. Norepinephrine should be initiated at a dose of approximately 0.050 μg per kilogram per minute and the infusion titrated to achieve the desired hemodynamic effect. Upper recommended limits of infusion are approximately 1.0 μg per kilogram per minute. Norepinephrine is rapidly cleared from the circulation with a half-life of 2 to 3 minutes, although this is variable. It is enzymatically degraded in the liver and kidney and is also cleared by regional reuptake into sympathetic nerve terminals.

If hypoxia, hypovolemia, and acidosis have been corrected, the lack of a response to norepinephrine is probably an indication of significant myocardial damage. Prolonged infusions of norepinephrine, or infusions of large doses, are associated with major end-organ (e.g., liver and kidney) ischemic necrosis. It is a potent vasoconstrictor of the pulmonary circulation and should be used with caution in patients with pulmonary hypertension.

Dopamine. This is one of the most commonly used drugs to treat many forms of shock, probably related to its unique dose-dependent pharmacologic effects. Dopamine is the naturally occurring precursor of norepinephrine. When administered in low doses (1 to 3 μg per kilogram per minute), dopamine activates dopaminergic (DA) vasodilatory receptors in the renal, mesenteric, cerebral, and coronary circulations. DA-1 receptors are located on postsynaptic membranes and mediate vasodilation, and presynaptic DA-2 receptors prevent the release of endogenous norepinephrine, thereby potentiating the vasodilating effects in these circulations. In infusion ranges of 3 to 10 μg per kilogram per minute, dopamine activates β_1-adrenergic receptors and increases heart rate, myocardial contractility, and cardiac output. In doses >20 μg per kilogram per minute, dopamine produces vasoconstriction by activating α-adrenergic receptors in the arteries and veins of most vascular beds. Thus, at the upper infusion ranges, dopamine may distribute blood flow away from the extremities and toward the kidney, gut, heart, and brain. However, it is necessary to administer moderate to large doses to maintain arterial pressure and coronary blood flow, particularly following myocardial infarction. These larger doses oppose the dopaminergically mediated vasodilation in some vascular beds.

Epinephrine. Epinephrine is an endogenous catecholamine that is produced and released primarily from the adrenal medulla. Epinephrine activates myocardial β_1 receptors and vasoconstrictor α receptors in most vessels except in skeletal muscle and coronary vessels, where it activates β_2 receptors when administered in low doses. It increases cardiac output but redistributes blood flow away from the kidney and splanchnic circulations toward skeletal muscle. At low doses (0.005 to 0.02 μg per kilogram per minute in adults), epinephrine primarily stimulates β-adrenergic receptors and produces peripheral vasodilation and increases in heart rate and contractility. As the infusion rate is increased, α-vasoconstrictor effects become more prominent. Epinephrine also has important respiratory effects, with β_2 receptor–mediated bronchodilation and inhibition of mast cell degranulation. Epinephrine is a potent renal artery vasoconstricting agent in humans, even at low doses, and this limits its clinical utility.

Epinephrine is rapidly cleared from the circulation by the liver and kidney and has a half-life of approximately 2 minutes. Metabolism is via the enzymes catechol-O-methyl transferase and monoamine oxidase. Epinephrine is also well absorbed from the tracheobronchial tree, and this agent may be injected through an endo-tracheal tube during initial resuscitation of patients in cardiac arrest or those in whom venous access is not yet available.

Isoproterenol. Isoproterenol is a synthetic nonselective β-adrenergic agonist that activates primarily vascular β_2 receptors, resulting in vasodilation, and myocardial β_1 receptors, resulting in an increase in heart rate, contractility, and cardiac output. The magnitude of the vasodilator effect of isoproterenol varies in different vascular beds, depending on the density of β_2 receptors and the affinity of the drug for them. The major vasodilator action of isoproterenol is in skeletal muscle beds.

Isoproterenol is *not* recommended for cardiogenic shock because it significantly increases myocardial O_2 demands, and despite the increase in coronary blood flow, the ischemic region of the myocardium may be hypoperfused, as indicated by increased lactate production. Use of isoproterenol for shock should probably be limited to the temporary treatment of hemodynamically significant, atropine-resistant, high-grade AV block until a temporary pacemaker can be inserted. Even in this condition, the potential for inducing vasodilatory hypotension and increasing ventricular arrhythmias must be recognized. In addition, by overcoming hypoxia-induced pulmonary vasoconstriction in some patients, isoproterenol may increase intrapulmonary shunting of blood and result in a worsening of arterial oxygenation.

Dobutamine. Dobutamine is the preferred agent for managing low-output states with heart failure in the setting of an acute myocardial infarction. This synthetic sympathomimetic amine has predominant β_1 activity. In contrast to dopamine, dobutamine has much less α-vasoconstricting activity but equal positive inotropic effects. Thus, in equal inotropic doses, dobutamine tends to lower the pulmonary capillary wedge pressure, while dopamine tends to increase it. Dobutamine is reported to have a lower incidence of cardiac arrhythmias. In experimental models of myocardial infarction, dobutamine resulted in significantly smaller infarcts than did dopamine, possibly owing to the intracardiac release of norepinephrine produced by dopamine. Thus, especially in the setting of acute myocardial infarction with pump failure but without significant hypotension, dobutamine may be a preferred agent over dopamine for improving cardiac output.

Dobutamine is usually initiated at an infusion rate of 2 to 5 μg per kilogram per minute and titrated to desired hemodynamic effect. The usual infusion rate is 5 to 15 μg per kilogram per minute. The plasma half-life of dobutamine is approximately 2 to 3 minutes in patients with heart failure, with clearance achieved via catechol-O-methyl transferase.

Amrinone. Amrinone is a bipyridine that differs from the sympathomimetic amines and digitalis glycosides with respect to its mechanism of action. Amrinone has phosphodiesterase-inhibiting action that is thought to be (at least in part) the mechanism of its inotropic effect. It possesses positive inotropic and, to a lesser extent, chronotropic actions and is a potent vasodilator. In patients with heart failure, amrinone augments cardiac dP/dt without significant increases in heart rate or blood pressure and reduces left heart filling pressures as well as systemic vascular resistance. There is, however, wide variability in responses of individual patients to amrinone which makes dosing guidelines difficult to apply.

The recommended dosage for amrinone is an initial intravenous loading dose of 0.75 mg per kilogram over 3 to 5 minutes, followed by a continuous infusion of 5 to 10 μg per kilogram per minute and a second loading dose of equal magnitude 30 minutes after the initial load. The total daily dose of amrinone should not exceed 10 mg per kilogram.

Amrinone has a relatively long half-life. It is not approved for children. Intravenous amrinone has been associated with thrombocytopenia in approximately 4% of patients, and elevation of liver enzymes is reported with long-term infusion. This agent may be considered as an alternative to dobutamine in patients with severe cardiogenic low-output syndromes. In addition, the combined use of amrinone and dobutamine or dopamine may be considered in some patients who fail to respond to one agent alone.

Digitalis Glycosides. In general, digitalis glycosides are not indicated as inotropic agents for managing most forms of cardiogenic shock. This is related to the narrow therapeutic-to-toxic ratio and the difficulty in titrating the dose. In addition, the vasoconstrictor actions of digitalis may exacerbate splanchnic ischemia in the shock patient. The one possible role of digitalis in management of the shock patient may be heart rate control in patients with atrial fibrillation who cannot be successfully electrically cardioverted. However, even in this condition, digitalis must be given very carefully and the patient monitored closely for adverse effects, particularly if there is superimposed renal impairment.

VASODILATOR AGENTS IN CARDIOGENIC SHOCK. While at first glance use of vasodilator agents in patients in shock may seem contradictory, the clinical utility of these agents in certain disorders of low cardiac output emphasizes the critical relationship between the contractile state of the ventricle and the afterload against which it must contract. In general, the beneficial effects of vasodilators are to (1) decrease myocardial metabolic demands by decreasing cardiac preload and cardiac size, (2) to decrease ventricular afterload and increase cardiac output without adversely affecting mean perfusion pressure, and (3) to dilate microcirculatory vessels. An important point that must be stressed is that the beneficial effects of vasodilator agents in the therapy of severe heart failure and/or shock depend on the presence of adequate (e.g., not reduced) cardiac filling pressures and the ability of the ventricle to respond to changes in preload or afterload (e.g., absence of fixed obstructions to cardiac flow, such as is seen with critical aortic stenosis).

Reduction in Preload. Patients in cardiogenic shock may require a high preload and filling pressure to maintain an adequate stroke volume. However, an excessive elevation of filling pressure is detrimental because of pulmonary congestion and increased myocardial oxygen demand. A reduction in myocardial O_2 demand without a significant reduction in stroke volume can be achieved by decreasing ventricular volume and size in patients who have abnormally elevated cardiac filling pressures (e.g., pulmonary capillary wedge pressures of ≥ 18 mm Hg) and evidence of pulmonary congestion. Reduction in cardiac size decreases myocardial wall tension, which is a major determinant of myocardial O_2 requirements. Preload may be reduced by diuretic agents or venodilating drugs. The goal of venodilator therapy is to decrease cardiac preload and cardiac size without altering arterial blood pressure. As previously noted, the efficacy of such an approach depends on the compliance of the ventricle. A reduction in excessively high cardiac preload may be of benefit not only in reducing myocardial O_2 demands, but also in relieving pulmonary venous congestion and pulmonary edema. In some patients with marked increases in preload, in association with marked impairment of contractile performance and borderline hypotension, it may be desirable and necessary to combine a vasodilator agent with an inotropic agent so as to maintain mean arterial pressure within acceptable bounds.

Reduction in Afterload. It is possible to reduce afterload on a failing ventricle without adversely altering mean arterial pressure by nature of the increase in cardiac output that usually follows the reduction in impedance to ventricular emptying. However, such an approach requires close hemodynamic monitoring, and systemic hypotension is always a potentially catastrophic side effect of afterload reduction in patients with severely compromised hemodynamic status. During administration of afterload-reducing vasodilators, the systolic arterial pressure should not fall more than 10 mm Hg (unless the patient is being treated for hypertension), and the diastolic arterial pressure (coronary perfusion pressure) should be maintained at or above 60 to 65 mm Hg in most patients. Reduction in ventricular afterload is ideal in the patient with severe heart failure, marked pulmonary venous hypertension with pulmonary edema and impaired cardiac output, but without systemic arterial hypotension of significant degree.

Arteriolar vasodilators are particularly effective for managing shock due to acute intracardiac left-to-right shunts or regurgitant lesions. Examples of these conditions include acute ventricular septal rupture, acute mitral insufficiency due to papillary muscle rupture, and acute aortic insufficiency due to flail aortic valve leaflet complicating bacterial endocarditis. By acutely reducing impedance to ventricular ejection, nitroprusside may limit the degree of left-to-right shunt in the setting of a septal defect or the degree of mitral insufficiency or aortic insufficiency by reducing resistance to ventricular ejection. However, this effect is frequently achieved at the expense of an increase in heart rate due to unloading of arterial baroreceptors by this agent.

Microcirculatory Vasodilation. In some patients, despite prolonged administration of dopamine or norepinephrine, tissue perfusion is not improved. The reason may be that extensive myocardial damage has occurred. It is also possible that constriction of microcirculatory vessels may prevent perfusion of exchange capillaries.

Nitroprusside. Nitroprusside is a cyanide-containing, direct-acting, smooth-muscle–vasodilating agent that relaxes both arteries and veins. It is the classic "balanced" vasodilator, with effects on both capacitance and resistance vessels. The mode of action of nitroprusside is believed to involve activating soluble guanylate cyclase, consequently elevating cGMP in vascular smooth-muscle cells, leading to activation of cGMP-dependent protein kinase activity. It does not depend on the sympathetic nervous system or adrenergic receptors. Its onset of action is within seconds of administration, and its duration of effect is 1 to 3 minutes. Nitroprusside can be initiated as an intravenous infusion at approximately 10 μg per minute, with the rate increased every 5 to 10 minutes by 10 μg per minute increments until the desired hemodynamic effect is achieved.

In the setting of power failure following myocardial infarction, nitroprusside should be administered only to patients who are instrumented with indwelling systemic and pulmonary arterial catheters, as the clinician needs to follow arterial and cardiac filling pressures closely during infusion of this very potent vasodilator.

The principal complications associated with nitroprusside infusion include the possibility of hypotension, thiocyanate/cyanide toxicity with prolonged (≥ 72 hour) infusions of high doses, and a reduction in arterial oxygen tension due to pulmonary vascular vasodilating effects and consequent increase in ventilation-perfusion mismatching.

Nitroglycerin. This is also a very effective vasodilator with predominant effects on the venous capacitance vessels and lesser effects on arteriolar resistance vessels. When therapy is initiated, nitroglycerin can be started as an intravenous infusion of 10 μg per minute and then titrated upward in 10 μg per minute increments every 3 to 5 minutes as indicated by hemodynamics. Nitroglycerin is particularly effective for managing acute pulmonary edema complicating myocardial infarction. Adverse side effects include headache, hypotension, and occasional nausea and vomiting.

INTERVENTIONAL THERAPY

Recent advances in the management of patients with acute myocardial infarction have included use of intracoronary and intravenous thrombolytic agents (e.g., streptokinase and tissue plasminogen activator) within the early hours following the onset of a myocardial infarction. Unequivocal evidence is now available that thrombolytic therapy reduces the mortality and improves ventricular function following acute myocardial infarction. While early intervention with salvage of ischemic, jeopardized myocardium would presumably reduce the incidence of cardiogenic shock, this has not been demonstrated conclusively. Indeed, the incidence and prognosis of cardiogenic shock have remained essentially unchanged for the past two decades.

More recently, noncontrolled studies have suggested that emergency coronary angioplasty may improve the prognosis of patients with an acute myocardial infarction complicated by cardiogenic shock as compared with patients treated with thrombolytic therapy alone. However, whether these beneficial results can be demonstrated in controlled, prospective studies remains to be determined. Pending such studies, such invasive interventional therapy directed at mechanical reperfusion of occluded coronary arteries in patients with cardiogenic shock complicating a myocardial infarction due to profound power failure (in the absence of a mechanical regurgitant lesion) can be considered a heroic measure, of probable but unproven efficacy.

MECHANICAL CARDIOPULMONARY ASSISTANCE IN SHOCK. Recent advances have made available various mechanical support devices for temporarily managing patients with medically refractory shock of various etiologies. While clinical experience is limited and controlled clinical trials often are not available, it is appropriate to consider such devices in certain subgroups of patients. The decision to proceed with mechanical circulatory support and other heroic efforts should be made as rapidly as possible after the shock state is recognized and the patient fails to respond to more traditional pharmacologic and supportive therapy. The decision to entertain mechanical circulatory support should be based on the desires of the patient (see Ch. 2) and his/her family, the overall underlying condition of the patient, the likelihood of achieving reasonable functional recovery, and the presence of reversible or correctable cardiac lesions (as defined by diagnostic procedures such as echocardiography and cardiac catheterization).

Before or concomitant with initiating mechanical circulatory support, the patient with cardiogenic shock should undergo a complete diagnostic cardiac catheterization. This includes right- and left-sided hemodynamic and oximetric studies, left ventricular angiography, and coronary arteriography. These studies are indicated to define the extent of cardiac disease and the presence of potentially reversible or correctable cardiac lesions. Mechanical circulatory support may be required before or during the procedure in some patients with profound hemodynamic compromise in order to provide optimal support during the diagnostic studies.

Intra-aortic Balloon Counterpulsation. The intra-aortic balloon pump (IABP) has been used for 20 years in the management of certain types of cardiogenic shock. Currently, the device can be inserted percutaneously through a femoral artery and advanced under fluoroscopic guidance to the thoracic aorta just distal to the left subclavian artery. The balloon is mechanically inflated with CO_2 or helium during diastole and rapidly deflated at the onset of ventricular systole. The primary effects of the balloon are therefore (1) an increase in diastolic aortic root (coronary perfusion) pressure and (2) a mechanical reduction in aortic root blood pressure and volume (impedance) at the onset of systole. The desired hemodynamic effects of the intra-aortic balloon pump are increased coronary perfusion pressure, reduced ventricular afterload, increased forward cardiac ejection fraction, and reduced left-to-right or backward cardiac flow.

The IABP is most useful for managing patients with cardiogenic shock due to acute ventricular septal rupture or acute papillary muscle rupture or dysfunction with mitral insufficiency. In contrast to similar afterload-reducing effects achieved with nitroprusside, the IABP can reduce impedance to ventricular ejection without causing an increase in heart rate (myocardial O_2 demand). At the same time, the mechanical increase in peak augmented diastolic arterial pressure provides an increase in myocardial O_2 supply. The IABP also may temporarily benefit patients with ischemia-induced ventricular depression in the setting of high-grade coronary artery lesions until revascularization can be achieved (i.e., coronary angioplasty or coronary artery bypass surgery) or following cardiopulmonary bypass.

The IABP should be considered only a temporary support device and should be used only in patients who have a correctable cardiac lesion or reasonable likelihood of recovery from an acute cardiac insult. Despite optimal technique, a major complication rate of approximately 10 to 30% is reported with the device, most notably secondary to distal limb ischemia, vascular damage, or infection. The IABP is contraindicated in patients with aortic insufficiency, severe peripheral vascular disease, or inability to tolerate systemic anticoagulation. The IABP may be a useful support device for patients undergoing major surgery (cardiac or otherwise) in the presence of severe impairment of cardiac function.

Cardiac Assist Devices and Artificial Heart. Significant progress has been made over the past four decades since the first heart-lung machine was used in 1957 to support a patient with cardiogenic shock following acute myocardial infarction. In selected patients with refractory cardiogenic shock, external left and/or right cardiac assist devices have been used to "bridge" patients to cardiac transplant or permit patient survival for a long enough period to allow recovery of intrinsic myocardial function (e.g., in certain patients with severe inflammatory myocarditis). These assist devices require surgical thoracotomy for insertion of large vascular conduits involving the great vessels or the atria and ventricles themselves. Major complications including infection, bleeding, and thrombosis with systemic embolization have been reported with these devices. However, they have been successfully used as a bridge to successful cardiac transplantation in selected patients.

Implantable mechanical heart devices have been reported in a small number of patients, but no long-term success has been achieved and major complications are associated with these devices. Implantable artificial hearts have been utilized for up to 243 days in patients awaiting cardiac transplantation.

Extracorporeal Membrane Oxygenator and Bedside Cardiopulmonary Bypass. Additional recent experience has been reported with emergent bedside initiation of full cardiopulmonary bypass via percutaneous femoral arterial and venous approaches, using a portable cardiopulmonary bypass machine with membrane oxygenator. Limited experience has been reported with this technique in patients with refractory shock or cardiac arrest.

NUTRITIONAL SUPPORT OF THE SHOCK PATIENT

A frequently overlooked but extremely important aspect of caring for the shock patient is nutritional support. In many cases, wound healing, tissue repair, weaning from ventilator support, and therefore long-term survival may be adversely influenced by failure to appreciate the metabolic stresses of the shock state and to provide adequate nutritional support during the early as well as later phases of treatment. Time is a crucial element in the nutritional support of the shock patient. The physician must not allow his/her attention to other traditional details of management to prevent or delay attention to this important aspect of the patient's care. In general, most patients developing shock have suffered major metabolic insults and can rapidly develop catabolic states. This is particularly true of the intubated patient or the patient maintained NPO for extended periods of time following resuscitation. In the case of intubation, placement of an endotracheal tube should routinely be followed with a nasogastric tube for initial gastric decompression and then conversion to a gastric feeding tube. Potential contraindications to nasogastric tube placement include midline craniofacial and head trauma, suspected or potential esophageal perforation, and known obstruction of the esophagus.

As soon as possible, patients should begin receiving nutritional support via enteral or parenteral routes. Close monitoring should be performed on a routine basis with daily determinations of calorie intake and biweekly determinations of serum albumin, electrolytes, total lymphocyte count, transferrin level, liver function studies, and prothrombin time. Estimations of carbohydrate, protein, and fat requirements should be based on the patient's nitrogen balance, nature of insult, and associated medical problems. Continuing assessment of vitamin and essential trace metal levels is important in the long-term care of these patients.

Abboud FM, Heistad DD, Mark AL, Schmid PG: Reflex control of the peripheral circulation. Prog Cardiovasc Dis 18:371, 1976. *Review of the major factors of autonomic circulatory control operative in both healthy human subjects and under various disease states.*

Bernton EW, Long JB, Holaday JW: Opioids and neuropeptides: Mechanisms in circulatory shock. Fed Proc 44:290, 1985. *Reviews potential roles of endogenous opioids, thyrotropin-releasing hormone, and other neuropeptides in central cardiovascular regulatory mechanisms during shock.*

Colucci WS, Wright RF, Braunwald E: New positive inotropic agents in the treatment of congestive heart failure, 2 parts. N Engl J Med 314:290–299 and 349–358, 1986. *Reviews the mechanisms of action and recent clinical developments of newer positive inotropic agents in severe heart failure and cardiogenic shock.*

Gacioch GM, Ellis SG, Lee L, et al.: Cardiogenic shock complicating acute myocardial infarction: The use of coronary angioplasty and the integration of the new support devices into patient management. J Am Coll Cardiol 19:647, 1992. *Reviews one center's experience with treatment of cardiogenic shock complicating acute myocardial infarction in 68 patients using aggressive application of coronary angioplasty and various cardiovascular support devices.*

Goldberg LI, Rajfer SI: Dopamine receptors: Applications in clinical cardiology. Circulation 72:245, 1985. *Reviews the cardiovascular and renal actions of dopamine and emphasizes the unique effects of this agent on dopaminergic receptors.*

Goldberg RJ, Gore JM, Alpert JS, et al.: Cardiogenic shock after acute myocardial infarction: Incidence and mortality from a community-wide perspective, 1975–1988. N Engl J Med; 325:1117, 1991. *Observational, community-wide study examining the incidence and prognosis of cardiogenic shock complicating acute myocardial infarction.*

Joyce LD, Johnson KE, Toninato CJ, et al.: Results of the first 100 patients who received symbion total artificial hearts as a bridge to cardiac transplantation. Circulation 80(suppl III):III-192, 1989. *Reviews the clinical results of use of total artificial heart as a bridge to cardiac transplantation in 100 patients at 22 centers, including 27 patients with acute cardiogenic shock.*

Lefer AM: Interaction between myocardial depressant factor and vasoactive mediators with ischemia and shock. Am J Physiol 252 (Regulatory Integrative Comp. Physiol. 21):R193, 1987. *This excellent review discusses a variety of vasoactive mediators produced in ischemia and shock states, with particular emphasis on myocardial depressant factor, and reviews new pharmacologic approaches to the blockade of these mediators.*

Moosvi AR, Khaja F, Villanueva L, et al.: Early revascularization improves survival in cardiogenic shock complicating acute myocardial infarction. J Am Coll Cardiol 19:907, 1992. *Reviews a 5-year experience in managing patients with cardiogenic shock following acute myocardial infarction using emergent coronary revascularization with coronary angioplasty, coronary artery bypass surgery, or both.*

Mueller HS, Cohen LS, Braunwald E, et al.: Predictors of early morbidity and mortality after thrombolytic therapy of acute myocardial infarction: Analyses of patient subgroups in the thrombolysis in myocardial infarction (TIMI) trial, phase II. Circulation 85:1254, 1992. *Contemporary study of the prognosis of 3339 patients treated with acute thrombolytic therapy with either invasive (early cardiac catheterization) or conservative strategies. A strong independent correlation of pulmonary edema and/or cardiogenic shock with death suggests that thrombolysis alone is not sufficient to improve survival.*

Oliva PB, Hammill SC, Edwards WD: Cardiac rupture, a clinically predictable complication of acute myocardial infarction: Report of 70 cases with clinicopathologic correlations. J Am Coll Cardiol 22:720, 1993. *A retrospective and prospective study of 70 patients with acute myocardial infarction complicated by left ventricular free wall rupture. Results suggest that this catastrophic complication of infarction, and one cause of cardiogenic shock, can be suspected by a complex of signs and symptoms.*

Shapiro BA, Cane RD: Blood gas monitoring: Yesterday, today, and tomorrow. Crit Care Med 17:573, 1989. *Reviews the history of blood gas determination and provides an up-to-date assessment of new monitoring techniques.*

Tcheng JE, Jackman JD Jr, Nelson CL, et al.: Outcome of patients sustaining acute ischemic mitral regurgitation during myocardial infarction. Ann Intern Med 117:18024, 1992. *Prospective study of 50 patients with acute myocardial infarction complicated by moderately severe or severe mitral regurgitation out of 1480 consecutive patients undergoing emergent cardiac catheterization within 6 hours of onset of infarction. Physical examination failed to identify significant mitral regurgitation in 50%. Moderately severe to severe mitral regurgitation complicating acute myocardial infarction had a grave prognosis. Acute reperfusion therapy did not appear to reduce mortality or reliably restore valvular competence.*

Tobin MJ: Respiratory monitoring in the intensive care unit. Am Rev Respir Dis 138:1625, 1988. *Extensive review of recent advances in monitoring ventilation/respiration parameters in the intensive care environment.*

Zehender M, Kasper W, Kauder E, et al.: Right ventricular infarction as an independent predictor of prognosis after acute inferior myocardial infarction. N Engl J Med 328:981, 1993. *Prospective study of 200 patients admitted with acute inferior wall myocardial infarction, indicating that right ventricular involvement is a strong, independent predictor of major complications and in-hospital mortality.*

70 SHOCK SYNDROMES RELATED TO SEPSIS

Joseph E. Parrillo

Sepsis refers to the systemic response to serious infection. Patients with sepsis usually manifest fever, tachycardia, tachypnea, leukocytosis, and a localized site of infection. Microbiologic cultures from blood or the infection site are frequently, though not invariably, positive. When this syndrome results in hypotension or multiple organ system failure (MOSF), the condition is called *septic shock.*

INCIDENCE AND EPIDEMIOLOGY. The incidence of sepsis and septic shock has been increasing since the 1930's, and all recent evidence suggests that this rise will continue. The reasons for this increasing incidence are many: increased use of invasive devices such as intravascular catheters, widespread use of cytotoxic and immunosuppressive drug therapies for cancer and transplantation, increased longevity of patients with cancer and diabetes who are prone to develop sepsis, and an increase in infections due to antibiotic-resistant organisms. Septic shock is the most common cause of death in intensive care units, and it is the thirteenth most common cause of death in the United States. The precise incidence of the disease is not known because it is not reportable; however, a reasonable annual estimate for the United States is 400,000 bouts of sepsis, 200,000 cases of septic shock, and 100,000 deaths from this disease.

ETIOLOGY. Gram-negative and gram-positive organisms, as well as fungi, can cause sepsis and septic shock. Certain viruses and rickettsiae probably can produce a similar syndrome. Compared with gram-positive organisms, gram-negative bacteria are somewhat more likely to produce septic shock. Culture-positive gram-negative bacteremia produces shock in approximately 50%, whereas gram-positive bacteremia produces shock in 25% of such patients.

Any site of infection can result in sepsis or septic shock. Frequent causes of sepsis are pyelonephritis, pneumonia, peritonitis, cholangitis, cellulitis, or meningitis. Many of these infections are nosocomial, occurring in patients hospitalized for other medical problems. In patients with normal host defenses, a site of infection is identified in most patients. However, in neutropenic patients, a clinical infection site is found in less than half of septic patients,

probably because small, clinically inapparent infections in skin or bowel can lead to bloodstream invasion in the absence of adequate circulating neutrophils.

DEFINITIONS. Recently, considerable effort has been directed toward identifying septic patients early in their clinical course, when therapies are most likely to be effective. Definitions have incorporated manifestations of the systemic response to infection (fever, tachycardia, tachypnea, and leukocytosis) along with evidence of organ system dysfunction (cardiovascular, respiratory, renal, hepatic, central nervous system, hematologic, or metabolic abnormalities). The most recent definitions (Table 70–1) use the term *systemic inflammatory response syndrome* (SIRS), emphasizing that sepsis is one example of the body's inflammatory responses that can be triggered not only by infections but also by noninfectious disorders, such as trauma and pancreatitis (Fig. 70–1).

Sepsis is severe and has a poorer prognosis when it is associated with organ dysfunction, hypoperfusion (lactic acidosis, oliguria, or altered mental status), or hypotension (septic shock). *Septic shock* is defined as sepsis-induced hypotension, persisting despite adequate fluid resuscitation, along with the presence of hypoperfusion abnormalities or organ dysfunction. In clinical practice, many of these patients are receiving vasopressor and/or inotropic agents and are no longer hypotensive when they manifest hypoperfusion abnormalities or organ dysfunction, but they would still be considered as having septic shock.

PATHOGENESIS. A summary of the pathogenetic steps leading to septic shock is diagrammed in Figure 70–2. Microorganisms proliferate at a nidus of infection. The organisms may invade the bloodstream, resulting in positive blood cultures, or they may grow locally and release a variety of substances into the bloodstream. These consist of structural components of the microorganisms, such as teichoic acid antigens from staphylococci or endotoxins from gram-negative organisms or exotoxins (e.g., toxic shock syndrome

TABLE 70–1. DEFINITIONS OF SEPSIS

Infection: A microbial phenomenon characterized by an inflammatory response to the presence of microorganisms or the invasion of normally sterile host tissue by those organisms.

Bacteremia: The presence of viable bacteria in the blood.

Systemic inflammatory response syndrome: The systemic inflammatory response to a variety of severe clinical insults. The response is manifested by two or more of the following conditions:
Temperature > 38° C or < 36° C
Heart rate > 90 beats per minute
Respiratory rate > 20 breaths per minute or Pa_{CO_2} < 32 mm Hg (< 4.3 kPa)
White blood cell count > 12,000 cells per cubic millimeter, < 4000 cells per cubic millimeter, or > 10% immature (band) forms

Sepsis: The systemic response to infection. This systemic response is manifested by two or more of the following conditions as a result of infection:
Temperature > 38° C or < 36° C
Heart rate > 90 beats per minute
Respiratory rate > 20 breaths per minute or Pa_{CO_2} < 32 mm Hg (< 4.3 kPa)
White blood cell count > 12,000 cells per cubic millimeter, < 4000 cells per cubic millimeter, or > 10% immature (band) forms

Severe sepsis: Sepsis associated with organ dysfunction, hypoperfusion, or hypotension. Hypoperfusion and perfusion abnormalities may include, but are not limited to, lactic acidosis, oliguria, or an acute alteration in mental status.

Septic shock: Sepsis with hypotension, despite adequate fluid resuscitation, along with the presence of perfusion abnormalities that may include, but are not limited to, lactic acidosis, oliguria, or an acute alteration in mental status. Patients who are on inotropic or vasopressor agents may not be hypotensive at the time that perfusion abnormalities are measured.

Hypotension: A systolic blood pressure < 90 mm Hg or a reduction > 40 mm Hg from baseline in the absence of other causes for hypotension.

Multiple organ system failure: Presence of altered organ function in an acutely ill patient such that homeostasis cannot be maintained without intervention.

Adapted from American College of Chest Physicians/Society of Critical Care Medicine Consensus Conference: Definitions for sepsis and organ failure and guidelines for the use of innovative therapies in sepsis. Crit Care Med 20:864, 1992.

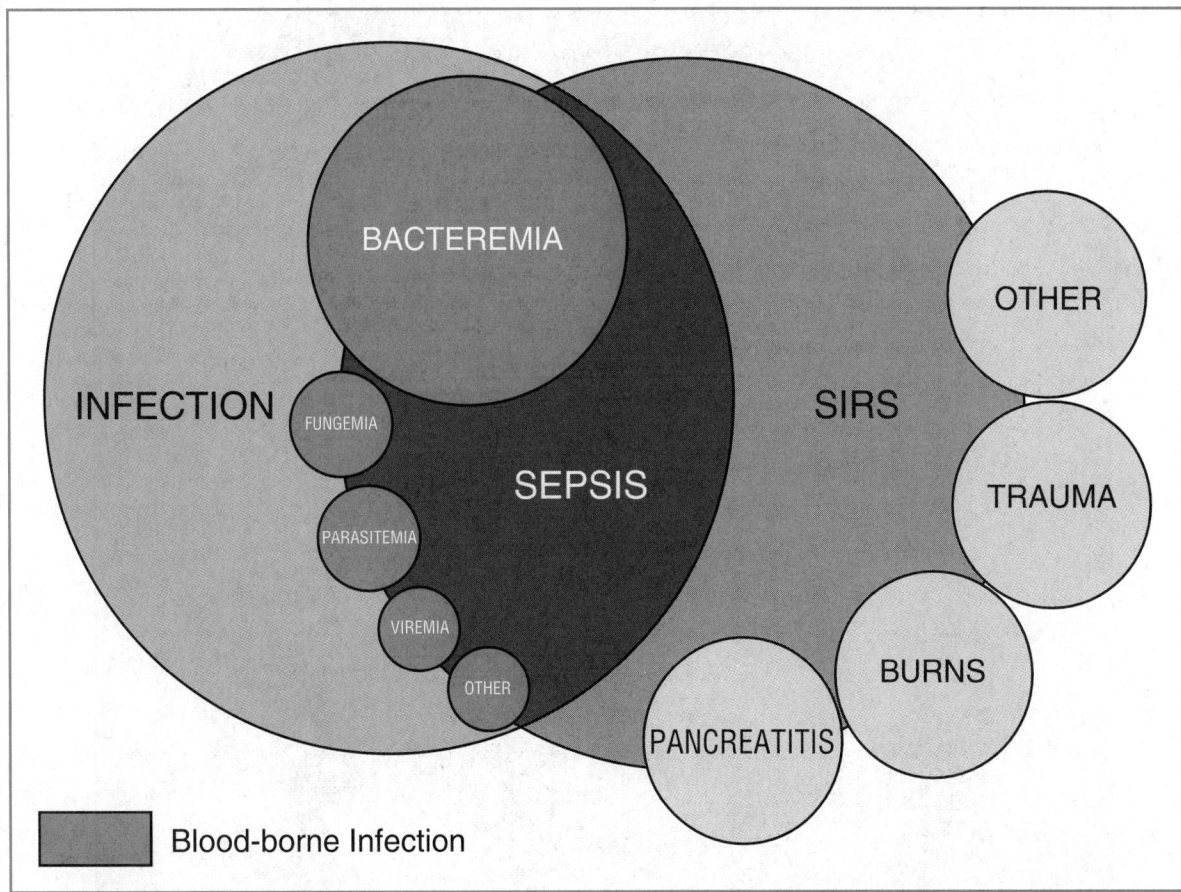

FIGURE 70–1. Interrelationships among systemic inflammatory response syndrome (SIRS), sepsis, and infection. (From American College of Chest Physicians/Society of Critical Care Medicine Consensus Conference: Definitions for sepsis and organ failure and guidelines for the use of innovative therapies in sepsis. Crit Care Med 20:864, 1992.)

toxin-1, or TSST-1) synthesized and released by the microorganisms. These organism-derived products can stimulate the release of a large number of endogenous host-derived mediators from plasma protein precursors or cells (monocytes/macrophages, endothelial cells, neutrophils, and others).

The endogenous mediators can produce profound physiologic effects on vasculature and organ systems. Some of these effects stem from direct mediator-induced injury to end organs. However, a portion of the organ dysfunction is probably due to mediator-induced abnormalities in vasculature, resulting in abnormalities of systemic and regional blood flow. Although certain mediators are undoubtedly more important than others in producing sepsis, probably dozens of organism- and host-derived mediators interacting, accelerating, and inhibiting one another, are responsible for the pathogenesis of septic shock.

Approximately 50% of patients with hypotension secondary to sepsis admitted to an intensive care unit will survive. The other 50% will develop refractory hypotension or MOSF and will die from progressive septic shock. Early and throughout the course of most of these patients, cardiovascular evaluation reveals a low systemic vascular resistance and a high cardiac output—the hyperdynamic response to sepsis. Despite this elevated cardiac output, cardiac performance is abnormal, with decreased ventricular ejection fraction and a dilated ventricle. In approximately 20% of patients, progressively diminished cardiac performance results in an abnormally low cardiac output. In nonsurvivors, organ system dysfunction progresses to MOSF, manifested by further myocardial dysfunction, adult respiratory distress syndrome (ARDS), acute renal failure, hepatic failure, and disseminated intravascular coagulation (DIC). Death results from progressive hypotension or complete failure of one or more organ systems.

Microorganism-Derived Mediators. A number of molecules can initiate the pathway leading to septic shock (Fig. 70–2). Certain microorganisms synthesize and release exotoxins that can

activate the cascade. Examples include toxin A produced by *Pseudomonas aeruginosa* and TSST-1 produced by staphylococci. More frequently, the structural components of the microorganism initiate the sequence. The polysaccharide surface of *Candida albicans,* the teichoic acid antigens of staphylococci, and the polysaccharide capsule of *Streptococus pneumoniae* can all initiate the sepsis pathway.

However, endotoxin—the distinctive lipopolysaccharide (LPS) associated with the cell membrane of the gram-negative organism—represents the classic example of an initiator of the septic shock pathogenetic cascade. The endotoxin molecule consists of an outer core with a series of oligosaccharides that are antigenically and structurally diverse, an inner oligosaccharide core that has similarities among common gram-negative bacteria, and a core lipid A that is highly conserved across bacterial species. The lipid A is responsible for many of the toxic properties of endotoxin, and this has led to the synthesis of nonactive analogues and inhibitors of the lipid A molecule.

Administering endotoxin to a variety of animals results in a cardiovascular response very similar to human septic shock. Administering a very small dose of purified endotoxin to normal humans results in fever, mild constitutional symptoms, and a cardiovascular pattern qualitatively similar to that of spontaneous sepsis: tachycardia, decreased systemic vascular resistance, and depressed ventricular ejection fraction. In septic patients, detectable plasma levels of endotoxin are correlated with positive blood cultures, decreased systemic vascular resistance, depressed ventricular ejection fraction, and lactic acidemia. In patients with positive blood cultures and septic shock, detectable plasma endotoxin is associated with increased mortality (39%, versus 7% for those without endotoxemia). Thus endotoxin is an important mediator in many (though not all) septic shock patients; however, routinely measuring circulating plasma endotoxin is not prognostically reliable enough to be used clinically.

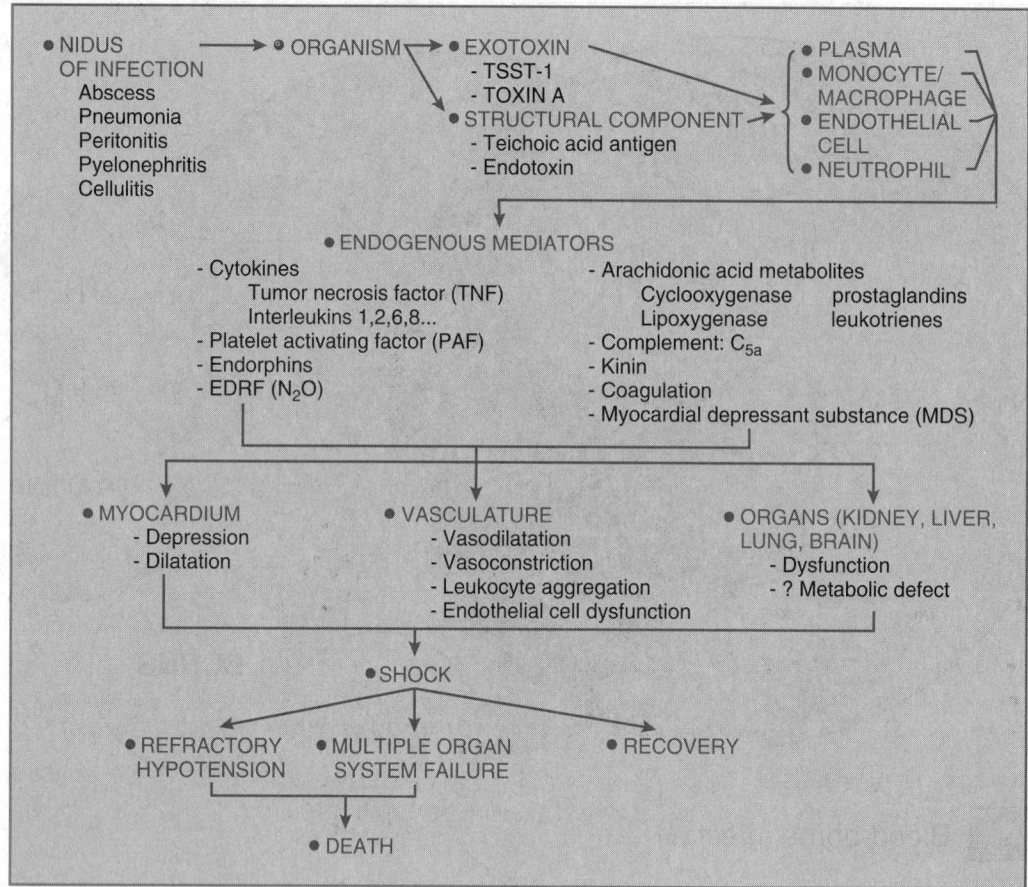

FIGURE 70-2. Pathogenetic sequence of the events in septic shock. (Used with permission from Parrillo JE: Mechanisms of disease: Pathogenetic mechanisms of septic shock. N Engl J Med 328:1471, 1993. Copyright Massachusetts Medical Society.)

Cytokines. The monocyte/macrophage plays an important role in the body's response to infection or endotoxin. Endotoxin can stimulate monocytes to produce tumor necrosis factor (TNF), interleukin-1 (IL-1), and other cytokines. Serum contains a protein, the LPS-binding protein, or LBP, that can bind the lipid A portion of endotoxin. When complexed with LBP, LPS can bind the CD14 receptor and stimulate the monocyte to produce cytokines at concentrations far below those required for stimulation by LPS alone.

Cytokines are 15- to 30-kilodalton (kDa) polypeptides that have profound immune regulatory and physiologic effects. Considerable evidence suggests that cytokines can enhance host defense mechanisms (e.g., stimulating lymphocyte progenitor cells, enhancing neutrophil oxidative burst) but also can produce harmful effects. In animal models, administering TNF results in a cardiovascular pattern of shock that is very similar to clinical sepsis. Anti-TNF antibodies have prevented shock and death from endotoxin and live organism challenge in animals. TNF produces vascular dilation and myocardial cell depression in biologic models, suggesting its involvement in these sepsis-associated physiologic abnormalities. Although TNF probably has a central role in mediating sepsis-induced injury, it may not work alone. TNF and IL-1 have been shown to work synergistically to produce hypotension in animals, and additive or synergistic actions among a number of cytokines probably account for many sepsis-associated abnormalities.

Myocardial Depressant Substance(s). A number of animal models suggest the presence of a circulating myocardial depressant as the possible cause of ventricular dysfunction during sepsis. Human studies have documented the presence of circulating myocardial depressant activity that correlates temporally with the reduced ventricular ejection fraction (Table 70-2). Recent data suggest that this depression may result from the effect of several cytokines on myocardial cell contraction.

Endothelial Cells and Neutrophils. A number of mediators, including LPS and TNF, can cause endothelial cells to express ad-

hesion receptors (selectins) and also can activate neutrophils to express ligands for these receptors. Neutrophils must adhere to the endothelial cell surface for adherence, margination, and migration of neutrophils into tissue inflammatory foci. Blocking the adhesion process with monoclonal antibodies prevents tissue injury and improves survival in certain animal models of septic shock.

Nitric Oxide. In response to LPS, TNF, and other mediators, endothelial cells and macrophages can release a potent vasodilator agent, endothelial-derived relaxing factor (EDRF), which has recently been identified as nitric oxide. This molecule causes smooth-muscle cell relaxation and potent vasodilatation. Inhibiting nitric oxide production with competitive inhibitors of nitric oxide synthase results in increased blood pressure in animals with endotoxin shock. This suggests that nitric oxide may be partially responsible for the hypotension associated with sepsis (see Ch. 37). Although inhibition of nitric oxide restores blood pressure, such inhibition may reduce tissue blood flow. More studies are needed to define the potential beneficial or harmful role of nitric oxide inhibition in sepsis.

Complement, Kinin, and the Coagulation System. Endotoxin can activate the complement cascade, usually via the alternative pathway. This results in the release of the anaphylotoxins C3a and C5a, which can induce vasodilation, increased vascular permeability, platelet aggregation, and activation and aggregation of neutrophils. These complement-derived mediators may be responsible in part for the microvascular abnormalities associated with septic shock. Further, endotoxin can result in the release of bradykinin via the activation of Factor XII (Hageman factor), kallikrein, and kininogen. Bradykinin is a potent vasodilator and hypotensive agent. LPS activation of factor XII also leads to intrinsic and (through macrophage and endothelial cell release of tissue factor) extrinsic coagulation pathway activation. This may result in consumption of coagulation factors and DIC. TNF also activates the extrinsic pathway and may contribute to these coagulation abnormalities.

TABLE 70–2. CARDIOVASCULAR RESPONSE TO SEPTIC SHOCK: A REPRESENTATIVE EXAMPLE

	Acute Phase (Hypotension and Reduced Systemic Vascular Resistance)	Recovery Phase (Normotension)
Mean arterial pressure (mm Hg)	40	75
Central venous pressure (mm Hg)	2	5
Cardiac output (liters per minute)	11.25	5.25
Heart rate (beats per minute)	150	70
Stroke volume (ml)	75	75
Systemic vascular resistance (dyne $\cdot$ sec $\cdot$ cm^{-5})	270	1067
Left ventricular volumes (ml):		
Diastole	225	125
Systole	150	50
Ejection fraction (%)	$\dfrac{225\ ml\ -\ 150\ ml}{225\ ml} = 33$	$\dfrac{125\ ml\ -\ 50\ ml}{125\ ml} = 60$

Arachidonic Acid Metabolites. Different metabolites of the arachidonic acid cascade are known to cause vasodilation (prostacyclins), vasoconstriction (thromboxanes), platelet aggregation, or neutrophil activation. In experimental animals, inhibiting cyclo-oxygenase or thromboxane synthase has protected against endotoxin shock. Elevated levels of thromboxane B_2 (TBX_2) and 6-keto-prostaglandin $F_{1\alpha}$ (the end-product of prostacyclin metabolism) are present in patients with sepsis. A number of cytokines can cause release of these arachidonic acid metabolites from endothelial cells or leukocytes.

Opioid Peptides. In certain animal models of endotoxin challenge, administering an endogenous opioid antagonist, such as naloxone, can reverse hypotension. The role of endogenous opioids in clinical septic shock is unclear.

CARDIOVASCULAR DYSFUNCTION. Shock is classically defined as inadequate perfusion of tissues resulting in cell dysfunction and, if prolonged, cell death. This definition adequately describes shock due to the hypovolemic, cardiogenic, and vascular obstructive mechanisms that result in reduced cardiac output and poor tissue perfusion. In these forms of shock, systemic vascular resistance is elevated as a compensatory mechanism to maintain blood pressure, and pulmonary artery oxygenation is reduced, reflecting enhanced extraction of oxygen from erythrocytes by hypoperfused tissues.

However, sepsis results in a much more complex form of shock. The onset of sepsis is frequently accompanied by hypovolemia due to both leakage of plasma (capillary leak) into the intravascular space and arterial and venous vasodilation. If this hypovolemia is corrected by aggressive volume replacement, it will result in a decreased systemic vascular resistance, increased or normal cardiac output, tachycardia, and an elevated oxygen content in the pulmonary artery blood—the hyperdynamic shock syndrome. This hemodynamic pattern has been termed *distributive shock* to indicate the presumed maldistribution of systemic blood flow leading to the high blood oxygen content returning to the right side of the heart. Prior to volume resuscitation, patients with septic shock may manifest features of both hypovolemic and distributive shock, that is, a mixed form of shock.

Despite the elevated or normal cardiac output in volume-resuscitated septic shock, ventricular function is abnormal (see Table 70–2), as reflected by decreases in ventricular ejection fraction and stroke work and increases in end-diastolic and end-systolic volumes. In survivors, this cardiovascular dysfunction is reversible and returns to normal by 5 to 10 days following septic shock (see Table 70–2). Certain hemodynamic patterns have prognostic implications. At disease onset, a lower heart rate predicts survival, probably reflecting less severe disease. Serial hemodynamics demonstrate that normalization (within 24 hours) of either the elevated cardiac index or tachycardia is associated with survival, whereas persistence of the hyperdynamic state correlates with nonsurvival.

Vascular dysfunction is one of the most prominent physiologic and pathologic findings in septic shock. Patients usually manifest an overall decrease in systemic vascular resistance, reflecting widespread systemic vasodilatation; however, some localized vascular beds are constricted. The decreased extraction of oxygen in the systemic circulation suggests that oxygen is not reaching or not being used by cells. One hypothesis argues that vascular abnormalities (vasodilation, vasoconstriction, leukocyte aggregation, and endothelial cell dysfunction induced by complex interactions among the mediators summarized above) result in decreased tissue perfusion. A second hypothesis argues that a direct mediator-induced cellular metabolic abnormality causes the oxygen uptake failure. A central question in the pathogenesis of sepsis is whether decreased perfusion due to microvascular dysregulation is a primary cause or only an associated event in sepsis-induced organ failure.

Another method to judge whether a vascular perfusion abnormality is important in septic shock is to evaluate the relationship between oxygen delivery and oxygen consumption. In patients with cardiogenic or hypovolemic shock, when tissue hypoperfusion clearly occurs, increases in oxygen delivery result in increased consumption until hypoperfusion is reversed and oxygen consumption plateaus. Some investigators have argued that septic shock (especially with ARDS) is characterized by a pathologic delivery-consumption relationship in which consumption continues to increase (and not plateau) with increased delivery, suggesting the presence of a perfusion abnormality that can be overcome by increasing delivery to a supranormal range. This observation is controversial. Animal experiments have yielded conflicting results. Although some clinical studies have reported improved outcomes when oxygen delivery is increased, flaws in selecting and randomizing patients make these trials impossible to interpret.

CLINICAL MANIFESTATIONS AND DIAGNOSTIC EVALUATION. Sepsis and septic shock produce three categories of clinical manifestations, as outlined in Table 70–3. First, the patient usually will manifest symptoms and signs related to the primary focus of infection. If this is pneumonia, then the patient usually has cough, dyspnea, and productive sputum; if a urinary tract infection is the focus, then flank pain and dysuria would be expected. A careful history, physical examination, and directed laboratory studies will reveal the probable infection focus in most patients. However, elderly, debilitated, and immunosuppressed patients may not provide the usual localizing clinical signs. In some patients, especially those with severe neutropenia, no site is identified. Second, as discussed in above, patients usually manifest one or more signs of the systemic inflammatory response. Fever is the most characteristic and is frequently accompanied by shaking chills. A significant proportion of patients (perhaps 15%) will be hypothermic ($< 36.5°$ C or $97.6°$ F) or normothermic, especially the elderly, debilitated, or immunosuppressed. Elderly patients may present with tachypnea-induced respiratory alkalosis and mental status changes as the only signs of sepsis. Third, septic patients may develop evidence of shock, such as hypotension, lactic acidemia, and progressive organ system dysfunction. Frequently involved organs and their characteristic abnormalities are listed in Table 70–3.

The diagnosis of sepsis is confirmed by culturing pathogenic organisms from blood or from the likely site of infection. Blood cul-

TABLE 70-3. CLINICAL MANIFESTATIONS OF SEPSIS AND SEPTIC SHOCK

I. **Site of infection**
  A. Pneumonitis, empyema
  B. Urinary tract infection
  C. Cellulitis
  D. Peritonitis
  E. Cholangitis
  F. Abscess (peritoneum, skin, brain, paraspinal)
  G. Sinusitis
  H. Meningitis
  I. No identifiable site (especially in neutropenic patients)
II. **Systemic inflammatory response**
  A. Fever or hypothermia; chills
  B. Tachycardia
  C. Tachypnea
  D. Leukocytosis or leukopenia
III. **Shock-induced organ dysfunction**
  A. Cardiovascular: hypotension; myocardial depression; lactate production
  B. Respiratory: adult respiratory distress syndrome (ARDS)
  C. Renal: acute renal failure (ARF), oliguria
  D. Hepatic: hyperbilirubinemia
  E. Coagulation: thrombocytopenia; disseminated intravascular coagulation (DIC)
  F. Central nervous system: confusion, stupor, obtundation

tures are positive in only 40 to 60% of patients with clinical manifestations of septic shock, probably due to the intermittent nature of the bacteremia and the high incidence of prior antibiotic administration. A Gram stain from an abscess, empyema, or other usually sterile site can provide invaluable early diagnostic information.

TREATMENT. One can effectively manage septic shock at three points along the pathogenetic sequence (Fig. 70–2 and Table 70–4). First, the infection site can be eradicated with antimicrobials, surgical drainage, or both. Second, the serious disturbances in cardiovascular, respiratory, and other organ system physiology can be reversed in an intensive care unit. Third, the toxic mediators of sepsis can be inhibited or modulated.

Antimicrobial Therapy. Shock secondary to sepsis is a very serious disease that should be treated aggressively. When the diagnosis is seriously entertained, blood cultures (usually three) and cultures of relevant body fluids and exudates should be obtained rapidly. Several large retrospective trials have provided convincing evidence that early appropriate antimicrobial therapy (i.e., the pathogen has *in vitro* sensitivity to the chosen antibiotic regimen) is associated with significantly improved patient survival. Once a specific pathogen is isolated, the antimicrobial spectrum can be narrowed.

When considering the choice of antibiotics, a number of issues must be considered. A broad-spectrum regimen with activity against gram-positive and gram-negative organisms should be chosen. Generally, drugs should be administered intravenously at maximum recommended dosages, and bactericidal agents are preferred over bacteriostatic agents. Knowing the most likely organisms to infect a given site and the local bacteriologic sensitivity and resistance patterns is important in choosing the best initial antimicrobial regimen. In neutropenic patients with gram-negative pneumonia, many physicians favor using at least two effective antimicrobial agents. Many authorities advocate a two-drug synergistic combination when treating serious enterococcal infection (see Ch. 297). Anaerobes are likely pathogens in intra-abdominal infections, aspiration pneumonia, and abscesses. Intravascular catheter infection should raise the possibility of methicillin-resistant staphylococcal infection and the need for vancomycin therapy. In up to one third of patients, especially those who are neutropenic, no organism or source will be identified. Such patients require a broad-spectrum regimen effective against gram-positive and gram-negative organisms such as vancomycin, gentamicin and metronidazole, or cephtazidine and gentamicin. The need for early antifungal therapy with amphotericin B should be considered in neutropenic immunosuppressed patients and those unresponsive to antibacterial regimens.

Therapy for Shock. Prior to the general availability of intensive care units, gram-negative bacteremic shock had a >90% mor-

tality. Now, about 50% of such patients survive, largely due to treatment in intensive care units, where cardiac rhythm, blood pressure, cardiac performance, oxygen delivery, and metabolic derangements can be monitored and abnormalities can be corrected (see Table 70–4). Adequate oxygenation and ventilatory support are critical goals of therapy and can be achieved with supplemental oxygen and, if necessary, mechanical ventilation and positive endexpiratory pressure (PEEP). Although no prospective trial has evaluated outcomes with and without intensive care unit support, two retrospective studies have reported a significantly reduced septic shock mortality when patients were managed with aggressive hemodynamic support by critical care personnel. A controlled, prospective trial of intensive care unit support has been conducted in dogs with gram-negative sepsis. Survival was increased only in the animals that received both antibiotic therapy and cardiovascular support. This argues that these two therapies work synergistically.

Patients with septic shock who remain hypotensive after a 1- or 2-liter volume resuscitation should have arterial and pulmonary artery catheters placed to allow serial evaluations of blood pressure, ventricular filling pressures, cardiac output, and oxygen delivery. Initial emphasis should be placed on restoring mean blood pressure to greater than 65 mm Hg. Aggressive volume resuscitation using blood (if hemoglobin < 10 grams per 100 ml), colloid (if serum albumin < 2 grams per 100 ml), or crystalloid (in all other patients) should be instituted to raise pulmonary artery wedge mean pressure to 15 to 18 mm Hg. If hypotension persists, dopamine (low-dose and then, if necessary, higher doses up to 20 μg per kilogram per minute) should be administered. In dopamine-unresponsive patients, norepinephrine should be infused to raise mean blood pressure to >65 mm Hg. Patients requiring high doses of norepinephrine may

TABLE 70-4. GUIDELINES FOR THE CARE OF PATIENTS WITH SEPTIC SHOCK

Abnormality	Intervention	Therapeutic Goal
Infection	Appropriate antibiotics and surgical drainage, if necessary	Eradication of infection
Cardiovascular and organ dysfunction		
Hypotension	ICU monitoring, volume expansion, vasopressor agents	Mean arterial pressure of at least 60 mm Hg Pulmonary-artery wedge pressure of 14–18 mm Hg
Tissue hypofusion	ICU monitoring, volume expansion, inotropic agents, vasopressors	Hemoglobin level >10 g/dl Oxygen saturation >92% Normal blood lactate concentrations Cardiac index >2.2 liters/min/m² in non-septic shock and >4.0 liters/min/m² in septic shock
Organ-system dysfunction	ICU monitoring, volume expansion, inotropic agents, vasopressors, mechanical ventilation	Normal values or reversal of evidence of dysfunction in the following systems: Renal—blood urea nitrogen, serum, creatinine, urinary output Hepatic—serum bilirubin Pulmonary—alveolar-arterial oxygen gradient Cardiovascular—mean arterial pressure, cardiac index Central nervous system—mental status
Mediators producing effect	Mediator inhibitor*	Reversal of toxic effect

ICU = intensive care unit.
* This therapy is still in the experimental phase.
Adapted with permission from Parrillo JE: Pathogenetic mechanisms of septic shock.
N Engl J Med 328:1471, 1993. Copyright by the Massachusetts Medical Society.

benefit from concomitantly administered low-dose dopamine to enhance renal blood flow. Once blood pressure is adequate, attention should be turned to cardiac output and oxygen delivery. Although the role of achieving very high levels of oxygen delivery and consumption is controversial, since myocardial depression is known to occur in sepsis, most authors favor inotropic support (with dobutamine, if necessary) to maintain a cardiac index in the high normal range (> 4.0 liters per minute per square meter). Serial measures of lactate, urine output, and organ function (see Table 70–4) provide good measures of patient prognosis.

Mediator Inhibitors. Treatments that inhibit the action or formation of mediators are being developed. High-dose corticosteroids can inhibit mediator release and improve survival in some animal models of endotoxemia. However, three prospective, randomized clinical trials have demonstrated convincingly that corticosteroids do not improve survival in human septic shock. Small trials in certain diseases—meningococcal meningitis in children and typhoid fever—suggest that they may have a therapeutic role in these specific infections but are not indicated in the usual patient with septic shock.

Another therapeutic strategy has been to inhibit endotoxin. Large, controlled clinical trials using a polyclonal antisera and monoclonal antibodies raised against endotoxin reveal a survival benefit in some subgroups receiving the anti-endotoxin. These results support the pathogenic importance of endotoxin in the many patients with septic shock. However, the patients in whom the treatment is likely to be effective (e.g., patients with blood cultures positive for gram-negative organisms) cannot be identified early in the course of infection, when therapy must be initiated. Further, the clinical characteristics of the patients who benefited from the treatment varied in the different trials. For these reasons, none of these anti-endotoxin preparations have been approved in the United States. More potent pharmacologic inhibitors of endotoxin may prove efficacious in future trials.

Monoclonal antibodies to TNF have the theoretical advantage of efficacy against gram-positive and fungal as well as gram-negative infections. TNF inhibitors are presently undergoing clinical trials. Using recombinant technology, an IL-1 receptor antagonist has been synthesized in large quantities and has shown therapeutic efficacy in animal models of sepsis. In preliminary clinical trials, certain subgroups of sepsis patients appear to benefit from IL-1 receptor blockade. Inhibitors of nitric oxide synthesis have been shown to raise blood pressure in animal models of septic shock. All these mediator inhibitors show some promise in reducing the toxic effects of the sepsis cascade. However, none has proved to have clear efficacy in prospectively defined groups of sepsis patients.

A word of caution is warranted regarding mediator inhibitor therapy. The pathways of septic shock pathogenesis are very complex and highly interdependent, and many mechanisms represent the body's compensatory response to sepsis and therefore have salutary effects. For example, in dogs with gram-negative sepsis, plasma exchange increases mortality, presumably because removing all circulating mediators is more harmful than beneficial. All these mediator inhibitors must be evaluated carefully with rigorous animal and human trials to ensure that they improve morbidity and mortality.

Selective mediator inhibition holds the greatest promise for managing septic shock in the future. A greater understanding of the complex interrelationships among the mediators of sepsis should allow effective interruption of the pathogenetic sequence and reduce mortality from this very serious disease.

American College of Chest Physicians/Society of Critical Care Medicine Consensus Conference: Definitions for sepsis and organ failure and guidelines for the use of innovative therapies in sepsis. Crit Care Med 20:864, 1992. *A consensus conference panel summarizes definitions of sepsis, septic shock, and related syndromes.*

Beutler B, Milsark IW, Cerami AC: Passive immunization against cachectin/tumor necrosis factor protects mice from lethal effect of endotoxin. Science 229:869, 1985. *Documents the importance of TNF as a mediator of endotoxin shock by demonstrating protection from endotoxin challenge using an anti-TNF antibody.*

Danner RL, Elin RJ, Hosseini JM, et al.: Endotoxemia in human septic shock. Chest 99:169, 1991. *Describes the frequency and prognostic significance of endotoxemia in septic shock.*

Dantzker DR, Foresman B, Gutierrez G: Oxygen supply and utilization relationships: A re-evaluation. Am Rev Respir Dis 143:675, 1991. *Provides a thoughtful review of the conflicting data regarding oxygen supply and utilization.*

Natanson C, Danner RL, Reilly JM, et al.: Antibiotics versus cardiovascular support in a canine model of human septic shock. Am J Physiol 259:H1440, 1990. *Describes a controlled trial of antibiotics versus cardiovascular (ICU) support in a canine model of gram-negative bacteremia documenting the synergistic therapeutic effect of these interventions.*

Parker MM, Shelhamer JH, Bacharach SL, et al.: Profound but reversible myocardial depression in patients with septic shock. Ann Intern Med 100:483, 1984. *Describes the characteristic cardiovascular profile of hyperdynamic sepsis with myocardial depression in septic shock.*

Parrillo JE, moderator: Septic shock in humans: Advances in the understanding of pathogenesis, cardiovascular dysfunction, and therapy. Ann Intern Med 113:227, 1990. *A review of pathogenetic pathways and mechanisms of cardiovascular dysfunction in sepsis.*

Reynolds HN, Haupt MT, Thill-Baharozian MC, et al.: Impact of critical care physician staffing on patients with septic shock in a university hospital medical intensive care unit. JAMA 260:3446, 1988. *Describes improved survival that results from staffing an ICU with fill-time critical care physicians.*

Suffredini AF, Fromm RE, Parker MM, et al.: The cardiovascular response of normal humans to the administration of endotoxin. N Engl J Med 321:280, 1989. *Describes the characteristic hemodynamic profile when normal volunteers are challenged with a small dose of endotoxin.*

Ziegler EJ, Fisher CJ Jr, Sprung CL, et al.: Treatment of gram-negative bacteremia and septic shock with HA-1A human monoclonal antibody against endotoxin: A randomized, double-blind, placebo-controlled trial. N Engl J Med 324:429, 1991. *Describes the results of a multicenter trial in sepsis patients using a human monoclonal antibody to endotoxin.*

71 DISORDERS DUE TO HEAT AND COLD

Ernest Yoder

TEMPERATURE HOMEOSTASIS. Humans as homeothermic organisms depend on a highly integrated neuroendocrine system to maintain their thermal homeostasis. Equilibrium between heat gained and lost must be maintained to prevent the organism from becoming either hyperthermic or hypothermic. Thus body temperature is normally maintained at $36.5 \pm 0.7°$ C ($97.7 \pm 1.3°$ F). Mechanisms of heat transfer to the environment, largely dependent on a temperature gradient between the body and its milieu, are radiation, conduction, convection, and evaporation.

Information from peripheral and central receptors is integrated by the hypothalamus, which effects changes in autonomic tone and endocrinologic function, to maintain stable body temperature. Voluntary responses, also important in preventing hypo- and hyperthermia, include moving to a cooler or warmer environment, removing or adding clothing, decreasing or increasing activity level, and increasing or decreasing exposed skin areas.

HYPERTHERMIC SYNDROMES. Hyperthermia is present when core body temperature is $>37.2°$ C. Heat injury syndromes may result in body temperatures in $>40°$ C ($104°$ F) (Table 71–1). When temperatures are $>41°$ C, enzymes are denatured, mitochondrial function is disturbed, cell membranes are destabilized, and oxygen-dependent metabolic pathways are disrupted. Multisystem failure regularly occurs concomitantly with heat injury syndromes, with significant associated mortality and morbidity. Patients with heat illness frequently need to be admitted to the intensive care unit.

Painful spasm of major muscle groups is the hallmark of *heat cramps.* Typically seen in young, unacclimatized athletes or laborers who exert themselves excessively in a hot climate, heat cramps are related to excessive losses of sodium, chloride, and water. Patients complain of nausea, vomiting, and fatigue in addition to muscle cramps, with onset of symptoms typically occurring several hours after they stop exercising.

Heat exhaustion, the most common heat injury syndrome seen in athletes, may be preceded by heat cramps and is due to severe dehydration and electrolyte loss. In the young, heat exhaustion usually occurs following strenuous activity by unacclimatized individuals in a hot, humid environment. In the elderly, the problem is usually related to inadequate cardiovascular response to heat with disruption of normal compensatory mechanisms. Patients frequently complain of cramps, headache, fatigue, nausea, and vomiting. They appear listless, with pallor of the skin and profuse sweating. Other clinical findings include orthostatic hypotension, core temperatures of 37.5 to 39° C (99.5 to 102.2° F), altered mental status, incoordination, and diffuse weakness.

TABLE 71-1. FACTORS PREDISPOSING TO HYPERTHERMIA

Patient factors	Medical conditions
Lack of acclimatization	Alcoholism
Dehydration	Neurologic lesions/events
Exercise when poorly trained	Cardiovascular disease
Fever/infection	Skin/sweat gland diseases
Obesity	Diabetes mellitus
Fatigue/exhaustion	Thyrotoxicosis
Excessive clothing	Hypokalemia
Advanced age	COPD
Upper floors of buildings	Psychiatric illness
Environmental factors	**Drugs**
High ambient temperature	Amphetamines
High humidity	Anticholinergics
Lack of wind	Antidepressants
	Antihistamines
	Anti-Parkinson's drugs
	Barbiturates
	Beta blockers
	Butyrophenones
	Diuretics
	Ethanol
	Hallucinogens
	Phenothiazines

Heatstroke, classified as *exertional* or *nonexertional,* is a syndrome due to acute disruption of thermoregulatory mechanisms manifested by central nervous system depression, hypohidrosis, core temperatures $\geq 41°$ C, and severe physiologic and biochemical abnormalities. Exertional heatstroke occurs in people working or exercising in a warm environment with an overwhelmed but unimpaired central thermoregulatory center. Nonexertional heat stroke occurs most frequently in elderly, debilitated, schizophrenic, intoxicated, or paralyzed individuals. These people have impaired central and/or peripheral thermoregulatory mechanisms (*physiologic* or *drug-induced autonomic impairment*), impaired awareness of or inability to leave a hot environment, poor acclimatization, and inadequate ability to increase cardiac output in response to heat.

Consequences of heat-induced cell damage are rhabdomyolysis, cardiac failure and arrhythmias, vasodilation, cytotoxic cerebral edema, hypotension, acute renal failure, adult respiratory distress syndrome (ARDS), gastrointestinal hemorrhage, and acute hepatic

TABLE 71-2. INITIAL DIAGNOSTIC STUDIES: HYPERTHERMIC AND HYPOTHERMIC STATES

ECG
Chest x-ray
CBC
Platelet count
WBC with differential
Serum studies
    Lactate dehydrogenase
    Transaminases
    Alkaline phosphatase
    Bilirubin
    Creatine kinase
    Blood urea nitrogen
    Creatinine
    Phosphate
    Calcium
    Glucose
    Electrolytes
    Uric acid
    Lactate*
    Cortisol*
    TSH, T_3, T_4*
PT and PTT
Fibrin split products
Fibrinogen
Arterial blood gases
Urinalysis
Toxicology screen

* Necessary only in hypothermic states.

failure. Concomitant laboratory abnormalities include hyperkalemia, hypocalcemia, hyperphosphatemia or hypophosphatemia, rising creatinine, hemoconcentration, stress leukocytosis, thrombocytopenia, consumptive coagulopathy, lactic acidosis, hypoglycemia, proteinuria, and an active urinary sediment. Table 71-2 lists diagnostic studies that should be obtained in pathologic states of altered core temperature.

MANAGEMENT. The primary goal of therapy is rapid cooling. Three initial steps include removal from the hot environment, inhibition of thermogenesis, and active cooling. Table 71-3 describes a management protocol. In the emergency room, the patient should be placed on continuous core temperature and electrocardiographic (ECG) monitors. The severity of the patient's clinical condition dictates the aggressiveness of cooling techniques.

Initial therapy may require central venous access, infusing room-temperature glucose/saline or colloidal solutions. For hypotension, fluids should be provided and in emergent situations small doses of isoproterenol may be cautiously infused. Because they impede heat loss, α agonists should be avoided. If hypotension persists, arterial and pulmonary arterial catheters should be inserted to determine cardiac output, ventricular filling pressures, and vascular resistance. Bicarbonate, if indicated, should be supplied as an isotonic infusion with frequent pH monitoring. Blood pH should be maintained at approximately 7.30. Phosphate should be replaced if the level approaches 1 mg per deciliter. If tetany occurs or ionized calcium is low, calcium should be infused. Corticosteroids and antibiotics are not routine therapy and should be used only when concurrent clinical conditions dictate. Supraventricular tachycardia is common with severe hyperthermia, is resistant to therapy, and usually resolves spontaneously as core temperature declines toward normal. Digoxin should be avoided because hyperkalemia is frequent in these patients and the risk of heart block is high.

Heat cramps and exhaustion rarely result in permanent sequelae, and in heatstroke, mild to moderate neurologic, hepatic, and renal dysfunction usually resolves after return to normothermia. Muscle weakness may persist for several months when rhabdomyolysis has been severe. The greater the severity of injury, the greater is the likelihood of permanent sequelae. Mortality for heatstroke may approach 50% and is usually associated with advanced age and severe organ failure.

Neuroleptic malignant syndrome (NMS) is a complex of extrapyramidal muscular rigidity (see Ch. 407-412), high core temperature, altered level of consciousness, and elevated creatine kinase levels occurring as an acute or subacute reaction to therapy with neuroleptic medications.

Malignant hyperthermia (see Ch. 457) is a hypermetabolic, myopathic syndrome, chemically or stress induced, and is manifested by an abrupt rise in core temperature, vigorous muscle contractions, metabolic and respiratory acidosis, and ventricular arrhythmias, usually when inducing anesthesia.

HYPOTHERMIC SYNDROMES. *Hypothermia,* defined as a core body temperature $< 35°$ C ($95°$ F), is classified as *accidental* (primary) or *secondary.* The accidental form is defined as a spontaneous decrease of core temperature to $< 35°$ C, usually in a cold

TABLE 71-3. MANAGEMENT OF HYPERTHERMIA

1. Protect the airway
2. Insert at least two large-bore IVs
3. Monitor core temperature
    a. PA catheter
    b. Rectal probe
    c. Esophageal probe
4. Actively cool the skin until core temperature reaches $39°$ C
    a. Exposure to cool environment
    b. Wetting with water (avoid alcohol rubs)
    c. Continuous fanning
    d. Ice baths/immersion ($22°$ C)
    e. Axillary/perineal ice packs
    f. Infuse of room-temperature saline
    g. Gastric/colonic iced saline lavage
    h. Peritoneal lavage with cool saline
5. If shivering occurs, administer chlorpromazine, 10 to 25 mg intramuscularly
6. Monitor for seizures
7. Monitor ECG for dysrhythmia
8. Obtain serial diagnostic studies (see Table 71-2)

TABLE 71-4. FACTORS PREDISPOSING TO HYPOTHERMIA

Patient factors	Medical conditions
Inadequate clothing	Alcoholism
Extremes of age	Burns, severe
Mental impairment	Cancer chemotherapy
Immobility	Cardiac failure
Altered level of consciousness	CNS lesions/events
Debility and exhaustion	Dementia
Wet clothing	Encephalopathy
Drugs	Diabetes, complications
Alcohol	Hypoadrenalism
Anesthetics	Hypoglycemia
Antidepressants	Hypopituitarism
Antithyroid agents	Malnutrition
Cannabis	Myxedema
Hypoglycemic agents	Prolonged CPR
Major tranquilizers	Prolonged surgery
Narcotics	Sepsis
Paralyzing agents	Shock
Sedative/hypnotics	Uremia

TABLE 71-5. MANAGEMENT OF HYPOTHERMIA

Mild hypothermia (34-36° C)
1. Remove from cold environment, replace wet clothing, cover with blankets or equivalent, use gentle passive rewarming techniques.
2. Give warm oxygen through a mask or an endotracheal tube.
3. Give warm dextrose/saline intravenous fluids.
4. Warm the environment (thermostat, overhead lights).
5. Monitor ECG, respiratory status, core temperature.
6. Obtain initial diagnostic studies (see Table 71-2).

Moderate to severe hypothermia (≤ 33° C)
1. Admit to intensive care unit.
2. Peripheral active rewarming: heating blankets, heating pads, hot-water bottles, warming lights, warm-water immersion.
3. Actively warm central core: inhale heated, humidified oxygen, gastric lavage, colonic irrigation, and warmed intravenous fluids.
4. Consider special beds, and protect against pressure necrosis.
5. If core temperature is not rising 0.5 to 1.0° C per hour, consider peritoneal dialysis, bladder lavage, hemodialysis, or bypass.
6. Anticipate multiorgan dysfunction and secondary infection.

environment, often but not necessarily associated with an acute medical problem, and without a primary disturbance of the temperature-regulating center.

Secondary hypothermia is characterized by dysfunction of hypothalamic thermoregulation. An underlying illness or drug is often the predisposing factor. Table 71-4 lists conditions and factors related to hypothermia.

Hypothermia affects virtually every body system due to generalized slowing of enzymatic activity, peripheral vasoconstriction, and uncoupling of oxygen-dependent metabolism. Alterations in cardiovascular physiology include an early catecholamine-mediated increase in heart rate, cardiac output, and mean arterial pressure. Later, negative inotropic and chronotropic effects of hypothermia and decreased effective blood volume cause diminished cardiac output and tissue perfusion.

Patients may present with tachypnea, but as hypothermia becomes pronounced, there is depression of the respiratory center. Shivering increases oxygen consumption. Because alveolar ventilation is decreased, Pa_{O_2} may decline to subnormal levels. Hypoxemia also may result from aspiration pneumonia, pulmonary edema, or ARDS.

The ECG may demonstrate sinus bradycardia and slowing of conduction with atrioventricular block, prolonged QT interval, widened QRS complex, and T-wave inversion. P waves may be absent. After core temperature reaches 32° C, the classic Osborne (or J) wave appears (Fig. 71-1). The cold heart is highly irritable, and any physical stimulation may lead to ventricular fibrillation.

Due to enzyme damage, renal concentrating ability is lost, resulting in very dilute (cold diuresis) urine and systemic hyperosmolarity. Later, with decreased perfusion, acute tubular necrosis may develop. Laboratory abnormalities include metabolic acidosis, hyperkalemia, hyponatremia, hyperglycemia, and hyperphosphatemia. Complications of hypothermia also include rhabdomyolysis, gastric dilatation, ileus, upper gastrointestinal bleeding, acute pancreatitis, and severe hepatic dysfunction. Hematologic alterations include hemoconcentration, increased blood viscosity, thrombocytopenia, granulocytopenia, and consumptive coagulopathy. Infection is a frequent sequela of hypothermia.

Hypothermia should be considered in the differential diagnosis of any hypotensive, comatose patient. Initial evaluation (see Table 71-2) should be directed toward identifying predisposing conditions such as those listed in Table 71-4.

MANAGEMENT (Table 71-5). The goals of management are to prevent further heat loss, increase core temperature, and anticipate and prevent complications. If the person is without vital signs, cardiopulmonary resuscitation should be initiated and continued until the patient is normothermic. Hospital management depends somewhat on the severity of hypothermia and should follow recommendations made in Table 71-5.

Due to liver impairment and cardiac irritability, all drugs must be used with caution. Digitalis should be avoided. If myxedema or panhypopituitarism is suspected, proper hormonal replacement therapy should be initiated. Dysrhythmias can be treated safely with lidocaine, propranolol, and bretylium. Electrocardioversion is rarely successful. Vasoactive agents may be required for severe hypotension. Intravenous sodium bicarbonate should be used only in severe acidosis (pH <7.1) and with extreme caution.

Gibb WRG, Lees AJ: The neuroleptic malignant syndrome—a review. Q J Med 56:421, 1985. *A detailed review of NMS, including pathogenesis, epidemiology, clinical characteristics, complications, and management. Also includes 96 references.*

Nelson TE, Flewellen EH: The malignant hyperthermia syndrome. N Engl J Med 309:416, 1983. *A very concise review of this rare condition, including causes, diagnostic criteria, clinical characteristics, and basics of management.*

Simon HB: Hyperthermia. N Engl J Med 329:483, 1993. *A complete review of hyperthermia, including pathophysiology, clinical presentation, and details of management.*

Weinberg AD: Hypothermia. Ann Emerg Med 22:370, 1993. *An up-to-date review of hypothermia with emphasis on management, including recent advances.*

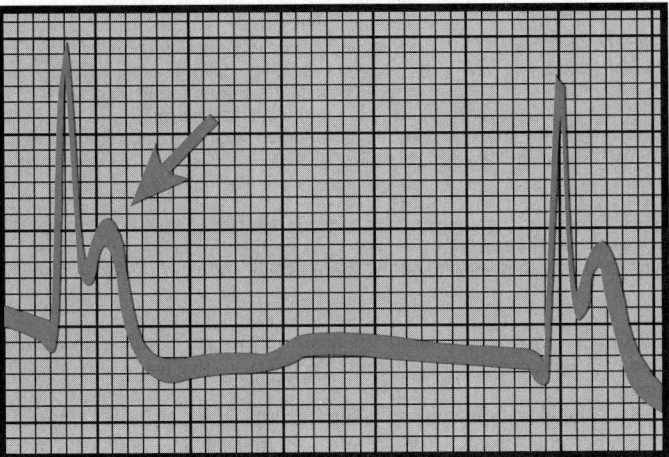

FIGURE 71-1. J (Osborne) wave.

72 ACUTE POISONING*
Lester M. Haddad

Defining the extent of human poisoning is not easy, since the three major sources of data have different viewpoints and surely overlap. The Toxic Exposure Surveillance System (TESS) of the American Association of Poison Control Centers tabulates information phone calls and in 1992 recorded 1,864,188 exposures with 705 deaths, cyclic antidepressants being the leading cause.

* The author wishes to thank James F. Winchester, M.D., and the many contributors to the textbook *Clinical Management of Poisoning and Drug Overdose,* edited by LM Haddad and JF Winchester.

TABLE 72–1. COMMON EMERGENCY ANTIDOTES

Poison	Antidote	Adult Dosage*	Comments
Acetaminophen	N-Acetylcysteine	140 mg/kg initial oral dose, followed by 70 mg/kg q4h × 17 doses	Most effective within 16 hours; may be useful up to 24 hours; IV NAC protocols available
Atropine	Physostigmine	Initial dose 0.5–2 mg (IV)	Can produce convulsions, bradycardia
Benzodiazepines	Flumazenil	0.2 mg (2cc) (IV) over 15 seconds; repeat 0.2 mg (IV) every minute as necessary; initial dose not to exceed 1 mg	Recommended *only* for reversal of pure benzodiazepine sedation; competitive GABA antagonist
β blockers	Glucagon	1 mg/ml ampule; 5–10 mg (IV) initially	Stimulates cyclic AMP synthesis, increasing myocardial contractility
Calcium channel blockers	Calcium	Calcium chloride 10% 1 gram (10 ml) (IV) over 5 minutes as initial dose; repeat as necessary in critical patients	Each syringe contains 1 gram or 10 ml of 10% calcium chloride; each milliliter contains 100 mg of calcium chloride or 1.4 mEq of Ca^{2+}
Carbon monoxide	Oxygen		Hyperbaric oxygen may be indicated
Cyanide	Amyl nitrate, *then* sodium nitrite	Pearls every 2 minutes; 10 ml of 3% solution over 3 minutes (IV); 0.33 ml (10 mg 3% solution)/kg initially for children	Methemoglobin cyanide complex; causes hypotension; dosage assumes normal hemoglobin
	Sodium thiosulfate	25% solution 50 ml (IV) over 10 minutes; 1.65 ml/kg for children	Forms harmless sodium thiocyanate
Digitalis	Digibind FAB antibodies	IV dose of Digibind in critical patients with unknown ingestion = 800 mg (20 vials); dosage if serum digoxin and patient's weight (in kg) are known: the number of vials to administer = [concentration (in ng/ml) × 5.6 × kg]/600	FAB (antigen-binding fragments); IV dose of Digibind should be equimolar to total body load of digoxin; one vial of Digibind contains 40 mg of FAB fragments, which neutralizes 0.6 mg digoxin; the number of milligrams of digoxin ingested divided by 0.6 is the number of vials required; indicated for life-threatening cardiac arrhythmias, hyperkalemia, serum digoxin level > 10 ng/ml
Hydrofluoric acid	Calcium	Calcium gluconate gel or calcium carbonate paste; 10% calcium gluconate 10 ml in 40 ml D_5W via intra-arterial infusion over 4 hours may be indicated for significant digital hydrofluoric acid burns	A single intra-arterial infusion of 10% calcium gluconate provides 84 mg (4.7 mEq) of elemental calcium to bind fluoride ion, preventing cellular injury and tissue necrosis
Iron	Deferoxamine	Initial dose: 40–90 mg/kg (IM) not to exceed 1 gram; 15 mg/kg/hr (IV)	Deferoxamine mesylate forms excretable ferrioxamine complex
Lead	DMSA (Succimer), 2,3-dimercaptosuccinic acid	5-day course of 30 mg/kg/day in 3 divided doses; then 14-day course of 20 mg/kg/day divided in 2 doses	Succimer 100-mg capsule; oral congener of chelator dimercaprol, indicated for blood lead levels > 45 μg/dl
Mercury (arsenic, gold)	BAL British Anti-Lewisite	5 mg/kg (IM) as soon as possible	Each milliliter of BAL in oil has dimercaprol, 100 mg, in 210 mg (21%) benzyl benzoate and 680 mg peanut oil; forms stable, nontoxic, excretable cyclic compound
Methyl alcohol (ethylene glycol)	Ethyl alcohol in conjunction with dialysis	1 ml/kg of 100% ethanol initially in glucose solution; dilute ethanol to 10%; maintain blood level of 100 mg/dl; maintenance dose 0.15 ml/kg/hour (double during dialysis)	Competes for alcohol dehydrogenase; prevents formation of formic acid, oxalates
Nitrites	Methylene blue	0.2 ml/kg of 1% solution (IV) over 5 minutes	Often exchange transfusion is needed for severe methemoglobinemia
Opiates, Darvon, Lomotil	Naloxone	2.0 mg (IV); 0.1 mg/kg (IV) for children; repeat as needed	Naloxone; no respiratory depression (0.4 mg/1 ml ampule)
Organophosphates	Atropine	Initial dose: 0.5–2 mg (IV); 0.05 mg/kg (IV) initially for children	Physiologic: blocks acetylcholine; cardiac monitoring and proper oxygenation are indicated
	Pralidoxime (2-PAM chloride) (Protopam)	Initial dose: 1 gram (IV); children: 25–50 mg/kg (IV)	Specific: breaks alkyl phosphate–cholinesterase bond; up to 500 mg every hour may be necessary in the critical adult patient
Tricyclic antidepressants	Sodium bicarbonate	Sodium bicarbonate 1–2 ampules (IV); (1 mEq/kg) (IV) bolus for initial dose; (IV) drip to maintain arterial pH of 7.5	One ampule of 50 cc sodium bicarbonate contains 50 mEq $NaHCO_3$ in 50 cc or 1 M sodium bicarbonate; (IV) bolus for life-threatening cardiac arrhythmias

* Dosages listed may require modification according to specific clinical conditions; see each specific chapter for details.

Updated and adapted from Haddad LM, Winchester JF (eds): Clinical Management of Poisoning and Drug Overdose (2nd ed.). Philadelphia, WB Saunders, 1990; and the American College of Emergency Physicians poster on poisoning, Dallas, Texas, 1980.

Ninety-nine percent of all significant poisoning presents directly to a hospital emergency department. The National Institute of Drug Abuse surveys emergency room visits through the Drug Abuse Warning Network (DAWN) and in 1991 reported a total of 15,570 deaths (including trauma victims) in which drugs were at least implicated and 6601 deaths in which the major cause of death was overdose, most commonly cocaine. The National Center of Health Statistics reviews primarily medical examiner death certificates and yearly reports carbon monoxide (CO) as the leading cause of death.

Poisoning is defined as "to injure or kill with poison, a chemical substance that usually kills, injures, or impairs an organism." The terms "poisoning" and "drug overdose" often are used interchangeably, especially with prescription drugs, although, by definition, a drug overdose does not produce poisoning unless it causes clinical symptoms.

The modern era of clinical treatment of poisons began in the specialty of pediatrics, with the development of safety caps for St. Joseph's aspirin in 1959. Deaths by overdose became almost commonplace in the early 1960's, dramatized by the tragic death of Marilyn Monroe from an overdose of barbiturates. Dialysis to remove drugs was subsequently introduced as a therapeutic regimen. The nationwide growth of hospital emergency departments and the proliferation of street drugs (see Ch. 12) such as quaaludes, LSD, PCP, and subsequently cocaine necessitated rapid involvement in toxicology by emergency physicians.

The most common causes of poisoning death in the United States have been CO, cocaine, and tricyclic antidepressants. Analgesics remain a leading cause. Calcium channel blocker overdose has surpassed digitalis as the most common cause of cardiovascular drug death.

DIAGNOSIS AND EMERGENCY MANAGEMENT. The general approach to the poisoned patient may be divided into seven phases: (1) emergency management, (2) clinical evaluation, (3) eliminating poison from the gastrointestinal tract, skin, and eyes or removal from the site of exposure in inhalation poisoning, (4) administering an antidote, (5) elimination of absorbed substance, (6) supportive therapy, and (7) observation and disposition.

Emergency Management. Since overdose patients often present moribund, resuscitation with airway establishment, adequate ventilation and perfusion, and maintaining all vital signs (including temperature) must first be accomplished. Continuous cardiac and pulse oximetry monitoring is essential. Rapid-sequence intubation may be indicated. Naloxone 2 mg (IV), thiamine 100 mg (IV), and 50% glucose 50 cc (IV) (if the patient by Dextrostix is hypoglycemic) are given to all patients in coma after inserting an intravenous (IV) line and drawing appropriate blood samples. Maintaining blood pressure and tissue perfusion may require adequate volume replacement, correcting acid–base disturbance, antidotal therapy (e.g., IV calcium with calcium channel blocker overdose, sodium bicarbonate with tricyclic antidepressant overdose), and pressor agents. Table 72–1 lists the common emergency antidotes. Cardiac arrhythmias and seizures should be treated appropriately if possible.

Clinical Evaluation. Any patient presenting with multisystem involvement should be suspected of poisoning until proved otherwise. A thorough history and physical examination are essential. While the initial manifestations of poisoning are legion, a patient with acute poisoning often presents with *coma, cardiac arrhythmia* (Table 72–2), *seizures* (Table 72–3), *metabolic acidosis,* and/or *gastrointestinal disturbances,* either together as symptom complexes or as isolated events. Symptom complexes, or *toxic syndromes,* may give clues to an unknown poisoning. For example, a patient with a history of depression who presents in coma with seizures, a widened QRS complex or dysrhythmia on electrocardiogram (ECG), and dilated pupils suggests tricyclic antidepressant overdose. *Hepatic, renal, respiratory,* and *hematologic* disturbances are generally delayed manifestations of poisoning. Table 72–4 lists important clues on physical examination. Laboratory evaluation generally supports the assessment. Table 72–5 lists specific blood studies which may direct therapy.

Elimination of Poison. In the event of *inhalation,* such as smoke, CO, hydrogen sulfide, or chlorine gas, removing the patient from the site of exposure and administering 100% oxygen is indicated. Caustic alkalis, acids, and other chemicals should be removed from the *eye* with copious irrigation by normal saline, at least 30 minutes for caustic alkalis. Ophthalmologic consultation is emergently indicated for caustic alkali exposure. *Skin* exposure requires 30-minute irrigation as well.

The majority of poisoning occurs via the gastrointestinal tract. Gastric decontamination is indicated to reduce absorption of the poisonous substance. Principal modalities in historical order include syrup of ipecac, gastric lavage, activated charcoal, and whole-bowel irrigation. Controversy has raged over which modality is most effective, and several experimental and clinical studies have sought to find a solution. There has been no resolution of the issue, since with each individual patient the exact amount ingested and the exact amount remaining after each procedure is never known.

Syrup of ipecac is still indicated for home use. Dosage recommendations include ages 6 to 12 months, 10 ml; ages 1 to 12 years, 15 ml; and age 12 years to adulthood, 30 ml. Contraindications to ipecac include caustic or petroleum distillate ingestion, impending or frank coma, and seizures. Because both gastric lavage and activated charcoal have each demonstrated superiority over ipecac in recent studies, ipecac is seldom used in the hospital emergency room today, although it is still useful in the child who will not drink charcoal and whose parents will not allow a nasogastric tube.

Gastric lavage has been shown to be effective within the first hour of ingestion, and with proper airway management, it is indicated for the critical patient with a recent life-threatening ingestion such as theophylline, tricyclic antidepressants, calcium channel blockers, digoxin, salicylate, or unknown substance. Use the largest-bore tube possible, such as a 36 French Ewald with gravity drainage. Activated charcoal may be beneficial prior to lavage and is indicated after lavage. Gastric lavage is contraindicated in caustic ingestion.

Activated charcoal is considered safe and adequate treatment for the majority of overdoses, especially for those patients who are awake or have ingested only a mildly toxic substance. The dose is 1 gram per kilogram, or 50 to 100 grams in an adult. Commercial preparations of charcoal usually include sorbitol as a cathartic, and while this has never been proven effective, it is safe except for the very young. Table 72–6 lists toxins not effectively absorbed by charcoal. Serially administered activated charcoal (50 grams every four hours) has a role in inpatient management of overdose of drugs that enter the hepatobiliary circulation (digitoxin, tricyclic antidepressants, glutethimide) or diffuse into the gastrointestinal lumen (theophylline and phenobarbital).

Whole-bowel irrigation with a nonabsorbable osmotically active compound such as polyethylene glycol (GoLYTELY) is a new means of catharsis. In adults, 240 ml by mouth or nasogastric tube every 10 to 15 minutes is given until the gallon container is emp-

TABLE 72–3. COMMON TOXIC CAUSES OF SEIZURES

Amoxapine	LSD
Anticholinergics	Oral hypoglycemics
Camphor	Parathion
Carbon monoxide	Phencyclidine
Cocaine	Phenothiazines
Ergotamine	Propoxyphene
Insulin	Propranolol
Isoniazid	Strychnine
Lead	Theophylline
Lindane	Tricyclic antidepressants
Lithium	

TABLE 72–2. COMMON TOXIC CAUSES OF CARDIAC ARRHYTHMIA

Tricyclic antidepressants	Digitalis
Arsenic	Dinitrophenols
β blockers	Fluoroacetate
Calcium channel blockers	Phenol
Carbon monoxide	Phenothiazines
Chloral hydrate	Phosphorus
Chloroquine	Physostigmine
Clonidine	Quinine
Cocaine	Succinylcholine
Cyanide	

TABLE 72–4. IMPORTANT CLUES ON PHYSICAL EXAMINATION

Clinical Finding	Diagnostic Example
Needle tracks	IV drug abuse
Characteristic odor of breath	Gasoline
Destruction of nasal mucosa/cartilage	Cocaine
New significant heart murmur	Infective endocarditis
Pulmonary edema	Heroin
Boardlike abdomen	Black widow spider bite
Changes in neurologic status	Organophosphates

TABLE 72-5. TOXICOLOGIC BLOOD STUDIES WHICH MAY DIRECT THERAPY

Acetaminophen
Digoxin
Dilantin
Ethylene glycol
Iron
Lithium
Methanol
Salicylate
Theophylline

TABLE 72-7. TREATMENT METHODS FOR ELIMINATION OF ABSORBED SUBSTANCE

Forced diuresis	Hemodialysis
Phenobarbital	Lithium
Salicylate	Methanol
Alkalinization of urine	Ethylene glycol
Salicylate	Salicylate
Barbiturates	**Hemoperfusion**
	Theophylline
	Barbiturates

tied or the rectal effluent becomes clear. Whole-bowel irrigation is probably useful for awake, functional patients who have ingested iron tablets, sustained-release preparations such as theophylline or calcium channel blockers, or "crack" vials or cocaine packets.

Other modalities include milk for caustic ingestion and as a general demulcent; potassium permanganate for quinine, strychnine, and nicotine poisoning; sodium polystyrene sulfonate for lithium overdose; and sodium bicarbonate for iron poisoning.

Antidotes. With the development of sophisticated new antidotes and the changing spectrum of clinical poisoning, the use of emergency antidotes has become the primary treatment method in clinical toxicology. Table 72-1 lists the common emergency antidotes. With known poisoning, early use is indicated to provide emergency stabilization, often within the first hour. Admission to an intensive care unit following antidotal therapy is often indicated.

Elimination of Absorbed Substance. Table 72-7 outlines treatment methods and indications for elimination of absorbed substances, such as charcoal hemoperfusion and hemodialysis. Hemodialysis is also indicated for any drug overdose patient who has severe intractable metabolic acidosis, electrolyte abnormalities, or renal failure.

Supportive Therapy. Observation and prudent medical care are the mainstay of therapy for the toxic patient and may be all that is necessary for the majority of patients. Indiscriminately using drugs, antidotes, and gastric lavage should be avoided. Hospitalization in an intensive care unit is often indicated for the serious poisoning.

SPECIFIC AGENTS. *Acetaminophen* is one of the three leading over-the-counter analgesics (Tylenol, Panadol, and Tempra) and thus is one of the leading causes of drug overdose in the United States and the leading cause in the United Kingdom. It is also a leading cause of liver failure. Acetaminophen is metabolized in the liver and is relatively safe in therapeutic doses. A small fraction of each administered dose is converted to a reactive metabolite, *N*-acetyl-*p*-benzoquinoneimine (NAPQI), by the cytochrome P450–dependent mixed-function oxidase hepatic enzymes. With therapeutic doses, glutathione stores can detoxify NAPQI by conjugation. Glutathione stores are depleted in overdoses, however, and NAPQI covalently binds to cellular proteins, producing hepatocellular necrosis.

The therapeutic dose of acetaminophen is 10 to 20 mg per kilogram every four hours. Toxicity is likely to occur after a minimum acute ingestion of 140 mg per kilogram, or about 10 grams in an adult. Acetaminophen poisoning clinically produces only nausea, vomiting, and anorexia 12 to 24 hours after ingestion. Hepatic coma and coagulopathy do not occur until 48 to 96 hours after ingestion, after irreversible hepatic necrosis has occurred. *N*-Acetylcysteine (NAC, Mucomyst) is the drug of choice for acetaminophen overdose. NAC effectively prevents hepatotoxicity if given within 8

TABLE 72-6. TOXINS NOT EFFECTIVELY ABSORBED BY CHARCOAL

Acids	Heavy metals
Alcohols	Hydrocarbons
Alkalis	Iron
Carbamates	Lithium
Cyanide	Organophosphates
Ethylene glycol	

hours; it is strongly effective if given within 16 hours and may be effective up to and perhaps beyond 24 hours. NAC therapy should be instituted when a 4-hour acetaminophen level ≥ 150 μg per milliliter, an 8-hour level of 75 μg per milliliter, or a 12-hour level of 37.5 μg per milliliter. Because NAC therapy may be effective 24 hours after ingestion, the presence of any measurable acetaminophen or biochemical evidence of hepatic injury at 24 hours is an indication to start NAC therapy. The oral dose of NAC is 140 mg per kilogram initially and then 70 mg per kilogram every 4 hours for 17 doses. Both 20- and 48-hour intravenous NAC protocols are available but are presently under investigation.

The *salicylates* (aspirin) remain a leading cause of analgesic drug overdose. The association of Reye's syndrome with aspirin and introduction of the safety cap have produced a dramatic fall in use and accidental poisoning in the pediatric age group. Salicylates inhibit the cyclo-oxygenase enzyme of the prostaglandin synthetase complex, uncouple oxidative phosphorylation, and produce respiratory alkalosis and a high anion gap metabolic acidosis. Salicylates are metabolized by first-order kinetics and are conjugated with glycine and glucuronic acid; as plasma concentrations rise in overdose and glycine stores are depleted, zero-order kinetics prevail, and renal excretion of salicylate becomes prominent.

Clinical presentation includes tinnitus, hearing loss, diaphoresis, facial flushing, hyperpyrexia, and hyperventilation. With severe salicylate poisoning, patients progressively develop dehydration, hypernatremia, pulmonary edema, purpura and gastrointestinal bleeding, and death. A plasma salicylate level of > 30 mg per deciliter indicates salicylate toxicity, and a level of 80 to 100 mg per deciliter indicates critical salicylate poisoning.

The treatment of choice for salicylate poisoning is a forced alkaline diuresis with sodium bicarbonate; correcting fluid, electrolyte, and acid–base disturbances; vitamin K supplementation; and supportive care. Hemodialysis is indicated for patients whose salicylate level is > 100 mg per deciliter, patients who do not respond to a trial of bicarbonate therapy, or patients whose condition is critical.

Ibuprofen is the leading nonsteroidal anti-inflammatory drug (NSAID) and has become a common prescription and over-the-counter product. While a common cause of overdose, ibuprofen produces only mild toxicity, primarily gastroenteritis. Supportive care is all that is generally indicated.

The incidence of *anticholinergic* poisoning has dramatically decreased since atropine, scopolamine, and hyoscyamine have been removed from over-the-counter sleep medications. Overdoses of benztropine, amantadine, and prescription sinus, gastrointestinal, and eye medications are still seen occasionally, as well as abuse of Jimson weed, the plant *Datura stramonium*, and the mushroom *Amanita muscaria*. Emergency rooms still have victims of theft present psychotic and delirious after being poisoned by scopolamine eye drops.

The classic anticholinergic syndrome is produced by blockade of acetylcholine with central and peripheral effects: psychosis, delirium, seizures, flushing, dry mucous membranes and skin, hyperpyrexia, dilated pupils, and urinary retention.

The antidote *physostigmine* should be reserved only for severe cases of pure anticholinergic poisoning. Physostigmine should *not* be used for agents with anticholinergic properties such as cyclic antidepressants. The initial dose of physostigmine is 0.5 to 2 mg (IV) slowly in adults (0.02 mg per kilogram for children). The maximum dose is not to exceed 4 mg in 30 minutes in adults. Cardiac monitoring is essential, since physostigmine has caused asystole, bradycardia, and seizures.

Barbiturates still comprise a major source of overdose and mortality. Largely replaced as prescription sleep medication by the benzodiazepines, barbiturates still present in headache prescriptions such as butalbital (Fiorinal and Esgic), and the sleep medications such as secobarbital (Seconal) are common drugs of abuse. Phenobarbital is one of the leading anticonvulsant medications. Thiopental is an essential intravenous anesthetic for in-hospital rapid-sequence intubation or as a sedative prior to cardioversion and surgery.

The barbiturates have been classified as long-acting (phenobarbital), intermediate-acting (butabarbital), short-acting (secobarbital), and ultra-short-acting (thiopental). Phenobarbital is excreted primarily unchanged by the kidney, whereas most barbiturates are metabolized by the liver. The barbiturates are the classic sedative-hypnotics and in overdose produce depression of the central nervous (CNS) and cardiovascular systems, with coma, hypotension, loss of reflexes, hypothermia, respiratory arrest, and death. A characteristic of a barbiturate overdose is the persistence of the pupillary light reflex even with stage IV coma. Bullous skin lesions often occur over pressure areas.

Treatment of the critical patient involves gastric lavage and activated charcoal after securing the airway, mechanical ventilation, resuscitation of cardiovascular status, and supportive care in an intensive care unit. Forced alkaline diuresis is specifically indicated for phenobarbital, since it is a weak acid that is excreted unchanged in the urine. Charcoal hemoperfusion and hemodialysis have a role in barbiturate overdose for those critical patients who do not respond to conservative therapy.

The *benzodiazepines* have become extremely popular, and the 13 now available have virtually replaced other sedative-hypnotics. All benzodiazepines are effective anxiolytics and sedatives, and they have varying properties as muscle relaxants, anticonvulsants, and amnestics. In addition, diazepam (Valium), lorazepam (Ativan), and midazolam (Versed) have major therapeutic roles as intravenous drugs for in-hospital use as anticonvulsants, preanesthetics, and sedatives.

While the benzodiazepines are common agents involved in overdose, they generally cause only coma and ataxia; mortality is rare, and supportive care is all that is usually necessary. The new antidote flumazenil is reserved only for reversing in-hospital benzodiazepine sedation. Its use in the general overdose patient or patient with head injury or coma of unknown etiology is *not* recommended, since flumazenil has been reported to cause seizures in patients who have co-ingested benzodiazepines and cyclic antidepressants and has caused increased intracranial pressure in patients with head injury.

The *calcium channel blockers* are now the most common antihypertensive agents in the United States and also are now the most common cause of cardiovascular drug death by overdose. They are marketed as 9 pharmacologic agents primarily to treat hypertension and angina in the 13 commercial preparations listed in Table 72–8.

The calcium channel blockers are highly toxic in overdose with significant mortality. A special problem is presented by the sustained-release preparations, which allow for continued absorption. Persistent hypotension, bradycardia with atrioventricular block (especially with verapamil), coma, the development of pulmonary edema, and cardiac arrest may comprise the clinical picture. Treatment must be aggressive if these patients are to survive, and high-dose IV calcium is the therapeutic drug of choice. Whole-bowel irrigation with polyethylene glycol is indicated if sustained-release preparations have been ingested. IV 10% calcium chloride 1-gram bolus (over 5 minutes) may be lifesaving, and 1 gram (IV) every 15 minutes over the first hour may be necessary in critical patients. This is followed by 10% calcium chloride via continuous IV infusion until blood pressure stabilizes, the dosage and rate depending on the clinical condition. For those patients who do not respond to

high-dose calcium therapy, dopamine, dobutamine, amrinone, epinephrine, and/or glucagon have been employed with varying results. Glucagon is indicated in those patients with concomitant β-blocker overdose. Pacing may be necessary, especially with verapamil overdose. Symptomatic patients and those patients who have ingested sustained-release preparations should be admitted to the critical care unit for continuous ECG monitoring for at least 24 hours after stabilization.

Carbon monoxide is the leading cause of death from poisoning in the United States. CO is a colorless, odorless, tasteless gas produced by incomplete combustion of carbon materials. CO has a 200 times greater affinity for hemoglobin than oxygen and thus produces cellular hypoxia and death. New research suggests that CO produces injury by other mechanisms. Fires, smoke, wood-burning stoves, gas space heaters, and engine exhaust are sources of unintentional poisoning. Since the heart and brain are the most sensitive to hypoxic insult, clinical presentation usually involves CNS or cardiac symptoms—headache, altered mental status, convulsions, chest pain, cardiac arrhythmia, and/or acute myocardial infarction.

Since most patients receive oxygen on the way to the emergency room, the carboxyhemoglobin level is usually an unreliable indicator of the extent of poisoning. In general, the deeper the level of coma of the patient, the greater is the chance of neuropsychiatric sequelae.

Treat CO poisoning with oxygen. Breathing room air, it takes a patient 6 hours to halve his/her carboxyhemoglobin level ($T_{1/2}$); breathing 100% oxygen, the CO $T_{1/2}$ is 90 minutes; hyperbaric oxygen at 2.5 atmospheres of pressure absolute (ATA) reduces the CO $T_{1/2}$ to less than 1 hour. Because of this and because hyperbaric oxygen has been demonstrated to reduce the incidence of neurologic sequelae, hyperbaric oxygen has become the standard of care for treating CO patients with coma and altered mental status. Table 72–9 lists specific indications for hyperbaric oxygen therapy of CO poisoning.

Fortunately, the incidence of *caustic alkali* ingestion has fallen dramatically thanks to the reduction of lye in liquid products to ≤5%. Clinitest tablets, button batteries >20 mm in diameter, and intentional ingestion are the major causes of morbidity. Because solid crystals adhere to the tongue and cause burning, they uncommonly produce esophageal burn. While the extent of burn cannot be determined by symptoms, drooling in children and inability to swallow are highly suggestive. Mouth burns are suggestive; the absence of mouth burns does not exclude esophageal burn. Milk is the only possible home antidote but must be given immediately. There are those who claim they can detect all significant burns by performing esophagoscopy within 12 hours, but others prefer to wait 24 to 72 hours following ingestion. A 3-week course of methylprednisolone 2.5 mg per kilogram per day to prevent esophageal stricture has been the mainstay of therapy, but this has recently come into question. Esophageal dilation and, if necessary, gastric tube esophageal replacement are indicated for treating esophageal stricture.

Cocaine is the leading cause of death from illicit drug abuse in the United States. Cocaine is an alkaloid of the plant *Erythoxylon coca* which grows in the Andes Mountains. Cocaine alkaloid benzolymethylecgonine is metabolized to benzoylecgonine and ecgonine methyl ester and is excreted in the urine for 24 to 36 hours following administration. Cocaine in the acid form as the hydrochloride can be inhaled nasally or injected intravenously. Cocaine HCl can be converted to basic form and smoked as crack or as free base from a water pipe (see Ch. 12).

Cocaine is a powerful sympathomimetic and CNS stimulant and increases both heart rate and blood pressure, as well as social activ-

---

TABLE 72–8. THE CALCIUM CHANNEL BLOCKERS

Diltiazem (Cardizem, Dilacor)
Nifedipine (Procardia, Adalat)
Verapamil (Calan, Isoptin, Verelan)
Amlodipine (Norvasc)
Bepridil (Vascor)
Felodipine (Plendil)
Isradipine (Dynacirc)
Nicardipine (Cardene)
Nimodipine (Nimotop)

TABLE 72–9. CARBON MONOXIDE POISONING: SPECIFIC INDICATIONS FOR HYPERBARIC OXYGEN THERAPY

All comatose patients
Patients with neurologic impairment by examination or psychometric testing
Patients with carboxyhemoglobin levels >40%
Cardiovascular involvement (chest pain, ECG changes, arrhythmias)
Pregnant patients with CO levels >15%
Patients who do not respond to 100% oxygen
Patients with recurrent symptoms up to 3 weeks after exposure

ity. In overdose, cocaine induces primarily cardiac, neurologic, and psychophysiologic effects. Cardiac effects include palpitations, chest pains, ischemia, acute myocardial infarction, cardiac arrhythmia, and/or cardiac arrest. Neurologic events include altered mental status, seizures often progressing to status epilepticus, focal neurologic signs, and ischemic stroke. The obstetric and neonatal complications must be kept in mind when appropriate. Suicide attempts and violent behavior are often part of the acute cocaine experience.

Cocaine toxicity should be suspected in all young patients who present to the emergency room with chest pain, palpitations, cardiac arrhythmia, or cardiac arrest; altered mental status, seizures, or other neurologic signs; or any bizarre illness inappropriate for the patient's age.

Emergency management consists of supportive therapy, cardiac monitoring, and management of complications. The common presentation of the patient with palpitations (secondary to sinus tachycardia), hypertension, and excitability is generally managed with observation, although judicious use of IV labetalol—which has both α- and β-blocking effects—may be clinically helpful. Patients with chest pain are often admitted because they may have either coronary vasospasm or acute myocardial infarction. Nitrates and/or calcium channel blockers may be warranted if angina is present. Thrombolytic therapy may be indicated for acute myocardial infarction. Grand mal seizures are common, and standard therapy with IV benzodiazepines, phenytoin, or phenobarbital may not be successful because these patients often progress to status epilepticus. Should status epilepticus occur, paralysis with pancuronium bromide and pentobarbital- or thiopental-induced coma with electroencephalographic (EEG) monitoring may be warranted. Correction of the high anion gap metabolic acidosis is indicated, and observation and treatment for rhabdomyolysis may be necessary. In addition to psychiatric follow-up, those patients who used cocaine intravenously must be screened for hepatitis, HIV, and other complications of IV drug use.

The *stimulants* amphetamine and phenylpropanolamine produce effects clinically similar to those of cocaine but generally more benign and of shorter duration.

The most common cause of *cyanide* poisoning is smoke inhalation. A source to the public is acetonitrile in the form of acrylic nail remover. Hydrogen cyanide gas is a fumigant rodenticide. Prolonged administration of nitroprusside can result in elevated cyanide levels. Cyanide poisoning produces cellular hypoxia by binding with the ferric iron of mitochondrial cytochrome oxidase, disrupting the electron transport chain and the ability of cells to use oxygen. Patients who inhale cyanide rapidly develop coma, shock, seizures, lactic acidosis, and respiratory and cardiac arrest. Mild exposures following smoke inhalation are now being described. Diagnosis may be difficult in these patients. Emergency administration of antidote may be lifesaving. Patients with smoke inhalation who have evidence of lactic acidosis should be suspected of cyanide poisoning. The Lilly cyanide antidote kit contains amyl nitrite pearls, 12.5-gram ampules of sodium thiosulfate, and 300-mg ampules of sodium nitrite. The body has a natural enzyme rhodanese which can complex cyanide and sulfur to form thiocyanate, which is only mildly toxic. IV administration of sodium thiosulfate 12.5 grams provides the sulfur necessary to produce thiocyanate and is relatively safe. Because sodium nitrite causes hypotension and methemoglobinemia, its use is reserved for the most critical cases only. Once the new antidote hydroxocobalamin (initial adult dosage 5 grams IV) is approved, a safer alternative for cyanide poisoning will be available.

Digitalis intoxication is still common. Patients who suffer yellow or blurred vision, nausea or vomiting, and sinus bradycardia may respond by simply stopping the drug. Significant digitalis intoxication is heralded by hyperkalemia and major cardiac rhythm disturbances. Virtually every cardiac arrhythmia has occurred with digitalis intoxication. Digoxin-specific FAB antibodies (Digibind) offer a definitive means of therapy and are indicated for life-threatening cardiac arrhythmia, hyperkalemia, a serum digoxin level of 10 ng/ml, or massive overdose of 10 mg or greater in adults or 4 mg in children. Table 72–1 lists three means of calculating dosage. Antidotal therapy should be instituted before conventional therapy in life-threatening situations.

The most common *drugs of abuse* are *alcohol,* the leading cause of drug-related emergency department visits, cocaine (already described), and the *opiates* (see Ch. 11 and 12). The legal definition of intoxication by alcohol is a blood level of 100 mg per deciliter; a lethal blood level is 500 mg per deciliter. However, because of tolerance to alcohol, the patient's mental state may not correlate with the alcohol level. Supportive therapy for acute alcohol intoxication includes restoring fluid, electrolyte, and acid–base balance, and thiamine and magnesium replacement are indicated.

Respiratory arrest and noncardiogenic pulmonary edema are common presentations of IV abuse of heroin and other opiates. The antidote to opiate toxicity is naloxone, which is relatively safe, and it is administered to all patients who present in coma of unknown etiology. The adult dose is 2 mg (IV) repeated as needed up to a total of 10 mg. It is effective against all opiate derivatives, including codeine, propoxyphene, methadone, fentanyl, and diphenoxylate. Naloxone blocks the mu, kappa, and sigma opiate receptors; its effect on the delta receptor is unknown. Because the duration of action of some opiates may exceed that of naloxone, such as methadone, IV naloxone by continuous infusion may be indicated. Supportive therapy for pulmonary edema and complications attendant to IV drug abuse are warranted.

The most common *hallucinogens* are listed in Table 72–10. The synthetic chemical LSD is actually a derivative of woodrose. LSD (100 μg) can produce a full-scale "trip." LSD is not addictive, but it can produce "flashbacks." Phencyclidine (PCP), commonly known as "angel dust," was first produced as a human anesthetic but, because of emergent hallucinosis, was restricted to veterinary use. Its milder analogue ketamine is now used for human anesthesia. Street preparations usually use 1 to 2 mg PCP to produce the desired hallucinogenic effects. While LSD trips are usually self-limiting, phencyclidine and its many synthetic derivatives in overdose cause a serious clinical picture, including nystagmus, hypertensive crisis, sensory anesthesia, hyperpypexia, seizures, and respiratory arrest.

Treating the hallucinating patient involves placing him/her in a quiet room, "talking down" the patient, and sedating him/her with benzodiazepines. Haloperidol may be necessary for prolonged toxic psychosis. While acidification with ascorbic acid markedly increases excretion of phencyclidine, this has fallen into disfavor because acidification in the presence of rhabdomyolysis can precipitate renal failure. Intensive supportive care may be indicated for the critical phencyclidine patient.

Iron poisoning remains a source of mortality to children because their mothers' iron tablets are available to toddlers. Iron poisoning has a direct corrosive action on the stomach and proximal small bowel, and once absorbed, iron produces shock, metabolic acidosis, liver failure, and death. Initially, gastrointestinal symptoms prevail with persistent vomiting, abdominal pain, and hemorrhage. A quiescent phase may be observed, followed by shock, coma, metabolic acidosis, and liver failure. Laboratory data may reveal leukocytosis, hyperglycemia, and radiopaque tablets on a flat plate of the abdomen. A serum iron level should be determined (during peak levels) at 2 to 4 hours after ingestion: > 300 μg per deciliter indicates mild intoxication, and > 500 μg per deciliter indicates serious intoxication. It has been shown recently that a serum iron level in excess of the total iron-binding capacity does not serve as a useful predictive indicator of iron poisoning.

Managing iron poisoning includes gastric lavage with a moderate volume of 1% sodium bicarbonate, which converts iron to insoluble ferrous carbonate salt. Whole-bowel irrigation may be indicated with ingestion of sustained-release capsules. The treatment of choice is the antidote deferoxamine, which chelates free serum iron in the plasma to form ferrioxamine, which is readily excreted and imparts a vin rosé color to the urine. Deferoxamine is indicated for

TABLE 72–10. HALLUCINOGENS

LSD (lysergic acid diethylamide)
PCP (phencyclidine)
Mescaline (the active chemical from the peyote cactus)
Nutmeg
Psilocybin (mushrooms)
Psychotomimetic amphetamines
Woodrose (the active chemical from the morning glory seed)

all critical patients who present with coma, shock, or hemorrhage, for all patients with a serum iron level > 500 μg per deciliter, and for patients who are symptomatic with a serum iron level > 300 μg per deciliter. IV deferoxamine at a rate of 15 mg per kilogram per hour is the preferred initial rate of administration; up to 6 grams may be given in 24 hours. Chelation therapy should continue until the patient becomes stable for at least 24 hours, until the vin rosé urine (when present) becomes clear, and until the serum iron level has fallen below 300 μg per deciliter. Exchange transfusion may be indicated for the unusual patient who is critical and does not respond to chelation therapy.

Lithium intoxication may occur from either acute overdose or chronic administration of lithium carbonate in treating manic depressive psychosis. Lithium has a narrow therapeutic index, and patients who do not have serial blood levels determined during treatment frequently become toxic. Lithium displaces sodium, potassium, magnesium, and calcium in that order. Lithium intoxication produces altered mental status, parkinsonism, and ataxia; gastroenteritis following acute overdose; hypotension, cardiac arrhythmia, and myocarditis; nephrogenic diabetes insipidus; and renal insufficiency. Treatment involves withdrawing the drug and correcting fluid and electrolyte abnormalities in mild intoxication (serum lithium level of 1.5 to 2.5 mEq per liter). Gastric lavage with sodium polystyrene sulfonate is indicated for acute lithium overdose. Patients with moderate acute lithium intoxication (2.5 to 3.5 mEq per liter) who have normal renal function and are asymptomatic may respond to an IV infusion of normal saline to reduce the lithium level. Since lithium is the most dialyzable toxin known, the treatment of choice for lithium intoxication is hemodialysis. Hemodialysis should be used for patients with a serum lithium level > 3.5 mEq per liter or for those who are symptomatic or have impaired renal function and whose level may be ≥ 2.5 mEq per liter or whose condition clinically warrants such treatment.

Methanol and *ethylene glycol* poisoning comprise true medical emergencies. Methanol is most commonly found as the active ingredient in windshield washer fluid, and ethylene glycol constitutes antifreeze; both are also found in many commercial and marine products.

Methanol, or wood alcohol, is converted by alcohol dehydrogenase to formaldehyde and then to formic acid. Signs and symptoms develop over a 24-hour period and include those listed in Table 72–11. Infarction of the putamen noted on magnetic resonance imaging has been described in methanol poisoning. Severe high anion gap metabolic acidosis occurs with an increase in the osmolal gap.

Table 72–11 shows therapy of methanol poisoning.

Metabolism of ethylene glycol by alcohol dehydrogenase causes poisoning by producing severe metabolic acidosis due to aldehyde, glycolate, and lactate formation and the deposition of oxalate crystals in the lungs, heart, and kidneys. Patients show symptoms listed in Table 72–11. Hemodialysis is the treatment of choice for ethylene glycol poisoning and should be instituted as early as possible once the diagnosis is made (Table 72–11).

Isopropanol, or rubbing alcohol, is a common source of ingestion. Approximately 15% of isopropyl alcohol is converted by alcohol dehydrogenase to acetone. Its clinical manifestations are similar to those of ethanol ingestion. Treatment is generally conservative. Although both isopropanol and acetone are readily dialyzable, hemodialysis is seldom necessary in management.

The *organophosphate insecticides* are the insecticides of choice in the agricultural world and are the most common cause of insecticide poisoning. The organophosphates (Table 72–12) are highly popular because they are effective and disintegrate within days of application and do not persist in the environment. Despite educational efforts, these products remain a source of toxicity and death, and the public persists in being unaware that even minute quantities can penetrate the skin and be lethal.

The organophosphates irreversibly inhibit acetylcholinesterase, resulting in an overabundance of acetylcholine at synapses and the myoneural junction, which initially excites and then paralyzes the CNS, the parasympathetic nerve endings and the sweat glands (muscarinic effects), and the somatic nerves and ganglionic synapses of autonomic ganglia (nicotinic effects).

Initial symptoms resemble a flulike syndrome with abdominal pain, vomiting, headache, and dizziness. The full-blown picture generally develops by 24 hours and includes coma, convulsions, confusion, or psychosis; fasciculation and weakness or paralysis; dyspnea, cyanosis, and pulmonary edema; and in some pancreatitis. Torsades de pointes ventricular tachycardia has been described outside the United States.

Emergency management includes decontamination of the skin, if necessary, and removal of clothes; establishing an airway and ensuring proper ventilatory support and cardiac monitoring; and administering the specific antidote pralidoxime and the physiologic antidote atropine. A 25% reduction in red cell cholinesterase confirms organophosphate poisoning.

IV pralidoxime is the treatment of choice for organo-phosphate poisoning and should be begun on clinical grounds prior to return of any blood studies. Pralidoxine must be given in the first 48 hours in order to be effective before irreversible binding of acetylcholinesterase occurs. The initial dose is 1 gram IV given over 15 to 30 minutes; the effect may be dramatic. Pralidoxime by continuous infusion of up to 500 mg per hour may be necessary in critical patients. Using pralidoxime seems to obviate the need for high-dose atropine therapy and reduces the incidence of late-onset paralysis. Atropine is useful as a physiologic antidote to reverse the muscarinic effects and will help to dry the excessive pulmonary secretions seen in patients with respiratory distress. Atropine use requires cardiac monitoring and proper oxygenation of the patient.

The *carbamate insecticides* include carbaryl, methomyl, and propoxur and are reversible cholinesterase inhibitors. They produce clinical effects similar to those of the organophosphates but without CNS signs; they are considerably more benign and of much shorter duration. Atropine is the drug of choice for carbamate poisoning. Pralidoxime is not indicated because the carbamate–cholinesterase complex is quite reversible.

Paraquat, a bipyridyl herbicide, is a highly lethal concentrate that accounts for roughly 1000 deaths a year in Japan alone. The

TABLE 72–11. POISONING WITH METHANOL OR ETHYLENE GLYCOL

	Methanol	Ethylene Glycol
Signs and symptoms	Altered mental status; coma; seizures; gastrointestinal disturbance with abdominal pain; pancreatitis in some; visual disturbances: blurred vision, diplopia, photophobia, sensation of "being in a snowstorm," blindness (end result)	*Early* Altered mental status; seizures; hypocalcemic tetany *12 hrs after ingestion* Congestive heart failure *24–72 hrs after ingestion* Profound renal failure
Treatment	Aggressively prevent methanol conversion by infusing IV ethanol (see Table 72–1 for dose) Correct metabolic acidosis with: sodium bicarbonate; hemodialysis to remove methanol/metabolites indicated for patients with visual disturbance; serum methanol > 50 mg/dl, or with intractable metabolic acidosis	Treat ethylene glycol with: aggressive gastric lavage; ethanol infusion; sodium bicarbonate Correct hypocalcemia with calcium chloride Hemodialysis

TABLE 72-12. THE ORGANOPHOSPHATE INSECTICIDES

Highly toxic agricultural insecticides
    Parathion
    Mevinphos
Moderately toxic animal insecticides
    Coumaphos
    Dursban
    Ronnel
    Trichlorfon
Mildly toxic products for household and garden use
    Acephate
    Diazinon
    Malathion

TABLE 72-13. THE TRICYCLIC ANTIDEPRESSANTS

Amitriptyline (Elavil)
Amoxapine (Asendin)
Clomipramine (Anafranil)
Desipramine (Norpramin)
Doxepin (Sinequan)
Imipramine (Tofranil)
Nortriptyline (Pamelor)
Protriptyline (Vivactil)
Trimipramine (Surmontil)

lung is the primary target organ for paraquat toxicity. Paraquat reduces oxygen to form superoxide radicals which cause alveolar cell injury and death. Extensive pulmonary fibrosis ensues, preventing gas exchange and causing subsequent hypoxic death. Patients who ingest >30 mg per kilogram die within a few hours to days of multiple organ system failure. Ingesting smaller amounts produces esophagitis with possible perforation, pulmonary edema with subsequent development of pulmonary fibrosis, and renal failure.

Aggressive intervention within the first 2 hours following ingestion may be the only hope of preventing the clinical picture. If the patient arrives within the first hour, gastric lavage should be performed immediately. Paraquat is absorbed by a 15% solution of Fuller's earth or a 7% solution of bentonite, the diatomaceous clays. Soil or clay in a slurry of water may be substituted at home if the patient is found within minutes of ingestion. Activated charcoal and kayexalate also may be effective. Beyond early gastric decontamination, supportive care may be all that one can afford the patient. Because oxygen is converted to superoxide radicals by paraquat to produce cellular injury, oxygen is withheld until it becomes mandatory.

Theophylline is widely used primarily for treating asthma. Theophylline intoxication and mortality from both plain theophylline and sustained-release preparations occur from acute overdose and chronic unintentional intoxication from therapy. Vomiting is often the first symptom, and sinus tachycardia is the most common sign in both acute and chronic toxicity. Seizures may be common when the serum concentration of theophylline is >40 μg per milliliter in chronic toxicity or >80 to 100 μg per milliliter in acute overdose. Likewise, cardiac arrhythmia, cardiovascular collapse, and respiratory arrest are seen infrequently unless the serum theophylline concentration is >50 μg per milliliter in chronic toxicity or >100 μg per milliliter in acute overdose. Profound hypokalemia, hyperglycemia, and metabolic acidosis are also seen. Serum theophylline concentrations are considerably higher in acute overdose as compared with chronic toxicity.

Treatment of theophylline toxicity includes withdrawing the drug, cardiac monitoring, and supportive care. Gastric lavage and activated charcoal are indicated for acute overdose. The serum half-life of theophylline can be reduced by serially administering activated charcoal, since theophylline diffuses into the gastrointestinal lumen; dosage is 1 gram per kilogram every 4 hours. Whole-bowel irrigation may be indicated for ingestion of sustained-release capsules.

Cardiac arrhythmias are often difficult to manage but may respond to IV propranolol. Correcting hypokalemia, metabolic acidosis, and fluid–electrolyte balance is indicated. While seizures may respond to intravenous diazepam, status epilepticus and rhabdomyolysis may occur and generally signify a poor outcome.

Charcoal or resin hemoperfusion is the treatment of choice for significant theophylline toxicity. A delay in therapy because of a lack of diagnosis is not uncommon. Charcoal hemoperfusion is most beneficial for those patients with a serum theophylline concentration >80 to 100 μg per milliliter in acute overdose, >40 μg per milliliter in chronic toxicity (especially in the elderly or patients with hepatic disease or other conditions that delay theophylline clearance), or those patients in critical condition.

Tricyclic (or *cyclic*) *antidepressant* overdose is the leading cause of prescription drug death in the United States. The tricyclic antidepressants (Table 72–13) derive their names from their three-ring structure. The name "cyclic antidepressant" was introduced when maprotiline (Ludiomil), the first tetracyclic antidepressant, was marketed. Because all the agents have similar pharmacologic and toxic effects, the name "tricyclic antidepressants" (TCA's) has persisted.

Newer antidepressants that are not structurally related to the cyclic agents include the serotonin reuptake inhibitors fluoxetine (Prozac), sertraline (Zoloft), and paroxetine (Paxil), which generally cause only sedation in overdose.

Cardiovascular toxicity (primarily cardiac arrhythmia and hypotension), CNS effects (especially coma and seizures), and anticholinergic signs are seen with TCA overdose. The cardiotoxic effects are seen with ingestion of ≥1 gram (10 to 20 mg per kilogram) and account for the high mortality rate. The hallmark of TCA toxicity on ECG is prolongation of the QRS complex. A QRS complex longer than 100 ms is a sign of severe toxicity and generally correlates with a plasma drug level >1000 ng per milliliter. While sinus tachycardia and anticholinergic signs are evident with mild toxicity, QRS complex prolongation is associated with the development of ventricular arrhythmias, seizures, and death. Ventricular tachycardia is the most common ventricular rhythm, although ventricular bigeminy, slow ventricular rhythms, and torsades de pointes ventricular tachycardia also have been described. Ventricular fibrillation and sudden cardiac arrest are not uncommon.

The treatment of choice for TCA overdose is intravenous sodium bicarbonate. Alkalinization of blood via continuous infusion to maintain a blood pH of 7.5 appears to reduce the incidence of cardiac arrhythmia, and an IV bolus of sodium bicarbonate (1 to 2 mEq per kilogram) is the treatment of choice for the sudden onset of ventricular tachycardia, ventricular fibrillation, and cardiac arrest. Sodium bicarbonate also may be useful for correcting hypotension, although vasopressors may be necessary. Airway establishment, proper oxygenation and ventilation, fluid replacement at maintenance levels (to avoid pulmonary edema), gastric lavage with serially administered activated charcoal, and supportive therapy are indicated. Phenytoin (Dilantin) has been reported to reverse QRS complex prolongation in TCA overdose, but it is generally reserved for managing seizures. Prophylactic IV phenytoin (15 mg per kilogram) before the onset of seizures may be given in cases of amoxapine overdose, which has a high incidence of status epilepticus. Diazepam is quite effective in controlling seizures, although intensive therapy including pentobarbital and pancuronium bromide may be necessary to manage status epilepticus. Physostigmine no longer has a role in TCA overdose, since by itself it can cause seizures, bradycardia, and asystole. Death generally occurs within the first 24 hours after overdose. Because sudden death has occurred after apparent stabilization, prolonged cardiac monitoring for at least 24 hours after stabilization and normalization of the QRS complex is indicated.

The following medical journals are especially useful:
The American Journal of Emergency Medicine. This journal has excellent articles on toxicology and publishes yearly the annual report of the American Association of Poison Control Centers Toxic Exposure Surveillance System.
The Annals of Emergency Medicine. Published by the American College of Emergency Physicians, this journal publishes many case reports of acute toxic emergencies.

PART X

73 APPROACH TO THE PATIENT WITH RENAL DISEASE

Juha P. Kokko

A compulsive history and physical examination are crucial in the approach to the patient with renal disease. While it is well accepted that significant variability exists in the presentation of renal disease patients, there nevertheless are historical, physical, and laboratory findings that require emphasis.

Historically, it should be recognized that patients may be relatively asymptomatic for long periods even though they may have relatively far advanced renal disease. On the other hand, less advanced but rapidly progressive renal disease may be associated with severe symptoms. When taking a history from a patient with renal disease, specific emphasis should be placed on history of gross hematuria, dysuria, polyuria, the presence and nature of flank pain, nocturia, and signs and symptoms of uremia (see Ch. 77).

Likewise, the physical examination needs to be complete, but emphasis should be placed on carefully measuring the blood pressure in both the supine and upright positions, evaluating both the circulatory and interstitial blood volume status, examining the cardiovascular system, palpating the kidneys together with listening for potential renal-vascular bruits, and palpating potentially enlarged bladder or prostate gland.

Certain minimal laboratory evaluations are necessary, including a complete urinalysis, hematocrit and hemoglobin, and an SMA-6 determination that includes measuring serum levels of sodium, potassium, chloride, bicarbonate, glucose, and serum creatinine or blood urea nitrogen (BUN). The history, physical examination, and the laboratory findings will provide sufficient initial information to determine if any additional examinations are necessary for complete evaluation of a patient with renal disease.

APPROACH TO RENAL FAILURE

For the kidney to maintain normal volume, electrolyte, and acid–base homeostasis, it is necessary that it receives normal amounts of substrate (normal blood flow) to form urine, has normal glomerular filtration rate (GFR) and tubular function to form urine, and has a normal excretory path for urine. Thus renal failure may be broadly classified as prerenal (those conditions in which the kidney does not receive adequate blood flow), renal (those conditions in which components of the kidney *per se* do not function normally), and postrenal (those processes which impair normal excretion of urine after it has been formed) (Table 73–1). Renal failure is also classified according to the rate of progression of functional abnormality as being either *acute* (see Ch. 76) or *chronic* (see Ch. 77). "Acute" generally refers to states where an identifiable decrease in function occurs within days (often reversible), whereas "chronic" is a more insidious process in which the decline in GFR is progressive over weeks or months, often progressing through years to end-stage renal disease (ESRD) that requires dialysis or transplantation (see Ch. 78).

"Prerenal failure" refers to a state where the kidney is underperfused. In the broadest terms, this is the result of either contraction of true circulatory volume or decrease in effective arterial blood volume (EABV). The term "effective arterial blood volume" is a dynamic concept that cannot be measured directly but reflects the amount of blood reaching volume-sensitive organs, mainly the kidney and hypothalamus. Often the true circulatory volume may be increased as measured by red cell dilution techniques such as in congestive heart failure, but the blood flow reaching the kidney is actually decreased. Thus in these states the homeostatic mechanisms sense that the circulation is decreased (states referred to as decrease in EABV), while the true circulatory volume is actually increased. Other examples of decrease in EABV besides congestive heart failure include states with decreased systemic vascular resistance, as seen in sepsis and vascular shunts, hepatorenal syndrome, and bilateral renal artery stenosis, thrombosis, or renal vasoconstriction, and occasionally, as seen in circumstances where prostaglandin synthesis is inhibited. Measures of decrease in EABV include increases in antidiuretic hormone, renin, or aldosterone, but clinically, the most useful measure of decrease in EABV is a decrease in fractional excretion of sodium to values of $< 1\%$.

"Renal failure" is a term reserved for those conditions which are associated with abnormalities of the renal parenchyma. These may be primarily glomerular diseases (states with decreased GFR or increased protein leakage or both), primarily tubular lesions, or disease processes of the interstitium (interstitial nephritis). These abnormalities may occur as discreet events, but often the abnormalities are combined involvements of the aforementioned renal components. However, it is convenient to consider renal diseases either as primarily glomerular, tubular, or interstitial, since then it is easier to consider various etiologies and therapeutic approaches that are common to these renal components.

"Postrenal failure" is a term that refers to structural and/or functional impairment to normal urine flow which may be due to intrinsic obstruction of the ureter or urethra or secondary to extrinsic obstruction of multiple etiologies to compress the upper or lower urinary tract. By far the most common of these diseases is benign prostatic hyperplasia and ureteral calculi. While the etiologies of postrenal failure may be multiple, many patients present with hydronephrosis and pain. Anuria is not a feature of urinary obstruction unless there is complete bilateral ureteral obstruction. Similarly, functional acute renal failure secondary to obstruction does not occur unless there is bilateral ureteral obstruction or unless unilateral obstruction is superimposed on pre-existing parenchymal renal failure.

STUDIES OF RENAL FUNCTION

URINALYSIS. Urinalysis is an inexpensive, often informative laboratory procedure that should be a component of any initial evaluation. A number of important parameters may be measured. These will be described sequentially.

Specific Gravity. Specific gravity is the weight of an equal volume of urine to water. It therefore is a measure of the weight of solutes in water. Thus urine with a specific gravity of 1.010 is 10% heavier than water. In practical terms, clinicians have used specific

TABLE 73–1. MAJOR GROUPINGS OF RENAL FAILURE

Prerenal	(Ch. 76)
Renal	
Acute	(Ch. 76)
Chronic	(Ch. 77)
Postrenal	(Ch. 81)

TABLE 73–2. FACTORS INTERFERING WITH URINE DIPSTICK INTERPRETATION*

	False Negative	False Positive	Comments
Glucose	Elevated urinary ascorbate concentrations	Oxidizing agents in urine containers	Ketone bodies reduce sensitivity of test Reactivity of test decreases as specific gravity increases Newer preparations minimize false-negative with ascorbate
Bilirubin	Elevated urinary ascorbate concentrations	Phenazopyridine Etodolac	Sensitivity lowered by ascorbate Sensitivity lowered by elevated urine nitrite Indoxyl sulfate interferes with both negative and positive
Ketone		Pigmented urine (trace or less) Large amount levodopa metabolites in urine 2-Mercaptoethane sulfonic acid (MESNA)	No reaction with β-hydroxybutyrate or acetone Colors red to red-orange colors with phenylketone or phthalein compounds, distinguishable from ketone color
Specific gravity		Significant glycosuria Radiocontrast media	Note some new indicators not affected as previously by nonionic particles or radiocontrast Very alkaline urine may read low Elevated values may occur with significant proteinuria (>100 mg/dl)
Blood	Formalin urine preservation	Oxidizing agents in urine container Microbial peroxidase with UTI	
pH			False lowering of pH if urine spills from protein region of dipstick
Protein	Bence Jones protein, globulin not detected	Highly alkaline urine Urine contamination with quaternary ammonium compounds (skin cleansers, chlorhexidine), Phenazopyridine Polyvinylpyrrolidone infusion (blood substitute) Gross hematuria	
Urobilinogen	Formalin	p-Aminosalicylic acid, sulfonamides, PABA Phenazopyridine (with non-Ehrlich reagent)	The absence of urobilinogen cannot be determined with this test
Nitrite	Infecting organisms lacking nitrate → nitrite reductase Short bladder transit time limiting nitrate → nitrite reduction Ascorbate concentrations ≥ 25 mg/dl	Meds discoloring urine red or which make red in acid medium	
Leukocytes	High urine tetracycline levels		Decreased activity with high glucose concentration (>3 grams/dl), high specific gravity, high oxalic acid concentration Interference from nitrofurantoin, gentamicin, cephalexin, and high albumin concentrations (>500 mg/dl)

* This table incorporates data drawn from several commercially available dipsticks. Individual preparations may differ in terms of test reagents used, and therefore, clinical settings in which false or ambiguous readings occur may vary. The package insert always should be reviewed in each individual instance.

Data from Ames, Multistix reagent strips, tests for glucose, bilirubin, ketone, specific gravity, blood, pH, protein, urobilinogen, nitrite, and leukocytes in urine, Boehringer Mannheim Diagnostics, Chemstrip, urinalysis tests for leukocytes, nitrite, pH, protein, glucose, ketones, urobilinogen, bilirubin, and blood in urine, Rose BD: Pathophysiology of Renal Disease. New York, McGraw-Hill, 1986.

gravity of urine to estimate urine osmolality and thus the patient's state of hydration. This is especially important to pediatricians, whose patients can change their volume status rapidly. Indeed, low urine specific gravity of (<1.015) always indicates hypotonic urine with corresponding urine osmolalities below 220 mOsm per kilogram of H_2O. However, values above this do not necessarily reflect normal concentrating ability, since substances such as glucose, protein, and radiocontrast material highly increase the specific gravity. Thus, in adult patients with episodes of albuminuria and glucosuria, specific gravity has less limited significance than in pediatric patients. However, a real limitation of measuring specific gravity in pediatric patients is that using a hydrometer requires more urine than often is available. Therefore, alternate measures of urinary specific gravity have been developed. These include using a refractometer that measures the refractive index of urine and various reagent strips that change color in response to ionic (electrolyte) strengths of urine and not to undissociated solutes (mainly urea). However, the strip tests do not reflect urine concentration accurately and are mainly useful if the specific gravity is < 1.015 (Table 73–2). Under these conditions, urine has been found to be hypotonic. The refractometer is more useful and a better index of urinary osmolality, but it is mainly accurate at both extremes. Values

< 1.008 predict hypo-osmolality, while values > 1.020 predict hyperosmolality. Still the most accurate measure of urine concentration is measuring urine osmolality by freezing-point depression or by vapor-pressure techniques, but unfortunately, these measurements require a technician and more complex equipment.

Urine pH. Calorimetric pH reagents strips measure urine pH in freshly voided specimens with satisfactory accuracy for clinical use. The more cumbersome glass electrodes with special techniques to collect urine are necessary to evaluate renal tubular acidosis or other abnormalities of acid–base metabolism that require sophisticated evaluation of urinary acid excretion. It should be pointed out that urinary pH does not measure net acid excretion but only the unbuffered ion concentration. This, in turn, is affected by many variables, including diet.

Glucose. Glucose oxidase reagent strips measure urinary glucose (see Table 73–2). Once the serum glucose concentration exceeds 160 to 200 mg per deciliter, then it is routine to exceed renal capacity to reabsorb glucose with resultant glycosuria. Glucose measured in urine is used as a presumptive indicator of diabetes mellitus except in rare cases of renal glycosuria.

Protein. Urinary protein concentrations are commonly measured by colorimetric reagent strips (see Table 73–2). These are quite qualitative but can measure concentrations as low as 10 mg per deciliter (trace) to values > 500 mg per deciliter (4+). Clearly, the measurement of 24-hour urinary protein excretion rate correlates better with disease processes than urinary concentration; however, using reagent strips can alert the physician that further studies are needed if the rest of the clinical picture so dictates.

Normal urinary protein excretion rates are < 40 mg per 24 hours. However, many nephrologists have accepted protein excretions of up to 150 mg per 24 hours as "normal" in nondiabetic patients. The reason for this more liberal upper limit is that in the absence of any other disease processes these patients generally do not develop progressive renal disease. Consensus exists that urinary excretion rates > 150 mg per 24 hours are abnormal and reflect either renal or extrarenal causes (Table 73–3). "Overflow proteinuria" refers to those conditions in which increased quantities of low-molecular-weight protein are present in the circulation and the amount that is filtered exceeds the tubular capacity to reabsorb it, e.g., light chain proteinuria of multiple myeloma. "Selective proteinuria" refers to a primary increase in albumin excretion, with the predominant pathophysiologic change being the loss of a negative charge from the endothelial surface of the glomerular basement membrane that would normally reject the permeation of negatively charged albumin, e.g., "minimal-change" nephrotic syndrome. "Nonselective glomerular proteinuria" refers to proteinuria with severe disruption of the glomerular capillary wall. In these cases, the urinary proteins reflect the concentrations of circulating proteins to a first approximation. A typical example of this type of proteinuria is diabetic nephropathy. "Tubular proteinuria" refers to conditions with a defect in normal endocytic reabsorption of filtered protein. In these conditions, the urine contains a disproportionate amount of light-molecular-weight proteins, such as β_2-microglobulin, in contrast to albumin. An example of this is various heavy metal poisons or tubular interstitial diseases. "Functional proteinuria" refers to common sources of proteinuria that do not indicate primary renal disease, e.g., high fever, exercise, congestive heart failure, and orthostatic proteinuria. It is for these reasons that urine collections should be done under standardized conditions. While 24-hour urine collections without undue exercise are preferable, it is acceptable to collect a shorter 8-hour urine if it is done overnight. Functional proteinuria usually is transient and reversible.

All patients with abnormal excretion of protein must be evaluated. Indeed, persistent microalbuminuria in a 24-hour urinary specimen of a diabetic has prognostic significance and suggests development of diabetic nephropathy in the future. If proteinuria is noted, then one should consider obtaining two or three 24-hour urinary protein excretion rates because the coefficient of variance between these 24-hour samples can be quite high. If these measurements document that proteinuria is persistent, then efforts should be made to establish the etiology. The degree of proteinuria is only of limited value. However, the protein excretion rates seldom exceed 2 grams per 24 hours in interstitial nephritis, whereas protein excretion rates vary widely in primary glomerular diseases. Protein excretion rates > 3.5 grams per 24 hours per 1.73 square meter of body surface area are known as "nephrotic-range proteinuria" and almost always reflect primary glomerular disease. Patients with significant and persistent proteinuria > 150 mg per 24 hours are at risk for developing functional renal insufficiency without appropriate therapy. Thus these patients must undergo a thorough investigation (described later in this chapter), including further blood studies for evidence of specific systemic disease, urinary electrophoresis to determine the nature of proteinuria, various radiologic studies, and/or renal biopsy in those patients in whom there is reasonable chance of obtaining therapeutically relevant information. There exists some difference of opinion as to how aggressively a patient should be worked up if he/she is nondiabetic and has a protein excretion rate between 40 to 150 mg per 24 hours. A reasonable approach is to follow these patients on an annual basis if urinalysis is otherwise normal ("isolated proteinuria") and they do not have evidence of any systemic disease. While an occasional patient is at increased risk of developing hypertension and renal disease in the future, in most, the long-term prognosis is good and does not justify further evaluation by a renal biopsy.

MICROSCOPIC. *Hematuria.* Hematuria may be macroscopic (red in color) or microscopic (more than two to three cells per high-power field in a button of sediment over a 12-ml spun urine sample). While the quantitative count of microscopic hematuria is of little or no value, it is important to differentiate between glomerular hematuria, renal nonglomerular hematuria, and extrarenal causes of hematuria. In general, red cells in glomerular hematuria tend to be spiculated and have many sizes and shapes, while in nonglomerular hematuria the red blood cells are nonspiculated and uniform in size. It should be recognized, however, that in very dilute urine with specific gravities of < 1.006, the red blood cells of any origin may be hemolyzed.

Pyuria. A number of techniques have been developed to establish the presence of pyuria: calculating excretion rate of leukocytes, examining the button of a spun sediment, using a hemocytometer on an unspun urine specimen, and using the leukoesterase dipstick method. The simplest is the routine microscopic examination on a spun specimen, or even more simple is the leukoesterase dipstick method. More than three white blood cells per high-power field and a positive leukoesterase dipstick measurement are abnormal values. These observations are a cost-effective way (with a relatively high degree of sensitivity) to suggest the presence of a urinary tract infection. However, it is important to recognize that wide variation in specificity in leukoesterase determination has been reported. This variation is due in part to spectrum bias of the patient population and in part to variations in test performance. The test must be done according to the directions that are provided with the specific dipsticks. Indeed, it is reasonable to initiate treatment for cystourethri-

TABLE 73–3. TYPES OF PROTEINURIA*

Type	Mechanism	Quantity†	Molecular Weight	Examples
Overflow	Increased filtration of abnormal plasma proteins across normal glomeruli	Variable (0.2 to >10 grams)	Low (<40,000)	Bence Jones proteinuria, myoglobinuria
Glomerular‡	Defective			Minimal-change
Selective	glomerular retention of	>3 grams	60,000	nephrotic syndrome
Nonselective	normal plasma proteins	>3–5 grams	High (>68,000)	Glomerulonephritis, diabetes
Tubular	Defective reabsorption of normally filtered plasma proteins	<2 grams	Low (<40,000)	Interstitial nephritis, antibiotic injury, heavy metals
Hemodynamic	Increased filtration and possibly decreased reabsorption	<2 grams	Variable (20,000–68,000)	Transient proteinuria, congestive heart failure, fever, seizures, exercise

* Values > 150 mg per 24 hours.
† Quite variable—values given are characteristic.
‡ Molecular weight of proteinuria is a function of impairment of change and structural integrity.

tis in noncomplicated sexually active females without cultures based simply on the finding of more than three white blood cells per high-power field or leukoesterase-positive urine if symptoms of urinary tract infection exist. However, the more costly urine cultures are necessary if patients are diabetic, elderly, pregnant, or have recurrent urinary tract infections. It should be noted that not all patients with pyuria have bacteriurea and may reflect tuberculosis, viral infections, or fungal or other nonbacterial pathogens. Also, the presence of significant eosinophiliuria may suggest allergic interstitial nephritis.

Urine also should be examined microscopically for bacteria, yeasts, fungi, crystals, casts, and other components in the sediment that may be of diagnostic importance.

Once the urine has been examined, then further laboratory testing of renal function becomes an important component of nephrologic evaluation. However, the physician must be aware of sensitivity, specificity, and predictive values of each test. Table 73–2 lists circumstances where certain clinical situations cause false-positive and false-negative results. Evaluating volume, electrolyte, and acid-base homeostasis will be covered in Ch. 75, but a routine SMA-6 that includes measurements of sodium, potassium, chloride, bicarbonate, glucose, and either BUN or creatinine will offer useful information concerning metabolic abnormalities caused by abnormal renal function. Many of the above-mentioned variables are highly dependent on GFR.

Glomerular Filtration Rate. While many sophisticated techniques for measuring GFR exist, such as inulin clearance and radioactive iothalamate clearance tests, in most clinical circumstances the endogenous creatinine clearance is a sufficient estimate of a patient's GFR. Because there is some creatinine secretion, the creatinine clearance actually overestimates GFR as measured by more exact techniques. Also, drugs such as cimetidine, trimethoprim, triamterene, spironolactone, and amiloride inhibit tubular secretion of creatinine and therefore may cause a falsely low estimate of GFR. Nevertheless, measuring GFR by collecting a 24-hour urine specimen is adequate in most circumstances and can give a good estimate by

$$C_{Cr} = \frac{U_{Cr} \cdot V}{P_{Cr}}$$

where C_{Cr} is a measure of creatinine clearance, U_{Cr} is urinary concentration of creatinine, V is urine volume for 24 hours, and P_{Cr} is plasma concentration of creatinine.

Serum creatinine is a much better index than BUN of renal function. Indeed, isolated measurements of BUN should not be used because synthetic rates of urea (primary end-products of protein metabolism) are influenced by protein intake as well as liver function, and urea excretion rates from the kidney are influenced by renal tubular flow rates. In conditions with decreased tubular flow rates such as exist in prerenal failure, there is increased tubular reabsorption of urea and therefore a disproportionate rise in BUN with respect to creatinine. In these cases, the high BUN might falsely suggest a lower than actual GFR, while anorexia with poor protein intake with a low BUN would actually suggest the presence of a higher GFR. BUN is at best a rough index of renal function.

URINARY ELECTROLYTES. The significance of urinary electrolyte measurement has recently become more apparent. Measuring urinary sodium or chloride excretion is especially useful in attempting to differentiate between etiologies of hyponatremia, as seen in volume contraction (whether a decrease in total circulatory volume or a decrease in effective arterial blood volume) versus conditions associated with increased salt loss, as seen with the syndrome of inappropriate antidiuretic hormone secretion (SIADH), salt-losing nephropathy, or adrenal insufficiency. If metabolic alkalosis is present in its early generation phase, as seen with vomiting, then urinary chloride, as will be discussed later, becomes a more important measure of volume status than urinary sodium. A measure of urinary potassium is also important to differentiate between etiologies of both hypo- and hyperkalemia.

Measuring the 24-hour urine excretion rate of electrolytes is both cumbersome and does not provide as much significant information as a spot urinary measurement of fractional secretion of these ions. The reason for this is that the 24-hour urine reflects total intake in a steady-state condition (higher sodium intakes are associated with higher sodium excretion rates), while fractional excretion of ions reflects the sum of regulatory factors on a more acute basis. Fractional excretion *(FE)* does not depend on accurate timed volume collections and is easy to calculate:

$$FE_X = \frac{U_X/P_X}{U_{Cr}/P_{Cr}} \cdot 100$$

where urinary (U) to plasma (P) concentrations of given electrolytes (X) are measured and divided by simultaneously measured urinary and plasma concentration of creatinine.

FE_{Na} generally has a value of <1 in prerenal failure, while in SIADH, acute tubular necrosis, or salt-losing nephropathy the values are $>1\%$ and tend to be $>3\%$ (Table 73–4). The clinical utility of values in the intermediate range is less, but in general, values >1 suggest disease processes other than states where the kidney is underperfused. Exceptions to this are those pure glomerular diseases, especially acute poststreptococcal glomerular nephritis, where tubular function and renal blood flow are well maintained but the tubule has low flow rates as a result of an isolated decrease in GFR. In these cases, the FE_{Na} also will be decreased, as it will occasionally with radiocontrast-induced nephropathy, but in general, $FE_{Na} < 1$ indicates renal underperfusion, whether secondary to decreases in EABV or due to true volume depletion. A decrease in FE_{Na} is especially useful in patients who have increases in total-body fluid volume but decreases in EABV. Examples include congestive heart failure and hypoalbuminemic states, whether secondary to renal or hepatic etiologies.

There is one clinical scenario worthy of special comment where volume contraction is associated with a high FE_{Na}—the generation phase of metabolic alkalosis related to vomiting. As a patient develops metabolic alkalosis with vomiting, the plasma bicarbonate concentration rises to levels that exceed renal capacity for reabsorption, and therefore, urinary bicarbonate concentration rises. This bicarbonate must be associated with a cation, either sodium or potassium. In these circumstances, the urine sodium excretion is elevated, but it is essentially free of chloride. FE_{Cl} thus becomes a better index of volume status than FE_{Na}. However, without increases in nonreabsorbable anion in the urine, the FE_{Na} is a good index of functional status of renal perfusion.

FE_K normally rises with decreases in renal function (Fig. 73–1). It is thus important to interpret the significance of FE_K in this context. FE rates below normal indicate aldosterone deficiency or renal tubular defects for K secretion, while values above normal suggest increased concentration of aldosterone or other factors that stimulate K secretion. However, one of the most important uses of FE_K is determining the etiology of hypokalemia. Extrarenal losses or a decrease in dietary intake of K is associated with low FE_K, while renal losses are associated with an increase in FE_K. Generally, a U_K of 40 mEq per liter suggests renal losses of K, as seen with primary aldosterone secretion, diuretics, Bartter's syndrome, renal artery stenosis, and other causes with increased stimulus for K secretion.

Once the history, physical examination, and laboratory values have been interpreted, there are certain patients who require further evaluation to fully determine the nature of abnormalities in renal function. The next subsection describes the indications, use, and predictive value of various additional studies.

TABLE 73–4. URINARY FINDINGS IN OLIGURIC* PRERENAL VERSUS ACUTE PARENCHYMAL RENAL FAILURE

	Prerenal	Parenchymal
U_{osm},† mOsm/kg H_2O	>500	<350
Urine sodium, mEq/liter	<20	>40
Fractional excretion of sodium	<1	>1

* Urinary indices are of less significance in nonoliguric renal failure, though U_{Na} and FE_{Na} tend to be lower in nonoliguric versus oliguric acute intrinsic renal failure.

† Significant amount of overlap exists between these two groups if urine osmolality is between 350 and 500 mOsm/kg or urine Na is between 20 and 40 mEq/liter for these indices to be of diagnostic significance.

From Miller TR, Anderson KJ, Linas SL, et al.: Urinary diagnostic indices in acute renal failure: A prospective study. Ann Intern Med 89:47, 1978.

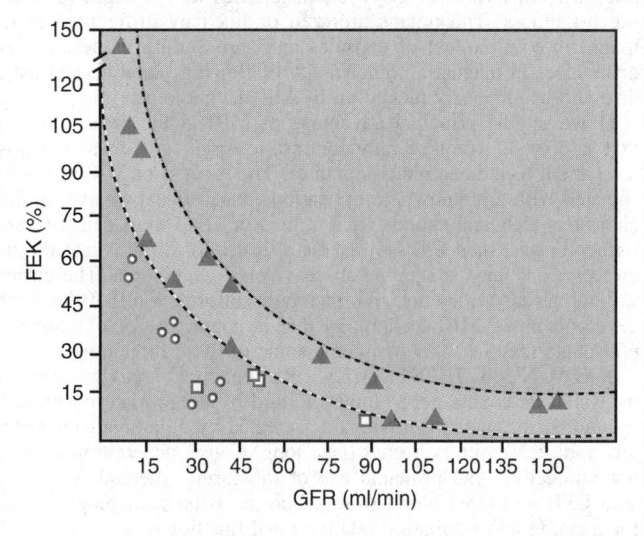

FIGURE 73–1. The relationship between fractional excretion of potassium (FE_K) and glomerular filtration rate (GFR) in patients with normal adaptive increase in FE_K with progressive decrease in GFR (area inside broken lines with individual patients depicted with solid triangles). The open circles and squares refer to patients with renal tubular secretory defects and aldosterone deficiency, respectively. (Reprinted with permission from Batlle DC, Arruda JAL, Kurtzman NA: Hyperkalemic distal renal tubular acidosis associated with obstructive uropathy. N Engl J Med 304:373, 1981. Copyright the Massachusetts Medical Society.)

RADIOLOGIC STUDIES

Modern departments of radiology have a number of different diagnostic techniques that are useful in evaluating patients with renal abnormalities.

ULTRASOUND EXAMINATION. Ultrasonography (US) is a noninvasive, relatively inexpensive diagnostic tool that does not depend on renal function and gives information in "real-time" format. It has no complications and can be done at the bedside if necessary. In this technique, the US transducer is both a transducer and a receiver where images are created from differences in acoustic impedance of different tissues containing various quantities of water, fat, collagen, and other substances. It is important to recognize that high-frequency sound waves are transmitted through solid tissues and water but not through air or calcified structures. Thus collections of air (lungs, bowel gas, and bones) severely impair penetration of sound waves and result in poor-resolution imaging. In general, more aqueous media have better sound wave transmission and appear darker, while less aqueous tissues appear less dark. The white hyperechogenic images arise from calcified structures or free air.

While US often contributes to a correct diagnosis, its main use diagnostically is to rule out hydronephrosis and polycystic renal disease (Table 73–5). In circumstances of anuria, with resultant acute renal failure, US can be used rapidly to determine whether hydronephrosis exists—either unilaterally or bilaterally. US is not sensitive to etiologies of hydronephrosis, but it may suggest the diagnosis of benign prostatic hypertrophy, nephrolithiasis, or any extrinsic or intrinsic cause of obstruction. In hydronephrosis, the central caliceal system is dilated and appears darker because it is filled with fluid (Fig. 73–2).

US can be used to help differentiate between benign and malignant cysts. Benign cysts have smooth walls without internal septa or mural nodules. Classically, benign cysts do not need further eval-

TABLE 73–5. INDICATIONS FOR RENAL ULTRASONOGRAPHY

Rule out hydronephrosis
Define the nature of renal cysts
Localize calculi
Guide needles

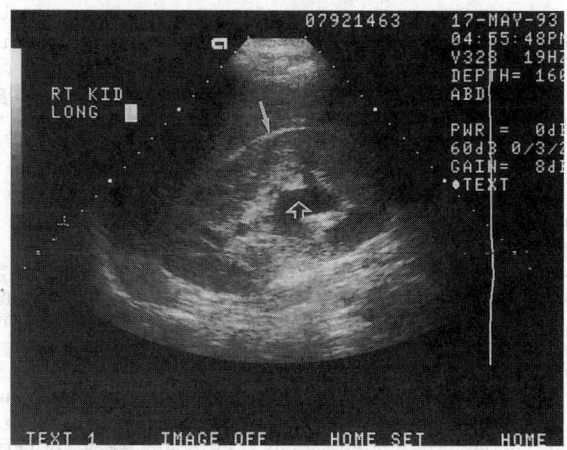

FIGURE 73–2. Ultrasonography of a hydronephrotic kidney. The kidney is surrounded by echogenic renal capsule *(closed arrow),* while the dark anechoic area located centrally *(open arrow)* represents dilated renal pelvis.

uation, but cysts that do not meet these criteria need additional workup. However, US is not particularly sensitive nor specific in evaluating solid renal masses. Primary renal carcinomas, renal metastases, lymphomas, and various benign tumors are not uniformly picked up until they are >3 cm, and then their echogenicity is highly variable. US also is not very helpful in posttransplant evaluations, with the exception of ruling out hydronephrosis, but the technique is very beneficial for guiding diagnostic needles into appropriate anatomic spaces.

INTRAVENOUS PYELOGRAPHY. Intravenous pyelography (IVP) is used predominantly to evaluate anatomic features of the renal excretory system. After preliminary plain x-ray films, the radiologist injects one of various types of iodinated contrast materials, followed by serial x-rays. The contrast material is filtered by the glomeruli, after which it follows the normal flow of urine. Initial films (≤1 minute) after injecting the dye are known as "nephrograms," where general radioopacity of the kidney is seen. Nephrograms initially can be used to measure the size of the kidney by measuring the maximum distance from the cephalad to the caudad margins. However, plain nephrotomography also can be used to estimate renal size without having to administer contrast material. The left kidney is normally somewhat larger than the right, with normal kidneys being somewhere between 11.5 to 12.5 cm. However, because of size differences in patients, some investigators feel that expression of renal size with respect to vertebral height is a more accurate measure of normal renal size. In adults, mean kidney length to height of the second lumbar spine is 3.7. After the nephrogram, calyces, pelvis, ureters, and bladder are sequentially viewed. The radiologist needs to be flexible to modify views and timing of the IVP to tailor his/her approach to suspected findings. IVP can be helpful in the kidney to define scars, cysts, and other anatomic abnormalities, while in the renal pelvis it is used to evaluate hydronephrosis, calyceal deformities, and stones; in the ureter it is used to evaluate obstruction, dilation, and abnormal course due to extrinsic factors; in the bladder it can be used to examine for intrinsic or extrinsic masses that cause either filling defects or extrinsic displacement of bladder opacification.

Special note should be taken with respect to radiocontrast-induced nephropathy. The incidence of radiocontrast nephropathy is most frequent in patients with chronic renal failure, diabetes mellitus, or multiple myeloma. Incidences as high as 50% have been reported in some patients receiving high doses of radiocontrast material for cardiac catheterization, but the incidence of renal failure secondary to IVP is relatively rare if the patient is adequately volume expanded. Regretfully, there are no proven methods to prevent prophylactically radiocontrast-induced nephropathy except volume repletion and good clinical judgment with respect to patients with risk factors for acute renal failure (see Ch. 76).

RETROGRADE PYELOGRAPHY. If adequate definition of the urinary collecting system is not achieved by IVP, then the physician may consider a retrograde pyelogram. It should be recognized that indications for retrograde pyelography are steadily decreasing with improvements in IVP technology. In this technique, the ureters are catheterized by cystoscopy, and contrast material is injected. This technique does not give information concerning the renal parenchyma but is used to define anatomically the calyces, renal pelvis, and remainder of the excretory system.

RENAL ARTERIOGRAPHY. Renal arteriography may be performed by a skilled radiologist, introducing vascular catheters percutaneously into the femoral artery and advancing them above the renal arteries to indicate their exact number and takeoff points. Subsequently, the catheters may be selectively advanced into a specific renal artery under fluoroscopic control. Contrast dye then is injected into the renal artery, and the branches subsequently will be opacified. A number of magnification techniques can be used to improve visualization, and vasoconstrictive agents occasionally will be helpful to define normal vessels that constrict to epinephrine from tumors or inflammatory changes that are not as vigorously constricted by epinephrine. Renal arteriography is especially useful for defining the extent and type of fibromuscular dysplasia and is diagnostically helpful in differentiating other stenotic lesions such as arteriosclerosis, arteriodissections, emboli, thromboses, various types of vasculidities, and effects of trauma. There are no well-accepted criteria for choosing patients for renal arteriography, but the technique should be considered in those in whom therapeutically useful information is reasonably expected: patients with moderately severe hypertension, especially if they are young and have renal bruits on physical examination, and patients in whom renal arteriography can help define the nature of suspected tumors or help in the differential diagnosis of specific types of vasculitis.

A modification of traditional renal arteriography is intravenous digital subtraction arteriography. In this technique, radiocontrast material is injected into either the inferior or superior vena cava, and digital subtraction imaging and filming are done later when the radiocontrast material circulates over the renal arteries. The technique has the advantage of using a lower contrast material dose, but the disadvantage is that it is mainly useful for diseases of the main renal artery and not its subsequent segments.

COMPUTED TOMOGRAPHY. Since the introduction of computed tomography (CT) technology in the mid-1970's, the technique has undergone significant advances to the point where the contrast and spatial resolutions have enormous diagnostic utility. The principle of this technique is that a computer constructs images mathematically from multiple x-ray absorption measurements from different projections of the body. To enhance the renal image, the studies are usually done with the aid of contrast material, except in circumstances where the nature of renal calculi is being evaluated. Although CT scanning is not a primary modality to evaluate the kidney, it is especially useful to evaluate renal masses, study perirenal anatomy, and evaluate a nonfunctioning kidney, and recently it is being used more and more frequently in the biopsy of renal masses, where exact localization of small lesions is mandatory.

MAGNETIC RESONANCE IMAGING. While nuclear magnetic resonance has been a routine tool of the chemist since the 1950's, magnetic resonance imaging (MRI), which uses the principles of nuclear magnetic resonance, has only recently become a routine diagnostic tool for the clinician. However, whereas MRI is an excellent tool in neuroimaging, the current generation of MRI should be considered only as an expensive and complementary modality to examine the kidney.

In the simplest phenomenologic terms, the signal in the MRI is produced by protons that flip from a lower energy state to a higher one and again return to the lower energy state. Protons can be considered as small magnets with a north and a south pole that rotate about a static magnetic field (as applied by an MRI machine). These protons can absorb energy at only a very specific combination of local magnetic strength and the applied radiofrequency. Once the applied radiofrequency is stopped, the protons (small magnets) return to their previous lower energy orientation in the magnetic field. The process of changing magnetic vector orientation (relaxation) creates a small electric current that is interpreted by the receiving coils. The signal is dependent on unique magnetic surroundings of protons in tissue, and the ultimate image is constructed by complicated computer technology from evaluating the proton signals in three separate magnetic field axes. The resulting images from tissues of given characteristics form images of differing brightness. The organs are well outlined by differences in the magnetic environment of capsules and surrounding tissues. Indeed, differences in magnetic homogeneity of flowing blood in contrast to thromboses are easily picked up by MRI technology.

However, the principal advantage of MRI at the present time is that it does not require radiocontrast material, nor does it expose the patient to radioactive compounds. The process of MRI is not associated with any known complications, but it is expen-sive, rquires enormous technical support, and at present gives more sensitive soft tissue contrast than CT. Nevertheless, it cannot differentiate the nature of renal masses such as abscess versus carcinoma. The current technology also does not give metabolic information, but the future development of MRI technology that is coupled with simultaneous phosphate imaging may overcome some of these limitations.

RADIONUCLIDE STUDIES. Radionuclide activity can be measured as counts per volume of fluid by appropriate counters or by number of energy emissions as detected by a gamma camera (alpha and beta emittors do not have long enough penetration to be of use clinically). The principal use of the former method is to measure GFR and renal blood flow, while the latter technology is used for imaging and estimating relative renal function.

Glomerular Filtration. GFR may be measured by clearance techniques or by disappearance rates of radiotracer from blood. In each case, an ideal tracer is one that is only cleared from the body by glomerular filtration.

The clearance of radionuclide is much easier to measure than the time-honored measure of GFR by clearing inulin. In this technique, stable blood concentrations of radionuclide must be achieved by either continuous infusion techniques or by single subcutaneous injections with suitable equilibration periods (usually 40 to 60 minutes). Urine must be collected for a known time period, and GFR can be calculated as

$$GFR = \frac{U_X \cdot V}{P_X}$$

where U_X and P_X are counts per minute and per milliliter of radionuclide in urine and plasma, respectively, and V is volume of urine per minute. Many centers use the single subcutaneous method because of its ease. There are a number of good tracers for measuring GFR, and one currently in favor is ^{125}I-iothalamate. If the rate of disappearance of radiotracer from blood is used to estimate GFR, a radioactive material is injected and samples of blood are obtained at fixed intervals, e.g., 3, 4, 5, and 24 hours. The GFR may then be calculated from disappearance rates of the compound from blood. While the technique is not easy, it is useful in situations where collecting urine is difficult, such as in pediatric populations or patients with urinary diversions.

Renal Blood Flow. Renal blood flow is measured by the same technology as GFR except in this case the patient is injected with a radiotracer that is extracted as completely as possible by a single pass through the kidney. Clinically, the most effective compound that is available is radiolabeled *para*-aminohippurate, which has an extraction efficiency of 87%. Other compounds have been developed with both lower and higher extraction efficiencies. The renal blood flow can be calculated from the clearance of radioactive nuclide from blood at short intervals up to 2 hours. The renal blood flow can be calculated from the rate of decrease of the compound from blood and corrected for the extraction efficiency.

Radionuclide Imaging. Radiopharmaceuticals may be used to obtain general images of the kidney. These are only rough estimates of renal anatomy but have some advantage in that allergic reactions or induced nephropathy is essentially nonexistent to radioactive compounds as compared with radiocontrast materials. In this technique, radiopharmaceuticals that are taken up by the kidney are injected. Images are then collected at 30-second intervals for 2 minutes and then at 5-minute intervals. The technique is useful to compare the function of one kidney versus the other and gives a general outline of renal size and shape.

Relative Renal Function. One of the most important uses of radionuclides in nephrology is to measure the function of one kidney relative to that of the other when nephrectomy is considered. The technique is similar to imaging, but in this circumstance the uptake of radiopharmaceuticals by one kidney is compared with the other. It is important to start images only after adequate mixing of radionuclide has occurred in circulation—usually within $2\frac{1}{2}$ to 3 minutes.

1. Nephrotic syndrome
2. Systemic disease
   a. Systemic lupus erythematosus
   b. Goodpasture's syndrome*
   c. Wegener's granulomatosis*
   d. Diabetes mellitus only if atypical course
3. Hematuria if persistent for >6 months
4. Acute renal failure†
5. Transplanted kidney‡

* If etiology of process cannot be determined with a renal biopsy.
† If unknown cause and not acute tubular necrosis.
‡ To help manage posttransplant state.

RENAL BIOPSY. If the preceding approaches fail to give a diagnosis or are not indicated for clinical reasons, then one might consider the potential of a renal biopsy. In broadest terms, renal biopsy is indicated for diagnostic information and as an aid in a rational approach to treatment. It is of limited prognostic use, and only rarely is it indicated for monitoring progression of renal disease. Table 73–6 lists the indications for renal biopsy, but it should be recognized that wide variations exist among nephrologists for indication of a renal biopsy, and therefore, it regretably often becomes a matter of personal preference. However, each patient should be evaluated carefully to choose those patients in whom diagnostic yield is thought to be high while complication rates are minimized. In general, it is rare that a renal biopsy is indicated in chronic renal failure with small kidneys. Similarly, renal biopsy is not required to confirm diabetic nephropathy if the presentation of diabetic nephropathy is classic. However, in cases of persistent hematuria (if glomerular), proteinuria, acute renal failure, various systemic diseases with renal failure, and after renal transplant in patients with unexplained deterioration of renal function, a renal biopsy is indicated to obtain a diagnosis or to initiate or modify therapy. However, renal biopsy should not be done if the patient cannot cooperate, if he/she has bleeding abnormalities with platelets that are below 60,000 and a prothrombin time >3 seconds from control, and/or if bleeding time is prolonged. Also, renal biopsy should not be done if a solitary kidney exists or before diastolic blood pressure has been brought to <90 mm Hg.

The biopsy may be performed percutaneously or by open technology. The percutaneous approach is much more inexpensive and, when performed by a skilled nephrologist, yields adequate tissue in >90% of cases. Open biopsy should be reserved for uncooperative patients and those who are at risk for uncontrolled bleeding or have solitary kidneys. Clearly, in the latter case, the index of suspicion for therapeutically relevant information must be high. Adequately sized samples should be obtained for electron microscopy, immunofluorescence, and light microscopy. If minimal tissue is present, then electron microscopy should be done alone, followed by electron microscopy and immunofluorescence, and both of these should be done with light microscopy if adequate tissue is present. While renal biopsy gives only histologic information, it nevertheless often will allow a correct clinical diagnosis that could not be made otherwise when interpreted in the context of other clinical information.

Blum RN, Wright RA: Detection of pyuria and bacteriuria in symptomatic ambulatory women. J Gen Intern Med 7:140, 1992. *Evaluating accuracy and cost-effectiveness of dipstick urinalysis and standard microscopic urinalysis to predict significant bacteriuria.*

Lachs MS, Nachamkin I, Edelstein PH, et al.: Spectrum bias in the evaluation of diagnostic tests: Lessons from the rapid dipstick test for urinary tract infection. Ann Intern Med 117:135, 1992. *A careful determination of sensitivities and specificities of leukocyte esterase and bacterial nitrate dipstick tests for urinary tract infections.*

Madaio MP: Renal biopsy. Kidney Int 38:529, 1990. *A complete discussion of indications, safety, and value of renal biopsy.*

Miller TR, Anderson RJ, Linas SL, et al.: Urinary diagnostic indices in acute renal failure: A prospective study. Ann Intern Med 89:47, 1978. *A nice prospective analysis of the significance in fractional excretion of filtered sodium as a predictor of a prerenal versus a renal cause of azotemia.*

Mogensen CE: Microalbuminuria as a predictor of clinical diabetic nephropathy. Kidney Int 31:673, 1987. *A complete discussion of the significance of microalbuminuria.*

Rowe MI, Lloyd DA, Lee M: Is the refractometer specific gravity a reliable index for pediatric fluid management? J Pediatr Surg 21:580, 1986. *A study to examine the accuracy of the refractometer to determine the osmolarity of urine in pediatric patients.*

74 STRUCTURE AND FUNCTION OF THE KIDNEYS

C. Craig Tisher

The complex multicellular composition of the kidney reflects the complicated nature of its functional properties. This organ is responsible for maintaining both the volume and ionic composition of the body fluids, excreting fixed or nonvolatile metabolic waste products such as creatinine, urea, and uric acid, and eliminating exogenous drugs and toxins. The kidney is a major endocrine organ, since it produces renin, erythropoietin, 1,25-dihydroxycholecalciferol, prostaglandins, and kinins, and it also serves as a target organ for many hormones. The kidney also catabolizes small-molecular-weight proteins and is responsible for a host of metabolic functions, e.g., ammoniagenesis and gluconeogenesis.

DEVELOPMENT. The kidney originates from two sources: (1) the ureteral bud, which gives rise to the ureter, pelvis, calyces, and collecting ducts; and (2) the metanephric blastema, which gives rise to the glomerulus and tubules. During embryogenesis, three successive sets of excretory organs develop: the pronephros, mesonephros, and metanephros. The permanent kidney evolves from the metanephros. Cellular and molecular mechanisms that underlie renal morphogenesis include cell proliferation, expression of nuclear proto-oncogenes and homeobox genes, the actions of peptide growth factors, and alterations in both cell adhesion and the composition of the extracellular matrix.

GROSS ANATOMY. The kidneys are located in the retroperitoneal space and extend from the twelfth thoracic to the third lumbar vertebrae. The right organ usually is more caudad, while the left organ tends to be slightly larger. Each adult human kidney weighs 115 to 170 grams, measures approximately 11 × 6 × 2.5 cm, and is surrounded by a tough, fibroelastic capsule.

The cut surface of a bisected kidney reveals a darker inner region, the medulla, and a pale outer region, the cortex. The human kidney has a multipapillary configuration in which the medulla is divided into 8 to 18 striated conical masses called *pyramids* (Fig. 74–1). The base of each pyramid is positioned at the corticomedullary junction, and the apex extends toward the renal pelvis, forming a papilla. On the tip of each papilla there are numerous small openings that represent the distal ends of the collecting ducts (of Bellini). Extending downward between the pyramids are portions of cortex, the septa of Bertin. Close examination of the cut

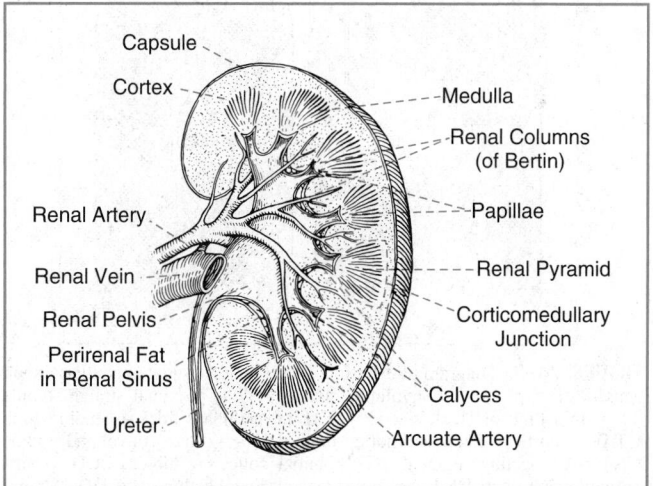

FIGURE 74–1. Sagittal section of human kidney illustrating gross anatomic features.

surface reveals fine longitudinal striations, the medullary rays (of Ferrein), which extend into the cortex. Despite their name, the medullary rays actually represent part of the cortex and are formed by the straight segments of the proximal tubule, the thick ascending limbs, and the collecting ducts.

The renal pelvis is the saclike dilatation of the upper ureter. Two or three major calyces extend from the pelvis and divide into the minor calyces which surround individual papillae.

THE NEPHRON. Each human kidney contains about 0.8 to 1.2×10^6 nephrons—the functional units of the kidney. A nephron consists of the glomerulus or renal corpuscle, the proximal tubule, the thin limbs of Henle, and the distal tubule, all of which originate from the metanephric blastema (Fig. 74–2). The connecting tubule, a transitional segment also derived from the metanephric blastema, joins the nephron to the collecting duct system. Although not anatomically precise, the term "nephron" is commonly used to also include the entire collecting duct.

ARCHITECTURE. In the renal cortex, two architectural regions can be distinguished, the *cortical labyrinth* and the *medullary rays* (Fig. 74–1). The cortical labyrinth is a continuous zone of parenchyma that surrounds the medullary rays. Glomeruli, proximal and distal convoluted tubules, connecting tubules, initial collecting tubules, interlobular veins, and a rich capillary network are located in the cortical labyrinth. Ascending connecting tubules of juxta-medullary nephrons fuse to form arcades within the cortical labyrinth. The medullary rays contain the proximal and distal straight tubules and collecting ducts that all enter the medulla.

In the medulla, specific nephron segments are found at precise levels and divide the medulla into an inner and an outer zone, with the latter subdivided into an inner and an outer stripe (Fig. 74–2). In the outer stripe of the outer medulla are the terminal portions of the proximal straight tubules, the thick ascending limbs, and the collecting ducts. The thicker inner stripe of the outer medulla contains thin descending limbs, thick ascending limbs, and collecting ducts. The thin descending and thin ascending limbs of long loops and the collecting ducts are located in the inner medulla. This intricate arrangement of the parenchyma in the cortex and medulla provides an anatomic basis for integration of the various complex functions of the kidney.

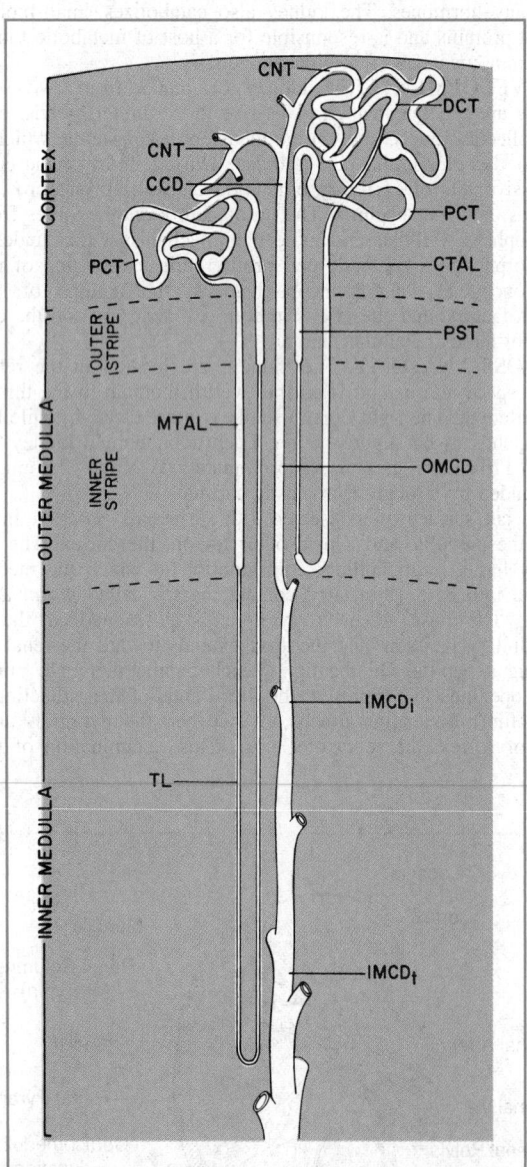

FIGURE 74–2. Diagram illustrating superficial and juxtamedullary nephrons. PCT = proximal convoluting tubule; PST = proximal straight tubule; TL = thin limb of Henle's loop; MTAL = medullary thick ascending limb; CTAL = cortical thick ascending limb; DCT = distal convoluted tubule; CNT = connecting segment; ICT = initial collecting tubule; CCD = cortical collecting duct; OMCD = outer medullary collecting duct; IMCD = initial inner medullary collecting duct; and IMCD = terminal inner medullary collecting duct. (Modified from Madsen KM, Tisher CC: Structural-functional relationships along the distal nephron. Am J Physiol 250:F1, 1986.)

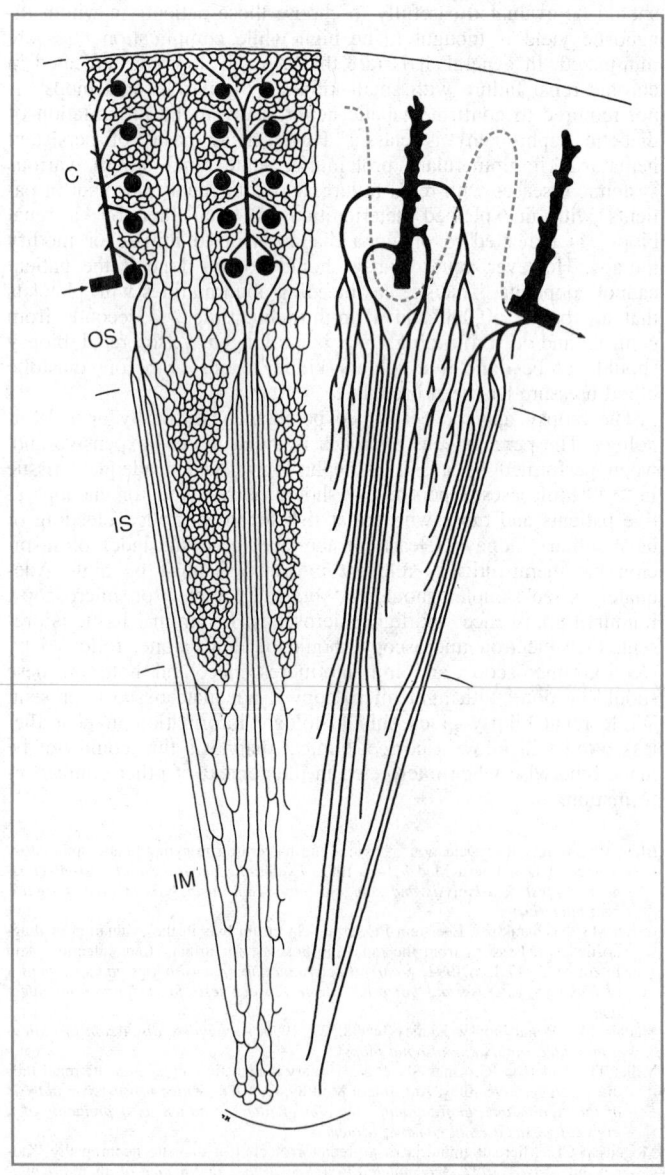

FIGURE 74–3. Diagram illustrating the vascular arrangement in the renal cortex and medulla. (Reproduced with permission from Kriz W, Kaissling B: Structural organization of the mammalian kidney. *In* Seldin DW, Giebisch G [eds.]: The Kidney: Physiology and Pathophysiology. 2nd ed. New York, Raven Press, 1992, p 709.)

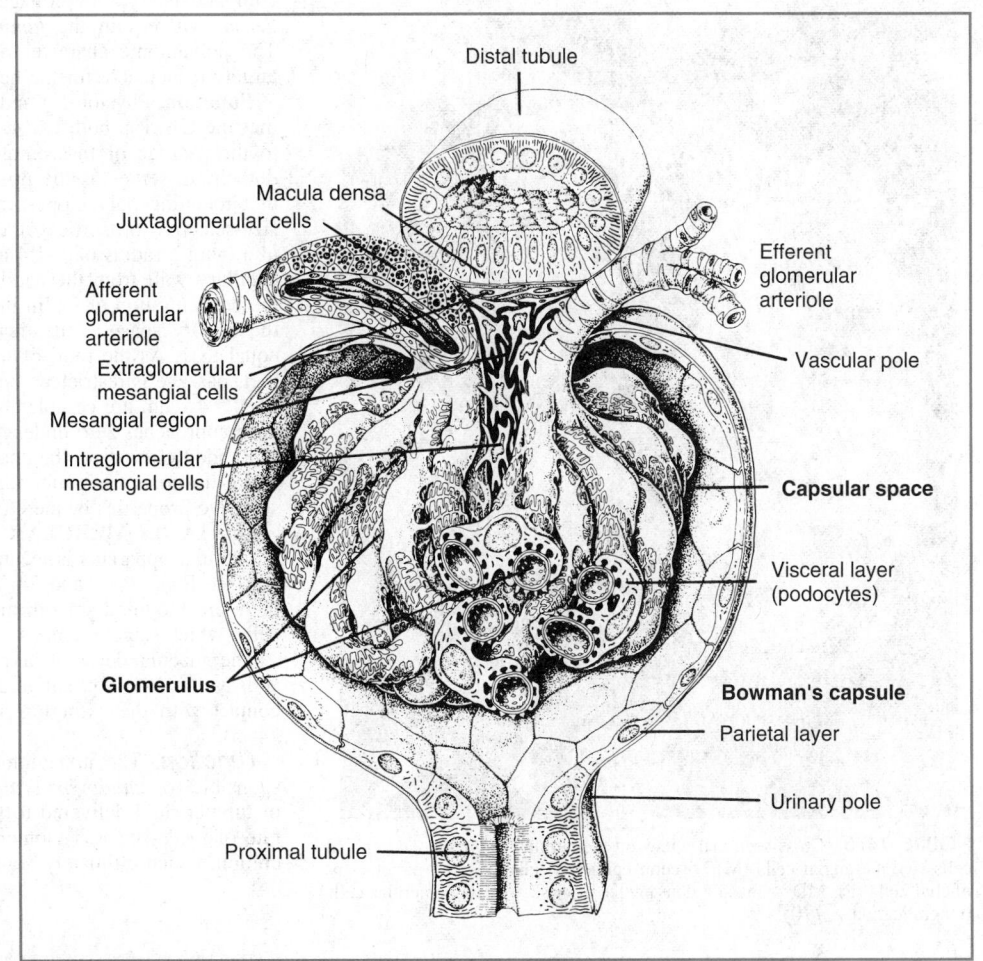

Distal tubule

Macula densa

Juxtaglomerular cells

Efferent glomerular arteriole

Afferent glomerular arteriole

Vascular pole

Extraglomerular mesangial cells

Mesangial region

Intraglomerular mesangial cells

Capsular space

Visceral layer (podocytes)

Glomerulus

Bowman's capsule

Parietal layer

Urinary pole

Proximal tubule

FIGURE 74–4. Schematic three-dimensional depiction of the glomerulus. (From Bargmann W: Histologie und Mikronscopische Anatomie des Menschen. Stuttgart, Georg Thieme Verlag, 1977, p 86.)

VASCULATURE. *Structure.* The kidney has an extensive vasculature that accommodates 20 to 25% of the cardiac output. The main renal artery branches to form anterior and posterior divisions, which in turn divide into five segmental arteries. The *segmental arteries* traverse the renal sinus to divide into the *interlobar arteries.* The latter pierce the parenchyma and course toward the cortex along the septa of Bertin between adjacent renal pyramids (Fig. 74–1). At the corticomedullary junction, the interlobar arteries branch into the *arcuate arteries,* which follow a gently curved course along the base of the pyramids. The arcuate arteries give rise to the *interlobular arteries* that ascend in the cortex toward the renal surface.

Afferent arterioles are branches of the interlobular arteries, and each supplies a single glomerulus (renal corpuscle) (see Fig. 74–3). The *efferent arterioles* exit the glomeruli and divide to form an intricate peritubular microcirculation. The capillary networks formed by the efferent arterioles of superficial and midcortical glomeruli supply the cortical labyrinth and medullary rays, while the efferent arterioles of the juxtamedullary glomeruli are responsible for the entire medullary blood supply. In the outer stripe of the outer medulla these vessels divide to form the *descending vasa recta,* which are located in vascular bundles. At various levels in the medulla the descending vasa recta exit the bundles to form capillary networks. The *ascending vasa recta* drain the medulla.

Function. In a 70-kg person, renal blood flow (RBF) amounts to one fourth to one fifth of the resting cardiac output or 1.2 liters per minute. The renal cortex receives approximately 85 to 90% of this flow compared with 10% for the outer medulla and 1 to 2% for the inner medulla including the papilla. With one kidney removed, blood flow to the remaining kidney will nearly double within a few weeks.

RBF and glomerular filtration rate (GFR) remain relatively constant over a wide range of perfusion pressures, a process that is termed "autoregulation." An intrinsic property of smooth muscle cells in the renal vasculature—the myogenic reflex—permits instantaneous alterations in the tone of the vessel wall to main-

tain RBF and GFR constant over a pressure range of 80 to 180 mm Hg.

There are a host of hormonal and neural factors that can alter RBF. Renal vasoconstrictors that reduce RBF include endothelin, angiotensin II, thromboxane, stimulation of the α-adrenergic system, vasopressin, and catecholamines. Vasodilating agents include the prostaglandins PGI_2 and PGE_2 and atrial peptides, bradykinin, and endothelial-derived relaxing factor or nitric oxide.

GLOMERULUS. *Structure.* The anatomically correct name for the glomerulus is the *renal corpuscle.* However, because of common usage, this structure is usually called the *glomerulus.* The glomerulus, or renal corpuscle, includes the glomerular tuft and Bowman's capsule (Fig. 74–4). The glomerular tuft contains three specialized cells, a basement membrane, and a supporting framework, the mesangium. The specialized cells include the *endothelial cells* that line the lumina of the capillaries, the *mesangial cells* located in the centrilobular region of the glomerular tuft, and the *visceral epithelial cells* that are situated on the outer surfaces of the capillaries (Fig. 74–5). A fourth cell type, the *parietal epithelial cell,* lines Bowman's capsule. At the vascular pole where the afferent and efferent arterioles enter and exit the glomerulus, respectively, the visceral epithelium is continuous with the parietal epithelium. Thus the glomerulus resembles an epithelial-lined sac invaginated by a tuft of capillaries. Bowman's space, also called the "urinary space," represents the expanse between the visceral epithelial cells and the parietal epithelial layer lining Bowman's capsule. It receives the glomerular filtrate and at the urinary pole leads into the proximal tubule (see Fig. 74–4). A filtration barrier is formed between the blood and the urinary space by the fenestrated endothelium, the peripheral glomerular basement membrane (GBM), and the overlying visceral epithelial cell (Fig. 74–6). In humans, the mean area of the filtration surface per glomerulus is approximately 0.136 sq mm.

Function. Ultrafiltration. In a 70-kg person, the kidney forms approximately 180 liters of glomerular filtrate each day via a process termed "ultrafiltration." This represents the initial step in

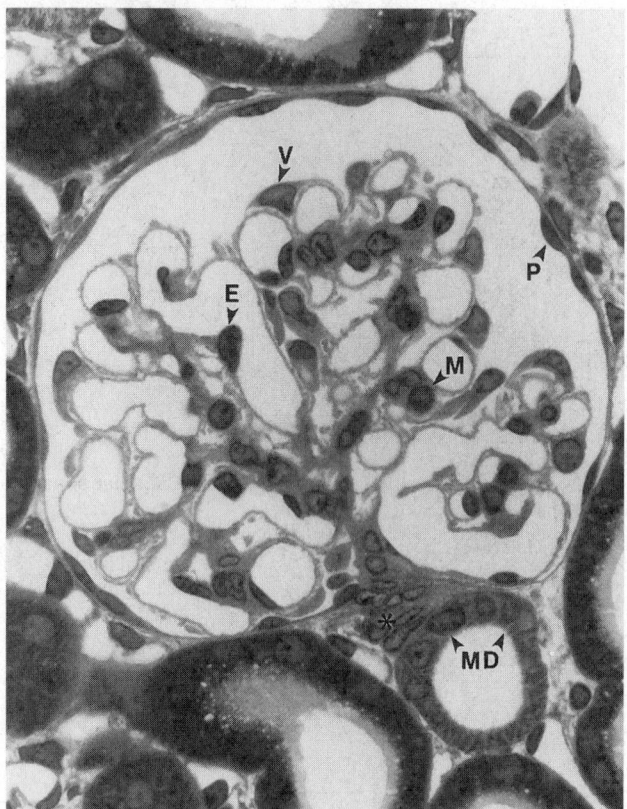

FIGURE 74–5. Cross-sectional view of glomerulus depicting endothelial cells (E), mesangial cells (M), visceral epithelial cells (V), and parietal epithelial cells (P). MD = macula densa cells; asterisk = juxtaglomerular cells (magnification × 770).

urine formation. The driving force to move fluid from the glomerular capillaries across the glomerular capillary wall to the urinary space (Bowman's space) is derived from the hydraulic pressure that is generated by the pumping action of the heart. Each glomerulus has a filtration rate (single nephron glomerular filtration rate [SNGFR]) of 60 nl per minute, which is much higher per unit surface area than other capillary beds in the body. The rate of filtration is proportional to the net ultrafiltration pressure (P_{UF}) that is present across the glomerular capillary wall and is determined by the balance of hydraulic *(P)* and oncotic (Π) pressures (Starling forces) that are operative between the glomerular capillary lumen and Bowman's space. The intrinsic water permeability of the capillary wall *(k)* and the surface area *(A)*, which together define the ultrafiltration coefficient *(K_f)*, are also important determinants of ultrafiltration. Thus

$$\begin{aligned} \text{SNGFR} &= K_f \cdot \overline{P}_{UF} \\ &= K_f \cdot [(\overline{P}_{GC} - P_T) - (\Pi_{GC} - \Pi_T)] \\ &= k \cdot A(\overline{\Delta P} - \overline{\Delta \Pi}) \end{aligned}$$

where GC and T refer to glomerular capillary and Bowman's space, respectively, and the overbar denotes mean values.

Since under normal circumstances there is virtually no protein in the ultrafiltrate, the oncotic pressure in the urinary space (Π_T) approaches zero and therefore does not affect ultrafiltration. Increasing the oncotic pressure in the glomerular capillary (as in multiple myeloma with its characteristic hyperproteinemia), increasing the hydraulic pressure in Bowman's space (via ureteral obstruction), and lowering glomerular capillary hydraulic pressure (as in hypotension) all reduce SNGFR.

Glomerular Basement Membrane. Structure. The GBM is a hydrated gel containing cross-linked molecules that form a complex, three-dimensional lattice-like network (see Fig. 74–6). Biochemical and immunocytochemical studies have revealed that the GBM is composed of type IV and type V collagen, laminin, hepa-

ran sulfate proteoglycans, and nidogen or entactin, as well as other components. Type IV collagen is the main component in the *lamina densa,* whereas in the *laminae rarae* other proteins predominate. The polyanionic character of the heparan sulfate proteoglycans is largely responsible for the net negative charge of the GBM.

Function. Physiologic and ultrastructural studies have established that the GBM is both a *size-selective* and a *charge-selective* barrier to the passage of macromolecules. The GBM, along with the endothelium, serves as the principal functional barrier to the passage of circulating polyanions across the glomerular capillary wall. The size-selective properties of the GBM allow molecules such as inulin, with a radius of ∼ 1.4 nm, to pass freely across the glomerular capillary wall from the capillary lumen to the urinary space. Since the concentration of inulin in both the plasma water and the fluid in the urinary space is identical, the fractional clearance of inulin is equal to 1. As the radii of macromolecules increase above 2.0 nm, their passage is restricted across the GBM, and molecules with a radius >4.2 nm are completely restricted. Thus their fractional clearance approaches zero under normal circumstances.

In addition to size, the charge of a molecule can greatly affect its ability to cross the glomerular capillary wall. The size and charge-selective properties of the GBM are summarized in Figure 74–7.

JUXTAGLOMERULAR APPARATUS. Structure. The juxtaglomerular apparatus is located at the vascular pole of the glomerulus (see Figs. 74–4 and 74–5). In the wall of the afferent arteriole there are modified smooth muscle cells, the so-called myoepithelial cells, which secrete renin.

The macula densa is a plaquelike configuration of specialized cells within the cortical thick ascending limb of Henle that is in contact with the extraglomerular mesangium (see Figs. 74–4 and 74–5).

Function. The juxtaglomerular apparatus is believed to be responsible for *tubuloglomerular feedback,* in which the composition of tubular fluid delivered to the macula densa changes the filtration rate of the associated glomerulus, presumably by altering renin secretion, which ultimately regulates glomerular hemodynamics.

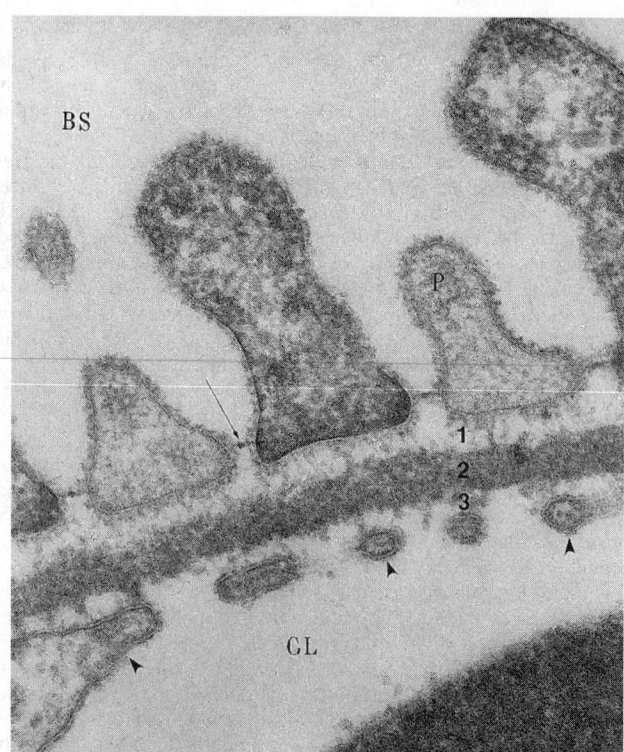

FIGURE 74–6. Cross section of glomerular capillary wall illustrating the pedicels (P) of the visceral epithelial cells, the fenestrated endothelium *(arrowheads),* and the three layers of the GBM that include the lamina rara externa (1), the lamina densa (2), and the lamina rara interna (3). BS = Bowman's space; CL = capillary lumen; arrow = filtration slit diaphragm (magnification × 120,000). (From Tisher CC, Madsen KM: Anatomy of the kidney. *In* Brenner BM, Rector FC Jr [eds.]: The Kidney. 4th ed. Philadelphia, WB Saunders, 1991, p. 14.)

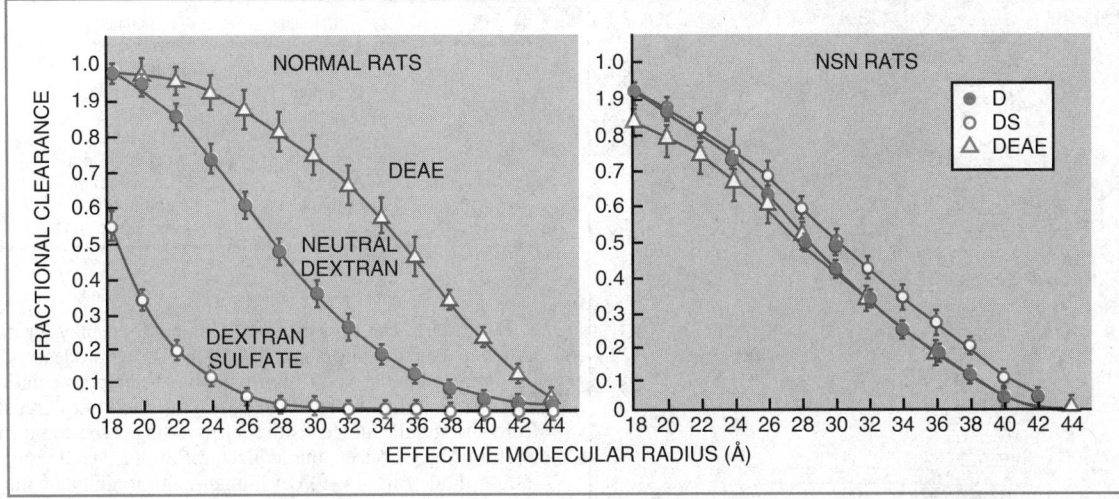

FIGURE 74–7. Fractional clearances of diethylaminoethyl (DEAE) dextran, neutral dextran, and dextran sulfate, plotted as a function of effective molecular radius in normal rats (left) and in rats with nephrotoxic serum nephritis (NSN, right). Values are expressed as means ± 1 SEM. (From Bohrer MP, Baylis C, Humes HD, et al.: Permselectivity of the glomerular capillary wall: Facilitated filtration of circulating polycations. J Clin Invest 61:72, 1978, by copyright permission of the American Society for Clinical Investigation.)

PROXIMAL TUBULE. Structure. The proximal tubule includes an initial convoluted portion, the *pars convoluta,* located in the cortical labyrinth, and a straight portion, the *pars recta,* located in the medullary ray. Proximal tubule cells are tall and possess a prominent brush border that markedly increases the surface area of the luminal membrane. The cells contain a well-developed endocytic-lysosomal apparatus that has an important role in the absorption and degradation of macromolecules such as albumin from the glomerular filtrate.

The basolateral plasma membranes are markedly amplified due to extensive interdigitations of basal and lateral cytoplasmic processes between adjacent cells. The localization of Na$^+$-K$^+$-ATPase (the sodium pump) to the basolateral membranes explains the active transport of sodium characteristic of this tubule segment. Numerous elongated mitochondria are located close to the interdigitating basolateral membrane processes, providing a source for the cellular energy required for active transport. There is an excellent correlation along the length of the proximal tubule between the elaborate basolateral membrane expressed as surface area, the high Na$^+$-K$^+$-ATPase activity localized to this membrane, and the capacity to transport sodium and other ions. Therefore, the intrinsic rates at which solutes and fluid are transported decrease along the proximal tubule from S$_1$ to S$_3$.

Function. The proximal tubule is the first component of the nephron that modifies the volume and ionic composition of the glomerular ultrafiltrate. Through isosmotic fluid reabsorption, fluid volume is reduced by ≥60% under normal conditions. The principal driving force for the reabsorption of solutes is Na$^+$-K$^+$-ATPase located along the basolateral plasma membrane. By maintaining a low intracellular sodium concentration, there is passive entry of Na$^+$ into the cell across the luminal plasma membrane and down its electrochemical gradient. In the early proximal tubule this leads to a small electrical potential difference *(PD)* that is lumen-negative. Sodium is pumped out of the cell actively at the basolateral surface

via Na$^+$-K$^+$-ATPase. This process also creates a slight osmotic gradient which facilitates the reabsorption of fluid. The balance between osmotic and hydraulic pressures (Starling's forces) in the peritubular capillaries and the surrounding interstitium determines the extent of the backleak of sodium and water to the tubule lumen via the intercellular space through the nonoccluding tight junction and thus the net reabsorption of sodium and water and other solutes.

Reabsorption of glucose, amino acids, citrate, lactate, acetate, and phosphate also occurs early in the proximal tubule via sodium-coupled active transport processes. Other ions are listed in Table 74–1.

The critical elements of bicarbonate reabsorption are depicted in Figure 74–8.

The proximal tubule is also an important site for *ammoniagenesis,* where glutamine serves as the substrate. Ammonia combines with protons, forming the ammonium ion (NH$_4^+$) , which is then secreted into the tubule lumen. This process is enhanced in metabolic acidosis and hypokalemia.

Secretion. The proximal tubule also modifies the composition of the tubular fluid through a number of well-defined secretory processes. The liver produces a number of cationic and anionic organic waste products such as urate, hippurate, oxalate, and bile salts that must be eliminated by the kidney. Certain exogenous compounds and drugs are also removed from the plasma in a single pass through the kidney. The S$_2$ segment of the proximal tubule represents the prime, although not exclusive, site for organic ion secretion. The initial step in the secretory process involves active transport against a concentration gradient at the basolateral surface of the cell followed by passive diffusion across the luminal plasma membrane into the tubule fluid. Table 74–2 lists several of the more common drugs that are secreted by the proximal tubule.

THIN LIMBS OF HENLE'S LOOP. Structure. There is an abrupt transition from the terminal proximal tubule to the descending thin limb of Henle's loop at the junction between the outer and inner stripes of the outer medulla (see Fig. 74–2). Short-looped

TABLE 74–1. RESORPTION OF IONS IN THE PROXIMAL TUBULE

Anion	Site of Resorption	Process
Potassium	Freely filtered in glomerulus	70% reabsorbed by passive, parallels Na$^+$ + H$_2$O regulated by transepithelial potential difference.
Bicarbonate	Proximal tubule	90 of 4500 mEq HCO$_3^-$ filtered daily by sodium-hydrogen exchange in brush border secondary to hydrogen ion secretion.
Hydrogen	Proximal tubule	65% reabsorbed: mediated by Na$^+$/H$^+$ antiporter; 35% reabsorbed by electronic Na$^+$-independent H$^+$-ATPase.
Chloride	S$_2$ segment of proximal tubule	Couples to active transport of Na$^+$; passive transport driven by favorable lumen-to-peritubular concentration grade for Cl$^-$.
Calcium	Proximal tubule	Passive transport: exits tubular lumen by voltage-dependent diffusion. Active transport: Na$^+$-Ca^{2+} exchanger and Ca^{2+} ATPase.

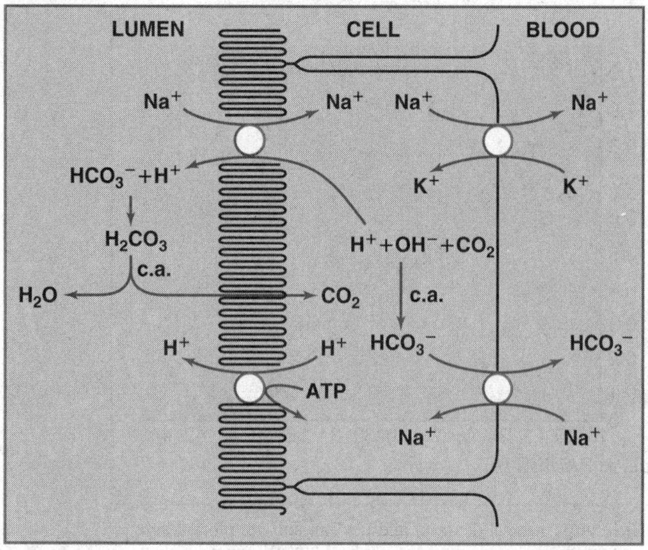

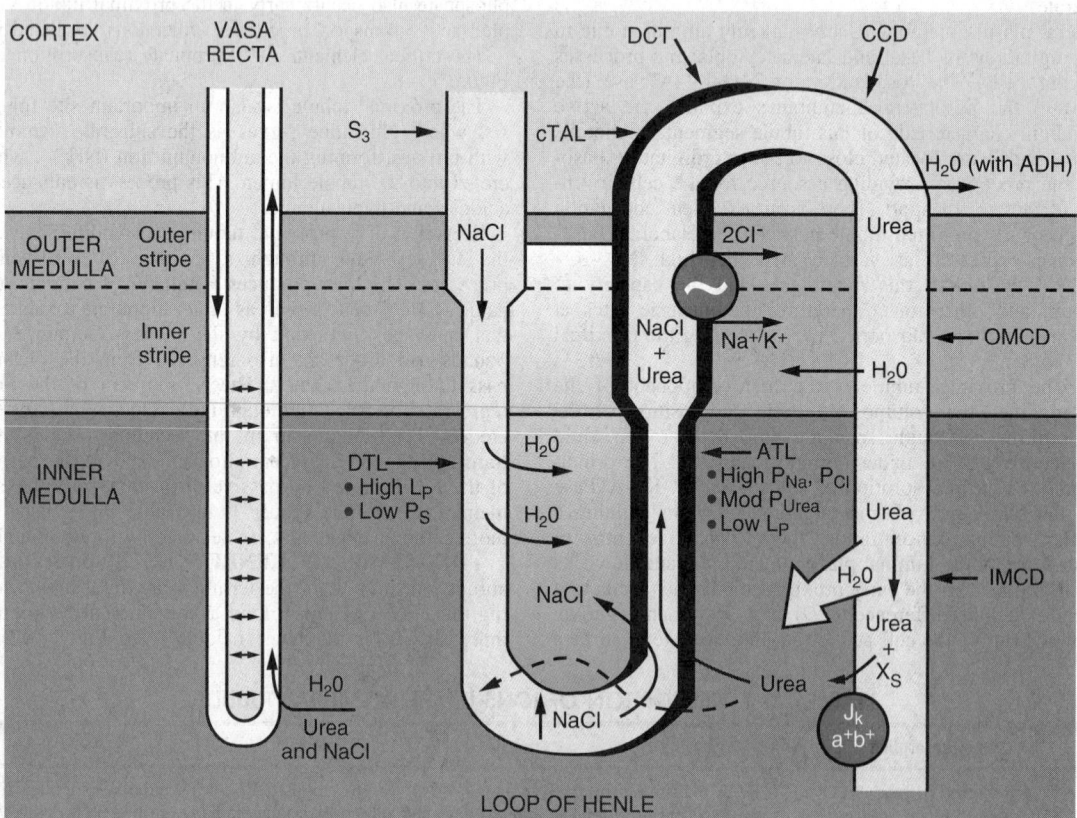

FIGURE 74–8. Diagram depicting the major mechanism for bicarbonate reclamation in the proximal convoluted tubule. c.a. = carbonic anhydrase.

nephrons have a short descending thin limb that continues into the thick ascending limb near the bend in the loop. Long-looped nephrons have a long descending thin limb that enters the inner medulla, forms a bend, and returns as a long ascending thin limb. The thin limbs are lined with a low-lying simple epithelium.

TABLE 74–2. COMMON DRUGS SECRETED BY THE PROXIMAL TUBULE

Cationic	Anionic
Cimetidine	Penicillin
Paraquat	Furosemide
Quinine	Probenecid
Morphine	Salicylates
Trimethoprim	Acetazolamide
Atropine	Chlorothiazides
Epinephrine	Cephalothin
	Ethacrynic acid

Function. The thin limbs of Henle's loop play an important role in urine concentration and dilution. The thin descending limb in the inner medulla has a high osmotic water permeability (L_p) but a low permeability to solutes (P_S). This facilitates transfer of water from the tubule lumen to the surrounding hypertonic medullary interstitium and raises the concentration of NaCl and urea in the tubule fluid (Fig. 74–9). In humans, the tonicity of the tubule fluid can reach 1200 mOsm per kilogram of H_2O with severe water restriction.

The thin ascending limb of Henle has a low osmotic water permeability, a moderate permeability for urea, and a high permeability for NaCl. The surrounding interstitium has an NaCl concentration that is lower and a urea concentration that is higher than the tubule fluid at the hairpin turn. These characteristics favor formation of a dilute tubule fluid, since the passive movement of NaCl out of the tubule exceeds the passive entry of urea into the tubule. Thus, at any given level in the inner medulla, the tonicity of the surrounding interstitial fluid is greater than that of the tubule fluid in the thin ascending limb of Henle (see Fig. 74–9). Overall, the thin limbs of

FIGURE 74–9. Diagram illustrating the essential components of the countercurrent multiplication and exchange systems in the kidney (see text for explanation). The heavy black line indicates water-impermeable segments of the nephron, and shading denotes progressive increase in tonicity of the medullary interstitium. S_3 = third segment of proximal tubule; DTL = descending thin limb; ATL = ascending thin limb; cTAL = cortical thick ascending limb; DCT = distal convoluted tubule; CCD = cortical collecting duct; OMCD = outer medullary collecting duct; IMCD = inner medullary collecting duct; L_p = osmotic water permeability; P_S, P_{Na}, P_{Cl}, P_{ure} = permeability to solutes, Na^+, Cl^-, and urea, respectively; X_S = nonreabsorbable solutes; and $J_K a^+ b^+$ = Kidd antigen and urea transporter. (Modified from Brenner BM, Coe FL, Rector FC Jr [eds]: Renal Physiology in Health and Disease. Philadelphia, WB Saunders, 1987, pp 53 and 160.)

the loop of Henle reabsorb about 15% of the glomerular ultrafiltrate and up to 25% of the sodium and chloride.

DISTAL TUBULE. *Structure.* The distal tubule includes three morphologically distinct segments: the *thick ascending limb* (TAL) of Henle's loop, the *macula densa,* and the *distal convoluted tubule* (DCT) (see Fig. 74–2). The TAL traverses the outer medulla upward into the cortex near its glomerulus of origin to end just beyond the macula densa. Thus the TAL can be divided into a medullary and a cortical segment.

The *TAL* is composed of cuboidal cells with extensive basolateral plasma membrane invaginations and interdigitations between adjacent cells which enclose elongated mitochondria. These ultrastructural features are typical of epithelial cells involved in active solute transport.

The *DCT* represents the terminal part of the distal tubule and begins at a variable distance beyond the macula densa. The cells of the DCT resemble those of the TAL.

Function. The TAL actively reabsorbs NaCl, which is mediated by an $Na^+-K^+-2Cl^-$ co-transport mechanism in the apical plasma membrane (see Fig. 74–9). The energy for this process is provided by the N^+-K^+-ATPase localized on the basolateral plasma membrane. The principal function of the medullary TAL is to generate and maintain a hypertonic medullary interstitium that permits a maximally concentrated urine to form, while the cortical segment continues to dilute the tubule fluid, permitting the formation of a maximally dilute urine. Thus the tubule fluid that exits the cortical TAL has an osmolality of < 150 mOsm per kilogram of H_2O. At this point, the total volume of the original glomerular ultrafiltrate in the nephron has been reduced by 85%.

The TAL also reabsorbs *calcium* from the tubular fluid. Throughout the TAL, a significant component of calcium transport is passive and driven by the transepithelial potential difference (PD_t). Active transport has been identified in the cortical TAL, which is independent of Ca^{2+}-ATPase activity, Na^+ transport, and anerobic metabolism. Calcium transport is enhanced in the cortical TAL by parathyroid hormone (PTH) and cAMP and in the medullary TAL by calcitonin and cAMP.

Bicarbonate transport is present along the entire TAL via a sodium-coupled HCO_3^- transport mechanism located on the basolateral plasma membrane. Active and passive transport of NH_4^+ out of the lumen and into the interstitium for subsequent transport in the form of NH_3 into the lumen of the collecting duct also occurs in the TAL. Thus this region of the nephron also plays a role in acidification of the tubule fluid.

The cortical TAL is a major site for reabsorbing *magnesium.* The passive component of magnesium transport is facilitated by the $Na^+-K^+-2Cl^-$ co-transport mechanism that establishes a favorable lumen-positive electrochemical gradient, while the active magnesium transport mechanism is incompletely understood.

In the DCT, *sodium chloride* continues to be reabsorbed via a ouabain-sensitive Na^+-K^+-ATPase–driven active transport process. Because the DCT is also impermeable to water, there is further dilution of the tubule fluid to an osmolality of approximately 100 mOsm per kilogram of H_2O. This segment is also a site for *calcium* reabsorption stimulated by calcitonin and PTH.

CONNECTING TUBULE. *Structure.* The connecting tubule or connecting segment joins the DCT with the collecting duct system (see Fig. 74–2). Representing a transitional segment in the human kidney, the connecting tubule is composed of four specific cell types resulting from an intermixing of cells from the adjacent DCT and the initial collecting tubule (ICT). The most characteristic cell type is the connecting tubule cell, which is intermediate in appearance between the DCT cell and the principal cell of the collecting duct. Intercalated cells involved in proton and bicarbonate transport vary considerably in structure in the connecting tubule.

Function. PTH affects *calcium* transport in this segment, while vasopressin (ADH) has no effect on adenylate cyclase activity or water permeability. This segment is responsible for reabsorbing *sodium* and secreting *potassium.* The latter is believed to be at least partially controlled by mineralocorticoids. The connecting segment is also involved in *proton* and *bicarbonate* transport and is a major site for kallikrein production and secretion in the kidney.

COLLECTING DUCT. *Structure.* The collecting duct begins in the cortex and descends through the medulla to the tip of the papilla. It can be divided into cortical, outer medullary, and inner medullary segments (see Fig. 74–2). There is remarkable cellular heterogeneity along the collecting duct.

The *cortical collecting duct* (CCD) can be subdivided into the ICT and the medullary ray portion. The CCD is composed of both principal cells and intercalated cells. The principal cells, which represent approximately two-thirds of the total cell population, have a light-staining cytoplasm and relatively few organelles but prominent infoldings of the basal plasma membrane. The intercalated or "dark" cells comprise approximately one-third of the cells in the CCD. There is now evidence for the presence of two distinct configurations of intercalated cells, type A and type B, in the CCD. Type A cells have prominent microprojections on the apical plasma membrane and extensive tubulovesicular structures in the apical cytoplasm. Type B cells have a more dense cytoplasm, more mitochondria, more spherical vesicular structures in the cytoplasm, and a larger basolateral membrane surface area. The type B cell is localized to the CCD.

The *outer medullary collecting duct* (OMCD) is lined by principal cells and intercalated cells. The latter comprise one-third of the cells in the OMCD and resemble the type A cells in the CCD.

The *inner medullary collecting duct* (IMCD) is subdivided into two regions: the initial IMCD, located in the outer third of the inner medulla, and the terminal IMCD, situated in the distal two-thirds of the inner medulla (see Fig. 74–2). The initial IMCD is composed mainly of principal cells and a few intercalated cells, while the terminal IMCD is composed of one cell type, the IMCD cell.

Function. The collecting duct represents the final site in the renal tubule that modifies the volume and solute composition of the tubule fluid.

Water Transport. In all segments of the collecting duct the osmotic water permeability is controlled largely by vasopressin or antidiuretic hormone (ADH). In the absence of vasopressin, only the papillary collecting duct manifests some residual permeability. With vasopressin, the principal cells and all cells in the terminal IMCD are highly permeable to water (see Fig. 74–9). However, in vasopressin-induced antidiuresis, the bulk of the tubule fluid is reabsorbed in the CCD.

Proton and Bicarbonate Transport. The entire collecting duct is involved in proton transport and hence the fine tuning of acid secretion by the kidney. The presence of high levels of carbonic anhydrase II in the intercalated cells suggested initially that they were involved in urine acidification. Immunocytochemical studies have localized a vacuolar type H^+-ATPase in the apical membrane and a Cl^-/HCO_3^- exchanger in the basolateral membrane of type A intercalated cells (Fig. 74–10A). These findings implicate the type A cell in proton or hydrogen ion secretion in the CCD. The immunolocalization of H^+-ATPase to the basolateral membrane of type B cells and the functional evidence for an apical Cl^-/HCO_3^- exchanger in these cells provide evidence that type B intercalated cells are involved in bicarbonate secretion (Fig. 74–10B).

The intercalated cells in the OMCD are responsible for hydrogen ion secretion, which is an active mineralocorticoid-stimulated, sodium-independent process driven in part by H^+-ATPase. The IMCD is also involved in urine acidification. Acid-secreting intercalated cells are present in the initial IMCD, while microcatheterization studies have documented a decrease in luminal pH along the IMCD.

Urea Transport. The cortical and outer medullary segments of the collecting duct are largely impermeable to urea in both the presence and absence of vasopressin. In the terminal IMCD, urea reabsorption occurs via a vasopressin-sensitive, phloretin-inhibitable, facilitated transport pathway that helps to maintain a high urea concentration in the deep inner medulla to facilitate urea recycling, which is important for maximum urine concentration (see Fig. 74–9).

Sodium and Potassium Transport. Virtually all sodium transport and much of the potassium transport in the collecting duct is controlled by aldosterone. While it is this region of the renal tubule that "fine tunes" sodium excretion, it is estimated that < 10% of the filtered load of sodium is actually controlled by aldosterone. The target cell for aldosterone is the principal cell. Aldosterone increases sodium reabsorption by increasing the number of sodium channels in the apical plasma membrane of the principal cell. The sodium channels permit electrogenic sodium entry down a concentration gradient, creating a lumen-negative potential difference. The increase in intracellular sodium concentration stimulates basolateral

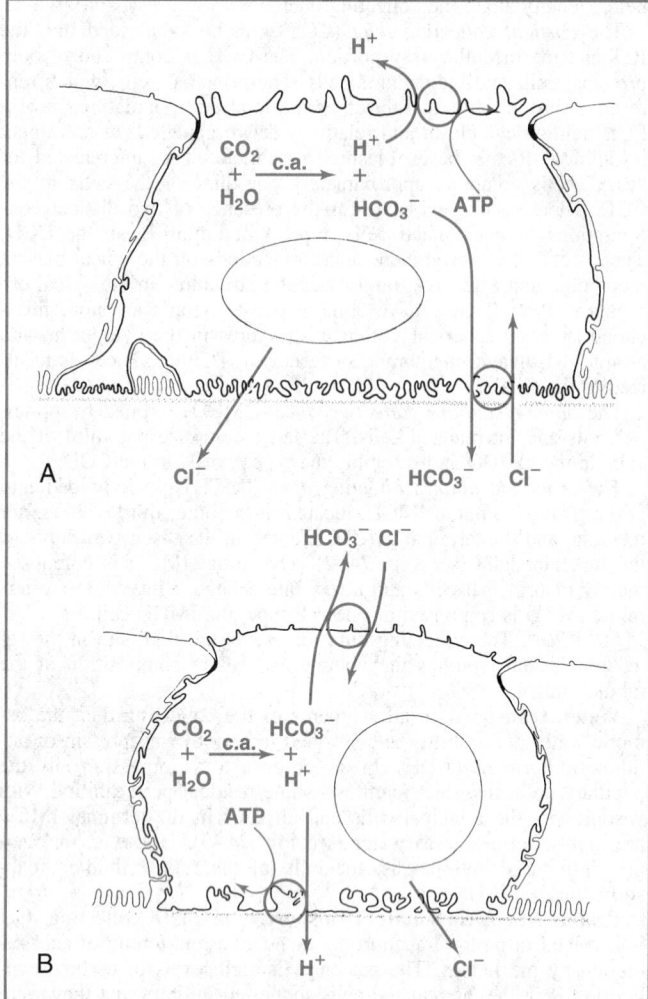

FIGURE 74-10. Diagrams illustrating transport characteristics of type A *(above)* and type B *(below)* intercalated cells of the CCD. (Used with permission from Madsen KM, Verlander JW, Kim J, Tisher CC: Morphological adaptation of the collecting duct to acid-base disturbances. Kidney Int 40(Suppl 33):S57, 1991.)

Na^+-K^+-ATPase activity to maintain a concentration gradient for sodium entry while at the same time increasing the intracellular potassium concentration. Potassium secretion across the luminal membrane through aldosterone-sensitive potassium channels is also enhanced by the lumen-negative potential difference. Thus conditions that increase plasma aldosterone levels will enhance sodium absorption and potassium secretion.

Intercalated cells also help maintain potassium balance by the collecting duct. During states of potassium deprivation, an H^+-K^+-ATPase located in the intercalated cell facilitates reabsorption in exchange for hydrogen ions throughout the CCD and OMCD.

INTEGRATION OF NORMAL NEPHRON FUNCTION.
Sodium Homeostasis. Each day approximately 25,000 mEq of sodium (140 mEq per liter × 180 liters) is filtered, while <1% is actually excreted in the urine by a euvolemic individual. Thus the bulk of filtered sodium is reabsorbed along the nephron. Normally, about 65% of the filtered sodium is reabsorbed by the proximal tubule, 20% by the TAL, 7 to 10% by the DCT, and the remainder by the collecting duct. With a salt load, there is a progressive increase in urine sodium excretion until a new steady state is achieved where output matches intake. Until a steady state is attained, however, the individual goes into positive sodium balance, retains water, and gains weight. Restricting sodium intake will produce the opposite effect until the kidney fully compensates over a 3- to 5-day period.

Several factors influence normal sodium balance. For instance, the kidney is extremely sensitive to changes in effective arterial blood volume. Dehydration or acute volume depletion secondary to blood loss leads to a fall in RBF and GFR secondary to a decrease in cardiac output, activation of the renin-angiotensin-aldosterone system, and an increase in renal sympathetic nerve activity. As the filtered load of sodium decreases, the proximal tubule increases sodium reabsorption. Because the vasoconstrictive effect of angiotensin II affects the efferent glomerular arteriole to a greater degree than the afferent arteriole, the filtration fraction is increased, thereby increasing the oncotic pressure in the peritubular capillaries. This, in turn, enhances proximal tubule sodium and fluid reabsorption. An increase in the plasma level of aldosterone from activation of the renin-angiotensin-aldosterone system stimulates sodium reabsorption in the collecting duct. Expansion of the effective arterial blood volume, as occurs with excessive sodium intake or administering intravenous saline, has the opposite effect.

Other factors also control renal sodium excretion. Several hormones lead to retention of sodium by acting at the tubular level (e.g., growth hormone, cortisol, insulin, and estrogen). On the other hand, PTH, progesterone, and glycogen inhibit the tubular reabsorption of sodium. Atrial natriuretic peptide—a 28–amino acid peptide produced in the atria of the heart and released in the circulation in response to atrial stretch from, for example, expansion of the central blood volume—also enhances sodium excretion, in part by inhibiting sodium reabsorption by the collecting duct.

Potassium Homeostasis. The kidney is chiefly responsible for maintaining potassium homeostasis. The total-body potassium content of a 70-kg individual is estimated at approximately 3500 mEq, 98 to 99% of which resides in the intracellular compartment at a concentration of 125 mEq per liter. The concentration of potassium in the extracellular fluid ranges between 3.5 and 4.5 mEq per liter. Each day approximately 720 mEq of potassium (4.0 mEq per liter × 180 liters) is filtered, while only 10 to 15% is excreted in the urine by an individual with normal body potassium stores. In general, potassium excretion equals potassium ingestion. With a normal potassium intake of approximately 100 mEq per day, the kidney will excrete all but about 10 mEq. Approximately 70% of the filtered load of potassium is reabsorbed in the proximal tubule and another 15 to 20% in the loop of Henle. The kidney can respond quickly to increase potassium excretion by as much as 10-fold when potassium intake is increased. However, with potassium deprivation, it takes up to 14 days to reach a new steady state, a period of time sufficient to develop a considerable potassium deficit.

It is the collecting duct that is responsible for "fine tuning" potassium excretion. In general, the principal cells secrete potassium under the control of mineralocorticoids, while intercalated cells reabsorb potassium. Most of the potassium that appears in the urine is secreted by the collecting duct. Several factors influence renal potassium secretion. These include the rate of distal tubule fluid flow, acid–base balance, aldosterone, and the electronegativity of the distal tubule. The flow dependence of potassium secretion in the collecting duct is well documented. With an increase in flow (such as that induced by diuretics), there is a parallel increase in sodium delivery to the collecting duct, which facilitates sodium reabsorption and potassium secretion. With metabolic acidosis, and to a lesser extent with respiratory acidosis, potassium secretion is suppressed. An opposite effect is observed in metabolic alkalosis. With an increase in the circulating aldosterone level (such as that induced by hyperkalemia), there is a parallel increase in the exchange of sodium for potassium by the principal cells, leading to enhanced potassium secretion. Finally, an increase in the lumen-negative potential, a decrease in the luminal potassium concentration, an increase in the intracellular potassium concentration, and an increase in the luminal membrane permeability to potassium all favor potassium secretion by the principal cell.

The kidney also can protect against *hypokalemia*. Recently, the presence of H^+-K^+-ATPase has been documented in the intercalated cell of the collecting duct, and data suggest that with potassium deprivation there is enhanced reabsorption of potassium in exchange for protons in these cells.

Acid–Base Balance. (See Ch. 75.)
Calcium, Phosphorus, and Magnesium Homeostasis. (See Ch. 211 and 212.)
Urine Concentration and Dilution. (See Ch. 75.)

Alpern RJ, Stone DK, Rector FC Jr: Renal acidification mechanisms. *In* Brenner BM, Rector FC Jr (eds.): The Kidney. 4th ed. Philadelphia, WB Saunders, 1991, p 318. *A detailed and up-to-date review of acidification in the kidney.*

Clapp WL, Abrahamson DR: Development and gross anatomy of the kidney. *In* Tisher CC, Brenner BM (eds.): Renal Pathology with Clinical and Functional Correlations. 2nd ed. Philadelphia, JB Lippincott, 1994, pp 3–59. *One of the most detailed and current discussions of kidney development.*

Gonzalez-Campoy JM, Knox FG: Integrated responses of the kidney to alterations in extracellular fluid volume. *In* Seldin DW, Giebisch G (eds.): The Kidney: Physiology and Pathophysiology. 2nd ed. New York, Raven Press, 1992, pp 2041–2098. *An elegant presentation of the mechanisms that control sodium excretion by the kidney.*

Tisher CC, Madsen KM: Anatomy of the kidney. *In* Brenner BM, Rector FC Jr (eds.): The Kidney. 4th ed. Philadelphia, WB Saunders, 1991, pp 3–75. *A detailed and lucid review of kidney structure.*

Wright FS, Giebisch G: Regulation of potassium excretion. *In* Seldin DW, Giebisch G (eds.): The Kidney: Physiology and Pathophysiology. 2nd ed. New York, Raven Press, 1992, pp 2209–2240. *A thorough discussion of how the kidney handles potassium.*

75 DISORDERS OF FLUID VOLUME, ELECTROLYTE, AND ACID-BASE BALANCE

*Juha P. Kokko**

Disorders of fluid, electrolyte, and acid-base metabolism are encountered frequently. While efficient homeostatic mechanisms exist that regulate these metabolic parameters under relatively narrow limits, the capacity of these regulatory mechanisms can be exceeded with derangements of renal, pulmonary, and/or cardiovascular function. These abnormalities are generally reflected in changes in body weight or altered laboratory values or both. It thus has become standard to weigh all patients and to obtain certain laboratory tests such as SMA-7 if alterations in fluid, electrolyte, and acid-base metabolism are suspected. This chapter addresses these areas by sequentially considering disorders of volume, osmolality, potassium, and acid-base metabolism.

75.1 Volume Disorders

PHYSIOLOGIC CONSIDERATIONS

Considering that total body water is distributed into distinct compartments, the volumes of these compartments can be measured relatively accurately. However, to understand fluid homeostasis, one must recognize the significance of the term "effective arterial blood volume." This is discussed in Ch. 73, but in its broadest sense it refers to the volume of blood delivered to the volume-sensitive organs, predominantly brain and kidney.

The Body Fluid Compartments

In healthy adults, body water comprises about 60% of body weight and exists in two compartments: The intracellular compartment (ICF) contains two thirds of body water, or 40% of body weight; the extracellular compartment (ECF) contains the remaining one third of total body water; and total blood volume, that is, plasma plus formed elements, constitutes one third of the total ECF volume. This "rule of thirds" for the body fluid compartments is useful in assessing most clinically encountered fluid and electrolyte disorders. Thus, in a healthy 70-kg man, total body water comprises about 40 liters, of which 25 liters is intracellular. The functional extracellular fluid volume is 15 liters, 5 liters of which is blood, and since the normal hematocrit is 40 to 45%, total plasma volume is approximately 2.75 to 3.0 liters (Fig. 75–1).

More than 95% of total body sodium is extracellular, and sodium and its associated anions, primarily chloride and bicarbonate, con-

* This chapter is revised and modified from the chapter by Thomas E. Andreoli in the preceding edition.

stitute the principal solutes of the ECF. Albumin and other macromolecules present in plasma are restricted to the vascular bed and constitute 5% of plasma volume, so plasma is about 95% water. Since capillaries are freely permeable to water and small solutes, interstitial fluid is a protein-poor, but not entirely protein-free, ultrafiltrate of plasma.

While principal anions of intracellular fluid vary among different cells, Figure 75–1 summarizes the approximate concentrations of various intra- and extracellular cation and anion concentrations.

Regulation of Fluid Transfer Among Compartments

The transfer of fluid between vascular and interstitial compartments occurs at the capillary level and is governed by the balance between hydrostatic pressure gradients and plasma oncotic pressure gradients. This relation may be stated by the familiar Starling equation:

$$J_v = K_f(\Delta P - \Delta \pi)$$

where J_v is rate of fluid transfer between vascular and interstitial compartments, K_f is the water permeability of the capillary bed, ΔP is the hydrostatic pressure difference between capillary and interstitium, and $\Delta \pi$ is the oncotic pressure difference between capillary and interstitial fluids. Under normal circumstances, interstitial tissue pressure is low, and the ΔP term in the Starling equation represents the integrated hydrostatic pressure gradient from arteriolar to venular ends of a capillary. Since interstitial fluid is protein poor, the $\Delta \pi$ term in the Starling equation represents the oncotic pressure of plasma proteins, principally albumin; 5 grams of albumin per deciliter of plasma exerts an oncotic pressure of about 15 mm Hg.

Protection of Fluid Balance

As noted earlier, protection of the circulatory volume is the single most fundamental characteristic of body fluid homeostasis. This primacy is underscored by the fact that, in circumstances in which multiple physiologic variables are threatened simultaneously, the homeostatic response invariably protects ECF volume even at the expense of aggravating another electrolyte disorder. For example, a volume-contracted patient replenished with water, and not sodium, will retain water and become hyponatremic in an attempt to avoid circulatory collapse. Likewise, maintaining metabolic alkalosis in patients who have vomited and are not repleted with salt depends, in part, on an elevated renal absorptive capacity for sodium bicarbonate. The latter maintains fluid balance at the expense of pH homeostasis.

Two cardinal mechanisms protect ECF volume: alterations in systemic hemodynamic variables and alterations in external sodium and water balance. Both mechanisms maintain filling of the arterial tree and consequently are activated by external fluid losses, by inability to transfer fluid from the interstitium to the venous system, for example, in ascites, or by impaired fluid transfer from venous to arterial systems, for example, in congestive heart failure, pericardial tamponade, or constrictive pericarditis.

The combination of alterations in systemic hemodynamic variables and alterations in external water and solute balance has been termed the "integrated volume response" (Table 75–1). Increases in pulse rate and blood pressure are modulated not only by antidiuretic hormone (ADH), catecholamines, and angiotensin II but also by a series of factors derived from vascular endothelial cells. These factors include endothelin 1, a 21-residue peptide with potent vasoconstrictor properties, and thromboxane A_2 and prostaglandin H_2, both derived from the cyclo-oxygenase pathway in vascular endothelial cells. The major inactivators of these systemic hemodynamic changes include prostaglandin E_2 and atriopeptin, both of which are discussed below, and nitric oxide, an endogenous vasodilator released by vascular endothelial cells.

There are differences in the two response systems, indicated in Table 75–1. Tachycardia, peripheral arteriolar vasoconstriction, and peripheral venoconstriction occur within minutes of external fluid losses, whereas renal salt and water conservation lag behind by 12 to 24 hours. The sensitivities of the two limbs also differ. For example, a 2 to 3% decrease in extracellular fluid volume, which amounts to the loss of 40 to 60 mEq of sodium, results in the virtual elimination of sodium from the urine but produces negligible changes in systemic hemodynamic factors, such as heart rate, blood

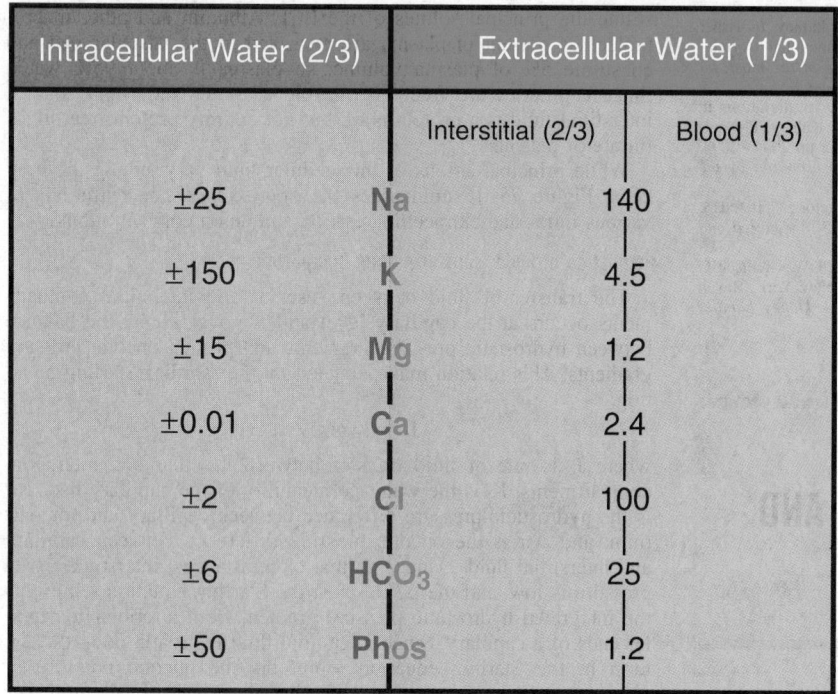

FIGURE 75–1. Relative volumes of various body fluid compartments. In a normally built individual, the total body water content is roughly 60% of body weight. Since adipose tissue has a low concentration of water, the relative water to total body weight ratio is lower in obese individuals. The intracellular electrolyte concentrations are in millimoles per liter and are typical values obtained from muscle.

pressure, or systemic vascular resistance. Since there is 2500 to 3000 mEq of exchangeable sodium in the ECF, the system for conserving renal sodium is remarkably sensitive.

Renal Volume Regulation

Figure 75–2 provides a schematic summary of the renal factors regulating volume homeostasis. In general, the system is characterized by a positive limb, activated by volume contraction, and by negative feedback, activated by volume repletion. The separate details of this mechanism are as follows.

SENSING AND EFFECTOR ELEMENTS. Changes in effective ECF volume that exceed acceptable physiologic limits are sensed by baroreceptors located in both the high- and the low-pressure regions of the circulation. The low-pressure baroreceptors are located primarily in the left atrium and in major thoracic veins, whereas the arterial high-pressure baroreceptors are located in the sinus body and aortic arch. Both sets of baroreceptors respond to pressure and stretch stimuli associated with changes in ECV. Activation of these extrarenal baroreceptors by slightly reducing effective circulating volume results in increased sympathetic nerve activity and in rises in plasma catecholamine activity.

This catecholamine response raises blood pressure by increasing arteriolar resistance and heart rate while simultaneously decreasing venous capacitance. Increases in arteriolar resistance also reduce capillary hydrostatic pressure and therefore promote fluid transfer from interstitial fluid to the vascular compartment. Within the kidney this increase in arteriolar resistance results in renal hypoperfusion. Moreover, adrenergic nerve terminals are in direct contact with proximal renal tubular epithelial cells, and direct stimulation of renal sympathetic nerves increases proximal tubular sodium absorption.

A second effector mechanism activated by stimulation of extrarenal baroreceptors is release of ADH. When blood volume is isotonically contracted by more than 8 to 10%, afferent stimuli carried by the ninth and tenth cranial nerves result in nonosmotic ADH release by the neurohypophysis. In turn, ADH enhances renal water conservation and, because the hormone also has potent vasoconstrictor activity, reduces renal perfusion.

In addition to these extrarenal baroreceptors, the renal juxtaglomerular apparatus serves as an intrarenal baroreceptor system. Sympathetic nerve stimulation, reductions in afferent arteriolar blood pressure, or reductions in the rates of distal tubular sodium delivery enhance renin release by the juxtaglomerular apparatus. Renal renin release into plasma accelerates the formation of angiotensin II according to the following general scheme:

$$\begin{array}{l} \textit{Renin Substrate} \\ \quad \downarrow \text{renin} \\ \textit{Angiotensin I} \\ \quad \downarrow \text{pulmonary converting enzyme} \\ \textit{Angiotensin II} \\ \quad \downarrow \text{circulating angiotensinase} \\ \textit{Angiotensin III} \end{array}$$

The octapeptide angiotensin II has three major effects on volume conservation: (1) It is a potent pressor agent; on a molar basis, angiotensin II is a more potent vasoconstrictor than norepinephrine. (2) Angiotensin II is the major stimulus to aldosterone secretion and consequently is a key factor modulating renal sodium conservation. (3) The angiotensin II formed in the central nervous system (CNS) is a potent stimulus to thirst. Recently it has become evident that angiotensin II may be synthesized locally in the vessels. At this writing it is not clear what effect locally synthesized angiotensin II has on vasoconstriction with respect to renally synthesized angiotensin II. The heptapeptide angiotensin III is also a potent vasoconstrictor but is not as potent a stimulator of aldosterone secretion as is angiotensin II; angiotensin III also stimulates thirst.

Finally, as indicated in Table 75–1, factors produced and released by vascular endothelial cells also play a major role in modulating systemic hemodynamics. The vasoconstricting factors include the potent vasoconstrictor peptide endothelin 1. Moreover, endothelin 1 is also released from the posterior pituitary and may play a role in modulating ADH release. The vasoconstrictor agents derived from

TABLE 75–1. THE INTEGRATED VOLUME RESPONSE

	Systemic Hemodynamic Changes	External Salt and Water Balance
Response	Tachycardia ↑ Peripheral resistance ↓ Venous capacitance	Thirst Renal Na$^+$, water retention
Onset	Minutes	Hours

Major activators	Catecholamines
	ADH
	Angiotensin II
	Endothelin 1
	  Prostaglandin H$_2$
	  Thromboxane A$_2$
		Catecholamines
		Aldosterone
		ADH

Major inactivators	Prostaglandin E$_2$ Atriopeptin Nitric acid	Prostaglandin E$_2$ Atriopeptin

ADH = Antidiuretic hormone.

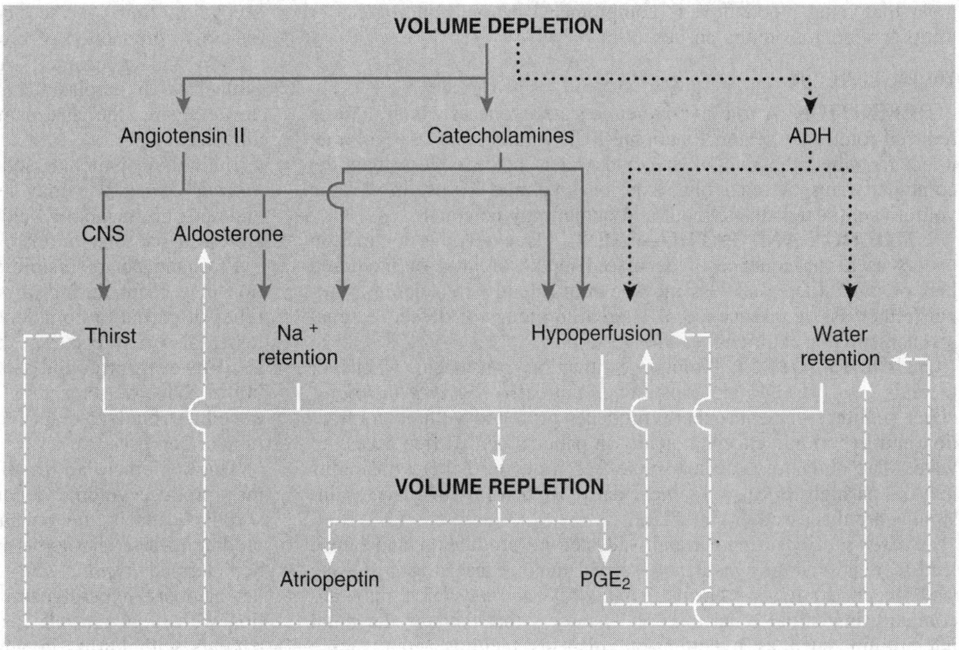

FIGURE 75-2. The volume repletion reaction. The solid and dotted lines originating from "volume depletion" indicate positive mechanisms activated when volume depletion is either modest or severe, respectively. The dashed lines originating with "volume repletion" indicate negative feedback mechanisms.

the cyclo-oxygenase pathway in vascular endothelial cells include thromboxane A_2 and prostaglandin H_2. Nitric oxide produced by vascular endothelial cells is the major endogenous nitrovasodilator.

RENAL ELEMENTS. The kidneys respond to slight reductions in extracellular volume (ECV) by increasing the rate of proximal tubular sodium absorption without disturbing either the glomerular filtration rate (GFR) or osmoregulatory mechanisms. In normal circumstances, approximately 70% of filtered sodium is absorbed by the proximal nephron. As long as euvolemia persists, the fractional rate of proximal sodium absorption remains constant when the GRF is varied; this constant relation is referred to as *glomerulotubular balance.*

A number of factors modulate glomerulotubular balance in association with changes in ECV. In empirical terms, this modulation includes a downsetting of glomerulotubular balance in volume-expanded states and an increase in the rate of fractional proximal sodium absorption when arterial tree filling is impaired. Among these factors, the hemodynamic regulation of oncotic pressure in peritubular capillaries seems to have a dominant role. At relatively low concentrations, angiotensin II has a vasoconstricting effect on efferent, but not afferent, glomerular arterioles. Therefore, this agent, by increasing the glomerular filtration fraction, can increase peritubular capillary oncotic pressure and thereby enhance proximal tubular rates of sodium absorption. At high concentrations, angiotensin II, like norepinephrine, produces afferent glomerular arteriolar constriction, resulting in reductions in GFR and in renal ischemia.

The kidney responds to modest sodium depletion by increasing the rate of tubular sodium absorption without altering the GFR. Glomerulotubular balance is reset upward so that a greater fraction of glomerular filtrate is absorbed in the proximal nephron; both direct stimulation of renal nerves and the effect of angiotensin II on efferent glomerular arterioles contribute in part to this resetting of glomerulotubular balance. Angiotensin II also provides a second mechanism for conserving renal sodium by increasing the rate of aldosterone secretion, which enhances sodium absorption in the cortical collecting tubule. When volume contraction becomes severe, the vasoconstrictive effects of high levels of norepinephrine and angiotensin II tend to reduce both the GFR and the rate of renal sodium excretion.

NEGATIVE FEEDBACK. As indicated in Figure 75-2, atriopeptin and E series prostaglandins (PGE) constitute the principal negative-feedback elements of the renal volume regulatory response. The major features of these negative feedback mechanisms are as follows.

Prostaglandins, particularly of the E series, are potent vasodilators. Within the kidney, two cardinal loci of PGE_2 production include renal glomeruli, where angiotensin II activates eicosanoid production and release, and renal medullary interstitial cells, which produce and release PGE_2 in response to increases in medullary osmolality.

As indicated in Figure 75-2, E series prostaglandins suppress renal volume conservation by at least three effects: (1) These agents are natriuretic due to both changes in renal hemodynamics and a direct inhibition of tubular sodium absorption. (2) Prostaglandins are potent renal vasodilators and consequently play a major role in protecting the kidneys from ischemia in circumstances such as volume depletion, when levels of the vasoconstrictor agents angiotensin II and norepinephrine are increased. (3) PGE_2 is a direct antagonist of the renal tubular effects of ADH and thus impairs renal water conservation.

An important therapeutic principle follows from considering the renal vasodilatory effects of prostaglandins. Specifically, the use of aspirin and other nonsteroidal anti-inflammatory agents (NSAID's) should be avoided in circumstances characterized by a high degree of sodium avidity, that is, by a reduction in ECV. These agents inhibit prostaglandin synthesis and thus reduce the rate of prostaglandin production. Consequently, in sodium-avid states, use of aspirin or other NSAID's increases the rate of development of renal ischemia and hence azotemia.

Atriopeptin, or atrial natriuretic peptide, is the second negative-feedback element in the renal volume regulatory response. This hormone is released from cardiac atrial storage granules in response to atrial distention; immunoreactive atriopeptin also has been identified within the CNS. Atriopeptin is discussed in detail in Ch. 200. In the present context, three actions of atriopeptin have particular pertinence: (1) Centrally released atriopeptin suppresses pituitary ADH release and angiotensin II–mediated thirst. (2) Atriopeptin of cardiac origin inhibits aldosterone secretion and hence renal Na^+ conservation; atriopeptin also may block collecting duct Na^+ and water absorption directly. (3) Atriopeptin is a potent vasodilator that increases renal blood flow strikingly. The last-named effect also accounts in part for the natriuretic effects of this peptide.

SUMMARY. When considered in an overall context, two features of the volume repletion reaction illustrated in Figure 75–2 are noteworthy. First, redundant mechanisms protect ECV. Thus angiotensin II release, catecholamine release, and ADH release all produce overlapping results. Second, the magnitude of the volume repletion reaction varies depending on the degree of volume contraction. In modestly volume-contracted states, peripheral vasoconstriction and renal sodium conservation occur, but renal blood flow, GFR, and osmoregulation are unaffected. When volume contraction becomes advanced, nonosmotic ADH release, angiotensin II–mediated thirst, and reductions in the rate of salt delivery to the loop of Henle act in concert to produce hyponatremia. Finally, when catecholamine release and angiotensin II release become sufficiently great that renal blood flow is compromised beyond autoregulatory limits, prerenal azotemia ensues.

VOLUME DEPLETION

DEFINITION. A true hypovolemic state is one in which there is reduced total body water, functional ECF volume, and ICF volume; it occurs when the rate of salt and water intake is less than the combined rates of renal plus extrarenal volume losses. In chronic volume-contracted states, input and output may be equal.

ETIOLOGY AND PATHOGENESIS. True volume contraction occurs as a consequence of decreased intake of fluid or increased loss of fluid. Increased loss may be conveniently considered as renal (either as a consequence of altered hormones or defective renal mechanisms) or extrarenal (Table 75–2).

Hormonal Deficit. Volume contraction can occur whenever there is loss of ADH or aldosterone. Untreated *diabetes insipidus,* either pituitary or nephrogenic, produces profound volume contraction and hypertonic encephalopathy in patients denied free access to water. The obligatory loss of solute-free water in diabetes insipidus may be as high as 10 to 18 liters daily. Both forms of diabetes insipidus are discussed in Ch. 202.2.

Addison's disease may impair aldosterone production and hence lead to renal sodium wasting. A second major cause of aldosterone lack occurs in *hyporeninemic hypoaldosteronism,* which may accompany interstitial renal disease. Disorders that damage the renal interstitium, such as hypertension, diabetes mellitus, gout, sickle cell disease, chronic ingestion of lead-containing illicit alcohol, and analgesic abuse, can suppress the ability of the juxtaglomerular apparatus to produce renin. In turn, the low rate of renin secretion results in low rates of aldosterone secretion. Thus hyporeninemic hypoaldosteronism represents a disorder in which impaired aldosterone production results in renal salt wasting, hyperkalemia, and metabolic acidosis. It is not yet known why hyperkalemia, which is a potent stimulus to aldosterone secretion, fails to enhance rates of aldosterone secretion in patients with hyporeninemic hypoaldosteronism.

Renal Deficits. A number of disorders impairing renal tubular sodium or water conservation can lead to volume contraction. For convenience, these derangements may be grouped into three classes. First, various tubular nephropathies are characterized by specific deficits in salt or water absorption. As mentioned earlier, nephrogenic diabetes insipidus and interstitial renal disease may produce water or sodium wasting, respectively. Because interstitial renal disease often results in hyperchloremic, hyperkalemic metabolic acidosis, the term "renal tubular acidosis, type IV" is often applied to this disorder. However, the general term "renal tubular acidosis" also includes other sodium-wasting disorders accompanied by hyperchloremic acidosis, such as proximal tubular acidosis, a specific proximal defect in bicarbonate reabsorption, and gradient-limited distal renal tubular acidosis, a specific defect in distal tubular sodium bicarbonate regeneration (see Ch. 82).

TABLE 75–2. MAJOR CAUSES OF VOLUME DEPLETION

Renal Losses	Extrarenal Losses
Hormonal Deficit	**Hemorrhage**
Pituitary diabetes insipidus	
Aldosterone insufficiency	**Cutaneous Losses**
Addison's disease	Sweating
Hyporeninemic hypoaldosteronism	Burns
Renal Deficits	
Specific Tubular Nephropathies:	**Gastrointestinal Losses**
Renal tubular acidosis	Vomiting
Proximal	Diarrheal disorders
Distal, gradient-limited	Gastrointestinal fistulas
Bartter's syndrome	Tube drainage
Nephrogenic diabetes insipidus	
Diuretic abuse	
Postobstructive diuresis	
Excessive Filtration of Nonelectrolytes:	
Osmotic diuresis	
Generalized Renal Disease:	
Chronic renal failure	
Interstitial nephritis	

Alternatively, Bartter's syndrome is a specific tubular nephropathy that results in failure of sodium chloride absorption by the thick ascending limb of the nephron; the disorder is accompanied by excessive production of prostaglandins by the renal medullary interstitium and is characterized by sodium chloride wasting, juxtaglomerular hyperplasia, high renin levels, and secondary hyperaldosteronism; the last-named results in hypokalemic metabolic alkalosis.

Inhibition of tubular sodium absorptive processes due to *chronic diuretic abuse* also may lead to salt wasting, volume contraction, and specific metabolic acid-base abnormalities. These abnormalities are discussed later in this chapter.

Profound but reversible defects in tubular salt and water absorption may occur during *postobstructive diuresis,* that is, shortly after relief of partial or complete urinary tract obstruction. Salt and water losses also may occur in the *diuretic phase* of acute tubular necrosis. However, profound salt and water losses associated with the diuretic phase of acute tubular necrosis are seen uncommonly if extracellular fluid volume is carefully controlled during oliguric acute tubular necrosis.

Third, glomerular filtration of large amounts of nonelectrolytes may produce volume deficits by overwhelming renal tubular reabsorptive capacity for salt and water; in this instance, water losses predominate so that hypernatremia generally occurs. This phenomenon, termed *osmotic diuresis* or *solute diuresis,* occurs in diabetic ketoacidosis, hyperglycemic hyperosmolar coma, or hyperalimentation with large glucose loads in chronically debilitated patients; in patients with burns, in whom there are abnormally high rates of urea production; and during mannitol or glycerol administration to those with CNS disorders requiring reductions of intracranial pressure.

Finally, in *chronic renal failure* of any cause, an obligatory loss of sodium occurs. The extent of obligatory sodium loss in chronic renal failure is most pronounced in cystic renal diseases, notably medullary cystic disease and polycystic kidney disease (see Ch. 89).

Extrarenal Losses. In addition to hemorrhage, two other classes of extrarenal losses account for volume contraction. Simple dehydration may result from increased insensible water loss in *excessive sweating* due to high ambient temperatures or to fever. Because sweat usually contains < 50 mEq per liter of sodium, the ICF and the ECF share the water loss, and body water osmolality rises while ECF volume loss is modest. *Burns* allow the loss of large amounts of plasma and interstitial fluid through affected areas and therefore can lead rapidly to profound ECF losses.

Finally, gastrointestinal volume losses occur when portions of the 8 to 10 liters of normal gastrointestinal secretions are lost, particularly in secretory diarrheas. Volume depletion is most commonly the consequence of vomiting, gastric drainage, or diarrhea but may occur with any type of bowel fistula. Loss of hydrochloric acid from the stomach may produce metabolic alkalosis, whereas loss of sodium bicarbonate from pancreatic secretions lost through the lower gastrointestinal tract, as in diarrhea, may produce metabolic acidosis.

CLINICAL MANIFESTATIONS. The clinical findings in states of true volume contraction are due both to underfilling of the arterial tree and to the subsequent renal and hemodynamic responses. In mild or partially compensated volume contraction, particularly when the latter has occurred gradually, the patient may exhibit nothing more than mild postural giddiness, postural tachycardia, and weakness, while in severe volume contraction, life-threatening circulatory collapse may occur. The lack of physical findings does not exclude the presence of mild to moderate volume contraction in a given patient. In the postoperative period, 7 to 10% blood volume losses in patients are often accompanied by normal vital signs and by only slight decreases in the central venous pressure or the pulmonary capillary wedge pressure. Skin turgor and the moistness of mucous membranes are valuable indices to the volume of body water in infants but are unreliable in adults. In young adults, reductions in skin turgor do not occur unless profound volume contraction is present, and normal loss of skin elasticity makes skin turgor difficult to assess in older patients. Similarly, mouth breathing and other factors affect the oral mucosa independently of external volume balances.

The signs and symptoms of volume contraction, regardless of cause, are referable to a reduction in ECV. Consequently, the clinical findings in volume contraction depend primarily on the interplay among four major factors: the magnitude of the volume loss; the rate of volume loss; the nature of the fluid loss, that is, whether the fluid loss is primarily water, a combined sodium plus water loss, or a blood loss; and finally, the responsiveness of the vasculature to volume reduction. Some simple considerations illustrate these relations.

The clinical manifestations of volume contraction are obviously related intimately to the volume and rate of fluid loss. For example, an acute gastrointestinal hemorrhage of 1 liter of blood can easily result in oliguria, coupled with the signs and symptoms of circulatory collapse, while the hematocrit remains constant. In other words, the hemorrhage is sufficiently acute that fluid flux from the interstitial to the vascular bed makes a negligible contribution to expanding the vascular bed. However, the same amount of gastrointestinal blood loss occurring more slowly—for example, over a 1-day period—permits a partial transfer of fluid from the interstitium to the vascular bed and consequently produces a fall in hematocrit; but since the ECV is at least partially restored by this fluid shift, the volume of urine flow and the hemodynamic response to volume contraction may be minimally affected.

Second, the kind of fluid loss significantly affects the clinical findings in volume contraction. Consider, for example, a 1-liter loss of different kinds of body fluids in a 70-kg man with a total body water of 40 liters and a hematocrit of 45%. The acute loss of 1 liter of predominantly solute-free water, as in diabetes insipidus, reduces the blood volume by 2.5%; urine flow and systemic hemodynamics are minimally affected. The acute loss of 1 liter of predominantly extracellular fluid reduces blood volume by 6.6%, since sodium is confined to the ECF; in this circumstance, modest oliguria and tachycardia while the patient is recumbent ensue. Lastly, the acute loss of 1 liter of blood by hemorrhage reduces blood volume by 20%, thus resulting in profound oliguria and near circulatory collapse.

Finally, peripheral vasoconstriction and tachycardia represent important physiologic responses to volume losses. Consequently, even modest signs and symptoms of volume contraction are amplified appreciably in patients with diminished myocardial reserve or reduced sympathetic nervous system function. The former occurs commonly in cardiomyopathies of any cause or in pericardial tamponade or pericardial constriction. The latter occurs commonly in patients on prolonged bed rest, in diabetic patients with autonomic neuropathy, and as a consequence of therapy with certain antihypertensive drugs.

DIAGNOSIS. The pulse, blood pressure, and changes of these variables with position, together with a clinical estimate of the venous pressure and skin temperature, provide an initial assessment of circulatory dynamics. Because these findings may be inconclusive in moderate degrees of volume contraction, a fluid challenge is useful to evaluate critically ill patients in whom a volume deficit is thought to contribute to a reduced cardiac output. A convenient way of achieving this goal is to administer 500 ml of normal saline over 1 to 3 hours.

In patients with a normal cardiac reserve, the effect of a fluid challenge may be monitored safely by evaluating the pulse, blood pressure, and urine flow. In patients with impaired cardiac function, using a flow-directed Swan-Ganz catheter to measure the pulmonary capillary wedge pressure or cardiac output, as estimated by thermal dilution, provides a more precise indicator to early volume overload secondary to a fluid challenge. Because volume contraction is associated with vasoconstriction, both in the venous and the arterial circuits, transient changes in the pulmonary capillary wedge pressure may not accurately reflect volume status. During volume expansion, the wedge pressure rises and subsequently falls. The initial pressure elevation is due to fluid infusion into a vasoconstricted, low-capacity vascular bed and should not be misinterpreted to indicate adequacy of volume repletion. The subsequent reduction in wedge pressure coincides with decreases in arterial resistance coupled with increases in venous capacitance. Finally, central venous pressure measurements provide unreliable estimates of pulmonary vascular volume.

The cardinal laboratory findings associated with volume contraction follow directly from the volume repletion mechanism summarized in Figure 75-2. The kidney initially responds to a decrease in effective circulating blood volume by reducing urine volume and sodium excretion. Severe degrees of volume contraction also reduce

filtration rate and result in prerenal azotemia and a decrease in fractional excretion of sodium (see Ch. 73).

TREATMENT. The major goal of treating volume contraction is to expand the ECV by replacing fluid deficits. The type of fluid, the route and rate of fluid administration, and the total amount of fluid to be given will vary with the particular circumstance. For example, a mild, nonpersisting upper gastrointestinal hemorrhage may be treated appropriately by infusing normal saline, whereas a major, persisting upper gastrointestinal hemorrhage will generally require replacement with whole blood.

The degree to which a given volume of crystalloid solution expands the ECV depends on solution composition. If glucose metabolism is normal, infusing 5% dextrose in water (D_5W) is equivalent to administering solute-free water, which distributes uniformly in total body water. Since <10% of total body water is in the intravascular compartment, infusing 1 liter of D_5W expands the intravascular volume by 75 to 100 ml, that is, by about 2%. Thus expansion of ECV by D_5W cannot be suggested except when used principally in hypertonic volume-contracted states such as diabetes insipidus and excessive sweating.

Solutions containing sodium as the principal solute preferentially expand the extracellular fluid volume. Infusing 1 liter of a normal saline solution increases blood volume by about 300 ml, or about 6%; the remaining portion is distributed in the interstitial compartment. Hypotonic sodium-containing salt solutions expand intravascular volume in a manner intermediate between that of D_5W and normal saline. Sodium-containing crystalloid solutions are indicated primarily in volume-contracted states secondary to renal or gastrointestinal sodium losses (see Table 75-2). They are also useful adjuncts to therapy in burns and in hemorrhage.

Colloid-containing solutions, such as iso-oncotic albumin solutions and plasma, preferentially expand the intravascular compartment, since large molecules like albumin are mainly restricted to the intravascular space. This kind of fluid replacement is most helpful in burns, in which cutaneous protein losses are appreciable, and in circulatory collapse, in which rapid intravascular expansion is critical. In most other instances of volume contraction, using colloid-containing solutions is difficult to justify, since the half-life of infused albumin in ill patients is relatively short, only 4 to 6 hours, and the cost of colloid solutions such as iso-oncotic albumin is more than 50 times greater than that of an equal volume of crystalloid solution.

Finally, blood—which contains formed elements—is the most potent expander of the intravascular space. A unit of packed red blood cells will remain entirely in the vascular bed. In most hemorrhagic situations, the combination of packed red blood cells with either normal saline solutions or colloid solutions is adequate for volume replacement. Few circumstances occur in modern practice, with the possible exception of massive hemorrhagic shock, in which whole-blood therapy for volume expansion is used.

CIRCULATORY COMPROMISE WITHOUT EXTERNAL FLUID LOSSES

DEFINITION. In the preceding section we considered those disorders characterized by inadequate filling of the arterial tree that occurred because of true volume deficits. Clearly, the cardinal signs and symptoms of these disorders are referable to responses accompanying the integrated volume repletion reaction (see Fig. 75-2). There are also disorders in which inadequate arterial filling occurs in the absence of external fluid losses and which indeed are often associated with increased total body water. However, the signs and symptoms of these disorders mimic closely those which characterize true volume contraction.

ETIOLOGY AND PATHOGENESIS. Table 75-3 lists three commonly encountered classes of derangements that may manifest clinically with tachycardia, acute hypotension, oliguria, azotemia, and a reduced FE_{Na}.

Impaired Cardiac Output. A profound collapse of cardiac output, due to acute myocardial infarction with pump failure (cardiogenic shock) or to acute pericardial tamponade, may clearly result in circulatory collapse. In this instance, failure to fill the arterial tree and to maintain an ECV occurs because the heart fails to translocate blood adequately from venous to arterial beds.

Increased Vascular Capacitance. Circulatory collapse with its attendant signs and symptoms occurs when there is a sud-

TABLE 75–3. CIRCULATORY COMPROMISE WITHOUT EXTERNAL FLUID LOSSES

I. **Impaired Cardiac Output**
 Acute myocardial infarction
 Pericardial tamponade
II. **Increased Vascular Capacitance**
 Septic shock
 Cirrhosis
III. **Vascular → Interstitial Fluid Shifts**
 A. Hypoalbuminemia
  Nephrotic syndrome
  Liver failure
  Malnutrition
  Cytokine-mediated
 B. Normal plasma albumin
  Acute pancreatitis
  Bowel infarction
  Rhabdomyolysis
  Noncardiogenic pulmonary edema

den increase in the capacitance of the vascular bed, most notably in the venous part of the circulation. This kind of increase in ratio of vascular capacitance to vascular volume occurs most commonly in sepsis and cirrhosis with increased A-V shunts and decreased systemic vascular resistance. Increased vascular capacitance also may be seen in circumstances in which peripheral vasodilators, particularly those having a postarteriolar locus of action, are administered injudiciously.

Vascular-Interstitial Fluid Shifts. Profound hypotension, tachycardia, progressive oliguria, and azotemia are also encountered when there is a translocation of fluid from vascular to interstitial compartments, presumably because of a sudden, profound increase in the permeability characteristics of peripheral capillaries or when there is decreased circulatory oncotic pressure such as in any disease process with hypoalbuminemia. Some common causes of increased translocation of vascular fluid without hypoalbuminemia having an etiologic role include infarction of the small or large intestine, extensive tissue trauma, acute pancreatitis, and rhabdomyolysis. An analogous mechanism—namely, a marked increase in the permeability of pulmonary capillaries—is also presumed to account for the formation of noncardiogenic pulmonary edema in the adult respiratory distress syndrome.

DIAGNOSIS AND THERAPY. The diagnosis and therapy of acute myocardial infarction with circulatory collapse and of acute pericardial tamponade are considered in detail in Part VII. It is, however, worth citing certain factors particularly germane to managing fluid therapy in such patients. In individuals affected either by right ventricular infarction or by pericardial tamponade, maintaining adequate filling of the systemic arterial tree depends critically on providing a relatively high venous preload to the right side of the heart. Attempts at volume contraction in patients with right ventricular infarcts or pericardial tamponade may exacerbate systemic hypotension. Thus treating these disorders generally requires concomitant hemodynamic monitoring with a flow-directed Swan-Ganz catheter to avoid excessive preload to the left side of the heart.

In patients with left ventricular infarction and systemic hypotension, particular attention should be directed to excluding the possibility that antecedent true volume depletion—for example, with prolonged diuretic therapy and salt restriction prior to the myocardial infarction—may be a significant contributor to what otherwise might be mistaken for true cardiogenic shock. The combined findings of acute left ventricular infarction, systemic arterial hypotension, the absence of pulmonary edema on the chest radiography, a reduced pulmonary capillary wedge pressure, and an antecedent history of prolonged diuretic therapy, when taken together, indicate that improved systemic hemodynamics may be achieved by cautious attempts to expand volume while also measuring—serially—the cardiac output and the pulmonary capillary wedge pressure.

The distinction between hypotension as being due either to true volume contraction or to an increase in the capacitance-volume ratio of the vascular bed, as occurs in sepsis, is often difficult. This distinction is particularly difficult in individuals who have been in

intensive care units for prolonged periods of time and in those at high risk for developing sepsis, such as cancer patients treated with potent chemotherapeutic agents. A useful clue to the presence of septic circulatory collapse is the occurrence of warm extremities coupled with hypotension and oliguria, since true hypovolemia, particularly when advanced, is ordinarily accompanied by profound peripheral vasoconstriction and hence cool and often cyanotic extremities.

True hypovolemia and sepsis also may coexist. In such a circumstance, invasive hemodynamic monitoring may be helpful. Both in true hypovolemia and in sepsis, the pulmonary capillary wedge pressure is reduced, but in septic circulatory collapse, the calculated systemic vascular resistance falls, because of peripheral vasodilation, whereas in true hypovolemia, peripheral vasoconstriction ordinarily raises the systemic vascular resistance. The diagnosis of disorders producing rapid transfer of fluids from the vascular bed to the interstitium, such as trauma, acute pancreatitis, or rhabdomyolysis, is generally evident from clinical appraisal.

Treating patients with sepsis and an increased vascular capacitance-volume ratio, as well as those with rapid vascular to interstitial fluid shifts, has as a mainstay the administration of sufficient sodium-containing fluids, generally isotonic saline, to permit adequate filling of the arterial tree. This therapy necessarily expands total body water, particularly in the vascular and interstitial compartments. Consequently, during recovery from the underlying disorder, care must be taken to avoid unnecessary expansion of the vascular bed and consequently the risk of volume-mediated cardiac decompensation.

VOLUME EXCESS

DEFINITION. Volume-expanded states are characterized by an increase in total body water, which is usually accompanied by an increase in total body sodium. Total body salt and water may be increased while the ECV is decreased. In other words, certain volume-expanded states are characterized by dissociation between total body salt and water and the ECV.

ETIOLOGY AND PATHOGENESIS. Volume expansion occurs whenever the rate of salt or water intake exceeds the rate of renal plus extrarenal losses; in chronic volume expansion, the external salt and water balance may be normal. A convenient way of considering volume-expanded states is to view them in the context of three different classes of physiologic explanations (Table 75–4).

Disturbances in Starling Forces. The most common diseases encountered in which both volume expansion and edema occur are those in which derangements in the Starling forces regulating fluid transfer between capillaries and interstitium tend to expand the interstitial compartment at the expense of the ECV. Consequently, renal sodium retention and edema occur. By definition, this group of disorders is characterized by increases in capillary hydrostatic pressure, by decreases in capillary oncotic pressure, or by a combination of these two factors.

Four groups include most edematous states characterized by abnormal Starling forces (Table 75–4). First, the systemic venous

TABLE 75–4. DISORDERS OF VOLUME EXCESS

I. **Disturbed Starling Forces** (Reduced effective circulating volume; edema formation)	II. **Primary Hormone Excess** (Increased effective circulating volume)
Systemic venous pressure increases	Primary aldosteronism
Right heart failure	Cushing's syndrome
Constrictive pericarditis	SIADH
Local venous pressure increases	III. **Primary Renal Sodium Retention** (Increased effective circulating volume)
Left heart failure	Renal failure
Vena cava obstruction	
Portal vein obstruction	
Reduced Oncotic Pressure	
Nephrotic syndrome	
Decreased albumin synthesis	
Combined disorders	
Cirrhosis	

SIADH = Syndrome of inappropriate antidiuretic hormone production.

pressure may be increased because of primary cardiac disorders, such as right-sided heart failure or constrictive pericarditis. Second, local elevations in pulmonary or systemic venous pressure may occur, as in left-sided heart failure, vena caval obstruction, or portal vein obstruction. Third, a reduction in plasma oncotic pressure, and consequently a net increase in the tendency for fluid to transudate from capillaries to interstitium, accounts plausibly for edema formation in the nephrotic syndrome. Circulatory albumin concentrations of < 3.2 grams per deciliter are usually insufficient to prevent transudation of fluid across capillary beds. Finally, a combination of these factors may be responsible for edema. For example, both hypoalbuminemia and portal hypertension are major contributory factors to developing ascites in hepatic cirrhosis.

Plasma renin activity and aldosterone concentrations in these disorders tend to be elevated, although the results also tend to be variable. In advanced cases of disorders characterized by increases in local or systemic venous pressure, most notably in severe congestive heart failure and in cirrhosis, hyponatremia may occur; this finding represents an ominous prognostic sign. Finally, edema formation due to such derangements of Starling forces may result in the "third space" phenomenon, namely, large volumes of interstitial fluid sequestered in regions such as the pleural or peritoneal cavities.

Primary Hormonal Excess. These disorders include those disturbances with unregulated production of mineralocorticoids or ADH. The volume expansion that occurs in states of mineralocorticoid excess, such as primary hyperaldosteronism, is due to sodium retention and is accompanied by a primary, preferential expansion of the ECF and consequently by hypertension. The serum sodium level is generally normal. In the syndrome of inappropriate ADH production (SIADH), primary water retention occurs. Consequently, the volume expansion involves both the ICF and ECF; dilutional hyponatremia is the hallmark of SIADH, whereas hypertension is uncommon. Edema is not characteristic in either of these two disorders. Instead, patients with primary aldosteronism or SIADH reach a volume-expanded steady state in which output equals input.

Primary Renal Sodium Retention. The kidneys also may retain sodium abnormally when the ECV is normal and there is no effector excess. For example, in acute glomerulonephritis, unidentified renal mechanisms are primarily responsible for edema. Patients with acute glomerulonephritis retain salt and water and become hypertensive without reductions in the GFR or in ECV. Furthermore, sodium retention and edema may develop when intake exceeds renal capacity for excretion with a decrease in GFR of any cause.

DIAGNOSIS AND TREATMENT. The recognition and management of volume-expanded states depend on proper identification and treatment of the underlying disorder. Clearly, the cornerstones of therapy in volume-expanded states characterized by sodium excess include salt restriction and diuretics. Table 75-5 provides a summary of some of the major diuretics used commonly and certain of their properties, while Figure 75-3 summarizes the sites of action of the various families of diuretics. For convenience, these drugs have been classified according to their sites of action in the nephron.

Proximal Tubule Diuretics. The cardinal example of a proximal tubule diuretic is acetazolamide, a carbonic anhydrase inhibitor that blocks proximal reabsorption of sodium bicarbonate. Consequently, prolonged use of acetazolamide may lead to hyperchloremic acidosis, in contrast to all other diuretics that act at loci prior to the late distal nephron. Metolazone, a congener of the thiazide class of diuretics, blocks sodium chloride absorption in two nephron sites by unknown mechanisms. Specifically, in addition to an action on the early distal tubule, metolazone also inhibits proximal tubular sodium chloride absorption. Since the major locus for phosphate absorption is in the proximal nephron, the phosphaturia accompanying metolazone administration exceeds considerably that observed with other thiazide class diuretics.

Proximal tubule diuretics are rarely used as primary diuretic therapy in modern practice. More commonly, these diuretics, particularly metolazone, are used as supplements to loop diuretics in instances where loop diuretics alone are ineffective in producing diuresis.

Mannitol also inhibits proximal tubule reabsorption. It is mainly used to prevent acute tubular necrosis.

Loop Diuretics. Loop diuretics, such as furosemide, bumetanide, and ethacrynic acid, produce diuresis by inhibiting the coupled entry on Na^+, Cl^-, and K^+ across apical plasma membranes in the thick ascending limb of Henle. The latter is responsible for the reabsorption of approximately 25% of filtered sodium. The natriuretic dose-response characteristics of these diuretic agents are considerably more linear than those of all other currently used diuretics. Consequently, the loop diuretics are, for practical purposes, the most potent diuretics currently available; therefore these drugs are commonly referred to as "high-ceiling" diuretics.

Distal Tubule Diuretics. Distal tubule diuretics, such as thiazide and metolazone, interfere primarily with sodium chloride absorption in the earliest segments of the distal convoluted tubule. The thiazide diuretics appear to exert their effect by blocking the NaCl cotransport mechanism across apical plasma membranes.

With the exception of acetazolamide (which impairs bicarbonate absorption), hypokalemia and metabolic alkalosis may complicate the administration of proximal diuretics, loop diuretics, and distal tubular diuretics. This occurs because the rate of sodium delivery to the collecting duct, in which a significant fraction of potassium and proton secretion occurs, is a major factor promoting these two processes. Consequently, increase in salt delivery to the late distal nephron, occasioned by inhibition of sodium reabsorption in the proximal tubule, the ascending limb of Henle, or the distal tubule and collecting duct, leads to accelerated rates of proton and potassium secretion and consequently to hypokalemia and metabolic alkalosis.

In general, distal tubule diuretics are used for the same circumstances as loop diuretics. The major exception occurs in chronic renal failure and in disorders of calcium metabolism. Loop diuretics are calciuric and therefore are valuable for managing acute hypercalcemia. In contrast, thiazide diuretics promote hypocalciuria and

TABLE 75-5. CHARACTERISTICS OF COMMONLY USED DIURETICS

	Diuretic	Primary Effect	Secondary Effect	Complications
I.	**Proximal Diuretics**			
	Acetazolamide	↓ Na^+/H^+ exchange	↑ K^+ loss, ↑ HCO_3^- loss	Hypokalemic, hyperchloremic acidosis
	Metolazone	↓ Na^+ absorption	↑ K^+ loss, ↑ Cl^- loss	Hypokalemic alkalosis
II.	**Loop Diuretics**			
	Furosemide			Hypokalemic alkalosis
	Bumetanide	↓ $Na^+ : K^+ : 2Cl^-$ absorption	↑ K^+ loss, ↑ H^+ secretion	
	Ethacrynic acid			Hearing deficits
III.	**Early Distal Diuretics**			
	Thiazide	↓ Na^+ absorption	↑ K^+ loss, ↑ H^+ secretion	Hypokalemic alkalosis
	Metolazone			Hyperglycemia, hyperuricemia
IV.	**Late Distal Diuretics**			
	Aldosterone antagonists			
	Spironolactone			
	Nonaldosterone antagonists	↓ Na^+ absorption	↓ K^+ loss, ↓ H^+ secretion	Hyperkalemic acidosis
	Triamterene			
	Amiloride			

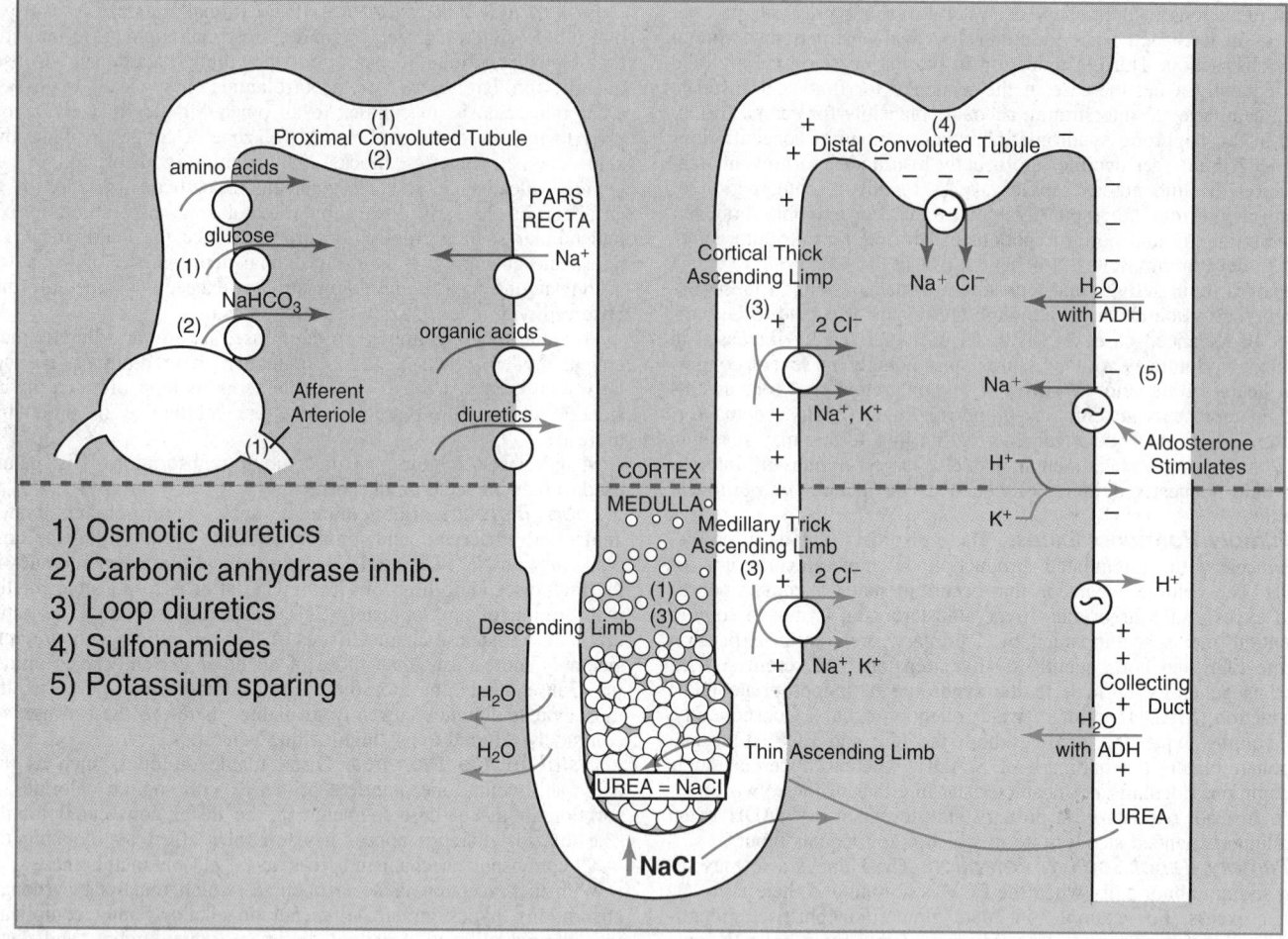

FIGURE 75-3. Major transport processes along the nephron segment and the primary sites of action of the diuretics. The numbers next to diuretics in the insert refer to sites of action along the nephron. (From Kokko JP: Diuretics. *In* Schlant RC, Alexander RW [eds.]: The Heart. 8th ed. New York, McGraw-Hill, 1994.)

calcium retention and are therefore useful in managing hypercalciuric states, but not hypercalcemia. Loop diuretics are much more effective in chronic renal failure than are thiazide diuretics.

Collecting Duct Diuretics. Finally, a group of agents inhibit sodium absorption in the collecting duct and concomitantly suppress indirectly potassium secretion and proton secretion. Spironolactone competes with aldosterone; the primary use of this agent is restricted to conditions of aldosterone excess, either primary or secondary. Alternatively, both triamterene and amiloride operate independently of aldosterone. These agents directly block sodium uptake by collecting duct cells and concomitantly suppress indirectly both potassium and proton secretion. Accordingly, hyperkalemic, hyperchloremic metabolic acidosis may complicate the injudicious use of spironolactone, triamterene, or amiloride. These diuretics are useful especially in managing disorders characterized by secondary hyperaldosteronism, such as cirrhosis with ascites, and in promoting diuresis in hypokalemic patients.

One factor common to treatment of disorders with reduced ECV's and expanded ECF volumes merits particular consideration. A major factor in edema formation is an increase in the Starling forces promoting fluid translocation from the vascular to interstitial spaces. When potent diuretics are given to patients with portal hypertension or with hypoalbuminemia, urinary sodium excretion may exceed the rate at which salt and water are transferred from the interstitium to the vascular bed. As a result, vigorous diuretic therapy may result in volume contraction, reduced salt delivery to diluting segments, nonosmotic ADH release, and consequently hyponatremia. Hyponatremia occurs most commonly with the thiazide group of diuretics, because these diuretics inhibit free water formation. In advanced cases of diuretic abuse, hypotension, hemoconcentration, and azotemia also occur.

Dzau VJ: Circulating versus local renin-angiotensin system in cardiovascular homeostasis. Circulation 77(suppl I):1, 1988. *A comprehensive review demonstrating that renin and angiotensinogen genes are expressed in many tissues. Studies also have shown that cardiac vascular cells can synthesize angiotensin II in vitro. Current data further suggest that angiotensin antagonists affect vascular contractility by their effects on angiotensin produced by either the kidney or local vascular mechanisms.*

Johnston CI, Hodsman PG, Kohzuki M, et al.: Interaction between atrial natriuretic peptide and the renin, angiotensin, aldosterone system. Am J Med 87(Suppl 6B):24S, 1989. *A review of the renin-angiotensin system and the interaction with atriopeptin.*

King AJ, Brenner BM, Anderson SH: Endothelin: A potent renal and systemic vasoconstrictor peptide. Am J Physiol 256:F1051, 1989. *A description of the physiology of endothelin.*

Kokko JP: Diuretics. *In* Schlant RC, Alexander RW (eds.): The Heart. 8th ed. New York, McGraw-Hill, 1994, pp 595–609. *Complete overview of site of action, indications, and complications of diuretics.*

Nonoguchi H, Sands JM, Knepper MA: ANF inhibits NaCl and fluid absorption in cortical collecting duct of rat kidney. Am J Physiol 256(Renal Fluid Electrolyte Physiol 25):F179, 1989. *Carefully conducted* in vitro *study examining how atrial natriuretic factor increases urinary sodium and water excretion.*

Weinman EJ, Andreoli TE (eds.): Diuretics: I. Physiology, biochemistry and pharmacology. Semin Nephrol 8:197, 1988. *A complete issue devoted to the physiology of diuretics.*

75.2   Osmolality Disturbances

PHYSIOLOGIC CONSIDERATIONS

In normal individuals, the serum osmolality as determined by freezing-point depression is virtually constant from day to day. It is useful to define "effective ECF osmolality," since the osmoregulatory mechanisms that adjust water balance in normal individuals are determined primarily by changes in cell volume that result from variations in effective ECF osmolality. "Effective ECF osmolality" is that osmolality which is "sensed" across a specific membrane. In dilutional states, the measured and effective ECF osmolalities are approximately equal, since ECF dilution also produces ICF dilution and, at least acutely, cell swelling. Osmoregulatory mechanisms are activated when ECF hypertonicity is due to a solute that is excluded from cells and therefore produces, at least acutely, cell shrinkage; in this case, the measured and effective ECF osmolalities are approximately equal. If the ECF osmolality is increased by solutes such as urea, which penetrate cell membranes readily, acute cell shrinkage does not occur and osmoregulatory mechanisms are not activated. In this case, the measured ECF osmolality is greater than the effective ECF osmolality.

The freezing-point serum osmolality can be approximated from the following formula:

$$\text{Osmolality} = 2[\text{Na}^+] + \frac{[\text{glucose}]}{18} + \frac{[\text{BUN}]}{2.8}$$

where the glucose and blood urea nitrogen (BUN) concentrations are expressed as milligrams per deciliter and the serum sodium concentration is expressed as milliequivalents per liter. In normal circumstances, glucose contributes 5.5 mOsm per kilogram of H_2O to the serum osmolality. When hyperglycemia occurs, the effective ECF osmolality rises because glucose entry into cells is limited. When azotemia occurs, the effective ECF osmolality does not rise because urea enters cells readily.

Cell Volume Regulation

Starling forces regulate fluid transfer between the ICF and the ECF. Because plasma membranes cannot tolerate even small hydrostatic gradients, the operational Starling forces between ICF and ECF are almost entirely osmotic. Significant changes in cell volume, particularly in the CNS, are by themselves potentially lethal. Thus the goals of fluid transport between the ECF and ICF are to maintain constancy of cell volume and to maintain a negligible hydrostatic pressure gradient between cells and the ECF. Since most cell membranes are freely permeable to water, these two goals are achieved when the ECF osmolality is normal and intracellular and extracellular osmolalities are identical.

Since cell membranes are partially permeable to sodium and potassium, there is a tendency for sodium to leak into cells and for potassium to leak out of cells. Because impermeant macromolecules account for a large fraction of intracellular anions, passive sodium and potassium movements tend toward a Donnan distribution, in which total intracellular cations would exceed total interstitial cations, in precise analogy to the way in which total plasma water cations exceed total interstitial cations. If these passive cation movements across cell membranes were unopposed, osmotic water movement into cells would tend to produce cell lysis. Consequently, active transport mechanisms are required to balance intracellular and interstitial cation concentrations.

Specifically, both sodium leakage from the ECF into cells and potassium leakage out of cells into the ECF are counterbalanced exactly by active outward sodium transport coupled to active inward potassium transport. These active transport events maintain the intracellular cation (and therefore osmolar) content equal to that of extracellular fluid and also maintain the predominant extracellular and intracellular distributions of sodium and potassium, respectively. Thus, because cellular cation pumps balance cellular cation leaks, cells are *operationally* impermeable to sodium and to potassium. Active sodium efflux coupled to active potassium influx is mediated by membrane-bound Na^+-K^+-ATPase, and the activity of these cellular cation pumps accounts for >50% of the basal caloric consumption.

Cation transport mediated by Na^+-K^+-ATPase is the major factor regulating cell volume when the effective ECF osmolality is normal. When the effective ECF osmolality is increased or decreased, additional processes are required to maintain the constancy of cell volume. These auxiliary mechanisms are particularly important in minimizing potentially lethal changes in brain volume because of osmotic water shifts into or out of brain cells.

In chronic hypotonic disorders, cell swelling is offset by the loss of potassium chloride from cells. This potassium chloride efflux mechanism appears to be activated by small increases in cell volume produced by ECF dilution. In chronic hypernatremia, brain shrinkage is minimized by the accumulation of additional solutes within brain cells. These latter solutes, often called "idiogenic osmoles," include amino acids and other solutes, including myoinosi-

tol betaine, and urea. As will be discussed in the section on Treatment, these auxiliary transport processes affect significantly the therapeutic approach to patients with osmoregulatory failure.

Water Balance

The key elements regulating water balance are summarized in Figure 75–4. The osmoreceptors, both for ADH release and for thirst, respond to small changes in effective ECF osmolality, while baroreceptors respond to changes in ECV. As little as a 2% increase in effective ECF osmolality shrinks osmoreceptor cells and stimulates both ADH release from the posterior pituitary and thirst. A second way of stimulating both ADH release and thirst involves volume-mediated stimuli that can operate independently of changes in plasma osmolality. When the ECV volume is reduced by approximately 10%, these volume-dependent mechanisms stimulate ADH release.

SENSORS AND EFFECTORS. Three kinds of *sensor* elements adjust water balance. Two of these, osmoreceptors and the thirst center, respond to small changes in effective ECF osmolality, whereas baroreceptors respond to changes in ECV. The osmoreceptors are situated in the supraoptic and paraventricular nuclei of the hypothalamus, whereas the thirst center is in the organum vasculosum of the anterior hypothalamus. As little as a 2% increase in effective ECF osmolality produced by solutes such as sodium chloride, but not urea, shrinks osmoreceptor cells and thirst center cells. The osmoreceptors stimulate the release of the *effector* hormone ADH from storage sites in the posterior pituitary gland. The stimulation of thirst by the thirst centers depends on centrally produced angiotensin II.

Endothelin 1 is also released from the posterior pituitary in response to water deprivation. Moreover, administered endothelin 1 increases plasma ADH levels. Thus endothelin 1 may have a central role in modulating ADH release.

When the ECV is reduced by more than 10%, volume-dependent blood volume produces afferent signals, carried by the ninth and tenth cranial nerves, which result in nonosmotic ADH release. Vol-

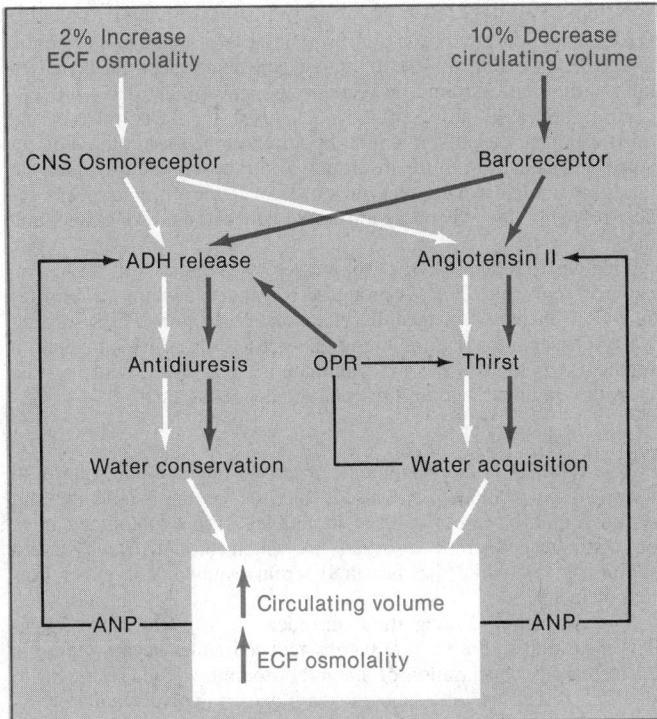

FIGURE 75–4. The water repletion reaction. The white lines are positive water conservation processes activated by osmolality. The red lines are water conservation processes that are volume activated. The black lines indicate negative feedback. OPR = oropharyngeal reflex. (From Reeves WB, Andreoli TE: The posterior pituitary and water metabolism. *In* Wilson JD, Foster DW [eds.]: Williams Textbook of Endocrinology. 8th ed. Philadelphia, WB Saunders, 1992.)

ume contraction also acts as a potent stimulus to thirst via angiotensin II.

THE ANTIDIURETIC RESPONSE. The cardinal characteristics of the antidiuretic response depend primarily on the integrated activity of two nephron regions: the medullary thick ascending limb of Henle, which concentrates the medullary interstitium, and the collecting duct, which, with ADH present, allows water reabsorption from this segment.

The medullary thick ascending limb absorbs much, possibly as much as 25%, of the filtered load of sodium. Some of this reabsorbed sodium is trapped in the renal medullary interstitium, thus accounting largely for the hypertonicity of the renal medullary interstitium. However, the medullary thick limb of Henle is also impermeable to water. Consequently, salt abstraction from the thick limb of Henle accounts simultaneously for the development of medullary hypertonicity, thus permitting—in the presence of ADH—maximal antidiuresis, and the appearance of maximally dilute urine in early distal convolutions, thus permitting—in the absence of ADH—maximal water diuresis.

In normal individuals, approximately 18 liters daily of tubular fluid reaches the early distal tubule; the osmolality of this fluid is quite dilute, approximately 50 mOsm per kilogram of H_2O. Thus, in the total absence of ADH and volume contraction, maximal rates of water diuresis include a urinary volume of 18 liters per day having an osmolality of 50 mOsm per kilogram of H_2O. During antidiuresis, ADH increases the water permeability of collecting ducts (see Ch. 202.2). Tubular fluid equilibrates osmotically with the hypertonic medullary interstitium, reducing urinary volume, concentrating the urine, and conserving body water. When ADH is absent, the water permeability of collecting ducts is low, and absorption of tubular fluid is reduced, so it escapes unchanged as hypotonic urine.

Finally, since collecting ducts are partially permeable to water in the absence of ADH, a reduced volume of hypotonic fluid reaching collecting ducts equilibrates partially with the medullary interstitium, thereby limiting the ability to dilute urine maximally. In some experimental circumstances, sufficiently significant reductions in the rate of solute excretion result in formation of a hypertonic urine when ADH is absent.

NEGATIVE FEEDBACK. Water repletion activates a negative feedback of water conservation by at least two systems, atriopeptin and OPR (see Fig. 75–2). Immunoreactive atriopeptin is released both within the CNS and by secretory granules in cardiac atria. The centrally released atriopeptin can suppress by ADH release and thirst. Oropharyngeal stimulation by water suppresses both ADH release and thirst prior to absorbing water or producing a fall in plasma osmolality. This mechanism, termed the *oropharyngeal reflex,* probably depends on neural traffic between the oropharynx and the CNS.

Finally, intrarenal PGE_2 suppresses the effects of ADH on nephron segments. PGE_2 is produced by renal interstitial cells in response to increases in medullary osmolality. In turn, PGE_2 impairs water conservation by inhibiting the actions of ADH on nephron segments involved in the antidiuretic response, namely, the medullary thick ascending limb and the collecting duct.

HYPOTONIC DISORDERS

DEFINITION. In a hypotonic disorder, the ratio of solutes to water in body fluids is reduced, and the serum osmolality and serum sodium are both reduced in parallel. True hypotonicity must be distinguished from disorders in which the *measured* serum sodium is low while the measured serum osmolality is either normal or increased.

The distinction among these disorders is listed in Table 75–6. The measured serum sodium can be reduced either because there is an increased concentration of small, nonsodium solutes restricted to the ECF or because of a laboratory artifact. In hyperglycemia or excessive mannitol administration, these solutes, which are restricted to the ECF, draw water from the cellular compartment. The serum sodium level is therefore reduced, even though the serum osmolality may be increased. When a small, nonsodium solute is distributed in total body water, as in ethanol intoxication or in azotemia, the serum osmolality rises but the serum sodium concentration remains normal, resulting in an "osmolar gap." The latter is a useful

TABLE 75–6. DISTINCTION BETWEEN APPARENT AND REAL HYPOTONICITY

Condition	Measured Serum (Na)	Measured Serum Osmolality
True hypotonicity	↓	↓
Increased nonsodium ECF solutes		
Hyperglycemia	↓	↑
Mannitol administration	↓	↑
Increased nonsodium ECF and ICF solutes		
Ethanol	Normal	↑
Ethylene glycol	Normal	↑
Methanol	Normal	↑
Isopropyl alcohol	Normal	↑
Laboratory artifact		
Hyperlipemia	↓	Normal
Hyperproteinemia	↓	Normal

diagnostic aid in intoxication with the different alcohols shown in Table 75–6.

Instances of spurious hyponatremia due to hyperlipemia or hyperproteinemia are becoming less common as more laboratories use ion-selective electrodes to measure the serum sodium concentration.

ETIOLOGY AND PATHOGENESIS. Hyponatremia and simultaneous body water hypotonicity develop whenever water intake exceeds the sum of renal plus extrarenal water losses; in chronic hyponatremia, the net water intake and net water output may be equal. Thus hyponatremia and body fluid hypotonicity occur when there is a primary increase in water ingestion, when the ability of the kidney to dilute urine maximally is limited, or when a combination of these factors is operative.

The kidney regulates serum sodium concentration by increasing or decreasing free water excretion. The term "free water" refers to that amount of solute-free water that has to be added or subtracted from urine to leave it isosmolar to blood. Thus adding free water to blood, either by failure to generate free water or by increased reabsorption of free water, will decrease serum sodium concentration. Free water is generated by the kidney across the diluting segments by absorbing salt without water. Thus free water is formed and excreted. Failure to generate free water occurs in those clinical circumstances in which less salt is delivered to the diluting segments.

Free water is absorbed in the collecting duct. The rate of free water reabsorption is regulated in large part by ADH. Thus, the higher the ADH concentration, the greater is the rate of free water reabsorption, assuming that other driving forces for water reabsorption remain constant. Conditions with increased ADH concentrations are generally associated with hyponatremia. The collecting duct can maintain large osmotic gradients; however, this capacity is limited, and the minimal osmolality of the urine is approximately 50 mOsm per kilogram of H_2O. If more dilute fluid is delivered to the collecting duct, this water will be reabsorbed even in the absence of ADH, as occurs in psychogenic polydipsia and in beer potomania. These conditions are described below.

Reduced Solute Delivery to Distal Nephron Segments. These disorders may occur because of decreased sodium delivery to the diluting segment or decreased solute delivery to the collecting duct. Decreased sodium delivery generally occurs in a setting of decreased effective arterial blood volume, e.g., congestive heart failure, hypoalbuminemic states, and decreases in systemic vascular resistance, as in sepsis and cirrhosis. These conditions often are also associated with ADH increases.

An example of decreased solute delivery to the collecting duct is *beer potomania.* Without beer, a normal individual on a normal diet produces roughly 1000 mOsm of solute for urinary excretion. Because maximally dilute urine is 50 mOsm per kilogram, each 50 mOsm of solute can capture no more than 1 liter of free water. Thus, on a normal diet, an individual can consume up to 20 liters of fluid without becoming hyponatremic. However, beer has a low concentration of salts and other solutes, except it has a relatively high carbohydrate content that prevents metabolic generation of solutes by preventing protein catabolism. Indeed, it has been estimated that total urinary osmolal clearance is no more than 200 mOsm. Thus beer drinkers who get most of their calories from beer cannot drink more than 4 liters of free water (most of which will be consumed as beer) without becoming hyponatremic.

Hyponatremia due to reduced solute intake is not restricted to individuals with beer potomania but may occur during starvation, when intake may be dramatically reduced without parallel reductions in water intake. This form of hyponatremia occurs with increasing frequency in elderly patients in nursing homes who are inadequately supervised.

Primary Effector ADH Excess. **The Syndrome of Inappropriate ADH Production (SIADH).** In SIADH, hyponatremia occurs as a result of sustained endogenous production and release of ADH or ADH-like substances; the ECV is normal or increased, and there are no other physiologic or pharmacologic stimuli to ADH release. Table 75–7 lists the major causes of SIADH. A similar process may account in part for the hyponatremia seen in myxedema.

ADH, or a peptide having comparable biologic activity, is produced by tumors. Increased ADH levels, estimated by either bioassay or radioimmunoassay, also have been noted in patients with cranial disorders such as skull fractures, subdural hematomas, subarachnoid hemorrhage, and brain tumors; in acute intermittent porphyria; and possibly in myxedema. Four different patterns of plasma ADH concentrations have been described in patients with SIADH. Figure 75–5 illustrates three of these patterns; the shaded area in the figure illustrates the normal relation between plasma ADH levels and serum osmolality. The pattern denoted "erratic ADH release" in Figure 75–5 accounts for about 37% of patients with SIADH; the hormone is released completely independently of osmotic control. About one-third of patients with SIADH have a "reset osmostat"; there is an abnormally low threshold for ADH secretion, but if sufficiently hyponatremic, these patients with SIADH can produce a maximally dilute urine. About 16% of patients with SIADH exhibit the "ADH leak" pattern, namely, sustained ADH production below the osmotic threshold, and normal increases in serum ADH levels with osmotic challenge (Fig. 75–5). Finally, about 14% of patients with SIADH have no detectable abnormality in ADH levels; they fail, for reasons not yet understood, to dilute urine maximally.

The typical features of SIADH are listed in Table 75–8. The cardinal results of the sustained water conservation in SIADH are twofold: hyponatremia and volume expansion. In fact, patients with SIADH who are allowed free access to water generally gain about 3 kg in water weight or, in other words, nearly 10% of body water. In that respect, patients with SIADH differ from those with hyponatremia secondary to salt depletion, Addison's disease, or diuretic excess, since patients with the latter disorders are volume contracted. However, patients with SIADH, although volume expanded, do not develop edema and thus differ in that respect from patients with congestive heart failure or cirrhosis.

When total body water is expanded by about 10% by water conservation in SIADH, a natriuresis occurs even with hyponatremia. Thus the patient with SIADH reaches a steady state when body water is expanded by water retention and when natriuresis, even with hyponatremia, prevents edema formation.

The causes for the natriuresis that is characteristic of SIADH are multiple. First, volume expansion will result in enhanced release of atriopeptin, which enhances urinary sodium wasting both by en-

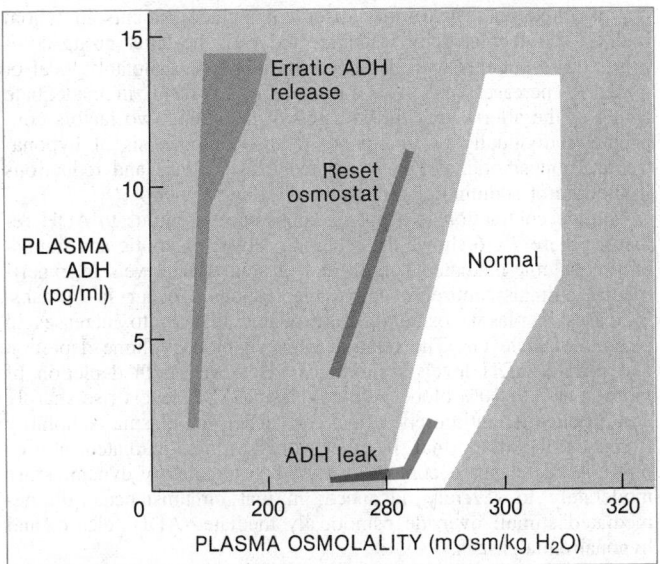

FIGURE 75–5. The patterns of serum ADH abnormalities in SIADH. The shaded areas indicate the normal relation between increases in effective ECF osmolality and ADH levels; the normal osmotic threshold is lower than the normal serum osmolality. The three shaded areas indicate ADH patterns in SIADH. (Adapted from Zerbe R, Strope L, Robertson G: Vasopressin function in the syndrome of inappropriate diuresis. Annu Rev Med 31:315, 1980.)

hancing glomerular filtration and by suppressing tubular sodium absorption. Second, the volume expansion of SIADH also reduces the rate of proximal tubular sodium absorption, as well as the rate of proximal uric acid absorption.

In short, SIADH is a disorder in which hormone-stimulated water conservation results in hyponatremia, volume expansion, and consequently an increased GFR, tubular sodium wasting, and reduced net tubular absorption of creatinine and uric acid, but no edema formation. These characteristics are summarized in Table 75–8. Finally, as indicated in connection with Figure 75–5, the urinary osmolality in patients with SIADH may be either inappropriately high for the level of serum osmolality or maximally dilute.

Other Causes of Excessive ADH Production and/or Release. There are other circumstances in which an increased level of ADH is the primary factor responsible for hyponatremia. A number of commonly used drugs stimulate ADH release: vincristine, cyclophosphamide, carbamazepine, phenothiazines, morphine, barbiturates, chlorpropamide, amitriptyline, thiothixene, and clofibrate. Chlorpropamide also potentiates the effect of ADH on the water permeability of collecting ducts. The posterior pituitary peptide oxytocin (Pitocin) also has an antidiuretic action, although oxytocin is a much less potent antidiuretic agent than is vasopressin. Thus intravenous hypotonic solutions containing oxytocin given to induce labor may result in profound hyponatremia. Trauma or surgical stress also stimulates ADH release.

Ordinarily, diuretic-induced hyponatremia is related to volume contraction; this kind of body fluid dilution will be discussed below. Chronic severe potassium depletion induced by diuretics can also result in ADH release, although the mechanisms by which potassium depletion stimulates ADH release are unknown.

Mixed Disorders. Hyponatremia occurs commonly in true volume contraction and in edematous states when filling of the arterial

---

TABLE 75–7. MAJOR CAUSES OF SIADH

Malignant Neoplasia
  Carcinoma: bronchogenic, pancreatic, duodenal, ureteral, prostatic, bladder
  Lymphoma and leukemia
  Thymoma and mesothelioma
Central Nervous System (CNS) Disorders
  Trauma
  Infection
  Tumors
  Porphyria
Pulmonary Disorders
  Tuberculosis
  Pneumonia
  Fungal infections
  Lung abscesses
  Ventilators with positive pressure

TABLE 75–8. MAJOR CHARACTERISTICS OF SIADH

Hyponatremia
Volume expansion without edema
Natriuresis
Hypouricemia
Normal or reduced serum creatinine level
Normal thyroid and adrenal function

tree is impaired. The former disorders include patients in whom both ECF and total body water are reduced; the latter group comprises those patients with deranged Starling forces, notably local or systemic increases in venous pressure, which result in inadequate filling of the arterial tree. In both sets of disorders, two factors contribute, individually or in unison, to the pathogenesis of hyponatremia: nonosmotic, volume-mediated ADH release and reductions in the rate of sodium delivery to the diluting segment.

Volume contraction is a potent nonosmotic stimulus to ADH release. Figure 75–6 shows the relations between osmotic and nonosmotic, volume-mediated stimuli and plasma ADH levels in experimental animals; entirely comparable responses occur in humans. Increases in plasma osmolality are related linearly to increases in plasma ADH levels. The relation between blood volume depletion and plasma ADH levels is nonlinear. However, with depletion of more than 7 to 10% blood volume, plasma ADH levels rise sharply and produce an antidiuretic effect even when the plasma osmolality is reduced below normal. In other words, volume-mediated, nonosmotic ADH release occurs primarily when circulatory dynamics are moderately to severely advanced; in that circumstance, volume-mediated stimuli override osmotically mediated ADH release, and hyponatremia ensues.

A second factor that accounts for hyponatremia in volume-contracted states is an inability to dilute urine maximally because the rate of sodium delivery to diluting segments in the thick ascending limb is reduced. This situation occurs because increased rates of proximal tubular sodium absorption are stimulated by reduced sodium intake or by inadequate filling of the arterial tree in conditions with combined ECF volume expansion and reduced arterial tree filling.

Hyponatremia is a common feature of untreated Addison's disease and occurs because of a combination of circumstances. In min-eralocorticoid deficiency, ECF volume contraction, glomerular filtration reduction, enhanced proximal tubular salt absorption, and volume-mediated, nonosmotic ADH release appear to be the major factors responsible for an inability to excrete water loads. Glucocorticoid deficiency also impairs the ability to excrete water loads. One of the factors responsible for water retention in Addison's disease is nonosmotic ADH release, which results from impaired cardiac function.

Hyponatremia occurs commonly in advanced stages of disorders characterized by edema formation and a reduced ECV, particularly in intractable heart failure and advanced hepatic cirrhosis with ascites. Reduced rates of salt delivery to diluting segments of the renal tubule clearly contribute to impaired water excretion in these disorders. In patients with heart failure or severe ascites, the plasma concentrations of ADH tend to be inappropriately high with respect to plasma osmolality so that nonosmotic ADH release secondary to contraction of the effective arterial blood volume may contribute to the development of hyponatremia in these disorders. Furthermore, since nonosmotic ADH release occurs only with profound reductions in blood volume (Fig. 75–6), the occurrence of hyponatremia in congestive heart failure or cirrhosis indicates profound arterial underfilling. This observation correlates well with the ominous prognosis of hyponatremia in these disorders.

CLINICAL MANIFESTATIONS. The clinical manifestations of hyponatremia are produced by brain swelling and are primarily a function of the rate of fall of serum sodium concentration and not the absolute level. The early symptoms include lethargy, weakness, and somnolence, which proceed rapidly to seizures, coma, and death as hyponatremia worsens. Untreated acute water intoxication is nearly uniformly fatal and represents a medical emergency. In chronic hyponatremia, CNS manifestations are far less common, even when the serum sodium concentration is as low as 100 mEq per liter, because the loss of brain solutes, principally potassium chloride, minimizes brain cell swelling for a given reduction in body water osmolality.

DIAGNOSIS. Hyponatremia should be considered whenever there is a sudden deterioration in CNS function, particularly in circumstances such as intractable heart failure, hepatic cirrhosis with ascites, or when large volumes of intravenous fluids are administered. The hyponatremic patient should be evaluated to determine the underlying condition that produced body fluid dilution. This evaluation should include a careful history and physical examination; measurement of the serum creatinine, BUN, and electrolytes; measurement of the urinary sodium concentration, or the FE_{Na}; measurement of serum and urinary osmolalities; and, when appropriate, evaluation of thyroid and adrenal function.

The history and physical examination are generally adequate for recognizing disorders such as beer potomania or compulsive water ingestion or for noting the ingestion of drugs that stimulate ADH release or enhance ADH action. The presence of edema is characteristic of individuals in whom hyponatremia occurs because of a reduced effective arterial blood volume coupled to ECF volume expansion. In myxedema or Addison's disease, the typical clinical or laboratory findings of these disorders are generally present (see Ch. 203 and 204.1).

The most difficult differential diagnosis among hyponatremic disorders involves the distinction between patients who are modestly volume contracted and those who have SIADH. In both circumstances, the serum sodium and the serum osmolality are reduced, whereas the urinary osmolality is inappropriately high with respect to the reduced serum osmolality. Nonosmotic water conservation in SIADH and in volume contraction is recognized by the presence of a urinary osmolality >120 to 150 mOsm per kilogram of H_2O in association with a reduced serum osmolality. The distinction between the two disorders therefore depends on a clinical and laboratory assessment of effective arterial blood volume.

Patients who are volume contracted may provide a history of volume losses or of diuretic ingestion and may exhibit the signs of ECF volume contraction discussed previously in the section on Volume Depletion. When the volume losses are due to extrarenal causes, the urinary sodium concentration is <10 to 15 mEq per liter and the FE_{Na} is generally <1%. Uric acid concentration is influenced by volume status of the patient. In volume expansion, there is increased urinary excretion of uric acid and therefore a tendency toward hypouricemia. Conversely, the presence of hyperuricemia suggests effective arterial volume contraction. Prerenal

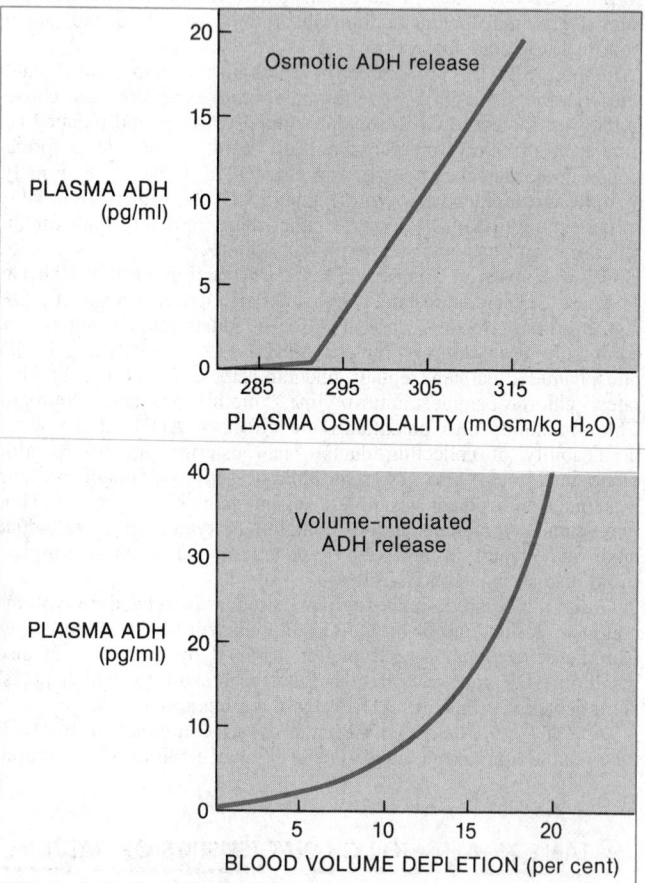

FIGURE 75–6. Relation between plasma ADH concentrations and either effective ECF osmolality *(upper plot)* or the percentage of blood volume depletion *(lower plot)*. (Adapted from Dunn FL, Brennan TJ, Nelson AE, et al.: The role of blood osmolality and volume in regulating vasopressin secretion in the rat. J Clin Invest 52:3212, 1973, by copyright permission of the American Society for Clinical Investigation.)

azotemia may occur if the volume contraction is severe. Patients with SIADH are generally normovolemic or slightly volume expanded and therefore exhibit none of the signs of volume contraction. The serum BUN and creatinine levels are normal, and the serum uric acid level is generally reduced. The urinary sodium concentration is usually >30 mEq per liter, and the FE_{Na} is >1%. Tests of adrenal function yield normal results (Table 75–9).

The above studies usually discriminate between SIADH and extrarenal volume contraction. When ECF volume contraction is due to renal salt wasting, urinary sodium losses generally persist unless volume contraction is profound. Moreover, as noted previously (see Volume Depletion), the blood pressure and pulse may be normal in states of modest volume contraction. A useful diagnostic and therapeutic maneuver in this situation is to observe the results of water restriction. When water intake is restricted to 600 to 800 ml daily, patients with SIADH exhibit a highly characteristic response: A 2- to 3-kg weight loss is accompanied by correction of hyponatremia and cessation of salt wasting, usually over 2 to 3 days. If weight loss fails to correct both hyponatremia and urinary sodium wasting simultaneously, the diagnosis of SIADH is doubtful. Rather, renal sodium wasting with ECF volume contraction, due to Addison's disease or the other renal salt-losing disorders listed in Table 75–2, is the more probable diagnosis.

TREATMENT. Neurologic symptoms secondary to osmotic swelling of the brain are much more common when hyponatremia develops rapidly, but the most severe neurologic complications of acute treatment of hyponatremia are more common if existing hyponatremia is longstanding and developed chronically. Patients with CNS manifestations of hyponatremia require immediate therapy to prevent death, while too-rapid hyponatremia correction may be associated with osmotic demyelination syndrome, which is the result of the selective loss of myelin (with sparing of neurons and axial cylinders). These histologic findings may occur in any part of the brain but are more common in the central areas of the pons. The symptoms of osmotic demyelinating syndrome often occur several days after too-rapid hyponatremia correction and include behavioral disturbances, fluctuating levels of consciousness, ataxia, pseudo-bulbar palsy, difficulty in speaking, and other varying features. In non-fatal cases, the recovery is slow, often taking weeks, and recovery may not be complete with residual sequelae. Thus differing opinions exist as to the ideal rate for correcting hyponatremia. The rate and magnitude of this correction can be considered conveniently as a two-step process: acute correction of symptomatic hyponatremia and chronic correction of asymptomatic or residual hyponatremia.

Acute Correction of Hyponatremia. Acute hyponatremia associated with a serum sodium concentration <120 mEq per liter and with CNS manifestations requires immediate therapy. In volume-contracted states, the treatment of choice is to raise the serum sodium concentration by 10 mEq per liter or to levels of 120 to 125 mEq per liter over a 6-hour interval by administering hypertonic 3 to 5% saline. As was discussed, elevating serum sodium too quickly to values >125 mEq per liter may be hazardous. Since the desired effect is to correct total body water osmolality, the amount of sodium administered must be sufficient to raise total body water osmolality to approximately 250 mOsm per kilogram of H_2O, i.e., to approximately twice the desired serum sodium concentration. A convenient formula for calculating this sodium requirement is as follows:

$$[125 - \text{measured serum } Na^+] \times 0.6 \text{ body weight}$$
$$= \text{required mEq of } Na^+$$

The serum sodium level is in milliequivalents per liter, and the body weight is in kilograms. Since 60% of body weight is water, the formula allows an estimate of the amount of sodium required to raise total body water osmolality to 250 mOsm per kilogram of H_2O. However, if one cannot remember this formula, a useful practice is to administer 250 ml of either 3 or 5% saline over 4 to 6 hours. This will usually raise the serum sodium concentration by 10 to 15 mEq per liter and abate the neurologic symptoms. Once the acute corrective phase of hyponatremia is complete, one can initiate the principle of chronic correction of hyponatremia.

Chronic Correction of Hyponatremia. The most important aspect in managing asymptomatic, non–volume-depleted hyponatremia is to restrict electrolyte-free water intake. If water intake is restricted to <1 liter per day, the serum sodium concentration will rise regardless of its cause. Fluid intake restriction should be coupled with high dietary salt intake. Since this approach is clinically unacceptably slow in certain patients, an alternative is to use normal saline in combination with a loop diuretic. The diuretic induces urinary salt loss and therefore reduces the risk of ECF volume expansion. It should be emphasized that isotonic saline infusion without a loop diuretic may actually lower the serum sodium concentration in patients with SIADH. Thus one must use a loop diuretic with intravenous saline if this approach is taken.

Another approach to correcting chronic hyponatremia in SIADH is to use lithium carbonate or demeclocycline. These two compounds block the effect of ADH at the level of the collecting duct and, therefore, increase the excretion of free water. However, both these drugs may have complications and should only be used if the patient cannot adequately comply with water restriction and high dietary salt intake.

HYPERTONIC DISORDERS

DEFINITION. A hypertonic disorder is one in which the ratio of solutes to water in total body water is increased. All hypernatremic states are hypertonic. In some hypertonic disorders, such as uncontrolled hyperglycemia, the increase in effective ECF osmolality is due to nonsodium solutes.

ETIOLOGY AND PATHOGENESIS. Hypernatremia develops whenever water intake is less than the sum of renal and extrarenal water losses; in chronic hypertonic states, net water balance may be zero. The most common causes of clinically significant hypernatremia occur as a consequence of three pathogenic mechanisms: impaired thirst, solute or osmotic diuresis, excessive losses of water, either via the kidneys or extrarenally, and combinations of these derangements. These disorders are grouped in Table 75–10 according to the primary pathogenic mechanism. There is also a group of miscellaneous disorders, such as hypokalemia, hypercalcemia, and interstitial renal disease, as well as chronic renal failure, which either partially impair renal urinary concentrating ability or partially blunt the responsiveness of collecting ducts to ADH. These disorders rarely cause significant hypernatremia and are not discussed further.

Inadequate Intake of Water. This problem occurs in patients who are comatose or who are otherwise unable to communicate thirst. Because of the exquisite sensitivity of thirst mechanisms to changes in effective body water osmolality, hypernatremia due to inadequate water intake is rare in conscious patients allowed free access to water. Rarely, patients will have a primary thirst deficiency. Patients with Cushing's syndrome or primary hyperaldosteronism commonly have slight elevations in the serum sodium level for unknown reasons.

TABLE 75–9. DISTINGUISHING FEATURES OF APPROPRIATELY VERSUS INAPPROPRIATELY INCREASED ADH CONCENTRATIONS

Appropriate		Inappropriate
↓	Plasma sodium	↓
↑	Urine osmolality	↑
↓	Urine sodium	↑
↑	Plasma uric acid	↓

TABLE 75–10. MAJOR CAUSES OF HYPERNATREMIA

I. **Impaired Thirst**
   Coma
   Essential hypernatremia
II. **Solute Diuresis**
   Osmotic diuresis: diabetic ketoacidosis, nonketotic hyperosmolar coma, mannitol administration
III. **Excessive Water Losses**
   Renal
     Pituitary diabetes insipidus
     Nephrogenic diabetes insipidus
   Extrarenal
     Sweating
IV. **Combined Disorders**
   Coma plus hypertonic nasogastric feeding

Finally, "essential hypernatremia" is characterized by a slightly elevated serum sodium level that occurs in the conscious state. The defect in patients with essential hypernatremia appears to be an insensitivity of thirst centers and osmoreceptors to osmotic stimuli. However, both thirst and antidiuresis occur when these patients are volume contracted. Consequently, it has been inferred that volume-mediated stimuli to thirst and ADH release are intact in patients with essential hypernatremia. This disorder may be either congenital or acquired, sometimes in association with histiocytic infiltration of the CNS.

Osmotic Diuresis. This is another mechanism for producing renal water losses in excess of sodium losses and therefore hypertonicity. Osmotic diuresis occurs commonly in uncontrolled glycosuria and may occur when mannitol is given. Since these solutes are restricted to the ECF, the serum sodium level is generally reduced in the early stages of osmotic diuresis, and the effective ECF osmolality is increased primarily by the impermeant nonsodium solute. In prolonged osmotic diuresis, net water losses may be sufficiently great that hypernatremia develops. In this circumstance, the increase in effective ECF osmolality is due to the combined effects of hypernatremia and the nonsodium solute. Hypernatremia due to an osmotic urea diuresis can occur if large amounts of protein and amino acids are administered by nasogastric tube, or if tissue catabolism is great, as in burns. In this circumstance, hypernatremia is entirely responsible for the increased effective ECF osmolality.

Hypernatremia also may complicate use of normal saline solutions when the endogenous osmolar solute load is high and renal concentrating ability is limited. Patients with diabetic ketoacidosis, who are generally young, have sufficient urinary concentrating ability that hypernatremia does not occur when normal saline solutions are used to treat ketoacidosis. In contrast, the nonketotic hyperglycemic syndrome generally occurs in elderly patients, who can have partial impairment of urinary concentrating power. In this setting, hypernatremia can occur during therapy with normal saline solutions. This complication can be avoided by treating with half-normal saline and thus providing sufficient solute-free water for urinary elimination of the osmolar glucose load.

Excessive Water Losses. Impairment of ADH production, release, or action, as in pituitary or nephrogenic diabetes insipidus, respectively, can lead to profound water deficits and to hypernatremia. In such circumstances, the urine volumes are large, the urinary osmolality is low, and the net rate of solute excretion is low, in contrast to individuals undergoing osmotic diuresis, in whom rates of urinary solute excretion are elevated. The diabetes insipidus syndromes are considered in detail in Ch. 202.2.

Striking water losses also may occur with excessive sweating, particularly during rigorous physical activity by untrained individuals exercising in high humidity. This phenomenon plays a major role in the evolution of heat stroke.

Combined Disorders. Finally, hypertonic dehydration may occur as a combination of these events. A common example in modern clinical practice involves injudiciously administering large amounts of carbohydrate or amino acids by nasogastric tube, coupled with limited amounts of water, to stroke patients unable to communicate thirst.

CLINICAL MANIFESTATIONS AND DIAGNOSIS. Because two-thirds of body water is intracellular, primary water losses tend to have modest effects on circulating volume unless fluid losses are profound. Rather, the clinical manifestations are produced by brain shrinkage that results from increases in effective ECF osmolality. Thus the symptoms of hypertonicity produced either by hypernatremia or by impermeant nonsodium solutes such as glucose are referable to the CNS and range from somnolence and confusion to coma, respiratory paralysis, and death. The degree of symptomatology varies with the degree of hypertonicity and with the rate at which hypertonicity develops. In acute hypertonicity, symptoms generally appear when the effective ECF osmolality exceeds 320 to 330 mOsm per kilogram of H_2O, and coma and respiratory arrest may occur when the ECF osmolality exceeds 360 to 380 mOsm per kilogram of H_2O. Chronic hypertonicity generally produces fewer CNS manifestations, because brain cells accumulate idiogenic osmoles, which minimize the tendency for brain shrinkage.

TREATMENT. To treat acute hypernatremia, normal saline solutions are initially given intravenously. These factors should be considered when treating acute hypernatremia: In the highly volume-contracted patient with severe hypernatremia, administering isotonic saline solutions has two advantages. It provides fluid resuscitation in impending cardiovascular collapse. Moreover, the isotonic salt solution, which is hypotonic with respect to the hypertonic patient, avoids an unnecessary rapid fall in the serum sodium level.

Rapid correction of hypertonicity to a normal serum osmolality is hazardous. Since accumulation of idiogenic osmoles by brain cells is a compensatory mechanism for preserving brain volume in hypertonic disorders, a normal serum osmolality may be relatively hypotonic to brain cells that have accumulated idiogenic solutes. Hence, if the serum osmolality is reduced rapidly, CNS damage due to brain swelling may occur. A useful guide to circumventing this difficulty is to reduce the serum sodium level by no more than 1 mEq per liter during every 2 hours of the first 2 days of treatment.

Ayus JC, Krothapalli RK, Arieff AI: Treatment of symptomatic hyponatremia and its relation to brain damage: A prospective study. N Engl J Med 317:1190, 1987. *A prospective study showing little relation between the rate of correction of hyponatremia and the occurrence of central pontine myelinolysis.*

Cheng J-C, Zikos D, Skopicki HA, et al.: Long-term neurologic outcome in psychogenic water drinkers with severe symptomatic hyponatremia: The effect of rapid correction. Am J Med 88:561, 1990. *Study of patients with hyponatremia secondary to compulsive water drinking demonstrating that it is safe to reverse the neurologic sequelae by rapid correction of serum sodium level by 15 mEq per kilogram of H_2O followed by more gradual correction of the remaining hyponatremia.*

DeVita MV, Michelis MF: Perturbations in sodium balance. Clin Lab Med 13:135, 1993. *Discusses the pathophysiology, assessment, and treatment of hypo- and hypernatremia syndromes.*

Goldman MB, Luchins DJ, Robertson GL: Mechanisms of altered water metabolism in psychotic patients with polydipsia and hyponatremia. N Engl J Med 318:397, 1988. *An account of factors causing hyponatremia in hospitalized patients with affective disorders.*

Sonnenblick M, Friedlander Y, Rosin AJ: Diuretic-induced severe hyponatremia: Review and analysis of 129 reported patients. Chest 103:601, 1993. *Literature review of severe diuretic-induced hyponatremia showing that severity of hyponatremia as well as too-rapid correction was associated with higher mortality. Thiazide diuretics were associated with severe hyponatremia much more frequently than loop diuretics.*

Sterns RH: Severe symptomatic hyponatremia: Treatment and outcome. Ann Intern Med 107:656, 1987. *An extensive retrospective analysis of acute symptomatic hyponatremia that argues that rapid correction of hyponatremia is hazardous.*

Tang WW, Kaptein EM, Feinstein EI, Massry SG: Hyponatremia in hospitalized patients with the acquired immunodeficiency syndrome (AIDS) and the AIDS-related complex. Am J Med 94:169, 1993. *A well-conducted prospective study showing that hyponatremia is common in AIDS patients and is usually associated with gastrointestinal losses with hypovolemia, but euvolemia with SIADH was also a common association. Hyponatremia of either cause was associated with increased morbidity and mortality.*

Zerbe R, Strope L, Robertson G: Vasopressin function in the syndrome of inappropriate diuresis. Ann Rev Med 31:315, 1980. *The patterns of ADH response in SIADH.*

75.3 Disturbances in Potassium Balance

PHYSIOLOGIC CONSIDERATIONS

Hypokalemia ($K^+ < 3.5$ mEq per liter) and hyperkalemia ($K^+ > 5.5$ mEq per liter) are common in the practice of medicine. While the plasma potassium concentration is influenced by total body potassium stores, it should be recognized that factors influencing the distribution of potassium between extra- and intracellular spaces are important determinants of plasma potassium concentration.

Transfer Between ICF and ECF

The intracellular compartment acts as a large potassium reservoir in series with the small ECF potassium pool. In potassium-depleted states with normal acid-base status, a 1 mEq per liter fall in the serum potassium level reflects the loss of about 300 mEq of potassium; hence the bulk of external potassium loss comes from the cellular compartment. Conversely, if large amounts of potassium are administered acutely, the rise in serum potassium level is less than would be expected if the administered potassium were distributed solely in the ECF. In this situation, cellular uptake of potassium obviously occurs and prevents greater increases in the serum potassium concentration. This ability of cells to accumulate potassium can be enhanced strikingly by chronic administration of high-potassium diets.

A number of *effector* mechanisms regulate the partition of potassium between the ICF and ECF. These include active and passive ionic transcellular transport processes.

ACTIVE TRANSPORT PROCESSES. The cardinal transport process regulating K^+ distribution between ICF and ECF is cell membrane–bound Na^+-K^+-ATPase, which actively transports potassium into cells and therefore counterbalances the passive leak of potassium from cells into interstitial fluid. Insulin is a second effector that promotes potassium transfer from ECF to ICF. This hormone promotes cellular uptake of potassium independently of cellular glucose uptake by increasing Na^+-K^+-ATPase activity. Insulin also reduces sodium permeability; the resultant cellular hyperpolarization of cells produces a passive driving force for potassium accumulation within cells. Furthermore, hyperkalemia augments insulin release. Thus hyperkalemia may be the sensor that stimulates release of insulin, which then serves as an effector for potassium entry into cells. β-Adrenergic agents, particularly β_2 agonists such as terbutaline, also promote cellular potassium uptake by enhancing Na^+-K^+-ATPase activity; it is not yet known whether hyperkalemia can provoke β-agonist release, as it does for insulin release. Finally, mineralocorticoids such as aldosterone, in addition to enhancing renal potassium excretion (see below), also enhance cellular potassium uptake; the mode of aldosterone action in the latter instance is not understood.

PASSIVE TRANSPORT PROCESSES. A number of passive effector mechanisms also regulate the partition of potassium between the ICF and the ECF. First, alterations in the pH of ECF reproducibly shift potassium between the ICF and the ECF. Systemic acidosis, whether metabolic or respiratory, promotes potassium efflux from cells, whereas systemic alkalosis, either metabolic or respiratory, promotes cellular potassium uptake. As a general rule, a reduction in plasma pH of 0.1 unit in metabolic acidosis raises the serum potassium level by 0.6 mEq per liter, whereas a plasma pH increase of 0.1 unit produces a similar reduction in serum potassium. The magnitude of transcellular potassium shifts is not as great in response to acid-base balance changes due to respiratory causes as it is in those due to metabolic causes.

Second, cellular shrinkage produced by increases in effective ECF osmolality raises the intracellular potassium concentration and thereby increases the driving force for passive potassium leakage from the ICF to the ECF. This leakage may result in hyperkalemia when large glucose loads are administered to insulin-deficient diabetic patients who also have hyporeninemic hypoaldosteronism; the insulin lack limits cellular reentry of potassium, and the aldosterone deficiency limits renal potassium excretion. Increases in cellular potassium concentrations produced by cellular shrinkage also contribute significantly to the hyperkalemia of diabetic ketoacidosis, because hyperglycemia raises cellular potassium levels by cell shrinkage and insulin lack prevents accelerated potassium reentry into cells.

Finally, brain cells and renal tubular cells lose potassium when exposed to chronic ECF hypotonicity. However, muscle cells, which are the largest component of ICF potassium, do not appear to participate in this process. Consequently, hypotonic disorders, by themselves, have little effect on the serum potassium level or on external potassium balance.

Renal Handling of Potassium

The kidney is responsible for the excretion of approximately 90% of dietary potassium. While the stool potassium concentration is quite high (75 to 90 mEq per liter of stool water) under normal circumstances, only roughly 10% of dietary potassium is excreted by the gastrointestinal tract. Thus factors that cause an increase in renal excretion of potassium are of importance (Table 75–11).

Almost all the potassium excreted in urine gains access to the urinary space by secretory mechanisms that are located across distal convoluted and collecting duct segments. These transport processes are described in Ch. 74, but for the purposes of this chapter, it is important to identify these factors in clinical situations that cause increased excretion of potassium. Of the factors listed in Table 75–11, increased plasma aldosterone is most important, with a higher resultant kaliuresis occurring by the other factors if they are superimposed on a baseline of higher aldosterone concentration.

TABLE 75–11. FACTORS CAUSING INCREASED URINARY LOSS OF POTASSIUM

Increased mineralocorticoids
Increased delivery of Na^+ to collecting duct
Increased fluid flow to distal tubule
Metabolic and respiratory alkalosis
Increased excretion of nonreabsorbable solutes

The rate of urinary potassium excretion in any given clinical circumstance depends on the interplay between these factors.

The rate of renal tubular adaptation to factors regulating urinary excretion of potassium is relatively slow. However, the renal adaptation to excess loads occurs over a 24- to 36-hour period, and therefore, hyperkalemia from the ingestion of large oral potassium loads is uncommon in normal individuals. But the renal response to dietary potassium restriction is more sluggish and requires 7 to 10 days for full development. Even under the latter circumstances, urinary potassium losses are rarely <20 mEq per day.

HYPOKALEMIA AND POTASSIUM DEPLETION

DEFINITION. Chronic hypokalemia generally reflects a reduction in total body potassium. A 1-mEq reduction in serum potassium level generally implies the net loss of 300 mEq of potassium from the body. In extreme body potassium depletion, the serum potassium level may be as low as 1.5 to 2.0 mEq per liter. Acute reductions in serum potassium level without parallel reductions in total body potassium occur when potassium is shifted from the ECF to the ICF.

ETIOLOGY AND PATHOGENESIS. Hypokalemia and simultaneous potassium depletion occur whenever renal plus extrarenal potassium losses exceed potassium intake. In advanced body potassium depletion, intake and output of potassium may be equal. The four major causes for hypokalemia are given in Table 75–12.

Excessive Renal Losses. Many of the causes for renal potassium wasting can be analyzed in terms of factors that modulate the common effector system for potassium secretion. *Mineralocorticoid excess* accelerates distal tubular potassium secretion. Consequently, hypokalemia occurs regularly in primary hyperaldosteronism, in Cushing's syndrome, and in secondary hyperaldosteronism. *Chronic European licorice ingestion* produces a syndrome that mimics primary hyperaldosteronism, because glycyrrhizic acid, a component of licorice extract, has physiologic properties similar to those of aldosterone.

The primary pathophysiologic defect in Bartter's syndrome is incomplete reabsorption of NaCl by the thick ascending limb of Henle. This causes increased delivery of Na^+ to the collecting duct and net salt wastage. The resulting volume contraction results in increased renin and aldosterone concentrations. These hormonal changes, together with increased delivery of Na^+ to the collecting duct, cause increased excretion of potassium.

TABLE 75–12. MAJOR CAUSES OF HYPOKALEMIA

I. Excess Renal Loss	**II. Gastrointestinal Losses**
Mineralocorticoid excess	Vomiting
Bartter's syndrome	Diarrhea, particularly secretory
Diuresis	diarrheas
Diuretics with a pre-late	**III. ECF → ICF Shifts**
distal locus	Acute alkalosis
Osmotic diuresis	Hypokalemic periodic paralysis
Chronic metabolic alkalosis	Barium ingestion
Antibiotics	Insulin therapy
Carbenicillin	Vitamin B_{12} therapy
Gentamicin	Thyrotoxicosis (rarely)
Amphotericin B	**IV. Inadequate Intake**
Renal tubular acidosis	
Distal, gradient-limited	
Proximal	
Liddle's syndrome	
Acute leukemia	
Ureterosigmoidostomy	

Most diuretics having a locus of action before the late distal tubule (see Fig. 75–3) increase urinary potassium losses. Enhanced sodium delivery to distal nephron segments is the major factor responsible for the kaliuresis produced by these diuretics, and sodium restriction or volume depletion tends to minimize diuretic-induced potassium losses. Carbonic anhydrase inhibitors such as acetazolamide inhibit proximal bicarbonate absorption and thereby accentuate potassium losses. Distal tubular segments are relatively impermeable to bicarbonate; consequently, increased delivery of bicarbonate to distal nephron regions has an impermeant anion effect that increases luminal electronegativity in these nephron regions.

Osmotic diuresis is commonly associated with increased renal potassium losses, because increased tubular flow rates enhance net potassium secretion. In diabetic ketoacidosis, renal potassium losses are common. Yet patients with diabetic ketoacidosis and a reduced total body potassium commonly present with hyperkalemia because metabolic acidosis tends to promote potassium shifts from the ICF to the ECF. Consequently, profound hypokalemia may develop if body potassium is not replenished concomitantly with insulin therapy and ECF volume expansion (see Ch. 205).

Potassium depletion is seen frequently in *chronic metabolic alkalosis*. When the alkalosis is associated with volume contraction, secondary hyperaldosteronism results in renal potassium losses. Potassium depletion in chronic metabolic alkalosis is also enhanced if bicarbonaturia is present, because of the impermeant anion effect produced by bicarbonate delivery to collecting duct segments. In fact, the hypokalemia associated with upper gastrointestinal fluid losses, as in vomiting or nasogastric suction, is primarily the result of the renal potassium losses produced by secondary hyperaldosteronism or bicarbonaturia or both. The potassium losses from the upper gastrointestinal tract are small, since upper gastrointestinal tract fluid contains only about 10 mEq of potassium per liter.

Hypokalemia may develop during therapy with certain *antibiotics*. Carbenicillin or other penicillin-like antibiotics exist as sodium or potassium salts of impermeant anions and promote kaliuresis because they increase net sodium excretion and because of an impermeant anion effect. Amphotericin B increases the permeability of luminal membranes to potassium and therefore promotes potassium secretion. Gentamicin produces potassium losses by unknown mechanisms.

Hypokalemia and potassium depletion are common findings in both type II proximal tubular acidosis and type I *distal, gradient-limited renal tubular acidosis* (see Ch. 82). Increased distal sodium delivery and the impermeant anion effect produced by bicarbonate wasting account for most of the potassium losses seen in proximal renal tubular acidosis. Consequently, salt restriction, which enhances the rate of proximal sodium bicarbonate absorption in this disorder, also tends to correct potassium depletion. In gradient-limited distal renal tubular acidosis, hypokalemia may be accentuated by volume losses and secondary hyperaldosteronism. Other factors, not yet understood, also contribute to hypokalemia in this disorder. Hyperkalemia, rather than hypokalemia, commonly accompanies the hyperchloremic acidosis of interstitial disease (type IV acidosis) or of voltage-dependent renal tubular acidosis (see below).

Liddle's syndrome is a rare tubular disorder characterized by hypokalemia, metabolic alkalosis, hypertension, and normal aldosterone secretion rates. Therapy with triamterene, but not with aldosterone antagonists such as spironolactone, ameliorates the disorder. These findings suggest that collecting duct sodium avidity and potassium secretion independent of aldosterone are major factors in the pathogenesis of Liddle's syndrome. Thus, in operational terms, Liddle's syndrome may be described as distal nephron hyperfunction, in regard to Na^+ absorption and H^+ and K^+ secretion.

Gastrointestinal Losses.
These provide the major route for potassium depletion, other than the kidney. As indicated above, potassium depletion associated with vomiting is referable primarily to renal potassium losses. Diarrhea produces significant potassium losses, since normal stool water potassium concentration is 70 to 90 mEq per liter and voluminous diarrheal fluid contains 30 mEq per liter of potassium. The most striking diarrheal potassium losses occur in secretory diarrheas, such as with non–beta islet cell tumors of the pancreas, which produce vasoactive intestinal polypeptide, and in laxative abuse. In both secretory diarrheas and chronic laxative abuse, hypokalemia is probably caused by increased rates of K^+ secretion through apical membrane K^+ channels. Villous adenomas of the colon produce potassium depletion because of excessive colonic K^+ secretion from the adenoma. Hypokalemia is uncommonly seen in inflammatory bowel disease.

ECF-ICF Shifts.
Acute hypokalemia with a normal total body potassium may occur because of *potassium shifts* from the ECF to the ICF. In *hypokalemic periodic paralysis,* acute shifts of potassium from the ECF to the ICF produce limb and trunk paralysis. The periodic attacks are often precipitated by high-carbohydrate meals. Patients with the disorder often can abort attacks by exercising affected muscles. The chronic use of acetazolamide can prevent attacks. A condition resembling hypokalemic periodic paralysis occurs with the ingestion of *barium salts* and is endemic in China, where the disorder is referred to as *Pa-Ping*. Barium appears to produce hypokalemia by blocking K^+ channels in skeletal muscle and thus blocking efflux of potassium from the ICF to the ECF. *Insulin* therapy and *vitamin B_{12}* therapy also promote potassium shifts from the ECF to the ICF. Hypokalemia also can result rarely from thyrotoxicosis, especially in Asian males, for reasons that are unclear.

Inadequate Intake.
Reduced potassium intake may result in potassium depletion and hypokalemia because maximal renal conservation of potassium requires, as indicated previously, 7 to 10 days. During this interval, the net renal potassium loss may be as much as 150 to 200 mEq.

CLINICAL MANIFESTATIONS. The clinical effects of potassium deficiency are manifest in one or more organ systems, including skeletal muscle, heart, kidneys, and the gastrointestinal tract. The most serious disturbances are those affecting the neuromuscular system. At serum potassium concentrations in the range of 2.0 to 2.5 mEq per liter, muscular weakness is likely to occur; with more severe hypokalemia, the patient may develop areflexic paralysis, in which case respiratory insufficiency is an immediate threat to survival. The severity of the neuromuscular disturbance tends to be proportional to the speed with which the potassium level has declined.

Losses of large amounts of potassium from skeletal muscle may contribute to the development of rhabdomyolysis and myoglobinuria. Hence rhabdomyolysis sometimes occurs in athletes and in military recruits subject to severe exercise, sweating, and ECF volume contraction. The secondary hyperaldosteronism that follows excessive salt loss produces urinary potassium wasting and consequently potassium depletion. Potassium and phosphate depletion secondary to malnutrition and alcoholism is also a pathogenic mechanism in the development of rhabdomyolysis in these conditions.

The electrocardiographic abnormalities of potassium depletion, shown in Figure 75–7, affect primarily repolarization segments of the electrocardiogram, in keeping with the effects of hypokalemia on the action potential. The common electrocardiographic manifestations of hypokalemia include sagging of the ST segment, depression of the T wave, and elevation of the U wave. With marked hypokalemia, the T wave becomes progressively smaller and the U waves show increasing amplitude. In some cases the merging of a flat or positive T wave with a positive U wave may erroneously be interpreted as a prolonged QT interval. Ordinarily, there are no serious clinical consequences from the abnormalities in cardiac excitation. In patients treated with digitalis, hypokalemia may precipitate serious arrhythmias.

Longstanding potassium depletion may produce renal tubular damage, referred to as "hypokalemic nephropathy." Potassium deficiency also affects smooth muscle of the gastrointestinal tract and can result in paralytic ileus.

TREATMENT. The treatment of potassium depletion involves replacement therapy with potassium salts and attempts to correct the underlying disorder. It is useful to remember that a decrease in plasma potassium concentration of 1 mEq per liter with normal acid-base balance is roughly equivalent to 300 mEq of total body potassium deficiency.

Except in extreme circumstances, oral rather than parenteral potassium replacement is prudent. However, when gastrointestinal function is impaired, or when neuromuscular manifestations of hypokalemia are present, parenteral therapy with potassium may be advisable. Since potassium deficits involve both the ICF and the ECF, their correction requires the transfer of administered potas-

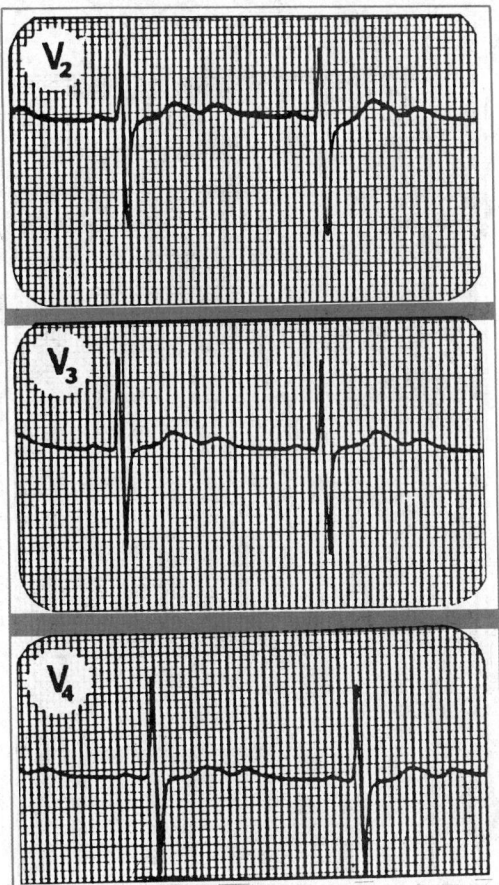

FIGURE 75-7. The electrocardiographic manifestations of hypokalemia. The serum potassium was 2.2 mEq per liter. Note that the ST segment is prolonged, primarily because of a U wave following the T wave, and that the T wave is flattened.

sium from the ECF into the ICF. The major problem in parenteral therapy is to avoid intravenous administration of potassium at rates sufficiently great to produce hyperkalemia. A prudent protocol to follow is to add potassium chloride to intravenous solutions at a final concentration of 40 to 60 mEq per liter and to administer no more than 10 to 20 mEq of potassium per hour. Except in unusual circumstances, the total amount of potassium administered daily should not exceed 200 mEq. The serum potassium level should be monitored at appropriate intervals; the frequency of monitoring should be determined by the patient's clinical condition, by the initial serum potassium, by the rate at which the serum potassium changes in a given patient, and by the patient's renal function. Because the electrocardiographic manifestations of hypokalemia are subtle, the electrocardiogram should not be used as a guide to replacement therapy.

Although potassium chloride is the salt of choice for intravenous potassium replacement, oral potassium chloride solutions are not well tolerated because of gastrointestinal irritation. Enteric-coated potassium chloride tablets are to be avoided, because they may produce small bowel ulcerations. Oral potassium is administered most conveniently in the form of organic salts such as gluconate or citrate. This form of therapy is, however, not effective in hypokalemic metabolic alkalosis with hypochloremia. In this circumstance, chloride supplementation is required together with potassium replacement and is most easily achieved by administering sodium chloride supplementation.

HYPERKALEMIA AND POTASSIUM EXCESS

DEFINITION. Chronic hyperkalemia (> 5.5 mEq per liter) can occur with little or no increase in total body potassium. However, acute increases in serum potassium concentrations, produced by potassium shifts from the ICF to the ECF, can occur even when total body potassium is normal or reduced.

ETIOLOGY AND PATHOGENESIS. Hyperkalemia develops whenever the rate of potassium intake or the rate of potassium ef-

flux from cellular to extracellular fluids exceeds the sum of renal plus extrarenal potassium losses. The renal mechanisms for potassium excretion adapt efficiently to increases in the rate of potassium influx to extracellular fluid, particularly from dietary sources. Hence acute or chronic hyperkalemia due to exogenous potassium intake is uncommon, unless renal mechanisms for potassium excretion are compromised. In the latter setting, injudicious potassium administration may result in hyperkalemia. This occurs most commonly when intravenous potassium chloride is administered too rapidly, when potassium salts of antibiotics such as pencillin are administered, when transfusions are given with blood that has been stored for long periods, or when salt substitutes containing potassium are used. The occurrence of hyperkalemia in these settings usually requires that renal potassium excretion be impaired.

Acute or chronic hyperkalemia occurs most commonly either because of diminished *renal excretion* or because there is a sudden *transcellular shift* of potassium from the ICF to the ECF. The major causes for hyperkalemia listed in Table 75-13 follow this format.

Diminished Renal Excretion. Hyperkalemia may occur in *acute oliguric renal failure* of any cause. In *chronic renal failure,* hyperkalemia generally does not occur until the GFR has reached markedly low levels, usually not until the GFR is < 15 ml per minute. Hyperkalemia may be precipitated in chronic renal failure, however, either by the development of acidosis or, as indicated above, by the injudicious administration of potassium salts. Hyperkalemia also occurs with little or modest reduction in the GFR, if there is impairment of potassium secretion by collecting duct segments. This occurs in *Addison's disease,* in *hyporeninemic hypoaldosteronism,* and with injudiously administering *potassium-sparing diuretics,* such as triamterene or spironolactone. Hyperkalemia also may be seen with angiotensin-converting enzyme (ACE) inhibitors and NSAID's.

Hyperkalemia also characterizes *voltage-dependent renal tubular acidosis.* The latter is a specific defect in sodium transport of distal nephron segments. This blockade of distal sodium absorption reduces luminal electronegativity and consequently impairs both proton secretion and potassium secretion. Thus voltage-dependent renal tubular acidosis, like hyporeninemic hypoaldosteronism, is characterized by sodium wasting and hyperkalemia. In hyporeninemic hypoaldosteronism, the urine is acidic, and plasma levels of aldosterone are reduced even during volume contraction, whereas in voltage-dependent renal tubular acidosis there is impaired urinary acidification but a normal plasma aldosterone response to volume contraction.

Finally, in each of the disorders characterized by diminished renal potassium excretion, hyperkalemia can be aggravated by ECF volume contraction, which reduces sodium delivery to collecting duct segments, or by acidosis, which promotes cellular potassium efflux.

Transcellular Shifts. The second class of disorders causing acute hyperkalemia includes situations when there is an abrupt shift of potassium from the ICF to the ECF. This shift occurs in acidosis or in circumstances that result in *cell destruction;* in the former, the serum potassium level rises by 0.6 mEq per liter with a metabolic decrease in plasma pH of 0.1 unit, while the latter occurs commonly with tissue trauma, burns, rhabdomyolysis, or hemolysis, as well as with lysis of large masses of tumor cells. As indicated pre-

TABLE 75-13. MAJOR CAUSES OF HYPERKALEMIA

I. Diminished Renal Excretion	II. Transcellular Shifts
Reduced GFR	Acidosis
Acute oliguric renal failure	Cell destruction
Chronic renal failure	Trauma, burns
Reduced tubular secretion	Rhabdomyolysis
Addison's disease	Hemolysis
Hyporeninemic hypoaldosteronism	Tumor lysis
	Hyperkalemic periodic paralysis
Potassium-sparing diuretics	Diabetic hyperglycemia
Voltage-dependent renal tubular acidosis	Insulin dependence plus aldosterone lack
	Depolarizing muscle paralysis
	Succinylcholine

GFR = glomerular filtration rate.

viously, hypokalemia predisposes to rhabdomyolysis. Thus the sudden occurrence of hyperkalemia in potassium-depleted patients is a diagnostic clue to the development of rhabdomyolysis.

Hyperkalemic periodic paralysis is an autosomal dominant disorder in which sudden increases in the serum potassium level result in muscle paralysis. The hyperkalemia is often provoked by excessive dietary potassium intake or by exercise. Myotonia occurs commonly in the disorder and appears either between attacks or immediately preceding attacks. The pathogenesis of the disorder is not understood. The acute paralytic attack can be treated by intravenous administration of calcium gluconate or glucose and insulin. Chronic treatment with diuretics such as acetazolamide minimizes the frequency of attacks.

Paradoxical hyperkalemia occurs when *sudden hyperglycemia* develops in insulin-dependent diabetics who also have interstitial renal disease and associated hyporeninemic hypoaldosteronism. The sudden increase in ECF osmolality draws water from cells, raises intracellular potassium concentrations, and therefore promotes passive potassium efflux from cells. The insulin lack minimizes cellular reentry of potassium, and the aldosterone deficiency blunts renal potassium excretion. Insulin therapy promptly corrects the hyperkalemia. Finally, anesthetic agents or other drugs that cause a *depolarizing muscle paralysis*, such as succinylcholine, promote potassium efflux from muscle cells. The loss of cell electronegativity in this situation increases passive potassium efflux from muscle cells.

Pseudohyperkalemia may occur in thrombocytosis or leukocytosis, because clotting of blood promotes potassium release from these cells and may be identified by noting that the *serum* potassium level is elevated while the *plasma* potassium level is normal. This kind of artifact occurs most commonly in patients with myeloproliferative disorders.

CLINICAL MANIFESTATIONS. The most important clinical manifestations of hyperkalemia relate to alterations in cardiac excitability. For this reason, the electrocardiogram is the single most important guide in appraising the threat posed by hyperkalemia and in determining how aggressive a therapeutic approach is necessary.

The electrocardiographic manifestations of hyperkalemia, shown in Figure 75–8, follow directly from the effects of hyperkalemia on cardiac action potentials. The earliest manifestation of hyperkalemia is the development of peaked T waves, which become evident when the serum potassium level exceeds 6.5 mEq per liter. This peaking of the T waves is a manifestation of the accelerated repolarization of the cardiac action potential produced by hyperkalemia. When the potassium concentration exceeds 7 to 8 mEq per liter, diminished cardiac excitability results in prolongation of the PR interval, followed by a loss of P waves and widening of the QRS complex. These changes indicate progressive inexcitability of cardiac muscle and are referable to hyperkalemia-induced inactivation of sodium permeability during the initial spike of the action potential. When the serum potassium level exceeds 8 to 10 mEq per liter, the electrocardiogram may develop a sine wave pattern and cardiac standstill can occur.

The correlation between serum potassium concentrations and electrocardiographic abnormalities is approximate at best; in a given patient, progression from peaked T waves to a sine wave pattern may occur rapidly, particularly if the serum potassium concentration rises rapidly. Therefore, the development of peaked T waves in conjunction with hyperkalemia should be viewed as a serious disorder; more advanced electrocardiographic manifestations of hyperkalemia should be treated as life-threatening medical emergencies.

TREATMENT. Three kinds of maneuvers are used to treat hyperkalemia: agents such as glucose plus insulin, sodium bicarbonate, or β agonists, which promote the transfer of potassium from the ECF to the ICF; maneuvers that enhance potassium elimination from the body, such as diuretics, exchange resins, or dialysis; and the use of calcium, which does not alter serum potassium concentrations but counteracts the effects of hyperkalemia on cardiac excitability.

Both insulin and sodium bicarbonate promote potassium entry into cells. Administering 25 grams of glucose, together with 10 units of regular insulin, is an effective way of reducing the serum potassium level rapidly. The glucose should be administered over 30 minutes as a 10% solution. Using a 50% glucose solution may actually worsen the hyperkalemia transiently if given rapidly. In-

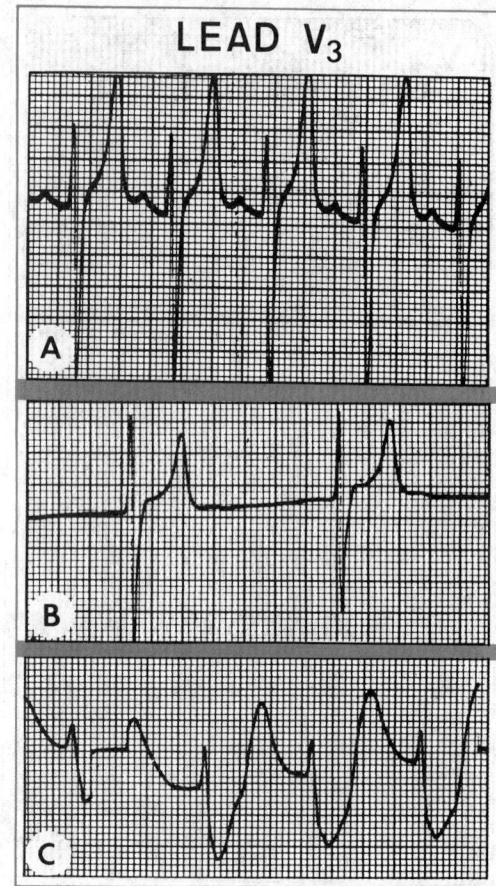

FIGURE 75–8. The effects of progressive hyperkalemia on the electrocardiogram. All of the illustrations are from lead V_3. *A,* Serum K^+ = 6.8 mEq per liter; note the peaked T waves together with normal sinus rhythm. *B, C,* Serum K^+ = 8.9 mEq per liter; note the peaked T waves and absent P waves. *C,* Serum K^+ = 8.9 mEq per liter; note the classic sine wave with absent P waves, marked prolongation of the QRS complex, and peaked T waves.

sulin promotes potassium entry into cells, and glucose is administered to prevent hypoglycemia. In insulin-dependent diabetic patients in whom sudden hyperglycemia has precipitated the hyperkalemia, insulin administration alone suffices to reduce the serum potassium concentration.

Administering 40 to 150 mEq of sodium bicarbonate intravenously over a 30- to 60-minute interval also promotes potassium entry into cells, particularly if acidosis is also present. This maneuver should be used with caution in patients with compromised renal function because of the risks of hypernatremia and of ECF volume overload.

Potassium shifts from extracellular to intracellular fluids also may be enhanced by using aerosolized specific β_2 agonists; albuterol is a commonly used agent of this kind. Agents such as albuterol are most helpful in managing mild hyperkalemia in chronic disorders such as chronic renal failure and hyperkalemic periodic paralysis.

In settings of extreme hyperkalemic cardiotoxicity, when P waves are absent and the QRS complexes are widened, calcium gluconate, 10 to 30 ml of a 10% solution given over a 10- to 20-minute interval, may be life-saving. This approach should be undertaken with constant electrocardiographic monitoring and should be used with extreme caution in patients who have received digitalis. In the latter circumstance, calcium administration may unmask digitalis intoxication, especially if other agents are used simultaneously to reduce the serum potassium level. Calcium salts should not be added to bottles of intravenous fluids containing bicarbonate, because water-insoluble calcium salts will form.

The influence of calcium salts in minimizing the cardiotoxic effects of hyperkalemia may be understood by noting that depolarization of excitable tissues by elevating serum K^+ concentrations inactivates sodium channels and that the extracellular sides of these sodium channels are electronegative. Divalent cations such as calcium provide a remarkably effective way of screening these electronegative sites. Thus calcium salts raise the voltage gradient across sodium channels by screening electronegative surface charges of these channels on their extracellular fluid sides and consequently restoring the voltage-dependent excitability of these channels.

None of the maneuvers described removes potassium from the body. Gastrointestinal potassium losses may be produced by the use of cation exchange resins in the sodium cycle, such as sodium polystyrene sulfonate (Kayexalate). Each gram of the resin contains approximately 1 mEq of sodium and exchanges for about 1 mEq of potassium. This stoichiometry is not precise, since the sodium form of the resin also exchanges for other cations in gastrointestinal secretions, including calcium. In chronic hyperkalemia, 20 grams of Kayexalate may be given three or four times a day in a 70% solution of sorbitol. The sorbitol creates an osmotic diarrhea and enhances resin passage through the gastrointestinal tract. In acute circumstances, Kayexalate may also be administered by enema, generally as 100 grams of resin suspended in 200 ml of 20% sorbitol. The use of chronic Kayexalate therapy in patients with chronic renal failure carries with it the risk of sodium overload.

Finally, acute hemodialysis or peritoneal dialysis provides another mechanism for potassium removal from the body. This approach is particularly advantageous in acute renal failure, when patients are volume expanded and sodium administration may produce congestive heart failure, or when there is a continued efflux of large amounts of potassium from the ICF to the ECF, as in burns or rhabdomyolysis.

Allon M, Dunlay R, Copkney C: Nebulized albuterol for acute hyperkalemia in patients on hemodialysis. Ann Intern Med 110:426, 1989. *A description of the use of β agonist nebulization in hyperkalemia.*

Clausen T, Everts ME: Regulation of the Na, K-pump in skeletal muscle. Kidney Int 35:1, 1989. *A description of the Na⁺-K⁺-ATPase in skeletal muscle and its regulation by insulin and β agonists.*

Kupin WL, Narins RG: The hyperkalemia of renal failure: Pathophysiology, diagnosis and therapy. Contrib Nephrol 102:1, 1993. *Pathophysiology and treatment of patients with hyperkalemia and renal failure.*

Kurtzman NA, Gonzalez J, DeFronzo R, et al.: A patient with hyperkalemia and metabolic acidosis. Am J Kidney Dis 15:333, 1990. *A concise account of the renal tubular disorders causing hyperkalemia.*

Whang R, Whang DD, Ryan MP: Refractory potassium repletion: A consequence of magnesium deficiency. Arch Intern Med 152:40, 1992. *Data review showing that refractory K⁺ repletion is often associated with total body Mg²⁺ deficiency.*

Wingo CS, Cain BD: The renal H-K-ATPase: Physiological significance and role in potassium homeostasis. Annu Rev Physiol 55:323, 1993. *Reviews the role of the collecting duct and renal H⁺, K⁺-ATPase on potassium homeostasis.*

75.4 Disturbances in Acid-Base Balance

PHYSIOLOGIC CONSIDERATIONS

Much of the confusion and apparent complexity in understanding disturbances in acid-base balance comes from failure to appreciate basic terminology in the field and is due to a lack of understanding of the simple principles of the Henderson-Hasselbalch equation.

"Acidemia" and "alkalemia" refer to blood hydrogen concentration and therefore to the pH of the blood. These terms do not refer to the mechanism by which a disturbance in pH is reached. "Acidosis" and "alkalosis," on the other hand, refer to the mechanism by which a given acid-base disturbance is reached. "Primary" refers to the initiating process of acid-base disturbance, while "secondary" refers to a compensatory process. Mixed acid-base disturbances are combinations of two or more primary acid-base disturbances. These terms are defined early in this chapter for the sake of clarity and are developed in more detail later.

The pH of arterial blood and interstitial fluid normally ranges between 7.38 and 7.42 despite wide variations in dietary intake of acids or alkali. The arterial pH range over which cardiac function, metabolic activity, and CNS function can be maintained is narrow; the widest range of pH values compatible with life is from 6.8 to 7.8, or an interval of 1 pH unit.

The major buffer system in ECF is the bicarbonate–carbonic acid pair. The relation between pH, bicarbonate, and carbonic acid con-

centrations in ECF may be expressed according to the familiar Henderson-Hasselbalch equation:

$$pH = pK + \log \frac{HCO_3^-}{H_2CO_3}$$

where pK is the carbonic acid dissociation constant, HCO_3^- is the plasma bicarbonate concentration, and H_2CO_3 is the plasma carbonic acid concentration. The H_2CO_3 concentration is given by αPa_{CO_2}, where α is the CO_2 solubility constant and has a value of 0.0301, and Pa_{CO_2} is the arterial carbon dioxide tension. Therefore, the Henderson-Hasselbalch equation becomes

$$pH = 6.1 + \log \frac{HCO_3^-}{0.03 \, P_{CO_2}}$$

Primary changes in the numerator (blood bicarbonate concentration) refer to primary metabolic changes, while primary changes in the denominator (blood carbon dioxide tension) refer to primary respiratory changes.

Proton shifts between the ECF and ICF stabilize the plasma pH against acute fluctuations. But the ultimate maintenance of pH balance requires that input of acid or base into the body be matched by output of acid or base so that the HCO_3^-/H_2CO_3 ratio and the total bicarbonate content in the ECF remain constant. The cardinal systems involved in these external processes are the kidneys, for bicarbonate balance, and the lungs, for CO_2 balance.

Carbon Dioxide Production and Elimination

VOLATILE ACID INPUT. The largest source of endogenous acid production is from combustion of glucose and fatty acids to carbon dioxide and water or, in other words, to a volatile acid. During aerobic glycolysis, that is, cellular respiration, glucose oxidation involves oxygen utilization and carbon dioxide production according to the following reaction:

$$C_6H_{12}O_6 + 6O_2 \longrightarrow 6CO_2 + 6H_2O$$

Since red blood cells contain carbonic anhydrase (c.a.), carbon dioxide hydration in erythrocytes yields the following:

$$CO_2 + H_2O \overset{c.a.}{\rightleftharpoons} H_2CO_3 \rightleftharpoons H^+ + HCO_3^-$$

The protons formed from carbonic acid dissociation are buffered by hemoglobin, whereas bicarbonate leaves red blood cells in exchange for chloride. In other words, the CO_2 generated is equivalent to the carbonic acid formed, and the bulk of hydrogen ion formed is buffered intracellularly.

A simple way of calculating the daily rate of nonvolatile acid production is to note, from the preceding reactions, that producing 1 mole of metabolic water and 1 mole of carbon dioxide represents, through dissociation of carbonic acid, the formation of 1 mole of hydrogen ions.

Since the molecular weight of water is 18, 1 liter of water contains about 55 moles of water. Consequently, the average rate of metabolic water production, about 400 ml daily, yields 22,000 mmol of water and an equal number of CO_2 molecules. Thus the rate of volatile acid production amounts to about 22,000 mEq of hydrogen ion daily. The cellular combustion of carbohydrates and fatty acids to CO_2 and water is remarkably efficient. Under normal circumstances, organic anions such as lactate and keto acids, which derive from incomplete combustion of carbohydrates and fatty acids, have plasma concentrations of approximately 5 mEq per liter.

VOLATILE ACID OUTPUT. Pulmonary ventilation excretes the CO_2 formed by cellular respiration. During blood transit through the lungs, bicarbonate reenters red blood cells and combines with protons to form carbonic acid, which dissociates to CO_2 and water. The CO_2 so formed diffuses freely through red blood cells and alveolar epithelium so that the rate of CO_2 excretion is governed primarily by the rate of minute ventilation.

MODULATION OF RESPIRATION. The prime factors normally regulating alterations in the rate of minute ventilation are subtle changes in cerebrospinal fluid (CSF) pH or arterial pH. Sensor chemoreceptors in central medullary centers or in the carotid body are activated by small reductions in CSF pH or arterial pH, respectively; the pH reduction can result either from CO_2 accumulation or from nonvolatile acid accumulation, which reduces the plasma bicarbonate concentration. In most circumstances, central medullary chemoreceptors provide the major impetus to altering ventilatory response, and the carotid body chemoreceptors serve as relatively minor stimuli to ventilation. The medullary respiratory centers therefore serve as the major *effector* mechanism for regulating CO_2 output by increasing ventilation rate.

The ventilatory response for CO_2 removal involves an increase in both tidal volume and respiratory rate. On average, for every 1 mEq per liter reduction in plasma bicarbonate produced by metabolic acidosis, increased minute ventilation will produce a 1.0 to 1.2 mm Hg fall in the Pa_{CO_2}. In most circumstances, the maximum reduction in Pa_{CO_2} produced by the hyperventilatory response to severe metabolic acidosis is to a Pa_{CO_2} in the 10 to 12 mm Hg range, but hyperventilation to Pa_{CO_2} values < 10 mm Hg in severe chronic metabolic acidosis is rare but may occur. Conversely, an increase in arterial pH reduces the rate of minute ventilation and therefore results in CO_2 retention. For increases in plasma bicarbonate concentrations to 35 mEq per liter, the Pa_{CO_2} usually remains <50 mm Hg. When profound metabolic alkalosis occurs, the Pa_{CO_2} may rise further but virtually never exceeds 65 mm Hg.

Renal Bicarbonate Processing

In addition to volatile acid production due to CO_2 formation, cellular metabolism also results in the formation of a number of nonvolatile acids. The major source for nonvolatile acid production is the metabolism of sulfur-containing amino acids, such as cysteine and methionine, which results in sulfuric acid formation. Consequently, the daily rate of nonvolatile acid production is closely related to dietary protein intake and to the rate of endogenous protein catabolism. Nonvolatile acids also derive from oxidation of phosphoproteins and phospholipids, which results in phosphoric acid formation; nucleoprotein degradation, which yields uric acid; and incomplete combustion of carbohydrates and fatty acids, which produces lactic acid and the keto acids.

The daily rate of nonvolatile acid production under normal conditions is about 1 mEq per kilogram of body weight. Thus daily nonvolatile acid production would consume the total body fluid buffering capacity in about 2 weeks, were it not for the fact that the kidneys excrete nonvolatile acids and, in so doing, regenerate bicarbonate. Since the minimal urinary pH ordinarily attainable is 5.0 and the amount of nonvolatile acid to be excreted is about 70 mEq per day, renal hydrogen ion excretion, which is equivalent to renal bicarbonate regeneration, occurs mainly as protons trapped in an undissociated form by urinary buffers.

The kidneys also filter large quantities of bicarbonate daily: For a normal plasma bicarbonate concentration of 24 mEq per liter and a glomerular filtration of 180 liters per day, the net amount of bicarbonate filtered daily is approximately 4300 mEq, or about four times the total body buffering capacity. Thus, in addition to generating new bicarbonate, the renal tubules must also absorb filtered bicarbonate.

BICARBONATE REABSORPTION. Virtually all filtered bicarbonate is absorbed, together with sodium, by the proximal tubule. Within renal tubular cells, CO_2 is hydrated to H_2CO_3. Apical membrane Na^+ exchange permits H^+ secretion into urine and Na^+ entry into cells, with subsequent absorption of sodium bicarbonate to blood.

The rate of proximal bicarbonate reabsorption is modulated by the same *effectors* that regulate proximal sodium absorption. Among these, the ECV exerts a central effect. Volume expansion, which resets glomerulotubular balance downward, reduces the fractional rate of proximal bicarbonate reabsorption. Conversely, volume contraction raises the bicarbonate threshold by increasing the fractional rate of proximal tubular sodium bicarbonate reabsorption.

Two other *effectors* regulate, in operational terms, the rate of bicarbonate reabsorption. One of these is the arterial Pa_{CO_2}: High Pa_{CO_2} values raise the apparent bicarbonate threshold, whereas low Pa_{CO_2} values reduce the rate of bicarbonate reabsorption. This factor accounts for the compensatory increase in plasma bicarbonate concentrations in respiratory acidosis. Second, hypokalemia also increases the rate of bicarbonate reabsorption, presumably by raising the intracellular hydrogen ion concentration. This factor accounts for the fact that in hypokalemic, hypochloremic metabolic alkalosis associated with volume contraction, alkalosis can persist after vol-

ume deficits are restored. In this circumstance, correcting potassium deficits is required to correct the alkalosis.

BICARBONATE REGENERATION. The excretion of nonvolatile acids and the simultaneous renal regeneration of bicarbonate occur principally in distal nephron segments. Distal renal tubular cells hydrate CO_2 to carbonic acid, which dissociates to protons, which are secreted into urine, and bicarbonate anions, which are absorbed into blood. The major mode of proton secretion in terminal nephron segments, particularly collecting tubules, involves an apical membrane proton–ATPase.

The secreted protons titrate urinary buffers, principally phosphate, while sodium is absorbed. Thus the overall reaction is as follows:

$$\underset{\text{(filtered)}}{Na_2HPO_4} + H^+ + HCO_3^- \longrightarrow \underset{\text{(excreted)}}{NaH_2PO_4} + \underset{\text{(absorbed)}}{NaHCO_3}$$

Titratable acid formation normally accounts for about one-third of renal acid excretion. The remaining two-thirds of acid excretion is accounted for by ammonia (NH_3) secretion by the following sequence:

$$\underset{\text{(filtered)}}{NaR} + NH_3 + H^+ + HCO_3^- \longrightarrow \underset{\text{(reabsorbed)}}{NaHCO_3} + \underset{\text{(excreted)}}{NH_4R}$$

where NaR is the filtered sodium salt of a nonvolatile acid, NH_3 is ammonia produced by renal tubular cells, and the protons and bicarbonate come from CO_2 hydration by tubular cells.

Distal acid excretion and bicarbonate absorption are accompanied by sodium absorption. Consequently, *effector* systems that enhance distal sodium absorption, such as aldosterone or increased rates of sodium delivery to terminal nephron segments, also promote terminal nephron hydrogen ion excretion. Three other *effector* mechanisms also increase the rate of hydrogen ion excretion: (1) Delivery of sodium to terminal nephron segments in association with impermeant anions such as sulfate favors proton movement from tubular cells to lumen. (2) Hypokalemia enhances hydrogen ion excretion, particularly in sodium-acquisitive states, presumably because hypokalemia is accompanied by a fall in intracellular pH. (3) Acidosis stimulates ammoniagenesis by renal tubular cells; consequently, in metabolic acidosis, increases in the rate of renal acid excretion are referable primarily to increased rates of ammonium excretion. In other words, these last-named three effector systems enhance renal acid excretion by creating a favorable situation for proton transfer from tubular cells to urine. Conversely, aldosterone deficiency, alkalosis, or reduced rates of salt delivery to terminal nephron segments reduce renal capacity for acid excretion.

pH Disequilibria Between Plasma and CSF

Central rather than arterial chemoreceptors are the prime sensors for pH-mediated changes in respiration. The ventilatory responses to pH changes mediated by respiratory processes or by metabolic processes therefore differ. The blood-brain barrier is freely permeable to CO_2. Consequently, pH changes produced exclusively by hyperventilation or hypoventilation occur almost simultaneously in arterial plasma and in the CSF, and the respiratory response to primary increases or decreases in Pa_{CO_2} occurs almost instantaneously. The blood-brain barrier imposes a lag, however, in the rate at which arterial bicarbonate equilibrates with the CSF. Thus, in metabolic acidosis, the arterial pH and bicarbonate concentration fall more rapidly than they do in the CSF, and in metabolic alkalosis, the CSF pH and bicarbonate concentration rise more slowly than they do in arterial plasma. Consequently, in the early stages of acute metabolic acidosis, there may be a 1- to 3-hour delay in the development of a maximal hyperventilatory response. Conversely, when metabolic acidosis is corrected rapidly, hyperventilation may persist for a few hours because of a delay in the rise of CSF pH.

An unusual situation relating to this effect occurs in diabetic ketoacidosis and in certain other metabolic acidoses associated with impaired CNS function. In these situations, carotid body chemoreceptors, rather than central medullary chemoreceptors, provide the major stimulus to respiration driven by a reduced arterial pH. The rapid correction of ECF acidosis by administering bicarbonate reduces the rate at which carotid body chemoreceptors drive ventilation. When this occurs, Pa_{CO_2} levels in plasma and in the CSF rise almost simultaneously, but because of a lag in the rate of bicarbonate entry into the CSF, the CSF bicarbonate/carbonic acid ratio tends to fall. In severe diabetic ketoacidosis, this situation can result in an actual fall in CSF pH simultaneously with a rise in arterial pH produced by intravenous bicarbonate administration.

DEFINITION OF ACID-BASE ABNORMALITIES

The arterial pH is determined by the ratio of the bicarbonate/carbonic acid buffer system, as expressed in the Henderson-Hasselbalch equation. These data also provide an index to total body acid-base balance, because, as indicated in the preceding section, the majority of body buffering occurs within cells. As stated earlier, acid-base disturbance can therefore occur either by altering the serum bicarbonate concentration, referred to as a "metabolic" disorder, or by altering arterial CO_2 tension, referred to as a "respiratory" disorder. A convenient way for considering these disturbances is illustrated in Figure 75–9, which illustrates pH isobars (for pH 7.0, 7.4, and 7.8) calculated according to the Henderson-Hasselbalch equation for the bicarbonate concentrations and Pa_{CO_2} values listed on the ordinate and abscissa, respectively.

TYPES OF ACID-BASE ABNORMALITIES. The left-hand panel in Figure 75–9 shows the directional changes in Pa_{CO_2} and bicarbonate concentrations that initiate the four primary types of acid-base abnormalities. *Respiratory acidosis* results from hypoventilation and reduces pH by raising the Pa_{CO_2}. *Respiratory alkalosis* results from hyperventilation and raises pH by reducing the Pa_{CO_2}. *Metabolic alkalosis* occurs when increases in the plasma bicarbonate concentration raise pH, and *metabolic acidosis* occurs when reductions in plasma bicarbonate decrease pH.

Any of these initial acid-base disturbances activates *compensatory responses,* illustrated in the right-hand panel of Figure 75–9, that tend to minimize the pH changes produced by the initial acid-base abnormality. By comparing the directional arrows in the left- and right-hand panels of Figure 75–9, it becomes evident that the initial disturbance in any of these four acid-base abnormalities tends to displace the arterial pH away from the pH 7.4 isobar and that the compensatory response partially restores arterial pH values toward the pH 7.4 isobar. The arterial pH, Pa_{CO_2}, and plasma bicarbonate concentrations illustrated in the right-hand panel of Figure 75–9 are the values usually observed clinically in the four primary acid-base disturbances.

TABLE 75–14. RELATIONSHIPS BETWEEN HCO_3^- AND P_{CO_2} IN SIMPLE ACID-BASE DISORDERS

Condition	Primary Disturbance	Predicted Response
Metabolic acidosis	$\downarrow HCO_3^-$	$\Delta P_{CO_2} (\downarrow) = 1\text{--}1.4\Delta HCO_3^-$*
Metabolic alkalosis	$\uparrow HCO_3^-$	$\Delta P_{CO_2} (\uparrow) = 0.4\text{--}0.9\Delta HCO_3^-$*
Respiratory acidosis	$\uparrow P_{CO_2}$	Acute: $\Delta HCO_3^- (\uparrow) = 0.1\Delta P_{CO_2}$ Chronic: $\Delta HCO_3^- (\uparrow) = 0.25\text{--}0.55\Delta P_{CO_2}$
Respiratory alkalosis	$\downarrow P_{CO_2}$	Acute: $\Delta HCO_3^- (\downarrow) = 0.2\text{--}0.25\Delta P_{CO_2}$ Chronic: $\Delta HCO_3^- (\downarrow) = 0.4\text{--}0.5\Delta P_{CO_2}$

* After at least 12 to 24 hours.
From Hamm L: Mixed acid-base disorders. *In* Kokko JP, Tannen RL (eds.): Fluids and Electrolytes. 2nd ed. Philadelphia, WB Saunders, 1990, p 487.

The Compensatory Responses. Renal and pulmonary mechanisms aggressively protect the body from changes in pH of arterial blood and interstitial fluid against primary acid-base disturbances that would threaten the optimal activity of various pH-dependent organ functions. These are known as "compensatory mechanisms" that blunt the effect of the initial insult or pH homeostasis (see Fig. 75–9). While the magnitude and rate of the compensatory responses vary among individual patients and do not provide complete compensation for the initiating abnormality, they nevertheless are relatively predictable. The predicted compensatory responses to the primary acid-base disturbances are listed in Table 75–14.

THE SERUM ANION GAP. Sodium is the principal cation in extracellular fluids. The sum of plasma chloride plus bicarbonate concentrations is less than the serum sodium concentration; the remaining anions required for electroneutrality, generally not reported

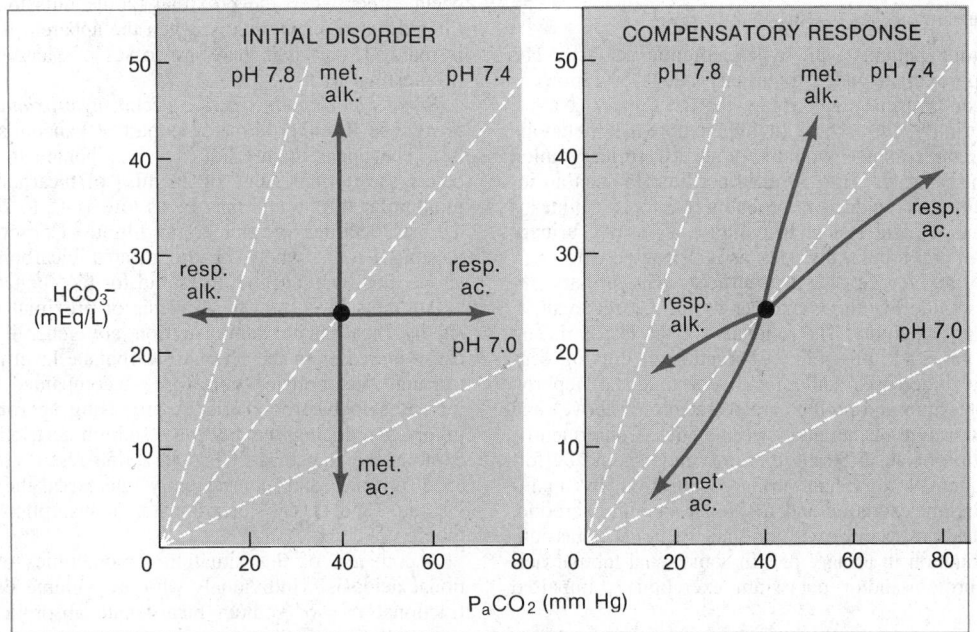

FIGURE 75–9. Schematic frame of reference for considering acid-base disturbances. The dotted lines are the pH isobars for pH values of 7.8, 7.4, and 7.0 computed from the Henderson-Hasselbalch equation for given combinations of arterial bicarbonate values (vertical axes) and arterial carbon dioxide tensions (horizontal axes). The graph on the left shows the initial derangement in HCO_3^- concentrations in metabolic acidosis and metabolic alkalosis and the initial Pa_{CO_2} derangement in respiratory acidosis and respiratory alkalosis. Note that each of the four changes in either HCO_3^- or Pa_{CO_2} tends to displace the arterial pH from the pH 7.4 isobar. The graph on the right, labeled compensatory response, indicates the general trend of pH, HCO_3^-, and Pa_{CO_2} changes actually observed in the four primary acid-base disturbances: respiratory acidosis, respiratory alkalosis, metabolic acidosis, and metabolic alkalosis. Respiratory acidosis and alkalosis are accompanied by compensatory renal bicarbonate retention and loss, respectively. Metabolic acidosis and alkalosis are accompanied by compensatory hyperventilation and hypoventilation, respectively. Note that the compensatory response in each of the four acid-base disorders tends to restore arterial pH values toward the pH 7.4 isobar.

with routine serum electrolyte measurements, are referred to as unmeasured anions, or as the serum anion gap. A convenient formula for calculating the serum anion gap is the following:

$$Serum\ anion\ gap = Na^+ - (Cl^- + HCO_3^-)$$

where Na^+, Cl^-, and HCO_3^- are the serum sodium, chloride, and bicarbonate concentrations, respectively. The anion serum gap includes primarily phosphates and sulfates derived from tissue metabolism, lactate and keto acids arising from incomplete combustion of carbohydrates and fatty acids, and negatively charged protein molecules, principally albumin. The normal value for unmeasured anions, or the serum anion gap, is 10 to 12 mEq per liter; albumin and other proteins normally account for about half the anion gap.

An *increased* serum anion gap generally indicates the presence of metabolic acidosis. The factors responsible for this kind of metabolic acidosis are discussed in the next section.

A *reduced* serum anion gap provides an index to certain other disorders. The anion gap will be reduced if the sodium concentration falls while the chloride plus bicarbonate concentrations are unchanged or, in other words, when the concentration of another cation in serum is increased while the serum osmolality remains normal. This may occur in multiple myeloma of the immunoglobulin G (IgG) variety if the myeloma proteins are cationic at pH 7.4. Hyperviscosity syndromes also may result in a reduced anion gap because of a laboratory artifact: When serum is excessively viscous, automatic pumps deliver decreased volumes of serum to a flame photometer, producing artifactual reductions in sodium concentrations. Rarely, lithium intoxication, hypermagnesemia, and hypercalcemia raise nonsodium cation concentrations sufficiently high to reduce the anion gap.

The serum anion gap also will be decreased if the serum sodium concentration remains normal while the serum chloride plus bicarbonate concentrations are increased. This situation occurs most commonly in hypoalbuminemia. A low serum anion gap also occurs in bromide intoxication, since colorimetric techniques for serum chloride determinations give spuriously high values for chloride plus bromide when bromide is present in relatively high concentrations in serum.

The Urinary Anion Gap. The urinary anion gap, defined as:

$$Urinary\ anion\ gap = (Na^+ + K^+) - Cl^-$$

is useful in evaluating patients with hyperchloremic acidosis. The test provides an approximate index to urinary NH_4^+ excretion, as measured by a negative urinary anion gap, that is, urinary ($Na^+ + K^+$) is less than urinary Cl^-. Thus, in hyperchloremic metabolic acidosis, a normal renal response would be a negative urinary anion gap, generally in the range of 30 to 50 mEq per liter. In such an instance, the hyperchloremic acidosis is probably due to gastrointestinal losses rather than a renal lesion. In contrast, a positive urinary anion gap implies a renal tubular disorder, as is discussed below.

Urinary Response to Oral Furosemide. The urinary response to oral furosemide loading is another useful test for evaluating tubular acidifying capability. The rationale for the test is that in normal individuals blockade of sodium absorption in diluting segments by furosemide increases sodium delivery to distal nephron segments where potassium and protons are secreted (see above) and increases the excretion rate of the latter two moieties. Consequently, the oral administration of 40 to 80 mg of furosemide should be followed, in a subsequent 4- to 6-hour urinary collection, by an increase in urinary sodium excretion and fractional sodium excretion, an increase in urinary potassium excretion and fractional potassium excretion, and a reduction in urinary pH. In some renal tubular acidosis syndromes, proton and/or potassium excretion is impaired (Table 75–15).

TABLE 75–16. MAJOR CAUSES OF METABOLIC ACIDOSIS

Normal Anion Gap	Increased Anion Gap

I. Renal Causes
  A. Bicarbonate Loss
    Proximal RTA, type II
    Dilutional acidosis
    Carbonic anhydrase inhibitors
    Primary hyperparathyroidism
  B. Failure of Bicarbonate
    Regeneration
    Distal RTA, type I
    Distal RTA, type IV
    Diuretics: amiloride, spiro-
    lactones, triamterene
II. Gastrointestinal Causes
  Diarrheal states
  Small bowel drainage
  Ureterosigmoidostomy
III. Acidifying Salts
  Ammonia chloride
  Lysine hydrochloride
  Arginine hydrochloride
  Parenteral hyperalimentation
	I. Endogenous Causes
	  A. Uremic acidosis
	  B. Lactic acidosis
	  C. Ketoacidosis
	  D. β-Hydroxybutyric
	    acidosis
	
	II. Exogenous Causes
	  A. Salicylates
	  B. Paraldehyde
	  C. Methanol
	  D. Ethylene glycol

METABOLIC ACIDOSIS

ETIOLOGY AND PATHOGENESIS. A convenient way to consider the metabolic acidoses is to divide them into two groups: normal anion gap and increased anion gap metabolic acidoses (Table 75–16). The pathogeneses of these two groups differ appreciably.

NORMAL ANION GAP METABOLIC ACIDOSIS. The metabolic acidoses having a *normal anion gap* result whenever there are abnormally high net bicarbonate losses. This situation may occur because the kidneys fail to reabsorb or regenerate bicarbonate, because there are extrarenal losses of bicarbonate, or because excessive amounts of substances yielding hydrochloric acid have been administered.

RENAL CAUSES. *Bicarbonate Losses.* Bicarbonate losses occur either when the proximal tubule fails to absorb virtually all filtered bicarbonate, that is, when the apparent bicarbonate threshold is reduced, or when there are losses of bicarbonate from the gastrointestinal tract.

Renal bicarbonate wasting occurs in *proximal renal tubular acidosis* type II, either alone or as part of Fanconi's syndrome (see Ch. 82). The apparent threshold for bicarbonate in this disorder is set below the normal value of 26 mEq of bicarbonate per deciliter of glomerular filtrate and may be as low as 15 to 20 mEq of bicarbonate per deciliter of glomerular filtrate. Consequently, bicarbonate wasting occurs whenever the plasma bicarbonate level is raised above the apparent renal threshold for bicarbonate.

Attempts to correct the acidosis of proximal renal tubular acidosis by bicarbonate administration are generally unrewarding, because increases in the plasma bicarbonate level produced by administering bicarbonate salts are accompanied by corresponding increases in bicarbonaturia. A promising approach to this disorder involves reducing the ECV by sodium restriction. This maneuver exploits the fact that ECF contraction resets glomerulotubular balance upward and consequently increases the fractional rate of sodium, and hence bicarbonate, reabsorption by the proximal tubule.

A converse of this situation is sometimes referred to as "dilutional acidosis." Individuals who are volume expanded reduce the fractional rate of sodium bicarbonate absorption by the proximal

TABLE 75–15. CHARACTERISTICS OF DISTAL TUBULAR ACIDOSIS (RTA) SYNDROMES

Condition	Urinary pH	Serum K+	Urinary Anion Gap	Response to Furosemide		Aldosterone Secretion
				Urinary pH	*Urinary K+*	
Gradient-limited RTA	>5.5	↓	Positive	Unchanged	↑	Normal
Hyporeninemic hypoaldosteronism	<5.5	↑	Positive	↓	↑	Reduced
Voltage-dependent RTA	>5.5	↑	Positive	Unchanged	Unchanged	Normal

tubule and consequently develop mild reductions in plasma bicarbonate concentrations. *Carbonic anhydrase inhibitors* such as acetazolamide inhibit proximal sodium bicarbonate absorption, resulting in metabolic acidosis. *Primary hyperparathyroidism* also reduces the apparent bicarbonate threshold in the proximal tubule; mild degrees of hyperchloremic acidosis are commonly noted in patients with this disorder.

Failure of Bicarbonate Regeneration. The second major group of disorders producing hyperchloremic acidosis includes those disorders in which the ability of the distal nephron to regenerate bicarbonate is impaired. Three different tubular disorders account for the majority of cases of renal hyperchloremia encountered clinically. *Classic gradient-limited renal tubular acidosis* type I is a tubular disorder in which proton secretion may be normal, but because the collecting duct is unable to maintain a steep urine to blood proton concentration gradient, secreted protons are recycled back to blood. Administering large quantities of phosphate salts permits the excretion of large amounts of titratable acid in this disorder, because the pH of the phosphate buffer system is 6.8, i.e., relatively high. Potassium wasting and hypokalemia are common in distal gradient-limited renal tubular acidosis owing at least in part to secondary hyperaldosteronism stimulated by sodium wasting.

In *hyporeninemic hypoaldosteronism* type IV renal tubular acidosis, which generally occurs in association with interstitial disease and diabetes mellitus, the distal tubular derangements include diminished rates of sodium absorption and diminished rates of proton and potassium secretion. Aldosterone secretion is impaired. Consequently, sodium wasting and hyperkalemic, hyperchloremic acidosis are the hallmarks of this disorder. Diuretics such as *triamterene, spironolactone,* and *amiloride,* which interfere with distal tubular sodium absorption, proton secretion, and potassium secretion, also result in hyperkalemic, hyperchloremic metabolic acidosis (see Table 75–5).

Finally, *voltage-dependent renal tubular acidosis,* also known as *hyperkalemic tubular acidosis,* is characterized by an impaired ability of the distal nephron to absorb sodium and by an inability to secrete either potassium or protons. The latter two secretory deficits appear to be secondary to the defect in sodium absorption, which diminishes the magnitude of the lumen-negative transepithelial voltage in those nephron segments. Aldosterone secretion is normal.

Table 75–15 provides a summary of the distinguishing features of the three renal tubular acidosis syndromes. It should be noted that when hyporeninemic hypoaldosteronism is associated with extensive interstitial disease, the ability to increase urinary potassium excretion or decrease urinary pH in response to furosemide may be blunted.

Gastrointestinal bicarbonate wasting can occur in several circumstances. First, since stool water is rich in bicarbonate, diarrheal states result in significant bicarbonate losses. Both pancreatic and small bowel secretions are rich in bicarbonate; pancreatic fluid, for example, has a pH of approximately 8.0. Hence *ileal drainage* also can result in significant bicarbonate losses. *Ureterosigmoidostomy* results in metabolic acidosis because the colon can secrete bicarbonate in exchange for chloride. Thus in these patients urine reaching the colon is alkalinized by bicarbonate exchange for chloride, thereby producing a net bicarbonate loss.

GASTROINTESTINAL CAUSES. Acidifying Salts. The third major group of conditions producing hyperchloremic acidosis includes those that result from administering *acidifying salts,* such as ammonium hydrochloride, lysine hydrochloride, or arginine hydrochloride. In each instance, metabolism of the ammonium or of the amino acids leads to hydrochloric acid formation. *Parenteral hyperalimentation* without administering adequate amounts of bicarbonate or bicarbonate-yielding solutes (such as lactate or acetate) also can produce hyperchloremic metabolic acidosis. The acidosis occurs because the synthetic amino acids used in hyperalimentation mixtures contain positively charged amino acids, such as arginine, lysine, and histidine, which yield proton equivalents when metabolized.

INCREASED ANION GAP METABOLIC ACIDOSIS. Metabolic acidoses characterized by an increased anion gap occur either because the kidneys fail to excrete inorganic acids, such as phosphate or sulfate, or because there is net accumulation of organic acids (Table 75–16).

Reduced Acid Excretion. Renal failure, either acute or chronic, results in metabolic acidosis with an increased anion gap

due to retention of sulfates and phosphates. In chronic renal failure, metabolic acidosis occurs because the net amount of ammonium excreted daily falls as functional renal mass diminishes. The plasma bicarbonate concentration in most patients with chronic renal failure ranges between 16 and 20 mEq per liter. Although this degree of acidosis appears relatively modest, the daily acid load is buffered by bone salts; this buffering may contribute to the osteopenia of chronic renal failure (see Ch. 216). In acute tubular necrosis, acidosis occurs because of generalized tubular dysfunction, including impaired net acid excretion. The plasma bicarbonate level generally remains above 16 mEq per liter unless sepsis, profound hypoxia, or extensive tissue necrosis complicates the disorder. In chronic renal failure, the anion gap generally does not exceed 22 to 24 mEq per liter. Thus, if the anion gap exceeds this value, then other superimposed causes of metabolic acidosis must be sought.

Organic Acid Accumulation. Accumulation of organic acids represents the second major cause for metabolic acidosis with an increased anion gap and is the most common cause for acute metabolic acidosis. Normally, the complete combustion of carbohydrates and fatty acids to CO_2 and water is highly efficient and results in the production of approximately 22,000 mEq of hydrogen ion per day. Thus the lungs eliminate, as expired CO_2, more than 300 times as much acid as the 70 mEq of fixed acid excreted daily by the kidneys as titratable acid plus ammonia. Processes that impair cellular respiration and therefore result in nonvolatile rather than volatile acid production lead to profound metabolic acidosis. In these circumstances, the interplay of four cardinal factors determines the magnitude of the anion gap acidosis.

The first two of these factors are insulin and glucagon and the interplay between these two hormones. In disorders such as diabetic ketoacidosis or starvation, insulin lack accelerates lipolysis while aerobic glycolysis is impaired. Concomitantly, glucagon increases augment ketogenesis by the liver.

The third variable is the rate of cellular respiration, which in practical terms is determined by the rate of tissue perfusion with oxygen and the functional state of mitochondria. Lactic acidosis due to hypoperfusion or phenformin thereby is an anion gap acidosis caused by impaired cellular respiration.

The last factor determining the magnitude of the anion gap for such conditions is the extent of renal perfusion, which in turn regulates the proximal renal tubular threshold for organic acid excretion. Thus, in diabetic ketoacidosis, volume expansion with normal saline can convert a large anion gap acidosis to a normal anion gap acidosis, not by correcting the underlying metabolic derangement, which requires insulin, but simply by increasing the rate of renal organic acid excretion.

The syndrome of *lactic acidosis* results from impaired cellular respiration. Lactic acid is produced in muscle, red blood cells, and other tissues as a consequence of anaerobic glycolysis. Lactic acid oxidation involves reduction of nicotine adenine dinucleotide (NAD) by lactic acid dehydrogenase (LDH) according to the following reaction:

$$\text{Lactate} + \text{NAD} \xrightleftharpoons{LDH} \text{pyruvate} + \text{NADH}$$

Cellular respiration involves mitochondrial oxidation of pyruvate and NADH to CO_2 and water. When lactic acidosis occurs because of impaired cellular respiration, the lactate/pyruvate ratio rises, as does the NADH/NAD ratio. Thus glycolysis in a setting of impaired cellular respiration results in increased production of nonvolatile lactic acid. Lactic acidosis should not be confused with states in which serum lactate levels are elevated with normal lactate/pyruvate and NADH/NAD ratios, as, for example, in vigorous exercise. Lactic acidosis is also characterized by negative serum nitroprusside (Acetest) reactions, since Acetest tablets react only with ketone bodies such as acetoacetic acid and acetone, but not with lactic acid or β-hydroxybutyric acid. β-Hydroxybutyric acid does not have a ketone group and therefore does not react in nitroprusside reactions. In lactic acidosis the β-hydroxybutyric acid/acetoacetic acid ratio is elevated in parallel with the increased NADH/NAD ratio.

Lactic acidosis occurs most commonly in disorders characterized by inadequate oxygen delivery to tissues, such as shock, septicemia, and profound hypoxemia. Drug-induced lactic acidosis may occur with phenformin therapy and isoniazid toxicity; in both circumstances, oxygen utilization by tissues is thought to be impaired. Lactic acidosis also occurs in association with leukemia and diabetes mellitus. There is also a spontaneous, idiopathic form of lactic acidosis in debilitated patients, which is almost uniformly fatal.

A second group of disorders characterized by an anion gap metabolic acidosis includes those disorders in which cellular respiration may not be impaired, but accelerated rates of organic acid production, particularly from lipolysis, result in an increased anion gap. *Alcoholic ketoacidosis* occurs in patients with chronic alcoholism and a recent history of binge drinking, little or no food intake, and recurrent vomiting. Hypoglycemia may be present. The major pathogenic mechanism for alcoholic ketoacidosis is accelerated lipolysis and hepatic ketoacid production because of relative decreases and increases in the secretion rates for insulin and glucagon, respectively (Fig. 75–10). The Acetest reaction is variably positive, and the β-hydroxybutyrate/acetoacetate ratio is elevated. Lactate utilization is diminished in this disorder. Patients with alcoholic ketoacidosis have β-hydroxybutyric acid, rather than lactic acid, as the principal nonvolatile acid. *Diabetic ketoacidosis* is the most common cause of metabolic acidosis with an increased anion gap and occurs because of increased rates of ketogenesis due to insulin lack and inadequate carbohydrate combustion. *Starvation* produces metabolic acidosis by essentially the same mechanism: increased hepatic ketogenesis with reduced caloric intake. Thus in a general sense, alcoholic ketoacidosis, diabetic ketoacidosis, and starvation share at least one common feature: accelerated lipolysis and ketogenesis due to a relative insulin lack coupled with a relative glucagon excess.

Finally, a number of ingested substances result in severe metabolic acidosis with a large anion gap. *Salicylism* produces a complex set of acid-base abnormalities. Salicylates stimulate ventilation through central mechanisms; the decrease in Pa_{CO_2} then results in reductions in plasma bicarbonate concentrations. Since salicylate is a relatively strong acid, the ingestion of large quantities of salicylate can, by itself, contribute to metabolic acidosis and an increased anion gap. Salicylates also interfere with mitochondrial function. As a consequence, a number of as yet unidentified organic acids accumulate in serum and are the major factors responsible for the anion gap acidosis of salicylism.

A number of other agents, including *paraldehyde, methanol,* and *ethylene glycol,* also produce severe metabolic acidosis with organic acid accumulation. In methanol poisoning, formic acid (an endproduct of methanol metabolism) accounts in large part for the reduction in serum bicarbonate concentration. In ethylene glycol intoxication, glycolic and lactic acid accumulation accounts for the majority of the reduction in plasma bicarbonate level; however, oxalate deposition in tissues is clearly a major factor in ethylene glycol toxicity. The organic acids responsible for an increased anion gap in paraldehyde intoxication have not been identified.

DIAGNOSIS AND TREATMENT. The diagnosis of metabolic acidosis requires analyzing serum electrolytes and measuring arterial pH and Pa_{CO_2}. A cardinal clinical manifestation of metabolic acidosis is hyperventilation, which, when severe, is manifest as Kussmaul's respiration. In patients with chronic metabolic acidosis, however, hyperventilation may be difficult to detect clinically.

Severe metabolic acidosis exerts a negative inotropic effect on the heart, which depends, at least in part, on the fact that acidosis diminishes tissue responsiveness to catecholamines. Thus, in lactic acidosis, negative inotropy sets the stage for a potentially lethal chain of events: poor tissue perfusion $\rightarrow$ lactic acidosis $\rightarrow$ decreased cardiac function $\rightarrow$ further reduction in tissue perfusion.

Acidosis also affects the delivery of oxygen to tissues. In acidosis, the Bohr effect shifts the oxyhemoglobin dissociation curve to the right. This compensatory mechanism permits oxygen delivery to inadequately perfused tissues. However, the protective characteristics of the Bohr effect may be offset by the effect of pH variation on red blood cell 2,3-diphosphoglycerate (2,3-DPG). Increases in red cell 2,3-DPG also shift the oxyhemoglobin dissociation curve to the right. However, acidosis tends to reduce red blood cell 2,3-DPG; this may offset partially the compensatory Bohr effect and therefore aggravate inadequate tissue oxygenation in acidosis.

Since metabolic acidosis is a manifestation of a variety of different diseases, the treatment of metabolic acidosis varies, depending on the underlying process and on the acuteness and severity of the acidosis. Certain general principles serve as useful guidelines for therapy. Those disorders characterized by *failure of bicarbonate regeneration* or *reduced excretion of inorganic acids* represent acidoses in which the kidneys fail to excrete a normal load of nonvolatile acid or, in other words, fail to regenerate approximately 70 mEq of bicarbonate daily. Thus the treatment of these metabolic acidoses requires administering relatively modest amounts of bicarbonate. In chronic renal failure, alkali therapy is generally not required unless the plasma bicarbonate level falls below 16 to 18 mEq per liter. If the acidosis is more severe, bicarbonate supplementation in the form of Shohl's solution (see below) may be instituted. Caution should be exercised to avoid sodium overload or the appearance of tetany, if overalkalinization occurs.

In distal, gradient-limited renal tubular acidosis, administering 30 to 60 mEq of bicarbonate daily, either as sodium bicarbonate tablets or as Shohl's solution, usually corrects the acidosis. A 650-mg sodium bicarbonate tablet provides 7.7 mEq of bicarbonate. Shohl's solution is a mixture of sodium citrate and citric acid; 1 ml of Shohl's solution yields the equivalent of 1 mmol of sodium bicarbonate. The cost of sodium bicarbonate, either as tablets or as common baking soda, is considerably less than that of Shohl's solution.

Potassium supplementation is also required in the disorder. In children with distal renal tubular acidosis, greater quantities of bicarbonate, in the range of 5 to 14 mEq of alkali per kilogram per day, are usually required to avoid growth retardation.

The therapy of patients with metabolic acidosis due to *external bicarbonate loss* varies with the nature of the disorder. In acute metabolic acidosis due to gastrointestinal losses, the net bicarbonate deficit may be roughly calculated from the reduction in "bicarbonate space," or total body buffering capacity, as follows:

$$(24 \text{ mEq/L} - \text{measured plasma HCO}_3^-) \times 0.6 \text{ body weight (kg)}$$

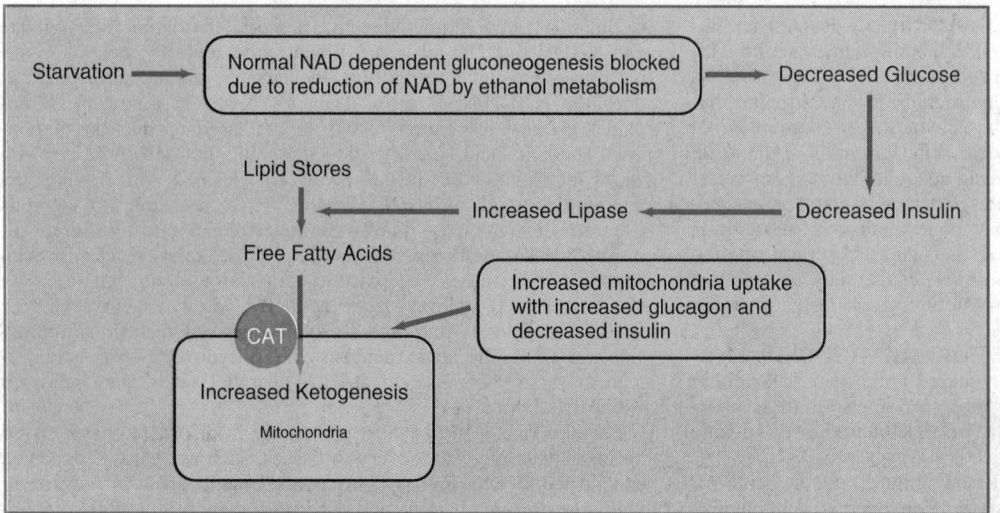

FIGURE 75–10. Pathophysiology of alcoholic ketoacidosis. Hypoglycemia develops due to decreased nicotine adenine dinucleotide (NAD)–dependent gluconeogenesis. This results in hypoglycemia and a compensatory decrease in insulin and an increase in glucagon concentrations. Decreased insulin activates free fatty acid formation by increasing lipolysis from adipose tissue. Free fatty acids in turn are transported into mitochondria for ketogenesis by carnitine acyltransferase (CAT), which is activated in part by increased glucagon content. Alcohol also may increase ketogenesis directly by being metabolized to acetate and thus providing substrate for ketogenesis.

Bicarbonate therapy should be instituted when the arterial pH falls below 7.1. It is prudent to administer sufficient sodium bicarbonate intravenously to raise the plasma bicarbonate concentration to 16 mEq per liter over a 12- to 24-hour interval, rather than to repair the entire bicarbonate deficit. Calculating the bicarbonate deficit in this manner is valid only if there are no further bicarbonate losses. If the latter persist, as in cholera or other types of secretory diarrhea, the daily amount of bicarbonate given to maintain the plasma bicarbonate concentration in the range of 16 mEq per liter may actually exceed the calculated bicarbonate space.

The treatment of acidoses due to *accumulation of organic acids* varies with the disorder. In *lactic acidosis,* therapy should be directed toward improving tissue perfusion. Because the disorder results from a failure of lactic acid and other organic acids to convert to CO_2 and water, large amounts of sodium bicarbonate, sometimes in excess of 1000 mEq per 24-hour period, have been used in attempts to avoid lethal acidosis.

The treatment is complicated by the fact that the response to alkali therapy is not predictable. In experimental lactic acidosis, dichloroacetate can raise arterial pH by suppressing endogenous lactic acid production, but bicarbonate therapy worsens the disorder by increasing the rate of splanchnic bed lactate production. Moreover, large amounts of sodium bicarbonate (in the form of ampules containing 44.5 mmol of sodium bicarbonate per 50 ml) can produce cellular shrinkage due to hypertonicity and circulatory overload due to ECF volume expansion. Finally, in controlled clinical trials in patients with lactic acidosis, sodium bicarbonate therapy has failed to improve circulatory dynamics when compared to equimolar sodium chloride therapy.

The treatment of *alcoholic ketoacidosis* generally requires only administering saline solutions and glucose. Since blood insulin values are generally decreased in alcoholic ketoacidosis–associated hypoglycemia, insulin is contraindicated in this condition because it may induce life-threatening hypoglycemia. Alkali therapy should not be used unless the metabolic acidosis is in the lethal range. The same considerations apply to starvation ketosis. The insulin release provoked by administering glucose suppresses lipolysis and consequently the overproduction of keto acids.

In *diabetic ketoacidosis,* insulin therapy promotes glucose utilization and, consequently, complete oxidation of ketoacids; simultaneously, ketogenesis is reduced. Therefore, alkali therapy is ordinarily not required in the disorder. Furthermore, because the hyperventilatory response to acidosis in some diabetic patients is governed by arterial rather than central medullary chemoreceptors, intravenous sodium bicarbonate administration may result in arterial alkalinization, a reduction in the rate of minute ventilation, and a fall in CSF pH.

However, there is no consensus that a transient fall in CSF pH may change mental status or otherwise be detrimental. Also, it has been postulated that bicarbonate therapy may adversely effect the oxygen-releasing capacity of hemoglobin. Furthermore, some authors have noted that late metabolic alkalosis may develop with vigorous use of bicarbonate, once the ketone bodies are metabolized to bicarbonate. Thus, while good reasons exist to administer bicarbonate with severe depression of arterial pH, there also are reasons to not administer bicarbonate. It seems prudent to give parenteral bicarbonate to all diabetics in ketoacidosis with an arterial pH of ≤6.95, to not give bicarbonate if arterial pH is ≥7.15, and to use clinical judgment, largely based on the cardiovascular status of the patient, in those with an intermediate arterial pH.

Finally, because *salicylates, methanol,* and *ethylene glycol* are by themselves tissue toxins, appropriate therapy for these disorders includes not only alkalinization but also hemodialysis for removing the offending agent. When the blood levels are at potentially lethal range, hemodialysis should be used to treat patients with salicylate levels of > 100 mg per deciliter, and hemodialysis may be beneficial in the early course of all patients with ethylene glycol or on methanol poisoning. However, hemodialysis should be performed all those with ethylene glycol or methenol poisoning if the serum HCO_3^- concentration falls below 15 mEq per liter, because mortality rates rise to unacceptable levels without hemodialysis. Also, ethanol should be infused first as in initial bolus of 0.6 grams per kilogram body weight and then as a sustaining solution to maintain blood alcohol levels at approximately 100 mg per deciliter, since ethanol competes effectively for alcohol dehydrogenase against metabolism of ethylene glycol and methanol to their toxic products.

METABOLIC ALKALOSIS

ETIOLOGY AND PATHOGENESIS. Maintaining the plasma bicarbonate concentration depends on renal bicarbonate reabsorption and renal bicarbonate regeneration (i.e., net acid excretion). Consequently, although metabolic alkalosis may be *initiated* by hydrogen ions lost from the body—for example, during gastric drainage—the *maintenance* of a sustained metabolic alkalosis requires that the net rate of renal bicarbonate reabsorption or renal bicarbonate generation, or both, be greater than normal. In other words, a steady-state elevation of plasma bicarbonate concentrations to levels greater than 24 mEq per liter requires increased activity of one or more of the effector mechanisms regulating bicarbonate handling by renal tubules. In normal individuals it is therefore difficult to produce metabolic alkalosis by simple alkali loading.

Table 75–17 lists the major clinical causes of increased serum bicarbonate concentrations. The table includes three disorders in which the apparent threshold for proximal bicarbonate reabsorption is increased, namely, volume contraction, potassium depletion, and increased Pa_{CO_2}, and disorders that increase net bicarbonate regeneration, including increased rates of distal salt delivery and mineralocorticoid excess, either primary or as a consequence of volume contraction. It should be noted that all factors that increase serum bicarbonate concentrations in Table 75–17 are associated with metabolic alkalosis except increased Pa_{CO_2}, in which the rise in serum bicarbonate concentration is a compensatory mechanism for increased Pa_{CO_2}. The latter is included in Table 75–17 for the sake of completeness, even though the arterial pH is acidemic with rises in Pa_{CO_2}.

Volume contraction can sustain metabolic alkalosis because of an increase in the apparent rate of bicarbonate reabsorption by the proximal tubule. The most common cause for initiating this kind of alkalosis is hydrochloric acid loss because of vomiting or gastric suction. In the early stages of gastric fluid losses, there is a modest sodium bicarbonate diuresis, but urinary sodium chloride excretion is reduced. As volume contraction becomes increasingly severe, sodium conservation occurs and potassium bicarbonate is excreted in an attempt to maintain pH homeostasis. Finally, when potassium depletion becomes severe, urinary sodium plus potassium excretion is sharply reduced and paradoxical aciduria occurs: The urine is acidic while the plasma bicarbonate level and pH are both elevated. "Contraction alkalosis" is a frequently misunderstood term; the designation should be reserved for those patients in whom metabolic alkalosis has developed and volume contraction maintains the alkalosis by increasing the apparent proximal tubular threshold for bicarbonate reabsorption. Thus contraction alkalosis is a mirror image of dilutional acidosis.

Potassium depletion from any cause, when sufficiently severe, can sustain metabolic alkalosis initiated by acid loss, for example, during gastric drainage. Presumably, potassium loss from cells is accompanied by increased hydrogen ion concentrations within cells, including renal tubular cells. Thus potassium depletion, when sufficiently severe, can raise the rate of renal tubular bicarbonate reabsorption and hence maintain a metabolic alkalosis. Consequently, when serum potassium concentrations are reduced to about 2 mEq per liter, metabolic alkalosis due to gastric fluid loss becomes saline resistant but responsive to potassium chloride administration.

Acute increases in Pa_{CO_2} initiate renal compensatory mechanisms almost immediately, whereby the kidney increases acid excretion and thereby increases bicarbonate regeneration. The cumulative effect of these renal responses is increased net bicarbonate addition to the circulation. While the compensatory changes begin immediately, they are not complete for several days.

TABLE 75–17. MAJOR CAUSES FOR INCREASED PLASMA BICARBONATE CONCENTRATION

ECF volume contraction
Potassium depletion
Hypercapnia
Increased distal salt delivery
Mineralocorticoid excess

Situations in which there occurs *enhanced delivery of sodium chloride* to terminal nephron segments enhance renal acid excretion and therefore lead to metabolic alkalosis by increasing the rate of renal bicarbonate generated. This effect occurs with loop diuretics (see Table 75–5), such as furosemide, ethacrynic acid, or bumetanide, and with the proximal tubular diuretic metolazone. These diuretics also contribute to the maintenance of metabolic alkalosis by contracting ECF volume and by promoting potassium depletion. Salt wasting is common in *Bartter's syndrome;* metabolic alkalosis due to renal bicarbonate generation is therefore a common feature of the disorder. Administering large amounts of *impermeant anions* such as carbenicillin also favors distal hydrogen ion secretion. Thus carbenicillin therapy is one of the few circumstances in which an increased anion gap and metabolic alkalosis can be produced simultaneously by the same agent.

Mineralocorticoid excess, either primary or secondary, also can result in metabolic alkalosis because of renal bicarbonate generation. The disorder can occur in volume-expanded patients, as, for example, in primary hyperaldosteronism, in which the alkalosis is unresponsive to sodium chloride loading, and in patients with a reduced ECV and secondary hyperaldosteronism. The alkalosis of mineralocorticoid excess occurs primarily because of increased generation of bicarbonate by collecting duct segments (or, in other words, by increased renal acid excretion) and is clearly accentuated by potassium depletion. *Liddle's syndrome* is a disorder that is due to collecting duct sodium channels being more conductiveThis syndrome is characterized by metabolic alkalosis, hypokalemia, and hypertension that occurs because of an increase in sodium avidity by collecting duct segments, which can be blocked by triamterene therapy. This disorder metabolically simulates a mineralocorticoid excess state but one in which aldosterone measurements are normal.

In normal circumstances it is nearly impossible to produce metabolic alkalosis by increasing dietary alkali intake. In certain situations, however, *bicarbonate loading* can produce either a transient or a steady-state alkalosis. One such circumstance is *posthypercapnic alkalosis.* Patients with chronic hypercapnia develop compensatory increases in plasma bicarbonate concentrations: On an average, chronic hypoventilation results in a 0.3 to 0.5 mEq per liter rise in serum bicarbonate level for each 1.0 mm Hg increase in excess of a Pa_{CO_2} of 40 mm Hg. If ventilatory status is improved acutely, the Pa_{CO_2} will fall quickly but the plasma bicarbonate level will remain elevated, particularly if the patient is salt acquisitive because of congestive heart failure or ECF volume contraction. A common way to accentuate posthypercapnic alkalosis is to maintain patients on ventilators having high positive end-expiratory pressures (PEEP), which causes a central tourniquet effect that reduces cardiac output.

Delayed conversion of *accumulated organic acids* is a second mechanism for producing transient metabolic alkalosis. This may occur after insulin therapy for diabetic ketoacidosis, during the recovery phase of lactic acidosis, and following high-efficiency hemodialysis. In the last-named circumstance, acetate in the dialysis bath is taken up rapidly during dialysis. The accumulated acetate, which represents "potential bicarbonate," is then converted to bicarbonate after dialysis has been completed. Prolonged metabolic alkalosis because of alkali loading is a common feature of the *milk-alkali syndrome.* The alkalosis occurs because of prolonged ingestion of absorbable alkali in patients with impaired renal function due to hypercalcemic nephropathy. Frequent vomiting and attendant ECF volume contraction may also contribute to alkalosis in this disorder.

CLINICAL FEATURES AND DIAGNOSIS. There are no specific signs or symptoms of metabolic alkalosis. Relatively severe metabolic alkalosis can result in cardiac arrhythmias. Severe metabolic alkalosis also can result in severe hypoventilation, especially in patients with reduced renal function. Tetany and increased neuromuscular irritability, which are quite common in acute respiratory alkalosis, are very rare in chronic metabolic alkalosis. Rather, since hypokalemia generally accompanies metabolic alkalosis, muscular weakness and hyporeflexia are often seen in chronic metabolic alkalosis.

The diagnosis is inferred in most cases by routine measurements of serum electrolytes and can be confirmed by arterial blood gas analysis. Hypokalemia is generally present.

The urinary chloride concentration is a useful index for distinguishing metabolic alkalosis due to volume contraction from that due to primary mineralocorticoid excess. In volume-contracted states, the urinary chloride concentration is generally < 10 mEq per liter. Volume-contracted patients with Bartter's syndrome or volume-contracted patients taking diuretics generally have elevated urinary chloride concentrations. The combination of postural hypotension, hypokalemic metabolic alkalosis, and a urinary chloride concentration >20 mEq per liter is therefore suggestive of diuretic abuse or Bartter's syndrome.

TREATMENT. Some authorities have classified metabolic alkalosis patients by response to treatment. Two broad classifications are chloride-responsive patients, who have urinary chlorides < 10 mEq per liter, and chloride-resistant patients, with urinary chlorides > 20 mEq per liter.

Examples of chloride-responsive patients include those with gastric fluid loss, after diuretic therapy, and after hypercapnea. Treatment in these patients should focus on intravenously administering 0.9% NaCl at rates sufficient to correct tachycardia and hypotension. Many are also potassium deficient, so simultaneous repletion with potassium salts is indicated. If the metabolic alkalosis is sufficiently severe that significant hypoventilation is present (Pa_{CO_2} > 60 mm Hg), it may be necessary to administer dilute hydrochloric acid or other acidifying salts, such as lysine hydrochloride or arginine hydrochloride. The use of these amino acid salts carries with it the risk of hyperkalemia that is in excess of that expected simply from the change in arterial pH, presumably because these agents promote potassium efflux from cells. Ammonium chloride, lysine hydrochloride, or arginine hydrochloride should not be used in patients with significant liver disease.

Chloride-resistant alkaloses are characterized by urinary chlorides > 20 mEq per liter and normal or expanded ECF volume. Patients with excessive mineralocorticoid states are common examples, although other causes include Bartter's syndrome, Liddle's syndrome, hypercalcemia, and selective dietary potassium depletion. Metabolic alkalosis in these circumstances is best handled by treating the underlying disease process.

MIXED METABOLIC DISORDERS

Mixed metabolic derangements occur commonly. Consequently, the evaluation of metabolic acid-base abnormalities depends on history and physical examination with a simultaneous assessment of the anion gap, serum electrolytes, and, when appropriate, arterial blood gases. Electroneutrality requires that the sum of the principal anions in serum ($Cl^- + HCO_3^- +$ anion gap) equals the serum sodium level. Thus unless the serum sodium level changes, a change in the serum concentration of one or more of these principal anions necessitates a reciprocal change in the remaining anions.

Table 75–18 indicates the pattern of serum anion concentrations in single and mixed acid-base disorders. In the single acid-base disturbances, the change in the concentration of one anion is usually balanced by a reciprocal change in one other anion. For example, in hyperchloremic acidosis, the increase in chloride concentration equals the decrease in bicarbonate concentration.

TABLE 75–18. ANION PATTERNS IN METABOLIC ACID-BASE DISORDERS

Condition	Serum Anion Concentrations		
	HCO_3^-	Cl^-	Anion Gap
Simple Disorders			
Hyperchloremic acidosis	↓	↑	nl
Anion gap acidosis	↓	nl	↑
Metabolic alkalosis	↑	↓	nl
Mixed Disorders			
Metabolic alkalosis + anion gap acidosis	nl, ↑, or ↓	↓	↑
Anion gap acidosis + hyperchloremic acidosis	↓	↑	↑
Metabolic alkalosis + hyperchloremic acidosis	nl	nl	nl

nl = normal.

In mixed disorders, the anion patterns are more complex. In a mixed metabolic alkalosis combined with an anion gap acidosis (e.g., diabetic ketoacidosis complicated by vomiting), the identifying pattern is an increased anion gap offset partially or entirely by a reduction in chloride; the serum bicarbonate level is variable. In an anion gap plus hyperchloremic acidosis, the reduction in bicarbonate is offset by increases in both chloride and the anion gap. Finally, in metabolic acidosis combined with hyperchloremic acidosis (e.g., vomiting combined with interstitial nephritis), offsetting changes in serum bicarbonate and chloride concentrations may result in normal anion concentrations.

RESPIRATORY ACIDOSIS

ETIOLOGY AND PATHOGENESIS. Respiratory acidosis occurs whenever the rate of alveolar ventilation is impaired. CO_2 elimination involves the following sequence: transfer of CO_2 from tissues to the lungs in the form of venous bicarbonate, formation of CO_2 within red blood cells, perfusion of the lungs with systemic venous blood, diffusion of CO_2 from pulmonary capillaries to alveoli, and alveolar ventilation. Under normal circumstances, the rate of CO_2 hydration within red blood cells and the rate of CO_2 diffusion from pulmonary capillaries into alveoli are sufficiently rapid that CO_2 accumulation is virtually synonymous with hypoventilation.

Acute respiratory acidosis may result from a number of different causes in which the common denominator is failure of pulmonary excretion of CO_2. In the broadest terms, these causes may be classified into three general categories: primary failure in the CNS drive to ventilation (e.g., anesthesia, sleep apnea, or sedative overdose), primary failure in transport of CO_2 from alveolar space (e.g., obstructive defects, restrictive defects or neuromuscular defects as in myasthenic crises, severe hypokalemia, Guilain-Barré syndrome), and primary failure in the transport of CO_2 from tissues to alveoli (e.g., severe heart failure).

Chronic respiratory failure may occur essentially from the same causes except that the duration of CO_2 retention is longer and thus the renal compensation in plasma bicarbonate concentrations may be to higher levels. While individual differences exist, Table 75–14 provides the general predicted responses to both acute and chronic changes in Pa_{CO_2}.

These concepts are also useful in evaluating the possibility of mixed acid-base disorders occurring in association with respiratory acidosis. For example, since the rate of compensatory bicarbonate retention is delayed in acute respiratory acidosis, the presence of an elevated plasma bicarbonate concentration in a setting of acute CO_2 retention should be an index to the simultaneous occurrence of acute respiratory acidosis and metabolic alkalosis. Similarly, because renal bicarbonate reabsorption is an effective compensatory mechanism for chronic CO_2 retention, plasma bicarbonate concentrations below 28 to 30 mEq per liter in patients having chronic Pa_{CO_2} values >50 mm Hg should alert one to the possible coexistence of acute metabolic acidosis and chronic respiratory acidosis.

Since hypercapnia is synonymous with alveolar hypoventilation, patients with CO_2 retention are invariably hypoxemic. A compensatory polycythemia occurs commonly in chronic hypercapnic states.

CLINICAL MANIFESTATIONS. The clinical manifestations of respiratory acidosis vary, depending on the severity of the disorder and on the rate at which CO_2 retention has occurred. Acute increases in Pa_{CO_2} values result in somnolence, in confusion, and ultimately in *CO_2 narcosis.* Asterixis may also be present. Because CO_2 is a cerebral vasodilator, the blood vessels in the optic fundi are often dilated, engorged, and tortuous; in severe hypercapnic states, frank papilledema may occur.

TREATMENT. The only practical treatment for acute respiratory acidosis involves treating the underlying disorder and ventilatory support. The possibility of drug abuse should always be considered in otherwise healthy patients who suddenly develop acute respiratory depression; consequently, naloxone (Narcan) therapy should be considered in all comatose patients seen in the emergency room in whom no apparent cause for respiratory depression can be identified.

In patients with chronic hypercapnia who develop sudden increases in Pa_{CO_2} values, attention should be directed toward identifying factors such as pneumonia which may have aggravated the underlying disorder. It should be emphasized again that oxygen therapy in patients with chronic hypercapnia should be instituted with extreme caution and in the lowest possible concentration to avoid serious tissue hypoxia, since hypoxemia may be the primary stimulus to respiration in this setting. Consequently, in such patients, sudden increases in the arterial Pa_{CO_2} produced by oxygen administration may result in cessation of respiration. Under such severe circumstances, mechanically assisted ventilation should be considered. Care must be exercised to prevent posthypercapnic alkalosis. Administering alkalinizing salts has no place in the management of chronic respiratory acidosis.

RESPIRATORY ALKALOSIS

ETIOLOGY AND PATHOGENESIS. Respiratory alkalosis occurs when hyperventilation reduces the arterial Pa_{CO_2} and consequently increases arterial pH. There are divergent causes. Acute respiratory alkalosis generally is a consequence of increased stimulation of the CNS or secondary to tissue hypoxia. Increased CNS stimulation may be voluntary, as in anxiety hyperventilation syndrome, or involuntary, as occurs secondary to neurologic disorders (e.g., trauma, infections, CNS malignancies, or CVA's), pharmacologic agents (e.g., salicylates, nicotine, methylxanthines), or various heat-related causes (e.g., heat stroke, fever, or sepsis). Chronic respiratory alkalosis may have the same causes in addition to being a commonly associated finding in pregnancy, hepatic encephalopathy, severe anemia, and chronic exposure to high altitudes.

The predicted changes in plasma bicarbonate concentrations in response to acute and chronic decreases in Pa_{CO_2} are listed in Table 75–14. It is difficult to achieve Pa_{CO_2} values of <15 to 17 mm Hg acutely, while Pa_{CO_2} values of <10 mm Hg may be achieved in young individuals as a compensatory response to chronic metabolic acidosis, such as diabetic ketoacidosis.

CLINICAL MANIFESTATIONS AND TREATMENT. Chronic hyperventilation may be asymptomatic. The acute hyperventilation syndrome is characterized by light-headedness, paresthesias, circumoral numbness, and tingling of the extremities. Tetany occurs in severe cases. Both the acute letabolic alkalosis and the reduction in ionized calcium and magnesium contribute to the increased neuromuscular excitability.

The treatment of acute respiratory alkalosis involves correcting the underlying disorder. When severe anxiety provokes the hyperventilation syndrome, air rebreathing with a paper bag generally terminates the acute attack. If this maneuver fails, sedation may also be required. If an individual is to be exposed to high altitude, 2 days of pretreatment with acetazolamide, 500 mg daily, will produce a mild metabolic acidosis that will offset the initial respiratory alkalosis on exposure to high altitude and thus minimize symptoms due to hyperventilation on initial exposure to high altitude.

Androguée HJ, Rashad MN, Gorin AB, et al.: Assessing acid-base status in circulatory failure. Differences between arterial and central venous blood. N Engl J Med 320:1312, 1989. *A comparison of arterial blood gases with central venous blood measurements.*

Batlle DC, Hizon M, Cohen E, et al.: The use of the urinary anion gap in the diagnosis of hyperchloremic metabolic acidosis. N Engl J Med 318:594, 1988. *An account of the urinary anion gap in renal tubular disorders. The data in Table 75–15 are adapted in part from this paper.*

Cooper DJ, Walley KR, Wiggs BR, et al.: Bicarbonate does not improve hemodynamics in critically ill patients who have lactic acidosis. Ann Intern Med 112:492, 1990. *This paper compares the effects of sodium chloride versus sodium bicarbonate on pH balance and hemodynamics in critically ill patients with lactic acidosis.*

Gabow PA: Disorders associated with an altered anion gap. Kidney Int 27:472, 1985. *A good summary of anion gap acidosis.*

Haber RJ: A practical approach to acid-base disorders. West J Med 155:146, 1991. *Shows that acid-base disturbances are easy to analyze if approached systematically.*

Kitabchi AE, Murphy MB: Diabetic ketoacidosis and hyperosmolar hyperglycemic nonketotic coma. Med Clin N Am 72:1545, 1988. *A clinical summary of these two disorders.*

Krapf R, Beller I, Hertner D, Hulter HN: Chronic respiratory alkalosis. The effect of sustained hyperventilation on renal regulation of acid-base equilibrium. N Engl J Med 324:1394, 1991. *Study in normal patients showing that chronic hypocapnia decreases plasma bicarbonate concentration; however, plasma bicarbonate concentration decrease is not low enough to prevent increases in arterial pH.*

Kurtzman NA, Gonzalez J, DeFronzo R, et al.: A patient with hyperkalemia and metabolic acidosis. Am J Kidney Dis 15:333, 1990. *A concise account of the renal tubular disorders causing hyperkalemia and the diagnostic approach to these disorders.*

Preuss HG: Fundamentals of clinical acid-base evaluation. Clin Lab Med 13:103, 1993. *Excellent review on evaluating disturbances in acid-base homeostasis.*

76 ACUTE RENAL FAILURE
William E. Mitch

The problems associated with failure of kidney function arise from the patient's reduced capacity to achieve a balance between the intake and excretion of water and minerals plus the accumulation of metabolic by-products (chiefly from protein) that cause the symptoms of uremia. These two problems account for the serious complications of acute renal failure (ARF), including pulmonary edema, hyponatremia, hyperkalemia, acidosis, hyperphosphatemia, anorexia, nausea, vomiting, and other uremic symptoms. The severity of these problems depends on how much function is lost and on how successfully the treatment plan keeps a patient close to a zero balance between intake and excretion. Compared with chronic renal failure (see Ch. 77), the consequences of ARF are invariably more severe because ARF patients have not had time to activate adaptive mechanisms to blunt the consequences of accumulated waste products.

SCOPE OF THE PROBLEM

Some degree of ARF can be found in about 5% of hospitalized patients, usually as a complication of other illnesses or surgery or both. How serious is ARF? It has a 60 to 65% mortality—a risk that has not changed substantially since the 1950's. Despite the almost universal availability of dialysis, only in obstetric patients with ARF has a sharp decline in mortality to about 1.2% been achieved. The reason for persistently high mortality is unknown, but it cannot be blamed on loss of kidney function, because dialysis can replace the excretory capacity of the kidney. Undoubtedly, illnesses associated with ARF (e.g., sepsis) and especially the degree of hypercatabolism are important factors; mortality rates are higher in older patients and in those with more severe renal damage or with serious underlying disorders (e.g., infection, cancer).

A SYSTEMATIC APPROACH TO DIAGNOSIS

Diagnosing the cause of an acute decline in kidney function is crucial because some conditions are remediable (Table 76–1). The diagnosis should be approached systematically, and it must be remembered that patients with ARF have impaired function of *both* kidneys (unless the patient initially has only one functioning kidney). This concept is emphasized because few or no clinical signs of renal insufficiency are seen in subjects with only one kidney who have donated a kidney for transplantation.

The steps in a systematic approach are shown in Table 76–2. After a urine sample is collected for evaluation of clinical renal function (Tables 76–3 and 76–4), a bladder catheter should be placed to exclude obstructing lesions in the urethra or bladder. The urine is obtained first to avoid diagnostic problems caused by catheter-induced urethral or bladder trauma (e.g., hematuria). A systematic approach should be used to assign ARF to one of three causes: prerenal obstruction, postrenal obstruction, or intrarenal intrinsic damage. Understanding the pathophysiology of each cause helps establish the diagnosis.

PRERENAL ACUTE RENAL FAILURE. Causes of renal insufficiency not associated with histologic damage of the kidney are referred to as "prerenal" or "prerenal azotemia" (azotemia means the accumulation of nitrogenous waste products). Prerenal azotemia from various causes (Table 76–1) is characterized by decreased perfusion of the kidney leading to positive balance of water and minerals because of reduced glomerular filtration rate (GFR) and limited excretory capacity. The crucial point is that prerenal ARF is potentially reversible because no histologic kidney damage has occurred. Fortunately, it is unusual for prerenal ARF to progress to intrinsic kidney damage if perfusion of the kidney is restored. Protection against intrinsic damage is afforded by autoregulation, a response that preserves renal blood flow despite systolic blood pressures as low as 70 to 80 mm Hg. Although autoregulation depends on relaxation of the preglomerular arterioles, the exact mechanism for this phenomenon is still debated.

TABLE 76–1. CAUSES OF ACUTE RENAL FAILURE

Location of Primary Disorder	Clinical Examples
Prerenal	
Hypovolemia	Hemorrhage, skin losses (burns, sweating), gastrointestinal losses (diarrhea, vomiting), renal losses (diuretics, glycosuria), extravascular pooling (peritonitis, burns)
Ineffective arterial volume	Congestive heart failure, cardiac dysrhythmias, sepsis, anaphylaxis, liver failure
Arterial occlusion	Bilateral arterial thromboembolism, thromboembolism of solitary kidney, aortic or renal artery aneurysm
Postrenal	
Ureteral obstruction	Bilateral or in a solitary kidney (calculi, neoplasm, clot, retroperitoneal fibrosis, iatrogenic)
Urethral obstruction	Prostatitis, clot, calculus, neoplasm, foreign object
Venous occlusion	Bilateral or solitary kidney (renal vein thrombosis, neoplasm, iatrogenic)
Intrarenal/Intrinsic	
Vascular	Vasculitis, microangiopathy, malignant hypertension, vasopressors, eclampsia, hyperviscosity states, hypercalcemia, iodinated radiocontrast agents
Glomerulus	Acute glomerulonephritis
Tubular injury	
Ischemia	Profound hypotension, postrenal transplant, vasopressors, microvascular constriction, sepsis
Endogenous proteins	Hemoglobinuria, myoglobinuria, light-chain myeloma
Intratubular crystals	Uric acid, oxalate, sulfonamides, pyridium
Tubulointerstitial inflammation	Interstitial nephritis due to drugs, infection, radiation
Nephrotoxins	Antibiotics (aminoglycosides, cephaloridine, amphotericin B); metals (mercury, bismuth, uranium, arsenic, silver, cadmium, iron, antimony); solvents (carbon tetrachloride, ethylene glycol, tetrachloroethylene); iodinated contrast agents; streptozotocin, cisplatin

Another type of prerenal ARF is termed "ineffective perfusion" or "ineffective arterial volume." In these conditions, extracellular fluid volume is, in fact, normal or expanded (such patients usually have edema or ascites or both), but the kidneys respond as if the blood volume were inadequate. In these conditions as well (e.g., heart or liver failure), histologic kidney damage is unusual; however, certain prerenal conditions can progress to histologic damage of the kidney (e.g., sepsis, anaphylaxis). In fact, kidneys from patients with terminal ARF from liver failure function normally when transplanted into chronically uremic patients. Bilateral renal artery occlusion from emboli originating in the heart or from atheromata in the aorta (especially following difficult surgical procedures) can

TABLE 76–2. A SYSTEMATIC APPROACH TO DIAGNOSING THE CAUSE OF ACUTE RENAL FAILURE

1. Medical history: Clinical setting, medications
2. Physical examination: Evaluation of hemodynamic status, skin rash, signs of systemic diseases
3. Urinalysis with evaluation of sediment
4. Chemical analysis of blood and urine: serum bicarbonate, potassium, uric acid, calcium, phosphorus, urine osmolality, urine and serum urea, creatinine, and sodium
5. Bladder catheterization
6. Fluid-diuretic challenge
7. Radiologic studies to exclude obstruction:
   Ultrasonography
   CT scan
   Retrograde pyelography
8. Renal biopsy

TABLE 76–3. URINARY INDICES IN ACUTE RENAL FAILURE

	Prenatal	Acute Tubular Injury
Urinary osmolality, mOsm/kg H_2O	>500	<350
Urinary sodium, mEq/liter	<20	>40
Urinary/plasma creatinine ratio	>40	<20
Fractional sodium excretion*	<1	>1

* $\dfrac{\text{Urine [Na]/Serum [Na]}}{\text{Urine [creatinine]/Serum [creatinine]}} \times 100$

also cause prerenal ARF. In this setting, severe, sudden compromise of renal blood flow causes ischemic damage to the kidney.

The term *prerenal azotemia* is applied when the serum urea nitrogen concentration (SUN) relative to the serum creatinine concentration exceeds 10 to 1. The SUN is excessively high because tubular function is unimpaired and there is avid reabsorption of filtered sodium and water, which creates a high concentration of urea in tubular fluid and raises urea reabsorption. These responses decrease urea clearance. The pathophysiology of prerenal azotemia, then, includes reduced perfusion of the kidney with high plasma levels of renin, aldosterone, and antidiuretic hormone resulting in avid tubular reabsorption of water and ions. The urine is concentrated and contains small amounts of sodium. The latter finding has been refined by correcting sodium excretion for the amount of functioning renal tissue (i.e., the fraction of filtered sodium that is excreted, or FE_{Na}). When tubular function is intact, the FE_{Na} is low (<1%) (see Tables 76–3 and 76–4).

Because there is no histologic damage to the tubules, no erythrocytes, inflammatory cells, or granular casts should be present in the urine. Although a strict definition of prerenal ARF excludes patients with damaged renal tubules, reduced renal perfusion from heart failure can decrease the function in patients with established renal disease, leading to a diagnosis of "acute or chronic renal failure."

POSTRENAL OBSTRUCTION. Bilateral ureteral obstruction is caused by blood clots, calculi or necrotic papillae (e.g., with diabetes or analgesic nephropathy), neoplasms closing both ureters (e.g., retroperitoneal lymphoma), and iatrogenic factors affecting both ureters and/or urethra. In obstructive nephropathy, urine flow may decrease rapidly or cease, but this is unusual for the following reasons: (1) if only one kidney is obstructed, the other kidney will compensate for the loss; and (2) even if a solitary kidney is obstructed (or both kidneys are obstructed simultaneously), filtration continues and tubular pressure rises to overcome the obstruction and increase urine flow.

The causes of postrenal ARF are listed in Table 76–1. In hospitalized patients with indwelling urinary catheters, the catheter should always be checked for correct placement and patency. Obstruction, like prerenal ARF, does not make the urine sediment abnormal, unless a coexisting infection produces pyuria and bacteria. Because there are no characteristic features, obstruction should be suspected in all patients with ARF.

INTRARENAL HISTOLOGIC DAMAGE. The different types of acute vasculitis and glomerulonephritis fall in this category, as do scleroderma, malignant hypertension, eclampsia, and microangiopathies. Vascular damage leads to infarction and/or ischemic

TABLE 76–4. CONDITIONS ASSOCIATED WITH A FRACTIONAL SODIUM EXCRETION (FE$_{Na}$) LESS THAN 1% DESPITE INTRINSIC RENAL DAMAGE

Intense Intrarenal Vasoconstriction

1. Liver disease
2. Congestive heart failure
3. Norepinephrine, dopamine administration
4. Severe burns, sepsis
5. Nonsteroidal anti-inflammatory drugs
6. Acute bilateral ureteral obstruction
7. Iodinated radiocontrast agents

Vascular Inflammation

1. Acute glomerulonephritis
2. Acute vasculitis
3. Renal transplant rejection

damage to glomeruli. Glomerular inflammation (i.e., acute glomerulonephritis, see Ch. 79) can cause ARF by the sharp reduction of blood flow to, and hence function of, glomeruli. Finally, ischemic glomerular damage can result from the infusion of α-adrenergic agonists (e.g., norepinephrine, dopamine) or use of nonsteroidal anti-inflammatory drugs (NSAID's) or iodinated radiocontrast agents (especially in patients with pre-existing renal vasoconstriction associated with hypovolemia).

Whenever glomerular damage occurs, it will be reflected in abnormalities of clinical function and the urinalysis. Clinical abnormalities in renal function include a high SUN to creatinine ratio, and a concentrated urine that contains very little sodium, presumably because the tubules are less severely damaged. Urinalysis reveals proteinuria, generally with hematuria; in classic cases, red cell casts are seen. Proteinuria and hematuria result from loss of the barrier function of the glomerular basement membrane. Interestingly, urinary erythrocytes may appear to be irregular or crenated because their membranes are damaged and hemoglobin is lost as erythrocytes pass through the inflamed glomerular capillaries.

Casts result from aggregation of Tamm-Horsfall proteins secreted by cells of the ascending limb of the loop of Henle (plus proteins filtered through the damaged glomerulus). Normal subjects constantly excrete Tamm-Horsfall proteins, but when prerenal azotemia and a low urine flow coexist, Tamm-Horsfall proteins aggregate to form casts of the tubule lumen and are excreted as hyaline casts. Hyaline casts do not signify pathology, because they do not arise from histologic damage to the kidney. With ischemic glomerular damage from vasculitis involving smaller arteries, arterioles, or capillaries (see Ch. 244 and 245), or in glomerulonephritis, erythrocytes filtered through the glomerulus are trapped in the aggregating Tamm-Horsfall protein, producing red cell casts that are excreted when tubular fluid flow increases to flush them into the urine.

ARF can also be caused by disorders damaging renal tubules. This most common clinical form of ARF is often designated as *acute tubular necrosis* (ATN). Clinically, urine flow slows dramatically or ceases, and casts containing damaged tubular cells are formed. If casts remain in the kidney for only a short period, they appear as tubular cell casts, but more commonly the cells are partly degraded to form "coarsely granular casts" (Fig. 76–1). Because of the severity of injury, it is not surprising that red cells and inflammatory cells are also present in the urine.

Ischemic injury to tubules occurs with hypotension during sepsis or surgery (especially in elderly patients), producing loss of tubular cells (especially in the loop of Henle), or even irreversible necrosis of the kidney cortex. Cells in the loop of Henle appear to be especially prone to ischemic damage because blood flow to this region is low, and the cells have a high ATP requirement. Other causes of ischemic damage include powerful vasoconstrictors (e.g., norepinephrine) and sepsis. In ATN, it has been suggested that tubule cell damage results from loss of cell membrane integrity because of insufficient ATP and/or the excessive production of reactive oxygen metabolites or "free radicals" released during oxidative processes. Free radicals are implicated because they can damage cell membranes directly.

It is interesting that ATN does not occur more frequently, considering the number of patients who experience hypotension from heart disease or during surgery. Presumably, the autoregulatory response protects the kidney. Alternative explanations are that tubular cell damage does occur but is not clinically important because sufficient reserve capacity exists to achieve water and mineral balance and to excrete waste products. It is also possible that hypovolemia and/or hypotension by themselves are not sufficient to cause kidney damage unless one or more vasoactive agents that depress renal blood flow profoundly are released concomitantly. The need for a "second insult" is consistent with the widely held notion that acute tubular injury is usually not clinically significant except in susceptible patients (e.g., elderly or patients with infection or other serious illnesses).

Besides ischemia, renal tubule cells are susceptible to injury from nephrotoxic drugs, chemicals, and high levels of endogenous proteins that are filtered after hemolysis or muscle damage (i.e., hemoglobinuria and myoglobinuria, respectively) or certain proteins produced by multiple myeloma (i.e., the κ and λ light chains). Damage to renal tubules can also occur following occlusion of tubules by

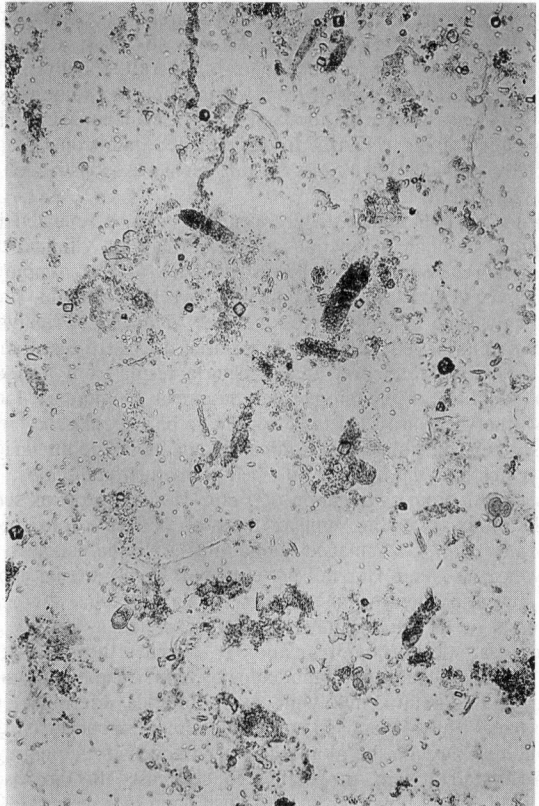

FIGURE 76-1. The urine sediment of a patient with acute intrinsic renal failure from sepsis. Pigmented coarsely and finely granular casts of different sizes plus erythrocytes and clumps of cells are seen. The larger cells are probably renal tubular cells and the crystals are talc from gloves worn to protect the examiner.

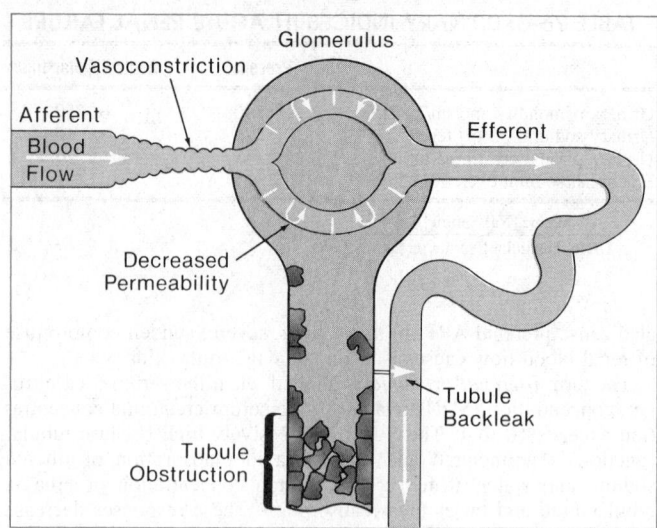

FIGURE 76-2. Potential mechanisms causing oliguria in patients with acute renal failure.

CLINICAL MANIFESTATIONS

Following initiation of ARF, four factors depress renal function (Fig. 76–2): vasoconstriction, decreased glomerular permeability, tubular obstruction, and backleak of filtrate. Clinical evidence of recovery may not be observed for days or weeks (average 10 to 14 days). Recovery of function is generally better in younger individuals who have no serious disease.

The most common problems in ARF are positive sodium and water balance with weight gain and edema. Kidney pain is uncommon (except with acute pyelonephritis, urolithiasis, or tumors). Although serum creatinine and urea nitrogen rise steadily, their ratio should remain at 10:1 unless prerenal ARF is present or there is gastrointestinal bleeding, hypercatabolism, and/or excessive protein intake (or infusion of amino acids in hyperalimentation regimens). If renal function is stable, these possibilities can be separated by the urinalysis and a 24-hour urine collection. In urine of patients in the prerenal classification inflammatory cells, erythrocytes, or casts should not be present (Table 76–5). The 24-hour urine is used to measure

uric acid, oxalate, sulfonamide, or pyridium crystals. Filtration of toxic proteins or endogenous compounds causes more severe renal damage in patients who are hypotensive or hypovolemic.

Nephrotoxic compounds are concentrated in tubular fluid when water is reabsorbed, establishing a concentration gradient to reabsorb the toxins by a passive process, or there may be transport mechanisms that actually reabsorb toxins to increase their uptake into tubule cells. Exogenous nephrotoxic agents include heavy metals (e.g., lead), certain antibiotics (e.g., aminoglycosides, cephaloridine, amphotericin), and chemotherapeutic drugs (e.g., cisplatin). Generally, nephrotoxicity occurs only with high blood levels (from high doses or with a "usual dose" in a patient with impaired drug clearance). However, lower doses of certain compounds can damage renal tubules when they are given in combinations (e.g., aminoglycosides and certain cephalothin drugs). Likewise, the nephrotoxic potential rises when two classes of drugs are given simultaneously (e.g., cisplatin plus aminoglycosides). Nephrotoxic damage is more frequent in hypotensive or hypovolemic patients and in patients with impaired kidney function from other diseases. Radiocontrast agents are more likely to damage the kidneys of patients with diabetic nephropathy, systemic lupus erythematosus, or multiple myeloma.

Interstitial nephritis also falls into the intrarenal damage classification. Inflammatory cells (lymphocytes, mononuclear cells, and/or eosinophils) are present in the kidney interstitium when ARF results from immunologic or allergic damage. Whenever clinical findings suggest a hypersensitivity reaction (e.g., ARF associated with a rash following treatment with methicillin or allopurinol) or there is a kidney infection, acute interstitial nephritis is likely to be present. Acute interstitial nephritis can cause a urinary sediment similar to that in Figure 76–1; more commonly, abundant polymorphonuclear leukocytes and especially eosinophils are found in the urine. Whenever acute interstitial nephritis is suspected, it has been suggested that a Hansel stain rather than a Wright stain of the urine sediment be made because it detects eosinophils more easily.

TABLE 76-5. DIAGNOSTIC CLUES TO THE CAUSE OF ACUTE RENAL FAILURE

Primary Disorder	Urinalysis	Clinical Findings
Prerenal		
Hypovolemia	Hyaline casts, no RBC or WBC, low FE_{Na}	Rapid weight loss, postural hypotension
Ineffective arterial volume	Hyaline casts, no RBC or WBC, low FE_{Na}	Weight gain, edema, normal or low blood pressure
Arterial occlusion	Hyaline casts, rare to many RBC's	Occasional flank or low back pain
Postrenal		
Ureteral obstruction	WBC's if infected, crystals or RBC's	Flank pain radiating into groin
Urethral	WBC's and RBC's	Urethral pain
Venous occlusion	Proteinuria, hematuria	Occasional flank pain
Renal		
Vascular	Granular casts, proteinuria, RBC's and WBC's	Systemic illness suggesting vasculitis, hypertension
Glomerulus	RBC casts, granular casts, RBC's, WBC's, proteinuria	Systemic illness, hypertension
Tubular	Granular casts, tubular cells, RBC's, WBC's	Hypotension, sepsis

urea and creatinine clearances. Since the ratio of urea to creatinine clearances should be about 0.6, patients in the prerenal category have a ratio of 0.3 or less because the high SUN to serum creatinine ratio results from selective depression of the urea clearance. As a further check, the 24-hour excretion of urea nitrogen must be less than nitrogen intake. If this is not the case, the extra nitrogen must have come from gastrointestinal bleeding or hypercatabolism. In short, a high SUN to serum creatinine ratio should always prompt a search for other causes, since the diagnosis of prerenal ARF is made by excluding other causes.

Another use of the 24-hour urine values is to estimate the rate of rise of serum creatinine. It is often said that the serum creatinine should rise at a rate of about 1.0 to 2.0 mg per deciliter per day in ARF and that a more rapid rise means the patient has myoglobinuric ARF. It is not wise to rely on this guideline, because the 1 to 2 mg per deciliter per day guideline is based on results obtained from Vietnam war patients who had varying degrees of kidney damage. In fact, the rise in serum creatinine depends on both the creatinine clearance and the rate of creatinine production. If renal failure is stable (i.e., body weight and serum creatinine are relatively constant), the 24-hour production rate of creatinine can be estimated from urinary creatinine excretion and compared with average values for patients of the same age and gender: in males, creatinine production per kg ideal body weight is $28 - 0.2 \times$ age, while in females, the value is $22 - 0.17 \times$ age. The maximal rate of rise of serum creatinine can then be calculated as creatinine production $\div$ total body water ($0.6 \times$ ideal body weight plus weight from edema). If the rise in serum creatinine is too high, myoglobinuria may be present.

Clinical problems caused by ARF include hyperkalemia and metabolic acidosis from impaired renal excretion of potassium and hydrogen ions, respectively. If no attention is given to maintaining balance, hyponatremia can occur in ARF patients given too much water by mouth or as dextrose in water intravenously, whereas excessive sodium intake will cause edema. Hyperphosphatemia, hypocalcemia, hyperuricemia, and anemia usually develop after several days, or more rapidly in patients with rhabdomyolysis or hemolysis. Hypercalcemia can occur in some patients recovering from myoglobinuric ARF, and hypercalcemia associated with any disease can cause ARF because hypercalcemia directly depresses glomerular function. Finally, the accumulation of unexcreted waste products can cause the uremic syndrome, which affects virtually every organ and is manifested by progressive anorexia, nausea, vomiting, nervous irritability, hyperreflexia, asterixis, seizures, and coma. Disorders of coagulation can cause ecchymoses and gastric hemorrhage.

TREATMENT

Treatment of ARF includes correction of reversible causes, prevention of additional injury, use of metabolic support during the maintenance and recovery phases of the syndrome, and attempts to convert oliguric to nonoliguric renal failure (Table 76–6).

CORRECTION OF REVERSIBLE CAUSES. In all ARF patients, drugs that interfere with renal perfusion or are directly nephrotoxic should be stopped and radiocontrast agents avoided. In fact, dosages of all drugs should be adjusted according to guidelines for renal failure; plasma drug levels should be monitored because the guidelines provide only average dosing recommendations. For hypovolemic, hypotensive patients in the prerenal classification, the blood pressure should be restored by discontinuing antihypertensive drugs and administering blood (if there is bleeding or anemia) or isotonic saline to expand the extracellular volume. In elderly patients with longstanding hypertension, a blood pressure of 100/70 may, in fact, be inadequate to maintain GFR. If doubt exists about the adequacy of the plasma volume, an intravenous challenge of

TABLE 76–6. GUIDELINES FOR TREATING ACUTE RENAL FAILURE

General	Avoid drugs that reduce renal blood flow (e.g., NSAID's and/or nephrotoxic [e.g., radiocontrast agents])
Prerenal	Restore blood pressure and vascular volume
Postrenal	Urologic evaluation
Intrinsic	Prevent hypotension and try to convert oliguria to nonoliguria; if edematous, try 2 to 10 mg furosemide per kg, but if nonedematous, try 500 ml saline intravenously

isotonic saline (500 to 1000 ml) is warranted. Saline should not be given to patients with edema and/or ascites because, in these cases, the low perfusion of the kidney is due to intrarenal vasoconstriction, which is not counteracted by intravenous fluids. Moreover, the presence of edema and ascites means that the patient is in positive sodium balance, and the infused saline will merely increase edema and/or ascites. Obstructed patients require urologic consultation plus careful attention to maintenance of zero fluid balance.

Not all patients with intrinsic kidney damage and ARF are oliguric, even though the clearance function of the kidney is low and waste products accumulate. The physiologic basis for nonoliguric ARF is not understood; it may represent a milder, less extensive form of tubular damage, but these patients do not necessarily regain renal function more rapidly. Because fluid balance is less of a problem, it is worthwhile to attempt to convert oliguric patients to the nonoliguric state of ARF, since fluid balance in such patients is more easily managed. For example, in conditions (see Table 76–4) associated with a low fractional sodium excretion and no edema, a challenge with 500 ml of saline combined with 40 to 80 mg of intravenous furosemide may reverse an oliguric to a nonoliguric state and, in some cases, prevent the maintenance phase of ATN. A trial of 2 to 10 mg furosemide per kg can be used in edematous patients in the attempt to convert oliguric to nonoliguric renal failure. If urine flow does increase to exceed 20 to 30 ml per hour, furosemide can be used to achieve fluid balance. Infusion of low doses (1 to 3 μg per kg per minute) of dopamine has become popular because it can cause renal vasodilatation and, if urine flow increases, within hours dopamine or furosemide or both can be continued. If not, dopamine or furosemide should not be continued, because there is no evidence that either drug increases rate or extent of recovery of renal function.

GENERAL SUPPORT. Indwelling urinary catheters should be avoided in uncomplicated cases; intermittent catheterization using careful sterile technique usually suffices even in oliguric obtunded patients and reduces the risk of infection. In all patients, maintaining fluid balance is crucial. The simplest and most accurate estimate of fluid balance is a compulsive daily weight measurement; fluid intake and output records are more cumbersome and less accurate. To approximate the required fluid intake, patients can be given fluids (water, tea) equal to 500 ml plus the amount of urine excreted in the preceding 24 hours. In febrile patients this limit can be increased as long as weight does not increase. Severely catabolic patients can be expected to lose about 0.5 kg per day.

Extra sodium, potassium, and chloride besides that in food should not be given to patients with ARF. If weight increases sodium should be restricted, but as long as the serum sodium is normal, water restriction is unnecessary. If serum sodium falls, water should be restricted. Dietary protein should be limited to 0.8 gram per kg of body weight per day, unless there is hypercatabolism, and energy intake (carbohydrates plus fats) should supply 35 kcal per kg per day. In patients who cannot eat, an intravenous infusion of essential amino acids and glucose may be necessary. On the other hand, this requires a considerable fluid intake and may lead to the need for dialysis.

Besides daily weights, serial determinations of blood pressure (supine and upright), serum electrolytes, creatinine, SUN, and hematocrit are needed. Hyperkalemia exceeding 6 mEq per liter is potentially serious and can be treated by ingesting sodium polystyrene sulfonate exchange resin (25 to 50 grams) in a solution containing sorbitol to ensure excretion of potassium polystyrene resin. Electrocardiographic abnormalities such as widened QRS complexes or atrioventricular dissociation demand immediate treatment with intravenous calcium gluconate or calcium chloride, because this is the most rapidly acting method of correcting the cardiac conduction abnormality. Glucose and insulin (25 units regular insulin per liter of 10% glucose) or hypertonic sodium bicarbonate (for acidotic patients) can reduce the serum potassium within 30 to 60 minutes. However, none of these measures removes excess potassium, and dialysis is usually required. (See Ch. 75 for a discussion of hyperkalemia.)

Hemodialysis should be considered for hyperkalemia that is unresponsive to the polystyrene exchange resins or that causes cardiac abnormalities. Hemodialysis is also required for severe metabolic acidosis that cannot be managed by sodium bicarbonate; hemodialysis is necessary to treat pulmonary edema, progressive azotemia (urea nitrogen > 100 mg per dl), encephalopathy, seizures, bleeding, pericarditis, and/or uremic enteropathy. Peritoneal dialysis may be the most suitable method of treatment for patients with severe heart failure, if the patient does not require rapid removal of potassium or waste products. Peritoneal dialysis avoids the rapid shifts in blood volume and components of the blood that occur with hemodialysis. Moreover, anticoagulants are not needed for peritoneal dialysis.

RECOVERY OF RENAL FUNCTION. ARF due to prerenal causes is potentially reversible if the underlying disease is treated. In postrenal, obstructive ARF, renal function may be expected to stabilize or improve significantly if the obstruction is relieved. Intrarenal, intrinsic ARF has a variable outcome. Glomerulonephritis and vasculitis may respond to immunosuppressive therapy with complete recovery of renal function. Renal tubular injury from ischemia or toxins is usually reversible; recovery to nearly normal renal function seems to be more likely in nonoliguric than in oliguric patients. Whereas a major improvement in renal function usually appears in the second week, mild defects in renal function can persist for months or years after acute tubular injury.

PREVENTION

Every effort should be made to prevent ARF. Patients should be given intravenous saline before receiving iodinated radiocontrast material and before surgical procedures, especially those with poor kidney function or those in whom renal blood flow will be interrupted (e.g., repair of abdominal aortic aneurysm). Intravenous saline is also given with cisplatin and other nephrotoxic drugs. Pretreatment with allopurinol can decrease uric acid production when leukemia or massive tumors are being treated. NSAID's should be avoided in patients with renal disease, and nephrotoxic antibiotics should be avoided or carefully monitored in ARF patients.

Druml W: Nutritional support in acute renal failure. *In* Mitch WE, Klahr S (eds.): Nutrition and the Kidney. Boston, Little, Brown, 1993, pp 314–345. *A review of metabolic abnormalities associated with acute renal failure that affect nutritional therapy. Guidelines for providing adequate nutrition are provided.*

Faber MD, Kupin WL, Krishna GG, et al.: The differential diagnosis of acute renal failure. *In* Lazarus JM, Brenner BM (eds.): Acute Renal Failure. New York, Churchill Livingstone, 1993, pp 133–192. *A comprehensive discussion of clinical abnormalities associated with acute renal failure and the interpretation of commonly used tests of kidney function.*

Finn WF: Recovery from acute renal failure. *In* Lazarus JM, Brenner BM (eds.): Acute Renal Failure. New York, Churchill Livingstone, 1993, pp 553–596. *Discusses the prognosis of acute renal failure and how it varies with age and severity of associated illnesses. Possible causes of the persistently high mortality are also discussed.*

Molitoris BA: Ischemia-induced loss of epithelial polarity: Potential role of the actin cytoskeleton. Am J Physiol 260:F769, 1991. *Discusses potential mechanisms of tubular cell damage in ischemia. Damage to the cytoskeleton results in loss of cellular integrity.*

Myers BD, Morna SM: Hemodynamically-mediated acute renal failure. N Engl J Med 314:97, 1986. *Covers the changes in renal blood flow that appear to play such a large role in the development of acute renal failure.*

Weinberg JM: The cell biology of ischemic renal injury. Kidney Int 39:476, 1991. *The generation of oxygen radicals is discussed. The ability of these compounds to damage cell membranes provides a clue to the mechanism of extensive loss of tubular cells in ischemic and toxic acute renal failure. If these compounds are important causes of cellular damage in patients, treatment strategies could be devised.*

77 CHRONIC RENAL FAILURE
David G. Warnock

Chronic renal failure (CRF) is a functional diagnosis characterized by a progressive and generally irreversible decline in glomerular filtration rate (GFR). It is caused by a large number of diseases. Over 165,000 in the United States were treated for end-stage renal disease (ESRD) during 1990. The prevalence in 1977 was only 45,000 patients, so it is apparent that the ESRD programs are expanding. Approximately 12% of the U.S. population was black in 1990, while nearly 32% of the patients in the Medicare ESRD program were black; it is clear that renal failure disproportionately af-

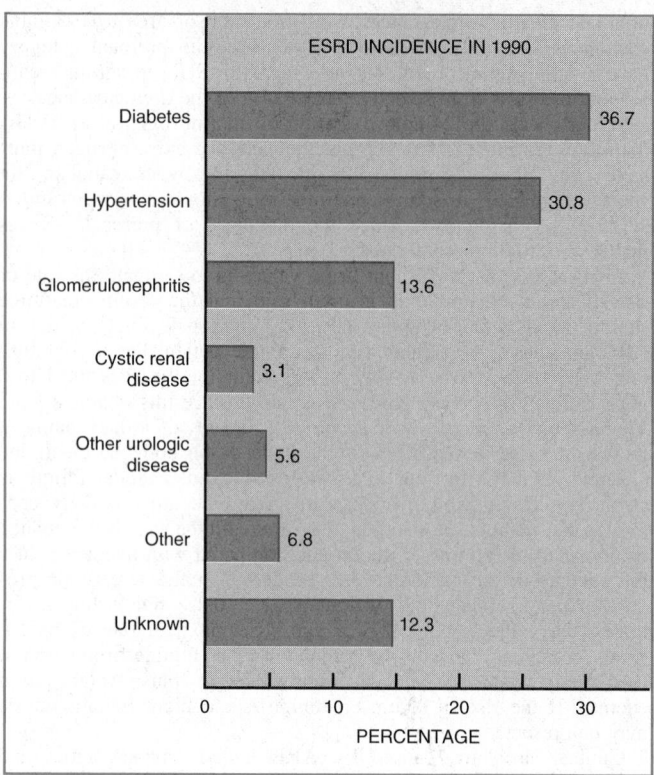

FIGURE 77–1. Histogram of primary renal diseases leading to end-stage renal disease. (Data based on U.S. Renal Data System, 1988.)

fects blacks compared with whites. Figure 77–1 summarizes the incidence of CRF for 1990 according to causes (U.S. Renal Data System Report). Diabetes and hypertension are now recognized as the leading causes of CRF in the United States.

This chapter considers the pathophysiology and clinical manifestations of CRF, an approach to the patient with CRF, and principles of management.

PATHOPHYSIOLOGY AND CLINICAL MANIFESTATIONS

The clinical constellation of signs and symptoms of end-stage renal failure is known as the "uremic syndrome." Unfortunately, patients often seek medical attention only when their disease has progressed to the uremic stage. Normally, the adult patient is unaware of advancing renal failure until the GFR has decreased to less than 15 ml per minute. When conservative medical management is no longer adequate, alternative approaches, such as dialysis or transplantation (see Ch. 78), must be considered.

The uremic syndrome results from functional derangements of many organ systems, although the prominence of specific symptoms may vary from patient to patient (Table 77–1). *Azotemia* refers to the retention of nitrogenous waste products as renal insufficiency develops. *Uremia* refers to the final stages of progressive renal insufficiency when the complex, multiorgan system derangements become clinically manifest. A variety of metabolites of proteins and amino acids have been considered possible uremic toxins, but the clinical symptoms of uremia correlate to their blood levels rather poorly. Uremia generally results from the accumulation of such metabolites and from the progressive failure of renal catabolic, metabolic, and endocrinologic processes.

WATER, ELECTROLYTE, AND ACID-BASE METABOLISM IN UREMIA. Renal and extrarenal compensatory mechanisms maintain electrolyte and water metabolism in a nearly normal state until the late stages of renal failure. However, characteristic changes develop as renal function declines.

Potassium. The normal human dietary intake of potassium is 1 mEq per kilogram of body weight per day, more than 90% of which is excreted by the kidneys. The potassium excreted in the urine has been largely secreted by distal nephron segments beyond the macula densa. Both normal and uremic subjects adapt to high-potassium diets by increasing potassium excretion per

TABLE 77–1. THE UREMIC SYNDROME

77 CHRONIC RENAL FAILURE / 557

1. Electrolyte disorders
    a. Potassium: hyperkalemia, total body depletion
    b. Sodium: salt-losing nephropathy, sodium retention
    c. Acidosis: metabolic acidosis with high "anion gap," type IV renal tubular acidosis (hyporeninemic hypoaldosteronism)
    d. Calcium (see Table 216–1): tendency toward hypocalcemia—phosphate retention and secondary hyperparathyroidism, with vitamin D deficiency
    e. Phosphate: hyperphosphatemia contributes to disorders of calcium metabolism
    f. Magnesium: accumulation due to excessive intake
    g. Aluminum: accumulation due to excessive intake
2. Cardiovascular abnormalities
    a. Accelerated atherosclerosis
    b. Hypertension
    c. Pericarditis
    d. Myocardial dysfunction
3. Hematologic abnormalities
    a. Anemia: erythropoietin deficiency, iron deficiency
    b. Leukocyte dysfunction: infection
    c. Hemorrhagic diathesis: defective platelet function
4. Gastrointestinal disorders
    a. Anorexia, nausea, vomiting, gastroparesis
    b. Gastrointestinal bleeding
    c. Disorders of taste
5. Renal osteodystrophy (see Table 216–1)
    a. Osteomalacia
    b. Osteitis fibrosa (secondary hyperparathyroidism)
    c. Osteosclerosis
    d. Osteoporosis
6. Neurologic abnormalities
    a. Central nervous system: insomnia, fatigue, psychological symptoms, asterixis
    b. Peripheral neuropathy: stocking-glove sensory neuropathy
7. Myopathy: especially of proximal muscles
8. Endocrine and metabolic disorders
    a. Glucose intolerance: insulin resistance, insulin degradation, hypoglycemia
    b. Other endocrine disorders: fertility, sterility
    c. Hypothermia
9. Hyperuricemia: clinical gout is rare; pseudogout occurs
10. Pruritus, soft tissue calcification, uremic frost

nephron. In addition, the gut can increase its ability to secrete potassium and serves as an important adjunct for potassium adaptation in CRF.

In spite of these adaptive processes, potassium homeostasis in patients with CRF is not normal. In advanced CRF, the serum potassium concentration tends to be higher than normal, even though body stores of potassium may be reduced. Hyperkalemia can be accentuated by oliguria, trauma, surgery, anesthesia, blood transfusion, acidosis, or increased dietary intake. It can produce serious cardiac abnormalities, but many patients are asymptomatic until cardiac arrest occurs. Occasional patients complain of muscle weakness or paresthesias. The major warning signs are detected by electrocardiography and include peaked T waves and prolongation of the PR interval and QRS complex.

Sodium. The kidney has a remarkable ability to maintain total body sodium within normal limits even with advanced CRF. As renal disease progresses, the remaining nephrons must excrete a proportionately greater quantity of dietary sodium to maintain total body sodium balance. This observation has led to a search for hormonal factors that might be responsible for the increased natriuresis per nephron observed in CRF.

Sodium Wasting. Some patients with CRF have salt-losing nephropathy and may lose sodium chloride to the point of extracellular volume contraction and hypotension. These patients will require dietary salt supplementation to prevent their hypotensive symptoms. A variety of renal diseases may be associated with salt wasting, including pyelonephritis, medullary cystic disease, hydronephrosis, interstitial nephritis, and milk-alkali syndrome. The collecting ducts are damaged in these conditions and cannot regulate the final urinary excretion of sodium chloride.

Sodium Retention. Many patients with CRF are unable to rapidly increase sodium chloride excretion to appropriate levels with increases in dietary intake and come to a new steady state with increased total body weight. These patients often have expanded extracellular fluid volume: hypertension, peripheral edema, pulmonary vascular congestion, and cardiomegaly. The clinical picture may suggest heart failure, and valvular heart disease or cardiomyopathy may be suspected. Volume overload worsens hypertension and thus accelerates all forms of CRF.

Acid-Base Balance. The kidney normally regulates blood pH within narrow limits by reabsorption (proximal tubule) and regeneration (distal tubule) of bicarbonate by secretion of protons into the urinary fluid. A maximally acidic urine has a pH of 4.5 to 5.0. The total quantity of acid that can be excreted is a function of the amount of buffer that is excreted and the net rate of proton secretion. The excreted buffers may be filtered or generated; the most important filtered buffer is phosphate, and the most important buffer generated within the kidney is ammonia.

In chronic renal disease, net ammonia secretion is reduced progressively. While the urinary pH may be maximally acid in CRF, the total amount of acid secretion is reduced owing to the limitation on buffer delivery to the distal tubule. Metabolic acidosis develops when exogenous intake and endogenous production of acid exceed renal net acid excretion. In chronic metabolic acidosis, extrarenal buffering mechanisms become involved, including bone salts and intracellular buffers. These buffering mechanisms allow for maintenance of relatively stable, but reduced, blood bicarbonate concentrations when the urinary net acid excretion rate cannot keep up with endogenous production of acid. Loss of bone buffer stores contributes to the development of osteomalacia and renal osteodystrophy. As the GFR falls below 10 ml per minute, there is retention of various organic anions and a progressive rise in the "anion gap" $[Na^+ - (Cl^- + HCO_3^-)]$ to around 20 to 24 mEq per liter, with a reciprocal fall in plasma bicarbonate concentration ("uremic acidosis"). The serum bicarbonate concentration does not usually fall below 12 to 15 mEq per liter. The overall buffer reserve is limited, however, so that acute acid-base challenges (ketoacidosis, sepsis) can cause severe metabolic acidosis.

Another form of renal acidosis, distinct from the uremic acidosis described above, is type IV renal tubular acidosis (RTA), or hyporeninemic hypoaldosteronism with hyperkalemia and hyperchloremic acidosis. This condition can occur in the early stages of CRF when the GFR is only moderately depressed. At this stage the kidney still has the capacity to excrete various organic acids, and therefore patients with type IV RTA, in contrast to those with uremic acidosis, have normal anion gaps. Type IV RTA is often seen in all forms of CRF but is most characteristically seen in diabetic patients with progressive renal disease or those with predominantly tubulointerstitial disease. It is described further and compared with other types of RTA in Ch. 82. Potassium retention and overt hyperkalemia are the most significant manifestations of hyporeninemic hypoaldosteronism in CRF.

Calcium. The total serum calcium concentration in patients with CRF is often significantly lower than normal. Patients with CRF tolerate the hypocalcemia quite well, and rarely is a patient symptomatic from the decreased calcium concentration. Tetany is occasionally precipitated by the infusion of sodium bicarbonate, but the usual muscle twitching and cramping of CRF are primary neuromuscular disorders unrelated to hypocalcemia.

CRF patients have decreased intestinal absorption of calcium, and consequently fecal calcium loss exceeds that of normal subjects. Jejunal and ilial malabsorption of calcium in CRF can be corrected by administration of active vitamin D analogues. In addition, patients with either acute renal failure or CRF are resistant to the normal calcemic action of parathyroid hormone (PTH). The mechanism of resistance may be secondary to a decreased permissive effect of 1,25-$(OH)_2D_3$ on the bone action of PTH.

Phosphate retention develops as renal insufficiency progresses. With increases in serum phosphate level, calcium phosphate is deposited into soft tissues and serum calcium concentration (both total and ionized) falls. The decrease in serum calcium levels is a potent stimulus to PTH secretion and leads to hyperplasia of the parathyroid glands. In addition, the kidney is a major site for catabolism of PTH, so CRF is often associated with secondary hyperparathyroidism and elevated circulating levels of PTH.

A subgroup of CRF patients develops hypercalcemia owing to persistent secretion of PTH from glands that have previously undergone hyperplasia. Occasionally, these patients become symptomatic with bone pain or exhibit signs of metastatic calcification. Parathyroidectomy may be indicated if other causes of hypercalcemia are ruled out. Measurements of serum levels of intact PTH are very helpful in this setting.

Phosphate. The most important determinant of serum phosphate level is the relationship between net reabsorption of phosphate from the gut and excretion of phosphate by the kidney. The serum phosphate concentration is higher than normal in patients with a GFR below 20 ml per minute, but retention of phosphate can be documented with even less severe declines in GFR.

The retained phosphate is a major cause of the development of secondary hyperparathyroidism in CRF. Adaptive mechanisms will maintain a normal serum phosphate concentration until GFR has fallen to approximately 20% of normal. However, if dietary phosphorus intake is not reduced in patients with advancing renal disease, these adaptive mechanisms cannot compensate fully, and hyperphosphatemia ensues. If hyperphosphatemia can be prevented, the expected rise in serum PTH will be blunted. In addition to dietary restriction, intestinal absorption of phosphate can be reduced by nonabsorbable phosphate binders. Calcium carbonate is an effective phosphate binder when taken with meals, and it enhances gut calcium absorption and provides a base equivalent for treating metabolic acidosis. This approach avoids the potentially toxic effects of aluminum (dementia, anemia, bone disease) that can result from use of aluminum-containing antacids and phosphate binders in patients with CRF.

Magnesium. Patients with CRF tend to have modest elevations in serum magnesium concentration. The urinary excretion of magnesium is diminished, and intestinal magnesium absorption continues normally. Most CRF patients with hypermagnesemia have no associated symptoms or findings. Nevertheless, it is prudent to discontinue magnesium-containing antacids and cathartics in patients with a GFR below 20 ml per minute.

CARDIOVASCULAR ABNORMALITIES. Cardiovascular complications are common in patients with CRF and can be classified into three main categories: atherosclerosis and hyperlipidemia, hypertension, and pericarditis. There also may be a primary myocardial dysfunction in uremia that responds to acute dialysis.

Atherosclerosis. Accelerated atherosclerosis is one of the major factors limiting the longevity of patients with CRF. The most characteristic lipid abnormality is elevated triglyceride concentrations with normal or slightly elevated plasma cholesterol levels. A positive relationship appears to exist between the elevation of plasma triglyceride levels and the increased incidence of occlusive coronary disease. The cause of hypertriglyceridemia in CRF is unknown, but current evidence favors a defect in triglyceride removal rather than an increase in triglyceride production.

Hypertension. At least two factors contribute to the high incidence of hypertension in CRF: (1) The tendency toward sodium retention and volume expansion is perhaps the most important. Patients with volume-sensitive hypertension may have increasing problems with blood pressure control as they progress into renal failure. (2) Alterations of the renin-angiotensin axis are also important contributors to the pathogenesis of hypertension. Angiotensin-converting enzyme (ACE) inhibitors effectively control hypertension in CRF and can be used as long as hyperkalemia is not a problem. A small number of patients with hypertension can be controlled only by bilateral nephrectomy. The vast majority of patients with CRF will have much better control of their hypertension once fluid volume is controlled by dialysis.

Brenner and colleagues have focused their attention on glomerular capillary hypertension rather than systemic arterial pressure. It is known that reduction in renal mass in rats causes functional and structural hypertrophy of the remaining intact nephrons. Increases in glomerular capillary pressures and blood flow may be a central factor in this adaptive hypertrophy. The role of adaptive glomerular hyperfiltration in the progression of chronic renal disease in humans must be viewed as somewhat controversial but does provide a therapeutic approach that emphasizes the use of antihypertensive agents effective at the level of the glomerular capillary for treating progressive renal insufficiency.

Pericarditis. "Uremic pericarditis" is a term that refers to pericarditis of unknown etiology occurring in association with uremia. Conventionally, pericarditis is classified as "uremic" or "dialysis associated." However, the pathophysiologic characteristics are similar in both settings. Uremic pericarditis was originally described in nondialyzed patients, whereas it is now most commonly observed in patients who are not dialyzed adequately. Characteristically, the pericardial fluid is hemorrhagic. The onset of pericarditis is usually signaled by pain, often on the left side of the chest with respiratory accentuation, and is frequently associated with a friction rub. The friction rub can be loud and even palpable but also may be evanescent. Tamponade can occur with signs of falling blood and pulse pressures, raised jugular venous pressure, and poorly perfused extremities. It is recognized that in previously nondialyzed patients uremic pericarditis responds to dialysis more rapidly than in patients who develop pericarditis during dialysis. However, the pericarditis in this latter group usually responds to intensification of hemodialysis. Pericarditis should be viewed as potentially lethal, and it may require surgical intervention if tamponade becomes evident. Two-dimensional echocardiography can be very helpful in documenting the magnitude of the pericardial effusion and assessing its functional significance. If "diastolic collapse" can be demonstrated with this technique, emergent surgical drainage is indicated.

HEMATOLOGIC ABNORMALITIES. Hematologic abnormalities are among the most consistent manifestations of uremia. These abnormalities include anemia, bleeding, and platelet dysfunction.

Anemia. Many patients with CRF have severely reduced hematocrits. Hematocrits in the 15 to 20% range are not uncommon. The manifestations of anemia include pallor, tachycardia, a wide pulse pressure with accentuation by exercise, a systolic ejection murmur best heard over the pulmonary area, and the precipitation of angina pectoris in patients with underlying coronary artery disease.

The primary cause of anemia in CRF is a deficiency of erythropoietin, which is a glycoprotein normally produced in the kidney in response to hypoxia. It is responsible for normal red blood cell differentiation from stem cells. Decreased erythropoietin production results primarily from destruction of renal parenchyma and causes normochromic, normocytic anemia. Other factors may contribute to anemia. Many patients on maintenance hemodialysis are iron deficient. Inadequate iron intake is very common in CRF, and iron deficiency may develop in dialyzed patients because of frequent blood sampling and accidental losses during the course of dialysis. Red blood cell survival is shortened in uremia, probably owing to mechanical factors and changes in the red blood cell membrane composition. In addition, patients with CRF may have additional factors that contribute to anemia.

Erythropoietin therapy has greatly increased the well-being of CRF patients. A target hematocrit of 30 to 33% is generally accepted, and use of erythropoietin in predialysis patients with severe CRF is worthwhile. Worsening hypertension and even seizures have occurred if the initial rise in the hematocrit is too rapid. Iron supplementation is essential, and monitoring of total-body iron stores is mandatory. Iron saturation (serum iron/total iron-binding capacity) is a better index of available iron than serum ferritin levels. The importance of erythropoietin in minimizing transfusions in CRF cannot be overemphasized with respect to parenteral transmission of viruses, pretransplant sensitization, and blood banking requirements.

Hemorrhagic Diathesis. A hemorrhagic tendency, manifested by epistaxis, menorrhagia, or excessive bleeding or bruising after trauma, is common in CRF. Whole-blood clotting time and prothrombin time are usually normal. Bleeding time may be prolonged, perhaps related to the associated abnormalities of platelet function. Platelets are often decreased in number owing to increased peripheral destruction. In addition, functional defects exist, such as decreased adhesiveness and aggregation. These abnormalities are often rapidly corrected by hemodialysis and may be secondary to a dialyzable uremic toxin (e.g., guanidinosuccinic acid). The abnormal bleeding time is not rapidly corrected by dialysis and, as such, may not be a reliable prospective guide to the risk of bleeding complications. The utility of desmopressin (DDAVP), cryoprecipitates, and even estrogens has not been established.

INFECTIONS. Most patients with CRF develop serious infections during the course of their disease. The increased susceptibility to infection could be due to deranged or deficient humoral or cellular immunity, impaired inflammatory reaction, leukocyte dysfunction, or increased exposure to pathogenic bacteria and viruses. Humoral immunity is, in general, intact. Most patients have normal humoral responses to vaccines, but more aggressive immunization may be required, as demonstrated by the difficulty in achieving full responses to hepatitis B vaccine in patients with CRF. The neutrophil count is usually normal in CRF, and it rises appropriately in response to infection. However, leukocytes of uremic subjects have a decreased phagocytic function. The chemotactic response of polymorphonuclear leukocytes is also depressed; this function improves with hemodialysis. In addition, patients on hemodialysis are often exposed to bacterial and viral infections. Staphylococcal sepsis is commonly due to cutaneous contamination through the arteriovenous hemodialysis access. Gram-negative sepsis also occurs with greater frequency. The frequency of hepatitis is increased in dialysis patients that is related to multiple blood transfusions. The incidence of hepatitis has been diminished with erythropoietin therapy, effective hepatitis screening, and vaccinations.

GASTROINTESTINAL DISORDERS. Gastrointestinal disorders are common in patients with uremia. The most common early symptom is loss of appetite. Uremic patients may develop nausea and vomiting, sometimes severe enough to cause volume depletion and negative caloric balance, which results in weight loss. These symptoms quickly resolve with the institution of dialysis, and even with erythropoietin therapy in the predialysis setting.

Gastrointestinal bleeding is also common in uremic patients and may be the result of scattered petechiae, ulceration, or angiodysplasia. There is also an increased incidence of peptic ulcer disease in CRF. The platelet defects contribute to the increased frequency of gastrointestinal bleeding characteristic of uremic patients, but structural abnormalities must not be overlooked.

OSTEODYSTROPHY. "Renal osteodystrophy" is an all-inclusive term for the skeletal changes in uremia, which include osteitis fibrosa, osteomalacia, osteoporosis, and osteosclerosis. Osteitis fibrosa is almost universal in advanced CRF. A number of patients complain of actual bone tenderness or muscle weakness. Renal osteodystrophy becomes a major limitation for patients on long-term dialysis. Spontaneous fractures and bone pain, due to osteitis fibrosa and osteomalacia, can have severe functional consequences. Even in the absence of aluminum intake, a small subset of patients has low-turnover bone disease marked by low alkaline phosphatase and intact PTH levels.

NEUROPATHY. Many patients with CRF have abnormalities in central and peripheral nervous system function. Tiredness, insomnia, and psychological symptoms, including agitation, irritability, depression, regression, and rebellion, are common. Patients with secondary hyperparathyroidism have abnormal electroencephalograms (EEG's) characterized by increased frequency of slow wave activity. Patients with secondary hyperparathyroidism caused by CRF may show improvement in their EEG's and psychological symptoms after parathyroidectomy. The mechanism by which PTH exerts these effects on the central nervous system is not known, but a variety of mechanisms may be involved, including changes in brain calcium content, abnormal neuroendocrinologic responses, and alterations in ion transport systems involved in normal neurotransmission.

Peripheral neuropathy is also common in CRF. Clinical manifestations include painful paresthesias of extremities, twitchings, "restless leg syndrome," loss of deep tendon reflexes, muscular weakness, and occasional sensory deficits. Lower extremities are involved much more frequently than upper extremities. Diminished deep tendon reflexes and vibratory sense may be found, but the most common presentation is sensory loss in a stocking-glove distribution. Diabetic patients can develop peripheral neuropathy as part of their underlying disease processes, which only worsens as their CRF progresses.

MYOPATHY. Muscular weakness and wasting develop slowly but are common in patients with end-stage renal failure. Proximal muscles are affected more than distal muscles. Nutritional factors obviously play a central role in the development and treatment of uremic myopathy. The resting transmembrane potential difference of skeletal muscle cells is abnormally low, and the average mean duration of the action potential is significantly shortened in uremic individuals. These findings are consistent with either increased permeability of the muscle membrane to these ions or decreased active efflux of sodium. These abnormalities can be corrected by dialysis and have been used as an index of the adequacy of hemodialysis. Polymyositis syndromes with elevated creatinine phosphokinase

levels have been observed in patients with CRF, especially in conjunction with various drugs, including colchicine, clofibrate, and lovastatin.

ENDOCRINE AND METABOLIC DISORDERS. *Carbohydrate Metabolism.* Fasting blood glucose values are normal or slightly elevated, but glucose tolerance may be abnormal. Severe hyperglycemia does not occur unless the patient receives a large load of glucose, e.g., during peritoneal dialysis with hypertonic glucose solutions. Nevertheless, the requirement for exogenous insulin decreases in insulin-dependent diabetics as renal failure progresses. At least two different mechanisms are responsible for the simultaneous coexistence of abnormal glucose tolerance and a decreased requirement for exogenous insulin: (1) enhanced peripheral resistance to insulin and (2) a decreased renal clearance of insulin.

A number of possibilities may explain the insulin resistance in uremia. First, some uremic substances may interfere with the action of insulin, since aggressive hemodialysis decreases exogenous requirements for insulin. Second, potassium deficiency may alter the nature of insulin released from the pancreas. Indeed, proinsulin-insulin ratios rise in nonuremic patients who are potassium deficient. Third, there is decreased binding of insulin to peripheral receptors in CRF.

Insulin is filtered and metabolized by the kidney. With progressing CRF, blood insulin concentrations rise owing to decreased extraction of insulin by renal proximal tubular cells. These observations explain the decrease in insulin requirements of diabetics with progressing CRF, but it is also necessary to postulate a degree of peripheral resistance to insulin to explain the carbohydrate intolerance ("uremic pseudodiabetes") of nondiabetic subjects with CRF. A small number of patients with CRF will not manifest insulin resistance and may in fact develop severe, life-threatening hypoglycemia.

Other Endocrine Disturbances. Pituitary, thyroid, and adrenal function is relatively normal in CRF. Sexual function is often compromised in CRF, with amenorrhea and infertility occurring in women and impotence and oligospermia occurring in men. Reduced estrogen and testosterone levels can often be observed, and prolactin excess may be of pathogenetic importance.

Hypothermia. Patients with CRF often have reduced basal metabolic rates and abnormalities in temperature regulation. The reduced activity of Na^+-K^+-ATPase may play a central role in the reduced rate of metabolism. Overt hypothermia is very common in CRF, with a resetting of the normal temperature from 37° C to as low as 35.5° C. This observation is of practical importance in assessing fever in patients with CRF; a temperature of 37.5° C may denote a serious, acute infection.

Elevation of Uric Acid Level. Hyperuricemia is a consistent finding once GFR has decreased to 20% of normal. However, the correlation between the rise of the serum uric acid level and the severity of CRF is poor. Only rarely does the serum uric acid concentration rise above 10 mg per deciliter unless dehydration is superimposed. Whether or not the elevated serum uric acid levels hasten the development of ESRD is not known. Symptomatic gout occurs in patients with CRF, as well as other forms of arthritis, including "pseudogout" due to crystalline deposits other than uric acid, and deposition of amyloid and beta$_2$-microglobulin.

Pruritus. Generalized pruritus is a frequent symptom of CRF and is occasionally severe and intractable. Causal factors include dialyzable products of uremia, a high calcium-phosphorus product in extracellular fluid with deposition of calcium salts in the dermal structures, and abnormalities in nerve end-plates. Symptomatic relief has been reported with more frequent dialysis, parathyroidectomy, dietary protein restriction, and correction of secondary hyperparathyroidism. Other dermatologic conditions include a sallow, yellow discoloration due to deposition of "urochromes," bronze discoloration due to hemochromatosis, uremic frost due to deposition of urea crystals on the skin surface, and metastatic calcifications.

APPROACH TO THE PATIENT WITH UREMIA

A detailed clinical history is imperative, with special emphasis on urinary tract symptoms, such as nocturia, hematuria, dysuria, polydipsia, and polyuria. Also of special importance is a complete history of systemic diseases, of exposure to toxins and infections, and of renal diseases in the family. The medical history will often be of diagnostic significance. The physical examination should emphasize the blood pressure, retina, cardiovascular system, renal examination with auscultation for bruits and palpation of size, rectal examination for size of prostate in men, gynecologic examinations for pelvic masses in women, extremity examination for edema and nailbed findings, and neuroskeletal examination for evidence of myopathy, neuropathy, and osteodystrophy. Laboratory tests should include a complete blood count and urinalysis.

Additional studies should determine whether a patient has acute reversible renal failure, acute worsening of CRF resulting from aggravating factors, or a chronic progressive disease. It is unlikely that a patient with acute renal disease is asymptomatic with elevations of serum creatinine and blood urea nitrogen (BUN) above 10 and 100 mg per deciliter, respectively. On the other hand, patients with slowly progressing CRF are often asymptomatic with much higher elevations of serum creatinine and BUN. In CRF, the hematocrit tends to be lower, the phosphate concentration is higher, and the urinary sediment is usually benign. However, none of these tests is specific enough to differentiate with certainty between acute renal failure and CRF.

Renal sonograms can be used to estimate renal size and identify hydronephrosis or cystic masses. If the kidneys are significantly reduced in size, this almost always indicates chronicity and irreversibility. Normal kidney size tends to favor an acute process, although exceptions exist: polycystic kidney disease, amyloidosis, scleroderma, and diabetes mellitus. The sonogram may reveal asymmetrical renal size, which may be due to unilateral renal agenesis, or renal arterial disease processes, which would suggest a need for arteriography to assess the renal arteries directly.

It is important to differentiate between renal and extrarenal causes of azotemia. Extrarenal causes of progressive azotemia may be either prerenal or postrenal. Prerenal causes are those disease processes that decrease the blood flow the kidneys. It is also imperative to rule out postrenal causes of azotemia, including lower or upper urinary tract obstruction. Lower urinary tract obstruction may be diagnosed by having the patient void completely and then measuring the residual urine volume in the bladder via catheterization. By far the most common cause in men is an enlarged prostate. Any time anuria is seen, it is imperative that lower urinary tract obstruction be ruled out, especially if accompanied by symptoms such as hesitancy in initiating the urinary stream, slow urinary stream, and incontinence. Upper urinary tract obstruction can be established by ruling out residual urine in the bladder and demonstrating dilated renal calices, pelvis, and ureters above the obstruction with sonography. The most common causes of upper urinary tract obstruction include renal stones, congenital obstruction, and bladder cancer. Superimposed volume depletion can limit the usefulness of sonography in diagnosing upper urinary tract obstruction.

Once it has been determined that uremia is secondary to renal parenchymal disease and not due to prerenal or postrenal causes, the physician must ascertain whether a treatable form of parenchymal disease is present. The most common forms of treatable renal disease are listed in Table 77–2. Renal biopsy and arteriography are often considered. In general, renal arteriography is of limited diagnostic value in patients with uremia. It may be helpful in patients suspected of having polyarteritis nodosa, tumors (although uremia

TABLE 77–2. TREATABLE TYPES OF PARENCHYMAL RENAL DISEASE

Acute hypertensive nephropathy
Analgesic nephropathy
Hemolytic-uremic syndrome
Hypercalcemic nephropathy
Intestinal nephritis
Lupus nephritis
Multiple myeloma
Oxalate nephropathy
Pyelonephritis
Rapidly progressing glomerulonephritis with crescents
Renal vein thrombosis
Wegener's granulomatosis

TABLE 77–3. AGGRAVATING FACTORS FOR PROGRESSION OF RENAL DISEASE

1. Vascular volume depletion
   a. Absolute: aggressive use of diuretics, gastrointestinal fluid losses, dehydration
   b. Effective: low cardiac output, renal hypoperfusion with atheroembolic disease, ascites with liver disease, nephrotic syndrome
2. Drugs: aminoglycosides, prostaglandin synthesis inhibitors in a setting of renal hypoperfusion, diuretics in dosage to cause volume depletion
3. Obstruction
   a. Tubular: uric acid, Bence Jones protein, and so on
   b. Post-tubular: prostatic hypertrophy, necrotic papillae, ureteral stones
4. Infections: sepsis with hypotension, urinary tract infections
5. Toxins: radiographic contrast material
6. Hypertensive crises
7. Metabolic: hypercalcemia, hyperphosphatemia

is an uncommon association), and renal disease secondary to severe hypertension. Asymmetry in renal size in the setting of severe hypertension suggests renal artery stenosis and should be evaluated by arteriography.

Renal biopsy may give a definitive histologic diagnosis, provided it is performed before the disease has progressed to such a degree that the only possible morphologic interpretation is ESRD. Renal biopsy can be performed by a percutaneous route with local anesthesia or as an open biopsy with the patient under general anesthesia. The associated morbidity and mortality are low, but the possibility of complications nevertheless exists. For these reasons, renal biopsy is probably indicated in only a small number of patients with uremia; on the other hand, an argument can be made for an aggressive approach to renal biopsy in those patients who have not yet progressed to end-stage renal failure. Biopsy should not be done unless the physician has strong feelings that the information to be gained will influence management. In that light, serious consideration of any of the treatable renal diseases listed in Table 77–2 should be pursued with renal biopsy. Contraindications to renal biopsy include uncorrectable bleeding tendencies, severe hypertension, bacteriuria, suspicion of perinephric abscess, hydronephrosis, and extreme obesity. Biopsy is often most useful in patients with normal-sized kidneys and progressive renal disease if they have (or are suspected of having) nephrotic syndrome, collagen vascular disease (especially systemic lupus erythematosus), tubulointerstitial disease, or rapidly progressive glomerular disease.

MANAGEMENT

The management of patients with CRF can be divided conveniently into three separate categories: treatment of aggravating factors, treatment of specific complications of uremia, and consideration of optimal diet and general principles in the long-term care of patients with CRF.

Aggravating Factors

Patients with CRF are highly susceptible to factors that may cause a deterioration of renal function. These must be treated immediately so that the underlying renal failure will not be worsened permanently. Table 77–3 lists factors that may rapidly worsen renal function in a patient with previously stable CRF.

VOLUME DEPLETION. One of the most common causes of worsening renal function in a patient with CRF is vascular volume depletion. Vascular volume depletion can be the result of either absolute volume depletion or contraction of the effective arterial blood volume. Common causes of volume depletion include the aggressive use of diuretics coupled with salt and water restriction and gastrointestinal loss of fluid from either vomiting or diarrhea. Vascular volume depletion also can be "effective" and associated with decreases in renal blood flow. Therefore, aggravating factors that cause decreases in renal blood flow can produce rapid rises in serum creatinine concentrations (Table 77–3). Physical signs of volume depletion should thus be sought. In addition, urinary electrolyte measurements often suggest volume depletion. Patients with CRF may rapidly and irreversibly decrease their GFR with volume depletion, so it is imperative for treatment, either oral or intravenous fluid replacement, to be started as soon as possible.

DRUGS. Patients with CRF are often treated with a variety of drugs, many of which are nephrotoxic. Of these, the aminoglycoside antibiotics are a common cause of worsening renal failure. In addition, prostaglandin synthesis inhibitors can decrease the creatinine clearance in patients with CRF, especially in a setting of volume depletion. It is prudent to obtain a detailed drug ingestion history whenever a CRF patient with an accelerating rate of renal failure is seen. In addition, drug dosing appropriate to the level of renal function is important to avoid superimposed nephrotoxicity (Table 77–4).

OBSTRUCTION. Obstruction of the urinary tract can occur from multiple causes in patients with CRF. Urinary tract obstruction is conveniently divided into that from tubular causes and that from posttubular causes. The more common etiologies for tubular obstruction include acute uric acid crystal deposition (as observed with malignancies) and Bence Jones protein deposition (in association with multiple myeloma). More common causes of posttubular obstruction include prostatic hypertrophy and/or prostatism; necrotic papillae, especially in patients with diabetes; and ureteral stones. When the clinical symptoms suggest urinary tract obstruction, it is important that prompt diagnostic and therapeutic measures are undertaken. Rapid in-and-out catheterization rules out bladder obstruction, whereas ultrasonography is useful in ruling out ureteral obstruction. If any doubt persists, then retrograde pyelography should be performed. These measures are simple and safe, and appropriate intervention often prevents progression of azotemia.

INFECTION. Urinary tract infections are significantly worsened when obstruction is present. The rate of infection rises especially after repeated catheterization. Although infection limited to the urinary tract rarely causes progression of renal failure, specific attention should be directed toward evaluating proteinuria, pyuria, and bacteriuria. Increased proteinuria and exaggerated pyuria suggest urinary tract infection. If infection is documented, specific antibiotics are indicated. Care must be exercised to adjust the drug dosage for the degree of renal failure. Uremic patients are also more prone to other infections, such as pneumonia and sepsis, on a *de novo* basis. These systemic infections, if present, in turn may compromise renal blood flow and result in worsening uremia. The index of suspicion should be high for sepsis in hypotensive CRF patients with urinary tract infection in whom the serum creatinine level is rising.

TOXINS. The list of potential nephrotoxins is long. Therefore, it is important to obtain a good exposure history in patients with CRF. In a hospitalized patient with CRF, when the serum creatinine level starts to rise rapidly, one must consider exposure to radiocontrast materials, nephrotoxic antibiotics, and vasodilators. Patients with CRF, especially diabetics and individuals with multiple myeloma, may experience worsening renal disease because of volume depletion. Fortunately, the prognosis is quite good if the patients are adequately hydrated; it appears that the incidence and severity of contrast dye nephrotoxicity have been reduced with this approach.

HYPERTENSIVE CRISIS. Many patients with CRF are hypertensive, and hypertension is one of the factors that may accelerate the rate of progression of renal disease. Thus strict attention must be paid to adequate control of blood pressure in patients with CRF. Occasionally, patients with CRF develop malignant hypertension with rapidly deteriorating renal function. It is imperative that the blood pressure be quickly controlled in these patients. Even so, the restoration of renal blood flow may be delayed if significant vascular abnormalities are seen secondary to accelerated hypertension. This recovery phase can take months, with only gradual improvement in the renal function.

METABOLIC FACTORS. Of the metabolic abnormalities that worsen the progression of renal disease, the rises in calcium-phosphorus products are among the most common. The rise in the calcium-phosphorus products not only causes soft tissue calcification but also may be a precipitating factor in the progression of renal disease. This is especially true in patients with multiple myeloma. Vitamin D supplementation and using calcium carbonate as a phosphate binder provide reasonable control of the calcium-phosphorus products. Carefully monitoring the serum calcium level and restricting dietary phosphate are also important adjuncts to the care of patients with CRF.

Complications of Uremia

WATER AND ELECTROLYTE ABNORMALITIES. *Hyper-kalemia.* The mean serum potassium concentration is higher than normal, whereas the total-body potassium contents lower than normal in CRF. Serum potassium concentrations up to 6 mEq per liter are well tolerated in patients with CRF. However, patients with CRF have difficulty in excreting an acute potassium load. Therefore, potassium concentrations above 6 mEq per liter require treatment. One should initially determine whether the hyperkalemia is a result of some aggravating factor, such as volume depletion, tissue breakdown, transient worsening of acidosis, drugs (spironolactone, amiloride, triamterene, trimethoprim, continued oral potassium supplements, converting enzyme inhibitors, nonsteroidal anti-inflammatory agents, β-blockers), fever, or high intake of potassium. If hyperkalemia is of modest degree and due to some aggravating factor, the therapy should be directed toward correcting the source of hyperkalemia. Dietary potassium restriction is a rational first step. However, if hyperkalemia is severe, skeletal muscle weakness and electrocardiographic changes may be present. This situation represents a medical emergency and requires immediate intracellular transfer of potassium and rapid removal of potassium from the body. The treatment of hyperkalemia is described in detail in Ch. 75.

Abnormalities of Sodium Balance. Although the fractional excretion of sodium per nephron increases as renal disease progresses, patients with CRF are nevertheless susceptible to both volume contraction and volume expansion. Since even mild volume depletion may adversely affect renal function in patients with CRF, it is prudent to maintain these patients in a somewhat volume-expanded state. Volume-sensitive hypertension and pulmonary edema are limiting factors, but it is even more hazardous to keep a patient completely free of edema. If a patient should develop orthostatic hypotensive symptoms, salt intake should be liberalized. Some of the sodium may be given as sodium bicarbonate to correct metabolic acidosis. If the patient is poorly compliant and becomes volume expanded, the use of diuretics, such as furosemide alone or in combination with a thiazide, is indicated, assuming that there is a satisfactory clinical response to these drugs. is seen. If volume expansion does not respond to conventional techniques, acute peritoneal dialysis or hemodialysis is indicated. Hyponatremia and hypernatremia are treated with the same general principles of water restriction or free water administration as in any other patients. Neurologically symptomatic, life-threatening hyponatremia may require the administration of hypertonic sodium chloride, but the resultant volume expansion may then require acute dialysis.

TABLE 77–4. ANTIBIOTIC DOSAGE IN CRF

Major Reduction in Dosage	Moderate Reduction in Dosage	Minor or No Reduction in Dosage	Agents That Should Not Be Used
Flucytosine	Ampicillin	Amphotericin B	Bacitracin
Gentamicin	Carbenicillin	Cefotaxime	Chlortetracyline
Kanamycin	Cefazolin	Cefoperazone	Nitrofurantoin
Oxytetracycline*	Cephaloridine	Chloramphenicol	
Streptomycin	Cephalothin	Clindamycin	
Tetracycline*	Cloxacillin	Deoxycycline	
Tobramycin	Co-trimoxazole	Erythromycin	
Vancomycin	(trimethoprim-sulfameth-oxazole)	Isoniazid	
		Lincomycin	
	Methicillin	Nafcillin	
	Moxalactam		
	Oxacillin		
	Penicillin G		
	Ticarcillin		

* Although tetracyclines are not significantly nephrotoxic *per se,* their dosage should be reduced in CRF because of their hepatotoxicity with increased blood levels (especially with chlortetracyline) and because their antianabolic actions cause an increase in blood urea nitrogen disproportionate to the degree of renal failure. If tetracyclines are indicated in renal failure, doxycycline is the drug of choice because it is cleared by hepatic routes.

CARDIOVASCULAR ABNORMALITIES. Hypertriglyceridemia and hypertension are the primary risk factors leading to accelerated atherosclerosis and high cardiovascular mortality in CRF. It is not clear whether the course of atherosclerotic vascular disease in patients with CRF can be altered. Even patients who have undergone successful renal transplantation seem to have an increased incidence of cardiovascular deaths. Nevertheless, it seems advisable to adhere to the same dietary principles in patients with hypertriglyceridemia and CRF as in patients without CRF (see Ch. 173). If clofibrate or cholesterol synthesis inhibitors are used, the dose should be decreased proportionately to the degree of renal failure to prevent adverse side effects.

Hypertension is most commonly volume dependent and volume sensitive in CRF. Decreasing intravascular volume is sufficient to control hypertension in most patients. If the patient has an adequate urinary volume, the judicious use of diuretics together with a decrease in the dietary intake of salt and water is indicated. Of the available diuretics, furosemide and thiazides are preferred because of their effectiveness. Excess fluid also can be removed in patients on dialysis by ultrafiltration. If volume contraction is not sufficient, then the same general principles apply to the treatment of hypertension as in any other patient (see Ch. 38). Additional drugs, such as clonidine, calcium channel blockers, and β-blockers, may be required. Oral inhibitors of ACE have been shown to be particularly useful in some patients. These agents and "tight control" have been shown to slow the progression of CRF in type I diabetics. Minoxidil, a direct smooth muscle vasodilator, also has been advocated in patients with otherwise refractory hypertension. There still exists an extremely small number of patients with malignant hypertension that cannot be controlled by any medical regimen. These patients may respond to bilateral nephrectomy.

The diagnosis of uremic pericarditis requires hospitalization and treatment of impending cardiac tamponade. The best initial therapy is daily dialysis for approximately a week. Indomethacin is not effective in uremic pericarditis. If pericarditis remains refractory to increased frequency of dialysis, drainage and intrapericardial injection of nonabsorbable steroids may prove therapeutic. Some patients will require partial pericardiectomy if they develop circulatory impairment that does not respond to medical management.

HEMATOLOGIC ABNORMALITIES. Besides achieving the best possible metabolic status of the patient with CRF, two general considerations exist for treating anemia: long-term medical management and transfusion. The general aim of medical treatment is to increase the hematocrit to reasonable levels without secondary side effects. Because patients with CRF, especially those on maintenance hemodialysis, are iron deficient, supplemental iron should be given. Iron can be given daily as a ferrous salt or on a periodic basis as intravenous iron dextran. Oral iron supplementation is inexpensive and is associated with very few side effects. Unfortunately, some patients do not absorb iron normally in spite of hemodialysis and require periodic intravenous iron dextran. Most patients with CRF do not have folate deficiency unless they are receiving maintenance dialysis treatment; routine folate supplementation is advisable.

Clinical trials have been recently carried out with recombinant human erythropoietin for treatment of uncomplicated anemia in patients with ESRD. Gratifying and dose-dependent rises in the hematocrit occurred in response to intravenous erythropoietin. The phase III trial confirms that recombinant erythropoietin represents a major breakthrough in treating the anemia of ESRD. The use of erythropoietin has changed the indications for transfusions and androgen therapy in CRF. Many patients with CRF tolerate extraordinarily low hematocrits surprisingly well. This tolerance may be due to increased release of oxygen from hemoglobin during chronic anemia. Substantial increases in overall well-being are observed when the hematocrit is maintained between 30 and 33%. Higher levels are associated with side effects, including hypertension, headaches, and occasionally seizures.

INFECTIONS. The general approach to the use of antibiotics should be the same in CRF as in nonuremia patients. Ideally, the antibiotic dose should be adjusted by monitoring the serum concentration of the antibiotic. This often is not feasible, and after an initial normal loading dose, dosage levels must be adjusted for the degree of renal failure if the antibiotic is excreted by the kidney (Table 77–4). Some antibiotics are more nephrotoxic than others,

and nephrotoxicity is potentiated in CRF. If drug sensitivities allow a choice in the treatment of a given infection, the physician should choose the least nephrotoxic antibiotic that is therapeutic.

RENAL OSTEODYSTROPHY. Hyperparathyroidism, decreased amounts of active vitamin D metabolites, and chronic metabolic acidosis all contribute to the development of renal osteodystrophy, as noted above. The goals of treatment are to normalize these abnormalities to the greatest extent possible. Aggressive use of calcium carbonate as a phosphate binder and pharmacologic dosing with calcitriol have greatly improved the control of secondary hyperparathyroidism. Routine monitoring of circulating intact PTH levels in CRF patients has supplanted radiographic surveys for detecting secondary hyperparathyroidism; intact PTH levels are elevated long before radiographic changes become apparent. In addition, aggressive correction of metabolic acidosis by base supplementation has an important role in the treatment of renal osteodystrophy.

NEUROPATHY. No specific treatment exists for either central or peripheral neuropathy. However, both objective and subjective improvement may occur by prolonging the periods of dialysis and by using dialyzers with a larger surface area. A gratifying improvement in peripheral neuropathy has been noted following successful renal transplantation, even in patients who were well dialyzed before transplantation.

MYOPATHY. Patients may improve dramatically with adequate dialysis. Some patients have shown improvement of myopathy following treatment with active vitamin D analogues and aggressive nutritional supplementation. Erythropoietin has a generalized anabolic effect, which may be useful in this setting. Some patients with secondary hyperparathyroidism may benefit from parathyroidectomy.

CARBOHYDRATE METABOLISM. Abnormalities of carbohydrate metabolism in the nondiabetic patient are of no or minimal clinical significance. In the diabetic patient, insulin dosages must be adjusted to maintain serum glucose values at normal levels. Often, smaller insulin doses will be adequate as CRF progresses. Overt hypoglycemia may develop in a small number of patients with CRF.

URIC ACID. Although uric acid levels are consistently elevated in CRF, they are rarely much above 10 mg per deciliter. Little evidence exists to suggest that asymptomatic hyperuricemia should be treated. Elevated uric acid levels in uremic patients should be treated only when there are tophaceous deposits or symptomatic gout. If treatment is elected, allopurinol is the drug of choice, since patients with CRF do not respond to uricosuric agents. Because of potential toxic side effects, the allopurinol dose should be decreased to no more than 100 mg per day in patients with chronic uremia. Chronic suppressive therapy with cholchicine (0.6 mg per day) also may be beneficial in patients with gout.

PRURITUS. No specific therapy has withstood the test of time in the treatment of pruritus. A few patients get relief from topical emulsified oils or oral antihistamine agents. Some patients have benefited from lowering the serum phosphate concentration by more effective dialysis and phosphate restriction. Parathyroidectomy has sometimes relieved intractable pruritus. The most general approach is the aggressive treatment of secondary hyperparathyroidism.

Diet

An appropriate diet can be crucial in managing patients in CRF. Although nutritional and caloric intake should be individualized for obese and malnourished patients, some general principles are applicable to all. In general, the higher the amount of protein in the diet, the higher is the serum urea concentration. This is because amino acids are metabolized to form urea in addition to all other nitrogenous waste products that have been implicated by factors causing the uremic syndrome. Reducing the amount of protein in the diet lowers the BUN and reduces symptoms. Moreover, the difficulties in controlling serum phosphorus and acidosis are overcome, since a high protein intake is always associated with a high intake of phosphates as well as other inorganic ions. However, if dietary protein intake is too low, protein malnutrition will occur, with loss of strength, body weight, and muscle mass. This condition can be avoided if the protein requirements are met by providing 0.6 gram of protein per kilogram of body weight per day, of which at least 60% contains proteins rich in essential amino acids, e.g., eggs, lean meat, and milk. A high-calorie intake can improve nitrogen utilization at very low nitrogen intakes, so a diet of adequate calories manifests a protein-sparing (anticatabolic) effect. Providing about 30 kcal per day generally suffices, although this figure may be lowered for obese patients or raised for patients weighing less than their ideal body weight. Accumulated waste products can be reduced even further by lowering the daily protein intake to approximately 20 grams of protein per day, but only if the diet is supplemented with essential amino acids or a mixture of essential amino acids and their alpha-ketoanalogues. Furthermore, it does not appear that aggressive protein restriction slows the rate of progression of CRF in predialysis patients. The emerging consensus is that adequate nutritional intake is essential in CRF and that the provision of adequate dialytic support and excellent nutrition will minimize morbidity and mortality in those patients.

Diets should be supplemented with the water-soluble B vitamins plus vitamin C and folic acid; there is no need to supply additional vitamin A or E. Vitamin D should be reserved for treating severe renal osteodystrophy. In general, dietary sodium does not need to be severely restricted unless hypertension or edema is present. Most patients with CRF can readily excrete sodium until renal function is markedly impaired (creatinine clearance less than 10 ml per minute), but they cannot rapidly reduce salt excretion when dietary sodium is markedly restricted. As long as the amount of urine excreted is greater than 1 liter per day, it is unusual to have to restrict potassium in the diet. Renal potassium excretion is promoted by increasing the dietary salt content. Using these guidelines, uremic symptoms and the consequences of renal insufficiency can be controlled for most patients. Once chronic hemodialysis becomes necessary, the diet should be altered to meet the added requirements related to dialysis therapy.

General Principles of Follow-Up

Patients with CRF should be seen regularly to monitor the progress of their disease. The frequency of these visits depends on the presence of other diseases, e.g., hypertension and heart failure, and on how rapidly residual renal function is being lost. All patients should be seen at least every 3 months, at which time a medical history is taken and a physical examination performed. In addition, laboratory values, including hematocrit, white blood cell count, serum urea nitrogen and creatinine concentrations, and electrolyte values, should be obtained. Monitoring the progress of renal insufficiency is generally accomplished by measuring the serum creatinine concentration as an indirect index of the GFR. Alternatively, 24-hour urine collections can be obtained to measure creatinine and urea clearances, as an approximation of the GFR and a general indication of dietary protein intake. For most patients, the loss of residual renal function proceeds at a constant rate; this rate is different for each patient, although generally patients with polycystic kidney disease have a slower rate of loss of renal function than do those with diabetic nephropathy. When the reciprocal of serum creatinine concentration reaches 0.1 or less (a creatinine concentration of 10 mg per deciliter), the patient is close to the time when dialysis becomes necessary. It must be emphasized that the serum creatinine level is a reflection of muscle mass, which decreases as CRF progresses. In addition, creatinine secretion may be relatively well maintained as the GFR falls, so that creatinine clearance and serum creatinine will progressively overestimate the "true" GFR. Therefore, wide variations exist between individual patients with CRF when serum creatinine values are compared with the GFR. These considerations eliminate any absolute relationship between the serum creatinine level and the need for dialysis. Nevertheless, in the individual patient, the serum creatinine concentration provides the most immediately available marker for following the progression of renal insufficiency.

Allon M: Treatment and prevention of hyperkalemia in end-stage renal disease. Kidney Int 43:1197, 1993. *An authoritative review with specific treatment guidelines.*

Bricker NS: Sodium homeostasis in chronic renal disease. Kidney Int 21:886, 1982. *This article examines factors regulating sodium homeostasis in normal persons and patients with CRF.*

The Diabetes Control and Complications Trial Research Group: The effect of intensive treatment of diabetes on the development and progression of long-term complications in insulin-dependent diabetes mellitus. N Engl J Med 329:977, 1993. *Large treatment group demonstrating the utility of an insulin pump or regular insulin administration three times per day.*

Eschbach JW, Abdulhadi MH, Browne JK, et al.: Recombinant human erythropoietin in anemic patients with end stage renal disease: Results of a phase III multicenter clinical trial. Ann Intern Med 111:992, 1989. *This is an important report of results from the phase III clinical trial using recombinant human erythropoietin to treat uncomplicated anemia in patients with end-stage renal failure undergoing hemodialysis. The authors demonstrate a remarkable dose-dependent rise in hematocrit in response to intravenous erythropoietin, which eliminates transfusions, reduces iron overload, and improves quality of life.*

Klahr S, Levy A, Beck GJ, et al.: The effects of dietary protein restriction and blood pressure control on the progression of chronic renal disease. N Engl J Med 330:877, 1994. *The modification of diet in renal disease (MDRD) study; no clear-cut effect of protein restriction, but antihypertensive treatment was clearly worthwhile.*

Lewis EJ, Hunsicker L, Bain RP, et al.: The effect of angiotensin-converting-enzyme inhibition on diabetic nephropathy. N Engl J Med 329:1456, 1993. *Dramatic protective effect in hypertensive type I diabetics with serum creatinine levels >13 mg per deciliter and >500 mg urinary protein per day at entry into the study.*

Rostand SG, Brown G, Kirk K, et al.: Renal insufficiency in treated essential hypertension. N Engl J Med 320:684, 1989. *Despite acceptable blood pressure control, renal function may continue to deteriorate in approximately 15% of treated patients. Black patients were twice as likely as white patients to have elevations in serum creatinine concentrations, even though diastolic blood pressure was maintained at 90 mm Hg.*

Slatapolsky E, Weerts C, Norwood K, et al.: Long-term effects of calcium carbonate and 2.5 mEq/liter calcium dialysate on mineral metabolism. Kidney Int 36:897, 1989. *Calcium carbonate was shown to be an effective phosphate binder in large doses (10.5 grams per day). Hypercalcemia was prevented by lowering dialysate calcium concentration, thus obviating phosphate binders that contain aluminum.*

US Renal Data System: USRDS 1993 Annual Report. The National Institutes of Health, National Institute of Diabetes and Digestive and Kidney Diseases, Bethesda, Md., March 1993.

Warnock, DG: Uremic acidosis. Kidney Int 34:278, 1988. *A review of the renal responses to chronic acidosis, with an emphasis on the adaptations that develop during chronic renal insufficiency. The importance of chronic metabolic acidosis in the development of renal osteodystrophy is emphasized.*

Young EW, Mauger EA, Jiang K-H, et al.: Socioeconomic status and end-stage renal disease in the United States. Kidney Int 45:907, 1994. *Provocative analysis of the U.S. Renal Data System reports for 1983–1988.*

78 TREATMENT OF IRREVERSIBLE RENAL FAILURE
John J. Curtis

78.1 Dialysis

As early as 1861, chemists applied the techniques of dialysis to remove solutes from solution. Indeed, the first solution used for dialysis in the 1800's was urine—from which urea could be extracted. Nearly a century passed, however, before dialysis moved from the chemistry laboratories into clinical medicine. Two seemingly unrelated events occurred. Heparin was discovered by workers not focused on dialysis, and cellophane was invented for use in the meat packing industry. These developments and the genius of men such as Abel, Thalheimer, and Kolff resulted in applying dialysis as a treatment—first for poison ingestion and ultimately for acute and chronic renal failure (see Ch. 76 and 77). It was humanity's first attempt at simulating the function of a then vital organ system. *It worked!* In 1960, in Seattle, Washington, the first patient was treated for chronic renal failure with long-term dialysis.

Today, there are over 200,000 chronic renal failure patients treated with dialysis in the United States, and the number grows each year (more rapidly than expected). Much to the chagrin of health care planners, no plateau in the number of patients is in sight. Many of these patients have survived without natural kidney function for more than 20 years. In 1972, the Congress of the United States was approached with a trial of dialysis. Physicians performed hemodialysis on a renal failure patient in front of the legislators. This clinical trial convinced Congress that the therapy of dialysis worked. The performance won Medicare financial coverage for end-stage renal failure patients in the United States. Nephrology is the only medical subspecialty that has dealt with a "single-payer" reimbursement system since 1973. It has been both a good and a bad experience. It is impossible to separate the clinical aspects of dialysis from its unique (in the United States) form of financing.

ARTIFICIAL KIDNEYS. The dialysis procedure is based on two scientific principles—diffusion and ultrafiltration. Diffusion is *not* how the normal kidney works, yet it plays a critical role in dialysis. Ultrafiltration (which is more akin to normal kidney function) plays a less crucial role in dialysis.

Small particles of differing concentrations in two different solutions will, with time, equalize their concentration when separated by a thin, semipermeable membrane. Cellophane is the classic semipermeable membrane. The peritoneal membrane is a natural semipermeable membrane. The smaller the particle, the more brownian movement there is, and the more quickly it will move across the semipermeable membrane. The direction of net movement the particle (or solute) takes is from the solution of higher concentration to the solution of lower concentration. Larger particles will move across the membrane, but more slowly. Particles larger than the pores in the membrane will not move. The cellophane membranes were replaced by cuprophan or cuprophane, which, like cellophane, is derived from cellulose. Moreover, synthetic membranes (polymethyl methacrylate, polycarbonate, etc.) are in use in newer dialysis devices. Human blood is exposed to a solution in a hollow-fiber dialyzer (Fig. 78–1). This device allows blood and solution (dialysate) to be separated by a large surface area of semipermeable membrane.

Important, then, in dialysis by diffusion are the membrane (its pore number and size), the time that solutions are exposed to the membrane, and the concentration of the particles in the solutions. Small molecules, such as urea, are effectively cleared by diffusion. The difference in concentration gradient between blood and the dialysate is important, and thus the flow rate of blood and dialysate consequentially influences clearance of small molecules. Rapid flow ensures a large concentration difference. Larger molecules are not as sensitive to flow rates of blood and dialysate. They require more time for diffusion. The normal kidney does not employ diffusion and is quite effective in removing both small molecules such as urea and larger molecules. If larger molecules are responsible for uremia, this may be a problem in assessing how well artificial kidneys function.

Ultrafiltration, on the other hand, depends on pressure to move particles or water across a membrane. The pressure is either hydrostatic or osmotic in nature. In the normal kidney, pressure generated by the heart is transmitted to the glomerular capillary and, with the proper resistance, can force fluid across the capillary into Bowman's space. This forced fluid moves (drags) small and relatively large molecules (up to a point) equally well. In dialysis, pressure from the heart and specially designed extracorporeal blood pumps (Fig. 78–2) can be used to move fluid and solutes out of the circulation and across membranes. Large particles that move slowly or not at all across the semipermeable membrane attract water to move in their direction. This is osmotic pressure, which, like the pressure

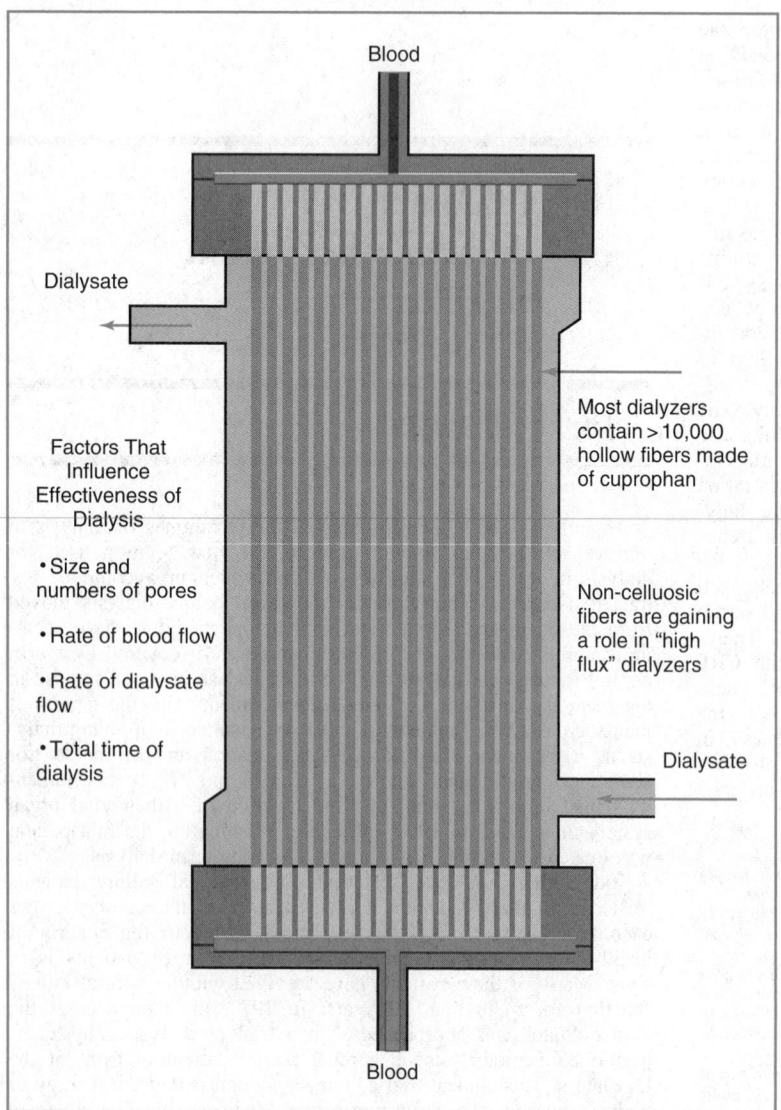

Blood

Dialysate

Factors That
Influence
Effectiveness of
Dialysis

• Size and
numbers of pores

• Rate of blood flow

• Rate of dialysate
flow

• Total time of
dialysis

Most dialyzers
contain > 10,000
hollow fibers made
of cuprophan

Non-celluosic
fibers are gaining
a role in "high
flux" dialyzers

Dialysate

Blood

FIGURE 78–1. Most dialyzers in clinical use today are hollow-fiber types. Some use of parallel-plate dialyzers continues, but coil dialyzers have almost disappeared from clinical use.

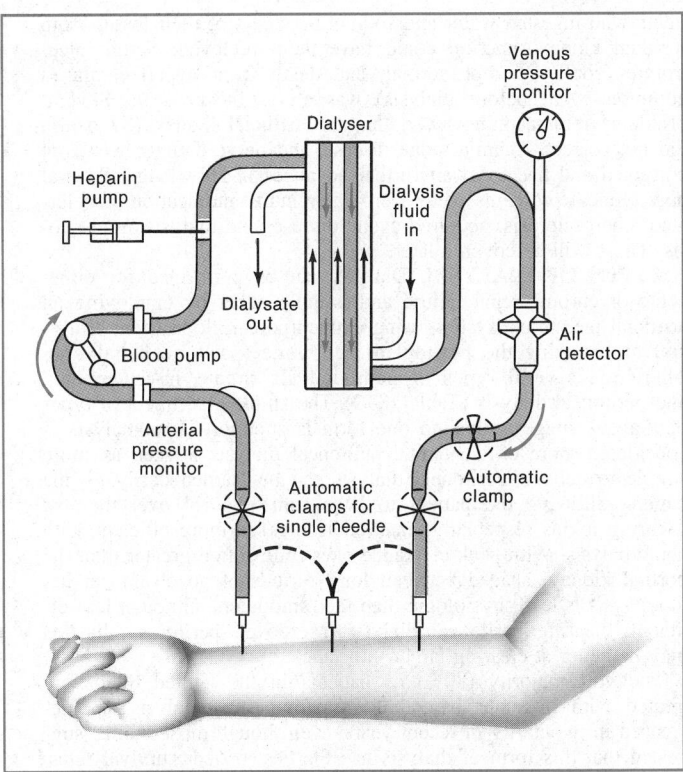

FIGURE 78–2. Essential components of a dialysis delivery system, which, together with the dialyzer, makes up an "artificial kidney." (From Keshaviah PR, Shaldon S: Hemodialysis monitors and monitoring. *In* Drukker W, Parsons FM, Maher FJ [eds.]: Replacement of Renal Function by Dialysis. 3rd ed. Boston, Martinus Nijhoff Publishers, 1988.)

generated by pumps, can be used in dialysis (especially peritoneal dialysis) to produce ultrafiltration.

The normal kidney, however, does more than ultrafilter. It reclaims from the ultrafiltrate exactly those solutes which are needed and excretes (and secretes) those which are toxic and not needed. This is critical. Without the tubular function of reclamation, we would all quickly die of ultrafiltration. Just how the kidney "knows" what to keep and what to discard is the question that has created the entire branch of medicine called "nephrology."

REMOVING SUBSTANCES THAT CAUSE UREMIA. It is not known for certain, however, what substances are responsible for the uremic syndrome and uremic death when the kidneys fail (see Ch. 77). Without this knowledge, it might seem that an artificial kidney would be impossible to develop—even with an understanding of diffusion and ultrafiltration and their ability to remove and replace solutes and water. The genius of the early pioneers of dialysis was their ability to put aside (for the moment) the unknown but to continue the thought process. Without knowing the toxic substance(s), one can make a nontoxic solution with the known concentration of solutes in a normal person's serum. Dialysis of this solution against a solution with unknown toxic substances should result in moving these unknown toxic substances into the normal solution. This assumes that the toxic substances are small enough to pass the membrane pores, not tightly bound to huge proteins, and located in the blood. The clinical success of dialysis suggests that the assumptions are correct.

The solutions (dialysate) that are usually used in hemodialysis and peritoneal dialysis are described in Table 78–1. Before dialysis, neither solution has urea, creatinine, or the toxic substances associated with uremia. At the end of dialysis, these solutions have urea, creatinine, and presumably many of the toxic substances of uremia. They are discarded. The patient has lost urea, creatinine, and many of the toxic substances associated with uremia, and the uremic symptoms disappear.

Two points need to be made about the dialysate solutions. First, note that neither solution contains bicarbonate (the solutions have a low pH of approximately 5). This is unlike human plasma, which has a pH of 7.4 and a bicarbonate concentration of 22 to 25 mmol per liter. The reason that some dialysate solutions do not contain bicarbonate is to keep calcium and magnesium in solution. At the concentrations listed, they could precipitate out of solution, combining with bicarbonate. Dialysate without bicarbonate has a low pH

and is bacteriostatic. Acetate and lactate are often used as substitutes for bicarbonate because they are quickly converted by the liver into bicarbonate. Quickly is sometimes not fast enough—especially with newer high-efficiency (large surface areas) and high-flux dialyzers (dialyzers with special membranes designed to be exceptionally porous). In some patients, acetate has been associated with dialysis hypotension. In the last few years, high-efficiency dialysis machines have used "bicarbonate dialysis" with water and concentrate of dialysate mixed with complex-proportioning units to prevent calcium bicarbonate insolubility. Bicarbonate dialysis has advantages for some patients. It is believed to cause less hypotension; clinical problems associated with severe metabolic acidosis are often better managed with bicarbonate dialysis. Bicarbonate dialysis is becoming much more common.

Second, note that the solution for peritoneal dialysis contains considerable glucose—more than 10 times that of hemodialysis dialysate. Hemodialysis uses blood pumps for ultrafiltration, while peritoneal dialysis uses the osmotic forces of high concentrations of glucose to remove water. This glucose load has the advantage of providing nutrition to patients but the disadvantage of occasionally leading to severe hyperglycemia and hypertriglyceridemia.

Using diffusion and ultrafiltration, nephrologists had made life without kidneys possible. Blood urea nitrogen (BUN) and creatinine levels could be corrected and the uremic toxins removed. Pa-

TABLE 78–1. COMPARISON OF TYPICAL MAKEUP OF DIALYSATE USED IN DIALYSIS

Solutes	Hemodialysis (mEq/L)	Peritoneal Dialysis (mEq/L)
Sodium	135	132
Potassium	0–4.0	0
Calcium	2.5–3.5	3.5
Magnesium	0.5–1.0	1.5
Chloride	100–119	102
Acetate or lactate	35–38 acetate	35–40 lactate
Bicarbonate	0	0
Dextrose	200 mg/dl	1.5% (1500 mg/dl) or 2.5% (2500 mg/dl) or 4.25% (4500 mg/dl)
Urea-Creatinine-toxins	0	0

tients who ingested water and sodium in excess of their losses from residual kidney function could have them removed. Serum electrolytes could be kept normal, and death from hyperkalemia (a common event before dialysis) was almost never seen. Several problems remained, however, that the artificial kidney (by itself) did not correct. Anemia, bone disease, and nerve damage were not corrected and had to await further advances in knowledge. Several new clinical problems were seen—aluminum intoxication, accelerated atherosclerosis, acquired cystic disease, and dialysis amyloidosis. These will be covered later.

TYPES OF DIALYSIS. Dialysis can be performed for either acute or chronic renal failure and is done either by employing an artificial membrane system using extracorporeal blood (hemodialysis) or by using the peritoneal membrane (peritoneal dialysis). There are several types of hemodialysis (home, in-center, etc.) and peritoneal dialysis (Table 78–2). The ample assortment of types of dialysis suggests that no one form is superior. Hemodialysis is considered more efficient, and peritoneal dialysis is seen as more simple to deliver. Peritoneal dialysis can be learned easily by the patient, allowing the patient to have some control over therapy. Clearing toxins (especially small molecules) is more efficient with hemodialysis. With peak clearance rates (rates often greater than the normal kidney) spaced between long periods of no clearance, hemodialysis is less physiologic than the "smoother," although less efficient, clearing peritoneal dialysis. Moreover, peritoneal dialysis may be better at clearing larger molecules.

The vast majority (80%) of patients in the United States are treated with in-center hemodialysis. Home hemodialysis has decreased in popularity in recent years, even though most studies suggested that this form of dialysis had the best patient survival rates. Chronic ambulatory peritoneal dialysis (CAPD) has increased to nearly 12% of patients on chronic dialysis. Patients on peritoneal dialysis are slightly younger than those on hemodialysis. They have fewer co-morbid conditions. On the other hand, patients whose renal failure is due to diabetes mellitus often are placed on peritoneal dialysis because insulin delivery can be simplified by infusing it with the dialysate. There are no controlled trials that compare survival rates between hemodialysis and peritoneal dialysis. Patient selection for these two different forms of treatment is usually decided by special needs of the patient and the nephrologist's clinical judgment of which treatment will be best tolerated. There is more long-term experience with hemodialysis, and clearly, many patients who start peritoneal dialysis switch to hemodialysis before they finish a year of treatment. Nonetheless, CAPD currently is the fastest growing form of dialysis. Decisions based primarily on clinical judgment, of course, will result in differences of opinion about the relative merits of peritoneal and hemodialysis.

RECENT ADVANCES IN DIALYSIS. Advances in access to both the vascular circulation and the peritoneal cavity have been made in the last decade. Indeed, new medical industries have grown from these technical advances. Using arteriovenous (A-V) fistulas is best for hemodialysis patients. It requires the nephrologist's skilled timing to have a functioning A-V fistula placed at the proper time. If it is constructed (surgical connection of the radial artery to the forearm venous system) too soon, it may clot; if late, however, the patient may need dialysis before the fistula is ready to use. A good A-V fistula may make the difference between long-term success and failure of dialysis. Using longer-lasting temporary access procedures (subclavian catheters, etc.) has helped make timing slightly easier. Artificial grafts (polytetrafluoroethylene, bovine) have been used with success when A-V fistulas cannot be placed. Permanent peritoneal catheters also have advanced in construction. Those with double cuffs seem to provide the best protection against peritonitis. Tubing connectors (another new growth industry) also have reduced infections for the patient on peritoneal dialysis.

Replacing only the excretory functions of the kidney ignores the fact that the kidney also manufactures and adds substances to the systemic circulation. Thus the kidney plays a major role in blood and bone production, and lack of normal kidney function can lead to anemia and bone disease (see Part XIII and Part XVIII). Recently, the complication of anemia in dialysis patients has been nearly resolved by the development of recombinant human erythropoietin, and most dialysis patients now receive erythropoietin regularly. The quality of life for dialysis patients has improved as their anemias have diminished. Recent work suggests that correcting anemia also had an unexpected beneficial effect on neurologic problems in dialysis patients.

Nephrologists have advanced the knowledge of bone disease greatly in the last decade. Bone disease in dialysis patients is much better understood and relates in part to another product that is created (not excreted) by the kidney, 1,25-dihydroxyvitamin D (see Ch. 212). Impaired production of this vitamin increases the production of parathyroid hormone (PTH). Now, most patients can have secondary hyperparathyroidism controlled medically by supplementing 1,25-dihydroxyvitamin D (which results in decreases in PTH and increases in calcium absorption) and adjusting serum calcium and phosphate levels. The bone disease of renal failure, however, is not entirely due to secondary hyperparathyroidism. Aluminum poisoning (which may be due to trace quantities of aluminum in the dialysate and aluminum antacids) may be responsible for some portion of the bone disease. Bone biopsy has become a common procedure to assess the type and degree of bone disease in dialysis patients.

Newer, more efficient membranes have been made—"high-flux" and "high-efficiency" dialyzers. These newer membranes have allowed nephrologists to remove more urea and water in shorter time periods. High-flux membranes remove larger-molecule toxins more efficiently. The newer machines allow careful control of ultrafiltration and use of bicarbonate dialysis. Thus artificial kidneys now are more efficient in replacing the kidney's excretory and fluid-control functions. The failed kidney's inability to produce erythropoietin

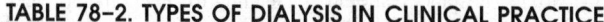

TABLE 78–2. TYPES OF DIALYSIS IN CLINICAL PRACTICE

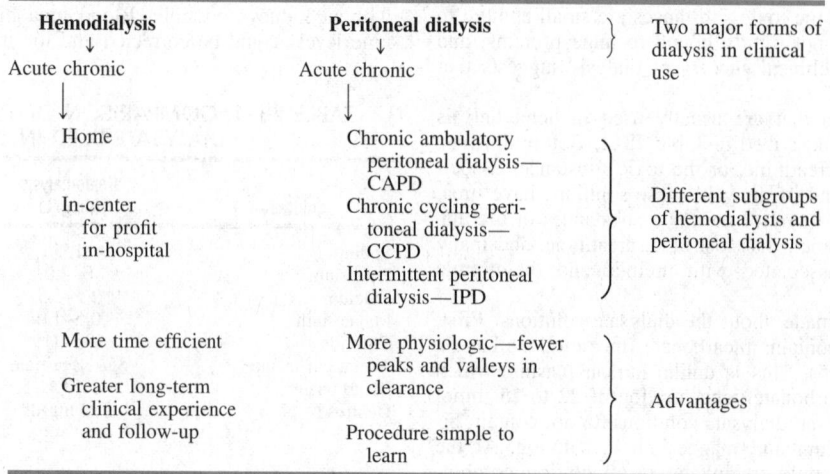

Hemodialysis	Peritoneal dialysis	
↓	↓	} Two major forms of dialysis in clinical use
Acute chronic	Acute chronic	
↓	↓	
Home	Chronic ambulatory peritoneal dialysis—CAPD	
In-center for profit in-hospital	Chronic cycling peritoneal dialysis—CCPD	Different subgroups of hemodialysis and peritoneal dialysis
	Intermittent peritoneal dialysis—IPD	
More time efficient	More physiologic—fewer peaks and valleys in clearance	
Greater long-term clinical experience and follow-up	Procedure simple to learn	Advantages

and 1,25-dihydroxyvitamin D has been overcome. Advances in vascular and peritoneal access have been dramatic.

BETTER TECHNOLOGY BUT DECLINING SURVIVAL. Despite these modern techniques, new drugs, and extra emphasis on urea kinetics, a rather worrisome trend toward decreased patient survival has been noted in the United States that has not been seen elsewhere. Convincing arguments have been made that the reason for this difference has to do (at least in part) with the method of financing dialysis in the United States and thus the amount of time that patients are dialyzed.

The federal program that finances dialysis grossly underestimated the numbers of patients and thus the cost of chronic dialysis. A program that was estimated to cost $100 million (at most) when first proposed now is estimated to cost $7 billion. To hold down expenditures of tax money, the cost of a dialysis procedure has not increased since 1972—it is the only medical procedure that has decreased in cost (nearly a 50% decrease when inflation is considered) over the last 15 years. Today, a dialysis procedure in the United States costs less than in a number of other countries. This cost consciousness has been responsible (in part) for two widely practiced procedures in the United States that are not seen elsewhere: (1) reuse of dialyzers and (2) shorter dialysis time with fewer, less experienced staff.

Most do not believe that reusing dialyzers has been harmful. Even without the cost savings, most nephrologists would favor reusing dialyzers to eliminate the so-called first-use syndrome. This is a syndrome of chest and back pain seen immediately after onset of dialysis with a new dialyzer. It has, on occasion, been more severe, with an anaphylactic type of clinical picture. This is rare, but it appears to be eliminated by reusing dialyzers. Nonetheless, reuse is not standard procedure in Europe and Japan.

Shorter dialysis has been correlated with decreasing reimbursement. While efforts to maintain urea kinetics with high-efficiency dialysis have been instituted, it is possible that larger molecules (those more affected by time of treatment) are the more important measure of adequacy of dialysis and that the 20 to 25% longer times that patients spend on dialysis in Europe are responsible for better survival. In Japan, reimbursement for dialysis (which is also higher than U.S. reimbursement) is linked to time of dialysis. If dialysis lasts less than 4 hours per treatment, reimbursement is decreased. In the United States, time of treatment averages 3 hours. Many people believe that the failure of some U.S. patients "to thrive on dialysis" is due to underdialysis. It is, of course, possible that all the difference seen in dialysis survival in the United States and other countries is due to patient selection. At any rate, decreasing patient survival rates have resulted in a re-examination of both dialysis prescription and the means of dialysis reimbursement in the United States.

NEW CLINICAL PROBLEMS UNCOVERED WITH LONG-TERM DIALYSIS. Nephrologists with large numbers of patients surviving on dialysis therapy have called attention to four disease concepts that were previously unknown. Dialysis dementia, or aluminum intoxication, was seen in nearly epidemic proportions in some dialysis units. Its pathogenesis was debated at first, but now, all agree that both aluminum from the dialysate and that used for phosphate binders are responsible. The syndrome usually occurs in patients who have been on dialysis for a number of years. It is characterized by intermittent speech disturbance, stuttering, personality changes, seizures, myoclonus, and auditory and visual hallucinations. The symptoms progress until patients become mute and unable to perform useful motions—followed by coma and death.

Patients dying of dialysis dementia were found to have elevated levels of brain aluminum. Epidemiologic studies demonstrated that those dialysis units with high rates of dialysis dementia also had high concentrations of aluminum in the water used for their dialysate. Removing aluminum using deionizers and reverse-osmosis devices from dialysate water halted dialysis dementia. Understanding that dialysis dementia is caused by aluminum intoxication has decreased the incidence in patients. Nonetheless, it is seen occasionally in dialysis units, and aluminum bone disease (see Ch. 216) remains a common complication.

Myocardial infarction and cerebral vascular accidents account for nearly 50% of deaths in dialysis patients. This rate and the age of deaths are strikingly different from those of the general population. Some nephrologists have even suggested that chronic dialysis *per se* may cause a syndrome of "accelerated atherosclerosis." Hypertension, which is common in dialysis patients, is a major risk factor for cardiac problems. Left ventricular hypertrophy is also common and can lead to cardiac arrhythmias. Anemia, increased cardiac preload, and A-V fistulas all lead to increased cardiac output that may contribute to left ventricular hypertrophy. Abnormal lipid metabolism also has been incriminated (heparin may lead to the high rates of hypertriglyceridemia seen in dialysis patients) as increasing cardiac risks. Hyperparathyroidism may induce vascular calcification. Acetate in the dialysate may be toxic to the myocardium. All these factors then might contribute to the high rate of cardiac mortality seen in dialysis. On the other hand, it has been suggested that the dialysis procedure may not have any deleterious effects on atherosclerosis but that chronic renal disease results in patients arriving at dialysis settings with well-established cardiac and cerebral vascular disease. The kidney transplantation (see Ch. 78.2) experience (of high mortality from the same vascular events) supports this view.

While it occurs with chronic renal failure (before dialysis), acquired cystic disease was first noted in long-term dialysis patients. The number of patients who have cysts develop in their kidneys increases with time on dialysis and total time of uremia. The presence of at least four cysts in each native kidney is usually used to diagnose acquired cystic kidney disease. It is easily differentiated from polycystic kidney disease because the kidneys are small and there is no family history of cystic disease. Unlike polycystic kidney disease, the cysts are limited to the kidneys. The clinical importance of this new entity is that some have reported that 2 to 10% of patients will have malignant tumors develop in the acquired cysts. On the other hand, death from renal malignancies does not appear to be greater for dialysis patients than for the nondialysis population. There remains controversy about the need to screen for the problem of acquired cystic disease.

The fourth new complication is hemodialysis-related amyloidosis. β_2-Microglobulin is an amyloid material that becomes deposited in the bones and joints of long-term dialysis patients. It can cause carpal tunnel syndrome and the severe problem of erosive spondyloarthropathy. Amyloidosis is becoming an increasingly difficult problem for long-surviving patients on hemodialysis—by 20 years on dialysis, the majority of patients have evidence of amyloidosis (see Ch. 248).

Along with the new clinical problems that long-term survival of patients with end-stage renal disease (ESRD) on dialysis has created, both hemodialysis and peritoneal dialysis have their own set of specific complications and share a set of long-term complications that are quite similar (Table 78–3). It is interesting that the long-term difficulties of both forms of dialysis and of long-surviving transplant patients are similar, involving vascular disease and infections.

Ahmad S, Blagg CR, Scribner BH: Center and home chronic hemodialysis. *In* Schrier RW, Gottschalk CW (eds.): Diseases of the Kidney. 5th ed. Boston, Little, Brown 1993, p 3031. *This is an in-depth chapter written by authors who were responsible for many of the clinical successes of dialysis.*

Nuhad I, Hakim RM, Oreopoulos DG, et al.: Renal replacement therapies in the elderly: I. Hemodialysis and chronic peritoneal dialysis. Am J Kidney Dis 22:759, 1993. *This report is an in-depth review of dialysis and the changes in the demographics of the end-stage population in the United States.*

United States Renal Data System. USRDS 1993 Annual Data Report. Bethesda, MD, U.S. Department of Health and Human Services, National Institutes of Health, National Institute of Diabetes and Digestive and Kidney Diseases, August 1993. *This is the best source of data concerning dialysis outcome available in the United States.*

TABLE 78–3. DIALYSIS COMPLICATIONS

Peritoneal Dialysis	Hemodialysis
Peritonitis	Hypotension
Abdominal hernias	Hypoxia
Diminished peritoneal ultrafiltration	Nausea, vomiting, and headache
Hyperglycemia	Air embolism
Protein malnutrition	Trace metal intoxication

Complications Common to Both Types of Dialysis

Hepatitis, infection, osteodystrophy, heart disease

78.2 Renal Transplantation

In the 1920's, Alexis Carrel developed the technique of vascular anastomoses. This momentous surgical breakthrough made possible David Hume's and Joseph Murray's human allograft attempts in the early 1950's. Similarly, Willem Kolff fashioned dialysis techniques and machinery that set the stage for George Thorn's group at Harvard Medical School to advance clinical dialysis to a viable and familiar therapy. Both accomplishments eventually joined, with synergistic results, to effect truly dramatic changes in managing chronic renal disease.

Those involved in other forms of organ transplantation envy the advantages produced by combining dialysis techniques with allograft transplantation. Because of the combination of these two effective renal replacement therapies, the volume of kidney transplant operations is vastly greater than that of other transplantation procedures. Patients can freely move back and forth between dialysis and transplantation so that life does not depend on only one form of treatment. Kidney transplantation leads the field of organ replacement therapies by a large and growing margin.

Other advances in knowledge flow from these milestone developments. Peter Medawar's description of second-set reactions and his insights into cellular immunology were pre-eminent advances in thinking. Both ideas are still actively advancing our understanding of human life. The close collaboration of pharmaceutical companies and clinical researchers resulted in azathioprine, which made kidney transplantation possible in nonrelated individuals. The advance in kidney transplantation is perhaps medicine's success story of the 1980's.

IMMUNOLOGIC ASPECTS OF KIDNEY TRANSPLANTATION. In kidney transplantation, the translation of understanding of the human immune system into clear-cut clinical advances is dramatic. Small lymphocytes are central to the problem of kidney allograft rejection. Both T and B lymphocytes are important players in kidney allograft rejection. B lymphocytes make circulating antibodies. The T lymphocyte, however, is critical: Acute rejection depends on the presence of T lymphocytes.

T lymphocytes constitute a heterogeneous group (see Ch. 221): helper, suppressor, cytotoxic, and natural-killer (NK) T lymphocytes are recognized by the presence of characteristic antigens on their cell membranes. The helper T lymphocyte is required for the rejection process. It participates in initial recognition of foreign antigen on transplanted tissue. Foreign antigens stimulate the T helper lymphocyte to release lymphokines that produce both growth and differentiation of other T and B lymphocytes.

Newly developed immunosuppressive agents target T lymphocytes and the lymphokines they produce. These new agents may be

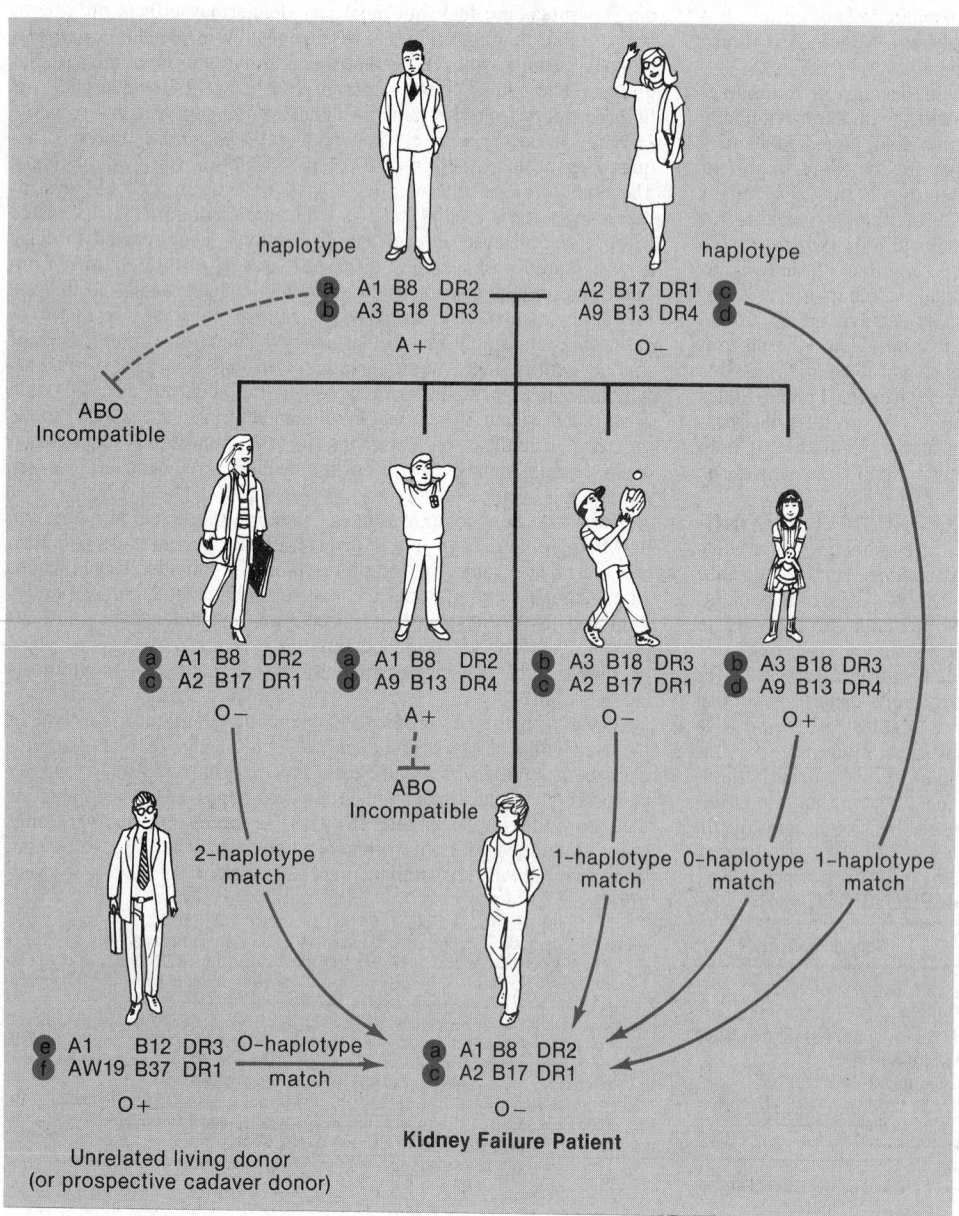

FIGURE 78–3. Family tree of HLA genotypes and unrelated HLA genotype.

both more potent and more specific than those used in the past. Further understanding of the methods by which foreign antigens are presented to lymphocytes and the lymphokine communication network (in which the T helper cell is central) will yield more specific immunosuppression.

The major histocompatibility complex (MHC) (see Ch. 229), which in humans is on chromosome 6, codes for two classes of antigens (class I [A, B, and C] and class II [D, DR, DQ, DP, and DO]) on cell membranes. Inheritance of these cell antigen markers is co-dominant. Each parent transmits one set of HLA antigens (haplotype) to his/her child. Nearly all cells, except red blood cells, express class I antigens, while B lymphocytes, monocytes, and endothelial cells express class II antigens. These antigens are pivotal in the rejection process.

Transplantation usually succeeds if all known class I and class II antigens between donor and recipient are identical. Unfortunately, from a matching perspective, the MHC is the most polymorphic coding system known in human biology. Most donors and recipients cannot be matched perfectly for MHC-coded antigens unless the organ comes from a close family member. Figure 78–3 shows that siblings of a given patient with end-stage renal disease (ESRD) may be either two-haplotype matches (25% likelihood), one-haplotype matches (50% likelihood), or zero-haplotype matches (25% likelihood). True parents are usually a one-haplotype match. As noted in Figure 78–3, ABO blood groups also must be compatible to ensure successful transplantation.

In animals and human recipients of kidney allografts, matching for both class I and class II antigens correlates with successful graft outcomes. The source of most human kidney transplants, however, is a cadaveric donor (a donor who has died but whose kidneys are still viable). Finding a good HLA match is more difficult from cadavers than from blood relatives. Although retrospective analysis of cadaveric transplantation data shows the benefit of class I and class II matching, the benefit is not as dramatic as for kidneys from relatives. Recently, new methods of identifying cell antigens using "DNA typing" have shown that the previous typing was not as accurate as thought. This improvement in technology may increase the benefit of typing in cadaver transplants.

Transplantation centers in the United States currently follow a policy of mandatory sharing of six-antigen (both class I and class II) matches for cadaveric kidneys. Organ banks consider other factors besides HLA match (e.g., the patient's age and length of time on a waiting list) in distributing cadaveric kidneys.

Unquestionably important for both living-related transplantation and cadaveric transplantation is the "crossmatch" test. Tissue-typing laboratories perform this test before all kidney transplant operations. Technicians incubate leukocytes from the potential donor (living-related or cadaveric) with serum from the potential recipient and serum complement. If the serum of the recipient destroys the membranes of the leukocyte of the potential donor, the laboratory reports the test as positive.

The surgeon usually cancels the transplant operation if the crossmatch is positive. Such a result signifies circulating antibodies against the HLA antigens. A positive crossmatch predicts nearly immediate and severe ("hyperacute") allograft rejection if the transplant is done. Investigators are testing modifications of the crossmatching procedure to find a more sensitive yet more specific test. The current tests, however, have all but eliminated hyperacute rejections. More sensitive tests could decrease other types of early rejection ("accelerated rejections").

Currently, many patients on waiting lists for kidney transplants have developed broad anti-HLA sensitization. Exposure to blood transfusions, failed previous transplants, or pregnancy causes such sensitization to HLA antigens. Nearly one-third of patients awaiting transplantation fall into this "highly sensitized," difficult-to-transplant category. Such patients benefit from receiving the best HLA antigen match possible.

Physicians have tried other strategies such as plasmapheresis and extracorporeal immunoadsorption to find a suitable method of overcoming the problem of circulating preformed antibodies. These trials offer promise but are not yet established practice. The more common use of erythropoietin in patients awaiting transplantation will reduce the exposure to blood transfusions. Introducing this new therapy to dialysis promises to decrease the rate of development and degree of circulating antibodies in patients with ESRD.

INDICATIONS FOR KIDNEY TRANSPLANTATION. The most common diseases that result in referring patients for transplantation are (1) diabetes mellitus with renal failure, (2) hypertensive renal disease, and (3) glomerulonephritis. These three causes of ESRD account for nearly 75% of candidates.

No specific cause of intrinsic and irreversible renal failure is considered a contraindication to kidney transplantation. Nonetheless, all patients still should have reversible causes of renal dysfunction excluded (e.g., incomplete obstruction) before considering renal replacement therapy. Most patients undergo a period of chronic dialysis prior to receiving an allograft. Table 78–4 lists select diseases that can cause renal failure and need special consideration before choosing renal transplantation as a therapy. The listed diseases are not contraindications for transplantation, yet the outcome may be less satisfactory for patients with these diseases as compared with other renal diseases.

Patients with renal failure induced by diabetes (Kimmelstiel-Wilson disease) make up the greatest population of patients currently referred for transplantation. A decade ago such patients were not routinely considered for kidney transplantation, but today many nephrologists consider this the treatment of choice. The change in medical practice for this condition has resulted in a major extension of the life expectancy of patients whose kidneys fail from diabetes.

The long-term outcome for patients with diabetes is less likely to result in full rehabilitation than for patients with forms of renal disease that do not have other organ involvement. Although allograft replacement restores normal renal function to such patients, kidney transplantation does not correct the diabetes. Long-term complications of diabetes do not reverse, and new complications develop. Eventually, other organ involvement with diabetic disease limits both survival and rehabilitation in diabetic recipients of renal allografts.

Today, living-related transplantation offers patients with diabetic renal failure the highest likelihood of prolonged survival. Most centers perform transplantations earlier in diabetic patients than in those referred for other forms of renal disease. If diabetic patients can undergo transplantation before extensive damage occurs in other organs, such as the eye and heart, rehabilitation will be more satisfactory. Late referral of diabetic patients is not in their best interest. Such patients may develop severe neurologic and cardiovascular disease to a degree that excludes them from transplantation.

Hypertension is better treated than in the past, yet the incidence of end-stage renal failure due to hypertension has not decreased. It ranks second only to diabetes as a cause of renal failure in patients sent to renal transplant units. Such patients often have suffered from a malignant phase of hypertension. It is more common for elevated blood pressure to destroy the kidneys of black patients than white patients. Kidney transplantation in this group of patients often restores normal renal function and normal blood pressure control. The reason the numbers of patients referred to transplant centers with end-stage failure due to hypertension are not decreasing is unclear and deserves intensive investigation. Black patients tend to have slightly poorer success with renal transplants than white patients.

The various forms of glomerulonephritis usually progress

TABLE 78–4. FACTORS LIMITING SUCCESS OF RENAL TRANSPLANTATION IN CERTAIN DISEASES

Disease	Comment
Hemolytic uremic syndrome	Disease can recur and cause graft failure rapidly; cyclosporine may increase the risk of recurrence.
Sickle cell disease	Improved hematocrit can result in increased incidence of sickle crises.
Scleroderma	Long-term vascular and gastrointestinal problems of scleroderma can limit rehabilitation.
Oxalosis	Recurrence of stone disease can be severe.
Cystinosis and Fabry's disease	Disease activity continues.
Focal glomerulosclerosis	Graft loss from recurrence is common.

(slowly) to end-stage function (see Ch. 79). Patients with these diseases are ideal candidates for kidney transplantation. They often have no medical problems other than their kidney disease, and replacing kidney function restores them to normal health. Rehabilitation can be excellent in this group of patients.

However, there is one form of glomerulonephritis (see Table 78–4) that causes continuing difficulty in renal transplant centers. Focal glomerulosclerosis (FGS) is an idiopathic form of glomerulonephritis that (like many other forms of glomerulonephritis) can recur in the allograft. Patients with FGS have a rate of graft loss from recurrent disease (20 to 30%) that is greater than in other forms of glomerular disease. The problem of recurrence of disease should be discussed with patients and prospective family kidney donors. The histologic lesion of focal sclerosis can occur in other circumstances (e.g., reflux nephritis), and recurrence in the allograft does not appear to be a problem in such cases.

Age is never an absolute contraindication for kidney transplantation. Although infants have had successful transplantations, most centers maintain infants on dialysis until body size is increased to 10 to 20 kg. Older patients are becoming more numerous in transplant clinics. Older age (>60 years) never precludes transplantation, but it increases the risk of complications. Transplant centers usually encourage older patients who have multiple medical problems (rather than isolated kidney failure) to remain on dialysis. On both ends of the age spectrum, however, transplantation is becoming more common.

Malignancy is considered a contraindication for kidney transplantation, as is severe atherosclerotic or pulmonary disease. Patients with active liver disease are also usually excluded. Both hepatitis B and C can result in eventual liver failure in some patients after transplantation. How best to screen patients infected with these agents and who to avoid transplanting are problems currently under active investigation. Infection with the HIV virus is a relative contraindication. Case reports suggest that such patients progress more rapidly from carrier status to clinical AIDS when given immunosuppressive therapy. Social circumstances (inability to take medications or arrange follow-up) also can make kidney transplantation an impossibility.

EVALUATING THE DONOR AND RECIPIENT OF THE KIDNEY TRANSPLANT.

The transplant team that will perform the surgery and follow-up should evaluate the donor (living-related) and potential recipient of the transplant. This is best done at the transplant center, before the actual transplantation date. The evaluation team usually includes a transplant surgeon, nephrologist, transplant nurse, urologist, social worker, and psychiatrist.

Evaluating the living donor focuses on three issues. Physicians must document that the patient does not have significant medical problems that would increase the risk of surgery. The donor's motives should be appraised to ensure that they are altruistic. Finally, the renal function and anatomy of the donor's renal arteries need to be defined, usually with a renal arteriogram. This evaluation is best performed in the hospital.

Evaluating the recipient also has three goals. Physicians should assess the patient's overall medical status, since the recipient may face both major surgery and potent immunosuppression in the future. Emphasis should be placed on the recipient's cardiovascular risks and urologic status. The recipient's original disease often is uncertain, and the transplant center should attempt to clarify the diagnosis. Knowledge of the original kidney disease is important in managing the patient after the transplant. Finally, the recipient needs to discuss the risks and benefits of transplantation surgery.

The patient's social circumstances need evaluation. A discussion that explores the patient's understanding of the disease process and the planned intervention is part of the evaluation. Both audiovisual aids and personal discussions with nurses, physicians, and other kidney transplant patients are key to preparing the patient.

Potential recipients found to have correctable cardiovascular or urologic lesions are encouraged to have them repaired before transplantation. Bilateral nephrectomy of native kidneys before transplantation is rarely done. In the past, this was a more common procedure to control severe hypertension. A nephrectomy is also suggested if the native kidneys are infected in such a fashion that only by removing them will the patient be protected from serious infections after transplantation. Occasionally, patients excrete such large amounts of protein from diseased native kidneys that nephrectomy is recommended because of protein malnutrition.

Preparing the recipient with deliberate blood transfusions was a common procedure before routine use of cyclosporine. It is no longer as popular as in the past. An understanding of the mechanism by which such blood transfusions altered rejection, however, promises to increase our understanding of immune responses.

THE ADMISSION FOR KIDNEY TRANSPLANTATION.

Cadaveric transplant operations are more "planned" than in the past. Improved allograft harvesting has removed some (but not all) of the urgency from the procedure. It is not elective surgery, however, and time remains an important factor. The pretransplantation evaluation of the recipient prepares the patient for the actual day of the transplantation.

During this admission, the transplant surgeon places a kidney allograft into the recipient's iliac fossa. An anastomosis is created between the donor renal artery and the hypogastric artery. The surgeon also must connect the donor renal vein to the iliac vein and implant the ureter to the recipient's bladder. These three connections all have variations, and all need skillful surgical technique.

On return from the operating room, three issues face the patient. If the kidney is not working immediately ("immediate nonfunction"), the reasons need to be identified. If the kidney is working, careful observation for possible rejection is begun. In either case, a new immunosuppressive regimen starts.

Immediate nonfunction of the allograft is less common with improvement of techniques for procurement and storage. It is due, most often, to an acute tubular necrosis (ATN)–like syndrome in which there is reversible ischemic damage to the allograft that will heal, given time. Recent evidence suggests that this phenomenon, while similar to classic ATN, differs in that the immune system plays a major role.

Obstruction, vascular thrombosis, and ureteral compression from hematoma should be considered in cases of primary nonfunction. Renal scans and ultrasound tests, as well as the patience of the managing physician, are indicated. Occasionally, immediate return to the operating room is required. Most patients with immediate nonfunction, however, have reversible renal impairment that does not require surgical intervention.

Allografts that work immediately after releasing the vascular clamps engender immediate optimism. Observation is key in the postoperative management. It is usually in the first three months after transplantation that reversible acute rejections occur. Many of these rejections will occur during the initial hospital stay. All patients should have daily assessment of renal function, and when physicians notice impairment, a rapid diagnosis of cause (rejection versus other causes) is in order. Despite pressures to cut costs, early discharge is not in the best interest of the kidney transplant patient.

During the first hospital stay, patients are given potent immunosuppressive agents. Immunosuppressive regimens remained stable from the 1960's through the early 1980's. Azathioprine and prednisone were the two drugs used. Physicians became experienced with these two agents and with their predictable complications.

The Food and Drug Administration (FDA) approved cyclosporine in 1983. Since then, the transplant community has developed a frenzy for new and different immunosuppressive protocols. Transplant centers often change to new protocols before research groups test the older protocols with controlled, randomized trials. Nonetheless, as transplant groups have experimented with new and different immunosuppressive agents, results have improved markedly over the results seen in previous years.

Currently, many centers in the United States use sequential or "induction" therapy. Initially, either antilymphocyte globulin (ALG) or monoclonal antibody (OKT3) is given as the primary immunosuppressant agent. These anti–T lymphocyte agents are continued until the allograft functions well. Then, cyclosporine, azathioprine, and prednisone are added, and ALG or OKT3 is discontinued shortly thereafter. Other groups begin with a regimen of cyclosporine, azathioprine, and prednisone immediately preceding the transplant operation ("triple-drug therapy"). Some groups believe that a combination of cyclosporine and prednisone or cyclosporine alone is adequate therapy.

Adding cyclosporine and routinely using anti–T lymphocyte agents, while credited with improved allograft success rates, makes management more complex. Cyclosporine can result in impaired renal function that is difficult to distinguish from rejection. OKT3 and

ALG can cause febrile reactions (so-called first-dose reactions) and may result in renal dysfunction.

Cyclosporine has revolutionized organ transplantation. Transplant groups have achieved a 10 to 15% improvement in initial and long-term allograft survival rates with cyclosporine. Some investigators believe that the added immunosuppression of this agent overcomes the risks of rejection with poorly matched allografts. Others suggest that preparing of recipients with pretransplant blood transfusions is no longer necessary.

Unfortunately, one of cyclosporine's major side effects is nephrotoxicity. Investigators have shown acute, "reversible," and chronic kidney damage. Cyclosporine slows recovery from ATN and potentiates nephrotoxicity due to other substances. Cyclosporine is difficult to monitor, and clinical toxicity is common even in experienced hands. Besides nephrotoxicity, cyclosporine commonly causes tremor, palmar and plantar paresthesia, hyperglycemia, hepatotoxicity, hypertrichosis, gingival hypertrophy, and hyperkalemia. Currently, OKT3 is the only monoclonal antibody commercially available. The antibody is directed against the T lymphocyte receptor for antigen and is thus a "pan" T lymphocyte agent. More specific monoclonal antibodies remain in investigational status. OKT3 is effective for the treatment of acute rejection. Patients who do not respond to traditional acute rejection therapy (bolus methylprednisolone) usually respond to OKT3. OKT3 is also used in the immediate posttransplant period as part of some sequential protocols. It is one of the most potent agents available for reversing and preventing T lymphocyte–mediated rejection.

Like cyclosporine, however, OKT3 has several drawbacks. Antibodies against this murine antibody develop and may limit its effectiveness. After a single course of treatment, many patients will not respond to further therapy.

OUTPATIENT FOLLOW-UP. If the transplant admission is uncomplicated, it is possible for patients to be discharged as early as a week after surgery. Unless arrangements can be made for daily outpatient visits after discharge, however, most centers keep patients in the hospital for longer periods. Complications can lengthen this first admission to months. Geography, financial resources of patients, facilities of the center, and clinical judgment of physicians involved result in initial hospital stays that vary markedly in length. Nonetheless, whether patients are in the hospital or are outpatients, the two major problems faced are infection and rejection.

Two forms of rejection have been alluded to previously: hyperacute rejection and accelerated rejection. Both, by definition, occur before the end of the first week. Hyperacute rejection is rare with current crossmatch techniques. Accelerated rejections are less well understood, are more common, and often do not respond to therapy. More sensitive crossmatch techniques might decrease the frequency of accelerated rejections.

Acute and chronic rejections are more common. These episodes usually occur after the first week and can occur at any time, even years after the transplant. Mediated by T lymphocytes, such rejections are often associated with marked cellular infiltration of the allograft with edema. Kidney vascular lesions also occur and suggest a poor prognosis.

Most acute rejection episodes, if diagnosed early, will respond to therapy with increased dosages of immunosuppressive agents. Diagnosis is suggested by a sudden impairment of function. Confirmation of acute rejection is obtained with renal scans and allograft biopsies.

Chronic rejection is a phenomenon less well understood than acute rejection. Most cadaveric allografts eventually show histologic changes of rejection. These changes are vascular and are similar to the histology of nephrosclerosis. Eventually, the allograft develops fibrosis and glomerular lesions that appear secondary to ischemia. There is neither a good understanding of chronic rejection nor an accepted effective therapy.

Serial "flowsheet" measurements of serum creatinine concentration reveal a gradual trend for slow but progressive impairment of allograft function. The renal scan reveals a more marked loss of renal blood flow than of glomerular filtration rate (GFR), and renal biopsy reveals fibrosis and vascular narrowing. Patients are generally asymptomatic. Recurrence of original kidney disease and cyclosporine toxicity are two other causes of allograft impairment that can mimic chronic rejection.

Renal scans and isotope measurements of renal blood flow (^{131}I-orthoiodohippurate) and GFR (^{99m}Tc-diethylenetriamine) are used frequently to provide additional functional assessment of renal function. Ultrasound has proven useful to visualize the structure of the allograft and to rule out obstruction. Arteriography of the transplant renal artery is useful to diagnose stenosis. Although an invasive procedure, an arteriogram of the allograft also can provide information about the small vessels of the allograft in a more global fashion than renal biopsy. Biopsy of the allograft is also an invasive procedure. Transplant physicians believe that it gives the most useful assessment of the allograft and helps differentiate the causes of allograft dysfunction. When other clinical assessment leaves considerable doubt in the mind of the managing physician concerning the cause of impaired function, a biopsy is indicated. More recently, the technique of fine-needle biopsy has gained popularity. This technique is considerably safer than the percutaneous core biopsy, yet its sensitivity and specificity remain controversial.

Infections during the first few weeks after transplantation cause fever and can impair allograft function. They may be confused with rejection. Wound, intravenous line, and catheter-related infections are common and not usually due to opportunistic organisms when they occur within a few weeks of transplantation.

Opportunistic infections usually occur a month or more after the transplant operation. While *Aspergillus, Nocardia,* and *Toxoplasma* were once common, newer immunosuppressive protocols have resulted in a change in the spectrum of opportunistic infections. Viral infections, especially cytomegalovirus, have become dominant. Many investigators believe this is a result of using more specific anti–T lymphocyte preparations, such as OKT3. Infection with cytomegalovirus can be asymptomatic or can be so severe as to cause coma and death. Fortunately, most of these infections after transplantation, characterized by spiking fevers, leukopenia, and general malaise, last only 1 to 2 weeks and then resolve without sequelae.

Immunosuppressed kidney transplant patients believed to be infected should be hospitalized and aggressively managed. Infections in this group are the leading early cause of mortality, and aggressive management can reverse the process without need of sacrificing the allograft.

LONG-TERM FOLLOW-UP. Long-term immunosuppression is surprisingly well tolerated by most kidney transplant recipients. Nonetheless, it is this therapy that accounts for most of the posttransplant morbidity and mortality. Vascular disease, infections, malignancy, and chronic liver disease pose the most serious problems for recipients of kidney transplants. Immunosuppressive agents either cause or aggravate these four medical problems. Table 78–5 lists some of the more common medical problems that are seen in kidney transplant clinics.

Like the general population, kidney transplant patients are most likely to die of atherosclerotic vascular disease. Kidney transplant patients, however, die of myocardial infarctions and cerebral vascular accidents at an earlier age. The reason for this precocious onset of vascular disease is not understood.

Kidney transplant patients experience a high incidence of hypertension, which is multifactorial in nature. Some immunosuppressive drugs (cyclosporine and prednisone) can cause hypertension, as does kidney disease. Even if the allograft is normal, the diseased native kidneys can maintain elevated blood pressure. Stenosis of the artery of the transplanted kidney is another cause of such hypertension. Abnormal lipid profiles in kidney transplant patients are a risk factor for atherosclerotic death. These abnormal lipid patterns are believed to be an effect of the immunosuppressive drugs. Besides hypertension and abnormal lipid profiles, there is convincing evidence that renal transplant patients usually have vascular disease even before the transplant. This vascular disease is associated with their chronic renal failure.

Most successful recipients of renal transplants enjoy a quality of life superior to that achieved on dialysis. Women frequently give birth after transplantation, and men can father children. It is unusual for patients with successful transplants not to return to employment. Many return to a lifestyle similar to that preceding the onset of kidney disease. On the other hand, the experience of chronic disease, frequent hospitalizations, disability financing, and fear of allograft failure with long-term complications of transplant immunosuppression limit full rehabilitation for some patients.

In the United States in 1989, the average 1-year allograft survival rate was 79% for recipients of cadaveric kidneys. This is a remark-

TABLE 78–5. MEDICAL COMPLICATIONS AFTER KIDNEY TRANSPLANTATION

Cardiovascular events
 Myocardial infarction
 Cerebrovascular accident
Hypertension
 Stenosis of transplant renal artery
 Native kidney–induced
 Drug-induced
 Renal impairment of the allograft
Malignancies
 Skin carcinomas
 Lymphomas
Erythrocytosis
 Induced by native kidneys (?)
 Thromboembolic disease
Bone disease
 Osteoporosis
 Aseptic necrosis
 Persistent hyperparathyroidism
Infections
 Listeria monocytogenes
 Pneumocystis carinii
 Cryptococcus
 Aspergillus
 Nocardia
 Toxoplasma
 Mycobacterium
 Legionella pneumophila
 Cytomegalovirus (CMV)
 Herpes simplex virus (HSV)
 Varicella-zoster virus (VZV)
 Hepatitis viruses
 Papovaviruses
 Human immunodeficiency virus (HIV)
 Epstein-Barr virus (EBV)
Gastrointestinal problems
 Peptic ulcer
 Pancreatitis
 Diverticulitis
 Hepatitis
Glucocorticoid-induced complications
 Obesity
 Cataracts
 Hyperglycemia
 Myopathy
Endocrine and metabolic disorders
 Secondary hyperparathyroidism
 Proximal and distal types of renal tubular acidosis
 Asymptomatic hyperuricemia and gout
 Mild hyperkalemia
 Glycosuria without an increased serum glucose concentration
 Hypophosphatemia
Miscellaneous
 Idiopathic polyarthritides
 Hirsutism
 Lymphocele
 Warts
 Psychiatric affective disorders

able advance compared with survival rates of 50% for cadaveric kidneys just a few years ago. Mortality and morbidity continue to decrease as allograft survival rates increase. It seems likely that even these rates of success will improve in the near future. New immunosuppressive agents that are currently in clinical trials, such as FK-506, rapamycin, and RS-61443 (mycophenolic acid), hold promise of improving allograft success and patient survival rates.

Success can create problems. The number of patients on waiting lists for kidney transplantation is growing faster than the number of transplant operations that are possible. The shortage of donor kidneys is the most consequential limitation of kidney transplantation.

Alexander JW: The cutting edge: A look to the future of transplantation. Transplantation 49:237, 1990. *A review of the growth of kidney transplantation and predictions about future growth.*

Class FHJ, van Rood JJ: The hyperimmunized patient: From sensitization toward treatment. Transplant Int 1:53, 1988. *The reasons that patients develop antibodies against HLA antigens and current strategies for dealing with this problem are reviewed.*

Combined Report on Regular Dialysis and Transplantation in Europe, XIX, 1988. Nephrology Dialysis Trans 4(Suppl 4):5, 1989. *A review of recent trends in immunosuppressive regimens in Europe.*

Kahan BD: Cyclosporine. N Engl J Med 321:1725, 1989. *A detailed description of cyclosporine from pharmacology to future prospects.*

Shapiro ME, Reed MH, Strom TB, et al.: The role of a primate model of renal transplantation in the development of new monoclonal antibodies. Am J Kidney Dis 14(Suppl 2):58, 1989. *A brief description of testing of new monoclonal antibodies.*

79 GLOMERULAR DISORDERS
Gerald B. Appel

Glomerular diseases affect many millions of persons in the United States and worldwide. In 1990, in the United States >200,000 person were in end-stage renal disease (ESRD) programs, largely as a result of renal involvement by glomerular diseases. One form of glomerular damage alone, diabetic glomerulonephropathy, affects millions of persons in the United States with a cost to the government of billions of dollars annually. Worldwide, glomerular disease associated with infectious agents such as malaria and schistosomiasis are major health problems. In both this country and elsewhere the recent emergence of glomerular diseases linked to viral causes, such as human immunodeficiency virus (HIV) and hepatitis B and C, have focused new attention on the patterns and mechanisms of glomerular injury. The manifestations of glomerular injury may be as subtle as the asymptomatic presence of microhematuria and albuminuria or as dramatic as the abrupt onset of oliguria and severe renal failure. Other patients develop massive fluid retention with peripheral and periorbital edema as presenting symptoms and signs of glomerular damage, whereas still others present only with the slow insidious signs and symptoms of chronic renal failure.

The mechanisms of the glomerular injury are quite varied. Although certain common mechanisms may underlie the hematuria and proteinuria (e.g., loss of the glomerular charge barrier), the nature of the processes initiating this damage differ. Immune-mediated renal injury is a major pathogenetic mechanism of glomerular damage. In diabetic nephropathy and amyloidosis, other mechanisms clearly are at work.

The Normal Glomerulus (see also Ch. 73 and 74)

Each glomerulus, the basic filtering unit of the kidney, consists of a tuft of anastomosing capillaries formed by the branchings of the afferent arteriole. Approximately 1 million glomeruli comprise about 5% of the kidney weight and provide almost 2 square meters of glomerular capillary filtering surface. The glomerular basement membrane (GBM) provides both a size and charge selective barrier to the passage of circulating macromolecules.

Histopathologic Terms

Renal processes involving all glomeruli are called "diffuse" or "generalized"; if only some glomeruli are involved, the process is called "focal." When dealing with the individual glomerulus, a process is "global" if the whole glomeruler tuft is involved and "segmental" if only part of the glomerulus is involved. The terms "proliferative," "sclerosing," and "necrotizing" are often used (e.g., focal and segmental sclerosing glomerulonephritis; diffuse global proliferative lupus nephritis). Extracapillary proliferation or crescent formation is caused by the accumulations of macrophages, fibroblasts, proliferating epithelial cells, and fibrin within Bowman's space. In general, crescent formation in any form of glomerular damage conveys a serious prognosis.

Clinical Manifestations of Glomerular Diseases

Several findings are common to many glomerular diseases and focus the differential diagnosis of unknown parenchymal renal diseases toward a glomerular origin. They include the findings of erythrocyte casts and/or dysmorphic erythrocytes in the urinary sediment and the presence of large amounts of albuminuria. In a normal person, the urinary excretion of albumin is <50 mg daily. Although increases in urinary protein excretion may come from the filtration of abnormal circulating proteins (such as light chains in multiple myeloma) or from the deficient proximal tubular reabsorption of normal filtered small-molecular-weight proteins (such as β_2-microglobulin), the most common cause of proteinuria and specifically albuminuria is glomerular injury. Proteinuria associated with glomerular disease may range from several hundred milligrams to >30 grams daily. In some diseases such as minimal change nephrotic syndrome, albumin is the predominant protein found in the urine. In others, such as focal sclerosing glomerulonephritis and diabetes, the proteinuria, although still largely composed of albumin, contains many larger molecular weight proteins as well and is said to be "nonselective." Proteinuria >3 to 3.5 grams daily is seen in the nephrotic syndrome (see below).

Although a small number of erythrocytes may appear in the urine of normal individuals, urinary excretion of >500 to 1000 erythrocytes per milliliter defines abnormal hematuria. Red blood cell casts, which form when erythrocytes pass the glomerular capillary barrier and become enmeshed in a proteinaceous matrix in the tubules, are also highly suggestive of glomerular disease.

THE NEPHROTIC SYNDROME

The nephrotic syndrome is classically defined by proteinuria in amounts >3 to 3.5 grams daily accompanied by hypoalbuminemia, edema, and hyperlipidemia. In clinical practice many nephrologists refer to "nephrotic range" proteinuria regardless of whether their patients have the other manifestations of the full syndrome because the latter are consequences of the proteinuria.

Hypoalbuminemia is in part a consequence of urinary protein loss. It is also due to the catabolism of filtered albumin by the proximal tubule as well as to redistribution of albumin within the body. This, in part, accounts for the inexact relationship between urinary protein loss, the level of the serum albumin, and other secondary consequences of heavy albuminuria.

The salt and volume retention in the nephrotic syndrome may occur through at least two different major mechanisms. In the classic theory, proteinuria leads to hypoalbuminemia, a low plasma oncotic pressure, and intravascular volume depletion. Subsequent underperfusion of the kidney stimulates the priming of sodium-retentive hormonal systems such as the renin-angiotensin-aldosterone axis, causing increased renal sodium and volume retention. In the peripheral capillaries with normal hydrostatic pressures and decreased oncotic pressure, the Starling forces lead to transcapillary fluid leakage and edema. In some patients, however, the intravascular volume has been measured and found to be increased along with suppression of the renin-angiotensin-aldosterone axis. An animal model of unilateral proteinuria shows evidence for primary renal sodium retention at a distal nephron site, perhaps due to altered responsiveness to hormones such as atrial natriuretic factor. Here only the proteinuric kidney retains sodium and volume and at a time when the animal is not yet hypoalbuminemic. Thus local factors within the kidney may account for the volume retention of the nephrotic patient as well.

A recent epidemiologic study has strongly supported an increased risk of atherosclerotic complications in the nephrotic syndrome. Moreover, many nephrotic patients have additional risk factors besides hyperlipidemia for cardiovascular disease, including hypertension, smoking, and left ventricular hypertrophy. Most nephrotic patients have elevated levels of total and LDL cholesterol with low or normal HDL cholesterol.

Initial evaluation of the nephrotic patient includes a variety of simple laboratory tests to define whether the patient has primary, idiopathic nephrotic syndrome or a secondary cause related to a systemic disease. Commonly used screening tests include the fasting blood sugar to exclude diabetes, an antinuclear antibody test to exclude collagen vascular disease, and the serum complement, which screens for many immune complex–mediated diseases (Table 79–1). In selected patients cryoglobulins, hepatitis B and C serology, antineutrophil cytoplasmic antibodies, anti-GBM antibodies, and the Venereal Disease Research Laboratory (VDRL) test may be useful. Once secondary causes have been excluded, treating the adult nephrotic patient often requires a renal biopsy to define the pattern of glomerular involvement. In adults the nephrotic syndrome is a common condition leading to renal biopsy. In many studies patients with heavy proteinuria and the nephrotic syndrome have been a group highly likely to benefit from renal biopsy in terms of a change in specific diagnosis, prognosis, and therapy. Selected adult nephrotic patients such as the elderly have a slightly

TABLE 79-1. SERUM COMPLEMENT LEVELS IN GLOMERULAR DISEASES

Diseases with a reduced complement level
Poststreptococcal glomerulonephritis
Subacute bacterial endocarditis–visceral abscess–shunt nephritis
Systemic lupus erythematosus
Cryoglobulinemia
Idiopathic membranoproliferative glomerulonephritis

Diseases associated with a normal serum complement
Minimal change nephrotic syndrome
Focal segmental glomerulosclerosis
Membranous nephropathy
IgA nephropathy
Henoch-Schönlein purpura
Anti-GBM disease
Pauci-immune rapidly progressive glomerulonephritis
Polyarteritis nodosa
Wegener's granulomatosis

different spectrum of disease, but once again the renal biopsy is the best guide to treatment and prognosis (Tables 79–2 and 79–3).

Idiopathic Nephrotic Syndrome

MINIMAL CHANGE DISEASE. Minimal change disease, also known as "nil disease" and "lipoid nephrosis," is the most common pattern of idiopathic nephrotic syndrome in children and comprises up to 20% of idiopathic nephrotic syndrome in adults. A similar histologic pattern may be seen as an adverse reaction to certain medications (nonsteroidal anti-inflammatory drugs [NSAID's], lithium) and associated with certain tumors (Hodgkin's disease and leukemias). Patients typically present with periorbital and peripheral edema related to the proteinuria. Proteinuria is usually well into the nephrotic range. Additional findings in adults are hypertension and microscopic hematuria, each in about 30%. However, active urinary sediment with erythrocyte casts is not found. Many adult patients have mild to moderate azotemia, which may be related to hypoalbuminemia and intravascular volume depletion. Complement levels and serologic tests are normal in minimal change disease.

In true minimal change disease histopathology typically reveals no glomerular abnormalities in the light microscopy (LM) (see Color Plate 4A). The tubules may show lipid droplet accumulation from absorbed lipoproteins (hence the older term "lipoid nephrosis"). Immunofluorescence staining (IF) and electron microscopy (EM) (Fig. 79–1) show no immune-type deposits. By EM the GBM is normal, and effacement or "fusion" of the visceral epithelial foot processes is noted along virtually the entire distribution of every capillary loop.

The course of minimal change nephrotic syndrome is often one of remissions and relapses and responses to additional treatment. When treated with corticosteroids for 8 weeks, 90 to 95% of children experience a remission of the nephrotic syndrome. In adults the response rate is somewhat lower, with 75 to 85% of patients responding to regimens of daily (60 mg per day) or alternate day (120 mg q.o.d.) prednisone therapy, tapered after 2 months of treatment. The time to clinical response may be slower in adults, and they should not be considered steroid-resistant until they have failed to respond to 16 weeks of treatment. Tapering of the steroid dose should begin one to several weeks after complete remission and should continue gradually over 1 to 2 months. Both children and adults are likely to have a relapse of their minimal change disease once steroids have been discontinued. Approximately 30% of adults relapse by 1 year, and 50% by 5 years. Most clinicians treat the

TABLE 79-2. CAUSES OF THE NEPHROTIC SYNDROME

Idiopathic or Primary Nephrotic Syndrome	Incidence (%)
Minimal change disease	20
Focal segmental glomerulosclerosis	15–20
Membranous nephropathy	25–30
Membranoproliferative glomerulonephritis	5–10
Other proliferative and sclerosing glomerulonephritides	15–30

TABLE 79–3. NEPHROTIC SYNDROME ASSOCIATED WITH SPECIFIC CAUSES ("SECONDARY" NEPHROTIC SYNDROME)

I. Systemic diseases
  A. Diabetes mellitus
  B. Systemic lupus erythematosus and other collagen diseases
  C. Amyloidosis (amyloid AL or AA associated)
  D. Vasculitic-immunologic diseases (mixed cryoglobulinemia, Wegener's granulomatosis, RPGN, polyarteritis, Henoch-Schönlein purpura, sarcoidosis, Goodpasture's syndrome)

II. Infections
  A. Bacterial (post-streptococcal, congenital and secondary syphilis, subacute/acute bacterial endocarditis, shunt nephritis)
  B. Viral (hepatitis B, hepatitis C, HIV, infectious mononucleosis, cytomegalovirus)
  C. Parasitic (malaria, toxoplasmosis, schistosomiasis, filariasis)

III. Medication-related
  A. Gold, mercury, and the heavy metals
  B. Penicillamine
  C. Nonsteroidal anti-inflammatory drugs
  D. Lithium
  E. Paramethadione, trimethadione
  F. Captopril
  G. "Street" heroin
  H. Others—probenecid, chlorpropamide, rifampin, tobutamide, phenindione

IV. Allergens, venoms, and immunizations

V. Associated with neoplasms
  A. Hodgkin's lymphoma and leukemia-lymphomas (with minimal change lesion)
  B. Solid tumors (with membranous nephropathy)

VI. Hereditary and metabolic disease
  A. Alport's syndrome
  B. Fabry's disease
  C. Sickle cell disease
  D. Congenital (Finnish type) nephrotic syndrome
  E. Familial nephrotic syndrome
  F. Nail-patella syndrome
  G. Partial lipodystrophy

VII. Other
  A. Pregnancy-related (includes preeclampsia)
  B. Transplant rejection
  C. Serum sickness
  D. Accelerated hypertensive nephrosclerosis
  E. Unilateral renal artery stenosis
  F. Massive obesity—sleep apnea
  G. Reflux nephropathy

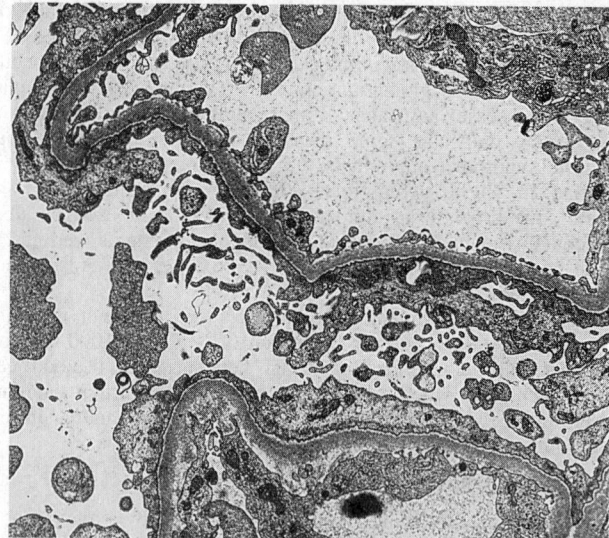

FIGURE 79–1. Minimal change disease. Electron micrograph showing widespread effacement of foot processes with microvillous transformation of the visceral epithelium. No electron-dense deposits are present (uranyl acetate, lead citrate, ×6000).

first relapse similarly to the initial nephrotic syndrome. Patients who relapse a third time or who become steroid-dependent (unable to tolerate decrease in the prednisone dose beyond a certain level without proteinuria recurring) may be treated with a 2-month course of an alkylating agent. Cyclophosphamide at a dose of 2 mg per kilogram per day has been used successfully, as has chlorambucil. Up to 50% of these patients have a prolonged remission of the nephrotic syndrome (at least 5 years). The response rate is lower in steroid-dependent patients. An alternative to an alkylating agent is low-dose cyclosporine (4 to 6 mg per kilogram per day for 4 months), but this carries the risk of nephrotoxicity and a high potential relapse rate.

FOCAL SEGMENTAL GLOMERULOSCLEROSIS.
From 15 to 20% of adults with idiopathic nephrotic syndrome are found on biopsy to have focal segmental glomerulosclerois (FSGS). FSGS is especially common in blacks with idiopathic nephrotic syndrome. This histologic diagnosis may be either idiopathic or secondary to a number of different causes (e.g., heroin abuse, HIV disease, sickle cell disease, obesity, reflux of urine from the bladder to the kidneys, and lesions associated with single or remnant kidneys.)

Patients with idiopathic FSGS typically present with either asymptomatic proteinuria or edema. Although the nephrotic syndrome is present in two thirds of patients at presentation, proteinuria may vary from <1 to 30 grams per day and is typically nonselective. Hypertension is found in 30 to 50% and microscopic hematuria in about one half of these patients. The glomerular filtration rate (GFR) is decreased at presentation in 20 to 30% of patients. Complement levels and other serologic tests are normal in FSGS.

By IF staining IgM and C3 are commonly found in the areas of glomerular sclerosis (see Color Plate 4*B*). As renal function declines, repeat biopsies show many glomeruli with segmental sclerosing lesions and increased numbers of globally sclerotic glomeruli.

Although variable, the course of untreated FSGS is usually one of progressive proteinuria and declining GFR. Only a minority of patients experience a spontaneous remission of proteinuria. Eventually most patients develop ESRD in 5 to 20 years from presentation.

The therapy of FSGS is controversial. There have been few randomized, controlled trials, and newer studies with promising results remain uncontrolled. In general, patients with a sustained remission of their nephrotic syndrome are unlikely to progress to ESRD, whereas those with unremitting nephrotic syndrome are likely to progress. Recent studies using more intensive and more prolonged immunosuppressive regimens (6 to 12 months) with steroids and cytotoxics have achieved up to a 40 to 60% remission rate of the nephrotic syndrome with preservation of long-term renal function. Low-dose cyclosporine (4 to 6 mg per kilogram per day for 2 to 6 months) has also been used with success even in patients who have been steroid- and cytotoxic-unresponsive.

MEMBRANOUS NEPHROPATHY.
Membranous nephropathy is the most common pattern of idiopathic nephrotic syndrome in white Americans. Membranous nephropathy may also be associated with infections (lues, hepatitis B and C), with systemic lupus, with certain medications (gold salts, trimethadione [Tridione]), and with certain tumors (solid tumors and lymphomas). It typically presents with the onset of proteinuria and edema. Hypertension and microhematuria are not infrequent findings, but the renal function and the GFR are usually normal at presentation. Despite the finding of complement in or within the glomerular immune deposits, serum complement levels are normal in membranous nephropathy. Membranous nephropathy is the most common pattern of the nephrotic syndrome to be associated with thrombotic events, especially renal vein thrombosis. The presence of sudden flank pain, deterioration of renal function, or symptoms of pulmonary disease in a patient with membranous nephropathy should prompt an investigation for renal vein thrombosis and pulmonary emboli.

On LM the glomerular capillary loops often appear rigid or thickened, but there is no cellular proliferation (see Color Plate 4*C*). EM shows subepithelial electron-dense deposits all along the glomerular capillary loops (Fig. 79–2).

In most large series renal survival is >75% at 10 years. There is

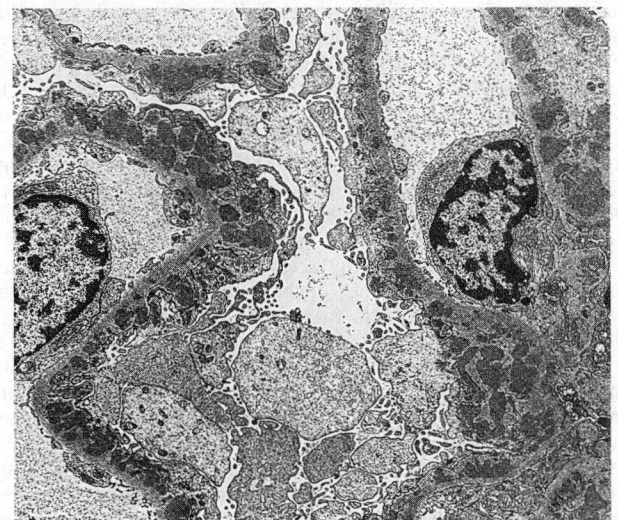

FIGURE 79–2. Membranous glomerulopathy. On ultrastructural examination, there are numerous, closely apposed epimembranous electron-dense deposits separated by basement membrane spikes (uranyl acetate, lead citrate, ×2500).

also a spontaneous remission rate of 20 to 30%. Both the slow progression and spontaneous remission rate have confounded clinical treatment trials. Several studies suggested that short-term corticosteroid therapy reduced the progression to renal insufficiency in membranous nephropathy, and another study found that longer corticosteroid therapy led to preservation of renal function and remissions of proteinuria. However, the design of these studies has been criticized, and other studies have shown no benefit of corticosteroid regimens. Recent trials with cytotoxic agents have shown promising results. A controlled trial of pulse methylprednisolone followed by oral prednisone for 1 month alternating with 1 month of oral chlorambucil has given a greater number of total remissions and better preservation of renal function. Recent controlled studies using only corticosteroids by a similar regimen have shown similar beneficial results. Once again, others believe that the good results in the treatment arms are not significantly better than the natural history of the disease. Finally, several recent studies that focus just on those membranous patients who are progressing to renal failure suggest that cyclophosphamide plus steroids can reverse progressive renal failure and cause remission of heavy proteinuria.

Idiopathic Membranoproliferative Glomerulonephritis

Membranoproliferative or mesangiocapillary glomerulonephritis (MPGN) is an uncommon glomerular disease that comprises only a small percentage of renal biopsies. By LM, similar patterns of glomerular damage have been seen in association with certain infectious agents (hepatitis B and C), autoimmune disease (systemic lupus erythematosus [SLE]), and diseases of intraglomerular coagulation. All of these stimuli have been proposed to incite the glomerular mesangial cells to grow out along the capillary wall and split the GBM. Type II MPGN, dense deposit disease, has been called an autoimmune disorder with an autoantibody (an IgG, C3 nephritic factor) directed against C3bBb, the alternate pathway C3 convertase (see Ch. 222). By preventing degradation of the enzyme, there is increased activation and consumption of complement noted in dense deposit disease.

Most patients with MPGN present with the nephrotic syndrome. Others may present with asymptomatic microhematuria and proteinuria or with an acute nephritic picture with active urinary sediment, renal insufficiency, and hypertension. Presenting findings that correlate with a poor prognosis include hypertension, a reduced GFR, and the nephrotic syndrome. A low serum complement level is found intermittently in type I MPGN, whereas the C3 level is always reduced in type II MPGN. Glomerular crescent formation and severe tubulointerstitial changes have been correlated with a poor prognosis. Most studies have found a similar course and prognosis for the various patterns of MPGN. Attempts to treat MPGN have included using corticosteroids and other immunosuppressive medications; anticoagulants and antiplatelet agents to minimize

glomerular damage from coagulation; and NSAID's. No therapy has proven to be effective in adults with MPGN.

ACUTE GLOMERULONEPHRITIS

Pathophysiology

Known inciting causes of acute glomerulonephritis include a variety of infectious agents such as upper respiratory and dermal streptococcal infections and bacterial endocarditis as well as the deposition of immune complexes in autoimmune diseases such as SLE, or the damaging effect of circulating antibodies directed against the GBM as in Goodpasture's syndrome. Regardless of the inciting cause, acute glomerulonephritis is characterized on LM by hypercellularity of the glomerulus. This may be secondary to infiltrating inflammatory cells, proliferation of resident glomerular cells, or both. Both invading inflammatory neutrophils and monocytes, as well as resident cells, can damage the glomerulous through a number of mediators, including a host of oxidants, chemoattractants, proteases, cytokines, and growth factors. Some factors, such as transforming growth factor-β, have been related to eventual glomerulosclerosis and chronic glomerular damage.

Patients with acute glomerulonephritis often present with a nephritic picture characterized by a decreased GFR and azotemia, oliguria, hypertension, and an active urinary sediment. The hypertension is caused by intravascular volume expansion, although renin levels may not be appropriately suppressed for the degree of volume expansion. Patients may note dark, smoky, or cola-colored urine in association with the active urinary sediment. This sediment is composed of erythrocytes, leukocytes, and a variety of casts, including erythrocyte casts, as damage to the glomerular capillaries allows cellular elements to exit into Bowman's space and the proximal tubule. Although many patients with acute glomerulonephritis have proteinuria, sometimes even in the nephrotic range, most patients have lesser degrees of albumin leakage into the urine, especially when the GFR is markedly reduced.

IgA Nephropathy

IgA nephropathy was originally thought to be an uncommon and benign form of glomerulopathy (Berger's disease). It is now recognized as the most frequent form of idiopathic glomerulonephritis worldwide (comprising 15 to 40% of primary glomerulonephritides in parts of Europe, Asia, and Japan) and clearly can progress to ESRD. In geographic areas where renal biopsies are commonly performed for milder urinary findings, a higher incidence of IgA has been noted. In the United States some centers report this diagnosis in up to 20% of all primary glomerulopathies. Males outnumber females, and the peak occurrence is in the second to third decade of life.

The diagnosis of IgA nephropathy is established by finding glomerular IgA deposits either as the dominant or co-dominant immunoglobulin on IF microscopy (see Color Plate 4D). Deposits of C3 and IgG are also often found. The LM picture varies from mild mesangial proliferation to crescentic glomerulonephritis. The most common picture is mesangial hypercellularity. By EM, immune-type dense deposits are typically found in the mesangial and paramesangial areas. In IgA nephropathy the predominant antibody appears to be composed of polymeric IgA1 originating in the secretory-mucosal system, but the antigen—whether viral, dietary, or other—to which it is directed is unknown in the vast majority of cases.

IGA nephropathy often presents either as asymptomatic microscopic hematuria and/or proteinuria (most common in adults), or episodic gross hematuria following upper respiratory and other infections or exercise (most common in children). The course of IgA nephropathy is variable, with some patients showing no decline in GFR over decades and others developing the nephrotic syndrome, hypertension, and renal failure. Hypertension is present in 20 to 50% of all patients. Increased serum IgA levels, noted in one third to one half of cases, do not correlate with the course of the disease.

Factors predictive of a poor outcome in IgA nephropathy have included (1) older age at onset, (2) absence of gross hematuria, (3) hypertension, (4) persistent and severe proteinuria, (5) being male, (6) an elevated serum creatinine, and (7) the histologic features of severe proliferation and sclerosis and/or tubulointerstitial damage and crescent formation. Renal survival is estimated at 85 to 90% at

10 years and 75 to 80% at 20 years. A significant percentage of patients transplanted have a morphologic recurrence in the allograft, but graft loss due to the disease is uncommon.

Because the pathogenesis of IgA nephropathy is thought to involve abnormal antigenic stimulation of mucosal IgA production and subsequent immune complex deposition in the glomeruli, treatment has been directed at these sites. Efforts to treat the disease by preventing antigenic stimulation, including broad-spectrum antibiotics (e.g., doxycycline), tonsillectomy, and dietary manipulations (e.g., gluten elimination), have been generally unsuccessful. The benefit of glucocorticoids and cytotoxic agents is far from clear; however, they have been recommended for patients with crescentic IgA nephropathy. Recent trials with fish oils have given conflicting results. With no proven therapy, many physicians choose to treat only those patients at highest risk for progression to renal failure.

Henoch-Schönlein Purpura

Henoch-Schönlein purpura (HSP) is characterized by a small-vessel vasculitis with arthralgias, skin purpura, and abdominal symptoms along with a proliferative acute glomulonephritis that has similar histopathologic features to IgA nephropathy. HSP is predominantly a disease of childhood, although cases do occur in adults. The incidence of HSP has been estimated to be as high as 18 cases per 100,000 in the pediatric age group but < 1 case per 100,000 in adult populations. Despite the finding of circulating IgA-containing immune complexes, no infectious agent or allergen has been defined as causative.

The renal histopathology of HSP is similar to that of IgA nephropathy. In the skin there is a small vessel vasculitis, a leukocytoclastic angiitis, and immune deposition of IgA.

The clinical manifestations of HSP (see Ch. 243) include dermatologic, gastrointestinal, rheumatologic, and renal findings. Skin involvement typically starts with a macular rash on the ankles that extends to the legs and occasionally the arms and buttocks. The macules darken and coalesce into purpuric lesions that are often palpable. Gastrointestinal symptoms include cramps, diarrhea, and less frequently nausea and vomiting. Melena and bloody diarrhea are present in the most severely involved cases. Although arthralgias of the knees, wrists, and ankles are common, true arthritis is uncommon. Symptoms of different organ system involvement may occur concurrently or separately, and recurrent episodes during the first year are not uncommon.

Like IgA nephropathy, HSP has no proven therapy. Episodes of rash, arthralgias, and abdominal symptoms usually resolve spontaneously. Some patients with severe abdominal findings have been treated with short courses of high-dose corticosteroids. Patients with severe glomerular involvement may benefit by modalities used to treat patients with severe IgA nephropathy. Although most patients with HSP recover fully, patients with a more severe nephritic or nephrotic presentation and more severe glomerular damage on renal biopsy have an unfavorable long-term prognosis.

Post-Streptococcal Glomerulonephritis

Acute post-streptococcal glomerulonephritis (PSGN) may present as an acute nephritic syndrome or with isolated hematuria and proteinuria. It may occur in either an epidemic form or as sporadic cases. PSGN is largely a disease of childhood, but well-documented cases of severe disease do occur in adults. The disease is most common in winter following episodes of pharyngitis, but it can occur after streptococcal infections at any site, and subclinical cases greatly outnumber clinical cases.

The exact pathogenesis of PSGN remains unknown. It is clearly an immune complex disease in its acute phase and is characterized by the formation of antibodies against streptococcal antigens, and the localization of immune complexes with complement in the kidney. PSGN occurs only after infection with certain strains of group A β-hemolytic streptococci, the so-called nephritogenic strains. Typical nephritogenic strains, characterized by antibodies to antigenic M components of their cell wall, include M types 1, 2, 4, 12, 18, 25, 49, 55, 57, and 60. Despite a number of theories relating to the immune deposition in PSGN, it remains unclear how this immune insult may lead to progressive glomerular inflammation and eventual glomerulosclerosis.

On LM, glomeruli are markedly enlarged and often fill Bowman's space. They exhibit hypercellularity due to both an infiltration of monocytes and especially polymorphonuclear cells during the early weeks of the disease and a proliferation of the glomerular cellular elements. The capillary lumina are often compressed by the glomerular hypercellularity. Some cases demonstrate extracapillary proliferation with crescent formation. By IF microscopy there is coarse granular deposition of IgG, IgM, and complement, especially C3, along the capillary wall. EM shows the classic dome-shaped, electron-dense subepithelial deposits resembling the humps of a camel at isolated intervals along the GBM.

Most cases are diagnosed by detecting hematuria and proteinuria and only some of the findings of the nephritic syndrome following a latency period of 10 days to several weeks after a stretococcal pharyngitis or a longer interval after a streptococcal skin infection. Hypertension is present in most patients, but severe hypertension and hypertensive encephalopathy are uncommon. Throat cultures and skin cultures of suspected sites of streptococcal involvement may often not be positive for group A β-hemolytic streptococci. A variety of antibodies, e.g., ASLO (anti–streptolysin O), AHT (anti-hyaluronidase), and a streptozyme panel of antibodies against streptococcal antigens (which includes ASLO, AHT, antistreptokinase, and anti-DNAse) often show high titers, but a change in titer over time is more indicative of a recent streptococcal infection. More than 95% of patients with PSGN secondary to pharyngitis and 85% of patients with streptococcal skin infections have positive antibody titers. The serum total hemolytic complement levels and C3 levels are decreased in >90% of patients during the episode of acute glomerulonephritis. C4 levels are usually normal.

In the classic case of an acute nephritic episode following a latency period after a streptococcal infection and associated with both a change in streptococcal antibody titer and a depressed serum complement level, a renal biopsy adds little to the diagnosis. In less classic cases a biopsy may prove valuable to confirm or refute the diagnosis. In most patients PSGN is a self-limited disease, with recovery of renal function and disappearance of hypertension in several weeks. Proteinuria and hematuria may resolve more slowly over months. Therapy is symptomatic and directed at controlling the hypertension and fluid retention with antihypertensives and diuretics.

Glomerulonephritis with Endocarditis and Visceral Abscesses

A variety of glomerular lesions has been found in patients suffering from acute and chronic bacterial endocarditis (see Ch. 278). Although embolic phenomena can lead to glomerular ischemia and infarcts, a common finding is an immune complex pattern of glomerular damage. In the preantibiotic era with most cases of endocarditis due to *Streptococcus viridans,* both focal and diffuse proliferative glomerulonephritides were seen in many patients. More recently the incidence of acute endocarditis associated with *Staphylococcus aureus* has markedly increased, especially in the drug-addicted population. From 40 to 80% of patients with staphylococcal endocarditis have clinical evidence of a proliferative glomerulonephritis. Glomerulonephritis is now more common with acute rather than subacute bacterial endocarditis, and the duration of illness is not an important determinant of the renal disease.

Patients often have hematuria and erythrocyte casts in urinary sediment, proteinuria ranging from < 1 gram daily to nephrotic levels, and progressive renal failure. Serum total complement and C3 levels are usually reduced. Renal insufficiency may be mild and reversible with appropriate antibiotic therapy or progressive, leading to dialysis and irreversible renal failure.

A proliferative glomerulonephritis with similar pathology has also been noted in patients with deep visceral bacterial abscesses and infections such as empyema of the lung and osteomyelitis. With appropriate antibiotic therapy most patients' glomerular lesions heal and they recover renal function. Immune complex forms of acute glomerulonephritis have also been noted in patients with pneumonias associated with many bacterial organisms as well as mycoplasma. Patients with chronically infected cerebral ventriculoatrial shunts for hydrocephalus have also had renal damage associated with immune deposits in the glomeruli. Many have nephrotic-range proteinuria and only mild renal dysfunction.

Rapidly Progressive Glomerulonephritis (RPGN)

RPGN comprises a group of glomerulonephritides that have in common progression to renal failure in a matter of weeks to months

TABLE 79-4. CLASSIFICATION OF RAPIDLY PROGRESSIVE ("CRESCENTIC") GLOMERULONEPHRITIS

Primary
Type I   Anti–glomerular basement membrane antibody disease (with pulmonary disease—Goodpasture's syndrome)
Type II   Immune complex mediated
Type III   Pauci-immune (usually anti-neutrophil cytoplasmic antibody-positive)

Secondary
Membranoproliferative glomerulonephritis
IgA nephropathy—Henoch-Schönlein purpura
Post-streptoccoccal glomerulonephritis
Systemic lupus erythematosus
Polyarteritis nodosa, hypersensitivity angiitis

and the presence of extensive extracapillary proliferation, i.e., crescent formation. RPGN thus includes renal diseases with different causes, pathogeneses, and clinical presentations (Table 79–4). Patients with RPGN have been divided into three patterns defined by immunologic pathogenesis: type I, with anti-GBM disease (e.g., Goodpasture's syndrome); type II, with immune complex deposition (e.g., SLE, post-streptococcal); and type III, without immune deposits or anti-GBM antibodies, so-called pauci-immune. Most of the latter patients fall into the category of antineutrophil cytoplasmic antibody (ANCA)–positive RPGN. In the past, with the exception of postinfectious RPGN, prognosis was generally poor for most patients regardless of pathogenesis. This prognosis has dramatically changed for some patterns of RPGN.

Anti-GBM Disease (Table 79–5)

Anti-GBM disease is caused by circulating antibodies directed against the noncollagenous domain of type 4 collagen which damages the GBM. This leads to an inflammatory response, breaks in the GBM, and the formation of a proliferative and often crescentic glomerulonephritis. If the anti-GBM antibodies cross-react with and damage the basement membrane of pulmonary capillaries, the patient develops pulmonary hemorrhage and hemoptysis. The association of anti-GBM antibody–mediated damage to the kidneys and lungs is called Goodpasture's syndrome (see Ch. 54). The disease most commonly affects young adults, and males are far more commonly affected than females. The patient presents with a nephritic picture. Renal function may deteriorate from normal to dialysis-requiring levels in a matter of days to weeks. Patients with pulmonary involvement may have life-threatening hemoptysis. The course of the disease, once it has progressed to renal failure, is usually one of permanent renal dysfunction. If treatment is started early in the course of the disease, patients may regain considerable kidney function.

The pathology of anti-GBM disease shows a proliferative glomerulonephritis, often with severe crescentic proliferation in Bowman's space (see Color Plate 4E). There is linear deposition of immunoglobulin along the GBM by IF, but EM does not show any electron-dense deposits (see Color Plate 4F).

The treatment of anti-GBM disease is unproven, with no significant controlled trials of this least-common form of crescentic glomerulonephritis. For patients with pulmonary hemorrhage, high-dose oral or intravenous corticosteroids have successfully halted the

TABLE 79-5. COMMON RENAL DISEASES WITH ASSOCIATED PULMONARY DISEASES

Disease	Marker
Goodpasture's syndrome	+ Anti-GBM antibodies
Wegener's granulomatosis, polyarteritis	+ Anti–neutrophil cytoplasmic antibodies
Systemic lupus erythematosus	+ Anti-DNA antibodies, low complement
Nephrotic syndrome, renal vein thrombosis, pulmonary embolus	+ Lung scan
Pneumonia with immune complex glomerulonephritis	− Low complement, circulating immune complexes
Uremic lung	− Elevated BUN-creatinine

pulmonary bleeding. They have usually not proven effective in treating the renal lesions. Intensive therapy to reduce the production of anti-GBM antibodies (immunosuppressive agents such as cyclophosphamide and corticosteroids) combined with plasmapheresis to remove circulating anti-GBM antibodies has proven effective for the renal lesion in many cases. Rapid intensive therapy is necessary to prevent irreversible renal damage.

Immune Complex RPGN

Type II RPGN, associated with immune complex–mediated damage to the glomeruli, may occur with a spectrum of diseases from primary glomerulopathies such as IgA nephropathy and MPGN to disease of known origin such as postinfectious glomerulonephritis and SLE. The therapy of IgA nephropathy and MPGN is discussed above. Most cases of crescentic postinfectious glomerulonephritis resolve with successful treatment of the underlying infection. The treatment of severe SLE is considered later.

Pauci-immune RPGN and Vasculitis-associated RPGN

Pauci-immune type III RPGN includes patients with and without evidence of systemic vasculitis. A large retrospective analysis found no difference in prognosis between the patients with or without small artery or medium-sized renal artery vasculitis along with crescentic and focal segmental necrotizing glomerulonephritis (polyateritis-like) (see Ch. 243 and 244). Patients often present with progressive renal failure and a nephritic picture. Many patients have circulating antibodies directed against components of neutrophil primary granules, ANCA. Patients who are P-ANCA positive (antibodies usually directed against granulocyte myeloperoxidase) more often have a clinical picture akin to microscopic polyarteritis with arthritis, skin involvement with leukocytoclastic angiitis, and constitutional and systemic signs. Patients who are C-ANCA positive (antibodies usually directed against a granulocyte serine proteinase) more likely have granulomatous disease associated with their glomerulonephritis as in Wegener's granulomatosis (see Ch. 245). There is considerable overlap between these groups. As in all forms of RPGN, renal function may deteriorate rapidly. Using oral cyclophosphamide in addition to corticosteroids in disease such as Wegener's granulomatosis and polyarteritis nodosa has led to markedly improved patient and renal survival rates. For example, in a series of 158 patients with Wegener's granulomatosis, >90% experienced marked improvement and 75% experienced a complete remission. These excellent results include patients with true crescentic glomerulonephritis. More recently, steroids plus cytotoxic agents have produced successful results in both oliguric and dialysis-dependent patients.

ASYMPTOMATIC URINARY ABNORMALITIES

Some patients have the asymptomatic urinary abnormalities of microhematuria and/or proteinuria discovered through routine evaluations. Microscopic hematuria associated with deformed erythrocytes and/or erythrocyte casts is likely to be glomerular in origin. Levels of proteinuria less than the nephrotic range may be due to orthostatic proteinuria, hypertension, and tubular disease as well as glomerular damage.

In patients with a glomerular cause for their asymptomatic urinary abnormality, the underlying glomerular lesion is either the early phase of one of the progressive glomerular diseases (discussed in other sections) or due to a benign, nonprogressive glomerular lesion. Most such patients have a lesion with mild proliferation limited to the mesangial areas of the glomeruli. Some patients have mesangial IgA immune deposits and hence IgA nephropathy, whereas others have deposition of IgM or complement only. Some patients, often with a history of similar findings in siblings and other relatives, have a hereditary nephritis or a lesion with areas of focal thinning of the GBM, so-called thin basement membrane disease. In general, for patients with <1 gram of proteinuria daily and/or glomerular microhematuria if the GFR (as measured by the creatinine clearance) is normal, most clinicians would not proceed to a renal biopsy to confirm a diagnosis. Because the vast majority of these patients need no therapy, they prefer to follow the patient closely and perform biopsy only on patients with progressive increasing proteinuria or evidence of a decreasing GFR.

GLOMERULAR INVOLVEMENT IN SYSTEMIC DISEASES

Systemic Lupus Erythematosus (SLE) (see Ch. 240)

Renal involvement may greatly influence the course and therapy of SLE. The incidence of clinically detectable renal disease varies from 15 to 75%. Histologic evidence of renal involvement by immune deposits is found in the vast majority of biopsies, even in the absence of clinical renal disease.

The WHO classification of lupus nephritis has been used successfully for both clinical and research activities (Table 79–6). It has the advantages of using LM, IF, and EM to classify each biopsy rather than only one form of microscopy; of separating the milder mesangial forms of lupus nephritis from the true focal and diffuse proliferative forms; and of using well-defined criteria allowing different groups to compare results (see Color Plate 4G; Fig. 79–3). The WHO classes correlate well with the clinical picture and subsequent course of SLE patients.

In general, all patients with class IV lesions on biopsy deserve vigorous therapy for their lupus nephritis. Many class III patients (especially those with active necrotizing lesions and large amounts of subendothelial deposits) also would benefit from such therapy. The optimal therapy for class V patients is less clear; some clinicians treat all membranous lupus nephritis patients vigorously, whereas others reserve such therapy for those with serologic activity or more severe nephrotic syndrome. Vigorous lupus nephritis therapy may include intravenous pulse steroids, plasmapheresis, oral azathioprine or cyclophosphamide, intravenous cyclophosphamide, and cyclosporine. Intravenous pulse methylprednisolone is most effective in patients with a recent decline in GFR, with diffuse proliferative lesions, and with greater serologic activity. It is clearly not effective in all patients, and recent studies at the NIH have shown it to be less effective than intravenous cyclophosphamide in preventing long-term renal failure in patients with severe lupus nephritis. Plasmapheresis, reported to be successful anecdotally, has recently proven unsuccessful in a major clinical controlled trial. Patients treated with steroid-cytotoxics and plasmapheresis had no improvement in clinical activity or renal or patient survival compared with a control group at a mean follow-up period of 80 weeks.

A series of well-performed studies have reviewed the results of lupus nephritis patients randomized to one of five treatment protocols: oral prednisone, oral azathioprine, oral cyclophosphamide (Cytoxan), oral azathioprine plus oral Cytoxan, and every third month high doses of intravenous Cytoxan (1 gram per square meter). Patients treated with any of the cytotoxic agents had less renal failure

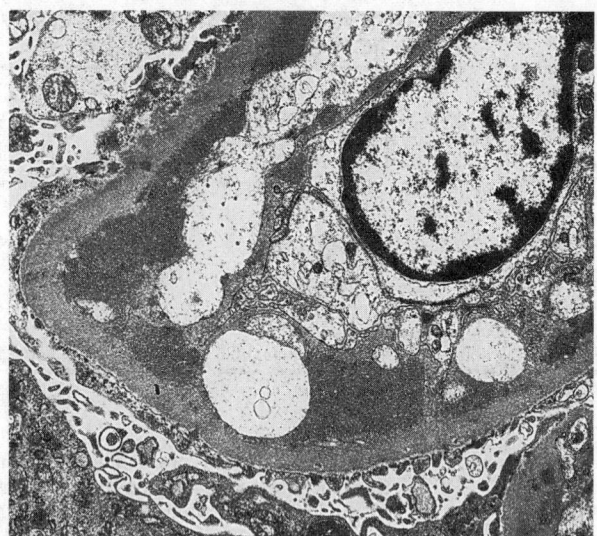

FIGURE 79–3. Lupus nephritis. At the ultrastructural level, wire-loop deposits correspond to large subendothelial electron-dense deposits (uranyl acetate, lead citrate, × 5000).

at 10 years than those with steroid treatment. Extended long-term follow-up at 20 years shows the azathioprine group to be no different from the prednisone groups. Intravenous Cytoxan appeared to be a most effective form of therapy in preventing progressive renal failure. The side effects were no worse in the cytotoxic treatment group than in the steroid group and were lowest in the intravenous Cytoxan group. Recent studies document the efficacy of monthly high-dose intravenous cyclophosphamide therapy in severe lupus nephritis. Initial uncontrolled trials with cyclosporine and intravenous gamma globulin have been promising.

Many patients with lupus nephritis (40 to 75%) produce autoantibodies against certain phospholipids, including anticardiolipin antibodies and lupus anticoagulant. Some of these patients have renal thrombotic microangiopathy with evidence of coagulation in the glomeruli and arterioles and require treatment with anticoagulation and/or antiplatelet agents as well as immunosuppressive medications.

Diabetes Mellitus (see Ch. 205)

Diabetic nephropathy is probably the most common form of glomerular damage seen in developed countries. Currently 30 to 40% of insulin-dependent diabetics develop nephropathy and eventually progressive renal failure. Many patients with non–insulin-dependent diabetes also have progressive renal involvement. Diabetes is already the leading cause of renal disease for new patients entering ESRD programs in this country.

The histopathologic changes in the kidneys of diabetics involve all components of the kidney, including the glomeruli, vessels, tubules, and interstitium. In the glomeruli there are thickening of the GBM, mesangial sclerosis, nodular intercapillary glomerulosclerosis (the so-called Kimmelsteil-Wilson or KW nodules), lesions due to insudation of plasma proteins along the glomerular capillary walls, and microaneuryms of the glomerular capillaries (see Color Plate 4H).

A current goal of treatment in diabetics is to prevent diabetic nephropathy by controlling hyperglycemia and blood pressure and reducing intracapillary glomerular pressures (by ACE inhibition). Survival in diabetics with renal transplantation may approach that of the nondiabetic population.

Amyloidosis (see Ch. 248)

Amyloid deposits—whether due to AL or to AA amyloid—are predominantly found within the glomeruli, often appearing as amorphous eosinophilic extracellular nodules (see Color Plate 4I). They also may be found deposited in the tubular basement membranes, the interstitium, and the vessels. They stain positively with Congo red and, under polarized light, display apple-green birefringence. Under EM amyloid appears as nonbranching rigid fibrils 8 to 10 nm in diameter.

TABLE 79–6. WHO CLASSIFICATION OF LUPUS NEPHRITIS

	Class	Clinical
I.	Normal glomeruli (LM, IF, EM)	No renal findings
II.	(a) Mesangial disease normal by LM with mesangial deposits by IF and/or EM	Mild clinical renal disease; minimally active urinary sediment; mild to moderate proteinuria (never nephrotic) but may have active serology.
	(b) Mesangial hypercellularity with mesangial deposits	
III.	Focal proliferative glomerulonephritis	More active sediment changes; often active serology; increased proteinuria (about 25% nephrotic); hypertension may be present; some evolve into class IV pattern.
IV.	Diffuse proliferative glomerulonephritis	Most severe renal involvement with active sediment, hypertension, heavy proteinuria (frequent nephrotic syndrome), often reduced GFR; serology very active.
V.	Membranous glomerulonephritis	Significant proteinuria (often nephrotic) with less active lupus serology

Although almost 80% of patients with AL amyloid have renal disease, amyloidosis is a disease with multisystem involvement and hence patients may present with symptoms referable to other organ involvement as well as renal symptoms. Diagnosis may be made from organ biopsy other than the kidney, e.g., gingival biopsy, rectal biopsy, or fat pad biopsy. Common renal manifestations are albuminuria and renal insufficiency found in almost one half of patients. Approximately 25% of patients with AL amyloid present with the nephrotic syndrome, and this is eventually found in up to one half of patients. Amyloid is rarely found in association with light chain cast nephropathy.

Light Chain Deposition Disease (see Ch. 149)

Light chain deposition disease (LCDD), like AL amyloidosis, is a systemic disease caused by the overproduction and extracellular deposition of a monoclonal immunoglobulin light chain. However, the deposits do not form β-pleated sheets, do not stain Congo red, and are granular rather than fibrillar in nature. LCDD affects predominantly older males, and most patients have a lymphoplasmacytic B cell disease compatible with multiple myeloma.

On LM most glomeruli have eosinophilic mesangial glomerular nodules. Others are either normal or have sclerosing or proliferative features. By IF a single class of immunoglobulin light chain (kappa in 80% of cases) stains in a diffuse linear pattern along the GBM's, in the nodules, and along the tubular basement membranes with little or no staining for complement components.

Moderate albuminuria is common, and the nephrotic syndrome is found in one half at presentation, often accompanied by hypertension and renal insufficiency. Some patients may present with acute renal failure, classic Bence Jones cast nephropathy, and the changes of LCDD.

The treatment for most patients with LCDD is chemotherapy similar to that for myeloma, which has led to significant renal and patient survival.

Fibrillary Glomerulopathy—Immunotactoid Glomerulopathy

Some patients with renal disease have glomerular lesions with deposits of nonamyloid fibrillar proteins ranging in size from 12 to 49 nm. In the past these lesions were called fibrillary glomerulopathy, immunotactoid glomerulopathy, amyloid-like glomerulopathy, Congo red–negative amyloid-like glomerulonephritis, and nonamyloiditic fibrillary glomerulopathy. Recently patients with these lesions have been divided into two groups: fibrillary and immunotactoid glomerulonephritis. In fibrillary glomerulonephritis the fibrils are approximately 20 nm in diameter and are typically deposited in the GBM. Immunotactoid glomerulonephritis, a much rarer disease in which the fibrils are much larger in size (30 to 50 nm), is often associated with a plasma cell dyscrasia. Although the ultrastructural finding of typical fibrils defines both fibrillary and immunotactoid glomerulonephritis by LM the glomeruli of both may exhibit a variety of changes including mesangial proliferative, membranous, membranoproliferative, and crescentic glomerulonephritis. By IF there is evidence for glomerular deposition of immunoglobulins and complement in a similar distribution within the glomeruli. Proteinuria is found in almost all patients, and hematuria, the nephrotic syndrome, and renal insufficiency are eventually found in the majority. Patients progress to ESRD in a mean of 2 to 4 years. Corticosteroid therapy has not proved successful, but some patients with a crescentic pattern on LM have been treated successfully with cyclophosphamide plus corticosteroids.

HIV Nephropathy (see Ch. 370)

Infection with HIV has been associated with a number of patterns of renal disease, including acute renal failure and a unique form of glomerulopathy now called HIV nephropathy. The most common precipitating factors for acute renal failure include medications (pentamidine, aminoglycosides, trimethoprim-sulfamethoxazole, NSAID's), and pyrexia and dehydration superimposed on sepsis-hypotension-respiratory failure. HIV-infected patients with acute renal failure often regain renal function if supported by dialysis through the renal failure.

Several histologic patterns of glomerulopathy seen in HIV-infected patients have included minimal change pattern, mesangial hyperplasia, glomerulopathies associated with immune complex deposition and/or IgA deposition and, most important, HIV nephropathy. HIV nephropathy is a unique pattern of glomerulopathy charac-

terized by heavy proteinuria and rapid progression to renal failure. "HIV nephropathy" is a better term than "AIDS nephropathy" because this glomerulopathy may occur in patients with AIDS as well as in asymptomatic carriers.

Both clinical and histologic data suggest that HIV nephropathy differs from the older entity of heroin nephropathy. The latter is a form of FSGS, occurring in intravenous heroin users associated with proteinuria and often the nephrotic syndrome and renal insufficiency. HIV nephropathy may occur in nonaddicted patients and has a more fulminant course to renal failure than heroin nephropathy. The pathology of HIV nephropathy also shows several features distinct from heroin nephropathy or classic FSGS. In HIV nephropathy on LM, diffuse global glomerular sclerosis and glomerular collapse are common. There are severe tubulointerstitial changes with interstitial inflammation, edema, microcystic dilatation of tubules, and severe tubular degenerative changes. On EM tubuloreticular inclusions are prevalent in the glomerular endothelium.

Mixed Cryoglobulinemia

Cryoglobulinemia refers to a pathologic condition caused by the production of circulating immunoglobulins that precipitate upon cooling and resolubilize on warming. Cryoglobulinemia may be found associated with many types of diseases, including infections, collagen-vascular disease, and lymphoproliferative diseases such as multiple myeloma and Waldenström's macroglobulinemia (see Ch. 149). Recently many patients with what was originally described as glomerulonephritis due to essential mixed cryoglobulinemia have been found to have hepatitis C–associated renal disease.

Up to one quarter to one third of patients develop an acute nephritic picture and acute renal insufficiency. Most patients have proteinuria, and about 20% present with the nephrotic syndrome. The majority with renal disease have a slow, indolent renal course characterized by proteinuria, hypertension, hematuria, and renal insufficiency. Hypocomplementemia, especially of the early components Clq-C4, is a characteristic and often helpful finding in cryoglobulinemic GN.

Thrombotic Microangiopathies

A number of systemic diseases with prominent glomerular involvement are characterized by microthromboses of the glomerular capillaries and small arterioles. These include hemolytic-uremic syndrome, thrombotic thrombocytopenic purpura, and the antiphospholipid syndrome (see Ch. 152), as well as microangiopathy associated with using drugs such as mitomycin and cyclosporine. The renal findings may be either the most salient features of the disease or only part of a more generalized picture of microangiopathy.

The histologic findings in all of the microangiopathies resemble each other. Glomerular capillary thromboses are noted in some glomeruli, whereas others downstream from thrombosed arterioles may show only ischemic damage. Arterioles and small arteries show intimal proliferation with luminal narrowing by thrombus.

The renal manifestations of the thrombotic microangiopathies may include gross or microscopic hematuria, proteinuria that is typically < 2 grams daily but may reach nephrotic levels, and renal insufficiency. The patient may have oliguric or nonoliguric acute renal failure. Treatment of the thrombotic microangiopathies includes correcting hypovolemia, controlling hypertension, and using dialytic therapy for those with severe renal failure. In the antiphospholipid syndrome anticoagulation with heparin and then warfarin (Coumadin) has been used for patients with thrombotic microangiopathy.

Renal Vasculitis—Polyarteritis, Wegener's Granulomatosis, Hypersensitivity Angiitis (see Ch. 243 and 244)

A number of systemic vasculitic disease processes can involve the kidney. In many cases of polyarteritis nodosa, hypersensitivity angiitis, and Wegener's granulomatosis, renal involvement is predominant and overshadows other manifestations of the systemic vasculitis. The renal lesions of these disorders typically range from focal and segmental necrotizing glomerulonephritis to severe necrotizing crescentic glomerulonephritis. Therapy for the microscopic form of polyarteritis and Wegener's granulomatosis is discussed under the therapy of RPGN.

Appel GB, Valeri A: The course and treatment of lupus nephritis. Ann Rev Med 45:525, 1994. *Reviews clinical features, histopathology, course, and treatment options in lupus nephritis patients.*

Boumpas DT, Austin HA, Vaughn EM, et al.: Controlled trial of pulse methylprednisolone versus two regimens of cyclophosphomide in severe lupus nephritis. Lancet 340:741, 1992. *A randomized controlled trial of monthly high-dose intravenous methylprednisolone versus monthly intravenous cyclophosphamide treatment of two different durations in patients with severe lupus nephritis.*

D'Agati V: The many masks of focal segmental glomerulosclerosis. Kidney Int 46:1223, 1994. *Discusses various histologic patterns of focal sclerosis and their course and therapy.*

D'Amico G, Ferrario F: Mesangiocapillary glomerulonephritis. J Am Soc Nephrol 2:S159, 1992. *Reviews the course, prognosis, and treatment.*

Glassock R: Treatment of immunologically mediated glomerular disease. Kidney Int 42:S38, 1992. *A review of therapeutic options in IgA nephropathy, membranoproliferative glomerulonephritis and membranous nephropathy.*

Heilman RL, Velosa JA, Holley K, et al.: Long-term follow-up and response to chemotherapy in patients with light chain deposition disease. Am J Kidney Dis 20:34, 1992. *Long-term experience at one center treating 17 patients with LCDD.*

Hoffman G, Kerr G, Leavitt R, et al.: Wegener's granulomatosis: An analysis of 158 patients. Ann Intern Med 116:488, 1992. *The long-term NIH experience with treatment of Wegener's granulomatosis, emphasizing improved survival with cytotoxic agents.*

Iskander SS, Falk RJ, Jennette JC: Clinical and pathologic features of fibrillary glomerulonephritis. Kidney Int 42:1401, 1992. *Describes the clinical features, pathology, and course of patients with this unique glomerulopathy.*

Johnson RJ, Gretch DR, Yamabe H, et al.: Membranoproliferative glomerulonephritis associated with hepatitis C virus infection. N Engl J Med 328:465, 1993. *A series of patients with membranoproliferative glomerulonephritis associated with hepatitis C–related cryoglobulinemia documents the relationship of the virus to the cryoprecipitate and the glomerular lesions.*

Korbet S, Schwartz M, Lewis E: Primary focal segemental glomerulosclerosis: Clinical course and response to therapy. Am J Kidney Dis 23:773, 1994. *Analysis of available data on the course and various treatment studies of focal glomerulosclerosis.*

Ponticelli C, Passerini P: Treatment of nephrotic syndrome associated with primary glomerulonephritis. Kidney Int 46:595, 1994. *Reviews the immunosuppressive treatment of the various patterns of idiopathic nephrotic syndrome plus the therapy of manifestations of the nephrotic syndrome.*

Ponticelli C, Zucchelli P, Passerini P, et al.: Methylprednisolone plus chlorambucil as compared with methylprednisolone alone for the treatment of idiopathic membranous nephropathy. N Engl J Med 327:599, 1992. *A randomized controlled treatment trial in idiopathic membranous nephropathy showing equivalent efficacy of two immunosuppressive regimens.*

Rock GA, Shumak KH, Buskard NA, et al.: Comparison of plasma exchange with plasma infusion in the treatment of thrombotic thrombocytopenic purpura. N Engl J Med 325:393, 1991. *Shows the superiority of plasma exchange to plasma infusion in patients with thrombotic thrombocytopenic purpura.*

Schieppati A, Mosconi L, Perna A, et al.: Prognosis of untreated patients with idiopathic membranous nephropathy. N Engl J Med 329:85, 1993. *A long-term follow-up of idiopathic membranous nephropathy showing favorable prognosis without specific immunosuppressive therapy.*

Tarshish P, Bernstein J, Tobin J, Edelmann C: Treatment of mesangiocapillary glomerulonephritis with alternate-day prednisone: A report of the International Study of Kidney Disease in Children. Pediatr Nephrol 6:123, 1992. *A randomized controlled trial showing the benefits of long-term alternate-day prednisone therapy in children with membranoproliferative glomerulonephritis.*

Valeri A, Radhakrishnan J, Estes D, et al.: Intravenous pulse cyclophosphamide treatment of severe lupus nephritis: A prospective five-year study. Clin Nephrol 42:71, 1994. *Long-term follow-up of patients with severe lupus nephritis treated with intravenous cyclophosphamide documenting its safety and efficacy.*

80 TUBULOINTERSTITIAL DISEASES AND TOXIC NEPHROPATHIES

T. Dwight McKinney

COMMON FEATURES OF TUBULOINTERSTITIAL DISEASES

"Tubulointerstitial disease" (tubulointerstitial nephritis or nephropathy, interstitial nephritis) refers to a diverse group of acute and chronic disorders that primarily affect the renal tubules and interstitium. In contrast, in other primary renal diseases, most notably glomerulonephritis, the tubules and interstitium are only secondarily involved. Approximately 30% of all cases of chronic renal insufficiency in the United States result from tubulointerstitial diseases; usually the cause can be identified. Renal function may improve or stabilize with appropriate therapy.

CLINICAL MANIFESTATIONS. In tubulointerstitial diseases, functional renal tubular defects, which are present to some degree

in advanced renal insufficiency of any cause, are frequently out of proportion to the degree of renal insufficiency, as measured by reduction in glomerular filtration rate (GFR). In fact, the finding of such a disproportional loss of tubular compared with glomerular function should lead one to suspect the diagnosis of tubulointerstitial disease (Table 80–1). Urinary concentration in response to water deprivation or exogenous antidiuretic hormone may be reduced, particularly in chronic interstitial nephritis. This may result in decreased maximal urinary osmolarity, polyuria (generally < 3 liters per day), and nocturia. Concentration defect, an acquired form of nephrogenic diabetes insipidus, may result from interference with the action of antidiuretic hormone on the collecting ducts or anatomic damage or disruption of the medullary structures involved in the urinary concentrating mechanism (see Ch. 202.2). Damage to the proximal tubules may result in excessive urinary excretion of substances normally reabsorbed in this location. Bicarbonaturia (proximal renal tubular acidosis), phosphaturia, aminoaciduria, uricosuria, glycosuria, kaliuresis, and low-molecular-weight proteinuria may occur. These losses may cause low plasma levels of some of these substances, particularly phosphate, bicarbonate, and urate. The presence of multiple proximal tubular defects is referred to as "Fanconi's syndrome" (see Ch. 82). In addition to proximal renal tubular acidosis, failure of the distal nephron to acidify the tubular fluid maximally results in classic distal renal tubular acidosis. Hyperkalemic (type IV) distal renal tubular acidosis also may occur. All these cause a hyperchloremic (normal anion gap) metabolic acidosis (see Ch. 75). Hyperkalemia may result from a primary failure of potassium secretion by the distal nephron but more commonly results from decreased renal production of renin and subsequent secondary hypoaldosteronism. Patients with tubulointerstitial disease also may fail to conserve sodium normally. In some, this is due to the hyporeninemic hypoaldosteronism noted above. Renal sodium wasting may result in signs of extracellular fluid volume depletion when sodium intake is restricted and may worsen renal function. With acute and, to a lesser extent, chronic interstitial nephritis, these tubular defects may be accompanied or, indeed, overshadowed by other signs, symptoms, and laboratory abnormalities of renal failure (see Ch. 76 and 77).

DIAGNOSIS. A specific diagnosis of tubulointerstitial renal disease often can be made or inferred from historical information, physical examination, or laboratory tests. Renal biopsy is the most definitive method, but this is not always necessary. Pathologic features are discussed below. Radiographic, ultrasonographic, and radionuclide examinations generally show only evidence of acute or chronic renal insufficiency but may provide a specific diagnosis, such as urinary tract obstruction or polycystic kidney disease.

PROGNOSIS AND TREATMENT. The prognosis usually depends on the specific cause of tubulointerstitial renal disease, as discussed below. General supportive therapy, such as treatment of electrolyte disorders, and management of acute and chronic renal failure are discussed in Ch. 76 and 77.

TABLE 80–1. MANIFESTATIONS OF RENAL TUBULOINTERSTITIAL DISEASES

1. Tubular dysfunction disportionate to reduction in GFR
2. Tubular abnormalities
   a. Reduced maximal urinary concentrating ability (polyuria, nocturia)
   b. Renal tubular acidosis (hyperchloremic metabolic acidosis)
   c. Partial or complete Fanconi's syndrome
      | Phosphaturia | Uricosuria |
      | Bicarbonaturia | Glycosuria |
      | Aminoaciduria | |
   d. Sodium wasting
   e. Hyperkalemia
3. Renal endocrine deficiencies
   a. Hyporeninemic hypoaldosteronism (hyperkalemia, metabolic acidosis)
   b. Calcitriol deficiency (renal osteodystrophy)
   c. Erythropoietin deficiency (anemia)
4. Urinalysis
   a. May be normal but usually contains cellular elements
   b. Proteinuria is usually modest (< 3.5 grams per day) and consists largely of low-molecular-weight "tubular" proteins, such as lysozyme and β_2-microglobulin

The term toxic nephropathy refers to those renal disorders resulting directly or indirectly from the kidneys being exposed to exogenous chemicals and physical factors, including both drugs and environmental agents, and abnormal concentrations of substances normally present in the body fluids, such as calcium and uric acid. Drug-related renal disease is the most important cause of toxic nephropathy. Toxic nephropathy often results in tubulointerstitial disease, but it is not synonymous with it.

Several factors predispose the kidneys to toxic injury: (1) The kidneys receive approximately 20% of the resting cardiac output and, therefore, are exposed to more blood-borne materials than any other organ except the lungs. (2) The high metabolic rate of the renal tubules required for active transport processes makes them particularly vulnerable to toxic insults. (3) The large glomerular capillary surface area is a major site for trapping immune complexes or for antigen-antibody reactions *in situ.* (4) Some substances (e.g., aminoglycosides) are selectively concentrated in the renal cortex because of specific transport processes located in the proximal tubules, whereas others (e.g., phenacetin) are concentrated in the medulla owing to the renal countercurrent system. This selective concentration accounts, in part, for the anatomic distribution of damage by some nephrotoxins. (5) Certain substances are converted to less soluble forms resulting in precipitation (e.g., urate to uric acid) consequent to acidification of tubular fluid in the distal nephron. This may lead to tubular obstruction.

Nephrotoxins injure the kidneys in a variety of ways, both direct and indirect (Fig. 80–1). Indirect injury may result from immunologic reactions or from secondary effects, such as drug-induced hypotension or hemolysis. These mechanisms, alone or in concert, may cause an array of renal disorders, ranging from isolated functional tubular defects to reversible acute renal failure to progressive end-stage renal disease.

ACUTE INTERSTITIAL NEPHRITIS

PATHOLOGY AND PATHOGENESIS. Characteristically, in acute interstitial nephritis (AISN), mononuclear cells infiltrate the interstitium, particularly in the cortex. Eosinophils, especially in cases of drug-related AISN, and occasionally small numbers of polymorphonuclear leukocytes also may be present. Inflammatory cells may invade the tubule walls and, in severe cases, may be associated with areas of tubular necrosis. The infiltrate may be diffuse or patchy; the extent of the infiltrate corresponds in general to the degree of renal functional impairment. In addition to the cellular infiltrate, the renal tubules are separated by interstitial edema, but no fibrosis is present. With prolonged AISN, interstitial fibrosis may develop, and the pathologic picture may merge into that of chronic interstitial nephritis. In primary AISN, the glomeruli are generally normal, although there may be some mesangial prominence. The predominant mononuclear inflammatory cells in infiltrates are T cells. Both helper/inducer and suppressor/cytotoxic T cells are present. These observations suggest that both T-cell–mediated delayed hypersensitivity reactions and cytotoxic T-cell injury may be involved in AISN. In some cases immunoglobulins and complement components are demonstrable in the interstitium and/or tubular basement membrane by immunofluorescence. Rarely, electron microscopy may reveal electron-dense deposits in these areas, suggestive of immune complexes. Finally, in occasional cases immunoglobulins and complement may linearly deposit in the tubular basement membrane, which indicates anti–tubular basement membrane antibodies. There is, therefore, considerable evidence that immune injury mediated by cellular and humoral mechanisms causes AISN. Usually, however, the immunopathogenetic mechanisms involved in a given case of AISN remain unknown.

ETIOLOGY. Acute interstitial nephritis may result from a variety of causes (Table 80–2). Drug-related AISN is becoming more frequently recognized as an important cause of acute renal insufficiency, probably because of (1) the more widespread use of renal biopsy, (2) the increasing number of drugs being used, and (3) the characteristic clinical presentation.

Drug-Induced Acute Interstitial Nephritis. The list of drugs that have been implicated as etiologic in AISN continues to expand (Table 80–3). AISN is a rare complication of drug therapy, but because of the frequency with which these agents are used, drugs account for a substantial portion of all cases of acute renal failure.

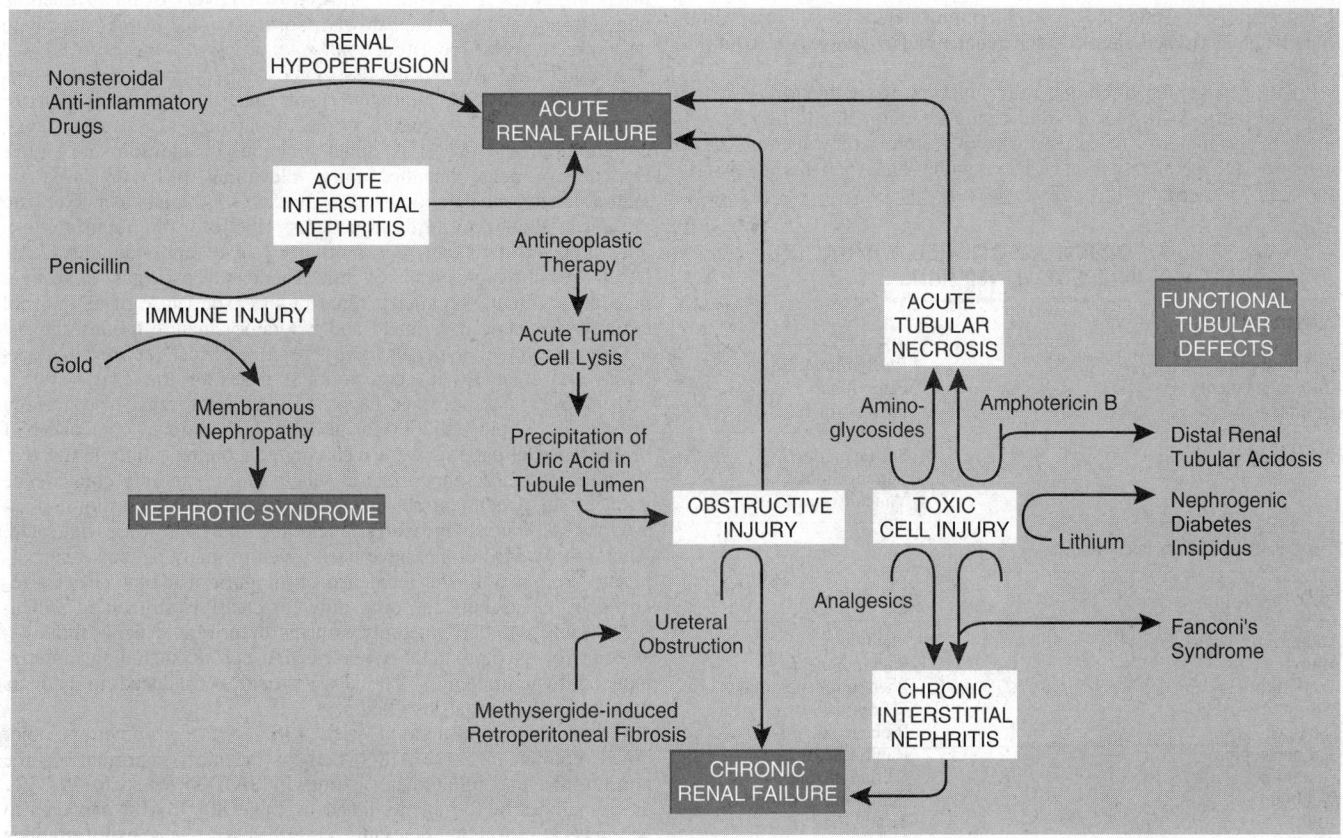

FIGURE 80–1. Types of toxin-induced renal disease.

TABLE 80-2. CAUSES OF ACUTE INTERSTITIAL NEPHRITIS

1. Drug-related (see Table 80–3)
2. Systemic infections
   Brucellosis
   Cytomegalovirus
   Diphtheria
   Infectious mononucleosis
   Legionnaires' disease
   Leptospirosis
   Mycoplasmal pneumonia
   Polyomavirus
   Rocky Mountain spotted fever
   Streptococcal infections
   Syphilis
   Toxoplasmosis
3. Primary renal infections
   Bacterial pyelonephritis (see Ch. 84)
   Renal tuberculosis
   Fungal nephritis
4. Immune disorders
   Acute glomerulonephritis associated with anti-tubular basement membrane antibodies and/or secondary interstitial nephritis (see Ch. 79)
   Systemic lupus erythematosus
   Acute rejection of a renal transplant (see Ch. 78.2)
   Necrotizing vasculitis
5. Other conditions
6. Idiopathic

Penicillins. Several penicillin congeners may cause AISN, including amoxicillin, ampicillin, carbenicillin, methicillin, mezlocillin, nafcillin, oxacillin, and penicillin G. Methicillin has been responsible for most reported cases, but the clinical syndrome is similar for the other penicillins. It is reasonable to presume that AISN may occur with any penicillin. Typically, penicillins have been taken for about 2 weeks prior to the onset of signs and symptoms of AISN, but this time interval has varied from 2 days to several weeks. The disorder appears to be more frequent in men and children. There is no correlation between drug dosage and subsequent development of AISN. The most frequent manifestations are hematuria (which may be gross and associated rarely with red cell casts in the urinary sediment), proteinuria (usually less than nephrotic range), pyuria (eosinophiluria is frequently present and strongly suggests the diagnosis of AISN), fever, eosinophilia (this may be evanescent), azotemia (often associated with oliguria), and skin rash. Serum immunoglobulin E (IgE) levels may be elevated. Renal sodium wasting and hyperchloremic metabolic acidosis with hyperkalemia (hyperkalemic distal renal tubular acidosis) also may occur.

For treatment, the offending drug must be discontinued, and another appropriate drug for the underlying infection should be substituted. In the majority of cases, this will restore renal function. Recovery may require several weeks, with some patients needing

TABLE 80-3. DRUGS ASSOCIATED WITH ACUTE INTERSTITIAL NEPHRITIS

Antimicrobial Drugs

Cephalosporins	Para-aminosalicylic acid
Chloramphenicol	Penicillins*
Ciprofloxacin	Polymyxin B
Erythromycin	Rifampin*
Ethambutol	Sulfonamides*
Isoniazid	Tetracyclines
	Vancomycin

Nonsteroidal Anti-inflammatory Drugs*

Miscellaneous

Allopurinol*	Methyldopa
Antipyrene	Phenindione
Azathioprine	Phenylpropanolamine
Bismuth	Phenytoin
Captopril	Probenecid
Carbamazepine	Ranitidine
Cimetidine	Sulfinpyrazone
Clofibrate	Sulfonamide diuretics*
Gold	Triamterene

* Most frequent or clinically important.

interval dialysis. A short course of high-dose corticosteroids (1 mg per kilogram per day of prednisone for 1 to 2 weeks) may accelerate recovery, but the added risk in patients with underlying infections must be weighed against possible benefits.

Sulfonamides. Both antimicrobial sulfonamides and sulfonamide diuretics (thiazides, furosemide, chlorthalidone, acetazolamide) have been implicated in AISN. Although frequently these are prescribed in combination with other drugs (e.g., sulfamethoxazole plus trimethoprim as antimicrobials and hydrochlorothiazide plus triamterene as diuretics), it is most likely that the sulfonamide moiety of these combinations is responsible for AISN. Typically, evidence for AISN develops several days after therapy is begun, but rechallenging a patient with a past history of sulfonamide-induced AISN may result in signs and symptoms within hours of exposure. The clinical presentation is in many ways similar to that described for the penicillins. Pyuria, hematuria, eosinophilia, and azotemia are frequent. A skin rash is present in a minority of patients. Renal failure may be severe and may require temporary dialysis, but recovery is the rule when the offending drug is discontinued. A brief course of corticosteroids may hasten recovery if no contraindications exist.

Drug-induced AISN should be particularly considered in patients with underlying renal disease, such as nephrotic syndrome, treated with sulfonamide diuretics who experience a more rapid decline in renal function than expected or other manifestations, such as eosinophilia, that suggest an allergic reaction. If diuretic therapy is required in a patient in whom a diagnosis of AISN is made by renal biopsy or presumed to be present based on characteristic clinical findings, a nonsulfonamide diuretic, such as ethacrynic acid, should be prescribed.

Antituberculous Drugs. A number of patients have developed AISN while receiving chemotherapy for tuberculosis, usually with more than one agent. Although rifampin, isoniazid, ethambutol, and para-aminosalicylic acid have all been incriminated as causing AISN, the evidence is most compelling for rifampin. AISN appears to occur more often and to be more severe with intermittent therapy with rifampin or after reinstituting therapy following a drug-free interval than during continuous therapy. Fever, chills, flank pain, and anuria may develop after readministering a single dose of rifampin. In contrast to other types of acute renal failure, transient hypercalcemia of unknown cause has been reported in several patients developing AISN during therapy for tuberculosis. Discontinuing the offending drugs is generally followed by recovery of renal function, although sometimes rather slowly. Corticosteroids do not appear to hasten recovery of renal function.

Allopurinol. Allopurinol-associated AISN generally develops after several days of treatment (mean interval of 3 weeks). Most patients have an exfoliative maculopapular skin rash, fever, eosinophilia, and decreased renal function. In addition, most have evidence of acute hepatic injury. Elevations of serum aspartate aminotransferase, sometimes to values >1000 units per liter, are present in about two thirds of patients. This form of allopurinol toxicity is severe and carries a mortality rate of approximately 20%. Deaths result from severe systemic reactions, sepsis, gastrointestinal bleeding, or acute hepatic or renal failure. The cause of allopurinol toxicity is uncertain. Clinical and laboratory manifestations suggest a severe systemic hypersensitivity reaction. Most reported patients have been treated with conventional doses of the drug (200 to 400 mg per day), but most have had underlying renal insufficiency prior to developing allopurinol toxicity. In addition, about one half of the reported patients were receiving concomitant diuretic therapy. Whether this represents a causal relationship or merely coincidence is uncertain. Treatment consists of discontinuing allopurinol and instituting supportive measures, including dialysis, when indicated. Although corticosteroids have been given to many patients, their efficacy is unproved. The incidence of allopurinol toxicity can be reduced by prescribing the drug only for clearly documented indications, such as recurrent gouty arthritis or uric acid nephrolithiasis, and not for asymptomatic hyperuricemia per se (including diuretic-induced hyperuricemia). The dose should be reduced in patients with underlying renal insufficiency.

Other Drugs Associated with AISN. Of the numerous other drugs reported to cause AISN, perhaps the most important are the nonsteroidal anti-inflammatory drugs (NSAID's) (see Ch. 19). For the remainder of the agents listed in Table 80–3, AISN appears to be a very rare complication. Nevertheless, when manifestations characteristic of AISN occur in patients receiving these drugs (or other drugs not listed), the diagnosis of AISN should be entertained. In this setting it may be simplest to discontinue the suspected drug and replace it with an alternative agent. On the other hand, in patients for whom no suitable alternative exists, it may be necessary to confirm or exclude the diagnosis of AISN by renal biopsy.

AISN Associated with Infection. Systemic bacterial, viral, rickettsial, mycoplasmal, and parasitic infections have been associated with AISN. Infections with group A beta-hemolytic streptococci are perhaps the most frequent, especially in children. The pathogenesis of AISN related to systemic infection is uncertain. Many patients with AISN associated with systemic infections have received antibiotic therapy and may have drug-induced AISN (see above). Therapy consists of treating the underlying infection and supportive measures. The prognosis for recovery of renal function is usually quite favorable.

Acute bacterial pyelonephritis is a common cause of AISN. The clinical presentation with fever, chills, flank pain, and bacteriuria is characteristic (see Ch. 84). Similarly, renal parenchymal fungal and mycobacterial infections may acutely inflame the renal interstitium. All these can result in renal scarring but only rarely cause acute renal failure.

AISN Associated with Immune Disorders. Varying degrees of acute and chronic interstitial nephritis may accompany numerous renal or systemic diseases of presumed immune origin. Several types of glomerulonephritis are associated with interstitial inflammation that may be out of proportion to the degree of glomerular injury (see Ch. 79). In some, there may be antibodies to the tubular basement membranes. Although glomerulonephritis is generally the primary renal lesion in systemic lupus erythematosus, interstitial nephritis is the predominant finding in some patients (see Ch. 79 and 240). Acute and chronic interstitial inflammation is the hallmark of renal transplant rejection (see Ch. 78.2). Renal involvement with necrotizing vasculitis generally manifests as a focal segmental glomerulonephritis, but in some patients, particularly those with Wegener's granulomatosis, there may be prominent interstitial involvement.

Other Conditions Associated with AISN. Sarcoidosis (see Ch. 61) may involve the kidneys in a number of ways, including acute (granulomatous) interstitial nephritis, chronic interstitial nephritis (often associated with hypercalcemia and hypercalciuria), and primary glomerulonephritis. Rarely, AISN may cause acute renal failure in sarcoidosis. There have been isolated case reports of AISN following therapy with recombinant leukocyte interferon.

Idiopathic AISN. In occasional patients with AISN, a specific cause cannot be identified. Some of these have evidence, such as eosinophilia, suggesting a hypersensitivity reaction to an unknown antigen. In addition to acute interstitial inflammation, renal biopsies sometimes demonstrate evidence for anti–tubular basement membrane antibodies. Others have granulomatous interstitial nephritis in the absence of an obvious etiology. The course of idiopathic AISN is variable, with some patients recovering spontaneously or in response to corticosteroid therapy and others progressing to renal insufficiency.

CLINICAL MANIFESTATIONS. In AISN the GFR may decline abruptly, often with oliguria. The urinary sediment typically contains numerous leukocytes. In cases of drug-induced AISN, eosinophils are frequently present as well. Hematuria is ordinarily present, and red blood cell casts, although rare, may be observed. Proteinuria is usually present but modest (< 3.5 grams per day), except in AISN due to NSAID's (see below). The fractional excretion of sodium tends to be high, as it is in most cases of acute tubular necrosis (see Ch. 76). A spectrum of renal tubular defects may be present (see Table 80–1). In cases of drug-induced AISN (see above), other manifestations of drug allergy, such as fever, skin rash, and eosinophilia, are frequent. In AISN occurring as part of a systemic process, such as systemic lupus erythematosus, clinical and laboratory manifestations of the primary disease may dominate the clinical presentation. The diagnosis of AISN is established by examining renal tissue obtained by biopsy (or autopsy). In drug-induced AISN, the diagnosis is often inferred from characteristic clinical and laboratory findings. The outcome of AISN depends on the underlying disease process. In drug-induced disease, renal function generally improves once the offending drug is stopped. Corticosteroid therapy may be beneficial, as discussed above. With prolonged and severe AISN, variable degrees of chronic renal insufficiency may result.

CHRONIC INTERSTITIAL NEPHRITIS

PATHOLOGY. Chronic interstitial nephritis (CISN) is characterized pathologically by interstitial fibrosis with atrophy and loss of renal tubules. The glomeruli may be normal but frequently are contracted. There is generally a patchy interstitial infiltrate of chronic inflammatory cells. The renal vasculature may show evidence of associated hypertension. In addition to these general findings, there may be others that suggest a specific disease, such as casts typical of multiple myeloma.

ETIOLOGY (Table 80–4). CISN may result from persistence or progression of many of the acute forms of interstitial nephritis (see Table 80–2) or may evolve without an obvious preceding phase of acute injury. Many of the specific causes of CISN are discussed subsequently; some of the remainder are commented on briefly below.

Urinary tract obstruction (including vesicoureteral reflux), the single most important cause of CISN, is discussed in Ch. 81. Perhaps the second most important group of disorders comprises those caused by nephrotoxins, most of which are discussed later as toxic nephropathies. In addition to exogenous toxins, certain endogenous chemical abnormalities may result in CISN. The major renal complication of *chronic hypokalemia* is nephrogenic (vasopressin-resistant) diabetes insipidus, which results in mild polyuria, but chronic interstitial nephritis with modest renal insufficiency may rarely occur as well. *Hypercalcemia* also produces mild polyuria due to nephrogenic diabetes insipidus. Acute hypercalcemia also acts on the glomeruli and renal vasculature to reduce GFR in a manner largely reversible with correction of hypercalcemia. Chronic hypercalcemia results in nephrocalcinosis and chronic interstitial nephritis with reduced GFR that may be only slowly and incompletely reversible. In addition, nephrocalcinosis may cause distal renal tubular acidosis (see Ch. 82). In the absence of urinary tract obstruction, *chronic bacterial pyelonephritis* rarely causes severe renal failure. Renal *tuberculosis* can result in acute and chronic tubulointerstitial disease. Tuberculous ureteral strictures may cause hydronephrosis.

A variety of *immune disorders* may be associated with both acute and chronic interstitial nephritis, including several types of glomerulonephritis (see Ch. 79), chronic renal transplant rejection (see Ch. 78.2), and systemic lupus erythematosus. Renal involvement in *Sjögren's syndrome* is usually in the form of CISN. The most common functional abnormalities are distal renal tubular acidosis and urinary concentrating defects.

Neoplastic and *paraproteinemic* disorders may be associated with CISN. In patients with lymphomas and leukemias, particularly acute lymphoblastic leukemia, neoplastic cells may infiltrate the renal in-

TABLE 80–4. CAUSES OF CHRONIC INTERSTITIAL NEPHRITIS

1. Persistence or progression of acute interstitial nephritis (see Table 80–2)
2. Chronic urinary tract obstruction (see Ch. 81)
3. Nephrotoxins
   Drugs: analgesics, nitrosoureas
   Endogenous substances: hypercalcemia, hypokalemia, oxalate, uric acid
   Metals: cisplatin, copper, lead, lithium, mercury
   Radiation
4. Chronic bacterial pyelonephritis (see Ch. 84) or renal tuberculosis (see Ch. 311)
5. Immune disorders
   Chronic glomerulonephritis with interstitial nephritis (see Ch. 79)
   Chronic rejection of a renal transplant (see Ch. 78.2)
   Systemic lupus erythematosus (see Ch. 240)
   Sjögren's syndrome (see Ch. 242)
6. Associated with neoplasia or paraproteinemias
   Leukemia
   Lymphoma
   Amyloidosis (see Ch. 248)
   Waldenström's macroglobulinemia (see Ch. 149)
   Cryoglobulinemia (see Ch. 79)
   Multiple myeloma (see Ch. 149)
7. Cystic diseases
   Medullary cystic disease
   Polycystic kidney disease (see Ch. 89)
8. Miscellaneous
   Diabetes mellitus
   Sickle cell hemoglobinopathies
   Vascular diseases
   Advanced renal failure
   Idiopathic

terstitium and cause renal enlargement. Adjacent renal tubules may be compressed and destroyed, but renal function is rarely compromised. Renal disease in patients with *amyloidosis* (see Ch. 248), *Waldenström's macroglobulinemia* (see Ch. 149), and *mixed cryoglobulinemia* (see Ch. 79) usually involves the glomeruli, but rarely, there may be prominent tubulointerstitial involvement. Renal failure is a common cause of death in patients with *multiple myeloma*, especially in those with Bence Jones proteinuria (monoclonal immunoglobulin light chain paraproteins). CISN, often associated with cast nephropathy, is the most important cause of renal failure in multiple myeloma. Large, dense eosinophilic casts occur within the tubule lumina, surrounded by a chronic interstitial infiltrate. Renal failure appears to result both from obstruction of the renal tubules by these casts and/or from direct toxic effects of the Bence Jones proteins. In addition to renal insufficiency, multiple myeloma may cause proximal and distal renal tubular acidosis, Fanconi's syndrome, urinary concentrating defects, and the nephrotic syndrome. The last is usually associated with renal amyloidosis. Recovery from renal failure due to CISN with cast nephropathy is rare in contrast to that occurring from other abnormalities in these individuals, particularly hypercalcemia.

MISCELLANEOUS FACTORS. In *diabetes mellitus* and *sickle cell hemoglobinopathies,* CISN may be accompanied by papillary necrosis. Hyperkalemia and hyperkalemic distal renal tubular acidosis may occur in both. In diabetic patients, this is generally due to hyporeninemic hypoaldosteronism. Urinary concentrating defects are particularly common in sickling disorders. Chronic reduction in renal blood flow from a variety of *renovascular disorders* causes atrophy of both the renal tubules and the glomeruli, along with interstitial fibrosis. *Advanced renal disease* of any etiology results in interstitial fibrosis with mild interstitial inflammation, tubular atrophy, and glomerulosclerosis characteristic of the "end-stage" kidney. Cysts of varying size also may be present. In many cases, these changes are so severe that it is not possible to determine whether the underlying cause of renal failure was tubulointerstitial, glomerular, or vascular in origin. In occasional cases of CISN, sometimes accompanied by granulomas, no recognized cause can be identified.

CLINICAL AND LABORATORY MANIFESTATIONS. The clinical manifestations may be primarily those of renal tubular functional defects (see Table 80–1) or may primarily reflect those of advanced renal failure. Sterile pyuria may be seen, but in contrast to AISN, eosinophilia and eosinophiluria are not. Historical and laboratory findings may suggest a specific diagnosis, e.g., flank pain, and radiographic or ultrasonographic evidence of hydronephrosis suggesting obstructive nephropathy. Clinical presentations unique to certain entities are discussed elsewhere.

TOXIC NEPHROPATHIES (Table 80–5)

Drug-induced AISN, an important type of nephrotoxic renal injury, is discussed in the preceding section with other causes of AISN. Other important toxic nephropathies are discussed below.

TABLE 80-5. PROMINENT OR COMMON NEPHROTOXINS

Anticonvulsants: paramethadione, phenytoin, trimethadone
Antihypertensive drugs: angiotensin-converting enzyme inhibitors, methyldopa
Antimicrobials: aminoglycosides, amphotericin B, cephalosporins, ethambutol, isoniazid, *para*-aminosalicylic acid, penicillins, rifampin, sulfonamides, tetracyclines, pentamidine, acyclovir
Antineoplastic agents: cisplatin, methotrexate, mitomycin C, nitrosoureas, radiation
Sulfonamide diuretics: acetazolamide, chlorthalidone, furosemide, thiazides
Endogenous substances: Bence Jones proteins, calcium, hemoglobin, myoglobin, oxalate, uric acid
Halogenated alkanes, hydrocarbons, and solvents: carbon tetrachloride, ethylene glycol, paraquat, toluene
Iodinated radiographic contrast media
Metals: arsenic, bismuth, cadmium, copper, gold, lead, lithium, mercury
Nonsteroidal anti-inflammatory drugs
Miscellaneous compounds: acetaminophen, allopurinol, amphetamines, azathioprine, cimetidine, cyclosporine, heroin, methoxyflurane, methysergide, D-penicillamine, phenacetin, phenindione, silicon

CISN leading to chronic renal failure may result from excessive consumption of certain analgesic agents. In the United States, 2 to 10% of all cases of end-stage renal disease are thought to be due to analgesic nephropathy (AN). In some other countries, AN is an even more important cause of chronic renal failure. The drugs most commonly associated with AN are phenacetin or acetaminophen (phenacetin is largely converted to acetaminophen soon after ingestion), usually in combination with aspirin. Generally, the offending agents are taken in the form of proprietary drugs, but sometimes they are obtained by prescriptions from physicians. In most countries the availability of phenacetin in proprietary drugs is now greatly restricted. Acute acetaminophen poisoning may cause acute renal failure due to acute tubular necrosis (see Ch. 76).

PATHOGENESIS AND PATHOLOGY. Although phenacetin, acetaminophen, and aspirin may be nephrotoxic when consumed in large quantities over extended periods, there is some debate about which of these may be the most noxious to the kidney. The combination of acetaminophen or phenacetin with aspirin appears to be more nephrotoxic than either drug alone. Prospective epidemiologic studies show a convincing correlation between the amount of phenacetin or acetaminophen consumed and the development of renal disease. The generally accepted requirement for the presumptive diagnosis of AN is a cumulative ingestion of 3 kg or more of these drugs or daily consumption of 1 gram for 3 or more years. In most reported cases of AN, consumption has far exceeded these amounts.

The pathogenesis of AN is still uncertain. Both aspirin and acetaminophen are concentrated within the kidney, and for acetaminophen, and perhaps aspirin, a concentration gradient exists within the kidney from the renal cortex to the medulla. Phenacetin and acetaminophen are metabolized to reactive species that covalently bind to proteins and result in oxidative tissue damage by depleting reducing equivalents such as glutathione. Aspirin may exacerbate this toxicity by inhibiting glutathione production. In addition, aspirin is a potent inhibitor of prostaglandin synthesis. This latter action may reduce renal medullary blood flow and result in ischemic damage. In addition to aspirin, other NSAID's that also inhibit prostaglandin synthesis have been associated with papillary necrosis and chronic renal disease in a small number of individuals.

In the initial stages of AN, there is patchy necrosis of interstitial cells, loops of Henle, and capillaries in the inner medulla, with calcium deposition and lipid accumulation in the involved areas. With continued exposure to these drugs, the process progressively involves the outer medulla and often results in total papillary necrosis. In advanced stages, the renal cortex is thin, and the renal tubules are atrophic. Interstitial fibrosis is accompanied by a round cell infiltrate. The glomeruli are initially spared, but later they and the arterioles become sclerotic. If AN is complicated by bacterial infection, focal collections of acute inflammatory cells are evident. The necrotic papillae may remain *in situ,* often with cavities in them, or they may totally detach from the medulla and slough into the renal pelvis.

CLINICAL AND LABORATORY MANIFESTATIONS. AN is usually associated with a characteristic group of signs, symptoms, and laboratory findings. The diagnosis of AN is often overlooked because patients frequently do not admit to taking analgesics or, if they do, will not provide a true estimate of the amount consumed. When the diagnosis is suspected, therefore, the possibility of AN should be vigorously pursued by discussions with family members or physicians who have cared for the patient previously. AN occurs more frequently in women (usually middle age) with a female/male ratio of 3:1 to 6:1. Although patients may consume analgesics for a variety of complaints, especially headaches, more often than not there is no disease that warrants taking large amounts of analgesics. In many patients there is a psychological component to the clinical presentation. Some patients have a family history of heavy analgesic use. Anemia is present in most patients and is frequently more severe than can be attributed to the degree of renal insufficiency. In addition to renal insufficiency, anemia may result from hemolysis or gastrointestinal blood loss due to peptic ulcer disease or gastritis, which also occur commonly. Hypertension is present in about half of patients but generally appears after renal disease is obvious. Malignant hypertension occasionally develops. Finally, AN is associated with an increased incidence of atherosclerosis, particularly coronary artery disease and renal artery stenosis.

Urinalysis frequently reveals pyuria. Urinary tract infections are present in approximately half of patients at some point and may be associated with leukocyte casts in the urinary sediment. Sloughing of a necrotic papilla into the urinary tract may be associated with gross hematuria, flank pain (ureteral colic), passage of tissue in the urine, and an abrupt decline in renal function. Proteinuria is generally modest (< 2 grams per day), but as the disease progresses, occasional patients develop focal sclerosing glomerulopathy with heavy proteinuria. Generally, progression to end-stage renal failure occurs over several years. Renal tubular abnormalities may be reflected by hyperchloremic metabolic acidosis due to decreased renal acidification, mild polyuria with an inability to concentrate the urine above the osmolality of blood due to nephrogenic diabetes insipidus, and an inability to appropriately reduce urinary sodium excretion with sodium deprivation (renal salt wasting).

Early in the disease course, the kidneys may be of normal size and contour when evaluated radiographically or by ultrasonography. In the late stages, the kidneys are small with a thin cortex and an irregular surface. A variety of findings on intravenous urography or retrograde pyelography—including caliceal clubbing, papillary cavities, and caliceal filling defects due to the presence of a sloughed papilla (ring sign)—may suggest papillary necrosis. Demonstration of papillary necrosis in the absence of its more common causes (e.g., diabetes mellitus, urinary tract obstruction, often with infection, or sickle cell disease) should suggest AN. Finally, patients with AN are at increased risk for developing transitional cell carcinoma of the urinary tract, particularly of the renal pelvis. The appearance of hematuria should lead to prompt evaluation to exclude a uroepithelial neoplasm. This evaluation should generally include examination of the urine for neoplastic cells, cystoscopy, and retrograde pyelograms.

PREVENTION AND THERAPY. Obviously, avoiding drugs implicated as causes of AN will prevent the disorder. Public education about the dangers of excessive analgesic consumption is important. The most important factor in the treatment of established AN is cessation of analgesic use. For individuals who habitually abuse analgesics, this requires a great deal of education and encouragement. Often psychological counseling is needed. For patients with diseases requiring analgesics—e.g., rheumatoid arthritis—alternative forms of therapy are indicated. Once analgesics are stopped, renal function will generally stabilize or improve. If renal disease is clearly established and drug use continues, renal function inexorably declines, often to the point of end-stage renal disease, over a period of several years. Urinary tract infections, ureteral obstruction from sloughed papillae, hypertension, and dehydration are conditions that may cause a more rapid decline in renal function, and all should be treated promptly.

Nonsteroidal Anti-Inflammatory Drugs

Several drugs that inhibit production of the various prostaglandins are now available. These agents are referred to collectively as "nonsteroidal anti-inflammatory drugs" (NSAID's) (see Ch. 19). With more widespread use of these drugs, several renal and electrolyte complications have been recognized.

The functions of renal prostaglandins have yet to be completely elucidated. Vasodilator prostaglandins (PGE_2, PGI_2) are important in maintaining renal blood flow in states of sodium depletion or when "effective" arterial blood volume is low. These states are generally associated with elevated levels of circulating angiotensin II and catecholamines. By causing renal vasodilation, prostaglandins preserve renal blood flow while angiotensin II and catecholamines maintain systemic blood pressure by increasing systemic vascular resistance. Prostaglandins also cause a natriuresis, stimulate renin release, and antagonize the effect of antidiuretic hormone. Many of the renal and electrolyte complications of prostaglandin inhibition by NSAID's (Table 80–6) are predictable, based on these recognized functions of the prostaglandins.

HEMODYNAMICALLY MEDIATED (VASOMOTOR) ACUTE RENAL FAILURE. This has been reported in several patients receiving NSAID's, most notably indomethacin. Renal failure results from renal hypoperfusion and occurs shortly after drug therapy is instituted. Patients at risk are those with sodium depletion (e.g., from diuretic therapy) or low "effective" arterial blood volumes (e.g., nephrotic syndrome, congestive heart failure, and hepatic cirrhosis with ascites), older individuals, and patients with underlying renal disease. Individuals receiving triamterene may be

TABLE 80–6. RENAL AND ELECTROLYTE COMPLICATIONS OF NONSTEROIDAL ANTI-INFLAMMATORY DRUGS

1. Renal failure
   a. Hemodynamic (major risk factors are sodium depletion, low "effective" arterial blood volume, and underlying renal disease)
   b. Acute interstitial nephritis with or without the nephrotic syndrome
   c. Glomerulonephritis associated with diffuse vasculitis
   d. Papillary necrosis with chronic interstitial nephritis
2. Sodium and fluid retention
3. Hyperkalemia, metabolic acidosis (occurs more often in patients with renal insufficiency, sodium depletion, or other factors predisposing to hyperkalemia)

especially at risk. This type of acute renal failure is usually associated with oliguria and low fractional excretion of sodium and thus resembles prerenal azotemia (see Ch. 76). The urinary sediment is generally unremarkable. Renal biopsies have shown evidence of acute tubular necrosis. Azotemia generally resolves promptly after discontinuation of the offending drug. Occasional patients, however, require temporary dialysis.

ACUTE INTERSTITIAL NEPHRITIS. AISN resulting in acute renal failure has been described in several patients in association with NSAID's, particularly fenoprofen. Heavy proteinuria, often in the nephrotic range, is peculiar to this form of drug-induced AISN. In addition to copious proteinuria, there are other features of AISN due to NSAID's that differ from those associated with other drugs. For example, eosinophilia, eosinophiluria, and skin rashes are uncommon. As with other types of drug-induced AISN, however, urinalysis frequently reveals microscopic hematuria and pyuria. In addition to histopathologic changes of AISN (described earlier), electron microscopy of the glomeruli reveals fusion of podocyte foot processes. Unlike hemodynamically mediated acute renal failure, AISN usually appears only after the offending drug has been administered for several days to several months. The disorder usually resolves when the drug is discontinued, but recovery may not occur until several months later, and interval dialysis may be required. Corticosteroid therapy is believed by many to hasten recovery, and in the absence of contraindications, it is reasonable to prescribe a short course of high-dose corticosteroids (1 mg per kilogram per day of prednisone) if renal failure is severe and spontaneous recovery does not occur within several days of stopping the drug.

OTHER RENAL COMPLICATIONS OF NSAID's. In addition to the preceding causes of acute renal insufficiency, systemic vasculitis with glomerulitis and papillary necrosis with CISN may occur rarely in association with NSAID's.

RETAINING SODIUM (AND FLUID). This is perhaps the most common renal side effect of NSAID's. Although this retention may not present a problem in persons with normal cardiovascular and renal function, it may result in worsening of pre-existing congestive heart failure or hypertension. Finally, inhibition of prostaglandin synthesis may result in hyperkalemia and metabolic acidosis largely due to inhibition of renin secretion and secondary hypoaldosteronism. Underlying renal insufficiency, sodium depletion, or concomitant administration of other drugs that predispose to hyperkalemia (e.g., potassium-sparing diuretics) increases the risk for developing the latter electrolyte abnormalities.

Antimicrobial Drugs

Renal damage from penicillin, sulfonamide, and antituberculous antimicrobials usually results from AISN, described earlier. Additional antibiotics may cause renal disease manifested in other ways.

AMINOGLYCOSIDES. The aminoglycosides, excreted primarily by glomerular filtration, accumulate in the renal cortex at higher than serum levels. They may cause several renal tubular functional abnormalities, the most clinically relevant of which are potassium and magnesium wasting, which may result in hypokalemia and hypomagnesemia. The most important manifestation of aminoglycoside renal toxicity, however, is acute renal failure. This results from both a direct effect of these drugs on glomerular filtration and tubular toxicity, causing acute tubular necrosis. Up to 10% of patients receiving aminoglycosides develop some degree of acute renal failure, accounting for 10 to 15% of all cases of this disorder in the United States. Generally, this failure is manifested by a rise in the serum creatinine level after several days of therapy with one of the aminoglycosides. At times, renal failure may become evident only after the drug has been discontinued. Acute renal failure is usually mild and of the nonoliguric variety. However, oliguria and severe renal failure requiring dialysis may be seen.

The most nephrotoxic aminoglycoside is neomycin, which is therefore not administered parenterally. It may rarely cause acute renal failure when given orally or by enema to decrease the bowel flora. The least nephrotoxic is streptomycin. Tobramycin and netilmicin are perhaps less nephrotoxic than gentamicin and amikacin. Risk factors for developing aminoglycoside toxicity include the dose of drug administered, the length of therapy, simultaneous administration of other potential nephrotoxins, particularly cephalosporins, renal insufficiency, advanced age, extracellular fluid (ECF) volume depletion, liver disease, and possibly potassium depletion. In older individuals the GFR normally declines, although this is unaccompanied by an elevated serum creatinine level. Failure to consider this variable when calculating the maintenance dose of aminoglycosides is a major (and preventable) factor in the production of acute renal failure.

Management of acute renal failure following aminoglycoside administration consists of discontinuing the drug and substituting another appropriate antibiotic if continued treatment is necessary. When no alternative antibiotic can be found, aminoglycosides may be continued in appropriately reduced doses. In this setting, serum aminoglycoside levels should be monitored. Supportive measures are similar to those indicated with acute renal failure of other causes (see Ch. 76). The prognosis for recovery of renal function after several days is excellent.

CEPHALOSPORINS. Renal failure due to acute tubular necrosis and AISN may rarely accompany treatment with the cephalosporins. The combination of a cephalosporin and an aminoglycoside carries a risk higher than for either drug alone, requiring close monitoring of renal function when this combination of agents is used.

TETRACYCLINES. Tetracyclines inhibit protein synthesis and, therefore, shunt amino acids into urea. The enhanced synthesis of urea elevates the blood urea nitrogen (BUN) without a concomitant elevation of serum creatinine or a reduction in GFR. In normal individuals this is of little consequence. In patients with underlying renal insufficiency, however, the increase in BUN may be dramatic. With the exception of doxycycline and minocycline, which do not accumulate in renal failure and which require only minor dosage adjustments, tetracyclines should be avoided in individuals with significant renal insufficiency. Demeclocycline causes a dose-related nephrogenic diabetes insipidus. This property has been used to treat some hyponatremic patients, particularly those with the syndrome of inappropriate secretion of antidiuretic hormone (see Ch. 75). Demeclocycline has been reported to cause acute renal failure, however, when given to hyponatremic patients with hepatic cirrhosis. Although the renal failure is reversible, demeclocycline (and other tetracyclines) should be avoided in these patients. Outdated tetracyclines can cause Fanconi's syndrome.

AMPHOTERICIN B. Most patients receiving more than 2 grams of this antifungal agent develop one or more renal abnormalities. Defects in distal nephron function are the first to appear: distal renal tubular acidosis, nephrogenic diabetes insipidus, and renal potassium wasting. These alterations may occur without a reduction in GFR and are generally reversible with discontinuation of the drug. Metabolic acidosis and hypokalemia should be treated with supplemental alkali and potassium salts. Acute renal insufficiency, which may be progressive and incompletely reversible, is a major side effect of amphotericin B. This side effect is dose-related and appears to result both from direct renal tubular toxicity and ischemia due to renal vasoconstriction. Acute renal failure is more likely to occur in patients who are sodium depleted from whatever cause—diuretics, vomiting, and so on—and in patients with underlying renal insufficiency. Sodium repletion may protect against amphotericin B nephrotoxicity. Once moderate azotemia is present (BUN > 50 mg per deciliter), consideration should be given to prescribing the drug on alternate days or to temporarily discontinuing therapy until renal function improves. The risk of renal insuffi-

ciency has to be weighed, of course, against the severity of the underlying infection and whether alternative antifungal therapy is available.

Radiographic Contrast Agents

Acute renal failure resulting from acute tubular necrosis is an uncommon but important complication of iodinated radiographic contrast agents used, for example, in intravenous urography, arteriography, or contrast-enhanced computed tomography. The incidence of acute renal failure associated with these agents has varied in large series from 0 to 13% but is much higher in certain groups of patients. Risk factors include underlying renal insufficiency, diabetes mellitus, older age, dehydration, history of prior acute renal failure following use of contrast agents, multiple contrast procedures in a short period, concomitant exposure to other nephrotoxins, and, perhaps, multiple myeloma. In addition, acute renal failure is more likely after administration of larger doses of these agents. Clearly, individuals at highest risk are diabetic patients with renal insufficiency. The incidence of acute renal failure following exposure to these agents in this population of patients may be as high as 75%. In the absence of other risk factors, diabetes *per se* does not appear to pose a major risk.

Pathogenetic factors in radiocontrast-induced acute renal failure may include ischemia resulting from renal arteriolar vasoconstriction due to the hypertonicity of these agents, tubular obstruction due to precipitation of proteins, and direct tubular toxicity. In addition, as with any drug, anaphylaxis with hypotension is a rare cause of acute renal failure. Patients who develop acute renal failure generally have an elevation in serum creatinine level within 24 hours of exposure to radiocontrast agents. The peak in creatinine elevation typically occurs within 7 days. Renal insufficiency is usually moderate and resolves in a few days, but it may be severe and necessitate temporary dialysis. With advanced underlying renal disease, the acute insufficiency may be irreversible. In patients at risk, the serum creatinine concentration should be measured the day after exposure to these agents to determine if nephrotoxicity has occurred. A persistent nephrogram at this time also suggests renal injury.

Prevention of renal failure in patients at high risk includes avoiding dehydration, minimizing the amount of contrast administered (no more than 0.88 mg of iodine per kilogram of body weight), and using alternative diagnostic methods such as ultrasonography, if possible. Nonionic agents appear to be minimally, if at all, less nephrotoxic than ionic ones. Hypertonic mannitol (25 to 50 grams given over 1 hour) immediately following exposure to radiographic contrast agents may reduce the incidence of acute renal failure in high-risk patients. Treatment of acute renal failure due to contrast agents is similar to that resulting from other etiologies (see Ch. 76).

Nephropathies Resulting from Antineoplastic Therapy

Several drugs used in the treatment of neoplasia may produce renal toxicity. Some of these may cause isolated abnormalities in renal tubular function, whereas others may produce acute or chronic renal insufficiency. For some of these compounds, renal damage represents the dose-limiting toxicity.

CISPLATIN. Cisplatin and its metabolites are eliminated primarily by urinary excretion. Acute tubular necrosis, which may occur after intravenously administering the drug, is dose-related, being uncommon with single doses < 50 mg per square meter but occurring in most patients with doses > 100 mg per square meter. The cause of cisplatin toxicity is uncertain, but it appears similar to that produced by other heavy metals (see below). Concomitant administration of cisplatin and other nephrotoxins, such as aminoglycosides, increases the risk of acute renal failure. Generally, azotemia appears a few days after administration of the drug and is usually reversible over a period of 2 to 4 weeks. With severe acute renal failure and/or repeated administration of cisplatin, chronic renal insufficiency due to CISN may develop. The incidence of acute renal failure due to cisplatin can be reduced by ensuring adequate hydration and establishing a saline diuresis prior to and during administration of the drug and by continuously infusing the drug slowly over several hours or a few days. Hypomagnesemia due to renal magnesium wasting may occur in as many as 50% of patients treated with cisplatin. Hypomagnesemia may be severe, may develop in the absence of renal insufficiency, and may persist for several weeks following cisplatin therapy. Other renal tubular abnormalities, such as potassium wasting, decreased urinary concentrating ability, and low-molecular-weight proteinuria also may be observed but are generally of little clinical importance. A new analogue, carboplatin, appears to be less nephrotoxic than cisplatin.

METHOTREXATE. This folic acid antagonist is eliminated principally by urinary excretion. Nephrotoxicity is rare with low doses (5 to 60 mg per square meter). With high-dose therapy (500 to 7500 mg per square meter), the drug precipitates in the renal tubule lumina and causes acute renal failure from tubular obstruction. Direct tubular toxicity may also play a role. Nephrotoxicity may be reduced by vigorous (intravenous) hydration to maintain a urine flow of >100 ml per hour for several days following high-dose therapy. In addition, the urine pH should be kept above 7 by alkali administration, since methotrexate is more soluble in alkaline solutions. Development of renal insufficiency prolongs the half-life of methotrexate and increases the likelihood of systemic toxicity.

NITROSOUREAS. A number of nitrosoureas used in cancer chemotherapy, including streptozocin, carmustine (BCNU), lomustine (CCNU), and methyl CCNU, may produce several types of renal toxicity. Streptozocin may cause proteinuria, sometimes resulting in nephrotic syndrome, due to glomerular injury; acute tubular necrosis leading to acute renal failure; and a variety of renal tubular abnormalities, including proximal renal tubular acidosis, glycosuria, phosphaturia, and aminoaciduria. Proteinuria is generally the first manifestation of renal toxicity. Should this occur, therapy should be withheld and only cautiously restarted if this resolves. Azotemia developing after streptozocin should lead to permanent discontinuation of the drug. The other nitrosoureas given in multiple courses over several weeks have been associated with a very high incidence of chronic renal insufficiency. The principal pathologic findings are CISN and glomerulosclerosis. Any nitrosoureas generally should be discontinued at the first sign of an otherwise unexplained decrease in renal function.

MITOMYCIN C. There is a 5 to 40% incidence of nephrotoxicity following mitomycin C therapy. Toxicity is dose related and generally appears after repeated courses and/or a cumulative dose of 60 mg per square meter. Renal injury is manifested by proteinuria (usually mild) and azotemia. Renal insufficiency may develop gradually or abruptly. In the latter instance, the clinical features are similar to those of the hemolytic uremic syndrome (see Ch. 79) and include thrombocytopenia, microangiopathic hemolytic anemia, and acute renal failure. Renal pathologic findings consist of glomerular alterations (mesangial fragmentation, capillary thrombi, and hemorrhage) and thrombosis and fibrinoid necrosis of the arterioles. There is no established therapy except for supportive measures for renal failure developing after administration of mitomycin C. Renal function should be monitored closely in patients receiving this drug, and therapy should probably be discontinued if otherwise unexplained azotemia occurs.

MISCELLANEOUS ANTINEOPLASTIC AGENTS. Nephrotoxicity has occasionally been reported with other cancer chemotherapeutic agents, including 5-azacytidine, daunorubicin, doxorubicin, ifosfamide, mithramycin, dacarbazine, and recombinant leukocyte A interferon. Administration of recombinant interleukin-2 to patients with advanced cancer is commonly associated with acute renal insufficiency, probably resulting from severe prerenal azotemia. Finally, therapy resulting in massive acute killing of neoplastic cells may cause the tumor lysis syndrome (see below).

RADIATION NEPHRITIS (Also see Ch. 13.1). Exposure of the kidneys during abdominal irradiation for cancer may subsequently result in damage of varying degree. Manifestations range from mild proteinuria, urinary concentrating defects, and benign hypertension with a reduced GFR to malignant hypertension with end-stage renal failure. Evidence for renal damage occurs several months to years after renal irradiation, and the severity bears a general relationship to the amount of irradiation received. Clinically evident renal injury is uncommon with less than 1000 to 2000 cGy but develops in approximately 50% of patients receiving doses higher than this. In the early stage of radiation nephritis, tubular necrosis, medial and intimal thickening of the small renal arteries, and damage to the glomerular endothelium are present. Later, glomerulosclerosis, collagenous thickening of the small renal arteries, and interstitial fibrosis are prominent. The incidence of radiation nephritis can be minimized by limiting the total dose of abdominal irradiation in a single course to 2000 cGy over 2 weeks and by shielding the kidneys as much as possible. Malignant hypertension resulting from unilateral radiation nephritis can be cured by nephrectomy.

URIC ACID AND THE TUMOR LYSIS SYNDROME. Patients with certain hematologic malignancies, particularly acute lymphoblastic leukemia and poorly differentiated lymphomas, may rarely develop spontaneous acute renal failure from obstruction of the renal tubules by uric acid. More frequently, this complication follows aggressive chemotherapy or radiation therapy, which kills cells and releases massive amounts of purine uric acid precursors. The resulting hyperuricemia greatly increases the filtered load of urate. Its solubility is exceeded in acidified tubular urine, and uric acid precipitation occurs in the renal tubules, often resulting in acute obstructive renal failure. A ratio of urinary uric acid/creatinine concentrations >1:1 suggests the diagnosis of acute uric acid nephropathy. During massive cell lysis, phosphate is also released in large amounts, and hyperphosphaturia with intrarenal precipitation of calcium phosphate may contribute to the renal failure. Hyperkalemia due to release of intracellular potassium also may be observed. Prevention of acute renal failure secondary to massive tumor cell killing includes establishing a urinary output of ≥3 liters per 24 hours and treatment with high-dose allopurinol (300 to 400 mg per square meter per day) before beginning cytotoxic therapy. The role of urinary alkalinization is uncertain. Although this will increase the solubility of uric acid, a high urinary pH will favor precipitation of phosphate salts in the renal tubules. If renal failure occurs despite the foregoing precautions, hemodialysis is indicated for supportive therapy and for removing uric acid and other cellular products. This practice allows renal function to recover, generally in a few days. Chronic interstitial nephritis (gouty nephropathy), a complication of chronic hyperuricemia and gout, is discussed in Ch. 251.

Metal Nephropathies

The diagnosis and treatment of intoxication with trace metals are discussed in detail in Ch. 13.3. Only certain aspects of this subject related to the kidney are discussed below. Acute intoxication with some metals may cause both acute renal injury with a reduction in GFR and renal tubular dysfunction. With chronic intoxication, the most common form of injury is chronic interstitial nephritis manifested by renal tubular abnormalities with or without reduction in GFR. In certain instances glomerular injury also may occur. Metal intoxication is often treated by chelation therapy. Unfortunately, some of the drugs used for this purpose, e.g., penicillamine, also may be nephrotoxic, as discussed below.

LITHIUM. Lithium carbonate, used in the treatment of affective disorders, causes a variety of renal abnormalities. The most frequent is a form of vasopressin-resistant nephrogenic diabetes insipidus. This is of little consequence in most patients. Polyuria (urine volumes >3000 ml per day) may result but usually abates when lithium therapy is stopped. The diuretic amiloride may significantly reduce the polyuria associated with lithium. Incomplete distal renal tubular acidosis and mild renal sodium wasting may also result from lithium therapy. CISN occurs in some lithium-treated patients. However, since CISN is more frequent in individuals with affective disorders than in the general population, the importance of lithium is debated. However, a history of acute lithium intoxication may predispose to development of chronic renal insufficiency.

LEAD. Lead poisoning may result from acute exposure, such as from ingestion of lead-containing paint, but more often from chronic exposure, such as in foundry and battery workers or from consumption of illicit alcoholic beverages ("moonshine"). Acute intoxication, more common in children, is manifested primarily by abdominal colic, hemolytic anemia, and encephalopathy. AISN with eosinophilic inclusions in the proximal tubular cells, tubular necrosis with a reduction in GFR, and Fanconi's syndrome also may occur. Whether acute lead intoxication without further exposure results in chronic renal disease in later years is unclear. Chronic lead intoxication causes interstitial nephritis with variable reductions in GFR and renal tubular dysfunction. Some patients develop gout and hypertension as a result of chronic lead intoxication ("saturnine gout"). Chronic lead intoxication should be considered in individuals with the triad of gout, hypertension, and chronic renal insufficiency. A history of exposure to lead should be sought and a $CaNa_2$-ethylenediaminetetra-acetic acid (EDTA) infusion carried out to evaluate lead stores. Treatment of acute lead intoxication consists of preventing further exposure to the metal, supportive care, and chelation with dimercaptopropanol (BAL) or CaNa₂-EDTA. Chronic renal insufficiency resulting from lead may sometimes improve during chelation therapy but also may progress despite this therapy.

MERCURY. Acute intoxication with mercurial salts may cause tubular necrosis and severe renal failure. The strong affinity of mercury for sulfhydryl groups, along with the hypotension that frequently accompanies acute intoxication, probably accounts for the acute renal injury. Acute exposure may occur rarely in industrial settings or with intentional ingestion of mercurial salts. Treatment of acute poisoning from mercurial salts consists of chelation therapy with dimercaptopropanol or penicillamine and supportive care. Chronic exposure to organomercurials may result in subtle renal damage manifested by increased urinary excretion of low-molecular-weight proteins and renal tubular enzymes (tubular proteinuria). Chelation therapy is ineffective in removing organomercurials. Chronic exposure to mercurial compounds also may cause the nephrotic syndrome as a result of glomerular damage, most commonly from membranous nephropathy. The pathogenesis of this disorder is uncertain, as mercury is not demonstrable in the glomeruli.

GOLD. Proteinuria may complicate the treatment of rheumatoid arthritis with gold salts, more frequently with parenteral than with oral administration. Proteinuria may develop at any time but usually after several months of therapy. Rarely, it may be severe enough to result in the nephrotic syndrome associated with membranous nephropathy. It is unlikely that gold *per se* is directly responsible for the glomerular injury, since the metal can be demonstrated in the renal tubules, but not in the glomeruli. Gold may in some way modify an intrinsic protein so that it becomes antigenic and elicits the immune reactions that produce membranous nephropathy. Membranous nephropathy also may occur in patients with rheumatoid arthritis who have not been treated with gold. If proteinuria appears, promptly discontinue the drug. This practice generally results in disappearance of the proteinuria, but this disappearance may occur only several months later.

ARSENIC. Arsenic is used in a number of industrial applications and is present in several commercial products, such as insecticides. In addition, illicit alcohol may be contaminated with the metal. Gastrointestinal symptoms and peripheral neuropathy are the most prominent manifestations of acute arsenic poisoning but acute tubular necrosis may also occur. Like mercury, arsenic has a high affinity for sulfhydryl groups of proteins. Cellular damage resulting from this interaction and from hypotension are the most likely causes of acute renal damage. Treatment of arsenic poisoning includes supportive measures and chelation therapy with dimercaptopropanol. Arsine gas may cause acute renal failure secondary to hemoglobinuria from acute hemolysis and from hypotension.

CADMIUM. With chronic low-level exposure—for example, in alkaline battery workers—cadmium accumulates in the renal cortex. This may result in mild proteinuria, of both glomerular and tubular origin, and in early renal insufficiency. The incidence of proteinuria increases with the length of exposure.

MISCELLANEOUS METALS. *Bismuth* has been reported to cause both acute tubular necrosis and the nephrotic syndrome. Acute *copper* poisoning may produce acute tubular necrosis, most likely resulting from hemolysis with hemoglobinuria and from hypotension. Chronic copper accumulation in Wilson's disease (see Ch. 188) may be associated with proximal renal tubular acidosis and other components of Fanconi's syndrome and mild renal insufficiency. In rare instances, renal injury has been reported with *antimony, thallium,* and *uranium* intoxication. *Platinum* nephrotoxicity is discussed under cisplatin.

Oxalate

End-stage renal failure from CISN and from recurrent nephrolithiasis is the major complication of primary hyperoxaluria and may rarely occur in enteric hyperoxaluria as well (see Ch. 172).

Acute intoxication with ethylene glycol is the major cause of acute renal failure due to oxalate. Ethylene glycol is the principal component of antifreeze and is usually ingested by desperate alcoholics, by children accidentally, or in a suicide attempt. Ethylene glycol is metabolized to several toxic substances, one of which is oxalic acid. Intoxication with ethylene glycol causes acute renal

failure, profound metabolic acidosis of the anion gap variety (see Ch. 75), and acute central nervous system and pulmonary dysfunction. Renal failure results from massive deposition of oxalate within the renal tubules. This is usually accompanied by large numbers of calcium oxalate crystals in the urinary sediment. Ethylene glycol intoxication is managed by (1) administration of ethyl alcohol to slow the metabolism of ethylene glycol by competing for alcohol dehydrogenase; (2) hemodialysis to remove the parent compound, to allow treatment with sodium bicarbonate therapy, which may be required in amounts that would otherwise result in pulmonary edema and hypernatremia, and to treat acute renal failure; and (3) administration of pyridoxine and thiamine to help shunt ethylene glycol into other metabolic pathways that result in less toxic metabolites. If patients survive acute intoxication, chances for recovery of renal function are good, but many will require temporary dialysis for several days prior to functional renal recovery.

Angiotensin-Converting Enzyme (ACE) Inhibitors

Acute renal failure may occur (in the absence of hypotension) following treatment with ACE inhibitors. Frequently, but not always, this develops in the presence of bilateral renal artery stenosis or stenosis of the artery supplying a solitary kidney. Usually, ACE inhibitor–associated acute renal failure is thought to be hemodynamic in origin, resulting from loss of autoregulation of renal blood flow and GFR. Sometimes, however, acute renal failure following captopril therapy has been accompanied by skin rash, eosinophilia, and eosinophiluria, a constellation of findings strongly suggesting allergic interstitial nephritis. Acute renal failure in both the preceding settings generally resolves with discontinuation of the ACE inhibitor but may recur upon rechallenge. Membranous nephropathy with the nephrotic syndrome also may occur in association with captopril therapy. This complication may resolve slowly after discontinuation of the drug. Membranous nephropathy occurring during therapy with captopril and penicillamine (see below) may possibly be related to the active sulfhydryl group that they contain.

D-Penicillamine

Therapy with this drug for metal chelation, rheumatoid arthritis, scleroderma, or cystinuria is complicated by proteinuria in 4 to 7% of patients, often sufficiently severe to result in the nephrotic syndrome. Proteinuria, which may be associated with mild azotemia, usually results from membranous nephropathy (see Ch. 79). Rarely, rapidly progressive glomerulonephritis accompanied by pulmonary hemorrhage occurs. Proteinuria generally resolves or decreases when D-penicillamine therapy is discontinued, but usually only after several months.

Methoxyflurane

This fluorinated anesthetic agent may cause a dose-related postoperative nephrogenic diabetes insipidus and acute renal failure. Similar complications have rarely been reported with enflurane. The initial polyuric acute renal failure may progress to oliguria in severe cases. Renal function may recover after several days, but persistent renal failure, which has required long-term dialysis, may develop. The pathogenesis of methoxyflurane-induced acute renal failure is uncertain. The drug is metabolized to fluoride and oxalate. Although oxalate is nephrotoxic (see above), it is believed that the major toxic product is fluoride, since nephrotoxicity correlates with blood levels of this ion and fluoride produces nephrotoxicity in experimental animals. Volume depletion due to the urinary concentrating defect may also contribute to acute renal failure.

Miscellaneous Nephrotoxins

Exposure to *hydrocarbons,* frequently in the form of paint or glue sniffing, has been associated with a variety of (generally) reversible abnormalities, including azotemia, renal tubular acidosis, Fanconi's syndrome, proteinuria, hematuria, and pyuria. Similar findings may result from exposure to halogenated alkane solvents, such as *carbon tetrachloride,* and insecticides, such as *paraquat. Silicon* exposure—for example, in sandblasters—has been implicated in a connective tissue–like disease with multiple serologic abnormalities and progressive renal failure associated with both glomerular and renal tubular pathologic changes that appear to be immune mediated.

Heroin abuse is associated with a variety of glomerular lesions, including amyloidosis, and glomerulonephritis due to bacterial endocarditis or hepatitis B infection. In some patients, however, these etiologies cannot be implicated. Most commonly, focal sclerosing glomerulopathy is found, often resulting in the nephrotic syndrome. Recently, it has been found that many of these patients have human immunodeficiency virus (HIV) infections with or without full-blown acquired immunodeficiency syndrome (AIDS) (see Ch. 370). Heroin-associated nephropathy generally results in progressive renal failure unless abuse of the drug is stopped.

The nephrotic syndrome may occur as a rare complication of *trimethadione* and *methimazole*. *Sulfonamides* and intravenous *amphetamines* may cause systemic vasculitis that results in renal damage from segmental renal infarction or glomerulonephritis (see Ch. 79 and 243). Acute renal insufficiency is a major complication of cyclosporin A therapy of organ transplantation (see Ch. 78.2). Administration of cyclosporin A for several months may be associated with occlusion of renal arterioles, CISN, and a reduced GFR. The antiviral drug acyclovir may cause acute renal failure because of precipitation of the agent in the tubular lumina with resultant intrarenal obstruction. A similar process may occur in patients treated with high-dose sulfadiazine. Pentamidine used to treat *Pneumocystis carinii* and other protozoal diseases results in acute renal insufficiency in approximately 25% of cases. *Nifedipine,* like many other drugs, may cause prerenal azotemia because of hypotension but, in addition, also may rarely cause reversible acute renal failure in the absence of a fall in blood pressure and without abnormalities in the urinary sediment.

Retroperitoneal fibrosis as a complication of long-term treatment of migraine headaches with *methysergide* may obstruct the ureters. *Anticoagulant therapy* may cause ureteral obstruction from intraluminal blood clots or from ureteral compression by a retroperitoneal hematoma.

Acute and Chronic Interstitial Nephritis

Bennett WM, Elzinga LW, Porter GA: Tubulointerstitial disease and toxic nephropathy. *In* Brenner BM, Rector FC Jr (eds.): The Kidney. 4th ed. Philadelphia, WB Saunders, 1991. *A comprehensive review (831 references).*

Cameron JS: Immunologically mediated interstitial nephritis: primary and secondary. Adv Nephrol 18:207, 1989. *A detailed review emphasizing drug-induced interstitial nephritis (228 references).*

Eknoyan G: Chronic tubulointerstitial nephropathies. *In* Schrier RW, Gottschalk CW (eds.): Diseases of the Kidney. 5th ed. Boston, Little, Brown and Company, 1993. *A detailed review of this topic (93 references).*

Hande KR, Noone RM, Stone WJ: Severe allopurinol toxicity. Am J Med 76:47, 1984. *This report describes 7 patients with allopurinol toxicity treated by the authors and reviews another 78 cases from the literature. Dosage guidelines for allopurinol for patients with varying degrees of renal insufficiency are proposed.*

Toto RD: Review: Acute tubulointerstitial nephritis. Am J Med Sci 299:392, 1990. *A good general review of this subject (114 references).*

Toxic Nephropathy (General References)

Bernard A, Lauwerys RR: Proteinuria: Changes and mechanisms in toxic nephropathies. Crit Rev Toxicol 21:373, 1991. *Particular emphasis on mechanisms of nephrotoxicity and on occupational/environmental exposure to a variety of nephrotoxins (425 references).*

Weinberg JM: The cellular basis of nephrotoxicity. *In* Schrier RW, Gottschalk CW (eds.): Diseases of the Kidney. 5th ed. Boston, Little, Brown and Company, 1993. *This chapter provides an exhaustive review of the pathophysiology of nephrotoxic renal injury (974 references).*

Analgesic Nephropathy

De Broe ME, Elseviers MM: Analgesic nephropathy—Still a problem? Nephron 64:505, 1993. *Includes summaries of several case-control studies indicating the magnitude of renal disease due to analgesic nephropathy in various parts of the world.*

Kincaid-Smith P, Nanra RS: Lithium-induced and analgesic-induced renal diseases. *In* Schrier RW, Gottschalk CW (eds.): Diseases of the Kidney. 5th ed. Boston, Little, Brown and Company, 1993. *This recent chapter contains a thorough review of these disorders (382 references).*

Nonsteroidal Anti-Inflammatory Drugs

Henrich WL: Nephrotoxicity of nonsteroidal antiinflammatory agents. *In* Schrier RW, Gottschalk CW (eds.): Diseases of the Kidney. 5th ed. Boston, Little, Brown and Company, 1993. *This chapter contains a thorough discussion of the renal, fluid, and electrolyte complications of NSAID's (173 references).*

Schlondorff D: Renal complications of nonsteroidal anti-inflammatory drugs. Kidney Int 44:643, 1993. *Emphasizes the effects of NSAID's on glomerular filtration and electrolyte excretion (113 references).*

Antimicrobial Drugs

Kaloyanides GJ: Aminoglycoside nephrotoxicity. *In* Schrier RW, Gottschalk CW (eds.): Diseases of the Kidney. 5th ed. Boston, Little, Brown and Company, 1993. *A comprehensive review that particularly emphasizes pathophysiology (316 references).*

Sawyer MH, Webb DE, Balow JE, et al.: Acyclovir-induced renal failure. Am J Med 84:1067, 1988. *This report describes four patients with intrarenal obstruction and crystalluria resulting from acyclovir.*

Velázquez H, Perazella MA, Wright FS, Ellison DH: Renal mechanism of trimethoprim-induced hyperkalemia. Ann Intern Med 119:296, 1993. *In this report of 39 consecutive AIDS patients treated with high-dose trimethoprim (given in association with sulfamethoxazole or dapsone), the serum potassium level increased by an average of 0.6 mmol per liter and to levels >6 mmol per liter in three patients. Studies in rats indicated that trimethoprim blocked potassium secretion in the distal nephron in a manner similar to that produced by amiloride.*

Radiocontrast-Induced Nephrotoxicity

Goldfarb S, Spinler S, Berns JS, Rudnick MR: Low-osmolality contrast media and the risk of contrast-associated nephrotoxicity. Invest Radiol 28(suppl 5):S7, 1993. *Several recent trials and a meta-analysis indicate a similar low risk of nephrotoxicity with the two types of agents in individuals with normal renal function. However, in patients with pre-existing renal insufficiency, nephrotoxicity was greater with the low-osmolality media.*

Nephrotoxicity Associated with Antineoplastic Therapy

Anand AJ, Bashey B: Newer insights into cisplatin nephrotoxicity. Ann Pharmacother 27:1519, 1993. *A recent review of the clinical and experimental aspects of this subject.*

Hande KR, Garrow GC: Acute tumor lysis syndrome in patients with high-grade non-Hodgkin's lymphoma. Am J Med 94:133, 1993. *In this report of 102 patients, 42% developed laboratory and 6% clinical evidence for tumor lysis syndrome after combination chemotherapy. Clinical tumor lysis occurred more frequently in patients with pretreatment renal insufficiency and correlated with pretreatment serum lactate dehydrogenase concentrations.*

Jorkasky DK, Singer I: Drug-induced tubulo-interstitial nephritis: Special cases. Semin Nephrol 8:62, 1988. *This paper concisely reviews nephrotoxicity associated with several drugs, including methotrexate, cisplatinum, and the nitrosoureas (118 references).*

Rieselbach RE, Garnick MB: Renal diseases induced by antineoplastic agents. *In* Schrier RW, Gottschalk CW (eds.): Diseases of the Kidney. 5th ed. Boston, Little, Brown and Company, 1993. *Provides a thorough review of this topic (207 references).*

Metal Nephropathies

Bautman V: Lead nephropathy, gout and hypertension. Am J Med Sci 305:241, 1993. *Succinctly reviews the frequent association of the triad of gout, hypertension, and renal insufficiency with increased body burden of lead.*

Järup L, Persson B, Edling C, Elinder CG: Renal function impairment in workers previously exposed to cadmium. Nephron 64:75, 1993. *In this long-term follow-up study of 16 workers exposed to cadmium, renal tubular damage was shown to be irreversible. Glomerular dysfunction also may be irreversible and progressive even after cadmium exposure ceases.*

Wedeen RP: Heavy metals. *In* Schrier RW, Gottschalk CW (eds.): Diseases of the Kidney. 5th ed. Boston, Little, Brown and Company, 1993. *This chapter reviews the renal complications that may accompany intoxication with several heavy metals (163 references).*

Toxic Nephropathy (Miscellaneous References)

Baldwin DS, Gallo GR, Neugarten J: Drug abuse with narcotics and other agents. *In* Schrier RW, Gottschalk CW (eds.): Diseases of the Kidney. 5th ed. Boston, Little, Brown and Company, 1993. *Provides a good discussion of the several renal complications that may result from drug abuse, along with representative photographs of histopathologic findings (147 references).*

Hricik DE, Dunn MJ: Angiotensin-converting enzyme inhibitor-induced renal failure: Causes, consequences and diagnostic uses. J Am Soc Nephrol 1:845, 1990. *A good review of these clinically important issues (112 references).*

McDiarmid SV, Colonna JO II, Shaked A, et al.: A comparison of renal function in cyclosporine and FK-506–treated patients after primary orthotopic liver transplantation. Transplantation 65:847, 1993. *This report indicates that the nephrotoxicity of these two immunosuppressive drugs is similar. After 1 year of therapy, glomerular filtration rate had fallen by 35% and 51% in the cyclosporine and FK-506 groups, respectively.*

Walker RG: Lithium nephrotoxicity. Kidney Int 44(suppl 42):S-93, 1993. *Reviews the several renal abnormalities associated with lithium therapy.*

81 OBSTRUCTIVE UROPATHY
Saulo Klahr

"Obstructive uropathy" refers to the structural or functional changes in the urinary tract that impede the normal flow of urine. It occurs in a variety of settings and is a relatively common cause of impaired renal function (obstructive nephropathy). Obstructive uropathy also may cause dilation of the urinary tract (hydronephrosis). Since the consequences of obstructive uropathy are potentially reversible, prompt diagnosis and appropriate treatment are important to prevent permanent loss of renal function, which is directly related to the degree and duration of the obstruction.

INCIDENCE. A relatively common disorder, obstructive uropathy is seen in all age groups. Hydronephrosis has been found at autopsy in 3.5 to 3.8% of adults and in 2% of children. Urolithiasis occurs predominantly in young adults (ages 25 to 45) and is three times more common in men than in women. In patients older than 60 years, obstructive uropathy is seen more frequently in men than in women owing to benign prostatic hyperplasia and prostatic carcinoma. Each year, approximately 166 patients per 100,000 population are hospitalized with a presumptive diagnosis of obstruction, and about 387 patient visits per 100,000 population are related to obstructive uropathy. Approximately 450,000 surgical procedures for benign prostatic hyperplasia are performed annually in the United States.

ETIOLOGY. Obstruction can occur anywhere in the urinary tract from the renal tubules (uric acid nephropathy) to the urethral meatus (phimosis) (Table 81–1). Clinically, it is helpful to divide the causes of obstruction into *upper urinary tract* (lesions located above the ureterovesical junction) and *lower urinary tract* (below the ureterovesical junction). The causes of upper urinary tract obstruction can be divided into *intrinsic* (intraluminal or intramural) and *extrinsic* (Table 81–1). Intraluminal obstruction is due to stones, clots, or sloughed papillary tissue. Intramural causes are ei-ther anatomic (tumors, strictures) or functional (defects in peristalsis: pyeloureteral or vesicoureteral junctions). Extrinsic causes of obstruction can be classified based on the system of origin of the obstructing lesion (Table 81–1).

Clinically, the age and gender of the patient are helpful in narrowing the differential diagnosis. In children, congenital causes of obstructive uropathy are common (stenosis at the ureteropelvic or ureterovesical junction, urethral valves, and so on). In middle-aged women, cervical cancer is a common cause of extrinsic ureteral or ureterovesical junction obstruction. In elderly men, benign prostatic hyperplasia and prostatic carcinoma are frequent causes of obstruction.

PATHOLOGY AND PATHOPHYSIOLOGY. The effects of obstructive uropathy on renal function are due to several factors with complex interactions. Following the onset of obstruction, pressures in the renal pelvis and tubules increase, resulting in dilatation of these structures. Renal damage is probably initiated by high intraureteral and high intratubular pressures. Decreases in renal blood flow cause ischemia, cellular atrophy, and necrosis. In addition, parenchymal infiltration by macrophages and T lymphocytes may cause scarring of the kidney. Superimposed infection may accelerate kidney destruction in this setting.

Normal urine flow from the renal pelvis to the bladder depends on ureteral peristalsis and a progressive decrease in hydrostatic pressure from Bowman's space to the renal pelvis. Impaired urine flow in the urinary tract leads to a rise in the pressure and volume of urine proximal to the obstruction. In this setting, high intra-ureteral pressures are transmitted to the kidney. This results in increased intratubular pressure. The rise in intratubular pressure without a similar rise in intraglomerular pressure decreases the net hydrostatic filtration pressure across glomerular capillaries, resulting in a fall in the glomerular filtration rate (GFR) (Fig. 81–1).

After the onset of complete obstruction, there is a transient renal vasodilatation, which is followed by progressive vasoconstriction of the renal circulation. This vasoconstriction leads to a decrease in renal blood flow, a fall in intraglomerular pressure, and a decrease in the GFR (Fig. 81–1). The vasoconstriction is mediated by angiotensin II and thromboxane A_2. These two compounds, through their effects on mesangial cell contraction, also may decrease the glomerular surface area available for filtration. This may explain the greater decrease in the GFR than in renal plasma flow observed in obstruction.

Due to increased intrarenal levels of angiotensin II, there is augmented synthesis of prostaglandin E_2 (PGE_2) and prostacyclin. These eicosanoids are vasodilatory substances that also antagonize the effects of angiotensin II on mesangial cell contraction. Hence, in the setting of obstruction, the increased synthesis of both PGE_2 and prostacyclin tends to prevent the GFR and renal blood flow from decreasing further. After the obstruction is released in experimental animals, administering inhibitors of prostaglandin synthesis, such as nonsteroidal anti-inflammatory agents or inhibitors of nitric oxide, decreases the GFR and renal blood flow.

Partial obstruction of the urinary tract also may decrease renal blood flow and the GFR. In addition, functional tubular defects are prominent. There is an inability to concentrate the urine and a decreased excretion of hydrogen ions and potassium. The concentrating defect is due in part to decreased osmolality of the renal medulla, probably related to decreased sodium reabsorption in the thick ascending limb of Henle's loop, and to the removal of medullary solutes (sodium, urea) as a consequence of the initial increase in medullary blood flow seen in obstruction. A decrease in the hydro-osmotic response of the cortical collecting duct to vasopressin also contributes to the concentrating defect. The decreased hydrogen ion and potassium excretion is due to impaired secretion of these ions in distal segments of the nephron, presumably as a consequence of a diminished response to the action of aldosterone.

CLINICAL MANIFESTATIONS. The clinical manifestations of urinary tract obstruction depend on the location (upper or lower urinary tract), degree (complete or partial), and duration (acute or chronic) of the obstruction (Table 81–2).

The symptoms of upper and lower urinary tract obstruction differ. Patients with acute complete obstruction may present with acute renal failure. Patients with chronic partial obstruction (chronic hydronephrosis) may be asymptomatic, may have intermittent pain, or may have symptoms and laboratory findings of impaired renal func-

TABLE 81–1. CAUSES OF URINARY TRACT OBSTRUCTION

Upper Urinary Tract	Lower Urinary Tract
A. Intrinsic Causes	1. Phimosis, meatal stenosis, paraphimosis
1. Intraluminal	2. Urethra: strictures, stones, diverticulum, posterior or anterior urethral valves, periurethral abscess, urethral surgery
a. Intratubular deposition of crystals (uric acid, acyclovir)	3. Prostate: benign hyperplasia, abscess, carcinoma
b. Ureter: stones, clots, renal papillae	4. Bladder
2. Intramural	a. Neurogenic bladder: spinal cord defect or trauma, diabetes, multiple sclerosis, cerebrovascular accidents, Parkinson's disease
a. Ureteropelvic or ureterovesical junction dysfunction	b. Bladder neck dysfunction
b. Ureteral valve, polyp, stricture, or tumor	c. Bladder calculus
B. Extrinsic Causes	d. Bladder cancer
1. Vascular system	5. Trauma
a. Aneurysm: abdominal aorta, iliac vessels	a. Straddle injury
b. Aberrant vessels: ureteropelvic junction	b. Pelvic fracture
c. Venous: retrocaval ureter	6. Drugs: spinal anesthesia, anticholinergics, smooth muscle depressants
2. Reproductive system	
a. Uterus: pregnancy, prolapse, tumors, endometriosis	
b. Ovary: abscess, tumors, ovarian remnants	
c. Gartner's duct cyst, tubo-ovarian abscess	
3. Gastrointestinal tract: Crohn's disease, diverticulitis, appendiceal abscess, tumors, pancreatic tumor, abscess, or cyst	
4. Retroperitoneal disease:	
a. Retroperitoneal fibrosis (idiopathic, radiation, drugs)	
b. Inflammatory: tuberculosis, sarcoidosis	
c. Hematomas	
d. Primary tumors (lymphoma, sarcoma, and so on)	
e. Metastatic tumors (cervix, bladder, colon, prostate, and so on)	
f. Lymphocele	
g. Pelvic lipomatosis	

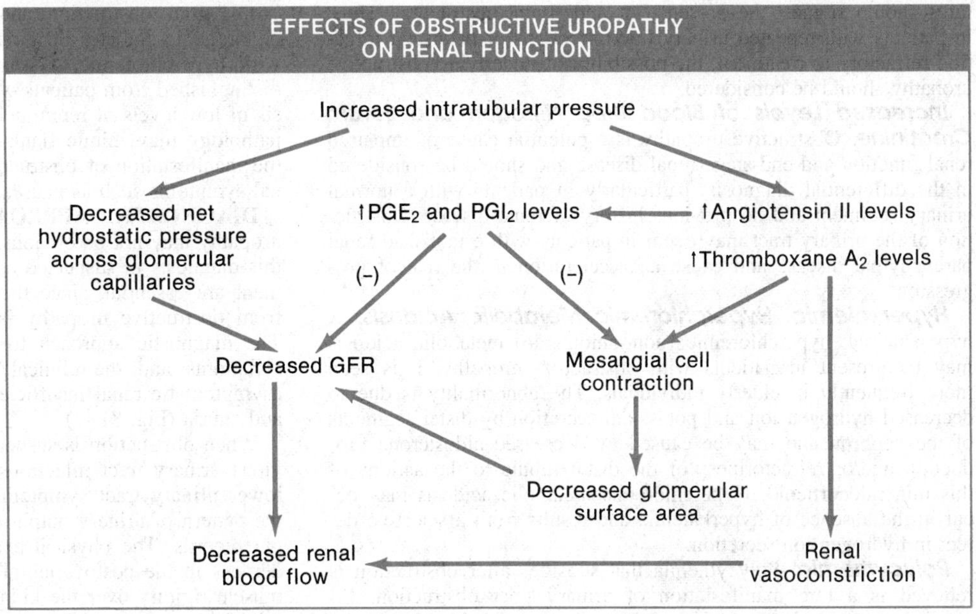

EFFECTS OF OBSTRUCTIVE UROPATHY ON RENAL FUNCTION

FIGURE 81–1. Increased levels of prostaglandin E_2 (PGE_2) and prostacyclin (PGI_2) tend to antagonize (−) the effects of angiotensin II and thromboxane A_2 on mesangial cell contraction and renal vasoconstriction. Hence they tend to prevent GFR from decreasing further.

tion, including inability to concentrate the urine, manifested as nocturia and/or polyuria, with or without elevated levels of blood urea nitrogen (BUN) and serum creatinine.

Pain and Renal Colic. Pain, due to distention of the bladder or to stretching of the collecting system or the renal capsule, is a common presenting symptom in obstructive uropathy, particularly in patients with ureteral calculi. Classic "renal colic" is a steadily increasing severe pain located in the flank (in the case of stones lodged in the upper third of the ureter) or radiating to the labia, testicles, or groin (stones in the lower two-thirds of the ureter) and may be associated with sweating and vomiting. The acute attack may last < 30 minutes or as long as a day. Pain radiating into the flank during micturition is said to be pathognomonic of vesicoureteral reflux. Chronic partial obstruction may cause intermittent flank pain. Pain may be elicited in some of these patients by administration of diuretics and/or excessive fluid intake. Physical examination may be normal or may reveal flank tenderness in patients with acute upper urinary tract obstruction. In patients with lower

urinary tract obstruction, a distended, palpable, and occasionally painful bladder may be found. Careful rectal examination in men or pelvic examination in women should be performed, since it may reveal prostatic enlargement or pelvic masses.

Changes in Urinary Output. Anuria and acute renal failure occur in patients with complete bilateral ureteral obstruction, with complete lower urinary tract obstruction, or with unilateral ureteral obstruction when there is a solitary kidney. In patients with partial or incomplete obstruction of the urinary tract, the urinary output may be normal or increased (polyuria). Occasionally, such patients may develop marked polyuria and increased thirst (a diabetes insipidus–like syndrome). This condition may cause hypernatremia. A pattern of oliguria or anuria alternating with polyuria or the acute onset of anuria strongly suggests the presence of obstructive uropathy.

Hematuria. Gross hematuria may be seen in obstruction, particularly when it is due to stones. In the presence of gross hematuria, clots may cause ureteral obstruction.

Palpable Masses. Longstanding obstructive uropathy may increase kidney size. Such patients may have increased abdominal girth or a palpable flank mass. Hydronephrosis is a common cause of a palpable abdominal mass in children. In patients with lower urinary tract obstruction, particularly that due to benign prostatic hyperplasia, a suprapubic mass may be caused by a distended bladder. This part of the physical examination should not be neglected in patients with anuria and suspected obstructive uropathy. This type of obstruction is readily reversed by placing a catheter in the bladder.

Hypertension. Hypertension is commonly associated with renal disease of diverse causes. Patients with obstructive uropathy may have hypertension due to (1) fluid retention and expansion of the extracellular fluid volume, (2) increased renin secretion, and (3) possibly decreased synthesis of medullary vasodepressor substances. In some patients with obstructive uropathy, hypertension may be coincidental, occurring in about one third of patients with acute unilateral obstruction and usually, but not always, renin-dependent. Release of acute obstruction should alleviate the hypertension when the two are causally related.

In patients with chronic bilateral obstruction, the hypertension is usually due to impaired sodium excretion and expansion of the extracellular fluid volume (volume-dependent hypertension). In such patients, the circulating levels of renin are usually suppressed.

Urinary Tract Infections or Infection That Is Refractory to Treatment. Repeated urinary tract infections without apparent cause suggest obstruction. Infection is more common in patients with lower urinary tract obstruction. This may be due to decreased bacterial "washout" and increased bacterial adherence to the mucosa of the bladder. Moreover, in the presence of obstruction, eradicating the infection is difficult. In noninstrumented patients, the finding of unusual organisms (*Proteus, Pseudomonas*) in urine cul-

TABLE 81–2. CLINICAL MANIFESTATIONS AND LABORATORY FINDINGS IN URINARY TRACT OBSTRUCTION

1. No symptoms (chronic hydronephrosis)
2. Intermittent pain (chronic hydronephrosis)
3. Elevated levels of BUN and serum creatinine with no other symptoms (chronic hydronephrosis)
4. Renal colic (usually due to ureteral stones or papillary necrosis)
5. Changes in urinary output
   a. Anuria or oliguria (acute renal failure)
   b. Polyuria (incomplete or partial obstruction)
   c. Fluctuating urinary output
6. Hematuria
7. Palpable masses
   a. Flank (hydronephrotic kidney; usually in infants)
   b. Suprapubic (distended bladder)
8. Hypertension
   a. Flank (hydronephrotic kidney; usually in infants)
   b. Suprapubic (distended bladder)
9. Hypertension
   a. Volume dependent (usually due to chronic bilateral obstruction)
   b. Renin dependent (usually due to acute unilateral obstruction)
10. Repeated urinary tract infections or infection that is refractory to treatment
11. Hyperkalemic, hyperchloremic acidosis (usually due to defective tubular secretion of hydrogen and potassium)
12. Hypernatremia (seen in infants with partial obstruction and polyuria)
13. Polycythemia (increased renal production of erythropoietin)
14. Lower urinary tract symptoms: hesitancy, urgency, incontinence, postvoid dribbling, decreased force and caliber of urinary stream, nocturia

tures should suggest the presence of underlying obstruction. Thus, in patients with repeated urinary tract infections or persistent infection refractory to treatment, the possibility of underlying obstructive uropathy should be considered.

Increased Levels of Blood Urea Nitrogen and Serum Creatinine. Obstructive uropathy is a potential cause of impaired renal function and end-stage renal disease and should be considered in the differential diagnosis, particularly in patients with a normal urinary sediment and no previous history of renal disease. Obstruction of the urinary tract may occur in patients with established renal parenchymal disease and cause an acceleration in the rate of progression.

Hyperkalemic, Hyperchloremic Metabolic Acidosis. A hyperkalemic, hyperchloremic (non–anion gap) metabolic acidosis may be present in patients with obstructive uropathy. It is seen more frequently in elderly individuals. The abnormality is due to decreased hydrogen ion and potassium secretion by distal segments of the nephron and may be caused by decreased aldosterone production and/or refractoriness of the distal tubule to the actions of this mineralocorticoid. Hyperchloremic metabolic acidosis may occur in the absence of hyperkalemia and results from a selective defect in hydrogen ion secretion.

Polycythemia. Polycythemia that subsides after obstruction is relieved is a rare manifestation of urinary tract obstruction. Increased renal production of erythropoietin, presumably due to ischemia, may account for the development of polycythemia.

Lower Urinary Tract Symptoms. Patients with obstruction of the lower urinary tract may develop symptoms such as decreased force and caliber of the urine stream, intermittency, incontinence, postvoid dribbling, hesitancy, and urgency. Alterations in the process of micturition due to neurogenic bladder disease also may result in urgency, frequent urination, and urinary incontinence (overflow incontinence).

DIFFERENTIAL DIAGNOSIS. The differential diagnosis varies depending on the clinical presentation and clinical symptoms.

Patients presenting with anuria and acute renal failure should be evaluated for other potential causes of acute renal failure (see Ch. 76). Partial obstruction and polyuria may mimic the entity of nephrogenic diabetes insipidus. Patients with obstruction presenting with hyperchloremic, hyperkalemic metabolic acidosis should be distinguished from patients who have the same syndrome on the basis of low levels of renin and aldosterone secretion. Gastrointestinal pathology may mimic flank pain due to renal stones. In children, the manifestation of obstructive uropathy can include gastrointestinal symptoms such as nausea, vomiting, and abdominal pain.

DIAGNOSTIC APPROACH. The presence of obstructive uropathy may not be obvious. Definitive tests are needed to exclude this diagnosis in suspected cases. Early diagnosis and prompt treatment are essential, since the degree of renal impairment resulting from obstructive uropathy is related to its severity and duration. The diagnostic approach to obstructive uropathy depends on the symptoms and the clinical findings of patients presenting with asymptomatic renal insufficiency, renal colic, or acute renal failure and anuria (Fig. 81–2).

When obstruction is suspected, the history may be of value: previous urinary tract infections, drugs ingested, and the presence of lower urinary tract symptoms (see above). In the hospital setting, the pattern of urinary output can be ascertained from input and output records. The physical examination may yield some clues: tenderness in the costovertebral angle, a mass in the flank area, and muscle rigidity over the kidney area. Abdominal distention and diminished peristalsis accompany acute renal colic. A suprapubic mass may be due to bladder outlet obstruction. The urinalysis may yield important clues: Is there hematuria, bacteriuria, or a urinary pH >7.5 to indicate stones and/or infection with urea-splitting organisms? The urinary sediment should be examined carefully for the presence of crystals (uric acid, cystine, and so forth). Laboratory studies should include an assessment of renal function (BUN, serum creatinine).

The tests used to diagnose obstructive uropathy are summarized in Table 81–3. *Ultrasound* is a noninvasive diagnostic test used as the initial procedure in suspected obstruction. The main finding de-

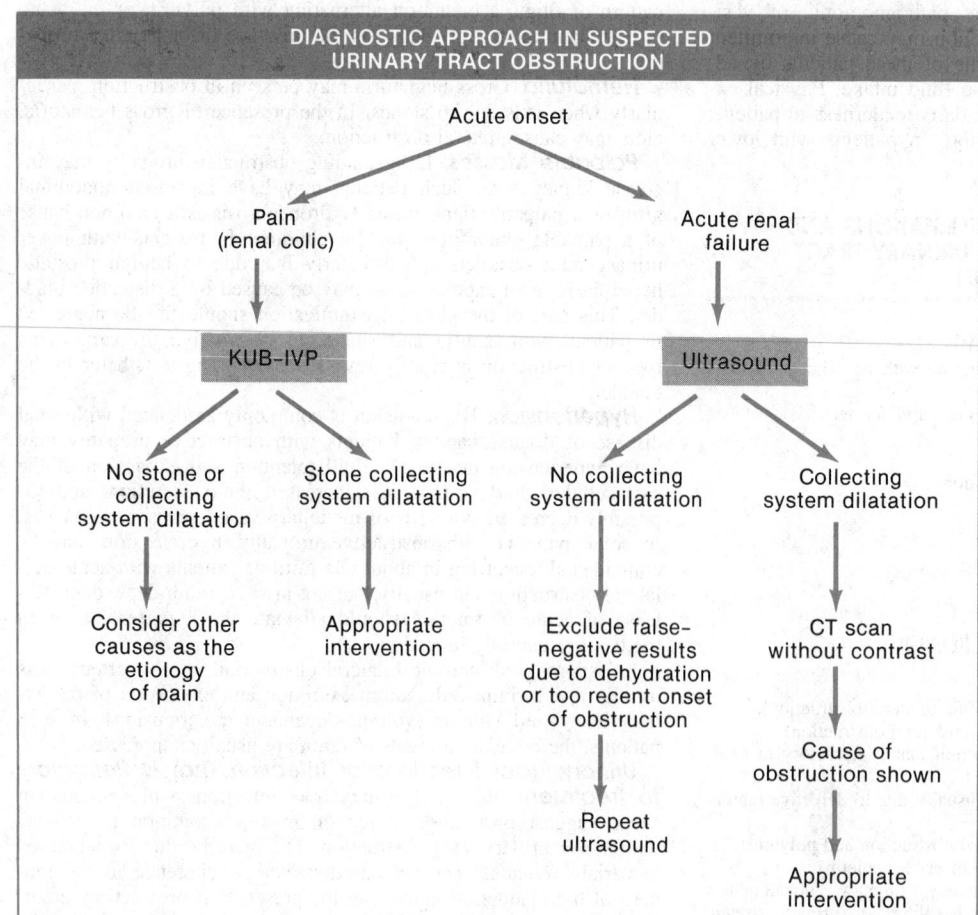

FIGURE 81–2. Scheme of diagnostic approach to urinary tract obstruction. KUB (kidney, ureter, bladder) = a flat film of the abdomen without contrast material; IVP = intravenous pyelography; CT = computed tomography.

TABLE 81-3. DIAGNOSTIC TESTS UTILIZED IN OBSTRUCTIVE UROPATHY

Upper Urinary Tract Obstruction

Sonography (ultrasound)
Plain films of the abdomen (KUB)
Excretory or intravenous pyelography (IVP)
Retrograde pyelography
Isotopic renography
Computed tomography
Magnetic resonance imaging
Pressure flow studies (the Whitaker test)

Lower Urinary Tract Obstruction

Some of the tests listed above
Cystoscopy
Voiding cystourethrogram
Retrograde urethrogram
Urodynamic tests
    Debimetry
    Cystometrography
    Electromyography
    Urethral pressure profile

Reproduced by permission from Klahr S: Obstructive uropathy. *In* Jacobson HR, Striker GE, Klahr S (eds.): The Principles and Practice of Nephrology. Toronto, B. C. Decker, 1991, pp 432–441. By permission of Mosby-Year Book.

tected by ultrasound is dilation of the urinary tract. In a few instances, the ultrasound may give false-negative results because dilation does not occur as a consequence of dehydration or too recent an onset of obstruction (Fig. 81–2). *Plain films of the abdomen (kidneys, ureter, bladder [KUB])* are particularly useful in patients with renal colic because ureteral calculi may be visualized (Fig. 81–2). They also provide information on renal and bladder morphology, such as size differences between the two kidneys or an enlarged bladder that suggests outlet obstruction. The *intravenous pyelogram (IVP)* is suggested to investigate acute renal colic (Fig. 81–2). The excretion of contrast media may be delayed in patients with a low GFR because of a decrease in the filtered load of the dye. In such patients, the procedure should be extended until the collecting system and the site of obstruction are identified. This identification may require obtaining delayed films. The IVP is not useful in patients with compromised renal function, particularly those with serum creatinine levels >3 to 4 mg per deciliter. It also has the risk of potential nephrotoxicity. *Retrograde pyelography* requires the retrograde injection of radiocontrast material and is used to visualize the ureter and collecting system when the IVP cannot be done or is not justified because of a history of allergic reaction to contrast material or other contraindications. This procedure can identify both the site and the cause of the obstruction. *Isotopic renography* can be used to diagnose upper urinary tract obstruction. It requires the intravenous injection of a radionuclide and subsequent imaging with a gamma scintillation camera. This imaging can be combined with intravenous furosemide administered 20 to 30 minutes after the isotope is injected. Other diagnostic procedures for obstructive uropathy include *computed tomography* and *magnetic resonance imaging.* Computed tomography is particularly useful to diagnose causes of obstruction. Occasionally, upper urinary tract obstruction is difficult to diagnose using the techniques described above, and *pressure flow studies* (the Whitaker test) may be required. This test consists of measuring pressure differences between the renal pelvis and the bladder during the infusion, at a known rate, of fluid into the renal pelvis.

A number of tests are useful in diagnosing lower urinary tract obstruction. These include a *voiding cystourethrogram,* which is used to investigate the presence of vesicoureteral reflux as a cause of dilation of the urinary tract. *Cystoscopy* allows visual inspection of the entire urethra and bladder during the same procedure. However, this procedure requires the use of anesthesia in children and young adults. The anterior urethra can be assessed by *retrograde urethrography,* performed by occluding the urethral meatus using a syringe or a catheter and injecting contrast medium. However, a retrograde urethrogram is not adequate to evaluate the posterior urethra. This anatomic area is best examined by an *excretory or retrograde cystogram.* The two tests combined usually provide a complete study of the urethra. *Urodynamic tests* with measurements

of urine flow rate per unit time are useful to evaluate bladder outlet obstruction. Measurement of *urine flow rate (debimetry)* is a noninvasive test that examines the interplay between the expulsive force of the detrusor muscle and urethral resistance. *Cystometrography* can be used to assess the force of the detrusor muscle in the bladder, and it quantifies the pressure-volume relationships of this organ. "Dyssynergy" of the bladder sphincter refers to the inability of the sphincter to relax during contraction of the detrusor muscle and is seen in patients with neurologic disorders. This type of resistance is better analyzed by *electromyography* and *urethral pressure profiles.* About 25% of children with spina bifida have detrusor sphincter dyssynergia at birth.

TREATMENT. After establishing a diagnosis of obstructive uropathy, it is necessary to decide whether or not surgery or instrumentation is required. The goals of therapy are (1) restoring and/or preserving renal function, (2) relieving pain and/or other symptoms of obstruction, and (3) preventing or eradicating infection.

Acute Obstruction (Complete). Obstructive uropathy presenting as acute renal failure requires prompt intervention. The site of obstruction determines the approach in these patients. If the obstruction is distal to the bladder, the placement of a urethral catheter may suffice. In some cases a suprapubic cystostomy is required. If the obstruction is located in the upper urinary tract, placement of percutaneous nephrostomy tubes or passage of a retrograde ureteral catheter may be necessary. Nephrostomy tubes not only provide drainage of the urine but also can be used for the local infusion of pharmacologic agents to treat infection, calculi, and so on. In patients with urinary tract infection and generalized sepsis, prompt relief of the obstruction is necessary, and appropriate antibiotic therapy is indicated. Sometimes dialysis may be required prior to instrumentation or surgery in patients with obstruction and acute renal failure.

Acute Obstruction (Partial). Calculi are the most common cause of ureteral obstruction. Their treatment includes relieving pain, eliminating obstruction, and treating the infection. Pain can be relieved by injecting a narcotic analgesic intramuscularly. Stones <5 mm in diameter do not usually require surgical intervention or instrumentation. About 90% of these stones are passed spontaneously. If the stones are 5 to 7 mm, however, only about half will pass, and stones >7 mm usually are not passed spontaneously. High fluid intake to increase the urinary volume to at least 2 liters per day may help to mobilize the stone. The urine must be strained through a gauze sponge to recover the calculi for analysis. If the stone completely occludes the ureter and does not move, surgical treatment is necessary. "Endourology" refers to the closed controlled manipulation of the entire urinary tract. Endourologic methods can be used to successfully treat stones obstructing the ureter in about 98% of patients. In addition, this approach shortens the hospital stay to 3 to 4 days and the convalescence period to only 4 to 7 days. Extracorporeal shock wave or ultrasound lithotripsy involves focusing of electrohydraulic or ultrasonically generated shock waves to disintegrate the stone. The method is effective for ureteral calculi of 7 to 15 mm that lie above the pelvic brim. The stone is disintegrated in 90% of patients, and all particulate matter passes within a 3-month period. Morbidity is low. However, all patients should be followed up for stone recurrence and should be given preventive therapy. In addition, there is a question of posttreatment hypertension, which requires follow-up. In selected individuals, the procedure can be done on an outpatient basis. Most patients are back at work 2 to 3 days after shock wave therapy. Calculi located distal to the pelvic brim can be approached from below. Antibiotics are useful when infections complicate renal calculi. The choice of antibiotic depends on appropriate urine cultures and sensitivity studies.

Chronic Partial Obstruction. Surgical intervention can be delayed sometimes for weeks or even months in patients with low-grade obstruction or partial chronic obstruction. However, prompt relief of partial obstruction is indicated when (1) there are repeated episodes of urinary tract infection, (2) the patient has significant symptoms (dysuria, voiding dysfunction, flank pain), (3) urinary retention exists, or (4) evidence of recurrent or progressive renal damage is present.

Lower Urinary Tract Obstruction. Urethral and bladder neck obstruction requires surgery in patients with recurrent infections who are ambulatory, particularly when reflux, renal parenchymal damage, marked urinary retention, repeated bleeding, or other symptoms are present. Obstruction secondary to benign prostatic hyperplasia is not always progressive. Therefore, patients with minimal symptoms, no infection, and a normal upper urinary tract may be followed safely until patient and physician agree that surgery is desirable. Urethral strictures in men can be treated by dilation or direct visual internal urethrotomy. The incidence of bladder neck and urethral obstruction in women is low. Hence urethral dilation, internal urethrotomy, meatotomy, and revision of the bladder neck in women are seldom indicated.

When obstruction is the result of neuropathic bladder function, dynamic studies are essential to determine therapy. The main goals of therapy should be (1) to establish the bladder as a urine storage organ without causing renal injury and (2) to provide a mechanism for bladder emptying that is acceptable to the patient. Patients fall into two categories, those with atonic bladders secondary to lower motor neuron injury and those with unstable bladder function due to upper motor neuron disease. The neurogenic bladder seen in diabetes mellitus is usually the result of lower motor neuron disease. Requesting these patients to void at regular intervals achieves satisfactory emptying of the bladder. Occasionally, these individuals respond to cholinergic agents, such as bethanechol chloride (Urecholine). α-Adrenergic blockers relax urethral sphincter tone but have only limited success because of side effects. The best treatment for patients with significant residual urine and recurrent urosepsis is to establish clean, intermittent, regular self-catheterization. The goal is to catheterize four or five times per day so that the amount of urine drained from the bladder does not exceed 400 ml. This technique may be successful but requires patient acceptance and adequate training. In patients with a hypertonic bladder, the major goal is to improve its storage function. Anticholinergic agents may be indicated. Occasionally, long-term, clean, intermittent self-catheterization is necessary. In all patients with neurogenic bladders, long-term use of indwelling catheters should be avoided if possible, owing to risk of infection and other complications.

POSTOBSTRUCTIVE DIURESIS. "Postobstructive diuresis" refers to the marked natriuresis and diuresis that occasionally follow the relief of obstruction. This diuresis is characterized by excretion of large amounts of sodium, potassium, magnesium, and other solutes. Although usually self-limited, the losses of solutes and water may result in hypokalemia, hyponatremia or hypernatremia, hypomagnesemia, and marked volume depletion. In many patients, a brisk diuresis after relief of obstruction may represent a physiologic response to expansion of the extracellular fluid volume occurring during the period of obstruction. This postobstructive diuresis is appropriate and does not compromise the volume status of the patient. Postobstructive diuresis in this setting can be prolonged by overzealous replacement of salt and water after relief of obstruction.

Fluid replacement is justified only when excessive losses of sodium and water occur that are inappropriate for the volume status of the patient and are presumably due to an intrinsic tubular defect in sodium and water reabsorption. Fluid replacement in these patients is guided in large part by what is excreted. Intravenous fluid administration may be necessary, but urinary losses should be replaced only to the extent necessary to prevent extracellular fluid volume contraction or electrolyte imbalance.

PROGNOSIS. The return of renal function after relieving obstruction is variable and is influenced by the severity and duration of obstruction. Other events that condition the degree of recovery of renal function include the presence of infection, stones, pre-existing renal disease, and/or the underlying cause of the obstruction. Renal cortical thickness is a prognostic indicator of residual renal function in patients with chronic hydronephrosis. Patients with a very thin cortex have lost considerable renal function.

Klahr S: Obstructive uropathy. *In* Glassock RJ (ed.): Current Therapy in Nephrology and Hypertension. St. Louis, Mosby–Year Book, 1992, pp 81–87. *Discusses the therapeutic approach to the patient with urinary tract obstruction and postobstructive diuresis.*

Klahr S, Harris KPG: Obstructive uropathy. *In* Seldin DW, Giebisch G (eds.): The Kidney: Physiology and Pathophysiology. 2d ed. New York, Raven Press, 1992, pp 3327–3369. *An extensive chapter on pathophysiology and pathogenesis of obstructive nephropathy. Numerous references.*

Wilson D, Klahr S: Urinary tract obstruction. *In* Schrier RW, Gottschalk CW (eds.): Diseases of the Kidney. Boston, Little, Brown, 1993, pp 657–687. *A recent detailed discussion of clinical, pathologic, and diagnostic issues in obstructive nephropathy.*

82 SPECIFIC RENAL TUBULAR DISORDERS
Russell W. Chesney

Renal tubular disorders represent a group of conditions wherein the renal tubular reabsorption of either ions or organic solutes is diminished, resulting in excessive amounts of either substance in the urine. The defect can be characterized by the nephron segment affected. The functions of each segment will influence the type of substance lost as well as the rate of loss. As noted in Ch. 74, the proximal nephron is responsible for reclaiming most of the filtered glucose, amino acids, uric acid, phosphate, bicarbonate, and low-molecular-weight proteins. Henle's loop reabsorbs over half the filtered sodium chloride as well as divalent cations. The distal nephron (including the cortical and medullary collecting ducts), under the influence of aldosterone, reabsorbs the final amount of sodium and secretes hydrogen and potassium ions. The terminal collecting ducts are influenced by antidiuretic hormone to permit water reabsorption and hence lead to urinary concentration.

Many tubular disorders are inherited and appear to involve the loss or formation of a defective transport protein ("carrier") and represent an inborn error of transport. Acquired conditions also can perturb transport function (Table 82–1). These conditions include (1) a single selective transport defect, (2) a class-specific defect (e.g., dibasic amino acids in cystinuria), or (3) those solutes whose transport is influenced by a specific hormone, which can arise from hormone deficiency or resistance (e.g., in hypoaldosteronism or diabetes insipidus). Perturbation of tubular energy production or direct structural alteration is more likely to result in a global disorder, such as the generalized tubular dysfunction found in Fanconi's syndrome. Luminal, intracellular, or peritubular components of the net transport process can be affected in each situation. Here described are several of the more usual transport defects of individual nephron segments.

DISORDERS OF THE PROXIMAL TUBULE FUNCTION

The proximal tubule is the site of reabsorption of 80 to 99% of filtered solutes, including glucose, amino acids, and phosphates. Urinary wastage of bulk quantities of these solutes implies a disorder of proximal tubular function.

RENAL GLYCOSURIAS. The renal glycosurias are caused by inherited or acquired defects in proximal tubule glucose reabsorption such that glycosuria is evident at normal serum glucose concentrations.

Pathophysiology. D-Glucose is actively reabsorbed across the luminal surface of the proximal tubule by a stereospecific carrier that requires sodium. The quantity of glucose reabsorbed changes, depending on the filtered glucose load, until a maximal reabsorptive capacity, or T_m, is achieved. Before saturation, glucose reabsorption is incomplete, and a "splay" is evident (Fig. 82–1). The initial point in the splay represents that filtered glucose concentration (the "threshold") at which reabsorption no longer equals filtration and glucose appears in the urine. Normally, the threshold concentration, 200 to 240 mg per deciliter, is far above the plasma values; thus scant glucose (< 125 mg daily) appears in the urine. The kinetics of D-glucose reabsorption have been compared with classic enzyme kinetics. The T_m is likened to the V_{max}, while the degree of splay represents the K_m. In the two main forms of renal glucosuria, either the capacity (type A, V_{max}, or K_m mutation) or the affinity (type B, K_m, or extent-of-splay mutation) of glucose reabsorption is affected. Consistent with this view, the genes encoding the high affinity (SGLT 1) and low affinity (SGLT 2) are found on different chromosomes: SGLT 1 is at chromosome 22q13.1, and SGLT 2 is on chromosome 16. SGLT 1 alone also transports galactose. Either way, the

TABLE 82–1. CLINICAL SYNDROMES ASSOCIATED WITH NEPHRON TRANSPORT DEFECTS

Proximal Nephron

I. *Selective transport defects*
  A. Renal glycosurias
    1. Primary
    2. Combined
      a. Glucose/galactose malabsorption
      b. Glucoglycinuria
  B. Renal aminoacidurias
    1. Basic aminoacidurias
      a. General: cystinuria (cystine, lysine, arginine, ornithine)
      b. Specific: hypercystinuria, dibasic aminoaciduria (lysine, arginine, ornithine), lysinuria
    2. Neutral aminoacidurias
      a. General: Hartnup disease
      b. Specific: methioninuria, tryptophanuria, histidinuria
    3. Iminoglycinuria
      a. General (proline, hydroxyproline, glycine)
      b. Specific: glycinuria
    4. Dicarboxylic aminoaciduria
      a. General (glutamic, aspartic acids)
  C. Proximal renal tubular acidosis
    1. Primary: idiopathic or genetic
    2. Transient (infants)
    3. Carbonic anhydrase deficiency, inhibition, alteration
      a. Drugs: acetazolamide, sulfanilamide, mafenide acetate
      b. Idiopathic?
  D. Renal uric acid disorders (see Ch. 80, 181, 251)
  E. Phosphate and calcium disorders (see Ch. 213, 214)
II. *Nonselective transport defects: Fanconi's Syndrome*
  A. Primary: idiopathic or genetic
  B. Genetically transmitted systemic diseases
    1. Cystinosis
    2. Lowe's syndrome
    3. Wilson's disease
    4. Tyrosinemia
    5. Hereditary carboxylase deficiency
    6. Pyruvate carboxylase deficiency
  C. Dysproteinemic states
    1. Multiple myeloma
    2. Monoclonal gammopathy
  D. Secondary hyperparathyroidism with chronic hypocalcemia
    1. Vitamin D deficiency or resistance
    2. Vitamin D dependency
  E. Drugs and toxins
    1. Outdated tetracycline
    2. Methyl-3-chromone
    3. Streptozotocin
    4. Glue
    5. Gentamicin
    6. Ifosfamide
  F. Heavy metals
    1. Lead
    2. Cadmium
    3. Mercury
  G. Tubulointerstitial diseases
    1. Sjögren's syndrome
    2. Medullary cystic disease
    3. Renal transplantation
  H. Other diseases
    1. Nephrotic syndrome
    2. Amyloidosis
    3. Osteopetrosis
    4. Paroxysmal nocturnal hemoglobinuria

Loop of Henle

I. *Bartter's syndrome*
II. *Drugs*
  A. Furosemide
  B. Bumetanide
  C. Ethacrynic acid

Distal Nephron

I. *Selective transport defects*
  A. Classic distal RTA
    1. Primary: genetic or idiopathic
    2. Genetically transmitted systemic diseases
      a. Ehlers-Danlos syndrome
      b. Hematologic disorders: hereditary elliptocytosis, sickle cell anemia, carbonic anhydrase I deficiency or alteration
      c. Medullary cystic disease
      d. With nerve deafness
      e. Glycogenosis type III
    3. Autoimmune diseases
      a. Hypergammaglobulinemia: hyperglobulinemic purpura, cryoglobulinemia, familial
      b. Sjögren's syndrome
      c. Thyroiditis
      d. Pulmonary fibrosis
      e. Chronic active hepatitis
      f. Primary biliary cirrhosis
      g. Systemic lupus erythematosus
    4. Diseases associated with nephrocalcinosis
      a. Primary hyperparathyroidism
      b. Vitamin D intoxication
      c. Hyperthyroidism
      d. Hypercalciuria: idiopathic or genetic
      e. Hereditary fructose intolerance
      f. Medullary sponge kidney
      g. Fabry's disease
      h. Wilson's disease
    5. Drug or toxic nephropathies
      a. Amphotericin B
      b. Toluene
      c. Glue
      d. Analgesics
      e. Cyclamate
    6. Tubulointerstitial diseases
      a. Chronic pyelonephritis secondary to urolithiasis
      b. Obstructive uropathy
      c. Renal transplantation
      d. Leprosy
      e. Hyperoxaluria
    7. Miscellaneous
  B. RTA of glomerular insufficiency
  C. Hypermineralocorticoid and other potassium secretory disorders (see Ch. 204.1)
II. *Nonselective transport defects: generalized distal RTA, hyperkalemia, and renal salt washing*
  A. Primary mineralocorticoid deficiency (see Ch. 204.1)
  B. Hypoangiotensinemia
    1. Converting enzyme inhibitors: captopril, enalapril
    2. Angiotensin receptor blockers
  C. Hyporeninemic hypoaldosteronism
    1. Diabetic nephropathy
    2. Tubulointerstitial nephropathies
    3. Nephrosclerosis
    4. Nonsteroidal anti-inflammatory agents
    5. Acquired immunodeficiency syndrome (AIDS)
  D. Mineralocorticoid-resistant hyperkalemia
    1. Without salt wasting: genetic
    2. With salt wasting
      a. Childhood forms
      b. Tubulointerstitial nephropathies: methicillin, obstructive nephropathy, transplantation, sickle cell disease, cyclosporine
      c. Other drugs: spironolactone, amiloride, triamterene

Loop and Medullary Collecting Ducts

I. *Diabetes insipidus* (see Ch. 202.2)
II. *SIADH* (see Ch. 202.2)
III. *Other concentrating and diluting disorders*

---

threshold is influenced so that glucose is lost in the urine at a normal plasma glucose concentration. Glucosuria becomes marked after intravenous infusion of D-glucose.

Symptoms and Etiologies. Renal glucosuria is uncommon, with a prevalence of 0.2 to 0.6%. Inheritance is autosomal recessive, and heterozygotes have more marked glucosuria. Usually, but not always, V_{max} and K_m variants are inherited separately, as would be anticipated with two separate genes. Renal biopsy samples reveal no consistent pathologic features. Unlike the aminoacidurias, no intestinal transport defects are found. Renal glucosuria is completely asymptomatic.

Intermittent glucosuria is not uncommon during the third trimester of pregnancy (see Ch. 86) and in terminal chronic renal insufficiency. In each instance, the functional change in glucose transport kinetics relates to an increase in tubular flow rate from an increase in total single-nephron glomerular filtration rate (GFR). In

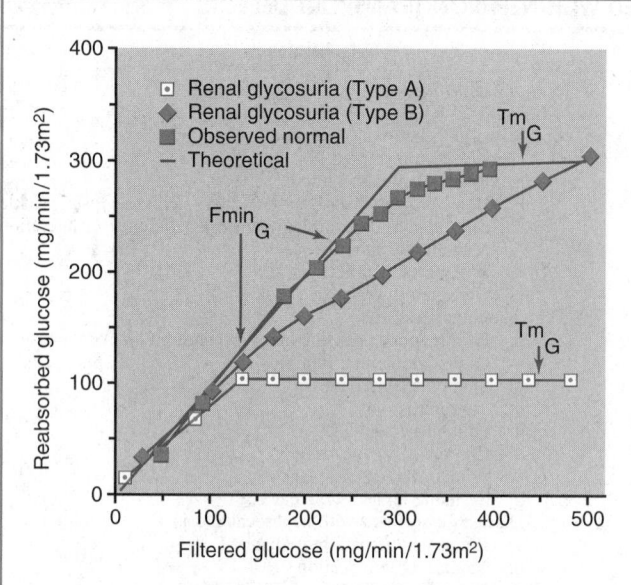

FIGURE 82–1. Glucose titration curves demonstrating the maximal transport rate (T_{m_G}) on the ordinate and the venous plasma threshold (F_{min_G}) on the abscissa. This depicts both the normal pattern and the pattern in the two variants of renal glucosuria (type A and type B).

a rare disorder in children, markedly decreased SGLT 1 results in both gut and renal malabsorption of both glucose and galactose, which results in diarrhea and melliituria.

Diagnosis and Treatment. Diagnosis should be based on finding glucosuria of more than 500 mg per 24 hours (on a diet containing 50% carbohydrate) without hyperglycemia (serum glucose < 140 mg per deciliter). To confirm the excreted sugar as glucose, the glucose oxidase method should be used; this will exclude other melliituric conditions (pentosuria, fructosuria, sucrosuria, maltosuria, galactosuria, and lactosuria). Appropriate tests should be performed to exclude coexistent tubular transport defects (of amino acids, bicarbonate, phosphorus, and uric acid) such as Fanconi's syndrome, as well as diabetes. If desired, differentiation of the V_{max} or K_m variants can be made by glucose loading (see Fig. 82–1).

This condition is completely benign, and therapy is unnecessary.

RENAL AMINOACIDURIAS. The renal aminoacidurias represent inborn errors of renal tubular transport in which a single or group of amino acids are hyperexcreted and are often accompanied by intestinal malabsorption of the same amino acid(s) (see Table 82–1).

General Characteristics. The 20 L-amino acids are predominantly reabsorbed by the proximal tubule at a rate of reabsorption exceeding 95 to 98% of the filtered load. Stereospecific amino acid transport occurs across the luminal membrane of the proximal tubule, accompanied by sodium and driven by the lumen-to-cell sodium concentration gradient. Reabsorptive kinetics are similar to those of D-glucose. Amino acid transport systems for at least five groups or classes of amino acids have been described: *basic*—lysine, arginine, ornithine, and cystine; *acidic*—aspartic and glutamic acid; *neutral amino group*—glycine, proline, hydroxyproline, and sarcosine; *neutral (Hartnup) group*—alanine, serine, threonine, valine, leucine, isoleucine, phenylalanine, glutamine, histidine, asparagine, tyrosine, tryptophan, and citrulline; and *β-amino acids*—taurine, β-amino acids, and β-aminoisobutyrate. Inherited dysfunction of a carrier results in urinary loss of the entire amino acid group: cystinuria (basic aminoaciduria), dicarboxylic aminoaciduria, Hartnup disease (neutral aminoaciduria), and iminoglycinuria. There are at least 25 selective amino acid carriers that transport a single or few numbers of a given amino acid group. Human disorders of these carriers result in even more selective aminoaciduria: hypercystinuria, histidinuria, and lysinuria.

Many proximal nephron amino acid carriers are also expressed within the luminal (brush border) membrane of gastrointestinal epithelial cells. Defective gut absorption occurs concomitantly with

renal hyperexcretion of the amino acid(s) in question. Di- and tripeptides can be absorbed normally by the gut; hence nutritional problems arising from amino acid malabsorption are unusual.

To diagnose a renal aminoaciduria, an elevated plasma level of the amino acids must be excluded. Whenever the filtered load of an amino acid exceeds the transport capacity of the renal tubule, an "overload" or "prerenal" aminoaciduria can occur. Most inborn errors of amino acid metabolism exhibit this type of aminoaciduria because the plasma concentration of individual amino acids that are poorly metabolized rises sharply. By contrast, the renal aminoacidurias are associated with low or normal levels of plasma amino acid concentrations, since the aminoaciduria is due to an inborn error of proximal tubule transport.

CYSTINURIA. *Cystinuria* is the term used to designate a group of renal transport disorders that have in common the excessive excretion of the highly insoluble amino acid cystine and the formation of urinary calculi. An autosomal recessive disease is estimated to affect 1 in 7000 individuals (between 1 in 1000 and 1 in 20,000, depending on the population examined). Urinary losses of lysine, arginine, and ornithine are asymptomatic. Cystine loss leads to cystine urolithiases, which accounts for 1 to 2% of all urinary calculi. Stone formation usually becomes evident during the second and third decades of life, though presentation may occur from infancy to the ninth decade, and males are more severely affected. Cystine stones are radiopaque, can create staghorn calculi, and often form a nidus for calcium oxalate stone formation. Symptoms include renal colic, which may be associated with obstruction or infection or both. Evidence associating cystinuria with central nervous system (CNS) disorders has been tenuous. A more general discussion of nephrolithiasis can be found in Ch. 88.

The diagnosis of cystinuria should be considered in any patient with renal calculus, even if the stone is composed primarily of calcium oxalate. Typical hexagonal crystals may be recognized by urinalysis, particularly in a concentrated, acidic, early-morning specimen. A useful screening test is the cyanide-nitroprusside test, which detects a cystine concentration of > 75 to 150 mg per liter. Because of false-positive tests, a definitive diagnosis requires thin-layer or ion-exchange chromatography. Excretion ratios in an adult > 18 mg cystine per gram of creatinine confirm the diagnosis. Homozygous individuals usually excrete > 250 mg cystine per gram of creatinine.

Medical therapy of cystinuria is aimed at reducing the urinary concentration below the solubility limit of 300 mg cystine per liter. The production of a high-volume alkaline urine (pH > 7.5) will increase the solubility of cystine to this level. Since cystine excretion may be as high as 1 gram per 24 hours, a total of 4 liters of water should be ingested. The most effective means of converting cystine to a more soluble compound follows the therapeutic administration of D-penicillamine, which by way of a disulfide exchange reaction produces cysteine-penicillamine. Pyridoxine also should be given, since penicillamine can deplete this cofactor. The compound mercaptopropionylglycine (XMPG) may prove to be more efficacious, since it is more effective in disulfide exchange reactions and its side effects appear to be fewer than those of D-penicillamine.

HARTNUP DISEASE. Hartnup disease, a neutral aminoaciduria, is a rare autosomal recessive disorder (1 in 26,000 births) in which the clinical presentation is dominated by nicotinamide deficiency. Since up to 50% of nicotinamide is normally supplied by metabolism of tryptophan, malabsorption and renal loss of tryptophan contribute to nicotinamide deficiency, especially when dietary nicotinamide is insufficient. Hence this disorder demonstrates the importance of both the intestinal and renal transport defects. Clinical evidence of nicotinamide deficiency is intermittent and often worse in children and includes pellagra in sun-exposed areas, cerebellar ataxia, and sometimes psychiatric disturbances.

Hartnup disease should be suspected in a patient with pellagra or cerebellar symptoms without a history of niacin deficiency. The diagnosis can be confirmed by chromatography of the urine. Sibs of an affected individual should be examined for heterozygosity. Supplemental nicotinamide (40 to 250 mg per day) will prevent pellagra and neurologic problems.

OTHER AMINOACIDURIAS. Less common aminoacidurias that are asymptomatic include iminoglycinuria, isolated hypercystinuria (without hyperexcretion of other basic amino acids), isolated glycinuria, and dicarboxylic aminoaciduria. Mental retardation predominates in the rare disorders of hyperdibasic aminoaciduria, isolated lysinuria, histidinuria, and methioninuria.

PROXIMAL RENAL TUBULAR ACIDOSIS (RTA). Proximal (type II) RTA is a hyperchloremic, hypokalemic metabolic acidosis caused by a selective defect in proximal acidification and defined by a normally acidic urine during acidosis but marked bicarbonate wasting after normalization of plasma bicarbonate concentrations.

Pathophysiology. Between 85 and 90% of the filtered bicarbonate load occurs in the proximal nephron, mainly by Na^+/H^+ exchange and the degradation of H_2CO to CO_2 plus H_2O by carbonic anhydrase (Fig. 82–2). Interference with a normal Na^+/H^+ exchange or carbonic anhydrase activity results in excessive delivery of bicarbonate to the distal nephron. Due to limited bicarbonate reabsorptive capacity, excessive bicarbonate is wasted into the urine. The loss of 15% or more of filtered bicarbonate at a normal plasma bicarbonate concentration is pathognomonic of proximal RTA. Excess delivery of bicarbonate to the distal nephron also results in accelerated potassium secretion and hypokalemia with defective proximal bicarbonate reabsorption. The plasma bicarbonate concentration and filtered load fall, and absolute bicarbonate delivery to the distal nephron decreases progressively. After a certain time, usually when plasma bicarbonate is between 15 to 18 mm, the distal nephron can cope with excessive delivery from the proximal nephron. At this point bicarbonaturia ceases, urinary pH can be lowered normally, and net acid excretion equals endogenous acid production. Acid-base homeostasis is re-established at the expense of metabolic acidosis.

Symptoms and Etiologies. Clinical features of proximal RTA are related to acidemia (growth failure, anorexia and malnutrition,

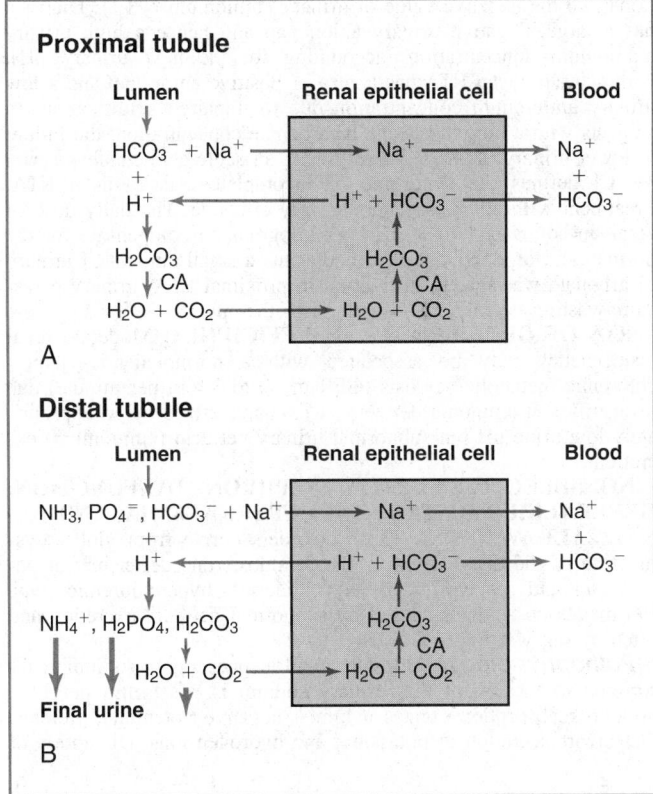

FIGURE 82–2. *A,* Proximal tubule bicarbonate reabsorption. Sodium hydrogen exchanges hydrogen ion for the formation of H_2CO_3, which is rapidly broken down to $H_2O + CO_2$ by the enzyme carbonic anhydrase (CA). $H_2O + CO_2$ are both translocated into the proximal tubule, where carbonic anhydrase rapidly catalyzes the reverse reaction to form H_2CO_3 and then $H^+ + HCO_3^-$. Na^+ and HCO_3^- are then returned to the circulation. *B,* Distal tubule secretion of hydrogen ion occurs via sodium-dependent and voltage-dependent transport processes. The absence of CA on the luminal membrane of the distal tubule results in a delay in the formation of $H_2O + CO_2$ from H_2CO_3. CO_2 is "trapped" in the urine, raising the urinary P_{CO_2}. H^+ ion is also excreted in the form of titratable acids such as H_2PO_4 or NH_4^+. The process does result in the regeneration of some bicarbonate, which is ultimately returned to the circulation.

volume depletion), hypokalemia and potassium depletion (muscular weakness, polyuria, nocturia, polydipsia), and disordered mineral, parathyroid, and vitamin D metabolism (osteomalacia and rickets). Proximal RTA is quite rare, usually due to defective carbonic anhydrase activity or in association with the complete Fanconi's syndrome (see Table 82–1).

Diagnosis and Treatment. Laboratory evidence of proximal RTA consists of a hyperchloremic, hypokalemic metabolic acidosis. When the patient is acidemic, the urine is acidic, and net acid excretion equals endogenous acid production. If bicarbonate is infused to normalize plasma bicarbonate concentrations, massive bicarbonaturia ensues ($\geq$ 15% of the filtered load). Proximal RTA is not usually an isolated diagnosis but part of Fanconi's syndrome. Therapy of the underlying disease should be undertaken if possible (e.g., multiple myeloma) or offending drugs or toxins removed (e.g., heavy metals). When this is not feasible, proximal RTA is treated with large quantities of sodium and potassium bicarbonate. Potassium wasting is enhanced as plasma bicarbonate rises after therapy, which raises the requirement for potassium supplements because bicarbonate alone cannot correct the disorder. Volume contraction using diuretics (particularly thiazides) is also attempted to stimulate fractional proximal bicarbonate reabsorption. Therapy with vitamin D analogues is indicated when clinically relevant.

GENERALIZED PROXIMAL TUBULE DYSFUNCTIONS: THE FANCONI'S SYNDROME. In Fanconi's syndrome, the entire panoply of proximal tubule transport functions is impaired, resulting in glucosuria, generalized aminoaciduria, proximal RTA phosphaturia, and uricosuria. The lumen-to-cell sodium gradient provides the driving force in the proximal tubular epithelium for the reabsorption of these respective compounds. Collapse of the sodium gradient could arise by several mechanisms: a primary disturbance of the Na^+-K^+-ATPase, increased permeability of the cell to sodium, or reduced metabolic energy due to an abnormality in the redox potential or in the intracellular phosphate supply. Recently, Fanconi's syndrome has been associated with depletion of mitochondrial DNA, particularly in a mitochondrial myopathy associated with generalized tubulopathy.

In addition to the solutes previously described, there exists impaired reabsorption and frequently reduced serum concentrations of calcium, magnesium, citrate, and low-molecular-weight ($<$ 50 kDa) proteins. Since the proximal tubular mitochondria is the site of conversion of 25-(OH) vitamin D to 1,25-(OH)$_2$ vitamin D, the circulating value of this latter compound may be reduced (see Ch. 212).

Symptoms and Etiologies. As a result of the complex disorders of mineral and vitamin D metabolism, the most frequent clinical finding is metabolic bone disease, either rickets in children or osteomalacia in adults (see Ch. 213). Nausea, episodic vomiting, anorexia and marked growth failure are common in children. Other features include polyuria and muscle weakness secondary to potassium depletion.

Causes of Fanconi's syndrome are listed in Table 82–1. The most common is the inherited disease cystinosis, in which cystine accumulates in cells, specifically in lysosomes of the kidney, liver, gut, lymphoid tissue, conjunctivae, thyroid gland, cornea, and bone marrow. Cystinosis may present as Fanconi's syndrome after the first birthday or with renal failure in childhood (infantile nephropathic form) or during adolescence. An adult form, which is generally benign, may involve corneal and conjunctival cystine crystal deposition. The defect represents a failure in the lysosomal cystine efflux process. A form of Fanconi's syndrome that can be induced by diet is *hereditary fructose intolerance* due to a deficiency of fructose aldolase B (see Ch. 171). Ingestion of fructose by affected patients causes acute symptoms, including nausea, vomiting, abdominal pain, and neurologic dysfunction, as well as profound hypophosphatemia. In adults, acquired Fanconi's syndrome is most often due to dysproteinemias, heavy metal exposure (especially chronic cadmium or acute lead), and immunologic disorders (see Table 82–1). An older adult presenting with Fanconi's syndrome should be assumed to have multiple myeloma unless proven otherwise.

Diagnosis and Treatment. Diagnosis is established by finding evidence for global tubular dysfunction. Underlying causes of Fanconi's syndrome should be sought. Serum and urine electrophoresis are indicated in adults.

Therapy includes sodium and potassium supplements (up to 10 to 15 mEq per kilogram per day), potassium, phosphate, magnesium, and vitamin D analogues. Therapy of the underlying disorder is also important. Efficacy has been shown for cysteamine in cystinosis, D-penicillamine in Wilson's disease (see Ch. 188), fructose restriction in hereditary fructose intolerance, and removal of heavy metals by environmental changes or chelation (for lead).

DISORDERS OF FUNCTION OF THE ASCENDING LIMB OF THE LOOP OF HENLE

The thick ascending limb of the loop of Henle reabsorbs sodium chloride by means of a luminal Na^+-K^+-$2Cl^-$ system. A lumen-positive potential difference and parallel transport system affect potassium, calcium, and magnesium reabsorption. Defective reabsorption by the thick ascending limb of Henle occurs during diuretic therapy or in Bartter's syndrome.

BARTTER'S SYNDROME. Bartter's syndrome includes hypokalemia, metabolic alkalosis, and hyperreninemic hyperaldosteronism. Hypertension and edema are absent.

Pathophysiology. Mild extracellular volume depletion causes hyperreninemic hyperaldosteronism and the juxtaglomerular hyperplasia evident in renal biopsy. Enhanced sodium chloride delivery to the collecting duct stimulates potassium secretion (exacerbated by concurrent hyperaldosteronism), resulting in marked hypokalemia.

Symptoms and Etiology. Bartter's syndrome usually presents during childhood. Inheritance is autosomal recessive with more affected males. Adult cases are described. Presenting features relate mainly to hypokalemia, including growth failure, muscle weakness, and vasopressin-resistant polyuria consisting of polyuria, nocturia, and enuresis. Divalent cation (calcium and magnesium), wasting, and metabolic alkalosis may result in hypocalcemia with Trousseau and Chvostek signs. These electrolyte abnormalities also can present as paralytic ileus or growth failure in children.

Diagnosis and Treatment. Other conditions associated with hypokalemia, metabolic alkalosis, and secondary hyperreninemic hyperaldosteronism must be excluded before making the diagnosis of Bartter's syndrome. Surreptitious vomiting, chronic diarrheal states, or surreptitious diuretic or laxative abuse can cause symptoms and laboratory findings indistinguishable from those of Bartter's syndrome. The diagnosis must be preceded by determination that urinary chloride concentration is > 20 ml per liter and by negative screening test results for diuretics in the urine and for laxatives in the stool (phenolphthalein test). In general, other states of primary hyperreninism or hypermineralocorticoidism can be readily excluded, since they are normally associated with hypertension.

Therapy involves amelioration of hypokalemia by disrupting the renin-angiotensin-aldosterone and the kinin-prostaglandin axes. Potassium supplementation, magnesium repletion, propranolol, spironolactone, prostaglandin inhibition (in the form of aspirin or indomethacin), and captopril have all been used.

DISORDERS OF DISTAL NEPHRON FUNCTION

Distal nephron, including the distal convoluted tubule and collection ducts, absorbs the final quantity of sodium in the tubular fluid and is the site for potassium and hydrogen ion secretion. Inherited and acquired defects exist for selected and combined disorders of sodium, potassium, and acid-base regulation.

CLASSIC DISTAL RENAL TUBULAR ACIDOSIS (RTA) (see also Ch. 75). Classic distal (type I) RTA is a hypokalemic, hyperchloremic metabolic acidosis related to a selective defect in distal acidification.

Pathophysiology. The distal nephron (especially the cortical and medullary collecting ducts) usually can lower the urinary pH fully 2 to 3 pH units below that of blood in order to hydrate the filtered buffers (mainly phosphate) to form titratable acids and endogenously produced ammonia to form ammonium (see Fig. 82–2). If the distal nephron is incapable of lowering the luminal pH below 5.5 after challenge by metabolic acidosis, classic distal RTA is present. Due to the inappropriately high urinary pH, net acid excretion (titratable acid plus ammonium minus bicarbonate) is reduced and is below total acid production by the body. Enhanced potassium secretion occurs, presumably because there is reduced competition by proton secretion for the electrochemical driving forces in the distal nephron. The acidification defect may result from an insufficient number of proton-secreting pumps in the distal nephron. Alternately, a back leak of acid across the luminal membrane may exist so that establishment of a pH gradient is prevented even when proton secretion is normal.

Symptoms and Etiologies. Distal RTA is evident in infants, children, and adults; symptoms are those of acidosis or hypokalemia, as noted above. Nephrocalcinosis and nephrolithiasis are common, either as a cause or result of classic distal RTA. However, bone disease is not as frequent as in proximal RTA. Classic distal RTA also may be genetic (usually autosomal dominant) or due to autoimmune diseases, drugs and toxins, and various tubulointerstitial diseases (see Table 82–1).

Diagnosis and Treatment. The findings of hyperchloremic, hypokalemic metabolic acidosis with an inappropriately high urine pH (> 5.5) and diminished net acid excretion confirm the diagnosis. Diagnosis is facilitated by measuring the urinary anion gap (defined as urinary sodium plus potassium minus chloride, which is proportionate to the negative value of urinary ammonium NH_4^+). Diarrhea has a large, negative urinary anion gap and hence a high urinary ammonium concentration (accounting for the high urinary pH), while classic distal RTA has a zero or positive anion gap and a low urinary ammonium concentration due to impaired acidification. In subjects with a normal plasma bicarbonate concentration, the failure to lower urinary pH to < 5.5 following an acute acid challenge with NH_4Cl defines the syndrome of incomplete classic distal RTA. Treatment with alkali is generally very effective. The daily dose of alkali in adults is 1 to 3 mEq per kilogram, to compensate for the normal acid production by the body plus a small amount of urinary bicarbonate wastage. In distinction to proximal RTA, urinary potassium wasting is ameliorated with alkali therapy.

RTA OF GLOMERULAR INSUFFICIENCY. Moderate renal insufficiency may be associated with a normokalemic, hyperchloremic metabolic acidosis (GFR of 20 to 30 ml per minute) due to insufficient ammonia delivery. It is characterized by an appropriately low urine pH but subnormal urinary net acid (ammonium) excretion.

NONSELECTIVE DISTAL NEPHRON DYSFUNCTION: GENERALIZED DISTAL RTA, HYPERKALEMIA, AND RENAL SALT WASTING. These disorders derive from global dysfunction of the distal nephron due to aldosterone deficiency or antagonism and are typified by hyperkalemic, hyperchloremic (type IV) metabolic acidosis caused by subnormal net acid excretion and often by salt wasting.

Pathophysiology. Aldosterone influences distal sodium reabsorption to the extent that urinary sodium is < 10 mEq per liter. Sodium reabsorption creates a lumen negative potential difference that favors secretion of potassium and hydrogen ions. Disruption of

TABLE 82–2. RENAL TUBULAR ACIDOSES

Type	Renal Defect	GFR	Plasma [K+]	Proximal Acidification HCO_3^- Reabsorption (During HCO_3^- Loading)	Distal Acidification Minimal Urinary pH (During Acidosis)	$UAG \approx -Urine[NH_4^+]$ (During Acidosis)
Proximal (type II)	⇓ Proximal acidification	N	⇓	⇓	<5.5	0 or +
Classic distal (type I)	⇓ Distal pH gradient	N	⇓	N	>5.5	0 or +
Glomerular insufficiency	⇓ NH_3 production	⇓	N	N	<5.5	0 or +
Generalized distal (type IV)	⇓ Aldosterone action	⇓	⇑	N	<5.5	0 or +

N = normal; UAG = urinary anion gap = $[Na^+] + [K^+] - [Cl^-] \approx - [NH_4^+]$; GFR = glomerular filtration rate.

sodium reabsorption and of potassium and hydrogen ion secretion may be ascribable to a defect in the integrity of the distal nephron cell, reduced aldosterone production or action, diminished sodium reabsorption, or blunting of the lumen negative potential to enhanced chloride reabsorption. Any of these processes can diminish total hydrogen and potassium excretion, resulting in hyperkalemic metabolic acidosis. This hyperkalemia also serves to depress renal ammoniagenesis independently, which enhances the defect in renal acidification. The ability of the distal nephron to lower urine pH remains intact.

Diagnosis and Treatment. Generalized distal RTA is unique among the hyperchloremic metabolic acidoses in being a hyperkalemic disorder (Table 82–2). GFR is invariably reduced in hyporeninemic or tubulointerstitial nephropathy but may be at levels (≥ 30 ml per minute) above those typically found in the RTA of glomerular insufficiency. Treatment of the hyperkalemia and generalized distal RTA is effected with 9α-fluorocortisone, 0.1 mg per day, when mineralocorticoid is deficient. When hyporeninemia is the cause, high doses of the synthetic mineralocorticoid are necessary (up to 0.5 mg per day) because of associated mineralocorticoid resistance. Hypertension can be precipitated with this treatment. A loop diuretic (furosemide or ethacrynic acid) is also useful, especially when hypertension precludes administration of mineralocorticoid, because it augments urinary potassium excretion even when endogenous aldosterone is reduced. Useful adjuncts to diuretic therapy include dietary potassium restriction (< 50 mEq per deciliter), alkali therapy to compensate for daily acid generation (sodium bicarbonate, 1 to 3 mEq per kilogram per day), and sometimes short-term use of cation-exchange resin.

Chesney RW, Kurtz F: Renal tubular disorders. *In* Gonick H (ed.): Current Nephrology. Vol. 16. Chicago, Mosby–Year Book, 1992, p 1. *This review relates recent progress made in the understanding of renal Fanconi's syndrome and distal RTA.*

Chesney RW, Novella AC: Defects of renal tubular transport. *In* Massry SG, Glassock R (eds.): Textbook of Nephrology. Baltimore, Williams & Wilkins, 1994, pp 513. *This review discusses the major aminoacidurias of humans.*

Friedman AL, Chesney RW: Isolated renal tubular disorders. *In* Schrier RW, Gottschalk CW (eds.): Diseases of the Kidney. Boston, Little, Brown, 1993, p 611. *This comprehensive article describes in-depth the various isolated renal tubular disorders.*

Kanai Y, Lee W-S, You G, et al.: The human kidney low affinity Na$^+$/glucose co-transporter SG-T2: Delineation of the major renal reabsorptive mechanism for D-glucose. J Clin Invest 93:397, 1994. *Knowledge of the structural and functional properties of this transporter advances our understanding of familial renal glucosuria pathophysiology.*

83 DIABETES AND THE KIDNEY
Thomas H. Hostetter

Diabetes is not only the leading cause of chronic renal failure in the United States, it is one of the most serious long-term complications for the individual diabetic patient. Approximately one third of patients who develop chronic renal failure in the United States do so because of diabetes. At present, about half these patients have had longstanding insulin-dependent diabetes mellitus (IDDM) and the other half non–insulin-dependent diabetes mellitus (NIDDM), at least in the initial presentation of their metabolic disorder. However, not all patients with diabetes develop serious renal complications. Although the fraction of patients with IDDM who develop renal failure seems to have been declining over the last several decades, between 20 and 40% still suffer this complication. On the other hand, for patients with NIDDM, a somewhat lower fraction, perhaps as low as 10 to 20%, develop uremia due to diabetes, and therefore their nearly equal contribution to the total number of diabetic patients developing kidney failure results from the much larger total number of patients with NIDDM than IDDM (5- to 10-fold more cases of the former than the latter). The lower cumulative incidence of renal failure and NIDDM may reflect different aspects of the disease but also likely reflects the more advanced age of these patients and their susceptibility to death from other cardiovascular events such as myocardial infarction and stroke before renal failure occurs.

NATURAL HISTORY. While the renal disease of IDDM and NIDDM is in many regards similar, the natural history follows somewhat different paths. Following the initial polyuria and ketoacidosis that usually announce the abrupt onset of IDDM, by clinical standards renal function is generally normal. However, careful measurements of glomerular filtration rates (GFR) have demonstrated that a substantial fraction, 25 to 50%, of patients with IDDM will have a GFR well in excess of the normal range (Fig. 83–1). In addition, in the early phases of IDDM, patients tend to have enlarged kidneys commensurate with the heightened filtration rate. This hyperfiltration depends somewhat on the degree of glycemic control. Over the succeeding several years, renal function by standard laboratory testing as well as arterial pressure tends to be no different than that for aged-matched normal individuals. However, beginning toward the end of the first decade of IDDM, a certain fraction of patients will begin to demonstrate urinary abnormalities which bespeak the underlying structural and functional renal alterations of early diabetic nephropathy. The earliest finding is usually a small but abnormal amount of urinary albumin detectable only by sensitive antibody-based techniques. This "microalbuminuria" precedes the later development of larger rates of albumin excretion detectable by standard dipstick technology or other chemical assays. The lag time between the appearance of microalbuminuria and full-blown proteinuria is typically in the range of 1 to 5 years. However, recent advances in therapy seem likely to prolong this interval, forestalling the appearance of the more overt phases of the disease (see below). In addition to serving as an early marker for the nephropathic complications, the presence of microalbuminuria also marks those patients who are more likely to develop serious extrarenal cardiovascular disease as a consequence of IDDM. Without effective treatment (see below), the albuminuria tends to progressively worsen, and arterial hypertension usually supervenes in this subgroup during the transition between microalbuminuria and greater degrees of proteinuria. Finally, with the presence of dipstick-positive proteinuria and arterial hypertension, GFR begins to decline below normal values and serum creatinine rises. Prior to effective intervention, the rate of decline in filtration rate in these individuals was quite variable but averaged about 1 ml per minute of GFR per month. Thus, from the first evidence of standard dipstick-positive proteinuria and numerically only modest elevations of serum creatinine above the normal range, the time to end-stage renal disease has been about 3 to 8 years.

As with IDDM, patients with NIDDM also tend to have elevated GFR in the early period after being diagnosed with diabetes. The degree of increase in GFR is usually not so striking, however. In contrast to the IDDM patients, those with NIDDM have a higher prevalence of microalbuminuria and arterial hypertension when their diabetes is first identified. As many as 10 to 25% will have such abnormalities. That this relatively early appearance of hypertension and urinary abnormalities presents a fundamentally different aspect of the disease is possible, but this difference seems more likely to represent the effects of the much longer periods of asymptomatic hyperglycemia before formal diagnosis in NIDDM. Nevertheless, microalbuminuria in NIDDM also reflects an underlying predisposition to developing progressive kidney disease as well as serving as a marker of predilection for generalized cardiovascular disease. The progression of the renal complications in NIDDM generally thereafter essentially follows the same course as for IDDM.

CLINICAL PRESENTATION. During the period of declining GFR, patients often remain asymptomatic until they have lost 70 to 90% of their normal filtration rate. However, during this interval, arterial hypertension is prevalent, if asymptomatic, and protein excretion rates can rise to the levels of a nephrotic syndrome with the usual clinical and biochemical consequences of edema, hypoalbuminemia, and hypercholesterolemia. When the decay in filtration rate reaches the last 10 to 30% of baseline levels, uremic symptoms begin to appear. However, as with other progressive renal diseases, considerable individual variability exists in the development and severity of uremic symptoms. Furthermore, several elements of diabetes and its complications may exacerbate uremic symptoms or be indistinguishable from them. The nausea and vomiting that mark the uremic phase may be complicated by diabetic autonomic neuropathy with poor gastric emptying due to gastroparesis. Distinguishing between gastroparesis and uremic nausea and vomiting is often difficult. Furthermore, diabetic peripheral neuropathy in its sensory disturbance may to some degree mimic uremic neuropathy,

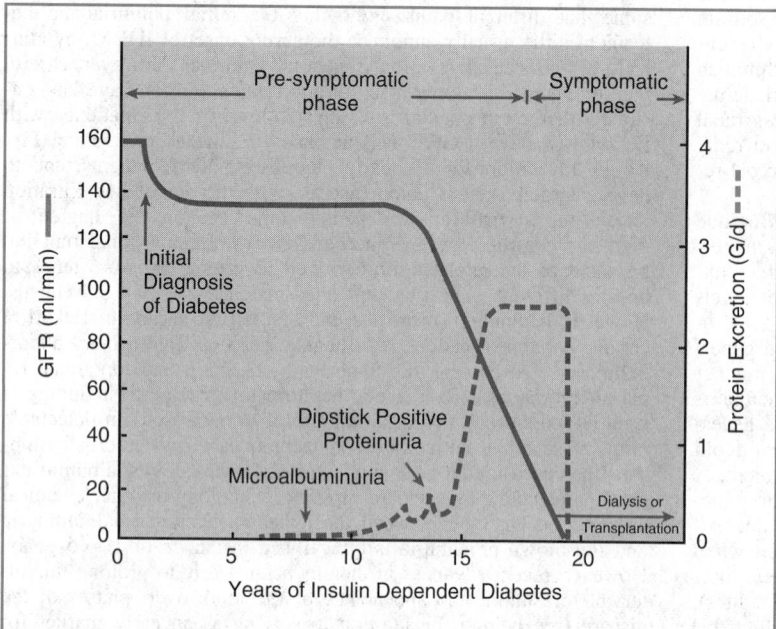

FIGURE 83–1. Course of diabetic nephropathy.

although in general the painful and hypesthetic neuropathic symptoms are more attributable to long-standing diabetes than to uremia in most patients. The presence of autonomic neuropathy also may make it harder to manage arterial hypertension in some patients. Specifically, the propensity to orthostatic hypotension with certain drugs may be exaggerated in the presence of autonomic neuropathy, and for some patients, their arterial pressure may be quite elevated when supine but below normal when standing. Diabetic retinopathy is nearly universally present in patients with IDDM who develop renal disease, but for patients with NIDDM, a sizable fraction, perhaps as large as 30 to 40%, manifests significant renal dysfunction without retinopathy. Cardiovascular complications commonly accompany renal disease both for NIDDM and IDDM, although they are generally more severe in the patients with NIDDM. However, for both categories of diabetes, myocardial infarction, stroke, and progressive peripheral vascular disease often requiring amputation seem to occur disproportionately in diabetic patients with renal failure compared with those spared from kidney disease.

PATHOLOGY. The heightened filtration and an enlarged overall renal size of early diabetes are matched by increases in glomerular and tubular size. With microalbuminuria and yet greater degrees of proteinuria and hypertension, the more characteristic glomerular changes become ever more prominent (Fig. 83–2). Increases in the mesangial compartment of the glomerulus are produced by increases in matrix and probably in the number of mesangial cells. These expansions can manifest as diffuse enlargement of this portion of the glomerulus as well as nodular increases in extracellular matrix material. These latter lesions have been termed Kimmelstiel-Wilson nodules but probably represent simply a different geometric arrangement of the generalized mesangial expansion. As the mesangium expands, the density of capillaries and their area for filtration progressively decline, and these abnormalities are thought to play an important role in the falling filtration rate. The glomerular basement membrane also progressively thickens, although this change does not clearly bear a relationship to the decline in filtration. Hyaline-like material (a presumed protein of uncertain type) can deposit in the arterioles about the glomerulus as well as in droplets along the capillary loops themselves. As with most progressive renal diseases, a prominent tubulointerstitial pathology develops *pari passu* with the glomerular abnormalities. The tubular basement membranes thicken, and occasional glycogen droplets appear in tubular epithelium. However, these tubulointerstitial abnormalities have few particular diagnostic features for diabetes but may be important in occluding vascular and tubular structures and contributing to the demise of renal function. In the main, the tubulointerstitial lesions comprise progressive fibrosis and mononuclear cell infiltrates surrounding atrophic tubules, some containing proteinaceous casts. These lesions are essentially identical in IDDM

and NIDDM patients sustaining renal complications. However, roughly similar patterns of nodular expansion can develop in the glomerulus in nondiabetic renal disease.

Amyloidosis, membranoproliferative glomerulonephritis type II, and light chain nephropathy may all demonstrate nodular patterns, and specific staining and other histologic techniques, as well as clinical data, are necessary to distinguish them from diabetes. In addition to glomerular and nonspecific tubular disease, diabetic patients will more rarely develop sufficient compromise of the circulation to the medullary regions to cause papillary necrosis. This abnormality, although potentially serious, is relatively unusual compared with the progressive glomerular and tubular interstitial lesions of the cortex.

PATHOGENESIS. The degree of glycemic control determines the appearance of diabetic nephropathy. Multiple lines of evidence indicate that better glucose control leads to a lower incidence of this complication. The mechanism whereby poorly controlled diabetes injures the kidney is less certain, however. The chemical consequences of an elevated glucose level have received the most consideration. Glucose reacts with amino groups on proteins to form covalently bonded glycated products. An example of such a product is the glycated hemoglobin used to monitor the long-term control of glucose in patients with diabetes. However, multiple other circulating and structural proteins also are modified.

Glycation by itself can substantially alter functions of numerous proteins, including changing their permeability through vascular walls and reducing their rates of normal catabolism. The simple glycation product is nevertheless reversible such that with better glucose control the glucose is removed from the protein. However, with sustained hyperglycemia, further and more complicated reactions occur, yielding what are generally termed advanced glycosylation end-products. These complex compounds often include several glucose or glucose-derived products that are covalently bound to proteins, and they also can encompass the binding of several proteins through bridging glucose products. These advanced glycosylation products are nearly irreversibly formed and, hence, once created, respond very little to improvements in metabolic control.

As with simple glycation, these alterations can importantly change the functions of the affected proteins, and such products may even interact with receptors on cells such as macrophages, which can in turn liberate cytokines and other factors that scar or restructure the renal parenchyma. Glucose reduced to sorbitol through the aldose reductase pathway also may perturb the oxidation states of cells with pathophysiologic consequences. However, blockers of this pathway have as yet shown only modest effects on the diabetic kidney.

In addition to the more direct chemical effects of hyperglycemia on renal structures, diabetes is associated with renal vasodilation early in the course of the disease, leading to the heightened GFR in a subset of diabetic patients, as noted above. Studies in experimental animals have demonstrated that this hyperfiltration is associated with elevations in glomerular capillary pressures, and such elevations also may occur in nonrenal capillaries as well. The elevations in glomerular capillary pressure may in their own right, or perhaps through interacting with the effects of glycation or the structural glomerular enlargement, induce pathologic glomerular capillary changes, including mesangial proliferation matrix expansion and basement membrane thickening. Maneuvers designed to reduce these capillary pressures in experimental animals, and more recently in clinical reports, have successfully mitigated damage to the kidney.

In addition to the renal hemodynamic alterations that lead to hyperfiltration and glomerular capillary hypertension, patients with overt diabetic nephropathy (dipstick-positive proteinuria and decreasing GFR) generally develop systemic hypertension. Hypertension is an adverse factor in all progressive renal diseases and seems especially so in diabetic nephropathy. The deleterious effects of hypertension are likely directed at the vasculature and microvasculature. Furthermore, the renal vasodilation noted above allows for greater transmission of systemic elevations in pressure to the glomerulus and may further exaggerate the glomerular capillary hypertension.

In addition to the hemodynamic and metabolic factors contributing to the appearance of diabetic nephropathy, familial or perhaps even genetic factors also appear to play a role. Evidence for this possibility derives from studies demonstrating familial clustering of diabetic nephropathy such that siblings who are both diabetic are more likely to either be concurrent for this renal complication or to avoid it entirely. Furthermore, certain ethnic groups, particularly American blacks, Hispanics, and Native Americans, may be particularly disposed to renal disease as a complication of diabetes. Obviously, their ethnic and familial risks also may include a complex set of social and economic factors.

TREATMENT. Prevention of diabetic nephropathy has not yet been achieved but may be possible by use of several approaches. First, control of glucose by careful insulin administration diminishes the risk of nephropathy in patients with IDDM. Whether assiduously maintaining near euglycemia would be equally effective in NIDDM is less certain but seems a highly desirable goal. Since animal experiments suggest that maintaining euglycemia could prevent the renal complications, it seems likely that the nearer to euglycemia a patient can be reasonably maintained, the better. In addition to glycemic control, antihypertensive treatment is a crucial element in preventing diabetic nephropathy or at least in forestalling its progression. Indeed, initiating converting enzyme inhibitors at the stage of microalbuminuria, even without significant arterial hypertension, appears to delay and perhaps prevent more substantial degrees of proteinuria. Whether such therapy will prevent the decline in the filtration rate is yet uncertain. Nevertheless, patients with IDDM should be screened regularly for microalbuminuria with antibody-based tests that either use special antibody-impregnated dipsticks or immunoassays for albumin on urine collection. If there are abnormal rates of albumin excretion even before the standard dipstick is positive, converting enzyme inhibitors should be prescribed. Even though such patients are often normotensive, they do not suffer adverse hemodynamic consequences of treatment with a converting enzyme inhibitor. With more advanced degrees of nephropathy and dipstick-positive proteinuria and a diminution in GFRs reflected in even modest elevations in creatinine, arterial hypertension is more frequently present. Therapy with converting enzyme inhibition has proven more effective than other types of antihypertensive agents in slowing the progression of renal disease at this point as well. The efficacy of this class of antihypertensives has been extended to patients with both IDDM and NIDDM. However, particularly in the latter group, special care must be exercised to ensure that hyperkalemia does not occur in the first few days to weeks of converting enzyme inhibition. Also, because of the potential for renal artery stenosis, particularly in the older NIDDM group, careful monitoring of serum creatinine level in the first 1 to 2 weeks of a converting enzyme inhibitor regimen is necessary to screen for the occasional patient who may have a serious decline in GFR based on renal vascular disease. The level of blood pressure sought is not entirely certain, but probably levels of < 130 mm Hg systolic and < 90 mm Hg diastolic would be desirable using a regimen based on converting enzyme inhibitors. Dietary protein also should be restricted at this stage of disease. The value to the kidney of intensified glycemic control and lipid-lowering agents in these more advanced phases is unknown. But because of the high rates of extrarenal cardiovascular disease in this group, such efforts seem justified.

For those patients who either progress despite therapy or are noted at advanced stages of their diabetic nephropathy, the criteria used to initiate dialysis or recommend transplantation do not differ substantially from those used for patients with other types of chronic progressive renal diseases. However, because of their propensity to multiple other systemic lesions, particularly those of cardiovascular and autonomic nervous system, patients with diabetic nephropathy may tolerate uremia less well than patients with isolated kidney diseases of other sorts. For example, hyperkalemia may supervene more rapidly because of the predisposition to hyporenonemic hypoaldosteronism. Symptoms of gastroparesis and uremic gastrointestinal disturbance may adversely interact. As yet another example, patients with ischemic or diabetic cardiomyopathies may tolerate hypertension and extracellular fluid volume overload less readily than do nondiabetic uremic patients. For these sorts of reasons, patients with diabetes may often require treatment for their end-stage renal disease at somewhat earlier phases in the decline of GFR than do other subjects. However, as with chronic renal disease in general, the decision to initiate such therapy is generally based on the patients' symptoms rather than the biochemical indices of uremia *per se*.

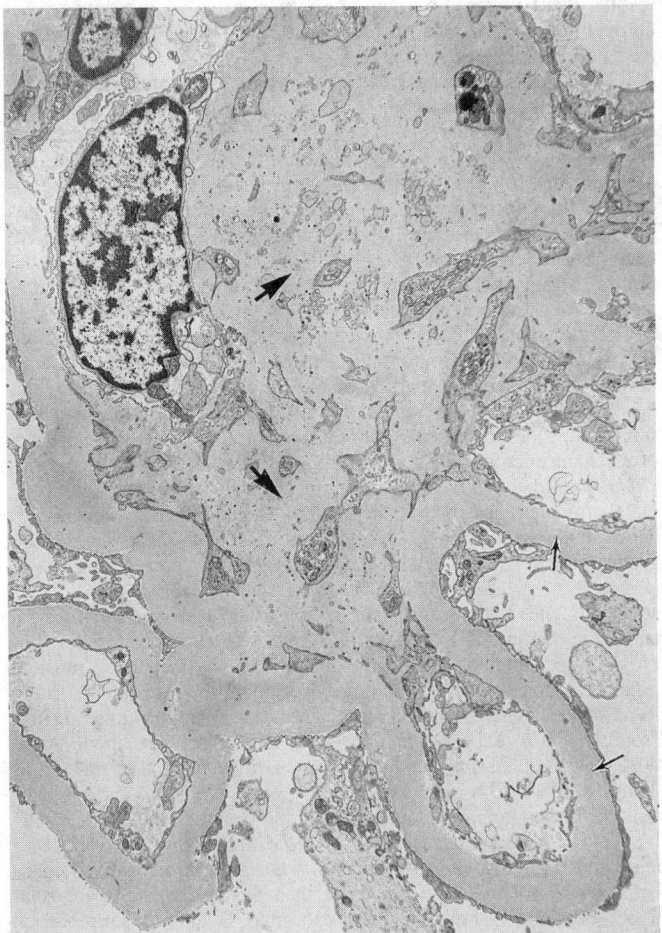

FIGURE 83–2. Electron photomicrograph of a portion of a glomerulus from a patient with proteinuric, diabetic glomerulopathy (magnification × 5000). A striking increase in collagenous components has resulted in (1) widening of the basement membrane of peripheral capillary loops *(small arrows),* and (2) expansion of the matrix of the glomerular mesangium *(large arrows).* The latter alteration is responsible for compressing and ultimately obliterating the glomerular capillary network.

Patients with diabetes do less well with both transplantation and dialysis than nondiabetic patients. The poorer outcomes with therapy of end-stage renal disease rest mainly on the associated cardiovascular mortality, with stroke, myocardial infarction, and periperal vascular disease that requires amputation representing significant co-morbid risks. However, efforts to prevent, screen for, and prophylactically treat these other complications seem to be rewarded by improved outcomes for these patients.

Borch-Johnsen K, Norgaard K, Hommel E, et al.: Is diabetic nephropathy an inherited complication? Kidney Int 41:719, 1992. *This original article confirms earlier work and outlines the status of familial clustering of diabetic renal disease.*

Brownlee M: Glycosylation products as toxic mediators of diabetic complications. Annu Rev Med 42:159, 1991. *This review considers some of the pathologic consequences of glycation and advanced glycation products.*

Diabetes Control and Complications Trial Research Group: Effective intensive treatment of diabetes on the development and progression of the long-term complications in insulin-dependent diabetes. N Engl J Med 329:977, 1993. *The first large-scale population trial demonstrating the efficacy of careful glycemic control.*

Hostetter TH: Diabetic nephropathy: Metabolic versus hemodynamic considerations. Diabetes Care 15:1205, 1992. *Reviews the hemodynamic risk factors and their physiology.*

Lewis EJ, Hunsicker LG, Bain RP, et al.: The effect of angiotensin converting enzyme inhibition on diabetic nephropathy. N Engl J Med 329:1456, 1993. *This study compares the efficacy of standard antihypertensives with converting enzyme inhibition and establishes that the latter more effectively slows renal failure progression.*

Messent JWC, Elliott TG, Hill RD, et al.: Prognostic significance of microalbuminuria in insulin-dependent diabetes mellitus: A 23-year follow-up study. Kidney Int 41:836, 1992. *This group of investigators summarizes a very long-term survey of microalbuminuria.*

84 URINARY TRACT INFECTIONS AND PYELONEPHRITIS

Calvin M. Kunin

DEFINITION. *Urinary tract infection* (UTI) is a broad term that encompasses both asymptomatic microbial colonization of the urine and symptomatic infection with microbial invasion and inflammation of urinary tract structures. Epithelial surfaces of the urinary tract are contiguous, extending from the renal postglomerular filtrate to the urethral meatus. In the absence of infection, these structures are bathed in a common stream of sterile urine. The infectious process may involve the kidney, renal pelvis, ureters, bladder, and urethra, as well as the adjacent structures, such as the perinephric fascia, prostate, and epididymis. Bacteria are by far the most common invading organisms, but yeasts, fungi, and viruses also may produce UTI. *Invading microbe(s) and inflammatory cells present in the urine are the laboratory hallmarks of the disease.* Urine may be sterile when the infection site does not contact the stream (such as when the ureter is blocked by a stricture or stone, during treatment with an antimicrobial drug, soon after metastatic infection to the kidney, or with perinephric or prostatic abscesses).

The concept of *significant bacteriuria* distinguishes colonization and growth of microorganisms in the urine from contaminants collected during voiding, particularly in females. The standard criterion of $\geq 10^5$ colony-forming units (CFU) per milliliter takes into account that most microorganisms which cause UTI grow well in urine. The quantitative count is an excellent guide to diagnosing and evaluating therapy, since infection may persist even when symptoms are no longer present. Lower counts of 10^3 to 10^4 CFU per milliliter (with "uropathogens"; see definition below) may be clinically meaningful when voided specimens are obtained from males, under conditions of brisk diuresis and suppressive antimicrobial therapy, and for relatively slow-growing organisms such as staphylococci. The suprapubic aspiration (SPA) of urine from the bladder is considered the diagnostic "gold standard." SPA also may detect transient colonization in the bladder by commensal urethral and vaginal microbes without true infection. Low bacterial counts with "uropathogens" are found in about a third to a half of females who present with pyuria and dysuria. This condition, termed the "pyuria/dysuria (urethral) syndrome," appears to be an early phase of UTI. It is often clinically indistinguishable from urethritis caused by *Chlamydia trachomatis, Neisseria gonorrhoeae,* or herpes simplex.

Asymptomatic bacteriuria is a common condition, particularly in females, where large numbers of bacteria are present in the urine despite a lack of symptoms. It is considered to be an *asymptomatic infection* when accompanied by pyuria. Clinical conditions such as *urethritis, cystitis, prostatitis,* and *pyelonephritis* reflect the symptomatology manifest by the involved organ, but the infection may be more widespread.

Acute pyelonephritis is a pyogenic, focal infection of the renal parenchyma usually involving one or more wedge-shaped segments of the kidney accompanied by local and systemic symptoms of infection. "Chronic pyelonephritis" refers to the pathologic and radiologic findings of chronic cortical scarring, tubulointerstitial damage, and deformity of the underlying calyx. Chronic pyelonephritis may be *active,* with persistent infection, or *inactive,* with focal sterile scars of a past infection.

Noninfectious diseases can produce renal lesions that mimic chronic pyelonephritis. Identical changes on radiographic studies may be seen in patients who suffered severe vesicoureteral reflux during childhood. The entity, "reflux nephropathy," refers to the radiologic triad of intrarenal reflux, vesicoureteral reflux, and scarring with loss of parenchymal mass. In the absence of infection it can lead to end-stage renal failure with scarred, shrunken kidneys. There is evidence that reflux nephropathy may result from autoimmune renal damage rather than bacterial infection of the kidney. Since reflux is usually detected by radiologic studies in patients with recent infection, it may be difficult to determine whether renal scarring was produced by reflux alone or in combination with infection. Sensitive methods such as radionuclide scanning may help resolve these issues. Longstanding *hypertension* may produce renal cortical scars similar to pyelonephritis, and *analgesic nephropathy* may produce papillary necrosis.

ETIOLOGY. The nature of the invading microbe depends, for the most part, on history of infection, underlying host factors, receipt of antimicrobial drugs, and instrumentation of the urinary tract. The term *uropathogen* is used commonly to describe the microorganisms found most frequently in patients with UTI. These include Enterobacteriaceae, *Pseudomonas* species, *Staphylococcus* species, enterococci, and other gram-negative and gram-positive bacteria and yeasts that grow well in urine. *Lactobacillus,* α-hemolytic streptococci, and anaerobes are considered to be contaminants if found in voided urine.

The clinical distinction between uncomplicated and complicated UTI is of paramount importance. Host factors are the key in determining the invasive properties of the microorganisms and localization of infection; the extent of renal damage, bacteremia, and dissemination; therapeutic and prophylactic strategies; the development of resistant microorganisms; and the ultimate prognosis.

Uncomplicated infections occur in otherwise healthy individuals, most often females, with intact voiding mechanisms. There is evidence that susceptibility to infection is related to several blood group antigens (see Ch. 138), including Lewis nonsecretor status [Le (a + b −)] and [Le (a − b −)], P1, and B, rather than to personal hygiene. Patients may suffer considerable morbidity from recurrent symptomatic infections but almost never develop renal failure. Acute, uncomplicated pyelonephritis may produce transient functional abnormalities and leave residual renal scars but rarely leads to permanent renal damage. The most common invading microorganism is *Escherichia coli,* which is present in about 80 to 90% of cases. *Staphylococcus saprophyticus* may account for as many as 10 to 20% of cases in young adult women occurring during the late summer and fall. Occasionally, other members of the family Enterobacteriaceae, such as *Klebsiella, Enterobacter, Proteus,* and rarely, *Salmonella* and *Shigella,* may be causative organisms. Gram-positive bacteria other than *S. saprophyticus* are relatively uncommon but may include group B and D streptococci. Most uncomplicated infections respond readily to antimicrobial agents.

Complicated infections occur in individuals of both sexes who have structural or functional abnormalities of the voiding mechanism (Table 84–1). Complicated infections are exceedingly difficult to eradicate without correcting the underlying defect or removing a foreign body. Patients with complicated infections are at increased

TABLE 84-1. CHARACTERISTICS OF COMPLICATED URINARY TRACT INFECTIONS

1. Host factors
   a. Structural abnormalities of the voiding mechanism
      Calculi (renal, bladder, or prostatic)
      Strictures (urethra or ureter)
      Prostatic obstruction (benign or neoplastic)
      Vesicoureteral reflux
      Neurogenic bladder (diabetics, paraplegics)
      Indwelling urinary catheters
   b. Common underlying diseases
      Diabetes mellitus
      Sickle cell anemia
      Polycystic renal disease
      Renal transplantation
2. Common microorganisms*
   a. Gram-negative bacteria
      Escherichia coli
      Klebsiella pneumoniae
      Enterobacter aerogenes
      Proteus mirabilis
      Pseudomonas aeruginosa
      Acinetobacter species
      Serratia marcescens
      Providencia stuartii and *rettgeri*
   b. Gram-positive bacteria
      Staphylococcus aureus
      Coagulase-negative staphylococci
      Groups B and D streptococci
   c. Yeasts
      Candida albicans

* See text.

risk of developing severe renal damage, bacteremia, sepsis, and increased mortality. The organisms tend to be less susceptible to antimicrobial drugs (see Table 84–1). *Candida albicans* and even *Cryptococcus neoformans* may be significant and produce disease in diabetics and in patients treated with corticosteroids and immunosuppressive agents.

INCIDENCE AND PREVALENCE. UTI's are among the most common conditions encountered in office practice, hospitals, and extended-care facilities. There are about 6,200,000 physician office visits each year (about two-thirds are females) for acute symptomatic infection. About 40 to 50% of adult women report that they had a UTI at some time. UTIs are important complications in pregnancy, diabetes, polycystic renal disease, renal transplantation, and structural and neurologic conditions that interfere with urine flow. UTIs are the leading cause of gram-negative sepsis in hospitalized patients. About half of all hospital-acquired infections originate in the urinary tract in association with the urinary catheter and urologic procedures. Urinary catheters are used in about 10% of patients admitted to hospitals and long-term care facilities. Catheter-associated UTIs have been shown to increase mortality threefold in a general hospital and to be an independent risk factor for death in long-term care facilities.

EPIDEMIOLOGY. The quantitative bacterial count has proven useful for detecting asymptomatic infections and defining the frequency of underlying infection in large populations. The frequency of bacteriuria is about 1 to 2% in newborns, as determined by SPA or meticulously clean urine samples. Newborn males are more often infected than females, and uncircumcised males are at higher risk. After the first year of life, infections are more common in females. During the ages 5 to 18 years, the prevalence is 1.2% in girls and 0.03% in boys. The incidence in girls is 0.4% per year, is linear with time throughout the school years, and is unaffected by menarche. The cumulative frequency of asymptomatic infection in girls during the school years is about 5%. Bacteriuria in girls is independent of socioeconomic status and race and is not increased in diabetics. The prevalence of bacteriuria in females rises about 1% per decade and may be as high as 10% in elderly women. Women with asymptomatic bacteriuria appear to be prone to symptomatic infections when they become sexually active or pregnant. The frequency of bacteriuria during pregnancy varies from 2 to 6%, depending on age, parity, and socioeconomic group. Detecting and treating bacteriuria early in pregnancy prevents acute pyelonephritis during the third trimester.

Role of Instrumentation. Following a single catheterization, about 1 to 2% of healthy individuals will develop persistent bacteriuria; the risk is increased at the time of delivery, in the debilitated patient, or in males with prostatic obstruction. With open indwelling catheter drainage, >90% of patients will develop infection within 3 to 4 days. Catheter-associated infection may be prevented by avoiding using instruments whenever possible, removing the catheter when it is no longer needed, and using aseptic closed drainage.

PATHOGENESIS. The urinary tract is ordinarily sterile except at the distal urethra and meatus. These regions are colonized by staphylococci, diphtheroids, and other commensal organisms that do not grow well in urine. In contrast, in females prone to recurrent infections, the urethra and vaginal introitus are more likely to be colonized with small numbers of enteric gram-negative bacteria, which do grow well in urine. Urine is a variable culture medium. High concentrations of urea, low pH, hypertonicity, and dietary organic acids produce unfavorable conditions for bacterial growth. Enteric gram-negative bacteria overcome hypertonic conditions by taking up the osmoprotectants glycine betaine and proline betaine that exist in urine. Important defense mechanisms include the dynamics of urine flow (washout) and the antibacterial properties of the membrane lining the urinary tract.

Urinary infections arise most commonly by an ascending route. Gram-negative enteric bacilli and other microorganisms normally present in the large bowel colonize the distal urethra, enter the bladder intermittently, and become established when conditions are favorable. The bladder defense mechanism is usually highly effective. Most women suffer only an occasional episode, and men rarely develop infection spontaneously. The higher rate of urinary infections in females appears to be due to their shorter urethra. Homosexual males who engage in anal intercourse are at increased risk. The role of sexual intercourse in acquiring urinary infection in females is controversial but may be important for a subpopulation prone to recurrent infections. Vaginal diaphragms increase the risk of UTI apparently by mechanical effects and by altering the vaginal flora.

Other less common pathways include the hematogenous and possibly the lymphatic routes. Staphylococcal bacteremia from a distant site can produce multiple microabscesses in the kidney (renal carbuncles). These may extend to the perinephric fascia and produce perinephric abscesses. A similar but more insidious process may occur with tuberculosis. Disseminated *C. albicans* infections in the immunocompromised, leukopenic host can involve the kidney. Occasionally, bacteremia arising from an infected kidney may produce metastatic abscesses to bone and back to the kidney. Septic emboli, particularly in the setting of infective endocarditis, can produce extensive infection in the kidney. A rare but striking finding in diabetics is the occurrence of pneumaturia or urinary flatulence due to the production of gas by fermentation.

Hematogenous infection in experimental models requires antecedent structural damage to the kidney. The renal medulla is much more susceptible to infection than is the cortex. In experimental pyelonephritis, as few as 10 to 100 *E. coli* can produce infection in the medulla, whereas 100,000 are required to infect the cortex. The increased susceptibility of the renal medulla is thought to be due to its unique hypertonicity, which impairs leukocyte mobilization and phagocytosis. Ascending infections begin in the renal fornices and extend in a segmental fashion to the papilla, medulla, and cortex.

Microbial virulence factors are also important (see Ch. 297). Strains of *E. coli* isolated from patients with pyelonephritis are more likely to contain capsular polysaccharides (K antigens), which resist phagocytosis, and to possess P-fimbriae (pili). These are hairlike surface structures with a lectin at their tip that recognizes complementary structures on the surface of host epithelial cells. P-fimbriated strains bind to α-D-Gal-($-$ 4)-β-D-Gal (P blood group) receptors on urothelial cells and are more commonly recovered from the blood and urine of patients with acute uncomplicated pyelonephritis. Type 1 (mannose-sensitive) fimbriae appear to help initiate infection in the bladder. They are recognized by phagocytic cells and bound by Tamm-Horsfall mucoprotein in the urine. Fimbriated *E. coli* convert to nonfimbriated forms (phase variation), possibly to avoid recognition by phagocytic cells. Other less well established virulence factors include the O antigens and production of hemolysin and aerobactin. Virulent strains are found more often in patients with uncomplicated rather than complicated infections, presumably because of the greater need to overcome host resistance. Urease-producing bacteria such as *Proteus, Providencia, Morganella, S. saprophyticus,* and *Corynebacterium* D2 are particularly virulent because they can produce ammonia, which is toxic to the kidney, and form infection (struvite) stones, which may block the urinary tract and urinary catheters.

CLINICAL MANIFESTATIONS. Symptoms and laboratory findings in acute urinary infection and pyelonephritis are shown in Table 84–2. It is usually not possible to distinguish on clinical grounds whether the patient has urethritis, cystitis, or the pyuria/dysuria syndrome. Otherwise healthy females may have an occasional isolated episode of uncomplicated UTI, but some suffer from highly recurrent infections. Recurrence is usually due to reinfection with a new bacterial strain (about 80% of the time) rather than to relapse with the same strain.

Acute pyelonephritis is easy to recognize and is seldom confused with any other renal disease. Renal colic and hematuria due to passage of urinary calculi may mimic pyelonephritis, but patients are usually afebrile. Pyelonephritis at times presents with symptoms that do not point to the urinary tract. Dysuria and fever may be absent. There may be only backache, without demonstrable flank tenderness. Some patients have pain in either the upper or the lower abdomen, together with symptoms of disturbed gastrointestinal function. Others complain only of general fatigue. Clues to the diagnosis include a past history of infection, underlying host abnormalities such as diabetes, the presence of a urinary catheter, fever of uncertain etiology, and unexplained pyuria, bacteriuria, and gram-negative bacteremia. Uroradiographic studies are often helpful to demonstrate a specific lesion. There are usually no changes in renal function other than a transiently decreased ability to concentrate urine, and secondary hypertension is unusual.

A number of tests have been developed to differentiate "upper" (kidney) from "lower" (bladder) infection. Ureteral catheterization and bladder washout maneuvers are considered as research studies. The antibody-coated bacteria test has insufficient sensitivity and specificity for clinical use. The most useful guide is clinical assessment. Patients with complicated infections are more likely to have upper tract infection.

The symptoms and signs of acute, uncomplicated pyelonephritis usually resolve within several days after instituting adequate antimicrobial therapy. More severe forms of pyelonephritis or urinary tract obstruction should be suspected if fever, leukocytosis, and flank pain persist. Diabetics are prone to widely destructive, emphysematous pyelonephritis and renal papillary necrosis. Other conditions that should be considered are renal carbuncle or perinephric abscess, xanthogranulomatous pyelonephritis, and metastatic abscess in the vertebrae. Surgical drainage may be required for perinephric and large renal abscesses. Patients with chronic active pyelonephri-

tis may have persistent smoldering infections and gradual progression to end-stage renal failure. This process may persist for many years and be complicated by generalized debility, anemia of chronic infection, and secondary amyloidosis and eventually result in proteinuria and severe hypertension and its complications.

Patients subjected to urethral instrumentation, especially the indwelling catheter, are at increased risk for bacteremia and acute pyelonephritis. The urinary catheter is an independent risk factor for about a threefold increase in mortality among patients in short-term general hospitals and extended-care facilities. The infectious process is often subclinical but in some individuals may take a sudden fulminating course, with bacteremia, septic shock, and death. Gram-negative sepsis and bacteremic shock are described in Ch. 70.

DIAGNOSIS. *Microscopic and Dipstick Methods.* Rapid diagnostic methods include examining a Gram stain of unsedimented urine with an oil-immersion lens or the centrifuged urinary sediment using the high-dry objective under reduced light, with or without adding methylene blue. The presence of one or more organisms on the Gram stain correlates about 90% with quantitative culture (10^5 CFU per milliliter). Examining the unstained sediment is very helpful and can be done with the routine examination for formed elements. The criterion is the presence of many (preferably more than 20) obvious bacteria regardless of motility. "Pyuria" is usually defined as 10 or more leukocytes per high-powered field in the centrifuged specimen or 5 or more when uncentrifuged. The leukocyte esterase test correlates well with chamber counts of >10 to 20 leukocytes per cubic millimeter. "Sterile pyuria" may be due to vaginal leukorrhea. The nitrite test is highly specific but relatively insensitive unless performed on a first morning urine. Microscopic hematuria is common in acute infections, but proteinuria is rare.

Urologic and Radiologic Investigations. Searching for important structural abnormalities such as urethral valves (in male infants), severe vesicoureteral reflux, malformations, and obstructive and neurogenic lesions is indicated for young children of both sexes. Urologic studies are rarely productive in adult females, even with recurrent infections. Ultrasonography of the kidneys with bladder-voiding studies and radionuclide examinations have reduced the need to use more invasive procedures routinely such as intravenous urograms, cystoscopy, and voiding cystourethrograms. Computed tomography is particularly helpful for detecting renal abscesses. There usually is no need to repeat normal studies. Cystoscopy should be reserved for demonstrating anatomic defects, interstitial cystitis, and bladder tumors and should not be used as a guide to measure response to therapy.

MANAGEMENT. The goals are to eradicate bacteria from the urinary tract, relieve symptoms, prevent renal damage, and diminish the likelihood of spreading infection to other sites. Prophylaxis is used to prevent recurrent symptomatic infection. Suppression, although rarely effective, may be used to diminish the number of bacteria in the urine or tissues. Indications for therapy depend on the potential of infection to produce symptoms or damage the urinary tract and the likelihood that treatment will be effective.

Asymptomatic Bacteriuria. Asymptomatic bacteriuria need not be treated in otherwise healthy or elderly females without underlying structural or neurologic lesions, since the likelihood of renal damage is slight and the toxicity and expense of therapy often outweigh the risk of disease. Furthermore, reinfection is common following successful eradication of bacteriuria, and little is accomplished in the long term. Urease-producing bacteria (see above) should be eradicated whenever possible because of their potential to produce urinary calculi. *Antimicrobial therapy is usually ineffective in patients with indwelling catheters and should not be used. It will result in superinfection with more resistant microorganisms.*

Treatment is recommended for patients who are at high risk for developing symptomatic infections or have complicating conditions. These include patients with diabetes, polycystic kidneys, anatomic or neurologic abnormalities, or those scheduled for urologic procedures or renal transplantation. Treating asymptomatic bacteriuria early in pregnancy quite successfully prevents acute pyelonephritis in the third trimester.

Acute Symptomatic Urinary Tract Infection. The initial attack of UTI is usually by *E. coli.* Treatment should be started before the results of susceptibility tests are available. The choice of drug is based on the likelihood that the organism will be susceptible. The choice of an oral or parenteral agent depends on the sever-

TABLE 84–2. COMMON MANIFESTATIONS OF URINARY TRACT INFECTIONS

Clinical	Laboratory
1. Urethritis or cystitis	
Frequent urination	Leukocyte esterase test positive
Burning on urination	Nitrite test may be positive
Suprapubic discomfort	Gram stain of uncentrifuged urine
Lassitude	Leukocytes (≥ 5/hpf)
Cloudy or blood-tinged urine	Gram-negative rods or gram-positive cocci (≥ 1/hpf)*
Occasional low-grade fever	Urine culture ($\geq 10^5$ CFU/ml*)
	Low-count bacteriuria*
	(10^3–10^4 CFU/ml*)
2. Acute pyelonephritis	
Sudden onset of fever	Same findings as above *plus*
Shaking chills	Leukocytosis
Flank pain (may radiate)	Blood cultures positive (about 20%)
Leukocytosis	Minimal effect on serum creatinine
Urinary symptoms may be absent	Decreased concentration ability

* See text.

ity of the infection and the patient's ability to take the oral agent. Drugs are selected on the basis of cost, side effects, and antibacterial spectrum.

Microscopic examination of urine and urine cultures ensure an accurate diagnosis of UTI. Pretreatment urine cultures are desirable, but not essential, in young women with acute dysuria and pyuria, in whom the probability of uncomplicated bacterial cystitis is high. These patients usually respond to short-course empirical therapy. Response to therapy can be determined by disappearance of bacteria on microscopic examination by 24 to 48 hours, but pyuria may persist for up to a week. It is important to recognize bacteriologic failure early and to change antibiotics. Pretreatment urine cultures should be obtained in symptomatic infants, children, men, and the elderly; patients with suspected pyelonephritis or complicated infection; patients with relapsing infections; those with *symptomatic* catheter- or instrument-associated nosocomial infection; and pregnant women to detect covert bacteriuria.

Acute uncomplicated episodes of symptomatic infection (bacterial cystitis or urethritis) are treated most effectively with a short course of oral therapy (Table 84–3). Three-day treatment is recommended because it is more effective than single-dose therapy and is as effective as 7 to 10 days of treatment. Single-dose therapy usually fails to eradicate either renal bacteriuria or complicated infections and, if used, should be started early in the course of infection. Patients with complicated infections should be treated for 7 to 14 days or even longer, provided that the drug is effective in eradicating bacteriuria (Fig. 84–1). Effective drugs are listed in Table 84–3. Symptomatic urethritis caused by *Chlamydia trachomatis* should respond to oral doxycycline (100 mg twice daily) or tetracycline (500 mg four times per day) for 7 days.

Acute uncomplicated pyelonephritis should be treated for 7 to 14 days. Parenteral agents such as trimethoprim-sulfamethoxazole, ampicillin-sulbactam, a cephalosporin, or an aminoglycoside may be required when the patient is too ill to receive an oral agent. There is usually no need for more than one drug. Oral agents may be used on an outpatient basis, provided that the patient is not nauseated. Patients treated with parenteral agents should be converted to oral therapy as soon as they are stable. Patients with active chronic pyelonephritis may not respond to antimicrobial therapy, even when the organism is susceptible, unless an obstruction or foreign body is removed or an abscess is drained. Hematogenous pyelonephritis requires specific therapy directed at the invading organism. A follow-up culture 1 week after completion of antimicrobial therapy is recommended to document a cure.

Recurrent Infections. Recurrent infection within a week or two after treatment is usually due to persistence of the same focus, whereas recurrence after several weeks is more often a result of reinfection, especially in women. Relapses in diabetics, transplant recipients, and elderly men should be treated for up to 4 to 6 weeks. Frequently recurrent infections may be managed either by repeated short courses for each symptomatic episode (these can be self-administered by the reliable patient) or by long-term prophylaxis with

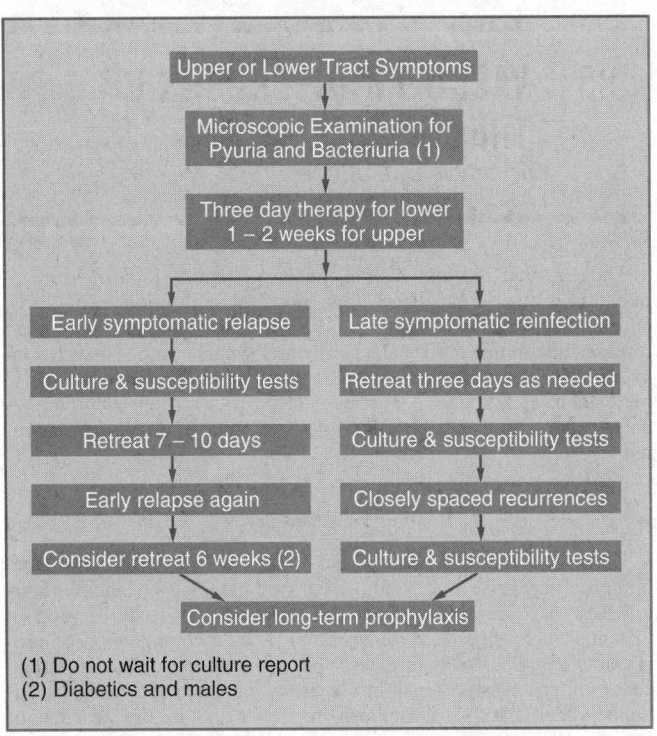

FIGURE 84–1. Management of urinary tract infections.

trimethoprim, trimethoprim-sulfamethoxazole, or nitrofurantoin as a single bedtime dose. Resistant strains infrequently emerge with these drugs. Prophylaxis, when given for 6 months or longer, is highly effective for recurrent infections. There is still a high risk of recurrence once prophylaxis is stopped, and it may need to be resumed. Urinary antiseptics, such as methenamine mandelate or hippurate, require an acidic urine, preferably at pH 5.5, and are relatively ineffective unless given with agents that consistently lower urinary pH such as a high-protein diet, ammonium chloride, ascorbic acid, or methionine. Methenamine and its salts may be used for prophylaxis when no other drug is active. Infection should be eradicated first by a more potent drug before beginning prophylaxis with these drugs.

Some women take high volumes of fluids when they develop acute urinary symptoms. This may be helpful at times, but antimicrobial drugs are much more effective. Double voiding in patients with vesicoureteral reflux is recommended. Voiding after sexual intercourse is felt by some to decrease the chance of recurrent infection, but postcoital use of prophylactic agents is far more effective.

Complicated Infections. Complicated urinary infections are exceedingly difficult to eradicate. The key to management is to relieve obstruction and remove foreign bodies combined with the use of effective antimicrobial drugs. It is important to recognize failure early and not to continue using an ineffective drug. This will only lead to superinfection with more resistant microorganisms and increase costs unnecessarily. It is often best to leave the infection untreated except to manage acute episodes. Suppressive therapy should be abandoned unless it can be shown that the bacterial populations in the urine are markedly reduced.

Johnson JR: Virulence factors in *Escherichia coli* urinary tract infection. Clin Microbiol Rev 4:80, 1991. *A well-written, comprehensive review of a complex field.*

Kass EH, Svanborg Eden C (eds.): Host-Parasite Interactions in Urinary Tract Infections. Chicago, University of Chicago Press, 1989. *An international symposium that provides an excellent overview of both basic and clinical aspects of urinary tract infections.*

Kunin CM: Detection, Prevention and Management of Urinary Tract Infections. 4th ed. Philadelphia, Lea & Febiger, 1987. *A comprehensive text that describes the pathogenesis, management, and prevention of urinary tract infections.*

Kunin CM: Urinary tract infections in females. Clin Infect Dis 18:1, 1994. *A state-of-the art clinical article dealing with recent advances in the field.*

Sheinfeld J, Schaeffer AJ, Corrdon-Cardo C, et al.: Association of the Lewis blood-group phenotype with recurrent urinary tract infections in women. N Engl J Med 320:773, 1989. *An explanation for the remarkable susceptibility of some women to undergo recurrent urinary tract infections.*

Stamm WE, Hooton TM: Management of urinary tract infections in adults. N Engl J Med 329:1328, 1993. *A recent comprehensive review of the current recommendations for therapy.*

TABLE 84–3. ORAL ANTIMICROBIAL DRUGS FOR TREATMENT OF UNCOMPLICATED URINARY TRACT INFECTIONS*

Drug	Dose	Comments
Trimethoprim	100 mg every 12 hours† ⎤	About equally
Trimethoprim-sulfamethoxazole	80/400 mg every 12 hours† ⎦	effective
Nitrofurantoin	100 mg every 6 to 8 hours‡	Take with food
Amoxicillin-clavulanate	500 mg every 6 to 8 hours	Check for penicillin allergy; expensive
Norfloxacin	400 mg every 12 hours	Expensive§
Ciprofloxacin	250 mg every 12 hours	Expensive§
Ofloxacin	200 mg every 12 hours	Expensive§
Lomefloxacin	400 mg once daily	Expensive§
Enoxacin	200 mg every 12 hours	Expensive§
Carbenicillin indanyl	Two 382-mg tablets every 6 hours	For *Pseudomonas*

* Ampicillin, amoxicillin, cephalexin, or a tetracycline may be used if the bacteria are susceptible, but resistance to these drugs is common.

† Many clinicians prefer to use a double dose of these drugs.

‡ Contraindicated in patients with elevated serum creatinine levels.

§ The quinolones may fail to eradicate *S. saprophyticus*. Bacteria resistant to one quinolone are often resistant to all others.

85 VASCULAR DISORDERS OF THE KIDNEY

Thomas D. DuBose, Jr.

The fact that the kidneys depend on systemic blood pressure to maintain normal renal blood flow, glomerular filtration rate (GFR), and tubular function underscores the vulnerability of the kidneys to diseases involving the renal vasculature. Renal vessels may be involved by thrombosis, emboli, atherosclerosis, inflammation, or hypertension. Renal vascular disease can be classified according to anatomic location: arteries, arterioles and microvasculature, and renal veins.

ARTERIES

Thromboembolic Occlusion of the Renal Arteries

CAUSES. Thrombosis of the renal arteries and segmental branches may arise as a result of intrinsic pathology of the renal arteries or as a complication of embolization of thrombi arising in distant vessels. *In situ* thrombosis occurs as a complication of progressive atherosclerosis in elderly patients and may be an important cause of progressive renal insufficiency in this population. In patients under age 60, thrombosis rarely occurs in the absence of trauma. Blunt trauma and the deceleration injury may cause acute thrombosis. Trauma to the renal pedicle may result in an intimal tear with thrombosis in the middle third of the renal artery. Thrombosis may arise in the setting of dissection of the renal artery or as a complication of renal arteriography, angioplasty, or stent placement. Finally, thrombosis may occur as a consequence of inflammatory disorders that involve the large arteries (Takayasu's arteritis, syphilis, systemic vasculitides, and thromboangiitis obliterans), as well as structural lesions of the renal arteries such as fibromuscular dysplasia or renal artery aneurysms. Embolization is a more common cause of renal artery occlusion than *in situ* thrombosis and is usually unilateral (bilateral in 15 to 30%). Total infarction of the kidney is much less common than segmental infarction or ischemia. Approximately 90% of thromboemboli to the renal arteries originate in the heart, and a common cause is left atrial thrombi in patients with atrial fibrillation. Valvular heart disease, bacterial endocarditis, nonbacterial (aseptic) endocarditis, and atrial myxomas are other sources of emboli originating in the heart. The diverse causes of occlusion of the renal artery or its segmental branches are summarized in Table 85–1.

CLINICAL MANIFESTATIONS. The manifestations of thromboembolic occlusion of the renal arteries depend on the extent and time course of the occlusive event, as well as the pre-existing status of the renal circulation. Occlusion of a primary or secondary branch of the renal artery in a patient with pre-existing disease and established collateral circulation, such as longstanding renal artery stenosis, may produce little or no infarction and minimal symptoms. Acute thrombosis and infarction may result in sudden onset of flank pain (which resembles renal colic), fever, nausea, vomiting, and on occasion, hematuria. Pain may be localized to the abdomen or back or even the chest, but in more than half the cases, pain is absent. If infarction occurs, leukocytosis usually develops, and serum enzymes may be elevated (aspartate aminotransferase [AST], lactate dehydrogenase, and alkaline phosphatase); urinary lactate dehydrogenase and alkaline phosphatase also may increase. The urinalysis usually reveals microscopic hematuria. The blood urea nitrogen (BUN) and creatinine levels typically increase transiently with unilateral infarction, but more severe and protracted renal dysfunction may follow bilateral renal infarction or infarction of a solitary kidney. Hypertension, which usually occurs with infarction, is the result of release of renin from the ischemic area or renal parenchyma.

DIAGNOSIS. The diagnosis of renal artery occlusion is most reliably established by renal arteriography. Newer radiographic procedures are being used increasingly with success and include computed tomography (CT), magnetic resonance imaging (MRI) with angiography, and duplex Doppler studies.

TABLE 85–1. CAUSES OF RENAL ARTERY OCCLUSION

Thrombosis
Progressive atherosclerosis
Trauma, blunt
Aortic or renal artery aneurysm
Aortic or renal artery dissection
Aortic or renal artery angiography
Superimposed on inflammatory disorders
  Vasculitis
  Thromboangiitis obliterans
  Syphilis
Superimposed on structural lesions
  Fibromuscular dysplasia

Thromboembolism
Atrial fibrillation
Mitral stenosis
Mural thrombus
Atrial myxoma
Prosthetic valve
Septic or aseptic valvular vegetations
Paradoxical emboli
Tumor emboli
Fat emboli

Atheroemboli (Cholesterol Embolization)
Elderly patients with advanced atherosclerosis
Surgery of the abdominal aorta
Trauma, blunt
Angiographic catheters
Angioplasty, or stint placement
Excessive anticoagulation

MANAGEMENT. Managing acute arterial thrombosis usually includes surgical revascularization, controlling hypertension, adequate hydration, anticoagulation, and dialysis when needed. Alternative approaches, such as thrombolytic therapy, are being used more frequently. Traumatic renal artery thrombosis is associated with poor salvage of renal function unless surgery is accomplished within 12 hours after injury. Nontraumatic unilateral occlusion is more often treated conservatively. In chronic ischemic renal disease, surgical revascularization appears to offer advantages, particularly with pre-established renal insufficiency, when improved circulation might be expected to stabilize or improve the progression of renal insufficiency. Hypertension may develop as a late sequela of renal artery occlusion and may be treated by angiotensin-converting enzyme (ACE) inhibitors or, if refractory, by balloon angioplasty. Mortality remains high in these conditions, particularly because of underlying and associated conditions.

Renal Artery Stenosis and Azotemic-Ischemic Renal Disease

CAUSES. The prevalence of renal artery stenosis as the etiology of hypertension in the general population is only 2 to 4%. In selected subgroups of patients (accelerated hypertension with renal insufficiency), the prevalence increases to 30 to 40%. Atherosclerosis causes approximately 60 to 70% of cases in middle-aged and elderly patients. In younger women, renal artery stenosis is usually the result of fibromuscular dysplasia. Atherosclerosis of one or both renal arteries is being recognized more frequently among the elderly, in whom it may or may not be associated with hypertension. It is often associated with generalized atherosclerotic peripheral vascular disease, and may progress to cause progressive loss of renal function with or without renal infarction. This entity has been referred to as "azotemic," or "ischemic," renal disease. There is a striking association between the number of peripheral vessels involved (more than five) with peripheral vascular disease and the presence of renal artery stenosis. Renal artery stenosis due to atherosclerosis is more prevalent among heavy smokers and those with high cholesterol levels.

CLINICAL MANIFESTATIONS. Renal artery stenosis should be suspected when hypertension develops in a previously normotensive patient over age 55 or under 30 or when accelerated hypertension develops in a patient with previously established, controlled hypertension. Features that suggest renal artery stenosis include persistent hypokalemia, metabolic alkalosis, symptoms or signs of peripheral vascular disease, unexplained progression of renal insufficiency with or without hypertension (especially in the elderly patient), recurrent pulmonary edema, disparate renal size, and the presence of an epigastric bruit on physical examination.

DIAGNOSIS. The captopril renal scintigram (scan) is an excellent noninvasive function test for screening patients with suspected renal artery stenosis. It has been most useful in patients with unilateral renal artery stenosis associated with hypertension. This test is based on the assumption that angiotensin II–dependent constriction of the efferent arteriole is a physiologic prerequisite for maintaining GFR and renal blood flow in significant renal artery stenosis. ACE inhibition is usually associated with decreased uptake of the nuclide, prolonged retention, or a longer peak uptake on the affected side. Three-dimensional phase-contrast MRI has been reported to achieve sensitivities and specificities of >90%. Duplex scanning or Doppler flowmetry relies on combined techniques to localize the renal arteries and estimate blood flow but is less reliable. While no single screening test is sufficiently sensitive and specific, in patients in whom stenosis is suspected, renal arteriography is often required to confirm the diagnosis and define the vascular anatomy prior to surgical or nonsurgical intervention. The risk for contrast nephropathy, as well as the risks of catheterization, must be considered, especially in the older patient with renal insufficiency. Peripheral vein renin determinations are not helpful in the diagnosis or management of renal artery stenosis. Renal vein renin determinations are not usually helpful for screening or diagnosis but may assist with planning the approach to therapy. In unilateral renal artery stenosis, the expected finding for clinically significant disease is a ratio of renin from the affected side versus the contralateral renal vein of >1.5.

MANAGEMENT. The goal of therapy in renal artery stenosis is to control the blood pressure and to stabilize renal function by restoration of renal perfusion. Therapeutic options include percutaneous transluminal angioplasty, surgical revascularization, and conservative medical management. Conservative medical management is clearly inferior to either form of interventional therapy and should be reserved for patients with definite contraindications to surgery or angioplasty. Angioplasty is generally considered to be the initial treatment of choice in both fibromuscular dysplasia and atherosclerotic renal artery stenosis. Angioplasty has been effective in approximately 50% of patients with fibromuscular dysplasia and is at least as effective in atherosclerotic renal artery stenosis. Angioplasty is also particularly useful in elderly patients who are considered at high risk for surgical intervention. It has been suggested by uncontrolled studies that angioplasty may be helpful in elderly patients with renal functional impairment due to renal artery stenosis. Stabilization of or improvement in renal function has been observed in patients with bilateral renal artery stenosis. In the event that angioplasty fails, surgical revascularization should be considered, but the patient's age and suitability as a surgical candidate must be considered. Operative mortality has been reported to be as low as 2% but as high as 7%.

ARTERIOLES AND MICROVASCULATURE

Atheroembolic Disease of the Renal Arteries

CAUSES. Embolization of cholesterol crystals as a cause of renal artery occlusion occurs almost exclusively in elderly patients with widespread atherosclerosis. Atheroemboli also may occur as a complication of abdominal aorta or renal artery manipulation or surgery or as a consequence of angiography or transluminal angioplasty. This entity is frequently overlooked because patients at risk for this complication often have other chronic illnesses associated with renal failure, hypertension, and atherosclerosis.

CLINICAL MANIFESTATIONS. Renal insufficiency and hypertension or both disorders occur regularly with atheroembolization to the renal vasculature. Evidence of cholesterol embolization in the retina, muscles, or skin (associated with livedo reticularis) can be helpful and obviate the need for a renal biopsy. There may be evidence of embolization to other organs resulting in cerebrovascular events, acute pancreatitis, ischemic bowel, and gangrene of the extremities. Urinalysis may not be helpful, since cholesterol crystals are not usually present, but mild proteinuria, eosinophiluria, and increased cellularity are more often observed.

MANAGEMENT. Therapy for this disorder is often disappointing, since cholesterol embolization leads to structural changes in the microvasculature without inflammation. Anticoagulants have not been proven to be of value and may delay healing or ulcerating ath-

erosclerotic lesions. Dialysis, treating the hypertension with attention to avoiding hypotension, and adequate hydration are the mainstays of treatment.

Hypertensive Arteriolar Nephrosclerosis (see Ch. 37)

CAUSES. Although autoregulation of renal blood flow and GFR occurs throughout a wide range of systemic blood pressure, the renal vasculature is exquisitely sensitive to damage incurred by systemic hypertension when it is transmitted to the glomerular capillary bed. Unopposed or sustained increases in glomerular capillary hydrostatic pressure result eventually in sclerosis. In *benign nephrosclerosis,* the kidney is the victim of the adverse effects of chronic hypertension over a prolonged period and does not appear to participate in the pathogenesis of the disorder. The vascular injury in the kidney is nonspecific but more pronounced than vascular changes observed systemically. When advanced, such changes can result in end-stage renal disease (ESRD). In *malignant* or *accelerated hypertension,* the vascular changes are unique and severe and lead to renal ischemia, renin production, and exacerbation of the disease which may terminate in acute renal failure and, if not treated successfully, ESRD. In contrast to benign nephrosclerosis, in which the principal lesion is in the media of the vessels, malignant or accelerated hypertension is characterized by a unique lesion of the intima. Renal vascular lesions similar to those seen in malignant hypertension are also observed in scleroderma, thrombotic microangiopathy, and renal transplant rejection.

CLINICAL MANIFESTATIONS. Patients with benign hypertensive nephrosclerosis have been hypertensive for many years (more than 10 to 15 years). Kidney size is usually reduced, and the urine sediment is unremarkable except for proteinuria, which is usually <1.5 grams per day. The sudden development of malignant or accelerated hypertension, in either patients with previously established mild to moderate hypertension or patients not previously diagnosed as hypertensive, is evidenced by an abrupt increase in blood pressure (diastolic usually >130 mm Hg). Papilledema may develop, and renal function may decline rapidly. The kidneys may be enlarged, or the urinary sediment is active, with gross or microscopic hematuria, and proteinuria is often in the nephrotic range. Microangiopathic hemolytic anemia may be present. Abnormalities in the central nervous system (CNS) are usually evident, ranging from headaches to generalized seizures to coma. Malignant hypertension may coexist with cerebral vascular accidents.

The availability of effective antihypertensive medication has sharply reduced the occurrence of this devastating disorder. However, both benign and malignant hypertensive renal disease and the sequelae of these disorders appear to be more prevalent in African-Americans.

MANAGEMENT. For either benign or malignant hypertension, the primary goal is to control the blood pressure. In benign hypertensive nephrosclerosis, the renal outcome is dependent on timely initiation of effective therapy, patient compliance, and careful follow-up. Inadequate treatment may result in glomerular sclerosis, as well as end-organ damage in the cardiovasculature and CNS. Antihypertensives that provide renal protection usually include ACE inhibitors and calcium channel blockers. Malignant hypertension, by contrast, represents a medical emergency and must be approached aggressively. Controlling the blood pressure can reverse the major manifestations, including the renal functional impairment, in most patients. Parenteral antihypertensives such as nitroprusside, infused in the critical care setting, may be necessary initially. The blood pressure should be controlled smoothly and gradually but be into the normal range by 36 to 48 hours. Antihypertensives should be continued even if renal function continues to deteriorate and renal replacement therapy is required. Some patients experience partial reversal of vascular lesions and return of renal function to levels compatible with nondialytic, conservative management.

Hemolytic-Uremic Syndrome (HUS) and Thrombotic Thrombocytopenic Purpura (TTP)

CAUSES. Renal failure is a common consequence of both hemolytic-uremic syndrome (HUS) and thrombotic thrombocytopenic purpura (TTP). For additional information, see Ch. 79 and 152. These conditions are characterized by platelet and fibrin thrombi within the renal microvasculature, accompanied by thrombocytopenia and a microangiopathic hemolytic anemia. Although the vascular lesions are identical, central venous system involvement predominates in TTP, while renal involvement is predominant in HUS.

CLINICAL MANIFESTATIONS. TTP is suggested by the co-occurrence of hemolysis, thrombocytopenia, fever, purpura, and alternating mental status changes. HUS may be associated with acute renal failure, thrombocytopenia, and microangiopathic hemolytic anemia, most commonly in children following an acute diarrheal illness. Either disorder may be observed in the setting of cancer, infections, and while administering chemotherapeutic agents.

MANAGEMENT. Renal replacement therapy acutely has significantly improved survival. The oliguria and degree of renal failure, as well as severity of hypertension, are more pronounced in HUS. Early diagnosis and initiation of dialysis, antihypertensives, supportive transfusions, and control of seizures are essential to a good outcome. Up to 85% of children with typical HUS recover with supportive care. In TTP, plasma exchange combined with antiplatelet therapy is recommended and may be required for 1 to 2 weeks.

Scleroderma (see Ch. 241)

CLINICAL MANIFESTATIONS. The presentation and progression of scleroderma is highly variable. The various limited skin and systemic manifestations of scleroderma are considered in more detail in Ch. 241. While it is widely appreciated that the mortality in scleroderma increases as a function of the number of organ systems involved, significant renal involvement (which has been reported in 50% of patients with systemic sclerosis of 20 years or more) is the most dreaded complication and is associated with the poorest prognosis. When the kidneys are involved, the typical manifestation is intimal proliferation, medial thinning, and increased collagen deposition in the adventitial layer of small renal arteries. An increase in vasomotor tone at the level of the renal vasculature is likely a renal manifestation of Raynaud's phenomenon and contributes to the reduction in renal blood flow, hypertension, and progressive renal functional impairment. The increase in renin and angiotensin II elaboration contributes to the development of worsening hypertension and hypertensive nephrosclerosis. Most patients with renal scleroderma display mild proteinuria with or without hypertension. Once azotemia develops, hypertension may become more difficult to manage, and dialysis is required within 1 to 2 years. Conversely, patients may present with a "renal crisis" manifested by the abrupt onset of malignant hypertension and renal failure. This manifestation, which occurs in 10 to 25% of patients with type 3 scleroderma, usually of several years' duration, represents a medical emergency requiring aggressive antihypertensive therapy.

MANAGEMENT. Therapy in scleroderma with renal involvement should be directed primarily toward controlling hypertension in an attempt to slow progression of the renal failure. Adequate control may require several drugs in combination, such as ACE inhibitors, calcium channel blockers, and vasodilators (such as minoxidil) and other agents. For patients with manifestations of a "renal crisis," intravenous antihypertensive therapy in the critical care setting may be indicated because of the high mortality without therapy. With aggressive management, particularly with ACE inhibitors, there is evidence that progression to ESRD may be slowed significantly. Indeed, even in the event that long-term maintenance dialysis is required, there is evidence that with continued aggressive management of hypertension, a small but significant percentage of patients will regain sufficient renal function to allow cessation of renal replacement therapy.

Sickle Cell Nephropathy (see Ch. 137)

CAUSES. The hypoxemic and hypertonic environment of the renal medulla (vasa recta) encourages the sickling of red blood cells circulating through this region. When sickle hemoglobin desaturates, polymerization of hemoglobin can impair or interrupt capillary flow. The major manifestations of sickle cell nephropathy can all be explained by the development of papillary infarction.

CLINICAL MANIFESTATIONS. A defect in urinary concentration resulting in a tendency toward volume depletion is one of the best-characterized abnormalities in sickle cell nephropathy. Obliteration of the vasa recta compromises the operation of the medullary countercurrent system and impairs the ability to generate and maintain medullary solute gradients. The concentrating defect is also observed in sickle trait. A defect in urinary acidification is common and is manifest as type 4 distal renal tubular acidosis with hyperkalemia and hyperchloremic metabolic acidosis. The acidification defect is not usually observed in patients with sickle trait. Painless gross hematuria has been estimated to occur in up to 50% of patients with sickle cell nephropathy. It also occurs in patients with Hgb SA or Hgb SC. With recurrent papillary infarction, papillary necrosis can occur and progress. Sickle cell "crisis," dehydration, hypoxemia, and the use of nonsteroidal anti-inflammatory drugs (NSAID's) predispose to papillary necrosis. Renal papillary necrosis is often "silent" but may progress to chronic renal insufficiency and may predispose the patient to repeated urinary tract infections. Nephrotic syndrome may occur in approximately 4% of patients with sickle glomerulopathy. Findings on renal biopsy usually indicate membranoproliferative glomerulopathy with segmental and global sclerosis. As this disorder progresses, glomerulopathy results in sclerosis and progressive loss of glomerular function, while papillary infarction can result in persistent hematuria.

MANAGEMENT. Volume depletion should be corrected by isotonic or hypotonic saline intravenously, as dictated by the serum sodium concentration. Hyperkalemia may require potassium exchange resin (sodium polystyrene, Kayexalate) per rectum or orally. When acidosis accompanies the hyperkalemia, alkali may help correct the hyperkalemia and the acidosis. Long-term administration of Shohl's solution or sodium bicarbonate tablets may be necessary, and loop diuretics may be helpful. Potassium-sparing diuretics, NSAID's, or potassium supplements should be strictly avoided. Attempts to increase medullary blood flow and reduce medullary tonicity may alleviate the hematuria, including distilled water, sodium bicarbonate, and diuretics, such as mannitol or loop diuretics. Rarely, small doses of epsilon-aminocaproic acid may be necessary but can result in thrombosis and ureteral obstruction.

RENAL VEINS

Renal Vein Thrombosis

CAUSES. Unilateral or bilateral thrombosis of the major renal veins or their segments is a common but often subtle disorder that may develop in a variety of conditions. The serious risk for thromboembolic complications and vascular occlusion underscores the need for accurate and timely diagnosis and therapy. The disparate causes of renal vein thrombosis are outlined in Table 85–2. The reported incidence of renal vein thrombosis in patients with nephrotic syndrome is striking, ranging from 5 to 62%. Although some series emphasize a stronger association with membranous nephropathy, a prospective study of 26 patients with nephrotic syndrome demonstrated an association of renal vein thrombosis with a variety of glomerulopathies, including membranoproliferative, membranous, proliferative glomerulonephritis and focal glomerular sclerosis. Renal vein thrombosis also has been reported in sickle cell nephropathy, amyloidosis, diabetic nephropathy, renal vasculitis, and lupus nephritis, as well as allograft rejection. Predisposing factors include abnormalities in coagulation or fibrinolysis, and attention has focused on components of clotting parameters in the blood or urine of patients with nephrotic syndrome. Antithrombin III levels are depressed as a result of loss in the urine of nephrotic patients, and the association between low antithrombin III levels and renal vein thrombosis has been reported in some but not all studies. Circulating levels of protein S and C also may be altered in nephrotic syndrome and contribute to the tendency toward thromboembolic complications. Renal vein thrombosis in infancy usually occurs in the setting of severe volume depletion and impaired renal blood flow. Extrinsic compression from retroperitoneal processes such as lymph nodes, retroperitoneal fibrosis, abscess, aortic aneurysm, or tumor may lead to renal vein thrombosis as a result of sluggish renal ve-

TABLE 85–2. CAUSES OF RENAL VEIN THROMBOSIS

Nephrotic syndrome
Renal cell carcinoma with invasion of renal vein
Pregnancy or estrogen therapy
Volume depletion (especially in infants)
Extrinsic compression (lymph nodes, tumor, retroperitoneal fibrosis, aortic aneurysm)

nous flow. Acute pancreatitis, trauma, and retroperitoneal surgery also may predispose to renal vein thrombosis. Renal cell carcinoma characteristically invades the renal vein and compromises venous flow, resulting in renal vein thrombosis.

CLINICAL MANIFESTATIONS. The manifestations of renal vein thrombosis depend on the extent and rapidity of development of renal venous occlusion. Patients with *acute renal vein thrombosis* may present with nausea, vomiting, flank pain, leukocytosis, hematuria, renal functional compromise, and an increase in renal size. Adult nephrotic patients with *chronic renal vein thrombosis* may have more subtle findings such as a dramatic increase in proteinuria or evidence of tubule dysfunction such as glycosuria, aminoaciduria, phosphaturia, and impaired urinary acidification.

DIAGNOSIS. Supportive data may be provided by noninvasive studies such as MRI with angiography. Doppler ultrasonography is not adequately sensitive for segmental thrombosis. Diagnosis is established by selective renal venography. Evidence of parenchymal edema, stretching of calyces, and notching of the ureters on intravenous pyelography is much less reliable.

MANAGEMENT. The most widely accepted form of therapy for both acute and chronic renal vein thrombosis is anticoagulation with heparin, which can be converted to oral warfarin (Coumadin) after 7 to 10 days and maintained long term. Therapy is usually continued for at least 1 year. In patients with recurrence or continued risk factors, anticoagulation might be continued indefinitely. In the pediatric patient with volume depletion and acute renal vein thrombosis, attention to restoration of fluid and electrolyte balance is essential. Fibrinolytic therapy might be considered in patients with acute renal vein thrombosis associated with acute renal failure.

Breyer JA, Jacobson HR: Ischemic nephropathy. Curr Opin Nephrol Hypertens 2:216, 1993. *Emphasizes "ischemic nephropathy" as an important cause of progressive renal failure, particularly in elderly patients with atherosclerotic peripheral vascular disease.*

Ives HE, Daniel TO: Vascular diseases of the kidney. *In* Brenner BM, Rector FC (eds.): The Kidney. 4th ed. Philadelphia, WB Saunders, 1991, p 1497. *An exhaustive compendium with an authoritative section on vascular biology and pathogenesis; the major and most comprehensive reference in this area.*

Missouris CG, Buckenham T, Cappuccio FP, et al.: Renal artery stenosis: A common and important problem in patients with peripheral vascular disease. Am J Med 96:10, 1994. *Demonstrates the strong association between peripheral vascular disease and renal artery stenosis.*

86 HYPERTENSION AND RENAL DISEASE IN PREGNANCY

Thomas F. Ferris

Hypertension is the most common medical complication of pregnancy; a blood pressure of 140 systolic and 90 diastolic or higher occurs in approximately 10% of pregnant women. Hypertension during pregnancy virtually always indicates one of four conditions: (1) pre-eclampsia (toxemia), (2) pre-eclampsia superimposed on chronic hypertension or renal disease, (3) chronic essential hypertension, or (4) gestational hypertension. An understanding of the changes in cardiovascular and renal physiology during pregnancy is necessary to differentiate between these four conditions, which is imperative because each has a different prognosis and treatment.

CARDIOVASCULAR AND RENAL PHYSIOLOGY IN PREGNANCY. A striking feature of pregnancy is that blood pressure and peripheral vascular resistance fall soon after conception. Therefore, the upper limit of blood pressure in nonpregnant individuals (140 systolic and 90 diastolic, which is based on survival statistics in nonpregnant individuals) is of little significance in pregnancy. One criterion used to assess blood pressure in pregnancy is fetal survival. A study of over 24,000 pregnancies demonstrated that blood pressure > 125 and 75 prior to the thirty-second week of gestation or 125 and 85 thereafter was associated with a significant increase in fetal risk. A trend toward increased perinatal mortality is found when mean arterial blood pressure (MAP, diastolic blood pressure plus one third the pulse pressure) is > 82 mm Hg at midpregnancy or > 92 mm Hg at the beginning of the third trimester. Since a blood pressure of 120 systolic and 80 diastolic is an MAP

of 93 mm Hg, one can appreciate how differently blood pressure must be viewed in pregnancy. Although blood pressure tends to increase in late pregnancy, any rise in systolic pressure > 30 mm Hg or diastolic pressure > 15 mm Hg should be of concern regardless of the absolute values attained.

The reduction in arterial blood pressure in pregnancy is thought to be due to increased synthesis of vasodilating prostaglandins, particularly PGI_2, which antagonize the pressor effects of circulating vasoconstrictors such as angiotensin II and norepinephrine. The stimulus for increased prostaglandin synthesis during pregnancy is not known, but resistance to angiotensin II, norepinephrine, and arginine vasopressin occurs early in pregnancy.

Cardiac output also increases in the first trimester of pregnancy, reaching a maximum of 30 to 40% above the nonpregnant level by the twenty-fourth week. Blood volume increases approximately 50% in pregnancy beginning in the first trimester with a rise in both plasma and red cell volume. The greater increase in plasma than in red cell volume causes the physiologic anemia of pregnancy. Expansion of extracellular volume frequently causes edema, which is benign; there is no association of edema with increased perinatal mortality or poor fetal development.

Renal blood flow and glomerular filtration rate (GFR) increase early in pregnancy due to both an increase in cardiac output and a decrease in renal vascular resistance. The rise in GFR in pregnancy results in a mean serum creatinine level of 0.45 ± 0.06 mg per 100 ml in pregnant women compared with 0.67 ± 0.17 mg per 100 ml in nonpregnant women and a mean blood urea nitrogen level of 8.7 ± 1.5 mg per 100 ml compared with 13 ± 3 mg per 100 ml. Since there is evidence in animals that the increase in single-nephron GFR that occurs following reduction in renal mass causes glomerulosclerosis, the effect of increasing GFR in pregnancy has been of concern. Unlike the increase in GFR that follows reduction in renal mass from an increase in glomerular hydrostatic pressure, the increase in GFR in pregnant animals is caused by an increase in glomerular plasma flow without an increase in glomerular hydrostatic pressure. The rat, which is particularly prone to developing glomerulosclerosis with increases in glomerular pressure, demonstrates no evidence of glomerulosclerosis despite repeated pregnancies.

Plasma osmolality falls 10 mOsm per kilogram of H_2O in late pregnancy, with sodium concentration approximately 5 mEq per liter lower than normal. A reduced threshold for secreting antidiuretic hormone (ADH) in pregnancy maintains the lower serum osmolality. A chronic respiratory alkalosis occurs in late pregnancy with Pa_{CO_2} approximately 30 mm Hg compared with normal values of 40 mm Hg in nonpregnant women. Hyperventilation in pregnancy is thought to be caused by elevated plasma progesterone acting on the respiratory center. The hypocapnia increases renal excretion of bicarbonate, with plasma bicarbonate level in pregnancy ranging from 16 to 20 mEq per liter. This compensated respiratory alkalosis has little clinical significance unless a superimposed metabolic acidosis occurs, i.e., ketoacidosis or lactic acidosis, in which the low bicarbonate level decreases total buffering capacity.

PATHOGENESIS AND PATHOLOGY OF PRE-ECLAMPSIA (TOXEMIA). *Pre-eclampsia* describes the disease unique to pregnancy that is manifested by hypertension and evidence of multiple organ dysfunction. The term implies that "eclampsia," a synonym for a seizure, is the ultimate manifestation of the disease. Historically, convulsions have been the most dramatic expression of the disease, but life-threatening pre-eclampsia may occur without seizures. The disease usually occurs after the thirty-second week of pregnancy, but it may occur earlier in patients with underlying renal disease. When it occurs in the first trimester, it is virtually always associated with hydatidiform mole. The hypertension that occurs with pre-eclampsia is caused by an increase in peripheral vascular resistance and is associated with proteinuria and a fall in GFR. Hyperuricemia occurs with pre-eclampsia due to decreased renal clearance and is a valuable marker to differentiate pre-eclampsia from other causes of hypertension during pregnancy. A serum urate level > 5.5 mg per deciliter is a strong indicator of pre-eclampsia, and when it exceeds 6 mg per 100 ml, the disease is usually severe. Decreased urate clearance may be caused by the decreased plasma volume that occurs in pre-eclampsia that decreases tubular secretion of urate. Although plasma volume contraction occurs in all hypertensive states, volume contraction in pre-eclampsia precedes the onset of hypertension and may be due to increased capillary permeability to protein. There is increased disappearance of Evans blue dye from the vascular space and higher protein concentration in edema fluid in pre-eclamptic women.

With pre-eclampsia there is decreased synthesis of vasodilating prostaglandins, particularly 6-keto PGF_1—the metabolite of PGI_2—which precedes the development of hypertension (see Ch. 19). An increase in sensitivity to angiotensin can be detected as early as the eighteenth week in women destined to develop pre-eclampsia that may be caused by decreased PGI_2 synthesis. The balance that exists normally in pregnancy between the increased synthesis of PGI_2 in endothelial cells becomes deranged with pre-eclampsia, since the fall in urinary PGI_2 metabolites is accompanied by increased urinary excretion of thromboxane metabolites. This may predispose to the fibrin deposits seen in the kidney, liver, and heart of women with pre-eclampsia. Renal biopsies in pre-eclamptic women demonstrate the glomerular capillaries to be bloodless, with swollen endothelial and mesangial cells and lipid accumulation in glomerular cells. Immunofluorescent staining demonstrates fibrin deposits without evidence of immunologically mediated damage to the glomerulus. Liver biopsies demonstrate histologic evidence of patchy necrosis with fibrin deposits in sinusoids and microvesicular fat in hepatic cells. Acute fatty liver of pregnancy is a hepatic manifestation of pre-eclampsia (see Ch. 121). In one woman with pre-eclampsia cardiac catherization with an endocardial biopsy demonstrated a similar change in endothelial cells with lipid accumulation. Fibrin deposits in the brain may cause central nervous system (CNS) excitability and convulsions. Cerebral hemorrhage is a major cause of maternal mortality with either petechial hemorrhages or large cerebral hematomas. Fulminant pre-eclampsia can cause a consumptive coagulopathy owing to widespread endothelial cell damage and fibrin deposits. Clinical findings in humans and experimental studies of uterine ischemia in pregnant animals suggest that reduced uterine blood flow is the proximate cause of pre-eclampsia. Development of hypertension with endothelial cell damage occurs in pregnant animals with reduced uterine blood flow, and sera from pre-eclamptic women have been demonstrated to have several effects on endothelial cells in tissue culture. It decreases PGI_2 and endothelin synthesis and causes rapid lipid accumulation within endothelial cells similar to that described in renal, myocardial, and hepatic cells obtained from biopsies.

Incidence. Pre-eclampsia occurs in approximately 7% of pregnant women in the United States. The disease has a familial prevalence with a higher incidence in women from a poor socioeconomic status, probably related to inadequate prenatal care with little attention to monitoring of blood pressure and weight gain during pregnancy. The disease has a bimodal distribution, occurring predominantly in primigravidas but also in multiparous women bearing children in their 30's. Primiparous women are six to eight times more susceptible than multiparous women to develop pre-eclampsia.

Clinical Manifestations. Pre-eclampsia can be differentiated from gestational and essential hypertension by evidence of generalized endothelial cell dysfunction which may mimic other diseases (Table 86–1). Thrombocytopenia may be prominent and suggest idiopathic thrombocytopenic purpura, and when accompanied by neurologic findings, it is reminiscent of thrombotic thrombocytopenic purpura. CNS involvement is manifested by hyperexcitability, which is assessed by determining the deep tendon reflexes. Abdominal pain is frequently present that may be pancreatic in origin, and

TABLE 86–1. DISTINGUISHING FEATURES OF PRE-ECLAMPSIA

Clinical
Weight gain with puffy edema of face and hands, headache, abdominal pain, anxiety, hyperreflexia
Laboratory
Proteinuria with reduced renal function
Creatinine > 1.0 mg/dl, BUN > 12 mg/dl, urate > 5.0 mg/dl
Elevated SGOT, LDH
Microangiopathic anemia
Thrombocytopenia

if the serum amylase level is elevated, a diagnosis of acute pancreatitis may be made. The so-called HELLP syndrome, an acronym for severe pre-eclampsia with *h*emolysis, *e*levated *l*iver enzymes, and *l*ow *p*latelet count, is a particularly fulminant form of pre-eclampsia. Jaundice may be severe, particularly when hemolysis occurs. In some patients, hepatic abnormalities may be more prominent than either hypertension or proteinuria. Renal manifestations of pre-eclampsia are prominent with proteinuria, usually under 2 grams per 24 hours but occasionally in the nephrotic range, without microscopic hematuria.

Treatment. The most important feature in treating pre-eclampsia is recognizing the disease. A rise in blood pressure in late pregnancy accompanied by proteinuria must be presumed to be pre-eclampsia, which always warrants admission to the hospital. If the disease is mild, i.e., blood pressure < 140 systolic and 90 diastolic, proteinuria under 500 mg per 24 hours, normal renal function, serum urate < 4.5 mg per deciliter, normal platelet count, and no evidence of hemolysis or hepatic involvement, bed rest is usually sufficient therapy to lower the blood pressure and allow time to estimate fetal size and maturation. If fetal size and maturation are thought to be adequate, delivery is the definitive treatment for pre-eclampsia. If fetal size and maturation are of concern, continuing the pregnancy and controlling blood pressure are indicated. If any worsening of the disease occurs, delivery should be accomplished, particularly if the pregnancy is at 32 weeks or longer, since fetal survival at that age in a neonatal unit is close to 100%. When renal function is decreased, proteinuria is > 500 mg per 24 hours, and hyperuricemia is present, delivery is indicated in pregnancies of 32 weeks' duration. Convulsions or the HELLP syndrome is always an indication for delivery (see Ch. 121).

There is clinical evidence that antihypertensive therapy is beneficial in pre-eclampsia. Aldomet and hydralazine have been relied on historically, but newer agents such as nifedipine, atenolol, or labetolol have proven more effective. Obstetricians use magnesium sulfate as an antihypertensive agent in pre-eclampsia, but the therapeutic levels of magnesium, approximately 6 to 8 mEq per liter, can cause respiratory depression. The only antihypertensive agents contraindicated in pregnancy are the angiotensin-converting enzyme (ACE) inhibitors, which reduce uterine blood flow in pregnant animals and increase fetal mortality and morbidity in humans. If anticonvulsant therapy is needed, Dilantin can be used, and to control seizures, diazepam is the drug of choice.

Low-dose aspirin has been given to correct the potential imbalance in endothelial PGI_2 and platelet thromboxane synthesis in pre-eclampsia (see Ch. 19). Low-dose aspirin inhibits platelet thromboxane synthesis more than endothelial PGI_2 synthesis. In large studies of women, the incidence of pre-eclampsia is lower in the aspirin-treated group without significant difference in the incidence of gestational hypertension. In those women with a greater risk for developing pre-eclampsia, i.e., systolic blood pressure of 120 to 134 mm Hg in the second trimester, or with underlying essential hypertension or renal disease, aspirin is particularly effective.

ESSENTIAL HYPERTENSION. The evidence is overwhelming that antihypertensive therapy should be continued in women with essential hypertension throughout pregnancy. Therapy results in fewer exacerbations of hypertension, lowers the incidence of proteinuria and pre-eclampsia, and improves perinatal outcome. All antihypertensive agents—except the ACE inhibitors—can be continued throughout pregnancy. Approximately half of women with essential hypertension have a spontaneous reduction in blood pressure in the second trimester, which may allow for lowering the dose or discontinuing the antihypertensive medication. Provided blood pressure is controlled throughout pregnancy, women with essential hypertension do not have the increased risk of pre-eclampsia, abruptio placentae, or intrauterine growth retardation that was a major problem for hypertensive women before antihypertensive therapy was available.

GESTATIONAL HYPERTENSION. Hypertension that appears in late pregnancy, not associated with signs of pre-eclampsia, and that disappears postpartum is termed *gestational hypertension.* Women with gestational hypertension are usually multiparous, frequently overweight, and have a positive family history of hypertension. Many ultimately develop essential hypertension. The hypertensinogenic and diabetogenic effects of pregnancy may be related, since, although resistance to insulin occurs in all pregnant women, greater antagonism occurs in hypertensive pregnant women. Obstetricians usually recommend treating gestational hypertension with bed rest, which lowers blood pressure, but this is an inconvenience, particularly in working women or those with household responsibilities. Hydrochlorothiazide with either nifedipine or an adrenergic blocker such as atenolol or labetalol is quite effective.

RENAL DISEASES COMPLICATING PREGNANCY. Pregnancy predisposes to pyelonephritis, particularly in women with bacteriuria, owing to the increased capacity of the urinary collecting system, slowed emptying, and vesicoureteral reflux which occurs in all pregnant women. Women with bacteriuria should be treated with antibiotics either for 5 to 10 days or single-dose therapy to prevent pyelonephritis. Acute renal failure due to bilateral ureteral obstruction from a gravid uterus can occur rarely in primigravid patients with multiple gestations or polyhydramnios.

Although proteinuria indicates renal disease, urinary excretion of albumin increases in pregnancy because of the increase in GFR and an increase in glomerular capillary permeability to albumin. However, proteinuria should not exceed 200 mg per 24 hour in normal pregnancy. When underlying renal disease is present, as manifested by proteinuria >300 mg per 24 hours early in pregnancy, there is increased incidence of fetal loss, intrauterine growth retardation, and prematurity owing to the high incidence of hypertension during pregnancy in these women. The presence of renal insufficiency or the nephrotic syndrome is an additional fetal risk factor. The cause of the underlying renal disease is not as important as whether hypertension or loss of renal function is present. Women with underlying renal disease have an increased incidence of pre-eclampsia that can be difficult to diagnose when proteinuria is present throughout the pregnancy. If renal function is normal, the incidence of pre-eclampsia is approximately 12%, and perinatal mortality is around 10%, a rate three to four times greater than in normal pregnant women. With a decrease in renal function and hypertension, fetal loss is around 20%, and 20 to 40% of women develop superimposed pre-eclampsia in late pregnancy.

Since a common feature of all chronic renal disease is increased glomerular blood flow and pressure, the effect of pregnancy on progression of renal disease has always been a concern. The fall in renal vascular resistance in pregnancy is caused by dilation of the afferent arteriole, so any rise in systemic blood pressure is transmitted to the glomerulus. The potential adverse effect of pregnancy on underlying renal disease is due to an increase in glomerular pressure that results in increased glomerular damage. It is imperative in women with underlying renal disease that urinary protein excretion be followed carefully during pregnancy and any increase in proteinuria accepted as presumptive evidence of increased glomerular pressure. Although ACE inhibitors are usually used to lower glomerular pressure in nonpregnant patients, in pregnant patients, calcium channel blockers can be used.

When renal function is normal or only minimally depressed, pregnancy does not have a deleterious effect on renal function. In one study of over 200 pregnancies in women with GFR's >70 ml per minute, blood pressure remained below 140 and 90 throughout pregnancy, and the underlying renal disease was not adversely affected. In contrast, about a third of women with renal insufficiency (serum creatinine >1.8 mg per deciliter) experience some decline in renal function either during or following pregnancy. However, these findings were made before the importance of rigorous treatment of hypertension or increase in proteinuria during pregnancy with antihypertensive agents was recognized. No adequate trial has been done of vigorous control of hypertension during pregnancy in women with moderate renal insufficiency to determine if the acceleration of a downhill course could be prevented.

Systemic lupus erythematosus frequently affects women of childbearing age. There is no evidence that pregnancy worsens its activity, provided that the disease has been quiescent for at least 6 months before the pregnancy (see Ch. 240).

In normotensive women with diabetic nephropathy, >50% will become hypertensive during pregnancy, and approximately 70% develop proteinuria in the third trimester. Whether aggressive treatment of hypertension with calcium channel blockers throughout pregnancy would prevent proteinuria in these women has not been evaluated. Fetal survival in women with diabetic nephropathy is approximately 90%, and following delivery, hypertension and proteinuria return to prepregnancy levels.

There have been over 2000 successful pregnancies in women following renal transplantation, with fetal survivals >90%. Similar to women with renal disease, hypertension or pre-eclampsia develops in approximately one third of the patients if there is diminished renal function before pregnancy. Cyclosporine does not seem to affect pregnancy, and there is no evidence that pregnancy adversely affects the renal allograft. Women on dialysis have occasionally become pregnant, although only about 25% have a live birth.

Ferris TF: Hypertension and pre-eclampsia. *In* Burrow GN, Ferris TF (eds.): Medical Complications During Pregnancy. 4th ed. Philadelphia, WB Saunders, 1994. *A comprehensive review of hypertension during pregnancy.*
Paller MS: Renal diseases. *In* Burrow GN, Ferris TF (eds.): Medical Complications During Pregnancy. 4th ed. Philadelphia, WB Saunders, 1994. *A complete coverage of the effect of pregnancy on various renal diseases.*

87 HEREDITARY CHRONIC NEPHROPATHIES*

Manuel Martinez-Maldonado

Several genetically transmitted renal disorders of unknown pathogenesis may fall under this heading. This chapter will discuss two of these disorders: Alport's syndrome and the nail-patella syndrome. Some hereditary disorders of renal tubular function are described in Ch. 82. Other genetic disorders that may be associated with renal disease are listed in Table 87–1 and discussed in the section on metabolic diseases (Part XV).

ALPORT'S SYNDROME

DEFINITION. Alport's syndrome, or chronic hereditary nephritis, is characterized by the familial occurrence in successive generations of a progressive nephritis, more severe in males, manifested invariably by hematuria and frequently associated with a sensorineural hearing deficit.

GENETICS. The mode of transmission in most kindreds is consistent with X-linked dominant inheritance; mutations of *COL4A5*, a gene located in Xq22 that codes for the α_5 chain of type IV collagen, are responsible. Deletions also occur and tend to result in more severe renal disease and more severe hearing loss. Genetic heterogeneity is suggested because autosomal recessive and autosomal dominant inheritances are found in certain kindreds. Alport's disease is termed "juvenile" when early onset occurs in males and "adult" when renal failure occurs in middle age. Juvenile kindreds tend to be small and frequently arise from new mutations; adult kindreds are large and exhibit few new mutations.

INCIDENCE AND PREVALENCE. Several hundred kindreds of all races and geographic origins exist. Incidence is approximately 1 in 5000 people; Alport's syndrome accounts for nearly 5% of patients with end-stage renal disease.

PATHOLOGY AND PATHOGENESIS. Kidneys may be normal or large size at the onset, but they shrink as the disease progresses. While glomeruli may be normal (as seen under light microscopy), there may be hypertrophy of epithelial cells and an increase in mesangial matrix. Later changes consist of mesangial cell proliferation, thickening and splitting of glomerular and tubular basement membranes, thickening of Bowman's capsule, tubular cell atrophy, interstitial fibrosis, and the presence of foam cells. Glomerular crescents may be found in the juvenile form. Electron microscopy characteristically reveals both thinning and irregular thickening of the glomerular and tubular basement membranes, with splitting of the lamina densa into several lamellae separated by lucent zones containing electron-dense round granulations ("basketweave" appearance).

The etiology of Alport's syndrome appears to be the absence of a 28-kD peptide component of the noncollagenous (NC1) domain of the α_3 chain of type IV collagen in glomerular basement membrane (GBM). This peptide is also known as the "Goodpasture antigen" (see below).

---

* Revised and updated from chapter by Wadi N. Suki, M.D., in the preceding edition.

TABLE 87-1. INHERITED RENAL DISEASES*

Disorders of Tubular Function
Proximal tubule
    Cerebro-oculorenal syndrome of Lowe
    Cystinosis (Fanconi's syndrome)
    Cystinuria
    Galactosemia
    Glycogen storage (von Gierke's) disease
    Glycinuria
    Hartnup disease
    Hepatolenticular degeneration (Wilson's disease)
    Hereditary fructose intolerance
    Hypophosphatemic vitamin D–resistant rickets
    Iminoaciduria
    Proximal renal tubular acidosis
    Pseudohypoparathyroidism
    Renal glucosuria
Distal/collecting tubule
    Distal renal tubular acidosis
    Nephrogenic diabetes insipidus

Disorders of Renal Structure
Agenesis
Cystic disorders
    Hepatocerebrorenal syndrome of Zellweger
    Medullary sponge kidney
    Medullary cystic disease
    Polycystic kidney disease, adult type
    Polycystic kidney disease, infantile type
    Renal retinal dysplasia
Duplication
Renal malformations with extrarenal anomalies

Biochemical Disorders
Alkaptonuria
Cystinosis
Diabetes mellitus
Glycosphingolipidosis (Fabry's disease)
Hepatolenticular degeneration (Wilson's disease)
Hyperuricemia
Primary hyperoxaluria (oxalosis)
Xanthine oxidase deficiency

Systemic Disorders
Amyloidosis
Asphyxiating thoracic dystrophy (Jeune's disease)
Charcot-Marie-Tooth disease
Laurence-Moon-Biedl syndrome
Osteo-onychodysplasia (nail-patella syndrome)

Hereditary Chronic Nephropathies
Benign recurrent hematuria
Hereditary chronic nephritis
Hereditary chronic nephritis with hyperprolinemia
Hereditary chronic nephritis with thrombocytopathy
Hereditary immune nephritis
Infantile nephrosis

* Includes diseases that affect the kidney secondarily.

CLINICAL MANIFESTATIONS. The disease is discovered in 70% of patients by age 6, the rest of the cases being discovered at any age thereafter up to and well into adulthood. Table 87–2 lists the major clinical findings. Persistent or intermittent microscopic hematuria and proteinuria are common. Sensorineural hearing loss and ocular disorders are typical of the syndrome.

In several kindreds, patients with classic Alport's syndrome have been reported to have thrombocytopenia with giant platelets manifested clinically by bruising, epistaxis, gastrointestinal bleeding, and prolonged bleeding time. A few cases also have been associated with hyperprolinemia, leiomyomatosis, and a variety of other disorders.

DIAGNOSIS. The basis for diagnosing Alport's syndrome is the presence of progressive renal disease in a patient with hematuria with or without proteinuria, azotemia, or hypertension in one family member younger than age 50 other than the proband, and the pres-

TABLE 87-2. CLINICAL MANIFESTATIONS OF ALPORT'S SYNDROME

Hematuria
Microscopic: Persistent or intermittent, ~ 100%; dysmorphic erythrocytes are common
Gross: Especially after exercise or respiratory infections, 60% affected children; rarely in adults

Proteinuria
Mild, ~ 70% of patients
Nephrotic range, 30–40%

Sensorineural Hearing Loss*
High-frequency range, 4000–8000 Hz, 40–60% of patients, predominantly in males

Ocular Disorders
15% of patients, especially anterior and posterior lenticonus, and spherophakia

Renal Disease
Mild and nonprogressive, especially in women; those affected may experience decline of renal function during pregnancy
Severe and progressive, predominantly in males; hypertension, chronic renal failure, azotemia (uremia), predilection for those with massive proteinuria, deafness, and lenticonus

* May require audiometric testing, and may progress to clinical deafness. Tinnitus is present in some cases.

ence of neural hearing loss in the patient or a relative. The major differential diagnosis is shown in Table 87–3.

TREATMENT. There is no specific treatment that will alter the course of Alport's syndrome. Control of hypertension is necessary. Conventional management of progressive renal disease such as peritoneal dialysis or hemodialysis and related or cadaveric donor kidney transplantation have been used with degrees of success that at least match those obtained in other renal disorders. Improvement of hearing deficit, but not recurrence of the renal lesion, has been observed after transplantation. Several patients have developed Goodpasture's syndrome in the renal graft caused by an antibody directed against the basement membrane antigen absent in Alport's syndrome (see above). Genetic counseling may be useful but complicated in view of genetic heterogeneity.

NAIL-PATELLA SYNDROME

An autosomal dominant trait, nail-patella syndrome is also known as "osteo-onychodysplasia." This disorder of mesenchymal tissue is characterized by atrophic or absent fingernails, hypoplasia or aplasia of the patella, accessory conical iliac horns, thickening of the scapula, and subluxation of the radial heads at the elbow. In 40% of patients, kidney involvement is manifested by mild proteinuria and, rarely, hematuria. The nephrotic syndrome and progression to renal failure (27%) may be observed occasionally. Light microscopy shows glomerular, cellular proliferation, mesangial sclerosis, and basement membrane thickening. Electron microscopy reveals areas of rarefaction in the lamina densa of the glomerular basement membrane filled with bundles of curvilinear fibrils having the typical periodicity of collagen ("motheaten" appearance). No specific therapy exists for this disorder. Renal transplantation has been carried out without evidence of recurrence of the disease in the transplanted organ.

TABLE 87-3. DIFFERENTIAL DIAGNOSIS OF ALPORT'S SYNDROME

Condition	Characteristics
Benign familial hematuria	Nonprogressive disorder, uniformly thin GBM
Berger's disease	IgA nephropathy; mesangial proliferation glomerulonephritis with mesangial deposits of IgA and variable amounts of C_3, IgM, or IgG; strong IgA immunofluorescence in mesangial regions

Kashtan CE, Michael AF: Alport syndrome: From bedside to genome to bedside (In-depth Review). Am J Kidney Dis 22:627, 1993. *An excellent review of the biochemical defect in and the genetic transmission of Alport's syndrome.*

Noël LH, Gubler MC, Bobrie G, et al.: Inherited defects of renal basement membranes. Adv Nephrol 18:77, 1989. *A good review of the genetics of hereditary chronic nephropathies including the nail-patella syndrome.*

88   RENAL CALCULI
(Nephrolithiasis)
Keith Hruska

EPIDEMIOLOGY. Nephrolithiasis is a common disorder defined as the development of stones within the urinary tract. It is a major cause of morbidity in the United States, and it is becoming an increasingly greater problem in Western Europe and Japan. Approximately 12% of the US population will have a kidney stone at some time. The economic impact of the morbidity associated with kidney stones is > $2 billion per year; most of the costs relate to surgical extraction or fragmentation and loss of productivity. Kidney stones are two to three times more common in men than women and are distinctly uncommon in African-Americans and Asians. There is also a geographic distribution of nephrolithiasis, with the highest incidence in the southeastern United States.

GENERAL CLINICAL CONSIDERATIONS. The pain associated with passing a kidney stone is referred to as *renal colic.* It begins suddenly and quickly becomes an unbearable pain that may cause nausea and vomiting. The distribution of the pain resembles that of the path of the stone to the bladder, beginning in the flank and curving anteriorly toward the groin. Urinary frequency and dysuria occur as the stone reaches the ureterovesical junction. When the stone passes into the bladder or moves in the ureter to decompress the urinary system, the pain vanishes. Unique symptoms develop when the stone passes into the urethra.

Hematuria from nephrolithiasis is common and disturbing to patients. Occasionally, the hematuria is associated with flank pain without detectable obstruction. Nephrolithiasis may be associated with obstructive uropathy (see Ch. 81), especially if the stone is not painful and remains undetected for long periods. Obstruction predisposes to infection, especially in women.

Radiologic techniques are used to diagnose stone disease. The radiographic appearance of stones may help identify stone type and guide further evaluation. Calcium phosphate and calcium oxalate stones are radiodense, and struvite (magnesium ammonium phosphate), when it complexes with calcium carbonate or phosphate, is also visible. Cystine stones are usually poorly visualized, and uric acid stones are radiolucent, requiring computed tomographic (CT) scanning, ultrasonography, or intravenous urography for detection.

Intravenous urography is usually the first step in evaluating patients with renal colic, although there is concern regarding use of this test in patients with renal insufficiency. It is the most useful test to define the degree and extent of urinary tract obstruction. Renal ultrasonography, which is the safest approach, is useful to rule out significant hydronephrosis or hydroureter; however, it may not detect stones unless they are relatively large. Ultrasonography does not delineate the site of obstruction. Retrograde pyelography allows visualization of the urinary tract without intravenously administering contrast dye. This test requires cystoscopy and is usually performed during endourologic procedures or when the intravenous pyelography is contraindicated (in patients with renal insufficiency or contrast dye allergy).

CT scanning is the modality most useful for defining radiolucent stones not detectable by other means. Pure uric acid stones and, in some cases, cystine stones can be identified by CT scanning with or without contrast material.

Treating Renal Colic. Treatment should focus on relieving pain and urinary tract obstruction. A stepwise scheme for management of patients with renal colic is presented in Figure 88–1. Careful analgesic therapy, hydration, and radiologic assessment are the cornerstones. If significant obstruction is detected, the patient is ob-

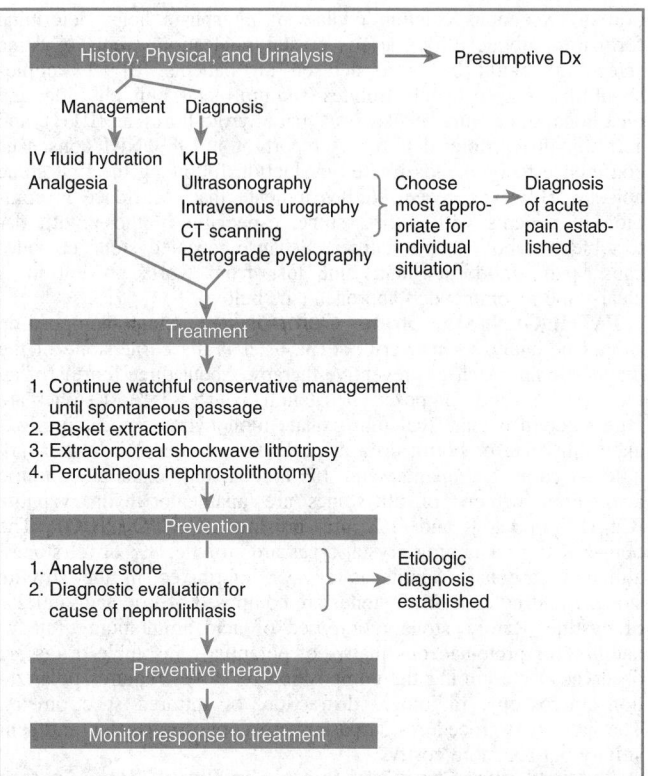

FIGURE 88–1. Flow diagram for management of renal colic. See text for the description of the approach to patients with acute stone episodes.

served during hydration for movement of the stone. If evidence does not suggest that the stone will pass within 2 to 3 days, urologic intervention is indicated. Stones lodged in the ureteropelvic junction or in the proximal ureter are best pushed into the renal pelvis and disrupted by extracorporeal shockwave lithotripsy (ESWL). Moving the stone backward requires cystoscopy and passing a catheter up the ureter. If the stone cannot be pushed back, it can be bypassed with a stent to provide drainage and disrupted *in situ* with ESWL. Percutaneous nephrolithotomy is required if lithotripsy fails. Surgical ureterolithotomy is largely an operative procedure of the past.

Stones that are < 2 cm but > 5 mm in diameter are best treated with ESWL alone. Stones > 2 cm, or those > 1 cm and in the lower poles, may be best treated with percutaneous nephrostolithotomy, because with lithotripsy alone residual stones are left in 35 to 50% of cases. Percutaneous nephrostolithotomy succeeds in most cases. Asymptomatic kidney stones < 5 mm in diameter should be left untreated. The guidelines for ESWL and percutaneous nephrostolithotomy hold for struvite and uric acid stones. Because lithotripsy disrupts cystine stones poorly, often percutaneous nephrostolithotomy is required.

Preventing Recurrent Nephrolithiasis. Careful correlation of stone counts with the clinical history and information from hospital emergency room and past office records determines whether a stone is a new episode or the passage of an existing stone. Renal stone prevention requires accurate diagnosis of the cause of nephrolithiasis. Diagnosis requires a battery of urine and blood tests that are begun after the patient has fully recovered from an episode of renal colic and has resumed normal activity and diet for approximately 2 weeks. Because of inherent day-to-day variation, repeated sampling of 24-hour urine specimens from patients on their normal diets and following test diets is required. The most useful test diet is a 400-mg calcium diet used for 1 week prior to a calcium challenge test in order to carefully define hypercalciuria. The analyses performed on urine specimens include determining volume, pH, creatinine, calcium, phosphorus, magnesium, uric acid, urinary urea nitrogen, potassium, sodium, citrate, and oxalate. Adding ammonia, chloride, and sulfate allows calculation of relative supersaturation. The addition of exogenous calcium oxalate or phosphate helps determine formation products for various crystal nucleation events. Cystine screening should be performed on all patients. Blood samples should be assayed for electrolytes (sodium, potassium, chloride, and bicarbonate), calcium, phosphorus, parathyroid hormone (PTH), and 1,25-dihydroxycholecalciferol. A report of a 1989 NIH consensus conference recommends limited evaluation following the first stone episode. However, recent studies indicate that recurrence is common in patients with a first stone, especially in those with detectable metabolic abnormalities. Because repeated stone episodes cause pain, morbidity, and time loss from work, prevention is clearly the recommended approach (see below).

PATHOGENESIS. Stone Composition. Stone composition should be analyzed in every patient, as it is the cornerstone of the diagnostic approach to preventive therapy. About three-fourths of all kidney stones are composed of calcium oxalate: 35% of stones are pure calcium oxalate (calcium oxalate monohydrate or calcium oxalate dihydrate or both); 40% are calcium oxalate with hydroxyapatite or carbonate apatite; and 1% are calcium oxalate with uric acid. Four percent of all stones are apatite or hydroxyapatite $[Ca_{10}(PO_4)_6(OH)_2]$ and 1% are brushite $(CaHPO_4 \cdot 2H_2O)$. The non–calcium-containing crystal types are struvite, 8% of all stones, although carbonate apatite is always intermixed in the struvite stone. Eight percent of all stones are composed of uric acid and 2% of cystine. Rarely, stones composed of acid ammonium urate or xanthine or proteinaceous matrix of potentially insoluble drugs are observed. Determining the composition of stones requires polarization microscopy, radiologic diffraction, or infrared spectrometry. The latter two procedures surpass microscopy in precision and sensitivity but are more costly.

Physical and Chemical Factors in Renal Stone Formation. Formation of kidney stones results from (1) initial formation of crystals (nucleation), (2) reduced effects of normal urinary constituents that inhibit crystal growth and aggregation, (3) the presence of substances promoting crystal growth and aggregation, and (4) the processes that determine crystal attachment to the surface of renal papillary epithelial cells (Table 88–1). Attachment allows time for crystal growth and/or aggregation to the size of a clinically symptomatic stone in high urinary solute concentrations. Much of the current approach to evaluating, treating, and preventing nephrolithiasis is centered on identifying excessive urinary excretion of salts that precipitate (nucleate) when units of metastable supersaturation are exceeded. Supersaturation can result from (1) too little urine output; (2) an absolute increase in the amount of stone constituent excreted over a period of time, such as calcium, oxalate, or uric acid; or (3) altered urine pH. Low urinary pH (< 5.5) decreases solubility of uric acid, whereas high urinary pH decreases that of calcium phosphate and magnesium ammonium phosphate.

Deficient Urinary Inhibitors. Although most recurrent stone formers tend to have an increased risk of nucleation, 1% or more of stone formers exhibit no detectable abnormality. Many healthy subjects, patients with cancer, and normal pregnant women exhibit hypercalciuria but do not form kidney stones. Thus, factors beside supersaturation are crucial in the pathogenesis of kidney stones. Macromolecular inhibitors of crystal growth and aggregation, particularly the growth and aggregation of calcium oxalate, have recently been identified (Table 88–1). Nephrocalcin is a powerful inhibitor of calcium oxalate crystal growth and appears to act by binding to crystal surfaces. This substance is apparently defective when isolated from the urine of calcium stone formers. Urinary osteopontin (uropontin) is perhaps the most potent calcium oxalate crystal growth inhibitor. Tamm-Horsfall mucoprotein may inhibit crystal growth but at times promotes calcium oxalate crystal aggregation. Some patients with recurrent nephrolithiasis produce Tamm-Horsfall mucoprotein that self-aggregates and loses its ability to inhibit aggregation of calcium oxalate crystals.

Crystal Attachment. Crystal attachment to epithelial surfaces is also crucial for forming at least some stones. Normal subjects often have crystalluria without forming stones. Crystal binding appears to depend on the physicochemical structure of urothelial cell surfaces because the chemically injured urinary bladder binds more calcium oxalate than the uninjured bladder. In addition, there exist specific calcium oxalate crystal receptors on renal tubular epithelial cells.

PATHOGENESIS OF CALCIUM, OXALATE, AND APATITE STONES. Hypercalciuria. After low urinary volumes, hypercalciuria is the most frequently observed abnormality of the urine from stone formers (Fig. 88–2). The definition of hypercalciuria varies with body size and diet. In general, the normal upper limits for urinary calcium is 4 mg of calcium per kilogram of body weight per day (280 mg per day, males; 240 mg per day, females) on a diet containing 1000 mg of calcium per day. Total excretion may drop to 200 mg per day on a diet of 400 mg of calcium and 100 mEq or less of sodium. Dietary sodium is important because calcium reabsorption parallels that of sodium in the proximal nephron, such that high rates of sodium excretion are calciuric. Hypercalciuria can result from (1) enhanced absorption from dietary intake; (2) primary renal transport defects leading to excess calcium excretion and secondary enhanced calcium absorption; (3) excessive resorption from storage in bone; or (4) a combination of the above (Table 88–2).

Since the late 1980's, a consensus has emerged that the hypercalciuria of nephrolithiasis is a more uniform defect than was previously thought. The basis for this change is the fact that hypercalciuria is the most frequent abnormality found in patients with a family history of nephrolithiasis, suggesting a genetic basis for hypercalciuria. In addition, it has been found that fasting hypercalciuria, observed in 20 to 30% of patients who have nephrolithiasis and hypercalciuria, is not due to a renal transport defect (renal leak) as previously thought (Table 88–3). The source of fasting hypercalciuria has been shown to be bone, and in many patients is associated with a decrease in bone mineral density. This presumed increase in skeletal remodeling is a transient defect and does not persist throughout the clinical course of nephrolithiasis. Patients with nephrolithiasis and hypercalciuria uniformly exhibit an increase in intestinal calcium absorption. (See Fig. 88–3 and Ch. 214 for a discussion of calcium homeostasis.)

The pathogenesis of intestinal hyperabsorption of calcium in nephrolithiasis is unclear. Approximately 30 to 40% of the patients have abnormally high $1,25(OH)_2D_3$ levels compared with a population of non–stone-formers. In the other patients, an abnormally active vitamin D receptor exhibiting either a high affinity or an increase in receptor number may contribute to intestinal calcium hyperabsorption. Finally, there appears to be a subset of patients whose intestinal hyperabsorption is independent of vitamin D action.

The finding of hypercalciuria that persists on a low calcium diet or the presence of fasting hypercalciuria increases the likelihood of associated reductions in bone mineral density with nephrolithiasis. Hence, the wisdom of low calcium diets in nephrolithiasis is most certainly questioned by the observed reductions in bone mineral density associated with the disease.

Hyperoxaluria. Dietary Hyperoxaluria. Oxalate is the anion most frequently associated with calcium in the precipitation of salts leading to crystal formation, growth, retention, and stone formation. Normal people excrete 20 to 40 mg (222 to 444 μmol) of oxalate daily. A reasonable upper limit of excretion is 45 mg (500 μmol) daily for men and 40 mg for women. A simple dietary excess of oxalate from foods such as spinach, rhubarb, swiss chard, cocoa, beets, peppers, wheat germ, pecans, peanuts, okra, chocolate, and lime peel commonly increases urinary oxalate to 50 to 60 mg (556 to 667 μmol) daily. This form of hyperoxaluria is frequently observed in nephrolithiasis (Fig. 88–3), and treatment consists of altering the diet to avoid an excess of oxalate. However, no clinical trials have proven the efficacy of avoiding oxalate for treating nephrolithiasis.

Enteric Hyperoxaluria. Malabsorption by the small bowel from any cause, including resection, intrinsic disease, and jejunal ileal bypass, often leads to hyperoxaluria. The pathogenesis is exposure of the colonic mucosa to detergents—in the form of bile salts—and

TABLE 88–1. PHYSICAL-CHEMICAL FACTORS IN THE FORMATION OF RENAL STONES

High urinary solute concentration	$\uparrow$ Ca, $\uparrow$ Ox, $\downarrow$ UV
Deficient inhibitor	Citrate, uropontin, nephrocalcin
Excess promoter	Uric acid
Crystal attachment	Epithelial crystal receptors

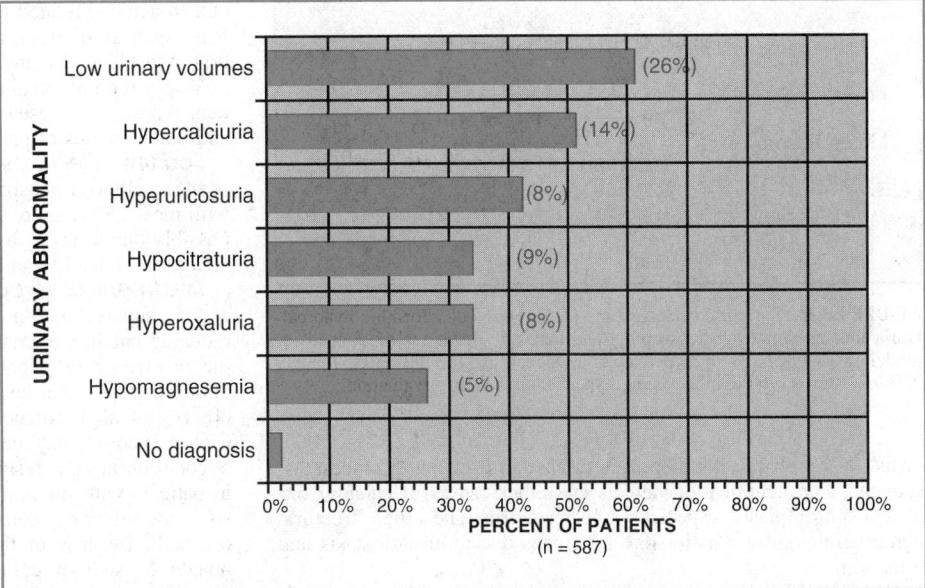

FIGURE 88-2. Causes of urinary supersaturation in patients with nephrolithiasis: 587 consecutive patients seen in the stone center of St. Louis, Missouri, from 1987 to 1992 were evaluated with a standardized approach described in the text section Preventing Recurrent Nephrolithiasis. Numbers in parentheses indicate sole occurrence of abnormality. (Data taken from Seltzer J, Winborn K, Hruska K [unpublished observation].)

fatty acids, which nonselectively increase the permeability to numerous molecules, including oxalate. These detergents also bind calcium and magnesium, making oxalate more available for transport. The hyperoxaluria from small bowel malabsorption often exceeds 100 mg (1111 μmol) daily, provoking frequent stone formation and even tubulointerstitial renal disease from intrarenal calcifications. A consistent metabolic pattern is observed in the urine of patients with enteric hyperoxaluria, consisting of low urinary volumes, a tendency toward hypocalciuria, hypocitraturia, and hyperoxaluria. Treatment includes reducing dietary oxalate and fat, oral calcium supplements, cholestyramine, oral citrate supplements, and high fluid intake (see below).

Primary Hyperoxaluria (see Ch. 172). Two genetic disorders lead to hyperoxaluria. Type I primary hyperoxaluria, an autosomal recessive trait, results from molecular abnormalities that reduce the activity of hepatic peroxisomal alanine glyoxylate aminotransferase, thereby increasing the availability of glyoxylate, which is irreversibly converted to oxalic acid. The second form, resulting from a deficiency of D-glycerate dehydrogenase or glyoxylate reductase (type II), is much rarer than type I. Both forms cause a high level of oxalate production and corresponding urinary oxalate excretion above 135 to 270 mg (1523 μmol) daily. Stone formation often begins in childhood.

Hypocitraturia. Reductions in urinary citrate excretion are a common trait among patients who form stones. This hypocitraturia may be (1) idiopathic; (2) due to defective urinary acidification; (3) due to small bowel malabsorption; (4) due to hypokalemia, especially iatrogenic. Hypocitraturia, defined as < 300 mg per day in women and 200 mg per day in men, was observed in approximately 40% of patients with nephrolithiasis (see Fig. 88-2). More women than men exhibited hypocitraturia. Hypocitraturia often overlaps with hypercalciuria owing to the high prevalence of idiopathic hypercalciuria in nephrolithiasis. In patients who do not spontaneously acidify urine (especially in the early morning) to 5.5 or less, an ammonium chloride load test should rule out an acidification defect as the cause of hypocitraturia. The hypocitraturia associated with small

bowel malabsorption is due to a metabolic acidosis and stimulation of citrate transport in the proximal nephron. The metabolic acidosis stems from bicarbonate lost in the stool. Treating nephrolithiasis with thiazides may induce hypokalemia and a secondary hypocitraturia.

Hyperuricosuria (see Ch. 251). Hyperuricosuria is a common finding associated with hypercalciuria in patients with calcium oxalate nephrolithiasis. The relationship between hyperuricosuria and calcium oxalate precipitation remains controversial. Some evidence suggests that urate crystals increase the nucleation of calcium oxalate by the process of heterogeneous nucleation and epitaxial growth. However, urate crystals are uncommon in urine compared with the frequency of calcium oxalate crystallization, and the epitaxial theory remains to be proven. However, well-controlled studies demonstrate that allopurinol, a drug that decreases urate synthesis, significantly reduces the rate of recurring calcium oxalate stones. Because allopurinol has no direct effect on calcium oxalate crystallization, it is likely that this effect was produced by reduced urinary uric acid excretion. Because an excess of purine in the diet causes hyperuricosuria, normal levels of dietary purine should also be protective.

New Protein Inhibitors of Calcium Oxalate Stone Formation. See discussion of various inhibitors of calcium oxalate stone formation in the section on the physical chemistry of nephrolithiasis (above).

Renal Structural Abnormalities. Were they not retained within the kidney, the forming and passing of crystalline particles would be no more than a common urologic curiosity. Crystal adherence promoting crystal growth and aggregation, especially in areas of relatively diminished urinary flow, is crucial in the development of urinary stones. Little is known regarding the process of crystal growth attachment. The role of urinary stasis has not been quantified. Other structural abnormalities, such as medullary sponge kidney, ectopic kidney, polycystic kidney, and horseshoe kidneys, may be associated with nephrolithiasis. Medullary sponge kidney probably is a process that occurs or develops as a result of nephrocalci-

TABLE 88-2. POTENTIAL MECHANISMS OF HYPERCALCIURIA

Increased intestinal calcium absorption
  Direct
  Excess 1,25(OH)$_2$D$_3$
Decreased renal mineral reabsorption
  Calcium
  Phosphorus
Enhanced bone demineralization

TABLE 88-3. PATHOGENESIS OF HYPERCALCIURIA IN NEPHROLITHIASIS

	Frequency (%)
Idiopathic absorptive ± skeletal remodeling defect	95
Primary hyperparathyroidism	3
Sarcoidosis	< 1
Renal tubular transport defects	
Calcium	1–2
Phosphorus	< 1

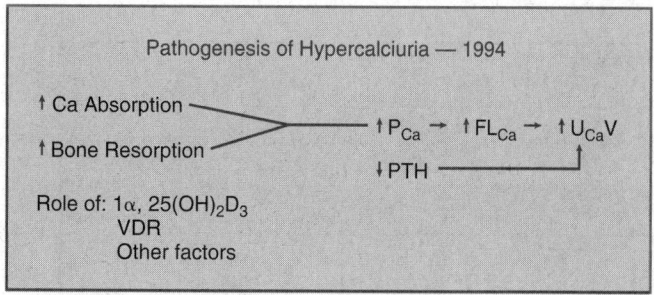

FIGURE 88–3. Current concepts of the pathogenesis of idiopathic hypercalciuria link intestinal hyperabsorption and transient elevations of skeletal remodeling as the basis of hypercalciuria, accounting for the approximately 20% of patients who exhibit fasting hypercalciuria during evaluation.

nosis. It is probably not a specific disease in itself but a process associated with acidification defects and other causes of calcium oxalate nephrolithiasis, especially hypercalciuria. The other structural abnormalities pose a major risk for stones due to urinary stasis and infection.

DIAGNOSIS. Prevention of nephrolithiasis requires a diagnosis of the cause of the stone. Especially for calcium oxalate/apatite stone formers, this is accomplished by the use of urine and blood chemistry measurements and stone analysis. Repeated testing of urine samples is necessary in order to correct for day-to-day variability as a result of diet. We have established a standard evaluation that consists of two 24-hour urine samples from outpatients following their normal diets and a third 24-hour urine sample following 1 week of a low-calcium, salt-restricted, purine- and oxalate-controlled diet. Following the week of special diet, the patients receive a calcium tolerance test and, depending upon earlier results, possibly an oxalate tolerance test or an ammonium chloride load test. All urine samples are measured for volume, pH, creatinine, calcium, phosphorus, uric acid, magnesium, urinary urea nitrogen, sodium, potassium, oxalate, and citrate. A serum profile consisting of calcium, phosphorus, electrolytes, uric acid, creatinine, 1,25-dihydroxycholecalciferol, and PTH levels is also performed at the end of 1 week on the test diet.

TREATMENT OF CALCIUM OXALATE OR APATITE STONES. The first tenet of therapy for preventing nephrolithiasis is an increase in the urinary volume. Urinary volumes between 2 and 3 liters must be maintained. Helpful clues to assist the patient with increasing urinary volume include avoiding urinary concentration at night and taking a metered amount of water to the work place.

Diet. With careful attention to diet, most calcium oxalate stones could be prevented, but long-term dietary compliance is essential (Table 88–4). Recurrent calcium nephrolithiasis should be considered a disease of dietary excess superimposed on the genetic predispositions of hypercalciuria, renal tubular acidosis, gout, and cystinuria. In patients with calcium oxalate stones, reduced sodium and calcium diets may be effective. In patients with idiopathic hypercalciuria, diets containing 700 to 800 mg of calcium contain sufficient calcium to prevent further bone loss during therapy.

Thiazide Diuretics. Thiazide diuretics are the mainstay of the pharmacologic approach to preventing nephrolithiasis. They lower urinary calcium excretion by increasing calcium reabsorption in the proximal nephron due to volume contraction. They also directly stimulate calcium reabsorption and actions in the distal nephron. The relative importance of the two actions is heavily weighted toward the proximal nephron/volume contraction effects. Thus, an adequate response to thiazide diuretics requires controlling sodium intake. Retention of calcium by the kidney results in a secondary suppression of intestinal calcium hyperabsorption. Some reports suggest that this secondary action on the intestine is lost after a period of 2 to 3 years on therapy. This may result in thiazide resistance during long-term treatment of absorptive hypercalciuria. Thiazide diuretics tend to improve calcium balance, and the result is observed as an increase in bone mineral density due to increased bone formation (Table 88–4).

Oral Phosphate. In patients with absorptive hypercalciuria, 1500 mg of neutral potassium phosphate per day in three to four di-

vided doses lowers urinary calcium excretion in some trials as effectively as thiazide diuretics. However, compliance is more difficult to achieve related to frequency of dosing and intestinal side effects such as diarrhea and bloating. Studies estimating efficacy of oral phosphate therapy (Table 88–4) reported relapses of 9 and 25%, but the only available controlled trial used acid phosphate and demonstrated increased frequency of stones. New formulations and additional studies of phosphate therapy are needed.

Sodium Cellulose Phosphate. A calcium-binding resin, sodium cellulose phosphate, reduces calcium absorption when taken with meals. This approach has not demonstrated a high success rate, possibly due to reflex hyperoxaluria. In addition, a negative calcium balance may lead to additional bone mineral loss.

Treatment of Hypocitraturia. Because citrate lowers calcium oxalate supersaturation by binding calcium and, to some extent, by reducing calcium excretion, correcting hypocitraturia should reduce the recurrence of nephrolithiasis. No carefully controlled trials of citrate therapy have been reported. Uncontrolled studies suggest an efficacy of approximately 88% over a 2-year period (Table 88–4). Citrate therapy may be very useful for patients who demonstrate hypocitraturia as a result of thiazide diuretic therapy. Furthermore, in patients with inflammatory bowel disease or renal tubular acidosis, citrate therapy seems a very rational replacement for the losses of alkali. Because of the volume expansion effects, sodium bicarbonate or sodium citrate does not have the required actions of potassium citrate to lower urinary calcium and improve calcium balance.

Treating Hyperoxaluria. **Dietary.** Normal people excrete 20 to 40 mg (222 to 444 μm) of oxalate daily. A simple dietary excess of oxalate from foods may increase urinary oxalate, and a low-calcium diet may further increase excretion. Treating this mild form of dietary hyperoxaluria associated with calcium oxalate stones consists of altering the diet to avoid foods that contain high concentrations of oxalate. However, no carefully controlled trials have proven the efficacy of this approach.

TABLE 88–4. SUMMARY OF TREATMENT OPTIONS FOR DIFFERENT TYPES OF RENAL STONES

Indication	Treatment	Expected Results (% Successful Treatment)
All stones	High fluid intake	Unknown—probably less than 50
CaOx/CaHPO$_4$ stones		
Idiopathic hypercalciuria	1. Controlled protein, Na and Ca diets	Unknown
	2. Thiazide diuretics and related drugs	85–90
	3. Oral phosphate	
	4. Na cellulose phosphate	Unknown
Hypocitraturia	Potassium citrate	
Renal tubular acidosis	Potassium citrate	88
Ileostomy or small bowel malabsorption	Potassium citrate	Unknown
Hyperoxaluria		
Dietary	Reduced oxalate diet	Unknown
Enteric	Low-fat diet	Unknown
	Ca supplement	Unknown
	Cholestyramine	Unknown
Primary	Pyridoxine	Only in a small fraction
Hyperuricosuria	Allopurinol	86
	Potassium citrate	Unknown
Uric acid stones	Allopurinol	Unknown
	Potassium citrate	88
Struvite stones	Extracorporeal shockwave lithotripsy or percutaneous nephrostolithotomy	30–40 with stones < 2 cm
	Acetohydroxamic acid	Control of stone growth if tolerated
Cystine stones/cystinuria	Tiopronin	Unknown
	Penicillamine	Unknown

Each type of renal stone is listed under indication, and the expected success rate per 100 patients is listed under expected results and described in the text.

Enteric. Hyperoxaluria observed in patients with inflammatory bowel disorders and intestinal bypass is usually associated with hypocitraturia. Patients exhibiting hypocalciuria should be treated with a low-fat diet in addition to calcium supplements. Cholestyramine, a nonresorbable resin that binds fatty acids, bile acids, and oxalate (4 to 16 grams daily in four divided doses with meals), oral citrate supplements, and high fluid intake are the mainstays of therapy. These patients may also exhibit magnesium deficiency and hypomagnesuria. Magnesium replacement may be important to increase urinary citrate excretion in response to exogenous potassium alkali.

Primary Hyperoxaluria. Type I primary hyperoxaluria occasionally responds to pyridoxine supplement (2 to 200 mg daily). High urinary volume and supplemental citrate, thiazide diuretics, and possibly oral phosphate supplements can also be used. Following renal transplantation, a special protocol is required to avoid accelerated renal oxalosis. Liver transplantation restores the missing enzymes, and many patients with hyperoxaluria have been treated in this manner.

Hyperuricosuria. Because an excess of purine in the diet causes hyperuricosuria, normal levels of dietary purine should prevent stones. However, careful studies documenting a response to low purine diets are not available. Compelling evidence that hyperuricosuria contributes to the formation of calcium oxalate stones comes from a prospective double-blind trial that demonstrated a reduction in stone formation with allopurinol compared with placebo (see Table 88–3).

URIC ACID STONES. A persistently acid urine decreases the solubility of fully protonated uric acid. Half of the uric acid is fully protonated at pH 5.35, making uric acid supersaturation inevitable at normal excretion rates of 600 to 800 mg (3.6 to 4.8 mM) because the solubility of fully protonated uric acid in urine is 96 mg per liter. Acidic urine is a common finding in patients with uric acid stones, and many of these patients also have gout. Attempts to alkalinize the urine by raising urinary pH to 6 to 6.5 with potassium alkali salts may be effective. However, avoidance of temporary periods of acidification sufficient to nucleate uric acid or uric acid and calcium oxalate is difficult. Because of the general tolerance and safety of allopurinol, which is very effective in reducing urinary uric acid excretion rates, it is the mainstay of therapy.

STRUVITE STONES. Struvite, or magnesium ammonium phosphate, crystals are produced when the urinary tract is colonized by bacteria, producing high concentrations of ammonia. *Proteus, Pseudomonas,* and enterococci usually cause struvite stones. Patients who produce only struvite stones generally present with large stones that cause bleeding, obstruction, and infection without stone passage. These patients rarely have idiopathic hypercalciuria and often have reduced renal function. Patients who pass struvite stones have a higher frequency of idiopathic hypercalciuria because the stone is usually a calcium stone that became secondarily infected, resulting in the struvite. Contralateral spread of struvite stones due to urinary tract infection is frequent.

Struvite stones must be removed. ESWL and percutaneous nephrostolithotomy are used to reduce the damage incurred by growth and spread of these stones. Prolonged use of antibiotics in patients with struvite stones amounts to treatment of an infected foreign body. Once patients are free of stones, they benefit from antibiotics directed against the predominant urinary organism, although no controlled studies support this reasonable approach. Acetohydroxamic acid has limited use because of patient intolerance of side effects.

CYSTINE STONES. Approximately 2% of patients attending renal stone clinics exhibit a hereditary defect of amino acid transport leading to excessive amounts of cystine in the urine. Cystine is the disulfide of cysteine, which is soluble in the urine to the level of only 20 to 48 mg per deciliter (1 to 2 mM per liter). The rate of cystine excretion in patients with cystinuria ranges from 480 to 3600 mg (2 to 15 mM per day) so that high fluid intake can prevent stones in only some patients. Most patients require treatment with penicillamine or tiopronin. Both combine with cysteine to form a soluble salt that reduces, through competition, the formation of cystine. The ability of these treatments to reduce stone frequency is not quantitatively known, although they are effective. However, they exhibit a high rate of intolerance due to severe side effects, which require careful surveillance.

Breslau NA, Preminger GM, Adams BV, et al.: Use of ketoconazole to probe the pathogenetic importance of 1,25-dihydroxyvitamin D in absorptive hypercalciuria. J Clin Endocrinol Metab 75:1446, 1992. *Establishes the roles of the 1α,25(OH)₂D₃/vitamin D receptor complex in at least two thirds of patients with idiopathic hypercalciuria.*

Coe FL, Parks JH, Asplin JR: The pathogenesis and treatment of kidney stones. N Engl J Med 327:1141, 1992. *Very good recent review by an established leader in nephrolithiasis, on pathogenesis of hypercalciuria, bone mineral density in nephrolithiasis, and treatment options.*

Consensus Conference: Prevention and treatment of kidney stones. JAMA 260:977, 1988. *An NIH conference establishing standards to consider in the approach to nephrolithiasis.*

Hess B: Tamm-Horsfall glycoprotein—inhibitor or promoter of calcium oxalate monohydrate crystallization processes? Urol Res 20:83, 1992. *Current studies on the dual potential of Tamm-Horsfall glycoprotein in nephrolithiasis.*

89 CYSTIC DISEASES OF THE KIDNEY
Patricia A. Gabow

Renal cystic diseases encompass numerous disorders that share the characteristic of epithelial-lined cavities filled with fluid or semisolid debris within the kidneys. The cysts may be single or multiple, inherited or acquired, occurring in infancy or old age, clinically silent or symptomatic, producing renal insufficiency. This discussion focuses on simple cysts, the polycystic kidney diseases, acquired cystic disease, and medullary cystic disorders.

Certain clinical settings suggest specific cystic disorders (Fig. 89–1 and Table 89–1). The presence of abdominal masses in a neonate or infant should raise the consideration of either autosomal dominant (ADPKD) or autosomal recessive polycystic kidney disease (ARPKD), tuberous sclerosis, or one of the many congenital syndromes. Renal failure in adolescence suggests ARPKD or medullary cystic disease (MCD). The finding of a solitary cyst in a 50-year-old is most compatible with a simple cyst. A history of renal disease in a family raises the possibility of ADPKD, ARPKD, or MCD. Renal stones can recur in ADPKD or medullary sponge kidneys. The onset of gross hematuria in a patient undergoing chronic hemodialysis raises the possibility of acquired cystic disease (ACD). The accompanying nonrenal manifestations provide other important diagnostic clues.

SIMPLE CYSTS

Simple renal cysts, the most common and clinically least important of all the cystic disorders, increase in frequency with age from 0.1 to 4% in children to as great as 30% of the population over age 70. Often, simple cysts are asymptomatic and are an incidental finding during abdominal imaging studies. Occasionally, patients with simple cysts present with hematuria or flank pain, thereby raising the question of malignancy within the cyst. With renal ultrasonography (US), a simple cyst will demonstrate smooth walls, good sound transmission, and no intracystic debris. If the US pattern differs

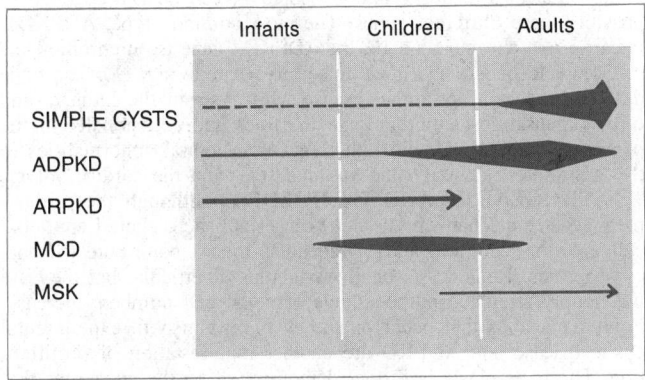

FIGURE 89–1. Ages of renal cystic disease patients.

TABLE 89–1. CHARACTERISTICS OF RENAL CYSTIC DISORDERS

Feature	Simple Cysts	ADPKD	ARPKD	ACD	MCD	MSK
Inheritance pattern	None	Autosomal dominant	Autosomal recessive	None	Often present, variable pattern	None
Frequency	Common, increasing with age	1/200 to 1/1000	Rare	100% in long-term dialysis patients	Rare	Common
Age of onset	Adult	Usually adults	Neonates, children	Usually older adults	Adolescents, young adults	Adults
Presenting symptom	Incidental finding, hematuria	Pain, hematuria, infection, family screening	Abdominal mass, renal failure, failure to thrive	Hematuria	Polyuria, polydipsia, enuresis, renal failure, failure to thrive	Incidental, urinary tract infections, hematuria, renal calculi
Hematuria	Occurs	Common	Occurs	Occurs	Rare	Common
Recurrent infections	Rare	Common	Occurs	No	Rare	Common
Renal calculi	No	Common	No	No	No	Common
Hypertension	Rare	Common	Common	Present from underlying disease	Rare	No
Method of diagnosis	Ultrasound	Ultrasound, gene linkage analysis	Ultrasound	CT scan, ultrasound	None reliable	Excretory urogram
Renal size	Normal	Normal to very large	Large initially	Small to normal, occasionally large	Small	Normal

Note: ADPKD = autosomal dominant polycystic kidney disease; ARPKD = autosomal recessive polycystic kidney disease; ACD = acquired cystic disease; MCD = medullary cystic disease; MSK = medullary sponge kidney.
From Fick G, Gabow P: Hereditary and acquired cystic disease of the kidney. Kidney Int 46:951, 1994.

from this, computed axial tomography (CT) should be performed. Information from the two modalities permits accurate differentiation of benign from malignant lesions in almost all cases. When simple cysts are associated with pain or renin-dependent hypertension, they can be punctured with US guidance, drained, and sclerosed with alcohol instillation into the cyst. For another discussion of renal masses, see also Ch. 91.

Bosniak M: The current radiological approach to renal cysts. Radiology 158:1, 1986. *A comprehensive review of the subject.*
Ozgur S, Cetin S, Ilker Y: Percutaneous renal cyst aspiration and treatment with alcohol. Int Urol Nephrol 20:481, 1988. *A discussion of the role of sclerotherapy of simple cysts.*
Ravine D, Gibson RN, Donlan J, et al.: An ultrasound renal cyst prevalence survey: Specificity data for inherited renal cystic diseases. Am J Kidney Dis 22:803, 1993. *A large study that describes frequency of simple cysts in adult population.*

POLYCYSTIC KIDNEY DISEASE

The polycystic kidney diseases include four disorders, three of which display dominant inheritance: ADPKD, which is the most common, tuberous sclerosis (TS), and von Hippel-Lindau (VHL) disease. All three are systemic disorders, and like ADPKD, TS demonstrates genetic heterogeneity, and both have genes on chromosome 16 (see Ch. 23, 24, and 26). Since ARPKD, ADPKD, and TS can be detected with renal imaging in infancy and childhood and ARPKD and ADPKD can appear ultrasonographically similar *in utero,* misdiagnosis among these three diseases occurs. Thus, in early-onset cystic disease, the pattern of inheritance and the associated abnormalities must be assessed carefully.

Autosomal Dominant Polycystic Kidney Disease (ADPKD)

ADPKD has a worldwide occurrence, with 1 in 200 to 1 in 1000 people affected, and it is the most common hereditary disease in the United States, affecting 500,000 people. It can be caused by two, possibly three, different genes. The most common type, ADPKD1, is carried on chromosome 16; the ADPKD2 gene is on chromosome 4. Complete penetrance is estimated to occur by age 90. The gene defects produce a systemic disease with cysts in the kidneys and other organs, most commonly in the liver and occasionally in the pancreas and ovaries, and with frequent structural abnormalities in the gastrointestinal tract, the vascular tree, and the cardiac valves.

PATHOGENESIS AND PATHOLOGY. Although the primary pathogenetic mechanism has not been established, altered epithelial cell growth, secretion, and extracellular matrix contribute to renal cystogenesis. Renal cysts begin as tubular diverticula, but they are not simply stretched outpouchings of cells; cell numbers increase. Polypoid lesions that occur on the cyst walls in both experimental cystic disease and ADPKD are another manifestation of proliferation. The hyperplasia is further demonstrated by the adenomas that occur in 21% of ADPKD kidneys. However, unlike the hyperplasia in VHL, TS, and ACD, which can result in renal cell carcinoma,

this malignancy does not seem to be increased in ADPKD. Secretion also must occur to form a fluid-filled cyst. Interestingly, ADPKD cyst fluid itself contains substances that promote cyst epithelial secretion. In keeping with this observation, intact renal cysts that are drained rapidly reaccumulate fluid unless the epithelium is altered with alcohol sclerosis. In addition, the renal basement membrane appears abnormal even early in the course of the disease, and ADPKD cyst epithelium in culture elaborates an abnormal basement membrane.

CLINICAL MANIFESTATIONS. Individuals usually present for either screening because of a family history of the disease or evaluation of symptoms. Early in the course of ADPKD, the kidneys can be normal in size with only a few cysts. Ultimately, the kidneys enlarge and may attain the size of a football, weighing as much as 8 kg. The end-stage kidney appears to be virtually replaced by cysts (Figs. 89–2 and 89–3). This enlargement produces many of the renal symptoms, including flank and back pain and hematuria (Table 89–2). The pain can be chronic or acute, mild or severe and disabling. Chronic pain tends to occur in patients with kidneys larger than 15 cm. Acute pain requires considering upper urinary tract infection, cyst or retroperitoneal hemorrhage, or nephrolithiasis. As many as 36% of ADPKD patients can have renal stones of either urate or calcium composition. Both microscopic and gross hematuria occur. One third of patients will have microscopic hematuria on a random urinalysis, and approximately 40% of patients will have at least one episode of gross hematuria. Hematuria is more common in patients with larger kidneys and hypertension.

The extrarenal manifestations of ADPKD are detailed in Table 89–2. Hepatic cysts occur in 40 to 60% of patients. As with renal cysts, hepatic cysts increase in number and/or size over time; however, unlike renal cysts, hepatic cysts rarely occur before puberty, appear to increase in size and number due to pregnancy, and very rarely produce functional impairment. Hepatic cysts also can become infected. Colonic diverticulosis appears to be another clinically important gastrointestinal manifestation, especially in patients with end-stage renal disease (ESRD), and may be complicated by perforation and intra-abdominal abscess.

Hypertension in ADPKD begins in childhood, occurs in 60% of patients with normal renal function, and is present in 80% of those with renal insufficiency. The hypertension results in part from the activation of the renin-angiotensin system. Intracranial aneurysms occur in about 10% of affected persons. Aneurysms in ADPKD appear to cluster in certain families, are often multiple, can recur in some patients, and rupture at a younger age than in the general population. Cardiac valve abnormalities are common; 26% of all ADPKD patients have mitral valve prolapse, often accompanied by palpitations and atypical chest pain. Myxomatous degeneration requiring valve replacements occurs in some patients.

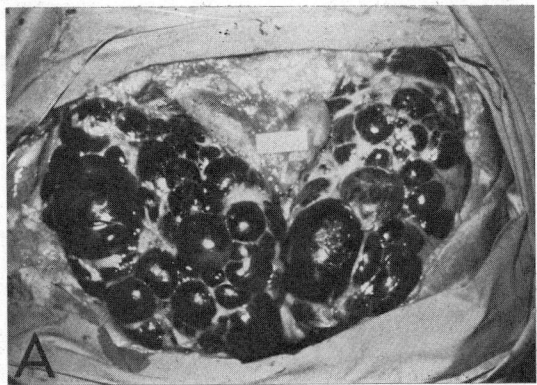
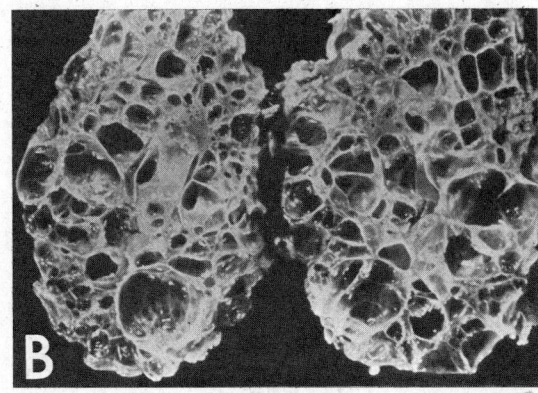

FIGURE 89–2. Autosomal dominant polycystic kidney disease (ADPKD) *in situ (A)* and on cut section *(B).* Note diffuse, bilateral distribution of cysts. (Courtesy of FE Cuppage, Kansas City, KS; from Brenner BM, Rector FC Jr [eds.]: The Kidney. 3d ed. Philadelphia, WB Saunders, 1986, p 1346.)

The natural history of renal functional impairment with ADPKD is variable. However, renal failure rarely occurs before age 40, except in children who were diagnosed *in utero* or in the first year of life. Approximately 50% of patients have well-preserved renal function at age 60, suggesting that factors other than the gene itself have an important modulating role in renal function. Those factors that have been associated with a worse renal outcome include the ADPKD1 gene, being male, and having hypertension, episodes of gross hematuria, urinary tract infections in males, and larger kidneys.

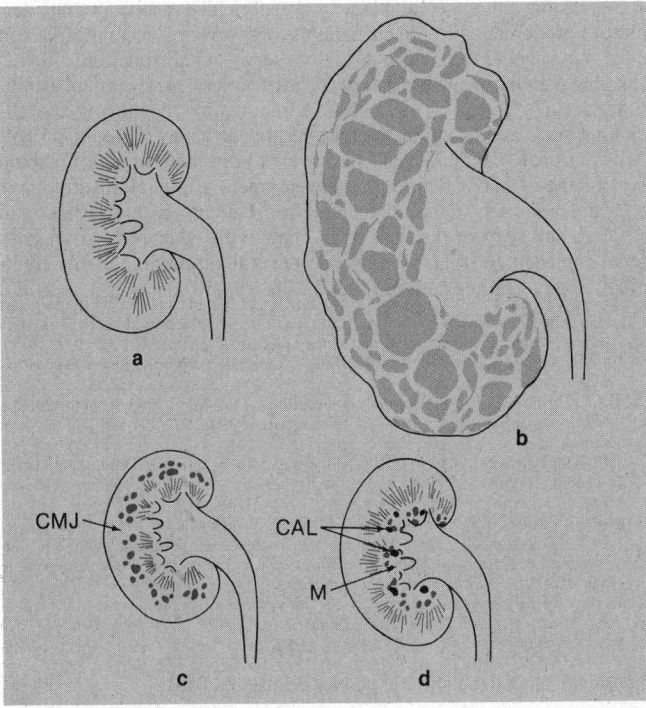

FIGURE 89–3. Schematic drawing of a cut section of *(a)* a normal kidney, measuring 12 cm with normal papilla, cortex, medulla, and corticomedullary junction. *(b)* Kidney from a patient with ADPKD. The kidney is large, measuring 29 cm, and contains cysts throughout the cortex and medulla which vary in size from 1 mm to 5 cm. *(c)* Kidney from a patient with medullary cystic disease. The kidney is small, measuring 8 cm, with a scarred surface. The cysts are at the corticomedullary junction (CMJ) and are small, measuring 1 to 5 mm across. *(d)* Kidney from a patient with medullary sponge kidney; these are multiple ductal dilations measuring 1 to 5 mm in diameter and giving the medulla (M) a porous appearance. Some dilations contain calculi (CAL). (*c* and *d* from Spence HM, Singleton R: What is sponge kidney disease and where does it fit in the spectrum of cystic disorders? J Urol 107:176, 1972; © by Williams & Wilkins, 1972.)

TABLE 89–2. FREQUENCY OF MANIFESTATIONS OF AUTOSOMAL DOMINANT POLYCYSTIC KIDNEY DISEASE IN ADULTS

Extrarenal Manifestations	Frequency
Gastrointestinal	
Hepatic cysts	Approximately 50%; increases with age
Cholangiocarcinoma	Rare
Congenital hepatic fibrosis	Rare
Pancreatic cysts	Approximately 10%
Colonic diverticula	80% of patients with ESRD
Cardiovascular	
Cardiac valvular abnormalities	26%
Intracranial aneurysms	5 to 10%
Thoracic and abdominal aortic aneurysms	Unknown
Genital	
Ovarian cysts	Unknown
Testicular cysts	Unknown
Seminal vesicle cysts	Unknown
Miscellaneous cysts	
Arachnoid cysts	5%
Pineal cysts	Rare
Splenic cysts	Rare

Renal Manifestations	Frequency
Anatomic	
Renal cysts	100%
Renal adenomas	21%
Cyst calcification	Common
Functional	
Decreased renal concentrating ability	Affects potentially all adults
Decreased urinary citrate excretion	67% (10/15 subjects)
Impaired renal acidification	Unknown
Hormonal alterations	
Increased renin production	Probably affects all hypertensive adults
Preserved erythropoietin production	Probably affects all patients with ESRD

Complications	Frequency
Hypertension	Affects > 80% of patients with ESRD*
Hematuria and/or hemorrhage	50%
Acute and chronic pain	60%
Urinary tract infection–bladder, interstitium, cysts	Common
Nephrolithiasis	20–36%
Nephromegaly	100% of adults
Renal failure	Affects 50% of patients by age 60

ESRD = end-stage renal disease.
* This complication also affects 30% of children with polycystic kidney disease.
From Gabow PA: Autosomal dominant polycystic kidney disease. N Engl J Med 329:332, 1993. Copyright the Massachusetts Medical Society.

DIAGNOSIS. The method of ADPKD diagnosis depends on the level of certainty needed, the patient's symptoms, the need for anatomic information, and the presence of renal cysts (Table 89–3). Imaging studies remain the mainstay for diagnosis, but they depend on detectable cysts. Demonstrating the characteristic bilateral renal cystic involvement is best accomplished by renal US. US screening studies of at-risk children under age 18 identify a majority of gene carriers, but unilateral cysts occur in 18% and bilateral cysts with only one or two cysts in each kidney occur in 5% of these children. This pattern may be seen in some adults as well. In adults, a CT scan with contrast material occasionally will reveal more cystic involvement than does US. Imaging studies which reveal only a few cysts require differentiation of early ADPKD from multiple simple cysts (Table 89–4). The patient's age and the presence of extrarenal involvement are helpful in this instance (see Fig. 89–1). Since simple cysts are uncommon in children, the finding of any cysts in a child in an ADPKD family strongly suggests the disorder. However, in an individual over 50 with similar US findings, the diagnosis is much less certain. In these older patients, the presence of bilateral involvement and extrarenal involvement, particularly hepatic cysts, lends support to the diagnosis of ADPKD. If definitive diagnosis is needed, gene linkage analysis can be used in many families and can predict gene status with 99:1 likelihood at any age, even in fetuses. Because gene linkage analysis is expensive, requires the cooperation of other family members, and supplies no anatomic information, it is probably best reserved for patients with nondiagnostic imaging studies in whom the diagnosis has major clinical significance, such as occurs with a potential renal transplant donor to a family member.

It is not necessary to establish the presence of extrarenal involvement in all ADPKD patients. Currently, neither total abdominal US to detect extrarenal cysts nor echocardiography to diagnose cardiac valve lesions nor a search for intracranial aneurysm is recommended in ADPKD patients without specific clinical indications. Current recommendations for investigating aneurysms are that asymptomatic patients should be examined only if there is a positive family history of aneurysms, an occupation in which sudden loss of consciousness would place the patient or others at great risk, pending elective surgery in which hemodynamic instability with severe hypertension may occur, or the patient demands investigation for peace of mind. If screening is to be done, either dynamic CT or magnetic resonance angiography can be used.

TREATMENT. Treatment for patients with ADPKD is aimed at preventing complications of the disease and preserving renal function. Patients and family members should be educated about the inheritance and manifestations of the disease. Episodes of gross hematuria should be managed conservatively with bed rest, analgesics, and hydration. Urinary tract instrumentation, including Foley catheter placement, should be avoided because of the increased risk of serious urinary tract and renal cyst infections after such instrumentation. Patients suspected of having a urinary tract infection

TABLE 89–3. METHODS OF DIAGNOSIS IN ADPKD

Method	Limitations
Ultrasonography	May miss 2 to 6% of patients with cysts
	Highly operator- and reader-dependent
	Will not identify precystic gene carriers; this may be as high as 20% under age 20
CT scan	May miss rare patient with small cysts
	Radiation and contrast exposure
	Difficult to perform in children
	Expense
	Will not identify precystic gene carriers; slightly more sensitive than ultrasonography
Gene linkage analysis	Requires other family members to participate
	Requires that physician understand interpretation of results
	Expense
	Provides no anatomic information of organs involved

Modified from Gabow PA: Autosomal dominant polycystic kidney disease—More than a renal disease. Am J Kidney Dis 16:403, 1990.

TABLE 89–4. COMPARISON OF MULTIPLE SIMPLE CYSTS AND EARLY ADPKD

Feature	Multiple Simple Cysts	ADPKD
Family history	No	60%
Ultrasonographically demonstrable cysts in other family member(s)	No	90%
Sex distribution	M > F	M = F
Renal size	Normal	Normal to mildly enlarged
Kidney involvement	Usually unilateral, rarely bilateral	Usually bilateral, may be unilateral early
Cyst distribution	Cortical	Cortical and medullary
Cyst size	Usually < 2 cm, occasionally larger	< 2 cm early
Blood in cysts	Rare	Common
Hepatic cysts	No	40–60%; likelihood increases with age
Intracranial aneurysm	No	10%
Mitral valve prolapse	No	26%
Hypertension	Rare	60%
Gene linkage analysis for chromosome 16 or 4	No	> 90%

should have urine and blood cultures obtained. The presumed site of infection influences selection of antibiotic therapy. Bladder and renal parenchymal infections can be treated as they are in other patients. Failure to respond to appropriate antibiotic treatment suggests cyst infection. In this instance, the antibiotic must be one that enters cyst fluid. These include chloramphenicol, trimethoprim-sulfamethoxazole, or the fluoroquinolones. Infected hepatic cysts appear to require both drainage and antibiotics for successful treatment.

Hypertension should be treated aggressively. Although cyst decompression either percutaneously or surgically results in considerable improvement in pain in patients with severe, disabling pain, it does not appear to improve or preserve renal function. Repeat imaging studies need not be performed unless new clinical symptoms occur. CT scan is the method of choice for diagnosing complications such as intracystic or retroperitoneal hemorrhage, renal calculi, or renal malignancy. A serum creatinine determination should be obtained yearly before the development of renal insufficiency and at least every 6 months thereafter. Patients with ADPKD and renal failure respond as well as patients with other renal disease to renal replacement therapy. A more general discussion of the treatment of renal failure is found in Ch. 78.

Chapman AB, Johnson A, Gabow PA, et al.: The renin-angiotensin-aldosterone system and autosomal dominant polycystic kidney disease. N Engl J Med 323:1091, 1990. *A comprehensive study of the role of the renin-angiotensin mechanism in ADPKD hypertension.*

Gabow PA: Autosomal dominant polycystic kidney disease. N Engl J Med 329:332, 1993. *A comprehensive review of genetics, pathogenesis, and clinical features with a large reference list.*

Gardner KD, Bernstein J [eds.]: Cystic Kidneys and Their Diseases. Dordrecht, Klower Academic Publishers, 1990. *Addresses the genetic, clinical, and pathogenetic aspects of all types of cystic disease.*

Huston J 3d, Torres VE, Sullivan PP, et al.: Value of magnetic resonance angiography for the detection of intracranial aneurysm in autosomal dominant polycystic kidney disease. J Am Soc Nephrol 3:1871, 1993. *A prospective study exemplifying uses of MRL angiography and characteristics of the abnormality.*

Kimberling WJ, Pieke-Dahl SA, Kumar S: The genetics of cystic diseases of the kidney. Semin Nephrol 11:596, 1991. *A discussion of the genetics of ADPKD with case examples exemplifying the utility of gene linkage techniques.*

Autosomal Recessive Polycystic Kidney Disease (ARPKD)

ARPKD is rare, occurring in 1 in 10,000 to 1 in 50,000 live births. It has been classified into perinatal, neonatal, infantile, or juvenile types based on age of onset. The responsible gene has been located on chromosome 6. Animal models have supported a role for growth factors in proliferation as well as altered differentiation in the cystogenesis. The clinical manifestations include failure to thrive, abdominal masses, hypertension, and urinary tract infections. The kidneys are large early in life and may diminish in size with time. The cut surface of the kidney reveals radially oriented fusiform cysts. As in ADPKD, US is the diagnostic method of choice. Examining the parents and in some instances liver biopsy of the affected child are necessary to distinguish ARPKD from the childhood presentation of ADPKD. Normal renal US in the parents, especially if they are age 30 or older, strongly suggests ARPKD. All children with ARPKD have some hepatic involvement, but it is clinically most apparent in older children with the juvenile form, who may have severe enough hepatic fibrosis to have portal hypertension and its complications. As with other forms of renal disease, aggressive, early treatment of hypertension may be important in preserving renal function. Children with ARPKD usually progress to ESRD before adolescence; in the perinatal form, this occurs within the first few weeks of life. Among children who survive the first year of life, 79% are alive at age 15. Treatment of the chronic renal failure of ARPKD is similar to that for other childhood renal diseases.

McDonald RA, Avner ED: Inherited polycystic kidney disease in children. Semin Nephrol 11:632, 1991. *Reviews findings of ARPKD and ADPKD in children.*

ACQUIRED CYSTIC DISEASE (ACD)

"Acquired cystic disease" refers to the development of cysts in previously noncystic kidneys in patients with ESRD from a disease other than a renal cystic disease. Reported frequencies range from 7 to 22% in patients with long-term renal insufficiency before dialysis to almost 90% in patients with 10 years or more of dialysis (see Ch. 78.1). Males and black patients appear to have a higher frequency. Although most patients have no symptoms from the cysts, others develop retroperitoneal or intrarenal bleeding or bleeding into the pelvicaliceal system with hematuria. Renal tumors, both adenomas and carcinomas, complicate this disorder. This latter complication prompts screening in high-risk groups. US can establish the diagnosis, but the small size of the kidneys and cysts makes the CT scan more sensitive. Episodes of hematuria can be treated as in ADPKD. Severe, recurrent hematuria can be treated with renal arterial embolization, because it is not crucial to preserve renal parenchyma in dialysis patients. Renal tumors of <3 cm can be followed with a yearly CT scan; larger tumors require surgery because of their greater propensity for malignancy.

Ishikawa I: Acquired cystic disease: Mechanisms and manifestations. Semin Nephrol 11:671, 1991. *A comprehensive discussion of the pathogenetics and clinical aspects of this disorder.*

MEDULLARY CYSTIC DISORDERS

Medullary cystic disease (MCD) and medullary sponge kidney (MSK) make up the majority of the medullary cystic disorders. MCD is an uncommon disorder that also has been labeled familial juvenile nephronophthisis (FJN); the latter is treated as a somewhat distinct subset. A familial pattern is present in a majority of cases, with autosomal recessive inheritance in FJN and autosomal dominant in MCD. FJN presents in childhood and is associated with extrarenal involvement, including retinal defects. MCD more frequently occurs in adults. Preliminary information places the recessive gene on chromosome 2.

PATHOGENESIS AND PATHOLOGY. No pathogenetic theory has been defined. The kidneys are small and generally display some cysts at the corticomedullary junction and in the medulla (see Fig. 89–3c). An acystic form of the disorder occurs. The glomeruli are hyalinized, and the tubules vary in appearance from atrophic to tortuous. The tubular basement membrane is often irregular, with some areas thickened and others thinned and split; in addition, the composition of the tubular basement membrane appears abnormal. The interstitium reveals fibrosis and mononuclear cell infiltrate.

CLINICAL MANIFESTATIONS AND DIAGNOSIS. A majority of patients present in childhood or early adolescence with polydipsia, polyuria, and enuresis; this constellation presumably reflects a defect in urinary concentrating ability and secondary polydipsia. Often the children demonstrate growth retardation and anemia. Renal salt wasting has been suggested to occur in the disorder in excess of the impaired sodium conservation that accompanies any ESRD.

Diagnosis of the disorder is often difficult. The urinalysis is unremarkable, and proteinuria is minimal. Imaging studies reveal small end-stage kidneys. Some patients are simply labeled "chronic renal failure" or "chronic pyelonephritis." The disorder should be considered in children or young adults with renal insufficiency, small kidneys, and a family history of renal disease. No specific treatment exists. Management is that appropriate for any child with renal insufficiency, including attention to growth, bone disease, and sodium

balance. The possibility of a retinal abnormality also must be considered in initial evaluation.

Chagnac A, Zevin D, Weinstein T, et al.: Combined tubular dysfunction in medullary cystic disease. Arch Intern Med 146:1007, 1986. *A report of a patient with proximal and distal renal tubular acidosis and medullary cystic disease.*
Cohen AH, Hoyer JR: Nephronophthisis: A primary tubular basement membrane defect. Lab Invest 55:564, 1986. *Presents data supporting abnormal basement membrane composition.*
Gretz N, Scharer K, Waldher R, et al.: Rate of deterioration of renal function in juvenile nephronophthisis. Pediatr Nephrol 3:56, 1989. *A study of the rate of decline of renal function in patients with familial juvenile nephronophthisis.*

MEDULLARY SPONGE KIDNEY

MSK is a relatively common disorder affecting between 1 in 5000 and 1 in 20,000 individuals. There is no known pathogenetic mechanism. Tubular dilations occur within the medullary collecting ducts (see Fig. 89–3d). Patients present with recurrent hematuria, urinary tract infections, or renal calculi. The diagnosis is established with an excretory urography that reveals normal-sized kidneys with medullary ductal ectasia, which has been described as a "bouquet of flowers" or a "paintbrush" appearance. Often a plain film of the abdomen will reveal renal calculi or calcification in the cystic areas. Coincident hypercalciuria as well as hyperparathyroidism has been reported in MSK; therefore, both serum calcium and 24-hour urinary calcium determinations should be obtained and, if indicated, a serum parathyroid hormone level (see Ch. 214). Conversely, as many as 20% of patients presenting with nephrolithiasis may have MSK. Other clinical manifestations of MSK reflect the structural alterations in the renal papillae with a consequent decreased renal concentrating ability, impaired acidification with an incomplete renal tubular acidosis, and an impairment in renal potassium excretion in response to acute potassium loading. Despite these defects, serum electrolyte concentrations are almost always normal. Treatment includes appropriate management of renal infections and renal calculus disease (see Ch. 88). Urinary tract obstruction must be considered during acute episodes of renal colic. In the absence of obstruction, renal function remains normal.

Ginalski JM, Portmann L, Jaeger PH: Does medullary sponge kidney cause nephrolithiasis? AJR 155:299, 1990. *This study examines the frequency of medullary sponge kidney in a large number of patients with and without nephrolithiasis.*
Ginalski JM, Schnyder P, Portmann L, et al.: Medullary sponge kidney on axial computed tomography: Comparison with excretory urography. Eur J Radiol 12:104, 1991. *Defines the uses of excretory urography in establishing the diagnosis.*

90 ANOMALIES OF THE URINARY TRACT
Jay Bernstein

Developmental abnormalities of the urinary tract are relatively common, believed to affect 10% of newborns and to account for almost one third of all congenital malformations. Many are asymptomatic and inconsequential, but major malformations are important causes of early infantile death and of later morbidity and renal failure. The congenital malformations that cause renal and urinary tract disease in adolescents and adults are the subject of this chapter.

RENAL PARENCHYMAL DEFICIENCY. *Renal agenesis* is a failure of embryogenesis that, when unilateral, results in a solitary kidney. Bilateral agenesis, the more common abnormality, is fatal to newborns. *Renal hypoplasia* signifies a small kidney with otherwise normal renal parenchyma, resulting from deficient nephrogenesis or reduced postnatal growth, whereas *renal dysplasia,* regardless of renal size, indicates abnormal metanephric differentiation resulting in abnormally and incompletely differentiated renal elements and in abnormal metanephric structure. Small dysplastic kidneys are commonly referred to as "aplastic." Large dysplastic kidneys are often cystic, the most common type being *multicystic dysplasia.*

Renal Agenesis. Unilateral agenesis in adults occurs both as an isolated abnormality and as a component of several heritable disorders, e.g., Turner's syndrome (see Ch. 207). Its most important association is in the syndrome of hereditary renal adysplasia (HRA), an autosomal dominant condition with variable penetrance. Unilateral and bilateral renal agenesis, renal dysplasia, and congenital hydronephrosis all may occur in a family, and the recurrence risk is for any of the defects. First-degree relatives of infants with bilateral renal agenesis carry a 12% risk of HRA, and conversely the offspring of either affected or obligate heterozygotes carry a 15 to 20% empirical risk of bilateral renal maldevelopment. Unilateral agenesis occurs in approximately 1 in 1000 births. Males predominate, approximately 2:1. More than one third of patients with unilateral agenesis have other congenital defects, e.g., cardiovascular and gastrointestinal. Almost 70% have genital anomalies. Because renal agenesis is a developmental field defect, unilateral agenesis is commonly associated with müllerian defects in women (e.g., absent ipsilateral oviduct) and with wolffian defects in men (e.g., absent ipsilateral ductus deferens), which are sometimes clues to the renal abnormality. The solitary kidney is not ordinarily at increased risk of acquired disease, except that one serious but uncommon complication is compensatory hypertrophy with hyperfiltration, glomerular sclerosis, and renal insufficiency.

Renal Hypoplasia. Bilateral hypoplasia, in which small kidneys contain a reduced complement of nephrons and in which the glomeruli and tubules individually undergo hypertrophy, has been called *oligoméganéphronie,* or *oligonephronic hypoplasia.* Patients often survive into the second decade with slowly progressive renal insufficiency and are good candidates for renal transplantation. The abnormality is characterized by the early onset of a urinary concentrating defect, often with salt wasting, and hypertension occurs late, if at all. This abnormality is a sporadic, usually isolated maldevelopment that must be differentiated from acquired renal atrophy, particularly segmental atrophy in reflux nephropathy, and from nephronophthisis–medullary cystic disease. Unilateral hypoplasia may be recognized in imaging studies that show unirenicular and birenicular kidneys, often with contralateral hypertrophy.

Renal Dysplasia. Unilateral dysplasia may be asymptomatic well into adult life. Small aplastic and large multicystic dysplastic kidneys are nonfunctioning, but modern imaging studies differentiate these abnormalities from renal agenesis. The ipsilateral ureter is typically atretic, and contralateral malformations, among them obstruction and reflux, are common and increase morbidity if left untreated. Unilateral multicystic kidneys involute over time and sometimes disappear almost completely, to become indistinguishable from renal agenesis. Unilateral aplasia and multicystic dysplasia may, as noted above, be manifestations of the HRA syndrome.

RENAL AND URETERAL DUPLICATION AND ECTOPY. Duplex kidneys with partial ureteral duplication are harmless, relatively common abnormalities. Renal duplication with complete ureteral duplication, on the other hand, is a more serious malformation because of associated ureteral ectopy (Fig. 90–1). The ureter arising from the cephalad portion of the duplicated kidney typically enters the bladder below the normal ureterovesical junction, e.g., in the lower trigone or proximal urethra, where it often terminates in an ectopic ureterocele—a cystlike dilation of the terminal ureter in the bladder submucosa. Stenosis of the ectopic ureteral orifice results in varying degrees of urinary obstruction. High-grade obstruction is associated with maldevelopment and nonfunction of the upper part of the kidney, and enlargement of the ureterocele may impinge on and mildly obstruct the lower-pole ureter. This malformation, commonly discovered during childhood because of reflux and urinary tract infection, may not become symptomatic until adulthood, also because of urinary tract infection.

Simple intravesical ureteroceles arising in single ureters may be mildly obstructed. Ureteral ectopy in the urethra or vagina is associated with incontinence and an increased risk of ascending infection. Ectopic ureters in the seminal vesicle become symptomatic at the onset of sexual activity. The ipsilateral kidneys in these circumstances may be small and dysplastic.

Renal ectopy is often unilateral, e.g., a pelvic kidney located at the pelvic brim with its blood supply from pelvic or iliac vessels. Pelvic kidneys are occasionally injured during parturition and are susceptible to infection and lithiasis because of stasis and reflux. Bilateral renal ectopia is often associated with fusion of the two kidneys, the most common type being the horseshoe kidney (Fig. 90–2). It occurs in about 0.25% (1 in 400) of the population, with

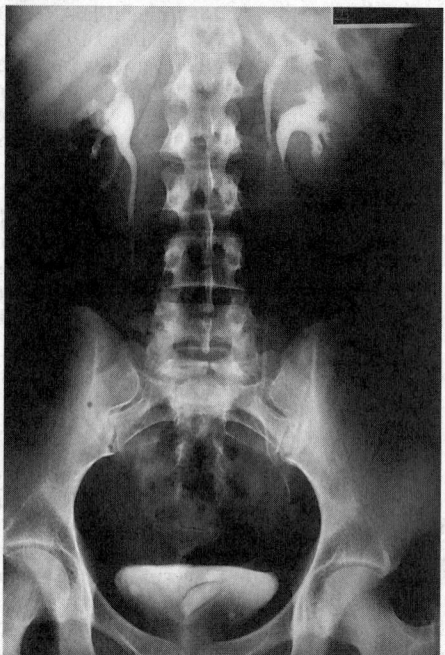

FIGURE 90–1. Urographic demonstration of left renal duplication with ectopic ureterocele in bladder. (Copyright © Jay Bernstein, M.D.)

a 2:1 male predominance. Crossed ectopia occurs with and without fusion. Supernumerary (extra) kidneys are also ectopic, varying in location.

CONGENITAL LOWER URINARY TRACT OBSTRUCTION AND MALDEVELOPMENT. Ureteropelvic obstruction in the adult is less often congenital and more often acquired as a result of ureteritis and pyelitis. Extrinsic ureteropelvic and upper ureteral obstruction has sometimes been attributed to aberrant blood vessels that appear to kink and to constrict the ureter, but intrinsic ureteral abnormalities may underlie this association. Hydrocalicosis, secondary to infundibular stenosis, and caliceal diverticula in early life are probably congenital, although the same abnormalities later in life are of uncertain pathogenesis. Both become symptomatic because of infection and lithiasis. Diverticula and mucosal folds and valves are rare, presumably congenital causes of low ureteral obstruction.

Abnormal insertion of the ureter into the bladder is arguably the basis of vesicoureteral reflux. Nonetheless, reflux gradually diminishes in frequency and severity during childhood. Extreme ureteral dilation in association with severe vesicoureteral reflux (refluxing megaureter) is associated with obstructive maldevelopment of the lower urinary tract, e.g., posterior urethral valves, functional bladder outlet obstruction, and prune-belly syndrome. Some boys with

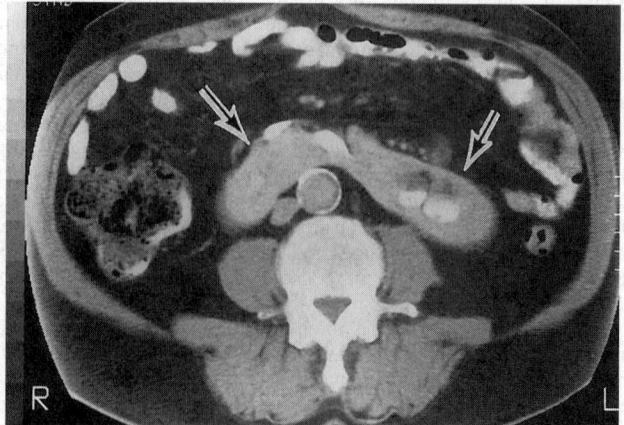

FIGURE 90–2. Horseshoe kidney, fused across the midline (*arrows*), demonstrated by enhanced computed tomography. The pelvis of the right kidney faces anteriorly. (Copyright © Jay Bernstein, M.D.)

posterior urethral valves and reasonably functioning urinary tracts survive into adulthood with little impairment of renal function. Posterior urethral valves are only occasionally familial. The *prune-belly syndrome* comprises a distended abdominal wall with deficient abdominal musculature, cryptorchidism, dilated bladder and ureters, and hypoplastic prostate. The major factor in survival is preserving renal function. The lax, wrinkled anterior abdominal wall, from which the syndrome derives its name, smoothes out with growth into a prominent pot belly. Only about 3% of patients are female. Siblings are at some risk of recurrence; surviving males have been sterile. Anterior urethral diverticula related to mucosal folds that function as flap valves partially obstruct the urethra and become complicated by local infection and lithiasis. In megalourethra, the penile urethra distends during micturition because of partial or complete absence of the corpus spongiosum. Severe forms of the abnormality are usually accompanied by other malformations, but milder forms involve only the distal urethra.

Vesical exstrophy and epispadias are ordinarily treated in early childhood and rarely neglected into adolescence. Late repair of exstrophy is associated with a greatly increased risk of bladder cancer. Repair may be followed by vesicoureteral reflux, and inguinal hernias are commonly present in males. Although complete epispadias causes incontinence, the less severe balanic and penile forms are usually continent. Hypospadias, with a short and curved penis (chordee), is rarely allowed to persist into adulthood. Urethral duplication and vesical septation are rare abnormalities.

Bauer SB, Perlmutter AD, Retik AB: Anomalies of the upper urinary tract. *In* Walsh PC, Retik AB, Stamey TA, Vaughan ED (eds.): Campbell's Urology. 6th ed. Philadelphia, WB Saunders, 1992, pp 1357–1442. *A comprehensive urologic discussion of renal and upper urinary tract malformations.*

Bernstein J, Churg J: Urinary Tract Pathology: An Illustrated Practical Guide to Diagnosis. New York, Raven Press, 1992, pp 3–35. *A concise and heavily illustrated description of common and important developmental abnormalities of the upper and lower urinary tracts.*

Bernstein J, Gilbert-Barness E: Congenital malformations of the kidney. *In* Tisher C, Brenner B (eds.): Renal Pathology. 2d ed. Philadelphia: JB Lippincott, 1994, pp 1355–1386. *A clinicopathologic evaluation of renal maldevelopment.*

91 TUMORS OF THE KIDNEY, URETER, AND BLADDER

Charles L. Shapiro, Marc B. Garnick, and Philip W. Kantoff

RENAL CELL CARCINOMA

EPIDEMIOLOGY AND ETIOLOGY. Renal cell carcinoma is typically diagnosed during the sixth and seventh decade. The male to female ratio is 2:1. Approximately 26,500 new cancers are diagnosed annually, and there are 10,700 cancer deaths. Risk factors for renal cell carcinoma include cigarette smoking, obesity, excessive ingestion of phenacetin analgesics, acquired cystic kidney disease in dialysis patients, adult polycystic kidney disease, exposure to Thorotrast contrast medium, and occupational exposure to asbestos, cadmium, leather tanning, and petroleum products. Rare familial forms of renal cell carcinoma include von Hippel-Lindau (VHL) disease. VHL is an autosomal dominant disorder characterized by the development of multiple tumors of the central nervous system, pheochromocytomas, and bilateral renal cell carcinomas.

A putative tumor suppressor gene for renal cell cancer has recently been identified. Over 90% of nonhereditary renal cell carcinomas, and renal cell carcinomas occurring in patients with VHL disease are associated with structural deletions or alterations of 3p, the short arm of chromosome 3. A gene for VHL was mapped to the 3p region using genetic linkage studies and has recently been cloned and partially sequenced. Loss of one copy of the VHL gene through deletion and a mutation in the remaining copy of the gene has been found in the majority of nonhereditary renal cell carcinomas. These data suggest that the loss of the function of the VHL gene is a crucial step in the development of renal cell carcinoma.

PATHOLOGY. Renal cell carcinomas arise from the proximal renal tubular epithelium. Although most are solitary, 7% are multicentric. The histopathologic subtypes of renal cell carcinoma are the clear cell, the granular cell, and the spindle cell or sarcomatoid variant. The clear cell subtype is the most common form (75% of cases), and the less frequent sarcomatoid variety (1 to 6% of cases) is associated with a poorer prognosis. Oncocytomas are rare variants of renal cell carcinoma thought to arise from the distal tubule. These are well differentiated tumors of low malignant potential. In contrast to the common forms of renal cell carcinoma, 3p deletions are not found in oncocytomas.

CLINICAL MANIFESTATIONS AND DIAGNOSIS. Hematuria is the most frequent presenting symptom of renal cell carcinoma. Pain and an abdominal mass are also common, but the "classic triad" of hematuria, pain, and abdominal mass occurs in <10% of patients. Systemic symptoms, including fever, weight loss, anemia, polycythemia, hypercalcemia, and nonmetastatic hepatic dysfunction, occur frequently in patients with renal cell carcinoma and may represent the sole manifestation of the cancer. Cytokines and hormones such as interleukin-6, transforming growth factor α and β, erythropoietin-like substances, and parathyroid hormone–like substances are produced by renal cell carcinomas and may be responsible for some systemic symptoms. Systemic symptoms may be relieved by surgical removal of the primary tumor.

Routine use of computed tomography (CT) and ultrasonography (US) has led to increased detection of incidental renal masses. The majority of these are benign and include cysts, inflammatory process, pseudotumors, and benign tumors. Cysts are the most frequent renal masses, and several radiographic features help to distinguish benign renal cysts from renal cell carcinomas. The thickness and contour of the wall, the presence and thickness of septa, the extent and location of calcifications, the density of the fluid, and the presence of solid components are used to categorize lesions into those that are benign and do not require surgical evaluation and those in which the suspicion of carcinoma is high and surgery is required.

An algorithm for the workup of an incidental renal mass is presented in Figure 91–1. US is particularly useful to determine whether masses imaged on excretory urography are either cystic or solid. If the US appearance suggests a complex or solid mass, contrast-enhanced CT is the most sensitive imaging method for renal cell carcinoma. CT also provides important information regarding perirenal tumor extension, regional nodal involvement, renal vein involvement, and local and regional spread of cancer. In comparative studies, magnetic resonance imaging (MRI) provides information similar to CT. Although controversial, there is generally no need for selective renal arteriography unless nephron-sparing surgery is planned (see below).

A variety of tumors may spread to the kidney, the most common being lung cancer. Metastases to the kidney are often multiple and typically occur in the setting of other disseminated disease. A solitary renal mass in a patient with a prior history of malignant disease without evidence of metastases suggests a new primary renal cell carcinoma and should prompt a diagnostic evaluation. Lymphoma of the kidney usually is found with other evidence of systemic lymphoma and often occurs with multiple masses or more diffuse infiltration of the kidney.

STAGING AND PROGNOSIS. The Robson and TNM (Tumor, Nodes, Metastases) staging systems for renal cell carcinoma are described in Table 91–1. Renal vein invasion *per se* does not adversely affect prognosis, and tumor thrombus in the vena cava that can be completely removed also does not adversely affect prognosis, even if the thrombus extends above the diaphragm. About 18% of patients with surgically staged renal cell carcinoma have regional lymph node metastases. Regional nodal metastases provide direct evidence of the metastatic potential of the tumor, and virtually all such patients subsequently develop overt metastases. Other prognostic factors include nuclear grade, tumor size, histologic pattern, and flow cytometry, but currently these have little impact on routine clinical decisions.

One third of patients with renal cell carcinoma have distant metastases at the time the primary tumor is diagnosed. The most common sites are the lung (50%), bone (49%), skin (11%), liver (8%), and brain (3%). In patients with newly diagnosed renal cell carcinoma, radiographic staging evaluation with chest radiograph or CT and bone scan must be done to determine whether metastases are present before definitive surgical treatment of the primary tumor.

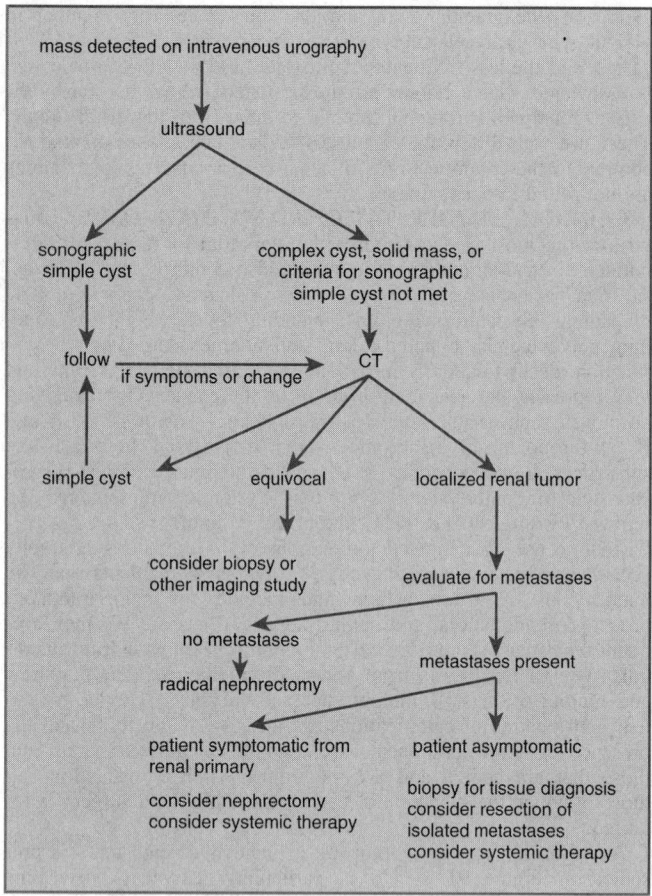

FIGURE 91–1. Algorithm for workup of incidental renal mass.

TREATMENT. The standard treatment for localized renal cell carcinoma is radical nephrectomy, including removal of the kidney, Gerota's fascia, the ipsilateral adrenal gland, and often the regional hilar nodes. The value of extended regional lymph node dissection is unproven, and it cannot be routinely recommended. Removal of the ipsilateral adrenal gland may not be necessary unless the primary renal tumor is located in the mid or upper pole of the kidney. Radiation therapy either before or after nephrectomy is of no proven benefit.

Indications for nephron-sparing surgery, which removes the tumor and leaves the rest of the normal kidney, are situations in which a radical nephrectomy would result in an anephric patient requiring dialysis. Examples include bilateral renal cell carcinomas and renal cell carcinoma in a solitary functioning kidney. In carefully selected patients with stage I renal cell carcinomas the long-term prognosis after nephron-sparing surgery is favorable and exceeds that of patients after nephrectomy and dialysis. Experience with nephron-sparing surgery in patients who would otherwise be candidates for radical nephrectomy or in patients with stage IV renal cell carcinoma is more limited.

The definitive indication for nephrectomy in patients with documented stage IV disease is symptom palliation. Pain, hemorrhage, and systemic symptoms may be relieved after nephrectomy. In the asymptomatic stage IV patient, a so-called adjunctive nephrectomy is controversial. It has been suggested that nephrectomy improves patient survival or increases the possibility of response to immunotherapy. However, it is not possible to separate the therapeutic benefits of nephrectomy from the patient selection factors for nephrectomy, which are likely to identify patients with inherently more favorable prognoses or greater chances of responding to immunotherapy. Prospective randomized controlled trials of the value of adjunctive nephrectomy in stage IV patients are under way. Except for a clinical trial, nephrectomy cannot be routinely recommended for asymptomatic patients with stage IV renal cell carcinoma.

Patients with renal cell carcinoma may have a solitary metastasis at the time of the initial diagnosis, or they may develop it after nephrectomy. After resection of a solitary metastasis, particularly in the lung, long-term disease-free survival has been observed in some patients. This approach may be advocated for selected patients.

Following nephrectomy there is no established role for additional systemic forms of therapy (called adjuvant therapy) to reduce the risks of relapse. Treatment options for patients with stage IV disease include immunotherapy and chemotherapy, and in selected patients surgical removal of metastatic deposits. Interferons possess limited activity in renal cell carcinoma with objective tumor regressions of 12 to 14%. Recombinant human interleukin-2 (rh IL-2) induces partial tumor regression in about 13% of patients and complete tumor regression in 7%. Occasionally, patients experiencing complete tumor regression have remained free of disease for more than 5 years. rh IL-2 toxicity can be severe. The vascular leak syndrome characterized by a generalized increase in capillary permeability, fluid retention, and hypotension can be life threatening. Lowering the dose of rh IL-2 may lessen the toxicity but preserve the antitumor activity.

Adding lymphokine-activated killer cells (LAK) to rh IL-2 does not provide additional benefits over rh IL-2 alone. Outpatient combinations of rh IL-2 and interferon appear to offer benefits similar to rh IL-2 alone, although the toxicity of outpatient regimens may be lower. Tumor-infiltrating lymphocytes isolated from primary renal cell carcinomas can be expanded and activated *ex vivo* and reinfused into the patient. Too few patients with renal cell carcinoma have been treated with tumor-infiltrating lymphocytes to determine whether this therapy is superior to rh IL-2 alone. New therapeutic approaches for metastatic renal cell carcinoma, including autologous tumor vaccines and new cytokines such as IL-12, are being evaluated in the clinic.

Most chemotherapy drugs have little or no activity in renal cell carcinoma. Two drugs with limited activity are vinblastine and floxuridine, which induce objective tumor regression in about 10 and 16% of patients respectively. Normal proximal tubules and renal cell carcinomas express high levels of the p-glycoprotein, which mediates multidrug resistance. Calcium channel blockers and other drugs that interfere with the function of the p-glycoprotein are being tested in clinical trials. The hormones medroxyprogesterone acetate and tamoxifen induce objective tumor regression in 1 to 2% and < 10% of renal cell carcinoma patients, respectively.

WILMS' TUMOR (NEPHROBLASTOMA). Wilms' tumors are rare malignant tumors of the kidney occurring predominantly in children younger than 4 years of age. A gene located on chromosome 11 is abnormally mutated in Wilms' tumor. Signs and symptoms of Wilms' tumor in decreasing order of frequency are abdominal mass, pain, hematuria, hypertension, and fever. CT or MRI is useful in identifying the tumors and assessing the extent of disease. In 5% of patients the tumors are bilateral, and in 15% of patients metastases are present at the time of the initial diagnosis. The most common sites of metastases are the lung and liver. Neuroblastoma, another common malignant pediatric tumor that may involve the kidney, may be distinguished from Wilms' tumor by the production

TABLE 91–1. STAGING OF RENAL CELL CARCINOMA

Robson Stage	Robson Description	TNM Stage	T	N	M	5-Year Survival (%)
I	Tumor confined to renal parenchyma	I II	T1 T2	No	Mo	66–88
II	Tumor invades perinephric fat	III	T3a	No, 1	Mo	47–68
IIIa	Tumor invades renal vein or vena cava	III	T3b	No, 1	Mo	35–60
IIIb	Tumor in regional lymph nodes	III	T1–3	N1–3	Mo	15–30
IV	Tumor in adjacent or distant organs	IV	T4 Any T	N1–3 Any N	Mo M1	2–13

Modified from Robson CJ, Churchill BM, Anderson W: The results of radical nephrectomy for renal cell carcinoma. J Urol 101:297, 1969; and Linehan WM, Shipley WU, Longo DL: Cancer of the kidney and ureter. *In* Devita VT, Hellman S, Rosenberg SA (eds.): Principles and Practice of Oncology. Philadelphia, JB Lippincott, 1993, pp 1023–1051.

of urinary vanillylmandelic acid and homovanillic acid, which are increased in over 90% of neuroblastoma patients. Treatment involves surgical excising of the tumor, followed by multiagent chemotherapy for all patients, and radiation for patients with tumor in a more advanced stage. In selected instances, bone marrow transplantation may be used. The combined method treatment approach cures nearly 90% of patients.

Latif F, Tory K, Gnarra J, et al.: Identification of the von Hippel-Lindau disease tumor suppressor gene. Science 28:1317, 1993. *The cloning of the von Hippel-Lindau gene.*

Olsson CA, Sawczuk IS (eds.): Urol Clin North Am vol. 20, no. 2, 1993. *Excellent chapters on pathology of benign and malignant kidney tumors, problems in the radiologic diagnosis of renal parenchymal tumors, renal-sparing surgery for renal cell carcinoma, surgery of renal cell carcinoma, and cytotoxic chemotherapy for advanced renal cell carcinoma.*

Pizzo PA, Horowitz ME, Poplack DG, et al.: Solid tumors of childhood. *In* Devita VT, Hellman S, Rosenberg SA (eds.): Principles and Practice of Oncology. Philadelphia, JB Lippincott, 1993, p 1744. *A review of Wilms' tumor.*

Rosenberg SA, Yang JC, Topalian SL, et al.: Treatment of 283 consecutive patients with metastatic melanoma or renal cell cancer using high-dose bolus interleukin 2. JAMA 271:907, 1994. *A large experience with high-dose interleukin-2 treatment of renal cell carcinoma and melanoma.*

BLADDER CANCER AND OTHER UROTHELIAL CANCERS

EPIDEMIOLOGY AND ETIOLOGY. Tumors that arise from the transitional cell lining of the urinary tract are referred to as urothelial cancers. Over 90% of these tumors are transitional cell carcinomas; the remainder are squamous cell carcinomas and adenocarcinomas. These tumors may arise from any location where urothelium exists, including the collecting system of the kidney (i.e., the calices and renal pelvis), the ureter, the bladder, and the urethra, and from within the urothelial-lined ducts of the prostate. The most common malignant urothelial tumor is bladder cancer, accounting for 51,200 new cases and 10,600 deaths in 1994. Urothelial cancers arising in the renal pelvis are histologically and clinically distinct from the more common renal parenchymal tumors. These latter tumors, called renal cell carcinomas, are usually adenocarcinomas. Similarly, the rare transitional cell carcinomas that arise from within the prostate are distinct from the much more common prostatic adenocarcinomas.

Urothelial cancers have long been recognized as attributable to environmental toxins (see Ch. 13). Studies 100 years ago determined that exposure to aromatic amines caused an increased likelihood of developing transitional cell carcinomas of the bladder. Workers within the dye industry in Germany, particularly those who distilled 2-naphthylamine, had a strikingly high incidence of bladder cancer. Since that time, numerous other aromatic amines have been associated with bladder cancer, as have the industries in which these chemicals are used, such as the rubber, electric, cable, paint, and textile industries. In today's workplace the relative risk of developing urothelial cancers due to environmental exposures is low. Tobacco use, however, is probably the most important etiologic factor with respect to bladder cancer in the United States; it may account for one half the cases currently diagnosed (see Ch. 9.4). Worldwide, infection with *Schistosoma haematobium (Bilharzia)* accounts for a large proportion of bladder cancer cases, particularly in endemic areas such as the Nile River delta in Egypt (see Ch. 385). Bladder cancer occurring as a result of *S. haematobium* frequently is squamous cell carcinoma, although transitional cell carcinomas may occur. Two other factors associated with an excess risk of urothelial cancers are long-term administration of cyclophosphamide, an alkylating agent used in treating many malignant diseases, and chronic excessive use of the analgesic phenacetin. Transitional cell carcinoma of the renal pelvis and ureters are more likely to occur with analgesic abuse.

Our understanding of the molecular basis of bladder cancer over the past few years has increased. Chromosome 9 abnormalities, particularly monosomy, is a common early event in bladder cancer, and abnormalities of 11p and 17p, including mutations in the P-53 gene, may be found in more advanced tumors.

The majority of urothelial cancers are confined to the transitional cell epithelial layer and do not invade into the lamina propria or muscularis layers. Such tumors tend to be polypoid in appearance and papillary in configuration. With invasion beyond the transitional cell layer, the potential for metastatic spread increases dramatically. Higher-grade cancers tend to have a greater propensity for invasion and metastatic spread, as do tumors that possess P-53 mutations. Urothelial cancers have a high propensity for multifocality, i.e.,

multiple simultaneous tumors and polychronotropism, i.e., recurring over time. Tumors arising in the bladder most commonly recur elsewhere in the bladder and rarely in the renal pelvis or ureter, whereas tumors that arise from the renal pelvis or ureter frequently (25% of the time) recur in the bladder. Recent studies have supported the concept that these multifocal and polychronotropic tumors are clonal in origin, suggesting a common malignant stem cell abnormality and/or reimplantation of tumor cells as a dominant mechanism for tumor recurrence. Although tumors confined to the epithelial layer may recur and require treatment because of bleeding or other problems, it is tumors that invade the deeper layers of the wall that may compromise survival.

BLADDER CANCER

PATHOLOGY AND STAGING. Bladder cancer, the most common urothelial malignant tumor, is diagnosed three times as frequently in men as in women. Death occurs in a fraction of patients and is largely attributable to the uncontrolled growth of metastatic deposits of tumor. Fortunately the majority of patients with bladder cancer have superficial bladder tumors confined to the transitional cell layer, which have low potential for metastatic spread. One particularly troublesome type of superficial bladder cancer is carcinoma *in situ* (CIS), a multifocal disease that can persist despite treatment. If persistent, CIS may progress to invasive bladder cancer. Although superficial tumors are very common, few patients ultimately succumb to their disease. The staging of bladder cancer is shown in Table 91–2.

CLINICAL MANIFESTATIONS AND DIAGNOSIS. Hematuria and irritative bladder symptoms such as dysuria or urinary frequency are the most common presenting symptoms of bladder cancer. Most patients have hematuria, frequently gross but occasionally microscopic. The hematuria can be episodic. Irritative urinary symptoms such as the urgency, dysuria, frequency without hematuria, particularly in the absence of infection, should lead to an evaluation for bladder cancer. Larger tumors may cause bladder outlet obstruction or ureteral obstruction resulting in hydronephrosis. Bilateral ureteral obstruction leading to azotemia is rare. Bladder tumors may cause pelvic pain by infiltrating regional nerves or bone, may cause lymphedema as a result of lymphatic obstruction from lymph node metastasis or may present as manifestations of metastatic disease to bone, lungs, or liver. If bladder cancer is suspected an intravenous pyelogram (IVP) should be obtained to locate filling defects in the bladder and in the upper tracts. In addition, cystoscopy should be performed to locate the tumor and to facilitate biopsy for pathologic confirmation and to determine depth of invasion. Urinary cytology is a useful adjunct in the initial assessment and follow-up evaluation of treatment in patients who have tumors that are invasive into the muscular layer of the bladder or beyond. Evaluation of metastatic sites is essential, including abdominal pelvic CT, chest radiograph, and bone scan.

TREATMENT AND PROGNOSIS. Bladder tumors confined to the transitional cell layer are generally treated only with transurethral excision. These tumors tend to recur, and current practice dictates frequent cystoscopy and removal of recurrent tumors, although the value of this practice is uncertain. Higher-grade tumors

TABLE 91–2. STAGING OF BLADDER CANCER

	Marshall-Jewett	TNM*
Confined to mucosa	0	Ta
Carcinoma *in situ*	0	Tis
Infiltration of submucosa	A	T1
Infiltration of superficial muscle	B1	T2
Infiltration of deep muscle	B2	T3a
Perivesical infiltration	C	T3b
Adjacent organ		
Prostate	D1	T4a
Uterus/Vagina	D1	
Fixed to pelvic or abdominal wall	D1	T4b
Nodes positive (pelvic only)	D1	T (any), N+
Distant metastases or nodes positive above aortic bifurcation	D2	T (any), N (any), M1

* (Tumor, Nodes, Metastasis)

confined to the transitional cell layer and high-grade flat tumors, so-called CIS, may be treated with intravesical chemotherapy or immunotherapy with bacille Calmette-Guérin (BCG), since use of intravesical agents may deter or prevent the development of more deeply invasive cancers that have greater metastatic potential. Bladder tumors that invade into the deeper layers of the bladder wall, in general, require more definitive therapy. The preferred treatment is radical cystectomy (i.e., total removal of the bladder), with urinary diversion in the form of an ileal loop, a continent reservoir, or an orthotopic neobladder. Alternative strategies include attempts to preserve bladder function with either partial cystectomy or chemotherapy coupled with radiation therapy. Such treatments may be appropriate for a subset of patients. For patients with tumors that have invaded into the deeper layers of the bladder wall, the likelihood of occult distant spread and future recurrence at metastatic sites is quite high and may be diminished with the use of chemotherapy after cystectomy. For patients with metastatic bladder cancer, polyagent chemotherapy may be life prolonging and under rare circumstances curative.

TRANSITIONAL CELL CARCINOMAS OF THE RENAL PELVIS, CALICES, AND URETER

Similar to bladder tumors, upper tract tumors frequently present as gross or microscopic hematuria. However, these tumors may present with ureteral obstruction and pain due to renal colic. The diagnosis is strongly suspected with the finding of a filling defect in a calix, infundibulum, renal pelvis, or ureter, but cystoscopy with retrograde pyelography with cytology or ureteroscopy may be required to document the lesion.

TREATMENT AND PROGNOSIS. Many of these lesions are superficial in nature, i.e., are confined to the transitional cell layer and are low grade. Selected cases may be treated with less radical therapy, i.e., segmental resection, particularly in patients with solitary kidneys. Higher-grade and/or tumors that invade more deeply into the wall of the ureter or renal pelvis are associated with a greater likelihood of metastatic spread. With definitive treatment, which is nephroureterectomy and removal of a cuff of bladder, the prognosis for such tumors is excellent. The role of chemotherapy as an adjunct to surgery in such cases is less well documented. Before surgery, it is essential to evaluate other areas in the urothelium by IVP, cystoscopy, and retrograde pyelography because of the high likelihood of contralateral kidney involvement and simultaneous or subsequent bladder involvement. Invasive transitional cell carcinomas of the renal pelvis, calices, and ureter have a high propensity for metastatic spread. The pattern of spread is similar to that of bladder cancer to lymph nodes, liver, lung, and bone. Multiagent chemotherapy under such circumstances may be of benefit.

Kaufman DS, Shipley WU, Griffin PP, et al.: Selective bladder preservation by combination treatment of invasive bladder cancer. N Engl J Med 329:1377, 1993. *Documents utility of chemotherapy used with radiation for invasive bladder cancer.*

Macfarlane MT, Figlin RA, deKernion JB: Neoplasms of the bladder. *In* Holland JF, Frei E, Bast RC, et al. (eds.): Cancer Medicine, 3rd ed. Philadelphia, Lea & Febiger, 1993, p 1546. *A comprehensive view of bladder neoplasms.*

Richie JP, Kantoff PW: Neoplasms of the renal pelvis and ureter. *In* Holland JF, Frei E, Bast RC, et al. (eds.): Cancer Medicine, 3rd ed. Philadelphia, Lea & Febiger, 1993, p 1539. *A good general review of these unusual tumors.*

Sternberg CN, Yagoda A, Scher HI, et al.: M-VAC (methotrexate, vinblastine, docorubicin and cisplatin) for advanced transitional cell carcinoma of the urothelium. J Urol 139:461, 1988. *Describes utility of combination chemotherapy in urothelial cancers.*

PART XI

GASTROINTESTINAL DISEASES

92 INTRODUCTION TO GASTROINTESTINAL DISEASES

Robert K. Ockner

Because of its obvious importance in the digestion and assimilation of nutrients, and the consequences of fluid and electrolyte losses resulting from vomiting, diarrhea, and other disturbances of gastrointestinal function, the important role of the digestive system in nutrition and fluid balance has long been recognized. More recent advances, however, have demonstrated that this organ system plays an equally fundamental role in other systemic phenomena. For example, its neural pathways and mediators comprise a specialized component of the nervous system, and studies of the intestinal immune system have contributed substantially to elucidating the mechanisms involved in development of and resistance to diseases caused by infectious agents, from viral to metazoan. Similarly, accumulating evidence indicates that the gastrointestinal system, including the liver, is crucial in the regulation of intermediary metabolism, i.e., nutrition at the cellular level. Finally, elucidation of the mechanisms involved in regulation of normal and abnormal cell growth, differentiation, and tumorigenesis have been especially impressive in regard to the digestive system and liver, and have provided significant insights into these broadly important processes. Fundamentally scientific advances such as these have spawned equally profound changes in medical practice, ranging from application of molecular approaches to disease prevention, diagnosis, and treatment, to breakthroughs in nonoperative radiographic and endoscopic therapeutic intervention, minimally invasive surgery, and organ transplantation.

Despite these impressive advances, however, and those which are certain to follow, the cornerstone of medicine will remain the thoughtful, compassionate, and efficient care of the patient. This, in turn, continues to depend on a careful and thorough history and physical examination, upon which a sound differential diagnosis and selection of appropriate diagnostic and therapeutic options must be based.

HISTORY

A carefully obtained history almost always provides information important to understanding the basis for the patient's symptoms and to planning diagnostic studies. Systemic symptoms, such as anorexia, weight loss, fatigue, fever, and emotional changes, are nonspecific but may be prominent. When caused by digestive disorders, these symptoms are usually associated with other evidence, such as abdominal pain, diarrhea, or jaundice, that more directly links them to digestive disease. Occasionally, however, systemic symptoms may be the only clinical manifestations of such processes as inflammatory bowel disease, abdominal lymphoma, and pancreatic cancer. Similarly, systemic diseases that secondarily involve the digestive organs, such as sarcoidosis and vasculitis, may be manifested only by general and constitutional symptoms. In these settings, special diagnostic studies, such as laboratory tests, abdominal angiography, and liver biopsy, may be needed to document digestive system involvement. As in all branches of clinical medicine, the investigation and assessment of symptoms, through discussions with the patient and others, require a careful, systematic, and, to the extent possible, quantitative approach.

Abdominal pain or discomfort is one of the most important and common presenting symptoms, and its accurate interpretation requires careful analysis. It is discussed in greater detail below. Among the other symptoms that must be specifically addressed are *dysphagia* (difficulty in swallowing), *odynophagia* (painful swallowing), *heartburn, nausea, vomiting, hematemesis, melena, diarrhea,* and *constipation.* For all symptoms, it is necessary to be as quantitative as possible (e.g., with respect to frequency, duration, or severity of a symptom, volume of stool or vomitus, and interval between aggravating or mitigating factors and the onset of their effects).

Mood and emotional stress may aggravate or even seem to produce many digestive symptoms. Because of the substantial role that emotions may play, digestive complaints are often more difficult to interpret than are symptoms referable to other organ systems. While emotional factors within the range of "normal" may influence many gastrointestinal functions and symptoms, certain eating disorders, such as anorexia nervosa and bulimia (see Ch. 195), and some cases of morbid obesity (see Ch. 196), are more often associated with clinically significant psychopathology. A patient's psychological profile may sometimes be helpful in suggesting a diagnosis of irritable bowel syndrome, for example, which otherwise depends entirely on exclusion of demonstrable "organic" pathology. Notably, disorders of swallowing are almost always attributable to demonstrable organic disease, unlike other complaints such as abdominal discomfort or change in bowel habit. Although emotional factors may profoundly influence digestive function and the management of digestive diseases, there is no evidence that they alone account for the cause or pathogenesis of diseases that in the past have been so represented, such as peptic ulcer disease or ulcerative colitis. Nor does convincing evidence exist that certain personality types are predisposed to these disorders.

The *background upon which a symptom occurs* is also quite important. Thus, abdominal pain or melena in a patient with a documented history of peptic ulcer suggests ulcer recurrence. Pain, bilious vomiting, or diarrhea in a patient with previous ulcer surgery, on the other hand, may be evidence of a complication of the surgery itself. Jaundice in a patient with chronic ulcerative colitis could be consistent with any of several possible explanations, including medication-induced hemolysis or liver injury, viral hepatitis transmitted by blood transfusion, or primary sclerosing cholangitis. Finally, a history of alcohol abuse may provide the crucial information needed to account for any of several manifestations of digestive disease, including jaundice, gastrointestinal hemorrhage, and severe abdominal pain caused by acute pancreatitis.

In the initial evaluation of the patient with manifestations of digestive disease, the medical history must not be limited to matters directly related to gastroenterology. For example, epigastric pain or gastrointestinal hemorrhage in a patient taking nonsteroidal anti-inflammatory agents suggests gastric erosions induced by the medication. Sudden onset of severe abdominal pain in a patient with known systemic vasculitis or advanced atherosclerosis immediately raises the possibility of intestinal ischemia. In many instances, patients and those close to them are unable to provide sufficient detail or documentation. In such cases, diagnosis and management may depend critically on access to medical records, including previous clinical and laboratory findings, biopsy and imaging studies, diagnoses, and treatments.

PHYSICAL EXAMINATION

A thorough physical examination is also an essential part of the initial evaluation of the patient with apparent digestive disease. It may provide crucial information about the patient's general health, for example, to determine suitability for urgent surgery. It may also provide clues to a systemic explanation for abdominal complaints. For example, severe abdominal pain may be a manifestation of sickle cell disease, while intestinal pseudo-obstruction may develop in a patient with progressive systemic sclerosis. Significant weight loss may reflect anorexia, dysphagia, malabsorption, or the catabolic effects of inflammatory or neoplastic disease. Finally, the general physical examination may provide clues to the extent or severity of newly recognized digestive disease, e.g., cutaneous spider angiomata or asterixis in a patient with liver disease, or uveitis or erythema nodosum in a patient with inflammatory bowel disease.

Examination of the abdomen may disclose distention caused by ileus, intestinal obstruction, ascites, or mass, or may demonstrate the abdominal venous collaterals associated with portal hypertension or inferior vena cava obstruction. On palpation, the patient may intentionally tense the muscles of the abdominal wall in order to mitigate the actual or feared discomfort resulting from pressure of the examiner's hand on a tender organ or mass ("voluntary guarding"), or the musculature may be reflexly and involuntarily in spasm or rigid because of peritonitis-induced irritation of nerve endings in the parietal peritoneum. Midline tenderness in the epigastrium is typical of peptic ulcer disease or pancreatitis, whereas right upper quadrant tenderness suggests disease of the liver or biliary tract. If the tenderness is well localized to the region of the midclavicular line below the right costal margin, inflammation of the gallbladder is suggested, whereas tenderness just below and along much of the costal margin, especially if associated with the liver edge, suggests hepatic inflammation or a distended liver capsule. Tenderness in the right lower quadrant, possibly associated with guarding or spasm, is consistent with acute appendicitis, whereas a tender mass in this area suggests Crohn's disease or other chronic inflammatory or neoplastic process involving the ileocecal area, such as tuberculosis or lymphoma. Similar findings in the left lower quadrant, on the other hand (i.e., suggestive of a "left-sided appendicitis") are consistent with sigmoid diverticulitis.

Examination of the liver should include an attempt not only to identify its lower edge but also to characterize the edge with regard to form (e.g., sharp and nontender as in normal individuals, or rounded and possibly irregular as in cirrhosis) and consistency (firm as in cirrhosis or hard as in cancer), to determine whether it is tender, and to measure its cephalad-caudad span by defining its upper and lower borders. The clinical detection of ascites is often possible by demonstrating flank dullness, shifting dullness, or fluid wave, but if the volume of ascites is small, the relative nonspecificity of these signs makes their interpretation uncertain, in which case sonography may be necessary. Auscultation may detect hepatic friction rub, suggesting malignancy. Abdominal bruits indicate turbulent vascular flow, usually in the mesenteric, splenic, or renal arteries, but their correlation with intestinal ischemia is poor. Abdominal aortic aneurysms can be detected by deep palpation in the epigastrium. Their size and the presence or absence of symptoms are important determinants of their prognosis with respect to the probability of rupture and the possible need for elective resection. An abdominal mass also may be found in association with pancreatic pseudocyst, Crohn's disease, abscess, and malignancy.

LABORATORY EVALUATION AND SPECIAL TESTS

Certain tests, such as routine blood counts and tests for fecal occult blood, are sufficiently informative and inexpensive that they may be considered standard for evaluating virtually all patients with digestive disease. Other studies, including those to assess intestinal absorption or the status of the liver, are employed as indicated. (Laboratory tests for the liver are discussed in Ch. 116.) Endoscopy and the various methods for imaging play an essential role in the diagnosis of certain disorders, and therapeutic endoscopy, interventional radiology, and minimally invasive surgery are increasingly contributing to treatment of some conditions, replacing more conventional surgical approaches (see Ch. 93 and 94). Rapid scientific and technologic progress in these areas will require continuing evolution of clinical decision making with respect to their use. Various biopsy and fine-needle aspiration techniques are available for the histopathologic characterization of known or suspected disease, and esophageal manometry may be useful in the diagnosis of certain esophageal diseases (see Ch. 97). The decision to use these options may be straightforward or complex. Without exception, such decisions must involve assessment of their documented efficacy or accuracy, available alternatives, safety, cost, and possible impact on management.

SELECTED SYMPTOMS OF DIGESTIVE DISEASE

The symptoms discussed in the following section may occur in many digestive diseases. The reader is referred to other chapters as indicated for discussions of heartburn and dysphagia (see Ch. 97), diarrhea (see Ch. 102), constipation (see Ch. 101), malabsorption (see Ch. 103), and jaundice (see Ch. 115).

ABDOMINAL PAIN. Abdominal pain, or a variant of it, such as indigestion, is one of the most important symptoms of digestive disease, often providing the patient the first hint that something is wrong and providing the physician with information helpful in diagnosis. Abdominal pain can be characterized in terms of its location, quality, severity, and temporal pattern. Because it is, by definition, "subjective," the significance of pain in relation to other symptoms and to underlying disease processes can be evaluated only by thoughtful and systematic discussions with the patient.

Empiric observations have related specific pain patterns to a particular organ or other site of origin. Esophageal pain, such as occurs in spasm or esophagitis, is located retrosternally, usually at or above the level of disease. If the pain is severe, it may be felt in the back. Pain arising from the stomach or duodenum is also midline and usually perceived in the epigastrium; if severe, it too may be felt in the back, a phenomenon that does not necessarily imply perforation of an ulcer. Small intestinal pain, as occurs with obstruction or ischemia, is usually periumbilical, and if severe, may also be felt in the back. Right lower quadrant pain suggests involvement of the cecum or appendix, and pain in the lower midabdomen suggests colon and rectum. Pain arising from the liver, gallbladder, or common bile duct is usually felt in the right upper quadrant. Pancreatic pain is localized to the mid- to left side of the epigastrium but may also be felt in the back or the left shoulder, depending on its severity and on whether there is involvement of diaphragmatic nerves, e.g., during acute pancreatitis.

Abdominal pain is diverse in type, and its quality is an important characteristic that reflects the dual nature of pain fibers and pathways that serve the intra-abdominal structures: *(1) Visceral fibers,* largely type C, are present in the muscular walls of the hollow viscera and in the capsule of the solid organs; they conduct afferent impulses from these sources via the vagus nerve. Innervation is usually bilateral. Pain conducted by these fibers is often perceived as midline in location, poorly localized but generally dull, cramping, or burning in quality, gradual in onset, prolonged in duration, and associated with autonomic manifestations such as nausea, vomiting, and diaphoresis. *(2) Somatic fibers,* largely type A-delta present in skin and muscle, innervate principally the parietal peritoneum and enter the spinal cord via the intercostal nerves. Pain conducted by these fibers tends to be sharper, more intense, more sudden in onset, and far more precisely localized than visceral pain. For example, the pain associated with intestinal obstruction, early acute cholecystitis, or uncomplicated peptic ulcer is typically visceral, whereas that associated with acute peritonitis resulting from ulcer perforation is usually somatic.

Abdominal pain can be caused by (1) tension, stretching, or forceful contraction of the musculature of a hollow viscus, such as the intestine or gallbladder; (2) ischemia, presumably mediated by the local accumulation of metabolic intermediates, and chemical mediators of inflammation; (3) local or generalized inflammation of the parietal peritoneum; (4) neoplastic or fibrotic involvement of nerve fibers; or (5) extra-abdominal causes, such as certain metabolic disorders (e.g., acute intermittent porphyria) or extra-abdominal pain referred to an intra-abdominal location.

Significant information may be obtained by assessing the temporal characteristics of the pain, its possible intermittency, its relationship to certain events such as eating or sleeping, and factors that precipitate or alleviate it, such as its relationship to eating, bowel pattern, sleep, or emotional state. For example, duodenal ulcer pain is not usually present in the morning on arising but typically begins 30 minutes to 1 hour after meals or during the night, when it may awaken the patient and elicit the desire for food or antacid. Atypical manifestations of digestive disorders are common, especially among older patients and those taking certain medications such as corticosteroids. In both of these settings, for example, acute cholecystitis may be painless.

DISORDERS OF APPETITE AND FEEDING BEHAVIOR. The control of feeding behavior is complex and is often disturbed as an early manifestation of digestive disease. Subjectively, several sensations are involved. *Appetite* is the desire to ingest food, whether or not there is a physiological need for nutrient. *Hunger,* in contrast, is the perceived need for nutrient replacement and is usually associated with a particular epigastric sensation of food craving ("hunger pangs"). *Satiety* is the diminished sensation of appetite and of hunger produced by feeding, whereas *anorexia* is the absence of appetite and hunger, usually because of illness, physiological or pharmacological factors, or emotion. "Feeding" and "satiety" centers in the hypothalamus and the neuroendocrine tracts associated with them play an important role in the regulation of feeding behavior. These centers appear to respond to changes in plasma levels of glucose, free fatty acids, and amino acids and are influenced directly or indirectly by concentrations of humoral or paracrine mediators, such as insulin, glucagon, cholecystokinin, α_2-agonist sympathomimetic amines, opioids, growth hormone–releasing factor, somatostatin, gastrin, bombesin, pancreatic polypeptide, and possibly other neuropeptides.

The pathophysiologic basis for the appetite-suppressant effects of many illnesses and of digestive diseases in particular is not well understood, although presumably the regulatory factors just noted and possibly other factors as well are involved. Anorexia nervosa, bulimia, and hyperphagia seem to represent instances of a predominantly emotional basis for abnormal feeding behavior, but the

pathophysiology of these illnesses is not known. Rarely, hyperphagia may reflect hypothalamic disease.

NAUSEA AND VOMITING. The unpleasant triad of nausea, retching, and vomiting serves teleologically as a method to eliminate potentially harmful substances from the upper gastrointestinal tract. The process also can occur as a result of various chemical, humoral, or physical influences or disease states. *Nausea,* an undefinable and unmistakable sensation mediated via unknown neural pathways, is associated with hypersalivation, diminished gastric tone and peristalsis, increased duodenal tone, and duodenal-gastric reflux. *Retching* is characterized by spasmodic respiratory movements against a closed glottis with contractions of the abdominal musculature, during which the pyloric sphincter is closed and the lower esophageal sphincter relaxed (Fig. 92–1). Repeated herniations of the abdominal esophagus and gastric cardia during this phase may account for the occasional occurrence of Mallory-Weiss tears or the Boerhaave syndrome (see Ch. 97). During *vomiting* itself, a sustained contraction of the abdominal musculature associated with the status of the gastric sphincters noted above results in a forceful expulsion of gastric contents. Other physiological phenomena may accompany the process, including changes in cardiac rate and rhythm and in intestinal and colonic motility.

The initiation and coordination of these events depend on two specialized areas of the brain, i.e., the vomiting center in the lateral reticular formation and the chemoreceptor trigger zone (CTZ) in the area postrema in the floor of the fourth ventricle. The vomiting center, which is excited by visceral afferent fibers from the gastrointestinal tract, serves to coordinate other medullary centers in producing the patterned response to the variety of noxious stimuli and disease processes that affect the digestive tract, mesentery, peritoneum, and ureters and that are associated with vomiting. An intact vomiting center is also required for the CTZ to cause vomiting. Because the CTZ is in a region in which the blood-brain barrier is poorly developed, it is influenced by a wide variety of endogenous and exogenous substances in plasma, including various chemical agents and transmitters. It also mediates radiation sickness and, in some species, motion sickness.

In approaching the patient with vomiting, its timing and the characteristics of the vomitus should be noted. For example, psy-

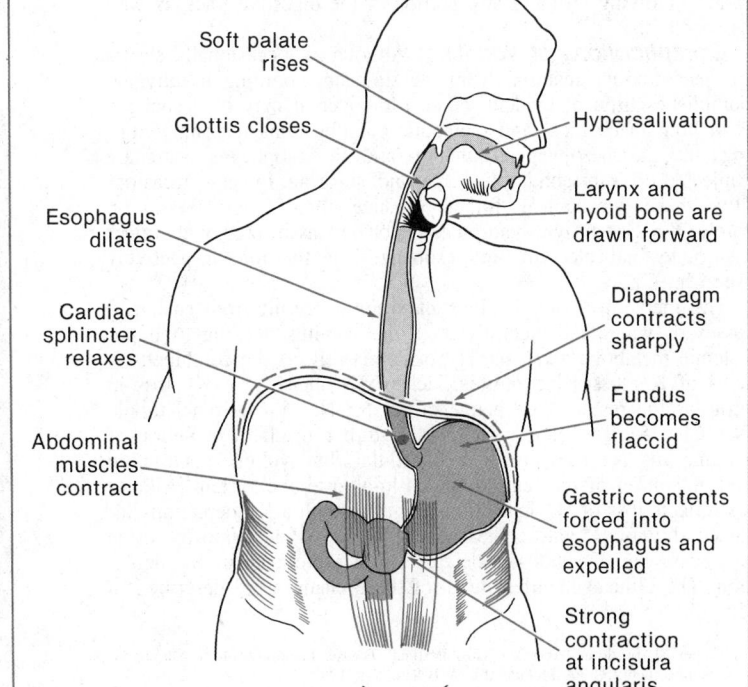

FIGURE 92–1. A diagrammatic summary of the act of vomiting. (From Feldman M: Nausea and vomiting. *In* Sleisenger M, Fordtran J [eds.]: Gastrointestinal Disease: Pathophysiology, Diagnosis, Management. 4th ed. Philadelphia, WB Saunders, 1989.)

TABLE 92–1. MAJOR CAUSES OF VOMITING

Psychogenic (including anorexia nervosa and bulimia)
Pain (including cardiac and abdominal)
Intracranial disease
Drugs and toxins
Pregnancy (including hyperemesis gravidarum and acute fatty liver of pregnancy)
Metabolic disorders
Cyclic vomiting of childhood
Gastric retention (including gastric dysmotility and pyloric obstruction)
High small intestinal obstruction
Visceral inflammation, ischemia, or perforation
Peritonitis

chogenic vomiting typically occurs during or soon after a meal and rarely if ever is delayed as long as 12 hours. Conversely, vomiting due to gastric outlet obstruction or impaired motility tends to be somewhat delayed and usually occurs more than an hour after a meal. Vomiting that occurs in the morning before breakfast is typical of pregnancy and may also be associated with alcohol ingestion, uremia, or increased intracranial pressure. The presence of old food suggests impaired gastric emptying, whereas undigested food may possibly have come from an esophageal or Zenker's diverticulum. The presence of bile in vomitus excludes obstruction at the gastric pylorus or in the proximal duodenum. A feculent odor suggests prominent bacterial overgrowth, as may occur in intestinal obstruction, gastrocolic fistula, or longstanding intestinal stasis syndrome.

The causes of vomiting are many and not limited to the digestive system or the abdomen (Table 92–1). Psychogenic vomiting is often associated with anorexia nervosa or bulimia. Intracranial diseases, especially those associated with increased pressure, are typically associated with "projectile" vomiting, but ordinary emesis also occurs. Many drugs and toxins cause vomiting, either through a direct effect on the CTZ or indirectly through their effects on the digestive tract, for example, the gastric mucosa. Vomiting is frequently a problem confined to the first trimester of pregnancy but in severe cases (hyperemesis gravidarum) may persist through the third trimester. The mechanism for cyclic vomiting of childhood is unknown. Certain metabolic diseases, including disorders of fatty acid and amino acid metabolism, may be associated with episodic vomiting and possibly stupor or coma. The intra-abdominal causes of vomiting include inflammation, obstruction, ischemia, and perforation involving virtually any portion of the digestive tract, as well as peritonitis.

Complications of Vomiting. Although it occasionally serves to eject noxious material from the stomach, vomiting usually accomplishes little of evident value. Moreover, it may be associated with both mechanical and metabolic complications. During vomiting, the gastroesophageal junction and the esophagus itself are subjected to substantial pressures and shearing forces. Occasionally, these mechanical forces produce the Mallory-Weiss or, rarely, the Boerhaave syndrome, which are associated with upper gastrointestinal bleeding and esophageal perforation, respectively (see Ch. 97).

The metabolic complications of vomiting result from sustained losses of water and electrolytes in the vomitus, leading to hypokalemic metabolic alkalosis. Hypokalemia reflects the combined effects of K^+ losses in vomitus, lack of K^+ intake, and K^+ loss in urine as the result of exchange of K^+ for Na^+ in the renal tubule (see Ch. 75). The latter process is in turn a result of depletion of volume and Na^+, leading to extracellular fluid volume contraction and activation of the renin-angiotensin-aldosterone system. Alkalosis reflects loss of H^+ in vomitus, together with a K^+ depletion–induced shift of H^+ into cells in exchange for K^+ and into the urine in response to the aldosterone effect in the presence of K^+ depletion. The clinical manifestations of these changes are described in Ch. 75.

Sleisenger M, Fordtran J (eds.): Gastrointestinal Disease: Pathophysiology, Diagnosis, Management. 5th ed. Philadelphia, WB Saunders, 1993.
Zakim D, Boyer T (eds.): Diseases of the Liver. 3rd ed. Philadelphia, WB Saunders, 1995.

Two recent, authoritative, and extensively referenced texts.

93 DIAGNOSTIC IMAGING PROCEDURES IN GASTROENTEROLOGY
Susan D. Wall

With the development of increasingly complex diagnostic imaging procedures in gastroenterology, the importance of direct communication with the consulting radiologist has increased. Clinical information regarding each diagnostic question is essential to tailoring the studies; none is "routine." In addition to conventional plain films of the abdomen and barium examination of the gastrointestinal tract, radiographic procedures of interest to the gastroenterologist include computed tomography, ultrasonography (including endoscopic and transrectal), endoscopic retrograde cholangiopancreatography, percutaneous transhepatic cholangiography, enteroclysis, radionuclide scanning, and magnetic resonance imaging.

Interventional radiology plays an important role in the management of some problems in gastroenterology. Interventional radiology procedures of the biliary tract include percutaneous transhepatic biliary drainage, stone extraction, and internal stenting, as well as percutaneous cholecystostomy. Balloon dilatation of the esophagus can be performed for benign stricture, and esophageal stenting is in the early stages of development. Transjugular intrahepatic portosystemic shunt (TIPS) (Fig. 93–1) can be life-saving in the acute management of esophageal hemorrhage particularly when varices have been unresponsive to sclerotherapy. TIPS is also being evaluated as treatment for portal hypertensive ascites that is recalcitrant to medical management. TIPS is a less invasive means of reducing portal hypertension than is the alternative, surgical shunting. Its long-term efficacy is still being evaluated, but it has been established as a means of palliative decompression of portal hypertension while awaiting liver transplantation. Furthermore, interventional radiology provides minimally invasive management of complications related to liver transplantation, gastrointestinal and biliary surgery, and, in particular, the recently developed laparoscopic cholecystectomy.

COMPUTED TOMOGRAPHY

The faster scan time (2 to 3 seconds) and higher spatial resolution available with current computed tomography (CT) have improved greatly the images of the alimentary tract as well as of the pancreas (Fig. 93–2), liver, and gallbladder. CT continues to be an

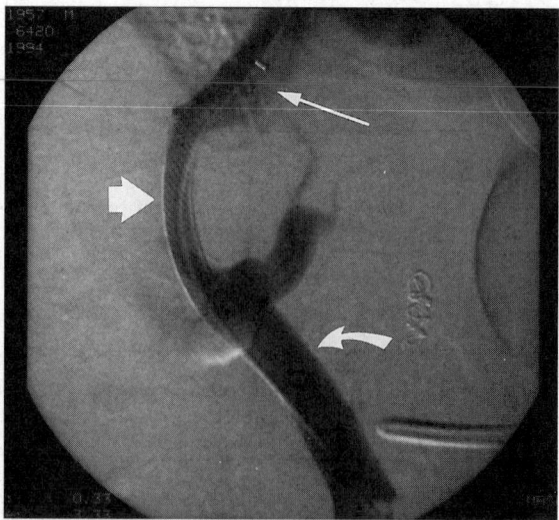

FIGURE 93–1. TIPS (Transjugular intrahepatic portosystemic shunt). Portal venography demonstrates a patent shunt *(solid arrow)* connecting the portal vein *(curved arrow)* with the right hepatic vein *(straight arrow)*. There has been decompression of large esophageal varices which do not fill. The TIPS was performed percutaneously via right internal jugular vein access by the interventional radiologist using conscious sedation.

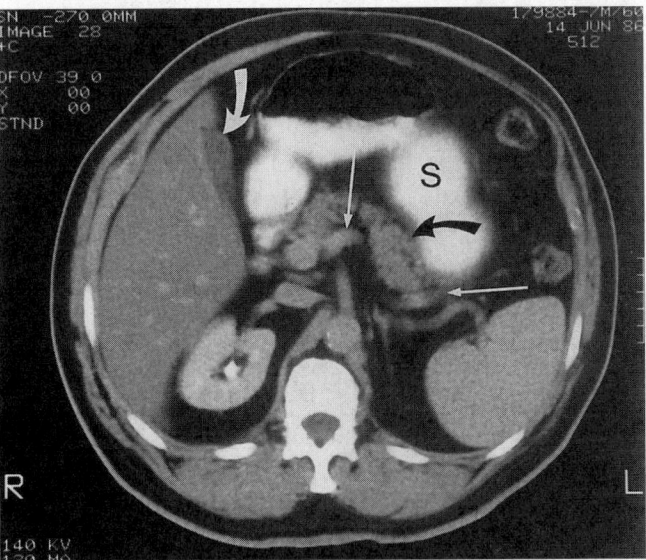

FIGURE 93–2. Normal CT. One-cm thick transverse image (supine, patient's right to reader's left) is at the level of the pancreas *(black arrow)*, which is behind the contrast-filled stomach (S). The splenic artery is posterior to the splenic vein *(straight white arrows)*, which abuts the posterior margin of the tail and neck of the pancreas. The density of the right kidney is enhanced because of intravenous contrast material. *Curved white arrow* points to gallbladder.

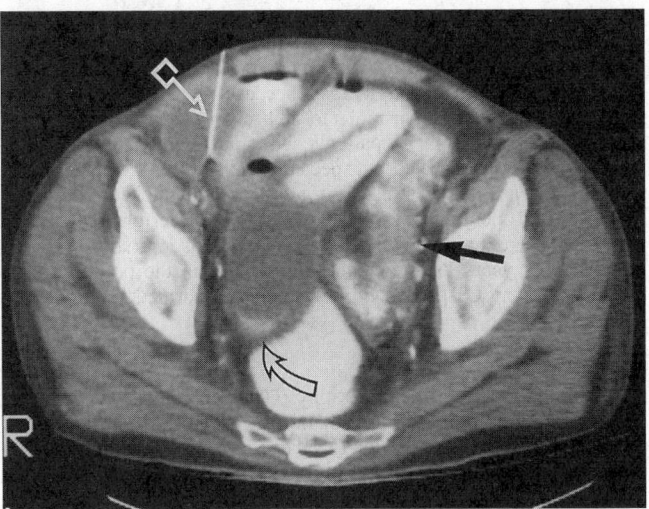

FIGURE 93–4. CT of diverticular abscess. Percutaneous fine-needle aspiration *(boxed white arrow)* of pelvic fluid collection diagnosed abscess in this patient with thickening of the wall of the sigmoid colon *(straight black arrow)* and diverticulitis. Note second fluid collection with small amount of contrast material *(curved open white arrow)* extravasated from the diseased colon. Abscesses were drained percutaneously until the patient was well enough for surgery.

important modality for investigating possible hepatic tumor, pancreatic carcinoma, and retroperitoneal adenopathy. Increasingly recognized is its contribution in evaluating the acute abdomen. When the diagnosis is unclear, CT is helpful in evaluation for possible pancreatitis (Fig. 93–3), perforated viscus, and subdiaphragmatic abscess, and in assessing the extent of Crohn's disease or bowel ischemia. CT can diagnose bowel obstruction, and it can demonstrate the site and often the cause. It can detect extraluminal abscess associated with appendicitis and diverticulitis (Fig. 93–4) and can sometimes help in the decision regarding surgical versus nonsurgical management. CT also can detect free intra- or retroperitoneal air and small amounts of contrast material that have extravasated from the gastrointestinal tract (Fig. 93–4); it provides excellent visualization of the mesentery. It is the modality of choice for evaluation of suspected complications of pancreatitis, such as necrosis, abscess, pseudocyst, and colonic or mesenteric inflammation (see Ch. 107). It is the best imaging study for diagnosis of aortoenteric fistula in

the patient with gastrointestinal bleeding and a history of aortofemoral bypass graft.

Percutaneous fine needle aspiration (PFNA) with CT guidance can diagnose pancreatic carcinoma, primary and metastatic tumor of the liver, and sometimes tumor involvement of enlarged lymph nodes. False-negative results occur, but this procedure usually obviates the need for diagnostic laparotomy. Furthermore, PFNA can diagnose a suspected abscess (see Fig. 93–4), which can be variable and nonspecific in its radiographic appearance. Percutaneous drainage of intra-abdominal or pelvic abscess with CT guidance is a nonsurgical treatment option for selected patients; it can palliate others until surgery is performed.

CT sometimes replaces barium contrast examination as the initial study of the gastrointestinal tract. Barium examination, which provides mucosal detail and delineation of the intraluminal contour, cannot demonstrate thickening of the wall and causes severe artifacts on CT images, precluding the possibility of a diagnostic study. Moreover, even unsuspected disease in the gastrointestinal tract, both primary and secondary, often is detected initially with CT. Assessment of thickening of the esophageal, gastric, and bowel wall is possible with current CT (Fig. 93–5), and surrounding organs may

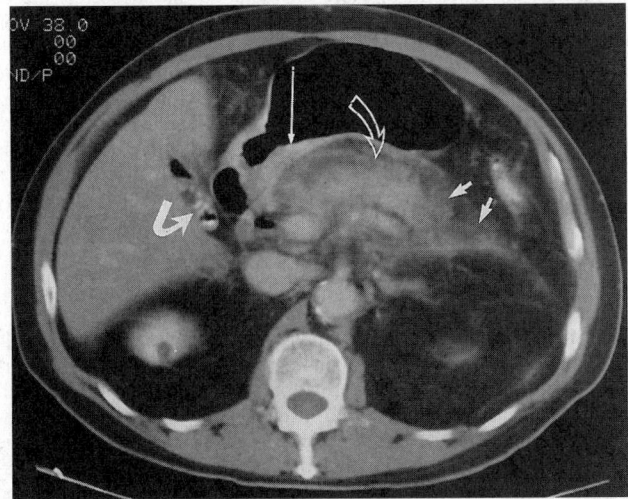

FIGURE 93–3. CT of acute pancreatitis. Abnormally dense fat surrounds the swollen pancreas *(open curved arrow)*. Free pancreatic fluid *(short arrows)* is present in the left anterior pararenal space, and the air-distended stomach has a thickened antral wall *(straight arrow)*. Note cholelithiasis *(closed curved arrow)*.

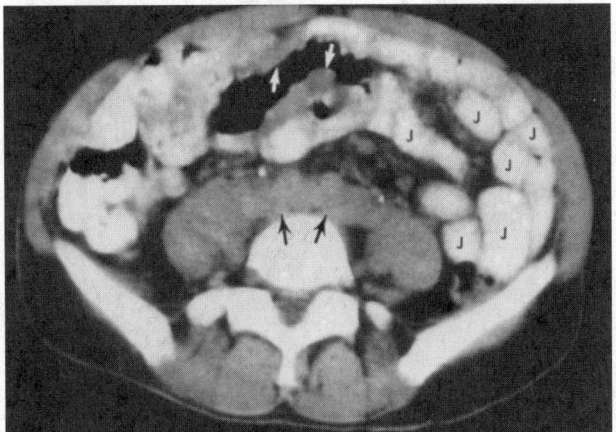

FIGURE 93–5. Small bowel Kaposi's sarcoma. Focal thickening *(white arrows)* of a single segment of small bowel is due to Kaposi's sarcoma in this patient with acquired immunodeficiency syndrome. Note the normal jejunum (J) proximal to the tumor and the retroperitoneal lymphadenopathy *(black arrows)* anterior to the spine.

also be evaluated, especially regarding inflammatory processes, such as diverticulitis, appendicitis, Crohn's disease, pancreatitis, and possible perforated ulcer. CT has limited value in the regional staging of gastrointestinal malignancies because of its limited accuracy in determining tumor invasion into adjacent tissues. Indications for preoperative evaluation of patients with rectosigmoid colon carcinoma, for example, include suspected extensive disease or complications such as perforation. CT is more helpful in determining recurrence postoperatively. A baseline study is performed 2 to 4 months after resection, with follow-up comparison studies every 6 months for 2 years. New or enlarging masses in the pelvis suggest recurrent tumor; CT-guided biopsy can be performed for tissue diagnosis.

ULTRASONOGRAPHY

Abdominal-pelvic ultrasonography (US) is noninvasive and inexpensive, requires no ionizing radiation, and can be performed with a portable unit. US is superior to other modalities in differentiating cystic from solid lesions and is highly sensitive in detecting ascites. Because of the superb ability to demonstrate gallstones (Fig. 93–6), US has replaced oral cholecystography for the diagnosis of cholelithiasis. US is an effective and efficient first examination of suspected liver tumors (see Ch. 124). It is the primary screening examination for hepatobiliary disease and often is the only study needed. Dilatation of the intra- and extrahepatic biliary system can be detected (Fig. 93–7), but the distal common bile duct often is not seen adequately with US. Similarly, the tail or body of the pancreas or both are well visualized less often than the head, principally because of interference by the overlying gas-filled bowel. US, which plays a complementary role with CT in many diseases, often is the preferred modality when follow-up examination is needed, as in pancreatic pseudocyst, abdominal aortic aneurysm, and drained fluid collections. Percutaneous fine needle aspiration and some drainage procedures can be performed with US guidance with greater ease and less cost than with CT.

Recent advances in US involve the application of a transducer to an exposed organ at surgery or through an endoscope. US has facilitated the intraoperative search for pancreatic islet cell tumor and occasionally demonstrates unsuspected multiple tumors. Endosonography requires an end-viewing fiberoptic gastroscope, which is modified to incorporate a transducer. This new imaging procedure can demonstrate the wall thickness of the esophagus, stomach, and duodenum and identify both diffuse and focal intramural lesions. It may also be valuable for diagnosis of early pancreatic lesions. Preoperative assessment of rectal carcinoma with a high-frequency, 7.5 to 10 MHz endorectal transducer is reported to be at least as accurate as CT and magnetic resonance imaging in local staging of tumor.

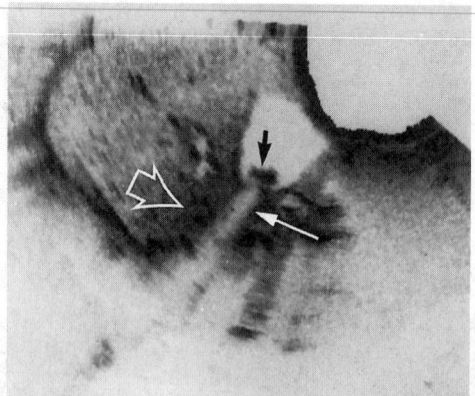

FIGURE 93–6. US of cholelithiasis. Sagittal image (patient's head to reader's left) demonstrates a single gallstone *(black arrow)*. The sound waves easily pass through the fluid (bile) in the gallbladder—hence the "posterior acoustical enhancement" *(open arrow)* characteristic of a cystic structure. The echogenic stone impedes the sound waves—hence the "posterior shadowing" *(straight white arrow)* characteristic of a gallstone. This "static" ultrasound image produces black echoes on white background.

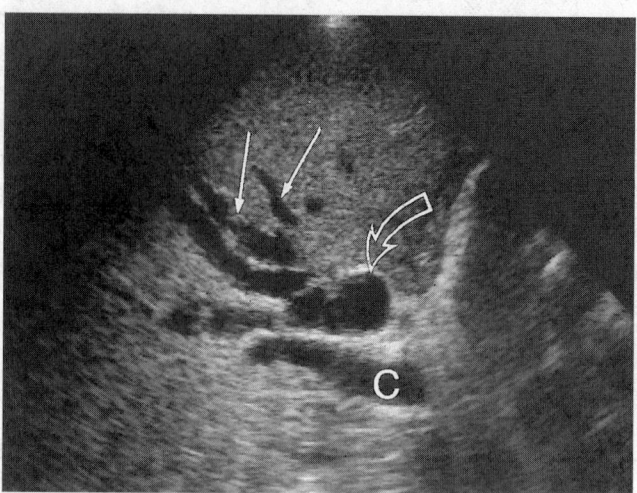

FIGURE 93–7. US of dilated bile ducts. Dilatation of the intrahepatic *(straight arrows)* and extrahepatic *(curved arrow)* bile ducts is well demonstrated on the sagittal ultrasound image of a patient with distal biliary obstruction. (C indicates the inferior vena cava.) This real-time ultrasound image produces white echoes on black background.

ENDOSCOPIC RETROGRADE CHOLANGIOPANCREATOGRAPHY

Endoscopic retrograde cholangiopancreatography (ERCP) is performed with the fluoroscopic guidance of the radiologist. The papilla of Vater is visualized through a fiberoptic endoscope, and the common bile duct or the pancreatic duct or both are cannulated. Water-soluble iodinated contrast material is injected, and images are taken of the opacified biliary tree or pancreatic duct (Fig. 93–8). ERCP is performed specifically to evaluate the pancreatic duct or follows US or CT in demonstrating distal biliary obstruction. When a constricting or obstructing lesion is seen in the distal common bile duct, biopsy or papillotomy can be performed. A further discussion of ERCP is contained in Ch. 107. When retrograde extraction of biliary stones is unsuccessful, a transhepatic route is attempted.

TRANSHEPATIC CHOLANGIOGRAPHY

Percutaneous transhepatic cholangiography is used to visualize the intra- and extrahepatic biliary tree following CT, US, or ERCP that has demonstrated proximal obstruction of the common hepatic or common bile duct. It is performed by injecting water-soluble iodinated contrast material through a flexible 22-gauge needle introduced percutaneously into the intrahepatic biliary tree under fluoroscopic guidance. After the biliary tree is opacified, multiple radiographs are taken in order to characterize the suspected site of blockage or narrowing (Fig. 93–9). This study provides the surgeon with the best demonstration of possible anastomotic sites of the biliary tree in the porta hepatis. Serious complications such as bile peritonitis or intraperitoneal hemorrhage occur in <2% of cases. Biliary obstruction can be treated in patients who are poor surgical risks by several interventional procedures, including percutaneous stricture dilatation, percutaneous drainage, or insertion of a biliary stent. The last procedure can be performed percutaneously or via an ERCP in conjunction with a percutaneous transhepatic procedure.

ENTEROCLYSIS

Procedures used to study the small bowel include the "dedicated" small bowel follow-through, single- and double-contrast enteroclysis, and the peroral pneumocolon. Examination of the small bowel should not accompany most studies of the esophagus, stomach, and/or duodenum because the high-density barium used for the latter interferes with visualization of detail of the small bowel, especially the jejunum. Consequently, lesions that are present may be seen poorly or may be missed, and often it is nearly impossible to exclude abnormality. Hence, the traditional "upper gastrointestinal series with small bowel follow-through" is no longer the examination for small intestinal disease. An exception to this is the patient

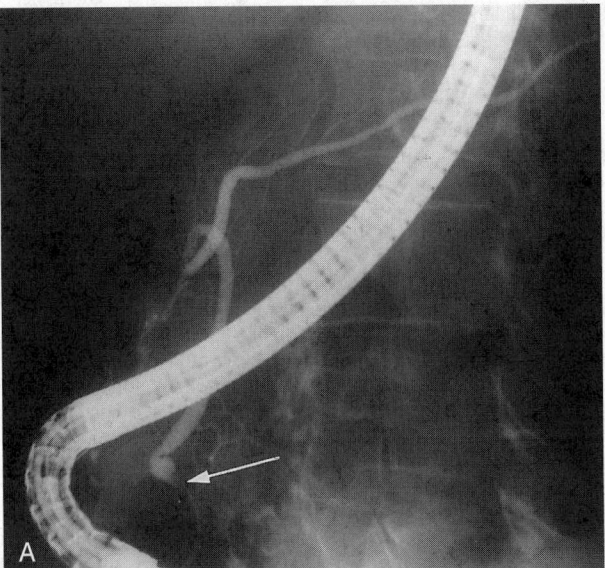

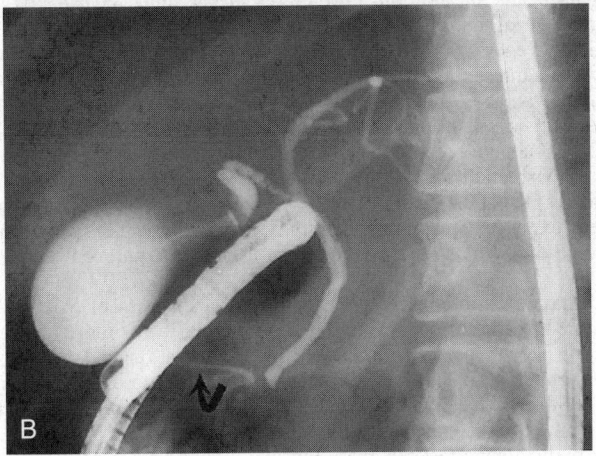

FIGURE 93–8. Normal ERCP. *A,* Normal pancreatogram. The cannula *(arrow)* at the tip of the fiberoptic endoscope has been inserted into the papilla of Vater under direct visualization and the pancreatic duct opacified. *B,* Normal cholangiogram. The gallbladder, cystic duct, common hepatic duct, and common bile duct are visible. *Arrow* indicates cannula in the papilla of Vater.

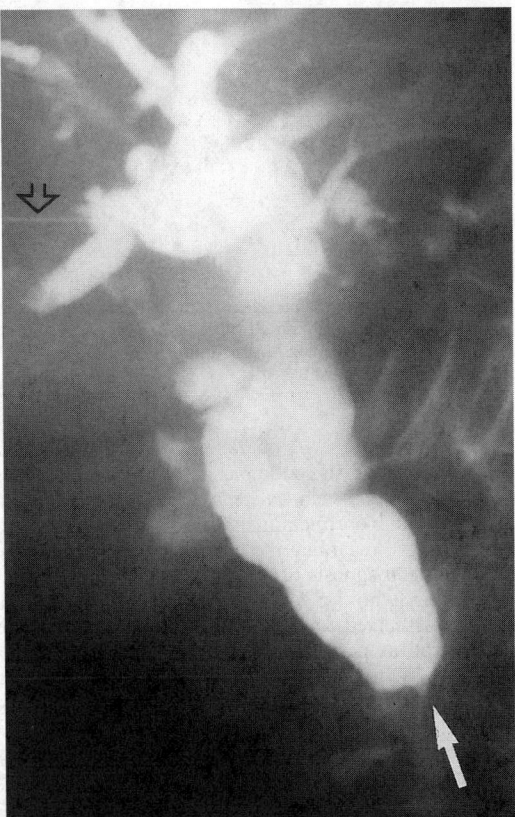

FIGURE 93–9. Percutaneous transhepatic cholangiogram. Dilatation of the biliary tree is demonstrated after percutaneous puncture and opacification of a dilated intrahepatic duct with a long 23-gauge needle *(open black arrow).* The distal common bile duct is abruptly narrowed and obstructed *(white arrow)* owing to cholangiocarcinoma.

RADIONUCLIDE IMAGING

Acute cholecystitis is usually due to obstruction of the cystic duct by a calculus. Scanning with technetium-labeled iminodiacetic acid (^{99m}Tc HIDA), which is excreted by the hepatobiliary system, is valuable when such a diagnosis is in question. Visualization of the liver, bile ducts, gallbladder, and bowel occurs within 60 minutes of injection in normal, fasting patients (Fig. 93–10). Visualization of the gallbladder excludes the diagnosis of obstruction of the cystic duct. Nonvisualization of the gallbladder with normal visualization of the common bile duct and bowel indicates cystic duct obstruction (Fig. 93–11). Nonvisualization of both the gallbladder

in whom the terminal ileum is the only suspected site of involvement. In this case, the peroral pneumocolon is the most precise approach. It is performed when insufflated air is introduced rectally after orally administered thin barium has reached the cecum. With reflux of air across the ileocecal valve, double-contrast images of the terminal ileum are obtained.

Enteroclysis, also known as small bowel enema, refers to the direct introduction of contrast material after peroral intubation of the first loop of jejunum or, less optimally, the distal duodenum. It allows for controlled delivery of contrast material independent of gastric emptying and thus optimizes luminal distention. The double-contrast method uses air or methylcellulose to provide fine detail to the folds of the small bowel. Enteroclysis has been advocated as the most accurate method for detecting focal lesions in the small bowel. However, it is comparable to a dedicated (tubeless) small bowel study for detecting lesions due to Crohn's disease and tumor and is only slightly more sensitive for adhesions. A dedicated small bowel study does not immediately follow examination of the esophagus, stomach, or duodenum; it is performed with frequent, intermittent spot films by the radiologist. Enteroclysis, which is more lengthy and requires more expertise by the radiologist, is tolerated less well by the patient and, most importantly, involves a much greater radiation exposure. Preparation requires colon cleansing as well as 24 hours of clear liquid diet in order to clear the small bowel of particulate matter.

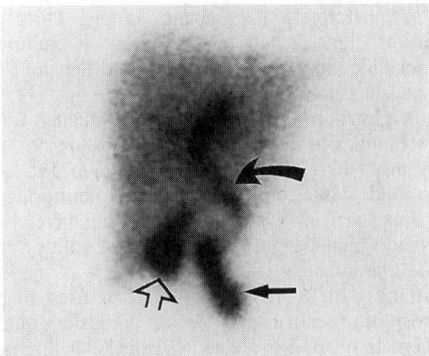

FIGURE 93–10. Normal Tc HIDA scan. Technetium-99m–labeled iminodiacetic acid (HIDA) has been excreted by the liver in this normal, fasting patient. Within 60 minutes of intravenous injection, there is visualization of the common bile duct *(curved arrow),* gallbladder *(open arrow),* and duodenum *(straight arrow).*

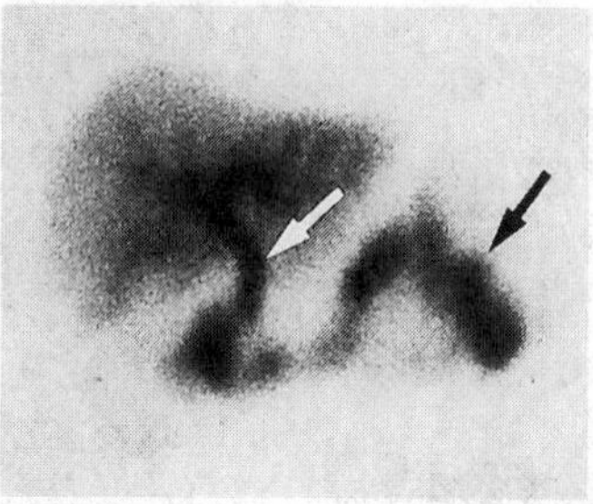

FIGURE 93–11. Tc HIDA of acute cholecystitis. Visualization of the common bile duct *(white arrow)* and small bowel *(black arrow)* without visualization of the gallbladder indicated obstruction of the cystic duct in this fasting patient with acute cholecystitis.

and the bowel can occur in conditions involving cholestasis without cystic duct obstruction, such as hepatocellular disease, total parenteral nutrition, and obstruction of the distal common bile duct. US is more sensitive regarding the detection of cholelithiasis, but is less accurate in the diagnosis of acute cholecystitis. However, cross-sectional imaging with US or CT is excellent when acalculous cholecystitis is suspected, as both can demonstrate gallbladder wall thickening as well as pericholecystic fluid and/or air. Percutaneous cholecystostomy by the interventional radiologist provides nonsurgical treatment for the acutely ill patient.

Gastric mucosa secretes intravenously administered ^{99m}Tc pertechnetate. It can be used to detect ectopic gastric mucosa, especially in Meckel's diverticulum and sometimes in Barrett's esophagus. Ectopic gastric mucosa is present in most symptomatic Meckel's diverticula and in nearly all that bleed, but only half of the bleeding Meckel's diverticula in adults are detected by this study. False-positive results are common. This method of detecting Meckel's diverticulum is far more useful in children.

There are two nuclear medicine procedures available for detecting acute and chronic gastrointestinal bleeding sites, both of which rely upon the extravasation of the radionuclide into the intestinal lumen. Injected ^{99m}Tc sulfur colloid remains in the circulation only briefly, and therefore its use requires active bleeding (approximately 2 ml per minute) at the time of the study. This disadvantage, which is shared with angiography, does not apply to ^{99m}Tc-labeled autologous erythrocytes because they remain in circulation. With the latter procedure, intermittent bleeding of 10 to 20 ml per hour may be detected on delayed views. Both procedures are far more reliable for the colon and small bowel than for the esophagus, stomach, and duodenum because of overlapping structures in the upper abdomen. *Angiography* for gastrointestinal hemorrhage is used when the site of bleeding cannot be identified by endoscopy or radionuclide imaging or when transcatheter embolization therapy is indicated. Visceral angiography of most abdominal pathologic conditions has been replaced by other diagnostic procedures, but it is indicated still in the evaluation of vascular occlusive disease, in polysystemic vasculitis, and preoperatively for hepatic tumors. Direct chemoembolization of the right or left hepatic artery is useful in treating some nonresectable hepatic tumors such as hepatocellular carcinoma and metastatic colon cancer.

Disorders of gastric motility are not well evaluated by barium radiographic techniques because these techniques are not quantitative, are relatively insensitive, and are not physiologic. Procedures using radiolabeled food with continuous gastric monitoring can yield quantitative data, such as gastric half-emptying time. Furthermore, with radionuclide imaging gastric emptying of solids versus liquids can be assessed simultaneously.

Liver scanning with ^{99m}Tc sulfur colloid is used to assess size, shape, and position; identify space-occupying lesions such as tumor, abscess, or hematoma; and evaluate hepatocellular disease. Sensitivity for the detection of primary and metastatic tumor is comparable to that of CT (which is slightly more accurate) and that of US (which is slightly less sensitive). The newer technique of liver scanning with SPECT (single photon emission computed tomography) imaging produces three-dimensional cross-sectional tomographic images and eliminates the overlapping influences of the surrounding

radioactivity (see Ch. 22). Thus, the sensitivity for small (2 cm) space-occupying lesions is increased.

MAGNETIC RESONANCE IMAGING

A very brief and simplified summary of the physics of magnetic resonance (MR) imaging is presented here as a background. Hydrogen nuclei (protons) have a dipole moment and therefore behave as would a magnetic compass. In MR scanning, the protons align with the strong magnetic field but are easily disturbed by a brief radiofrequency (rf) pulse of very low energy and then are altered in their alignment. As the protons return to their orientation with the magnetic field, they release energy of an rf that is strongly influenced by the biochemical environment. T_1 and T_2 relaxation times are a description of the released energy, which is detected, mathematically analyzed, and displayed as a two-dimensional proton-density map according to the "signal intensity" of each tissue. Because the water molecule contains two hydrogen nuclei, changes in distribution of water in tissue, as well as its overall concentration, strongly influence the "intensity" of the MR signal. Hence, MR can provide superior contrast differentiation of tissues with varying amounts of water compared with conventional radiographic modalities, which depend only upon the attenuation of the roentgenographic beam. In addition, fat emits a strong signal because of the abundance of lipid protons. Other advantages of MR include its noninvasiveness, lack of ionizing radiation, and ability to image directly in transaxial, sagittal, coronal, and nonorthogonal planes. Its disadvantages include cost, limited availability, slow scanning time, and problems associated with the powerful magnetic field. The last-named precludes imaging patients with a cardiac pacemaker or metallic clips on intracranial blood vessels. Moreover, critically ill patients cannot easily be monitored because of limited access to the patient during the study and because the strong magnetic field prohibits the presence of resuscitative equipment made of metal.

Physiologic motion limits the diagnostic capability of MR in the abdomen. With current imaging times of minutes for most scanners (as opposed to a few seconds for CT), respiration and peristalsis cause blurring and artifact, especially of pancreatic and bowel images. Several recently developed techniques have decreased the scan time to seconds and sometimes milliseconds. This makes it possible to image the pancreas (Fig. 93–12) and the mesenteric alimentary tract with MR in addition to the fixed segments as in the rectum (Fig. 93–13) and distal esophagus. MR imaging may have a greater sensitivity to primary and metastatic liver tumors compared with CT, US, and nuclear medicine; but whether it has greater specificity has not been established. The very long T_2 value of most cavernous hemangiomas makes it possible to noninvasively differentiate this common, incidentally noted, benign liver tumor from hepatic malignancy, either primary or metastatic in most cases. MR

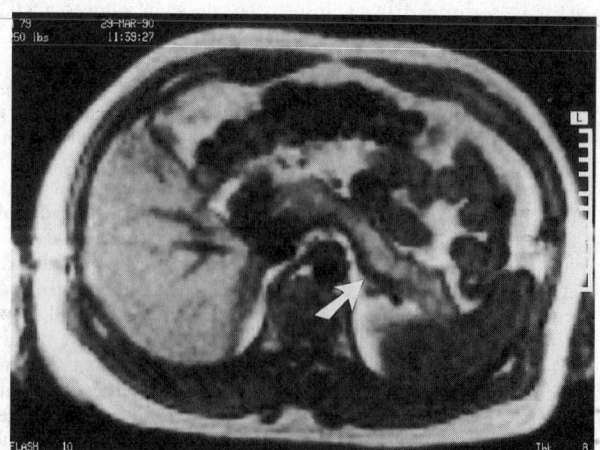

FIGURE 93–12. Normal abdominal magnetic resonance. TurboFlash (Seimens, Magnetom Imager, 1.5 Tesla) (TR = 507 msec, TE = 4 msec) transaxial image of the upper abdomen was acquired in .1 second. The tail of the pancreas abuts the splenic hilum and the body is seen anterior to the splenic vein *(arrow)*. Multiple segments of small bowel are seen posterior to the transverse colon.

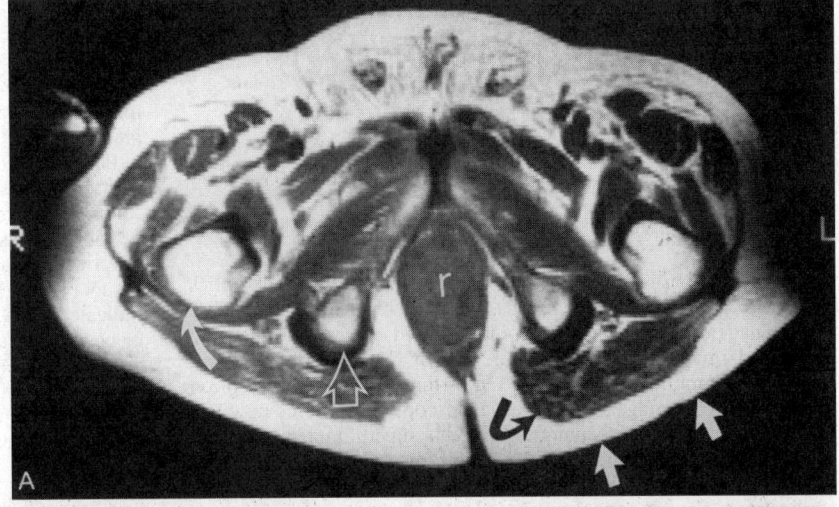

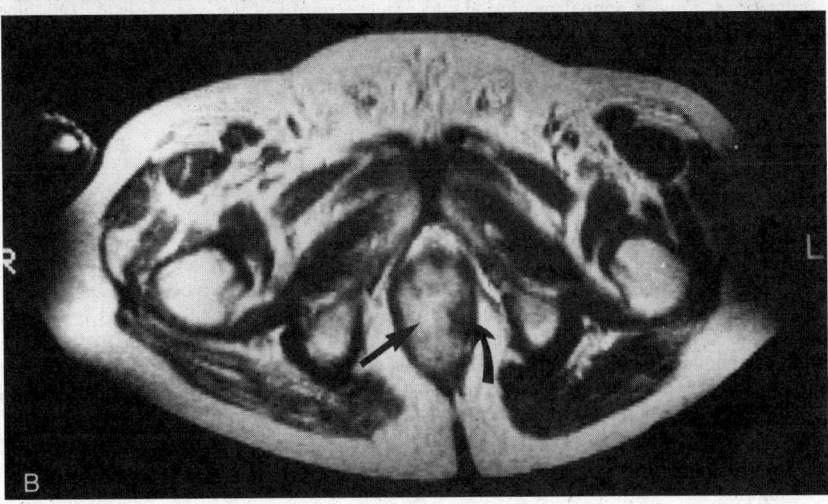

FIGURE 93-13. Magnetic resonance of rectal tumor. *A,* Transverse T_1- weighted image (TR = 0.5 sec, TE = 30 msec) demonstrates thickening of the rectum (r) due to cloacogenic carcinoma, which is isointense with the surrounding uninvolved muscle. Normal structures demonstrated include the gluteus muscle *(curved black arrow),* which is emitting a low-intensity signal, subcutaneous fat *(white arrows),* which is emitting a high-intensity signal, the right ischium *(open arrow),* and the right femoral head *(curved white arrow). B,* T_2-weighted image of the same area demonstrates a relative increase in the signal intensity of the tumor *(straight arrow)* because of prolongation of its T_2 relaxation time. It now can be differentiated from the adjacent, noninvolved muscle *(curved arrow),* which has retained a normal low-intensity signal. (Courtesy of Diasonics, San Francisco, CA.)

can also image blood vessels noninvasively, and as such may be useful to evaluate the patency of surgical shunts for portal hypertension. The effect of the presence of a paramagnetic substance, such as ferric iron, on the T_1 and T_2 relaxation times alters the MR signal intensity of involved tissue. Hence, MR can detect hemosiderosis and hemochromatosis (see Ch. 189) and intravenously introduced ferric iron can enhance the detection of hepatic and splenic metastases. Similarly, paramagnetic substances such as gadolinium-DTPA can be used as contrast-enhancing agents. MR can image the gallbladder, detect cholelithiasis, and differentiate concentrated from nonconcentrated bile. With further development, it may become the procedure of choice for assessing not only morphology but also function of the gallbladder and for diagnosing acute cholecystitis.

Magnetic resonance spectroscopy (MRS) of tissue specifically localized by imaging techniques is a new procedure that is still in the research stage of development. It has not yet achieved clinical applicability in the abdomen, but early work indicates some promise of diagnostic value in the study of high-energy phosphate metabolism (^{31}P) and in imaging sodium (^{23}Na), fluorine (^{19}F), and carbon (^{13}C). Such a procedure, which would facilitate the *in vivo* study of the biochemistry of normal and diseased organs, is technically more demanding than proton imaging. Because of great potential clinical impact, research is progressing rapidly.

Balthazar EJ, Birnbaum B, Yee J, et al.: Acute appendicitis: CT and US correlation in 100 patients. Radiology 190:31, January 1994. *Excellent description of the uses of cross-sectional imaging of this entity.*

Balthazar EJ, Robinson DL, Megibow AJ, et al.: Acute pancreatitis: Value of CT in establishing prognosis. Radiology 174:331, 1990. *A prospective study of 88 patients demonstrating radiographic findings predictive of serious complications.*

Frager D, Medwid S, Baer J, et al.: CT of small-bowel obstruction: Value in establishing the diagnosis and determining the degree and cause. AJR 162:37, 1994. *Important paper detailing the cross-sectional imaging of bowel obstruction as opposed to the more traditional imaging with barium fluoroscopy.*

Hamm B, Thoeni R, Goulld R, et al.: Focal liver lesions: Characterization with nonenhanced and dynamic contrast material-enhanced MR imaging. Radiology 190:417, 1994. *Good discussion of MRI of liver lesions, both benign and malignant.*

LaBerge J, Ring EJ, Gordon RL, et al.: Creation of transjugular intrahepatic portosystemic shunts with the Wallstent endoprosthesis: Results in 100 patients. Radiology 187:413, 1993. *Describes the first large series of an important new percutaneous procedure for life-threatening hemorrhage of esophageal varices due to portal hypertension. TIPS is also currently being used to manage portal hypertensive ascites.*

Lang EK, Brown CL Jr: Colorectal metastases to the liver: Selective chemoembolization. Radiology 189:417, 1993. *Current data demonstrates efficacy of this treatment for patients with colorectal metastases to the liver, a resectable primary, and no evidence of other metastatic disease.*

Levine MS, Laufer I: Perspective. The upper gastrointestinal series at a crossroads. AJR 161:1131, 1993. *A superb up-to-date summary of the use of this valuable diagnostic study.*

McAtee JG, Kopecky RT, Frymoyer PA: Nuclear medicine comes of age: Its present and future roles in diagnosis. Radiology 174:609, 1990. *An overview of current uses of radionuclide imaging with up-to-date references.*

McLean GK, Burke DR: Role of endoprostheses in the management of malignant biliary obstruction. Radiology 170:961, 1989. *State-of-the-art review of endoscopic versus percutaneous approaches to biliary drainage.*

Muller MF, Meyenberger C, Bertschinger P, et al.: Pancreatic tumors: Evaluation with endoscopic US, CT, and MR imaging. Radiology 190:745, 1994. *Recent comparison of these modalities showing increased accuracy of endoscopic ultrasound.*

Pykett IL: NMR imaging in medicine. Sci Am 246:78, 1982. *An excellent, understandable review of the physical principles of MRI.*

Semelka RC, Ascher SM: MR imaging of the pancreas. Radiology 188:593, 1993. *Addresses the clinically important roles for MR imaging and emphasizes the detection of islet cell tumors, non–organ-deforming pancreatic ductal adenocarcinomas, and the distinction between chronic pancreatitis and cancer.*

Sugarbaker PH: Surgical decision making for large bowel cancer metastatic to the liver. Radiology 174:621, 1990. *A superb summary of the current radiologic, laboratory, and medical considerations regarding this issue.*

Taourel P, Baron MP, Pradel J, et al.: Acute abdomen of unknown origin: Impact of CT on diagnosis and management. Gastrointest Radiol 17:287, 1992. *A helpful discussion of the utility of CT in this frequently difficult clinical evaluation.*

Zuckerman DA, Bocchini TP, Birnbaum EH: Massive hemorrhage in the lower gastrointestinal tract in adults: Diagnostic imaging and intervention. AJR 161:703, 1993. *Analyzes the use of scintigraphy, angiography, and interventional techniques in diagnosis and treatment of this entity.*

94 GASTROINTESTINAL ENDOSCOPY

(See Color Plates 1A–H; 2A–H and Fig. 94–1A–I)

Jeffrey M. Rank and Jack A. Vennes

Remarkable progress in optical engineering and in fiberoptics during the past two decades has basically altered the understanding and management of many gastrointestinal disorders. Advances in digitalized imaging have been achieved. In fact, this development has been so rapid that the last edition of this text made no mention of digitalized imaging. Virtually all endoscopic procedures now use this video endoscopy technique, with its superb imaging in real time. Endoscopic techniques were initially used primarily for diagnosis, but increasingly they have been used in important therapeutic applications. Superb optical resolution and precise control of the endoscope tip permit direct visualization of mucosal abnormalities in the esophagus, stomach, and duodenum. Alternatively, the entire colon may be seen; remote reaches of the small bowel are being visualized. Internal channels permit routine aspiration, air insufflation, mucosal biopsy, or cytologic examination. Therapeutic devices can be precisely directed. Side-viewing instruments are used for visualizing the ampulla of Vater and for cannulation of the biliary and pancreatic ductal systems for contrast visualization, and often for therapy.

It has been a fascinating time. Coincident with the evolution of endoscopic techniques, diagnostic and therapeutic modalities have been developed using radiography, ultrasound, and nuclear scanning. Thus the problem is often deciding which of these diagnostic and therapeutic alternatives is best and most cost-effective for patients. Proper sequencing of these diagnostic tools requires some understanding by both the referring physician and the consultant of their relative procedural strengths.

Procedural indications may be influenced by factors of cost and locally available skill. Diagnostic accuracy and therapeutic success of most procedures are dependent on operator competence. Rare complications do occur; they can be minimized by ensuring that procedures are carried out by trained and credentialed endoscopists. The frequency of an erroneous diagnosis bears a direct relationship to operator experience. Endoscopic training programs are required and should be integrated with the disciplines of gastroenterology and colorectal or general surgery. Fairly clear and precise indications for various gastrointestinal endoscopic procedures have gradually evolved. Indications are prominently clustered in Tables 94–1 and 94–2 to underline the importance of this information for those caring for patients with gastrointestinal disease.

Endoscopic procedures are generally contraindicated if a perforated viscus is suspected or if the diagnostic results are unlikely to affect management. Endoscopic procedures should be discussed carefully with the patient in advance to provide reassurance and help in decision making. Procedures done by trained personnel are generally well tolerated after light parenteral sedation and analgesia. Topical pharyngeal anesthesia usually improves acceptance of upper tract endoscopy and indeed is often the only medication required for safe, minimally uncomfortable examinations with modern small-caliber endoscopes. Discussions in this chapter focus on the clinical attributes and capacities of endoscopic procedures and only secondarily on the diseases being investigated.

ESOPHAGOGASTRODUODENOSCOPY (EGD)

Endoscopic examination of the entire esophagus, stomach, and duodenum is accomplished with routine examination to the deep descending duodenum. All mucosal surfaces are visualized, and photographic still or video records are made of recognized abnormalities. Histologic and cytologic diagnosis can be made as necessary. When occasionally indicated, the examination with special instruments called push enteroscopy can be carried out to visualize more of the small bowel beyond the ligament of Treitz. This is most often useful in the discovery and evaluation of mucosal lesions associated with chronic blood loss.

Routine EGD is most frequently used to evaluate possible acid peptic disease, malignancy, or gastrointestinal bleeding. Endoscopy used "just in case" disease is present can lead to *overutilization;* however, managing a presumed disease without diagnostic confirmation often leads to *underutilization.* Both extremes are often cost-*in*effective.

Patients frequently seek medical help for upper abdominal discomfort and associated dyspeptic symptoms of recent onset. If other findings indicating serious disease are absent, a trial of therapy may be indicated as a first diagnostic test. Most respond to a trial of appropriate therapy directed toward presumed acid peptic problems. In about 30% of patients with dyspeptic symptoms, endoscopy is indicated because the test of therapy does not produce a diagnosis, or because of early recurrence of symptoms. Clinical conditions that do not generally require endoscopy include irritable bowel syndrome, intermittent dyspepsia, heartburn responding to medical therapy, asymptomatic or uncomplicated hiatus hernia, and uncomplicated duodenal bulb ulcer seen radiographically that responds to therapy.

Acid Peptic Disease

Acid peptic disease, i.e., reflux esophagitis, gastric ulcer, or duodenal ulcer, can be strongly suspected on the basis of the history, but one cannot confidently predict the specific site or pathologic condition. Although symptoms of reflux esophagitis are often quite specific, other gastrointestinal lesions frequently coexist (see Ch. 97). The presence of esophageal reflux symptoms correlates well with the presence of endoscopic findings and less well with histologic findings. Local symptoms in the mid- or lower esophagus usually predict disease location, whereas high substernal symptoms may be due to disease anywhere in the esophagus. Gastric or duodenal ulcers are usually symptomatic, but in patients with previous gastric or duodenal ulcer, asymptomatic recurrences are discovered in 5% or more of those who have had endoscopy in long-term investigational studies.

EGD is more sensitive and specific than radiographic studies in evaluating disease of the upper gastrointestinal tract, although neither is infallible. Radiographs may be required for evaluation of specific complex situations such as motility disorders, suspected obstructing lesions beyond the reach of the endoscope, and diffuse submucosal infiltration or extrinsic compression on a hollow viscus. Radiographic studies are least sensitive in evaluating lesions without apparent depth, such as flat stomal postgastrectomy ulcers, bleeding mucosal arteriovenous malformations or giant duodenal ulcers involving the entire wall of the duodenal bulb, and erosive esophagitis.

Cancer

Malignant lesions of the upper gastrointestinal tract are generally evident as exophytic masses protruding into the lumen (see Ch. 100). Flat, infiltrative lesions do occur occasionally, and in the esophagus such lesions may resemble a benign stricture. In the stomach, the flat lesions of linitis plastica are primarily evident as stiffness and poor distensibility, although the mucosa is usually demonstrably abnormal. Since malignancy may occasionally present as ulceration, accurate evaluation of all gastric ulcers is mandatory and challenging. More than 75% of malignant gastric ulcers are correctly identified by endoscopic visual criteria alone, as asymmetric folds or nodules that randomly form the crater rim and extend irregularly into surrounding mucosa. Malignant tissue is often seen as multihued. Benign ulcers are typically smoother with more crater depth and with more symmetry and less randomness, and a zone of erythema is usually present at the junction of the crater and the rim.

Histologic and cytologic data should be added to the endoscopic evaluation of all suspicious lesions and of most gastric ulcers. This results in a sensitivity (positive when disease is present) and specificity (negative when disease is absent) of 95%. Brush cytology is a particularly important adjunct in evaluating the smooth, infiltrative esophageal stricture, the linitis plastica gastric lesion, or the occasional superficial, spreading, flat gastric cancer, because these lesions may be firm enough to hinder efforts at obtaining adequate capsule biopsy material. Primary gastric lymphoma may present as an ulcer, ulcerated mass, or large, asymmetric folds. Specific histologic features are frequently present only in submucosal tissue.

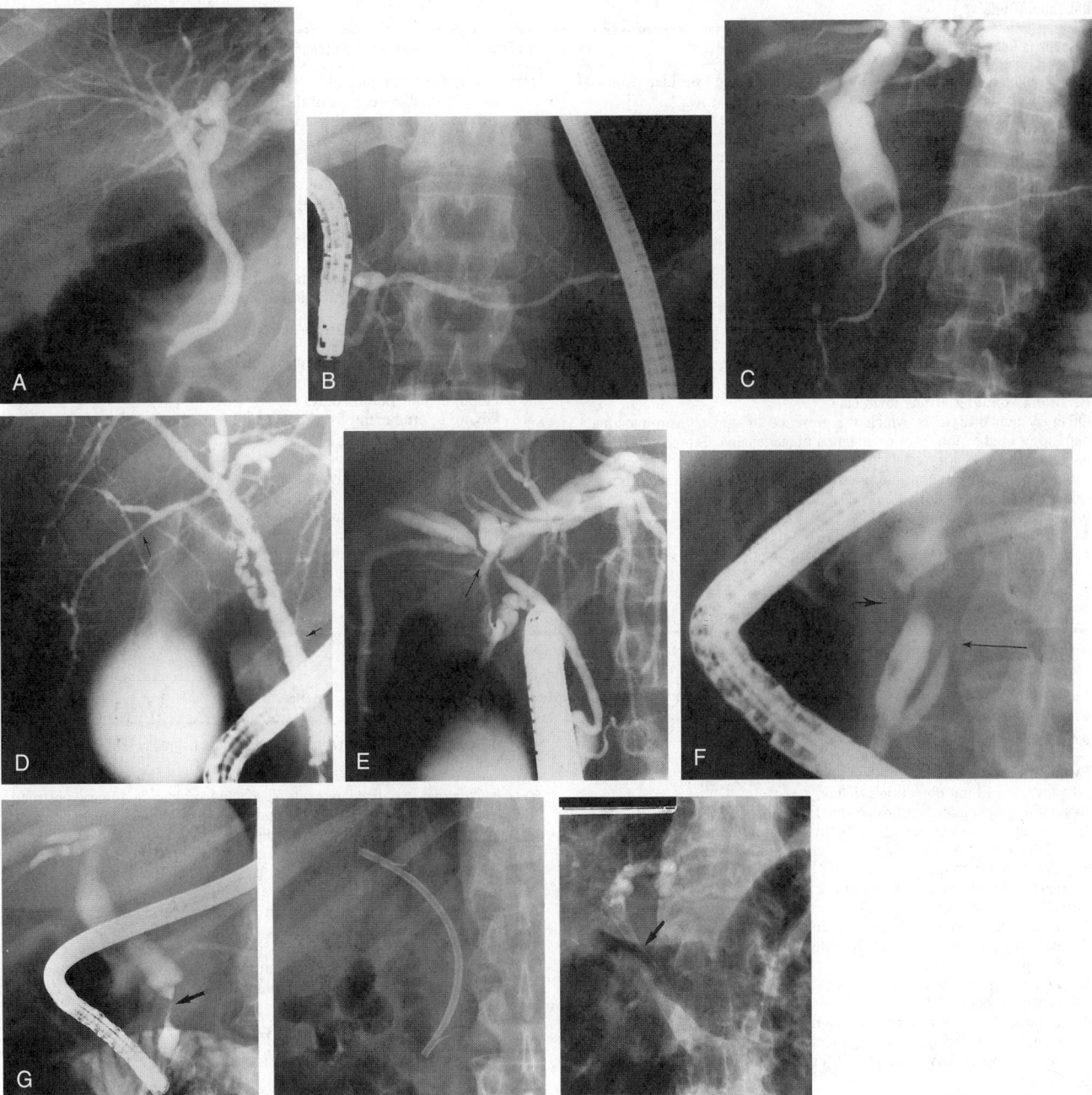

FIGURE 94–1. *A,* Normal cholangiogram. Note the patent cystic duct is beginning to fill. *B,* Normal pancreatogram. Note the abundant normal lateral branches. There is a normal bifurcation of the tail of the gland. *C,* Biliary system is greatly dilated and at least two calculi are seen, one of them very large. Stone was removed during ERCP with sphincterotomy and mechanical lithotripsy. *D,* Primary sclerosing cholangitis. The patient had ulcerative colitis. Note the pleating of the common bile duct *(small arrow).* Alternate dilation and constriction of the intrahepatic duct are characteristic *(long arrow). E,* Retrograde cholangiogram: bile duct cancer. Multiple strictures at the bifurcation of the common hepatic duct *(arrow)* are due to a primary bile duct cancer (Klatskin tumor). Intrahepatic ducts are dilated and partially obstructed. The extrahepatic ductal system distal to the tumor is of normal caliber, here seen coursing medial to the endoscope. *F,* Double-duct sign in pancreatic cancer. Pancreatogram and cholangiogram: pancreatic cancer. Both ducts are outlined by retrograde instillation of contrast at the bottom of the picture. Both the common bile duct *(large arrow)* and the pancreatic duct *(small arrow)* are strictured in the classic "double duct sign" of pancreatic cancer. *G,* The initial panel on the left demonstrates malignant stricture of the common bile duct *(arrow).* In the middle panel a plastic stent has been placed across the stricture, relieving symptoms of severe pruritus and deepening jaundice. In the final panel on the right, the plastic stent has been replaced by a metal sleeve stent for permanent installation and prolonged patency *(arrow).*

Mucosal polyps are rare in the stomach and rarer still in the duodenum and esophagus. Submucosal or intramucosal polypoid defects with normal overlying mucosa are usually pancreatic rests or leiomyomas and can be left in place. Adenomatous polyps have premalignant potential, which increases with size. All polypoid lesions should be endoscopically visualized and biopsied or removed with snare cautery. Multiple small, hyperplastic polyps are not premalignant and need not all be removed; no surveillance is indicated. Adenomas > 1 cm should be excised endoscopically when feasible. Very large lesions may require surgical removal. Surveillance is indicated after removal of gastric adenomatous polyps. Other upper

gastrointestinal malignancies originating in the pancreas or biliary tree do not usually extend into gastric or duodenal mucosa, and they require other diagnostic studies (see below). Ampullary carcinoma is usually visible *if* the papilla of Vater is adequately seen via a conventional end-viewing endoscope or a side-viewing instrument.

Upper Gastrointestinal Bleeding (see Ch. 95)

Using therapeutic endoscopic techniques to control gastrointestinal hemorrhage has revolutionized treatment of this difficult clinical problem. Most bleeding ceases without therapeutic intervention. It

TABLE 94-1. GENERAL AND SPECIFIC INDICATIONS FOR VARIOUS GI ENDOSCOPIC PROCEDURES

GENERAL INDICATIONS

GI Endoscopy Is Generally Indicated:

A. If a change in management is probable or is being considered based on results of endoscopy
B. After an empiric trial of therapy for a suspected benign digestive disorder has been unsuccessful
C. Often as the initial method of evaluation as an alternative to x-rays

GI Endoscopy Is Generally Contraindicated:

A. When the risks to patient health or life are judged to outweigh the most favorable benefits of the procedure
B. When adequate patient cooperation cannot be obtained
C. When a perforated viscus is known or suspected

SPECIFIC INDICATIONS

Diagnostic Esophagogastroduodenoscopy (EGD) Is Generally Indicated For Evaluating:

A. Upper abdominal distress persisting despite an appropriate trial of therapy
B. Upper abdominal distress associated with symptoms and/or signs suggesting serious organic disease (e.g., anorexia and weight loss)
C. Dysphagia or odynophagia
D. Esophageal reflux symptoms persisting or recurring despite appropriate therapy
E. Persistent vomiting of unknown cause
F. Other system disease in which the presence of upper gastrointestinal pathology might modify other planned management. Examples include patients with a history of gastrointestinal bleeding who are scheduled for organ transplantation; long-term anticoagulation; chronic nonsteroidal therapy for arthritis
G. Familial polyposis coli
H. X-ray findings of:
1. Suspected neoplastic lesion, for confirmation and specific histologic diagnosis
2. Gastric or esophageal ulcer
3. Evidence of upper tract stricture or obstruction

I. Gastrointestinal bleeding:
1. In most actively bleeding patients
2. When surgical therapy is contemplated
3. When rebleeding occurs after acute self-limited blood loss
4. When portal hypertension or aorta-enteric fistula is suspected

Therapeutic EGD Is Generally Indicated For:

A. Treating bleeding from lesions such as ulcers, tumors, vascular malformations (e.g., with electrocoagulation, heater probe, laser photocoagulation, or injection therapy)
B. Giving sclerotherapy for esophageal or proximal gastric variceal bleeding
C. Removing foreign bodies
D. Removing selected polypoid lesions
E. Placing feeding tubes (peroral, percutaneous endoscopic gastrostomy, percutaneous endoscopic jejunostomy)
F. Dilating stenotic lesions (e.g., with transendoscopic balloon dilators or dilating systems employing guidewires)
G. Palliative therapy for stenosing neoplasms (e.g., with laser, bipolar electrocoagulation, stent placement)

Adapted from Appropriate Use of Gastrointestinal Endoscopy. American Society for Gastrointestinal Endoscopy, 1989.

TABLE 94-2. INDICATIONS FOR COLONOSCOPY AND ERCP

Diagnostic Colonoscopy Is Generally Indicated For:

A. Evaluating an abnormality on barium enema likely to be clinically significant (e.g., filling defect or stricture)
B. Evaluating unexplained gastrointestinal bleeding
1. Hematochezia not thought to be from rectum or perianal source
2. Melena of unknown origin
3. Fecal occult blood
C. Unexplained iron deficiency anemia
D. Surveillance of colonic neoplasia
1. Examination to evaluate entire colon for synchronous cancer or neoplastic polyps in a patient with a treatable cancer or neoplastic polyp
2. Follow-up in 1 year, then at 3- to 5-year intervals after colorectal cancer resection
3. Follow-up for noncancerous neoplastic polyps in 3 years and if examination negative, 5-year intervals. (Earlier and more frequent colonoscopies may be indicated for large sessile polyps and multiple polyps.)
4. In chronic ulcerative colitis patients colonoscopy every 1–2 years with multiple biopsies to detect cancer and dysplasia in patients with
   a. Pancolitis >7 years' duration
   b. Left-sided colitis of >15 years (no surveillance needed for disease limited to rectosigmoid)
E. Chronic inflammatory bowel disease of colon if more precise diagnosis or determination of extent of activity of disease will influence immediate management
F. Clinically significant diarrhea of unexplained origin
G. Intraoperative identification of site of a lesion that cannot be detected by palpation or gross inspection at surgery (e.g., polypectomy site, location of a bleeding source)

Therapeutic Colonoscopy Is Generally Indicated For:

A. Treating bleeding from such lesions as vascular anomalies, ulceration, neoplasia, and polypectomy site (e.g., electrocoagulation, heater probe, laser or injection therapy)
B. Removing foreign bodies
C. Excising colonic polyps
D. Decompressing acute nontoxic megacolon
E. Balloon dilation of stenotic lesions (i.e., anastomotic strictures)
F. Palliatively treating stenosing or bleeding neoplasms (e.g., laser, electrocoagulation)
G. Decompressing colonic volvulus

Diagnostic Endoscopic Retrograde Cholangiopancreatography (ERCP) Is Generally Indicated For:

A. Evaluating jaundiced patients suspected of having biliary obstruction
B. Evaluating patients without jaundice whose clinical presentation suggests pancreatic or biliary tract disease
C. Evaluating signs or symptoms suggesting pancreatic malignancy when results of indirect imaging (e.g., US, CT, MRI) are equivocal or normal
D. Evaluating recurrent or persistent pancreatitis of unknown cause
E. Preoperatively evaluating chronic pancreatitis patients
F. Evaluating possible pancreatic pseudocyst undetected by CT or US and for known pseudocyst prior to planned surgical therapy
G. Evaluating sphincter of Oddi and bile duct by biliary and pancreatic manometry

Therapeutic ERCP Is Generally Indicated For:

A. Endoscopic sphincterotomy
1. Choledocholithiasis (e.g., in postcholecystectomy patients or patients with intact gallbladders who are not candidates for surgery)
2. Papillary stenosis or sphincter of Oddi dysfunction
3. Placing biliary stent or balloon dilation of biliary stricture
4. Sump syndrome
5. Choledochocele
6. Ampullary carcinoma in patients who are not candidates for surgery
B. Placing a stent across benign or malignant strictures or biliary fistula, or in "high risk" patients with large, unremovable common duct stones
C. Balloon dilation of biliary strictures
D. Nasobiliary drain placement for preventing or treating acute cholangitis or infusing chemical agents to dissolve common duct stones

Diagnostic Flexible Sigmoidoscopy (FS) Is Generally Indicated For:

A. Screening asymptomatic patients at risk for colon neoplasia
B. Evaluating suspected distal colonic disease with no indication for colonoscopy
C. Evaluating the colon in conjunction with barium enema studies

Adapted from Appropriate Use of Gastrointestinal Endoscopy. American Society for Gastrointestinal Endoscopy, 1989.

is important to identify those who continue to bleed or rebleed, as they are candidates for emergency endoscopic therapy. Recognition of clinical conditions associated with poor outcome in the face of gastrointestinal hemorrhage has led to better understanding of the situations in which early endoscopic intervention is prudent. The most important indicator is the severity of the initial bleeding. Signs of hemodynamic instability, the need for multiple transfusions, and the presence of bright red blood on gastric lavage are obvious indicators of the need for early intervention. Likelihood of continued or subsequent bleeding in the patient with portal hypertension is great, and if this is clinically suspected and varices are present, emergency endoscopy and sclerotherapy or esophageal banding is justified. Bleeding that begins in the hospital—especially rebleeding—probably calls for intervention. A history of abdominal aortic aneurysm repair several years earlier requires early endoscopy to view the distal duodenum for signs of graft erosion. Other conditions are associated with increased morbidity or mortality when gastrointestinal bleeding is present, including cardiac and respiratory disease. Patient age over 60 also increases the complications of gastrointestinal bleeding. These comorbid conditions should be considered when a decision is made as to which patients will benefit from early endoscopic intervention.

Once it is decided to examine the upper gastrointestinal tract to locate the bleeding site, a therapeutic plan is necessary to deal with the findings. Endoscopic treatment of gastrointestinal hemorrhage requires a highly skilled operator. Surgical backup should be available as a primary, or, if endoscopic therapy is undertaken, a secondary treatment option. Endoscopic findings can predict potential for further hemorrhage quite well. Varices are associated with continued and recurrent bleeding and increased mortality and require endoscopic intervention. Conversely, it is important to rule out any other potential sources of bleeding if varices are present but not actively bleeding, because some patients with portal hypertension have concomitant peptic disease.

Objective criteria associated with a decreased probability of continued bleeding in peptic ulcers include a clean ulcer base and a base with a flat pigmented area. These findings indicate a very small potential for further bleeding, and thus monitoring in the intensive care setting can be discontinued. Active bleeding at the time of endoscopy is an ominous sign, requiring emergency endoscopic, surgical, or radiologic intervention. A raised pigmented spot in the ulcer base indicates an intermediate risk, and should most often lead to intervention. An adherent clot also indicates an intermediate risk, and the decision to intervene in this setting should be based on clinical indicators of potential rebleeding. The finding of a protruding clot or actual graft in the duodenum of a patient with an old aortic aneurysm requires immediate surgical attention.

The technology to deal with gastrointestinal bleeding has advanced incredibly in the last decade. Multiple studies have shown cost-effectiveness of sclerotherapy for bleeding varices. Although endoscopic banding offers promise in this setting, it is difficult to perform in the presence of acute bleeding. Multiple endoscopic therapies have been shown to decrease the potential for rebleeding, to lower transfusion needs, and to decrease costs. Among the technologies are bipolar electrocoagulation, heater probe coagulation, injection therapy, and laser therapy. The choice of one modality over another is determined by the resources available as well as the skill of the endoscopist. Therapeutic endoscopy has decreased the need for surgical intervention. The source of chronic gastrointestinal blood loss or iron deficiency anemia in men and postmenopausal women is usually discovered in the colon. EGD may be indicated by history suggesting upper tract sources or after negative findings on colonoscopy in patients with chronic blood loss.

Therapeutic Applications of Esophagogastroduodenoscopy

Therapeutic endoscopic procedures commonly carried out in the upper gastrointestinal tract include removing foreign bodies, dilating benign or malignant esophageal strictures, sclerotherapy or banding of bleeding esophageal varices, placing percutaneous gastrostomies, and controlling focal bleeding lesions. Foreign bodies in the esophagus or stomach can be removed by techniques that use snares or forceps as grasping devices. A protective overtube may be used to prevent soft tissue injury or aspiration. Food may become impacted because of an underlying esophageal abnormality. Careful esophagoscopy after removal of the food may reveal a benign or malignant stricture. Esophageal motility studies may be required to

evaluate a possible motility disorder as the underlying reason for the impaction.

Esophageal strictures found to be benign on careful evaluation can be successfully dilated. If a stricture is too tight to admit the endoscope, wire is passed and dilation is done under fluoroscopic control. If the esophagus pursues a tortuous course or if epiphrenic diverticula are present, safety dictates that the dilator be passed over an endoscopically placed wire. Tapered bougies or inflatable balloons of progressively increasing diameter may also be passed over the wire. Following this, endoscopy and biopsy are done to assess whether a malignant lesion is present. After initial endoscopy, less complex strictures with full luminal view may be safely dilated with tapered bougies without wire guidance and without further endoscopy. Generally no more than three bougies of successive diameter are passed in a single session. Maintenance dilation can be scheduled with intervals tailored to the patient's needs. Once an inflammatory stricture is dilated and the inciting cause of reflux and inflammation has subsided, dilation intervals can be lengthened out to weeks or months, or eventually discontinued.

Management of malignant esophageal strictures is directed at reducing tumor mass and allowing the unobstructed passage of food, liquids, and oral secretions by surgical resection or bypass, with or without radiation therapy. Endoscopic procedures include repeated esophageal dilation, maintenance of oral alimentation, dilation and endoscopic placement of a stent across the malignancy (or across a tracheoesophageal fistula), and use of laser energy to restore the lumen by destroying the tumor. All of these latter procedures have good reported results; all require skill for success and safety; and all can be done without prolonged hospitalization or discomfort. Quality survival time is usually brief, but 85 to 90% of patients can be helped, with a complication rate of about 5%.

Percutaneous endoscopic gastrostomy (PEG) provides selected patients with long-term enteral feeding. Candidates are those with a functioning gut and inadequate oral intake. Some may have recurrent aspiration secondary to upper esophageal sphincter dysfunction. Specific indications include neurologic disorders that affect the swallowing mechanism or that result in diminished food intake secondary to a decreased sensorium. Other indications include cancer of the pharynx or upper esophagus that does not totally obstruct (so that an endoscope can be passed). The decision to initiate chronic enteral feeding can be a difficult one, involving the wishes of patient and family and the gravity of the underlying disease. Once the decision is made, however, PEG is a simple and safe method.

COMPLICATIONS. Complications from EGD are rare with modern small-caliber flexible instruments, but they do occur. A morbidity of 0.13% and a mortality of 0.0004% have been reported. During or following endoscopic examination, perforation has occurred in the upper esophagus near the cricopharyngeus, through Zenker's diverticula, and through areas of tumor. Use of sedative or analgesic drugs may transiently suppress respiration, especially in elderly patients or those with severe obstructive pulmonary disease. Aspiration during endoscopy is very unlikely unless vomiting due to massive bleeding or gastric outlet obstruction occurs. Cardiovascular complications, sepsis, prolonged bleeding, and thrombophlebitis from intravenous medications occur rarely.

COLONOSCOPY AND FLEXIBLE SIGMOIDOSCOPY

The entire colon is now routinely accessible to high-resolution viewing with biopsy, brush cytology, polypectomy, and photography of observed lesions. Much has been learned of the polyp-cancer progression, and significant control of colon cancer is within cost-effective reach of the endoscopist.

INDICATIONS. The indications for colonoscopy are listed in Table 94–2. As with EGD, colonoscopic examination is primarily used to evaluate possible cancer, inflammation, and bleeding. The procedure is contraindicated in the presence of fulminant colitis, acute, severe diverticulitis, and probable perforated viscus. Colonoscopy is generally not indicated for stable irritable bowel syndrome, acute diarrhea, upper gastrointestinal bleeding, or rectal bleeding from an anorectal source on anoscopy or sigmoidoscopy. Other nonindications include routine follow-up of inflammatory bowel disease (except as noted in Table 94–2) and routine preoperative examination of patients undergoing elective abdominal surgery for noncolonic disease.

Flexible fiberoptic sigmoidoscopy (FFS) is usually carried out with 60-cm instrumentation. Training requirements are less rigorous than those for colonoscopy. Indications for FFS are listed in Table 94–2. At least 60% of colon cancers and potential colon cancers (neoplastic polyps) are located in the rectosigmoid and lower descending colon and thus are in reach of the "screening" FFS. FFS has the same contraindications as colonoscopy and is generally not indicated when colonoscopy is indicated (see Table 94–2). FFS is specifically not indicated for polypectomy because colonoscopy is needed, and full colonic preparation is necessary to prevent possible explosions during electrocautery. FFS preparation is simple, using two enemas, whereas colonoscopy requires a two-day liquid diet preparation or total gut lavage with large volumes of an isotonic solution. FFS is a more comfortable, more informative replacement for rigid proctosigmoidoscopy at nearly equivalent cost.

Polyps and Cancer of the Colon (see Ch. 106)

Colonoscopy to evaluate the possibility of colon cancer or its precursor polyps is usually indicated after an abnormality is detected by barium enema or proctosigmoidoscopy or when there is unexplained lower gastrointestinal bleeding. If occult blood is detected in the interior of a passed stool, colonoscopy will identify an age-related 20 to 30% incidence of adenomatous polyps and 8 to 15% incidence of cancers. During active bleeding, colonoscopy may present technical difficulties in accurately locating the bleeding source. Repeat colonoscopy may be necessary after bleeding stops to accurately assess the colon.

After endoscopic removal of neoplastic polyps or after resection of colon cancer, continued surveillance is indicated, since the patient is now identified as being at risk for later colon cancer. A full colonoscopy is necessary once the diagnosis of colon cancer has been made to rule out synchronous polyps or cancer. This would optimally be performed prior to surgical intervention to allow the appropriate procedure to be done. Once an adequate view of the colon has been obtained, a repeat colonoscopy between 1 and 3 years afterward is reasonable. Because this patient is at increased risk for developing colonic cancer in the future, screening is mandatory. If two postsurgical colonoscopies with a complete mucosal view have been performed and do not reveal any neoplasms, surveillance may reasonably be done at 5-year intervals. If an adequate view is not obtained due to a poor bowel preparation or other technical problems, or if new neoplasms are seen and resected, then a 3-year wait is reasonable.

Neoplastic polyps found with flexible sigmoidoscopy or barium studies require a full colonoscopy with polypectomy to clear the colon of possible synchronous lesions. Patients with small polyps found during flexible sigmoidoscopy should have biopsy performed to determine whether the lesions are hyperplastic. The hyperplastic polyp does not require further follow-up. Once all polyps are resected during colonoscopy, a repeat procedure is generally warranted every 3 years. If no further polyps are noted, this interval may be increased to 5 years. Several factors influence the timing of repeat colonoscopies. A large sessile polyp may not be adequately excised during polypectomy and may require a repeat surveillance in 6 months to a year. Similarly, when multiple polyps are resected, an earlier repeat colonoscopy may be warranted. Clearly, if an adequate view of the entire colon is not obtained owing to technical troubles, the time interval to repeat screening should be shortened or an air contrast barium enema performed. It is important to point out that these recommendations pertain to patients without other risk factors for developing colon cancer such as family cancer syndrome or inflammatory bowel disease. Surveillance recommendations for these conditions are listed in Table 94–2.

Most colonic polyps are hyperplastic and are not premalignant. In neoplastic polyps, cancer risk increases with increasing dysplasia and villoglandular transformation and also with size. Pedunculated polyps with an uninvolved stalk and with cancer confined to the mucosa can be cured by snare cautery removal. Most colonoscopists remove all polyps > 5 mm in diameter. Polyps < 5 mm may be neoplastic; coagulation or a coagulation biopsy technique during colonoscopy is used to remove them.

Polypectomy is the main therapeutic use of colonoscopy. Endoscopic control of bleeding is not usually feasible. Electrocautery of bleeding angiodysplastic lesions in the cecum and ascending colon has been successful, but new lesions may appear within months. Dilation of anastomotic strictures by balloons passed over a guide wire or through the endoscope is occasionally useful.

Inflammatory Bowel Disease (see Ch. 104)

Most patients with inflammatory bowel disease do not require colonoscopy for diagnosis. At times, however, colonoscopy may provide unique and important information. Differentiation between granulomatous colitis (Crohn's disease) and ulcerative colitis is usually possible with colonoscopy and multiple biopsies. The anatomic extent of disease can be determined. The presence or absence of inflammatory bowel disease can be determined more accurately when clinically suspected despite absence of radiographic or sigmoidoscopic findings. Diagnostic colonoscopy in ulcerative colitis is at times necessary to evaluate a stricture or a mass seen on barium enema. Occasionally, strictures are malignant with submucosal tumor spread. Pseudopolyps are not premalignant and need not be histologically examined. In surveillance examinations of patients with ulcerative colitis, multiple biopsies are obtained throughout the involved colon. When moderate to severe dysplasia is consistently found, colectomy is usually recommended.

COMPLICATIONS. Diagnostic colonoscopy has a complication rate of 0.5%, which rises to 1% when polypectomy is added, with hemorrhage and perforation being the principal complications.

ENDOSCOPIC RETROGRADE CHOLANGIOPANCREATOGRAPHY (ERCP)

Utilizing side-viewing endoscopes, the ERCP technique is now widely available for identifying and cannulating the ampulla of Vater. Diagnostic-quality radiographs are obtained with selective instillation of contrast medium in the common bile duct and/or pancreatic ductal system in 90% of attempts. Failure may result from anatomic distortion resulting from prior surgery, tumor infiltration, or duodenal edema of acute pancreatitis. Pancreatic and biliary ductal systems and their diseases are no longer accessible only by surgical means. ERCP and radiographic techniques now combine and precisely characterize problems. When surgical management is required, decisions are based on precise preoperative evaluation. As clinical experience has been massively collated and shared, these two hitherto remote ductal systems have given up their secrets, both in terms of disease and in terms of normal anatomy, physiology, and function.

INDICATIONS. Indications for ERCP are listed in Table 94–2. ERCP is generally not helpful for evaluating abdominal pain of obscure origin in the absence of objective findings that suggest pancreatic or biliary tract disease. Known or suspected gallbladder disease is not an indication for ERCP without evidence for bile duct involvement. Detailed ductal study of patients after acute pancreatitis is usually deferred until a second episode has established its recurrent nature, unless there is evidence to suggest gallbladder disease as a possible cause of the pancreatitis. Pancreatic malignancy clearly demonstrated on preoperative computed tomographic (CT) scans and ultrasonography need not be further evaluated with ERCP, if no metastases are evident and if cytologic findings on CT-guided examination are positive. Other tests provide diagnostic evidence of pancreatic and biliary disease, including percutaneous transhepatic cholangiography (PTC). Transabdominal fine-needle aspiration cytology with CT guidance is helpful; malignant cells are found in 60 to 85% of patients with malignancy when meticulous technique is used.

Ultrasonography and CT have greatly improved in their ability to detect pancreatic malignancy (see Ch. 108). Equivocal results at times require confirmation by ERCP. Cutoff or stenosis of the pancreatic duct and often of the bile duct (double-duct sign) is a reliable ERCP finding of carcinoma (see Fig. 94–1F). Patients with chronic pain and suspected chronic pancreatitis who are surgical candidates should have preoperative pancreatography and cholangiography to assess patency of the main pancreatic duct and possible stricture of the intrahepatic bile duct. Choice of surgical methods may be altered or dictated by these ductal findings. Differentiating chronic pancreatitis from pancreatic cancer may be impossible because the pancreatic duct is often dilated and tortuous with dilated, stubby lateral branches in both diseases. Downstream ductal stricturing in the pancreatic head is the hallmark of malignancy, however.

In evaluating suspected biliary obstruction, a cholangiogram is indicated before deciding on therapy. When Charcot's triad of fever, pain, and icterus is present, these clinical findings alone strongly suggest choledocholithiasis. Cholangiography by PTC or preferably by ERCP may then be done if endoscopic sphincterotomy is planned. Ultrasonography may be performed to access ductal dilation, but this is of limited value because calculi often reside in undilated ducts.

Therapeutic Applications of ERCP

Endoscopic retrograde sphincterotomy (ERS) has a number of important therapeutic applications. Soft tissues and sphincter fibers of the papilla and intraduodenal portion of the common bile duct are divided with electrocautery to relieve ductal obstruction. ERS has assumed a major role in management of choledocholithiasis and offers a relatively safe and simple alternative to surgery.

Obstruction due to ductal calculi is relieved by ERS in 90% of attempts. ERS is now widely considered the therapy of choice for patients with symptomatic stones of the common bile duct when the procedure is available. ERS is often carried out immediately after ERCP as soon as the presence of stones in the duct is confirmed. It is safer and cheaper than surgery in these generally elderly patients and more successful than percutaneous transhepatic extraction. Cholangitis and gallstone pancreatitis usually respond dramatically to decompression in this manner. About 40% of patients with symptomatic choledocholithiasis have never had cholecystitis; therefore, their gallbladders are intact. Almost all contain calculi. After removal of duct calculi with ERS in elderly patients, the gallbladder may be left in place and removed only as future symptoms dictate. The probability of subsequent cholecystitis does not exceed 2 to 5% per year. For younger patients under age 60 or 65, it may be prudent to remove the gallbladder electively.

Papillary stenosis is a poorly defined disorder or group or disorders in which recurrent biliary colic and occasionally pancreatitis may result from papillary fibrosis or sphincter of Oddi dysfunction. Diagnostic criteria include a dilated bile duct, delayed ductal drainage after cholangiography, cholestasis following painful episodes as judged by liver function tests, and elevated sphincter of Oddi pressures during manometry. The problem arises most commonly in women who have had a cholecystectomy either for cholelithiasis or for biliary colic–like pain without stones. ERS is often curative for carefully selected patients with papillary stenosis. There remain a number of diagnostic and therapeutic questions unanswered in this troubling condition.

Placing plastic stents across biliary strictures is a major therapeutic extension of ERCP. Most strictures are caused by inoperable pancreatic or bile duct malignancy, and another treatment option is surgical or transhepatic decompression. A catheter containing a guide wire is introduced via the endoscope or via the percutaneous transhepatic route through the stricture, and a stent is passed over the catheter. The distal end is left in the duodenum, bile drainage is restored, and barbed flaps prevent dislodgment of the stent. Procedures are successful in 90% of cases. Present-day stents remain patent for up to 5 months and can be rather easily replaced. Several configurations of metal stents have been developed. Typically a metal mesh stent is deployed across the malignant stricture, maintaining long-term patency. The metal mesh stent—not currently retrievable—remains in place permanently. In a minority of patients, the tumor ingrowth results in reobstruction, which is managed by placement of a plastic stent through the metal one. Future developments may result in removable metal stents, thus making them adaptable for managing benign strictures.

Endoscopic therapy has been increasingly applied to other problems of pancreatic disease. Studies to date are largely uncontrolled and only preliminary results of clinical studies are available. ERCP-related techniques are promising in several spheres of pancreatic disease, however. Drainage of pancreatic secretions through a low-pressure run-off as sphincterotomy or endoprosthesis is a promising technique for closing draining pancreatic fistulas. The same principle holds and is successful for managing cystic duct or bile duct leaks postoperatively. In a frequent pancreatic anomaly, pancreas divisum, the major pancreatic duct drains through the lesser Santorini papilla. Placing sequential stents across the small, often stenotic lesser papilla is proving to be effective thus far in management of recurrent pancreatitis due to this entity. Similarly, pain due to chronic pancreatitis may selectively be treated with sequential stenting of the papilla. Ultimately, fibrosis may hold the duct open and unobstructed, or pain response to stenting may help identify those patients in whom decompressive surgery will be successful. Finally, pseudocysts or pancreatic duct disruption by trauma can be successfully managed by transpapillary ductal drainage.

COMPLICATIONS. In 1% of patients, acute pancreatitis follows ERCP, usually beginning within 2 hours of the procedure as a clinically mild complication. Biliary sepsis occurs less commonly but is more serious. Even a few bacteria introduced into a semi-closed space—bile duct, gallbladder, pancreatic pseudocyst—may occasionally have serious septic consequences. Organisms may be introduced from the unsterile gastrointestinal tract or from instruments. Stringent cleaning and disinfection techniques are mandatory. Sepsis is prevented by prompt decompression within 24 hours of ERCP, plus judicious use of appropriate parenteral antibiotics in patients with possible infectious problems.

LAPAROSCOPY

Laparoscopy is a term now applied to three dissimilar but important uses. Gynecologic laparoscopy, which is standard for both diagnostic and therapeutic indications, is well accepted. Second, laparoscopy has been adapted for general abdominal surgery, notably cholecystectomy but now other intra-abdominal procedures as well. Medical developments and clinical acceptance have moved ahead very rapidly, and laparoscopic cholecystectomy is now the standard approach in nearly 90% of patients requiring gallbladder removal.

Laparoscopy as practiced by endoscopists is largely a diagnostic technique. Direct inspection of the anterior abdominal space is afforded routinely. A pneumoperitoneum is created and a rigid or flexible laparoscope is introduced through a puncture in the abdominal wall, with use of local anesthesia and the patient under conscious sedation. The procedure is well tolerated; complications of bleeding or bowel perforation occur in only 0.1 to 0.2%. Two thirds of the liver and variable parts of the gallbladder, spleen, peritoneum, and diaphragm can usually be visualized. The colon and small bowel are variably available for inspection. Assessment of the endoscopic appearance and the results of a guided biopsy result in the 90% accuracy of diagnosis, substantially better than that for percutaneous blind liver biopsy. The major indications for laparoscopy are inspection and guided biopsy in suspected diffuse or focal liver disease. The presence of hepatic metastases is accurately assessed in this manner, information that is important in assessing operability. Evaluation of ascites is occasionally an indication for laparoscopy. The procedure is contraindicated in the presence of acute peritonitis, intestinal obstruction, severe coagulopathy, infection of the abdominal wall, and peritoneal adhesions resulting from prior peritonitis.

FUTURE OF ENDOSCOPY

Endoscopic instrumentation is approaching optimal size and optical resolution, in both fiberoptic and electronic digital imaging equipment. The number of skilled endoscopists has increased so that precise diagnostic studies are generally available to most patients. Endoscopy results are contributing enormously to assessment and management of gastrointestinal disease and will continue to do so. For example, the colon polyp-cancer progression is now worked out, demonstrably improving the discovery rate for colon cancer and reducing the mortality of colonic malignancy. Most cases of common bile duct stones and cholangitis or pancreatitis are being treated endoscopically, obviating surgery. Measures for successful control of gastrointestinal bleeding are greatly improving, and their influence on mortality should soon become clear. As additional anatomic sites are reached, and further therapeutic options are developed, the role of endoscopy continues to grow as a first-line clinical tool.

Bond JH: Polyp guideline: Diagnosis, treatment, and surveillance for patients with non-familial colorectal polyps. Ann Intern Med 119:836, 1993. *An important summary statement.*

Cotton PB: Nonsurgical palliation of jaundice in pancreatic cancer. Surg Clin North Am 69:613, 1989. *An acceptable alternative to surgery.*

Cook DJ, Fuller HD, Guyatt GH, et al.: Risk factors for gastrointestinal bleeding in critically ill patients. N Engl J Med 330:377, 1994. *Prophylactic therapy not routinely indicated.*

Fan S-T, Lai ECS, Mok FPT, et al.: Early treatment of acute biliary pancreatitis by endoscopic papillotomy. N Engl J Med 328:228, 1993. *Evolving management of a morbid disease.*

Proceedings of the consensus conference on therapeutic endoscopy in bleeding ulcers. Gastrointest Endosc Suppl 36, 1990. *An important position statement on the current role of endoscopy.*

Saeed ZA, Ramirez FC, Hepps KS: Endoscopic stent placement for internal and external pancreatic fistulas. Gastroenterology 105:1213, 1993. *Fistulas close with low-pressure stent drainage.*

Soper NJ, Brunt LM, Kerbl K: Laparoscopic general surgery. Med Prog 330:409, 1994. *Important surgical evaluation.*

Vaira D, Ainley C, Williams S, et al.: Endoscopic sphincterotomy in 1000 consecutive patients. Lancet 2:431, 1990. *A broad review of experience with endoscopic sphincterotomy for choledocholithiasis.*

Vennes JA: Management of calculi in the common duct. Semin Liver Dis 3:162, 1983. *Endoscopic observations add to understanding of disease.*

Winawer SJ, Zauber AG, Ho MN, et al.: Prevention of colorectal cancer by colonoscopic polypectomy. N Engl J Med 329:1977, 1993. *Landmark paper.*

95 GASTROINTESTINAL HEMORRHAGE

John. P. Cello

Bleeding from the gastrointestinal tract is one of the most common causes of hospitalization. While in some countries the number of patients admitted for peptic ulcer disease has gradually decreased, the overall mortality for gastrointestinal tract hemorrhage has remained largely unchanged over the past several decades. Many diseases cause bleeding from the gastrointestinal tract (Tables 95–1 and 95–2). Although the specific bleeding lesion and pathophysiology of hemorrhage may vary considerably, the initial therapeutic and diagnostic approach to the bleeding patient remains largely the same (Fig. 95–1).

SIGNS AND SYMPTOMS

Gastrointestinal tract hemorrhage usually produces dramatic clinical signs and symptoms that bring patients to the attention of physicians. *Hematemesis* is vomiting of gross blood. Usually, vomiting of bloody material indicates bleeding from the upper gastrointestinal tract, but blood passing into the gastrointestinal tract from anywhere proximal to the ligament of Treitz (duodenojejunal junction) can be vomited by the patient (Table 95–1). Hematemesis most frequently follows bleeding *from* the esophagus, stomach, or duodenum, but occasionally nasopharyngeal, pulmonary, and even pancreaticobiliary tract bleeding can be manifested initially by hematemesis. *Melenemesis*, or "coffee grounds" vomiting, occurs when blood has had an appreciable period of time in contact with gastric acid. Patients vomiting "coffee grounds" material are usually bleeding at a slower rate than those who have bloody emesis. As with hematemesis, "coffee grounds" emesis follows bleeding into the gastrointestinal tract from a site proximal to the duodenojejunal junction. As with hematemesis, however, it too can follow bleeding from the nasopharynx, tracheobronchial tree, liver, or pancreas. *Melena*, usually noted by patients with bleeding from the proximal gastrointestinal tract, is characterized by dark black, liquid, tarry, metallic-smelling stools. Melenic stools usually indicate upper gastrointestinal tract bleeding, but not infrequently mid- to distal small bowel and even proximal colonic bleeding can be manifested by dark black, liquid stools. *Hematochezia*, bright red stools, is usually a sign of distal small bowel or colonic hemorrhage (Table 95–2). Brisk hemorrhage from the proximal gastrointestinal tract with accelerated transit may, however, be the source of dark red blood in the stools. Up to 10% of patients with hemodynamically significant hematochezia are actually bleeding from an upper, not lower, gastrointestinal tract lesion. The remaining 90% of patients with hematochezia are bleeding from some site distal to the ileocecal valve, with the majority, particularly those without orthostatic signs or symptoms, bleeding from superficial mucosal lesions in the sigmoid, rectum, or anorectal junction. In addition to signs of gross blood loss, patients with hemodynamically significant gastrointestinal tract bleeding often have lightheadedness, dizziness, diaphoresis, or frank syncope if hypovolemia has occurred. Patients with

TABLE 95–2. ETIOLOGY OF HEMATOCHEZIA IN 72 HOSPITALIZED PATIENTS*

Source of Hemorrhage	Percentage
Colonic cancer	7
Colonic polyps	11
Diverticula	23
Colitis	11
Vascular ectasia	1
Large hemorrhoids only	12
Ulcer/tear (rectum)	10
Upper gastrointestinal or small bowel source	10
No site identified	15
	100

* Patients underwent colonoscopy (and endoscopy if colonoscopy was negative) at the San Francisco General Hospital.

TABLE 95–1. ETIOLOGY AND SEVERITY OF UPPER GASTROINTESTINAL TRACT HEMORRHAGE*

Source of Hemorrhage	Severity of Hemorrhage	
	Mild-Moderate (246 patients)	*Severe* (140 patients)
Esophagus		
Esophagitis	12%	7%
Ulcer	2%	2%
Mallory-Weiss tear	5%	19%
Esophageal varices	5%	31%
Total Esophagus	24%	59%
Stomach		
Gastric ulcer	15%	14%
Prepyloric ulcer	2%	4%
Pyloric channel ulcer	4%	2%
Gastric erosions	2%	0
Gastritis	7%	0
Varices	1%	2%
Portal-hypertensive gastropathy	2%	
Gastric cancer	2%	2%
Polyp	0	
Dieulafoy lesion	0	
Total Stomach	35%	24%
Duodenum		
Ulcer	31%	15%
Duodenitis	8%	
Diverticulum		
Aortoenteric fistula		
Pancreatic pseudocyst	2%	2%
Post-sphincterotomy		
Total Duodenum	41%	17%
	100%	100%

* All patients underwent diagnostic endoscopy at the San Francisco General Hospital over 3 years.

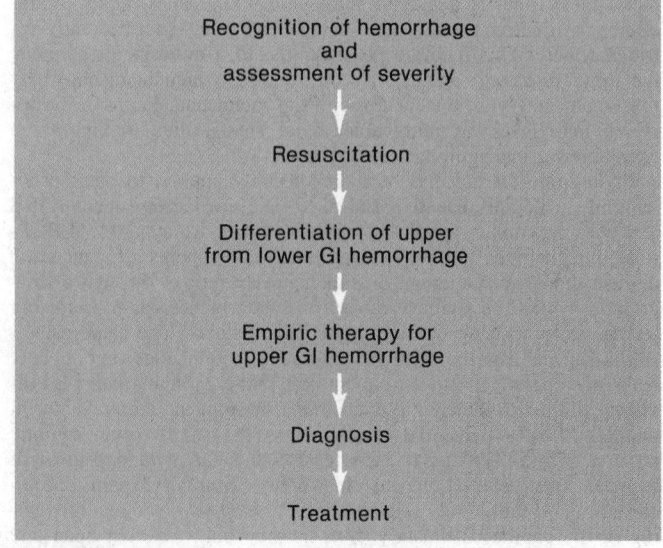

FIGURE 95–1. Approach to the patient with gastrointestinal hemorrhage.

slow but persistent gastrointestinal tract bleeding have signs and symptoms of profound iron deficiency anemia, including pallor, dyspnea, angina, and exertional weakness (Ch. 132).

DETERMINING SEVERITY OF THE HEMORRHAGE

Patients with gastrointestinal tract bleeding must be rapidly assessed and resuscitated. The most accurate noninvasive indicator of the severity of blood loss is the presence of *shock* or changes in *postural vital signs.* Shock indicates an acute blood volume loss of at least 15 to 20%. Postural vital sign changes, i.e., upright tachycardia, widening of the pulse pressure, and/or upright systolic hypotension, indicate acute intravascular volume loss of at least 10 to 15%. It is therefore essential to determine the blood pressure and pulse in the sitting and standing positions in patients who report signs and symptoms of gastrointestinal tract blood loss but who have normal *supine* vital signs.

Other bedside diagnostic findings indicate the severity of hemorrhage in patients with upper gastrointestinal tract bleeding. Brisk hemorrhage with hematemesis and/or "coffee grounds" emesis is usually associated with *increasing stool frequency, hyperactive bowel sounds,* and a *change in the color of the stools* from dark black to dark red color. With bleeding from a duodenal ulcer, relatively small amounts of blood may be vomited or lavaged by nasogastric tube, most passing distally into the gastrointestinal tract. *Nasogastric lavage* is helpful but highly inaccurate in estimating the severity of upper gastrointestinal tract bleeding. Young patients with duodenal ulcers in particular may exhibit a small amount of bloody emesis and/or "coffee grounds" on nasogastric tube lavage. However, the absence of significant blood by nasogastric lavage (particularly when the lavage does not contain bile) does not rule out upper gastrointestinal tract bleeding. With profuse hematemesis, the return of large amounts of clots or bright red blood obviously indicates vigorous active upper gastrointestinal tract hemorrhage. In the face of fresh bleeding, the *hematocrit and hemoglobin levels* are not reliable indicators of the severity of bleeding. For the hematocrit to fall, the blood plasma must have equilibrated with extracellular fluid or with administered intravenous fluids. Exsanguination can occur with a relatively normal hematocrit, and patients with extremely low hematocrits can be hemodynamically quite stable. For these reasons, one should avoid relying too heavily upon the initial hemoglobin concentration or hematocrit, particularly in those patients with other manifestations of brisk gastrointestinal tract hemorrhage.

INITIAL EVALUATION AND TREATMENT

Regardless of the site or etiology of hemorrhage, all patients with significant active blood loss from the gastrointestinal tract should be approached in a similar manner (Fig. 95–1). Initially, vital signs, including supine and upright blood pressure and pulse, must be measured to assess hemodynamic severity of blood loss. If blood loss is significant, intravenous fluids must be started immediately to restore intravascular volume. Saline or other balanced electrolyte solutions are most rapidly available, but there is no substitute for packed red blood cells in patients who are bleeding briskly. With brisk hemorrhaging, especially in patients with known cardiopulmonary disease, pulmonary artery and peripheral arterial catheters may be helpful in monitoring the severity of bleeding and the adequacy of resuscitation. Nasal oxygen should be administered to these patients to improve blood oxygen transport.

The history of the bleeding episode and of any previous gastrointestinal tract hemorrhage should be rapidly obtained after the initial evaluative and resuscitative measures noted above. A personal or family history of gastrointestinal tract illness, particularly from peptic ulcers, cancer, or vascular ectasias (e.g., Osler-Weber-Rendu syndrome) is helpful, as is a history of previously documented gastrointestinal tract disease as determined by radiography, endoscopy, or surgical procedures. Patients with alcohol abuse or known or suspected chronic active liver disease may present with painless hematemesis from esophageal varices. Substernal burning pain, regurgitation, or reflux symptoms may indicate longstanding reflux esophagitis. Patients with forceful, dry retching or multiple episodes of vomiting of food prior to the onset of hematemesis may be bleeding from Mallory-Weiss tears of the gastroesophageal junction. A history of epigastric burning pain promptly relieved by food or antacids or nocturnal pain suggests peptic ulcer disease, particularly

duodenal ulcer (see Ch. 99). Dyspepsia may not always occur in patients with bleeding from peptic ulcer disease, however.

A history of known diverticular disease supports the possibility of colonic diverticular hemorrhage in patients with brisk hematochezia (see Ch. 112). Colorectal malignancy is often suggested by a history of gradual weight loss, intermittent blood in the stools, or altered bowel habits (see Ch. 106). Patients with idiopathic inflammatory bowel disease often have longstanding mucous and bloody diarrhea (see Ch. 104). Hemorrhoidal bleeding is often suggested by the presence of bright red blood surrounding well-formed, normal-appearing stools.

The physical examination is sometimes helpful in suggesting the etiology of hemorrhage. Patients with stigmata of chronic liver disease (e.g., spider angiomata, ascites, gynecomastia) and upper gastrointestinal tract bleeding often bleed from esophageal varices, but almost half are found to be bleeding from lesions other than varices. Localized epigastric tenderness to palpation may indicate peptic ulcer disease or gastritis. Occasionally patients with lower gastrointestinal tract bleeding from a malignancy have a palpable lower abdominal mass, hepatomegaly, signs of obvious weight loss, or adenopathy. A rectal examination is essential to document stool color as well as to palpate for gross anorectal mass lesions such as polyps, cancers, or large hemorrhoids.

Following rapid resuscitation and an expedited history and physical examination, nasogastric tube lavage should be carried out, not only for obvious signs and symptoms of upper gastrointestinal tract hemorrhage but also for hemodynamically significant hematochezia. Blood or "coffee grounds" material in a nasogastric lavage may indicate that bright red blood per rectum is coming from an upper gastrointestinal tract site. Nasogastric tube lavage using room temperature water may also decrease the bleeding rate by vasoconstricting smaller gastric vessels.

Following the initial evaluation, the hematocrit or hemoglobin, the prothrombin time, and the partial thromboplastin time should be measured and a specimen of blood obtained for typing and cross-matching for transfusions. For patients with shock or postural vital sign changes, four to six units of packed red cells should be cross-matched immediately. A serum electrolyte and chemistry panel should likewise be requested. A disproportionate elevation of the blood urea nitrogen (BUN):creatinine ratio may indicate bleeding from a proximal gastrointestinal site. In addition, gross abnormalities of liver function tests may suggest the presence of varices as the cause of hemorrhage.

UPPER GASTROINTESTINAL TRACT BLEEDING

Peptic ulcer disease is the most common cause of upper gastrointestinal tract bleeding (see Color Plate 1*C*). It is responsible for 50% of moderately severe and 35% of severe bleeding episodes (Table 95–1). Bleeding from peptic ulcers may not always be associated with heartburn or epigastric burning pain, especially in older patients. *Hemorrhage from esophageal or gastric varices* (responsible for nearly one third of the episodes of massive upper gastrointestinal hemorrhage) is usually, but not always, associated with known or suspected chronic liver disease (see Color Plates 1*A* and 1*B*). Most patients with variceal hemorrhage due to alcohol abuse have physical stigmata of liver disease such as a large, firm liver, gross ascites, scleral icterus, palmar erythema, and evidence of peripheral muscle wasting. However, patients with postnecrotic cirrhosis due to viral hepatitis often lack overt peripheral stigmata of chronic liver disease. Variceal hemorrhage usually involves brisk bleeding, occasionally with regurgitation of large amounts of dark, clotted blood without emesis. However, variceal hemorrhage may occasionally be accompanied by only "coffee grounds" emesis and melena. *Mallory-Weiss tears* of the gastroesophageal junction (causing 5% of minor and 20% of severe upper gastrointestinal hemorrhage) are usually associated with antecedent, forceful retching. Nearly half of patients with Mallory-Weiss tears abuse alcohol and report "dry heaves" followed by small and then progressively larger amounts of bloody emesis. *Gastritis* due to alcohol or nonsteroidal anti-inflammatory agents is usually manifested by epigastric discomfort not relieved by food or antacids (see Ch. 98). The signs and symptoms of gastritis-associated bleeding may be identical to those of gastric ulcer disease. *Esophagitis* (see Color Plate 1*D*), particularly in the patient with longstanding reflux or regurgitation, is suggested by substernal burning pain occasionally relieved by ingestion of food or antacids (see Ch. 97). Alcohol abusers or patients with prolonged recumbency may sometimes have brisk bleeding from esophagitis without any antecedent substernal burning. *Gastrointestinal tract malignancies,* such as esophageal and gastric cancer or carcinoma of the ampulla of Vater, rarely cause hemodynamically significant upper gastrointestinal tract bleeding (see Table 95–1). Rare causes of upper gastrointestinal tract bleeding include (1) *aortoduodenal fistulas* in patients with atherosclerotic aneurysms of the abdominal aorta, usually following prosthetic grafting; (2) chronic renal disease and *acquired vascular ectasias;* and (3) ectasias associated with other systemic conditions, such as hereditary hemorrhagic telangiectasias (Osler-Weber-Rendu syndrome). Patients with trauma to the liver or with pancreatic pseudocysts may have signs and symptoms that suggest upper gastrointestinal tract bleeding but are actually bleeding from adjacent organs. Ectatic superficial arteries (Dieulafoy lesions), duodenal diverticula, and certain AIDS-related conditions (cytomegalovirus infection–related ulcers, Kaposi's sarcoma, and lymphoma) are occasionally encountered by clinicians (see Part XXII).

Diagnostic and Therapeutic Approach

ENDOSCOPY. Multiple diagnostic procedures are available to localize the site of hemorrhage in patients with upper gastrointestinal bleeding. For patients with hemodynamically significant upper gastrointestinal tract bleeding (bleeding associated with shock, postural vital sign changes, transfusion requirements of multiple units), endoscopy is the diagnostic procedure of choice because of its high accuracy and immediate therapeutic potential. Endoscopy, however, must be performed only following adequate resuscitation and clinical assessment of the patient (Fig. 95–1). If bleeding is severe, the patient should be transferred to an intensive care unit or an operating room where adequate monitoring and resuscitation can be maintained. Endoscopy can document the site of brisk hemorrhage in at least 95% of patients. In patients with significant cardiopulmonary disease, however, endoscopy is not without risk, since it does require sedation and analgesia. An endoscopic evaluation of a vigorously bleeding, unstable patient should be performed by an expert because it requires careful sedation, lavage, selection of instruments, and the use of accessory therapeutic endoscopic procedures. Although endoscopy is used in virtually all patients with manifestations of acute gastrointestinal tract hemorrhage, its urgent use is indicated primarily for patients with any of the following: postural vital sign changes or shock, multiple transfusions, hematocrits diluting below 30%, a high index of suspicion of variceal hemorrhage, recurrent hemorrhage from unknown sources, and high risk for surgery (prior to undertaking a surgical procedure). Contraindications to endoscopy include acute myocardial infarction, severe chronic lung disease, hemodynamic instability, patient agitation, and terminal malignancy.

In addition to documenting the site and probable cause of hemorrhage, endoscopy may provide definitive therapy for active bleeding. Acute variceal bleeding, for example, can be controlled with endoscopic sclerotherapy or varix band ligation in nearly 90% of patients and the likelihood of recurrent bleeding diminished. The long-term effect of this treatment on survival is less well established. Endoscopic multipolar (or bipolar or "Bicap") electrocoagulation, heater probe coagulation, and injection of dilute epinephrine solution are inexpensive, widely available, and highly reliable techniques for controlling upper gastrointestinal tract hemorrhage, particularly for patients with actively bleeding ulcers. These techniques, essentially comparable to one another in effectiveness, not only control acute hemorrhage but also decrease transfusion requirements, the necessity for surgery, and the duration and cost of hospitalization.

BARIUM RADIOGRAPHY. An "upper GI series," when performed with a double-contrast technique, identifies at least 70 to 80% of lesions confirmed to be associated with upper gastrointestinal tract bleeding. Barium radiography is noninvasive, costs less than endoscopy, and is readily available but has significant disadvantages, particularly in patients who are bleeding briskly. Large amounts of retained blood in the upper gastrointestinal tract impede the mucosal coating by barium and therefore the localization of superficial mucosal lesions. In patients who are briskly bleeding and

hemodynamically unstable, contrast radiography is also impractical. Moreover, on occasion, multiple lesions may be detected by barium radiography and the actual site of bleeding may be difficult to assess. Barium contrast radiography is an acceptable means of diagnosing upper gastrointestinal lesions, however, in patients who have not bled excessively, who have no stigmata of chronic liver disease, and who are not in need of endoscopic hemostasis.

ANGIOGRAPHY. The site of upper gastrointestinal tract bleeding may occasionally be missed on endoscopy. In these patients, angiography may localize the site of bleeding. In addition, selective infusion with vasopressin or coil embolization of actively bleeding arteries may control bleeding. In most instances, angiography localizes the bleeding site but does not establish its etiology. Bleeding must also be active because angiography detects only extravasation of contrast into the gastrointestinal tract. Angiography is expensive, time consuming, and invasive and requires transporting the patient to a specialized unit, but it is particularly helpful if bleeding is brisk in the face of a negative evaluation of the upper or lower gastrointestinal tract.

NUCLEAR SCINTIGRAPHY. For patients with less active blood loss, technetium red cell nuclear scintigraphy ("red cell scan") can be helpful in localizing the site of bleeding, with adequate sensitivity maintained with as little as 3 ml of blood loss per hour. Scintigraphy is noninvasive and can be performed with portable gamma cameras. As with angiography, the sensitivity of technetium scintigraphy is limited, since active hemorrhage is needed; therefore, frequent repeat scanning is necessary. Technetium red cell scanning is often performed prior to any angiographic evaluation to assist in the localization of the bleeding focus.

LOWER GASTROINTESTINAL TRACT BLEEDING (Table 95–2)

Colonic diverticula (see Color Plate 1G) are responsible for nearly one quarter of all episodes of hemodynamically significant bleeding from the lower gastrointestinal tract (Table 95–2). Diverticular hemorrhage is characteristically painless and associated with large-volume hematochezia. Patients with clinical diverticulitis rarely bleed significantly (see Ch. 112). *Colonic cancers and polyps* (see Color Plate 1E through 1H) often present as hematochezia, particularly with lesions in the distal sigmoid colon and rectum. Colonic neoplasms cause nearly 20% of lower gastrointestinal bleeding episodes. Proximal colonic polyps and cancers, however, often involve iron deficiency anemia and frequently dark black or bloody stools. Patients with *idiopathic ulcerative colitis and Crohn's colitis* commonly present with bloody diarrhea and tenesmus, and usually with a longstanding history of inflammatory bowel disease (see Ch. 104). Significant lower gastrointestinal tract bleeding also occurs from abnormal, superficial vessels called *vascular ectasias* (see Color Plate 1F). As noted above, up to 10% of cases of hemodynamically significant hematochezia are secondary to bleeding from upper gastrointestinal sites, particularly from duodenal bulbar ulcers (see Table 95–2). Other uncommon causes of "lower" gastrointestinal blood loss include aortoenteric fistulas, Meckel's diverticula of the ileum, and mesenteric varices.

Diagnostic and Therapeutic Approach

Proctoscopy (whether by rigid or flexible instruments) and careful evaluation of the anorectal junction is the initial diagnostic step for all patients with hematochezia. The anus and anorectal junction must be carefully examined for hemorrhoids or lacerations, since documented brisk bleeding from one of these sources can obviate the need for further invasive or noninvasive imaging. Blood from a very distal site in the rectum may retrogress into the colon and appear as blood coming from above the maximal depth of insertion of the proctoscope or sigmoidoscope. In addition to hemorrhoids, diverticula, and rectal lacerations, colitis and many polyps and cancers are found within reach of a sigmoidoscope.

Following anorectal and sigmoidoscopic examination, the evaluation of patients with lower gastrointestinal tract hemorrhage depends on the clinical presentation. If blood loss is modest (as evidenced by a normal hematocrit and vital signs), sigmoidoscopy may be followed by *double-contrast barium radiography,* which is highly accurate for detecting even smaller polyps and superficial mucosal abnormalities such as colitis. If signs and symptoms indicate lower gastrointestinal tract hemorrhage together with anemia, *colonoscopy* should be performed as the next step in evaluation. The colon can be rapidly cleansed within a few hours, using oral, nonabsorbable electrolyte solutions, in order to make colonoscopy technically feasible. Colonoscopic evaluation not only allows the site of hemorrhage to be accurately determined but also allows for biopsy of suspicious mass lesions, polypectomy for modest-sized polyps, and the use of coagulation techniques to control bleeding from vascular ectasias. If brisk bleeding continues, as evidenced by profuse hematochezia, *upper endoscopic evaluation* should be considered. Certainly this should be performed in all patients with "coffee grounds" nasogastric lavage and in patients with known or suspected peptic ulcer disease.

If bleeding is brisk, colonoscopy is usually not possible and other means of determining the site of hemorrhage are required. *Technetium red blood cell scintigraphy* can be used in patients in whom there is substantial active bleeding (at least 3 to 10 ml per hour for a positive scan). Frequent repeat scanning may be needed over the first several hours. Technetium red cell scintigraphy usually localizes the site but not the etiology of active hemorrhage. If bleeding continues at a rate exceeding 30 to 50 ml per hour, *angiography* can be extremely helpful in localizing the site of hemorrhage. In addition, angiographic therapy is possible with vasopressin or embolization techniques. An obvious advantage for technetium scintigraphy or angiographic localization is that surgical resection of the site of hemorrhage, regardless of etiology, is usually very effective.

Surgery

While the use of therapeutic endoscopy, interventional radiology, and potent antisecretory medications has dramatically reduced the need for emergency surgery, the clinician must consult surgical colleagues early. Approximately 10% of patients undergoing endoscopic coagulation or injection therapy continue to bleed despite repeat attempts at endoscopic hemostasis, thus necessitating operative intervention. A upper limit should be set on the number on units of blood transfused (perhaps as low as six to eight) and the number of sessions of therapeutic endoscopy (realistically no more than two) before surgery is undertaken, particularly for patients with peptic ulcers, colonic neoplasms, or diverticular hemorrhage. These lesions are easily amenable to standard surgical therapy, and the operations have low morbidity and mortality when performed in low-risk patients by skilled surgeons.

ACTIVE HEMORRHAGE OF UNKNOWN ORIGIN

Rarely patients continue to bleed from the gastrointestinal tract without detection of any lesion by upper gastrointestinal endoscopy or pancolonoscopy. In these cases bleeding is usually from a lesion distal to the inferior duodenal angle and proximal to the ileocecal valve. In such patients, technetium scintigraphy, often repeated frequently, can be extremely helpful in localizing the site of hemorrhage. In addition, angiography may determine the site of active blood loss. Other techniques that are sometimes useful in patients with persistent gastrointestinal tract blood loss are *small bowel enteroclysis* and *small bowel enteroscopy*. Enteroclysis, or small bowel enema, is performed by passing a nasoduodenal tube to facilitate the direct instillation of barium and methylcellulose. Radiographic evaluation of the entire small bowel can be completed by enteroclysis in less than 1 hour. Mass lesions such as polyps or cancers and diverticula such as Meckel's diverticula can thus be detected with a high degree of reliability. In patients who have bled repeatedly and profusely from the gastrointestinal tract and have negative evaluations by upper and lower tract endoscopy, enteroscopy should be considered. The small bowel may be examined well into the jejunum by this technique. This is most commonly employed in detecting lesions and treating patients with multiple vascular ectasias of the small bowel.

IRON DEFICIENCY ANEMIA

While most patients with gastrointestinal hemorrhage have obvious signs and symptoms of bleeding (i.e., hematemesis, melenemesis, melena, or hematochezia), a substantial number present solely with iron deficiency anemia. Some of these patients are asymptomatic while others, particularly the elderly, complain of lightheadedness, weakness, and dyspnea. Thorough evaluation of the gastrointestinal tract is mandatory when anemic patients are found to have occult blood in the stools and other obvious sites of hemorrhage are excluded. While the colon is widely thought to be the most frequent and important site of occult blood loss (especially from malignancies), the upper gastrointestinal tract also needs eval-

TABLE 95–3. GASTROINTESTINAL LESIONS IN 100 PATIENTS WITH IRON-DEFICIENCY ANEMIA*

Source of Hemorrhage	Percentage
Colon	
Cancer	11
Polyp	5
Vascular ectasia	5
Colitis	2
Cecal ulcer	2
Parasites	1
Total	26
Upper gastrointestinal tract	
Duodenal ulcer	11
Esophagitis	6
Gastritis	6
Gastric ulcer	5
Vascular ectasia	3
Anastomotic ulcer	3
Gastric cancer	1
Portal hypertensive gastropathy	1
Adenomatous polyp	1
Total	37

* Patients evaluated by colonoscopy followed by upper endoscopy under the same conscious sedation.

uation in iron-deficient anemic patients with negative colonoscopy studies (Table 95–3). The upper gastrointestinal tract may, in fact, be a more common site of blood loss anemia than the colon. Not infrequently, asymptomatic peptic ulcers, gastritis, and esophagitis will be found in these patients following normal colonoscopy.

Cello JP, Thoeni RF: Gastrointestinal hemorrhage—comparative values of double-contrast upper gastrointestinal radiology and endoscopy. JAMA 243:685, 1980. *Study of endoscopy and radiography in diagnosing sites of acute upper gastrointestinal hemorrhage.*

Jensen DM, Machicado GA: Diagnosis and treatment of severe hematochezia. The role of urgent colonoscopy after purge. Gastroenterology 95:1569, 1988. *Prospective study of 80 patients admitted with severe rectal bleeding.*

Laine L: Multipolar electrocoagulation in the treatment of active upper gastrointestinal tract hemorrhage. A prospective controlled trial. N Engl J Med 316:1613, 1987. *Endoscopic coagulation reduces rebleeding, transfusions, duration of hospitalization, and hospital costs.*

Laine L: Multipolar electrocoagulation in the treatment of peptic ulcers with nonbleeding visible vessels. A prospective controlled trial. Ann Intern Med 110:510, 1989. *Endoscopic treatment of nonbleeding vessels in ulcer bases decreases morbidity, hospital stay, and hospital costs.*

Lewis BS, Waye JD: Chronic gastrointestinal bleeding of obscure origin: Role of small bowel enteroscopy. Gastroenterology 94:1117, 1988. *Endoscopic examination of the small bowel discloses additional lesions missed by standard endoscopy and colonoscopy.*

Rockey DC, Cello JP: Evaluation of the gastrointestinal tract in patients with iron-deficiency anemia. N Engl J Med 329:1691, 1993. *Prospective study of upper and lower gastrointestinal endoscopy in 100 consecutive patients with severe anemia. A substantial number of upper gastrointestinal lesions were uncovered.*

96 DISEASES OF THE MOUTH AND SALIVARY GLANDS

Troy E. Daniels

More than 200 primary lesions or diseases occur in the oral mucosa, gingiva, teeth, jaws, and minor or major salivary glands. In addition, secondary abnormalities of the oral mucosa or salivary glands can be caused by systemic diseases or drugs. This chapter briefly discusses only the most common or important of the mucosal and salivary gland diseases because they may be observed during physical examination and are often part of a systemic process. It will provide a basis for developing a differential diagnosis and guiding treatment and referral. More complete coverage of these and other topics will be found in the references cited at the end of the chapter.

ORAL MUCOSAL DISEASES

Acute Ulcerations

Painful short-term ulcerations are usually caused by mechanical trauma, immunologic mechanisms, and bacterial or viral infections (Table 96–1). Soon after formation, ulcers in the mouth become covered by a white to gray pseudomembrane, analogous to the scab that forms on dry epidermis. Pseudomembrane-covered ulcers are distinguished from the white hyperkeratotic lesions described below by their clinical features of pain, a flat surface, and an erythematous periphery. Traumatic ulcers characteristically are located on the tongue or inside the cheeks or lips, are close to the chewing surfaces of the teeth, and have irregular borders.

APHTHOUS ULCERS. These idiopathic recurrent ulcers, which afflict about 20% of the population, are found on all areas of the oral mucosa except the hard palate, gingiva, and vermilion. They are well-defined circles and may be single or multiple. There are three clinical forms: (1) minor, which are flat and <1 cm in diameter, and last only 5 to 10 days; (2) major, which have raised borders, are >1 cm, and often last for weeks or months; and (3) herpetiform, which are usually clusters of very small ulcers that resemble recurrent herpetic lesions but are not preceded by vesicles and do not occur on keratinized mucosa. A viral pathogenesis has not been established for any of these forms. Lesions clinically identical to minor aphthous ulcers occur in Behçet's syndrome (see Ch. 249). Aphthous ulcers are occasionally associated with macrocytic anemias or gluten-sensitive enteropathy and may become more frequent and severe in association with human immunodeficiency virus (HIV) infection (Table 96–2).

Minor or herpetiform aphthous ulcers may not require treatment. Topical steroids, such as fluocinonide ointment in Orabase, can reduce the severity and duration of the lesions only if used with prodromal symptoms or early signs. Major aphthae usually require treatment by topical or systemic corticosteroids and occasionally are biopsied to rule out neoplasia.

VIRAL ULCERS. Several types of virus (most commonly herpes virus type 1, the cause of herpes simplex) may cause oral mucosal vesicles that last only a few hours or days and then become shallow ulcers. In the initial infection by herpes simplex virus, usually in children, numerous vesicles may appear on any oral mucosal site (primary herpetic gingivostomatitis), accompanied by malaise, headache, fever, and cervical lymphadenopathy. Patients previously exposed to this virus may develop recurrent lesions, most commonly as clusters of small vesicles on the lips (herpes labialis); only a few will develop intraoral recurrent herpes, as clusters of vesicles on the keratinized mucosa of the gingiva or hard palate. Such lesions tend to recur at the same site, but less frequently with age.

Similar mucosal vesicles may also accompany the initial infection by the varicella-zoster virus in children with chicken pox (see Ch. 336), and unilateral lesions may occur if herpes zoster (see Ch. 426) affects branches of the trigeminal nerve. Uncommonly, oral mucosal lesions may be caused by different types of coxsackievirus (see Ch. 343), appearing on any oral site in hand-foot-and-mouth disease (see Ch. 325) or on the soft palate or pharynx in herpangina. After infection by the measles (rubeola) virus, small ulcers (Koplik's spots) form on the inside of the cheeks 1 to 2 days before development of the skin rash (see Ch. 334).

ERYTHEMA MULTIFORME. In this potentially recurrent mucocutaneous disease, painful oral mucosal ulcerations develop rapidly in as many as half of the patients. The lesions may be confined to the mouth, with no skin involvement. The affected patients, usually young adults with minimal or no systemic symptoms, have irregularly shaped ulcers that can be small and few or involve large areas of the mucosa, most commonly the lower labial mucosa. These lesions can be distinguished from those of primary herpes by the absence of oral vesicles and systemic symptoms or by the presence of characteristic skin lesions (see Ch. 272). A major variant of this disease is the Stevens-Johnson syndrome.

VENEREAL INFECTIONS. Primary syphilis may present as a solitary, indurated, painless ulcer on the oral mucosa that resolves spontaneously in 4 to 6 weeks (see Ch. 318). Uncommonly, *Neisseria gonorrhoeae* may cause oral ulcers, usually in the pharynx, that may be confused with oral ulcers of other causes.

Oral Squamous Cell Carcinoma

About 4% of all cancers occur in the mouth, largely squamous cell carcinomas of the mucosal epithelium. Oral carcinoma occurs usually in the fifth decade or beyond, in men twice as frequently as in women, and with long-term use of tobacco (>80% of cases) (Table 96–1).

Oral carcinoma usually presents as a chronic, indurated, cratered ulcer, but early lesions of squamous cell carcinoma may appear as white or red macules (Table 96–2). About 15% of oral carcinomas arise within a pre-existing white plaque (leukoplakia). The overall 5-year survival is approximately 50%, but early treatment of small, localized lesions can lead to survival rates as high as 90%.

Other Chronic Ulcerations

Several mucocutaneous diseases can cause chronic multifocal oral mucosal lesions composed of ill-defined areas of erythema and ulceration. They are among the most difficult oral lesions to diagnose and are discussed below with the red lesions (Table 96–2). Several microbial infections can lead to indurated, chronic oral mucosal ulcerations with moderate symptoms (Table 96–1).

TABLE 96–1. ORAL MUCOSAL ULCERS

Type/Disease	Clinical Features
Insidious Onset, Chronic	
Multiple or bilateral	Shallow ulcers on mucosa, skin, or both
Pemphigus vulgaris	Begin as short-duration blisters
Mucous membrane pemphigoid	Begin as short-duration blisters
Lichen planus	Bilaterally symmetric lesions (associated with hyperkeratoses and/or erythema)
Lupus erythematosus	Asymmetric lesions, with or without systemic lupus (associated with hyperkeratoses and/or erythema)
Drug reaction	Variable lesions; appropriate history of drug use
Epidermolysis bullosa	Begin as blisters; life-long history
Solitary	Indurated or cratered ulcers
Squamous cell carcinoma	Most commonly on tongue, oropharynx, lip, mouth floor
Adenocarcinomas, various	Most commonly on palate, cheeks, mouth floor
Tuberculosis	Usually painful
Actinomycosis	Often associated with draining sinus
Deep mycoses (particularly histoplasmosis, coccidioidomycosis)	Associated with systemic infection
Midline granuloma	Associated with necrosis, may perforate palate
Acute Onset, Often Self-Limiting	
Clusters	Usually small and shallow ulcers; history of blisters
Primary herpes simplex	Any oral mucosal site, associated with fever, malaise
Recurrent herpes simplex	Only on gingiva, hard palate, or lip (keratinized mucosa)
Varicella-zoster	Unilateral lesions along neural distribution
Herpangina	Usually on oropharynx
Measles (rubeola)	Precede skin rash; associated with fever, malaise
Solitary or multiple (without clustering)	Variable, usually without history of blisters
Traumatic ulcers	Usually solitary; history of trauma
Recurrent aphthae	Circular, often multiple, only on non-keratinized mucosa
Behçet's syndrome	Oral lesions similar to recurrent aphthae
Erythema multiforme	Multiple lesions, often involve lower labial mucosa; can be recurrent or chronic
Drug reaction	Appropriate history of drug use
Necrotizing sialometaplasia	Usually on palate
Primary syphilis	Solitary, indurated, painless, any site
Gonorrhea	Painful, surrounded by erythema, any site

PLATE 1 GASTROINTESTINAL DISEASES

Endoscopy and colonoscopy in gastrointestinal hemorrhage.

A, Esophageal varices. Large serpiginous dilated submucosal veins *(arrows)* are noted coursing longitudinally down the distal esophagus.

B, Gastric varices. The endoscope has been turned around on itself to examine the gastric cardia, where large submucosal masses are seen projecting into the lumen *(arrows).*

C, Duodenal bulbar ulcer. A white excavated base is noted just inside the pylorus *(large arrows)* containing a dark red central artery oozing blood *(small arrow).*

D, Esophagitis. The normal pink esophageal mucosa is replaced by white exudate overlying extensive superficial erosions in a patient with reflux esophagitis.

E, Colonic cancer. Nearly all the lumen is obstructed by a fungating, bleeding colonic malignancy.

F, Vascular ectasia of the cecum. The normal delicate branching mucosal vessels are altered by a "coral reef" *(arrow)* telangiectatic lesion in an elderly patient with recurrent bouts of hematochezia.

G, Diverticulum of colon. Clotted blood can be seen within an outpouching of the colonic wall *(arrow)* in a patient with massive hematochezia.

H, Colonic polyp. An irregular fleshy mass on a pedicle *(arrow)* is noted projecting into the bowel lumen. Polypectomy subsequently removed and retrieved an adenomatous polyp.

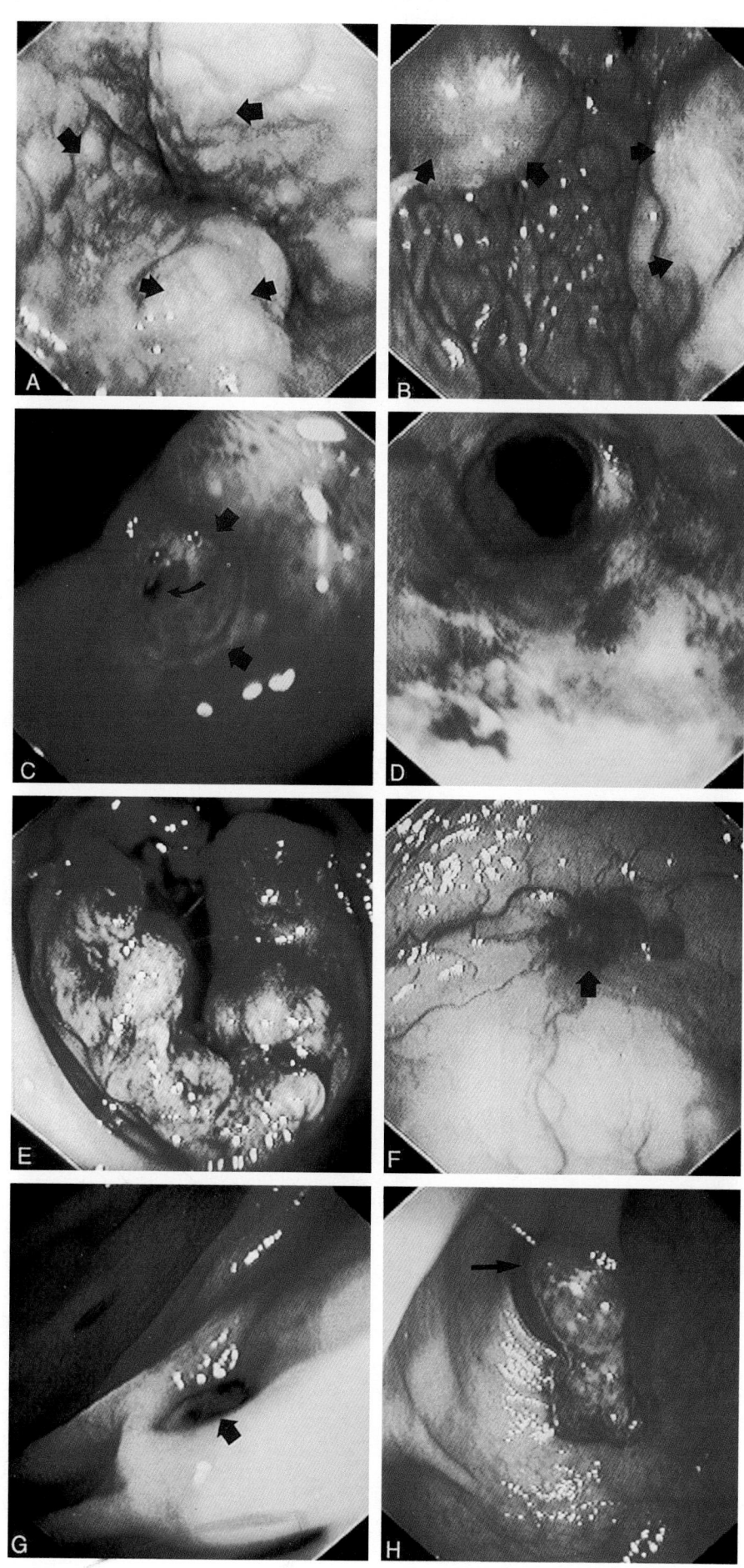

PLATE 2   GASTROINTESTINAL AND CARDIOVASCULAR DISEASES

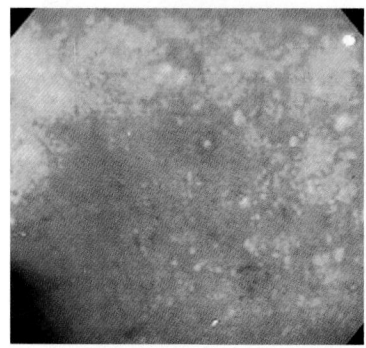

A, Endoscopic mild ulcerative colitis. Granular-appearing mucosa with friability and pinpoint ulceration.

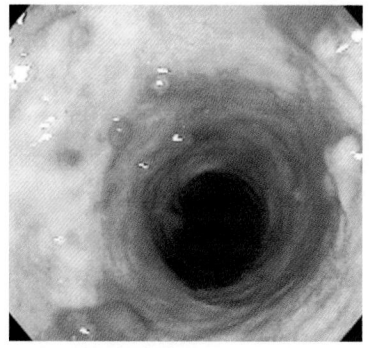

B, Endoscopic quiescent ulcerative colitis. Distorted vascular pattern with residual "pseudopolyps."

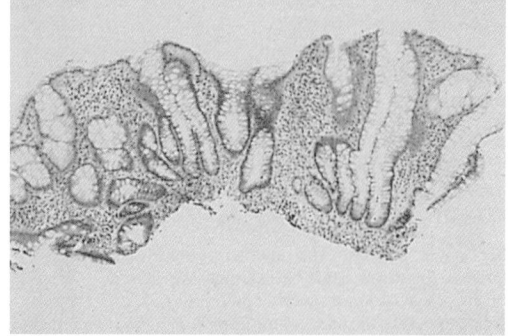

C, Mucosal biopsy of quiescent ulcerative colitis. Distorted, branching glands with reduced goblet cell mucus and minimal chronic inflammation.

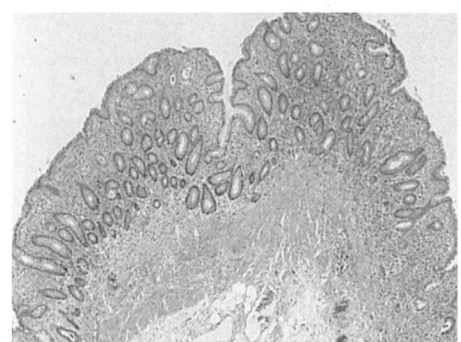

D, Mucosal biopsy of active ulcerative colitis. *Left,* Low power. Acute and chronic inflammation. *Right,* High power. Crypt abscess.

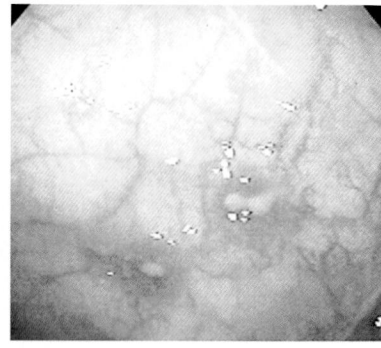

E, Aphthoid ulcer of Crohn's disease. Note normal surrounding mucosa.

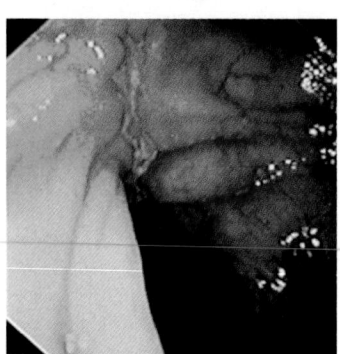

F, Crohn's disease. Linear ulceration.

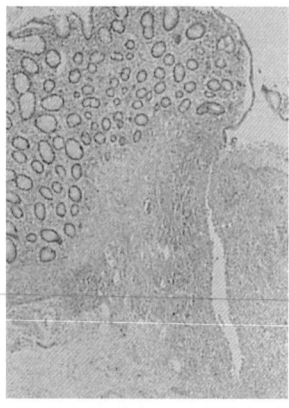

G, Mucosal biopsy of Crohn's disease. Focal inflammation with fissuring ulceration.

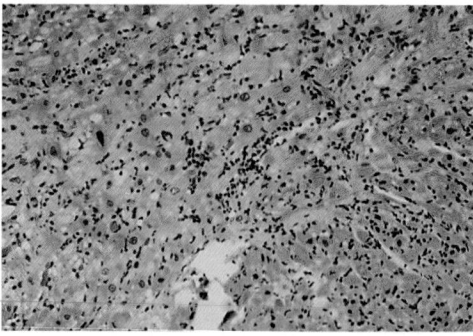

I, Endomyocardial biopsy specimen stained with hematoxylin-eosin demonstrating a severe lymphocytic infiltrate and myocyte necrosis with vacuolization in a 34-year-old woman with biventricular cardiomyopathy of 2 months' duration.

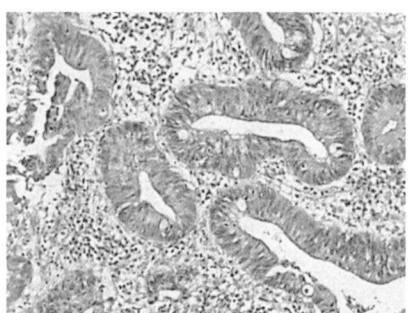

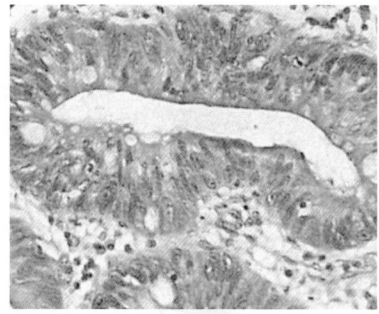

H, Low-power *(left)* and high-power *(right)* views of mucosal dysplasia with hyperchromatic epithelial cells and mucus depletion with stratification and loss of polarity.

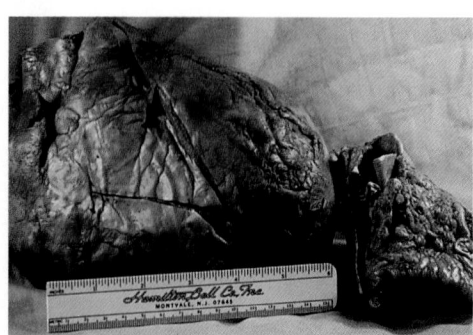

J, Comparison between an undiseased heart *(right)* and a dilated heart *(left)* removed from a transplant candidate with a 5-year history of idiopathic cardiomyopathy. (Courtesy of Mary Woo, DNSc.)

PLATE 3 CARDIOVASCULAR AND RHEUMATOLOGIC DISEASES

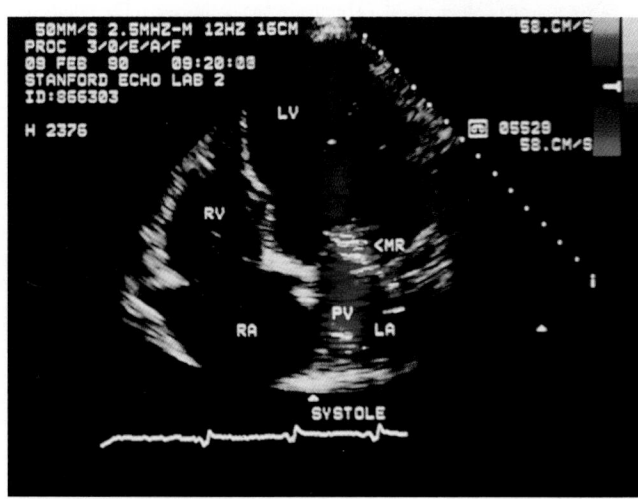

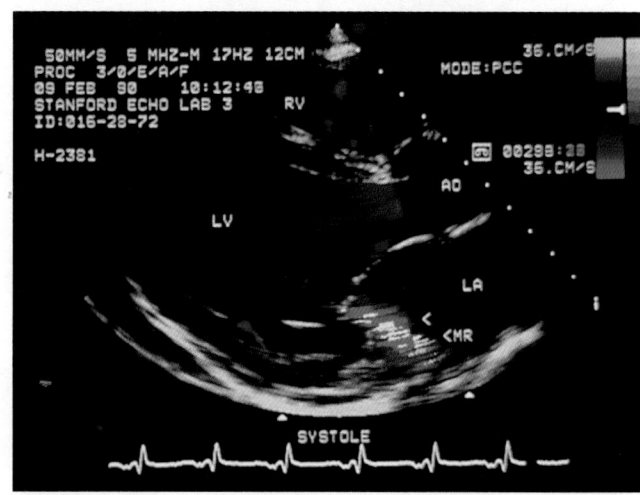

A, A two-dimensional echocardiographic image with Doppler color flow mapping superimposed to indicate blood flow. A portion of the image contains color-coded information regarding the direction and velocity of flow. Shades of orange represent flow toward the transducer, and shades of blue represent flow away from the transducer. Pulmonary venous (PV) flow into the left atrium is noted in orange during systole, while mitral regurgitation (MR) is indicated by the eccentric color at the lateral left atrial wall, extending from the area of the mitral valve. The mitral regurgitation signal contains blue, orange, and white, giving a mosaic pattern that is typical of high-velocity turbulent flow. LA = Left atrium; LV = left ventricle; RA = right atrium; RV = right ventricle.

B, A two-dimensional echocardiogram with Doppler flow mapping superimposed on a portion of the image. The color information is represented in the sector of the imaging plane extending from the apex of the triangular plane to the two small arrows at the bottom of the image plane. Mitral regurgitation (MR) is indicated *(open arrows),* extending from the mitral valve leaflets toward the posterior aspect of the left atrium (LA) during systole. The mosaic of colors representing the mitral regurgitant signal is typical of high-velocity turbulent flow. The low-intensity orange-brown signal represents flow directed away from the transducer on the chest wall, and the blue shades represent blood in the left ventricular outflow tract moving toward the transducer. AO=Aorta; LV=left ventricle; RV=right ventricle.

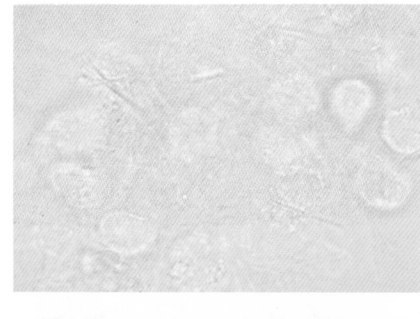
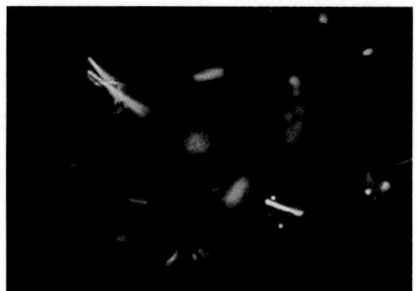
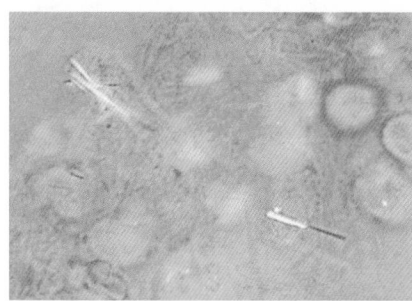
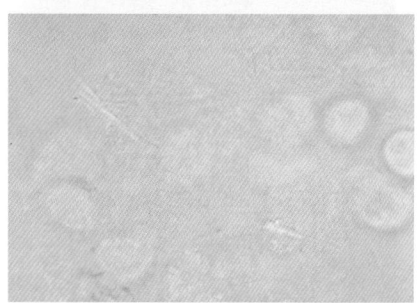

C, Monosodium urate crystals in synovial fluid aspirate. *Top left,* Plain light microscopy. *Top right,* Polarized light. *Bottom left,* First-order red compensator with axis of vibration perpendicular to crystals (2 o'clock to 7 o'clock). *Bottom right,* First-order red compensator with axis of vibration parallel to crystals (11 o'clock to 4 o'clock).

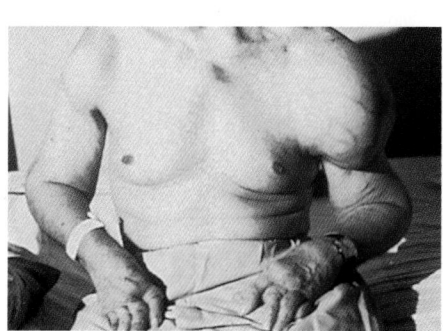

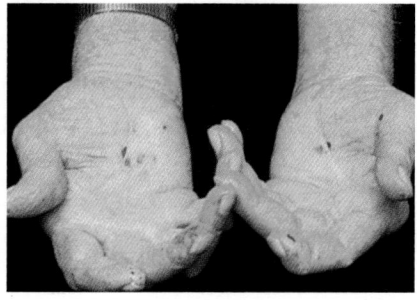

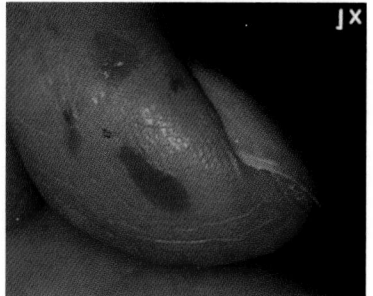

D, Large synovial cysts of the shoulders, especially on the left, in a patient with chronic deforming rheumatoid arthritis.

E, Left and *right,* Rheumatoid vasculitis with small brown infarcts of palms and fingers in chronic rheumatoid arthritis. (Courtesy of Dr. Martin Lidsky, Houston, Texas.)

PLATE 4   RENAL DISEASES

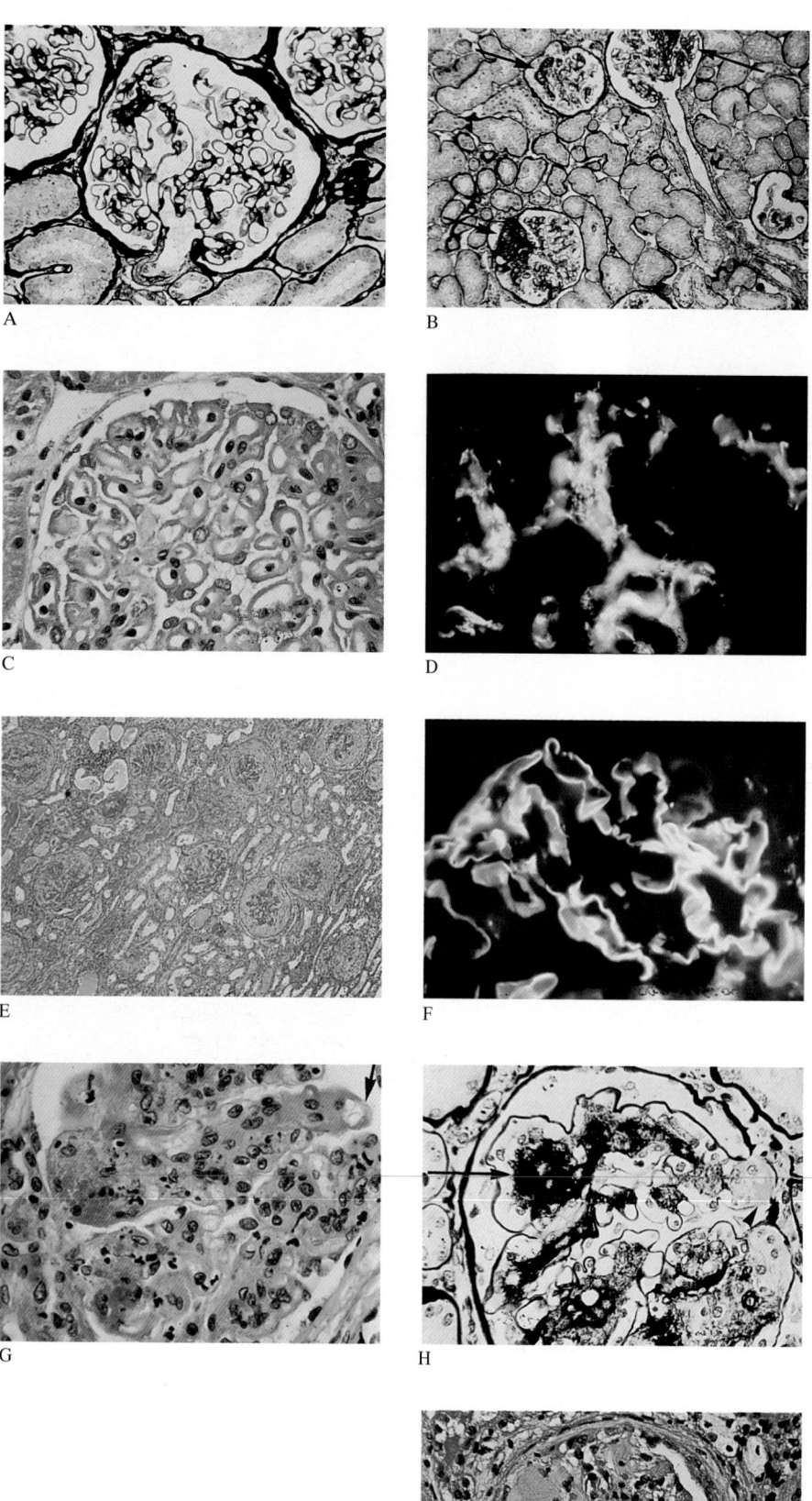

A, Minimal change disease. The glomeruli demonstrate no abnormalities at the light microscopic level (Jones methenamine silver, ×260).

B, Focal segmental glomerulosclerosis. The glomerular capillary lumina are segmentally obliterated by basement membrane material *(arrows).* The adjacent glomerular lobules are unremarkable (Jones methenamine silver, ×100).

C, Membranous glomerulopathy. The glomerular basement membranes are uniformly thickened and rigid. There is no hypercellularity of the glomerular tuft (H & E, ×400).

D, IgA nephropathy. Fluorescence micrograph showing intense staining of the mesangium with antisera to IgA (×600).

E, Anti–glomerular basement membrane disease. Low-power micrograph showing diffuse involvement of the glomeruli by crescents, which compress the glomerular tuft (PAS, ×40).

F, Anti–glomerular basement membrane antibody disease. Fluorescence micrograph showing intense linear reactivity of the glomerular basement membranes with antisera to IgG (×600).

G, Lupus nephritis. Diffuse proliferative lupus nephritis showing global occlusion of the glomerular capillary lumina by endocapillary and mesangial proliferation. There are numerous infiltrating mononuclear and polymorphonuclear leukocytes with focal pyknosis and karyorrhexis. The arrow denotes a "wire-loop" deposit (H & E, ×400).

H, Nodular diabetic glomerulosclerosis. The mesangium is expanded by matrix material forming nodules *(arrow).* The glomerular basement membranes are diffusely thickened. Inframembranous hyaline deposits are also present *(arrowhead)* (Jones methenamine silver, ×400).

I, Amyloidosis. The glomerular tuft is segmentally infiltrated by amorphous eosinophilic material with a hyaline appearance (H & E, ×260).

TABLE 96–2. WHITE AND RED ORAL MUCOSAL LESIONS

White Lesions (Plaques)
Squamous cell carcinoma (early)
Frictional keratosis
Leukoplakia (idiopathic)
Smokeless tobacco–associated lesions
Nicotine stomatitis (palate)
Lichen planus (reticular and plaque types)
Pseudomembranous candidiasis (thrush)
Hyperplastic candidiasis (candidal leukoplakia)
Hairy leukoplakia (HIV-associated; usually on lateral tongue)
Geographic tongue
Mucous patch or condyloma latum of secondary syphilis
Pseudomembrane-covered ulcers (see Table 96–1)

Red Lesions (Macular, Maculopapular)
Squamous cell carcinoma (early)
Erythroplakia (epithelial dysplasia)
Erythematous (atrophic) candidiasis
Median rhomboid glossitis
Mucocutaneous diseases (see Table 96–1)
Angular cheilitis
Telangiectasias and purpuras
Kaposi's sarcoma (blue to purple color)

White Lesions

White plaques are commonly found in the mouth but, like ulcerations, have a wide variety of causes and outcomes (Table 96–2). The term "leukoplakia" applies to a white plaque that does not rub off and whose appearance does not indicate another disease. Leukoplakia can occur in any area of the mouth and usually exhibits benign hyperkeratosis on biopsy. On long-term follow-up, 2 to 6% of these lesions will have undergone malignant transformation into squamous cell carcinoma. Areas of leukoplakia with a corrugated surface or mixed with areas of erythema are often found in the lower labial or buccal vestibule of those who use smokeless tobacco.

Frictional keratoses are often found posterior to the lower molar teeth as irregular white plaques and on the buccal mucosa as white lines adjacent to the dental occlusion. Unlike leukoplakia, these lesions rarely become malignant.

LICHEN PLANUS. Oral lesions of lichen planus occur in about 1% of the population, usually as multiple, bilaterally symmetric reticular white plaques, with or without adjacent areas of erythema (atrophy or erosion) or ulcers. The presence of mucosal atrophy, erosion, or ulceration usually causes pain or sensitivity to certain foods. Most lesions can be adequately controlled by frequent topical application of fluocinonide ointment mixed with an equal weight of Orabase for periods of several weeks to several months, although recurrence is common.

ORAL CANDIDIASIS. This fungal disease has three clinical forms: pseudomembranous (thrush), erythematous (atrophic), and hyperplastic (candidal leukoplakia). Pseudomembranous candidiasis, usually of relatively short duration, occurs on any site and consists of white fungal plaques that can be rubbed off, leaving a red or bleeding base. Lesions of hyperplastic candidiasis are white, have fungal hyphae within the surface layers of hyperkeratotic epithelium, do not rub off, and are most often found on the anterior buccal mucosa or on the tongue. Erythematous candidiasis is discussed below with the red lesions. All forms of oral candidiasis represent overgrowth or superficial infection by *Candida* species from the oral flora, induced by a variety of causes. These include suppression of bacterial flora by systemic antibiotics, chronic xerostomia, uncontrolled diabetes mellitus or anemia, and immunosuppression (especially in HIV-infected patients; Table 96–3).

HAIRY LEUKOPLAKIA. This recently identified lesion is a white plaque occurring most frequently on the lateral surfaces of the tongue bilaterally, mainly in HIV-infected persons. *Candida* may be present in the surface layers, but the lesion is not eliminated by effective antifungal therapy and contains large quantities of Epstein-Barr virus. Its diagnosis should be followed by an HIV antibody test.

GEOGRAPHIC TONGUE. Also called "benign migratory glossitis," this benign idiopathic condition affects the dorsal tongue of about 2% of the population. It is characterized by well-defined areas of atrophied filiform papillae bordered by arcs of normal or hyperplastic filiform papillae and by changes in the location of these lesions over time. Treatment is usually not necessary.

SECONDARY SYPHILIS. Secondary syphilis may manifest as a well-defined white plaque on the labial or palatal mucosa, called "condyloma latum" (or "split papule," because of their lobulated periphery).

Red Lesions

Solitary red macules or plaques ("erythroplakia") are less common in the mouth than white lesions but should be viewed with concern because they may exhibit microscopic dysplasia or represent carcinoma *in situ* (see Table 96–2). They may be associated with areas of leukoplakia. However, a red macule occurring in the midline of the posterior dorsal tongue, classified as median rhomboid glossitis, is an idiopathic but uniformly benign condition that is often associated with localized overgrowth of *Candida* species.

ERYTHEMATOUS (ATROPHIC) ORAL CANDIDIASIS. This chronic condition is characterized by erythema and atrophy of the filiform papillae on the dorsal tongue or by ill-defined erythema on the palate, tongue, or buccal mucosa. It is accompanied by symptoms of oral mucosal burning and sensitivity to certain foods and is often associated with salivary hypofunction. Patients who wear removable dentures often have mucosal erythema confined to the denture-bearing area.

Topical nystatin or clotrimazole or systemic ketoconazole can resolve these lesions and are usually administered for several months. In patients who have salivary hypofunction and remaining natural teeth, topical antifungal preparations containing sucrose or glucose must be avoided to prevent caries; slow oral dissolution of vaginal nystatin tablets is safe and effective. Systemic ketoconazole may not be effective in patients with severe xerostomia. Effective treatment significantly improves oral symptoms, regardless of the cause of the candidiasis. Treatment of denture-associated candidiasis also requires appropriate treatment of the denture.

ANGULAR CHEILITIS. Erythema or crusting of the labial angles is usually caused by *Candida*. It is usually associated with intraoral candidiasis and in such cases topical treatment of the angular cheilitis should be accompanied by intraoral or systemic antifungal treatment as described above.

MUCOCUTANEOUS DISEASES. The mucocutaneous diseases of pemphigus vulgaris, mucous membrane pemphigoid, atrophic or erosive lichen planus, and lupus erythematosus can cause similar-appearing oral lesions. Their diagnosis requires examination of a biopsy specimen by routine histopathology and usually also by direct immunofluorescence to identify characteristic deposits of immunoglobulins and complement components.

The first lesions of pemphigus vulgaris usually are oral mucosal vesicles that rapidly rupture, leaving painful erosions or ulcerations. These are followed by development of skin lesions. Rarely, the lesions remain confined to the mouth.

TABLE 96–3. ORAL LESIONS ASSOCIATED WITH HIV INFECTION

Kaposi's sarcoma
Candidiasis
  Pseudomembranous
  Hyperplastic
  Erythematous
Other opportunistic fungal infections (e.g., histoplasmosis or coccidioidomycosis)
Epithelial lesions
  Aphthous ulcers (increased frequency, duration, or size)
  Virus-associated epithelial hyperplasias
    Hairy leukoplakia
    Oral wart
    Focal epithelial hyperplasia (Heck's disease)
    Condyloma acuminatum
  Herpes zoster
Exaggerated forms of gingivitis and inflammatory periodontal disease
Decreased salivary gland function
Parotid gland enlargement (benign lymphoepithelial lesion)
Non-Hodgkin's lymphoma

Lesions of mucous membrane (cicatricial) pemphigoid are usually confined to the oral mucosa or conjunctivae and occur in patients over age 50. They begin as vesicles that quickly rupture, leaving ulcers and areas of atrophic epithelium that are chronic but only moderately symptomatic. Use of topical fluocinonide for several months, as described above for lichen planus, will sometimes be sufficient to treat the oral lesions, but some patients also need systemic treatment (see Ch. 475).

Oral mucosal lesions of lupus may occur in patients who have systemic lupus erythematosus (SLE), in patients who do not have SLE but later develop that disease, or in patients who do not develop SLE. In this latter group, the lesions of mucosal lupus may be analogous to the skin lesions of chronic discoid lupus. Lesions of oral lupus are usually solitary or bilaterally asymmetric. They take the form of reticular hyperkeratotic figures associated with erythema, often resembling atrophic lichen planus. The lesions can be controlled by topical fluocinonide or intralesional triamcinolone.

Lesions of Kaposi's sarcoma associated with HIV infection often appear first on the oral mucosa, especially the palate. They begin as macules with a blue or purple color, at which time they need to be distinguished from purpura. Later, they spread radially and expand vertically (Table 96–3).

Pigmentations

Brown or gray-black macules on the oral mucosa are relatively common and may be caused by localized increase in melanin production, proliferation of melanin-producing cells, or deposition of local or systemically distributed pigmented substances (Table 96–4). Mucosal pigmentation may occur after long-term administration of chloroquine, minocycline, nystatin, or cyclophosphamide. Malignant melanoma can occur at any oral mucosal site but develops most frequently on the mucosa or gingiva covering the maxilla. Diagnosis of any of these is usually established by biopsy and knowledge of relevant underlying conditions.

ORAL SOFT TISSUE TUMORS

In addition to the malignant neoplasms just described, a variety of observable benign soft tissue tumors exist that are usually treated by dentists or oral-maxillofacial surgeons.

Connective Tissue Hyperplasias

The most common oral soft tissue tumors are small, pedunculated masses of hyperplastic fibrous connective tissue covered by normal-appearing mucosa (Table 96–5). Solitary lesions are usually found on the inside of the cheeks or lips. Similar lesions may be present at the border of an ill-fitting denture or may occur in clusters on the hard palate under an ill-fitting denture ("palatal papillomatosis"); the latter is often associated with erythematous candidiasis.

Generalized enlargement of the gingiva may be caused by chronic administration of phenytoin, cyclosporine, diltiazem, verapamil, or nifedipine. It can also be associated with a hereditary defect or be caused by an infiltration of white blood cells in some

TABLE 96–4. PIGMENTATIONS OF THE ORAL MUCOSA (BROWN OR GRAY-BLACK IN COLOR)

Increased Melanin Production (Flat Lesions)
Oral melanotic macule
Ephelis (vermilion border)
Systemic diseases: Addison's disease, von Recklinghausen's disease of skin, Albright's syndrome, Peutz-Jeghers syndrome

Proliferation of Melanin-Producing Cells (Flat or Raised Lesions)
Pigmented cellular nevi (benign and premalignant types)
Atypical melanocytic hyperplasia, melanoma *in situ,* radial growth phase of melanoma
Malignant melanoma

Nonmelanin Pigmentation
Amalgam tattoo
Focal deposition of systemically distributed metal (lead, bismuth, mercury, others) usually at sites of chronic inflammation
Systemically administered drugs (chloroquine, minocycline, nizoral, cyclophosphamide)

TABLE 96–5. ORAL SOFT TISSUE TUMORS

Connective Tissue Hyperplasia (Normal-Appearing Overlying Mucosa)
Irritation fibroma
Denture-associated hyperplasia
Palatal papillomatosis
Generalized gingival hyperplasia
  Drug-induced (phenytoin, nifedipine, cyclosporine)
  Hereditary

Reactive Hyperplasia (Erythematous Overlying Mucosa)
Pyogenic granuloma/pregnancy tumor
Peripheral giant cell granuloma
Inflammatory gingival hyperplasia
Hyperplastic lingual tonsil

Epithelial Masses (Usually Irregular White Surface)
Papilloma/oral wart
Squamous cell carcinoma
Verrucous carcinoma
Focal epithelial hyperplasia (Heck's disease)
Condyloma acuminatum (venereal wart)
Keratoacanthoma (on lips)

Salivary Duct Obstruction (Minor Salivary Glands)
Mucocele/ranula (usually fluctuant)
Salivary stone (sialolith)

Subepithelial Neoplasms
Primary connective tissue or salivary gland tumors
Metastatic lesions, (especially in the mandible)
Lymphoma (especially in the palate or posterior mandible)
Focal or generalized leukemic infiltrates in the gingiva (especially with acute monocytic leukemia)

types of leukemia, especially acute monocytic. The drug-associated cases apparently represent an exaggerated response in susceptible patients to commonly occurring local irritants.

Reactive Hyperplasias

Small masses with surfaces that are ulcerated or only partially covered by normal-appearing mucosa usually represent reactive lesions in the form of pyogenic granulomas (whose frequency increases during pregnancy), peripheral giant cell granulomas, or lymphoid hyperplasia of the lingual or other tonsillar tissue. The granulomas are most often located on the gingiva. Rarely, such lesions may represent a metastatic neoplasm.

Epithelial Tumors

Small, white, wartlike epithelial masses are common and can occur in any area of the oral mucosa. They are occasionally classified as epithelial neoplasms, but most do not continue to grow. Human papillomavirus types 2, 6, 11, and 13 have been identified in some but not all of these wartlike lesions, which are usually classified generically as papillomas. A large wartlike lesion on the oral mucosa should raise the suspicion of verrucous carcinoma.

Mucus Retention Cysts (Mucoceles)

Mucoceles are small, chronic or recurring nodules that occur commonly on the inside of the cheeks and lips, the posterior palate, and the mouth floor. They are caused by injury to one of the many minor salivary glands, resulting in extravasation of mucus, which causes granulomatous inflammation or blockage of the excretory duct. Both types of lesions require conservative surgical excision.

SALIVARY GLAND DISEASES

Primary Diseases of Salivary Glands

Patients with enlargement of a major or minor salivary gland usually present a diagnostic challenge (Table 96–6). More than 20 types of benign or malignant salivary gland neoplasms may appear as unilateral enlargement of a major gland that is firm and nontender to palpation or as a firm submucosal nodule on the palate or the labial or buccal mucosa. Uncommonly, unilateral major gland enlargement may be reactive—e.g., benign lymphoepithelial lesion, or chronic sialadenitis from a sialolith or inadequately treated bacterial sialadenitis. Observation of any of these lesions should be followed by appropriate imaging and biopsy.

Unilateral major salivary gland enlargement that is markedly painful or tender to palpation and has a purulent exudate or nothing

Usually Unilateral

Benign or malignant salivary gland neoplasms (more than 20 different histopathologic types)
Bacterial infection
Chronic sialadenitis (single gland)

Usually Bilateral and Associated with Salivary Hypofunction

Viral infection (mumps, cytomegalovirus, influenza, coxsackie A)
Sjögren's syndrome (benign lymphoepithelial lesion)
Chronic granulomatous diseases (sarcoidosis, tuberculosis, leprosy)
Recurrent parotitis of childhood
Human immunodeficiency virus infection/AIDS

Bilaterally Symmetric, Soft, Nontender, Parotid Only

Sialadenosis (asymptomatic parotid enlargement), idiopathic or associated with:

Diabetes mellitus	Chronic pancreatitis
Hyperlipoproteinemia	Acromegaly
Hepatic cirrhosis	Gonadal hypofunction
Anorexia/bulimia	Phenylbutazone use

expressible from the duct suggests bacterial sialadenitis. Any exudate should be cultured, and initial treatment should be oral cephalexin or dicloxacillin.

Bilateral Salivary Gland Enlargement and Decreased Salivary Secretion Associated with Systemic Diseases

The best-known cause of bilateral salivary gland enlargement is infection by the mumps virus in children (Table 96–6). The incidence of mumps decreased in the United States by >90% after the introduction of an effective vaccine in 1967, but the number of cases began to rise again in the late 1980's, apparently as a result of reduced use of the vaccine. Uncommonly, a less acute, mumps-like illness may occur in adults in association with cytomegalovirus, influenza, or coxsackie A virus infection.

Sjögren's syndrome is characterized in about one third of patients by gradual development of firm, nontender or only slightly tender, bilateral enlargement of major salivary glands (see Ch. 242). The enlargement may slowly wax and wane. Salivary secretion decreases gradually, and, if hypofunction is severe and prolonged, the resulting dry mouth can impair speech and swallowing and be associated with rapidly progressive dental caries, symptomatic erythematous candidiasis, and difficulty in wearing dentures. In severe cases, the oral mucosa is dry and sticky and saliva is not expressible from the major ducts. About one third of patients show signs of erythematous candidiasis (see above).

The salivary component of Sjögren's syndrome should be diagnosed from a labial salivary gland biopsy specimen containing at least five glands. Examination must show focal lymphocytic sialadenitis in most or all of the specimen and exclude nonspecific chronic sialadenitis or abnormality indicative of another disease, such as noncaseating granuloma. A patient's symptoms of oral dry-

TABLE 96–7. CAUSES OF DECREASED SALIVARY SECRETION (XEROSTOMIA)

Temporary

Effects of short-term drug use (e.g., antihistamines)
Virus infections (e.g., mumps)
Dehydration
Psychogenic causes (fear, depression)

Chronic

Effects of chronically administered drugs (especially antidepressants, MAO inhibitors, neuroleptics, parasympatholytics, some combinations of drugs for treating hypertension)

Systemic Diseases (With or Without Gland Enlargement)

Sjögren's syndrome
Granulomatous diseases (sarcoidosis, tuberculosis, leprosy)
Amyloidosis
HIV infection
Diabetes mellitus (uncontrolled)
Graft-versus-host disease
Depression
Therapeutic radiation to the head and neck
Absent or malformed glands (rare)

ness are important, but, being subjective and nonspecific (Table 96–7), they are not diagnostic. Results from salivary functional or imaging studies are not specific to Sjögren's syndrome.

Several chronic granulomatous diseases, such as sarcoidosis, tuberculosis, and leprosy, can cause bilateral enlargement and decreased function of salivary glands. The clinical and serologic features of sarcoidosis may closely mimic those of Sjögren's syndrome, and the distinction must be made by salivary gland biopsy.

A few adult patients with HIV infection, and most children who are infected *in utero,* develop major salivary gland enlargement and reduced salivary secretion that are caused by lymphocytic infiltration. Parotid gland enlargement usually represents a solid or cystic benign lymphoepithelial lesion (see Table 96–3).

Recurrent parotitis of childhood includes episodes of unilateral or bilateral parotid enlargement. During flares of this illness, salivary secretion may be reduced, but usually without prominent secondary symptoms or signs. This condition, of unknown cause, usually subsides after puberty. Some serologic evidence suggests an association with Epstein-Barr virus infection.

Asymptomatic Parotid Enlargement (Sialadenosis)

Parotid glands can develop bilateral, symmetric enlargement that is soft and nontender to palpation and not associated with salivary hypofunction (see Table 96–6). Diagnosis is established by the clinical presentation and (if necessary to rule out Sjögren's syndrome or sarcoidosis) a normal labial salivary gland biopsy. Usually, results of sialography and salivary scintigraphy are within normal limits. Biopsy of the affected glands is not indicated for diagnosis.

This chronic, noninflammatory, and non-neoplastic condition is usually associated with a variety of systemic diseases, including diabetes mellitus, hyperlipoproteinemia, hepatic cirrhosis, anorexia/bulimia, chronic pancreatitis, acromegaly, and gonadal hypofunction. It can also result from use of phenylbutazone or be a reaction to iodine-containing contrast media.

Impaired Salivary Secretion Without Gland Enlargement

The very common symptom of dry mouth (xerostomia) is most often a side effect of chronically administered drugs. Many classes of drugs reduce unstimulated salivary secretion through anticholinergic or other mechanisms (Table 96–7). At least initially, most of these drugs do not interfere with salivary production in response to gustatory, olfactory, or masticatory stimuli. This means that patients will experience the symptoms soon after beginning to use the drug, but will produce enough saliva during a meal for normal chewing and swallowing. The effects are dose-dependent and are produced by most tricyclic antidepressants, most neuroleptics, monoamine oxidase inhibitors, and all anticholinergics. A combination of drugs for treatment of hypertension may cause symptoms of dry mouth, but usually not to the extent of the drugs listed above.

Several systemic diseases affect salivary secretion. As noted above, most patients with Sjögren's syndrome, some with sarcoidosis, and a few patients with HIV infection experience symptoms of dry mouth to various degrees, with or without salivary gland enlargement (Table 96–7). In addition, patients who have primary or secondary amyloidosis with salivary gland deposition may develop impaired secretion. Depressed patients who are not taking antidepressants apparently have decreased resting salivary secretion and complain more frequently of symptoms of dry mouth.

Irradiation of the head and neck region to treat a malignant tumor usually produces profound dry mouth before therapy is completed. Secretory capacity recovers only slightly in the months following treatment. Less severe dry mouth can accompany graft-versus-host disease following bone marrow transplantation. Secretory capacity usually recovers when the reaction resolves.

Clinical Management of Patients with Impaired Salivary Secretion

Significant chronic salivary hypofunction from any cause produces a risk for dental caries in approximate proportion to the secretory impairment. This caries can largely be prevented if appropriate measures are taken as soon as the hypofunction begins. Remaining teeth should be protected by a comprehensive dental caries prevention program, monitored by a dentist, that includes daily application of an appropriate topical fluoride and removal of dental plaque, counseling on control of cariogenic dietary carbohydrates, and placement of appropriate dental restorations as necessary.

Chronic erythematous oral candidiasis is a frequent sequela of chronic xerostomia, and its treatment and retreatment, as noted above, will improve the patient's oral symptoms.

Symptomatic treatment of mild to moderately severe salivary hypofunction can include sialogogues such as sugarless hard candies or chewing gum, frequent sips of water, and use of saliva substitutes at night. Severe hypofunction, especially that following irradiation, can be improved by systemic pilocarpine, 5 to 10 mg three times a day, if not contraindicated.

Daniels TE, Fox PC: Salivary and oral components of Sjögren's syndrome. Rheum Dis Clin North Am 18:571, 1992. *This review outlines the clinical features of the salivary component of Sjögren's syndrome and clinical management of patients with dry mouth.*

Daniels TE, Whitcher JP: Association of patterns of inflammation in labial salivary glands with keratoconjunctivitis sicca: analysis of 618 patients suspected of having Sjögren's syndrome. Arthritis Rheum 37:869, 1994. *This study confirms the current need for salivary biopsy to diagnose the salivary component of primary Sjögren's syndrome and reviews current controversies over diagnostic criteria.*

Ellis GL, Auclair PL, Gnepp DR (eds.): Major Problems in Pathology. Pathology of the Salivary Glands. Philadelphia, WB Saunders, 1991. *This recent text includes comprehensive discussion of neoplastic, infectious, and autoimmune salivary gland diseases.*

Jones JH, Mason DK (eds): Oral Manifestations of Systemic Diseases. 2nd ed. London, Bailliere Tindall/WB Saunders, 1990. *This international reference text provides comprehensive coverage of essentially all oral manifestations of systemic diseases.*

Regezi JA, Sciubba JJ: Oral Pathology: Clinical-pathologic Correlations. 2nd ed. Philadelphia, WB Saunders, 1993. *This useful and comprehensive text discusses and illustrates the clinical features, differential diagnosis, pathogenesis, and pathology of most diseases affecting the oral mucosa, jaws, and salivary glands.*

97 DISEASES OF THE ESOPHAGUS

Sidney Cohen and Henry P. Parkman

The esophagus, a relatively simple organ, is responsible for transporting materials from the mouth to the stomach and for preventing retrograde flow of gastric contents. Antegrade flow is achieved by the act of swallowing with the initiation of primary peristalsis. Gastroesophageal reflux is prevented by the physiologic lower esophageal sphincter.

Disorders of the esophagus occur when one or both of these major esophageal functions become impaired. Abnormalities in esophageal transport may be due to disruption of peristalsis by a neuromuscular disorder or by an organic obstructing lesion. The physiologic lower esophageal sphincter may contribute to transport disorders when relaxation of its tonically elevated pressure is impaired. Disorders of peristaltic function such as achalasia may occur together with abnormalities in sphincter relaxation. When the lower esophageal sphincter fails to function as an effective barrier to reflux, the patient develops gastroesophageal reflux with the associated complications of mucosal inflammation (peptic esophagitis).

The symptoms of esophageal disease relate closely to the abnormality in function. Disorders in transport lead to difficulty in swallowing or dysphagia. Abnormal esophageal contractions may cause chest pain. Gastroesophageal reflux leads to heartburn and postural regurgitation of food into the mouth.

The esophagus and its sphincters function through complex neural, humoral, and myogenic mechanisms. The pharynx, upper esophageal sphincter, and upper third of the esophagus are composed of skeletal muscle. Timing of upper esophageal events during swallowing is controlled by the central nervous system (CNS). The lower two thirds of the esophagus and the lower esophageal sphincter are smooth muscle. Disorders of skeletal muscle such as polymyositis affect the upper portions of the swallowing mechanism. Disorders of smooth muscle such as scleroderma affect the distal esophagus and the lower esophageal sphincter.

The neurohumoral control of the esophagus is incompletely understood. The initiation of peristalsis by swallowing involves both cholinergic and noncholinergic neural pathways as well as myogenic mechanisms. The relaxation of the lower esophageal sphincter during swallowing is initiated by nonadrenergic inhibitory nerves in the vagus. These nerves may release vasoactive intestinal peptide (VIP) and/or nitric oxide. The role of excitatory peptides such as gastrin, substance P, and motilin in the physiologic control of the sphincter is not clear, but they may cause the wide fluctuations in sphincter pressure that follow a meal.

DYSPHAGIA. Consciousness of food bolus arrest during swallowing, even if transient, indicates esophageal dysfunction. The patient usually uses the term "sticks," "pauses," or "hangs up" and often points to the subjective site of arrest with a finger.

Bolus arrest closely associated with the act of swallowing is dysphagia. The sensation of a substernal lump (globus) present one-half hour after eating is not dysphagia.

Dysphagia is never an expression of a purely psychiatric disorder; it is not a manifestation of hysteria. Some patients with well-established esophageal disease such as achalasia may report that their dysphagia is often worse at a time of severe emotional tension.

"Transfer dysphagia" occurs when the bolus cannot be propelled from the mouth or hypopharynx into the esophagus. This type of dysphagia is most commonly related to neurologic disease or to pharyngeal muscle weakness.

The sensation of dysphagia is localized to the suprasternal notch or substernal region. The exact location of the sensation is of little use in pinpointing the site of bolus arrest. Dysphagia for a liquid bolus usually indicates an esophageal motor disorder. Dysphagia for solids can occur either with an organic obstruction (stricture or cancer) or secondary to esophageal motor disorders. The patient's response to dysphagia can also provide useful information about the cause of dysphagia. If the bolus must be regurgitated, and if an attempt to force the bolus down with water is met by a sudden return of the fluid, then an organic obstruction should be suspected. If the patient is able to force the bolus down by posturing, by performing a Valsalva maneuver, by repeated swallowing, or by ingesting fluid, then a motor disorder is more likely. Inexorable progression of dysphagia over months usually signals the presence of organic narrowing, either a lumen-obliterating carcinoma or a stricture caused by active peptic esophagitis.

ODYNOPHAGIA. Pain upon swallowing, odynophagia, is another cardinal symptom of esophageal disease. Bolus arrest producing dysphagia can sometimes progress to a sensation of pain as esophageal obstruction continues. However, odynophagia usually occurs during the transit of the bolus and disappears once the swallowed material has left the esophagus. It may be mild in intensity so that the patient is merely aware of the location of the swallowed bolus. This is most commonly seen in patients with reflux disease. It can be of such intensity that the patient refuses to swallow any solids or liquids and expectorates saliva. Odynophagia can be seen after involvement of the mucosa by *reflux,* by *radiation,* or by *viral* or *fungal infections.* Odynophagia can be an uncommon manifestation of carcinoma or of a localized ulcer caused by a lodged tablet. Odynophagia thus localizes a process to the esophagus but gives no clue to pathogenesis.

HEARTBURN (PYROSIS). Heartburn or pyrosis is the most common manifestation of esophageal disease and may occur in up to 20% of "normal" subjects. The term "burning" rather than "pain" is usually used, although heartburn can increase in intensity until it is perceived as pain. Patients commonly illustrate heartburn with a movement of the open hand up and down the sternum. This is in contrast to the stationary tightly clenched fist of angina pectoris. Heartburn is usually relieved, even if only temporarily, by taking antacids. A constant burning, unrelieved by antacids, may well be of esophageal origin, but it does not represent heartburn. Heartburn is often worse after recumbency or lifting and may follow overeating or alcoholic indiscretion.

REGURGITATION. Regurgitation of fluid contents into the mouth often accompanies heartburn. Sometimes such regurgitation is associated with eructation; often it accompanies bending over, lifting, or lying down at night. The bitter regurgitated fluid is often described as yellow-brown or green. Regurgitation at night may lead to stridor or to wheezing, a hoarse voice, and other respiratory symptoms from unrecognized reflux. Less commonly, regurgitated fluid is not from the stomach or duodenum, but from fluid retained in an *achalasic esophagus* or in a large *pharyngeal diverticulum*. An uncommon but fascinating process that can be confused with regurgitation is *rumination*. In this condition, recently eaten food is propelled back into the mouth from the stomach by a strong contraction of the abdominal wall musculature. The food commonly is rechewed, reswallowed, and again returned to the stomach (see Ch. 195).

SPONTANEOUS ESOPHAGEAL CHEST PAIN (ESOPHAGEAL COLIC). In addition to the discomfort from severe reflux, which can advance from heartburn into pain, abnormal motor activity of the esophageal muscle can cause severe chest pain clinically indistinguishable from angina pectoris in terms of intensity, radiation, relationship to exercise, and even response to nitroglycerin. Chest pain of esophageal origin can radiate directly through to the back and is often found in patients who also notice dysphagia. Esophageal chest pain can last from several seconds to many hours.

HEMATEMESIS. Although vomiting blood is less specific for esophageal disease than are many of the symptoms listed above, hematemesis can signal the presence of esophageal varices, of mucosal ulceration resulting from esophageal reflux, of a mucosal tear in the lower esophagus, or, uncommonly, of an ulcerating carcinoma or leiomyoma of the esophagus. Although nonvariceal bleeding from the esophagus may be life threatening, more often it is a slow ooze, usually caused by esophageal reflux disease, which presents clinically as an iron deficiency anemia or occult blood–positive stool.

Haubrich W, Schaffner F, Berk JE (eds.): Bockus Gastroenterology. 5th ed. Philadelphia, WB Saunders, 1994. *Reference textbook chapters on esophagus.*

Richter, JE: Heartburn, dysphagia, odynophagia, and other esophageal symptoms. *In* Sleisenger MH, Fordtran JS (eds.): Gastrointestinal Disease. 5th ed. Philadelphia, WB Saunders, 1993. *Reference gastrointestinal textbook.*

GASTROESOPHAGEAL REFLUX DISEASE

DEFINITION. Gastroesophageal reflux disease (GERD) refers to the varied clinical manifestations of reflux of stomach and duodenal contents into the esophagus. It is preferable to the term "reflux esophagitis" because the latter expression tends to mean different things to the clinician, the endoscopist, and the pathologist. Although it may be associated with a sliding hiatus hernia, "symptomatic hiatus hernia" is a term that tends to put the emphasis on an anatomic entity and not the underlying pathophysiology. Gastroesophageal reflux disease can be characterized by any combination of symptoms and radiologic, endoscopic, or pathologic changes. In its milder manifestations, it is a common disease; its most florid state is uncommon but may be life threatening.

PATHOGENESIS. Several factors must work in concert to produce clinical effects of esophageal reflux. Normal subjects may have a few short duration reflux episodes. This reflux is seen postprandially and usually in the upright position. Those in whom reflux has produced symptoms or pathologic changes will demonstrate more frequent and prolonged episodes of reflux, which also tend to occur at night. The factor or factors that cause this difference are not known. However, important differences between persons with and without reflux might help explain these findings.

The *lower esophageal sphincter* (LES) is a specialized bundle of circular muscle at the lower end of the esophagus with different physical and pharmacologic characteristics when compared with the circular muscle above and below it. Although mean LES pressure is significantly lower in subjects with GERD than in normal persons, LES pressures are not very useful in predicting whether reflux is present in an individual patient unless the pressure is very low. The most common event associated with reflux appears to be an *inappropriate relaxation of the lower esophageal sphincter,* i.e., LES relaxation unassociated with either swallowing or the distention of the esophageal body by refluxed fluid. Thus, two abnormalities of LES may be associated with reflux: a sphincter with very low tone, as measured by LES pressure, or inappropriate relaxation of a normally competent sphincter.

Several factors are important in removing refluxed material. The upright position facilitates esophageal emptying by gravity. Peristaltic waves initiated by swallowing or by esophageal distention help remove the refluxed material. Acid placed within the esophagus is cleared less well by patients with GERD than by normal subjects, even though the manometric tracings seen in both groups

seem identical. Clearing occurs in two phases. The bulk of the fluid is returned to the stomach by a peristaltic contraction; the remainder of the acid film clinging to the esophageal wall is neutralized by swallowed saliva.

The composition and perhaps the quantity of the refluxed material also play a role in the production of GERD. Gastric acid and pepsin seem clearly important in the pathogenesis of GERD. Bile salts and possibly pancreatic enzymes may be responsible in those patients in whom acid is absent. The combination of bile salts plus acid is more injurious to the esophagus than either agent alone. Other less well-studied factors such as altered or abnormal esophageal mucus, swallowed saliva of high bicarbonate content, and diminished resistance of the esophageal mucosa to digestion may be important in determining the amount of mucosal damage in GERD.

Esophageal squamous epithelium reacts to reflux by an increase in the basal cell or germinative layer. The dermal pegs are increased in height and may become more vascular. If the process becomes more severe, the epithelial layer is destroyed, with the appearance of microulcers and classic signs of inflammation in the lamina propria, such as infiltration with polymorphonuclear leukocytes and edema. Even deeper lesions cause first submucosal and then muscular inflammation and fibrosis, resulting in an esophageal stricture. Why reflux is so common, yet inflammation and stricture formation are so relatively uncommon, is not known.

Other conditions can be associated with the pathogenesis of reflux. Reflux during pregnancy, once thought to be due to the increased abdominal pressure from the fetus, may be due mainly to diminished LES strength caused by increased estrogen and progesterone. Weight gain also tends to aggravate reflux through an unknown mechanism. As expected, resection of the lower esophageal area for cancer or myotomy for achalasia can lead to severe postoperative reflux (see below). Gastroesophageal reflux with stricture formation is especially severe in patients with progressive systemic sclerosis.

The crural diaphragm usually wraps around the gastroesophageal junction to augment the intrinsic LES. In a hiatus hernia, there is anatomic displacement of the LES and crural diaphragm. Although hiatus hernias may be associated with reflux, the presence of a hiatus hernia is now considered to be much less of a factor in GERD than previously thought, since it is present in a large percentage of normal subjects. It is not appropriate to spend time trying to define whether a hiatus hernia is present or absent in dealing with most patients with GERD; rather, the important entity to investigate is reflux.

SYMPTOMS OF GASTROESOPHAGEAL REFLUX DISEASE. *Heartburn* is the most common manifestation of GERD. It can vary from an occasional mild burning after overeating to an ever-present, severe discomfort that severely limits a patient's lifestyle. It may be accompanied by *regurgitation* of gastric contents either into the mouth or into the respiratory tree. This latter group of patients may complain of nocturnal wheezing, coughing, hoarseness, a need to clear the throat repeatedly, or a sensation of deep pressure at the base of the neck. This group of symptoms may be the primary clinical presentation and more prominent than the classic symptoms of GERD.

Dysphagia is often present in those with significant GERD. Although dysphagia may be severe and even mark the onset of stricture formation, it usually is mild and must be carefully sought. Dysphagia of GERD is for solids, and the dysphagia is usually overcome by swallowing repeatedly or by washing down the bolus with some water. Many patients with GERD do not complain of bolus arrest but rather of being aware of the location of each solid morsel as it travels down the esophagus.

Blood loss may result from esophageal erosion and shallow ulcers. Rarely producing life-threatening hemorrhage, the erosions are much more likely to weep quietly over a prolonged period of time, producing iron deficiency anemia. Some of these patients have very few other clinical manifestations of GERD, and the condition is discovered by endoscopy during evaluation of occult gastrointestinal bleeding. Persons who vigorously and repeatedly abuse alcohol seem prone to develop severe erosive esophagitis with bleeding; this lesion heals with abstinence from alcohol without other major antireflux therapy.

DIAGNOSIS. The history and clinical manifestations of GERD are the most important diagnostic aids in establishing the diagnosis; objective testing is used to quantify the extent and severity of the process. In the evaluation of an individual, questions to be answered dictate the appropriate test.

Does reflux exist and, if so, to what degree? This question might arise either if another condition such as pulmonary disease is present and a causal relationship is being sought, or if some idea of the frequency and extent of reflux is important. Reflux during a barium swallow in adults is uncommon unless vigorous provocative maneuvers are employed. When spontaneous reflux of barium is seen, it usually denotes free reflux. The absence of reflux seen radiographically does not, however, imply that the patient does not have GERD.

Twenty-four-hour esophageal pH monitoring can be performed with a portable unit, which allows the patient to follow an almost normal lifestyle. The pH probe is placed by nasal intubation and positioned 5 cm above the lower esophageal sphincter, as determined manometrically. During the prolonged monitoring period, the relationship between symptoms (heartburn, pain, wheezing) and episodes of reflux can be ascertained, and calculations can be made of the number of episodes of reflux and the amount of time the esophagus is acidified (pH < 4). A small amount of reflux, especially in the postprandial period, can be seen normally. Repeated and prolonged bursts of acid exposure suggest that abnormal gastroesophageal reflux is present.

Reflux can be measured noninvasively by scanning of the esophageal area with a gamma camera after placing a solution of ^{99m}Tc sulfur colloid in the stomach. An abdominal binder is used to increase intra-abdominal pressure and to stress the gastroesophageal junction if free reflux is not seen. This technique seems to be of most value in infants and children, who tolerate esophageal tubes very poorly.

Could reflux be responsible for the patient's symptoms? This question might be asked if pain is the predominant symptom rather than more classic heartburn. This question can be answered with the Bernstein test using the same catheter assembly used for esophageal manometry. After a 5-minute period of dripping normal saline through one of the pressure catheters whose opening has been localized to the mid-esophagus, this infusion is changed to 0.1 N hydrochloric acid. Reproduction of the symptoms during acid infusion (usually 4 to 5 minutes into the infusion), followed by rapid symptom disappearance with a switch back to saline infusion, suggests an esophageal cause of the discomfort.

As another approach, the patient is asked to signal the time of discomfort during prolonged pH monitoring of the esophagus. If the patient signals discomfort at the same time that reflux is demonstrated by the pH probe, then a causal relationship is made more likely. Prolonged pH monitoring has shown good correlation between periods of reflux and heartburn as well as other unexplained chest pain syndromes.

What has reflux done to the esophageal mucosa? A barium swallow detects gross changes such as stricture formation or a deep esophageal ulcer but misses the much more common shallow ulcerations and erosions. These are detected by direct inspection with the endoscope. Only discrete lesions such as erosions and ulcerations should be taken as proof of esophageal damage, since endoscopic findings such as erythema, edema, or friability are subject to wide interobserver variation. If the mucosa appears absolutely normal, as it is in approximately one third of patients with moderate to severe symptoms of GERD, a biopsy may demonstrate the changes of reflux.

A logic tree of how these tests might be used is shown in Figure 97–1. The algorithm can be modified depending on the individual patient. Endoscopy is indicated as an initial test if hematemesis is present, if symptoms are prolonged and do not respond to empiric treatment, or if systemic manifestations such as weight loss, anemia, and occult blood–positive stool are present. If the appearance of the esophageal mucosa is normal during endoscopy, biopsies can also be obtained to search for objective evidence of microscopic esophagitis. If dysphagia is present, starting with a barium swallow is appropriate. Uncommonly, reflux is demonstrated, a stricture found, or a deep ulcer seen. This might lead to immediate endoscopy for more complete evaluation. After first evaluation, it may be appropriate to begin empiric therapy (see Treatment, below). If

there is a poor response to therapy, esophageal pH monitoring should be used to confirm the diagnosis. At the same time, an esophageal manometry may be performed to estimate LES pressure and the presence or absence of peristaltic waves determined.

COMPLICATIONS OF GASTROESOPHAGEAL REFLUX DISEASE. *Esophageal Stricture.* Of the many who complain of symptoms of GERD, only a few develop esophageal strictures. Usually reflux-induced strictures begin at the lower end of the esophagus; however, they may migrate over years to the midesophagus or higher. Presumably patients who develop strictures have had deep circumferential ulceration of the esophageal mucosa due to reflux damage. Instead of healing with only minimal submucosal and muscular fibrosis, these patients develop esophageal obstruction with a narrowed esophageal lumen. If reflux can be controlled, these strictures may disappear.

Dysphagia is the clinical hallmark of esophageal stricture formation. Unlike the relatively mild dysphagia seen in uncomplicated GERD, the dysphagia in patients with strictures tends to be constant and slowly progressive, causing the patient to alter the type of food taken. If a bolus becomes arrested in the stricture, it is usually necessary for the bolus to be regurgitated back into the mouth before further intake of food or fluids is possible.

Strictures are most easily evaluated by barium swallow. Sometimes the extent of the strictured area is overestimated unless the esophagus below the stricture can be fully distended by barium. For mild strictures, the ingestion of barium-soaked bread or marshmallow bolus can draw attention to slight luminal narrowing when the bolus impacts there. Once this has been demonstrated, endoscopy with biopsy and/or brush cytology is in order to make certain that the stricture is benign.

Esophageal Ulcer. In addition to the more common shallow ulcerations, deep esophageal ulcers may complicate severe GERD. These ulcers, which retain barium and usually project outside the wall of the esophagus, characteristically produce severe and unrelenting pain, often with radiation of the pain through to the back. Brisk hemorrhage is another manifestation, from erosion through to an esophageal artery. The presence of an ulcer can be suspected on a barium swallow and confirmed endoscopically. The ulcer is usually found to reside in columnar (Barrett's) epithelium.

Barrett's Esophagus (Columnar Epithelium). In some patients who have suffered with chronic reflux esophagitis, the healing epithelium may be replaced not with squamous epithelium but with a specialized columnar epithelium. The junctional zone between squamous and columnar (Barrett's) epithelium can progress orad over years. Columnar epithelium is found at and below midesophageal strictures and around deep esophageal ulcers. The major clinical importance of Barrett's epithelium is not only as a marker for severe reflux but also as a precursor to adenocarcinoma of the esophagus (see under Esophageal Tumors).

Pulmonary Aspiration. If refluxed material breaches the upper esophageal sphincter, it may easily spill into the larynx and tracheobronchial tree. Some patients react to such a spill with intense respiratory stridor. Others seem to tolerate the presence of refluxed material in the larynx and tracheobronchial tree with milder laryngeal or respiratory symptoms. It is even possible that the gastric contents do not have to reach the larynx; instilling acid in the esophagus of susceptible individuals can be shown to cause closing of small bronchial airways by a vagal reflex.

None of the clinical features of pulmonary aspiration, such as wheezing, hoarseness, or coughing, is pathognomonic. Taken together they may point toward reflux and aspiration as a possible etiology. Diagnostic proof of the relationship may be difficult with current techniques. Dual esophageal pH monitoring with pH probes in both the lower and upper esophagus can help determine if acid reflux ascends into the upper esophagus. Correlation of symptoms with proximal esophageal reflux may be helpful. Correcting reflux with subsequent disappearance of pulmonary symptoms can help prove the relationship.

TREATMENT OF GASTROESOPHAGEAL REFLUX DISEASE AND ITS COMPLICATIONS. *Medical Management.* Most mildly symptomatic patients with reflux and some moderately afflicted individuals can be helped by manipulations designed to alter the frequency or type of esophageal reflux. Many patients respond to the simple measures outlined in Table 97–1. Elevating the head of the bed by 6 to 8 inches is a simple and effective form of therapy. Twenty-four-hour pH monitoring has shown that this simple measure decreases the frequency and length of reflux episodes.

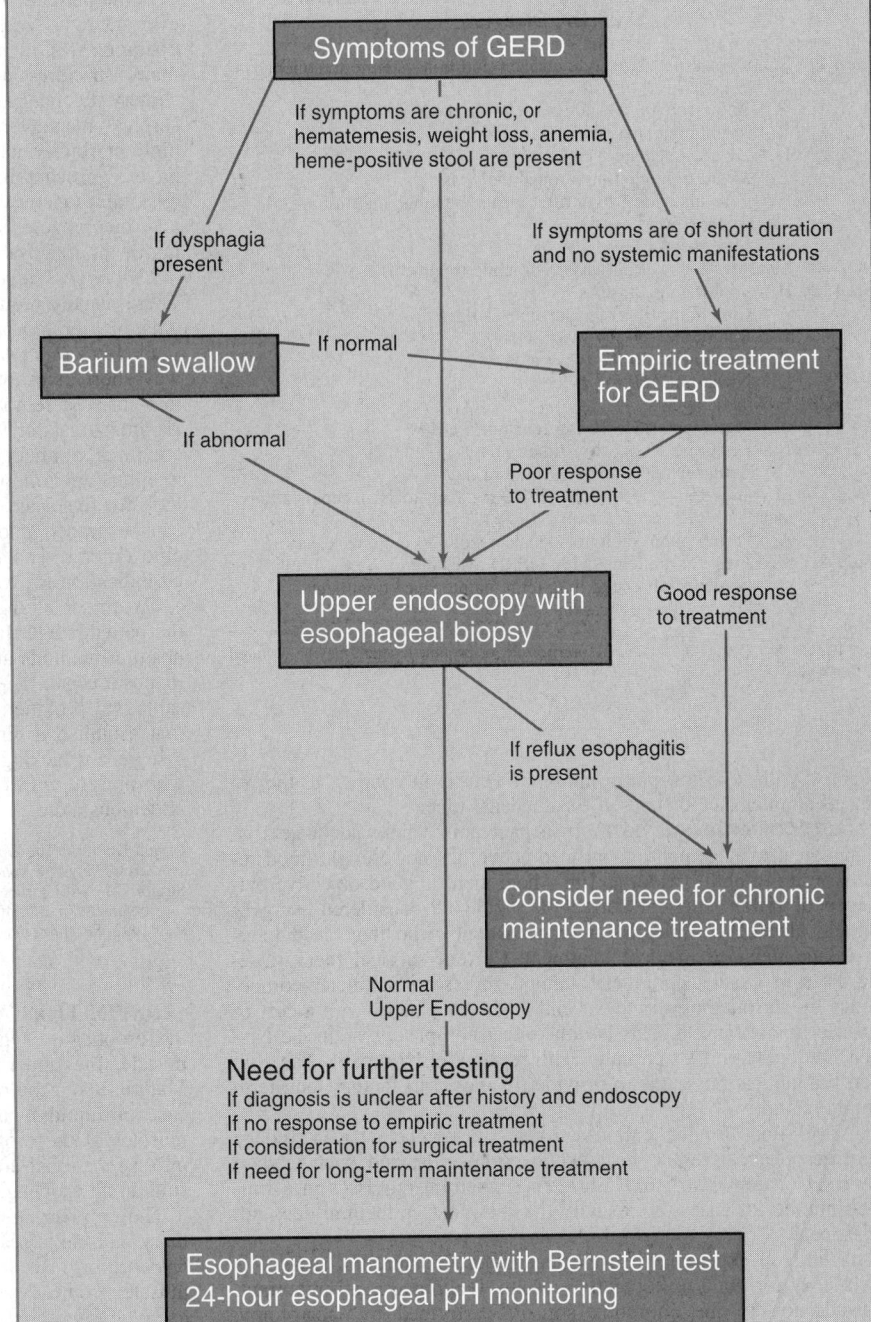

FIGURE 97-1. Diagnosis/evaluation of patients with possible GERD.

Pillows to elevate the thorax do not work well, as patients tend to roll off the pillows during the night. A foam rubber wedge can be used if the bed frame cannot be moved. Avoiding food and fluid for at least 3 hours before retiring decreases the amount of material available for reflux at night. Avoiding food that the patient finds distressing, such as fatty foods, chocolate, and onions, makes sense but has never been subjected to clinical trial.

Acid can be neutralized by taking 30 ml of aluminum hydroxide–magnesium hydroxide antacid 1 and 3 hours after meals and at bedtime. In recalcitrant cases, hourly antacids may be tried, with substitution of pure aluminum hydroxide gel to control diarrhea produced by the magnesium ion. Most patients do not tolerate such a regimen for long.

An attempt should be made to have the patient stop smoking, drinking alcohol, and overeating. Most patients, however, apparently prefer to suffer with reflux symptoms rather than to give up these mainstays of life.

If these simple measures are not effective, systemic medical treatment is indicated. The H_2-receptor antagonists in the usual dosage range for duodenal ulcer improve symptoms of heartburn better than placebo. Higher dosage regimens, cimetidine 800 mg, ranitidine 300 mg, or famotidine 40 mg, each twice per day, have been more effective for controlling symptoms and healing peptic esophagitis. Healing of esophageal erosions with H_2-receptor antagonists usually takes 12 to 16 weeks.

The proton pump inhibitor omeprazole, 20 mg once per day, can often give dramatic symptom relief and heal esophagitis in 4 to 8 weeks.

Prokinetic agents may also be useful, often given in addition to gastric acid suppressants. Metoclopramide, 10 mg three times a day, can be helpful, but CNS side effects, which may occur in 25%, may limit its usefulness. Cisapride 10 mg four times a day is effective primarily for nocturnal GERD and has fewer side effects than metoclopramide.

Once healing has been achieved with either an H_2 antagonist or a proton pump inhibitor, recurrence rates exceed 80% if no maintenance therapy is used. Maintenance therapy for esophagitis generally requires full dosage of an H_2-receptor antagonist or prolonged

TABLE 97-1. TREATMENT OF GASTROESOPHAGEAL REFLUX DISEASE

Step 1. Simple measures (lifestyle changes and nonsystemic treatment)
  A. Elevate head of bed
  B. Avoid food and fluid intake before bedtime
  C. Avoid cigarettes, coffee, alcohol
  D. Avoid chocolate, peppermint
  E. Avoid tight clothing around the waist
  F. Take antacids 1 hour after meals, bedtime, and prn
  G. Reduce fat in diet
  H. Lose weight
Step 2. Measures for resistant cases (systemic treatment)
Step 2a. H$_2$-receptor antagonists
  A. Cimetidine 300 mg four times a day*
  B. Ranitidine 150 mg twice a day*
  C. Famotidine 20 mg twice a day*
  D. Nizatidine 150 mg twice a day*
Step 2b. Prokinetic agents
  A. Metoclopramide 10 mg four times a day*
  B. Cisapride 10 mg four times a day*
  C. Bethanechol 10 mg four times a day*
Step 3. Measures for patients with GERD resistant to H$_2$-receptor antagonists
  A. Proton pump inhibitor—Omeprazole 20 mg once a day*
Step 4. Measures for patients with GERD resistant to Steps 1, 2, 3 or some patients who need long-term maintenance treatment
  A. Surgical fundoplication

* Higher doses of an H$_2$ antagonist, omeprazole, or prokinetic agent may be required in some cases.

therapy with a proton pump inhibitor. This is in contrast to the reduced maintenance dose used for duodenal ulcer.

Surgical Management. In a patient in whom adequate trial of medical management as outlined above has not brought good results in a 6-month period, and in whom there is good objective evidence of reflux, surgical correction should be considered. Surgery should also be considered for some patients who may need long-term maintenance medical treatment. Current surgical therapy, regardless of exact techniques, attempts to restore sphincter competence by surrounding the lower end of the esophagus with a cuff of gastric fundal muscle. This is done either completely, as in the Nissen fundoplication, or partially (Hill repair, Belsey repair). The Nissen fundoplication seems to provide the most satisfactory long-term improvement.

A well-done fundoplication can restore a competent LES, reduce gastroesophageal reflux, heal peptic esophagitis, and even lead to reversal of peptic stricture. Barrett's epithelium regresses in a limited number of cases, but usually the columnar epithelium does not disappear.

A surgeon experienced in the techniques of antireflux surgery is necessary for good postoperative results. Technique is all-important. In addition to the antireflux surgery performed by laparotomy, laparoscopic techniques are also being performed by experienced laparoscopic gastrointestinal surgeons. Although some individual surgeons have enviable postoperative results, antireflux surgery has a relatively poor reputation in many medical communities. Currently, a conservative approach toward antireflux surgery seems indicated.

Treatment of Complications. Esophageal strictures, if only mildly symptomatic, can be handled by careful attention to dietary intake, improvement of dentition, and use of medical therapy. Techniques of dilation have proliferated in recent years, but they still require an experienced operator. Short, simple strictures can be dilated with weighted rubber or Teflon dilators (Hurst, Maloney). Tortuous or angulated strictures are more easily approached over a previously placed guide wire passed through an endoscope or under radiographic control. Graded steel olives (Eder-Puestow), a dilator with graded increases of size (Celestin), or a balloon with a fixed maximal diameter (Cooke) can be passed over the previously placed wire. Alternatively, a balloon of fixed maximal diameter can be passed through the large channel of an endoscope during diagnostic endoscopy and dilated under direct vision. Once the lumen is restored to a diameter of 13 to 15 mm, most patients swallow without difficulty. If the stricture is stable and requires dilation only every 4 to 6 months, nothing else is necessary.

Some patients do not tolerate dilation or require vigorous dilation every 3 to 4 weeks. This is an indication for definitive antireflux operation, following which the stricture may regress. Unfortunately, many strictures persist after attempts at correction by antireflux surgery. Esophageal replacement by colon, jejunum, or stomach is a surgical maneuver of last resort; such procedures have relatively high morbidity and mortality. Patients afflicted by strictures may have significant lung and cardiovascular disease that makes them unsuitable operative candidates. High-dose H$_2$ antagonists or preferably omeprazole along with dilation of the stricture has led to healing of the mucosa and less need for repeated stricture dilation.

Esophageal ulcers also represent a major therapeutic problem. These usually require treatment with a high-dose H$_2$-receptor antagonist or a proton pump inhibitor.

Barrett's (columnar) epithelium may be premalignant. There is no way short of esophageal resection to make certain that the epithelium can be removed. Adequate antireflux therapy with high-dose H$_2$ antagonists or with a proton pump inhibitor causes regression of columnar epithelium in some patients. Patients with Barrett's epithelium are followed closely with periodic endoscopic biopsies to look for dysplasia and early changes of adenocarcinoma. Dysplasia can be graded into mild, moderate, or severe dysplasia using specific criteria. The persistence of confirmed high-grade dysplasia is an indication for esophagectomy.

Treatment of the pulmonary complications of reflux depends on the patient's age. Infants with recurrent bronchitis can be treated by postural methods and by thickening the formula. In adults, attention to posture at night is important (see above). Gastric acid suppressants and prokinetic agents may be used. Since diagnostic methods that establish a direct causal relationship between reflux and lung disease are lacking, caution is advised in offering surgery to those who present with primary pulmonary problems and in whom reflux is demonstrated.

Castell DO (ed): The Esophagus. Boston, Little, Brown, 1992. *Recent textbook devoted exclusively to esophageal physiology and pathophysiology.*
Streitz JM, Williamson WA, Ellis FH: Current concepts concerning the nature and treatment of Barrett's esophagus and its complications. Ann Thorac Surg 54:586, 1992. *Recent review on Barrett's esophagus.*

MOTOR DISORDERS OF THE ESOPHAGUS

DEFINITION AND PATHOGENESIS. The muscular tube of the esophagus is guarded at both ends by specialized bundles of muscle, the upper and lower esophageal sphincters (UES, LES). Material from the oropharynx is propelled at a high velocity (in the case of liquids), and precise coordination is required to link the muscles of the oropharynx, UES, body of the esophagus, and LES into a functional unit. Failure of any or all of these components results in an esophageal motor disorder.

The oropharyngeal and UES units can fail because of either primary muscle disease such as *myotonia dystrophica* or *dermatomyositis* or neurologic lesions involving the innervation of these muscle groups. *Brain stem infarcts, multiple sclerosis,* and *amyotrophic lateral sclerosis* serve as examples for the latter process.

The pathogenesis of motor abnormality of the esophageal body is less well understood. The striated muscle that constitutes the upper one quarter to one third of the body can be affected by primary muscle disease, such as *myotonia dystrophica,* or by metabolic disease affecting muscle function, such as *hypothyroidism.* The smooth muscle seems more resistant to muscular disease, but the intrinsic nervous network can be involved in *Chagas' disease* and *achalasia.* In the latter disorder, there is infiltration of Auerbach's plexus with lymphocytes or actual disappearance of the neuron cell bodies in the myenteric plexus.

The motor disorders of the body of the esophagus have historically been classified as *achalasia* or *diffuse spasm* (Table 97–2). In achalasia, dysphagia and esophageal retention predominate; the radiograph shows a dilated esophagus with a distal beak, and manometry reveals high LES pressure with no or incomplete relaxation as well as only simultaneous low-amplitude esophageal contractions in response to a swallow. Diffuse spasm has been characterized as a clinical syndrome of esophageal chest pain or dysphagia or both; segmental contractions seen by radiograph; and a manometric picture of some peristaltic waves interspersed with periods of simultaneous esophageal contractions. Another common manometric abnor-

TABLE 97-2. MANOMETRIC CLASSIFICATION OF ESOPHAGEAL MOTOR DISORDERS

Achalasia
Diffuse esophageal spasm
Sclerodema
Isolated LES dysfunction
    High pressure with normal relaxation
    Normal pressure with impaired relaxation
Nonspecific esophageal motor disorder
    High-amplitude peristaltic esophageal contractions ("nutcracker esophagus")
    Repetitive esophageal contractions
    Nontransmitted esophageal contractions
    Low-amplitude esophageal contractions

mality is high-amplitude, long-duration waves that are peristaltic and can be associated with either esophageal chest pain or dysphagia or both (nutcracker esophagus). There are many variations of these "classic" diseases, and progression from diffuse spasm to achalasia has been documented in some patients. Many nonspecific motor disorders of the esophagus do not fit these syndromes (see Table 97-2). The pathophysiology of these nonspecific disorders and how it relates to symptoms are not well understood.

SYMPTOMS. The type of symptom produced is a function of the level and extent of the problem. *Weakness of the oropharyngeal musculature* may cause *transfer dysphagia*—the inability to propel a solid or liquid bolus from the pharynx to the esophagus. Patients are aware usually that they cannot begin the act of deglutition. Solids are usually more trouble than liquids. Palatal weakness may lead to *nasal regurgitation* of fluids or to *laryngeal aspiration* because of muscular failure to seal off the larynx. Such weakness may be signaled by a nasal quality of the voice.

Incoordination of UES relaxation with pharyngeal contraction has been suggested as a cause of transfer dysphagia and for Zenker's diverticulum. Transfer dysphagia can be accompanied by a prominent cricopharyngeal impression on a barium swallow ("cricopharyngeal achalasia"); however, no defect in relaxing or in timing is seen with modern manometric methods.

Motor disorders in the body of the esophagus produce either *dysphagia* or *pain,* or both. This transport dysphagia may be intermittent or continuous. It may occur with both solids and liquids. It is rare for the arrested material to be regurgitated; often posturing (throwing the shoulders back and extending the neck) or a Valsalva maneuver helps the material pass into the stomach.

Chest pain or esophageal colic is the other major clinical presentation of esophageal motor disorders. The pain is usually substernal, described as a feeling of pressure or aching, radiating to the back as well as to the neck, jaw, and arms. It can range in intensity from a transient discomfort to an overwhelming, agonizing pain similar to that of a major myocardial infarction or dissecting aortic aneurysm. The pain may last for only several seconds or may be present for hours. The differentiation between angina pectoris and esophageal chest pain may be impossible on clinical grounds; both may be related to exercise, have the same intensity and distribution, and respond to sublingual nitroglycerin.

Failure of the LES may present as two separate symptom complexes. If the sphincter fails to relax on deglutition (as occurs in achalasia), dysphagia and retention of contents in the body of the esophagus occur. This failure, coupled with loss of peristalsis (achalasia), leads to marked esophageal retention, regurgitation, and overflow of esophageal contents into the tracheobronchial tree. If there is primary muscle failure of the sphincter, as occurs in *scleroderma,* massive reflux and the consequences of GERD follow.

DIAGNOSIS. A careful history is essential in choosing the correct diagnostic tools for evaluating esophageal motor disorders. If the difficulty is thought to be in the oropharynx and UES, a video-esophagram would offer the most information. The video film allows for slow-motion analysis of this rapidly moving portion of the gastrointestinal tract. Incoordination of tongue and palate, unilateral pharyngeal weakness, and aspiration of small amounts of barium into the trachea on swallowing can be shown. Air double-contrast examinations of the pharynx can elucidate an unsuspected hypopharyngeal carcinoma. A diverticulum or prominence of the cricophatyngeal muscle can also be seen. Manometric examination of the hypopharynx and UES are often not helpful.

Radiology of the esophageal body offers the best chance of diagnosis when the motor disorders are associated with relatively static changes. In achalasia the body of the esophagus commonly dilates with retention of food, secretions, and barium (Fig. 97-2). Special attention can be paid to the terminal end of the esophagus. In achalasia, there is a smooth, tapering beak. Any irregularity of this beak should lead to a vigorous search for an infiltrating neoplasm of the cardia, which can exactly mimic achalasia clinically and radiologically.

If the esophageal muscle is atonic, as is seen in far-advanced scleroderma, barium and even air are retained for long periods of time in the supine position. Assuming the upright position rapidly clears the barium from the esophagus and leaves a double-contrast view of a dilated esophagus.

The radiologist has more difficulty when the motor abnormality is more intermittent (Fig. 97-3). Simultaneous contractions can be occasionally detected fluoroscopically. Such a radiologic appearance is not always evidence for a clinically important motor disorder; elderly patients often show similar radiologic findings and yet are totally asymptomatic (presbyesophagus).

Manometric examination allows more prolonged evaluation of esophageal motor function and is the only method that allows LES function to be directly determined. Normally, a swallow causes a peristaltic wave to be detected sequentially by pressure detectors spaced along the esophagus. Aperistalsis (no peristaltic response to a swallow), simultaneous single or multiple contractions, prolonged contractions of high amplitude and low velocity, and spontaneous activity not related to swallowing can be recorded. Some of the "classic" patterns associated with diseases are shown in Figure 97-4.

Manometric examination can especially benefit the evaluation of chest pain if the patient happens to have an attack during the examination. If the chest pain is accompanied by motor activity that allows the manometrist to predict its onset, intensity, and disappearance by watching the manometric tracing, the diagnosis of an esophageal origin of chest pain is firmly established. Similarly, if pH is being simultaneously monitored and the episodes of chest pain correlate closely with drops in intraesophageal pH, an

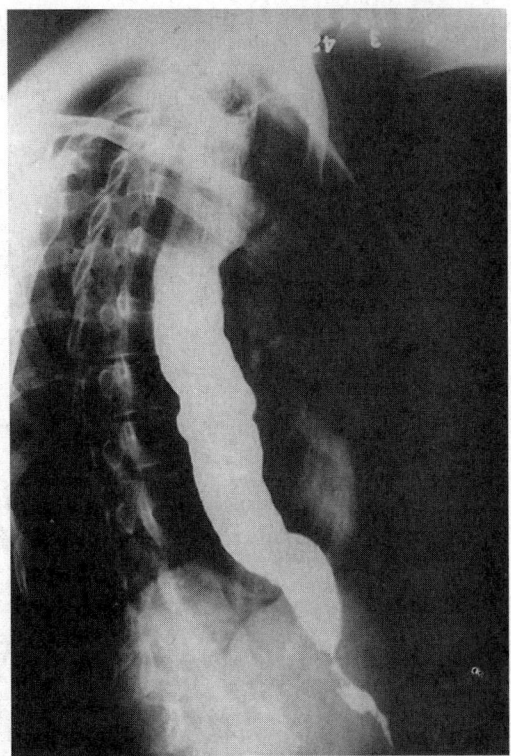

FIGURE 97-2. Radiologic appearance of achalasia. The esophageal body is dilated and terminates in a narrowed segment. (Courtesy of Dr. FE Templeton. From Pope CE II: *In* Sleisenger MH, Fordtran JS [eds.]: Gastrointestinal Disease. 3rd ed. Philadelphia, WB Saunders, 1983.)

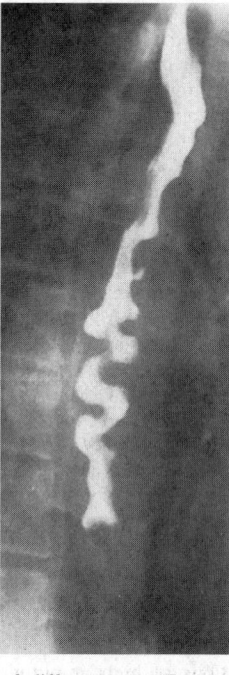

FIGURE 97–3. Radiologic appearance of diffuse spasm. Two spot films were taken within 10 seconds of each other. A fairly normal appearance on the left changes rapidly to an appearance of numerous contractions. (Courtesy of Dr. CA Rohrmann. From Pope CE II: *In* Sleisenger MH, Fordtran JS [eds]: Gastrointestinal Disease. 3rd ed. Philadelphia, WB Saunders, 1983.)

esophageal origin of pain is likely. Conversely, if typical chest pain occurs but there is no change in motor activity or pH over control values, an esophageal cause of pain is unlikely. Unfortunately, such definitive statements can be made only in a small minority of the patients examined.

Pharmacologic stimulation of the esophagus has been used for diagnostic purposes. Edrophonium (Tensilon) is the most widely used provocative agent for inducing chest pain along with simultaneous esophageal contractions. The cholinesterase inhibitor is short acting and extremely safe in clinical usage. Provocative testing has been helpful in delineating the cause of chest pain in patients with normal baseline esophageal manometry.

Endoscopy is useful for evaluating motor disorders, for inspecting the cardia with a retroflexed view from the stomach to rule out an infiltrating carcinoma, and for excluding inflammatory disorders.

Prolonged esophageal pH monitoring and pH/motility monitoring may help correlate symptoms of dysphagia or chest pain to reflux episodes or motility abnormalities.

TREATMENT. Of the various motor disorders of the esophagus, *achalasia* seems most amenable to relief. Since the problem in achalasia is one of obstruction at the lower end of the esophagus by a sphincter that does not relax, all forms of therapy are directed at relieving this obstruction. Short-term improvement in clinical symptoms and in scintigraphic esophageal emptying may occur with isosorbide dinitrate, a long-acting nitrate, or with nifedipine, a calcium channel blocker. A successful approach to long-term pharmacologic management of achalasia has not been established. Dilation with a large Hurst bougie may give temporary relief; a few patients have been maintained for long periods with weekly self-dilations, but this treatment is no longer recommended. Much more effective is dilation with a pneumatic bag under radiographic control. This should be performed by an expert, since perforation even in good hands may occur in about 5% of patients. Pneumatic dilation is preferable initially for almost all patients.

Surgery is reserved for those in whom bag dilation fails or those who do not wish to be exposed to the risk of perforation. Direct section of the LES muscle (myotomy) is carried out, sparing some gastric muscle fibers to prevent postoperative reflux (Heller esophagomyotomy). Many surgeons currently combine a "loose" fundoplication along with the Heller myotomy. Postoperative gastroesophageal reflux with esophagitis and peptic stricture of the esophagus may occur in patients if the myotomy abolishes all LES pressure and if no fundoplication is performed. Surgery is performed using either laparotomy or thoracotomy. Recently, Heller myotomies have been performed laparoscopically.

Treating most other motor disorders is much more difficult. Patients with diffuse spasm can be given nitroglycerin, anticholinergics, or calcium channel antagonists. Balloon dilation of the LES has also been suggested to be of benefit in diffuse spasm and has been helpful in those patients with abnormal lower esophageal function, high basal tone with impaired relaxation. Dividing all the circular muscle with a long myotomy has been tried, but the long-term results of this procedure have not been favorable.

Treating other nonspecific motor disorders such as nutcracker esophagus associated with chest pain can be equally frustrating. Prescribing sublingual nitroglycerin is justifiable. If it is ineffective, long-acting nitrate therapy will probably not work. Anticholinergic drugs benefit only a few. Calcium channel antagonists reduce the force of the esophageal contractions and relieve pain. Meperidine

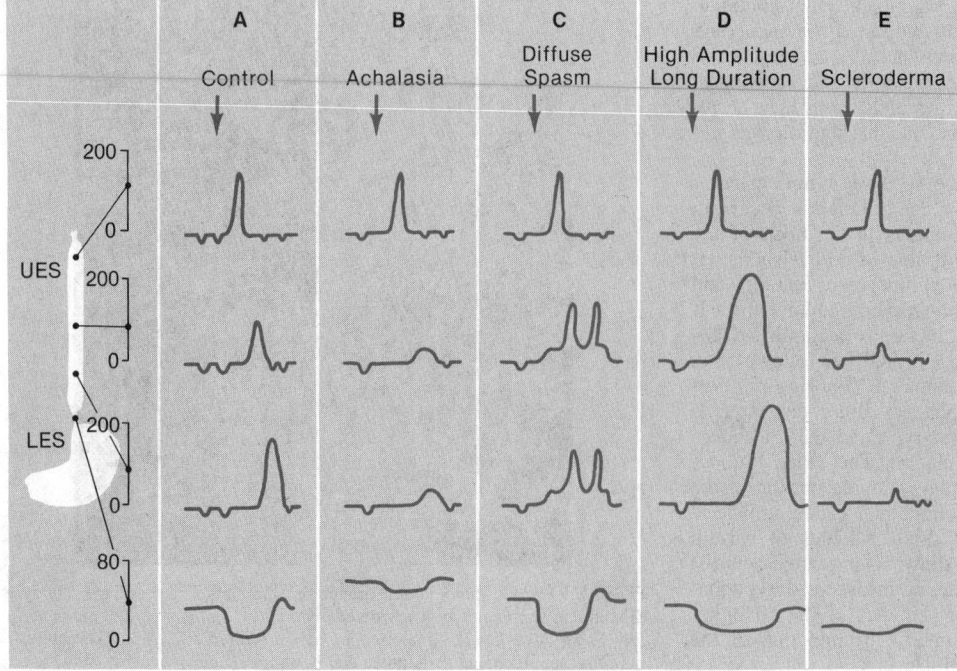

FIGURE 97–4. Idealized manometric patterns. *A,* The normal swallow consists of a progressive wave with a wave of short duration and rapid rise time in the striated upper esophagus. The lower esophageal sphincter shows a fall in pressure coincident with swallowing. *B,* In achalasia the striated muscle sometimes but not always produces a typical wave. The smooth muscle portion of the esophagus has a simultaneous low-amplitude contraction that follows the striated muscle contraction. The elevated pressure in the LES shows either incomplete or no relaxation. *C,* Diffuse spasm shows an elevation of the baseline after swallowing, on top of which are superimposed repetitive simultaneous contractions. LES pressure may be high and relaxation may terminate prematurely. *D,* High-amplitude, long-duration waves (nutcracker esophagus). The wave is peristaltic but of high amplitude. Duration is increased and velocity of propagation may be decreased. *E,* Scleroderma. Striated muscle contraction is normal, but the amplitude of contraction in the smooth muscle is reduced, or contraction may be absent. Sphincter pressure is low.

(Demerol) has been useful; however, this medication is not a good long-term solution to the problem. Some patients respond to gastric acid suppression, indicating that some of these nonspecific motility disorders may be secondary to gastroesophageal reflux. Recently, a form of microvascular coronary artery disease has been suggested as a cause of chest pain in patients with nutcracker esophagus.

The treatment of *scleroderma* and other conditions marked by aperistalsis revolves mostly around the associated reflux. If there is no obstruction at the lower end of the esophagus—either by a malfunctioning sphincter or by an organic narrowing—aperistalsis is amazingly well tolerated, usually with only mild dysphagia for solids. Antireflux surgery should be offered with caution to patients with scleroderma, as a tight fundoplication without any peristalsis in the body of the esophagus leads to severe dysphagia. Additionally, fundoplication has poor results because the disease progresses to severe muscle atrophy and collagen deposition in the esophageal wall.

Castell DO (ed.): The Esophagus. Boston, Little, Brown, 1992. *Devoted exclusively to esophageal physiology and pathophysiology.*

Clouse RE: Motor disorders. *In* Sleisenger MH, Fordtran JS (eds.): Gastrointestinal Disease. 5th ed. Philadelphia, WB Saunders, 1993. *Reference gastrointestinal textbook.*

ESOPHAGEAL TUMORS

ETIOLOGY AND PATHOGENESIS. Carcinoma of the esophageal epithelium, both squamous cell and adenocarcinoma, is by far the most common and important tumor of the esophagus. Benign neoplasms (leiomyoma, papilloma, and fibrovascular polyps) are rarer by far. Squamous cell cancer has an incidence of 5 per 100,000 in males (United States), rising to 130 per 100,000 in North China. It is associated with both alcohol intake and tobacco smoking. Esophageal cancer occurs more commonly in patients with squamous cancers of the head and neck, in those with lye strictures, and in patients with untreated or inadequately treated achalasia.

Adenocarcinoma of the esophagus arises in columnar (Barrett's) epithelium and appears to represent malignant degeneration in the metaplastic columnar tissue that arises in response to chronic inflammation. The actual incidence of adenocarcinoma in a patient with columnar epithelium is probably less than the original estimate of 10 to 15%, but the tumor still represents a significant problem.

SYMPTOMS. In Western countries, the most common clinical symptom of carcinoma is *progressive dysphagia* over a several-month period until only liquids can be taken. The obstruction reflects circumferential involvement of the esophageal wall by tumor and does not occur until the cancer is biologically far advanced. The dysphagia may be accompanied by a *steady, boring pain,* which often signals mediastinal involvement and inoperability. Unexplained persistent chest pain should always be investigated by a careful double-contrast radiographic view of the esophagus or by endoscopy.

More advanced lesions manifest themselves with *halitosis, weight loss,* and *coughing after drinking fluid.* The last-named symptom is caused either by nearly complete esophageal lumen obstruction with overspill into the larynx or by the development of a tracheo-esophageal fistula. Hoarseness from involvement of the recurrent laryngeal nerve by tumor and hematemesis are unusual symptoms. Nail bed clubbing can be seen with both benign and malignant tumors.

Since dysphagia is the most common presenting symptom of neoplasm of the esophagus, the physician is responsible for making absolutely certain that cancer is not the cause of dysphagia. Early diagnosis affords the only chance for cure. Early diagnosis allows the patient, family, and physician to plan better all aspects of the patient's future.

DIAGNOSIS. The clinical suspicion of cancer of the esophagus should lead immediately to an esophagogram, possibly with double-contrast techniques. Any irregularity, especially if it narrows the lumen, mandates further evaluation. If dysphagia is present, the radiologist should give a bolus of barium-soaked bread or marshmallow to discover any possible sites of arrest.

In the presence of suspicious symptoms but a normal barium swallow, endoscopy with biopsy and brushing of any suspicious lesion for examination of tissue is indicated. The endoscopist should always obtain a good retroflexed view of the cardia from below to make certain that an adenocarcinoma of the gastroesophageal junction has not been overlooked.

If narrowing has been seen by barium swallow, endoscopy with biopsy and cytologic brushings of the involved area must be done. With the fiberoptic endoscope, numerous blind biopsies from as deep in the lesion as possible will be most helpful. Biopsy of visible tissue will often reveal only inflammatory tissue. Sometimes as many as eight or nine biopsies must be obtained before tumor is recovered.

Once a tumor is identified, evaluation for local tumor spread, mediastinal nodal involvement, and liver metastases is essential for staging before a therapeutic decision is reached. Careful physical examination for lymphadenopathy, liver function testing, chest radiography, and computed tomographic (CT) scanning are usually performed. For upper and mid-esophageal tumors, bronchoscopy is indicated to evaluate for asymptomatic invasion of the tracheobronchial tree. Endoscopic ultrasound may be useful to detect the level of invasion and presence of mediastinal lymph node abnormalities.

TREATMENT. The ideal treatment of esophageal cancer, either for cure or for palliation, has not yet been developed. No series exists in which patients were carefully staged with the best noninvasive methods available and then randomized to different treatment modalities.

Surgical resection of squamous cell carcinoma and adenocarcinoma of the lower third of the esophagus is preferred in most centers if the patient does not have widespread metastases. Surgery offers the benefit of rapidly restoring esophagogastric continuity. Perhaps only one quarter of all patients coming to a medical-surgical center have a resectable tumor; of these patients 10 to 20% do not survive the operative period, and 5-year survival is only 5 to 20%, even with extensive resections. Long-term survival cannot be predicted in the individual case by the operative findings. There is growing enthusiasm for palliative resection with restoration of gastrointestinal continuity with stomach or colon.

Radiotherapy is employed in lesions of the upper third of the esophagus and often in middle third tumors as well. This form of therapy has little hospital mortality, although it carries some short-term and long-term morbidity. Approximately 40% of tumors cannot be destroyed with conventional 6000-rad therapy. Combination of pre- and postoperative radiation with resective therapy has been employed, but there is no good evidence that such combined therapy is better. Adenocarcinomas occasionally respond to radiotherapy but are not as radiosensitive as squamous cell carcinomas.

Chemotherapy with cisplatin-containing combinations has demonstrated objective tumor response. Preliminary evidence suggests that multimodality treatment with radiation therapy plus chemotherapy with cisplatin and fluorouracil is superior to radiation therapy alone.

When obvious extraesophageal spread is present, palliation with bougienage to restore and maintain an adequate esophageal lumen may be done. If performed with a guide wire under fluoroscopic guidance, such therapy is not hazardous in skilled hands. If dilation does not offer lasting relief, then a Silastic tube or metal stent can be placed perorally to relieve esophageal obstruction. Such tubes are also greatly beneficial in treating a malignant tracheoesophageal fistula. Destruction of intraluminal tumor and restoration of an adequate lumen may be performed by endoscopic laser therapy or an intraluminal heat-coagulating probe.

Choice of therapy will depend on the location and size of the lesion, presence or absence of spread, cell type, and the skills of the medical community. Until an adequate randomized trial after adequate staging is carried out, choice of treatment modality will continue to be a matter of preference.

Herskovic A, Martz K, Al-Sarraf M, et al.: Combined chemotherapy and radiotherapy compared with radiotherapy alone in patients with cancer of the esophagus. N Engl J Med 326:1593, 1992.

Boyce HW: Tumors of the esophagus. *In* Sleisenger MH, Fordtran JS (eds.): Gastrointestinal Disease. 5th ed. Philadelphia, WB Saunders, 1993. *Reference gastrointestinal textbook.*

OTHER CONDITIONS

RINGS AND WEBS. During early development, the lumen of the esophagus becomes completely obliterated and then is recanalized to form the adult hollow viscus. A failure of this process leads to atresia or a residual web. Such webs usually occur in the upper esophagus, often with eccentric openings; occasionally they are multiple. An acquired web located in the postcricoid area is sometimes associated with iron deficiency anemia (Plummer-Vinson syndrome). A much more common web or ring is located in the terminal esophagus, has a symmetric opening, and is usually at the junction between squamous and the normal transitional or columnar epithelium of the stomach (Fig. 97–5). This latter ring (Schatzki's ring) can be demonstrated in many individuals if video studies of the lower esophageal zone are used.

All these types of webs or rings cause dysphagia for solids, and the impacted bolus usually has to be regurgitated. The lower esophageal ring (Schatzki's ring) has a characteristic clinical presentation that allows the diagnosis to be made by history. Every 3 to 4 months, after a bolus of meat or bread, the patient complains of dysphagia and total inability to swallow solids or liquids. The bolus is regurgitated, and then the patient can continue to eat normally. Lower esophageal rings may be dilated using a through-the-endoscope balloon or a bougie. Rings of < 12.0 mm across their narrowest diameter cause symptoms and require rupture.

Treatment of all webs involves mechanical disruption either with a dilator or with the endoscope. Treating iron deficiency anemia may cause the postcricoid webs to disappear. Only very rarely is a surgical approach to a web or ring necessary.

DIVERTICULA OF THE ESOPHAGUS. Zenker's diverticulum of the pharynx is not anatomically an esophageal diverticulum, as its neck is above the UES muscle, but custom has dictated its inclusion in description of esophageal diverticula. An epiphrenic diverticulum usually occurs on the right side of the esophagus just above the LES. Other diverticula are at the level of the carina and are known as *traction diverticula,* although traction by scar tissue is rarely demonstrated. Scleroderma is occasionally associated with numerous wide-mouthed diverticula scattered along the length of the esophagus. Large-amplitude motor waves have been associated with midbody diverticula and either achalasia or motor incoordination with epiphrenic diverticula.

Symptoms vary widely; many diverticula are found by accident during barium examination of the esophagus. If a patient with dysphagia is found to have a diverticulum, it is difficult to tell whether the diverticulum or the associated motor disorder is the cause. Zenker's diverticulum often has a classic symptom complex, particularly when it becomes large. It retains saliva and food particles, which may either be aspirated or cause repeated postprandial throat clearing with production of liquid and food particles. Patients with this type of diverticulum can often press on the neck and empty the

diverticulum. The pouch can become so large that it can compress the esophagus anteriorly and obstruct it. In the presence of diverticula great caution must be exercised in passing tubes or endoscopes into the esophagus or stomach. Zenker's diverticulum is a special problem, since tubes naturally enter it rather than the esophageal opening, and the risk of perforation into the mediastinum is great. Traction and epiphrenic diverticula do not require treatment. Zenker's diverticulum, if large, may require diverticulectomy or diverticulopexy with coincident section of the cricopharyngeus muscle. Most techniques for diverticulectomy automatically accomplish cricopharyngeal section at the same time. If the diverticulum is small, it may regress after section of the cricopharyngeus.

INFECTIONS OF THE ESOPHAGUS. Infections afflicting the esophagus are usually fungal *(Candida)* or viral (cytomegalovirus [CMV], herpes simplex virus [HSV]). Although both are most common in immunocompromised hosts such as those on corticosteroids, undergoing cancer chemotherapy, or afflicted with AIDS, either or both can infect apparently healthy hosts. All can be found incidentally at autopsy or during endoscopy for other indications. Most commonly, infection of the mucosa leads to odynophagia of rather marked degree. Dysphagia for both solids and liquids usually accompanies the odynophagia and can be of such intensity that weight loss is rapid. Herpes esophagitis may present with hematemesis.

Although the radiograph occasionally reveals a shaggy mucosa in the case of monilial involvement, and occasionally even a stricture, endoscopy is the best method of detecting and confirming infectious involvement. *Candida* infection can present as isolated white plaques, which can be confused with glycogenic acanthosis or progress to form confluent ulcerations with an overlying membrane. Herpesvirus tends to produce vesicles or isolated superficial ulcers, but extensive involvement can produce confluent ulcerations. CMV lesions initially appear as serpiginous ulcers, but may coalesce to form giant ulcers. Biopsy of the ulcerated area usually shows either invasive hyphae of *Candida* or characteristic nuclear changes of the squamous cells when herpesvirus is present. Cytologic washings occasionally demonstrate the same change. Viral cultures of esophageal biopsies or brushings are useful for diagnosing HSV.

Treatment depends on correct identification of the etiologic agent. For *Candida* infection, an assessment of the degree of severity is needed. For mild noninvasive disease, topical therapy with nystatin (250,000 units every 2 hours) or clotrimazole (dissolved in the mouth 5 times per day) suffices. For more serious infections, systemic treatment with oral fluconazole or occasionally ketoconazole is used. Low-dose intravenous amphotericin may be needed for patients not responding to oral treatment and those unable to swallow medications. Herpesvirus infection is treated with parenteral acyclovir. Ganciclovir or foscarnet can be tried to treat CMV infection.

ESOPHAGEAL INJURIES. *Caustic Ingestion.* Caustic burns of the esophagus occur in children by accident; adults usually suffer such burns because of suicide attempts. Lye crystals, and especially liquid lye preparations for drain cleaning, are the most common cause. The speed of lye injury is so great that attempts to neutralize the caustic are futile. Detergents and Clorox also find their way into the esophageal lumens of both children and adults. The history is all-important, but the degree of esophageal injury still must be assessed endoscopically as an emergency. Significant esophageal damage has been seen even without oral burns; conversely, oral burns do not necessarily mean that the material has reached the esophagus. If there is no esophageal reaction after apparent caustic ingestion, further care directed toward the esophagus will not be necessary.

The accepted therapy of a definite lye or caustic burn remains unsupported by clinical trials. For burns with solid lye or other solid agents, corticosteroids have been recommended, at an initial dose of 80 mg per day, tapering to 20 mg per day until esophageal healing. Most clinicians also use broad-spectrum antibiotics. If liquid lye has been the damaging agent, serious consideration of emergency esophagogastrectomy is in order, as lesser measures have met with unacceptably high mortality.

Damage by Medication. Ingested pills may lodge in the esophagus and damage the mucosa in a localized area. Tetracycline, doxycycline, potassium tablets, ascorbic acid, quinidine, and nonsteroidal anti-inflammatory agents are the main medications that cause pill-induced esophagitis, but the list is long. Normal individuals can retain small capsules in the esophagus, even when swallow-

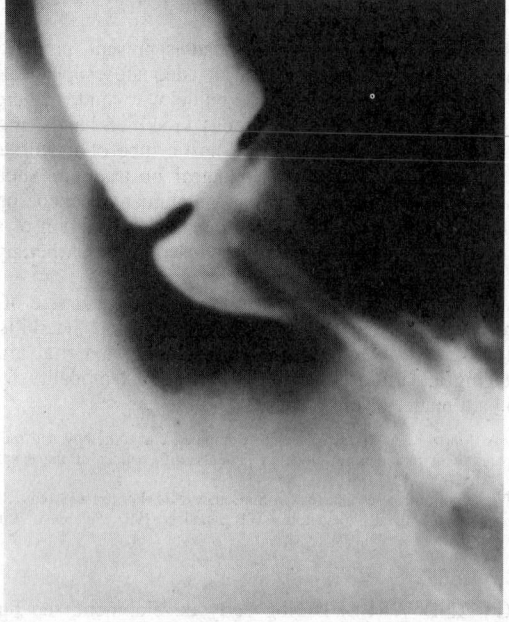

FIGURE 97–5. Lower esophageal ring (Schatzki's ring). This ring consists of a symmetric thin web located in the terminal esophagus. (From Pope CE II: *In* Sleisenger MH, Fordtran JS [eds.]: Gastrointestinal Disease. 3rd ed. Philadelphia, WB Saunders, 1983.)

ing in the upright position. The clinical syndrome consists of steady burning or chest pain, accompanied by local odynophagia, all occurring 4 to 6 hours after ingesting one of the offending capsules or tablets. Endoscopy usually shows a localized mucosal ulcer, which heals without a scar or may lead to a stricture requiring dilation. Symptomatic therapy is adequate, but prophylaxis seems to be a more practical idea. Pills of the offending class should be taken in the upright position with several swallows of water both before and after pill ingestion.

Esophageal Trauma. The esophagus is well protected by the thoracic cage but can be involved either by blunt trauma (automobile accidents) or by penetrating missiles (gunshots, knives). Often the surgeon's attention is directed toward more life-threatening damage to heart, lungs, or major blood vessels, and it is understandable that a rent in the esophagus may thus be overlooked. This unfortunate oversight, however, is followed by mediastinitis, which may worsen an already grave situation. Iatrogenic perforation with endoscope, dilator, or, very rarely, nasogastric tube leads to a similar complication.

Vomiting itself can cause esophageal injury, either mucosal (*Mallory-Weiss*) or through-and-through rupture (*Boerhaave's syndrome*). The mucosal lesion first described by Mallory and Weiss has been recognized much more frequently since the advent of emergency endoscopy with fiberoptic endoscopes. Classically, the patient has repeated attacks of retching, at first producing gastric contents and later bright red blood. One quarter of patients shown to have a Mallory-Weiss tear have no prior history of vomiting. The tear is usually in the gastric mucosa just below the gastroesophageal junction, although it can extend through the junction and up into the esophageal mucosa. Diagnosis of this condition is almost always made at endoscopy; the rent is usually seen as the endoscope is being withdrawn from the stomach into the esophagus. The majority of such lesions heal with conservative therapy. Angiographic or surgical therapy is necessary in <5%. Bleeding has been stopped by directly applying electrocoagulation through the endoscope.

Vomiting can also cause a complete tear in the esophageal wall. Unlike the Mallory-Weiss lesion, the tear in Boerhaave's syndrome is located above the gastroesophageal junction on the left side. It usually follows vomiting, but other marked increases in intra-abdominal pressure such as lifting a heavy weight or straining at stool have been associated with a tear. The clinical diagnosis can be extremely difficult; often patients with esophageal rupture are thought to have a myocardial infarct, pneumothorax, a perforated viscus, or pancreatitis. Air in the mediastinum or the rapid appearance of a hydrothorax on the left usually leads to the correct diagnosis.

The diagnosis of esophageal perforation can usually be established by a cautious radiographic examination with water-soluble material. Barium may be used only if a rent is not demonstrated by the water-soluble agent. Immediate surgical repair is the accepted method of treatment of esophageal perforation. In those too ill for surgery, treatment consists of nasogastric suction, antibiotics, and subsequent mediastinal drainage if necessary.

Baehr PH, McDonald GB: Esophageal infections: Risk factors, presentation, diagnosis and treatment. Gastroenterology 106:509, 1994. *Recent review on esophageal infections.*

Pope CE II: Rings, webs, diverticula. *In* Sleisenger MH, Fordtran JS (eds.): Gastrointestinal Disease. 5th ed. Philadelphia, WB Saunders, 1993. *Reference gastrointestinal textbook.*

98 GASTRITIS
Andrew H. Soll

The normal gastric mucosa has a remarkable ability to resist acid-peptic injury (see Ch. 99.1). Although "gastritis" was interpreted to be an effect of aging and lifelong exposure to various insults, it is now clear that this common inflammatory condition is due to infection with *Helicobacter pylori* (HP). Although much remains to be learned about pathogenesis and natural history, gastritis can be most readily classified by cause (Table 98–1). The term "nonerosive" has not been used because the most common form, HP gastritis, can also be associated with erosions and peptic ulcers.

TABLE 98–1. CLASSIFICATION OF "GASTRITIS" AND GASTROPATHY

A. *Helicobacter pylori*–induced gastritis (superficial, forms a spectrum from antral predominant, type "B" gastritis to pangastritis, type "AB")
B. Atrophic gastritis
  1. Pernicious anemia (fundal gland predominant, type "A," autoimmune markers)
  2. Atrophic pangastritis (involving antrum and fundal gland region, probably end-stage form of *Helicobacter pylori* gastritis.
C. Erosive/hemorrhagic gastropathy
  1. Nonsteroidal anti-inflammatory drug (NSAID) gastroenteropathy
  2. Stress-related mucosal disease
  3. Alcohol gastropathy
D. Unusual or specific forms of gastritis
  1. Phlegmonous gastritis
  2. Infections, usually in immunocompromised hosts
    Viral (CMV, herpes)
    Fungal (*Candida*, histoplasmosis)
    Tuberculosis, syphilis
  3. Chronic erosive (diffuse varioliform) gastritis
  4. Postoperative alkaline gastritis
  5. Gastric ischemia
  6. Radiation-induced gastritis
  7. Ingestion of corrosive substances
  8. Ménétrier's disease (giant hypertrophic gastritis)
  9. Eosinophilic gastritis
  10. Granulomatous gastritis
  11. Vascular ectasia: watermelon stomach (antral vascular ectasia)

Three conditions causing erosive or hemorrhagic damage have been traditionally included among disorders causing gastritis. However, these three disorders cause little if any inflammation; when inflammation is present, it is associated with HP infection.

HELICOBACTER PYLORI–INDUCED GASTRITIS

HP, a gram-negative microaerophilic organism, appears to be the most common worldwide human infection. This organism has three attributes that allow it to fill a unique ecologic niche (Table 98–2). The inflammation associated with HP is usually superficial, found in the foveolar or gastric pit region and upper portion of the lamina propria. Infiltration with polymorphonuclear leukocytes is characteristic and therefore the gastritis is called "chronic active." The antrum is consistently involved, whereas inflammation in the *acid-secreting fundic gland (gastric body and fundus) mucosa* is more variable (see below). Four arguments establish that this antral-predominant, superficial gastritis (type B) is due to HP: (1) HP is present in virtually all patients with superficial gastritis, (2) the gastritis resolves once the infection is cured, (3) gastritis has been induced in a few subjects by inadvertent or self-administration of HP, and (4) the epidemiologic and geographic patterns for the occurrence of HP and superficial gastritis are identical.

EPIDEMIOLOGY. No reservoir other than the human gastric mucosa has been identified. The epidemiology of HP reflects a pattern typical of fecal-oral transmission and is similar to hepatitis A or polio, with high prevalence at a young age in developing countries and in impoverished subpopulations in developed countries. Poor hygiene and poor sanitation are important variables. Transmission is most likely with exposure to gastric juice of infected indi-

TABLE 98–2. FEATURES OF THE UNIQUE ECOLOGIC NICHE FOR *HELICOBACTER PYLORI*

1. Colonization
  a. Motility
  b. Urease (and catalase)
  c. Adhesion to surface epithelial cells
2. Virulence (noninvasive, due to release of bacterial factors)
  a. Epithelial cytolysis and tight junction disruption by cytotoxins
  b. Induction of inflammatory/immune response: chemotaxins, lipopolysaccharide, immune modulators, antigenic stimulation, induction of epithelial cytokines
3. Persistence
  a. Inaccessibility
  b. Immune evasion

viduals (*oral-gastric*) but has occurred with contaminated nasogastric tubes and endoscopes. Overall, the *prevalence* of HP infection increases with age at an average rate of about 1% per year, but it appears that most acquisition of infection occurs in childhood or in families with young children. A large component of the increase in prevalence with age reflects an *age cohort* effect whereby older individuals, especially those over 60, acquired the infection at a young age when in the United States sanitization was less strict. HP infection appears to be decreasing in parallel with the decrease in the incidence of peptic ulcer and cancer of the gastric body and antrum.

ACUTE HP GASTRITIS. With acute HP infection, superficial gastritis develops in association with epigastric pain, nausea, and vomiting. Two "epidemics" of HP have been reported following common source exposure. Despite the absence of glandular gastritis and the presence of histologically robust parietal cells, acid secretion was markedly reduced, suggesting release of a factor inhibiting acid secretion. These epidemics occurred before the bacterium was recognized, but retrospective analysis revealed histology and serology consistent with HP infection in most of the patients. Occasionally, sporadic acute HP gastritis can be recognized.

DISTRIBUTION AND PROGRESSION: RELATION TO PEPTIC ULCER AND GASTRIC CANCER. In studies performed in the era before HP was recognized, gastritis involving predominantly the antrum was common in "normal" younger subjects. Follow-up over subsequent decades revealed progressive involvement of the fundic gland mucosa, resulting in pangastritis (type AB). However, in contrast to this progressive involvement of the acid-secreting mucosa, marked involvement of both the antrum and fundic gland regions has been observed in some young individuals, particularly in regions with high endemic rates and early onset of HP infection. A different pattern occurs in HP-positive duodenal ulcer patients; although modest to moderate superficial antral gastritis is invariably found (see Ch. 99), involvement of the fundic gland mucosa is usually minimal and progression occurs at a slower rate than in nonulcer subjects. The clinical correlate is that duodenal ulcer patients secrete acid at high-normal or high rates and have a lower risk of gastric cancer. In contrast to duodenal ulcer, patients with gastric ulcer tend to have more severe antral gastritis, more involvement with superficial fundic gland gastritis, and low-normal acid secretory rates. It is not known whether the variability in the distribution and progression of HP gastritis among individuals is due to age at acquisition of HP infection or host or environmental factors.

With time and increasing severity of pangastritis, fundic gland atrophy can occur accounting for the decrease in maximal acid secretion with age. Atrophy of antral glands can also occur. Pseudopyloric metaplasia (the parietal and chief cells of fundic glands are replaced by mucous glands indistinguishable from normal antrum) and intestinal metaplasia (mucin-containing goblet cells, absorptive cells, and occasionally rudimentary villi) often develop along with atrophic glandular change. Dysplastic epithelial change can develop subsequent to this metaplasia as part of the progression to gastric cancer induced by HP gastritis.

OTHER PATHOGENIC FACTORS. In the pre-HP era, many other factors were considered in the pathogenesis of chronic gastritis, including chronic trauma, gastric bacteria, toxins, thermal insult, dietary factors including dietary nitrosamines, and reflux of bile and pancreatic enzymes. It was hypothesized that lysolecithin—formed by the action of the pancreatic enzyme phospholipase A on biliary lecithin—was a component of bile reflux capable of disrupting the surface epithelial barrier to acid "back-diffusion," thus creating a chronic insult that could provoke an inflammatory response. Because curing HP infection rapidly resolves superficial gastritis, it is unlikely that these factors are involved in superficial gastritis, although they may affect progression to chronic atrophic gastritis, intestinal metaplasia, or gastric cancer.

DETECTING HP (see Ch. 99.3). HP can be detected using "noninvasive" modalities: serology with an ELISA assay for IgG or IgA antibodies and ^{13}C or ^{14}C-urea breath tests after an oral urea load. "Invasive" testing includes biopsy for histologic examination, urease test on antral biopsies, or culture (which is not routinely available). The optimal method depends on circumstances, local expertise, and availability. All have good sensitivity and specificity, but false determinations occur. Pathologists need to be educated to detect HP; we and they ignored the organism for decades. In tests that depend on the number of organisms (testing breath and gastric biopsies for urease activity, histology, and culture), false-negatives occur especially when the organism has been suppressed by antibiotics, omeprazole, or bismuth. Several weeks off therapy may be necessary before these tests become positive.

CLINICAL PRESENTATION AND TREATMENT. Individuals with gastritis are usually asymptomatic and a relation to dyspepsia is mired in the vagaries of visceral sensation (see Ch. 99.1). However, HP gastritis is found in patients with dyspepsia more frequently than in age-matched controls. In contrast to the clear indication for antibiotic therapy with HP-positive peptic ulcer, the causal relation and proper approach to HP in the setting of "nonulcer" dyspepsia is controversial. It is clear that this dyspepsia is frequently due to functional disorders that are independent of HP; therefore, it is not surprising that infection cure does not eliminate symptoms in many patients. However, some individuals with HP gastritis and upper abdominal symptoms improve once HP infection is cured, although benefit over placebo has not been established in controlled studies. Because antibiotic therapy for HP (see Ch. 99.3) is less expensive than additional diagnostic studies and ongoing maintenance "ulcer" therapy and usually free from serious side effects, cure of HP infection is a reasonable option for patients with persisting symptoms who do not respond to or require continued treatment.

ATROPHIC GASTRITIS

ATROPHIC PANGASTRITIS DUE TO HP. As noted above, HP-associated pangastritis can progress to fundic and antral gland atrophy. Sorting out pathogenesis can be quite difficult: (1) HP is frequently absent once hyposecretion of acid allows overgrowth of other bacteria and disruption of HP's unique ecologic niche in the acidic stomach; (2) the adhesion molecule for HP is present on the apical membrane of normal and metaplastic gastric-type but not intestinal-type cells; and (3) IgG and IgA antibodies to HP fall within months after loss of the organism. Immune markers are generally absent from HP pangastritis, and only a small (and undefined) proportion of subjects develop vitamin B_{12} deficiency. Contribution of other factors to pathogenesis and the overlap with "autoimmune" gastritis and pernicious anemia remain to be established.

PERNICIOUS ANEMIA (see Ch. 133). This "autoimmune" gastritis (type A) predominantly involves the fundic gland mucosa, is *deep* (encompassing the gastric glands that contain parietal and chief cells), and usually atrophic (with decreased or absent glandular elements and mucosal thinning). Superficial inflammation is minimal, and deep inflammatory changes are usually most prominent along the greater curvature of the fundus and body. Once glandular atrophy develops, the inflammatory infiltrate may be minimal. Even with sufficient fundic gland atrophy to produce histamine-fast achlorhydria, some patchy nests of parietal and chief cells may persist. The relative absence of glandular atrophy in the antrum accounts for the ability of many of these patients to develop marked hypergastrinemia as the feedback inhibition of acid on gastrin release is lost.

Immunologic mechanisms appear operative in pernicious anemia but not HP gastritis. About 90% of patients with pernicious anemia have antibodies against parietal cells, which appear to react with the parietal cell H^+-K^+-ATPase. Antibodies reacting with intrinsic factor also occur and block the vitamin B_{12} binding site, leading to depleted serum levels and body stores of B_{12} and a megaloblastic anemia. Sera from patients with pernicious anemia contain an antibody cytotoxic to canine gastric mucosal cells. Pernicious anemia is also associated with other immunologic disorders, Hashimoto's thyroiditis, hyperthyroidism, insulin-dependent diabetes mellitus, and vitiligo. Caution regarding "autoimmune" mechanisms is appropriate; before recognition of HP, type B gastritis was also hypothesized to reflect immune or genetic pathogenesis.

Genetic factors are important in pernicious anemia; family members of patients have an increased incidence of atrophic gastritis, achlorhydria, vitamin B_{12} malabsorption, and antibodies to parietal cells and intrinsic factor.

Clinical Presentation. Patients with pernicious anemia may develop symptoms secondary to vitamin B_{12} deficiency. Macroscopic endoscopic findings (erythema, petechiae, nodularity, pallor, and atrophy) are generally nonspecific. Diagnosis requires multiple biopsies because the histopathology may be patchy. The ratio of pepsinogen I (present in fundic chief cells) to pepsinogen II (present in both chief cells and surface epithelial cells) falls in proportion to glandular atrophy.

Enterochromaffin-like cells undergo hyperplasia in atrophic gastritis because the elevated gastrin levels exert trophic effects on enterochromaffin-like (ECL) cells. ECL cells are an endocrine population present in the fundic gland mucosa that contain histamine and are distinguished by characteristic granules and silver staining properties. ECL cells can form carcinoid tumors in atrophic gastritis. ECL cell hyperplasia also occurs in Zollinger-Ellison (gastrinoma) syndrome (see Ch. 99.6), but carcionoid tumors are largely restricted to patients with multiple endocrine neoplasia (MEN) type I. ECL cells do not contain serotonin, and thus these tumors do not produce the classic "carcinoid" syndrome found with tumors composed of serotonin-containing enterochromaffin (EC) cells (see Ch. 210.2). ECL carcinoids associated with hypergastrinemia can be metastatic; they are usually indolent, multifocal tumors that may respond to antrectomy and local excision. This setting provides a logical indication for a gastrin B receptor antagonist when one becomes available for clinical use. In contrast, gastric carcinoids found without hypergastrinemia are solitary, aggressive tumors.

Management. No specific therapy exists for pernicious anemia, beyond replacing vitamin B_{12}. It is reasonable to evaluate family members for gastritis and vitamin B_{12} deficiency. *Gastric adenocarcinomas* have been reported to occur with increased frequency with pernicious anemia, but the assessment of increased risk is variable, ranging from nil to threefold in different series. Endoscopy at the time of an initial diagnosis, with sufficient antral and fundic gland biopsies to assess the severity of intestinal metaplasia and epithelial dysplasia, is appropriate. Although imperfect, these features are the best indicators of the cancer risk; using this approach, only those patients with dysplasia warrant close follow-up and/or surgical intervention. Otherwise, no recommendations regarding screening have been established.

EROSIVE/HEMORRHAGIC GASTROPATHY

NSAID GASTROENTEROPATHY. (See Ch. 99.1.)
STRESS-RELATED MUCOSAL DAMAGE AND ULCERS. (See Ch. 99.1.)
ALCOHOL GASTROPATHY. Characteristic subepithelial (intramucosal) hemorrhages, with the endoscopic appearance of "blood under a plastic wrap," are commonly found in individuals abusing alcohol. Although termed "hemorrhagic gastritis," these lesions are composed of hemorrhage and edema in the interstitial space under the surface epithelium, without inflammation. Usually the bleeding is mild. If more severe bleeding is found, associated lesions, such as portal hypertension, peptic ulcer, or a Mallory-Weiss tear, should be sought (see Ch. 95).

UNUSUAL OR SPECIFIC FORMS OF GASTRITIS. *Phlegmonous Gastritis.* This rarely encountered, purulent process involves the gastric submucosa and wall. Alpha-hemolytic streptococci, but also staphylococci, *E. coli,* and *Proteus,* have been implicated. The course is usually fulminant and medical management ineffective, leaving surgery as the drastic, but unavoidable, last resort.

Other Infections. As with infections in all other sites, the spectrum of gastric infections is expanded and altered in the immunocompromised host. Gastric tuberculosis, diagnosed by finding caseating granulomas and positive cultures, occurs in AIDS. Secondary syphilis may involve the stomach with thickened folds and erosions. Despite the frequency of esophageal candidiasis, gastric ulcers appear to be secondarily colonized by these organisms. Mycelia may occur at the ulcer margin, but ulcer healing does not appear to be impaired and antifungal therapy does not accelerate healing, suggesting a lack of clinical importance. Cytomegalovirus can involve the stomach in the immunocompromised host. Herpes simplex virus type I has been implicated as a cause of ulcer disease in nonimmunocompromised hosts (see Ch. 99.1). The ascaris-like larva, *Anisakis,* present in raw fish, may infect the normal gastric mucosa, producing pain and dyspepsia. *Strongyloides stercoralis* involves the small intestine much more frequently than the stomach and can cause dyspepsia. Diagnosis is made by examining duodenal aspirates or stool specimens.

Chronic Erosive (Diffuse Varioliform) Gastritis. Lesions are multiple and consist of gastric erosions on top of small nodules,

usually involving the body and fundus more than the antrum. The multiplicity and chronicity distinguish this entity from occasional isolated antral erosions found without symptoms. The entity can be considered only after HP and use of NSAID's and alcohol have been excluded. Symptoms are nonspecific and include abdominal pain, nausea, vomiting, anorexia, weight loss, and sometimes bleeding. Lymphocytic gastritis may occur adjacent to the erosions.

Postoperative Alkaline Gastritis. Macroscopic gastritis with a dramatic red color may rapidly develop after gastric resection or pyloroplasty, but this endoscopic appearance does not correlate with symptoms, bile reflux, or histologic inflammation. The occurrence of this difficult-to-treat complication of surgery for peptic ulcer is another indication to do the least physiologically disruptive operation (i.e., highly selective vagotomy), whenever possible.

Gastric Ischemia. Ischemic gastric injury is rarely recognized, although erosive changes have been reported with vasculitis and atheromatous embolization. Whether chronic gastric ulcers have an ischemic component remains speculative.

Ménétrier's Disease. Ménétrier's disease is defined by four features: (1) giant folds in the gastric fundus and body; (2) diminished acid secretory capacity; (3) hypoalbuminemia secondary to protein-losing gastropathy; and (4) histologic features of foveolar hyperplasia (gastric pit region) and a marked increase in mucosal thickness combined with gland atrophy and cystic dilation. Tortuous gastric folds may resemble the cerebral cortex. Hypochlorhydria is generally present, but a hypersecretory variant (that may be an unrelated entity) has been described. Symptoms are variable and may include abdominal pain, nausea, vomiting, weight loss, and edema. The disease is more common in men than in women, generally presenting after age 50, although a childhood form exists. Typical biopsies confirm the diagnosis, but variant patterns warrant the less specific diagnosis of idiopathic hypertrophic gastropathy. Variant cases that do not include all of the typical features are more common than classic cases. The differential diagnosis includes gastrinoma syndrome, infiltrating carcinoma, lymphoma, and amyloidosis. Large gastric folds and a picture of hypertrophic gastritis have been reported associated with HP infection. If present, the organism should be treated, but the impact on gastric protein loss has not been established. Accompanying ulcers and erosions usually respond to standard antiulcer therapy if HP is not present. No increased risk of cancer has been established.

Eosinophilic Gastritis. Eosinophils may infiltrate the gastrointestinal mucosa and muscular layers, especially with antral involvement, in association with peripheral eosinophilia as an idiopathic syndrome. Thickening of gastric mucosal folds and wall rigidity are common. Antral motility may be altered, leading to gastric retention. Patients may present with eosinophilia, nausea, vomiting, or pain. Rarely, serosal involvement results in ascites. Milk-sensitive enteropathy of infancy, connective tissue disorders, and parasitic infections should be ruled out. Glucocorticoid therapy may be useful, and surgery may be needed if mechanical outlet obstruction occurs.

Granulomatous Gastritis. Granulomas in the gastric mucosa may occur associated with generalized diseases such as sarcoidosis, Crohn's disease, or infections. Crohn's disease may involve the duodenum, pylorus, antrum, and gastric body (in that order), usually in association with disease in the small intestine or colon. Mucosal granulomas may also be incidental findings or occur in eosinophilic granulomas or in isolated, idiopathic granulomatous gastritis. Involved portions of the stomach may be rigid or narrow or have thickened folds on radiographic examination; these findings must be distinguished from malignancy. The antrum is most often involved, and granulomas may occur in all layers of the stomach. Ulcerated lesions may perforate. Patients are often operated upon because of the difficulties in differentiating this entity from malignancy. Once the diagnosis is made, it is important to exclude potentially curable diseases (e.g., tuberculosis, histoplasmosis, syphilis) or treatable processes (e.g., sarcoidosis, Crohn's disease). With malignancy and associated diseases excluded, the patient can be followed because spontaneous resolution has been reported.

Watermelon Stomach. This entity, also known as gastric antral vascular ectasia, represents another nongastritic condition. At endoscopy, the antrum has erythematous folds or linear angioid streaks, the latter converging at the pylorus in a pattern reminiscent of a watermelon. Biopsy can be diagnostic, demonstrating dilated antral vasculature with intravascular fibrin thrombi and fibromuscular hyperplasia. This uncommon lesion can present with either acute gastrointestinal bleeding or chronic iron deficiency anemia. Corticosteroid therapy has been tried with uncertain success. Antrectomy is effective in eliminating bleeding; however, success has also been reported with repeated coagulation using endoscopic laser or heater probes. No relation to HP has been reported.

Lewin KJ, Riddell RH, Weinstein WM: Stomach and proximal duodenum: Inflammatory and miscellaneous disorders. *In* Gastrointestinal Pathology and its Clinical Implications. New York, Igaku-Shoin, 1992, p 506. *Definitive reference on gastritis and related conditions.*

Weinstein WM: Gastritis and gastropathies. *In* Sleisenger MH, Fordtran JS (eds.): Gastrointestinal Disease: Pathophysiology, Diagnosis, Management. 5th ed. Philadelphia, WB Saunders, 1993, p 545. *Detailed discussion of the common forms of gastritis.*

99 PEPTIC ULCER

99.1 Pathophysiology

Andrew H. Soll

Peptic ulcers are holes extending through the mucosa into the muscularis propria of the esophagus, stomach, or duodenum. Schwartz, who was credited with the "no acid: no ulcer" dictum, recognized in 1910 that "peptic ulcer (PU) was a product of self-digestion, resulting from an excess of autopeptic power in gastric juice over the defensive power of gastric and intestinal mucosa." Three lines of defense functioning at pre-epithelial, epithelial, and post-epithelial levels preserve mucosal integrity (Table 99–1). When these lines of defense are overwhelmed, epithelial repair mechanisms restore mucosal integrity (Table 99–1). When these defense and repair processes are overwhelmed and wounds form in the basement membrane, classic wound healing processes remodel the basement membrane and permit epithelial regrowth. Thus, peptic ulcers are a failure of wound healing. In the last decade it has become apparent that, with rare exception, these mucosal defense, repair, and healing mechanisms fail only when disrupted by exogenous factors. The two most common forms of peptic ulcer are associated with *Helicobacter pylori* (HP) infection and use of aspirin and other nonsteroidal anti-inflammatory drugs (NSAID's) (Table 99–2). In the absence of these factors, ulcers would be a rare disease. Another dictum is also valid: "No HP, no NSAID's: no ulcer" or "Normal mucosal defense, repair, and healing: no ulcer."

HELICOBACTER PYLORI AND PEPTIC ULCER

Even in the era before the HP revolution, peptic ulcer in the absence of NSAID's was recognized to be consistently associated with diffuse, chronic antral-predominant inflammation. Duodenal ulcer (DU) is also associated with duodenitis, but the distribution is patchy and variable among studies. The significance of this inflammation remained unknown until Marshall and Warren recognized that the very common superficial, antral-predominant (type B) form of gastritis was linked to HP (see Ch. 98). Two lines of evidence established HP as a crucial causal factor for development of both DU and gastrointestinal ulcer (GU): (1) The large majority of DU (>90%) and GU (>75%) are associated with HP. (2) Several well-designed, controlled studies and numerous other less rigorous trials have consistently indicated that successfully curing the HP infection predicts a markedly reduced rate of ulcer recurrence.

The challenging aspect of this pathophysiology is that HP is the most common infection in the world and only a small percentage (about 10 to 20%) of infected subjects develop peptic ulcer during a lifetime of infection. The ulcer diathesis that separates the few subjects destined to develop peptic ulcer disease (PUD) from those with HP infection without ulcer disease has not been defined. Factors have been identified that determine the virulence of HP for producing infection and gastritis (see Ch. 98). Organisms from DU patients have been distinguished from those occurring in nonulcer subjects by genetic homology and cytotoxin production, but no single pathogenic factor has been identified that is consistently and selectively associated with ulcer formation. Once the HP infection is cured, inflammation rapidly resolves and ulcer recurrence is infrequent, making it unlikely that autoimmunity contributes to pathogenesis.

ARE PEPTIC ULCERS STILL PEPTIC? Schwartz recognized that peptic activity is an indispensable component of ulcer pathogenesis; therefore, this dictum should read: "No acid/peptic activity: no ulcer." The persisting validity of this generalization is supported by the observation that very potent antisecretory agents heal the large majority of peptic ulcers.

ACID SECRETION. Maximal gastric acid output (MAO) is elevated in about one third of DU patients and in the high-normal range in the remaining patients. DU virtually does not occur with an MAO less than about 12 mEq per hour. It is agreed that acid secretion is "robust" (high-normal or elevated) in DU. No agreement exists regarding whether these changes are due to increased secretory mass, defective inhibitory mechanisms, or increased basal drive to acid secretion. About 80% of DU subjects also have an increased nocturnal acid secretion; this increased rate of acid secretion between 4 P.M. and midnight probably reflects an exaggeration of a normal circadian rhythm.

HP and the Secretion of Gastrin, Somatostatin, and Acid. Both ulcer and nonulcer subjects infected with HP demonstrate enhanced secretion of gastrin in response to food and other stimuli. Abnormalities of gastric somatostatin cells have also been identified in HP-infected subjects. Despite the elevation in serum

---

TABLE 99–1. THE MULTIPLE LINES OF MUCOSAL DEFENSE, REPAIR, AND HEALING

Lines of defense
First line: mucus and bicarbonate
  Adherent mucous layer excludes pepsin
  Bicarbonate output creates pH gradient stabilized by mucous layer
Second line: Epithelial cell mechanisms
  Barrier function of apical plasma membrane
  Intrinsic cell defense (e.g., glutathione and heat shock protein)
  Extrusion of "back-diffused" H^+ via basolateral carriers
Third line: Mucosal blood flow (removal of "back-diffused" H^+ and supply of energy substrate)

Lines of repair and healing
First line: Epithelial cell restitution (sliding of adjacent cells to fill gaps created by sloughed cells)
Second line: Epithelial cell replication
Third line: Classic wound healing (formation of granulation tissue, angiogenesis, and remodeling of basement membrane permitting ingrowth of epithelial cells)

TABLE 99–2. CAUSES AND ASSOCIATIONS OF PEPTIC ULCER

Common forms of peptic ulcer
1. *Helicobacter pylori*–associated
2. NSAID-associated
3. Stress ulcer

Uncommon specific forms of peptic ulcer
1. Acid hypersecretion
  a. Gastrinoma: inherited—MEN I, sporadic
  b. Increased mast cells/basophils
    Mastocytosis: inherited and sporadic
    Basophilic leukemias
  c. Antral G cell hyperfunction/hyperplasia
2. Other infections
  a. Viral infection: herpes simplex virus type I, CMV
  b. ? Other infections
3. Duodenal obstruction/disruption (congenital bands, annular pancreas)
4. Vascular insufficiency: Crack cocaine–associated perforations
5. Radiation-induced
6. Chemotherapy-induced (hepatic artery infusions)
7. ? Rare genetic subtypes
  a. ? Amyloidosis type III (Van Allen–Iowa)
  b. ? Tremor-nystagmus-ulcer syndrome of Neuhauser

Modified from Soll AH: Gastric, duodenal, and stress ulcer. *In* Sleisenger M, Fordtran J (eds.): Gastrointestinal Disease. 5th ed. Philadelphia, WB Saunders, 1993, p 580.

gastrin and the decrease in the paracrine (locally acting) inhibitor somatostatin, acid secretion is usually normal in nonulcer, HP-infected subjects. The robust acid secretion found in DU subjects appears to be a feature of the ulcer diathesis rather than of the HP infection *per se*. Three hypotheses are probably true regarding DU and acid secretion: (1) In *some* DU subjects acid secretion is decreased following successful cure of the HP infection, suggesting in this subset that acid secretion may be increased by either HP-induced hypergastrinemia or the perturbed inhibitory mechanisms. (2) In another subset of DU subjects, acid hypersecretion appears to reflect a predisposing condition that is independent of HP infection. (3) DU subjects may be "selected" from non-DU HP-infected subjects by the relative sparing from gastritis of the fundic gland mucosa and, therefore, preservation of acid secretion.

DUODENITIS, GASTRIC METAPLASIA, AND DU. Gastric metaplasia, the replacement of intestinal epithelium by cells with the staining properties of gastric surface mucous cells, may be a key pathogenic step in the duodenum. The importance of this metaplasia in the duodenum probably reflects the fact that HP binds only to a glycoprotein receptor on the surface of these gastric-type cells; gastric metaplasia therefore appears to be the carpet on which HP resides in the duodenum. Present evidence indicates that gastric metaplasia occurs as a function of exposure to the acid/peptic activity in gastric juice. Studies are needed to confirm the pathogenic role of gastric metaplasia in the duodenum. Another consistent pathogenic feature present in about 80% of DU subjects is a decrease in duodenal bicarbonate secretion, although the mechanisms and significance of this decrease remain to be established.

Many features of peptic ulcer remain enigmatic. No pathophysiologic variables have been identified to correlate with the tendency of ulcers to heal and recur spontaneously. Ulcer disease is a focal process, and ulcers tend to recur in the same region; while ulcers persist, nearby biopsies readily heal.

NONSTEROIDAL ANTI-INFLAMMATORY DRUGS (see Ch. 19)

The second common form of ulcer disease is that related to use of NSAID's. NSAID's can be delivered to the gastroduodenal mucosa via topical, systemic, or enterohepatic delivery. Although each of these routes may be important, parenterally administered ketorolac (Torodol) produces ulcer complications within a few days, leaving no doubt that the systemic route is sufficient for ulcerogenesis. Although this conclusion is still controversial, it is likely that clinically relevant GU's occur from inhibition of endogenous prostaglandin (PG) production by NSAID's. In turn PG-dependent mucosal defense and repair mechanisms are disrupted. All NSAID's inhibit the enzyme cyclo-oxygenase that catalyzes the formation of the PG precursor endoperoxide from arachidonic acid derived from cell membrane phospholipids. In animal models GU's are also produced by antibodies to PG's but not to inactive PG analogues, further supporting the conclusion that endogenous PG's are important elements in mucosal defense.

It is crucial to distinguish among three types of NSAID-induced lesions (Table 99–3): (1) superficial injury, which includes erosions and petechiae (punctate intramucosal hemorrhage); (2) "endoscopic ulcers," which are found in 10 to 25% of subjects taking NSAID's; and (3) "clinical ulcers," which present with significant bleeding, perforation, or obstruction at a rate of about 1 to 2% per patient year of NSAID use. Intramucosal hemorrhages are frequent but of little clinical significance. Erosions, unlike ulcers, are small, superficial breaks that do not extend deeper than the mucosa itself and therefore do not cause perforation or significant bleeding. Superficial gastric lesions from NSAID ingestion may occasionally lead to iron deficiency anemia from chronic blood loss or to active bleeding due to widespread involvement. Gastric erosions are often blamed for occult blood in the stool of patients taking NSAID's, but a thorough workup is appropriate because the probability of finding other lesions, such as colonic neoplasia, is similar in subjects who are not taking NSAID's. NSAID's also can cause very significant intestinal damage, ulceration, and weblike strictures presenting as chronic GI blood loss, obstruction, or perforation.

Most of the clinical investigation of NSAID pathogenesis or of the prevention of NSAID ulcers in fact involves endoscopic and not clinical ulcers. The definition of endoscopic ulcers varies among studies and is usually based on size alone. There is little doubt that flat lesions < 5 mm have a different natural history and response to therapeutic intervention than do lesions > 5 mm with visible depth.

TABLE 99–3. THREE TYPES OF NSAID-ASSOCIATED MUCOSAL LESIONS

Feature	Superficial Mucosal Injury	Endoscopic Ulcers	Clinical Ulcers
Onset	Acute (onset in minutes)	Subacute (onset days to months)	Chronic (persist for days to years)
Site	Fundus > antrum	Antrum > fundus	Antrum, duodenum > fundus
Depth	Involves mucosa only	Often indeterminate	Penetrate submucosa
Mode	Topical contact, pH partition	Probably systemic, secondary to decreased prostaglandins	Probably systemic, secondary to decreased prostaglandins
Size	Smaller	Arbitrary (> 3, > 5 mm)	Big enough
Enteric coating	Decreases acute injury	Probably some decrease	May not decrease ulcer incidence
Clinical importance	Usually trivial	A few probably evolve to clinical ulcers	Sometimes cause complications
Healing	Rapid	Probably rapid, little chronic change	Slower or slow
Adaptation	Occurs, especially at low doses	Uncertain	Probably not: ulcers reflect failed adaptation
Prostaglandin cyto-protection	Yes	Yes	Probable partial prevention

NSAID use is reported in about 40% of patients presenting with the ulcer complications of bleeding and perforation. Although the magnitude of the risk from NSAID's is controversial, in a controlled study aspirin (1 gram daily) caused about a nine- to tenfold increased risk of hospitalization for both DU *and* GU. The risk begins within days after treatment and, although it may be highest in the first 3 months of therapy, the risk persists for years. Ulcer risk also appears to be increased with one aspirin tablet (325 mg) daily; mucosal prostaglandin production is decreased with doses as low as a "baby" ASA tablet daily, although the ulcer risk with this dose has not been determined.

RISK FACTORS FOR NSAID ULCERS. The risk of NSAID-associated ulcer complications is higher in elderly women, probably because of the increased consumption of NSAID's by this group and the poor tolerance to complications because of associated diseases. However, the randomized study comparing 1 gram of aspirin daily to placebo indicated that age is an independent risk factor for hospitalizations due to ulcer complications. Corticosteroids alone cause little risk of ulcer disease, but combined with NSAID's, their added risk is significant.

Acid secretion has to be markedly inhibited to promote rapid healing of gastric ulcers in presence of continued NSAID use. Although the gastric mucosa may be very sensitive to the gastric acid/peptic activity in the presence of NSAID's, NSAID's should be considered along with cancer as a cause of ulcers in the face of achlorhydria. The ability of NSAID's to cause intestinal ulcers leaves no question about ulcerogenesis independent of acid-peptic activity.

RARE CONDITIONS ASSOCIATED WITH PEPTIC ULCERS

GASTRINOMA (ZOLLINGER-ELLISON SYNDROME). This uncommon form of ulcer disease is caused by excessive secretion of gastrin by a tumor, 80% of which occur in the "gastrinoma triangle" bounded by the junction of the cystic and common bile ducts, the junction of the second and third portions of the duodenum, and the junction of neck and body of the pancreas (see Ch. 99.6).

RETAINED ANTRUM. This is an unusual complication of peptic ulcer surgery (see Ch. 99.4 and 99.5).

ANTRAL G CELL HYPERFUNCTION. This is a rare form of DU disease in which acid hypersecretion is caused by enhanced secretion of antral gastrin. Fasting gastrin levels are usually only modestly elevated, but the response to a meal is greatly exaggerated. Unlike in patients with gastrinoma, secretin does not elevate gastrin secretion. Although controversial, this entity appears both in an HP-independent form and as the end of the spectrum of HP-induced hypergastrinemia and acid hypersecretion.

MASTOCYTOSIS AND BASOPHILIC LEUKEMIA. These unusual conditions can be associated with peptic ulcer, with the secretagogue being histamine rather than gastrin.

CONGENITAL DISORDERS OF THE DUODENUM. Disorders such as annular pancreas and congenital bands have been associated with DU and acid hypersecretion. The mechanisms accounting for these associations remain to be established.

"VIRO-PEPTIC" ULCERS. The presence of herpes simplex virus type I (HSV-I) has been documented in the mucosa near ulcers in 4 of 22 cases of ordinary peptic ulcer. Although the studies are intriguing, causality in ulcer pathogenesis needs to be established.

STRESS ULCERS

Superficial mucosal damage (petechiae and erosions) is found in most patients hours after major operation, such as cardiopulmonary bypass, or within 24 hours of the onset of major multisystem illness, such as hypotension, sepsis, or severe respiratory failure. However, this damage remains silent in the large majority of these patients. This superficial damage rarely results in clinically significant acute bleeding unless complicated by severe coagulopathy. Experience indicates that major bleeding in the setting of severe and prolonged physiologic stress occurs with discrete ulcers rather than with superficial mucosal lesions. Mechanical ventilation for more than 5 days and coagulopathy are the clearest predictors of major hemorrhage. Prolonged hospitalizations with serious multisystem disease, sepsis, and poor nutrition are probably also important predictors of stress ulcer risk. Ulcer complications have become much less frequent with improved management of seriously ill patients. No association with HP has been established.

Cover TL, Blaser MJ: *Helicobacter pylori* and gastroduodenal disease. Annu Rev Med 43:135, 1992. *Review of HP and pathogenesis.*

Graham DY: I. *Helicobacter pylori:* Its epidemiology and its role in duodenal ulcer disease. J Gastroenterol Hepatol 6:97, 1991. *Outlines pathogenesis and epidemiology of HP in relation to gastritis and peptic ulcer.*

Hentschel E, Brandstatter G, Dragosics B, et al.: Effect of a bismuth-free antibiotic regimen on eradication of *Helicobacter pylori* and duodenal ulcer relapse. N Engl J Med 328:308,1993. *The definitive double-blinded, controlled study of the effects of HP eradication on peptic ulcer recurrence, thereby providing the key indirect evidence establishing a causal role for HP in peptic ulcer.*

Lohr JM, Nelson JA, Oldstone MBA: Is herpes simplex virus associated with peptic ulcer disease? J Virol 64:2168, 1990. *Provides solid evidence linking HSV-1 infection with peptic ulcer in immunologically competent hosts.*

Soll AH: Gastric, duodenal, and stress ulcer. *In* Sleisenger M, Fordtran J (eds.): Gastrointestinal Disease. 5th ed. Philadelphia, WB Saunders, 1993, p 580. *Detailed reference for peptic ulcer pathogenesis and therapy.*

99.2 Epidemiology, Clinical Manifestations, and Diagnosis

Jon I. Isenberg and Andrew H. Soll

EPIDEMIOLOGY

THE PROBLEM. Peptic ulcer diseases (gastric and duodenal ulcer) represent serious medical problems largely due to their frequency and high economic costs. Each year in the United States there are approximately 500,000 new cases and 4 million recurrences with direct costs (physician visits, hospitalizations, medications) that are estimated at approximately $10 billion and equivalent indirect costs (time lost from work). The annual mortality rate due to ulcer disease is low ($< 15,000$), and deaths are due in large part to ulcer complications (see Ch. 99.5). Peptic ulcer diseases unrelated to taking nonsteroidal anti-inflammatory drugs (NSAID's) are

chronic, with a high recurrence rate (approximately 60 to 90% per year). In patients with NSAID-induced ulcer disease, recurrences are substantially diminished in those who can discontinue NSAID intake.

Two major recent observations that affect the epidemiology of ulcer diseases are (1) the association between chronic active antral gastritis secondary to *Helicobacter pylori* (HP) infection and ulcer disease (see Ch. 99.5) and (2) the association between NSAID's and gastrointestinal mucosal injury resulting in gastric and/or duodenal ulcer. HP affects the vast majority of patients, whereas NSAID's tend to be most common in elderly patients with degenerative joint diseases.

INCIDENCE, PREVALENCE, AND RISK RATIOS. In contrast to a disease such as cerebrovascular accidents (stroke), the diagnosis of ulcer disease is less precise, based only upon symptoms and physical examination (see below), and endoscopic surveys of large random US populations have not been conducted. However, time trends observed by separate groups in different populations reveal distinct and similar patterns. Also, ulcer complications (see Ch. 99.5; hemorrhage and perforation) require hospitalization and thereby their frequency can be assessed with greater accuracy.

Prior to 1900, gastric ulcer (GU) was considerably more common than duodenal ulcer (DU). At about the turn of the century, the incidence of DU began to increase, reaching a peak in about the 1950's, and then progressively decreased (Fig. 99–1). The reason for the greater prevalence of DU in the cohort born during the latter decades of the last century and first decade of this century is not fully understood. It was attributed to the urbanization of society and associated factors (e.g., cigarette smoking, stress). However, with the recognition of the role of HP in the pathogenesis of DU (see Ch. 98 and 99.1), the increased incidence of DU in those born near the turn of the century may have been secondary to poor sanitation associated with an increased HP infection rate.

The overall lifetime prevalence for peptic ulcer (combined GU and DU) is approximately 12% in males and about 9% in females; the 1-year "point prevalence" (percentage of the population with ulcer) in the United States is about 1.8%. Thus, assuming about 250 million adults in the United States, about 4.5 million suffer from ulcer disease each year; approximately 10% are new cases and 90% are ulcer recurrences. In the mid-1950's the male:female ratio for deaths due to DU was 5:1, but this ratio has decreased to about 1.3:1. The change in DU male:female ratio is due largely to a decrease in males, with little change in females. The explanation for the decreased frequency in males is not known. GU tends to occur with equal frequency in males and females. Hospitalization rates, physician visits, and surgery for ulcer disease also decreased from the mid-1970's to 1985. Age of onset for DU is most commonly between 25 and 55, whereas GU is most frequent between ages 40 and 70.

Risk, or odds, ratios have recently been applied to some of the factors involved in ulcer disease. Risk ratios estimate the risk of ulcer disease developing in those with a specific factor(s) versus a similar population free of this specific variable. Daily use of NSAID's significantly increases the risk of ulcer disease (risk ratio, RR = 10- to 20-fold), attributed to suppression of prostaglandin synthesis, whereas HP increases the risk of developing ulcer disease about five- to sevenfold, likely secondary to the release of chemotactic factors that activate and attract neutrophils, alter microvascular function, and cause tissue injury that results in chronic active gastritis in all and in ulcer disease in about 10 to 20% of infected subjects (see Ch. 99.1). Cigarette smoking increases the risk of ulcer disease about twofold.

GENETICS. Genetic factors play a role in the pathogenesis of ulcer disease. For example, in monozygotic twins in whom one twin develops ulcer, the concordant twin has about a 50% chance of ulcer. Also, first-degree relatives of ulcer patients have about a threefold greater chance of developing ulcer. Both DU and GU run independently in families. DU families have a greater risk of DU; the same applies to GU families. It is possible that members of these "genetic" families with ulcer may instead have had early infection with HP. This question requires additional study. If genetic factors do play a role in ulcer disease, they are likely polygenic, involving several genes acting in concert with environmental and pathophysiologic factors. Rare genetic syndromes associated with

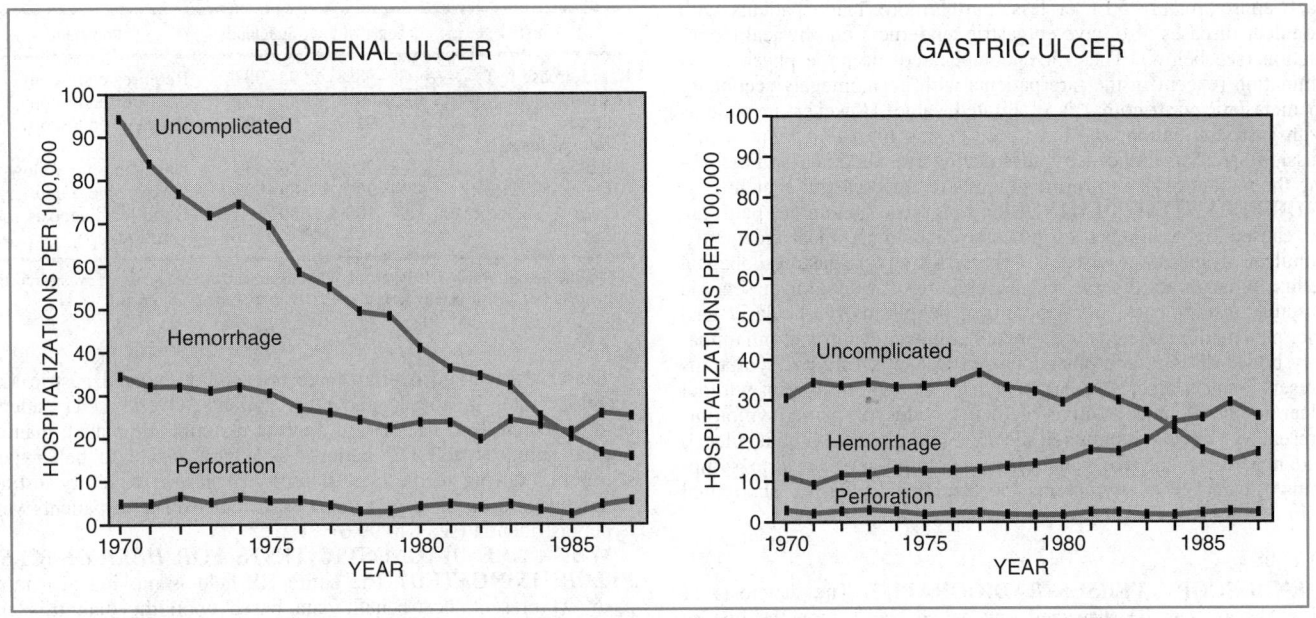

FIGURE 99-1. Hospitalization rates (100,000 population per year) for duodenal ulcer *(left panel)* and gastric ulcer *(right panel)*. There has been a marked decrease in hospitalization of uncomplicated DU since 1970. Of note is the increase in hospitalization for GU hemorrhage that is attributed to the increased intake of NSAID's. (From Kurata JH: Epidemiology of peptic ulcer disease. *In* Swabb EA, Szabo S [eds.]: Ulcer Disease: Investigation and Basis for Therapy. New York, Marcel Dekker, 1991, p 31.)

DU include multiple endocrine neoplasia type 1 (MEN 1), gastrin-secreting pancreatic tumor associated with another endocrine tumor (e.g., hyperparathyroidism), and systemic mastocytosis (increased circulating levels of histamine).

CLINICAL MANIFESTATIONS

ABDOMINAL PAIN. Classically, pain due to ulcer disease was considered likely when the pain was epigastric in location, burning in quality, occurred 1 to 3 hours after meals and at night, was relieved by antacids and/or meals, and tended to wax and wane over months. Furthermore, it was assumed that most patients with ulcer disease had epigastric abdominal pain. However, with the ready availability of upper gastrointestinal endoscopy, which permits an accurate diagnosis of ulcer, it is now recognized that the majority of patients (approximately 70%) with epigastric distress ("dyspepsia") do not have evidence of active ulcer disease; conversely up to 40% of patients with an active ulcer crater deny abdominal pain (Table 99–4). In addition, it is not uncommon for patients to present with an ulcer-related complication, particularly hemorrhage in chronic NSAID users, in the absence of antecedent symptoms. Thus, the presence of a history of epigastric abdominal pain, particularly after meals and at night, suggests the possibility of ulcer disease but is both insensitive and nonspecific.

The dissociation between organic pathology and symptoms highlights the marked individual variation in visceral sensitivity. Those with high visceral sensitivity may have one or more manifestations of functional bowel disease (see Ch. 92).

Clinical evaluation attempts to tease out patterns indicative of the four common functional manifestations of the "irritable" gut: (1) gastroesophageal reflux (including upright and supine reflux and noncardiac chest pain); (2) acid dyspepsia; (3) "dysgastria" (functional dyspepsia = symptoms of indigestion occurring with or shortly after eating and characterized by epigastric fullness and discomfort, belching, bloating, nausea, early satiety, and specific food intolerances); and (4) the irritable bowel syndrome (IBS) (see Ch. 101). Dysgastria can be associated with gastric dyskinesia (gastroparesis, slow gastric emptying) or with gastric dysesthesia (hypersensitivity to gastric distention or specific foods). Delayed gastric emptying can be secondary to diabetic neuropathy, drugs, or connective tissue diseases, although it is most commonly part of the spectrum of functional bowel disorders.

Although emphasis is usually placed on separating organic disease from "functional" disorders, the presentation of organic disease is based upon the level of visceral sensation. When visceral sensation is low, organic disease, such as peptic ulcer, may present "silently," even with life-threatening complications. If visceral sensation is high, the presentation may be confounded by the other functional manifestations such as functional bowel disease. For example, about one half of the patients evaluated for peptic ulcer also have symptoms indicative of gastroesophageal reflux, functional dyspepsia, or IBS, suggesting the presence of an "irritable gut." Somatic hyperalgesia may also be a confounding factor of peptic ulcer. Patients who have undergone surgery for "intractable" ulcer disease have a high recurrence of ulcer-type symptoms in the absence of recurrent ulcer, suggesting that the symptoms represent other manifestations of visceral hyperalgesia. The advantage of endoscopy, the ability to cure HP infection, and rapid ulcer healing with potent antiulcer therapy is that symptoms due to an active crater can be separated from symptoms due to other causes, thereby permitting appropriate clinical decisions.

PHYSICAL EXAMINATION. Physical examination is also of limited value in patients with uncomplicated ulcer. Epigastric tenderness on deep palpation has been suggested as a finding of active ulcer disease. However, when assessed in patients with dyspepsia prior to undergoing endoscopy, the sensitivity, specificity, and positive and negative predictive values of epigastric tenderness were

TABLE 99–4. DIAGNOSIS OF ULCER DISEASE BY SYMPTOMS ALONE IS IMPRECISE

Symptom	Prevalence (%)		
	Duodenal Ulcer	*Gastric Ulcer*	*Nonulcer Dyspepsia*
Epigastric pain	~70	~70	~70
Nocturnal pain	50–80	30–45	25–35
Food causes pain relief	20–65	5–50	5–30
Episodic pain	50–60	10–20	30–40
Belching/bloating	30–65	30–70	40–80

Ulcers occur without symptoms (10–40%), and ulcer symptoms occur without ulcer (30–60%).

Modified from Isenberg JI, Walsh JH, Johnson LR: Peptic Ulcer Diseases. AGA Undergraduate Teaching Project—Unit 23. Timonium, MD, Milner-Fenwick, Inc., 1991.

each approximately 50% or less. Furthermore, many patients with nonulcer diseases also have epigastric tenderness on physical examination (see below). Thus, in uncomplicated ulcer the physical examination (except in the rare patients with hepatomegaly secondary to metastatic gastrinoma) is of limited value. However, in patients with gastric retention who have been fasting for a few hours, a succussion splash (produced by auscultating the abdomen while rocking the patient back and forth) suggests retained gastric contents.

DIFFERENTIAL DIAGNOSIS. Epigastric abdominal pain can be caused by a number of processes including, most frequently, nonulcer dyspepsia ("visceral hypersensitivity"), gastroesophageal reflux, biliary tract disease, pancreatitis, coronary and/or mesenteric vascular insufficiency, intra-abdominal neoplasms (particularly gastric, pancreatic, and hepatic), functional bowel syndrome, inflammatory bowel disease, and others. Therefore, the sensitivity (symptoms present + ulcer/ulcer disease), specificity (symptoms absent without ulcer/no ulcer), and positive predictive value of pain ([symptoms present + ulcer]/[symptoms + ulcer] + [symptoms without ulcer]) and negative predictive value ([no symptoms, no ulcer]/[no symptoms + ulcer] + [no symptoms, no ulcer]) of epigastric abdominal pain as a marker for ulcer disease are low.

DIAGNOSIS

ENDOSCOPY VERSUS RADIOGRAPHY. The diagnosis of ulcer disease can be suspected only when based upon the history and physical examination. Diagnostic confirmation requires either upper gastrointestinal endoscopy or radiography. Current endoscopic instruments contain a wide-angle TV chip that permits careful examination of the esophagus, stomach, and duodenum, as well as directed biopsies and photographic documentation (see color plate 1C). Overall, endoscopy has a greater accuracy of establishing the diagnosis than does non–air contrast radiography but has approximately a three- to fourfold greater cost. Furthermore, endoscopy has a modest risk of untoward events (<1 in 1000 procedures). In centers with highly skilled radiologists, air-contrast radiography is reported to be as accurate as endoscopy. There is no justification for routinely using one procedure followed by the other. However, there are instances when a lesion observed on radiography (e.g., GU) requires endoscopic biopsies to ensure that it is nonmalignant.

DU's are always benign and therefore do not require biopsies or repeat endoscopy to ensure healing. However, ulcerating lesions within the stomach may be due to gastric cancer. Therefore, under almost all circumstances it is imperative to obtain multiple biopsies of GU's as well to ensure their complete endoscopic healing after 8 to 12 weeks of medical treatment. The only exceptions to performing repeated endoscopy to ensure complete GU healing are young GU patients with a history of regular NSAID intake and a benign (both in appearance and by biopsy) ulcer.

IS A PRECISE DIAGNOSIS OF ULCER REQUIRED? One of the major tenets of medicine has been to establish a precise diagnosis and thereby apply the appropriate and specific therapy. This principle has come into question as applied to ulcer disease. Most patients with dyspepsia who undergo endoscopy do not have active ulcer disease but instead have either "nonulcer dyspepsia" or evidence of esophagitis, gastritis, or duodenitis. In 1985, a policy statement by the American College of Physicians recommended that patients with uncomplicated dyspepsia be treated with antiulcer medications (e.g., histamine H_2-receptor antagonists). Further evaluation was recommended only in patients unresponsive to an empiric trial of medical therapy. This approach is appropriate in those under age 40 with mild, intermittent symptoms and in the absence of ulcer-related complications. However, in those requiring NSAID's on a regular basis, those older than 50, or those with persistent or systemic symptoms (e.g., anorexia, weight loss, back pain) the diagnosis should be established, usually by endoscopy. This not only permits the endoscopic diagnosis of the process but also provides an opportunity to obtain biopsies of the lesion for the presence of HP.

MEASURING SERUM GASTRIN AND GASTRIC SECRETORY TESTING. Determination of fasting and secretin-stimulated serum gastrin is indicated in those patients with intractable ulcer disease, those who will undergo elective DU surgery, and those in whom a diagnosis of Zollinger-Ellison (gastrinoma) syndrome is a consideration (see Ch. 99.6).

TABLE 99–5. DIAGNOSTIC TESTS FOR HELICOBACTER PYLORI

Test	Sensitivity	Specificity	Comments
Rapid urease test	89–98%	93–98%	Requires endoscopy
Histology	93–99%	95–99%	Requires endoscopy
Culture	77–92%	97–100%	Requires endoscopy
Serologic tests			
ELISA	88–99%	86–95%	Unsuitable for follow-up
Quick office test	94–96%	88–95%	Inexpensive, rapid
^{14}C- or ^{14}C-urea breath test	90–100%	89–100%	Good for diagnosis and follow-up

Modified from Walsh JH, Peterson WL: Treatment of *Helicobacter pylori* infection in the management of peptic ulcer diseases. N Engl J Med—in press.

There is a marked overlap in resting and stimulated gastric acid secretory rates in normal and ulcer patients. Overall, GU patients tend to secrete less gastric acid, both at rest and stimulated, than do normal subjects; and DU patients as a group tend to be "hypersecretors." Owing to the lack of utility of gastric secretory testing, it has become obsolete as a diagnostic tool except in patients with hypergastrinemia (see Ch. 99.6).

WHEN ARE DIAGNOSTIC TESTS FOR *HELICOBACTER PYLORI* INDICATED? The entire HP field is moving at a rapid pace. At present, cost-benefit data based upon the diagnosis and routine treatment of HP in all patients with dyspepsia, the major presenting symptom of ulcer, or ulcer disease are unavailable. Because HP produces urease, its presence can be determined by breath tests (^{14}C- or ^{13}C-urea), by gastric mucosal biopsies (Rapid Urease Test, CLOtest), or by histologic identification of the microorganism or culture. Because HP induces immunologic responses, it can also be diagnosed by ELISA or a rapid serologic test. However, at present these latter methods cannot be used with accuracy to determine HP eradication (Table 99–5).

HP TESTING IN ULCER PATIENTS. A recent NIH Consensus Conference on HP concluded that only those ulcer patients (DU and/or GU) in whom HP has been diagnosed by one of the sensitive and specific tests should be treated to eradicate the microorganism. Such a policy mandates that all ulcer patients undergo HP testing. Because approximately 90% of patients with DU harbor HP, an argument could be made for not routinely performing HP testing in uncomplicated DU patients and instead empirically prescribing anti-HP therapy. However, drug costs plus adverse effects need to be balanced with the costs of determining HP status and ultimate clinical outcomes. Approximately 70% of GU patients are infected with HP, and NSAID's are incriminated as causative in the remainder. As endoscopy is performed in almost all GU patients because of the potential for gastric cancer, it is appropriate to determine the HP status at the time of endoscopy. Those who harbor HP, even those with a history of NSAID intake, should be treated to eradicate HP (see Ch. 99.3).

HP TESTING IN PATIENTS WITH NONULCER DYSPEPSIA. Controversy, not only regarding pathogenesis but also regarding evaluation and treatment, continues to surround "nonulcer dyspepsia" (i.e., is it a single disease or a manifestation of more than one disease?) Most studies to date indicate that eradicating HP in patients with nonulcer dyspepsia fails to significantly alter dyspeptic symptoms. However, there may be a subgroup of patients with chronic dyspeptic symptoms related to HP infection and chronic active gastritis. Therefore, in those patients unresponsive to routine treatment for nonulcer dyspepsia, testing for HP is reasonable.

Dooley CP, Cohen H: *Helicobacter pylori* infection. Gastroenterol Clin North Am, 22:1, 1993. *A recent issue devoted entirely to Helicobacter pylori from microbiology to treatment.*

Isenberg J, McQuaid KR, Laine L, et al.: Peptic ulcer diseases. *In* Yamada T (ed.): Textbook of Gastroenterology. 2nd ed. Philadelphia, JB Lippincott, 1995. *A recent encyclopedic review of all aspects of peptic ulcer diseases.*

Soll AH: Gastric, duodenal and stress ulcer. *In* Sleisenger MH, Fordtran JS (eds.): Gastrointestinal Disease: Pathophysiology, Diagnosis, Management. 5th ed. Philadelphia, WB Saunders, 1993, p 580. *Encyclopedic review of current knowledge regarding peptic ulcer diseases.*

Talley NJ, Weaver AL, Tesmer DL, et al.: Lack of discriminate value of dyspeptic subgroups in patients referred for upper endoscopy. Gastroenterology 105:1378, 1993. *A careful analysis of dyspeptic subgroups (ulcer-like, dysmotility-like, and reflux-like), indicating the marked overlap between groups and difficulties in therapeutic interventions.*

99.3 Medical Therapy

David Y. Graham

Recently there has been a major change in thinking about peptic ulcers, which has resulted in a reconsideration of the basic concepts of therapy. Until recently, peptic ulcer disease was considered to be a heterogeneous disorder resulting from an imbalance between aggressive factors such as acid and pepsin and protective factors such as mucosal blood flow. Although this concept has not been entirely discarded, acid has been relegated to a supportive role. We now recognize that most peptic ulcers can be assigned to specific causes; the two most common causes are infection with the bacterium *Helicobacter pylori* and use of nonsteroidal anti-inflammatory drugs (NSAID's). *H. pylori* infection is the more common cause, accounting for >90% of duodenal ulcers and for 60 to 90% of gastric ulcers. NSAID use makes up the bulk of the remainder, with pathologic hypersecretory diseases such as the Zollinger-Ellison syndrome (see Ch. 99.6) and even less common causes accounting for <1%.

Knowledge that peptic ulcer disease could be categorized by causation led to a reappraisal of the approach to therapy. Most traditional therapies centered on reducing aggressive factors such as gastric acid. They resulted in rapid reduction or resolution of symptoms and were also effective in acceleration of ulcer healing. However, they did not change the natural history of peptic ulcer because ulcers recurred soon after therapy was discontinued. Recurrence could be delayed or reduced by continuing antisecretory therapy indefinitely; this practice also reduced the frequency of ulcer complications such as bleeding. Current practice is to tailor therapy to the underlying cause of the disease. We now ask, "What is the cause?" and then, "What is the therapy?"

DETERMINING THE CAUSE

Clues suggesting various causes of ulcer are shown in Table 99–6. A variety of methods are available to determine whether an *H. pylori* infection is present, ranging from those that require tissue obtained at endoscopy to serologic tests and simple urea breath tests. Because *H. pylori* infection is lifelong, detecting the presence of IgG antibodies against *H. pylori* is the simplest and least expensive method. Urea breath tests based on the very active *H. pylori* urease are particularly useful in assessing the results of antimicrobial therapy. If an ulcer is diagnosed at endoscopy, biopsy of normal-appearing gastric mucosa provides definitive proof of *H. pylori* infection, because histologically normal mucosa excludes the infection. Some NSAID users also have *H. pylori* infection and then it becomes impossible to distinguish the cause. Gastric ulcers still remain a special challenge, as 1 to 5% of endoscopically benign gastric ulcers are gastric cancers. Endoscopy still has a major role to play in excluding cancer in gastric ulcer patients and can be used to assess *H. pylori* status (Table 99–7).

ULCER THERAPY

The goals of ulcer therapy are to relieve symptoms, to heal the ulcer, and to cure the disease (*H. pylori* ulcers) or prevent recurrence (NSAID ulcers). A number of strategies are available to heal

TABLE 99–6. CLUES SUGGESTIVE OF SPECIFIC CAUSES OF PEPTIC ULCER

	Helicobacter pylori	NSAID	Zollinger-Ellison Syndrome
One or more			
Serology	Positive	Negative	Negative
Urea breath test	Positive	Negative	Negative
Histology	Positive	Negative	Negative
NSAID use			
History	Absent	Positive	Absent
Elevated serum salicylate	Absent	Positive	Absent
Unusual location	Absent	Absent	Present
Severe esophagitis	Absent	Absent	Present
Diarrhea	Absent	Absent	Present

TABLE 99–7. FACTORS INFLUENCING THE DECISION FOR EARLY AND FOR DELAYED ENDOSCOPY IN GASTRIC ULCER DISEASE

Early Endoscopy	Delayed Endoscopy
Advanced age	Young patient
Long history	Short history
Weight loss	No weight change
Anorexia	Normal appetite
Upper gastrointestinal (UGI) bleeding/anemia	Normal blood count
Significant vomiting	No vomiting
No ulcerogenic drugs	NSAID use and positive *H. pylori* serology
Equivocal UGI series	Unequivocal UGI series

ulcers, varying from antacids that directly neutralize acid to antisecretory agents such as receptor antagonists, prostaglandins, anticholinergics, and proton pump inhibitors, and surface active agents such as sucralfate.

ANTISECRETORY DRUGS. Antacids were the mainstay of therapy until the H_2-receptor antagonists were introduced (Fig. 99–2). Antacids are still useful, as they are available without prescription and provide rapid pain relief. Nevertheless, they are outmoded as primary therapy. Antisecretory therapy accelerates healing of ulcers regardless of cause. The H_2-receptor antagonists available in the United States include cimetidine (Tagamet), ranitidine (Zantac), famotidine (Pepcid), and nizatidine (Axid). The main difference is potency, not effectiveness. The trend has been toward full-dose therapy administered with or after the evening meal. Administered in this way, clinically equivalent doses are 800 mg of cimetidine, 300 mg of ranitidine or nizatidine, and 20 mg of famotidine. (Because the patent on cimetidine has expired, it may be the least expensive.) H_2-receptor antagonists as a class have been remarkably free of side effects and are among the safest drugs ever introduced. Cimetidine is associated with prolongation of the metabolism of warfarin, theophylline, and phenytoin, and the dosage of those drugs may have to be adjusted if they are administered with cimetidine.

Misoprostol is the only synthetic prostaglandin available in the United States. It is a relatively weak antisecretory drug; 200 μg of misoprostol is slightly less potent as an antisecretory drug than 300 mg of cimetidine. Although misoprostol is not a first-line therapy for treating peptic ulcers, it is the only drug that prevents both gastric and duodenal ulcers in NSAID users.

Although a number of anticholinergic agents are available, their ability to reduce acid secretion is poor and the frequency of side effects is high. Anticholinergic agents are also outmoded for ulcer therapy.

Acid-pump inhibitors are the most effective antisecretory agents available, as these agents block the H^+-K^+-ATPase responsible for

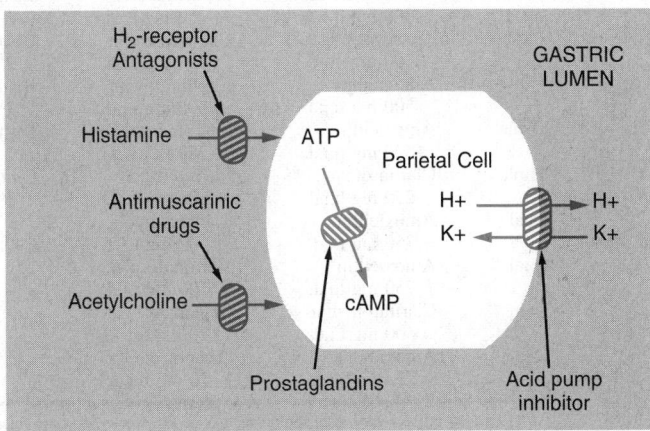

FIGURE 99–2. Sites of action of four drugs employed to inhibit acid secretion.

acid secretion. Despite the increased antisecretory activity, 20 mg of omeprazole is only slightly more effective than 300 mg of ranitidine when measured in terms of percentage of patients with healed duodenal ulcers after 4 weeks of therapy. Because the percentage of patients with healed ulcers is cumulative, this advantage is lost when healing percentage after 8 or 12 weeks is evaluated. Higher doses of acid-pump inhibitors lead to even more rapid ulcer healing, making them especially useful for "problem" cases. The main disadvantages of the acid-pump inhibitors are high cost and lack of a long history of usage. Early concerns about enterochromaffin cell–like hyperplasia resulting from long-term acid suppression appear to have been unfounded.

TOPICALLY ACTIVE AGENTS. Sucralfate is the aluminum hydroxide salt of sulfated sucrose. The mechanism of action is thought to be related to its ability to form a protective coat over the ulcer. Healing rates and time to pain relief with sucralfate are generally better than with H$_2$-receptor antagonists. Sucralfate must be given in multiple dosages per day and is probably another outmoded drug. In Europe and other countries outside the United States, bismuth subcitrate is available, usually in the colloidal form as DeNol. This drug also coats ulcers and in addition is an effective *H. pylori* antimicrobial.

ANTIMICROBIAL THERAPY. *H. pylori* is a gram-negative spiral bacterium that is sensitive *in vitro* to a variety of antimicrobials. Although *in vivo H. pylori* infection proved difficult to cure, a number of effective regimens are now available (Table 99–8). The best results have been obtained with combination therapies called triple therapy. The one with the highest success is a combination of bismuth subsalicylate (two Pepto-Bismol tablets four times a day, with each meal and at bedtime); tetracycline HCl (500 mg four times a day, with meals and at bedtime); and metronidazole (250 mg three times a day, with meals). Variations include substitution of amoxicillin (500 mg) for tetracycline and clarithromycin (500 mg) for metronidazole. Other effective therapies include dual therapies of amoxicillin (750 mg) and metronidazole (500 mg) or clarithromycin (500 mg) three times a day. Therapy is continued for 2 weeks and can be combined with or given after antisecretory therapy. The acid-pump inhibitors have a potential benefit over H$_2$-receptor antagonists in that they more effectively control pH and may also have some anti–*H. pylori* activity. Typically, antibiotics are more effective as the pH approaches 7.4. A number of studies of the combination of omeprazole and amoxicillin or omeprazole and clarithromycin have been done with varying results. Neither regimen has consistently achieved cure rates >80%, and they are possibly inferior to protocols using a second antimicrobial. The omeprazole/amoxicillin protocols with better success call for twice-a-day omeprazole and 2 or more grams of amoxicillin. Success as measured by cure of the *H. pylori* infection cannot reliably be determined until 4 or more weeks after the end of antimicrobial therapy.

Treating the Patient with an Ulcer and *H. pylori* Infection

The goals are to relieve symptoms, heal the mucosal defect, and cure the disease. To heal the ulcer, patients should receive full-dose antisecretory therapy once or twice a day. Cost and convenience are the major factors in deciding which H$_2$-receptor antagonist to use or whether to prescribe an acid-pump inhibitor. In general, because of the marginal benefit obtained with 20 mg of omeprazole compared with full-dose H$_2$-receptor antagonists, omeprazole is not recommended as first-line therapy. Now that we have a better understanding of the causes of ulcer, the simplest approach is to combine antisecretory therapy and give triple antimicrobial therapy for the first 2 weeks of therapy. Antisecretory therapy is then continued for 6 to 8 weeks and the effectiveness of the antimicrobial therapy is assessed (4 to 6 weeks after ending antimicrobial therapy).

Results of antimicrobial therapy can be assessed by urea breath test or by endoscopy with histologic examination of mucosal biopsies. Alternatively, one could wait to ascertain whether the ulcer recurred; although this may be acceptable for patients with truly mild peptic ulcer disease, it is not recommended. The titers of anti–*H. pylori* IgG fall after successful therapy, but the decline is slow, and effectiveness by this method cannot be reliably determined for 6 months to 1 year after therapy ends. The easiest noninvasive approach is to obtain both serology and a breath test at the outset and assess effectiveness with a urea breath test.

NSAID ULCER

The available data suggest and our own experience is that continued NSAID use delays ulcer healing. The steps are therefore to stop the NSAID and use traditional antisecretory therapy to heal the ulcer. Patients who are NSAID users and are also infected with *H. pylori* should also receive therapy for *H. pylori* infection. Many elderly patients with osteoarthritis receive potent anti-inflammatory drugs when they actually require only analgesia. Stopping the NSAID is a form of reverse therapeutic challenge that allows one to assess whether the NSAID was actually needed. In many instances the patient does just as well using acetaminophen or low doses of less potent over-the-counter NSAID's, such as 200 mg of ibuprofen or 220 mg of naproxen sodium. For patients with rheumatoid arthritis (see Ch. 237) who require active anti-inflammatory therapy, prednisone (5 to 10 mg daily) can be given without apparent adverse affect on ulcer healing. After ulcer healing, anti-inflammatory therapy can be restarted with misoprostol therapy.

Preventing Ulcer Recurrence

With cure of *H. pylori* infection, *H. pylori* ulcers are cured, and maintenance anti-secretory therapy is not needed. For patients with resistant infections, antisecretory therapy can be continued at ap-

TABLE 99–8. ANTIMICROBIAL THERAPIES FOR TREATMENT OF *H. PYLORI* INFECTION

Therapy	Hp Drug 1	Hp Drug 2	Hp Drug 3	Notes*	Success
Triple	Tetracycline HCl 500 mg q.i.d.	Metronidazole 250 mg t.i.d.	Bismuth subsalicylate† 2 tablets q.i.d.	With meals for 14 days plus an antisecretory drug	>90%
Triple	Tetracycline HCl 500 mg q.i.d.	Clarithromycin 500 mg t.i.d.	Bismuth subsalicylate 2 tablets q.i.d.	With meals for 14 days plus an antisecretory drug	>90%
Triple	Amoxicillin 500 mg q.i.d.	Clarithromycin 500 mg t.i.d.	Bismuth subsalicylate 2 tablets q.i.d.	With meals for 14 days plus an antisecretory drug	>90%
Triple	Amoxicillin 500 mg q.i.d.	Metronidazole 250 t.i.d.	Bismuth subsalicylate 2 tablets q.i.d.	With meals for 14 days plus an antisecretory drug	>80%
Triple	Clarithromycin 250 mg b.i.d.	Metronidazole 500 mg b.i.d.	Omeprazole 20 mg. b.i.d.	For 7 to 14 days	>90%
Dual	Amoxicillin 750 mg t.i.d.	Clarithromycin 500 mg t.i.d.		With meals for 14 days plus an antisecretory drug	>90%
Dual	Amoxicillin 750 mg t.i.d.	Metronidazole 500 mg t.i.d.		With meals for 14 days plus an antisecretory drug	>85%
Dual	Clarithromycin 500 mg t.i.d.	Omeprazole 40 mg q.A.M.		With meals for 14 days	70–80%
Dual‡	Amoxicillin 1 gram b.i.d.	Omeprazole 20 mg b.i.d.		With meals for 14 days	35–60%‡

* Generally antisecretory drug should be taken for 6 weeks to ensure ulcer healing.
† Bismuth subcitrate can be substituted.
‡ This outcome is based on author's impression and estimates based on review of the available data as well as on the results of clinical trials. This particular combination at these lower dosages is not recommended.

proximately half the healing dose. This reduces ulcer recurrence and prevents ulcer complications. Patients who have experienced NSAID ulcers and require continued NSAID therapy should also receive therapy with misoprostol, 200 μg either twice a day or four times a day.

Special Situations

Patients with a history of ulcer complications such as bleeding have a high probability of having another complication. It is important, therefore, not to discontinue antisecretory therapy until one is confident that *H. pylori* infection has been cured. In cases of very large ulcers, especially those that have recently bled, ulcers developing after balloon dilatation of gastric outlet obstruction, or ulcers in very old frail individuals with major comorbid disease, the considerations concerning cost may be outweighed by the potential increased effectiveness obtained with acid-pump inhibitors. For these patients an acid-pump inhibitor is recommended—for example, omeprazole 40 to 60 mg per day, in divided doses.

Graham DY: The relationship between nonsteroidal anti-inflammatory drug use and peptic ulcer disease. Gastroenterol Clin North Am 19:171, 1990. *Review of the relationship between NSAID use and peptic ulcer disease.*

Graham DY: Treatment of peptic ulcers caused by *Helicobacter pylori*. N Engl J Med 328:349, 1993. *Editorial defining the place of anti–*Helicobacter *therapy in the management of peptic ulcer disease.*

Graham DY, Lew GM, Klein PD, et al.: Effect of treatment of *Helicobacter pylori* infection on the long-term recurrence of gastric or duodenal ulcer. A randomized, controlled study. Ann Intern Med 116:705, 1992. *Results of randomized comparison of follow-up of ulcers after healing with ranitidine compared with ranitidine plus triple therapy. Eradication of* H. pylori *infection resulted in cure of duodenal and gastric ulcers. Also gives data on the effectiveness of this therapy for resistant ulcers.*

Penston JG, Wormsley KG: Review article: Maintenance treatment with H$_2$-receptor antagonists for peptic ulcer disease. Aliment Pharmacol Ther 6:3, 1992. *An extensive personal experience involving maintenance therapy; provides data on relapse rates and complications resulting from maintenance therapy with H$_2$-receptor antagonists.*

Soll AH: Gastric, duodenal, and stress ulcer. *In* Sleisenger M, Fordtran J (eds.): Gastrointestinal Disease. 5th ed. Philadelphia, WB Saunders, 1993, p 580. *Outstanding overview of peptic ulcer disease, including pathogenesis and therapy.*

Tytgat GNJ, Lee A, Graham DY, et al.: The role of infectious agents in peptic ulcer disease. Gastroenterol Int 6:76, 1993. *Excellent overview of the data concerning* H. pylori *and its therapy.*

Van Deventer GM, Elashoff JD, Reedy TJ, et al.: A randomized study of maintenance therapy with ranitidine to prevent the recurrence of duodenal ulcer. N Engl J Med 320:1113, 1989. *Excellent study of the benefits of maintenance therapy, especially for those with complicated ulcer disease.*

99.4 Surgical Therapy
Haile T. Debas and Susan L. Orloff

INDICATIONS

The advent of powerful antiulcer drugs (e.g., H$_2$-receptor antagonists, omeprazole) has made elective surgery for peptic ulcer a rare event. The need for surgery may be further decreased with the greater understanding of the role and treatment outcome of *Helicobacter pylori*. Despite the sharp decline in elective ulcer surgery, neither the incidence of nor the need for surgery for the emergent complications of ulcer (perforation, bleeding, and obstruction) has changed significantly over the past 15 years. The major cause of decline in elective ulcer surgery is that the condition in fewer and fewer patients is truly intractable to medical therapy. In patients who have "cimetidine-resistant" ulcers and have had a history of prior complications (bleeding, perforation) or have a "giant" (>2 cm diameter) ulcer, it is advisable to perform gastric acid secretory studies while the patient is on drug therapy. Even in this group of "blocker-resistant" ulcers, most ulcers could be healed safely and with minimal side effects with omeprazole, the potent proton-pump inhibitor.

A patient clearly needs surgery when presenting with acute peritonitis due to a perforated peptic ulcer. In the patient with equivocal peritoneal signs, some have advocated examination of the upper gastrointestinal tract with a water-soluble contrast medium. These authors advocate conservative management if the perforation is sealed but an operative approach under other circumstances. The patient who presents 48 or more hours after a perforation is a special problem. Here conservative management is indicated provided that the perforation is sealed and the patient is not septic.

TABLE 99–9. INDICATIONS FOR EMERGENT/URGENT OPERATIONS IN PEPTIC ULCER DISEASE

1. Perforation
2. Bleeding
   a. Exsanguinating hemorrhage
   b. Bleeding >6 units of blood
   c. "Visible vessel," especially if bleeding
   d. Rebleeding on medical therapy
   e. Slow, persistent bleeding over days
3. Gastric outlet obstruction

In >90% of patients admitted with bleeding duodenal ulcer, the bleeding stops spontaneously. The clinical situations that require emergent surgical interventions are listed in Table 99–9. The older the patient is, the more life-threatening the bleeding and the sooner a surgical consultation should be obtained.

Gastric outlet obstruction is the least common indication for emergent/urgent surgery. The clinical dilemma is whether the obstruction is due to inflammation and edema or fixed scarring. A period of 8 to 10 days of conservative management with nasogastric suction resolves inflammatory obstruction. Otherwise, operative intervention is required.

OPERATIVE PROCEDURES

Surgery for duodenal ulcer has evolved from simple gastroenterostomy to subtotal gastrectomy, to truncal vagotomy with drainage, and to more selective types of vagotomy. The most common operative procedures currently used are presented in Figure 99–3.

LAPAROSCOPIC ULCER SURGERY

A major recent advancement in the surgical treatment of peptic ulcer disease is videoscopic ulcer surgery using laparoscopy or thoracoscopy. This minimal access surgery has the advantages of less postoperative pain, a shortened hospital stay (1 to 3 days), earlier return to work (7 to 10 days), and no large scar. Table 99–10 lists the procedures that have been successful for treating peptic ulcer.

CHOICE OF OPERATIVE PROCEDURE
Duodenal Ulcer

ELECTIVE SURGERY. The elective procedure of choice for duodenal ulcer is highly selective vagotomy because it has few side effects and a mortality rate that approaches 0%. Although some surgeons in the United States still use truncal vagotomy and drainage, the authors believe that the practice is inappropriate in most patients.

EMERGENT/URGENT SURGERY *Perforation.* The primary goal of surgery is to close the perforation and prevent infection. Recent prospective, randomized clinical studies have shown that routinely adding highly selective vagotomy is associated with no increase in morbidity or mortality but a significant decrease in ulcer recurrence and subsequent need for operation. Highly selective vagotomy should not be performed if (a) the perforation is more than 24 hours old, (b) severe peritoneal contamination exists, and (c) the general condition of the patient is unstable.

TABLE 99–10. LAPAROSCOPIC SURGICAL PROCEDURES

Procedure	Comments
Laparoscopic closure of perforated peptic ulcer	Closure, omental patching, peritoneal toilet
Laparoscopic/thoracoscopic truncal vagotomy and endoscopic balloon dilation at pylorus	Suboptimal procedure
Laparoscopic/thoracoscopic truncal vagotomy with laparoscopic gastrojejunostomy	Adequate procedure
Posterior truncal vagotomy and anterior highly selective vagotomy (HSV) or seromyotomy (Taylor II)	Widely used, adequate results
HSV	Best elective antiulcer procedure

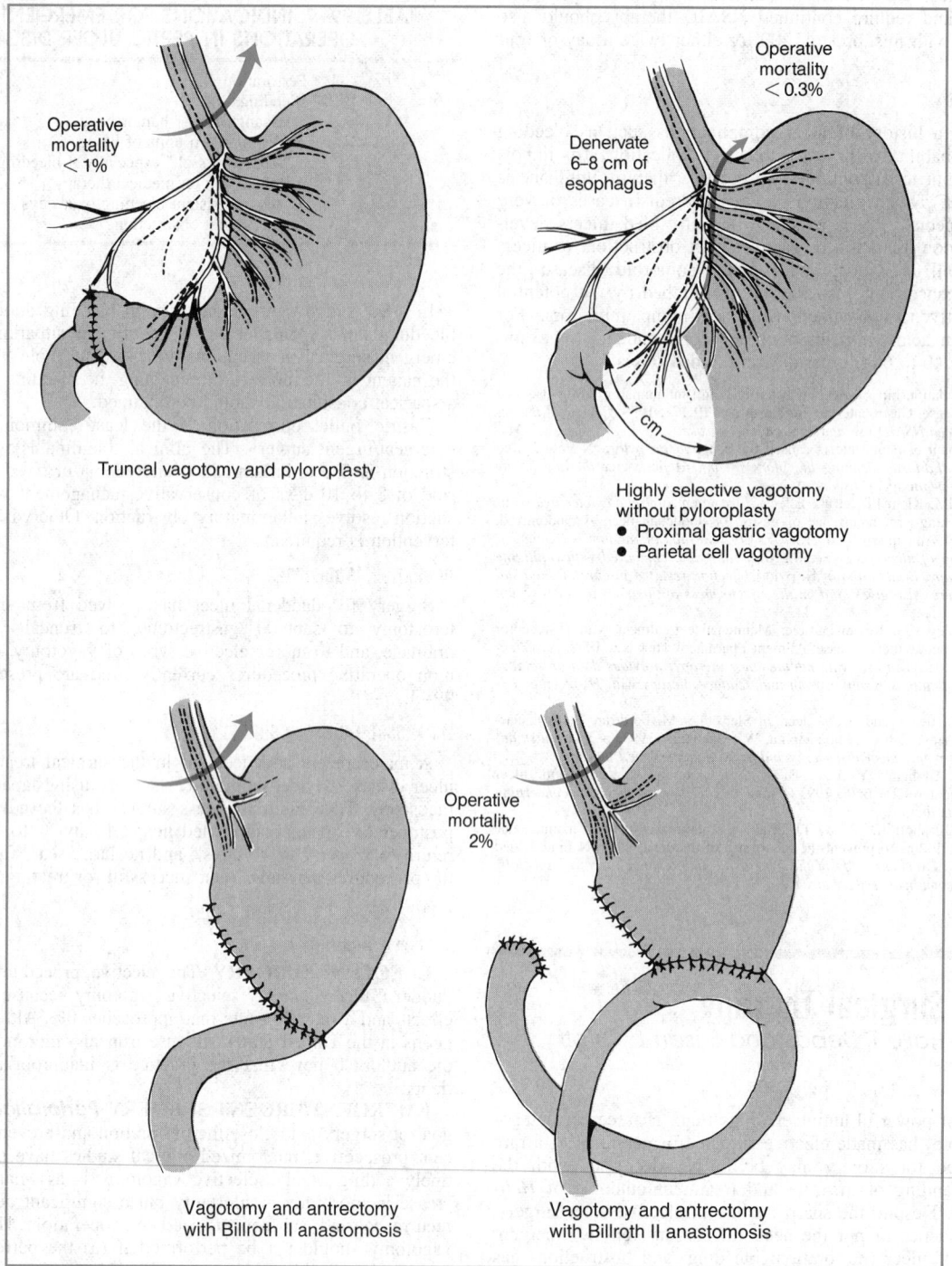

FIGURE 99–3. Model illustrating the most common surgical procedures currently used for peptic ulcer disease.

TABLE 99–11. SURGICAL OPTIONS FOR GASTRIC ULCER

Type	Location	Incidence	Treatment of Choice	Comments
I	Body (lesser curve)	55–60%	Antrectomy (Billroth I)	Ulcer resected with specimen. Mortality/recurrence rate of 2%
II	In association with duodenal ulcer	20–25%	Vagotomy and antrectomy	Acid reduction and ulcer excision accomplished
III	Prepyloric	20%	Vagotomy and antrectomy	Behaves like duodenal ulcer
IV	High-lying near gastro-esophageal junction	<5%	Resection and esophago-gastrojejunostomy (Csendes)	More common in South America

Bleeding. In the emergent operation for bleeding, the preferred procedure is suture control of bleeding and truncal vagotomy and pyloroplasty. However, the authors prefer suture control of bleeding via duodenotomy and highly selective vagotomy, except in the unstable patient.

Obstruction. The operation of choice when a duodenal ulcer has caused gastric outlet obstruction is truncal vagotomy and antrectomy with gastroduodenal anastomosis. This procedure is avoided if the duodenum is involved in an inflammatory mass or is otherwise severely distorted. In such situations, truncal vagotomy and gastrojejunostomy are performed, leaving the duodenum undisturbed.

Gastric Ulcer

ELECTIVE OPERATION. The elective operation depends on the type of gastric ulcer. There are four types of gastric ulcer, and the surgical options for these are given in Table 99–11.

The problem of an ulcerated cancer masquerading as a benign ulcer is more common than a benign gastric ulcer degenerating into a malignant one. With the advent of endoscopy, fewer patients diagnosed as having a benign ulcer have an ulcerated cancer. In the United States, carcinoma has been found in only 3% of resected gastric ulcers.

EMERGENT OPERATION. Bleeding. Bleeding is a more serious complication in gastric ulcers than in duodenal ulcers. The definitive treatment in a stable patient is distal gastrectomy that removes the ulcer and constructs a Billroth I anastomosis. However, the patient's condition may dictate a lesser operation, which may include ulcer excision alone or with vagotomy and pyloroplasty. If the ulcer cannot be excised, bleeding should be controlled by sutures, and biopsy may be done if deemed safe or postponed for subsequent endoscopy.

Perforation. Again the procedure of choice is distal gastrectomy with a Billroth I anastomosis. This operation is not indicated if the perforation is older than 24 hours, if the patient is frail or unstable, or if there is severe peritoneal contamination. In these situations, a lesser procedure may be considered, such as ulcer excision, closure, and vagotomy and pyloroplasty. In extremely ill patients, the ulcer may be patched with omentum after taking a biopsy sample from each quadrant, and no acid-reducing procedure is performed.

Recurrent Ulcer

Ulcers recurring after peptic ulcer surgery depend on both the type of primary ulcer, i.e., duodenal or gastric, and the type of surgical procedure used to treat the primary ulcer. The causes of postoperative ulcer recurrence are listed in Table 99–12. The incidence of ulcer recurrence is 6 to 10% after truncal vagotomy and drainage, 10 to 15% after highly selective vagotomy, and <1% after vagotomy and antrectomy.

The incidence of the Zollinger-Ellison syndrome (ZES) in patients with duodenal ulcer disease is only 1:1000, but rises to 1:50 in patients with postoperative recurrent ulcer. A thorough investigation for ZES is warranted in all patients with recurrent ulcer. The incidence of gastrinoma as a cause of recurrent ulcer could be minimized by measuring plasma gastrin concentration in all duodenal

TABLE 99–12. CAUSES OF POSTOPERATIVE ULCER RECURRENCE

Inappropriate primary operation
   Gastroenterostomy alone
   HSV for gastric and prepyloric ulcer
Inadequate operation
   Incomplete vagotomy
   Inadequate drainage
   Inadequate resection
   Retained antrum
Hypersecretory states
   Gastrinoma
   MEN I syndrome
   G cell hyperplasia
   Hypercalcemia
Ulcerogenic drugs
   Nonsteroidal anti-inflammatory drugs
   Steroids
   Reserpine

ulcer patients preoperatively. In addition, a gastrinoma should be ruled out with a secretin test preoperatively in duodenal ulcer patients with the following clinical features: (a) hypercalcemia or renal stones, (b) diarrhea, (c) multiple ulcers, (d) ulcer in distal duodenum or jejunum, and (e) family history of endocrinopathy, particularly of the multiple endocrine neoplasia (MEN I) syndrome.

The diagnosis of recurrent ulcer is based on recurrence of ulcer pain (95%), hemorrhage or anemia due to occult bleeding (20 to 63%), obstruction (5 to 19%), and free perforation (1 to 9%). Endoscopy is the most useful method of establishing the diagnosis. Once this is done, the cause of recurrence must be identified. If the recurrence has occurred after vagotomy, modified sham feeding is performed to determine completeness of vagotomy. Investigation for the ZES includes measuring plasma gastrin in the fasting state in response to intravenous secretin and after ingesting a meal. Elevated fasting plasma gastrin may result from vagotomy. However, a paradoxical rise in plasma gastrin after secretin is characteristic of ZES and not of postvagotomy hypergastrinemia. On the other hand, plasma gastrin elevation is only modest after a meal in ZES, but exaggerated in G cell hyperplasia that may follow vagotomy or may very rarely be primary. In the retained antrum syndrome, neither secretin nor a meal causes further elevation from the basal level of hypergastrinemia. Technetium pertechnetate radioisotope scan may be used to confirm the presence of retained antrum.

Before the introduction of cimetidine, postoperative recurrent ulcer was considered a surgical disease. However, H_2-receptor antagonists have been shown to be effective in treating recurrent ulcer, particularly after vagotomy. With the increased understanding of the role of *H. pylori* in peptic ulcer disease, indications for surgical treatment of recurrent ulcer will likely be further diminished. In the absence of a surgically treatable cause of the recurrence (retained antrum, gastrinoma), medical treatment should be attempted and surgery considered only if medical therapy fails.

Which type of operative procedure to use depends both on the cause of the recurrence and on the type of the primary ulcer operation. If gastrinoma is diagnosed and identified by localization studies, the tumor should be resected. If the tumor cannot be identified by localization studies, including thorough surgical exploration of the pancreas, duodenum, and retroperitoneum, the treatment of choice is omeprazole. Total gastrectomy is reserved for omeprazole failure or intolerance to its use.

In most patients, however, none of these causes are identified, and the treatment should be a more extensive antiulcer operation, to include re-vagotomy and resection or re-resection of the antrum.

CHRONIC POSTOPERATIVE COMPLICATIONS

Ulcer operations disrupt, to a greater or lesser degree, both the secretory functions and the motility of the stomach, sometimes resulting in postgastrectomy syndromes, which include the following.

DUMPING SYNDROME. When the antropyloric mechanism is either destroyed (resection, pyloroplasty) or bypassed (gastrojejunostomy), large quantities of hyperosmolar chyme can be "dumped" into the upper small intestine. This results in (a) distention and activation of the distention reflex, leading to stimulation of motility; (b) osmotic shift of fluid from the intravascular compartment into the gut lumen, further aggravating the distention and leading to relative hypovolemia and hemoconcentration; and (c) release of vasoactive substances (substance P, neurotensin, vasoactive intestinal peptide, bradykinin, serotonin) that may cause peripheral vasodilatation and flushing. These mechanisms cause the *early dumping syndrome,* which has abdominal and systemic manifestations and occurs within 1 hour of eating. The abdominal symptoms include pain, borborygmi, and diarrhea. Systemic manifestations include weakness, sweating, flushing (rarely), tachycardia, and palpitations. With chyme rapidly entering the intestine, rapid absorption of glucose results in hyperglycemia, causing hyperinsulinemia. Secondary hypoglycemia develops in the second hour after eating because the hyperinsulinemia lasts longer than the hyperglycemia. These hypoglycemic symptoms are responsible for the *late dumping syndrome.* When the pylorus and its innervation are preserved, as occurs in proximal gastric vagotomy, dumping can be prevented. Dietary manipulation is usually effective in controlling symptoms. This includes a low carbohydrate diet (which has a low osmolality), delaying liquid intake for 30 minutes after eating (so that hyperosmolar contents are not washed out of the stomach), and reclining for 20 to 30 minutes (to avoid gravitational acceleration of emptying). Medical treatment includes pectin, ephedrine, and the long-acting somatostatin analogue octreotide. Somatostatin inhibits the release and action of vasoactive peptides from the intestine and inhibits the release of insulin, thereby preventing the late dumping symptoms of hypoglycemia. Surgery is reserved for intractable cases; however, corrective operations are not always successful. Possible operations include the construction of a Roux-en-Y gastro-jejunostomy (Fig. 99–4), conversion of Billroth I to Billroth II or vice versa, or the insertion of a 10-inch reversed jejunal segment between the pylorus and the duodenum.

DIARRHEA. Chronic diarrhea may occur after both vagotomy and subtotal gastrectomy, and its cause is largely unknown. Possible etiologic factors include (1) rapid gastric emptying, (2) rapid small intestinal transit, (3) increased ileal fluid and bile acid delivery to the colon, (4) carbohydrate wastage with delivery to the colon, and (5) colonization of the upper gastrointestinal tract by bacteria causing malabsorption. It is often called *postvagotomy diarrhea* because it occurs more frequently after vagotomy. The diarrhea usually occurs 1 to 2 hours after eating and tends to be episodic. Following truncal vagotomy, 20 to 30% of patients develop loose bowel movements; however, only 5% have frank diarrhea and 1% develop intractable diarrhea. Dietary treatment of diarrhea includes avoiding certain foods such as milk, bananas, sweetened juices, and carbonated drinks. Medical treatment has had limited success and includes cholestyramine and broad-spectrum antibiotics. Surgical correction has not been uniformly successful.

ALKALINE REFLUX GASTRITIS. Excessive reflux of bile and pancreatic and intestinal secretions into the stomach may result from gastric resection or ablating or bypassing the pylorus. Characteristic symptoms include burning, midepigastric pain unresponsive to antacids and aggravated by eating and recumbency. Bilious vomiting, anemia, and significant weight loss may also occur. The stomach contains little or no acid, and endoscopic biopsy shows poorly defined gastritis. The diagnosis is difficult to make and is often one of exclusion and uncertainty. Surgical correction has been unsuccessful in 40 to 70% of cases (because of difficulty in diagnosis).

MALDIGESTION. Maldigestion is rarely a severe problem and probably occurs to some degree after all types of ulcer operations, excluding proximal gastric vagotomy. Potential etiologic factors include accelerated gastric emptying; delivery of large food particles

into the intestine; small intestine rapid transit; impaired pancreatic enzyme response and gallbladder contractility to food following truncal vagotomy; bacterial colonization of the upper gastrointestinal tract; and, in procedures with gastrojejunostomy, arrival of food in the intestine earlier than that of biliary-pancreatic secretions. Maldigestion may become an aggravating factor in patients with other postgastrectomy problems.

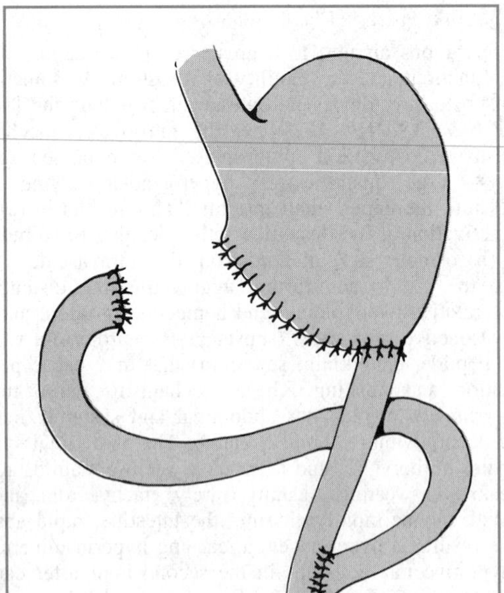

ANEMIA. Deficiencies in iron, vitamin B_{12}, and folate absorption are largely responsible for the chronic anemia developing after major gastric resection. Iron deficiency is the main cause of anemia and occurs because there is less available ferric iron for absorption from food with the reduced postoperative acid secretion. In addition, because digestion is the major source of dietary iron, maldigesting meals contributes to iron deficiency. Treatment with ferrous iron supplements is effective. In general, anemia occurs less often after vagotomy than after gastric resection. Megaloblastic anemia secondary to vitamin B_{12} deficiency rarely develops except in patients who have had radical subtotal or total gastrectomy. Monthly parenteral administration of vitamin B_{12} prevents and treats the anemia.

WEIGHT LOSS. Weight loss occurs frequently after surgery, but severe weight loss is usually seen only after gastrectomy. The cause is multifactorial and includes inadequate food intake, malabsorption, and maldigestion. Weight loss is frequently accompanied by large fecal fat and nitrogen losses. Ulcer surgery can unmask gluten-sensitive enteropathy (sprue).

BONE DISEASE. Bone disease is more common in older patients and occurs more commonly after gastrectomy than after vagotomy. Defective calcium absorption and malabsorption of vitamin D lead to bone demineralization, which takes many years to become clinically apparent.

Debas HT, Orloff SL: Surgery for peptic ulcer disease. *In* Yamada T (ed.): Textbook of Gastroenterology. 2nd ed. Philadelphia, JB Lippincott, 1994. *A detailed overview of the indications, surgical treatment, and management of the complications of duodenal, gastric, and recurrent ulcers.*

Laws HL, McKernan JB: Endoscopic management of peptic ulcer disease. Ann Surg 217:548, 1993. *A review of the authors' experience with endoscopic treatment of duodenal ulcer and ulcers occurring after previous drainage procedure. The indications, techniques, advantages, and limitations of laparoscopic and thoracoscopic procedures are discussed.*

Stabile BE: Current surgical management of duodenal ulcers. Surg Clin North Am 72:335, 1992. *An update on the epidemiology, pathophysiology, and surgical management of ulcers and their complications.*

Stabile BE, Passaro E: Recurrent peptic ulcer. Gastroenterology 70:124, 1976. *A complete description of the pathophysiology and treatment of ulcer recurrence after previous surgery.*

FIGURE 99–4. Model illustrating a Roux-en-Y gastrojejunostomy.

99.5 Complications
David Y. Graham

Approximately 1% of ulcer patients per year experience a complication; the likelihood of a complication sometime during the life history of peptic ulcer disease is in the range of 20 to 30%. Once a complication has occurred, the risk of a subsequent complication increases remarkably and identifies a group with clinically severe peptic ulcer disease.

INTRACTABILITY

Modern definitions of intractability might include failure of an ulcer to heal despite successfully treating *Helicobacter pylori* infection and adequate antisecretory therapy or rapid ulcer recurrence because of inability to cure the infection. Intractability is now a rare indication for surgery in peptic ulcer disease. The presence of a difficult-to-heal ulcer in a patient without *H. pylori* infection or after successful cure of the *H. pylori* infection is one of the most difficult management problems in ulcer disease. An ulcer that fails to respond to the combination of antisecretory and anti–*H. pylori* therapy suggests a complicating factor such as Zollinger-Ellison syndrome (see Ch. 99.6), concomitant and often covert nonsteroidal anti-inflammatory drug (NSAID's) use, or diseases such as Crohn's disease masquerading as peptic ulcer. Evaluation should include determining the serum gastrin and calcium levels and requestioning about drug use, especially over-the-counter medications that contain aspirin.

The incidence of major upper gastrointestinal (UGI) bleeding is 150 per 100,000. The mortality rate of major UGI bleeding ranges from 5 to 10% and has not changed significantly over the past 50 years despite major improvements in intensive care, resuscitation with blood products, and new endoscopic and surgical techniques. One reason mortality rate fails to fall may be that the population has grown older and a higher percentage of patients are at risk for mortality. Peptic ulcer disease is the most common cause of major UGI bleeding. Between 15 and 20% of ulcer patients experience hemorrhage during the course of their disease. Recently, NSAID's have become responsible for an increasingly large percentage of UGI bleeding.

Approximately 80% of patients relate a history of symptomatic ulcer disease prior to the onset of bleeding. About one third have suffered a previous hemorrhage, and about 10% of patients have bled more than once. At presentation, hematemesis, melena, or a combination of both is evident in more than 95%; 15% present in shock. Clinical features that suggest a poor outcome are being older than 60, hematemesis, the presence of shock, severe bleeding requiring multiple transfusions, and/or the presence of clinically active comorbid disease (particularly of cardiovascular, respiratory, hepatic, or malignant origin). Physical examination should assess circulatory status, search for presence of comorbid disease, and look for features suggesting the cause of hemorrhage such as the presence of chronic liver disease or cutaneous telangiectasis.

MANAGEMENT. The management steps are resuscitation, diagnosis, therapy, and planning long-term management (Table 99–13). Outcome is best if initial management is in an intensive care unit and decisions are made by a team experienced in managing gastrointestinal hemorrhage. One of the first steps for the patient with significant bleeding is to begin to restore the vascular and the oxygen-carrying capacity of the blood. A systolic blood pressure < 100 mm Hg or pulse > 100 per minute is indicative of volume depletion of at least 20%. A positive Tilt test (defined as a systolic blood pressure drop > 10 mm Hg or an increase in pulse rate > 20 per minute upon standing or sitting) suggests an acute blood loss of more than 1 liter. An intravenous line should be inserted in all patients, and 0.9% saline should be infused as rapidly as the patient's cardiopulmonary status allows. Blood should be obtained for a complete blood count, assessment of coagulation status, serum electrolytes, blood urea nitrogen (BUN), and creatinine. In most instances it is prudent to also send blood for typing and crossmatching. Transfusions should generally be given in order to maintain the hemoglobin around 10 grams per deciliter; avoid overtransfusion. The response of the blood pressure to postural changes usually provides a reasonably reliable indication of whether the intravascular volume is unstable. The hematocrit is not reliable following acute hemorrhage. The presence of an elevated BUN and a normal serum creatinine in the presence of melena strongly suggests a UGI site of bleeding of significant proportions. The decrease and rate of normalization in the BUN are gauges of effectiveness of volume replacement because correcting the deficit in the vascular volume rapidly returns the BUN to normal. Most physicians would insert a nasogastric tube to ascertain whether fresh blood or clots are present within the stomach.

Bleeding from a peptic ulcer is usually self-limited; 5% continue to bleed. Rebleeding occurs in 20 to 25%, with 80 to 90% of rebleeding episodes occurring within 48 hours of entry. After the patient's condition has stabilized, the site of bleeding can be identified. One cannot rely on the history, and endoscopy is required. Endoscopically applied therapy has now largely replaced surgery as the method of choice for initially managing bleeding ulcers. All patients with clinical evidence of major bleeding, such as hemodynamic instability, transfusions, or decreasing hematocrit, should undergo early endoscopy, and those with endoscopic evidence of active bleeding, adherent clot, or visible vessel should receive endoscopic therapy. Most would also begin ulcer therapy with an H_2-receptor antagonist administered intravenously by continuous infusion.

MANAGEMENT AFTER BLEEDING. Patients who have bled should be investigated for *H. pylori* status and for NSAID use. Maintenance antisecretory therapy markedly reduces subsequent complications and should not be withdrawn until successful treatment of the *H. pylori* infection has been confirmed. If the patient was receiving NSAID's (including aspirin) such medications should be prohibited in the future, if at all possible. If not, cotherapy with the synthetic prostaglandin misoprostol (200 μg two or three times a day) should be considered, as well as use of the least amount of NSAID that yields the desired therapeutic benefit. Maintenance therapy with H_2-receptor antagonist is recommended only if the patient cannot tolerate misoprostol and the ulcer was duodenal in location.

Recognizing that peptic ulcer disease can be cured has led to a reassessment of the role of surgery for ulcer disease (see Ch. 99.4). Traditional gastric surgery is no longer an acceptable first-line therapy. Ulcer surgery for bleeding should now be used primarily as a second-line form of homeostasis. If an operation is required to control hemorrhage, simple oversewing of the ulcer and, if possible, a highly selective vagotomy are the treatment of choice. One should be hesitant to introduce a new disease—gastrectomy—for a potentially curable problem.

PERFORATION

The incidence of ulcer perforation is 7 to 10 per 100,000 population per year. Perforation is more common in men than in women (4 to 8:1), although that ratio appears to be changing as the frequency of gastric perforation is increasing in association with NSAID use in elderly women. The most common presentation is an abrupt onset of severe abdominal pain, followed rapidly by signs of peritoneal inflammation. The typical patient appears to be acutely and seriously ill, lying immobile in bed with grunting and shallow respirations; abdominal tenderness is usually most pronounced in the epigastrium, with spasm of the abdominal musculature usually approaching boardlike rigidity. Loss of hepatic dullness, if present, is a valuable clue to the correct diagnosis. Leukocytosis appears rapidly. The blood chemistries are usually normal with the exception of the serum amylase, which may be slightly increased. The suspected diagnosis can be confirmed by identifying free intraperitoneal air, which is demonstrable in about 80% of cases. An erect chest radiograph or a left decubitus film of the abdomen is better than a plain abdominal film for detecting the presence of free air. When the diagnosis is suspected and the radiographs are negative, it is worthwhile to repeat the radiographic evaluation after several hours. The diagnosis may be confirmed by a UGI series using Gastrografin, especially if combined with computed tomographic scanning to enhance the ability to identify the perforation and exclude other pathology. One aid to increased diagnostic accuracy may be to include perforated viscus in the differential diagnosis of patients with unexplained shock.

Initial management is to prepare the patient for surgery. The steps include resuscitation by correcting fluid and electrolyte abnormalities, treatment of complications, use of continuous nasogastric suction and parenterally administered broad-spectrum antibiotics (ampicillin-sulbactam and gentamicin), and, if a tension pneumoperitoneum is present, needle aspiration of the peritoneal cavity. Nasogastric suction is one of the mainstays of therapy, and it is important to confirm that the aspirating ports of the nasogastric tube are positioned in the most dependent portion of the stomach.

Both the perforation and the underlying disease must be considered when planning long-term treatment. A randomized trial comparing nonoperative treatment with emergency surgery showed that

---

TABLE 99–13. PRINCIPLES OF MANAGEMENT OF UPPER GASTROINTESTINAL HEMORRHAGE

1. Preventing exsanguination takes priority over everything.
   a. Resuscitation takes priority over diagnosis of bleeding site.
   b. Initial care for most patients should be in an intensive care unit.
   c. Therapeutic endoscopic and surgical consultations should be obtained early.
   d. Specific and beneficial therapy is available for most causes of hemorrhage.
   e. There is no place for diagnostic endoscopy in the management of bleeders.
2. Comorbid disease (e.g., chronic lung, liver, kidney, or heart) adversely influences outcome.
3. There is no right way to do the wrong thing.

an initial period of nonoperative treatment with careful observation produced a similar outcome, and the decision not to operate should be based on the age and clinical condition of the patient. If there is evidence of increasing peritoneal irritation after 6 hours of treatment, it is best to declare nonoperative therapy a failure and to proceed to surgery. Simple closure of the perforation and proximal selective gastric vagotomy is the preferred operation.

The long-term plan for a patient who survived the perforation and is ready to be discharged from the hospital depends on whether the patient received a definitive ulcer operation, had simple closure of the perforation, or was managed with conservative medical therapy, or whether the perforation was a complication of concomitant NSAID use. In general, *H. pylori* status should be determined and if present the infection should be treated. Because treating *H. pylori* infection cures peptic ulcer disease, we presume that it also prevents this complication from recurring; this hypothesis has not yet been studied. Even if the patient received a definitive ulcer operation, *H. pylori* should be eradicated if present. As with bleeding, if the perforation is possibly related to NSAID use, further use should be prohibited unless the patient requires them. For those patients misoprostol prophylaxis is recommended.

OBSTRUCTION

Approximately 2% of ulcer patients develop gastric outlet obstruction; 90% are caused by previous or coexistent duodenal or channel ulcers. Inflammatory swelling surrounding the ulcer, muscular spasm associated with nearby ulcer, and cicatricial narrowing with fibrosis are the factors responsible for the obstruction. Conservative medical management with decompression of the obstructed stomach; correcting fluid, electrolyte, and acid-base abnormalities; and use of intravenous H_2-receptor antagonist are the mainstays of initial resuscitation and therapy. Two events have occurred to reduce the need for surgery of obstruction—endoscopic balloon dilatation and treating *H. pylori* infection. Intraoperative dilatation of the stenotic segment combined with highly selective vagotomy is often successful in managing patients with pyloric stenosis longterm. One would presume that the combination of therapy that cures the disease (*H. pylori* therapy) and endoscopic dilatation of the pyloric ring should be equally effective. The author's approach to these patients is resuscitation followed by balloon dilatation of the pylorus and antisecretory therapy (e.g., omeprazole 40 to 60 mg daily) followed by treating the *H. pylori* infection. For those in whom the therapy is not successful, one should consider missed cancer.

Boey J, Wong J: Perforated duodenal ulcers. World J Surg 11:319, 1987. *A scoring system separates those with essentially no risk from those with a high risk of dying. Those with all three risk factors have a very high risk of dying.*

Crofts TJ, Park KGM, Steele RJC, et al.: A randomized trial of nonoperative treatment for perforated peptic ulcer. N Engl J Med 320:970, 1989. *A randomized trial of nonoperative treatment compared with emergency surgery showed that an initial period of nonoperative treatment with careful observation produces similar outcome.*

Graham DY: Ulcer complications and their nonoperative treatment. *In* Sleisenger M, Fordtran J (eds.): Gastrointestinal Disease. 5th ed. Philadelphia, WB Saunders, 1993, p 698. *Comprehensive review of peptic ulcer complications and the impact of the new approach to ulcer causation on choosing therapy.*

Laine L: Rolling review: Upper gastrointestinal bleeding. Aliment Pharmacol Ther 7:207, 1993. *Excellent review of management of upper gastrointestinal bleeding with up-to-date references.*

99.6 Zollinger-Ellison Syndrome
Robert T. Jensen

The Zollinger-Ellison syndrome (ZES) is a clinical syndrome caused by a gastrin-releasing endocrine tumor located, usually, in the pancreas or duodenum and characterized by clinical symptoms/signs due to gastric acid hypersecretion (ulcer disease, diarrhea, esophageal reflux disease).

HISTORY AND EPIDEMIOLOGY. In 1955, Zollinger and Ellison described two patients with severe peptic ulcer disease, marked increases in basal gastric acid output (hyperchlorhydria), and a non-β islet cell tumor of the pancreas. Subsequently, in the 1960's these tumors were shown to release the gastrointestinal hormone gastrin, and elevated levels of gastrin were found in the circulation (hypergastrinemia). The gastrin-containing tumors are therefore called gastrinomas. The incidence of ZES is one patient per million population per year, and gastrinomas are one-half as common as insulin-secreting tumors (insulinomas).

CLINICAL FEATURES. ZES occurs most frequently between ages 35 and 65 and is slightly more common in males (60%). Abdominal pain resulting from a peptic ulcer is the most common symptom (>80%). The majority of ulcers occur in the duodenum (>85%), but they occasionally occur in the postbulbar area, jejunum, or stomach and are occasionally in multiple locations. The pain is usually similar to that of patients with typical peptic ulcers, especially early in the disease course. With time the symptoms become persistent and, in general, respond poorly to conventional doses of H_2-receptor antagonists, to conventional surgical treatments, or to treatments aimed at eliminating the bacterium *Helicobacter pylori*, which are commonly used for routine duodenal ulcer disease. Pain due to reflux of gastric acid into the esophagus (heartburn) is also common (20%). Diarrhea (60 to 70%) occurs frequently and may precede the peptic ulceration in some patients (10 to 20%). A proportion of patients (20 to 25%) have ZES as part of the multiple endocrine neoplasia type 1 (MEN 1) syndrome, an autosomal dominant inherited disease (see Ch. 210.1 and 215). These patients have hyperplasia or tumors of multiple endocrine glands and most commonly have parathyroid hyperplasia (>90%), pituitary tumors (60%), and pancreatic endocrine tumors (80%). ZES is the most common functional pancreatic endocrine tumor syndrome these patients develop. These patients typically first develop renal stones due to hypercalcemia from hyperparathyroidism or have elevated prolactin levels due to pituitary tumors and later develop ZES.

PATHOLOGY AND PATHOPHYSIOLOGY. In older studies, gastrinomas were found primarily in the pancreas. In recent large surgical series, gastrinomas are found as frequently in the duodenum as in the pancreas. Duodenal gastrinomas are generally small (< 1 cm), whereas pancreatic gastrinomas are generally larger. Occasionally ZES is due to a gastrinoma in the splenic hilum, mesentery, stomach, or only in a lymph node or to a gastrin-releasing tumor of the ovary. Approximately one third of patients have metastatic liver disease at presentation. The gastrinoma characteristically metastasizes first to regional lymph nodes, later to the liver, and very late, more distally, especially to bone. The exact percentage of malignant gastrinomas is unclear. In older series, 60 to 90% of patients had metastatic disease. However, at present, of the 70% of patients who do not have metastatic disease to the liver at the initial evaluation, < 20% develop metastatic disease to the liver during a 10-year follow-up period. This demonstrates that in most patients the time course of progression is long. Gastrinomas are histologically similar to carcinoid tumors, demonstrating characteristically monotonous sheets of small round cells with uniform nuclei and cytoplasm, with mitotic figures being uncommon. Malignancy can be reliably determined only by demonstrating the presence of metastatic disease, and no light microscopic or ultrastructural finding can clearly establish malignant behavior. In most gastrinomas 74 to 80% of the gastrin is heptadecapeptide gastrin (gastrin-17), with most of the remainder being gastrin-34. In contrast, gastrin-34 comprises 60% of the total serum gastrin, similar to normal subjects. In addition to gastrin-34 and gastrin-17, smaller and larger precursor forms circulate in abnormal amounts in patients with gastrinomas. Similar to other pancreatic endocrine tumors, by immunocytochemistry, gastrinomas frequently contain numerous other gastrointestinal hormones such as insulin, pancreatic polypeptide, glucagon, and ACTH or ACTH fragments. In 60% of patients, an increased plasma concentration of another gastrointestinal hormone is found, but these peptides are almost always clinically silent except for ACTH. Up to 5% of patients with ZES develop Cushing's syndrome (see Ch. 204.1) due to ACTH secretion by the gastrinoma. These patients usually have metastatic gastrinoma in the liver, have ZES without MEN 1, and have a poor prognosis.

Gastrin stimulates parietal cells to secrete acid and also has a growth effect (trophic) on cells of the gastric mucosa. Chronic hypergastrinemia thus leads to increased gastric mucosal thickness, prominent gastric folds, and increased numbers of parietal cells and gastric enterochromaffin-like cells (ECL cells). Patients with gastrinomas have increased basal acid output and an increased maximal acid output, which is a measure of the total number of parietal

TABLE 99–14. CLINICAL FINDINGS SUGGESTING ZOLLINGER-ELLISON SYNDROME

1. Peptic ulcer disease with diarrhea
2. Peptic ulceration in unusual locations
3. Multiple peptic ulcers
4. Nonhealing peptic ulcer
5. Peptic ulcer disease with complications (bleeding, obstruction, esophageal stricture)
6. Recurrent peptic ulcer after surgery
7. Large gastric folds
8. Family history of peptic ulcer disease
9. Peptic ulcer disease with renal stones or other endocrinopathies
10. Duodenal ulcer with no *H. pylori* present
11. Peptic ulcer with hypercalcemia
12. Fasting hypergastrinemia

cells. Almost all of the symptoms are due to the effects of gastric acid hypersecretion except for those late in the course of the disease in patients with metastatic disease, in whom the symptoms can be due to the extensive tumor bulk (cachexia, weight loss, pain). Peptic ulcers are thought to be due to the increased acid and pepsin release. In contrast to patients with routine peptic ulcers, the bacterial pathogen *H. pylori* appears not to be important in the pathogenesis of the ulcer disease in ZES. Diarrhea is due to the large-volume gastric acid output, leading to small intestinal structural damage (inflammation, blunted villi, edema), interference with fat transport, inactivation of pancreatic lipase, and precipitation of bile acids. These same mechanisms, if prolonged, can lead to steatorrhea. If acid hypersecretion is controlled either medically, surgically, or with nasogastric suction, the diarrhea stops at once.

DIAGNOSIS AND DIFFERENTIAL DIAGNOSIS. ZES should be suspected in any patient with the findings listed in Table 99–14. The initial measurement if the diagnosis is suspected is a fasting serum gastrin determination. The fasting serum gastrin level is elevated in 99 to 100% of patients with ZES. However, there are other causes of hypergastrinemia. Therefore, the most important initial determination is to establish that the hypergastrinemia is not physiologic in that it is secondary to achlorhydria or hypochlorhydria. Pernicious anemia, atrophic gastritis, renal failure, and *H. pylori* infections can all cause physiologic hypergastrinemia and are much more common than ZES. If the serum gastrin level is elevated, the fasting gastric pH should be determined. If the serum gastrin is >1000 pg per milliliter (normal is <100) and the pH is <2.5, the patient almost certainly has ZES; this is the case in 40% of patients. If the gastrin is elevated less than 10-fold and the pH <2.5, then basal acid output should be measured. Basal acid output is increased in patients with ZES (>10.6 mEq per hour in males and >5.6 mEq per hour in females) and >95% have a value >15 mEq per hour.

A number of conditions can mimic ZES and are listed in Table 99–15. To exclude these causes, a secretin stimulation test should be done. Normal individuals show an increase in serum gastrin level of <200 pg per milliliter after intravenous secretin, whereas 87% of patients with ZES with an elevated fasting gastrin <10-fold increased have a positive test. No false positives have been reported except in patients with achlorhydria. The MEN 1 syndrome should be sought in all patients with ZES by assessing if there is a family history of endocrinopathies and excluding hyperparathyroidism and pituitary adenomas.

THERAPY. Therapy needs to be directed both at controlling the gastric acid hypersecretion and at the gastrinoma itself. The H^+-K^+-ATPase inhibitor, omeprazole, is now the drug of choice. Because of its long duration of action, acid hypersecretion can be controlled in all patients with once or twice a day dosing. H_2-receptor antagonists are also effective but frequent dosing (every 4 to 6 hours) and high doses are needed. The recommended starting dose for omeprazole is 60 mg once a day. In 30% of patients a higher dose is needed. Higher doses are particularly needed by patients with MEN 1, previous gastric surgery, or a history of severe esophageal reflux disease. Patients need to remain on the omeprazole indefinitely, unless cured; however, long-term therapy appears safe, with patients being treated for up to 9 years without side effects or complications. Surgical treatment for gastric acid hypersecretion is now performed only for patients who cannot or will not take oral antisecretory medications (see Ch. 99.4). Total gastrectomy, the classic treatment for this disease, is the recommended procedure for these rare patients. Selective vagotomy effectively reduces the acid secretory rate, but almost all patients continue to require a low dose of drug. Parathyroidectomy in patients with hyperparathyroidism, ZES, and MEN 1 can have a dramatic effect on reducing acid secretion and increasing the sensitivity to antisecretory drugs and thus should be done in these patients. To manage the tumor, all patients need careful imaging studies. The CT scan is generally performed first and identifies most primary tumors ≥ 3 cm in diameter and 70% of patients with liver metastases. Magnetic resonance imaging (see Ch. 93) is better for detecting liver metastases and identifies 90% of such patients. Selective angiography is the most sensitive study for the primary tumor and identifies tumors in 40% of all patients. Routine surgical exploration for cure is now recommended in all patients without liver metastases, MEN 1, or complicating medical conditions limiting life expectancy. Tumors are currently found in 95% of patients, with a 5-year cure rate of 30%. Surgical resection has been shown to decrease the metastatic rate. Patients with metastatic gastrinoma in the liver have a poor prognosis with a 5-year survival rate of 30%. If the metastatic disease is increasing in size or is symptomatic, treatment with chemotherapeutic agents (streptozotocin, 5-fluorouracil, doxorubicin) is usually the first treatment. Treatment with α-interferon or octreotide is

TABLE 99–15. DIFFERENTIAL DIAGNOSIS OF HYPERGASTRINEMIA AND ELEVATED BASAL ACID OUTPUT (HYPERCHLORHYDRIA)

Diagnosis	Occurrence	Symptom(s)/Sign(s)	Technical Findings	Comments
Zollinger-Ellison syndrome	Uncommon—1 case/million population/year	Abdominal pain Diarrhea Heartburn	Peptic ulcer disease	1. Positive secretin test 2. 50% have tumor on imaging
H. pylori infection	Common	Abdominal pain Asymptomatic	Mild hypergastrinemia; peptic ulcer disease	Negative secretin test
Retained gastric antrum syndrome	Rare	Abdominal pain	Mimics ZES	1. Negative secretin test 2. Positive ^{99M}Tc-pertechnetate gastric scan 3. History gastric resection
Antral G cell hyperfunction/hyperplasia	Unknown	Abdominal pain	1. Peptic ulcer disease 2. Mild hypergastrinemia	1. Negative secretin test 2. Increased numbers of G cells (hyperplasia) 3. Frequently associated with *H. pylori*
Chronic renal failure	>50% of patients with serum creatinine >266 μM/liter	Abdominal pain	Peptic ulcer disease	1. Most (85%) have low acid output 2. Negative secretin test
Gastric outlet obstruction	2 to 5% of all patients with peptic ulcers	Vomiting Abdominal pain	Secondary to malignant or peptic ulcer disease	Negative secretin test

reported to be effective in a small percentage of patients if chemotherapy fails.

del Valle J, Yamada T: Zollinger-Ellison syndrome. *In* Yamada T, Alpers DH, Owyang C, et al. (eds.): Textbook of Gastroenterology. Philadelphia, JB Lippincott, 1991, p 1340. *An excellent general chapter on all aspects of this disease.*

Jensen RT, Fraker DL: Zollinger-Ellison syndrome: Recent advances in management of the gastric hypersecretion and the gastrinoma. JAMA 271:1, 1994. *A summary of recent advances for treating gastric acid hypersecretion and gastrinomas, with the most recent references in each of these areas.*

Jensen RT, Gardner JD: Gastrinoma. *In* Go VLW, DiMagno EP, Gardner JD, et al. (eds.): The Pancreas: Biology, Pathobiology and Diseases. 2nd ed. New York, Raven Press, 1993, p 931. *An in-depth treatment of all aspects of the disease, including the pathology, pathophysiology, diagnosis, tumor localization, and treatment of both acid secretion and gastrinoma.*

100 NEOPLASMS OF THE STOMACH
Robert C. Kurtz and Sidney J. Winawer

The majority of gastric neoplasms are malignant, in contrast to the colon, where the reverse is true. Although gastric carcinoma is steadily decreasing in the United States, it still represents a major public health problem throughout the world. In some countries it is the most frequent cancer and the leading cause of death from cancer. In the United States gastric carcinoma is responsible for 90 to 95% of malignant disease of the stomach. Approximately 5% of all primary gastric malignancy is non-Hodgkin's lymphoma. Hodgkin's disease rarely involves the stomach as a primary site. The sarcomas, including leiomyosarcoma, liposarcoma, neurogenic sarcoma, and fibrosarcoma, are all relatively rare malignant tumors that may involve the stomach. Leiomyosarcoma of the stomach represents about 1% of gastric tumors.

CARCINOMA OF THE STOMACH

EPIDEMIOLOGY. The incidence of gastric cancer varies markedly in different areas of the world. It is extremely common in Japan, Latin America west of the Andes, some parts of the Caribbean, and Eastern Europe; moderately common in Finland, Austria, and Czechoslovakia; and uncommon in the United States, Australia, New Zealand, and other Anglo-Saxon countries. Colorectal cancer tends to be rare where gastric cancer is common and vice versa. The low incidence in the United States is a recent development (Fig. 100–1), since gastric cancer was the most common known cancer 50 to 60 years ago. Other countries that previously had a high incidence have also begun to show a decrease. This is particularly noteworthy because the incidence of proximal gastric and esophagogastric junction adenocarcinomas is rising in the United States and in Western Europe. The reasons for this are unknown. Environmental factors are considered important in the etiology of gastric cancer, as evidenced by populations migrating to areas of either low or high risk and taking on the risk of the area of migration. Japanese moving to Hawaii have a decreased incidence of gastric cancer in subsequent generations, and there is a further reduction with migration to the mainland.

ETIOLOGY. *Dietary influences* are thought to be important, but without direct proof. Barbecued meals, smoked or pickled fish and sauces, and alcohol and deficiencies of magnesium and vitamin A have all been postulated but unproved as causes of gastric cancer (Table 100–1).

Nitrosamines are powerful carcinogens for animals. They can be formed easily from common, secondary, tertiary, and quaternary amines by combining these with nitrite (the nitrosation reaction). This reaction can take place under varying conditions of pH and temperature, so that nitrosamines may be formed in the soil, under conditions of food storage, during food preparation such as frying bacon, or in the body. Bacteria may play a role by catalyzing the amine nitrite union or by reducing nitrate to nitrite. Thus the achlorhydric stomach is considered a favorable site for nitrosamine

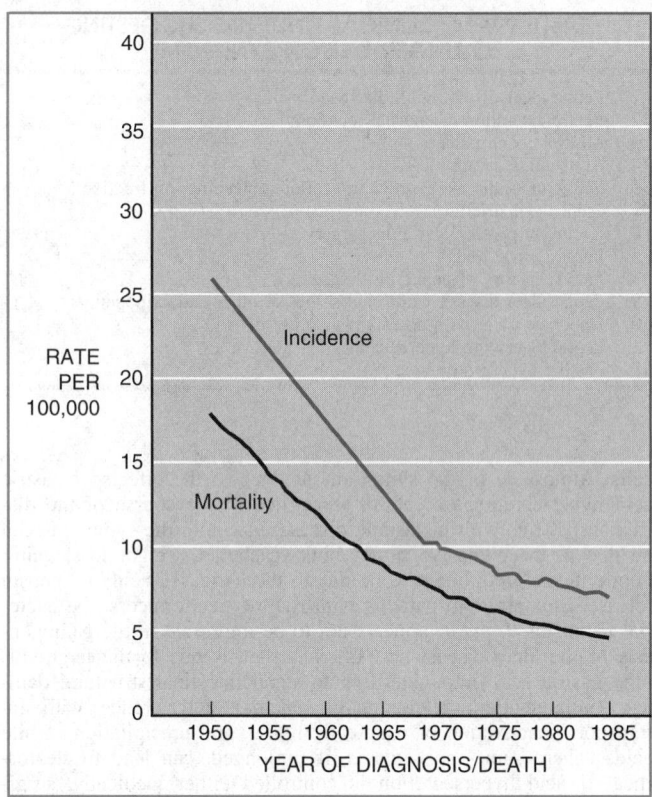

FIGURE 100–1. Incidence and mortality of gastric adenocarcinoma in the United States. (Data obtained and modified from the NCI Annual Cancer Statistics Review including Cancer Trends: 1950–1985 and is representative of the United States population.)

synthesis. The necessary amines can be found in many foods and medications, whereas nitrate and nitrite are found naturally in food and water and are present in food preservatives. Ascorbic acid (vitamin C) blocks the nitrosation reaction in the test tube. Increased intake of vitamin C and refrigeration have been postulated to be responsible for the decrease in gastric cancer in this country over the last few decades, but the nitrite hypothesis itself remains to be validated.

Blood group A is associated with a higher incidence of gastric cancer even in areas of the world where gastric cancer is rare. This fact and the threefold increase in gastric cancer among first-degree relatives, (parents, siblings, children) of gastric cancer patients has raised the possibility of a genetic component. *Helicobacter pylori,* an organism affecting the stomach and associated with a high rate of duodenal ulcer recurrence, has also been found in epidemiologic studies to be associated with gastric adenocarcinoma and some gastric lymphomas.

Pernicious anemia had been considered a premalignant condition, but the prior high incidence of gastric cancer once seen in this disease is no longer seen. This may be a reflection of the progressively decreasing incidence of gastric cancer being observed worldwide. Although atrophic gastritis is usually seen in association with gas-

TABLE 100–1. DIETARY FINDINGS FROM CASE CONTROL STUDIES OF GASTRIC CANCER*

Positive Association	Negative Association
Salted fish	Vegetables
Pickled vegetables	Fruit
Salty foods	Milk
Smoked fish	Meat
Starchy foods	Squash
Cabbage, potatoes	Eggplant
Cooked cereals	Lettuce
Bacon	Celery
Animal fat	

* United States (including Hawaii), Japan, Norway, England, and Israel.

tric cancer, this disorder is extremely common, and the vast majority of such patients never develop cancer.

Adenomatous polyps of the stomach, especially those larger than 2 cm, may occasionally give rise to carcinoma. Most stomach polyps, however, are hyperplastic and do not become malignant.

Subtotal resection for benign disease results in chronic atrophic gastritis from either bile reflux or removal of the gastrin trophic factor. This has been shown to produce gastric cancer in animals. It has also been shown to result in gastric cancer after a 10-year interval in persons living in countries at increased risk for gastric cancer, especially in men, who are at higher risk than women.

Immunologic deficiencies, particularly the common variable type, may cause a predisposition to gastric cancer.

Gastric ulcer does not transform into cancer. Cancer foci may be present in association with an ulcer, however. All gastric ulcers must be suspected of having small areas of malignancy even when the ulcer appears benign by radiography or endoscopy. Biopsy and cytologic examination reveal the true nature of the lesion.

INCIDENCE AND PREVALENCE. It is estimated that there were 23,000 new cases of gastric cancer and 14,000 deaths from gastric cancer in the United States in 1991. Although this is a substantial number, a dramatic decline in the incidence of stomach cancer has occurred here and in many other countries (Fig. 100–1). The magnitude of the decline varies. In the United States the age-adjusted mortality rate for males and females of all races decreased 25% from 1973 to 1985. Carcinoma of the stomach occurs most frequently between the ages of 50 and 70 and is rare in patients younger than 30. The incidence and mortality rise steeply with age. Rates are higher in males than females by 2 to 1. The 5-year survival is <20%.

PATHOLOGY. Carcinoma of the stomach is adenocarcinoma that usually is manifested pathologically in one of four ways (Fig. 100–2): (1) Most often it appears as a bulky mass with deep central ulceration projecting into the lumen and invading the wall. (2) The tumor may infiltrate and narrow a portion of the lumen, most often in the antrum. Less commonly, the infiltration extends throughout the entire stomach, resulting in *linitis plastica*—a fixed, nondistensible stomach with absence of normal folds and a narrowed lumen. (3) Polypoid or exophytic carcinoma may occur and be difficult to distinguish from a benign polyp on radiograph. (4) More rarely, carcinoma of the stomach may occur as a superficially spreading tumor involving only the mucosal surface and producing a granular appearance. This is unlike linitis plastica, which extends through the entire thickness of the wall. *Early gastric cancer* is a term used to characterize very superficial cancer that is often detected in high-

TABLE 100–2. STAGING OF GASTRIC CANCER*

	Stage	Tumor, Nodes, Metastasis
0	(T_{is}, N_0, M_0)	T_{is}—Limited to mucosa
I	(T_1, N_0, M_0)	T_1—Limited to mucosa and submucosa
II	$(T_{2,3}; N_0, M_0)$	T_2—To but not through serosa
		T_3—Through serosa but not adjacent structures
III	$(T_{4a}, N_0, M_0; T_{1-4}, N_{1-2}, M_0)$	T_{4a}—Through serosa and involves adjacent structures
		N_1—Perigastric nodes within 3 cm of tumor
		N_2—Perigastric nodes more than 3 cm from tumor (within celiac group)
IV	$(T_{4b}, N_{0-3}, M_0; T_{1-3}, N_3, M_0;$ Any T, Any N, $M_1)$	T_{4b}—Involves liver, diaphragm, pancreas, abdominal wall, retroperitoneum, small bowel, or duodenum via serosa
		N_3—Other intra-abdominal nodes (retroperitoneal, mesenteric, etc.)
		M_1—Distant metastasis

* From American Joint Committee on Cancer: Manual for Staging of Cancer, Philadelphia, JB Lippincott, 1983.

risk areas of the world by screening radiography or endoscopy. This has the same anatomic and male-female distribution as the more advanced stage. Prognosis is excellent even with lymph node involvement (Table 100–2).

Gastric carcinomas may be well-differentiated adenocarcinomas or may be so anaplastic as to resemble diffuse histiocytic lymphoma or sarcoma. A true carcinoma *in situ* is rarely found and is confined entirely to the glands. This is more commonly seen at the surface of large adenomatous polyps of the stomach.

CLINICAL MANIFESTATIONS (Table 100–3). Early carcinoma of the stomach is frequently asymptomatic. *Anorexia* and *weight loss* are nonspecific symptoms and not well correlated with the size of the tumor. *Early satiety* (particularly with linitis plastica), *bloating, dysphagia, epigastric distress,* or more severe epigastric boring pain may be later symptoms. *Vomiting* is commonly a later symptom that may be caused by pyloric obstruction but may occur with other levels of obstruction. Vomiting also occurs without obstruction and may be secondary to the motility disturbance that a fixed mass in the wall produces. The pain is similar to that of peptic ulcer in about one fourth of patients, particularly when the tumor has ulcerated. In most patients, however, the pain usually occurs after eating and is not relieved by foods or antacids. Boring pain radiating to the back may indicate penetration of the tumor into the pancreas.

Dysphagia may occur with more proximal lesions, particularly when they have invaded the area around the esophagogastric junction or spread submucosally to the esophagus, which is common in fundal lesions. Weakness and fatigue from *anemia* caused by chronic occult blood loss are common, although acute massive bleeding and hematemesis are unusual. Angina pectoris, congestive heart failure, and rarely cerebral ischemia may occur because of the

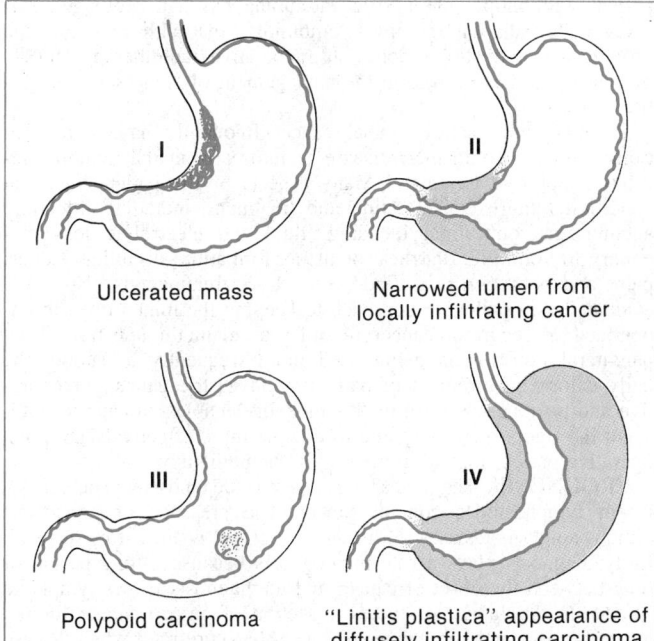

FIGURE 100–2. Diagrammatic representation of various presentations of gastric carcinoma.

TABLE 100–3. ADENOCARCINOMA OF THE STOMACH

Associated With	Clinical Manifestations
Environment–geographical differences	Anorexia, early satiety, weight loss
Diet–? nitrosamines	Dysphagia, vomiting, weakness
Blood group A–genetic	Epigastric distress to severe, boring pain
Atrophic gastritis	Anemia, occult blood in stools
Adenomatous polyps (>2 cm)	Epigastric mass, signs of metastases
Subtotal resection for benign ulcer disease in high-risk countries	Rare–Virchow's node, Blumer's shelf, Trousseau's syndrome, acanthosis nigricans

anemia. Perforation occurs in a very small percentage of patients and can simulate peptic ulcer. When the tumor metastasizes, additional symptoms may include jaundice or right upper quadrant pain from liver metastases, cough from lung metastases, hiccups, and vague abdominal discomfort and bloating from peritoneal seeding and ascites.

Physical examination during the early stages of gastric carcinoma may be completely normal. Later there may be signs of weight loss and anemia. When the tumor has disseminated, hepatomegaly from metastases, jaundice, or ascites may be present. Splenomegaly may occur if the portal or splenic vein is invaded. A palpable *epigastric mass* is present in less than one half of patients and usually, but not always, indicates extensive involvement. Rarely, left supraclavicular adenopathy (Virchow's node), a nodular perirectal wall (Blumer's shelf), or umbilical nodules give evidence of metastatic spread.

Several extragastric signs may precede the detection of an underlying malignancy. These include recurrent thrombophlebitis (Trousseau's syndrome); acanthosis nigricans, a verrucous, hyperpigmented, elevated skin lesion involving primarily the flexor spaces of the body; neuromyopathy characterized by localized sensory and/or motor disturbances; and profound central nervous system involvement with abrupt onset of confusion, memory defects, hostility, or ataxia. More detailed descriptions of the paraneoplastic syndromes are contained in specific chapters in Part XIV.

Laboratory studies may disclose iron deficiency, or megaloblastic anemia if the tumor is associated with untreated pernicious anemia. *Occult blood in the stool* is present in less than half of the patients. Most patients have gastric acid present but in reduced amounts. A few have achlorhydria after maximal stimulation with pentagastrin. A few have hypersecretion, especially with antral tumors. Therefore the presence of acid does not ensure that carcinoma is not present. Abnormalities in liver function, particularly a markedly elevated alkaline phosphatase and $5'$ nucleotidase level, suggest liver metastases. Microangiopathic hemolytic anemia has been reported in several patients with gastric cancer. Rarely, protein-losing enteropathy occurs with ulcerated carcinomas of the stomach. Elevated carcinoembryonic antigen is a late finding, usually in the presence of metastatic disease.

DIAGNOSIS. Roentgenologic Diagnosis. Most gastric cancers will be suspected on roentgenologic examination. The standard upper gastrointestinal series has been refined to include barium contrast studies that can detect very small lesions. With the gastric mucosa covered by a thin layer of barium and distended with air or gas, multiple projections are taken, which outline almost the entire stomach surface. Technique can be refined by using high-density barium, CO_2, simethicone for gas dispersion, and glucagon to induce gastroparesis. With such methods films showing fine detail may be produced and small mucosal lesions visualized.

The radiologist is usually able to define the characteristics of a benign versus malignant lesion and suggest a histologic diagnosis. For example, lymphoma of the stomach may be suspected by the extensive involvement, multiple shallow ulcerations, and giant rugal hypertrophy caused by infiltrative disease, and by the fact that the duodenum may be involved in the neoplastic process. A gastric ulcer often gives difficulty, but radiologic accuracy is in the range of 80%. Characteristic radiographic signs that suggest a malignant lesion are the presence of an ulcer in a mass, irregular folds stopping short of the ulcer crater, and an irregular ulcer base. It is essential, however, to determine the nature of the ulcer by endoscopy with biopsy and cytology. Generally the location of an ulcer is not important in determining malignancy. Ulcers on the greater and lesser curvatures have about equal frequency of malignancy. Rigidity, loss of distensibility, unchanging contour, and irregular peristalsis are characteristic of a malignant lesion; when extensive infiltration from linitis plastica is present, a "leather bottle" appearance may result.

Endoscopy with Biopsy and Cytology. Fiberoptic endoscopy has increased the diagnostic yield over radiology alone. When combined with biopsy and brush cytology, the diagnostic accuracy ranges from 95 to 99% in various series. About one half of early gastric cancers present as small ulcerations; some have slight elevation or depression of the adjacent mucosa. The next most common type is a small polyp. Appearance at endoscopy may be misleading. Directed tissue-sampling techniques, such as biopsy or brush cytology, should be used on any suspicious area, whether it is raised, depressed, or ulcerated. With more advanced carcinoma a specific tissue diagnosis can also be achieved with high accuracy by directed biopsy and cytology. Endoscopy is now being used also to stage and treat gastric cancer. Endoscopic ultrasonographic probes are highly accurate in evaluating depth of penetration of the cancer through the wall and extension to lymph nodes. This information can complement CT scans or standard ultrasonography in defining the extent of the tumor. The use of endoscopy to diagnose malignancies of the stomach is described in greater detail in Ch. 94.

TREATMENT. At present *surgery* provides the only satisfactory curative treatment for gastric cancer. The high frequency of regional node metastases plays a major role in the choice of surgical procedure and the results of various therapeutic efforts. When the tumor is localized in the distal portion of the stomach, the omentum as well as nodes in the region of the porta hepatis and the pancreatic head are dissected, and a generous subtotal gastrectomy is performed. For tumors in the pars media and the proximal stomach, total gastrectomy may be indicated to obtain an adequate margin and for dissection of the predictable lymphatic spread in all directions. Distal pancreatectomy and splenectomy are usually necessary. There is little doubt that operative mortality is greater after total gastrectomy than after subtotal resection, and the procedure should be avoided whenever possible.

With extensive bleeding or obstruction, a palliative limited subtotal gastric resection can be done even in the presence of residual cancer. Palliative total gastrectomy should rarely be done. Resection of recurrent cancer in the gastric remnant may be palliative even when a cure is not obtained.

Chemotherapy is often suggested for unresectable gastric adenocarcinoma in an effort to decrease symptoms and prolong survival. The most widely used drug has been 5-fluorouracil (5FU), with an overall partial response rate of 15 to 20%. Other agents such as mitomycin-C, doxorubicin (Adriamycin), and the various nitrosoureas have also been used as single agents with varying response. Combined use of several agents such as 5FU, doxorubicin, and methotrexate (FAMTX), has resulted in some studies in a better response rate but has not improved survival.

Adjuvant chemotherapy following apparently curative surgery is an attractive concept for gastric carcinoma because of its high recurrence rate. Micrometastases are undoubtedly frequently present after surgery, and it has been postulated that chemotherapy might be most effective against such minimal disease. However, multiple trials with single agents and combinations have not been universally successful.

Radiation therapy is generally unsatisfactory, since gastric carcinomas are not very radiosensitive. Occasionally palliation may be obtained for persistent bleeding, obstruction, or pain. An occasional patient with inoperable gastric carcinoma has had prolonged survival with radiation therapy. Combining 5FU with radiation can provide a synergistic response. Intraoperative radiotherapy (IORT) may prove to have a role in the management of some selected gastric cancers.

Patients with gastrointestinal cancer frequently have complications associated with their disease or its treatment that require vigorous supportive treatment. Many aspects of the patients' general condition require consideration and treatment, including infection; anemia; gastrointestinal bleeding; fluid and electrolyte loss secondary to vomiting, diarrhea, or fistula formation; disabling ascites; pain; and poor nutrition. Endoscopic laser treatment is also being evaluated as a palliative approach to keeping the lumen open in unoperated or recurrent cancer in order to maintain nutrition. Total parenteral nutrition is being used more frequently to supply the daily caloric requirement of patients with gastric cancer. Preoperative and postoperative use of this modality enables patients to withstand the rigors of surgery and to tolerate more effectively the postoperative period, including the use of chemotherapy.

PROGNOSIS. The 5-year survival rate depends on whether adjacent lymph nodes contain cancer. The presence of perigastric lymph node metastases indicates a $<15\%$ chance for survival. Early diagnosis plays a role in prognosis because a long period of time between the onset of cancer and its diagnosis favors lymphatic spread. In the Japanese studies, resection of gastric cancer limited to the mucosa and submucosa had a $>80\%$ cure rate; when disease was limited to the mucosa, cure rate was 90 to 95%. Linitis plastica and infiltrating lesions have a very poor prognosis compared with polypoid or exophytic disease.

PREVENTION. Until more is learned about the causes of gastric carcinoma, we cannot practice primary prevention. We can only practice limited secondary prevention, i.e., detect the disease at an earlier stage in minimally symptomatic people in order to prevent its devastating consequences. The mass survey approach used in Japan is not practical in the United States because of the relatively low incidence of gastric cancer.

LYMPHOMA OF THE STOMACH (see Ch. 145 and 146)

Primary lymphoma represents about 5% of all primary malignant tumors of the stomach, and non-Hodgkin's lymphoma accounts for most of these. It is extremely rare for Hodgkin's disease to involve the stomach as a primary lesion. Patients with lymphoma are generally about a decade younger than those with carcinoma of the stomach, and males are affected more frequently. There are reports of non-Hodgkin's lymphoma of the stomach occurring in patients positive for HIV-1. Pain is the most frequent symptom, and mild anemia is common, owing to gastrointestinal bleeding (which on occasion can be massive). A palpable mass is the most common presenting physical finding. Studies of maximal stimulation of gastric acid secretion have not been done in a large group of patients, but achlorhydria seems to be unusual. Secondary lymphoma involving the stomach is common in the course of disseminated lymphoma but is difficult to diagnose.

Lymphoma of the stomach frequently presents radiographically as a bulky mass and less frequently as a diffusely infiltrating tumor—the most common form of secondary lymphoma—giving the appearance of large folds on upper gastrointestinal series, frequently associated with multiple nodular defects and ulcerations. Lymphoma of the stomach often resembles superficially spreading carcinoma, linitis plastica, or solitary adenocarcinoma. Gastroscopy with directed biopsy and brush cytology gives a higher yield than was previously appreciated. Exophytic lesions provide a diagnosis in about 88% of cases; the infiltrative type does not yield as high an accuracy.

Pseudolymphoma is a gastric lesion that may be confusing. This diffuse or discrete lesion is an atypical inflammatory response in the region of benign gastric ulcers. It is frequently difficult for the pathologist to differentiate pseudolymphoma from a true lymphoma.

Patients with lymphoma of the stomach have a significant incidence of nontumorous lesions such as stress ulcer, hemorrhagic gastritis, monilial gastritis, and esophagitis. Therefore in such patients with upper gastrointestinal bleeding or other symptoms referable to the stomach, it is important that a careful diagnostic approach be undertaken to determine the possible nontumor cause of the sign or symptom.

Treatment of primary lymphoma of the stomach is usually surgical resection followed by radiotherapy and/or chemotherapy, particularly if lymph nodes are involved. Some have advocated radiotherapy alone because of the marked sensitivity of lymphoma to radiation. The 5-year survival following surgery for primary lymphoma of the stomach is in the range of 50% for non-Hodgkin's lymphoma and less for Hodgkin's disease, suggesting that it is already disseminated when initially found in the stomach. HIV-1-associated gastric lymphoma carries a poor diagnosis. The best prognosis for primary tumors occurs with small lesions confined to the stomach, differentiated into tumor follicles without lymph node involvement and with only superficial infiltration of the wall.

OTHER MALIGNANT TUMORS OF THE STOMACH

Leiomyosarcoma of the stomach represents about 1% of gastric cancers and may present with a large intramural mass with central ulceration. Systemic symptoms are minimal, but massive bleeding or a palpable mass of which the patient is aware may be the presenting complaints. The tumor may be slow growing; 5-year survival following resection is in the range of 50%. Metastases to the liver and nodes are common, but these patients have a better prognosis than those with other metastatic tumors. Liposarcoma, fibrosarcoma, myxosarcoma, and neurogenic sarcoma are extremely rare and cause symptoms similar to those of leiomyosarcoma. Neurogenic sarcoma can be associated with von Recklinghausen's disease.

Metastatic disease to the stomach from other sites is not common but may simulate primary gastric cancer. Malignant melanoma and breast and lung carcinomas are the most frequent offenders. In breast cancer the metastatic lesions may be ulcerative, of linitis plastica type, or polypoid.

LEIOMYOMAS AND BENIGN TUMORS

Leiomyomas are commonly found at postmortem examination but are rarely of clinical significance. They occur equally in men and women, and are usually found in the midportion and antrum of the stomach. They may grow toward the mucosa, encroach on the lumen, and cause mucosal effacement and secondary ulceration. They may grow in the direction of the serosa, producing a mass that is predominantly extrinsic. Simultaneous inward and outward growth results in a dumbbell shape. These features are also characteristic of leiomyosarcomas, and differentiation on radiography or gastroscopy is difficult. Bleeding is common and epigastric pain may simulate peptic ulcer disease. On roentgen examination the findings are usually an intramural filling defect with or without secondary ulceration. Gastroscopic examination reveals effaced but normal mucosa overlying the mass. Central ulceration may be seen.

Asymptomatic leiomyomas need not be removed while symptomatic lesions are excised locally.

Neurofibroma occasionally associated with von Recklinghausen's disease, neuroma, lymphangioma, ganglioneuroma, lipoma, carcinoid, and hamartoma associated with Peutz-Jeghers syndrome all may involve the stomach. About 10% of hamartomas of the stomach and duodenum in Peutz-Jeghers syndrome become malignant.

ADENOMAS

Adenomas of the stomach are relatively rare lesions. Most polyps of the stomach are hyperplastic, not neoplastic, and do not become malignant. Adenomatous polyps are the usual neoplastic type of polyp. These are more frequent in men than in women and are generally seen in patients over 50. Patients with familial adenomatous polyposis or Gardner's syndrome (see Ch. 106) have a 30% probability of having polyps in the upper gastrointestinal tract. These are usually hyperplastic in the stomach and adenomatous in the duodenum. Patients with Peutz-Jeghers syndrome occasionally have similar findings. Bleeding, dyspepsia, and nausea are the most common symptoms, but most patients are asymptomatic. The diagnosis may be strongly suspected when a rounded smooth defect in the stomach on upper gastrointestinal series or a mass covered by mucosa with or without a stalk is detected by radiography or endoscopy.

The size of polyps strongly influences management. It is rare for a polyp <2 cm to show malignant change. In view of their potential for malignancy (present and future), polyps >2 cm or polyps of any size causing significant symptoms should be removed. Pedunculated polyps can now be safely removed by cautery-snare technique through the fiberoptic endoscope. For sessile polyps >2 cm in diameter, a segmental gastric resection may be necessary. If carcinoma is diagnosed histologically at the time of surgery, subtotal gastric resection should be done. Multiple gastric polyps are usually hyperplastic and of no significance.

TUMORS OF THE DUODENUM

Adenocarcinoma of the duodenum is rare but is more common than lymphoma, which, in turn, arises more commonly in the jejunum and ileum. The second and third portions of the duodenum are the usual sites of adenocarcinoma except when associated with Crohn's disease, in which it is in the ileum. Cancer in the duodenal bulb is exceedingly rare. Adenocarcinoma of the duodenum more frequently affects men and develops at a younger age than carcinoma of the stomach or colon. The tumor tends to grow into the lumen or to invade the wall of the duodenum. Cramping abdominal pain, anorexia, weight loss, vomiting, and melena are common. Jaundice or fever may result from obstruction of the ampulla of Vater or the common bile duct when the carcinoma involves the second portion of the duodenum. The tumor may simulate benign postbulbar ulceration. The diagnosis is usually made by radiologic examination and confirmed by endoscopy. Pancreaticoduodenectomy is necessary. Five-year survival ranges between 4 and 15%.

Lymphoma, leiomyosarcoma, carcinoid, metastatic cancer, and benign tumors may involve the duodenum, and these are discussed in more detail in Ch. 106. In general, these lesions are manifested as an intramural and submucosal mass with the exception of lymphoma and metastatic cancer, which frequently are exophytic and ulcerate. Any tumor, benign or malignant, may occur in a diverticulum at the descending portion of the duodenum. Aberrant pancreatic tissue may produce a submucosal filling defect in the duodenum, which may resemble a neoplastic lesion. Also, hyperplasia or adenoma of Brunner's glands may produce multiple polypoid defects in the duodenal bulb and is frequently associated with hypersecretion, duodenal ulcer and, rarely, Zollinger-Ellison syndrome. A prominent ampulla of Vater may resemble a neoplastic lesion radiographically. Endoscopy may be necessary to clarify the situation.

Blot WJ, Devesa SS, Kneller RW, Fraumeni JF: Rising incidence of adenocarcinoma of the esophagus and gastric cardia. JAMA 265:1287, 1991. *Demonstration of the rising incidence of proximal gastric cancers and esophagogastric cancers predominantly in white middle-aged men.*

Botet JF, Lightdale CJ: Preoperative staging of gastric cancer. Comparison of endoscopic ultrasound and dynamic CT. Radiology 181:426, 1991. *A prospective study of endosonography and CT scanning in staging gastric cancer, demonstrating a significantly greater concordance of endosonography with surgical pathology and CT scanning, especially in T staging.*

Kelsen D: Adjuvant therapy of upper gastrointestinal tract cancers. Semin Oncol 18:543, 1991. *A review of studies applying adjuvant chemotherapy to gastric and esophageal cancers.*

Kurtz RC, Lightdale CJ, Winawer SJ, et al.: Endoscopy and gastrointestinal neoplasm: Diagnosis and management. Curr Probl Cancer 5:4, 1980. *This monograph describes the techniques and applications of endoscopy in cancer of the gastrointestinal tract, including the stomach.*

Kurtz RC, Sherlock P: The diagnosis of gastric cancer. Semin Oncol 12:11, 1985. *A review of the sequencing of diagnostic tests to detect gastric cancer.*

Le Chevalier T, Smith FP, Harter WK, et al.: Chemotherapy and combined modality therapy for locally advanced and metastatic gastric carcinoma. Semin Oncol 12:46, 1985. *An overview of therapeutic results. Response rates are still disappointing, and combination protocols have not as yet been dramatically better.*

Parsonnett J, Friedman GD: *Helicobacter pylori* infection and the risk of gastric cancer. N Engl J Med 325:1127, 1991. *A large epidemiologic study of H. pylori antibodies in serum; demonstrates a significantly higher odds ratio associated with gastric cancers and lymphoma.*

Shiu MH, Moore E, Sanders M, et al.: Influence of the extent of resection on survival after curative treatment of gastric carcinoma. Arch Surg 122:1347, 1987. *Surgery varies with the size and location of the gastric cancer. This paper presents data and concepts underlying a rational operative approach.*

101 DISORDERS OF GASTROINTESTINAL MOTILITY

William J. Snape, Jr.

NORMAL MOTILITY IN STOMACH, SMALL INTESTINE, AND COLON

Motility of the gastrointestinal tract regulates the orderly movement of ingested material through the gut to ensure adequate absorption of nutrients, electrolytes, and fluid. Transit of intraluminal contents through the stomach, small intestine, and colon depends on the coordination of regional control of intraluminal pressure. Sphincters, interposed at several discrete areas along the length of the bowel, not only regulate the forward movement of intraluminal contents but impede the retrograde flow of intestinal contents. Coordinated gastrointestinal motility depends on neural and hormonal control of sphincter and longitudinal and circular smooth muscle contraction and relaxation.

SMOOTH MUSCLE. Changes in tension of the smooth muscle wall control regional intraluminal pressures, which in return regulate movement of intraluminal contents through the bowel. Movement of luminal contents from the stomach to the distal colon requires coordination between phasic and tonic contractions and relaxation of the intrinsic smooth muscle tone (peristaltic reflex), since luminal contents move from a high-pressure zone to a lower one. Differences in the physiologic control of contraction or relaxation of the muscle in each region determine the local pressure gradients. Myoelectric activity, including slow waves and spike potentials, coordinates regional intestinal smooth muscle contractions by controlling their frequency and by electrically linking neighboring smooth muscle cells (Fig. 101–1). The slow wave is a cyclic

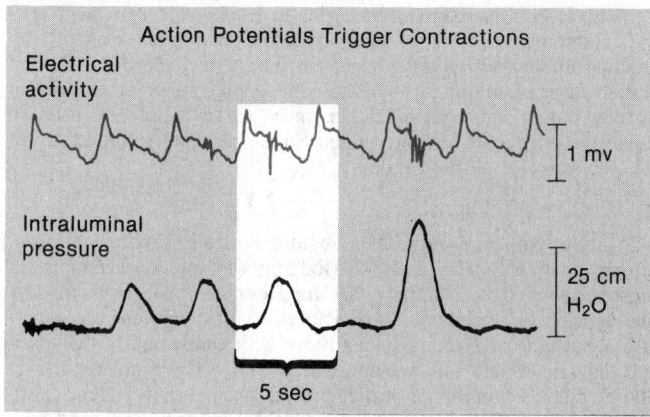

FIGURE 101–1. Simultaneous electrical and mechanical activity in the canine jejunum. The electrical signal was recorded from an extracellular electrode in the tunica muscularis; it shows a regular cycle of depolarization-repolarization at 12 to 14 cycles per minute. Superimposed on some of these cycles (basic electrical rhythm, slow wave, or pace-setter potential) are more rapid oscillations (fast waves, spikes). When spiking occurs, the smooth muscle contracts, causing intraluminal pressure to rise (lower tracing).

change in membrane potential that occurs in smooth muscle from the stomach, small bowel, and colon. The slow wave frequency of a smooth muscle cell is intrinsic to the cell, but it can be modified by the activity in neighboring cells. A pacemaker region sets the dominant frequency of each region of the gastrointestinal tract. Calcium influx during spike potentials, superimposed upon the slow waves, results in smooth muscle cell contraction.

Tight electrical coupling of gastric smooth muscle cells is responsible for progressive propagation of the slow waves, oral to caudal, along the proximal to distal slow wave gradient. Therefore, without a change in the slow wave frequency, contractions also propagate in an oral to caudal direction. In the small intestine and colon, in addition to tight intercellular coupling, regional differences in slow wave and contraction frequency maintain the forward movement of intraluminal contents. A higher contraction frequency elevates mean pressure, stimulating movement of intraluminal contents distally into the lower pressure area. Higher intraluminal pressure in the descending colon creates a pressure gradient that regulates the movement of intraluminal contents back to the transverse colon and forward to the sigmoid colon. Therefore, a pressure amplitude gradient, rather than a frequency gradient, determines colonic transit. In the colon the dominance of contractions in the proximal descending colon and splenic flexure mixes the intraluminal contents and is responsible for a storage area in the transverse colon. Another motility pattern, the propagating contraction, is under neural control and propagates the fecal content distally from the transverse colon for further storage in the sigmoid colon.

Circular and longitudinal muscles have different functions. Circular contractions throughout the gut segment the lumen, mixing the contents to expose the mucosa to continually different contents. The longitudinal muscle shortens the bowel, moving intraluminal contents forward.

Sphincters are high-pressure zones interposed through the gastrointestinal tract. The upper esophageal and external anal sphincter are localized bands of skeletal muscle. The lower esophageal sphincter is not an anatomically distinct structure; in contrast, the pylorus is a localized collection of smooth muscle. The ileocecal valve, a valvelike structure separating the colon and the ileum, responds like a sphincter. The internal anal sphincter is a localized collection of circular smooth muscle surrounded by the external anal sphincter. Sphincter contraction or relaxation is controlled by enteric neurotransmitters or by circulating peptide hormones, in response to changes in pressure in the surrounding bowel or physiologic stimuli, such as eating and emotional stress. In general, proximal distention relaxes all sphincters; distal distention contracts sphincters.

Contraction of gastrointestinal smooth muscle requires an increase in the intracellular calcium concentration. Regulation of intracellular calcium begins at the smooth muscle cell membrane.

When receptors are activated, inositol triphosphate is produced, which releases calcium from the sarcoplasmic reticulum or stimulates opening of voltage or receptor-operated calcium channels. Each of these mechanisms increases intracellular calcium, which is necessary to phosphorylate the myosin light chain, required to form cross-bridges with actin. The rapid actin-myosin cross-bridge formation is associated with a rapid increase in the velocity of smooth muscle shortening. Cross-bridge cycling slows during a prolonged contraction, which conserves muscle energy use.

Relaxation of smooth muscle is equally important for transporting intraluminal contents through the gastrointestinal tract. Cyclic AMP production, initiated by ligand activation of receptors on the smooth muscle cell membrane, decreases intracellular calcium concentration by moving calcium into sarcoplasmic reticulum or out of the cell.

Enteric Nervous System. Enteric neurons contain many different excitatory and inhibitory neurotransmitters (Table 101–1). Many nerve cells release more than one neurotransmitter when stimulated. The complex interaction among inhibitory and excitatory neurotransmitters coordinates bowel activity. Although some neurotransmitters are generally stimulating (e.g., acetylcholine) and others inhibitory (e.g., vasoactive inhibitory polypeptide [VIP]), some neurotransmitters may control the motility pattern through different effects on nerve and muscle (opiates stimulate muscle and inhibit acetylcholine release) or by different regional effects (neurotensin relaxes gastric muscle and stimulates small intestinal and colonic muscles). Nitric oxide (NO) is the prime contender for the final mediator of gastrointestinal smooth muscle relaxation by inducing intracellular cyclic guanosine monophosphate (cGMP). In addition to the efferent neurons, afferent neurons provide important signals for control of motility through relaying sensations from one region of the gut to other regions or to the central nervous system (CNS).

The intrinsic enteric neurons of the gastrointestinal tract have numerous interconnections (Fig. 101–2). Input comes from the CNS, internuncial neurons, and interaction with afferent neurons via the prevertebral ganglia. Sympathetic and cholinergic fibers, which originate in the CNS and travel in the vagus, splanchnic, lumbar colonic, or sacral nerves, regulate the output of neurotransmitters from the myenteric plexus. Control of the myenteric plexus is mediated by intestinal afferent neurons and CNS neurons, interacting in the celiac, superior mesenteric, and inferior mesenteric ganglia. The interaction of interneurons within the myenteric plexus controls neural output to the gut. Each site of neural interconnection may be a potential target for future therapeutic intervention.

Enteric Peptide Hormones. Peptides, released from the gastrointestinal mucosa into the blood after eating, act as hormones and affect gastric, small intestinal, and colonic smooth muscle contractions. As in the enteric nervous system, a counterbalance between stimulating peptides (gastrin, cholecystokinin, and motilin) and inhibitory peptides (enteroglucagon and peptide yy) controls motility. Further flexibility is gained as peptide hormones modulate motility by regional variation in response to a peptide (e.g., cholecystokinin stimulates gallbladder emptying and inhibits gastric emptying). Blood levels of the enteric hormonal peptides reach their maximum approximately 30 to 60 minutes after eating. In contrast to the enteric neurotransmitters, which affect motility soon after the stimulus, the hormones may mediate a delayed gastrointestinal response to eating.

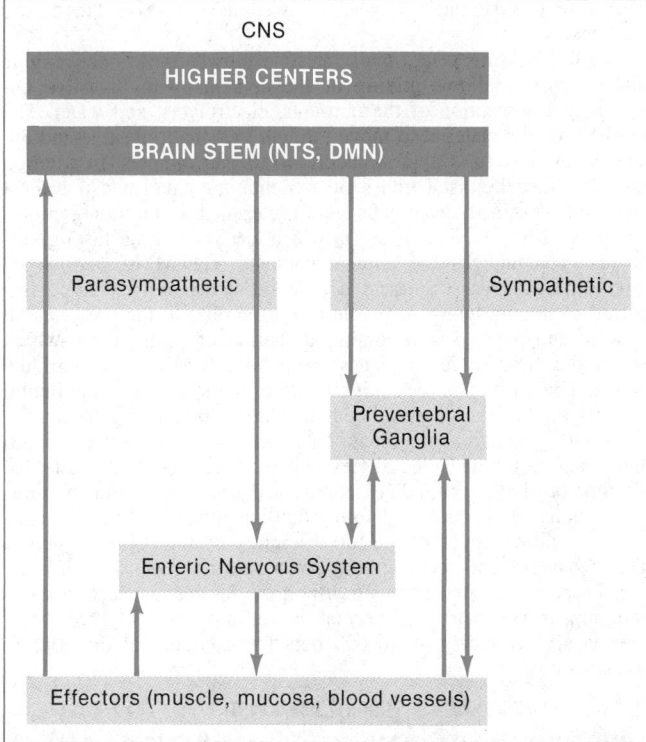

FIGURE 101–2. Schematic diagram showing control levels for neural regulation of gastrointestinal effector function. The enteric nervous system integrates information from the periphery and the central nervous system and modulates effector function. In prevertebral ganglia, afferent inputs from the gut and descending inputs through the sympathetic branch of the autonomic nervous system are integrated into output that has primarily inhibitory effects on gut motility. Autonomic nuclei of sympathetic and parasympathetic nerves located in the brain stem integrate inputs from the periphery and the cortex. Output reaches the gut via the parasympathetic and sympathetic nerves. NTS = Nucleus tractus solitarius; DMN = dorsal motor nucleus. (Adapted from Mayer EA, Raybould H: Role of neural control in gastrointestinal motility and visceral pain. *In* Snape WJ Jr. [ed.]: Pathogenesis of Functional Bowel Disease. New York, Plenum, 1989, pp 13–35.)

In summary, the neurohumoral control of gastrointestinal smooth muscle involves interactions among the CNS, local neural reflexes, and circulating hormones. This control mechanism modulates smooth muscle contraction and regulates the coordinated movement of intraluminal contents through the entire gastrointestinal tract.

Gastrointestinal Transit. Regulated smooth muscle contractions result in coordinated changes in gut intraluminal pressure, which control the transit of chyme through the gastrointestinal tract. Each of the major sections of the gastrointestinal tract has a specific function that requires a different transit pattern. Different transit patterns exist during fasting and after eating. Eating ends the fasting motility pattern and initiates a postprandial transit pattern in each segment of the alimentary tract. Emotional stress and physical exercise modulate these patterns but are not the primary controls.

Stomach. As an initial response to eating, the proximal stomach relaxes to accommodate the volume of a meal. The distal stomach grinds the masticated chunks of food to < 1 mm diameter and regulates the delivery of the processed gastric contents to the intestine synchronous with the release of digestive enzymes. Gastric emptying adjusts to the different physical and chemical characteristics of the food. Liquids are emptied faster ($T_{1/2}$ = 6 to 12 min) than solids ($T_{1/2}$ = 45 to 70 min). Specific chemoreceptors regulate gastric emptying of different substances. Gastric emptying of glucose solutions is regulated so that approximately 2 kcal of glucose is emptied per minute; an equiosmolar solution of saline empties more rapidly. The gastric fundal tone regulates liquid emptying, whereas antral contractions control the rate of solid food emptying.

TABLE 101–1. ENTERIC NEUROTRANSMITTERS AND PEPTIDES AFFECTING GASTROINTESTINAL MOTILITY

Excitatory	Inhibitory
Acetylcholine	Vasoactive inhibitory polypeptide (VIP)
	Nitric oxide
Neurokinins	Calcitonin gene-related peptide
Gastrin-releasing peptide	Adenosine triphosphate
Neurotensin	Neurotensin
Enkephalin	Enkephalin
Cholecystokinin	Somatostatin (high dose)
5-Hydroxytryptamine	Neuropeptide Y
Somatostatin (low dose)	Peptide YY

Therefore, the stomach prepares as well as transports the gastric contents.

Small Intestine. The small intestine slowly moves the chyme distally, which allows mixing of the contents with digestive enzymes and absorption of the nutrients, electrolytes, and water. The transit time for material to move through the small intestine and appear in the cecum is approximately 40 to 180 minutes. In addition to controlling the distal transit of nutrients, the small intestine must clear the extruded dead cells and bacteria. The migrating motor complex (MMC) (Fig. 101–3), which occurs during fasting, removes these indigestible luminal contents. The MMC consists of three different phases: Phase 1 is a period of inactivity; phase 2 is a period of intermittent phasic contractions similar to the postprandial pattern; and phase 3 is a continuous period of contractions, which are at the slow wave frequency indigenous for that region of the bowel. The entire complex migrates from the stomach to the ileum. Phase 3 propels the intestinal contents that remain during fasting.

Colon. Regulation of colonic transit allows the colon to absorb additional water and electrolytes and to store the fecal waste for elimination. Eating stimulates aboral and orad movement of luminal contents. This back and forth shuttling mixes the luminal contents and allows greater time for absorption by the colonic mucosa. The transverse and rectosigmoid colons are separate sites of storage. Propagating contractions transport the luminal contents distally and appear necessary for normal bowel movements. The transit time is approximately 40 to 60 hours for excretion of the colonic content.

CLINICAL ASSESSMENT OF GASTROINTESTINAL MOTILITY

HISTORY AND CLINICAL EXAMINATION. Although symptoms can originate from disturbances of any part of the gastrointestinal tract, particular symptoms may suggest dysfunction of a specific site. In motility disturbances of each of the distinct organs (stomach, small intestine, colon), cramping abdominal pain occurs frequently, often after eating. The pain location can indicate the most likely source—epigastric for stomach, periumbilical or generalized for small intestine, or lower quadrants for the colon. In fact, pain referred from the anatomic location of the colon may occur in any of the abdominal quadrants. Colonic pain resolves after a bowel movement or passing flatus.

Early satiety or postprandial vomiting occurs in patients with delayed transit through the stomach and upper small bowel. Both symptoms can also result from organic nonmotility disorders (e.g., gastritis), which are not discussed in this chapter. Because receptive relaxation of the stomach is usually intact, postprandial vomiting secondary to an obstructed gastric outlet is characteristically voluminous and may not occur until after eating several meals. When disturbed motility causes either symptom, the pathophysiologic defect may be secondary to reduced receptive relaxation, a low threshold for sensory nerve recognition of gastric distention, or uncoordinated antroduodenal contractions. Rapid gastric emptying causes symptoms of the "dumping syndrome," which include sweating, weakness, occasional orthostasis, tachycardia, and diarrhea (see Ch. 99.5).

If massive gastric retention (>750 ml) is present, findings include a soft mass in the left upper quadrant. In a fasting patient, recovery of >150 ml of gastric contents via nasogastric tube, especially if old food is present, suggests gastric retention. An abdominal radiograph shows a large fluid-filled viscus in the left upper quadrant. If the patient is vomiting acutely, nasogastric suction should be initiated for therapy and the hypovolemia and metabolic alkalosis should be treated.

Intestinal pseudo-obstruction may present with symptoms that are difficult to differentiate from those of true obstruction. Abdominal distention and pain occur in both anatomic and functional disorders of the gastrointestinal tract. Distention is an objective physical sign in patients with pseudo-obstruction, but in patients with the irritable bowel syndrome, a bloating sensation may be secondary to a defect in sensory recognition. Tightly fitting clothes are uncomfortable to these patients. There is no increase in bowel gas in patients with the irritable bowel syndrome complaining of abdominal bloating.

Bowel sounds are loud with high-pitched rushes in patients with obstruction. If the obstruction has been present a long time the bowel sounds are quieter or absent. In acute ileus or pseudo-obstruction the bowel sounds are quiet but usually present. If the ileus is associated with a severe abdominal insult, such as peritonitis or surgery, the bowel sounds are absent.

Vomiting is a common symptom of intestinal pseudo-obstruction, acute ileus, and a high anatomic obstruction. If the obstruction is in the distal small intestine, distention is a more prominent complaint than vomiting. In distal obstructions the vomitus, when present, has a feculent odor. An abdominal radiograph usually shows a cut-off between dilated and nondilated bowel in a true obstruction. In acute ileus or pseudo-obstruction the bowel is dilated throughout, with air visible in the rectum.

An alteration in bowel habit (diarrhea or constipation) is the cardinal symptom of motor disorders of the gastrointestinal tract, but these alterations do not specifically identify the pattern of motility. In the absence of a defect in mucosal absorption, diarrhea results from more rapid transit of intestinal contents through either the small intestine or the colon (see Ch. 102). The mechanism of rapid transit through the small intestine is unclear, but diarrhea due to altered colonic motility is associated with an increased frequency of propagating contractions. Constipation generally results from slow colonic transit due to either colonic inertia or increased segmenting contractions, which impede the forward movement of the intraluminal contents. Propagating contractions are markedly decreased or absent in patients with constipation.

The frequency, character, and volume of bowel movements should be carefully defined in each patient. More than three bowel movements a day defines excessive frequency. Stool volume is increased in small bowel–mediated diarrhea, whereas low-volume stools result from disordered colonic motility. Stools may vary in consistency from liquid to merely soft. Constipation is defined as fewer than three bowel movements each week. The constipated stool generally has a lower volume (weight) and is firmer than normal stools, since more water has been absorbed. These strict definitions may exclude the patient complaining of constipation who has stools of normal size and consistency but who strains to defecate. The patient who has only increased straining may have a functional anal outlet obstruction.

MOTILITY TESTS. Regional differences in anatomy and physiologic controls in the gastrointestinal tract require distinct proce-

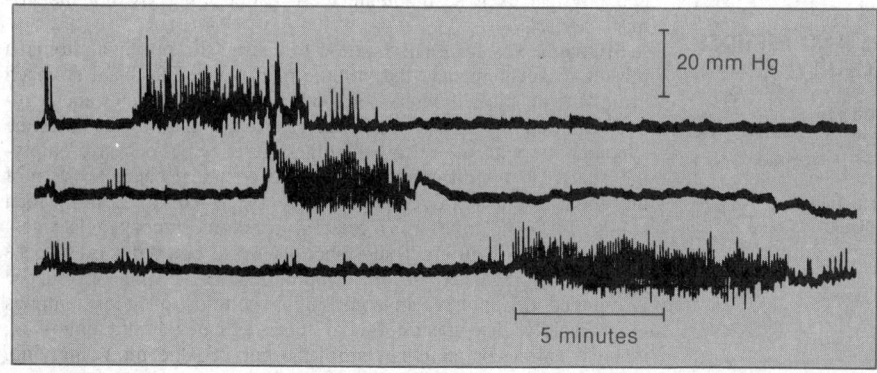

FIGURE 101–3. The activity front of the interdigestive motor complex is characterized on manometric tracings by a burst of rhythmic contraction waves that progress down the intestine. The top tracing is in the distal duodenum. The pressure ports are 25 cm apart. (From Van Trappen G, Janssen SJ, Hellmans J, et al.: The interdigestive motor complex of normal subjects and patients with bacterial overgrowth of the small intestine. J Clin Invest 59:1158, 1977, by copyright permission of the American Society for Clinical Investigation.)

dures to measure motility and transit. In addition to identifying the motility disturbance responsible for the patient's symptoms, standardized motility tests allow objective assessment of response to treatment.

Gastric emptying of liquids and solids must be measured independently to provide a full description of the organ's function. Gastric emptying can be performed simultaneously using different radionuclides to tag the liquid and the solid phases. Bedside assessment of the gastric transit of a bolus of isotonic saline may be a useful and inexpensive screening test. After 30 minutes, the residual should be <40% of an oral volume of 750 ml administered. Estimating gastric emptying from an upper gastrointestinal barium study often does not provide useful information. Changes in gastric fundic pressure can be measured by placing a large balloon in the fundus and measuring the tone before and after a meal. Correlation of the results of the radionuclide emptying with measurement of the antroduodenal motility provides an estimate of the duodenum's contribution to slow gastric emptying. In addition, the presence or absence of the MMC and the amplitude of the phasic contraction may suggest a neuropathic or myopathic cause of the motility disorder. Thus, with an enteric neuropathy, the MMC is absent, whereas with a myopathy, contractions are present but their amplitude is decreased.

Small intestinal transit is measured by different techniques. Breath tests estimate small intestinal transit by reflecting (1) the bacterial metabolism of nonabsorbable carbohydrate marker to H_2, or (2) the bacterial release of a radionuclide label from a bile salt conjugate, both of which increase in the breath after the substrates reach the colon. These tests are invalid if the patient has small intestinal bacterial overgrowth resulting from the motility dysfunction or a blind loop of intestine, since the bacteria release the marker proximal to the ileocecal valve. The appearance in the right lower quadrant (cecum) of a radionuclide-labeled nonabsorbable marker ingested with a meal also provides an estimate of small intestinal transit. Intraluminal pressures measured in the small intestine may document abnormalities in the fasting MMC and the postprandial motility response. As in the stomach, concomitant use of transit and manometric studies allows the contribution of the enteric nerves and smooth muscle to the motility disorder to be estimated objectively.

Global colonic transit can be easily measured by orally administering radiopaque markers and measuring the distribution of the markers throughout the colon 5 days later. If no markers are then present within the colon, the patient probably is not constipated. In the constipated patient localization of the markers to the rectosigmoid region suggests a rectoanal outlet dysfunction. If the markers are distributed throughout the colon, a colonic motility disturbance exists. Regional emptying times can be calculated from this test. Release of radionuclides in the cecum allows regional measurement of colonic transit. Once the motility defect has been localized to the colon, more specific transit and motility tests, measuring increases in intraluminal pressure and segment transit times with radionuclide markers, are available in specialized centers. The absence of a postprandial increase in segmenting contractions suggests a neural lesion, whereas low amplitude or absent postprandial contraction suggests a disturbed smooth muscle function. Anorectal manometry shows whether the anal sphincter contributes to outlet dysfunction. The internal anal sphincter relaxes and the external anal sphincter contracts after the rectum is distended. If this spinal reflex is absent, an abnormality of the enteric neurons controlling the internal anal sphincter is suggested.

Meyer JII: Motility of the stomach and gastroduodenal junction. *In* Johnson LR (ed.): Physiology of the Gastrointestinal Tract. 2nd ed. New York, Raven Press, 1987, pp 613–630. *Comprehensive review of physiology of the region; contains all major references and basic mechanism.*

Rand MJ: Nitric oxide as a mediator of nonadrenergic, noncholinergic neuroeffector transmission. Clin Exp Pharmacol Physiol 19:147, 1992. *Excellent review of nitric oxide's inhibitory role.*

Sarna SK, Otterson MF: Small intestinal physiology and pathophysiology. Gastroenterol Clin North Am 18:375, 1989. *Excellent review of pathophysiology of intestinal motility disorders.*

Willenbucher RF, Snape WJ Jr: Pathophysiology of colinic motility disorders. *In* Haubrich WS, Schaffner F, Berk JE (eds.): Bockus Gastroenterology, 5th ed. Philadelphia, WB Saunders, 1995. *Complete review of associations between alterations in physiology and presentation of colonic disease.*

DISORDERS OF GASTRODUODENAL MOTILITY
Delayed Gastric Emptying

Delayed gastric emptying is a more frequent source of symptoms than is excessively rapid emptying. The only significant cause of excessively rapid emptying, resulting in the "dumping syndrome," is partial gastric resection, the incidence of which is decreasing as the indications for gastric surgery diminish (see Ch. 99.5). Chronic delayed gastric emptying (gastroparesis) is caused most often by an intrinsic disturbance in gastric or upper gastrointestinal motility and requires specific therapy of the underlying neuromuscular disorder. Acute gastroparesis, which is most frequently associated with an electrolyte disturbance, ketoacidosis, systemic infection, or an acute abdominal insult, is managed by treating the underlying disease, not the gastric motility disorder.

Delayed gastric emptying may be associated with other systemic diseases or may be due to a primary dysfunction of the stomach (Table 101–2). The typical symptoms of delayed gastric emptying include early satiety, nausea, and vomiting. Phytobezoars sometimes occur in these patients as well, especially if the MMC is absent.

DELAYED GASTRIC EMPTYING COMPLICATING GASTRIC SURGERY. Delayed gastric emptying not infrequently complicates gastric surgery for peptic ulcer disease. Vagotomy, with the exception of the highly selective vagotomy (parietal cell vagotomy), decreases fundic relaxation, antral contractions, and coordinated relaxation of the pylorus. The expected physiologic response to vagotomy is rapid emptying of liquids, possibly predisposing the patient to dumping syndrome, and slow emptying of solids. Although most often patients have no gastric symptoms following abdominal vagotomy, approximately 5 to 10% have delayed gastric emptying. This complication is more likely to occur if the patient had gastric outlet obstruction caused by a primary disease. Antral contractions are poorly coordinated owing to irregular antral slow wave activity. Gastric MMC activity is often absent, although intestinal MMC remains normal.

Metoclopramide, a putative dopamine receptor antagonist, improves symptoms in many patients with delayed gastric emptying after a vagotomy. The usual dose of metoclopramide (10 mg orally, four times a day) can cause anxiety, fatigue, or sedation in about 15% of patients. Domperidone, also a dopamine antagonist, does not cross the blood-brain barrier and has fewer CNS side effects but is investigational in the United States. Cisapride, which releases acetylcholine from the enteric neurons, may be useful in gastroparesis. Erythromycin, a macrolide antibiotic, initiates phase 3 in the stomach, improving gastroparesis symptoms.

Roux-en-Y anastomoses after gastric resection occasionally cause poor gastric emptying, especially of solids (see Ch. 99.4). The MMC and the postprandial motor response are abnormal in the roux limb. Delayed gastric emptying of solids is the major functional disturbance; liquid gastric emptying may be normal. Patients with severe vomiting can be treated with subcutaneous bethanechol, further gastric resection, or elimination of the roux loop. The patient's symptoms may be recalcitrant to other prokinetic agents, such as metoclopramide or cisapride. Leuprolide may reduce symptoms in some patients.

TABLE 101–2. GASTRIC MOTILITY DISORDERS

Delayed gastric emptying
Postvagotomy
Diabetes mellitus
Viral infections
Reflux esophagitis
Brain stem lesions
Anorexia nervosa
Tachygastria
Rapid gastric emptying
Dumping syndrome
Pancreatic insufficiency
Celiac sprue
Zollinger-Ellison syndrome
Duodenal ulcer

DIABETIC GASTROPARESIS. Delayed gastric emptying complicating diabetic ketoacidosis resolves as the patient improves, but the stomach is sometimes massively distended, exhibits mucosal bleeding, and may require decompression by nasogastric tube. Chronic delayed gastric emptying, associated with longstanding insulin-dependent diabetes mellitus, is a greater clinical problem. Such patients have frequent episodes of nausea and vomiting, which affect food intake and complicate insulin requirements. Retinopathy, nephropathy, peripheral neuropathy, and other complications are commonly present. Absence of the gastric MMC, necessary for emptying of nondigestible material >1 mm, predisposes the diabetic patient to bezoars, causing abdominal discomfort, early satiety, and vomiting. Vagal neuropathy is thought to be the pathogenesis of gastric stasis in diabetes mellitus, although a demonstrable autonomic neuropathy is not always present. Early in the patient's course gastric emptying of liquids may be rapid, although in many patients emptying of liquids is slow from the onset of symptoms. Gastric emptying of solids is slow throughout the disease.

Metoclopramide improves the symptoms of gastric stasis in patients with diabetes mellitus both by increasing gastric emptying and decreasing the CNS recognition of nausea and distention. Gastric emptying is rarely normalized after treatment with metoclopramide, even though symptoms may be completely alleviated. Bethanechol also stimulates an increase in gastric motility and improves symptoms in patients with diabetic gastric stasis. Cisapride, which has no demonstrated CNS effect, improves both symptoms and gastric emptying. Cisapride also improves the emptying of nondigestible solids and may prevent the occurrence of bezoars. Erythromycin improves symptoms of gastroparesis.

ANOREXIA NERVOSA. This psychiatric disorder, which occurs predominantly in young women, is characterized by excessive weight loss (see Ch. 195). The gastric emptying of solids, but not of liquids, is slowed in patients with anorexia nervosa, but not in patients with bulimia. The delayed gastric emptying is associated with antral dysrhythmia, fundal hypotonia, decreased postprandial plasma concentrations of norepinephrine and neurotensin, and impaired autonomic function (decreased resting diastolic blood pressure and skin conductance). The mechanism causing delayed gastric emptying is unclear. Patients with equal weight loss but without the psychiatric disorder do not have delayed gastric emptying. Interestingly, gastric emptying in obese patients is more rapid than in healthy subjects.

Repleting the patient's calories improves gastric emptying in the absence of prokinetic medicine. Bethanechol, metoclopramide, and cisapride increase the emptying of solids by stimulating antral motility. The ultimate success of prokinetic drugs for anorexia nervosa is unclear, since they treat only the peripheral symptom of gastric emptying. Reversal of the underlying psychiatric disturbance appears necessary for complete resolution of symptoms.

MISCELLANEOUS CAUSES. *Tachygastria* is a condition of unknown etiology which presents as intractable vomiting that causes failure to thrive in infants and vomiting in young adults. Tachygastria is caused by rapid slow wave activity in the antral smooth muscle segment, which becomes the dominant pacemaker initiating orad propagating contractions. Parvovirus-like agents (Norwalk or Hawaii viruses) can slow gastric emptying. The decreased gastric emptying associated with an acute viral infection usually resolves quickly. Up to 25% of patients with reflux esophagitis, associated with an incompetent lower esophageal sphincter, have delayed gastric emptying, which must be corrected in order to treat the reflux esophagitis adequately. Lesions such as tumors, infarction, or viral encephalitis that affect the vagal complex in the medulla can delay gastric emptying.

Rapid Gastric Emptying

Rapid gastric emptying occurs in some patients with duodenal ulcer disease and Zollinger-Ellison syndrome as a result of duodenal insensitivity to an acid load. Rapid liquid emptying occurs in patients with pancreatic insufficiency and possibly with celiac sprue because of poor feedback inhibition of gastric motility by fat due to a maldigestion or malabsorption. The dumping syndrome is discussed in Ch. 99.5.

Malagelada JR, Azpiroz F, Mearin F: Gastroduodenal motor function in health and disease. *In* Sleisenger MH, Fordtran JJ, et al. (eds.): Gastrointestinal Disease. 5th ed. Philadelphia, WB Saunders, 1993, pp 486–508. *Comprehensive review of pathophysiology of gastroduodenal motility disorder; complete bibliography.*

DISORDERS OF SMALL INTESTINAL MOTILITY

Motility disorders of the small intestine can be most usefully categorized by their respective motility patterns, although some symptom complexes (e.g., postprandial bloating) foil simple categorization. Small intestinal motility may be hypoactive, hyperactive, or uncoordinated. Decreased intestinal motility reflects either absent or fewer contractions of phase 3 of the MMC during fasting or a minimal increase in postprandial motility in the different regions of the small bowel. Conversely, increased motility is reflected in increased numbers of fasting MMC's or an augmented intraluminal pressure response to eating. Uncoordinated intestinal motility can be caused by retrograde MMC's and clustered contractions. For rational therapy it is important to determine if the decreased intestinal motility is due to a neuropathy or a myopathy. In general, increased or uncoordinated motility is secondary to neural dysfunction. A disease may affect both the enteric nerves and smooth muscle and may involve different abnormalities in motility during its course (e.g., progressive systemic sclerosis). Table 101–3 lists the conditions associated with chronic disordered small intestinal motility.

In patients with motility disorders, qualitatively similar transit patterns may result in different symptoms. For example, patients with the irritable bowel syndrome may have delayed small intestinal transit that results in constipation. In contrast, a patient with pseudo-obstruction may have a greater delay in intestinal transit that results in diarrhea due to bacterial overgrowth. Therefore, symptoms may not be helpful in determining the cause of a disease.

Patients with slow intestinal transit tend to complain of nausea, vomiting, abdominal distention, and periumbilical abdominal cramps. Although constipation can occur with delayed intestinal transit, diarrhea is more common. Phase 3 of the MMC—in which bacteria and sloughed, dead epithelial cells are propelled from the small intestine into the colon—is often absent or severely deranged by an enteric neuropathy. Bacterial overgrowth due to a diminished number of MMC contractions deconjugates bile salts, causing steatorrhea and diarrhea. The absence of postprandial motility impedes the normal transit through the small intestine.

Diarrhea is generally the result of rapid intestinal transit because of decreased time of contact of the luminal contents with the mucosa. The patients also may have maldigestion and malabsorption due to poor mixing of the dietary material with the digestive enzymes and bile salts. Accentuated borborygmi may also disturb the patient.

Decreased Intestinal Motility

HOLLOW VISCERAL MYOPATHY (PRIMARILY INTESTINAL PSEUDO-OBSTRUCTION). This disorder is the prototype for myopathic diseases of the small intestine. The disease generally displays vacuolized and degenerated smooth muscle in the

TABLE 101–3. SMALL INTESTINAL MOTILITY DISORDERS

Decreased motility
Hollow visceral myopathy (primary intestinal pseudo-obstruction)
Progressive systemic sclerosis (late)
Amyloidosis
Muscular dystrophy
   Duchenne's
   Myotonic
Hypothyroidism
Jejunal diverticulosis
Jejunoileal bypass
Increased or uncoordinated motility
Primary visceral neuropathy
Carcinoma-associated visceral neuropathy
Progressive systemic sclerosis (early)
Irritable bowel syndrome
Diabetes mellitus
Infectious diarrhea
Mass lesion of brain stem
Amyloidosis
Hyperthyroidism
Carcinoid syndrome
Shy-Drager syndrome

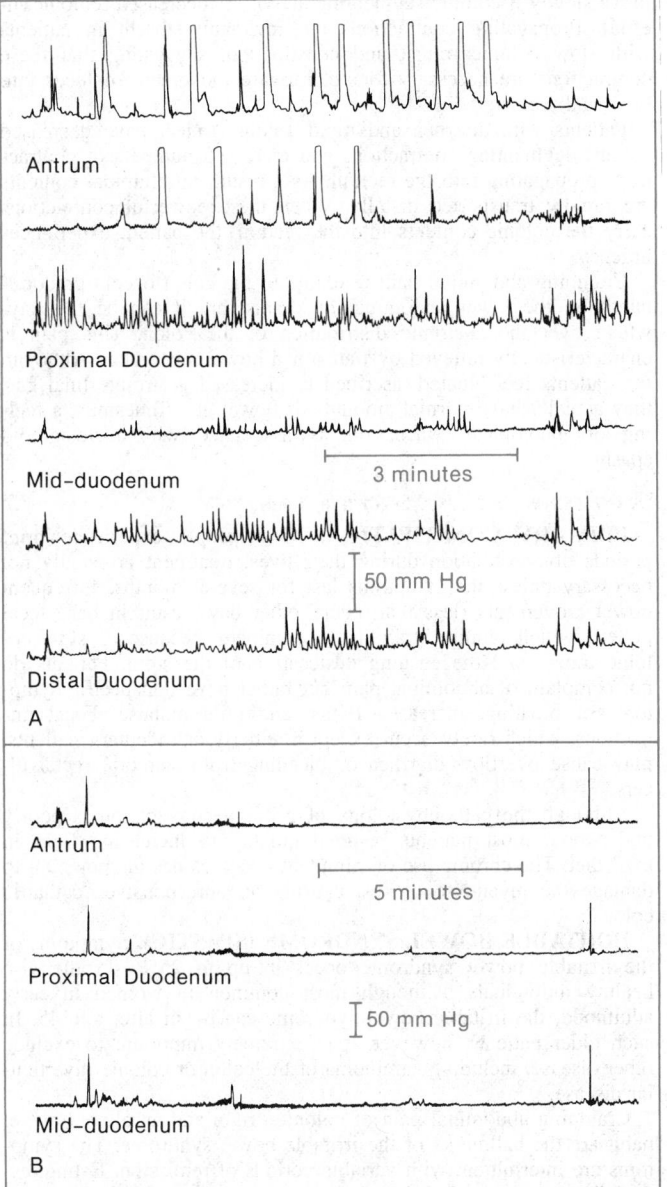

FIGURE 101–4. Postprandial gastroduodenal manometry recordings from a healthy subject *(A)* and a patient with myopathic pseudo-obstruction *(B)*. The postprandial response is decreased in the patient with pseudo-obstruction. (From Hyman PE: Absent postprandial duodenal motility in a child with cystic fibrosis: Correction of the symptoms and manometric abnormality with Cisapride. Gastroenterology 90:1274–1279, 1986.)

circular or longitudinal layers, separately or together, without affecting the enteric nerves. In some cases the muscle is not histologically altered. Defective slow wave generation or actin-myosin cross-bridge formation may cause the decreased muscle contraction. The contractions are decreased in amplitude and number, but usually the MMC is present because the nerves are unaffected (Fig. 101–4). The MMC may function poorly, however, because of the low-amplitude contractions. The motility pattern differs from that associated with a partial small bowel obstruction in which 3 to 10 clustered contractions occur regularly, separated by 1-minute intervals of quiescence.

Patients usually present with symptoms and signs of small intestinal stasis without evidence of an anatomic obstruction or of a secondary cause for pseudo-obstruction (Table 101–3). Hollow visceral myopathy is familial, but random, nonfamilial cases are probably more common. With familial primary intestinal pseudo-obstruction, parts of the urinary system (bladder, renal pelvis) may also be dilated as a result of abnormal smooth muscle contraction. Familial visceral myopathy is also associated with a high incidence of intestinal malrotation.

Anatomic bowel obstruction or acute ileus must be excluded be-

fore the diagnosis of pseudo-obstruction is made. Acute adynamic ileus occurs most frequently after abdominal surgery, peritonitis, intra-abdominal vascular accidents, or a severe electrolyte imbalance. Ileus or obstruction can cause hypovolemia or third-space accumulation of fluid. The signs and symptoms of acute ileus are similar to those of chronic disorders of decreased intestinal motility, but in contrast treatment of the initiating cause resolves the symptoms. Acute ileus or obstruction is treated by decompression via a nasogastric tube, replacement of fluid volume, and correction of electrolyte and acid-base imbalances.

The therapy of hollow visceral myopathy is generally highly unsatisfactory. Metoclopramide has little efficacy in treating patients with pseudo-obstruction, but the newer prokinetic agent cisapride shows promise for treating severe small intestinal motility disorders, especially in those patients with postprandial hypomotility with a normal fasting pattern. Intestinal bypass surgery should be avoided in patients with pseudo-obstruction. Occasionally antibiotics may be of help if a blind loop syndrome with bacterial overgrowth is present.

PROGRESSIVE SYSTEMIC SCLEROSIS (see Ch. 241). This is the most common "collagen vascular disease" to cause disordered intestinal motility, although polymyositis and systemic lupus erythematosus may rarely do so. Approximately 40% of patients with progressive systemic sclerosis have defects in both neural and smooth muscle of the intestine. Early in the course of the disease, signs of neuropathy predominate, whereas collagen later replaces smooth muscle and myopathy becomes the major component of the disease. In symptomatic patients, characteristically postprandial motility is markedly reduced. Since a neuropathy is often present, the MMC's are absent. In general patients become symptomatic only after extensive replacement of the smooth muscle with collagen. In contrast to hollow visceral myopathy, muscle cells in progressive systemic sclerosis are decreased in number but morphologically normal. Since the number of functional smooth muscle cells is decreased, pharmacologic stimulation with prokinetic drugs is generally unsuccessful. However, low doses of the somatostatin analogue octreotide stimulate phase 3 of the MMC and improve symptoms in systemic sclerosis.

OTHER CONDITIONS. *Amyloidosis* of the small intestine may cause either a myopathy or a neuropathy, depending on its distribution. Several of the *muscular dystrophy* syndromes may affect the intestinal smooth muscle in addition to skeletal and cardiac muscle. *Hypothyroidism* decreases the slow wave frequency and amplitude of contraction of the intestine, which may result in atony. *Jejunal diverticulosis* is secondary to pseudo-obstruction, which predominantly involves the small intestine. The histologic pattern is similar to that of progressive systemic sclerosis in most patients, although some patients have neuropathy.

Increased or Uncoordinated Motility

VISCERAL NEUROPATHY. Intestinal motility can be increased, as well as uncoordinated, in patients with visceral neuropathy because of a decrease in neural inhibition. The hallmark of visceral neuropathy is a patchy loss of nerve tracts, a decreased number of neurons, or fragmentation and dropout of axons. Specialized silver stains are needed for the accurate histologic diagnosis of an enteric neuropathy.

Primary visceral neuropathy can be familial or random. Familial cases may be associated with other neural lesions, including mild autonomic insufficiency, mental retardation, altered sensory recognition of position, and absent deep tendon reflexes. Random cases may be secondary to injury from a viral infection or an environmental toxin or to carcinomatous neuropathy (see Ch. 160). The motility patterns associated with visceral neuropathy vary, probably because different disease complexes have not been separated at this time. In general, during fasting a neuropathy disrupts either the propagation or configuration of the MMC. In some patients the MMC may be absent. Eating may initiate no contractions, or uncoordinated contractions, or may fail to inhibit MMC's in patients with neuropathy.

IRRITABLE BOWEL SYNDROME. In this common disorder, to be discussed more fully under colonic disorders, symptoms of abdominal pain and an altered bowel habit consistent with the irritable bowel syndrome may be associated with abnormal motility in the small intestine as well as in the colon. Balloon distention of the small intestine provokes characteristic abdominal pain in some patients. Two patterns of contractions, "discrete clustered contractions" and "prolonged propagated contractions," are associated with abdominal pain more frequently in patients with the irritable bowel syndrome than in healthy control subjects.

DIABETES MELLITUS. The diarrhea associated with diabetes mellitus is most likely due to small intestinal motility disturbances. Abnormal manometric patterns in diabetics, who also have gastroparesis, include decreased motility or uncoordinated bursts of small intestinal contractions. The MMC's can be present, deranged, or absent in diabetic patients. Patients with a central autonomic nervous system disturbance, Shy-Drager syndrome, have similar findings to patients with diabetes (see Ch. 402). Diabetic diarrhea may respond to treatment with the α_2-adrenergic agent clonidine.

OTHER DISORDERS. *Infectious diarrhea* (e.g., due to enterotoxigenic *E. coli* or *Shigella*) initiates a significant motility disorder, characterized experimentally by powerful aborad migrating contractions. *Brain stem mass lesions* can either slow the small intestinal MMC or initiate an activity front simultaneously at different levels of the small intestine, by affecting the vagal motor complex and the autonomic nuclei in the medullary reticular formation. *Amyloid* can affect the enteric nerves of the small intestine as well as replace smooth muscle. *Hyperthyroidism* increases the slow wave frequency of the bowel, which is a possible cause of the frequently associated diarrhea. *Carcinoid syndrome* with increased 5-hydroxytryptamine (5-HT) production increases the migration velocity of the MMC and increases the cycling frequency.

Lynn RB, Friedman LS: Irritable bowel syndrome. N Engl J Med 329:1940, 1993. *Up-to-date review of the syndrome; 71 references.*
Malagelada J-R, Camilleri M, Stanghellini V: Manometric Diagnosis of Gastrointestinal Motility Disorders. New York, Thieme-Stratton, 1986. *A monograph on the diagnosis of motility disorders but dealing also with normal physiology and the pathophysiology of the common and uncommon disorders of motility. The bibliography is extensive and will guide the reader into any area.*
Kellow JE, Phillips SF: Functional disorders of the small intestine. In Snape WJ Jr. (ed.): Pathogenesis of Functional Bowel Disease. New York, Plenum, 1989, pp 171–198. *Extensive discussion of pathophysiology of small intestinal motility disturbance; extensive bibliography.*

DISORDERS OF COLON MOTILITY

Orderly transit of contents through the colon "fine tunes" the absorption of salt and water. If the transit is too slow, the mucosa can extract too much water and the stool becomes hard, resulting in constipation. Rapid transit causes frequent, soft stools. Diarrhea caused by colonic motility disorders is low in volume (< 400 ml per day), since most intestinal fluid is absorbed in the small intestine (see Ch. 102). Table 101–4 lists the diseases or syndromes that cause disordered colonic motility. Many of the systemic diseases that affect gastric and small intestinal motility also alter colonic motility.

Either increased or decreased segmenting contractions can slow transit through the colon. A functional partial obstruction results from increased segmenting contractions, since the segmentation impedes movement of colonic contents. The colonic contents also

TABLE 101–4. PATHOGENESIS OF COLONIC MOTILITY DISORDERS

Slow transit
  Increased segmenting contraction
    Primary constipation
    Irritable bowel syndrome (spastic)
    Diverticular disease
    Anal outlet obstruction
      Congenital—Hirschsprung's disease
      Acquired
  Decreased segmenting contractions
    Irritable bowel syndrome (inertia)
    Primary colonic pseudo-obstruction
    Ogilvie's syndrome
    Diabetes mellitus
    Progressive systemic sclerosis
    Spinal cord injury
Rapid transit
  Functional diarrhea
  Bile salt diarrhea
  Surreptitious abuse of laxatives

move slowly if colonic segmenting activity is decreased (colonic inertia). Propagating contractions are invariably absent in patients with slow colonic transit and constipation, suggesting that these contractions are necessary for net forward movement of feces into the distal rectosigmoid.

Patients with diarrhea and rapid colonic transit have decreased colonic segmenting contractions and increased numbers of contractions propagating into the rectum. As a result, intraluminal contents are rapidly transported distally. When these powerful contractions carry the colonic contents into the rectum, the patient experiences urgency.

Cramping abdominal pain referable to the colon occurs predominantly in the lower abdominal quadrants, but it can be felt anywhere over the anatomic distribution of the colon. This pain is characteristically relieved by flatus or a bowel movement. Although the patients feel bloated, ascribed to increased gastrointestinal gas, they actually have normal amounts of bowel gas. Tenesmus, a feeling of incomplete evacuation, is associated with rectosigmoid spasm.

Slow Transit with Increased Segmenting Contractions

PRIMARY CONSTIPATION. Most people experience brief periods of constipation during their lives; treatment is usually not necessary unless the symptoms last for several months. Infrequent bowel movements (less than every other day) result in hard fecal pellets, which require straining to eliminate, because of slow colonic transit and the ensuing desiccation of the stool. Patients do not complain of abdominal pain but rather have nonspecific symptoms of bloating, increased flatus, and mild malaise. Fecal impactions, which rarely occur except in elderly or sedentary patients, may cause overflow diarrhea or bleeding from stercoral rectal ulcers.

Although the pathophysiology of primary constipation is poorly understood, most patients respond quickly to increasing fiber in their diet. The chronic use of stimulant laxatives has the potential to damage the myenteric plexus, causing an unresponsive "cathartic colon."

IRRITABLE BOWEL SYNDROME (SPASTIC). Symptoms of the irritable bowel syndrome occur in up to 25% of otherwise healthy individuals. Although most common in women in early adulthood, the irritable bowel syndrome can begin after age 45. In such older patients, however, it is extremely important to exclude other disease, including carcinoma of the colon or colonic diverticular disease.

Cramping abdominal pain of colonic origin and an altered bowel habit are the hallmarks of the irritable bowel syndrome. The symptoms are intermittent with variable periods of remission. Eating, especially a large meal with a high fat content, or episodes of emotional stress increase the pain. Constipation alternating with an increased frequency of low-volume stools is the "classic" bowel pattern, although patients may have more frequent looser stools at the onset of an attack or may complain only of constipation. A perception of uncomfortable abdominal distention as well as increased fecal mucus are common adjunctive symptoms.

Patients with constipation-predominant irritable bowel syndrome have an increased prevalence of colonic slow waves at a frequency of 3 cycles per minute compared with normal individuals. In approximately 60% of patients with constipation-predominant irritable bowel syndrome, segmenting contractions are increased after a meal, whereas in the remainder no increase in motility and little mixing movement of the fecal contents in the colon occur. The increased segmenting contractions shuttle the colonic contents back and forth in the transverse and descending colon. When present, the normal increase in postprandial motility is delayed. Subtle differences exist in symptoms in the two groups of patients; nausea and vomiting are more prominent symptoms in patients with little postprandial motility (colonic inertia). Propagating contractions are absent in both groups of patients.

Balloon distention of the rectum or other regions of the colon causes abdominal pain at a lower threshold in patients with the irritable bowel syndrome than in healthy people. This is not a generalized increase in pain perception because the patients generally feel less somatic pain. The abnormal pathophysiology in visceral sensory nerves and in colonic motility combines to cause the classic symptoms of the irritable bowel syndrome.

The diagnosis of the irritable bowel syndrome requires exclusion of other diseases. Functional diarrhea, variably lumped into the irritable bowel syndrome, is discussed in detail later in reference to rapid transit. The rigor used to exclude the diagnosis of other diseases should depend on the age and clinical presentation of the patient. The major differential diagnoses include carcinoma of the colon, diverticulitis, and inflammatory bowel disease. After a careful history and physical examination, the stool should be examined for occult blood. Patients over age 40 should have colonoscopy or barium enema to exclude anatomic colonic disease. If the symptoms persist, especially that of diarrhea, the terminal ileum should be visualized to exclude inflammatory bowel disease (see Ch. 104).

Once organic disease is excluded, the irritable bowel syndrome is best treated by reassuring the patient, explaining the cause of symptoms, and instituting some alterations of the diet. Decreasing dietary fat reduces colonic intraluminal pressure. Increasing soluble and insoluble dietary fiber decreases water net absorption and intraluminal pressure, respectively. Pharmacologic agents should be used only if counseling and dietary changes do not affect symptoms. Anticholinergics, the next line of therapy, decrease the colonic contractions and may relieve symptoms. Combined therapy with dietary fiber supplements and anticholinergics has enhanced efficacy. Low-dose tricyclic antidepressants increase the sensory afferent nerve threshold, decreasing pain. Octreotide or certain of the 5-HT$_3$ antagonists (ganisetron) also decrease pain. Diarrhea and fecal continence may improve following a dietary fiber supplement owing to increased bulk. Anxiolytics or antidepressants should be used only after documenting a psychoneurosis.

ACQUIRED DIVERTICULAR DISEASE OF THE COLON. Diverticular disease, mucosal outpouchings through the colonic wall that occur with aging, results in a spectrum of abnormalities extending from no symptoms to diverticulitis.

Acquired diverticula, which occur most frequently in the left colon, result from increased intraluminal pressure pushing sleeves of mucosa through perivascular weaknesses in the wall of the colon juxtaposed to the taeniae coli. The predilection for the left colon results from the decreased colonic diameter there leading to increased pressures, as predicted by Laplace's law: Intraluminal pressure is directly correlated with wall tension and inversely correlated with bowel diameter. Decreased dietary fiber and distal colonic smooth muscle hypertrophy contribute to elevation in distal colonic intraluminal pressure.

The symptoms of *painful colonic diverticular disease* are similar to those of irritable bowel syndrome but are more likely to be localized in the left lower quadrant. When *diverticulitis* occurs as a complication, the patient may have similar symptoms as well as fever, left lower quadrant mass, leukocytosis, and occult blood in the stool (see Ch. 112). Gross hematochezia is more frequent in asymptomatic patients with diverticula. Diverticula can be diagnosed by barium enema or colonoscopy. Muscular hypertrophy gives a saw-tooth pattern visible on barium enema. Narrowing due to diverticular inflammation can be difficult to differentiate from carcinoma of the colon.

Painful diverticular disease of the colon is best treated by decreasing the intraluminal pressure, similar to the therapy in the irritable bowel syndrome. Narcotics, especially morphine, should be avoided because of an exaggerated increase in smooth muscle contraction.

ANAL OUTLET OBSTRUCTION. Constipation may result from a disturbance in the elimination of stool through the anal sphincter. Elimination normally begins by the involuntary relaxation of the internal anal sphincter after distention of the rectum. The patient uses voluntary control to open the rectoanal angle and relax the external anal sphincter. A disturbance of any component of this mechanism leads to constipation.

Hirschsprung's disease is the congenital absence of enteric neurons in the submucosal and myenteric plexuses, due to an arrest of the embryonic caudad migration of the enteric neurons along the gut. The aganglionic segment remains contracted, dilating the proximal normal bowel. The severity of symptoms and the age at diagnosis are related to the length of the aganglionic segment. Involvement of the rectum or additional parts of the colon results in constipation or obstipation in infancy, requiring emergent resection of the aganglionic bowel and a pull-through anastomosis to the anus.

Abnormalities in anal physiology are a significant cause of constipation; impaired anal sphincter relaxation occurs relatively frequently in adults. The absent rectoanal reflex may be secondary to a short aganglionic segment (short-segment Hirschsprung's disease),

to chronic distention with a fecal impaction, or to an insufficient distention stimulus due to an enlarged rectal vault. In acquired megacolon, relaxation of the internal anal sphincter may be impaired if a large volume is not used to distend the rectum. Some patients have subtle histologic abnormalities in the myenteric plexus, suggesting that an acquired neuropathy may also account for the abnormal sphincter response. In the spastic pelvic floor syndrome (animus) the external anal sphincter and the puborectalis relax poorly or the levator ani contracts poorly, leading to impaired opening of the rectoanal angle. This acquired condition, which occurs more often in multiparous women, can prevent normal stool evacuation. Anal outlet dysfunction can be diagnosed as a cause of constipation by observing the accumulation of the fecal markers in the rectum and impaired anal sphincter relaxation after rectal distention or attempted defecation.

Impaired internal anal sphincter relaxation in an adult may respond to a posterior anal sphincter myomectomy. Patients who have difficulty in opening the rectoanal angle or who have animus may sometimes respond to biofeedback training.

Slow Transit With Decreased Segmenting Contractions

Patients with decreased segmenting contractions have symptoms similar to those in patients with increased contractions. The colonic inertia form of the irritable bowel syndrome and primary colonic pseudo-obstruction may be a similar pathophysiologic disturbance. Postprandial increases in colonic motility are absent in both, but the colon is dilated in primary intestinal pseudo-obstruction, explaining the increased incidence of abdominal distention. Constipation is a major symptom in both conditions. Ogilvie's syndrome is a form of primary colonic pseudo-obstruction, often paraneoplastic.

Constipation is present in many patients with longstanding, insulin-requiring diabetes mellitus, progressive systemic sclerosis, or thoracic spinal cord lesions. Colonic motility is not increased postprandially in these patients. In the patients with diabetes or spinal cord lesions, colonic smooth muscle can be stimulated with exogenous drugs, suggesting a neural lesion, not a myopathy. In progressive systemic sclerosis the colon cannot increase intraluminal pressure after drug stimulation, as expected in a neuropathy.

It is difficult to treat patients with decreased colonic motility. In patients with neuropathy and normal smooth muscle function, prokinetic drugs have had some success. In myopathy it is unlikely that pharmacologic stimulation will have much effect.

Rapid Transit

FUNCTIONAL DIARRHEA. Some patients have functional, painless diarrhea with fecal urgency but with no associated anatomic or histologic abnormality of the gastrointestinal tract. These patients present with small frequent stools, consistent with a large bowel abnormality, and fecal incontinence is relatively frequent because their anal sphincters cannot retard evacuation of liquid stool. Lactose intolerance must be excluded either by history or by a lactose tolerance test. The diarrhea is greater than that in the spastic irritable colon syndrome, and abdominal pain may be absent.

Segmenting postprandial contractile activity is decreased in functional diarrhea. Propagating contractions are increased and propagate into the rectum, possibly accounting for the increased urgency and fecal incontinence in these patients. The lack of segmenting contractions to impede forward movement or transit may exacerbate the urgency. Specific foods may stimulate increased prostaglandin E$_2$ production by the colon, which could initiate the diarrhea. Increased concentrations of fecal bile salts, which occur in some patients, may also contribute to the functional diarrhea. Bile salts irritate colonic sensory nerves and thereby stimulate frequent propagating contractions in the colon by irritating sensory nerves.

Microscopic or collagenous colitis presents as functional diarrhea without obvious anatomic abnormalities. The diagnoses can be made by histologic examination of the rectal biopsy.

In treating functional diarrhea, antidiarrheal agents such as the opioid analogues, loperamide, and diphenoxylate are used to decrease symptoms. Fecal continence improves as the stool consistency becomes firmer. Some patients may require biofeedback training to maintain continence. If excess bile salts contribute to the diarrhea, low doses of cholestyramine may decrease the diarrhea.

Microscopic and collagenous colitis may respond to 5-aminosalicylic compounds. 5-HT$_3$ antagonists decrease fluid content of stool.

Surreptitious Laxative Abuse. Surreptitious laxative abuse is a common cause of functional diarrhea (see Ch. 102). Oxyphenisatin and bisacodyl stimulate increased numbers of propagating contractions and diarrhea. Patients may take these or other laxatives as a manifestation of a psychiatric disorder. It is a challenge to the physician to make the correct diagnosis.

Ulcerative Colitis. Rapid transit of colonic contents, in addition to increased mucosal secretion, occurs in patients with active ulcerative colitis. As in the other colonic causes of diarrhea, propagating contractions are increased in number and propagate into the rectum, accounting for the significant incidence of fecal incontinence. The rapid transit improves as the mucosal inflammation decreases after therapy for the underlying inflammation (see Ch. 104).

Devroede GJ: Constipation. *In* Sleisenger MH, Fordtran JS (eds.): Gastrointestinal Disease. 4th ed. Philadelphia, WB Saunders, 1993, pp 837–887. *This is a complete examination of the pathophysiology and treatment of constipation.*

Snape WJ Jr: Irritable bowel syndrome. *In* Haubrich WS, Schaffer F, Berk JE (eds.): Bockus Gastroenterology. 5th ed. Philadelphia, WB Saunders, 1995. *Summary of the field with extensive reference list.*

DRUGS THAT AFFECT GASTROINTESTINAL MOTILITY

As understanding of the pathophysiology of gastrointestinal motility disorders grows, the number and the diversity of the drugs that are available for therapy increases (Table 101–5). Drugs that stimulate motility may indiscriminately increase smooth muscle contractions or increase a specific motility function, such as MMC initiation. Many of the drugs on the list, used to treat other systemic diseases, may precipitate gastrointestinal symptoms as a side effect.

Excitatory Agents

Drugs that excite the gastrointestinal tract should be used to treat decreased motility when the smooth muscle can functionally contract. In general, patients who benefit from these agents have an enteric neuropathy with decreased release of endogenous stimulatory neurotransmitters or an increased release of inhibitory neurotransmitters. When the smooth muscle is absent or severely damaged, the prokinetic drugs are rarely helpful. Acetylcholine analogues, such as bethanechol, stimulate both longitudinal and circular gastrointestinal smooth muscle by directly binding to the M$_2$ muscarinic receptor to release inositol triphosphate or to open receptor-operated or voltage-dependent calcium channels. Drugs that block acetylcholinesterase increase endogenous acetylcholine concentration at the myoneural junction. These drugs have a theoretical advantage in regulating as well as in increasing motility, since the distribution of acetylcholine release is predetermined by the autonomic nervous system.

Dopamine antagonists can variably increase motility throughout the gastrointestinal tract. Metoclopramide, a centrally and peripherally acting dopamine antagonist, increases gastric emptying and transit through the small intestine and the colon. Metoclopramide is useful in diabetic gastroparesis, in the placement of small intestinal tubes in patients with ileus, and in diabetic constipation. It has little therapeutic value in symptomatic patients with progressive systemic sclerosis or in many patients with pseudo-obstruction. Domperidone, a peripherally acting dopamine antagonist, mainly increases gastric emptying and has little therapeutic effect in small intestinal or colonic motility disorders.

Cisapride may stimulate motility through agonism of a serotonin 5-HT$_4$ receptor in the bowel. Cisapride stimulates gastric emptying, increases small intestinal transit, and stimulates colonic contractility. Cisapride may improve symptoms in patients with decreased gastric emptying, small intestinal pseudo-obstruction, or colonic inertia.

Erythromycin stimulates MMC activity by binding at the motilin receptor on the small intestinal smooth muscle cell. Normal MMC activity is absent in many patients with neuropathic pseudo-obstruction. Octreotide in a low dose (< 100 μg) initiates phase 3 of the MMC, which makes it useful in patients with pseudo-obstruction.

Leuprolide acetate may improve symptoms secondary to functional disturbances of small intestinal motility. This drug is believed to work by decreasing the concentrations of the smooth muscle inhibitory hormones progesterone and relaxin.

Inhibitory Agents

Inhibitory drugs should be most useful for treating patients whose symptoms result from increased motility, which causes uncoordinated movement of the intestinal contents. The inhibitory drugs may block the receptors for excitatory neurotransmitters or block the increase in intracellular calcium necessary for normal smooth muscle contraction.

Anticholinergic drugs, which inhibit muscarinic receptor stimulation, are sometimes effective for the small intestinal or colonic variants of the irritable bowel syndrome. The anticholinergics must be used with care in patients who may develop urinary retention (e.g., prostatism) or glaucoma.

Calcium channel blockers inhibit the increase in intracellular calcium that is necessary for smooth muscle contraction. Several classes of calcium channel blockers, including verapamil and the dihydropyridines, are available. The dihydropyridine, nifedipine, decreases smooth muscle contraction and may be used in some patients with increased small intestinal or colonic motility.

Nitrate compounds inhibit smooth muscle contraction, probably by increasing the intracellular concentration of cGMP and decreasing calcium influx into the smooth muscle cell.

Peppermint oil relaxes smooth muscle, which improves symptoms in some patients with the irritable bowel syndrome. Cholecystokinin antagonists may prove useful for treating multiple gastrointestinal motility disorders.

Burks TF: Actions of drugs on gastrointestinal motility. *In* Johnson LR (ed.): Physiology of the Gastrointestinal Tract. 2nd ed. New York, Raven Press, 1987, pp 723–744. *Extensive references are provided for the background of drug action.*

Camilleri M, Malagelada JR, Abell TL, et al.: Effect of six weeks of treatment with Cisapride in gastroparesis and intestinal pseudo-obstruction. Gastroenterology 96:704, 1989. *Report of efficacy for the class of prokinetic drugs.*

TABLE 101–5. EFFECTS OF DRUGS ON SMALL AND LARGE INTESTINAL CONTRACTILITY

Drug	Effect on Stomach	Effect on Small Intestine	Effect on Colon	Mechanism of Action
Acetylcholine analogues	Excitatory	Excitatory	Excitatory	Agonist of muscarinic receptors on muscle cells
Neostigmine	Excitatory	Excitatory	Excitatory	Acetylcholine esterase inhibitor
Metoclopramide	Excitatory	Excitatory	Excitatory	Dopamine antagonist (central, peripheral)
Domperidone	Excitatory	Excitatory	No effect	Dopamine antagonist (peripheral)
Cisapride	Excitatory	Excitatory	Excitatory	5-HT$_4$ agonist
Macrolide antibiotic	Excitatory	Excitatory	?	Binds to motilin receptor
Octreotide (low dose)	No effect	Excitatory	?	Possible block of inhibitory neurons
Leuprolide acetate	?	Excitatory	?	Reduces progesterone and relaxin
Atropine	Inhibitory	Inhibitory	Inhibitory	Antagonist of muscarinic receptor
Secoverine	?	Inhibitory	Inhibitory	Antagonist of M$_2$ muscarinic receptors on muscle cells
Papaverine	?	?	Inhibitory	Unknown
Calcium channel blockers	Inhibitory	Inhibitory	Inhibitory	Blocks voltage-operated calcium channels
Nitrate compounds	?	Inhibitory	Inhibitory	Blockade of receptor-operated calcium channels; Increase of intracellular cGMP
Peppermint oil	?	Inhibitory	Inhibitory	Possible block of calcium channels
Cholecytokinin antagonists	?	?	?	Blocks CCK receptors

102 DIARRHEA
Guenter J. Krejs

Diarrhea is defined as the presence of stool liquidity (instead of formed or soft stool) and an increase in daily stool weight, the upper normal limit of which is 200 grams in industrialized societies. Diarrhea is usually associated with increased stool frequency (more than three bowel movements per day) and is often accompanied by urgency, perianal discomfort, and incontinence. Some patients may have increased frequency and liquidity of stools, however, when daily stool weights are < 200 grams. Since diarrhea results from a disturbance in the normal flow and transport of gut fluids, the normal physiology of absorption in the digestive tract is first considered.

NORMAL PHYSIOLOGY

DELIVERY, FLOW, AND ABSORPTION RATES. During fasting, the intestine contains very little fluid, but when three normal meals per day are eaten, about 9 liters of fluid are delivered to the proximal duodenum. Approximately 2 liters of this fluid are from ingested food and liquids, the rest being digestive secretions.

The volume of chyme that passes through different segments of the small bowel depends on the type of food that has been eaten. For example, meals containing high concentrations of sugar are hypertonic, and when such meals are ingested, the volume of material passing through the jejunum is even greater than the volume that enters the proximal duodenum. On the other hand, after isotonic or hypotonic meals (such as a meal of steak, potatoes, and tea), the volume of fluid traversing the jejunum is much less than that which was delivered to the duodenum. (These considerations are especially important in patients' who have had gastric surgery or intestinal resection.) In either case, the osmolality of chyme is adjusted toward that of plasma as fluid travels through the duodenum and upper jejunum, and by the time chyme reaches the ileum, most of the dietary sugars, amino acids, and fats have been absorbed. Fluid arriving at the ileum is mainly an isotonic salt solution and therefore similar in its ionic composition to plasma. The ileum absorbs much, but not all, of this salt solution. About 1 liter per day of this isotonic unabsorbed ileal fluid enters the colon. Although ileal fluid resembles plasma with regard to its sodium (Na^+) and potassium (K^+) concentrations, the concentrations of chloride (Cl^-) and bicarbonate (HCO_3^-) are quite different, being approximately 70 and 60 mEq per liter, respectively.

The colon can absorb 2 to 4 liters of isotonic salt solution per day (even more in patients with secondary hyperaldosteronism associated with salt depletion). The presence of nonabsorbable and osmotically active solutes from the diet and from bacterial action, a relatively slow rate of absorption from the rectosigmoid, and timely bowel movements prevent complete fluid absorption and desiccation of the fecal mass. About 100 ml of fluid is excreted in the feces; its Na^+ and Cl^- concentrations are about 50 mEq per liter, while the K^+ concentration is about 90 mEq per liter. This fluid also contains a high concentration of volatile fatty acids (from bacterial action on nondigestible carbohydrates), which dissipate most of the unabsorbed or secreted HCO_3^- ions and which often cause stool fluid to be hypertonic to plasma. Since the gastrointestinal tract does not have a diluting mechanism, the osmolality of fecal fluid is never less than the osmolality of plasma.

To summarize, daily volumes of fluid traversing the duodenum are 9 liters, traversing the ileocecal valve area are 1 liter, and traversing the anal sphincter are 0.1 liter. Stated in another way, the small bowel absorbs 8 liters of fluid per day and empties 1 liter into the colon, and the colon absorbs 0.9 liter. Theoretically 2 to 4 liters of fluid would have to be delivered to the colon per day before diarrhea would ensue, provided that delivery rates were steady, the fluid contained no abnormal solutes, and colon function was normal. Unfortunately, the latter qualifications do not apply in many gastrointestinal diseases.

TRANSPORT PHYSIOLOGY. The mechanisms responsible for fluid absorption differ in different regions of the gut and in different species. According to the model for the ileum shown in Figure 102–1, the brush border membrane contains a carrier that facilitates the simultaneous entry of Na^+ and glucose into the cells; Na^+ cannot enter without glucose. A separate pair of exchange carriers work together to facilitate the simultaneous and electrically neutral entry of Na^+ and Cl^-. Na^+ enters in exchange for H^+, and Cl^- enters in exchange for HCO_3^-. If these two exchange carriers operate at the same rate, Na^+ and Cl^- are absorbed in equal amounts, and H^+ and HCO_3^- are secreted in equal amounts and react in the lumen to form CO_2 and water. However, the anion carrier usually operates more rapidly than the cation carrier, and there is a net secretion of HCO_3^-. (This accounts for the high concentration of HCO_3^- and the low concentration of Cl^- in fluid that the ileum delivers to the colon.) Once inside the cell (via either the Na^+-H^+ exchange or the Na^+-glucose carrier), Na^+ is pumped out of the cell across the basolateral membrane by a pump that is probably an Na^+-K^+ adenosine triphosphatase (ATPase). Cl^- and glucose exit the basolateral membrane by facilitated or passive diffusion.

Na^+ pumping at the basolateral membrane causes a potential difference (PD) across the mucosa (serosal side positive). However, the tight junctions between small bowel mucosal cells (the "shunt pathway") are "leaky," and passive diffusion of anions (in the absorptive direction from lumen to plasma) or cations (in the secretory direction) readily dissipates the PD. Therefore, the residual PD across small bowel mucosa is only 2 to 4 mV.

Colonic cells and colonic transport are somewhat different. The brush border membrane apparently has a carrier for Na^+ that is not

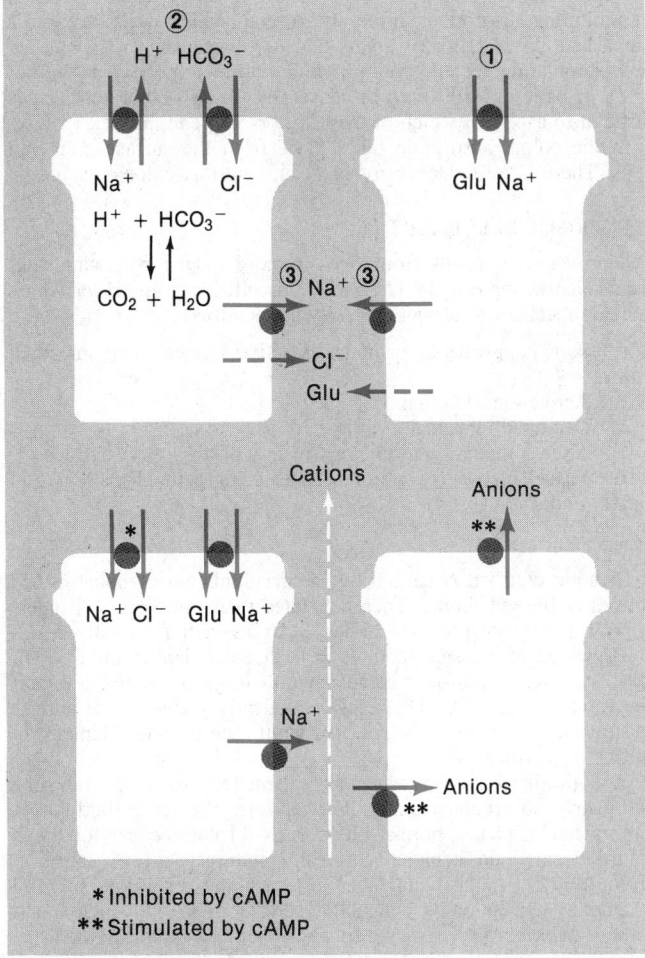

FIGURE 102–1. *Top,* Active transport mechanisms in the human ileum. *1,* Brush border glucose-sodium carrier. *2,* Double exchange carriers for neutral NaCl entry. *3,* Basolateral membrane sodium pump. *Bottom,* Model of cyclic AMP–mediated change in intestinal transport. Active anion secretion is stimulated (**), and there is inhibition of neutral NaCl entry across the brush border membrane (*). The glucose-sodium entry carrier and the basolateral membrane sodium pump are intact. Cations are secreted passively via the tight junction pathway.

influenced by glucose or other actively absorbed nonelectrolytes (glucose is not absorbed in the colon). There is no convincing evidence for Na^+-H^+ exchange, but the brush border membrane appears to have an anion exchange carrier that facilitates chloride absorption and HCO_3^- secretion. The tight junctions are "tight," so the electrical gradient generated by the basolateral membrane pump is sustained. The PD is, therefore, about 30 mV (serosal side positive).

K^+ movement in all regions of the gut is passive, in response to electrochemical gradients. Thus, passive K^+ absorption in the colon is retarded (owing to the high lumen-negative PD), and the K^+ concentration in fecal fluid is much higher than in plasma (up to 100 mEq per liter). Water movement throughout the gut is passive, secondary to osmotic pressure gradients generated by active solute transport.

NORMAL SMALL BOWEL SECRETION. Small intestinal cells normally secrete as well as absorb electrolytes and water, with the secretory rate normally being of less magnitude than the absorptive rate, so that the net effect of small bowel transport processes is absorption of fluid. (Although it is possible that the same cell might both absorb and secrete, the putative small bowel secretion probably originates in crypt cells, whereas absorption takes place from villous cells.) This is an extremely important concept, because it means that a hormone or toxin might reduce net absorption rate in either of two ways: (1) by stimulating secretion, or (2) by inhibiting absorption. In either case, the observed effect is reduced absorption. Similarly, a hormone or a toxin might cause small bowel secretion by stimulating active secretion, so that it overwhelms the normal absorptive process; or a hormone or a toxin could cause secretion by inhibiting absorption, so that the normal small bowel secretion is unmasked. In fact, many toxins and hormones appear capable of both stimulating secretion and inhibiting normal absorption (see below). In patients with diarrhea caused by toxins or hormones, it is difficult to ascertain which of these factors is predominant.

In the colon, absorption takes place from the surface epithelial cells. There is no evidence for or against normal colonic secretion.

PATHOPHYSIOLOGY OF DIARRHEA

Diarrhea may result from one or more of the following four mechanisms. There is, in addition, a miscellaneous group for which a single mechanism cannot currently be identified:

1. Poorly absorbable, osmotically active solutes in the intestinal lumen.
2. Active ion secretion.
3. Deranged intestinal motility.
4. Altered mucosal morphology or loss of absorptive surface.
5. Miscellaneous (several mechanisms or pathophysiology not clearly understood).

Osmotic Diarrhea

Osmotic diarrhea is caused by the accumulation of nonabsorbed solutes in the gut lumen. There are three main subtypes: (1) ingestion of poorly absorbable solutes, such as saline purgatives; (2) maldigestion of ingested food, as in lactase deficiency; and (3) failure of a mucosal transport mechanism, as in glucose-galactose malabsorption (Table 102–1). Being osmotically active, these solutes cause water and salts to be retained within the intestinal lumen, resulting in diarrhea.

Osmotic diarrhea stops when the patient fasts (or stops ingesting the poorly absorbable solute). Furthermore, the fecal fluid has a large solute gap; i.e., normal electrolytes do not account for much of the fecal fluid osmolality (fecal solute gap = [osmolality] − $2[(Na^+) + (K^+)]$; the factor of 2 is to account for anions in stool water). An exception is congenital chloridorrhea, in which unabsorbed chloride prevents water absorption. In chloridorrhea the chloride concentration in fecal fluids exceeds the sum of the concentration of sodium and potassium. Such fecal fluid analysis is performed on supernatant stool water following centrifugation of a stool sample in a test tube (30 minutes at 2000 g). In most instances, electrolytes and osmolality will provide meaningful information only if the stools are liquid enough that at the end of centrifugation the supernatant stool water constitutes at least one third of the total sample. In osmotic diarrhea resulting from carbohydrate

TABLE 102–1. CAUSES OF OSMOTIC DIARRHEA

Ingestion of poorly absorbable solutes
  Magnesium sulfate, sodium sulfate, citrate-containing laxatives
  Some antacids—$Mg(OH)_2$
  Mannitol, sorbitol (chewing gum, diet candy)

Maldigestion
  Disaccharidase deficiencies (lactose, sucrose-isomaltose, trehalose intolerance)
  Gastrocolic fistula, jejunoileal bypass, short bowel syndrome
  Postgastrectomy, postvagotomy state
  Chronic intestinal ischemia
  Lactulose therapy

Mucosal transport defects
  Glucose-galactose malabsorption
  Chloridorrhea
  Congenital sodium diarrhea
  General malabsorption in diffuse disease of small bowel mucosa

malabsorption, the concentration in stool of short-chain fatty acids is high, and thus the pH is low (pH 4.0 to 6.0). In some instances it is necessary to measure magnesium (Mg^{2+}) (normal < 12 mM), sulfate (normal < 5 mM), and phosphate (normal < 12 mM) in stool water to identify the cause of osmotic diarrhea, especially in surreptitious laxative abuse.

Normal fecal fluid, which can be isolated from stool by dialysis methods, often has a modest solute gap (mainly because of unabsorbed carbohydrates and their bacterial products). Therefore, the presence of a solute gap is suggestive of osmotic diarrhea only if stool volume losses are substantially higher than normal. For example, a modest osmotic gap with a stool weight of only 200 grams per 24 hours would not by itself be suggestive of osmotic diarrhea.

Secretory Diarrhea

The net effect of a secretory stimulus on intestinal mucosa can be either inhibition of absorption or a net luminal gain (secretion) of water and electrolytes. This sequence of net movement changes may follow a dose-response curve, with a low secretagogue dose (e.g., circulating vasoactive intestinal polypeptide [VIP] concentration) inhibiting intestinal water and ion absorption and a high dose causing net secretion. On a cellular level, both processes can occur at the same time, with inhibited villus absorption and enhanced crypt secretion in the small bowel.

Secretory diarrhea is recognized clinically by certain features: Stools are large in volume and watery (>1 liter per day), and diarrhea persists with fasting. The stool osmolality can be totally accounted for by normal ionic constituents: $([Na^+] + [K^+]) \times 2$ equals stool osmolality, which is close to the osmolality of plasma. Table 102–2 gives the major causes of secretory diarrhea. A few examples are discussed in detail.

ENTEROTOXIN-INDUCED SECRETION. The classic disease in this category is Asiatic cholera (see Ch. 296). Intestinal secretion is caused by cholera toxin; the intestinal mucosa, however, appears normal. An increase in intracellular cyclic adenosine monophosphate (cAMP) in cholera mediates active ion secretion by the enterocytes (Fig. 102–1B). Patients may lose 10 to 20 liters of watery stool per day. Mortality was high before oral rehydration solutions were introduced. This therapy is successful because glucose-stimulated Na^+ absorption remains normal despite ongoing secretion.

Enterotoxigenic *Escherichia coli* strains can produce one or more of at least three types of toxins (one heat-labile and two heat-stable toxins). Intestinal secretion caused by these toxins is responsible for many episodes of acute diarrhea, including traveler's diarrhea (see Ch. 298). Enterotoxin is produced by a large number of other bacteria, some of which are also capable of tissue invasion (*Campylobacter jejuni, Yersinia enterocolitica, Salmonella, Shigella, Clostridium difficile, Staphylococcus aureus, Klebsiella pneumoniae, Aeromonas, Plesiomonas*).

PANCREATIC CHOLERA SYNDROME (see Ch. 206.2). High circulating levels of VIP cause intestinal water and electrolyte secretion that results in large-volume diarrhea. In adults, VIP production usually comes from tumors originating in pancreatic islet cells, whereas in children these tumors are often ganglioneuromas or ganglioneuroblastomas. The disease can be mimicked by pro-

TABLE 102-2. INTESTINAL SECRETION: DIARRHEAL SYNDROMES AND CORRESPONDING SECRETORY STIMULI

Diarrheal Syndromes	Secretory Stimulus
Traveler's diarrhea, Asiatic cholera	Enterotoxins (Escherichia coli., Vibrio cholerae)
Laxative abuse	Laxatives (phenolphthalein, senna, bisacodyl)
Pancreatic cholera syndrome	Vasoactive intestinal polypeptide
Medullary carcinoma of the thyroid	Calcitonin
Carcinoid syndrome	Serotonin, substance P
Zollinger-Ellison syndrome	Gastrin
Secreting villous adenoma of the rectum	Prostaglandins
Small intestinal obstruction	Intestinal distention
Diarrhea in patients with portal hypertension plus severe hypo-albuminemia	Increased hydrostatic vascular pressure and tissue pressure
Congenital chloridorrhea (intestinal secretion in some instances); lethal familial protracted diarrhea	Congenital mucosal ion transport defects
Giardiasis, strongyloidosis, ame-biasis	Unknown mechanism activated by protozoa
Idiopathic chronic secretory diar-rhea (pseudopancreatic cholera syndrome)	Unknown
Collagen vascular diseases (sclero-derma, systemic lupus erythema-tosus, mixed connective tissue disease)	Unknown
Intestinal lymphoma	Unknown

longed intravenous VIP infusion in healthy subjects. This syndrome is also known as Verner-Morrison syndrome, VIP-oma syndrome, or watery diarrhea-hypokalemia-hypochlorhydria (WDHH) syndrome. Diarrhea disappears when plasma VIP levels return to normal following tumor resection. Fifty percent of patients have metastatic disease at diagnosis, however, so that resection is not possible.

In one study of patients with pancreatic cholera, mean daily stool weights averaged 4224 grams during a regular diet and 1817 grams during fasting. Hypokalemia and metabolic acidosis due to large fecal potassium and bicarbonate losses are prominent features, whereas hypochlorhydria is variable. Cosecretion of calcitonin, pancreatic polypeptide, PHM (peptide histidine methionine), or helodermin by these tumors has been found in a number of patients.

IDIOPATHIC SECRETORY DIARRHEA. Patients with this syndrome have large-volume secretory diarrhea and other clinical features of pancreatic cholera, but no evidence of tumor or an abnormally elevated concentration of a circulating secretagogue. These patients undergo extensive negative investigations that often include exploratory laparotomy. Autopsy may also be unrevealing, and the etiology remains unknown. Both the severity of this syndrome and the prognosis vary widely. Spontaneous resolution of the diarrhea may occur after several months. A few patients respond to opiates.

CARCINOID SYNDROME (see Ch. 210.2). Diarrhea is a common manifestation of the carcinoid syndrome, occurring in about 70 to 80% of patients. In most patients, intestinal secretion can be demonstrated. Serotonin and substance P elicit intestinal water and ion secretion in experimental animals, and these agents are often increased in the plasma of patients with the carcinoid syndrome. In other patients, the diarrhea appears episodic and possibly associated with the hypermotility that can be demonstrated when serotonin is given intravenously to normal volunteers. In addition, other contributing causes for diarrhea may be (1) bile salt catharsis if ileal resection was required for tumor removal, (2) lymphatic obstruction due to tumor mass, and (3) subacute intestinal obstruction as a consequence of bowel wall fibrosis induced by the tumor.

MEDULLARY CARCINOMA OF THE THYROID (see Ch. 203). Diarrhea occurs in 30% of patients with medullary carcinoma of the thyroid and may precede the presence of a palpable thyroid mass. Circulating calcitonin is the major mediator of intestinal secretion in this syndrome. Since this tumor may be part of multiple endocrine neoplasia syndromes (see Ch. 210.1), first-degree rela-

tives need to be investigated by measuring basal and postprovocation (intravenous pentagastrin) plasma calcitonin concentrations. Other than in medullary carcinoma of the thyroid, calcitonin is also found in high concentrations in the plasma and tumor tissue of a number of patients with endocrine pancreatic tumors (VIPoma, somatostatinoma), but usually it is not the predominant peptide.

ZOLLINGER-ELLISON SYNDROME (see Ch. 99.6). The secretory diarrhea that occurs in gastrinoma (Zollinger-Ellison syndrome) has a unique pathophysiology. Owing to the gastric hypersecretion caused by high concentrations of circulating gastrin, an excessive load of acidic fluid enters the small bowel and overwhelms the intestinal absorptive capacity. In such patients, daily delivery of up to 24 liters of acidic fluid to the jejunum can occur in the fasting state. Although the percentage of decrease in luminal flow rates in the intestine is similar to that in healthy subjects, the remaining fecal volume is often still in excess of 1 liter per day. Other factors that may play a role in causing diarrhea in gastrinoma are the functional or morphologic impairment of the mucosal brush border by the abnormal acid milieu, the direct effect of excessive gastrin on the small bowel mucosa (reducing absorption), and inactivation of pancreatic lipase by the acidic fluid, causing a mild degree of steatorrhea. Low intraluminal pH may also cause some of the primary bile acids to become insoluble, leading to a reduction of micelle formation and a mild degree of steatorrhea.

BILE ACID DIARRHEA. Watery diarrhea in choleric enteropathy results from the secretory effect of malabsorbed bile acids on colonic mucosa. Interruption of the normal enterohepatic circulation of bile acids can be caused by three types of bile acid malabsorption. Type I is due to ileal disease or resection. Type II, which is less common, consists of a selective ileal transport defect for bile acids. Type III is bile acid malabsorption in the postcholecystectomy and postvagotomy state. Cholestyramine is the treatment of choice for type I and type II bile acid diarrhea. Patients with type III are rarely found to have secretory concentrations of fecal bile acids and rarely respond to cholestyramine.

Deranged Intestinal Motility

Three major derangements might cause diarrhea: (1) Abnormally reduced peristalsis may allow bacterial overgrowth in the small bowel. (2) "Intestinal hurry" may reduce contact time between the small bowel mucosa and its contents and thus result in delivery of abnormally large and qualitatively abnormal fluid loads to the colon. This occurs despite the fact that absorption in the small bowel is normal per unit of time. (3) Premature emptying of the colon caused by an abnormality of its contents, or by intrinsic colonic "irritability" or inflammation, results in reduced contact between luminal contents and colonic mucosa and therefore increased volume and liquidity of the stools.

Some diarrheal diseases due, at least in part, to deranged motility are irritable bowel syndrome (IBS), malignant carcinoid syndrome, postvagotomy diarrhea, diarrhea resulting from diabetic neuropathy, diarrhea resulting from thyrotoxicosis, and the diarrhea associated with postgastrectomy dumping syndrome. Abnormal motility may also contribute to acute diarrhea caused by infections. Stool analysis in diarrhea due to a motility disturbance may be consistent with that in osmotic diarrhea if nutrient absorption is impaired in the small bowel or may resemble that in secretory diarrhea, if, following nutrient absorption, the ileocecal transit volume remains largely unabsorbed. Alternatively, a mixed pattern can exist, with electrolytes accounting for an osmolality equal to that of plasma and an additional component making stool water hyperosmolar, owing mainly to bacterial metabolism of malabsorbed carbohydrates in the collection unit following passage of the stool. IBS and fecal incontinence are discussed in more detail.

IRRITABLE BOWEL SYNDROME. In the United States, up to 50% of all patients seen by primary care physicians for digestive tract problems have IBS. Diarrhea is usually referred to as functional diarrhea, since no obvious cause can be found on extensive routine clinical testing. On special investigations, altered myoelectric activity in the large bowel and significant acceleration in small bowel transit have been demonstrated in patients with IBS and diarrhea. At present, however, it is unclear what clinical relevance these findings may have in the diagnostic and therapeutic management of such patients.

Although functional diarrhea as part of the IBS is generally considered a diagnosis by exclusion, this does not mean that extensive testing is necessary when one is initially confronted with such a patient. Rather, a positive diagnosis can often be made at the first interview. This is based mainly on a typical history: abdominal pain of long duration (often for several years), discomfort and pain in different areas of the abdomen, bloating associated with various so-called food intolerances, and alternating diarrhea and constipation. Functional diarrhea may show a temporal relation to meal intake, and nocturnal diarrhea is typically absent. Furthermore, signs of systemic disease, such as weight loss, are usually absent. Classically, patients are female and in their 20's and 30's, and a history of emotional conflict, stress, or anxiety is common.

In functional diarrhea, stool weight is rarely > 500 grams per day (normal < 200 grams). In a patient who complains of increased frequency of defecation, normal or nearly normal 24-hour stool weight may be the first clue to fecal incontinence, a diagnosis often confused with functional diarrhea.

INCONTINENCE. Most patients whose major disability is due to fecal incontinence present to their physician with "diarrhea." Either they are embarrassed to mention the incontinence, or they interpret it as a manifestation of severe diarrhea. If patients do mention incontinence, the physician also usually attributes it to voluminous diarrhea. In most instances, however, these patients are suffering primarily from a defect in the continence mechanisms rather than from severe diarrhea. As a matter of fact, quantitative stool collections usually reveal rather small fecal volumes, even though stools are soft to liquid in consistency. In any case, the major problem in most such patients is in the anal continence mechanisms. The most frequent causes for sphincter dysfunction are previous anal surgery for fissures, fistulas, or hemorrhoids; episiotomy or tear during childbirth; anal Crohn's disease; and diabetic neuropathy.

Anal sphincter training may improve sphincter function and reduce the frequency of incontinent episodes. It is also important to establish the cause of diarrhea if possible, since effective therapy of the diarrhea usually prevents further incontinence. Symptomatic therapy with opiate drugs is helpful in some patients. There is recent interest in surgical treatment for incontinence, but no good prospective studies have been done. No therapy for incontinence in patients with diarrhea, whether involving drugs, biofeedback, or surgery, has included objective data that convincingly establish its benefit.

Morphologic Alterations

Efficient intestinal absorption requires that the intestinal mucosa be intact with a well-functioning blood supply and intact neural connections. A large number of diseases can cause diarrhea by disrupting the normal anatomy of the intestine (Table 102–3).

VIRAL GASTROENTERITIS. It is estimated that every year 5 million children under age 2 die in developing countries as a consequence of acute diarrhea. Rotavirus is responsible for at least 50% of these infections. The pathogenesis of viral diarrhea is thought to

TABLE 102–3. DIARRHEA DUE TO DISRUPTION OF STRUCTURAL INTEGRITY OF THE INTESTINE

Viral gastroenteritis
Bacterial infection with tissue invasion
Sprue (tropical, nontropical, collagenous)
Whipple's disease
Radiation enteritis
Drugs (e.g., chemotherapeutic agents)
Amyloidosis
Collagen vascular diseases (systemic lupus erythematosus, scleroderma, mixed connective tissue disease)
Inflammatory bowel disease (Crohn's disease, ulcerative colitis, microscopic and collagenous colitis)
Eosinophilic gastroenteritis
Intestinal lymphoma
Ileocecal tuberculosis
Intestinal ischemia, mesenteric vasculitis
Diverticulitis
Pelvic inflammatory disease
Acquired immunodeficiency syndrome (AIDS)

be as follows: The virus enters the absorptive epithelial cells on the tip of the villus, and these cells are sloughed off. Crypt cells then move quickly to replace the lost enterocytes. These cells, however, are immature and cannot absorb effectively. Their sucrase and lactase activities are low, whereas adenylate cyclase activity and cAMP content are normal (in contrast to cholera, in which sucrase and lactase activities are normal and adenylate cyclase activity and cAMP content are increased). There is no enhanced water and electrolyte secretion in viral gastroenteritis; however, sodium-stimulated glucose absorption is markedly diminished. Malabsorption of water, electrolytes, and nutrients results until the infection subsides and mature enterocytes again coat the surface of the villus.

SPRUE (see Ch. 103). The changes associated with sprue involve villous atrophy and marked diminution in the effective absorptive surface of the bowel. When studied with intestinal perfusion techniques, such patients demonstrate jejunal secretion. This can be expected from the observation that the mucosa in total villous atrophy consists only of crypts, and crypts normally secrete fluid and electrolytes. Diarrhea is a result of fat and carbohydrate malabsorption. Typically there is no diarrhea when these patients fast, suggesting that the colon reabsorbs the small bowel secretions. In rare cases patients with sprue have severe secretory diarrhea; a stool output as high as 5 liters a day has been observed.

RADIATION ENTERITIS. Acute radiation enteritis usually occurs within the initial weeks of radiation exposure and is characterized by abdominal cramping, diarrhea, nausea, and vomiting. With time, symptoms abate, and a quiescent period ensues. The average onset of further symptoms is 1 year, but symptoms may occur at any time. Malabsorption of varying degree for bile acids, fat, carbohydrate, and vitamin B_{12} is observed. Interference with absorption occurs owing to infiltration of the mucosa by inflammatory cells and luminal narrowing of the submucosal arterioles with fibrin plugs. Disturbances in motility due to the effects of radiation on the muscularis propria can also contribute to the diarrhea. Late-appearing structural changes with intermittent obstruction, mucosal ulceration, and fistula formation may also lead to diarrhea. Medical therapy with antidiarrheal agents, broad-spectrum antibiotics for bacterial overgrowth, and prednisone rarely provides total control of symptoms. Ultimately, 15% of patients require surgical intervention, such as segmental resection or fistula closure.

LOSS OF ABSORPTIVE SURFACE. The diarrhea that results from intestinal resection may be on the basis of the region removed (e.g., ileum, with its special transport sites for active bile acid absorption) or of the length of bowel resected. At least 50% of the small bowel is required to avoid diarrhea and malnutrition associated with the short bowel syndrome.

AIDS (ACQUIRED IMMUNODEFICIENCY SYNDROME). Small intestinal morphologic alterations and consequent malabsorption and diarrhea are common among patients with AIDS. Infectious agents (*Giardia, Salmonella, Cryptosporidium,* and *Stronglyoides*) and Kaposi's sarcoma can cause gastrointestinal disturbances in AIDS (see Ch. 366). There remains a group of patients, however, who do not have identifiable infectious or parasitic agents or Kaposi's sarcoma but who still manifest diarrhea, malabsorption, and weight loss. Such patients have abnormal D-xylose and fat absorption. Duodenal biopsies reveal blunting of the villi and an inflammatory infiltrate in the lamina propria. This condition is referred to as AIDS enteropathy. Other patients with AIDS may demonstrate a histiocytic infiltrate (pseudo-Whipple's disease) containing numerous acid-fast organisms. *Mycobacterium avium-intracellulare* has been isolated in these patients.

MICROSCOPIC COLITIS. Some patients with chronic diarrhea demonstrate inflammation of colonic mucosa despite normal appearance of the colon on barium enema and colonoscopy. The histologic changes consist of excess neutrophils and round cells in the lamina propria, cryptitis, and reactive changes of surface epithelial cells. When colonic absorption is measured in these patients by perfusion techniques, water and electrolyte absorption is either abolished or abnormally low. Thus, the normal ileocecal transit volume (1 liter per day) remains largely unabsorbed, and stool weights are typically in the range of 400 to 800 grams per day.

Miscellaneous Causes of Diarrhea

Table 102–4 lists diseases in which several of the discussed mechanisms may cause diarrhea or in which the pathophysiology is not clearly understood.

TABLE 102-4. MISCELLANEOUS CAUSES OF DIARRHEA

Drugs
Diuretics, cardiac glycosides, propranolol, quinidine, colchicine, antibiotics, methotrexate, 6-mercaptopurine, 5-fluorouracil, guanethidine, ethanol
Endocrine disorders
Addison's disease, hypoparathyroidism
Neurologic diseases
Tabes dorsalis, multiple sclerosis, myelitis, encephalitis, heat stroke, Charcot-Marie-Tooth disease, myotonia dystrophica, orthostatic hypotension
Toxicologic disorders
Lead poisoning
Immunoglobulin deficiency
Allergy
Systemic mastocytosis

DIAGNOSIS

Although the cause of diarrhea is obvious in many clinical situations, in many others it is not. Here we are concerned with a diagnostic approach to the patient with diarrhea in whom the cause is unknown.

History and Physical Examination

When the stools are consistently large in volume, the underlying cause of diarrhea is likely to be located in the small bowel or in the proximal colon. By contrast, in small-volume diarrhea, in which the patient has frequent urges to defecate but passes only small amounts of feces or mucus, the disorder is usually in the left portion of the colon and rectum. Passage of blood mixed in with the diarrheal stool usually indicates inflammation of the mucosa, less often a neoplasm. Passage of nonbloody mucus suggests IBS, as does a history of small-volume diarrhea alternating with constipation. Frothy stools and excessive flatus suggest fermentation of unabsorbed carbohydrates. Excessively foul stools suggest putrefaction of unabsorbed amino acids. Visible oil or fat indicates severe steatorrhea. Fecal soiling (incontinence) suggests an anal sphincter defect. Diarrhea in a patient with features of anorexia nervosa suggests laxative abuse.

There are, of course, many other pertinent facts obtainable from the history, including previous surgery, drug intake (Table 102–4), symptoms of systemic illness, travel, and related illnesses in family members. In chronic and recurrent diarrhea, an association of exacerbation of diarrhea with emotional stress should be sought, an association that may suggest IBS. The patient's sexual history should be discussed, as male homosexuals have a high incidence of shigellosis, giardiasis, other intestinal infections, and the usually recognized venereal diseases. Diarrhea may be the presenting manifestation of AIDS.

The physical examination may provide clues to the cause of diarrhea. Some physical findings, as well as other clinical associations that may assist in the diagnosis of diarrhea, are listed in Table 102–5.

Diagnostic Tests

ROUTINE EXAMINATION OF STOOL. Unless the diagnosis is readily apparent from the history and physical examination, certain relatively simple studies on the stool should routinely be performed. Regardless of the clinical classification, the information obtained usually narrows the diagnostic possibilities.

Stain for Pus. The presence or absence of intestinal inflammation can often be ascertained by examination of a stained stool specimen. Wright's or methylene blue stains are satisfactory. The presence of large numbers of white blood cells is diagnostic of inflammation. The presence of rare, scattered white cells is within normal limits.

In patients with acute or traveler's diarrhea, pus in the stool suggests invasion of the mucosa by *Shigella, Escherichia coli, Entamoeba histolytica, Salmonella, Campylobacter,* gonococci, or other invasive organisms. In general, shigellosis and invasive *E. coli* infections cause more pus than do *Salmonella* and *E. histolytica* infections. Antibiotic-related colitis may or may not be associated with pus. Diarrhea caused by noninvasive organisms that produce enterotoxins (toxigenic *E. coli,* for example), viruses, and *Giardia* is not associated with pus in the stool.

TABLE 102-5. CLUES TO DIAGNOSIS OF DIARRHEA FROM OTHER SYMPTOMS, SIGNS, AND LABORATORY TESTS

Symptom or Sign Associated with Diarrhea	Diagnoses to Be Considered
Arthritis	Ulcerative colitis, Crohn's disease, Whipple's disease
Liver disease	Ulcerative colitis, Crohn's disease, malignant bowel disease with metastasis to liver
Fever	Ulcerative colitis, Crohn's disease, amebiasis, lymphoma, tuberculosis
Marked weight loss	Malabsorption, inflammatory bowel disease, cancer, thyrotoxicosis
Eosinophilia	Eosinophilic gastroenteritis, parasitic disease
Lymphadenopathy	Lymphoma, Whipple's disease, AIDS
Neuropathy	Diabetic diarrhea, amyloidosis
Postural hypotension	Diabetic diarrhea, Addison's disease, idiopathic orthostatic hypotension
Flushing, large liver	Malignant carcinoid syndrome
Proteinuria	Amyloidosis
Perianal disease or right lower quadrant abdominal mass	Crohn's disease
Purpura	Celiac disease
Peptic ulcer	Zollinger-Ellison syndrome, antacid therapy, gastrocolic fistula
Following cholecystectomy	Bile acid malabsorption
Frequent infections	Immunoglobulin deficiency, AIDS
Immunodeficiency	Giardiasis, nodular lymphoid hyperplasia, celiac sprue
Hyperpigmentation	Whipple's disease, celiac disease, Addison's disease
Good response to corticosteroids	Ulcerative colitis, Crohn's disease, Whipple's disease, Addison's disease, pancreatic cholera, eosinophilic enteritis
Good response to antibiotics	Bacterial overgrowth in small intestine, tropical sprue, Whipple's disease, celiac disease

In patients with chronic and recurrent diarrhea or diarrhea of unknown etiology, pus suggests colitis of some type—idiopathic ulcerative colitis, Crohn's colitis, antibiotic-associated colitis, amebic colitis, ischemic colitis, or tuberculous colitis. Pus is especially abundant in idiopathic ulcerative colitis and tends to be less so in amebic colitis. It is usually absent in microscopic colitis. Absence of pus on a single examination does not, of course, absolutely rule out any of these entities. Radiation-induced disease of the large or small bowel and Crohn's disease limited to the small intestine may or may not be associated with pus in the stool. Pus is not present in the stools of patients with IBS, most causes of malabsorption syndrome, laxative abuse, viral gastroenteritis, and giardiasis.

Occult Blood. Occult (or gross) blood in association with diarrhea usually indicates inflammation and therefore usually has the same significance as pus in the stools (see above). When blood is present in diarrheal stools that do not contain pus, one should consider neoplasms of the colon, heavy metal poisoning, and acute ischemic damage to the gut.

Sudan Stain for Fat. If excess fat is evident on Sudan stain, steatorrhea is probably present, and the various causes of malabsorption syndromes should be considered (see Ch. 103). Most such patients have chronic and recurrent diarrhea; steatorrhea in a patient with acute or traveler's diarrhea suggests giardiasis.

Alkalinization. A pink color following alkalinization of a stool or urine sample indicates phenolphthalein ingestion as the cause of diarrhea. The test is so easily and quickly done, and the significance of a positive result is so great, that it should be carried out routinely in female patients with chronic diarrhea. Surreptitious laxative ingestion is rarely seen in males.

OTHER TESTS. Evidence of systemic illness has obvious implications in the etiology of diarrhea (Table 102–5). For instance, a history of flushing and diarrhea leads to determination of urinary 5-hydroxyindoleacetic acid (see Ch. 210.2). The order in which tests are carried out, assuming that further tests are necessary, varies according to the physician's intuition regarding a particular patient. Certain of the diagnostic tests deserve brief discussion here.

Search for Infectious and Parasitic Organisms. It is important to complete the examination for parasites and to have adequate bacterial cultures in progress before examining the patient with radiologic contrast media because barium interferes with successful demonstration of pathogens. Failure to find *Giardia* in stool samples is not strong evidence against giardiasis; sometimes it is necessary to examine duodenal fluid to demonstrate this organism. *Cryptosporidium* can be revealed by acid-fast stain of feces subjected to a flotation technique for concentration. Special culture methods are required if the presence of infection by *Gonococcus, Campylobacter,* or *Yersinia* is to be established. A microimmunofluorescent test with monoclonal antibodies can be used on a rectal mucosal smear to assess for chlamydial proctitis. Serologic tests for amebae and lymphogranuloma venereum may assist in the diagnosis in some patients. Finally, tests for clostridial toxin in fecal fluid help in the diagnosis of pseudomembranous colitis.

Proctosigmoidoscopy. Proctosigmoidoscopy is helpful in establishing the presence or absence of mucosal inflammation. In antibiotic-associated diarrhea, it may reveal pseudomembranes. Proctosigmoidoscopy is often essential in patients with chronic and recurrent diarrhea and in patients with diarrhea of unknown etiology. The findings are especially apt to be abnormal in those whose stools contain pus or blood or both; they are usually normal in patients with diarrhea caused by the various malabsorption syndromes.

Proctosigmoidoscopy to investigate diarrhea should be done without enemas, laxatives, or suppositories. Such preparation may wash away exudate, distort the mucosa, induce trauma, and possibly obscure evidence of disease or create the false impression of disease. In almost all instances, fecal matter can easily be aspirated or pushed aside, and since most abnormalities are diffuse, fecal matter does not interfere greatly with a satisfactory examination. The presence of solid stool in the rectum of a patient who supposedly has diarrhea is also revealing, suggesting that an acute diarrhea is subsiding, that the patient may have IBS, that the diarrhea is an illusion, or that the diarrhea is secondary to fecal impaction.

Since proctitis may not be evident grossly, even to the experienced eye, mucosal smears should always be obtained and stained for pus. The mucosa should be carefully examined for melanosis coli, although melanosis may be present microscopically even if it is not present grossly.

Rectal Biopsy. Biopsy can often be helpful in evaluating diarrhea. The main disorders that might be detected by biopsy, but not by smears and stool examination, are amyloidosis, Whipple's disease, microscopic colitis, granulomatous inflammation, melanosis coli, intestinal spirochetosis (other than that caused by *Treponema pallidum*), and schistosomiasis. Biopsy is indicated in patients with diarrhea of unknown origin, especially in a search for melanosis coli and unsuspected colitis that may not have been evident grossly. It is my opinion that IBS should not be diagnosed until after a rectal mucosal smear has shown that pus is not present and a rectal biopsy is found to reveal no abnormality. The biopsy should be taken from the posterior wall of the rectum on a valve. Although the risk is uncertain, some clinicians believe that a rectal biopsy with large forceps predisposes to a colonic perforation if a barium enema is done within 10 days of the biopsy.

Quantitative Fecal Fat. Collected stools (usually for 72 hours) should be quantitatively analyzed for fat content (1) when malabsorption is suggested by the history and physical examination, (2) when the qualitative test for fecal fat is positive, or (3) routinely in patients with diarrhea of unknown origin. If steatorrhea is present, the differential diagnosis of malabsorption syndrome can be pursued (see Ch. 103). Of course, the results of this test must be interpreted with knowledge of the approximate intake of dietary fat. Stool weight in grams (which is equivalent to stool volume in milliliters) should also be noted and recorded (see below).

Twenty-four-Hour Stool Volume. For reasons indicated under History and Physical Examination above, knowing stool volume helps localize the region of the intestine that is most likely responsible for diarrhea, and in several instances specific information on stool volume is of great diagnostic help. For example, stool volumes > 500 ml per day are rarely seen in patients with IBS, and

stool volumes < 1000 ml per day provide evidence against pancreatic cholera syndrome. In addition, very large measured stool volumes will alert the physician to the need for vigorous fluid replacement therapy.

Collection of 24-hour stool specimens is easy in the initial phases of a diarrhea workup, prior to barium radiography or administration of enemas or other preparations. With a little effort, it can be accurately done on an outpatient basis. If a record of stool frequency is kept, the average volume of each stool can be calculated, and the results may give useful insight.

In special instances, e.g., in diarrhea of unknown origin, it is useful to measure stool electrolytes and osmolality and to determine whether or not the diarrhea persists during a 48-hour fast (while the patient is given glucose and salt solutions intravenously). These results help establish whether the diarrhea is secretory or osmotic in type (see Pathophysiology, above). If the osmolality of stool water is < 250 mOsm per kilogram, water has been added to the stool to simulate diarrhea. A sodium concentration in fecal water that is higher than that of plasma indicates contamination by urine.

Vasoactive Intestinal Polypeptide (VIP) and Other Circulating Agents. The pancreatic cholera syndrome should be considered if diarrhea of unknown origin has lasted longer than 4 weeks, is secretory in type, and is severe (>1 liter per day and/or associated with hypokalemia and salt and water depletion), and if surreptitious laxative abuse and organic disease of the gastrointestinal tract have been excluded. The incidence of this syndrome is 1 in 10 million population per year. Only in this rare subgroup of patients is serum assay for VIP, PHM, and calcitonin likely to be helpful. Other gastrointestinal hormones such as pancreatic polypeptide (PP) may be increased in plasma and serve as markers of endocrine pancreatic malignant disease.

Therapeutic Trials. In some instances therapeutic trials are indicated as diagnostic tests. (Obviously, in most instances, the results must be considered suggestive rather than conclusive.) These trials may include pancreatic enzymes, antibiotics (also as part of the Schilling test), metronidazole or quinacrine (for giardiasis), cholestyramine (for bile acid malabsorption), indomethacin (for prostaglandin synthetase inhibition), and various diets (lactose free, carbohydrate free, low fat, and avoidance of any specific food to evaluate the unlikely possibility of food allergy).

THERAPY

The most satisfactory therapy is to cure the underlying disease. When this is not possible, certain drugs may ameliorate the disease and thus reduce the severity of diarrhea (prednisone for inflammatory bowel disease is an example). In a few instances, the disease cannot be ameliorated, but there is fairly specific therapy for the diarrhea, such as cholestyramine for bile acid malabsorption.

At present, unfortunately, in many patients the disease process responsible for diarrhea cannot be satisfactorily suppressed, and specific therapy is lacking. Supportive and symptomatic therapy is required in such instances.

Fluid Replacement

The most important aspect of therapy in acute and traveler's diarrhea, and in some patients with chronic diarrhea, is prevention or correction of salt and water depletion. This can be done by oral ingestion of liquids and salty foods, oral glucose-saline solutions, or intravenous fluid therapy, as dictated by the clinical situation. Two points deserve emphasis: First, soft drinks, tea, and citrus juices contain little, if any, sodium chloride (even Gatorade contains only 23 mEq per liter of sodium chloride). Second, oral glucose-saline solutions or liquids plus salty foods will actually worsen the diarrhea (in terms of stool volume) as they help correct fluid depletion. The oral rehydration solution recommended by the World Health Organization contains the following in millimoles (grams) per liter: glucose, 111 (20); NaCl, 60 (4); KCl, 20 (2); NaHCO$_3$, 30 (2); and osmolality is 331 mOsm per kilogram. In some patients, particularly those with short bowel syndrome, a high Na$^+$ concentration is needed in the oral rehydration solution to achieve a positive Na$^+$ and fluid balance. To prevent hypertonicity of such a solution, glucose is best given as a polymer.

Avoidance or Treatment of Perianal Discomfort

Helpful therapy consists of the following: (1) avoidance of soap, toilet paper, washcloths, and towels; (2) gentle washing with warm water on absorbent cotton after each bowel movement, followed by gentle, thorough drying with absorbent cotton; (3) if seepage is present, absorbent cotton retained next to the anal orifice and held in place by snug underwear; (4) sitz baths for 10 minutes two or three times a day; and (5) hydrocortisone creams (1%). In addition to these measures, patients may obtain relief by additional gentle cleaning with soft pads containing witch hazel (Tucks). Locally applied anesthetic ointments may be transiently helpful, but ointments restrict perspiration and anesthetics may irritate the perianal skin, so these agents should be used only for short periods. It is important to recognize specific treatable conditions, such as perianal moniliasis.

Opiates

Codeine, diphenoxylate with atropine (Lomotil), and loperamide reduce urgency, bowel movement frequency, and stool volume in many acute or chronic diarrheal illnesses. This is not to say that they have a beneficial effect in every patient; but they do in most, so that when groups of patients are studied, both stool frequency and volume are reduced to a statistically significant extent. Of the three drugs, loperamide and codeine are usually somewhat superior to diphenoxylate; loperamide may have less tendency than codeine to cause addiction. Codeine, however, is much less expensive. In chronic diarrhea, the drugs may be given once a day in a maximally tolerated dose or several times daily in smaller doses.

Opiate drugs are generally thought to reduce diarrhea by reducing the propulsive activity of the gut and thereby reducing stool frequency. This mechanism might also enhance contact time between intestinal mucosa and luminal contents. Assuming that at least part of the gut mucosa is in an absorbing and not a secretory state, this would allow greater absorption of fluid and thereby reduce stool volume. *In vitro* opiates have also been reported to stimulate NaCl absorption and to have antisecretory action against several secretagogues. These effects cannot be demonstrated in clinical situations using therapeutic doses of opiate drugs.

Opiates should not be used in patients with severe ulcerative colitis with impending toxic megacolon, and there is evidence suggesting that they may prolong the diarrhea in shigellosis and perhaps in diarrheal diseases caused by other invasive bacteria and in antibiotic-associated diarrhea. These reservations notwithstanding, opiates are often of benefit in the symptomatic relief of diarrhea in patients with less severe ulcerative colitis and with many acute infectious diarrheal illnesses. Obviously they should be prescribed only when diarrhea is causing significant disability.

There are rare case reports suggesting that opiate drugs can be a cause of paradoxical diarrhea.

Bismuth Subsalicylate

Bismuth subsalicylate may prevent infection with enterotoxin-producing *E. coli* organisms. In addition, this agent brings mild symptomatic relief in patients with acute infectious diarrhea, whether bacterial or viral. The mechanism of the effect is unknown. The dose is 30 to 60 ml every 30 minutes for eight doses. Patients should be warned that this medication may turn their stools black. If the patient is taking other medications, possible drug interaction should be considered.

Antibiotics in Acute and Traveler's Disease (see Ch. 298)

For at least two reasons, antibiotics should not usually be used: First, in most patients they do not shorten the duration of illness. Second, their use risks the development of antibiotic-associated diarrhea or colitis, superimposed on whatever was causing the diarrhea initially. This greatly confuses the problem if the diarrhea becomes chronic.

In mild disease (small-volume diarrhea, no chills or fever, no blood or pus in the stool), antibiotics should not be prescribed unless a specific indication emerges from the bacteriology and parasitology laboratory. In patients who are severely ill, especially if they have blood or pus in the stool, antibiotic therapy aimed at shigellosis is reasonable, pending the result of stool culture.

Antisecretory Drugs

A specific and potent inhibitor of intestinal secretion is not available. On the basis of *in vitro* observations and individual case reports, a number of agents can be tried on an empiric basis. Phenothiazines inhibit secretion caused by cholera toxin and *E. coli*

enterotoxins; aspirin, indomethacin, and other nonsteroidal anti-inflammatory agents reduce secretion mediated by prostaglandins (inhibition of prostaglandin synthesis); glucocorticoids decrease mucosal inflammation and enhance NaCl absorption (increase in Na^+-K^+-ATPase activity); nicotinic acid, clonidine, and lithium carbonate may increase intestinal NaCl absorption (inhibition of adenylate cyclase); and cromoglycate may inhibit release of mediators of allergic reaction in the intestine. When diarrhea is due to circulating agents (VIPoma, carcinoid), a somatostatin analogue given subcutaneously may abolish diarrhea by decreasing secretagogue release from tumor tissue.

Bo-Linn GW, Vendrell DD, Lee E, et al.: An evaluation of the significance of microscopic colitis in patients with chronic diarrhea. J Clin Invest 75:1559, 1986. *First description of microscopic colitis as a separate disease entity. Patients reveal abolished water and electrolyte absorption during colonic perfusion studies.*

Brunt LM, Mazoujian G, O'Dorisio TM, Wells SA, Jr: Stimulation of vasoactive intestinal peptide and neurotensin secretion by pentagastrin in a patient with VIPoma syndrome. Surgery 115:362, 1994. *Results emphasize the importance of comprehensive biologic evaluation in patients with VIPoma syndrome to detect the production of a range of peptide hormones. Intravenous pentagastrin appears to stimulate release of VIP, but requires further evaluation.*

Field M, Fordtran JS, Schultz SG (eds.): Secretory Diarrhea. Bethesda, Md., American Physiological Society, 1980. *Sixteen chapters by different experts on various aspects of the pathophysiology of secretory diarrhea. The emphasis is on basic research, although there is a highly original chapter on the pharmacology of antidiarrheal drugs.*

Fine KD, Krejs GJ, Fordtran JS: Diarrhea. *In* Sleisenger MH, Fordtran JS (eds.): Gastrointestinal Disease, 5th ed. Philadelphia, WB Saunders, 1993, p1043. *A detailed description of the physiology of the human intestinal tract with regard to water and electrolyte movement and the pathophysiology of chronic diarrhea.*

Gallagher DM: Gastrointestinal manifestations of HIV/AIDS. Crit Care Nurs Clin North Am 5:121, 1993. *Reviews potential problems in the HIV-infected patient specific to the gastrointestinal tract and discusses current available therapy.*

Krejs GJ (ed.): Diarrhoea. Clin Gastroenterol 15, No 3, 1986. *Thirteen chapters on the pathophysiology and clinical investigation of diarrhea. Contains re-evaluation of criteria for defining secretory diarrhea and extensive description of* diarrhée motrice *(diarrhea due to motility derangement).*

103 MALABSORPTION
Phillip P. Toskes

The malabsorption syndrome refers to a clinical condition in which a number of nutrients and minerals are not normally absorbed; almost always, however, lipids fail to be normally absorbed. At times the absorption of a single nutrient may be selectively impaired. A sound knowledge of normal absorptive processes allows the physician to pursue a logical approach to the patient with malabsorption.

NORMAL ABSORPTION OF NUTRIENTS

Absorption is the integration of those processes whereby the products of digestion pass from the lumen of the intestine through the small intestinal enterocyte to appear in the general circulation via the lymphatics or the portal vein. Although the digestive process is initiated by acid and pepsin within the stomach, the exocrine pancreas has the major role in digesting fat, carbohydrate, and protein by its secretion of lipase, amylase, and proteases. Fat is eventually broken down to monoglycerides and fatty acids; carbohydrate, to disaccharides and monosaccharides; and proteins, to peptides and amino acids. These forms of nutrients are absorbed through the intestinal enterocyte. The villi and microvilli of the small intestine provide an enormous area for absorption. The motility of the intestine and the contraction of the microvilli allow molecules to pass through an "unstirred layer" adjacent to the microvilli.

Nutrients pass through the enterocyte by several processes: active transport, passive diffusion, facilitated diffusion, and endocytosis. Active transport and passive diffusion are the main mechanisms whereby nutrients pass through membranes. *Active transport* moves nutrients against a chemical or electrical gradient, requires energy, is carrier mediated, and is subject to competitive inhibition. *Passive diffusion* does not require energy and allows nutrients to pass through a membrane according to chemical concentration and electrical gradients. Passive diffusion, best typified by water absorption, is not carrier mediated and does not demonstrate competitive inhibition. *Facilitated diffusion* is similar to passive diffusion but may be carrier mediated and may be subject to competitive inhibition. *Endocytosis* is a process whereby nutrients are engulfed by parts of the cell membrane. Although endocytosis may be most important in the neonatal period, this absorptive mechanism may also occur to some extent in the adult and may be involved in the absorption of antigens.

Absorption of nutrients may be regionalized (Table 103–1). Although many nutrients can be absorbed throughout the small intestine, each nutrient has a major site of absorption. When areas of the intestine are damaged or resected, the remaining intestine usually adapts effectively to absorb the nutrients that would normally have been absorbed by those areas. Two noteworthy exceptions to this adaptation process are cobalamin (vitamin B_{12}) and bile salts. If the distal ileum has been resected, the patient can *never* again actively absorb these two nutrients. This has important clinical implications, especially for cobalamin. Patients who have had distal ileum resection must receive monthly parenteral cobalamin or they will develop macrocytic anemia and neuropathy secondary to cobalamin deficiency (see Ch. 133).

FAT ABSORPTION. Dietary fat is ingested largely as long-chain triglycerides, the absorption of which is a complex process involving the pancreas, liver, small intestine, and lymphatics (Fig. 103–1). Nevertheless, the process is efficient; the coefficient of fat absorption is >93%, i.e., <7% of ingested fat escapes absorption and appears in the stool per day. A breakdown in any one of these steps (Fig. 103–1) leads to malabsorption of fat (steatorrhea). A thorough knowledge of this physiologic process allows a logical approach to evaluation of steatorrhea.

Some triglyceride digestion begins in the stomach by lingual and gastric lipases. Triglyceride is emulsified in the stomach, and fat is slowly emptied into the duodenum, where its entry and that of acid release cholecystokinin and secretin. As a result, the pancreas secretes enzymes and bicarbonate, and the gallbladder contracts to release bile salts. Bicarbonate maintains the pH of the intestinal lumen above 4, allowing pancreatic lipase to effect hydrolysis of triglycerides to yield free fatty acids and monoglycerides. Another pancreatic protein, colipase, facilitates the interaction between lipase and triglyceride for effective lipolysis. Fatty acids and monoglyceride interact with conjugated bile salts to form molecular aggregates or micelles (Fig. 103–1). A crucial concentration of bile salts for micelle formation (5 to 15 μmol per milliliter) is maintained by a very efficient enterohepatic circulation of bile salts. Although the total bile salt pool is only 2 to 4 grams, 95% of bile salts is actively absorbed in the ileum and returned to the liver by the portal venous system. Each day 20 to 30 grams of bile salts recirculate in this enterohepatic circulation. Only about 200 to 600 mg of bile salts is excreted in the feces per day and must be replaced by hepatic biosynthesis from cholesterol.

Micellar fat passes through the "unstirred" water layer covering the surface of the enterocyte. Because of their solubility in the lipid-rich surface membrane, the fatty acids and monoglycerides are released and diffuse into the enterocyte. Inside the enterocyte, fatty acids and monoglycerides are re-esterified to form triglyceride. Absorbed cholesterol is also largely esterified with fatty acids for opti-

mal transport. The intestine must also synthesize phospholipids and specific proteins (apoproteins) in order to incorporate these nonpolar lipids into lipoproteins, the major transport vehicles for fat transport in lymph and plasma (see Ch. 173). These polar components are added to the surface of the lipid droplet, producing lipoproteins called *chylomicrons*. Chylomicrons are concentrated in the Golgi apparatus and then discharged through the lateral basal portion of the cell to the interstitium and mesenteric lymph to be delivered via the thoracic duct to the vena cava.

Medium-chain triglycerides (C-6 to C-12 fatty acids) are absorbed quite differently and more effectively than are long-chain triglycerides (C-16 to C-18 fatty acids) described above. Medium-chain triglycerides (MCT) (1) are more completely hydrolyzed by pancreatic lipase, (2) do not require bile salts for absorption, (3) can be directly taken up into the enterocyte and hydrolyzed by a mucosal lipase to fatty acids, (4) do not need to be re-esterified, (5) are not incorporated into lipoproteins, and (6) can pass directly into the portal venous system, transported as fatty acids bound to albumin. These characteristics of MCT allow it to improve fat absorption in a number of diseases in which dietary triglyceride absorption is impaired.

Fat-soluble vitamins (A, D, E, K) are absorbed after micellar solubilization and are transported into lymph with chylomicrons. In the case of vitamin A, the free vitamin is esterified within the enterocyte with palmitic acid, transported via chylomicrons in the lymph and stored as retinol palmitate in the liver. Vitamin metabolism is described more fully in Ch. 192.2.

CARBOHYDRATE ABSORPTION. Carbohydrate is ingested in the form of starch, sucrose, and lactose. Salivary and pancreatic amylases hydrolyze starch to oligosaccharides and disaccharides. All carbohydrate must be digested to a final monosaccharide product before it can be absorbed. Disaccharides are split by membrane-bound disaccharidases located on the microvilli of the enterocyte. Lactose is digested by lactase to glucose and galactose; sucrose, by sucrase to glucose and fructose; and maltose by maltase to two molecules of glucose. These monosaccharides are then transported through the enterocyte to the portal blood. Glucose and galactose are absorbed by active transport requiring sodium. Fructose is transported by facilitated diffusion. Glucose is transported into the enterocyte, probably bound along with sodium (Na^+) to a protein carrier. These monosaccharides are transported out of the cell by active sodium extrusion across the basolateral aspect of the enterocyte via a sodium pump.

PROTEIN AND AMINO ACID ABSORPTION. The digestion of dietary protein is initiated in the stomach by acid and pepsin but is largely completed by pancreatic proteases, both endopeptidases (trypsin, chymotrypsin, elastase) and exopeptidases (carboxypeptidase). Pancreatic proteases secreted in inactive forms (zymogens) must be activated. Enterokinase from the small intestinal mucosa activates trypsin from trypsinogen, and trypsin then activates all of the other protease precursors. The digestive products of pancreatic proteases are peptides containing two to six amino acids as well as single amino acids. Peptidases on the microvillus membrane or in the cytosol of the enterocyte further hydrolyze oligopeptides to free amino acids, which are directly absorbed in the portal vein.

The L forms of amino acids are actively transported in the enterocyte by specific energy-requiring, sodium-dependent processes. There are several specific transport systems for amino acids: (1) the dibasic amino acid system, which is often abnormal in cystinuria; (2) the neutral amino acid system, which is abnormal in Hartnup disease; (3) the iminoglycine system; and (4) the dicarboxylic acid system. Intact di- and tripeptides are also actively transported across the enterocyte membrane without hydrolysis by peptidases on the microvillus membrane. These peptides are hydrolyzed in the cytosol of the enterocyte to amino acids, which are then released into the circulation.

WATER AND ELECTROLYTE ABSORPTION. Over 7 liters of water (both ingested and reabsorbed from intestinal secretion) is absorbed by the small intestine per day through the process of passive diffusion. Absorption of water often follows that of glucose and electrolytes in order to maintain isotonicity of intraluminal contents.

Na^+ is actively transported linked to an exchange with H^+ in the jejunum and ileum and with Cl^- and HCO_3^- in the ileum. Na^+ transport is enhanced by glucose absorption in the jejunum (via the glucose-Na^+ carrier on the microvillus membrane) and by solvent

TABLE 103–1. REGIONALIZATION OF NUTRIENT ABSORPTION

Nutrient	Major Site of Absorption
Fat	Proximal small intestine
Protein	Mid small intestine
Carbohydrate	Proximal and mid small intestine
Iron	Proximal small intestine
Calcium	Proximal small intestine
Folic acid	Proximal and mid small intestine
Cobalamin (vitamin B_{12})	Distal small intestine (ileum)
Other water-soluble vitamins	Proximal and mid small intestine
Bile salts	Distal small intestine (ileum)
Water and electrolytes	Small intestine and colon (especially cecum)

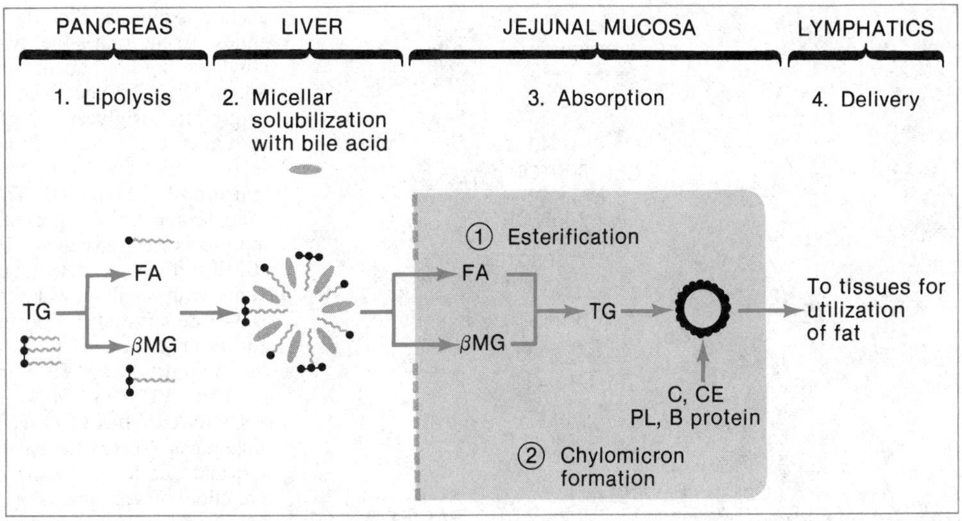

FIGURE 103-1. Schematic of intestinal absorption, showing the participation of the pancreas, liver, and intestinal mucosal cell in fat absorption. (From Wilson FA, Dietschy JM: Gastroenterology 61:911, 1971. Copyright 1971, The Williams & Wilkins Company, Baltimore.)

(water) drag. Some Na^+ also moves down a gradient across the mucosa, i.e., by passive diffusion. Changes in the concentration of Na^+ in the lumen depend on relative rates of exchange of both Na^+ and water between blood and lumen. Potassium passively diffuses from the lumen of the proximal small intestine and into the lumen of the distal small intestine.

CALCIUM ABSORPTION. Calcium is actively absorbed in the duodenum largely regulated by the active form of vitamin D_3-1,25-dihydroxycholecalciferol (calcitriol). Vitamin D_3 from the diet is metabolized first by the liver (25-hydroxylation) and then by the kidney (1-hydroxylation) to form 1,25-dihydroxycholecalciferol $(1,25[OH]_2D_3)$(see Ch. 212). This process is influenced by parathyroid hormone levels, which are regulated by plasma levels of ionized calcium. Calcitriol stimulates the synthesis of calcium-binding protein, alkaline phosphatase, and a calcium-activated ATPase—all involved in active calcium transport. Absorption of vitamin D, a fat-soluble vitamin, is often impaired in the malabsorptive syndromes such that calcium absorption is diminished. Fatty acids within the lumen of the intestine may also directly impair absorption by binding calcium. In turn, the unavailability of ionized calcium in the lumen leads to excessive absorption of oxalate and a resulting propensity to form calcium oxalate kidney stones.

IRON ABSORPTION (see Ch. 130). The average intake of iron from dietary sources is 15 to 25 mg per day, of which 0.5 to 2.0 mg is normally absorbed. Iron is absorbed as inorganic iron (cereals, vegetables) or as heme iron (meat). For optimal absorption, inorganic iron must be released from dietary components to soluble iron complexes in the intestinal lumen. Gastric acid enhances the absorption of inorganic iron (both Fe^{3+} and Fe^{2+}) by facilitating its chelation with sugars, amino acids, bile, and ascorbic acid. Such iron complexes remain in solution at the alkaline pH of the duodenum—the major site of iron absorption. Inorganic iron is absorbed from the intestinal lumen by the mucosa and then transported to the blood by mechanisms that are unclear. A mucosal regulatory system keeps much of the iron trapped within the enterocyte, to be excreted into the feces depending on the need for iron, as determined by body stores of iron or by the rate of erythropoiesis. Organic iron (heme iron) is absorbed more efficiently than is inorganic iron. Heme is split from globin and absorbed as an intact metalloporphyrin at an alkaline pH. Iron is released from heme by heme oxygenase intracellularly. In plasma, iron is transported bound to transferrin, a specific globulin, to various tissues for use or storage.

Iron absorption is increased in iron deficiency, pregnancy, idiopathic hemochromatosis, and any conditions in which there is active erythropoiesis. Absorption is decreased in chronic infection and after large amounts of iron are ingested. Diffuse disease of the duodenum as nontropical sprue may impair iron absorption and lead to iron deficiency.

FOLIC ACID ABSORPTION. Dietary folic acid is conjugated with glutamyl peptides; prior to its absorption, these polyglutamates must be deconjugated to monoglutamates by folic deconjugase, an enzyme found on the microvillus membrane. Folate monoglutamates are absorbed by active transport at low concentrations of folate and by passive diffusion at high concentrations of folate. Folic acid undergoes an enterohepatic circulation. Since its body stores are limited, the major cause of folate deficiency is diet poor in fresh fruits and vegetables. Folic acid deficiency may also occur if there is extensive damage to the proximal small intestine (e.g., nontropical sprue) or secondary to the use of a number of medications (sulfasalazine, phenytoin, trimethoprim) that inhibit its absorption. Other causes of folate deficiency are discussed in Ch. 133.

COBALAMIN (VITAMIN B_{12}) ABSORPTION (Ch. 133). The current concept of cobalamin absorption and transport is depicted in Figure 103-2. Cobalamin, found in animal protein, is released from protein in the stomach by the synergistic action of both acid and pepsin. Cobalamin initially binds to a cobalamin-binding protein (R binder or cobalophilin), also secreted by the stomach. The cobalophilin-cobalamin complex is degraded by pancreatic proteases within the duodenal lumen, with release of cobalamin to bind with gastric intrinsic factor (a glycoprotein secreted by the parietal cells). After intrinsic factor binds cobalamin, the intrinsic factor–cobalamin complex passes down the small intestine until it reaches the distal 60 cm of the ileum, where it binds to a specific receptor of the brush border. In the absence of the terminal ileum, intrinsic factor–mediated cobalamin absorption ceases, although large doses of cobalamin (milligram in contrast to microgram amounts) may lead to adequate absorption by passive diffusion throughout the gastrointestinal tract.

Intrinsic factor does not enter the ileal cell and is not absorbed. Transcobalamin II (TCII), the most important transport protein for cobalamin, picks up cobalamin in the ileal mucosa and promotes its uptake by tissues throughout the body. The TCII-cobalamin complex enters tissues via endocytosis, with cobalamin being released by lysosomal proteolysis.

At equilibrium, the majority of circulating cobalamin is attached to cobalophilin, which is also found in saliva, gastric secretions, intestinal secretions, semen, and tears. It also moves continuously in an enterohepatic circulation. The function of the ubiquitous cobalophilins is unclear, but they may prevent or retard the absorption and dissemination of a variety of cobalamin analogues, either produced by bacteria or even found within multivitamin supplements.

CLASSIFICATION AND CLINICAL MANIFESTATIONS OF MALABSORPTION

CAUSES. Table 103-2 divides the causes of the malabsorption syndrome into nine categories, based on its pathophysiology (see Fig. 103-1). Some conditions have multiple reasons for malabsorption but are arbitrarily classified under one major category. The differential features and management of important types of this syndrome are detailed later in the chapter.

CLINICAL MANIFESTATIONS. Patients with the malabsorption syndrome usually have diarrhea, weight loss, and malnutrition.

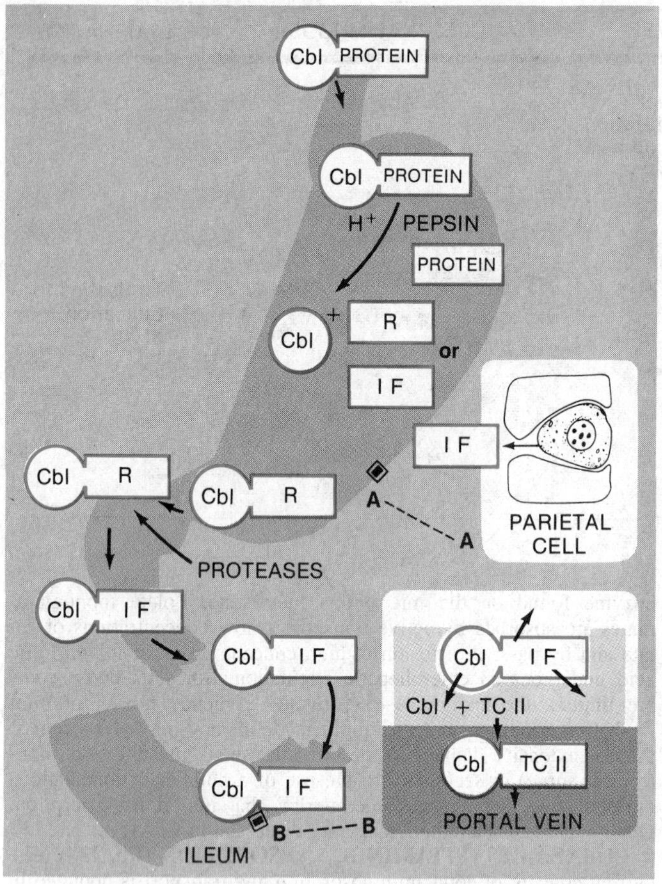

FIGURE 103-2. Cobalamin absorption and transport. Cbl = Cobalamin, R = R-protein or cobalophilin, IF = intrinsic factor, TC II = transcobalamin II. (From Toskes PP: J Clin Gastroenterol 2:287, 1980.)

They often complain that their stools are bulky, greasy, and excessively malodorous and that they float and are difficult to flush down the toilet. Steatorrheal stools float not because of their fat content but because of their high gas content. Patients with severe malabsorption, as exemplified by that secondary to pancreatic insufficiency, may complain of oil seeping out of the rectum. The symptoms and signs of malabsorption are varied and involve a number of organ systems. Patients may demonstrate one or more of these manifestations depending on the severity of the malabsorption. Causes of these different symptoms and signs are detailed in Table 103-3. These aspects of the history and physical examination are crucial in evaluating such patients.

DIAGNOSIS OF MALABSORPTION

Although there may be selective malabsorption of nutrients, most patients with clinically relevant malabsorption have steatorrhea. Consequently, documentation of steatorrhea is important and is the cornerstone of diagnostic evaluation. The only truly reliable means to document steatorrhea is quantitative chemical analysis of fat in a 72-hour stool collection while the patient is ingesting a high-fat diet (at least 100 grams per day). On such a diet normal subjects excrete <7 grams of fat per day (coefficient of absorption of >93%). Unfortunately, the quantitative fecal fat determination is cumbersome to perform and difficult to obtain in most hospitals. Furthermore, the documentation of steatorrhea indicates only that the patient has the malabsorption syndrome—it does not indicate the pathophysiology or confer a specific diagnosis.

Table 103-4 details some alternative tests (other than the quantitative fecal fat determination) that can be used to detect the presence and the cause of malabsorption. They are categorized into screening tests and those more specific in localizing the malabsorption site. It is usually necessary to use a number of malabsorptive tests to establish the cause of the malabsorption.

QUALITATIVE STOOL FAT. The microscopic examination of stool for fat is helpful if performed properly and if the patient is ingesting a high-fat diet. Two specimens of stool are placed on two slides. To the first slide, two drops of water and two drops of 95% ethyl alcohol are added, followed by two drops of a fat stain (e.g., Sudan III). The specimen is microscopically examined for orange neutral fat (triglyceride) globules. The globules should be larger than a red cell and should be numerous per high-power field. To the second slide, several drops of 36% acetic acid are added, then several drops of Sudan III. The slide is heated until it begins to boil. Microscopically, the presence of large orange globules or spicules represents free fatty acids. Part 1 is positive in patients with pancreatic insufficiency, detecting undigested triglyceride; part 2, in patients with small bowel disease, detecting free fatty acids. Figure 103-3 demonstrates a positive part 1 test in a patient with pancreatic insufficiency. There is a 25% false-negative rate when steatorrhea is mild, i.e., <10 grams per 24 hours. The false-positive rate is about 15%. This test is simple to perform and inexpensive.

URINARY D-XYLOSE TEST. The urinary xylose excretion test distinguishes between malabsorption due to small intestinal disease and that due to pancreatic exocrine insufficiency. A 5-hour urinary excretion of ≥5 grams is normal after oral administration of 25 grams of D-xylose to a well-hydrated subject. Decreased xylose ab-

TABLE 103-2. CLASSIFICATION OF THE MALABSORPTION SYNDROME

1. Impaired digestion
   a. Primary pancreatic exocrine insufficiency
   b. Gastric surgery (Billroth I and II, vagotomy, and pyloroplasty)*
   c. Gastrinoma*
2. Reduced bile salt concentration
   a. Liver disease
   b. Small intestine bacterial overgrowth (scleroderma, diabetes mellitus, primary motility disturbances, postgastrectomy, achlorhydria)*
   c. Ileal disease or resection*
3. Abnormalities of intestinal mucosa
   a. Disaccharidase deficiency
   b. Impaired monosaccharide transport
   c. Folate or cobalamin deficiency
   d. Nontropical sprue
   e. Nongranulomatous ileojejunitis
   f. Amyloidosis
   g. Crohn's disease*
   h. Eosinophilic enteritis
   i. Radiation enteritis*
   j. Abetalipoproteinemia
   k. Cystinuria
   l. Hartnup disease
4. Inadequate absorptive surface
   a. Short bowel syndrome
   b. Jejunoileal bypass*
5. Infection
   a. Tropical sprue
   b. Whipple's disease*
   c. Acute infectious enteritis
   d. Parasitic infections
6. Lymphatic obstruction
   a. Lymphoma*
   b. Tuberculosis
   c. Lymphangiectasia
7. Cardiovascular disorders
   a. Congestive heart failure
   b. Constrictive pericarditis
   c. Mesenteric vascular insufficiency
8. Drug-induced
   a. Cholestyramine
   b. Neomycin
   c. Colchicine
   d. Phenindione
   e. Irritant laxatives
9. Unexplained
   a. Carcinoid syndrome
   b. Diabetes mellitus*
   c. Adrenal insufficiency
   d. Hyper- and hypothyroidism
   e. Mastocytosis
   f. Hypogammaglobulinemia

* = Multiple reasons for malabsorption

TABLE 103–3. SYMPTOMS AND SIGNS OF MALABSORPTION

History	Pathophysiology	Physical Examination	Pathophysiology
Diarrhea	Increased secretion and impaired absorption of water and electrolytes, unabsorbed dihydroxy bile acids, unabsorbed fatty acids	Pallor	Anemia secondary to iron, folate, or cobalamin deficiency
		Glossitis, stomatitis, cheilosis	Iron, folate, cobalamin, and other vitamin deficiencies
Greasy, bulky, malodorous stools that are difficult to flush	Increased fat in stool		
Oil seeping from rectum	Unabsorbed triglyceride (pancreatic insufficiency)	Ecchymosis, purpura	Vitamin K malabsorption
		Acrodermatitis	Zinc and fatty acid deficiency
Weight loss despite good appetite	Loss of calories from malabsorption	Dehydration, hypotension	Water and electrolyte malabsorption
Excessive flatus	Fermentation of unabsorbed carbohydrates by colonic bacteria	Edema	Protein malabsorption (decreased serum albumin)
Diffuse abdominal pain	Inflammation or infiltration of tissue (pancreatic insufficiency, Crohn's disease, lymphoma)	Peripheral neuropathy	Cobalamin deficiency
Postprandial (30 minutes after eating) midabdominal pain	Intestinal ischemia		
Abnormal bruisability	Vitamin K malabsorption		
Weakness and fatigue	Protein, electrolyte, fat, iron, folate, cobalamin malabsorption		
Milk intolerance	Lactase deficiency		
Bone pain	Calcium and protein malabsorption		
Tetany, paresthesias	Calcium and magnesium malabsorption, cobalamin deficiency (paresthesias only)		
Night blindness	Vitamin A malabsorption		
Nocturia	Delayed absorption of water, hypokalemia		
Amenorrhea	Protein malabsorption		

sorption and excretion are found in patients with damage to the proximal small intestine and in bacterial overgrowth in the small intestine (the bacteria catabolize the xylose). Patients with pancreatic steatorrhea usually have normal xylose absorption. As with any urinary excretion test, decreased renal function or incomplete collection of the urine may invalidate the test. Impaired renal function is most important when evaluating an elderly patient who may not have obvious renal disease but whose creatinine clearance may be low. Decreased urinary xylose values may also be seen in ascites. Although a blood level of ≥ 30 mg per deciliter 1 hour after ingesting xylose may indicate normal absorption, overlap may exist between control subjects and those with malabsorption.

BENTIROMIDE URINARY EXCRETION TEST. Bentiromide is a synthetic peptide attached to para-aminobenzoic acid (PABA). The bond between the peptide and PABA is easily split by chymotrypsin. Following oral administration of 500 mg of bentiromide, PABA is absorbed in the proximal small intestine, partially conjugated in the liver, and excreted in the urine as arylamines. A cumulative 6-hour arylamine excretion of $< 50\%$ of that ingested as bentiromide is virtually diagnostic of pancreatic insufficiency. In a patient with symptomatic diarrhea or steatorrhea or both, a normal bentiromide test result virtually excludes pancreatic disease as the cause of the symptoms. The use of bentiromide offers a simple, reliable confirmatory test (high specificity, few false-positive results) for diagnosis of pancreatic insufficiency. The test is not accurate when the serum creatinine level exceeds 2.0 mg per deciliter.

SERUM TRYPSIN-LIKE IMMUNOREACTIVITY (TLI). TLI, a radioimmunoassay, measures serum levels of this pancreas-derived protein. Although not as sensitive as the bentiromide or secretin tests, a decreased value appears to be completely specific for pancreatic insufficiency.

SECRETIN TEST. The most sensitive tests of impaired pancreatic function are direct measurements of its exocrine function; unfortunately, these are the most complex to perform. The patient swallows a tube that is fluoroscopically placed, with the aspiration site within the second part of the duodenum near where the pancreatic duct enters the duodenum. A hormone is given intravenously, and a component of pancreatic secretion (bicarbonate after secretin; trypsin, amylase, or lipase after cholecystokinin) is measured. False-positive tests are virtually nonexistent if the tube has been properly positioned, and false-negative tests are not relevant because the secretin test will invariably be abnormal if the steatorrhea is secondary to pancreatic insufficiency.

TESTS FOR COBALAMIN (VITAMIN B₁₂) ABSORPTION (see Ch. 133). In the Schilling test, 1.0 μg of ^{57}Co-cyanocobalamin is administered orally, followed by 1000 μg of nonlabeled cobalamin given intramuscularly to help "wash out" that fraction of the isotope that has been absorbed. If the subsequent 24-hour urinary excretion of the radioactivity is $< 8\%$ of that administered, cobalamin malabsorption is present. There are four common clinical causes of cobalamin malabsorption, which can be sorted out by a differential Schilling test (Table 103–5). If an abnormal test result improves with concomitant administration of hog intrinsic factor or pancreatic extract (six to eight conventional tablets or three enteric-coated microsphere capsules), the cobalamin malabsorption is secondary to pernicious anemia or exocrine pancreatic insufficiency, respectively. If cobalamin malabsorption still persists, the tests should be repeated after 4 days of antimicrobial therapy (metronidazole, 250 mg three times daily). If the malabsorption of labeled cobalamin is corrected by this therapy, bacterial overgrowth was the cause. Metronidazole is the antimicrobial agent of choice because anaerobes such as *Bacteroides* are usually responsible for the cobalamin malabsorption. If the malabsorption still persists, damage to the ileal receptor (Crohn's disease, ileal resection, lymphoma, Imerslund's syndrome) is probably present and the patient must always receive a monthly injection of cobalamin (100 μg). In the face of renal impairment, 4 ml of plasma may be obtained 8 hours after the administration of labeled cobalamin. A value $> 0.6\%$ of the orally administered dose is considered normal.

There are two caveats concerning the Schilling test: (1) Severe cobalamin deficiency itself may damage the ileum such that the ileal receptors may not bind the intrinsic factor-cobalamin complex. This may confuse its interpretation. Thus, it is advisable to wait until 1 week of cobalamin therapy (100 μg per day intramuscularly) has been completed before performing the differential Schilling test. (2) Two other clinical conditions are associated with cobalamin deficiency—cobalamin deficiency secondary to lack of intake (as in complete vegetarians) and the failure to absorb food-bound cobalamin because of decreased acid secretion—that are not associated with an abnormal Schilling test (Table 103–5). The patient's history is the key to the former, and a test of protein-bound cobalamin absorption detects the latter.

BREATH TESTS. Two breath tests are reliable enough to receive routine clinical use—the lactose-H₂ breath test for detecting lactase deficiency and the ^{14}C-xylose breath test for the diagnosis of small intestine bacterial overgrowth.

TABLE 103–4. TESTS FOR MALABSORPTION

Test	Normal Values	Comments Relevant to Patients with Malabsorption
Screening Tests		
1. Serum carotene	>0.06 mg/dl	Decreased; very good test if poor oral intake has been excluded
2. Serum calcium	9.0 to 10.5 mg/dl	Decreased, not very sensitive
3. Serum cholesterol	150 to 250 mg/dl	Decreased, not very sensitive
4. Serum albumin	4.0 to 5.2 mg/dl	Decreased, not very sensitive
5. Serum magnesium	1.7 to 2.0 mEq/liter	Decreased, not very sensitive
6. Prothrombin time	Control value	Increased, not very sensitive
7. Qualitative stool fat	No fat globules per hpf*	Numerous fat globules per hpf; part 1 for neutral fats, part 2 for split fats (see text)
Specific Tests		
1. Serum iron	80–150 μg/dl	Malabsorbed in proximal small bowel disease
2. Serum folate	5–21 ng/ml	Decreased in proximal small bowel disease, may be increased in bacterial overgrowth
3. Serum cobalamin (vitamin B_{12})	200–900 pg/ml	Malabsorbed in distal small bowel disease, pernicious anemia, bacterial overgrowth, chronic pancreatitis
4. Urinary D-xylose	>5 grams/5 hr	Decreased in small bowel disease and bacterial overgrowth, normal in pancreatic disease
5. Bentiromide test	Arylamine excretion >57% in 6 hr	A value of <50% is diagnostic of pancreatic insufficiency
6. Serum trypsin–like immunoreactivity (TLI)	29–80 ng/ml	A value of <20 ng/ml is specific for pancreatic insufficiency
7. Secretin test	HCO_3^- conc >80 mEq/liter Vol >1.8 ml/kg/hr	Most sensitive test of pancreatic function
8. ^{37}Cyanocobalamin urinary excretion test	>8% 24 hr	Decreased in pernicious anemia, chronic pancreatitis, bacterial overgrowth, ileal disease
9. Urine 5-HIAA	1.7–8.0 mg/24 hr	Markedly elevated in carcinoid syndrome, minimally elevated in any kind of malabsorption
10. Breath tests		
a. ^{14}C-xylose	<0.0013% of administered dose as breath $^{14}CO_2$ at 30 min	Elevated in bacterial overgrowth
b. cholyl-1-^{14}C-glycine	<1% of administered dose as breath $^{14}CO_2$ at any interval over 4 hr	Elevated in bacterial overgrowth or bile acid malabsorption
c. Lactulose H_2	<10 ppm rise in breath H_2 over baseline at any interval for 120 min	Elevated in bacterial overgrowth; increase in fasting breath H_2 suggests bacterial overgrowth; up to 27% of subjects may not have flora that produces H_2
d. Lactose-H_2	<20 ppm rise in breath H_2 over baseline at any interval for 180 min	Elevated in lactase deficiency
11. Small intestinal culture	$\leq 10^5$ organisms per ml jejunal secretions	>10^5 organisms per ml jejunal secretions indicates bacterial overgrowth
12. Small intestinal biopsy	See Figure 103–4	See Table 103–7

* hpf = High-power field; 5-HIAA = 5-hydroxyindoleacetic acid.

The *lactose-H_2 breath test* has superior sensitivity and specificity. Lactose (1 gram per kilogram) is administered orally, and an increase in breath H_2 of more than 20 ppm over basal breath H_2 indicates lactose malabsorption. This test depends on release of H_2 from unabsorbed lactose by bacterial metabolism.

The ^{14}C-*xylose breath test* is a sensitive and specific test for bacterial overgrowth. Following oral administration of xylose (1 gram, 5 to 10 μCi), breath $^{14}CO_2$ concentration is monitored at 30 and 60 minutes, with an increase of $^{14}CO_2$ at 30 minutes being the most reliable assessment. Neither false-negative nor false-positive results

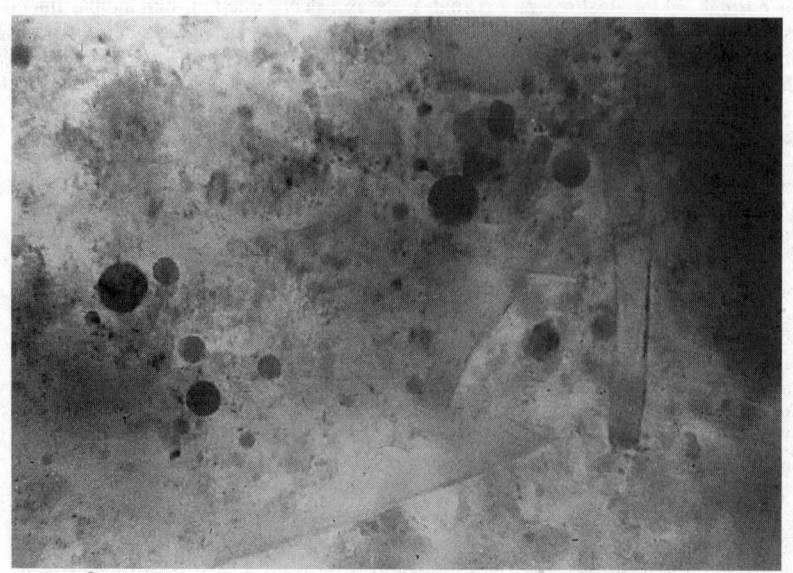

FIGURE 103–3. Positive fecal fat stain. Note the many globules of undigested triglycerides.

TABLE 103-5. THE DIFFERENTIAL SCHILLING (^{57}CO-CYANOCOBALAMIN) TEST

	Stage 1: Free Cobalamin	Stage 2: Free Cobalamin and Intrinsic Factor	Stage 3: Free Cobalamin and Pancreatic Extract	Stage 4: Free Cobalamin and Antibiotics	Comment
Pernicious anemia	Abnormal	Normal	Abnormal	Abnormal	In face of severe cobalamin deficiency, test should be performed only after a week of cobalamin therapy
Chronic pancreatitis	Abnormal	Abnormal	Normal	Abnormal	Although cobalamin malabsorption is common, cobalamin deficiency is rare
Bacterial overgrowth	Abnormal	Abnormal	Abnormal	Normal	Anaerobicidal antibiotic is needed
Ileal disease	Abnormal	Abnormal	Abnormal	Abnormal	Once receptor is permanently damaged, cobalamin malabsorption is permanent
Complete vegetarian* (vegan)	Normal	Normal	Normal	Normal	Cobalamin deficiency secondary to poor intake, absorption normal
Hypo- or achlorhydria*	Normal	Normal	Normal	Normal	Absorption of cyanocobalamin (free B$_{12}$) does not depend on acid; food B$_{12}$ (protein-bound) does; must employ protein-bound cobalamin absorption test.

* Cobalamin deficiency with normal Schilling test.

appear to be a clinically significant problem. Xylose is catabolized by gram-negative aerobes, which are always part of the overgrowth flora, whereas other breath tests often use substrates that are catabolized by gram-negative anaerobes, which may or may not be present in bacterial overgrowth. The small dose of xylose (1 gram) is either catabolized by the overgrowth flora or absorbed in the proximal bowel, leaving very little xylose to "dump" into the colon, causing a possible false-positive result. An abnormal xylose breath test indicates, similar to a culture, the presence of increased numbers of bacteria within the lumen of the proximal small intestine. Whether the abnormal test indicates that therapy is necessary is a decision the clinician must make. Table 103-6 lists two other breath tests used to diagnose bacterial overgrowth, both of which suffer from inadequate sensitivity and specificity.

A ^{14}C-triolein breath test has received some use as a test of fat absorption, but it does not appear to separate control subjects from those with malabsorption very reliably, especially if the steatorrhea is not severe.

CULTURE OF THE SMALL INTESTINE. The proximal small intestine of normal subjects has < 10^5 organisms per milliliter of jejunal fluid—usually < 10^3, largely streptococci and staphylococci, and only an occasional coliform or *Bacteroides*. The ileocecal area is a transition zone with both a qualitative and a quantitative change toward the pattern that is found in the colon. In the colon, there is a marked increase in both aerobes (> 10^7 organisms per milligram of stool) and anaerobes (> 10^{10} organisms per milligram of stool). The qualitative change is also remarkable, with a preponderance of anaerobes (*Bacteroides, Clostridium,* enterococci) and coliforms (*Escherichia coli, Klebsiella*). In small intestine bacterial overgrowth, the small intestine becomes populated with a colon-like flora. Cultures should be considered suspicious if > 10^3 organisms per milliliter are present (especially when anaerobes are identified) and clearly abnormal when > 10^5 organisms per milliliter are present.

BIOPSY OF THE SMALL INTESTINE. Biopsy of the small intestine is important in evaluating malabsorption presumed to be secondary to disease of the small intestine itself. Most instruments (Rubin's tube, Crosby's capsule, Carey's capsule) use a blind suction biopsy technique, but biopsies can be obtained endoscopically as well. Figure 103-4 illustrates the findings of a normal biopsy,

with long, frondlike villi. The lining columnar epithelium is regular with basal orientation of the nuclei. There is not much cellular infiltration of lamina propria. The villus/crypt ratio favors the villus, with villus height normally being three to four times the height of the crypts.

For contrast, Figure 103-5 represents a biopsy from a patient with nontropical sprue (adult celiac disease). There is total villus atrophy, elongated crypts, and a dense infiltration of chronic inflammatory cells in the lamina propria, and at higher magnification the surface epithelial cells are cuboidal, not columnar. Total villus atrophy, as shown in Figure 103-5, is almost always nontropical sprue (adult celiac disease), but it is not a specific lesion, since it may occasionally be observed in other diseases such as lymphoma, Whipple's disease, tropical sprue, ileojejunitis, or bacterial overgrowth. Table 103-7 lists disorders associated with abnormalities in the biopsy of the small intestine and points out that in few disorders and multiple biopsies consistently abnormal and diagnostic, i.e., a diagnostic diffuse lesion.

GASTROINTESTINAL RADIOLOGY. With the possible exception of pancreatic calcification on plain film of the abdomen, radiographs of the intestinal tract do not play a primary role in the diagnostic evaluation of malabsorption. Function tests as described previously are more sensitive and more specific and afford the patient little, if any, radiation exposure. The radiation exposure received from a small bowel series may be considerable. The traditional signs of malabsorption on small bowel radiographs—segmentation or clumping of the barium (moulage sign)—were noted when thick barium was used in contrast to the thin barium commonly employed now. Small bowel radiographs are most frequently used now to determine why bacterial overgrowth has occurred (e.g., the presence of diverticula or dilation of the small intestine in scleroderma) or to confirm a clinical diagnosis of Crohn's disease.

ALGORITHM FOR EVALUATION OF MALABSORPTION. An algorithm presented in Table 103-8 complements a thorough history and physical examination. A serum carotene determination and a microscopic fat stain of the stool are the best screening tests and together detect the presence of steatorrhea about 85% of the time, especially if the patient is excreting > 15 grams of fat per day. Once steatorrhea has been confirmed, the clinician should ask whether the steatorrhea is secondary to pancreatic disease or to

TABLE 103-6. BREATH TESTS FOR BACTERIAL OVERGROWTH

Procedure	Simplicity	Sensitivity	Specificity	Safety
^{14}C-xylose	Excellent	Excellent	Excellent	Good
Cholyl-1-^{14}C-glycine	Excellent	Fair	Poor	Good
Lactulose-H$_2$	Excellent	Fair–good	Fair	Excellent

Modified from King CE, Toskes PP: The use of breath tests in the study of malabsorption. Clin Gastroenterol 12:591, 1983.

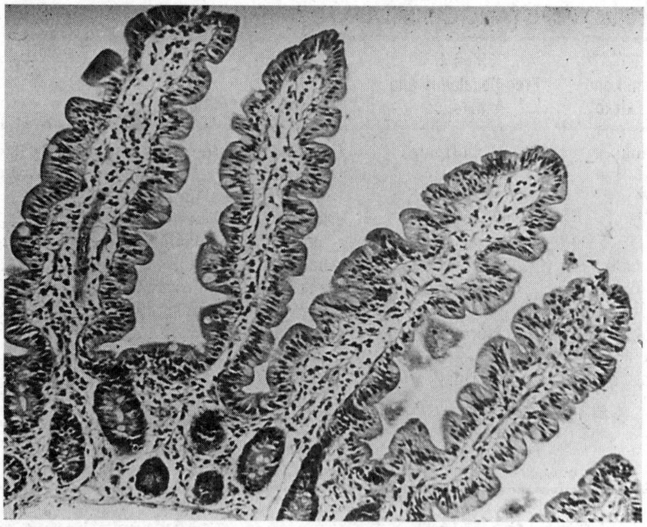

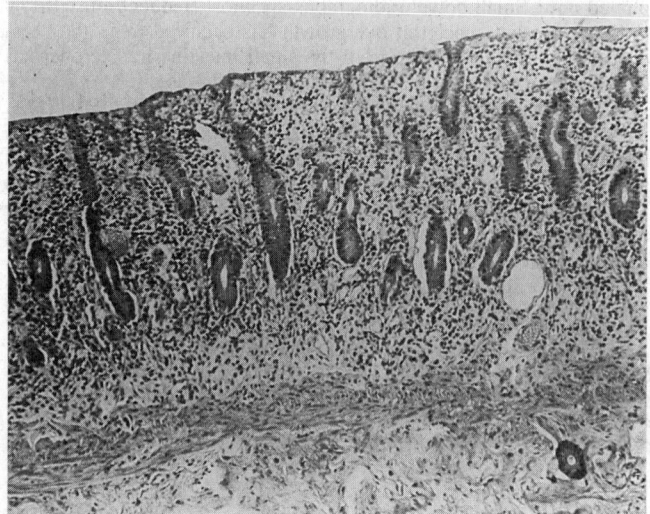

FIGURE 103–4. Appearance of normal small intestine on biopsy.

small bowel disease. The urinary xylose test helps differentiate between these two categories. If xylose absorption is normal, tests of pancreatic function should be pursued. If diffuse calcification of the pancreas is present on a plain film of the abdomen, there is likely to be approximately 80% damage to the exocrine pancreas. The bentiromide test has about the same sensitivity as plain film calcification and is abnormal 80 to 90% of the time if the steatorrhea is pancreatic. A serum trypsin level complements the bentiromide test, adding specificity to the evaluation. If these simple tubeless tests of pancreatic function are not diagnostic, a direct tube test like the secretin test should be performed.

If the xylose test is abnormal, small bowel tests should be performed. A breath test (^{14}C-xylose, lactulose H_2) detects bacterial overgrowth. If normal, a small bowel radiograph, culture, and biopsy should be done, with the radiograph suggesting the site to be biopsied. If steatorrhea is not present, tests designed to detect selective malabsorption of single nutrients can be pursued (lactose H_2 breath test, the Schilling test, and so on).

The algorithm is logical and cost effective, emphasizing inexpensive, noninvasive outpatient evaluation. A specific diagnosis can often be made for less than $700 with minimal or no discomfort to the patient. If more complicated tests are needed, such as the secretin test or small bowel biopsy, the expense and discomfort to the patient increase. The algorithm also emphasizes initial testing for the more common causes of malabsorption (pancreatic insufficiency,

TABLE 103–7. VALUE OF SMALL INTESTINAL BIOPSY

I. Conditions in which the biopsy is consistently abnormal and diagnostic:
Abetalipoproteinemia
Immunodeficiency syndrome
Whipple's disease

II. Conditions in which the biopsy is diagnostic but the lesion is often patchy:
Amyloidosis
Capillariasis
Coccidiosis
Crohn's disease
Cryptosporidiosis
Eosinophilic enteritis
Giardiasis
Lymphangiectasia
Lymphoma
Mastocytosis
Strongyloidiasis

III. Conditions in which the biopsy is often abnormal but not diagnostic:
Bacterial overgrowth
Cobalamin (vitamin B_{12}) deficiency
Celiac sprue (nontropical)
Drug enteritis
Folate deficiency
Infectious gastroenteritis
Protein-calorie malnutrition
Radiation enteritis
Tropical sprue
Unclassified sprue
Zollinger-Ellison syndrome

IV. Conditions in which the biopsy is invariably normal:
Functional bowel disease
Liver disease
Pancreatic disease
Primary disaccharidase deficiency
Ulcerative colitis

bacterial overgrowth) and delayed testing for less common disorders (nontropical sprue, Whipple's disease, and so on).

DIFFERENTIAL FEATURES AND TREATMENT OF INDIVIDUAL FORMS OF THE MALABSORPTION SYNDROME

Numerous disorders can be associated with malabsorption (see Table 103–2). Although specific therapy can be given for individual disorders (gluten-free diet for nontropical sprue, pancreatic enzymes for pancreatic insufficiency), many nonspecific therapies exist for malabsorption (Table 103–9).

Impaired Digestion

PANCREATIC EXOCRINE INSUFFICIENCY (see Ch. 107). Pancreatic exocrine insufficiency is a relatively common cause of severe malabsorption. It is not rare to note steatorrhea in excess of 50 grams of fat per day. Steatorrhea in pancreatic disease is relatively well treated with pancreatic extract. Large doses of pancreatic extract are required: six to eight conventional tablets (Viokase, Cotazym) or three enteric-coated, microsphere preparations (Creon, Pancrease MT) with each meal. Adjuvant therapy (sodium bicarbonate, H_2-receptor antagonists) along with conventional tablet therapy may lead to the best results by raising duodenal pH. The adjuvant of choice is sodium bicarbonate (650-mg tablet before and after each meal) because of its effectiveness, low cost, and lack of side effects at this dose. Antacids containing calcium or magnesium are not to be used as adjuvant therapy because they may increase steatorrhea. Adjuvant therapy is not recommended with enteric-coated preparations, for it may cause the enteric coat to open up within the stomach and the released enzymes may then be destroyed by gastric acid before they can enter the duodenum.

POSTGASTRECTOMY STATES (see Ch. 99.4). The pathogenesis of the malabsorption noted in patients with gastric surgery (Billroth I, Billroth II, vagotomy and antrectomy, vagotomy and pyloroplasty) is multifactorial: (1) loss of reservoir function with rapid emptying and dispersion of food through the small intestine, thereby diluting the normal output of pancreatic enzymes; (2) postcibal asynchrony, i.e., in a patient who has undergone a Billroth II

FIGURE 103–5. Small intestinal biopsy from a patient with nontropical sprue showing total villus atrophy.

TABLE 103-8. ALGORITHM FOR EVALUATION OF MALABSORPTION

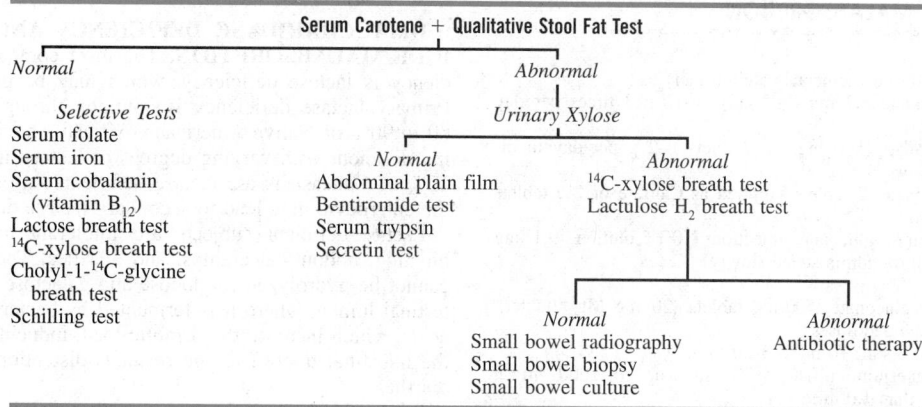

procedure, food may get to the jejunum before bile salts and pancreatic enzymes do; and (3) occurrence of stasis, leading to bacterial overgrowth of the small intestine. Postgastrectomy steatorrhea is usually mild (< 10 grams of fat per day) but occasionally may be marked. Severe steatorrhea in this setting is usually the result of bacterial overgrowth or rarely is secondary to pancreatic insufficiency. Because the duodenum (the major site for calcium and iron absorption) is bypassed when a Billroth II procedure is performed, clinically significant problems related to calcium and iron malabsorption may result.

GASTRINOMA (see Ch. 99.6). Multiple mechanisms contribute to the malabsorption observed in patients with a gastrinoma (Zollinger-Ellison syndrome). The extreme hypersecretion of acid irreversibly inactivates lipase, causing a secondary pancreatic insufficiency. In addition, this acid environment precipitates bile salts and may cause abnormal small bowel histologic findings. All of these abnormalities have been shown to revert to normal after effective therapy with large doses of H_2-receptor antagonists.

Reduced Concentration of Bile Salts

LIVER DISEASE. Steatorrhea (usually mild) may occur in acute or chronic liver disease, presumably owing to impaired synthesis and excretion of conjugated bile salts. Patients with liver disease who manifest clinically significant steatorrhea should have their pancreatic function evaluated, since they often have pancreatic exocrine insufficiency responsive to pancreatic extract therapy. Metabolic bone disease (bone pain, spontaneous pathologic fractures) resulting from malabsorption of calcium and vitamin D may occur, particularly in those with biliary cirrhosis (see Ch. 213).

BACTERIAL OVERGROWTH. Overgrowth of bacteria within the small intestine accompanied by nutrient malabsorption is called the stasis, stagnant loop, or blind loop syndrome. The normal subject usually has sparse bacterial growth in the proximal small intestine (see section on Diagnosis—Culture of the Small Intestine). In the stasis syndrome, the proximal small intestinal flora resembles that of the colon and the overgrowth flora competes with the human host for ingested nutrients. The resultant malabsorption is due to a disturbed intraluminal environment (catabolism of carbohydrate by gram-negative aerobes, deconjugation of bile salts by anaerobes, binding of cobalamin by anaerobes) and patchy damage to the small intestinal enterocyte, perhaps secondary to toxins secreted by the overgrowth flora.

In healthy persons, bacteria within the small intestine are controlled by the cleansing motion of the small intestine, gastric acid secretion, and luminal immunoglobulins. Any alteration of these protective factors may lead to bacterial overgrowth (Table 103–10). Bacterial overgrowth was once thought to be related largely to blind loops and other structural abnormalities. Now the emphasis is on motor disturbances, often with no structural abnormality, and on states of decreased acid secretion. Indeed, bacterial overgrowth is one of the major, if not the major, cause of clinically significant malabsorption in the elderly, who often have both decreased acid secretion and a motility disturbance of the small intestine.

The diagnosis has become much more practical with the development of noninvasive breath tests (see section on Diagnosis—Breath Tests, Tables 103–4 and 103–6). This has greatly increased the awareness of this syndrome. Intestinal cultures have been expensive, awkward to perform, and usually not used extensively in clinical practice.

In the past, treatment was often empiric, not based on a firm diagnosis but dictated by a clinical impression. Broad-spectrum antibiotics (tetracycline) were prescribed for 7 to 10 days and the clinical response monitored. Up to 60% of the anaerobes (Bacteroides) now may be resistant to tetracycline. It behooves the physician to establish the diagnosis firmly, for the antibiotics needed may have serious side effects.

The mainstays of therapy are antimicrobial therapy and nutritional support. If there is a surgically correctable cause of the overgrowth, surgery should be performed if possible. Most patients with overgrowth do not have a surgically correctable cause (e.g., they have scleroderma, diverticulosis, or diabetes) and must receive lifelong antimicrobial and nutritional therapy.

A 10-day course of a cephalosporin (Keflex), 250 mg four times a day, and metronidazole (Flagyl), 250 mg three times a day, is very effective in suppressing the flora and correcting malabsorption, as is the clavulonic acid derivative Augmentin, 250 mg three times a day. Tetracycline is an alternative, resistance may be a problem. If these fail, chloramphenicol (50 mg per kilogram per day in four divided doses) is also very effective. Anaerobicidal agents by themselves (metronidazole, clindamycin) do not seem to be as effective as the combination of an aerobicidal and an anaerobicidal agent.

Three therapeutic patterns occur. Usually a 10-day course of an effective antimicrobial program corrects the malabsorption for months; some patients may need cyclic therapy (1 week out of every 6); rarely a patient may need continuous therapy for several months. Antibiotic sensitivity assays of the overgrowth flora are not recommended because of the multitude of organisms present. Octreotide has recently been demonstrated to stimulate small intestine motor activity in patients with scleroderma and bacterial overgrowth. Octreotide cleared the bacterial overgrowth and decreased nausea, vomiting, bloating and abdominal pain in these patients. Only a small dose of Octreotide was used (50 μg sq) and only at bedtime so as not to impair the motor response to feeding. This may be an exciting new alternative to antimicrobial therapy.

Nutritional therapy (especially with medium-chain triglyceride oil or the liquid diet Lipisorb) is very important but often ignored. Medium-chain triglyceride administration is ideal therapy for this condition, since this form of fat does not need bile salts for absorption. Other agents such as cobalamin, vitamin D, and calcium are given in doses detailed in Table 103–9.

ILEAL DISEASE OR RESECTION. Disease of the distal ileum leads to an interruption of the enterohepatic circulation of conjugated bile acids, resulting in a diminished bile acid pool and steatorrhea. The degree of steatorrhea is proportional to the amount of diseased or resected intestine. When < 100 cm of intestine is damaged or resected, proximal to the ileocecal valve, the steatorrhea is mild and choleretic diarrhea tends to be the most frequent

TABLE 103-9. AGENTS USED IN THE TREATMENT OF MALABSORPTION

1. **Calcium**
   Oral: Requires 1200 mg elemental calcium daily as
   a. Calcium gluconate (91 mg Ca^{2+}/gm), 5–10 g 3 times per day *or*
   b. Calcium carbonate (500 mg Ca^{2+}/tablet) 1–2 g per day in divided doses *or*
   c. Calcium carbonate, 2 tablets supplied as Caltrate or 2½ tablets as Os-Cal 500
   Intravenous: Calcium gluconate injection (10% solution, 9.1 mg Ca^{2+}/ml), 10–30 ml administered slowly)

2. **Magnesium**
   Oral: Magnesium gluconate, 500-mg tablets (20 mg Mg^{2+}/tablet), 1–4 g daily in divided doses
   Intramuscular: (20% sol.) 10 ml 2–3 times daily
   Intravenous: Magnesium sulfate, 0.5% sol., up to 1000 ml at a rate not faster than 1.0 mEq/min

3. **Iron**
   Oral: Ferrous sulfate, 325 mg (65 mg elemental iron) 3 times daily
   Intramuscular: Imferon must be calculated according to severity of anemia; detailed instructions accompany preparation

4. **Cyanocobalamin (vitamin B_{12})**
   Intramuscular: 100 μg daily for 2 weeks, then 100 μg monthly

5. **Folic acid**
   Oral: 5 mg daily for 1 month; maintenance 1 mg daily

6. **Vitamin B complex**
   Any multivitamin preparation that contains US RDA amounts; use 2 tablets daily; intramuscular preparations are available for severe deficiencies

7. **Fat-soluble vitamins**
   a. Vitamin A
      Vitamin A capsules (25,000 units per capsule), 100,000–200,000 units daily in severe deficiencies; maintenance, 25,000–50,000 units daily. *Caution:* Vitamin A toxicity can occur with recommended doses if hypertriglyceridemia is present
   b. Vitamin D
      Vitamin D (as vitamin D_2 or D_3), 30,000 units daily; dosage varies considerably depending on response as determined by level of serum calcium and urinary calcium
   c. Vitamin K
      Oral: Menadione, 4–12 mg daily; vitamin K tablets (Mephyton), 5–10 mg daily
      Intravenous: Acute bleeding episodes: vitamin K (Mephyton), 50-mg ampule administered slowly over 10-min period; repeat in 8–12 hr if prothrombin time has not returned to normal

8. **Cholestyramine**
   4-g pk, 1–2 pk before breakfast and lunch

9. **Medium-chain triglyceride (MCT oil)**
   Administer 60% of fat intake as MCT oil or Lipisorb, 40% as dietary long-chain triglyceride

10. **Human albumin, salt poor (0.25 g/ml)**
    Intravenous administration of 50–100 g daily for 3–7 days to elevate a severely depressed serum albumin level

11. **Immune serum globulin (0.165 g/ml)**
    Intramuscular injection of 0.05 ml/kg each 3–4 wk in patients with hypogammaglobulinemia and recurrent infection

12. **Adrenocorticosteroids**
    Prednisone, 40–60 mg daily for 2 wk, then decrease by 5 mg each week to maintenance of 5–15 mg daily

13. **Antidiarrheal agents**
    Oral: Diphenoxylate hydrochloride (Lomotil), 5.0 mg (2 tablets) initially and after each loose bowel movement, not to exceed 8 tablets daily; loperamide hydrochloride (Imodium), 2-mg capsules, 2 capsules initially and then 2 capsules after each loose bowel movement, not to exceed 8 capsules daily

14. **Drugs for parasites**
    Oral: Metronidazole (Flagyl), 250-mg tablet 3 times daily for 1 wk, or quinacrine hydrochloride (Atabrine), 100-mg tablet 3 times daily for 1 wk for *Giardia lamblia.* Thiabendazole (25 mg/kg/day): strongyloidiasis, 2–3 days; *Capillaria phillipinensis,* 30 days; *A. duodenale, N. americanus,* 25 mg/kg/day twice daily for 2 days.

problem. The malabsorbed bile acids dump into the colon and impair water and electrolyte absorption. When > 100 cm of small intestine is resected, the steatorrhea is large owing to a number of factors, including a diminished bile acid pool, loss of the absorptive function of the ileum, and bacterial overgrowth (loss of the ileoce-

cal valve). Choleretic diarrhea can usually be managed with cholestyramine (see Table 103–9).

Abnormalities of the Intestinal Mucosa

DISACCHARIDASE DEFICIENCY AND MONOSACCHARIDE MALABSORPTION. The most common disaccharide deficiency is lactase deficiency, which may be primary or secondary. Primary lactase deficiency is common throughout the world, with 60 to 90% of Native Americans, African Americans, and Asians being deficient with varying degrees of lactose intolerance. Only 5 to 15% of Caucasians are lactase deficient. Any disease that damages the enterocyte may lead to secondary lactase deficiency.

Lactase-deficient subjects are intolerant to milk, experiencing bloating, abdominal cramps, and diarrhea. The lactose within milk cannot be hydrolyzed to glucose and galactose. It remains in the intestinal lumen, where it is fermented by bacteria, producing organic acids, which increase the osmotic load, inducing shifts of water into the intestinal tract. The end result is distention of the intestine and diarrhea.

Primary lactase deficiency may not manifest itself until adulthood, yet the reason for this delayed appearance is not clear. Subtotal gastrectomy or pyloroplasty and vagotomy may unmask the condition by increasing the load of ingested lactose on the jejunal mucosa. Although the diagnosis is often made by taking a history, the lactose-H_2 breath test is the best way to document lactose intolerance (see Diagnosis section and Table 103–4). Treatment of primary lactase deficiency is avoidance of milk products or the ingestion of one to two capsules of Lactrase when dairy products are ingested. Lactrase, derived from *Aspergillus oryzae,* is commercially available.

Sucrase deficiency is quite rare. In afflicted patients, diarrhea occurs after ingesting sucrose. Elimination of sucrose, dextrins, and starches from the diet is effective.

Monosaccharide (glucose-galactose) malabsorption is a rare disorder present from birth. All sugars metabolized to glucose or galactose cannot be tolerated. Therapy consists of using fructose as a source of sugar.

NONTROPICAL SPRUE (ADULT CELIAC DISEASE, CELIAC SPRUE, GLUTEN-SENSITIVE ENTEROPATHY). Nontropical sprue is a disease of unknown cause characterized by malabsorption resulting from gluten-induced damage to the differentiated villus epithelial cells of the small intestine. Gluten is a high molecular weight protein found in wheat, rye, oats, and barley. The mechanism for this toxic effect is not known, but the most accepted theory is that metabolites of gluten initiate an immunologic reaction in the enterocyte. The enterocyte is often strikingly damaged, and biopsy of the small intestine demonstrates characteristic changes

TABLE 103-10. CLINICAL CONDITIONS ASSOCIATED WITH BACTERIAL OVERGROWTH

I. Gastric proliferation of bacteria
Hypo- or achlorhydria, especially when combined with motor or anatomic disturbances

II. Small intestinal stagnation
Anatomic
 Afferent loop of Billroth II partial gastrectomy
 Duodenal or jejunal diverticulosis
 Surgical blind loop (end-to-side anastomosis)
 Surgical recirculating loop (side-to-side anastomosis)
 Obstruction (stricture, adhesion, inflammation, cancer)
Motor
 Scleroderma
 Idiopathic intestinal pseudo-obstruction
 Derangements of interdigestive motor complex
 Diabetic autonomic neuropathy

III. Abnormal communication between proximal and distal gastrointestinal tract alignments
Gastrocolic or jejunocolic fistula
Resection of ileocecal valve

IV. Miscellaneous
Hypogammaglobulinemia
Chronic pancreatitis

Modified from King CE, Toskes PP: Small intestine bacterial overgrowth. Gastroenterology 76:1035, 1979.

(see Fig. 103–5 and discussion of small bowel biopsy in Diagnosis section). Malabsorption is secondary to the impaired transport of nutrients through the damaged enterocyte. In addition, a net secretory state for water and electrolytes has been noted in the jejunum, and pancreatic exocrine function may be secondarily diminished owing to a decreased release of secretin and cholecystokinin from the damaged small bowel mucosa.

Genetic factors appear important in this disease. Nontropical sprue is closely linked to two histocompatibility antigens, HLA-B8 and HLA-DRw3. These antigens are present in 60 to 90% of patients with this disease and in only 20 to 30% of the general population. An additional antigen has been found on the surface of B lymphocytes in 70 to 80% of patients with nontropical sprue and in 15% of normal controls. The same antigen is present in 100% of the patients' parents. Perhaps these antigens evoke antibodies to gluten, which result in the binding of gluten to the enterocyte with subsequent mucosal damage.

Patients with nontropical sprue usually have severe malabsorption—steatorrhea, diarrhea, weight loss, and many of the other symptoms and signs detailed in Table 103–3. Symptoms typically begin in infancy, disappear in late childhood, and reappear in the third to sixth decade of life. The proximal small intestine is usually the most severely damaged, and the symptoms, signs, and laboratory evaluation reflect this (Tables 103–3 and 103–4). At times, the clinical presentation may be quite subtle, e.g., anemia secondary to iron deficiency or bone pain from osteomalacia without obvious diarrhea or steatorrhea. Small bowel biopsy is essential in this disease, for a diagnosis of nontropical sprue commits the patient to a very restricted diet indefinitely. Evidence is accumulating that increased levels of serum antibodies to gliadin may be of considerable diagnostic benefit. Elevated serum IgA antigliadin may spare patients unnecessary small bowel biopsies.

The cornerstone of therapy is the withdrawal of all gluten from the diet, i.e., all grains must be eliminated except rice and corn. Most patients respond to dietary restriction with a remarkable decrease in symptoms and signs within a few days to a week. In some patients, however, it may take months before significant improvement is noted. Function tests such as urinary xylose excretion return to normal within a few weeks of gluten withdrawal. Post-treatment biopsies demonstrate marked improvement in most patients and completely normal histologic findings in many. The patient with the characteristic syndrome and biopsy findings who does not respond to gluten withdrawal is usually not adhering to the diet. Some patients may have the characteristic clinical picture and flat biopsy and in reality are not responding because they have another disease such as Whipple's disease, nongranulomatous ileojejunitis, giardiasis, lymphoma, or collagenous sprue. Collagenous sprue, a variant of nontropical sprue, demonstrates not only the characteristic changes in the small intestinal biopsy but also masses of eosinophilic hyaline material in the lamina propria. Such patients have a poor prognosis. Corticosteroid therapy (see Table 103–9) or parenteral hyperalimentation may be needed in some.

Small bowel lymphoma and carcinoma in general seem to be increased in patients with nontropical sprue. Abdominal pain in a patient with sprue should suggest lymphoma. Whether or not these complications are fewer in those who adhere strictly to a gluten-free diet is controversial.

Two other associated abnormalities in patients with sprue are (1) ulcers of the jejunum and ileum with abdominal pain, bleeding, and perforation, which are unresponsive to therapy, and (2) dermatitis herpetiformis. Some patients with this skin lesion may have latent sprue. The dermatitis is pruritic, vesicular, and papular and responds to sulfone treatment. Sulfone does not improve the intestinal lesion, but some of the skin lesions may respond to gluten withdrawal.

NONGRANULOMATOUS ILEOJEJUNITIS. This disease has features of both Crohn's disease and nontropical sprue, even a flat small intestinal biopsy. There is an abrupt onset with fever, abdominal pain, at times splenomegaly, and elevated white count—all suggesting lymphoma. Malabsorption may be profound, resulting in a therapeutic trial of steroids and a gluten-free diet—often to no avail.

CROHN'S DISEASE (see Ch. 104). Malabsorption in Crohn's disease results from several problems: (1) decreased absorptive surface from active disease or surgical resection, (2) bile salt depletion from ileal disease, and (3) bacterial overgrowth secondary to dilatation of the bowel and resection of the ileocecal valve.

EOSINOPHILIC ENTERITIS. Peripheral blood eosinophilia and infiltration of the gastrointestinal tract by eosinophils characterize this disease. Three patterns of involvement are seen: (1) involvement of the muscle layers of the stomach and small intestine causing obstruction, (2) involvement of the mucosa of the small intestine causing malabsorption, and (3) involvement of the subserosa causing ascites. Most patients have no evidence of allergy or food sensitivity. Corticosteroids and occasionally surgery are employed successfully.

RADIATION ENTERITIS (see Ch. 13.1 and 112). Radiation injury to the intestine may lead to malabsorption from (1) extensive mucosal damage, (2) lymphangiectasia from lymphatic obstruction, and (3) bacterial overgrowth. Malabsorption may occur shortly after exposure to radiation or years later. Most patients with clinically significant malabsorption appear to respond to therapy for bacterial overgrowth.

ABETALIPOPROTEINEMIA (see Ch. 173). This rare disease represents a defect in chylomicron formation. The intestinal cells are lacking apoprotein B, and therefore fat absorption cannot occur normally. Biopsy of the small intestine shows the epithelial cells to be engorged with fat even after an overnight fast. The clinical manifestations are steatorrhea, neurologic disease (ataxia, retinitis pigmentosa), very low serum cholesterol and triglyceride levels, and "spiny red cells" (acanthocytes). Therapy consists of substitution of dietary fat with medium-chain triglyceride and administration of fat-soluble vitamins, especially vitamin E.

Inadequate Absorptive Surface

SHORT BOWEL SYNDROME. Extensive resection of the small intestine is usually performed for Crohn's disease, intestinal infarction, or trauma. Acute hyperalimentation in these patients has been life-saving, and the ability of the remaining gut to adapt for increased nutrient absorption by hypertrophy of residual small intestinal villi is remarkable. Patients do rather well despite extensive resection if approximately 90 to 100 cm of duodenum and jejunum and the terminal ileum (intact ileocecal valve) remain.

Treatment consists of parenteral hyperalimentation for weeks to months until evidence exists that the remaining gut is functional. Gradual introduction of oral feedings, high in protein content, vitamins, and minerals, as well as medium-chain triglyceride (MCT), forms the basis for maintenance therapy. Antidiarrheal agents and cholestyramine may help (see Table 103–9). Occasionally, pancreatic extract therapy and H_2-receptor antagonists are necessary to treat the transient acid hypersecretion and secondary pancreatic insufficiency that may occur. Steroids may increase water absorption. Some patients must receive hyperalimentation at home indefinitely. Diarrhea resistant to all other therapy may respond to somatostatin analogues (Sandostatin).

JEJUNOILEAL BYPASS. Some patients with morbid obesity have had a surgical procedure performed (14 inches of proximal jejunum is anastomosed to 4 inches of terminal ileum) that induces malabsorption. In addition to many of the problems detailed above in the short bowel syndrome, other serious complications occur, such as oxalate kidney stones, intestinal pseudo-obstruction, cirrhosis, and arthritis. Because of these complications, the operation has been abandoned.

Infection

TROPICAL SPRUE. The pathogenesis of this malabsorptive disorder occurring in tropical regions (Far East, India, Caribbean) is poorly understood. An overgrowth of coliforms within the jejunum has been demonstrated in these patients. Such organisms have been shown to elaborate an enterotoxin that induces fluid secretion. Tropical sprue is not a true bacterial overgrowth, since anaerobes (particularly *Bacteroides*) are conspicuously absent. Malabsorption of many nutrients occurs, especially folic acid, cobalamin, and fat. The intestinal biopsy does not demonstrate total villus atrophy, but rather nonspecific changes in the villi (shortening, thickening) and cellular infiltration of the lamina propria. Successful therapy has been achieved with cobalamin, folic acid, or antibiotics. A 2-month course of a broad-spectrum antibiotic (e.g., tetracycline, 250 mg orally four times daily) and folic acid, 5.0 mg daily, is most effective. In those patients with cobalamin deficiency, 1000 μg of cobalamin should be given intramuscularly for 2 consecutive days. Improvement of malabsorption following therapy with folic acid or cobalamin alone casts doubt upon infection as the sole etiology.

WHIPPLE'S DISEASE. Patients (usually male) with Whipple's disease manifest steatorrhea, weight loss, abdominal pain, nondeforming arthritis, fever, peripheral lymphadenopathy, and neurologic abnormalities (nystagmus, ophthalmoplegia, cranial nerve defects). Protein-losing enteropathy may be present because of lymphatic obstruction.

Small bowel biopsy is diagnostic, demonstrating heavy infiltration of the mucosa and lymph nodes by macrophages that stain positive with periodic acid-Schiff reagent (PAS). Biopsy of the small intestine also shows blunting of villi and dilated lymphatics. The macrophages are filled with rod-shaped bacilli, which disappear after antibiotic therapy and reappear prior to an exacerbation of the disease. Although these rodlike structures resemble bacilli, no bacteria have been consistently cultured from patients with this disease. Polymerase chain reaction (PCR) amplification of tissues containing Whipple bacilli indicates that the Whipple bacillus is an actinobacter. It has been provisionally named *Tropheryma whippleii*.

Untreated, this is a fatal disease. These patients should be treated for at least a year and probably indefinitely. The antibiotic of choice appears to be trimethoprim-sulfamethoxazole, 500 mg given orally four times daily.

Lymphatic Obstruction

LYMPHOMA (INTESTINAL). Malabsorption occurs in patients with intestinal lymphoma from (1) mucosal invasion, (2) lymphatic obstruction, and (3) bacterial overgrowth secondary to dilatation of the bowel with stasis. Antibiotic therapy often completely corrects the clinical manifestations of malabsorption (diarrhea, steatorrhea), suggesting that bacterial overgrowth is an important cause of malabsorption in these patients. Abdominal pain, fever, and steatorrhea are principal complaints; lymphadenopathy and hepatosplenomegaly are uncommon. The small bowel biopsy may mimic nontropical sprue but not respond to a gluten-free diet. The diagnosis is usually made by finding malignant lymphoid cells in the mucosa or submucosa via small bowel biopsy or by full-thickness biopsy at surgery. As many as 10% of patients with nontropical sprue may develop lymphoma.

LYMPHANGIECTASIA. Primary or congenital lymphangiectasia is characterized by diarrhea, mild steatorrhea, edema, enteric loss of protein (protein-losing enteropathy), and abnormal dilated lymphatic channels on small intestinal biopsy (Fig. 103–6). The main clinical feature of this disorder, affecting primarily children and young adults, is asymmetric edema secondary to the hypoplastic peripheral lymphatics and chylous effusions. Lymphocytopenia and depressed serum protein levels are a result of the protein-losing enteropathy. The hypoplastic lymphatics lead to an obstruction in lymph flow, increased pressure within lymphatics, dilated lymphatic channels in the intestine, and finally rupture of the lymphatic channels, discharging lymph into the bowel lumen. Therapy is directed to decreasing lymph flow via a low-fat diet and substitution of dietary fat with MCT's, which are transported by the portal venous system rather than the lymphatic system.

Although protein-losing enteropathy is a hallmark of intestinal lymphangiectasia, many other disorders can also cause enteric protein loss. The mechanisms are multifactorial: (1) exudation of protein through inflamed or engorged mucosa (gastric cancer, hypertrophy of gastric mucosa, ulcerative colitis), (2) loss of protein because of abnormal enterocytes (nontropical sprue, scleroderma), and (3) passage of proteins into the intestine secondary to increased pressure within lymphatics (lymphangiectasia, constrictive pericarditis, lymphoma).

Enteric protein loss can be detected by intravenously administering various labeled macromolecules and measuring the radioactivity in the feces. These tests are cumbersome to perform and not readily available. Recently, α_1-antitrypsin has been used as a marker for this disorder. α_1-Antitrypsin (similar size as albumin) can be measured in the feces by immunodiffusion.

Other Causes

CARDIOVASCULAR DISORDERS. Any disorder causing poor perfusion of the intestine may lead to steatorrhea. Atherosclerosis and vasculitis may both affect the mesenteric blood supply.

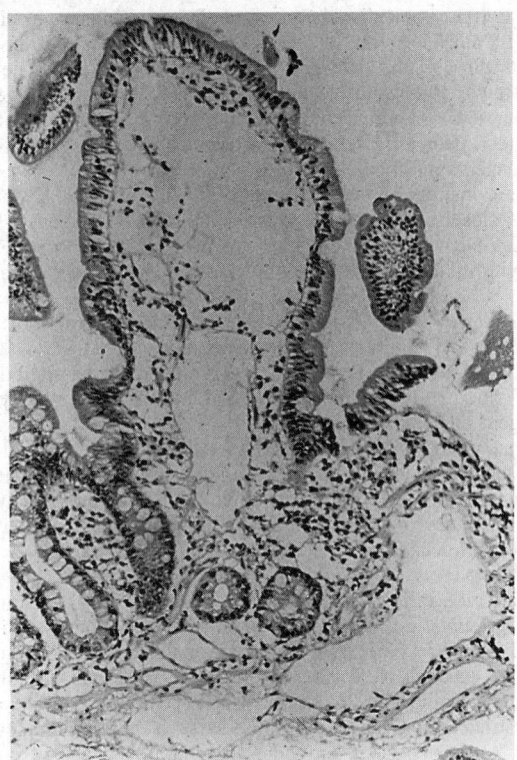

FIGURE 103–6. Small intestinal biopsy from a patient with intestinal lymphangiectasia. Note the dilated lymph channels (clear spaces).

DRUG-INDUCED MALABSORPTION. This entity is not very common and usually produces clinically insignificant malabsorption. Steatorrhea secondary to therapy with cholestyramine and neomycin is thought to be a result of precipitation of bile salts. The mechanism or mechanisms of most drug-induced malabsorption is not well understood.

UNEXPLAINED MALABSORPTION. Other than that in diabetes and perhaps in the carcinoid syndrome, the malabsorption occasionally observed in endocrine disorders (adrenal insufficiency, thyroid disease) is not at all understood. In diabetes, malabsorption may result from neuropathic changes (diarrhea) or bacterial overgrowth (steatorrhea). In systemic mast cell disease, there may be massive infiltration of the small intestine with mast cells, blunting of intestinal villi, and marked acid hypersecretion (see Ch. 231). Malabsorption, however, does not appear to correlate well with any of these abnormalities. Hypogammaglobulinemia is at times associated with severe malabsorption. Although the pathogenesis is not well defined, such patients may have giardiasis, bacterial overgrowth, and histologic abnormalities of the small intestine (patchy villus atrophy, nodular lymphoid hyperplasia). Plasma cells are absent within the intestine.

MALABSORPTION IN THE ELDERLY. Elderly patients may develop malabsorption from any of the disorders listed in Table 103–2, but bacterial overgrowth appears to be the most common cause of clinically significant steatorrhea in this population. The elderly often have decreased gastric acid secretion and abnormalities in intestinal motility that predispose them to malabsorption from bacterial overgrowth. The hypo- or achlorhydria may lead to cobalamin (vitamin B_{12}) deficiency from malabsorption of food-bound cobalamin (see Table 103–5). Such patients may be treated effectively just with tablets of cyanocobalamin (unbound B_{12}), because they have intrinsic factor in adequate amounts. Recognition of this problem may avoid parenteral administration of cobalamin.

MALABSORPTION IN THE ACQUIRED IMMUNODEFICIENCY SYNDROME (AIDS) (Ch. 366). Patients with AIDS often have diarrhea, malabsorption, and weight loss. A number of infectious agents, including *Giardia lamblia, Mycobacterium avium-intracellulare, Cryptosporidium, Microsporidium, Strongyloides stercoralis,* and *Isospora belli,* may cause malabsorption in these patients. Although these patients often have enteric infections and intestinal involvement with Kaposi's sarcoma, many with AIDS have malabsorption without these two abnormalities. In some AIDS patients, small intestinal biopsy demonstrates large numbers of histiocytes within the lamina propria. Although such biopsy findings may be confused with Whipple's disease, in patients with AIDS these histiocytes contain acid-fast bacilli, representing *M. avium-intracellulare*. Still other AIDS patients have malabsorption with the only abnormality found being that of a nonspecific mild to moderate chronic inflammatory response in the small bowel biopsy. The malabsorption in this last group of patients may be due to bacterial overgrowth or other unidentified enteric infections.

Brasitus TA, Sitrin MD: Intestinal malabsorption syndrome. Ann Rev Med 41:339, 1990. *New developments in malabsorption associated with AIDS, celiac sprue, bacterial overgrowth, and old age.*

Goggins M, Kelleher D: Celiac disease and other nutrient related injuries to the gastrointestinal tract. Am J Gastroenterology 89:S2, 1994. *Current review of celiac disease.*

Keinath RD, Merrell DE, Vlistra R, et al.: Antibiotic treatment and relapse in Whipple's disease. Long-term follow-up of 88 patients. Gastroenterology 88:1867, 1985. *Current discussion of therapy in this disease.*

Ladefoged IK, Christensen KC, Hegnhoj J, et al.: Effect of a long-acting somatostatin analogue SMS 201-995 on jejunostomy effluents in patients with severe short bowel syndrome. Gut 30:943, 1989. *Somatostatin analogues offer new therapy for intractable diarrhea of short bowel syndrome.*

Relman DA, Schmidt TN, MacDermott RP, Falkow S: Identification of the uncultured bacillus of Whipple's disease. N Engl J Med 317:293, 1992. *Identification of the bacterium that causes Whipple's disease using molecular biological methodology.*

Rich EJ, Christie DL: Anti-gliadin antibody panel and xylose absorption test in screening celiac disease. J Pediatr Gastroenterol Nutr 10:174, 1990. *Role of serum antibodies to gliadin in the diagnosis of celiac disease.*

Sleisenger MH, Fordtran JS (eds.): Gastrointestinal Disease. 5th ed. Philadelphia, WB Saunders 1993, *Normal absorption and malabsorption in well-referenced text on gastroenterology.*

Soudah HC, Hasler WL, Owyang C: Effect of octreotide on intestinal motility and bacterial overgrowth in scleroderma. N Engl J Med 325:1461, 1991. *A potential novel means to treat bacterial overgrowth.*

Toskes PP: The bentiromide test for pancreatic endocrine insufficiency. Pharmacotherapy 4:74, 1984. *Review of the worldwide experience with this noninvasive test of pancreatic function.*

Toskes PP, Donaldson RM Jr: Enteric bacterial flora and bacterial overgrowth syndrome. *In* Sleisenger MH, Fordtran JS (eds.): Gastrointestinal Disease. 5th ed. Philadelphia, WB Saunders, 1993, p. 1106. *Complete review of pathophysiology, diagnosis, and treatment of small intestine bacterial overgrowth.*

104 INFLAMMATORY BOWEL DISEASE

Stephen B. Hanauer

The term "inflammatory bowel disease" applies to the idiopathic, chronic inflammatory bowel diseases (IBD): Crohn's disease (CD) and ulcerative colitis (UC). These are distinguished from IBD of established origin such as viral, bacterial, and parasitic infections; diverticulitis; radiation enteritis or colitis; drug- or toxin-induced enterocolitis; and vasculitis of the intestinal tract. CD and UC are disorders of unknown cause involving genetic and immunologic influences on the gastrointestinal tract's ability to distinguish foreign from self-antigens and/or to down-regulate the mucosal immune response. They share many overlapping epidemiologic, clinical, and therapeutic features. Both are chronic, medically incurable conditions. Whereas a proctocolectomy cures UC, surgery for CD is limited to treatment of complications.

Ulcerative colitis encompasses a spectrum of diffuse, continuous, superficial inflammation of the colon, which begins within the rectum and extends to a variable proximal level. The inflammatory features are constant within the involved segment of the colon and, once established, the upward margin of inflammation usually remains constant in the same individual. Occasionally, the disease progresses to more proximal areas, usually within the first several years after diagnosis. The condition never involves the small intestine except when the distal terminal ileum is inflamed in a similar, superficial manner (backwash ileitis) in patients with inflammation throughout the colon (pancolitis). The inflammation extends beneath the lamina propria only in severe cases, when submucosal involvement produces a thinning of the circular and longitudinal muscles leading to colonic distention (toxic megacolon). UC is primarily a mucosal process, and removal of the entire mucosa is curative.

Crohn's disease is characterized by focal, asymmetric, transmural inflammation affecting any portion of the gastrointestinal tract from the mouth to the anus. The ileum and right colon are most often involved, but any segment of the gastrointestinal tract can be inflamed. The focal, transmural inflammation and the potential for proximal gastrointestinal tract involvement distinguish CD from UC. The presence of noncaseating granuloma also distinguishes CD from UC but is not necessary for the diagnosis. Microscopic changes are present throughout the gastrointestinal tract, distant from grossly involved segments of intestine.

The cause(s) of UC and CD is not known. Although genetic, biochemical, and immunologic patterns are recognized in patients, a definitive etiopathogenesis remains elusive. The absence of an appropriate animal model for chronic IBD has hampered progress in determining pathogenesis. No infectious agent has been linked to UC or to CD, although it is speculated that exposure to a common bacterial antigen stimulates an autoimmune reaction against a shared host antigen via molecular mimicry.

EPIDEMIOLOGY (Table 104–1)

UC and CD occur among all age groups but have a peak incidence in the second and third decades. CD incidence has risen over the past 20 years; CD now shares incidence and prevalence rates with UC of 5 per 100,000 and 50 per 100,000, respectively. The combined prevalence of the two diseases is approximately 100 per 100,000 population. These disorders are seen most commonly in Northern Europe and North America and in relatives of European immigrants in the cities of South Africa, Australia, and New Zealand. IBD is rare in Central America, South America, Africa, the Middle East, and Asia. Although IBD can be seen in all ethnic groups, there is an increased prevalence in Jews who have immigrated from Northern Europe. This Jewish predisposition is not seen in Sephardic (Mediterranean or Middle-Eastern) Jews. Although less common in the nonwhite population, more cases are being recognized in black, Hispanic, and Asian immigrants to western cities.

A presumed genetic influence is derived from family studies, in which approximately 20% of individuals with IBD have a relative with UC or CD. The pattern of inheritance is more complicated than that of a simple mendelian trait, and the risk is spread across families. In children with IBD the likelihood of another family member having the diagnosis is >40%. Although the risk to a child of a parent with IBD is <5%, when both parents have IBD the risk to offspring is >50%. A stronger concordance exists within families and in twin studies for CD than for UC. The only epidemiologic difference between UC and CD pertains to cigarette smoking. Cigarette smoking appears to protect against UC and is associated with CD. More than 80% of patients with UC are nonsmokers, whereas 80% of patients with CD smoke cigarettes. Often, UC begins after a "predisposed" individual stops smoking.

Attempts have been made to implicate a number of environmental factors in the development of IBD, including atypical mycobacterium, diets high in refined sugar (including corn flakes), increased consumption of polyunsaturated fats (margarine), and oral contraceptive pills, but none has been proven.

PATHOGENESIS

The absence of an etiologic factor leaves a gap in our understanding of the pathogenesis of IBD. Although a number of potential factors may influence the *initiation* of the inflammatory response, a popular view is that a defect exists in the "down-

TABLE 104–1. EPIDEMIOLOGY OF INFLAMMATORY BOWEL DISEASE

More common in whites than nonwhites
Increased frequency among European stock
More common among Jews (especially Ashkenazic) than non-Jews (3 to 6 times)
Most frequent age of onset: 15 to 30 years
Aggregation in families (25–40%)
Concordance for Crohn's in twins
Cigarette smokers—Crohn's disease
Nonsmokers—ulcerative colitis

regulation" of immune events (see Part XIX), allowing persistent *amplification* of the tissue-damaging process. The inflammatory reaction in IBD closely mimics infectious enterocolitis with the exception of the failure to halt progressive tissue destruction. Subtle differences exist between the immunologic findings of UC and CD, such as the production of immunoglobulin heavy-chain allotypes or neutrophil-cytoplasmic antibodies; however, pathognomonic findings to classify these disorders remain elusive. Nosology is currently based on descriptive clinical, endoscopic, and histologic criteria, and misclassification often is recognized as the clinicopathologic process evolves over time. When the diagnosis changes, it is almost always from UC to CD and virtually never the converse.

Potential initiating events in IBD include increased intestinal permeability, aberrant epithelial processing of antigen, improper epithelial utilization of short-chain fatty acids, and molecular mimicry between a luminal antigen and components of intestinal mucosa. There is evidence of increased intestinal permeability to small or medium-sized molecular particles in patients and relatives of patients with IBD, which may be affected by qualitative differences in intestinal mucus glycoprotein. Similar alterations in colonic mucin fraction IV from patients with UC are present in cotton-top tamarins with spontaneous colitis. Cigarette smoking can also influence mucin production and intestinal permeability, and nonsteroidal anti-inflammatory drugs (NSAID's) damage proximal and distal intestinal epithelium, increase intestinal permeability, and tend to exacerbate IBD.

Intestinal epithelial cells stimulated by interferon express class II major histocompatibility complexes and become antigen-presenting cells. The processing and presentation of antigens to T8 (suppressor T cells) are altered in patients with IBD such that the presentation of antigen is preferentially directed toward the T4 (helper T cell) system. This could be a primary, genetically mediated event that stimulates the gut immune system rather than induces tolerance.

A defect in the ability of the gut epithelium to metabolize short-chain fatty acids derived from the intestinal lumen or injury to the epithelium by an infectious or toxic injury may alter or expose cell proteins that are perceived as foreign by the mucosal immune system. A conclusive target antigen has not been identified for either UC or CD. A variety of antibodies to epithelial cell components, some of which cross-react with enterobacterial antigens, are present but are not specific for IBD. In addition, serum antibodies against enteric bacteria or food-related antigens (e.g., milk protein) are increased nonspecifically. Also, evidence exists of autoimmune lymphocyte-mediated cytotoxicity against epithelial cells, but a consistent abnormality in mucosal or systemic immune regulation has not been identified. Most of the local (mucosal) or systemic immunologic parameters represent secondary rather than primary changes.

Once initiated, many of the pathophysiologic events in IBD are related to amplification of the inflammatory process (see Ch. 235). When antigens are presented to mucosal macrophages, cytokines and other inflammatory mediators are activated and released. IL-1 is released and induces T-cell activation and proliferation. Activated T cells become cytotoxic and/or release IL-2, which induces clonal expansion of helper T cells, B-cell proliferation, and antibody synthesis. IgG production by B cells activates complement and subsequently the kinin system. The arachidonic acid cascade of inflammatory mediators is shifted toward the proinflammatory, lipoxygenase pathway with enhanced production of leukotriene B_4, a potent chemotactic agent for neutrophils, and platelet-activating factor (PAF) is produced. When neutrophils accumulate and are stimulated, they further damage tissue by releasing reactive oxygen species, amplifying the inflammatory process by recruiting additional acute inflammatory cells, whether or not the primary initiating sequences have been halted.

The release of inflammatory mediators, including prostaglandins and leukotrienes, histamine from mast cells, and neuropeptides such as substance P or vasoactive intestinal peptide, alters epithelial function and contributes to the intestinal secretory process, including diarrhea. The enteric nervous system helps regulate the local and systemic immune system, linking the association of "stress" and psychological factors with disease flare-ups.

PATHOLOGY

UC and CD encompass a spectrum of clinicopathologic findings. Most of the macroscopic and microscopic changes are not specific and overlap with those of acute and chronic infectious enterisides, toxin or radiation-induced damage to the intestine, ischemic changes, and, rarely, malignancy.

ULCERATIVE COLITIS. UC, primarily a mucosal disease, begins in the anorectum and involves a variable contiguous proximal segment of colonic mucosa. In approximately one quarter of patients the disease is limited to the rectum (proctitis); in another 25 to 50% the rectum and sigmoid (proctosigmoiditis) or the descending colon (left-sided colitis) is involved. In approximately one third of patients the inflammation extends proximal to the splenic flexure (extensive colitis) or involves the entire colon (pancolitis). The small intestine occasionally is involved by superficial inflammation (backwash ileitis) in a small group of patients with pancolitis. Once the upper demarcation of disease has been identified, it usually remains constant. Up to 40% of patients develop proximal extension of colonic involvement, usually within the first few years after diagnosis. Some patients with proctitis have patches of endoscopic or histologic changes in the cecum or right colon. The prognostic implications of these findings are uncertain.

The gross or endoscopic appearance of the colonic mucosa in UC ranges from normal-appearing mucosa to complete denudation. Mild inflammatory changes include absence of the mucosal vascular pattern, fine granularity of the mucosa, pinpoint hemorrhage to mucosal swabbing, and exudation of mucopus (see Color Plate 2A). Moderate changes include coarse granularity and pinpoint ulceration, confluent hemorrhage, confluent mucopus that progresses to gross ulcerations, spontaneous hemorrhage, and exudation of pus (see Color Plate 2A). With healing the mucosal vascular pattern remains distorted. Islands of postinflammatory "pseudopolyps" may appear as filamentous projections or mucosal bridges that may be quite friable or indistinguishable from adenomatous polyps (see Color Plate 2B).

In the active phase of inflammation, acute inflammatory cells, primarily polymorphonuclear leukocytes, accumulate near the epithelium, invade the crypts, and are concentrated within the crypt lumen (crypt abscess) (see Color Plate 2D). Progressive changes include degeneration or necrosis of the crypt epithelium with coalescence of crypt abscesses to produce shallow ulcerations extending to the lamina propria. Only rarely, in severe UC or toxic megacolon, do inflammation and necrosis extend below the lamina propria to involve the submucosa and circular or longitudinal muscles. Then the bowel wall may become "tissue paper" thin with a significant risk of spontaneous perforation. With healing and regeneration of the epithelium, depletion of epithelial goblet cell mucus (see Color Plate 2C) occurs.

Typically with acute disease, reversible changes in the colonic musculature lead to loss of haustrations, thickening of the smooth muscle of the colon, and the "lead pipe" appearance of the colon or, occasionally, the appearance of a stricture on radiographic examination.

Epithelial dysplasia may occur in longstanding UC and is highly associated with the presence of colonic malignancy as a long-term complication (see below).

CROHN'S DISEASE. CD involves any segment or combination of segments of the alimentary tract from the mouth to the anus. Unlike UC, microscopic changes often are identified distant from sites of macroscopic disease. These focal changes and the tendency of CD to recur after segmental resection suggest that subtle changes of CD exist throughout the alimentary tract. Most commonly the distal ileum and right colon are macroscopically inflamed (ileocolitis). The colon is involved, exclusively, in about 20% of patients (Crohn's colitis or granulomatous colitis); approximately 15 to 20% have gross disease limited to the small bowel (ileitis or regional enteritis). The stomach or duodenum is involved in < 10% of patients and usually in association with more distal disease. Disease of the anal canal, including deep fissures, fistulas, and prominent "hemorrhoidal" skin tags, are common and distinguish CD confined to the colon from UC. Unlike UC, the mucosa in CD is involved in a focal, discontinuous manner, both microscopically and macroscopically. Rarely, lesions indistinguishable from those of CD occur in the skin or urogenital mucosal surfaces (miliary CD).

The earliest macroscopic lesion of CD is the minute aphthoid ulcer (see Color Plate 2E), invariably occurring over a lymphoid aggregate. These ulcerations extend linearly (see Color Plate 2*F*), often isolating normal islands of mucosa to produce a "cobblestone appearance," or extend deep throughout the layers of the bowel wall, producing a fissure that can become a fistula into the mesentery or a contiguous organ. Inflammatory changes in CD are typically transmural, accounting for the thickening of the bowel wall and narrowing of the lumen. As CD heals, fibrotic changes replace acute inflammation, creating permanent focal strictures. In gross specimens, changes include thickened, sausage-shaped bowel with serosal hyperemia, "creeping fat" along the antimesenteric border, and thickening and lymphoid hyperplasia of the adjacent mesentery. The inflammatory process is focal in all layers of the bowel (see Color Plate 2*G*). Acute and chronic inflammatory cells invade isolated or contiguous single crypts (including the production of crypt abscesses) with normal adjacent glands. Lymphoid aggregates are common throughout all layers of the mucosa, submucosa, and serosa, with characteristic aggregations of histiocytes forming non-caseating granulomas in up to 50% of resected specimens. Mucosal biopsies, however, reveal granuloma formation in <20% of patients. The presence of granulomas differentiates CD from UC, but they are not necessary to distinguish the two diseases. Rather, the focal, transmural involvement of CD associated with aphthoid or linear ulcers, fissures, fistulas, perianal disease, or small intestinal involvement morphologically distinguishes CD from UC. In approximately 20% of patients with colitis, "indeterminate" features do not allow classification between UC and CD. Response to therapy and repeated observations over the course usually allow eventual classification.

CLINICAL MANIFESTATIONS

ULCERATIVE COLITIS. The symptoms of UC depend upon the extent and severity of inflammation. Patients with proctitis have rectal bleeding, tenesmus, and the passage of mucopus. The consistency of stools is variable, and many patients with ulcerative proctitis are constipated. The greater the extent of colon involved, the more likely the patient is to suffer from diarrhea. Rectal urgency reflects reduced compliance of the inflamed rectum. Abdominal cramping is common, but abdominal pain or tenderness, reflecting transmural disease and stimulation of serosal or peritoneal pain receptors, is not typical due to the superficial (mucosal) nature of UC.

As the severity of inflammation increases, the patient is more likely to suffer from systemic symptoms. Low-grade fever, malaise, occasional nausea and vomiting associated with defecation, night sweats, and arthralgias are frequent complaints. With severe UC, patients present with fever, dehydration, tachycardia, and symptoms of abdominal tenderness, reflecting progressive inflammation into deeper layers of the colon. A distended abdomen and tympanic bowel sounds accompanied by fever, tachycardia, and vomiting are ominous signs of fulminant colitis or toxic megacolon.

Patients with UC in remission have normal bowel habits, although many patients suffer from an accompanying irritable bowel syndrome with occasional cramping, irregular bowel habits, and the passage of mucus without blood or pus.

Laboratory studies reflect the severity of colitis. Iron deficiency anemia secondary to chronic blood loss is the most common abnormality. A low serum ferritin confirms the presence of iron deficiency anemia and better documents iron stores than do serum iron and iron-binding capacity, which are reduced by chronic disease (see Ch. 129). Elevated erythrocyte sedimentation rate and other acute phase reactants are inconstant features in UC and are of no value in the evaluation of individual patients. A low serum albumin occurs with extensive colitis as a manifestation of protein exudation from the inflamed colon. Serum alkaline phosphatase and GGTP may be modestly elevated (less than twice normal) in patients with pericholangitis; greater changes in bilirubin or hepatocellular enzymes suggest sclerosing cholangitis or chronic hepatitis.

CROHN'S DISEASE. The symptoms and signs of CD also are determined by the site and extent of inflammation. Gastroduodenal CD mimics peptic ulcer disease, with nausea, vomiting, and epigastric pain. Patients with small intestinal involvement have abdominal cramping, diarrhea, and abdominal tenderness. The pain and tenderness of CD are due to transmural inflammation. Transmural inflammation leads to fibrosis and narrowing of the intestinal lumen, which produce symptoms of obstruction: nausea, vomiting, waves of abdominal pain, and a reduced output of stool on physical examination. This is appreciated as a thickened, tender loop of bowel or

an abdominal mass, if the mesentery is involved. Patients with colonic CD present with abdominal pain, cramping or localized pain, rectal bleeding, and diarrhea.

Weight loss is more common in CD than in UC because of small bowel–related malabsorption or a reduced intake of food to minimize postprandial symptoms. Systemic symptoms, including fever, night sweats, malaise, and arthralgias, are common.

Laboratory features in CD reflect blood loss, malabsorption, protein-losing enteropathy, and elevation of acute phase reactants. Anemia may be due to a deficiency in iron (blood loss or malabsorption), folic acid, or vitamin B_{12}. Serum albumin and total protein are reduced with either malnutrition or protein-losing enteropathy. Electrolyte abnormalities reflect the severity of diarrhea, and lowered serum calcium may reflect reduced serum albumin, calcium malabsorption, or vitamin D deficiency. Patients with ileal disease often malabsorb fat-soluble vitamins (A, D, E, and K), deficiency of which can produce clinically significant symptoms or signs.

COMPLICATIONS

INTESTINAL COMPLICATIONS. *Rectal bleeding* is a common manifestation of both UC and CD. In UC the superficial inflammation induces capillary hemorrhage, manifested as bright red coating of stool or blood-tinged mucopus. In severe UC the bleeding can be more prominent and on rare occasions is profuse. Iron deficiency anemia is a common secondary association due to the chronic blood loss. In CD, hemorrhage may be profuse as a result of deeper inflammation and ulceration into larger vessels. Recurrent bleeding occurs in a small subset of patients with CD and is rarely the single indication for surgery.

Toxic megacolon, once thought to occur only with UC, also occurs in CD and infectious colitis. Toxic megacolon develops in seriously ill individuals when transmural inflammation extends into the muscular layer, thinning the intestinal wall. The entire colon, or segments of the colon, can dilate as a result of disruption of the neural and muscular elements that maintain normal tone. Dilatation of the diameter of the colon on a plain abdominal radiograph to >6 cm (see Color Plate 2*H*), associated with clinical symptoms of increasing abdominal pain, distention, rebound tenderness, and signs of fever, tachycardia, and dehydration, indicates the condition. Even without prominent dilatation, similar symptoms and signs are sufficient to diagnose severe colitis with an identical risk of perforation and the hazard of peritonitis. Precipitating circumstances include severe colitis, instrumentation with barium studies or endoscopic procedures in severe inflammation, potassium depletion, anticholinergic medications, or narcotics, which are thought to reduce neuromuscular activity of the gut. Associated laboratory findings include leukocytosis, hypokalemia, anemia, and hypoalbuminemia.

Toxic megacolon should be anticipated in any patient with severe colitis, including segmental colitis, and these individuals require careful monitoring of vital signs, abdominal examinations for rebound tenderness, flat-plate abdominal radiographs for dilatation or free air, and laboratory studies to maintain an adequate hematocrit and electrolyte status. Toxic megacolon should be treated with intensive medical therapy, and failure to improve within 12 to 24 hours is an indication for colectomy. Early colectomy can prevent the morbidity and mortality of a perforation, which may exceed 20%.

CD, being transmural, is associated with additional intestinal complications. Thickened segments of inflamed bowel become fibrotic, and stricturing is common. Whereas bowel narrowing in UC is due to reversible muscular hypertrophy, the scarring in CD is largely irreversible. Transmural fissures extend into adjacent structures, producing an inflammatory mass, abscess, or fistula. Enteroenteric, -vesicular, -mesenteric, or cutaneous fistulas are common, as are rectovaginal fistulas, perianal fistulas, and abscesses.

CANCER (Table 104–2, also Ch. 106). Cancer of the colon is a long-term complication of UC. Its development depends on two factors: the extent of mucosal involvement (pancolitis greater than left-sided colitis) and the duration of disease. Severity of the initial attack, subsequent course, and specific medical therapies are not related to the cancer risk. Colonic adenocarcinomas may occur in patients who have had quiescent UC for decades. Indeed, these may be the patients at highest risk. In Europe, where colectomy is performed earlier, the risk of cancer is reduced.

TABLE 104-2. CANCER IN ULCERATIVE COLITIS

Risk factors
Extent of colon involved
Duration of disease after 10 years
Surveillance
Begin after 10 years
Increase frequency of surveillance with increased duration of disease
Warning
Indefinite dysplasia: requires follow-up 3–6 months and/or confirmation by experienced pathologist
Surgical indication
Confirmed dysplasia, or dysplasia-associated lesion or mass (DALM)

Mucosal dysplasia is a precursor of cancer. Dysplasia can be identified with colonoscopic biopsies by experienced pathologists and must be distinguished from inflammatory or regenerative epithelial changes. Repeat biopsies and aggressive medical therapy should be considered when pathologic interpretation is in doubt. Confirmed epithelial dysplasia is an indication for colectomy, as malignancies are often identified separate from the dysplastic foci. Routine screening for dysplasia and neoplasia is now recommended in longstanding UC. Surveillance colonoscopies and biopsies throughout the length of the colon should be initiated after 8 to 10 years of extensive colitis and repeated at 1- to 2-year intervals. The finding of dysplasia warrants confirmation by an experienced pathologist or repeat examination. Dysplasia in a nodular or polypoid lesion has an extremely high (>50%) association with concurrent malignancy. Dysplasia and cancers in UC can occur in normal flat mucosa, with ulceration or stricture formation, or within a polyp or mass.

CD also increases the incidence of adenocarcinomas of the intestine. The same risk factors (extent and duration) probably apply but have not been as clearly established for CD. Patients with inactive CD should be monitored for a change in symptoms, bleeding, or obstruction; endoscopic or radiographic evaluation should be pursued for a change in an otherwise inactive phase. There is also a small increased risk of leukemia, lymphoma, and bile duct carcinomas in patients with IBD.

EXTRAINTESTINAL COMPLICATIONS (Table 104-3). The extraintestinal manifestations of IBD can be divided into complications of gastrointestinal inflammation or diseases associated with IBD. The latter occur most often with "colitis" but can occur in either UC or CD when the colon is inflamed.

Nutritional and metabolic abnormalities occur with chronic disease, inadequate intake of calories, maldigestion, and malabsorption. Blood and protein loss contribute to iron deficiency anemia and hypoalbuminemia. Deficiencies of calcium, magnesium, or zinc are most often noted with small intestinal CD in the presence of active inflammation or extensive surgical resections. Calcium deficiency may be aggravated by milk-free diets or vitamin D deficiency. Deficiency of folic acid can be secondary to inadequate intake, proximal small bowel disease, or competitive inhibition of folate absorption by sulfasalazine. Treatments for these nutritional deficiencies require appropriate diagnosis, treatment of the underlying inflammation, and enteral or parenteral repletion. Deficiencies in fat-soluble vitamins (vitamin A, D, E, and K) are most often produced by ileal disease or resection. Low vitamin D levels can aggravate metabolic bone disease and calcium malabsorption. Vitamin B_{12} deficiency can be avoided by regular replacement intramuscular injections (see Ch. 133).

Diarrhea is aggravated by malabsorption of fat or bile salts due to ileal disease or resection. Diarrhea due to fat malabsorption is diagnosed by increased fecal fat (greater than 5 grams per day) and treated with a low-fat diet (see Ch. 102). Additional calories can be supplied by medium-chain triglycerides, which are absorbed more proximally and do not require bile salts. Ileal resection also can deplete the bile salt pool owing to inadequate reabsorption and recirculation. Bile salt malabsorption induces diarrhea after bile salts are converted into bile acids in the colon, which stimulate secretion. Bile acid–induced diarrhea can be treated with small amounts of cholestyramine, which binds to bile salts and prevents the conversion to bile acids. Malabsorption of fat and bile salts in CD in-

creases gallstone and kidney stone incidence. Gallstones form because cholesterol levels are more saturated in the gallbladder secondary to a reduced bile salt pool. Fat malabsorption also increases the risk of calcium oxalate kidney stones. Normally dietary oxalate binds to calcium within the lumen of the small intestine and is excreted as insoluble calcium oxalate in the feces. With fat malabsorption, calcium binds to long-chain fatty acids rather than oxalate. Free oxalate is then hyperabsorbed from the colon and excreted in the urine (enteric hyperoxaluria). In addition, patients with IBD have low levels of urinary citrate, a nonspecific solubilizer that reduces mineral saturation in the urine. The treatment of calcium oxalate kidney stones includes reduction of fat intake to reduce fat malabsorption; maintenance of fluid intake and hydration; a low-oxalate diet; supplementation of citrate; supplementation with oral calcium as an intestinal oxalate binder, and the addition of cholestyramine as an alternative binder for intestinal oxalate. Enteric hyperoxaluria is discussed further in Ch. 88.

Skin and mucous membrane changes are common in IBD. Oral aphthae occur in CD, and fissuring of the lips or mouth may be due to zinc deficiency or *Candida* infection. Inflammatory skin disorders associated with IBD, pyoderma gangrenosum and erythema nodosum, tend to correlate with the disease activity in the colon, although, on occasion, skin changes may precede symptomatic colitis. Erythema nodosum presents as a painful, tender, erythematous, or violaceous nodule, most commonly on the leg. The lesions may be multiple, may develop on an extremity, and may be induced by minor trauma. Erythema nodosum usually responds to treatment of the underlying inflammation in the bowel but may respond more rapidly to topical or systemic steroids. The course of pyoderma gangrenosum, a more serious, necrotizing ulceration, occasionally runs independent from that of intestinal inflammation. It also typically occurs on the lower extremities but can also appear anywhere on the skin and occasionally on surgical incisions or adjacent to a soma. These lesions should not be biopsied, since this may lead to cutaneous breakdown and ulceration. Effective treatment of the underlying IBD, as well as topical antibiotics and potent topical steroids, should be implemented immediately. Resistant lesions may require systemic steroids, cyclosporine, or oral sulfone therapy.

Ocular complications of IBD share many inflammatory components with the intestinal inflammation. Conjunctivitis, episcleritis,

TABLE 104-3. EXTRAINTESTINAL MANIFESTATIONS OF THE INFLAMMATORY BOWEL DISEASES

Nutritional and metabolic abnormalities
Weight loss, growth retardation in children
Hypoalbuminemia—nutritional, protein-losing enteropathy
Vitamin deficiencies*
Deficiencies of calcium, magnesium, or zinc*
Hematologic abnormalities
Anemia—Fe, folate, B_{12}* deficiency
Leukocytosis, thrombocytosis
Skin and mucous membranes
Pyoderma gangrenosum
Erythema nodosum
Stomatitis with multiple aphthous ulcers
Musculoskeletal
Ankylosing spondylitis, sacroiliitis (HLA-B27 associated)
Peripheral arthritis of large joints
Osteoporosis
Osteomalacia*
Hepatic and biliary manifestations
Fatty liver
Pericholangitis
Sclerosing cholangitis
Gallstones*
Carcinoma of the bile ducts
Renal complications
Kidney stones
Uric acid
Calcium oxalate*
Obstructive uropathy*
Fistulas to urinary tract*
Amyloidosis (rare)
Eye complications
Conjunctivitis, episcleritis, iritis
Uveitis (HLA-B27)

* Crohn's disease.

and iritis often occur in conjunction with active intestinal inflammation and respond to topical steroids. Uveitis, an HLA-B27–associated complication, may run an independent course from the IBD.

Hepatic and biliary complications of IBD are frequent. Gallstones are related to bile salt malabsorption in CD, and steatosis may be secondary to malnutrition, corticosteroid therapy, or excessive carbohydrates from parenteral nutrition solutions. The spectrum of bile duct inflammation ranges from pericholangitis to sclerosing cholangitis and associated biliary cirrhosis. Pericholangitis (portal triaditis) is a nonprogressive inflammation of intrahepatic bile ductules manifested as a minor elevation of the alkaline phosphatase and GGTP with minimally elevated serum transaminases. Bilirubin remains normal, and inflammation is confined to the portal triads. Sclerosing cholangitis is a progressive form of bile duct inflammation involving the intrahepatic and/or extrahepatic biliary tree. Elevations of serum alkaline phosphatase and GGTP are greater than two times normal, and transaminase elevation can occur. Intermittent cholangitic episodes or asymptomatic jaundice may be the first manifestation. Visualization of the biliary tree via ERCP or transhepatic cholangiography confirms the extent of bile duct abnormalities. No proven therapies can limit the biliary inflammation, although preliminary studies using ursodeoxycholic acid or methotrexate are encouraging. Occasionally, endoscopic dilatation of a prominent stricture can relieve obstruction, although the disease is typically multifocal. Rarely, carcinoma of the bile duct mimics sclerosing cholangitis limited to the extrahepatic biliary system.

Kidney stones are a common complication of IBD. Hyperoxaluria and calcium oxalate stones are related to steatorrhea, whereas uric acid stones are more commonly associated with dehydration in patients with diarrhea or ileostomies. Obstructive uropathies can occur as a complication of an inflammatory mass in CD. Fistula to the bladder occurs with ileal CD associated with ileo-sigmoid-bladder communication, manifested as urinary frequency, dysuria, sterile pyuria, or recurrent cystitis. Amyloidosis is a rare, occasionally reversible complication of longstanding intestinal inflammation.

The metabolic bone diseases, osteoporosis and osteomalacia, occur commonly in chronic IBD. Osteoporosis is a frequent complication of long-term steroid therapy. Reduced bone mineralization also is a complication of malabsorption of vitamin D and calcium. Clubbing of the fingers and two distinct syndromes of enteric arthropathy may occur: (1) Peripheral arthritis frequently involves larger joints (knees, elbows, ankles) asymmetrically with swelling, erythema, and an inflammatory synovial analysis. It precedes or coincides with bowel symptoms and usually responds to treatment of the intestinal inflammation. Joint destruction does not occur, and serologic studies for rheumatoid factors are negative. (2) Central arthritis of the spine, ankylosing spondylitis, and sacroiliitis are HLA-B27–associated arthropathies that run a course independent from the bowel disorders. Progressive calcification and joint fusion proceed despite treatment of the IBD and require independent therapy (physical therapy and anti-inflammatory drugs). NSAID's must be used with caution in patients with IBD because they can potentially aggravate intestinal inflammation.

Children are susceptible to several unique complications of IBD. Often the initial manifestations of IBD occur without intestinal symptoms. Growth retardation, delayed sexual maturation, peripheral arthritis, fevers of undetermined origin, or anemia can precede abdominal symptoms. Impaired growth and development usually are associated with inadequate nutritional status. Improved caloric intake can reverse growth failure in conjunction with treatment of intestinal inflammation. Surgical resection is sometimes necessary to reverse growth failure. Children also are susceptible to delayed psychological development because of chronic illness and may require additional supportive therapy from the physician and other health care providers. Family counseling can also provide an important service to the patient and family. Patient support groups and education material from the Crohn's and Colitis Foundation of America have offered substantial benefit to patients and their families.

Fertility, pregnancy, and lactation are important aspects for young adults with IBD. In general, IBD does not reduce fertility. Women with active IBD or high-dose steroid therapy, however, often have anovulatory menstrual cycles or secondary amenorrhea, which temporarily impairs fertility. Women with active IBD are more likely to miscarry, but usually fetal development is normal in those carried to term. Medicinal and nutritional support for the pregnant woman should be continued throughout pregnancy. Corticosteroids and sulfasalazine should not be discontinued if they are successful in managing the mother's intestinal symptoms. Metronidazole should be avoided in the first trimester. Immunosuppressive therapies with 6-mercaptopurine or azathioprine are controversial in pregnancy but have been used with success based on the experience following transplantation. Approximately one third of women with quiescent IBD experience flare-ups during the postpartum period. Corticosteroids and sulfasalazine are secreted in small quantities in breast milk, but nursing is generally safe.

DIAGNOSIS

There are no pathognomonic clinical, endoscopic, or histologic features of the idiopathic IBD's. The physician must therefore consider the entire clinical picture and the evolution of the illness. It is particularly important to exclude other disorders that may mimic the broad range of IBD symptoms and findings. First it is important to establish the presence of intestinal inflammation. A cardinal feature is the exudation of inflammatory cells into the lumen, manifested by fecal leukocytes or red blood cells on stool examination. Symptoms of rectal bleeding, tenesmus associated with the passage of pus, nocturnal pain and diarrhea, fever, night sweats, weight loss, or extraintestinal symptoms or signs generally exclude an uncomplicated "irritable bowel syndrome." The presence of anemia, electrolyte disorders, hypoalbuminemia, or an elevated erythrocyte sedimentation rate of C-reactive protein is sufficient, but not necessary, to suggest IBD. On physical examination, evidence of significant weight loss or extraintestinal signs, a palpable abdominal mass or tenderness, or significant perianal disease suggests IBD. When suspicion of the diagnosis warrants, endoscopic and radiographic studies, in conjunction with histologic interpretation of biopsy specimens, confirm the diagnosis; the degree of illness at presentation should determine the aggressiveness of the diagnostic workup. Acutely ill patients should be stabilized before invasive studies are pursued.

ENDOSCOPY. Patients presenting with colitic symptoms of rectal bleeding, cramping, tenesmus, mucopus, or watery diarrhea in conjunction with fecal leukocytes warrant a colonic examination. A proctoscopic examination or flexible sigmoidoscopy reveals the presence and pattern of distal colonic inflammation. In the absence of perianal disease, diffuse, continuous mucosal changes with a distinct upper boundary to adjacent normal-appearing mucosa are typical of ulcerative proctitis or proctosigmoiditis. Focal inflammation with aphthoid ulcers, linear or stellate ulcers with normal intervening mucosa, or inflammatory changes beginning above the rectum (rectal sparing) in previously untreated patients suggest CD. If the patient is not acutely ill, colonoscopy demonstrates more proximal colonic changes and allows examination and intubation of the ileocecal valve to evaluate terminal ileal findings. Patients with upper abdominal symptoms can be diagnosed with upper gastrointestinal endoscopy when typical mucosal changes of CD involve this area. Findings can be correlated with mucosal biopsy studies and radiographic evaluation of the small and large intestine.

RADIOGRAPHY. Radiographic examination should begin with a supine and upright view of the abdomen. Associated findings of nephrolithiasis, cholelithiasis, or arthritis of the spine or sacroiliac joints may be identified. Intestinal dilatation or air-fluid levels suggesting obstruction preclude aggressive barium studies until the patient's clinical condition is stabilized. In colitis, a plain view of the abdomen often demonstrates a tubular, ahaustral segment of colon in the presence of distal UC with fecal matter proximal to diseased mucosa. Intestinal edema, ulceration, or thumb-printing may give a gross estimate of disease activity. Air-contrast barium studies of the colon reveal diffuse, contiguous granularity, superficial ulceration, and absent haustration in active UC. Pseudopolyps or a tubular-appearing "lead pipe" colon may be found in chronic UC. Focal, asymmetric ulceration with linear or fissuring ulcers, the presence of fistulas, rectal sparing, or a diseased terminal ileum with reflux of the barium define the radiographic extent and severity of colonic CD. A small bowel follow-through or enteroclysis (small bowel enema) demonstrates the extent of small intestinal involvement in CD and is normal in the absence of backwash ileitis in UC.

Specialized diagnostic imaging studies are occasionally useful to diagnose the extent or complications of IBD. Ultrasonography (US) or a computed tomography (CT) examination can clarify the presence of thickened bowel wall and mesentery versus an abscess cavity in an abdominal mass. Perineal CT scan or rectal US demonstrates the degree of involvement and the complexity of anorectal fistulas. Occasionally, US- or CT-guided aspiration of a cavity can reduce the morbidity of abdominal or retroperitoneal suppuration. Injected indium- or technetium-labeled leukocytes localize in sites of intestinal inflammation, and fecal excretion of radiolabeled leukocytes can be a measure of inflammatory activity.

DIFFERENTIAL DIAGNOSIS. Patients with irritable bowel syndrome rarely present with "inflammatory" features. Persistent symptoms despite therapy for presumed irritable bowel syndrome (especially in the presence of weight loss), bleeding attributed to "hemorrhoids," or a family history of IBD deserve a more comprehensive evaluation to exclude IBD. Most enteric infections are self-limited. Viral gastroenteritis typically lasts 1 to 4 days without rectal bleeding or fecal leukocytes. Most bacterial pathogens produce self-limited disease lasting less than 7 to 14 days, despite intermittent rectal bleeding, fevers, fecal leukocytes, and a mucosal appearance that may be indistinguishable from that of UC or CD. Occasionally, *Campylobacter jejuni* produces protracted symptoms and *Clostridium C. difficile* toxin–induced colitis can mimic the symptoms, signs, and endoscopic appearance of UC or CD. When a patient with IBD presents with new or exacerbated symptoms, stool cultures for enteric pathogens and studies for *C. difficile* toxin should be obtained, especially if the patient has been recently treated with antibiotics. In Northern Europe and Canada, *Yersinia enterocolitica* infection can mimic terminal ileitis. If the clinical suspicion warrants, cultures and serologic studies for *Yersinia* should be obtained. Similarly, tuberculosis of the gastrointestinal tract may mimic CD in geographic areas where intestinal tuberculosis is edemic, and, rarely, *Actinomycosis* simulates fistulizing CD.

Chronic intestinal infections usually are parasitic. Amebiasis may cause diarrhea, rectal bleeding, and a sigmoidoscopic appearance similar to that of idiopathic IBD. Deep "collar button" ulcerations are similar to focal ulcerations of CD. Fresh stool specimens should be examined repeatedly for amebic cysts or trophozoites; biopsies may be indicated in patients who have been exposed to endemic environments (e.g., nursing home residents and homosexual men). Syphilis, gonorrhea, and lymphogranuloma venereum also induce proctitis in gay men. HIV diarrhea should be excluded by serologic studies in patients with suspected exposure.

Occasionally, with an acute onset, Crohn's ileitis is diagnosed at laparotomy performed for presumed appendicitis. Likewise, in young individuals with acute right lower quadrant pain, mesenteric adenitis may mimic the symptoms of CD. In the older population, ischemic bowel disease, especially chronic mesenteric ischemia, or recurrent diverticulitis can mimic Crohn's colitis.

Persistent rectal bleeding should not be attributed to hemorrhoids unless a flexible sigmoidoscopy has excluded IBD. In older people, colonic carcinomas also can produce chronic symptoms and intermittent rectal bleeding. Intestinal lymphoma may be difficult to distinguish from CD and often requires a surgical diagnosis when suspected. Radiation enteritis is limited to patients with a history of that therapy. Some patients receiving chemotherapy or gold develop diarrhea and mucosal ulceration. Eosinophilic gastroenteritis presents with diarrhea, malabsorption, and protein-losing enteropathy, but the associated peripheral blood eosinophilia and biopsies are distinguishing. The diffuse, proximal malabsorptive pattern of celiac sprue, associated with diffuse villous atrophy, is distinct from the focal, distal small bowel changes of CD. Table 104–4 outlines the distinguishing features between UC and CD confined to the colon.

NSAID-induced ulceration of the ileum and colon is the most commonly encountered drug-related enterocolitis owing to prevalent NSAID use. The incidence of subclinical NSAID-induced damage to the gut mucosa is high (over one-third of exposed individuals). Diffuse or focal ulceration including aphthous ulcers is common and may complicate the predisposed vulnerability of mucosa in the elderly resulting from ischemia or diverticular disease. NSAID exposure may also predispose to newer variants of colitis such as *collagenous colitis* and *microscopic colitis*. The latter are recently described colitides causing diarrhea and epithelial or subepithelial

TABLE 104–4. A COMPARISON OF THE CLINICAL AND PATHOLOGIC FEATURES OF CROHN'S COLITIS AND ULCERATIVE COLITIS

Feature	Crohn's Colitis	Ulcerative Colitis
Clinical		
Smoker	+ +	+/ −
Malaise, fever	+ +	+
Rectal bleeding	+ +	+ + +
Abdominal tenderness	+ + +	+
Abdominal mass	+ +	−
Abdominal pain	+ + +	+
Perianal disease	+ + +	−
Endoscopic		
Rectal disease	+	+ + +
Diffuse, continuous symmetric involvement	+	+ + +
Aphthous or linear ulcers	+ + +	−
Cobblestoning	+ +	−
Friability	+ +	+ + +
Radiologic		
Continuous disease	+	+ + +
Ileal involvement	+ +	−
Asymmetry	+ + +	−
Strictures	+ +	+
Fistulas	+ +	−
Pathologic		
Discontinuity	+ +	−
Transmural involvement	+ + +	+/ −
Lymphoid aggregates	+ + +	−
Crypt abscesses	+ + +	+ + +
Granulomas	+ +	−
Sinus tract/fistula	+ + +	−

+ + + = Always; + + = common; + = occasional; − = never.

histologic findings in the absence of identifiable endoscopic lesions. When suspected as a causative factor or in the setting of IBD, NSAID's should be discontinued and avoided.

TREATMENT

The therapy of either UC or CD depends on the extent and severity of intestinal involvement (Table 104–5). The patient/physician team must embark upon treatment carefully considering the entire clinical picture and the chronic nature of the illness. Both the patient and the family should participate in the decision-making; this requires education and support. Although the therapies for UC and CD overlap in many ways, they are considered separately to clarify the differences. A primary difference is that UC can be cured by removing the colon and all colonic mucosa. CD is not cured by surgery and has a predictable tendency to recur after removal of an involved segment of intestine. Medical alternatives are discussed first, followed by specific IBD syndromes.

Medical Alternatives

AMINOSALICYLATES. Sulfasalazine was developed more than 50 years ago to combine a known antibiotic (sulfapyridine) with a salicylate (5-aminosalicylic acid, mesalamine) for delivery into the connective tissue of the colon. It is now recognized that the

TABLE 104–5. INFLAMMATORY BOWEL DISEASE: SEVERITY CRITERIA

	Mild	Severe	Fulminant/Toxic
Bowel frequency	< 4/day	> 6/day	> 10/day
Blood in stool	+/ −	+ +	Continuous
Fever	Normal	> 37.5°C	> 37.5°C
Pulse	Normal	> 90/min	> 90/min
Hemoglobin	Normal	< 75%	Transfusion required
ESR	< 30 mm/hr	> 30 mm/hr	> 30 mm/hr
Abdominal x-ray		Colonic edema, thumbprinting, air-fluid levels	Dilated colon or small bowel
Clinical sign		Abdominal tenderness	Rebound tenderness, distention, diminished bowel sounds

azo bond between sulfapyridine and 5-aminosalicylic acid is split by colonic bacteria, relating both components in the colon. Most of the sulfapyridine is absorbed from the colon, acetylated by the liver in a genetically determined manner, and excreted in the urine. The majority of the mesalamine remains within the colon and is excreted within the feces. Mesalamine delivered into the colon has therapeutic efficacy similar to that of sulfasalazine, but without the potential adverse consequences of the sulfa moiety.

Sulfasalazine is effective in a dose-dependent manner for treating acute UC and for maintaining remission of quiescent UC. Sulfasalazine also has been effective for mild to moderate CD when the colon is involved. It has not been clearly shown that sulfasalazine maintains remission in CD, although patients with CD who respond symptomatically to sulfasalazine may have flare-ups when the drug is discontinued.

Many patients develop side effects from sulfasalazine before achieving therapeutic doses. Nausea, malaise, headache, and myalgias are common side effects that reduce patient compliance. Sulfa-induced hemolysis, allergic reactions, and toxic pancreatitis, pneumonitis, hepatitis, or colitis are rare, but reversible abnormalities of sperm motility and morphology are seen in up to 80% of males taking sulfasalazine. Sulfasalazine also competitively inhibits intestinal absorption of folate, occasionally producing folate deficiency (see Ch. 133). Folic acid supplementation (1 mg daily) is therefore recommended for patients on long-term therapy. Sulfasalazine seems to be safe for both the mother and the infant during pregnancy and with breast feeding.

Because 5-ASA (mesalamine) is an active moiety of sulfasalazine, topical mesalamine has been used as a substitute for sulfasalazine to treat distal colitis. Mesalamine enemas are effective for active UC confined to the left colon when administered nightly, and they prolong remissions of left-sided UC if therapy is maintained. Mesalamine suppositories (500 mg administered two to three times daily) are also effective for ulcerative proctitis, and nightly therapy with 500 mg suppositories maintains remissions.

Free mesalamine is rapidly absorbed from the proximal gastrointestinal tract. Several delayed or sustained-release preparations are currently under development in the United States. Asacol, which contains 400 mg of mesalamine coated with a resin that breaks down at pH 7, supplies the same amount of mesalamine present in 1 gram of sulfasalazine. Pentasa, which contains mesalamine encapsulated into microgranules of ethylcellulose, releases mesalamine throughout the small and large intestine. Dipentum (olsalazine), an azo-bonded dimer of two 5-ASA molecules, releases two molecules of mesalamine in the colon in a manner similar to sulfasalazine.

Mesalamine has fewer side effects than sulfasalazine. Except for topical therapy with mesalamine enemas in distal UC, mesalamine has no therapeutic advantage over sulfasalazine. Mesalamine preparations are tolerated in 80% of patients who cannot tolerate sulfasalazine. The sperm abnormalities associated with sulfasalazine are reversed with mesalamine treatment. Olsalazine may increase intestinal secretion to produce diarrhea severe enough to stop therapy in approximately 6% of patients. Diarrhea can be minimized or avoided by gradual titration of the therapeutic doses.

CORTICOSTEROIDS. Corticosteroids are indicated to induce remission in either UC or CD, but they should not be used for maintenance therapy because of their inability to prevent relapse and their associated side effects (see Ch. 18). In UC, hydrocortisone enemas are useful for treating distal colonic symptoms, and hydrocortisone foam or suppositories can be applied for the relief of rectal inflammation. Oral prednisone is indicated for moderate to severe UC at doses of 40 mg daily initially, followed by gradual tapering according to the clinical course. Severe UC should be treated with parenteral corticosteroids in intravenous daily doses comparable to 40 mg of prednisone. Alternatively, intravenous ACTH may be administered for patients who have not previously received steroid therapy. In CD, corticosteroids are useful in similar doses for acute disease and, again, are not recommended for maintenance therapy.

Corticosteroid therapy is also limited by its well-recognized adverse effects. Cushingoid features, acne, facial hair, and elevated blood pressure are common early side effects. Cataract formation, osteoporosis (aggravated by vitamin D deficiency and calcium malabsorption in CD), and aseptic necrosis limit high-dose or long-term therapy. In children, corticosteroid therapy may further aggravate growth retardation.

ANTIBIOTICS. Antibiotic therapy for UC is limited to the presurgical treatment of severe or toxic colitis. Antibiotics have not been useful for less severe UC or to prevent relapse. In CD, metronidazole is as effective as sulfasalazine for colonic CD and may be more beneficial for small intestinal disease and perianal complications of CD. Metronidazole (10 to 20 mg per kg administered orally in divided doses) can relieve symptoms of CD, reduce acute phase reactants, and heal perianal disease. Metronidazole therapy is limited by coating of the tongue, nausea, alcohol intolerance, and peripheral neuropathy. The latter may be most troublesome, with documented abnormalities on neurologic examination and nerve condition studies before clinical symptoms arise. Alternative antibiotics have not been adequately studied in CD, although many clinicians continue to use broad-spectrum antibiotics, such as ciprofloxacin, sulfa-trimethoprim, and cephalexin, for symptomatic therapy of mild to moderate CD.

IMMUNOSUPPRESSIVES. 6-Mercaptopurine (6-MP) and azathioprine are effective in the long-term therapy of UC and CD. In both settings, these agents are useful in doses (50 to 150 mg per day) that are not immunosuppressive but probably have anti-inflammatory activity. There has been a reluctance to use these agents in UC because immunosuppressives have been found to be carcinogenic in patients receiving organ transplants. These medications, which require 3 to 6 months for maximal therapeutic effect, are largely useful for patients who are steroid-dependent, for disease refractory to standard medical therapies, for healing some intestinal and perianal fistulas, and as maintenance therapy for patients in whom treatment fails or who cannot tolerate mesalamine. Allergic pancreatitis occurs in up to 15% of patients receiving these drugs (see Ch. 107). Blood counts should be monitored every 2 to 3 months, indefinitely, once a stable dose has been achieved, because of the short- and long-term risk of neutropenia or bone marrow suppression.

Recently, intravenous cyclosporine has been used in severe UC as an adjunct to parenteral steroids. It has not been determined whether this regimen alters the long-term course. Likewise, use of parenteral methotrexate has increased for chronic steroid-dependent CD with optimistic results that need to be compared with 6-MP or azathioprine therapy.

Specific Syndromes

ULCERATIVE COLITIS

The medical therapy of UC depends on the extent and severity of mucosal ulceration. It is advisable early in the course to define the colonic extent of disease with either colonoscopy or a combination of proctosigmoidoscopy and air-contrast barium enema. UC treatment can be divided into that for acute disease and that for maintaining remission (Table 104–6). Maintenance therapy is indicated because 80% of patients who improve as shown by endoscopic or histologic examination experience an exacerbation of their disease within a year after cessation of active therapy.

ULCERATIVE PROCTITIS. Mild ulcerative proctitis can be treated with topical corticosteroids or topical mesalamine. Hydrocortisone enemas (Cortenema) or foam (Cortifoam), administered intrarectally at night, generally provide prompt relief. Patients should be treated until the symptoms resolve and the mucosa has healed (absence of granularity, friability, and mucopus at proctoscopy). After healing, the topical corticosteroids should be discontinued and used intermittently for mild relapses, or an oral aminosalicylate should be substituted for maintenance therapy. Some patients prefer oral sulfasalazine or mesalamine therapy as initial treatment for mild disease. Patients with more severe symptoms of proctitis with profound urgency, tenesmus, and frequent stooling may require a combination of topical corticosteroids and oral aminosalicylate or a combination of oral and topical aminosalicylates. Rarely, systemically active steroids are required for distal proctitis.

PROCTOSIGMOIDITIS. Proctosigmoiditis also responds to hydrocortisone or mesalamine enemas but more often requires combination therapy with oral aminosalicylates. Patients with severe symptoms should receive oral corticosteroids at a dose equivalent to 40 mg of prednisone daily. As the inflammation resolves and the mucosa heals, the steroids should be tapered with maintenance by either oral or topical aminosalicylate. Steroids generally can be

TABLE 104–6. ULCERATIVE COLITIS: MEDICAL THERAPY

Therapy	Mild/ Moderate	Severe†	Fulminant†	Maintenance
Diet	Symptomatic	PO + PN	NPO/TPN	Symptomatic
Oral anti-inflammatory	(−)	(−)		
Sulfasalazine	2–6 g/day	2–6 g/day	—	2–4 g/day
Olsalazine	1.5–3.0 g/day	1.5–3.0 g/day	—	0.75–1.5 g/day
Mesalamine	1.5–4.8 g/day	1.5–4.8 g/day	—	1.5–3.0 g/day
Topical anti-inflammatory				
Mesalamine enema or suppository	1–4 g/day	—	—	—
Corticosteroid enema or foam	80–200 mg/day	100–200 mg/day	—	—
Systemic anti-inflammatory*				
Prednisone	20–60 mg/day	40–60 mg/day IV	40–60 mg/day	—
ACTH	—	80–120 U/day IV	80–120 U/day	—
Antibiotics	—	—	+	—
Surgical consultation	—	+	+ +	

* Not warranted for proctitis; † avoid anticholinergics, antidiarrheals, narcotics, invasive procedures.

withdrawn according to the acuteness of symptoms. A reduction by 5 to 10 mg per week from 40 to 20 mg, followed by a reduction for 2.5 mg per week, is a reasonable approach that should be modified according to the individual's response. Again, aminosalicylate maintenance therapy is beneficial.

EXTENSIVE COLITIS. Patients with extensive colitis but mild symptoms should be treated with oral aminosalicylates. More severe symptoms (e.g., more than 5 to 10 bowel movements per day, weight loss, abdominal tenderness, night sweats) require adding corticosteroids, with an aminosalicylate as a maintenance therapy.

SEVERE COLITIS OR TOXIC MEGACOLON. Either of these conditions is a medical emergency. Patients presenting with more than 10 bowel movements per day accompanied by fever, leukocytosis, anemia, and tachycardia should be hospitalized. Appropriate fluid and electrolyte resuscitation should be instituted, and patients with significant anemia should receive transfusions to keep up with continued blood loss until the inflammation is stabilized. Patients who have not received prior corticosteroid therapy may be treated with parenteral ACTH or corticosteroids. Rectal application of steroid enemas or foam provides relief from severe tenesmus in conjunction with systemic steroids. Less severely ill patients with no nausea or vomiting may continue an oral intake of elemental feedings or a light diet, as tolerated. Parenteral nutrition should be added for malnourished patients. Severely ill patients require constant monitoring because of the potential of toxic megacolon. Abdominal flat-plate examination should be performed at 12- to 24-hour intervals if there is evidence of colonic dilatation or any worsening. Patients with evidence of transmural disease, such as abdominal tenderness, fever, and leukocytosis, should receive broad-spectrum antibiotic treatment (e.g., metronidazole and an aminoglycoside) as if they had a bowel perforation. Failure to improve, evidence of rebound tenderness, or free air under the diaphragm requires surgical intervention.

MAINTENANCE THERAPY. Corticosteroids are not useful for the maintenance therapy of UC because they do not prevent relapse and they have many long-term adverse effects. Sulfasalazine, olsalazine, and mesalamine are effective as maintenance therapies and should be continued "indefinitely" at the lowest dose that prevents relapse, with any withdrawal being carried out at a very gradual pace. Any recurrent symptoms require resuming therapeutic doses.

SUPPORTIVE THERAPY. Dietary therapy has a limited role in treating inflammation in UC, but diet should not be ignored as symptomatic therapy. Patients having constipation improve with an increase in the fiber content of their diet. Patients with abdominal cramping or diarrhea have symptomatic improvement with a low fiber diet with the exclusion of nonabsorbed carbohydrates (sorbitol, fructose, and lactose in lactose-intolerant patients). Iron replacement is necessary for patients with continued blood loss, and folic acid should be supplemented in patients taking sulfasalazine. In patients with mild disease, antispasmodics or antidiarrheal agents improve associated symptoms of bowel "irritability," but these should be

used cautiously in severe disease because of the potential of inducing toxic megacolon.

SURGERY. UC can be cured by colectomy, which alleviates the symptoms, lessens medication requirements, and can prevent potential long-term complications of colitis (cancer). Indications for surgery include toxic megacolon, perforation, intractable hemorrhage, complications of medical therapy, failure to improve with medical therapy, and evidence of confirmed dysplasia or cancer.

Surgical alternatives include proctocolectomy and ileostomy, and sphincter-saving operations, which remove the abdominal colon and rectal mucosa (saving the distal rectal musculature) and create an ileal pouch and ileoanal anastomosis. This surgical approach is performed satisfactorily in one to three stages with an expected outcome of four to eight liquid bowel movements per day and full continence in 80% of patients. The operation is limited to patients with confirmed UC and may be complicated by inflammation of the ileal pouch ("pouchitis"), which often requires therapy with metronidazole or aminosalicylates. The cause of pouchitis is not yet known, although it occurs only in patients with ileoanal anastomoses performed for IBD.

CROHN'S DISEASE

Medical therapy for CD must be individualized according to the disease location, severity, and complications. Unlike in UC, nutritional therapies have a more prominent role in treatment of CD and prevention of complications. Furthermore, it has been difficult to prove any maintenance therapy effective in CD clinical trials. Corticosteroids should not be continued once clinical benefit has been obtained, because of their severe long-term sequelae and their lack of benefit in preventing relapse. Many patients who respond to sulfasalazine or mesalamine worsen upon withdrawal, and chronic therapy has a much larger benefit/risk ratio. Metronidazole has unique long-term toxicity (neuropathy), and other antibiotics can induce vitamin K deficiency or growth of *C. difficile*. Immunosuppressives have the best record in maintaining remission, but their long-term risks have not been established.

Symptomatic *gastroduodenal* CD is uncommon and usually responds to short-term corticosteroid therapy in conjunction with acid reduction with an H_2-receptor antagonist or omeprazole (see Ch. 99.3). Gastric outlet obstruction unresponsive to corticosteroids requires surgical diversion with a gastrojejunostomy. *Jejunoileitis* often presents with diarrhea and protein-losing enteropathy. Mild symptoms respond to oral mesalamine or alternating antibiotics, which control associated small bowel bacterial overgrowth. Corticosteroids or an elemental diet have equal beneficial effects on persistent symptoms and laboratory studies. Immunosuppressives are sometimes necessary to control this diffuse form of small intestinal CD when steroids cannot be withdrawn. *Ileitis* and *ileocolitis* are more common variants of CD. Mild symptoms respond to diet adjustments to control diarrhea and abdominal cramping. If a low-residue diet is not sufficient, elemental feedings can reduce symptoms. Sulfasalazine, mesalamine, or antibiotics control mild symptoms, but patients presenting with fever, abdominal tenderness, or the presence of an inflammatory mass usually require short-term corticosteroids. Immunosuppressives or total parenteral nutrition can be useful for patients who cannot be tapered off steroids or whose condition remains refractory with active disease. Colonic CD also responds to sulfasalazine, mesalamine, antibiotics, or, if necessary, corticosteroids. Immunosuppressives should be reserved for steroid-dependent or -refractory patients.

NUTRITION IN CROHN'S DISEASE. The panenteric nature of CD can lead to a variety of nutritional deficiencies. Besides the enhanced requirements for iron due to blood loss and protein due to inflammatory exudation from the digestive tract, patients with small bowel CD who malabsorb calcium and magnesium, folic acid, and water-soluble vitamins require supplementation. Ileal CD requires monitoring and therapy for malabsorption of fat-soluble vitamins and vitamin B_{12}.

In addition to treatment of symptoms with dietary alterations (e.g., fiber avoidance in patients with intestinal narrowing or diarrhea, the adding of fiber for constipation, fat avoidance for fat malabsorption, lactose avoidance for lactose intolerance), dietary modifications can reduce the inflammatory features of CD. Elemental diets and corticosteroid therapy have equal therapeutic benefit. Elemental feedings can be administered by nasoenteric tube at night and are most beneficial for children with impaired growth. Total parenteral nutrition also benefits patients who cannot tolerate elemental feedings, who have a short bowel syndrome, or who have refractory symptoms despite medical therapy. Bowel rest does not affect the natural history of CD after therapy is discontinued.

SURGERY IN CROHN'S DISEASE. Active CD recurs at a predictable rate at the margines of a surgical resection. Virtually all patients develop some endoscopic and microscopic inflammation at an anastomotic site by 1 year after an operation. Usually, the course of a recurrence is similar to the initial manifestations; e.g., inflammatory or suppurative CD tends to recur as an inflammatory mass or fistula, whereas chronic, fibrosing CD recurs at a slower rate, evolving to intestinal obstruction. The recurrence rate is lower after exteriorization of the bowel with an ileostomy or colostomy than after reanastomosis.

Since surgery does not cure CD, the indications for surgery are for treating complications rather than as a "cure." Surgery is indicated for recurrent intestinal obstruction, complicated fistulas, intractable hemorrhage, disease refractory to medical therapy or complicated by inability to withdraw corticosteroids, growth retardation that does not respond to medical or nutrition intervention in children, and cancer. Unfortunately, the recurrence of CD cannot be prevented after resection, although mesalamine or immunosuppressives may possibly delay the time to recurrence.

PROGNOSIS

ULCERATIVE COLITIS. The course of UC depends upon the severity of the initial attack and the response to medical treatment. Less than 5% of patients succumb to fulminant UC or require immediate colectomy, and a small percentage of patients have a single attack without recurrence. The majority of patients have periods of remission maintained by medical therapy interrupted by spontaneous, acute exacerbations induced by stress, intercurrent illness, pregnancy, infectious diarrhea, or the injudicious use of NSAID's. Noncompliance or cessation of maintenance therapy may lead to recurrence. Approximately 15% of patients have refractory UC with continuous symptoms, despite all attempts at medical therapy, and 20% of patients in the United States require a colectomy at some time. Advances in medical and surgical therapies have greatly improved the prognosis for patients with UC. Patients who are properly managed rarely succumb to acute disease, and supportive long-term treatment can reduce chronic morbidity and mortality. Death, when it occurs, is usually due to complications of colonic perforation when surgery is deferred, to postoperative complications after colectomy, or to colonic carcinoma. The life expectancy after recovery from an initial attack of UC is no different from that of the general population. Long-term morbidity from UC is usually due to complications of medical therapy, especially when chronic corticosteroid therapy is required or abused. In general, an improvement in well-being occurs after colectomy undertaken for protracted or complicated illness. Patients who have undergone the sphincter-saving operations prefer to accommodate to frequent stooling and the

occasional need for medical treatment of pouchitis rather than to life with a stoma.

CROHN'S DISEASE. The prognosis for CD depends on the site and extent of intestinal involvement, as well as on complications of the disease. Approximately 50% of patients require surgical intervention, the risk being higher for patients with small intestinal disease than large bowel CD. Fifty per cent of patients undergoing operation require a second operation, and 50% of these, a third. Periodic remissions and exacerbations are common, although disease-free intervals may extend for years or decades after surgery for chronic, fibrotic strictures. Relapses after acute inflammatory CD are more common and occur earlier. The tendency for recurrence is a frustrating psychosocial feature. Additionally, physical changes associated with surgical or medical therapy can greatly affect self-image, especially in adolescence or in socially active patients. Perianal disease can be an especially troublesome feature.

Fortunately, advances in medical and supportive therapy have limited mortality in CD to that of the general population. Death usually occurs as a complication of surgical therapy, related to pulmonary emboli or sepsis. Morbidity, however, may be significant in patients requiring dietary modifications, frequent medical therapy, or recurrent operations or in individuals troubled by refractory diarrhea or perianal disease. The quality of life with CD is lower than with UC, often because of uncertainties related to recurrence after operations. Corticosteroid therapy adds significant morbidity to the long-term treatment of CD, and the increasing recognition of intestinal cancer as a long-term complication may become important as patients survive longer.

Bayless TM: Current Therapy in Gastroenterology and Liver Disease. Philadelphia, BC Decker, Inc., 1990. *Individual aspects of medical and surgical management are discussed by experts.*

Hanauer SB: Medical therapy of ulcerative colitis. Lancet 342:412, 1993. *A brief review of therapeutic options for ulcerative colitis.*

Hanauer SB, Kirsner JB: Inflammatory Bowel Disease: A Guide for Patients and Their Families. New York, Raven Press, 1985. *A helpful text for patient and family information.*

Peppercorn M: Therapy of Inflammatory Bowel Disease: New Medical and Surgical Approaches. New York, Marcel Dekker, 1990. *A thorough review of medical therapies for IBD.*

Targan SR, Shanahan F: Inflammatory Bowel Disease: From Bench to Bedside. Baltimore, Williams & Wilkins, 1994. *A comprehensive text composed of basic and clinical information on all aspects.*

105 VASCULAR DISORDERS OF THE INTESTINE

Lawrence J. Brandt

ISCHEMIC DISORDERS

Three major vessels supply almost all of the blood to the gastrointestinal (GI) tract, albeit with incredible variation in vascular anatomy. The *celiac axis* (CA) and its branches supply the liver, biliary structures, spleen, stomach, duodenum, and pancreas; the *superior mesenteric artery* (SMA) gives off branches to the duodenum and pancreas and then supplies the entire small intestine as well as the ascending colon and a variable portion of the transverse colon; the *inferior mesenteric artery* (IMA) delivers blood to the rectum and descending colon and then anastomoses with the superior mesenteric artery to supply the transverse colon. In some areas— e.g., the stomach, duodenum, and rectum—collateral circulation is abundant and ischemia is unusual; in other regions, such as the splenic flexure and sigmoid, anastomoses are more limited and segmental ischemic damage is common.

Ischemic injury of the bowel is influenced by the health of the general circulation, the potential for collateral flow, the response of the vasculature to autonomic stimuli and circulating vasoactive substances, local modulation of blood flow, and a host of exogenous agents causing vasoconstriction (digitalis glycosides, vasopressin and α-adrenergic agonists) or vasodilation (β-adrenergic agonists, papaverine, calcium channel blockers, aminophylline).

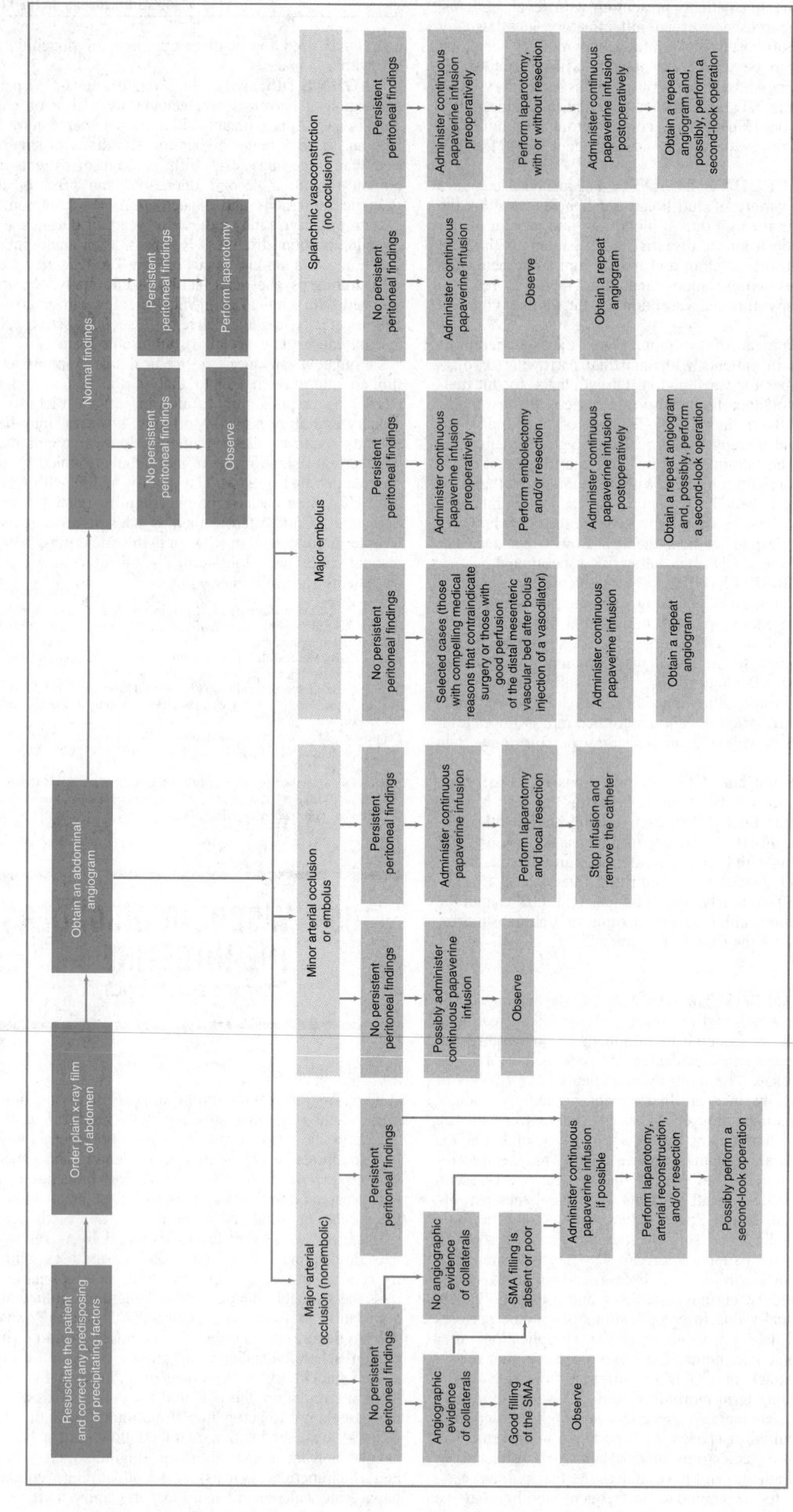

FIGURE 105–1. Algorithm for managing patients with suspected acute mesenteric ischemia.

The types of intestinal ischemia and their approximate incidences are colonic (60%), acute mesenteric (30%), focal segmental (5%), and chronic mesenteric (5%). Ischemic injury may be viewed in the broadest sense as occlusive (due to an anatomic obstruction to blood flow) or nonocclusive (mediated by vasoconstriction); however, these two processes often coexist. When a major vessel is suddenly occluded, collaterals open immediately in response to the fall in arterial pressure. Increased blood flow through these collaterals continues as long as the pressure in the vascular bed distal to the obstruction remains below systemic pressure. However, after several hours of ischemia, vasoconstriction develops in the involved vascular bed, elevating its pressure and reducing collateral flow. If the ischemia and vasoconstriction are sustained for long enough, the vasoconstriction can persist even after the cause of the ischemia is corrected. The bowel can tolerate a remarkable reduction in blood flow without damage. Normal O_2 consumption can be maintained with only 20 to 25% of normal blood flow because only one fifth of the mesenteric capillaries is open at any time. When blood flow is reduced, O_2 extraction is increased, allowing constant O_2 consumption over a wide range of blood flow. Below a critical level of flow, O_2 consumption falls because increased oxygen extraction can no longer compensate for diminished blood flow.

Acute Mesenteric Ischemia

Intestinal ischemia can be acute (AMI) or chronic (CMI) and of venous or arterial origin. AMI is much more common than CMI, and ischemia of arterial origin is much more frequent than venous disease. Forms and incidences of AMI are superior mesenteric arterial embolus (50%), nonocclusive mesenteric ischemia (25%), superior mesenteric artery thrombosis (10%), focal segmental ischemia (5%) resulting from atheromatous emboli or vasculitides, and acute mesenteric venous thrombosis (10%).

ARTERIAL FORMS OF ACUTE MESENTERIC IS-CHEMIA. *Superior mesenteric artery emboli (SMAE)* are responsible for 40 to 50% of AMI episodes. Emboli usually originate from a left atrial or ventricular thrombus and lodge distal to the origin of a major branch. Many patients with SMAE have had previous peripheral emboli, and approximately 20% have synchronous emboli to other arteries. *Nonocclusive mesenteric ischemia (NOMI)* causes 20 to 30% of AMI episodes and usually results from splanchnic vasoconstriction hours to days following some cardiovascular event, e.g., acute myocardial infarction, congestive heart failure, arrhythmia, or shock. Patients with chronic renal diseases, especially those requiring hemodialysis, and those undergoing major cardiac or intra-abdominal operations are also at risk. *Superior mesenteric artery thrombosis (SMAT)* occurs at areas of severe atherosclerotic narrowing, most often at the SMA origin. The acute episode is commonly superimposed on chronic ischemia, and 20 to 50% of these patients have a history suggesting intestinal angina during the weeks to months preceding the acute event.

CLINICAL ASPECTS OF ACUTE MESENTERIC IS-CHEMIA. Sudden abdominal pain developing in a patient with heart disease and arrhythmias, longstanding and poorly controlled congestive heart failure, recent myocardial infarction, or hypotension should suggest the possibility of AMI. Early on, the pain is accompanied by a paucity of physical findings. Increasing abdominal tenderness and muscle guarding reflect the progressive loss of intestinal viability and indicate infarcted bowel. Rightsided abdominal pain associated with passing of maroon or bright red blood in the stool, although characteristic of colonic ichemia, also suggest the diagnosis of AMI because the blood supply to both the right colon and small bowel originates from the SMA.

Leukocytosis, metabolic acidemia, elevated serum phosphate, amylase, lactate dehydrogenase, creatine phosphokinase, and intestinal alkaline phosphatase have been described with advanced ischemic bowel injury, but the sensitivity and specificity of these and other markers of intestinal ischemia have not been established. Plain films of the abdomen are usually normal before infarction. Later, formless loops of small intestine, ileus, or "thumbprinting" of the small bowel or right colon due to submucosal hemorrhage may develop. Selective mesenteric angiography is the mainstay of diagnosis and initial treatment of both occlusive and nonocclusive forms of AMI.

The approach to diagnosing and managing AMI is based on several observations: (1) if the diagnosis is not made before intestinal infarction, the mortality rate is 70 to 90%; (2) both occlusive and

nonocclusive forms of AMI can be diagnosed by angiography; (3) vasoconstriction may persist even after the cause of the ischemia is corrected and is the basis of NOMI as well as a contributing factor in the other forms of AMI; and (4) vasoconstriction can be relieved by vasodilators infused into the SMA. Early and liberal use of angiography and the incorporation of intra-arterial papaverine are therefore the cornerstones in the treatment of both occlusive and nonocclusive mesenteric ischemia.

Initial management of patients suspected of having AMI includes resuscitation, abdominal plain films, and selective angiography. Resuscitation includes relieving acute congestive heart failure and correcting hypotension, hypovolemia, and cardiac arrhythmias. Mesenteric blood flow cannot be improved if low cardiac output, hypovolemia, or hypotension persists. Broad-spectrum antibiotics are begun immediately. Plain films of the abdomen are obtained, not to establish the diagnosis of AMI but to exclude other causes of abdominal pain. A normal plain film does *not* exclude AMI. If no alternative diagnosis is made on the abdominal films, selective SMA angiography is performed. Based on the angiographic findings and the presence or absence of peritoneal signs, the patient is treated according to the algorithm in Figure 105–1.

Even when the decision to operate has been made based on clinical grounds, a preoperative angiogram should be obtained. Relief of mesenteric vasoconstriction is essential in treating emboli, thromboses, and "low flow" states and is accomplished by infusing papaverine at 30 to 60 mg per hour through the indwelling SMA angiography catheter (Fig. 105–2).

Laparotomy is performed in AMI to restore arterial flow after an embolus or thrombosis and/or to resect irreparably damaged bowel. Except in the case of mesenteric venous thrombosis, heparin probably should not be used immediately postoperatively. However, late thrombosis following embolectomy or arterial reconstruction occurs frequently enough that anticoagulation 48 hours postoperatively is advisable. With the approach described above, survival is in the range of 55%; 90% of patients with AMI diagnosed angiographically before the development of peritonitis have survived.

MESENTERIC VENOUS THROMBOSIS (MVT). MVT is an infrequent form of intestinal ischemia accounting for 5 to 10% of AMI. Underlying causes have been identified in >80% of patients and include antithrombin III, protein S and C deficiencies, and hypercoagulable states associated with polycythemia vera, myeloproliferative disorders, pregnancy, and neoplasms; oral contraceptive–related MVT accounts for <10% of patients. As many as 60% of patients with MVT have a history of peripheral vein thromboses. MVT can have an acute, subacute (weeks to months), or chronic onset; the latter is unaccompanied by symptoms unless and until late complications occur. *Acute MVT* resembles arterial forms of AMI as it presents with abdominal pain which, early on, is typically out of proportion to the physical findings. However, the tempo of illness is slower than that with arterial forms of AMI, and the mean duration of pain before admission is 5 to 14 days. Nausea and vomiting are common, and lower gastrointestinal bleeding or hematemesis indicating bowel infarction is found in 15%. Abdominal plain film signs of MVT are similar to those of other forms of AMI and almost always reflect the presence of infarcted bowel. Characteristic findings on small bowel series include luminal narrowing from congestion and edema of the bowel wall, separation of loops due to mesenteric thickening, and "thumbprinting" due to submucosal hemorrhage and edema. Selective mesenteric arteriography can differentiate venous thrombosis from arterial forms of ischemia, but ultrasonography, computed tomography (CT), and magnetic resonance imaging (MRI) are more commonly used to demonstrate thrombi in the SMV and portal vein. In the few patients with no physical findings of intestinal infarction in whom a diagnosis of MVT is made by ultrasonography, CT, or MRI, a trial of anticoagulant or thrombolytic therapy is worthwhile. All other patients should have prompt laparotomy, resection of nonviable bowel, and heparinization. The mortality of acute MVT is lower than that of the other forms of AMI, varying from 20 to 50%. Recurrence rates of 20 to 25% fall to 13 to 15% if heparin is begun promptly.

Subacute MVT is a condition in which patients have abdominal pain for weeks to months but have no intestinal infarction. Subacute MVT can be due either to extension of thrombosis at a rate rapid enough to cause pain but slow enough to allow collaterals to de-

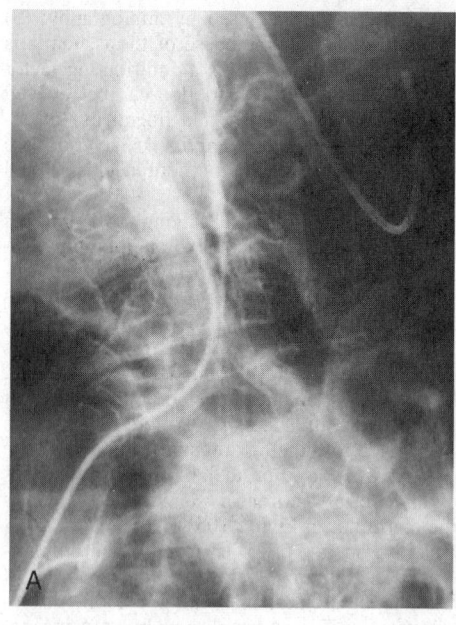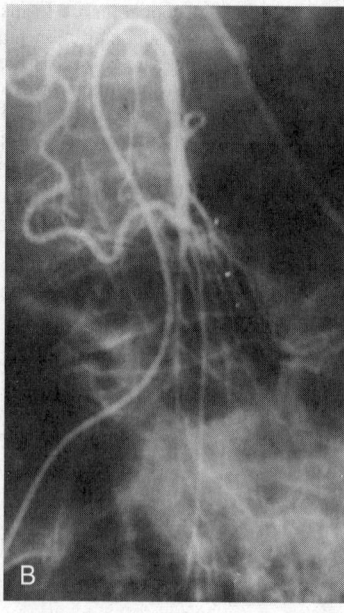

FIGURE 105–2. Selected films from a superior mesenteric angiogram revealing (*A*) diffuse vasoconstriction characteristic of nonocclusive mesenteric ischemia. *B*, Intra-arterial infusion of papaverine (30 to 60 mg per hour) resulted in vasodilation.

velop before infarction occurs or to acute thrombosis of only enough venous drainage to permit recovery from ischemic injury. Diagnosis usually is made on imaging studies done for other suspected diagnoses. Nonspecific abdominal pain is usually the only symptom of subacute MVT, and physical examination and laboratory tests are normal. In *chronic MVT,* there are no symptoms when the thrombosis occurs, and the patient may remain asymptomatic or may develop gastrointestinal bleeding, usually from esophageal varices. If the portal vein is involved, physical findings are those of portal hypertension, but if only the SMV is involved, there may be no abnormal findings. Laboratory studies may show hypersplenism with pancytopenia or thrombocytopenia. Treatment of chronic MVT is aimed at controlling bleeding, which is usually from esophageal varices. No treatment is indicated for patients with asymptomatic chronic MVT. The natural history of chronic MVT is not known, but from postmortem studies, it appears that almost 50% of patients with MVT have no bowel infarction, and most are without symptoms.

Focal Segmental Ischemia of the Small Bowel (FSI)

Vascular insults to short segments of small bowel produce a broad spectrum of clinical features without the life-threatening complications associated with more extensive ischemia. FSI is caused by atheromatous emboli, strangulated hernias, vasculitis, blunt abdominal trauma, radiation, and oral contraceptives. With FSI there is usually adequate collateral circulation to prevent transmural infarction, and patients present with one of three clinical patterns: acute enteritis often simulating appendicitis, chronic enteritis resembling Crohn's disease, and intestinal obstruction often with bacterial overgrowth and a "blind loop" syndrome. Treatment of FSI is resection of the involved bowel.

Colon Ischemia (CI)

CI is the most common ischemic injury to the GI tract. A spectrum of colon ischemic injury is recognized, including (1) reversible colopathy (submucosal or intramural hemorrhage) (30 to 40%); (2) transient colitis (15 to 20%); (3) chronic ulcerating colitis (20 to 25%); (4) stricture (10 to 15%); (5) gangrene (15 to 20%); and (6) fulminant universal colitis (<5%). In most cases, no specific cause for CI is identified, and what finally triggers the presenting episode is usually unknown. However, colonic blood flow is lower than that of any other intestinal segment, decreases with functional motor activity, and is greatly affected by autonomic stimulation—a combination that may make the colon especially susceptible to ischemia. More than 90% of patients with CI are over age 60, although CI has been documented in young individuals with vasculitis (especially systemic lupus erythematosus), sickle cell disease, coagulopathies, medication-induced reactions (estrogens, danazol, vasopressin, gold, psychotropic drugs), cocaine abuse, and long distance running. Approximately 15% of patients with CI have had a distal and potentially obstructing colonic or rectal lesion including carci-

noma, diverticulitis, stricture, or fecal impaction. CI is a complication of elective aortic surgery in 1 to 7% of cases, but following surgery for ruptured abdominal aortic aneurysm it may be as high as 60%.

Pathologic abnormalities in CI are varied. Mildest changes include mucosal and submucosal hemorrhage and edema with or without partial mucosal necrosis. Hemorrhages are subsequently resorbed or the overlying mucosa sloughs, forming an ulcer. Multiple ulcers manifest clinically as a transient segmental colitis. With more severe injury, the mucosa and submucosa are replaced by granulation tissue. Later, the mucosa may regenerate over the edematous submucosa, which contains granulation and fibrous tissue and iron-laden macrophages. Moderately severe CI can produce chronic ulcerations separated by normal bowel, a picture that mimics inflammatory bowel disease. With more severe and prolonged ischemia, the muscularis propria is damaged and replaced by fibrous tissue, thus forming a stricture. The most severe cases show transmural infarction with gangrene and perforation.

In contrast to AMI, most CI is not associated with either a major vascular occlusion or a period of low cardiac output. CI usually presents with sudden, crampy, mild, left lower abdominal pain, an urge to defecate, and passage of bright red or maroon blood mixed with the stool within 24 hours. Bleeding is not vigorous, and blood loss requiring transfusion suggests another diagnosis. Physical examination usually reveals only mild to moderate abdominal tenderness over the involved segment of bowel. Any part of the colon may be affected, but the splenic flexure, descending colon, and sigmoid are most commonly involved. Systemic low flow states usually involve the right colon; local nonocclusive ischemic injuries involve the "watershed" areas of the colon, i.e., the splenic flexure and rectosigmoid; ligation of the inferior mesenteric artery produces changes in the sigmoid.

If CI is suspected and the patient has no signs of peritonitis and an unrevealing abdominal plain film, colonoscopy or the combination of sigmoidoscopy and a gentle barium enema should be performed on the unprepared bowel within 48 hours of the onset of symptoms; colonoscopy is more sensitive in diagnosing mucosal abnormalities, and biopsy specimens may be obtained. Hemorrhagic nodules seen at colonoscopy represent submucosal bleeding and appear as filling defects called "thumbprints" on barium enema examination (Fig. 105–3). The initial diagnostic study should be performed within 48 hours, because thumbprinting disappears as the submucosal hemorrhages are resorbed or the overlying mucosa sloughs. Studies performed 1 week after the initial study should reflect evolution of the injury: normalization of the colon or replacement of the thumbprints with segmental ulceration. Mesenteric angiography is usually *not* indicated in CI, because by the time of presentation, colonic blood flow has returned to normal. Angiography may be indicated, however, when the clinical presentation does not allow a clear distinction between CI and AMI, or if only the right side of the colon is involved, a situation indicating disease in the distribution of the SMA and thus implying coincident AMI. In such situations, because untreated AMI rapidly becomes irreversible, and optimal management requires angiography, AMI must be excluded prior to barium studies, which would preclude an adequate angiographic examination.

Symptoms of CI usually subside within 24 to 48 hours, and healing is seen within 2 weeks. Two thirds of patients with reversible disease exhibit intramural and submucosal hemorrhage (reversible colopathy), whereas one third manifest a transient colitis. More severe reversible damage may take 1 to 6 months to resolve. In almost 50% of patients with CI, irreversible damage results; approximately two thirds of these develop gangrene with or without perforation. The prognosis of patients with CI complicating shock, congestive heart failure, myocardial infarction, or severe dehydration is particularly poor, perhaps due to associated AMI.

When physical examination does not suggest gangrene or perforation, the patient is treated expectantly. The bowel is placed at rest, broad-spectrum antibiotics are given, cardiac function is optimized, and medications that cause mesenteric vasoconstriction, e.g., digitalis and vasopressors, are withdrawn if possible. Serial roentgenographic or endoscopic evaluations of the colon and continued monitoring of the hemoglobin, white blood cell count, and electrolytes are performed. Increasing abdominal tenderness, guarding, rising temperature, and paralytic ileus indicate colonic infarction and mandate expedient laparotomy and colon resection. If, as usual, CI completely resolves within 1 to 2 weeks, no further therapy is indicated. When segmental colitis develops, corticosteroid therapy does not appear to be beneficial and may predispose to perforation. Asymptomatic patients with evidence of persistent disease should have frequent examinations to determine if the colon is healing, has persisting inflammation, or is developing a stricture. Recurrent fevers, leukocytosis, and septicemia in otherwise asymptomatic patients with unhealed segmental colitis are usually caused by the diseased bowel, and elective resection is indicated. Because patients with diarrhea or rectal bleeding for more than 2 weeks usually develop irreversible disease, often with colonic perforation, early resection is indicated. CI may not produce symptoms during the acute insult but still cause a chronic colitis frequently misdiagnosed as inflammatory bowel disease (see Ch. 104). Involvement is segmental, resection is not followed by recurrence, and the response to steroid therapy is usually poor. Local steroid enemas may be helpful, but parenteral steroids should be avoided. Ischemic strictures that produce no symptoms should be observed; some disappear over 12 to 24 months with no specific therapy. Of course, resection is required for those that cause obstruction. A rare form of fulminant CI involving all or most of the colon and rectum recently has been identified; its management is similar to that of other fulminant colitides.

Chronic Mesenteric Ischemia (CMI)

Atherosclerosis is almost always the cause of CMI or "abdominal angina." Although autopsy and angiographic studies have demonstrated frequent partial or complete occlusions of the major splanchnic vessels, CMI is rare. Moreover, many patients with occlusion of two or even all three of these vessels remain asymptomatic. Hence, the clinical significance of an angiogram demonstrating an occlusion of one or more of these vessels in an individual patient varies. The lack of available and reliable means to determine the inadequacy of intestinal blood flow before morphologic changes of ischemia occur has been the major obstacle to identifying patients with CMI.

The one consistent clinical feature of CMI is abdominal discomfort or pain, which most commonly occurs 10 to 30 minutes after eating, gradually increases in severity, reaches a plateau, and then slowly abates over 1 to 3 hours. The pain is usually dull, gnawing, or cramping and is located periumbilically or in the epigastrium. Initially the pain only follows a large meal but characteristically increases in frequency and severity, so the patient reduces the meal size ("small meal syndrome"), becomes reluctant to eat, and often loses significant weight. Bloating, flatulence, constipation, and diarrhea are not infrequent. Physical findings are limited and nonspecific. Patients with advanced disease appear chronically ill with marked weight loss. The abdomen is usually soft and nontender even during episodes of pain. A systolic bruit is usually present in the upper abdomen but is nonspecific. Many patients have cardiac, cerebral, or peripheral vascular insufficiency.

There has been no specific reliable diagnostic test for abdominal angina, so the diagnosis has been based on clinical symptoms, arteriographic demonstration of splanchnic arterial occlusions, and the exclusion of other GI disease. Conventional examinations of the GI tract usually are unremarkable. Studies for malabsorption often show increased fecal fat and decreased D-xylose excretion. Angiographic evaluation includes flush aortography and selective injections of the SMA, CA and, if possible, the IMA. The presence of stenosis of a major vessel with prominent collateral vessels indicates that the stenosis is hemodynamically significant and chronic.

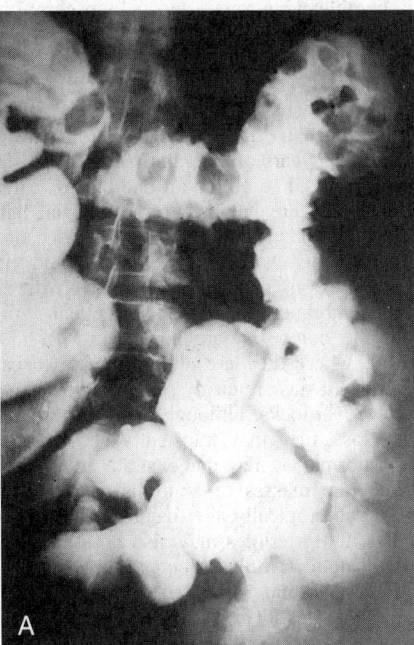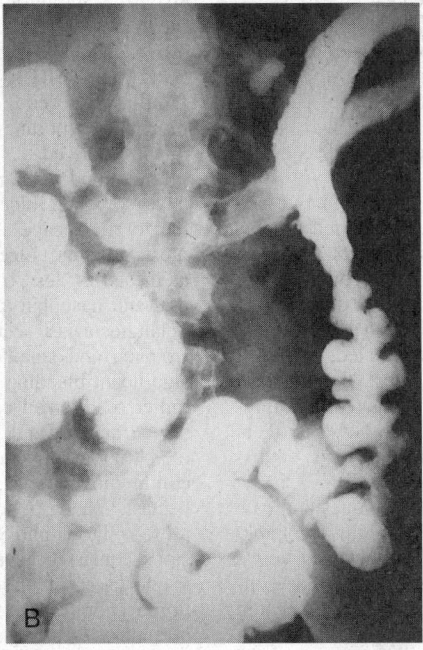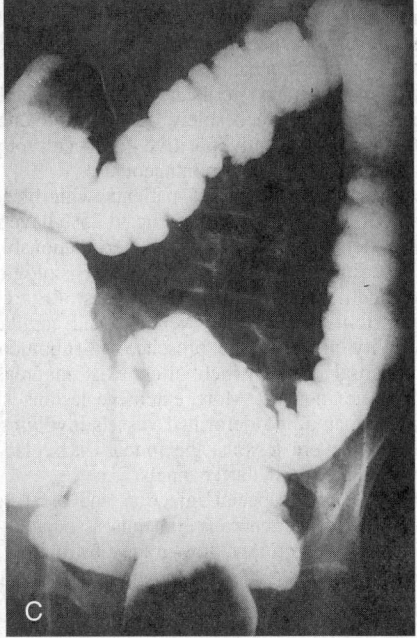

FIGURE 105–3. Ischemic changes in the transverse colon and splenic flexure. *A,* Initial study shows dramatic thumbprints throughout the involved area. *B,* Eleven days later thumbprints have resolved and a segmental colitis has developed. *C,* Five months after onset there is complete return to normal. Patient was asymptomatic 3 weeks after her illness. (From Boley SJ, Schwartz SS, Williams FL [eds.]: Vascular Disorders of the Intestine. New York, Appleton-Century-Crofts, 1971.)

However, *stenosis or occlusion of one or two or all of the major vessels does not by itself establish the diagnosis of CMI, and patients with even three occluded vessels may be asymptomatic.* Intestinal blood flow has been assessed by determining hepatic blood flow with indocyanine green. Patients with CMI failed to increase their splanchnic blood flow after a test meal, but after arterial reconstruction, the postprandial increase was similar to that of a control group. The complexity and invasiveness of this procedure have limited its use. Balloon tonometers have been used to determine intestinal intramural pH (pH$_I$), which is a measure of the adequacy of oxygenation in relationship to metabolic demands. *Intestinal angina probably results from a meal-induced increase in gastric blood flow which, with fixed splanchnic arterial inflow, is achieved by stealing from the blood flow to the intestines.* The decrease in intestinal blood flow is reflected in a fall in intestinal pH$_I$; hence, tonometric determination of small bowel pH$_I$ before and after eating offers another means of diagnosing intestinal ischemia.

A patient with typical pain and unexplained weight loss, whose diagnostic evaluation has excluded other GI disease and whose angiogram shows occlusion of at least two of the three major arteries, should have the benefit of surgical revascularization. Tests of the adequacy of blood flow described above may identify patients who should have mesenteric angiography and who may benefit from revascularization procedures. A variety of surgical procedures exist to revascularize the mesenteric circulation with reasonable operative risk and a good long-term prognosis. The infrequency of fatal acute mesenteric infarction after a successful revascularization operation suggests that such procedures may prevent a major intestinal ischemic episode.

VASCULAR LESIONS

Through the widespread use of endoscopy and angiography, vascular lesions of the GI tract are being recognized with increasing frequency as causing hemorrhage. They may be solitary or multiple, exist as isolated abnormalities, or be part of a syndrome or systemic disorder.

Colonic vascular ectasia (VE) (angiodysplasia or arteriovenous malformation) is the most common vascular abnormality of the GI tract. VE's are degenerative lesions associated with aging and are not associated with other cutaneous or visceral lesions. They almost always are confined to the cecum or ascending colon, are usually multiple, and rarely can be identified at operation or on routine histologic sections; they usually can be diagnosed by angiography or colonoscopy.

VE's are probably the most common cause of recurrent lower GI bleeding in the elderly. The type of bleeding frequently varies: Patients may have bright red blood, maroon-colored stools, and melena on separate occasions. Bleeding is usually low grade, but about 15% of patients present with massive hemorrhage. In 20 to 25% of episodes, only tarry stools are passed, and in 10 to 15% of patients, bleeding is evidenced solely by iron deficiency anemia with stools that are intermittently positive for occult blood. In >90% of instances bleeding stops spontaneously.

Approximately 50% of patients with bleeding VE's have evidence of cardiac disease, and up to 25% have been reported to have aortic stenosis. However, the inter-relationships of aortic stenosis, GI bleeding, and VE's are obscure. Histologic identification of VE is difficult without special techniques. VE's consist of dilated, distorted, thin-walled veins, venules, and capillaries. The earliest abnormality noted is the presence of submucosal dilated, tortuous, submucosal veins, which often exist in areas where the mucosal vessels are normal. More extensive lesions show increasing numbers of dilated and deformed vessels involving the mucosa until, in the most severe lesions, the mucosa is replaced by a maze of distorted, dilated vascular channels.

Studies using special injection and clearing techniques indicate that VE's are degenerative lesions associated with aging, probably caused by intermittent, low-grade obstruction of submucosal veins, where they pierce the colonic muscle layers during muscular contraction and distention of the cecum. Conceivably, repeated episodes of transiently elevated pressure over many years result in dilation and tortuosity of the submucosal vein, and later the venules and capillaries of the mucosal units draining into it. Finally, the capillary rings dilate, the precapillary sphincters lose their compe-

tency, and a small arteriovenous fistula is produced. The latter is responsible for the "early filling vein," which was the original angiographic hallmark of this lesion. The prevalence of VE's in the right colon can be attributed to the greater tension in the cecal wall than in other parts of the colon, according to Laplace's principle: $T = DP$ (where T = tension, D = diameter, P = intraluminal pressure).

Angiography was formerly the primary method to identify ectasias, but currently colonoscopy is preferable. The endoscopist's ability to diagnose the specific nature of a vascular lesion, however, is limited by the similar appearance of many disparate lesions, e.g., spider angiomata, hereditary hemorrhagic telangiectasia, angiomas, and the focal hypervascularity of various colitides. Biopsies of vascular lesions obtained during endoscopy are usually nonspecific; therefore, the risk of biopsying these abnormalities is not justified. The appearance of vascular lesions is influenced by blood pressure, blood volume, and state of hydration; VE's may not be evident in patients with severely reduced blood volumes or those who are in shock; thus, accurate evaluation may not be possible until red cell and volume deficits are corrected. Angiography can determine the site and nature of lesions during active bleeding and can identify some vascular lesions even when bleeding has ceased if a slowly emptying and tortuous vein, a vascular tuft, or an early filling vein is present.

The natural history of VE's is not known precisely. It has been estimated that < 10% of patients with such lesions eventually bleed, data that further support the recommendation not to treat incidently observed VE's. Although some colonoscopists remain eager to treat VE's, almost half the patients may not bleed again after the initial episode. Laser therapy, sclerosis, electrocoagulation, and the heater probe all have been used to ablate VE's. None has been established as superior, but the heater probe and bipolar coagulation are most commonly used. Moreover, no data prove that endoscopic ablation of colon VE's changes their natural history. Under emergent conditions, angiographic methods have been used to arrest bleeding from VE's, and intra-arterial (SMA) vasopressin infusions stop hemorrhage in > 80% of patients in whom extravasation is demonstrated. Right hemicolectomy is performed if the bleeding continues, if an experienced endoscopist is not available, or if endoscopic ablation has been unsuccessful. The extent of colonic resection is not altered by the presence or absence of diverticulosis in the left colon; only the right half of the colon is removed. Because up to 80% of bleeding diverticula are located in the right side of the colon, the risks of leaving a left colon containing diverticula are far outweighed by the increased morbidity and mortality of the larger, subtotal colectomy. Recurrent bleeding can be expected in up to 20% of patients so treated. Subtotal colectomy should be performed only as a last resort—that is, in the patient in whom active colonic bleeding persists, the angiogram is completely normal, and colonoscopy either yields negative findings or is not helpful.

HEREDITARY HEMORRHAGIC TELANGIECTASIAS (OSLER-WEBER-RENDU DISEASE). This autosomal dominant familial disorder is characterized by telangiectasias of the skin and mucous membranes and recurrent GI bleeding. Lesions are frequently noticed in the first few years of life, and recurrent epistaxis in childhood is characteristic. By age 10, about one half of patients have some GI bleeding, but severe hemorrhage is unusual before the fourth decade and has a peak incidence in the sixth decade. In most patients, bleeding presents as melena; epistaxis and hematemesis are less frequent. Lesions are usually present on the lips, oral and nasopharyngeal membranes, tongue, or periungual regions. Telangiectasias occur in the colon but are more common in the stomach and small bowel, where they are also more apt to cause significant bleeding. Telangiectasias are easily seen on endoscopy as millet seed–sized cherry red hillocks, although, in the presence of severe anemia and blood loss, they may transiently become invisible. Angiography may be normal or may demonstrate arteriovenous communications, conglomerate masses of abnormal vessels, phlebectasias, and aneurysms. Pathologically, the major changes involve the capillaries and venules, but arterioles may also be affected. Lesions consist of irregular ectatic tortuous blood spaces lined by a single layer of endothelial cells and supported by a fine layer of fibrous connective tissue. No elastic lamina or muscular tissue is present in these vessels, so they cannot contract, perhaps explaining why they tend to bleed. Arterioles show intimal proliferation, often with thrombi. Many forms of treatment have been recommended for these vascular lesions, including estrogens, endoscopic ablation, and resection of involved bowel. Long-term follow-up studies are needed to evaluate the ultimate efficacy of the various forms of therapy.

PROGRESSIVE SYSTEMIC SCLEROSIS (see Ch. 241). Vascular lesions are a prominent feature of progressive systemic sclerosis, especially in the CREST variant with calcinosis, Raynaud's phenomenon, esophageal dysmotility, scleroderma, and telangiectasias. These tiny lesions may be the source of occult and/or clinically significant bleeding and are best treated, if possible, by endoscopic ablation.

WATERMELON STOMACH. This term describes an unusual vascular lesion of the antrum consisting of tortuous dilated vessels radiating outward from the pylorus like spokes from a wheel and resembling the dark stripes on the surface of a watermelon. It produces both acute and chronic occult bleeding, but its cause is unknown; it has been proposed that gastric peristalsis causes prolapse of the loose antral mucosa with consequent elongation and ectasia of the mucosal vessels. The lesion is seen particularly in middle-aged or older women and is associated with achlorhydria, atrophic gastritis, and cirrhosis. Finding cirrhosis and portal hypertension in almost half the reported cases of watermelon stomach suggests an association. Microscopic features include dilated capillaries with focal thrombosis, dilated tortuous submucosal venous channels, and fibromuscular hyperplasia. Iron therapy, transfusions, and brief trials with steroids were unsuccessful in early attempts to diminish the bleeding episodes, and antrectomy was usually required. Transendoscopic therapy offers an attractive therapeutic alternative to antrectomy and is being used with increasing success.

DIEULAFOY'S ULCER. An increasingly diagnosed cause of massive GI hemorrhage, this lesion is usually found in the stomach and sometimes in the small or large bowel. Dieulafoy's lesion is twice as common in men as in women and presents at a mean age of 52. The abnormality is the presence of an artery of extramural caliber in the submucosa, and in some instances the mucosa, typically with a small overlying mucosal defect. It is believed that focal pressure from this large "caliber-persistent" vessel erodes the overlying mucosa, destroying the exposed vascular wall and resulting in hemorrhage. There is sudden onset of massive hematemesis or melena, usually followed by intermittent bleeding over several days. The bleeding site is usually 6 cm distal to the cardioesophageal junction, where the arteries are largest. The mortality rate for elderly patients with this lesion has been high, but with present angiographic and endoscopic techniques to localize and treat bleeding lesions, thus decreasing the need for emergent surgery, prognosis for this lesion is likely to improve.

HEMANGIOMAS. These are the second most common vascular lesions of the colon although they occur throughout the GI tract. Hemangiomas may be of cavernous, capillary, or mixed types. Most are small and appear as polypoid, reddish purple mounds, ranging from a few millimeters to 2 cm; larger lesions do occur, especially in the rectum, where they may be associated with phleboliths. Bleeding from hemangiomas is usually slow, producing occult blood loss with anemia or melena. Hematochezia is less common, except in large cavernous hemangiomas of the rectum. Diagnosis is best established by endoscopy, including enteroscopy, because roentgenologic studies, including angiography, are frequently normal. Small hemangiomas that are solitary or few in number and can be approached endoscopically are locally ablated. Large or multiple lesions usually require resection of either the hemangioma alone or the involved segment of colon.

BLUE RUBBER BLEB NEVUS SYNDROME. This term describes a particular type of cutaneous vascular nevus associated with intestinal lesions and GI bleeding. A familial history is infrequent, although a few cases of transmission in an autosomal dominant pattern have been reported. The lesions are distinctive: blue and raised, varying from 0.1 to 5.0 cm, and leaving a characteristic wrinkled sac when the contained blood is emptied by direct pressure. Lesions may be single or innumerable and are usually found on the trunk, extremities, and face but not on mucous membranes; they are most common in the small intestine. They are infrequently detected by barium or angiographic studies and are seen best by endoscopy. These lesions are cavernous hemangiomas composed of clusters of dilated capillary spaces lined by cuboidal or flattened endothelium with connective tissue stroma. Resection of the involved segment of bowel is recommended for recurrent hemorrhage. Endo-

scopic laser coagulation may be dangerous because these lesions may involve the full thickness of the bowel wall.

CONGENITAL ARTERIOVENOUS MALFORMATIONS (AVM's). These are developmental anomalies found mainly in the extremities but potentially located anywhere in the vascular tree. They may be small and resemble ectasias or involve a long segment of bowel. AVM's are persistent communications between arteries and veins located primarily in the submucosa. Characteristically there is "arterialization" of the veins, i.e., tortuosity, dilatation and thick walls with smooth muscle hypertrophy, and intimal thickening or sclerosis. Angiography is the primary means of diagnosis. Patients with significant bleeding should have resection of the involved segment.

KLIPPEL-TRENAUNAY-WEBER SYNDROME. This syndrome consists of (1) a vascular nevus involving the lower limb, (2) varicose veins limited to the affected side and appearing at birth or in childhood, and (3) hypertrophy of all tissues of the involved limb (especially the bones), probably due to venous hypertension and stasis. Edema of the involved leg is common, and if the thigh is involved, a variety of lymphatic abnormalities is usually present, e.g., chylous mesenteric cysts, chlyoperitoneum, and protein-losing enteropathy. Symptomatic GI or genitourinary involvement is rare and manifests with hemorrhage. Bleeding may be recurrent, mild or severe, and is usually due to a rectal or vaginal hemangioma, localized rectovaginal varices due to an obstructed internal iliac system, or portal hypertension with varices. Physical examination is diagnostic, and a variety of imaging techniques are used to define the anatomy and to plan surgical repair. Plain films showing calcified pelvic phleboliths in a child suggest pelvic hemangiomatosis.

Boley SJ, Brandt LJ: Intestinal ischemia. Surg Clin North Am 72:1, 1992. *An entire volume devoted to gastrointestinal ischemia, including pathphysiology, pathology, radiographic diagnosis, clinical presentations, and therapies.*

Boley SJ, DiBiase A, Brandt LJ, et al.: Lower intestinal bleeding in the elderly. Am J Surg 137:57, 1979. *Review of the causes of major and minor lower intestinal bleeding in subjects older than age 50, providing evidence that vascular ectasias and diverticula are the two most common causes of major bleeding in this age group.*

Boley SJ, Sammartano RJ, Adams A, et al.: On the nature and etiology of vascular ectasias of the colon: Degenerative lesions of aging. Gastroenterology 72:650, 1977. *Classic reference describing stages in development of colonic vascular ectasias; postulates chronic intermittent obstruction of submucosal veins as the initial step in their formation. Beautifully illustrated with color stereomicrographs of silicon-injected, cleared, and transilluminated specimens.*

Foutch PG: Angiodysplasia of the gastrointestinal tract. Am J Gastroenterol 88:807, 1993. *A recent article reviewing colon vascular ectasias and angiodysplasia of the upper GI tract; includes a discussion of hormonal and endoscopic therapy.*

Richter J, Christensen M, Colditz G: Angiodysplasia: Natural history and efficacy of therapeutic interventions. Dig Dis Sci 37:1542, 1989. *Compares medical (transfusion), endoscopic, and surgical therapy, showing that only surgical treatment significantly improves outcome over the "natural" history of these lesions.*

106 NEOPLASMS OF THE LARGE AND SMALL INTESTINES

Bernard Levin

Neoplasms of the Large Intestine

Cancer of the large bowel (colon and rectum) is the most common malignancy of the gastrointestinal tract and together with breast and lung cancer is one of the three most frequent malignancies in the United States. It is also a worldwide health problem of great importance, particularly in other Western countries. Approximately 160,000 cases of cancer of the colon and rectum were diagnosed in the United States in 1994, only one half of whom will survive 5 years or longer. The mortality from colorectal cancer has slowly declined over the past 10 years while the incidence has been stable. New understanding about the genetics and molecular biology of this neoplasm has been recently gained, and advances have also been made in methods of prevention, diagnosis, and treatment.

The large bowel also may be involved by other malignant tumors. These include anal carcinoma (squamous or transitional types), lymphoma, leiomyosarcoma, malignant carcinoid tumor, and Kaposi's sarcoma. The large bowel may also be involved through direct invasion by malignancies from adjacent sites such as prostate, ovary, uterus, and stomach. The most frequent tumors that occur in the large intestine are benign adenomas (adenomatous polyps). Except for lipomas of the ileocecal valve, other benign tumors are very unusual.

POLYPS OF THE COLON

A polyp is any lesion that arises from the surface of the gastrointestinal tract and protrudes into the lumen. In the large intestine polyps, noted at sigmoidoscopy or colonoscopy or during barium enema, may be single or multiple, pedunculated or sessile, and sporadic or part of an inherited syndrome. They become significant because of bleeding or because of their potential for malignant transformation.

PATHOLOGY. In addition to adenocarcinoma, which may present as a polypoid mass, three distinct types of benign polyps arise from colonic epithelium: hyperplastic (metaplastic), inflammatory, and neoplastic (adenomatous). Hyperplastic polyps, which tend to be small and asymptomatic, account for about one fifth of all polyps in the colon and for most of the polyps in the rectum and distal sigmoid. They are not considered neoplastic. Inflammatory polyps occur in chronic ulcerative colitis and also are not neoplastic (see Ch. 104). Juvenile polyps are hamartomas of the lamina propria and may be single or multiple and occur most commonly in the rectum. They are susceptible to hemorrhage and autoamputation.

Adenomatous Polyps

PREVALENCE AND DISTRIBUTION. The incidence of colonic adenomas increases with age in countries with a high or intermediate risk for colorectal cancer, occurring in 40 to 50% of individuals over age 60 in the United States. Adenomas are uncommon in areas where the incidence of cancer is low; for example, the prevalence of adenomas varies from almost zero among black South Africans to 10% in Japan and in Cali, Colombia. The presence of adenomas does not necessarily convey a high risk because the propensity for neoplastic transformation is related to size. The low incidence of cancer in some countries, such as Japan, is probably related to the small number of large adenomas as well as to the total number of adenomas.

MACROSCOPIC AND MICROSCOPIC APPEARANCES. Adenomas may be separated into tubular, villous, and intermediate tubulovillous types. The typical tubular adenoma is small and spherical and has a stalk. Its surface is roughly separated into lobules by intercommunicating clefts. In contrast, the villous adenoma may be large and sessile with a velvety surface. Histologically the tubular adenoma consists of closely packed tubular glands that divide and branch. In the villous adenoma, finger-like projections of neoplastic epithelium project toward the bowel lumen. The tubulovillous lesions consist of a mixture of tubular and villous patterns. About 60% of adenomas are tubular, 20 to 30% are tubulovillous, and about 10% are villous. All adenomas are dysplastic, and dysplasia in adenomas may be graded into mild, moderate, and severe. This classification is based on the presence of cytologic (mainly nuclear) abnormalities and glandular architectural changes.

DEVELOPMENT OF ADENOMAS. In the normal adult, the epithelial tissue of the colon actively renews itself with a turnover of about 3 to 8 days. DNA synthesis occurs primarily in cells in the lower one third of crypts. Normally cells replicate and migrate up the crypt to be subsequently exfoliated from the mucosal surface. In adenomas immature cells are found higher up the colonic crypt than normal, associated with unrepressed DNA synthesis, representing abnormal cell renewal along the surface of the crypt and the entire length of the crypt. DNA-synthesizing cells can accumulate on the luminal surface, thus forming new adenomatous tissue.

RELATIONSHIP OF COLONIC ADENOMAS TO CANCER. Colonic adenomas appear to have malignant potential:

(1) The epidemiology of adenomas and carcinoma is similar; (2) adenocarcinomas and adenomas occur in the same anatomic distribution in the colon; (3) residual adenomatous tissue is observed quite commonly in small cancers; (4) the incidence of cancer increases as the size of the adenoma increases; (5) the adenoma-to-cancer transition has been observed in familial polyposis and in experimental animals treated with a carcinogen; (6) the risk for colorectal cancer is higher in patients with a history of adenomas and may be lessened if the adenoma is removed; (7) a period of approximately 5 years elapses between the diagnosis of adenoma and the development of carcinoma.

Less than 5% of adenomas develop into carcinomas. Several important factors in this transformation can be identified, especially size, histologic type, and epithelial dysplasia. The frequency of cancer in adenomas under 1 cm is 1 to 3%, those between 1 to 2 cm have a rate of 10%, whereas those over 2 cm have a rate of malignancy over 40%. The highest malignancy rate is associated with a villous growth pattern. Invasive neoplasm has been found in 40% of the villous tumors, in < 5% of the tubular ones, and in 23% of the tubulovillous variety. The malignant potential of adenomas increases with increasing degrees of dysplasia. Most adenomas smaller than 1 cm show only mild dysplasia and have a low malignant potential. With severe dysplasia, the rate of malignant transformation rises to 27%.

Cancer in adenomas is usually well differentiated and occurs most commonly in the tip of a pedunculated adenoma without invasion of the muscularis mucosae. These lesions are usually satisfactorily treated by polypectomy. Occasionally cancers in adenomas invade the muscularis mucosae, grow down the stalk, invade lymphatics and adjacent lymph nodes, and metastasize. The roles of autocrine factors, tumor suppressor genes, and oncogenes in the development of adenomas and their malignant transformation are currently under study.

CLINICAL MANIFESTATIONS. Most adenomatous polyps are asymptomatic but may cause hematochezia. Some adenomatous polyps are diagnosed by detecting occult blood loss in asymptomatic individuals being screened for colon cancer. Adenomas may also be detected by double contrast barium enema examination or by fiberoptic sigmoidoscopy or colonoscopy.

MANAGEMENT AND FOLLOW-UP. Because of the association of adenomas with the development of adenocarcinomas, colonic polyps should usually be removed or destroyed. In individual clinical circumstances (e.g., age of patient, location of lesion) this rule may rarely have to be modified. Pedunculated polyps, even if large, can be removed by electrocautery snare while small sessile polyps (1 to 8 mm in size) should be biopsied and destroyed with the "hot biopsy" forceps. For sessile polyps with a wide-based attachment to the colonic wall, several electrocautery sessions may be required for complete excision. Endoscopic removal may not be safe or possible if a sessile lesion is larger than 3 cm or if it is in a relatively inaccessible location. In general, benign-appearing polyps are removed by electrosurgery and not biopsied and the entire lesion is submitted for histopathologic examination.

The endoscopic appearance of a polyp that suggests carcinomatous invasion includes ulceration, an irregular surface contour, firm consistency, and friability. If a diagnosis of malignancy is made after polypectomy, a decision has to be made about the adequacy of the polypectomy. In the presence of a poorly differentiated histology, penetration of the muscularis mucosa, vascular or lymphatic invasion, and a resection margin containing cancer, the risk of regional lymph node involvement is approximately 5%. The mortality from surgical resection is <2% in patients aged 50 to 69 and 4.4% for those over 70, so any decision to recommend surgical resection must take into account individual operative risk.

FOLLOW-UP AFTER COLONOSCOPIC POLYPECTOMY. Ideally, the colon should be cleared of all synchronous adenomas at the time of the initial examination. A follow-up colonoscopy is appropriate at 3 years to evaluate for the presence of any lesions missed at the time of the previous procedure as well as new lesions that may have arisen. If this examination is normal, an interval of 3 years is appropriate for the next colonoscopy. Chemotherapeutic strategies aimed at preventing adenoma recurrence are being studied, including diet and nonsteroidal anti-inflammatory drugs (NSAID's).

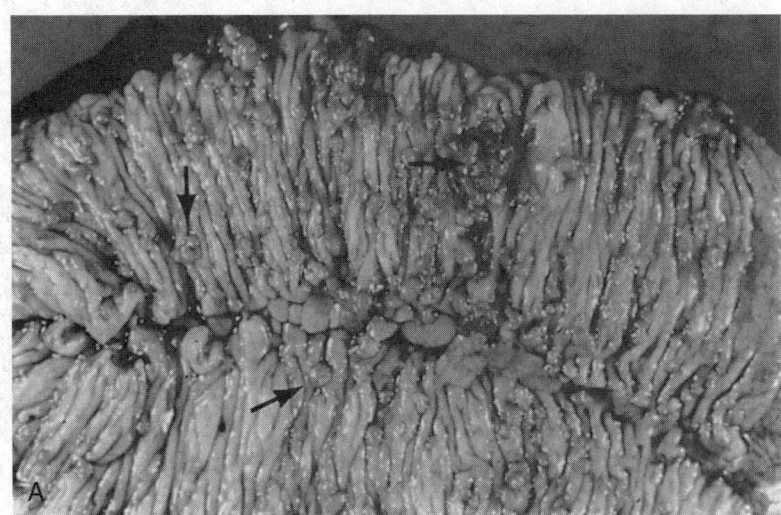

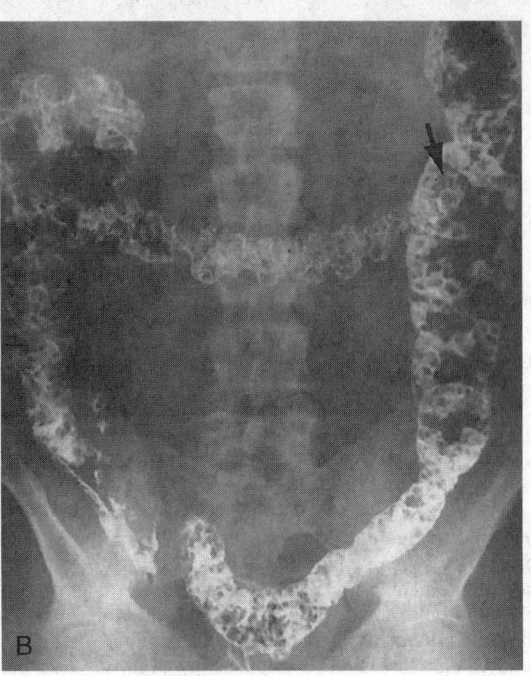

FIGURE 106–1. *A,* Patients with familial polyposis have multiple adenomatous polyps carpeting the colon, as demonstrated in this gross specimen. Note that the colon is diffusely studded with sessile and occasional pedunculated adenomatous polyps *(arrows).* Many of the larger polyps contain villous elements, and occasionally villous adenomas are found. Although no carcinoma was seen in this patient, nearly all patients eventually develop colorectal carcinoma if surgery is not performed. *B,* This barium enema examination of a patient with familial polyposis represents diffuse studding of the large bowel with adenomatous polyps. Note the marked variation in size of these polyps. Although this patient did not have osteomas or soft tissue tumors, the barium enema is similar to that seen in Gardner syndrome. (From Boland CR, Kim YS: *In* Sleisenger MH, Fordtran JS [eds.]: Gastrointestinal Disease. 3rd ed. Philadelphia, WB Saunders, 1983.)

Inherited Polyposis Syndromes

Recent advances in genetics and molecular biology have accentuated our interest in the inherited risk of colorectal cancer. The polyposis syndromes account for approximately 1% of colorectal cancer, whereas the nonpolyposis inherited conditions may be responsible for up to 6%.

ADENOMATOUS POLYPOSIS SYNDROMES

The adenomatous polyposis syndromes include familial adenomatous polyposis and Gardner syndrome; in both hereditary disorders hundreds to thousands of colonic adenomas are present (Fig. 106–1). The adenomas begin to appear early in the second decade of life. Gastrointestinal symptoms occur in the third or fourth decade. Almost all patients with familial polyposis develop carcinoma of the colon by age 40 if the colon has not been removed. Some cases occur without a family history and may represent spontaneous mutations.

Gardner syndrome differs from familial adenomatous polyposis in that affected individuals exhibit benign extraintestinal growth, including osteomas (especially mandibular) and soft tissue tumors (lipomas, sebaceous cysts, fibrosarcomas). Other associated features include supernumerary teeth, desmoid tumors, and mesenteric fibromatosis (Fig. 106–2). The colonic adenomas are similar to those of familial adenomatous polyposis and have the same potential for malignancy.

In both familial adenomatous polyposis and Gardner syndrome, upper gastrointestinal polyps are commonly found. Gastric polyps are hyperplastic and rarely cause symptoms. Adenomatous duodenal polyps are present in up to 80% of individuals with familial adenomatous polyposis or Gardner syndrome, and approximately 10% develop periampullary cancer. Adenomas occur in the small bowel distal to the duodenum but rarely undergo malignant transformation.

Familial adenomatous polyposis and Gardner syndrome are inherited as autosomal dominant disorders with incomplete penetrance. The mutant gene for both conditions is on the long arm of chromosome 5. Different mutations at that locus may account for the phenotypic differences between the syndromes. The APC (adenomatous polyposis coli) gene mutations lead to the formation of a truncated protein. Gene abnormalities can be detected by a blood test in 87% of affected individuals, thereby enabling screening within affected families to be much more accurate.

SCREENING RECOMMENDATIONS. Flexible proctosigmoidoscopy should be performed annually in all first-degree relatives, from age 12 until age 40, and every 3 years thereafter. This screening is appropriate for those with the mutant gene. Until gene markers are 100% specific and sensitive, screening is also indicated for those without the mutant gene, although considerably less often. Surveillance with a side-viewing endoscope for gastric and duodenal polyps should begin when the diagnosis of colonic polyposis is made and should continue every 2 to 3 years thereafter.

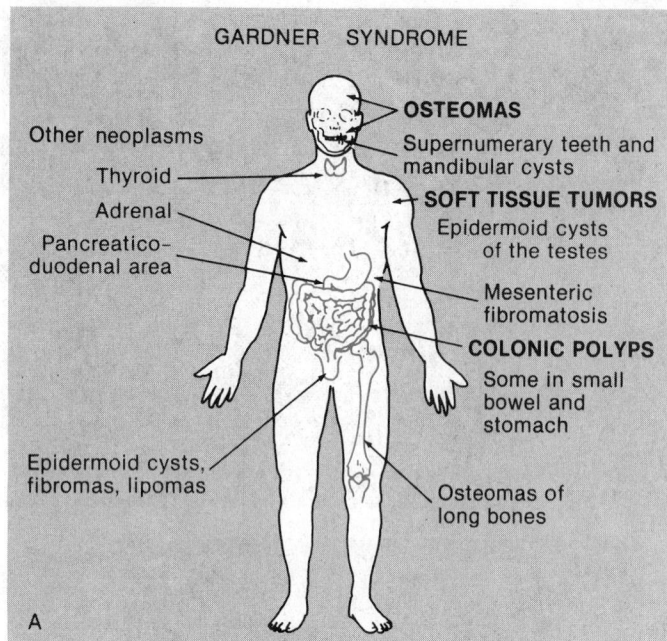
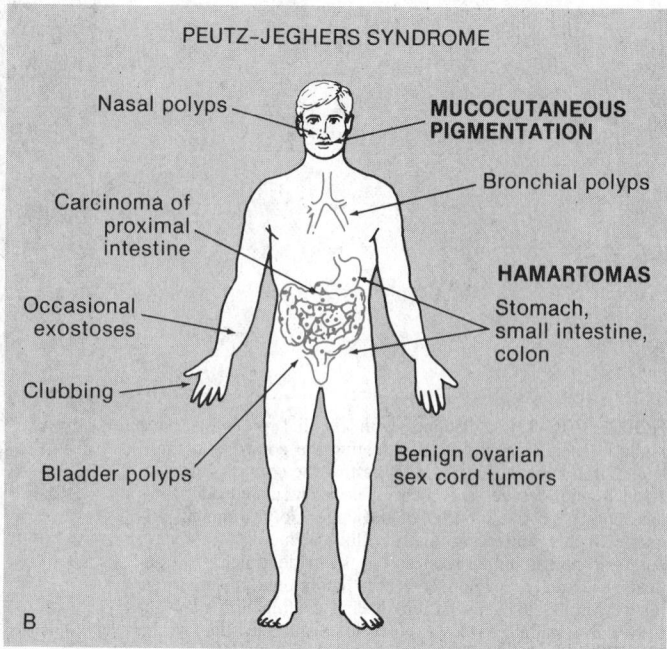

FIGURE 106–2. *A,* Schematic representation of Gardner syndrome. The triad of colonic polyposis, bone tumors, and soft tissue tumors (heavy print) constitutes the primary features; other features are indicated in lighter print. *B,* Schematic presentation of Peutz-Jeghers syndrome. Mucocutaneous pigmentation and benign gastrointestinal polyposis (heavy print) are the primary features of this syndrome. Lighter print shows the secondary features. (From Boland CR, Kim YS: *In* Sleisenger MH, Fordtran JS [eds.]: Gastrointestinal Disease. 3rd ed. Philadelphia, WB Saunders, 1983.)

Hereditary Nonpolyposis Colorectal Cancer (HNPCC; Lynch Syndromes I and II)

HNPCC is caused by germline mutations in one of a group of genes involved in DNA nucleotide mismatch repair.

In both of the Lynch syndromes, colon cancer is inherited in a highly penetrant, autosomal dominant manner. Several adenomas, which are occasionally flat, may be present (in spite of the name), but myriad adenomas are not found. The average age of diagnosis of cancer is the mid 40's, and it is characteristic to find a majority of lesions proximal to the splenic flexure as well as multiple synchronous cancers. In Lynch syndrome I (site-specific colon cancer) only inherited colonic neoplasms occur, whereas Lynch syndrome II (cancer family syndrome) includes female genital (uterine, ovarian) and breast cancer. Individuals in families with hereditary nonpolyposis colorectal cancer should have colonoscopy every 2 years beginning at an age 5 years younger than the age of the earliest colon cancer diagnosed in the family. Mammography (at an earlier age than the general population) and ovarian ultrasonography are also appropriate in Lynch syndrome II families in whom there is a preponderance of breast or ovarian malignancies (see Ch. 208).

The *Peutz-Jeghers syndrome* is characterized by melanotic spots on the lips, buccal mucosa, and skin and by multiple hamartomatous polyps throughout the gastrointestinal tract from the stomach to the rectum (Fig. 106–3). It is generally believed to be inherited in an autosomal dominant fashion but with variable expressivity. Usually polyps are fewer in number than in familial adenomatous polyposis. Microscopically, these polyps consist of elongated branching glands lined by benign epithelium native to the location of the polyps. The most distinctive feature is the presence of an arborizing proliferation of smooth muscle in the lamina propria. Rarely, malignancies have been described in the intestine with a preponderance in the small intestine. Other manifestations include ovarian sex cord stromal tumors and polyps of the gallbladder, ureter, and nose. Intestinal symptoms of recurrent, colicky abdominal pain may appear in adolescence, and intussusception may require surgical removal of a polyp. Gastrointestinal bleeding may occur, causing iron deficiency anemia.

Turcot's syndrome, inherited as an autosomal recessive or dominant condition, is rare and is characterized by hereditary adenomatous polyposis with a low number of polyps (20 to 300) and tumors of the central nervous system. These neoplasms include medulloblastoma, glioblastoma, and ependymoma. Recent evidence impli-

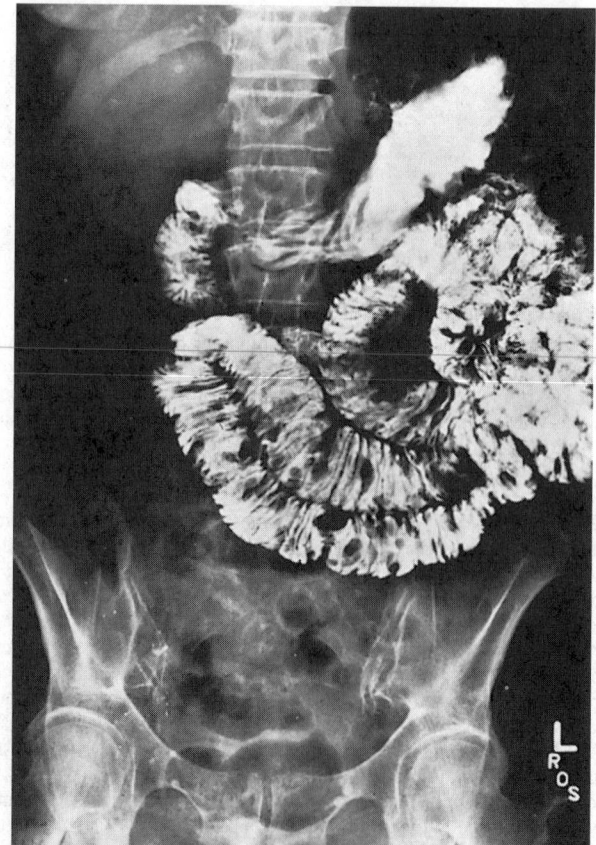

FIGURE 106–3. Barium study of the upper gastrointestinal tract showing multiple polyps of the small bowel in a patient with Peutz-Jeghers syndrome.

cates abnormalities of both APC and nucleotide mismatch repair genes in the pathogenesis of this condition.

Juvenile polyposis is inherited as an autosomal dominant trait, with an occasional case occurring spontaneously. The number of polyps is less than in familial adenomatous polyposis, averaging 25 to 40. Polyps may be found throughout the gastrointestinal tract or may be restricted to the colon. Symptoms may begin in childhood or adolescence with rectal bleeding, anemia, abdominal pain, or intussusception. A variety of extraintestinal symptoms including congenital abnormalities and pulmonary arteriovenous malformations have been described in association with juvenile polyposis. Foci of adenomatous epithelium may be present in these polyps, or adenomas may coexist. The true risk of malignancy in these patients is unknown, but 10% of the reported patients with juvenile polyposis have developed carcinoma of the gastrointestinal tract. Subtotal colectomy may occasionally be warranted in those with severely dysplastic adenomas.

Cronkite-Canada syndrome is a nonfamilial disorder of adults characterized by diffuse gastrointestinal polyposis, alopecia, dystrophy of the fingernails, and cutaneous hyperpigmentation. The polyps resemble juvenile polyps and are in greatest density in the stomach and colon. Watery diarrhea, anorexia, abdominal pain, cachexia, protein-losing enteropathy, and carcinoma of the gastrointestinal tract (in up to 14% of cases) have been reported.

Cowden's syndrome (multiple hamartoma syndrome) is transmitted in an autosomal dominant manner and is characterized by multiple facial tricholemmomas, oral papillomas, keratoses of the hands and feet, and a high rate of associated systemic malignancies, particularly of thyroid and breast. The polyps are not dysplastic, and the risk of gastrointestinal malignancy is not increased.

ADENOCARCINOMA OF THE LARGE BOWEL

Carcinoma of the colon and rectum varies widely in frequency in different parts of the world. Large bowel cancers occur commonly in North America, northwestern Europe, and New Zealand, whereas in South America, southwest Asia, equatorial Africa, and India the risk is much less. The incidence varies from 3.5 per 100,000 in India to 32.3 per 100,000 in Connecticut. Colorectal cancers display regional differences within the United States, with the highest incidence in the Northeast. Rectal cancer is more common in men in most, but not all, areas of the world. In the United States rectal cancer incidence has declined over the past 50 years. Overall mortality from colorectal cancer has also declined in the United States over the past 20 years.

Migrants from parts of the world with a low incidence to regions with a higher risk, such as the United States or Canada, show a rapid increase in incidence. This is also exemplified by the higher incidence in Puerto Ricans who have migrated to the mainland compared with those in Puerto Rico and in first- and second-generation Chinese and Japanese immigrants to Hawaii and the mainland United States compared with Japanese in Japan and Chinese in the Peoples' Republic of China.

ETIOLOGY. Both inherited predisposition and environmental factors seem to be implicated in carcinogenesis in the colon and rectum, but in ways yet to be clearly delineated. Of the environmental factors, diet has been the most extensively studied. Fat intake, not only the amount, but also the type of fat, has been correlated with the risk for colorectal cancer in many but not all studies. Consumption of saturated fat (with a high content of animal fat) has been reported to be positively correlated with colon cancer incidence. Other studies suggest that monounsaturated fatty acids may exert a protective effect against the development of colon cancer. In countries with a high incidence of colon cancer, the average fat content in the diet is about 40% of total calories, in contrast to the dietary fat content of 15 to 20% or less of total calories in countries with a low cancer incidence. If fat in the colon does in fact promote cancer, the effect might be related to increased biliary sterol excretion, leading to increased colonic epithelial proliferation, to modification of cell membranes, or to stimulation of the synthesis of prostaglandins that induce cellular proliferation. The possible role of *dietary fiber* in reducing colonic carcinogenesis has been suggested but not firmly established. Fiber is not a single chemical substance. Certain components of fiber found in cereals, fruits, and vegetables may be helpful in reducing the risk of cancer by diluting and binding carcinogens in the lumen, by modifying colonic bacterial flora, and by acidifying the colonic lumen by short-chain fatty

acids. Naturally occurring anticarcinogens found in fruits and vegetables (indoles, thioethers, dithiothiones, retinoids) are being investigated. Other factors that have been postulated to play a role in colonic carcinogenesis are excess caloric intake and obesity and inadequate intake of calcium and vitamin D. Aspirin and NSAID's appear to protect against the development of colorectal neoplasms.

AGE. Risk factors for colorectal cancer are listed in Table 106–1. The relationship of age to adenomas has been previously discussed. The risk of colorectal cancer begins to increase from the age of 50 and rises sharply at age 60; with each succeeding decade the risk doubles, reaching a peak by age 75.

INFLAMMATORY BOWEL DISEASE (see Ch. 104). Among all patients diagnosed as having a large bowel adenocarcinoma, only about 1% give an antecedent history of inflammatory bowel disease. In chronic ulcerative colitis, carcinoma of the colon occurs more commonly (approximately 10 to 20 times) than in the general population. The duration of disease and the extent of colonic involvement correlate with the subsequent development of colon cancer. Approximately 2 to 4% of all patients with chronic ulcerative colitis develop colorectal carcinoma, with a cumulative incidence of about 12% after 25 years. Patients with ulcerative proctitis have no increase in risk, and the risk for patients with left-sided colitis may be delayed until approximately 10 years later. In ulcerative colitis mucosal dysplasia, defined as an unequivocal neoplastic alteration of the colonic epithelium, is the recognized precursor for developing carcinoma. Dysplastic epithelium may itself overlie an area of malignancy associated with direct invasion into the submucosa. The dysplastic area may be flat or proliferative, and the likelihood of carcinoma increases significantly in the presence of a dysplasia-associated lesion or mass. Whether routine colonoscopic surveillance is useful in patients with inflammatory bowel disease is not settled. Nevertheless, many authorities favor periodic colonoscopy with multiple biopsies for dysplasia in individuals with more than 8 years of symptoms and extensive colonic involvement. The availability of newer surgical procedures, such as ileoanal pouches, favors a trend toward earlier colectomy in high-risk individuals. The demonstration of high-grade dysplasia or a dysplasia-associated lesion or mass, even in the presence of low-grade dysplasia, warrants prophylactic colectomy because the risk of an associated carcinoma may be as high as 50 or 60%. Newer epithelial markers, such as flow cytometry, oncogene, and tumor suppressor gene mutations and deletions, are being studied in an attempt to define the biology of neoplastic transformation and to identify individuals at high risk before cancer develops.

Patients with Crohn's colitis are also at higher risk (approximately four to seven times that of the general population) for the development of colorectal cancer, but this is probably lower than in ulcerative colitis. Colonic surveillance has not been widely used.

HEREDITY AND COLONIC CANCER. Inherited risk has become very important in colonic cancer screening. The adenomatous polyposis syndromes and hereditary nonpolyposis colorectal cancer, previously discussed, together account for approximately 7% of colon cancers. The remainder of colon cancers are referred to as "sporadic," but this term may be a misnomer. Population studies have demonstrated a two- or threefold increased risk for colon can-

TABLE 106–1. RISK FACTORS FOR COLORECTAL CANCER

Standard Risk: Age over 50 in men and women
Higher Risk
Associated disease
   Ulcerative colitis
   Crohn's colitis
Personal history
   Colorectal cancer
   Colorectal adenomas
   Female genital or breast cancer
Family history
   Familial polyposis syndromes
   Hereditary nonpolyposis colorectal cancer
     (Lynch syndromes I and II)
   Sporadic colorectal cancer

cer in first-degree relatives of individuals with colon cancer. A similar risk is present in first-degree relatives of individuals with adenomatous polyps. In fact, as many as 50% or more of "sporadic" adenomas and cancers may exhibit a partially penetrant autosomal dominant inheritance.

MOLECULAR GENETICS OF COLORECTAL CANCER. The genetic events surrounding the development of colorectal cancer are now being studied with increasing sophistication (Fig. 106–4). The gene for familial adenomatous polyposis has been mapped to chromosome 5. Deletions of DNA sequences at the same locus are also frequently observed in adenocarcinomas from "sporadic" cases. This may be the earliest change in the neoplastic process. K-*ras* mutations follow the chromosome 5 changes and are observed more commonly in larger adenomas and cancers (see Ch. 156). Chromosome 17 (p53 gene) and chromosome 18 (DCC gene) deletions are often present and may be important in malignant transformation. Mutations of the four nucleotide mismatch repair genes have been identified in both inherited and sporadic colorectal cancers. Overexpression of the c-*myc* gene has also been reported in colonic cancers. The total accumulation of genetic changes (allelic deletions, oncogene mutations) may be more important than a particular sequence of events in the development of invasive cancer.

PATHOLOGY. The vast majority of colorectal cancers are adenocarcinomas. The tumors exhibit varying degrees of glandular differentiation and produce variable amounts of mucin. Gross morphologic features may be divided into two major groups, polypoid and annular constricting lesions. The polypoid lesion is most commonly found on the right side, and the annular constricting lesion is more common on the left side of the colon. Adenocarcinomas of the rectum may be sessile or polypoid. Approximately 75% of colorectal cancers occur in the descending colon, rectosigmoid, and rectum. Approximately 50% are within the reach of the 60-cm fiberoptic sigmoidoscope. The cecum and ascending colon are involved in 15% and the transverse colon in 10% (Fig. 106–5). Carcinoma of the colon spreads by direct extension through the wall of the bowel into the pericolonic fat and mesentery, by invasion of surrounding organs, by way of the lymphatics to the regional lymph nodes, and via the portal vein to the liver. Additionally, the tumor may spread throughout the peritoneal cavity and to the lungs and bones. Rectal cancers may directly invade the perirectal fat, vagina, prostate, bladder, ureters, and bony pelvis and may metastasize to the lungs and liver.

CLINICAL MANIFESTATIONS. The major symptoms of colorectal cancer are *rectal bleeding, pain,* and *change in bowel habit.* The clinical presentation in an individual patient is related to the size and location of the tumor. Those on the right side are often asymptomatic, and bleeding may be occult. Tumors of the cecum and ascending colon rarely obstruct early. Changes in bowel habit, with reduction in stool caliber or progressive constipation, and hematochezia are more common with left-sided lesions. Adenocarcinomas of the colon may present with a localized perforation and with signs of peritonitis. An abdominal mass or symptoms and signs of liver metastasis may be the earliest clinical manifestations of an underlying colorectal cancer.

Rectal or anal cancers may present with rectal bleeding, perineal pain, or change in bowel habit. Presenting symptoms may also include those referable to invasion of adjacent organs, including hematuria, renal insufficiency (obstructive uropathy), and vaginal fistulas.

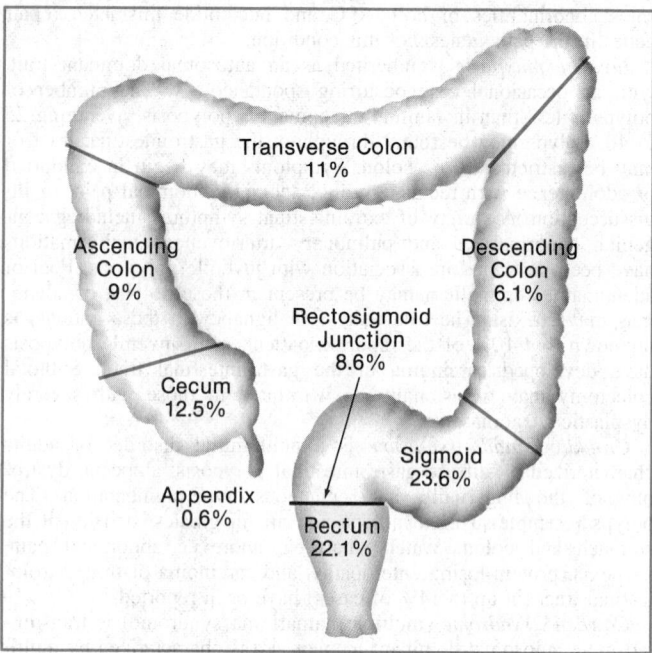

FIGURE 106–5. Distribution of large bowel cancer by anatomic segment according to the third national cancer survey (segment unspecified). (Based on data from Shottenfeld D, Fraumeni J Jr [eds.]: Cancer Epidemiology and Prevention. Philadelphia, WB Saunders, 1982, p 703.

Colorectal cancer must be suspected when patients present with rectal bleeding, a change in bowel habit, decrease in stool caliber, iron deficiency anemia, or unexplained abdominal pain. Rectal bleeding may be caused by other conditions, including hemorrhoids, angiodysplasia, diverticulosis, and other benign and malignant tumors (see Ch. 95). Over the age of 40, the frequency of neoplasia increases significantly. Unexplained iron deficiency in both older men and women always requires a thorough evaluation to exclude gastrointestinal cancer (see Ch. 132).

METASTATIC COLON CANCER. Metastases may be clinically apparent before or after resection of the primary colorectal cancer. Massive hepatomegaly may occur with pain due to distention of the liver capsule. Spread within the abdomen may cause small and large bowel obstruction and ascites. Pelvic spread may cause bladder dysfunction, sacral or sciatic nerve pain, and vaginal discharge or bleeding. Distant spread to lungs and bone may be silent until very advanced. Intestinal recurrences are uncommon and usually result from tumor implants related to the original resection growing from the serosa into the lumen.

DIAGNOSIS. A careful history, physical examination, and selected use of laboratory and radiologic tests facilitate the diagnosis of colorectal cancer. The history includes the patient's symptoms, prior removal of an adenoma or cancer, previous or present inflammatory bowel disease, or a family history of one of the inherited colorectal cancer syndromes. Special emphasis should be paid to first-degree relatives with a history of colorectal neoplasia. Physical examination may reveal evidence for Peutz-Jeghers or Gardner syndrome and may provide substantiation of spread to lymph nodes, liver, or peritoneal cavity. A digital rectal examination is essential in determining the presence of a distal rectal cancer or of perineal or

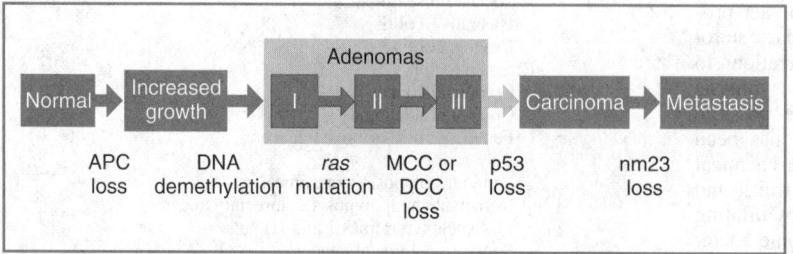

FIGURE 106–4. Correlation between stages of progression of colorectal carcinoma and recognized mutational events affecting specific colon cancer–associated genes. Although a preferred sequence of mutational events is apparent, the accumulation of genetic abnormalities is more important than the order in which they occur. APC, adenomatous polyposis coli tumor suppressor gene; DCC, deleted in colon cancer tumor suppressor gene; MCC, mutated in colon cancer tumor suppressor gene; nm23, nm23 metastasis suppressor gene; p53, p53 tumor suppressor gene; *ras,* Ki-*ras* oncogene. (Adapted from Vogelstein B, Kinzler KW: The multistep nature of cancer. Trends Genet 9:138, 1993.)

pelvic spread. A complete pelvic examination should not be omitted. Laboratory tests may reveal iron deficiency anemia or an abnormality of liver enzymes. Radiologic studies may include a chest roentgenogram or computed tomographic (CT) scan of the abdomen and pelvis.

In evaluating patients with symptoms or signs of colorectal cancer, the digital rectal examination is followed by colonoscopy or double-contrast barium enema following sigmoidoscopy. Endoscopic ultrasonography is being used with increasing frequency to help in the staging of rectal cancers. Depth of invasion can often be accurately determined. Flexible sigmoidoscopy has replaced rigid proctoscopy and is particularly useful in evaluating a patient with a rectosigmoid neoplasm or an individual who presents with rectal bleeding and in whom active inflammatory bowel disease is suspected. In the latter case a barium enema or even colonoscopy may be undesirable.

Colonoscopy is more sensitive than double-contrast barium enema in detecting small adenomas and cancers and is also valuable for evaluating patients who have had an abnormality detected by barium enema. In addition, the presence or absence of synchronous cancers and adenomas can be determined. Colonoscopy can be used to remove adenomas, to biopsy suspected cancers, and to obtain brush biopsy for cytology of suspected malignancies and colonic strictures.

MANAGEMENT. The modern approach to management is a multidisciplinary one and includes not only consideration of the immediate clinical problem but also a long-term approach to the patient. This may include postoperative adjuvant treatment, future plans for assessment of local recurrence or distant metastasis, and attention to family members at increased risk.

Surgery. The most important goal of treatment for primary malignancies of the colon and rectum is complete removal. Surgical resection of the affected segment, including omentum and lymph nodes, is performed. Increasingly, laparoscopic resections are being used, although long-term follow-up data are lacking. Cancers of the right and left colon are treated by hemicolectomies; cancers of the sigmoid and upper rectum above 6 cm from the anal verge are resected anteriorly with removal of a margin of normal colon above and below the tumor. Stapling techniques have facilitated anastomoses within the pelvis. While 3-cm proximal and distal margins have been previously emphasized, an adequate radial margin is equally important.

Lesions within 5 cm of the anal verge are usually treated by a combined abdominoperineal resection and permanent colostomy. Newer approaches for small, early rectal cancers include sphincter-saving procedures using local excision followed in some instances by radiation therapy to the pelvis. Preoperatively, combined radiation therapy and chemotherapy may facilitate resection, including sphincter-saving procedures.

For anal cancers the standard approach is to use a combination of radiation and chemotherapy, which usually shrinks or obliterates the cancer. It is unknown whether HIV-infected patients or those with AIDS are more susceptible to treatment-related toxicity. Surgical resection is now usually reserved for lesions that do not respond to chemoradiation and for those that recur.

Surgery may be required for palliation as well as for cure. Colonic obstruction may necessitate a palliative colostomy, although a primary resection and colostomy can often be accomplished at the same operation. A perforated carcinoma is usually managed by primary resection and colostomy with later closure of the colostomy. For selected medically fit patients with one to three hepatic metastases, surgical resection of part of the tumor-bearing liver is often possible. Careful preoperative radiologic staging as well as intraoperative ultrasonography of the liver facilitates these technically demanding procedures. Laser photoablation is being increasingly used to relieve colonic or rectal obstruction or bleeding in patients with unresectable tumors or extensive metastatic disease.

Radiation Therapy. Radiation therapy plays an important role in the postoperative management of rectal cancer. The combination of radiation (50 Gy) and chemotherapy, 5-fluorouracil (5-FU), is now standard therapy and has been shown to decrease local recurrence and distant metastasis. Biochemical modulation of 5-FU by leucovorin is also being incorporated. Preoperative radiation therapy decreases postoperative local recurrence but does not prolong overall survival. It may also be used to reduce tumor size and enable otherwise unresectable lesions to be resected. Radiation therapy is

useful in palliating recurrent rectal cancer (pain or bleeding) or bone or brain metastases.

Chemotherapy. Patients with resected colonic cancer with lymph node spread may have improved survival if treated with the combination of 5-FU and levamisole for a period of 1 year or 5-FU and leucovorin for 6 or 12 months. For patients with metastatic spread, the combination of 5-FU and leucovorin increases tumor shrinkage compared with 5-FU alone. New drugs such as topoisomerase I inhibitors (camptothecins) are promising.

In patients with liver metastases, hepatic arterial therapy with implantable pumps or via injection ports using floxuridine (FUDR) alone or in combination with other drugs such as leucovorin produces an enhanced tumor shrinkage in the liver, but increased duration and quality of survival have not yet been convincingly demonstrated.

PROGNOSIS AND FOLLOW-UP. The 10-year survival for patients with colorectal cancer after surgical resection is approximately 50%. The survival correlates well with the stage of the disease: cancer confined to the mucosa, 80 to 90% 10-year survival; cancer extending through all areas of the bowel wall, 70 to 80%; and cancer involving the regional lymph nodes, 30 to 55%. Cancers of the distal rectum with lymph node involvement have a poorer prognosis. Several histopathologic staging systems (e.g., Dukes' or TNM) are in use to describe the extent of the malignancy (Table 106–2).

Prior to surgical resection, the entire colon should be examined, preferably by colonoscopy, for the presence of synchronous adenomas. If not possible preoperatively, colonoscopy should be performed postoperatively, usually within 2 to 3 months of the surgical procedure. Colonoscopy should be repeated a year later and every 3 years thereafter because new adenomas require 3 years or more to develop into large adenomas with malignant potential.

After surgical resection, patients without known systemic metastases are evaluated for adjuvant therapy. Patients with colonic cancer and lymph node involvement should receive 5-FU and levamisole, or 5-FU and leucovorin, and those with rectal cancer and spread through the wall or with lymph node involvement should receive radiation plus chemotherapy. While receiving chemotherapy or radiation therapy, patients are followed very carefully according to protocol guidelines. For those not receiving any specific therapy, periodic follow-up including interim history, physical examination, and laboratory tests (liver enzymes, hematocrit) are performed every 6 months for the first 3 years, then every 6 months until the fifth year. Controversy exists concerning the cost-effectiveness of obtaining periodic chest radiographs or CT scans of the abdomen and pelvis as part of routine follow-up care in the absence of symptoms or laboratory test abnormalities.

Carcinoembryonic Antigen (CEA). CEA levels in the blood may rise before symptoms or other laboratory test abnormalities are evident in patients with recurrent or metastatic colonic cancer. Some authorities favor periodic CEA determinations (e.g., every 3 months) after colorectal cancer resection, but this is very expensive and helpful only in a minority of patients. Occasionally, a rising CEA may detect a localized, surgically resectable metastasis. In conjunction with conventional radiologic techniques (CT scan or MRI), radiolabeled monoclonal antibodies to CEA may be helpful

TABLE 106–2. AMERICAN JOINT COMMITTEE ON CANCER: CLASSIFICATION OF COLON/RECTAL CANCER

Stage 0	Carcinoma *in situ;* the cancer does not extend beyond the smooth muscle that separates the mucosa from the submucosa. (T_{ix}, N_0, M_0)
Stage I	Cancer confined to the mucosa, submucosa, or external muscle; the cancer does not extend through the bowel wall. (T_1 or T_2, N_0, M_0)
Stage II	Cancer that penetrates all layers of the bowel wall, with or without invasion of adjacent tissues. (T_3, N_0, M_0)
Stage III	Cancer involving regional lymph nodes or extending into nearby tissues or organs without spread to lymph nodes. (Any T, N_1–N_3, M_0; or T_4, N_0, M_0)
Stage IV	Cancer that has spread to distant sites, usually the liver or lungs. (Any T, any N, M_1)

T = Tumor size; N = lymph node involvement; M = degree of metastasis.

in localizing such metastases. In the absence of defined lesions, a "second look" laparotomy based on a rising CEA has not been shown to prolong survival.

PREVENTING COLORECTAL CANCER

Many colorectal cancers are first brought to medical attention by the patient's recognition of symptoms. For improved survival, the diagnosis should ideally be made earlier, in an asymptomatic phase. A greater emphasis is now being placed on preventive measures. Primary prevention is identifying factors, either genetic or environmental, responsible for colorectal cancers. Secondary prevention refers to identifying and eradicating premalignant lesions and detecting and resecting cancer while still curable.

Although definitive evidence of effectiveness is still lacking, the National Cancer Institute has issued certain dietary guidelines to try to reduce the risk of colorectal cancer: (1) reduce fat intake to <30% of calories; (2) increase dietary fiber to 20 to 30 grams per day; (3) include a variety of vegetables and fruits in the diet; (4) avoid obesity; (5) consume alcohol in moderation, if at all; and (6) avoid cigarettes and tobacco. In addition, regular exercise may also reduce risk. Chemopreventive measures such as aspirin or NSAID's are being studied.

Implicit in the concept of secondary prevention is the need for improved techniques for screening for early cancer or premalignant adenomas. Effective screening requires the availability and application of simple and economic measures to a large number of asymptomatic individuals to identify those with these lesions. Screening for colorectal cancer can be classified as follows: general screening of patients at average risk and screening of patients in high-risk groups. (For discussion of high-risk groups see *Polyposis Syndromes* and *Ulcerative Colitis*.)

AVERAGE-RISK PATIENTS. Currently, testing for fecal occult blood and flexible sigmoidoscopy in asymptomatic individuals are used for detecting early colorectal cancer. Testing for occult blood using guaiac-based methods seems to detect earlier lesions in those screened compared with controls, and in one major US trial, colorectal mortality was significantly reduced by annual testing for fecal occult blood and appropriate colonoscopic follow-up. Newer immunochemical tests for human hemoglobin in the stool, currently under clinical trial, are likely to be more specific. Randomized controlled trials of flexible sigmoidoscopy have not been performed on a large scale. Case-control studies have demonstrated significant effectiveness of flexible sigmoidoscopy in reducing mortality from distal colorectal cancer. Flexible sigmoidoscopy can not only identify and eradicate premalignant and malignant lesions in the area examined but also can identify individuals who may have more proximal synchronous adenomas and carcinomas.

Current guidelines for screening patients by physicians are: (1) annual digital rectal examination after age 40; (2) testing for fecal occult blood annually after age 50; and (3) flexible sigmoidoscopy every 3 to 5 years after age 50. Patients with abnormal findings require careful diagnostic evaluation, including colonoscopy. A critical evaluation of a mass screening program for colorectal cancer requires that important issues be addressed: (1) What are the expected benefits in terms of survival of patients whose disease is discovered by screening tests and treated? (2) Is there a mortality reduction from colorectal cancer in the entire screened population? (3) What are the psychological, economic, and other factors influencing patient compliance? (4) Are adequate health resources available for the diagnostic workup and treatment of patients with a positive screening test? (5) What are the costs and risks of such screening?

Neoplasms of the Small Bowel

Benign and malignant tumors of the lining epithelium and mesenchymal tissues may arise in the small intestine, or these areas may be secondarily involved by direct invasion from surrounding structures or by metastases. The small bowel represents almost 90% of the mucosal surface of the gut, but small intestinal cancers ac-

count for only 1 to 2% of all gastrointestinal neoplasms. Only about 2000 cases occur in the United States each year.

RISK FACTORS. Patients with regional enteritis, especially those who have had segments of intestine surgically bypassed, have an increased incidence of small bowel carcinoma. Individuals with Gardner syndrome have an increased risk of periampullary adenocarcinoma. In patients with Peutz-Jeghers syndrome, the relative risk of small intestinal adenocarcinoma is 16 times that expected, with a lifetime incidence of 2%. Patients with celiac disease of long duration have an increased incidence of intestinal lymphoma, as do patients with the AIDS and other immunodeficiency states. Mediterranean abdominal lymphoma (immunoproliferative small intestinal disease) has been widely reported among Arabs and Jews of Middle Eastern origin and also occurs sporadically throughout the world, including in blacks in southern Africa.

Why small bowel neoplasms, especially adenocarcinomas, are so uncommon compared with large bowel cancers is uncertain. It is possible that the rapid transit time with a resultant decreased exposure time to carcinogens, lower numbers of bacteria, and dilution of potential carcinogens by the large volume of enteric liquids may contribute.

PATHOLOGY. *Benign.* These lesions include adenomas, leiomyomas, lipomas, and angiomas. Brunner's gland adenomas are not neoplastic but represent a hyperplasia or hypertrophy of submucosal duodenal glands. These appear as small nodules in the duodenal mucosa detected at endoscopy or on barium radiographs.

Malignant. Adenocarcinomas, carcinoids, lymphomas, and leiomyosarcomas account for >90% of malignant small bowel tumors. Adenocarcinomas are most common in the proximal small intestine, whereas lymphomas and carcinoids are most common in the distal small intestine.

CLINICAL MANIFESTATIONS. More than half of all benign bowel tumors remain asymptomatic and may only be discovered incidentally at laparotomy or autopsy. Lack of symptoms is attributible to the liquid contents of the small intestine and distensibility of the small intestine. Large tumors may lead to partial or complete mechanical obstruction from intussusception or volvulus. Adenocarcinomas account for about half of the malignant tumors of the small intestine, with a peak incidence in the sixth and seventh decades. The duodenum is the most frequently affected site. When postbulbar in location, adenocarcinoma may simulate peptic ulcer disease; when in the periampullary region, it may cause obstructive jaundice. More distally, adenocarcinomas may remain silent until symptoms of intestinal obstruction or gastrointestinal hemorrhage occur.

Carcinoids are the most frequent small intestinal neoplasm, with over half found incidentally either at autopsy or at operation for other diseases. Small carcinoid tumors may be asymptomatic, but larger carcinoid tumors can obstruct the lumen or bleed. Once metastasis occurs to the liver, features of the carcinoid syndrome become apparent (see Ch. 210.2). Weight loss, intestinal obstruction, fever, bleeding, and evidence of malabsorption syndrome are features of lymphoma. Massive hemorrhage and intestinal perforation may be the presenting symptoms of large sarcomas.

SIGNS. Physical examination may be unremarkable in patients with benign tumors, unless the neoplasms are large enough to present with a mass. Loud borborygmi, visible peristalsis, and abdominal distention may be present in intestinal obstruction. In patients with malignant small bowel neoplasms, more obvious physical findings may be evident. Cachexia, hepatomegaly, ascites, and jaundice may be found. Peripheral lymphadenopathy or splenomegaly may be found in those with extensive lymphoma.

DIFFERENTIAL DIAGNOSIS. The initial symptoms may be vague and poorly defined. Once bleeding occurs, causes such as peptic ulceration, Meckel's diverticulum, and vascular anomalies need to be considered (see Ch. 95). Obstructive jaundice may occur with periampullary neoplasms, bile duct cancer, impacted common duct stones, pancreatitis, and pancreatic cancer (see Ch. 108). Intestinal obstruction may be due to adhesions, particularly in patients who have had prior abdominal operations, internal hernias, volvulus, or intussusception.

LABORATORY AND RADIOLOGIC STUDIES. A hypochromic, microcytic anemia is quite common. Elevation of alkaline phosphatase and bilirubin may recur if the ampulla of Vater is obstructed or if liver metastases are present. Elevated levels of plasma serotonin or urinary 5-hydroxyindoleacetic acid occur in the carcinoid syndrome (see Ch. 210.2). Dysproteinemia is a typical feature of Mediterranean lymphoma and is characterized by the presence of abnormal fragments of IgA in the serum and urine that is devoid of light chains (see Ch. 149).

Upper gastrointestinal barium radiographs and selective nasoenteric intubation (enteroclysis), which permits the introduction of barium and air into a relatively localized segment, may be useful in localizing tumors. Abdominal ultrasonography and CT may determine the extent of hepatic involvement, aid in the workup of jaundice, and assess intra-abdominal and retroperitoneal spread. Intestinal lymphoma may occasionally be diagnosed by peroral intestinal biopsy, but the disease mainly involves the lamina propria and usually requires a full-thickness surgical biopsy. A thorough staging of lymphoma involves bone marrow biopsy, laparotomy with splenectomy, and biopsies of regional lymph nodes and liver.

ENDOSCOPIC EVALUATION. Front-viewing and side-viewing fiberoptic endoscopes are used to examine the duodenum; suspicious lesions can be biopsied and brushed. Periampullary lesions can be well visualized; the pancreatic and biliary trees can be studied by contrast radiography after endoscopic cannulation. The terminal ileum can also be viewed at colonoscopy. Small bowel enteroscopy, a relatively new technique, is sometimes helpful in localizing a small bleeding lesion.

THERAPY. Treatment is primarily surgical for symptomatic benign tumors, adenocarcinomas, leiomyosarcomas, malignant carcinoids, and those with secondary involvement of the small intestine. Duodenal carcinomas or large villous adenomas are treated by pancreaticoduodenal resection (Whipple procedure). In patients with localized lymphoma (stage I) surgical excision is recommended. Combination chemotherapy is used for more extensive lymphoma (see Ch. 145). Radiation therapy may be helpful for bulky tumors or localized recurrences.

PROGNOSIS AND PREVENTION. The prognosis for benign tumors of the intestine is good if surgical resection can alleviate bleeding and obstruction. The prognosis of small intestinal adenocarcinomas is generally poor. The prognosis for leiomyosarcomas and primary lymphomas is good if surgical resection is complete, but this is rarely possible. Patients with malignant carcinoid tumors may survive for long periods even in the presence of extensive hepatic involvement (see Ch. 210.2).

Primary small intestinal lymphomas occurring in the Middle East could possibly be decreased by public health measures that decrease parasitic infestation. Earlier diagnosis and adequate treatment of celiac disease (gluten-free diet) may reduce the frequency of malignancy. Surgical bypass should not be performed in patients with Crohn's disease. In patients with familial polyposis syndromes, duodenal and periampullary adenomas should be monitored periodically. Prophylactic endoscopic or surgical removal may be appropriate.

Epidemiology

Greenwald P: Colon cancer overview. Cancer 70:1206, 1992. *A concise review covering epidemiology, prevention, and screening strategies.*
Potter JD: Reconciling the epidemiology, physiology and molecular biology of colon cancer. JAMA 268:1573, 1992. *A comprehensive overview.*

Screening and Early Detection

Levin B, Lennard-Jones J, Riddell RH: Surveillance of patients with chronic ulcerative colitis. Bull WHO 64:121, 1991. *A practically oriented article on managing patients at high risk.*
Levin B, Murphy GP: Revision in American Cancer Society recommendations for the early detection of colorectal cancer. CA: Cancer J Clin 42:296, 1992. *Guidelines for standard-risk individuals.*
Mandel JJ, Bond JH, Church TR, et al.: Minnesota colon cancer control study: Reducing mortality from colorectal cancer by screening for occult blood. N Engl J Med 328:1365, 1993. *The first large-scale study to show an effect of fecal occult blood testing on colorectal cancer mortality.*
Selby JF, Friedman GD, Quesenberry CPJ, et al.: A case-control study of screening sigmoidoscopy and mortality from colorectal cancer. N Engl J Med 326:653, 1992. *An important study demonstrating a long-term benefit of rigid sigmoidoscopy.*

Molecular Biology/Genetics

Aaltonen LA, Peltomaki P, Leach PS, et al.: Clues to the pathogenesis of familial colorectal cancer. Science 260:812, 1993. *The identification of widespread alterations in short repeated DNA segments in chromosome 2.*
Vogelstein B, Kinzler KW: The multistep nature of cancer. Trends Genet 9:138, 1993. *A concise modern review of new information about molecular biology.*

Adenomas and Their Management

Atkin WS, Morson BC, Cuzick J: Longterm risk of colorectal cancer after excision of rectosigmoid adenomas. N Engl J Med 326:658, 1992. *An important description of the natural history of adenomas.*

Ransohoff DF, Lang CA, Kho HS: Colonoscopic surveillance after polypectomy: Considerations of cost effectiveness. Ann Intern Med 114:177, 1991. *A discussion of the implications of adenoma discovery and subsequent management.*

Therapy

Cohen AM, Winawer SJ (eds.): Cancer of the Colon, Rectum and Anus. New York, McGraw-Hill, 1995. *A detailed and comprehensive text.*
Hart R, Levin B: Neoplasms of the Small Bowel. *In* Calabresi P, Schein PS (eds.): Medical Oncology. 2nd ed. New York, McGraw-Hill, 1993, p 741. *A comprehensive overview.*
Moertel CG: An odyssey in the land of small tumors. J Clin Oncol 5:1503, 1989. *An insightful description of the clinical biology of carcinoid tumors.*

107 PANCREATITIS
Konrad H. Soergel

ANATOMY AND PHYSIOLOGY OF THE PANCREAS

The pancreas first appears as ventral and dorsal budding evaginations of the primitive foregut at 5 weeks' gestation. The right portion of the ventral bud, including the common bile duct, migrates posteriorly with rotation of the duodenum. Both anlagen and their ducts fuse by the seventh week of gestation, with the ventral anlage forming the pancreatic head and uncinate process and the dorsal anlage the body and tail. Incomplete fusion results in two separate pancreatic ducts: the dorsal duct of Santorini draining through the minor papilla and a short ventral duct (Wirsung) ending at the major papilla of Vater. This anomaly, termed *pancreas divisum,* is present in 5 to 10% of the population. Fixation of the ventral bud while the duodenum rotates results in a band of pancreatic tissue encircling the descending duodenum; the resulting *annular pancreas* is very rare and may cause duodenal obstruction or pancreatitis.

The retroperitoneal location and the absence of a capsule surrounding the pancreas are important to the understanding of how pancreatitis evolves. Pancreatic inflammation and fibrosis may spread unimpeded by anatomic barriers to involve the spleen, the splenic artery and vein, the duodenum and distal common bile duct, the mesocolon and small bowel mesentery, the diaphragm and pararenal spaces, the lesser omental sac, and the celiac and superior mesenteric ganglia. The acinar cells of the exocrine pancreas synthesize approximately 20 digestive enzymes, colipase, a secretory trypsin inhibitor (PSTI), and lithostathine S_{2-5}, a protein that inhibits the precipitation of $CaCO_3$ from pancreatic juice. These secretory proteins are sorted into condensing vacuoles, which then become zymogen granules. The granules fuse with the apical cell membrane and discharge their contents into the acinar lumen by exocytosis. This secretory step is controlled by cholecystokinin (CCK) and by stimulation via central vagal pathways and gastropancreatic and enteropancreatic cholinergic reflexes. CCK is released from endocrine I cells in the duodenal and proximal jejunal mucosa during fat and protein digestion. All digestive enzymes, except α-amylase, lipase, ribonuclease, and deoxyribonuclease, are secreted as inactive zymogens. Trypsinogen is activated by enterokinase, which is secreted by the duodenum; trypsin then activates all other zymogens within the duodenal lumen. The centroacinar, ductular, and pancreatic duct epithelial cells represent a functional unit that exchanges HCO_3^- for Cl^-, with increasing flow rates of pancreatic secretion. This process involves the intracellular generation of carbonic acid by carbonic anhydrase and the actions of a Cl^-/HCO_3^- exchanger and a Cl^- channel, the cystic fibrosis transmembrane regulator (CFTR), at the luminal cell border. The excess intracellular H^+ ions are removed by a basolaterally located Na^+/H^+ exchanger. Secretion of alkaline, bicarbonate-rich pancreatic juice is stimulated by acetylcholine and by the hormone secretin, which is released from mucosal S cells when the duodenal pH decreases to ≤ 4.5. Premature activation of zymogens within the pancreas is the key event in the pathogenesis of acute pancreatitis. Protein and $CaCO_3$ precipitates within the pancreatic duct system play a major role in the development of chronic pancreatitis.

ACUTE PANCREATITIS

DEFINITIONS. Acute pancreatitis is an acute inflammatory process with variable involvement of adjacent and remote organs. Although pancreatic function and structure eventually return to normal, the risk of recurrent attacks is nearly 50% unless the precipitating cause is removed. Initial manifestations and exacerbations of chronic pancreatitis may be indistinguishable from attacks of acute pancreatitis, and they should be treated as such. The inflammation begins in the perilobular and peripancreatic fatty tissue, manifested by edema and spotty fat necrosis. The disease may progress to the peripheral acinar cells, pancreatic ducts, blood vessels, and bordering organs. In severe cases, patchy areas of the pancreatic parenchyma become necrotic. Local complications are defined as follows: (1) *Acute fluid collections:* these are common and frequently multiple; they occur early in the course and lack a defined wall. The majority of these collections resolve spontaneously. (2) *Pancreatic necrosis:* focal or diffuse necrosis of pancreatic parenchyma, frequently associated with peripancreatic fat necrosis. The necrotic tissue may be sterile or infected. (3) *Pancreatic abscess:* a rare complication that arises late in the course of acute pancreatitis. Several traditional descriptive terms have become ambiguous and should be discarded. These include pancreatic phlegmon, acute and infected pseudocysts, and edematous and hemorrhagic acute pancreatitis.

The annual incidence of acute pancreatitis is close to 10 per 100,000 in the adult population.

PATHOGENESIS. Premature activation of zymogens and the escape of activated enzymes from acinar cells and pancreatic ducts set the stage for the autodigestive process that represents acute pancreatitis (Fig. 107–1). Proteases released into the blood are inacti-

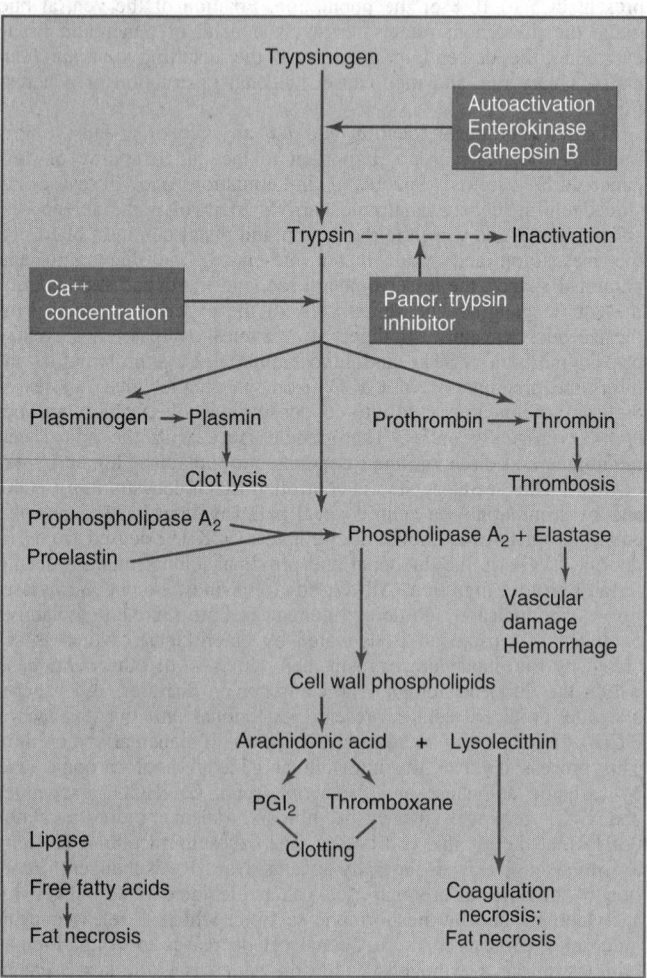

FIGURE 107–1. The pathophysiology of pancreatic autodigestion. (From Sleisenger MH, Fordtran JS [eds.]: Gastrointestinal Disease. 5th ed. Philadelphia, WB Saunders, 1993, p 1631.)

vated by circulating inhibitors, including α_2-macroglobulin, α_1-antitrypsin, and the C_1-esterase inhibitor. In addition, trypsin activates kallikrein, a peptidase, which then cleaves several peptides, including bradykinin and kallidin, from their inactive precursors in blood plasma. These peptides, termed kinins, have various deleterious effects including vasodilatation, increased vascular permeability, pain, and neutrophil accumulation.

Animal models of acute pancreatitis revealed two mechanisms that may trigger pancreatic autodigestion: (1) *Zymogen activation* within the pancreatic acinar cell (Fig. 107–2): The rate of exocytosis is decreased while acinar protein synthesis continues undiminished, leading to intracellular accumulation of zymogens. A variety of errors in intracellular traffic result in co-localization of zymogens and lysosomal enzymes in large autophagic vacules. Lysosomal enzymes and the acidic pH within these vacuoles activate the zymogens, which then undergo misdirected secretion across the basolateral wall of the acinar cell. (2) *Increased pancreatic duct permeability.* Raising the intraductal pressure, acute hypercalcemia, and orally administered acetylsalicylic acid or ethanol make the pancreatic duct epithelium permeable to molecules of up to 25,000 Da. Severe pancreatitis results when the pancreatic duct is then perfused with active pancreatic enzymes, particularly when microvascular permeability is increased by the actions of histamine or prostaglandins. Thus, pancreatic zymogen activation and increased pancreatic duct permeability may act sequentially in initiating acute pancreatitis.

Based on clinical and experimental observations, several mechanisms have been proposed to initiate acute pancreatitis. Among these, reflux of duodenal contents or bile into the pancreatic duct is no longer considered to play a role. Obstruction of the pancreatic duct near the ampulla of Vater remains a plausible mechanism that may explain many, although not all, episodes of acute pancreatitis.

ASSOCIATED FACTORS. Clinical conditions, medications, and toxins known to precipitate acute pancreatitis are listed in Table 107–1. Among these, choledocholithiasis and ethanol abuse account for 70 to 80% of all cases. The number attributed to the idiopathic type varies with the clinician's astuteness in identifying one of the factors listed. All remaining causes combined account for 10% or less of the total. *Alcoholic and familial* pancreatitis are discussed under "chronic pancreatitis."

Gallstones. They may cause pancreatitis by impacting in the ampulla of Vater. The stones usually pass spontaneously into the duodenum, and small gallstones can be found in the stools of 92% of patients with gallstone pancreatitis. Persistent stone impaction can cause severe pancreatitis combined with ascending cholangitis. The incidence of gallstone-associated pancreatitis parallels that of cholelithiasis: It peaks at ages 50 to 70 and women outnumber men by 2 to 1. As with other types of acute pancreatitis, chronic pancreatitis does not result from multiple episodes of pancreatitis associated with gallstones. Pancreatitis during *pregnancy* usually occurs during the third trimester and is caused by gallstones in approximately 90% of instances.

Drug-Induced Pancreatitis. This complication characteristically occurs within the first 2 months of exposure; it is not dose-related and the pancreatitis usually is mild. Most commonly implicated are azathioprine/6-mercaptopurine, valproic acid in children, sulfur-containing diuretics, and pentamidine and ddI in patients with AIDS.

Hypertriglyceridemia. The presence of lipemia, with serum triglyceride levels > 1000 mg per deciliter, represents a cause, not an effect, of pancreatitis. Causes include estrogen therapy, alcoholism, intravenous lipid infusions, and primary hyperlipidemias (see Ch. 114).

Miscellaneous Factors. *Acute hypercalcemia* may trigger acute pancreatitis. This may occur with intravenous calcium infusions, during cardiopulmonary bypass, and with vitamin D poisoning. Blunt abdominal *trauma* causes pancreatitis by disrupting the duct; it is the most common cause of pancreatitis in children. *Postoperative* pancreatitis may follow intra- and extra-abdominal surgery and carries a high mortality rate of 25 to 50%. Pancreatitis following *endoscopic retrograde cholangiopancreatography (ERCP)* is usually mild unless it is complicated by duodenal perforation during endoscopic sphincterotomy. *Pancreatic infections* are an exceedingly rare and poorly documented cause of pancreatitis. Whether *pancreas divisum* predisposes to recurrent acute pancreatitis remains controversial. The available evidence favors the decision

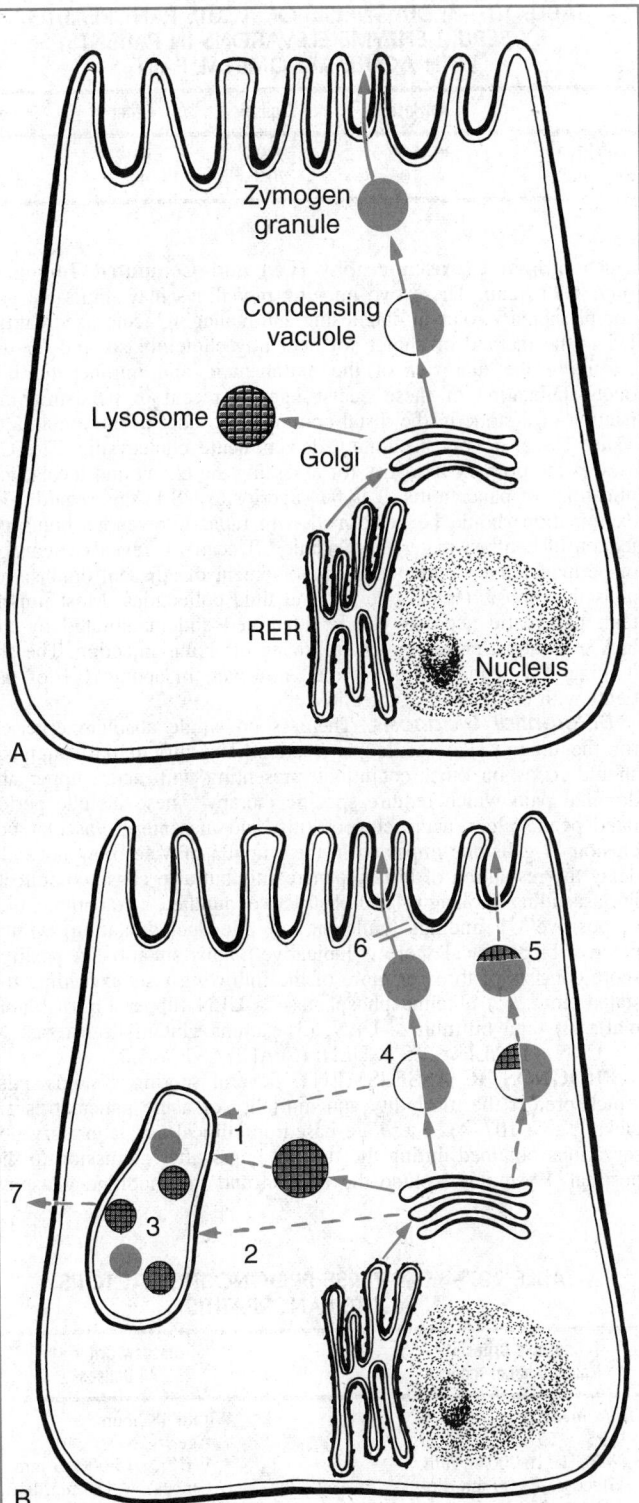

FIGURE 107–2. Synthesis, sorting, and secretion of hydrolytic enzymes and zymogens in the pancreatic acinar cell. *A,* Normal. *B,* Abnormalities observed in various models of experimental pancreatitis; (1) crinophagy: condensing vacuoles and lysosomes coalesce; (2) absent compartmentalization; (3) autophagic vacuole; (4) autoactivation; (5) increased lysosomal hydrolase secretion; (6) exocytosis block; (7) secretion across basolateral cell wall. Interrupted lines indicate abnormal events. (From Sleisenger MH, Fordtran JS [eds.]: Gastrointestinal Disease. 5th ed. Philadelphia, WB Saunders, 1993, p 1630.)

to proceed with surgical or endoscopic decompression of the dorsal pancreatic duct in these patients.

CLINICAL PRESENTATION. Steady, dull, or boring mid-epigastric pain associated with nausea and vomiting is the classic presentation of acute pancreatitis. The pain reaches peak intensity

TABLE 107–1. FACTORS ASSOCIATED WITH ACUTE PANCREATITIS

Obstructive causes
  Choledocholithiasis
  Ampullary obstruction by tumor or sphincter of Oddi hypertension
  Choledochocele
  Periampullary duodenal diverticulum
  Pancreas divisum(?); annular pancreas
  Primary or metastatic pancreatic tumor
  Parasites in pancreatic duct: *Clonorchosis ascaris*
Toxins
  Ethanol
  Methanol
  Organophosphorus insecticides
  Scorpion venom (*Tityus trinitatis*)
Drugs
  Definite association: Azathioprine/6-mercaptopurine; valproic acid; estrogens; metronidazole; loop diuretics, including thiazides, furosemide, bumetanide; pentamidine; sulfonamides; methyldopa; L-asparaginase; tetracyclines, cytarabine, cimetidine
  Probable association: chlorthalidone; mesalamine; ddI (2′ 3′ dideoxyinosine); ethacrynic acid; phenformin; ACE inhibitors; nitrofurantoin; cocaine and amphetamine abuse; acetaminophen
Metabolic causes
  Hypertriglyceridemia
  Hypercalcemia
Trauma
  Blunt abdominal trauma
  ERCP procedures
  Abdominal operations, cardiopulmonary bypass
Infections
  Viral: mumps, coxsackie B, hepatitis A and B
  Bacterial: mycoplasma, *Salmonella, Campylobacter jejuni*
Vascular
  Shock-hypoperfusion
  Vasculitis
  Cholesterol emboli
Miscellaneous
  Penetrating duodenal ulcer
  Organ transplantation
  Crohn's disease of duodenum
  Familial pancreatitis
Idiopathic

within 15 minutes to 1 hour from onset, in contrast to the more abrupt onset of pain with a perforated viscus. It radiates straight to the midline of the lower thoracic vertebral region in about 50% of patients and is usually worse in the supine position. Painless acute pancreatitis is very rare but carries a grave prognosis because the patients frequently present in shock.

Initial physical examination reveals mild fever and tachycardia; hypotension is present in 30 to 40% of patients. There is marked tenderness to deep palpation of the upper abdomen, but signs of peritoneal irritation such as abdominal wall rigidity and rebound tenderness are absent. Bowel sounds are diminished; paralytic ileus with abdominal distention may develop during the first few days, signifying extension of the inflammatory process into the small intestinal and colonic mesentery. One to 2 weeks after the onset, large ecchymoses rarely appear in the flanks (Grey Turner's sign) or the umbilical area (Cullen's sign); these represent blood dissecting from the retroperitoneally located pancreas along fascial planes. Similarly, inflammatory masses, large fluid collections, or a pancreatic abscess may become palpable later in the course of the disease.

DIAGNOSIS. The diagnosis of acute pancreatitis rests on a combination of clinical, laboratory, and radiologic findings, none of which is infallible. The goals of diagnostic studies are (1) to exclude other acute conditions that may require urgent surgical management; (2) to assess the prognosis; (3) to detect local and systemic complications early; (4) to identify a precipitating cause.

***Laboratory Tests.* Amylase.** Total serum amylase activity is the test most frequently used to diagnose acute pancreatitis. The level rises 2 to 12 hours after onset of symptoms and remains elevated for 3 to 5 days in most cases. Values >5 times the upper limit of normal are highly specific for acute pancreatitis, but these are found in only 80 to 90% of cases. The magnitude of the rise in serum amylase does not correlate with the severity of the attack, nor does prolonged hyperamylasemia indicate developing complications. Marked hypertriglyceridemia, sufficient to give the serum a lipemic appearance, masks elevations in serum amylase and lipase; dilution of these sera lead to a paradoxical rise in the reported enzyme values. Separation of total serum amylase into its pancreatic (P) and salivary (S) isoenzymes and measurements of urinary amylase output add little to the diagnostic information. The amylase-creatinine clearance ratio (ACR) (the ratio of amylase concentration in urine over plasma, divided by the corresponding values for creatinine) is useful in diagnosing asymptomatic macroamylasemia only when aggregates of circulating amylase escape glomerular infiltration and the ACR is abnormally low. Serum amylase may be elevated in many other clinical conditions (Table 107–2), illustrating the fact that the diagnosis of acute pancreatitis should not be based solely on laboratory results.

Lipase. Serum lipase assays, especially those using colipase, have similar specificity and sensitivity as serum amylase. The serum lipase tends to remain elevated longer than amylase during the healing phase of pancreatitis.

Combinations of Serum Enzyme Tests. The combination of serum amylase and lipase determinations is more accurate than either test alone (Table 107–3). The diagnostic accuracy can be improved further by calculating cut-off values that lie above the upper limit of normal. Additional measurements, such as serum immunoreactive trypsin (IRT), elastase, and phospholipase A_2, do not improve the diagnostic information obtained from serum amylase and lipase values.

Other Blood Tests. Leukocytosis of up to 25,000 cells per cubic millimeter is present in 80% of patients; the hematocrit is frequently elevated due to hemoconcentration. Hypocalcemia occurs in up to 30% of patients due to a combination of hypoalbuminemia and calcium precipitation in areas of fat necrosis. The ionized calcium concentration remains normal, and symptoms of tetany are extremely rare. Pre-existing hypercalcemia may, however, be obscured by the calcium-lowering effect of pancreatitis. Transient, mild hyperglycemia is common and does not require insulin treatment. Serum triglyceride levels should be obtained in all patients because of their etiologic implications and to help interpret unexpectedly normal serum amylase and lipase levels. Elevated alanine aminotransferase (ALT) and alkaline phosphatase values suggest gallstone-associated pancreatitis (see below). The serum aspartate aminotransferase (AST) is elevated in approximately 50% of patients owing to alcoholic liver disease or to the pancreatic inflammation itself.

Imaging Tests. **Plain Films of the Abdomen.** These should be obtained routinely to rule out the presence of free air caused by perforation of a viscus and "thumbprinting" of the intestinal wall, suggesting mesenteric infarction. Changes caused by pancreatitis include localized ileus of a loop of jejunum ("sentinel loop"), generalized paralytic ileus, spasm of the transverse colon with absent colonic gas beyond ("colon cut-off sign"), and calcifications indicating the existence of underlying chronic pancreatitis.

Chest Radiographs. These frequently show pleural effusion and basilar atelectasis. Such findings indicate diaphragmatic involvement by acute pancreatitis but are not necessarily confined to the left side. Interstitial fluffy infiltrates are the hallmark of the adult respiratory distress syndrome (see below). Barium contrast studies of the upper gastrointestinal tract may show nonspecific abnormalities but are of little diagnostic value.

TABLE 107–2. ADDITIONAL CAUSES OF ELEVATIONS IN SERUM PANCREATIC ENZYMES

Levels may be similar to those in acute pancreatitis
  Chronic pancreatitis; pancreatic pseudocyst; carcinoma of the pancreas; perforation of stomach, duodenum, jejunum; mesenteric infarction.
Minor amylase and lipase elevations
  Acute cholecystitis; burn injury; end-stage renal disease; acute and chronic alcohol abuse.
Isolated amylase elevation
  Salivary adenitis; ovarian neoplasm; tubal pregnancy; metabolic acidosis; admission to an ICU; acute hepatitis; anorexia nervosa; upper gastrointestinal endoscopy; incidental finding.

TABLE 107–3. DIAGNOSIS OF ACUTE PANCREATITIS BY SERUM ENZYME ELEVATIONS IN PATIENTS WITH ACUTE ABDOMINAL PAIN

	Amylase	Lipase	Either	Both
Sensitivity	80–90%	90%	95%	—
Specificity	70%	70%	—	90%

Abdominal Ultrasonography (US) and Computed Tomography (CT) Scan. These two imaging modalities play important and complementary roles in diagnosing and managing acute pancreatitis. US is the method of choice for detecting cholelithiasis and for determining the diameter of the extrahepatic and intrahepatic bile ducts. Dilatation of these ducts suggests recent or persisting impaction of a stone in the distal common bile duct or the ampulla of Vater. US also very accurately detects acute cholecystis. The CT scan is the primary modality for assessing the extent and local complications of pancreatitis. It is far superior to US in this regard. The examination should be performed with rapid intravenous bolus injection of contrast material (dynamic CT scan). It reveals extension of peripancreatic inflammation, involvement of adjacent organs, venous thrombosis (splenic vein!), and fluid collections. Most important, pancreatic necrosis can be identified and quantitated by the lack of contrast enhancement following the bolus injection. The abdominal CT scan may be normal, however, in about 10% of patients with early, mild pancreatitis.

Differential Diagnosis. There is no single absolute criterion for the diagnosis of acute pancreatitis. The differential diagnosis should focus on other conditions presenting with acute upper abdominal pain which require specific therapy. These include perforated peptic ulcer, acute cholecystitis, and mesenteric vascular occlusion. A gallstone impacted in the ampulla of Vater may not only delay the resolution of biliary pancreatitis but also cause complicating ascending cholangitis and obstructive jaundice. The combination of positive US findings (gallstones or bile duct dilatation) with a positive biochemical score is indicative of this situation. A positive score consists of three or more of the following tests exceeding the stated limit: (1) alkaline phosphatase > ULN (upper limit of normal); (2) total bilirubin > ULN; (3) gamma glutamyltransferase > 2× ULN; (4) ALT > 1.5 × ULN; (5) ALT/AST > 1.0.

PROGNOSTIC ASSESSMENT. Several scoring systems exist which predict the morbidity and mortality of acute pancreatitis attacks (Table 107–4). These are based on clinical and laboratory observations obtained during the first 48 hours after admission to the hospital. Examples include the Ranson and the modified Glasgow

TABLE 107–4. ADVERSE PROGNOSTIC FACTORS IN ACUTE PANCREATITIS

Ranson's Criteria* Mainly Ethanol-Induced	Glasgow Criteria† All Causes

On Admission:
  Age > 55
  WBC > 16,000/cu mm
  Glucose > 200 mg/dl‡
  LDH > 350 IU/L
  AST > 250 IU/L
	Within 48 hours:
	  Age > 55
	  WBC > 15,000/cu mm
	  Glucose > 180 mg/dl‡
	  LDH > 600 IU/L
	  BUN > 45 mg/dl
	  Albumin < 3.2 gm/dl
	  Calcium < 8 mg/dl
	  Arterial PO$_2$ < 60 mmHg

Within 48 hours:
  Hematocrit decrease > 10%
  BUN rise > 5 mg/dl
  Calcium < 8 mg/dl
  Arterial PO$_2$ < 60 mmHg
  Base deficit > 4 mEq/L
  Fluid deficit > 6 L	

Three or more positive criteria predict a complicated clinical course; mortality rises when ≥4 criteria are met.
* Ranson JHC, Rifkind KM, Turner JW: Prognostic signs and nonoperative peritoneal lavage in acute pancreatitis. Surg Gynecol Obstet 143:209, 1976.
† Blamey SL, Imrie CW, O'Neill WH, et al.: Prognostic factors in acute pancreatitis. Gut 25:1340, 1984.
‡ No pre-existing hyperglycemia.
Abbreviations: LDH = lactic dehydrogenase; AST = aspartate aminotransferase; BUN = blood urea nitrogen.

criteria developed specifically for pancreatitis and the APACHE II (Acute Physiology and Chronic Health Evaluation) and SAPS (Simplified Acute Physiology) scores established for patients admitted to intensive care units (ICU's) are established for patients admitted to intensive care units (ICU's). These scoring systems are only 70 to 80% accurate in predicting a mild or a severe course. Their use cannot replace the careful observation of the individual patient. Recent reports indicate that elevations of serum C-reactive protein to > 120 mg per liter, and of polymorphonuclear elastase are accurate predictors for the development of pancreatic necrosis.

CLINICAL COURSE AND THERAPY. *Mild Pancreatitis.* Mild acute pancreatitis is defined by the absence of systemic and local complications. About 80% of patients belong to this category and require < 1 week of hospitalization. Treatment consists of general supportive care and close monitoring for signs of systemic complications; local complications tend to manifest during the second and third week of illness. There is no evidence that any medication is specifically beneficial. The intravascular volume deficit may exceed 30% due to peripancreatic fluid sequestration and vomiting. Volume restoration must be rapid and efficient in order to maintain regularly monitored urine output of > 40 ml per hour. The patient receives nothing by mouth, with the goal of resting the pancreas. Nasogastric aspiration is indicated in the presence of vomiting or developing ileus; it need not be initiated routinely. The patient should receive sufficient analgesic medications to alleviate pain. Meperidine HCl, 75 to 125 mg intramuscularly or intravenously, may be given every 3 to 4 hours. Neither total parenteral nutrition nor prophylactic antibiotic therapy is indicated. Small feedings of a high carbohydrate diet are begun once the pain has subsided and bowel sounds have reappeared.

Systemic Complications (Table 107–5). Most systemic complications occur during the first week of illness. They are treated by standard medical measures. Close patient monitoring is the key to their timely recognition. *Circulatory shock* arises by a combination of volume depletion and a hyperdynamic circulatory state with decreased peripheral vascular resistance. The management includes transfer to an ICU, volume replacement, and vasopressor substances. The occurrence of shock is frequently followed by pancreatic necrosis. *Acute renal failure* may be caused by circulatory shock and a selective increase in renal vascular resistance. The treatment is that of acute tubular necrosis arising in any setting (see Ch. 76). The leading cause of respiratory insufficiency during acute pancreatitis is the *adult respiratory distress syndrome* (ARDS), although respiratory depression caused by opiate medications, pleural effusions, intravascular volume overload, and shallow respirations due to abdominal "splinting" may contribute. The pathogenesis probably involves damage to the pulmonary surfactant layer by circulating phospholipase A and free fatty acids. *Sepsis* is most commonly caused by infection of the bile ducts, of areas of pancreatic necrosis, or of peripancreatic fluid collections (see below).

Local Complications. *Ascending cholangitis* and severe biliary pancreatitis present overlapping features and may coexist. Gram-negative bacteremia and spiking fevers are more common with infection of the biliary tract, whereas hyperbilirubinemia may be mild or absent in both situations. Appropriate antibiotic therapy should be instituted, e.g., gentamicin, ampicillin, and metronidazole (see Ch. 126). The main therapeutic objective is to clear the choledochus of gallstones without delay.

Pancreatic Necrosis. Pancreatic necrosis (PN) is found by dynamic CT scanning in approximately 80% of patients (16% of the total) with clinically severe disease, usually during the second or

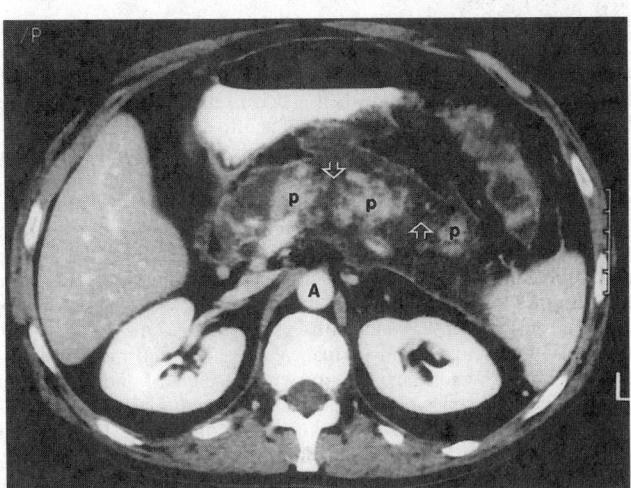

FIGURE 107–3. Dynamic CT scan of patient with pancreatic necrosis. Interposed between normally perfused portions of the pancreas (p) are nonperfused necrotic areas *(open arrows)*. The pancreas is surrounded by fluid in the retroperitoneum, which extends into the small bowel mesentery. A = Contrast-enhanced aorta. Failure of tissue enhancement during bolus injection with rapid scanning outlines areas of necrosis. (From Stewart ET: *In* Sleisenger MH, Fordtran JS [eds.]: Gastrointestinal Disease. 5th ed. Philadelphia, WB Saunders, 1993, p 1642.)

third week of illness (Fig. 107–3). PN, however, is present in approximately 40% of patients within 4 days of symptom onset. It follows that PN resolves without incident in nearly 60% of patients who develop it. Therapy and prognosis of the severely ill patient with PN depend crucially on the presence of necrotic tissue (Fig. 107–4). This question should be answered by fine-needle aspiration of necrotic areas under CT guidance before the patient leaves the CT suite. A Gram stain of the aspirate is > 95% accurate in predicting the final results of bacterial cultures. The bacteria represent enteric flora that gained access to mesenteric lymphatics by translocating across the colonic mucosa. Antibiotics with high penetration into pancreatic tissue include the fluoroquinolones, imipen/cilastatin, and metronidazole. The mortality of patients with *infected PN* treated conservatively is 60 to 100%. Immediately removing necrotic tissue (necrosectomy), combined with continued lavage of the necrotic space, lowers the mortality to about 20%. The patients frequently require re-operation for continuing necrosis and other local complications, such as bleeding and fistula formation. The management of patients with *sterile PN* remains controversial. Repeat CT scan with fine-needle aspiration reveals the later development of infection in 40% of these patients. The prognosis of the remainder is poor if shock had occurred at any time during the illness.

TABLE 107–5. COMPLICATIONS OF ACUTE PANCREATITIS

Systemic	Local
Circulatory shock	*Impacted common bile duct stones*
Respiratory insufficiency	Pancreatic necrosis ± *infection*
Acute renal failure	Fluid collections ± *infection*
Sepsis	*Pancreatic abscess*
Coagulopathy (DIC)	*Colonic necrosis*
Hyperglycemia	*Bleeding*
Hypocalcemia	Splenic vein thrombosis
	Splenic necrosis

Conditions in italics are life-threatening; they require prompt recognition and management.

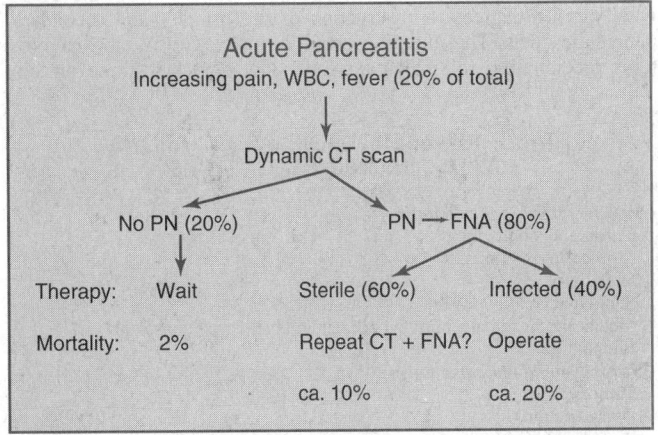

FIGURE 107–4. Management and prognosis of severe acute pancreatitis. PN = Pancreatic necrosis. FNA = fine-needle aspiration of necrotic areas under CT guidance with Gram stain and culture of aspirate.

Fluid Collections. These occur within or around the pancreas in up to 50% of patients with severe pancreatitis. The majority resolve spontaneously; collections that persist for >6 weeks develop a wall of granulation tissue and are then called pseudocysts (see "Chronic Pancreatitis"). Collections that continue to expand or become infected require drainage. *Pancreatic abscesses* contain liquid pus and may be considered to represent infected fluid collections. The presence of extraluminal gas bubbles on radiographs or CT films is a specific but rare clue to their presence. *Pancreatic ascites* reflects involvement of peritoneal surfaces by the inflammatory process and, rarely, the rupture of a pancreatic duct with pancreatic juice entering into the peritoneal cavity. There are several causes of *bleeding* during acute pancreatitis. Hemorrhage may occur into necrotic intrapancreatic and peripancreatic tissue and into fluid collections. Brisk hemorrhage occurs with erosion of the splenic or gastroduodenal arteries. At times, the blood gains access to a disrupted pancreatic duct and empties into the duodenum. Diffuse mucosal bleeding from antrum and duodenum is common but rarely severe. Finally, bleeding may signal perforation of peripancreatic inflammation into any portion of the gastrointestinal tract from esophagus to colon. The spleen may become involved by direct extension of the inflammatory process or, secondarily, by splenic vein thrombosis. The latter complication leads to gastric fundic varices.

PREVENTING RECURRENCES. The search for the precipitating cause begins during the acute attack. Serum calcium and triglyceride levels are determined and the medication list is reviewed for drugs listed in Table 107–1. An abdominal US examination is performed routinely. If gallstones are detected, the patient should undergo early cholecystectomy, preferably before discharge from the hospital. The absence of choledocholithiasis must be ascertained before or during this surgical procedure. At this stage, approximately 20% of patients are assumed to have idiopathic pancreatitis. ERCP with sphincter of Oddi manometry identifies correctable obstructive causes of the pancreatitis attack (see Table 107–1) in approximately one third of these patients. Bile aspirated from the common bile duct or the duodenum from the remaining patients should undergo microscopic analysis. Cholesterol crystals, Ca bilirubinate granules, or microspheroliths are present in up to 70% of these patients, and the majority develop biliary "sludge" or gallstones on serial US examinations. Treatment options include cholecystectomy, endoscopic papillotomy, or oral dissolution therapy with bile acids. This systematic search for obstructive causes of acute pancreatitis leaves only 5 to 10% of patients designated as having "idiopathic pancreatitis."

CHRONIC PANCREATITIS

DEFINITION AND PATHOGENESIS. Chronic pancreatitis is marked by progressive fibrosis, leading to loss of exocrine and endocrine (islets of Langerhans) tissue and irregular dilatation of pancreatic ductal structures. Episodes of acute pancreatitis may be interspersed, especially during the early years of alcoholic pancreatitis. There are two major categories of this disease (Table 107–6): *Chronic calcifying pancreatitis* is the most common form, by far. It is characterized by irregular distribution within the gland with varying degrees of obstruction of the primary and secondary pancreatic ducts. The initiating event is believed to be fibrillar proteins precipitating in small pancreatic duct branches; these protein

TABLE 107–6. ETIOLOGIC ASSOCIATIONS WITH CHRONIC PANCREATITIS

Chronic calcifying pancreatitis
  Chronic alcoholism
  Tropical pancreatitis
  Hereditary
  Senile/pancreatic atrophy
  Metabolic: hypercalcemia, hyperlipemia, post–renal transplant
  Idiopathic
Obstructive chronic pancreatitis
  Tumors
  Duct strictures
  Pancreas divisum(?)

Note: Hereditary isolated pancreatic enzyme deficiencies, congenital pancreatic insufficiency with neutropenia, and cystic fibrosis are separate nosologic entities.

plugs calcify by surface accretion. Later on, similar lamellar protein precipitates form in the major pancreatic duct which, subsequently, calcify as well. The plugs and concretions cause acinar atrophy, chronic inflammation with metaplasia of the ductal epithelium, periductal fibrosis, and irregular dilatation of major and secondary pancreatic ducts. The initiating event may be deficient acinar secretion of lithostathine (formally called pancreatic stone protein), a protein that inhibits calcium precipitation from the supersaturated pancreatic juice. Alternatively, lithostathine may undergo proteolytic cleavage that yields an insoluble residue, termed LH_1, that forms fibrillar precipitates and no longer keeps calcium in solution. Pancreatic citrate secretion may be reduced as well, resulting in reduced chelation of calcium. *Chronic obstructive pancreatitis* is caused by obstruction of the main pancreatic duct and leads to uniform dilatation of the duct system, rarely accompanied by protein plugs and intraductal calcifications.

ETIOLOGIC ASSOCIATIONS. *Alcohol.* Fully 70 to 80% of patients with chronic pancreatitis are chronic alcohol abusers. Alcoholic pancreatitis, even when it presents as an acute episode, is a chronic, progressive disease. Typically, the initial symptoms appear at ages 35 to 45, but some patients may experience their first attack before age 25. Alcoholic liver disease develops in 40 to 50% of patients and frequently becomes manifest 5 to 10 years after the onset of pancreatitis. Alcohol abstinence offers moderate and unpredictable benefits in terms of pain relief and the later development of diabetes mellitus but does not alter the progression of pancreatic fibrosis and exocrine insufficiency. The mechanism of alcohol-induced pancreatic injury remains unknown.

Tropical Pancreatitis. Calcific chronic pancreatitis occurs in children and young adults in certain tropical areas, including Southern India, Indonesia, and Central Africa. Although abdominal pain is common, the diagnosis is frequently made on the basis of newly discovered diabetes or pancreatic calcifications. Although malnutrition is suspected to play a role, this form of chronic pancreatitis is not found in other areas where malnutrition is equally common. There is no relationship to alcohol consumption.

Hereditary Pancreatitis. Pancreatitis can be inherited as an autosomal dominant trait with 40 to 80% penetrance; it accounts for approximately 2% of patients with chronic pancreatitis. Episodes of abdominal pain usually start at ages 10 to 12. An increased incidence of pancreatic adenocarcinoma has been observed in some affected families.

Senile Pancreatitis/Atrophy. Ten to 20% of patients with chronic pancreatitis are older than 60 at initial presentation. Pancreatic calcifications and malabsorption are common, but pain is commonly absent. Smoking and obesity, but not alcohol abuse, have been implicated. Senile atrophy and lipomatosis of the pancreas probably represent the same poorly understood entity. The clinical course is benign and generally nonprogressive.

Metabolic Causes. Chronic pancreatitis develops in up to 15% of patients with primary hyperparathyroidism and frequently is clinically silent. Hyperlipidemic conditions and renal transplantation have been reported as rare causes of chronic pancreatitis, but this has not been well documented.

Obstruction. Obstruction of the pancreatic duct by tumors, post-traumatic strictures, pancreatic duct calculi, or a "tight" minor papilla in patients with pancreas divisum may lead to chronic pancreatitis. The progression of the disease is halted when the obstructing lesion can be removed.

Idiopathic. The remaining 10 to 25% of patients are placed in the "idiopathic" category. They present the full spectrum of the disease, from mild functional disturbances to advanced calcific disease. Notably, gallstone-associated acute pancreatitis is not a cause of chronic pancreatitis.

CLINICAL PRESENTATION AND COURSE. Chronic pancreatitis initially presents with episodes that are indistinguishable from acute pancreatitis in approximately 40% of patients. Insidious onset of pain heralds the disease in another 40%, and the appearance of malabsorption, diabetes, or complications of chronic pancreatitis lead to the diagnosis in the remainder. Pain is minor or absent in 7 to 15% of patients during the course of the disease.

Pain. Pain is intermittent or chronic; it is boring and dull, often accompanied by nausea and vomiting. It is perceived in the epigastrium and/or the left and right subcostal areas and radiates straight through to the back in approximately one half of patients. Pain may be aggravated by eating and on the day after a drinking bout. Pancreatic pain fibers pass through the celiac plexus and the paravertebral sympathetic ganglia. Events that may trigger the pain of chronic pancreatitis are raised intraductal and pancreatic parenchymal pressure due to ductal obstruction and perineural inflammation with fibrosis. Pain is the predominant symptom of this disease; it may keep the patient from work, impair social and family relationships, and frustrate attempts at abstaining from alcohol. Spontaneous pain relief occurs in approximately 60% of patients, 6 to 9 years after the onset of symptoms. Pancreatic calcifications, diabetes mellitus, and malabsorption frequently appear when the patient's pain begins to diminish.

Weight Loss. Weight loss is common during the course of the disease. Contributing causes include anorexia caused by pain or using analgesics, funds being spent on alcohol rather than food, untreated diabetes, and malabsorption due to pancreatic exocrine insufficiency. Malabsorption develops in about 40% of patients, usually 5 to 10 years after the onset of pain. Most patients can compensate for weight loss due to malabsorption by increasing their food intake.

Diabetes Mellitus. Progressive loss of islets of Langerhans eventually leads to diabetes in 70% of patients, half of whom require insulin treatment. Patients with chronic pancreatitis and diabetes are at increased risk of hypoglycemia because of concomitant glucagon deficiency, poor dietary habits, and the hypoglycemic effects of alcohol.

Mortality. The 10-year survival is 65% in alcoholics and 80% in patients with nonalcoholic chronic pancreatitis. Only 10 to 20% of deaths are directly related to the disease. Major contributors to the excess mortality are extrapancreatic and pancreatic carcinoma, hypoglycemia, and the effects of alcoholism.

DIAGNOSIS. Imaging Studies. Plain anteroposterior and oblique views of the abdomen may reveal localized or diffuse calcifications of the pancreas. Abdominal CT scans may detect small calcifications missed on plain radiographs, dilatation of the main pancreatic duct, and pseudocysts. Differentiation from cancer of the pancreas may be difficult. Early in the course, ERCP may show blunting and dilatation of pancreatic duct branches, but the pancreatogram may be normal in up to 10% of patients. The main value of ERCP lies in its identifying potentially correctable lesions, such as large ductal stones, pseudocysts, and duct strictures.

Blood Tests. Serum amylase and lipase concentrations frequently remain normal during attacks of pain. Serum levels of pancreatic isoamylase and trypsin may be decreased, but these changes are not sufficiently reliable for the early diagnosis of chronic pancreatitis.

Pancreatic Function Tests. The so-called secretin test is the most sensitive test for chronic pancreatitis. Duodenal contents are aspirated after the intravenous administration of secretin $\pm$ cholecystokinin or cerulein. The calculated pancreatic output of bicarbonate and enzymes is decreased in approximately 85% of patients and the test accuracy is 87%. In the simpler Lundh test, trypsin concentration is determined in the proximal jejunum after a liquid test meal. Both tests are time-consuming, and neither is widely used.

Other Tests. The bentiromide (NBT-PABA) test assesses intestinal tryptic activity by quantitating the urinary excretion of *p*-amino benzoic acid following oral dosing with the test compound. This test, as well as determining stool chymotrypsin concentration, is reliably abnormal only with advanced pancreatic insufficiency. Vitamin B_{12} absorption may be impaired due to decreased liberation of this vitamin bound to gastric R-proteins by duodenal trypsin (see Ch. 103). An abnormal Schilling test of vitamin B_{12} (cobalamin) absorption that corrects with administration of pancreatic enzymes is a specific, but not a sensitive, test for chronic pancreatitis. Clinical vitamin B_{12} deficiency develops rarely.

Sequence of Tests. Diagnosing chronic pancreatitis rests on symptoms, tests of pancreatic function, and radiologic studies, including ERCP. In general, the documentation of any two of these three manifestations is sufficient for making the diagnosis. An example is the presence of pancreatic calcifications on a plain film of the abdomen in a patient with chronic upper abdominal pain. An abdominal CT scan frequently provides additional information regarding the presence and possible complications of chronic pancreatitis. Two diagnostic dilemmas generally require expert consultation: (1) to rule out early, mild chronic pancreatitis. Because neither the duodenal secretin test nor the ERCP examination is 100% sensitive, both invasive tests may have to be performed; (2) to differentiate chronic pancreatitis from adenocarcinoma or a cystic tumor of the pancreas. When imaging methods and cytologically examining percutaneously obtained aspirates from a pancreatic mass fail to provide the answer, surgical exploration and resection may be required. The diagnostic approach to the patient presenting with steatorrhea is described in Ch. 103.

THERAPY. Pain. Controlling abdominal pain is the most important and difficult task in treating chronic pancreatitis. Narcotics are frequently required and should not be withheld because of concerns about evolving addiction and concomitant alcoholism. Acute attacks of pain require hospitalization with no oral intake, parenteral analgesics, and renewed efforts at achieving abstinence from alcohol. The rationale for a trial of administering pancreatic enzymes is the inhibition of cholecystokinin release by intraduodenal trypsin, leading to decreased meal-stimulated pancreatic secretion. Conventional preparations of pancrelipase should be used, such as Viokase, Cotazyme, or Ilozyme, at doses of 6 tablets per meal. Concomitant suppression of gastric acid secretion with an H_2-receptor blocker is advisable to minimize the destruction of the enzyme supplement at low gastric pH. Pain relief has been reported in some patients with mild idiopathic pancreatitis—that is, without pancreatic calcifications or steatorrhea. Ongoing studies are exploring the possibility that suppressing pancreatic secretion by octreotide (Sandostatin), an analogue of somatostatin, may provide pain relief. Percutaneous destruction of the celiac plexus by alcohol or phenol injection reduces pain in approximately 60% of patients, but the effect is transient and the procedure has potential complications.

Patients with intractable chronic or intermittent pain should be considered for a surgical procedure based on ERCP and CT evaluation of the duct system. When the pancreatic duct is dilated to ≥ 8 mm in diameter, decompression may be attempted by endoscopically placing a stent across the ampulla of Vater. Most patients, however, require permanent duct decompression by longitudinal pancreaticojejunostomy. In the absence of a dilated pancreatic duct, partial pancreatectomy can be performed, such as pancreaticoduodenectomy (Whipple procedure), when severe changes are confined to the head of the pancreas. When expertly performed and limited to patients who abstain from alcohol, these operations relieve pain in approximately 70% of patients.

Malabsorption. Malabsorption is a late manifestation of chronic pancreatitis and occurs when pancreatic secretion of digestive enzymes is reduced by $\geq 90\%$. Fat malabsorption due to lipase deficiency is the predominant abnormality. The condition is documented by a stool fat content > 7 grams per day (steatorrhea). The indication for treatment is weight loss that cannot be corrected by increasing the caloric intake. Reducing or eliminating steatorrhea is difficult to achieve due to the low potency of available porcine pancreatic extracts and their irreversible denaturation at gastric pH values of < 4. Enzymes can be taken as described above. Alternatively, enteric-coated enzyme preparations such as Pancrease or Creon, which are released only in the alkaline milieu of the duodenum, can be prescribed in doses of two to three capsules per meal.

COMPLICATIONS. Pseudocysts. Pancreatic pseudocysts contain high concentrations of pancreatic enzymes and are encapsulated by a rim of chronic inflammation and fibrosis; they are without an epithelial lining. Pseudocysts may represent fluid collections that developed during acute pancreatitis but failed to resolve over a period of 6 to 8 weeks. More commonly, they result from obstruction of small pancreatic ducts, a type of retention cyst formed during the course of chronic pancreatitis. Pseudocysts are located within or around the pancreas, but may dissect retroperitoneally to the mediastinum or pelvis; pseudocysts in the head of the pancreas may compress the common bile duct. They can be diagnosed by abdominal US, CT, or endoscopic US, but their differentiation from rare uniloculated pancreatic cystic neoplasms is difficult. One or more pseudocysts appear in up to 60% of patients with chronic pancreatitis. Life-threatening but rare complications include infection, hemorrhage into the cystic space, and rupture of the pseudocyst. The contribution of a pseudocyst to the pain of chronic pancreatitis is difficult to assess. Treatment should be considered for large pseudocysts (> 5 cm in diameter). While surgical excision is rarely possible, internal drainage into stomach, duodenum, or jejunum shows excellent results. Successful treatment by percutaneous or endoscopic aspiration and drainage for several weeks has also been reported.

Pancreatic Ascites. Ascites and pleural effusions during the course of chronic pancreatitis are the result of leakage from a disrupted pancreatic duct. The amylase and lipase content is many times higher than in the blood. The majority of these patients require surgical correction of the leak by providing drainage into a loop of jejunum or by partial pancreatectomy.

Obstruction of Adjacent Organs. Several structures adjacent to the pancreas may become obstructed by fibrosis or a developing pseudocyst. *Common bile duct obstruction* with slowly developing jaundice requires a biliary-enteric drainage procedure to prevent the development of secondary biliary cirrhosis and ascending cholangitis. *Gastric outlet obstruction* can be bypassed by a gastrojejunostomy; a vagotomy should be added because the incidence of duodenal ulcer is increased in chronic pancreatitis. *Compression or thrombosis of the splenic vein* leads to gastric fundic varices that may bleed. Splenectomy is curative.

Bradley EL III: A clinically based classification system for acute pancreatitis. Arch Surg 128:586, 1993. *This international consensus statement describes the terms currently used for the diagnosis and complications of acute pancreatitis.*

Lebenthal E, Rolston DDK, Holsclaw DS Jr: Enzyme therapy for pancreatic insufficiency: Present status and future needs. Pancreas 9:1, 1994. *A review of pancreatic enzyme substitution therapy of malabsorption caused by pancreatic exocrine insufficiency.*

Lee SP, Nicholls JF, Park HZ: Biliary sludge as a cause of acute pancreatitis. N Engl J Med 326:589, 1992. *This important paper documents that many patients with "idiopathic" acute pancreatitis are forming small gallstones and should, therefore, be considered to have biliary pancreatitis.*

Steer ML, Waxman I, Freedman S: Chronic pancreatitis. N Engl J Med 332:1482, 1995. *Documents chronic pancreatitis and its control: pathology and pathogenesis, natural and medical history, the physical examination, laboratory and function tests, imaging, and differential diagnosis and treatment. 108 references.*

Wilson C, Heath DI, Imrie CW: Prediction of outcome in acute pancreatitis: A comparative study of APACHE II, clinical assessment and multiple factor scoring systems. Br J Surg 77:1260, 1990. *A critical comparison of several scoring systems proposed to predict the course of acute pancreatitis.*

108 CARCINOMA OF THE PANCREAS

Eugene P. DiMagno

DEFINITION. Ductal adenocarcinoma, compromising 90% of pancreatic cancers, is a relentlessly progressive and fatal disease. Most tumors are moderately well-differentiated mucinous carcinomas arising from the cuboid epithelium of pancreatic ducts. The remaining 10% of pancreatic cancers are endocrine tumors (see Ch. 206); acinar cell, giant cell, and epidermoid cancers; adenocanthomas; sarcomas; and cystadenocarcinomas.

INCIDENCE AND EPIDEMIOLOGY. In the past generation, the incidence of pancreatic cancer has increased from < 5 to between 11 and 12 per 100,000 population. Currently, pancreatic cancer kills more Americans than any other neoplasm except breast, colorectal, lung, and prostate cancers. Each year approximately 27,000 Americans develop pancreatic cancer and 25,000 die. Median survival after diagnosis is 4 to 8 months. Overall 5-year survival is < 1%. Resecting the tumor improves median survival to 17 to 20 months, but 5-year survival remains < 10%.

Pancreatic cancer is associated with certain demographic characteristics and risk factors (Table 108–1). Pancreatic cancer occurs more frequently in men (1.5 : 1). Eighty per cent occur between ages 60 and 80; the disease is unusual under age 40. Patients with chronic pancreatitis and members of families with the nonpolyposis colon cancer syndrome are at increased risk. Those with chronic pancreatitis have more than a ninefold risk of developing pancreatic cancer, and the cumulative risk increases 2% per decade and is independent of gender, nationality, and type of pancreatitis. Major environmental factors are associated with an increased risk of pancreatic cancer (Table 108–1), but it is unlikely that coffee consumption, alcohol abuse, diabetes mellitus, previous cholecys-

TABLE 108–1. RISK FACTORS FOR PANCREATIC CANCER

Definite
   Age > 60
   Male sex
   Cigarette smoking
   Chronic pancreatitis
   Nonpolyposis colon cancer syndrome
Probable
   High cholesterol and fat diet with high linoleic acid content
   Chemical exposure (coal tar derivative, coke, benzidine, β-naphthylamine)
Unlikely
   Diabetes mellitus
   Coffee
   Alcohol
   Prior cholecystectomy, gastrectomy

tectomy, or gastrectomy increases the risk. Eliminating cigarette smoking and eating a diet low in cholesterol with olive oil and fish as the main sources of fat may reduce the risk.

The most common molecular abnormalities in human cancer, including pancreatic cancer, are deletions and mutations that occur in many codons of the p53 gene. Gene mutations result in loss of function, failure of inactivation, and intranuclear accumulation of the p53 protein. A high proportion of pancreatic cancers also have mutations in the codon 12 of the k-*ras* gene, which is likely involved in cancer growth. EGF and *erb* B-2 receptor pathways also are altered and may have a role in pathogenesis of pancreatic cancer.

PATHOPHYSIOLOGY AND CLINICAL MANIFESTATIONS. In pancreatic ductal adenocarcinoma, well-differentiated to poorly differentiated duct glands are embedded in a dense network of fibrous tissue. As it extends in the pancreas and surrounding tissue, the tumor envelopes and fixes vessels and invades fat, lymph channels, and perineural areas. Symptoms and signs of pancreatic cancer are related to the location of the tumor within the gland and to the extension of the tumor to stomach, duodenum, bile duct, retroperitoneum, and porta hepatis. The presenting symptoms are nonspecific and consist of pain, jaundice, weight loss, and, rarely, diabetes mellitus.

Pain occurs in 90% of patients. It may be vague and rather nonspecific and may occur up to 3 months before the onset of jaundice. Early in the course the pain may be ignored by both the patient and the examining physician. The tumor most commonly extends to the retroperitoneal space, producing visceral pain variously described as persistent, disagreeable, aching, increased by lying supine or by eating, and causing the patient to waken at night. Relief is sometimes obtained by bending forward, lying on the side and drawing the knees to the chest or chin, and sometimes by crouching forward on all four extremities.

Jaundice secondary to obstruction of the common bile duct occurs early in the course of the disease in 60 to 70% of carcinomas of the head of the pancreas. When carcinomas of the head of the pancreas arise in its central part or in the uncinate process, jaundice is not an early presentation. In cancer of the body and tail, jaundice presents late and occurs secondary to hepatic metastases or obstruction of the bile duct at the porta hepatis by lymphadenopathy. Painless jaundice does not occur.

Weight loss of > 10% of ideal body weight, almost universal, is usually due to both malabsorption and decreased food intake. Seventy-five per cent of patients malabsorb fat and 50% malabsorb protein. Malabsorption occurs in patients who have a carcinoma of the head of the pancreas that obstructs the pancreatic duct, thereby producing pancreatic exocrine insufficiency (see Ch. 103).

Glucose intolerance due to increased plasma levels of islet amyloid polypeptide (IAPP) producing insulin resistance may be present in up to 80% of patients with pancreatic cancer, but in most patients diabetes is mild. Less than 5% of patients have hyperphagia, polydipsia, and polyuria.

Other symptoms and signs include *depression, light-colored stools* (60% of patients with carcinoma of the pancreatic head), *constipation,* and *emotional lability* (27% of patients with carcinoma of the pancreatic tail). *Vomiting* and *weakness* occur in one third of patients. More rarely patients exhibit superficial thrombophlebitis (Trousseau's syndrome) or gastrointestinal bleeding due either to direct extension of the tumor into the stomach or duodenum or to varices secondary to splenic vein obstruction.

Rarely, metastases from pancreatic cancer of the body and tail to the testicles, temporal bone, or esophagus may cause testicular enlargement and pain, sudden profound hearing loss, or dysphasia, respectively.

Hepatomegaly and *jaundice* are present in 80 and 30% of patients with carcinoma of the head and body and tail, respectively. A palpable gallbladder (Courvoisier's sign) is present in 30% of patients with carcinoma of the head of the pancreas. An abdominal mass or ascites is present in <20% of patients. Ascites, splenomegaly, and peripheral edema may occur secondary to occlusion of the portal vein by tumors, whereas compression of the aorta or splenic artery may produce an abdominal bruit.

DIAGNOSIS. After identifying patients suspected of having the disease based on their symptoms, a routine battery of tests is performed that include chemistry and hematology groups, chest and abdominal roentgenograms, and serum and urine pancreatic enzymes. As a group, patients with pancreatic cancer have higher values for serum lipase, amylase, and glucose than do other patients, but these tests do not distinguish between pancreatic cancer and pancreatitis. Similarly, serum alkaline phosphatase, aspartate aminotransferase, and bilirubin are commonly elevated, but these tests lack specificity to exclude hepatic disorders. Nonspecific findings on the chest radiograph and abdominal films may be present in patients with pancreatitis or pancreatic cancer. Pancreatic calcifications have a sensitivity of 95% for diagnosing chronic pancreatitis, but primary ductal carcinomas, mucosal pancreatic cancers such as a mucinous cystadenocarcinoma (curvilinear calcification), and solid and papillary epithelial neoplasms can calcify. If obvious pulmonary or bony metastases are found, one may opt not to perform further diagnostic tests.

If the diagnosis of pancreatitis is not apparent and no metastases are seen, a computed tomography (CT) scan is done. This test is usually the only additional test needed to make the diagnosis and to stage the tumor. Other tests that may be needed are ultrasonography (US) or endoscopic retrograde cholangiopancreatography (Table 108–2). Rarely is it necessary to perform an invasive pancreatic function test, in which either secretin or cholecystokinin is administered intravenously and pancreatic secretion is obtained through a tube placed into the duodenum. Patients with pancreatic cancer have low volume but normal bicarbonate concentration after secretin or reduced enzyme outputs after cholecystokinin. If the cancer is deemed resectable, laparoscopy or endoscopic US should be considered to determine if there is peritoneal seeding, small liver metastases, vascular invasion, and lymph node metastases.

New tests that have appeared in the last 5 to 10 years are magnetic resonance imaging (MRI), positron emission tomography (PET), and endoscopic US. The role of these tests in the diagnosis of pancreatic cancer is evolving. MRI may be as accurate as CT but is not widely used. The accuracy of PET is not known, and of all the tests it is the least available. Availability of endoscopic US is increasing, and it may be as useful to stage tumors preoperatively as is laparoscopy. Laparoscopy correctly identifies 85% of unresectable tumors. The accuracy of endoscopic US for T staging is 92% and 74% for N staging. Compared with US, CT, and angiography, endoscopic US is more sensitive for detecting portal vein involvement and lymph node metastasis. Aspiration cytology of the pancreatic mass with US or CT guidance is 90% sensitive but should not be performed unless the cancer is clearly unresectable because the procedure may cause intra-abdominal seeding of tumor cells.

TABLE 108–2. DIAGNOSTIC ACCURACY (IN %) OF IMAGING TESTS IN DIAGNOSIS OF PANCREATIC CANCER

	Sensitivity	Specificity	Predictive Value Positive	Predictive Value Negative
Ultrasonography	74	84	78	79
Computed tomography	79	64	76	78
Endoscopic retrograde cholangiopancreatography	95	90	87	97

TABLE 108–3. DIFFERENTIAL DIAGNOSIS OF PANCREATIC CANCER

Benign conditions
Chronic pancreatitis
Extrahepatic jaundice
  Common bile duct stones
  Bile duct stricture (secondary to previous biliary tract surgery or sclerosing cholangitis)
  Cholecystitis
Intrahepatic cholestatic jaundice
  Alcoholic hepatitis
  Toxins
  Cysts
  Abscess
Posterior penetrating duodenal or gastric ulcers
Depression
Functional bowel disorders
Malignant conditions
Retroperitoneal lymphomas
Bile duct cancer
Ampullary cancer
Gynecologic malignancies
Carcinoma of the duodenum or small intestine

No sensitive serologic marker (see Ch. 158.2) with tumor and organ specificity has been established as a routine diagnostic or screening test for pancreatic cancer. Currently available serologic tests include carcinoembryonic antigen (CEA), galactosyltransferase, monoclonal antibodies CA 19-9, CA-50, and DU-PAN-2, pancreatic oncofetal antigen, and pancreatic cancer–associated antigen. These tests have ranged in sensitivity from 50 to 85%, but positive tests occur in up to 46% of patients with benign diseases and in up to 65% of those with other malignancies.

DIFFERENTIAL DIAGNOSIS (Table 108–3). The presenting symptoms and signs of pancreatic cancer are nonspecific. Indeed, most patients presenting with weight loss and abdominal pain, with or without jaundice, do not have pancreatic cancer. In patients without jaundice, the abdominal pain and weight loss of pancreatic cancer may be difficult to distinguish from extensive list of disorders (Table 108–3). In jaundiced patients it is extremely important to differentiate pancreatic cancer from potentially treatable benign conditions, such as chronic pancreatitis obstructing the common bile duct and causes of extrahepatic and intrahepatic cholestasis (Table 108–3).

TREATMENT. Only *surgical resection* of pancreatic cancer offers any chance of cure. Unfortunately, only 10% of all pancreatic cancers are resectable and the 5-year survival after resection is only 10%. In Japan, however, resected tumors ≤2 cm in diameter were associated with a 37% 5-year survival. Pancreaticoduodenectomy is the surgical procedure of choice. In experienced hands, surgical mortality is 2 to 5%. Other surgical procedures such as total pancreatectomy and regional pancreatectomy are not commonly performed because of higher operative mortality and morbidity and 5-year survival rates that do not exceed those of pancreaticoduodenectomy. The pylorus-preserving pancreaticoduodenal resection is performed in patients with cancer of the lower duodenum or ampulla, but not for cancer of the pancreas, because the surgical margins may include pancreatic cancer.

Palliative procedures are performed to relieve symptoms of biliary obstruction, duodenal obstruction, or both. To relieve biliary obstruction, cholecystojejunostomy is the surgical procedure of choice, unless the cystic duct enters the common duct close to the tumor. In this case, choledochojejunostomy should be performed. To decompress the biliary tree, endoscopic stenting is preferable to percutaneous stenting. It is as successful as surgical decompression and may have lower morbidity, but jaundice is more likely to recur late in the disease. Thus, a stent should be placed endoscopically if the patient has a high surgical risk or a short life expectancy (1 to 3 months). In contrast, double bypass surgery should be performed if an unresectable tumor is found at the time of surgery or if the patient has a life expectancy of 6 to 7 months, because complete duodenal obstruction occurs in 5 to 15% of patients—usually as a preterminal event. Incomplete or functional obstruction occurs in 40 to 60% of patients. In such patients, a combination of a cholinergic (bethanechol, 25 mg three times a day) and a prokinetic agent (metaclopramide or cisapride, 10 mg four times a day) may alleviate symptoms of gastric stasis by enhancing gastric emptying.

No single agent or combination of *chemotherapeutic drugs* prolongs or enhances the quality of life. 5-Fluorouracil (5-FU) produces a partial response rate in 10 to 15% of patients, but its use is associated with a median survival of <20 weeks. Other agents have a similar effect (mitomycin-C), less effect (streptozotocin, doxorubicin, Epirubicin, ifosfamide, methyl-CCNU, and high-dose methotrexate), or no effect (actinomycin D, doxorubicin, BCNU, standard-dose methotrexate, cisplatin, melphalan, and L-asparaginase).

The combination of 5-FU or SMF (streptozotocin, mitomycin-C, and 5-FU) and external-beam radiation improves survival compared with radiation or chemotherapy alone. Intraoperative electron beam radiation and ^{125}I implants do not improve survival compared with external beam radiation. Even though these modalities may limit local tumor extension, they do not control liver and peritoneal metastases.

Pain can usually be successfully managed if analgesics are prescribed on a regular basis, adequate doses are used, and adjuvant drugs are used when necessary. Mild to moderate pain can be controlled with aspirin, acetaminophen, and nonsteroidal anti-inflammatory agents. If these drugs fail to relieve pain, opioid analgesics should be used (codeine or morphine). Adding an antihistamine or an amphetamine to an opiate increases analgesia. Intraoperative or percutaneous neurolytic celiac plexus block is remarkably effective in controlling pain. If patients have intolerable pain, subcutaneous patient-controlled analgesia or epidurally administered narcotics afford pain relief.

Malabsorption can be reasonably well controlled by ingesting 8 tablets of pancreatin with meals (total dose of lipase should be 30,000 IU). Two tablets should be taken immediately after eating a few bites, two tablets at the end of the meal, and four tablets interspersed during the meal (see Ch. 103).

DiMagno EP: Pancreatic adenocarcinoma. *In* Yamada T (ed.): Textbook of Gastroenterology. Philadelphia, JB Lippincott, 1991, p 1893. *A general overview of pancreatic cancer that includes over 170 references.*

Gullo L, Pezzilli R, Morselli-Labate AM: Diabetes and the risk of pancreatic cancer. Italian Pancreatic Cancer Study Group. N Engl J Med 331:81, 1994. *Diabetes is not a risk factor for pancreatic cancer; it is caused by the tumor.*

Korc M, Chandrasekar B, Yamanaka Y, et al.: Overexpression of the epidermal growth factor receptor in human pancreatic cancer is associated with concomitant increases in the levels of epidermal growth and transforming growth factor alpha. J Clin Invest 90:1352, 1992. *Possible molecular bases for pancreatic cancer.*

Lowenfels AB, Maisonneuve P, Cavillini G, et al., and the International Pancreatitis Study Group. Pancreatitis and the risk of pancreatic cancer. N Engl J Med 328:1433, 1993. *Definite evidence that there is an increased risk of pancreatic cancer in persons with chronic pancreatitis.*

Permert J, Larsson J, Westermark GT, et al.: Islet amyloid polypeptide in patients with pancreatic cancer and diabetes. N Engl J Med 330:313, 1994. *Plasma islet amyloid concentrations are elevated in pancreatic cancer, the likely cause of insulin resistance and diabetes.*

Riela A, Zinsmeister AR, Melton LJ, et al.: Increasing incidence of pancreatic cancer among women in Olmsted County, Minnesota, 1940 through 1988. Mayo Clin Proc 67:839, 1992. *Documentation of increasing incidence of pancreatic cancer, particularly in women.*

Rösch T, Braig C, Gain T, et al.: Staging of pancreatic and ampullary carcinoma by endoscopic ultrasonography. Comparison with conventional sonography, computed tomography, and angiography. Gastroenterology 102:188, 1992. *A staging strategy for pancreatic cancer.*

Warshaw AL, Gu Z, Wittenberg J, et al.: Preoperative staging and assessment of resectability of pancreatic cancer. Arch Surg 125:230, 1990. *Another staging strategy for pancreatic cancer.*

109 FOOD POISONING
Martin F. Heyworth

Food poisoning falls into three categories: (1) infections or parasitic infestations acquired by eating food contaminated with infectious microorganisms or parasites; (2) clinical problems that result from eating food contaminated with toxins; (3) clinical sequelae from eating inherently poisonous animals, plants, or mushrooms. Some overlap occurs between these different categories.

FOOD-BORNE MICROORGANISMS AND PARASITES

Bacteria (Table 109–1)

STAPHYLOCOCCUS AUREUS. Staphylococcal food poisoning is caused by eating food containing one or more heat-stable polypeptide enterotoxins of *S. aureus*. Food is contaminated by *S. aureus* when food is prepared nonhygienically by individuals who are carriers of this organism (cutaneous or nasal). Subsequent growth of *S. aureus* in the food (and enterotoxin production) occurs if the food is not cooked at a temperature sufficient to kill the bacteria or is not refrigerated. Staphylococcal food poisoning is manifested as nausea, vomiting, abdominal cramps, and diarrhea 2 to 6 hours after eating food contaminated by enterotoxin.

CLOSTRIDIUM SPECIES. Two species of *Clostridium* cause food poisoning, i.e., *C. perfringens* and *C. botulinum*. *C. perfringens* type A is a common cause of food poisoning in the United States and Europe. Food-borne botulism (see Ch. 288) is caused by eating food that contains *C. botulinum* toxin.

C. perfringens type A is ubiquitous. Food poisoning occurs after ingesting food that is heavily contaminated with vegetative forms of the bacterium. These organisms develop from *C. perfringens* spores contaminating the food; refrigeration inhibits their proliferation. After the contaminated food has been ingested, *C. perfringens* organisms sporulate in the small intestinal lumen. The bacterial cells then lyse, releasing spores and enterotoxin, a protein responsible for the symptoms of this type of food poisoning. These symptoms include diarrhea and abdominal cramps and occur 8 to 24 hours after contaminated food has been eaten. This condition is rarely fatal, although it has caused death among elderly, debilitated individuals.

SALMONELLA SPECIES (see Ch. 293). Nontyphoidal *Salmonella* serotypes (particularly *S. enteritidis* and *S. typhimurium*) are major causes of food poisoning. Clinical features of *Salmonella* food poisoning result from the causative bacteria proliferating in the intestine of affected individuals. The clinical picture is characterized by diarrhea, nausea, vomiting, abdominal cramps, fever, headache, and myalgia. These symptoms begin 12 to 48 hours after eating incriminated food and last for up to several days in otherwise healthy individuals. The mortality in such individuals is low, but hospital admission for rehydration is sometimes necessary. Nontyphoidal *Salmonella* infections are hazardous in infants, elderly persons, and immunodeficient patients. Prevention of foodborne *Salmonella* infections depends on hygienically preparing food, adequate cooking, and refrigerating cooked food.

Recent food-borne outbreaks of typhoid and paratyphoid fever (see Ch. 292) have occurred in the United States and Britain.

VIBRIO SPECIES. Three *Vibrio* species are mainly implicated as causes of food poisoning, i.e., *V. cholerae, V. parahaemolyticus,* and *V. vulnificus*.

V. cholerae, the cause of cholera (see Ch. 296), has traditionally been spread by water. In recent years, food-borne cholera caused by *V. cholerae* O1, El Tor biotype, has become increasingly frequent. Responsible foods include raw or incompletely cooked seafood. Non–O1 *V. cholerae* causes a disease that is usually milder than that caused by *V. cholerae* O1. Raw oysters are a source for non–O1 *V. cholerae* infection.

V. parahaemolyticus infection is a worldwide hazard of eating uncooked seafood. It is a halophilic bacterium that lives in sea water and is concentrated by oysters.

V. vulnificus is another halophilic organism that lives in sea water. Food-borne *V. vulnificus* infection is a devastating disease with a mortality rate that approaches 100%. The typical clinical presentation is an abrupt onset of fever and chills, 24 to 48 hours after eating raw seafood (usually oysters). These features of primary septicemia are rapidly followed by the development of a bullous hemorrhagic rash, hypotension, renal failure, and death in most instances. Nearly all the reported patients with this infection have had an underlying chronic condition (including cirrhosis, hemochromatosis, and/or diabetes mellitus).

LISTERIA MONOCYTOGENES (see Ch. 304). This gram-positive bacillus is transmitted in contaminated food—including raw meat, poultry, and milk. Several groups of individuals have an increased risk of developing this infection, including pregnant women, neonates, elderly persons, diabetics, and immunocompromised individuals.

TABLE 109-1. BACTERIAL CAUSES OF FOOD POISONING

Organism	Major Food Source(s)	Pathophysiologic Mechanism		Comments
		Toxin in Food	Ingestion of Bacteria	
Staphylococcus aureus	Cooked meat, cheese, pasta, cream buns, custard pies	Yes	No	
Clostridium perfringens type A	Cooked meat, vegetable soup (prepared in bulk)	No	Yes (bacteria release enterotoxin in intestine)	
Clostridium botulinum	Uneviscerated cured fish, preserved or fermented meat, home-preserved vegetables	Yes	No	Highest U.S. prevalence in Alaska
Salmonella enteritidis/ Salmonella typhimurium	Raw eggs, mayonnaise, incompletely cooked meat and poultry	No	Yes	
Salmonella dublin	Raw milk, unpasteurized cheese	No	Yes	
Salmonella typhi/ Salmonella paratyphi	Food contamination by infected food handlers	No	Yes	
Vibrio cholerae O1	Raw seafood	No	Yes	
Vibrio cholerae non-O1	Raw oysters	No	Yes	
Vibrio parahaemolyticus	Raw seafood	No	Yes	
Vibrio vulnificus	Raw seafood (especially oysters)	No	Yes	See text for predisposing conditions
Listeria monocytogenes	Soft cheese	No	Yes	See text for predisposing factors
Shigella species	Food contamination during preparation	No	Yes	
Escherichia coli O157:H7	Ground beef	No	Yes	
Campylobacter jejuni/ Campylobacter coli	Incompletely cooked poultry and other meats, raw milk	No	Yes	
Bacillus cereus				
Heat-stable toxin	Fried rice	Yes	No	
Enterotoxin	Meat products	Yes	No	
Yersinia enterocolitica	Pork, raw milk	No	Yes	

SHIGELLA SPECIES (see Ch. 294). *Shigella* infections are spread by the fecal-oral route and occur mainly in crowded, unhygienic conditions. Food-borne outbreaks of shigellosis have been linked to lack of hand-washing by food handlers.

ESCHERICHIA COLI (see Ch. 297). *E. coli* O157:H7 is an important food-borne pathogen; this organism causes hemorrhagic colitis, which is complicated by the hemolytic uremic syndrome (HUS) in up to 10% of cases. Most of the documented cases of *E. coli* O157:H7 infection have occurred from eating incompletely cooked hamburgers made from ground beef contaminated with the organism. This bacterium is pathogenic in individuals of any age; young children and the elderly are at highest risk of death from the infection. Uncomplicated infection with *E. coli* O157:H7 is characterized by diarrhea (frequently with blood in the stools), abdominal cramps, fever, and vomiting. Clinical features of HUS include hemolytic anemia, thrombocytopenia, and acute renal failure; this syndrome can be fatal.

CAMPYLOBACTER SPECIES (see Ch. 295). *C. jejuni* infection is acquired by eating incompletely cooked poultry and other meat and by drinking raw milk. The clinical picture is characterized by a febrile prodrome (with headache and vomiting), abdominal pain, and bloody diarrhea. Food-borne *C. jejuni* infection is preventable by thoroughly cooking food. *C. coli* is spread similarly to *C. jejuni* and produces an essentially identical clinical picture.

BACILLUS CEREUS. Two distinct food-poisoning syndromes are caused by this organism. In one, attributable to a heat-stable toxin, nausea and vomiting occur approximately 6 hours after eating toxin-contaminated food. The other type of *B. cereus*–induced food poisoning is caused by consuming food that is contaminated with a heat-labile enterotoxin. In this type of food poisoning, diarrhea occurs approximately 12 hours after eating toxin-containing food. Both of these syndromes result from initial contamination of food by *B. cereus* spores, subsequent growth of *B. cereus* in the food, and toxin produced by the organism. Growth of *B. cereus* in food can usually be inhibited by refrigeration, although some strains of the organism can grow slowly at 4°C.

YERSINIA ENTEROCOLITICA. Meat that has been incompletely cooked (especially pork) and milk are vehicles for food-borne *Y. enterocolitica* infection. The organism causes diarrhea (with or without fecal blood), fever, vomiting, and mesenteric adenitis, which is characterized by pain in the right lower abdomen. *Y. enterocolitica* in food or milk is killed by cooking or pasteurization, respectively.

Viruses

Raw shellfish (clams and oysters) are a well-documented vehicle of food-borne Norwalk virus (see Ch. 344) and hepatitis A virus infections. Shellfish are contaminated with these viruses in sewage-polluted sea water. Viruses in shellfish are killed by cooking.

Protozoan Parasites

Food is not a major vehicle for transmitting protozoan parasite infections. However, cysts of *Giardia intestinalis* (*G. lamblia*) have been detected on salads and fruit, and food-borne outbreaks of giardiasis have been described.

Helminth Parasites (see Ch. 373)

Many species of helminth parasites can be transmitted via uncooked food, including *Taenia* species tapeworms (raw pork or beef), *Diphyllobothrium latum* (raw fish), *Trichinella spiralis* (raw pork), and flukes, such as *Fasciola hepatica* (watercress).

Immature nematode worms of the species *Anisakis simplex*, which cause acute gastric anisakiasis, are transmitted to humans by eating raw fish. After raw infested fish is eaten, these worms emerge in the human gastric lumen and then burrow into the gastric (or occasionally intestinal) mucosa, causing sudden, severe abdominal pain. This pain characteristically occurs 1 to 12 hours after consuming the infested fish. Upper gastrointestinal endoscopy can be used to visualize the worm partially embedded in the gastric mucosa, and treatment consists of removing the worm with transendoscopic biopsy forceps. *A. simplex* in fish is killed by cooking or freezing.

Baird-Parker AC: Foodborne salmonellosis. Lancet 336:1231, 1990. *A concise review that covers the clinical features, sources, and prevention of food-borne* Salmonella *infections.*

Bean NH, Griffin PM, Goulding JS, et al.: Foodborne disease outbreaks, 5-year summary, 1983–1987. Centers for Disease Control. CDC Surveillance Summaries, March 1990. MMWR 39, No. SS-1:15, 1990. *Summarizes information about outbreaks of food poisoning reported to the United States Centers for Disease Control during 1983 to 1987. The frequency and food source(s) of each type of food poisoning are documented.*

Fang G, Araujo V, Guerrant RL: Enteric infections associated with exposure to animals or animal products. Infect Dis Clin North Am 5:681, 1991. *Surveys food-borne intestinal infections and parasitic infestations from milk, fish, shellfish, eggs, and meat.*

Koenig KL, Mueller J, Rose T: *Vibrio vulnificus*—Hazard on the half shell. West J Med 155:400, 1991. *The epidemiology, pathophysiology, clinical features, and management of* Vibrio vulnificus *infection.*

Labbé RG: *Clostridium perfringens.* J Assoc Official Analytical Chemists 74:711, 1991.

A concise review of the epidemiology, clinical features, diagnosis, and prevention of Clostridium perfringens*–induced food poisoning.*

Tranter HS: Foodborne staphylococcal illness. Lancet 336:1044, 1990. *Focuses on the epidemiology of* Staphylococcus aureus*–induced food poisoning and on the biologic effects of* S. aureus *enterotoxins.*

POISONING BY FOOD-BORNE TOXINS (also see Ch. 391)

AMNESIC SHELLFISH POISONING (ASP). So far, only one outbreak of this condition has been described. It occurred in 1987, in people who had eaten mussels collected on the east coast of Canada. These mussels had accumulated a diatom, *Nitzschia pungens,* which contains domoic acid (a nonphysiologic neurotransmitter that was responsible for ASP). Affected individuals developed gastrointestinal and neurologic symptoms, including vomiting, abdominal cramps, diarrhea, severe headache, confusion, disorientation, and persistent or permanent loss of short-term memory.

MYCOTOXINS. Mycotoxins are defined as toxins produced by fungi that grow on foods or on animal feeds. Ergot alkaloids are mycotoxins produced by *Claviceps purpurea,* a fungus that contaminates cereal grains. In humans, ingesting ergot alkaloids causes arterial spasm and thrombosis, with consequent ischemic necrosis of the extremities. Aflatoxins are mycotoxins produced by *Aspergillus flavus,* a fungus that can grow on cereal grains, legumes, nuts, and dried figs. The possibility that aflatoxins cause human hepatocellular carcinoma remains unproven.

ANTHROPOGENIC TOXINS. Methylmercury contamination of seafood caused serious food-borne neurologic disease in Japan during the 1950's and 1960's (Minamata disease). Contamination of cooking oils with polychlorinated biphenyls and with an aniline-like substance has caused multisystem disease and deaths in East Asia and Spain, respectively. Food poisoning has been caused by contamination of foods with the insecticides aldicarb (a cholinesterase inhibitor) and endrin (a chlorinated hydrocarbon, now banned from agricultural use in the United States).

POISONOUS ANIMALS, PLANTS, AND MUSHROOMS

POISONOUS PLANTS. Red kidney beans (*Phaseolus vulgaris*) contain hemagglutinin, a lectin that is removed and inactivated by soaking and boiling the beans in water. If these beans are eaten raw or after insufficient cooking, symptoms of hemagglutinin poisoning can occur (nausea, vomiting, and diarrhea).

Neurolathyrism is a chronic condition that results from eating the seeds of the grass pea, *Lathyrus sativus,* for a long time. Features of this condition include a spastic gait, urgency and frequency of micturition, and spastic paraplegia. Neurolathyrism is widespread in Asia and occurs in the Middle East and southern Europe. It appears to be caused by a toxic amino acid in *L. sativus* seeds, β-N-oxalyl-amino-L-alanine.

Pyrrolizidine alkaloids are present in plants of the genera *Senecio* and *Crotalaria,* which are used for making herbal infusions in various parts of the world. Because of these alkaloids, people drinking such infusions can develop hepatic veno-occlusive disease (see Ch. 118).

POISONOUS MUSHROOMS. It has been estimated that approximately 80 species of mushroom that grow in the United States can cause serious poisoning. Around 95% of the deaths from mushroom poisoning in the United States are due to a single species, *Amanita phalloides.* This lethal fungus contains cyclic octapeptides (amatoxins), which include α-amanitin, an inhibitor of RNA polymerase II. Amatoxins are not inactivated by cooking. The clinical picture of *A. phalloides* poisoning is characterized by vomiting and watery diarrhea (approximately 8 hours after eating the mushroom), followed by apparent improvement and then by hepatocellular necrosis, acute liver failure, and death in most instances. Liver transplantation is the only therapeutic option in most people with *A. phalloides* poisoning and has greatly increased the chances of survival.

Huxtable RJ: The harmful potential of herbal and other plant products. Drug Safety 5 (Suppl 1):126, 1990. *Focuses on hazards of ingesting herbal products, with particular reference to plants that contain pyrrolizidine alkaloids.*

Morgan MRA, Fenwick GR: Natural foodborne toxicants. Lancet 336:1492, 1990. *Reviews food-borne toxins that are present in plants, fish, and shellfish. This article includes a concise discussion of mycotoxins.*

Pinson CW, Daya MR, Benner KG, et al.: Liver transplantation for severe *Amanita phalloides* mushroom poisoning. Am J Surg 159:493, 1990. *Discusses the clinical course of patients with* Amanita phalloides *poisoning who were treated by liver transplantation.*

110 DISEASES OF THE RECTUM AND ANUS
Theodore R. Schrock

ANATOMY

The rectum and anus fuse over a zone several centimeters long, and together these structures are termed the "anorectum" (Fig. 110–1). The distal anal canal is lined by modified skin (anoderm), the epithelium of the upper anal canal is columnar, and the transitional zone (cuboidal epithelium) lies between the two. The anoderm is exquisitely sensitive, but the upper anal canal is relatively insensitive.

At the dentate line, an important site of pathologic problems, anal papillae project into the lumen. Flaps of skin connecting anal papillae are termed anal valves; behind these valves lie anal crypts, each containing in its depths an anal gland.

The internal anal sphincter is the thickened lower portion of the circular smooth muscle layer of the gut. This involuntary muscle is encircled by skeletal muscle bundles comprising the external sphincters. The levators ani form the muscular floor of the pelvis. One of the levators, the puborectalis, passes around the rectum as a sling and is easily palpable posteriorly on digital rectal examination.

EXAMINATION OF THE ANORECTUM

The anorectum is examined with the patient in the left lateral decubitus position or in the prone jackknife position, if a special table is available for that purpose. Good lighting is essential. The buttocks are retracted to expose the anal orifice. Digital rectal examination is performed. Anoscopy is required to thoroughly evaluate the anal canal. Rigid or flexible sigmoidoscopy completes the examination in some patients, but others (e.g., those with bleeding) need colonoscopy or a barium enema.

HEMORRHOIDS

Hemorrhoids are masses of areolar tissue containing numerous small arteries and veins. These congenital vascular cushions are located above the dentate line and are termed "internal hemorrhoids." External hemorrhoids are dilated vessels below the dentate line; they rarely cause symptoms by themselves, but they are enlarged in association with prolapsing internal hemorrhoids.

Intrarectal pressure pushes hemorrhoids downward, the anchoring fibromuscular structures attenuate, and the tissues congest, bleed, and eventually prolapse. Small hemorrhoids that protrude a short distance into the anal canal are first-degree hemorrhoids. Second-degree hemorrhoids prolapse but reduce spontaneously. Third-degree hemorrhoids must be manually reduced, and fourth-degree hemorrhoids are irreducible. Internal hemorrhoids occur in three primary locations: right posterior, right anterior, and left lateral.

Bleeding and *prolapse* are the most common symptoms of internal hemorrhoids. Blood is typically bright red, and it may spurt or drip from the anus. Nonspecific discomfort is noted, but pain is usually caused by some other associated condition such as fissure or abscess.

Anoscopy reveals a mass of tissue above the dentate line; large hemorrhoids prolapse to the outside as the anoscope is withdrawn. Differential diagnosis includes skin tags, hypertrophied anal papillae, and rectal prolapse.

Acute prolapse and thrombosis of internal hemorrhoids are severely painful. The entire circumference of the anus appears to protrude, and there is extreme pain from the edema and inflammation.

Initial treatment of internal hemorrhoids involves a high-bulk diet and avoiding prolonged sitting at stool. Proprietary remedies have little benefit. Small bleeding hemorrhoids can be treated by a "fixation procedure" that promotes adherence of the vascular cushions to the underlying sphincter. These outpatient procedures require no anesthetic. One popular method is injecting a sclerosing agent (e.g., 5% phenol in oil) into the submucosa of the hemorrhoid above the

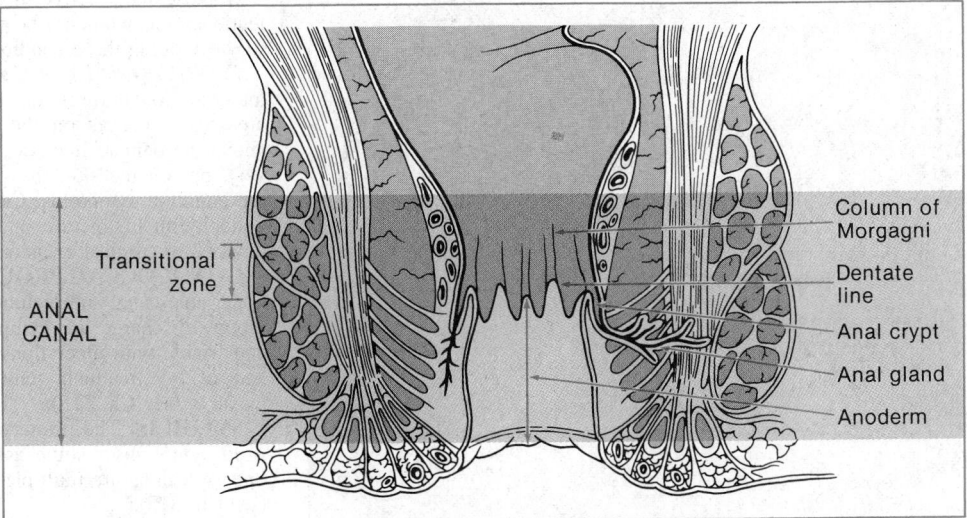

FIGURE 110–1. The lining of the anal canal. (Redrawn from Goldberg SM, Gordon PH, Nivatvongs S: Essentials of Anorectal Surgery. Philadelphia, JB Lippincott, 1980. Used by permission.)

dentate line. This painless injection evokes fibrosis and eventual adherence of the sliding mucosa. Another method is rubber band ligation, in which tiny bands are slipped over each internal hemorrhoid using a special instrument. The banded tissue sloughs and fixation results. Photocoagulation using an infrared device is also effective. Lasers can be used for the same purpose, but they are more expensive and more hazardous. Electrocoagulation with a bipolar electrode or a direct current device and thermocoagulation with a "heater probe" are alternatives. All of these procedures have the same objective, and they are similarly effective.

Fourth-degree hemorrhoids with large external components do not respond to fixation procedures, and if the symptoms warrant, hemorrhoidectomy is advised. Surgical excision can be performed in an outpatient setting. Results are good, although the operation is painful, and there is loss of time from work. Complications are uncommon and recurrences are unusual.

Thrombosed external hemorrhoid is a blood clot within a complex of subcutaneous external veins. This problem develops in young adults, often related to heavy exercise. A painful bluish mass is present at the anal verge. If pain does not subside after 48 hours, the thrombosed hemorrhoid can be excised under local anesthesia.

ANAL FISSURE

Anal fissure (fissure in ano, anal ulcer) is a tear in the anoderm just inside the anal verge. Acute fissures are common, but in some patients the tiny laceration does not heal and it becomes chronic. Severe pain with defecation and spots of blood on the toilet tissue are the symptoms.

The diagnosis is made by inspection. Pain is so severe that the patient may not tolerate digital rectal examination. Lateral traction on the buttocks exposes the fissure in nearly every instance. Acute fissures are red, but chronic fissures may have eroded completely through the anoderm to expose the white fibers of the internal sphincter in the base. The fissure triad seen in chronic lesions includes the fissure, an edematous sentinel tag at the anal verge, and a hypertrophied anal papilla at the dentate line.

Fissures are located in the posterior midline in 98% of men and 90% of women. The remaining fissures are in the anterior midline. A fissure off the midline should raise a suspicion of cancer, Crohn's disease, or a sexually transmitted infection.

Measures to improve bulk and softness of stools are important, and sitz baths are soothing. Acute fissures usually heal. Chronic fissures may require lateral subcutaneous internal anal sphincterotomy. This simple procedure reduces pressure in the anal canal and allows the fissure to heal. The long-term cure rate is >95%.

ANORECTAL ABSCESS

Infections arising in anal glands at the dentate line may develop into abscesses in the adjacent tissue spaces (Fig. 110–2). Abscesses near the skin surface cause throbbing pain that is worse with walking. Deeper abscesses may produce insidious symptoms including abdominal pain. Patients with large abscesses are febrile. An indurated tender mass is apparent on examination in a patient with a perianal or ischiorectal abscess, and the anus is pushed to one side. Intersphincteric abscesses are invisible on the outside, but they are palpable as a firm, tender area on digital rectal examination. Supralevator abscesses are also palpable.

Prompt surgical incision and drainage are required. A neglected abscess may extend, and necrotizing infections can be lethal. Abscesses in immunocompromised patients pose special problems, and standard treatment may not be appropriate.

ANORECTAL FISTULAS

A hollow fibrous tract lined by granulation tissue develops after an anorectal abscess is spontaneously or surgically drained. The primary orifice is usually at the dentate line where the infection originated. The secondary orifice is most often external at the site of drainage. The patient has pus, blood, mucus, and discomfort. One or more reddish papules on the perianal skin mark the sites of secondary openings. Gentle pressure may produce a drop of pus from the orifice. A firm tract may be palpated with a well-lubricated finger as it travels from the secondary orifice toward the anal verge.

Anoscopy reveals the primary opening; a hooked probe confirms

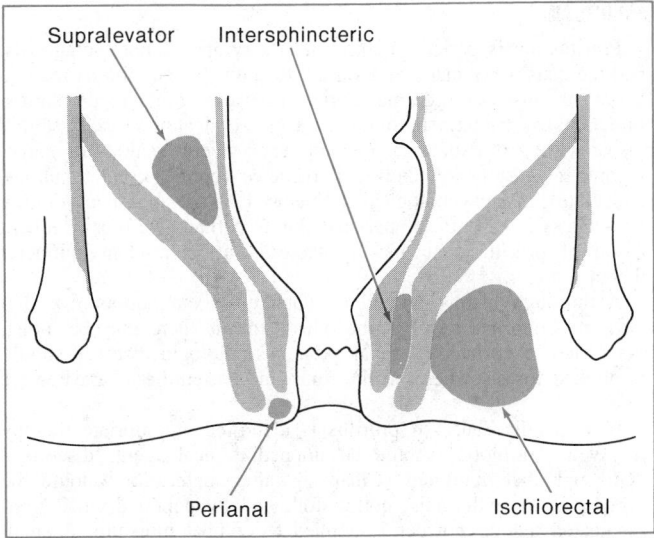

FIGURE 110–2. Classification of anorectal abscesses. (Redrawn from Gordon PH: Management of anorectal abscesses and fistulous disease. *In* Kodner IJ, Fry RD, Roe JP [eds.]: Colon, Rectal and Anal Surgery. St. Louis, CV Mosby, 1986.)

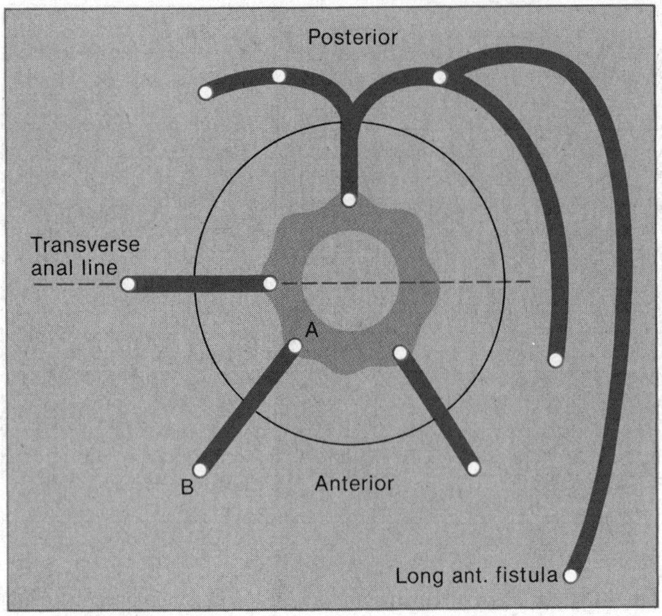

FIGURE 110-3. Goodsall's rule indicates the usual relationship of primary (A) and secondary (B) fistula orifices. The long anterior fistula is an exception to the rule. (Redrawn from Schrock TR: *In* Fromm D [ed.]: Gastrointestinal Surgery. New York, Churchill Livingstone, 1985. Used by permission.)

its patency. At times it is difficult to identify the primary orifice. Goodsall's rule describes the usual relationship of primary and secondary fistula orifices (Fig. 110-3). Crohn's disease, carcinoma, tuberculosis, and chlamydial infections should be considered in the differential diagnosis. Proctosigmoidoscopy is done routinely, and barium studies or even colonoscopy may be indicated in some cases.

Fistulas do not heal spontaneously, and operation is required (fistulotomy). The tissue overlying the tract is incised and the base is curetted. The defect heals secondarily. High fistulas encompass important sphincters and require special techniques.

Rectovaginal fistulas most commonly result from childbirth injuries. Fecal incontinence may be associated. The patient complains of passage of flatus and occasionally feces through the vagina. Surgical repair is usually successful.

PRURITUS ANI

Pruritus ani is perianal itching. It is a symptom, not a diagnosis, and the causes are many and varied. Responsible conditions include anorectal diseases, dermatologic diseases, contact dermatitis, infections by bacteria or fungi, parasites, oral antibiotics, systemic diseases (e.g., diabetes), poor or excessively zealous hygiene, warmth and moisture, dietary intolerance (coffee, cola, tomatoes, chocolate), and psychological problems. Leakage of mucus or tiny amounts of stool onto the perianal skin is perhaps the most frequent cause of pruritus, and usually there is no significant sphincter defect.

A thorough history should be obtained. Examination may disclose no abnormality, or at the other extreme there may be moist, macerated, excoriated perianal skin. Dermatologic diseases should be looked for elsewhere on the trunk and extremities. Parasites are rare.

If a specific cause of pruritus is identified, appropriate therapy is given. Antibiotics should be stopped, topical agents discontinued, and diet modified. Cleansing after defecation should be accomplished with moist cotton followed by gentle drying. Nonmedicated talcum powder is applied to combat moisture. A small bit of cotton applied to the anal verge may absorb excess moisture. More severe cases may require application of corticosteroid creams.

SEXUALLY TRANSMITTED DISEASES

Homosexually active men have a high incidence of anorectal infections, and women who practice anal intercourse also are at risk for developing these conditions.

CONDYLOMATA ACUMINATA. These are warts caused by human papillomaviruses, usually types 6 and 11. They are small, discrete excrescences on the perianal skin, on the anoderm, or just above the dentate line. In the latter location they are pink and velvety, but on the skin they are pearly white. Pruritus and bleeding are common symptoms. Condylomata are treated by applying 25% podophyllin in tincture of benzoin, fulguration with electrocautery devices, or surgical excision.

GONOCOCCAL PROCTITIS. This involves the mucosa of the upper anal canal and rectum. Pain, frequent defecation, and purulent bloody discharge are symptoms. The rectal mucosa is edematous and friable with ulcerations and thick pus. Cultures confirm the diagnosis but treatment may be warranted even if the cultures are negative (see Ch. 315).

SYPHILIS. The primary lesion of anorectal syphilis is an ulcer. Mild symptoms resolve as the lesion heals in a few weeks. Secondary lesions are multiple plaques with a white odorous discharge (see Ch. 318).

CHLAMYDIA TRACHOMATIS PROCTITIS. *Chlamydia trachomatis* is the most common sexually transmitted bacterial pathogen in the United States today (see Ch. 323). Three immunotypes of this organism cause lymphogranuloma venereum, which resembles Crohn's disease. Tetracycline is the treatment of choice after culture confirms the organism.

DISORDERS OF THE PELVIC FLOOR

Disorders of the pelvic floor are a group of conditions arising from abnormal structure or function of the levators ani and anal sphincters.

FECAL INCONTINENCE. Fecal incontinence has many causes (Table 110-1). Partial incontinence is occasional loss of flatus or loose stool, and major incontinence is abnormal control of stool of normal consistency. Thorough history should be obtained. The anus may be deformed and gaping, and an obvious anatomic defect may be visible and palpable. In other instances the structures seem intact but function is inadequate. Special investigations include anorectal manometry and electromyography.

The underlying systemic intestinal disorder, if any, should be treated. Loose stools are managed with bulk agents and constipating drugs. Elderly patients who soil because of fecal impaction may need regular laxatives and/or enemas. Biofeedback may improve

TABLE 110-1. CAUSES OF FECAL INCONTINENCE

Normal sphincters and pelvic floor
  Diarrhea
  Fistula
Abnormal function of sphincters and/or pelvic floor
  Minor incontinence
    Deficient internal sphincter
      Trauma
      Rectal prolapse
      Third-degree hemorrhoids
    Fecal impaction
      Advanced age
      Neurologic disorders
    Minor external sphincter and pelvic floor denervation
  Major incontinence
    Congenital anomalies
    Trauma
    Complete rectal prolapse
    Rectal carcinoma
    Anorectal infection
    Idiopathic
    Drug intoxication
    Neurologic
    Upper motor neuron
      Cerebral
      Spinal
    Lower motor neuron

Modified from Henry MM, Swash M (eds.): Coloproctology and the Pelvic Floor. Pathophysiology and Management. Boston, Butterworths, 1985.

patients with organic neuromuscular impairment. Surgical repair is successful for traumatically disrupted sphincters.

SOLITARY RECTAL ULCER SYNDROME. Solitary rectal ulcer syndrome is a chronic, benign condition characterized by anal pain, bleeding, mucous discharge, and obsessive straining to defecate. It affects mainly young women. Excessive straining forces the anterior rectal mucosa downward where it becomes traumatized.

On examination the anterior rectal mucosa 8 to 10 cm above the anal verge is indurated and may be grossly ulcerated. Biopsies confirm the diagnosis. Treatment should be directed toward avoiding straining by educating the patient and using bulk agents. Unfortunately, current methods of therapy are often disappointing, and patients must live with the chronic condition. Surgical repairs are unsatisfactory unless the patient has a true rectal prolapse.

DESCENDING PERINEUM SYNDROME. Some patients, mostly parous women, complain of a sense of incomplete evacuation and a constant desire to defecate. They are, in effect, attempting to evacuate their own rectal mucosa. The diagnosis is made if the patient strains and the plane of the perineum balloons downward below a line connecting the ischial tuberosities. Education, bulk agents, and occasionally local surgical procedures are helpful.

RECTAL PROLAPSE. Partial prolapse is protrusion of the mucosa alone, and complete rectal prolapse (procidentia) is protrusion of the entire thickness of the rectum. Prolapse is much more common in women than in men, and it appears with increasing frequency after age 40. Surgical or other traumatic injuries are causative in a few patients, but laxity of the pelvic musculature as a result of aging or neurologic disease is more commonly responsible.

With the patient sitting on the edge of the examining table or, even better, on a toilet seat, straining produces the prolapse. Mucosal prolapse is a small symmetric projection 2 to 4 cm long with radial folds. True procidentia may protrude as much as 12 cm from the anus, and the mucosal folds are concentric. Palpation reveals a large mass of tissue anteriorly. Proctosigmoidoscopy and barium enema are required.

Procidentia must be repaired surgically to avoid further weakening of the anal sphincters. Repairs can be accomplished abdominally or through the perineum, depending on the circumstances. Mucosal prolapse is managed by fixation procedures or excision, as described for hemorrhoids.

MALIGNANT TUMORS OF THE ANUS

Epidermoid carcinomas of the anus are uncommon (2% of cancers of the large bowel). Human papillomavirus is etiologically linked to anal cancer. Anal carcinoma may extend directly into the sphincters, perianal tissues, vagina, or prostate, and it tends to metastasize to lymph nodes behind the rectum and in the groins. Bleeding, pain, and a mass are the usual complaints. Often symptoms are mistakenly attributed to hemorrhoids until examination reveals the lesion. Biopsy provides proof. A combination of radiation therapy and chemotherapy is the first line of treatment, and it is followed by local or radical surgical excision if the tumor is not controlled. Overall 5-year survival rates of 60% are expected.

Bowen's disease is chronic squamous cell carcinoma *in situ.* Local excision is required to prevent progression to invasive cancer. Extramammary *Paget's disease* is an intraepithelial mucinous adenocarcinoma. It is treated by wide local excision. It tends to recur locally and can metastasize.

Gordon PH, Nivatvongs S: Principles and Practice of Surgery for the Colon, Rectum, and Anus. St. Louis, Quality Medical Publishing, 1991. *A beautifully illustrated, concise, authoritative textbook on the full range of topics in the field.*

Henry MM, Swash M: Coloproctology and the Pelvic Floor. Oxford, Butterworth Heinemann, 1992. *This recently updated monograph is the latest word on the subject. The importance of the pelvic floor in the pathogenesis of anorectal disease is emphasized.*

Schrock TR: Hemorrhoids: Nonoperative and interventional management. *In* Barkin J, O'Phelan CA (eds.): Advanced Therapeutic Endoscopy. New York, Raven Press, 1991, p 91. *Management of hemorrhoids is discussed in detail.*

Schrock TR: Examination of anorectum and diseases of anorectum. *In* Sleisenger MH, Fordtran JS (eds.): Gastrointestinal Disease: Pathophysiology/Diagnosis/Management. 5th ed. Philadelphia, WB Saunders, 1993, p 1494. *Details of the examination of the anorectum are described.*

111 DISEASES OF THE PERITONEUM, MESENTERY, AND OMENTUM

Michael R. Lucey

PERITONEAL DISORDERS

Abdominal pain and ascites are characteristic clinical features in disorders of the peritoneum.

Ascites

Ascites, the accumulation of serous fluid in the peritoneal cavity, has many causes (Table 111–1). More than 90% of cases of ascites are due to portal hypertension, usually as a result of cirrhosis (see Ch. 122). Perhaps half of the remainder, i.e., 5% of all cases of ascites, are due to peritoneal disease.

CLINICAL FEATURES OF ASCITES. Increasing abdominal girth and rapid weight gain are the most common symptoms associ-

TABLE 111–1. CAUSES OF ASCITES

Causes of Ascites	Comments
Portal hypertension	
Cirrhosis	Accounts for 80% of ascites in United States
Fulminant hepatic failure	Rarely causes ascites
Hepatic outflow obstruction	Ascites is a characteristic clinical feature of hepatic outflow obstruction
Congestive heart failure	
Constrictive/restrictive cardiomyopathy	
Budd-Chiari syndrome—hepatic vein and/or IVC occlusion	Most commonly associated with underlying thrombotic disorder
Veno-occlusive disease	Important cause of ascites in bone marrow transplant recipients
Portal vein occlusion	Rarely causes ascites
Malignancy	Accounts for 10% of ascites in United States. Peritoneal carcinomatosis causes 50% of malignant ascites.
Infection	
Peritoneal tuberculosis	See Tables 111–6 and 111–7
Fitz-Hugh–Curtis syndrome	Perihepatitis associated with fibrous perihepatic exudate usually due to *Neisseria gonorrhoeae* or *Chlamydia trachomatis*
Infectious peritonitis in HIV infected patients	
Renal	
Nephrotic syndrome	Covert cirrhosis should be excluded
Nephrogenous in hemodialysis recipients	Covert cirrhosis should be excluded
Endocrine	
Myxedema	
Meig's syndrome	
Struma ovarii	
Ovarian overstimulation syndrome	
Pancreatic ascites	Associated with pancreatitis, raised ascitic amylase concentration
Biliary leak	Previous surgery, including laparoscopic cholecystectomy, gangrenous gallbladder, trauma, percutaneous liver biopsy
Urine ascites	Urinary leak into peritoneum
Systemic lupus erythematosus	
Miscellaneous	Idiopathic chronic nonspecific peritonitis in HIV-infected patients
Mixed causes	See text.

ated with new-onset ascites. Dullness in the flanks when the patient is supine, shifting dullness during percussion of the abdomen, and a fluid wave are useful clinical signs to detect ascites. Small volumes of ascites (< 1500 ml) are often clinically undetectable. Older clinical signs such as the "puddle sign" are of no value. When it is clinically important to confirm the presence of suspected ascites, sonography or computed tomography (CT) scanning of the abdomen is advisable.

Investigating new-onset ascites which is unexplained by standard clinical examination and tests should always include paracentesis (Table 111–2). Ascitic fluid can be examined for biochemical content and cytology and sent for culture. In specific cases, such as suspected tubercular peritonitis, biopsy of the peritoneum during laparoscopy is valuable (see below).

The mechanism of ascites formation in portal hypertension is complex (see Ch. 122), including such factors as altered Starling forces in the portal circulation (increased portal venous hydrostatic pressure, reduced portal venous oncotic pressure), altered renal sodium handling, increased hepatic and possibly splanchnic lymph formation. Portal oncotic pressure is reduced in cirrhotic patients because of hypoalbuminemia, which in turn is due to hepatic synthetic failure. In contrast, obstructed outflow of normal lymphatics appears to be a principal causative factor in the development of ascites due to peritoneal carcinomatosis or malignant chylous ascites.

In the past, portal hypertensive ascites was distinguished from other forms of ascites by determining whether the ascitic fluid was a transudate or an exudate. This concept assumes that in portal hypertension, protein-poor ascitic fluid *transudes* from the normal peritoneal surface, whereas in peritoneal disease, such as peritoneal inflammation or malignancy, protein-rich ascitic fluid *exudes* from the abnormal peritoneal surface. Consequently, ascitic fluid with a protein content of ≥ 2.5 grams per deciliter is designated an exudate and fluid with a protein content of < 2.5 grams per deciliter is a transudate. More recently, it has been shown that the transudate-exudate characterization is flawed when applied to a large series of ascitic samples. This is because many samples from patients with spontaneous bacterial peritonitis, in which ascitic fluid is infected, nonetheless have low ascitic fluid protein rather than the expected high protein content (see below), and many samples of ascites due

to portal hypertension secondary to cardiac failure have a high protein content rather than the expected low protein.

An alternative method to distinguish ascites associated with portal hypertension from other forms of ascites is the serum-ascites albumin gradient. This is calculated by subtracting ascitic albumin concentration from serum albumin concentration. Ascites associated with portal hypertension has a serum-ascites albumin gradient of > 1.1 grams per deciliter, whereas ascites due to peritoneal inflammation or malignancy has a serum-ascites albumin gradient of < 1.1 grams per deciliter (Table 111–3). Many patients have more than one potential cause of ascites—so-called mixed ascites. An example would be a patient with cirrhosis and peritoneal tuberculosis. The serum-ascites albumin gradient usually reflects the presence of portal hypertension even when concomitant causes of nonportal hypertensive ascites are present.

A particular value of recognizing portal hypertension as a cause of ascites is that medical management using diuretics and salt restriction is often effective in portal hypertensive patients. Conversely, ascites due to peritoneal inflammation or malignancy alone does not respond to salt restriction and diuretics.

MALIGNANT ASCITES. Malignant ascites constitutes a small fraction of all cases of ascites and represents a heterogeneous group of disorders and mechanisms of ascites formation. Peritoneal carcinomatosis, the most common form of malignant ascites, arises from primary peritoneal disease such as mesothelioma or from the metastatic spread of a wide variety of malignant processes (Table 111–4). On occasion, in addition to malignant studding of the peritoneum, the primary tumor produces massive hepatic metastases sufficient to cause portal hypertension. Whenever ascites is due to malignant infiltration of the peritoneum, either alone or accompanied by massive hepatic metastases, shedding of malignant cells into the ascites is almost invariable (see Table 111–2). In contrast, massive hepatic metastases without peritoneal studding or multilocular primary hepatocellular carcinoma arising in a cirrhotic liver rarely causes shedding of malignant cells into the ascitic fluid. Thus, cytology of the ascitic fluid in extremely valuable when attempting to identify peritoneal malignancy. Mesothelioma is an exception to this rule because it produces cytologic results that are often difficult to interpret.

The serum-ascites albumin gradient in malignant ascites reflects the presence or absence of portal hypertension. Therefore, the

TABLE 111–2. DIAGNOSTIC TESTS IN ASCITES

	Diagnosis	Ascitic White Blood Cell Count (per mm³)	Ascitic Red Blood Cell Count	Cytology (% Positive Neoplastic Cells)	Biochemical Analysis	Serum-Ascites Albumin Gradient (g/dl)	Comments
Portal hypertension	Cirrhosis	<250 PMN*	Few or none	0	Protein usually <2.5 g/dl	>1.1	—
	SBP	>250 PMN	Few or none	0	Albumin <1 g/dl	>1.1	—
	Cardiac ascites	<250 PMN	Few or none	0	Protein >2.5 g/dl	>1.1	—
Malignancy	Peritoneal carcinomatosis	75% have >500	Few or none	100	Protein usually >2.5 g/dl	<1.1	—
	Massive hepatic metastases (MHM)	Usually <500	Few or none	0	Protein variable	>1.1	Serum alkaline phosphatase ≥350 mU/ml
	Peritoneal carcinomatosis plus MHM	Variable, usually elevated	Few or none	~80	Protein content variable	>1.1	Serum alkaline phosphatase ≥350 mU/ml
	Malignant chylous ascites	Often >300	Few or none	0	Triglycerides >200 mg/dl	Usually <1.1	—
	Hepatoma plus ascites	Often >500	Commonly increased	0		>1.1	Elevated serum α-fetoprotein
Infection	Tuberculous peritonitis	80% >500 predominantly lymphocytes	Frequently present	0	Ascitic adenosine deaminase ≥32.3 U/L	50% have >1.1 (i.e., many have cirrhosis)	See Table 111–7
Miscellaneous	Pancreatic ascites	Frequently increased		0	Ascitic amylase greatly increased	Variable	—

* PMN = Polymorphonuclear leukocytes.

TABLE 111-3. CLASSIFICATIONS OF ASCITES BY SERUM-ASCITES ALBUMIN CONCENTRATION GRADIENT

High Gradient (>1.1 g/dl)	Low Gradient (<1.1 g/dl)
Cirrhosis	Peritoneal carcinomatosis
Alcoholic hepatitis	TB peritonitis (without cirrhosis)
Congestive/restrictive heart failure	Pancreatic ascites (without cirrhosis)
Massive hepatic metastases	Bile leak
Fulminant hepatic failure	Nephrotic syndrome
Budd-Chiari syndrome	Systemic lupus erythematosus
Veno-occlusive disease	Bowel obstruction or infarction
Portal vein occlusion	
Acute fatty liver of pregnancy	
Myxedema	

serum-ascites gradient is low in patients with peritoneal carcinomatosis with normal portal pressure, whereas ascites associated with massive hepatic metastases irrespective of peritoneal studding or primary hepatocellular carcinoma arising in a cirrhotic liver are associated with a serum-ascites albumin gradient are >1.1 grams per deciliter, reflecting the presence of portal hypertension (see Tables 111–2 and 111–3). The underlying cause of malignant ascites is determined after a thorough clinical evaluation, which often includes laboratory tests and imaging procedures; e.g., massive hepatic metastases are invariably associated with a marked elevation of serum alkaline phosphatase, usually >350 IU per milliliter.

The presence of ascites with positive neoplastic cytology, indicating peritoneal carcinomatosis, signifies an expected survival of 6 months or less. Therapy is palliative. In certain instances, such as treating mesothelioma, instilling antitumor agents into the peritoneal cavity may be part of a therapeutic program directed against the underlying tumor. Diuretics and salt restriction are ineffective in controlling ascites due to peritoneal carcinomatosis. Serial paracentesis is the simplest method to control symptomatic malignant ascites. Occasionally a peritoneovenous shunt may provide valuable, albeit temporary, palliation. In contrast, when malignant ascites is associated with portal hypertension, salt restriction, and diuretics may effectively control ascites. The prognosis for patients with malignancy associated with portal hypertension is always poor. When diuretics are ineffective, serial paracentesis is often the best method to offer rapid palliation.

CHYLOUS ASCITES. This is milky ascites in which the triglyceride concentration is markedly elevated, always >200 mg per deciliter, and often >1000 mg per deciliter. It is due to leakage of lymph into the peritoneal cavity. New-onset chylous ascites is most often due to underlying malignancy, especially lymphoma. Occasionally, chylous ascites occurs after trauma, intra-abdominal surgery, and peritoneal infection such as tuberculosis. Rarely it occurs as an incidental unexplained finding in cirrhotic patients. Except in cases of known trauma, investigation is focused on identifying an underlying malignant process. However, malignant chylous ascites rarely contains malignant cells (see Table 111–2). Appropriate tests include abdominal CT scans and bone marrow aspiration. Lymphangiography does not identify intra-abdominal

TABLE 111-4. CAUSES OF PERITONEAL CARCINOMATOSIS

Primary disorders of peritoneum
  Mesothelioma
Metastatic spread from
  Gastrointestinal tumors
    Stomach
    Colon
    Pancreas
  Other intra-abdominal organs
    Ovary
    Pseudomyxoma peritonei
  Extra-abdominal primary tumors
    Breast
    Lung
  Hematologic malignancy
    Lymphoma

lymphadenopathy when CT scanning has failed to do so. Chylous ascites, whether of malignant or benign origin, responds poorly to salt restriction or diuretics, except in rare idiopathic cases associated with cirrhosis and portal hypertension. Paracentesis offers simple palliative therapy. In the majority of cases, treatment is directed at the underlying lymphoma. Fat in the diet can be replaced with medium-chain triglycerides in selected cases because medium-chain triglycerides are absorbed directly into the portal bloodstream and bypass the lymphatics. Occasional patients may be placed on total parenteral nutrition to reduce formation of chylous ascites.

PANCREATIC ASCITES. This is due to the leakage of pancreatic juice into the peritoneal cavity. It occurs in patients with pseudocyst formation following pancreatitis in whom the pseudocyst ruptures into the peritoneum, causing pancreatic ascites (see Ch. 107). Because alcohol is a frequent cause of pancreatitis and is the most common cause of chronic liver failure, it may be difficult to distinguish pancreatic ascites due to alcoholic pancreatitis from ascites due to alcoholic cirrhosis in someone with concomitant alcoholic pancreatitis. In these patients paracentesis is valuable in two ways. First, a high serum-ascites albumin gradient indicates the presence of portal hypertensive ascites, suggesting cirrhosis rather than pancreatitis as the source of ascites; and second, pancreatic ascites has a very elevated amylase concentration, usually considerably greater than the serum level (see Table 111–2). In pancreatic ascites, the ascitic amylase remains elevated even after the serum level declines toward normal limits. Endoscopic retrograde cholangiopancreatography (ERCP) is useful in pancreatic ascites, especially in trauma cases, to identify a disrupted pancreatic duct. Surgery to drain the pseudocyst and repair the duct is necessary in traumatic pancreatic ascites, but a conservative approach is often adopted in alcoholic and other nontraumatic cases.

ENDOCRINE ASCITES. In rare circumstances, ascites is a principal manifestation of an endocrine disorder. Examples include myxedema (which causes an elevated serum-ascites albumin gradient), struma ovarii, Meig's syndrome (see Ch. 63) (ascites and pleural effusion caused by benign ovarian neoplasms), and ovarian overstimulation syndrome, which occurs in women receiving fertility-enhancing drugs—clomiphene citrate, human chorionic gonadotropin (hCG), human menopausal gonadotropin (hMG), follicle-stimulating hormones, and luteinizing hormone–releasing hormone.

RENAL ASCITES. Nephrotic syndrome is another rare cause of ascites. It is reported that ascites may occur in the absence of liver disease when serum albumin falls below 2.0 grams per deciliter. However, whenever this diagnosis is considered, a careful search for underlying liver disease should be undertaken, including measuring hepatitis B surface antigen (see Ch. 119) and anti–hepatitis C antibodies (see Ch. 117). This is because hepatitis B or C may produce glomerulonephritis in addition to cirrhosis, so ascites may be due to any combination of portal hypertension, poor albumin synthesis, and renal albumin wasting. Similar considerations apply to the reported unexplained development of ascites in patients with chronic hemodialysis (nephrogenous ascites), especially because clandestine hepatitis B or C infections are common in chronic renal failure patients who require hemodialysis.

CONNECTIVE TISSUE DISORDERS. Occasionally systemic lupus erythematosus (see Ch. 240) is associated with the development of ascites in the absense of liver disease and portal hypertension. This is said to respond to prednisone therapy.

ASCITES IN HIV-INFECTED PATIENTS. When new-onset ascites occurs in patients with acquired immunodeficiency syndrome, causes of portal hypertension such as alcoholism or chronic viral hepatitis should be sought. Other sources of ascites in these patients include abdominal lymphoma or peritoneal infection. Among the infections reported to cause ascites in HIV-infected patients are cryptococcosis, tuberculosis (see below), and coccidioidomycosis. In addition, a group of HIV-infected patients has been described in whom chronic nonspecific peritonitis caused ascites for which no infectious or malignant cause could be identified.

Acute Peritonitis

DEFINITION. Acute inflammation of the peritoneum or peritoneal fluid due to intestinal contents (including gastric acid, gastrointestinal luminal contents, bile, or pancreatic juice) or bacteria entering into the peritoneal cavity. Acute peritonitis may result from perforation of a viscus owing to acute appendicitis or diverticulitis, perforation of an ulcer (peptic ulcer, Crohn's disease, malignancy), and trauma including iatrogenic intervention (e.g., surgery, needle biopsies). Primary peritonitis refers to peritonitis arising without a recognizable preceding cause, a particular form of which is spontaneous bacterial peritonitis (see below). When there is a definite antecedent event such as perforation or surgery, this is referred to as secondary peritonitis. Finally, some authorities refer to tertiary peritonitis as persistence of intra-abdominal sepsis without a discrete focus of infection, generally following surgical treatment of prior severe peritonitis. This often occurs in the setting of a severely ill patient in the intensive care unit and includes patients who are solid organ transplant recipients or are otherwise immunosuppressed.

PROGNOSTIC FACTORS. The antecedent events have prognostic implications for patients with secondary peritonitis. Peritonitis after acute appendicitis or perforated peptic ulcer occurring in an otherwise healthy patient has a low mortality, whereas peritonitis after elective operation, trauma, or pancreatitis has a high mortality, irrespective of the patient's overall clinical setting. The prognosis for severe peritonitis has not changed in the past 50 years despite the advent of broad-spectrum antibiotics, critical care units, and radical approaches to eliminate bacterial contamination of the peritoneal cavity. This suggests that the outcome in severe peritonitis is dictated by the overall health of the host, including his/her nutritional status, immunocompetence, and systemic factors such as cardiac and renal function.

CLINICAL PRESENTATION. The classic features of acute peritonitis are abdominal pain, abdominal tenderness, and the absence of bowel sounds. Severe, sudden-onset abdominal pain suggests a ruptured viscus. The clinical signs of peritoneal irritation include abdominal tenderness, rebound tenderness, and, eventually, abdominal rigidity. In the florid cases, these signs and symptoms are accompanied by fever, hypotension, tachycardia, and acidosis. Although this clinical pattern is characteristic, it is important to stress that acute peritonitis may frequently lack these features. Thus, for example, spontaneous bacterial peritonitis arising in ascites is often very subtle in presentation (see below). Acute peritonitis arising in elderly or immunosuppressed patients may lack the features of peritoneal irritation or systemic decompensation. Similarly, in patients with tertiary peritonitis, classic signs and symptoms may be absent or suppressed and the diagnosis suggested by persistent leukocytosis or fever only. In these circumstances, a high index of suspicion is necessary.

DIAGNOSIS. Investigating acute peritonitis includes plain abdominal radiographs to determine whether there is free air in the abdominal cavity. This is characteristic of perforation of viscus. CT scanning and/or ultrasonography is very important in identifying the presence of free fluid or abscesses. Where peritonitis is associated with ascites, paracentesis is mandatory (see Table 111–2).

THERAPY. The three key elements of therapy for acute peritonitis are resuscitation, laparotomy, and antibiotics. Resuscitation with intravenous fluids and correcting metabolic and electrolyte disturbances are the initial steps.

Laparotomy is a cornerstone of therapy for secondary or tertiary acute peritonitis, in order to identify and repair the cause of the acute catastrophe, to evacuate pus, and to irrigate the peritoneal cavity. This includes acute chemical peritonitis which occurs after perforation of a peptic ulcer or the gallbladder and biliary tree. The latter biliary peritonitis occurs after hepatobiliary surgery or occasionally liver biopsy. In some patients, when bilary peritonitis is accompanied by little systemic disturbance, careful conservative management with intravenous fluids and broad-spectrum antibiotics is adequate and laparotomy is avoided. However, there should be a low threshold for proceeding to laparotomy even in these circumstances.

Finally, systemic broad-spectrum antibiotics are mainstays of therapy. It is important to be alert for unexpected organisms as a cause of peritonitis. For example, in severe secondary and tertiary peritonitis, the typical organisms may include *Candida* species, enterococci, *Enterobacter*, and *Staphylococcus epidermidis*. Thus, antifungal agents (such as amphotericin B or fluconazole) may be appropriate even as empirical agents when peritonitis persists despite all standard measures.

Spontaneous Bacterial Peritonitis

DEFINITION. Bacterial infection of ascites in a patient with liver disease in whom there is no precipitating cause of peritonitis. Spontaneous bacterial peritonitis (SBP) occurs almost exclusively in cirrhotic patients but occasionally may complicate acute hepatic failure. SBP is a marker of severe hepatic failure. The most important predictor of the first episode of SBP is a low ascitic protein content and elevated serum bilirubin. Approximately 25% of patients with ascitic fluid total protein content of < 1 gram per deciliter develop SBP during 3 years of subsequent observation. The mechanism for SBP development is related to deficient opsonic activity in ascitic fluid. The offending organisms are almost always enteric gram-negative aerobes such as *Escherichia coli* or *Klebsiella pneumoniae* or gram-positive aerobes, particularly *Streptococcus pneumoniae*. Anaerobes rarely cause SBP.

CLINICAL PRESENTATION. The clinical presentation of SBP is often subtle. Consequently, SBP must be suspected whenever a cirrhotic patient with ascites develops a sudden deterioration in hepatic or renal function, worsening malaise, encephalopathy, or unexplained persistent leukocytosis, even in the absence of abdominal signs or symptoms typical of acute peritonitis. Conversely, SBP should be considered whenever a cirrhotic patient presents with fever and abdominal pain more typical of acute peritonitis. Finally, a high index of suspicion is necessary whenever a patient with known established liver disease presents with features of sepsis or hepatic deterioration despite the absence of clinical ascites. Small pockets of infected ascites may be present which are detectable only by sonography or CT scanning. In such cases, a presumptive diagnosis of SBP and instituting antibiotic therapy may be the wisest course.

DIAGNOSIS. The key to diagnosing SBP is diagnostic paracentesis. The diagnosis of SBP is made by finding ≥ 250 polymorphonuclear cells (PMN) per cubic millimeter. A very elevated PMN count in ascites (for example, > 5000 per cubic millimeter) suggests an intra-abdominal abscess or a secondary cause of peritonitis. Demonstrating an organism in the ascitic fluid is not required for the diagnosis but is helpful. The chances of identifying an organism in ascites are enhanced by directly transferring ascitic fluid to blood culture media bottles prior to incubation. Nonetheless, no organism is identified in 30 to 50% of cases. SBP is usually caused by a single species. A culture of multiple organisms from ascites suggests a perforated viscus. Measuring ascitic fluid pH or LDH is of secondary importance in making a diagnosis of SBP. In addition to inspecting and culturing ascitic fluid, all patients suspected of harboring SBP should undergo blood cultures, chest radiography, and urine microscopy and culture to identify blood-borne sepsis and to look for additional sites of infection.

THERAPY. Antibiotics are the cornerstone of managing of SBP. Contrary to other forms of peritonitis referred to above, laparotomy has no place in the SBP therapy. Cefotaxime, 2 grams IV every 6 hours, with dose reduction for renal function, is currently the best treatment for SBP in cirrhotic patients. The most important negative predictors of resolving an episode and of patient survival are the presence of renal failure, acquiring SBP while in the hospital, and elevated serum aminotransferases. Five days of treatment are usually adequate. At that point, efficacy can be determined by estimating the ascitic fluid PMN count, and intravenous antibiotics can be stopped if the count is < 250 per cubic millimeter.

SBP recurs in 70% of patients in the first year after their initial episode unless they are placed on prophylactic antibiotics. The frequency of recurrence is greatest in patients with a low ascitic fluid total protein content and impaired hepatic synthetic function. The incidence of SBP can be markedly reduced, in both patients who are at risk of a first episode and those who have already had SBP, by prophylactically administering antibiotics that cleanse the gut microflora. The quinolone norfloxacin (400 mg once a day) has been the most extensively studied. However, although the incidence of SBP is markedly reduced, mortality, which is related to underlying hepatic dysfunction, is not affected.

Peritoneal Tuberculosis

Tuberculosis (TB) is an important cause of peritonitis worldwide and since the advent of the AIDS epidemic has re-emerged in the developed world also. The risk factors for intra-abdominal tuberculosis are shown in Table 111–5. Patients with peritoneal TB fre-

TABLE 111-5. RISK FACTORS FOR INTRA-ABDOMINAL TUBERCULOSIS

HIV infection
Immunosuppressive therapy
Advanced age
Intravenous drug use/alcoholism/cirrhosis
Immigration from an endemic area
Poverty
Incarceration/long-stay care
Peritoneal dialysis

TABLE 111-7. DIAGNOSTIC TESTS OF PERITONEAL TUBERCULOSIS

Diagnostic Test	Comment
Paracentesis	
With smear	<3% positive
With culture	<20–80% positive
With ascitic ADA* measurement	≥32.3 U/l highly sensitive and specific. Low ascitic protein (i.e., cirrhosis) may cause false negatives. Not validated in HIV-infected persons.
Laparoscopy with biopsy	Best test Up to 100% positive
Needle biopsy of peritoneum	Largely replaced by laparoscopy
Diagnostic laparotomy	Should be considered if laparoscopy not available

* ADA = Adenosine deaminase.

quently have concomitant cirrhosis, which may be implicated incorrectly as the source of ascites, thereby obscuring the presence of TB peritonitis. The serum-ascites albumin gradient is high in cirrhotic patients with TB and low in patients with peritoneal TB without portal hypertension or cirrhosis (see Tables 111–2 and 111–3). TB in HIV infection is characterized by newly acquired infection rather than a recrudescence of quiescent infection; a high degree of acquisition of TB among at-risk persons who are exposed to TB; a high rate of clinical rather than quiescent TB; rapidly progressive TB that frequently has extrapulmonary involvement; and, finally, the emergence of TB strains that are resistant to one or more of the standard antituberculosis chemotherapeutic agents.

CLINICAL PRESENTATION. The clinical features of peritoneal TB are shown in Table 111–6. Ascites is almost invariable. Abdominal swelling and pain are common. Many patients have accompanying systemic effects such as fever, weight loss, and anemia.

DIAGNOSIS. Diagnostic tests for peritoneal TB are shown in Table 111–7. Paracentesis reveals a lymphocytosis but rarely shows acid-fast bacilli on smear. Culture of ascitic fluid has a somewhat higher diagnostic yield but at the expense of a 4- to 6-week delay. The potential impact of molecular diagnostic methods on identifying TB organisms in ascites has not yet been defined. Recently many groups have reported that an elevated ascitic concentration of adenosine deaminase (ADA)—a marker of T lymphocyte and macrophage activation—is a sensitive and specific diagnostic test for TB peritonitis. This test may be particularly helpful in Third World countries where laparoscopy and other diagnostic tests are scarce. However, the value of ADA in diagnosing TB peritonitis in HIV-infected persons has not been evaluated. Definitive diagnosis of peritoneal TB is best made by laparoscopy and directed peritoneal biopsy. Peritoneal biopsy using a Cope needle has been abandoned where laparoscopic procedures have become available. The laparoscopic appearance of the peritoneum, showing tubercles, is often a helpful clinical sign. Occasional patients without ascites—so-called fibroadhesive tubercular peritonitis—should not undergo laparoscopy.

THERAPY. Treatment of TB peritonitis involves standard protocols using two or three drugs, usually for 9 months. It is important to test all TB isolates for drug susceptibility. HIV-infected persons who are co-infected with a strain of TB that is susceptible to first-line chemotherapeutic agents usually respond well to standard therapeutic protocols. Managing resistant strains of TB is difficult, however, and relies on a combination of first- and second-line agents. Infection with resistant strains of TB among HIV-infected persons is associated with high mortality.

Peritonitis in Continuous Ambulatory Peritoneal Dialysis (CAPD)

Infection developing in the washout dialysate is common in patients on CAPD. It often is not accompanied by systemic disturbance or presents with mild abdominal pain and low-grade fever only. It is recognized by a cloudy effluent. Cytology of the infected dialysate shows that it has a high white cell count. The great majority of causative organisms are gram-positive. *Staphylococcus epidermidis* is the most common, followed by *S. aureus* and streptococci. Treatment should be begun promptly upon recognizing cloudy effluent before the availability of culture results. Treatment consists of infusing broad-spectrum antibiotics into the peritoneum with activity against gram-positive and aerobic gram-negative organisms. The antibiotics are infused through the abdominal wall catheter, which is not removed, and dialysis is not interrupted. Admission to the hospital, converting to intravenous antibiotics, and removing the catheter are necessary in a minority of patients who fail to respond to prompt outpatient therapy.

Miscellaneous Forms of Peritonitis

In familial Mediterranean fever, the most common recurring feature is peritonitis, which affects >90% of symptomatic patients. It presents as episodic abdominal pain and fever. Colchicine may reduce the frequency and severity of attacks.

DISEASES OF THE MESENTERY

Diseases of the mesentery are classified in Table 111–8. All are rare.

Mesenteric panniculitis and *retractile mesenteritis* may represent different manifestations of the same idiopathic disorder. Mesenteric panniculitus consists of diffuse fatty infiltration of the mesentery, which is then replaced by fat necrosis, fibrosis, and calcification. Retractile mesenteritis is at the fibrotic end of this spectrum. Patients with these conditions present with intermittent abdominal pain, abdominal swelling, and abdominal mass. However, many patients are asymptomatic. The diagnosis is usually made at laparot-

TABLE 111-6. CLINICAL CHARACTERISTICS OF PERITONEAL TUBERCULOSIS* (%)

Ascites	80–100
Abdominal swelling	65–100
Abdominal pain	36–93
Weight loss	37–87
Fever	56–100
Diarrhea	9–27
Abdominal tenderness	65–87
Anemia	48–68
Positive PPD† test	55–100

* The percentages represent the frequency with which these features have been observed in peritoneal tuberculosis. These data, which are based on Marshall, antedate studies of TB in HIV-infected persons.
† PPD = Purified protein derivative.

TABLE 111-8. DISORDERS OF THE MESENTERY

Primary inflammatory diseases
    Mesenteric panniculitis
    Retractile mesenteritis
Mesenteric cysts
    Embryonic
    Traumatic/acquired
    Neoplastic
    Infective
Mesenteric tumors
    Benign: Lipoma, hemangioma, leiomyoma, ganglioneuroma, fibroma (Gardner's syndrome)
    Malignant: Various sarcomas; metastatic tumors
Mesenteric vascular insufficiency
    Acute
    Chronic

TABLE 111-9. DISORDERS OF THE OMENTUM

Tumor
Benign: Fibroma, lipoma, hemangioma, neuroma, lymphangioma, leiomyoma, mesothelioma
Malignant: Primary
              Metastases—especially ovary, stomach, colon
Cysts
Vascular insufficiency
  Torsion
  Infarction
Inflammation: Usually secondary to peritonitis

omy, and once recognized, surgical resection should not be undertaken unless fibrosis is causing intestinal obstruction.

Cysts and tumors of the mesentery are listed in Table 111–8. Of note are the desmoid mesenteric fibromas, which are part of the syndromic complex of Gardner's syndrome.

DISEASES OF THE OMENTUM

These are categorized in Table 111–9. They are rare disorders that can be subdivided into mass lesions, acute vascular insufficiency due to torsion or infarction, and inflammatory processes.

Andreu M, Sola R, Sitges-Serra A, et al.: Risk factors for spontaneous bacterial peritonitis in cirrhotic patients with ascites. Gastroenterology 104:1133, 1993. *Prospective study of 110 cirrhotics with sterile ascites with average follow-up of 46 weeks.*

Christou NV, Barie PS, Dellinger EP, et al.: Surgical Infection Society intraabdominal infection study. Prospective evaluation of management techniques and outcome. Arch Surg 128:193, 1993. *Large uncontrolled data gathering study on 239 surgical patients with severe acute peritonitis. Indicates the importance of host factors (nutrition, age, cardiac status, APACHE II score), dictating need for reoperation and mortality.*

Marshall JB: Tuberculosis of the gastrointestinal tract and peritoneum. Am J Gastroenterol 88:989, 1993. *Excellent up-to-date review with 166 references.*

Runyon BA, Hoefs TC, Morgan TR: Ascitic fluid analysis in malignancy-related ascites. Hepatology 8:1104, 1988. *Prospective study of 45 patients with ascites and intra-abdominal malignancy.*

Runyon BA, Montano AA, Akriviadis EA, et al.: The serum-ascites gradient is superior to the exudate-transudate concept in differential diagnosis of ascites. Ann Intern Med 117:215, 1992. *Outstanding study of 901 paired serum and ascites samples which demonstrates the utility of the serum-ascites albumin gradient.*

Wilcox MC, Forsmark CE, Darragh T, et al.: High-protein ascites in patients with the acquired immunodeficiency syndrome. Gastroenterology 100:745, 1991. *Largest series to date of noncirrhotic ascites in HIV-infected persons.*

112   MISCELLANEOUS INFLAMMATORY DISEASES OF THE INTESTINE

C. Mel Wilcox

ACUTE APPENDICITIS (Including the Acute Abdomen)

DEFINITION. Appendicitis is an acute inflammatory disorder of the vermiform appendix. It is uncommon at the extremes of age, with the highest incidence in the second and third decades of life. Because of its prevalence, varied presentations mimicking other intra-abdominal diseases, and curability, an appreciation of this disorder provides a framework for an understanding of the causes and approach to the acute abdomen.

ETIOLOGY AND PATHOGENESIS. Although not demonstrable in all cases, obstruction of the appendiceal lumen by a fecalith is the usual inciting event. Less common causes include neoplasms (carcinoid tumors, adenocarcinoma, Kaposi's sarcoma) and infections (*Enterobius vermicularis,* cytomegalovirus). With appendiceal obstruction, a sequence of pathophysiologic events occurs: Normally secreted mucus becomes impacted, causing appendiceal distention, thrombosis, and subsequently, bacterial invasion of the wall; the end result is gangrene and perforation.

CLINICAL PRESENTATION. The clinical manifestations follow a stereotypical course paralleling these pathologic events. Almost invariably, abdominal pain is the first manifestation. Initially mild pain may be discounted as indigestion. It is often poorly localized to the periumbilical area or epigastrium; appendiceal distention results in this poorly localized visceral type of periumbilical discomfort. The pain is at first colicky, then steady, and increases in severity as the inflammatory process progresses. When the parietal peritoneum becomes inflamed, usually hours after the initial onset of symptoms, the pain becomes localized in the right iliac region. Right iliac pain is typical for appendicitis; however, pelvic pain (pelvic appendix) or right upper quadrant pain may result, depending on the location of the appendix. Anorexia is frequent and the urge to eat argues against the diagnosis of appendicitis. Vomiting is not a prominent symptom.

PHYSICAL EXAMINATION. Physical findings depend on the stage of the inflammatory process, location of the appendix, and in some cases, the age of the patient. Acute abdominal conditions notoriously present atypically in the elderly and in patients receiving corticosteroid therapy. The most consistent physical finding is tenderness in the right iliac region at McBurney's point (one fingerbreadth from the anterosuperior iliac spine toward the umbilicus). The area of tenderness, however, corresponds to the location of the inflamed appendix. With a retrocecal appendix, tenderness may be mild. Rectal examination may disclose tenderness anteriorly with a pelvic appendix or a bulge in the pelvic wall from an abscess. An inflamed parietal peritoneum results in localized rebound tenderness and rigidity. Only with generalized peritonitis are diffuse rebound tenderness and peritoneal signs elicited. Rarely a mass is palpable in the right lower quadrant. Rotating a flexed right hip when supine (obturator sign) or raising a straightened leg against resistance (psoas sign) may elicit pain. Bowel sounds can be heard unless peritonitis and ileus are present. Fever occurs only in the later stages of inflammation; fever at the onset of abdominal pain should suggest another diagnosis.

LABORATORY STUDIES. Leukocytosis with increased polymorphonuclear leukocytes is a consistent finding only in the later stages of appendicitis. Urinalysis is usually normal. Standard abdominal roentgenography is frequently normal, although it may demonstrate localized loops of bowel, obliteration of the psoas shadow, or soft tissue mass; however, these latter findings represent abscess formation. Less than 10% of patients have a calcified fecalith seen in the region of the appendix by abdominal imaging.

DIFFERENTIAL DIAGNOSIS OF APPENDICITIS AND THE ACUTE ABDOMEN

Although the differential diagnosis of acute appendicitis and the acute abdomen is broad, a systematic history and physical examination, combined with selected laboratory tests and abdominal imaging studies, in most cases lead to a diagnosis. For the acutely ill patient, early surgical consultation is mandatory. Although a firm diagnosis before laparotomy is the rule today, surgical exploration when the appendix is normal is entirely acceptable given the increase in morbidity and mortality with appendiceal rupture. Indeed, 5 to 10% of patients with suspected acute appendicitis have a normal appendix at the time of laparotomy.

A variety of disorders cause a subacute to acute right lower quadrant pain syndrome mimicking acute appendicitis (Table 112–1). In young children bacterial infections may result in a mesenteric adenitis or terminal ileitis or involve the right colon. Crohn's ileitis or ileocolitis frequently masquerades as acute appendicitis. Meckel's or cecal diverticulitis may be impossible to distin-

TABLE 112-1. CAUSES OF RIGHT LOWER QUADRANT PAIN SYNDROMES

Inflammatory Disorders	Neoplasms	Other
Appendicitis	Carcinoid	Gynecologic disorders
Crohn's ileitis/colitis	Lymphoma	
Cecal diverticulitis	Cecal adenocarcinoma (perforated)	
Meckle's diverticulitis		
Yersinia ileocolitis		
Amebic colitis		
Tuberculous colitis		

guish from acute appendicitis. Special consideration should be given to the female patient. Pelvic inflammatory disease is infrequently unilateral but may mimic appendicitis. Ectopic pregnancy, ruptured endometrioma, or torsion of an ovarian cyst may cause unilateral pain. A ruptured graafian follicle would occur in the midcycle and without fever and leukocytosis. Appendicitis may be difficult to diagnose during pregnancy because the appendix moves toward the right upper quadrant.

CHARACTERISTICS OF PAIN. Acute severe abdominal pain most often results from perforation of an abdominal viscus (peptic ulcer), small bowel obstruction, choledocholithiasis, nephrolithiasis, or rupture and dissection of an abdominal aortic aneurysm. Subacute onset of pain is more typical for intestinal ischemia, cholecystitis, pancreatitis, diverticulitis, Crohn's disease, and appendicitis. Pain of a constant nature is seen with cholecystitis, pancreatitis, intestinal ischemia, and other inflammatory disorders. Colicky pain occurs with nephrolithiasis or intestinal obstruction. Although more typical for nephrolithiasis, pain radiating to the groin may rarely be seen in appendicitis. Radiation of pain to the back suggests pancreatitis, peptic ulcer disease, or biliary tract disease. Shoulder pain results from diaphragmatic irritation (pancreatitis, cholecystitis). Significant vomiting is seen with pancreatitis or obstruction of the stomach or small bowel.

PHYSICAL EXAMINATION. Careful observation of the patient may provide clues to the cause. With peritonitis, the patient attempts to lie quietly. In contrast, patients with intermittent visceral type pain (nephrolithiasis or choledocholithiasis) are restless during the attack. Tachycardia is nonspecific. Hypotension suggests bleeding (ruptured aneurysm), sepsis, or severe pancreatitis. Low-grade fever occurs with any inflammatory process, including acute pancreatitis. Abdominal inspection should include attention to scars that may suggest hernias, or masses (aneurysm, abscess). Absence of bowel sounds suggests ileus, whereas "rushes and tinkles" occur with small bowel obstruction. Abdominal palpation should begin opposite the point of subjective pain to minimize voluntary guarding, which may limit the examination. Coughing may cause local pain with peritonitis. Diffuse abdominal rigidity, unequivocal rebound tenderness, or severe localized tenderness with rebound represents generalized peritonitis, indicating the need for urgent surgical exploration. Involuntary guarding or referred rebound suggests a focal peritoneal process. Abdominal ischemia causes subjective pain disproportionate to the findings on examination until infarction and perforation occur. Abdominal distention and tympany are found with dilation of either large or small bowel. Femoral artery or abdominal bruits suggest vascular disease (ischemic disease or aneurysms). Rectal and pelvic examinations may help evaluate for a pelvic appendix and peritonitis or gynecologic disorders.

LABORATORY STUDIES. In the patient with an acute abdomen, the following studies should be performed: complete blood cell count with differential, serum electrolytes, blood urea nitrogen and creatinine, serum amylase, liver chemistry tests, urinalysis, and a pregnancy test in women of childbearing potential. Elevated polymorphonuclear leukocyte count points to infection (appendicitis, cholecystitis), tissue necrosis (bowel infarction), or other inflammatory processes (pancreatitis). Anemia may result from gastrointestinal bleeding due to carcinoma or peptic ulcer. Pyuria and bacteriuria indicate a urinary tract infection, and microscopic or gross hematuria suggests nephrolithiasis. Fecal white blood cells or blood in the stool are seen with colitis (ischemia, inflammatory bowel disease, infection); fecal white cells are not present in acute appendicitis. Mildly elevated serum amylase (less than two times upper limit of normal) is nonspecific, occurring with a variety of intra-abdominal disorders (see Ch. 107).

ABDOMINAL IMAGING. Roentgenographic films of the chest and supine/upright abdominal series are useful to evaluate for free peritoneal air, bowel gas pattern, and presence of calculi (nephrolithiasis, 80%; gallstones, 15%; appendicolith, 5%; or pancreatic calcification). A pneumonia or other basilar pulmonic process may mimic an abdominal syndrome. Abdominal sonography may demonstrate gallstones and a thickened gallbladder wall (acute cholecystitis), dilated common bile duct (choledocholithiasis), or pancreatic calcifications (chronic pancreatitis). Recent studies suggest a sensitivity and specificity of sonography in diagnosing acute appendicitis of >90% in experienced hands.

Abdominal ultrasound or computed tomographic (CT) scanning has been invaluable for evaluation of patients with the acute ab-

domen. Localized inflammatory processes of the right lower quadrant may suggest appendicitis, or Crohn's disease if the terminal ileum and/or right colon is thickened; however, overlap between these two entities may occur. CT also helps exclude diverticulitis, acute pancreatitis, biliary obstruction, luminal disorders such as small bowel or colonic infarction, and aortic dissection, as well as unsuspected processes of the liver and spleen.

A variety of other nonsurgical conditions may cause an acute abdominal pain syndrome. Disorders "above the diaphragm" include myocardial infarction, bacterial pneumonia, and acute pericarditis. Severe right heart failure and a distended liver may cause mild to moderate right upper quadrant pain. Acute hepatitis rarely results in severe abdominal pain and should be suspected by marked elevations of the serum aminotransferases. Marked transient elevations of serum aminotransferases, however, are commonly seen with acute biliary obstruction (choledocholithiasis). Systemic disorders with abdominal manifestations include sickle cell crisis, acute intermittent porphyria, diabetic neuropathy, heavy metal poisoning, and cutaneous herpes zoster.

TREATMENT. Surgical therapy is curative. Mortality is minimal when the diagnosis is rapidly established and appendectomy performed. Mortality rates increase significantly with frank perforation, particularly in the elderly. For the patient with a typical history, no confirmatory studies may be necessary before surgical exploration. When the diagnosis is in doubt, careful observation over 6 to 12 hours may be diagnostic. Broad-spectrum antibiotics directed toward gram-negative rods and anaerobes should be given before surgery or at the time of CT drainage. In some patients acute appendicitis resolves with localized perforation alone; however, subsequent relapse is frequent (chronic appendicitis), so elective appendectomy should be performed.

Alvarado A: A practical score for the early diagnosis of acute appendicitis. Ann Emerg Med 15:557, 1986. *Presents predictive factors for diagnosis in order of importance.*

Jeffrey RB Jr, Laing FC, Townsend RR: Acute appendicitis; sonographic criteria based on 250 cases. Radiology 167:327, 1988. *A new compression technique shows a diagnostic accuracy of about 90%.*

Lau WY, Fan ST, Yiu TF, et al.: Acute appendicitis in the elderly. Surg Gynecol Obstet 161:157, 1985. *A prospective study of 104 patients older than 60 with appendicitis.*

Ridge JA, Way LW: Abdominal pain and the acute abdomen. *In* Sleisenger MH, Fordtran JS (eds.): Gastrointestinal Disease. 5th ed. Philadelphia, WB Saunders, 1993. *An excellent chapter containing complete information on diagnosis of the acute abdomen.*

Schrock TR: Acute appendicitis. *In* Sleisenger MH, Fordtran JS (eds.): Gastrointestinal Disease. 5th ed. Philadelphia, WB Saunders, 1993. *A concise yet comprehensive article on every aspect of the subject. A useful reference.*

DIVERTICULITIS OF THE COLON

Colonic diverticuli are mucosal outpouchings occurring where arteries penetrate the muscularis to reach the submucosa and mucosa. Because these areas are inherently weak, and under stress, prolapse of mucosa and submucosa may occur. Diverticuli form throughout the entire colon although more commonly in the left colon, particularly the sigmoid. Diverticulitis results when a fecalith becomes impacted in a diverticulum with erosion through the serosa, resulting in perforation.

CLINICAL PRESENTATION. This disorder typically affects patients aged 50 and older because the prevalence of diverticulosis increases with age. The pain is usually subacute and constant and located in the left lower quadrant (sigmoid diverticulitis). However, the location of pain depends on the involved colonic segment. Fever is almost invariably present. High-grade fever and sepsis occur when the perforation is not contained or with generalized peritonitis. Constipation or loose stools may be reported. Rectal bleeding is distinctly unusual.

DIFFERENTIAL DIAGNOSIS. Constant left lower quadrant pain and fever in the elderly are highly suggestive of acute diverticulitis. Lower abdominal pain, fever, and bloody diarrhea suggest a bacterial colitis (*Shigella, Salmonella, Campylobacter*), ischemic colitis, or other inflammatory bowel disease. With generalized peritonitis, the differential diagnosis becomes that of the acute abdomen (see above). Gynecologic disorders may be localized to left lower quadrant and should always be considered in females.

DIAGNOSTIC STUDIES. Leukocytosis is common although nonspecific. Urinalysis may demonstrate nonspecific findings such as protein or rare white blood cells. If significant diarrhea is reported, fecal leukocytes should be searched for.

Abdominal radiographs may indicate a displaced colon, extraluminal gas, or colonic mucosal abnormalities. These studies are probably more helpful in excluding other potential causes of left lower quadrant pain.

Diagnostic barium enema has been used for many years and is safe when carefully performed. Typical findings include spiculation of the mucosa, spasm, or frank perforation and abscess. These findings are relatively specific for acute diverticulitis but may be difficult to differentiate from carcinoma. Abdominal CT, which has become the test of choice, may demonstrate bowel wall thickening, abscess formation, and diverticuli (Fig. 112–1). Barium enema and CT are complementary because each is neither 100% sensitive nor specific.

Endoscopic examination is contraindicated with diverticulitis given the theoretical potential to exacerbate perforation; however, when carcinoma or inflammatory bowel disease is highly suspected, sigmoidoscopy is appropriate.

TREATMENT. Initial therapy includes broad-spectrum antibiotics such as a third-generation cephalosporin combined with anaerobic coverage (metronidazole). For mild disease, oral antibiotics and bowel rest can be used in the outpatient setting. Early surgical consultation is important, especially when there is more significant pain or an acute abdomen. If a large abscess is identified by CT imaging, percutaneous catheter drainage can be a temporary measure before subsequent definitive surgical therapy.

Complications of diverticulitis include colonic stricture, bleeding, or fistula formation to the small bowel, colon, bladder, or vagina.

Chappins CW, Cohn I Jr: Acute colonic diverticulitis. Surg Clin North Am 68:301, 1988. *A comprehensive review of the disease with a good summary of the modern tools for diagnosis and of the evolving relationship of CT scanning, percutaneous drainage, and surgery to manage complications.*

Johnson CD, Baker ME, Rice RP, et al.: Diagnosis of acute colonic diverticulitis: Comparison of barium enema and CT. AJR 148:541, 1987. *A careful analysis of the sensitivities of barium enema and CT to diagnose this disease and its complications.*

RADIATION ENTEROCOLITIS

Although radiation is commonly used to palliate abdominal and pelvic malignancies, clinically significant radiation injury in the gastrointestinal tract is unusual. Injury usually develops when the total dosage exceeds 5000 rads.

PATHOGENESIS. Given the high turnover rate of gastrointestinal epithelium, it is not unexpected that the gut, particularly replicating cells in the crypts, would be affected by radiation. If the dose of radiation does not exceed 5000 rads, minor mucosal injury (edema, erosions) may be temporary. With more intense therapy, submucosal blood vessels are damaged, resulting in an arteritis and secondarily, mucosal ischemia. Late complications include fibrosis and strictures, and diffuse vascular ectasias in the affected segments.

CLINICAL PRESENTATION. During the early phases of radiation therapy, patients may report nausea, vomiting, and diarrhea, which may be bloody. Symptoms representing the complications of high-dose radiation are not seen for months or even years following therapy (intestinal ulcerations with bleeding, obstruction from fibrosis and stricture, fistula to other pelvic organs or abscess, or chronic gastrointestinal bleeding and anemia from vascular ectasias.) If a significant amount of small bowel is in the radiation field, malabsorption may be noted.

DIAGNOSIS. In the appropriate setting, diagnosis is relatively straightforward. Symptoms early in the course of therapy suggest acute injury. Endoscopic features include mucosal edema, ulceration (early), and diffuse vascular ectasias and stricture (late). Although nonspecific, barium enema may demonstrate mucosal edema, fistula formation, and strictures. In the older patient with a stricture, carcinoma must be excluded.

TREATMENT. Treatment options are limited. Iron deficiency anemia from bleeding (vascular ectasias) should be treated with chronic iron therapy. For symptomatic distal colonic strictures, dilation may be attempted, although surgery is usually required. Diarrhea can be treated with antimotility agents. Abscess and fistula formation require surgical resection. Surgery should be performed only when necessary given the potential for further complications after anastomosis owing to involvement of adjacent bowel segments.

Earnest DH, Trier JS: Radiation enteritis and colitis. In Sleisenger MH, Fordtran JS (eds.): Gastrointestinal Disease. 5th ed. Philadelphia, WB Saunders, 1993. *A comprehensive discussion of radiation damage to the intestines.*

Hasling H, Balislev I: Long term prognosis of patients with radiation enteritis. Ann J Surg 155:517, 1988. *An important follow-up of 136 patients with radiation enteritis over nearly 5 years.*

Yeoh E, Horowitz M, Russo A, et al.: Effect of pelvic irradiation on gastrointestinal function: A prospective longitudinal study. Am J Med 95:397, 1993. *This longitudinal study of 27 patients undergoing abdominal and/or pelvic radiation documents the persistent changes in intestinal function.*

INTESTINAL AND COLONIC ULCERATION

Small intestinal and colonic ulceration are uncommon. Ulcerations may be isolated or diffuse and may be located anywhere throughout the small bowel. The location of disease and the character of the ulcers suggest the underlying cause. Isolated proximal small bowel ulcerations are most commonly caused by medications such as slow-release potassium pills or nonsteroidal anti-inflammatory drugs (NSAID's). Other disorders include infections, collagen-vascular diseases (Behçet's disease, systemic lupus erythematosus), and ulcerated neoplasms.

Because of the small size, these ulcers are difficult to identify by routine small bowel barium radiographs. Enteroclysis (see Ch. 93) is more sensitive in defining these abnormalities. Small bowel enteroscopy is time consuming and not widely available, although it is the best method to directly visualize the small bowel. Diffuse

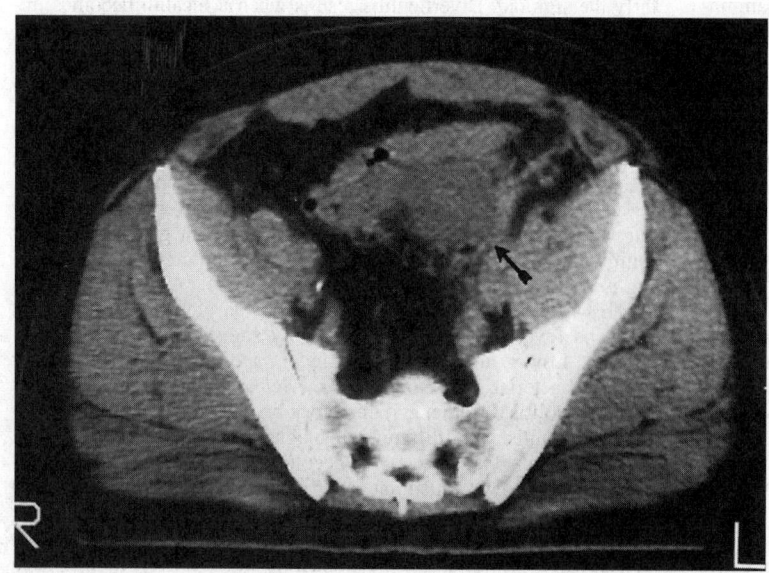

FIGURE 112–1. CT scan showing air-filled diverticula in a contracted segment of sigmoid colon lying just anterior to a paracolic abscess, indicated by a circumscribed area of uniform low density *(arrow)*. (From Sleisenger MH, Fordtran JS [eds.]: Gastrointestinal Disease. 5th ed. Philadelphia, WB Saunders, 1993, p 1357.)

processes (celiac sprue, lymphoma, or Crohn's disease) are more reliably identified by these radiographic studies.

Ulceration(s) in the right colon has been recently documented to result from NSAID's. Infections such as tuberculosis, amebiases, or rarely bacterial infections may produce right colonic ulceration. Ischemia usually produces diffuse segmental ulceration. Distal colonic ulcers result from ischemia, infections, or inflammatory bowel disease, particularly Crohn's colitis. Rectal ulcers, when solitary, may be seen with chronic constipation (stercoral ulcer) or trauma or may be idiopathic.

Barium enema may suggest Crohn's disease or ischemia. Colonoscopy with ulcer biopsy may demonstrate characteristic histopathologic changes in Crohn's disease or the solitary rectal ulcer syndrome.

Allison MC, Howatson AG, Torrance CJ, et al.: Gastrointestinal damage associated with the use of nonsteroidal anti-inflammatory drugs. N Engl J Med 327:749, 1992. *A large postmortem study documents the importance of NSAID's in causing ulcerative lesions in the small intestine.*

Bayless TR: Small intestinal ulcers: Isolated and diffuse. *In* Sleisenger MH, Fordtran JS (eds.): Gastrointestinal Disease. 4th ed. Philadelphia, WB Saunders, 1988. *Excellent clarification and description of isolated and diffuse ulceration of the small intestine.*

PART XII

DISEASES OF THE LIVER, GALLBLADDER, AND BILE DUCTS

113 CLINICAL APPROACH TO LIVER DISEASE

Robert K. Ockner

The liver plays a central and varied role in many essential physiologic processes. It is the sole source of albumin and many other plasma proteins and of blood glucose in the postabsorptive state; it is the major site of lipid synthesis and source of plasma lipoproteins; and it is the principal organ in which a variety of endogenous and exogenous substances such as ammonia, steroid hormones, drugs, and toxins undergo biotransformation. To the extent that biotransformation "detoxifies" or inactivates a substance, the liver may be viewed as serving a regulatory or protective function for the whole organism. To the extent that such biotransformation results in the formation of toxic products, as in the case of certain drugs, the liver may bear the brunt of their adverse effects.

The clinical manifestations of liver diseases are also varied. Moreover, the clues by which the clinician may be first alerted to the existence of liver disease, even when advanced, may be subtle, consisting of seemingly trivial information gleaned during a careful history (e.g., increased fatigue, or the reversal of sleep pattern or personality change of early hepatic encephalopathy), physical examination (e.g., prominence of breast tissue and small testes in a man with cirrhosis, or excoriation reflecting pruritus), or routine laboratory screening tests (e.g., mild decreases in one or more of the formed elements of the blood because of portal hypertension–associated hypersplenism). Careful assessment is equally important in the patient with obvious liver disease, to address more complex questions. For example, does what seems to be acute hepatitis in fact represent relapse of previously subclinical chronic hepatitis, or hepatitis D superinfection in a hepatitis B carrier? (see Ch. 117). Or does the deteriorating course of a patient with known cirrhosis represent the natural progression of the disease or a superimposed common bile duct stone, adverse drug reaction, or hepatocellular carcinoma?

HISTORY. Some very *nonspecific symptoms* may be important evidence of liver disease, including fatigue, malaise, fever, change in sleep pattern or behavior, diminished libido, anorexia, weight loss, nausea, and vomiting. *Pruritus* is an important symptom of *cholestasis* (impaired bile secretion) and may be present in the absence of jaundice. *Jaundice* is often first noted by family members or friends, and, especially in dark-skinned individuals, may appear first as a yellow discoloration of the conjunctivae ("scleral icterus"). Because jaundice in most forms of liver and biliary disease reflects cholestasis (see above), such patients often observe that stool color lightens and urine gets darker as the excretory route of "bile pigments" is diverted from bile to urine. Right upper quadrant abdominal discomfort or pain may reflect a rapidly enlarging liver with distention of Glisson's capsule because of acute hepatic inflammation or congestion, an acutely inflamed gallbladder, common bile duct obstruction by an impacted gallstone, or abscess or tumor in the liver or adjacent areas.

The history may provide important clues to the presence of complications of liver disease, especially those reflecting *portal hypertension* and *portal-systemic shunting.* Early hepatic *encephalopathy* may cause subtle changes in affect or sleep pattern. More overt symptoms include episodic somnolence, confusion, combativeness, ataxia, incoordination, or obtundation. A history of *abdominal swelling* suggests ascites and may be most easily recalled by the patient as a change in the fit of clothing, possibly associated with leg *edema.* Ascites may also occur in many other conditions, including hepatic vein or inferior vena caval occlusion, congestive cardiac failure, and constrictive pericarditis, and a wide variety of neoplastic and inflammatory processes (see Ch. 111). A history of *gastrointestinal bleeding* in a patient with liver disease may suggest esophageal varices or portal hypertensive gastropathy but can also reflect other lesions such as *gastritis, Mallory-Weiss syndrome,* and *peptic ulcer.*

The history is of major importance in identifying potentially significant *etiologic* or *predisposing factors.* Viral hepatitis is suggested by a history of contact with jaundiced persons, exposure to persons known to have hepatitis or to a common source of hepatitis, ingestion of uncooked or partially cooked shellfish, prior blood transfusion, work with subhuman primates, employment in certain health professions (especially in dialysis or transplantation units), accidental inoculation, sexual promiscuity (especially in the male homosexual community), sharing of needles, and travel to and consumption of water or uncooked vegetables in geographic areas with inadequate public health programs. Foreign travel may also suggest parasitic disease such as amebic liver abscess. Q fever hepatitis may occur in individuals in proximity to livestock. Exposure to drugs, ethanol, and other potential dietary, occupational, or environmental toxins must be reviewed in detail. The information obtained may require supplementation or corroboration by family members or other close associates, especially with regard to ethanol consumption. It is often possible to document previous liver function through recourse to medical records, and this is particularly useful in evaluating the chronicity of liver disease. A family history of jaundice or liver disease may suggest an inherited disorder such as Wilson's disease, α_1-antitrypsin deficiency, or hemochromatosis.

PHYSICAL EXAMINATION. Scleral *icterus* may be detected at a serum bilirubin concentration as low as 2.0 to 2.5 mg per deciliter. Although *spider telangiectasias,* most prominent around the shoulders and upper trunk, and *palmar erythema* are nonspecific and may be present to a limited extent in normal subjects (especially pregnant women), they are potentially important signs of liver disease and usually imply chronicity. Excoriations reflect pruritus and suggest significant cholestasis, not necessarily accompanied by jaundice. *Xanthomas* and *xanthelasmas* are not specific for hepatobiliary disease but may be a sign of prolonged cholestatic hypercholesterolemia. Changes in hair pattern, gynecomastia, and small or soft testes may reflect the *hormonal changes* that accompany cirrhosis in men. Prominence of cutaneous veins in the epigastrium or around the umbilicus may indicate a *portal-systemic collateral circulation* and therefore portal hypertension.

Examination of the heart and lungs may provide evidence of congestive cardiac failure, constrictive pericarditis, or disease of the lungs or pleura that may be associated with liver dysfunction, cause pain referred to the abdomen, or reflect processes involving the subdiaphragmatic regions such as tumor or abscess.

Examination of the *liver* should include documentation of its size and is best recorded both as the distance to which the lower edge extends below the costal margin and its overall vertical span as determined by percussion. These dimensions should be related to a reproducible landmark such as the midclavicular line. The form and consistency of the liver should be noted—e.g., smooth, with sharp edges; nodular and rock-hard; firm with a rounded and irregular edge. A rapidly decreasing liver size during the course of severe acute hepatitis may be a sign of massive hepatic necrosis. An abdominal mass, tenderness, or muscular spasm may suggest secondary involvement of the liver or biliary passages by a neoplastic or inflammatory process. Ascites, most readily detected as dullness or bulging in the flanks, fluid wave, or shifting dullness, may be caused by advanced liver disease and/or by infectious or neoplastic processes. Unfortunately, physical findings of ascites may be unreliable and in equivocal cases abdominal ultrasonography may be helpful.

A diffusely tender and enlarged liver suggests hepatitis or congestion, whereas tenderness in a relatively limited area at or below the lower margin in the region of the interlobal fissure may reflect acute cholecystitis. A visible or palpable gallbladder is abnormal and may be an important sign of primary gallbladder pathology or of cystic or common bile duct obstruction, the latter usually neoplastic in jaundiced patients (Courvoisier's sign). Splenomegaly may be the first evidence of portal hypertension of any cause or may reflect primary splenic pathology such as neoplasm or infection.

Neurologic evaluation is of particular importance with respect to signs of hepatic encephalopathy. These are discussed in detail in Ch. 123, but, as noted, they may be very subtle, consisting initially of a personality change, a mild confusional state, or lethargy. A *flapping tremor* (asterixis), characteristic of metabolic encephalopathy of any cause, is usually present in more obvious cases. In advanced hepatic encephalopathy, almost any form of neurologic abnormality may be present, including seizures, lateralizing signs, and abnormal posturing. Despite this, it is essential in patients with liver disease to consider other causes of central nervous system pathology such as the effects of ethanol, sedatives or other toxins, hypoglycemia, trauma, hemorrhage, infection, and primary or secondary neoplasms.

LABORATORY AND IMAGING STUDIES. These special studies, which may play an essential role in the evaluation and management of diseases of the liver and biliary tract, are discussed in Ch. 116 and 126.

Dooley J, Sherlock S: Diseases of the Liver and Biliary System. 9th ed. Oxford, Blackwell Scientific, 1993.

McIntyre N, Benhamou J-P, Bircher J, et al.: Oxford Textbook of Clinical Hepatology. New York, Oxford University Press, 1993.

Schiff L, Schiff E (eds.): Diseases of the Liver. 7th ed. Philadelphia, JB Lippincott, 1993.

Zakim D, Boyer T (eds.): Hepatology: A Textbook of Liver Disease. 3rd ed. Philadelphia, WB Saunders, 1995.

Four current and comprehensive textbooks that serve to introduce the topic and provide literature references dealing with the broad field of hepatobiliary structure, function, and disease.

114 HEPATIC METABOLISM IN LIVER DISEASE
Richard A. Weisiger

Intermediary metabolism may be profoundly disturbed in liver disease. In some instances, the resulting changes may overshadow the underlying disease process.

CARBOHYDRATE METABOLISM. Except during the absorption of dietary carbohydrate, maintenance of normal blood glucose levels depends entirely on the liver. Two distinct mechanisms are involved; *glycogenolysis* and *gluconeogenesis.* In glycogenolysis, glucose is released from hepatic glycogen by activated glycogen phosphorylase. The process is triggered by the action of glucagon or epinephrine on specific liver cell surface receptors, which activate glycogen phosphorylase kinase via the calcium messenger system. Conversely, insulin stimulates the incorporation of glucose into hepatic glycogen. Normal hepatic glycogen stores are sufficient to sustain blood glucose levels for only about 24 hours. Beyond that, maintenance of blood glucose in the fasting state depends entirely on hepatic gluconeogenesis: the *de novo* synthesis of glucose from precursors including lactate, pyruvate, and amino acids. This process is stimulated by glucagon and epinephrine and inhibited by insulin.

The normally functioning liver continually responds to changes in its nutritional and hormonal milieu. In the fed state (relative excess of insulin and glucose), glucose production by gluconeogenesis and glycogenolysis is minimal. Instead, dietary glucose is either stored as glycogen or converted to fatty acids *(lipogenesis),* largely to be secreted from the liver in the form of triglyceride-rich lipoproteins and destined for storage in adipose tissue. In the fasting state the process is reversed, resulting in mobilization rather than storage of energy substrates. High glucagon levels relative to insulin trigger glycogenolysis and gluconeogenesis. The resulting glucose is no longer diverted to lipogenesis but is released into the plasma. The decrease in fatty acid synthesis is associated with increased fatty acid oxidation, which becomes the principal energy source for the liver.

Failure of these homeostatic mechanisms in liver disease may produce *hypoglycemia* or *glucose intolerance.* Mild hypoglycemia (blood glucose concentrations between 45 and 60 mg per deciliter) occurs in about 50% of patients with uncomplicated acute viral hepatitis. As a rule, these patients are not hyperinsulinemic. Instead, hypoglycemia may reflect several metabolic abnormalities, including diminished glycogen stores, diminished glycogenolytic response to glucagon, diminished gluconeogenesis, and impaired repletion of hepatic glycogen during the fed state. In most cases, the hypoglycemia is not clinically significant, but in severe acute liver injury of any cause, such as virus- or toxin-induced necrosis, hypoglycemia may be profound and life threatening. Hepatic hypoglycemia may also occur in the absence of overt liver damage. For example, *alcoholic hypoglycemia* classically occurs in persons whose only source of calories over a period of days is ethanol, which cannot be metabolically converted to glucose and may inhibit gluconeogenesis. Hypoglycemia should be considered in the differential diagnosis of altered mental status in any patient with significant acute liver disease or exposure to ethanol or other toxins.

Glucose intolerance, on the other hand, is more typically associated with chronic liver disease and cirrhosis. Plasma insulin concentrations tend to be high, suggesting a state of *insulin resistance.* Both the number of insulin receptors and their binding affinity may be diminished in peripheral blood monocytes in liver disease, suggesting a more generalized receptor defect. In addition, insulin resistance may in part reflect increased plasma glucagon concentrations and in part a diminished insulin effect on the liver due to insulin diverted from the liver by portal-systemic shunts. Regardless of the mechanism, the glucose intolerance associated with chronic liver disease is rarely of clinical significance. Occasionally, patients with chronic liver disease may also have other disorders such as *hemochromatosis* (see Ch. 189) and *chronic pancreatitis* (see Ch. 107), in which *diabetes mellitus* may contribute to glucose intolerance.

LIPID METABOLISM. The liver plays a central role in the metabolism of fatty acids and other lipids and lipoproteins. Of the total daily turnover of plasma nonesterified (free) fatty acids derived from adipose tissue, about one third enter the liver, where they are esterified to triglycerides or other esters or undergo oxidation. The balance between esterification and oxidation is closely regulated, as is the rate of *de novo* fatty acid synthesis. In the fasting state, fatty acid synthesis is inhibited, whereas fatty acid oxidation is increased at the expense of the esterification pathways. In the fed state, *de novo* fatty acid synthesis and esterification are favored, whereas oxidation is diminished. Exclusive of dietary sources and *de novo* synthesis, a total of approximately 60 to 70 grams of plasma nonesterified fatty acid (> 200 mmol) is taken up by the liver each day in the average adult. This provides the major energy source for the liver in the fasting state. Interference with hepatic fatty acid metabolism may either cause or be caused by clinically significant abnormalities of hepatic structure and function.

Fatty liver usually reflects excess accumulation of triglyceride, which may be deposited as large vacuoles displacing the nucleus or as small droplets surrounding a central nucleus. It usually reflects an imbalance between the rate of triglyceride biosynthesis and secretion into the plasma, primarily as very low density lipoproteins (VLDL). This imbalance may result from many factors that can affect synthesis, secretion, or both. Conditions associated with large fat droplets in liver cells include obesity, protein-calorie malnutrition (e.g., kwashiorkor, jejunoileal bypass), diabetes mellitus, corticosteroid therapy, and ethanol ingestion (see Ch. 118). Small droplet fat accumulation (see below) is characteristic of acute fatty liver of pregnancy, Reye's syndrome, Jamaican vomiting sickness, and tetracycline and valproic acid hepatotoxicity but is occasionally ethanol related. Triglyceride accumulation in the liver cell is usually associated with hepatomegaly and reflects abnormal liver function but does not *by itself* appear to cause severe, progressive, or lasting liver damage.

Conversely, interference with fatty acid oxidation at any of several stages may have profound consequences. For example, *alcoholic ketosis* is attributed to an ethanol- or acetaldehyde-mediated impairment of the tricarboxylic acid cycle, resulting in incomplete oxidation of the products derived from β-oxidation of fatty acids. Metabolites of hypoglycin—a low molecular weight compound present in the unripened fruit of the ackee tree and the cause of *Jamaican vomiting sickness*—are converted to coenzyme A thioesters and to carnitine derivatives. Because these cannot be metabolized further, they effectively sequester the cellular carnitine pool. Fatty acid oxidation is inhibited, and there is a corresponding decrease in ATP production and gluconeogenesis. Continuing fatty acid esterification under these conditions leads to a form of fatty liver characterized by *small-droplet fat* deposition, associated in severe cases with liver failure and hypoglycemia. This entity is clinically similar to *Reye's syndrome, obstetric fatty liver,* and *tetracycline and valproic acid hepatotoxicity,* but in none of these latter conditions has the pathogenesis been fully elucidated.

The liver is the major source of endogenously synthesized cholesterol (approximately 0.5 gram per day). Together with cholesterol of dietary origin, this newly synthesized cholesterol enters a "metabolically active" hepatic cholesterol pool, the source of cholesterol destined for secretion into bile or into plasma (in lipoproteins), for synthesis of liver cell membranes, and for conversion to bile acids. Approximately half of the total daily turnover of cholesterol goes into synthesizing bile acid and, as such, is an important determinant of body cholesterol stores. Relative rates of secretion of bile acids, cholesterol, and phosphatidyl choline (lecithin) into bile are important factors in the pathogenesis of cholesterol gallstones (see Ch. 126), but the mechanism(s) by which the secretion of these substances is effected and controlled is incompletely understood.

AMINO ACID AND PROTEIN METABOLISM. Except for the immunoglobulins, most plasma proteins, including albumin, clotting factors, transferrin, α_1-antitrypsin, and the nonalimentary lipoproteins, are synthesized in the liver. The synthesis of each is controlled by specific regulatory mechanisms. In all cases, however, synthesis and secretion depend on the integrity of many aspects of cell function, including the transcriptional mechanisms in the nucleus, the translational mechanisms in the rough endoplasmic reticulum, and the secretory mechanisms in the Golgi apparatus. Despite these common features, individual proteins are affected differently in liver disease. This nonuniformity may result from several factors such as the availability of an essential *nutritional* component (e.g., the vitamin K–dependent clotting factors), *hormonal* influences (e.g., VLDL), *genetic* determinants (e.g., ceruloplasmin or α_1-antitrypsin), the effects of drugs or toxins (e.g., the warfarin-like anticoagulants or ethanol), or the response of selected proteins such as fibrinogen (and other "acute phase reactants," including C-reactive proteins, ceruloplasmin, haptoglobin, and transferrin) to inflammatory processes. In addition, the *kinetics* of synthesis and turnover of a particular protein are major determinants of how its plasma concentration responds to acute liver injury. In general, plasma concentrations of proteins with rapid turnover (e.g., clotting factors,

plasma half-time of hours to days) are more likely to be depressed by severe acute liver injury than are those proteins that turn over more slowly (e.g., albumin, plasma half-time about 3 weeks). Finally, *catabolism* of certain plasma proteins may be accelerated (e.g., clotting factors in *disseminated intravascular coagulation,* or albumin in *protein-losing enteropathy*). For these reasons, although liver disease generally tends to depress the plasma concentration of proteins of hepatic origin, plasma concentrations of such proteins may not accurately reflect the severity of the liver disease in a given patient. Interpretation of the prothrombin time, partial thromboplastin time, and serum albumin concentrations in the evaluation of liver disease is discussed in Ch. 116.

Amino acids, in addition to their obvious importance in protein synthesis, also participate in other reactions in the liver. Of special significance is the role of certain amino acids as precursors for gluconeogenesis, as discussed above. Amino acids may undergo *transamination,* in which the α-amino group is transferred to an α-keto group, as in the alanine transaminase (ALT)-mediated deamination of alanine to pyruvate; the resulting transfer of the amino group to α-ketoglutarate converts this acceptor to glutamate. Alternatively, amino acids may undergo *oxidative deamination.* In this case, an α-keto acid is formed as the amino group is converted to ammonium ion and, ultimately, to urea (see below).

BIOTRANSFORMATION AND DETOXIFICATION. The liver is the major site of chemical modification of a variety of exogenous drugs and toxins, as well as endogenous substances such as hormones. The reactions potentially involved are numerous and, in many instances, involve the cytochrome P-450–dependent microsomal mixed function oxidase system. The basic principles of drug disposition are discussed in Ch. 118, but several aspects warrant special emphasis in the context of liver function and disease. First, although biotransformation of an endogenous or exogenous substance may *inactivate* it or render it more suitable for urinary or biliary excretion, many examples exist of compounds that are rendered toxic by this process. A number of clinically significant hepatotoxins are *activated* in this way, and some "idiosyncratic" drug reactions may reflect individual differences in drug metabolism rather than an immunologic response (see Ch. 118). Second, diseases of the liver may seriously impair the biotransformation of exogenous substances, thereby resulting in an *increased sensitivity* to certain drugs (e.g., sedatives and opiates), or may enhance the biologic effect of endogenous hormones (e.g., contributing to the feminizing effects of chronic liver disease) or toxins (e.g., diminished hepatic conversion of ammonia to urea in hepatic encephalopathy). Finally, one substance may significantly influence the hepatic biotransformation of another. Examples of this particular form of *drug-drug interaction* include the well-recognized induction of the microsomal drug-metabolizing system by prior administration of phenobarbital and its inhibition by various toxins.

A particularly important hepatic detoxification pathway converts *ammonium ion* to urea via the Krebs-Henseleit *urea cycle,* in which ornithine, citrulline, argininosuccinate, and arginine are intermediates and which involves both mitochondrial and cytosolic components (see Fig. 178–1). Glutamate, formed from NH_4^+ and α-ketoglutarate, is the principal NH_2 donor. Ammonium ion is produced in abundance in the intestinal tract, especially the colon, by the bacterial degradation of luminal proteins and amino acids and of endogenous urea, 25% of the daily production of which diffuses into the intestinal lumen. The NH_4^+ diffuses into the portal circulation and is transported to the liver, where it is converted to urea by the mechanism described above. *Hepatic encephalopathy* in part reflects the failure of this important detoxification process (or of analogous pathways for other *enterogenous toxins*) owing to extensive acute liver cell necrosis or direct entry of portal blood into the peripheral circulation via spontaneous or surgically created portal-systemic shunts (see Ch. 123).

Arias IM, Jakoby WB, Popper H, et al. (eds.): The Liver: Biology and Pathobiology. New York, Raven Press, 1988. *An in-depth and well-referenced presentation of many basic aspects of normal and abnormal hepatic structure and function.*

Arky RA: Hypoglycemia associated with liver disease and ethanol. Endocrinol Metab Clin North Am 18:75, 1989. *Comprehensive review of this important clinical complication.*

Howden CW, Birnie GG, Brodie MJ: Drug metabolism in liver disease. Pharmacol Ther 40:439, 1989. *Includes practical information on adjusting drug dosages in liver disease.*

Zakim D, Boyer T (eds.): Hepatology: A Textbook of Liver Disease. 2nd ed. Philadelphia, WB Saunders, 1990. *A comprehensive and well-written clinical text with a good foundation in basic metabolism.*

115 BILIRUBIN METABOLISM, HYPERBILIRUBINEMIA, AND APPROACH TO THE JAUNDICED PATIENT

Bruce F. Scharschmidt

This chapter begins with a review of bilirubin metabolism and a summary of the hereditary disorders that lead to hyperbilirubinemia. The subsequent summary of the clinical approach to the patient with jaundice is complemented by other chapters in this section of the book describing specific hepatic disorders that may cause jaundice.

BILIRUBIN METABOLISM (Fig. 115–1)

BILIRUBIN FORMATION. Bilirubin is formed from the breakdown of heme. Daily bilirubin production in adults averages about 4 mg per kilogram body weight. About 70% is derived from the heme moiety of hemoglobin in senescent erythrocytes that are sequestered and degraded in the mononuclear phagocytic cells of the spleen, liver, or bone marrow. Most of the remainder results from the breakdown of nonhemoglobin hemoproteins in the liver, principally the cytochromes P-450. A minor fraction of bilirubin production results from ineffective erythropoiesis, i.e., premature destruction of newly formed erythrocytes in the bone marrow or circulation.

Microsomal heme oxygenase, the heme-cleaving enzyme, is most abundant in the liver, spleen, and bone marrow and exhibits substrate-mediated induction by heme or hemoglobin. The conversion of heme to biliverdin, which is rate limiting for bilirubin formation, is followed by reduction of biliverdin to bilirubin by cytosolic biliverdin reductase. Tinprotoporphyrin, a synthetic metalloporphyrin, is a potent competitive inhibitor of heme oxygenase. This compound may prove useful in reducing bilirubin production and preventing kernicterus in selected infants with hyperbilirubinemia. Mammals, unlike birds, reptiles, and amphibia, convert nontoxic, water-soluble biliverdin to water-insoluble bilirubin. This may reflect the fact that biliverdin, unlike bilirubin, is not able to cross the placenta.

BILIRUBIN CHEMISTRY. Bilirubin consists of four pyrrole rings linked by three carbon bridges. Unconjugated bilirubin is virtually water-insoluble at physiologic pH because its -COOH and -NH groups are involved in strong intramolecular hydrogen bonds and are therefore unable to interact with water. These bonds are disrupted by conjugation of the -COOH groups with glucuronic acid as occurs in the liver cell, thus greatly enhancing the aqueous solubility of the molecule and altering its biologic properties. In contrast to the more polar water-soluble conjugates, relatively nonpolar unconjugated bilirubin diffuses across most biologic membranes such as the blood-brain barrier, placenta, and intestinal and gallbladder epithelium. It is excreted in bile in only trace amounts. Thus, hepatic conjugation permits bilirubin to be eliminated from the body, thereby preventing damage to the central nervous system. Exposure of unconjugated bilirubin to light causes the formation of polar photoisomers and "lumirubin," which results from intramolecular cyclization. These compounds are excreted by the liver without conjugation; their formation is the mechanism by which phototherapy lowers serum bilirubin concentration in neonatal hyperbilirubinemia.

BILIRUBIN BINDING TO PLASMA PROTEINS. Unconjugated bilirubin is bound reversibly to albumin at a primary high affinity site (10^8 M^{-1}). At plasma concentrations exceeding its molar equivalence with albumin (about 35 mg per deciliter), bilirubin also binds to at least two low-affinity sites. A variety of compounds, including certain sulfonamides, penicillin derivatives, furosemide, and radiographic contrast media, may displace bilirubin from its albumin-binding sites and increase the risk of kernicterus in neonates. Presumably because of its tight albumin binding and low water solubility, unconjugated bilirubin is not excreted in urine. Conjugated bilirubin is somewhat less tightly bound to albumin than is bilirubin. It is filtered to a greater extent at the glomerulus, is incompletely reabsorbed by the renal tubules, and therefore appears in the urine in small amounts in patients with conjugated hyperbilirubinemia.

In addition to the reversible binding to albumin just described, another bilirubin fraction binds very tightly, perhaps covalently, to albumin. This pigment fraction has a serum half-life of about 17 days, similar to that of albumin. It has been detected only in patients with conjugated hyperbilirubinemia, in whom it accounts for a varying (8 to 90%) fraction of total bilirubin (see below). This protein-bound fraction helps explain the occasionally slow resolution of hyperbilirubinemia in patients convalescing from hepatitis or in whom biliary obstruction has been relieved, as well as the disappearance of bilirubinuria in these patients prior to the resolution of jaundice.

HEPATIC BILIRUBIN TRANSPORT. Uptake of bilirubin and other substances tightly bound to protein is facilitated by large fenestrations in the cells of the sinusoidal lining that permit plasma proteins to enter the space of Disse and directly contact the hepatocyte plasma membrane. Uptake of bilirubin and other organic anions such as sulfobromophthalein is mediated by a recently cloned carrier protein with a molecular weight of 74 kD. Once inside the liver cell, bilirubin and other organic anions appear to bind to cytoplasmic proteins such as ligandin. Ligandin, which constitutes 2% of cytoplasmic protein in human liver, may alter net uptake by re-

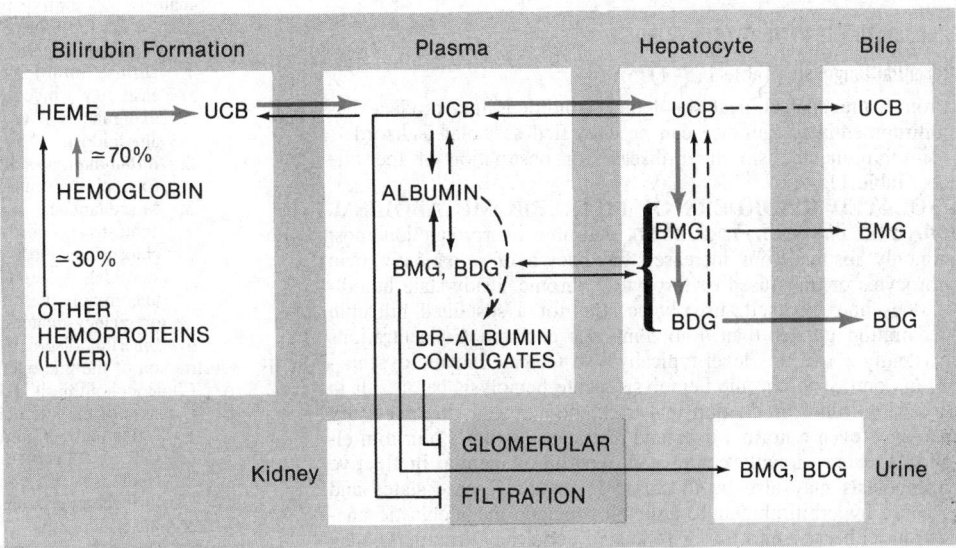

FIGURE 115–1. Overview of bilirubin metabolism. Unconjugated bilirubin (UCB) formed from the breakdown of hemoglobin heme and other hemoproteins is transported in plasma reversibly bound to albumin and is converted in the liver to bilirubin monoglucuronide (BMG) and diglucuronide (BDG), the latter being the predominant form secreted in bile. BMG and BDG together normally account for <5% of serum bilirubin. In the presence of hepatobiliary disease, BMG and BDG accumulate in plasma and appear in urine. Bilirubin glucuronides in plasma also react nonenzymatically with albumin and possibly other serum proteins to form protein conjugates, which do not appear in urine and have a plasma half-life similar to that of albumin.

ducing bilirubin efflux back into plasma. In addition to transport through the cytoplasm, bilirubin may be directly transferred from the plasma membrane to the membranes of the endoplasmic reticulum, where conjugation occurs.

In the process of conjugation, the carboxyl groups of one or both propionic acid side chains of bilirubin are esterified, usually with glucuronic acid. Glucose and xylose conjugates are formed in trace amounts only. Formation of bilirubin monoglucuronide and diglucuronide is catalyzed by microsomal UDP-glucuronyl-transferase. Secretion of conjugated bilirubin from the hepatocyte into the bile canaliculus occurs predominantly via an ATP-dependent process which also appears to mediate the transport of other amphipathic 400 to 1000 kD organic anions, including sulfobromophthalein, glutathione conjugates, sulfate and glucuronide conjugates of bile acids, and certain cysteinyl leukotrienes. Mutant rats defective for this carrier exhibit a disorder that closely mimics the human *Dubin-Johnson syndrome.* Excretion and/or conjugation, but not uptake, appears to be rate limiting for overall bilirubin transport from blood to bile. Bilirubin diglucuronide predominates in human bile (70 to 80%), with the isomeric monoglucuronides present in small amounts.

ENTEROHEPATIC CIRCULATION. Absorption of conjugated bilirubin from the gallbladder and small intestine is negligible. In the terminal ileum and colon, conjugated bilirubin is hydrolyzed by bacterial enzymes to form unconjugated bilirubin, which is converted into colorless urobilinogens and related products, including urobilins. Most urobilinogen absorbed from the intestine is re-excreted in bile and ultimately in feces; a small fraction appears in urine. Urobilinogen is absent from the bile and urine of patients with complete biliary obstruction; however, fecal and urinary urobilinogen levels correlate poorly with bilirubin production rate and are of little clinical utility. In addition to urobilins, the normal brown color of stool may reflect the presence of nonbilirubin pigments, perhaps of plant origin, which are also excreted in bile and undergo enterohepatic circulation.

CONCENTRATION IN PLASMA. Plasma bilirubin concentration, which ranges normally between 0.3 and 1.0 mg per deciliter, varies directly with bilirubin production and inversely with hepatic bilirubin clearance. About 95% of circulating bilirubin in healthy adults is unconjugated. In contrast, circulating bilirubin in patients with hepatocellular or biliary tract disease consists predominantly of monoconjugates and diconjugates. The conventional diazoassay, which is employed in most clinical laboratories, tends to overestimate the conjugated fraction, particularly at low concentrations of total bilirubin. The tightly, perhaps covalently bound conjugated bilirubin fraction reacts directly with the diazoreagent but is often removed by the deproteinizing step used in many laboratories. Nonetheless, for practical clinical application, conventional laboratory techniques are generally adequate. While more accurate methods to measure conjugated and unconjugated serum bilirubin have been developed, they are not readily automated and therefore not widely available.

APPROACH TO THE PATIENT WITH JAUNDICE

Differential Diagnosis (Table 115–1)

From a practical clinical standpoint, conditions that produce hyperbilirubinemia or jaundice can be classified as isolated disorders of bilirubin metabolism, liver disease, or obstruction of the bile ducts (Table 115–1).

ISOLATED DISORDERS OF BILIRUBIN METABOLISM. *Increased Bilirubin Production.* Bilirubin overproduction most commonly results from increased breakdown of a patient's own erythrocytes or transfused erythrocytes. Chronic steady-state hemolysis does not, by itself, usually account for a sustained bilirubin concentration greater than 4 to 5 mg per deciliter. Concentrations consistently above this level typically also indicate hepatic dysfunction. In contrast to chronic hemolysis, acute hemolysis can result in a rate of bilirubin production that transiently exceeds the excretory capacity of even a normal liver and may cause striking bilirubin elevation and occasionally conjugated hyperbilirubinemia. Ineffective erythropoiesis may also be increased in certain disease states and can cause hyperbilirubinemia. Examples include megaloblastic anemia from either vitamin B_{12} or folic acid deficiency, iron deficiency

anemia, sideroblastic anemia, thalassemia minor, polycythemia vera, aplasia, and lead poisoning. Markedly increased ineffective erythropoiesis is the basis of the rare disorder known as *shunt hyperbilirubinemia* or *idiopathic dyserythropoietic jaundice.* Bilirubin overproduction may also result from the resorption of large hematomas in patients who have suffered major trauma.

Decreased Hepatic Bilirubin Clearance (Table 115–2). The hereditary disorders of hepatic bilirubin metabolism are characterized by impaired ability of the liver to transport or conjugate bilirubin. The common, benign entity of *Gilbert's syndrome* and the rare, almost uniformly lethal type I *Crigler-Najjar syndrome* represent opposite ends of this spectrum. Routine tests of liver function are generally normal in all these disorders, but a variety of abnormalities in the hepatic handling of bilirubin and other compounds such as sulfobromophthalein have been described. Many of these disorders, including Gilbert's syndrome, the *Dubin-Johnson syndrome,* and *Rotor's syndrome,* may be mistaken for acquired hepatobiliary disease.

Gilbert's Syndrome. Because of its frequency (up to 7% of the population), Gilbert's syndrome is the disorder most likely to be encountered by the clinician. Mild unconjugated hyperbilirubinemia is recognized most commonly during the second and third decades of life because of the presence of scleral icterus, often first noted with fasting or as an incidental laboratory finding. Although a variety of nonspecific symptoms have been described, it is unlikely that any significant symptoms are attributable to Gilbert's syndrome itself. Gilbert's syndrome results from a decrease in the hepatic clearance of unconjugated bilirubin, probably due to impaired conjugation. Up to one half of patients with Gilbert's syndrome have a very slight decrease in red cell survival detectable by ^{51}Cr labeling. The principal clinical importance of this disorder is that it may be confused with more serious acquired hepatobiliary disease. From a practical standpoint, the diagnosis of Gilbert's syndrome is made by demonstrating low-grade unconjugated hyperbilirubinemia in a patient with a normal physical examination and otherwise normal biochemical tests who has no biochemical or clinical evidence of hemolysis. Liver biopsy to demonstrate normal histology is usually

TABLE 115–1. DIFFERENTIAL DIAGNOSIS OF JAUNDICE

I. Isolated disorders of bilirubin metabolism
   A. Increased bilirubin production. Examples: hemolysis, blood transfusion, resorption of hematomas, ineffective erythropoiesis
   B. Decreased hepatic bilirubin clearance.
     1. Decreased uptake or conjugation of bilirubin. Examples: Gilbert's syndrome, Crigler-Najjar syndrome, physiologic jaundice of the newborn
     2. Decreased canalicular secretion of bilirubin. Examples: Dubin-Johnson syndrome, Rotor's syndrome
II. Liver disease
   A. Acute or chronic hepatocellular disease. Examples: viral hepatitis, hepatotoxins (e.g., ethanol, acetaminophen), drugs (e.g., isoniazid, methyldopa), ischemia (e.g., hypotension, vascular occlusion), metabolic or inherited disorders (e.g., Wilson's disease, hemochromatosis, α_1-antitrypsin deficiency), pregnancy-related disorders (e.g., acute fatty liver of pregnancy, pre-eclampsia)
   B. Hepatic disorders with prominent cholestasis
     1. Diffuse infiltrative disorders. Examples: granulomatous disease (e.g., mycobacterial infections, sarcoidosis), infiltrative malignancies (e.g., lymphoma, malignant histiocytosis), amyloidosis
     2. Inflammation of intrahepatic bile ductules and/or portal tracts. Examples: primary biliary cirrhosis, graft-versus-host disease
     3. Miscellaneous conditions. Examples: benign recurrent cholestasis, postoperative hyperbilirubinemia, drugs (e.g., chlorpromazine, estrogen-containing compounds, anabolic steroids), systemic bacterial infections, parenteral nutrition, uncommon presentations of viral or alcoholic liver disease, pregnancy-related (e.g., cholestasis of pregnancy)
     4. Inherited disorders. Examples: arteriohepatic dysplasia
III. Obstruction of the bile ducts
   A. Choledocholithiasis. Examples: cholesterol or pigment gallstones
   B. Diseases of the bile ducts
     1. Inflammation/infection. Examples: primary sclerosing cholangitis, AIDS cholangiopathy, hepatic arterial chemotherapy
     2. Neoplasms. Example: cholangiocarcinoma
   C. Extrinsic compression of the biliary tree. Examples: neoplasms, chronic pancreatitis

not necessary. An exaggerated hyperbilirubinemic response to fasting, lipid withdrawal, or nicotinic acid has been found to be helpful by some investigators, but these tests are neither sensitive nor specific enough to warrant routine use. In patients with overt hemolysis, direct measurement of hepatic bilirubin clearance may be necessary to establish the diagnosis.

Fasting and Hyperbilirubinemia. Fasting increases the plasma concentration of unconjugated, indirect-reacting bilirubin owing primarily to a decrease in hepatic bilirubin clearance. This effect may be particularly marked in patients with Gilbert's syndrome and the type II Crigler-Najjar syndrome. Both dietary composition and total caloric intake are important because a normocaloric but lipid-free diet produces a response similar to that observed with complete fasting, and the effect of complete fasting is reversed by feeding small amounts of lipid. The mechanism of the decrease in hepatic bilirubin clearance with fasting is unclear. A slight increase in bilirubin production contributes to fasting hyperbilirubinemia.

LIVER DISEASE. Jaundice is a common manifestation of acute or chronic hepatic disease of nearly all types. The differential diagnosis is extensive and is outlined briefly in Table 115–1. These disorders are described in more detail in other chapters in this section. Although an accurate diagnosis is possible in most patients based upon clinical findings and biochemical studies (see below), certain hepatic disorders may be associated with cholestasis as their major manifestation, and these disorders are most likely to cause diagnostic confusion. These include infiltrative disorders, disorders that particularly affect the intrahepatic biliary tree, and certain other inflammatory or neoplastic conditions (Table 115–1).

Benign Recurrent Cholestasis. This familial syndrome of unknown cause is associated with intermittent and recurrent episodes of malaise, pruritus, and jaundice. These episodes of cholestasis last from days to months and are separated by asymptomatic periods with normal biochemical hepatic function.

Postoperative Hyperbilirubinemia. Jaundice in the postoperative patient is likely multifactorial in origin, with both increased

bilirubin production (e.g., breakdown of transfused erythrocytes, resorption of hematomas) and decreased hepatic clearance (e.g., bacteremia, parenteral nutrition, perioperative or postoperative hypoxia) as contributing factors. Hyperbilirubinemia is the most prominent biochemical manifestation and may be accompanied by a several-fold elevation of alkaline phosphatase or gamma-glutamyl transpeptidase. Transaminases are minimally elevated, and synthetic function is typically normal. The differential diagnosis includes biliary obstruction or liver disease due to shock, anesthetic injury, or post-transfusion hepatitis. Postoperative jaundice in the liver transplant patient presents a special problem, as the differential diagnosis also includes liver injury during organ preservation, rejection, and lymphoproliferative disorders. Postoperative jaundice *per se* does not pose a threat to the patient and typically resolves in 1 to 2 weeks as the overall condition of the patient improves.

OBSTRUCTION OF THE BILE DUCTS. Obstruction of the biliary tree can be caused by gallstones, neoplastic or inflammatory disorders of the biliary tree, or extrinsic compression. These disorders are summarized briefly in Table 115–1 and are described in more detail in other chapters in this section (see Ch. 126).

DIAGNOSTIC APPROACH TO THE PATIENT WITH JAUNDICE. The diagnostic approach (Fig. 115–2) to the jaundiced patient begins with a careful patient history, physical examination, screening laboratory studies, and formulation of a differential diagnosis. The multiplicity of currently available tests for imaging the biliary tree represents a major advance. However, if tests are employed indiscriminately or redundantly, the patient is exposed to unnecessary discomfort, risk, and expense. The rational selection of these tests is based on the initial differential diagnosis and the likelihood that further evaluation will yield beneficial information.

History and Physical Examination. A serum bilirubin of ≥ 3 mg per deciliter is usually required for jaundice or scleral icterus to be clinically evident. In evaluating a patient with jaundice, the dis-

TABLE 115–2. THE HEREDITARY DISORDERS OF HEPATIC BILIRUBIN METABOLISM

	Gilbert's Syndrome	Type I Crigler-Najjar Syndrome	Type II Crigler-Najjar Syndrome	Dubin-Johnson Syndrome	Rotor's Syndrome
Incidence	Up to 7% of population	Very rare	Uncommon	Uncommon	Rare
Inheritance	? Autosomal dominant	Autosomal recessive	? Autosomal dominant	Autosomal recessive	Autosomal recessive
Defect(s) in bilirubin metabolism	Decreased hepatic UDP-glucuronyl-transferase activity, (?) slow hepatic bilirubin uptake, associated mild hemolysis in up to 50% of patients	Absence of hepatic UDP-glucuronyltransferase activity	Markedly decreased or undetectable UDP-glucuronyltransferase activity	Impaired ATP-dependent canalicular secretion of conjugated bilirubin	Impaired biliary excretion of conjugated bilirubin
Plasma bilirubin concentration (mg/dl)	≤ 3 in absence of fasting or hemolysis, predominantly unconjugated	17–50, usually > 20, all unconjugated	6–45, usually < 20, all unconjugated	1–25, usually < 7, about 60% conjugated	1–20, usually < 7, about 60% conjugated
Clinical sequelae	None	Death in infancy from kernicterus in almost all cases	Usually none, rarely kernicterus	Probably none	Probably none
Plasma sulfobromophthalein disappearance rate	Mildly abnormal in some patients (45-minute retention <15%)	Usually normal	Usually normal	Slow initial disappearance with frequent secondary rise (45-minute retention < 20%)	Markedly slowed, no secondary rise (45-minute retention 30–50%)
Oral cholecystography	Normal	Normal	Normal	Faint or nonvisualization	Usually normal
Hepatic histology (light microscopy)	Normal, occasionally increased lipofuscin	Normal	Normal	Coarse pigment in centrolobular cells	Normal
Reduction of plasma bilirubin concentration by phenobarbital	Yes	No	Yes	Minimal	Unknown
Diagnosis	Clinical and laboratory findings, response to fasting occasionally helpful, liver biopsy not usually necessary	Clinical and laboratory findings, lack of response to phenobarbital	Clinical and laboratory findings, response to phenobarbital	Clinical and laboratory findings, sulfobromophthalein disappearance, urinary coproporphyrin excretion	Clinical and laboratory findings, sulfobromophthalein disappearance, urinary coproporphyrin excretion
Treatment	None necessary	Liver transplantation; other measures not uniformly effective	Phenobarbital if bilirubin concentration markedly elevated	None available, avoid estrogens (may worsen jaundice)	None available

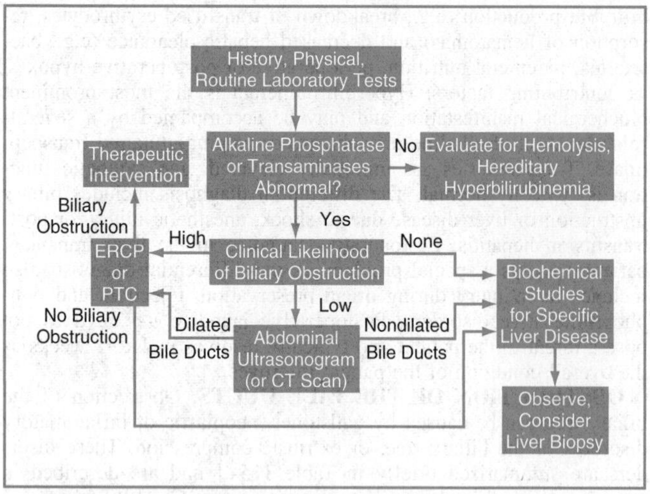

FIGURE 115–2. Approach to the patient with jaundice. (From Lidofsky SO, Scharschmidt BF: Jaundice. *In* Sleisenger MH, Fordtran JS, Scharschmidt BF, Feldman M (eds.): Gastrointestinal Disease. 5th ed. Philadelphia, WB Saunders, 1993, p 759.)

tinction between liver disease and extrahepatic obstruction is generally the most difficult and important aspect of the differential diagnosis. Potentially helpful clinical clues are listed in Table 115–3. Fever and rigors and pain in the right upper abdominal quadrant suggest cholangitis and hence biliary obstruction, as do past biliary surgery or an abdominal mass. Certain causes of jaundice such as gallstone disease and malignant neoplasm are more common in the elderly. Risk factors for liver disease (e.g., hepatitis exposure, transfusions, intravenous drug use, alcohol use) or physical evidence of cirrhosis (e.g., spider angiomata, gynecomastia, ascites, splenomegaly) should all raise the possibility of intrinsic liver disease.

Initial Laboratory Studies. Initial studies should include a complete blood count as well as measurement of serum bilirubin concentration, activities of alkaline phosphatase and transaminases (AST and ALT), and prothrombin time. If hepatic tests other than bilirubin are normal, one should consider an isolated disorder of bilirubin metabolism (see Table 115–1). Patterns of abnormalities that help distinguish intrinsic liver disease from biliary obstruction are summarized in Table 115–3. However, many exceptions to these general patterns exist, and hepatic disorders associated with prominent cholestasis (see Table 115–1) may mimic biliary obstruction. It is also worth emphasizing that both gamma-glutamyl transpeptidase and alkaline phosphatase are typically elevated in patients with cholestasis. The combination of an elevated alkaline phosphatase and normal gamma-glutamyl transpeptidase suggests

that the alkaline phosphatase is from bone. Conversely, an isolated elevation of gamma-glutamyl transpeptidase may result from using certain drugs (e.g., phenytoin) or alcohol even in the absence of liver disease.

IMAGING STUDIES. If extrahepatic obstruction is suspected, further evaluation should determine its site and nature (Fig. 115–2; Table 115–4). A reasonable next step is the use of a noninvasive study such as *ultrasonography* or *computed tomography* (CT) to determine whether the intra- and/or extrahepatic biliary system is dilated, thereby implying mechanical obstruction.

The accuracy and comparative advantages and disadvantages of these two imaging techniques as well as those of endoscopic retrograde cholangiopancreatography (ERCP) and percutaneous cholangiography (PTC) are summarized in Table 115–4. Because of its lesser experience, lack of radiation exposure, portability and convenience, ultrasonography is often used as a first procedure when obstruction is considered. CT may be preferred when precise definition of anatomic structure and information about the level of obstruction are desired. Both studies may occasionally fail to identify dilated ducts in obstructed patients with cirrhosis and poorly compliant hepatic parenchyma or in patients with primary sclerosing cholangitis. On the other hand, the presence of dilated ducts in a patient who has previously undergone cholecystectomy does not necessarily signify obstruction.

If dilated ducts are identified, it is generally appropriate to directly visualize the biliary tree by ERCP or PTC. ERCP involves passing an endoscope into the duodenum, introducing a catheter into the ampulla of Vater, and injecting contrast medium into the distal common bile duct and/or pancreatic duct. PTC involves percutaneous passage of a needle through the hepatic parenchyma and injection of contrast into the proximal biliary tree via a peripheral bile duct. The choice between these two procedures depends on factors including the suspected location of the obstruction (proximal versus distal); the presence of a coagulation disorder or prior gastroduodenal surgery that might preclude, respectively, PTC or ERCP; anticipation of a therapeutic maneuver such as stent placement or sphincterotomy; and the availability of skilled personnel.

Selection of Imaging Tests. The choice of which imaging technique to use depends on the likelihood of biliary obstruction based on the initial clinical evaluation (Fig. 115–2). If the likelihood of obstruction is judged negligible (e.g., clinical findings and biochemical and serologic tests consistent with viral hepatitis), no imaging studies are necessary. Conversely, if the likelihood of obstruction is judged to be very high (e.g., fever and rigors in a patient with recent biliary tract surgery), direct cholangiography may be an appropriate initial choice. If obstruction is considered possible but not highly likely, noninvasive imaging with ultrasonography or CT is a reasonable first study.

Other Imaging Studies. Magnetic resonance imaging (MRI) can detect dilated ducts in patients with obstruction. However, it

TABLE 115–3. CLINICAL CLUES IN THE DIFFERENTIAL DIAGNOSIS OF JAUNDICE

	Suggests Biliary Obstruction	Suggests Liver Disease
History	Abdominal pain, fever and rigors, prior biliary surgery, older age	Symptoms suggestive of viral prodrome, known hepatitis exposure, receipt of blood products, use of alcohol or intravenous drugs, exposure to hepatotoxins
Physical examination	High fever, abdominal tenderness, abdominal mass, or surgical scar	Stigmata of liver disease (e.g., ascites, gynecomastia, spider angiomata, dilated periumbilical veins), asterixis, encephalopathy
Laboratory studies	Predominant elevation of bilirubin and alkaline phosphatase, elevated serum amylase, prolonged prothrombin time corrects with vitamin K	Predominant elevation of serum transaminases, tests indicative of specific liver disease (e.g., hepatitis serologies)

TABLE 115–4. IMAGING STUDIES IN THE EVALUATION OF JAUNDICE

Test	Advantages	Disadvantages
Ultrasonography	Noninvasive, portable, least expensive	May be difficult in presence of bowel gas or obesity, not as sensitive or specific as ERCP or PTC
Computed tomography	Noninvasive, high resolution	Not portable, costly, typically requires contrast, not as sensitive or specific as ERCP or PTC
ERCP	Direct visualization of bile ducts with contrast, endoscopic examination, and biopsy may permit therapy (e.g., stenting of distal lesions; papillotomy for stone removal)	Invasive, may not be possible in patients with surgically altered anatomy (e.g., Billroth II or Roux-en-Y gastrojejunostomy)
PTC	Direct visualization of bile ducts with contrast, may permit therapy (e.g., stenting of proximal lesions)	Invasive, difficult in absence of dilated bile ducts

has been studied less extensively than ultrasonography or CT, it is more expensive, and it is uncertain whether it offers any advantage over these other techniques. *Hepatobiliary scintigraphy,* while occasionally helpful in the diagnosis of cholecystitis, is not sufficiently accurate to be used in most patients with suspected obstruction. *Intravenous cholangiography* and *oral cholecystography* currently have little or no role in the evaluation of biliary obstruction. *Liver biopsy* is not indicated in the routine evaluation of suspected obstruction, because findings diagnostic of obstruction are often absent even in the presence of biliary disease, and the biopsy usually provides no information about the type or location of the obstruction. Liver biopsy should generally be reserved for the differential diagnosis of difficult or confusing cases of intrahepatic cholestasis (Fig. 115–2).

Treatment

The treatment of hyperbilirubinemia, of course, depends on the cause. Apart from liver transplantation or phenobarbital for types I and II Crigler-Najjar syndrome, respectively, no specific therapy is available or necessary for hereditary disorders of bilirubin metabolism (see Table 115–2). Therapy in patients with increased bilirubin production should be directed at the underlying disorder, typically hemolysis. Little specific therapy is available for patients with cholestasis due to hepatic parenchymal disease. Offending agents such as drugs or alcohol should be withdrawn when possible, and transplantation is appropriate for patients with progressive cholestasis and hepatic dysfunction due to primary biliary cirrhosis or other disorders.

In patients with prolonged cholestasis and fat malabsorption, orally or parenterally administered fat-soluble vitamins may be necessary, as well as alteration of the amount or type (e.g., medium-chain triglycerides) of dietary fat. *Pruritus* can be a disabling manifestation of cholestasis and may be improved by bathing less frequently and using skin softeners. *Cholestyramine* should be tried in patients with more severe pruritus. The choleretic bile acid, *ursodeoxycholic acid,* has been shown to produce biochemical improvement in patients with certain cholestatic disorders (e.g., primary biliary cirrhosis, possibly primary sclerosing cholangitis). However, this agent does not consistently improve pruritus and it is unknown whether it alters the course of these disorders. Other agents (antihistamines, charcoal, rifampin, plasma exchange) are not of established benefit.

Arias IM, Che M, Gatmaitan A, et al.: The biology of the bile canaliculus. Hepatology 17:318, 1993. *A thorough yet concise review focusing on new information regarding the secretion of bilirubin by hepatocytes.*

Jacquemin E, Hagenbuch B, Stieger B, et al.: Expression cloning of a rat liver Na(+)-independent organic anion transporter. Proc Natl Acad Sci USA 91:133, 1994. *A concise article illustrating the impact of molecular biologic techniques in defining mechanisms of bilirubin transport.*

Scharschmidt BF: Bilirubin metabolism, bile formation, and gallbladder and bile duct function. *In* Sleisenger MH, Fordtran JS, Scharschmidt BF, Feldman M (eds.): Gastrointestinal Disease. 5th ed. Philadelphia, WB Saunders, 1993. Lidofsky SD, Scharschmidt BF: Jaundice. Ibid. p 1765. *Two thoroughly referenced contemporary reviews.*

Tiribelli C, Ostrow JD: New concepts in bilirubin chemistry, transport and metabolism: Report of the Second International Bilirubin Workshop, April 9–11, 1992, Trieste, Italy. Hepatology 17:715, 1993. *A review focusing on emerging concepts and controversies regarding the transport and metabolism of bilirubin.*

116 LABORATORY TESTS IN LIVER DISEASE
Richard A. Weisiger

Common liver tests fall into two categories—liver injury tests such as release of hepatic enzymes (often incorrectly called "liver function" tests) and true tests of liver function. Specific functions of the liver include clearance of toxic substances from the blood (including drugs, metabolites, and bacterial toxins), synthesis of plasma proteins and lipoproteins, and intermediary metabolism (e.g., glucose and ammonia) (see Ch. 114). Depending on the disease process, some of these functions may be highly compromised

while others remain nearly normal. Most liver tests provide only indirect evidence of hepatic integrity, and some may be abnormal for reasons other than liver disease. For these reasons, liver tests are most valuable when they are carefully selected and interpreted within the total clinical context. In most cases, serial determinations are required to assess the evolution of the disease.

ENZYME ASSAYS

A number of disorders, including inflammation, necrosis, and biliary obstruction, result in the release of hepatic enzymes into the blood. Enzyme release is an indirect indication of disease activity and does not measure liver function. Nevertheless, these tests are often useful for screening and for following the level of disease activity in a given patient.

TRANSAMINASES. *Transaminases (aminotransferases)* catalyze the transfer of the α-amino group from aspartate or alanine to the α-keto group of ketoglutarate; they are named according to the amino donor group. Serum levels of aspartate transaminase (AST, formerly SGOT) and alanine transferase (ALT, formerly SGPT) are typically below 40 IU per liter in normal patients but may exceed 1000 IU in acute viral or toxic injury. Different isozymes of AST are present in liver cell mitochondria and cytoplasm, whereas ALT is confined to the cytoplasm. Transaminases are not cleared from the blood by excretion into urine or bile. Serum levels of AST and ALT are elevated in most hepatic diseases; the height of the transaminase activity in general reflects the current activity of the disease process. However, transaminase levels correlate poorly with disease severity and prognosis. Moreover, there are important exceptions. Even the most severe forms of *alcoholic hepatitis,* for example, rarely increase transaminase levels above 200 to 300 IU per liter (see Ch. 118). In contrast, serum transaminase activities of 1000 IU or more are often present in mild acute *viral hepatitis* or shortly after acute *biliary obstruction,* as may occur during passage of a gallstone. Conversely, serum transaminase levels may fall during the clinical course of massive hepatic necrosis, suggesting that the liver is so severely damaged that little enzyme activity remains (see Ch. 123).

Despite these caveats, serum transaminase activities are helpful in many circumstances. Transaminase determination is a relatively specific *screening test* for hepatobiliary disease. Although AST levels may be increased in diseases of other organs (e.g., myocardium and skeletal muscle), values more than 10 times the upper limit of the normal range usually reflect hepatic or biliary pathology. In the context of other clinical and laboratory findings, identification of the source of increased serum transaminase activity is not usually difficult. Transaminase values are also useful in *monitoring the course of acute or chronic parenchymal liver disease,* although they may be misleading in certain cases, as noted earlier. Finally, they may be useful diagnostically. It is distinctly uncommon for the AST to exceed 15 times the upper limit of normal in chronic bile duct obstruction without cholangitis. Because hepatic ALT is a cytoplasmic enzyme while most AST is sequestered in mitochondria, a high ratio of AST to ALT often indicates severe hepatocellular necrosis (such as *alcoholic hepatititis*). Milder insults that cause leakage of cytoplasmic enzymes commonly produce a ratio of 1 or less.

ALKALINE PHOSPHATASE. *Alkaline phosphatases,* present in many tissues (e.g., liver, bile ducts, intestine, bone, kidney, placenta, and leukocytes), catalyze the release of orthophosphate from ester substrates at alkaline pH. The normal serum activity in adults is 25 to 85 IU per liter, although higher levels are normal in children and in pregnancy. The biologic function of alkaline phosphatase is unknown, except for an apparent role in the deposition of hydroxyapatite in osteoid to form bone. Normally, serum alkaline phosphatase activity reflects mainly the hepatic and bone isozymes, although occasionally the intestinal form may account for 20 to 60% of the total. In the later stages of pregnancy, the placental contribution may be substantial. A less common variant, called the *Regan isozyme,* is associated with tumors (especially hepatoma and lung cancer) and appears identical to the placental form (see Ch. 125).

Serum alkaline phosphatase activity may be increased in many conditions not associated with hepatobiliary disease, including bone disorders (e.g., Paget's disease, osteomalacia, metastases to bone), pregnancy, normal growth, and occasionally the presence of malignancy not involving bones or liver. In some cases, the source is obvious because of other clinical and laboratory findings. When the source is less apparent, methods such as heat stability and electrophoretic separation are available to differentiate hepatobiliary from other isozymes. However, it is usually more practical to measure serum levels of *5'-nucleotidase* (5'-NT), *leucine aminopeptidase* (LAP), or *gamma-glutamyl transpeptidase* (GGTP), which tend to parallel alkaline phosphatase in hepatobiliary disease but do not usually increase in bone disease (see next section). The increased serum activity in liver disease reflects increased enzyme synthesis rather than decreased biliary excretion or leakage from damaged cells and may be triggered by high tissue bile salt concentrations.

Slight to moderate increases in serum alkaline phosphatase activity (up to twice normal) occur in many parenchymal disorders of the liver such as *hepatitis* and *cirrhosis*. In the absence of bone disease, larger increases (3 to 10 times normal) usually indicate obstruction of bile flow. Although the highest levels usually occur with extrahepatic bile duct obstruction, very high levels may also be seen with *intrahepatic cholestasis* and with infiltrative or mass lesions (primary or metastatic *cancer, lymphoma, leukemia,* or *sarcoidosis*). The serum alkaline phosphatase level rarely remains normal in the presence of significant bile duct obstruction. Increased alkaline phosphatase may be the only clinically apparent abnormality in bile duct stricture or in lesions that produce obstruction of a single hepatic lobe or segment. Its measurement, therefore, offers a relatively sensitive screening test for primary or metastatic tumors of the liver. As many as one third of patients with isolated elevations of serum hepatobiliary alkaline phosphatase activity have no demonstrable liver or biliary disease.

OTHER HEPATIC ENZYMES. LAP is a ubiquitous cellular peptidase, while 5'-NT is a plasma membrane enzyme that cleaves orthophosphate from the 5' position on the pentose sugar of adenosine or inosine phosphate. The serum activity of both enzymes usually increases in cholestasis, and their major clinical value is to help determine if an elevated serum alkaline phosphatase activity originates from the liver. A parallel elevation of the serum activity of either of these enzymes suggests a hepatobiliary origin of the alkaline phosphatase, but the converse is not true. Serum levels of liver alkaline phosphatase may occasionally be increased while LAP and 5'-NT levels remain normal. Because both of these enzymes may be increased in late pregnancy, they are most useful in the nonpregnant patient.

GGTP, present in many tissues, increases in serum not only in hepatobiliary disease but also after myocardial infarction, in neuromuscular diseases, in pancreatic disease (even in the absence of biliary obstruction), in pulmonary disease, in diabetes, and during the ingestion of ethanol and other inducers of microsomal enzymes. The measurement of GGTP has been proposed as a sensitive screening test for hepatobiliary disease and for monitoring the abstinence from ethanol, but its high sensitivity ensures that many who test positive will have no identifiable liver disease on further study. It offers no clear advantage over LAP or 5'-NT for identifying the source of increased serum alkaline phosphatase activity except in pregnancy.

Lactate dehydrogenase (LDH) is often elevated in liver disease but is usually not helpful in diagnosis because it is also found in most other body tissues.

CLEARANCE OF METABOLITES AND DRUGS

A major function of the liver is to remove various metabolites and absorbed toxins from the blood (see Ch. 118). In liver disease, clearance of these compounds may be impaired owing to loss of parenchymal cells, obstruction of bile flow, reduced cellular uptake, or reduced hepatic blood flow. When a metabolite is produced at a relatively constant rate (as is usually true for bilirubin), its serum level can be a sensitive indicator of liver function. The removal rate of certain exogenous drugs and dye compounds from plasma can be used similarly.

BILIRUBIN. The metabolism of bilirubin and its measurement are discussed in detail in Ch. 115. Serum bilirubin is usually elevated in significant liver disease but may be elevated in benign disorders such as Gilbert syndrome and nonhepatic diseases such as hemolysis and ineffective erythropoesis.

BILE ACIDS. Bile acids, absorbed from the ileum in an active recycling process, are nearly completely removed by the liver before they reach the systemic circulation. Impaired hepatic uptake or reflux from blocked bile ducts can lead to high plasma levels of bile acids and result in severe pruritus. Quantitation of serum bile acids has little proven clinical utility at present, however.

AMMONIA. The liver clears ammonia from blood by converting it to urea via the Krebs-Henseleit cycle for excretion by the kidney (Fig. 178–1). In the setting of severe hepatic dysfunction (e.g., fulminant hepatic failure) or portosystemic shunting, serum ammonia levels rise. The level of serum ammonia is widely used to confirm the diagnosis of hepatic encephalopathy and to monitor the success of therapy, but the correlation of the ammonia level with the degree of encephalopathy is only approximate (see Ch. 123). Elevated ammonia levels may also be seen when ammonia production is increased by intestinal flora (e.g., following a high protein meal or gastrointestinal bleeding), by the kidney (in response to metabolic alkalosis or hypokalemia), or in certain rare genetic diseases affecting the pathway of urea synthesis (see Ch. 178). Arterial or cerebrospinal fluid levels of ammonia have little advantage over venous levels for clinical purposes.

DRUG CLEARANCE. The liver is primarily responsible for clearing many drugs from blood, particularly those that are poorly filtered by the kidney owing to binding to albumin or to other blood components. Clearance of certain drugs has therefore been used to quantitate this function. Indocyanine green (ICG) clearance provides a useful estimate of hepatic blood flow. The retention of sulfobromophthalein (BSP) in blood 45 minutes following bolus injection is normally 5% or less but is increased by even mild hepatic dysfunction. Unfortunately, this drug has produced occasional anaphylactic reactions and it is no longer routinely available in the United States. Other drugs that have been used to quantitate hepatic function include antipyrene, caffeine, and rose bengal.

SYNTHETIC FUNCTIONS

PROTHROMBIN TIME. The prothrombin time, usually performed by the one-stage (Quick) method, measures the rate at which prothrombin in citrated plasma is converted to thrombin in the presence of added calcium, tissue thromboplastin, and activated clotting factors (see Ch. 153). This test depends on the plasma concentration not only of prothrombin, but also of other clotting factors synthesized in the liver, including V, VII, IX and fibrinogen. Results may be expressed in seconds, percentage of a standardized control sample, or prothrombin content. The test is abnormal in the setting of reduced synthesis (e.g., liver failure, vitamin K deficiency), increased consumption (e.g., disseminated intravascular coagulation), or both.

Synthesis of fibrinogen, prothrombin, and Factors II, V, IX, X, XI, XII, and XIII occurs in the liver. Synthesis of prothrombin and Factors VII, IX, and X depends on an adequate supply of *vitamin K,* which activates certain hepatic polypeptides by stimulating the synthesis of the calcium-binding residue, γ-carboxyglutamic acid. An abnormal prothrombin time is commonly caused by *vitamin K deficiency, liver disease,* or both and may rarely be seen with *inherited abnormalities.* Vitamin K, a fat soluble vitamin that is found in many foods, is also produced by intestinal bacteria (see Ch. 192.2). Deficiency is most commonly seen in *malabsorption syndromes,* including failure to absorb dietary fat due to biliary obstruction or other causes of cholestasis (see Ch. 103). It may also be seen with antimicrobial suppression of intestinal bacteria, especially when the patient is receiving inadequate oral or parenteral vitamin K replacement.

Any acute or chronic liver disease may cause an abnormal prothrombin time if the synthesis of essential clotting factors is impaired. The plasma half-life of these factors is typically less than 1 day; the prothrombin time therefore responds rapidly to changes in hepatic synthetic function. This property makes the prothrombin time particularly useful for following the course of acute liver diseases; significant elevation often indicates an unfavorable prognosis.

An abnormal prothrombin time may be of diagnostic value in evaluation of the jaundiced patient. In general, when it is prolonged on the basis of vitamin K deficiency alone (as in fat malabsorption due to cholestasis), it will return to normal within hours of parenteral administration of vitamin K. In contrast, when the synthesis of clotting factors is diminished because of parenchymal liver disease, response to vitamin K may be slight or absent. Both factors may coexist, however. In severe liver failure, elevation of prothrombin time may also reflect disseminated intravascular coagulation (see Ch. 153). Because of these shortcomings, the prothrombin time must be interpreted in the context of all available information.

The *partial thromboplastin time* is used to assess the "intrinsic" clotting mechanism, and reflects the activity of all clotting factors except for platelet factor 3, Factor VII, and Factor XII. For this reason, the test is complementary to the prothrombin time and may indicate deficiencies of other clotting factors or the presence of a circulating anticoagulant (see Ch. 153).

ALBUMIN. *Albumin,* synthesized exclusively in the liver at a rate of 100 to 200 mg per kilogram of body weight per day, has a long half-life in plasma (about 3 weeks in healthy adults). The synthetic rate is influenced by many factors, including nutritional state, the presence of systemic and/or liver disease, thyroid and glucocorticoid hormones, plasma colloid osmotic pressure, and toxins such as alcohol and carbon tetrachloride. The normal mechanism of albumin turnover is not well understood, although losses are increased in nephrotic syndrome, protein-losing enteropathy, severe burns, exfoliative dermatitis, and gastrointestinal bleeding.

The serum albumin concentration reflects a balance between synthesis and loss and is therefore not specific for the functional state of the liver. Because the serum half life is long, abnormalities are slow to develop and may persist for weeks after correction of the underlying problem. On the other hand, when other factors can be excluded, hypoalbuminemia may be an important indicator of chronic liver disease. In patients with cirrhosis and ascites, hypoalbuminemia commonly reflects diminished synthesis; but in some, synthesis is normal and hypoalbuminemia is caused by a redistribution into ascitic fluid.

SERUM LIPIDS AND LIPOPROTEINS. Parenchymal liver disease and bile duct obstruction may produce significant abnormalities in serum lipids and lipoproteins. In acute parenchymal liver disease, the serum electrophoretic band of α_1-lipoprotein may be lost, reflecting an abnormal composition and altered physical properties of the high density lipoproteins. A transient hypertriglyceridemia may also occur because of the presence in serum of abnormal low-density lipoproteins rich in triglycerides. These changes appear attributable in part to deficient activity of plasma lecithin-cholesterol acyltransferase (LCAT), an enzyme of hepatic origin that esterifies plasma cholesterol. The changes are transient, and with resolution of the acute liver injury, plasma lipids and lipoproteins return to their previous state.

The liver is primarily responsible for removing cholesterol from the body by its direct secretion into bile or its conversion to bile acids. In cholestasis, the serum concentrations of unesterified cholesterol and phospholipids increase, and *xanthomas* and *xanthelasma* may develop if these abnormalities are severe and sustained. A major fraction of the increased plasma unesterified cholesterol is accounted for by an abnormal low-density lipoprotein, designated LPX. LPX consists mainly of unesterified cholesterol and phosphatidyl choline (lecithin) with a small amount of protein, largely albumin and C apolipoproteins. LPX is not of value in the differential diagnosis of jaundice, but it may contribute to an elevated plasma cholesterol concentration in patients with liver disease.

IMMUNOLOGIC TESTS

GLOBULINS. *Serum globulins* are of limited diagnostic use in hepatobiliary diseases. As a group, they are heterogeneous with respect to site and regulation of production, physical properties, and physiologic function. Their concentration, as measured by serum protein electrophoresis or salt fractionation, may be influenced by a variety of hepatic and extrahepatic factors and disease states. The mechanism of their increased serum concentration in liver disease is not fully understood, but it may include stimuli to increased antibody production resulting from decreased removal of bacterial antigens from the portal blood or release of antigenic material from damaged liver cells. An important exception is a diminished concentration of the α_1-globulin fraction as demonstrated by serum protein electrophoresis. Since approximately 85% of this fraction is accounted for by α_1-antitrypsin, a decrease in its concentration may be an important sign of α_1-antitrypsin deficiency, an inherited disorder associated with neonatal hepatitis, cirrhosis, and pulmonary emphysema (see Ch. 121). Elevated IgM concentrations are common in primary biliary cirrhosis, but other clinical, laboratory, and imaging procedures are of greater diagnostic value. Diffuse increases in globulin concentrations are commonly seen in cirrhosis and may be especially pronounced in chronic active hepatitis in the absence of serum markers for active infection by hepatitis B or C viruses.

MITOCHONDRIAL ANTIBODY. In approximately 90% of patients with primary biliary cirrhosis, the serum contains antibodies directed against a lipoprotein component of the inner mitochondrial membrane (see Ch. 122). The antibodies are neither organ nor species specific and are demonstrated by immunofluorescent techniques employing rat kidney, liver, and stomach and human thyroid, stomach, and kidney. These antibodies include the three main immunoglobulin classes, are complement fixing, and bind to at least seven different components of the inner and outer mitochondrial membranes. In patients with primary biliary cirrhosis, the titer is not related to the increased level of serum IgM or the stage or severity of the disease.

Mitochondrial antibodies are also present in up to 25% of patients with chronic active hepatitis and postnecrotic cirrhosis and in 7 to 8% of asymptomatic relatives of patients with primary biliary cirrhosis. They are rarely present in extrahepatic biliary obstruction. A small percentage of patients with nonhepatic diseases may also exhibit positive tests; these include the collagen-vascular disorders, thyroiditis, myasthenia gravis, Addison's disease, autoimmune hemolytic anemia, and chronic biologic false-positive reactions for syphilis. Of the several types of mitochondrial antibodies thus far identified, M_2 is the type usually found in primary biliary cirrhosis. Mitochondrial antibodies are demonstrable in only 0.4 to 0.7% of the general population.

The mitochondrial antibody is useful in the differential diagnosis of jaundice for two reasons. First, a negative result renders the diagnosis of primary biliary cirrhosis unlikely, although it does not exclude it. Second, because of its rarity in extrahepatic biliary obstruction, a positive result helps confirm parenchymal disease. Since the incidence of gallstones in patients with primary biliary cirrhosis is approximately 40% and is also increased in other forms of cirrhosis, the mitochondrial antibody test does not reliably exclude extrahepatic obstruction.

ANTINUCLEAR AND SMOOTH MUSCLE ANTIBODIES. Either or both of these tests are positive in a variable percentage of patients with chronic active hepatitis, usually in cases not associated with hepatitis B or C infection. These antibodies also occur in a minority of patients with primary biliary cirrhosis. As is true of the mitochondrial antibody, these factors are neither organ nor species specific. They probably do not play a role in pathogenesis. The presence of these antibodies in serum does not exclude bile duct obstruction.

TESTS FOR HEPATITIS VIRUS INFECTION. These tests and their clinical significance are discussed in Ch. 117.

EXAMINATIONS OF URINE AND STOOL

The presence of bilirubin in urine indicates that a significant fraction of plasma bilirubin is conjugated and is strong evidence for hepatobiliary disease. Jaundice in the absence of bilirubinuria indicates an exclusively unconjugated hyperbilirubinemia, usually reflecting hemolysis, ineffective erythropoiesis, or an inherited disorder of bilirubin conjugation. Urine and fecal urobilinogen determinations rarely provide useful information. Testing of stool for occult blood may provide the first evidence of an alimentary tract lesion related to hepatobiliary disease (e.g., tumors metastatic to liver, ulcerative colitis associated with sclerosing cholangitis) and may explain the onset or exacerbation of hepatic encephalopathy. In certain clinical circumstances, stool culture or examination for ova and parasites may provide information important in the diagnosis of liver disease.

HEMATOLOGIC TESTS IN LIVER DISEASE

Diseases of the liver may be associated with a wide variety of hematologic abnormalities, including qualitative and quantitative changes in the formed elements and in clotting function. The abnormalities depend not only on the etiology of the liver disorder but also on whether it is acute or chronic or associated with complications such as liver failure or portal hypertension.

In acute liver disease not associated with liver failure, major changes in the formed elements are uncommon and consist primarily of mild anemia, reflecting either low-grade hemolysis or marrow depression. Slight leukopenia is not uncommon and is often associated with atypical lymphocytes.

Severe aplastic anemia may sometimes complicate acute viral hepatitis, especially following liver transplantation for fulminant hepatitis C infection. In other forms of acute liver disease, hematologic abnormalities such as marrow suppression may be caused by toxins such as ethanol or drugs. In the alcoholic, Zieve's syndrome, consisting of hemolytic anemia and hypertriglyceridemia, may rarely be found. Coagulopathy may complicate massive hepatic necrosis, reflecting depressed hepatic synthesis of clotting factors and, frequently, disseminated intravascular coagulation.

In chronic liver disease, erythrocytic target cells, often associated with cholestasis, result from an expansion of the cell membrane with relative preservation of the cholesterol-phospholipid ratio. Spur cells (acanthocytes), most often found in advanced alcoholic cirrhosis, reflect a more profound relative and absolute increase in membrane cholesterol.

Red cells, white cells, and platelets may be decreased in patients with portal hypertension, primarily because of hypersplenism (see Ch. 150). A number of other abnormalities may be present, but to a large extent these are caused by associated nutritional, pathologic, or pharmacologic influences. Examples include iron deficiency, megaloblastic, and sideroblastic anemias.

LIVER BIOPSY

Liver biopsy is of value in the diagnosis of diffuse or localized parenchymal diseases, including cirrhosis, chronic hepatitis, and mass lesions. It is commonly performed by the blind percutaneous technique, but it may be done under direct visualization during laparoscopy or with sonographic or radiologic guidance when specific areas must be sampled. Because the histologic changes are usually nonspecific in acute hepatitis or acute cholestatic jaundice, the value of liver biopsy in this setting is primarily prognostic. Liver biopsy requires the cooperation of the patient, except in infants, and normal clotting function. Relative or absolute contraindications include the presence of biliary sepsis or high grade biliary obstruction, ascites, severe coagulopathy, and right pleural disease.

IMAGING TECHNIQUES AND CHOLANGIOGRAPHY

These techniques are discussed in detail in Ch. 126.

McKenna JP, Moskovitz M, Cox JL: Abnormal liver function tests in asymptomatic patients. Am Fam Physician 39:117, 1989. *Many enzyme abnormalities are detected during routine screening, such as for blood donation. Here is a cost-effective method for evaluating these patients.*

Reichling JJ, Kaplan MM: Clinical use of serum enzymes in liver disease. Dig Dis Sci 33:1601, 1988. *Comprehensive review of the use of serum enzymes for diagnosis and monitoring liver disease. Over 150 references.*

Zakim D, Boyer TD (eds.): Hepatology: A Textbook of Liver Disease. 2nd ed. Philadelphia, WB Saunders, 1990. *A comprehensive and well-written text covering all aspects of liver function and dysfunction.*

Zaloga GP, Prough DS: Monitoring hepatic function. Crit Care Clin 4:591, 1988. *Lucid review with an emphasis on clearance tests.*

117 ACUTE VIRAL HEPATITIS
Robert K. Ockner

GENERAL INTRODUCTION

DEFINITION. Acute viral hepatitis comprises a spectrum of syndromes ranging from entirely subclinical and inapparent to rapidly progressive and fatal. In most cases it is self-limited and uncomplicated, but depending on the viral agent involved, there is a variable incidence of clinically significant extrahepatic manifestations or progression to chronic liver disease. After a variable incubation period, viral replication in the liver cell approaches a maximum, leading to the appearance of viral components in body fluids and/or excreta, liver cell necrosis with an associated inflammatory response, changes in liver laboratory tests, and symptoms and signs of liver damage. The immunologic response of the host appears to play an important but not fully defined role in pathogenesis.

ETIOLOGY. Viral hepatitis is caused by at least five major agents and several minor agents with relative or absolute predilection for the hepatocyte, which differ in structure and in the epidemiology and natural history of the diseases they cause. The vast majority of cases in the United States are accounted for by hepatitis viruses A, B, C, and D. Hepatitis E has been identified as a cause of endemic and severe epidemic disease in Asia, Africa, and Mexico. Selected characteristics are summarized in Table 117–1, and each is considered in greater detail below. Other viral agents that cause an acute hepatitis syndrome include the Epstein-Barr virus (infectious mononucleosis), cytomegalovirus, herpes simplex, yellow fever, and rubella; the clinical disorders caused by these agents are considered in greater detail elsewhere in the text.

PATHOLOGY. The lesion of acute hepatitis consists of necrosis of individual hepatocytes associated with a mononuclear (lymphocytic) lobular and portal inflammatory response and increased prominence of bile ducts (bile duct "proliferation"). There may be a variable (usually minor) necrosis of hepatocytes bordering the portal areas (so-called periportal hepatitis or piecemeal necrosis). Necrosis of an individual liver cell, whether periportal or within the lobule, is usually reflected in its replacement by a cluster of mononuclear cells, or it may be represented by balloon degeneration or as a shrunken cell with homogeneously eosinophilic cytoplasm and a condensed pyknotic nucleus ("acidophil body"). The regular pattern of the cords of hepatocytes is disrupted, mitotic figures and cholestasis are more common, and Kupffer cells are prominent. Although these features are characteristic of typical acute viral hepatitis, they are not specific, individually or collectively. Thus, the same overall pattern of injury is seen in certain forms of drug-induced liver disease, and its individual components are seen in many processes of diverse cause and duration. Mononuclear cell portal infiltrates, periportal hepatitis, and bridging or confluent necrosis may be especially prominent in chronic forms of hepatitis.

More severe variants of the process include "bridging" necrosis, "confluent" or "submassive" necrosis, and massive necrosis. In these, the necrotic process simultaneously involves contiguous cells rather than single cells in isolation. As a result, there may be variable collapse or condensation of stroma. Bridging necrosis, so named because continuous zones of necrosis extend between (i.e., "bridge") adjacent portal and/or central areas, may be a necessary if not sufficient antecedent to evolution to a subacute form of hepatitis, with progressive deterioration of liver function leading over several months to death in liver failure, or to chronic hepatitis or cirrhosis. However, as bridging necrosis is compatible with complete recovery it does not *per se* constitute evidence of chronic or progressive liver disease.

Submassive and massive forms of hepatic necrosis are reflected in a more severe clinical course and a less favorable prognosis. Massive necrosis, in which broad areas of hepatocytes are destroyed, with condensation of stromal elements and portal structures (bile ducts and vessels), is usually manifested clinically as fulminant hepatic failure (see Ch. 123). This syndrome is characterized by severely deranged liver function, hepatic encephalopathy, and a high fatality rate. In survivors, however, a chronic course is unusual, and liver microscopic anatomy typically returns essentially to normal.

The recovery phase of acute viral hepatitis is characterized by regeneration of hepatocytes and largely complete restoration of normal lobular architecture. It is distinctly uncommon for the healing that follows a circumscribed acute hepatitis to be accompanied by fibrous scar formation or by nodular regeneration. In the latter, hepatocytes cluster in an abnormal configuration lacking a central vein and other components of the normal lobular architecture. These two manifestations of an *abnormal* healing process (fibrosis and nodular regeneration) are the essential components of cirrhosis, a form of chronic liver disease that almost always reflects ongoing injury and repair rather than a single acute event.

CLINICAL AND LABORATORY MANIFESTATIONS. The earliest symptoms of acute viral hepatitis typically are nonspecific, predominantly constitutional and gastrointestinal. They may include malaise, fatigue, anorexia, nausea, vomiting, and arthralgias and may suggest a "flu" or upper respiratory syndrome to both patient and physician. Classically, the patient may describe a loss of taste

TABLE 117–1. CHARACTERISTICS OF COMMON CAUSATIVE AGENTS OF ACUTE VIRAL HEPATITIS

	Hepatitis A	Hepatitis B	Hepatitis C	Hepatitis D	Hepatitis E
Causative agent	27-nm RNA virus	42-nm DNA virus	32-nm pestivirus-like RNA virus	36-nm, incomplete RNA virus, with HBsAg coat	27–34 nm nonenveloped RNA virus
Transmission	Fecal-oral; water-, food-borne	Parenteral inoculation, or equivalent; direct contact	Similar to HBV; uncertain in many cases	Similar to HBV	Similar to HAV
Incubation period	2–6 weeks	4 weeks–6 months	5–7 weeks	Similar to HBV	2–9 weeks
Period of infectivity	2–3 weeks in late incubation and early clinical phases	During HBsAg positivity (occasionally with anti-HBc positivity alone)	During HCV-RNA or anti-HCV positivity	During HDV-RNA or anti-HDV positivity	Similar to HAV
Massive hepatic necrosis	Rare	Uncommon	Rare, if ever	Yes	Yes
"Carrier" state	No	Yes	Yes	Yes	No
Chronic hepatitis	No	Yes	Yes	Yes	No
Prophylaxis (see text)	Hygiene; immune serum globulin, vaccine (pending)	Hygiene; hepatitis B immune globulin; vaccine	Hygiene; ? immune serum globulin	Hygiene; prevention of HBV infection	Hygiene, sanitation

for coffee or cigarettes. Fever, if present, is usually mild. Abdominal discomfort may reflect an enlarged tender liver.

After a period of several days to a week or more, the prodromal phase may lead to an icteric (jaundiced) phase. The earliest clinical manifestation of a rising serum concentration of direct-reacting bilirubin (reflecting impaired hepatic excretion) is bilirubinuria, followed by a lightening of stool color, scleral icterus, and, in light-skinned individuals, frank jaundice. Constitutional symptoms often abate during the icteric phase, especially in children, in whom the disease is characteristically less severe. In adults, the gastrointestinal components of the prodrome may persist or even increase for a time. If cholestasis worsens, pruritus may cause increasing discomfort.

Physical findings are variable and depend on the stage of the illness. The only objective finding during the prodrome, apart from mild fever, may be an enlarged and tender liver, associated in perhaps 20% with splenomegaly. Jaundice may or may not appear; indeed, it is likely that the majority of cases remain anicteric, especially among children with hepatitis A. Excoriations reflect the intensity of pruritus. Spider nevi occasionally develop during an acute hepatitis, but since this is unusual, it should suggest the possibility of a more chronic process.

Laboratory studies are highly variable, but almost by definition the clinical onset is accompanied by rising activities of serum aminotransferases; usually the alanine aminotransferase (ALT) exceeds the aspartate aminotransferase (AST). An elevated serum bilirubin is predominantly direct reacting; very high concentrations, e.g., > 15 to 20 mg per deciliter, indicate a severe lesion or may reflect associated hemolysis. The alkaline phosphatase is usually moderately increased, and serum albumin concentration may decrease slightly. A diffuse hyperglobulinemia is common. Prothrombin time is prolonged in more severe cases, and a persisting or increasing prolongation is an unfavorable prognostic sign. Mild and clinically insignificant hypoglycemia occurs in perhaps 50% of cases; more profound hypoglycemia may complicate fulminant hepatic failure. Hematologic tests are also quite variable. Usually the total leukocyte count is normal or slightly decreased and atypical lymphocytes may be present. In more severe cases, total leukocytes may be increased, with relative or absolute neutrophilia. Hemoglobin and hematocrit are usually relatively normal, but occasionally there may be a coincidental hemolytic process, and rarely the course is complicated by aplastic anemia especially following non-A, non-B hepatitis. (HCV does not appear to account for this phenomenon.) Urinalysis is usually nonspecific except for the presence of bilirubin.

An important aspect of the laboratory approach to acute viral hepatitis is serodiagnosis. Although establishing a specific etiologic diagnosis may not influence management, it may have a bearing on prognosis and is particularly useful epidemiologically and for preventing transmission. These tests are considered below, in discussions of the various forms of viral hepatitis and their prevention, and in Table 117–2.

After an icteric phase that usually lasts from several days to several weeks, the patient enters a convalescent phase of gradual improvement in symptoms and laboratory tests. The healing process may require several weeks to a few months, during which time residual weakness and malaise are common. Normalization of laboratory tests is usually complete within 4 to 6 months. Persistence of abnormalities beyond 6 to 12 months suggests that for hepatitis B, C, or D, the process may have become chronic; in this circumstance, further investigation including liver biopsy may be indicated if there is no evidence of continuing improvement.

COMPLICATIONS AND EXTRAHEPATIC MANIFESTATIONS. The two most important complications of acute viral hepatitis are massive hepatic necrosis (fulminant hepatic failure) and progression to chronic hepatitis. Fortunately, these are uncommon, especially in hepatitis A, in which chronicity does not occur and massive necrosis is less common and more favorable in its prognosis than in hepatitis B, C, and D.

Massive hepatic necrosis with fulminant hepatic failure occurs in fewer than 1% of cases of acute viral hepatitis; in some cases of hepatitis B, mutant viruses have been implicated (see below). It is usually signaled by deepening jaundice, increasing prothrombin time, and hepatic encephalopathy. Serum aminotransferase levels may remain high, but in many cases will fall, often associated with a decrease in liver size. These changes are assumed to reflect extensive loss of parenchymal mass and, in the presence of other evidence of a deteriorating course, are unfavorable prognostic signs suggesting a possible need to consider urgent orthotopic liver transplantation. The diagnosis and management of acute hepatic failure and encephalopathy are considered in greater detail in Ch. 123.

Evolution to chronic hepatitis is a more common complication of acute hepatitis B, C, and D than is massive necrosis. It is suggested by persistence of abnormal serum aminotransferase activities, with or without other laboratory abnormalities and clinical symptoms, beyond an arbitrarily selected endpoint. Authorities differ as to where that endpoint belongs; guidelines range from 4 to 12 months, but most would accept 6 months as reasonable. Clearly, however, judgments must be individualized as to when an acute process becomes chronic (or, more pragmatically, when additional investigations such as liver biopsy should be undertaken). For example, as long as the patient continues to show evidence of clinical and laboratory improvement, little is to be gained from a more vigorous diagnostic or therapeutic approach. Conversely, evidence suggesting chronic liver disease (e.g., signs of portal hypertension or progressive deterioration of laboratory tests) that appears before 6 months may justify earlier diagnostic intervention. Because many of the histopathologic features associated with chronic hepatitis also may be components of an acute process, however, liver biopsies obtained too early in the course may be difficult to interpret and potentially misleading. Chronic hepatitis is also considered in the following discussions of hepatitis B, C, and D, and in greater detail in Ch. 119.

The syndrome of *cholestatic hepatitis* occurs occasionally as a complication of acute viral hepatitis, especially hepatitis A. Patients

TABLE 117-2. SEROLOGIC TESTS IN VIRAL HEPATITIS

Agent	Terminology	Definition	Significance
Hepatitis A (HAV)	Anti-HAV IgM type IgG type	Antibody to HAV	Current or recent infection, or convalescence Current or previous infection; indicates immunity
Hepatitis B (HBV)	HBsAg	Surface antigen	Positive in most cases of acute or chronic infection
	HBcAg	Core (capsid) protein	Not usually tested for in serologic assays
	HBeAg	e Antigen; secreted separately from complete virion	Transiently positive during active virus replication in acute and some chronic cases; reflects virion concentration and infectivity
	Anti-HBc (IgM or IgG)	Antibody to core protein	Positive in all acute and chronic cases and in carriers; thus, marker of HBV infection; not protective; IgM anti-HBc reflects active virus replication
	Anti-HBe	Antibody to e antigen	Transiently positive during convalescence and in some chronic cases and carriers; not protective; reflects low infectivity
	Anti-HBs	Antibody to surface antigen	Becomes positive late in convalescence in most acute cases; protective
Hepatitis C (HCV)	Anti-HCV	Antibody to cloned HCV peptide epitopes	Becomes positive 5–6 weeks after clinical onset; not protective; seropositive patients should be regarded as infectious
Hepatitis D (HDV)	Anti-HDV (IgM or IgG)	Antibody to HDV antigen	Indicates infection; not protective
Hepatitis E (HEV)	Anti-HEV IgM type IgG type	Antibody to HEV antigen	Current or recent infection; or convalescence Current or previous infection; indicates immunity

may, for several months, have cholestatic features, including pruritus, dark urine, light stools, direct-reacting hyperbilirubinemia, and elevated alkaline phosphatase. Almost without exception, the prognosis is favorable. The major problem in management posed by this variant is the occasional need to exclude disorders such as biliary stones, stricture, and tumors by means of appropriate imaging and cholangiographic techniques. Brief corticosteroid therapy has been found to be useful symptomatically in those cases associated with hepatitis A, but only with definitive exclusion of other causes.

Aplastic anemia may very rarely complicate the icteric or convalescent phase of acute viral hepatitis. HCV has been excluded as a causative factor, which thus remains unknown, and possibly is an as yet unidentified viral or toxic agent. Its pathogenesis is unknown, and its prognosis is poor. Among the relatively few survivors, there is no clear evidence of a beneficial effect of glucocorticoids or anabolic steroid treatment. Other formed elements may also be depressed, and pancytopenia, agranulocytosis, and thrombocytopenia have been reported. Bone marrow transplantation should be considered early in the course.

Extrahepatic manifestations of acute viral hepatitis also include *arthralgias* and *arthritis, uticaria,* and *cutaneous vasculitis.* These are more likely to occur during the prodromal phase, are associated with immune complex formation, and may complicate any type of acute viral hepatitis. Other vasculitic manifestations such as cryoglobulinemia, polyarteritis nodosa, and glomerulonephritis are more likely to occur in chronic hepatitis B and C, and are discussed in Ch. 119. *Pancreatitis* is found in 12 to 40% of cases of fatal acute viral hepatitis, and serum amylase activity is elevated in up to 30% of nonfatal cases; the true overall incidence and pathogenesis of pancreatitis in viral hepatitis are not known. Myocarditis, pneumonitis, and other extrahepatic manifestations are rare, and in their presence other systemic disorders should be considered.

SPECIFIC ETIOLOGIC CATEGORIES OF VIRAL HEPATITIS

HEPATITIS A. This form of hepatitis also has been referred to as infectious or short-incubation hepatitis. The causative agent (hepatitis A virus, HAV) is a 27-nm diameter RNA virus that is readily and almost exclusively transmitted via the fecal-oral route (see Table 117–1). In this important respect it differs significantly from other forms of hepatitis except E (see below). Accordingly, when the cause of water-borne, point-source, food-handler-related, and institutional hepatitis outbreaks in North America and Europe has been defined, hepatitis A almost invariably has been implicated. In addition, hepatitis A occurs sporadically and is spread by direct person-to-person contact; there appears to be an increased incidence

among promiscuous homosexuals. Transfer of infectious doses of virus in both directions between fingertips and environmental surfaces has been documented. Spread of hepatitis A in day care centers may involve not only children but also the staff and the families of affected children. As a corollary, the incidence of the disease appears to correlate in a general way with personal hygiene and the efficacy of public health measures, as suggested by the apparent influence of socioeconomic status on the prevalence of hepatitis A antibodies (anti-HAV), which averaged 45% in one study of an urban population in the United States and approximated 90% in residents of Costa Rica. Parenteral transmission is rare but has been documented in transfusion-associated outbreaks in neonatal intensive care units, affecting newborns, nursing staff, and their respective household and family contacts. Also, an outbreak among hemophiliac patients was linked to the use of a Factor VIII concentrate prepared with an organic solvent-detergent mixture intended to inactivate viruses. There is no evidence for the existence of a chronic form of hepatitis A or a carrier state. The "reservoir" for the virus appears to consist of clinically inapparent acute cases, in which the disease is not recognized at the time of viral shedding. In the United States, incidence has varied cyclically over the past 40 years, ranging between 10 and 40 cases per 100,000 per year.

Hepatitis A infection typically has an incubation period of 2 to 6 weeks. Fecal shedding of virus occurs over a 2- to 3-week period beginning during the final week of the incubation period and the prodromal phase, and declines as serum transaminases reach maximal levels (Fig. 117–1 and Table 117–1) and antibody (anti-HAV) appears in serum. Although a transient viremia occurs during this interval, parenteral transmission of the disease is rare, as noted. Initially, serum antibody is predominantly of the IgM class, but an IgG antibody soon appears. The IgG antibody persists in serum for many years; its exclusive presence indicates prior exposure and immunity to the hepatitis A virus. The presence of the IgM antibody, on the other hand, almost always indicates infection within the past few months (see Table 117–2), although occasionally this antibody may persist for up to 1 year or more after the acute onset. An IgA antibody to HAV appears in the feces of patients at about the time fecal shedding of virus ceases and persists for several weeks.

The acute illness itself is diverse in its clinical manifestations and course. The majority of cases are clinically inapparent, especially in children, or are perceived as a nonspecific "flu" syndrome. Jaundice, when it occurs, is usually mild. Symptoms usually subside, and serum aminotransferase activities return to normal within 3 to 4 months. Hepatitis A virus infection has been implicated in some cases of acute cholestatic hepatitis and may exhibit a relapsing or

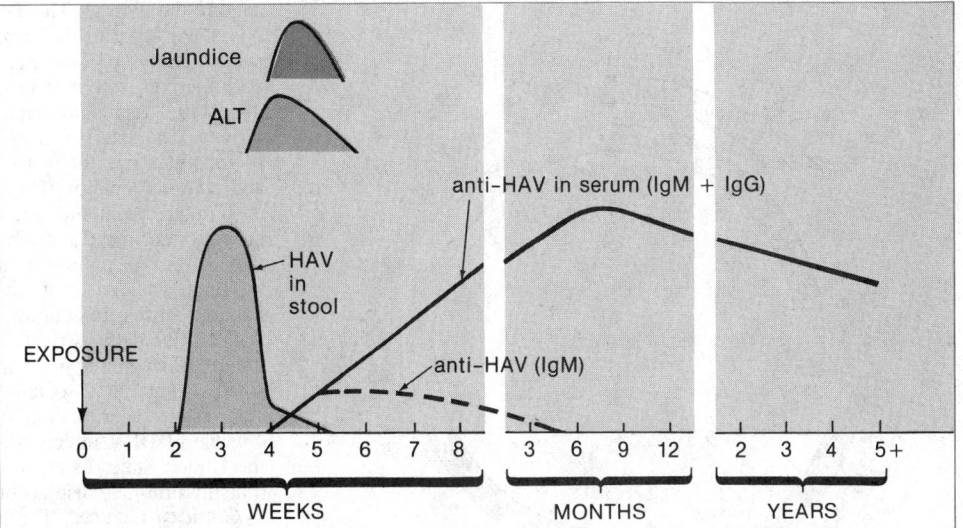

FIGURE 117–1. Sequence of clinical and laboratory findings in a patient with hepatitis A. Fecal shedding of virus is brief in duration and ends with the appearance of anti-HAV in serum. IgM anti-HAV, usually present for a few months, may persist in serum for a year or more after the acute illness. (From Krugman S, Gocke DJ: Viral Hepatitis. Philadelphia, WB Saunders,

protracted course lasting several months. In the latter cases, ongoing HAV infection has been documented by the presence of virus in stool and HAV RNA in serum. Systemic immune phenomena have been described including cryoglobulinemia, rheumatoid factor, purpura, leukocytoclastic vasculitis, and nephritis. Rarely, hepatitis A causes massive hepatic necrosis and fulminant hepatic failure, but this complication is less common and more favorable in prognosis than that in hepatitis B and C.

The ease with which hepatitis A is transmitted among contacts and via water and food, as well as the demonstrated efficacy of immune serum globulin in preventing or ameliorating the disease, underscores the value of individual hygiene and public health measures to control the spread of infection. Applying these to the management of the individual patient and his or her contacts is discussed below.

HEPATITIS B. In contrast to hepatitis A, hepatitis B virus infection may cause a variety of acute or chronic hepatic and extrahepatic diseases, as well as a chronic "carrier state." Its presentation as an acute hepatitis is typical of those cases that were previously designated serum hepatitis or long-incubation hepatitis, although it is now apparent that many of these cases represented hepatitis C infection (see below).

The hepatitis B virus (HBV) differs in almost every respect from hepatitis A (see Tables 117–1 and 117–2; Figs. 117–2 to 117–4). The complete infective virion, or *Dane (HBV) particle*, is a DNA virus of 42 nm diameter, consisting of antigenically distinct surface and core components. The HBV genome (Fig. 117–2) encodes four recognized products: (1) surface proteins (pre-S1, pre-S2, and S); (2) core and e proteins; (3) DNA polymerase/reverse transcriptase; and (4) X protein. The HBV *surface coat* is largely lipid and protein, and its protein components may exist in serum or other body fluids either in association with the complete virion or as separate 20 nm diameter spheres or cylinders. Its major antigenic determinant, the hepatitis B surface antigen (HBsAg) consists of three coterminal components, the S, pre-S1, and pre-S2 proteins (Fig. 117–3); pre-S1 and pre-S2 are important in virion attachment to and penetration of the cell and are relatively more abundant in the complete virion than in the HBsAg particles (Figs. 117–2 and 117–3). HBsAg includes a major antigenic ("a") determinant and several subtypes (d, y; w, r); it can be detected in the serum of at least 75% of infected persons during the acute disease (Fig. 117–4). The hepatitis B virus *core* consists of a nucleocapsid formed of aggregated hepatitis B core protein (HBcAg) dimers, containing incompletely double-stranded circular DNA, and the DNA polymerase/reverse transcriptase. HBeAg is a protein formed via specific self-cleavage of the pre-core/core gene product; unlike HBcAg an intramolecular disulfide bond renders HBeAg unable to participate in capsid formation and it is exported separately from the cell. The function of HBeAg is not fully defined, but it may serve to induce a state of relative host tolerance to HBV. HBcAg remains an intrin-

sic part of the complete virion. Each elicits a humoral immune response (anti-HBc and anti-HBe, respectively) during the course of the hepatitis B infection. The product of the *DNA polymerase* gene is a multifunctional enzyme protein that catalyzes several steps in DNA replication and virion assembly. *X protein* is a promiscuous transactivator of several viral and host genes, but its role in HBV replication and infection are not fully known. HBV-DNA can be detected in serum by molecular hybridization techniques, including polymerase chain reaction (PCR), and is the most sensitive indicator of the presence of infective virus.

In recent years, several HBV mutants have been identified (see Fig. 117–2). One category, affecting the "a" determinant of the surface protein (the principal target of the HBV vaccine), has caused infection despite active immunization against the wild-type agent ("vaccine escape"). A second mutant category affects the pre-core/core gene, often as the result of a stop codon just prior to the core protein open reading frame. This usually results in a failure to express HBeAg, although the host produces antibodies to HBe (anti-HBe). The core protein open reading frame itself is intact, permitting HBcAg formation and thus viral replication. Mutant viruses are thought to emerge and prevail during the course of infection by wild-type virus under the selective pressure of the host immune response. The pre-core mutants have been associated with more aggressive acute or chronic clinical courses, but this appears to be less common in the United States and a definite causal connection has not been established. Other much less common mutations, affecting the DNA polymerase/reverse transcriptase and X genes, have also been described.

HBV is believed to cause hepatocellular injury and necrosis as the result of a host immune attack on hepatocytes expressing HBV antigens, especially HBcAg, in conjunction with class I HLA determinants on their surface. Evidence in support of this concept includes the fact that active and ongoing viral replication may occur in the absence of overt hepatitis, e.g., in apparently healthy "carriers," as well as in the absence of serologic markers of the infection. In contrast, an unusually severe form of hepatitis B, attributed to a cytopathic effect, may occur in liver transplant recipients in whom HBV replication is exceptionally active, presumably as a result of iatrogenic immune suppression.

Transmission. Hepatitis B is transmitted primarily via parenteral routes, as the virus is present in virtually all body fluids and secretions. Therefore, it usually requires either overt inoculation (e.g., transfusion or injection via a contaminated needle) or intimate personal contact (e.g., between sexual partners, and mother and newborn infant). Unlike hepatitis A, transmission of hepatitis B by the fecal-oral route is relatively unimportant; infection may follow oral ingestion, but large doses appear necessary. The disease occurs with an increased frequency among sexual partners of acutely infected individuals, as well as among chronically exposed persons, including health professionals and patients exposed to blood and blood

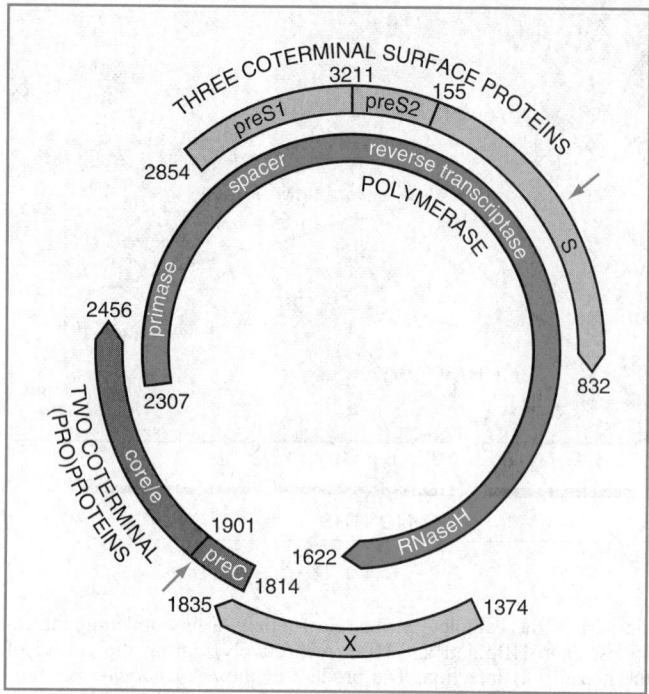

FIGURE 117–2. Schematic representation of the HBV open reading frames for the four established gene product categories. Solid black bars are transcription start sites; thin red arrows indicate approximate locations of most common mutations; numbers are those of nucleotides at various sites. (Adapted from Gerlich WH, Thomssen R: *In* McIntyre N, et al. [eds.]: Oxford Textbook of Clinical Hepatology. Oxford, Oxford University Press, 1993.)

products (e.g., workers and patients in clinical laboratories, dialysis, and oncology units), the sexually promiscuous (especially male homosexuals), drug users who share needles, and handlers of primates (which are susceptible to infection). In urban centers, hepatitis B may account for up to 50% of sporadic cases of acute hepatitis, even in the absence of documented parenteral inoculation. This attests to the importance of person-to-person contact in the spread of this disease.

Less than 1% of the general populations of the United States and Western Europe are HBsAg-positive. This low incidence contrasts with incidence of anti-HBs of about 10% in the same population, consistent with the fact that in most patients with acute hepatitis B the infection is self-limited and followed by immunity, only infrequently leading to chronic liver disease or a carrier state. The prevalence of HBsAg positivity is much higher in less-developed geographic areas (up to 15%) and among certain subpopulations with increased exposure and/or impaired immunity, such as patients with Down syndrome, leprosy, or lymphoproliferative disorders; substance abusers; and patients undergoing dialysis. In addition to acute cases, these chronically infected individuals constitute the "reservoir" that perpetuates the virus. Historically, it is likely that transmission of the disease has occurred not so often via overt parenteral inoculation but rather via close personal and sexual contact and from mother to newborn. In the latter instance (perinatal or "vertical" transmission), i.e., in infants born to mothers with acute or chronic infection, there is a high probability that the neonate will acquire the disease. This is especially likely when the mother develops acute hepatitis B in late pregnancy or in the early postpartum period or has chronic hepatitis. Transmission appears to correlate with the presence of HBeAg in maternal serum, reflecting the activity of viral replication and, therefore, the concentration of infective virions. Characteristically, these infants remain chronically infected for many years, either as "carriers" or with a persisting low-grade and chronic hepatitis. They are at increased risk of developing hepatocellular carcinoma (see Ch. 125). Perinatal transmission may be an important mechanism by which the reservoir of the virus is sustained from generation to generation and has been a major factor in the high incidence of chronic HBV infection in Asia. In sub-Saharan Africa, in contrast, the documented high incidence of HBV is not principally perinatal, but rather appears to occur most often among older children ("horizontal" transmission), possibly via personal contact in association with eczematous, abrasive, and other skin lesions, scarification, or human or insect bites. A significant incidence of HBV infection among Asian immigrant children born in the United States to HBV-negative mothers suggests that horizontal transmission may also account for many of these cases.

Clinical Course. The *incubation period* of acute hepatitis B, as defined by the appearance of clinical symptoms, varies between 4 weeks and 6 months, with an average of about 50 days. The first *serologic* evidence of viremia, however, may occur as soon as 2 weeks, especially after exposure to large parenteral doses. Two weeks to 2 months prior to the clinical onset, HBsAg becomes detectable in serum (see Fig. 117–4 and Table 117–2). At about the time of the clinical onset and the rise in serum aminotransferase activities, anti-HBc becomes detectable. Initially, an IgM anti-HBc is present in high titer and persists for several months to 1 year; thereafter IgG anti-HBc predominates. In chronic HBV infections, IgM anti-HBc may become detectable during periods in which the virus is actively replicating. IgG anti-HBc persists for up to several years after acute hepatitis and is present in all chronic carriers. It appears to play no role in host defenses; rather, it serves as a marker of prior hepatitis B infection. The markers of active replication (HBeAg, DNA polymerase, and HBV-DNA) usually become detectable in serum prior to the increase in aminotransferase activity. The duration of HBsAg positivity is highly variable. It may persist for a few days to 2 to 3 months; persistence beyond a few months may indicate a chronic course. Characteristically, HBsAg becomes undetectable before anti-HBs appears. This antibody can be demonstrated in 80 to 90% of patients, usually late in convalescence, and indicates relative or absolute immunity. Its appearance suggests a successful response to the infection, but there are exceptions to this in certain patients with chronic hepatitis (see Ch. 119).

Several important qualifications should be noted in interpreting the results of hepatitis B serologic tests. First, in a significant number of patients with acute hepatitis B the serum is negative for HBsAg, presumably because the antigen is very low in titer or evanescent. For this reason, a single negative HBsAg test does not exclude the diagnosis. Anti-HBc is more sensitive in this regard and may be the only serologic indication of hepatitis B infection. A negative test for anti-HBc effectively excludes the diagnosis. On the other hand, a positive test for anti-HBc in an HBsAg-negative serum could merely reflect a prior episode of hepatitis B. These HBsAg-negative, anti-HBc–positive patients may be classifiable on the basis of the anti-HBs: A positive test for anti-HBs early in the course of an acute hepatitis is evidence against the diagnosis of acute hepatitis B. Detection of IgM anti-HBc suggests either recent acute hepatitis B or chronic hepatitis B during a phase of active

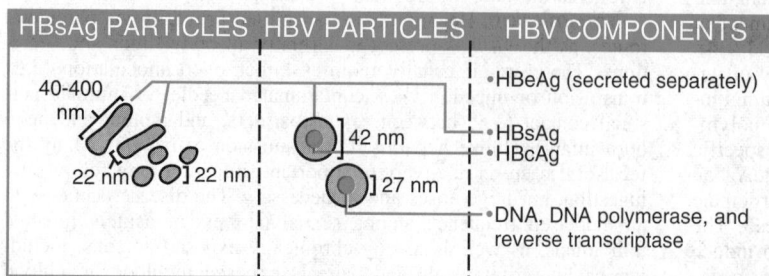

FIGURE 117–3. Forms of HBV in plasma, showing location of the various components and antigenic determinants. HBeAg, not an integral component of the complete virus particle, is not shown. (Adapted from Koff RS: *In* Sanford JP, Luby JP [eds.]: The Science and Clinical Practice of Medicine. Vol. 8. Infectious Diseases. New York, Grune & Stratton, 1981.)

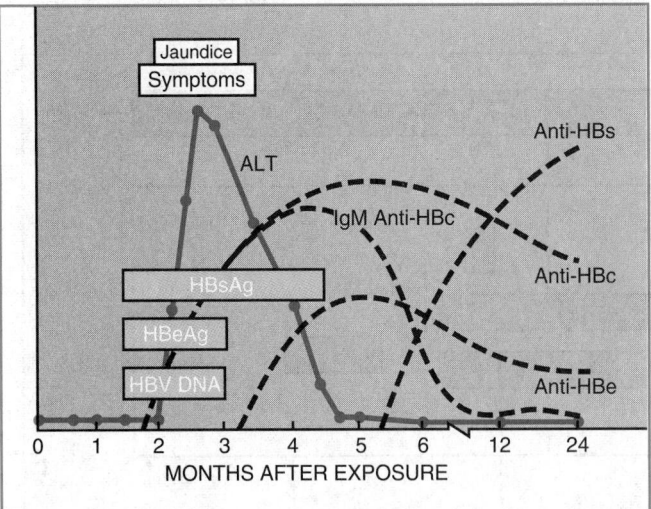

FIGURE 117–4. Sequence of clinical and laboratory findings in a patient with acute hepatitis B, followed by recovery. HBsAg-emia is the initial manifestation. Markers of the complete virion (HBeAg and HBV DNA) precede the ALT rise and are transient. Anti-HBc (IgM, then IgG) appears during the acute illness; after the disappearance of HBsAg and before the appearance of anti-HBs, anti-HBc may be the only marker of hepatitis B infection. Specific timing of the detection of a given variable depends to some extent on the method used. (Adapted from Hoofnagle J, Schafer DF: Serologic markers of hepatitis B virus infection. Semin Liver Dis 6:4, 1986.)

virus replication, as noted above. In those IgM-anti-HBc–negative subjects in whom HBV infection appears to have antedated an acute hepatitis syndrome, the possibility of superimposed infection by hepatitis D or other viral or nonviral causes of the illness must be considered. A positive test for HBeAg or HBV-DNA provides unequivocal evidence of ongoing HBV replication.

The *course* of acute hepatitis B is more variable and usually more prolonged than that of hepatitis A. It may be associated with extrahepatic manifestations, including urticaria and other rashes, arthritis, and much less commonly, glomerulonephritis and vasculitis. The immune complexes that appear to mediate these extrahepatic manifestations consist of HBsAg, anti-HBs, and complement components. Glomerulonephritis and vasculitis are also associated with chronic hepatitis B infection and are not necessarily accompanied by apparent liver disease. Indeed, up to one third of all cases of polyarteritis nodosa may be associated with HBV infection.

At least 95% of otherwise healthy adult patients with acute hepatitis B recover completely and become HBsAg negative. Fewer than 1% develop massive hepatic necrosis, but this complication is more common than in hepatitis A. The somewhat larger number (at most 5 to 10%) of patients who remain HBsAg positive beyond 6 to 12 months are at risk of developing chronic hepatitis (see Ch. 119).

HEPATITIS D (HDV, "DELTA-AGENT"). Infection with this unusual agent may be regarded as a complication of hepatitis B. HDV is an incomplete RNA virus most closely related to plant viroids and satellite viruses. Its closed circular genome of 1700 nucleotides is enclosed in a 35-nm particle, the coating of which is the hepatitis B surface antigen. Infection with HDV requires antecedent or simultaneous infection with hepatitis B, which acts thus as a helper virus. Although the HBsAg coating of the particle undoubtedly contributes to the hepatotropism and cellular uptake of HDV, its composition differs from that of the complete HBV virion in its relative lack of the pre-S1 and pre-S2 peptides, which are thought to be of particular importance in HBV virion association with and uptake by the hepatocyte, and more closely resembles that of the smaller particles of HBsAg alone that are produced in excess during HBV infection (see Fig. 117–3). The HDV genome replicates via a "rolling circle" mechanism, and its enzymatic properties (i.e., it is a ribozyme) account for the cleavage and ligation reactions necessarily involved. A single protein (HDAg) is encoded, which may be either 195 or 214 amino acids long, depending on the presence or absence of a stop codon in the open reading frame. The short form of HDAg is essential for replication, whereas the long form inhibits replication and is required for viral assembly;

possibly, the relative amounts of these two proteins influence the course and severity of the clinical illness.

Transmission. Five per cent or more of the 300 million HBV cases worldwide are infected with HDV as well. Because HDV depends on HBV, the epidemiologies of the two agents are generally parallel, but with important regional variations. In areas of high prevalence (>20% of chronic HBV carriers infected with HDV, e.g., Africa, southern Italy, South America), transmission is largely via person-to-person contact, whereas in the areas of lowest prevalence (0 to 2% of carriers, e.g., United States), transmission is principally among groups with high exposure to blood products or contaminated needles (e.g., hemophiliacs and intravenous drug abusers). The incidence among male homosexuals, dialysis patients, and institutional inmates is unexpectedly low. The disease exists endemically, but discrete outbreaks are well-documented, especially in high prevalence areas where transmission occurs chiefly among young people as the result of open skin lesions or sexual contact. Perinatal transmission does not appear to be important.

Clinical Course. HDV infection is reflected by the presence of anti-HDV antibody (IgM acutely; IgG chronically) or HDV-RNA in serum. Almost invariably, the serum is positive for HBsAg and anti-HBc and, in most, anti-HBe. In subjects who are acutely and simultaneously infected with HBV and HDV there is no apparent increase in the probability that chronic hepatitis will ensue, but the likelihood of fulminant hepatic failure is greater than for acute hepatitis B alone. In individuals chronically infected with HBV, however, superimposed acute HDV infection usually also becomes chronic and is associated with the histopathologic findings of chronic active hepatitis. Although it was previously thought not to be associated with hepatocellular carcinoma, recent evidence suggests otherwise.

HEPATITIS C. The ability to document hepatitis A and B virus infection made it clear that many cases of acute hepatitis were caused by one or more other agents, designated "non-A, non-B." One of these, hepatitis C virus, has been characterized and accounts for the great majority of such cases, especially those that are transmitted parenterally. Accordingly, the designation hepatitis C, as used here, includes most cases previously referred to as non-A, non-B (except for the enterically transmitted disease now referred to as hepatitis E—see below). It remains a possibility that some cases of non-A, non-B, non-C hepatitis may ultimately be attributed to one or more as yet unidentified agents.

Hepatitis C virus (HCV) was identified by a novel and painstaking application of the concepts and techniques of molecular biology, initially using the sera of chimpanzees known to carry post-transfusion non-A, non-B hepatitis infection in high titer. Nucleic acid sequences from chimpanzees' sera were cloned and screened for *in vitro* expression of a polypeptide antigen recognized by antibodies present in the sera of patients with well-characterized post-transfusion non-A, non-B hepatitis. These efforts led to an assay for an antibody to one viral epitope (C 100-3) and to the characterization of the virus itself (Fig. 117–5). HCV is an RNA agent related to the virus family which includes flaviviruses (e.g., Dengue, yellow fever) and pestiviruses (e.g., hog cholera, bovine viral diarrhea). It consists of an RNA genome of approximately 10 kilobases in length, encoding a polyprotein product, the cleavage of which generates several structural (capsid, envelope) and nonstructural (helicase, protease, and RNA-dependent RNA polymerase) viral proteins. The degree of variability in the HCV genome appears to be substantially greater than that of the other major hepatitis viruses, such that at least six distinct genotypes have been recognized worldwide. Some of these appear to be limited in distribution to a particular geographic area, whereas others are more widespread. Moreover, within a genotype, there may be considerable variation among isolates, predominantly affecting a portion of the E2/NS1 region (so-called hypervariable region) (Fig. 117–5), whereas other portions of the genome, especially within the 5'-untranslated region, are more highly conserved. These genotypic variations appear to be generated rapidly during the course of acute and chronic infections and are of importance in that they may lead to false-negative testing for either host antibody to HCV or for viral RNA by means of PCR assays, in which the primers and probes used may fail to recognize the nucleotide sequences of the particular isolate. Genomic variability may also account in part for the fact that naturally ac-

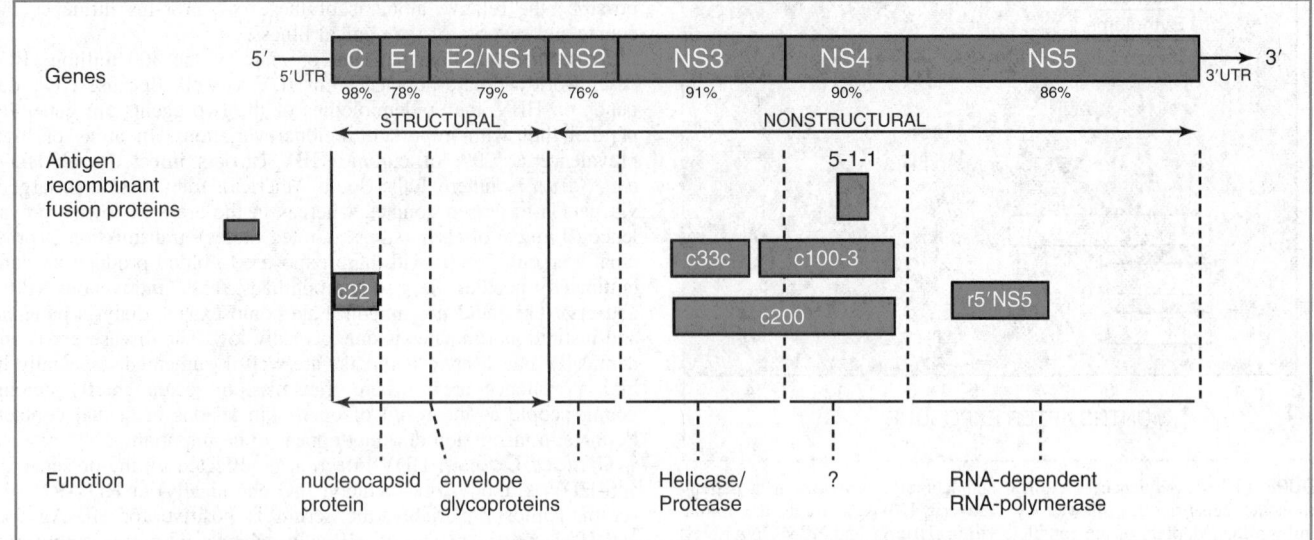

FIGURE 117–5. Structure of HCV genome, showing regions encoding envelope (E) and nonstructural (NS) portions of the polyprotein gene product. Percent homology among various strains is indicated for each portion; lowest homology in the E2/NS1 portion reflects presence of the hypervariable region. Location of epitopes represented by various recombinant proteins used in diagnostic tests are shown. Functions of various protein products of the viral genome are indicated where known. (Adapted from Esteban J, et al.: Hepatitis C: Molecular biology, pathogenesis, epidemiology, clinical features, and prevention. *In* Boyer J, Ockner R [eds.]: Progress in Liver Diseases, Vol X. Philadelphia, WB Saunders, 1992.)

quired HCV infection apparently does not lead to immunity against reinfection and that multiple infections with different HCV strains may occur. These characteristics of the infection may impede HCV vaccine development and may influence responsiveness of chronic HCV infection to antiviral and immunomodulatory therapy (see Ch. 327).

Transmission. HCV-RNA is readily detected in serum of infected individuals, but at much lower concentrations than are generally found with hepatitis B; HCV concentrations in other body fluids, e.g., saliva, semen, urine, stool, and vaginal secretions are even lower or undetectable. Thus, while the agent is readily transmitted by means of large-volume inocula, e.g., transfusion, it is much less likely than HBV to be spread via perinatal or sexual contact or among family members. The risk to health care workers of accidental needle stick, documented to be HCV-contaminated, is from 4 to 10%. It is a frequent complication of intravenous drug abuse with needle sharing, among renal dialysis patients, and in recipients of untreated commercial preparations of clotting factor concentrates. It may infect recipients of organ transplants from HCV-positive donors. Approximately 0.5% of healthy blood donors in the United States are positive for HCV antibodies by second-generation assays (see below). The fact that 40% or more of acute sporadic HCV cases were previously not associated with recognized risk factors such as those noted above indicates the importance of interpersonal transmission, but the mechanism(s) involved are not known with certainty.

HCV has been the major cause of post-transfusion hepatitis, the incidence of which has declined dramatically in the past two decades as a result of eliminating commercial (paid) donors, screening for HBsAg, screening for surrogate markers of non-A, non-B hepatitis, and finally screening for antibodies to HCV itself. Thus, in selected studies, the incidence of post-transfusion non-A, non-B hepatitis was 10 to 13% in 1981, 3.8% in 1985, 1.5% from 1986 to 1990, and 0.57% in 1992, or about 3 cases per 10,000 transfused units.

Clinical Course. After exposure, there is an incubation period of 5 to 7 weeks, when the serum aminotransferase activities rise and other clinical manifestations become evident. It remains unclear to what extent the acute hepatic injury may be cytopathic, immunologically mediated, or both. Although the first-generation enzyme-linked immunoassays (EIA-1) for HCV usually became positive only after 12 weeks or more, second-generation assays (EIA-2, and recombinant immunoblot assay, or RIBA) may become positive as early as 2 weeks, but more often 5 to 6 weeks, after infection, i.e., before the end of the clinical incubation period (Fig. 117–6). The

EIA-2 and the supplemental RIBA, both more sensitive and more specific than the original EIA-1, are positive in nearly all cases of post-transfusion hepatitis. A third-generation assay is expected to become available in the near future. Assays for HCV-RNA by PCR may be positive as early as 2 weeks after infection; newer PCR assays also provide quantitative results but are somewhat less sensitive.

The acute illness is not distinguishable on clinical or general laboratory grounds from other causes of acute hepatitis, although liver biopsy in hepatitis C is more likely to show evidence of lymphoid aggregates, hepatocellular microvesicular fat, or bile duct injury. Accordingly, diagnosis depends on demonstrating a positive second-generation serologic assay and/or a positive PCR assay for HCV-RNA. The latter may be useful in equivocal cases, but in most instances RIBA positivity correlates well with the presence of HCV-RNA. PCR assays, however, may be helpful in assessing the activ-

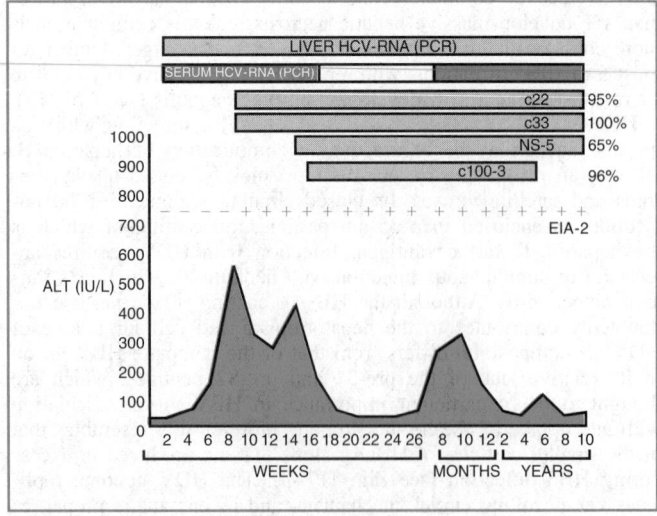

FIGURE 117–6. Course of acute hepatitis C infection. Intervals after infection at which various tests become positive are shown in relation to the clinical course as indicated by the aminotransferase elevation. (Adapted from Esteban J, et al.: Hepatitis C: Molecular biology, pathogenesis, epidemiology, clinical features, and prevention. *In* Boyer J, Ockner R [eds.]: Progress in Liver Diseases, Vol X. Philadelphia, WB Saunders, 1992.)

ity of viral replication, e.g., in an individual in whom several etiologic factors may be responsible for hepatic dysfunction.

Despite initial expectations, acute HCV infection appears to be associated only rarely if ever with massive hepatic necrosis and the syndrome of fulminant hepatic failure. Although evidence suggests that some of these cases of non-A, non-B massive hepatic necrosis may be caused by inapparent HBV infection, the cause of most remains unknown and could, conceivably, be an as yet uncharacterized viral agent.

In contrast, it has been recognized for some time that non-A, non-B hepatitis, including HCV infection, has a much greater propensity to become chronic than hepatitis B, even in otherwise healthy individuals. Based on the more sensitive diagnostic methods now available, it appears that persisting infection, whether active or quiescent, in fact follows the acute illness in the majority of patients. Moreover, it is now also clear that persisting HCV infection may be present in a given patient despite normalization of serum aminotransferase activity, negative second-generation tests for HCV antibodies, and even negative PCR assays for HCV-RNA. In the latter instance, HCV-RNA may be found in liver tissue or possibly in extrahepatic sites. Recognizing and managing chronic hepatitis C and its chronic complications and sequelae are discussed in Ch. 119.

HEPATITIS E. In recent years, an epidemic form of non-A, non-B hepatitis has been described, associated with outbreaks in India, Central Asia, Pakistan, China, Southeast Asia, North Africa and the Middle East, the former Soviet Union, and Mexico. The responsible agent is a 27- to 34-nm nonenveloped, single-stranded RNA agent distinct from HAV and the picornaviridae. On the basis of its genetic organization and expression strategy, hepatitis E virus (HEV) may represent a new form of nonenveloped agent infecting humans. Among the isolates obtained, there is substantial homology worldwide.

Transmission. HEV is transmitted almost exclusively via the fecal-oral route. In addition to the large-scale outbreaks that first called attention to this agent and led eventually to its isolation and characterization, it is also endemic in certain areas where it has been associated with sporadic cases, e.g., among school children in Egypt and the Sudan. Although the disease is apparently rare in Europe, the United States, and Canada, cases have been reported among travelers returning from areas where prevalence is higher. Moreover, approximately 2% of healthy blood donors in the United States and comparable percentages of those in Germany and the Netherlands have serum antibodies to HEV, possibly reflecting previous inapparent infection or cross-reactivity with an as yet unidentified agent. Significantly, the disease has been confirmed in three health care workers in Cape Town, a very low-incidence geographic area, who were attending an affected returning traveler, indicating the importance of routine precautionary measures in the care of such patients.

Clinical Course. The acute illness affects chiefly adolescents and young adults, ages 15 to 40, but younger children may also be affected. Following exposure, there is an incubation period of 2 to 9 weeks, averaging 6 weeks. Virus begins to appear in blood, bile, and feces before the end of the incubation period, as in hepatitis A. Virus in serum begins to decline within 10 days of clinical onset and disappears from stool after 14 days. The clinical presentation of the illness is typical for acute hepatitis except that there appears to be a higher frequency of icteric cases; subclinical disease has been documented, especially in children. Skin rash and arthralgia may occur. The histopathology is also typical for acute viral hepatitis or may be predominantly cholestatic. The illness is entirely acute and self-limited, with no evidence to suggest chronicity. However, the case-fatality rate for epidemic hepatitis E is significantly greater than that for other forms of acute viral hepatitis, approaching 1 to 2% overall, and as high as 20% for pregnant women, especially those in the third trimester. The reason for this is unknown.

The diagnosis can be suspected in epidemic situations in individuals with acute, usually icteric, non-A, non-B hepatitis. Serodiagnosis has recently become possible using specific enzyme-linked immunoassays for IgM and/or IgG anti-HEV; they are expected to become commercially available in the near future. IgM antibodies are present in serum for 2 to 24 weeks after the acute onset. IgG anti-HEV also appears at about 2 weeks and usually begins to decline in titer after about 2 years, although significant titers may persist for many years. Recovery from the acute illness appears to confer lifelong immunity.

GENERAL APPROACHES TO DIAGNOSIS AND MANAGEMENT

DIAGNOSIS. In its classic presentation, acute viral hepatitis is readily suggested by a compatible history and physical examination, in association with laboratory evidence of hepatocellular injury, especially significantly increased serum aminotransferase activities. Because all of these features are nonspecific, however, it is essential that other possible causes of an acute hepatitis syndrome be considered, such as use of medications or illicit drugs, alcohol, exposure to environmental or industrial toxins, and the possible acquisition of unusual infections as suggested by travel or residence in rural or less well-developed areas. Exposure to viral hepatitis itself is suggested by contact with jaundiced persons or persons known to have developed hepatitis, sexual promiscuity (especially among male homosexuals), transfusion of blood or blood products, or sharing of needles by drug users. Among health professionals, workers in dialysis and oncology units, surgeons, dentists, and clinical laboratory technicians are at increased risk, as is anyone in direct contact with blood, blood products, or other body fluids. Despite the importance of a careful inquiry into these possible risk factors, many patients with acute viral hepatitis report no significant exposures.

A careful and complete physical examination may help establish the diagnosis (tender hepatomegaly is the most common finding) and exclude other processes that occasionally mimic acute viral hepatitis, such as acute hepatic congestion, disseminated sepsis or liver abscess, or biliary tract disease with or without cholangitis.

Serodiagnosis of viral hepatitis is an important part of the initial evaluation. A positive test for the IgM class of anti-HAV or a rising titer of total anti-HAV is strong evidence for acute hepatitis A. Conversely, if the test for anti-HAV is negative well into the convalescent phase, the diagnosis is excluded. A single positive test for unfractionated anti-HAV is of little diagnostic value because this could reflect a previous infection.

Acute hepatitis B is suggested by positive tests for HBsAg (in approximately 75% of cases) and IgM anti-HBc (almost invariably). A single negative test for HBsAg does not definitely exclude acute hepatitis B. Even in those cases in which HBV-DNA is demonstrated, however, the possibility of chronic hepatitis B in reactivation or with superimposed hepatitis caused by another agent must be considered (see Ch. 119). The presence of anti-HBs early in the course of acute hepatitis tends to suggest chronic rather than acute HBV infection. Medical records, if available, may provide information about prior liver laboratory tests, hepatitis serologies, or blood donation. Because donated blood has been screened routinely for HBsAg since 1972, such information may be quite helpful in evaluating the chronicity of hepatitis B serologies.

As noted above, the second-generation EIA and RIBA-2 tests for acute hepatitis C are not usually reactive until an average of 5 to 6 weeks after the clinical onset, although HCV-RNA is detectable as early as 2 weeks. Hepatitis D may be documented by a positive test for serum anti-HDV.

A *liver biopsy* may demonstrate the pathologic features of acute viral hepatitis. However, these are nonspecific, and in the vast majority of cases biopsy is not indicated. Its use should be reserved for patients in whom the diagnosis is uncertain or in whom there is concern regarding chronicity or a deteriorating course, or any circumstance in which documentation of the histopathology may influence management. In the most severely ill patients, biopsy may be relatively or absolutely contraindicated because of abnormal clotting function.

DIFFERENTIAL DIAGNOSIS. Acute viral hepatitis may be mimicked by a large number of other acute infectious and noninfectious processes. Infections include other viruses such as cytomegalovirus, Epstein-Barr virus (infectious mononucleosis), and yellow fever virus and nonviral processes such as Q fever, secondary syphilis, leptospirosis, salmonellosis, pyogenic and amebic liver abscess, malaria, and toxoplasmosis. A number of drugs and toxins may injure the liver and cause a clinical syndrome that can resemble viral hepatitis (see Ch. 118). Inborn errors of metabolism such as Wilson's disease may also lead to acute hepatic necrosis. Acute hepatic congestion secondary to cardiac failure or venous occlusion, cholecystitis, and acute biliary obstruction should also be excluded. Finally, the possibility that what appears to be acute hepatitis may in fact represent the exacerbation of chronic hepatitis should be considered (see Ch. 119).

MANAGEMENT. No specific treatment is available for acute viral hepatitis. Major emphasis is placed on symptomatic and supportive care and on preventing transmission. Most patients with acute viral hepatitis do not require hospitalization and are appropriately managed at home. Rest is advisable, but strict confinement to bed is not necessary beyond what is dictated by the patient's own sense of fatigue and malaise. No specific dietary measures are indicated, but most patients find a low-fat, high-carbohydrate diet more palatable. During the most severe phase of the illness, anorexia and nausea may be so extreme that oral intake of any kind is minimal. In such instances, attention to fluid balance is important, and it may be necessary to advise the intake of small amounts of clear fluids at frequent intervals. Although there is an appropriate reluctance to administer medication to the patient with liver disease, judicious use of small doses of antinausea agents such as hydroxyzine, trimethobenzamide, and even prochlorperazine is occasionally necessary and usually well tolerated. As the patient's symptoms decrease and appetite improves, intake can be liberalized, usually according to taste. Alcoholic beverages should be avoided throughout the course of the acute illness. Ambulation and activity may be increased as symptoms and laboratory tests improve; the most useful advice is that such activity should be limited so as to avoid causing fatigue. The decision to return to employment or school must take into consideration the patient's symptoms, the strenuousness of the work, and the potential for transmission of the disease; this, in turn, is a function of the viral origin and the closeness of contact with others. In general, transmission is quite unlikely after 2 to 3 weeks in hepatitis A, whereas spread of hepatitis B or C ordinarily requires direct person-to-person contact.

Hospitalization is indicated for those patients in whom severe nausea and vomiting prevent maintenance of adequate fluid balance or in whom invasive diagnostic studies are indicated. In patients who are progressively deteriorating, especially with encephalopathy or a prolonged prothrombin time, arrangements should be made for urgent transfer to a facility where they can be evaluated for and emergency liver transplantation performed, should that become necessary.

Except for the unusual patient with prolonged cholestasis in hepatitis A, no convincing evidence justifies using corticosteroids in acute hepatitis, regardless of its severity. The management of fulminant hepatitic failure poses special problems in patient monitoring and support and should take place in a center that provides for the option of liver transplantation if that becomes necessary. Fulminant hepatic failure is discussed in detail in Ch. 124.

PREVENTION. The entire approach to hepatitis prophylaxis has been dramatically changed by the availability of an effective vaccine for hepatitis B and by the imminent availability of a vaccine for hepatitis A. Pending the advent of effective vaccines for all of the viral causes of acute hepatitis, however, prevention will continue to depend to a large extent on personal hygiene and public health measures directed at minimizing the exposure of potentially susceptible individuals and on the appropriate use of passive immunization.

Public health and hygienic measures rest on the premise that body fluids, secretions, and excreta of infected individuals are potentially infective. Clearly there are certain exceptions, depending on the specific virus involved, the clinical stage of the infection, the amount of potentially infective material involved, and the nature of the exposure. For example, because of the ease with which hepatitis A and E are spread via the fecal-oral route, contact of such patients with others should be minimized, and their excreta and essentially all materials handled by them during their brief period of infectivity should be disposed of carefully. In contrast, hepatitis B, C, and D are not commonly spread via the fecal-oral route. Although excreta are to be regarded as infective in these patients, the more important concern is transmission via puncture by contaminated needles (or equivalent exposure to infective material) or intimate personal (e.g., sexual) contact, especially during the period of HBsAg positivity. Because of the differences among the agents and differences in the approach to passive immunization, serologic diagnosis of the acute

viral hepatitis case is important, even though most patients with these disorders may be expected to do well. In practice, rapid serodiagnosis is not always possible, and for this reason certain generalizations apply to the early management of patients and their contacts and are discussed below, along with measures for specific agents.

Hepatitis A. Because the infection is spread primarily via the fecal-oral route, including transmission by handling food, in drinking water, and by fomites, strict attention to hygiene by patients and their attendants, whether in home or hospital, is of utmost importance during the period of viral shedding. Direct body contact should be limited to that necessary for care; attendants should wear gloves, and careful handwashing is appropriate. Food, utensils, clothing, linen, needles, and excreta should be handled separately and carefully, also by gloved attendants. The virus is readily inactivated by boiling or by exposure to formalin, chlorine, or ultraviolet irradiation. In the hospital setting, strict isolation is not usually required for cooperative and informed patients with hepatitis A. In the home, similar measures should be implemented to the extent possible.

Close contacts of patients with hepatitis A should receive passive immunization with immune serum globulin as soon as possible, preferably within the first few days. The official recommended dose is 0.02 ml per kilogram up to a maximum of 2 ml, although up to 5 ml has been advocated. This applies to immediate family members, sexual contacts, or others with whom the patient has been in close contact during the presumed period of infectivity. Casual contacts in the workplace or school probably do not require passive immunization unless there is reason to suspect mutual handling of food, beverages, or contaminated items. On the other hand, it is important to inquire about other possible cases among work or classroom associates. If there is reason to suspect a possible point-source outbreak, then all similarly exposed persons should receive immune serum globulin and appropriate epidemiologic information should be obtained.

The mode of transmission of hepatitis A also renders its prevention a matter of concern for those who intend to travel in areas where public health and sanitation measures may be suboptimal. In such circumstances, drinking water, fresh fruits and vegetables, and shellfish may be contaminated and should be avoided if possible. For these persons, a standard dose (0.02 ml per kilogram) of immune serum globulin may be expected to afford protection for up to 3 months; for longer periods a dose of 0.06 ml per kilogram is recommended and should be repeated at 4- to 6-month intervals.

A formalin-inactivated virus HAV vaccine has been developed and shown to be safe and effective. It elicits titers of serum anti-HAV apparently sufficient to provide immunity for 5 to 10 years, but not secretory anti-HAV. One preparation has been licensed for use in Europe. At the time of this writing, licensing in the United States and specific recommendations for its use in various settings and population groups are pending.

Hepatitis B. Although this agent is not readily transmitted via the fecal-oral route, due consideration should be given to the general hygienic measures outlined for hepatitis A, in both home and hospital. Transmission ordinarily requires direct contact with the patient or the equivalent of a parenteral inoculation of infective material. Thus, in the home, children are significantly less likely than the spouse to acquire hepatitis B from an acutely infected adult. In the hospital, strict isolation may not be necessary if excreta, needles and other medical supplies, and personal utensils are identified, carefully handled, and discarded.

Hepatitis B Vaccine. Safe and effective vaccines have been developed for preventing hepatitis B, consisting either of highly purified and triple-inactivated HBsAg obtained from the serum of chronic carriers or a recombinant preparation using HBsAg synthesized in microorganisms. The vaccine is administered in three doses, initially and 1 month and 6 months later, and elicits production of anti-HBs in 90% or more of healthy recipients. Intramuscular injection is important and is more likely effective in the deltoid than gluteal muscles. (Smaller doses are used for children, and larger doses for dialysis and immunocompromised patients.) The recombinant vaccine is safe for pregnant women. Although most subjects who have completed the three-dose immunization are protected against hepatitis B infection, there are important exceptions, especially among immunosuppressed subjects. The duration of this protection varies but probably is at least 5 years or more. No official recommendations have been made regarding booster doses.

The vaccine initially was recommended only for use in high-risk groups and individuals. These include, but are not limited to, health professionals (especially those with high exposure risk such as surgeons, dentists, and dialysis workers), susceptible dialysis patients, and those subject to multiple transfusions (e.g., hemophiliacs), certain residents and staff of custodial care institutions, parenteral illicit drug users, heterosexual and household contacts of HBsAg carriers, Alaskan Eskimos, and sexually active and promiscuous male homosexuals. Available evidence suggests that it is also effective when the first vaccine dose is combined with high-titer anti-HBs (i.e., hepatitis B immune globulin, or HBIG), in the passive-active immunization of health professionals after accidental needle stick and of infants born to HBsAg-positive mothers. The cost-effectiveness of screening of potential vaccine recipients (e.g., anti-HBs determination) varies with the circumstance. In general, in those groups in which prevalence of hepatitis B is relatively low, screening is not cost effective, whereas it may be useful in groups with a high prevalence (e.g., the homosexual community). For most health professionals, screening is marginally cost effective and depends on the prevalence of hepatitis B infection in the particular subgroup. In any case, it is established that administering the vaccine to individuals already infected or immune is not harmful.

These initial recommendations for using the vaccine in selected high-risk groups remain valid and have been expanded to include certain international travelers and immigrees from high prevalence areas. However, the incidence of hepatitis B in the United States continued to increase after the vaccine was introduced. Presumably, this reflected inability to immunize sufficient numbers of individuals in recognized high-risk groups as well as the fact that an estimated 30% of acutely infected individuals fall outside of these groups and therefore would not have been targeted in a selective immunization program. As a result, newer recommendations in the United States include universal screening of women in pregnancy, universal immunization of newborn infants, and immunization of high-risk adolescents. Although the benefits of such a program in terms of health and health care costs will not be fully realized for decades, it marks the beginning of an effort that could lead to eradicating the virus and its acute and chronic effects.

Post-exposure Prophylaxis and Passive Immunization. Exposure of unprotected persons to HBV may occur in several settings, including the following:

1. Inoculation of material known to be contaminated with the hepatitis B virus, e.g., inadvertent puncture of a health professional by a needle from an HBsAg-positive patient or accidental transfusion of HBsAg-positive blood or blood products.
2. Splash of HBsAg-positive material into the eye or on an open skin wound or eruption, as may occur in a laboratory accident or during a surgical or diagnostic procedure.
3. Ingesting HBsAg-positive material, as may occur during a laboratory pipetting accident.
4. Sexual partners of patients with *acute* hepatitis B (partners of patients with chronic hepatitis B presumably have been previously exposed) within 14 days of contact.
5. Infants born to HBsAg-positive mothers, especially those who have had acute hepatitis B during the final trimester of pregnancy or first 2 months postpartum or who are positive for both HBsAg and HBeAg at the time of delivery.

Because most persons so exposed, health professional or not, are likely to be at risk for future exposure, the recommended general approach is to institute as early as possible passive immunization with hepatitis B immune globulin (HBIG, 0.06 ml per kilogram) combined with simultaneous initiation of active immunization using HBV vaccine, administered intramuscularly at a separate site.

The rational approach to postexposure prophylaxis depends on two essential components. First, it must be documented that the material to which the person has been exposed contains HBsAg, and this requires identifying the source and appropriate serologic confirmation. For example, accidental puncture of the skin by one of several used needles in a disposal container effectively precludes meeting this requirement and, therefore, the use of HBIG. Second, the exposed person must actually be at risk. If, at the time of exposure, he/she is already positive for HBsAg (i.e., infected) or anti-HBs (i.e., immune if the s/n value by radioimmunoassay exceeds 10), nothing will be gained from administering HBIG or vaccine. Ideally, therefore, the serologic status of both "donor" and "recipient"

should be documented before the decision to administer HBIG and vaccine is made. In practice, however, this may not be possible within the few days' interval after exposure in which postexposure prophylaxis appears to be most effective. In this situation, serum should be immediately obtained from both the "donor" and the person at risk. Pending results of the serologic assays, the exposed person should initiate active immunization with the vaccine.

For sexual contacts of individuals with acute hepatitis B, available evidence suggests that HBIG is effective for up to 14 days after exposure and should be combined with initiation of active immunization with the vaccine. Infants under age 12 months whose primary caregiver has acute hepatitis B should receive both passive and active immunization. Other household contacts require no prophylaxis unless there has been sexual exposure or shared use of toothbrushes or razors. If the acutely infected member of the household becomes chronically infected (chronic hepatitis or "carrier"), all household contacts should receive the vaccine.

In all circumstances, if the exposed individual has completed hepatitis vaccination, additional immunization is unnecessary if it can be shown that the titer of anti-HBs is "protective" (10 mIU per milliliter). If vaccination has been initiated but not completed or if the level of anti-HBs is too low, a single dose of HBIG should be given and the vaccination series completed or a booster dose of vaccine given.

Hepatitis C. Hepatitis C appears to be transmitted in a manner more closely resembling that of hepatitis B than hepatitis A. Thus, close personal contact and parenteral inoculation appear necessary, suggesting that prophylactic measures suitable for hepatitis B are appropriate, although available evidence suggests that it is not as readily transmitted to sexual and household contacts.

A problem largely confined to hepatitis C at present is post-transfusion hepatitis. The single most effective means of reducing the incidence of this disorder has been excluding blood obtained from commercial (paid donor) sources. There is a correlation between both elevated aminotransferase activity and anti-HBc positivity in donor unit plasma and the probability of post-transfusion hepatitis in a recipient; exclusion of such units is desirable. The advent of widescale screening of donor units for anti-HCV has further diminished the incidence of post-transfusion hepatitis. The possible role of pre-exposure (i.e., pretransfusion) immune serum globulin in preventing the disorder remains unclear and, because there is no evidence for a neutralizing (protective) antibody to HCV, at present immune serum globulin is not officially recommended for this purpose. For the same reason, immune serum globulin is not recommended after accidental needlestick exposure to a source infected only with HCV.

Hepatitis D. There is no established method for active or passive immunization. Because HDV infection requires simultaneous or antecedent HBV infection, prevention of HBV, e.g., by the vaccine, protects against HDV. Because previously infected HBV subjects are at risk for HDV infection, care should be taken to minimize their exposure to materials that might contain HDV, e.g., HBV-positive serum or secretions.

Hepatitis E. Neither passive nor active immunization is available at this time

General

Dienstag JL (ed.): Viral hepatitis. Semin Liver Dis Vol 11, May 1991. *A minisymposium in which recognized experts critically review clinically relevant aspects of acute and chronic hepatitis.*

Dusheiko GM: Rolling review—the pathogenesis, diagnosis and management of viral hepatitis. Aliment Pharmacol Ther 8:229, 1994. *A current and concise overview.*

Favero MS, Maynard JE, Leger RT, et al.: Guidelines for the care of patients hospitalized with viral hepatitis. Ann Intern Med 91:872, 1979. *Specific recommendations that provide a useful guide.*

Hepatitis A

Gocke D: Hepatitis A revisited. Ann Intern Med 105:960, 1986. Glikson M, Galun E, Oren R, et al.: Relapsing hepatitis A. Review of 14 cases and literature survey. Medicine 71:14, 1992. Lemon SM: Type A viral hepatitis. New developments in an old disease. N Engl J Med 313:1059, 1985. Siegl G, Weitz M: Pathogenesis of hepatitis A: Persistent viral infection as basis of an acute disease? Microb Pathogen 14:1, 1993. *Four reports summarizing more recently recognized clinical features of the disease.*

Lemon SM: Inactivated hepatitis A vaccines [editorial]. JAMA 271:1363, 1994. Sjogren MH: The success of hepatitis A vaccine [editorial]. Gastroenterology 104:1214, 1993. *Concise status reports on the vaccine.*

Hepatitis B

Advisory Committee on Immunization Practices: Hepatitis B virus: A comprehensive strategy for eliminating transmission in the United States through universal childhood vaccination. MMWR 40:1, 1991. *A statement of current recommendations.*

Carman W, Thomas H, Domingo E: Viral genetic variation: Hepatitis B virus as a clinical example. Lancet 341:349, 1993. Lau JYN, Wright TL: Molecular virology and pathogenesis of hepatitis B; and Clinical aspects of hepatitis B infection. Lancet 342:1335 and 1340, 1993. *Succinct and timely reviews of various virologic and clinical aspects of hepatitis B.*

Kiire CF: The epidemiology and prophylaxis of hepatitis B in sub-Saharan Africa. *In* Boyer JL, Ockner RK (eds.): Progress in Liver Diseases, Vol XI. Philadelphia, WB Saunders, 1993, p 167. *Evidence for nonperinatal ("horizontal") transmission to children.*

Hepatitis C

Alter MJ: Transmission of hepatitis C virus—route, dose, and titer [editorial]. N Engl J Med 330:784, 1994. Donahue JG, Muñoz A, Ness PM, et al.: The declining risk of post-transfusion hepatitis C virus infection. N Engl J Med 327:369, 1992. *A summary of various aspects of epidemiology.*

Esteban JI, Genesca J, Alter HJ: Hepatitis C: Molecular biology, pathogenesis, epidemiology, clinical features, and prevention. *In* Boyer JL, Ockner RK (eds.): Progress in Liver Diseases, Vol X. Philadelphia, WB Saunders, 1992, p 253. Simmonds P, Alberti A, Alter HJ, et al.: A proposed system for the nomenclature of hepatitis C viral genotypes. Hepatology 19:1321, 1994. *Reviews of HCV biology, disease, and proposed classification.*

Wright TL: Hepatitis C virus infection and organ transplantation. *In* Boyer JL, Ockner RK (eds.): Progress in Liver Diseases, Vol XI. Philadelphia, WB Saunders, 1993, p 215. *A comprehensive review of epidemiologic, diagnostic, and therapeutic aspects.*

Hepatitis D

Polish LB, Gallagher M, Fields HA, et al.: Delta hepatitis: Molecular biology and clinical and epidemiological features. Clin Microbiol Rev 6:211, 1993. Smedile A, Rizzetto M, Gerin JL: Advances in hepatitis D virus biology and disease. *In* Boyer JL, Ockner RK (eds.): Progress in Liver Diseases, Vol XII. Philadelphia, WB Saunders, 1994, p 157. *Two reviews covering virtually all aspects of the agent and the syndromes it causes.*

Hepatitis E

Reyes GR: Hepatitis E virus (HEV): Molecular biology and emerging epidemiology. *In* Boyer JL, Ockner RK (eds.): Progress in Liver Disease, Vol XI. Philadelphia, WB Saunders, 1993, p 203. Krawczynski K: Hepatitis E. Hepatology 17:932, 1993. *Comprehensive summaries.*

118 TOXIC AND DRUG-INDUCED LIVER DISEASE

Nathan M. Bass

In clearing and biotransforming xenobiotics, the liver is exposed to a large variety of potentially toxic chemical agents and metabolites: naturally occurring plant alkaloids and mycotoxins, industrial chemicals, and, most commonly, pharmacologic agents used in treating disease. The manifestations of toxic and drug-induced liver disease also constitute a spectrum of clinical, laboratory, and histopathologic changes and prognoses virtually as broad as the entire range of acute and chronic hepatobiliary disorders. The severity may range, at one extreme, from asymptomatic abnormalities in liver function tests to fatal massive liver necrosis at the other. Viral hepatitis and biliary obstruction may be closely mimicked by hepatotoxic drug reactions, and exposure to certain agents may also lead to chronic hepatitis, cirrhosis, and liver tumors.

PATHOGENESIS

It is rare for a parent chemical to be directly responsible for drug- and toxin-induced liver disease; more commonly a toxic metabolite(s) formed by the drug-metabolizing enzymes within the liver is the immediate causative agent. Drug biotransformation appears to be a common requirement in the pathogenesis of many different types of drug-induced liver injury. Individual susceptibility to the injury produced by some drugs varies considerably. Potentially hepatotoxic agents are therefore conventionally divided into two categories based on the predictability with which they produce liver disease: *intrinsic hepatotoxins* and *idiosyncratic hepatotoxins.*

Intrinsic hepatotoxins typically produce acute liver damage after a relatively brief latent period (usually a few days) in a predictable, dose-dependent fashion that is largely independent of host susceptibility factors and that is readily reproducible in experimental animals. Examples of this group include the industrial solvents *carbon tetrachloride, 2-nitropropane, trichloroethane,* the octapeptide toxins of the *Amanita* mushroom species, and the antipyretic *acetaminophen.* In most instances, toxic metabolites formed from the parent compound by the cytochrome P-450 drug-metabolizing enzymes produce liver damage by covalently modifying liver macromolecules, or by generating reactive oxygen species and subsequent peroxidation of cell membrane lipids.

Idiosyncratic hepatotoxins, in contrast, produce liver disease in an infrequent, unpredictable fashion after a variable latent period, often only after several months of administration of the drug. A large number of therapeutic agents are capable of producing idiosyncratic hepatotoxic reactions in a small proportion of patients who receive them (e.g., halothane, isoniazid, phenytoin, and chlorpromazine). Although severe liver disease occurs infrequently with these drugs, milder hepatic dysfunction may occur frequently (e.g., with isoniazid and chlorpromazine), or toxic liver disease may be reproduced in animal models (e.g., halothane). Many of these agents may therefore be "intrinsic hepatotoxins" that lead to severe "idiosyncratic" liver disease in a few susceptible individuals, possibly because of variations in the pathways of drug biotransformation, immune-mediated hypersensitivity ("drug allergy"), or both. In a given individual, genetic polymorphism in drug-metabolizing enzymes may increase activity of subsidiary pathways that form toxic metabolites and thereby increase the risk of severe toxicity from drugs that are processed in part via these pathways. In idiosyncratic drug-induced liver disease, fever, arthralgias, rash, and eosinophilia are often prominent, indicative of a hypersensitivity-based mechanism. Furthermore, in some cases of drug-induced hepatitis (e.g., halothane), antibodies that recognize liver cell macromolecules covalently modified by metabolites of the implicated drug antibodies have been detected. Adducts formed on the liver cell surface between drug metabolites and liver cell membrane proteins may therefore constitute neoantigens that can provoke immune-mediated liver damage.

MORPHOLOGIC PATTERNS OF DRUG-INDUCED LIVER DISEASE

Drugs and toxins produce a variety of pathologic lesions in the liver (Table 118–1). Some agents may injure the liver in more than one way. For example, isoniazid may produce a nonspecific focal hepatitis, an acute viral hepatitis-like lesion, or chronic active hepatitis, whereas oral contraceptives may cause cholestasis or liver cell adenoma and have been implicated in hepatic vein thrombosis and other vascular lesions.

ZONAL NECROSIS. Intrinsic hepatotoxins typically cause liver cell necrosis, largely confined within a particular zone of the liver lobule. Centrilobular necrosis, the most common pattern of zonal injury, is produced by *carbon tetrachloride, acetaminophen,* and *Amanita toxins* (see Ch. 123). This pattern of injury is explained in part by the greater abundance of cytochrome P-450 drug-metabolizing enzymes in the central region of the liver lobule and possibly also by the relative hypoxemia of the centrilobular region. *Halothane,* despite its classification as an idiosyncratic hepatotoxic agent, also frequently produces centrilobular necrosis. Periportal zonal necrosis, a much rarer lesion, is produced by *allyl alcohol* and *yellow phosphorus.* Extremely high elevations of serum aminotransferases usually accompany this type of liver injury, and in severe cases, acute liver failure may result. Acute zonal necrosis is either fatal or is followed by complete recovery.

NONSPECIFIC FOCAL HEPATITIS. Nonspecific focal hepatitis consists of scattered foci of liver cell necrosis with mononuclear cell infiltrates, without the characteristic features of viral hepatitis. Nonspecific hepatitis may result from many forms of drug injury including the dose-dependent, intrinsic hepatotoxicity of *aspirin* and *oxacillin.* This lesion has an excellent prognosis and resolves completely when the responsible drug is discontinued.

VIRAL HEPATITIS-LIKE REACTIONS. Diffuse hepatocellular degeneration and necrosis with variable inflammatory infiltration and acidophil bodies, resembling the acute pathologic lesion and the clinical manifestations of viral hepatitis, is another common pattern of idiosyncratic injury. In severe cases this lesion may progress to bridging, submassive or massive liver necrosis, and fulminant

TABLE 118–1. CLASSIFICATION OF DRUG-INDUCED LIVER DISEASE

Category	Examples
Zonal necrosis	Acetaminophen, carbon tetrachloride
Nonspecific hepatitis	Aspirin, oxacillin
Viral hepatitis–like reactions	Halothane, isoniazid, phenytoin, diclofenac
Chronic hepatitis	
Autoimmune hepatitis–like	Methyldopa, dantrolene, diclofenac
Viral hepatitis–like	Isoniazid, halothane
Cholestasis	
Noninflammatory	Estrogens, 17α-substituted steroids
Inflammatory	Amoxicillin-clavulanate, piroxicam
Ductal	Flucloxacillin, thiabendazole
Sclerosing cholangitis	FUDR
Fatty liver	
Large droplet	Ethanol, corticosteroids
Small droplet	Tetracycline, valproic acid, didanosine
Phospholipidosis ±	
pseudoalcoholic hepatitis	Amiodarone, perhexiline maleate
Granulomas	Phenylbutazone, allopurinol
Fibrosis	Methotrexate, hypervitaminosis A
Tumors	
Adenoma	Estrogens
Angiosarcoma	Vinyl chloride
Vascular lesions	
Hepatic vein thrombosis	Estrogens
Veno-occlusive disease	Anticancer agents, azathioprine
Peliosis hepatis	Anabolic steroids, estrogens
Hepatic arteritis	Allopurinol, FUDR
Nodular regenerative	
hyperplasia	Azathioprine, anticancer agents

liver failure. Drugs producing viral hepatitis-like reactions include *halothane, isoniazid, ketoconazole, methyldopa, sulfonamides,* and *phenytoin.* In some instances, the presence of fever, rash, and serum and tissue eosinophilia, as well as other evidence of immunologic dysfunction, are important clues in the diagnosis of drug-induced disease and also implicate a hypersensitivity-based mechanism. In other examples, such as halothane and isoniazid, features of hypersensitivity are highly variable or distinctly rare.

CHOLESTASIS. Cholestasis is characterized by clinical symptoms of pruritus and jaundice and biochemically by elevated serum alkaline phosphatase and minimal or modest increases in serum aminotransferases. Four distinct forms of this common manifestation of drug-induced liver injury are recognized. In the first, caused principally by *natural and synthetic estrogens* and by *17 α-substituted androgenic and anabolic steroids,* there is usually little or no evidence of hepatocellular necrosis or inflammation. The injury is most simply viewed as the impaired secretion of bile by the liver cell, probably reflecting a direct steroid effect on the physical properties of cellular membranes or the function of canalicular proteins involved in bile secretion. The lesion is completely and rapidly reversible.

In the second form of cholestatic injury, there is significant hepatocellular necrosis and portal and lobular inflammation; acidophil bodies and eosinophils are variably present. Systemic features, including fever, rash, and arthralgias, are not uncommon. This form of injury is produced by a broad group of agents, including the *phenothiazines, amoxycillin-clavulanic acid, oral hypoglycemic* and *antithyroid* agents, and the *macrolide antibiotics* (e.g., erythromycin estolate). Its prognosis is generally favorable and complete recovery may be expected.

The third form of drug-induced cholestatic injury is characterized histologically by a progressive inflammatory destruction of the interlobular bile ducts, producing a clinical syndrome similar to primary biliary cirrhosis. Deep jaundice, pruritus, and xanthelasma develop during the course of this disease, which may persist for months to years prior to resolving. In a few patients, cholestasis has progressed to secondary biliary cirrhosis. This drug-induced ductal lesion, or vanishing bile duct syndrome, is an unusual variant of the cholestatic injury produced by *phenothiazines, carbamazepine,* and *sulfonylureas,* but is typical of the liver injury associated with *flucloxacillin.*

A fourth, unique type of drug-induced cholestatic lesion is the injury to the major hepatic ducts produced by intrahepatic arterial in-

fusion chemotherapy with *5-FUDR.* This lesion resembles the diffuse ductal strictures of primary sclerosing cholangitis and results from ischemic injury following drug-induced arteritis.

FATTY LIVER. Triglycerides may accumulate within hepatocytes in two forms. Most commonly, fat accumulates as large droplets that displace the liver cell nucleus and confer an adipocyte-like appearance. Hepatomegaly and mildly elevated aminotransferases are typically found, but liver function is usually well preserved. This form of fatty liver typically occurs with direct hepatotoxins including *ethanol, halogenated hydrocarbons, acetaminophen,* and also with *corticosteroids* and is similar in appearance to the fatty liver seen in other systemic conditions such as protein-calorie malnutrition, obesity, and uncontrolled diabetes mellitus.

A much less common pattern usually associated with significant, occasionally fatal, hepatic dysfunction, is seen in association with *tetracycline* or *valproic acid* hepatotoxicity, and occasionally with alcoholic liver disease, and resembles that seen in *Reye's syndrome, obstetric fatty liver,* and *Jamaican vomiting sickness.* It consists of fat deposited in smaller droplets throughout the liver cell, the nucleus remaining central. This pattern of liver injury, accompanied by profound, often fatal lactic acidosis, has been produced by several antiviral *nucleoside analogues,* including didanosine (ddI), fialuridine (FIAU), and zidovudine (AZT). Curiously, in the case of AZT, the hepatic morphologic lesion has been large-droplet rather than small-droplet fat. A distinctive type of hepatic lipid accumulation in the form of lysosomal phospholipid storage occurs as a direct effect of the drugs *amiodarone* and *perhexilene maleate.*

GRANULOMAS. Therapeutic agents are probably responsible for up to one third of cases of granulomatous hepatitis. Drug-induced granulomas are typically noncaseating and are often associated with extrahepatic granulomas and prominent systemic features of hypersensitivity. Responsible agents include *phenylbutazone, quinidine, allopurinol, phenytoin, hydralazine, sulfonamides,* and *sulfonylurea derivatives.*

CHRONIC HEPATITIS. Chronic hepatitis has been associated with an increasing number of drugs, including *amiodarone, dantrolene, isoniazid, methyldopa, nitrofurantoin, oxyphenisatin, perhexilene maleate, phenytoin, propylthiouracil, sulfonamides,* and *diclofenac.* Although these agents more often cause acute liver injury, prolonged use may occasionally result in a chronic progressive process leading in some instances to cirrhosis. The histologic and clinical abnormalities usually resemble those seen in idiopathic autoimmune or viral chronic active hepatitis. In the case of amiodarone, a lesion strikingly similar to that of alcoholic hepatitis with prominent Mallory bodies may be produced. In many cases, the lesion is largely or completely reversible, but in severe cases this may require many months after the drug is discontinued. Rarely, progressive liver failure and death may ensue despite stopping the drug.

FIBROSIS. Chronic liver injury from some agents increases collagen deposition, often with minimal or absent evidence of hepatocellular necrosis or inflammatory response. Fibrosis may progress to cirrhosis and portal hypertension, although the latter may occur as a result of hepatic portal fibrosis even in the absence of cirrhosis. This type of injury may occur following the chronic administration of *methotrexate* in treating psoriasis or exposure to *inorganic arsenicals* and in *hypervitaminosis A.*

TUMORS. Tumors caused by drugs and other chemical agents may be of several types, including *hepatic adenoma* (and possibly *hepatocellular carcinoma*) associated with *oral contraceptive* use, and *angiosarcoma* caused by prolonged exposure to *vinyl chloride* monomer or Thorotrast. The mechanisms by which these tumors are produced are not known, but their clinical and laboratory features generally resemble those of similar tumors occurring "spontaneously." A possible exception is the apparently greater size, vascularity, and tendency to sudden hemorrhage of hepatic adenomas associated with oral contraceptive use (see Ch. 125).

VASCULAR LESIONS. Vascular lesions of several kinds occasionally are caused by drugs. Oral contraceptives have been implicated as a cause of hepatic vein thrombosis. Hepatic *veno-occlusive disease,* a process that affects the smaller tributaries of the hepatic vein, has been associated with the use of *antitumor agents,* including *6-thioguanine, cytarabine,* and *azathioprine,* as well as with ingestion of *pyrrolidizine alkaloids,* e.g., from plants of *Senecio* and *Crotalaria* species ("bush tea poisoning"). *Oral contraceptives* and *anabolic steroids* have been identified as causes of *peliosis hepatis,* a condition in which the liver lobule contains extrasinusoidal blood-filled spaces; this lesion is also seen in certain chronic wasting neoplastic and inflammatory diseases.

PRINCIPLES OF DIAGNOSIS AND MANAGEMENT

A causal relationship between using a drug and liver injury may be difficult to establish. Drugs may produce abnormalities very similar to those of other common disorders such as viral hepatitis or biliary disease, and some drugs may produce more than one kind of lesion. A detailed drug history is essential, and information about past exposure and the response to a suspect agent may be of considerable value in diagnosis. Because a number of industrial chemicals are potential hepatotoxins, details of the patient's occupation and work environment should be routinely obtained. The diagnosis of drug-induced liver disease ultimately depends on (a) a history of exposure; (b) consistent clinical, laboratory, and occasionally liver biopsy findings; and (c) resolution of the liver injury after the presumed toxin is discontinued. In some instances, when only a single agent is involved and a characteristic histologic type of injury is found, the diagnosis based on laboratory and biopsy findings is relatively straightforward. Examples include the small-droplet fatty liver caused by tetracycline or the centrilobular necrosis produced by acetaminophen (usually associated with significant blood levels of the drug). Conditions are more complex when several drugs are being used, any one of which or even the underlying disorder for which the drugs were prescribed may be responsible for a nonspecific or viral hepatitis-like liver injury. The causal role of a particular drug in idiosyncratic liver disease can usually be established through rechallenge with the drug. Rechallenge is rarely justified, however, because of the risk of a severe or even fatal outcome. Furthermore, it is not necessary to incriminate the drug unambiguously if alternative drugs are available.

Drug-induced liver disease is managed by discontinuing the implicated drug(s) and giving supportive care for acute hepatitis and hepatic failure as needed. In the case of severe, acute drug- or toxin-induced liver failure, urgent liver transplantation may be lifesaving (see Ch. 124). Specific pharmacologic intervention is generally limited to the administration of *N*-acetylcysteine in acetaminophen overdosage (see below). Corticosteroids have no established value in treating drug-induced liver disease, although they may suppress the serum sickness-like syndrome associated with certain idiosyncratic reactions.

SELECTED EXAMPLES OF DRUG-INDUCED LIVER DISEASE

ACETAMINOPHEN. This readily available analgesic and antipyretic is a classic example of an intrinsic, dose-dependent hepatotoxin causing zonal necrosis and acute liver failure, often associated with renal failure. Significant liver injury usually occurs with doses > 10 to 15 grams, most frequently taken in a suicide attempt. Inadvertent therapeutic overdose has also occurred from frequent dosing with over-the-counter and prescription combination drugs that contain acetaminophen, e.g., Nyquil and Vicodin. Within a few hours, patients develop nausea, vomiting, and diarrhea. These initial symptoms soon subside and are followed by a relatively asymptomatic phase. Clinical and laboratory signs of liver damage become evident 24 to 48 hours following ingestion. Serum aminotransferase levels > 5000 U per liter are common, whereas severe liver injury may lead to progressive liver failure with encephalopathy, coagulopathy, hypoglycemia, and lactic acidosis.

The liver injury is caused by a toxic metabolite of acetaminophen formed by the cytochrome P-450–dependent drug-metabolizing system. Below threshold doses, this metabolite is efficiently detoxified by conjugation with glutathione. In the toxic dose range, glutathione stores are rapidly exhausted and the metabolite reacts with essential cellular constituents, leading to cell dysfunction and death. The rate at which reactive acetaminophen metabolites are formed is influenced not only by the dose ingested but also by the activity of the cytochrome P-450 enzymes (which may be stimulated by inducers such as phenobarbital and ethanol) and by the availability of glutathione, which may be reduced by fasting and ethanol. A combination of both enzyme induction and glutathione depletion may underlie the particular susceptibility of patients with chronic alcoholism to acetaminophen hepatotoxicity. In such individuals, doses of acetaminophen within the therapeutic range may produce significant liver damage.

The initial treatment of acetaminophen overdose consists of supportive measures and gastric lavage. *N*-Acetylcysteine should be administered to high-risk patients, in whom it may significantly reduce the severity of liver necrosis and its attendant mortality. The plasma level of acetaminophen is the most reliable means for assessing prognosis. Levels in excess of 200 mg per liter at 4 hours, 100 mg per liter at 8 hours, or 50 mg per liter at 12 hours after ingestion are predictive of severe liver damage and are indications for treatment with *N*-acetylcysteine. This agent appears to act mainly by providing cysteine for glutathione synthesis and is most effective when given within 10 hours of acetaminophen ingestion. *N*-Acetylcysteine may afford some benefit after 10 hours, but its benefit after 24 hours is not established. Intravenous preparations have been used in Britain, but only the oral form of *N*-acetylcysteine is currently available in the United States. The recommended oral dose is 140 mg per kilogram initially, followed by maintenance doses of 70 mg per kilogram every 4 hours for 72 hours.

Survivors of acute acetaminophen toxicity usually recover completely without progressive or residual liver damage.

AMIODARONE. A number of patients who receive amiodarone develop mild increases in serum aminotransferase levels, which may normalize despite continuation of therapy, accompanied by engorgement of lysosomes with phospholipid. Between 1 and 3% of patients receiving amiodarone develop a more severe liver injury that histologically resembles acute alcoholic hepatitis, with fat infiltration of hepatocytes, focal necrosis, fibrosis, polymorphonuclear leukocyte infiltrates, and Mallory bodies. This lesion may progress to micronodular cirrhosis, with portal hypertension and liver failure. The pseudoalcoholic lesion and its progression to cirrhosis often occur in a clinically insidious manner, with minimal elevation of serum aminotransferases. Hepatomegaly may be found, but jaundice is rare. Evidence of hepatotoxicity may persist for several months after the drug is discontinued.

Liver biopsy is helpful in diagnosis and should be considered in patients receiving amiodarone who develop persistent or significant (greater than twofold) elevation of serum aminotransferases or hepatomegaly. The decision to discontinue amiodarone in the presence of histologic evidence of hepatotoxicity is often difficult in view of the more ominous risk of sudden death from cardiac arrhythmias which may be increased by abrupt withdrawal of the drug.

AMOXICILLIN-CLAVULANIC ACID. Amoxicillin *per se* has little hepatotoxic potential, but in combination with the β-lactamase inhibitor clavulanic acid (Augmentin), has resulted in cholestatic liver injury often delayed for several weeks after treatment has ended. Elderly men are most frequently affected. Jaundice is a consistent feature, and liver histology shows cholestasis with minimal necrosis or inflammation. Hypersensitivity manifestations are unusual. The clinical course has been benign in the majority of cases, with complete recovery within 4 to 6 months.

ERYTHROMYCIN. A cholestatic reaction with components of inflammatory cell infiltration and liver cell necrosis may complicate the use of erythromycin. In most instances, this has occurred with erythromycin estolate; other erythromycins including the ethylsuccinate and lactobionate have been less frequently implicated. Hepatotoxicity typically presents as an acute syndrome of right upper quadrant pain, fever, and variable cholestatic symptoms. The clinical picture may closely mimic acute cholecystitis or cholangitis and has prompted surgical exploration in some instances. The prognosis is uniformly excellent, but the reaction may recur within days of readministering the drug.

FLUCLOXACILLIN. The biliary epithelium is selectively targeted in the idiosyncratic cholestatic liver injury that has affected several hundred individuals treated with this semisynthetic penicillin. Older patients treated for longer than 2 weeks seem to be at greatest risk, with the onset of jaundice and pruritus usually between 1 and 3 weeks after therapy is completed. Although clinical symptoms usually resolve within 2 months, abnormalities in serum liver enzymes may persist for months to years. Furthermore, in a minority of patients, the injury has pursued a progressive course characterized by damage to and depletion of interlobular bile ducts (vanishing bile duct syndrome), with secondary biliary cirrhosis developing over a period of years.

HALOTHANE. This halogenated alkane anesthetic rarely causes a viral hepatitis-like reaction which, in severe cases, may progress to fatal massive hepatic necrosis. Susceptibility to halothane hepatitis appears to be increased in older persons, women, and obese individuals, and severe reactions usually occur after previous or multiple exposures to this anesthetic. Symptoms usually indistinguishable from viral hepatitis occur between 7 and 10 days after anesthesia, but this interval may shorten considerably after repeated exposure. Fever, which may be hectic, with chills and sweats, commonly precedes the onset of jaundice; rash and eosinophilia are less consistent features. The course may terminate fatally within days, or recovery occurs, which is usually rapid and complete. Some patients run a more protracted course before either recovering or developing liver failure. Metabolites of halothane formed by the cytochrome P-450 system are clearly important in the mechanism of the hepatic injury. Some of these metabolites may be directly toxic; others may form haptens with cell membrane proteins, provoking an immune-mediated attack on the liver. Cross-sensitization may occur between halothane, methoxyflurane, and enflurane, although hepatic injury appears to be less common with the latter two anesthetic agents.

ISONIAZID (INH). Among persons taking INH for single-drug chemoprophylaxis against tuberculosis, there is approximately a 10 to 20% incidence of subclinical liver injury. This manifests during the first few weeks of therapy as a mild to moderate increase in serum aminotransferase levels. These laboratory abnormalities, which reflect a focal nonspecific hepatitis, subside in the majority of patients despite continued administration of the drug. About 1% of patients receiving INH develop significant liver injury, which clinically and histologically resembles the wide spectrum of viral hepatitis. The liver disease may present as a relatively mild, acute process, a subacute or chronic hepatitis, or fatal massive liver necrosis. The onset usually occurs within 2 to 3 months after starting the drug, and initial symptoms are often nonspecific, with malaise and anorexia preceding signs of liver disease. Clinical features of "drug allergy" are distinctly unusual. Age influences the incidence of severe INH liver injury, which increases significantly after age 35, and probably exceeds 2% among persons over age 50.

INH appears to injure the liver by forming a toxic metabolite, acetylhydrazine. The conversion of acetylhydrazine to the nontoxic diacetylhydrazine may be impaired in slow acetylators of the drug, thus favoring the formation of a toxic derivative of acetylhydrazine via the cytochrome P-450-dependent drug-metabolizing system. Induction of P-450 enzymes by rifampin may account for occurrences of a precipitous and severe form of isoniazid hepatitis in patients receiving both drugs.

Patients receiving INH should be followed at regular intervals and advised to report intercurrent symptoms. If these are associated with evidence of disturbed liver function, the drug should be discontinued, pending further evaluation. Because liver enzyme abnormalities are common early in the course of INH treatment and reflect, in the vast majority (especially in younger patients), a transient and self-limiting event, routine monitoring of liver function tests in patients taking INH is not generally recommended. The risk:benefit ratio of INH chemoprophylaxis rises rapidly after the age of 35, however, warranting a conservative approach to instituting chemoprophylaxis in this group. A several-fold elevation in aminotransferases in a patient over age 35, even in the absence of symptoms, should be regarded as potentially serious and may justify discontinuation of the drug.

METHYLDOPA. This antihypertensive drug is similar to INH in that minor and apparently inconsequential abnormalities in liver function occur in up to 6% of treated patients. Clinically overt hepatotoxicity is much less common and usually resembles acute viral hepatitis or chronic active hepatitis, as a rule developing within 20 weeks after methyldopa is started. The Coombs' test is not infrequently positive in users of this drug but does not correlate with the occurrence of hepatic injury. Furthermore, clinical manifestations of drug hypersensitivity are unusual in methyldopa-induced liver disease, which may be mediated by a toxic drug metabolite. Hepatitis usually abates when the drug is discontinued, but full recovery may be delayed by months, and progression to a fatal outcome despite stopping the drug has occurred in some cases.

ORAL CONTRACEPTIVES. These hormonal agents produce several adverse effects on the hepatobiliary system: (a) hepatocellular cholestasis, (b) liver cell neoplasms, (c) increased predisposition to cholesterol gallstone formation, and (d) hepatic vein thrombosis (Budd-Chiari syndrome). In many cases of hepatic vein thrombosis associated with oral contraceptives, a latent myeloproliferative disorder appears to be present and undoubtedly predisposes to the thrombogenic disorder.

The cholestatic effects of oral contraceptives are largely attributable to the estrogenic component. Estrogens appear to affect directly several aspects of bile formation. Indeed, most users of oral contraceptives exhibit subtle disturbances in hepatic excretory function as evidenced, for example, by impaired plasma clearance of sulfobromophthalein. A small number of patients develop clinical cholestasis with pruritus and jaundice in a matter of weeks to months after commencing the pill. Manifestations of drug hypersensitivity are absent, and histologically, cholestasis without inflammation or liver cell necrosis is found. This condition is highly analogous to the clinical syndrome of *intrahepatic cholestasis of pregnancy*, which manifests as subclinical to overt cholestasis in the later stages of gestation, resolving rapidly in the postpartum period. Women with either a personal or family history of cholestasis occurring during pregnancy are particularly susceptible to cholestasis induced by estrogenic preparations. A genetic predisposition to estrogen-induced cholestasis is also suggested by the high incidence of this disorder in certain populations (e.g., Scandinavian and Chilean women).

Treatment of oral contraceptive-induced cholestasis consists of discontinuing the drug and providing symptomatic support (e.g., cholestyramine for pruritus) as needed. Complete resolution within 2 to 3 months is the rule.

PHENYTOIN. This anticonvulsant has been rarely associated with a severe, viral hepatitis-like liver injury with pronounced hypersensitivity features. The onset, usually within 6 weeks of starting the drug, is characterized by malaise, marked fever, lymphadenopathy, and a striking rash. Leukocytosis may be marked, with atypical lymphocytosis and eosinophilia. Liver histology resembles that of acute viral hepatitis except with a greater abundance of eosinophils. In the most severe cases, progressive liver failure and death has ensued. In spite of the marked serum sickness-like syndrome that characterizes phenytoin hepatotoxicity, a toxic metabolite may participate in its pathogenesis. Phenytoin is partly converted in the liver to highly reactive arene oxides. A genetically determined impairment in the ability to detoxify arene oxides may underlie individual susceptibility to toxicity from these metabolites via their covalent and hence immunologic modification of hepatic macromolecules.

SODIUM VALPROATE. This branched, medium-chain fatty acid used principally in the treatment of petit mal epilepsy may produce severe hepatotoxicity, most commonly in children younger than 10. Similar to INH, sodium valproate treatment is accompanied by a high incidence of transient, slight, and asymptomatic increases in serum aminotransferase activity, usually after several weeks of therapy. In rarer cases of severe liver injury, nonspecific systemic and digestive symptoms are followed by jaundice and evidence of liver failure, including encephalopathy and coagulopathy. Rash and eosinophilia are absent. The liver injury is characterized histologically by centrilobular necrosis and small-droplet fat infiltration, and bile duct injury may also be evident. The clinical and histologic features of sodium valproate hepatotoxicity are, to a degree, reminiscent of Reye's syndrome, although the former is distinguished by a greater frequency of jaundice, bile duct injury, and liver necrosis. The mechanism of sodium valproate-induced liver disease is uncertain, but available evidence has implicated the impairment of mitochondrial oxidation of long-chain fatty acids by a metabolite of the drug. Underlying inherited abnormalities in mitochondrial β-oxidation and urea synthesis may also predispose to valproate hepatotoxicity. Spontaneous recovery after stopping sodium valproate is the rule; fatalities are rare.

Dossing M, Sonne J: Drug-induced hepatic disorders. Incidence, management and avoidance. Drug Safety 9:441, 1993. *A concise and lucid overview of the incidence, diagnosis, and prevention of drug-induced liver disease.*

Farrell GC: Drug-Induced Liver Disease. New York, Churchill Livingstone, 1994. *The most up-to-date, comprehensive text on drug- and toxin-induced liver disease. This authoritative reference work is meticulously researched and very readable.*

Kaplowitz N, Berk PD (eds.): Recent advances in drug metabolism and hepatotoxicity. Semin Liver Dis 10:233, 1990. *The nine articles in this issue devoted to hepatotoxicity provide in-depth reviews covering the molecular mechanisms of drug-in-*

duced liver disease, the pathogenesis and clinical features of drug-induced cholestasis, and an update on reports of hepatotoxicity produced by drugs in common use.

Perry MC: Chemotherapeutic agents and hepatotoxicity. Semin Oncol 19:551, 1992. *A focused and useful summary of the growing array of cancer chemotherapeutic agents implicated in the production of hepatotoxicity and the wide variety of different types of liver injury they may produce.*

Rabinovitz M, Van Thiel DH: Hepatotoxicity of nonsteroidal anti-inflammatory drugs. Am J Gastroenterol 87:1696, 1992. *A timely overview of the hepatotoxicity of NSAID's for which the elderly population appears to be most at risk. Discusses both the various types of hepatotoxic reactions produced by these widely used drugs and compares them with respect to their relative risk of producing liver disease.*

Thomas SHL: Paracetamol (acetaminophen) poisoning. Pharmac Ther 60:91, 1993. *A comprehensive review of the important topic of acetaminophen-induced hepatotoxicity, including mechanisms, diagnosis, and management.*

119 CHRONIC HEPATITIS
Robert K. Ockner

DEFINITION. Chronic hepatitis, a syndrome characterized by liver cell necrosis and inflammation lasting longer than 6 months to 1 year, encompasses a spectrum of disorders differing in cause, pathogenesis, histopathology, and clinical manifestations. Patients with chronic hepatitis may be entirely asymptomatic and exhibit only minimal abnormalities on routine laboratory tests or may be incapacitated by progressive liver failure and the complications of portal hypertension. At any given time, there may be little correlation among clinical and laboratory features, histopathology, and long-term prognosis. On biopsy, hepatocellular necrosis varies and the inflammatory response may be predominantly portal, periportal, or lobular in its distribution. When severe, this lesion may include collapse of stromal elements, distortion of the lobular architecture, and a reparative process consisting of fibrosis and nodular regeneration (i.e., cirrhosis). These disorders may be classified on the basis of both cause and histopathology.

ETIOLOGIC CLASSIFICATION (Table 119–1). In all cases of chronic hepatitis, it is important to establish a specific cause, if possible. Chronic hepatitis can be caused by hepatitis B virus (HBV), with or without superimposed hepatitis D virus (HDV) and hepatitis C virus (HCV) infection, one or more as yet unidentified viral agents ("non-ABC"), drugs and toxins (see below and Ch. 118), and inborn errors of metabolism, such as Wilson's disease (see Ch. 188) and α_1-antitrypsin deficiency (see Ch. 121). Exposure to drugs and toxins usually can be identified by means of a careful history, including, when appropriate, questioning of family members or friends. Wilson's disease should be excluded in any patient with chronic hepatitis who is under 40. In addition, the cause of some cases of chronic hepatitis is not known. In some of these, clinical and laboratory features may suggest but do not prove an immunologically mediated process (termed "autoimmune"), whereas others (termed "cryptogenic") lack these features. The relative prevalence of these categories of chronic hepatitis depends in part on the prevalence of hepatitis virus infection in the general population. The differential diagnosis of chronic hepatitis also includes

TABLE 119–1. ETIOLOGY OF CHRONIC HEPATITIS

Autoimmune
Hepatitis viruses
 Hepatitis B virus (HBV)
 HBV with superimposed hepatitis D virus (HDV)
 Hepatitis C virus (HCV)
 Hepatitis "non-A, non-B, non-C"
Drugs and toxins
 Acetaminophen, amiodarone, aspirin, dantrolene, ethanol, isoniazid, methyldopa, nitrofurantoin, oxyphenisatin, perhexilene maleate, phenytoin, propylthiouracil, sulfonamides
Wilson's disease
α_1-Antitrypsin deficiency
Cryptogenic

some cases of primary biliary cirrhosis in which clinical and pathologic features may resemble those of chronic hepatitis. Genetic hemochromatosis, although not typically associated with biopsy findings of chronic hepatitis, is a more common cause of chronic liver disease than had been appreciated and deserves consideration in the differential diagnosis.

HISTOPATHOLOGY AND HISTOPATHOLOGIC CLASSIFICATION. Because the clinical and laboratory features are nonspecific, a diagnosis of chronic hepatitis cannot be established with certainty without liver biopsy. In most forms of chronic hepatitis, hepatic portal areas are infiltrated by mononuclear cells, especially small lymphocytes and plasma cells. Necrosis and inflammation may also involve hepatocytes immediately adjacent to the portal area. In this *periportal hepatitis* (or *"piecemeal necrosis"*), the inflammatory process involves the peripheral portions of the hepatic lobule, so that individual liver cells or nests of cells become isolated. Periportal hepatitis is not specific for chronic hepatitis and often is present in uncomplicated acute hepatitis and several other processes. For this reason it does not necessarily reflect a chronic or progressive process, and its significance can be judged only in the context of associated histopathologic, laboratory, and clinical findings.

The lobular architecture may be substantially disrupted. The portal inflammatory and necrotic process may extend into the lobule to a depth sufficient to span adjacent portal and/or central areas, i.e., *"bridging necrosis."* Although bridging necrosis can occur as part of an otherwise uncomplicated and self-limited acute hepatitis, it suggests a more severe injury that may have a greater propensity to lead to progressive deterioration over a period of weeks to months (*"subacute hepatic necrosis"*) or to chronic hepatitis and cirrhosis. Thus, in patients with liver disease lasting more than 6 to 12 months, the presence of bridging or of submassive necrosis or significant fibrosis suggests a chronic and progressive process. Paradoxically, among survivors of the most severe form of acute liver injury (i.e., massive hepatic necrosis), chronic progressive liver disease is distinctly uncommon.

At the time of this writing, the nomenclature and classification of chronic hepatitis are undergoing active review, and any current classification could be supplanted. That which follows reflects to some extent accustomed usage, with important caveats. In this author's view, a *comprehensive* classification of any individual case of chronic hepatitis must address five areas: (1) cause, (2) histopathology, (3) clinical status of the patient, (4) functional status of the liver, and (5) prognosis and treatment. Unfortunately, any given cause of chronic hepatitis can encompass a spectrum of severity in any or all of the other four areas, and no single classification system can adequately characterize all patients while remaining convenient and clinically useful.

It has proved useful to have a classification based on histopathology alone, given uncertainties about cause in many cases, but it is important to recognize that no single histopathologic category can address the other variables that characterize the disease in a given patient. In this respect, the terms *chronic persistent hepatitis* and *chronic active hepatitis* are neither more nor less valid than other terms commonly used to describe liver histopathology, such as acute hepatitis or cirrhosis. None of these descriptive terms *per se* indicates cause, functional status, or prognosis. Rather, their utility resides in the fact that, properly used, they permit succinct communication of the severity of the process in morphologic terms.

The following is a description of idealized stages in a continuum of histopathologic severity. However, it is important to recognize that chronic persistent hepatitis (CPH) or chronic lobular hepatitis (CLH) may seem not to progress to chronic active hepatitis (CAH) or CAH to cirrhosis, that cirrhosis may develop in the apparent absence of antecedent CPH or CAH, and that CPH and CAH may evolve over time from one to the other and back again, apparently related in some situations to changes in host-virus interactions.

Chronic Persistent Hepatitis. CPH, the most common form of chronic hepatitis, is an inflammatory process largely confined to the portal areas. There is little or no periportal or lobular hepatitis; significant fibrosis and cirrhosis are absent. Of the small number of patients with acute hepatitis B and the larger number with acute hepatitis C whose illness becomes chronic, most are found to have this lesion. By definition, the diagnosis of CPH is not appropriate if significant fibrosis exists. The histologic picture of chronic persistent hepatitis may be found in those patients with chronic active hepatitis in whom medical treatment has induced a remission, if the disease had not already progressed to cirrhosis (see below).

CPH is usually associated with mild or nonspecific symptoms, such as fatigue, anorexia, abdominal discomfort, or jaundice. Extrahepatic manifestations such as arthritis, glomerulonephritis, and vasculitis are less common than in chronic active hepatitis. Physical findings are usually limited to palmar erythema, a few spider telangiectasias, and mildly tender hepatomegaly; the spleen occasionally is slightly enlarged. By definition, complications of advanced liver disease and portal hypertension, such as evidence of a collateral circulation, ascites, and encephalopathy, are absent. Laboratory abnormalities, including increases in serum aminotransferase activities, bilirubin, and globulins, usually are also mild, whereas albumin concentration and prothrombin time are usually normal.

Although progression of CPH to chronic active hepatitis, cirrhosis, or liver failure can occur, it is uncommon. However, the syndrome may last for 10 years or more and may cause continuing or intermittent discomfort or disability. Because of the uncertainties inherent in the biopsy diagnosis of this group of disorders, continuing observation is important. Significant clinical deterioration may occur, indicating the presence of a more serious process such as chronic active hepatitis, cirrhosis, or hepatocellular carcinoma, and would be reason to consider repeat liver biopsy. In chronic hepatitis B infection, for example, increased activity of virus replication ("reactivation") may be associated with clinical and histopathologic deterioration (see below).

Symptomatic and nutritional support is appropriate, and exposure to potential hepatotoxins should be avoided. For patients in whom alcohol has been excluded etiologically, small amounts of alcoholic beverages are permissible if these do not cause worsening of symptoms or laboratory tests. The role of antiviral therapy in chronic hepatitis B, C, and D has been examined in recent clinical trials (see below).

Chronic Lobular Hepatitis.
This is a less well-defined category of chronic hepatitis in which the predominant lesion is a scattered single-cell necrosis in the lobule, with a relatively minor portal inflammatory component. It is, in effect, a variant of chronic persistent hepatitis, appearing not to progress to cirrhosis or liver failure except in those subjects in whom the underlying disease becomes more active (e.g., associated with increased viral replication in chronic hepatitis B).

Chronic Active Hepatitis.
This most histologically severe form of chronic hepatitis has the greatest potential for progression to cirrhosis and liver failure. It is characterized by expansion of portal areas, which are infiltrated by lymphocytes and plasma cells; by periportal hepatitis; and by a variable degree of bridging necrosis, collapse, and fibrosis. In one third or more of patients, macronodular cirrhosis is present at the time of diagnosis. Except for the characteristic features of α_1-antitrypsin deficiency, which can be demonstrated histochemically, the various causes of chronic active hepatitis cannot be differentiated on the basis of routine histopathology.

In the United States, approximately 20% of cases of CAH are associated with, and presumably caused by, *chronic HBV* infection, with or without superimposed *HDV* infection. CAH may also follow post-transfusion or community-acquired *hepatitis C*, which accounts for nearly 50% of cases of chronic hepatitis. Many drugs can also cause CAH, as shown in Table 119–2. Long-term use of acetaminophen and aspirin occasionally may cause similar changes, as may *Wilson's disease* and *α_1-antitrypsin deficiency*. Ethanol substantially accelerates the progression of chronic hepatitis C. In a large number of cases, the cause is unknown, although many patients in this group exhibit clinical features and serologic abnormalities suggestive of autoimmunity (see below).

The course of CAH may be highly variable. The onset is usually insidious but in perhaps one third of cases may initially resemble an acute hepatitis. It may affect all age groups and both genders. Patients may be asymptomatic or may exhibit a wide range of local or constitutional symptoms typical of liver disease, such as fatigue, malaise, fever, anorexia, jaundice, or ascites. *Extrahepatic manifestations* are often quite prominent, especially in young females with the autoimmune type. These include amenorrhea, various skin rashes, glomerulonephritis, polyserositis, thyroiditis, vasculitis, Sjögren's syndrome, pneumonitis, depression of the formed elements of the blood, and an apparently increased incidence of ulcerative colitis.

Physical findings may also be quite variable. Patients may exhibit only a few spider telangiectasias, possibly with mild enlargement of liver and/or spleen, and may or may not be jaundiced. In advanced cases with cirrhosis, patients may have ascites, evidence of collateral circulation, or encephalopathy. In young women, acne and hirsutism may reflect the hormonal effects of chronic liver disease. Evidence of other extrahepatic manifestations may also be prominent, as noted above.

Serum aminotransferase activities are usually increased and may range from minimally abnormal to >1000 IU/L. Serum globulins usually are diffusely increased, and the albumin concentration often is low. The alkaline phosphatase activity is usually only slightly to moderately increased; major increases should suggest the possibility of biliary tract disease or infiltrative or mass lesions. Prothrombin time generally reflects the severity of the disease but may also be influenced by vitamin K deficiency. Because of their variability, the laboratory tests often poorly reflect the pathologic process; for this reason they may not provide a reliable basis for assessing natural history or response to treatment. Serologic tests, including autoantibodies and viral antigen/antibody markers, and measurement of viral nucleic acids, are discussed below in relation to specific etiologic categories, as are therapeutic options, which now include orthotopic liver transplantation.

CHRONIC HEPATITIS SYNDROMES

AUTOIMMUNE HEPATITIS. The general characteristics of this syndrome, including its propensity to affect young women and to be associated with extrahepatic manifestations, have been noted above. The syndrome has been characterized in addition by moderate to marked hyperglobulinemia, a feature not usually present in viral or genetic types, and by the presence in serum of several autoantibodies, of uncertain role in cause and pathogenesis (Table 119–2). These include smooth muscle antibodies, positive in approximately two thirds of patients; antinuclear antibodies in about one half; and anti–double-stranded DNA and antimitochondrial (AMA) antibodies in about one third each. These autoantibodies also occur with increased frequency in family members, although there is no evidence of a simple genetic basis for this phenomenon. A high incidence of HLA-A1, B8, DR3, and DR4 has also been noted.

Additional variants of the syndrome of autoimmune hepatitis have been described, based on recognition of novel autoantibodies and, to a variable extent, distinctive clinical features (Table 119–2). These autoantibodies include an anti–liver/kidney microsomal (anti-LKM1) antibody in a variant of autoimmune hepatitis, an anti-LKM2 associated with tricrynafen hepatitis, and an anti-LKM3 associated with chronic hepatitis D. Anti-LKM1 and anti-LKM2 are directed against the hepatic microsomal drug-metabolizing enzymes cytochrome P-450 2D6 and P-450 2C9, respectively; the significance of this is unknown, but sequence homologies between P-450 2D6 and herpes simplex virus have been implicated. Anti-LKM3 is directed against UDP-glucuronyltransferase in some patients with hepatitis D. Antibodies to an antigen of unknown significance (anti-GOR) are present in some patients with chronic hepatitis C (see below). Also identified in some patients with autoimmune hepatitis have been antibodies to a liver microsome antigen identified as P-450 1A2, soluble liver antigen (anti-SLA), liver-pancreas antigen, and liver cytosol antigen (anti-LC1).

Although some clinical differences exist among the syndromes associated with these autoantibodies, no clear evidence indicates that the latter either reflect the cause of the disease or are involved in its pathogenesis. In fact, the syndrome of chronic hepatitis with autoimmune features can be caused by chemical agents such as nitrofurantoin. Moreover, an unexpectedly high incidence of anti-measles antibodies and of persistent measles virus nucleic acid in peripheral blood mononuclear cells has been reported in patients with autoimmune hepatitis, raising the possibility that some of these cases represent a host response to a persistent viral infection. Finally, it is clear that chronic hepatitis C infection is present in some patients whose serologic tests suggest autoimmune hepatitis. In some instances, this association is the erroneous result of a false-positive test for anti-HCV, apparently reflecting hyperglobulinemia; in these cases RIBA-2 and tests for HCV-RNA are negative. It is also clear, however, that documented cases of chronic HCV infec-

TABLE 119–2. SERUM AUTOANTIBODIES IN CHRONIC HEPATITIS SYNDROMES

Autoantibody	Target Antigen	Etiology	Syndrome Designations Suggested
Smooth muscle	F actin, other cyto-skeletal components	Multiple	Type 1 autoimmune hepatitis (also present in some cases of chronic HBV, HCV, alcoholic liver disease, primary biliary cirrhosis)
Antinuclear (ANA)	Histones, lamins, double-stranded DNA	Multiple	
Antimitochondrial	*Pyruvate dehydrogenase complex	Multiple	
Anti–liver/kidney microsomal			
Anti-LKM1	†cyp 2D6	Unknown (U.S.)	Type 2a autoimmune hepatitis: younger, females, severe
		HCV‡	Type 2b autoimmune hepatitis: older, males, mild
Anti-LKM2	cyp 2C9	Ticrynafen	Ticrynafen-induced hepatitis
Anti-LKM3	UDP-glucuronosyl-transferase	HDV	Hepatitis D
Anti-GOR	Unknown	HCV	Chronic hepatitis C
Anti-liver microsome (anti-LM)	cyp 1A2	Dihydralazine	Dihydralazine-induced hepatitis
Anti–soluble liver antigen (anti–SLA)	Cytokeratins 8, 18	Unknown	? Type 3 autoimmune hepatitis
Anti–liver-pancreas (anti-LP)	Cytokeratins ?	Unknown	? Type 3 autoimmune hepatitis
Anti–liver cytosol antigen (anti-LC1)	Unknown	Unknown	?

* Nonspecific in some non-PBC cases
† cyp = cytochrome P-450
‡ HCV infection present in most anti-LKM1–positive cases in France and Italy; and < 10% in Britain and Germany

tion may be associated with autoantibodies of the same kind found in autoimmune hepatitis. This overlap may pose important problems in diagnosis and management and is discussed below (see Chronic Hepatitis C). Whether any cases of CAH are truly the result of a primary immune attack on a previously normal liver remains to be determined.

Treatment. In treating autoimmune hepatitis, *corticosteroids,* with or without low-dose azathioprine, usually reduce symptoms, improve laboratory test results, suppress the inflammatory process seen on biopsy, and decrease short-term and long-term morbidity and mortality.

Despite this seemingly beneficial overall response, several factors that importantly influence the natural history and response to treatment must be considered in making the decision to institute a chronic treatment plan with potentially significant adverse effects. First, this type of chronic hepatitis does not usually progress to cirrhosis or liver failure in the absence of bridging necrosis on liver biopsy; the absence of such changes would weigh significantly against using corticosteroids. Second, no evidence exists that corticosteroids are beneficial in asymptomatic autoimmune hepatitis. Third, in the Mayo Clinic series, the presence or absence of autoimmune features seemed to be unimportant in regard to prognosis or response to treatment. Finally, because many patients with CAH would fail to meet the criteria for inclusion in some of the published series, any decision regarding their treatment is necessarily an extrapolation from a selected study population.

In view of the uncertainty concerning the value of corticosteroids in certain subsets of patients with autoimmune hepatitis, it is difficult to make broadly applicable recommendations concerning their use. In general, however, an initially favorable response would most likely be expected in a young symptomatic female with progressive disease and no recent transfusion or other exposure to or evidence for hepatitis B or C. This also applies to those mostly young female patients who are positive for anti-LKM1 and negative for anti-HCV. The mostly older anti-LKM1–positive males who are also anti-HCV positive respond less well to immunosuppression.

The following regimen has been found to be effective: an initial daily dose of 60 mg of prednisone or 30 mg of prednisone combined with 50 mg of azathioprine, tapered gradually over several weeks to months to a daily maintenance dose of 20 mg of prednisone or 10 mg of prednisone plus 50 mg of azathioprine. Azathioprine was of no value when given alone but permitted use of the lower prednisone dose, thereby reducing the incidence of significant steroid-related complications, which otherwise approximated 60%. Alternate-day treatment was less effective. If a favorable response is not observed within 2 to 3 months, treatment should be discontinued.

Patients should be examined and have liver tests periodically.

The possible side effects of drug treatment should be monitored, and liver biopsies may need to be repeated at intervals of 6 months to 1 year, depending on the circumstances. Repeated biopsies serve little purpose in a stable patient. Return of liver enzymes to a level less than twice the upper limit of normal, together with a liver biopsy showing subsidence of the inflammatory and necrotic process to a picture similar to that of CPH, is considered a successful response and warrants an attempt gradually to discontinue treatment. In about 50% of patients, this attempt succeeds and additional corticosteroid treatment is not needed. In the remainder, evidence of relapse may suggest the need to reinstitute therapy.

Unfortunately, the disease may eventually progress to cirrhosis or liver failure despite an apparently favorable initial clinical response, especially in those patients in whom repeated recurrences of activity require treatment over a period of 3 years or more. Over these longer intervals, the advisability of continued corticosteroid therapy must be judged not only on the basis of symptoms and laboratory and biopsy findings but also in recognition of the successful treatment of many of these patients with orthotopic liver transplantation (see Ch. 124).

CHRONIC HEPATITIS B. From 2 to 10% of otherwise healthy adults remain chronically infected with HBV after acute hepatitis caused by this agent (see Ch. 117). Approximately two thirds of these are found to have the lesion of CPH and the remainder CAH. Chronicity is more common in men than women, is predisposed to by immune suppression, and is in general a clinically more subdued disease process than autoimmune hepatitis. Nevertheless, chronic hepatitis B clearly may evolve to cirrhosis, liver failure, and hepatocellular carcinoma. The severity of the course largely depends on the activity of virus replication in the hepatocytes and the response of the host immune system. In somewhat simplified terms, the process can be described as follows: Active replication of episomal (i.e., nonintegrated) viral DNA leads to biogenesis and secretion of complete HBV virions, as indicated by the presence of DNA polymerase and HBV DNA in serum. HBeAg is also present in serum; although not secreted as a component of the virion, it too is an indicator of replication. Viral antigens are also expressed on the surface of the hepatocyte in association with Class I HLA determinants, thereby eliciting lymphocyte cytotoxicity and a resulting immunologically mediated hepatitis. When replication subsides, fewer virions are produced; HBeAg gives way to anti-HBe (seroconversion); and a brief flare in the hepatitis ushers in a period of relative clinical and histopathologic quiescence. This may occur in 10 to 30% of patients each year. The reverse may also occur, if an increase in viral replication and/or a change in the host immune response leads to increased severity of the hepatitis (i.e., "reactivation").

This dynamic host-virus interaction has important diagnostic implications. Thus, an HBsAg-positive patient with a syndrome of apparent acute hepatitis may in fact have chronic hepatitis B undergoing either seroconversion or reactivation. The latter may occur spontaneously or may be precipitated by immunosuppressive or antitumor therapy and may result in a severe and even fatal acute hepatitis syndrome. Other factors, such as superimposed viral or drug-induced hepatitis, may lead to similar confusion. Active HBV replication and chronic hepatitis B are suggested by positive tests for HBsAg, HBeAg, and anti-HBc, and by anti-HBs negativity. (In a small number of patients, usually with active disease, heterotypic anti-HBs may be present simultaneously with HBsAg.) Definitive evidence of active replication is provided by demonstrating HBeAg, DNA polymerase, or HBV DNA in serum. In general, histopathologic features consistent with CPH tend to be associated with a less severe clinical course and longer survival, whereas the lesions of CAH and cirrhosis reflect a more aggressive process with shorter survival. As noted, however, these patterns may evolve from one to the other depending on the status of viral replication and the host immune response.

Treatment. The treatment of chronic hepatitis B remains frustrating. Corticosteroids are not beneficial and may be harmful, possibly in part reflecting their demonstrated enhancement of HBV replication. In trials of antiviral therapy, patients selected have usually exhibited active viral replication (i.e., HBeAg, DNA polymerase, and HBV DNA positivity). Recombinant interferon-α_{2b}, 5 million units daily or 10 million units three times weekly for 16 weeks, with or without a brief antecedent course of corticosteroids, has been effective in inducing a clinical and histologic response in approximately 40% of patients, as reflected by loss of serum markers of viral replicative activity (serum HBeAg and HBV DNA), in 90% of whom serum aminotransferase activities become normal. In approximately 10 to 15% of successfully treated patients, tests for serum HBsAg may also become negative, suggesting that the virus has been eradicated. Although at least a few individuals in whom all serum markers of the infection have become negative retain HBV DNA in the liver, its significance in regard to possible future HBV replication or disease recrudescence remains unknown. Although the great majority of responses to interferon appear to be sustained in chronic hepatitis B, reactivation may occur in a small minority (approximately 5%) of responders. Treatment of chronic HBV mutant virus infections (see Ch. 327) has been less successful in that there appears to be a higher rate of relapse after completion of therapy. Interferon treatment may also improve certain extrahepatic manifestations of chronic hepatitis B, including glomerulonephritis and vasculitis. Although patients with advanced cirrhosis caused by chronic hepatitis B have been studied less extensively, recent evidence suggests that selected individuals may benefit from lower dose interferon treatment.

Factors predisposing to a favorable response to interferon include low serum HBV DNA levels, high serum aminotransferase activity, being female, a clinically mild course, relatively brief duration, and immune competence (e.g., HIV negativity), whereas less favorable results have been obtained in male homosexuals, HIV-positive and Asian subjects, and individuals with perinatally acquired infections. It remains to be seen whether apparently successful treatment alters the longer-term course of the disease. Other antiviral and immunomodulatory agents are undergoing clinical trials.

Liver transplantation has been used to manage end-stage liver disease caused by hepatitis B (see Ch. 124). Results thus far indicate virtually universal reinfection of the transplanted liver in patients transplanted for chronic hepatitis B, whereas this is significantly less common among patients with fulminant hepatic failure, those with combined HBV and HDV infection, and those treated after transplantation with high-dose hepatitis B immune globulin (HBIG). Post-transplant recurrence of HBV infection presumably results from viremia at the time of surgery or viral replication in extrahepatic tissues of the recipient. It may exhibit an accelerated course, and in a few patients is associated with a syndrome, designated fibrosing cholestatic hepatitis, characterized by development of liver failure over weeks to months. In most centers, liver failure in chronic hepatitis B in association with active viral replication is considered to be a relative contraindication to liver transplantation.

CHRONIC HEPATITIS D. HDV infection depends on antecedent or simultaneous infection with HBV. When HDV infection is superimposed on pre-existing chronic hepatitis B, it also becomes chronic in most cases. Simultaneous infection with both HBV and

HDV does not increase the probability of chronic disease but is associated with an increased incidence of fulminant hepatic failure. Trials involving interferon-α treatment of chronic HBV with HDV infection have met with limited temporary success and a high probability of relapse after stopping treatment, although some encouraging results have been obtained with high-dose treatment over a period of 1 year. Patients with end-stage liver disease caused by chronic HBV and HDV appear to have a more favorable outcome after liver transplantation than those with HBV alone, presumably reflecting an inhibitory effect of HDV on HBV replication.

CHRONIC HEPATITIS C. Availability of specific molecular and serologic markers for HCV infection has contributed importantly to an understanding of the natural history of this illness, which has accounted for most cases of chronic non-A, non-B hepatitis and nearly half of all cases of chronic viral hepatitis in the United States. It has also provided evidence that at least one additional as yet unidentified agent may account for some cases. As suggested by earlier studies of post-transfusion hepatitis, chronicity of the infection is the rule rather than the exception, occurring in 50 to 80% of cases. Of these, approximately 20% have chronically elevated serum aminotransferase activities, and approximately half of those who undergo liver biopsy are found to have CAH or cirrhosis. For the group of chronically infected individuals as a whole, biopsy evidence of cirrhosis is eventually found in 20%, from 1.5 to 16 years after the implicated transfusion. However, most patients studied at an average of 18 years after infection are asymptomatic (including many of those with significant histopathologic abnormalities), with no clinical evidence of liver disease and with no greater mortality than a matched control population of transfused but uninfected subjects.

It has also become evident, however, that HCV infection has effects on the virus as well as the host. Apparently under the pressure of immune surveillance, the dominant viral subtype may evolve, reflecting changes predominantly in the hypervariable E2/NS1 envelope region (see Ch. 117). Furthermore, acute superinfection of patients with chronic hepatitis C by a different subtype has been documented, with reversion to the pre-existing chronic subtype after the superinfecting strain is cleared. These observations, in addition to the apparent failure of natural infection to confer immunity to the agent, indicate that HCV poses a challenge to the immune system and to the development of effective immunoprophylaxis that is far more complex than for the other major hepatitis viruses.

Typically, chronic hepatitis C exhibits an intermittent course in which episodes of increased symptoms and laboratory abnormalities are separated by periods of relative quiescence. As noted, however, 10 to 20% of patients develop cirrhosis or progressive liver failure. Furthermore, depending on the geographic region, a high percentage of patients with primary hepatocellular carcinoma test positive for anti-HCV, and it is regarded as the major predisposing factor for this malignancy in Japan.

The histopathologic manifestations of chronic hepatitis C are generally similar to those associated with other causes of chronic hepatitis, but with some distinctive features that may be useful in differential diagnosis and, possibly, in understanding the pathogenesis of the process. Thus, unlike both chronic hepatitis B and autoimmune hepatitis, it is more likely to include bile duct damage or even disappearance, portal lymphoid aggregates, and steatosis, whereas autoimmune hepatitis usually is associated with more severe periportal and lobular injury and inflammation.

Chronic Hepatitis C and "Autoimmunity." The consequences of chronic HCV infection may interface with processes considered to be "autoimmune" in two general areas. In the first, a number of extrahepatic manifestations occur in chronic hepatitis C and can be understood in terms of the host's immunologic response. For example, it is now clear that chronic HCV infection is present in a substantial majority of patients with type II cryoglobulinemia, and in some cases of type III, as evidenced by the presence of HCV RNA in serum and especially in cryoprecipitates. Hepatitis B may also be associated with cryoglobulinemia, but much less commonly. That the association of HCV is probably causal is suggested by the observation that in several cases, interferon-α–induced decreases in HCV RNA concentrations and anti-HCV titers (see below) have been associated with decreases in serum concentrations of cryoglobulins, rheumatoid factor, serum creatinine (in those with renal involvement), and the manifestations of cutaneous vasculitis. Unfortunately, in virtually all cases, stopping interferon therapy has led to a recrudescence of both HCV viremia and the manifestations of cryoglobulinemia. Membranous glomerulonephropathy has also been described, as has polyarteritis nodosa, Sjögren's syndrome, urticaria, erythema nodosum, and a higher than expected incidence of thyroid autoantibodies and of Hashimoto's thyroiditis.

The second area in which chronic hepatitis C interfaces with "autoimmunity" involves the frequent expression of autoantibodies in these patients, in whom liver damage is presumably the result of the viral infection and/or the host response to it. Thus, antinuclear antibodies are found in > 20% of patients, and anti–smooth muscle antibodies in > 50%, although the titers tend to be lower than in autoimmune hepatitis. In addition, among patients with autoimmune hepatitis characterized by autoantibodies to microsomal cytochrome P-450 2D6 (anti–liver-kidney microsomal antibody, anti-LKM1, i.e., so-called type 2 autoimmune hepatitis), most members of a subset of predominantly older male patients ("type 2b") have chronic hepatitis C, whereas patients in the subset that are predominantly younger and female ("type 2a") do not (Table 119–2).

Finally, an autoantibody to a host protein of unknown significance ("anti-GOR") is present in some chronic hepatitis C patients (Table 119–2) and may be present in patients who are also anti-LKM1 positive. Anti-GOR is absent or uncommon in chronic hepatitis B and in patients with chronic putatively autoimmune hepatobiliary diseases, including autoimmune hepatitis (other than HCV-positive anti-LKM1), primary biliary cirrhosis, and primary sclerosing cholangitis. Significantly, the presence or absence of this apparently HCV-specific autoantibody has no influence on any clinical, laboratory, or histopathologic characteristic of the illness or its response to medical treatment, either in a given patient or in general. The presence of these autoantibodies thus raises questions about the pathophysiologic significance of such phenomena in liver disease in general. Although it has been suggested that a limited region of sequence homology between HCV and P-450 2D6 may account for the generation of anti-LKM1 antibodies in some chronic HCV patients via "molecular mimicry," the antigen targeted by anti-GOR lacks such homology and the mechanism that leads to the generation of other autoantibodies in these patients is unknown.

Treatment. Treatment of chronic hepatitis C is still being defined. Interferon-α has been used with limited success and with an unknown overall effect on the natural history of the disease. Thus, normalization or near normalization of the serum aminotransferase activity was achieved in 46% of patients with chronic post-transfusion hepatitis C treated with 3 million units three times weekly for 24 weeks, as compared with untreated controls, and was associated with histologic improvement. Unfortunately, 51% of the responders relapsed within 6 months after treatment ended. The possibly beneficial effects of changes in dose or duration of drug treatment in this setting are under investigation. Furthermore, initial evidence suggests that viral subtypes may differ in their response to interferon treatment, a factor that may need to be considered either in the initial therapeutic decision or in assessing therapeutic response or disease recurrence. Also, newer methods for quantifying and characterizing the infection, apart from subtype analysis and newer therapeutic agents, require ongoing evaluation in carefully designed clinical protocols. Finally, the use of interferon in patients with chronic hepatitis C who also have autoantibodies (other than anti-LKM1 or anti-GOR) has occasionally resulted in a flare in the disease, presumably resulting from augmentation of an immunologically mediated process. For all these reasons, and despite the general licensing of recombinant interferon-α for treatment of chronic hepatitis C, it appears desirable for such patients to be managed in settings that provide access to, and continued monitoring under, established protocols that permit development of the additional knowledge required if the state of this particular art is to advance.

End-stage chronic hepatitis C is an accepted indication for orthotopic liver transplantation under appropriate circumstances. Although the probability is high that hepatitis C will recur in the engrafted liver, in most cases the recurrent disease is relatively mild and readily managed. The use of interferon in these patients is under investigation. A minority of cases of recurrent hepatitis C after transplantation, however, are severe and may lead to chronic active hepatitis, cirrhosis, or liver failure.

SPECIAL CLINICAL PROBLEMS

Two circumstances are encountered in clinical practice with sufficient frequency that they deserve particular comment with reference to diagnostic approach and management.

ASYMPTOMATIC ELEVATION OF SERUM AMINOTRANSFERASE ACTIVITY. With the advent and common use of multiphasic laboratory screening techniques we can now identify individuals in whom serum aminotransferase activities are abnormal but who lack clinical evidence of liver disease. If the abnormal finding is confirmed, and if it does not reflect muscle or other extrahepatic disease, it may have either of two possible implications: (1) it may reflect a subclinical acute process (e.g., acute viral hepatitis), or (2) it may reflect a chronic process (e.g., chronic toxic or viral hepatitis, or nonalcoholic steatohepatitis). If the patient is asymptomatic or nearly so, a period of observation is appropriate, and follow-up studies and hepatitis serologies should be obtained. Alcohol and potentially hepatotoxic drugs and toxins should be avoided. Improvement would presumably reflect resolution of a self-limited process or the response to removal of a toxin (e.g., ethanol). Worsening test results during observation may herald the onset of overt disease; its proper evaluation depends on the circumstances. Persistence of the abnormality beyond 6 to 12 months may reflect a chronic hepatitis and may justify liver biopsy.

HBsAg AND/OR ANTI-HCV POSITIVITY. Approximately 0.2% of the population of the United States are positive for HBsAg, and approximately 0.5% of otherwise healthy blood donors are positive by second-generation tests for anti-HCV. At any given time, most of these persons exhibit no overt evidence of liver disease and may be designated "carriers." The meaning of the term *carrier* is imprecise, however, as it has been used to include all chronically positive individuals or limited to those who have no apparent liver disease.

The practical question of significance concerns the management of the otherwise apparently healthy patient with a positive test. If the result is confirmed, it could indicate (1) a subclinical acute viral hepatitis, (2) chronic hepatitis or cirrhosis, or (3) a "healthy" carrier state. Although differentiation of these conditions may require liver biopsy, HBsAg-positive persons who have no other clinical or laboratory evidence of liver disease usually have normal or nonspecific biopsy findings, whereas the significance of a positive test for anti-HCV depends on other evidence for liver disease. Thus, in an individual in whom clinical and laboratory evaluation (e.g., serum aminotransferase activities) is otherwise negative, a positive second-generation test for anti-HCV could be a false positive, as suggested by negative supplemental antibody testing (RIBA-2). Those HBsAg-positive or anti-HCV–positive persons who do have clinical and/or laboratory signs of liver disease should be managed in accordance with the severity and duration of the process. Persistence of the abnormality beyond 6 months may suggest chronic hepatitis and the need to consider liver biopsy and, in selected cases, interferon therapy.

General and Histopathology

Czaja AJ: Chronic active hepatitis: The challenge for a new nomenclature. Ann Intern Med 119:510, 1993. Ludwig J: The nomenclature of chronic active hepatitis: An obituary. Gastroenterology 105:274, 1993. Desmet VJ, Gerber M, Hoofnagle JH, et al.: Classification of chronic hepatitis: Diagnosis, grading and staging. Hepatology 19:1513, 1994. *Two commentaries on current issues in the classification of chronic hepatitis, and a proposed new classification.*

Czaja AJ, Carpenter HA: Sensitivity, specificity, and predictability of biopsy interpretations in chronic hepatitis. Gastroenterology 105:1824, 1993. *Comparisons among chronic hepatitis C and "autoimmune" and "cryptogenic" chronic hepatitis.*

Maddrey WC: Chronic hepatitis. *In* Zakim D, Boyer T (eds.): Hepatology: A Textbook of Liver Disease. Philadelphia, WB Saunders, 1989, p 1025. *A comprehensive and well-referenced review, emphasizing clinical aspects.*

Autoimmune Hepatitis

Bianchi FB: Autoimmune hepatitis: The lesson of the discovery of hepatitis C virus [editorial]. J Hepatol 18:273, 1993. Maddrey WC: How many types of autoimmune hepatitis are there? [editorial]. Gastroenterology 105:1571, 1993. *Two summaries of the knowns and unknowns in "autoimmune" chronic hepatitis.*

Czaja AJ, Hay JE, Rakela J: Clinical features and prognostic implications of severe corticosteroid-treated cryptogenic chronic active hepatitis. Mayo Clin Proc 65:23, 1990. *In a large series, demonstration of the apparent lack of effect of autoimmune features on disease severity, histopathology, response to treatment, and survival.*

Manns M: Autoantibodies in chronic hepatitis: Diagnostic reagents and scientific tools to study etiology, pathogenesis and cell biology. *In* Boyer JL, Ockner RK (eds.): Progress in Liver Diseases, Vol XII. Philadelphia, WB Saunders, 1994. *A critical review of the nature and significance of various autoantibodies.*

Chronic Hepatitis B

Carman W, Thomas H, Domingo E: Viral genetic variation: Hepatitis B virus as a clinical example. Lancet 341:349, 1993. Lau JYN, Wright TL: Clinical aspects of hepatitis B infection, and molecular virology and pathogenesis of hepatitis B. Lancet 342:1335 and 1340, 1993. *Succinct and timely reviews of various virologic and clinical aspects of hepatitis B.*
Perrillo RP: Interferon in the management of chronic hepatitis B. Dig Dis Sci 38:577, 1993. *Review of issues and progress in this field.*

Chronic Hepatitis C

Esteban JI, Genesca J, Alter HJ: Hepatitis C: Molecular biology, pathogenesis, epidemiology, clinical features, and prevention. *In* Boyer JL, Ockner RK (eds.): Progress in Liver Diseases, Vol X. Philadelphia, WB Saunders, 1992, p 253.
Wright TL: Hepatitis C virus infection and organ transplantation. *In* Boyer JL, Ockner RK (eds.): Progress in Liver Diseases, Vol XI. Philadelphia, WB Saunders, 1993, p 215. *A comprehensive review of epidemiologic, diagnostic, and therapeutic aspects.*

Chronic Hepatitis D

Farci P, Mandas A, Coiana A, et al.: Treatment of chronic hepatitis D with interferon α-2a. N Engl J Med 330:88, 1994. *Recent experience in medical treatment.*
Rizzetto M, Gerin JL: Advances in hepatitis D virus biology and disease. *In* Boyer JL, Ockner RK (eds.): Progress in Liver Diseases, Vol XII. Philadelphia, WB Saunders, 1994. Polish LB, Gallagher M, Fields HA, et al.: Delta hepatitis: Molecular biology and clinical and epidemiological features. Clin Microbiol Rev 6:211, 1993. *Two authoritative reviews covering virtually all aspects of the agent and the syndromes it causes.*

---

120 PARASITIC, BACTERIAL, FUNGAL, AND GRANULOMATOUS LIVER DISEASES

Willis C. Maddrey

The liver is affected by a number of local and disseminated infections; their frequency and types vary considerably around the world. Parasitic disorders are more prevalent in developing countries, especially those in tropical and subtropical regions. Infectious agents reach the liver through the portal or arterial blood or arrive directly by spread from neighboring organs. Often hepatic involvement in an infectious process is manifest only by mild to moderate elevations in aminotransferase and alkaline phosphatase levels. Occasionally clinically apparent jaundice is noted. In these patients, jaundice may result from combinations of the effects of focal inflammation, endotoxemia, hemolysis, and bile duct obstruction. In patients with shock, hypoperfusion also contributes. The prognosis for infections involving the liver depends on the type of infection, the availability and early institution of appropriate therapy, and the underlying status of the patient. As would be expected, poor outcomes are more likely to occur in the elderly and in those with impaired immunocompetence as in AIDS or in those with an underlying malignancy. Only a few of the many infections that at one time or another affect the liver are discussed.

PYOGENIC LIVER ABSCESS

DEFINITION. Pyogenic liver abscesses are focal areas of infection within the hepatic parenchyma. These abscesses may be single or multiple and result from liver invasion by a variety of bacteria.

ETIOLOGY. Nowadays, pyogenic liver abscesses are more often found in individuals of middle age or older, especially those who have underlying biliary tract diseases with obstruction and bile stasis that favor infection. In this setting, multiple abscesses are frequent. Before antibiotics, appendicitis with bacterial seeding of the liver through the portal vein was a frequent cause. Pyogenic liver abscesses secondary to intestinal diseases are well recognized in patients with a variety of disorders including Crohn's disease and diverticulitis. Penetrating wounds to the liver may also lead to abscesses. In many patients (up to one half), no definite cause for the abscess is found, and often the presumption is made that an episode of septicemia or occult biliary tract disease has occurred.

A remarkable array of bacteria has been found to cause liver abscesses. Gram-negative enteric bacteria, especially *Escherichia coli, Klebsiella pneumoniae, Streptococcus fecalis,* and *Proteus vulgaris,* are major contributors. Gram-positive staphylococci cause abscess in many patients. The role of anaerobic organisms, especially bacteroides and clostridial species, has been increasingly recognized as culture techniques have improved. Infection by multiple organisms is frequent.

CLINICAL MANIFESTATIONS AND DIAGNOSIS. The presence of a bacterial liver abscess may be suspected when a patient develops fever, leukocytosis, and right upper quadrant abdominal pain. Often the presentation is subtle and involves an indolent process with loss of appetite, intermittent or low-grade fever, and dull abdominal pain. Anemia and hypoalbuminemia are often present, especially in patients who have longstanding abscesses. Imaging studies, especially ultrasonography and computed tomography (CT) scanning, have shortened the time from suspicion of the presence of liver abscess to confirmation (Fig. 120–1). Ultrasonographic examination usually is reliable in differentiating liver abscess from hepatic cysts.

Pyogenic liver abscess should be considered in any patient who has presumptive or definite evidence of septicemia in association with biochemical abnormalities of the liver. The liver is usually enlarged and is often tender when palpated. Most liver abscesses occur in the right lobe. If the abscess is high in the liver, the hemidiaphragm may be elevated and immobile (usually on the right), along with a pleural effusion. Rales and percussion dullness may be noted at the base of the compressed right lung.

Directed aspiration of the abscess with culture and cytologic examination usually accurately identifies the causative organism or organisms. Endoscopic cholangiography is useful to determine if there is underlying obstruction in the biliary tract. Bacterial cultures of the aspirate which include special attention to detection of anaerobics are positive in 90% of patients.

TREATMENT. The cornerstones of treating bacterial liver abscesses are antibiotics and drainage. The choice of antibiotics is determined by the results of blood cultures of and aspirates from the abscess. Occasionally an indwelling drainage catheter is placed into a single abscess. Surgical drainage of liver abscesses is rarely required. If multiple abscesses are present, the larger accessible ones should be aspirated. Broad-spectrum antibiotics, including coverage for anaerobes, should begin immediately following aspiration with later adjustments of treatment based on culture results. Metronidazole should be included in the initial therapeutic regimen if amebic abscess is being considered. If there is evidence of biliary tract obstruction, endoscopic or surgical approaches to relieve these determine in large measure how rapidly (or if) the abscesses resolve.

PROGNOSIS. The prognosis for patients with solitary bacterial liver abscesses is better than for those with multiple abscesses. The patient's underlying health status, age, the presence of immune compromising illnesses including AIDS and malignancy, the rapid-

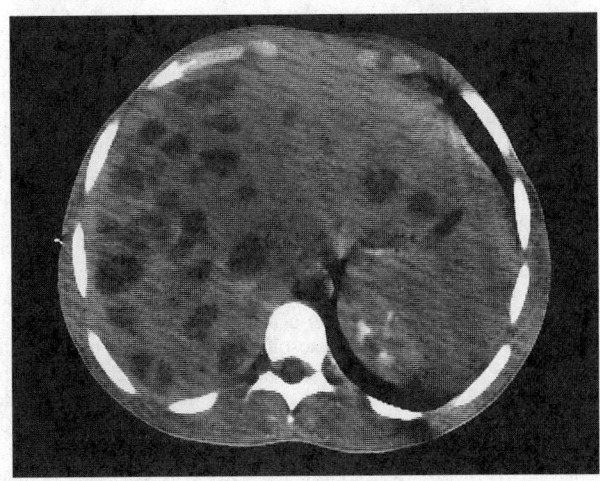

FIGURE 120–1. CT demonstrating multiple pyogenic liver abscesses in a 25-year-old man.

ity with which the diagnosis is established, and the effectiveness of draining the abscess, and, if necessary, the obstructed biliary tract all influence the likelihood of complete recovery.

Actinomycosis (see Ch. 306)

Actinomycosis is a chronic suppurative bacterial infection that may involve the liver directly from adjacent infected organs or via the portal vein from cecal and appendiceal infection. Solitary or multiple intrahepatic masses may develop. Sinuses from the liver and adherent viscera to the abdominal wall are frequent. The finding of characteristic sulfa granules containing branched filaments establishes the diagnosis. Once considered, the diagnosis is usually straightforward after examining sinus tract drainage. The treatment is large doses of intravenous penicillin.

FUNGAL INFECTIONS OF THE LIVER

Major fungal infections that affect the liver include actinomycosis, histoplasmosis, and coccidioidomycosis. A careful history emphasizing travel, places of residence, and lifestyle likely to affect immune status is often helpful for diagnosis. A variety of fungal infections have occurred in transplanted livers.

Granulomas are often found in patients with many fungal infections, including histoplasmosis, coccidioidomycosis, North American blastomycosis, and cryptococcosis. These infections may occur in patients who are immunocompetent. Several other types of fungal infections, including candidiasis, aspergillosis, and mucormycosis, are more likely to be found in patients with AIDS and other disorders that impair immunocompetence. Diagnosis of fungal diseases is based on identifying the organism on liver biopsy or occasionally from culture of the hepatic tissue. Serologic tests are generally not helpful. Treatment depends on the responsiveness of the underlying fungal agent and the immune status of the patient.

SPIROCHETAL DISEASES

SYPHILIS (see Ch. 318). The liver is involved in several stages of syphilis. In congenital syphilis, diffuse hepatitis occurs secondary to massive transplacental infection. In secondary syphilis, diffuse granulomatous changes are frequent. In tertiary syphilis, single or multiple gummas may be found. The treatment for all types of hepatic syphilis is penicillin.

PARASITIC DISEASES (Table 120–1)

Parasitic diseases often have distinctive geographic distributions. In part because of international travel and the occurrence of unusual infections in patients who are immunocompromised, clinicians need to be aware of the manifestations of these disorders.

HELMINTHIC INFECTIONS (see Ch. 373). *Pathogenesis.* An array of helminths with often complex life cycles either in larval or adult stages affect the human liver. The response to larvae is quite variable. The larvae of ascariasis cause little tissue damage, whereas in toxocariasis there is an intense inflammation reaction (visceral larva migrans). In few areas of medicine is it as important to understand the impact of environment on the diseases likely to be encountered.

ASCARIASIS. In ascariasis, the adult worm (*Ascaris lumbricoides*) may migrate into the common bile duct, become lodged, and obstruct the flow of bile. Some of the worms die in the bile duct and calcify. Occasionally, worm ova proceed up the bile duct, lodge in the liver, and lead to giant cells and granulomas. Effective treatment may require extracting the worms from the bile duct by endoscopic cholangiography and using piperazine citrate to kill any remaining worms.

SCHISTOSOMIASIS (see Ch. 385). Infections with several types of human blood flukes (schistosomiasis) are leading causes of liver disease worldwide, especially in the Far East, Middle East, and Africa. *Schistosoma mansoni* and *S. japonicum* regularly affect the liver. The life cycle of schistosomes is complex. Eggs excreted in human feces hatch in water, becoming swimming embryos that enter the snail's body, where they develop into motile, fork-tailed cercariae that are then released into water. The cercariae penetrate human skin and migrate via the bloodstream, taking up residence in the mesenteric capillaries. In the mesenteric vessels, the schistosomes reach adult status, then lay eggs which are taken via portal blood and delivered to the small presinusoidal intrahepatic portal

veins. The eggs elicit an immune response with a granulomatous reaction (Table 120–1). Subsequently, fibrosis and portal hypertension with esophagogastric varices develop. Identifying eggs in a stool examination is the preferred method to diagnose schistosomiasis. Liver biopsy changes include granulomas (some containing remnants of ova) and fibrosis, which often contains arteriolar clefts. Antischistosomal drugs including praziquantel are available. Portasystemic shunt surgery may be required if bleeding from esophagogastric varices occurs.

CLONORCHIASIS. The Chinese liver fluke (*Clonorchis sinensis*) is a parasite affecting fish-eating mammals, including humans. Snails are intermediate hosts in which cercariae develop and affect freshwater fish. The most important problems in humans with clonorchiasis are obstructed bile ducts and chronic cholangitis caused by flukes that have matured inside the bile ducts. Cholangiohepatitis and cholangiocarcinoma are known consequences. The diagnosis is based on finding characteristic eggs in the feces. Praziquantel is the drug of choice.

ECHINOCOCCOSIS (HYDATID DISEASE). *Echinococcus granulosa* is a tapeworm living in dogs that acquire the infection from eating infected sheep viscera. Humans, sheep, and cattle are intermediate hosts. The worms excrete ova that adhere to the dog's coat and may be passed to humans who have close contact with the dogs and ingest contaminated food. After the chitinous cover breaks down, the ova burrow into the intestinal mucosa and reach the liver via the portal vein. Complex cysts gradually develop in the liver and other organs. The rim of the cyst may calcify. The echinococcal cyst may remain asymptomatic or continue to expand. Most of these cysts occur in the right lobe of the liver. In some patients, rupture into bile ducts or the peritoneal cavity, lungs, and other organs occurs. Indirect hemagglutination and ELISA tests are helpful for diagnosis. Ultrasonography, CT, and magnetic resonance imaging are useful to diagnose the presence of a cyst and may be highly suggestive of the echinococcal origin (Fig. 120–2). If feasible, surgical removal of the cyst is indicated. Diagnostic aspiration is dangerous and may lead to dissemination of the infection. Mebendazole or albendazole is of some limited benefit.

PROTOZOAN INFECTIONS

Protozoa commonly infect the liver; some affect visceral reticuloendothelial cells (leishmaniasis and trypanosomiasis) and others the hepatocytes (toxoplasmosis and malaria). *Entamoeba histolytica* is one of the most important causes of liver abscess.

The clinical manifestations of protozoan infection are usually nonspecific and may resemble viral hepatitis (e.g., in toxoplasmosis and malaria). Hepatosplenomegaly, anemia, emaciation, and many general symptoms may be encountered. In certain infections, extrahepatic manifestations predominate (e.g., cardiomyopathy with chronic trypanosomiasis). Extrahepatic features may be prominent early in the course (e.g., amebic colitis), and hepatic symptoms predominate later (e.g., with hepatic abscess formation). Cryptosporidiosis has received increasing attention as an opportunistic infection in patients with AIDS. Cryptosporidial cholecystitis and bile duct changes that suggest sclerosing cholangitis have been found. Hepatic changes appear to be secondary to the biliary tract and gallbladder invasions.

In contrast to helminthic infections, serologic tests are often useful in making a specific diagnosis in protozoan infections. In visceral leishmaniasis (kala azar), the organisms may be identified in tissue or isolated in culture, with bone marrow a favored site.

AMEBIC LIVER ABSCESS

ETIOLOGY. *Entamoeba histolytica* (see Ch. 381) is an important worldwide cause of liver abscess. Amebiasis in all its forms is predominantly a disease of tropical and subtropical regions. The liver is invaded by the protozoan amebae, which have been ingested as cysts and have passed to the colon where vegetative trophozoites enter the intestinal mucosa, causing colonic ulcers. Amebae then enter the portal vein and are swept to the liver. In the liver, the amebae block small portal radicles, release enzymes, and cause focal inflammatory lesions. The term *amebic hepatitis* is a misnomer. Single or multiple abscesses may be formed, although in most patients a single abscess is found. The preferred site for abscess formation is superoanteriorly in the right lobe of the liver (Fig. 120–3*A*). The right hemidiaphragm may be elevated and fixed. Pleural effusion is quite frequent (Fig. 120–3*B*). For unknown rea-

TABLE 120-1. IMPORTANT PARASITIC DISEASES OF THE LIVER AND BILIARY TRACT

Disorder (Organism)	Predisposition to Infection*	Nature of Hepatic Involvement		
		Pathophysiology	*Manifestations*	*Diagnosis*
Schistosomiasis (*Schistosoma mansoni, japonicum*) (flatworm)	Exposure to water in which appropriate snail hosts reside	Host immune response to ova delivered via portal vein, resulting in granulomas and fibrosis	*Acute:* eosinophilic infiltrate *Chronic:* hepatosplenomegaly, complications of portal hypertension, granuloma formation	Ova identified in stool or on liver biopsy
Echinococcosis (*Echinococcus granulosa, E. multilocularis*) (tapeworm)	Exposure to sheep, cattle, and dogs	Larval migration to liver leading to hydatid cyst	*Asymptomatic:* symptoms of hepatic mass lesions, biliary tract obstruction, cyst rupture	Serologic tests (indirect hemagglutination, ELISA); CT scans
Ascariasis (*Ascaris lumbricoides*) (round worm)	Eating raw vegetables	Larval migration via portal vein to liver; later adult invasion of biliary tract with egg production	Abdominal pain, fever, jaundice during larval migration; bile duct obstruction, cholangitis; granuloma may form around eggs	Ova or adult worm in stool; worms in duodenum on contrast studies or endoscopic examination. Demonstration of ascaris in bile duct; may be calcified
Clonorchiasis (*Clonorchis sinensis*) (flatworm)	Ingesting raw freshwater fish	Worm migration through ampulla of Vater; eggs deposited in bile ducts	Bile duct obstruction, cholangitis, choledocholithiasis, cholangiocarcinoma	Ova in stool; multiple bile duct stones on ERCP
Fascioliasis (*Fasciola hepatica*) (flatworm)	Ingesting infected freshwater plants	Larval migration through liver, penetration of bile ducts	*Acute:* fever, abdominal pain, jaundice, hemobilia *Chronic:* asymptomatic hepatomegaly, choledocholithiasis	Eosinophilia; elevated liver tests; ova in stool; adult flukes in bile ducts on ERCP
Toxocariasis (*Toxocara canis, T. cati*) (round worm)	Contact with dogs and cats	Larval migration in hepatic parenchyma (visceral larva migrans)	Granulomas with eosinophilia	Larvae in tissue; serology; ELISA
Strongyloidiasis (*Strongyloides stercoralis*)	Immunodeficiency (AIDS, organ transplant, malignancy)	Penetration of larvae through intestinal wall into liver	Hepatomegaly, occasional jaundice, larvae in portal tract and liver lobule	Larvae in stool or duodenal aspirate; serologic tests not useful
Protozoan disorders Amebiasis (*Entamoeba histolytica*)	Poor sanitation	Hematogenous spread with tissue invasion; abscess formation	Fever, right upper quadrant pain, peritonitis, elevated right hemidiaphragm, pleural effusion	Cysts in stool; serologic test (counterimmunoelectrophoresis, indirect hemagglutination); ultrasonography, CT scan
Malaria (*Plasmodium vivax, falciparum, ovale, malariae*)	Blood transfusion, parenteral drug use. Travel to endemic areas	Sporozoites cleared from circulation by hepatocytes; exoerythrocytic replication in liver	Tender hepatomegaly; rarely hepatic failure (*P. falciparum*)	Identification of organism on blood smear
Cryptosporidiosis (*Cryptosporidium*)	Immunodeficiency (AIDS)	Unknown; biliary tract involvement thus far only in immunodeficient patients	Fever, right upper quadrant pain	Elevated serum alkaline phosphatase; bile duct dilatation on ERCP
Toxoplasmosis (*Toxoplasma gondii*)	Intrauterine infection; immunodeficiency (AIDS, organ transplant)	Multiplication in liver causing necrosis and inflammation	Fever, hepatosplenomegaly	Aminotransferase elevation; isolation of organism from tissue; Sabin-Feldman dye test
Visceral leishmaniasis (*Leishmania donovani*)	Immunodeficiency (AIDS, organ transplant)	Infection of reticuloendothelial cells of liver	Fever, leukopenia, hepatosplenomegaly	Organism in bone marrow; immunoserologic tests
Trypanosomiasis (*Trypanosoma cruzi, rhodesiense, gambiense*)	*Acute:* parasites in reticuloendothelial cells of liver *Chronic:* passive congestion secondary to heart failure	*Acute:* fever, hepatosplenomegaly *Chronic:* hepatomegaly	Organisms in blood, tissue; immunofluorescent tests	

* Travel in endemic areas predisposes to specific infections.

sons, amebic liver abscesses are far more likely to occur in males. There is scant correlation between the appearance of the liver abscess and evidence of active colonic infection. Long latent intervals to the onset of an abscess have been documented.

CLINICAL MANIFESTATIONS AND DIAGNOSIS. The gradual onset of fever, malaise, and right upper quadrant abdominal pain is the usual presentation for a patient with an amebic abscess of the liver. Occasionally the onset is abrupt with fever and repeated rigors. Almost all patients with amebic abscess have hepatic tenderness and dull aching right upper quadrant abdominal pain. Jaundice is unusual and, if present, suggests that the abscess has compressed a major bile duct. Leukocytosis and anemia may be present. If the abscess affects the hemidiaphragm, pain may be referred to the shoulder and may be worsened by deep breathing or coughing. Only a few patients have concomitant evidence of amebic colitis, and cysts are found in the stool in a minority of patients. Occasionally the diagnosis is first suspected following intraperitoneal or intrathoracic rupture into the pleura or pericardium. Amebic abscesses should be considered in any patient who has resided in or traveled to an endemic area and in whom a hepatic filling defect is found on an imaging study. The indirect hemagglutination test indicates tissue invasion by amebae and is almost always indicative, although not diagnostic, of liver involvement. An elevated right hemidiaphragm and pleural effusion are often found. Aspiration is generally not required to establish the diagnosis.

TREATMENT. Metronidazole is the drug of choice. Aspiration may prove useful for patients who have large abscesses or those in whom there has been little response to 5 days of metronidazole therapy. Aspiration is also used if an abscess is likely to rupture. A course of a luminal amebicide such as diiodoquine may add to overall treatment.

GRANULOMATOUS LIVER DISEASE

ETIOLOGY. Granulomas represent a specific form of inflammatory response found in a wide variety of conditions and present a reaction pattern involving stimulation of macrophages and lymphocytes. Granulomas of diverse causes may appear identical. Large, pale-staining epithelioid cells are characteristic. Evidence of

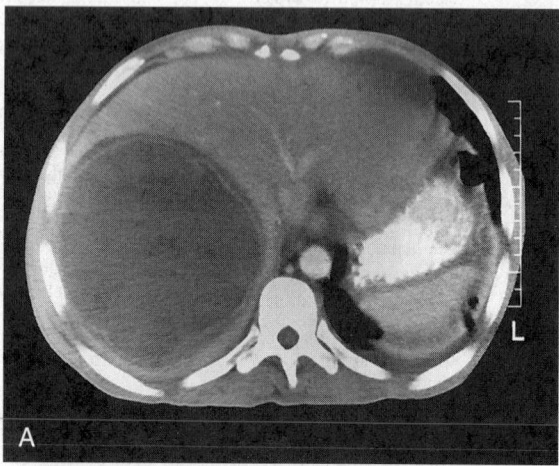

FIGURE 120–2. CT scan of an echinococcal cyst in a 25-year-old man demonstrating the complex structure of the wall and the interior.

caseation and necrosis may also be found. Macrophages, the predominant cells in granulomas, often fuse to form characteristic multinucleated giant cells. Most granulomas are found in or near the portal tract. Granulomas have been found in 2 to 10% of all liver biopsies, and often no specific cause is identified.

Major disorders in which hepatic granulomas are frequent include sarcoidosis, tuberculosis, histoplasmosis, and schistosomiasis. There

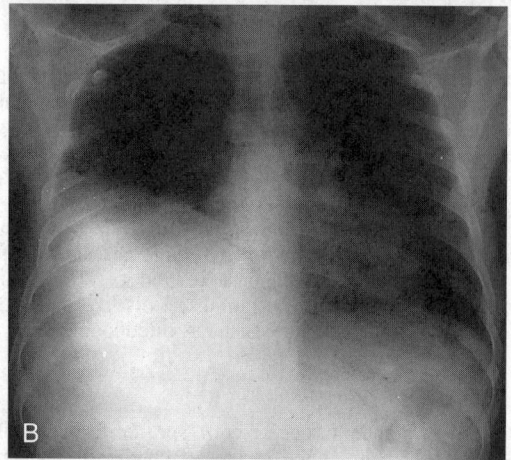

FIGURE 120–3. *A,* CT scan of a large amebic liver abscess in a 36-year-old man. *B,* Chest radiograph demonstrating elevated right diaphragm with compression of right lung and pleural effusion.

are considerable geographic variations in frequency of causes. A number of disorders associated with hepatic granuloma formation are listed in Table 120–2. Knowledge of a patient's profession, lifestyle, and travel may yield important clues. For example, coccidioidomycosis is a well-established cause of granulomas in the western United States. *Mycobacterium avium-intracellulare* has come to the fore as an important granulomatous disease in patients with AIDS. A variety of therapeutic drugs including phenylbutazone, allopurinol, and carbamazepine are well documented to cause granulomas. In addition, granulomas are characteristically found in the early stages of primary biliary cirrhosis.

CLINICAL MANIFESTATIONS. In most patients, the presence of granulomas does not adversely affect the liver and may be detected when a liver biopsy is being performed for some other reason, especially when evaluating an increase in serum alkaline phosphatase. Many patients with even extensive granulomatous inflammation in the liver are asymptomatic. Occasionally, however, the liver is enlarged and tender. In a few, a chronic active hepatitis—apparently related to the granuloma—has been associated and, in some, progression to cirrhosis with portal hypertension has occurred.

PATHOLOGY. Only occasionally are the histologic features of the granulomas specific enough to help in the search for a cause. Schistosomiasis ova may be found within the granuloma. Special stains may identify *Mycobacterium tuberculosis* or *M. avium-intracellulare.* Occasionally, birefringent granules of starch are identified. A rather characteristic type of inflammation with a fibrinoid ring is characteristic of Q fever.

DIAGNOSIS. Granulomas in the liver often direct diagnostic attention toward identifying a generalized disease process. Travel, profession, and lifestyle must all be considered. Even with exhaustive searching, the cause of granulomas in many is never identified. Culture of liver tissue rarely yields the diagnosis.

TABLE 120–2. MAJOR CAUSES OF HEPATIC GRANULOMAS

Disease	Diagnosis
Sarcoidosis	Paratracheal or hilar lymph node enlargement found on chest radiograph
	Elevated serum angiotensin-converting enzyme level
	Conjunctival granulomas
Tuberculosis (*Mycobacterium tuberculosis*)	Isolation/culture of sputum bronchitis-alveolar lavage, bone marrow, liver
Mycobacterium avium-intracellulare	Tuberculin skin tests
	HIV positive
	Sputum cultures
Histoplasmosis	Complement fixation test (limited value)
	Chest radiograph
	Sputum cultures
Brucellosis	Agglutinin titer
	Blood culture
Lymphomas	Chest radiograph
Hodgkin's disease	CT scan
	Biopsy of lymph nodes
Schistosomiasis	Demonstration of parts of ova in granulomas
	Schistosomal eggs in rectal biopsy
Primary biliary cirrhosis	Antimitochondrial antibodies
	Female with cholestatic liver disease
Leprosy	Skin test for lepromin
	Country of origin
Drug reactions (Allopurinol, procainamide, hydralazine, sulfonamides, phenylbutazone, carbamazepine, quinidine)	History of use of a drug known (or suspected) to cause granulomas
Berylliosis	Occupational exposure
	Chest radiograph
Q fever	Serologic tests
	Characteristic fibrinoid ring
Syphilis (secondary)	Serologic test (STS)
Lipogranulomas	Demonstration of mineral oil in a granuloma
Talc	Birefringent inclusions

TREATMENT. Because granulomas represent a reaction pattern rather than a disease, the treatment depends on the diagnosis established.

SARCOIDOSIS (see Ch. 61)

Sarcoidosis is a granulomatous disease of unknown cause which almost always involves the liver. Most patients have no symptoms from the granulomas. A few patients develop a chronic active liver disease that may progress to cirrhosis. There is no specific diagnostic test for sarcoidosis. Most patients have an elevated serum angiotensin-converting enzyme (ACE) level associated with elevated serum alkaline phosphatase levels. There is no treatment for sarcoidosis affecting the liver. Corticosteroids have not been proven to have any major effects on the liver disease. Patients who have features indicating an overlap of sarcoidosis and primary biliary cirrhosis have been described.

INFECTIONS OF THE LIVER IN PATIENTS WITH AIDS (see Part XXII)

Patients who have AIDS are at high risk of acquiring hepatic infections. Concomitant hepatitis B and hepatitis C are the most frequently associated infections. *M. avium-intracellulare* and *M. tuberculosis* both represent major problems in these immunocompromised patients. Other problems include infection with cytomegalovirus, herpes simplex, *Cryptococcus neoformans,* coccidioidomycosis, histoplasmosis, and Epstein-Barr virus. Hepatotoxicity from one or more of the drugs used to treat AIDS and its complications may cause liver injury.

Cello JP: Human immunodeficiency virus–associated biliary tract disease. Sem Liver Dis 12:213, 1992. *A comprehensive review of HIV infection and biliary tract disease.*

Elliott DL, Tolle SW, Goldberg L, et al.: Pet-associated illness. N Engl J Med 313:985, 1985. *Review of parasitic, bacterial, and rickettsial illnesses acquired from cats and dogs.*

Greenstein AJ, Sachar DB: Pyogenic and amebic abscesses of the liver. Sem Liver Dis 8:210, 1988. *Excellent summary and comparison of features of these types of abscesses.*

Kamath PS, Joseph DC, Chandran R, et al.: Biliary ascariasis: Ultrasonography, endoscopic retrograde cholangiopancreatography, and biliary drainage. Gastroenterology 91:730, 1986. *Complete description of the effects of ascariasis on the biliary tract.*

Maddrey WC: Granulomatous liver disease: Clinical aspects. *In* Current Perspectives in Hepatology, 1989, p 309. *Comprehensive review of pathogenesis and causes of granulomatous liver disorders.*

121 INHERITED, INFILTRATIVE, AND METABOLIC DISORDERS INVOLVING THE LIVER

Jacquelyn J. Maher

This chapter focuses on the hepatic manifestations of inherited, infiltrative, and metabolic diseases. Because many of the disorders mentioned herein involve multiple organs, the reader is also referred to other chapters for further details.

ALPHA₁-ANTITRYPSIN DEFICIENCY

Alpha₁-antitrypsin (A_1AT) is a circulating glycoprotein whose primary function is to inhibit neutrophil elastase (see Ch. 52). This 52-kD protein, which comprises the α_1 globulin fraction of serum, is synthesized primarily by hepatocytes. Deficiencies in circulating A_1AT are caused by mutations in the A_1AT gene that lead either to single amino acid substitutions or more extensive frameshifts or deletions. These mutations can block protein synthesis, cause its premature degradation in hepatocytes, prevent its secretion from liver cells, or alter its activity toward neutrophil elastase.

Because A_1AT production is controlled by codominant alleles, the protease inhibitor (Pi) phenotype of an individual is designated by the allelic pair. The normal allele is M, with the most common abnormal alleles being S and Z. Individuals who are PiMM have circulating levels of antitrypsin in the range of 200 mg per deciliter; those who are PiZZ have only 15% of this amount. Heterozygous combinations of 75 or more alleles permit a wide range of A_1AT

levels in serum. Pulmonary disease in patients with A_1AT deficiency is directly linked to the amount of functional enzyme in the serum. Liver disease, by contrast, is caused by retention of abnormal A_1AT within the endoplasmic reticulum of hepatocytes. Liver involvement occurs almost entirely with the Z allele, which encodes a protein that is improperly folded and incompletely glycosylated. One or both of these defects prevent the translocation of A_1AT to Golgi and its ultimate secretion by the hepatocyte. That liver disease is related to the presence of abnormal A_1AT in the hepatocyte and not to a deficiency of the circulating enzyme has been demonstrated in experiments with transgenic mice, in which overexpression of the human Z allele causes liver disease despite normal serum levels of A_1AT. This conclusion is further supported by the fact that patients homozygous for null mutations (in which A_1AT is absent from both serum and liver) do not develop liver injury. Only homozygotes for the Z allele are at clear risk of liver injury. Liver disease has been reported in Z heterozygotes, but cause and effect have not been clearly established. This correlates well with the transgenic mouse model in which liver disease is most severe in animals with multiple copies of the human gene.

Approximately 10% of PiZZ individuals develop clinical liver disease in infancy. This manifests as neonatal cholestasis, which often resolves by age 4 months. One in five infants with neonatal cholestasis (2% of all PiZZ individuals) progresses to childhood cirrhosis; the risk of progression exists even if the initial cholestasis was self-limited. PiZZ homozygotes who escape liver disease in childhood have a 10% chance of developing cirrhosis as adults. Males are at higher risk for adult-onset cirrhosis than are females; why females, and indeed why the majority of PiZZ adults, avoid chronic liver injury is uncertain. Patients who do develop liver disease have an unusually high incidence of liver cancer.

A_1AT deficiency should be suspected in adults with cirrhosis of unknown etiology. Emphysema need not be present to entertain the diagnosis. A_1AT deficiency can be detected by measuring the enzyme in serum or by directly analyzing protease inhibitor phenotype. Liver biopsy in individuals inheriting a Z allele reveals globular deposits of abnormal A_1AT within the rough endoplasmic reticulum of hepatocytes. Because the inclusions are present in heterozygotes as well as homozygotes, however, their presence alone is not pathognomonic of A_1AT-induced liver disease.

The only treatment for hepatic cirrhosis due to A_1AT deficiency is liver transplantation (see Ch. 124). Although gene replacement holds promise for correcting the enzyme deficiency, current strategies do nothing to suppress overproduction of the Z protein that provokes liver injury. With liver transplantation, the A_1AT in serum assumes the phenotype of the donor.

WILSON'S DISEASE

Wilson's disease is an autosomal recessive disorder characterized by accumulation of copper in multiple organs, including the liver (see Ch. 188). The specific molecular defect resides within a copper-transporting ATPase encoded by a gene on chromosome 13. Affected patients exhibit impaired biliary excretion of copper; this leads to copper accumulation in the liver, and in later stages, to its release into the circulation, permitting deposition in the brain, cornea, and kidneys. Patients with Wilson's disease begin to accumulate hepatic copper in infancy. Despite this, symptoms of disease rarely develop before adolescence.

Symptoms of liver disease are the presenting complaint in roughly half of affected individuals. The most common syndrome is that of postnecrotic cirrhosis with hepatic dysfunction and portal hypertension. A small proportion (10 to 30%) of patients have chronic active hepatitis. Rarely the disease manifests as fulminant hepatic failure; in patients with massive liver necrosis, coincident hemolysis may provide an important clue to the diagnosis.

No single biochemical test can establish the diagnosis. A useful screening test is serum ceruloplasmin, which is < 20 mg per deciliter in 85% of patients. If Kayser-Fleischer rings are found in a patient with a low ceruloplasmin level, the diagnosis is confirmed. However, because 15% of patients with symptomatic Wilson's disease have normal ceruloplasmin levels, and because asymptomatic patients (e.g., children) and those with hepatic presentations such as chronic active hepatitis or fulminant hepatic failure may lack Kayser-Fleischer rings, the diagnosis may be difficult to establish noninvasively. In this event a liver biopsy should be obtained to quantify total hepatic copper. Patients with > 250 μg copper per gram of dry liver tissue who have either Kayser-Fleischer rings or a low level of serum ceruloplasmin are considered to have Wilson's disease. Occasionally children with chronic liver disease who lack Kayser-Fleischer rings and have a normal ceruloplasmin level present a problem in diagnosis. In this case, measurement of urinary copper excretion in response to oral penicillamine challenge may be useful.

Copper chelation (discussed in Ch. 188) improves survival but does not reverse cirrhosis. Once initiated, therapy must be continued for life; discontinuation can result in rapid deterioration of liver function. In patients with fulminant hepatic failure or decompensated cirrhosis, liver transplantation provides effective therapy by correcting the primary metabolic defect.

HEMOCHROMATOSIS

Hereditary hemochromatosis (see Ch. 189) is an autosomal recessive disorder characterized by iron overload in the liver, heart, pancreas, pituitary gland, and joints. Although the specific inherited defect remains uncertain, the gene responsible for hemochromatosis has been mapped to chromosome 6 near the human leukocyte antigen-A (HLA-A) allele. The homozygote frequency is estimated from $1:400$ to as high as $1:100$. Patients with the disease absorb excessive amounts of iron from the gut and deposit the metal in many organs, where it injures cells. Only homozygotes develop clinically significant hepatic iron overload; heterozygotes exhibit increased hepatic iron stores, but do not develop liver injury.

Iron accumulation is progressive from birth but rarely leads to symptoms before age 40. The onset of disease is delayed even further in females, because of loss of iron in menstrual blood and a lower intake of dietary iron. Presenting symptoms are often vague, with abdominal pain reported in as few as 16% or as many as 58% of patients. Despite the variability of symptoms, signs of liver disease (particularly hepatomegaly) can be found in $> 75\%$ of patients.

Biochemical abnormalities that suggest hereditary hemochromatosis in symptomatic individuals include elevations in transferrin saturation ($> 62\%$ in males; $> 50\%$ in females) and ferritin (more than twice normal). It must be noted, however, that both of these parameters are prone to false-positive elevations and must be interpreted with caution. Transferrin saturation can be falsely elevated in nonfasting patients, in those with active liver necrosis, and even in heterozygotes for hemochromatosis. Ferritin also increases nonspecifically with hepatocellular necrosis and may cause particular confusion in patients with alcoholic liver disease. To diagnose hereditary hemochromatosis with certainty, a liver biopsy must be obtained to quantify total hepatic iron. Patients with hereditary hemochromatosis who have clinical evidence of liver disease will have $> 10,000$ μg iron per gram of dry liver tissue. Younger patients who have less pronounced increases in total hepatic iron can be distinguished from heterozygotes and from patients with alcoholic liver disease by measuring the "hepatic iron index" (micro-*moles* hepatic iron $\div$ age; a ratio of greater than 2 indicates hereditary hemochromatosis). More than 22,000 μg iron per gram dry liver is required to establish a diagnosis of cirrhosis.

Phlebotomy (discussed in Ch. 189) is the mainstay of therapy and can prevent or even reverse hepatic fibrosis. Fully developed cirrhosis is not usually reversible, although phlebotomy can enhance the survival of patients with cirrhosis. Unfortunately, patients with cirrhosis are at high risk of developing hepatocellular carcinoma, whether or not they undergo iron depletion. Hepatocellular carcinoma is currently the leading cause of death among patients with hereditary hemochromatosis.

Family members of probands are screened by HLA typing and by serial measurements of transferrin saturation and ferritin. Because of the high frequency of the genetic defect, screening the general population with iron studies is under review but has not been advocated to date. HLA typing has no role in population screening.

PROTOPORPHYRIA

Protoporphyria is an inherited disorder marked by a profound reduction in ferrochelatase, the final enzyme in the pathway of heme synthesis. The mode of inheritance is debated. The primary clinical features of protoporphyria are cutaneous photosensitivity and scarring of sun-exposed skin; patients can also develop pigment gallstones, frequently at a young age. Parenchymal liver disease has been reported in fewer than 30 patients.

Protoporphyria can be diagnosed by measuring elevated protoporphyrin levels in erythrocytes or feces. Patients with the highest levels of protoporphyrin ($> 1,000$ μg per deciliter in erythrocytes) may be predisposed to liver disease and should undergo liver biopsy. Histology reveals birefringent deposits of protoporphyrin in hepatocytes and Kupffer cells. Development of jaundice predicts rapid deterioration and demise.

Treating liver disease in protoporphyria is aimed at reducing production and increasing excretion of protoporphyrin. Hematin appears to decrease protoporphyrin production and has been useful in selected patients. Cholestyramine and activated charcoal both bind protoporphyrin in the gut, preventing enterohepatic recirculation and promoting excretion. For patients with severe liver disease and jaundice, liver transplantation should be considered.

CYSTIC FIBROSIS

Cystic fibrosis (see Ch. 58) manifests rarely in infants as a syndrome of obstructive jaundice. Older children and adolescents are more likely to develop liver disease, although the reported incidence varies from 2.2 to 16%. Patients usually have established hepatic fibrosis at the time of diagnosis. Biochemical tests often fail to predict liver injury; indeed, a catastrophe such as variceal hemorrhage is sometimes the first sign of hepatic disease. Because chronic liver disease may be the initial manifestation of cystic fibrosis, the diagnosis should be considered in any child or adolescent with hepatic fibrosis of unknown etiology. Therapy for portal hypertension follows that for other liver diseases.

GLYCOGEN STORAGE DISEASES

Most of the glycogen storage diseases, discussed in detail in Ch. 170, are accompanied by hepatic glycogen accumulation and hepatomegaly. Only four of these (types O, I, III, and IV) result in clinical liver disease. Type O (glycogen synthetase deficiency) is extremely rare. Type IV (α-1, 4 glucan-6-glycosyl transferase deficiency) leads to mortality from cirrhosis in early childhood. Types I and III are the two most likely to be encountered in adults.

Type I glycogenosis (glucose-6-phosphatase deficiency) is characterized not only by hepatic glycogen accumulation but also by marked hepatic steatosis. Biochemical studies reveal profound hypoglycemia and hypertriglyceridemia. Transaminases are only mildly increased. Patients treated with a high glucose diet can survive to adulthood but are at extremely high risk for developing hepatic adenomas. These tumors, which can undergo malignant transformation, are present in over 50% of patients by age 25. Rigorous therapy designed to maintain blood glucose above 75 mg per deciliter at all times may prevent or reverse adenoma formation.

Type III glycogenosis (debrancher enzyme deficiency) differs from type I in that hypoglycemia and hyperlipidemia are much milder. Liver biopsy does not reveal steatosis but frequently demonstrates fibrosis. Hepatic fibrosis rarely progresses to cirrhosis or portal hypertension. Supplemental feedings are recommended for patients with progressive liver injury.

AMYLOIDOSIS

Hepatic involvement is common in patients with systemic amyloidosis (see Ch. 248). Localized disease in the liver is rare but has been reported. Features of hepatic amyloidosis include hepatomegaly and increased serum alkaline phosphatase (each found in 60% of patients with biopsy-proven liver involvement); clinical liver disease, however, is rarely encountered. A small number of patients with hepatic amyloidosis develop severe intrahepatic cholestasis with jaundice. This syndrome portends a poor prognosis, although death results from extrahepatic (primarily renal) disease.

Liver biopsy is not required to confirm hepatic involvement in patients with known systemic amyloidosis. If the diagnosis is uncertain, however, liver biopsy may be useful and can be performed safely as long as clotting parameters are normal and any history of a bleeding disorder is excluded.

SARCOIDOSIS

Sarcoidosis is one of the most common granulomatous diseases affecting the liver. Hepatic granulomas can be identified in approximately two thirds of patients with sarcoidosis, placing the liver behind only the lung and lymph nodes as the primary sites of involvement (see Ch. 120). Despite this, clinical symptoms of liver disease in sarcoidosis are rare. Liver involvement is usually recognized because of hepatomegaly or an elevated alkaline phosphatase level. A small minority of patients can develop a cholestatic syndrome characterized by pruritus and jaundice or can have hepatic failure and portal hypertension in the event the disease progresses to cirrhosis.

Liver biopsy can be useful in establishing a diagnosis of sarcoidosis, because granulomas are so numerous as to be sampled even with a random needle core. Occasionally, portal granulomas can destroy intrahepatic bile ducts, mimicking primary biliary cirrhosis. The latter can be distinguished by the presence of antimitochondrial antibodies in serum. When sarcoidosis progresses to hepatic fibrosis, connective tissue deposition is more extensive than around the granulomas alone.

Corticosteroids alleviate the symptoms of sarcoidosis but have not been proven to alter liver histology or the tendency toward hepatic fibrosis. Therapy should therefore be reserved for symptomatic patients in whom tuberculosis and other infectious diseases have been excluded.

TOTAL PARENTERAL NUTRITION

The most common hepatobiliary complication of total parenteral nutrition (TPN) is hepatic steatosis. This is true despite careful preparation of solutions to contain a balance of glucose, amino acid, and lipid. Fatty liver occurs in 25 to 100% of patients receiving TPN; the lesion is heralded by an increase in serum transaminases with a smaller increase in alkaline phosphatase. Enzymes peak at around 2 weeks of therapy and then decline even if TPN is continued without modification. Steatosis is completely reversible upon cessation of the infusion.

Adults receiving TPN for more than 30 days are at risk of forming biliary sludge and gallstones. Fifty percent of patients develop sludge after 6 weeks, and virtually 100% of patients are affected after 3 months. Acalculous and calculous cholecystitis can both occur. Although the pathophysiology of sludge and stone formation in the setting of TPN is due in part to decreased bile flow, gallbladder stasis plays an important role. Stasis may be ameliorated by cholecystokinin, by pulsed infusions of amino acids, or by small enteral feedings.

Long-term TPN poses a risk of chronic liver injury in adults. The most common abnormality is steatohepatitis; cholestasis and hepatic fibrosis have also been observed. Because steatohepatitis and cholestasis can both progress to hepatic fibrosis, their development is considered by many an indication to discontinue therapy. Chronic liver injury may be prevented by avoiding caloric excess, by infusing TPN cyclically, and by providing small amounts of enteral nutrition when possible.

LIVER DISEASE IN PREGNANCY

Pregnant women are susceptible to the full range of hepatic diseases. For the most part, pregnancy does not pose an increased risk of acute liver disease, nor does it alter the natural history of hepatic illnesses contracted during gestation. Notable exceptions to this are viral hepatitides caused by the herpes simplex, herpes zoster, and hepatitis E viruses. Herpes simplex hepatitis has a higher incidence in pregnant women than in the population at large. All three agents can provoke severe illness in pregnant women, with mortality rates as high as 20% in the case of hepatitis E. Liver diseases that are not unique to pregnancy are not discussed here. Below is a summary of hepatic disorders that occur only in pregnant women, followed by a brief discussion of pregnancy in the setting of chronic liver disease.

LIVER DISEASES UNIQUE TO PREGNANCY (Table 121–1). Transient elevations in hepatic transaminase levels may accompany *hyperemesis gravidarum.* Biochemical *cholestasis,* defined as an increase in circulating bile acids, can be detected in as many as 10% of normal gestations. Symptomatic cholestasis occurs in only 1 to 5% of pregnant women and is generally confined to the second and third trimesters. Most patients complain only of pruritus ("pruritus gravidarum"); a minority exhibit a more severe syndrome with disabling pruritus, jaundice, and steatorrhea. The latter may have an inherited predisposition toward cholestasis, with women of South American Indian and Swedish descent being at high risk. Cholestasis of pregnancy is a self-limited syndrome, resolving spontaneously after delivery. Whereas mild disease poses no risk to either mother or fetus, severe cholestasis places women at increased risk of premature delivery and fetal death. Treatment of gestational cholestasis is supportive. Antihistamines may relieve pruritus, and drugs such as *S*-adenosylmethionine may improve cholestasis. Patients should be counseled that the syndrome often recurs with future pregnancies.

Acute fatty liver of pregnancy is a disorder characterized by microvesicular fat accumulation in hepatocytes and hepatic necrosis. The pathogenesis of the disease may be related to an impairment in mitochondrial fatty acid oxidation. The incidence is estimated from 1 in 6000 to 1 in 13,000 gestations. Roughly half of women are primiparas, and 14% have twin fetuses. Manifestations of the disease are listed in Table 121–1. A specific diagnosis can be made histologically only by demonstration of microvesicular fat droplets in hepatocytes; liver biopsy is not essential for management, however, and may be precluded by coagulopathy. Because acute fatty liver almost always resolves spontaneously post partum, prompt delivery of the fetus is the treatment of choice. Patients deteriorating despite delivery should be considered for liver transplantation. Fatty liver of pregnancy tends not to recur with subsequent gestations.

HELLP syndrome is the name given to a disorder of pregnancy characterized by Hemolysis, Elevated Liver enzymes, and Low Platelets. It is a microangiopathic disorder of the liver that occurs in the setting of severe preeclampsia or eclampsia with a frequency of 2 to 12%. Older, multiparous patients are at increased risk of HELLP syndrome; of note is that the classic triad of hypertension, proteinuria, and edema need not be present to make the diagnosis. Patients can develop HELLP syndrome in the second or third trimester or even post partum. Symptoms are similar to those of acute fatty liver of pregnancy, including abdominal pain, nausea, and vomiting. In rare instances subcapsular hematomas can occur, leading to hepatic rupture and circulatory collapse. Laboratory abnormalities are not specific but often include anemia (hematocrit < 30%), increased transaminases, and depressed platelet count (< 100,000 per cubic millimeter). Lactate dehydrogenase is commonly above 600 U per liter. Prothrombin time, partial thromboplastin time, and fibrinogen are usually normal and may provide some distinction from acute fatty liver of pregnancy. Blood smear

TABLE 121–1. LIVER DISEASES UNIQUE TO PREGNANCY

	Trimester of Onset	Symptoms	Laboratory Abnormalities	Recurrence with Future Pregnancies
Hyperemesis gravidarum	1	Nausea, vomiting	Elevated AST/ALT (60–1000 U/L), occasional hyperbilirubinemia	
Cholestasis	2, 3	Pruritus	Bile acids > 8 μM, elevated AST/ALT and bilirubin in more severe cases	Common
Acute fatty liver	3	Nausea, vomiting, abdominal pain	Elevated AST/ALT (100–1000 U/L), bilirubin > 5 mg/dl, prolonged prothrombin time*	Rare
HELLP syndrome	2, 3 or post partum	Abdominal pain, nausea, vomiting	Elevated AST/ALT (60–1500 U/L), platelets < 100,000/cu mm, LDH > 600 U/L, microangiopathic anemia	3–25%

* Useful diagnostic distinction from HELLP syndrome, in which PT, PTT, and fibrinogen are usually normal.

should suggest intravascular hemolysis. Liver biopsy, when performed, reveals focal hepatocellular necrosis and fibrin deposits within the sinusoids.

Prompt delivery is the treatment of choice. In gestations of less than 34 weeks, steroids can be given to promote fetal lung maturity, followed by delivery. The syndrome usually resolves rapidly post partum; in patients with persistent thrombocytopenia, plasmapheresis has been used successfully. The recurrence rate of HELLP syndrome in two large series varied between 3 and 25%.

PREGNANCY WITH CHRONIC LIVER DISEASE. Fertility is reduced in women with chronic liver disease and particularly in those with cirrhosis. Nevertheless, pregnancies can occur in women with advanced liver disease and are encountered with some frequency in mild to moderate liver disease. In general, pregnancy does not alter the course of underlying liver disease. Nevertheless, severe underlying liver disease places the mother at risk of gestational complications such as variceal hemorrhage and fetal death. Prophylaxis of gastrointestinal bleeding is not warranted in patients with cirrhosis. Patients receiving specific medications, however, such as corticosteroids for autoimmune chronic active hepatitis or copper chelators for Wilson's disease should continue them throughout gestation.

Adams PC, Kertesz AE, Valberg LS: Clinical presentation of hemochromatosis: A changing scene. Am J Med 90:445, 1991. *Study emphasizing increased frequency of detection in women and in asymptomatic patients.*

Barton JR, Sibai BM: Care of the pregnancy complicated by HELLP syndrome. Gastroenterol Clin North Am 21:937, 1992. *One article from an entire volume devoted to liver disease in pregnancy.*

Crystal RG: α1-Antitrypsin deficiency, emphysema, and liver disease. J Clin Invest 85:1343, 1990. *Clear and comprehensive review of the genetics, pathophysiology, and treatment of the disorder.*

Quigley EMM, Marsh MN, Shaffer JL, et al.: Hepatobiliary complications of total parenteral nutrition. Gastroenterology 104:286, 1993. *Current review emphasizing the different complications that affect children and adults.*

Yarze JC, Martin P, Munoz SJ: Wilson's disease: Current status. Am J Med 92:643, 1992. *Succinct review with 147 references.*

122 CIRRHOSIS OF THE LIVER AND ITS MAJOR SEQUELAE

Scott L. Friedman

OVERVIEW

DEFINITION AND GENERAL FEATURES. Cirrhosis consists of fibrosis of the hepatic parenchyma resulting in nodule formation. It represents the consequences of a sustained wound-healing response to chronic liver injury from a variety of causes (Table 122–1), including toxins (e.g., alcohol), chronic viral infection, cholestasis, and metabolic disorders. The clinical consequences of cirrhosis vary widely, from lack of symptoms to liver failure, and are determined by both the nature and severity of the underlying liver disease as well as the extent of fibrosis. Clinical manifestations can be broadly classified into those resulting from impaired hepatocellular function, such as jaundice and coagulopathy, and those that result from physical disruption of the parenchyma, such as gastroesophageal varices and ascites.

EPIDEMIOLOGY. Up to 40% of patients with cirrhosis are asymptomatic. In these individuals, cirrhosis may be discovered during routine examination or at autopsy. The overall incidence of cirrhosis in the United States is estimated at 360 per 100,000 population, or approximately 900,000 total patients. Of these, the large majority have either alcoholic liver disease or chronic viral infection.

Cirrhosis is the most common non-neoplastic cause of death among hepatobiliary and digestive diseases in the United States, accounting for approximately 30,000 deaths per year. An additional 10,000 deaths occur due to liver cancer, the majority of which involve underlying cirrhosis. Mortality in patients with alcoholic disease is considerably higher than in patients with other

TABLE 122–1. CLASSIFICATION OF HEPATIC FIBROSIS AND CIRRHOSIS

1. Presinusoidal fibrosis
   Schistosomiasis
   Idiopathic portal fibrosis
2. Parenchymal (sinusoidal) fibrosis (true cirrhosis)
   A. Drugs and toxins
      Alcohol
      Methotrexate
      Isoniazid
      Vitamin A
      Amiodarone
      Perhexiline maleate
      α-Methyldopa
      Oxyphenisatin
   B. Infections
      Chronic hepatitis B or C
      Brucellosis
      Echinococcus
      Congenital or tertiary syphilis
   C. Autoimmune
      Autoimmune chronic hepatitis—types 1, 2, and 3
   D. Vascular abnormalities
      Chronic passive congestion due to right-sided heart failure, pericarditis
      Hereditary hemorrhagic telangiectasias (Osler-Weber-Rendu)
   E. Metabolic/genetic diseases
      Wilson's disease
      Hemochromatosis
      α₁-Antitrypsin deficiency
      Carbohydrate disorders (e.g., fructose intolerance, galactosemia, glycogen storage diseases)
      Lipid disorders (e.g., Wolman's disease, abetalipoproteinemia)
      Urea cycle defects (e.g., ornithine transcarbamylase)
      Porphyria
      Amino acid disorders (e.g., tyrosinosis)
      Bile acid disorders (e.g., Byler's disease)
   F. Biliary obstruction
      Primary biliary cirrhosis
      Secondary ("mechanical") biliary obstruction
         Primary sclerosing cholangitis
         Neoplasm of bile ducts or pancreas
         Iatrogenic or inflammatory biliary stricture
      Cystic fibrosis
      Biliary atresia/neonatal hepatitis
      Congenital biliary cysts
   G. Idiopathic/miscellaneous
      Nonalcoholic steatonecrosis (including JI bypass, obesity)
      Indian childhood cirrhosis
      Granulomatous liver disease
      Polycystic liver disease
3. Post-sinusoidal fibrosis
   Veno-occlusive disease

forms of cirrhosis. Death rates are also higher in men than in women. In the 1980's overall cirrhosis mortality decreased by 25% in the United States, possibly reflecting decreasing alcohol consumption and, to a lesser extent, the advent of hepatitis B vaccination, improved supportive care, and availability of liver transplantation (see Ch. 124).

CLASSIFICATION AND ETIOLOGY. Cirrhosis has traditionally been classified as either macronodular (>3-mm nodules) or micronodular (<3 mm). There is, however, no etiologic, functional, or prognostic value to the nodule size. A rare exception is in the cirrhotic patient with a massive "regenerative" nodule, which must be distinguished from a neoplasm.

Current classification of cirrhosis is based on cause (Table 122–1). The chemical composition of the scar tissue in cirrhosis is similar regardless of etiology and consists of the extracellular matrix (ECM) molecules, collagen types I and III (i.e., "fibrillar" collagens), sulfated proteoglycans, and glycoproteins. These scar constituents accumulate from a net increase in their deposition in liver and not simply collapse of existing stroma. While the cirrhotic bands surrounding nodules are the most easily seen form of scarring, it is actually the early deposition of matrix molecules in the subendothelial space of Disse—so-called capillarization of the sinusoid—that more directly correlates with diminished liver function (Fig. 122–1).

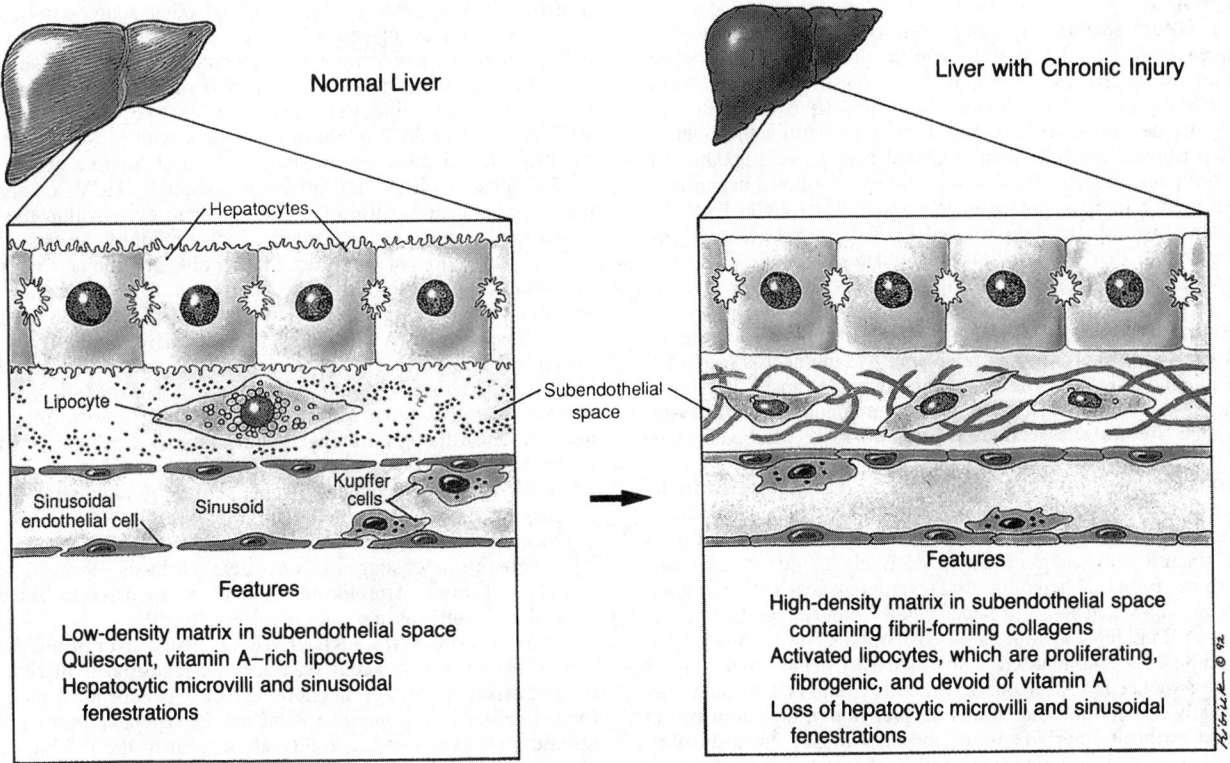

FIGURE 122–1. Cellular and pathologic alterations in the hepatic sinusoid during chronic liver injury and fibrosis. (From Friedman SL: The cellular basis of hepatic necrosis. (Reprinted by permission of the New England Journal of Medicine, 328:1829, 1993. Copyright 1993, Massachusetts Medical Society.)

Efforts to identify the cellular source of scar constituents in cirrhosis have established that the lipocyte, or stellate cell, is the main producer of matrix. In both human disease and animal models, these mesenchymal cells undergo characteristic activation from a resting perisinusoidal cell rich in vitamin A to a proliferating and fibrogenic cell type with reduced vitamin A content. Lipocyte activation is common to all forms of experimental liver injury studied to date, including chronic biliary obstruction. Increased matrix produced by lipocytes in liver injury results from increased cell numbers as well as enhanced matrix production per cell. Cell proliferation is regulated primarily by the cytokine platelet-derived growth factor (PDGF), whereas fibrogenesis is stimulated by transforming growth factor beta (TGFβ), whose mRNA levels are markedly increased in human cirrhosis. Activated lipocytes can also contract and secrete proteases, which can remodel the hepatic ECM. At present there is no established treatment to arrest or reverse scar formation in chronic liver injury. Rather, removing the primary insult when possible remains the most effective way to prevent irreversible scarring.

DIAGNOSIS AND PROGNOSIS OF CIRRHOSIS. Liver biopsy remains the gold standard for documenting cirrhosis, identifying a cause, and assessing the extent of scar formation. Biopsy specimens should be large enough to identify portal tracts and central areas. Sections should be examined with both hematoxylin-eosin and a connective tissue stain such as Masson's trichrome or reticulin. Special stains may be appropriate as well to identify metals (e.g., iron, copper) lipids, carbohydrates, and/or protein accumulation associated with inborn errors of metabolism (Table 122–1; also see Ch. 121).

In the clinical setting, prognosis is best determined by the Pugh modification of the Child-Turcotte classification, which includes the variables of ascites, encephalopathy, serum albumin, serum bilirubin, and prothrombin time. Both the Child-Turcotte and Pugh classifications correlate closely with albumin synthesis rates. Several noninvasive markers of cirrhosis have been advocated that measure fragments of matrix molecules in serum (e.g., collagen propeptides). In general, however, these assays reflect inflammatory activity and may be falsely normal in established, quiescent cirrhosis. By reflecting inflammatory activity they may indirectly have prognostic value but do not discriminate in all cases between different stages of injury and fibrosis.

ALCOHOLIC LIVER DISEASE

OVERVIEW, EPIDEMIOLOGY, AND RISK FACTORS. Alcoholic liver disease (ALD) encompasses a spectrum of abnormalities ranging from fatty liver, a reversible consequence of acute ingestion, to irreversible cirrhosis (Laënnec's cirrhosis). It is the leading cause of cirrhosis in the United States and Europe. While many patients who drink heavily develop hepatic enlargement and fatty accumulation, only a minority (~20%) of cases will progress to alcoholic hepatitis or cirrhosis. *Risk factors* for developing these more severe sequelae include: *(1) Duration and magnitude of alcohol ingestion.* An average total intake required for development of cirrhosis has been estimated as the regular consumption of 80 grams of ethanol per day for 20 years, but the relative risk of chronic liver disease increases substantially with as little as 40 to 60 grams daily (80 grams of ethanol equals eight 12-oz beers, a liter of wine, or a half-pint of spirits). Only the total dose and not the type of alcoholic beverage or pattern of intake influences progression. *(2) Gender.* In females there is greater likelihood of progression to cirrhosis than in males ingesting the same relative amount of alcohol. *(3) Hepatitis B or C infection.* Concurrent liver disease of any type may be an accelerant to hepatic injury in the patient who drinks heavily. In particular, a strikingly high incidence of anti-HCV (hepatitis C virus) (10 to 40%) has been reported in patients with alcoholic cirrhosis; HCV acquired in this population is not solely explained by either prior transfusion or intravenous drug use, which are known risk factors for HCV infection. *(4) Genetic factors.* An inherited predisposition to alcoholism has been clearly established, but genetically determined increased susceptibility to liver damage in heavy drinkers is less certain. Increased susceptibility to organ injury may also be associated with certain isoenzymes of alcohol dehydrogenase, the principal metabolizing enzyme of ethanol. *(5) Nutritional status.* Protein-calorie malnutrition is extremely common in alcoholics. Malnutrition may be due not only to poor intake but also to abnormal nutrient metabolism. While poor nutrition may contribute to the evolution of alcoholic liver disease, adequate nutrition does not prevent its development.

PATHOLOGY

Fatty Liver. Steatosis, or fatty liver, is a reversible short-term consequence of alcohol toxicity. Large fat droplets fill hepatocytes, distorting the nuclei and enlarging the acinus. The lesion occurs even in well-nourished alcoholics and results from enhanced production and decreased oxidation of fatty acids within the liver, as well as peripheral lipolysis with increased hepatic lipid uptake. The lesion does *not* predict the development of alcoholic hepatitis or cirrhosis. Fatty liver is not pathognomonic of alcoholic liver disease; it may be seen in drug-induced liver disease, obesity, hypertriglyceridemia, diabetes mellitus, malnutrition, Reye's syndrome, fatty liver of pregnancy, and during therapy with parenteral nutrition.

Perivenular Fibrosis. Connective tissue deposition around the central vein, also referred to as sclerosing hyaline necrosis, predicts a high likelihood of progression to panlobular cirrhosis. The lesion may develop in the absence of severe inflammation. Progressive perivenular fibrosis can lead to obliteration of central veins and postsinusoidal portal hypertension.

Alcoholic Hepatitis. Several obligatory features define the lesion of alcoholic hepatitis: liver cell necrosis, perivenular distribution, pericellular fibrosis, infiltration by neutrophils, and Mallory's hyaline. Neutrophil accumulation is relatively unique to alcoholic injury (most forms of hepatitis display mononuclear cells predominantly) and may contribute to hepatocellular injury (see Pathogenesis, below). Mallory's hyaline is an eosinophilic intracellular inclusion composed of condensed cytoskeletal filaments. While most typically associated with alcoholic hepatitis, Mallory's hyaline may occasionally be seen in other forms of liver injury, including Indian childhood cirrhosis, morbid obesity, primary biliary cirrhosis, Wilson's disease, and following jejunoileal bypass. Other common pathologic findings of alcoholic hepatitis include steatosis, bridging necrosis, bile duct proliferation, cholestasis, and mitochondrial enlargement within hepatocytes.

Alcoholic Cirrhosis. Perivenular fibrosis often progresses to panlobular cirrhosis, which may be either micronodular or macronodular. As scarring continues, the organ shrinks because of contraction of fibrous bands by activated lipocytes. At the ultrastructural level, loss of sinusoidal fenestrations may contribute to impaired nutrient exchange across the subendothelial space between sinusoidal blood and hepatocytes, contributing to the decay in liver function. In the cirrhotic patient who continues to drink, pathologic elements of both fatty liver and hepatitis may persist. It is unsettled whether hepatitis is a necessary precursor to cirrhosis.

PATHOGENESIS. The mechanism of alcoholic liver injury is not established. In fact, the most compelling evidence for an etiologic role of ethanol in alcoholic hepatitis is epidemiologic, not biochemical.

Theories of alcoholic liver injury invoke three complementary mechanisms: *(1) centrilobular hypoxia,* which proposes that metabolism of ethanol acetaldehyde increases lobular oxygen consumption, leading to relative hypoxemia and cell damage in regions furthest from oxygenated blood (i.e., pericentral zones); *(2) neutrophil infiltration/activity,* which may occur because of release of neutrophil chemoattractants by hepatocytes metabolizing ethanol. Tissue injury could ensue from neutrophils releasing reactive oxygen intermediates, proteases, and cytokines; *(3) formation of acetaldehyde-protein adducts,* which serve as neoantigens, generating sensitized lymphocytes and specific antibodies that attack hepatocytes bearing these antigens. The pathogenesis of alcoholic fibrosis involves many of the cytokines prominent in other forms of liver injury, including tumor necrosis factor, interleukin-1, PDGF, and TGFβ. Acetaldehyde may have minor fibrogenic activity toward activated lipocytes but is not a major pathogenic factor in alcoholic fibrosis.

CLINICAL PRESENTATION. *Fatty liver* is associated with moderate to marked hepatomegaly and occasionally with right upper quadrant tenderness and epigastric discomfort. Liver test results are generally normal or only modestly elevated, and jaundice is unusual. The lesion may develop after a single binge of alcohol, in contrast to hepatitis, which requires more extensive alcohol intake.

Alcoholic hepatitis may lead to anorexia, fever, hepatomegaly, and jaundice. Alcoholic hepatitis generally requires several weeks to months of alcohol ingestion to develop. Associated stigmas of

chronic liver disease (e.g., spider angiomas, palmar erythema, ascites) suggest underlying cirrhosis. The fever of alcoholic hepatitis is generally low grade (<38.3° C), and other sources must be excluded, such as spontaneous bacterial peritonitis, urinary infection, and pneumonia. Liver tests characteristically reveal elevations of aspartate aminotransferase (AST) and alanine aminotransferase (ALT) to <500, with AST values one to two times greater than ALT. An AST or ALT >500 in the patient with presumed alcoholic hepatitis should raise the possibility of an alternative or additional hepatic insult such as viral infection (especially HCV) or drugs. In particular, concurrent use of acetaminophen, even within the therapeutic range, may lead to marked hepatic injury because of enhanced production of toxic drug metabolites, combined with a diminished capacity to neutralize them due to hepatic glutathione depletion. In the hospitalized patient with acute alcoholic hepatitis, acute elevations of AST and ALT resolve over several days, followed by more persistent and sometimes marked elevation of bilirubin up to 20 times normal. Elevations of hepatic alkaline phosphatase may also persist, but to a lesser extent (two to three times normal). Even though prolonged cholestasis in alcoholic hepatitis is common, extrahepatic obstruction from common bile duct disease or tumor should be excluded in this setting by abdominal imaging (ultrasound [US] or computed tomography [CT]).

Evidence of liver dysfunction is common in patients with alcoholic hepatitis and suggests concurrent cirrhosis. Typical features include elevations of prothrombin time unresponsive to vitamin K, hypoalbuminemia, ascites, and/or encephalopathy.

PROGNOSIS AND TREATMENT. Fatty liver resolves completely within 4 to 6 weeks once alcohol ingestion is discontinued. In contrast, prognosis of alcoholic hepatitis is dependent on at least four variables: *(1) Continued drinking.* Persistent, progressive liver disease and accelerated mortality are certain in the patient with alcoholic hepatitis who continues to drink. In contrast, in up to two thirds of patients who stop drinking function will return to normal provided there is little underlying fibrosis. *(2) Degree of inflammation.* Peripheral leukocytosis in the absence of concurrent infection correlates with both increased tissue leukocytosis and mortality. Ten to 20% of cases with persistent blood leukocytosis (e.g., 15,000 to 25,000 per cubic millimeter) progress to subfulminant hepatic failure despite withdrawal of alcohol. *(3) Perivenular fibrosis.* As noted above (see Pathology), this lesion portends likely progression to panlobular fibrosis. *(4) Indices of liver failure.* Evidence of coagulopathy, ascites, hepatorenal syndrome, or encephalopathy is a poor prognostic sign.

Abstinence is the crucial component in treating alcoholic hepatitis. Recognizing alcoholism and maintaining sobriety require family and social support. Ongoing studies are attempting to optimize strategies of behavioral and pharmacologic intervention. These include 12-step programs (Alcoholics Anonymous) and use of disulfiram, which inhibits acetaldehyde metabolism, leading to marked flushing and discomfort when alcohol is ingested (see Ch. 11).

In the hospitalized patient, sedation with benzodiazepines may be indicated if signs of withdrawal are present such as tachycardia, hypertension, and agitation. Multivitamins (including thiamine, folate, vitamin K, and pyridoxine), fluids, and replacement of minerals (phosphate, magnesium) are usually warranted. In the patient with severe life-threatening alcoholic hepatitis, therapy with methylprednisolone (32 to 40 mg per day for 28 days), will lessen the chance of short-term mortality. Patients likely to respond to corticosteroids have evidence of liver failure with an elevated bilirubin level, prolonged prothrombin time, and encephalopathy. In one study, patients who benefited from steroids were those with either spontaneous hepatic encephalopathy or a discriminant function value greater than 32, calculated by the formula: 4.6 (prothrombin time − control time) + serum bilirubin·(in micromoles per liter)/17.1. The drug is not appropriate in patients with mild hepatitis or with either gastrointestinal bleeding or concurrent bacterial infection. Several other approaches have shown benefit in clinical trials but are not yet established for clinical practice, including propylthiouracil (PTU), invasive nutritional support, and androgenic steroids.

In patients with established cirrhosis, abstinence remains a crucial determinant of prolonged survival. In abstinent patients in whom there is progression to decompensated liver failure, orthotopic liver transplantation is a viable option (see Ch. 124). Survival of patients with alcoholic cirrhosis following transplantation is as high as for other forms of cirrhosis, and recidivism rates are <15%

if patients have maintained documented abstinence for at least 6 months prior to surgery.

POSTVIRAL CIRRHOSIS

Chronic hepatitis B virus (HBV) and hepatitis C virus (HCV) infections are the second leading cause of cirrhosis in the Western World and the leading cause in Asia and Africa (see Ch. 119). The identification of HCV in 1989 as the major cause of "non-A, non-B" hepatitis has dramatically reduced the percentage of patients classified with truly "cryptogenic" cirrhosis.

In chronic HBV infection, the rate of progression to cirrhosis is influenced by the degree of inflammation and lobular distortion. These parameters in turn are determined by the replicative activity of the virus (i.e., e-antigen positive) and whether there has been superinfection by hepatitis delta virus (HDV). Concurrent liver injury from other causes (e.g., alcohol) may also amplify the degree of inflammation and hasten the onset of cirrhosis. Similarly, in chronic HCV, progression to cirrhosis is influenced by the degree of liver damage at initial biopsy, as well as the age of exposure and duration of infection. Although the development of cirrhosis in most patients with chronic HBV or HCV is insidious over many years, rapid progression within 1 year has been seen in cases with aggressive inflammation. Particularly rapid progression to cirrhosis has also been seen in patients with recurrent HBV or HCV after liver transplantation. Overall, at least 25% of cases of chronic HCV will progress to cirrhosis within 10 years.

PATHOLOGY. Although the extent of inflammation is a determinant of severity, distinguishing between chronic persistent and chronic active hepatitis is less meaningful in predicting progression to cirrhosis than previously thought. In either HBV or HCV, evidence of bridging necrosis and fibrosis is a harbinger of likely progression. As in other forms of cirrhosis, the activated lipocyte is likely to be responsible for fibrogenesis. Cirrhosis from HBV or HCV may be either micronodular or macronodular.

CLINICAL FEATURES AND ROLE OF BIOPSY. Clinical features in patients with postviral cirrhosis may span the spectrum from completely asymptomatic to evidence of liver failure. In general, typical hepatitis symptoms of fatigue, malaise, and anorexia correlate more closely with disease activity in chronic HBV than in HCV. It is not unusual for HCV to be first recognized by routine laboratory screening, yet biopsy will reveal marked inflammation and tissue distortion. Moreover, in chronic HCV, AST and ALT do not correlate well with the degree of inflammation on liver biopsy, so that modest elevations of laboratory test findings do not exclude the possibility of advanced liver disease. Thus, liver biopsy is an important tool to determine the type and extent of fibrosis. Biopsy may also determine the need and response to therapy. Improvement in liver histology following treatment with interferon-α is associated with diminished fibrosis and reduced tissue mRNA levels of fibrogenic cytokines. Once cirrhosis is well established in the patient with chronic viral infection, sequelae of liver failure are indistinguishable from other forms of end-state liver disease.

CRYPTOGENIC CIRRHOSIS

Although HCV testing has substantially reduced the percentage of patients with unexplained cirrhosis, there remains a subset who develop progressive liver disease in the absence of viral infection, cholestasis, or genetic liver disease. This subset is a heterogeneous group of patients, about 75% of whom have features of autoimmunity (see Ch. 119). In autoimmune hepatitis, bridging necrosis and fibrosis predict a high likelihood of cirrhosis. Approximately 40% of patients with autoimmune hepatitis will develop cirrhosis within 10 years. Survival in cirrhotics with autoimmune hepatitis is 65%, which is greater than in those with cryptogenic cirrhosis lacking autoimmune features.

CIRRHOSIS IN GENETIC DISEASES

Several inborn errors of metabolism associated with accumulation of either metals or metabolites can lead to cirrhosis (see Ch. 121). Mechanisms of cirrhosis are not well understood in these conditions. Abnormal accumulation of a metal or metabolite is the common link, yet inflammation is often minimal. Most common is *hemochromatosis,* in which the cirrhotic liver is greatly enlarged and stained reddish brown as a result of iron infiltration. Microscopically, late-stage liver disease is characterized by extensive pigmentation and dense fibrous septa progressing to complete nodule for-

mation. Cirrhosis usually develops over decades. Early diagnosis is critical because removing excess iron in the precirrhotic stage prevents cirrhosis and its complications from developing. *Wilson's disease* often occurs with evidence of inflammatory liver disease or cirrhosis. Similar to hemochromatosis, cirrhosis can be averted by copper chelation with D-penicillamine in the precirrhotic phase. Onset of cirrhosis is generally more rapid and occurs at a younger age than in hemochromatosis. *Alpha₁-antitrypsin deficiency* is associated with cirrhosis as early as 2 weeks in homozygotes, and as late as the ninth decade. In addition to these more common disorders, a large number of rarer genetic diseases are also associated with cirrhosis (Table 122–1). These include errors in the metabolism of carbohydrates, amino acids, lipids, bile acids, or porphyrins.

BILIARY CIRRHOSIS

Biliary cirrhosis refers to nodular fibrosis due to bile duct obstruction, which may be intrahepatic or extrahepatic. *Primary biliary cirrhosis* is a well-defined inflammatory disease of intrahepatic bile ducts. *Secondary biliary cirrhosis* encompasses other causes of fibrosing biliary obstruction, including longstanding mechanical obstruction, sclerosing cholangitis, and genetic or developmental diseases in which cholestasis is prominent (e.g., cystic fibrosis, biliary atresia, and congenital biliary cysts).

PRIMARY BILIARY CIRRHOSIS. Primary biliary cirrhosis (PBC) is an immune-mediated disorder of unknown cause characterized by progressive destruction of intrahepatic bile ducts and the presence of antimitochrondrial antibodies. The disease has a strong female preponderance (10:1). Although it is most common in Caucasians from North America and Europe, cases have occurred in all races. The reason why prevalence appears to be increasing in Western populations is unknown. The disease is commonly associated with other autoimmune disorders, including sicca complex, CREST syndrome, rheumatoid arthritis, thyroiditis, pernicious anemia, and renal tubular acidosis.

Pathology. The pathologic progression of PBC is divided into four successive stages: Stage I: Florid duct lesion, characterized by marked periductular inflammation and injury to septal and interlobular bile ducts. The inflammation is predominantly mononuclear cell and may be associated with granuloma formation. These pathognomonic features may be spotty and can coexist with features of later-stage disease. Stage II: Ductular proliferation, marked by bile duct proliferation in portal tracts and early cholestasis, combined with periportal inflammation of the type also seen in chronic hepatitis. Stage III: Fibrosis, marked by waning inflammation but increasing septal fibrosis and distortion of the normal architecture. Cholestasis may be prominent. Stage IV: Cirrhosis, features possibly distinguishing PBC-related cirrhosis from other types include the absence of bile ducts, continued mononuclear cell infiltration, and cholestasis.

Pathogenesis. An autoimmune attack against the bile duct is probably an important pathogenetic element, but the precipitating event and contribution of genetic and environmental factors are not known. The antigens against which antimitochondrial antibodies are directed have been recently identified as components of the E2 subunits of the 2-oxo-acid dehydrogenase enzyme family (M2 antigen). It is not known why these antibodies develop or whether they are critical to the disease's pathogenesis.

Clinical Features and Diagnosis. The disease typically occurs in middle-aged females, either as an incidental three- to fourfold elevation of alkaline phosphatase or in evaluating complaints of fatigue and pruritus. Mild (two- to three-fold) elevation of transaminases is common. Identifying antimitochondrial antibodies (AMA) in serum usually leads to liver biopsy, which establishes the diagnosis. Atypical presentations in several patterns may occur, including in patients with negative AMA but compatible biochemistry and biopsy ($\sim 5\%$), those with positive AMA and compatible biopsy but normal liver biochemistry ($\sim 15\%$), and disease in men ($\sim 10\%$).

Insidious onset of pruritus is the most characteristic symptom. Its etiology is uncertain, and it may appear at any stage of the disease. Fatigue is also common. Symptoms resulting from malabsorption of fat-soluble vitamins may be evident, including those due to vitamin A, D, E, or K deficiency. There may be symptoms attributable to other autoimmune diseases, especially dry eyes or mouth and arthritis. Physical findings are subtle in the patient with asymptomatic or early disease. As the disease progresses, however, jaundice develops, the skin becomes dry, xanthomas appear, and liver and spleen enlarge but are nontender. Once cirrhosis develops, symptoms of portal hypertension and liver failure may predominate.

In addition to AMA, characteristic laboratory abnormalities include increased serum IgM (95%), hypercholesterolemia, and other autoantibodies, including rheumatoid factor (70%), anti-smooth muscle (65%), and thyroid-specific or antinuclear antibodies. Impaired sulfoxidation of sulfur-containing compounds is common (84%) in PBC, unlike in other forms of cirrhosis. Increasing prothrombin time and decreasing albumin characterize the late stages of disease.

The presence of AMA and a compatible biopsy establish the diagnosis of PBC. Extrahepatic ductal disease should be excluded with an abdominal imaging procedure, but ERCP is not required unless there are atypical laboratory or clinical features. Rare cases of progressive bile duct injury due to drugs may clinically resemble PBC but are distinguishable by the lack of AMA.

Prognosis. PBC is a slowly progressive disease usually leading to liver failure over 5 to 10 years. Survival is impaired even in asymptomatic patients, emphasizing the need to consider therapy in hopes of delaying the onset of late-stage disease. Prognosis can be predicted more accurately than in most other types of chronic liver disease by using time-dependent multivariate analyses based on age, bilirubin, serum albumin, prothrombin time, presence of gastrointestinal bleeding, and severity of edema; biopsy findings may also be incorporated. Alternatively, serum bilirubin > 10 mg per deciliter by itself is a remarkably accurate indicator of impending liver failure. These indices are important for determining optimal timing for liver transplantation (see Ch. 124).

Treatment. Ursodeoxycholic acid (UDCA), a hydrophilic bile acid, has shown early success in slowing the progression of PBC (13 to 15 mg per kilogram per day), possibly by reducing the concentration of toxic bile acids in the hepatic pool. The drug is well tolerated. No specific antifibrotic effect of the UDCA has been observed, however, and long-term follow-up (i.e., > 2 years) is lacking. Cyclosporine has shown promise in a small controlled trial, but larger long-term trials should be awaited before using the drug outside of clinical investigations. Other immunosuppressive agents have met with modest success in some patients, including azathioprine, methotrexate, chlorambucil, and prednisone. In addition to specific agents against the disease, management should include correcting vitamin A, D, E, and K deficiencies and using antipruritics, including cholestyramine (8 to 12 grams per day). In rare cases of intractable pruritus, opioid antagonists and plasmapheresis may be beneficial. Liver transplantation offers excellent quality of life in most patients with end-stage disease. Although transplantation is usually curative, rare cases of disease have recurred after transplant.

SECONDARY BILIARY CIRRHOSIS. Secondary biliary cirrhosis occurs in response to chronic biliary obstruction from a variety of causes (see Ch. 126). Neither the mechanism of scarring nor the duration and severity of obstruction required for irreversible fibrosis are established. In general, however, at least 6 months of obstruction are required for cirrhosis to develop, but shorter intervals have been reported.

Etiology. Cholestasis may be intrahepatic or extrahepatic, the latter also referred to as "mechanical" cholestasis. *Primary sclerosing cholangitis* is the most common cause of intrahepatic cholestasis besides PBC (see Ch. 126). Cholestasis in this condition is incomplete but progressive and leads to cirrhosis in most but not all patients within 10 years. Patients with associated inflammatory bowel disease who have undergone bowel resection may develop peristomal varices. In *cystic fibrosis,* intrahepatic cholestasis with focal biliary cirrhosis may complicate up to 25% of patients by the time of death, although liver disease is often asymptomatic. The precirrhotic lesion is marked by biliary proliferation and ductal occlusion. *Cholestatic syndromes of infancy and childhood* are frequently complicated by rapid progression of fibrosis within 10 to 12 weeks of birth even when recognized promptly. These disorders represent a spectrum of pathologic changes often involving atresia of either intrahepatic or extrahepatic ducts. There is overlap both clinically and histologically with neonatal hepatitis. Fibrosis often progresses even after successful biliary decompression and normal-

ization of bilirubin, with biopsy specimens revealing a pattern resembling congenital hepatic fibrosis.

Extrahepatic cholestasis in adults most commonly results from structural or mechanical obstruction. Common lesions include choledocholithiasis, biliary or pancreatic cancer, iatrogenic stricture, or chronic pancreatitis. A variant form of cholangiohepatitis in Asians is characterized by intrahepatic obstruction from biliary sludge, which can lead to recurrent cholangitis and secondary cirrhosis; the cause is unknown.

Pathology. The progression of histologic changes in chronic cholestasis has been well characterized. Hepatocyte degeneration with formation of cellular rosettes and ductular proliferation may be followed by inflammatory biliary necrosis and early periductal fibrosis. Inspissated bile within ductal lumens, formation of bile lakes, and periductular bile infarcts are classic late features. Early ductular changes are reversible, but persistent obstruction ultimately leads to portal-central septa and nodule formation typical of irreversible fibrosis.

Clinical and Laboratory Features. Clinical consequences of secondary biliary cirrhosis will initially be determined by the underlying disease. With progression, jaundice may become the prominent symptom. Pruritus is variable in severity. Fat malabsorption with steatorrhea and deficiencies of vitamins A, D, E, and K occur in longstanding obstruction. Osteomalacia or osteoporosis may occur because of vitamin D malabsorption and calcium deficiency.

Disproportionately increased hepatic alkaline phosphatase (four- to fivefold increase) relative to other liver tests is typical of secondary biliary cirrhosis. Other results of serum tests of biliary injury may be similarly elevated, including gamma glutamyl transpeptidase and 5′-nucleotidase. Transaminases are increased less than twofold. Hypercholesterolemia is common. Associated markers of immunologic disease or bacterial cholangitis may be evident in patients with sclerosing cholangitis or mechanical obstruction, respectively.

Treatment. Recognizing and treating the underlying cause of cholestasis is the mainstay of therapy. For extrahepatic obstruction this usually requires biliary decompression, either by surgical drainage or via placement of a biliary stent for neoplasms. Intrahepatic cholestasis is less amenable to surgical drainage, with management limited to treating complications. Pruritus can be controlled with cholestyramine (4 grams three times a day) or in severe cases, opioid antagonists (e.g., naloxone, nalmefene). Calcium and vitamin D supplementation may be required for bone disease. Parenteral replacement of vitamins A, E, and K is sometimes required. Regular exposure to sunlight enhances the conversion of 7-dehydrocholesterol to vitamin D and can reduce the development of osteomalacia. Current single-agent medical therapy for primary sclerosing cholangitis is not effective. For example, ursodeoxycholic acid improves biochemical parameters but does not retard disease progression; future approaches may use combination therapy (e.g., ursodeoxycholic acid and methotrexate). Liver transplantation is highly successful in most patients with secondary biliary cirrhosis and deteriorating liver function (see Ch. 124).

VASCULAR DISORDERS ASSOCIATED WITH CIRRHOSIS

CHRONIC RIGHT-SIDED HEART FAILURE. Longstanding right-sided heart failure due to cardiomyopathy, tricuspid valve insufficiency, pulmonary disease, or pericardial constriction can lead to hepatic fibrosis; however, this late sequela is uncommon. The clinical picture is usually dominated by cardiac or pulmonary dysfunction. Liver abnormalities may be typical of hepatic congestion, with disproportionate elevation of bilirubin (up to tenfold) and prothrombin time (2 to 6 seconds prolonged) yet modest transaminase elevations (less than threefold). Gross inspection of affected liver characteristically reveals focal areas of congestion (nutmeg liver).

HEPATIC VENO-OCCLUSIVE DISEASE. This syndrome occurs most commonly as a complication of bone marrow transplantation and/or pyrrolizidine alkaloid therapy and is characterized clinically by rapid onset of hepatomegaly, weight gain, and ascites. Hyperbilirubinemia and increased transaminases are typical. There is deposition of a fibronectin-rich matrix around terminal hepatic (central) veins, with evidence of endothelial cell injury. Because of its characteristic presentation, however, biopsy is rarely necessary to establish the diagnosis. The lesion is not a true cirrhosis, yet the clinical consequences are rapid and profound because the deposition of extracellular matrix occurs in a critical site of sinusoidal outflow.

BUDD-CHIARI SYNDROME.

BUDD-CHIARI SYNDROME. Like veno-occlusive disease, Budd-Chiari syndrome is not a true cirrhosis but rather an acute or subacute obstruction to hepatic venous outflow. Fibrous webs are one of the many causes of the disorder, but these are usually extrahepatic, and parenchymal fibrosis is uncommon.

MISCELLANEOUS DISORDERS ASSOCIATED WITH CIRRHOSIS

A variety of poorly understood chronic liver diseases are associated with cirrhosis. *Nonalcoholic steatonecrosis* is a clinicopathologic syndrome remarkably similar to alcoholic liver disease, but it occurs in the absence of alcohol use. The disorder, which is often identified incidentally, is found with several conditions, including diabetes mellitus, morbid obesity, jejunoileal bypass surgery, Weber-Christian disease, and abetalipoproteinemia. Amiodarone, diethylstilbestrol, perhexilene maleate, total parenteral nutrition, and synthetic estrogens have also been implicated. Cirrhosis develops in at least one third of patients if the precipitant is not removed. *Indian childhood cirrhosis* is a significant cause of preschool pediatric morbidity, occurring in up to 1 in 4000 live births in the Indian subcontinent. Marked hyaline accumulation, increased copper deposition, and extensive fibrosis are typical histologic features. The underlying defect is unknown. D-Penicillamine has been used to slow progression in some patients. *Polycystic liver disease* is usually associated with renal cysts and is characterized by macroscopic or microscopic hepatic cysts associated with fibrosis. *Granulomatous liver diseases, including sarcoidosis* (see Ch. 120), may progress to cirrhosis in some patients.

In addition to medications associated with nonalcoholic steatonecrosis, drug-induced hepatic fibrosis may also be seen in patients taking isoniazid or antimetabolites, especially methotrexate. The latter is associated with dose-dependent fibrosis in patients treated for psoriasis or rheumatoid arthritis for at least 2 years. Continuous therapy is more fibrogenic than intermittent dosing, and coexisting liver disease or heavy alcohol intake amplifies the risk of fibrosis. Surveillance liver biopsies are required in patients whose cumulative dose exceeds 1.5 to 2 grams, as considerable fibrosis may develop in the absence of symptoms.

Major Sequelae of Cirrhosis (Table 122–2)

PORTAL HYPERTENSION. *Features of the Portal Circulation and Classification of Portal Hypertension.* The portal circulation is a low-pressure system (< 10 mm Hg) formed by the venous drainage from intraperitoneal viscera, including the luminal gastrointestinal tract, spleen, gallbladder, and pancreas. Veins collecting from these sites form the splenic vein and superior and inferior mesenteric veins, which in turn merge to create the portal vein. *Portal hypertension* occurs when portal venous pressure exceeds the pressure in the nonportal abdominal veins (e.g., inferior vena cava) by at least 5 mm Hg; portal-systemic collateral vessels develop in an effort to equalize pressures between these two venous systems. These collateral vessels, or varices, most commonly develop in the esophagus and proximal stomach and can cause clinically significant bleeding. Altered portal hemodynamics can also lead to the development of ascites (see below) and contribute to hepatic encephalopathy (see Ch. 123).

Increased portal pressure in cirrhosis primarily results from increased resistance to blood flow through the shrunken, fibrotic liver. Increased intrahepatic resistance results both from fixed obstruction to flow by extracellular matrix and from dynamic organ and sinusoidal contraction by activated lipocytes (also referred to as myofi-

TABLE 122–2. SEQUELAE OF CIRRHOSIS

1. Portal hypertension: bleeding from varices in esophagus/stomach (most common), duodenum, rectum, or surgical stomas; bleeding from congestive gastropathy; splenomegaly with hypersplenism
2. Ascites: spontaneous bacterial peritonitis; hepatic hydrothorax, abdominal hernia
3. Hepatorenal syndrome
4. Hepatic encephalopathy
5. Synthetic dysfunction/coagulopathy
6. Hepatopulmonary syndrome
7. Hepatocellular carcinoma
8. Feminization
9. Altered drug metabolism
10. Hepatic osteodystrophy

---

broblasts). Since pressure is a function of both resistance and flow, independent increases in portal inflow due to the hyperdynamic circulation of cirrhosis and splanchnic arteriolar vasodilation also contribute to portal pressure elevation.

In cirrhosis, which is the most common cause of portal hypertension, the lesion is intrahepatic and primarily *sinusoidal*. Portal hypertension may also arise from *presinusoidal* obstruction, either outside (e.g., portal vein thrombosis) or within (e.g., schistosomiasis) the liver. Similarly, lesions leading to portal hypertension may be *postsinusoidal*, either within the liver (e.g., veno-occlusive disease) or distal to it (e.g., Budd-Chiari syndrome, right-sided heart failure). In rare circumstances, portal hypertension can result in a normal liver from markedly increased inflow beyond the capacity of the compliant portal vessels to absorb. Examples include arterial-portal fistulas and massive splenomegaly due to infection or neoplasm.

Clinical Presentation. The cirrhotic with portal hypertension will often have variceal hemorrhage (Fig. 122–2), ascites, encephalopathy, or some manifestation of hepatic dysfunction such as coagulopathy or infection. Splenomegaly and/or distention of abdominal wall veins (caput medusae) may be initial or associated findings. Patients with noncirrhotic portal hypertension generally have well-preserved liver function so that clinical manifestations primarily reflect altered hemodynamics. In patients with presinusoidal lesions such as schistosomiasis or portal vein thrombosis, variceal hemorrhage and splenomegaly are prominent. In postsinusoidal obstruction, such as veno-occlusive disease or Budd-Chiari syndrome, hepatomegaly and rapid onset of ascites and weight gain are typical presenting symptoms. When portal abnormalities are a manifestation of infection or neoplasm, there may be specific associated nonhepatic findings, such as a hypercoagulable state, anemia, or evidence of heart failure.

Diagnosis. Portal hypertension should be suspected in any patient with ascites, splenomegaly, encephalopathy, or gastroesophageal varices. Assessment should include liver chemistry, prothrombin time, serum albumin, and complete blood count. Noninvasive abdominal imaging using US with Doppler probe can assess the hepatic parenchyma and patency/flow characteristics of the portal and hepatic veins. Varices may also be visualized using either this technique or abdominal CT or may be seen directly by upper endoscopy. It is important to remember that the presence of varices does not establish whether the lesion is intrahepatic or extrahepatic, as varices can develop with presinusoidal and postsinusoidal lesions. If abdominal US with Doppler is not conclusive, portal hemodynamics may be measured more directly by hepatic

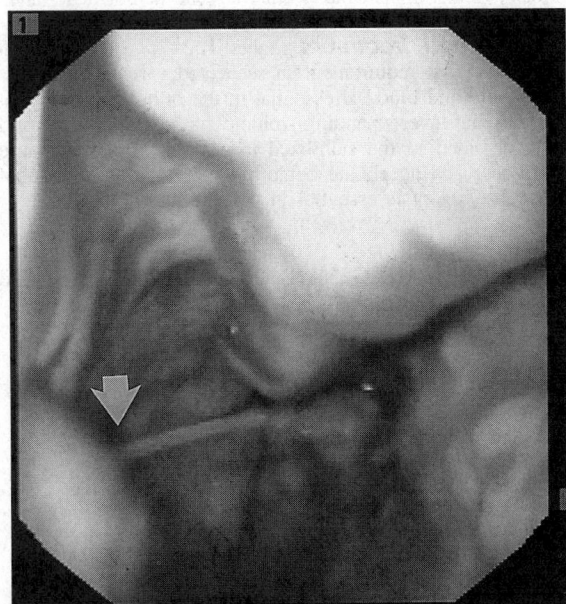

FIGURE 122–2. Active hemorrhage from an esophageal varix. An endoscopic view of hemorrhage in a patient with esophageal varices; a stream of blood across the esophageal lumen is evident *(arrow).* (Courtesy of Dr. Timothy Davern and Dr. Johannes Koch.)

vein catheterization with a ballon-tipped catheter within the liver attached to a pressure transducer. When deflated, the catheter measures systemic venous (i.e., IVC) pressure. When inflated within the liver this "wedged" hepatic vein pressure (WHVP) reflects the pressure distal to the balloon (i.e., within the hepatic parenchyma). The differences between these two measurements (WHVP − IVC) or the wedged hepatic venous gradient (WHPG) is normally < 5 mm Hg. Once this difference exceeds 12 mm Hg, variceal hemorrhage is possible; however, the risk of hemorrhage does not correlate with the extent of elevation beyond this threshold. Mesenteric angiography may be useful to directly visualize portal vessels, either when an extrahepatic cause of portal hypertension is suspected or in anticipation of elective short surgery in which definition of the anatomy is required.

VARICEAL HEMORRHAGE. Hemorrhage from gastroesophageal varices is often the initial complication of portal hypertension (Fig. 122–2). Less commonly, variceal hemorrhage occurs from other sites of portal-systemic collateral vessels, including the duodenum, rectum, or sites of prior abdominal surgery.

Esophageal variceal hemorrhage typically occurs as painless, large-volume hematemesis or melena with minimal abdominal pain. Signs of significant volume depletion, including orthostasis and pallor, are common. Mortality from variceal hemorrhage is more a function of underlying liver disease than severity of hemorrhage *per se*.

In a patient with known varices, risk factors that correlate with increased likelihood of bleeding include (1) variceal size (large varices have increased wall tension and thus greater thinning of the vessel wall); (2) endoscopic signs known as red wales or cherry red spots overlying the varix, which are believed to represent hemorrhage within the vessel wall; (3) WHPG >12 mm Hg; (4) poor liver function with ascites and/or jaundice. Gastric acid plays little role in the pathogenesis of bleeding.

Patients with esophageal varices may bleed from associated *gastric varices*. A gastric variceal hemorrhage is more difficult to diagnose than an esophageal one because gastric varices are not easily distinguished from prominent rugae. A rare cause of gastric variceal hemorrhage that should not be overlooked is splenic vein thrombosis due to pancreatic or retroperitoneal disease. In this setting, localized obstruction of short gastric veins leads to hemorrhage from gastric varices in the absence of esophageal varices. Splenectomy and splenic vein resection are curative. Hemorrhage from *portal hypertensive gastropathy*, also known as *congestive gastropathy*, refers to bleeding in the proximal stomach from submucosal veins engorged as a result of portal hypertension. Bleeding from this lesion is clinically indistinguishable from variceal hemorrhage and responds to portal decompression.

Diagnosis and Treatment (Table 122–3). Stabilizing blood pressure is the first requirement in suspected variceal hemorrhage. Replacing fluid and blood is essential in the orthostatic or hypotensive patient, but overexpanding volume with fresh-frozen plasma should be avoided in the stabilized individual, as it may increase portal pressure and accelerate hemorrhage. Endotracheal intubation to protect the airway is essential in the obtunded or inebriated patient to avoid aspiration and facilitate emergent endoscopy. Hemodynamic monitoring within the intensive care unit may require placing intra-arterial or pulmonary artery catheters.

Once the patient's condition is stabilized, vigorous gastric lavage followed by emergent endoscopy is necessary to establish the source of hemorrhage, even if acute bleeding has subsided. Approximately 30 to 50% of bleeding episodes in patients with varices originate from nonvariceal sources, particularly Mallory-Weiss tears, esophagitis, gastritis, or peptic ulcers. Bleeding from more than one lesion is not unusual.

Initial Control of Variceal Hemorrhage. Two thirds of variceal hemorrhage episodes will cease spontaneously, but rapid onset of rebleeding is significant. Thus, endoscopic hemostasis is required, either when varices are actively bleeding or when they display endoscopic evidence of recent bleeding (i.e., a visible punctum). Two endoscopic methods are equally effective in arresting active hemorrhage in >95% of patients: (1) direct or paravariceal injection with 1 to 2 ml of a sclerosant (ethanolamine oleate or sodium tetradecyl) or (2) band ligation, in which a rubber ligature is placed around the varix. Band ligation is associated with a lower incidence of esophageal ulceration and more rapid variceal obliteration than sclerotherapy; this technique awaits final approval by the FDA.

Pharmacologically controlling acute hemorrhage may be achieved using either a combination of intravenous vasopressin (0.4 μg per minute) and nitroglycerin (40 μg per minute, increased by 40-μg per-minute increments to a maximum of 400 μg per minute) or a somatostatin analogue (octreotide, 50 μg bolus, then 50 μg per hour intravenously; this drug is not yet FDA approved for this indication). While more costly, somatostatin analogues carry less systemic hemodynamic side effects than vasopressin (e.g., vasoconstriction).

In patients who continue to bleed after endoscopic or pharmacologic therapy, a Minnesota or Sengstaken-Blakemore tube can be used for balloon tamponade of vessels at the gastroesophageal junction. Intubation prior to placing the tube will reduce the risk of pulmonary aspiration. Only the gastric balloon should be inflated (250 ml for Sengstaken tube, 450 ml for Minnesota tube); inflating the esophageal balloon or using these devices in patients with hiatus hernias is associated with significant risk of esophageal perforation.

Emergent surgical portal decompression is an option in the rare patient in whom hemodynamic stabilization is not possible because of persistent hemorrhage. Optimal surgical options include esophageal staple-transection or portacaval shunt (end-to-side or mesocaval). Emergent abdominal surgery to control variceal hemorrhage should be undertaken with the recognition that subsequent liver transplantation may become much more technically difficult.

In the patient who is a potential candidate for liver transplantation, placing a *transjugular intrahepatic portasystemic shunt* (TIPS) is an attractive alternative to surgery. The shunt is placed under fluoroscopic guidance, creating an intrahepatic channel that decompresses the portal circulation nonselectively. TIPS is physiologically similar to a side-to-side surgical shunt. In experienced hands, placement is successful in >90% of patients, and bleeding is controlled in 90 to 95%.

Preventing Initial or Recurrent Variceal Hemorrhage. In the patient with moderate or large varices and well-preserved liver function, prophylactic use of β blockers (propranolol or nadolol) to reduce resting heart rate by 25% will lessen the risk of first variceal hemorrhage. β blockers will also reduce the risk of bleeding from congestive gastropathy and gastric varices associated with portal hypertension. Despite this efficacy in portal hypertension, the agents have no effect on mortality. In contrast to β blockers, prophylactic sclerotherapy has not been shown consistently to reduce the likelihood of initial bleeding.

In patients who have already survived an episode of hemorrhage from varices or congestive gastropathy, β blockers reduce the risk of rebleeding, but are discontinued in up to 25% of patients because of adverse effects (e.g., bronchoconstriction, impotence, lethargy, heart failure). In those in whom β blockers fail or who are intolerant of β blockers, obliterating varices by endoscopic sclerotherapy is equally effective; multiple sessions are required to initially eliminate varices, followed by regular endoscopic surveillance every 3 to 6 months. There is no synergistic effect of β blockers and long-term sclerotherapy. Studies attempting long-term control by endoscopic band ligation are anticipated.

TABLE 122–3. MANAGEMENT OF GASTROESOPHAGEAL VARICEAL HEMORRHAGE

1. Hemodynamic stabilization
2. Emergent diagnostic endoscopy
3. Initial control of hemorrhage (options)
   Endoscopic sclerotherapy
   Endoscopic variceal band ligation
   Intravenous vasopressin/nitroglycerin or octreotide
   Balloon tamponade
   Transjugular intrahepatic portacaval shunt (TIPS)
   Surgery: esophageal transection or nonselective portacaval shunt
4. Prevention of initial or recurrent variceal hemorrhage (options)
   Prophylactic β blockers in high-risk patients who have not bled
   β blockers after initial bleeding episode
   Chronic obliterative endoscopic sclerotherapy or band ligation
   Portacaval shunt surgery
   Liver transplantation

Elective portacaval shunt surgery is more effective at eliminating rebleeding than long-term sclerotherapy but is associated with higher initial transfusion requirement and cost. Like nonsurgical treatments, there is no improvement in survival afforded by portacaval shunts. In experienced surgical hands, the optimal operation is a distal splenorenal shunt that selectively decompresses the short gastric veins draining the varices. The procedure is time consuming and usually requires preoperative angiography. Because portal flow is preserved, however, it is associated with a lower rate of encephalopathy and ascites. The role of TIPS is uncertain in long-term management of patients with variceal hemorrhage; randomized trials are under way. A significant risk of shunt occlusion or encephalopathy is emerging in longer follow-up of patients treated by TIPS, which may confine its use to those awaiting liver transplantation.

ASCITES. Ascites is the accumulation of excess fluid in the abdomen. Cirrhosis is the underlying cause in at least 80% of patients, but other etiologic factors in addition to liver disease must always be considered.

Pathogenesis. Multiple factors contribute to ascites formation in chronic liver injury: *(1) sinusoidal hypertension,* which develops because of increased outflow resistance from matrix deposition and possibly lipocyte contraction. (Initially, albumin traverses the porous sinusoidal endothelium along with fluid, but as fibrosis progresses, only protein-free fluid can escape the sinusoid, from where it enters hepatic lymphatics. Continued accumulation of lymph overcomes the capacity for lymphatic drainage, and the excess fluid "weeps" from the liver into the peritoneal cavity); *(2) hypoalbuminemia,* which worsens with advancing liver dysfunction and decreases oncotic pressure; *(3) fixed capacity to resorb ascites,* despite its increasing accumulation; *(4) increased sodium reabsorption by the kidneys,* possibly due to humoral factors; *(5) splanchnic arteriolar vasodilation,* which may independently stimulate sodium and free water retention by increasing sympathetic tone. The roles of antidiuretic hormone (ADH) and atrial natriuretic peptide (ANP) are not clearly established despite extensive study.

Diagnostic Evaluation of Ascites (Table 122–4). All patients with new-onset ascites or those requiring hospitalization because of ascites should undergo diagnostic paracentesis with cell count, ascites albumin determination, Gram stain, and culture. US guidance may be necessary if ascites is minimal or fluid is loculated. Directly inoculating ascites into blood culture broth at the bedside is essential because the low bacterial count of infected ascites may otherwise lead to false-negative culture results. The status of all patients with new ascites should be evaluated by abdominal US.

The serum-ascites albumin gradient (SAAG), calculated by subtracting the ascites albumin concentration from the serum value, is the most accurate method to classify ascites. A SAAG value of ≥ 1.1 gram per deciliter predicts a portal hypertensive cause with >95% accuracy. Values <1.1 gram per deciliter are associated with neoplasms, tuberculosis, pancreatitis, or bile leak. SAAG values <1.1 gram per deciliter indicate the ascites fluid needs additional testing, which may include amylase, cytology, mycobacterial culture.

Treatment. Most patients with cirrhotic ascites respond to dietary sodium restriction (40 to 60 mEq per day) and a diuretic. Spironolactone should be started at 100 mg per day and can be advanced up to 400 mg to achieve a daily weight loss of 0.5 to 0.75

kg in patients without peripheral edema; more rapid weight loss is safe if peripheral edema is present. Furosemide can be used instead of or in combination with spironolactone, beginning at a dose of 40 mg per day, although there is a greater incidence of azotemia than with spironolactone. Patients treated with two diuretics must be monitored carefully because weight loss may be rapid, even when one diuretic alone has been ineffective. In patients with alcoholic liver disease, abstinence may be effective therapy if cirrhosis has not yet developed.

Ten percent of patients with ascites fail to respond to standard therapy, either because fluid cannot be mobilized or there is associated prerenal azotemia. In these patients, therapeutic paracentesis is safe and can remove 4 to 6 liters or more per visit in those with peripheral edema. In nonedematous patients safe paracentesis requires infusing 6 to 8 grams of albumin per liter of ascites removed. This option is quite costly; cost may be reduced by substituting for albumin with other plasma expanders such as dextran 70, although experience with nonalbumin expanders is less extensive. Repeated paracentesis may increase the risk of bacterial peritonitis. *Peritoneovenous shunting,* performed by surgically placing a subcutaneous catheter between the superior vena cava and peritoneum, is as effective as therapeutic paracentesis in treating refractory ascites. However, low-grade disseminated intravascular coagulopathy, catheter infection, and shunt occlusion are frequent complications that reduce long-term efficacy substantially. Like other therapy for complications of portal hypertension, neither paracentesis nor peritoneovenous shunts prolong survival. Instead, survival is a function of the severity of liver disease. TIPS has been proposed as an alternative to the peritoneovenous shunt in treating refractory ascites. Preliminary results are encouraging in small numbers of patients, but long-term follow-up in larger study groups is required. *Liver transplantation* remains the most definitive therapy for liver disease underlying ascites and should be considered first when ascites develops. The urgency for transplantation is increased if complications of ascites appear, particularly spontaneous bacterial peritonitis.

Complications of Ascites. Spontaneous bacterial peritonitis (SBP) is an ominous complication of late-stage liver disease because it portends a 2-year survival rate of <50%. The pathogenesis is uncertain but is thought to reflect altered gut wall permeability to bacteria, impaired capacity of hepatic and splenic macrophages to clear portal bacteremias, and/or the presence of a large volume of peritoneal fluid conducive to bacterial growth. The clinical presentation is subtle, and frank peritoneal pain or tenderness is uncommon. Thus, clinicians must have a high index of suspicion to recognize SBP before it is fatal. Typical findings include fever, signs of sepsis, or decompensation of previously stable liver function manifested by new encephalopathy or azotemia. Common causative organisms include *Escherichia coli, Pneumococcus, Klebsiella,* and anaerobes. Because ascites Gram stain is rarely positive, if ascites PMN count is ≥ 250 per cubic millimeter, a presumptive diagnosis should be made and empiric antibiotics (e.g., cefotaxime, 2 grams intravenously every 6 to 8 hours, or ceftriaxone, 500 to 1000 mg intravenously every 12 hours) given for 5 to 7 days. Adequate response to therapy should be documented by demonstrating a 50% reduction in ascites white blood cell (WBC) count. Culture-negative neutrocytic ascites (i.e., ascites WBC ≥ 250 per cubic millimeter) is common, especially if ascites has not been promptly inoculated into blood culture broth; these patients should be treated for presumed SBP and response to antibiotics documented with repeat paracentesis. The recurrence rate of SBP is >70% in 1 year, but can be reduced if patients are treated prophylactically with norfloxacin, 400 mg per day. Prophylaxis may be appropriate for high-risk patients even before the first episode of SBP (i.e., those with gastrointestinal bleeding or low-protein ascites), especially if the patient is a candidate for liver transplantation.

Other complications of ascites include hepatic hydrothorax, abdominal wall hernias with rupture, and tense ascites with leakage (especially after paracentesis). Conservative management consists of appropriate initial therapy for most of these except hernia rupture, which requires surgical reduction.

HEPATORENAL SYNDROME. Hepatorenal syndrome, also known as *functional renal failure,* is defined as renal failure associated with severe liver disease without an intrinsic abnormality of

---

TABLE 122–4. DIAGNOSTIC EVALUATION OF ASCITES

1. Paracentesis
   A. Fluid analysis: cell count, albumin, Gram stain
   B. Calculate serum-ascites albumin gradient (SAAG):
      SAAG ≥ 1.1 gm/dl: portal hypertension very likely
      SAAG < 1.1 gm/dl: suspect other causes
   C. Direct bedside inoculation of ascites into blood culture broth
   D. Optional: amylase, bilirubin, triglycerides, cytology, mycobacterial culture
2. Abdominal US with Doppler
   A. Assess patency/flow in portal, hepatic, and splenic veins
   B. Examine hepatic and splenic parenchyma
   C. Exclude neoplasm or peritoneal disease
   D. Assess biliary ductal size

the kidney. Ascites is typically present. The cause is unknown, but reductions in renal blood flow, cortical perfusion, and glomerular filtration rate are consistent features. Elevated circulating levels of endothelin-1, a potent vasoconstrictor, may play an important role. The diagnosis is established in patients with cirrhosis by documenting very low urine sodium (< 10 mEq per liter) and oliguria in the absence of intravascular volume depletion. The syndrome must therefore be distinguished from prerenal azotemia. To exclude this possibility, measuring pulmonary wedge pressure may be necessary or alternatively an empiric fluid challenge (1000 ml saline) can be administered. Other likely causes of renal failure must be excluded, such as acute tubular necrosis or renal impairment from aminoglycosides and contrast agents, although these typically lead to high sodium excretion. Patients with liver disease are especially sensitive to inhibition of renal vasodilation by nonsteroidal anti-inflammatory agents (NSAID's). The prognosis of hepatorenal syndrome is very poor, in part because onset of the syndrome denotes end-stage liver disease. The most effective treatment for hepatorenal syndrome is correcting the underlying liver disease, by liver transplantation if appropriate. Treating any underlying infections and optimizing volume status are important adjunctive measures. Potentially nephrotoxic drugs, especially NSAID's, should be withdrawn. Isolated responses to peritoneovenous shunt or TIPS have been reported, but no randomized trials have been conducted to confirm these treatments. There are no effective pharmacologic agents.

HEPATIC ENCEPHALOPATHY (see Ch. 123).

SYNTHETIC DYSFUNCTION AND COAGULOPATHY. Broad defects in protein synthesis and/or secretion characterize the cirrhotic liver. Clinically apparent defects include hypoalbuminemia, which can reduce oncotic pressure and accentuate edema formation, and reduced concentrations of plasma clotting factors. All clotting factors except Factor VIII are synthesized in the liver and may be defective both qualitatively and quantitatively. Fibrinolysis is also affected. In addition, Factors II, VII, IX, and X are vitamin K dependent, and thus may have reduced activity if deficient because of cholestasis-related fat malabsorption. Thrombocytopenia can result from bone marrow hypoplasia induced by alcohol or due to *hypersplenism* associated with splenomegaly in portal hypertension. Platelet sequestration by the congested spleen often leads to significant thrombocytopenia, yet clinically significant bleeding almost never occurs; platelet transfusions are therefore not indicated in this setting unless there is an additional platelet defect. Similarly, portacaval decompression or splenectomy is usually curative, but is not appropriate unless required to manage variceal hemorrhage.

HEPATOPULMONARY SYNDROME. Hepatopulmonary syndrome refers to the triad of liver disease, pulmonary vascular dilation, and reduced arterial oxygenation. While marked manifestations of the syndrome are unusual in patients with chronic liver disease, more subtle abnormalities of oxygenation are common. The abnormalities have been attributed to right-to-left shunts through pulmonary arteriovenous fistulas and development of bronchial varices in association with pulmonary hypertension. The syndrome occurs in chronic liver disease of all types and is more common in those with severe liver disease (i.e., Child's C cirrhosis). As a result, the prognosis is poor, on the basis of both the pulmonary and hepatic disease. Affected patients complain of exertional dyspnea, with pulmonary function tests demonstrating normal lung volumes but markedly reduced diffusing capacity. Hypoxemia and dyspnea are usually worse in the standing than the supine position. Oxygen can improve symptoms but does not reverse the defects. Resolution of the syndrome has been seen in many but not all patients following liver transplantation.

HEPATOCELLULAR CARCINOMA (see Ch. 125).

OTHER SEQUELAE. *Feminization* in men with end-stage cirrhosis is particularly common in alcoholics and has been associated with increased estrogen and diminished testosterone levels. Hypogonadism can be an independent consequence of alcohol abuse. *Altered drug metabolism* (see Ch. 118) is an important consideration in prescribing drugs to those with end-stage liver disease, either because of impaired clearance leading to enhanced activity or toxicity, reduced sulfoxidation, or decreased protein binding. *Bone disease*

manifested as thinning and spontaneous fractures is a major complication of late-stage cholestatic or alcoholic liver disease, especially primary biliary cirrhosis. Hepatic osteodystrophy can be due to osteoporosis (see Ch. 217), osteomalacia (see Ch. 213), or both.

Cirrhosis—General

Friedman SL: The cellular basis of hepatic fibrosis. N Engl J Med 328:1828, 1993. *Review of the cellular and molecular events underlying hepatic fibrosis, and cirrhosis.*
Infante-Rivard C, Esnaola S, Villeneuve J-P: Clinical and statistical validity of conventional prognostic factors in predicting short-term survival among cirrhotics. Hepatology 7:660, 1987. *Analysis of current methods for assessing prognosis in patients with cirrhosis.*

Alcoholic Liver Disease

Carithers RL, Herlong F, Diehl AM, et al.: Ann Intern Med 110:685, 1989. *One of the first multicenter randomized trials showing efficacy of methylprednisolone in severe alcoholic hepatitis; used a discriminant function value to identify patients most likely to respond to therapy.*
Lieber CS: Alcoholic liver disease. Semin Liver Dis 13:109, 1993. *Entire multiauthor issue devoted to all aspects of alcoholic liver disease, including epidemiology, pathology, etiology, and treatment.*
Lucey MR, Merion RM, Henley KS, et al.: Selection for and outcome of liver transplantation in alcoholic liver disease. Gastroenterology 102:1736, 1992. *Clinical series emphasizing the efficacy of liver transplantation in appropriately selected patients with end-stage alcoholic liver disease.*

Primary Biliary Cirrhosis

Poupon RE, Balkau B, Eschwege E, et al.: A multicenter, controlled trial of ursodiol for the treatment of primary biliary cirrhosis. N Engl J Med 324:1548, 1991. *One of largest trials demonstrating some efficacy of ursodeoxycholic acid in slowing progression of primary biliary cirrhosis.*
Van De Water J, Cooper A, Surh CD, et al.: Detection of autoantibodies to recombinant mitochondrial proteins in patients with primary biliary cirrhosis. N Engl J Med 320:1377, 1989. *Report that identified major antigens detected by antimitochondrial antibodies in patients with primary biliary cirrhosis.*
Wiesner RH, Porayko MK, Dickson ER, et al.: Selection and timing of liver transplantation in primary biliary cirrhosis and primary sclerosing cholangitis. Hepatology 16:1290, 1992. *Review of current models for determining prognosis in primary biliary cirrhosis and sclerosing cholangitis to determine optimal timing for liver transplantation.*

Variceal Hemorrhage

Laine L, el-Newihi HM, Migikovsky B, et al.: Endoscopic ligation compared with sclerotherapy for the treatment of bleeding esophageal varices. Ann Intern Med 119:1, 1993. *Comparison between two widely used methods of endoscopic therapy of variceal hemorrhage, demonstrating an advantage of band ligation in time required to obliterate varices and frequency of complications.*
Poynard T, Cales P, Pasta L, et al.: Beta-adrenergic-antagonist drugs in the prevention of gastrointestinal bleeding in patients with cirrhosis and esophageal varices: An analysis of data and prognostic factors in 589 patients from four randomized clinical trials. N Engl J Med 324:1532, 1991. *Large clinical series supporting use of prophylactic β blockers to prevent variceal hemorrhage in selected patients with chronic liver disease.*
Rossle M, Haag K, Ochs A, et al.: The transjugular intrahepatic portasystemic stent-shunt procedure for variceal bleeding. N Engl J Med 330:165, 1994. *Large trial demonstrating efficacy of TIPS to treat patients with cirrhosis and variceal hemorrhage, which documents reduction in portal venous pressure gradient and cites incidence of complications.*
The North Italian Endoscopic Club for the Study and Treatment of Esophageal Varices: Prediction of the first variceal hemorrhage in patients with cirrhosis of the liver and esophageal varices: A prospective multicenter study. N Engl J Med 319:983, 1988. *Detailed analysis of those endoscopic features of esophageal varices that predict a high likelihood of subsequent hemorrhage.*

Ascites—Diagnosis and Management

Gines P, Arroyo V, Quintero E, et al.: Comparison of paracentesis and diuretics in the treatment of cirrhotics with tense ascites: Results of a randomized study. Gastroenterology 93:234, 1987. *Large series demonstrating efficacy and safety of large-volume paracentesis in selected patients with cirrhotic ascites.*
Runyon B: Care of patients with ascites. N Engl J Med 330:337, 1994. *Practical review of diagnostic and therapeutic issues in management of ascites.*
Runyon BA, Montano AA, Akriviadis EA, et al.: The serum-ascites albumin gradient is superior to the exudate-transudate concept in the differential diagnosis of ascites. Ann Intern Med 117:215, 1992. *Clinical series demonstrating the advantage of measuring SAAG over conventional transudate/exudate analysis of ascites.*

Hepatorenal Syndrome

Moore K, Wendon J, Frazer M, et al.: Plasma endothelin immunoreactivity in liver disease and the hepatorenal syndrome. N Engl J Med 327:1774, 1992. *Clinical series demonstrating elevated levels of the potent vasoconstrictor endothelin-1 in patients with hepatorenal syndrome, raising the possibility that this compound has an etiologic role.*

123   ACUTE AND CHRONIC HEPATIC FAILURE AND HEPATIC ENCEPHALOPATHY

Bruce F. Scharschmidt

Severe acute or chronic liver disease is associated with a variety of manifestations that reflect decompensated disease or liver failure. The spectrum and frequency of these complications differ for acute and chronic disease. Certain complications most characteristic of chronic liver disease, including variceal hemorrhage, ascites, and other manifestations of portal hypertension, are discussed in the preceding chapter. This chapter begins with a discussion of hepatic encephalopathy and other neurologic manifestations of acute or chronic liver disease. The chapter then focuses on acute hepatic failure, a highly lethal disorder that differs from chronic liver disease in terms of its pathogenesis, manifestations, and clinical approach.

HEPATIC ENCEPHALOPATHY

DEFINITION AND SIGNIFICANCE. Hepatic encephalopathy (also called hepatic coma or portal-systemic encephalopathy) is a reversible neuropsychiatric syndrome that can accompany advanced, decompensated liver disease of all types and/or extensive portal-systemic shunting. Recognition of the signs and symptoms of encephalopathy provides an important clue to the presence of deteriorating liver function or superimposed complications. In addition, repeated evaluation of the neurologic status of the encephalopathic patient provides valuable information regarding the course and prognosis.

PATHOGENESIS. The pathogenesis of hepatic encephalopathy is likely multifactorial, and possible mechanisms are outlined in Table 123–1. The encephalopathy is at least partially attributable to toxic materials that are derived from the metabolism of nitrogenous substrate in the gut and that bypass the liver through anatomic or functional shunts. This is the origin of the term *portal-systemic encephalopathy.* Ammonia and *mercaptans* are produced by the degradation of urea or protein and sulfur-containing compounds, respectively, and mercaptans in the breath of some encephalopathic patients probably account for the characteristic sweetish musty odor termed *fetor hepaticus.*

Gamma-aminobutyric acid (GABA), the principal inhibitory neurotransmitter in the mammalian brain, is also produced in the gut. GABA, or GABA-like substances such as endogenous benzodiazepines that act as agonists at the GABA-receptor, are reported to be present in increased amounts in the blood or brain of patients and animals with hepatic failure. A role for GABA or GABA-like substances is supported by experimental studies (Table 123–1), as well as anecdotal reports of improvement in some patients after administration of the benzodiazepine receptor antagonist flumazenil.

A separate hypothesis holds that accelerated entry of *aromatic amino acids* into the central nervous system results in decreased synthesis of normal neurotransmitters such as norepinephrine and enhanced synthesis of *false neurotransmitters* such as octopamine. Other compounds such as short-chain *fatty acids* are also present in blood in increased amounts and have been proposed as potentially toxic. Finally, there is impaired integrity of the *blood-brain barrier* in animals with acute hepatic failure. Current evidence suggests that none of these abnormalities individually accounts for the syndrome of hepatic encephalopathy, which likely reflects the synergistic effects of a number of toxins acting on an unusually susceptible nervous system.

NEUROLOGIC MANIFESTATIONS. Patients with hepatic encephalopathy display a characteristic spectrum of mental and motor changes. These are frequently divided into stages (Table 123–2). However, individual variations occur, and many patients do not show an orderly progression of symptoms. Moreover, the clinical grading scale is relatively insensitive. Standardized testing has revealed psychomotor abnormalities in a high proportion of patients with cirrhosis in whom conventional neurologic examination is normal. Such *subclinical encephalopathy* is potentially important inasmuch as it may be associated with impaired functional capacity, including job performance and ability to drive an automobile.

In addition to the acute, reversible signs and symptoms already mentioned, rare patients with longstanding liver disease and portal-systemic shunting develop *irreversible neurologic dysfunction.* Acquired *hepatocerebral degeneration* is characterized by tremor, rigidity, dysarthria, oral-facial dyskinesia, choreoathetosis, and ataxic gait. *Myelopathy* is another rare manifestation of advanced chronic liver disease and portal-systemic shunting and may be manifested by spastic paraparesis, hyperreflexia, and incontinence.

As with other types of metabolic encephalopathy, asymmetric neurologic findings are unusual, and brain stem reflexes such as the pupillary light response, oculovestibular response, and oculocephalic response are typically preserved. Thus, asymmetric neurologic signs or abnormal brain stem reflexes may suggest a structural

TABLE 123–1. HEPATIC ENCEPHALOPATHY: PROPOSED PATHOGENIC MECHANISMS

Mechanism	Hypothesis	Evidence For	Evidence Against	Therapeutic Implications
Toxins (ammonia and mercaptans)	Produced by action of intestinal bacteria on urea, protein; decreased clearance from portal blood by diseased liver; enhanced brain synthesis of glutamine causes osmotic swelling and depletion of the neurotransmitter glutamate	Increased levels of these substances or their metabolites in blood, CSF; administration can produce coma	Poor correlation of plasma levels with encephalopathy; EEG changes produced by administration of these agents differ from those in hepatic encephalopathy	Oral administration of poorly absorbable antibiotics, lactulose
False neurotransmitters (increased brain octopamine and phenylephrine; decreased dopamine and noradrenaline)	Increased brain influx of aromatic amino acid precursors for false neurotransmitters	Increased ratio of plasma aromatic amino acids to branched-chain amino acids	Inconsistent findings regarding brain levels of neurotransmitters; lack of effect of false neurotransmitter administration on neurologic function	Administration of branched-chain amino acids (no consistent benefit in clinical trials)
Enhanced GABA (-ergic) neurotransmission	Decreased hepatic clearance of gut bacteria-derived GABA, which enters brain and inhibits neurotransmission	Increased plasma or brain levels of GABA or GABA-like substances such as benzodiazepines; visual evoked responses in encephalopathy mimic those produced by GABA; increased brain GABA receptors	Inconsistent evidence regarding serum GABA levels and GABA receptor density in brain	Administration of poorly absorbable antibiotics; administration of benzodiazepine receptor antagonists undergoing evaluation

TABLE 123–2. STAGES OF HEPATIC ENCEPHALOPATHY

Stage	Mental Status	Motor Changes
Subclinical	No changes on routine examination; may be associated with impaired work performance or driving ability	Impaired performance on standardized psychomotor tests or bedside tests such as figure drawing or number connection
I	Mild confusion, apathy, agitation, anxiety, euphoria, restlessness, sleep disorder	Fine tremor, slowed coordination, asterixis
II	Drowsiness, lethargy, disorientation, inappropriate behavior	Asterixis, dysarthria, primitive reflexes (suck and snout), ataxic paratonia
III	Somnolent but rousable, marked confusion, incomprehensible speech	Hyperreflexia, extensor plantar response, incontinence, myoclonus, hyperventilation
IV	Coma	Decerebrate posturing; brisk oculocephalic reflexes; response to painful stimuli present early; may progress to flaccidity and absence of response to stimuli

lesion of the central nervous system such as a subdural hematoma. Seizures are also uncommon in the absence of alcohol withdrawal and should alert the clinician to the possibility of a structural lesion or hypoglycemia. The disappearance of pupillary reactivity, of the oculocephalic or oculovestibular response, or of deep tendon reflexes is associated with a very poor prognosis. Electroencephalographic changes are sensitive indicators of hepatic encephalopathy, being present in most patients with subclinical disease (Table 123–2), but are not specific for this disorder. They include symmetric slowing observed initially over the frontal areas with later spreading laterally and posteriorly.

DIAGNOSIS. The diagnosis of hepatic encephalopathy is based upon the presence of compatible neurologic signs and symptoms in a patient with advanced liver disease and exclusion of other possible causes of the neurologic abnormalities. The diagnosis is most difficult when liver disease is not obvious. Routine laboratory studies, including electrolytes, calcium, blood urea nitrogen, creatinine, glucose, and standard liver function tests, primarily help exclude other causes of metabolic encephalopathy and evaluate the presence and severity of hepatic disease. Toxicologic screening is also appropriate when ingestion of sedatives or toxins capable of altering neurologic function is suspected. Blood ammonia and cerebrospinal fluid levels of glutamine correlate only roughly with mental status and are therefore of limited value in most circumstances. Structural lesions such as a subdural hematoma are often a consideration and may require special radiologic studies. Other causes of encephalopathy such as the Wernicke-Korsakoff syndrome, sepsis, or meningitis must also be excluded, depending on the clinical circumstances.

TREATMENT. The management of patients with hepatic encephalopathy is largely supportive and has as its goals (1) improvement, when possible, of hepatic function; (2) prevention or correction of factors that may precipitate or aggravate encephalopathy (Table 123–3); and (3) decreasing the production of putative toxins that result from enteric bacterial metabolism of nitrogenous substrates. All nonessential drugs should be stopped—particularly sedatives and potentially hepatotoxic agents. For the occasional patient who demonstrates manic disorientation as an early manifestation of encephalopathy, soft restraints are preferable to sedative hypnotic agents.

Decreasing Production and Absorption of Enteric Toxins. Gut cleansing should be accomplished by enema and oral administration of cathartics or lactulose (see below). It is also generally appropriate to restrict dietary protein to about 40 grams per day in mildly encephalopathic patients and eliminate it in patients with more advanced or progressive encephalopathy. *Vegetable protein* has been reported to be marginally less likely to induce encephalopathy than animal protein and may be useful in the long-term management of patients with chronic or recurrent encephalopathy. While anecdotal reports suggest that benzodiazepine

TABLE 123–3. HEPATIC ENCEPHALOPATHY— COMMON PRECIPITATING FACTORS

Deterioration in hepatic function
Drugs (sedative or potentially hepatotoxic agents)
Gastrointestinal hemorrhage
Increased dietary protein
Azotemia
Hypokalemia
Infection
Constipation
Anesthesia and surgery
Hypoxia
Diuretics (hypokalemia, alkalosis, and hypovolemia)

receptor antagonists produce transient neurologic arousal, there is no controlled evidence that they are beneficial, and their use should be regarded as experimental. *Branched-chain amino acids* have not been shown to be beneficial and are not recommended (Table 123–1).

In addition to these measures aimed at decreasing nitrogenous substrate, production of enteric toxins should be further inhibited by oral administration of a poorly absorbable antibiotic (such as neomycin in a dose of 1 to 2 grams every 6 hours) or lactulose. Lactulose is neither metabolized nor absorbed in the upper small bowel and is metabolized by ileal and colonic bacteria to organic acids. It is as effective as neomycin in lowering blood ammonia and reversing encephalopathy in patients with chronic liver disease. Because prolonged neomycin administration may produce ototoxicity or malabsorption, lactulose is preferable as long-term therapy. Lactulose may increase bacterial assimilation of ammonia, decrease ammonia production, and possibly trap ammonia as NH_4^+ in the bowel lumen. Therapy is commonly initiated by administering 30 to 45 ml of the syrup orally every 2 hours until diarrhea ensues. Thereafter, the dose is decreased to that amount necessary to produce two to four soft stools per day. Lactulose can also be given by retention enema. Concomitant administration of neomycin and lactulose may be useful in selected patients.

FULMINANT HEPATIC FAILURE

DEFINITION. *Fulminant hepatic failure* is defined as hepatic failure with encephalopathy developing in less than 8 weeks in a patient without pre-existing liver disease. *Subacute* or *late-onset hepatic failure* refers to a slower-paced illness, also occurring in patients without pre-existing disease, in whom the time from jaundice to onset of encephalopathy ranges from 8 weeks to 6 months.

ETIOLOGY. Two-thirds or more of cases of fulminant hepatic failure in most reported series result from acute hepatitis B (with or without coexistent hepatitis D), hepatitis A, or acetaminophen poisoning or are of uncertain etiology (Table 123–4). These latter cases had been presumed to be due to viral hepatitis and have often been referred to as non-A, non-B. However, newer serologic tests indicate that hepatitis C (and in developed countries, hepatitis E) rarely cause fulminant hepatic failure. Hepatitis B virus DNA has been found in some of these patients, despite the absence of serologic markers of hepatitis B virus infection. The term *non-A, non-B hepatitis* is therefore no longer appropriate. The remaining cases are due to a variety of less common causes (Table 123–4).

The time course and prognosis of the illness differ depending on the etiology. Acetaminophen poisoning, *Amanita phalloides* ingestion, and toxic injury typically represent a one-time insult and produce a fulminant illness leading to death or recovery in a period of days. The combined presence of hepatic and renal failure often represents a clue to the presence of toxic exposure. The etiology of most cases of late-onset hepatic failure, by contrast, is unknown.

DIAGNOSIS. The diagnosis of fulminant hepatic failure requires the presence of encephalopathy in a patient with severe, acute liver disease. Synthetic function of the liver as reflected by the prothrombin time is nearly always markedly abnormal. Serum bilirubin concentration is less helpful, since some patients may become very ill rapidly and progress to coma before the serum bilirubin is markedly elevated. Serum transaminase levels are usually elevated early in the illness, but do not reliably distinguish between fulminant hepatic failure and acute hepatitis without encephalopathy.

TABLE 123–4. CAUSES OF FULMINANT HEPATIC FAILURE

Common	Uncommon

Viral hepatitis
  A
  B
  D (as coinfection or superinfection with B)
Acetaminophen
Idiopathic (also called non-A, non-B)
	Drugs (other than acetaminophen):
	  Necrosis (e.g., halothane, isoniazid, methyldopa)
	  Steatosis (e.g., tetracycline, valproate)
	Toxins (e.g., *Amanita phalloides,* chlorinated hydrocarbons, phosphorus)
	Ischemia
	Occlusion of large (Budd-Chiari syndrome) or small hepatic veins
	Hyperthermia
	Malignant infiltration
	Wilson's disease
	Fatty liver of pregnancy
	Reye's syndrome
	Viral infection (hepatitis C, hepatitis E, herpes simplex)

TREATMENT. The immediate objectives are to initiate supportive measures and to assess prognosis. If the prognosis with supportive care alone appears poor or is uncertain (see below), prompt contact with a liver transplant center is essential.

Supportive Measures. A thorough search should be made to detect and correct factors that may precipitate encephalopathy (see Table 123–3) or complicate hepatic failure (Table 123–5); several points merit emphasis. Encephalopathy in fulminant hepatic failure primarily reflects the severe nature of the underlying liver injury, and correcting potential precipitating factors is less likely to produce neurologic improvement than in patients with encephalopathy complicating chronic liver disease. For example, administration of lactulose by enema or nasogastric tube to comatose patients with fulminant hepatic failure is unlikely to produce benefit, complicates nursing care, and may increase the risk of aspiration. Aspiration is an important hazard in these patients as a result of encephalopathy and ileus, which may jeopardize survival as well as transplant candidacy. Endotracheal intubation is therefore essential in patients unable to protect their airway. *Cerebral edema* is present in most comatose patients, and intracranial herniation is a major cause of death. Because the clinical manifestations of cerebral edema are insensitive and CT of the head is both unreliable and cumbersome in these critically ill patients, invasive monitoring of intracranial pressure has been advocated by several centers, both for diagnosis and monitoring of therapy with osmotic agents or barbiturates. However, use of such monitors has been associated with up to a 5% incidence of fatal intracranial hemorrhage, and decisions regarding intracranial pressure monitoring must be carefully individualized. Coagulation abnormalities must be corrected before insertion of the monitor. *Infection* in these patients is common and cannot be reliably diagnosed by clinical criteria such as fever, leukocytosis, or chest radiography. Cultures of blood, urine, and other sites as appropriate must therefore be routinely obtained and empiric therapy instituted in the presence of clinical deterioration or if infection is suspected. Empiric antibiotics have been shown to decrease the occurrence of infection, but have not influenced survival.

Liver Transplantation. The survival of patients with fulminant hepatic failure who undergo transplantation ($\geq 70\%$ at 1 year) compares favorably with that of supportive care alone, and transplantation is the appropriate therapy for patients judged unlikely to survive with supportive care alone. Because lethal complications or complications precluding transplantation occur rapidly and unexpectedly, early consultation with a transplant center is appropriate, as is a prompt assessment of prognosis (see below) and transplant candidacy.

Experimental Measures. Because the mortality of fulminant hepatic failure is high even with optimal supportive care, a variety of other forms of therapy have been tried. These include administration of *corticosteroids, L-dopa, prostaglandins,* selected *amino acids,* or *hepatitis B hyperimmune globulin* (for hepatitis B). Additional strategies include measures to remove putative circulating toxins (e.g., *exchange transfusion, plasmapheresis*) or extracorporeal circulation through an intact liver (human donor liver not suitable for transplantation or animal liver) or liver-assist device, generally comprised of hepatocytes or liver-derived cell lines. While the need to support these critically ill patients until a donor organ can be identified has reawakened interest in these measures, they are still undergoing evaluation. None has yet been shown to be of benefit, and use should be restricted to controlled trials.

PROGNOSIS. The short-term prognosis for patients with fulminant hepatic failure that progresses to coma is poor, the average reported survival being 10 to 40%. In contrast to the poor overall short-term prognosis, the long-term outlook for those patients who do survive is excellent. Virtually all patients have returned to their previous state of health within 2 to 3 months, and follow-up liver biopsies have usually demonstrated no or minimal abnormalities. Patients with persistent biochemical or histologic abnormalities have frequently been found to have had pre-existing liver disease or to have continuing exposure to toxic or infectious agents.

Identification of those patients who are or are not likely to survive with supportive care alone is critical. The presence of complications, in particular the presence of advanced encephalop-

TABLE 123–5. HEPATIC FAILURE: COMPLICATIONS AND MANAGEMENT

Complications	Pathophysiology	Management
Aspiration	Decreased mental status, emesis	Endotracheal intubation with onset of coma
Azotemia	Volume depletion, acute tubular necrosis, hepatorenal syndrome	Assess volume (may require invasive monitoring or fluid challenge), fluid administration if appropriate
Cerebral edema	?Altered vascular permeability, circulating toxins	Clinical assessment insensitive; intracranial pressure monitoring advocated by some, but entails risk and not of proven value; elevation of head of bed; hyperventilation; mannitol; barbiturates
Encephalopathy	See Table 123–1	See Table 123–1
Gastrointestinal bleeding	Stress gastritis aggravated by coagulopathy and portal hypertension	Prophylaxis (e.g., with H_2-receptor antagonists, antacids or sucralfate); fresh frozen plasma if overt bleeding occurs
Hypoxemia	Right to left shunting, noncardiogenic pulmonary edema	Increased inspired O_2; intubation with positive end-expiratory pressure
Hypotension	Decreased vascular resistance, sepsis, gastrointestinal bleeding	Identify and treat underlying cause, pressors if necessary
Infection	Via intravenous lines, enteric origin	Surveillance cultures, empiric treatment if infection suspected
Metabolic		
Acidosis	Decreased perfusion, decreased hepatic clearance of organic acids	Identify and treat underlying cause; administration of HCO_3^-
Alkalosis	Hyperventilation, presumably central	No treatment necessary
Hypoglycemia	Decreased glycogenolysis and gluconeogenesis	Frequent glucose monitoring, intravenous glucose administration
Hypokalemia	Renal or gastrointestinal K^+ loss	KCl administration
Hyponatremia	Decreased renal free water clearance, fluid administration	Minimize administration of free water

athy (see Table 123–2), is associated with a poor outcome. Additional clinical and biochemical variables indicative of a poor prognosis, based upon the very large experience at the Royal Free Hospital in London and selected U.S. centers, are summarized in Table 123–6.

CHRONIC LIVER DISEASE WITH ENCEPHALOPATHY

ETIOLOGY. Hepatic encephalopathy may also occur in patients with chronic liver disease, usually cirrhosis with portal-systemic shunting due to spontaneous collaterals or shunts created surgically or via a transvenous approach (TIPS, see preceding chapter) to prevent variceal hemorrhage. Some patients with cirrhosis may be chronically encephalopathic. In most, however, encephalopathy tends to occur acutely and intermittently. In this latter group, the occurrence of encephalopathy reflects a worsening of hepatic function and/or the presence of one or more precipitating factors (see Table 123–3).

DIAGNOSIS. As with fulminant hepatic failure, diagnosis requires signs and symptoms compatible with hepatic encephalopathy in a patient with underlying chronic liver disease. Routine tests of liver function are typically abnormal, but are of little value in differential diagnosis. Unlike fulminant hepatic failure, encephalopathy in patients with chronic liver disease may be accompanied by only minimally abnormal liver function tests. A markedly elevated or rising prothrombin time in an encephalopathic patient with known chronic liver disease suggests superimposed acute hepatocellular necrosis. It is extremely important in patients with chronic alcoholic liver disease to exclude other causes of metabolic encephalopathy (e.g., hypoglycemia, alcohol intoxication, Wernicke-Korsakoff syndrome), meningitis, or structural lesions such as subdural hematoma.

TREATMENT. Supportive Measures. Unlike fulminant hepatic failure, encephalopathy in the patient with chronic liver disease frequently results from one or more potentially reversible precipitating factors. These should be sought and, when possible, corrected (see Table 123–3). Additional general measures as outlined earlier for the treatment of hepatic encephalopathy should be undertaken.

The complications and additional supportive care required for these patients are outlined in the preceding chapter. Overall, however, the severity and frequency of complications (e.g., cerebral edema, hypoglycemia) are less than with fulminant hepatic failure. The various forms of experimental therapy that have been tried in fulminant hepatic failure also have no established role in the management of patients with chronic liver disease with encephalopathy.

Liver Transplantation. Patients with chronic, progressive liver disease of all types may be candidates for transplantation. The presence of encephalopathy or other complications should prompt the physician to consider this option and contact a transplant center (see Ch. 124).

PROGNOSIS. Because encephalopathy in patients with chronic liver disease is frequently precipitated by potentially reversible factors, the short-term prognosis is better than in fulminant hepatic failure, particularly if the encephalopathy is not attributable to sudden deterioration of hepatic function. However, because the underlying chronic liver disease is commonly irreversible and slowly progressive, the long-term prognosis is guarded.

TABLE 123–6. ADVERSE PROGNOSTIC FACTORS IN PATIENTS WITH FULMINANT HEPATIC FAILURE

Acetaminophen Poisoning

Prothrombin time (international normalized ratio >6.5, or still rising on the fourth day after ingestion)
Creatinine >3.4 mg/dl

Acute Liver Failure Not Caused by Acetaminophen

Age <10 or >40
Cause unknown or related to drugs or toxins
Prothrombin time (international normalized ratio >3.5)
Serum bilirubin concentration >18 mg per deciliter
Slow-paced illness (>1 week from jaundice to encephalopathy)

Lidofsky SL: Liver transplantation for fulminant hepatic failure. Gastroenterol Clin North Am 22:257, 1993. *Concise summary of key management issues in patients with fulminant hepatic failure in era of liver transplantation.*
Morgan, MY: The treatment of chronic hepatic encephalopathy. Hepato-Gastroenterology 38:377, 1991. *Review focusing on practical aspects of management from a world's leading center.*
O'Grady J, Alexander GJM, Hayllar KM, et al.: Early indicators of prognosis in fulminant hepatic failure. Gastroenterology 97:439, 1989. *Very important article summarizing information on nearly 600 patients, representing the world's largest experience.*

124 LIVER TRANSPLANTATION
John P. Roberts

In the last 25 years liver transplantation has moved from an experimental procedure to accepted medical therapy for patients with acute liver failure and patients with chronic liver failure. Survival following liver transplantation has improved from approximately 30% in the 1970's to 85 to 90% or better at the end of the 1980's. The procedure is currently underwritten by many states and most private insurance companies, and recently Medicare decided to pay for liver transplantation for specific indications. Although liver transplantation is still an expensive procedure, the cost has decreased such that it now offers a better outcome and lower cost than many treatments for acute and chronic liver failure.

A total of 3650 liver transplantations were carried out in the United States during 1994. The improvement in patient and graft survival following liver transplantation has resulted from changes in patient selection, operative techniques, and immunosuppressive drugs and their use. As newer immunosuppressive medications become available, it appears likely that the morbidity, mortality, and costs of liver transplantation will continue to decrease. With improvement in survival and with more patients undergoing liver transplantation, availability of donor organs has become rate limiting in its use.

PATIENT SELECTION

The indications for liver transplantation have broadened with improved postoperative survival. Predictability for survival based on natural history data has been reasonably well established for primary biliary cirrhosis and for fulminant liver failure; however, the natural histories of other liver diseases vary widely, making it difficult to accurately predict survival. It may still be possible to make predictions based on the development of complications of the liver disease—for example, an episode of spontaneous bacterial peritonitis suggests a 1-year survival of approximately 50%.

With the marked improvement in survival after liver transplantation it has been possible to broaden the criteria and to include quality-of-life issues in making the decision for liver transplantation. These issues include extreme fatigue or pruritus in patients with chronic liver disease, recurrent cholangitis in patients with sclerosing cholangitis, portal-systemic encephalopathy, ascites refractory to medical management, and correction of certain metabolic diseases.

Liver transplantation has also changed the indications for or replaced many of the operations previously done for complications of chronic liver disease, such as portal-systemic shunting for recurrent variceal hemorrhage, peritioneovenous shunting for intractable ascites, and radical biliary tract surgery for patients with sclerosing cholangitis. These operations, which were once the only option for the patient with liver disease, are now assuming a secondary role. As an example, portacaval shunting has a poor outcome in patients with severe liver dysfunction, whereas these patients can do well following liver transplantation. It is therefore important that patients who would otherwise be suitable candidates for transplantation and in whom another surgical procedure is contemplated discuss the appropriateness of the planned procedure with a liver transplantation center.

Early referral is extremely important in patients with *fulminant liver failure* (see Ch. 123). This diagnosis can be made only in patients with evidence of hepatic failure, including stage III or IV encephalopathy developing less than 8 weeks after onset in the absence of pre-existing liver disease. Viral hepatitis is the most common cause of fulminant liver failure, but other causes include toxins (e.g., *Amanita phalloides*), medications (e.g., acetaminophen), or metabolic disorders (e.g., fulminant Wilson's disease). These patients are at high risk for developing cerebral edema followed by brain herniation if not properly managed. Pretransplantation management includes elevating the head, monitoring intracranial pressure, and aggressive therapy using mannitol, hyperventilation, and barbiturate coma for increased intracranial pressure.

The diseases for which transplantation is commonly performed are shown in Table 124–1. Contraindications to liver transplantation include systemic sepsis, active substance abuse (including ethanol), extrahepatic malignant disease, and advanced cardiopulmonary disease. Transplantation for cholangiocarcinoma is controversial because survival of these patients following transplantation is poor, although disease limited to the extrahepatic ducts without lymph node involvement may have a more favorable prognosis. Although liver transplantation seems to be logical therapy for hepatocellular carcinoma, effective adjuvant chemotherapy is lacking, and hepatic and systemic relapse of the disease is common. Thus, only 20% of patients with large hepatocellular carcinomas survive 3 years following liver transplantation. The fibrolamellar variant of hepatocellular carcinoma carries a much better prognosis. It does appear that patients with small hepatomas (3 to 5 cm) may have survival similar to patients without hepatoma. End-stage liver disease caused by chronic ethanol abuse has been increasingly recognized as an appropriate indication for transplantation; results in these patients are the same as those for patients with chronic liver failure of other causes. The 6- and 12-month actuarial survival is given for different disease entities in Table 124–1. The overall patient survival is given in Figure 124–1.

DONOR SELECTION

Selecting the appropriate organ donor for liver transplantation is primarily based on ABO blood type and body size compatibility between donor and recipient. In general, donors for large non-O recipients tend to be more available than for small O recipients. This discrepancy reflects a higher accident rate for young adult males and the use of type O livers in recipients of other blood types. In October 1987, a nationwide organ-sharing system was instituted in the United States. In this system, potential organs are first offered to local transplantation programs; if no local recipient is available, the organs are then offered regionally and then nationally. Recipient selection is based on criteria that include the level of care that potential recipients currently require. Those in intensive care are assigned the highest priority—those at home, the lowest.

POST-TRANSPLANTATION COMPLICATIONS

Complications of liver transplantation are primarily vascular (e.g., thrombosis of the anastomosed hepatic artery or portal vein), biliary (relating to reconstruction of the biliary tract), infectious, or those relating to organ rejection. Early postoperative hepatic artery thrombosis requires retransplantation, because it usually results in necrosis of the liver and/or biliary tree. Portal vein thrombosis can be asymptomatic or occur with complications of portal hypertension. Biliary tract complications usually appear as strictures within the biliary tree or as bile leaking from the biliary reconstruction.

Renal failure may complicate the post-transplantation period, resulting from pre-existing renal dysfunction, intraoperative renal ischemia, postoperative cyclosporine toxicity, or a combination of these factors.

Postoperative infections are common (see Ch. 431). The average patient develops at least one episode of bacterial infection and has a 40 to 50% chance of developing a fungal or viral infection following liver transplantation. As one of the major complications of immunosuppression is infections, use of prophylactic anti-infectives improves the therapeutic index of the immunosuppressive agents. Bacterial infections appear in the early post-transplant period and may involve the biliary tree, intra-abdominal abscesses, or pneumonia or may be related to central venous catheters. Fungal infections include systemic candidiasis, usually occurring during the early transplant period, and are related to intravascular catheters or intra-abdominal candidal abscesses. Other opportunistic fungal infections, such as aspergillosis, predominate later, and all can represent a serious threat to the patient's life. Viral infections following liver transplantation are most often caused by herpesviruses. Mucocutaneous herpes simplex and varicella-zoster can occur following transplantation, and prophylactic or therapeutic acyclovir is effective in preventing or treating these infections. Post-transplantation cytomegalovirus (CMV) infections represent either a reactivation of disease in a previously infected, immunosuppressed recipient or a primary infection arising from transmission of the agent via the donor liver or a blood transfusion. In general, primary disease appears to be more serious than reactivation. In renal transplantation recipients, high doses (3200 mg per day) of acyclovir are effective prophylaxis for CMV infections, and this approach is also effective in liver transplantation recipients. Ganciclovir, a congener of acyclovir, appears to effectively prevent *and* treat systemic CMV disease in liver recipients. *Pneumocystis carinii* infection was previously a problem in all forms of solid organ transplantation, but with prophylactic use of trimethoprim-sulfamethoxazole, morbidity and mortality related to this agent have been eliminated in transplantation recipients.

IMMUNOSUPPRESSION

Immunosuppression in the liver transplant recipient was largely based on the use of cyclosporine, but it is expected that FK506 (tacrolimus) may play an important role in preventing rejection. Both drugs interfere with the production of interleukin-2 (IL-2) by T helper cells; this in turn prevents cell proliferation and the generation of cytotoxic T cells. Both drugs are usually started in the early post-transplantation period and are continued indefinitely. Because intestinal absorption of oral cyclosporine depends on the presence of bile, external biliary diversion or postoperative liver dysfunction can interfere with this process. Absorption of FK506 appears to be independent of the presence of bile. Both are metabolized by the cytochrome P-450–dependent mono-oxygenases, and therefore systemic levels can be decreased by drugs that induce this pathway, such as rifampin, barbiturates, or phenytoin. Major side effects of both drugs include neurotoxicity manifested by headache

TABLE 124–1. INDICATIONS FOR LIVER TRANSPLANTATION AND POSTOPERATIVE SURVIVAL*

Disease	Group	% of Patients	(n)	Actuarial Patient Survival (Months)				
				6	12	24	36	48
Chronic active hepatitis/cryptogenic cirrhosis	6	27	153	91	89	85	82	82
Alcoholic liver disease	2	19	108	94	93	90	90	90
Primary biliary cirrhosis	10	8	47	93	88	81	81	81
Fulminant liver failure	8	8	43	90	90	90	90	90
Sclerosing cholangitis	11	7	37	97	94	94	90	90
Chronic active hepatitis B	5	6	36	80	72	64	58	58
Autoimmune hepatitis	1	4	24	100	100	100	89	89
Extrahepatic biliary atresia	7	4	23	91	80	73	73	73
α-Antitrypsin disease	3	1	8	88	88	68	68	68
Subacute fulminant liver failure	12	1	8	100	100	100	100	100
Hemochromatosis	9	1	6	100	100	100	100	100
Cancer	13	1	3	100	100	100	—	—
Miscellaneous	4	11	63	71	66	66	61	61

* Based on 559 patients who underwent liver transplantation at the University of California, San Francisco, between January 31, 1988, and February 1, 1994.

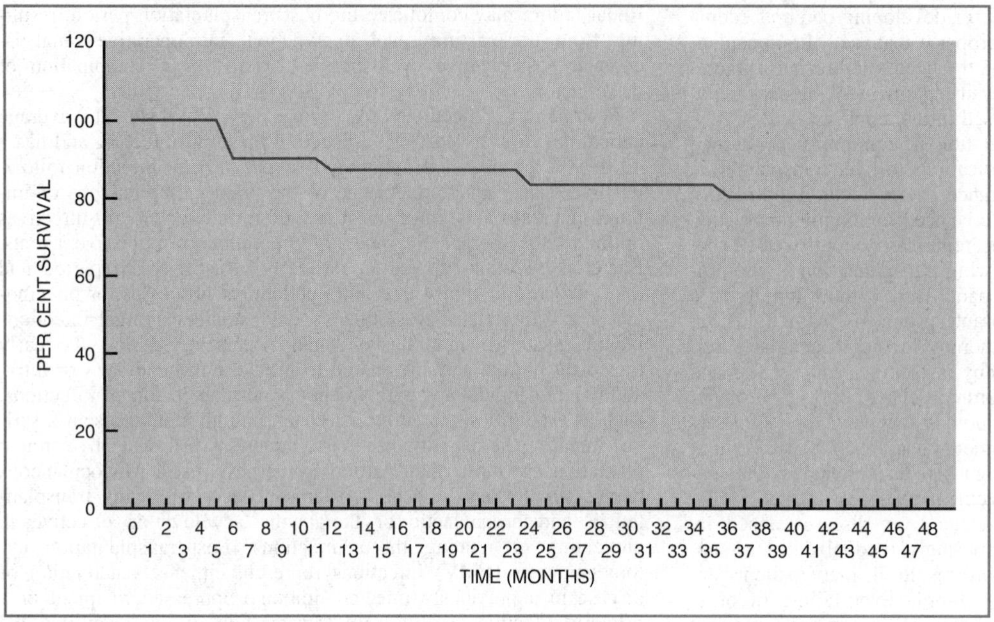

FIGURE 124-1. UCSF liver transplants: actuarial survival analysis.

and tremor, nephrotoxicity manifested by increase in blood urea nitrogen (BUN) and creatinine and sensitivity to volume depletion, hyperkalemia, and glucose intolerance. Both drugs appear to increase the risk of post-transplantation lymphoproliferative disorders.

Prednisone is generally used in combination with cyclosporine or FK506 to prevent rejection. Prednisone reduces the release of interleukin-1 (IL-1) by macrophages, and in this fashion inhibits amplification by IL-1 of IL-2 production. The complications of using glucocorticoids are well known, but in particular the pretransplant bone loss associated with cholestatic liver disease is exacerbated by posttransplant corticosteroid use and may lead to significant disability in the early post-transplant period.

Azathioprine, a third agent used for post-transplantation immunosuppression, blocks proliferation of white blood cells and thereby decreases the proliferative or amplification response of the rejection process. The major adverse effect of azathioprine is marrow depression.

Rejection occurs commonly after liver transplantation, but with prompt diagnosis and treatment it is less important as a cause of graft loss. Its histologic features include periportal infiltrate, bile duct epithelial damage, and endotheliitis. Treatment for rejection includes use of additional steroids or antilymphocyte preparations. A change from cyclosporine to FK506-based immunosuppression may result in an improved rate of salvage from ongoing rejection.

Kusne S, Dummer JS, Singh N, et al.: Infections after liver transplantation. An analysis of 101 consecutive cases. Medicine 67:132, 1988. *Compilation of infectious complications at the University of Pittsburgh.*

Lake JR (ed.): Advances in liver transplantation. Gastroenterol Clin North Am 22:213, 1993. *Recent review of liver transplantation in monograph form.*

Starzl TE, Demetris AJ, Van Thiel DH: Liver transplantation. N Engl J Med 321:1014, 1989. *Comprehensive review of the history of clinical liver transplantation and a summary of advances in the field.*

125 HEPATIC TUMORS
Bruce F. Scharschmidt

The differential diagnosis and management of suspected hepatic tumors represent a challenging problem that must take into account the clinical and biochemical findings and operative candidacy of an individual patient. Characteristic features of specific neoplasms are summarized below and in Table 125–1. Principles that guide the approach to the patient are summarized at the end of the section.

BENIGN HEPATIC TUMORS

Hemangioma

Cavernous hemangioma is probably the most common benign hepatic tumor, occurring in up to 7% of necropsies with a predominance in females. The great majority are asymptomatic and are found incidentally by imaging studies or at surgery or necroscopy. These lesions can, however, present with signs and symptoms of an abdominal mass, infarction, rupture, or thrombocytopenia and hypofibrinogenemia. Because of the accuracy of current imaging techniques in distinguishing hemangioma from other tumors (Table 125–1), resection is not usually necessary to establish a diagnosis and is appropriate only for large symptomatic lesions. There are also case reports of regression following radiotherapy or hepatic artery ligation.

Hepatocellular Adenoma

Hepatocellular adenomas occur almost exclusively in women. These tumors are most frequently detected during the third and fourth decades of life, but are occasionally found in postmenopausal women as well. Adenomas most commonly occur in the right lobe of the liver, are frequently solitary, and are often quite large, with up to one half being ≥10 cm in diameter. Hepatocellular adenomas are usually well circumscribed, may be surrounded by a pseudocapsule, and often show areas of bile stasis, hemorrhage, and necrosis. Microscopically, these tumors consist of a monotonous sheet of normal to slightly atypical hepatocytes without portal tracts or bile ducts. Kupffer cells are markedly reduced in number or absent, and a few arteries and thin-walled veins are present.

The preponderance of this tumor in women suggests a hormonal role in its pathogenesis, and there is strong evidence implicating oral contraceptives. Nearly 90% of cases are associated with oral contraceptive use, and some adenomas have regressed in a period of months to years after use of oral contraceptives was discontinued. The annual incidence is estimated to be 3 to 4 per 100,000 in women who have taken oral contraceptives continuously for several years. Glycogen storage disease also predisposes to hepatocellular adenoma. Although not generally regarded as a premalignant lesion, there are instances in which hepatocellular carcinoma appears to have arisen in a hepatocellular adenoma.

Symptomatic patients with hepatocellular adenomas have signs and symptoms of an abdominal mass, tumor infarction, intratumor hemorrhage (pain, fever, leukocytosis), or, in about one third of cases, tumor rupture (pain, hemoperitoneum, circulatory collapse). The mortality in this last group is approximately 20%. Because the true incidence of these tumors is unknown, the actual proportion that ruptures cannot be determined.

TABLE 125–1. CHARACTERISTICS OF HEPATIC NEOPLASMS

	Predisposing Factors	M/F Ratio	Manifestations and Complications	Imaging/Diagnostic Studies	Treatment
Benign tumors					
Hepatocellular adenoma	Oral contraceptives; glycogen storage disease type I	<1:10	Abdominal mass; intratumor or intraperitoneal hemorrhage; rare transition to malignancy	Detectable by US, CT, or MRI and may show areas of hemorrhage or necrosis; cold spot on colloid scan; typically hypervascular on AG; may be difficult to diagnose on biopsy	Must be individualized: discontinue oral contraceptives and observe if no symptoms; resection if symptomatic or diagnosis uncertain
Focal nodular hyperplasia	None established	1:2–7	Typically none; occasionally mass effect and rarely portal hypertension	Detectable by US, CT, or MRI and may show central scar; has Kupffer cells and may not be visible on colloid scan; typically hypervascular on AG; may be difficult to diagnose on biopsy	Usually none; resection if symptomatic
Hemangioma	None established	<1:1	Typically none; occasionally mass effect, rarely infarction, rupture, or thrombocytopenia	Characteristic appearance on MRI, CT with bolus contrast, or radionuclide blood pool scan; typically hyperechoic on US; biopsy not necessary if imaging studies show typical findings and probably associated with increased risk of hemorrhage	None if asymptomatic; resection if symptomatic; radiotherapy or hepatic artery ligation in unusual circumstances
Malignant tumors					
Hepatocellular carcinoma	Cirrhosis; hepatitis B or C virus infection; hemochromatosis; mycotoxin exposure; α_1-antitrypsin deficiency; androgenic steroids; Thorotrast; possibly oral contraceptives or alcohol; tyrosinemia; glycogen storage disease types I and II	3:1	Abdominal mass; pain; tumor infarction, intratumor or intraperitoneal hemorrhage; portal or hepatic vein occlusion; rarely hypercalcemia, hypercholesterolemia, carcinoid syndrome, hypoglycemia, acquired porphyria	Detectable by US, CT, MRI, or colloid scan (cold spot); often multicentric with vascular invasion; takes up gallium; biopsy or aspiration cytology often diagnostic; elevated or rising α-fetoprotein suggestive	Resection if technically feasible and permitted by hepatic function; transplantation curative in less than one third of even selected cases; tumor ablation by chemoembolization or ethanol injection undergoing investigation; palliative chemotherapy
Fibrolamellar carcinoma (variant of hepatocellular carcinoma)	None established	About equal	Mass effect	Detectable by US, CT, MRI (may show calcifications on CT and central scar); cold spot on colloid scan; α-fetoprotein typically not elevated	As for hepatocellular carcinoma; resection or transplantation more likely to result in cure
Cholangiocarcinoma	Primary sclerosing cholangitis; clonorchiasis or opisthorchiasis	—	Mass effect; obstructive jaundice	Direct cholangiography often helpful in jaundiced patients; also detectable by US or CT, which may show dilated biliary radicles; aspiration cytology may be diagnostic	As for hepatocellular carcinoma; resection or transplantation rarely curative; biliary bypass or stenting via surgery, interventional endoscopy, or radiology may produce palliation
Angiosarcoma	Exposure to vinyl chloride, arsenic, or Thorotrast	>1:1	Mass effect; intraperitoneal hemorrhage; thrombocytopenia	Detectable by US, CT; MRI or AG particularly helpful; biopsy	As for hepatocellular carcinoma; resection or transplantation rarely curative

Abbreviations: US = ultrasonography; CT = computed tomography; MRI = magnetic resonance imaging; AG = angiography

The management of hepatocellular adenomas is debated. In patients taking oral contraceptives that can be discontinued, a several-month period of observation with repeated imaging studies is justifiable, particularly if the location, size, or number of tumors would make resection hazardous. Surgery is appropriate for most persistent or symptomatic resectable lesions.

Focal Nodular Hyperplasia

Focal nodular hyperplasia, which shows a female to male predominance of 2:1 to 7:1, has also been referred to as pseudotumor, focal cirrhosis, and hepatic hamartoma. Focal nodular hyperplasia generally is a solitary tumor in the right lobe measuring ≤5 cm in diameter. It has a characteristic grossly lobulated appearance on cut section, which is produced by a central fibrous core with septa radiating in a stellate pattern. Hemorrhage and necrosis are rare. Microscopically these fibrous septa contain bile ductules and inflammatory cells and are surrounded by normal or slightly atypical hepatocytes as well as Kupffer cells.

Unlike hepatocellular adenomas, focal nodular hyperplasia does not usually produce symptoms and is generally found incidentally by imaging studies or at surgery or necropsy. In up to 20% of the cases, it presents as an upper abdominal mass. Portal hypertension has been reported in association with multiple lesions, and rupture is rare. Since focal nodular hyperplasia has no known malignant potential, asymptomatic lesions can be followed nonoperatively. If the lesion is encountered unexpectedly at surgery, simple wedge biopsy is appropriate if complete excision would be difficult.

Other Benign Tumors

A variety of less common benign liver tumors may also occur in adults. They usually produce no symptoms unless they are very large or located so as to produce bile duct obstruction. Included in this group are *bile duct adenomas, bile duct cystadenomas, fibromas, lipomas, leiomyomas, mesotheliomas, teratomas,* and *myxomas.*

MALIGNANT HEPATIC TUMORS
Hepatocellular Carcinoma

EPIDEMIOLOGY. Hepatocellular carcinoma (hepatoma) is relatively uncommon (<2.5% of all malignant tumors) in the United States and Western Europe. In certain other areas of the world, including parts of sub-Saharan Africa, Southeast Asia, Japan, Oceania, and Greece, hepatocellular carcinoma is among the most frequent malignant tumors. Hepatocellular carcinoma occurs predominantly in males and usually arises in a cirrhotic liver. The risk appears to be greatest in cirrhosis associated with hemochromatosis and hepatitis B and C virus infection. Prospective epidemiologic studies suggest that the incidence of hepatocellular carcinoma increased about 100-fold in individuals with hepatitis B virus infection. Moreover, tumor tissue in patients with hepatitis B virus infection frequently has hepatitis B virus integrated into the genome, and woodchucks and ducks infected with viruses that are related to the human hepatitis B virus also develop hepatocellular carcinoma. Infection with hepatitis C virus is associated with a similarly increased prevalence of hepatocellular carcinoma.

Epidemiologic evidence suggests a link between hepatocellular carcinoma and ingestion of aflatoxins, mycotoxins produced by *Aspergillus flavus,* a mold that can grow in warm moist areas and contaminate peanuts and stored grains. Case reports also suggest a link between hepatocellular carcinoma and glycogen storage disease types I and II, α_1-antitrypsin deficiency and administration of androgenic steroids, Thorotrast (a long-lived radionuclide previously used for imaging) and possibly estrogenic steroids in the form of oral contraceptives (Table 125–1).

CLINICAL FEATURES. The most common presenting features of hepatocellular carcinoma are *abdominal pain,* the presence of an *abdominal mass,* and *weight loss.* Hepatocellular carcinoma may also present with rupture and hemoperitoneum, obstructive jaundice, unexplained deterioration in a patient with cirrhosis, or a variety of paraneoplastic syndromes, including erythrocytosis, persistent fever, hypercalcemia, and hypoglycemia. Hepatomegaly is present in about two thirds of patients. Other suggestive physical findings include the presence of a bruit, hepatic friction rub, or bloody ascites. Hepatocellular carcinoma may invade and obstruct the portal and hepatic veins and metastasizes most often to regional lymph nodes and the lungs. α-Fetoprotein levels in serum >1000 ng per milliliter or progressively rising levels highly suggest hepatocellular carcinoma. Unfortunately, only a minority of patients with asymptomatic hepatocellular carcinoma in most parts of the world, including the United States, have elevations of this magnitude. Elevations up to about 200 ng per milliliter are a more sensitive indicator of early tumors, but are also less specific. α-Fetoprotein and imaging studies such as ultrasound (US) can detect hepatic tumors at an early, preclinical stage. For this reason, screening of high-risk patients (e.g., with chronic hepatitis B or C and abnormal biochemical studies) with 3- to 6-monthly α-fetoprotein and US has been advocated by many experts. Unfortunately, such screening is time consuming and expensive and has not yet been shown to improve survival in populations at high risk for hepatocellular carcinoma.

TREATMENT AND PROGNOSIS. The results of current treatment for hepatocellular carcinoma are discouraging. In the United States, median survival from the time of diagnosis is about 6 months, and the therapy of choice is surgical resection. Unfortunately, because of the advanced stage of the disease at the time of diagnosis and the frequent coexistence of severe liver disease, <20% of patients are candidates for hepatic resection. The presence of coexisting cirrhosis in a patient with well-preserved hepatic function does not altogether preclude surgery; however, such patients may not tolerate more than limited resection of a localized tumor. Adriamycin alone or in combination with other agents has produced objective tumor response in up to 50% of patients, but has minimally affected survival. Radiation therapy has also yielded disappointing results. Uncontrolled or partially controlled studies suggest that treatment aimed at ablation of a large portion of the tumor mass (e.g., hepatic arterial embolization with material impregnated with chemotherapeutic agents, percutaneous intralesional injection of ethanol) may improve survival and decrease morbidity. While encouraging, such therapy is still experimental and should be restricted to controlled trials. Other approaches such as hormonal therapy or use of radiolabeled antibodies are also being investigated. As discussed in Ch. 124, liver transplantation for unresectable hepatocellular carcinoma is curative in only a minority of patients.

A variant of typical hepatocellular carcinoma termed *fibrolamellar carcinoma* differs from the typical form of the disease in that it usually occurs in young adults without underlying cirrhosis, lacks the usual male predominance, is associated with longer survival (32 to 68 months) when untreated, and has been cured surgically in 10 to 30% of cases.

Other Primary Hepatic Malignant Tumors

Cholangiocarcinoma occurs much less frequently than hepatocellular carcinoma and shows an association with sclerosing cholangitis and with clonorchiasis and opisthorchiasis in Eastern Asia. It may occur with obstructive jaundice when it involves major ducts in the area of the hepatic hilum. Truly mixed hepatocellular cholangiocarcinomas are rare. Angiosarcoma, an unusual tumor associated with vinyl chloride exposure as well as arsenic and Thorotrast administration, frequently causes thrombocytopenia and has a propensity to rupture, causing hemoperitoneum and circulatory collapse. Other unusual primary hepatic malignant tumors of adults include cystadenocarcinoma, squamous carcinoma, and hepatoblastoma.

As with hepatocellular carcinoma, treatment of these malignant hepatic tumors has been unsatisfactory. Resection is seldom possible. Of patients with cholangiocarcinoma who have undergone liver transplantation, the 3-year survival is less than among patients with hepatocellular carcinoma.

Tumors Metastatic to Liver

The liver and lung are the most frequent sites of metastatic cancer, and metastases constitute the largest group of hepatic tumors in adults. Necropsy studies have demonstrated hepatic metastases in more than half of patients with primary malignant tumors having portal venous drainage (e.g., stomach, colon, and pancreas). Other solid tumors that frequently metastasize to the liver include melanoma and tumors of the lung, oropharynx, and bladder. Next to the spleen, the liver is also the most common extranodal site of involvement by Hodgkin's disease, the non-Hodgkin's lymphomas, and malignant histiocytosis (histiocytic medullary reticulosis). Lymphoma is an important problem in immunosuppressed patients (e.g., following transplantation, AIDS). Such tumors are particularly likely to occur in extranodal sites, including the liver.

Pseudotumors and Miscellaneous Disorders

A variety of non-neoplastic lesions may mimic hepatic tumors. These include regenerative nodules, anomalous hepatic lobulation, cysts, focal fatty deposits, and inflammatory pseudotumors. Imaging studies may distinguish some of these lesions (e.g., low-density by computed tomography (CT) characteristic of focal fatty deposits, lack of internal echoes by US in cysts) from true neoplasms. *Nodular regenerative hyperplasia* (also called *nodular transformation* or *multiple adenomatosis*) typically is characterized by nodules of varying size composed of disordered liver plates that are two cells thick, occurring focally or throughout a noncirrhotic liver. It is reported in association with rheumatoid arthritis, Felty's syndrome, CREST syndrome, oral contraceptives, and certain other drugs. Detailed pathologic studies suggest that it may result from intrahepatic microvascular disease and occlusion.

DIAGNOSTIC APPROACH TO THE PATIENT WITH A SUSPECTED HEPATIC NEOPLASM

CLINICAL EVALUATION. Most hepatic neoplasms present as a right upper quadrant or epigastric mass. Additional clinical features that may provide clues regarding the specific type of tumor are summarized above and in Table 125–1. Cholangiocarcinoma and hepatocellular carcinoma can cause biliary obstruction, but this may potentially result from strategically located tumors of all types. Physical examination most commonly reveals hepatomegaly or a discrete mass. The presence of a bruit or friction rub may suggest hepatocellular carcinoma, but is not specific. Elevations of alkaline phosphatase and transaminase levels are the most common biochemical abnormalities; however, liver function tests are not particularly helpful in diagnosis and may be entirely normal in some patients. A markedly elevated and/or rising α-fetoprotein level is strongly suggestive of hepatocellular carcinoma.

IMAGING TECHNIQUES. The detection of hepatic neoplasms has been improved by modern imaging methods. US, CT, and magnetic resonance imaging (MRI) have gradually replaced hepatic scintigraphy. Unlike scintigraphy, these other studies visualize structures outside the liver, and US and CT can be used for directed biopsy. Because of its lesser expense and lack of radiation exposure, US is often a useful initial study. As compared with US, CT provides sharper definition of other abdominal structures, is not hindered by bowel gas, and probably detects smaller hepatic lesions. MRI appears comparable to CT, but its role in hepatic imaging is still being defined. Angiography, which entails more risk and discomfort for the patient, may be particularly helpful in planning surgical resection. Because of the rapidly evolving capabilities of current imaging methods, radiologic consultation is often appropriate.

METASTATIC TUMORS. In a patient with a known extrahepatic malignant tumor and clinical or biochemical evidence of hepatic metastases, US is a reasonable screening study. The finding of a single defect or multiple defects is consistent with metastatic disease, and a percutaneous biopsy can be expected to recover tumor in 50 to 75% of such cases. Two biopsies performed through the same skin site and cytologic examination of the tissue core and aspirated fluid appear to enhance the yield without increasing the risk of bleeding. In patients with lymphoreticular malignant disease, histologic evidence of hepatic involvement may be found even in the absence of clinical, biochemical, or imaging abnormalities.

PRIMARY TUMORS. The workup in suspected primary hepatic tumor must be individualized on the basis of the relative risks and benefits of establishing a diagnosis. Asymptomatic patients may not require additional evaluation if biochemical studies are normal and imaging studies yield findings characteristic of hemangioma (Table 125–1). In most other instances, however, examination of tissue is appropriate. In a patient who is a candidate for operation and who has an apparently resectable lesion of uncertain or suspicious nature based on imaging studies, preoperative biopsy may not be necessary. In the patient who is not a candidate for surgery or in whom information regarding tumor type will importantly influence decisions regarding further evaluation and therapy, biopsy is usually appropriate. Several factors should be considered in this regard. First, needle biopsy of lesions such as hemangioma, angiosarcoma, and possibly hepatocellular adenoma is probably associated with increased risk of hemorrhage, particularly when these lesions are large and superficial in location, and biopsy of a possible echinococcal cyst is contraindicated. Second, definitive diagnosis of hepatocellular adenoma and focal nodular hyperplasia, which consist predominantly of normal or minimally abnormal hepatocytes, may be difficult from examination of a needle biopsy specimen alone. Third, compared with percutaneous biopsy, laparoscopy permits directed biopsy of visible tumor deposits. Finally, a CT- or US-directed fine-needle percutaneous aspiration biopsy has yielded excellent results in many centers and appears to be associated with a lower risk of hemorrhage than standard biopsy. It is particularly helpful for lesions not accessible to blind percutaneous biopsy.

Okuda K: Hepatocellular carcinoma: Recent progress. Hepatology 15:948, 1992. *This authoritative review stresses the pathogenesis and biology of hepatocellular carcinoma.*

Piva A, DeFazio C, Covini G, et al.: Detection of preclinical hepatocellular carcinoma in patients with cirrhosis. J Surg Oncol 3:46, 1993. *This concise and balanced review of a controversial and important topic is but one article in an entire issue of this journal devoted to hepatocellular carcinoma.*

Tsukuma H, Hiyama T, Tanaka S, et al.: Risk factors for hepatocellular carcinoma among patients with chronic liver disease. N Engl J Med 328:1797, 1993. *Risk factors for hepatocellular carcinoma identified in this study are important considerations in screening as well as in the clinical approach to the individual patient with a mass lesion.*

126 DISEASES OF THE GALLBLADDER AND BILE DUCTS

Z. Reno Vlahcevic and Douglas M. Heuman

BILE

The liver is the human body's largest exocrine gland. Its exocrine secretion, bile, provides detergents (bile salts) needed to digest and absorb lipids, as well as bicarbonate to neutralize gastric acid. Secretion of bile also has an excretory function, serving as the major pathway for eliminating many waste products of metabolism as well as exogenous toxins. Bile is formed in bile canaliculi, a network of tubular structures within the hepatocyte plates. The walls of a canaliculus consist of specialized regions of the plasma membranes of two adjacent hepatocytes. The canalicular (biliary) domain of the hepatocyte plasma membrane is separated from the sinusoidal (plasma) domain by tight junctions that allow free passage of water but restrict movement of macromolecules. The composition of bile produced by the normal liver is illustrated in Figure 126–1. Bile salts are the most abundant organic solute of hepatic bile (*bile salts* are the ionized species of *bile acids;* these terms are often used interchangeably by the physiologist). Bile also contains large amounts of two lipids: phosphatidylcholine (also termed lecithin) and unesterified (free) cholesterol. Bilirubin is secreted into bile as mono- and di-glucuronides and is responsible for bile's yellow color. The total protein content of bile is low (about one fiftieth of the plasma protein concentration). A number of biliary proteins appear to stabilize biliary calcium salts or lipid aggregates, thus preventing crystal formation. Biliary electrolytes resemble those of plasma (bile is isotonic with plasma) and are responsible for most of the osmotic activity of bile, because bile salts and lipids are present largely in osmotically inactive forms (micelles and vesicles). Under physiologic circumstances bile flow averages about 500 to 1000 ml per day.

Bile salts, the major organic constituents of bile, have a unique spectrum of physical and biologic properties. Bile salts are biologic detergents. Their structure is amphophilic, with both hydrophilic

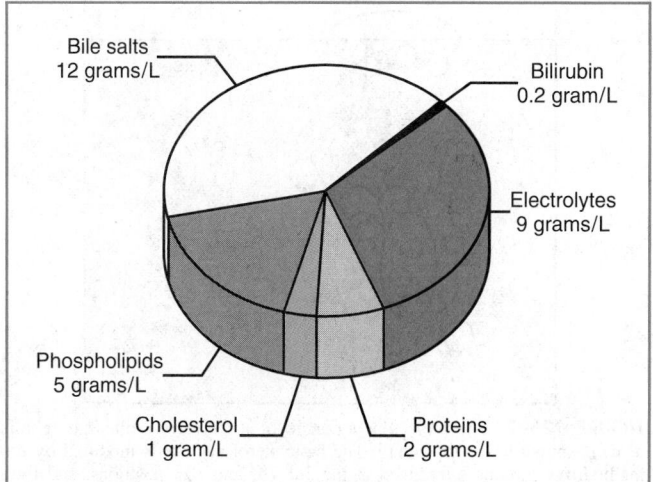

FIGURE 126–1. Solute composition of hepatic bile. Bile salts include principally glycine and taurine conjugates of cholic, chenodeoxycholic, and deoxycholic acids. More than 95% of biliary phospholipid is phosphatidylcholine (lecithin). Cholesterol is present exclusively in its unesterified form. Protein concentration in bile is only 2 to 4% of the plasma protein concentration. Biliary electrolyte composition resembles that of plasma.

and hydrophobic surfaces (Fig. 126–2). Above a threshold concentration, hydrophobic interaction leads to stable clusters in which the hydrophobic surfaces of the bile salt molecules huddle together, exposing only the hydrophilic surfaces to the aqueous environment. This structure is termed a micelle, and the threshold concentration of bile salt at which it forms is termed the critical micellar concentration, which is different for different bile salts. Bile salt micelles can incorporate a variety of lipophilic molecules, acting as "carriers" for these lipids in bile and in the intestine. Bile salt secretion represents the major driving force for bile flow and for biliary secretion of cholesterol and lecithin. Finally, bile salt synthesis from cholesterol is a major pathway for elimination of cholesterol from the body. Approximately 50% of cholesterol eliminated from the body each day occurs via its degradation to bile salts; most of the remaining 50% of daily cholesterol elimination occurs via bile salt–induced secretion of free cholesterol into the bile.

The term "primary bile salts" refers to those bile salts that are synthesized in the liver from cholesterol (in humans, *cholic* and *chenodeoxycholic acids*). Cholesterol's conversion to these bile acids takes place in the liver via a series of 14 enzymatic reactions in four different organelles (Fig. 126–3). Before leaving the hepatocyte, bile salts are conjugated (amidated via their carboxyl group) with glycine or taurine, which lowers the pKa and makes them more polar, thereby preventing their absorption from the biliary tree or the proximal intestine.

Bile salts are secreted into bile across the canalicular membrane via active transport. Although the movement of bile salts into the canaliculus is favored by electrochemical forces, it is also driven by ATP-dependent active transport. The osmotic activity of bile salts and their accompanying cations draws water along with electrolytes through the tight junctions, which are impermeable to bile salts. Some bile secretion is bile salt–independent, driven by secretion of other organic anions such as glutathione and possibly electrolytes. In some species such as guinea pig, bile salt–independent canalicu-

lar bile secretion is a large fraction of the total flow; in humans the bile salt–independent fraction is small. Bile salt secretion draws cholesterol and phospholipid into bile in the form of unilamellar vesicles about 80 nm in diameter, which subsequently are dissolved by bile salts to form mixed micelles. The mechanisms by which fluxes of bile salts through hepatocytes mobilize cholesterol and phospholipid and cause their secretion into bile are not well understood.

Canaliculi are surrounded by an actin network and can contract in response to various signals, propelling nascent bile toward larger biliary ductules. Bile ductules are lined by cuboidal epithelium, which is both absorptive and secretory. Bile ductular epithelial cells add bicarbonate to bile, stimulated by secretin; biliary bicarbonate contributes to neutralization of gastric acid in the duodenum. The ductules merge into bile ducts, hepatic ducts, and eventually the common hepatic duct. In the interdigestive period, a fraction of bile is diverted to the gallbladder, where it is stored and concentrated. Filling of the relaxed gallbladder is permitted by muscle tone of the sphincter of Oddi in the distal common bile duct, which provides resistance to outflow of bile into the intestine. The gallbladder concentrates bile as much as 10-fold by isotonically reabsorbing Na^+, Cl^-, and HCO_3^- with accompanying water. The gallbladder also secretes mucus and acidifies bile slightly. Following food ingestion, gallbladder evacuation is triggered by cholecystokinin, which is released from enterochromaffin cells in the duodenal mucosa in response to the presence of luminal fats and amino acids. Cholecystokinin causes gallbladder smooth muscle contraction, which reaches maximum over 10 to 20 minutes, and also simultaneously causes relaxation of the sphincter of Oddi. Between 50 and 90% of the gallbladder contents typically are expelled during normal postprandial gallbladder emptying.

Conjugated bile salts in the proximal intestine play a major role in fat digestion. All ingested lipids first undergo emulsification. Then pancreatic lipase breaks down triglycerides into monoglycerides, diglycerides, and free fatty acids, a process known as lipolysis. In combination with ingested and secreted phospholipids, bile salts form mixed micelles that can solubilize products of lipolysis, cholesterol, and fat-soluble vitamins. The mixed micelles deliver solubilized lipids across the unstirred mucous layer to the apical membranes of enterocytes, where lipid absorption occurs. Reducing the concentration of intestinal bile salts below their critical micellar concentration results in fat maldigestion. This situation can occur in diseases associated with bile salt wasting (Crohn's disease, ileal resection), conditions leading to small bowel bacterial overgrowth (Crohn's disease, scleroderma) in which deconjugation of bile salts permits passive reabsorption of free bile salts in the jejunum, and in cholestatic disorders in which delivery of bile salts to the intestine is impaired.

Only a small amount of conjugated bile salt normally is absorbed from the duodenum and jejunum by passive diffusion. Thus high luminal bile salt concentrations, adequate for micelle formation, normally are maintained throughout those segments of proximal intestine which mediate fat digestion and absorption. In the distal ileum, conjugated bile salts are reabsorbed by an efficient, active, carrier-mediated transport process. A small fraction of bile salt which escapes ileal absorption enters the colon. In the colon, the anaerobic bacteria deconjugate the bile salts and remove the 7-hydroxyl group from cholic or chenodeoxycholic acids to make the secondary bile salts, *deoxycholic* and *lithocholic acids* (Fig. 126–3), respectively. Secondary bile salts are strongly lipophilic and can be reabsorbed passively. This pathway salvages about half of the bile salts delivered to the colon. Overall >95% of the bile salts secreted into the duodenum are recaptured and returned to the liver via the portal blood. The liver takes up bile salts actively, clearing 70 to 90% of bile salts from portal blood on a single pass. Hepatic sinusoidal uptake of bile salts is a sodium- and energy-dependent, saturable, carrier-mediated process.

This cycle of biliary secretion followed by intestinal reabsorption and efficient hepatic uptake from the portal blood is termed the *enterohepatic circulation* (Fig. 126–4). Deoxycholic acid is conjugated by hepatocytes and accumulates in the enterohepatic circulation, comprising about 20% of the normal bile salt pool in humans. In contrast, lithocholic acid, which is strongly hydrophobic and cytotoxic, is sulfated by the liver, secreted into the bile, but poorly reabsorbed from the intestine. Thus, lithocholic acid does not accumulate in the enterohepatic circulation and normally represents <5% of the bile salt pool in normal humans. The total amount of

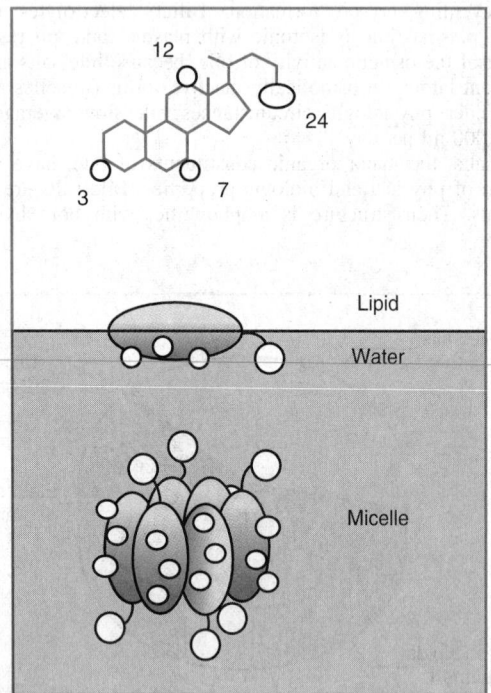

FIGURE 126–2. The molecular structure of a trihydroxy bile salt (cholic acid) is shown in the top figure. The basic sterol nucleus is modified by polar hydroxyl groups introduced at the 3α, 7α, and 12α positions, and by a terminal carboxylic acid moiety at position 24. Because these polar groups are distributed asymmetrically, bile salts are amphophilic molecules having both lipophilic and hydrophilic surfaces *(center)*. In aqueous solution at millimolar concentrations, bile salts self-aggregate to form micelles *(bottom)*. In bile, bile salt micelles incorporate phospholipid (lecithin) and cholesterol (mixed micelles). In the intestines, bile salts form micelles that solubilize cholesterol, fat-soluble vitamins (A, D, K, and E) and products of lipolysis (mono- and diglycerides, fatty acids).

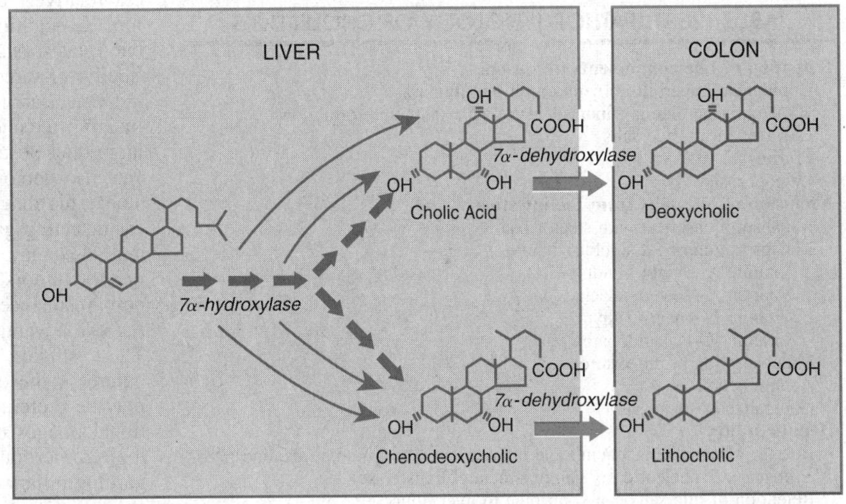

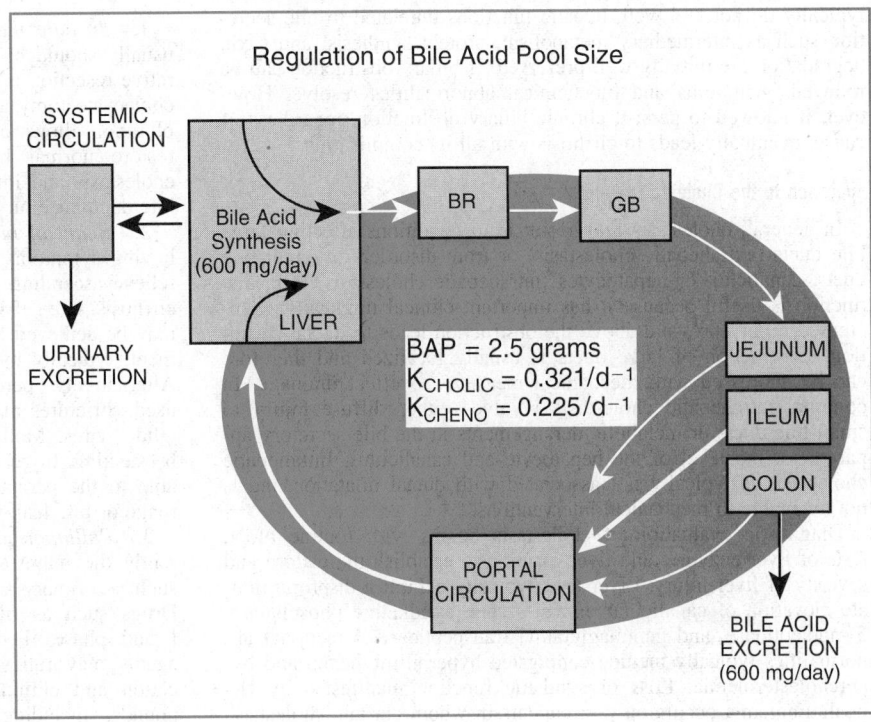

FIGURE 126–3. The primary bile salts of humans—cholic acid and chenodeoxycholic acid—are synthesized from cholesterol exclusively in the liver via a number of intermediary steps. In the colon, anaerobic bacteria deconjugate and 7α-dehydroxylate cholic and chenodeoxycholic acids form the corresponding secondary bile salts, deoxycholic acid, and lithocholic acid, respectively. All bile salts are conjugated by the liver with glycine or taurine. In humans, the ratio of glycine to taurine conjugates is 3:1.

all bile salts in the enterohepatic circulation ("bile salt pool") averages about 2 to 3 grams (5 to 8 mmol). It has been estimated that the entire bile salt pool recirculates six to eight times each day (i.e., two to three times with each meal). About 20 to 30% of the total bile salt pool (roughly 300 to 600 mg) escapes reabsorption each day and is excreted via the feces.

Bile salts in the colon act on epithelial cells to cause net sodium and water secretion. This phenomenon may play a role in normal bowel habits; administering bile salt–binding resins such as cholestyramine or colestipol frequently produces constipation. Bile salt malabsorption is observed in diseases of the ileum or after ileal resection ("bile salt diarrhea"); administering bile salt–binding resins relieves bile salt diarrhea in these patients. Massive resection of ileum (> 100 cm) results in bile salt losses that exceed the maximum capacity of the liver to synthesize bile salts, leading to diminution of the bile salt pool, decreased concentrations of intestinal bile salts, fat maldigestion, and steatorrhea.

CHOLESTASIS

Pathophysiology

Cholestasis is the clinical condition that results from failure of bile secretion. Pathophysiologic, chemical, and laboratory features of cholestasis are summarized in Table 126–1. Biochemically cholestasis is characterized by accumulation in plasma of compounds normally secreted into the bile (bilirubin, bile salts). Elevated levels of serum bile salts are the most sensitive indicators of cholestasis; this determination is not routinely available and therefore not used widely.

Exclusion of bile from the intestine in severe cholestasis has several consequences (Table 126–1). Urobilinogen normally is formed in the colon by bacterial metabolism of bilirubin and subsequently absorbed and excreted into urine. Disappearance of urobilinogen from the urine of a jaundiced patient is indicative of cholestasis.

Certain canalicular membrane enzymes, including alkaline phosphatase, 5′-nucleotidase, and gammaglutamyl transpeptidase, also commonly accumulate in plasma of cholestatic patients. These enzymes normally are present on the luminal surface of the canalicular plasma membrane. When canalicular pressure rises (as when flow of bile is obstructed), these enzymes are synthesized in increased amounts, accumulate on the sinusoidal membrane, and are released into the blood. Disproportionately elevated blood levels of these enzymes are useful in establishing the diagnosis of obstructive cholestasis. Acute obstruction of the common bile duct also can be associated with transient hepatocellular necrosis. For this reason el-

FIGURE 126–4. Enterohepatic circulation of bile salts. Bile salts are secreted by the liver in the biliary radicles and stored in the gallbladder. Following meals and release of cholecystokinin, bile salts are expelled from the gallbladder and into the intestines, where they participate actively in the intestinal digestion of lipids. Small amounts of bile salts are passively absorbed from the jejunum; they are actively absorbed in the ileum and return to the liver via portal circulation. Following uptake at the sinusoids, bile salts are transferred to the canalicular membrane through the cytosol by binding to bile salt binding proteins and secreted through the canalicular membrane. The total bile acid pool (BAP) circulating in the enterohepatic circulation is 2 to 3 grams in normal adults. In steady state, daily bile salt turnover (K) averages 20 to 30% of the bile salt pool.

TABLE 126–1. PATHOPHYSIOLOGY OF CHOLESTASIS

Retention of bile components in plasma
Conjugated hyperbilirubinemia with bilirubinuria
Hypercholesterolemia (lipoprotein X) with xanthoma formation
Elevated serum bile salts
Pruritus
Osteoporosis
Exclusion of bile salts from the intestine
Malabsorption of fat with steatorrhea
Malabsorption of fat-soluble vitamins
Vitamin A—night blindness
Vitamin D—osteomalacia
Vitamin E—neuropathy
Vitamin K—coagulopathy
Malabsorption of cholesterol
Acholic stools
Generalized osteoporosis
Hepatic injury
Release of canalicular membrane enzymes into the plasma (alkaline phosphatase, 5'-nucleotidase, gammaglutamyl transferase)
Retention of bile salts can contribute to liver injury
Biliary ductular proliferation
Cirrhosis

evations of serum aminotransferases and lactate dehydrogenase may predominate during the early hours following acute biliary obstruction. However, with time the levels of these enzymes decline, whereas alkaline phosphatase and other canalicular enzymes rise, producing the typical cholestatic pattern.

Patients with advanced cholestasis experience generalized malaise, weakness, easy fatigability, nausea, and anorexia and often complain of severe pruritus. The underlying cause responsible for pruritus in cholestasis is unknown. Although pruritus has been attributed to cutaneous toxicity of retained bile salts, its severity does not correlate with cutaneous bile salt concentrations, and treatment with cholestyramine is not invariably helpful in relieving the symptoms. Endogenous opiates acting on cutaneous neurons may produce pruritus, and in recent experimental trials the severity of pruritus was relieved with opiate antagonists.

Bacteria introduced into bile above an obstructing lesion can lead rapidly to purulent infection of the biliary tree and liver, termed ascending cholangitis. Contributing factors include high biliary pressure and stasis. Ascending cholangitis is discussed in detail in the section on gallstones. In the absence of infection, cholestasis may be well tolerated for very long periods of time. Although patients typically do not feel well, hepatic functions unrelated to bile secretion such as intermediary metabolism, protein synthesis, and toxin degradation are initially well preserved. If biliary obstruction can be relieved, symptoms and biochemical abnormalities resolve. However, if allowed to persist, chronic biliary obstruction, regardless of cause, eventually leads to cirrhosis with all its complications.

Approach to the Cholestatic Patient

In general, cholestasis may result from conditions affecting large bile ducts (extrahepatic cholestasis) or from disorders of small bile ducts, canaliculi, or hepatocytes (intrahepatic cholestasis). The distinction is useful because it has important clinical implications. Increased biliary pressure above the obstruction leads to ductal dilatation. Obstruction of large ducts is usually localized and therefore can be addressed with mechanical measures to effect drainage. In contrast, intrahepatic cholestasis involves either diffuse injury to small bile ducts or metabolic derangements in the bile secretory apparatus at the level of the hepatocyte and canaliculus. Intrahepatic cholestasis is typically not associated with ductal dilatation and is not amenable to mechanical interventions.

Diagnostic evaluation of cholestasis begins with routine blood tests of liver enzymes and liver function to establish the pattern and severity of liver injury. Liver tests typically exhibit a disproportionate elevation of canalicular enzymes such as alkaline phosphatase, 5'-nucleotidase, and gammaglutamyl transpeptidase. Functional abnormalities typically include conjugated hyperbilirubinemia and hypercholesterolemia. Loss of synthetic function manifested by hypoalbuminemia occurs only in patients in whom chronic cholestasis

has progressed to cirrhosis. An abnormal prothrombin time may occur relatively early in cholestasis because of malabsorption of vitamin K. Additional blood tests may indicate a specific cause for the cholestasis, such as primary biliary cirrhosis (antimitochondrial antibody) or sarcoidosis (serum angiotensin-converting enzyme).

Once a cholestatic pattern of liver disease has been established, imaging techniques such as ultrasonography (US) can determine if large duct obstruction with proximal ductal dilatation is present. US can also demonstrate the location and nature of the obstructing lesion. This diagnostic modality is a very sensitive and accurate test for detecting gallstones, a common cause of obstructive cholestasis, and also may detect focal mass lesions such as primary or secondary tumors in the liver. Computed tomography (CT) and magnetic resonance imaging (MRI) are expensive tests that currently offer no advantage over US for detecting large duct obstruction. These studies, however, provide additional information about the nature of the obstructing lesion. If cancer is strongly suspected, it may be preferable to image initially with CT or MRI to obtain sectional images of the entire abdomen with high-resolution views of the retroperitoneum and pancreas. The most precise information regarding biliary anatomy is obtained by direct *cholangiography* (percutaneous transhepatic cholangiography [PTC] or endoscopic retrograde cholangiopancreatography [ERCP]); these latter tests may be necessary if noninvasive methods are inconclusive. Some examples of cholangiographic appearance of the bile ducts in cholestatic disorders are shown in Figure 126–5.

If the large bile ducts appear normal with imaging studies, *liver biopsy* usually is indicated to look for evidence of a parenchymal process. In disorders that diffusely involve the small bile ducts, the pattern of tissue injury on liver biopsy may be diagnostic. Obstruction to bile flow produces a typical histologic pattern that includes retention of bilirubin granules in the hepatic cytoplasm and inspissated "bile plugs" in canaliculi, most prominent in the perivenular zone. Scattered hepatocyte injury, possibly attributable to bile salts, is manifested as feathery degeneration with focal necrosis. Mild edema and polymorphonuclear inflammation of portal tracts may be seen. With prolonged obstruction, the characteristic finding of proliferation of bile ductules is observed. If the duct obstruction is not relieved, an increasing amount of fibrosis occurs around the portal tracts, accompanied by atrophy of hepatocytes. True cirrhosis with regenerative nodules occurs after months to years of biliary obstruction. The small sample of liver tissue obtained on a percutaneous biopsy is not always representative of the entire liver, and information from a single biopsy must be interpreted with caution.

General principles for therapy of cholestasis include the following:

1. *Specific therapy to cure or control the underlying disorder* usually should be undertaken whenever possible. For example, curative resection is indicated if feasible for an obstructing neoplasm; cholecystectomy and, if clinically indicated, common bile duct exploration allows cure of gallstones; repair of biliary strictures may restore normal biliary drainage. Withdrawal of drugs causing cholestasis and immunosuppressive therapies for immune-mediated bile ductular injury are other examples of this approach.

2. *Relief of biliary obstruction* is generally worthwhile for relieving symptoms of cholestasis (pruritus, jaundice), to prevent or relieve ascending cholangitis, and to prevent progression to biliary cirrhosis, even if the underlying disease cannot be cured. Drainage may be achieved by surgical resection or bypass of obstructed segment, typically by means of a Roux-en-Y choledochojejunostomy. Alternatively, percutaneous and endoscopic approaches may be used. Strictures may be dilated using balloon catheters passed over guide wires. Malignant biliary obstruction commonly is managed by stenting. In general the endoscopic retrograde approach is preferable to the percutaneous approach because of the risk of hemorrhage or bile leak with liver puncture.

3. *Palliation of symptoms and supportive measures* are currently the mainstay of treatment for chronic cholestatic disorders such as primary sclerosing cholangitis or primary biliary cirrhosis. Drugs such as rifampin and phenobarbital induce hepatic phase I and phase II drug-metabolizing enzymes; therapy with these agents may relieve cholestasis somewhat by enhancing detoxification and elimination of a variety of retained lipophilic compounds, including bile salts. Bile salt–binding resins such as

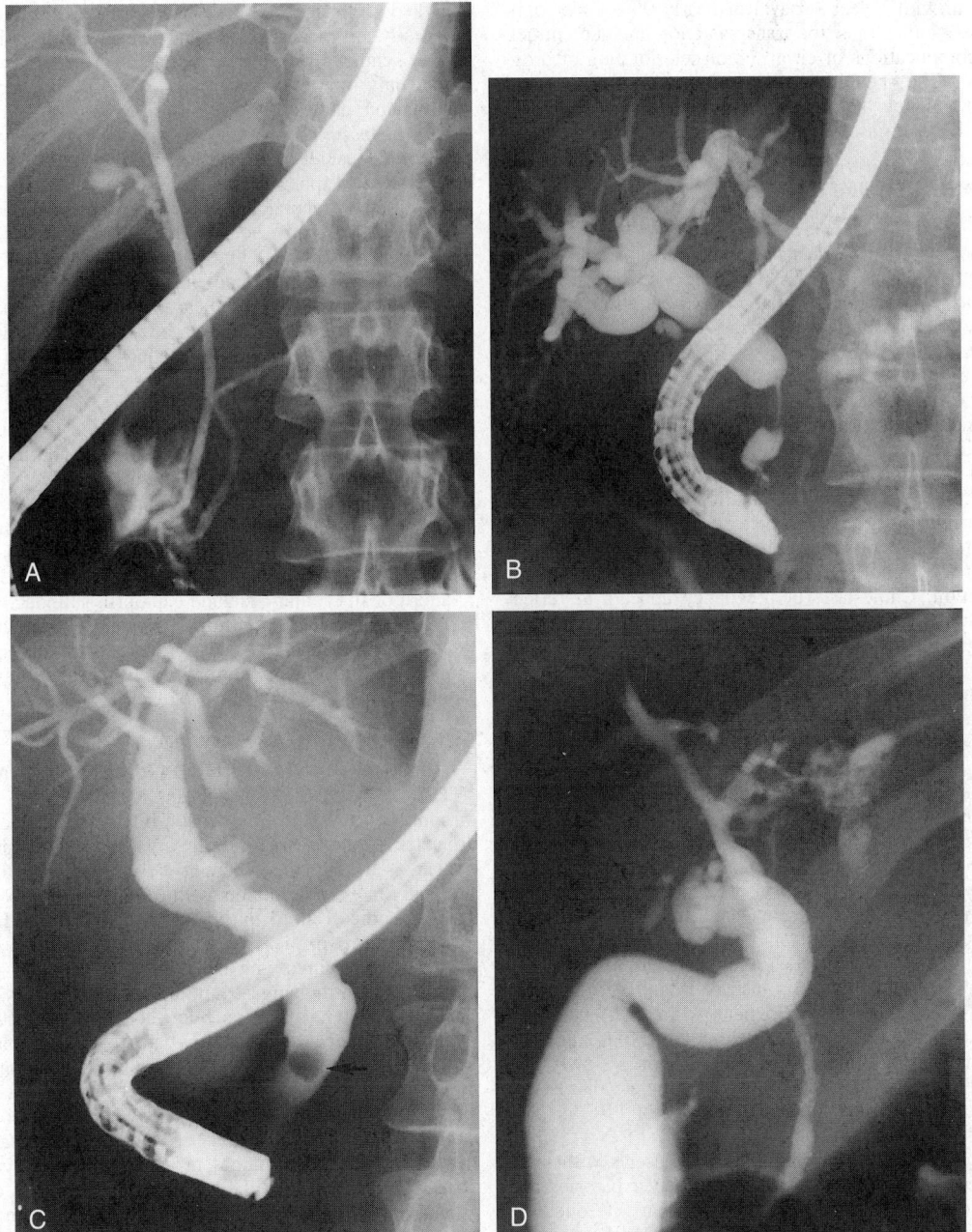

FIGURE 126–5. Cholangiographic appearance of cholestatic disorders. *A,* Normal cholangiogram and pancreatogram. *B,* Pancreatic cancer. The tumor is obstructing the common bile duct and the pancreatic duct, producing proximal dilatation of both (double duct sign). A cannula extending from the endoscope has been passed through the area of obstruction and its tip lies in the proximal common hepatic duct. *C,* Choledocholithiasis. A large cholesterol gallstone in the common bile duct appears as a radiolucent shadow outlined by radiodense contrast material. The common bile duct is dilated. *D,* Primary sclerosing cholangitis. Multiple strictures are present in both the intrahepatic and extrahepatic biliary tree. Intrahepatic ducts are attenuated and reduced in number. Beadlike areas of dilatation can be noted between areas of stricture, but the fibrotic process in the liver prevents generalized dilatation of the proximal biliary ducts. The gallbladder is filled with contrast material and appears normal.

cholestyramine offer symptomatic relief from pruritus, which may be a serious problem in the more advanced cases. Opiate receptor antagonists such as naloxone may be helpful for treating pruritus. Patients with chronic cholestasis and fat maldigestion also require dietary fat restriction, fat-soluble vitamin supplements, and calcium supplements.

Ursodeoxycholic acid, the 7β epimer of chenodeoxycholic acid, is a naturally occurring bile salt of the bear. In contrast to chenodeoxycholic acid, it is a poor detergent because its 7-hydroxyl group projects toward the hydrophobic surface of the molecule, impeding hydrophobic interactions with other lipids. Ursodeoxycholic acid is intrinsically nontoxic even at supraphysiologic concentrations. It was originally used to dissolve cholesterol gallstones (see

below) but was serendipitously found to improve cholestasis and liver injury in a variety of chronic cholestatic liver diseases. Reductions in serum bilirubin, aminotransferases, and alkaline phosphatase are well established, and improvement of clinical symptoms and liver histology has been reported. Ursodeoxycholic acid in various experimental models attenuates toxicity of more hydrophobic bile salts. Ursodeoxycholic acid also may directly protect the liver and may alter immunologic function. It is currently unclear whether ursodeoxycholic acid can slow the progression of cholestatic liver disease to biliary cirrhosis.

4. *Hepatic transplantation* in certain types of cholestatic diseases (primary biliary cirrhosis, sclerosing cholangitis, biliary atresia) is an excellent therapy for end-stage biliary cirrhosis in both

adults and children, with 1-year survival of nearly 90% under optimal circumstances. Indications for transplantation include intractable symptoms, complications of cirrhosis, or deterioration of prognostic indicators. The healthier the patient at the time of transplantation, the better the outcome; conversely, patients with complications of liver disease frequently die while awaiting transplantation.

DISORDERS ASSOCIATED WITH CHOLESTASIS

Intrahepatic Causes of Cholestasis

Intrahepatic cholestasis may occur because of diffuse obliteration of small bile ducts or generalized disorders affecting bile secretion at the level of the hepatocytes or canaliculi. Obliteration of small bile ducts usually leads to chronic progressive cholestasis and biliary cirrhosis. Small duct obliterative disorders are often collectively termed vanishing bile duct syndromes. Diseases in this category include infiltrating neoplasms (discussed below); granulomatous disorders such as sarcoidosis; immune-mediated bile duct destruction of primary biliary cirrhosis, hepatic allograft rejection, and chronic graft-versus-host disease; and congenital Alagille's syndrome in children. Cholestasis of metabolic origin may be seen commonly in severely ill patients, associated with trauma, surgery, sepsis, and parenteral hyperalimentation. Numerous drugs and hormones also can produce cholestasis either as a direct effect or as an idiosyncratic reaction. Cholestasis of pregnancy appears to reflect sensitivity to the direct cholestatic effects of estrogen.

Noncaseating granulomas are a common and nonspecific finding in the liver (see Ch. 120). In *sarcoidosis,* an idiopathic disease characterized by noncaseating granulomas in lung and other tissues, liver involvement is common. Usually these patients are symptom-free with mild abnormalities of liver function tests. Granulomas in the portal tracts may produce fibrotic obliteration of small bile ducts. Rarely, bile duct obliteration may be sufficiently severe to produce biliary cirrhosis.

Primary biliary cirrhosis (PBC) is a progressive cholestatic disorder characterized by autoimmune destruction of small interlobular bile ducts. Injury is thought to occur as a result of cytotoxic T cell–mediated immune attack directed against bile ductular epithelial cells. PBC is a disease of middle-aged women ($>10:1$ female/male ratio). It may be associated with other autoimmune disorders. A characteristic marker of this disease is antimitochondrial antibody, which is found in 90% of patients with PBC and only rarely in other disorders. Based on histologic criteria, four stages of disease have been described. PBC generally progresses slowly but relentlessly to cirrhosis and hepatic failure. A complete discussion of pathogenesis, clinical presentation, and therapy of PBC is presented in Ch. 122.

Paucity of intrahepatic bile ductules typically presents with mild to moderate cholestasis in infancy or childhood. Liver biopsies appear generally unremarkable except for the fact that bile ductules can be identified in $<50\%$ of portal tracts. The disorder may occur in a sporadic (nonsyndromatic) form or may be part of a hereditary condition termed Alagille's syndrome or arteriohepatic dysplasia. Severity and prognosis are variable; whereas some patients develop biliary cirrhosis requiring transplantation in childhood, others have an indolent course.

Chronic graft-versus-host disease occurs when T cells from an allogenic source are infused into an immunodeficient patient, most typically at the time of bone marrow transplantation. The allogeneic T cells attack host tissues, typically in the skin, liver, and intestine. Liver involvement is characterized by mononuclear infiltration of portal tracts with obliteration of small bile ductules, similar to that seen in PBC. Intensive immunosuppression may control the graft-versus-host reaction; if this fails, cholestasis typically progresses to biliary cirrhosis. Ursodeoxycholic acid may improve cholestasis in patients with this disorder. Following hepatic transplantation, *chronic hepatic allograft rejection* is associated with immunologic injury to biliary ductules and hepatic arterioles. Arterial intimal injury leading to intimal hyperplasia may compromise hepatic circulation and accelerate the progression of liver injury. Chronic rejection often is unresponsive to changes in immunosuppression, and retransplantation may be necessary.

A benign intrahepatic cholestasis of metabolic origin is seen commonly in severely ill patients. Predisposing factors include major trauma or surgery, severe infection, and parenteral hyperalimentation. The mechanism is unknown. Serum bilirubin often is markedly elevated, whereas elevations of the alkaline phosphatase typically are modest and aminotransferases usually are near normal. Liver synthetic function usually is well preserved. Liver biopsies reveal only minimal abnormalities. With the precipitating factors eliminated, cholestasis typically resolves over a few weeks.

Intrahepatic cholestasis of pregnancy is a relatively common disorder that usually appears late during the third trimester of pregnancy and disappears after delivery. In its usual form the only manifestation is generalized itching (pruritus gravidarum), but more severe cases may be accompanied by jaundice. The pathogenesis is uncertain, but several lines of evidence suggest that estrogens are involved; they may impair intracellular transport and/or canalicular excretion of bile salts. Cholestasis may also appear in some women taking contraceptives. There appears to be a familial predisposition to the development of intrahepatic cholestasis of pregnancy, and it can occur in subsequent pregnancies.

Drug-induced cholestasis may be a complication of treatment with a number of therapeutic agents. Cholestasis induced by steroids or cyclosporine is associated with little or no inflammation and is thought to result from metabolic effects at the level of the hepatocyte. Chlorpromazine typically produces an acute febrile illness accompanied by elevation of both aminotransferases and alkaline phosphatase. A hypersensitivity mechanism is thought to be responsible. Other common drugs that can produce a cholestatic pattern of liver injury include captopril, sulindac, and benoxaprofen. The recognition that drugs frequently can cause intrahepatic cholestasis is important because in most instances simply withdrawing offending agents normalizes liver function tests and clinical symptoms.

Diseases of the Large Bile Ducts and Gallbladder

PRIMARY AND SECONDARY NEOPLASMS INVOLVING THE BILE DUCTS. Neoplasms are among the most common and important causes of extrahepatic biliary obstruction. Primary malignancies of the liver, bile ducts, gallbladder, ampulla of Vater, and pancreas in aggregate account for $>50,000$ deaths annually in the United States, and patients with these cancers most typically present with jaundice caused by bile duct obstruction. Malignancies classically produce painless obstructive jaundice, but it is more typical for neoplasms involving the liver, bile ducts, or pancreas to cause vague pain in the epigastrium or back, which may precede the onset of jaundice. The common bile duct may be obstructed distally by pancreatic cancer or ampullary carcinoma, proximally by hepatocellular carcinoma or gallbladder carcinoma, or anywhere along its length by cholangiocarcinoma. Rare benign neoplasms that may obstruct the common bile duct distally include pancreatic cystadenoma and villous adenoma of the papilla of Vater. Metastatic tumor from any source to lymph nodes in the porta hepatis can also cause extrinsic compression of the proximal common bile duct, and this is a common cause of cholestasis in patients with cancers of the breast, lung, colon, or stomach. Not all cholestasis caused by malignancies is extrahepatic. Extensive tumor metastases within the liver parenchyma may produce intrahepatic cholestasis by obstructing smaller intrahepatic ducts. Diffuse infiltration of malignant cells along hepatic sinusoids with consequent cholestasis also may occur, especially in small cell carcinoma of the lung and lymphoma. Rarely a nonobstructive metabolic cholestasis may occur as a paraneoplastic syndrome complicating extrahepatic malignancies such as lymphoma or renal cell carcinoma (Stauffer's syndrome).

Cholangiocarcinoma is a form of adenocarcinoma arising from the intrahepatic or extrahepatic biliary epithelium. Cholangiocarcinoma occurs somewhat more commonly in men than women. There is a high incidence in the Far East, related to infestation by liver flukes (see Ch. 386) and Oriental cholangiohepatitis. In Western countries there is an increased incidence in patients with primary sclerosing cholangitis or choledochal cysts. Grossly, three patterns of growth are described: polypoid, sclerosing, and infiltrative. Most cancers of the extrahepatic ducts appear as poorly defined gray-white thickenings of the bile duct wall which narrow the lumen, often resembling fibrous strictures or sclerosing cholangitis radiographically. They tend to grow slowly, infiltrating the wall of the duct and dissecting along tissue planes. Perineural invasion and metastasis to regional nodes are common. Tumors at the bifurcation of the common hepatic duct (termed Klatskin tumors) commonly invade the liver by direct extension. The usual presentation of cholangiocarcinoma involving the common hepatic or common bile duct is progressive obstructive jaundice. More proximal lesions that produce localized obstruction of intrahepatic branches of the biliary tree may cause vague abdominal pain associated with marked elevation of the serum alkaline phosphatase without jaundice. US and CT typically reveal dilated intrahepatic bile ducts with focal narrowing of the biliary tree, sometimes accompanied by a mass. The most useful imaging study is cholangiography, which typically demonstrates segmental narrowing or obstruction. In patients with primary sclerosing cholangitis, diagnosis of cholangiocarcinoma is suggested by rapid worsening of jaundice with a new dominant stricture on cholangiography. Diagnosis may be confirmed by endoscopic brush cytology or needle aspiration, but in some cases the diagnosis can be established only at laparotomy. Only one-third of cholangiocarcinomas are resectable for cure at the time of presentation. The 5-year survival after attempted curative resection is about 20%. The best results are obtained with tumors of the distal bile duct and polypoid tumors; absence of lymph node metastases and clear surgical margins also indicate a better prognosis. Radical surgical attempts to cure intrahepatic cholangiocarcinoma by total hepatectomy with hepatic transplantation were disappointing because of a high risk of postoperative recurrence, and this approach has been abandoned by consensus. Response to chemotherapy or radiation is limited, although brachytherapy (intraductal radiation) holds promise as a palliative measure for some patients. Most patients die of local hepatic invasion rather than distant metastases. Overall survival for cholangiocarcinoma is < 10% at 5 years.

Gallbladder adenocarcinoma is an uncommon malignancy in the United States. Most patients are older than 70, and women are affected more than men by a 3:1 ratio. There is a strong association of gallstones with carcinoma of the gallbladder (80 to 90% of carcinomatous gallbladders have stones), and the risk factors for gallbladder carcinoma are largely the same as the risk factors for gallstones. In some groups of Native Americans who are genetically predisposed to develop gallstones with very high frequency at relatively young ages, gallbladder adenocarcinoma is 5 to 10 times more common than in the general population. The duration and severity of cholelithiasis appear to correlate with the risk of gallbladder carcinoma. Gallbladder cancer is especially associated with very large gallstones (>3 cm in diameter) or calcification of the chronically inflamed gallbladder wall (porcelain gallbladder), and these findings are therefore considered by many experts to be indications for cholecystectomy even in the asymptomatic patient. However, because the incidence of adenocarcinoma of the gallbladder in patients with cholelithiasis is < 1 in 1000 patient years, the prevention of gallbladder cancer currently is not considered a sufficient indication for cholecystectomy in most patients with asymptomatic gallstones. Early symptoms of gallbladder cancer are nonspecific and similar to those of cholelithiasis or cholecystitis; later patients develop persistent pain and *unremitting* jaundice as the tumor invades the liver and bile ducts. Imaging studies such as US, CT, and cholangiography can reveal features suggestive of gallbladder cancer such as thickening or mass of the gallbladder wall or extension of mass to involve the liver, but > 80% of gallbladder cancers are undiagnosed preoperatively. Lesions localized to the gallbladder may be cured by cholecystectomy, but these represent < 20% of all patients with gallbladder cancers. Extension to adjacent bile ducts or liver or metastasis to portahepatic lymph nodes or distant organs is common at initial presentation. By the time patients develop jaundice, 85% are unresectable. Chemotherapy and radiation therapy currently are of little benefit. Overall 5-year survival is <10%.

New onset of cholestasis over days to weeks in any adult, especially over age 50, is worrisome for cancer. Physical examination revealing a palpable, dilated, nontender gallbladder (Courvoisier's sign) suggests cancer obstructing the common bile duct. Laboratory studies most typically reveal a rapid and progressive increase in serum alkaline phosphatase and bilirubin. Because cancers are common and may sometimes present with atypical symptoms or laboratory findings, most adults with new onset of abnormal liver tests or jaundice should undergo imaging of the liver and bile ducts to look for masses or ductal dilatation. US is generally the first imaging procedure in a cholestatic patient, but it may be preferable to go directly to CT or MRI if the clinical picture strongly suggests cancer because these procedures provide more information about the nature

and level of the obstructing lesion and the presence of metastases. Further workup depends on the initial findings. In patients who appear to be candidates for surgical resection, it may be appropriate to proceed with surgery. The diagnosis of cancer can be established by intraoperative biopsy, and the surgeon at laparotomy can choose between a radical, potentially curative resection, a drainage procedure to palliate unresectable cancer, or correction of a benign obstructing process. Additional preoperative diagnostic techniques such as cholangiography (Fig. 126–5B), endoscopic US, and angiography may sometimes be helpful in determining resectability and in resolving diagnostic uncertainties. If patients are poor candidates for surgery or have unresectable disease, a diagnosis can be established by CT-guided needle aspiration biopsy of the primary lesion or a metastasis.

When obstructing malignancy is not resectable for cure, relieving the cholestasis becomes the main goal. Advances in therapeutic radiology and endoscopy over the past decade now permit relief of bile duct obstruction by placing internal stents without surgery in most patients. Commonly used stents are of two types: flexible plastic stents ranging in diameter from 7 to 14 F are inexpensive. Because they occlude over a period of months from accumulation of bacterial biofilm and minerals on their inner surface, they must be removed and replaced periodically. Permanently implanted self-expanding metallic mesh stents, introduced in the last few years, provide a much wider lumen (on the order of 1 cm) and occlude less commonly; however, they are expensive and ingrowth of tumor through the openings in the mesh can occur.

OTHER DISORDERS OF THE LARGE BILE DUCTS. *Choledochal cysts* are congenital anatomic malformations of the bile duct. Five forms of choledochal cysts are described: (1) type I (fusiform or saccular dilatation of the extrahepatic tree), type II (diverticular common bile duct cyst), type III (choledochocele), type IV (diffuse dilation of common bile duct and hepatic ducts), and type V (intrahepatic ductal dilatation [Caroli's disease]). Histologic examination demonstrates a thick-walled structure of very dense connective tissue with smooth muscle fibers. A pericystic inflammatory process or cholangitis frequently accompanies choledochal cyst. The mechanism of cyst formation is uncertain. If the common bile duct is blocked, patients may present with cholestasis in infancy, resembling patients with biliary atresia. If the common bile duct is patent, patients may remain asymptomatic into adulthood. About half of patients with choledochal cysts present after age 10. In the adult form, abdominal pain, jaundice, and palpable mass are the classic presentation. Fever may be present as a result of bile stasis with cholangitis. Complications include primary formation of brown pigment gallstones in the cyst and liver abscesses. Abdominal US and CT often demonstrate dilated bile ducts. However, the best test method to establish diagnosis is ERCP. Once the diagnosis of choledochal cyst is established, therapy is surgical. Simple cystenterostomy can provide drainage and prevent cholangitis. However, whenever possible, completely excising the cyst surgically is desirable because there is a high incidence of cholangiocarcinoma in choledochal cysts.

Benign biliary strictures are fibrotic narrowings of the large bile ducts. They occur as a result of trauma, inflammation, infection, or ischemia. Surgical injury to the bile ducts, although uncommon, is a major technical complication of cholecystectomy. Repair of bile duct injuries is technically difficult and postsurgical strictures are associated with significant chronic morbidity, including biliary cirrhosis. *Chronic pancreatitis* commonly produces fibrotic narrowing of the common bile duct where it passes through the head of the pancreas. Although proximal ductal dilatation and alkaline phosphatase elevation are common, significant cholestasis is unusual and liver failure from biliary cirrhosis is quite uncommon. In patients with chronic pancreatitis who have elevated serum alkaline phosphatase or common bile duct dilatation on US examination, periodic liver biopsy has been recommended to detect progressive hepatic fibrosis. Surgical drainage (choledochojejunostomy) usually is successful in relieving ductal obstruction and halting the progression of biliary cirrhosis in chronic pancreatitis in the few cases in which it is required. Strictures of the bile ducts have been noted following *hepatic irradiation,* possibly secondary to vascular endothelial injury and ischemia. Similarly, strictures have been reported following *chemotherapy* with intrahepatic arterial infusion of floxuridine or mitomycin C. Surgical drainage is preferred to endoscopic or percutaneous stenting in most patients with benign strictures because of uncertainties regarding long-term patency and late complications of stents.

Liver flukes (see Ch. 386) are trematode parasites that are ingested in food, taken up from the gut, travel through the circulation to the liver, and from there pass into bile. The adult flukes mature in the biliary tree, where they can reside for decades, releasing eggs into bile. Mild infections usually are asymptomatic; heavier infections may produce fever and eosinophilia initially and later may cause signs and symptoms of biliary obstruction. Chronically liver flukes may cause ductal fibrosis and strictures, and have been associated with cholangiocarcinoma. Liver flukes have also been implicated in the pathogenesis of *Oriental cholangiohepatitis,* a chronic inflammatory disorder of the biliary tree associated with bile duct strictures, recurrent episodes of obstructive jaundice and ascending cholangitis, development of brown pigment gallstones in the intrahepatic and extrahepatic bile ducts, and biliary cirrhosis. Long-term management includes eradicating parasites and eliminating stones and strictures. Intrahepatic stones that cannot be extracted may require resection of hepatic segments. The prognosis varies with the extent of involvement, but death from complications of sepsis and cirrhosis is common.

AIDS cholangiopathy is a term used to describe a number of biliary tract abnormalities associated with infection with the human immunodeficiency virus (HIV). Patients with advanced immunodeficiency may develop acalculous cholecystitis, focal distal biliary stenosis at the papilla of Vater, or multifocal stenoses of the biliary tree resembling primary sclerosing cholangitis. Although the pathogenesis of this complication is not known with certainty, AIDS cholangiopathy is strongly associated with colonization of bile with cryptosporidia or microsporidia. Patients typically complain of right upper quadrant abdominal pain and often have abnormal liver tests, particularly alkaline phosphatase. The diagnosis may be suggested by US examination of the gallbladder, revealing edema of the wall; ERCP demonstrates strictures and delayed emptying and may permit direct sampling of bile for pathogens. No specific therapy is of proven benefit. AIDS cholangiopathy is a late complication; although rarely fatal of itself, it portends a poor prognosis.

Biliary atresia is a disorder of infants. Typically the bile duct is normal at the time of birth but over the next 6 to 12 weeks its lumen gradually becomes obliterated and the duct becomes a fibrotic cord. The cause is unknown. Infants become jaundiced around 4 to 6 weeks of age. Without treatment, >90% of affected children die before age 1 of complications of biliary cirrhosis. If the diagnosis is established promptly, a surgical portoenterostomy (Kasai procedure) can benefit: a core of tissue is removed from the hilum of the liver and the ends of the transected bile ducts are allowed to drain into a loop of jejunum. The Kasai procedure improves cholestasis and prolongs survival if performed early in infancy. Even after this procedure, most affected children progress to cirrhosis over the next few years. Biliary atresia is the most common indication for hepatic transplantation in young children.

Primary sclerosing cholangitis (PSC) is a disorder characterized by a patchy obliterative inflammatory fibrosis of the large bile ducts. Chronic inflammation leads to extensive bile duct strictures, cholestasis, and gradual progression to biliary cirrhosis. Over half of patients with PSC also have idiopathic inflammatory bowel disease (ulcerative colitis or Crohn's disease). The cause of PSC is not known. Both genetic and immunologic abnormalities have been implicated. The frequency of HLA B8 and DR3 is higher in PSC than in normal subjects. HLA B8 and DR3 are associated with a number of autoimmune diseases. Also, humoral and cellular immune abnormalities (low suppressor T cells in serum and increase in suppressor and helper T cells in the portal tract) observed in these patients suggest that primary sclerosing cholangitis is an immunologically mediated disease. Autoantibodies directed against an epitope present on colonic and biliary epithelial cells have been described in some patients. Unlike other extraintestinal manifestations of ulcerative colitis, PSC shows little correlation with the severity of bowel inflammation and does not remit following colectomy. The definitive diagnostic study for PSC is ERCP, which in classic cases demonstrates multiple areas of irregular stricturing and beadlike dilatations of the intrahepatic and extrahepatic ducts (Fig. 126–5*D*). Because

the fibrotic process may diffusely involve both intrahepatic and extrahepatic ducts, it is not uncommon for US to reveal nondilated bile ducts. The diagnosis of PSC also may be suggested by liver biopsy, which shows portal and periportal inflammation with small and large lymphocytes and periductular inflammation with epithelial destruction. With the progression of the disease, concentric "onion-skin" fibrosis develops around disappearing bile ducts. Liver biopsy staging may be useful to characterize the stage and rate of progression of disease.

Patients with PSC typically present with insidious onset of chronic cholestasis, including jaundice, pruritus, fatigue, and malaise. The disease is often detected in a preclinical stage by routine blood tests revealing marked elevation of the serum alkaline phosphatase, although in some patients with early disease the alkaline phosphatase may be normal. About 15% of patients have manifestations suggestive of recurrent bacterial cholangitis, with episodes of fever, chills, night sweats, right upper quadrant pain, and jaundice. Often the associated inflammatory bowel disease dominates the clinical picture.

No specific therapy is available for sclerosing cholangitis. Corticosteroids, azathioprine, penicillamine, and antibiotics are ineffective. Ursodeoxycholic acid often improves liver function tests and sometimes may alleviate symptoms; ursodeoxycholic acid has not yet been demonstrated to retard progression of the disease. Immunosuppressive therapy with methotrexate and cyclosporine are under study. Antibiotics are indicated for recurrent bacterial cholangitis. Surgical therapy has been directed toward improving biliary drainage. In recent years endoscopic stenting or balloon dilatation of focal strictures has largely replaced surgery in this disease. Endoscopic drainage in selected cases may improve cholestasis and expedite clearing of biliary infections, but the long-term benefit is generally only marginal. PSC is a common indication for liver transplantation. Several large trials indicate that the mean interval from diagnosis of PSC to death from complications of biliary cirrhosis is 10 to 12 years. In the absence of hepatic transplantation, independent indicators of prognosis include age, serum bilirubin, histologic stage, and presence of splenomegaly. Statistical models using these parameters to determine optimal timing of hepatic transplantation have been developed and currently are undergoing validation.

Patients with PSC are at very high risk to develop cholangiocarcinoma. Approximately 20 to 30% of patients with advanced PSC may develop secondary cholangiocarcinoma, which is often very difficult to diagnose. Cholangiocarcinoma should be suspected in any patient with this disease who exhibits an abrupt worsening of cholestasis or in whom cholangiography indicates a single dominant stricture. Even with close evaluation and follow-up, cholangiocarcinoma currently is found incidentally in 10 to 15% of patients with PSC undergoing hepatic transplantation.

GALLSTONES. Gallstones are concretions that form in the biliary tree, usually in the gallbladder. They occur when certain biliary solutes (cholesterol, calcium) precipitate as solid crystals that subsequently grow and aggregate within the mucin layer lining the gallbladder. Roughly 10 to 20% of men and 20 to 40% of women in the United States develop gallstones during their lifetimes; gallstone disease is responsible for about 10,000 deaths annually, and over one-half million gallbladders are removed each year because of gallstone-related disease, at a cost >$6 billion.

Pathogenesis. The pathophysiology of gallstone formation involves several factors (Fig. 126–6). First, bile must become supersaturated with cholesterol or calcium. Second, the solute must nucleate from solution and precipitate as solid crystals. Third, crystals must aggregate and fuse to form stones. The growth and aggregation of crystals occur in a mucous gel along the wall of the gallbladder. Gallstone formation is favored in conditions in which gallbladder emptying is impaired.

There are two major categories of gallstones—cholesterol stones and pigment (calcium) stones. Cholesterol gallstones represent about 80% of all gallstones in the United States. They are yellow-brown in color, ranging in size from a few millimeters to 2 to 3 cm. More than 50% of their dry weight (often >90%) consists of crystalline cholesterol monohydrate, but variable amounts of other components, including mucin glycoproteins and calcium bilirubinate, are also present. Cholesterol gallstones can form when the amount of cholesterol secreted into bile exceeds the amount that can be held in stable micellar solution by the concentrations of bile salts

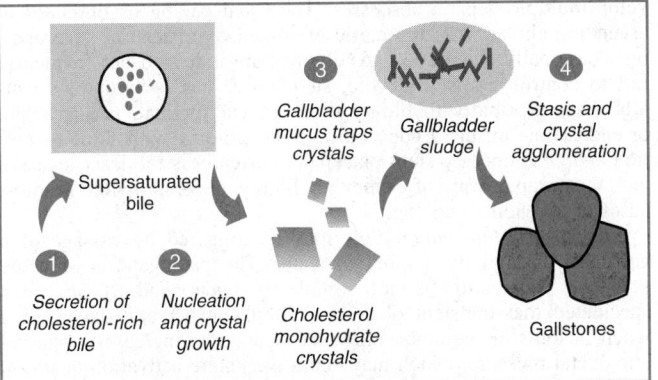

FIGURE 126–6. Pathogenesis of cholesterol gallstones. Canalicular secretion of bile containing excess cholesterol relative to bile salts and phospholipids (supersaturated bile) is necessary but not sufficient. Additional requirements for stone formation are nucleation and growth of crystals, trapping of crystals in a mucin gel, and gallbladder stasis with retention of sludge permitting gradual aggregation and fusion of crystals to form macroscopic stones. Abnormalities in each of these four areas have been noted in gallstone patients. In principle, elimination of any any of these four steps should prevent gallstone formation.

and lecithin present. In unsaturated bile, newly secreted vesicles containing cholesterol and lecithin are dissolved completely by bile salts as bile is concentrated in the gallbladder. In contrast, as supersaturated bile is concentrated, vesicles fail to dissolve completely and instead fuse to form large, cholesterol-rich multilamellar liquid crystals, from which excess cholesterol may precipitate as platelike cholesterol monohydrate crystals.

The causes of biliary cholesterol supersaturation generally can be divided into those associated with a primary increase in biliary secretion of cholesterol and those associated with deficiency of bile salts. Estrogens cause increased absolute rates of biliary cholesterol secretion, and this fact accounts for the twofold increased risk of cholesterol gallstones in women during their childbearing years and the increased risk of gallstones in multiparous women and women taking oral contraceptives. Obesity also is associated with increased biliary cholesterol secretion. Some hypocholesterolemic drugs, such as the fibric acid derivatives clofibrate and gemfibrizol, directly stimulate secretion of cholesterol into bile and are associated with increased risk of cholesterol gallstones. Bile salt deficiency is noted in patients with chronic intestinal bile salt losses resulting from ileal inflammation (Crohn's disease) or ileal resection. Many nonobese patients with cholelithiasis have a small bile salt pool and low rates of bile salt synthesis. Bile salt synthesis decreases and biliary cholesterol saturation increases with age, and this may account for the progressive increase in prevalence of gallstones with age. Genetic factors clearly are of importance in determining gallstone risk. Gallstones develop more commonly in first-degree relatives of cholesterol gallstone patients. The high risk of cholesterol gallstones in Native Americans of the southwestern United States (>80%) also appears to have a genetic basis.

Pigment gallstones account for about 20% of US gallstones. The predominant components of these gallstones are calcium salts of organic and inorganic anions, especially bilirubin. Ionized calcium is present in bile at concentrations similar to those of plasma. Unconjugated bilirubin has a low solubility product with calcium, and its presence in bile even in small amounts favors precipitation of calcium bilirubinate. Two subtypes of pigment gallstones have different composition, pathogenesis, and risk factors. *Black pigment gallstones* are hard, dense, brittle concretions composed of calcium bilirubinate with inorganic calcium salts of carbonate and phosphate. The bilirubin in these stones becomes oxidized and polymerized, producing a mixture of altered pigments that absorb light over the entire visible spectrum, thus giving these stones a characteristic jet-black color. The major predisposing factor appears to be an increased heme turnover leading to increased biliary secretion of unconjugated bilirubin, as occurs in hemolytic disorders, hypersplenism (cirrhosis), or disorders associated with ineffective erythropoiesis. *Brown pigment (earthy) gallstones* have a soft, clay-like consistency. In addition to calcium bilirubinate, they contain a substantial proportion of calcium soaps of fatty acids. Brown pig-

ment gallstones occur in chronically infected bile in areas of stasis, where bacterial cleavage of phospholipid and conjugated bilirubin releases unconjugated bilirubin and fatty acids. Factors predisposing to this type of stone include biliary strictures, biliary infestation with parasites, Oriental cholangiohepatitis, and choledochal cysts. Most stones forming primarily in the bile ducts are of the brown pigment type.

In addition to bile supersaturation, a variety of other abnormalities contribute to formation of both cholesterol and pigment gallstones. Precipitation of crystals from supersaturated bile requires the formation of an initial solid nidus (nucleation) with subsequent deposition of solute on the surface leading to crystal growth. Many individuals who secrete supersaturated bile have very slow nucleation and do not develop gallstones. Nucleation and growth of cholesterol crystals is much more rapid in bile of gallstone patients than in gallstone-free controls for equal degrees of cholesterol supersaturation. A number of proteins in bile can accelerate or retard the nucleation and growth of crystals, and abnormal levels of these proteins may account for the abnormally rapid crystal appearance in bile of gallstone patients. Nascent cholesterol crystals precipitating from vesicles or mixed micelles are trapped in a mucin gel lining of the gallbladder. Over time these crystals fuse to form macroscopic stones. Mucous secretion is stimulated by prostaglandins, and the prevention of excessive mucin secretion with cyclo-oxygenase inhibitors in animal models can prevent cholesterol gallstone formation. Lastly, many gallstone patients have defective gallbladder emptying and an abnormally high residual volume following administration of cholecystokinin. Conditions in which gallbladder stasis occurs such as parenteral alimentation, low-fat weight-reducing diets, and pregnancy are associated with a high rate of gallstone formation.

Clinical Manifestations. Gallstone disease can be divided conceptually into four stages (Table 126–2). In the first stage ("lithogenic"), no discrete stones have yet formed, but the necessary conditions for stone formation (bile supersaturated with cholesterol, rapid nucleation and crystal growth, mucus, gallbladder stasis) are in place. Identification of patients at high risk for gallstones in this early stage may allow targeted use of preventive therapies. In the second stage, the gallstones have already been formed but are still asymptomatic. Several epidemiologic studies have shown that the majority of gallstones are asymptomatic and may remain so for decades.

Onset of symptoms heralds the third stage of gallstone disease. The typical symptom complex associated with gallstones is termed *biliary colic*. Biliary colic is thought to result from increased wall tension in the gallbladder and/or bile ducts due to impaction of a stone in the cystic duct or distal common bile duct. It is characterized by continuous severe pain in the epigastrium or right upper quadrant, sometimes radiating to the back or scapula, and typically lasting for more than 30 minutes. The pain is unrelieved by changes in position and often causes the patient to seek emergent medical attention. Biliary colic is frequently associated with nausea and vomiting. Examination of the abdomen during attacks of biliary colic usually reveals no evidence of peritonitis, and the patient is afebrile. Transient elevations of bilirubin and alkaline phosphatase, AST, and ALT are sometimes noted. Biliary colic is the only pattern

TABLE 126–2. STAGES OF GALLSTONE DISEASE

Lithogenic bile (stage 1)
↓
Asymptomatic gallstones (stage 2)
↓
Symptomatic gallstones (stage 3)
↓
Severe complications of gallstones (stage 4):
  Acute
    Acute cholecystitis (localized peritonitis, perforation, abscess, sepsis)
    Choledocholithiasis (obstructive jaundice, acute pancreatitis, ascending cholangitis)
  Chronic
    Chronic cholecystitis
    Choledochoduodenal fistula with gallstone ileus
    Gallbladder adenocarcinoma

of pain consistently associated with gallstones; in large prospective studies, the frequency of nonspecific symptoms such as vague abdominal discomfort, bloating, and flatulence in individuals with gallstones has been no higher than in the general population. In patients who have experienced at least one attack of biliary colic, about two thirds experience additional attacks of pain during the next 2 years, and biliary colic therefore is commonly an indication for cholecystectomy.

The fourth and most serious stage of gallstone disease is marked by onset of complications. *Acute cholecystitis* (inflammation of the gallbladder) typically presents with acute onset of constant, dull, right upper quadrant pain, fever, shaking chills, nausea, and vomiting. Abdominal pain is often aggravated by coughing or moving; these symptoms are due to localized peritonitis over the area of the gallbladder. A characteristic physical finding is Murphy's sign, defined as tenderness of the gallbladder to palpation elicited when examining the abdomen. Patients with cholecystitis develop leukocytosis with marked shift to the left, but bilirubin and alkaline phosphatase are usually not elevated. In most cases, the cholecystitis develops as a result of impaction of a stone in the neck of the gallbladder. In about 10% of cases, however, no gallstones are present; such *acalculous cholecystitis* may result from impaction of mucus or sludge, from ischemia in vasculitic disorders, or from direct infection of the gallbladder. Some cases are sterile, but in the majority bacteria can be cultured from the gallbladder. The usual organisms present are *Escherichia coli* and other enteric gram-negative organisms. If untreated, the gallbladder may become empyematous, develop gangrene, and perforate, leading to peritonitis, subphrenic abscess, and septic shock. Sometimes infection with gas-forming anaerobic organisms may produce emphysematous cholecystitis with air in the gallbladder wall.

Patients with longstanding gallstone disease frequently develop *chronic cholecystitis*. The evolution of chronic cholecystitis is obscure. It may be the result of repeated bouts of acute cholecystitis in some cases, but many patients cannot relate a history of acute cholecystitis. Often patients note vague, poorly defined, nonspecific intermittent epigastric discomfort, and many are asymptomatic. The gallbladder is thickened, fibrotic, and contracted and frequently fails to visualize by oral cholecystography. A chronic inflammatory infiltrate is present, and mucosal pseudodiverticula termed Rokitansky-Aschoff sinuses are seen histologically. In longstanding cases, deposition of calcium in the fibrotic gallbladder wall may give an eggshell appearance on radiograph, termed *porcelain gallbladder*. Chronic cholecystitis, particularly with porcelain gallbladder, is thought to predispose to adenocarcinoma of the gallbladder. In an occasional patient, impaction of a large stone in the cystic duct with persistent obstruction of the cystic duct may gradually lead to distention of the gallbladder with clear mucus, a condition termed *gallbladder hydrops (mucocele)*. Calcium salts may become concentrated in the hydropic gallbladder, producing a limy or milk-of-calcium bile which may be visible on plain abdominal radiographs.

Rarely in chronic cholecystitis a large gallstone erodes through the wall of the gallbladder or common bile duct into the duodenum, producing a *choledochoduodenal fistula*. In the absence of prior biliary surgery, this unusual condition is strongly suggested by the finding of *air in the biliary tree on plain radiography*. The large stone frequently impacts in the ileum, and patients then present with small bowel obstruction, a phenomenon termed *gallstone ileus*. Fistulization also can occur into other structures adjacent to the gallbladder such as colon, stomach, or abdominal wall.

Gallstones in the common bile duct (choledocholithiasis) may impact at the level of the ampulla of Vater to produce obstructive jaundice and biliary colic (see Fig. 126–5C). Bacterial infection above an obstructing stone in the common bile duct is common and leads to *ascending cholangitis*. Patients with ascending cholangitis typically present with acute onset of high fever and signs of sepsis, associated with right upper quadrant pain and tenderness as well as jaundice (Charcot's triad). Leukocytosis with shift to the left, conjugated hyperbilirubinemia, abnormally high alkaline phosphatase, and elevated AST and ALT are commonly seen laboratory abnormalities. Bacteria often can be cultured from the blood. In severe cases, pus may be present in the biliary tree and patients may de-

velop multiple hepatic abscesses. The usual pathogens observed in ascending cholangitis are enteric gram-negative bacteria, anaerobes, or occasionally enterococci. Antibiotics are indicated but frequently fail to control sepsis in severe, suppurative cases. Symptoms usually respond rapidly to biliary drainage via surgical, radiographic, or endoscopic means. Endoscopic sphincterotomy with stone extraction and/or temporary stent placement currently is the least invasive and most rapid way of achieving biliary decompression in most cases of ascending cholangitis.

Attacks of *acute pancreatitis* may be triggered by passage of a gallstone through the papilla of Vater. The pathogenesis of acute gallstone pancreatitis is not completely understood. It has been speculated that transient obstruction of the pancreatic duct orifice where it joins the common bile duct leads to an increase in pancreatic ductal pressure, which may cause premature activation of proteolytic enzymes within the pancreatic acinar cells. Gallstones are responsible for most cases of pancreatitis in the nonalcoholic. Recent data suggest that episodes of recurrent acute pancreatitis previously thought to be idiopathic may be caused by small gallstones below the limits of detection with common imaging techniques. Gallstone-induced pancreatitis is among the most catastrophic complications of gallstones. A full discussion of gallstone pancreatitis is found in Ch. 107.

Diagnostic Studies in Gallstone Disease

A variety of diagnostic imaging studies are of value in patients with suspected gallbladder disease (Fig. 126–7). Plain radiographs may reveal calcium-containing (pigment) gallstones, which are usually radiopaque. Occasionally foci of calcification either in the core or around the rim also can be seen in predominantly cholesterol stones. Air in the biliary tree can be caused by gas-forming organisms or by fistulas between the bowel and biliary tract. Calcification of the gallbladder ("porcelain gallbladder") indicates chronic cholecystitis.

US is a sensitive, specific, noninvasive, and inexpensive test for diagnosing gallstones. In general, US is the only procedure needed to diagnose gallstones in the gallbladder. The typical gallstone on US appears as an echogenic focus that casts a sound "shadow." Biliary sludge also is diffusely echogenic and located in the dependent gallbladder but lacks acoustic shadowing. In acute cholecystitis US may reveal edema of the gallbladder wall and pericholecystic fluid. The accuracy of US in diagnosing gallstones is about 95%; however, it does not provide accurate information on the type of gallstone (cholesterol versus pigmented), number of gallstones, and cystic duct obstruction. US often fails to image stones in the common bile duct but may provide clues to the presence of choledocholithiasis such as dilatation of the major bile ducts.

The oral cholecystogram (OCG) is a diagnostic procedure in which patients are given an oral radiocontrast agent, iopanoic acid. The contrast is absorbed from the intestine, taken up by the liver, and secreted into the bile. When concentrated by the gallbladder overnight, the contrast agent outlines most of the gallbladder. Radiolucent gallstones appear as negative shadows within the gallbladder. Failure of the gallbladder to visualize generally suggests chronic cholecystitis with loss of gallbladder mucosal function or cystic duct obstruction. Acute and chronic liver disease may also be associated with failure to visualize the gallbladder. The size and type of stones can be estimated with reasonable accuracy by this test. Typical cholesterol gallstones are radiolucent and floating. Because of more extensive information provided by oral cholecystography on the type and size of gallstones and gallbladder visualization, this procedure should be used in evaluating patients for medical gallstone therapies.

Hepatobiliary radionuclide scans employ a variety of iminodiacetic acid (IDA) derivatives (for example, HIDA, DISIDA, or PIPIDA) to assess the patency of the cystic duct and the common bile duct. These organic anions are administered intravenously, taken up by the liver, and excreted rapidly into bile. Failure of these agents to enter the gallbladder or the intestine suggests obstruction of the cystic or common bile duct, respectively. This test is very useful in diagnosing cholecystitis with cystic duct obstruction.

Contrast material may be injected directly into the biliary tree via either a percutaneous, fluoroscopically guided approach (PTC), or a retrograde approach (ERCP). These tests represent the gold standard for examining the biliary tree and generally reveal stones or

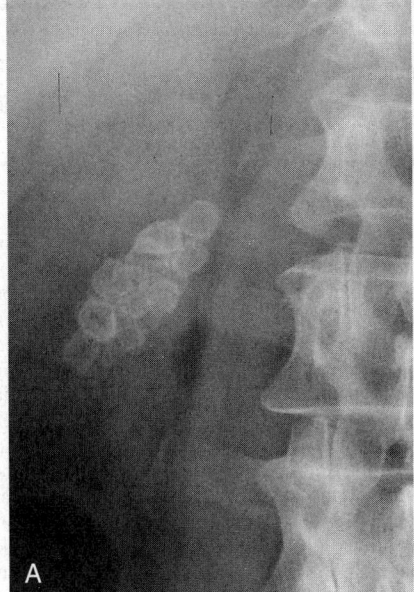
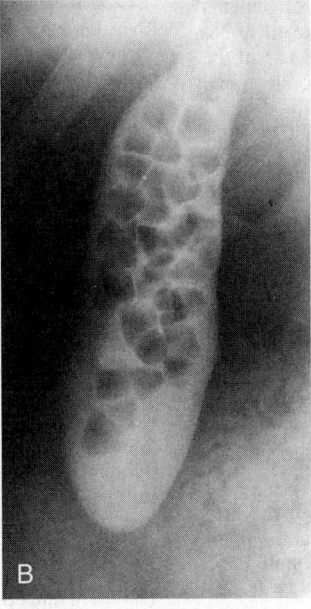
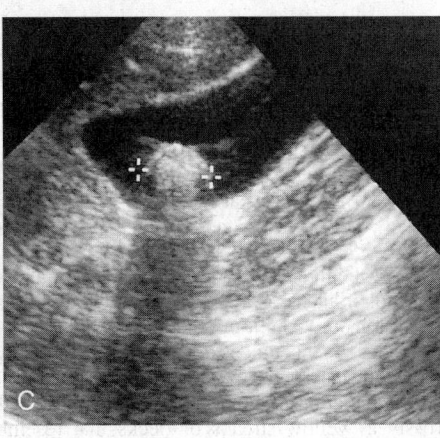

FIGURE 126–7. Images of gallstones. *A*, Plain radiograph reveals calcified pigment gallstones. The more common cholesterol gallstones are not detectable on plain radiography. *B*, Oral cholecystogram showing contrast material outlining multiple radiolucent cholesterol stones in a normally functioning gallbladder. *C*, Ultrasound examination showing a large gallstone as an echogenic focus in the gallbladder which casts a sonic "shadow."

narrowing (stenosis) in the common bile duct not detectable by other means. In occasional patients in whom gallstones are strongly suspected but all routine studies are negative, microscopic examination of a sample of bile aspirated at ERCP may reveal the presence of crystals of calcium bilirubinate or cholesterol.

Therapy

In general, no treatment is required for asymptomatic gallstones in most cases because of their low propensity to become symptomatic. Longitudinal studies have shown that conversion from asymptomatic to symptomatic stones takes place at the rate of no more than 1 to 2% per year, and risk-benefit analyses indicate that surgery for asymptomatic gallstones generally causes more morbidity than it prevents. Exceptions to this rule may include very large gallstones (>3 cm in diameter) and porcelain gallbladder, both of which have been associated with an increased risk of gallbladder carcinoma. Some experts also recommend prophylactic cholecystectomy for asymptomatic gallstones in patients with diabetes mellitus or spinal cord injury because gallstone complications such as acute cholecystitis may be more severe and more often life-threatening in these groups.

Symptomatic gallstones are cured by cholecystectomy. Surgically removing the gallbladder is indicated in all instances of acute cholecystitis or in symptomatic patients with nonvisualized gallbladder on OCG. Laparoscopic cholecystectomy in the last 5 years has largely replaced open cholecystectomy in most US hospitals. This therapy is now preferred because of shorter hospitalization time and quicker recovery. Serious bile duct injury, often requiring reconstructive surgery, occurs in about 0.5% of cases.

The surgeon may remove gallstones in the common bile duct at the time of cholecystectomy. In the past this required common bile duct exploration, which adds significantly to postoperative complications and recovery time. More recently, development of methods for direct choledochoscopy and stone extraction during surgery have reduced the need for common duct exploration. Alternatively, stones up to 1.5 cm in diameter can be extracted from the common bile duct by endoscopic methods following endoscopic sphincterotomy. Larger stones can be crushed and extracted in pieces. These techniques are valuable when patients are acutely ill with ascending cholangitis or acute pancreatitis, or when stones are inadvertently left in the common duct after cholecystectomy.

Ascending cholangitis is treated aggressively with antibiotics and endoscopic sphincterotomy, which removes the obstructed stones and allows for normalization of bile flow. The drainage of infected bile combined with appropriate antibiotic therapy results in quick

recovery, after which the patient ordinarily should have an elective cholecystectomy. In patients at high surgical risk, cholecystectomy can be deferred indefinitely after sphincterotomy and stone extraction with only a few percent per year risk of subsequent gallstone complications.

Cholesterol gallstones may also be treated medically. Oral administration of certain bile salts (chenodeoxycholic or ursodeoxycholic acid) reduces biliary cholesterol saturation. When bile becomes unsaturated, stones in the gallbladder may slowly dissolve. Bile salt therapy is most successful in patients with pure cholesterol gallstones and does not work with calcified stones. Other critical factors for success include small stones, a normally functioning gallbladder, and adequate bile salt dosage. In an ideal group of patients with small, radiolucent, floating stones, 75% complete dissolution of gallstones within 1 year has been observed. Chenodeoxycholic acid is moderately toxic; it may cause mild to moderate elevations of liver function tests and serum cholesterol. In therapeutic doses chenodeoxycholic acid is frequently associated with disabling diarrhea. Because of these side effects, the use of chenodeoxycholic acid in patients with gallstones has been abandoned in this country. Ursodeoxycholic acid is as efficacious in dissolving gallstones as chenodeoxycholic acid but has practically no side effects. Because oral dissolution therapy is slow and sometimes unsuccessful, it generally is reserved for patients with mildly symptomatic gallstones who are at high risk for surgery or who are otherwise reluctant to undergo cholecystectomy. Ursodeoxycholic acid is also effective for primary prevention of rapidly forming gallstones in patients with morbid obesity who are experiencing rapid weight loss after medical or surgical treatment. Prophylactic ursodeoxycholic acid during this period reduces gallstone incidence by >80%.

Experimental medical therapies for gallstones include solvent dissolution and extracorporeal shock wave lithotripsy (ESWL). Cholesterol gallstones can be dissolved rapidly (within hours) with organic solvents such as methyl-tert-butyl ether or ethyl propionate, instilled directly into the gallbladder by percutaneous transhepatic approach. The dissolution rate for noncalcified stones using this modality is close to 100% and the side effects are few. This approach has not gained wide acceptance because of its invasive nature and labor intensity. ESWL was first introduced with great success for treatment of renal stones and later, in the mid-1980's, was modified to permit shattering of stones in the gallbladder. Gallstone fragments following lithotripsy are eliminated with bile or can be dissolved with concurrent oral bile salt treatment. This therapy is particularly effective for solitary gallstones. Biliary colic following ESWL occurs relatively frequently as a result of elimination of small fragments of pulverized stones, and in about 1% of patients treated, passage of stone fragments causes acute pancreatitis. No gallstone lithotripsy device has been approved for general use in the United States, and with the advent of laparoscopic cholecystectomy, this technology has largely been abandoned. A major limitation of all medical treatments of cholesterol gallstones (bile salt dissolution, solvent dissolution, lithotripsy) is gallstone recurrence, which averages about 50% over 5 years.

Other Benign Disorders of the Gallbladder

A number of benign gallbladder wall abnormalities sometimes may mimic cholelithiasis. *Cholesterolosis* of the gallbladder is usually an asymptomatic condition in which cholesterol accumulates within histiocytes in the mucosa of the gallbladder. Aggregates of these lipid-laden macrophages distend and enlarge the mucosal folds. The accumulation of lipid at the tips of these folds is readily visible grossly as yellow streaks or flecks that resemble the seeds of a strawberry, hence the common name "strawberry gallbladder." There is usually no inflammation or calculi. Focal aggregation of cholesterol-laden macrophages may produce polyps that may be visible on US. Other benign gallbladder lesions that may produce polyps of the gallbladder wall include benign *adenomas* and *adenomyomatous hyperplasia*. In general, these lesions are asymptomatic and require no treatment.

Postcholecystectomy Disorders

A small fraction of patients develop generally mild diarrhea following cholecystectomy. Increased circulation of the bile salt pool with increased delivery of bile salts to the colon has been implicated in postcholecystectomy diarrhea, and patients with this syndrome often respond well to treatment with cholestyramine. More difficult is the problem of recurrent upper abdominal pain, noted in about 5% of patients following cholecystectomy. In some instances pain may be secondary to retained gallstones in the common bile duct, abscess, or other complications of surgery. In the absence of such a specific cause, biliary-type pain following gallbladder removal is termed "post-cholecystectomy syndrome." This term is a misnomer because in most cases pain probably is unrelated to gallstones or cholecystectomy but rather is due to an error in the original diagnosis. The prevalence of gallstones is so great that many patients with abdominal pain from other causes are coincidentally found to have gallstones. When these patients undergo cholecystectomy, persistence of symptoms is not surprising. Recurrence of abdominal pain following cholecystectomy should lead the physician to consider other, overlooked causes of pain such as irritable bowel syndrome, peptic ulcer, pancreatitis, and biliary dyskinesia.

Biliary Dyskinesia

Biliary dyskinesia refers to a syndrome of repeated attacks of biliary colic resulting from motor dysfunction of the sphincter of Oddi. The sphincter of Oddi is a major factor in regulating the delivery of bile into the duodenum. Bile flow is regulated by a combi-

TABLE 126–3. CRITERIA FOR DIAGNOSIS OF BILIARY DYSKINESIA

Right upper quadrant pain associated with transient elevation of alkaline phosphatase, bilirubin, AST, and ALT
Diameter of common bile duct >11 mm (ultrasound)
Delayed emptying of common bile duct (>45 min) after ERCP or quantitative hepatobiliary scintigraphy
Elevated basal sphincter of Oddi pressure (by manometry)

nation of phasic contractions superimposed on tonic pressure. The motor activity of the sphincter of Oddi is influenced by hormonal and neural factors. Cholecystokinin is the principal hormone that regulates the sphincter of Oddi (relaxes it) and gallbladder (contracts it). After cholecystectomy with loss of the gallbladder reservoir, modest increases normally have been noted in the sphincter of Oddi tone, bile ductal pressure, and common bile ductal diameter. Rarely patients may develop abnormalities of sphincter of Oddi function, including increased basal tone or increased amplitude and frequency of phasic contraction, which may episodically impede efflux of bile and trigger typical attacks of biliary colic. The association of sphincter of Oddi motor abnormalities with symptoms and signs of functional biliary obstruction is termed biliary dyskinesia. The criteria for diagnosis of biliary dyskinesia are shown in Table 126–3. Clinically, biliary dyskinesia produces episodic right upper quadrant abdominal pain mimicking an attack of choledocholithiasis. The diagnosis is suspected when symptoms and laboratory abnormalities suggest intermittent common bile duct obstruction at the level of the papilla of Vater (elevated alkaline phosphatase, AST and/or bilirubin, dilatation of the common bile duct), but cholangiography reveals no evidence of gallstones. Additional objective signs that support this diagnosis are delayed emptying of the common bile duct at ERCP and abnormal sphincter of Oddi manometry showing an increase in basal pressure to >40 mm Hg. Once the diagnosis is established, endoscopic sphincterotomy is the therapy of choice.

American College of Physicians: Guidelines for the treatment of gallstones. Ann Intern Med 119:620, 1993. *A concise summary of the natural history of gallstone disease with current recommendations for medical and surgical treatment.*

Bergash NV, Jones EA: The pruritus of cholestasis. Semin Liver Dis 13:319, 1993. *Reviews current theories regarding pathogenesis of pruritus in cholestasis, with particular emphasis on the role of endogenous opiates.*

Heuman DM, Moore EW, Vlahcevic ZR: Pathogenesis and dissolution of gallstones. *In* Zakim D, Boyer DT (eds.): Hepatology. 3rd ed. Philadelphia, WB Saunders, 1996. *A current review of gallstone science, with particular emphasis on determinants of cholesterol and calcium secretion and solubility in bile and medical approaches to gallstone dissolution.*

Reichen J, Simon FR: Cholestasis. *In* Arias IM, et al.: Liver: Biology and Pathobiology, New York, Raven Press, 1994. *Summarizes research findings regarding the pathophysiology of cholestasis.*

Wiesner RH: Selection and timing of liver transplantation in primary biliary cirrhosis and primary sclerosing cholangitis. Hepatology 16:1290, 1992. *Presents mathematical models based on clinical data which describe the natural history, key prognostic factors, and optimal timing of liver transplantation in these chronic cholestatic disorders.*

127 APPROACH TO THE PATIENT WITH HEMATOLOGIC DISEASE

David G. Nathan

This introduction provides a general background to diagnostic hematology and marrow function. The remaining chapters in Part XIII emphasize fundamental physiologic principles and provide descriptions of relatively common hematologic disorders. It is hoped that the entire part will influence the reader to consider such diseases broadly and systematically.

The nonmalignant disorders of erythrocytes, phagocytes, and platelets, including their precursors and progenitors, are initially discussed. Then follows a description of the acute and chronic proliferative disorders that involve the cells of the marrow and lymphoid systems, a series of chapters that ends with a discussion of bone marrow transplantation. The final chapters of Part XIII are devoted to a review of the disorders of the fluid phase of blood coagulation and the vascular purpuras.

DIAGNOSTIC HEMATOLOGY. The circulating blood cells are the products of the terminal differentiation of recognizable precursors. In fetal life, hematopoiesis occurs throughout the reticuloendothelial system. In the normal adult, terminal differentiation of the recognizable precursors of erythrocytes, granulocytes, and platelets occurs exclusively in the marrow cavities of the axial skeleton, with some extension into the proximal femora and humeri. The space is highly expandable, however, when the demand for blood cell production is accelerated.

Observations of differentiated blood cells by enumeration and relatively simple morphologic studies of properly prepared blood films provide the essential cornerstone of diagnostic hematology. Automated blood counts and cell sizing now provide both reproducibility and enhanced diagnostic capacity. For example, early failure of red cell production may be heralded by unexpected macrocytosis. Peripheral blood cell counts and morphology offer insight into the rate of effective hematopoiesis; the state of marrow nutrition with respect to vitamin B_{12}, folic acid, and iron; the presence of acquired and congenital disorders of the erythrocyte membrane; the energy metabolism of the hemoglobin of erythrocytes, which influences the rate of their destruction; the differential diagnosis of infections; the presence of allergic reactions; the acquired or congenital abnormalities of intracellular organelles; and the invasion of the marrow by malignant cells or infectious agents. The contributions of morphologic techniques to hematologic diagnosis depend entirely upon the adequacy of specimen preparation and the skill of the observer. Egregious errors are made when diagnostic pronouncements are based on inadequate material. The slavish enumeration of individual cells is rarely helpful without careful overall inspection and positive searches for diagnostic clues that are relevant to the case at hand. Morphology can be particularly misleading if the observer does not understand that many kinds of disorders induce similar changes in shape, particularly in the red cells.

Although circulating lymphocytes appear to be terminally differentiated cells, they are instead capable of rapid proliferative responses to appropriate stimuli, during which they resume the appearance of relatively undifferentiated precursors. At this stage, they are often called atypical. The functional subsets of lymphoid cells are not readily demonstrable by inspection, although "killer" lymphocyte function may be associated with larger cells that contain granules. Obtaining useful information about lymphocyte subsets requires studies of lymphocyte function and measurements with specially prepared antibodies reactive with lymphocytes.

Well-prepared marrow films and biopsy specimens also contribute important information, such as total marrow cellularity, the presence of invading malignant cells or infectious granulomas, the adequacy of the numbers of megakaryocytes, the ratio of myeloid to erythroid precursors, the state of marrow cell nutrition, the presence of abnormal storage cells, and even the deposition of abnormal crystals in metabolic diseases. In brief, the blood and marrow lend themselves to biopsy and to structural, chemical, and functional studies far more readily than do any other human organs. Their mature cellular elements are diverse, bearing in common only a joint ancestral cell, origin in the marrow, and the property of being transported through vessels suspended in plasma.

PRECURSORS OF CIRCULATING BLOOD CELLS. *Erythrocytes.* Much of the progress of differentiation of erythroid precursors can be appreciated morphologically, particularly the onset of hemoglobin synthesis and the maturation and extrusion of the nucleus. During this process, each proerythroblast may give rise to approximately eight erythrocytes. The transit time from proerythroblast to emergence of reticulocytes is approximately 5 days. The transit time may decrease during anemic stress to as few as 2 days by means of skipped divisions. The red cells that emerge under conditions of stress are macrocytic and may contain as much as 25% fetal hemoglobin (F cells). They may also bear additional fetal characteristics, particularly the presence of i antigen on their surfaces. More quantitative analyses of the transit of erythroid precursors during the process of maturation may be appreciated from the use of radioactive iron that, when injected intravenously, accumulates preferentially in the newly synthesized ferritin of proerythroblasts and ultimately emerges in peripheral blood incorporated into reticulocyte hemoglobin. The use of surface scanning following infusion of ^{59}Fe-labeled transferrin reveals the site as well as the rate of intramedullary erythropoiesis, and the rate of erythropoiesis may be estimated from the level of transferrin receptors in plasma. The use of ^{59}Fe transferrin is largely an investigative and not a clinical tool, except for cases in which the anatomic site of erythropoiesis needs to be determined, such as in myeloid metaplasia. A qualitative clinical assessment of erythroid precursor activity throughout the body may be gained from injection of indium chloride and marrow scintigraphy. Indium-111 binds to transferrin and is incorporated into immature marrow erythroid precursors. Body scanning then reveals the distribution of marrow.

Granulocytes. The process of intramedullary granulocyte maturation involves changes in nuclear configuration and the accumulation of specific intracytoplasmic granules. A model that describes the production and kinetics of neutrophils is shown in Figure 127–1 (see also Ch. 139). It is highly compartmentalized. The relatively small peripheral blood pool is divided into two compartments in equilibrium, the circulating and the marginated pools. These pools provide entrance into the tissues. The level of peripheral cells is buffered by an immense marrow reserve of identifiable precursors, some of which are in the mitotic compartment and some in the maturing and storage compartment. The kinetics of proliferation of these recognizable precursors have been studied using labeled

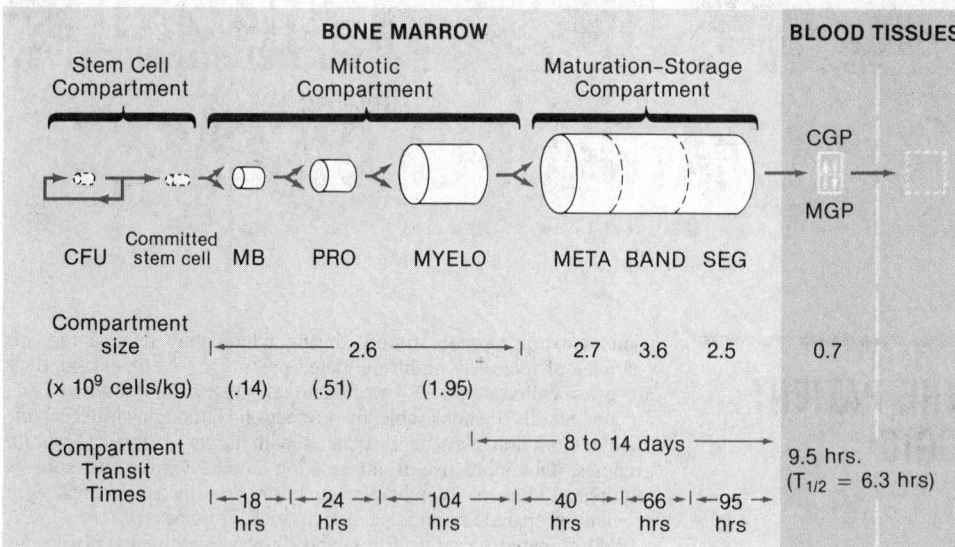

	BONE MARROW		BLOOD TISSUES

FIGURE 127–1. Model of the production and kinetics of neutrophils in humans. The marrow and blood compartments have been drawn to show their relative sizes. The compartment transit times, as derived from labeling studies with di-isopropyl phosphofluoridate ($DF^{32}P$) and tritiated thymidine, are shown on the next to last line and the last line. The less obvious symbols in the figure include CGP, the circulating granulocyte pool; MGP, the marginating granulocyte pool; CFU (colony-forming unit), the tripotential stem cell; MB, myeloblast; and PRO, promyelocyte. (From Wintrobe MM, Lee RG, et al.: Clinical Hematology. 7th ed. Philadelphia, Lea & Febiger, 1974, p 244.)

precursors of DNA. These so-called labeling indices, from which estimates of cell cycle times can be derived, have served as important approaches to the study of pharmacology and toxicity of chemotherapeutic agents.

Platelets. The differentiation of committed megakaryocytes, the precursors of platelets, involves a nuclear endoreduplication phenomenon that produces 16N and 32N megakaryoblasts. The endoreduplication ceases at the stage of the mature megakaryocyte. Platelet shedding from megakaryocytes is accomplished by the formation of multiple demarcation membranes within the cytoplasm of the cell, usually visible only by electron microscopy. Although the platelet appears to be a simple tissue fragment, its functions are diverse and hemostatically versatile. It must selectively adhere to abnormal surfaces and then sequentially secrete, aggregate, fuse, and retract to ensure a firm platelet-fibrin plug. In the process, it assists in the coagulation cascade, synthesizes prostaglandins, and releases adenosine diphosphate (ADP) and a variety of growth factors that stimulate vascular smooth muscle proliferation (see Ch. 152).

Lymphocytes. The geography of lymphocyte precursor maturation and differentiation is considerably more complex than that of the other hematopoietic cells. Primitive lymphoid precursors of B cell origin arise in the marrow, spleen, and lymph nodes, where they continue their maturation and differentiation. Primitive T cell precursors arise in the marrow; migrate to the thymus, where they undergo further differentiation; and are finally exported to the spleen, lymph nodes, and marrow, where they establish their final residence and perform many of their functions. Both T and B cells enter the peripheral blood circulation, which delivers them to tissue sites at which their functions may be required or their unbridled activity may cause disease. T cells previously "educated" in the thymus give rise to progeny that may survive for the life of the individual. Circulating lymphocytes represent only a tiny fraction of the total lymphocyte pool. Therefore, analysis of these circulating cells may not reflect the nature of the total pool.

THE HEMATOPOIETIC MICROENVIRONMENT. For clarity, we have separately described each class of blood precursor cells, but in reality they are closely packed together. The bone marrow is a vast mesh that is best described as millions of fronds of fibroblasts and endothelial cells (to be described below), which provide a lacy framework in which are embedded differentiating progenitor cells, developing precursors bound by adhesive proteins to the mesh, tissue macrophages, and T cells.

The fronds of developing marrow cells float in a bog of sluggishly moving venous blood, the so-called sinusoids. Figure 127–2 demonstrates one of the least understood, but most dramatic, aspects of hematopoiesis, the migration of completed blood cells in the fronds through gaps that exist between endothelial cells and fibroblasts to gain access to the sinusoids and on to the general circulation. Bone marrow aspiration disrupts the fronds and eliminates a view of this microanatomy, whereas marrow biopsy provides only a two-dimensional aspect that sacrifices cytology for a better, albeit imperfect, representation of architecture. The fronds of hematopoi-

etic tissue are lined by reticular cells that form the adventitial surfaces of the vascular sinuses and extend cytoplasmic processes to create a lattice for the mesh of endothelial cells and fibroblasts on which blood cells reside. The lattice is revealed by reticulin stains of marrow sections and scanning electron photomicrographs. To escape the fronds, the developing blood cells must lose their adhesiveness and do so, at least with respect to the erythroid system, by shedding fibronectin receptors to escape the sticky embrace of the microenvironment and pass into the circulation. Clumps of megakaryocytes are found adjacent to marrow sinuses. They shed platelets, the products of their cytoplasm, directly into the lumen. This situation avoids the requirement for movement of bulky megakaryocytes, a mobility characteristic of the granuloid and erythroid differentiated precursors as they approach the point at which they egress from the marrow.

KINETICS OF HEMATOPOIESIS. The marrow microenvironment supporting the progenitors and precursors must provide for the normal steady-state rates of renewal of the cellular elements of blood. Under homeostatic conditions, the production rates precisely equal destruction rates. The average lifespan of a human red cell is approximately 120 days. This means that approximately 5×10^4 red cells must be produced per day per microliter of blood in an adult. The average lifespan of platelets is 7 to 10 days, for a daily production rate of 2×10^4 platelets per microliter of blood. The white blood cell compartment exhibits more complex kinetics. Granulocytes are rapidly turned over, with an approximate intravascular lifespan of 6 to 12 hours in humans. To maintain a level of circulating granulocytes of 5×10^3 per microliter requires a daily production that is roughly comparable to that of red cells and platelets, approximately 2×10^4 cells per microliter of blood. At the opposite extreme in terms of lifespan are lymphocytes, some of which can exhibit lifetimes measured in months, or even years. This long lifespan of lymphocytes suggests that the daily renewal of certain lymphocyte progenitors occurs at a rate substantially lower than that of the progenitors of the other formed elements of blood. The various symptoms of complete marrow failure are closely related to the lifespan and the turnover of the peripheral cells of the blood. Thus, patients with complete marrow failure initially lose granulocytes and therefore usually present with enhanced susceptibility to infection. Bleeding caused by platelet deficiency rapidly follows, and finally pallor and symptoms of anemia occur. Loss of circulating lymphocytes and cellular immune function is an unusual event in such circumstances and represents severe and longstanding marrow failure.

The turnover of red cells and platelets can be measured for diagnostic purposes, using $Na_2^{51}CrO_4$ as a labeling agent. Both the red cell and the platelet lifespans can be estimated and the site of the red cell destruction determined. This is sometimes a useful maneuver in decisions regarding splenectomy.

HEMATOPOIETIC PROGENITORS. The recognizable marrow precursors of the differentiated peripheral blood cells tend to occupy the attention of hematologists, but they are rarely primary

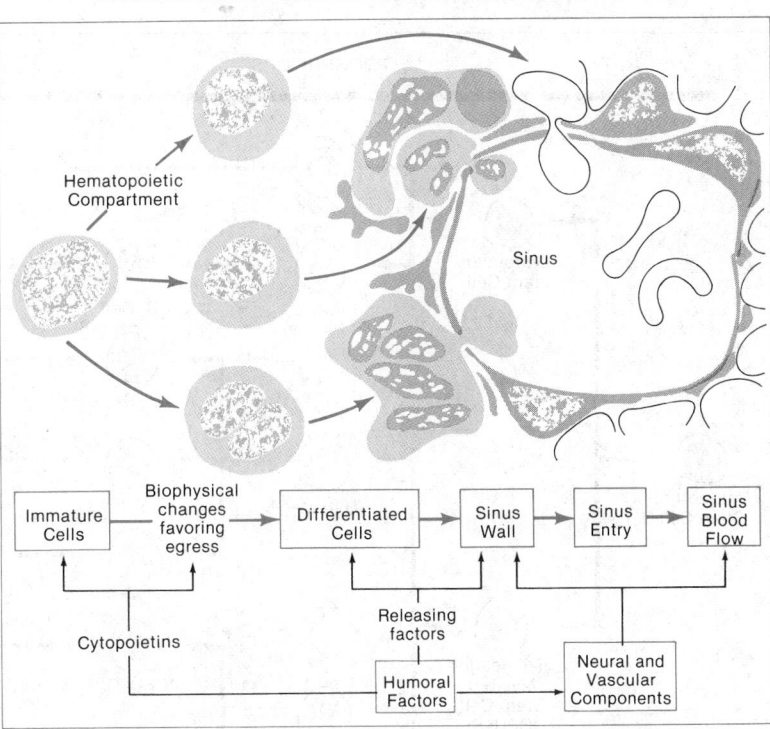

FIGURE 127–2. A schematic diagram of the factors that may be involved in controlling the release of marrow cells. The central relationship between the hematopoietic compartment and the marrow sinus is depicted. The drawing highlights the similarity of the egress process for the three major hematopoietic cells: reticulocytes in the top pathway, granulocytes and monocytes in the center pathway, and platelets in the lower pathway. Immature cells undergo biophysical changes under the influence of cytopoietins that favor egress. In the case of reticulocytes, enucleation precedes egress. This is shown by the solid black inclusion in the perisinal macrophage, representing nucleophagocytosis antecedent to digestion of the erythroblast nucleus. The cytoplasmic protrusion of the megakaryocyte presumably detaches itself from the cell and will further fragment into platelets in the circulation. (From Lichtman MA, Chamberlain JK, Santillo PA: *In* Silber R, LoBue J, Gordon AS [eds.]: The Year in Hematology, 1978. New York, Plenum Medical Book Company, 1978, p 274.)

causes of the hematopoietic cytopenias. It is true that various toxins, cytotoxic antibodies, or nutritional deficiencies can so seriously damage the orderly progression of precursor differentiation that effective production of fully differentiated cells is embarrassed. In general, however, deficient or excessive production of blood cells is due to abnormalities of *undifferentiated progenitor cells.* They must themselves undergo vital processes of maturation and amplification to give rise to the recognizable precursors of circulating differentiated blood cells.

Progenitor Maturation. The hematopoietic progenitor system can be envisaged as a continuum of functional compartments (Fig. 127–3). The most primitive compartment is made up of very rare cells with high self-renewal capacity. These are so-called pluripotent stem cells (PSC's). These PSC's randomly (or stochastically) give rise to more mature stem cells that are committed to either lymphoid or myeloid development. But the fidelity of these commitments is not absolute. Hence, lymphoid surface markers may be expressed on myeloid leukemic cells. Lymphoid stem cells give rise to T and B cell precursors and their mature progeny (see Ch. 221).

Trilineage myeloid stem cells are called CFU-S, for the spleen colony-forming unit described by Till and McCulloch in mice. They observed hematopoietic colonies in the spleens of lethally irradiated mice rescued with bone marrow cells of histoidentical donors. The spleen colonies contained megakaryocyte, granulocyte, and erythroid precursors. Following bone marrow transplantation in mice with a limited number of PSC's, a process of so-called clonal equilibration takes place, in which the progeny of some PSC's are extinguished while other PSC's begin to populate the marrow. A subset of the grafted pluripotent stem cells then dominates hematopoiesis.

Trilineage myeloid stem cells (CFU-S) eventually give rise to the committed single-lineage progenitors of the recognizable precursors through a random process of lineage restriction, shown in Figure 128–3 as a stepwise process. Actually, this represents a random set of choices that eventuate in progenitors that are restricted to single-lineage development. The restriction is probably due to the cell-surface expression of lineage-specific growth factor receptors. These single-lineage progenitors, including erythroid burst-forming units (BFU-E), erythroid colony-forming units (CFU-E), megakaryocyte colony-forming units (CFU-Meg), and basophil, granulocyte, monocyte, and eosinophil colony-forming units (CFU-Baso, CFU-G, CFU-M, and CFU-Eo, respectively), proliferate and differentiate to their respective precursors in response to the growth factors that bind to their unique receptors. The capacity of lineage-specific committed progenitors to proliferate and differentiate in response to demand constitutes the most important buffer of the hematopoietic system against increased requirement for mature blood cell production. Little is known about the cell biology of progenitors because their rarity makes their purification extremely difficult. Such purification has been recently accomplished to a considerable extent in mice, and the antibody to the cell-surface antigen CD-34 has been useful in achieving partial purification of progenitors in humans.

Hematopoietic Growth Factors. The proliferation, differentiation, and survival of immature hematopoietic progenitor cells are sustained by a family of glycoproteins, the hematopoietic growth factors (HGF's) (Table 127–1). In addition to their effect on the proliferation and differentiation of progenitors, these factors also influence the survival and function of mature blood cells. The HGF's are also known collectively as the colony-stimulating factors (CSF's), a term derived from the *in vitro* observation that they stimulate progenitor cells to form colonies of recognizable maturing cells. It is important to recognize that the lineage-specific HGF's, erythropoietin (EPO), G-CSF, M-CSF, and interleukin-5 (IL-5), are not active alone except in their interactions with the most mature committed progenitor cells. The majority of lineage-specific progenitors demand the presence of either IL-3 or GM-CSF in addition to a lineage-specific HGF to produce the colonies for which they are programmed. Hence, immature committed progenitors bear receptors for both IL-3 and GM-CSF. They differ from one another with respect to their lineage-specific receptors.

The genes for several human HGF's have been cloned, and this, in turn, has led to the production and purification of the respective recombinant proteins. This advance in molecular biology has allowed intensive investigations of the actions of purfied HGF's, their cellular origins, and their regulatory mechanisms (Fig. 127–4), while the availability of large quantities of highly purified HGF's has led to preclinical and clinical evaluation of their effectiveness *in vivo.* In general, IL-3 and GM-CSF stimulate the survival, proliferation, and differentiation of a broad range of progenitors, if lineage-specific HGF's are also present. Stem cells may also be stimulated by three other interleukins, IL-1, IL-4, and IL-6, but the actions of these factors may be indirect or may require the presence of other cytokines. Stem cell replication and differentiation are also influenced by Steel factor (SF), which additionally stimulates the growth of mature progenitors. Interleukin-6 is particularly interesting because in combination with IL-3 it reduces the time during which blast cells in culture begin to divide to form colonies, suggesting that the combination influences stem cell cycling. It may also synergize with IL-3 or GM-CSF to induce megakaryocyte differentiation. Figure 127–4 emphasizes the interaction of the most important

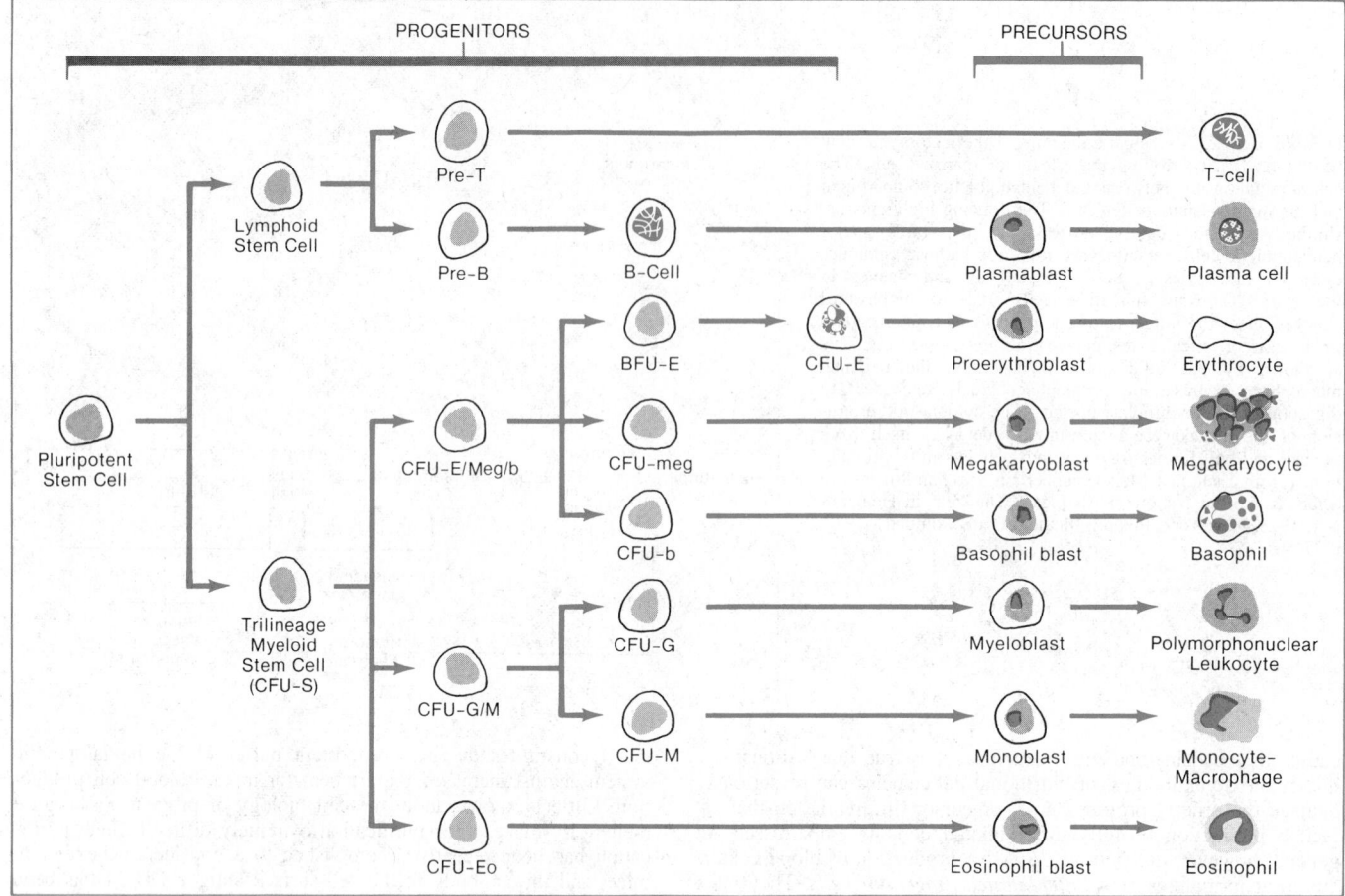

FIGURE 127–3. A schematic outline of the progenitor basis of hematopoiesis. Note the progressive restriction in the potential for terminal differentiation of the progenitors as they mature from left to right in the drawing. They finally form the recognizable marrow precursors from which the circulating blood cells, shown on the far right, are derived. Not shown in this outline is the process of self-renewal of fractions of the progenitor cell populations, particularly the immature progenitors. Also not shown is the progressive amplification of progenitors and precursors as they mature and differentiate. The bipotential erythroid-megakaryocyte progenitor shown in this drawing and referred to in the text has been demonstrated in the mouse, but not definitely in humans.

HGF's with progenitor cells. Note the requirement for combinations of IL-3 and/or GM-CSF with lineage-specific growth factors for the induction of specific precursors. The newest hematopoietic growth factor is thrombopoietin (TPO). It is the most potent stimulator of CFU-Meg and will soon be evaluated clinically.

The bottom of Figure 127–4 summarizes the cells of origin of the HGF's and demonstrates that the monocyte and T cell play an important role in progenitor differentiation. Monocytes produce IL-1 and tumor necrosis factor (TNF) in response to bacterial prod-

ucts. These in turn stimulate fibroblasts and endothelial cells to produce all of the HGF's except IL-3, IL-5, EPO, and TPO, the latter two of which are hormones made in the kidney and liver, respectively. Antigens of various kinds stimulate T cells to produce IL-3 and IL-5, as well as GM-CSF. All of these growth factors in turn interact with their specific progenitors to produce the developing blood cells. As mentioned above, fibroblasts and endothelial cells are not merely factories of growth factors. They also provide a critically important adherent layer on which progenitor differentiation

TABLE 127–1. CHARACTERISTICS OF SOME HUMAN HEMATOPOIETIC GROWTH FACTORS

Growth Factor*	Cellular Source	Progenitor Cell Target†	Mature Cell Target
SF (IL-3)	T lymphocytes	CFU-Blast, CFR-GEMM, CFU-GM, CFU-G, CFU-M, CFU-Eo, CFU-Meg, CFU-Baso, BFU-E	Eosinophils, monocytes
GM-CSF	T lymphocytes, monocytes, fibroblasts, endothelial cells	CFU-Blast, CFU-GEMM, CFU-GM, CFU-G, CFU-M, CRU-Eo, CFU-Meg, BFU-E	Granulocytes, eosinophils, monocytes
G-CSF	Monocytes, fibroblasts, endothelial cells	CFU-G	Granulocytes
M-CSF	Monocytes, fibroblasts, endothelial cells, uterus	CFU-M	Monocytes
EPO	Peritubular cells of the kidney, Kupffer cells	CFU-E, late BFU-E?, CFU-Meg	None
IL-5	T lymphocytes	CFU-Eo	Eosinophils
IL-11	Fibroblasts, endothelial cells	CFU-Meg	Platelets
TPO	Liver	CFU-Meg	Platelets

* SF = steel factor; IL-3 = interleukin-3; GM-CSF = granulocyte-macrophage colony-stimulating factor; G-CSF = granulocyte colony-stimulating factor; M-CSF = macrophage colony-stimulating factor; IL-5 = interleukin-5; IL-11 = interleukin-11; and TPO = thrombopoietin.

† CFU-Blast = Colony-forming unit—blast; CFU-GEMM = colony-forming unit—granulocyte, erythrocyte, monocyte, and megakaryocyte; CFU-GM = colony-forming unit—granulocyte and macrophage; CFU-Eo = colony-forming unit—eosinophil; CFU-Meg = colony-forming unit—megakaryocyte; BFU-E = burst-forming unit—erythroid; CFU-G = colony-forming unit—granulocyte; CFU-M = colony-forming unit—macrophage; CFU-E = colony-forming unit—erythroid; and CFU-Baso = colony-forming unit—basophil.

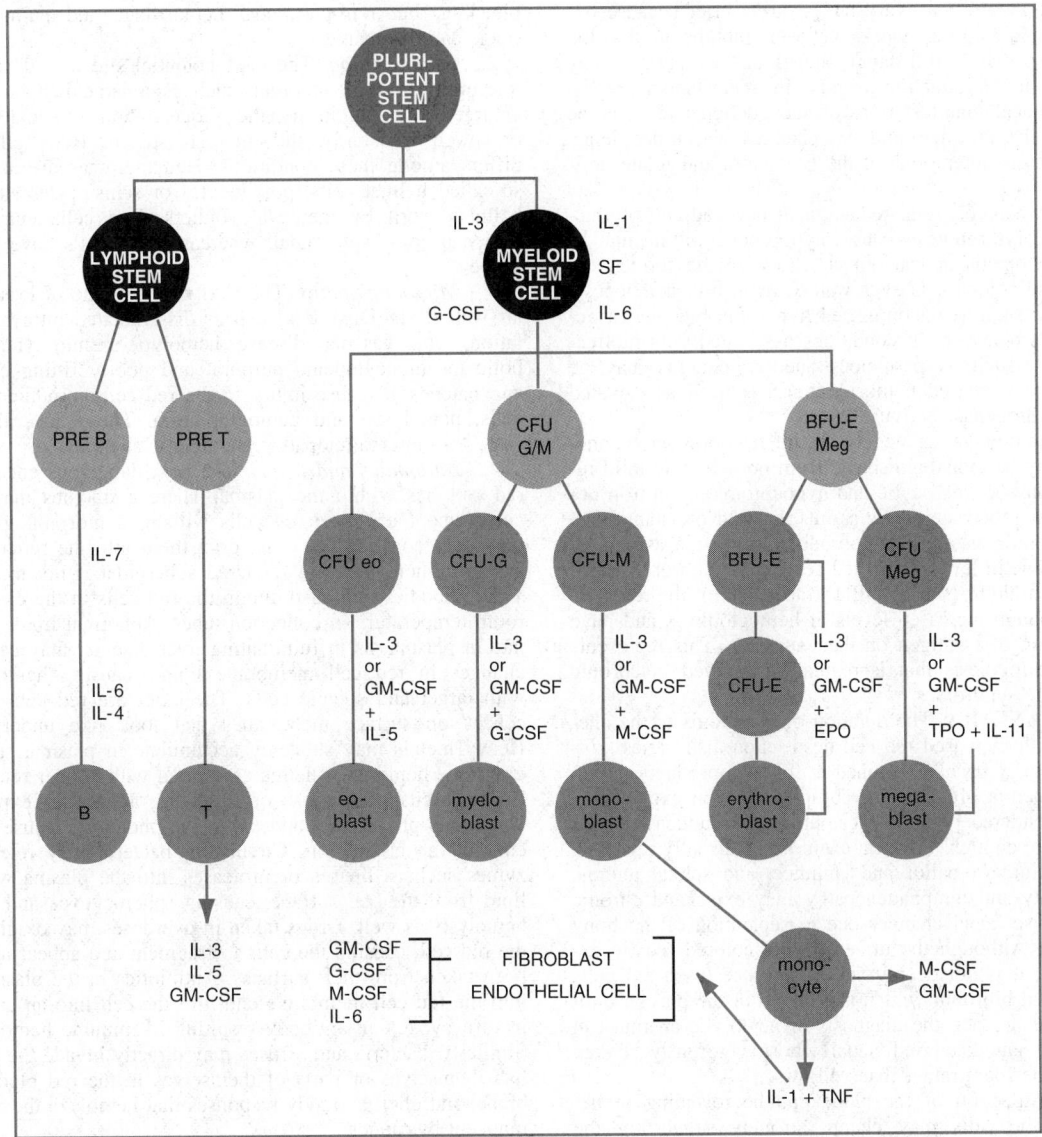

FIGURE 127–4. The hematopoietic progenitors and growth factors. The differentiation of hematopoietic progenitors is shown, beginning with the pluripotent stem cell. The myeloid stem cell differentiates randomly into the CFU-G/M, BFU-E/meg, and CFU-Eo lineages. The rate of differentiation is influenced by IL-3 (interleukin 3) and IL-6 and perhaps by G-CSF (colony-stimulating factor) and IL-1. The synergistic effects of IL-5, G-CSF, M-CSF, and IL-6 with either IL-3 or GM-CSF are shown. The production of growth factors is demonstrated at the bottom of the figure. See footnote to Table 127–1 for definition of the growth factors.

must take place. Fibronectin is a key component of the microenvironment because it binds progenitors to fibroblasts and endothelial cells through fibronectin receptors.

THERAPEUTIC APPLICATIONS. Thus far, three HGF's have shown promise in clinical trials. GM-CSF regularly elevates the granulocyte count in a dose-dependent fashion in patients with acquired immunodeficiency syndrome (AIDS) and shows promise as well in the management of aplastic anemia in children. It may also be useful in protocols involving autotransplantation following intensive chemotherapy, and GM-CSF and G-CSF stimulate the circulation of progenitors in the peripheral blood. G-CSF is also useful in granulocytopenia associated with chemotherapy and has shown distinct promise in the treatment of severe congenital neutropenia. Erythropoietin markedly reduces the transfusion requirements of patients undergoing chronic dialysis for renal failure. Its application in other disorders requiring red cell transfusion, including autotransfusion, is currently under study.

Bazan JF: Haemopoietic receptors and helical cytokines. Immunol Today 11:350, 1990.
Boulay J-L, Paul WE: Hematopoietin sub-family classification based on size, gene organization and sequence homology. Curr Biol 3:573, 1993.
Clark SC: The lymphohematopoietic cytokines. *In* Nathan DG, Oski FA (eds.): Hematology of Infancy and Childhood. Philadelphia, WB Saunders, 1993, p 1078.
Cosman D, Lyman SD, Idzerda RL, et al.: A new cytokine receptor superfamily. Trends Biochem Sci 15:265, 1990.
Metcalf D: Hematopoietic regulators—redundancy or subtlety? Blood 82:3515, 1993.
Ogawa M: Differentiation and proliferation of hematopoietic stem cells. Blood 81:2844, 1993.
Sieff CA, Nathan DG: The anatomy and physiology of hematopoiesis. *In* Nathan DG, Oski FA (eds.): Hematology of Infancy and Childhood. Philadelphia, WB Saunders, 1993, p 156.

128 HEMOLYTIC DISORDERS: INTRODUCTION
David G. Nathan

Anemia results from either a low production or an increased rate of destruction of red cells or a combination of both. The differential diagnosis of decreased production versus increased destruction is relatively easily made if one considers the following criteria.

HYPOPRODUCTION ANEMIA. (see also Ch. 129 to 133). Patients with decreased production of red cells are usually pale, with little evidence of jaundice or organomegly. The duration of their symptoms of fatigue may vary but is rarely brief because hypoproduction anemia requires weeks or even months to develop (the red cell life span is > 100 days). Nutritional deficiencies may be responsible for hypoproduction anemias in a substantial proportion of cases. Physical manifestations of such deficiencies may be evident, including the nail, hair, and skin changes of iron deficiency and the lip and tongue alterations of the B vitamin and folate deficiencies.

Irrespective of whether a total reduction in new red cell production or ineffective erythropoiesis causes hypoproduction anemia, an absolute reticulocytopenia appears in all cases. In the former, the serum has a normal color (or is even watery, as in iron deficiency), and lacks evidence such as unconjugated hyperbilirubinemia of accelerated red cell production. In conditions associated with ineffective erythropoiesis, such as pernicious anemia, patients may be jaundiced and have increased hemosiderinuria as well as elevated serum lactate dehydrogenase activity.

Red cell morphology varies widely in the hypoproduction anemias. The cells may be indistinguishable from normal as in mild renal failure; they may be microcytic and hypochromic as in iron deficiency; or they may be macrocytic as in folic acid or vitamin B_{12} deficiency. In chronic, sustained hypoproduction anemia associated with high erythropoietin levels (pure red cell anemia, chronic aplastic anemia or, in children, Diamond-Blackfan anemia), the red cells are macrocytic, contain increased levels of hemoglobin F, and have increased expression of i antigen on their surfaces. This represents the fetal-type erythropoiesis that is regularly observed in chronic bone marrow failure syndromes.

HEMOLYTIC ANEMIA. The duration of symptoms of the anemias associated with increased red cell destruction also varies. Unlike the gradual history usually obtained in the hypoproduction anemias, hemolytic anemia often begins abruptly or even explosively. Patients may be rendered prostrate in hours if the sudden red cell destruction is severe enough. Physical examination usually reveals a sallow hue, a mixture of pallor and jaundice, and scleral icterus. Hepatosplenomegaly and lymphadenopathy may exist, and chronic hemolysis may cause facial changes due to separation of the bony plates of the skull. Although the urine may be colored red by excreted hemoglobin, it is not deeply yellow because lysed red cells release unconjugated bilirubin, which is retained in the plasma until excreted in the bile. In fact, the diagnosis of hemolytic anemia can be inferred in any jaundiced individual whose vigorously shaken urine produces white foam rather than yellow.

Simple visual inspection of the blood can be revealing in hemolytic anemia. The cells may clump, strongly suggesting the presence of an agglutinating antibody that is active at room temperature. Unfortunately, measurement of hematocrit by centrifugation is rarely performed because automatic blood counting machines now dominate clinical laboratories. But inspection of an hematocrit tube following centrifugation can be diagnostically valuable. A dark layer of red cells at the bottom of the tube indicates sickle cell anemia, the most dehydrated of the cells having migrated to the bottom of the tube. The cells are dark because of their low oxygen affinity. The buffy coat is often increased in hemolytic anemia because platelet production may be stimulated. The color of the plasma may be revealing; a yellow hue suggests hyperbilirubinemia, a brown color indicates methemalbumin, and a red tint suggests red cell lysis. The microscopic appearance of polychromatophilic red cells and reticulocytosis often suggest a specific diagnosis.

The differential diagnosis of the specific causes of hemolytic anemia should always be considered in every case. Although long lists of inciting agents can be memorized by physicians with agile brains, such an approach usually fails. A broad consideration of the fate of red cells in the circulation brings better results.

1. *Bleeding.* If one looks at the body from the outside toward the red cells, the first danger to the cell is the integrity of the vascular wall itself. A hole in a large blood vessel allows a rapid loss of red cells. Therefore, the first differential point is to distinguish acute hemolytic anemia from acute bleeding. Both may be associated with normal red cell morphology and reticulocytosis with thrombocytosis and neutrophilia. The bleeding patient, however, shows no indirect hyperbilirubinemia and no increase in circulating

enzymes of red cell origin. One must evaluate all potential sites of bleeding. It is simple to exclude gastrointestinal and urinary tract bleeding, but retroperitoneal hemorrhage and pulmonary hemorrhage can be elusive.

2. *Sequestration.* The next potential site of red cell loss is sequestration within an organ such as a large hemangioma, a very enlarged liver as in hepatic sequestration in sickle cell anemia or, more frequently, an enlarged spleen. Red cell morphology differs among these conditions. Hemangiomas are associated with so-called helmet cells, poikilocytes or schistocytes shaped like the helmets worn by medieval soldiers. Red cells entrapped in the spleen become spheroidal, whereas sickle cells have their nominal shapes.

3. *Microangiopathy.* The next potential site of loss is the vascular wall itself. Disorders such as disseminated intravascular coagulation, renal vascular disease, hemolytic-uremic syndrome, thrombotic thrombocytopenic purpura, and poorly fitting cardiac valves and patches all cause injury to the red cells, producing helmet red cells, hemolysis, and hemoglobinuria. These are called "schistocytic" or "microangiopathic" hemolytic anemias.

4. *Antibodies and toxins.* The next dangerous encounter for the red cell lies within the plasma. There antibodies may directly fix complement and lyse red cells without a morphologic change, or they may coat red cells and drag them into the reticuloendothelial system, where they are rendered spheroidal if not totally ingested. The antibodies may also clump the red cells in the circulation or at room temperature in collection tubes. Abnormal lipids that accumulate in plasma, as in fulminating liver disease, may cause profound changes in red cell membrane lipids, causing hemolytic anemia with target and spicule cells. The latter are red cells with excrescences on surface membranes that look like underwater mines. Heavy metals may suddenly accumulate in plasma, such as in the explosive hemolytic anemia associated with copper release from the liver in Wilson's disease or following arsine gas exposure. These conditions produce a nondescript morphology because the lysis occurs in the circulation. Circulating bacteria may release lytic enzymes such as lipases or proteases into the plasma which remove lipid from the cell surface, causing spherocytosis and intravascular hemolysis as well. Drugs taken in overdoses may oxidize and injure the red cell, causing the cells to fragment and appear as if bites had been taken from their surfaces. Antibiotics in the plasma may soak into the red cell membrane and turn the cell into an antigen, which in turn evokes an antibody resulting in immune hemolytic anemia. Similarly, bacteria and viruses may directly invade the blood, establish themselves or parts of themselves in the red blood cell membrane, and elicit antibody responses that hemolyze the red cell as an innocent bystander.

5. *Intrinsic membrane disease.* The red cell may also be endangered by disorders of its own membrane. Most such conditions are inherited, such as hereditary spherocytosis, elliptocytosis, and the rare disorders of cation permeability. By contrast, paroxysmal nocturnal hemoglobinuria is an acquired disease of the red cell membrane due to the clonal loss of a protein that anchors other proteins to the red cell membrane by a phosphatidylinositol linkage. One such protein is decay accelerating factor (DAF). Loss of DAF allows complement to lyse the cell within the circulation. There is no morphologic defect.

6. *Internal defects.* The last site of danger for the red cell is its own internal milieu. The cell can be damaged by a paucity of its own enzymes. By far the most common is glucose-6-phosphate dehydrogenase deficiency, which renders red cells susceptible to standard doses of oxidant drugs. Pyruvate kinase deficiency is much less common and causes deficient glycolysis and ATP instability. A few enzyme deficiencies are so rare that they can be diagnosed only in special laboratories. Finally, the red cell may be damaged by its own hemoglobin, such as occurs in thalassemia, in which the hemoglobin chains are present in an imbalanced ratio or by an abnormal hemoglobin such as sickle hemoglobin, which distorts the cell and destroys it.

If this systematic approach to differential diagnosis is kept in mind and the history, physical examination, and study of the blood are directed toward these broad possibilities, nearly all causes of hemolytic anemia can be correctly diagnosed and appropriate treatment begun before the hematologist can arrive to make more expensive suggestions.

129 AN APPROACH TO THE ANEMIAS

John Lindenbaum

Anemia is one of the most common manifestations of disease worldwide. Indeed, in some developing countries the majority of apparently normal people in certain population groups are anemic. Even in technologically advanced nations, a third or more of patients admitted to the medical service of a hospital are anemic. Yet a low hematocrit is often ignored or is put aside to be dealt with at a later time while other, more pressing medical problems are managed on an urgent basis. This practice is frequently a mistake because anemia is usually a clue that should not be ignored. In fact, the clinician should almost always think of anemia in a manner similar to the way in which he or she regards symptoms like chest pain or diarrhea—as an indicator or a manifestation of an underlying disease, rather than an entity in itself.

Physicians often use laboratory tests inappropriately in the evaluation of anemic patients. In some instances, the small number of crucial tests needed to diagnose the cause of any anemia is not obtained. In others, blood is withdrawn for a long list of unnecessary tests, often worsening the anemia without elucidating it. This chapter advocates a logical and orderly approach to anemia. Commonly encountered diagnostic challenges receive greater emphasis than rare entities. The strategy outlined allows the clinician to diagnose the cause of anemia in the great majority of patients using a small number of laboratory tests, because most anemias are caused by only a handful of conditions. The strategy also furnishes clues to the less common or more esoteric causes of anemia.

DEFINITION OF ANEMIA

Table 129–1 lists normal ranges for the hematocrit, hemoglobin concentration, and red blood cell count in adults. Any of these three tests can estimate the presence or absence of anemia. Because the hemoglobin and hematocrit usually correlate strongly with each other in anemic patients, recording both values is unnecessary. The ranges shown are arbitrary estimates of normality (as is the case for the normal range for any laboratory test) based on the mean ± 2 standard deviations (SD's) of measurements made in a presumably healthy normal population. In a given individual, the values remain remarkably constant during health within a much narrower range than that for the population. Thus, in a man whose hematocrit normally is 48 to 50%, a decline to 40%—although still within the normal range—may indicate the presence of underlying disease. Therefore, if baseline values are available, they are often useful. Also, because the normal range excludes 2.5% of the normal population, some persons with hematocrits below the lower limits shown in Table 129–1 may not actually be "anemic." Because of erythropoietic effects of androgens, the normal ranges differ significantly between men and women.

The normal ranges for the hematocrit and the MCV are higher in newborns and lower in infants during the first 24 months of life. The ranges used to define anemia in adults chronically exposed to low ambient oxygen levels at higher altitudes are also higher than those shown. For unexplained reasons, the lower limits of normal for the hematocrit in black persons are 1 to 2% lower than those for white persons. Whether the hematocrit normally declines with aging

or the slightly decreased levels seen in the elderly are indicators of occult chronic disease remains controversial. When electronic counters are used, the hematocrit is a calculated rather than a measured value and is occasionally affected by artifacts; the most common is a spurious elevation caused by cold agglutinins.

Each of the tests used to define anemia is affected by changes in the *plasma volume*. Patients with an expanded plasma volume appear to be anemic, even though the total number of circulating red cells may be normal. Such hemodilution is frequently encountered in normal pregnancy; in fluid-retaining states, such as cirrhosis of the liver and, less commonly, congestive heart failure; and in patients with splenomegaly. The hematocrit may fall as low as 28% merely because of an expansion of the plasma volume. Conversely, in an anemic patient who has a decreased plasma volume (e.g., due to dehydration), the hematocrit may lie within the normal range. The total number of circulating red cells can be measured by a radioisotope dilution method, yielding a value known as the "red cell mass." As a rule, the test is unnecessary, and used only in the evaluation of polycythemia.

CARDIOVASCULAR ADJUSTMENTS TO ANEMIA

The circulating erythrocyte is a nonreplicating, differentiated cell with a normal average lifespan of 120 days. Its function is to deliver oxygen to the tissues. Therefore, the main consequence of anemia is tissue hypoxia. When anemia develops slowly, several adjustments tend to maintain tissue oxygenation. The plasma volume increases to maintain the total blood volume at a normal or only slightly reduced level. Early in the development of anemia, the glycolytic intermediate, 2,3-diphosphoglycerate (2,3-DPG), increases in erythrocytes. The 2,3-DPG binds to hemoglobin, causing a rightward shift in the oxyhemoglobin dissociation curve, which allows more oxygen to be unloaded from the erythrocyte at any given blood oxygen tension.

With more severe anemia, compensatory peripheral vascular dilatation increases blood flow to the tissues, through a fall in the systemic vascular resistance and an increase in the cardiac output. The latter mainly results from an increased cardiac stroke volume because the heart rate increases only slightly, if at all, in most anemic patients. An increase in cardiac output is usually seen only in severe anemia, when the hematocrit falls to levels of about 20% or less. As a result of the decrease in peripheral resistance, the blood pressure falls modestly, especially the diastolic component, leading to an increased pulse pressure. The systolic pressure, although often reduced from the baseline value of the patient, typically remains normal. Not infrequently, a patient with previous hypertension who develops severe anemia (due, for example, to deficiency of iron or vitamin B_{12}) becomes unexpectedly normotensive; hypertension then recurs after the anemia is corrected. Similarly, correction of anemia due to renal failure by treatment with erythropoietin may cause or exacerbate hypertension. In a minority of anemic patients (usually but not invariably those with underlying cardiovascular disease), the demands of the high output state coupled with impaired coronary oxygenation lead to circulatory congestion, in some cases without an associated fall in output ("high output failure").

The cardiovascular adjustments described above arise when anemia develops slowly. In patients with acute blood loss, however (e.g., massive gastrointestinal bleeding), there is no time for them to occur. Instead, the intravascular volume suddenly contracts, which may cause severe postural hypotension, a fall in cardiac output, the shunting of blood from the skin to central organs, sweating, restlessness, thirst, and air hunger (see Ch. 95). This life-threatening emergency must be managed by immediate restoration of intravascular volume, usually by transfusing red cells. In contrast, in the chronically anemic patient, who often has a relatively well maintained central intravascular volume, blood transfusions may expand the central blood volume and precipitate or worsen congestive heart failure, particularly in elderly patients with heart disease.

SYMPTOMS AND SIGNS OF ANEMIA

The complaints caused by anemia relate to tissue hypoxia. In patients with chronically developing anemia, the hematocrit level at which symptoms appear varies widely, influenced by the rate of development of anemia, the age of the patient, and the presence of underlying vascular disease. Frequent symptoms include dyspnea

TABLE 129–1. NORMAL RANGES* OF ERYTHROCYTE MEASUREMENTS IN ADULTS

Test	Females	Males
Hematocrit (%)	36–48	40–52
Hemoglobin (grams/dl)	12.0–16.0	13.5–17.7
Red blood cells ($\times 10^{6}/\mu l$)	4.0–5.4	4.5–6.0
Mean cell volume (fl)	80–100	80–100

* Ranges of values measured by Coulter electronic counting representing 2 SD's above and below the mean for healthy white adults living at sea level.

with exertion, dizziness, light-headedness, throbbing headaches, tinnitus, palpitations, syncope, easy fatigability, disruption of sleep patterns, decrease in libido, disturbances of mood, and impaired ability to concentrate. In elderly patients with vascular disease, angina pectoris may be a prominent complaint, even with only modest reductions in hematocrit. Anemia also frequently worsens or precipitates dementia or intermittent claudication. Anorexia is common and may be accompanied by significant weight loss. *Common physical findings* in severely anemic patients include pallor of the skin and mucous membranes (a sign of limited sensitivity and specificity), modest tachycardia and increased pulse pressure, systolic ejection murmurs, venous hums, and mild peripheral edema. Retinal hemorrhages, often flamelike, may occur in severe anemia, most commonly in association with thrombocytopenia.

THE HISTORY

A careful history usually provides information crucial to diagnosing the underlying cause of anemia. The duration and time of onset of anemia or its symptoms should be determined. Onset during childhood is seen with congenital hemolytic disorders, although when anemia is not severe, these conditions may first manifest in adult life. A history of scleral icterus or gallstones, or the presence of jaundice, gallstones, or anemia in a sibling or a parent, suggests hemolysis. A history of blood loss or blood donation should be sought. Onset of the anemia during or soon after pregnancy is consistent with iron or folate deficiency. Recurrences and remissions of anemia are frequent in iron, cobalamin (vitamin B_{12}), and folate deficiencies. Pica, or excessive craving for certain (sometimes bizarre) food items, occurs with lack of iron. A history of alcohol intoxication raises a number of diagnostic considerations (see below). Paresthesias or ataxia suggests cobalamin deficiency; a sore tongue may indicate lack of cobalamin, folate, or iron. If these deficiencies are caused by celiac or tropical sprue, diarrhea or other gastrointestinal symptoms are commonly present. The patient must be questioned closely about the possible intake of various medications (Table 129–2). Often the most important aspect of the history is to search for underlying disease such as renal, liver, or endocrine disturbances; the acquired immunodeficiency syndrome (AIDS), tuberculosis, or other infections; chronic inflammatory disorders, such as rheumatoid arthritis or lupus erythematosus; or malignancies.

THE PHYSICAL EXAMINATION

Findings on physical examination that point to specific underlying etiologic mechanisms include atrophy of the tongue (in cobalamin, folate, or iron deficiencies); abnormal gait or impaired vibration sense or other sensory modalities (in cobalamin lack); scleral icterus, splenomegaly, or leg ulcers (in certain hemolytic anemias); petechiae (with thrombocytopenia of any cause, e.g., acute leukemia); and the myriad signs of primary diseases (e.g., infec-

tions, malignancies, liver disorders, hypothyroidism) that may cause a secondary anemia.

THE INITIAL LABORATORY DATA BASE

A small number of tests should be obtained on every anemic patient: the complete blood count (CBC), including the white blood cell count and differential, a platelet count, or an estimate on the smear of the numbers of platelets; a careful evaluation of red blood cell morphology on the Wright-stained blood smear; the reticulocyte count; the mean cell volume (MCV); and some measure of iron stores—the serum ferritin (preferably) or the combined determination of the serum iron and total iron-binding capacity (Table 129–3). In at least three quarters of patients, the results of these tests, combined with the history, physical examination, and other diagnostic studies guided by complaints not caused by the anemia, will identify the cause of anemia.

THE BLOOD SMEAR. Careful, expert assessment of red cell morphology on the blood smear is essential to the diagnosis of many anemias and virtually always provides useful information, even when findings are unremarkable or normal. Proper identification of the full range of clinically useful abnormalities requires a certain expertise. Blood smears are subject to both *overinterpretation* (usually because of frequent artifacts in poorly prepared smears or in inappropriate areas of well-prepared ones) and *underinterpretation* (most frequently the result of hurried interpretation by an overwhelmed routine laboratory). Therefore, the clinician must take the time to develop expertise in this area or, in most instances, demand that the hospital laboratory provide an expert assessment of the blood smear.

Red cell abnormalities useful in the diagnosis of various anemias are listed in Table 129–4. The *context* in which a particular morphologic finding is noted must be emphasized. If red cell fragmentation is the most striking abnormality on the blood smear of a patient with a high reticulocyte count, hemoglobinuria, and a poorly functioning aortic valve prosthesis, the morphologic changes strongly support the diagnosis of a traumatic hemolytic anemia. In contrast, an occasional fragmented cell in the blood smear of a patient with marked hypochromia, microcytosis, a low reticulocyte count, and a history of recent blood loss is more likely to be caused by iron deficiency. The widely used term *poikilocytosis,* to indicate variation in cell shape, is of limited usefulness. The clinician needs to know specifically which abnormalities have been noted, e.g., sickle cells, oval macrocytes, elliptocytes, or fragments. Although *polychromasia* (see Color Plate 5F, left) indicates the presence of young reticulocytes (see below), the abundance of polychromatic cells is important. An occasional polychromatic cell is often seen in severe anemias due to bone marrow failure (e.g., megaloblastic anemia, marrow infiltration by tumor). The presence of blasts in the differential white count suggests acute leukemia as the cause of a patient's anemia. Decreased numbers of platelets or white cells point toward conditions in which anemia is associated with other cytopenias (e.g., megaloblastic anemia, hypersplenism, acute leukemia, aplastic anemia).

TABLE 129–2. DRUGS AND OTHER AGENTS THAT MAY CAUSE ANEMIA

Anemia	Type of Agent	Example
Marrow aplasias	Anticancer	Antimetabolites, alkylating agents
	Anti-inflammatory	Phenylbutazone, gold
	Antibiotic	Chloramphenicol, sulfonamides
	Anticonvulsant	Phenytoin
	Other	Benzene, insectides
Macrocytic or megaloblastic states	Dihydrofolate reductase inhibitors	Methotrexate, pyrimethamine, trimethoprim, triamterene, pentamidine
	Antiviral	Zidovudine
	Anticancer	Hydroxyurea, cytosine arabinoside, alkylating agents
	Immunosuppressive	Azathioprine
	Other	Alcohol, sulfasalazine
Hemolytic	Antibiotic	Penicillin,* cephalosporins,* sulfonamides *†
	Antiarrhythmic	Procainamide,* quinidine*
	Antihypertensive	Alpha-methyldopa*
	Antimalarial	Primaquine*
	Other	Fava beans,† naphthalene,† dapsone†
Blood loss	Anti-inflammatory	Aspirin, nonsteroidal drugs
	Anticoagulants	Warfarin, heparin

* Causes antibody-induced hemolysis.
† Causes hemolysis in glucose-6-phosphate dehydrogenase (G6PD)–deficient persons. Sulfonamides also cause hemolysis in patients with unstable hemoglobins.

TABLE 129–3. THE INITIAL LABORATORY DATA BASE IN THE EVALUATION OF ANEMIA

Hematocrit
Reticulocyte count (absolute)
MCV
Blood smear
Serum ferritin level
White blood cell count and differential
Platelet count (or estimate)

MCV = mean cell volume.

ERYTHROPOIETIC RESPONSE TO ANEMIA. As tissue hypoxia develops with increasing anemia, homeostatic systems attempt to return the number of circulating red cells to normal. Although several other hormones and growth factors may influence erythrocyte production, erythropoietin, a glycoprotein, is probably the most important. Erythropoietin appears to be predominantly produced by peritubular cells of the kidney (most likely capillary endothelial cells). Other cells, possibly including hepatocytes and macrophages, may be less important sources. A heme protein present in cells sensitive to hypoxia may undergo a conformational change that in some way activates the gene for erythropoietin production. Erythropoietin released into the circulation acts mainly to stimulate the differentiation of erythroid stem cells in the bone marrow, cells that are already committed to form red cells (so-called CFU-E, or colony-forming units–erythroid). The hormone also acts on later erythroid precursors. The result is the enhanced production and release of young red cells, or *reticulocytes* (see Color Plate 5F, right).

THE RETICULOCYTE COUNT. The initial workup of every anemic patient should include a reticulocyte count as a key test. The reticulocyte, a 1- to 2-day-old cell that is continuing to synthesize protein (unlike more elderly erythrocytes), contains aggregates of ribosomes, demonstrated by a supravital stain (new methylene blue). The reticulocyte count is the percentage of such cells per 500 or 1000 cells counted, rather than an absolute number. It therefore needs to be "corrected" to make it a better index of total production of young cells. This can be done by multiplying the reticulocyte percentage times the red blood cell count. Thus, for example, in a normal person with a reticulocyte count of 1% and a red cell count of 5 million per microliter, the absolute numbers of circulating reticulocytes would be $0.01 \times 5,000,000 = 50,000$ reticulocytes per microliter. The upper limit of normal is approximately 100,000 per microliter. In contrast, in an anemic patient with a red cell count of 2 million per microliter and a reticulocyte count of 1%, the number of circulating reticulocytes would be $0.01 \times 2,000,000$, or 20,000 per microliter; although the reticulocyte percentage is the same (1%), the absolute number is markedly below normal, indicating that the bone marrow has failed to respond to the severe anemia by increasing its production of young cells.

INITIAL EVALUATION OF ANEMIA

Calculation of the absolute numbers of reticulocytes allows the clinician to make an important early decision that will shape further diagnostic thinking (Table 129–5). Anemias can be divided into those in which the marrow response to the anemia is appropriate, that is, red cell production is increased, and those in which there is an inappropriate failure of the marrow to augment cell output. An anemia in which the absolute number of reticulocytes is not increased is due to *bone marrow failure* (Table 129–5). *In most anemic patients encountered in clinical medicine, the underlying cause of the anemia is marrow failure.* The subsequent evaluation of patients with marrow failure differs markedly from that of those in whom the reticulocyte count is elevated.

The classification shown in Table 129–5, although quite useful clinically, is an oversimplification. It emphasizes the *predominant* cause of the anemia. In many anemias, more than one mechanism is operative. Thus, for example, in the anemia of chronic disease, the red cell lifespan is modestly shortened, although the primary cause of the anemia is the failure of the bone marrow to increase the number of circulating reticulocytes. Similarly, in severe anemias due to deficiencies of iron, vitamin B_{12}, or folate, or in beta-thalassemia major, the red cell lifespan may be shortened, although the primary problem is one of cell production. In addition, in many chronic hemolytic anemias, even though the bone marrow has increased its output of new cells, the marrow response is less than maximal and an element of inadequate marrow compensation may contribute to the anemia. Furthermore, when acute hemolysis or blood loss develops, the maximal reticulocyte response may be delayed for several days or as long as a week. Thus, approximately 20% of patients with an acute episode of autoimmune hemolytic anemia do not have an elevated absolute reticulocyte count at the time of admission to the hospital, although reticulocytosis develops subsequently. In patients hospitalized for several weeks, the equivalent of a unit of whole blood is often obtained as part of the diagnostic workup for various disorders. Such acute blood loss caused by multiple venesections may be superimposed upon a marrow failure anemia, frequently without evoking an adequate reticulocyte response.

ANEMIA DUE TO BONE MARROW FAILURE

RED CELL SIZE IN PATIENTS WITH MARROW FAILURE. The first question that should be asked about a patient with a marrow failure anemia is, *what is the average size of the red cells?* The MCV is measured directly by electronic counters and is usually available as part of the initial hemogram. Although the mean cell hemoglobin (MCH) and mean cell hemoglobin concentration (MCHC) are also routinely provided, they add little information of diagnostic value. The MCH varies in the same direction as the MCV in microcytic or macrocytic anemias. Moreover, the MCHC is of limited value and often is normal in patients with frank microcytic anemias. The normal range for the MCV in adults is 80 to 100 fl (femtoliters), a better working range in the classification of anemias than the more narrow ones often reported by hospital laboratories. MCV determinations may be falsely elevated by laboratory artifacts, caused by cold agglutinins, marked hyperglycemia, and extreme leukocytosis.

On the basis of the MCV, anemias due to marrow failure should be classified as normocytic, microcytic, or macrocytic (Table 129–6). In normocytic or microcytic anemias, the subsequent diagnostic evaluation differs markedly from that in macrocytic anemias.

TABLE 129–4. ABNORMALITIES ON BLOOD SMEARS IN ANEMIC PATIENTS

Abnormality	Characteristic Disorder	Found Also in Other Conditions
Hypochromia, microcytosis	Iron deficiency, thalassemias	Anemia of chronic disease, sideroblastic anemias
Macro-ovalocytes	Cobalamin and folate deficiencies	Myelodysplasias, myelofibrosis, autoimmune hemolysis
Hypersegmented neutrophils	Cobalamin and folate deficiencies	Renal failure, iron deficiency, chronic myelocytic leukemia, congenital hypersegmentation
Teardrop cells, nucleated red blood cells	Myelofibrosis	Marrow replacement by tumor, autoimmune hemolysis, megaloblastic anemias, thalassemia major
Microspherocytes	Autoimmune hemolysis, hereditary spherocytosis	Microangiopathic hemolysis, hypophosphatemia
Sickle cells	Hemoglobin SS, SC, S-thalassemia	Hemoglobin C$_{\text{Harlem}}$
Red cell fragments (schistocytes)	Microangiopathic or traumatic hemolysis	Iron deficiency, megaloblastic anemias, cancer chemotherapy
Target cells	Hemoglobin C, SC, thalassemias, liver disease	Artifact, SS disease, iron deficiency, splenectomy
Elliptocytes	Hereditary elliptocytosis	Iron deficiency, myelofibrosis, megaloblastic anemias
Burr cells (echinocytes)	Renal failure	Artifact, pyruvate kinase deficiency
Spur cells (acanthocytes)	Liver disease, abetalipoproteinemia	

TABLE 129–5. CAUSES OF ANEMIA

Cause	Absolute Reticulocyte Count
Bone marrow failure	Low or normal
Acute blood loss	High
Hemolysis	High

Normocytic Anemias Due to Marrow Failure

Normocytic anemias due to marrow failure represent the most frequent anemia encountered in clinical practice. The most common causes of normocytic anemia due to decreased cell production (Table 129–7) are iron deficiency, the anemia of chronic disease, and anemias secondary to renal, hepatic, and endocrine disorders. Less frequently, a normocytic marrow failure anemia may result from one of a variety of "primary" marrow disturbances.

IRON DEFICIENCY ANEMIA (see Ch. 132). Iron deficiency anemia is usually considered microcytic and hypochromic. As iron deficiency develops, however, the hematocrit often falls before the MCV becomes subnormal. Therefore, iron lack (especially when the hematocrit is above 30%) must always be considered in patients with normocytic marrow failure anemia. In outpatient practice, iron deficiency is a frequent cause of such an anemia. Blood smears may be entirely normal except for mild anisocytosis; or there may be a minority of microcytic cells, even though the MCV is still normal. Because most of the iron in the body is found in red cells, loss of blood (commonly from gastrointestinal or uterine sources) is usually the underlying cause of iron deficiency. Imbalances between demand and dietary supply frequently cause iron deficiency anemia in normal pregnancy, infancy, and adolescence. Rare causes include loss of hemoglobin and hemosiderin in the urine in certain hemolytic anemias (e.g., with malfunctioning valve prostheses or in paroxysmal nocturnal hemoglobinuria), intrapulmonary hemorrhage (in idiopathic pulmonary hemosiderosis), and malabsorption of iron (usually secondary to gastrectomy or to celiac or tropical sprue). Iron deficiency anemia due to primary inadequacy of iron intake in the diet is an unusual cause of anemia in adults in industrialized countries. In many developing nations, in addition to blood loss, anemia may be caused by a diet that is adequate in total iron content but contains iron in poorly bioavailable forms.

ANEMIA OF CHRONIC DISEASE (see Ch. 132). Patients who have chronic infections (e.g., tuberculosis, lung abscess), chronic inflammation (e.g., rheumatoid arthritis, systemic lupus erythematosus, inflammatory bowel disease), or underlying malignancies that are not necessarily metastatic to the bone marrow, or who have recently had major trauma or surgery often develop a characteristic anemia that is gradual in onset and usually normocytic. Typically, the anemia is mild, although in 10% of patients (usually with very severe chronic illnesses) the hematocrit may be below 20%. Red cell morphology is little changed from normal, although there may be modest anisocytosis with a few microcytes. Marked anisocytosis, poikilocytosis, or nucleated red blood cells are absent. The primary problem is failure of cell production. Relative lack of erythropoietin, sequestration of iron in macrophages, and inhibitory effects of cytokines are among the postulated causes of the marrow failure. The anemia remits when the underlying disorder clears. The presence of one of the associated chronic disorders is usually obvious. Occasionally, however, the anemia of chronic disease is the only apparent illness, and a careful search for an occult disorder, such as a malignancy or polymyalgia rheumatica, is indicated. Not all chronic conditions, however, produce the anemia of chronic disease. Uncomplicated diabetes mellitus, hypertension, asthma, ischemic heart disease, or congestive heart failure should not be considered a satisfactory explanation for anemia.

TABLE 129–6. CLASSIFICATION OF ANEMIAS DUE TO MARROW FAILURE

Type	MCV (fl)
Normocytic	80–100
Microcytic	< 80
Macrocytic	> 100

TABLE 129–7. CAUSES OF NORMOCYTIC MARROW FAILURE ANEMIAS

Iron deficiency
Anemia of chronic disease
Renal failure
Liver disease
Endocrine disorders
"Primary" marrow disorders*
   Aplasias
   Myelodysplasias
   Myelofibrosis
   Hematologic or solid tumors
   Granulomas
   HIV infection

* Marrow aspiration and biopsy are useful.

DIFFERENTIATION OF IRON DEFICIENCY ANEMIA FROM THE ANEMIA OF CHRONIC DISEASE. Iron deficiency is usually accompanied by greater variation in red cell size than is seen in the anemia of chronic disease. Accordingly, a quantitative assessment of the degree of anisocytosis, as measured by electronic cell sizing (the "red cell distribution width," or RDW), has been considered helpful in distinguishing these two common causes of marrow failure anemia. This assessment has not proved reliable. The differentiation is often aided, however, by serum tests that are influenced by the amount of iron in body stores. The most useful screening measure is the *serum ferritin* level (see Ch. 132), which is low in most patients with iron deficiency and normal or elevated in the anemia of chronic disease. A low serum ferritin value nearly always indicates iron deficiency. Unfortunately, there is an overlap zone (of approximately 20 to 150 ng per milliliter) in the lower end of the normal range that is compatible with *either* condition. Other tests frequently used for estimating iron stores are the *serum iron* and the *serum total iron-binding capacity* (TIBC). The serum iron level is typically low in both disorders, however. In chronic disease, the TIBC (an indicator of circulating levels of the iron-binding protein transferrin) is usually depressed, and in iron deficiency it is often elevated. Unfortunately, many patients with iron deficiency anemia, especially if complicated by a chronic disease, may have normal or even low levels of the TIBC. In both conditions, *the percent saturation of serum transferrin* (i.e., the serum iron divided by the TIBC × 100) is low. The test is helpful only if the value is higher than 25%, which argues against iron deficiency. The interpretation of these laboratory measures is summarized in Table 129–8. If these tests are equivocal, one should obtain direct examination of the bone marrow with histochemical staining of iron stores in macrophages to exclude iron deficiency. Alternatively, a therapeutic trial of iron can be given, repeating the hematocrit after 3 to 4 weeks. This practice may be reasonable in a patient with uncomplicated iron deficiency anemia (for example, a menstruating woman who is otherwise well but has a serum ferritin level of 35 ng per milliliter). In a patient with an underlying chronic disorder, however, if iron is given at the same time as the chronic disease is treated or spontaneously improves, the "response" of the hematocrit to iron is difficult to interpret. It is preferable to assess marrow iron stores directly before treatment because once lack of iron is proved, a search for an underlying cause of blood loss is mandated.

The serum ferritin is an acute phase reactant; it is elevated out of proportion to the amount of iron in stores in acute and chronic inflammatory disorders or malignancies (as well as liver and kidney disease). Nonetheless, the presence of some iron in stores appears to be necessary for a marked increase in the serum ferritin level to occur in association with these conditions. *An elevated or high-normal ferritin value does not occur in iron-deficient patients suffering from inflammation, malignancy, liver disease, or renal failure.* Such a ferritin result rules out the presence of coexistent iron deficiency.

ANEMIAS SECONDARY TO OTHER SYSTEMIC CONDITIONS. In addition to iron deficiency and the anemia of chronic disease, normocytic marrow failure frequently accompanies renal failure, hepatic disease, and a variety of endocrine disturbances. The anemia in such patients often resembles the anemia of chronic disease but commonly has a multifactorial cause.

TABLE 129–8. RELIABILITY OF SERUM TESTS IN PREDICTING IRON STORES

Test	Interpretation
Definitive	
Low ferritin	Deficient
High TIBC	Deficient
High normal or high ferritin	Not deficient*
Equivocal	
Low normal ferritin	Uncertain
Low serum iron	Uncertain
Low or normal TIBC	Uncertain
Low percentage	Uncertain

* Even if inflammation, malignancy, liver disease, or renal failure is present.
TIBC = total iron-binding capacity.

Renal Failure. A normocytic marrow failure anemia occurs in chronic renal insufficiency with a severity roughly (but not invariably) proportional to the degree of renal failure. Erythrocyte survival is modestly decreased; absolute reticulocyte counts are not elevated. Serum iron levels and TIBC are low or normal, and the serum ferritin level typically increases. Red cells with scalloped outlines ("burr" cells) (see Color Plate 6*F*, right) may be noted on blood smears. Failure of the kidney to elaborate erythropoietin in amounts appropriate to the degree of anemia appears to be a major cause of the anemia. In most cases, the anemia responds completely to the parenteral administration of recombinant human erythropoietin, obviating blood transfusions. Resistance to erythropoietin also probably contributes to the marrow failure state, although circulating inhibitors of erythropoiesis have not been clearly identified. In some patients with renal failure, other mechanisms such as iron deficiency also contribute to anemia. A serum ferritin level below 60 ng per milliliter in the presence of renal insufficiency strongly suggests lack of iron. Anemia in renal disease may (seldom) be caused by folate deficiency; aluminum toxicity, in which case the anemia is typically *microcytic;* partial fibrous replacement of the bone marrow in patients with severe hyperparathyroidism and osteitis fibrosa, which may be associated with leukopenia and thrombocytopenia; hypersplenism, which occasionally develops with chronic hemodialysis; and "microangiopathic hemolytic anemia" accompanied by fragmentation on blood smears and an elevated absolute reticulocyte count (with malignant hypertension, vasomotor nephropathy, acute glomerulonephritis, thrombotic thrombocytopenic purpura, and the hemolytic-uremic syndrome).

Liver Disease. Any chronic liver disease may cause an associated anemia of the type seen in other chronic diseases, but additional mechanisms are also often important. For example, anemia caused by acute blood loss may occur, and iron deficiency may eventually supervene owing to continuing hemorrhage. A variety of hemolytic states are also seen, including "spur cell" anemia, in which irregularly contracted red cells, or *acanthocytes,* are seen on blood smears in tandem with brisk hemolysis in advanced liver disease; autoimmune hemolytic anemia accompanying acute viral or chronic active hepatitis; acute hemolysis caused by profound hypophosphatemia in alcoholics; and, rarely, acute hemolytic states associated with alcoholic hepatitis. Chronic alcoholics (regardless of the presence of liver disease) are highly prone to develop megaloblastic anemia due to folate deficiency, as well as sideroblastic anemia. Chronic infections, such as tuberculosis and lung abscesses, may cause an anemia of chronic disease. Anemic patients with liver disease require careful evaluation with particular attention to the MCV, reticulocyte count, and blood smear, to determine likely contributory factors. In alcoholics the anemia is *usually* multifactorial. The term "anemia of liver disease" should be abandoned in favor of more precise diagnostic thinking. Also, in many patients with portal hypertension and an expanded plasma volume, the hematocrit may be moderately decreased, even though the number of circulating red cells is normal ("hemodilution").

Endocrine Disorders. A mild normocytic anemia occurs in some patients with endocrine disturbances. One quarter of patients with *hypothyroidism* are anemic. The red cell lifespan is normal, and there is no reticulocytosis. In many patients the anemia responds to hormone replacement therapy. Such anemias are usually normocytic, although in a minority the MCV may be mildly elevated and may return to normal after treatment with thyroid prepa-

rations. Another cause of macrocytic marrow failure anemia in hypothyroidism is pernicious anemia due to associated autoimmune gastritis. When microcytic anemia occurs, iron deficiency is the rule. Ferritin synthesis may be depressed as a result of insufficient thyroid hormone action, and the serum ferritin level may not be a reliable indicator of iron stores in hypothyroid patients.

A mild normocytic marrow failure anemia is characteristic in *hypopituitarism* and also may occur in *primary adrenal insufficiency,* often masked by a contracted plasma volume due to dehydration. A normocytic marrow failure anemia is also encountered in a few patients with *thyrotoxicosis,* although some may have a low MCV. In either event, the anemia remits after suppression of thyroid hyperactivity. Occasional patients with *hyperparathyroidism* have a mild normocytic anemia due to marrow failure.

"PRIMARY MARROW DISORDERS." When iron deficiency and anemia related to systemic diseases have been excluded, there remains a minority of normocytic marrow failure anemias that are caused by primary disturbances of the bone marrow (see Table 129–7). These include rare disorders in which developing red cells are absent or markedly diminished in the bone marrow (aplastic anemia, pure red cell aplasia) or in which there are increased marrow erythroid precursors that fail to mature normally, so-called ineffective erythropoiesis (sideroblastic anemias, other myelodysplasias); replacement of the bone marrow by fibrosis or a variety of hematologic and solid tumors or granulomas; and a poorly understood marrow failure state that may be associated with AIDS. (Most patients with AIDS develop the anemia typical of chronic disease; in others ineffective erythropoiesis, often associated with neutropenia, occurs.) In most patients with these marrow disturbances, certain features of the initial laboratory data base strongly suggest that the problem is something other than iron deficiency, the anemia of chronic disease, or anemia secondary to renal, hepatic, or endocrine dysfunction. Clues include depression of the platelet count, white blood cell count, or both; abnormalities in the white cell differential; significant numbers of nucleated erythrocytes on the blood smear; marked abnormalities in red cell morphology, especially significant poikilocytosis; and a normal or increased serum iron level with an above-normal saturation of transferrin. In the normocytic anemias due to primary disturbances of marrow function, *bone marrow aspiration* and *biopsy* (see Color Plates 5 to 8) often provide highly useful diagnostic information, whereas in the previously discussed causes of normocytic anemia, marrow examination is rarely useful. These primary marrow disorders may, on occasion, also present as a *macrocytic* marrow failure anemia.

Microcytic Anemias Due to Marrow Failure

In contrast to the potentially complex considerations in normocytic anemias, the differential diagnosis of marrow failure associated with a low MCV is relatively straightforward (Table 129–9). Two major conditions commonly cause marrow failure with microcytic anemia—iron deficiency and the anemia of chronic disease. Although most patients with the anemia of chronic disease have a normal MCV, mean red cell size is slightly decreased in approximately 30%, with the MCV in the range of 70 to 80 fl. An MCV lower than 70 fl is almost always due to iron deficiency or thalassemia. With severe iron deficiency, the MCV may fall as low as 50 fl, and the smear may contain marked anisocytosis and poikilocytosis. Serum tests of iron status provide results similar to those found when iron deficiency and the anemia of chronic disease occur with a normal MCV (see Table 129–8).

THALASSEMIAS (see Ch. 136). In these disorders, decreased synthesis of either the alpha or the beta chain of hemoglobin occurs. The resultant imbalance in globin chain formation leads to a decreased rate of hemoglobin production as well as microcytosis. In

TABLE 129–9. CAUSES OF MICROCYTIC MARROW FAILURE ANEMIAS

Common	Rare
Iron deficiency	Aluminum toxicity
Anemia of chronic disease	Thyrotoxicosis
Thalassemias	Hereditary sideroblastic anemias

homozygous beta-thalassemia, which manifests in childhood, a severe microcytic anemia results owing to a combination of ineffective erythropoiesis and a shortened red cell lifespan. Reticulocytosis is modest, although grossly inadequate. In *heterozygous beta-thalassemia,* anemia is frequently absent, or only mild in degree, although the MCV is low. In some patients the blood smear may show target cells, basophilic stippling, anisocytosis, and poikilocytosis; in others the smear is unremarkable, with a uniform population of small red cells with little anisocytosis. The reticulocyte count is normal or minimally elevated, and the serum ferritin, iron, and TIBC values are normal. The disorder is usually detected when a CBC, including an MCV, is obtained during the evaluation of some other medical problem. *Alpha-thalassemia* is more varied because four genes contribute to alpha globin chain synthesis. When three alpha chain genes are deleted or abnormal, a moderate hemolytic anemia develops, with microcytosis and the formation of β_4 tetramers (hemoglobin H disease). This anemia sometimes occurs as an acquired disorder in association with acute leukemia or myelodysplastic states. Much more commonly, *heterozygous alpha-thalassemia* with two-chain deletion is encountered, particularly in American blacks, 3% of whom are affected. Typically, affected patients have a low MCV and a normal blood smear and iron studies and are not anemic. In some the hematocrit may be slightly decreased. A common error in attempting to diagnose heterozygous thalassemic states is to obtain a routine hemoglobin electrophoresis, which is normal. Instead, the conditions can be differentiated by specific measurement of the hemoglobin A_2 concentration, which is usually elevated in patients with beta-thalassemia but is normal or reduced in those with alpha-thalassemia. There is no readily available test for alpha-thalassemia. It should be suspected in blacks and patients from Southeast Asia with microcytosis. Family members also often have microcytosis without anemia.

RARE CAUSES OF MARROW FAILURE WITH MICROCYTIC ANEMIAS. *Aluminum toxicity* in patients with renal failure who receive aluminum-containing phosphate binders can result in a microcytic marrow failure anemia by an unknown mechanism. Aluminum overload may cause resistance to erythropoietin therapy in chronically hemodialyzed patients (even those with a normal MCV). *Thyrotoxicosis* may occasionally result in a mild microcytic anemia. Although the MCV is normal or elevated in the acquired sideroblastic anemias, mean red cell size is decreased in the rare *hereditary sideroblastic anemias,* which may appear in childhood or adult life.

Macrocytic Anemias Due to Marrow Failure (see Ch. 133)

Macrocytic anemias due to bone marrow failure (Table 129–10) are common. Major clinical clues include the recent use of alcohol, exposure to chemotherapeutic or immunosuppressive drugs, and evidence of liver disease, glossitis, or neurologic signs and symptoms. In most macrocytic anemias, the blood smear contains round macrocytes without multilobed granulocytes. On the other hand, *the combination of macro-ovalocytes and hypersegmented neutrophils strongly suggests the presence of cobalamin or folate deficiency.* Rarely this dual abnormality also may follow chemotherapy with methotrexate or cytosine arabinoside, or occur in myelodysplasias or acute myelocytic leukemia (see Color Plate 6*G* and *H*). The reticulocyte count is also a useful early test in patients with macrocytosis. Because of the slightly increased size of young erythrocytes, brisk *reticulocytosis* (an uncorrected count of ≥10%) caused by hemolysis or blood loss often causes a modest elevation of the MCV.

TABLE 129–10. CAUSES OF MACROCYTIC MARROW FAILURE ANEMIAS

Megaloblastic anemias
    Cobalamin and folate deficiencies
    Congenital disorders
Alcoholism
Drugs (see Table 129–2)
Liver disease
"Primary" marrow disorders (see Table 129–7)
Hypothyroidism
Artifactual MCV elevations

MEGALOBLASTIC ANEMIAS (see Ch. 133). Megaloblastic anemias due to a disturbance in DNA synthesis caused by cobalamin or folate deficiency account for only 5 to 10% of macrocytic anemias with marrow failure. Early recognition is important, because they respond promptly to treatment and if neglected lead to irreversible neurologic damage if there is lack of cobalamin. As with most other causes of macrocytic anemia, the MCV becomes elevated early in the development of cobalamin or folate deficiency, before a lowered hematocrit is evident. A distinction should be made between the hematologic and biochemical profiles of patients with *early* cobalamin or folate deficiency (with little or no anemia) and the classic textbook manifestations of severe megaloblastic anemia. With severe anemia, blood smears typically contain marked anisocytosis and poikilocytosis (often including teardrop erythrocytes, microcytes, and red cell fragments). The consequences of ineffective erythropoiesis (destruction of red cell precursors in the bone marrow) may simulate a hemolytic anemia, with decreased or absent plasma haptoglobin values, elevated serum unconjugated bilirubin levels, sometimes exceptionally high serum lactate dehydrogenase (LDH) levels, and an elevated serum iron level with an increased transferrin saturation. In such severely deficient patients, marrow failure often causes thrombocytopenia and (sometimes) neutropenia. In any moderately or severely anemic patient with pancytopenia, the presence of cobalamin and folate deficiency should always be considered. Patients with deficiency of cobalamin or folate who have little or no anemia often have minimal changes on the blood smear. A few macro-ovalocytes and only rare hypersegmented neutrophils in blood smears may be overlooked by routine hospital laboratories. In addition, there may be normal values for serum LDH, bilirubin, haptoglobin, white cell count, and platelet count. In cobalamin deficiency, severe involvement of the tongue or nervous system may occur early or late relative to the hematologic manifestations, so that patients with advanced neurologic impairment may not have developed anemia or even a clear-cut elevation of the MCV.

Radioisotopic assays of serum cobalamin and folate levels are valuable in diagnosis (see Ch. 133). A serum cobalamin level should be measured in any patient with neutrophil hypersegmentation, macro-ovalocytes, atrophic glossitis, or a neurologic disorder compatible with cobalamin deficiency, as well as in virtually all patients with an elevated MCV in the absence of reticulocytosis. Possible exceptions to this rule are those treated with drugs that interfere with DNA synthesis (e.g., zidovudine, azathioprine, methotrexate) in whom the MCV has been clearly documented to be normal immediately prior to beginning drug therapy. There are problems with both the specificity and the sensitivity of the vitamin assays. The serum cobalamin level is often low in patients who are not deficient in the vitamin, and it may also be depressed as a result of folate deficiency. At least 5% of patients with unequivocal clinical evidence of cobalamin deficiency have normal serum cobalamin concentrations (usually in the range of 200 to 350 pg per milliliter). The measurement of *methylmalonic acid* and *total homocysteine* in serum is very useful in the interpretation of low or low-normal serum cobalamin values when the presence of deficiency of the vitamin is not clinically obvious (see Ch. 133). There are similar problems with the *serum folate* level. The *red cell folate* concentration is a better indicator of tissue folate stores; however, it is diminished in 50% of patients with primary cobalamin deficiency and may be normal in some patients deficient in folate. Serum total homocysteine levels are almost always elevated in clinically significant folate depletion (as well as in cobalamin deficiency); however, the serum methylmalonic acid value remains normal in deficiency of folate. With the combined use of a careful history and physical examination, as well as examination of the blood smear, serum vitamin levels, and (if needed) serum metabolites, it is rarely necessary to perform a bone marrow examination to show the presence of a megaloblastic anemia. The determination of *antibodies to intrinsic factor* in serum is a useful early test in patients with cobalamin deficiency because it is positive in approximately half of those with pernicious anemia (the most common cause of lack of cobalamin) and is specific for that diagnosis, eliminating the need for a Schilling test when such antibodies are present.

Iron deficiency frequently coexists with lack of cobalamin (e.g., in patients with pernicious anemia) or folate (e.g., in pregnant patients or alcoholics). In such combined deficiency states, the MCV may be low, normal, or high, and macro-ovalocytes and hypersegmented neutrophils on blood smear may be the most important clues to the presence of a "masked" megaloblastic anemia when the MCV is low or normal.

MACROCYTOSIS OF ALCOHOLISM. The most common cause of an elevated MCV in chronic alcoholic patients is not folate deficiency, but the *macrocytosis of alcoholism.* The cause appears to be a direct effect of chronic alcohol intoxication not related to the presence of liver disease, reticulocytosis, or vitamin deficiency (which are all part of the differential diagnosis of an elevated MCV in an alcoholic). The macrocytosis does not respond to vitamin B_{12} or folic acid and disappears only after months of abstinence. The degree of MCV elevation is modest (usually ≤ 110 fl), and anemia is often absent. Round macrocytes are noted on blood smears. In many anemic patients with the macrocytosis of alcoholism, the anemia is due to some other cause (e.g., lung abscess, hepatic inflammation, or even iron deficiency), and the patient only apparently has a macrocytic anemia.

DRUG-INDUCED MACROCYTOSIS. In current clinical practice, this is the most common cause of an elevated MCV in nonalcoholic patients (see Table 129–2). Most of the drugs that cause macrocytosis interfere with DNA synthesis by erythroid precursors. These agents most commonly cause macrocytosis without anemia; a low hematocrit typically develops only after prolonged high dosage. The reticulocyte count is characteristically not increased, although slight elevations are not uncommon with sulfasalazine and azathioprine.

LIVER DISEASE. In patients with hepatic dysfunction, because of a poorly understood abnormality in serum lipoproteins, increased amounts of cholesterol and phospholipids are deposited on the membranes of circulating erythrocytes, causing an increase in surface area, which results in macrocytosis. Blood smears typically show round macrocytes and target cells. These morphologic abnormalities are benign and do not affect red cell survival.

PRIMARY MARROW DISTURBANCES. Most of the derangements involving the bone marrow that occasionally cause normocytic anemias from decreased cell production (see Table 129–7) may also cause a macrocytic marrow failure. The mechanisms underlying the macrocytosis in such diverse disorders as marrow aplasia, sideroblastic anemia, myelodysplasias, acute myeloblastic leukemia, and infiltration of the marrow by myeloma, lymphoma, or solid tumors have not been established. Macro-ovalocytes may be present in these conditions, but neutrophil hypersegmentation is extremely unusual. Aspiration and biopsy of the marrow are often crucial to establishing the cause of macrocytosis in this group of patients. Cytogenetic studies on material obtained by marrow aspiration may also be useful.

ANEMIAS ASSOCIATED WITH INCREASED RED CELL PRODUCTION

Assuming that recovery from marrow failure (e.g., pernicious anemia recently treated with an injection of vitamin B_{12}) has been excluded, patients with an absolute reticulocytosis usually have underlying blood loss or hemolysis. In these conditions, the MCV is normal or increased, although it rarely may be low in hemolytic anemias. Owing to the presence of reticulocytes, modest increments in red cell volume (usually MCV's in the range of 100 to 115 fl) are common in patients with increased cell production. Rarely, an even higher MCV is caused by artifactual clumping of red cells by a cold agglutinin. Elevations in the MCV are more common in hemolytic anemias than in acute blood loss. The diagnostic approach to the patient with an elevated reticulocyte count differs from that in patients with marrow failure. The first consideration is to rule out obvious or occult blood loss. In the absence of bleeding, evidence of an underlying hemolytic disorder must be sought utilizing a different set of diagnostic tests than in the patient with marrow failure. Even in the absence of reticulocytosis, a rapidly developing anemia cannot be due primarily to marrow failure, because of the long lifespan of the red cell. Thus, if a marked fall in hematocrit (e.g., 10% over a period of a few days) is noted, a search for blood loss or hemolysis should be initiated, regardless of the reticulocyte count. When the marrow fails, anemia develops gradually over many weeks.

HEMOLYTIC ANEMIAS (see Ch. 138)

Anemias primarily due to red cell destruction are much less common than those caused by marrow failure or blood loss. Nonetheless, after blood loss has been excluded, the possibility of a he-

molytic anemia takes center stage in the patient with an absolute reticulocytosis. At this point, a long list of laboratory tests might be ordered. Therefore, the clinician needs to make a fundamental distinction. One group of tests (Table 129–11) attempts to answer the question, *is hemolysis present?* An entirely separate, subsequent set of laboratory determinations addresses the question, *what is the cause of hemolysis?* Examples of the latter type include the Coombs test and hemoglobin electrophoresis. Such studies are often inappropriately ordered in the assessment of marrow failure or blood loss anemias. It is much more rational to obtain evidence first that the patient is actually hemolyzing before undertaking a search for various disorders that are known to cause hemolysis.

IS HEMOLYSIS PRESENT? Unfortunately, no one measure has been shown to be 100% sensitive in detecting clinically significant hemolysis. Therefore, to answer the first question, a number of tests should be obtained (Table 129–11). Hemoglobin liberated into the circulation after red cells are damaged forms a complex with circulating haptoglobin, which is rapidly removed by hepatocytes. If the capacity of the liver to compensate by synthesizing new haptoglobin is exceeded, the plasma concentration falls. Once the plasma haptoglobin reaches zero, free hemoglobin circulates and is filtered by the kidney. Modest amounts of filtered hemoglobin are taken up by renal tubular cells, which convert the iron in hemoglobin to a storage form, hemosiderin. This can be detected days later by histochemical staining of renal tubular cells that have been shed in the urine. If the amount of hemoglobin filtered exceeds the renal tubular uptake capacity, hemoglobin itself appears in the urine. This may be detected by specific laboratory assays or may be suspected when a routine urinalysis detects occult blood in the absence of hematuria. If the amount of hemoglobin excreted is great, the patient passes urine that is red, reddish-brown, or even black. In contrast, when red cells are engulfed by macrophages and digested intracellularly, the heme moiety of hemoglobin is processed to unconjugated bilirubin, which is transferred to the circulation (see Ch. 115). Lactate dehydrogenase is also released from hemolyzed cells. A distinction is sometimes made between *intravascular* and *extravascular* hemolytic states, but this is only occasionally useful. Acute intravascular hemolysis certainly occurs with a severe hemolytic transfusion reaction after ABO-incompatible blood is given. The plasma haptoglobin, however, is often decreased in states such as hereditary spherocytosis, in which red cell destruction is believed to occur primarily in splenic macrophages. Probably most hemolytic anemias reflect a combination of intravascular and extravascular events. The presence of hemoglobin or hemosiderin in the urine may reflect the *rate* of hemolysis as much as its location.

Any of the tests listed in Table 129–11 may be normal in patients with a clear-cut hemolytic anemia. In almost all patients with a hemolytic anemia, at least one of the tests listed in Table 129–11 is abnormal. Any of the findings also can be individually absent in such patients. The ability of the liver to clear a load of unconjugated bilirubin is greater in some individuals than in others. The plasma haptoglobin level is often normal in patients with acute hemolysis who have an associated illness because it is an acute-phase reactant and hepatic synthesis may be markedly stimulated. Many of the tests are also not specific for hemolysis. LDH may be released from many different injured organs; unconjugated bilirubin elevations are commonly due to Gilbert's disease; the plasma haptoglobin may be reduced on a genetic basis or due to liver dysfunction; myoglobin may cause a positive urine test for occult blood. It is rarely necessary to measure the red cell lifespan to diagnose a hemolytic anemia, because one or more of these tests will usually be positive.

TABLE 129–11. COMMONLY USED TESTS INDICATING THE PRESENCE OF HEMOLYSIS

Test	Result
Plasma haptoglobin	Decreased
Urine hemosiderin	Present
Urine hemoglobin	Present
Serum unconjugated bilirubin	Increased
Serum lactate dehydrogenase	Increased

WHAT IS THE CAUSE OF HEMOLYSIS? The list of possible causes of hemolytic states is formidably long. Many of these disorders are discussed in Ch. 134 to 136. Table 129–12 lists some hemolytic conditions that are likely to be encountered over the course of a year in an adult medical service. It is representative but not necessarily exhaustive. With so many possible causes of hemolytic anemia, the clinician must judiciously choose appropriate laboratory tests based on clues provided by the history, physical examination, and blood smear. For example, a young black man with a history of episodes of bone pain and sickle cells on the smear needs a hemoglobin electrophoresis, not a Coombs test or sucrose hemolysis determination. A previously healthy middle-aged woman who suddenly develops a severe anemia with many microspherocytes on the smear should have a Coombs test, not a hemoglobin electrophoresis, as part of the initial evaluation. In a man with malignant hypertension, evidence of hemolysis, and many red cell fragments on the blood smear, no further diagnostic studies may be required to conclude that a microangiopathic hemolytic anemia has developed secondary to damage to small blood vessels. Morphologic abnormalities (see Table 129–4) often provide highly useful clues, although in some hemolytic anemias (e.g., glucose-6-phosphate dehydrogenase [G6PD] deficiency, paroxysmal nocturnal hemoglobinuria), the blood smear may be unremarkable or nondiagnostic. In some cases, clinical judgment may supersede the laboratory results. About 10% of patients with autoimmune hemolytic anemias have a negative Coombs test, but this diagnosis may still be considered on the basis of clinical and morphologic findings.

Hemolytic anemias may appear in deceptive disguises. Hereditary spherocytosis, a common congenital disorder that can be caused by a variety of abnormalities of the major red cell skeletal protein, spectrin, is frequently so mild that little or no anemia results (see Ch. 134). Only an elevated reticulocyte count, microspherocytes on smear, and minimal splenomegaly may indicate a state of *compensated hemolysis*. Such a patient may present as an adult with bilirubin gallstones or may develop anemia for the first time when a parvovirus B19 infection of committed red cell marrow precursors (CFU-E) causes an *aplastic crisis* with a sudden loss of the compensatory reticulocytosis. This virus is the most common cause of aplastic crisis, which may occur in a number of hemolytic anemias, including sickle cell disease. The presence of continuing hemolysis no longer accompanied by reticulocytosis may rapidly lead to a life-threatening worsening of the anemia and require immediate transfusion. In the most common type of G6PD deficiency, the A variant seen in 11% of American blacks, there is no chronic hemolytic state. Anemia and hemolysis occur only acutely, after exposure to an oxidant stress, such as infection, acidosis, or certain drugs, e.g., antimalarials or sulfonamides.

TABLE 129–12. SOME RELATIVELY COMMON CAUSES OF HEMOLYTIC ANEMIA

Mechanism	Examples
Congenital	
Enzyme deficiency	Glucose-6-phosphate dehydrogenase, pyruvate kinase
Membrane skeletal protein abnormalities (e.g., spectrin)	Hereditary spherocytosis, hereditary elliptocytosis
Hemoglobinopathies	Hemoglobin SS, SC, CC, S-thalassemia
Acquired	
Antibody-induced	Autoimmune hemolysis (warm antibodies), cold agglutinin disease, hemolytic transfusion reaction
Mechanical fragmentation	Intravascular coagulation, malignant hypertension, cancer chemotherapy, malfunctioning valve prosthesis, thrombotic thrombocytopenic purpura
Membrane protein anchoring abnormality	Paroxysmal nocturnal hemoglobinuria

ANEMIA DUE TO ACUTE BLOOD LOSS

The causes and management of blood loss are discussed in other chapters. A few points are worth noting here. In the bleeding patient, a reticulocytosis is sustained until iron stores are depleted by continued chronic blood loss. In acute blood loss, however, a high reticulocyte count may not occur until a few days after the onset of bleeding. In most patients, the source of hemorrhage is clinically obvious, e.g., the gastrointestinal or genitourinary tract. The clinician must be alert to more occult sites of potentially massive blood loss, e.g., into a fractured hip or the retroperitoneal area, especially in patients with coagulation disorders or those receiving anticoagulants. Even though hemorrhage may be documented, it is worthwhile to obtain the entire initial laboratory base. The blood smear may reveal unexpected findings. It is not unusual in a bleeding alcoholic to find evidence of other coexistent causes of anemia (e.g., macro-ovalocytes and hypersegmented neutrophils). In the hemorrhaging patient with AIDS, absence of reticulocytosis may point to a coexistent marrow failure.

Because red cells are lost from the body in most bleeding patients, the tests used to demonstrate hemolysis are usually negative. With hemorrhage into an internal space, however (as with a hemothorax, hemoperitoneum, or hip fracture), the decomposed blood in the body cavity is handled in similar ways to red cells that are hemolyzed. The plasma haptoglobin may be absent and the LDH and unconjugated bilirubin elevated in patients bleeding internally. Combined with the increased reticulocyte count, these findings may lead the unwary clinician to misdiagnose a hemolytic anemia.

EXAMINATION OF THE BONE MARROW IN ANEMIC PATIENTS

In more than 90% of patients with anemia, it is unnecessary to obtain a bone marrow aspiration or biopsy if the approach advocated here is followed. In certain situations, however, the test is quite useful, such as in marrow failure anemias for definitive estimation of marrow iron stores when serum tests of iron status are equivocal. In all of the primary marrow disorders that cause normocytic and macrocytic marrow failure states (see Table 129–7), marrow aspiration and biopsy are often diagnostic. In a pancytopenia of unknown cause, it is wise to obtain an early marrow examination. If aplasia, marrow infiltration by tumor, myelofibrosis, or granulomatous infection is suspected, a greater diagnostic yield is obtained by biopsy than by aspiration (see Color Plate 5). A marrow aspirate may resolve diagnostic conundrums in patients suspected of having combined or dimorphic anemias (e.g., simultaneous iron and cobalamin deficiency, megaloblastic anemia accompanying the anemia of chronic disease). Marrow aspiration and biopsy are also indicated in monoclonal gammopathies and in any patient with a severe unexplained anemia.

BLOOD TRANSFUSION

In contrast to patients with acute hemorrhage, those with chronic anemia often have few symptoms, particularly while at rest in the hospital, and the physician should always think twice before exposing them to the risks of blood transfusion, some potentially fatal (see Ch. 138). There is no threshold level of hematocrit that mandates transfusion, and the decision to administer red blood cells must be based on the functional status and symptoms of the patient. Transfusion should never be used as a substitute for careful diagnostic evaluation that may lead to more definitive and less dangerous therapy. It may be necessary, however, to transfuse elderly anemic patients before they undergo rigorous procedures, such as colonoscopy or barium enema.

ABNORMAL MEAN CELL VOLUMES IN THE ABSENCE OF ANEMIA

With the widespread availability of electronic cell counting, patients frequently turn up with increased or decreased MCV's in the absence of anemia. Not uncommonly, an MCV elevation is ignored because the hematocrit is normal—a potentially dangerous practice, especially in patients with macrocytosis. In some instances, a minimal increase or decrease in the MCV may be compatible with no underlying disorder, because the normal range excludes 2.5% of healthy individuals at either extreme. An *elevated MCV* in the absence of anemia is most commonly a sign of chronic alcoholism (often in patients who deny it). Cobalamin or folate deficiency is another frequent cause of such an MCV increment; correct diagnosis may prevent subsequent hospitalization or avert serious nervous system damage. Drugs represent another common cause of nonanemic macrocytosis (see Table 129–2). An MCV elevation may precede the development of anemia in a patient with a myelodysplasia (e.g., a sideroblastic anemia or refractory anemia following antimetabolite therapy) or marrow aplasia (e.g., a congenital Fanconi anemia occurring in a young adult) (see Color Plate 6*I* and 6*J*). Occasionally, a modest rise in the MCV without anemia is caused by reticulocytosis in a compensated hemolytic state.

A *decreased MCV* associated with a normal hematocrit is almost always caused by heterozygous alpha- or beta-thalassemia. In some patients with polycythemia vera or polycythemia secondary to chronic hypoxia, iron stores may be outstripped by the expanding erythroid marrow. The previously elevated hematocrit then falls to the normal range as the MCV decreases. Studies of iron status are typically diagnostic of iron deficiency in these patients, and iron administration causes a return of the hematocrit to polycythemic levels. Blood loss should be ruled out before the iron depletion is merely attributed to increased internal demands. Occasionally, a patient with microcytosis and a normal hematocrit is recovering from a self-limited or treated episode of iron deficiency anemia.

Cook JK: Clinical evaluation of iron deficiency. Semin Hematol 19:6, 1982. *A clinically sophisticated review of the use of laboratory tests in the diagnosis of iron deficiency and related conditions.*

Erslev AJ, Schuster SJ, Caro J: Erythropoietin and its clinical promise. Eur J Hematol 43:367, 1989. *An excellent review of the physiology of erythropoietin and the therapeutic use of the recombinant hormone.*

Liesveld JL, Rowe JM, Lichtman MA: Variability of the erythropoietic response in autoimmune hemolytic anemia: Analysis of 109 cases. Blood 3:820, 1987. *An interesting series of antibody-induced anemias with a focus on the lag in the response of the erythroid marrow to hemolytic stress.*

Lindenbaum J: Hematologic complications of alcohol abuse. Semin Liver Dis 7:169, 1987. *A comprehensive review of the pathophysiology and clinical features of the effects of ethanol on blood cells and the hematologic syndromes seen in liver disease.*

Petz LD, Swisher SW (eds.): Clinical Practice of Transfusion Medicine. 2nd ed. New York, Churchill Livingstone, 1989. *A well-written text centered on the transfusion of blood components. Contains many nuggets of clinical wisdom and a number of interesting chapters on the pathophysiology and immunologic aspects of various anemias.*

Stabler SP, Allen RH, Savage DG, et al.: Clinical spectrum and diagnosis of cobalamin deficiency. Blood 76:871, 1990. *A large series of patients with clinically significant cobalamin deficiency as seen in current practice, including many with "atypical" presentations. Data are presented that support the use of serum metabolite values as ancillary tests in the diagnosis of deficiency of this vitamin.*

TABLE 130–1. CLASSIFICATION OF APLASTIC ANEMIA AND SINGLE CYTOPENIAS

I. Acquired aplastic anemia
Radiation
Drugs and chemicals
　Regular effects
　Idiosyncratic reactions
Viruses
　Epstein-Barr virus (infectious mononucleosis)
　Hepatitis (non-A non-B non-C hepatitis)
　Human immunodeficiency virus (AIDS)
Immune diseases
　Eosinophilic fasciitis
　Hypoimmunoglobulinemia
　Thymoma and thymic carcinoma
　Graft-versus-host disease in immunodeficiency
Paroxysmal nocturnal hemoglobinuria
Pregnancy
Idiopathic—the most frequent diagnosis

II. Inherited aplastic anemia
Fanconi's anemia
Dyskeratosis congenita
Schwachman-Diamond syndrome
Reticular dysgenesis
Amegakaryocytic thrombocytopenia
Familial aplastic anemias
　Preleukemia (e.g., monosomy 7)
Nonhematologic syndromes (Down's, Dubovitz's, Seckel's)

I. Acquired cytopenias
Anemias
　Pure red cell aplasia (see Table 130–3)
　Transient erythroblastopenia of childhood
Neutropenias
　Idiopathic
　Drugs, toxins
Thrombocytopenias
　Drugs, toxins

II. Inherited cytopenias
Anemias
　Congenital pure red cell aplasia
Neutropenias
　Kostmann's syndrome
　Schwachman-Diamond syndrome
　Reticular dysgenesis
Thrombocytopenias
　Thrombocytopenia with absence of radii
　Idiopathic amegakaryocytic thrombocytopenia

130 APLASTIC ANEMIA AND RELATED BONE MARROW FAILURE SYNDROMES

Neal S. Young

Blood counts may be low because cells are prematurely removed from the peripheral circulation or are inadequately produced in the bone marrow. Bone marrow failure occurs commonly, but is often classified by other dominant clinical or morphologic features (like the leukemias) or by specific etiology (like pernicious anemia). The term *bone marrow failure* is vague and inclusive, and it awaits redefinition with more precise understanding of pathophysiologic processes. By default, therefore, the disorders discussed in this chapter are currently defined by their marrow pathology: the fatty bone marrow of aplastic anemia, the disordered hematopoiesis of the myelodysplasias, and the fibrosis of myelofibrosis. Making inferences about disease processes from the appearance of the bone marrow is as misleading as it is inevitable, and an effort is made here to distinguish what is understood from what is conjecture.

APLASTIC ANEMIA

Definition (Table 130–1)

APLASTIC ANEMIA. Aplastic anemia is a disease of the young, with a median age at onset of about 25 years (excluding aplasia secondary to cancer chemotherapy). It must be a leading diagnosis in the pancytopenic adolescent or young adult. The bone marrow is usually readily aspirated but appears dilute on smear. The biopsy specimen (see Color Plate 5*G*), often grossly pale, shows mainly fat under the microscope, with hematopoietic cells occupying by definition less than 25% of the marrow space and, in the most serious cases, 0 to 5% (Fig. 130–1). Prognosis is determined by the degree of blood count depression. The commonly accepted standard for severe disease requires two of the following three values: (1) absolute neutrophil count (percentage of polymorphonuclear and band forms multiplied by the total white blood cell count) of less than 500 per cubic millimeter; (2) platelets less than 20,000 per cubic millimeter; and (3) reticulocyte count (corrected for hematocrit) in the presence of anemia of less than 1% (or an absolute reticulocyte count less than 40,000 per cubic millimeter).

BICYTOPENIA AND SINGLE-LINEAGE FAILURE STATES. Some patients have bone marrow hypocellularity and depression of only two of the three major blood lines; many cases progress to typical aplastic anemia. Failure of a single lineage also occurs, as in pure red blood cell aplasia (rare), amegakaryocytic thrombocytopenia (extremely rare), and agranulocytosis (not rare but usually an idiosyncratic drug reaction). Single-lineage failures show characteristic absence of a single set of recognizable precursor cells in otherwise cellular bone marrow, and in this way they are differentiated from the much more common causes of anemia (such as vitamin or iron deficiency and hemolysis) or thrombocytopenia (from peripheral destruction of platelets). The pathophysiology of the more restricted marrow failure states is probably similar to that of general bone marrow failure, but with a more mature target cell.

CONSTITUTIONAL (FANCONI'S) ANEMIA. Fanconi described children with inherited pancytopenia and marrow hypocellularity with associated anomalies of the skeletal and urogenital systems. Fanconi's anemia now is defined by specific chromosomal aberrations in cultured cells after clastogenic stress. Indeed, cytoge-

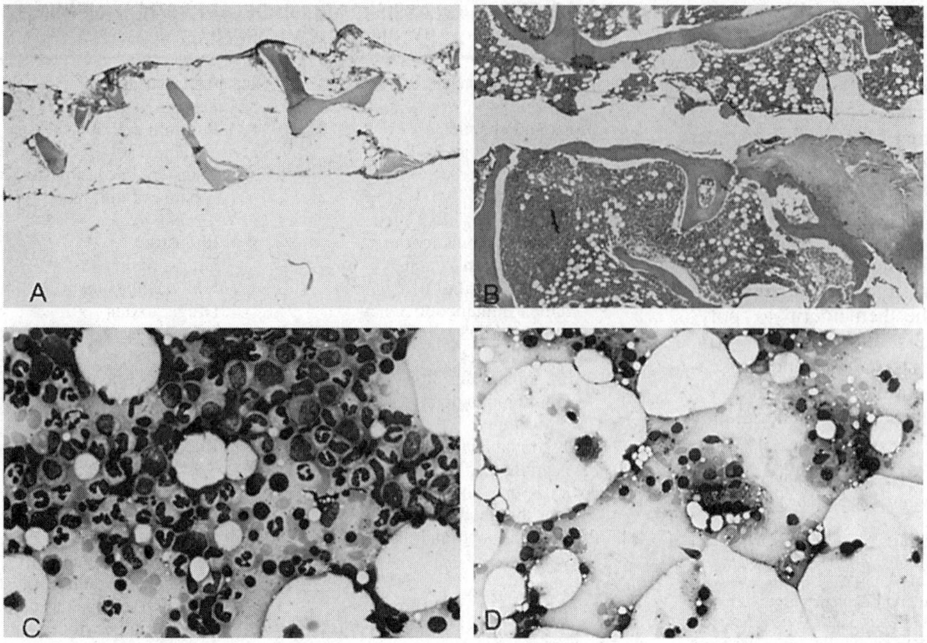

FIGURE 130-1. The bone marrow is normally 30 to 70% cellular, and there is a heterogeneous mix of myeloid, erythroid, and lymphoid cells. Marrow biopsies show (A) severe hypocellularity of aplastic anemia and (B) hypercellularity of myelodysplasia. Normal aspirate smear (C) shows a variety of hematopoietic precursor cell types, replaced in aplastic anemia (D) by fat and only residual stromal and lymphoid cells.

netic analysis of families of children with Fanconi's anemia has shown that the majority of patients lack associated anomalies and that the disease can manifest in adults, in the third and fourth decades or even later. Congenital pure red cell aplasia (Diamond-Blackfan syndrome) lacks a cytogenetic marker or associated physical abnormalities, and distinction from acquired aplastic anemia after infancy is possible only by family history. Isolated neutropenia or thrombocytopenia occurs in a number of pediatric syndromes.

Etiology

In the majority of patients, aplastic anemia is diagnosed as "idiopathic." There is little to distinguish these cases clinically from those with a presumed cause, like exposure to a drug or chemical. Even when clinical associations are established, they should not automatically be equated with etiology and pathophysiology: Association is not equivalent to cause, nor does it define a mechanism.

RADIATION. Marrow aplasia is a major acute sequela of radiation exposure. Radiant energy damages DNA. The bone marrow, as a tissue dependent on active mitosis, is particularly susceptible to its effects. Nuclear accidents and radiation injury can involve not only power plant workers but also employees of hospitals, laboratories, and industry (e.g., food sterilization, metal radiography, and so forth), as well as persons exposed to stolen, misplaced, or misused radiation sources. The radiation dose can be approximated from the rate and degree of decline in blood counts; dosimetry by reconstruction of the exposure can help to estimate the patient's prognosis and also to protect medical personnel from contact with radioactive tissue and excreta. Myelodysplasia and leukemia, but not aplastic anemia, are late effects of irradiation.

CHEMICALS (Table 130–2). Benzene has been clearly linked to bone marrow failure, being implicated in causing aplastic anemia, acute leukemias, and probably multiple myeloma. The occurrence of hematologic abnormalities is roughly correlated with cumulative exposure, but there must also be an important element of susceptibility, as only a minority of even heavily exposed workers develop evidence of benzene myelotoxicity. A history of past employment is important, especially in "open" industries in which benzene is used for a secondary purpose (usually as a solvent) rather than in "closed" industries for chemical production. Benzene-related blood diseases have declined with regulation of industrial exposure, and benzene is not generally available as a household solvent. The benzene content of gasoline increased with its unleading. The association of marrow failure with other chemicals that contain a benzene ring is much less well substantiated.

DRUGS (Table 130–2). Many of the common cancer chemotherapeutic drugs suppress the bone marrow. The mechanisms by which these drugs act offer useful clues to the pathophysiology of idiopathic aplastic anemia (see below). A very large and diverse group

of drugs is related to aplastic anemia by rare but serious idiosyncratic reactions. Some of these associations, which rest mainly on case reports, are tenuous at best. For example, some incriminated drugs may have been used to treat the first symptoms of bone marrow failure (antibiotics for fever or the preceding viral illness) or may have provoked the first symptom of a pre-existing disease (petechiae produced by nonsteroidal anti-inflammatory agents administered to a thrombocytopenic individual). In the context of total drug employment, idiosyncratic reactions, while individually devastating, are very rare events.

Chloramphenicol, the most infamous culprit, reportedly produced aplasia in only about 1 of 60,000 therapeutic courses, and even this number is almost certainly an overestimate. Chloramphenicol also consistently causes dose-related, rather modest marrow depression, mainly reticulocytopenia and altered marrow morphology and iron kinetics. This effect of chloramphenicol use is mechanistically unrelated to and clinically not predictive of the rare, severe reaction, which occurs 1 to 2 months or longer after its routine use. The introduction of chloramphenicol was thought to have produced a notable increase in the number of cases of aplastic anemia, but its diminished use has not been followed by reduced fre-

---

TABLE 130-2. SOME DRUGS AND CHEMICALS ASSOCIATED WITH APLASTIC ANEMIA

I. **Agents that regularly produce marrow depression as the major toxicity in commonly employed dose or normal exposures:**
   Cytotoxic drugs used in cancer chemotherapy: alkylating agents, antimetabolites, antimitotics
   Some antibiotics

II. **Agents that frequently but not inevitably produce marrow aplasia:**
   Benzene (and benzene-containing chemicals like kerosene, carbon tetrachloride, Stoddard's solvent, chlorophenols)

III. **Agents probably associated with aplastic anemia but with relatively low probability:**
   Insecticides
   Chloramphenicol
   Antiprotozoals: quinacrine and chloroquine, mepacrine
   Nonsteroidal anti-inflammatory drugs (including phenylbutazone, indomethacin, ibuprofen, sulindac, aspirin)
   Anticonvulsants (hydantoins, carbamazepine, phenacemide)
   Heavy metals (gold, arsenic, bismuth, mercury)
   Sulfonamides: some antibiotics, antithyroid drugs (methimazole, methylthiouracil, propylthiouracil), antidiabetes drugs (tolbutamide, chlorpropamide), carbonic anhydrase inhibitors (acetazolamide and methazolamide)
   Antihistamines (cimetidine, chlorpheniramine)
   D-Penicillamine
   Estrogens (in pregnancy and in high doses in animals)

quency of aplastic anemia. Chloramphenicol remains a popular antibiotic in less developed countries.

Suspected drug reactions account for only about 5% of cases of aplastic anemia, while virtually all instances of agranulocytosis in the adult are drug related. The drugs associated with agranulocytosis are similar but not identical to those related to generalized bone marrow failure. Myeloid cells may be uniquely susceptible because of their ability to metabolize drugs, often to toxic intermediate compounds. In contrast to drug-associated aplastic anemia, agranulocytosis should spontaneously resolve with removal of the drug, and the severely neutropenic patient should survive if infection is adequately treated.

INFECTIONS. Hepatitis is the most common infection preceding aplastic anemia, accounting for about 5% of Western cases and perhaps twice that proportion in Asian series. Typically, severe aplasia occurs in a young man who has recovered from a mild bout of hepatitis 1 to 2 months earlier. The hepatitis is most often non-A, non-B, and non-C by serologic testing. Aplastic anemia can rarely follow infectious mononucleosis, and Epstein-Barr virus has been found in the marrow of some patients with aplastic anemia, with or without a suggestive preceding history. Parvovirus B19 has not been associated with generalized bone marrow failure. Moderate marrow depression occurs commonly in the course of many viral and bacterial infections, but the primary disease is usually overt.

IMMUNOLOGIC DISEASE. Aplasia regularly occurs in immunodeficient children who develop graft-versus-host disease after infusion of unirradiated blood products. The syndrome eosinophilic fasciitis is associated with aplastic anemia. Pure red blood cell aplasia is associated with thymoma, and patients with red cell aplasia or pancytopenia may be hypoimmunoglobulinemic. Immunologic aspects of aplastic anemia are discussed in greater detail below.

OTHER ASSOCIATIONS. Aplastic anemia may occur during pregnancy and has sometimes resolved with delivery or with spontaneous or induced abortion. Pancytopenia occurs in about one third of patients with paroxysmal nocturnal hemoglobinuria (Ch. 135), and perhaps 5% of patients with aplastic anemia have a positive Ham test, often with hematopoietic recovery; a much larger proportion can show evidence of decreased glycophosphoinositol proteins on granulocyte or monoocyte cell surface membranes.

Pathophysiology

TYPES OF INJURY. Most bone marrow failure almost certainly results from damage to the hematopoietic stem cell compartment; little evidence exists that aplastic anemia results from defective stroma or from inadequate production of growth factors. Two different routes to stem cell damage are derived from animal experiments and models of the stem cell compartment. The paradigm for type I damage is the effect of drugs that directly damage DNA. The administration of busulfan in the mouse is followed by a long latent period and then severe aplasia. DNA damage is random and will affect late precursor cells and primitive stem cells alike; the consequences for the earlier cell may be graver, owing to its necessity to transit more mitotic cycles to mature. In humans, examples of type I aplasia are Fanconi's anemia, the result of defective DNA repair (the same chromosomal phenotype and recessive inheritance might result from genetic defects in different DNA repair enzymes), and aplasia caused by irradiation, benzene, and perhaps also chloramphenicol. Type I aplasia is associated with both early aplasia (immediate, direct cytotoxicity) and later myelodysplasia and leukemia (the sequelae of mutational events).

Type II aplasia is illustrated by the effect of a cycle-active agent like 5-fluorouracil, which mainly depletes later progenitor cells and leaves relatively intact the most quiescent and also most proliferatively capable stem cells. The drug- and virus-associated marrow failure syndromes are probably type II, mediated either by chemical injury to the hematopoietic cell's metabolic machinery or by immunologic injury to the cell membrane. The severity of injury in both types I and II is probably related to the duration, repetition, or specific type of the damaging agent.

METABOLIC DRUG INJURY. Many drugs and chemicals, especially if they are polar and have limited water solubility, are metabolized to highly reactive electrophilic intermediates that bind to cellular macromolecules. Excessive generation of such toxic intermediates or failure to detoxify them may be genetically determined and apparent only on drug challenge. The complexity and specificity of the pathways imply multiple susceptible loci. In one case

of phenytoin-associated aplastic anemia, a defect in detoxification of that drug's metabolites was detected in the patient after recovery, and cells from the patient's mother were intermediately susceptible; cells from both normally detoxified metabolites generated from closely related drugs.

IMMUNE-MEDIATED INJURY. The recovery of their own marrow function by some patients being prepared for bone marrow transplantation with immunosuppressive horse antilymphocyte globulin first suggested that aplastic anemia might be immune mediated. Blood and bone marrow of patients often suppress normal bone marrow growth in progenitor assays, and removal of T cells from the bone marrow of those with aplastic anemia can improve colony formation in vitro. Patients with aplastic anemia may have increased numbers of activated cytotoxic lymphocytes (CD8+ cells bearing HLA-DR and interleukin-2 [IL-2] receptors) that overproduce lymphokines (particularly gamma-interferon phototoxin), and the gamma-interferon gene is overexpressed in the marrow of most aplastic anemia patients. These abnormalities usually improve with successful immunosuppressive therapy. The clinical effectiveness of cyclosporine is further evidence that T cells play a pathogenic role in many cases of bone marrow failure.

The inciting cause of the immune response may be a particular viral infection or drug exposure. Presumably, disease is the result of genetically determined features of the immune response that convert a normal physiologic response to a sustained and abnormal pathologic process.

PURE RED BLOOD CELL APLASIA (Table 130–3). Like aplastic anemia, pure red blood cell aplasia results from diverse mechanisms. Immune mechanisms have been implicated when pure red cell aplasia is associated with thymoma, systemic lupus erythematosus, and chronic lymphocytic leukemia, but not in failed erythropoiesis secondary to myelodysplasia, myeloproliferative diseases, and distinct cytogenetic abnormalities. Antibodies to red blood cell precursors can be detected in the blood of some patients, but T cell inhibition is probably the more common mechanism. Cytotoxic lymphocyte activity restricted by histocompatibility locus or specific for cells infected by human T cell lymphotropic virus (HTLV1) has been demonstrated in a particularly well-studied case.

Parvovirus B19 (see Color Plate 5H, right) represents the best example of the interaction of virus, host hematologic target cell, and immune response. This common virus causes fifth disease, a benign exanthema of childhood and a polyarthralgia syndrome in adults. In persons with underlying hemolysis, parvovirus infection causes abrupt but temporary worsening of anemia resulting from failed erythropoiesis, a syndrome called transient aplastic crisis. Parvovirus B19 has extraordinary tropism for human erythroid progenitor cells. Direct cytotoxicity of the virus causes anemia if demands on erythrocyte production are high. In normal individuals, the temporary cessation of red cell production is not clinically apparent, and symptoms are entirely the result of immune complex deposition. In persons unable to mount an adequate antibody re-

---

TABLE 130–3. CLASSIFICATION OF PURE RED BLOOD CELL APLASIA

Self-limited
  Transient erythroblastopenia of childhood
  Transient aplastic crisis of hemolysis (B19 parvovirus infection)
Fetal red blood cell aplasia
  Nonimmune hydrops fetalis (in utero parvovirus infection)
Hereditary pure red cell aplasia
  Congenital pure red cell aplasia (Diamond-Blackfan syndrome)
Acquired pure red cell aplasia
  I. Thymoma and malignancy: thymoma, lymphoid malignancies (and more rarely other hematologic diseases), paraneoplastic to solid tumors
  II. Connective tissue disorders with immunologic abnormalities: systemic lupus erythematosus, juvenile rheumatoid arthritis, rheumatoid arthritis, multiple endocrine gland insufficiency
  III. Virus: especially persistent B19 parvovirus, more rarely hepatitis, adult T cell leukemia virus, Epstein-Barr virus
  IV. Pregnancy
  V. Drugs: especially phenytoin, azathioprine, chloramphenicol, procainamide, isoniazid
  VI. Idiopathic

sponse, parvovirus B19 can persist in the bone marrow and cause chronic anemia that resembles pure red blood cell aplasia. The presence of giant pronormoblasts (Fig. 130–2), the cytopathic sign of the infection, should suggest the diagnosis. Persistent parvovirus infection should be sought in anemic patients with congenital and acquired immunodeficiency syndromes and in patients iatrogenically immunosuppressed, because it can be effectively treated with immunoglobulin infusions.

Incidence and Epidemiology

The incidence of aplastic anemia is approximately 2 per million in Europe and Israel, but the disease is more frequent in Asia, being 4 per million in Bangkok and higher in rural Thailand. Mortality statistics indicate an equal sex ratio and a preponderance of older persons, but at referral centers the median age is about 25 years.

Agranulocytosis has an incidence of 3.4 per million. Pure red blood cell aplasia is a very rare disease, with only a few hundred reported cases, and amegakaryocytic thrombocytopenia is rarer still, with only a few dozen cases reported in the literature.

Clinical Description

HISTORY. Bleeding is the most common early symptom of aplastic anemia: A complaint of days to weeks of easy bruising, including oozing from the gums, nose bleeds, or heavy menstrual flow is made, and sometimes petechiae will have been noticed. With thrombocytopenia, massive hemorrhage is unusual, but small amounts of bleeding in the central nervous system can result in serious intracranial or retinal hemorrhage. In cases of more gradual onset, symptoms of anemia are also described, usually lassitude, weakness, shortness of breath, and a pounding sensation in the ears. Infection is unusual as a first symptom in aplastic anemia, in contrast to agranulocytosis, in which pharyngitis, anorectal infection, and frank sepsis may be presenting syndromes. A striking feature of aplastic anemia is the restriction of symptoms to the hematologic system. Patients often feel and look remarkably well despite drastically reduced blood counts; systemic complaints and weight loss should point to other causes of pancytopenia. Drug use, chemical exposure, and preceding viral illnesses must often be elicited with repeated questioning; prompt cessation of drug or chemical exposure is especially important in agranulocytosis, which is usually self-limited.

PHYSICAL EXAMINATION. Petechiae and ecchymoses are frequently present, and there may be retinal hemorrhages. Pelvic and rectal examinations should be performed infrequently and gently to avoid trauma; these examinations may show bleeding from the cervical os and blood in the stool. Pallor of the skin and mucous membranes is also common except in the most acute cases or in those patients who have received transfusions. Although infection on presentation is uncommon, by the time the patient reaches a referral center, fever and signs of systemic or local infection may well be present. Lymphadenopathy and splenomegaly are very unusual in aplastic anemia. Café au lait spots and short stature point to Fanconi's anemia; peculiar nails suggest dyskeratosis congenita.

Diagnosis and Differential Diagnosis

The diagnosis of aplastic anemia is usually straightforward (Table 130–4), based on the combination of pancytopenia with fatty, empty bone marrow. Prompt arrival at the appropriate diagnosis is part of the effective management of the patient with aplastic anemia.

BLOOD. The smear typically shows large erythrocytes and a paucity of platelets and granulocytes. Macrocytosis as determined by automated cell counting is very common. Lymphocyte numbers may be normal or also reduced. The presence of immature myeloid forms should suggest leukemia or myelodysplasia; nucleated red blood cells suggest marrow fibrosis or invasion; and abnormal platelets suggest either peripheral destruction or dysplasia.

BONE MARROW (see Fig. 130–2). "Watery" marrow can almost always be obtained, and a "dry tap" occurs in fibrotic or myelophthisic disease. In severe aplasia, the smear of the aspirated specimen shows only residual lymphocytes and stromal cells; in milder cases, the remaining hematopoietic cells can show "megaloblastoid" erythropoiesis. Megakaryocytes are invariably greatly reduced and usually absent. The areas adjacent to the spicule should be searched for myeloblasts, which are not increased in aplastic anemia. Total cellularity is assessed by biopsy (see Color Plate 5G) of a core more than 1 cm in length, which in the most severe cases is virtually 100% fat and in more moderate disease less than 20% cellular. Nonetheless, the correlation between marrow cellularity and severity is imperfect: Some patients with moderate disease according to blood counts have empty iliac crest biopsies, and there may be "hot spots" of hematopoiesis in severe cases. In single-lineage failure states, the bone marrow reflects the absence of a specific morphologic subtype, but in both pure red blood cell aplasia and agranulocytosis, early and midmature precursor cells may be present. Granulomas may indicate an infectious cause of the marrow failure.

ANCILLARY STUDIES. Cytogenetic studies of peripheral blood should be performed on patients younger than 35 years (at least) to exclude Fanconi's anemia. Testing for abnormal sensitivity of erythrocytes to complement (Ham test) establishes paroxysmal nocturnal hemoglobinuria; flow microfluorometry of granulocytes is much more sensitive for the characteristically underexpressed proteins of this syndrome (see Ch. 135). Serologic studies may show evidence of viral infection, especially antibodies to human immunodeficiency virus, Epstein-Barr virus, and hepatitis viruses. Parvovirus may be detected by DNA hybridization in chronic pure red cell aplasia. Hypoimmunoglobulinemia and thymoma are also associated with pure red blood cell aplasia; a thymoma should be sought by computed tomography, less because the hematologic disease remits with thymectomy (it often does not) than because a potentially malignant tumor must be removed. The size of the spleen

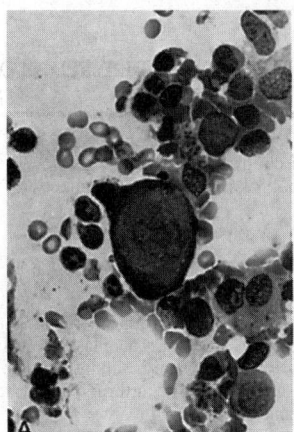
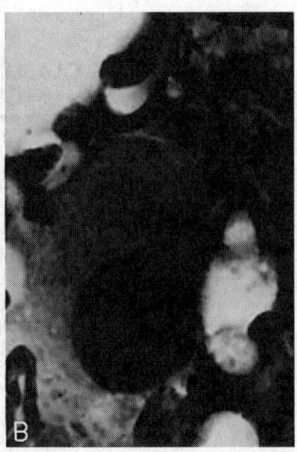
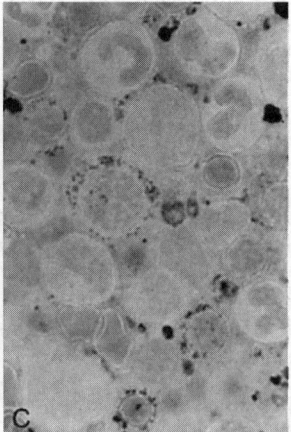
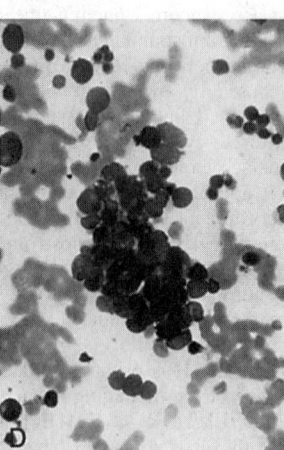

FIGURE 130–2. Four pathognomonic cells in the bone marrow. *A,* Giant pronormoblast, the cytopathic effect of B19 parvovirus infection of the erythroid progenitor cell. *B,* Uninuclear megakaryocyte and microblastic erythroid precursors typical of the 5q-myelodysplasia syndrome. *C,* Ringed sideroblast showing perinuclear iron granules. *D,* Clump of nonhematopoietic cells forming syncytium of metastatic tumor cells.

Pancytopenia with hypocellular bone marrow
  Acquired aplastic anemia
  Inherited aplastic anemia (Fanconi's anemia)
  Some myelodysplasia syndromes
  Rare aleukemic leukemia (acute myelogenous leukemia [AML])
  Some acute lymphoblastic leukemias in childhood
  Some lymphomas of bone marrow

Pancytopenia with cellular bone marrow
  Myelodysplasia syndromes
  Paroxysmal nocturnal
    hemoglobinuria
  Myelofibrosis   } Primary bone marrow diseases
  Some aleukemic leukemias
  Myelophthisis
  Bone marrow lymphoma
  Hairy cell leukemia

  Systemic lupus erythematosus
  Hypersplenism
  Vitamin B$_{12}$, folate deficiency
  Overwhelming infection
  AIDS   } Secondary to systemic diseases
  Alcoholism
  Brucellosis
  Sarcoidosis
  Tuberculosis

Hypocellular bone marrow ± cytopenia
  Q fever
  Legionnaires' disease
  Anorexia nervosa, starvation
  Mycobacterial infection

should be determined by scanning if the physical examination of the abdomen is suspicious or unsatisfactory.

DIFFERENTIAL DIAGNOSIS. Pancytopenia occurs in many diseases, but when secondary blood count depression rivals that of severe aplastic anemia, the primary diagnosis is usually obvious from either a history or the physical examination (e.g., the massive spleen of alcoholic cirrhosis, a history of metastatic cancer or systemic lupus erythematosus, or obvious miliary tuberculosis on the chest radiograph).

Treatment

BONE MARROW TRANSPLANTATION (see Ch. 151). This offers the best therapy for a young patient with a fully histocompatible sibling donor. Survival of patients younger than 20 years old following bone marrow transplantation is about 65 to 70%. Early consideration of the transplantation option in a child or adolescent can avoid unnecessary transfusions. Transfusions increase the risk of graft rejection, already peculiarly high in patients with aplastic anemia, and graft rejection is the major determinant of a successful clinical outcome. Survival of minimally transfused patients approximates that of patients who have had an identical twin as donor— 80% or better. Graft-versus-host disease increases progressively with age and occurs in the majority of adults over 30 years old. In older persons, marrow transplantation also carries significant risks from interstitial pneumonitis and opportunistic infections secondary to the conditioning regimen. As a result, it is usually not recommended for patients with aplastic anemia who are more than 45 years old. Management of patients in the intermediate range, 20 to 45 years old, depends on their transfusion history, on their general clinical condition, and, unfortunately, often on their medical insurance. Use of alternative donors, unrelated histocompatible volunteers or closely but not perfectly matched family members, remains experimental and largely unsuccessful; best results have been achieved in children employing intensive conditioning regimens.

IMMUNOSUPPRESSION. Most patients with aplastic anemia lack a suitable marrow donor. Antithymocyte globulin (ATG) therapy leads to recovery of autologous bone marrow function in about 50% of patients, usually with independence from transfusion and a leukocyte count adequate to prevent infection. About 50% of patients in whom therapy with ATG fails will respond to a 3- to 6-month course of cyclosporine. The combination of ATG and cyclosporine is superior to ATG alone as initial therapy for severe aplastic anemia, producing hematologic responses in about 70% of cases. Improvement in granulocyte number is generally apparent within 2 months of treatment. In most patients who recover with this treatment, the blood counts remain somewhat depressed, the mean corpuscular volume continues to be high, and the bone marrow cellularity returns only very slowly toward normal, if at all. Relapse can occur, and some patients may develop myelodysplasia, paroxysmal nocturnal hemoglobinuria, or acute leukemia years after successful immunosuppressive treatment of their aplastic anemia. Bone marrow examinations should therefore be performed annually or when there is an unfavorable change in blood counts, and a Ham test should be performed periodically.

ATG can be given intravenously in a regimen of 40 mg per kilogram per day for 4 days. Anaphylaxis is a rare but occasionally fatal complication of ATG treatment; allergy should be tested for by a prick test with an undiluted solution and immediate observation. ATG binds to peripheral blood cells, and therefore platelet and granulocyte numbers may fall further during active treatment. Serum sickness often develops about 10 days after initiation of treatment. Most patients receive methylprednisolone (1 mg per kilogram per day for 2 weeks) to ameliorate the immune consequences of heterologous protein infusion. Cyclosporine is administered orally at an initial dose of 12 mg per kilogram per day in adults and 15 mg per kilogram per day in children, with subsequent adjustment according to blood levels obtained every 2 weeks. Nephrotoxicity, hypertension, seizures, and opportunistic infections, especially *Pneumocystis carinii* pneumonia, are the most serious complications of cyclosporine treatment.

Immunosuppression is also effective in pure red blood cell aplasia and probably in amegakaryocytic thrombocytopenia as well. Immunosuppressive agents include corticosteroids, azathioprine, and cyclophosphamide, followed by ATG or cyclosporine.

OTHER THERAPY. Androgens have not been verified as effective in controlled trials, but occasional patients respond or even demonstrate blood count dependence on continued therapy. For patients with moderate disease or for those with severe pancytopenia in whom immunosupression has failed, a 3-month trial is appropriate: nandrolone decanoate at 5 mg per kilogram per week given intramuscularly (with firm pressure at the injection site to prevent hemorrhage) or oxymetholone at 150 mg per day by mouth.

Hematopoietic growth factors, GM-CSF and G-CSF, have not been shown to induce remissions in aplastic anemia, although they may increase the white blood cell count during the period of administration in some patients.

PRINCIPLES OF SUPPORT. Meticulous medical care is required so that the patient can survive to benefit from definitive therapy or, having experienced treatment failure, can maintain reasonable existence in the face of pancytopenia. First and most important, infection in the patient with severe neutropenia must be aggressively treated. Parenteral, broad-spectrum antibiotics should be started promptly, usually a combination of an aminoglycoside, cephalosporin, and semisynthetic penicillin (monotherapy with ceftazidime is a reasonable alternative). Therapy is empiric and must not await results of culture, although specific foci of infection, like oropharyngeal or anorectal abscesses, pneumonia, sinusitis, and typhlitis, should be sought on physical examination and with suitable radiographic studies. When indwelling plastic catheters become contaminated, vancomycin should be added. Persistent or recrudescent fever implies fungal disease; candidiasis and aspergillosis are common, especially after several courses of antibacterial antibiotics, and a progressive course may be averted by timely initiation of amphotericin. Granulocyte transfusions are not indicated. Handwashing, the single most effective method of preventing the spread of infection in the hospital, remains a neglected practice. Nonabsorbed antibiotics for gut decontamination may be helpful but are rarely tolerated because of their gastrointestinal side effects. Total reverse isolation is difficult, expensive, psychologically debilitating, inhibitory of nursing and medical attention, and not clearly beneficial in reducing mortality from infections.

Platelet and erythrocyte levels can be maintained by transfusion. Candidates for bone marrow transplantation should be transfused sparingly and, of course, never with blood products from a family member. Alloimmunization limits the usefulness of prophylactic platelet transfusions, and single-donor platelets from which leukocytes have been removed by filtration are the best product. There are no direct studies of the value of prophylaxis versus demand platelet transfusions in chronic bone marrow failure. Any rational regimen of prophylaxis requires transfusions once or twice weekly to maintain the platelet count above 10,000 per microliter (oozing from the gut, and presumably also from other vascular beds, increases precipitously at values lower than 5000 per microliter). About one third of patients become refractory to platelet transfusions, sometimes to HLA-matched as well as to random-donor platelets. Inhibitors of fibrinolysis, like aminocaproic acid, may help reduce mucosal oozing. Menstruation should be suppressed by either oral estrogens or nasal follicle-stimulating hormone (FSH)/luteinizing hormone (LH) antagonists. Aspirin and other nonsteroidal anti-inflammatory agents that inhibit platelet function must be avoided.

Red blood cells should be transfused to allow a normal level of activity, usually to a hemoglobin value of 70 grams per liter (90 grams per liter if there is underlying cardiac disease). A regimen of 2 units every 2 weeks replaces the normal loss of erythrocytes in a patient without functioning bone marrow. In chronic anemia, the iron chelator deferoxamine should be added at about the time the patient receives the fiftieth transfusion to avoid secondary hemochromatosis.

Prognosis

The natural course of untreated severe aplastic anemia is rapid deterioration and death resulting from infection or hemorrhage. Survival in patients with severe disease treated with transfusions only is poor, probably about 20% at 1 year. In most large unselected series, bone marrow transplantation leads to a 60 to 90% survival rate at 1 year. In Europe, immunosuppression has given overall results equivalent to marrow transplantation in adults. The physician has the responsibility of informing the patient of the relative values of bone marrow transplantation, which cures the hematologic disease but at great cost and often with significant morbidity, and immunosuppressive therapy, which is easier but often not completely effective.

Red cell aplasia is compatible with long life. Patients with congenital anemias have survived for decades with a combination of transfusions and iron chelation. Probably more than half of patients with acquired red cell aplasia can be cured by immunosuppression.

MYELODYSPLASIA

Definition

Myelodysplasia describes a heterogeneous group of hematologic disorders that are defined only broadly by cytopenias associated with dysmorphic or abnormal-appearing bone marrow (Table 130–5) (see Color Plates 6I and 6J). The classification scheme marks the convergence of two areas of investigation: preleukemia, the cytopenic phase sometimes observed to precede frank malignancy, and refractory anemia, states that resemble megaloblastic anemia but without evidence of vitamin deficiency. The French-American-British nomenclature, while based on morphologic features, has predictive value. (Sideroblastic anemia is also discussed in Ch. 132 as an example of hypochromic anemias.)

Etiology and Pathophysiology

The myelodysplastic syndromes are clonal disorders and have been convincingly linked to exposure to radiation, benzene, and many drugs employed in the treatment of cancer, particularly the radiomimetic alkylating agents. Cytogenetic abnormalities are common in patients with myelodysplasia. Some of the same specific chromosomal lesions also occur in frank leukemia and can be a transient stage in the development of a fully malignant phenotype. The presence and number of gross cytogenetic abnormalities in myelodysplasia are strongly correlated with the probability of leukemic transformation and therefore inversely with survival. One stereotypical karyotypic finding is deletion of a portion of the short arm of the fifth chromosome, or 5q− syndrome, particularly provocative because the genes for multiple hematopoietic growth factors and their receptors are found in the affected region (including granulocyte-macrophage and macrophage colony-stimulating factors; interleukins-3, -4, -5, and -9; and the cell-surface receptors for macrophage colony-stimulating factor [the c-fms gene] and platelet-derived growth factor). Mutations that activate the ras oncogene and the c-fms gene have also been implicated in other cases of myelodysplasia. The dysfunction measured in erythrocyte enzyme pathways for heme synthesis or in platelet aggregation in myelodysplasia is likely a secondary effect of mutations that dysregulate progenitor cell growth.

Incidence and Epidemiology

Idiopathic myelodysplasia is a disease of the elderly; the average mean age at onset is approximately 68 years, with slight male preponderance. The exact incidence of myelodysplasia is unknown, but this is not a rare syndrome in our aging population. Therapy-related myelodysplasia, which is not age-related, may occur in 10 to 15% of patients within a decade following intensive treatment, especially following a combination of irradiation and drugs like busulfan, nitrosourea, or procarbazine.

Clinical Description

Anemia dominates the early course. Most symptomatic patients complain of the gradual onset of fatigue and weakness, dyspnea, and pallor, but half are asymptomatic, with the myelodysplasia being discovered only incidentally. Previous chemotherapy or radiation exposure is an important historical fact. Fever and weight loss are more indicative of a myeloproliferative than of a myelodysplastic process. A family history may indicate a hereditary form of sideroblastic anemia. The physical examination is remarkable for signs of anemia and, in about 20% of cases, splenomegaly. In addition, some unusual skin lesions, like those of Sweet's syndrome (febrile neutrophilic dermatosis), have been associated with myelodysplasia.

Diagnosis and Differential Diagnosis

BLOOD. Anemia is present in the majority of cases, either alone or as part of bicytopenia or pancytopenia, but isolated neutropenia or thrombocytopenia is unusual. Macrocytosis is common, and the smear may be dimorphic with a distinctive population of large cells. Platelets are large and lack granules. Neutrophils may be hypogranulated, show Pelger-Huët, ringed, or abnormally segmented nuclei, and contain Döhle's bodies. Circulating myeloblasts usually correlate with the number of marrow blasts, and their quantitation is important for classification and prognosis. The total white blood cell count is usually normal or low, with the exception of the monocytosis observed in chronic myelomonocytic leukemia.

BONE MARROW. The bone marrow is usually normocellular or hypercellular, but in 20% of patients with myelodysplasia, it is

TABLE 130–5. CLASSIFICATION OF MYELODYSPLASIA

Subtype	Blood	Marrow	Percentage of Cases	Median Survival (mo)	Leukemic Evolution (%)
Refractory anemia	Blasts <1%	Blasts <5%	27	50	16
Refractory anemia with ringed sideroblasts	Blasts <1%	Blasts <5%	20	65	15
Refractory anemia with excess blasts	Blasts ≤5%	Blasts 5–20%	26	15	48
Refractory anemia with excess blasts in transformation	Blasts >1%	Blasts 20–30% or Auer rods	13	9	62
Chronic myelomonocytic leukemia	≥1 × 10^9/L monocytes	Any number	14	23	29

By definition, the bone marrow of acute myelogenous leukemia contains more than 30% blasts. Leukemic evolution refers to the percentage of cases that transform into acute myelogenous leukemia. Data derived from published series after Dunbar and Nienhuis.

sufficiently hypocellular to be confused with aplasia. No single characteristic feature of marrow morphology distinguishes myelodysplasia. Megaloblastoid and dyserythropoietic changes in the red blood cell precursors, hypogranulated polymorphonuclear cells, a left shift with an increase in myeloblasts, and abnormal megakaryocytes with reduced numbers of disorganized nuclei are common features. The specific diagnosis is based on the presence of ringed sideroblasts, the percentage of blasts, and increased immature myelomonocytic forms. Skilled assessment of morphology helps to delineate myelodysplasia from acute myelogenous leukemia on the one hand and aplastic anemia on the other. Analysis of chromosomes from cultured bone marrow cells should always be performed, as cytogenetic abnormalities are unusual in aplasia and common in myelodysplasia. Complex chromosomal abnormalities imply poor survival.

Treatment

Therapy for myelodysplasia has generally been unsatisfactory. Occasional patients with sideroblastic anemia respond to pyridoxine. Androgens and corticosteroids may improve blood counts but have not been shown to influence survival. Older patients suffer high mortality during induction with high-dose chemotherapy for leukemia and have a lower remission rate than do patients with acute myelogenous leukemia. Reported good responses using low-dose chemotherapy (in particular, cytosine arabinoside) or retinoids to induce marrow differentiation have not been widely confirmed.

A substantial proportion of patients with myelodysplasia have been found to respond with significant blood count improvement to granulocyte or granulocyte-macrophage colony-stimulating growth factors. Leukocytes almost always increase during factor therapy, and in some cases blast numbers have been significantly reduced and cytogenetic abnormalities have resolved. Platelet and reticulocyte numbers respond less consistently. No studies have yet demonstrated a survival benefit for growth factor therapy in myelodysplasia.

The same principles of supportive care described for aplastic anemia apply to myelodysplasia. Because many patients will be anemic for years, erythrocyte transfusion support should be accompanied by iron chelation to prevent hemochromatotic damage to the heart, liver, and pancreas.

Prognosis

The median survival for a patient with myelodysplasia is about 2 years, but survival varies with the specific subtype. Most patients die as a result of complications of pancytopenia and not because of leukemic transformation. Approximately one third succumb to other diseases unrelated to myelodysplasia. Precipitous worsening of pancytopenia, acquisition of new chromosomal abnormalities detected on serial cytogenetic determination, and increase in the number of blasts are all obviously poor prognostic indicators. The outlook in therapy-related myelodysplasia is particularly poor, with many cases rapidly progressing to refractory acute myelogenous leukemia.

MYELOPHTHISIC ANEMIAS AND MYELOFIBROSIS

Marrow fibrosis, usually accompanied by a characteristic blood smear presentation called leukoerythroblastosis (see Color Plate 7F, left), can occur as a primary hematologic disease, called myelofibrosis or myeloid metaplasia (see Color Plate 5J), and as a secondary process, called myelophthisis, which represents reaction to invading tumor cells (see Color Plate 5I), infectious agents like mycobacteria or fungi, intracellular lipid deposition in Gaucher's disease (see Color Plate 7E), and the granulomas of sarcoidosis (Table 130–6). In secondary fibrosis, the infectious or malignant underlying processes are usually obvious. The pancytopenia of human immunodeficiency virus may be associated with moderate marrow fibrosis. Modest degrees of fibrosis can also be a feature of a variety of other hematologic syndromes, especially chronic myelogenous leukemia, poorly differentiated lymphomas, myeloma, and hairy cell leukemia. Marrow fibrosis also occurs in the bony proliferative disease of childhood called osteopetrosis.

The pathophysiology of myelofibrosis has three distinct features: proliferation of fibroblasts in the marrow space; extension of hematopoiesis into the long bones and most peculiarly into extramedullary sites, usually the spleen, liver, and lymph nodes (myeloid metaplasia); and ineffective erythropoiesis. The etiology of fibrosis is unknown, but most likely involves dysregulated pro-

TABLE 130–6. CAUSES OF MYELOPHTHISIS

A. Neoplastic infiltration of the marrow
 1. Hematologic malignant diseases
    Leukemias—acute and chronic
    Lymphomas—Hodgkin's and non-Hodgkin's
    Plasma cell myeloma
    Hairy cell leukemia
 2. Nonhematologic malignant diseases
    Carcinomas—especially breast, prostate, lung, stomach
    Neuroblastoma
B. Myelofibrosis
 1. Primary (idiopathic)
 2. Secondary—chronic myeloid leukemia, cancers, vasculitis (lupus, rheumatoid arthritis)
C. Granulomatous infections
 1. Tuberculosis
 2. Fungal infections
D. Metabolic abnormalities
 1. Lipid storage diseases, e.g., Gaucher's disease
 2. Osteopetrosis

duction of growth factors. Many cell types in the marrow produce growth factors for fibroblasts: Platelet-derived growth factor is one example, and profuse megakaryocytopoiesis and thrombocytosis are often seen early in the course of idiopathic myelofibrosis. Abnormal regulation of other hematopoietins would lead to the localization of blood-producing cells in nonhematopoietic tissues and uncoupling of the usually balanced processes of stem cell proliferation and differentiation. Myelofibrosis is remarkable for pancytopenia despite extraordinarily large numbers of circulating hematopoietic progenitor cells.

Idiopathic (or agnogenic) myelofibrosis is one of the myeloproliferative syndromes, a category that also includes polycythemia vera, essential thrombocythemia, and chronic myelogenous leukemia. It is discussed in Ch. 141.2 in the context of the myeloproliferative disorders.

Dunbar C, Nienhuis A: The myelodysplastic syndromes. *In* Handin R, Lux S, Stossel T (eds.): Blood, Principles and Practice of Hematology. Philadelphia, J.B. Lippincott, 1995, p 373. *Good clinical descriptions and in-depth considerations of mechanisms.*

Young NS: B19 parvovirus. *In* Baillière's Clinical Haematology. London, Baillière-Tindall, 1995. *The story of this virus, from its discovery to the genetic engineering of a vaccine, should make good reading.*

Young NS, Alter BA: Aplastic Anemia, Acquired and Inherited. Philadelphia, W.B. Saunders Company, 1994. *Exhaustive review of aplastic anemia, both acquired and constitutional, and single-lineage failures.*

131 NORMOCHROMIC, NORMOCYTIC ANEMIAS
Thomas P. Duffy

An optimal red blood cell (RBC) mass is maintained within the body via a feedback loop whereby the hormonal stimulus for RBC production, erythropoietin (EPO), is released in response to the hemoglobin needs of the body. EPO is a glycoprotein secreted by renal interstitial cells that respond to the oxidative state of hematin in RBC perfusing the kidney. As anemia develops, this sensing device within the kidney causes an increased EPO secretion, with overdrive of the erythroid component of the marrow. EPO causes amplification of erythroid precursors within the marrow and hastens their differentiation and release from the marrow; under heightened EPO stimulation, a normal marrow responds with erythroid hyperplasia and accelerated release of young reticulocytes. The latter can be recognized on supravital staining of their residual, polyribosomal, reticulated network, which is the marker for these RBC in the peripheral blood.

Under normal conditions the marrow compensates for the 1 to 1.5% of the RBC mass that is lost each day through senescence by replacing it with reticulocytes. When anemia occurs, a physiologic "surge" in reticulocytes should follow if the marrow is capable of responding appropriately to EPO overdrive. This normal response is evidenced by an elevated reticulocyte count, significantly above the usual 1 to 1.5%. If an anemia has its origin within the marrow or secondary to inadequate EPO stimulation, an appropriate reticulocytosis is not mounted to compensate for the anemia. This reticulocytopenic response indicates that the anemia is due to problems in RBC production within the marrow rather than accelerated RBC loss or destruction in the periphery.

Knowledge of this feedback EPO loop and of the reticulocyte count permits a broad dissection of the cause(s) of anemia. Absence of an appropriate reticulocyte response in patients with anemia is the hallmark of hyporegenerative anemias; these conditions have myriad causes that include a lack of marrow precursors (stem cell or pure RBC aplasia), of necessary building blocks (iron, vitamin B_{12}, folate), and of adequate EPO stimulation as well as abnormalities in proliferation and differentiation of RBC (leukemia, myelodysplasias, infiltrative disorders of the marrow). The lesion in hyporegenerative anemias has its locus within the marrow, and bone marrow aspiration/biopsy are the definitive procedures for investigation of such anemias if serum measurements (iron, iron binding capacity, vitamin B_{12}, folate) do not provide any answer.

The presence of an elevated reticulocyte count has the opposite implications regarding the cause of anemia. Reticulocytosis indicates the presence of a hyperregenerative anemia, in which the marrow is able to respond appropriately to the stimulus of anemia. This lesion has its locus in the periphery with accelerated loss of RBC from either premature RBC destruction due to hemolysis or excessive loss of blood due to bleeding. The explanation for such anemias needs be looked for in hemolytic mechanisms or documentation of blood loss.

With knowledge of the reticulocyte count assigning the cause of anemia to the marrow or the peripheral blood, a second parameter permits further definition of the cause of a low RBC count. This measurement is the mean corpuscular volume (MCV) of RBC, a value derived from the electronic Coulter counter. Small, or microcytic, RBC (MCV < 80 fl) most commonly have iron deficiency as their cause. Large, or macrocytic, cells (MCV > 95 fl) have abnormalities in nucleic acid metabolism, with vitamin B_{12} or folate deficiency most commonly responsible for this alteration. Anemias with RBC of normocytic size (MCV 80 to 95 fl) have numerous causes, from faulty production to excessive loss or destruction; hypoerythropoietin states also result in normocytic anemias. The early stages of most anemias are also normochromic/normocytic because of the presence of the original normal RBC population manufactured before the new pathologic lesion appeared.

BLOOD LOSS ANEMIA

The hematologic manifestations of bleeding depend upon the interval that separates the acute event from the measurement of the hematocrit or hemoglobin concentration. Immediately following an acute bleed, the hematocrit is normal because there has not yet been time for hemodilution to occur to compensate for any reduction in blood volume; evidence for blood loss may be apparent in postural changes in blood pressure and pulse at this time. After about 24 hours, volume re-expansion corrects this defect by mobilization of extravascular fluid into the intravascular compartment; this results in a fall in hematocrit that parallels the degree of blood loss. After 3 to 5 days there is a rise in reticulocyte count to compensate for the anemia; such a reticulocytosis may lead to confusion of acute blood loss with hemolytic anemia. Both are normochromic, normocytic anemias with high reticulocyte counts; the MCV may actually be increased in both conditions because reticulocytes are polychromatophilic macrocytes that may elevate the mean corpuscular volume. Distinguishing the two anemias are the by-products of accelerated RBC breakdown in hemolytic anemias, in which hyperbilirubinemia is frequently the marker of hemolysis. The evidence of bleeding usually permits an easy differentiation of the two. However, when bleeding occurs into soft tissues or into a body cavity such as the retroperitoneum, resorption of this blood may be associated with hyperbilirubinemia. This may be a confusing picture until the hematoma extends to the surface as an ecchymosis or a radiographic study identifies a retroperitoneal bleed.

The normochromic, normocytic anemias of hemolysis and acute posthemorrhagic states are both accompanied by leukocytosis and thrombocytosis; these responses represent cytokine stimulation of all cell lines within the marrow in response to the stimulus of anemia.

OTHER NORMOCYTIC, NORMOCHROMIC ANEMIAS

ANEMIA OF CHRONIC RENAL INSUFFICIENCY. Chronic renal failure leads to anemia because of the progressive absence of adequate EPO production in the feedback loop for the maintenance of erythropoiesis. No strict correlation exists between the degree of azotemia and the severity of this anemia, although anemia usually supervenes once the creatinine clearance falls below 35 to 45 ml per minute. Many other factors also may contribute to the development of anemia in renal failure. Bleeding may occur from angiomatous malformations that develop in the gastrointestinal tract in uremia, and the hemostatic platelet defect of renal failure may exaggerate this threat. Significant iron loss also occurs as a byproduct of hemodialysis, and folate stores may be compromised by loss of this dialysable vitamin. Aluminum toxicity interferes with iron metabolism, and a microcytic anemia may develop in patients whose dialystate baths contain high concentrations of this metal. A microangiopathic process often develops with malignant hypertension, and this same RBC lesion is a hallmark of the hemolytic-uremic syndrome and thrombotic thrombocytopenia.

A modest shortening of RBC survival occurs as a result of a metabolic lesion incurred from uremia. However, this is only a very minor contribution to anemia in these states because the uncomplicated anemia of renal disease can be reversed with the administration of erythropoietin. EPO is usually administered three times weekly, either subcutaneously or intravenously following dialysis treatments. Treatment is initiated with EPO doses of 150 units per kilogram three times weekly and reduced to 50 to 100 units per kilogram per dose once the desired response has been obtained. With this therapy, this major co-morbid feature of renal failure has been eliminated.

ANEMIA OF LIVER DISEASE. RBC, once released from the marrow, undergo remodeling of their membranes by splenic macrophages, and the lipid constituents of the membrane remain in dynamic equilibrium with plasma lipoproteins. Advanced stages of liver disease are complicated by progressive lipoprotein abnormalities that result in the sequential transformation of normochromic, normocytic RBC into macrocytes, target cells, echinocytes, and the final and most severe stage, acanthocytes. Acanthocytes, or spur cells, are converted into spherocytes by the spleen with their lifespan significantly shortened because the lipid deposition interferes with the normal plasticity or deformability of RBC. In liver disease associated with portal hypertension, hypersplenism may shorten RBC survival even in the absence of any lipid-membrane lesion.

Anemia in liver disease may also have its origin in the several other insults that often accompany hepatic damage. Alcohol, with its effect upon folate metabolism, may create a macrocytic, megaloblastic anemia; the same toxin may interfere with heme metabolism and produce a sideroblastic anemia. A metabolic product of alcohol, acetaldehyde, is a direct inhibitor of erythropoiesis *in vitro*. Iron deficiency is also not uncommon in liver disease states because of blood loss from varices, alcohol-induced gastritis, and the coagulopathy resulting from defective synthesis of the coagulation factors. A rare form of liver disease, Wilson's disease, has hemolytic anemia as a feature; copper accumulation in this disorder is toxic to hepatic parenchymal cells and the RBC.

ANEMIA OF ENDOCRINE DISORDERS. The endocrine system maintains homeostasis of the body and dysfunction in hormonal regulation has systemic effects that include the production and survival of RBC. An anemia, usually normocytic but sometimes macrocytic, accompanies hypothyroidism as a physiologic downtuning in response to the decreased metabolic needs of this state. Erythrocytosis may be a feature of Cushing's disease secondary to androgen overdrive of the marrow; a reduction in RBC mass occurs in Addison's disease, but anemia is not usually evident because of a concomitant reduction in plasma volume due to mineralocorticoid deficiency. Hypopituitary states are complicated by mild anemias; growth hormone has a growth-stimulating effect upon RBC.

Anemia is not a feature of uncomplicated diabetes but usually occurs in the course of the disease as renal complications develop. A shortened RBC survival occurs in uncontrolled diabetes, attribut-

PLATE 5   HEMATOLOGIC DISEASES

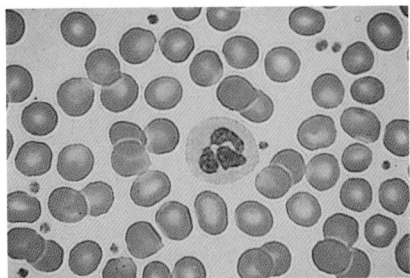

A, A normal peripheral blood smear. The red cells are normocytic with a good hemoglobin content. A normal segmented neutrophil is in the center of the field. A normal platelet is immediately adjacent. (L.O.)

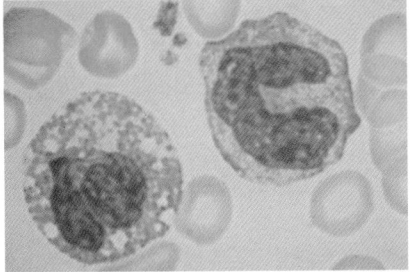

B, A normal eosinophil *(left)* and band *(right).* The eosinophil shows orange granules, vacuoles, and a segmented nucleus. The band has gray-pink cytoplasm and a reticular, horseshoe-shaped nucleus. (V.H.O.)

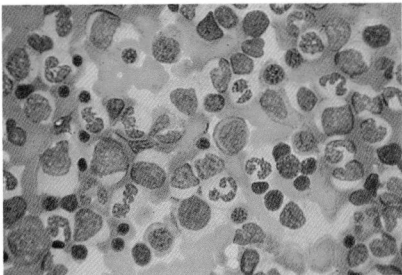

C, Normal bone marrow aspirate seen at low power. There is a 2:1 ratio between myeloid and erythroid precursors. The latter are identified by their shrunken, pyknotic ("coal black") nuclei. (L.P.)

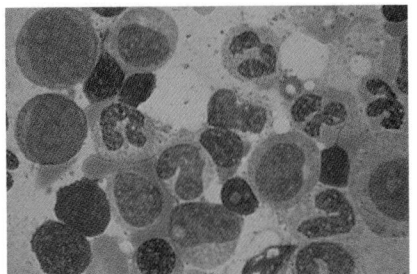

D, A bone marrow aspirate. Five erythroid precursors (with pyknotic nuclei) are present. The remaining cells are myeloid precursors in various stages of maturation, ranging from myeloblast to segmented neutrophil. (L.O.)

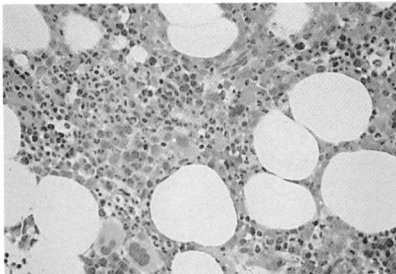

E, A hematoxylin and eosin (H & E)-stained normal bone marrow biopsy. Normal distribution and cellularity are seen. Several distinct megakaryocytes can be recognized because of their large size and multiple nuclear lobes. (L.P.)

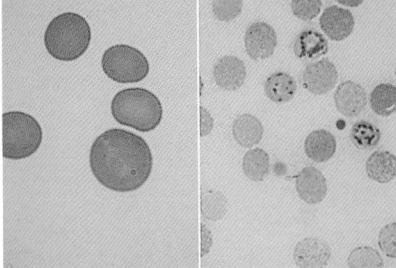

F, Left, The larger, gray-pink erythrocyte in the center of this field is called a polychromatophilic or "shift" cell. (H.O.) *Right,* Reticulocytes. The dark purple reticulin in red blood cells newly entering the blood is demonstrated by this new methylene blue stain. (L.O.)

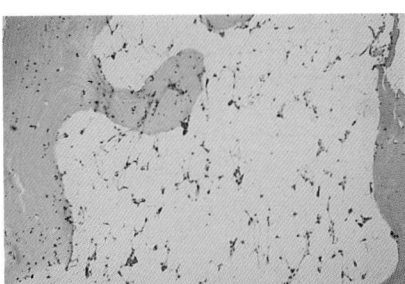

G, This low-power view of an H & E-stained bone marrow biopsy is from a patient with severe aplastic anemia. The virtually empty marrow can be appreciated by comparing with frame *E.* Even the marrow stroma is scanty. (L.P.)

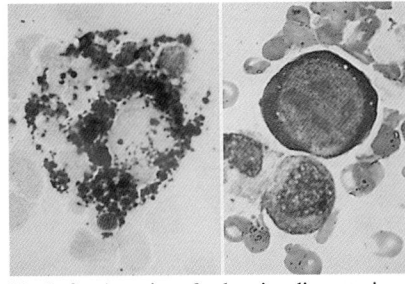

H, Left, Anemia of chronic disease; iron-stained bone marrow aspirate. Heavy dark blue granules of iron are seen in the storage cells. *Right,* This giant pronormoblast is from the bone marrow aspirate of a patient with red cell aplasia due to parvovirus infection. (H.O.)

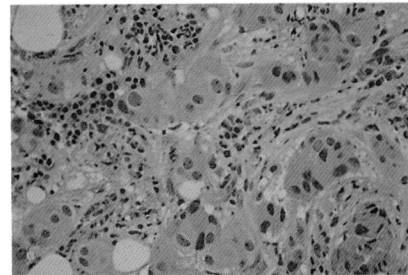

I, Metastatic breast carcinoma is seen in this view of an H & E-stained bone marrow biopsy. The malignancy has virtually replaced normal marrow elements. (L.P.)

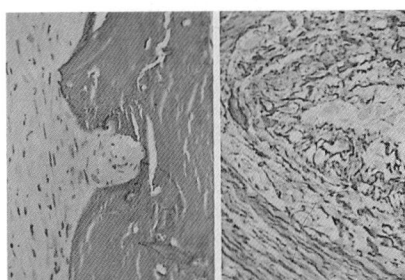

J, Agnogenic myeloid metaplasia with myelofibrosis. *Left,* This H & E-stained preparation shows virtual replacement of the marrow cavity with light pink-staining fibrous tissue. *Right,* A reticulin stain demonstrates the fibrosis as well. (L.P.)

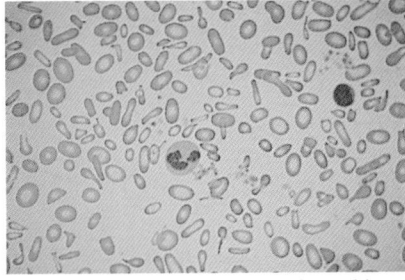

K, The peripheral blood in a patient with severe iron deficiency anemia. A normal lymphocyte is present (for comparison purposes) to the right of center. Marked anisocytosis and poikilocytosis can be appreciated, as can microcytosis and hypochromia. (L.P.)

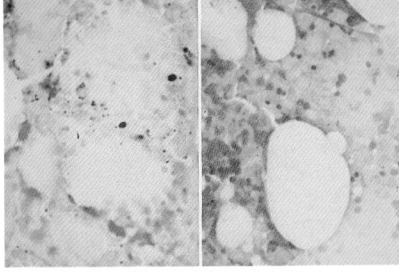

L, These are views of iron-stained bone marrow. *Left,* Normal iron stores are seen as dark blue-staining material. *Right,* The absence of iron is a characteristic finding in iron deficiency anemia. (L.P.)

PLATE 6 HEMATOLOGIC DISEASES

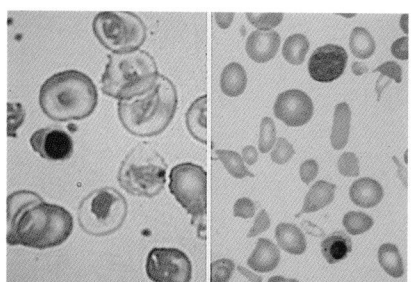

A, *Left,* Beta-thalassemia. Smear shows an orthochromic normoblast to the left. Also seen are targeting, hypochromia, and a Howell-Jolly body. (H.O.) *Right,* Alpha-thalassemia, E hemoglobinopathy. A normoblast and lymphocyte and anisocytosis are present. (L.O.)

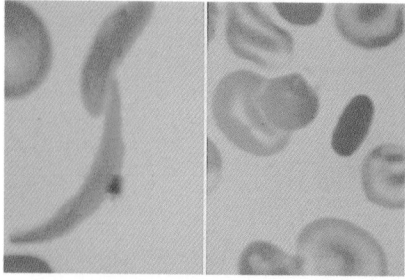

B, *Left,* Sickle cell disease. A classic sickle cell is seen in this field. *Right,* The cell to the right of center is a classic finding in hemoglobin C disease. It represents crystallized hemoglobin C. Also present are targeting and anisocytosis. (V.H.O.)

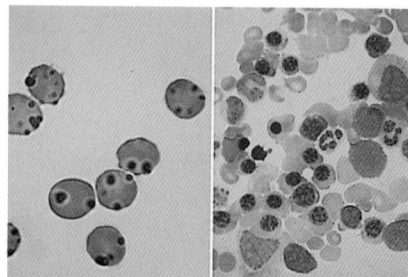

C, Hemolytic anemia. *Left,* Heinz body preparation showing dark-staining denatured globin intraerythrocytic particles. (H.O.) *Right,* Moderate bone marrow erythroid hyperplasia is often seen in hemolysis. (L.O.)

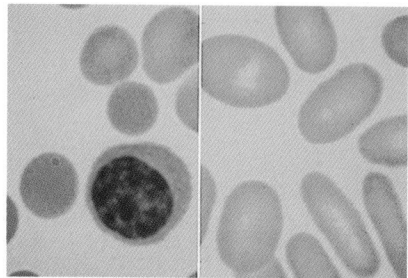

D, *Left,* This view of the peripheral blood in a patient with hereditary spherocytosis (HS) shows microspherocytes and a normal lymphocyte. *Right,* Hereditary elliptocytosis. Significant numbers of elliptocytes (oval erythrocytes) are seen in this field. (V.H.O.)

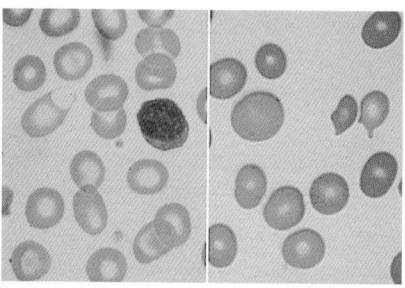

E, *Left,* G6PD deficiency. To the left of the normal lymphocyte is a red cell with a blistered appearance secondary to portions of denatured hemoglobin being "bitten" off. *Right,* Microangiopathy. A shift cell and fragments are seen centrally. (L.O.)

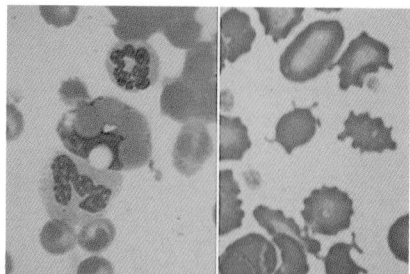

F, Hemolytic anemia. *Left,* Erythrophagocytosis. Four red blood cells (center) have been engulfed by a cell of the monocyte-macrophage line. *Right,* Marked red cell membrane abnormalities in severe hepatorenal failure, with burr cells and spur cells. (L.O., H.O.)

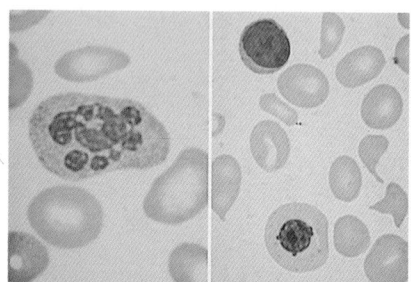

G, Pernicious anemia. *Left,* Marked neutrophil hypersegmentation. *Right,* Peripheral blood with large lymphocyte (top), macrocytosis, and orthochromic megaloblast (bottom). The latter has nuclear-cytoplasmic disproportion and beaded nuclear chromatin. (V.H.O.)

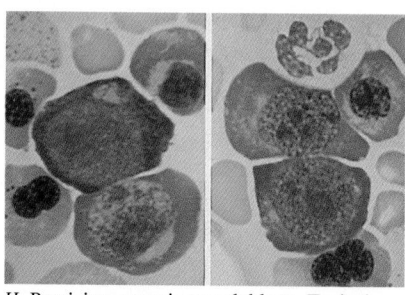

H, Pernicious anemia megaloblasts. Typical nuclear chromatin changes are seen in both frames. *Left,* Large central cell is a promegaloblast. *Right,* Large cell below is a basophilic megaloblast. Two cells above are polychromatophilic megaloblasts. (V.H.O.)

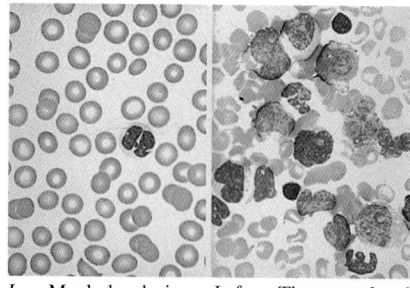

I, Myelodysplasia. *Left,* Therapy-related myelodysplasia. Dysmorphic red cells and a markedly abnormal granulocyte are seen. *Right,* Refractory anemia with excess blasts in transformation (RAEB-T). Several blasts and other dyspoietic changes are seen. (H.P.)

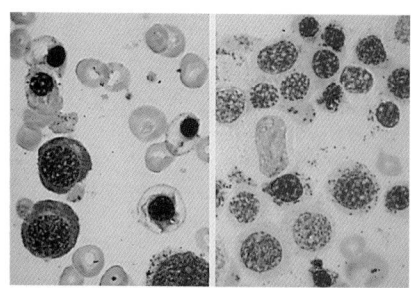

J, Myelodysplasia. *Left,* Marked erythroid dyspoiesis. Diagnosis was refractory anemia with ring sideroblasts (RARS). *Right,* An iron stain in the same patient showing perinuclear rings of iron-laden mitochondria. (L.O.)

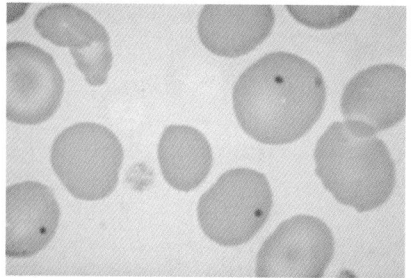

K, Postsplenectomy changes. This view of the peripheral blood shows three deeply basophilic granules peripherally in three different red cells: Howell-Jolly bodies. Targeting is also seen. (V.H.O.)

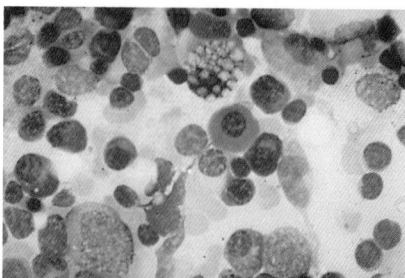

L, A bone marrow aspirate in a patient with Felty's syndrome. Maturation arrest is at the metamyelocyte stage. There is significant reactive plasmacytosis (30%). A "Mott cell" with grapelike inclusions is seen top center. (L.O.)

PLATE 7 HEMATOLOGIC DISEASES

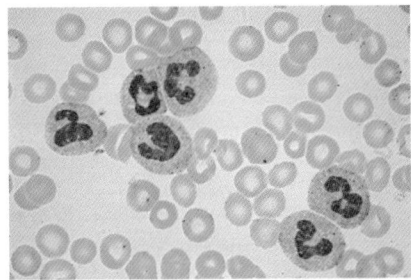

A, Neutrophilia. Four segmented and two band neutrophils are seen in this view of the peripheral blood. Some red blood cells are slightly hypochromic. (L.O.)

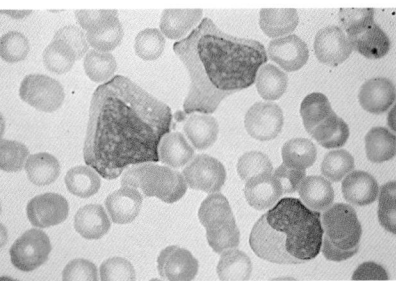

B, Infectious mononucleosis. Reactive (or atypical) lymphocytosis is seen in this peripheral blood smear. Pleomorphic reticular nuclei, peripheral basophilia of cytoplasm, and scalloped cell borders are characteristic. Slight rouleaux are also present. (H.O.)

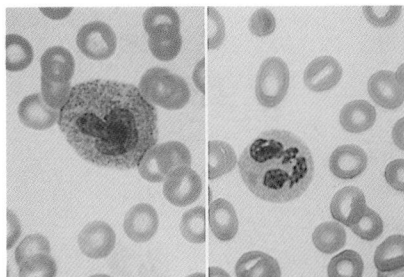

C, Left, This band neutrophil shows basophilic or toxic granulation. *Right,* This segmented neutrophil shows some toxic granulation and a grayish Döhle body at 7 o'clock. Both are blood changes seen in bacterial infection. (H.O.)

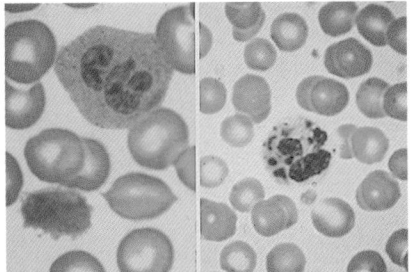

D, Left, May-Hegglin anomaly. The segmented neutrophil at the top of this field has a gray, spindle-shaped Döhle body at 4 o'clock. A giant platelet is seen at the bottom. (V.H.O.) *Right,* Chédiak-Higashi syndrome. Characteristic giant neutrophilic lysozymes are seen. (H.O.)

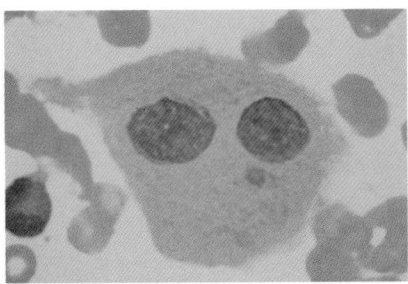

E, Gaucher's disease. This bone marrow aspirate shows a giant binucleate storage cell filled with glucocerebrosides. The fibrillar pattern is characteristic. (H.O.)

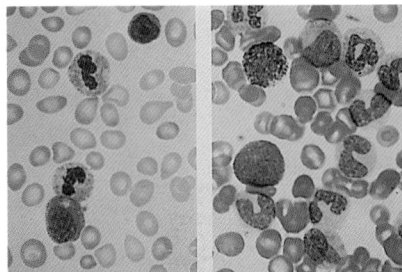

F, Left, Agnogenic myeloid metaplasia. This blood smear shows some teardrop-shaped red cells and a characteristic leukoerythroblastic reaction. *Right,* Chronic myelogenous leukemia (CML). Marked neutrophilia with left shift and two abnormal eosinophils are seen. (H.P.)

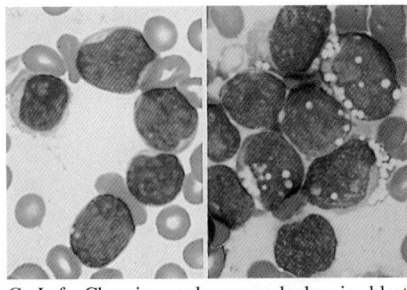

G, Left, Chronic myelogenous leukemia, blast crisis. The blasts have very immature nuclear chromatin. The patient was Ph[1] chromosome positive. *Right,* Ph[1] chromosome-positive acute lymphoblastic leukemia. These blasts are shown for comparison. (H.O.)

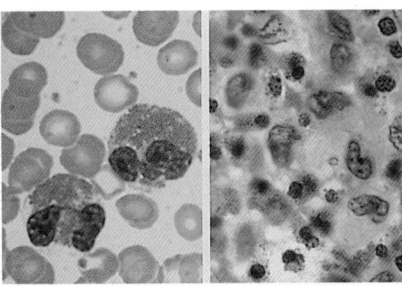

H, Left, Two eosinophils are shown from the peripheral blood of a patient with the hypereosinophilic syndrome. (H.O.) *Right,* Eosinophilic granuloma. In this lymph node, eosinophils and histiocytes are seen. (H.P.)

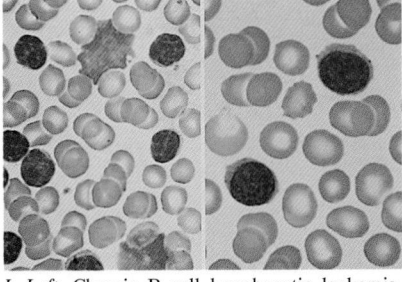

I, Left, Chronic B cell lymphocytic leukemia. The neoplastic lymphocytes are B cells. Two destroyed lymphocytes are in the center. (L.O.) *Right,* Chronic T cell lymphocytic leukemia. The neoplastic lymphocytes have been identified as T cells. (H.O.)

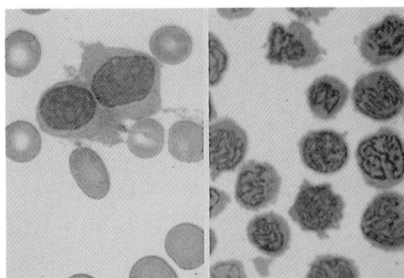

J, Left, Hairy cell leukemia (HCL). This frame shows two "hairy cells" with thin cytoplasmic projections and reticular nuclear chromatin. (H.O.) *Right,* Sézary's syndrome. This buffy coat preparation shows nuclear pleomorphism and convolutions.

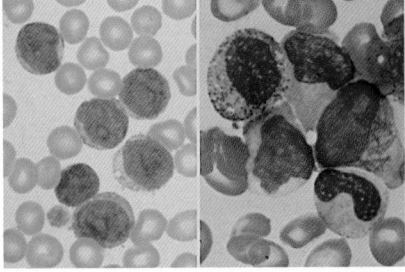

K, Acute nonlymphoblastic leukemia (ANLL). *Left,* M-1 type. The blasts have round or slightly indented nuclei, fine nuclear chromatin, and very little cytoplasmic granulation. *Right,* M-3 type. Three leukemic promyelocytes with multiple Auer rods and cytoplasmic inclusions are seen. (H.O.)

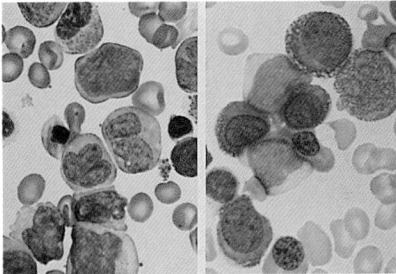

L, ANLL *(continued). Left,* M-4 type. Blasts in the center of this field have both monocytic and myeloid features. *Right,* M-6 type. This field shows abnormalities seen in erythroleukemia. Most blasts have marked nuclear dyspoiesis. The central blast could be myeloid. (H.O.)

PLATE 8   HEMATOLOGIC DISEASES

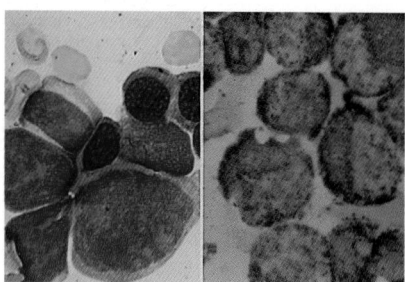

A, ANLL *(continued). Left,* M-7 type. This bone marrow aspirate shows characteristic large blasts. *Right,* The myeloperoxidase stain is often useful in identifying myeloid blasts. Dark granules are characteristic of a positive reaction. (H.O.)

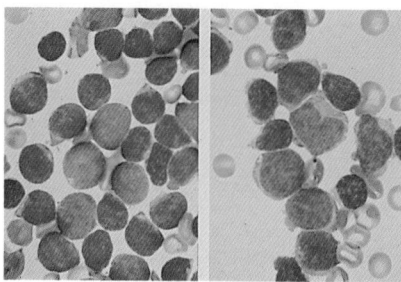

B, Acute lymphoblastic leukemia (ALL). *Left,* L-1 type. This bone marrow aspirate shows L-1 lymphoblasts that are moderately uniform in size. *Right,* L-2 type. In this bone marrow aspirate, the pleomorphism of the blasts is apparent. (H.O.)

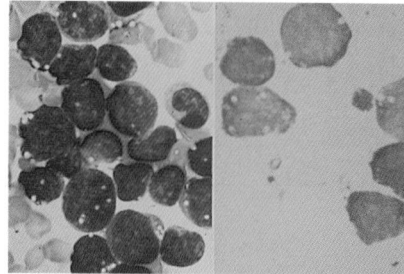

C, ALL *(continued). Left,* L-3 type. This bone marrow aspirate shows characteristic blasts. Cytoplasmic and nuclear vacuoles are seen. *Right,* Coarse, red-pink cytoplasmic granules characterize PAS-positive lymphoblasts.

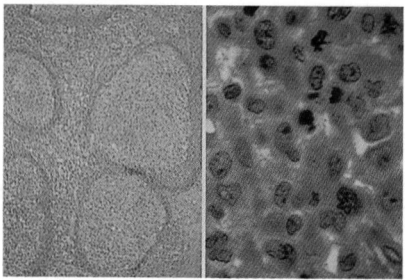

D, Left, Non-Hodgkin's lymphoma (follicular, small cleaved cell type). Lymph node. The follicular pattern is seen. (L.P.) *Right,* Non-Hodgkin's lymphoma (diffuse, T immunoblastic type). Lymph node, H & E stain. A diffuse pattern of large neoplastic cells is seen. (H.P.)

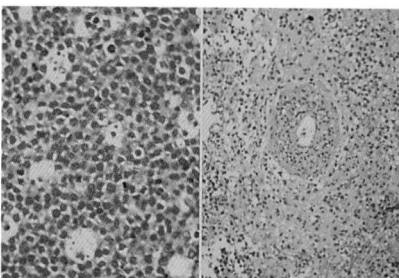

E, Left, Non-Hodgkin's lymphoma (B cell type) in a patient with AIDS. Lymph node biopsy, H & E stain. *Right,* Non-Hodgkin's lymphoma in a patient with AIDS. Brain involvement is present. (L.P.)

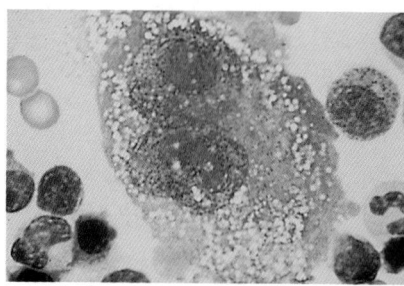

F, Hodgkin's disease. This bone marrow aspirate shows a classic Reed-Sternberg cell. The "mirror-image" nuclei are characteristic, as are the large nucleoli. It is unusual to find these cells in the bone marrow aspirate. (H.O.)

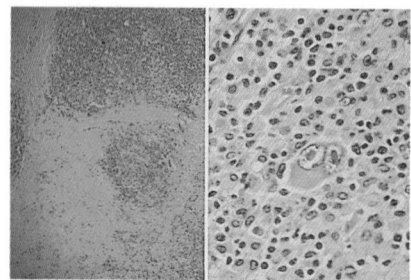

G, Left, Hodgkin's disease (nodular sclerosis type). Large fibrotic nodules enclose the cellular areas of Hodgkin's disease. (L.P.) *Right,* Hodgkin's disease (lymphocyte-depleted type). Lymph node biopsy. A Reed-Sternberg cell is near the center of the field. (H.P.)

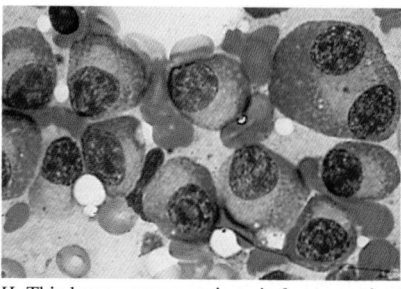

H, This bone marrow aspirate is from a patient with multiple myeloma. All plasma cells in this field are neoplastic myeloma cells. The nuclei are pleomorphic and eccentric, and the cytoplasm is gray-blue. One cell is binucleate. (H.O.)

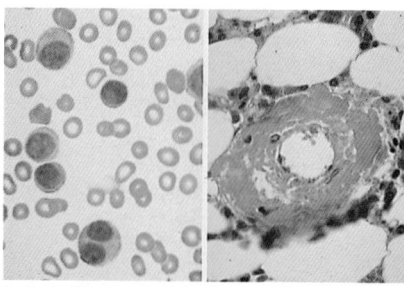

I, Left, Plasma cell leukemia. Five neoplastic plasma cells (one of which is binucleate) are seen in this field. (L.O.) *Right,* Amyloid. Bone marrow biopsy. A small blood vessel is heavily infiltrated with the pink-staining, waxy amyloid material. (H.P.)

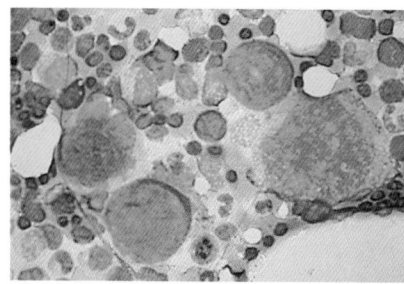

J, Immune thrombocytopenic purpura (ITP). Bone marrow aspirate. Megakaryocytosis is reflected in this field, where four are seen. These range from a megakaryoblast (top) to a mature megakaryocyte (middle right).

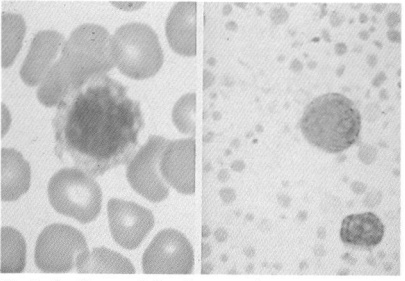

K, Left, Bernard-Soulier syndrome. A typical giant platelet is seen in the center of the field. *Right,* Essential thrombocythemia. Massive thrombocytosis is noted, as is variation in platelet size and a giant platelet. (H.O.)

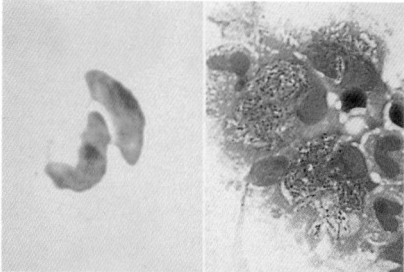

L, Left, Falciparum malaria. Peripheral blood showing two crescent-shaped gametocytes. *Right,* AIDS. *Mycobacterium avium–intracellulare* infection. Massive numbers of red, acid-fast organisms are seen in the macrophages of this marrow aspirate. (H.O.)

able to a poorly documented metabolic lesion in RBC metabolism. Severe hemolysis may occur in diabetic ketoacidosis when significant hypophosphatemia is unmasked following insulin treatment of this condition.

Berliner N, Duffy TP: Approach to the patient with anemia. *In* Hoffman R, Benz E, et al. (eds.): Basic Principles and Practice of Hematology. Edinburgh, Churchill Livingstone, 1991, p. 302.

Cambi V, David S: The hematopoietic system in renal failure. Contrib Nephrol 106:43, 1994.

Duffy TP: Hematologic aspects of systemic disease. *In* Handin R, Lux S, Stoessel T (eds.): The Principles and Practice of Hematology. Philadelphia, JB Lippincott, 1995.

Graber SE, Krantz SB: Erythropoietin: Biology and clinical use. Hematol Oncol Clin North Am 3:369, 1989.

Rotig A, Cormier V, Blanche S, et al.: Pearson's marrow-pancreas syndrome. A multisystem mitochondrial disorder in infancy. J Clin Invest 86:1601, 1990.

Solomon L: Hematologic complications of liver disease and alcoholism. *In* Hoffman R, Benz E, et al. (eds.): Basic Principles and Practice of Hematology. New York, Churchill Livingstone, 1994, p. 1684.

132 MICROCYTIC AND HYPOCHROMIC ANEMIAS
Thomas P. Duffy

Hemoglobulin synthesis for the needs of normal red blood cell (RBC) production requires an adequate supply of iron and intact metabolic pathways for the generation of heme and globin molecules. Any deficiency in this triad of iron, heme, or globin may result in RBC with a deficient hemoglobin concentration (mean corpuscular hemoglobin concentration: MCHC). Such hemoglobin-deficient RBC are usually microcytic with a reduced mean corpuscular volume (MCV), attributable to additional divisions in the RBC maturation sequence in the setting of a low hemoglobin concentration. This combination of small and hypochromic RBC can be detected on examination of the peripheral smear when the process is advanced and can be confirmed by indices generated from measurements of RBC size using electronic Coulter counters. An emerging population of microcytic RBC at an early stage of iron deficiency anemia can be recognized by studying a red cell distribution width (RDW), where any small cells constitute a peak separate from RBC of normal size.

Characterization of anemia as hypochromic and microcytic narrows the possible causes of the RBC deficiency to some abnormality in iron, heme, or globin metabolism. Low values for MCV and MCHC, generated by the electronic counter, delimit a small number of possible lesions as the causes of this type of anemia.

IRON DEFICIENCY ANEMIA

DEFINITION. Iron, as the core of the hemoglobin molecule responsible for the oxygen-carrying capabilities of blood, is the most precious element within the body; an efficient system of conservation and recycling of this valuable resource serves to guarantee the amount of iron necessary for daily hemoglobin synthesis. Storage depots of iron exist within the reticuloendothelial (RE) cells of the liver, spleen, and bone marrow and the parenchymal cells of the liver, and these stores are depleted before any restriction in hemoglobin synthesis occurs. Iron deficiency anemia therefore represents the final temporal development in the chronology of progressive iron deficiency within the body. Because this anemia does not supervene until iron stores are mobilized to maintain an optimal hemoglobin mass, absence of iron stores on examination of the marrow is a reliable confirmation that iron deficiency is contributing to any anemia that is present.

PREVALENCE. Iron deficiency is the most common cause of anemia throughout the world and one of the most common medical problems that confront the general physician. Its geographic distribution is determined by dietary deficiencies and intestinal parasitism, especially in Third World countries; hookworm infection has created the same lesion in the American South.

Its prevalence is much higher in women than in men because of the toll of menstruation and pregnancy on the iron stores of women.

The expansion of the blood pool that occurs during adolescence also leads to low iron stores in this group which may be further critically depleted as a result of inadequate dietary intake. The latter factor contributes to the iron deficiency state in many women, even in affluent societies, as they embark upon pregnancy.

IRON METABOLISM. Mechanisms exist within the body to ensure that the total iron content of the body is maintained within a defined range; exceeding these limits results in the condition recognized as hemochromatosis with organ damage created by the tissue accumulation of elemental iron. In specific contrast with other body constituents, the control of iron content is imposed by limiting its entrance into the body rather than by increasing the excretion of any excess, the usual pathway to maintain electrolyte balance. Once iron has entered the plasma after absorption from the gastrointestinal tract or from the breakdown of transfused red blood cells, it can be removed only by the withdrawal of blood or by the more laborious process of iron chelation therapy. The normal metabolism of iron is strictly weighted in favor of ensuring adequate iron reserves even at the cost of iron overload, which may result in pathologic states.

The major locus of iron within the body is the center of the hemoglobin molecule within RBC and as part of the myoglobin molecule in muscle; a smaller fraction is a constituent of important tissue-based enzymes. Storage pools of iron in the form of ferritin and hemosiderin are present within the liver, spleen, and bone marrow. These reserves of approximately 1000 mg in males and 500 mg in females are derived from the breakdown of senescent RBC within the RE system and from any surplus of absorbed iron beyond that needed for hemoglobin synthesis. The disparity in the size of these stores in men and women is attributable to the previously mentioned demands of menstruation and pregnancy in women.

The tiniest compartment of iron within the body is transport iron (7 mg), in which iron travels linked to the transport protein transferrin. Although this is the smallest compartment, it is kinetically the most active, turning over several times a day as iron is transported to its various destinations within the body. Transferrin picks up iron from the gastrointestinal cells and delivers it primarily to cells engaging in hemoglobin synthesis. Transferrin also picks up iron from the storage depots in the daily recycling of iron stores.

This system of conservation and recycling of iron serves to provide a constant supply of iron for the needs (30 to 35 mg) of daily hemoglobin synthesis. Only a tiny fraction of iron (1 mg) is lost each day via the pathway of sweating and epidermal shedding from the gut and urinary tracts; this minuscule amount can easily be replaced from the food in a normal diet. The major fraction is derived from the breakdown of RBC which, after a survival of 90 to 120 days in the peripheral blood, are phagocytosed by splenic macrophages and their contents re-enter the economy of the body. The iron released from senescent RBC is immediately available for the needs of hemoglobin synthesis, with the excess stored as ferritin and hemosiderin. The vector of iron transport is always in the direction of providing iron to fulfill the body's needs in maintaining an optimal RBC mass.

ABSORPTION. The normal diet in the United States contains approximately 15 to 30 mg of iron each day, with every thousand calories in the diet containing about 6 mg of elemental iron. Iron in food is present as a portion of the heme ring in meats and in a less easily absorbable form as ferric hyroxide complexes in other food. The acid environment of the stomach and its enzymatic secretions emulsify ingested food and liberate iron for its absorption within the small intestine; pancreatic secretions counter this pH alteration and help to control excessive absorption of iron.

Iron must be in the reduced or ferrous form for absorption to take place. Ingestion of reducing substances such as ascorbate or succinate enhances iron absorption because of their effect upon iron valency. Other substances such as phytates in cereals, tannates in tea, antacids, and certain antibiotics (tetracycline) may complex with iron and thereby hinder its absorption. Maximal absorption of iron occurs in the duodenum and upper portions of the jejunum. Malabsorptive states or bypass of these areas resulting from gastrojejunostomies may contribute to an iron deficiency state.

As outlined previously, iron absorption within the body can be adjusted over a broad range according to the body's needs. In the presence of iron deficiency, the body can increase its absorption efficiency at least fivefold, easily and rapidly compensating for any deficiency. This is a departure from the usual situation in which the body must guard itself against iron overload by absorbing only one tenth of iron available in the diet. The mechanism whereby such a limitation or "mucosal curtain" is imposed upon iron absorption is still not defined; it appears to be regulated by some aspect of dynamic iron turnover because hemolytic anemias, ineffective erythropoiesis, and hypoxemic states all have increased iron turnover and are all associated with increased iron absorption. The mucosal curtain is lowered by imposing a limit on the amount of iron that gets across the gastrointestinal membranes. Whatever iron is not needed by the body is diverted into a storage molecule within the gastrointestinal mucosal cells; this iron is lost from the body as these cells are exfoliated during the normal cycle of cell turnover. In iron deficient states in which iron needs are exaggerated, little of the iron is diverted to the storage form, with the majority of the absorbed iron passing directly through the cells for plasma transport linked to transferrin. When iron stores are adequate, much of the absorbed iron never reaches the plasma and is lost with the gastrointestinal shedding.

A failure to properly lower this mucosal curtain is thought to be the explanation for iron accumulation in primary hemochromatosis; such patients continue to absorb iron even in the face of total body iron overload. Increased iron absorption also occurs with pancreatic insufficiency because of the absence of the pH alteration contributed by normal pancreatic secretions; the absence of this restraint on iron absorption explains in part the iron overload that often occurs in chronic alcoholic states.

TRANSPORT. Transferrin is a glycoprotein of approximately 80,000 molecular weight which is produced by liver parenchymal cells in inverse proportion to the iron stores within these cells. This matching of transferrin production to iron needs explains in part the elevated transferrin or iron-binding capacity levels that characterize the iron deficiency state. Transferrin can bind one or two molecules of ferric iron, a process accompanied by the simultaneous attachment of an equal number of bicarbonate ions; the latter molecules facilitate the uncoupling of iron from the binding protein.

Transferrin binding of iron protects the body against the toxicity of elemental iron and increases the solubility of this molecule within plasma. Transferrin also imparts a preferential direction of flow of iron molecules to cells engaging in hemoglobin synthesis and, in the pregnant woman, to the trophoblastic cells of the placenta. The protein is measured in the plasma by quantitating the amount of iron-binding sites available, a measurement called the total iron-binding capacity (TIBC) of plasma. Under normal circumstances, the TIBC is only one third saturated, with the total amount of transferrin within the plasma being approximately 300 mg per 100 ml.

Iron levels vary diurnally, with the highest levels present in the morning: normal iron levels are usually within 60 to 180 mg per 100 ml. A small amount of iron is also present in plasma in the form of the storage molecule ferritin, with the concentration of this molecule mirroring the stores of iron within the marrow. Iron also complexes with lactoferrin, an iron-binding protein liberated from neutrophilic granules which is thought to play a role in defense against infection. Lactoferrin rapidly sequesters iron in RE cells, thereby depriving microorganisms of iron, which is an essential growth factor for most microorganisms.

IRON KINETICS. Ferrokinetic measurements using radiolabeled iron-59 can quantitate iron absorption, marrow transit time of iron, and plasma and erythrocyte iron turnover. These studies permit *in vivo* localization of any defect in the uptake, transport, or delivery of iron; such measurements are now primarily investigative tools that are not used in routine clinical situations.

PATHOGENESIS. Conservation and recycling of iron within the body provide an excellent buffer to fulfill the daily needs of iron for hemoglobin synthesis. Iron deficiency anemia therefore occurs only after an extended period of negative iron balance, a period during which the storage pool is exhausted of its reserves. Although this depletion may result from decreased ingestion or absorption of iron, the most common causes of iron deficiency have their source in blood loss from lesions in the gastrointestinal tract or from the demands of menstruation and pregnancy.

DECREASED IRON UPTAKE. To maintain iron balance within the body, the adult male needs to absorb only 1.0 to 1.5 mg

of iron each day, whereas an adult female needs to absorb a larger amount (2 to 3 mg) because of the iron losses sustained with menstruation. Each milliliter of blood contains approximately 0.4 mg of iron so that the monthly menstrual loss of approximately 60 ml creates the need for an additional 20 to 30 mg of iron absorption each month. Pregnancy with its expansion of the maternal blood pool and the additional needs for fetal hemoglobin synthesis frequently overwhelms an already marginal iron storage pool and requires supplemental iron as a prophylactic measure against the development of frank anemia.

Because the iron/calorie ratio of the normal U.S. diet is 6 mg iron for every 1000 calories, there is usually no shortage of dietary iron for males; the restricted diets of some women may not provide a comparable surfeit and may give rise to an iron deficiency state without frank anemia. The latter does not commonly have a dietary cause as the sole insult; gastric achlorhydria with its negative effect upon iron absorption may exaggerate the deficiency, but it too is not an acceptable isolated cause for iron deficiency anemia.

Gastrojejunostomies and sprue may both result in iron deficiency due to the loss of the necessary mucosal surface and/or increased intestinal transit time. The anemia seen with gastrojejunal bypass procedures has anastomotic mucosal lesions as a larger contribution to this deficiency.

Certain foods that complex with iron and hinder its absorption have already been discussed. Contributing somewhat to decreased uptake is the modern shift to non–iron-containing cooking utensils, eliminating this rich source of iron from the diet. The popularity of vegetarian diets may also lessen the amount of iron available from the diet.

A vicious circle may occur which is unique to patients with iron deficiency; such patients may develop an appetite for bizarre foods which is temporally and causally related to the iron deficiency. This phenomenon, pica, is the only known example of a compulsive appetite or behavior created by the lack of a normal body element. Its victims may ingest clay (geophagia), which in turn may potentiate the problem by chelating iron within the gut; ice (pagophagia) or starch (amylophagia) may be other targets of this appetite. Iron replacement corrects the problem, which may or may not be accompanied by anemia.

INCREASED IRON LOSS. The most common cause of iron deficiency anemia in both men and women is blood loss; this loss most frequently has its source in gastrointestinal bleeding in the former and menstrual bleeding in the latter. The implication of the discovery of iron deficiency anemia in men and postmenopausal women is the same; the gastrointestinal tract harbors the causal lesion until proven otherwise. Even in the absence of positive stool guaiacs or a history of melena, it is still imperative to examine the gastrointestinal tract because of its frequent involvement when iron deficiency is present. Iron deficiency may be the initial presentation of an otherwise occult carcinoma of the gut, with right-sided colon tumors not infrequently having this clinical picture. Multiple other gastrointestinal lesions such as large hiatal hernias, ulcer disease, inflammatory bowel disease, or angiodysplasias may all present with iron deficiency.

Ingestion of aspirin and nonsteroidal agents, often in the treatment of arthritic conditions, may be complicated by gastrointestinal blood loss. Less common causes of excessive iron loss include urinary tract bleeding and renal filtration of hemoglobin released from the breakdown of red blood cells; individuals with mechanical heart valves all have potential for this problem as a result of the traumatic rupture of RBC's as they flow across the artificial surfaces of these valves. Pulmonary sequestration of iron also occurs following some pulmonary hemorrhagic states, with no mechanism available to the body to recapture this closeted iron. The stores of iron may also be depleted in the act of frequently donating blood, a good samaritan cause of iron deficiency.

CLINICAL MANIFESTATIONS. Iron deficiency anemia is characterized by a degree of fatigue that may be disproportionate to the apparent severity of the anemia. This has been attributed to a depletion of essential tissue-based iron-containing enzymes with an attendant reduction in energy generation by muscle. Transfusion of RBC for correction of this anemia reverses only in part the symptoms of the condition; iron repletion is the definitive correction for this fatigue state.

Iron deficiency has several characteristic clinical manifestations, but all of them are rare relative to the high incidence of this condition. A sore tongue (glossitis), atrophy of the lingual papillae, and erosions at the corner of the mouth (angular stomatitis) are oral manifestations of iron deficiency; atrophy of the gastric mucosa with achlorhydria is a further extension of the same process. An atrophic rhinitis with a foul nasal discharge (ozena) may progress to anosmia in iron-deficient individuals. A greenish hue to the complexion (chlorosis) is an accompaniment of the same deficiency, especially in adolescent girls in Victorian literature. Brittle, fragile fingernails and spooning of the nails (koilonychia) are peripheral clues to the disorder.

Dysphagia, attributable to an esophageal web, occurs most frequently in elderly women with iron deficiency; this lesion, the Plummer-Vinson or Paterson-Kelly syndrome, may be later complicated by the development of esophageal carcinoma. The web may not disappear with iron replacement, and such patients may require dilatation for relief of the symptoms.

Splenomegaly has been described as an accompaniment of iron deficiency, although an independent or concomitant thalassemic trait may be the true cause of the enlargement. Pseudotumor cerebri has also been described as a very rare accompaniment of iron deficiency.

LABORATORY FINDINGS. The laboratory findings in full-blown iron deficiency anemia include a reduction in all three parameters (MCV, MCH, MCHC) that are generated from the Coulter counter. In contrast, early iron deficiency anemia has normochromic, normocytic indices because the iron-deficient population of RBC constitutes only a small percentage of the RBC mass. Only when the hematocrit falls below 31 to 32% do the RBC indices become microcytic; a normochromic, normocytic anemia is therefore the earliest form of anemia with iron deficiency.

The Coulter counter indices have replaced the examination of the peripheral blood smear in the recognition of hypochromia and microcytosis in most circumstances; the smear may still contain important clues to the presence of iron deficiency because an elevated platelet number is usually evident on the peripheral smear of the iron-deficient patient. Serum iron and transferrin levels help to confirm the diagnosis of iron deficiency, with a low serum iron and an elevated transferrin level resulting in a transferrin saturation of less than 10 to 15%; a low iron level is not in itself diagnostic of iron deficiency because many other systemic insults can alter the serum level of iron. Ferritin levels also permit recognition of iron deficiency with reduction in this serum protein to less than 10 ng per milliliter in uncomplicated iron deficiency. The final step in heme synthesis is the incorporation of iron into a protoporphyrin ring; deficient delivery of iron to the red cells results in elevated levels of free erythrocyte protoporphyrin as an additional marker of iron-deficient erythropoiesis.

Diagnosis of iron deficiency is usually possible using the combination of RBC indices and serum measurement of transferrin saturation or ferritin levels. However, because both these levels are altered by perturbations as broad as infection, inflammation, malignancy, and starvation, bone marrow iron stores remain the final arbiter when any uncertainty exists as to the presence of iron deficiency. The marrow in this state is devoid of macrophage iron, and less than 10% of the RBC precursors contain siderotic granules. Absence of iron stores categorically confirms the presence of iron deficiency and serves as the gold standard for making the diagnosis.

TREATMENT. Recognition and treatment of iron deficiency anemia require the identification and reversal, if possible, of its cause; the anemia is the only important sign of an underlying lesion that may be as benign as aspirin ingestion or as threatening as an occult malignancy. Treating the anemia without identifying its cause may mean loss of the only opportunity to discover a malignancy at a potentially curable stage.

The treatment of iron deficiency anemia is made somewhat difficult by its frequent induction of gastrointestinal distress manifested by nausea, dyspepsia, constipation, and diarrhea. These symptoms are usually proportional to the iron content of the prescribed oral iron preparation; the most commonly administered preparation is ferrous sulfate tablets, 300 mg, which contain 60 mg of elemental iron in each tablet. The drug is best absorbed on an empty stomach but, because it is better tolerated when ingested with meals, this is the manner in which it is most frequently prescribed. Starting with a once-daily dosing and escalating to a final dose of three times daily permits most patients to tolerate this optimal dose. Persistent intolerance can be addressed by switching to ferrous gluconate with

its lower content of elemental iron and the attendant need for a longer period of iron administration to correct the deficiency state.

Innumerable iron preparations are marketed, but there is little to recommend them over the cost-effective ferrous sulfate pills. Although ascorbate and succinate enhance the absorption of iron, the addition of these agents to iron preparations is costly and unnecessary in light of the body's efficiency in iron absorption under normal circumstances. Enteric coated iron tablets may actually be contraindicated because the coating may remain a shield against absorption in the upper portions of the small intestine where maximal iron absorption takes place. Liquid iron preparations are available and may be better tolerated by some patients. Because iron salts can stain the teeth, iron solutions should be ingested through a straw. Such preparations may be better absorbed in patients with gastrojejunostomies or rapid intestinal transit times.

At the time iron therapy is initiated, a baseline reticulocyte count and ferritin level should be obtained. With iron replacement there is usually an early improvement in the symptoms of fatigue and lassitude, although a maximal reticulocytosis does not occur for 7 to 10 days. The hemoglobin level does not rise for 2 to 2½ weeks, and it requires about 2 months of daily iron therapy for the hemoglobin level to return to normal. Measurement of ferritin levels allows one to determine when iron stores have been reconstituted and when iron therapy should be discontinued.

In the rare patient who cannot tolerate or cannot absorb iron from the gastrointestinal tract and in individuals who require large iron boluses to compensate for chronic blood loss, parenteral iron in the form of an iron-dextran complex is available. It should be used with restraint because of the threat of acute (anaphylaxis) and subacute (arthralgias, myalgias, and adenopathy) side effects. This parenteral preparation can be administered intramuscularly or intravenously, with the latter routine more advantageous because the total dose can be delivered in a single administration. No more than 2 ml of imferon, containing 50 mg iron per milliliter, can be administered at a single intramuscular site; staining of the skin may occur even though the recommended Z-track technique of injection is used.

A small test dose (0.25 ml) of the drug should be administered before intramuscular or intravenous injections to determine hypersensitivity to the agent. The dose to be infused for correction of iron deficiency can be calculated according to the following formula:

Dose (ml) = 0.0476 × wt (kg) × (normal hgb − observed hgb)
            + (1 ml/5 kg) to maximum of 14 ml to replete iron stores

This total dose can be diluted in normal saline at a 1:20 dilution and infused slowly over several hours while watching for any side effects.

PROGNOSIS. The prognosis in iron deficiency anemia is strictly related to the underlying cause of the anemia. Iron deficiency *per se* does not usually alter the prognosis because it is easily treated once it is recognized. The importance of the diagnosis is the recognition of the need to identify the underlying cause of the condition and to correct this lesion so that the anemia does not recur.

HYPOCHROMIC ANEMIAS NOT CAUSED BY IRON DEFICIENCY

Because characterization of an anemia as hypochromic restricts its cause to some abnormality in iron, heme, or globin metabolism, the elimination of iron deficiency as its cause narrows the choices to these other components of hemoglobin metabolism. Abnormalities in globin chain synthesis, the thalassemias, are a more prominent consideration when hypochromic anemia occurs in the appropriate ethnic groups; hemoglobin electrophoresis with quantitation of fetal and A_2 hemoglobin should be undertaken early when hypochromic indices are discovered in Mediterranean or black individuals. The sideroblastic anemias are iron-loading anemias due to abnormalities in heme synthesis; a clue to their presence is nearly total saturation of serum transferrin levels, a striking departure from the findings in iron deficiency. Confirmation of the diagnosis requires bone marrow documentation of ringed sideroblasts, the pathognomonic lesion in this condition.

Deficient delivery of iron to developing RBC occurs in the anemia of chronic disease (ACD) even in the presence of the increased iron stores that characterize this anemia. This lesion is easily confused with pure iron deficiency anemia because serum iron levels and transferrin saturation may overlap in the two conditions. The bone marrow iron stores distinguish the two because of the presence of marrow iron in ACD; iron deficiency anemia is the only cause of hypochromic, microcytic RBC when iron stores are absent from the marrow.

THE ANEMIA OF CHRONIC DISEASE. Although iron deficiency anemia is the most common anemia in general, ACD is the most common anemia in the hospitalized patient. This condition represents a shared hematologic response to systemic insults as varied as infection, inflammation, malignancy, and trauma. The anemia is moderate in degree, with the hematocrit usually in the range of 28 to 32%. The morphology is normochromic normocytic in 60 to 70% of such patients, with the remainder having a mild hypochromic microcytic anemia. Hypoferremia is characteristic of ACD in the face of marrow iron overload. Confusion of ACD with iron deficiency anemia results from the overlapping of microcytosis and hypoferremia in both disorders. In iron deficiency anemia, the lesion is secondary to iron lack; in ACD the lesion includes deficient delivery of iron to developing RBC in addition to other derangements in RBC production.

Etiology and Pathogenesis. At least three different pathophysiologic mechanisms contribute to ACD, an anemia that develops within a few weeks of the onset of systemic disease and is independent of any marrow involvement or specific hematologic complication of the systemic disease. Accelerated RBC breakdown, abnormalities in iron mobilization and delivery, and cytokine inhibition of erythropoiesis have all been implicated to various degrees in producing this picture. There is a modest shortening of RBC survival, likely due to extravascular sequestration by a stimulated RE system because RBC from individuals with ACD demonstrate an unimpaired survival when transfused into a normal individual. The degree of hemolysis in ACD is modest, and the failure of the host to mount an appropriate reticulocyte response to compensate for the anemia indicates that a hypoproliferative defect, rather than hemolysis, is the major lesion in ACD.

Iron studies reveal low serum iron and transferrin levels in ACD, a contrast with the findings in iron deficiency anemia, in which elevated transferrin levels are present. Nevertheless, the transferrin saturation levels in ACD may overlap with those of iron deficiency, further adding to the confusion of these two entities. The features that help to distinguish them have their source in the ACD as a sideropenic anemia in the face of RE iron overload. Serum ferritin levels and bone marrow iron stores are both increased in ACD in concert with its basic abnormality in iron mobilization; an elevated erythrocyte sedimentation rate is also an accompaniment of ACD, wherein the sedimentation rate and the anemia constitute sickness indices of the body.

The cause of the hypoferremia in ACD is not strictly defined. The disproportionate incorporation of iron into ferritin in storage depots may have its explanation in ferritin elevation as an acute-phase reactant in all the conditions associated with ACD. Another explanation for the hypoferremia in ACD is a form of nutritional immunity because microorganisms and malignancies require iron for growth and proliferation. In the face of infection and malignancies, normal iron metabolism is subverted to bolster the body's defenses against these assaults; lactoferrin, the product of polymorphonuclear leukocytes, redirects the vector of iron delivery away from RBC, which lack lactoferrin receptors, to cells of the RE system. Malignancies may themselves alter the vector of iron delivery because many tumors contain siderophores, which are molecules that can effectively extract iron from the surrounding plasma. This closeting of iron explains the fall in serum iron in the ACD, although hypoferremia is unlikely to be the primary cause of the anemia. Administration of iron to such patients does not correct the anemia and is not indicated in its management. The hypoferremia is considered an advantage to the body in restraining bacterial or tumor cell growth; the anemia is the cost of the body's defense against invasion.

Elevated ferritin production and lactoferrin linkage are not the only factors causing hypoferremia in ACD; the low serum iron level is now thought to be only part of a more generalized response to infection, malignancy, or inflammation. These systemic threats to the body start a cascade of cytokines initiated by interleukin-1 release from macrophages. Anabolic and catabolic responses result with elevation of the acute-phase reactants (C-reactive protein, haptoglobin, ceruloplasmin, fibrinogen, ferritin) and reduction in serum iron and hematocrit levels. Playing an important role in the production of anemia is the liberation of tumor necrosis factor or cachectin, a product of macrophages, as part of the cytokine network. Injection of these substances creates the anorexia, debilitation, and weight loss of chronic disease and also inhibits the growth of erythroid precursor cells; ACD represents "cachexia" of the marrow, a sharing by the marrow in the defense of the body against the threat of infection, malignancy, or inflammatory disorders.

Clinical Manifestations. ACD is not itself usually a cause of symptoms. The anemia is mild and well tolerated unless it is superimposed upon other threatening conditions. The importance of recognizing ACD is in identifying its underlying cause. ACD is not infrequently the initial evidence that otherwise occult disease is present.

Diagnosis. ACD is a moderate (Hct 28 to 32%), normochromic, normocytic anemia that supervenes during the early course of disorders as diverse as malignancy, infection, inflammation, or trauma. Iron indices usually reveal hypoferremia and a reduced iron-binding capacity. Confusion with iron deficiency anemia occurs because microcytic anemia occurs in 30 to 40% of such cases, and the transferrin saturation may be reduced to levels seen in iron deficiency. Distinguishing the two is an elevated ferritin level and erythrocyte sedimentation rate in ACD as well as the plentiful marrow iron stores in this condition.

Treatment. ACD is a secondary manifestation of an underlying disorder, and its successful reversal requires recognition and correction of that disorder. Although hypoferremia is present, iron therapy does not correct the anemia and only contributes to the iron overload in this condition. Blood transfusions are frequently not necessary because the anemia is modest and usually well tolerated. Because ACD results from a cytokine-induced hypoerythropoietin state, the defect can be overridden with EPO administration. This is not an appropriate intervention under most circumstances because the ACD is usually not severe.

SIDEROBLASTIC ANEMIAS. Sideroblastic anemias are uncommon causes of hypochromic anemias which have their origins in altered production of the heme component of the hemoglobin molecule. The final step in heme synthesis involves the incorporation of iron into the protoporphyrin ring, which is synthesized in and around the mitochondria of the developing RBC. Any defect in the multistep generation of protoporphyrin creates a mismatch between iron delivery and iron incorporation into heme. This results in iron overloading of the mitochondria because heme, the feedback inhibitor of further RBC iron uptake, is deficient related to globin synthesis. Such cells are designated "ringed" sideroblasts because the iron-laden mitochondria occupy a perinuclear distribution within the developing RBC; Prussian blue staining of the RBC within the marrow demonstrates these siderotic granules surrounding the nucleus. The siderotic granules of normal siderocytes are fewer in number and are distributed throughout the cytoplasma of the cell. The mitochondrial accumulation of iron is what distinguishes the sideroblastic anemias.

A clue to the presence of these anemias is the paradoxical finding of hyperferremia and a nearly total transferrin saturation in a patient with a hypochromic anemia. The hypochromia has its origin in deficient protoporphyrin ring synthesis, leading to a reduced hemoglobin complement in affected cells.

Pathogenesis and Classification. Protoporphyrin ring synthesis is a multistep process that depends upon several sequential enzymatic reactions occurring in and around the surface of cell mitochondria. A lesion at any stage in this sequence, whether due to an enzymatic deficiency or an abnormality in mitochondrial structure or function, may result in faulty protoporphyrin synthesis. These lesions may occur as inherited or acquired defects in the pathway. The inherited forms have both mitochondrial and nuclear genetic mutations as their cause. As with disturbances in other metabolic pathways within the body, drugs and toxins are the major causes of acquired sideroblastic anemia; a less common form of acquired sideroblastic anemia exists as a clonal disorder that is a subgroup of the myelodysplasias.

The primary lesion in sideroblastic anemia results in a mismatch between iron delivery and its incorporation into heme. The unincorporated iron accumulates on the mitochondria with oxidant damage to these critical organelles. Such iron loading of the mitochondria further contributes to ineffective erythropoiesis. Cautious phlebotomy of patients with sideroblastic anemia may improve their anemia by unloading iron from the mitochondria and correcting this secondary lesion.

The morphologic evidence in the peripheral blood for the sideroblastic process is a population of hypochromic RBC. Transferrin levels are saturated and ferritin levels are increased, although not usually to the same degree as in hemochromatosis. Rare RBC containing siderotic granules or Pappenheimer bodies may also circulate in the peripheral blood. The diagnosis of sideroblastic anemia is confirmed by the presence of ringed sideroblasts within the marrow which are nucleated RBC with a perinuclear collection of iron granules.

Acquired Sideroblastic Anemia.
Idiopathic Refractory Sideroblastic Anemia. A hypochromic anemia, frequently with slightly macrocytic indices, develops in elderly individuals as a predominantly erythroid manifestation of a myelodysplastic syndrome. The RBC population is often dimorphic, with a varying proportion of hypochromic and normochromic cells; the hypochromic cells have their origin in a clonal population of ringed sideroblasts within the marrow. The cause of the disorder is not known, although its occurrence following chemotherapy suggests that damage to chromosomal material responsible for normal erythroid development creates this picture.

The lesion is chronic and may remain restricted to the erythroid line with ineffective erythropoiesis in addition to the defect in heme synthesis. The lesion may also evolve into leukemia, but with no firm predictors of whether or when this transition will occur. Associated leukopenia, especially when accompanied by WBC developmental abnormalities (pseudo-Pelger-Huët anomaly), and alterations in platelet number are common antecedents to leukemia transformation.

Because the cause is not known with certainty, treatment of the disorder remains experimental. Pharmacologic doses of pyridoxine, a vitamin necessary for the initial step in heme synthesis, have been administered but with very limited success, and this therapy is usually of no benefit. Androgens and erythropoietin therapies also add little to its reversal. Because the condition remains refractory to therapy, blood transfusions contribute the only major intervention available. Prolonged support with RBC may lead to secondary hemochromatosis and require chelation therapy with deferoxamine. Fortunately, the process may be very chronic with no need for transfusion until late in its course.

Sideroblastic anemia may be discovered in the setting of a large variety of medical conditions, including rheumatoid disease, malignancies, and endocrine disorders. The relation to these disorders is not likely causal because treatment or correction of the underlying disorder does not correct the anemia. It is more likely that the medical condition serves to unmask an otherwise undetected anemia.

Sideroblastic Anemia Associated with Drugs or Toxins. Consumption of large amounts of alcohol over a several-week period can induce sideroblastic anemia in volunteers in the absence of any concomitant vitamin deficiency. The lesion is thought to have its origin in alcohol's interference with pyridoxine metabolism and its essential role as a coenzyme in the delta-aminolevulinic acid synthetase step in porphyrin synthesis. Alcohol is also a mitochondrial toxin, and the anemia may have its source in damage to mitochondrial function.

In alcoholics with sideroblastic anemia, the marrow lesion persists for 7 to 10 days following the withdrawal of alcohol. Other insults to this metabolic pathway include lead, chloramphenicol, and several antituberculous drugs. All of these agents interfere with the initial step in protoporphyrin ring synthesis, with lead also hindering a second site where heme synthesis catalyzes the incorporation of iron into the heme ring in the final step in this pathway.

Hereditary Sideroblastic Anemias.
Hereditary sideroblastic anemia is most commonly a moderate to severe hypochromic, normocytic anemia inherited in a sex-linked recessive fashion. A point mutation resulting in an amino acid change near the pyridoxal phosphate-binding site of the erythrocytic 5-amino-levulinate synthase isoenzyme is the underlying defect in kindreds with this disorder. The anemia does not usually become evident until early adulthood and responds to varying doses of pyridoxine, which are usually much larger than the daily requirements for this vitamin.

Mitochondrial cytopathies may also be responsible for congenital disorders when a sideroblastic anemia is linked to pancreatic, liver, and kidney dysfunction, as in Pearson's syndrome. These rare syndromes affect infants and are thought to be due to inherited mutations in mitochondrial DNA that result in defective oxidative phosphorylation in the organs involved.

Bottomley SS, Muller-Eberhard U: Pathophysiology of heme synthesis. Semin Hematol 25:282, 1988.
Brock JH (ed.): Iron Metabolism in Health and Disease. London, WB Saunders, 1994.
Cazzola M, Barosi G, Gobbi PG, et al.: Natural history of idiopathic sideroblastic anemia. Blood 71:305, 1988.
Conrad ME: Regulation of iron absorption. Progr Clin Biol Res 380:203, 1993.
Cox TC, Bottomley SS, Wiley JS, et al.: X-linked pyridoxine-responsive sideroblastic anemia due to a Thr388-to-Ser substitution in erythroid 5-aminolevulinate synthase. N Engl J Med 330:675, 1994.
Finch C: Regulator of iron balance in humans. Blood 84:1697, 1994.
Massey AC: Microcytic anemia: Differential diagnosis and management of iron deficiency anemia. Med Clin North Am 76:549, 1992.
Means RT Jr, Krantz SB: Progress in understanding the pathogenesis of the anemia of chronic disease. Blood 80:1639, 1992.
Rockey DC, Cello JP: Evaluation of the gastrointestinal tract in patients with iron-deficiency anemia. N Engl J Med 329:1691, 1993.
Spivak JL: Cancer-related anemia: Its causes and characteristics. Semin Oncol 21:3, 1994.

133 MEGALOBLASTIC ANEMIAS
Robert H. Allen

DEFINITION

Megaloblastic anemias are caused by various defects in DNA synthesis that lead to a common set of hematologic abnormalities of the bone marrow and peripheral blood. The term "megaloblastic" refers to a morphologic abnormality of cell nuclei that is readily recognizable but difficult to describe (see Color Plate 6*G* and 6*H*). The erythrocytic, granulocytic, and megakaryocytic cell lines are all involved, and pancytopenia may develop. Recognition of megaloblastic anemia is important because two of its most common causes, cobalamin (vitamin B_{12}) deficiency and folate deficiency, are completely corrected with appropriate therapy. The recognition of cobalamin deficiency is of particular importance because it also causes a wide variety of neurologic and psychiatric abnormalities that are preventable or reversible if the diagnosis is made at an early stage.

Etiology

The four major etiologic categories of megaloblastic anemia are (1) cobalamin deficiency, (2) folate deficiency, (3) drugs, and (4) miscellaneous, which includes rare enzyme deficiencies and unexplained disorders (Table 133–1). The etiology of cobalamin deficiency can be subdivided into causes of decreased ingestion, impaired absorption, or impaired utilization of the vitamin. Folate deficiency can also be caused by decreased intake, impaired absorption, impaired utilization, and, in addition, a number of conditions in which there is an increased requirement for folic acid or increased loss of folic acid. Drugs that cause megaloblastosis can be categorized as those that are purine or pyrimidine antagonists and those that inhibit some other aspect of DNA synthesis. The miscellaneous category includes enzyme defects and some cases of myelodysplastic syndrome and acute leukemia.

It is important to determine the correct etiologic factor in megaloblastic anemia. For example, if a myelodysplastic syndrome is misdiagnosed in a cobalamin-deficient patient, the use of chemotherapy might result in early death of a patient who could have been completely cured with cobalamin therapy. Similarly, some causes of cobalamin and folate deficiency require therapy for the underlying disease in addition to replacement therapy with the appropriate vitamin.

TABLE 133–1. ETIOLOGIC CLASSIFICATION OF THE MEGALOBLASTIC ANEMIAS

Category	Etiologic Mechanisms
I. Cobalamin deficiency	
A. Decreased ingestion	Poor diet, lack of animal products, strict vegetarianism
B. Impaired absorption	1. Failure to release cobalamin from food protein
	Old age
	Gastrectomy (partial)
	2. Intrinsic factor (IF) deficiency
	Pernicious anemia
	Gastrectomy (total)
	Destruction of gastric mucosa by caustics
	Congenital abnormal or absence of IF molecule
	3. Chronic pancreatic disease
	4. Competitive parasites
	Bacteria in diverticula of bowel, blind loops
	Fish tapeworm infestations (*Diphyllobothrium latum*)
	5. Intrinsic intestinal disease
	Ileal resection, Crohn's disease, radiation ileitis
	Tropical sprue, celiac disease
	Infiltrative intestinal disease (e.g., lymphoma, scleroderma)
	Drug-induced malabsorption
	Congenital selective malabsorption (Imerslund-Gräsbeck syndrome)
C. Impaired utilization	Congenital enzyme deficiencies
	Lack of transcobalamin II
	Nitrous oxide administration
II. Folate deficiency	
A. Decreased ingestion	Poor diet, lack of vegetables
	Alcoholism
	Infancy
B. Impaired absorption	Intestinal short circuits
	Tropical sprue, celiac disease
	Anticonvulsants, sulfasalazine, other drugs
	Congenital malabsorption
C. Impaired utilization	Folic acid antagonists: methotrexate, triamterene, trimethoprim, pyrimethamine, ethanol
	Congenital enzyme deficiencies
D. Increased requirement	Pregnancy, infancy
	Hyperthyroidism
	Chronic hemolytic disease
	Neoplastic disease, exfoliative skin disease
E. Increased loss	Hemodialysis
III. Drugs—metabolic inhibitors	Purine synthesis: methotrexate, 6-mercaptopurine, 6-thioguanine, azathioprine
	Pyrimidine synthesis: methotrexate, 6-azauridine
	Thymidylate synthesis: methotrexate, 5-fluorouracil
	Deoxyribonucleotide synthesis: hydroxyurea, cytosine arabinoside
IV. Miscellaneous	
A. Inborn errors	Lesch-Nyhan syndrome
	Hereditary orotic aciduria
	Others
B. Unexplained disorders	Pyridoxine-responsive megaloblastic anemia
	Thiamine-responsive megaloblastic anemia
	Some cases of myelodysplastic syndrome
	Some cases of acute myelogenous leukemia

INCIDENCE AND PREVALENCE

Cobalamin Deficiency

The term *pernicious anemia,* often used as a synonym for cobalamin deficiency, should be reserved for conditions in which a gastric mucosal defect results in insufficient intrinsic factor to facilitate absorption of physiologic amounts of cobalamin. It is by far the most common cause of cobalamin deficiency in the Western Hemisphere. Pernicious anemia was originally believed to be primarily a disease of elderly individuals of northern European ancestry. It is now clear that it also occurs in individuals in their 20's and in all ethnic groups, including blacks and Hispanics. Before the discovery of liver therapy in 1926, pernicious anemia was invariably fatal. About 1.0% of individuals in the United States will develop pernicious anemia at some time during their life. With a population of 250 million, an average lifetime of 75 years, and the assumption that cobalamin deficiency exists for an average of 5 years before it is treated or the patient dies, there should be about 150,000 patients at various stages of cobalamin deficiency in the United States at any point in time. Approximately 10% of the U.S. population over age 70 have low or low-normal serum cobalamin levels *and* metabolic evidence of cobalamin deficiency (elevated levels of serum methylmalonic acid and homocysteine that fall to normal with cobalamin therapy). The etiology and the hematologic and neu-

ropsychiatric significance of these findings are unknown at the present time. These estimates of the actual and potential incidence of cobalamin deficiency further emphasize the importance of recognizing this eminently treatable disease.

Folate Deficiency, Drugs, and Other Causes

The incidence of folate deficiency and of drug-related megaloblastic anemia is less well established. Through its association with alcoholism, folate deficiency is far from a rare condition. The marked increase in the use of chemotherapeutic agents to treat malignant disease and immune disorders suggests that these drugs may now be the most common cause of megaloblastic anemia in the Western Hemisphere.

PATHOGENESIS AND PATHOLOGY

Mechanism of Megaloblastosis

FOLATE DEFICIENCY. Folate functions to transfer one-carbon units, such as methyl, methylene, and formyl groups, to various substrates in a variety of enzymatic reactions that are intimately related to the synthesis of DNA, RNA, and proteins. In folate deficiency, all forms of folate are reduced within cells, which impairs the growth and maturation of rapidly growing cells, such as those in the bone marrow. For example, thymidylate synthase catalyzes the synthesis of thymidine (dTMP) from deoxyuridine (dUMP) and 5,10-methylenetetrahydrofolate. Inhibition of thymidylate synthase leads to increased intracellular concentrations of deoxyuridine triphosphate (dUTP), which is incorporated into DNA in positions that normally arise from deoxythymidine triphosphate (dTTP). Attempts to repair this abnormal DNA increase DNA fragmentation, which may play a major role in causing the abnormalities of cell growth and maturation that are present in folate deficiency.

COBALAMIN DEFICIENCY. Cobalamin functions as an essential cofactor for only two enzymes in human cells, methionine synthase and L-methylmalonyl-CoA (coenzyme A) mutase (Figs. 133–1 and 133–2). Methionine synthase catalyzes the recycling of homocysteine to methionine, using 5-methylcobalamin as a required coenzyme (Fig. 133–1). Methionine, an essential amino acid for protein synthesis, also serves in the form of S-adenosylmethionine as the major methyl donor in numerous important enzymatic reactions. In cobalamin deficiency, increasing amounts of intracellular folate are converted to 5-methyl-tetrahydrofolate in an attempt to prevent intracellular methionine deficiency. The "trapping" of intracellular folate as 5-methyl-tetrahydrofolate is augmented by the fact that this is the major component of plasma folate and is the form that enters cells and must be converted to tetrahydrofolate by methionine synthase before it can enter the folate pool. Thus cobalamin deficiency results in secondary intracellular deficiency of all forms of folate except for 5-methyltetrahydrofolate. As a result, the activities of all of the enzymes that utilize folate to transfer one-carbon moieties, including thymidylate synthase, are impaired. This concept of "methylfolate trapping" explains why cobalamin deficiency and folate deficiency produce indistinguishable hematologic abnormalities and why the hematologic abnormalities seen in cobalamin deficiency can be completely reversed by pharmacologic amounts of folic acid. The latter oxidized, nonphysiologic form of folate can be reduced directly to tetrahydrofolate without first being converted to 5-methyltetrahydrofolate. This concept also explains why the hematologic abnormalities caused by folate deficiency respond only slightly, if at all, to large amounts of cobalamin.

DRUGS AND OTHER CAUSES. Drugs that cause megaloblastic anemia inhibit a variety of enzymes involved in DNA synthesis. 5-Fluorouracil (5-FU) inhibits thymidylate synthase directly. The addition of 5-formyltetrahydrofolate (leucovorin) to 5-FU regimens actually increases the inhibition of thymidylate synthase, since 5-formyltetrahydrofolate is readily converted to 5,10-methylenetetrahydrofolate, which is involved in the formation of inhibitory ternary complexes between 5,10-methylene-tetrahydrofolate, 5-FU, and thymidylate synthase. Why megaloblastic changes occur in some cases of the myelodysplastic syndrome and acute leukemias is unknown, but this is probably due to a variety of mutations that alter DNA synthesis.

Mechanism of Neuropsychiatric Abnormalities in Cobalamin Deficiency

A wide variety of neuropsychiatric abnormalities are seen in cobalamin deficiency and appear to be due to an undefined defect involving myelin synthesis. These abnormalities are not seen in folate deficiency. It has therefore been tempting to ascribe them to deficient activity of the second cobalamin-dependent enzyme, L-methylmalonyl-CoA mutase, which is unrelated to any folate-dependent enzyme or pathway. This enzyme catalyzes the conversion of L-methylmalonyl-CoA to succinyl-CoA, utilizing adenosylcobalamin as a required coenzyme (Fig. 133–2). Abnormal odd-carbon and branched-chain fatty acids are formed when the mutase is impaired. The neuropsychiatric abnormalities of cobalamin deficiency are not seen, however, in individuals with genetic defects of the mutase reaction, caused either by primary defects in the enzyme itself or by defects in the formation of adenosylcobalamin. Impairment of methionine synthase has also been postulated as the cause of the neuropsychiatric abnormalities as a result of the importance of methionine and S-adenosylmethionine for the many methylation reactions that take place in the nervous system. As noted, however, the neuropsychiatric abnormalities caused by cobalamin deficiency are not seen in folate deficiency, even though methionine synthase appears to be equally impaired in both vitamin deficiencies (based on similar marked elevations in serum homocysteine concentrations). Genetic defects in which the synthesis of adenosylcobalamin and methylcobalamin are both impaired do lead to neuropsychiatric abnormalities of the kind seen in cobalamin deficiency. These observations suggest that both cobalamin-dependent enzymes must be impaired for the neuropsychiatric abnormalities to develop and that the two cobalamin-dependent enzymes or pathways are connected or interrelated in some way that has not yet been discovered.

Mechanisms of Cobalamin Deficiency

Cobalamin is not present in plants; until recently, humans obtained their cobalamin exclusively from animal products. Cobalamin is synthesized only by certain microorganisms. During the past 45 years, humans have received increasing amounts of their dietary cobalamin from multivitamin supplements taken in the form of pills and as additives to many food preparations. Most cobalamin in animal products is tightly bound to proteins, i.e., the two cobalamin-dependent enzymes, and is released from them in the stomach by the concerted action of HCl and pepsin. The stomach is also the site of synthesis of intrinsic factor (IF), which binds free cobalamin with high affinity and plays an essential role in cobalamin absorption. Gastric juice contains another cobalamin-binding protein that originates in saliva and has a more rapid or "R"-type electrophoretic mobility than does IF. R protein binds cobalamin with a higher affinity than does IF, particularly at an acid pH. Thus, under normal conditions of gastric acidity, dietary cobalamin enters the duodenum bound to R protein. Additional cobalamin bound to R protein enters the duodenum after it is secreted into bile by the liver (this is the only significant route by which cobalamin is lost from the body). Pancreatic proteases partially degrade salivary and biliary R protein-cobalamin complexes in the jejunum, and only after this occurs is cobalamin bound to IF. The IF-cobalamin complex remains intact until it reaches the distal ileum, where it binds with high affinity to specific receptors located on ileal mucosal cells. Cobalamin then enters these cells and reaches the portal plasma, which contains three cobalamin-binding proteins known as transcobalamin I (TC I), transcobalamin II (TC II), and transcobalamin III (TC III). Their roles are summarized in Table 133–2. Although it contains only about 10% of the plasma cobalamin, TC II is the important transport protein because of its rapid clearance and its ability to deliver cobalamin to all cells within the body. TC II-cobalamin is taken up by cells by endocytosis during a process in which the TC II moiety is degraded and the cobalamin is reduced and eventually converted to its two coenzyme forms, i.e., methyl-cobalamin and adenosylcobalamin. Cobalamin is not stored intracellularly; all of the intracellular vitamin is bound to the two enzymes, which are present in greater amounts than is cobalamin. Additional information concerning the gastrointestinal phase of cobalamin absorption is found in Ch. 103.

A large number of acquired and genetic diseases affect the pathway of cobalamin absorption and transport and result in cobalamin deficiency (see Table 133–1). Strict vegans, i.e., those who ingest neither meat nor other animal products, such as milk, cheese, and eggs, and who do not ingest multivitamin supplements, become cobalamin deficient on a dietary basis. Approximately 10 to 15 years are required for clinical signs to develop, since the absorption

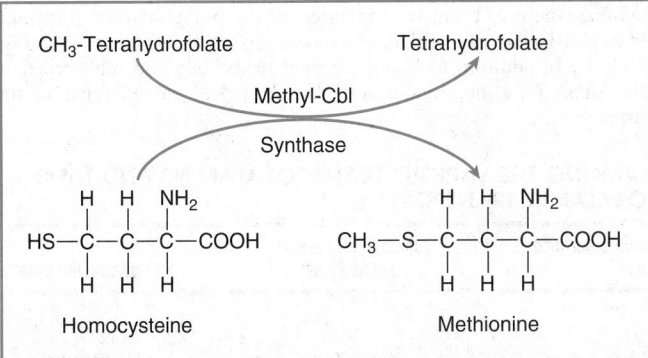

FIGURE 133–1. Reaction catalyzed by methionine synthase that requires methylcobalamin (methyl-Cbl) and transfers the methyl group of 5-methyltetrahydrofolate (CH₃-tetrahydrofolate) to homocysteine to form methionine and tetrahydrofolate. Homocysteine accumulates in cobalamin deficiency owing to a lack of methylcobalamin and in folate deficiency owing to a lack of 5-methyltetrahydrofolate.

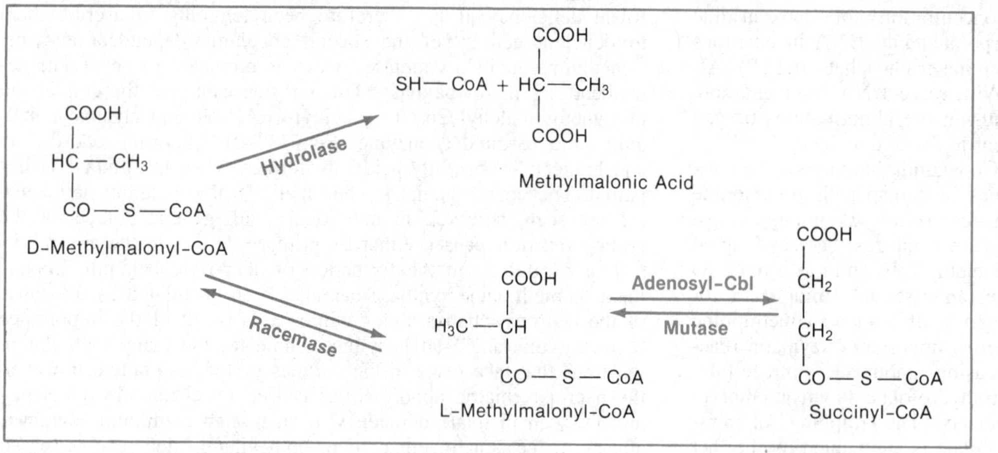

FIGURE 133–2. Reactions involved in the metabolism of D- and L-methylmalonyl-CoA. Methylmalonic acid accumulates in cobalamin deficiency owing to a lack of adenosylcobalamin (adenosyl-Cbl), which leads to an increase of L-methylmalonyl-CoA, which is converted to D-methylmalonyl-CoA and hydrolyzed to methylmalonic acid. (CoA = coenzyme A.)

of biliary cobalamin remains intact. The secretion of biliary cobalamin ranges from 5 to 10 μg per day, and approximately 90% is reabsorbed by strict vegans and other normal individuals. Thus, only 0.5 to 1.0 μg of the 5 to 10 μg of cobalamin present in a normal diet must be absorbed each day to maintain the total body content of cobalamin in the normal range of 2000 to 5000 μg.

Achlorhydria and the loss of pepsin secretion are very common in elderly subjects (>50% of individuals >age 70) and in those with partial gastrectomy. These individuals develop cobalamin deficiency because of inability to liberate cobalamin from its protein-bound form in foods of animal origin. Secretion of IF is reduced, but because it is normally formed in vast excess, sufficient IF usually remains for the reabsorption of biliary R protein-cobalamin, which is not dependent upon HCl and pepsin. The same time span of 10 to 15 years is required for these subjects to develop clinical signs of cobalamin deficiency as for those with dietary lack. Many of them never develop cobalamin deficiency, apparently because of the availability of free, nonprotein-bound cobalamin in multivitamin pills and supplements and because some natural animal products contain small amounts of free cobalamin.

A complete lack of IF occurs in individuals who have undergone total gastrectomy or who have pernicious anemia, in which there is idiopathic and essentially complete atrophy of the gastric mucosa in association with autoantibodies to parietal cells and IF. Only about 3 to 5 years are required for clinical signs of cobalamin deficiency to develop because in these individuals there is malabsorption of biliary as well as all forms of dietary cobalamin.

Cobalamin malabsorption occurs commonly in severe pancreatic exocrine insufficiency because of inability to degrade R protein-cobalamin complexes in the jejunum. Clinically evident cobalamin deficiency rarely occurs, however, probably because oral therapy with pancreatic extract is usually instituted in these patients during the 3 to 5 years that are necessary for the signs of cobalamin deficiency to develop.

The abnormal presence of high concentrations of bacteria and certain parasites in the small intestine can result in cobalamin malabsorption, since these organisms can avidly take up and retain cobalamin. Diseases that interfere with the integrity of the distal ileal mucosa can also result in cobalamin malabsorption, which occurs invariably after the surgical removal of the distal 100 cm of ileum.

A large number of genetic disorders involve the plasma transport of cobalamin, its intracellular conversion to its coenzyme forms, or its utilization by the two cobalamin-dependent enzymes. They usually manifest themselves within the first few weeks of life.

The general anesthetic nitrous oxide causes multiple defects in cobalamin utilization that include the following: (1) rapid (within minutes) inhibition of methionine synthase activity, with slow (over several days) recovery when nitrous oxide is stopped; (2) displacement of cobalamin from methionine synthase; (3) decrease in the level of methylcobalamin; (4) irreversible conversion of cobalamin to inactive and inhibitory cobalamin analogues; (5) gradual (over many weeks) development of cobalamin deficiency; (6) eventual decrease in L-methylmalonyl-CoA mutase activity; and (7) further decrease in methionine synthase activity.

Mechanisms of Folate Deficiency

Folate is widely distributed in plants and products of animal origin. Green vegetables are particularly rich sources of folate. Excessive cooking can destroy or remove a high percentage of folate in foods. Folate either is missing or is present in relatively small amounts (≤800 μg) in nonprescription multivitamin pills and supplements because of the justified concern that its presence in larger amounts could mask the diagnosis of cobalamin deficiency by correcting its hematologic abnormalities without having any beneficial effect on the neuropsychiatric abnormalities. Folates in natural foods are conjugated to chains of polyglutamic acid. Enzymes in the lumen of the small intestine convert the polyglutamate forms of folate to the monoglutamate and diglutamate forms, which are much more readily absorbed in the proximal jejunum. Absorption involves active and passive transport. Most of the folate in plasma is present as 5-methyltetrahydrofolate in the monoglutamate form. The majority is loosely bound to albumin, from which it is readily taken up by high-affinity folate receptors that are present on cells throughout the body. Once it enters the cell, the 5-methyltetrahydrofolate must be converted to tetrahydrofolate by the cobalamin-dependent enzyme methionine synthase before it can be converted to the polyglutamate form and take part in the other folate-dependent enzymatic reactions (see Fig. 133–1). In addition to being secreted in the bile and reabsorbed in the small intestine, folates are also degraded and excreted in the urine.

TABLE 133–2. DISTRIBUTION OF ENDOGENOUS COBALAMIN AMONG THE VARIOUS TRANSCOBALAMINS AND THEIR RELATIVE IMPORTANCE TO COBALAMIN TRANSPORT*

Cobalamin Transport Protein	Endogenous Cobalamin (pg/ml)	T½ for Cobalamin Clearance (hr)	Cobalamin Clearance (pg/ml/24 hr)	Site of Specific Uptake
R proteins:†				
Transcobalamin I	425–450	240.0	30	None
Transcobalamin III	0–25	0.1	0–4000	Hepatocytes
Transcobalamin II‡	50	0.1	8000	All cells

* In a typical normal subject with a serum cobalamin level of 500 pg per milliliter.

† In congenital R protein deficiency, the total serum cobalamin level is very low, but no hematologic abnormalities are present because R proteins do not transport cobalamin to rapidly dividing cells, such as those in the bone marrow.

‡ In congenital transcobalamin II deficiency, the total serum cobalamin level is well within the normal range, but severe megaloblastic anemia develops because only transcobalamin II transports cobalamin to rapidly dividing cells, such as those in the bone marrow.

Decreased intake is by far the most common cause of folate deficiency. Normal individuals have about 5000 to 20,000 μg of folate in body stores. Because folate is degraded within the body and is excreted in both the bile and the urine, approximately 50 to 100 μg must be absorbed each day from the average Western diet, which contains about 200 to 500 μg of folate. Clinical signs of folate deficiency develop in about 4 months of decreased intake, as can occur readily in chronic alcoholics.

Absorption of folate is impaired in a variety of diseases that affect the mucosa of the jejunum, including tropical sprue and celiac disease. Certain drugs, such as anticonvulsants and sulfasalazine, may impair folate absorption in some individuals. Ethanol and drugs such as triamterene impair the utilization of folate. Certain conditions associated with hypermetabolism or rapid cell growth lead to an increased requirement for folate that often cannot be met by a normal diet. These conditions include hyperthyroidism, pregnancy, chronic hemolytic disease, and various exfoliative skin diseases. An increased loss of folate from the body is caused by hemodialysis.

CLINICAL MANIFESTATIONS OF MEGALOBLASTIC ANEMIA

Hematologic Manifestations

All of the causes of megaloblastic anemia produce a common set of hematologic, laboratory, and other abnormalities that are summarized in Table 133–3. None of the abnormalities is specific for the various diseases that cause megaloblastic anemia. The abnormalities may also be present in any combination, which can vary greatly from patient to patient. In addition, none of the abnormalities is always seen in conditions that cause megaloblastic anemia, and the absence of any one or more of them cannot be used to exclude any of the diseases that cause megaloblastic anemia, including cobalamin or folate deficiency, in a given patient.

The anemia typically develops slowly over many months and may not cause symptoms until the hematocrit is less than 20%. The reticulocyte count is not elevated, in either absolute or relative (percentage) terms, even when the anemia is severe. The mean cell volume (MCV) is often increased (normal, 80 to 100 fl), and values as high as 140 fl may be seen. A review of previous blood counts often reveals a steady increase in the MCV over several months or years, often within the normal range. Neutropenia and thrombocytopenia occur less commonly than anemia and are usually not severe. On occasion, however, neutrophil counts of less than 1000 per microliter and platelet counts of less than 50,000 per microliter are seen. The peripheral blood smear frequently shows neutrophil hypersegmentation (Fig. 133–3 and Color Plate 6G, left), which can be documented by observing one or more of the following: (1) the presence of at least one neutrophil containing 6 or more lobes; (2)

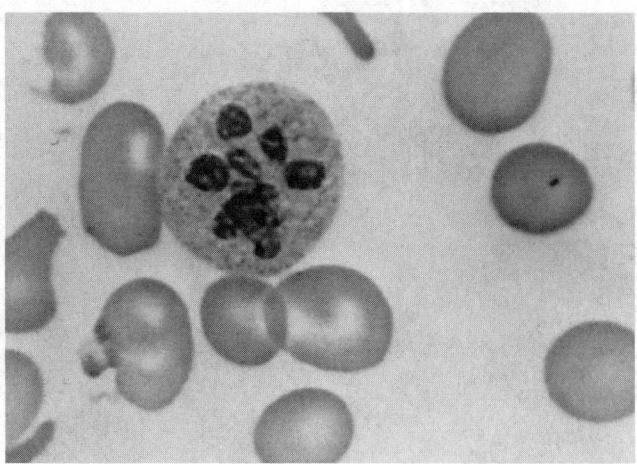

FIGURE 133–3. A hypersegmented neutrophil on a peripheral blood smear from a patient with megaloblastic anemia.

the presence of 5% or more of 5-lobe neutrophils; or (3) an increased neutrophil lobe average, which is normally fewer than 3.4 lobes per neutrophil. Erythrocytes often vary markedly in size and shape, and macroovalocytes—large, oval erythrocytes—are frequently present (Fig. 133–4 and Color Plate 6G, right). When the hematocrit is low, nucleated red cells may be seen on the peripheral smear, and then the megaloblastic morphology of the nuclei can be observed without performing a bone marrow aspiration or biopsy.

Although the reticulocyte count is normal or low, a number of serum abnormalities are often present that are usually seen and associated with hemolytic anemia. These include elevated serum levels of lactate dehydrogenase, indirect bilirubin, and iron and decreased levels of haptoglobin. Red cell production and destruction can be markedly increased in megaloblastic anemia, but both are confined to the bone marrow, described as intramedullary hemolysis or ineffective erythropoiesis.

The bone marrow is usually hypercellular with an increase in all cellular elements. Megaloblastic morphologic changes are often seen in all cells within the bone marrow, but are usually more prominent in the erythroid series. All cells in the erythroid series are larger than their normal counterparts, their cytoplasm appears more mature than their nuclei (nuclear-cytoplasmic asynchrony), and the nuclear chromatin has a distinctive open and fine-grained texture (Fig. 133–5 and Color Plate 6H). Similar abnormalities are seen in neutrophil precursors and are usually most striking at the metamyelocyte and band stage, in which "giant metamyelocytes" and "giant bands" are seen. All of these features are much more prominent in the Wright stain smear of bone marrow aspirates than in fixed sections from the bone marrow biopsy. The use of the latter alone can lead to disastrous clinical consequences because even the most experienced hematopathologist can, on the basis of fixed bone marrow sections only, have difficulty in distinguishing the hypercellularity and abnormal morphology of megaloblastosis from the changes seen in the myelodysplastic syndromes and some cases of acute leukemia. Coexisting iron deficiency may also cause diagnostic problems, since all of the erythroid megaloblastic changes may be absent even in the Wright stain smears of aspirated bone marrow. Thus the diagnosis of megaloblastic anemia should never be excluded after a bone marrow examination has been performed unless bone marrow aspirates have been examined and the presence of bone marrow iron has been established.

Megaloblastic abnormalities may occur in other proliferating body cells, all of which share the underlying defect in DNA synthesis. These changes have been documented in the epithelial cells of the buccal mucosa, stomach, intestine, and vagina and account for such phenomena as glossitis, stomatitis, and secondary malabsorption. Similar changes may account for the infertility that is sometimes seen.

Few, if any, patients with cobalamin or folate deficiency or other causes of megaloblastic anemia have all or even most of the hematologic and other abnormalities listed in Table 133–3. Even the classic abnormalities, such as anemia and increased MCV, are fre-

TABLE 133–3. HEMATOLOGIC AND OTHER ABNORMALITIES THAT MAY BE DUE TO ANY OF THE VARIOUS CAUSES OF MEGALOBLASTIC ANEMIA*

Hematologic	Other
Anemia	Glossitis
Reticulocytopenia	Stomatitis
Macrocytosis ($\uparrow$ MCV)	Gastrointestinal symptoms
Neutropenia	Hyperpigmentation
Thrombocytopenia	Infertility
Peripheral blood smear:	Orthostatic hypotension
Neutrophil hypersegmentation	Weight loss
Erythrocytes:	
Variation in size	
Variation in shape	
Macro-ovalocytes	
Serum:	
Elevated lactate dehydrogenase	
Elevated bilirubin	
Elevated iron	
Decreased haptoglobin	
Bone marrow:	
Hypercellular	
Megaloblastic morphology	
Giant bands and metamyelocytes	

* These abnormalities may be present in any number or combination in a given patient. The absence of any one or more of them occurs commonly in individual patients with all causes of megaloblastic anemia, including cobalamin deficiency and folate deficiency.

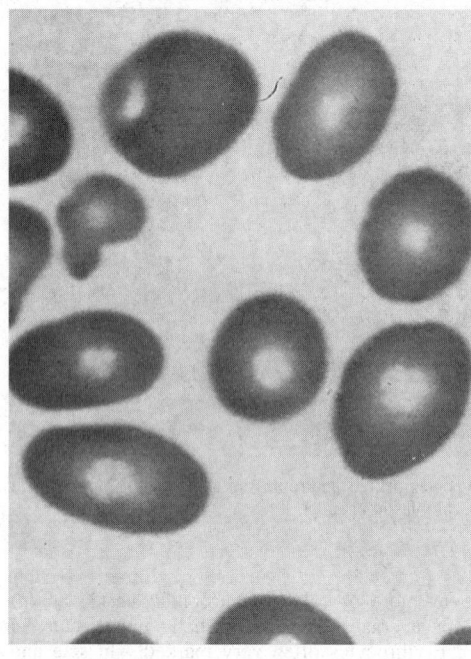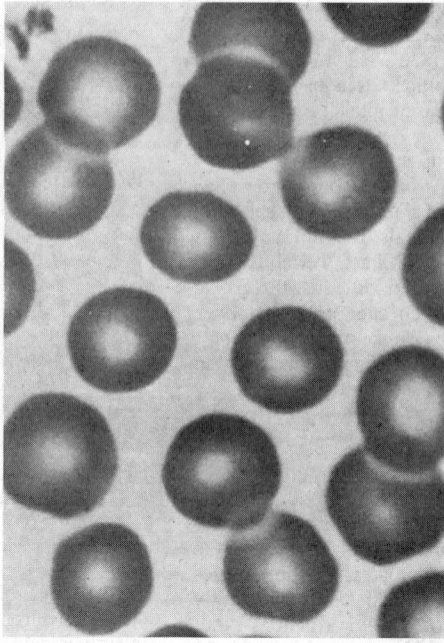

FIGURE 133-4. Peripheral blood smears from a patient with megaloblastic anemia *(left)* and from a normal subject *(right)*, both at the same magnification. The smear from the patient shows variation in the size and shape of erythrocytes and the presence of macro-ovalocytes.

quently absent, even in patients with otherwise severe deficiencies of cobalamin or folate. This point is often overlooked despite being well documented by several studies, including a prospective study of 86 consecutive patients with low serum cobalamin levels (< 200 pg per milliliter) *and* one or more objective hematologic and/or neuropsychiatric responses to cobalamin therapy. These patients failed to display the abnormalities listed in Table 133-3 with the following frequencies: (1) lack of anemia (44%); (2) MCV of 100 fl or less (36%); (3) normal white blood cell count (86%); (4) normal platelet count (79%); (5) normal peripheral smear on routine laboratory study (33%); (6) normal serum lactate dehydrogenase (43%); and (7) normal serum bilirubin level (83%).

Neuropsychiatric Abnormalities Caused by Cobalamin Deficiency

Cobalamin deficiency, unlike folate deficiency and other causes of megaloblastic anemia, produces a wide variety of neuropsychiatric abnormalities (Table 133-4). None of these abnormalities is specific for cobalamin deficiency. The abnormalities may be present alone or in any combination, which can vary greatly from patient to patient. In addition, none of the abnormalities is always seen in cobalamin deficiency, and the absence of any one or combination of them does not rule out cobalamin deficiency. The neuropsychiatric abnormalities may occur early or late in the course of cobalamin deficiency and with or without any of the hematologic or other abnormalities listed in Table 133-3. How the deficiency of a single substance, such as cobalamin, can produce a clinical picture with

such wide differences in the severity and dissociation of various hematologic and neuropsychiatric abnormalities is unknown.

Pathologic studies show loss of myelin with axonal degeneration, most frequently in the dorsal and lateral columns of the spinal cord but also in peripheral and cranial nerves and the cerebral cortex. *Combined systems disease* designates a spinal cord disorder marked by insidiously beginning and gradually progressing demyelination of, first, the dorsal (proprioceptive afferent) and, later, the lateral (corticospinal efferent) columns. Axonal degeneration affects the same pathways as a late, irreversible change. Demyelinative neuropathy of large peripheral fibers may precede or develop concurrently with the cord changes. Signs and symptoms are usually symmetric and often include paresthesias in the extremities, together with impaired vibration and position sense, which may progress to an abnormal gait, spastic ataxia, and quadriparesis. Urinary and fecal incontinence may be seen, as well as impotence. Cerebral and cranial nerve abnormalities include irritability, memory loss, disorientation, obtundation, and changes of taste, smell, and vision, with the last-named sometimes progressing to severe optic atrophy and

TABLE 133-4. NEUROPSYCHIATRIC ABNORMALITIES* THAT MAY BE CAUSED BY COBALAMIN DEFICIENCY

Neurologic Abnormalities	Psychiatric Abnormalities
Paresthesia	Depression
Impaired vibration sense	Paranoia
Impaired position sense	Listlessness
Impaired touch or pain perception	Acute confusional state
Ataxia	Hallucinations
Abnormal gait	Delusions
Fatigue	Insomnia
Memory loss	Apprehensiveness
Disorientation	Psychosis
Obtundation	Slow mentation
Decreased reflexes	Paraphrenia
Weakness	Mania
Decreased muscle strength	Panic attacks
Romberg's sign	Personality change
Increased reflexes	Suicide
Spasticity	
Babinski's sign	
Lhermitte's phenomenon	
Urinary or fecal incontinence	
Urinary urgency or nocturia	
Impotence	
Abnormal smell or taste	
Decreased vision or optic atrophy	

* These abnormalities may be present in any number or combination in a given patient. They are seen frequently with *or without* any of the hematologic or other abnormalities listed in Table 133-3.

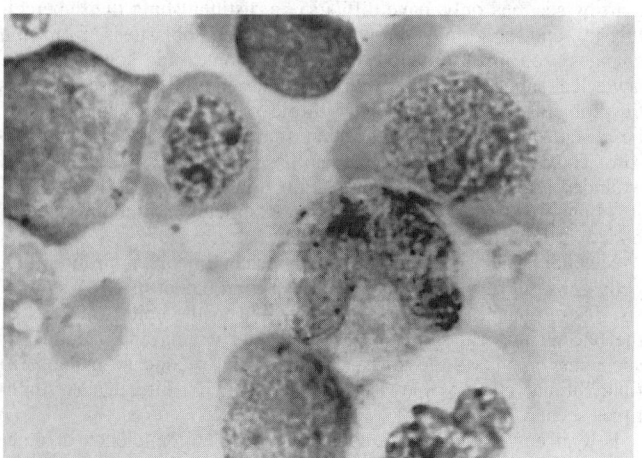

FIGURE 133-5. Erythroid precursors with marked megaloblastic features on a bone marrow smear from a patient with megaloblastic anemia.

near-blindness. Psychiatric abnormalities may be prominent and isolated. They include depression, hallucinations, agitation, marked personality change, abnormal behavior, and suicide.

The neuropsychiatric abnormalities caused by cobalamin deficiency frequently bear no relationship to the presence or degree of hematologic abnormalities. The severity of neuropsychiatric abnormalities actually bears a striking *inverse correlation* to the degree of anemia. The frequency with which hematologic and neuropsychiatric abnormalities are dissociated is often unappreciated. For example, several clinical studies document that a normal hematocrit, MCV, or both occur in at least 25 to 50% of patients with neuropsychiatric abnormalities that are caused by cobalamin deficiency *and* respond partially or completely to cobalamin therapy. Other hematologic and laboratory abnormalities of the kind outlined in Table 133–3 are lacking in a similar or even higher percentage of these patients.

DIAGNOSIS

INDICATIONS. If drugs are excluded as a cause, the differential diagnosis of megaloblastic anemia in adults is usually limited to the important task of distinguishing between cobalamin deficiency and folate deficiency and firmly establishing the presence of one or the other. The diagnostic approach to the patient with possible cobalamin or folate deficiency is outlined in Table 133–5. Patients should always be studied for these two conditions in the presence of any unexplained hematologic or other abnormality of the kind listed in Table 133–3. In addition, patients should always be investigated for cobalamin deficiency in the presence of any unexplained neuropsychiatric abnormality of the kind listed in Table 133–4, regardless of the presence or absence of hematologic abnormalities. The yield may be relatively low because of the nonspecific nature of the abnormalities in Tables 133–3 and 133–4, but such studies are clearly justified by the fact that all of the hematologic abnormalities caused by cobalamin or folate deficiency are completely corrected by safe and inexpensive therapy with the proper vitamin. In addition, the neuropsychiatric abnormalities caused by cobalamin deficiency are usually partially or completely corrected by cobalamin therapy, and in the small minority of patients who do not improve, cobalamin therapy always prevents them from getting worse. It is particularly important that the diagnosis of cobalamin deficiency be established with a high degree of certainty because parenteral cobalamin therapy must almost always be given for the lifetime of the patient. The distinction between cobalamin deficiency and folate deficiency is also very important because the treatment of cobalamin deficiency with folate does not improve the neuropsychiatric abnormalities, even though hematologic responses often occur.

SERUM COBALAMIN AND FOLATE. Radiodilution and nonisotopic assays for serum cobalamin and serum folate are used as the initial screening tests because they are widely available and relatively inexpensive. Essentially all serum cobalamin radiodilution assays today utilize cobalt-57-cobalamin and purified IF, which does not bind and measure the serum cobalamin analogues that caused problems with earlier assays. Radiodilution assays for serum folate utilize iodine-125-folate and a milk folate-binding protein. Because of the composition of commercial assay kits, and because cobalt-57 and iodine-125 are readily distinguished from each other, these assays for serum cobalamin and serum folate are almost always performed in the same test tube. Values for serum levels of both vitamins are thereby recorded by laboratories, even though they will report only the cobala-min or the folate level if only one was ordered by the physician. This point can be of practical importance because the physician can often obtain the value for the other vitamin many weeks or months later if questions arise about the possible deficiency of the other vitamin and the original serum is no longer available.

Normal ranges are defined as the mean ±2 standard deviations for normal subjects and thus include only 95% of normal individuals. Such normal ranges for serum cobalamin are approximately 200 to 900 pg per milliliter and for serum folate, approximately 2.5 to 20 ng per milliliter. By definition, 2.5% of normal subjects who have no evidence of cobalamin deficiency and who will not benefit in any way from cobalamin therapy have low values for serum cobalamin of less than 200 pg per milliter (false-positive readings). One can calculate that approximately 6,250,000 normal subjects in the United States have serum cobalamin levels lower than 200 pg per milliliter ($2.5\% \times 250,000,000 = 6,250,000$). This number is much greater than the estimate of approximately 150,000 cobalamin-deficient patients who are present in the United States at any point in time (see above). The number of false-positive readings will remain large even if cobalamin testing is restricted, as it should be, to individuals with one or more unexplained abnormalities of the kind contained in Tables 133–3 and 133–4. Similar calculations can be made with respect to serum folate values. Serum cobalamin and folate levels cannot, therefore, be used alone to establish unequivocally the diagnosis of cobalamin or folate deficiency. The problem is compounded by the fact that not all patients with clinically confirmed cobalamin or folate deficiency (defined as those who have objective clinical responses to appropriate therapy) have low values for serum cobalamin or folate (false-negative readings). The following distribution of serum cobalamin levels has been noted in clinically confirmed cobalamin-deficient patients: less than 100 pg per milliliter, approximately 50%; 100 to 200 pg per milliliter, approximately 40%; 200 to 350 pg per milliliter, approximately 10%; and higher than 350 pg per milliliter, approximately 0.1 to 1%. The distribution of serum folate levels in patients with clinically confirmed folate deficiency has been less well studied, but currently available data indicate that only about 75% of such patients have serum folate levels lower than 2.5 ng per milliliter, with almost all of the remaining 25% being in the 2.5 to 5.0 ng per milliliter range.

Perhaps it is not surprising that many patients with clinically confirmed cobalamin or folate deficiency have serum vitamin levels within the normal range. Both vitamins, after all, function within cells and not in plasma. In the case of cobalamin, furthermore, serum levels of the vitamin are greatly influenced by levels of plasma binding proteins, which bear no relationship to cellular cobalamin levels. In fact, TC I has no apparent function (see Table 133–2). Thus the assays for serum cobalamin and serum folate are useful as initial screening tests that allow the physician to exclude from consideration almost all patients with serum cobalamin levels of 350 pg per milliliter or higher and serum folate levels of 5.0 ng per milliliter or higher. Additional follow-up tests are required for serum cobalamin levels lower than 350 pg per milliliter, serum folate levels less than 5.0 ng per milliliter, or clinical conditions that are serious or very suggestive of cobalamin or folate deficiency. Examples of such conditions include (1) marked myelodysplasia in a patient who is about to start a regimen of chemotherapy; (2) incapacitating urinary and fecal incontinence of unknown cause in a young patient; (3) pancytopenia with an increased MCV and serum lactate dehydrogenase level; and (4) symmetric paresthesias in the hands and feet in a patient who also has spastic ataxia and a recent change in personality.

TABLE 133–5. DIAGNOSTIC APPROACH TO THE PATIENT WITH COBALAMIN OR FOLATE DEFICIENCY

I. Initial approach
  A. Indications
    1. Any unexplained hematologic or other abnormality of the kind listed in Table 133–3 (cobalamin and folate deficiency)
    2. Any unexplained neuropsychiatric abnormality of the kind listed in Table 133–4 (cobalamin deficiency)
  B. Initial tests
    1. Serum cobalamin (normal, 200–900 pg/ml)
    2. Serum folate (normal, 2.5–20 ng/ml)

II. Follow-up
  A. Indications
    1. Serum cobalamin < 350 pg/ml, *or*
    2. Serum folate < 5 ng/ml, *or*
    3. Clinical condition:
      a. Serious unexplained hematologic or neuropsychiatric abnormalities, *or*
      b. Very suggestive of cobalamin or folate deficiency
  B. Follow-up tests
    1. Serum methylmalonic acid (normal, 70–270 nM)—elevated in cobalamin deficiency
    2. Serum homocysteine (normal, 5–16 μM)—elevated in cobalamin and folate deficiency

SERUM METHYLMALONIC ACID AND HOMOCYSTEINE. The most useful follow-up tests for diagnosing and distinguishing between cobalamin and folate deficiency are serum levels of methylmalonic acid (normal, 70 to 270 nM) and homocysteine* (normal, 5 to 16 μM). These tests, which can be performed on serum that remains after cobalamin and folate levels have been determined, are now widely available in the United States through a number of laboratories, including all of the large national reference laboratories. The combined cost of the two tests, which are usually performed together, is similar to the cost of a Schilling test or a bone marrow examination. The serum methylmalonic acid level is elevated in more than 95% of patients with clinically confirmed cobalamin deficiency (see Fig. 133–2). Values as high as 2,000,000 nM have been observed, with a median value in the range of 3500 nM. Serum methylmalonic acid levels are not elevated in folate deficiency. In contrast, serum homocysteine concentrations are elevated in both cobalamin and folate deficiency (Fig. 133–1). Values as high as 500 μM have been observed in cobalamin deficiency, with a median value of 70 μM. Values as high as 250 μM have been observed in folate deficiency, with a median value of 50 μM. Except for rare inborn errors of metabolism involving cobalamin- and folate-dependent enzymes or pathways, the only other conditions that also give rise to elevations of serum methylmalonic acid or serum homocysteine are renal failure and intravascular volume depletion. Broad-spectrum antibiotics can lower an elevated serum methylmalonic acid level to normal in patients with cobalamin deficiency by inhibiting the gut microflora, an important source of precursors of methylmalonic acid. Antibiotics do not affect elevated homocysteine levels in these patients, nor do they change any clinical parameters.

Elevated levels of methylmalonic acid and homocysteine due to cobalamin deficiency return to normal within 5 to 10 days of starting cobalamin therapy. Elevated levels of homocysteine due to folate deficiency fall to normal during the same period following folate therapy. Elevations of serum methylmalonic acid and homocysteine due to cobalamin deficiency do not respond to pharmacologic doses of folate even in cobalamin-deficient patients in whom folate causes a marked hematologic improvement (together with no response or a worsening of neuropsychiatric abnormalities). Elevations of homocysteine due to folate deficiency do not respond to pharmacologic doses of cobalamin. Elevations of methylmalonic acid and homocysteine due to renal insufficiency or intravascular volume depletion are not corrected with therapy with either vitamin unless vitamin deficiency coexists. Thus, repeat determinations of serum methylmalonic acid and homocysteine levels after a short course of therapy with a single vitamin may provide additional information of diagnostic usefulness.

With few exceptions, patients with serum cobalamin levels lower than 350 pg per milliliter or serum folate levels less than 5.0 ng per milliliter do not show objective hematologic or neuropsychiatric responses to cobalamin or folate therapy if their serum levels of methylmalonic acid and homocysteine are normal. Thus the use of serum levels of cobalamin and folate as initial screening tests, together with the use of serum methylmalonic acid and homocysteine determinations as follow-up tests, makes it possible to diagnose cobalamin or folate deficiency and to distinguish between them in the vast majority of patients (Table 133–5). If in doubt, one can always start empiric therapy, but such therapeutic trials can be difficult to perform (see below) and should be monitored carefully in an attempt to establish a definitive diagnosis. As an alternative, patients can be observed carefully with repeat determinations of methylmalonic acid and homocysteine after 6 months or a year. The usual patterns of serum cobalamin, folate, methylmalonic acid, and homocysteine concentrations in cobalamin and folate deficiency are summarized in Table 133–6.

OTHER TESTS. A number of other tests have been used as diagnostic or follow-up tests in cobalamin deficiency. Serum antibod-

* What is actually measured is "total homocysteine," which consists of the sum of homocysteine and the homocysteine that is linked via disulfide bond formation in a variety of compounds that include homocystine (homocysteine-homocysteine disulfide), homocysteine-cysteine mixed disulfide, proteins via their cysteine moieties, and peptides such as glutathione via their cysteine moieties.

TABLE 133–6. TYPICAL SERUM FINDINGS IN MEGALOBLASTIC ANEMIA

	Normal Levels	Deficiency of Cobalamin	Folate
Cobalamin	200–900 pg/ml	↓ *	N
Folate	2.5–20 ng/ml	N	↓ *
Methylmalonic acid	70–270 nM	↑ ↑	N
Homocysteine	5–16 μM	↑ ↑	↑ ↑

* A significant number of patients with cobalamin deficiency will have serum cobalamin levels in the lower portion of the normal range (see text). The same is true with respect to folate deficiency and serum folate levels.

ies to IF are present in about 50% of patients with pernicious anemia and are highly specific for that condition. They fail to diagnose about 50% of such cases, however, as well as all cases with other causes of cobalamin deficiency. The standard Schilling test (see Ch. 103 for a complete description of this test) requires a reliable 24-hour urine collection, and since it uses free, i.e., non–protein-bound, cobalamin, it fails to diagnose cobalamin deficiency not only in patients who are strict vegans but also in the much more common patients who malabsorb cobalamin from food sources. Both the IF antibody test and the Schilling test actually provide information about the etiology of cobalamin deficiency rather than information about the presence or absence of cobalamin deficiency *per se.* The etiology of cobalamin deficiency (and of folate deficiency) should be pursued in unusual patients and those with gastrointestinal symptoms that do not respond to cobalamin therapy because such studies may disclose the presence of a disease that requires additional therapy. It is acceptable practice to institute lifetime cobalamin therapy in individuals with anti-IF antibodies or abnormal Schilling tests who lack evidence of current cobalamin deficiency, since they will likely become deficient in the future. A normal result with either test should never be used, however, to exclude the diagnosis of cobalamin deficiency or to withhold lifetime therapy.

RESPONSE TO THERAPY. Therapeutic trials with cobalamin or folate must be performed with physiologic levels of either vitamin (1 μg per day for cobalamin and 100 μg per day for folate), since larger amounts can give hematologic responses even if the incorrect vitamin is employed. Such trials may require months before responses can be completely evaluated. They can be particularly difficult to interpret in patients with neuropsychiatric abnormalities, since these do not always respond to even large doses of cobalamin, even if cobalamin deficiency is the cause of the abnormalities. Therapeutic trials with pharmacologic doses of folate are potentially dangerous, since partial or even complete hematologic responses may be seen in cobalamin-deficient patients. The continuation of folate therapy in such patients is extremely dangerous, since folate does nothing for the neuropsychiatric abnormalities, which may progress or develop during folate therapy.

THERAPY

COBALAMIN DEFICIENCY. Therapy consists of intramuscular or subcutaneous administration of either cyanocobalamin or hydroxocobalamin. Because cobalamin is inexpensive and free of any side effects, it is better to give too much than too little. The regimen used in our clinic consists of injections of 1000 μg of cyanocobalamin once a week for 8 weeks and then once a month for life. More frequent injections are often used in hospitalized patients or those with marked neuropsychiatric abnormalities, but there is no evidence that this is beneficial. Once the weekly injections are completed, one can often teach the patient or a family member or friend to give the injections. The absolute requirement of lifetime therapy must be well understood by the patient. Oral therapy with cobalamin in a dose of 10 μg per day can be used with strict vegans. In theory, such therapy could also be used in individuals who malabsorb food cobalamin, but this is not recommended, since their IF production is often precarious and may decrease further over the years. Oral therapy with cobalamin in doses of 500 to 1000 μg per day should be reserved for the occasional patient who, for some reason, cannot receive cobalamin injections. Future measurements of serum levels of methylmalonic acid and homocysteine under various treatment and maintenance regimens may lead to changes in these recommendations.

FOLATE DEFICIENCY. Therapy is usually administered orally in the form of 1-mg tablets of folic acid. Oral therapy is almost always satisfactory, even in the presence of intestinal malabsorption. The usual dose is 1 to 2 mg daily. Therapy limited to several weeks is usually adequate in an alcoholic who begins to eat a normal diet. In patients with chronic conditions, such as malabsorption, hemolysis, exfoliative skin diseases, or renal failure requiring hemodialysis, oral folate is continued indefinitely and usually given prophylactically.

COBALAMIN OR FOLATE DEFICIENCY. Red cell transfusions are rarely required because of the well-compensated state of moderately, and even severely, anemic patients. Such transfusions should be avoided if at all possible because of the cost and risk associated with them. If transfusions are required, they should be given very slowly, since fluid overload occurs commonly and can precipitate lethal congestive heart failure. The only additional therapy is that required for certain underlying causes of cobalamin or folate deficiency, such as antibiotics in bacterial overgrowth or dietary changes in celiac disease.

DRUGS OR OTHER CAUSES. When drugs are responsible, either they can be stopped or the dosages can be reduced if necessary. In other cases, pyridoxine or thiamine can be tried in pharmacologic doses, since an occasional patient will respond.

PROGNOSIS

The hematologic abnormalities due to cobalamin or folate deficiency respond rapidly to therapy with the appropriate vitamin. Reticulocytosis begins by day 5, followed shortly by an increase in the hematocrit, which returns to normal within several months. Neutrophil and platelet counts and other laboratory abnormalities usually return to normal within a week to 10 days. If a complete correction of all hematologic abnormalities does not occur, a search should be made for other conditions, such as iron deficiency or hypothyroidism.

The response of the neuropsychiatric abnormalities caused by cobalamin deficiency is less predictable. Cobalamin therapy always prevents such patients from getting worse and most often results in a partial or complete correction. Responses may be seen within several days, but may take as long as 12 or 18 months before improvement can be ruled out or is maximal. Patients with pernicious anemia have an approximately twofold increased risk of developing gastric carcinoma, an increased association with hyperthyroidism and hypothyroidism, and other manifestations of the polyglandular failure syndrome.

Allen RH, Stabler SP, Savage DG, et al.: Metabolic abnormalities in cobalamin (vitamin B_{12}) and folate deficiency. FASEB J 7:1344, 1993. *Review of multiple metabolic abnormalities that occur in cobalamin and folate deficiencies; 45 references.*

Carmel R, Sinow RM, Siegel ME, et al.: Food cobalamin malabsorption occurs frequently in patients with unexplained low serum cobalamin levels. Arch Intern Med 148:1715, 1988. *Provides a convincing explanation for the normal results that are frequently obtained with standard Schilling tests in patients with proven cobalamin deficiency and underscores the important point that a normal Schilling test should never be used to exclude the diagnosis of cobalamin deficiency.*

Healton EB, Savage DG, Brust JCM, et al.: Neurologic aspects of cobalamin deficiency. Medicine 70:229, 1991. *Detailed description of 143 patients seen from 1968 to 1985, together with an excellent review of the literature; 57 references.*

Hector M, Burton J: What are the psychiatric manifestations of vitamin B_{12} deficiency? J Am Geriatr Soc 36:1105, 1988. *Excellent review of psychiatric abnormalities that are caused by cobalamin deficiency and respond to cobalamin therapy, a though I disagree with the definition of and conclusions about dementia; 85 references.*

Joosten E, Van Den Berg A, Reizler R, et al.: Metabolic evidence that deficiencies of vitamin B_{12}, folate and vitamin B_6 occur commonly in the elderly. Am J Clin Nutr 58:468, 1993. *Intriguing message of this article is stated in its title.*

Lindenbaum J, Allen RH: Clinical spectrum and diagnosis of folate deficiency. In Bailey LB (ed.): Folate in Health and Disease. New York, Marcel Dekker, 1995, pp. 43-73. *Detailed review that includes discussion of clinical utility of serum folate versus red cell folate determinations; 130 references.*

Lindenbaum J, Healton EB, Savage DG, et al.: Neuropsychiatric disorders caused by cobalamin deficiency in the absence of anemia or macrocytosis. N Engl J Med 318:1720, 1988. *Detailed description of 42 patients with serious neuropsychiatric abnormalities that responded to cobalamin therapy despite the lack of one or more of the classic hematologic abnormalities that are also caused by cobalamin deficiency.*

Savage DG, Lindenbaum J, Stabler SP, et al.: Sensitivity of serum methylmalonic acid and total homocysteine determinations for diagnosing cobalamin and folate deficiencies. Am J Med 96:239, 1994. *Study of 406 patients with cobalamin deficiency and 119 patients with folate deficiency; 43 references.*

Stabler SP, Allen RH, Savage DG, et al.: Clinical spectrum and diagnosis of cobalamin deficiency. Blood 76:871, 1990. *A total of 145 patients with serum cobalamin levels lower than 200 pg per milliliter were studied before and after cobalamin therapy; 86 had objective clinical responses and 59 did not. The two groups are compared in detail.*

134 HEREDITARY DEFECTS IN THE MEMBRANE OR METABOLISM OF THE RED CELL

Samuel E. Lux

NORMAL RED CELL MEMBRANE

Structure

MEMBRANE LIPIDS. The red cell membrane, or *ghost,* is a mixture of phospholipids, unesterified cholesterol, and glycolipids, arranged in a bilayer, and traversed randomly by transmembrane protein channels and receptors. The phospholipids are asymmetrically arranged. Choline phospholipids (phosphatidyl choline and sphingomyelin) are found primarily in the outer half of the bilayer; amino phospholipids (phosphatidyl serine [PS] and phosphatidyl ethanolamine [PE]) and phosphatidyl inositols are confined to the inner half. In the case of the aminophospholipids this is accomplished by an adenosine triphosphate (ATP)-dependent translocase ("flippase"), which transports PS and PE from the outer to the inner bilayer. It is probably important to sequester amino phospholipids, because their exposure triggers coagulation and causes red cells to adhere to phagocytes.

MEMBRANE PROTEINS. The red cell membrane contains 10 to 15 major proteins and innumerable minor ones (Fig. 134–1). The proteins fall into two classes: (1) *Integral membrane proteins* traverse the bilayer, interact with the hydrophobic lipid core, and are tightly bound. They include functionally important transport proteins, such as protein 3 the anion exchange protein, and glycoprotein surface antigens, such as the glycophorins. (2) *Peripheral membrane proteins* are confined to the cytoplasmic membrane surface and include structural proteins, such as spectrin and actin, and some red cell enzymes (e.g., glyceraldehyde-3-phosphate dehydrogenase). These proteins bind to each other and to anchoring sites on integral proteins. The major peripheral membrane proteins form a two-dimensional protein network that laminates the cytoplasmic membrane surface (see Fig. 134–1). The principal components of this membrane skeleton are spectrin, actin, protein 4.1, and ankyrin. *Spectrin,* the major skeletal protein, is composed of two long, flexible chains, the α and β subunits. The chains are mostly a series of successive 106 amino acid repeats, the result of ancient gene duplications. The two subunits are aligned antiparallel and are twisted about each other. These heterodimers interact at their "head" end to

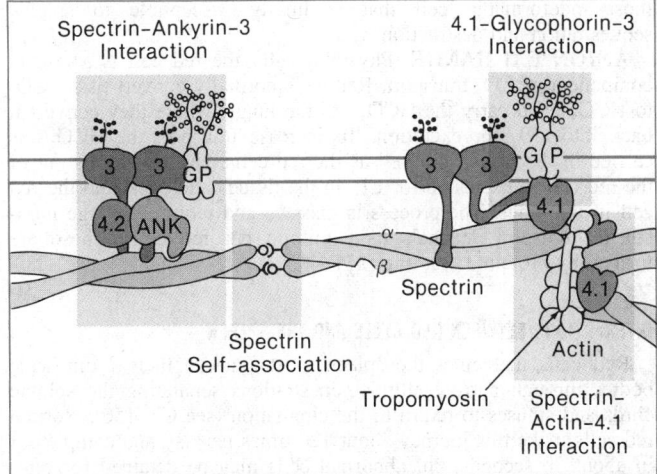

FIGURE 134–1. Organization of the major proteins of the red cell membrane and membrane skeleton. ANK, ankyrin; GP, glycophorin C.

form heterotetramers or higher-order oligomers (spectrin self-association) (Fig. 134–1). At the opposite ("tail") end, spectrin binds to short filaments of actin. This interaction is greatly strengthened by protein 4.1, which binds to both β-spectrin and actin. Because multiple spectrins can bind to each actin filament, the spectrin-actin-4.1 complex is a molecular junction that allows spectrin filaments to branch and form a two-dimensional membrane skeleton.

The skeleton is anchored to the overlying lipid bilayer by *ankyrin,* which binds to spectrin near the self-association site and links it to the cytoplasmic portion of protein 3, the anion exchange protein. Protein 4.2, which binds to both ankyrin and protein 3, may strengthen this interaction (Fig. 134–1). Interactions between protein 4.1 and glycophorin C and between various skeletal proteins and membrane lipids also occur but are less important functionally for skeletal stability.

Major Functions

MEMBRANE STRENGTH AND DURABILITY. In humans the red cell must be flexible enough to negotiate splenic and capillary channels less than half its diameter and still be strong and durable enough to survive the turbulent journey through the heart approximately 500,000 times during its 120-day lifespan. These properties are determined by the membrane skeleton. Mice with hereditary deficiencies of α- or β-spectrin or ankyrin have extremely fragile red cells that rapidly fragment in the circulation, leading to marked spherocytosis and severe hemolysis.

MAINTENANCE OF CELL VOLUME. The red cell controls its volume and water content by regulating its intracellular concentration of Na^+ and K^+. This is possible because the membrane is relatively impermeable to cations. Normally, small passive cation leaks are balanced by active transport of Na^+ outward and K^+ inward. These ion movements are powered by a pump that is fueled by the membrane enzyme Na^+,K^+-*ATPase.* Normally this system maintains intracellular Na^+ and K^+ at about 10 mEq per liter and 100 mEq per liter, respectively. The pump is regulated by the intracellular Na^+ concentration and has considerable ability to compensate for an increased leak of Na^+ into the cell. If this capacity is surpassed and the inward leak of Na^+ exceeds the K^+ leak out, red cells gain cations and water and swell. Unfortunately the pump does not compensate nearly as well to a decrease in intracellular K^+. Any increase in the outward leak of K^+ relative to Na^+ leads to loss of total monovalent cations and water and results in cellular dehydration.

CALCIUM HOMEOSTASIS. Excessive intracellular Ca^{2+} is very deleterious, and the red cell actively extrudes it with an efficient, calmodulin-regulated calcium pump that is driven by a Ca^{2+}-ATPase. Intracellular Ca^{2+} is normally almost undetectable (about 0.1 μM). If ATP levels fall below about 20% of normal or if Ca^{2+} leakage exceeds the capacity of the pump, Ca^{2+} accumulates and changes the red cell from a biconcave disc to an echinocyte—a spiculated sphere with numerous short, regular projections. Increased intracellular Ca^{2+} also causes selective loss of K^+ and water (the Gardos channel). The result is a crenated, dehydrated, almost indeformable cell that is highly susceptible to splenic sequestration and destruction.

ANION EXCHANGE. Physiologically the red cell is a crucial component of CO_2 transport. Red cells normally convert tissue CO_2 to HCO_3^- and carry the HCO_3^- to the lungs, where they convert it back into CO_2 for excretion. To increase transport the HCO_3^- is carried in the plasma as well as the red cells. HCO_3^- moves out of the red cell in exchange for Cl^- in the tissues and back into the red cell in the lungs. The process is massive and requires a large number of transport channels (≈ 1 million per red cell). These are formed by protein 3 (see Fig. 134–1).

INTERACTIONS BETWEEN RED CELLS AND THE SPLEEN

Red cells that enter the spleen must squeeze their 7-μm wide bodies through narrow elliptic fenestrations separating the splenic cords and sinuses to return to the circulation (see Ch. 150). Normal red cells make this journey about 120 times per day and complete it in about 30 seconds, but abnormal cells may be detained for minutes to hours in the hypoxic, acidic, hypoglycemic environment of the splenic cords. This taxing metabolic stress is often fatal for old or defective erythrocytes.

Red cells are detained in the spleen if they are rigid or if they are coated with proteins such as immunoglobulin G1 (IgG1), immunoglobulin G3 (IgG3), or the complement component C3b that bind to receptors on splenic macrophages. Probably other, less well defined changes in the red cell surface also attract phagocytes and lead to red cell death. Increased rigidity may result from (1) increased cytoplasmic viscosity (e.g., in sickled cells and other dehydrated red cells), (2) intracellular rubbish (e.g., Heinz bodies), and (3) a decrease in the red cell surface–volume ratio.

Surface-Volume Ratio: Osmotic Fragility Test

Spherocytes are caused by a decrease in the surface-volume ratio of the red cell. Target cells form when this ratio is increased. Because the area of the red cell membrane is fixed (i.e., the membrane is not stretchable), the cell becomes progressively more rigid as its spheroidicity increases. Surface-volume ratio is assessed clinically by the *unincubated osmotic fragility test.* This test measures the ability of red cells to swell in a graded series of hypotonic solutions. Spherocytes are osmotically fragile; that is, they can tolerate less osmotic swelling than normal cells before they hemolyze. Target cells are osmotically resistant.

MEMBRANE DISORDERS

Hereditary Spherocytosis (HS)

Hereditary spherocytosis is an inherited hemolytic anemia characterized by dense, osmotically fragile, partially spherical red cells that are selectively trapped by the spleen (see Color Plate 6D, left). The disease occurs in all races but is particularly common in northern Europeans, in whom the incidence is about 1 in 5000. There are at least two patterns of inheritance: 75% of the families show a classic autosomal dominant pattern. Most of the remainder are a combination of autosomal recessive disorders and new mutations.

PATHOGENESIS. Hereditary spherocytes transfused into normal subjects show impaired survival, demonstrating clearly that they are intrinsically defective. The primary molecular defects involve the "vertical" connections among spectrin, ankyrin, protein 4.2, and protein 3 that link the lipid bilayer and the membrane skeleton. Abnormalities in each of these proteins have been observed in HS. The precise mutations are an active topic of investigation. Initial studies suggest that many mutations exist and no single mutation is common.

Ankyrin defects are the most frequent (≈ 30 to 60% of cases). These occur in both dominant and recessive HS and are characterized by combined deficiency of ankyrin and spectrin (which binds to ankyrin) in roughly equivalent proportions. The degree of spectrin/ankyrin deficiency correlates with the degree of spherocytosis, as measured by osmotic fragility, and with the severity of hemolysis and response to splenectomy. In general, patients with dominant HS have only mild deficiency (spectrin/ankyrin content 70 to 90% of normal) and mild to moderate hemolysis. Patients with recessive HS often have a more severe deficit—occasionally so severe (spectrin/ankyrin content 30 to 50% of normal) that it produces life-threatening, transfusion-dependent hemolytic anemia.

Defects in protein 3 are also common (15 to 25% of patients). They are only seen in dominant HS and are characterized by selective deficiency of protein 3 (60 to 90% of normal) and mild to moderate hemolysis. Blood smears often contain a few mushroom-shaped red cells, which may be a distinguishing feature. Defects in α-spectrin (recessive HS), β-spectrin (dominant HS), and protein 4.2 (recessive HS, particularly in Japanese) also occur, but are less common (for each, less than 5 to 15% of patients).

It is thought that HS red cells gradually lose portions of the lipid bilayer and become progressively more spherocytic as they age in the circulation (Fig. 134–2). Eventually they are detained in the splenic cords where, for unknown reasons, their membrane loss is accentuated by the toxic cordal environment. This "splenic conditioning" can be mimicked *in vitro* by incubating red cells in the absence of glucose for 24 hours. Under these conditions, hereditary spherocytes lose membrane fragments more rapidly than do normal red cells. This is the basis of the *incubated osmotic fragility test. In vivo,* conditioned spherocytes are prevalent in the splenic pulp, and some escape into the peripheral circulation as the characteristic HS hyperchromic microspherocytes. These impaired cells form the hyperspheric tail on osmotic fragility curves. Undoubtedly, many HS red cells never escape the conditioning process. Those that do are especially susceptible to recapture and destruction by the spleen.

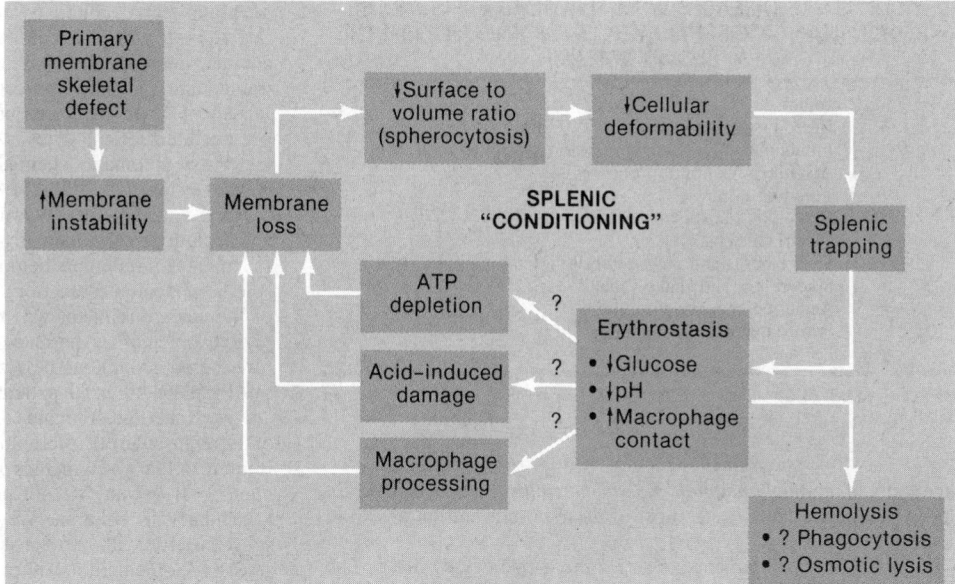

FIGURE 134-2. Currently favored model of the pathophysiology of hereditary spherocytosis. ATP = adenosine triphosphate.

CLINICAL FEATURES (Table 134-1). The hallmarks of HS are *anemia, jaundice,* and *splenomegaly.* The disease may occur at any age. In neonates, excessive jaundice is frequent ($\approx 50\%$) and sometimes requires an exchange transfusion. In addition, some HS infants respond sluggishly to their anemia during the first few months of life and require intermittent booster transfusions. After the neonatal period most patients develop partially compensated hemolysis with only mild to moderate anemia (hemoglobin [Hb] = 9 to 11.5 grams per deciliter), intermittent mild jaundice (especially during viral infections), and splenomegaly. *Clinical severity can vary widely,* presumably reflecting the wide variety of causative mutations and, in the case of dominant disorders, variable compensation by the normal allele. A small proportion of patients have life-threatening hemolysis and are transfusion dependent. A much larger proportion, about 25%, have unusually mild disease. In these patients marrow erythropoiesis is sufficient to balance the modest rate of spherocyte destruction, and there is no anemia, little or no jaundice, and minimal splenomegaly. However, severe hemolysis and anemia may develop with illnesses that cause the spleen to hypertrophy, such as infectious mononucleosis. Hemolysis may also be exacerbated by long-term intensive physical activity, possibly because of increased splenic blood flow. Finally, in old age, when bone marrow function becomes sluggish, previously well-compensated nonsplenectomized patients may become symptomatic.

COMPLICATIONS
Crises. The clinical course is interrupted in most patients by occasional crises, characterized by worsening anemia. *Hemolytic crises* are the most frequent but usually are mild and clinically insignificant. They are presumably secondary to the reticuloendothelial hyperplasia that accompanies many infections. *Aplastic crises* are less prevalent but are often severe enough to threaten heart failure and require transfusion. They are usually caused by parvovirus B19 (see Color Plate 5*H,* right) (see Ch. 130), which invades erythropoietic stem cells and inhibits their growth. The infection produces lasting immunity so patients rarely experience more than one aplastic crisis in a lifetime. Parvovirus B19 is contagious and is especially dangerous to the fetus. All patients with an aplastic crisis should be isolated from contact with pregnant women. *Megaloblastic crises* (see Color Plate 6*H*) occur when dietary intake of folic acid is inadequate for the increased needs of the erythroid bone marrow in HS or other hemolytic anemias. This need is particularly acute during pregnancy. To prevent megaloblastic crises, all HS patients should receive daily supplements of folic acid (1 mg per day).

Gallstones. Untreated older children and adults with HS often develop bilirubinate gallstones secondary to increased bilirubin production. Only 5% of children less than 10 years old are affected, but the incidence rises to 40 to 50% in the second to fifth decades and 55 to 75% thereafter. The frequency after age 30 parallels the frequency in the general population, which suggests that gallstones in HS patients form primarily in the second and third decades. Ultrasonography is the most reliable method for detecting bilirubin stones. Only 50% are radiopaque. Concern about cholecystitis and biliary obstruction is the major impetus for splenectomy in most patients. It is unfortunate, therefore, that there are no accurate data on the incidence of these complications in patients with bilirubin stones to help assess the indications (risk-benefit ratio) for operation.

Other Complications. Occasional adult patients with HS develop gout, indolent ankle ulcers, or chronic erythematous dermatitis on the legs. All of these complications disappear after splenectomy. Occasional adults also develop extramedullary tumors, usually in the thorax. These are most often seen in elderly adults with otherwise mild HS and may cause considerable diagnostic confusion. Diagnosis is best made by nuclear magnetic resonance because the tumors can bleed dangerously if biopsy is done. They undergo fatty metamorphosis following splenectomy but usually do not disappear. Rare but potentially interesting associations of HS with spinocerebellar degeneration and familial myocardiopathy have also been described.

DIAGNOSIS. Although many patients are not anemic, the reticulocyte count is always *increased* prior to splenectomy (except during an aplastic crisis). It is a much more dependable sign of hemolysis than is hyperbilirubinemia, since indirect bilirubin levels are elevated in only 50 to 60% of patients. *Spherocytosis,* the hallmark of the disease, is the other most reliable finding (see Color Plate 6*D,* left). However, spherocytes are a frequent artifact in normal blood smears, so the physician must take care to examine only areas of the smear in which the red cells are well separated and some cells with central pallor are evident. Spherocytosis is also observed in a variety of other conditions (Table 134-2); however, with the

TABLE 134-1. HEREDITARY SPHEROCYTOSIS

Clinical Manifestations	Laboratory Features
Anemia	Reticulocytosis
Splenomegaly	Spherocytosis
Intermittent jaundice	Elevated MCHC
From hemolysis	Increased osmotic fragility (especially
From biliary obstruction	incubated osmotic fragility) test
Aplastic crises	Normal Coombs' test
Often dominant inheritance	Decreased red cell spectrin or spectrin
	and ankyrin or protein 3 or protein 4.2
Rare manifestations	
Leg ulcers	
Spinal cord dysfunction	
Myocardiopathy	
Good response to splenectomy	

TABLE 134–2. DISEASES WITH SPHEROCYTOSIS AS THE PREDOMINANT MORPHOLOGIC ABNORMALITY ON THE BLOOD SMEAR

Common
    Hereditary spherocytosis
    Immunohemolytic anemias (warm antibody type)
    ABO incompatibility in neonates
Uncommon to rare
    Hemolytic transfusion reactions
    Clostridial sepsis
    Severe burns and other red cell thermal injuries
    Spider, bee, and snake venoms
    Acute red cell oxidant injury*
    Severe hypophosphatemia
    Bartonellosis

* Acute red cell oxidant injury is common, but spherocytosis is rarely the predominant morphology.

exception of certain *immunohemolytic anemias* (which can be excluded with a Coombs' test), most of these do not present any diagnostic difficulty.

In 20 to 25% of patients, classic microspherocytes are sparse, and it may be difficult to recognize spherocytosis from the blood smear alone. In these patients the unincubated osmotic fragility (OF) test is sometimes normal or only slightly increased, since it simply quantifies what is visible on the smear. The *incubated* OF, however, is almost always abnormal and is the most reliable available diagnostic test. HS red cells are quite dehydrated and therefore have an *increased mean corpuscular hemoglobin concentration (MCHC)*. An MCHC level of 36 or greater is present in 50% of HS patients, but all patients have some dehydrated cells. These are best revealed using instruments such as the Technicon H1 blood counter, which provides a histogram of MCHC's. Since deficiencies of spectrin, ankyrin, protein 3, or protein 4.2 appear to be the primary defects in HS, quantitation of these proteins should provide the most accurate diagnostic test; however, at present these measurements are available in only a few research laboratories.

Once HS is diagnosed, a careful search for the disease should always be made in all close relatives. It is tragic to see HS become symptomatic in elderly patients with a poor operative risk in whom this condition could have been discovered earlier.

TREATMENT. *Splenectomy.* Splenectomy cures almost all cases of spherocytosis—eliminating anemia and reducing the reticulocyte count to near-normal levels (1 to 3%). Patients with the most severe forms of the disease may not achieve complete remission, but will still benefit greatly from the operation.

However, the indications for splenectomy should be weighed carefully, as a small fraction of patients will die from overwhelming postsplenectomy infections or mesenteric/portal venous occlusion. The risk of postsplenectomy sepsis is very high in infancy and early childhood, and splenectomy should therefore be delayed until the age of 5 years or more if possible and to at least 2 to 3 years in all cases, even if repeated transfusions are required in the interim. It is difficult to estimate the risk later in life. The surveys of Schwartz and associates and Green and co-workers, the best available, are limited to adults and largely predate immunization against *Streptococcus pneumoniae* and other bacteria. They show an incidence of fulminant sepsis of 0.2 to 0.5 per 100 person-years of follow-up and a death rate of 0.1 per 100 person-years; in addition, other serious bacterial infections (e.g., pneumonia, meningitis, peritonitis, bacteremia) are much more common (4.5 per 100 person-years) than normal, particularly in the first few years after the operation.

The incidence of ischemic heart disease may also rise after splenectomy. In one careful study Robinette and Fraumeni observed that death from ischemic heart disease occurred 1.86 times as often in splenectomized men as in matched controls, a significant difference. The cause is unknown, although the chronically higher platelet count after splenectomy would be a good candidate.

In general, the indications for splenectomy have become more conservative during the past several decades. This trend will presumably accelerate as the threat of penicillin-resistant pneumococci (see Ch. 150) increases. We recommend splenectomy for all patients with severe HS (hemoglobin [Hb] ≤ 8 grams per deciliter, reticulocytes $\geq 10\%$) and for patients with moderate HS (Hb 8 to 11 grams per deciliter, reticulocytes $\geq 8\%$) if they suffer from reduced vitality or physical stamina due to anemia, or if, later in life, anemia compromises vascular perfusion of vital organs or extramedullary hematopoietic tumors develop. We defer splenectomy in patients with mild, compensated hemolysis (Hb 11 to 15 grams per deciliter, reticulocytes < 6 to 8%). Whether patients with moderate, asymptomatic anemia should undergo splenectomy remains controversial.

Recent studies of Tchernia and associates suggest that partial splenectomy may eventually be an effective compromise for many HS patients: relieving hemolysis while maintaining some residual splenic phagocytic function. Complications were low, and regrowth of the splenic remnant was not observed during a 4-year follow-up period, but more experience and longer follow-ups are needed before the procedure can be recommended.

All splenectomized patients must receive *polyvalent pneumococcal vaccine* (Pnu-Immune 23 or equivalent, 0.5 ml subcutaneously or intramuscularly), preferably given several weeks preoperatively. Immunization with meningococcal vaccines and *Haemophilus influenzae* B vaccine (if not previously given) is also recommended, particularly in children. We advocate prophylactic antibiotics after splenectomy, with emphasis on protection against pneumococcal sepsis (i.e., Penicillin-VK or equivalent, 125 mg orally twice daily in young children (< 7 years) and 250 mg orally twice daily in older children and adults), at least for the first 2 to 5 years after surgery, when the incidence of infection is greatest, and possibly for life. However, this is a controversial issue that depends on patient compliance, bacterial resistance in the local community, and a host of other factors.

Folic Acid. Prior to splenectomy, HS patients, like patients with other hemolytic disorders, should take folic acid (1 mg per deciliter orally) to prevent folate deficiency.

POSTSPLENECTOMY CHANGES. Spherocytosis persists following splenectomy because the basic red cell defect is unchanged, but conditioned microspherocytes disappear and changes typical of the postsplenectomy state (Howell-Jolly bodies, target cells, siderocytes, and acanthocytes) become evident on the blood smear (see Color Plate 6K). During the operation the surgeon must be careful to search for accessory spleens, which occur in 10 to 25% of patients. Recurrence of hemolysis due to regrowth of an accessory spleen is occasionally observed after years or even decades and should be suspected if reticulocytosis recurs or Howell-Jolly bodies disappear from the blood smear.

Hereditary Elliptocytosis (HE)

Although hereditary elliptocytosis is quite frequent (≈ 1 in 2500 in the white North European population and up to 1 in 150 in some parts of Africa), it is less important clinically than HS. Only about 10 to 15% of patients have significant hemolysis; however, in some cases this can be life-threatening. Four clinical phenotypes are distinguished: mild HE, hereditary pyropoikilocytosis (HPP), spherocytic HE, and Southeast Asian ovalocytosis (Table 134–3).

MILD HE

As its name implies, mild HE is little more than a morphologic curiosity in most heterozygous carriers; there is no anemia or splenomegaly and very mild hemolysis (reticulocyte counts $< 3\%$). The blood smear shows prominent elliptocytosis (usually $> 40\%$; normal $< 15\%$) (see Color Plate 6D, right). Osmotic fragility is normal. However, 10 to 15% of heterozygotes have more severe hemolysis, with a corresponding increase in elliptocytes and fragmented red cells, often due to coinheritance of spectrin α^{LELY} (see below). Patients with mild HE may also develop significant hemolysis if the spleen hypertrophies in response to various stimuli (e.g., infectious mononucleosis, cirrhosis).

PATHOGENESIS. In general, mild HE and HPP are caused by defects in the "horizontal" interactions that hold the membrane skeleton together. The most common defects affect spectrin self-association and lead to an increased fraction of spectrin heterodimers on the membrane (normal 5 to 8%). The fraction of heterodimers is assayed by extracting spectrin at low temperature (0 to 4° C), when the interconversion of spectrin heterodimers and heterotetramers is blocked, and separating the two species on nondenaturing polyacrylamide gels. Many mutations have been identified, particularly in

TABLE 134-3. HEREDITARY ELLIPTOCYTOSIS

Clinical Manifestations	Laboratory Features
Mild Hereditary Elliptocytosis	
Asymptomatic	Blood smear: elliptocytes, few or no poikilocytes
Dominant inheritance: one parent with HE	No anemia, little or no hemolysis (reticulocytes = 1 to 3 %)
Variants:	Normal osmotic fragility
Some neonates with moderately severe hemolytic anemia and HPP-like smear. Converts to typical mild HE by 1 to 2 years	Defect in α- or β-spectrin $\rightarrow$ decreased spectrin self-association, or deficiency of protein 4.1
Some patients with mild chronic hemolysis (often inherit α^{LELY} polymorphism in trans)	
Hereditary Pyropoikilocytosis	
Anemia	Blood smear: fragments, bizarre poikilocytes, spherocytes, ± elliptocytes
Splenomegaly	Reticulocytosis
Intermittent jaundice	Decreased MCV due to red cell fragmentation
Aplastic crises	Increased osmotic fragility
Recessive inheritance: both parents normal or one or both parents with HE	Decreased red cell heat stability
Good response to splenectomy	Marked defect in spectrin self-association
Spherocytic Hereditary Elliptocytosis	
Anemia	Blood smear: rounded elliptocytes, ± spherocytes
Splenomegaly	Reticulocytosis
Intermittent jaundice	Increased osmotic fragility
Dominant inheritance pattern	Some patients with β-spectrin mutations
Good response to splenectomy	
Southeast Asian Ovalocytosis	
Asymptomatic	Blood smear: rounded elliptocytes, some with transverse bar that divides central clear space
Dominant inheritance	Little anemia or hemolysis
Lowland aboriginal peoples of Melanesia, Malaysia, Indonesia, and Philippines	Very rigid red cells that resist invasion by malarial parasites
	Mutant protein 3

HE = hereditary elliptocytosis; MCV = mean corpuscular volume.

α-spectrin. The mutations cluster near the self-association sites: at the N-terminus of α-spectrin and the C-terminus of β-spectrin.

The other common horizontal mutations involve protein 4.1. Heterozygous deficiency of 4.1 or loss of its ability to strengthen the spectrin-actin bond causes mild HE. Homozygous defects result in severe poikilocytic anemias.

SPECTRIN-α^{LELY}. This important polymorphism alters α-spectrin mRNA splicing so that half of the α-spectrin molecules are defective (Sp α^{LELY}) and cannot pair with β-spectrin. By itself the mutation is harmless, since α-spectrin is made in excess. However, when paired, in trans, with an α-spectrin mutation that causes HE, the loss of normal alpha chains results in an increased proportion of spectrin dimers bearing the HE defect and greatly exacerbates the severity of the defect. The consequences are magnified because the α^{LELY} mutation is *very common* (20 to 30% gene frequency in several populations).

HEREDITARY PYROPOIKILOCYTOSIS

Patients with this rare recessive disease have moderately severe to life-threatening hemolytic anemia characterized by remarkable red cell fragmentation (mean corpuscular volume [MCV] 45 to 75 fl), bizarre poikilocytosis, and heat-sensitive red cells that fragment at 45° C to 46° C instead of the normal 49° C. The more severe variants also feature spectrin deficiency (20 to 40%) and spherocytosis. The hemolysis is diminished but not completely cured by splenectomy. HPP typically results from homozygosity or compound heterozygosity for α-spectrin defects that produce mild HE or from a combination of spectrin α^{LELY} with one of the more severe α-spectrin defects.

TRANSIENT INFANTILE POIKILOCYTOSIS. Interestingly, neonates with mild HE and an inherited spectrin self-association defect may begin life with an HPP-like syndrome: a severe poikilocytic, microcytic, hemolytic anemia that sometimes requires transfu-

sion. The condition converts to typical mild HE during the first 6 to 12 months, in parallel with the loss of fetal erythrocytes. It appears the high concentration of free 2,3-diphosphoglycerate in fetal cells weakens the spectrin-actin-4.1 interaction and aggravates the inherited defect in spectrin self-association.

SPHEROCYTIC HE

Spherocytic elliptocytosis is a relatively rare autosomal dominant condition with features of both HS and HE. Patients have mild to moderate hemolytic anemia characterized by rounded elliptocytes, occasional spherocytes, and a positive osmotic fragility test. The indications for splenectomy, which is curative, are the same as for HS. Some patients have β-spectrin defects that truncate the C-terminal end of the protein. The molecular cause in other cases is unknown.

SOUTHEAST ASIAN OVALOCYTOSIS

This curious autosomal dominant disorder is very prevalent (up to 30%) among the aboriginal peoples of Melanesia, Indonesia, Malaysia, and the Philippines but is rarely seen in other populations. Heterozygotes have rounded elliptocytes, some with unique morphology (a transverse bar that divides the central clear space), that are *extraordinarily rigid* and resist invasion by a variety of malarial parasites. The rigidity appears to be caused by increased binding of ankyrin to a mutant protein 3 or by aggregation of the mutant protein within the lipid bilayer. Surprisingly the red cells circulate freely, despite their rheology, and there is little or no hemolysis or anemia. In contrast, the homozygous state is apparently lethal, perhaps because the mutant protein 3 cannot transport anions.

TREATMENT

Splenectomy is indicated only in severe cases of HE or HPP and, especially because spontaneous regression occurs in some infants, should be postponed to at least the third year of life and preferably the fifth year or later.

Hereditary Defects In Membrane Permeability

HEREDITARY XEROCYTOSIS

In this rare autosomal dominant disorder of red cell membrane permeability, the ratio of K^+ loss to Na^+ gain exceeds the normal ratio of 2:3; as a result, total cation content and cell water decrease. This occurs as a secondary event in a variety of conditions (e.g., sickle cell disease, hereditary spherocytosis, and hemoglobin C disease). Morphologically, dehydrated red cells are typically either targeted or contracted and spiculated. Because dehydration increases intracellular viscosity, these cells are relatively rigid and risk splenic sequestration and hemolysis.

HEREDITARY HYDROCYTOSIS (HEREDITARY STOMATOCYTOSIS)

In this rare autosomal dominant disease, an inherited defect in Na^+ permeability causes massive Na^+ influx, which overwhelms the Na/K pump and leads to an increase in intracellular cations and water. In some families this results in severe hemolysis. In others, for unknown reasons, hemolysis is much milder. Patients with the severe variant respond well to splenectomy. The large, partially swollen red cells appear on blood smears as stomatocytes (i.e., red cells with a mouthlike band of pallor across the center of the stained cell). Stomatocytes are much more frequently seen as an acquired defect, without hydrocytosis, cation changes, or hemolysis, in patients with acute alcoholism or with various types of liver disease.

ENZYME DEFICIENCIES

Normal Red Cell Metabolism

Reticulocytes have no nuclei and lose their mitochondria and microsomes as they mature; consequently, mature red cells consume little oxygen and do not synthesize protein. Glucose, the main metabolic substrate of the cells, is metabolized via two major pathways: the *Embden-Meyerhof pathway* and the *pentose phosphate pathway* (hexose monophosphate shunt) (Fig. 134-3).

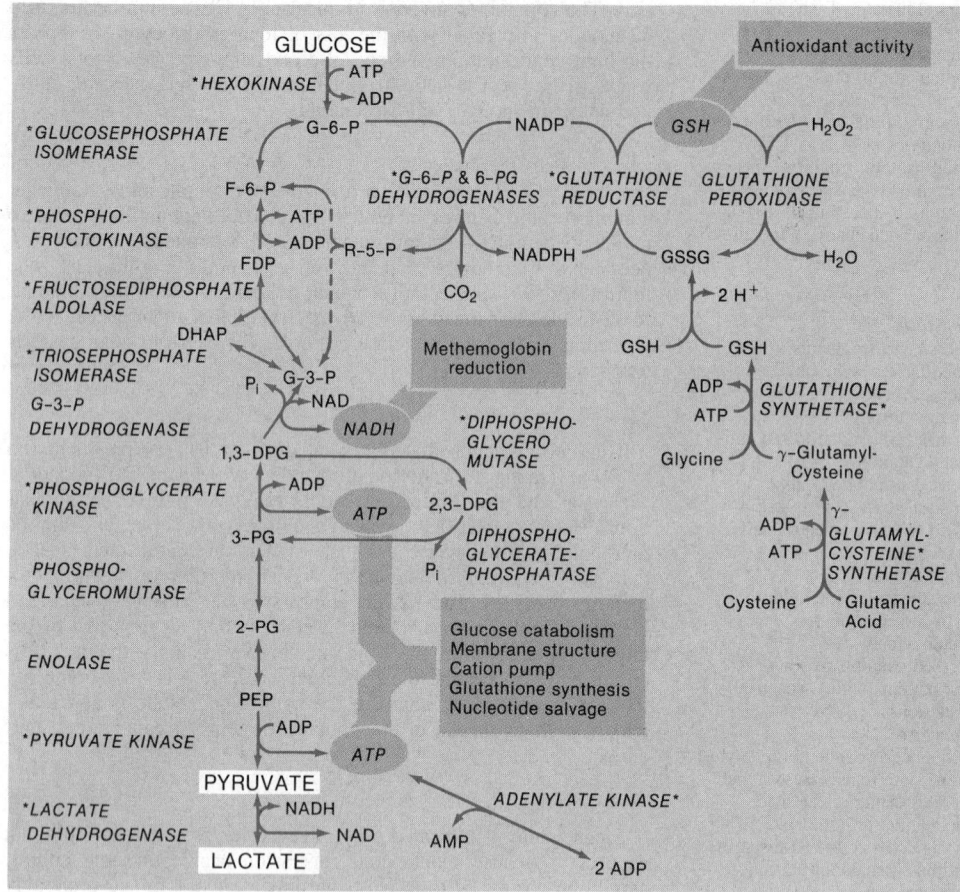

FIGURE 134-3. Glycolytic pathways and glutathione metabolism in the human erythrocyte. Asterisks indicate enzymes for which severe deficiency has been established. (From Valentine WN: Hemolytic anemia and inborn errors of metabolism. Blood 54:549, 1979.)

THE EMBDEN-MEYERHOF (EM) PATHWAY

Approximately 90 to 95% of metabolized glucose is converted to lactate via the EM pathway. This is the *major pathway of ATP synthesis in mature red cells.* Only 2 moles of ATP are generated from glycolysis per mole of glucose consumed, which is very inefficient compared with cells that possess mitochondria and an active Krebs cycle (that generates 38 moles of ATP per mole of glucose). Nevertheless, the meager amount of ATP produced permits renewal of 150 to 200% of the total red cell ATP every hour. Red cell ATP is used to transport monovalent cations and calcium, to phosphorylate various proteins, to synthesize glutathione, to salvage nucleotides, and to produce the hexose phosphates needed to fuel glycolysis. The EM pathway is also the major source of red cell nicotinamide adenine dinucleotide, reduced form (NADH). This cofactor is essential for maintenance of heme iron in the reduced state, an enzymatic process that is mediated by *NADH-methemoglobin reductase.* Oxidation of heme iron to Fe^{3+} produces methemoglobin, which does not transport oxygen (see Ch. 136).

Red cells have a uniquely high concentration of 2,3-diphosphoglycerate (2,3-DPG); only traces of this metabolic intermediate are present in other cells. This intermediate, formed by the Rapoport-Luebering shunt (Fig. 134–3), decreases the oxygen affinity of hemoglobin and increases oxygen delivery to peripheral tissues (see Ch. 136).

PENTOSE PHOSPHATE PATHWAY (PPP)

Approximately 5 to 10% of utilized glucose is normally directed through the PPP (also called the hexose monophosphate shunt). This pathway is the *major source of nicotinamide adenine dinucleotide phosphate, reduced form (NADPH),* in human red cells. Two moles of NADPH are produced for each mole of glucose metabolized. Under conditions in which the oxidation of NADPH is accelerated, diversion of glucose through the shunt can increase at least 10-fold.

The most important reactions associated with NADPH oxidation are those related to glutathione. Red cells contain relatively high concentrations (2 mM) of reduced glutathione (GSH), a tripeptide (gamma-glutamylcysteinylglycine) that is synthesized by mature red cells (Fig. 134–3). GSH protects red cells from injury by oxidants

such as superoxide anion (O_2^-), hydrogen peroxide (H_2O_2), and hydroxyl radical (OH·), which are produced continuously in normal red cells as by-products of the oxidation of heme by its dangerous oxygen cargo. Large amounts of oxidants are also generated by activated phagocytes (e.g., during infections) and by red cells in the presence of certain drugs. Injury to cell lipids and proteins occurs if these agents accumulate. Normally this is prevented by GSH. Detoxification of H_2O_2 can occur spontaneously, but it is enhanced by *glutathione peroxidase.* Catalase also degrades H_2O_2, but under physiologic conditions it is less important. In these reactions GSH is converted to *oxidized glutathione* (GSSG) and forms mixed disulfides with protein thiols (Fig. 134–3). GSH levels are restored by *glutathione reductase.* In the process, NADPH is oxidized to NADP, which stimulates the PPP, regenerating NADPH (a PPP inhibitor). This tight coupling of the PPP with glutathione metabolism normally protects red cells from oxidant injury.

Defects in the Pentose Phosphate Pathway or in Glutathione Metabolism

Almost all PPP defects are due to *glucose-6-phosphate dehydrogenase (G6PD) deficiency,* the most common enzyme abnormality associated with hemolytic anemia. It affects millions of people throughout the world. In contrast, pyruvate kinase deficiency, the most common glycolytic defect, affects only hundreds to thousands of patients.

GLUCOSE-6-PHOSPHATE DEHYDROGENASE (G6PD) DEFICIENCY

PATHOPHYSIOLOGY. Defects in the PPP or in glutathione metabolic pathways impair the ability of red cells to defend themselves against oxidative assault. Oxidants produced by infections or oxidant drugs are normally detoxified by GSH, but GSH levels are not maintained in G6PD deficiency because of diminished ability to generate NADPH. As a consequence, the oxidants are free to damage vital cell constituents. Oxidation of hemoglobin produces the functionless methemoglobin and intracellular precipitates of denatured hemoglobin that are known as Heinz bodies (see Color Plate 6C, left). Heinz bodies are not visible in ordinary Wright's-stained blood smears but are revealed with supravital stains such as *methyl violet.* They attach to the membrane and damage it in various ways. Among other things, they cause protein 3 molecules and immunoglobulin to cluster on the cell surface, opsonizing the cells for phagocytes. *In vitro,* they also increase membrane leakiness to cations and decrease osmotic fragility and cellular deformability. *In vivo,* Heinz bodies are "pitted" from circulating red cells by the spleen and thus are more plentiful in splenectomized patients. "Bite cells"—that is, red cells with localized invagination, possibly at the site of Heinz body damage or removal—appear in the circulation during acute hemolytic episodes. Red cells with a submembranous hemoglobin–free area, "blister cells," may also be seen (see Color Plate 6*E*, left). In addition to damage from Heinz bodies, G6PD-deficient red cells suffer oxidative crosslinking of spectrin and peroxidation of membrane lipids. Lipid damage may be responsible for the intravascular hemolysis seen during acute hemolytic episodes.

More than 400 G6PD variants are now known, but only a few of these are common. The normal enzyme is termed G6PD^B or Gd^B. It is present in about 70% of African Americans and in more than 99% of whites. Gd^{A+} is a normal variant found in about 20% of African Americans. It has greater electrophoretic mobility than does Gd^B because of substitution of an asparagine for an aspartic acid at position 126 in the amino acid sequence.

Gd^{A-}, the most common variant associated with hemolysis, is found in about 10% of African Americans and in many African black populations. It has the same electrophoretic mobility as Gd^{A+}, but its catalytic activity is decreased. Molecular analysis shows that Gd^{A-} has actually arisen at least three times, because of three different mutations (^{68}Val → Met, ^{227}Arg → Leu, or ^{323}Leu → Pro) superimposed on Gd^{A+}. The resulting enzymes are electrophoretically and functionally identical, and from the physician's point of view the related abnormalities constitute one disorder.

Gd^{Med} (^{188}Ser → Phe), the second most common abnormal variant, is found in peoples of the Mediterranean area (Italians, Greeks, Sardinians, Sephardic Jews, Arabs, and so forth), in India, and in Southeast Asia. Its electrophoretic mobility is normal, but its catalytic activity is markedly reduced.

As normal red cells age *in vivo,* the activity of intracellular Gd^B decays slowly, with a half-life of about 60 days (Fig. 134–4). Despite this loss of active enzyme, older normal red cells retain enough activity to produce NADPH and maintain GSH in the face of almost all oxidant stresses. The defect in Gd^{A-} results in a *labile enzyme* that disappears and has a half-life of about 13 days. *Young red cells thus have normal enzyme activity, while older red cells are grossly deficient.* As a consequence of this heterogeneity, hemolysis is self-limited in individuals with Gd^{A-}. This fact is shown graphically in Figure 134–5, which depicts the course of primaquine-induced hemolysis in an individual with Gd^{A-}. Acute he-

molysis with hemoglobinuria and decreased ^{51}Cr red cell survival develops when the drug is first administered, but this is followed by a recovery phase in which anemia and reticulocytosis abate and red cell survival improves despite continued administration of the drug. The reason is that once the oxidant-sensitive older red cells are destroyed, the remaining young cells are oxidant resistant. Since only about 50% of the cells are oxidant sensitive to begin with in Gd^{A-}, the bone marrow can compensate by simply doubling its output. This apparent drug resistance persists as long as the offending drug is continuously administered. Note, however, that if the drug is stopped for 2 to 3 months, older red cells will survive and accumulate, and the patient will again become drug sensitive.

Gd^{Med} is considerably more unstable than Gd^{A-} (Fig. 134–4). Very little activity is present in mature red cells. Despite this, chronic hemolysis does not occur, which must indicate that endogenous oxidant stresses are normally very low. When threatened by infections or oxidant drugs, however, these patients are at much greater risk because virtually their entire red cell population can be destroyed.

CLINICAL FEATURES (Table 134–4). The most dramatic clinical presentation is acute intravascular hemolysis. These patients typically develop hemoglobinemia (pink to brown plasma), hemoglobinuria (red-brown to black urine), and jaundice—acutely with an infection or within 1 to 3 days of exposure to an oxidant drug or fava beans. In severe cases, abdominal or back pain may be prominent. Symptoms of acute anemia (dizziness, headache, palpitations, dyspnea) may also develop, and if hemoglobinuria is severe, renal tubular necrosis and renal failure are risks (see Ch. 76). Heinz bodies and increased levels of methemoglobin appear in the red cells, and some bite cells and blister cells may be seen on the blood smear. In many cases, however, red cell morphology is relatively normal. More often, hemolysis is less dramatic, and a modest decline of hemoglobin (3 to 4 grams per deciliter) occurs, without hemoglobinuria or prominent symptoms. These episodes are easily overlooked unless the physician is alert. Between hemolytic episodes, patients with Gd^{A-} and Gd^{Med} are *entirely normal,* with no evidence of hemolysis and a normal blood smear.

The discovery of G6PD deficiency followed the observation that African American soldiers developed explosive hemolysis after receiving primaquine for malaria. Subsequently, numerous other oxidant drugs were implicated as causative agents, some of which are listed in Table 134–5. The most common cause of hemolysis, however, is *infection.* Virtually every type of infection has been associated. One speculation is that oxidants generated by warring phagocytes trigger hemolysis by impinging on neighboring G6PD-deficient red cells.

Severe hemolytic episodes occur in some patients following ingestion of *fava beans* (Italian broad beans), probably caused by divicine and isouramil, oxidant pyrimidine derivatives that are present in high concentrations in the beans. This dangerous phenomenon occurs mainly in individuals with Gd^{Med}. This, and the fact that not all patients with Gd^{Med} are susceptible, indicates that other unknown factors must be involved.

Neonatal jaundice is a common complication of G6PD deficiency. It typically develops at 1 to 4 days of age and may require an exchange transfusion. In most cases, however, the jaundice is adequately controlled with phototherapy.

In some patients with rare variants of G6PD, *chronic nonspherocytic hemolytic anemia* occurs in the absence of obvious oxidants. These cases vary from mild to life-threatening. They are characterized by enzymes that are unable to maintain basal NADPH production. Variants generally have low substrate affinity for G6P or nicotinamide adenine dinucleotide phosphate (NADP) and decreased affinity for the inhibitor, NADPH.

GENETICS. The gene for G6PD is located on the X chromosome, so its inheritance is sex linked. Males have one type of G6PD; females can have two types. For example, 70% of black males have Gd^B, 20% have Gd^{A+}, and 10% have Gd^{A-}. Black females, however, can be heterozygous for any two of these enzymes. According to the *Lyon hypothesis,* only one X chromosome is active in any somatic cell; thus any given red cell in heterozygous females is either normal or deficient. Mean enzyme activity in females who are heterozygous for G6PD deficiency may be normal,

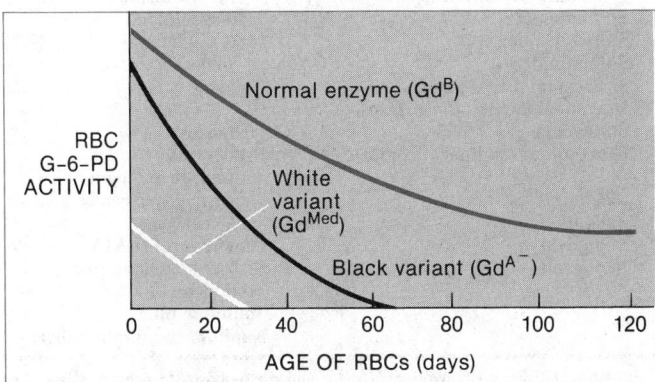

FIGURE 134–4. Intracellular decay of red cell G6PD as a function of cell age. The top curve shows the decay rate for Gd^B, the normal enzyme. The middle and lower curves show the greater than normal decay rates for the unstable Gd^{A-} and Gd^{Med} variants. Note that only the oldest Gd^{A-} red cells are markedly G6PD deficient and susceptible to hemolysis, whereas nearly all Gd^{Med} erythrocytes are vulnerable. Note also that after the most deficient Gd^{A-} red cells have been destroyed, the average G6PD level in the remaining cells will be near normal. This explains why G6PD assays after a hemolytic episode often fail to disclose the defect in Gd^{A-} males. (Modified from Lux SE: Hemolytic anemias. Metabolic disorders. *In* Beck WS [ed.]: Hematology, 4th ed. Cambridge, Mass, The MIT Press, 1985, p 223.)

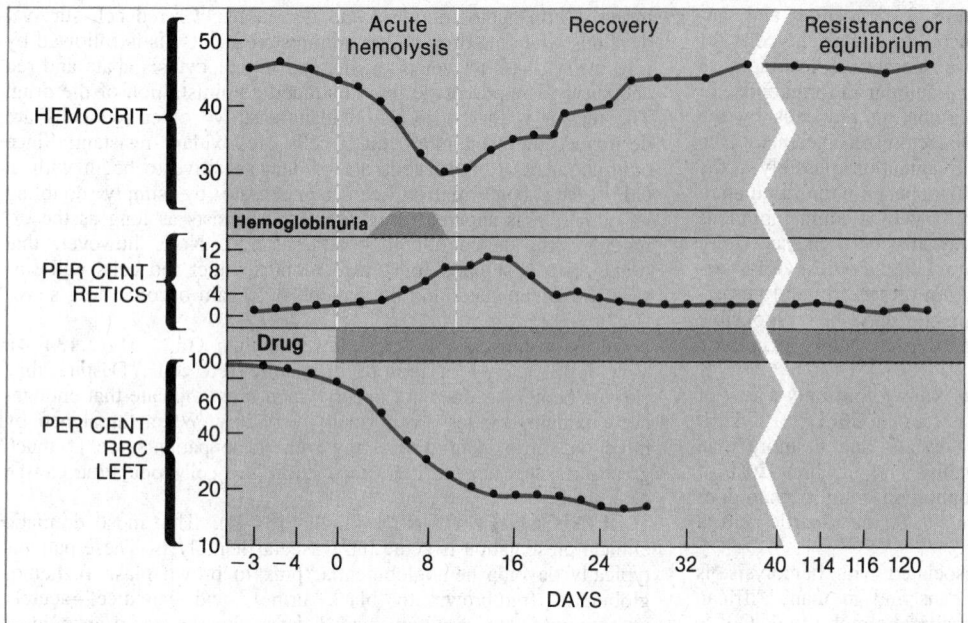

FIGURE 134–5. Course of drug-induced hemolysis in an individual with Gd^A−. Note that hemolysis abates and apparent resistance to the drug develops after the initial hemolytic episode owing to repopulation with young red cells. (Adapted from Alving AS: Bull World Health Organ 22:621, 1960.)

moderately reduced (usual), or grossly deficient, depending on the degree of lyonization. Deficient cells in heterozygous females are just as susceptible to oxidant injury as enzyme-deficient cells in males; however, the overall magnitude of hemolysis is less because of the smaller population of vulnerable cells.

Despite the disadvantages of a gene for G6PD deficiency, it remains common in many geographic areas. Its prevalence has been attributed to a selective advantage heterozygotes are believed to enjoy against malaria caused by *Plasmodium falciparum.* This proposal is supported by a large body of data, including epidemiologic studies, observations in heterozygous females demonstrating the resistance of cells containing the abnormal enzyme to malarial infection, and poor growth of *P. falciparum* parasites in G6PD-deficient red cells *in vitro.*

DIAGNOSIS. Several tests for the diagnosis of G6PD deficiency are currently available. Their sensitivity varies, and their usefulness is determined by the clinical situation (sex of patient, type of G6PD deficiency, and proximity to the hemolytic episode).

Commonly used screening tests are based on NADPH-mediated dye decolorization or on the reduction of methemoglobin in the presence of methylene blue. These tests are of limited sensitivity, since 30 to 40% of the cells must be abnormal for the deficient state to be detected. This criterion may not be met in patients with Gd^A− after a severe hemolytic episode, since most of their enzyme-deficient, older red cells will have been destroyed.

Definitive assay of the enzyme depends on direct spectrophotometric measurement of NADPH production. This test is more sensitive than the screening tests, but still requires 20 to 30% deficient cells for an abnormal result. The sensitivity can be enhanced by comparing the level of G6PD to other age-dependent enzymes. With this modification, diagnosis of G6PD deficiency can be made even after a hemolytic episode.

DEFECTS IN GLUTATHIONE METABOLISM

Abnormalities of GSH metabolism, the first line of defense against oxidants, can also be associated with hemolysis. Defects in either glutathione synthetase or *gamma-glutamylcysteine synthetase,* the two enzymes responsible for the synthesis of GSH, occur rarely. Erythrocytes lacking either of these enzymes have very low levels of GSH. Clinically the disorders are similar to G6PD deficiency; they are characterized by mild to moderate hemolytic anemia that is sensitive to drugs. Chronic neurologic disease also occurs in some patients with glutathione synthetase deficiency, but it

TABLE 134–4. CLINICAL COMPARISON OF THE TWO COMMON FORMS OF G6PD DEFICIENCY

	Gd^A−	Gd^Med
Frequency	Common in African populations	Common in Mediterranean populations
Chronic hemolysis	None	None
Degree of acute hemolysis	Moderate	Severe
G6PD defect	Old red cells	All red cells
Hemolysis with:		
Drugs	Unusual	Common
Infection	Common	Common
Need for transfusions	Rare	Sometimes

TABLE 134–5. DRUGS COMMONLY LEADING TO HEMOLYSIS IN G6PD DEFICIENCY*

Antimalarials	**Analgesics****
Primaquine†	Acetylsalicylic acid (aspirin)
Pamaquine‡	(can give moderate doses)
	Acetophenetidin (phenacetin)
Sulfonamides and Sulfones	
Sulfisoxazole (Gantrisin)	**Other Antibacterials**
Trimethoprin-sulfamethoxazole	
(Septra)	**Nitrofurans**
Salicylazosulfapyridine	**Nitrofurantoin (Furadantin)**
(Azulfidine, sulfasalazine)	**Nitrofurazone (Furacin)**
Sulfanilamide	**Furazolidone**
Sulfapyridine	Chloramphenicol
Sulfadimidine	*p*-Aminosalicylic acid
Sulfacetamide (Albucid)	Nalidixic acid††
Diaminodiphenylsulfone (Dapsone)§	
Sulfoxone§	**Miscellaneous**
Glucosulfone sodium (Promin)	Probenecid
	Vitamin K analogues (1 mg
Antihelminthics	menaphthone can be given to
β-Napthol	babies)
Stibophen	**Dimercaprol (BAL)**
Niridazole	Mepacrine (Quinacrine)
	Methylene blue
	Toluidine blue
	Naphthalene (moth balls)§

* Adapted from WHO Working Group: Glucose-6-phosphate dehydrogenase deficiency. Bull WHO 67:601, 1989. Drugs listed in bold print should be avoided by persons with all forms of G6PD deficiency; drugs in normal print should be avoided, in addition, by G6PD-deficient persons of Mediterranean, Middle Eastern, and Asian origin.

† Persons with Gd^A− may take this drug at reduced dosage (15 mg/dl or 45 mg twice weekly) under surveillance.

‡ Chloroquine may be used under surveillance when required for prophylaxis or treatment of malaria.

§ These drugs or chemicals may cause hemolysis in normal persons if given in large doses.

** Acetaminophen (paracetamol) is a safe alternative.

†† This drug applies only to individuals with Gd^A−.

is not certain that the enzyme disorder and neurologic defect are causally related.

Inherited deficiencies of *GSSG reductase* are thought to exist, but they are rare, and no case of hemolysis due to this disorder has been proved. Many individuals (including all newborn infants) are relatively deficient in *GSH peroxidase,* but they do not have excessive hemolysis. This probably reflects the fact that nonenzymatic reduction of peroxide by GSH occurs at a significant rate.

Defects in Glycolysis

GENERAL FEATURES. Abnormalities in most glycolytic enzymes have been described, but pyruvate kinase (PK) deficiency accounts for about 90% of the cases associated with hemolysis. Almost all of the glycolytic defects are inherited in an autosomal recessive pattern. Hemolysis is observed in homozygotes. Heterozygotes are normal, although their red cells contain less than normal amounts of enzyme. Phosphoglycerate kinase (PGK) deficiency is an exception, since this enzyme is located on the X chromosome.

Hemolysis caused by glycolytic defects is thought to be due to lack of ATP. However, red cell ATP concentrations are often not decreased because (1) the mean cell age is very young, and reticulocytes have high ATP levels; (2) defective cells with low ATP content are probably removed promptly from the circulation; and (3) ATP may be compartmentalized within reticulocytes, in which case a decline in ATP at one critical locus may be sufficient to cause cell injury.

CLINICAL FEATURES. Hemolysis is chronic and is not affected by drugs. *Splenomegaly* is usually present because of stagnation of red cells in the spleen. The acidic, hypoxic, and nutrient-poor environment of the spleen is an added insult to the metabolically abnormal cells. Thus the hemolytic rate often decreases after splenectomy. In most cases, red cell morphology is relatively unremarkable prior to splenectomy. After splenectomy the blood smear typically contains a small number of *dense, spiculated red cells,* but this is not invariable or unique to these disorders.

DIAGNOSIS. Definitive diagnosis requires spectrophotometric enzyme assays performed under a variety of conditions (i.e., with varying substrate and cofactor concentrations) to detect enzymes with abnormal kinetics. Measurements of glycolytic intermediates may reveal subtle enzyme abnormalities, since the concentration of an intermediate usually increases proximal to a defect and decreases distal to it.

PYRUVATE KINASE DEFICIENCY

Pyruvate kinase (PK) catalyzes one of the major reactions responsible for ATP production in glycolysis; it is not surprising, therefore, that deficiency of this enzyme causes hemolytic anemia. Hemolysis can be mild and completely compensated or severe enough to require frequent transfusions. The distal glycolytic block in PK deficiency causes a twofold to threefold increase in red cell 2,3-DPG, which enhances tissue oxygenation and may minimize some of the physiologic consequences of the anemia. In most cases, hemolysis improves following splenectomy, although the effect is not as dramatic as in diseases like hereditary spherocytosis. The improvement is related to the fact that PK-deficient reticulocytes depend on mitochondrial oxidative phosphorylation as an ATP source. In vitro incubation of PK-deficient reticulocytes under hypoxic conditions or with inhibitors of oxidative phosphorylation causes ATP levels to fall. The cells subsequently gain Ca^{2+}, lose K^+ and water, and become rigid. PK-deficient reticulocytes sequestered in the hypoxic splenic cords presumably undergo similar degeneration. Even when anemia improves following splenectomy, reticulocytes may rise to levels of 50 to 70%. This *paradoxical reticulocytosis* is due to increased reticulocyte survival once the adverse metabolic environment of the spleen is removed.

Defects in Red Cell Nucleotide Metabolism

Deficiency of *pyrimidine-5'-nucleotidase* also causes hemolysis. This enzyme degrades pyrimidine nucleotides to cytidine and uridine, which can diffuse out of the cell. Lacking this activity, red cells accumulate partially degraded messenger and ribosomal RNA, and up to 5% of the cells develop *prominent basophilic stippling.* Apparently the basophilic stippling in lead poisoning is produced by a similar mechanism, since pyrimidine-5'-nucleotidase is markedly inhibited by lead. Patients with an inherited (autosomal recessive) deficiency of this enzyme have chronic, moderately se-

vere hemolytic anemia. The mechanism of hemolysis is unknown. Splenomegaly is common, but splenectomy produces little discernible benefit.

Finally, a rare disorder characterized by *overproduction of adenosine deaminase* illustrates the importance of ATP in red cell integrity. In affected patients, excessive deamination of adenosine apparently reduces the amount of this purine sufficiently to impair ATP synthesis. Chronic hemolytic anemia results. The disorder seems to be caused by hyperefficient translation of an adenosine deaminase mRNA that is present in normal amounts and produces a qualitatively normal enzyme. This extraordinary result suggests that a defect will be found in the 5' untranslated region of the mRNA that enhances binding of the message to ribosomes or initiation factors.

Beutler E: Current concepts: Glucose-6-phosphate dehydrogenase deficiency. N Engl J Med 324:169, 1991. *Review of molecular defects responsible for G6PD deficiency and the insight they provide about structure and function of the normal enzyme.*

Green JB, Shackford SR, Sise MJ, Fridlund P: Late septic complications in adults following splenectomy for trauma: A prospective analysis in 144 patients. J Trauma 26:999, 1986. *Good prospective study of splenectomy complications in adults.*

Lux SE, Becker PS: Disorders of the red cell membrane skeleton: Hereditary spherocytosis and hereditary elliptocytosis. *In* Scriver CR, Beaudet AI, Sly WS, Valle D (eds.). The Metabolic Bases of Inherited Disease. 7th ed. vol III. New York, McGraw-Hill, 1995, pp 3513–3560. *Comprehensive review of etiology and clinical features of HS and HE.*

Lux SE, Palek J: Disorders of the red cell membrane. *In* Handin RI, Lux SE, Stossel TP (eds.): Blood: Principles and Practice of Hematology. Philadelphia, JB Lippincott, 1995, pp. 1701–1818. *Extensive (118 pages, 1534 references), up-to-date review of red cell membrane structure and membrane disorders, particularly HS and HE.*

Lux SE, Tse WT, Menninger JC, et al.: Hereditary spherocytosis associated with deletion of human erythrocyte ankyrin gene on chromosome 8. Nature 345:736, 1990. *First direct evidence that ankyrin deficiency causes HS.*

Palek J (ed.): Cellular and molecular biology of the red blood cell membrane proteins in health and disease. Pts. I–IV. Semin Hematol 29:229, 1992; 30:1, 85, 169, 1993. *Outstanding series of 18 reviews (340 pages, 2611 references) in four successive issues covers all aspects of red cell membrane structure and function, normal and abnormal, except for membrane lipids.*

Robinette CD, Fraumeni JF Jr: Splenectomy and subsequent mortality in veterans of the 1939–45 war. Lancet 2:127, 1977. *Provocative epidemiologic study that suggests splenectomy is associated with increased coronary artery disease.*

Schwartz PE, Sterioff S, Mucha P, et al.: Postsplenectomy sepsis and mortality in adults. JAMA 248:2279, 1982. *One of the only good epidemiologic studies of postsplenectomy sepsis. Indicates that the risk of serious infection is lower than previously thought.*

Tanaka KR, Paglia DE: Pyruvate kinase and other enzymopathies of the erythrocyte. *In* Scriver CR, Beaudet AL, Sly WS, Valle D (eds.): The Metabolic Bases of Inherited Disease, 7th ed. vol III. New York, McGraw-Hill, 1995, pp. 3485–3511. *Up-to-date review of inherited disorders of red cell glycolysis, glutathione metabolism, and nucleotide metabolism.*

Tchernia G, Gauthier F, Mielot F, et al.: Initial assessment of the beneficial effect of partial splenectomy in hereditary spherocytosis. Blood 81:2014, 1993. *Suggests that partial splenectomy is effective in relieving hemolysis while preserving some splenic phagocytic function. No evidence of splenic regrowth in a 4-year follow-up.*

135 AUTOIMMUNE HEMOLYTIC ANEMIA
Alan D. Schreiber

Immunologic mechanisms play a significant role in the pathophysiology of many disease processes. However, there are relatively few disorders in which it is possible to understand the ongoing mechanisms of immune damage in humans. Autoimmune hemolytic anemia is of particular interest in this regard, because it is possible to define many of the immunopathologic processes that occur in this disease in molecular and cellular terms. Autoimmune hemolytic anemia represents a group of disorders in which individuals produce antibodies directed toward one or more of their own erythrocyte membrane antigens. This leads to destruction of the antibody-coated erythrocytes by tissue macrophages. In this chapter the underlying mechanisms responsible for the immune clearance of red blood cells by antibodies are discussed. Also covered is the clinical syndrome of paroxysmal nocturnal hemoglobinuria, a complement-mediated hemolytic anemia characterized by intravascular hemolysis due to a red cell membrane defect. The clinical findings of this condition are contrasted with those in autoimmune hemolytic anemia, in which extravascular destruction of red blood cells predominates. Drug-induced immune hemolytic anemia is also a topic covered.

The most effective way to approach autoimmune hemolytic anemia is to determine which class of antibody is responsible for the hemolysis. In general, there are two major classes of antierythrocyte antibodies that produce hemolysis in humans: IgG and IgM. The pattern of red blood cell clearance, the site of organ sequestration, the response to therapy, and the prognosis all relate to the class of antierythrocyte antibody involved.

PATHOPHYSIOLOGY OF IMMUNE HEMOLYSIS

IgG-INDUCED IMMUNE HEMOLYTIC ANEMIA. Some years ago, an experimental model of immune hemolytic anemia was established in the guinea pig to examine the pathophysiology of erythrocyte destruction by antibodies. As with human erythrocytes, guinea pig erythrocytes are relatively resistant to the lytic action of complement, and their hemolysis, which is mediated by antibody and complement, is primarily extravascular. Each of the factors important in erythrocyte destruction defined in this model has been found to be important in the disease as it occurs in humans. This experimental model provides clearer understanding of many aspects of the human disease. IgG and IgM antiguinea pig erythrocyte antibodies were used to sensitize chromium 51-radiolabeled guinea pig erythrocytes. The radiolabeled antibody-coated erythrocytes were then injected intravenously into guinea pigs, and the rate and pattern of clearance as well as the site of organ sequestration of the antibody-sensitized cells were determined.

The number of antibody molecules on the erythrocytic surface was quantitated by both radiolabeling the antibody to directly assess the number of antibody molecules bound to the red cells and by using a sensitive complement fixation. With the latter test, antibody per erythrocyte could be expressed in terms of the number of complement or C1 (the first component of complement)-activating sites generated by the antibody. A single molecule of IgM antibody bound to an erythrocyte binds and activates a single molecule of C1 to initiate the classic complement pathway. In the case of IgG antibodies, two molecules of the IgG antibody need to be in proximity to one another on the erythrocyte surface for C1 binding and initiation of the classic pathway to occur. With antigens widely distributed on the erythrocyte surface, such as the antigens recognized by most antierythrocyte antibodies, many hundreds or thousands of IgG antibody molecules must be deposited on the erythrocyte membrane before two bind sufficiently close to each other to permit complement activation.

IgG-sensitized erythrocytes are removed progressively from the circulation and sequestered predominantly in the spleen (Fig. 135-1). Erythrocyte survival is determined by the number of antibody molecules per cell; increasing the number of IgG molecules per cell progressively increases the splenic sequestration of these cells.

IgG-coated erythrocytes are cleared from the circulation in an accelerated manner even in the absence of complement activation. This was evident from the studies performed in guinea pigs with IgG-coated erythrocytes deficient either in the fourth (C4) or third (C3) component of complement (Fig. 135-1). Complement-independent clearance of IgG-coated erythrocytes was predominantly by macrophages in the spleen, and a rather large number of antibody molecules per cell was required.

These studies indicated the importance of complement in accelerating clearance of IgG-coated red cells. C4-deficient guinea pigs have a complete block in their classic complement pathway, and complement is not activated beyond the C1 step. A comparison of C4-deficient and normal animals enabled the assessment of the role of antibody versus the role of antibody plus complement in altering erythrocyte survival. In addition, guinea pigs were depleted of the third component of complement, C3, as well as the later-acting components by treating the animals with cobra venom factor. In both animals genetically deficient in C4 and depleted of C3 by cobra venom factor, the complement activation sequence does not proceed through C3, and erythrocytes do not become coated with C3 in vivo. As shown in Figure 135-1, IgG-coated cells are cleared

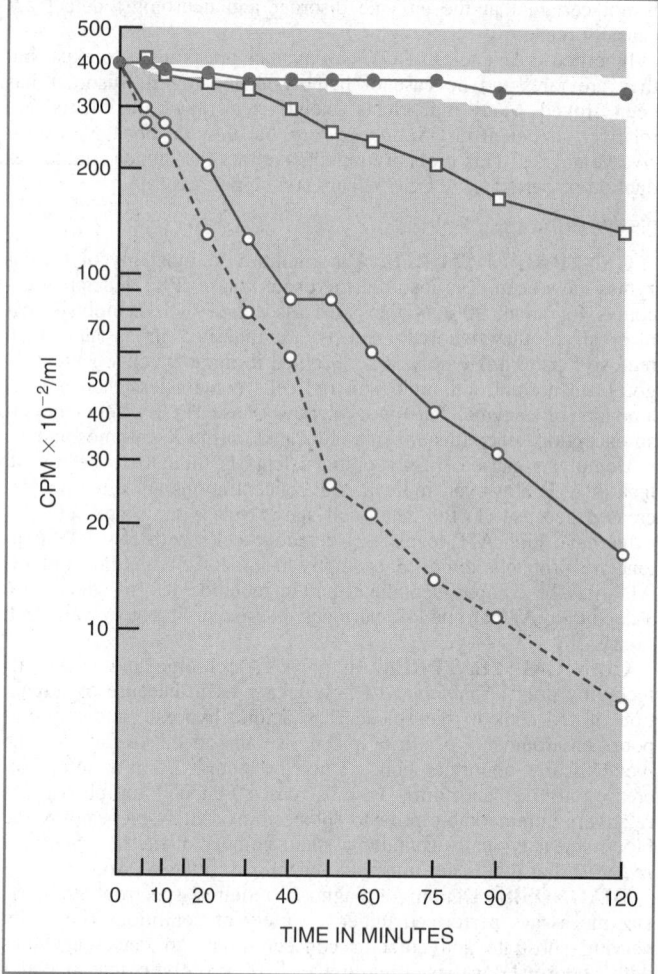

FIGURE 135-1. Survival of chromium 51-labeled guinea pig erythrocytes coated with IgG antibody in normal *(open circles)* and C4-deficient *(open squares)* guinea pigs. The survival of IgG-coated erythrocytes in C3-depleted guinea pigs was similar to that observed in C4-deficient guinea pigs. The *closed circles* represent the survival of chromium 51-unsensitized erythrocytes. (Shaded area = 95% confidence limits.) (From Schreiber AD, Frank MM: The role of antibody and complement in the immune clearance and destruction of erythrocytes: In vivo effects of IgG and IgM complement-fixing sites. The Journal of Clinical Investigation 51:575, 1972; by copyright permission of the American Society of Clinical Investigation.)

much more rapidly in normal animals compared with C4-deficient animals. The defect in the clearance of IgG-coated erythrocytes in both C4-deficient and C3-depleted animals resides in the failure of C3 to bind to the erythrocyte surface. The similar survival of IgG-coated erythrocytes in C4-deficient and C3-depleted guinea pigs suggests that the classic, rather than the alternative, complement pathway is of prime importance in the clearance of IgG-coated erythrocytes.

Thus these studies demonstrated that IgG-coated erythrocytes are cleared predominantly in the spleen regardless of whether complement activation occurs. When very large amounts of IgG are bound to the erythrocytes, the liver becomes the predominant organ of clearance. *In vitro* studies have shown that macrophages of the reticuloendothelial system have several classes of surface receptors for the Fc domain of IgG antibodies (Fcγ receptors). These receptors are responsible for the binding and phagocytosis of IgG-coated erythrocytes. One of the Fcγ receptor isoforms is a high-affinity receptor present on macrophages and monocytes, FcγRI. There are also two low-affinity receptors on macrophages: FcγRII and FcγRIII. These latter Fcγ receptors appear responsible, at least in part, for the clearance of IgG-coated cells, as they are not inhibited as efficiently by plasma concentrations of IgG. Erythrocytes coated with multiple IgG molecules interact with macrophages with multiple Fcγ receptors, leading to the binding of the erythrocytes to the macrophage surface, which in turn induces phagocytosis.

Macrophages can alter IgG- and/or C3b-coated erythrocytes in a manner that causes the red blood cells to form microspherocytes. These spherocytes are less able to pass through the splenic cords and sinuses and therefore have decreased survival. Their presence in the circulation is an indication of ongoing immune hemolysis. Macrophages also have receptors, designated CR1 and CR2, for the activated third component of complement, which recognize the C3b and iC3b forms of C3bi, respectively, and which are capable of binding C3b-coated erythrocytes. The receptors for the various C3 fragments do not recognize native C3; they recognize only fragments of C3 after C3 has undergone activation. Therefore they are capable of efficient function in the presence of normal plasma concentrations of C3. Fcγ receptors and C3b receptors can interact synergistically in their binding of IgG- and C3b-coated cells, and therefore the clearance of erythrocytes coated with IgG and C3b is greater than those coated with IgG alone.

IgM-INDUCED IMMUNE HEMOLYTIC ANEMIA. When erythrocytes are coated with IgM antibody and injected intravenously into guinea pigs, the pattern of clearance and site of organ sequestration are different from those of IgG-coated erythrocytes (Fig. 135–2). IgM-coated cells are cleared rapidly within the liver rather than the spleen. Erythrocyte survival is proportional to the number of IgM molecules per red blood cell.

There is an absolute requirement for complement in the clearance of IgM-coated cells. This was determined by examining the erythrocyte survival of IgM-coated cells in C4-deficient and C3-depleted guinea pigs. IgM-coated erythrocytes survive normally in complement-deficient animals, even when agglutinating concentrations of IgM antibody are employed. *In vitro* studies showed that macrophages did not bind IgM-coated erythrocytes in the absence of complement. This is because macrophages do not have receptors for the Fc domain of IgM antibodies, in contrast to their abundant receptors for the Fc domain of IgG antibodies. Activation of the complement sequence by IgM results in the deposition of C3b on the erythrocyte surface. Erythrocyte-bound C3b and iC3b leads to an interaction with hepatic macrophage C3b and iC3b receptors. This interaction with complement is responsible for the clearance of IgM-coated erythrocytes. Thus IgM-coated erythrocytes require complement for their clearance.

IgM- and C3b-coated erythrocytes are rapidly sequestered within the liver. Subsequently they are either phagocytized and destroyed,

or they are released from their hepatic macrophage C3b receptor attachment site back into the circulation where they then survive normally, even though they still are coated with IgM and antigenically detectable C3. Extensive *in vitro* and *in vivo* studies indicate that this release of IgM- and C3-coated erythrocytes from the macrophage C3 receptor attachment site is not due to elution of the antibody from the surface. Rather, the C3b/iC3b inactivator system, which involves several circulating plasma proteins, including factor I and factor H, causes the release of C3-coated erythrocytes from the macrophage C3b and iC3b receptor attachment sites. These released C3-coated cells have on their surface an antigenically altered form of C3 (C3d) that is no longer recognized by the macrophage C3b receptors. These C3d-coated erythrocytes then survive normally. Increasing the concentration of IgM per erythrocyte accelerates the sequestration by the liver macrophages and also decreases the number of erythrocytes released from the hepatic macrophage receptor binding sites. Pretreatment of IgM- and C3-coated erythrocytes with a source of serum C3 inactivator system proteins alters the erythrocyte cell-bound C3 and improves erythrocyte survival.

Thus these studies demonstrated that the two major classes of antibody that cause autoimmune hemolytic anemia, IgG and IgM, differ markedly in their biologic effects. IgG-coated erythrocytes are cleared predominantly in the spleen, whereas IgM-coated erythrocytes are sequestered predominantly within the liver. Splenic macrophage Fc receptors and C3 receptors are responsible for the clearance of IgG-coated cells. IgG-coated erythrocytes do not require complement for clearance. However, complement accelerates the clearance of IgG-coated erythrocytes in the spleen. Blood flow in the spleen is slower, with closer contact between sinusoidal macrophages and circulating red blood cells. This facilitates IgG-mediated splenic macrophage clearance.

The pattern of clearance of IgM-coated erythrocytes is entirely different from that of IgG-coated cells. IgM-coated cells are cleared rapidly by the hepatic macrophage C3 receptors. The clearance is entirely complement dependent, and in the absence of complement activation these cells survive normally. The C3 inactivator system serves as an important control mechanism for the clearance of IgM-coated cells, mediating the release of IgM- and C3-coated cells from their hepatic macrophage C3 receptor attachment sites. Furthermore, exposure of IgM- and C3-coated erythrocytes to C3 inactivator system proteins can attenuate the clearance of these C3-coated cells by hepatic macrophages.

CLINICAL FEATURES

IgG-INDUCED AUTOIMMUNE HEMOLYTIC ANEMIA. Autoimmune hemolytic anemia is most commonly caused by IgG antibody. The antigen to which the IgG antibody is directed is usually one of the Rh erythrocyte antigens, although often its precise specificity is not easily defined. This antibody usually has its maximal activity at 37° C, and thus this entity has been termed warm antibody–induced hemolytic anemia.

IgG-induced immune hemolytic anemia can occur without an apparent underlying disease (idiopathic autoimmune hemolytic anemia); however, it can also occur with an underlying immunoproliferative disorder, either malignant or nonmalignant, such as chronic lymphocytic leukemia, non-Hodgkin's lymphoma, and systemic lupus erythematosus. Certain patients with immunodeficiency such as agammaglobulinemia can develop autoimmune hemolytic anemia as well. Rarely, IgG-induced immune hemolytic anemia has also been observed in patients with an underlying malignant disease that is not an immunoproliferative disorder (Table 135–1). Such malignant disorders include ovarian tumors and myelofibrosis with myeloid hyperplasia. Additionally, bacterial infections such as tuberculosis, viral infections such as cytomegalovirus disease, and chronic inflammatory conditions such as ulcerative colitis have been described as associated conditions. The incidence of idiopathic IgG-induced autoimmune hemolytic anemia varies among different series. However, overall, approximately half of the patients with IgG-induced immune hemolysis do not have a detectable underlying disease at the time of diagnosis. The other half have an underlying disease, such as those mentioned above, or have a drug-induced immune hemolytic anemia. Both with the "idiopathic" disease and with that associated with an underlying immunoproliferative disorder, some patients have idiopathic thrombocytopenic purpura in

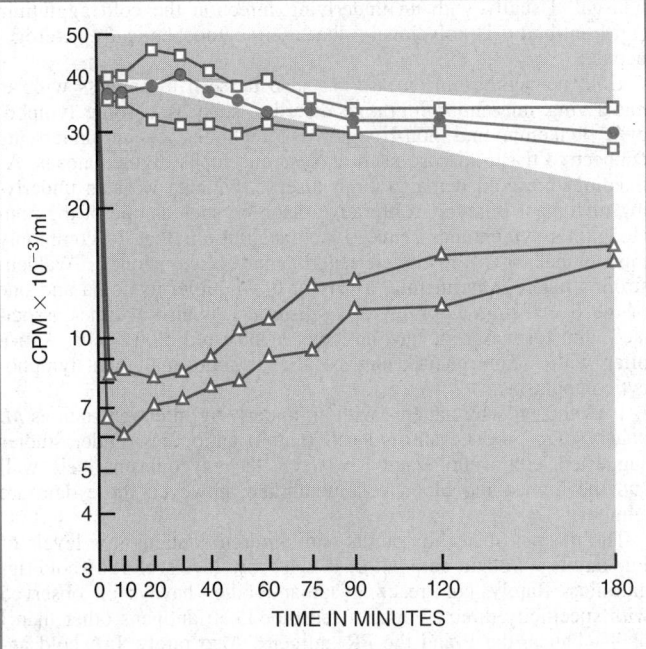

FIGURE 135–2. Survival of chromium 51-labeled guinea pig erythrocytes coated with IgM antibody in normal *(open triangles)* and C4-deficient *(open squares)* guinea pigs. The survival of IgM-coated erythrocytes in C3-depleted guinea pigs was similar to that observed in C4-deficient guinea pigs. (Shaded area = 95% confidence limits.) (From Nathan DG, Oski FA: Hematology of Infancy and Childhood, 4th ed. Philadelphia, WB Saunders, 1993, p. 497.)

TABLE 135-1. DISEASES ASSOCIATED WITH AUTOIMMUNE HEMOLYTIC ANEMIA

Infections

Viral infections, especially respiratory
Infectious mononucleosis and cytomegalovirus
Mycoplasma, especially pneumonia
Tuberculosis
Disorders associated with autoantibody production

Nonmalignant Disorders

Systemic lupus erythematosus
Rheumatoid arthritis
Thyroid disorders
Ulcerative colitis
Chronic active hepatitis

Immunodeficiency Syndromes

X-linked agammaglobulinemia
Dysgammaglobulinemia
Common variable hypogammaglobulinemia
IgA deficiency
Wiskott-Aldrich syndrome

Malignant Disorders

Non-Hodgkin's lymphoma
Hodgkin's disease
Acute lymphocytic leukemia
Carcinoma
Thymoma
Ovarian cysts and tumors

conjunction with IgG-induced autoimmune hemolytic anemia (Evans' syndrome). In addition, patients have been described with immune hemolytic anemia, immune thrombocytopenia, and immune granulocytopenia with antibodies directed toward erythrocytes, platelets, and granulocytes. It is not clear whether such IgG antibodies directed against each blood cell line recognize a common blood cell antigen or represent antibodies with different specificities.

In IgG-induced autoimmune hemolytic anemia, many IgG molecules on the erythrocyte surface are needed to bind and activate a single molecule of C1, the first component of complement, because two IgG molecules in proximity to each other (a doublet) are required. Once C1 is bound and activated, C4 and C2 activation occurs in a manner similar to that described for IgM antibody (see below), and C3 convertase is formed. C3 cleavage results, and C3b is deposited on the erythrocyte surface.

Macrophages within the reticuloendothelial system have receptors not only for C3b, but for the Fc fragment of IgG as well (Fcγ receptors). These macrophage Fcγ receptors bind IgG-coated erythrocytes and mediate spherocyte formation or phagocytosis. Thus, patients who have IgG on the erythrocyte surface in insufficient numbers or distributed in such a way to cause C1 binding and activation still have a substantial decrease in erythrocyte survival. However, once sufficient IgG is present on the erythrocyte surface so that C1 activation occurs, erythrocyte clearance is further accelerated. In such a circumstance, clearance is due to the macrophage Fcγ receptors and the macrophage C3b receptors. These receptors interact synergistically to induce the binding of erythrocytes coated with IgG and C3b. IgG-coated erythrocytes are cleared progressively from the circulation, primarily in the spleen, and hemolysis is almost always extravascular.

IgM-INDUCED AUTOIMMUNE HEMOLYTIC ANEMIA. In humans, IgM-induced autoimmune hemolytic anemia is caused by an IgM antibody that reacts most efficiently with erythrocytes in the cold. Thus, this disorder has also been called cold hemagglutinin disease. The IgM antibody in cold hemagglutinin disease is usually directed against the I antigen or related antigens on the human erythrocyte membrane. As with all IgM antibodies, agglutinating activity is particularly efficient because of the multiple antigen-combining sites on the IgM molecule. In this disorder the IgM antibody has particular affinity for its red cell antigen in the cold (0 to 10° C), and the affinity is lower at higher temperatures. Like warm antibody (i.e., IgG-mediated) autoimmune hemolytic anemia, cold agglutinin disease can be divided into those cases considered primary

or idiopathic and those associated with the presence of an underlying disease (secondary).

Chronic cold hemagglutinin is due to a clonal expansion of lymphocytes in which a monoclonal antibody that recognizes a polysaccharide antigen on red cells, termed I or i, is produced. The most common form of chronic cold agglutinin disease is the primary or idiopathic form. This is usually a disease of older persons, with a peak incidence in the 50's and 60's in some series. Most often it presents as fatigue, anemia, and occasionally jaundice in an elderly individual, but it may be associated with the development of acrocyanosis due to sludging of blood in peripheral vessels on exposure to cold or with acute hemolysis. This disease is associated with the presence of a monoclonal IgM antibody, usually exhibiting a high cold agglutinin titer ($>1:1000$). This IgM antibody binds to erythrocytes avidly in the cold but shows no binding activity at 37° C. In most, but not all, patients the antibody is of the κ light chain type and has specificity for the I antigen present on the erythrocytes of most adults. The I antigenic determinants are closely related to the ABO core antigenic determinants. Although present on the erythrocytes of almost all persons, the antigenic groupings recognized by the antibody develop during childhood and are not present in blood taken from the umbilical vein of the newborn. Thus, operationally, I specificity is established by the ability of the antibody to agglutinate the blood of almost all adults and its inability to agglutinate the erythrocytes of newborns. Although the monoclonal antibody responsible for the development of the cold hemagglutinin syndrome presumably reflects the expansion of a single clone of cells, these patients do not develop the symptom complex associated with multiple myeloma or Waldenström's macroglobulinemia. The monoclonal antibody appears to represent a highly restricted clonal response to the I antigen. Although each patient usually has only a single antibody with a single amino acid sequence, the antibodies among patients virtually always differ. Nevertheless, these antibodies tend to share idiotypic determinants consistent with their uniform recognition of the I antigen.

Secondary cold hemagglutinin disease, or IgM-induced immune hemolytic anemia, is most commonly associated with an underlying mycoplasma infection, particularly *Mycoplasma pneumoniae*, in which antibody with typical anti-I specificity is produced. However, it may also occur with other infections, such as infectious mononucleosis, cytomegalovirus, and mumps. With infectious mononucleosis anti-i (antibody to an antigen related to I but present on cord blood cells) cold agglutinins are produced, but overt hemolysis is unusual. Usually with an underlying infection the cold agglutinin (IgM antibody) is polyclonal—that is, immunochemically heterogeneous.

Cold hemagglutinin disease can also be seen in patients with an underlying immunoproliferative disorder, such as chronic lymphocytic leukemia and non-Hodgkin's lymphoma, or an underlying connective tissue disease such as systemic lupus erythematosus. As in idiopathic cold hemagglutinin disease, patients with an underlying malignant immunoproliferative disorder, such as one of the non-Hodgkin's lymphomas, have a cold agglutinin that is commonly monoclonal or of restricted heterogeneity (oligoclonal). Waldenström's macroglobulinemia, a variant of multiple myeloma and one of the B cell immunoproliferative disorders, is also at times associated with formation of IgM antibody against red blood cells. Anti-i, often with λ light chains, may be seen in more malignant lymphocytic neoplasias.

It is unclear why patients with an underlying infection such as *M. pneumoniae* produce anti-red cell (anti-I) antibodies. Older studies suggested cross antigenicity between the mycoplasma cell wall and the human red blood cell membrane; however, these data are tenuous.

The plasma of healthy adults and children contains low levels of IgM antierythrocyte antibodies, that is, low levels of IgM cold agglutinins. Rarely, cold-reacting autoantibodies have been observed with specificity directed against red blood cell antigens other than I or i—that is, the P and the PR antigens. Also rarely, IgA cold agglutinins have been observed.

The reason for the preferential reaction of cold agglutinin with the human red blood cell membrane in the cold is not completely understood. Most cold agglutinins have no measurable activity above 30° C. Although it has been postulated that either the antibody or the antigen may undergo a structural change on exposure to cold, most data suggest that the antigen on the erythrocyte surface is altered in the cold. This may represent a cold-dependent conformational change in the antigen recognized by the antibody-combining site or a cold-induced change in the erythrocyte surface, increasing antigen availability. When intact erythrocytes are studied, IgM anti-I interactions occur only in the cold. However, reactivity at 37° C is noted when the I antigen is isolated from the erythrocyte membrane.

As in all patients with autoimmune hemolytic anemia, erythrocyte survival is generally proportional to the amount of antibody on the erythrocyte surface. In cold hemagglutinin disease the extent of hemolysis is a function of the titer of the antibody (cold agglutinin titer), the thermal amplitude of the IgM antibody (the highest temperature at which the antibody is active), and the level of the circulating control proteins of the C3 inactivator system.

The factors that govern the survival of antibody- and complement-coated erythrocytes in humans are much the same as factors governing the clearance of these cells in animals. In cold hemagglutinin disease the IgM antibody in the circulation of patients with the disease interacts with the erythrocyte surface, where the cells circulate to areas below body temperatures, and activates the early steps of the classic complement pathway. Once C1, the first component of complement, is bound to the IgM molecule and activated, it sequentially binds and activates the fourth and second components of complement. The first of these two steps takes place at temperatures as low as 0° C. When the cells return to body temperature, activation proceeds, even though the cold agglutinin antibody can dissociate from the erythrocyte. The C3 convertase (C142) generated cleaves C3 into two antigenic fragments, one of which, C3b (and iC3b), binds to the erythrocyte surface. At this step there is considerable amplification of the IgM effect with a single C142 classic pathway (C3 convertase) capable of cleaving many C3 molecules and depositing many C3b molecules on the erythrocyte surface. In some cases the complement sequence of reactions may be completed with resulting hemolysis, but this is unusual because of the presence of membrane-bound proteins that restrict complement action. These C3b-coated erythrocytes are recognized by the hepatic macrophage complement receptors. The macrophage C3b and iC3b receptors bind, sphere, and may mediate phagocytosis of the C3b-coated erythrocytes. Extravascular sequestration usually predominates in patients with this disease. In humans, as in the guinea pig model, there are no receptors on macrophages capable of interacting with IgM-coated cells in the absence of complement; thus, in the absence of an intact classic complement pathway, through activation of C3, IgM-coated red cells have normal survival.

In humans, clearance of IgM-plus-complement–coated cells has been shown to be very rapid and takes place primarily in the liver. The human erythrocyte membrane, in contrast to the sheep erythrocyte membrane, is relatively resistant to the lytic action of complement. However, when large numbers of IgM molecules are present on the erythrocyte surface, sufficient terminal complement components (C5 to C9) are occasionally generated to lyse the erythrocytes in the intravascular space.

Control proteins involved in the C3 inactivator system are particularly important in cold hemagglutinin disease, because cell destruction is mediated entirely by C3 and the later complement components. Thus the level of the C3 inactivator proteins in plasma is thought to play an important role in determining hemolysis by regulating the number of active C3 fragments on the cell surface. The C3-coated erythrocytes interacting with C3 inactivator system proteins are degraded to C3dg or C3d. The C3dg- or C3d-coated erythrocytes are not bound by the macrophage C3 receptors and have normal survival. Thus the presence of C3 (C3dg or C3d)-coated erythrocytes in cold hemagglutinin disease explains the earlier observations of normal erythrocyte survival in patients who still have C3, as detected by the Coombs antiglobulin test, on their erythrocyte membranes.

The thermal amplitude of the IgM cold agglutinin is important in determining the extent of hemolysis in cold hemagglutinin disease. At a relatively low level of cold agglutinin sensitization, patients with higher thermal amplitude antibodies (those antibodies that possess activity at temperatures approaching 37° C) may still have considerable hemolysis. Such patients have been described as having a low-titer cold hemagglutinin syndrome with a high thermal amplitude antibody. The correct diagnosis in such patients is important, because they appear to respond to glucocorticoid therapy differently from the usual patient with high-titer cold hemagglutinin disease.

Furthermore, some unusual patients have an IgG cold agglutinin. The presence of such an IgG antibody is potentially important, as it appears to indicate responsiveness to steroids or splenectomy.

GENERAL FEATURES

There appears to be little genetic predisposition to the development of autoimmune hemolytic anemia. The occasional rare familial association of cases may be secondary to the familial predisposition to systemic lupus erythematosus or a similar underlying connective tissue disease. Thus there are patients with autoimmune hemolytic anemia who have a family history of other autoimmune diseases, such as autoimmune thrombocytopenia, rheumatoid arthritis, and glomerulonephritis.

Autoimmune hemolytic anemia is not an uncommon disease. In large centers 15 to 30 cases are seen yearly, with an annual incidence of approximately 1 case per 75,000 to 80,000 persons in the general population. As with any disease that may require careful serologic study for diagnosis, the level of sophistication and diagnostic capability of the institution influence the reported incidence. Nevertheless, autoimmune hemolytic anemia occurs considerably less commonly than does autoimmune thrombocytopenia. Autoimmune hemolytic anemia caused by either IgG or IgM antibody does not appear to be more prevalent in any particular racial group and can affect persons of any age. There is a general impression that autoimmune hemolytic anemia occurs more commonly in females, although in most series the incidence is about equal between sexes. Any increased incidence in females may be due to the increased incidence of systemic lupus erythematosus in women. Although warm antibody (IgG-induced) immune hemolytic anemia can occur at any age, there appears to be a peak incidence in the 50-year-old age group. In contrast, idiopathic cold agglutinin disease is a disease predominantly of the elderly.

The peak incidence of autoimmune hemolytic anemia in childhood is in the first 4 years of life. Children older than 10 years at onset are most likely to have a chronic course and most likely to have an underlying disorder. In a study of the prevalence of the disease in childhood, the incidence in those < 20 years old was slightly < 0.2 per 100,000. In contrast to the situation in adults, in the reported series in children there is a male preponderance. Patients with autoimmune hemolytic anemia vary considerably in mode of clinical presentation; the disease may be either indolent or fulminant. In general, the course of autoimmune hemolytic anemia is more acute in children than it is in adults, often ending in complete resolution of the disease. The fall in hemoglobin may occur over a period of hours to days, with resolution of the disease often within 3 months.

The Donath-Landsteiner cold hemolysin is an unusual IgG antibody with anti-P specificity that was originally noted in cases of congenital or acquired syphilis. The disease it causes is termed paroxysmal cold hemoglobinuria. Hemolysis in this syndrome most commonly occurs intravascularly, after the antibody has passed through a cell attachment phase in the lower temperatures of the peripheral circulation. The extravascular hemolysis is due to the unusual complement-activating efficiency of this IgG antibody. As its name implies, this antibody is associated with cold hemoglobinuria. This antibody, although uncommon, is most frequently found in children with viral infections. Hemolysis, although sometimes severe, is usually mild, and tends to resolve as the infection clears.

Mortality in the pediatric age group has ranged from 9 to 29%. Death during the acute stage is usually due to severe anemia or to hemorrhage from associated thrombocytopenia. Mortality in the chronic cases or in adults occurs more frequently, usually because of an underlying serious disorder such as Hodgkin's disease or non-Hodgkin's lymphoma or as a complication of therapy. Fatal sepsis has, of course, been observed following splenectomy.

CLINICAL AND LABORATORY FINDINGS

Many of the symptoms of autoimmune hemolytic anemia, such as weakness, malaise, and light-headedness, are caused by the presence of anemia. Patients who have underlying cardiovascular disease may have significant dyspnea on exertion and peripheral edema, as well as angina pectoris. If hemolysis is significant, mild jaundice may be noted, particularly in the presence of hepatic dysfunction. In addition, patients with an underlying disease often have the symptoms associated with that disease, for example, fever and weight loss with an underlying malignant disease or joint symptoms secondary to underlying systemic vasculitis. Physical findings are also generally referable to the underlying disease. For example, in patients with underlying non-Hodgkin's lymphoma, hepatosplenomegaly and lymphadenopathy are common. Mild splenomegaly may be present in patients with severe autoimmune hemolytic anemia. Massive splenomegaly suggests an underlying disorder such as lymphoma. Other signs that may result from the anemic state include those caused by congestive heart failure (edema, ascites, or pulmonary congestion). Severe jaundice is uncommon.

Thus the common presenting symptoms are pallor, jaundice, dark urine, abdominal pain, and fever. Pallor may precede the appearance of jaundice. The clinical status depends on the rapidity of the hemolysis and the severity of the anemia. In mild cases fatigue may be the only symptom. In severe cases the patient may appear acutely ill or even moribund, with tachycardia, tachypnea, signs of hypoxia, and even cardiovascular collapse. In severe IgM-induced cold agglutinin disease the skin may have a livedo reticularis pattern, and the patient may demonstrate acrocyanosis on exposure to the cold.

Laboratory data reveal the presence of anemia and, if bone marrow function is adequate, reticulocytosis. Diagnosis rests on the presence of anemia, reticulocytosis, and a positive result on direct Coombs' test. Examination of the peripheral blood smear may show spherocytes, polychromasia, nucleated red blood cells, and erythrophagocytosis. Rosetting of red cells around white cells may be visible in a buffy coat preparation.

Agglutination of the red cells may be evident in cold agglutinin disease. In severe cases, macroagglutination is visible on the microscope slide or in a capillary tube. The white cell count is usually normal or elevated. Autoimmune hemolysis is also associated with thrombocytopenia and/or leukopenia in a small number of patients. Indirect hyperbilirubinemia is common. It is the positive result on direct Coombs' test, however, that alerts the clinician to the correct diagnosis.

Reticulocytopenia may be observed, especially in children, in the first days of the anemia. In a small percentage of patients the reticulocytopenia may persist for weeks to months. Bone marrow aspiration usually shows erythroid hyperplasia, but hypoplasia is present in a few patients. Autoantibodies directed against burst-forming unit, erythroid (BFU-E) colonies are believed to be responsible for the reticulocytopenia in some patients. However, antibody directed at a blood cell antigen present primarily on reticulocytes is a theoretical possibility.

The diagnosis of autoimmune hemolytic anemia is most effectively established by directly examining the patient's circulating red blood cells for the presence of antibody and/or complement components on their surface. This is most easily done by a direct Coombs' antiglobulin test. Classically, in this test the patient's red blood cells are made to interact with a rabbit or goat anti-human serum globulin reagent, and agglutination of the patient's red blood cells is assessed. It is also possible to use antibody to human immunoglobulin or complement components as a more specific test reagent. In this case, agglutination induced by anti-IgG indicates the presence of IgG on the surface of the red blood cells, whereas agglutination with an anti-C3 or anti-C4 (a non-γ Coombs' test) is used to test for the presence of C4 and C3. In IgG-induced hemolytic anemia, IgG or IgG plus complement components is found on the surface of erythrocytes. Therefore such patients, while usually having a positive result on the γ Coombs' test, may have a nonpositive result on the non-γ Coombs' test as well. In IgM-induced hemolytic anemia (cold hemagglutinin disease), IgG is not found on the red cells, and the IgM cold agglutinin, because of its low affinity for red cell antigens at 37° C, is not found either; C3, stably bound at 37° C, is detected on the red cell membrane. Therefore, in cold hemagglutinin disease, usually only a positive result in the non-γ (C3) Coombs' test is observed. Rarely, patients with IgG-induced immune hemolysis have levels of IgG per erythrocyte undetectable by the standard Coombs' test, which requires the presence of hundreds of molecules of IgG on the erythrocyte surface for the result to be positive. When this phenomenon was originally described, the small amounts of red cell-bound IgG antibody were

detected with a complex antiglobulin consumption test. However, a Coombs' test using radiolabeled anti-IgG, which is 10 times more sensitive than the standard Coombs' test, also may be used to detect the antibody.

Testing with Coombs' antisera shows several patterns of reactivity. The red cells may be coated with IgG in the presence or absence of detectable complement (warm antibody IgG-mediated autoimmune hemolytic anemia) or with complement protein alone (IgM-induced hemolysis, i.e., cold hemagglutinin disease). Uncommonly, IgM is detected as well. In one large series of patients, IgG with or without complement was found on the red cells in 85 to 95% of patients with chronic disease, but in less (approximately 30%) of those with acute disease. Cold agglutinins (IgM-induced autoimmune hemolytic anemia) or the coating of red blood cells with complement alone were more common in the acute disease. Early studies suggested that the finding of IgG plus complement suggested a more guarded prognosis; however, it is now believed that it is not possible to predict chronicity or severity of autoimmune hemolytic anemia from the Coombs' testing pattern.

A cold agglutinin titer is also diagnostically helpful. This test is performed by examining the patient's plasma for agglutinating activity at 0° C directed against normal ABO-compatible erythrocytes containing the I antigen. The cold agglutinin titer is the highest dilution of antibody that still agglutinates normal red blood cells in the cold. Most patients with immune hemolysis secondary to cold hemagglutin disease have cold agglutinin titers greater than 1:1000.

THERAPY

In many patients with IgG- or IgM-induced immune hemolytic anemia, no therapeutic intervention is necessary, because the hemolysis is mild. If an underlying disease is present, control of this disease often brings the hemolytic anemia under control as well. However, if the patient is having significant anemia secondary to hemolysis, therapeutic intervention is in order.

GLUCOCORTICOIDS. We have studied the effect of glucocorticoids and other steroid hormones on the clearance of IgG-coated erythrocytes. Pretreatment of guinea pigs with glucocorticoids impairs the splenic clearance of IgG-coated erythrocytes. Pretreatment is necessary to observe this effect. Not all animals or individuals respond to steroids equally well, although the vast majority are steroid responsive. Glucocorticoids actually decrease the surface expression of splenic macrophage Fcγ receptors, probably by decreasing Fcγ receptor transcription.

Patients with IgG antibody-mediated autoimmune hemolytic anemia or immune thrombocytopenic purpura treated with glucocorticoids often respond within days of the onset of therapy. At the time of response, the cells remain antibody coated, and there may be no decrease in antibody synthesis. Furthermore, it has been observed that in some cases of IgG-mediated destruction of erythrocytes and platelets, the disease remains in clinical remission when patients are receiving steroid therapy, even when their cells remain antibody coated. These observations suggest that glucocorticoids affect the clearance mechanisms in humans. However, the data suggested that high doses of glucocorticoids might be effective in improving RBC survival in some patients with IgM-indirect immune hemolytic anemia whose RBC's are coated with limited amounts of IgM and C3. This observation led to studies in which patients identified with low-titer IgM (cold hemagglutinin)-induced immune hemolytic anemia, whose cells were coated with limited amounts of C3, were observed to respond to corticosteroids. However, very high concentrations of glucocorticoids were required to impair the clearance of IgM- and C3-coated cells in these patients.

More recently the capacity of other steroids and their analogues to modulate the clearance of the IgG-coated erythrocytes by splenic macrophages was examined. It was observed that estradiol, in contrast to cortisol, enhances the clearance of IgG-coated erythrocytes by splenic macrophages in a dose-dependent manner. On the other hand, estradiol does not alter the splenic macrophage clearance of heat-altered erythrocytes or the hepatic macrophage clearance of IgM- and C3b-coated erythrocytes. This suggests that the effect of estradiol is on the splenic macrophage Fcγ receptors responsible for the clearance of IgG-coated cells. These studies suggesting that the macrophage Fcγ receptors may be modulated *in vivo* by hormonal mechanisms were supported by studies demonstrating that splenic macrophages isolated from estradiol-treated animals exhibited remarkably enhanced Fcγ receptor expression, but not C3 receptor expression, when compared with control animals. These data may explain the alteration in the clinical status of patients with immune hemolytic anemia and immune thrombocytopenia during changes in hormonal states, such as pregnancy. During pregnancy estrogen levels rise to a level similar to that necessary to accelerate the clearance of IgG-coated erythrocytes. Similarly, during pregnancy the course of IgG-induced autoimmune hemolytic anemia is known to accelerate.

Patients with IgG-induced immune hemolytic anemia respond, in general, to glucocorticoid therapy in dosages equivalent to 1 to 2 mg of prednisone per kilogram of body weight a day. These drugs are believed to decrease hemolysis in IgG-induced hemolytic anemia by three major mechanisms: (1) They decrease the production of the abnormal IgG antibody. This is a common effect, is gradual, and can be expected to produce a gradual decrease in the strength of the Coombs' test result and a rise in hemoglobin within 2 to 6 weeks. (2) Glucocorticoids are reported to be associated with a fall in the amount of antibody detected by the direct Coombs' test and a rise in the amount detected by the indirect Coombs' test, as if they induced a decrease in antibody affinity. This has been associated with improved erythrocyte survival; it is probably an uncommon effect of glucocorticoid therapy. (3) Glucocorticoids have been shown *in vitro* and *in vivo* to interfere with the macrophage Fcγ receptors responsible for the erythrocyte clearance from the circulation. The effect is to improve erythrocyte survival despite the continued presence of IgG on the erythrocyte surface. Thus, the Coombs' test in some patients may remain positive in the face of improved erythrocyte survival and rising hemoglobin. This effect of glucocorticoids may be rapid and may be responsible for the rise in hemoglobin noted in some patients to occur with 1 to 4 days of glucocorticoid therapy. However, in a number of animal studies it was shown that glucocorticoids have no effect on erythrocyte survival until therapy has been continued for 5 to 7 days. Most patients respond to glucocorticoid therapy within 2 to 3 weeks. Although 4 to 6 weeks of therapy may be required for a response to be evident, in many of these delayed responders further therapy will be needed.

Once a therapeutic response is achieved and the patient's condition stabilizes, tapering of steroids should begin. This may take several months. Alternate-day steroid therapy can be effective in some patients after the clinical course stabilizes. Interestingly, alternate-day therapy may be less effective in autoimmune hemolytic anemia than in some of the inflammatory autoimmune diseases, and patients should be observed carefully for exacerbation. Great care should be taken in stopping glucocorticoids if the patient continues to demonstrate a positive result on the direct Coombs' test.

Approximately 80% of patients have an initial response to high-dose glucocorticoids. In many patients with acute autoimmune hemolytic anemia and in a small proportion of patients with chronic autoimmune hemolytic anemia the steroids can be tapered and stopped with the disease remaining in remission. In some patients there is control of the hemolytic process with continued low- to medium-dose steroid therapy. For those who are steroid dependent, the initial and long-term side effects of these drugs must be considered. These include exacerbation of diabetes and hypertension, electrolyte imbalance, increased appetite and weight gain, moonlike faces, osteoporosis, myopathy, and increased susceptibility to infection. The severity of these side effects relates both to duration of therapy and to dosage. Splenectomy should be considered in patients who are steroid unresponsive or require more than 10 to 20 mg of prednisone per day or substantial dosages of steroid every other day for maintenance. Each patient requires individual evaluation of underlying diseases, surgical risk, extent of anemia, and steroid intolerance. In some patients the presence of mild hemolytic anemia may be preferable to splenectomy or other treatment options. The initial goal of therapy is to return the patient to normal hematologic values and nontoxic levels of glucocorticoid therapy. However, in some patients, a modified goal of improvement in hemolysis to a clinically asymptomatic state with minimum glucocorticoid side effects is more realistic.

Glucocorticoids are not usually effective in cold hemagglutinin disease, probably because these patients generally have large amounts of IgM antierythrocyte antibody and many C3 molecules deposited on their red cells. Furthermore, macrophage C3b receptors, in contrast to the case with Fcγ receptors, are less responsive to glucocorticoid therapy. In addition, some of the hemolysis may

be intravascular, and glucocorticoids do not inhibit complement-mediated lysis. A few patients with a low-titer cold hemagglutinin disease syndrome, in which the antierythrocyte antibody has activity at temperatures approaching 37° C, do not respond to steroid therapy. In addition, the few patients described with an IgG cold agglutinin appear to be both steroid and splenectomy responsive. Patients with cold hemagglutinin disease respond best to the avoidance of cold and control of their underlying disease. Fortunately, in many patients hemolytic anemia is mild.

SPLENECTOMY. The spleen with its resident macrophages is the major site for sequestration of IgG-coated blood cells in humans as in animals. This appears to be due to the unique circulatory pathways in the spleen whereby hemoconcentration occurs in the splenic cords and erythrocytes make their way through fine fenestrations between macrophages. This results in intimate contact between macrophages (with their membrane Fcγ receptors) and IgG-coated blood cells, possibly in the presence of a minimal amount of plasma IgG.

The effect of splenectomy on the clearance of antibody- and complement-coated erythrocytes has also been studied in the experimental model. Splenectomy markedly decreases the sequestration of IgG-sensitized cells. However, as the antibody concentration was increased, splenectomy became less effective in preventing the clearance of IgG-coated cells, as the liver became the dominant organ in erythrocyte clearance. Splenectomy does not alter the clearance of IgM-coated cells.

Removal of this major site of red cell destruction is an effective therapeutic strategy in IgG-induced immune hemolytic anemia. The response rate to splenectomy is approximately 50 to 70%; however, the vast majority of the responses are partial remissions. Interestingly, before glucocorticoid therapy became available for the treatment of autoimmune hemolytic anemia, splenectomy was performed routinely. Remissions were common, but relapse usually occurred. Presumably, as the sensitized erythrocytes continued to circulate, they bound more and more antibody. They finally achieved a degree of sensitization at which the liver was able to mediate clearance. Probably those patients who are least responsive to splenectomy are those whose erythrocytes are coated with large amounts of IgG. In this circumstance the liver plays a larger role in clearance. The partial remissions that occur with splenectomy are often quite helpful in that they result in lessening of the hemolytic rate, with a rise in the hemoglobin value, and/or allow a reduction in the amount of glucocorticoid needed to control the hemolytic anemia. Because of the increased risk of sepsis, patients should be carefully selected. Those who are unresponsive to steroids, require moderate to high maintenance doses, or have developed glucocorticoid intolerance can be considered for splenectomy. Chromium-labeled red cell kinetic studies are probably not helpful, because the procedure is time consuming, expensive, and not a reliable indicator of response to splenectomy in most cases.

A second effect of splenectomy also has been suggested in autoimmune hemolytic anemia and shown to be important in autoimmune thrombocytopenia. Splenectomy may lead to a decrease in the production of the IgG antierythrocyte antibody, as the spleen contains a large B cell pool.

Splenectomy, like glucocorticoid therapy, is usually not effective in patients with cold hemagglutinin disease because IgM-coated erythrocytes are cleared predominantly in the liver. An occasional case in which a patient with apparent IgM-induced hemolytic anemia responded to splenectomy has been reported. This may be due to decreased production of IgM antibody by the spleen in these few patients or to the presence of an IgG cold agglutinin. Immunization with pneumococcal vaccine should be given before splenectomy to decrease the likelihood of postsplenectomy pneumococcal infection.

IMMUNOSUPPRESSIVE AGENTS. Several immunosuppressive agents have been used in the treatment of immune hemolytic anemia. The drugs most commonly used include the thiopurines (6-mercaptopurine, azathioprine, and thioguanine) and alkylating agents (cyclophosphamide and chlorambucil). Immunosuppressive agents act to decrease the production of antibody; therefore, it generally takes at least 2 weeks before any therapeutic result is observed. A reasonable clinical trial consists of 3 to 4 months of therapy. These drugs are rarely needed in childhood autoimmune hemolytic anemia.

Patients are selected for immunosuppressive therapy when a clinically unacceptable degree of hemolytic anemia persists following corticosteroid treatment and splenectomy. Alternatively, they may be corticosteroid resistant or intolerant and poor surgical candidates for splenectomy. Clinical benefit has been noted in about 50% of patients. Dosage of drug should be adjusted to maintain the leukocyte count >4000, the granulocyte count >2000, and the platelet count >50,000 to 100,000 per microliter. Although the side effects of these agents are not considered here, the use of alkylating agents, such as cyclophosphamide, may also have a long-term potential for increasing the incidence of malignant disease, particularly acute leukemia. Such side effects require that the clinical indications for an immunosuppressive trial be strong and that patient exposure to the drug be limited.

Immunosuppressive therapy has been effective in cold agglutinin disease. Alkylating agents (cyclophosphamide or chlorambucil) have been used and appear to help up to 60% of patients.

TRANSFUSION THERAPY. The majority of patients with autoimmune hemolytic anemia do not require transfusion therapy because the anemia has developed gradually and physiologic compensation has occurred. However, occasional patients experience acute and/or severe anemia and require transfusions for support until other treatment reduces the hemolysis. Transfusion therapy is complicated by the fact that the blood bank may be unable to find any "compatible" blood. This usually is due to the presence of an autoantibody directed at a core component of the Rh locus, which is present on the erythrocytes of essentially all potential donors, regardless of Rh subtype. The usual recommendation is for the blood bank to identify the most compatible units of blood of the patient's own major blood group and Rh type and to transfuse the most compatible units available. With this approach, it is unlikely that the donor blood will have dramatically shortened red blood cell survival.

In cold agglutinin disease it is important to prewarm all intravenous infusions, including whole blood, to 37° C, since a decrease in temperature locally in a vein can enhance the binding of the IgM antibody to red cells and accelerate the hemolytic process. Furthermore, agglutination of the transfused chilled or even room-temperature cells in small peripheral blood vessels can result in severe ischemic changes and vascular compromise.

MISCELLANEOUS THERAPY. Intravenous gamma globulin, which has been used extensively in the treatment of idiopathic thrombocytopenic purpura, may be effective in patients with autoimmune hemolytic anemia, probably by interfering with the clearance of the IgG-coated cells. Treatment regimens vary from 400 mg per kilogram per day for 5 days to 2 gm per kilogram, with additional treatment as needed to maintain the effect. Currently data are incomplete, but gamma globulin seems considerably less effective in autoimmune hemolytic anemia than in idiopathic thrombocytopenic purpura. Since autoimmune hemolytic anemia is usually very transient, prolonged treatment is rarely necessary.

Plasmapheresis or exchange transfusion has been used in patients with severe IgG-induced immune hemolytic anemia but has had limited success, possibly because more than half of the IgG is extravascular and the plasma contains only small amounts of the antibody (most of the antibody being on the red blood cell surface). However, plasmapheresis has been effective in IgM-induced hemolytic anemia (cold agglutinin disease), because IgM is a high-molecular-weight molecule that remains predominantly within the intravascular space, and at 37° C most of the IgM is in the plasma fraction. Obviously plasmapheresis is useful only as short-term therapy, but it may be life-saving in the rare patient with severe uncontrollable hemolysis.

Other measures that have been used effectively in some patients with IgG-induced immune hemolysis are vincristine, vinblastine infusions, and hormonal therapy. For example, there has been great interest in the use of the synthetic weak or impeded androgen danazol. Because of the limited side effects (limited masculinizing effects, mild weight gain), danazol may become an attractive additional agent for use in some patients with IgG-induced immune hemolytic anemia. The results with this agent in IgM-induced hemolysis suggest that it is ineffective.

IMMUNE PANCYTOPENIA

Evans' syndrome refers to autoimmune hemolytic anemia accompanied by thrombocytopenia. It occurs in a small percentage of adults and children with acute autoimmune hemolytic anemia; in even fewer patients it is also associated with marked neutropenia. Autoimmune hemolytic anemia in the presence of thrombocytopenia and/or neutropenia is more commonly associated with a chronic or relapsing course. Many patients have associated disorders, such as chronic lymphadenopathy or dysgammaglobulinemia. Some patients are hematologically normal between relapses, which may involve depressions in any of the three cell lines. Usually prednisone therapy is effective in controlling the acute episodes and is not needed between relapses. However, some patients have persistent immune cytopenia and require prolonged steroid treatment or more aggressive therapy. Splenectomy may result in improvement, but the risk of infection is probably higher in children and adults with pancytopenia than in those with autoimmune hemolytic anemia alone, and relapses are more common.

Antibodies directed against red cells, leukocytes, and platelets were demonstrated in some patients with immune pancytopenia. Suppression of hematopoietic cell maturation by T cells has been demonstrated in other patients.

PAROXYSMAL NOCTURNAL HEMOGLOBINURIA

This is an acquired disorder initially thought to consist of paroxysms of intravascular hemolysis reflected in nocturnal hemoglobinuria. It is now recognized that chronic intravascular hemolysis is the more frequent clinical presentation. Paroxysmal nocturnal hemoglobinuria (PNH) is a primary bone marrow disorder that not only affects the red cell lineage but also affects the platelet, leukocyte, and pluripotent hematopoietic stem cell lines. It is believed to be a disorder of stem cells of a clonal nature and can arise from or evolve into other dysplastic bone marrow diseases, including aplastic anemia, sideroblastic anemia, and myelofibrosis. Rarely, PNH may also evolve into acute leukemia.

A major clue to the etiology of this disease is provided by the recent findings that patients have a somatic mutation for a protein (phosphatidylinositol [PI] glycan class A) important in the pathway that controls the formation of the phosphatidylinositol anchor of several membrane proteins, including complement control proteins. PNH is often a disease of young adults, but it can occur at any age and in either sex. Chronic intravascular hemolysis of varying severity is the most common presentation. The severity of the hemolysis and the degree of hemoglobinuria depend on the number of circulating abnormal red cells and the degree of expression of the membrane abnormality among these cells. Two to three populations of abnormal red cells, termed PNH type I, II, and III cells, may be present simultaneously and differ in their lytic susceptibility. Patients commonly have iron deficiency anemia as well because of the large amount of iron lost in the urine during intravascular hemolysis with persistent hemoglobinuria and hemosiderinuria.

Other frequent clinical complaints include abdominal, back, and musculoskeletal pain. Such pain may be associated with intravascular hemolysis and hemoglobinuria, or it may be ischemic, secondary to the complication of thrombosis of major or minor vessels. Thromboses of the hepatic veins (Budd-Chiari syndrome) and of portal, splenic, mesenteric, cerebral, and other veins may occur and are common causes of death. Acute intestinal infarction requiring surgical resection has been reported, and thrombotic episodes are treated with anticoagulant therapy. Platelets and leukocytes also appear to have unusual susceptibility to lysis, and thrombocytopenia or granulocytopenia or both may be the initial manifestation(s) of the disease and are commonly present. The bone marrow is usually hyperplastic but may be hypocellular, consistent with aplastic anemia. The clinical course is variable and depends on the occurrence of the life-threatening complications of progressive bone marrow disease or venous thrombosis. The condition should be considered in everyone with aplastic anemia. In general, patients are not predisposed to the development of infection. At least half the patients live for many years.

Diagnosis rests on the clinical picture and the clinical laboratory measurement of a population of circulating cells with unusual sensitivity to complement-mediated lysis. This may be demonstrated in the sugar-water test; the patient's serum is mixed with 5% dextrose in water and incubated with the patient's cells. In PNH, hemolysis ensues. It has been shown that all individuals have antibody molecules that recognize their own cells under conditions of low ionic strength. These antibodies activate the classic complement pathway. Normal erythrocytes resist lysis, but PNH erythrocytes are susceptible to lytic attack. In Ham's test the patient's cells are incubated in acidified serum. Under these conditions the alternative complement pathway is triggered, and lysis of PNH, but not normal, cells follows. Ham's test result also is positive with some, but not all, normal sera from patients with a syndrome of congenital dyserythropoietic anemia (hereditary erythroblastic multinuclearity with a positive acid-hemolysis test).

PATHOGENESIS. Patients have unusual sensitivity of the erythrocytes, and often granulocytes and platelets, to the lytic action of complement. Activation of complement by either the classic or alternative pathway results in the deposition of many more C3 molecules on the PNH blood cell surface than on normal cells. The excessive binding of C3 to blood cells in PNH is due to more efficient alternative pathway C3-convertase activity on the cell surface. The surface of a PNH erythrocyte is a better acceptor for C3 than is the surface of a normal cell. This results in greater activation of the terminal complement components C5 to C9, causing more cell lysis than with normal cells. Furthermore, type II PNH cells are more effectively damaged by the C5b to C9 complex generated on the erythrocyte surface because the C5b to C9 lytic complex penetrates the PNH cell membrane more efficiently than the normal cell membrane. These patients lack the complement regulatory proteins present on the membranes of all normal blood cells, causing their increased susceptibility to complement lysis.

Many patients with PNH have several populations of abnormal erythrocytes. The complement lysis sensitivity test, which examines the susceptibility of antibody-sensitized erythrocytes to complement-mediated lysis, can be used to define the various PNH cell populations. PNH type II cells have a moderate increase in susceptibility to complement attack. These erythrocytes appear to have markedly decreased levels of DAF but do not have the membrane deficit that leads to sensitivity to attack by the C5b complex. PNH type III cells are highly susceptible to complement attack. They appear to lack phosphatidylinositol-linked control proteins completely. As noted, the platelets and leukocytes in PNH are also abnormally sensitive to complement-mediated lysis, and this abnormality is likely to have the same cause. This may relate to the pathogenesis of the venous thromboses.

THERAPY. Hemolysis is controlled in some patients with prednisone therapy. A dose of 15 to 40 mg every other day has been reported to decrease the rate of hemolysis in some adult patients, but a response is by no means certain. During acute episodes a higher dose given daily for a short period may help to control the hemolysis. In patients with anemia, androgens, including the anabolic steroid danazol, may be effective. A modest increase in platelet count was attained in several patients while they were receiving androgen therapy. Bone marrow transplantation has been successful in some patients, but in general the treatment of PNH has been unsatisfactory.

As discussed earlier, PNH patients may be iron deficient. Acutely, iron replacement may result in increased hemolysis because of the formation and release of a new cohort of sensitive red cells, and hemolysis on iron replacement has been noted. Oral replacement should be used if possible, but parenteral iron therapy may be necessary when iron losses are very large.

DRUG-INDUCED IMMUNE HEMOLYSIS

Drug-induced immune hemolytic anemia may be divided into three primary pathophysiologic entities. The clinical signs and symptoms are identical to those of autoimmune hemolytic anemia. Patients may have chronic hemolytic anemia or occasionally catastrophic intravascular hemolysis (quinidine type). The diagnosis is established primarily by history and *in vitro* assay.

METHYLDOPA TYPE. Methyldopa type and its derivatives (such as levodopa) produce a clinical syndrome virtually identical to IgG-induced immune hemolytic anemia. This is the most common type of drug-induced immune hemolytic anemia. The mechanisms of the IgG antibody formation are poorly understood. This drug stimulates production of IgG warm-reactive antibodies with anti-Rh specificity; it may also inhibit the splenic macrophage clearance of the IgG-coated cells. A primary mode of action of the drug in this disorder may be an alteration of immunoregulation, allowing B lymphocytes that produce Rh antibodies to escape from suppression.

It is of interest that 15% of patients receiving methyldopa therapy develop antinuclear antibodies. Many patients exposed to methyldopa, up to 25%, develop a positive result on Coombs' test

for IgG. Of diagnostic importance is that almost all patients have IgG antierythrocyte antibodies in their plasma as well. Most patients do not develop sufficient IgG coating for hemolysis; however, approximately 0.8% exposed to methyldopa do develop significant hemolysis and hemolytic anemia 3 to 37 months after the onset of therapy. Diagnosis can be made by examining the patient's red blood cells and plasma. *In vitro* it is not necessary to have the drug present for the patient's plasma to deposit IgG antibody on donor erythrocytes. The Coombs test result can remain positive in some patients up to 2 years after withdrawal of the drug. A similar syndrome has been reported with mefenamic acid.

Few patients receiving methyldopa therapy develop significant hemolysis. Probably the level of IgG per erythrocyte accounts for at least in part for this, because those patients with the highest amount of erythrocyte-associated IgG appear to have the most significant hemolysis. A second feature that may explain the high incidence of Coombs' positivity without hemolysis in this syndrome is a low-avidity antibody. The striking finding that almost all patients have antibody in their plasma, as well as on the erythrocytic surface, contrasts with the finding in most other patients with IgG-induced autoimmune hemolytic anemia, in which a positive result on indirect Coombs' test (plasma antibody) is less common. Second, the IgG antierythrocyte antibody appears to be easily elutable from the erythrocyte surface. These observations suggest that methyldopa-induced IgG antierythrocyte antibody may be an antibody having low avidity for its erythrocyte Rh antigen. This may partially explain its inefficiency in producing hemolysis.

HAPTEN TYPE. The hapten type of drug-induced immune hemolysis classically develops in patients exposed to high doses of penicillin. A portion of the penicillin molecule or its active metabolites combines with the erythrocyte surface, acting as a hapten. This induces an antibody response directed against the penicillin-coated erythrocyte membrane. This is usually an IgG response, and complement activation is common. The erythrocytes become coated with IgG and often with C3. This syndrome rarely develops unless patients have received 10 to 20 million units of penicillin a day. The diagnosis can be established by incubating the patient's serum with donor erythrocytes preincubated with penicillin. The deposition of IgG antibody occurs only in the presence of penicillin and can be detected with the Coombs test.

QUINIDINE TYPE. The quinidine type of autoimmune hemolytic anemia usually occurs with quinidine but has been reported with quinine, stibophen, chlorpromazine, and sulfonamides. Commonly called an innocent bystander reaction, it is thought to be due to an antibody directed against quinidine having a low affinity for the red cell surface. Presumably the drug binds weakly to the cell glycoprotein. The antibody recognizes the complex. This interaction results in activation of the classic complement pathway and deposition of C3 on the erythrocyte surface. It is believed that the immune complex transiently adheres to the red blood cell surface, activates complement, and then dissociates. With quinidine it has been shown that an IgM antiquinidine antibody appears to be involved. The diagnosis can be established *in vitro* by examining the complement deposition on donor erythrocytes by patient serum, which occurs only in the presence of the drug, for example, quinidine. The Coombs test is employed to detect the complement deposition on the erythrocyte surface.

Nonspecific coating of the erythrocyte surface has been observed with the antibiotic cephalothin, in which cephalothin becomes bound to the erythrocyte membrane and causes the red blood cell to be coated by many plasma proteins. The Coombs test is positive. Hemolytic anemia does not occur. Cephalothin, however, can cause hemolytic anemia by acting as a hapten by a mechanism similar to that of penicillin. In all these drug-induced processes, patients respond to withdrawal of the offending drug. If necessary, a brief course of corticosteroids can be given.

It should be noted that many autoimmune or drug-related hemolytic anemias are accompanied by thrombocytopenia and/or neutropenia and that this may result from similar pathophysiologic processes.

Indik ZK, Park JG, Hunter S, Schreiber AD: Structure/Function relationships of Fcγ receptors in phagocytosis. Semin Immunol 7:45, 1995.
LoBuglio AF, Cotran RS, et al.: Red cells coated with immunoglobulin G: Binding and sphering by mononuclear cells in man. Science 158:1582, 1967.

Schreiber AD, Frank MM: The role of antibody and complement in the immune clearance and destruction of erythrocytes; In vivo effects of IgG and IgM complement fixing sites. J Clin Invest 57:575, 1972.

Schreiber AD, Parsons J, et al.: Effect of corticosteroids on the human monocyte receptors for IgG and complement receptors. J Clin Invest 56:1189, 1975.

Schreiber AD, Rosse WF, Frank MM: Autoimmune hemolytic anemia. *In* Samter M, Austen KF, Clamans HN, Unanue ER, Frank MM (eds.): Immunological Diseases, 5th ed. Boston, Little, Brown and Co., 1995.

Silberstein LE, Berkman EM, et al.: Cold hemagglutinin disease associated with an IgG antibody. Ann Intern Med 106:238, 1987.

136 HEMOGLOBIN AND HEMOGLOBINOPATHIES

136.1 Structure, Function, and Synthesis of the Human Hemoglobins

Edward J. Benz, Jr.

The structure, genetics, physiology, and pathology of human hemoglobins are topics important for several reasons. First, hemoglobins and the erythrocytes in which they circulate are well characterized at the cellular, biochemical, and genetic levels. Second, hemoglobinopathies are extremely common disorders. Third, elucidation of the molecular basis of hemoglobinopathies has been the result of the most thorough and successful application to date of recombinant DNA technology. The derived principles have enhanced the understanding of many other clinical conditions. Finally, the mechanisms by which abnormal amounts or functions of hemoglobin derange other organ systems demonstrate uniquely well the pathophysiologic principles by which disordered function of a single gene can lead to multisystem disease.

THE STRUCTURE OF HEMOGLOBIN

Each human hemoglobin consists of a tetramer of globin polypeptide chains: a pair of "α-like" and a pair of "non-α" chains (Table 136–1). The major adult hemoglobin (Hb), Hb A, for example, has the following structure: $\alpha_2\beta_2$. Each chain enfolds a single heme moiety, consisting of a protoporphyrin IX ring complexed with a single ferrous ion atom (Fe^{2+}). The heme moiety resides within each polypeptide chain in a configuration optimal for reversible binding of oxygen. One heme moiety can bind a single oxygen molecule, so that every molecule of hemoglobin can transport up to four oxygen molecules. The α-like globin chains (α and ζ) are 141 amino acids long, whereas the non-α chains (ε, γ, δ, β) are 146 amino acids long.

TABLE 136–1. COMPOSITION OF NORMAL HUMAN HEMOGLOBINS

Name of Hemoglobin	Subunit Structure	Time of Expression
Hemoglobin Portland	$\zeta_2\gamma_2$	Embryonic life
Hemoglobin Gower I	$\zeta_2\epsilon_2$	Embryonic life
Hemoglobin Gower II	$\alpha_2\epsilon_2$	Embryonic life
Hemoglobin F	$\alpha_2 G\gamma_2$	Fetal life*
	$\alpha_2 A\gamma_2$	
Hemoglobin A₂	$\alpha_2\delta_2$	Adulthood (minor adult hemoglobin)
Hemoglobin A	$\alpha_2\beta_2$	Adulthood (major adult hemoglobin)

* Produced in small amounts in a limited subpopulation of cells (F cells) in adults.

Each globin has a largely helical *secondary structure*. About 80% of each polypeptide exists in the form of a helix. The non-α chains contain eight helical segments, designated A to H, separated from one another by short nonhelical stretches. The α-like chains contain seven helices; the D helix is absent. The helices fold into three-dimensional globular *tertiary structures* (Fig. 136–1).

Each globin chain folds in a manner that causes the exterior surface to be rich in polar (hydrophilic) amino acids that enhance solubility; the hydrophobic interior forms a cleft between the E and F helices into which the heme ring is deeply buried. This "heme pocket" excludes water from the vicinity of the heme, allowing numerous noncovalent hydrophobic "weak" bonds to form. These in turn stabilize the interaction between heme and globin chains. In particular, a histidine in the F helix forms a strong covalent bond with the iron atom; in the presence of oxygen, the iron also bonds with a histidine in the E helix. These histidine–iron-oxygen bonds are critical for reversible oxygenation.

The *quaternary structure* of normal adult Hb A is also complex and clinically important. The tetramer consists of two αβ dimers. The two α chains in the complete tetramer interact indirectly by means of numerous tight interactions ($\alpha_1\beta_1$ contacts) between the α and β chain within each dimer. The tetramer is held together by noncovalent bonds ($\alpha_1\beta_2$ contacts) between the α-like chain of one dimer and the non-α chain of the other dimer. These contact points undergo major conformational shifts during binding and release of oxygen.

Hemoglobin undergoes complex conformational changes within the heme groups, the globin chains, and the contact points between dimers during binding and release of oxygen. The hydrophilic surface amino acids, the hydrophobic amino acids lining the heme pocket, the F8 and E7 histidines, the $\alpha_1\beta_1$ and $\alpha_1\beta_2$ contact points, and the contacts between αβ dimers represent particularly critical regions within the globin polypeptide chains. Mutations in residues that influence these strategic sites tend to be the ones associated with significant changes in clinical phenotype.

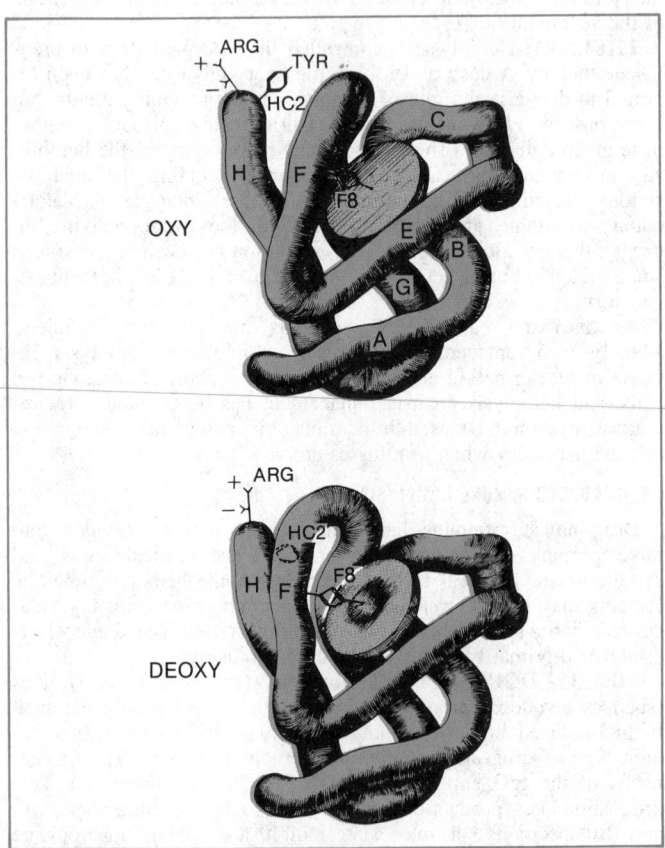

FIGURE 136–1. Structure of the oxy and deoxy states of a globin chain. Note that the amino acid sequence of globin dictates folding of eight helical segments (A–H) around the "heme" pocket in which the heme residue resides. In the deoxy state, the F8 histidine is bound to the heme group, but this bond is broken in the oxy state. Also shown is an allosteric effect of this change on the topology of the arginine and tyrosine residues in the H helix (not discussed in the text).

Hemoglobins bind avidly to oxygen at the Po_2 of the alveolar capillary bed, retain the bound oxygen as the red cells traverse the circulation, and unload the ligand to the tissues at the lower oxygen tensions of tissue capillary beds. Hemoglobins provide for the necessary amounts of oxygen acquisition and delivery over a relatively narrow range of oxygen tensions because of a property called cooperativity or heme-heme interaction. This property is inherent in the tetrameric arrangement of the heme and globin subunits.

Individual globin subunits acquire oxygen readily but cannot release it except at very low oxygen pressures incompatible with life. In contrast, complete hemoglobin tetramers exhibit an S-shaped oxygen dissociation curve (Fig. 136–2). At low oxygen tensions, the hemoglobin is deoxygenated. As the oxygen tension rises, oxygen binds to the tetramer; each heme group in the tetramer can bind one oxygen moiety. The binding of the first oxygen to deoxyhemoglobin requires considerable free energy (see below). Fully deoxygenated hemoglobin is thus said to be in the T (tense) state. As soon as one oxygen has been bound by the hemoglobin molecule, however, affinity for the binding of the remaining oxygen moieties increases, causing an increased slope in the binding curve. Oxyhemoglobin is said to be in the "R," or relaxed, state. In other words, oxygen binding begets more oxygen binding.

The oxygen affinity of normal hemoglobin is affected by many factors. Maintenance of the iron in the ferrous (Fe^{2+}) rather than the ferric (Fe^{3+}) form is crucial. Hemoglobin carrying ferric iron is called methemoglobin. The classic effect of pH on oxygen affinity, known as the Bohr effect, arises from the stabilizing action of protons on the deoxy confirmation. Deoxyhemoglobin binds protons more readily than oxyhemoglobin because it is a weaker acid. Protons tend to stabilize the salt bonds that make deoxyhemoglobin more resistant to oxygen binding. Hemoglobin thus has a lower oxygen affinity at lower pH.

Allosteric effectors are small molecules that bind hemoglobin and alter oxygen affinity. The best characterized of these is 2,3-diphosphoglycerate (2,3-DPG), generated and destroyed enzymatically as an intermediate of glycolysis in red cells. In its interaction with deoxyhemoglobin, 2,3-DPG stabilizes the deoxy state. High levels of 2,3-DPG or other conditions that increase the affinity of hemoglobin for 2,3-DPG tend to result in *lower* oxygen affinity.

The major adult hemoglobin, Hb A, has reasonably high affinity for 2,3-DPG. The oxygen affinity of Hb A is thus sensitive to the presence of 2,3-DPG. In contrast, Hb F, the major fetal hemoglobin, has very little ability to bind 2,3-DPG. Thus, Hb F and Hb A exhibit identical oxygen binding curves when analyzed as "stripped" hemoglobins in solution, but Hb F tends to have higher oxygen affinity than does Hb A *in vivo* because Hb F does not interact with 2,3-DPG very well. In brief, the structure-function features just outlined provide an exquisitely adaptive form of oxygen binding. Proper oxygen transport depends on the tetrameric structure of the proteins, the proper arrangement of charged and hydrophobic amino acids, and interaction with low molecular weight substances, such as protons or 2,3-DPG.

ONTOGENY OF HUMAN HEMOGLOBINS

Hemoglobin synthesis begins during the second month of gestation. Red cells first appear in yolk sac erythroblastic islands; these erythrocytes, called the primitive cell line, are large and nucleated. The predominant hemoglobins produced are Hb Portland ($\zeta_2\gamma_2$), Hb Gower I ($\zeta_2\epsilon_2$), and HB Gower II ($\alpha_2\epsilon_2$), but small amounts of Hb F and Hb A can be detected even at these early stages. At about 10 to 11 weeks of gestation, erythropoiesis moves to the liver and spleen. Coincidentally, the embryonic hemoglobins decline (Fig. 136–3), to be replaced by fetal hemoglobin (Hb F: $\alpha_2\gamma_2$), a mixture of two hemoglobins differing in the composition of the γ chain component. $^A\gamma$ chains have alanine and $^G\gamma$ chains have glycine at position 136. Red cell production shifts to bone marrow during the sixth to seventh month of gestation, but Hb F continues to predominate until late in the third trimester (about 38 weeks of gestation). At that time, a switch (Hb F $\rightarrow$ Hb A switch) to the predominant synthesis of Hb A (Hb A: $\alpha_2\beta_2$) occurs. The switch causes an abrupt increase in Hb A production accompanied by a reciprocal rapid decline in Hb F production (Fig. 136–3). Synthesis of a minor Hb A (Hb A_2: $\alpha_2\delta_2$) also commences at this time. Hb A (95 to 98%) predominates throughout the rest of life under normal conditions. Hb F is usually present in minute amounts of 0.5 to 1.5%, while Hb A_2 comprises 1.5 to 3.5% of total hemoglobin in normal subjects.

Fetal and adult erythrocytes differ from each other in several ways, in addition to hemoglobin content. Fetal red cells tend to be larger (macrocytes) and have shorter circulating lifespans. Fetal red cells express the i, rather than the I (adult), surface antigen; lack the β isozyme of carbonic anhydrase present in adult cells; and produce the $^G\gamma$ and $^A\gamma$ forms of Hb F at a $^G\gamma$:$^A\gamma$ ratio of 7:3, whereas the adult $^G\gamma$:$^A\gamma$ ratio is 2:3.

How hemoglobin switching is regulated is unclear. The potential of a given primitive erythroid stem cell (burst-forming unit–erythrocyte, or BFU-E) to express a particular globin gene is determined early in differentiation. By the time the stem cell has differentiated to the proerythroblast stage, when globin gene expression begins, the genetic program has been fixed and is not particularly susceptible to further modulation. The regulation of hemoglobin switching appears to result from a complex series of events. Changes in stem cell pools with varying potential for Hb F expression have profound effects, as does the chromatin configuration of the γ and β genes. Production of Hb F and Hb A is regulated largely at the stage of the primitive stem cell rather than the maturing erythroblast. Elevated Hb F levels in adults are thus often encountered in states of disordered erythropoiesis.

Small amounts of Hb F are produced during postnatal life but are confined to a small subpopulation of red cells called F cells. Both the numbers of F cells produced and the Hb F content of each F cell appear to be genetic polymorphisms. F cells are not truly fetal cells; they express other features of fetal cells incompletely. Changes in Hb F after birth result from altered stem cell dynamics. The most immature committed erythroid stem cell precursors (BFU-E) proceed through a series of proliferative and differentiating cell divisions before they actually form a pool of more fully differentiated progenitors (colony-forming units–erythrocyte, or CFU-E) ready to become proerythroblasts (Fig. 136–4). To a first approximation, the most immature or undifferentiated BFU-E's retain the highest potential to express Hb F in adult subjects. Under normal conditions of erythropoiesis, these cells continue to proliferate slowly and to differentiate into more mature BFU-E's before being "recruited" into the pool of maturing progenitors (CFU-E's and proerythroblasts). By this time, they have largely lost their ability to produce Hb F. Only a small number of "early" BFU-E's are actu-

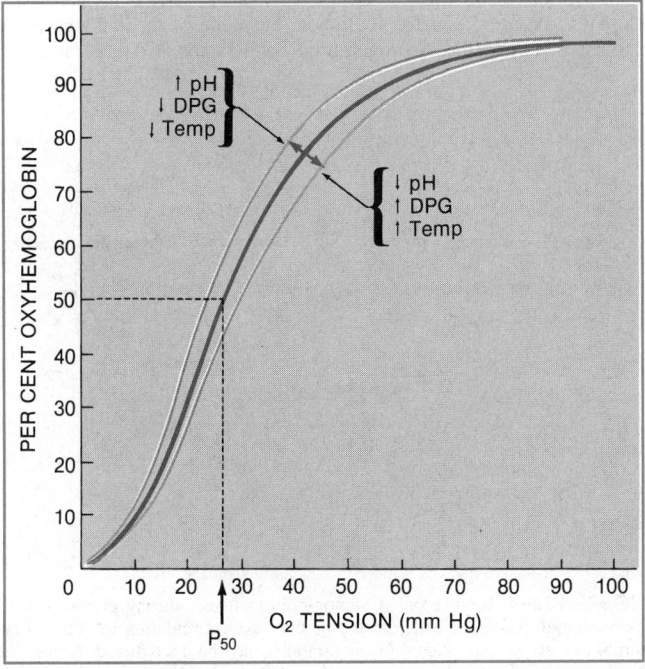

FIGURE 136–2. The oxygen binding curve for human hemoglobin A under physiologic conditions *(dark curve)*. The affinity will be shifted by changes in pH, diphosphoglycerate (DPG) concentration, and temperature as indicated. P_{50} represents the oxygen tension at half saturation. (From Bunn HF, Forget BG: Hemoglobin: Molecular, Genetic, and Clinical Aspects. Philadelphia, W B Saunders, 1986.)

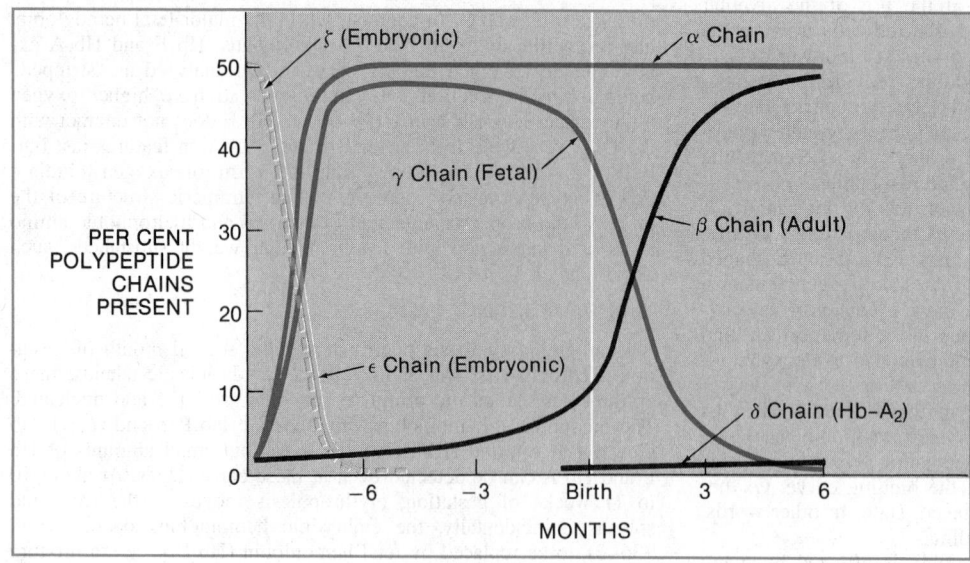

FIGURE 136–3. The relative abundance of various human globin chains during development. (From Bunn HF, Forget BG: Hemoglobin: Molecular, Genetic, and Clinical Aspects. Philadelphia, WB Saunders, 1986.)

ally recruited into the maturing pool, thus accounting for the small number of F cells produced under normal conditions.

Under conditions of marked erythroid stress or deranged erythropoiesis (e.g., as in chronic congenital hemolytic anemias, recovery from bone marrow transplantation or chemotherapy, or certain myelodysplastic syndromes), many BFU-E's are recruited into the pool of maturing progenitors before they have undergone their normal series of differentiating cell divisions. These cells still retain considerable potential to produce Hb F, resulting in higher than normal levels of F cells and Hb F. The molecular mechanisms mediating these complex events remain poorly understood.

GENETICS AND BIOSYNTHESIS OF HUMAN HEMOGLOBIN

The production of the various human hemoglobins is controlled by two tightly linked gene clusters (Fig. 136–5). The α-like globin genes are clustered on the short arm of chromosome 16, between band 13.2 and the telomere, and the non-α genes are found on chromosome 11 at band P15, near the terminus of the short arm. The α-like cluster consists of two α globin genes and a single copy of the ζ gene. The non-α gene cluster consists of a single ϵ gene, the $^G\gamma$ and $^A\gamma$ fetal globin genes, and the adult δ and β genes. The functional anatomy of globin genes is typical of most eukaryotic genes. Each globin gene contains three blocks of nucleotide sequences (exons) that ultimately code for mature messenger RNA (mRNA); these are arrayed in tandem with two intervening sequences (introns). The non-α globin genes contain a small (130 bases) and large (900 to 1100 bases) intervening sequence, whereas both of the intervening sequences in the α and ζ globin genes are small (100 to 200 bases).

Flanking sequences at each end of the globin genes are important for regulating their activity. Immediately upstream (30 to 70 base pairs [bp]) are typical eukaryotic promoter elements facilitating entry of mRNA polymerase (Fig. 136–6). Regions 100 to 500 bases upstream are important for proper developmental expression. Sequences in the 5' flanking region of the γ genes and the β genes influence, but do not exclusively control, the developmental regulation of these genes.

Important regulatory elements are also found in the 3' flanking regions. The regions in which these regulatory sequences exist exhibit the structural features of highly active genes in bulk chromatin, such as DNase hypersensitivity. The methylation state of the γ globin genes also changes during development. In fetal erythroblasts, the promoter regions are relatively devoid of methyl group modification of cytosines (hypomethylation). In general, this characteristic correlates with higher levels of gene activity. In adult erythroblasts, the genes are heavily methylated, a feature associated with inactivity. Whether this correlation is causally related to the level of γ gene expression in fetuses and adults is unclear.

In proerythroblasts, globin synthesis comprises at most 0.5 to 1% of total protein synthesis. During the subsequent maturation steps, globin gene expression increases enormously. For example, in reticulocytes generated during this 3- to 5-day period, globin mRNA and globin synthesis comprise 90 to 95% of total mRNA content and protein synthesis, respectively. To achieve this remarkable degree of activation, globin genes are highly adapted for expression in erythroid cells.

Tissue and developmental activation of individual globin genes depends in part upon short DNA sequences called enhancers. These are located in the 5' and 3' flanking sequences and possibly in the introns of the genes. An important enhancer activating the entire non-α gene complex (called the locus control region [LCR]) has been tentatively identified several thousand bases upstream of the ϵ gene. These regulatory DNA sequences are called *cis* acting elements. They achieve their biologic effects via their interaction with *trans* acting factors, i.e., nuclear DNA binding proteins that specifically bind to these sequences, thereby promoting or inhibiting transcription.

Several "transcription factors" have been found to bind the globin gene promoters and enhancers. Many of these protein factors appear to be nonspecific in that they can activate a number of genes in many tissues if they gain access to their binding sites. Several transcription factors (e.g., "GATA-1," NF-e2, EKLF-1) have been shown to be important for activation, but none of these is expressed exclusively in erythroid progenitors. Each factor also acts on an ar-

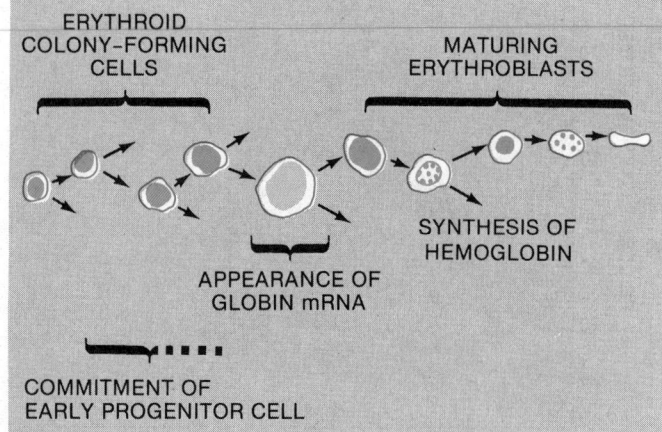

FIGURE 136–4. Regulation of hemoglobin synthesis during erythropoiesis. Two general classes of cells are the precursors of circulating red cells. Erythroblasts at various stages of maturation may be recognized within the bone marrow; these cells and circulating reticulocytes are engaged in hemoglobin synthesis. Erythroid stem cells, the progenitors of erythroblasts, are present within the bone marrow in very small numbers but may be detected by virtue of their ability to form colonies of erythroblasts in semisolid media *in vitro*. Current evidence suggests that commitment to expression of either the γ or the β globin genes occurs in erythroid stem cells prior to the initial appearance of globin messenger RNA (mRNA).

FIGURE 136–5. The arrangement of the clusters of human α-like and β-like globin genes on chromosomes 16 and 11 and the embryonic, fetal, and adult hemoglobins that result from the combinations of the various globin chains encoded by these genes. The ψ genes are similar to globin genes but do not code for protein. Distances along the chromosome are expressed in terms of 1000 nucleotide pairs (a kilobase).

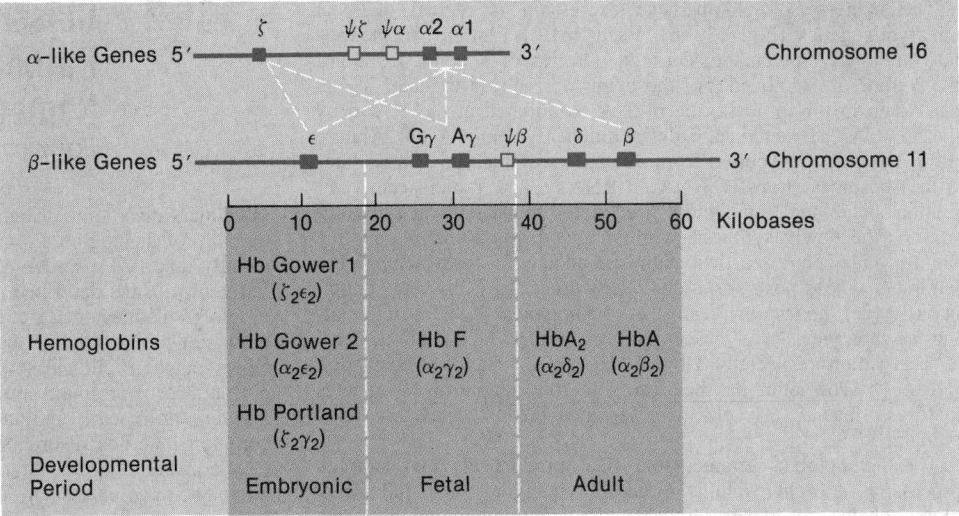

ray of genes. Specificity probably requires interactions among these factors and post-transcriptional modification of the apoproteins.

Each globin gene possesses structural features that are essential for the normal function of most genes (Fig. 136–6). These include the presence of a "CAP" site necessary to mark the beginning of transcription of the mRNA precursor; properly located initiation and termination codons to signal the beginning and end of translation of the mature mRNA; the presence in the appropriate locations, but nowhere else, of the donor (GT) and acceptor (AG) splicing sites that mark the points in the mRNA precursor at which the introns should be removed while the exons are ligated together; "consensus" sequences surrounding the donor and acceptor dinucleotides that form the functional splicing signal; and the presence of 5' and 3' untranslated sequences whose significance remains unclear. Like many other eukaryotic mRNA's, globin RNA's are polyadenylated. Their 3' untranslated sequences contain appropriate polyadenylation signals. As discussed in Ch. 136.4, these regions are mutated in various forms of thalassemia.

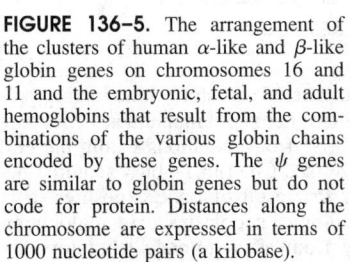

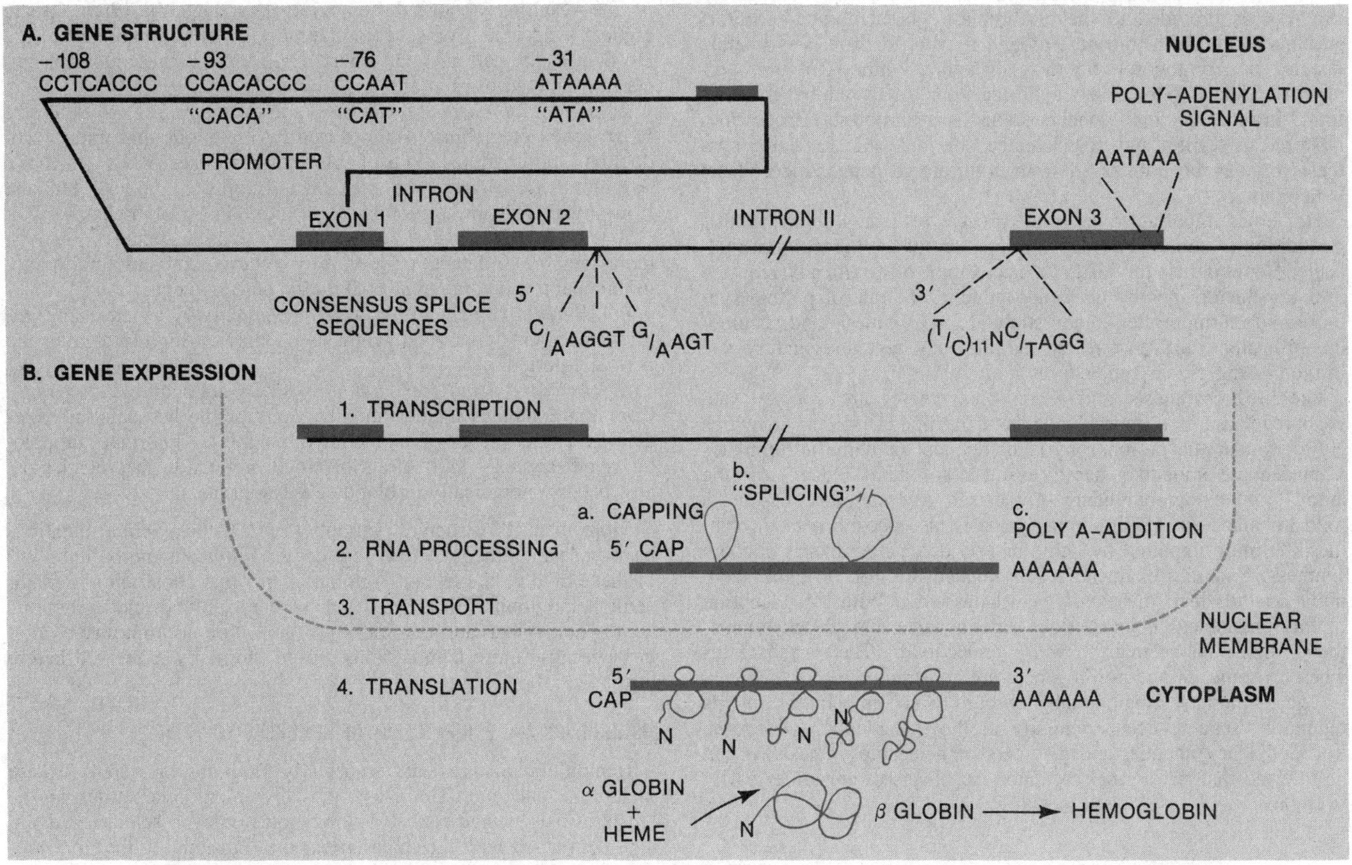

FIGURE 136–6. Structure and expression of the normal human β globin gene. The three exons encode for β globin; these coding sequences are interrupted by two introns or intervening sequences. Certain segments of the promoter region ("boxes") are conserved in many globin genes. The actual sequence of these boxes in the β globin gene promoter is shown. The splice sequences shown represent the consensus of those found at many exon-intron boundaries. Those actually found in the β globin gene resemble the consensus sequence but are not identical. The processes involved in gene expression include transcription of the gene, processing of the primary RNA transcript, transport of the mRNA from nucleus to cytoplasm, and translation of the mRNA into β globin. C = cytosine; T = thymine; A = adenine; G = guanine.

The pathway of globin gene expression is typical of most eukaryotic genes (Fig. 136–6). Each gene is initially transcribed into an mRNA precursor. Through a series of splicing reactions, the introns are removed and the exons are spliced together. At an early step in this process, the mRNA is modified at the 5' end by the "5' CAP" structure and the addition of a poly A tail. Mature mRNA is then transported from nucleus to cytoplasm. It associates with ribosomes, transfer RNA's (tRNA's), and proteinaceous initiation and elongation factors needed for translation on polyribosomes. The newly synthesized globin polypeptide chains combine rapidly with heme and then with one another to form hemoglobin tetramers. These posttranslational steps proceed rapidly and spontaneously (i.e., nonenzymatically). As hemoglobin "ages" in circulating erythrocytes, it is susceptible to further modification, such as acetylation (especially Hb F) and nonenzymatic glycosylation (Hb A_{1-C}). The latter has been used to follow control of diabetes mellitus, since A_{1-C} levels increase when the blood glucose level is high.

The hemoglobin tetramer, the final product of this complex process, is a highly soluble molecule. In contrast, the individual globin chains are rather insoluble. To prevent the globin chains from precipitating, it is essential that α and non-α globins be synthesized in approximately equal, or balanced, amounts. Each newly synthesized α or non-α globin chain will then have a "mate" with which to pair. The pathophysiology of severe thalassemia syndromes involves imbalance of globin chain synthesis and precipitation of the unpaired chains.

RELATIONSHIP OF IRON ACCUMULATION AND HEME SYNTHESIS TO HEMOGLOBIN PRODUCTION

The successful synthesis of hemoglobin requires coordination and regulation of the expression not only of the globin genes but also of the many genes responsible for heme and iron metabolism. The considerable amount of iron required for hemoglobin synthesis is provided to the erythroblast via membrane receptors specific for the iron transport protein transferrin. Iron is ultimately inserted into protoporphyrin to form heme. Synthesis of protoporphyrin IX occurs by a series of reactions catalyzed by enzymes found in relatively high concentrations in erythroblasts. Excess iron is stored as ferritin and may later become available for heme synthesis or may be transferred from erythroid to phagocytic cells in bone marrow.

Heme has important roles in the process of hemoglobin synthesis in addition to being an essential component of the hemoglobin molecule. Heme deficiency leads to inactivation of a critically required initiation factor, thereby markedly reducing the rate of protein synthesis. Furthermore, heme may stimulate the synthesis and accumulation of globin mRNA directly and thus may have a regulatory role in modulating globin gene expression.

Globin biosynthesis and heme biosynthesis are coupled and cross-regulated in a poorly understood fashion. Disorders in which either iron or the protoporphyrin component of heme accumulates in inadequate amounts generally result in secondary reduction in the amount of hemoglobin being synthesized. For complex reasons, a mild imbalance in globin chain synthesis also occurs: α chain synthesis is more impaired by heme or iron deficiency than is β chain synthesis. Anemias characterized by inadequate iron or heme accumulation thus tend to be *mildly* α-thalassemic. With the exception of this phenomenon, interactions among heme and globin biosynthetic pathways remain poorly understood. The mechanisms whereby heme, α, and non-α globin are constrained to be expressed in equal amounts remain totally obscure. Since imbalances in this regulatory scheme occur regularly in the thalassemic syndromes, iron deficiency anemia, and disorders of heme biosynthesis, it can be inferred that the normal regulatory mechanisms are rather easily overcome.

Benz EJ, Jr: Hemoglobin variants associated with hemolytic anemia, altered oxygen affinity and methemoglobinemia. *In* Hoffman R, Benz EJ, Jr, Cohen H (eds.): Hematology: Basic Principles and Practice. New York, Churchill Livingstone, 1994.

Steinberg MH, Benz EJ, Jr: Hemoglobin: structure and synthesis. *In* Hoffman R, Benz EJ Jr, Cohen H (eds.): Hematology: Basic Principles and Practice. New York, Churchill Livingstone, 1994.

136.2 Classification and Basic Pathophysiology of the Hemoglobinopathies

Edward J. Benz, Jr.

Clinical disorders attributed to altered structure, function, or production of hemoglobin are called hemoglobinopathies. They are usually inherited disorders that arise from mutations within the globin gene clusters described above (see Ch. 136.1), but "acquired hemoglobinopathies" can occur as the result of toxic exposures (e.g., methemoglobinemia) or hematologic neoplasms. Hemoglobinopathies range in clinical severity from asymptomatic laboratory abnormalities to profound multisystem syndromes that result in death *in utero* or in early childhood. Hemoglobinopathies are the most common inherited disorders in humans. In many geographic areas, they constitute significant public health problems because of their prevalence and chronicity. The hemoglobinopathies demonstrate extremely well the complex pathophysiologic consequences that can arise from deranged function of single genes. Hemoglobinopathies frequently manifest as clinical syndromes in childhood, but with improved supportive care, many of these patients now survive into adult life. The molecular basis, pathophysiology, epidemiology, and clinical features of the major hemoglobin disorders are therefore issues of increasing importance to internists.

CLASSIFICATION OF HEMOGLOBINOPATHIES

Hemoglobinopathies can be classified into five major groups:

1. *Structural hemoglobinopathies* are due to mutations altering the amino acid sequence and, thereby, the physiochemical properties of a particular globin polypeptide chain. The altered properties of the resulting abnormal hemoglobin produce the characteristic clinical syndrome. Some hemoglobins polymerize abnormally, e.g., Hb S in sickle cell anemia; others exhibit abnormal solubility; others have altered oxygen affinity.

2. The *thalassemia syndromes* are characterized by defective *biosynthesis* of globin chains, caused by mutations that impair production and/or translation of globin messenger RNA (mRNA). Symptoms result from the inadequate supply of hemoglobin and from imbalances in the production of individual globin chains.

3. *Thalassemic hemoglobin variants* exhibit features of both thalassemia, i.e., defective globin biosynthesis, and structural hemoglobinopathies, i.e., an abnormal amino acid sequence.

4. *Hereditary persistence of fetal hemoglobin,* as the name implies, represents continued synthesis of Hb F at high rates after the perinatal period.

5. *Acquired hemoglobinopathies* usually are acquired after birth. Common examples include modifications of the hemoglobin molecule by toxins (acquired methemoglobinemia). Abnormal hemoglobin synthesis, e.g., high levels of Hb F production in preleukemia, also occurs sporadically in blood cell dyscrasias.

More than 400 structural variants and 100 thalassemia mutations have been identified. Only a few cause significant morbidity. Most of these involve the α and β globin chains that constitute the major adult hemoglobin, Hb A ($\alpha_2\beta_2$). Disorders of fetal and embryonic hemoglobins that are not lethal *in utero* are asymptomatic after birth because these hemoglobins are not normally expressed before birth.

DISTRIBUTION AND EPIDEMIOLOGY OF HEMOGLOBINOPATHIES

Hemoglobinopathies are especially common in areas where malaria is endemic. The clustering of hemoglobinopathies in the "malaria belt" suggests that heterozygotes enjoy a selective advantage if infected with the malaria parasite. Presumably their erythrocytes provide a less hospitable environment during the obligate intraerythrocytic stages of the parasitic life cycle. For example, malarial parasites grow poorly in sickle cell trait erythrocytes. This selective advantage fixes the mutant genes in the population. One should thus be especially alert to the presence of hemoglobinopathies in Asians, blacks, and ethnic groups derived from the Mediterranean basin. Hemoglobinopathies do occur in every ethnic group, however.

INHERITANCE OF HEMOGLOBINOPATHIES

Hemoglobinopathies are "autosomal co-dominant" traits; thus, compound heterozygotes, who inherit a different abnormal globin allele from each parent, exhibit composite features of each abnormal allele. For example, patients inheriting a β-thalassemia gene from one parent and a β^s (sickle cell) allele from the other have sickle cell/β-thalassemia, which exhibits features of both β-thalassemia and sickle cell anemia. Each hemoglobinopathy is transmitted in families as a tightly linked allele of a globin gene. A thorough family history is thus an important part of the general approach to hemoglobinopathies, regardless of type.

Globin gene mutations behave like "co-dominant" traits in that some evidence of the abnormality, even if it be only laboratory evidence, can be detected in the heterozygote. The dominance of individual mutations with respect to clinical symptoms varies in different types of hemoglobinopathies. For example, patients with thalassemia trait and sickle cell trait are, for the most part, asymptomatic. In each case, the amount of normal hemoglobin (Hb) A generated by the normal β globin allele, coupled with the lessened impact of abnormal globin production from the affected allele, protects patients from the complications of these diseases under normal conditions. Certain provocative stresses, such as very high altitude (low partial pressure of oxygen [for the patient with sickle cell trait]) or pregnancy (for the patient with thalassemia trait), can occasionally produce symptoms characteristic of these disorders, i.e., sickling or anemia. Some hemoglobinopathies behave like dominant traits, especially the structural mutations, causing reduced solubility or profoundly altered oxygen affinity of the hemoglobin. In these cases, the absolute amount of the abnormal hemoglobin arising from the single affected allele is often sufficient to alter the behavior of the red cell.

In some hemoglobinopathies, the homozygous state is clinically benign, but compound heterozygous states are associated with severe disease. For example, homozygous hemoglobin C disease is only minimally symptomatic, but inheritance of β^s on one chromosome and β^c on the other (HbSC disease) behaves like a moderately severe form of sickle cell anemia, exhibiting certain distinctive features. Similarly, homozygous Hb E disease is very mild, but co-inheritance of Hb E and β-thalassemia produces a severe β-thalassemia–like syndrome. These considerations illustrate the complexity of hemoglobin genetics. The ultimate clinical phenotype is determined not only by the type of change resulting from the globin gene mutation but also by a composite effect of the altered properties of the abnormal chain, the amount produced (or the severity of the production deficit), and the interaction between the product of one abnormal allele and that of the normal allele or of a different type of abnormal allele present on the complementary chromosome. These principles, important for understanding individual syndromes, also offer the best existing examples of gene interactions in determining the ultimate clinical phenotype.

Spontaneous mutations occur at a measurable frequency within the globin gene cluster, producing symptomatic or asymptomatic hemoglobinopathies in patients with negative family histories. The unstable (insoluble) hemoglobin disorders seem especially prone to arise by de novo spontaneous mutation. Thus, while family history is an extremely important part of the evaluation in patients with potential hemoglobinopathies, a negative family history does not necessarily rule out the diagnosis.

BASIC PRINCIPLES OF PATHOPHYSIOLOGY

The α globin chains are duplicated; the β gene is a single-copy locus. In the diploid erythroblast, there are thus four copies of the α and only two copies of the β gene. Mutation of a single α globin gene thus affects only about 25% of the hemoglobin produced, while β mutations affect about 50%. Consequently, β chain mutations tend to be encountered more frequently than α variants as causes of symptomatic hemoglobinopathies.

Globin genes are expressed exclusively in developing erythroid cells. During the terminal stages of erythroid maturation, one might expect symptoms to be confined to the red cell compartment, e.g., anemia. The clinical manifestations of hemoglobinopathies are protean, however. In most cases, it has been possible to trace these

changes to the impact of specific mutations on particular properties of the hemoglobin molecule. Homeostasis of hemoglobin and the homeostasis of the red cells in which it circulates are closely linked. Deranged production or function of globin frequently deranges erythropoiesis, and the converse is also often true. Hemoglobin accumulates to extremely high concentrations within red cells, where it must remain soluble and chemically reduced. Individual globin chains are insoluble and have extraordinarily high oxygen affinities. If globin or hemoglobin molecules precipitate within red cells, the resulting inclusions cause premature destruction of the red cells (hemolytic anemia) with all of its attendant stigmata. Lesions affecting oxygen affinity perturb the erythropoietin circuit by which red cell production is regulated. The signal for release of erythropoietin is based upon *oxygen delivery* to cells within the kidney rather than to the *red cell mass*. Inappropriate secretion of erythropoietin as well as premature destruction of red cells can thus be caused by hemoglobinopathies. These consequences of deranged hemoglobin structures, amount, or structure-function relationships, rather than mere reduction in the amount or normal function of hemoglobin, tend to dominate the pathophysiology of the disorders.

The behavior of particular hemoglobinopathies is also influenced by the ontogeny of hemoglobin synthesis. Alpha chain hemoglobinopathies cause abnormalities of Hb A, Hb A_2, and Hb F, because the α chain is present in all of these hemoglobins. The α globin hemoglobinopathies are symptomatic both *in utero* and after birth because normal function of the α globin gene is required during gestation as well as adult life. In contrast, β globin gene expression is not abundant until after birth. Infants with β globin hemoglobinopathies thus tend to be asymptomatic until 3 to 9 months of age, the time at which Hb F is largely replaced by Hb A.

136.3 Hemoglobinopathies with Altered Solubility or Oxygen Affinity
Edward J. Benz, Jr.

Structural hemoglobinopathies are due to mutations that alter the amino acid sequence and thereby the functional properties of the hemoglobin molecule: (1) mutations causing abnormal polymerization, of which hemoglobin (Hb) S (sickle cell hemoglobin) is the most important example; (2) mutations causing altered solubility of hemoglobin within circulating erythrocytes; (3) mutations causing altered affinity of the hemoglobin molecule for oxygen; and (4) methemoglobinemia, which represents a subclass of hemoglobins with altered oxygen affinity. Sickle cell syndromes are so common, serious, and protean in their manifestations that they merit extended separate coverage (see Ch. 136.5). In this chapter, we consider hemoglobins exhibiting abnormal solubility and altered oxygen affinity. Methemoglobins are considered a separate category within this chapter, even though they could be considered a subclass of hemoglobins with altered oxygen affinity. The altered interaction with oxygen is far more severe in methemoglobin than in most other types of oxygen affinity mutations; moreover, methemoglobin is important as one of the few acquired hemoglobinopathies (carbon monoxyhemoglobin being another) that can develop by exposure to selected toxins. Finally, methemoglobins can arise by inherited mechanisms in other genes as well as globin genes. Therefore these syndromes receive special consideration.

HEMOGLOBINS EXHIBITING REDUCED SOLUBILITY—UNSTABLE HEMOGLOBINS

PATHOGENESIS AND CLINICAL MANIFESTATIONS. "Unstable" hemoglobins arise from amino acid substitutions that render the hemoglobin less soluble or more susceptible to oxidation of its amino acid residues (Fig. 136–7). Both α and β globin variants can cause this condition; about 100 such variants have been described. The mutations that produce insoluble hemoglobins tend

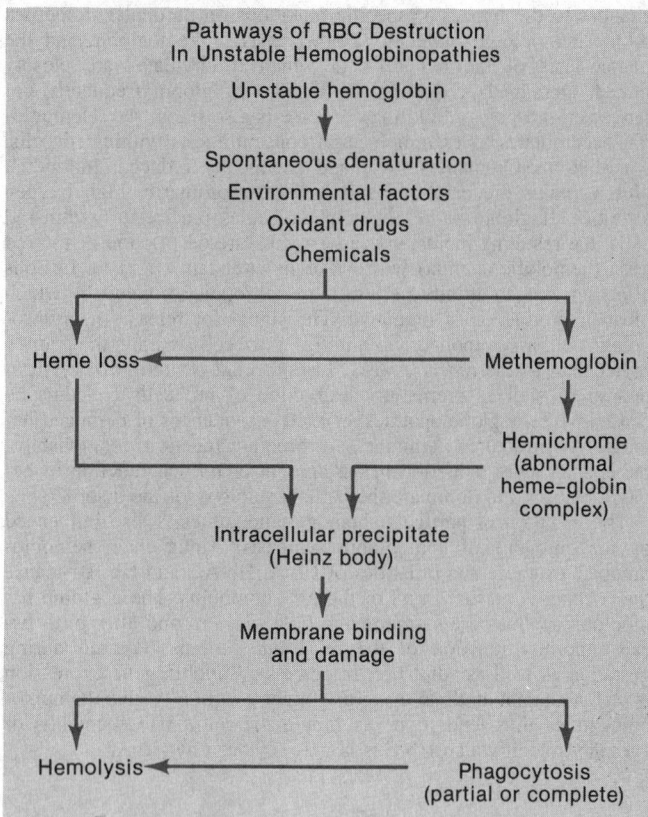

**Pathways of RBC Destruction
In Unstable Hemoglobinopathies**

Unstable hemoglobin

↓

Spontaneous denaturation
Environmental factors
Oxidant drugs
Chemicals

Heme loss ← Methemoglobin

Hemichrome
(abnormal
heme–globin
complex)

Intracellular precipitate
(Heinz body)

↓

Membrane binding
and damage

Hemolysis ← Phagocytosis
(partial or complete)

FIGURE 136–7. The presumed mechanisms by which denaturation of hemoglobin leads to erythrocyte destruction are outlined. The rate of travel through the various pathways probably differs for different hemoglobin variants and for a variety of stresses to which the protein is subjected.

to disrupt hydrogen bonding and hydrophobic interactions holding the tetramer together. Some alter the helical segments (Hb Geneva [$\beta^{28leu \rightarrow pro}$]); others disrupt contact points between the α- and β-subunits (Hb Philadelphia [$\beta^{35Tyr \rightarrow Pho}$]), while others disrupt interactions of the hydrophobic pockets of the globin subunits for heme (e.g., Hb Köln [$\beta^{98Val \rightarrow Met}$]). The most common biochemical basis for reduced solubility is reduced strength of the binding of heme to globin. An actual loss of heme groups can occur, e.g., in Hb Gun Hill, in which five amino acids, including the F8 histidine, are deleted.

Precipitation of hemoglobin in circulating red cells produces intracellular inclusions called Heinz bodies (Color Plate 6C, left). The spleen attempts to remove these inclusions, leading to formation of pitted, rigid cells that eventually become sequestered, thus producing hemolytic anemia. In severely affected patients, the anemia may require chronic transfusion therapy. Splenectomy is often effective for relief of anemia. Leg ulcers and premature gallbladder disease occur with high frequency.

Unstable hemoglobins are quite rare in comparison to sickle cell anemia and the thalassemias. They occur sporadically in many ethnic groups, often by spontaneous mutation. The heterozygous state is usually symptomatic ("dominant") because significant numbers of Heinz bodies form even when the unstable variant accounts for only half of the total hemoglobin. Most of the symptomatic unstable hemoglobins are β globin variants, since sporadic mutations affecting the α globin loci would usually involve only one of the four alleles, thus generating only 20 to 30% abnormal hemoglobin. The propensity of unstable hemoglobins to precipitate is exaggerated by "oxidative" stress, such as infection or exposure to oxidizing drugs (e.g., quinine). Indeed, some of these variants are symptomatic only when oxidant stress occurs.

DIAGNOSIS. The presence of an unstable hemoglobin should be suspected in individuals with chronic hemolytic anemia, unexplained jaundice, premature biliary tract disease (caused by bilirubin gallstones generated by excess red cell turnover), unexplained

reticulocytosis, or bouts of intermittent hemolysis that can be related to exposure to oxidant drugs or infections. Other suggestive symptoms include dark urine, transient jaundice, or leg ulcers. These findings are stigmata of chronic or intermittent hemolysis.

Laboratory diagnosis is based upon identification of a mutant hemoglobin that precipitates more easily than normal hemoglobin. The *in vivo* evidence for precipitated hemoglobin is the Heinz body, which is an intraerythrocytic inclusion body detectable by staining of a peripheral blood film with a supravital dye, usually brilliant cresyl blue or new methylene blue. Since the spleen can remove Heinz bodies efficiently, especially if hemolysis is not particularly acute or brisk, Heinz bodies may not be demonstrable at all times. Therefore, two provocative tests have been developed to unmask the tendency of unstable hemoglobins to precipitate: the heat instability test (heating of a hemoglobin solution to 50° C) or the isopropanol instability test (insolubility in 17% isopropanol).

Hemoglobin electrophoresis should be performed but not utilized as a sole diagnostic criterion for ruling in or ruling out a hemoglobinopathy. Many amino acid substitutions that can have a profound effect upon the heme pocket or chain-chain contacts do not change the overall charge on the hemoglobin molecule. Therefore these variants will not migrate to a new position on an electrophoresis gel. Demonstration of an abnormal band would clearly add strong evidence in support of the diagnosis. Failure to demonstrate an abnormal band, however, should never be regarded as strong evidence against the presence of a mutant hemoglobin, especially if the clinical picture or family history otherwise supports the diagnosis. A variety of more sophisticated analyses of hemoglobin can be obtained from reference laboratories.

In the case of unstable hemoglobin variants, the difficulties are further compounded by the selective precipitation of the unstable variant into Heinz bodies. Since most patients are heterozygotes, this phenomenon greatly reduces the apparent percentage of the variant in circulating blood. Thus, even a variant possessing altered electrophoretic mobility may be very difficult to detect.

The differential diagnosis of unstable hemoglobin variants is usually straightforward if the general category of diagnosis is suspected. Glucose-6-phosphate dehydrogenase (G6PD) deficiency can also manifest with bouts of intermittent or chronic hemolysis exacerbated by oxidant drugs or infection. This diagnosis should be considered, as should other causes of chronic or intermittent hemolytic anemia, such as red cell membrane disorders (e.g., hereditary spherocytosis) or immune hemolytic anemias. Spherocytes are relatively rare in unstable hemoglobin disorders; this is sometimes a useful discriminator.

MANAGEMENT. The severity of the clinical complications of unstable hemoglobins varies enormously. Many patients can be managed adequately by expectant monitoring and avoidance of drugs provoking hemolysis. Occasional patients may require transfusions during bouts of severe acute hemolytic anemia. Individuals who suffer significant morbidity because of chronic anemia or repeated episodes of severe hemolysis should be considered candidates for splenectomy, especially if hypersplenism has developed. Finally, the tendency of infection to exacerbate hemolysis should prompt one to monitor these patients closely during those episodes.

HEMOGLOBINS WITH INCREASED OXYGEN AFFINITY

Hemoglobin functions as a biologically useful oxygen transport pigment because of the sigmoidal shape of its oxygen affinity curve. In the transition from the fully deoxygenated (tense, or T) to the fully oxygenated (relaxed, or R) state, the initial oxygenation steps occur with difficulty. In fact, the act of binding the first oxygen molecule increases the affinity of the molecule for subsequent oxygen-binding events, thus creating the sigmoidal shape of the curve. The necessary intramolecular reorganization occurs only when the proper arrangement of hydrogen bonds, hydrophobic interactions, and salt bridges is broken and formed in the proper sequence during R-T transitions.

Mutant hemoglobins exhibiting altered oxygen affinity usually arise when amino acid substitutions occur at the interface between α and β chains or in regions affecting the hydrogen bonds, hydrophobic interactions, or salt bridges. A second major class of mutations comprises those affecting interaction with 2,3-diphosphoglycerate (2,3-DPG) (Ch. 136.1), which alters oxygen affinity when bound to hemoglobin.

PATHOGENESIS AND CLINICAL MANIFESTATIONS.

"High-affinity" hemoglobins exhibit higher avidity for oxygen, causing the oxygen dissociation curve to "shift to the left"; an example is Hb Zurich ($\beta^{63his} \rightarrow {arg}$). These hemoglobins bind oxygen more readily but are less able to deliver the oxygen to tissues at normal capillary oxygen pressures. Since the PO_2 in the lung (PO_2 = 90 to 100 mm Hg) is normally well above that needed to saturate hemoglobin fully with oxygen (60 mm Hg), these variant hemoglobins cannot acquire any additional oxygen in the lung despite their higher affinity. At capillary PO_2 (35 to 45 mm Hg), however, high-affinity hemoglobins deliver less oxygen. The resultant mild tissue hypoxia stimulates erythropoietin release and leads to inappropriately high red cell production and polycythemia (see Ch. 141). In extreme cases, hematocrits of 60 to 70% can be encountered.

High-affinity variants arise from several forms of mutations. Some alter interactions within the heme pocket, others disrupt the Bohr effect or the salt-bond site, and others impair the interaction of Hb A with 2,3-DPG. 2,3-DPG binding lowers the oxygen affinity of Hb A. Reduced 2,3-DPG binding results in an effective increase in oxygen affinity. As a good example of a high-affinity hemoglobin, a single amino acid substitution in Hb Kempsey blocks the hydrogen bond formation with the tyrosine at α^{42} needed to stabilize the T (deoxy) state. This and numerous other examples that have been analyzed at the molecular level have greatly aided our understanding of the molecular basis for reversible oxygen binding.

DIAGNOSIS. High-affinity hemoglobins should be considered in patients with unexplained erythrocytosis, especially if there is a positive family history. Oxygen affinity is usually measured as the P_{50}, the partial pressure of oxygen at which a hemoglobin preparation (either in the form of a red cell suspension or in the form of a hemoglobin solution) is 50% saturated with oxygen (Fig. 136–8). The hemoglobin preparation is exposed to increasing oxygen pressures in the laboratory, and the relative percentages of oxyhemoglobin and deoxyhemoglobin are determined optically, forming a curve from which the 50% saturation point is determined. A "shift to the left" means that the hemoglobin reaches 50% saturation at a *lower* partial pressure of oxygen. *High-affinity variants are thus associated with a lower than normal P_{50}* value. Hemoglobin electrophoresis should be performed but may not be revealing.

The most common cause of a low P_{50} value is carbon monoxide poisoning. Hemoglobin–carbon monoxide has an extremely "left-shifted" oxygen affinity curve, which reflects stabilization of hemoglobin in the R state without benefit of oxygen binding. The clinical impact is the same as that of a very high oxygen affinity hemoglobin. The most common cause of hemoglobin–carbon monoxide is cigarette smoking, although chronic carbon monoxide exposure in individuals such as caisson workers or tunnel toll booth collectors is encountered sporadically.

P_{50} curves should be determined with both whole-blood suspensions and isolated hemoglobin solutions. In the latter circumstance, the contribution of 2,3-DPG is eliminated. This can eliminate the potential confounding artifact and reveal those variants arising from abnormal interaction with this ligand.

MANAGEMENT. Most patients with high-affinity hemoglobins have mild erythrocytosis not requiring treatment. Very rarely, the hematocrit and, therefore, the blood viscosity are sufficiently elevated to warrant treatment by phlebotomy. Smoking cessation or a change in working environment will correct the effects of carbon monoxide.

HEMOGLOBINS WITH DECREASED OXYGEN AFFINITY

PATHOGENESIS AND CLINICAL MANIFESTATIONS.

Low-affinity variants, such as Hb Kansas ($\beta^{102Asn} \rightarrow {Thr}$), represent the pathophysiologic "mirror image" of the high-affinity hemoglobins. In Hb Kansas, the threonine position β^{102} cannot form a hydrogen bond with aspartic acid at position α^{94}, which normally stabilizes the R (oxy) state. Thus, Hb Kansas has less tendency to bind oxygen and exhibits a "right-shifted" P_{50} value (Fig. 136–8).

In all but the most severe examples of low-affinity variants, oxygen affinity remains high enough that the hemoglobin becomes fully saturated in the highly oxygen-abundant environment of the pulmonary capillary. At the PO_2 of the capillary bed in most tissues, however, these hemoglobins "dump" excessive amounts of oxygen and become more desaturated than normal hemoglobin. There are two pathophysiologic consequences of this higher than normal level of oxygen delivery. First, since tissue oxygen delivery is so efficient, the erythropoietin "thermostat" can be set lower, resulting in normal oxygen transport at lower than normal hematocrits. This situation produces a state of pseudoanemia. In other words, the hematocrit appears to be abnormally low, even though homeostasis of oxygen transport and the patient are completely normal. Second, the amount of desaturated hemoglobin circulating in capillaries can be greater than 5 grams per deciliter, producing clinically apparent cyanosis. In contrast to most other causes of cyanosis, this usually ominous finding is entirely benign in these individuals.

DIAGNOSIS. A low-affinity variant should be suspected in patients with unexplained anemia or cyanosis who, by all other criteria, appear to be entirely well, especially if there is a positive family history. Testing for the abnormal variant follows the same reasoning as that just described for high-affinity variants, except that the P_{50} value will be *higher* than normal.

MANAGEMENT. Patients with low-affinity hemoglobins are usually asymptomatic. No treatment is required. It is important to document that a low-affinity hemoglobin is the cause of apparent anemia and that this finding is only a physiologic response to the altered oxygen affinity. Cyanosis in some individuals can pose a cosmetic problem, but correction with transfusions is rarely, if ever, justified.

METHEMOGLOBINEMIAS

Methemoglobin is generated by oxidation of the iron moieties in hemoglobin from the ferrous (Fe^{2+}) to the ferric (Fe^{3+}) state. Oxygen transport by hemoglobin requires that iron be present in the ferrous state in deoxyhemoglobin. Yet oxygenation of hemoglobin causes partial transfer of an electron from the iron to the bound oxygen; iron in this state thus resembles ferric iron. The oxygen resembles superoxide (O_2^-). Deoxygenation returns the electron to the iron, with release of oxygen. When this electron return fails to occur, methemoglobin forms. Normally methemoglobin constitutes 3% or less of the total hemoglobin content. Indeed, reduction of methemoglobin levels to less than 1% is routinely accomplished *in vivo* by activity of an enzyme called methemoglobin reductase (nicotinamide adenine dinucleotide [NADH]-dehydratase, NADH-diaphorase, erythrocyte cytochrome b_5). This enzyme reduces hemoglobin iron by transfer of an electron from NADH to oxidize cytochrome b_5; cytochrome b_5 then converts ferric to ferrous iron by direct interaction with hemoglobin. The generation of NADH depends on the glycolytic pathway.

A second reducing enzyme, nicotinamide-adenine dinucleotide phosphate (NADPH)–dependent methemoglobin reductase, does not normally function in erythrocytes because there is no electron carrier available to interact with NADPH as the "go-between" with hemoglobin iron. Artificial electron carriers, such as methylene blue, can provide this missing link. As discussed later, methylene blue is therefore an important agent for the treatment of methemoglobinemia. Reduced glutathione and ascorbic acid can also reduce methemoglobin directly; however, these nonenzymatic reactions are considerably slower than the reductase pathways.

PATHOGENESIS AND CLINICAL MANIFESTATIONS. Methemoglobinemias of clinical import arise by one of three distinct mechanisms: (1) globin chain mutations that result in increased formation of methemoglobin; (2) deficiencies in the reductase pathways described above; and (3) "toxic" methemoglobinemia in which even normal red cells endowed with normal hemoglobin and normal methemoglobin reductase can be "overwhelmed" by exposure to substances that oxidize hemoglobin iron (Table 136–2).

Abnormal hemoglobins causing methemoglobinemia (M hemoglobins) tend to arise from mutations that alter the heme pocket in a fashion that favors stabilization of the iron in the ferric state. In the majority of these, a histidine is replaced by a tyrosine; the hydroxyl group of the tyrosine forms a complex that stabilizes the iron in the ferric state in a fashion resistant to reduction by the methemoglobin reductase system. A few of the variants tend to lose heme and thus also exhibit features of a mildly unstable hemoglobin disorder.

Methemoglobin is brownish to blue and does not become red upon exposure to oxygen. These individuals thus appear to be cyanotic. In contrast to truly cyanotic individuals, however, arterial PO_2 values are normal. These individuals are otherwise asymptomatic,

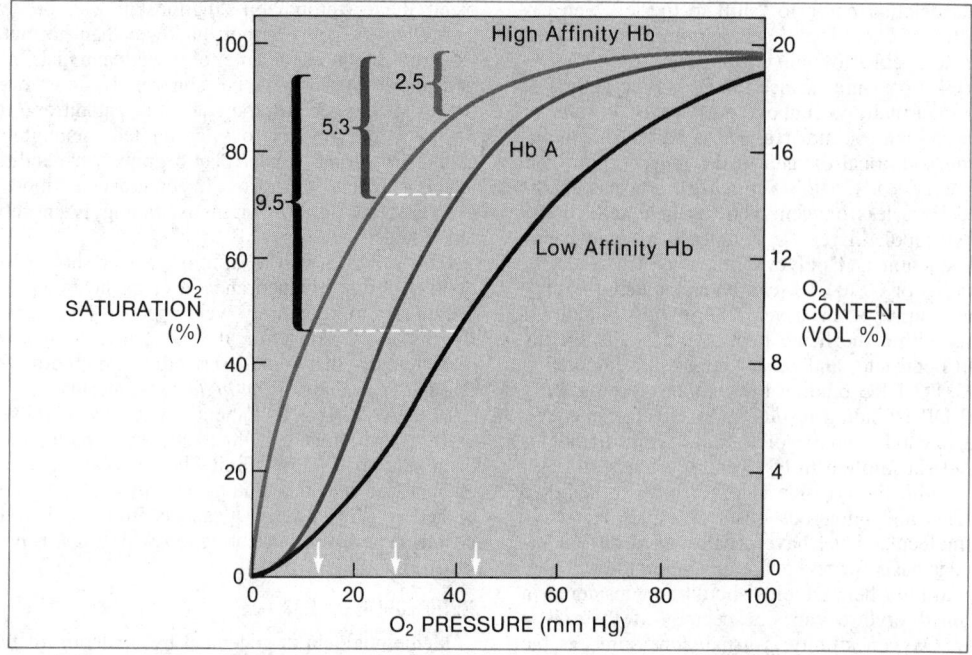

FIGURE 136–8. Hemoglobin-oxygen dissociation curves are illustrated for normal hemoglobin (Hb A) and for model abnormal hemoglobins with high and low oxygen affinities. On the abscissa the partial pressure of oxygen is indicated in millimeters of mercury. On the left ordinate the saturation of hemoglobin with oxygen is indicated as a percentage; on the right ordinate the oxygen content of the hemoglobin is expressed as volumes percent. As the partial pressure of oxygen drops from 100 (arterial) to 40 (tissues), hemoglobin desaturates, giving up a portion of its bound oxygen; the numbers on the brackets indicate the amount of oxygen unloaded by the three hemoglobin types, expressed in volumes percent. Note that the high-affinity hemoglobin delivers less than half the oxygen that Hb A gives to the tissues, resulting in tissue anoxia, increased erythropoietin secretion, and erythrocytosis. Conversely, the low-affinity hemoglobin is even more efficient than Hb A in supplying the tissues with oxygen, resulting in diminished erythropoietin production and anemia.

because methemoglobin is rarely above 30 to 50%, the levels at which symptoms become apparent.

Hereditary methemoglobinemia resulting from methemoglobin reductase deficiency is rare; 100 to 200 cases have been described. Numerous recessive mutations cause a variety of defects in the resulting variant enzymes, including catalytic activity, electrophoretic mobility, and structural stability. Hispanics, Eskimos, and Native Americans in particular are frequently affected. In some individuals, neurologic defects are also present, suggesting that the mutation affects isoforms of the enzyme common to both erythrocytes and other tissues, including brain. Other individuals exhibit only the methemoglobin abnormality.

Like patients with M hemoglobins, patients with methemoglobin reductase deficiency exhibit slight gray pseudocyanosis. Even homozygotes, however, rarely exhibit more than 25% methemoglobin, a level compatible with absence of symptoms. Heterozygotes often have normal methemoglobin levels but are especially susceptible to the effects of toxic agents that cause methemoglobinemia.

The third form of methemoglobinemia is caused by exposure to certain chemical agents and drugs that accelerate the oxidation of methemoglobin (Table 136–3). Nitrite compounds are especially notorious in this regard. Some of these agents also have a propensity to exacerbate G6PD deficiency and the precipitation of unstable hemoglobins.

Nitrates are a frequent environmental source of toxic methemoglobinemia, even though nitrates do not directly interact with either hemoglobin or the reductase system. Rather, nitrates are converted to nitrites in the gut. Well-water is the most frequently encountered source of excessive nitrates. In general, substantial intake of these agents is required before significant amounts of methemoglobin are generated. Very young infants are more susceptible to these agents than are adults, but all age groups are at risk if exposure is sufficient.

Toxic or acquired hemoglobinemia is virtually the only situation in which life-threatening amounts of methemoglobin accumulate. In general, the only symptom produced when methemoglobin comprises less than 30% of total hemoglobin is the cosmetic effect of cyanosis. As levels of methemoglobin rise above 30%, patients begin to exhibit symptoms of oxygen deprivation, such as malaise, giddiness, and other alterations of mental status. The symptoms reflect a true lack of oxygen availability at the tissue level, since a substantial number of hemoglobin molecules are no longer delivering oxygen to the tissues. At levels of methemoglobin greater than 50%, loss of consciousness, coma, and death can ensue rapidly. At this level of methemoglobin, "cyanosis" is severe, and the blood is chocolate brown.

DIAGNOSIS. Methemoglobinemia should be suspected in patients with unexplained cyanosis. One should be especially alert to the potential medical emergency inherent in a patient with cyanosis and altered mental status, despite a normal arterial P_{O_2}. The ingestion of nitrites as a suicide gesture, especially in individuals knowl-

TABLE 136–2. FORMS OF METHEMOGLOBINEMIA

I. Inherited
M hemoglobins
Methemoglobin reductase deficiency

II. Acquired
"Toxic" methemoglobinemia due to nitrates, etc.

TABLE 136–3. SOME AGENTS CAUSING METHEMOGLOBINEMIA

Nitrites
Nitrates (e.g., in well-water)
Aniline dyes
Phenacetin
Acetanilid
Menadione (vitamin K_3)
Acetaminophen
Dapsone
Phenazopyridine (Pyridium)
Sulfa drugs
Amyl nitrate
Nitroprusside
Benzocaine, procaine

edgeable with respect to chemistry, medicine, or pharmacology, is not uncommon. The diagnosis of methemoglobinemia can be suspected from the brownish color of blood when it is drawn. In the laboratory, methemoglobin exhibits characteristic peaks of absorption at 630 and 502 nm, rendering it easily distinguishable from normal hemoglobin. In addition, the inherited M hemoglobins are frequently detectable by altered electrophoretic mobility, especially if ferricyanide treatment *in vitro* is used to convert all of the hemoglobin solution to methemoglobin prior to electrophoresis.

In the case of toxic methemoglobinemia, recognition of exposure to an appropriate agent provides the most important historical clue. Acute poisoning can represent a life-threatening emergency; therefore, one should request laboratory evaluation for methemoglobin in any individual with atypical cyanosis or cyanosis occurring along with normal blood gas values. Methemoglobin due to deficiencies of the reductase system can be further evaluated in reference laboratories by direct analysis of these enzymes.

MANAGEMENT. Patients with M hemoglobins are usually asymptomatic and require no management. The secondary cyanosis can represent an unfortunate cosmetic problem, which cannot be reversed, since ascorbic acid and methylene blue (see below) are ineffective with most of these variants despite their utility in the treatment of methemoglobinemia due to other causes.

Patients with deficiency of the reductase system generally do not require treatment, but cyanosis can be improved by treatment with oral methylene blue, 100 to 300 mg per day, or 500 mg per day of oral ascorbic acid. Riboflavin (20 mg per day) has also been reported to be effective. Riboflavin treatment has been championed because methylene blue produces discolored (blue) urine, whereas ascorbic acid can generate sodium oxalate stones.

In the emergency treatment of high levels of toxic methemoglobinemia, 1 to 2 mg per kilogram of methylene blue is given as a 1% solution in saline, usually administered rapidly (10 to 15 minutes) intravenously. The dose may be repeated if necessary. This treatment is usually effective. As noted above, methylene blue acts via the NADPH reductase system, which in turn requires G6PD activity. The method is thus not effective in patients who also have G6PD deficiency. These patients, or patients who are severely affected, may require exchange transfusion. Oral ascorbic acid, at doses noted earlier, is not useful in emergency situations because it acts too slowly. Follow-up maintenance management, however, can be accomplished with either ascorbic acid or oral methylene blue.

Mild cases of methemoglobin intoxication do not require treatment. The patient can be monitored for 1 to 3 days, during which time methemoglobin levels will gradually return to normal if the offending agent is eliminated. The most important follow-up therapy of patients with toxic methemoglobinemia involves a thorough search for the offending agent and its removal from the environment.

Bunn HF, Forget BG: Hemoglobin: Molecular, Genetic and Clinical Aspects. Philadelphia, W.B. Saunders, 1986. *Chapter 13 discusses unstable hemoglobins; Chapter 14, hemoglobins with altered oxygen affinity; and Chapters 15 and 16, various forms of methemoglobinemia.*

Mansouri A: Methemoglobinemia. Am J Med Sci 289:200, 1985.

Weatherall DJ, Clegg JB, Higgs DR, et al.: The hemoglobinopathies. *In* Scriver CR, Beaudet AL, Sly WS, et al. (eds.): The Metabolic Basis of Inherited Disease, 6th ed. New York, McGraw-Hill, 1989.

136.4 The Thalassemias

Arthur W. Nienhuis and Edward J. Benz, Jr.

The thalassemias are hereditary anemias that occur because of mutations that affect the synthesis of hemoglobin. In β-thalassemia there is deficient synthesis of β globin, whereas in α-thalassemia there is deficient synthesis of α globin. Reduced synthesis of one of the two globin polypeptides leads to deficient hemoglobin accumulation, resulting in hypochromic and microcytic red cells. These red cell abnormalities are the most constant and characteristic features of this group of disorders. Table 136–4 contains a clinical classification of the thalassemias presented in the order in which they are discussed in this chapter.

TABLE 136–4. CLINICAL CLASSIFICATION OF THE THALASSEMIAS

I. Severe β-thalassemia (Cooley's anemia)	Severe anemia, growth retardation, hepatosplenomegaly, bone marrow expansion, and bone deformities
A. Thalassemia major	Transfusion dependent
B. Thalassemia intermedia	No regular transfusion requirement
II. Thalassemia trait (α or β)	Mild anemia with microcytosis and hypochromia
III. Hb H disease (α-thal)	Moderately severe hemolytic anemia, icterus, and splenomegaly
IV. Hydrops fetalis (α-thal)	Death *in utero* caused by severe anemia
V. Silent carrier (α or β)	Hematologically normal

The incidence and prevalence of these conditions are highly variable. Most common is thalassemia trait, a mild, clinically insignificant anemia that apparently protects individuals from malaria (see below), and therefore through natural selection it has become extremely common in certain parts of the world. Thalassemia trait generally represents the heterozygous form of either α- or β-thalassemia. Hence where thalassemia trait is common, homozygous, more severely affected patients will be found frequently. In the United States, the incidence of β-thalassemia is highest among ethnic groups originating from the Mediterranean area, parts of Africa, and Asia, whereas the incidence of α-thalassemia is highest among those from Asia. Generally the incidence of thalassemia trait in these ethnic groups is 3 to 5%. Approximately 1000 patients with more severe forms of thalassemia are known in the United States.

SEVERE β-THALASSEMIA (Cooley's Anemia)

Severe β-thalassemia occurs in patients who are homozygous for mutations that lead to a decrease in β globin synthesis. Because both β globin genes are affected, there is marked deficiency in β globin synthesis, but α globin synthesis continues at an approximately normal rate. Accumulation of a large excess of α chains for which there are no β chains with which to combine has several serious deleterious effects. Alpha globin is highly insoluble and forms large intracellular inclusions. These interfere with the cell cycle in the bone marrow, retard the passage of red cells from the bone marrow, and reduce the survival of red cells in the circulation by virtue of membrane damage and splenic trapping. Marked ineffective erythropoiesis is the hallmark of this disorder because α inclusions interfere with erythroblast maturation, leading to intramedullary death of many red cell precursors. Severe anemia stimulates erythropoietin production, leading to erythroid stem cell and erythroblast proliferation. The vastly expanded erythroid cell mass results in osteoporosis with a potential for pathologic fractures. Extramedullary hematopoiesis is also often seen, and compression of vital structures, particularly the spinal cord, may occur as a consequence. Because of marrow expansion and deformities of the skull and facial bones, patients with severe β-thalassemia often have an abnormal appearance with prominent epicanthal folds, referred to as a chipmunk facies.

Patients with severe β-thalassemia may be divided into two groups on the basis of their requirement for blood transfusion. Those with thalassemia major have an absolute requirement for blood without which severe anemia leads to death in infancy or early childhood. In contrast, patients with thalassemia intermedia are able to maintain their hemoglobin at 6 to 7 grams per deciliter without transfusion. This level is compatible with fairly normal growth and development, and many of these patients survive into adulthood. However, the hemoglobin level is maintained at the expense of expanded erythropoiesis, with its attendant bony abnormalities, excessive iron absorption, and hemolytic stigmata.

Thalassemia Major

CLINICAL FEATURES. At birth patients with thalassemia major are nearly normal hematologically, since γ globin synthesis is normal and hemoglobin (Hb) F production is therefore adequate. However, as the switch from Hb F to Hb A is completed during the first year of life, the deficiency in β globin production becomes evident. By 6 to 9 months of age, severe anemia reflected by pallor, poor growth, or inadequate food intake leads the anxious parents to bring the infant to the physician, at which time examination reveals the presence of marked hepatosplenomegaly. The hemoglobin may be 3 to 6 grams per deciliter, and the red cells exhibit the characteristic severe microcytosis, hypochromia, and fragmentation (Color Plate 6A, left). Demonstration of thalassemia trait (see below) in both parents is usually sufficient to establish the diagnosis. Study of the infant's blood shows absence of or low Hb A, a large amount of Hb F, and an increase in the amount of Hb A_2 to 4 to 10% of the total hemoglobin (normal < 2.5%). Biosynthetic studies, a tool of the research laboratory, may be employed to show the deficiency of β globin production.

CLINICAL COURSE. Prior to the use of regular blood transfusions, these children were grossly deformed because of expansion of the marrow spaces of the skull. Severe osteoporosis led to pathologic fractures, and anemia caused weakness and inanition. Death by 2 to 3 years of age was common. Blood transfusions were initially given infrequently for palliation, but gradually physicians interested in this condition came to recognize that regular transfusion to nearly normal hemoglobin levels could be used to suppress all disease manifestations. Growth and bone development are normal in children who have undergone hypertransfusion, and in fact they are virtually indistinguishable from other children if the hypertransfusion regimen is started at a very early age. If transfusions are given less frequently, the patient may exhibit some stigmata of the untreated disorder—bone deformities, growth retardation, and hepatosplenomegaly.

THE PROBLEM OF IRON OVERLOAD. Because humans have a very limited ability to excrete iron, regular blood transfusions inevitably lead to a vast accumulation of iron. Each unit of packed red cells contains approximately 200 mg of iron, so that by the age of 12 the average thalassemic, having received 125 to 150 units of packed cells, will have accumulated 25 to 30 grams of excess iron. This amount compares with the normal 3 to 4 grams found in adults, 75% of which is present in red cells as hemoglobin. Even the patient with thalassemia intermedia, who has not had transfusions, is susceptible. Excess iron absorption leads inevitably to the manifestations of hemochromatosis, although at a later age than in the patient with transfusion-dependent thalassemia. Excess iron deposition occurs in virtually all organs. Most cells have considerable ability to cope with this extra iron by making ferritin and its partial degradation product, hemosiderin. Nonetheless, cell damage occurs by virtue of iron-catalyzed peroxidation of membrane lipids and release of the enzymes from lysosomes rendered labile by their content of hemosiderin granules. Thus tissue hemosiderosis (excess iron) leads ultimately to the clinical condition of secondary hemochromatosis. The liver, endocrine glands, and particularly the heart are the primary target organs.

Liver dysfunction is mild in the thalassemic patient with secondary hemochromatosis. Typically the liver is enlarged several centimeters below the right costal margin, and the transaminases are two to four times above the normal limits. Despite a 20- to 30-fold increase in iron concentration over normal, liver biosynthetic function as reflected by the concentration of serum albumin and various clotting factors is preserved. Fibrosis, invariably present on liver biopsy, may progress to frank cirrhosis anatomically, but clinical evidence of cirrhosis is rare.

As noted above, the course of adequately transfused thalassemic patients is essentially normal until the age of 10 to 12. Growth failure then becomes a frequent and distressing complication for both the child and parents. The mechanism for this growth failure is not known; growth hormone levels are generally normal, but the serum somatomedin concentration may be low. Failure of growth is accompanied by lack of pubescence. Primary hypogonadism is exceedingly common. The mechanism is usually failure of the pituitary to produce adequate amounts of follicle-stimulating hormone (FSH) and luteinizing hormone (LH). Diabetes mellitus, hypothyroidism, and, rarely, hypoparathyroidism with tetany are additional complications that may occur, particularly in patients who are in their late teenage years or early 20's.

Cardiac disease in the patients with severe β-thalassemia may take three forms: pericarditis, congestive heart failure, and cardiac arrhythmias. Recurrent attacks of acute pericarditis are manifested by chest pain, often pleuritic and affected by a change of position, accompanied by fever and occasionally a pericardial friction rub. These attacks are usually self-limited, lasting 4 to 7 days. Treatment consists of bed rest, aspirin, and other anti-inflammatory agents, such as indomethacin in appropriate doses. Rarely, constrictive pericarditis may require pericardiectomy.

Congestive heart failure is to be expected ultimately in patients with secondary hemochromatosis unless death occurs early by virtue of cardiac arrhythmias. Careful echocardiographic studies have suggested that iron deposition begins by the age of 5 to 6 years. By 10 or 12 years, when the patient has received more than 100 units of blood, left ventricular dysfunction may be demonstrated by radionuclide cineangiography during the physiologic stress of exercise. Clinical congestive heart failure is usually a late complication; most patients die within 12 months of the onset of definite evidence of heart failure. Treatment with digoxin in doses adequate to achieve therapeutic blood levels may be helpful. Appropriate use of diuretics and vasodilator therapy may be useful in providing palliation and extending the lifespan of these patients.

Atrial and ventricular ectopy is present in 24-hour electrocardiographic recordings in virtually all patients who have received more than 150 units of packed red cells. High-grade ventricular ectopy with couplets, short runs of ventricular tachycardia, and multiple ventricular foci are of ominous prognostic significance. Ectopy may be extremely distressful to the patient, particularly at night, when it is often most severe. Tachyrhythmias such as ventricular tachycardia and/or ventricular fibrillation occur despite therapy and are frequent causes of death in patients with severe thalassemia who are undergoing regular transfusions. The pharmacologic treatment of cardiac arrhythmias is described in Ch. 35.

The prognosis in patients with thalassemia major is determined by the cardiac disease. The average age of death is 17 years, although a few patients may survive to their mid 20's. Because of this grim prognosis, considerable effort has been focused on attempts to reduce the iron burden in these patients.

THE ROLE OF SPLENECTOMY. Splenic enlargement is frequent and often causes functional hypersplenism as manifested by an increasing transfusion requirement. Careful documentation of the patient's needs often alerts the physician to the development of hypersplenism as the need for blood rises. An average patient on a hypertransfusion regimen designed to maintain the hemoglobin at a level greater than 10 grams per deciliter requires 250 ml of packed cells per kilogram per year. If substantially more blood is required, the spleen should be removed. Leukopenia and thrombocytopenia, if present, are indicators of the presence of hypersplenism and should lead to prompt splenectomy.

The complication of splenectomy in this patient population is a risk of sudden overwhelming sepsis by encapsulated organisms. For this reason, delay of splenectomy until after the age of 4 is highly desirable. Splenectomized patients should receive Pneumovax and may be placed on a regimen of daily penicillin prophylaxis. More important, each patient should be given a small supply of a broad-spectrum antibiotic, such as ampicillin, to be taken orally in appropriate doses if a high temperature develops and immediate medical attention cannot be obtained.

CHELATION THERAPY. The only drug available for use in removal of iron is deferoxamine (Desferal). This drug has an extremely high affinity for trivalent iron. Despite extensive clinical use it appears to be relatively free of serious toxicity. Its disadvantages are that it must be given parenterally and that it has a very short serum half-life. Thus, most of the drug, given as a single intramuscular injection, is rapidly excreted without binding any iron. To maximize the efficacy of the drug, a technique has been devised to administer it subcutaneously by using a small mechanical infusion pump. A needle is inserted into the subcutaneous tissue of the abdomen, and the drug is infused very slowly over a period of 8 to 12 hours. With 1.5 to 2.0 grams of deferoxamine, two to three times more iron may be removed than by a single daily intramuscular injection. Often, daily excretion of 30 to 40 mg of iron may be achieved in older patients and may lead to overall negative iron balance despite continued transfusion therapy, provided that the drug is used at least five times per week. This regimen retards the rate of iron accumulation in the liver and reduces liver fibrosis. Several chelators are under study. One has been shown to be effective in clinical trials. At this time, however, deferoxamine remains the only therapy with proven efficacy and safety.

Clinical evidence indicates that cardiac disease may be delayed. Indeed, reversal of established congestive heart failure with documented left ventricular dysfunction has been observed in patients treated intensively with intravenous deferoxamine. This may be accomplished by placement of a Hickman catheter. Well-motivated patients may be taught to administer the drug daily by the intravenous route in doses of 3 to 4 grams per day given over 18 to 20 hours. Gastrointestinal disturbances and reversible renal dysfunction have been observed. Reduction of dose eliminates these complications. The greatest probability of successfully preventing iron damage is in patients in whom treatment is begun early, preferably by the age of 5 years. Vitamin C in small doses (150 to 250 mg per day) given orally may increase the amount of iron excretion in response to deferoxamine infusions, although some evidence suggests that this agent may enhance tissue iron toxicity, particularly to the heart, and therefore it should be used with caution in older patients.

Thalassemia Intermedia

Those patients with severe β-thalassemia who maintain their hemoglobin levels above 6.0 to 7.0 grams per deciliter have a generally better prognosis. Individual patients with thalassemia intermedia generally have large amounts of Hb F, significant amounts of Hb A_2, and variable amounts of Hb A in their red cells. Iron accumulation may occur because of increased gastrointestinal absorption and ultimately may lead to secondary hemochromatosis with endocrine and cardiac dysfunction, but most patients with thalassemia intermedia survive into adulthood and many have children. Splenectomy may become necessary if evidence of hypersplenism is present. Osteoporosis may be severe, as the erythroid mass in these patients is not suppressed. A disabling form of arthritis has been described. Large masses of erythroid tissue in extramedullary sites may cause organ dysfunction. Particularly distressing is spinal cord compression with paraplegia, although usually local radiation reverses this condition. Any or all of these complications may ultimately lead to the use of a regular transfusion regimen in patients with thalassemia intermedia despite their marginally adequate hemoglobin levels. Such treatment has the added benefit of preventing the disfiguring facial abnormalities.

Genetically this condition is heterogeneous. Often the red cells of both parents exhibit stigmata of thalassemia trait, although frequently one parent may be a silent carrier of the thalassemia gene (see below). In such persons the impairment of β globin synthesis is so mild that the red cells are normal, but when the abnormal β gene is paired with another affected by a more severe β-thalassemia mutation, thalassemia intermedia results. Elucidation of many thalassemia mutations at the molecular level has revealed marked quantitative variability ranging from 50 to 100% reduction of β globin messenger RNA (mRNA) production (see below). Many patients are doubly heterozygous for two different mutations. The clinical heterogeneity of the β-thalassemias reflects the many combinations of mutations that may be present in individual patients. Other genetic modifiers of the β-thalassemia phenotype include α-thalassemia mutations and genetic variants characterized by increased Hb F production. Coinheritance of an α-thalassemia gene decreases α globin production, leading to partial correction of the highly deleterious imbalance in α and β biosynthesis. Increased γ globin synthesis, resulting in increased Hb F production, compensates directly for deficient β globin production.

THALASSEMIA TRAIT

CLINICAL CHARACTERISTICS. Common to both α- and β-thalassemia is a condition referred to as thalassemia minor or trait. This condition generally occurs in individuals who are heterozygous for a mutation affecting α or β globin synthesis (see below). Characteristically the red blood cells are small and contain less hemoglobin than normal; the mean corpuscular volume averages 65 μm^3 (range, 56 to 74), whereas the mean corpuscular hemoglobin averages 21 pg (range, 20 to 23). Normal values for these parameters are 88 ± 5 and 30 ± 2, respectively. The total red cell count is often increased to 10 to 20% above the normal range, so that anemia, if present, is mild. Rarely the packed cell volume may be as low as 30%; values of 32 to 38% are more typical. Splenomegaly is said to occur, but is distinctly unusual, and other causes should be sought if this physical finding is present. No clinical symptoms may be attributed solely to the presence of thalassemia trait.

DIFFERENTIAL DIAGNOSIS. A characteristic feature of β-thalassemia trait is elevation of the level of Hb A_2. This minor hemoglobin accounts for only 2 or 3% of the total in normal red cells, but in thalassemia trait it may be elevated in the range of 4 to 8% in more than 90% of persons with this condition. Similarly, the level of Hb F is often elevated to 1.5 to 2.5%, although in rare types of thalassemia trait it may be as high as 10 to 15%. In normal red cells, Hb F accounts for less than 1% of the total. The minor hemoglobins, Hb A_2 and Hb F, are either normal or slightly decreased in patients with α-thalassemia.

The differential diagnosis of thalassemia trait includes consideration of iron deficiency. This diagnosis can be excluded only by measurement of the serum iron, total iron-binding capacity, and serum ferritin. If these values are normal in patients whose red cells are severely microcytic, but in whom anemia, if present, is mild, the diagnosis of thalassemia trait can be considered established. The distinction between α- and β-thalassemia depends on the measurement of the minor hemoglobins. If these are normal, the diagnosis of α-thalassemia is most likely, although rare subjects with β-thalassemia also have normal levels of Hb A_2 and Hb F.

GENE FREQUENCY. Thalassemia trait is thought to protect persons from malaria, particularly during the early years of life when immunity is not yet established and fatal cerebral malaria caused by *Plasmodium falciparum* may occur. This selective advantage accounts for the high frequency of thalassemia genes in regions where malaria has been endemic for the past two millennia. These include the Mediterranean basin particularly, but also large parts of Asia and Africa. The gene frequency may be as high as 20% in certain populations.

HEMOGLOBIN H DISEASE

PATHOPHYSIOLOGY. Anemia of moderate severity characterized by hypochromia, microcytosis, striking red cell fragmentation, and the presence of a fast-migrating hemoglobin on electrophoresis occurs in patients who have a moderately severe deficiency in α globin production. The genetics of this condition are considered later in this chapter. The fast-migrating hemoglobin has the globin subunit composition β_4. It may account for up to 30% of the total hemoglobin in these patients. Because the β_4 tetramer exhibits no cooperativity and has an extremely high oxygen affinity, it is functionally useless in oxygen transport. Thus patients with a significant amount of Hb H functionally have more severe anemia than measurement of the hemoglobin concentration might suggest.

Hb H is an unstable tetramer. Thus as the red cell ages and loses its ability to withstand oxidative stress, Hb H may precipitate, forming inclusions that cause hemolysis. Oxidant drugs such as the sulfonamides may exacerbate hemolysis. Because the β_4 tetramer is soluble during the early phases of the red cell's lifespan, erythropoiesis in the bone marrow is effective and the anemia is generally not as severe as that seen in patients with β-thalassemia who have an equivalent impairment in β globin production.

CLINICAL FEATURES. The average patient with Hb H disease maintains gainful employment, marries, and reproduces. Usually the anemia is moderate, with a hemoglobin concentration of 7 to 10 grams per deciliter, although occasional patients may have more severe anemia. Moderate splenomegaly is often present. Splenectomy may be considered, but the occurrence of severe postoperative thrombocytosis with a propensity for recurrent pulmonary emboli makes this procedure inadvisable except in patients with unequivocal clinical evidence of hypersplenism, as manifested by leukopenia, thrombocytopenia, and worsening anemia or a transfusion requirement in a previously stable patient. Other therapeutic measures include prescription of folic acid, avoidance of oxidant drugs and iron salts, prompt treatment of infection, and judicious use of transfusions. Acquired Hb H disease has been described as a complication in patients with various forms of myeloproliferative and myelodysplastic disorders. In such patients, treatment and prognosis are related to the primary disorder.

HYDROPS FETALIS

The birth of stillborn infants from parents who both have α-thalassemia trait reflects the severest form of α-thalassemia. These infants are grossly edematous or hydropic because of the congestive heart failure that occurs as a result of severe anemia. Their failure to produce any α globin results in the production of only Hb Bart's (γ_4) and Hb H (β_4) during the later parts of gestation. Both these hemoglobins are nonfunctional in oxygen transport, so that once the embryonic hemoglobins disappear from the circulation early in fetal development, life is no longer possible. A high incidence of toxemia of pregnancy has been noted in mothers of hydropic infants. Prenatal diagnosis of this condition is possible with current methods (see below) and should be followed by prompt termination of the pregnancy.

SILENT CARRIER

The silent carrier state was first recognized among the α-thalassemia syndromes. One parent of a patient with Hb H disease usually has all the features of α-thalassemia trait, whereas the other has normal-appearing red cells with no anemia. Similarly, progeny of persons with Hb H disease fall into two groups: those having α-thalassemia trait and those with apparently normal hemoglobin production. In the silent carrier, the defect in α globin synthesis is so mild that no impairment in hemoglobin synthesis is evident, although when the mutation is paired genetically with a more severe impairment of globin synthesis, e.g., α-thalassemia trait, Hb H disease occurs. A similar silent carrier state has also been described among the β-thalassemia syndromes. Thalassemia intermedia occurs in those who inherit one thalassemia gene from a silent carrier and a second from a person with thalassemia trait.

THE GENETICS OF THE α-THALASSEMIA SYNDROMES

As described in Ch. 136.1, the α globin genes in humans are duplicated. Thus two genes are found on each chromosome 16, making a total of four in each diploid cell. Four clinical states are seen in α-thalassemia: silent carrier, thalassemia trait, Hb H disease, and hydrops fetalis. These conditions occur in persons who have, respectively, one, two, three, or four α globin genes affected by mutations that reduce α globin synthesis.

The most frequent mutation that leads to α-thalassemia is gene deletion. In the silent carrier one of the two genes on one chromosome 16 is missing, whereas the other two genes on the other chromosome 16 are normal. α-Thalassemia trait can occur by two mechanisms. Persons who have two chromosomes with only one α gene exhibit α-thalassemia trait. This form is most common in the black population. Hb H disease is distinctly uncommon in this population, since offspring of two persons, each of whom is homozygous for the one α gene chromosome, can have only α-thalassemia trait and not Hb H disease. In the Asian population, α-thalassemia trait occurs most commonly in those who lack both α genes on one chromosome and have the normal two on the other. Mating of such a person with a silent carrier who has one chromosome having only one α gene can lead to children with Hb H disease. Hydrops fetalis occurs among offspring of parents both of whom are heterozygous for chromosomes lacking both normal α globin genes. In Africans, a chromosome containing a deletion of only one locus is common, but deletion of both loci is almost never encountered. Therefore, α-thalassemia trait is thus very common, but hydrops fetalis is exceedingly rare.

In addition to the deletion mutations, many nondeletional types of α-thalassemia have been described. Molecular characterization of several has revealed a diversity of defects involving RNA splicing, polyadenylation, mRNA translation, or α globin stability. These mutations are similar to those in β-thalassemia globin genes; their effects on RNA metabolism are discussed in more detail in the next section.

THE MOLECULAR GENETICS OF THALASSEMIA

The β-thalassemia mutations may be separated into two classes: β^+-thalassemia, in which there is synthesis of a small amount of normal β globin, and β^0-thalassemia, which in the homozygote is manifested by no β globin production at all. Similarly, nondeletional types of α-thalassemia may abolish (α^0) or decrease (α^+) α globin production. Many mutations having specific effects on gene expression have been characterized by molecular cloning, DNA sequencing, and functional characterization. Each of the several steps in RNA metabolism—transcription, processing, transport, and mRNA translation—has been found to be affected by one or more individual mutations. The variable quantitative effect of the individ-

ual mutations on globin production has been clarified by these molecular studies.

MUTATIONS THAT AFFECT TRANSCRIPTION. Several mutations reduce promoter function to 20 to 25% of normal, but some β globin mRNA is produced from these genes; hence they cause β^+-thalassemia. Other mutations delete the LCR sequences (see Ch. 136.1) that switch on globin gene expression during erythropoiesis.

SPLICING AND POLYADENYLATION MUTATIONS. These are among the most common of mutations that cause thalassemia. Mutations that occur within the splice junction sequence decrease or abolish normal splicing at that site and often are accompanied by splicing at other sites that are not normally used. A substitution in the invariant GT abolishes splicing, making this a β^0 gene, whereas substitutions in consensus nucleotides at the splice junction have a quantitative effect on splicing and hence are β^+ mutations.

An interesting class of mutations consists of those that create an alternate site for splicing. These may occur within introns or within coding sequence (exons). These substitutions occur within regions of the precursor RNA molecule that resemble the consensus splice junction sequence (see Fig. 136–6) but lack some critical element necessary for splicing. Nucleotide substitutions that add that element to the potential splice junction sequence lead to its activation, causing abnormal splicing and hence a thalassemic effect. Substitution of A for T in codon 24 of the β globin gene does not alter the amino acid sequence (GGT and GGA both encode glycine) but creates an alternative splicing site. Two mutations, Hb E and Hb Knossos, alter both protein structure and the splicing pattern. Such structural mutations that are also characterized by decreased synthesis are referred to as *thalassemic hemoglobinopathies* (see Ch. 136.2).

A class of mutations that has interesting implications for control of splicing is made up of those that create an alternate site and also activate cryptic splice sites remote from the mutation. There is a potential or cryptic splice site in the β globin gene transcript that matches the consensus splice junction sequence nearly perfectly, and yet this site is used rarely, if ever, during normal splicing. Use of an alternative site, created by a thalassemia mutation, apparently alters the secondary structure of the precursor RNA molecule, leading to splicing at the otherwise cryptic site. Mutations that disrupt the AATAAA signal used for polyadenylation have also been described.

MUTATIONS THAT AFFECT mRNA TRANSLATION. Among the more common mutations in thalassemia genes are those that lead to premature termination of mRNA translation. Single nucleotide substitutions (or small deletions that alter the mRNA reading frame) introduce codons that signal the termination of protein synthesis on the abnormal mRNA. For example, substitution of thymine for cytosine in codon 39 introduces the stop codon UAG at that position. This abnormal β globin mRNA can be read only through codon 38, yielding a small, nonfunctional remnant of β globin. Premature termination mutations cause β^0- (or α^0-) thalassemia.

Common mutations that cause α-thalassemia are chain termination mutations. As described in Ch. 136.1, the completed globin molecule is released from the polyribosome when the protein synthetic apparatus encounters the normal terminator codon UAA. A single nucleotide change in this terminator codon converts it to a codon that is functional for the insertion of any one of several amino acids, depending on the exact nucleotide that is substituted. In this case, protein synthesis continues into the part of the mRNA that is usually untranslated, leading to the synthesis of a protein that may be as many as 30 amino acids longer than normal. Such an elongated α globin is found in Hb Constant Spring. This protein accounts for only 1 to 2% of the total α globin in the cells of patients with Hb Constant Spring, and their red cells exhibit the stigmata of thalassemia trait.

MUTATIONS THAT AFFECT GLOBIN STABILITY. Certain mutations may alter globin amino acid sequence and lead to instability and thus have a thalassemic effect despite a normal rate of synthesis of the mutant globin. Among the more dramatic of this class of mutations is one that leads to substitution of leucine for proline at position 125 of the α globin found in Hb Quong Sze. This mutation was discovered upon sequencing of the abnormal α gene and evidence of $\alpha^{\text{Quong Sze}}$ instability was subsequently obtained *in vitro*. Because of its marked instability, $\alpha^{\text{Quong Sze}}$ could not be detected in the red cells of the affected individual. Hb Quong Sze, like Hb E, is another of the thalassemic hemoglobinopathies characterized by both deficient net globin production and a structural abnormality.

DELETION MUTATIONS. Deletions causing α-thalassemia have been described earlier. Small deletions that leave one of the two α globin genes intact on a chromosome are classified as α^+ mutations, while large deletions that remove both α genes are considered α^0 mutations. In contrast to α-thalassemia, in which gene deletion is the most common mutation, gene deletion is rarely the mechanism for β-thalassemia. A few patients of Indian ancestry have been found to have a deletion that has removed the 3' half of the β globin gene and a small amount of flanking DNA. A special kind of deletion has resulted in the $\delta\beta$ fusion gene present in a few Italian patients who produce Hb Lepore. An unequal crossover during meiosis has led to the fusion gene that encodes for a globin that has the N-terminal sequence of δ globin and the C-terminal sequence of β globin. This globin is produced in very small amounts; hence this gene leads to thalassemia trait or thalassemia major in heterozygotes or homozygotes, respectively.

Several large deletions that have removed two or more genes from the β cluster have been characterized. The β-thalassemia mutations have resulted in loss of the δ and β genes; the $^A\gamma\delta\beta$-thalassemia deletions include the $^A\gamma$ gene in addition. Two interesting forms of $\gamma\delta\beta$-thalassemia have resulted in loss of all but the β gene, and yet this β gene does not function. These observations suggest that the DNA sequences remote from a gene can nonetheless influence its expression. Other deletions have resulted in loss of the entire β-like gene cluster.

MUTATIONS THAT INCREASE Hb F PRODUCTION. About 1% of the hemoglobin in adult blood is Hb F. This fetal hemoglobin is found in 2 to 10% of red cells; these cells—called F cells—contain roughly 4 to 8 pg of Hb F and 24 to 28 pg of adult hemoglobin. As discussed in Ch. 136.1, these F cells originate during the differentiation of erythroid progenitor cells. F cell number and therefore Hb F levels are genetically determined in humans.

Increased Hb F in individuals who are homozygous for β-thalassemia mainly reflects amplification of the F cell population. In the bone marrow, those erythroblasts producing small amounts of γ globin have less of an excess in α globin synthesis and therefore are more likely to survive and leave the bone marrow. By this mechanism, the 1% of γ synthesis in the bone marrow cell population may be amplified 10- to 40-fold in the peripheral blood. Of more interest from the aspect of gene control are those mutations that alter Hb F production by genetic mechanisms.

There are two general classes of deletion mutations that increase Hb F production in adults. The $\delta\beta$-thalassemia mutations are characterized by production of 5 to 12% of Hb F in heterozygotes, while *hereditary persistence of fetal hemoglobin* (HPFH) deletion mutations are characterized by production of 25 to 30%. Most of the red cells in heterozygous individuals with HPFH contain Hb F, whereas heterozygotes with $\delta\beta$-thalassemia mutations have Hb F in only 25 to 30% of their red cells. These mutations have been carefully characterized structurally in an attempt to define the basis at the DNA level for these differing phenotypes.

Another category of mutations that cause HPFH leave the β-like gene cluster intact and therefore are referred to as *nondeletion mutations*. Nondeletion HPFH mutations are characterized by a heterogeneous distribution of Hb F in red cells (heterocellular) in contrast to the pancellular distribution of Hb F in heterozygotes with the deletion types of HPFH. There may be many different heterocellular HPFH mutations; genetic studies indicate that at least some are not linked to the β-like gene cluster. Point mutations within the γ globin gene promoter region have been discovered in some individuals with nondeletion HPFH.

PRENATAL DIAGNOSIS. Because of the serious consequences of severe β-thalassemia (Cooley's anemia), prenatal diagnosis of this condition with subsequent therapeutic abortion is thought by many to be highly desirable. Two general strategies have made this a feasible undertaking. The first approach is based on the fact that small amounts of β globin synthesis may be detected in the early mid-trimester fetus (see Ch. 136.1). In fetuses who have inherited two genes for β-thalassemia, no β globin or very small amounts are produced at a time when normal fetuses are producing approximately 10% β globin. By using sophisticated obstetric techniques,

blood may be obtained from the umbilical vein and used for biosynthetic measurements of the globin synthetic pattern. Absence of or low β globin synthesis occurs in homozygous fetuses, whereas intermediate levels are found in heterozygotes. This strategy has been widely applied in parts of Greece and Italy and has led to significant reduction in the incidence of the severe form of β-thalassemia in certain populations.

A second strategy for prenatal diagnosis relies on the study of DNA prepared from amniotic fluid cells of potentially affected persons. The globin genes in such DNA samples may be characterized by the techniques referred to as restriction endonuclease mapping. The DNA is digested with an enzyme that cuts at a specific nucleotide sequence. Among the million or so fragments generated from human DNA are those few that include the globin genes. The DNA is resolved electrophoretically, transferred to a nitrocellulose paper, and annealed to a radioactive probe specific for globin gene sequences. Depending on the enzyme used, a characteristic set of fragments containing globin gene sequences is generated. In persons who have inherited a mutation reflected by deletion of all or part of a globin gene, a change in a position of a particular fragment serves to indicate the presence of such a mutation. Many cases of α-thalassemia and rare cases of β-thalassemia may be diagnosed in this way.

More widely applicable to the prenatal diagnosis of thalassemias are so-called restriction enzyme polymorphisms. A single nucleotide change, in an area within or remote from the globin gene, may result in loss of a restriction endonuclease site and therefore a change in the migration position of a particular fragment containing globin gene sequences. Most polymorphisms occur in association with both normal and abnormal β globin genes. Hence a different method of analysis is required rather than simple characterization of a single restriction endonuclease site. "Haplotype analysis" employs simultaneous analysis of several polymorphisms, but this strategy is also imperfect and requires extensive family studies.

An alternative approach utilizing DNA analysis for prenatal diagnosis is now feasible because several frequent mutations have been defined by DNA sequencing. Synthetic oligonucleotide probes, one specific for the normal gene and one specific for a particular abnormal gene, can be used to discriminate between the normal and abnormal genes in amniotic fluid DNA by rapid polymerase chain reaction (PCR)–based methods. This method is simple and direct but requires that several probes be available for each of the mutations that occur frequently in the population for whom prenatal diagnosis is offered.

The application of prenatal diagnosis requires appropriate screening and identification of persons at risk. Thalassemia trait usually can be identified readily by virtue of the morphologic changes in the red cells. Confirmation of the diagnosis depends on measurement of hemoglobin A_2 and Hb F.

EMERGING AND EXPERIMENTAL THERAPY

Chronic hypertransfusion therapy with early institution of iron chelation therapy has been convincingly shown to prolong survival and improve the quality of life of patients with severe thalassemia. Yet, as already noted, these treatments are self-limiting. Alloimmunization, blood-borne infections, and the long-term consequences of iron overload lead eventually to morbidity and mortality. Red cell transfusion and iron chelation require an infrastructure for the delivery of transfusion services, an adequate supply of blood donors, financial resources for the purchase of iron chelators, pumps, and transfusion care, and access to sophisticated medical facilities for the management of intercurrent complications. These assets are available in relatively few areas; many areas that are least well endowed are those in which the gene frequency is highest. These considerations have stimulated an ongoing search for improved therapy based upon better understanding of the globin genes and their regulation. Several experimental approaches are being actively investigated:

Allogenic bone marrow transplantation has been shown to be efficacious in patients with homozygous β-thalassemia, provided that a suitable HLA-compatible donor is available. Mortality ranges as high as 30%, but can be maintained at less than 15% if transplantation is done at an early age, most importantly before iron overload has begun. In areas of the world in which bone marrow transplantation is feasible, infants and young children with newly diagnosed homozygous β-thalassemia should be considered potential candidates. The benefits of possible long-term cure must be weighed against the expense and high risk of the procedure. In general, as of this writing, the outcomes among nearly 800 patients undergoing transplantation have been quite good.

Gene therapy has long been regarded as the ultimate, definitive solution for these diseases. Bone marrow transplantation replaces the defective genes with normal ones, in the form of the transplanted pluripotent hematopoietic stem cell. Introduction of normal β or γ globin genes into the pluripotent stem cells of the thalassemic patient should also correct the disorder, upon reinfusion of the genetically altered cells into the patient. A great deal has been learned about the structure of the globin genes and their regulation (see Ch. 136.1); these advances have identified DNA sequences that can be attached to globin genes and cause them to behave appropriately in the erythroid progenitors of transgenic animals. However, gene therapy for hemoglobinopathies remains a futuristic goal. Two major problems must first be solved: (1) Safe and effective means for delivery (e.g., viral vectors) must be developed. Progress toward this goal has been made in recent years. (2) The vector must be delivered into pluripotent stem cells from the patient. Since these appear to be nondividing cells, many of the preferred vectors, such as retroviral vectors, do not work. Intensive efforts designed to purify stem cells and allow them to divide in culture are under way.

Manipulation of the hemoglobin F to hemoglobin A switch is the most promising experimental therapy at the time of this writing. This therapy would be effective for β chain hemoglobinopathies, since both fetal and adult hemoglobin contain the α globin chain. The clinical well-being of patients with HPFH validates the rationale for this approach. Increased γ chain synthesis will increase the amount of functioning hemoglobin produced in erythroid progenitors and also reduce the burden of unpaired α globin chains, thus ameliorating the clinical phenotype. Early attempts to reactivate hemoglobin F synthesis in adult life were developed on the basis of the observation that the inactive γ globin gene in adult erythroblasts was modified by DNA methylation. 5-Azacytidine, an antineoplastic drug that also inhibits DNA methylation, was thus tried in a small group of adult patients after appropriate animal trials. The predicted effects were observed, and hematologic improvement occurred; however, 5-azacytidine is too toxic for widespread use. Moreover, subsequent work demonstrated that the beneficial effects of this drug were not due to its impact upon DNA methylation, but to alteration of the cytokinetics of the erythroid stem cell compartment. As noted in Ch. 136.1, disruption of these kinetics can cause primitive erythroid progenitors capable of synthesizing hemoglobin F to enter the cell cycle and increase the number of "F" cells. Other cytotoxic drugs, with more acceptable side effects, were thus tried. As of this writing, hydroxyurea is in widespread clinical trials; its efficacy in sickle cell anemia (which may be due in part to other effects of the drug) has been demonstrated recently. The utility of hydroxyurea for β-thalassemia remains in question. Butyrate compounds also stimulate Hb F production and are also being tested in preliminary clinical trials. Early results suggest that one or the other of these drugs, or both used in appropriate combinations, may eventually provide useful palliation for patients with thalassemia.

Brittenham GM: Disorders of iron metabolism: Iron deficiency and overload. *In* Hoffman R, Benz EJ, Jr., Shattil SJ, et al.: Hematology: Basic Principles and Practice, 2nd ed. New York, Churchill Livingstone, 1994. *Includes a detailed discussion of the pathophysiology of transfusional hemosiderosis, the approach to using iron chelators, and future development of more effective oral chelators.*

Ley TJ: The pharmacology of hemoglobin switching: Of mice and men. Blood 77:1146, 1991. *A concise and well-written summary of the rationale for pharmacologic manipulation of fetal to adult hemoglobin switching.*

Lucarelli G, Galimberti M, Polchi P, et al.: Bone marrow transplantation in adult thalassemia. Blood 80:1603, 1992. Lucarelli G, Galimberti M, Polchi P, et al.: Marrow transplantation in patients with thalassemia responsive to iron chelation therapy. N Engl J Med 329:840, 1993. *These references suggest that, with appropriate preparation, even adult patients with β-thalassemia might benefit from bone marrow transplantation.*

Thomas ED, Sanders JE, Buckner CD, et al.: Marrow transplantation for thalassemia. Ann NY Acad Sci 445:417, 1985. Lucarelli G, Polchi P, Izzi T, et al.: Marrow transplantation for thalassemia after treatment with busulfan and cyclophosphamide. Ann NY Acad Sci 445:428, 1985. *Two papers that represent accounts by leaders in this field of efforts to use bone marrow transplantation to achieve permanent cure in patients with severe β-thalassemia.*

Weatherall DJ: Bone marrow transplantation for thalassemia and other inherited disorders of hemoglobin. Blood 80:1379, 1992. *A succinct review of bone marrow transplantation.*

Weatherall DJ, Clegg JB: The Thalassemia Syndromes, 3rd ed. Oxford, Blackwell Scientific Publications, Ltd, 1981. *This superb monograph describes the clinical aspects, genetics, and interactions of the various thalassemia syndromes. It should be consulted by anyone with a serious interest in thalassemia.*

137 SICKLE CELL ANEMIA AND ASSOCIATED HEMOGLOBINOPATHIES

Stephen H. Embury

Sickle cell disease is an inherited disorder caused by the abnormal properties conveyed to sickle cell erythrocytes by mutant sickle cell hemoglobin (Hb S). The disease is complex, having as its cardinal features chronic hemolytic anemia and recurrent painful episodes. The illness is engendered by the interaction of the patient with this multisystem disease, the psychosocial impact of the chronic painful disorder, and the ethnic complexities of contemporary society. Traditional understandings of sickle cell disease attribute all disease features to a causative pathophysiologic cascade: an A → T nucleotide substitution in the sixth codon of the β globin gene; a Val → Glu β globin substitution on the surface of the Hb S tetramer; the reduced solubility and polymerization of deoxygenated Hb S; the impaired deformability and sickling of polymer-containing erythrocytes; and the occlusion of the microvasculature by poorly deformable red cells. The importance of these interdependent events notwithstanding, a contemporary understanding of sickle cell pathophysiology includes many polymerization-independent mechanisms (Fig. 137–1).

Different sickle cell syndromes result from distinct inheritance patterns of the sickle cell gene (β^S gene). These are divided into sickle cell disease and sickle cell trait. The former is associated with chronic anemia and recurrent pain, and the latter is associated with neither. Common varieties of sickle cell disease are inherited as homozygosity for the β^S gene (genotype = β^S/β^S) called sickle cell anemia, or as compound heterozygosity of the β^S gene with another mutant β globin gene—sickle cell/β^0-thalassemia (genotype = β^S/β^0-thalassemia), Hb SC disease (genotype = β^S/β^C), and sickle cell–β^+-thalassemia (genotype = β^S/β^+-thalassemia). Sickle cell trait is inherited as simple heterozygosity for the β^S gene (genotype = β^A/β^S).

Clinical management of these complex disorders is best accomplished by comprehensive approaches that address specific manifestations of the illness.

HISTORICAL BACKGROUND

In 1910 Dr. James Herrick published the first account of sickle cell anemia, in which he described sickle-shaped erythrocytes in the blood of a student from Granada who had recurrent pain and anemia (Fig. 137–2). Well before Herrick's report, African tribes had recognized the disorder and referred to it by various onomatopoeic terms that conveyed a sense of recurrent pain. The critical importance of deoxygenation to the pathobiology of sickle red cells derived from a description by Hahn and Gillespie in 1927 of red cell deformation, or "sickling," induced by deoxygenation. Sickling was reversed by reoxygenation, enhanced by acid pH, and presumed to rigidify sickle cells. These relationships provided the basis for the 1940 hypothesis by Ham and Castle of the now-celebrated "vicious cycle of erythrostasis." Direct evidence of deterimental rheologic effects of deoxygenation was not provided until 1956, when Harris reported deoxygenation-enhanced viscosity of sickle cell suspensions.

The notion that the hemoglobin within sickle cells is the effector of deoxygenation-associated changes was first suggested by the discovery of Sherman in 1940 that deoxygenation induces changes in the optical birefringence of sickle erythrocytes. After the 1949 discovery by Pauling, Itano, Singer, and Wells that sickle cell hemoglobin has abnormal electrophoretic mobility, it was possible to link the birefringence changes to the mutant Hb S. The critical importance of Hb S to cell sickling was established in 1950 by Harris

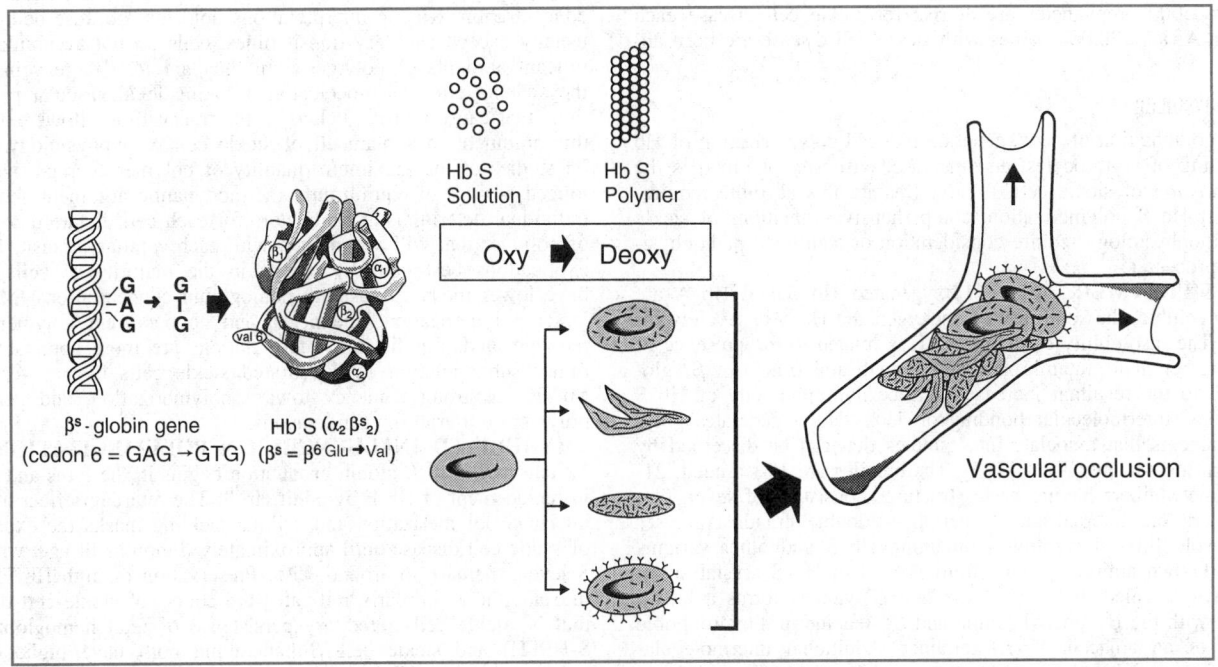

FIGURE 137-1. Schematic view of the pathophysiology of sickle cell disease. The double-stranded DNA molecule on the left represents a β-globin gene in which a GAG $\rightarrow$ GTG substitution in the sixth codon has created the sickle cell gene. The product of this gene is the β^S globin variant in which valine is substituted for glutamic acid as the sixth amino acid. The mutant hemoglobin tetramer $\alpha_2\beta^S_2$ is Hb S, which loses solubility and polymerizes when deprived of oxygen. Upon deoxygenation most sickle cells accumulate polymer and lose deformability; some cells sickle; a fraction of cells become dehydrated, irreversibly sickled, and poorly deformable; and a few cells retain or accrue cytoadherence molecules on their surface. Dehydrated and highly adherent cells also may be generated by polymerization-independent processes. Vaso-occlusion, shown on the right, is initiated by adherent cells sticking to the vascular endothelium, thereby creating a nidus that traps rigid cells and facilitates polymerization.

and by Perutz and Mitchison, who discovered independently the reversible, deoxygenation-induced insolubility of Hb S solutions. The 1957 report by Ingram of the substitution of valine for glutamic acid as the sixth amino acid of β globin unified the electrophoretic and solubility abnormalities of Hb S. Thus the paradigm of molecular polymerization and cellular sickling evolved. Only the 1939 observation by Diggs and Bibb of a population of irreversibly sickled cells (ISC) that did not revert to discocytes upon reoxygenation (Fig. 137–2) hinted that polymerization alone may not totally explain sickle cell pathophysiology.

GENETICS, EVOLUTION, AND MALARIA

The inherited nature of sickle cell anemia was confirmed independently in 1949 by Beet and by Neel, who found that sickle cell anemia results from the homozygous inheritance of a genetic determinant from heterozygous parents. This was verified in the same year by the discovery of Pauling and associates that erythrocytes

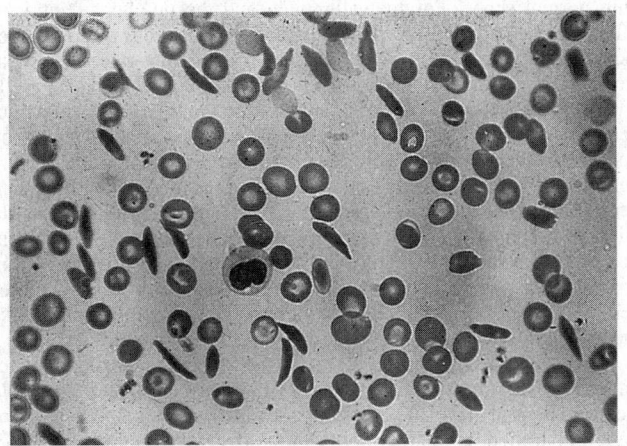

FIGURE 137-2. A peripheral blood smear showing the "peculiar elongated forms of the red corpuscles" originally reported by Herrick.

from patients with sickle cell anemia contain only Hb S and those from their parents contain both Hb S and Hb A. Consideration of the high frequency of both normal and sickle cell alleles in given populations led Allison to the concept of genetic polymorphism—the stable frequency of the sickle cell gene in areas of hyperendemic falciparum malaria was the result of balanced gene exclusion from early death of homozygotes and gene selection from protection of heterozygotes against death by malaria. The mechanism of this "heterozygous advantage" is not completely understood. Although children with sickle cell trait have a lower incidence of parasitemia, their red cells are parasitized at a normal rate. Thus, the inhospitable nature of Hb AS erythrocytes is manifest later in the symbiotic relationship. In this regard, replication of parasites is impaired by sickling and premature destruction of parasitized sickle cell trait red cells, cellular oxidation by iron released from denatured Hb S, depletion of cellular potassium, and deficient nutrition of parasites by Hb S. As a result of these influences, the worldwide distribution of sickle cell anemia mirrors the "malaria belt." In the United States, > 90% of patients are African American.

Near the β globin gene on chromosome 11 are a series of restriction fragment length polymorphisms (RFLP), combinations of which define ethnogeographic specific β globin haplotypes. The association of the sickle cell gene with five different haplotypes demonstrates the multiple occurrence of the sickle cell mutation among peoples of Senegal, Benin, Bantu, Cameroon, and Arab-Indian origins. No evidence suggests that these haplotypes have provided selective evolutionary pressures on the β^S gene. The effect of G6PD deficiency, another common African polymorphism, on the sickle cell gene remains controversial, but there is no apparent higher frequency of the mutant G6PD gene, greater hemolysis, or more frequent pain among males with coexistent sickle cell disease and G6PD deficiency.

PREVALENCE. The distribution and impact of the β^S gene have been influenced both by evolutionary pressures and by transmission via trade and slave routes. The prevalence of sickle cell trait is 8 to 10% among African-American newborns and as high as 25 to 30% in western Africa. Calculations based on the frequency among African Americans of the β^S (0.045), Hb C (β^C) (0.015), and β-thalassemia (0.004) genes indicate that in the United States

4000 to 5000 pregnancies are at risk for sickle cell disease each year. In Africa 120,000 babies with sickle cell disease are born annually.

PATHOPHYSIOLOGY

The combination of deoxygenation-induced polymerization of Hb S, sickling of erythrocytes, and increased viscosity of blood is the *sine qua non* of sickle cell disease. Despite this absolute requirement for Hb S polymerization, comprehensive valuations of sickle cell pathophysiology require consideration of additional pathophysiologic processes.

Hb S POLYMER. Although oxygenated Hb S and Hb A are equally soluble, the solubility of deoxygenated Hb S is severely reduced. The insolubility of deoxy-Hb S is related to the presence of valine rather than glutamic acid as the sixth amino acid of β^S globin and to the resultant increased surface hydrophobicity of Hb S molecules. Intermolecular bonding of deoxy-Hb S generates polymer filaments that associate into bundles that can be discerned by electron microscopy (Fig. 137–3). The bundles are 14-stranded, 21-nm-diameter fibers having basic structures consisting of seven filament pairs, one internal and six peripheral double strands. Analyses of the solubility of solutions containing Hb S and other variants having known amino acid substitutions and of Hb S crystal structure have revealed that one of the two β^6 valines forms a lateral contact with the β^{85} phenylalanine and β^{88} leucine in a hydrophobic pocket of an adjacent Hb S tetramer. Additional intermolecular bonds form axial and lateral contacts within double filaments and lateral contacts between double filaments. Differences in the surface hydrophobicities of Hb S and Hb F are responsible for the inhibitory effect of Hb F on Hb S polymerization.

POLYMERIZATION. The solubility of deoxy-Hb S is 17 grams per deciliter, far less than the usual 34 grams per deciliter concentration of hemoglobin within sickle erythrocytes. Upon deoxygenation, supersaturation, aggregation, and polymerization of deoxy-Hb S occur rapidly, with the progression from nuclear aggregation to polymer formation having a delay time inversely related to the 30th power of the deoxy-Hb S concentration. Resultant polymer fibers provide additional nuclei for further polymer formation. The effects of polymerization on sickle erythrocytes have been characterized using both kinetic and thermodynamic analyses, which concur that polymerization is detrimental and influenced by intracellular Hb S concentration. Kinetic interpretations hold that because delay times usually exceed capillary transit times, cells do not accumulate significant amounts of polymer until they are in a large vein where they cannot elicit vaso-occlusion. Evoking local vascular perturbations that cause unusual delays in the transit time allows extending this argument to explain all of sickle cell pathophysiology. Based on studies of the maximum quantity of polymer accrued over prolonged periods of equilibrium, thermodynamic arguments hold that individual deterministic parameters for each cell dictate the amount of polymer that will accumulate with each capillary transit. Kinetic explications best construe events in the majority of cells which have lower mean corpuscular hemoglobin concentrations (MCHC), lesser polymerization tendencies, and no persistent polymer when reoxygenated. Equilibrium interpretations are more applicable to a minor subpopulation of dehydrated sickle cells having very high MCHC, a strong tendency toward polymerization, and persistent polymer at arterial oxygen tensions.

INHERITED INFLUENCES ON POLYMERIZATION. The switch from γ to β globin production begins in the fetus and results in replacement of Hb F by adult Hb S. The retardant effect of Hb F on Hb S polymerization and cellular sickling masks the expression of sickle cell disease until approximately 6 months of age, when Hb S levels increase to around 75%. Preservation of high Hb F levels into adulthood similarly mitigates the course of sickle cell disease; that is, sickle cell–hereditary persistence of fetal hemoglobin (Hb S-HPFH) and sickle cell–β-thalassemia both have higher Hb F levels and milder clinical courses than sickle cell anemia. Polymerization is also influenced by elevated levels of Hb A_2 in sickle cell–β^0 or –β^+-thalassemia and by Hb A levels of 5 to 30% in sickle cell–β^+-thalassemia. Hb F inhibits polymerization 100 to 10,000 times more actively than Hb A does. This difference is accounted for by the exclusion of both Hb F and $\alpha_2\beta^S\gamma$ hybrid tetramers from polymer compared with the exclusion of Hb A and inclusion of $\alpha_2\beta^A\gamma$ hybrid tetramers. Another influence retarding polymerization in sickle cell–β-thalassemia is the lower intraerythrocytic Hb S concentration. Hematologic values for sickle cell anemia, the sickle cell–β-thalassemias, and Hb S-HPFH are shown in Table 137–1.

Alpha thalassemia also reduces the MCHC and influences certain aspects of sickle cell disease. The silent carrier of α-thalassemia syndrome (genotype $-\alpha/\alpha\alpha$) exists in about 30% of African Americans and α thalassemia trait (genotype $-\alpha/-\alpha$) in 2%. The lower intraerythrocytic concentrations of Hb S associated with either the $-\alpha/\alpha\alpha$ or the $-\alpha/-\alpha$ genotype modulate the hematologic, pathophysiologic, and clinical manifestations of disease, particularly the severity of anemia, which is diminished with either α thalassemia genotype after 7 years of age. Average hemoglobin levels associated with different α globin genotypes in adults are 7.9 grams per deciliter for $\alpha\alpha/\alpha\alpha$, 8.7 grams per deciliter for $-\alpha/\alpha\alpha$, and 9.0 grams per deciliter for $-\alpha/-\alpha$.

CELLULAR SICKLING. The increased viscosity of sickle cell suspensions when deoxygenated is associated with generation of deoxy-Hb S polymer and alteration of cellular morphology. Accrual of polymer is prompt and precedes changes in cell morphology during deoxygenation. With reoxygenation polymer is lost before cells regain normal shape. Polymer alignment and the number of intracellular polymer domains, which influence the rheologic properties of sickle cells, are affected by both deoxygenation rate and shear stress. During slow deoxygenation, classic crescent-shaped cells with a single domain of highly aligned polymer arise by homogeneous nucleation from a single nucleus; with faster deoxygenation holly-leaf–shaped cells with fewer and less-aligned domains are generated by heterogeneous nucleation from a few nuclei; and with very rapid deoxygenation granular cells with multiple poorly aligned domains are derived by heterogeneous nucleation from many nuclei. Shear stress during the delay period of polymerization creates more nucleation sites, shortens the delay time, and increases cell viscosity; shear applied after polymerization has begun breaks the polymer and diminishes viscosity.

IRREVERSIBLY SICKLED CELLS. Those cells that do not unsickle when reoxygenated, the ISC, are the least deformable sickle cells and have the shortest circulatory survival. Their rheologic impairment is related more to the effects of severe cellular dehydration on intraerythrocytic Hb S concentration, cytoplasmic viscosity, and polymerization tendency than to rigidly deformed

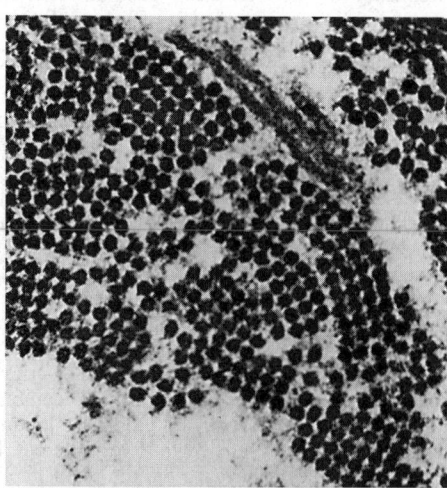
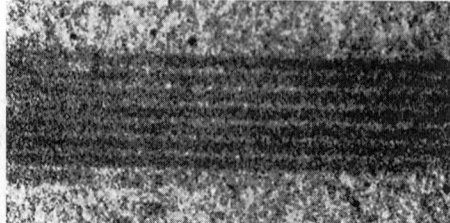

FIGURE 137–3. Electron micrographs of a centrifuge pellet of deoxy-Hb S ($\times$325,000). *Top,* Transverse section showing bundles of Hb S fibers. *Bottom,* Longitudinal section showing aligned fibers. (From Finch JT, et al.: Structure of sickled erythrocytes and sickle-cell hemoglobin fibers. Proc Natl Acad Sci USA 70:718, 1973.)

TABLE 137-1. HEMATOLOGIC VARIABLES ASSOCIATED WITH SICKLE CELL ANEMIA, THE SICKLE CELL-β-THALASSEMIA SYNDROMES, AND SICKLE CELL-HPFH

Genotype	Hb (gm/dL)	% Hb A	% Hb F	% Hb A$_2$	MCV	% Reticulocytes
Hb SS	7.83	0	4.56	2.87	85.9	10.18
Hb S-β^0-thal	8.85	0	5.86	5.02	69.3	7.2
Hb S-β^+-thal, type I	8.37	3–5	6.8	4.90	63.7	9.7
Hb S-β^+-thal, type II	10.28	8–14	5.2	4.68	70.0	6.6
Hb S-β^+-thal, type III	11.55	18–25	5.1	4.66	73.3	1.27
Hb S–HPFH	14.6	0	25.8	1.95	81.7	2.4

skeletal proteins. ISC had been assumed to be old cells damaged by repeated cycles of sickling and unsickling until Bertles and Milner found reticulocytes having very low Hb F contents among the ISC. Lacking the protective effects of Hb F against polymerization and sickling, these young RBC are predestined to rapid dehydration.

Sickled forms seen on the peripheral blood smear are ISC (see Fig. 137–2). Their number does not change with complications of disease such as the acute painful episode, is generally constant in individual patients, and correlates mainly with the degree of anemia. The presence of ISC on the peripheral smear is useful in diagnosing sickle cell syndromes; ISC exist in all sickle cell disease genotypes but not in sickle cell trait.

CATION HOMEOSTASIS AND CELL DEHYDRATION. During their brief survival in the circulation, sickle cells become dehydrated, some achieving MCHC > 50 grams per deciliter, which enhances polymerization materially. Several mechanisms contribute to sickle cell dehydration. The sodium-potassium pump, in attempting to restore the perturbations in cation homeostasis caused by deoxygenation-induced passive cation leaks, depletes cells of monovalent cations as a result of its fixed stoichiometry of three sodium ions pumped out for every two potassium ions pumped in. A more important cause of cell dehydration involves the interdependent actions of calcium-dependent potassium loss (Gardos pathway) and potassium-chloride cotransport on a population of calcium-sensitive reticulocytes. Gardos-mediated potassium efflux lowers the intracellular pH, thereby activating the volume-regulatory potassium-chloride cotransport activity, which further depletes cells of potassium and water.

Specific clinical complications demonstrate the importance of cell dehydration. First, the hematuria and diminished urine-concentrating ability of subjects with sickle cell trait demonstrate that even Hb AS cells sickle and occlude vessels when dehydrated in the 1300-mOsm environment of the renal medulla. Second, the clinical manifestations of Hb SC disease demonstrate that even heterozygous amounts of Hb S can cause clinical morbidity when the Hb S is sufficiently concentrated within the cell. The cellular dehydration effected by Hb C–induced potassium-chloride cotransport sufficiently increases intraerythrocytic Hb S concentration and polymerization that individuals with Hb SC disease, in contrast to those having sickle cell trait, have anemia and pain. Third, the interaction of α-thalassemia and sickle cell anemia is more important for broadening pathophysiologic interpretations than for recapitulating the polymerization principle. The less severe anemia associated with coexistent α thalassemia is related to better cell hydration, lower MCHC, fewer dense cells and ISC, and greater deformability of α-thalassemic sickle cells—all consistent with a retardant effect on polymerization. Yet, coexistent α-thalassemia is associated with more severe vaso-occlusion—more frequent pain and osteonecrosis and a higher mortality rate after the age of 20 years. These conflicting influences of α-thalassemia demonstrate the need for pathophysiologic understanding that includes polymerization-independent mechanisms and the fallacy of using polymerization formulae to predict clinical severity. Therapeutic strategies utilizing improved cellular hydration include pharmacologic preservation of sickle cell hydration using inhibitors of the Gardos phenomenon such as cetiedil citrate and clotrimazole.

OXIDATIVE DAMAGE. Besides having abnormal electrophoretic and solubility properties, Hb S is unstable. Its oxidation results in increased generation of methemoglobin, heme, and oxidative radicals. Resultant oxidative stresses affect RBC metabolism, membrane lipids, membrane proteins, and Hb S itself. Decreased

NADH redox potential, hexomonophosphate shunt activity, and GSH content contribute significantly to sickle cell pathobiology. Hemichrome aggregates on the cytoplasmic portion of band 3 initiate membrane coclustering of band 3 molecules, assembly of IgG and complement on their extracellular domains, and sickle cell adherence to macrophages and endothelial cells. Oxidative radicals oxidize spectrin, ankyrin, band 3, and band 4.1, disrupt membrane skeletons, and impair spectrin association into sickle cell membranes. Oxidative damage to membrane lipids causes their reduced lateral mobility in cell membranes and the loss of phosphatidylinositol-anchored complement-regulatory proteins of the membrane, such as DAF and MIRL.

SICKLE CELL ADHERENCE. The notion that vaso-occlusion is initiated by some process other than a stochastic polymerization happenstance is supported by two lines of evidence. First, severity of vaso-occlusive complications among patients correlates with the adhesivity of their sickle cells to vascular endothelial cells. Second, results of *ex vivo* flow studies indicate that vaso-occlusion is initiated by adherence of sickle cell reticulocytes to vascular endothelium and propagated by trapping of poorly deformable ISC (Fig. 137–4). The nidus provided by adherent sickle reticulocytes appears

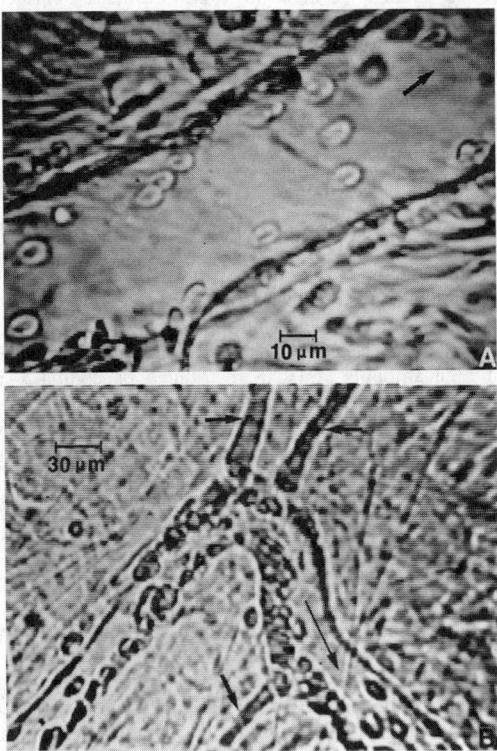

FIGURE 137–4. Adhesion of sickle erythrocytes in venules. *A*, Adherent discocytic sickle cells tethered to the endothelial wall of a venule and aligned in the direction of the flow *(arrow)*. *B*, Increased adherence of sickle cells at venule or bend and at junctions of smaller diameter postcapillary venules. The postcapillary vessels *(small arrows)* are totally blocked. Large arrow indicates flow direction. (From Kaul DK, et al.: Microvascular sites and characteristics of sickle cell adhesion to vascular endothelium in shear flow conditions: Pathophysiologic implications. Proc Natl Acad Sci USA 86:3356, 1989.)

sufficient for the prolonged transit time to exceed the delay time to polymerization. Sickle reticulocytes adhere to endothelial cells directly via $\alpha_4\beta_1$ integrins of reticulocytes and VCAM-1 of endothelial cells and indirectly through a variety of ligands, including unusually high molecular weight von Willebrand factor, immunoglobulin, fibronectin, fibrinogen, and thrombospondin. The most active ligand, thrombospondin, interacts with reticulocyte CD36 and both CD36 and the vitronectin receptor of endothelial cells. Increased endothelial expression of VCAM-1 and adhesivity of virus-infected endothelial cells may explain frequent painful episodes during viral illness.

COAGULATION ABNORMALITIES. The continuous perturbation and activation of the hemostatic system disease suggest that a steady state of normal vascular flow in sickle cells may be illusory. Ongoing platelet activation is demonstrated by chronically increased plasma levels of β-thromboglobulin and platelet factor 4, expression of activation-associated antigens on platelet membranes, reduced amounts of thrombospondin within circulating platelets, and increased urinary thromboxane levels. During acute vaso-occlusive episodes, reduced platelet counts, shortened platelet survival, and increased plasma thrombospondin levels evidence further platelet activation. Although findings of chronically abnormal levels of procoagulants, protein C, protein S, and antithrombin III have been inconstant, consistently high concentrations of fibrin degradation products suggest ongoing fibrinolysis.

One source of hemostatic activation specific for sickle cell disease is the phosphatidylserine contained in the outer membrane leaflet of ISC and deoxygenated reversibly sickled cells which is capable of activating the coagulation system. Phosphatidylserine-rich vesicles exovesiculated from sickle erythrocyte membranes during sickling are also capable of activating hemostasis. Activation of endothelial cells may also activate hemostasis. Increased thrombin levels stimulate endothelial cells to release von Willebrand factor, prostacyclin, plasminogen activators, and platelet-activating factor, to express tissue factor and cytoadhesive molecules, to promote vasoconstriction, and to activate thrombomodulin. Additional endothelial cell agonists germane to sickle cell disease further suggest the importance of endothelial cell pathobiology to sickle cell pathophysiology.

PATHOPHYSIOLOGY OF VASO-OCCLUSION. Polymerization of deoxy-Hb S is the *sine qua non* of sickle cell disease, and sickling of erythrocytes is its highly recognized accomplice. However, a critical assessment of polymerization and sickling as initiators of vaso-occlusion illustrates the need for a more comprehensive view of pathophysiology. Sickle cells become deoxygenated at least four times a minute, demonstrating that sickling is an assiduous, unrelenting process rather than a cataclysmic one. Moreover, the chronic activation of several processes involved in vaso-occlusion hints that the concept of a steady state in sickle cell disease is probably specious. Although the detrimental influence of high intraerythrocytic Hb S concentrations in Hb SC disease, the protective effect of high amounts of Hb F distributed pancellularly in sickle cell-HPFH, and the induction of vaso-occlusive complications by known precipitants of polymerization each supports the importance of polymerization, there are sufficient exceptions to this rule that polymerization may be regarded as necessary but not sufficient for vaso-occlusion. The "polymerization tendency" as a determinant of clinical severity is valid only as it predicts severity of anemia, as illustrated by the effect of α-thalassemia on sickle cell anemia wherein lower hemolytic rate improves the severity of anemia but resultant higher blood viscosity enhances vaso-occlusion. Furthermore, despite the considerable effect of high MCHC on polymerization within ISC, there is no greater frequency of pain in patients with high ISC number. Finally, *ex vivo* studies show that vaso-occlusion is initiated by low MCHC cells adhering to vascular endothelium (Fig. 137–4), not by the polymerization-prone ISC. Although polymerization tendencies provide a first approximation of sickle cell disease severity, transient changes in vascular flow are best understood in terms of a variety of pathophysiologic processes.

MECHANISMS OF HEMOLYSIS. Hemolysis of sickle cells is both extravascular and intravascular. The former is due to the effects of unstable Hb S and recurrent sickling on causing oxidative damage to cell membranes. Oxidatively denatured Hb S binds to the cytosolic portion of band 3, which induces adherence of IgG and complement to extracellular band 3, thereby promoting cell recognition by macrophages. Also, the very rigid ISC generated by recurrent sickling and by sickling-independent cell dehydration are trapped extravascularly, accounting for their short circulatory survival and correlation with the severity of anemia. Intravascular hemolysis accounts for one third of sickle cell destruction according to the levels of free plasma hemoglobin. One mechanism relates to sickling-induced exovesiculation of vesicles enriched in phosphatidylinositol-anchored membrane proteins, which depletes cells of complement-regulatory proteins and leaves them susceptible to complement-mediated lysis. A second mechanism relates to the mechanical fragility of cells, which accounts for accelerated hemolysis during exercise.

IMMUNE DEFICIT. The propensity of children with sickle cell disease to *Streptococcus pneumoniae* infection relates to their impaired splenic function and diminished serum opsonizing activity. The function of the spleen is deficient even before its eventual autoinfarction, but prior to the second decade function is restorable by transfusion. The greater the rate of hemolysis, the earlier the age at which splenic function is lost—sickle cell anemia > Hb SC disease > sickle cell–β^+-thalassemia. Opsonization defects and abnormalities of the alternate complement pathway coexist, but evidence of a causal relationship is lacking. The opsonic defect results from an abnormality in natural antibody response. The variable opsonic defects for different bacteria appear to depend on selective antibody requirements for their opsonization. The decreased titer of antibody against *S. pneumoniae* antigens following splenectomy in individuals without sickle cell disease suggests that splenic hypofunction may mediate opsonic deficiency in sickle cell disease.

CLINICAL MANIFESTATIONS

Clinical manifestations of sickle cell disease vary greatly between and among the disease genotypes. Even within the most severe genotype, sickle cell anemia, asymptomatic patients may be detected incidentally, whereas others are disabled by disease complications. The typical patient is anemic but asymptomatic except during painful episodes. Most organ systems are subject to vaso-occlusion, resulting in the characteristic acute and chronic multisystem failure. Important clinical features less directly related to vaso-occlusion are growth retardation, psychosocial problems, and susceptibility to infection. Therapeutic interventions are directed to the specific complications at hand.

LIFE EXPECTANCY. Decreased life expectancy is one of the original correlates of sickle cell disease. In contrast with the mean life-expectancy of 14.3 years posited by Diggs in 1973, the current survival is 42 years for men and 48 years for women with sickle cell anemia. This improved survival is more the result of better general medical care than of specific antisickling therapy. The effect of prophylactic penicillin therapy on preventing mortality from *S. pneumoniae* bacteremia is now influencing survival.

CHRONIC ANEMIA. Sickle cells are destroyed randomly, with a mean lifespan of 17 days. ISC survival is sufficiently shorter than the mean that the overall hemolytic rate reflects the fraction of ISC. The severity of anemia is most severe in sickle cell anemia and Hb S–β^0-thalassemia, milder in Hb S–β^+-thalassemia and Hb SC disease, and, among patients with sickle cell anemia, less severe in those who have coexistent α-thalassemia. In addition to hemolysis, inappropriately low erythropoietin levels contribute to anemia.

EXACERBATIONS OF ANEMIA. The rather constant level of hemolytic anemia may be exacerbated by any of several causes, most commonly aplastic crises. Aplastic crises are transient arrests of erythropoiesis characterized by abrupt falls in hemoglobin levels, reticulocyte number, and red cell precursors in the marrow. These episodes typically last only a few days, but the anemia may become severe as hemolysis continues in the absence of red cell production. Although general mechanisms that impair erythropoiesis in inflammation obtain in infections of all types, parvovirus B19 specifically invades proliferating erythroid progenitors, accounting for its importance in sickle cell disease. Parvovirus B19 infection accounts for 68% of aplastic crises in children with sickle cell disease, but the high frequency of protective antibodies in adults makes parvovirus a less frequent cause of aplastic crises in this age group. Bone marrow necrosis, with attendant fever, bone pain, reticulocytopenia, and leukoerythroblastic response, also causes aplastic crisis. It too may be due to parvovirus infection. High oxygen tensions associated with oxygen inhalation suppress erythropoietin production promptly and impair red cell production within 2 days. Red cell transfusion is the main therapeutic modality for aplastic crises. When cardiorespiratory symptoms indicate transfusion, a single transfusion usually suffices, as reticulocytosis soon resumes spontaneously. Transfusion sometimes may be avoided by enforcing bed rest and avoiding unnecessary oxygen therapy in the severely anemic.

Acute splenic sequestration is characterized by acute exacerbation of anemia, persistent reticulocytosis, a tender enlarging spleen, and sometimes hypovolemia. Those whose spleens have not undergone fibrosis are at risk—young patients with sickle cell anemia and adults with Hb SC disease or sickle cell–β^+-thalassemia. Thirty percent of children had splenic sequestration over a 10-year period, and 15% of the attacks were fatal. Transfusion is given to restore blood volume and red cell mass. Splenic sequestration recurs in 50% of cases, so splenectomy is recommended after the acute event. Acute sequestration may also occur in the liver.

Hyperhemolytic crisis is associated with a sudden exacerbation of anemia and increased reticulocytosis and bilirubin level. Apparent hyperhemolytic crises are usually occult splenic sequestration or aplastic crises detected during the resolving reticulocytosis. Actual hyperhemolysis may occur with coexistent G6PD deficiency.

Chronic exacerbations of anemia may be related to incipient renal insufficiency or lack of folic acid or iron. Inadequate erythropoietin production in renal failure limits compensation for hemolysis and has been treated using recombinant human erythropoietin. Chronic hemolysis consumes folic acid stores, which may result in megaloblastic crises. The combination of nutritional deficiency and urinary iron losses may result in iron deficiency. This diagnosis may be obscured by the elevated serum iron levels associated with chronic hemolysis and often depends upon finding low serum ferritin or elevated serum transferrin levels.

THE ACUTE PAINFUL EPISODE. The acute painful episode of sickle cell disease was originally called by Diggs "sickle cell crisis." Acute pain is often the first symptom of disease, is the most frequent complication after the newborn period, and is the most common cause of patients seeking medical attention. Although there is a general association between vaso-occlusive severity and genotype, tremendous variability exists within genotypes and in the same patient over time. One third of patients with sickle cell anemia rarely have pain, one third are hospitalized for pain two to six times per year, and one third have more than six pain-related hospitalizations per year. The frequency of pain is highest in the third and fourth decade, and after the second decade frequent pain is associated with increased mortality rates. High hemoglobin and low Hb F levels are associated with more frequent pain. Because 5% of patients account for one third of emergency room visits, emergency department personnel gain a biased view from a small minority of patients whose severe course is dictated by specific hematologic determinants.

Pain may be precipitated by cold, dehydration, infection, stress, menses, or alcohol consumption, but the cause of most episodes is indeterminate. Pain affects any area of the body, most commonly the back, chest, extremities, and abdomen. Severity varies from trifling to agonizing, and the duration is usually a few days. Although painful episodes are caused by vaso-occlusion, pain is an affect that consists of sensory, perceptual, cognitive, and emotional components. Frequent pain may cause despair, depression, and apathy, which predisposes to an existence that revolves around pain—a chronic debilitating pain syndrome.

Half of painful episodes are associated with objective clinical signs—fever, swelling, tenderness, tachypnea, hypertension, nausea, and vomiting. Potential laboratory indicators are a decline in the dense fraction of sickle cells and an increase in overall red cell deformability, acute phase reactants, serum lactate dehydrogenase (LDH), interleukin-1, tumor necrosis factor, and serum viscosity. Clinical application of these tests requires baseline data with which to compare acute variations.

PSYCHOSOCIAL ISSUES. Modern approaches to the psychosocial problems of patients with sickle cell disease often enable therapeutic intervention. Although most patients are generally well-adjusted, there exist risks of depression, low self-esteem, poor family relationships, and social isolation. Particular challenges to psychosocial adjustment are recurrent pain and the response to it, limitation of activity due to pain, misinterpretation of the meaning

of pain, and depression leading to learned helplessness. Some patients become addicted to narcotics, but this is uncommon and most often the result of social influences rather than analgesia therapy. Signs of good adjustment are active coping strategies and support from the family and the extended family unit common in African-American society. Interventional approaches stress recognizing and reinforcing individual strengths, confronting pathologic behavior, and establishing coping skills such as reinterpreting pain, diverting attention from pain, and using support systems. Attention to psychosocial welfare is critical to the health and integration into society of patients with sickle cell disease.

GROWTH AND DEVELOPMENT. Growth retardation affects weight more than height and has no clear gender difference. By adulthood normal height is achieved, but weight remains abnormally low. More severe growth delay is noted in children with sickle cell anemia and sickle cell–β^0-thalassemia than with Hb SC disease. Skeletal maturation is also delayed. Incidence of retarded sexual maturation is greater in sickle cell anemia and sickle cell–β^0-thalassemia than in Hb SC disease or sickle cell–β^+-thalassemia. It is associated with elevated gonadotropin levels for the stage of sexual development and, in girls, with delayed menarche. Retarded sexual maturation in males can be the result of primary hypogonadism, hypopituitarism, or hypothalamic insufficiency. Impaired development may be the effect of hemolysis on increasing basal metabolic requirements. In severe delayed growth and development, hormonal therapy may be tailored to the specific deficit.

INFECTIONS. Infectious complications of sickle cell disease are a major cause of morbidity and mortality. The specific organisms affecting different target organs are shown in Table 137–2.

S. pneumoniae, the most common cause of bacteremia in children with sickle cell disease, is accompanied by leukocytosis, a "left shift," aplastic crisis, sometimes disseminated intravascular coagulopathy (DIC), and a 20 to 50% mortality rate. The second most common cause of bacteremia, *Haemophilus influenzae* type b, affects older children, is less fulminant, but also may be fatal. Results of pneumococcal vaccination have been disappointing, but *H. influenzae* type b vaccination, prophylactic penicillin, and the long-acting, broad-spectrum antibiotic ceftriaxone have favorably impacted childhood bacteremia. Prophylactic penicillin beginning in infancy has reduced the incidence of *S. pneumoniae* bacteremia in newborns by 84%, and its use is standard. Disadvantages of this approach include impaired anti–*S. pneumoniae* antibody production, uncertainty regarding the safety of discontinuing prophylaxis, and the emergence of penicillin-resistant microorganisms. The efficacy of ceftriaxone for *S. pneumoniae* and *H. influenzae* infection has led to increased outpatient therapy in children with fevers. Urinary tract infections and bacteremia in older patients are more likely due to *Escherichia coli* and other gram-negative organisms.

Meningitis in sickle cell anemia is primarily a problem of infants and young children, and *S. pneumoniae* is the most frequent cause. Because meningitis occurs commonly in association with bacteremia, rapid administration of antibiotics for bacteremia has resulted in a much lower incidence of meningitis. *H. influenzae* type b is a less common cause of meningitis.

Bacterial pneumonia is one cause of the acute chest syndrome. Patients with any combination of dyspnea, cough, chest pain, fever, tachypnea, and leukocytosis, should be evaluated by chest radiography, arterial blood gases, blood and sputum culture, cold agglutinins, and serologic study for *Mycoplasma pneumoniae*, *Chlamydia*, and *Legionella*. *S. pneumoniae* and *H. influenzae* type b are uncommon causes of acute chest syndrome. *M. pneumoniae* and *C. pneumoniae* account for approximately 20%. Antibiotic therapy should cover these agents. General therapeutic approaches for the acute chest syndrome are presented in the section on pulmonary complications.

Osteomyelitis occurs more commonly in sickle cell disease, probably owing to infection of infarcted bone. Among sickle cell patients osteomyelitis is commonly caused by *Salmonella* species. *Staphylococcus aureus* accounts for < 25% of cases. Infection is often at multiple sites in long bones. Diagnosis is made by culture of blood or infected bone before parenteral antibiotics covering *Salmonella* and *S. aureus* are begun. Articular infection is less common and is often due to *S. pneumoniae.*

TABLE 137–2. ORGAN-RELATED INFECTION IN SICKLE CELL DISEASE

Primary Sites of Infection	Most Common Pathogens	Other Pathogens	Pathophysiology	Prevention	Management
Septicemia	S. pneumoniae	H. influenzae type b E. coli Salmonella spp.	Defective splenic function; deficiency of opsonic antibody	Vaccines* Prophylactic penicillin	Empiric intravenous antibiotics for fever
Meningitis	S. pneumoniae		————————————Same as for septicemia————————————		
Osteomyelitis and septic arthritis	Salmonella spp. S. pneumoniae	E. coli Proteus spp. S. aureus	Ischemic or infarcted tissue	—	Surgical drainage; prolonged course of intravenous antibiotics
Pneumonia	M. pneumoniae Respiratory viruses	C. pneumoniae S. pneumoniae	Concomitant infection and intrapulmonary vaso-occlusion leading to infarction and/or sequestration	Vaccines*	See Pulmonary and Therapy sections for management of chest syndrome

* Against S. pneumoniae and H. influenzae type b

From Buchanan GR: Infections. In Embury SH, Hebbel RP, Mohandas N, Steinberg MH (eds.): Sickle Cell Disease: Basic Principles and Clinical Practice. New York, Raven Press, 1994.

NEUROLOGIC COMPLICATIONS. Neurologic complications occur in 25% of patients with sickle cell disease, and common events are transient ischemic attacks (TIA), cerebral infarction, cerebral hemorrhage, seizures, and unexplained coma.

In patients with sickle cell disease cerebrovascular accident (CVA) may occur spontaneously or intercurrently with complications such as pneumonia, aplastic crises, painful episodes, or dehydration. Those at higher risk for CVA have more severe anemia, higher reticulocyte counts, lower Hb F levels, higher WBC counts, and sickle cell anemia rather than Hb SC disease or sickle cell–β thalassemia. Genetic markers of increased risk are the Central African Republic haplotype and the absence of α thalassemia. Cerebral thrombosis accounts for 70 to 80% of CVA and is due to large vessel occlusion rather than the microvascular occlusion commonly associated with sickle cell disease. CVA may be heralded by focal seizures or TIA, is fatal in approximately 20% of cases, recurs within 3 years in nearly 70%, and frequently causes motor and cognitive impairment.

Intracranial hemorrhage more commonly causes neck stiffness, photophobia, severe headache, vomiting, and altered consciousness. Coma is more frequently associated with hemorrhage than with thrombosis, and the combination of coma and seizures but no hemiparesis strongly suggests hemorrhage. The mortality rate with hemorrhage is 50%, but the morbidity of survivors is low. Many patients with sickle cell disease develop collateral vessels that appear as puffs of smoke ("moyamoya" in Japanese) on angiography. These friable pseudomoyamoya are vulnerable to both thrombosis and hemorrhage. The favorable neurosurgical outcome in subarachnoid hemorrhage from ruptured aneurysm justifies aggressive diagnosis, transfusion, vasodilatory therapy, and surgery.

Patients presenting with symptoms and signs of CVA are evaluated immediately by computed tomography scanning or magnetic resonance (MR) imaging to distinguish TIA, cerebral thrombosis, and hemorrhage. In hemorrhage, angiography is performed after a partial exchange transfusion to avoid complications associated with injected contrast material. In thrombosis, prompt partial exchange transfusion is performed; chronic direct transfusion to maintain the Hb S level below 30% is instituted to prevent recurrent thrombosis and promote resolution of arterial stenoses. Transfusion therapy provides the current best means of preventing recurrence. Transfusion may be required indefinitely for those with persistent flow abnormalities after 5 years of transfusion and for those whose flow abnormalities recur soon after discontinuing therapy.

MR imaging and transcranial Doppler flow studies are useful in detecting subclinical cerebral infarction and may be useful in predicting CVA. Neurodevelopmental abnormalities often result from silent cerebral infarcts, and the institution of transfusion therapy upon detection of premorbid lesions has been suggested.

PULMONARY COMPLICATIONS. The acute chest syndrome consists of dyspnea, chest pain, fever, tachypnea, leukocytosis, and pulmonary infiltrate on radiography. It affects approximately 30% of patients with sickle cell disease and may be life-threatening. The usual causes are vaso-occlusion, infection, and pulmonary fat embolus from infarcted marrow. Microbial pathogens are more commonly isolated in children. Often when common pathogens are not cultured one of the "atypical" agents—Mycoplasma, Chlamydia, or Legionella—is responsible, which suggests a therapeutic role for erythromycin. Pulmonary fat embolism has a severe clinical course and can be diagnosed by positive staining for fat in sputum macrophages. When patients have a progressive course associated with severely decreased arterial oxygen tension, intensive care may be required. When arterial oxygen tension cannot be maintained above 70 mm Hg using inhaled oxygen, partial exchange transfusion is indicated.

Evaluation of chronic pulmonary status in patients with sickle cell anemia may reveal restrictive lung disease, hypoxemia, and pulmonary hypertension singly or in combination, often preceded by a history of acute chest syndrome. Causes unrelated to prior acute episodes may relate to chronic vascular insufficiency. Blood gas and pulmonary function measurements should be obtained as baseline data.

HEPATOBILIARY COMPLICATIONS. Pigmented gallstones develop as a result of the chronic hemolysis of sickle cell disease and eventually occur in at least 70% of patients. Because of the advent of laparoscopic cholecystectomy, surgery for asymptomatic gallstones has become a feasible approach for avoiding subsequent confusion of gallbladder pain with acute painful episodes.

Chronic hepatomegaly and liver dysfunction caused by trapping of sickle cells, transfusion-acquired infection, and iron overload are associated with centrilobular parenchymal atrophy, accumulation of bile pigment, periportal fibrosis, hemosiderosis, and cirrhosis. In acute hepatic events the combination of hemolysis, hepatic dysfunction, and renal tubular defects often results in dramatically high serum bilirubin levels, sometimes exceeding 100 mg per deciliter. Acute hepatic complications may result from viral hepatitis; benign cholestasis, which causes severe hyperbilirubinemia but not fever, pain, or mortality; and ischemic "hepatic crisis," which causes severe hyperbilirubinemia, fever, pain, abnormal liver function tests, and hepatic failure.

OBSTETRIC AND GYNECOLOGIC ISSUES. The major reproductive concern in patients with sickle cell disease is pregnancy. Fetal complications of pregnancy relate to impaired placental blood flow and include spontaneous abortion, intrauterine growth retardation, low birth weight, preeclampsia, and death. Maternal complications include increased rates of painful episodes and infections, severe anemia, and death. Prophylactic transfusions do not improve fetal outcome, and their routine application is not recommended. Oral contraceptives containing low-dose estrogen are a safe and recommended method of birth control. Barrier methods and injections of medroxyprogesterone every 3 months may also be useful.

RENAL COMPLICATIONS. Renal complications result from medullary, distal tubular, proximal tubular, and glomerular abnormalities. Occlusion of the vasa rectae compromises blood flow to the medulla, causing impaired urinary concentrating ability, papillary infarction, hematuria, incomplete renal tubular acidosis, and abnormal potassium clearance. Isosthenuria is reversible with red cell transfusion up to the age of 15 years. Patients with sickle cell disease or trait who have hematuria should be evaluated by ultrasonography to exclude life-threatening causes. Therapeutic options include standard hydration, alkalization of the urine, and diuresis. In unresponsive cases ε-aminocaproic acid, triglycyl vasopressin, intravenous distilled water, and nephrectomy have been used.

Proximal tubular dysfunction may result in hyperuricemia and is aggravated by chronic use of analgesics.

Glomerular abnormalities result from vaso-occlusion, hyperperfusion, and immune complex nephropathy. Hypertension, proteinuria, hyperkalemia, and worsening anemia may herald chronic renal insufficiency, the average age of onset of which is 23 years in sickle cell anemia and 50 years in Hb SC disease. Angiotensin-converting enzyme inhibitors diminish hyperperfusion and proteinuria but do not increase glomerular filtration rate. Renal transplantation is effective therapy for end-stage renal disease.

PRIAPISM. Priapism, an unwanted painful erection, affects nearly two thirds of males with sickle cell disease and strikes most commonly between the ages of 5 and 13 years and 21 and 29 years. Its onset can be acute, recurrent, chronic, or "stuttering." In the priapism of sickle cell disease, the corpora cavernosa are usually engorged and the glans penis and corpus spongiosum are spared. In a minority of patients there is tricorporal priapism, which can be diagnosed using nuclear scanning of the penis. Priapism, particularly tricorporal priapism, may eventuate in impotence.

Therapy can be monitored by intercavernous pressure measurements. If there is no response to 12 hours of intravenous hydration and analgesia, partial exchange transfusion is employed. If there is still no resolution within 12 hours, corporal aspiration with saline and α-adrenergic agents is used. If there is no response within the next 12 hours, surgical creation of a fistula between the glans penis and the corpora cavernosa by inserting a large bore needle through the glans—the Winter procedure—is performed. Recurrences may be prevented using diethylstilbestrol. Forty-five percent of patients who develop priapism develop some degree of impotence.

OCULAR COMPLICATIONS. Ophthalmologic features include tortuosity of conjunctival vessels, anterior chamber ischemia, retinal artery occlusion, angioid streaks, proliferative retinopathy, and retinal detachment and hemorrhage. The earlier onset and greater frequency of proliferative retinopathy in Hb SC disease and sickle cell–β^+-thalassemia than in sickle cell anemia and sickle cell–β^0-thalassemia suggest that retinal vessels are more vulnerable to occlusion by more viscous blood. Regular retinal examination is part of routine health care maintenance. The retinopathy is often seen best using fluorescein angiography. Peripheral sickle retinopathy may require therapy with laser photocoagulation.

BONE COMPLICATIONS. Osteonecrosis may cause compression of vertebrae, shortening of cuboidal bones of the hands and feet, and acute "aseptic" or "avascular" necrosis. The painful bone infarction of the "hand-foot syndrome" is often the first symptom of sickle cell disease. Bone infarcts may be detected by nuclear medicine scintigraphy or MR imaging. Bone marrow infarction may be distinguished from osteomyelitis using scans that specifically idencity osteoclasts, bone marrow macrophages, and inflammatory cells, but cultures obtained directly from the affected tissue must be obtained before starting antibiotic therapy for osteomyelitis.

Osteonecrosis is most sensitively detected by MR imaging. Necrosis of femoral heads commonly progresses to joint destruction, which may be prevented by core decompression surgery to relieve increased intraosseous pressure. In advanced disease the options are to accept limited joint mobility or attempt major reconstructive therapy. Among the sickle cell syndromes, osteonecrosis occurs most frequently in sickle cell anemia with coexistent α thalassemia.

Arthritic pain, swelling, and effusion may be the result of periarticular infarction or gouty arthritis. Nonsteroidal anti-inflammatory agents are useful therapies.

Bone marrow infarction may cause reticulocytopenia, exacerbation of anemia, a leukoerythroblastic picture, and sometimes pancytopenia. It may also cause pulmonary fat embolism, which has a severe clinical course.

DERMATOLOGIC COMPLICATIONS. Leg ulcers begin spontaneously or as a result of trauma, arise near the medial or lateral malleolus, and frequently occur bilaterally. They may become infected and cause systemic infection, osteomyelitis, or tetanus. They rarely occur before the age of 10 years and are less frequent in those who have coexistent α thalassemia. Males have a threefold greater incidence. Ulcers are resistant to healing and recur in well over half the cases. Treatment requires weeks for healing. Initial therapy is intended to remove nonviable, superficial tissue using wet-to-dry dressings or Duoderm hydrocolloid dressings. After debridement, zinc oxide–impregnated Unna boots are applied. Bed rest, elastic wraps, and leg elevation control edema and facilitate healing.

The myofascial syndromes consists of soft tissue swelling and subcutaneous edema, which may cause a "peau d'orange" appearance. These may be large or only a few centimeters in diameter, are probably the result of dermal or subdermal vaso-occlusion, and are treated symptomatically.

CARDIAC COMPLICATIONS. Although no cardiomyopathy is specific for sickle cell disease, management of sickle cell patients often involves cardiac considerations. The high cardiac output compensation for anemia results in chamber enlargement and cardiomegaly even in childhood. Despite diminished exercise capacity and progressive loss of cardiac reserve, overt congestive heart failure is uncommon in sickle cell patients until they are stressed with volume overload, exacerbations of anemia, or hypertension. There are reports of acute myocardial infarction without coronary disease, and myocardial infarction was found in 17% of 70 consecutive autopsies. When the demand for oxygen exceeds the limited capacity for oxygen delivery, myocardial infarction may ensue despite normal coronary arteries.

VARIANT SICKLE CELL SYNDROMES

Sickle cell syndromes result from simple heterozygous inheritance of the sickle cell gene (i.e., sickle cell trait) and from its compound heterozygous inheritance with other mutant β globin genes (e.g., Hb SC disease, sickle cell–β-thalassemia). Sickle cell anemia with coinherited α-thalassemia and other sickle cell syndromes are reviewed in this section.

SICKLE CELL TRAIT. The approximate prevalence of sickle cell trait is 9% in African Americans and 25 to 30% in regions of western Africa. Those heterozygous for the sickle cell gene number approximately 2.5 million in the United States and 30 million in the world. Sickle cell trait is a benign carrier condition with no hematologic manifestations. Sickle forms (ISC) are not seen on the peripheral blood smear. The fractional partition of Hb A and Hb S is usually 60:40 due to a greater post-translational affinity of α chains for β^A than for β^S chains. Coinheritance of α thalassemia results in decreasing percentages of Hb S according to the number of α-globin genes deleted (i.e., 40%, 35%, 29%, and 21% Hb S, respectively, for the genotypes $\alpha\alpha/\alpha\alpha$, $-\alpha/\alpha\alpha$, $-\alpha/-\alpha$, and $--/-\alpha$), owing to the effect of fewer α chains on the preferential affinity for β^A.

Few clinical complications are associated with sickle cell trait. Splenic infarction at high altitude affects Caucasians with sickle cell trait more frequently than those of African ancestry. Sickle cell trait is a common cause of hematuria among African Americans. The impaired urine-concentrating ability is directly related to the intraerythrocytic concentration of Hb S, inversely related to the presence of α thalassemia, and reversed by transfusion up to age 8 years. There is no increased incidence of anesthetic complications. The 30-fold greater frequency of unexplained sudden death in military recruits during basic training is the result of exercise-induced vaso-occlusion and rhabdomyolysis.

Despite its known complications, the rare clinical events do not justify regarding sickle cell trait as anything but a benign carrier condition. Newborn screening programs identify infants with sickle cell trait whose parents require genetic counseling. Parents must understand that their child has a benign hereditary condition, not a disease, but that there may be a risk for a subsequent child to be born with sickle cell disease.

Certain individuals appear to have sickle cell trait but are symptomatic. In these the diagnosis must be verified. Rare hemoglobins other than S may polymerize and account for reports of symptomatic "sickle cell trait," such as heterozygous Hb S^Antilles and Hb Quebec–CHORI.

HB SC DISEASE. The prevalence of Hb SC disease among African Americans is one third that of sickle cell anemia, because the frequency of the Hb C gene ($\alpha_2\beta_2^{6Glu \rightarrow Lys}$, β^C) is approximately one third that of the β^S gene. Although oxy-Hb C forms crystals, Hb C does not participate in deoxy-Hb S polymerization. The fundamental contribution of Hb C to sickle erythrocyte pathobiology is the sustained potassium-chloride cotransport that induces cellular desiccation, thereby raising intraerythrocytic Hb S concentrations to levels that support polymerization, sickling, and clinical symptoms.

As a result of a longer circulatory survival of Hb SC red cells (27 days versus 17 days for Hb SS RBC), the degrees of anemia and reticulocytosis are frequently milder. Target cells predominate on the peripheral smear. ISC, folded (Pita bread) cells, "billiard ball" cells, and crystal-containing cells also are found. The clinical heterogeneity within the Hb SC genotype notwithstanding, the clinical course is generally milder than that of sickle cell anemia. The frequency of painful episodes is approximately half and the life expectancy 20 years longer than those of sickle cell anemia. The incidence of fatal bacterial infection is less than in sickle cell anemia, and leg ulcers are uncommon. There is a higher incidence of proliferative sickle retinopathy in Hb SC disease, but the reported higher incidence of osteonecrosis has been questioned.

SICKLE CELL–β-THALASSEMIA. The prevalence of compound heterozygous sickle cell–β-thalassemia among African Americans is one-tenth that of sickle cell anemia, because the frequency of β-thalassemia genes is one-tenth that of the β^S gene. Sickle cell–β-thalassemia is composed of sickle cell–β^+-thalassemia and sickle cell–β^0-thalassemia, which have, respectively, reduced amounts or no Hb A present. Sickle cell–β^+-thalassemia is subclassified according to the percentage of Hb A present: Type I has 3 to 5%, type II has 8 to 14%, and type III has 18 to 25% (see Table 137–1). Eighty per cent of African-American β-thalassemia is due to the -88 (C → T) and -29 (A → G) promoter region mutations that result in the type III phenotype.

Sickle cell–β-thalassemia red cells are hypochromic and microcytic. The ISC present on the peripheral blood smear are more numerous in sickle cell–β^0-thalassemia than in sickle cell–β^+-thalassemia. The hematologic severity is a function of the amount of Hb A inherited, as demonstrated in Table 137–1. The clinical nature of sickle cell–β^+-thalassemia is also more benign than that of sickle cell–β^0-thalassemia, as reflected by its threefold higher incidence of incidental diagnosis, later age of presentation, threefold less frequent leg ulcers, half as frequent acute chest syndrome, lower frequency of priapism and aplastic crisis, and less severe retardation of growth and development. Splenomegaly occurs in approximately one third of both groups. Proliferative retinopathy is more frequent in sickle cell–β^+-thalassemia, consistent with the notion that those sickle cell syndromes associated with higher hematocrits have more frequent ocular complications.

SICKLE CELL ANEMIA WITH COEXISTENT α-THALASSEMIA. The α globin gene deletion responsible for α-thalassemia among African Americans, the α-thalassemia-2 haplotype ($-\alpha$), has a frequency of 0.16 in this population. This high frequency combined with the powerful effect of Hb S concentration on polymerization originally suggested that the lower MCHC of thalassemia would influence a large number of patients with sickle cell anemia. This notion was substantiated by the finding of milder anemia in sickle cell anemia associated with the deletion of either one (genotype $-\alpha/\alpha\alpha$) or two (genotype $-\alpha/-\alpha$) α globin genes.

In addition to less rapid hemolysis and milder anemia, α-thalassemia is associated with fewer reticulocytes and ISC. Clear-cut clinical effects are less certain. There is a decreased incidence of leg ulcers and CVA but an *increased* incidence of osteonecrosis and frequency of acute painful episodes. The increased mortality rate associated with higher hemoglobin levels after the age of 20 years is the clearest detrimental effect associated with α-thalassemia and the best illustration of the invalidity of extrapolating from polymerization formulas to disease severity.

SICKLE CELL–δβ-THALASSEMIA. The δβ-thalassemia locus is one of several large deletions of the δ and β globin genes. It allows the switch from fetal to adult hemoglobin production, which in this case is an attempted switch in expression of γ globin genes to that of deleted genes. This is an uncommon compound heterozygous condition that is associated with Hb S, F, and A_2. The 15 to 25% Hb F is distributed heterocellularly. Anemia is mild and clinical complications are infrequent.

SICKLE CELL–HPFH. Hereditary persistence of fetal hemoglobin (HPFH) results from one of several large deletions of the δ and β globin genes which retard the switch from the production of Hb F to adult hemoglobin. Another type of HPFH is due to one of many nucleotide substitutions that upregulate the expression of the γ globin gene. The clinical expression of deletional and nondeletional HPFH differs in that heterozygosity for the former results in 15 to 35% Hb F distributed pancellularly and for the latter in 1 to 5% Hb F distributed heterocellularly. Certain mild varieties of HPFH do not express high Hb F levels in simple heterozygosity but do with erythropoietic stress, such as compound heterozygosity with the β^S gene. The gene frequency of deletional HPFH among African Americans is 0.0005, resulting in an incidence of sickle cell–deletional HPFH that is 1% that of sickle cell anemia. Individuals with the pancellular distribution of 25% Hb F associated with sickle cell–deletional HPFH are neither anemic (see Table 137–1) nor afflicted with vaso-occlusive manifestations—a finding that provided the first evidence that Hb F inhibits Hb S polymerization. Hemoglobin electrophoresis reveals only Hb S, F, and A_2, which resembles sickle cell anemia, sickle cell–β^0-thalassemia, and sickle cell–δβ-thalassemia, except for the pancellular distribution of 15 to 35% Hb F and Hb A_2 levels <2.5%.

SICKLE CELL–Hb LEPORE DISEASE. The Hb Lepore gene is a crossover fusion product of the δ and β globin genes, the product of which has the same electrophoretic mobility as Hb S. Thalassemic expression of the Hb Lepore gene results in only 12% Hb Lepore in simple heterozygotes. Compound heterozygous Hb S–Hb Lepore is similar to sickle cell anemia or sickle cell–β^0-thalassemia on electrophoresis, but the anemia is less severe. The combination of predominantly Hb S with microcytosis suggests sickle cell–β-thalassemia, but low to low-normal Hb A_2 levels due to crossover-incapacitation of one δ globin gene suggest Hb S–Hb Lepore. The peripheral smear reveals microcytosis, hypochromia, and ISC. Vaso-occlusive complications and splenomegaly occur.

SICKLE CELL–Hb D DISEASE. Hb SD disease was first reported as an unusual case of sickle cell anemia, because Hb D Punjab and Hb D Los Angeles ($\alpha_2\beta_2^{121Glu \rightarrow Gln}$) have alkaline electrophoretic mobility similar to that of Hb S. Hb D is distinguishable from Hb S by acid electrophoresis or isoelectric focusing. The peripheral smear shows marked anisocytosis and poikilocytosis, target cells, and ISC. There is moderately severe hemolytic anemia, and the clinical manifestations are similar to those of sickle cell anemia.

SICKLE CELL–Hb O ARAB DISEASE. Hb O Arab ($\alpha_2\beta_2^{121Glu \rightarrow Lys}$) was first described in an Israeli Arab family, but its distribution is widespread. On alkaline electrophoresis Hb S–O Arab disease resembles Hb SC disease, but either acid electrophoresis or isoelectric focusing distinguishes Hb O Arab from Hb C. There is moderately severe hemolytic anemia, and anisocytosis, poikilocytosis, and ISC are found on the peripheral smear.

SICKLE CELL–Hb E DISEASE. Hb E ($\alpha_2\beta_2^{26Glu \rightarrow Lys}$) is a β-thalassemic hemoglobinopathy found predominantly among Southeast Asians. Hb E has an electrophoretic mobility similar to Hb A_2, C, and O Arab under alkaline conditions but can be resolved by acid electrophoresis or isoelectric focusing. The codon 26 GAG → AAG mutation activates a cryptic splice site in the first exon, which decreases expression of the β^E gene. Hb E constitutes 30% of the hemoglobin in Hb SE disease. Although Hb SE disease has been reported to cause mild hemolysis, no vaso-occlusive complications, and no remarkable abnormality of red blood cell morphology, sufficient experience to the contrary indicates that Hb SE disease should be included among the sickle cell diseases.

DIAGNOSIS

Methods of diagnosing sickle cell syndromes and goals of diagnostic programs vary with developmental stage. In fetal and newborn periods the predominance of Hb F confounds characterization of the adult hemoglobins present. As Hb S increases and Hb F declines in infancy, clinical manifestations of sickle cell anemia emerge—ISC appear on the peripheral smear at 3 months of age, and by 4 months of age hemolytic anemia presents. Diagnostic methods include those that separate species having different amino acid compositions such as hemoglobin electrophoresis or thin-layer isoelectric focusing, solubility testing, and review of the peripheral blood smear (see Fig. 137–2).

OLDER CHILDREN AND ADULTS. The purpose of diagnosis is to identify those with disease or trait who need therapy or counseling. Hb S, G, and D have the same electrophoretic mobility by cellulose acetate electrophoresis at pH 8.4, the standard method of separating Hb S from other variants. However, Hb S has a different mobility than Hb D and G using citrate agar electrophoresis at pH

6.2. The Sickledex solubility test also distinguishes Hb S, which is not soluble, from Hb D and G, which are. Thin-layer isoelectric focusing separates Hb S, D, and G but also requires confirmatory solubility testing. The "sickle cell prep" using metabisulfite or dithionite currently is of historic interest only.

In sickle cell anemia and sickle cell–β^0-thalassemia nearly all the hemoglobin consists of Hb S—useful indicators of sickle cell–β-thalassemia are microcytosis or a parent without sickle cell trait. In Hb SC disease nearly equal amounts of Hb S and C are present. Sickle cell–β^+-thalassemia and sickle cell trait both have Hb A and Hb S; sickle cell trait has neither anemia nor microcytosis but an Hb A fraction that exceeds 50%; sickle cell–β^+-thalassemia has anemia, microcytosis, and an Hb A fraction between only 5 and 30%. Solubility tests are positive in both sickle cell–β^+-thalassemia and sickle cell trait, but sickled forms (ISC) occur on the peripheral smear only in sickle cell–β^+-thalassemia, not in sickle cell trait.

NEWBORN SCREENING. Prophylactic penicillin and comprehensive medical care in the first 5 years of life have reduced mortality to less than 3%, providing incentive for early identification of infants with sickle cell disease. Universal screening of newborns of all ethnic backgrounds is recommended. Tests used in newborn screening must distinguish Hb F, S, A, and C. Patterns of hemoglobins detected are listed, according to convention, in descending order according to their quantities. Sickle cell anemia has predominantly Hb F with small amounts of Hb S and no Hb A (FS pattern), which is also seen in sickle cell–β^0-thalassemia, sickle cell–HPFH, and sickle cell–Hb D or sickle cell–Hb G (i.e., Hb D and G have the same electrophoretic mobility as Hb S). Family studies, DNA-based testing, or repeat hemoglobin analysis at age 3 to 4 months can be used to establish difficult diagnoses.

Sickle cell trait and sickle cell–β^+-thalassemia have Hb F, Hb A, and Hb S. In the former, quantities of Hb A exceed those of Hb S (FAS pattern). In the latter quantities of Hb S exceed those of Hb A (FSA pattern). When it is not possible to distinguish FAS and FSA patterns in newborns, DNA-based testing or repeat hemoglobin testing at age 3 to 6 months is required.

PRENATAL DIAGNOSIS. The limited efficacy of current treatments for sickle cell disease emphasizes the importance of prenatal diagnosis, which is best performed by a comprehensive reproductive genetics team. The development of DNA-based testing methods led to the second trimester use of amniocentesis for obtaining fetal DNA for testing. The polymerase chain reaction (PCR) method of amplifying β globin DNA sequences *in vitro* allowed testing of minute quantities of DNA and motivated the development of new methods for detecting the sickle cell gene—restriction analysis (Fig. 137–5), allele-specific hybridization, reverse dot-blotting, and allele-specific fluorescence PCR. PCR-based diagnosis for Hb SC disease is possible using specific molecular methods for detecting the Hb C gene. The diagnosis of sickle cell–β-thalassemia can be made using reverse dot-blot methodology to screen the many African-American β-thalassemia mutations and the Hb S and Hb C mutations in a single hybridization reaction. Currently, fetal DNA samples are obtained by chorionic villus sampling at 8 to 10 weeks' gestation.

OTHER LABORATORY TESTING. The hemolytic anemia of sickle cell disease is associated with mildly to moderately reduced PCV, hemoglobin, and RBC levels; reticulocytosis of approximately 3 to 15%, unconjugated hyperbilirubinemia; elevated LDH levels; and low haptoglobin levels. The peripheral blood smear may reveal polychromasia related to reticulocytosis and Howell-Jolly bodies indicative of hyposplenia. Sickle cells are normochromic, except with coexistent thalassemia or iron deficiency. Hb F levels are slightly to moderately elevated, with average values of 5 to 6%. WBC and platelet counts tend to be elevated in sickle cell anemia but not in Hb SC disease or sickle cell–β^+-thalassemia. Serum bilirubin levels reflect the greater hemolytic rate in sickle cell anemia than in Hb SC disease and sickle cell–β^+-thalassemia.

THERAPY

HEALTH CARE MAINTENANCE. Routine clinical visits are important for patients with sickle cell disease to establish baseline clinical and laboratory findings for comparison at times of clinical exacerbations, relationships with health care professionals, and red cell phenotypes and individualized blood bank files. Counseling regarding the disease, genetics, and psychosocial issues is best accomplished during routine visits. Folic acid, 1 mg orally per day, is

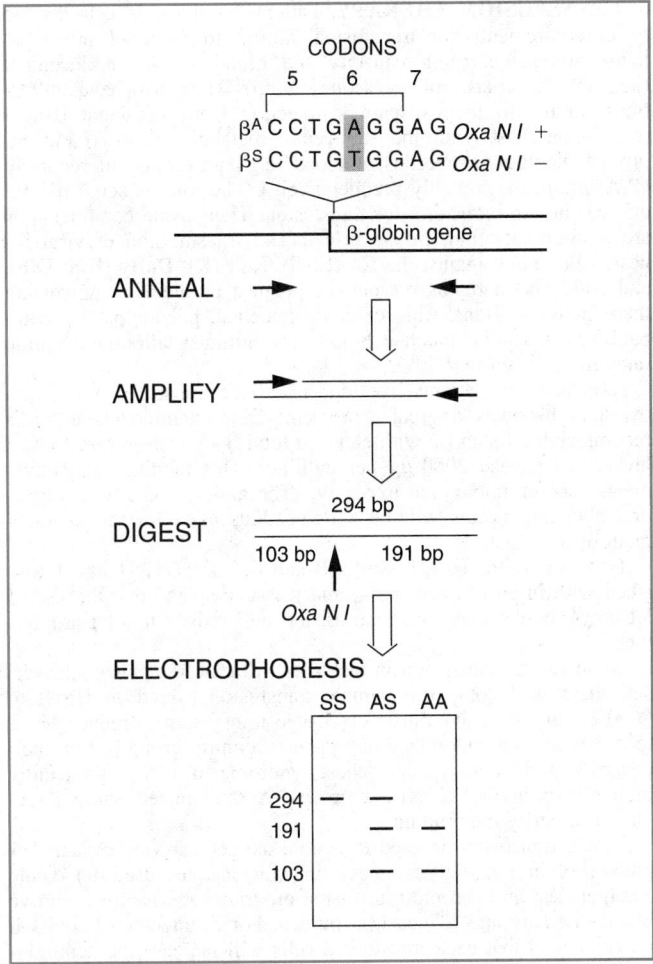

FIGURE 137–5. PCR-based restriction analysis for the sickle cell gene. The target β globin DNA containing the sixth codon, which is mutated in the sickle cell gene, is flanked by the two annealed PCR primers so that this codon is included in the PCR amplification product. The CCTNAGG cleavage site for the restriction enzyme *Oxa N I* found in normal β globin DNA is abolished by the GAG → GTG sickle cell mutation. The electrophoretic gel shows the *Oxa N I* digestion products of PCR amplified DNA with the sizes in base pairs shown at the left. The genotypes of the DNA samples tested are shown above the gel. The fragments from normal β globin DNA (AA) show complete *Oxa N I* cleavage; from sickle cell trait DNA (AS) show partial cleavage; and from sickle cell anemia (SS) show no cleavage. (Adapted with permission of YW Kan.)

administered. Retinal evaluation is begun at school age and continued routinely. Sexually active women receive routine pelvic examinations. Oral contraception with low-dose estrogen can be administered safely.

INFECTIONS. Owing to the high mortality rate of bacteremia in young children, hospitalization, obtaining blood and CSF cultures, and administration of parenteral antibiotics have been the standard of care for children with fevers greater than 38.5° C. However, the recent demonstration of the efficacy of ceftriaxone has led to the outpatient management of all but those who appear toxic, have temperatures > 40° C, or are not receiving prophylactic penicillin.

Treatment of meningitis should cover *S. pneumoniae* and *H. influenzae* type b and be continued for at least 2 weeks.

Antibiotic therapy for the acute chest syndrome should provide coverage for *S. pneumoniae*, *H. influenzae* type b, *M. pneumoniae*, and *C. pneumoniae*. Cefuroxime and erythromycin combinations are recommended.

The diagnosis of osteomyelitis is confirmed by culture of blood or infected bone, after which parenteral antibiotics that cover *Salmonella* and *S. aureus* are administered. Antibiotic therapy is tailored using culture and sensitivity results and continued for 2 to 6 weeks. Surgical drainage or sequestrectomy may be required.

TRANSFUSION THERAPY. Patients with sickle cell disease have requirements for transfusion similar to those of other patients—oxygen-carrying capacity and blood volume replacement (i.e., aplastic crisis, splenic sequestration). They also have indications unique to their disease—protection from imminent danger (e.g., acute chest syndrome, septicemia, metabolic acidosis) and improved rheologic properties of blood (e.g., prevention of recurrent CVA, priapism, probably preoperatively). The routine acute painful crisis is not an indication for transfusion. Transfusion complications are alloimmunization, iron overload, and transmission of viral illness. Antibodies against the Rh (E, C), Kell (K), Duffy (Fya, Fyb), and Kidd (Jk) antigens present the greatest problem in transfusing these patients. Transfusing extended-matched, phenotypically compatible, or racially matched blood may diminish alloimmunization rates from the current 30%.

As sickle cell patients live longer and are transfused more, iron overload becomes a greater problem. Deferoxamine chelation is recommended for those with elevated total body iron, serum ferritin levels that exceed 2000 μg per milliliter. This therapy is inconvenient, uncomfortable, and expensive. The anticipated availability of oral chelating agents will be a tremendous asset for the management of these patients.

Transmission of HIV, hepatitis B and C, and HTLV-1 has diminished with improved screening, and it is anticipated that the use of leukocyte-depleted red cell transfusion will reduce this hazard further.

Preoperative transfusion in sickle cell disease remains controversial. In a trial comparing simple transfusion to reduce Hb S to <60% and aggressive partial exchange transfusion to reduce Hb S to <30%, a nonrandomized untransfused control group had an incidence of perioperative acute chest syndrome of 13%, significantly higher than in the transfused groups. A randomized study is required to verify this finding.

Simple transfusion is used to restore oxygen-carrying capacity or blood volume; partial exchange transfusions are used for acute emergencies; and chronic transfusion programs are used to improve blood viscosity and reduce iron burden. For average-sized adults it is anticipated that each unit of red cells will increase the hemoglobin level approximately 1 gram per deciliter. Partial exchange transfusion in adults is accomplished by phlebotomizing 500 ml, infusing 300 ml of normal saline, phlebotomizing another 500 ml, and infusing 4 to 5 units of packed red cells.

PAIN MANAGEMENT. Acute painful episodes constitute the most common cause for sickle cell patients seeking medical care. The physician must rule out causes other than vaso-occlusion, maintain optimal hydration by oral or intravenous fluid administration, and make aggressive use of analgesics. Neither red blood cell transfusion nor oxygen inhalation is indicated in treating the routine acute painful episode, although oxygen should be administered to those who are hypoxemic. Health care providers must become familiar with the pharmacology of analgesia and overcome fears of narcotics addiction to treat pain optimally and to avoid prolonging the duration of pain, promoting a "drug-seeking" ("pain-relieving"?) behavior pattern and encouraging a pain-oriented personality.

Table 137–3 presents a description of analgesics and recommendations for their use in the treatment of the painful episodes of sickle cell disease. Optimal treatment of patients in pain occurs in a familiar setting that avoids the hectic environment of the emergency department. Hospitalization, intravenous fluid administration, and narcotics are necessary for the treatment of severe pain. Intravenous morphine is recommended for prompt pain relief, and patient-controlled analgesia is an excellent means of subsequent pain control. Patients with sickle cell disease metabolize narcotics more rapidly than normal, which may result in poor responses to conventional doses of analgesia. Comprehensive approaches to the biopsychosocial experience of pain include psychosocial support systems, local anesthetics, epidural anesthetics, combinations of nonsteroidal anti-inflammatory agents and narcotics, and antidepressive drugs. The chronic sickle cell pain syndrome is rare; its therapy may require approaches similar to those used for the management of terminal cancer pain—long-acting morphine and fentanyl patches.

NEW THERAPEUTIC MODALITIES

In the search for a cure for sickle cell disease many agents have been tested but no cure has been found. Because of the seminal importance of Hb S polymerization to sickle cell pathophysiology, attention has focused on agents that diminish polymerization of Hb S by increasing its solubility, either directly or by increasing its oxygen affinity. Such agents react with hemoglobin molecules noncovalently or covalently, and have stereospecific, left-shifting, hydrophobic bond–breaking, and electrostatic bond–breaking activities. In general, because of untargeted delivery to nonerythroid cells and attendant toxicity, inefficient transport into red cells, and perturbations to the red cell membrane which enhances hemolysis, these treatment options have been unsuccessful.

Membrane-active agents that improve sickle cell hydration, such as cetiedil citrate and imidazole compounds, such as clotrimazole, have shown therapeutic promise. Membrane-active compounds such as pentoxifylline generally are not efficacious. Pluronic F-68 or Poloxamer 188, a nonionic block copolymer, improves rheologic properties of sickle cells and inhibits adherence to endothelial cells by a "lubricating" effect on cell surfaces. Intravenous administration of the agent has the potential to terminate or shorten painful episodes. Vasodilating agents that improve membrane deformability have not been found effective. Systematic study of antioxidant agents has not been accomplished. This study would be complicated by the relative redox potentials of a panoply of intracellular molecules, which would influence the effects of potential reducing agents; that is, agents capable of reducing one component may oxidize another. It would be most challenging to design a study to dissect the complex interdependence of oxidation-reduction substrates.

Based on the inhibitory effect of Hb F on polymerization and sickling, the pharmacologic induction of Hb F has been investigated. Administration of 5-azacytidine increases Hb F production, but its potential carcinogenicity has discouraged its development. Hydroxyurea, an inhibitor of ribonucleotide reductase having minimal or no carcinogenic potential, also induces increased Hb F synthesis and improves rheologic properties of sickle cells independently of Hb F changes. Hydroxyurea's effects may be potentiated by recombinant human erythropoietin. Hydroxyurea has recently been found efficacious in reducing the incidence of pain in adult patients and will likely become a mainstay of management. The ability of butyric acid compounds to delay the switch from fetal to adult hemoglobin production has not been matched by therapeutic efficacy. Although arginine butyrate induces increased numbers of Hb F–containing reticulocytes, there has been no consistent improvement in levels of Hb F or hemolysis to justify the risk of its reported neurologic toxicity and severe nausea and vomiting. Valproic acid is a potent stimulant of Hb F production and may have therapeutic potential in selected patients with sickle cell disease.

In the 47 cases of sickle cell anemia treated with bone marrow transplantation (BMT), four deaths have been reported. A major challenge to BMT in this setting is identification of appropriate recipients. The increased life expectancy and large fraction of asymptomatic patients in sickle cell disease suggest that BMT be reserved for those destined to have severe disease and that it be used before patients become incapacitated by their disease. Current methods for selecting candidates for BMT are unsatisfactory; awaiting serious complications may result in disability prior to definitive therapy, and transplanting those predicted by DNA polymorphisms to be severe may result in unnecessary risks for the misidentified. Comparing the costs of $150,000 to $200,000 for uncomplicated BMT in the United States with up to $112,000 annually for conventional care suggests that BMT may be more cost-effective. The limited availability of suitable donors is further complicated in sickle cell disease; the usual one compatible donor per three siblings is lessened further by the presence of sickle cell disease in the family. Broadening the ethnic composition of the registry donor pool, using partially matched donors, and correcting the sickle cell gene in autologous marrow erythroid precursors may improve the outcome with BMT.

Recent advances in gene therapy technology provide promise for the future treatment of sickle cell disease. The sickle cell gene is an ideal candidate for this approach because of the thorough understanding available of a disease caused by a single nucleotide substitution. Gene transfer can be accomplished efficiently using replicative defective retroviral vectors, and high-level expression is attainable by including locus control region regulatory sequences in the vector and by inserting the normal gene into its native environment using homologous recombination, which also knocks out the mutant gene by inserting the normal sequence. Transfer of the nor-

TABLE 137–3. RECOMMENDED DOSE AND INTERVAL OF ANALGESICS FOR TREATING THE ACUTE PAINFUL EPISODE

	Dose/Rate	Comments
Severe/moderate pain		
Morphine	0.15 mg/kg q3–4h (IV, SC, IM, PCA*)	Drug of choice for pain; lower doses in aged, liver failure, and impaired ventilation
	0.6 mg/kg q4h (PO)	
Meperidine (Demerol)	1.5 mg/kg q2–4h (IM, IV)	Increased incidence of seizures, avoid in patients with renal or neurologic disease or those who receive monoamine oxidase inhibitors
	1.5 mg/kg q4h (PO)	
Hydromorphone (Dilaudid)	0.02 mg/kg q3–4h (IM, IV)	
	0.04 mg/kg q4h (PO)	
Oxycodone (Percodan)	5–10 mg q4h (PO)	
Mild pain		
Codeine	1.0 mg/kg q4h (PO)	Drug of choice for mild to moderate pain not relieved by aspirin or acetaminophen
Propoxyphene (Darvon)	65 mg q4h (PO) (100 mg as napsylate)	Not recommended for children; a narcotic with addiction potential; toxic metabolites accumulate with repetitive dosing
Aspirin	0.3–0.6 g (PO) q4h (adults) 8 mg/kg (children)	Often given with a narcotic to enhance analgesia, can cause gastric irritation
Acetaminophen (Tylenol)	0.3–0.6 g (PO) q4h (adults) 8 mg/kg (children)	Often given with a narcotic to enhance analgesia
Ibuprofen (Advil, Motrin)	300–400 mg q4h (PO)	Not FDA-approved for children; can cause gastric irritation
Naproxen (Naprosyn)	250 mg q12h (PO)	Long duration of action; can cause gastric irritation
Indomethacin (Indocin)	25 mg q4–8h (PO)	Contraindicated in psychiatric, neurologic, renal diseases; can cause gastric irritation; useful in gout

* Continuous intravenous or subcutaneous infusion and patient-controlled analgesic (PCA) devices are useful in pain control but should be performed only by those familiar with their use. Because of their risk of respiratory depression, vital signs should be monitored carefully.

Adapted from Vichinsky E and Lubin BH: Suggested guidelines for treatment of children with sickle cell anemia. Hematol Oncol Clin 1:483, 1987.

---

mal gene into self-replicating stem cells allows sustained expression of the corrected gene. The safety of gene therapy remains to be established.

Ballas SK: Treatment of pain in adults with sickle cell disease. Am J Hematol 34:49, 1990. *A comprehensive discussion of the scientific, ethnopsychosocial, and therapeutic aspects of treating pain in the sickle cell patient.*

Bunn HF, Forget BG: Hemoglobin: Molecular, Genetic and Clinical Aspects. Philadelphia, WB Saunders, 1986. *A scholarly classic discussing the historical development and modern concepts of hemoglobin function, structure, synthesis, inheritance, and disease.*

Eaton WA, Hofrichter J: Sickle cell hemoglobin polymerization. Adv Prot Chem 40:63, 1990. *A masterful presentation of polymerization and its importance to disease.*

Embury SH, Hebbel RP, Mohandas N, et al.: Sickle Cell Disease: Basic Principles and Clinical Practice. New York, Raven Press, 1994. *A recent comprehensive treatment of the scientific basis and clinical management of sickle cell disease.*

Hebbel RP: Beyond hemoglobin polymerization: The red blood cell membrane sickle cell disease pathophysiology. Blood 77:214, 1991. *A thoughtful expansion of sickle cell pathophysiology that includes important scientific considerations not encompassed by versions restricted to polymerization.*

Serjeant GR: Sickle Cell Disease. 2nd ed. Oxford, Oxford University Press, 1992. *The standard text on this subject, containing the perspectives of an author who has contributed much to the understanding of this disease.*

Stamatoyannopoulos JA, Nienhuis AW: Therapeutic approaches to hemoglobin switching: A treatment of hemoglobinopathies. Ann Rev Med 43:497, 1992. *An up-to-date review of an important strategy for treating sickle cell disease.*

Wayne AS, Kevy SV, Nathan DG: Transfusion management of sickle cell disease. Blood 81:1109, 1993. *A thorough review of the unique therapeutic considerations of transfusion therapy for sickle cell disease.*

138 BLOOD TRANSFUSION
Jay E. Menitove

A unit of whole blood contains 450 ml blood and 63 ml of an anticoagulant-preservative solution. Red blood cells (or packed cells) are prepared by separating the red cells from plasma by centrifugation. By supplying additional nutrients contained in a saline solution, the red cell concentrate is stored for up to 42 days at 1° to 6°C; the volume is approximately 325 ml and the hematocrit approximately 55%.

Blood donors are questioned extensively to determine if they have participated in activities that place them at risk for transmitting retroviruses and hepatitis. In addition, testing for HBsAg, syphilis, alanine aminotransferase, and antibodies against HIV-1/2, hepatitis C, hepatitis B core antigen, HTLV I/II and, if necessary, cytomegalovirus (CMV) is performed. Because all hazards cannot be eliminated, it is important to ensure that anticipated benefits of transfusion outweigh potential risks.

INDICATIONS FOR WHOLE BLOOD TRANSFUSION

The primary indication for whole blood (Table 138–1) is repletion of concomitant, symptomatic deficits of oxygen-carrying capacity and blood volume. Crystalloid or colloid solutions are administered to restore intravascular volume in patients with moderate hemorrhage. When blood loss approaches 25 to 30% of blood volume, there is a risk of hypovolemic shock; whole blood transfusion supplies red cell mass and plasma for volume expansion.

Factors V and VIII are labile and decrease during *ex vivo* blood storage. The activity of other coagulation factors is stable. Because a clinically significant isolated deficiency of Factor V or Factor VIII is unusual in massively transfused patients, whole blood transfusion is appropriate for patients with a documented coagulation factor deficiency who also require augmented oxygen-carrying capacity.

INDICATIONS FOR RED BLOOD CELLS

Red blood cells are indicated (Table 138–1) for symptomatic patients who require an increase in oxygen-carrying capacity. The hemoglobin/hematocrit level at which tissue oxygenation is compromised varies. Hence, the use of a preset value or "transfusion trigger" for ordering transfusions is suboptimal. Instead, in anemic patients, case-by-case monitoring is preferred for determining whether compensatory mechanisms for augmenting oxygen delivery to tissues are functioning adequately. These mechanisms include an increase in cardiac output by raising stroke volume or heart rate; a redistri-bution of blood to areas needing more oxygen; enhanced oxygen extraction by tissues; increased coronary artery blood flow, ventilatory volume, and respiratory rates; and augmented oxygen unloading as a result of elevated 2,3-diphosphoglycerate (2,3-DPG)

TABLE 138–1. INDICATIONS FOR RED BLOOD CELL COMPONENTS

Whole blood
  Symptomatic deficit in oxygen-carrying capacity and significant hypovolemia
Red blood cells (packed cells)
  Symptomatic deficit of oxygen-carrying capacity in anemic patients
Red blood cells, leukocyte reduced by "third-generation" filters
  Symptomatic anemia *and* prevention of recurrent febrile, nonhemolytic transfusion reactions, CMV transmission, or possibly HLA alloimmunization
Washed red blood cells
  Symptomatic anemia *and* prevention of severe urticarial reactions or anaphylaxis in IgA-deficient patients
Frozen/thawed red blood cells
  Inventory maintenance for rare blood types
Irradiated red blood cells
  Symptomatic anemia *and* prevention of graft-versus-host disease

levels. Patients become symptomatic when the hemoglobin concentration is between 7 and 10 grams per deciliter according to the patient's cardiac, respiratory, and cerebrovascular status; whether the anemia is acute or chronic; and whether there is localized anatomic pathology. Anemic patients are susceptible to fatigue, dyspnea on exertion, decreased exercise capacity, decreased mental acuity, and breathlessness. Tachycardia, tachypnea, congestive heart failure, angina, or confusion suggests that compensatory mechanisms are failing and that red cell transfusions may be indicated. Other factors to consider prior to ordering transfusions include the patient's activity level and fitness, the likelihood of ongoing blood loss, and the monitoring techniques being used. Myocardial ischemia may occur in the absence of clinical symptoms.

Transfusion is indicated in patients with acute anemia to alleviate signs or symptoms caused by blood loss that are not corrected by volume replacement with crystalloid or colloid solutions. With chronic anemia, symptomatic patients receive 2 to 3 units of blood at 2- to 3-week intervals, provided that correctable causes of anemia such as folate or vitamin B_{12} deficiency are not present. One unit of red cells raises the hemoglobin/hematocrit by approximately 1 gram per deciliter (or a hematocrit increase of 3%). A trial of recombinant erythropoietin therapy is an alternative to transfusion in some patients with chronic anemia.

LEUKOCYTE-REDUCED RED BLOOD CELLS. Leukocyte-reduced red blood cells are provided to patients with a history of two or more febrile, nonhemolytic transfusion reactions to prevent a recurrence. Several studies involving relatively small numbers of patients show reduced rates of HLA-alloimmunization in multitransfused oncology patients who receive red cells and platelets that are leukocyte-reduced by "third-generation" adhesion filters. Transfusion-transmitted CMV infection is reduced or prevented by use of these filters. Leukocyte content should be less than 5×10^8 per unit to avoid febrile reaction and less than 5×10^6 to reduce the incidence of alloimmunization. The level of white blood cell reduction needed for preventing CMV transfusion is less certain.

WASHED RED BLOOD CELLS. Washed red blood cells are used to prevent severe allergic or anaphylactic reactions. Saline is added to blood, followed by centrifugation. Subsequently the saline and plasma are decanted and the red cells resuspended in additional saline.

RED BLOOD CELLS STORED IN THE FROZEN STATE. Frozen red blood cells are stored in repositories of "rare" red blood cell units for patients with alloantibodies against red cell antigens that occur at high frequency.

Glycerol is used as a cryoprotective agent for storing red blood cells for up to 10 years. Prior to transfusion, red cells are thawed and washed to remove glycerol.

IRRADIATED RED BLOOD CELLS. Irradiated components are used to prevent graft-versus-host disease (GVHD). Patients at risk for this complication include bone marrow transplant recipients; patients with congenital immunodeficiency syndromes; infants weighing less than 1000 grams at birth; neonates who receive intrauterine transfusions; patients with Hodgkin's disease, non-Hodgkin's lymphoma, and hematologic and solid tumor malignancies who are profoundly immunosuppressed by chemotherapy; and recipients of transfusions from blood relatives or donors with homozygous HLA-haplotypes that are shared with the recipient. Components are exposed to a minimum of 2500 cGy to prevent transfusion-associated GVHD.

AUTOLOGOUS TRANSFUSION

Autologous transfusion involves collection and reinfusion of a patient's own blood to reduce allogeneic blood exposure. Blood donation may be performed as frequently as every 3 days—but at least 72 hours—before a scheduled surgical procedure. The hemoglobin concentration should be >11 grams per deciliter before each donation. Oral iron supplementation is given. Collections should begin at least 2 weeks before scheduled surgery. Autologous donations should be restricted to those likely to need a transfusion because only 50% of autologous units are returned to the donor and, in general, autologous units are not placed into the general blood supply. Perioperative blood salvage is another form of autologous transfusion. Blood lost during and immediately after surgery is collected and reinfused unless the operative field is contaminated with bacte-

ria. Acute normovolemic hemodilution is a third alternative to allogenic transfusion. Blood is removed before anesthesia induction, and blood volume is restored with crystalloid or colloid solutions. The removed blood is reinfused at the end of the procedure or to replace significant blood loss.

DIRECTED DONATIONS

A directed donation refers to blood provided by a donor (usually a family member or friend) selected by the patient. Available data do not support the contention that blood from these donors is "safer" than that from those donating for the general blood supply.

TRANSFUSION PRACTICE

In general, a reduction in the number of allogeneic donor exposures should decrease the risk of transfusion-associated infection. Exposures can be minimized by using whole blood from one donor instead of red blood cells from one person and fresh-frozen plasma from another or by using plateletpheresis to collect a platelet transfusion from one donor instead of an equivalent dose of pooled platelet concentrates from six to eight donors. Clinicians are responsible for obtaining informed consent and discussing alternatives to allogeneic transfusion with their patients. Physicians are responsible, also, for documenting and reporting suspected adverse transfusion reactions to the hospital transfusion service.

IMMUNOHEMATOLOGY

BLOOD GROUPS. The clinical importance of a particular blood group depends on its frequency in the population, the immunogenicity of the antigen, and whether alloantibodies directed against it are IgG, IgM, or activate complement.

Each of the 22 distinct blood group systems refers to red cell antigens controlled by a single gene or continuous homologous genes such as ABO, MNS, P, Rh, Lutheran (Lu), Kell (Kk), Lewis (Le), Duffy (Fy), and Kidd (Jk). Eight collections comprise specificities that have serologic, biochemical, or genetic connections; for example, Cost (Cs), Auberger (Au), Ii. In addition, two blood group series have determinants that are not assigned to systems or collections: one consists of 37 low-incidence (<1% in a random Caucasian population) and the other contains 11 high-incidence (>90% in a random Caucasian population) specificities. Examples of low-incidence antigens are Batty (By^a) and Christiansen (Chr^a); high-incidence markers include Vel, Langreis (Lan), JMH, and Sid (Sd^a).

Anti-A and anti-B are "naturally occurring" antibodies; that is, they are present in the absence of previous transfusion or pregnancy. Intravascular hemolysis may result if these antibodies are present at high titer and incompatible blood is infused. Approximately 70% of Rh-negative persons exposed to Rh-positive blood form anti-Rh antibodies. Anti-Rh antibodies are implicated in hemolytic reactions and cross the placenta to cause hemolytic disease of the newborn. Two genes code for three or more distinct membrane-associated proteins. One gene, Rh CcEe, encodes the C/c and E/e proteins. Another gene, RhD, encodes the principal antigen, D, that confirms Rh positivity.

A, B, and D are potent immunogens. Kell (K), c, and E are less immunogenic but are stronger antigenically than Fy^a and Jk^a. As a result of differences in antigenicity and frequency, anti-K, anti-D, anti-E, anti-Fy^a, anti-Jk^a, and other antibodies against Rh antigens comprise the majority of alloantibodies detected by hospital transfusion services. Generally, 1% of hospitalized patients have red cell alloantibodies, compared with 10 to 30% of multitransfused patients.

PRETRANSFUSION TESTING. Pretransfusion testing involves verification of ABO compatibility and detection of unexpected antibodies (i.e., antibodies other than anti-A and anti-B). Testing for ABO compatibility confirms the donor's and recipient's ABO groups and Rh types. Testing for unexpected antibodies includes antiglobulin reagents to detect nonagglutinating or coating antibodies in addition to agglutinating antibodies. Many transfusion services use a "type and screen" procedure in lieu of a major crossmatch. The patient's red cells are tested for ABO and Rh, and the serum is screened for unexpected antibodies. If blood is needed, the patient's serum is reacted with donor red cells and centrifuged briefly to detect ABO incompatibility (immediate spin crossmatch). If agglutination or hemolysis does not occur, the blood is released for transfusion. If unexpected antibodies are present, blood that does not contain the corresponding antigen is selected, and a major crossmatch performed that includes donor red cells, patient sera, and antiglobulin reagents. Pretransfusion testing also includes accurate identification and labeling, a review of previous records, and resolution of discrepancies.

Computerized crossmatching is used by some transfusion services instead of a serologic crossmatch, provided that steps are taken to ensure accuracy of blood typing results and records, and computer logic is present to detect ABO incompatibility.

Recipients of whole blood must receive blood from a donor with the same ABO group because infusion of plasma with anti-A and/or anti-B present may cause destruction of recipient red cells. For example, group O whole blood must be given only to group O patients, and group AB patients must receive only group AB whole blood. Because the amount of plasma is reduced in red blood cells (packed cells), recipients of this component may be compatible rather than identical to the donor; i.e., group O (universal donor) red blood cells may be given to group A, B, or AB patients, and group AB patients (universal recipients) may receive group O, A, or B red blood cells. Rh-negative patients should receive Rh-negative whole blood or red blood cells. Rh-positive recipients may receive either Rh-positive or Rh-negative blood.

If a patient's physician is concerned that a delay in transfusion will unduly jeopardize the patient, blood is issued without pretransfusion testing. If the ABO type of the recipient is not known, group O red cells should be provided. If the ABO group was determined by the transfusion service, ABO group-compatible red cells may be given. Whole blood must be ABO group identical. In these circumstances, the patient record should contain a statement from the attending physician explaining the urgent nature of the clinical situation and the requirement to transfuse blood before the compatibility testing is completed.

ADVERSE EVENTS ASSOCIATED WITH BLOOD TRANSFUSION

ACUTE REACTIONS (Table 138–2). Acute reactions caused by transfusion occur within minutes or hours after infusing red blood cells or components. Because of significant overlap in the presenting signs and symptoms, a laboratory investigation is required for making a definite diagnosis (Table 138–3).

Acute Hemolytic Transfusion Reactions. Antibody-associated complement activation results in intravascular red cell destruction, osmotic cell lysis, and release of free hemoglobin and antibody-coated red cell stroma into the plasma. The majority of acute hemolytic reactions involve ABO incompatibility; the mortality rate is approximately 5 to 10%. If antibodies coat red cells but complement is not fully activated, the opsonized red cells are removed by tissue macrophages. Antibodies directed against Rh, Kell, and Duffy antigens usually cause extravascular rather than intravascular hemolysis.

Fever is the most frequent sign of a hemolytic reaction. Nausea, vomiting, and chest pain occur less often. Wheezing and dyspnea, back pain, restlessness, and discomfort at the infusion site may occur. Hemoglobinuria, intravascular coagulation, hemolysis, renal failure, and hypotension are frequent clinical complications.

Most hemolytic reactions are a consequence of clerical error or blood given to the wrong patient. When a reaction is suspected, the blood infusion must be stopped and a laboratory investigation conducted to determine the cause. Treatment addresses correction of hypotension, control of bleeding, and prevention of renal injury. Intravenous fluids, mannitol, or other diuretics increase renal blood flow and maintain urine output.

Febrile Nonhemolytic Transfusion Reactions. Chills and temperature elevation of at least 1°C occur in the absence of hemolysis. Cytotoxic or agglutinating antibodies stimulated by previous transfusions or pregnancies react against antigens on donor lymphocytes, granulocytes, or platelets.

Approximately 1 hour after beginning a transfusion, the diastolic blood pressure increases and headache, chills, or frank rigors occur. The infusion should be stopped immediately and a laboratory investigation undertaken. Most febrile nonhemolytic reactions are self-limited and are treated with supportive measures and orally administered antipyretics. Fewer than 15% of patients suffer a recurrence when transfused subsequently. After a second reaction, further transfusions should be leukocyte-reduced by "third-generation" filters. Chills and/or fever may occur as a result of infusing cytokines accumulated during blood storage. This can be prevented by removing leukocytes from blood shortly after its collection.

TABLE 138–2. SIGNS AND SYMPTOMS OF ACUTE AND DELAYED ADVERSE CONSEQUENCES OF TRANSFUSION

Fever
Acute and delayed hemolytic transfusion reactions
Febrile nonhemolytic reactions
Acute lung injury
Anaphylaxis
Septic transfusions
Infusion of TNF, IL-1, 6, 8 (cytokines) released during blood storage

Chills/rigors
Acute hemolysis
Febrile nonhemolytic reactions
Anaphylaxis
Septic transfusions
Infusion of cytokines released during blood storage

Nausea/vomiting
Acute hemolysis
Anaphylaxis
Septic transfusions
Infusion of cytokines released during blood storage

Chest discomfort/pain
Acute hemolysis
Febrile nonhemolytic reactions
Acute lung injury
Anaphylaxis
Air embolus

Facial flushing
Brisk, acute hemolysis
Febrile nonhemolytic reactions
Anaphylaxis

Wheezing/dyspnea
Acute hemolysis
Acute lung injury
Anaphylaxis
Hypervolemia
Air embolus

Back/lumbar pain
Acute hemolysis
Anaphylaxis
Septic transfusions

Discomfort at infusion site
Acute hemolysis
Septic transfusions

Hypotension
Acute hemolysis
Anaphylaxis
Septic transfusions

Bleeding/disseminated intravascular coagulation
Acute hemolysis
Complication of massive transfusion

Hemoglobinuria
Acute hemolysis
Nonimmune hemolysis

Hives/pruritus
Allergic reactions

Transfusion-Related Acute Lung Injury. Passively infused donor antibody, including HLA and neutrophil-specific antibodies, reacts against recipient leukocytes. The symptom complex is marked by severe dyspnea, cyanosis, cough, blood-tinged sputum, hypoxemia, and fever within 6 hours after infusing plasma-containing components. The presentation resembles pulmonary edema, but hemodynamic measurements indicate a noncardiogenic cause. Rapid intervention with respiratory support and mechanical ventilation is required. If the pulmonary capillary wedge pressure is low and hypotension is present, fluid replacement may be indicated. Recovery usually ensues within 48 hours.

Allergic Reactions. Urticarial eruptions and pruritus are caused by an interaction between donor plasma proteins and recipient IgE antibody. The reactions are usually mild and respond to antihistamines. The transfusion may be continued after hives subside.

TABLE 138–3. FREQUENCY OF ADVERSE REACTIONS TO BLOOD TRANSFUSIONS

	Risk Per Unit Infused
Acute	
Hemolytic transfusion reactions	1:25,000
Febrile nonhemolytic transfusion reactions	1:200
Transfusion-related acute lung injury	1:5000
Allergic reactions (urticaria)	1:30–100
Anaphylactic reactions	1:150,000
Hypervolemia	Infrequent
Bacterial sepsis	Infrequent
Delayed	
"Hemolytic" transfusion reactions	
Serologic	1:300–1600
Hemolytic	1:1500–8000
Graft-versus-host disease	Infrequent
Iron overload	Following 60–210 units
Transfusion-transmitted infections	
Hepatitis A	Infrequent
B	1:200,000
C	1:6,000–50,000
D	Infrequent
E	Unreported
Retroviral infection	
HIV-1	1:420,000
HIV-2	Unreported
HTLV-I/II	1:70,000
Cytomegalovirus	Varies according to patient's status
Malaria	Infrequent
Chagas' disease	Unreported
Syphilis	Infrequent

Anaphylactic reactions develop in some IgA-deficient patients (approximately 1 per 500 to 1000 persons) who have anti-IgA antibodies against IgA in donor plasma. Facial flushing, generalized urticaria, laryngeal or facial edema with bronchospasm, hypotension, vomiting, or diarrhea occurs. Treatment with intravenous epinephrine may be indicated. If subsequent red cell transfusions are required, the components should be washed to remove IgA.

Hypervolemia. Patients with impaired myocardial reserve are at risk of hypervolemia and congestive heart failure. An average unit of whole blood contains 56 mEq of sodium, a unit of red cells 8 to 20 mEq, and a unit of red cells with additive solutions, 24 to 30 mEq of sodium.

Bacterial Sepsis. Septic transfusion reactions result from contamination of blood by skin flora or low level bacteremia at the time of phlebotomy. Bacteria proliferate during storage; for example, *Yersinia enterocolitica* grows preferentially at cold temperatures in iron-rich environments. After infusion of only 50 to 70 ml of blood, patients develop chills, frank rigors, or vomiting. Subsequently, fever, hypotension, shock, and disseminated intravascular coagulation may occur. The profound symptoms are related to endotoxin produced by gram-negative organisms. Less dramatic clinical presentations occur when gram-positive organisms are involved. The infusion must be stopped and a microbacteriologic examination, including a Gram stain or similar assessment and culture, of noninfused blood should be performed. Visualization of bacteria supports the diagnosis, but sepsis can occur despite a negative Gram stain. Broad-spectrum antibiotics must be started immediately.

DELAYED REACTIONS. Delayed or nonimmediate adverse consequences of blood transfusion occur days to years after the transfusion (Table 138–3).

Delayed Hemolytic Transfusion Reactions. Three to 8 days (range, 3 to 21 days) after transfusion anamnestic or newly formed antibodies are found that were not present or not detected at the time of pretransfusion testing. The direct antiglobulin test is positive, but fewer than 20% of patients develop clinical evidence of hemolysis. Specific therapy is rarely needed. Anti-E, anti-Jk^a, anti-K, anti-c, and anti-Fy^a are commonly associated with these reactions. Surprisingly, a positive direct antiglobulin test persists in many of these patients for months after the sensitized red cells are

expected to have been removed. Laboratory evaluation suggests that autoantibodies are present in addition to alloantibodies.

Graft-versus-host Disease. Transfused lymphocytes engraft, recognize, and react against the host (recipient). The pathogenesis involves transfer of immunocompetent T lymphocytes from donors who partially share HLA phenotypes with the patient. Transfusion-associated GVHD occurs 4 to 30 days after transfusion and affects the bone marrow, in contrast to marrow transplantation–associated GVHD. Pancytopenia, infection, and hemorrhage occur; the mortality rate is approximately 90%. Hence, prevention is a primary goal and is accomplished by subjecting blood and components to 2500 to 3000 cGy gamma irradiation. (See section on irradiated blood components, above.)

Iron Overload. Endocrine, cardiac, and liver dysfunctions occur in adults who receive 60 to 210 (mean 120) units of blood. Iron chelation therapy or in some instances exchange transfusion reduces iron stores or iron accumulation.

Post-transfusion Purpura. This infrequently occurring syndrome is manifested by profound thrombocytopenia 5 to 9 days after transfusion. The exact cause is uncertain. Therapy involves intravenous gamma globulin infusion or plasma exchange.

Immunomodulatory Effects of Transfusion. Several reports implicate blood transfusion as a cause of immunosuppression. Although the data are circumstantial and conflicting, some patients with malignancies given transfusions in the perioperative period have a greater recurrence rate and lower survival rate than nontransfused patients. Also, some studies found a higher incidence of postoperative infection in transfused than in nontransfused patients. Preliminary reports in humans and in animal models suggest that the immunomodulatory effect is abrogated when leukocyte-reduced components are transfused.

TRANSFUSION-TRANSMITTED DISEASES. These complications are among the most feared consequences of transfusion. Improved donor screening and laboratory testing procedures lessen the risk (Table 138–3).

Hepatitis. Screening tests to detect potential carriers of hepatitis C were introduced in 1990 and enhanced in 1992. Clinical signs and symptoms occur 7 to 8 weeks after transfusion in approximately 25% of those infected with hepatitis C. Although 50 to 65% of patients with hepatitis C develop chronic hepatitis, clinically significant liver failure does not occur until at least 10 years after infection. Subsequently, patients are at risk for cirrhosis and hepatocellular carcinoma. Hepatitis A, B, and D are less frequent complications of transfusion.

Retroviral Infections. Screening tests to detect HIV-1 carriers were introduced in 1985. Testing, combined with improved donor screening measures, reduced this risk to less than 1 per 420,000 components transfused.

Routine testing for antibodies against HIV-2 began in 1992. To date, no cases of transfusion-associated HIV-2 have been reported in the United States.

Human T-lymphotropic virus I (HTLV-I) induces adult T-cell leukemia/lymphoma and tropical spastic paraparesis. HTLV-II, a closely associated retrovirus, is not linked to a specific illness. Both of these viruses are transmitted by cellular blood components. Serologic tests for anti–HTLV-II were introduced in 1988; most blood donors detected by these tests are infected with HTLV-II.

Cytomegalovirus. This latent virus, present in polymorphonuclear leukocytes and lymphocytes, rarely causes symptomatic illness in immunocompetent patients. In contrast, CMV-seronegative patients who receive allogeneic bone marrow transplants from CMV-seronegative donors and infants weighing less than 1200 grams born to seronegative women have significant morbidity and mortality if they become infected with CMV as a result of transfusion. Cellular blood components from CMV antibody–negative donors or blood subjected to leukocyte-reduction by "third-generation" filters does not transmit the virus. Others at high risk of transfusion-transmitted CMV infection include CMV-seronegative pregnant women, CMV-seronegative AIDS patients, and possibly CMV-seronegative transplant recipients of solid organs from CMV-seronegative donors or CMV-seronegative candidates for bone marrow transplantation.

Malaria. Transfusion-induced malaria was reported in 45 patients between 1972 and 1988. Intermittent fever and chills occurred 1 to 3 weeks after transfusion in most of the infected patients. The risk of this complication is reduced by not accepting blood donations from persons who traveled to or emigrated from malarious areas within the previous 12 months.

Chagas' Disease. *Trypanosoma cruzi,* transmitted by transfusion, may cause fulminant illness in immunocompromised patients. Less severe disease may occur in immunocompetent patients. Methods for reducing the risk of transfusion-associated *T. cruzi* infection are under investigation.

Syphilis. Syphilis is an extremely uncommon complication of blood transfusion. *Treponema pallidum* loses viability within 96 hours in blood stored at 4°C, but not all units are kept for this length of time. Platelets are stored at room temperature. Serologic testing of donors is performed routinely.

Other Infectious Agents. Other infectious agents that are transmitted infrequently by blood transfusion include *Babesia, Bartonella,* Epstein-Barr virus, parvovirus, and *Toxoplasma.*

SUMMARY

Red blood cell transfusions increase oxygen-carrying capacity. Transfusion of one unit of red cells increases the hemoglobin concentration by 1 gram per deciliter and the hematocrit by 3%. The concept of a "transfusion trigger" is obsolete and should be replaced with a careful clinical assessment of the effectiveness of compensatory mechanisms for maintaining tissue oxygen delivery. However, the risk of decompensation increases as the hemoglobin concentration approaches 7 grams per deciliter. A decision to order red cell transfusions should include consideration of the patient's level of fitness and activity, whether the anemia is chronic or acute, the extent monitoring is available, and the expected response to alternative therapy such as replacement of vitamin deficiency or use of recombinant erythropoietin. The use of autologous transfusion in appropriate settings is encouraged.

American College of Physicians: Practice strategies for elective red blood cell transfusion. Ann Intern Med 116:403, 1992. *Description of clinical guidelines for red cell transfusion.*

Dodd RY: The risk of transfusion-transmitted infection. N Engl J Med 327:419, 1992. *This brief review summarizes the infectious disease risks associated with transfusion.*

Freedman JJ, Blajchman MA, McCombie N: Canadian Red Cross Society Symposium on leukodepletion: Report of proceedings. Transf Med Rev 8:1, 1994. *The benefits of leukocyte reduction to prevent febrile nonhemolytic reactions, alloimmunization, immunosuppression, and release of cytokines are discussed.*

Linden JV, Paul B, Dressler KP: A report of 104 transfusion errors in New York State. Transfusion 32:601, 1992. *One per 12,000 red cell transfusions were given to the wrong patient. The majority of errors involved a failure to properly identify the patient, the unit of blood, or the specimen obtained for testing.*

139 FUNCTION OF NEUTROPHILS AND MONONUCLEAR PHAGOCYTES

Laurence A. Boxer

Neutrophils and mononuclear phagocytes are essential components of the host defense system. Both cell types are made in the bone marrow, and both accomplish most of their purpose by protecting and maintaining the organism's internal biologic environment. Mononuclear phagocytes are versatile cells whose functions include the consumption and destruction of invading pathogens, the elimination of debris from the bloodstream and sites of tissue damage, the remodeling of normal tissue, the release of immune regulators, and the presentation of antigens to lymphocytes. Neutrophils remain dedicated primarily to the destruction of invading microbes.

THE NEUTROPHIL

ORIGIN. Like other cells in the circulation, neutrophils originate from pluripotential stem cells in the bone marrow. Depending on environmental influences, pluripotential stem cells may give rise to the committed progenitors of any of the blood cells (Fig. 139–1). Under the influence of certain colony-stimulating factors (CSF's), the stem cell generates a population of neutrophils. As outlined in Figure 139–1, myelopoiesis begins with about 10^6 stem cells in the bone marrow, which undergo both self-renewal and differentiation to produce all the individual types of blood cells. CSF's are proteins that control the proliferation and differentiation of particular types of cells. The mechanism that determines whether a stem cell simply self-renews or differentiates is not known, but it is strongly influenced by the CSF's, interleukins, and the local hematopoietic microenvironment defined by extracellular matrix proteins and other stromal elements. The CSF's are rarely lineage-specific and usually influence multiple steps in hemolymphopoiesis, often in synergy with as many as four or five other factors.

The terminal steps of neutrophil and monocyte differentiation are under the control of interleukin-3 (IL-3), granulocyte macrophage (GM)–CSF, and two relatively lineage-specific factors, granulocyte (G)-CSF and macrophage (M)-CSF. Based on kinetic studies, four cellular compartments containing myeloid cells are generally recognized: (1) the marrow mitotic compartment; (2) the marrow postmitotic and storage compartment; (3) the vascular compartment, which in the case of neutrophils is divided into a circulating pool and a marginating pool; and (4) the tissue compartments (Table 139–1). During infection, tissue macrophages can engage the invading microbes, release cytokines such as IL-1, IL-6, and tumor necrosis factor (TNF) that activate stromal cells, and activate T lymphocytes to produce additional growth factors (Fig. 139–1). Early progenitor cells in the marrow are then stimulated to proliferate and differentiate. This step markedly shortens the time of maturation of myeloid precursors through the postmitotic pool. Increased numbers of neutrophils are then released from the marrow storage compartment into the circulation. These same neutrophils are then primed by either G-CSF or GM-CSF for enhanced bactericidal activities.

STRUCTURE. The neutrophil is a terminally differentiated, nondividing cell that is well equipped for removing microorganisms. The cell is packed with granules whose contents kill and degrade target microorganisms (Table 139–2). The granules are primarily of three types. *Azurophil* granules contain proteases and other hydrolytic enzymes, defensins, other microbicidal peptides, and myeloperoxidase, a Cl⁻-oxidizing enzyme. *Specific* granules contain, among other things, apolactoferrin, collagenase, an as yet unidentified enzyme that releases C5a from complement component C5 and whose membranes contain receptors for chemoattractants, extracellular matrix proteins, and cytochrome b_{558}. *Tertiary* granules contain gelatinase, and the membranes bear the CD11/18 receptor essential to cell adhesiveness. The nucleus is a vestigial structure that can no longer replicate its DNA. The plasma membrane contains some of the neutrophil's killing equipment, sensors that locate the microorganisms against which the neutrophil responds, and adhesion molecules. The cytoskeleton of the neutrophil is a complex system of microfilaments and microtubules which is responsible for the orderly movement of this highly motile cell.

FUNCTION. Chemotactic factors generated by the interaction of plasma proteins with antigens or pathogens attract neutrophils from the blood to sites of infection. The diffusion of these factors creates a chemical gradient that directs the migration of neutrophils toward the source of the chemotactic factor (Fig. 139–2). Plasma, in addition to elaborating chemoattractants, provides antibodies and complement that coat microorganisms in a process called opsonization, from the Greek word for "providing victuals." Neutrophils ingest the opsonized microorganisms by surrounding them with moving pseudopodia, which fuse to enclose the microbe within a vesicle called the phagosome. The cytoplasmic granules of the neutrophil fuse with the phagosome and discharge their contents through the membrane, a process called degranulation. The neutrophil reduces molecular oxygen enzymatically to generate "activated" metabolites such as superoxide (O_2^-) and hydrogen peroxide (H_2O_2), which join with material discharged into the phagosome from the granules to destroy the ingested microbes. Granule contents and oxygen metabolites under certain circumstances may leak from the activated neutrophil into extracellular fluid, where they can injure surrounding tissue and engender tissue inflammation.

ADHESION. Because neutrophils move by crawling, they must adhere to surfaces to migrate through the tissues to an inflammatory site. A likely sequence of events leading to neutrophil activation during the acute inflammatory response *in vivo* is becoming better understood. As shown in Figure 139–3, activated neutrophils enter

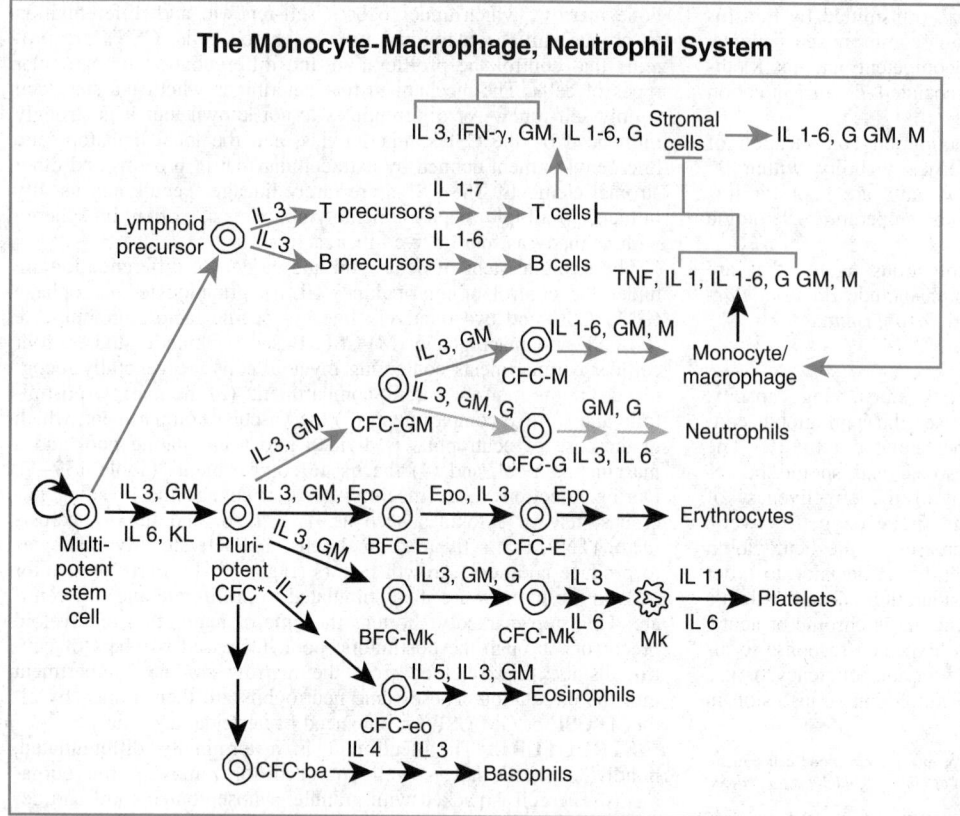

The Monocyte-Macrophage, Neutrophil System

FIGURE 139–1. Regulation of myelopoiesis. Schematic outline of hemolymphopoiesis, emphasizing the differentiation pathways for monocytes, macro-phages, and the various granulocytes as well as the key growth factors that regulate them. Designated in red are the pathways leading to monocyte-macro-phage formation, activation, and interaction with lymphocytes. Designated in black is the pathway leading to neutrophil formation. Abbreviations: CFC, colony-forming cell; CFC-GM, colony-forming cell for granulocytes and macrophages; CFC-G, colony-forming cell for granulocytes; CFC-M, colony-forming cell for monocytes; CFC-eo, colony-forming cell for eosinophils; CFC-ba, colony-forming cell for basophils; BFC-E, burst-forming cell, erythroid; BFC-Mk, burst-forming cell, megakaryocyte; T cell, T lymphocyte; B cell, B lymphocyte; IL, interleukin (1-7); GM, granulocyte-macrophage colony-stimulating factor; G, granulocyte colony-stimulating factor; M, macrophage colony-stimulating factor; TNF, tumor necrosis factor; IFN-γ, interferon-gamma; KL, kit ligand. The asterisk indicates that the pluripotent CFC may be equivalent to the CFC-GEMM (colony-forming cell for granulocyte-erythroid-macrophage-megakaryocyte) seen in in vitro experiments.

postcapillary venules adjacent to inflammatory foci and develop low-avidity, adhesive interactions with inflamed endothelium via specific classes of adhesion molecules that include the selectins—L-selectin, E-selectin (ELAM-1), and P-selectin (GMP-140) (Fig. 139–3A and B). Endothelial cells inducibly express selectins following exposure to inflammatory cytokines (TNF and IL-1). Specific oligosaccharide molecules expressed on neutrophil membrane glycolipids and glycoproteins serve as counterreceptors for E-selectin and P-selectin (sialyl Lewis X and Lewis X, respectively). In conjunction with neutrophil membrane L-selectin, which recognizes oligosaccharide molecules expressed by endothelial cells, the selectins promote low-affinity neutrophil-endothelial binding under flow conditions, termed neutrophil "rolling." Neutrophil rolling is a prerequisite for higher-affinity interactions with the inflamed endothelium. Subsequent to neutrophil rolling, high-affinity interactions are induced by a separate class of adhesion molecules (e.g., ICAM-1), whose functional affinity is increased by high and prolonged local concentrations of TNF and IL-1. ICAM-1 serves as a recognition receptor for neutrophil β_2 integrin counterreceptors, CD11/CD18. This latter agent's relative affinity for ICAM-1 is increased by neutrophil exposure to activating stimuli that include platelet-activating factor (PAF) expressed by the inflamed endothelium as well as by soluble chemotactic stimuli (formyl

bacterial peptides, C5a, IL-8, and LTB$_4$) (Fig. 139–3C). During neutrophil activation, a reciprocal relationship between the expression of L-selectin and the β_2 integrin on the plasma membrane leads to a release of L-selectin, followed by a dramatic increase in the number and affinity of surface CD11/CD18 receptors. Once the neutrophils adhere through their β_2 integrin receptors to the

TABLE 139–1. NEUTROPHIL AND MONOCYTE KINETICS

Neutrophils

Average time in mitosis (myeloblast to myelocyte)	7–9 days
Average time in postmitosis and storage (metamyelocyte to neutrophil)	3–7 days
Average T$_{1/2}$ in the circulation	6 hours
Average total body pool	6.5×10^8 cells/kg
Average circulating pool	3.2×10^8 cells/kg
Average marginating pool	3.3×10^8 cells/kg
Average daily turnover rate	1.8×10^{10} cells/kg

Mononuclear phagocytes

Average time in mitosis	30–48 hours
Average T$_{1/2}$ in the circulation	36–104 hours
Average circulating pool (monocytes)	1.8×10^7 cells/kg
Average daily turnover rate	1.8×10^9 cells/kg
Average survival in tissues (macrophages)	Months

TABLE 139–2. CONTENTS OF NEUTROPHIL GRANULES

Compound	Function
Azurophil granules	
Acid hydrolases (glycosidases, phospholipases, acid proteases)	Degradation of ingested material
Neutral proteases (cathepsin G, elastase)	Destruction of inflamed tissue?
Lysozyme	Digestion of bacterial cell wall
Defensins and bactericidal/permeability-increasing protein	Oxygen-independent bacterial killing
Myeloperoxidase	Oxygen-dependent bacterial killing
Specific granules	
Lysozyme	Digestion of bacterial cell wall
Cobalamin-binding protein	Binding of bacterial cobalamin analogues
Apolactoferrin	Binding of free iron
Collagenase	Digestion of connective tissue
C5-splitting enzyme	Release of C5a
Heparinase	Digestion of connective tissue
Extracellular matrix protein receptors (laminin, thrombospondin)	Adhesion to basement membrane
CD11/18 (C3bi) receptor	Adhesion to ICAM-1 on endothelium and phagocytosis of C3bi-coated particles
Cytochrome b$_{558}$	Component of NADPH oxidase
Tertiary granules	
Gelatinase	Digestion of connective tissue
CD11/18 (C3bi) receptor	Adhesion to ICAM-1 on endothelium and phagocytosis of C3bi-coated particles
Cytochrome b$_{558}$	Component of NADPH oxidase
FcRIII receptor	Phagocytosis of antibody-coated particles

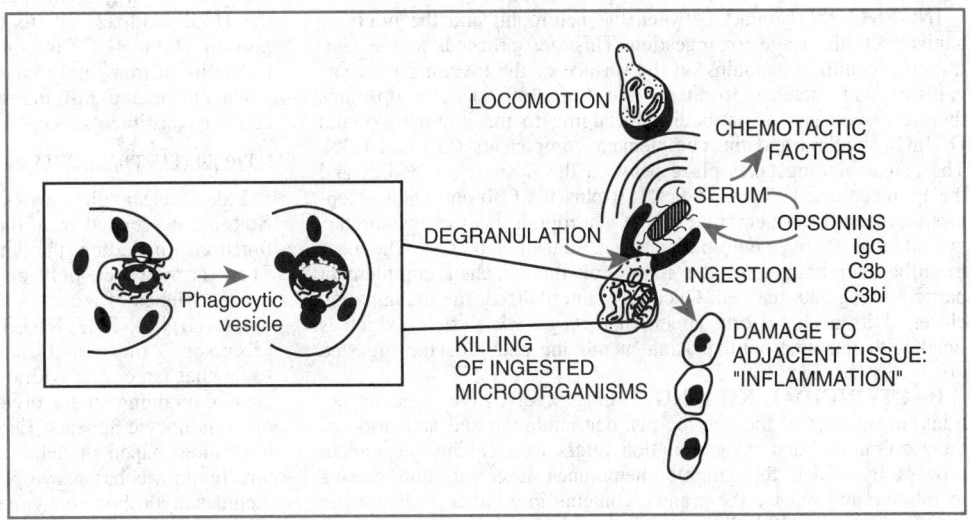

FIGURE 139–2. Functional activities of the neutrophil. The neutrophil is shown in a polarized shape responding to chemotactic factors. Subsequently opsonins, either IgG and/or C3b or C3bi, coat the bacteria for subsequent ingestion by the neutrophils. (The insert shows degranulation into a phagocytic vesicle. Granules migrate toward the phagocytic vesicle, eventually fusing with it. Upon fusion, the contents of the granule are released into the vesicle, and the granule membrane becomes incorporated into the vesicle wall.) Bacterial killing occurs following activation of the respiratory burst. Granule contents and oxygen metabolites (under certain circumstances before closure of the phagosome occurs) may leak from the activated neutrophil into the extracellular fluid, leading to inflammatory damage to adjacent tissue.

endothelium, subsequent transendothelial migration by neutrophils occurs in response to local gradients of chemotactic factors (Fig. 139–3D).

CHEMOTAXIS. The neutrophil finds its target through a chemical sensor that detects substances known as *chemotactic factors.* These factors are continuously released at sites where microorga-

nisms have invaded tissue, thereby establishing a concentration gradient. Circulating neutrophils recognize this gradient and travel toward its source, migrating between endothelial cells and penetrating the subendothelial basement membrane. Once outside the capillaries, they continue their directed migration, eventually reaching the microorganism-invaded site in which chemotactic factors originate.

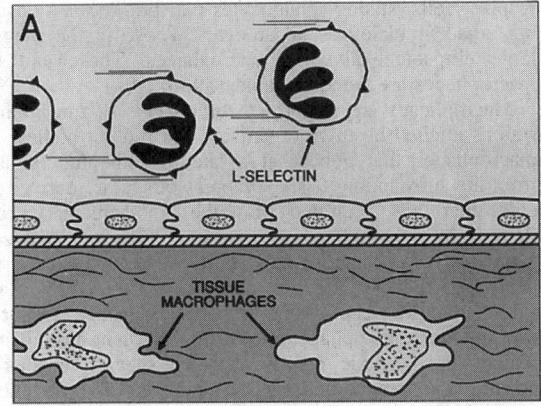
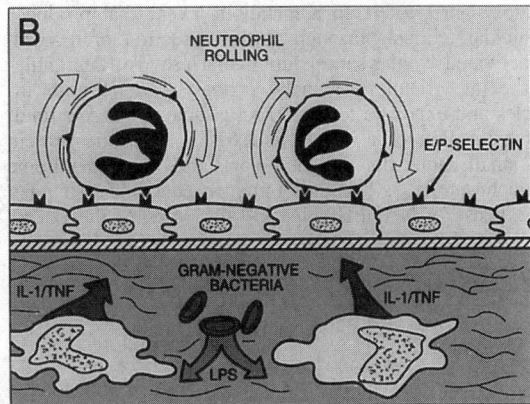
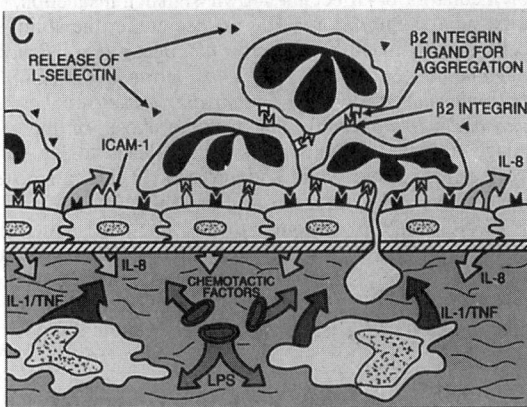
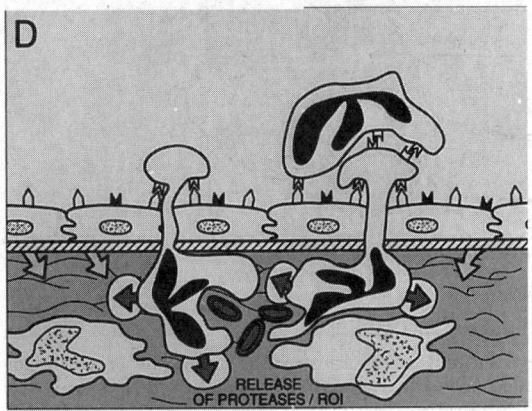

FIGURE 139–3. The neutrophil-mediated inflammatory response. *A,* Unstimulated neutrophils (expressing L-selectin) entering a postcapillary venule. *B,* Invasion of gram-negative bacteria with release of lipopolysaccharide stimulates tissue macrophages to secrete inflammatory monokines, IL-1 and TNF, which, in turn, activate endothelial cells to express E- and P-selectins. E- and P-selectins serve as counterreceptors for neutrophil sialyl Lewis X and Lewis X to cause low-avidity neutrophil rolling. *C,* Activated endothelial cells express ICAM-1, which serves as a counterreceptor for neutrophil β_2 integrin molecules, leading to high-avidity leukocyte spreading and the start of transendothelial migration. Transendothelial migration of activated neutrophils is stimulated by chemotactic factors such as endothelial cell–derived IL-8 and formylated bacterial factors. Chemoattractants promote neutrophil activation with the release of L-selectin and an increase in β_2 integrin affinity for ICAM-1 and for other counterreceptors promoting intravascular neutrophil aggregation. *D,* Neutrophils invade through the vascular basement membrane with the release of proteases and reactive oxidative intermediates, causing local destruction of surrounding tissue at sites of high concentrations of chemotactic factors. (Redrawn from Smolen JE, Boxer LA: Functions of neutrophils. *In* Williams WJ, Beutler E, Erslev AJ, et al. [eds.]: Hematology, 5th ed. New York, McGraw-Hill, 1994, p 779.)

INGESTION. Contact between the neutrophil and the microorganism sets the stage for ingestion. This step proceeds as the neutrophil recognizes opsonins on the surface of the invading microorganisms and attaches to them (see Fig. 139–2). The opsonins themselves consist of antibodies belonging to the immunoglobulin G (IgG) subclass and the complement components C3b and C3bi. The actual binding takes place between the opsonic antibodies and the Fc receptors, FcR11 and FcR111, plus the C3b and C3bi receptors on the surface membrane of the neutrophils. As the opsonic target attaches to the neutrophil surface, ingestion begins. The neutrophilic membrane and the region of the attached complement particle invaginate the cell. Once fully internalized, the invagination closes at its neck to form an internal *phagocytic vesicle*, which is lined with the neutrophil plasma membrane and kills the ingested organisms (see Fig. 139–2).

BACTERICIDAL KILLING. Killing involves two separate actions on the part of the neutrophils: degranulation and activation of the respiratory burst. Degranulation refers to a calcium-dependent process by which the granule membranes fuse with the plasma membrane and release the granule contents into either a phagocytic vesicle (see Fig. 139–2) or the external environment. Azurophil granules degranulate almost exclusively into the phagocytic vesicles, so that their microbicidal proteins destroy the ingested microorganisms; myeloperoxidase (MPO) reacts with H_2O_2 and a halide to produce hypochlorous acid (HOCl). Specific granules degranulate into both the phagocytic vesicles and the external environment to destroy their ingested microorganisms. Some of the constituents of each of these granules are listed in Table 139–2 together with their action.

The respiratory burst refers to a metabolic event that produces potent microbicidal oxidants through partial reduction of oxygen. The burst is activated by the same stimuli that provoke degranulation of the specific granules—namely, primary contact with ingestible particles and exposure to chemotactic factors. These stimuli initiate the translocation of a 47-kD and 67-kD cytosolic protein along with a small molecular weight G protein to the membrane containing cytochrome b_{558}. This step initiates reduction of oxygen to O_2^- at the expense of NADPH (Fig. 139–4). Most of the O_2^- re-

acts with itself to yield H_2O_2, and NADPH is regenerated concurrently by the way of the hexose monophosphate shunt. A portion of the H_2O_2 oxidizes Cl^- to the highly microbicidal HOCl. Another portion of the H_2O_2 is converted to the reactive hydroxyl radical ($\cdot$OH) in an iron-catalyzed reaction with O_2^-. These and related oxidants attack and kill ingested microorganisms by oxidizing their cellular constituents.

MONONUCLEAR PHAGOCYTES

Mononuclear phagocytes and neutrophils are closely related. Both are descended from the same progenitor, and both share many functions, including the unusual ability to ingest large particles. There is, however, only one type of neutrophil, whereas there are many varieties of mononuclear phagocytes.

ORIGIN AND STRUCTURE. The first recognizable monocyte precursor is the monoblast. The next stage is the promonocyte, a somewhat larger cell with cytoplasmic granules and an indented nucleus containing finely divided chromatin. Finally, the fully developed monocyte appears. Larger than the neutrophil and with a large horseshoe-shaped nucleus containing dispersed chromatin, the mature monocyte has a cytoplasm filled with granules whose content includes hydrolytic enzymes and other proteins necessary for the cell's activities. The transition from monoblast to mature circulating monocyte requires about 5 days.

Unlike neutrophils, monocytes contain a limited capacity to divide, and they undergo considerable further differentiation. After circulating in the bloodstream (see Table 139–1), they enter the tissues, where they differentiate into mature macrophages that live for weeks to months. Topologic factors seem to influence their final differentiation and to endow each type with particular metabolic and structural features. Those in the liver, for example, become Kupffer cells, spidery phagocytes that bridge the sinusoids separating adjacent plates of hepatocytes. Those in the lungs consist of large ellipsoidal alveolar macrophages. These and other tissue macrophages are listed in Table 139–3.

Macrophages are important components of the inflammatory reactions elicited by microorganisms and foreign bodies. Some of the macrophages that appear at a site of inflammation are recruited from the surrounding tissue, whereas others are derived from monocytes that have migrated from the bloodstream. Once at the inflamed site, macrophages can be stimulated by opsonized particles. Monocytes and macrophages share the receptors described for the neutrophils and, in addition, express other receptors (Table 139–4). The contact between a suitable particle and its receptor on the surface of the macrophage elicits the transient production of compounds that include reactive oxygen species, nitrous oxide, and arachidonate metabolites. Beside phagocytosable particles, a number of soluble substances can activate macrophages to release a number of mediators or affect their own signal transduction. Some activators, such as interferon-γ (IF-γ), also confer the ability to kill tumor cells and to inactivate specific pathogens (e.g., *Brucella, Listeria, Legionella, Salmonella, Mycobacterium, Coccidioides immitis, Histoplasma capsulatum, Chlamydia, Rickettsia, Leishmania, Trypanosoma, Toxoplasma*). The metamorphosis of the resting macrophage into the activated macrophage leads to the cell's ability to synthesize nucleic acids and proteins in addition to secreting the metabolites and cytokines listed in Table 139–4.

FUNCTIONS. Despite their functional specialization, the macrophages have at least three major functions in common: presentation of antigens, phagocytosis, and immunomodulation.

ANTIGEN PRESENTATION. The activation of mononuclear phagocytes by IF-γ is one of a series of mutually potentiating inter-

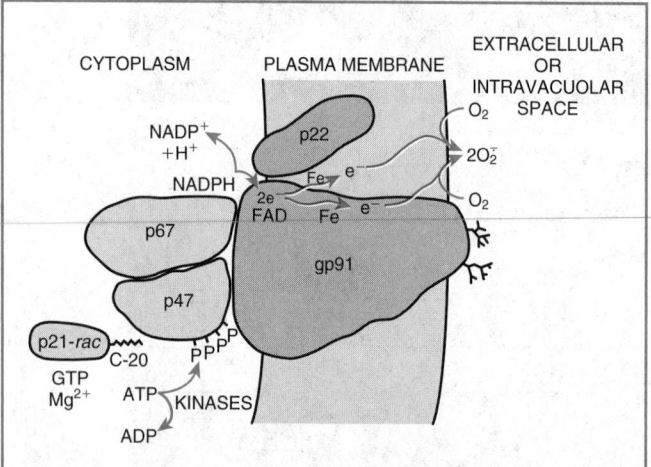

FIGURE 139–4. Possible mechanisms for the production of superoxide anion in polymorphonuclear leukocytes. Oxygen is reduced to superoxide (O_2^-) by an NADPH oxidase. The oxidase appears to be a composite of (1) a 47-kD cytosolic protein (p47); (2) a 67-kD cytosolic protein (p67); (3) one or more low molecular weight cytosolic G proteins, such as p21-*rac;* and (4) a membrane-bound cytochrome b_{558}. Cytochrome b consists of a 22-kD protein subunit and a 91-kD glycoprotein subunit, both of which contain heme. The gp91 subunit is an FAD-dependent flavoprotein that contains the NADPH binding site and ultimately shuttles electrons to the molecular oxygen, forming O_2^-. The p47 subunit can be phosphorylated to various extents, the significance of which is unclear. The low molecular weight G protein is also important in stabilizing the oxidase complex, a process that may be related to a C-20 polyisoprenoid hydrophobic "tail." (Courtesy of Dr. Robert Clark, University of Iowa.)

TABLE 139–3. TISSUE MACROPHAGES

Fixed
Kupffer cells
Microglial cells (central nervous system)
Macrophages of spleen, lymph nodes, and bone marrow sinusoids
Mesangial cells (kidney)
Osteoclasts

Wandering
Macrophages of serosal cavities (pleural, peritoneal, pericardial)
Alveolar macrophages

TABLE 139–4. MONONUCLEAR PHAGOCYTE SECRETORY PRODUCTS AND RECEPTORS

Enzymes
Plasminogen activator, urokinase, plasmin inhibitors
Plasminogen activator inhibitors, lipase, phosphatase, DNAse, RNAse, collagenase, elastase, angiotensin convertase, lysozyme, sphingomyelinase, phospholipase A_2, lipoprotein lipase

Oxidants
• OH, H_2O_2, $HOCl$, NO, O_2^-

Inflammation and immune modulation
Complement proteins: C1, 2, 3, 4, 5; factors B, D, H; properdin; C3b inactivator
Cytokines: interferon-α, β, γ, interleukin-1α, (IL)/IL-1β, IL-6, IL-8; tumor necrosis factor (TNF)
Growth factors: fibroblast growth factor (FGF), platelet-derived growth factor (PDGF), and transforming growth factor-β (TGF-β)
Colony-stimulating factors: G-CSF, GM-CSF, M-CSF

Coagulation
Factors V, VII, IX, and X and prothrombin
Prothrombinase

Cell adhesion
Fibronectin, thrombospondin, proteoglycans

Receptors
FcRI, II, III
CR1
CD11/18 (CR3)
β1: VLA$_2$, VLA-4, VLA-5, VLA-6
Factors VII and VIIa and thrombin
β-Endorphin
Lipoprotein: LDL, VLDL
Mannose-rich glycoprotein
CD4 for HIV
Colony-stimulating factors GM-CSF, M-CSF; IL-1, IL-3, IL-7, IL-10, IL-4, IL-8; interferon-γ, TGF-β
Monocyte chemotactic peptide-1

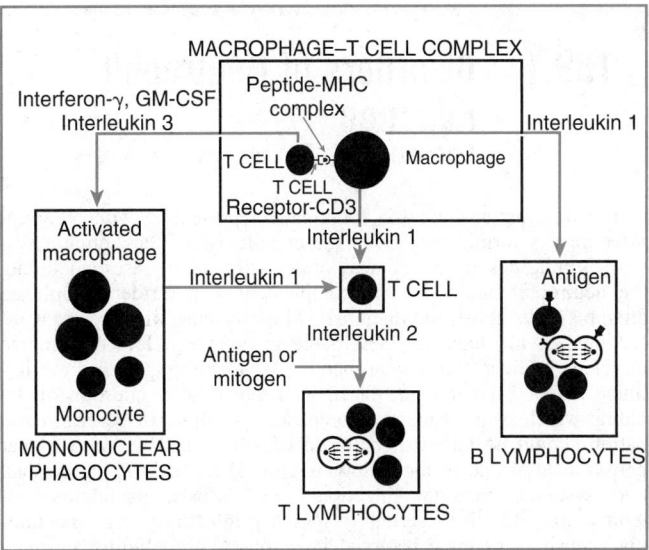

FIGURE 139–5. Macrophage-lymphocyte interactions. The macrophage, acting in its capacity as an "accessory cell," presents a peptide to a T cell equipped with specific receptors that recognize the complex between the peptide and a class II MHC molecule on the macrophage surface. The T cell to which the antigen has been presented undergoes activation and begins to secrete lymphokines. The lymphokines include interferon-γ, granulocyte-macrophage colony-stimulating factor (GM-CSF), and interleukin-3 (IL-3); they cause macrophages to accumulate and undergo activation at the site of the initial macrophage–T cell interaction. Macrophages so activated secrete IL-1, a potent mediator capable, among other things, of inducing the proliferation of both B and T cells. B cells are directly stimulated by IL-1 to proliferate and to differentiate into antibody-secreting plasma cells. T cells, however, proliferate under the influence of a mediator known as IL-2 (T-cell growth factors), itself a T-cell product. IL-1 promotes the proliferation of T cells indirectly by inducing them to secrete IL-2.

actions between these cells and lymphocytes which take place at sites of inflammation (Fig. 139–5). Both T and B lymphocytes participate in these interactions.

PHAGOCYTOSIS. Mononuclear phagocytes ingest for two purposes: to eliminate waste and debris (scavenging) and to kill invading pathogens. Mononuclear phagocytes play an important role as general scavengers. They dispose of effete cells, a process exemplified by destruction of aged red cells by splenic phagocytes or macrophagic destruction of cells that have not undergone programmed cell death (apoptosis). Similarly, phagocytes remove foreign materials from the bloodstream and clean up debris at sites of infection or tissue damage.

A dense network of resident macrophages lying chiefly in the liver and spleen removes material from the bloodstream. Bacteria and bacterial breakdown products such as lipopolysaccharide that enter the bloodstream from the large intestines are removed principally by the Kupffer cells of the liver during the process of gastrointestinal venous drainage. Similarly, macrophages recruited to the damaged area dispose of dead cells and tissue fragments at sites of infection or injury. Activated macrophages also secrete neutral proteases that break down damaged connective tissue and fibrin mesh, clearing the way for the reconstitution of injured tissues.

Mononuclear phagocytes also eliminate from the circulation denatured proteins, protein fragments, and activating clotting factors. Some proteins are eliminated through pinocytosis, a process in which the detritus is taken into the cell by invagination of the cell membrane that buds off and enters the cytoplasm as a pinocytotic vesicle. Other proteins are eliminated by receptor-mediated endocytosis. For instance, the lipids of atherosclerotic lesions are derived from lipoproteins that have been taken into the macrophage by receptor-mediated endocytosis. On occasion monocytes ingest oxidized lipoproteins, transforming the mononuclear cells into foam cells and contributing to the generation of atherosclerotic plaques.

KILLING. Mononuclear phagocytes can kill invading microorganisms. Like neutrophils, monocytes can adhere to endothelial

cells by multiple adhesion molecules, including the employment of the selectins and β_2 integrins. Monocytes differ importantly from neutrophils in that they express significant levels of β_1 (VLA) integrin receptors, including VLA-4, which binds to VCAM-1, on activated endothelial cells. Neutrophils are initially the predominant leukocyte at sites of acute inflammation, with the peak of immigration generally occurring in the first several hours. Subsequently, mononuclear phagocytes derived from blood monocytes become the most abundant cell type. These differences in the kinetics of immigration and accumulation can be explained by the elaboration of particular cytokines and chemoattractants in the inflamed tissue that alter the affinity of leukocyte integrin receptors or induce up-regulation or down-regulation of both leukocyte and endothelial cell adhesion molecules. Neutrophils generally find their targets by responding to chemotactic gradients, whereas fixed tissue macrophages have their targets brought to them by the bloodstream. Unlike neutrophils, monocytes and macrophages also express the CD4 antigen, involved in human immunodeficiency virus (HIV) uptake and infection.

IMMUNOMODULATION. As shown in Figure 139–1 and Table 139–4, activated monocytes also release interleukins IL-1 and IL-6, TNF, and interferon-α/β, cytokines that are involved in regulation of hematolymphopoiesis and in activation of endothelial cells and of the mononuclear cells themselves.

Adamson JW (ed.): Current Opinion in Hematology, vol 1. Philadelphia, Current Science, 1993. *A recent and excellent review of neutrophil function.*
Decker K: Biologically active products of stimulated liver macrophages (Kupffer cells). Eur J Biochem 192:245, 1990. *A clearly written review of macrophage function.*
Kuijpers TW, Harlan JM: Monocyte-endothelial interactions: Insights and questions. J Lab Clin Med 122:641, 1993. *A thorough review of processes underlying monocyte adhesion to endothelium.*
Smolen JE, Boxer LA: Function of granulocytes. *In* Williams WJ, Beutler E, Erslev AJ, et al. (eds.): Hematology, 5th ed. New York, McGraw-Hill, 1994, p 779. *Extensive review of neutrophil function.*
Stossel TP: On the crawling of animal cells. Science 160:1086, 1993. *An excellent review of the biochemistry underlying cell motility.*

139.1 Disorders of Neutrophil Function

Laurence A. Boxer

The differential diagnosis for a patient presenting with recurrent infections is formidable, given the complexity of the immune system. Similarities in the clinical presentation of diseases, including the neutrophil, antibody, and complement, can further complicate attempts to establish the diagnosis. Most patients with recurrent infections do not have an identifiable phagocyte defect or immune deficiency. Given the low probability of identifying a discrete immune defect, clinicians are faced with the difficult question of deciding which patients merit a complete evaluation. In general, evaluation should be initiated for those who have had within a 1-year period at least one of the following clinical features: (1) more than two systemic bacterial infections (e.g., sepsis, meningitis, osteomyelitis); (2) three serious respiratory infections (e.g., pneumonia, sinusitis), or three bacterial infections (e.g., cellulitis, draining otitis media, lymphadenitis); (3) the presence of an infection at an unusual site (e.g., hepatic or brain abscess); (4) infections with unusual pathogens (e.g., *Aspergillus* pneumonia, disseminated candidiasis, or infection with *Serratia marcescens, Nocardia* spp., or *Pseudomonas cepacia*); and (5) infections of unusual severity.

Neutrophils have a particularly important role in protecting the skin, mucous membranes, and lining of the respiratory and gastrointestinal tracts. As such, they form the first line of defense against microbial invasion. During the critical 2- to 4-hour period following invasion by microbial organisms, neutrophils must arrive at the site of invasion if infection is to be contained. In order to be effective, neutrophils must first arrive at the site of inflammation, where they *adhere* to the vascular endothelium. The neutrophils then traverse the vessel wall by diapedesis and move unidirectionally by *chemotaxis* toward the site. There they adhere to and *ingest* the offending organisms, simultaneously activating the biochemical pathways that destroy the intracellular microbes (e.g., *degranulation* and *oxidative metabolism*). Patients whose neutrophils have defects in adhesion or cell motility generally suffer cutaneous abscesses with common pathogens such as *Staphylococcus aureus* or have mucous membrane lesions due to microbes like *Candida albicans*. A profound defect in adhesion and chemotaxis is often reflected in a paucity of neutrophils at the site of inflammation. Disorders of phagocyte microbicidal activity, especially as is observed in chronic granulomatous disease (CGD), are also associated with cutaneous abscesses and pulmonary infections.

EVALUATING NEUTROPHIL FUNCTION

Once the decision is reached that a phagocyte evaluation is warranted, the algorithm presented in Figure 139–6 may be helpful in organizing the diagnostic evaluation. When coupled with a thorough clinical history and physical examination, the laboratory tests identified in Figure 139–6 should provide the diagnosis and help to formulate an appropriate therapeutic plan. Despite the rarity of the inherited disorders, the understanding gleaned from evaluating the molecular mechanisms underlying the inherited disorders has contributed immensely to our knowledge of normal neutrophil function.

ACQUIRED DISORDERS

Neutrophils may exhibit decreased adhesiveness and chemotaxis following exposure to a variety of drugs, the most common being corticosteroids and epinephrine. Clinically the diminished adhesiveness is manifested by a dramatic rise in the total neutrophil count in the blood as cells from the marginating pool are quickly released into the circulating pool. Although the mechanism by which corticosteroids alter adherence remains unknown, epinephrine exerts its effects indirectly by causing endothelial cells to release cyclic adenosine monophosphate (cAMP), which impairs the ability of the neutrophils to adhere to endothelium. In contrast, the adhesiveness of neutrophils can be dramatically enhanced in a variety of clinical conditions that generate biologically active complement fragments

(i.e., C5a) and the cytokine tumor necrosis factor (TNF). Disorders associated with gram-negative bacterial sepsis, severe thermal injury, pancreatitis, trauma, and exposure of neutrophils to artificial membrane surfaces during hemodialysis and cardiopulmonary bypass all can be associated with activation of neutrophils and in extreme cases may lead to the adult respiratory distress syndrome. In these various conditions, the generation of C5a and cytokines promotes enhanced neutrophil adhesiveness, possibly owing to enhanced expression of β_2-integrins. Under these conditions, neutrophils undergo increased aggregation with each other and become trapped within capillary beds of the lungs. It is believed that the aggregated neutrophils then generate toxic oxygen radicals and release proteases that damage structural proteins such as collagen and elastin.

Immune complexes are found in disorders such as rheumatoid arthritis and systemic lupus erythematosus and following bone marrow transplantation. The immune complexes can bind to Fc receptors on neutrophils and impair their motility. In turn, the diminished motility of the neutrophils may be associated with recurrent pyogenic infections. Some of the acquired disorders of adherence and chemotaxis are listed in Table 139–5.

INHERITED DISORDERS

CHEMOTAXIS. The *hyperimmunoglobulin E syndrome* (HIE; Table 139–6) is characterized by reduced neutrophil motility accompanied by markedly elevated levels of serum IgE, leading to chronic dermatitis and recurrent sinopulmonary infections. Skin infections in these patients are remarkable for their absence of surrounding erythema, leading to the formation of "cold abscesses." Neutrophils and monocytes from patients having this syndrome exhibit a variable but at times profound chemotactic defect that appears extrinsic to the neutrophil. The clinical manifestations of HIE can begin as early as 1 to 8 weeks of age. This syndrome is characterized by chronic eczematoid rashes, which are typically papular and pruritic and often involve the face and extensor surfaces of the arms and legs. Most frequently the offending pathogen is *S. aureus*. Patients have serum IgE levels exceeding 2500 IU per milliliter, but unlike atopic patients, who may have similarly elevated IgE levels, those with HIE syndrome have serum IgE antibodies directed against *S. aureus*. The molecular basis for the syndrome remains unknown. Some believe that the immunologic basis is a deficiency in the ability of suppressor T cells to inhibit IgE production. Alternatively, a predisposition to bacterial infections may arise from production of a chemotactic inhibitor released by mononuclear cells that inhibit normal neutrophil and monocyte chemotaxis. Preliminary studies indicate that some patients clinically improve following administration of interferon-γ (50 mg per square meter of body surface, given three times per week subcutaneously).

ADHESION (Tables 139–6 and 139–7). Leukocyte adhesion deficiency (LAD) is a rare autosomal recessive disorder of white cell function. About 75 cases have been reported worldwide. The disease is characterized clinically by recurrent soft tissue infections, delayed wound healing, and severely impaired pus formation despite a striking blood neutrophilia. The onset of clinical manifestation begins in the newborn period and is usually manifested by delayed separation of the umbilical cord, with patients often not surviving beyond the toddler age. Patients with moderate disease can survive into adulthood.

Etiology. Individuals with LAD have a decreased or absent expression of a family of structurally and functionally related leukocyte surface glycoproteins designated the CD11/CD18 complex (also referred to as the β_2-integrin family of leukocyte adhesive proteins) (Table 139–7). Molecules of the β_2-integrin family contain an α and β subunit noncovalently associated in α-β structure. The family members contain the same β subunit and are distinguished by their α subunit. In patients with LAD the expression of the β subunit is either absent or diminished, or the subunit is structurally abnormal, a condition caused by a distinct mutation in the gene encoding the β subunit. The lack of a β chain prevents active α-β dimers from forming. Diminished or absent surface expression of these proteins accounts for the failure of the patients' neutrophils to migrate to specific sites of inflammation. The impaired function of their neutrophils arises from the inability to adhere firmly to inflamed endothelial surfaces and to undergo transendothelial migration, a function dependent upon β_2-integrin binding to endothelial ICAM-1.

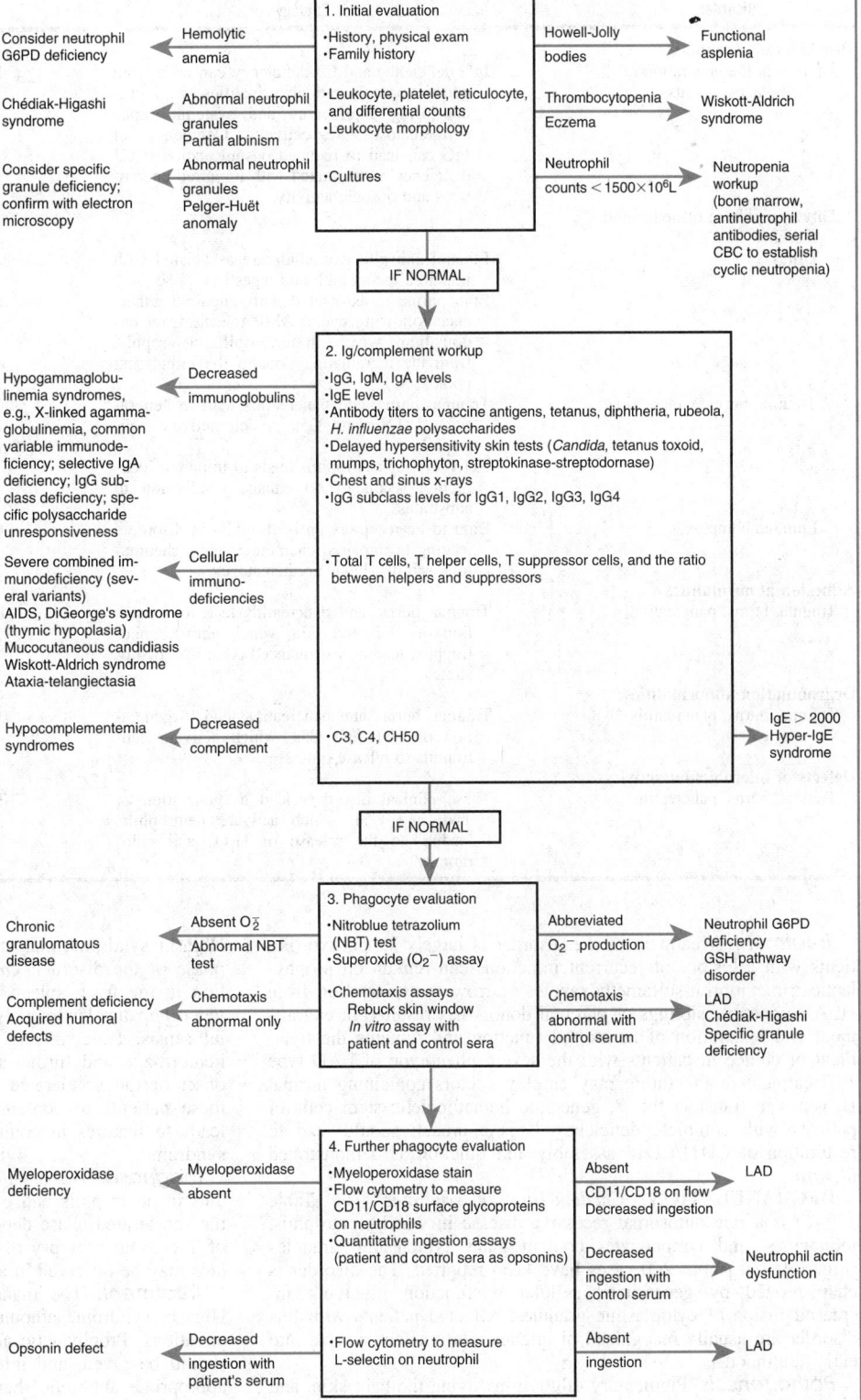

FIGURE 139–6. Algorithm for the workup of patients with recurrent infections. Abbreviations: CBC = complete blood count; Ig, immunoglobulin; G6PD = glucose-6-phosphate dehydrogenase; LAD = leukocyte adhesion deficiency syndrome. (Modified from Curnutte JT: Chronic granulomatous disease: Clinical and genetic aspects. Ann Intern Med 109:138, 1988.)

Clinical Manifestations. Patients with severe LAD involvement suffer from recurrent and gangrenous soft tissue infections of subcutaneous tissues or mucous membranes caused by *S. aureus*, *Pseudomonas* species, and other gram-negative enteric rods or *Candida* species. Patients with moderate involvement have fewer and less severe infections.

Diagnosis. The diagnosis is made most readily by flow cytometric measurement of surface CD11/CD18 in stimulated and unstimulated neutrophils using monoclonal antibodies directed against CD11/CD18. In contrast to those with true LAD, two patients have

been described with neutrophilia, recurrent bacterial infections, and an inability to form pus. Both patients also had Bombay blood phenotype, short-limbed dwarfism, and mental retardation. Functionally their neutrophils were unable to adhere to cytokine-activated endothelial cells expressing E-selectin. The neutrophils expressed normal levels of CD11/CD18 integrins but were deficient in the carbohydrate moiety of sialyl Lewis X, which renders the cells unable to adhere to E-selectin on activated endothelial cells. Thus, the neutrophils from the patients, categorized as LAD type 2, were unable to attach to inflamed venules for subsequent transendothelial migration.

TABLE 139–5. ACQUIRED DISORDERS OF NEUTROPHIL DYSFUNCTION

Disorder	Etiology	Clinical Consequence
Disorders of chemotaxis		
Defects in the generation of chemotactic signals	IgG deficiency and C3 deficiency can arise from genetic or acquired abnormalities, e.g., protein-losing enteropathy and systemic lupus erythematosus, respectively. Deficiency of IgG can lead to reduced opsonic activity. C3 deficiency is associated with impaired chemotaxis and opsonic activity.	Recurrent pyogenic infections
Direct inhibition of neutrophil mobility		
Drugs	Ethanol and glucocorticoids are associated with impaired locomotion and ingestion.	Possible cause of infection
	Epinephrine is associated with impaired adherence following cyclic AMP release from endothelium, which, in turn, shifts neutrophils from the marginating pool to the circulating pool.	Neutrophilia
Trauma, burns, pancreatitis	Trauma, burns, and pancreatitis lead to generation of TNF and C5a, which activate neutrophils. Activation of neutrophils leads to impaired locomotion secondary to enhanced adhesion to substrates.	Tissue damage and in severe situations the adult respiratory distress syndrome
Immune complexes	Bind to Fc receptors on neutrophils in disorders leading to impaired chemotaxis, e.g., rheumatoid arthritis, lupus erythematosus.	Recurrent infection
Adhesion abnormalities		
Trauma, burns, pancreatitis	Trauma, burns, and pancreatitis lead to generation of TNF and C5a, which activate neutrophils, leading to enhanced adhesion to substrates.	Enhanced accumulation of neutrophils at inflammatory sites
Degranulation abnormalities		
Trauma, burns, pancreatitis	Trauma, burns, and pancreatitis lead to generation of TNF and C5a, which activate neutrophils to release proteases.	Tissue damage and in severe situations the adult respiratory distress syndrome
Defects of microbicidal activity		
Trauma, burns, pancreatitis	These clinical disorders lead to generation of TNF and C5a, which activate neutrophils, leading to the release of H_2O_2 and chloramines.	Tissue damage and in severe situations the adult respiratory distress syndrome

Treatment. Treatment of the disorder is largely supportive. Patients with a history of recurrent infections can remain on prophylactic trimethoprim-sulfamethoxazole. Marrow transplantation from HLA-compatible siblings or parental donors has resulted in engraftment and restoration of neutrophil function and remains the treatment of choice in patients with the severe phenotype of LAD type 1. Treatment in the future may employ vectors containing normal β_2 genes to transfect the β_2 gene into hematopoietic stem cells of patients with complete deficiency. This approach should lead to restoration of CD11/CD18 assembly and function as demonstrated *in vitro.*

DEGRANULATION. *Chédiak-Higashi syndrome* (see Table 139–6) is a rare autosomal recessive disease in which neutrophils, monocytes, and lymphocytes contain giant cytoplasmic granules (Fig. 139–7). About 200 cases have been reported. The disorder is characterized by generalized cellular dysfunction involving increased fusion of cytoplasmic granules. Affected patients with this disorder are usually recognized in infancy. Only a few survive into early adulthood.

Pathogenesis. Pigmentary dilution involving the hair, skin, and ocular fundi results from pathologic aggregation of melanosomes. Patients with this syndrome exhibit an increased susceptibility to infection that can be explained in part by the presence of giant neutrophil granules. The granules alter cell motility by compromising the neutrophils' ability to traverse narrow passages between endothelial cells. The underlying molecular defect remains unknown.

Clinical Manifestations. Features of the disease include neutropenia arising from ineffective myelopoiesis, a platelet defect associated with a mild bleeding disorder, natural killer cell abnormalities, and peripheral neuropathies. The most serious clinical problem, however, is caused by abnormalities in neutrophil chemotaxis, degranulation, and bactericidal activity. Patients with the Chédiak-Higashi syndrome can at any time in life develop the accelerated phase of the disorder, characterized by polyclonal T-cell proliferation in the liver, spleen, and bone marrow. Typically patients develop hepatosplenomegaly and high fever in the absence of bacterial sepsis. Pancytopenia becomes pronounced and often leads to hemorrhage and further increased susceptibility to infections. The onset of the accelerated phase may be related to the inability of these patients to contain and control the Epstein-Barr virus and leads to features in common with virus-mediated hemophagocytic syndrome.

Diagnosis. The diagnosis is made by demonstrating giant granules in neutrophils and eosinophils (Fig. 139–7). The diagnosis of the accelerated phase depends on finding the characteristic infiltrate of T cells in a biopsy of involved tissue. Occasionally, giant granules may be observed in acute myelogenous leukemia.

Treatment. The management of the early stage of Chédiak-Higashi syndrome amounts to the management of infectious complications. Prophylactic antibiotics (trimethoprim-sulfamethoxazole) should be given, and infections should be treated vigorously with appropriate antibiotic therapy. Ascorbic acid (20 mg per kilogram per day) has corrected the microbicidal defect in some patients with Chédiak-Higashi syndrome. Treatment of the accelerated phase is unsatisfactory; splenectomy and chemotherapy are ineffective. Bone marrow transplantation remains the treatment of choice during progression to the accelerated phase.

RESPIRATORY BURST. *Chronic granulomatous disease* (CGD; Table 139–6) is a genetic disorder affecting 1 in 1 million humans. Neutrophils and monocytes from affected individuals ingest but do not kill catalase-positive microorganisms because of the inability to generate antimicrobial oxygen metabolites. Chronic granulomatous disease is caused by mutations involving one of several genes encoding the components of the nicotinamide adenine dinucleotide phosphate (NADPH) oxidase.

TABLE 139–6. INHERITED DISORDERS OF NEUTROPHIL DYSFUNCTION

Disorder	Etiology	Clinical Consequence
Disorders of chemotaxis		
Intrinsic defects of the neutrophil		
Chédiak-Higashi syndrome	Autosomal recessive; diminished ability to undergo diapedesis.	Mild propensity to develop pyogenic infections
Hyperimmunoglobin E syndrome	(?) Autosomal dominant; variable expression of a soluble inhibitor from mononuclear cells affecting neutrophil chemotaxis; high levels of antistaphylococcal IgE lead to impaired IgG opsonization of *Staphylococcus aureus.*	Recurrent skin and sinopulmonary infections
Adhesion abnormalities		
Leukocyte adhesion deficiency	Autosomal recessive; absence of CD11/CD18 surface adhesive glycoprotein (β_2 integrins) on leukocyte membranes arising from failure to express CD18 mRNA leads to decreased binding of C3bi to neutrophils and impaired adhesion of neutrophils to ICAM-1.	Neutrophilia; recurrent bacterial infections associated with a lack of pus formation
Leukocyte adhesion deficiency 2	Autosomal recessive (?); absence of neutrophil sialyl Lewis X, leading to decreased adhesion to inflamed endothelium.	Neutrophilia; recurrent bacterial infections associated with a lack of pus formation
Degranulation abnormalities		
Chédiak-Higashi syndrome	Autosomal recessive; disordered coalescence of lysosomal granules, leading to decreased neutrophil chemotaxis and degranulation bactericidal activity. Molecular basis remains unknown.	Neutropenia; recurrent pyogenic infections, propensity to develop marked hepatosplenomegaly in the accelerated phase
Defects of microbicidal activity		
Chronic granulomatous disease	X-linked and autosomal recessive; failure to express functional gp91phox in the phagocyte membrane in X-linked CGD; failure to express functional protein in the phagocyte membrane in p22phox (autosomal recessive). Other autosomal recessive CGD arises from failure to express protein p47phox or p67phox. The absence of either gp91phox, p47phox, or p67phox leads to failure to activate the neutrophil respiratory burst and failure to kill catalase-positive microbes.	Recurrent pyogenic infections with catalase-positive microorganisms
G6PD deficiency	Autosomal recessive; <5% of normal activity of G6PD leads to failure to activate NADPH-dependent oxidase.	Infections with catalase-positive microorganisms
Myeloperoxidase deficiency	Autosomal recessive; multiple causes; e.g., failure to process post-translationally modified precursor protein missense mutation; failure to express mRNA. The lack of myeloperoxidase leads to delay in microbial killing.	None

Abbreviations: G6PD = glucose-6-phosphate dehydrogenase; CGD = chronic granulomatous disease; CD = cluster designation; ICAM = intracellular adhesion molecule; phox=phagocytic oxidase; p = protein of a given molecular weight; NK = natural killer; C = complement.

Modified from Boxer, LA: Neutrophil disorders: Qualitative abnormalities of the neutrophil. *In* Williams WJ, Beutler E, Erslev AJ, et al. (eds.): Hematology, 5th ed. New York, McGraw-Hill, 1994, p 828.

Pathogenesis. The biochemical defect in CGD is now reasonably well understood. The inability of phagocytes to generate superoxide anion (O_2^-) is caused by the absence of one of the components of the NADPH oxidase system. Approximately two thirds of affected patients lack the membrane-bound component of the oxidase cytochrome b_{558}. The gene for this protein is located on the X chromosome. Not surprisingly, family histories of patients with the X-linked variety of CGD often include male maternal relatives who died of infections at a young age. Virtually all other patients with CGD lack one of two recently identified cytosolic factors, either a 47-kD protein or a 67-kD protein. These deficiencies are inherited in an autosomal recessive pattern. The manner in which the metabolic deficiency of the CGD neutrophil predisposes the host to infection is shown schematically in Figure 139–8.

Clinical Manifestations. Although the clinical presentation is variable, several clinical features suggest the diagnosis of CGD. Any patient with recurrent lymphadenitis should be considered to have CGD. Additionally, bacterial hepatic abscesses, osteomyelitis at multiple sites or in the small bones of the hands and feet, a family history of recurrent infections, or unusual catalase-positive microbial infections suggest the disorder. The onset of clinical signs and symptoms may occur from early infancy to young adulthood. The severity and frequency of infections vary widely. The most common offending organism is *S. aureus,* although any catalase-positive microorganism may be involved. Infection with *S. marcescens, Pseudomonas* species, *Aspergillus* species, or *C. albicans* occurs frequently. Pneumonias, lymphadenitis, and skin infections remain the most commonly encountered infections. Often the infections are characterized by microabscesses and granuloma formation. Patients may suffer from the sequelae of chronic infection, including the anemia of chronic disease, lymphadenopathy, hepatosplenomegaly, chronic purulent dermatitis, restrictive lung disease, gingivitis, hydronephrosis, and gastroenteral narrowing.

Diagnosis. The diagnosis is usually made using the nitroblue tetrazolium (NBT) test in which the yellow, water-soluble tetrazolium dye is reduced to a blue and soluble formazan pigment by O_2^- generated from activated normal phagocytes. Phagocytes from patients with CGD fail to reduce NBT because they cannot produce O_2^-. Because carriers of X-linked CGD are mosaics, only a fraction of their neutrophils are able to generate O_2^-; the NBT test stains only that fraction, leaving the rest of the cells unstained. Leukocytes from patients with CGD have normal glucose-6-phosphate dehydrogenase (G6PD) activity. A few individuals with apparent CGD, however, have neutrophils that lack almost all G6PD activity. Erythrocytes from these patients also lack G6PD, leading to chronic hemolysis. In cases of severe neutrophil G6PD deficiency, an atten-

TABLE 139–7. BIOLOGIC AND CLINICAL FEATURES OF LEUKOCYTE ADHESION DEFICIENCY

CD11/CD18 Family	Leukocyte Functional Abnormalities*	Clinical Features*
Mac-1 (CD11b/CD18): molecular mass of α chain 170 kD; found on monocytes, neutrophils, NK cells; receptor for C3bi (CR3) function, i.e., adherence, and antibody-dependent cellular cytotoxicity LFA-1 (CD11a/CD18): molecular mass of α chain 170 kD; found on all human leukocytes; adhesion-promoting molecule for leukocytes; facilitates NK binding, cytolytic T lymphocyte–mediated killing, and helper T-cell response p150,95 (CD11c/CD18): molecular mass of α chain 150 kD; found on monocytes and neutrophils; promotes neutrophil and monocyte adhesion	Neutrophils: adherence, spreading, aggregation, chemotaxis receptor CR3 activities (C3bi-binding phagocytosis, respiratory burst, and degranulation in response to C3bi-coated particles), antibody-dependent cellular cytotoxicity Monocytes: adherence, CR3 activities Lymphocytes: cytotoxic T-lymphocyte activities, NK activities, blastogenesis	Autosomal recessive; delayed umbilical cord separation, neutrophilia, defective neutrophil mobilization, recurrent bacterial infection without pus, impaired wound healing, recurrent (sometimes life-threatening) bacterial infections

* These functional abnormalities and clinical features are a consequence of lack of the CD11/CD18 complex, which includes CD11a, CD11b, and CD11c, markers of three different α chains, and the common β chain CD18 of molecular mass 95 kD.

From Boxer LA: Neutrophil disorders: Qualitative abnormalities of the neutrophil. *In* Williams WJ, Beutler E, Erslev AJ, et al. (eds.): Hematology, 5th ed. New York, McGraw-Hill, 1994, p 828.

uated respiratory burst progressively decreases owing to the depletion of intracellular NADPH, the primary substrate for the respiratory burst oxidase. G6PD deficiency and CGD can be distinguished from each other by the presence of hemolysis in G6PD deficiency.

Treatment. Management of CGD consists of long-term antibiotic prophylaxis (trimethoprim-sulfamethoxazole, 5 mg trimethoprim per kilogram per day), long-term interferon-γ (50 μg per square meter of body surface given three times per week), vigorous treatment of acute infections with antibiotics in adequate doses, and surgery if indicated. Families of patients with CGD should be investigated to ascertain the mode of disease transmission. Genetic counseling should be offered. Restoration of phagocyte oxidase activity by retrovirus-mediated gene transfer has been demonstrated using CGD-derived B-cell lines from patients deficient in either cytochrome b$_{558}$ or the 47-kD or 67-kD protein. These promising results suggest that eventually somatic gene therapy may be used to correct defective phagocyte oxidase function in selected patients with CGD.

MYELOPEROXIDASE DEFICIENCY (see Table 139–6). Deficiency of myeloperoxidase (MPO), an autosomal recessive disorder, is the most common inherited disorder of neutrophil function, with an incidence of 1 in 2000. The lack of MPO, an enzyme that cata-lyses the production of hydrochlorous acid in the phagosome, causes a delay in the microbicidal activity of neutrophils early after ingestion of microorganisms. Eventually, however, effective killing of bacteria occurs. Myeloperoxidase-deficient neutrophils accumulate more hydrogen peroxide than do normal neutrophils, which improves the bactericidal activity of affected neutrophils. Clinically, MPO deficiency is almost completely silent. The most frequent problem is an increase in *Candida* infections in occasional patients with coincident diabetes mellitus. The diagnosis is made from a peroxidase stain of the blood film. In MPO deficiency, peroxidase activity is missing from neutrophils and monocytes but is present in the eosinophils. Treatment is unnecessary for MPO deficiency.

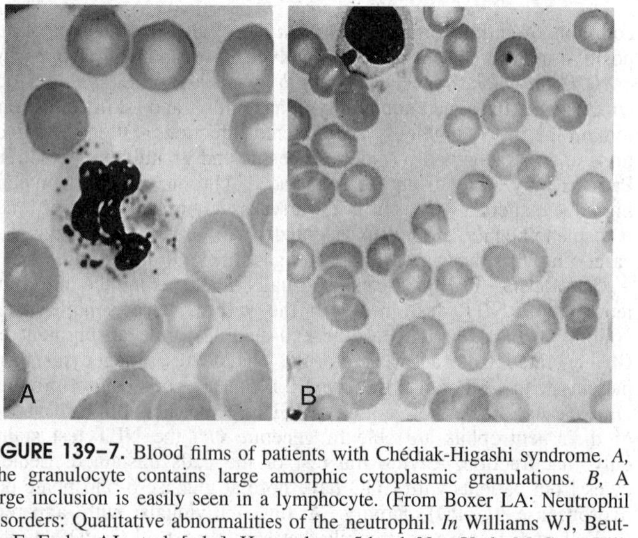

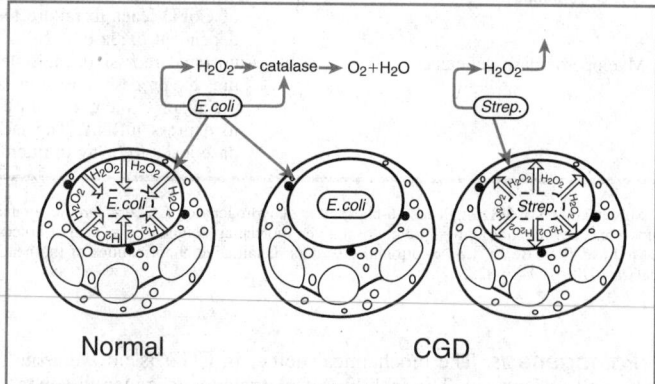

FIGURE 139–8. The pathogenesis of chronic granulomatous disease (CGD). The manner in which the metabolic deficiency of the CGD neutrophil predisposes the host to infection is shown schematically. Normal neutrophils accumulate hydrogen peroxide in the phagosome containing ingested *Escherichia coli*. Myeloperoxidase is delivered to the phagosome by degranulation, as indicated by the closed circles. In this setting, hydrogen peroxide acts as a substrate for myeloperoxidase to oxidize halide to hypochlorous acid and chloramines that kill the microbes. The quantity of hydrogen peroxide produced by the normal neutrophils is sufficient to exceed the capacity of catalase, a hydrogen peroxide–catabolizing enzyme of many aerobic microorganisms, including most gram-negative enteric bacteria, *Staphylococcus aureus, Candida albicans,* and *Aspergillus* species. When organisms such as *E. coli* gain entry into CGD neutrophils, they are not exposed to hydrogen peroxide because the neutrophils do not produce it, and the hydrogen peroxide generated by microbes themselves is destroyed by their own catalase. When CGD neutrophils ingest streptococci or pneumococci, these organisms, which lack catalase, generate enough hydrogen peroxide to result in a microbicidal effect. As indicated in the middle figure, catalase-positive microbes such as *E. coli* can survive within the phagosome of the CGD neutrophil. (From Boxer LA: Neutrophil disorders: Qualitative abnormalities of the neutrophil. *In* Williams WJ, Beutler E, Erslev AJ, et al. [eds.]: Hematology, 5th ed. New York, McGraw-Hill, 1994, p 828.)

FIGURE 139–7. Blood films of patients with Chédiak-Higashi syndrome. *A,* The granulocyte contains large amorphic cytoplasmic granulations. *B,* A large inclusion is easily seen in a lymphocyte. (From Boxer LA: Neutrophil disorders: Qualitative abnormalities of the neutrophil. *In* Williams WJ, Beutler E, Erslev AJ, et al. [eds.]: Hematology, 5th ed. New York, McGraw-Hill, 1994.)

Arnaout MA: Dynamics and regulation of leukocyte-endothelial cell interactions. Curr Opin Hematol 1:113, 1993. *Excellent review of the surface proteins on neutrophils and endothelial cells contributing to adhesion.*

Boxer LA: Neutrophil disorders: Qualitative abnormalities of the neutrophil. *In* Williams WJ, Beutler E, Erslev AJ, et al. (eds.): Hematology, 5th ed. New York, McGraw-Hill, 1994, p 828. *A thorough review of neutrophil disorders.*

Curnutte JT: Molecular basis of the autosomal recessive forms of chronic granulomatous disease. Immunodef Rev 3:149, 1992. *A thorough review of the genetics underlying CGD.*

Sibille Y, Reynolds HY: Macrophages and polymorphonuclear neutrophils in lung defense and injury. Am Rev Respir Dis 141:471, 1990. *An excellent review detailing the probable pathogenesis of the adult respiratory distress syndrome.*

Wilson JM, Ping AJ, Krauss JD, et al.: Correction of CD18-deficient lymphocytes by retrovirus-mediated gene transfer. Science 248:1413, 1990. *The initial paper describing the potential role of gene therapy for a phagocyte disorder.*

139.2 Familial Mediterranean Fever

Daniel G. Wright

DEFINITION. Familial Mediterranean fever (FMF) is an inherited, recurrent inflammatory disease of unknown cause. The disease is characterized by acute self-limited attacks of fever and peritonitis, sometimes accompanied by pleuritis, arthritis, and erythematous skin lesions. Among affected individuals in the Middle East and Europe, FMF is frequently complicated by amyloidosis and progressive renal failure. Familial Mediterranean fever has been given a number of other names: familial paroxysmal polyserositis, benign paroxysmal peritonitis, periodic peritonitis, and periodic disease. The first of these is descriptively accurate and an appropriate alternative name for the disease; the other terms, however, are misleading. Familial Mediterranean fever is not a benign condition, given the potentially lethal complication of amyloidosis. Moreover, attacks of acute serositis in FMF affect sites other than the peritoneum, and they recur at irregular, unpredictable intervals that do not reflect true periodicity.

INCIDENCE, PREVALENCE, AND GENETICS. Although FMF has been recognized in many parts of the world, it is largely restricted to ethnic groups originating in the eastern Mediterranean area. It is an uncommon disease, even in Israel, where the largest number of cases are seen. Half the reported cases of FMF are in patients of Sephardic Jewish ancestry; approximately 20% of patients are Armenian, and another 20% are of Turkish or Arabic descent. Most of the remaining patients are of Italian, Greek, or Ashkenazi Jewish ancestry. However, the disease has also been recognized rarely in individuals with Anglo-Saxon or northern European origins. The disease is familial, and in well-studied affected kindreds it appears to be inherited as an autosomal recessive trait. Nonetheless, nearly 50% of patients do not give a positive family history for the disease. Among reported cases males predominate by a ratio of 3:2. Recently, genetic studies of affected kindreds have mapped the gene that causes FMF (termed the MEF gene) to the short arm of chromosome 16 (in the region of 16p13). Despite variations in the clinical phenotype of patients with FMF from different ethnic groups, the disease has been linked to the same gene region in all affected populations studied. The carrier state for FMF in populations in which the disease is most commonly seen may be as high as 1 out of 6.

ETIOLOGY. Although many pathogenetic explanations have been suggested for the acute inflammatory episodes of FMF, the etiology of this disease remains unknown. Extensive studies have failed to establish an infectious or allergic basis for the disease, and no good evidence exists to support suggestions that FMF represents a hormonal or psychosomatic disturbance. Recently it has been proposed that FMF might be caused by a genetically determined defect in the normal regulation of acute inflammatory responses. Abnormalities of suppressor T lymphocytes, altered metabolism of lipoxygenase products of arachidonic acid, and absence of a normal inhibitor of the complement-derived anaphylatoxin C5a have been described in FMF. However, the possible etiologic significance of these observations remains to be clarified and confirmed. The recent identification of the chromosomal location of the gene associated with FMF should assist in the eventual elucidation of the biochemical defect that underlies this disease.

PATHOLOGY. Pathologic findings in FMF are those of nonspecific, acute inflammation. Neutrophilic infiltration predominates in exudates recovered from peritoneal, pleural, or joint spaces at the time of acute attacks. Serosal thickening and secondary adhesions may occur, which in the abdomen can lead to mechanical bowel obstruction. Amyloidosis is the most serious histopathologic finding in FMF. In affected individuals, amyloid is deposited in the intima and media of arterioles and in the subendothelium of venules in all major organs. There is also parenchymal deposition of amyloid, particularly in the renal glomeruli, adrenals, spleen, and alveolar septa of the lung, while the liver and heart are characteristically spared.

CLINICAL MANIFESTATIONS. In most patients the signs and symptoms of FMF begin during the first two decades of life, usually between the ages of 5 and 15 years. Rarely, however, the onset of the disease may occur in infancy or as late as the fifth or sixth decade. The duration and frequency of attacks vary considerably, even in the same patient. Acute attacks typically last 24 to 48 hours and recur once or twice a month. However, attacks may recur as frequently as several times a week or as infrequently as once a year, and symptoms may persist for as long as a week during individual episodes. Some patients experience spontaneous remission that persists for years, followed by recurrence of frequent attacks. Pregnancy is often associated with remission of attacks, which resume post partum. Some patients relate the occurrence of attacks to cold weather and find that they experience attacks more frequently during winter than summer. Recurrent attacks may also become less severe and/or less frequent as patients age or as they develop amyloidosis. Between attacks, patients typically feel entirely well.

Temperatures as high as 39° C to 40° C accompany almost all attacks. Fever may occur without concomitant evidence of serositis, but this is unusual. The rise in temperature is sometimes preceded by chills and typically peaks by 12 to 24 hours; diaphoresis frequently accompanies defervescence.

More than 95% of patients experience abdominal pain and signs of peritonitis during acute attacks. Pain often begins in one quadrant and then becomes diffuse, sometimes with distention, rigidity, rebound tenderness, and ileus with nausea and vomiting. Pain may radiate to the back or to the shoulders, and upright abdominal roentgenograms may show small air-fluid levels and edema of the bowel. Although these signs and symptoms are self-limited, they can be indistinguishable from those of an acute abdominal emergency, and patients may undergo one or more exploratory laparotomies before the true nature of their disease is recognized. Potential uncertainties about the clinical management of acute abdominal episodes have led to the recommendation that elective appendectomy be carried out during a symptom-free period so that acute appendicitis does not confuse a patient's subsequent care.

Pleuritic pain occurs during acute attacks in 75% of patients. Symptoms of pleuritis may sometimes precede abdominal pain, and a few patients experience pleuritic attacks without abdominal symptoms. Chest pain is usually one-sided and may be associated with diminished breath sounds, a friction rub, atelectasis, and transient pleural effusion.

Nonspecific, mild arthralgia is a common feature of febrile attacks, and acute, monoarticular, or oligoarticular arthritis may occur. Although arthritis is unusual among patients in the United States, it is a frequently observed manifestation of FMF among Israeli patients. Arthritis usually affects large joints, the knee in particular, and effusions are common. Although arthritis episodes are typically short lived, joint symptoms may also be protracted and follow a course distinct from that of the acute abdominal and/or pleuritic attacks. Roentgenographic findings are nonspecific.

As many as a third of patients experience transient, erysipelas-like skin lesions that appear typically on the lower leg, ankle, or dorsum of the foot. These lesions are well-circumscribed, painful, erythematous areas of swelling, 5 to 20 cm in diameter, that subside spontaneously within 24 to 48 hours.

Self-limited pericarditis with pericardial effusions, conjunctivitis, aseptic meningitis, and other forms of serositis have been reported as manifestations of this disease but are unusual. Migraine-like headaches and emotional lability have also been observed during acute attacks, but it is unclear whether these are primary or secondary manifestations.

The most serious complication of FMF is systemic amyloidosis of the AA type. The natural history of amyloidosis in this disease is one of relentless progression to renal failure and death, which may occur in adolescence or even earlier. While a substantial proportion of Turkish and Israeli patients develop amyloidosis, this complication has been very unusual among patients in the United States and in several well-studied Armenian and Arabic kindreds. The genetic and/or environmental factors that explain these differences in the incidence of amyloidosis remain unclear. In Israel, 90% of patients who develop amyloidosis (particularly common in Sephardic Jews) do so after experiencing typical attacks of FMF (phenotype I); however, amyloidosis may occur in asymptomatic siblings of FMF patients, or it may precede the onset of typical FMF attacks (phenotype II).

Laboratory findings in FMF are nonspecific. During acute attacks, prominent leukocytosis (up to 30,000 per cubic millimeter) is present, and the erythrocyte sedimentation rate and acute phase reactants are increased. These values return to normal between attacks. Elevated plasma dopamine beta-hydroxylase levels (which become normal during colchicine treatment) have been reported in patients with FMF, but confirmatory studies have yet to be done to determine whether this finding represents a specific diagnostic test for FMF. With amyloidosis, laboratory abnormalities reflect the associated nephrotic syndrome and renal failure.

DIAGNOSIS. The diagnosis of FMF is based primarily upon clinical presentation and history. In individuals of appropriate ethnic background with typical recurrent, self-limited attacks, diagnosis should not be difficult; in such individuals, delay in recognizing the disease is usually because the diagnosis is not considered. Chromosomal mapping studies that have determined the genomic location of the FMF gene have also identified microsatellite DNA markers that can be used for the preclinical diagnosis of the disease in most kindreds. Nonetheless, when a patient is first seen or when attacks are infrequent, a variety of other acute febrile conditions must be considered and excluded by appropriate diagnostic studies and follow-up—in particular, appendicitis, pancreatitis, cholecystitis, and intestinal obstruction. Familial hyperlipidemia and porphyrias associated with abdominal symptoms must also be considered.

The diagnosis is usually most elusive when patients have a limited or atypical symptom complex. Isolated pleural attacks may closely mimic acute infections or pulmonary emboli. Arthritis, when it is a prominent manifestation, can at first be clinically indistinguishable from various infectious and noninfectious arthritides, and skin lesions on the lower legs may resemble cellulitis or superficial thrombophlebitis. Rare patients have febrile episodes without serositis, and these may require orderly evaluation to determine their origin. Recently it has been reported that infusion of metaraminol diluted in normal saline provokes acute signs and symptoms of FMF with a high degree of specificity for the disease. However, the appropriate role of such a test in establishing the diagnosis remains unclear. At present, this procedure, which carries intrinsic risks from catecholamine effects and salt load, should be considered experimental and not for use in general practice.

Once FMF is diagnosed, a degree of diagnostic vigilance must be maintained, for patients are not immune to the more common acute illnesses that FMF mimics. Of note, these patients appear to be particularly prone to develop gallbladder disease.

TREATMENT. Colchicine treatment is effective in FMF. Several controlled clinical trials, together with extensive, uncontrolled clinical experience since the mid 1970's, have shown that prophylactic colchicine,* 0.6 mg orally two or three times a day, prevents or substantially reduces the acute attacks of FMF in 75 to 90% of patients. Treatment failures are often associated with noncompliance and/or intolerance to the drug. Some patients can abort attacks with intermittent courses of colchicine, beginning at the onset of attacks (0.6 mg orally every hour for 4 hours, then every 2 hours for 4 hours, and then every 12 hours for 2 days). In general, patients who benefit from intermittent colchicine therapy are those who experience a recognizable prodrome before developing fever and clear-cut acute symptoms. Colchicine does not alter fully developed attacks. Patients who experience gastrointestinal intolerance to colchicine

---

* This use of colchicine is not listed in the manufacturer's directive.

may benefit from reduced doses. Although definite chronic complications from colchicine have not become apparent with its long-term use in FMF, it is still recommended that a trial of intermittent colchicine therapy be attempted, particularly in young patients, before long-term colchicine prophylaxis is used. Azoospermia and chromosomal nondisjunctions have been associated with the use of this drug. This recommendation does not apply to individuals from ethnic groups and in geographic regions associated with a high risk of amyloidosis, for it is now evident that long-term colchicine therapy not only prevents the development of amyloidosis but may also arrest its progression in FMF.

Symptomatic and supportive treatment is indicated for patients who do not respond to colchicine. However, every effort should be made to avoid the use of narcotics. In the United States, addiction to narcotics has been a major long-term complication among FMF patients.

It has been estimated that patients with FMF and end-stage renal amyloidosis represent up to 6% of the candidates for renal transplantation in Israel. Many such patients have received successful renal grafts. Of note, it has been suggested recently that these patients may be particularly susceptible to gastrointestinal and other side effects of the immunosuppressive drug cyclosporine.

PROGNOSIS. The prognosis for normal longevity for patients in the United States with FMF is excellent, and since the recognition of colchicine's efficacy in this disease, most patients can be maintained almost entirely symptom-free. Except in very rare cases, this disease does not affect the physical growth and development of children. Long-term colchicine therapy has also clearly improved the prognosis of patients in the Middle East who are prone to develop amyloidosis, even those whose symptomatic attacks continue. However, among patients in whom amyloidosis has led to nephrotic syndrome or uremia and who are unable to receive a renal transplant or in whom renal transplantation has failed, the likelihood of eventual death from renal failure remains great.

Barakat MH, Karnik AM, Majeed HWA, et al.: Familial Mediterranean fever (recurrent hereditary polyserositis) in Arabs—a study of 175 patients and review of the literature. Q J Med 60:837, 1986. *Provides an extensive review of the clinical and pathologic manifestations of FMF and describes differences in the incidence of amyloidosis.*

Pras E, Aksentijevich I, Gruberg L, et al.: Mapping of a gene causing familial Mediterranean fever to the short arm of chromosome 16. N Engl J Med 326:1509, 1992. *The first report of the chromosomal location of the gene defect causing FMF.*

Zemer D, Pras M, Sohar E, et al.: Colchicine in the prevention and treatment of the amyloidosis of familial Mediterranean fever. N Engl J Med 314:1001, 1986. *A retrospective review of 1070 patients that provides convincing evidence that long-term colchicine therapy arrests the development of amyloidosis.*

140 DISORDERS OF NEUTROPHIL PRODUCTION
Grover C. Bagby, Jr.

140.1 Leukopenia

Circulating leukocytes consist of heterogeneous cell types (neutrophils, monocytes, basophils, eosinophils, and lymphocytes), each of which serves a unique purpose and represents a different fractional component of the total peripheral leukocyte population. Therefore, while the peripheral white blood cell (WBC) count ranges from 5.0 to 10.0×10^9 per liter in normal individuals, a rational approach to the leukopenic ($< 3.0 \times 10^9$ per liter) patient must focus on specific leukocyte types. A normal total WBC count does not assure against life-threatening deficiencies of specific leukocyte types. Patients may be severely neutropenic or lymphocytopenic despite having total WBC counts that fall within the normal range. If there is a reason to order a WBC count, that reason is generally sufficient to justify performance of a differential white count.

DEFINITION. Neutropenia exists when the peripheral neutrophil count is less than 2.0×10^9 per liter. Because the normal range in blacks and Yemenite Jews is somewhat lower, neutropenia in these populations is defined as counts less than 1.5×10^9 per liter. The obligation of the neutrophil in phagocytic defense of the host is generally met if the neutrophil count is above 1.0×10^9 per liter. If the neutrophil count drops further, particularly below 0.5×10^9 per liter, the incidence of serious, recurrent, and difficult-to-treat infections rises markedly.

ETIOLOGY AND PATHOGENESIS. The multiple pathophysiologic types of neutropenia are best described in the context of normal neutrophil kinetics. Such a description also simplifies initial diagnostic and therapeutic approaches to patients with neutropenia. Neutrophils arise from a pool of marrow precursor cells through serial divisions and synchronous maturation steps (Fig. 140–1). The rate of neutrophil production is astonishingly high; more than 10^{11} cells per day. The bone marrow component of the neutrophil's life consists of a mitotic pool and a storage pool, the latter containing mature neutrophils, cells that no longer divide. Released after a few days in the bone marrow, neutrophils circulate freely for only a matter of hours before crawling into the extravascular space looking for things to engulf and kill. For unknown reasons, half of the neutrophils in the peripheral blood are "marginated" along the endothelium and therefore are not measured in the WBC count. Accordingly, the true peripheral blood content of neutrophils, consisting of the circulating and the marginated pools, is ordinarily twice that measured by the neutrophil count (Fig. 140–1). Taking these kinetic considerations into account, a simple pathophysiologic classification of neutropenia can be derived from the three-compartment model: (1) the marrow compartment, (2) the peripheral blood compartment, (3) the extravascular compartment, or (4) combinations of the above (Fig. 140–2).

Abnormalities in the Marrow Compartment.

Bone marrow defects account for the majority of neutropenias in clinical practice. Failure of the marrow compartment can occur as a result of direct injury, in which case the marrow usually contains fewer than normal hematopoietic cells, or from maturation defects of hematopoietic cells, characterized principally by normal or increased numbers of morphologically abnormal hematopoietic cells. In either case, neutropenia most frequently occurs along with abnormalities in the number of platelets and red cells. Marrow injury can occur as a consequence of a variety of diseases (Fig. 140–2).

Drug-induced injury is most common (Table 140–1). Antineoplastic and immunosuppressive agents are generally designed to inflict injury on a proliferative population of cells (e.g., cancer cells); myelosuppressive toxicity is the rule but is generally predictable, as its intensity varies directly with the dose. Drugs that usually are not myelosuppressive and are well tolerated in the majority of patients can sometimes induce either marrow injury or peripheral neutrophil destruction in certain patients. These drug-induced reactions can result from direct drug-mediated cytotoxicity or from an immune mechanism in which (1) neutrophils are destroyed in extramedullary sites (e.g., the penicillins) or (2) the marrow compartment is injured (e.g., procainamide, chloramphenicol, dapsone).

Radiation may result in acute self-limited and chronic marrow injury. Chronic radiation-induced injury can also result in the later development of myelodysplasia and nonlymphocytic leukemia, both of which often present with neutropenia. Benzene toxicity can also result in acute or chronic neutropenia and, like radiation-induced marrow failure, is associated with a high risk of acute nonlymphocytic leukemia.

Immune-mediated bone marrow failure can be mediated by autoantibodies or by T lymphocytes that inhibit the growth of bone marrow precursor cells. Most patients with immune-mediated leukopenia have concurrent rheumatic or autoimmune diseases. Infection of the marrow *per se* is unusual and most often does not result in neutropenia; some exceptions include mycobacterial infection (especially those caused by *Mycobacterium tuberculosis* and *M. kansasii*) and certain viral infections.

Bone marrow invasion by abnormal cells can result in neutropenia. Carcinoma of the lung, breast, prostate, and stomach, as well as malignant hematopoietic disorders, can occupy enough of the medullary space to cause global marrow failure. Similarly, in certain of the myeloproliferative diseases and leukemias, bone marrow fibroblasts can proliferate in such excess that they dominate the marrow and contribute to bone marrow failure (Fig. 140–2).

Maturation arrest can result in functional bone marrow failure even though the bone marrow is full of granulocyte precursors. In the bone marrows of patients with folate or vitamin B_{12} deficiency, for example, are found numerous, morphologically abnormal, granulocyte precursors that, because of the effects of the vitamin deficiency state on nuclear replication, fail to mature normally and therefore suffer a high rate of intramedullary death (see Ch. 133). The marrow is hypercellular but packed with weird-looking cells exhibiting dysynchronous nuclear and cytoplasmic maturation (e.g., primitive nuclei and very differentiated cytoplasm [the hallmark of megaloblastic change]). Hematopoietic activity in the primitive cell

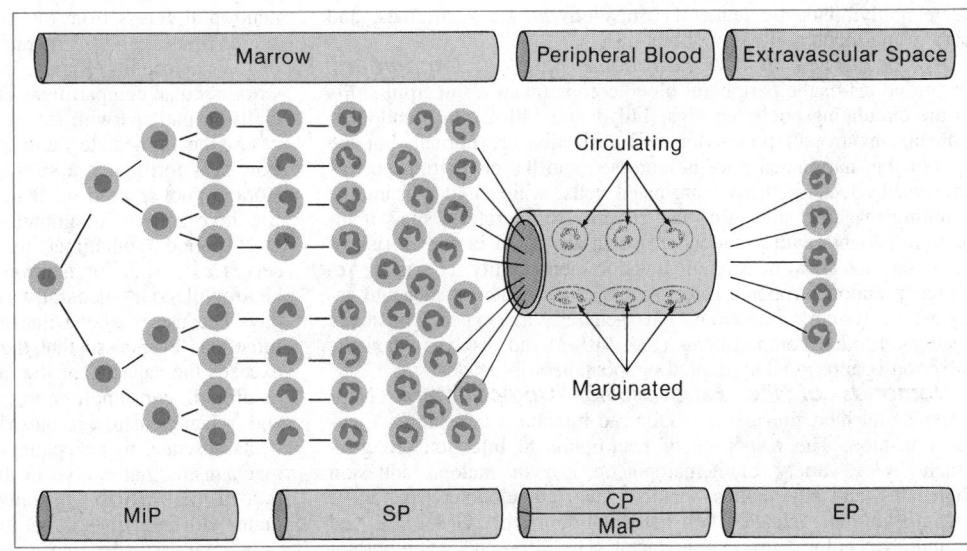

FIGURE 140–1. Production and distribution of neutrophils involve three compartments. Stem cells, committed progenitor cells, and morphologically recognizable bone marrow precursor cells proliferate and mature (differentiate) under the influence of a variety of humoral regulatory factors, including GM-CSF (granulocyte-macrophage colony stimulating factor) and G-CSF (granulocyte colony stimulating factor). These replicative responses occur in the "mitotic pool" (MiP). Once cells reach the intermediate maturation stage known as the metamyelocyte, they stop proliferating but continue differentiating to bands and segmented neutrophils. These cells, although capable of leaving the marrow if needed, generally spend about 5 days in the marrow in the "storage pool" (SP). The neutrophils then enter the bloodstream. Half of these circulating cells adhere to endothelial cells and compose the "marginated pool" (MaP). The nonmarginated cells make up the "circulating pool" (CP). After their brief sojourn in the peripheral blood, the neutrophils invade the extravascular compartments of most organs, where they are used as defenders or garbage disposal devices or die within 1 to 2 days.

Marrow

ABNORMALITIES IN THE BONE MARROW
COMPARTMENT

1. Bone Marrow Injury
   A. Drugs
      Cytotoxic and noncytotoxic agents
   B. Radiation
   C. Chemicals
      Benzene, DDT, dinitrophenol, arsenic,
      bismuth, nitrous oxide
   D. Certain congenital and hereditary
      neutropenias
   E. Immunologically mediated (largely seen
      in patients with rheumatic disorders)
      Cytotoxic T cell–mediated (T)
      Antibody-mediated (Ab)
      Mechanisms that require both T and Ab
   F. Infection
      Viral (hepatitis, parvovirus, AIDS)
      Bacterial (*M. tuberculosis, M. kansasii*)
   G. Bone marrow replacement (infiltrative
      diseases)
      Malignancies (lung, breast, prostate,
      stomach, lymphomas, and lymphoid leukemias)
      Fibrosis
      Agnogenic myeloid metaplasia
      Long-standing polycythemia vera
      Chronic myelogenous leukemia
      Radiation injury
      Injury from chronic cytotoxic drug therapy
      Acute megakaryocytic leukemia

2. Maturation Defects
   A. Acquired
      Folic acid deficiency
      Vitamin B_{12} deficiency
   B. Neoplastic and other clonal disorders
      Congenital neutropenias
      Acute nonlymphocytic leukemia
      Myelodysplastic syndromes
      Paroxysmal nocturnal hemoglobinuria

Peripheral Blood

ABNORMALITIES IN THE PERIPHERAL
BLOOD COMPARTMENT

1. Shift of neutrophils from the
   circulating to the marginated
   pool (known as pseudoneutropenia)
   A. Hereditary or constitutional
      benign pseudoneutropenia
   B. Acquired
      Acute: Severe bacterial
         infection, frequently
         associated with endotoxemia
      Chronic: Protein-calorie
         malnutrition, malaria
2. Intravascular
   sequestration
   A. In lung (complement–mediated
      leukoagglutination)
   B. In spleen (hypersplenism)

Extravascular

ABNORMALITIES IN THE EXTRAVASCULAR COMPARTMENT

1. Increased utilization
   A. Severe bacterial, fungal, viral, or
      rickettsial infection
   B. Anaphylaxis

FIGURE 140–2. The causes of neutropenia are arranged according to the compartment in which the abnormality usually resides. The approach to the neutropenic patient should begin by determining which of the three major compartments is likely the critical pathophysiologic point.

population is intensely active, but the activity is ineffective—the process is known as "ineffective hematopoiesis." Certain congenital neutropenias also represent maturation abnormalities, as do the acute nonlymphocytic leukemias, myelodysplastic syndromes, and paroxysmal nocturnal hemoglobinuria.

Abnormalities in the Peripheral Blood Compartment. Perturbations of the peripheral blood compartment result from shifts in the circulating pool (see Figs. 140–1 and 140–2). In pseudoneutropenia, neutrophil production and utilization are normal, but the size of the marginated pool is increased and the circulating pool is decreased. Because these marginated cells, while hidden from the counting machine, maintain their capacity to migrate to sites of infection, patients with pseudoneutropenia are not at increased risk of infection unless a neutrophil function abnormality coexists. Acquired pseudoneutropenia often occurs as an acute or subacute response to systemic infections. It is generally associated with acute changes in other compartments (Fig. 140–3) and resolves when the infection is appropriately treated or spontaneously abates.

Demands of the Extravascular Compartment. Neutrophils and their precursors respond to infections in a highly regulated fashion. The responses of neutrophils to infection are governed by a variety of hematopoietic growth factors, adhesion molecules, and interleukins, including two granulopoietic factors—granulocyte-macrophage colony stimulating factor (GM-CSF), and granulocyte colony stimulating factor (G-CSF)—and an important chemotactic factor, interleukin-8 (IL-8). These factors, along with IL-1, a cytokine that induces expression of many effector molecules of inflammation, account for (1) a prompt increase in the rate of production of neutrophils in the mitotic compartment, a response

mediated by a complex network of cellular and humoral regulatory interactions, (2) early release of neutrophils from the marrow storage pool to the peripheral blood pool, (3) an increase in the rate of neutrophil egress from the peripheral blood pool to the invaded tissue or tissues, and (4) increased phagocytic and bactericidal activity of the neutrophils. Rarely, increased demand for neutrophils in the extravascular compartment can lead to transient neutropenia, especially in patients with severe acute infections (Fig. 140–3). In such cases, the immediate demand for neutrophils in the zone of infection calls forth such a substantial release response that the marrow storage pool is used up before it can be restored by increased proliferative activity of granulocyte progenitor cells. Therefore, for a brief period (sometimes up to 5 to 6 days), the infected tissue serves as a sink for neutrophils. Even under these conditions, the neutrophil count generally rises well above normal within a few days because the bone marrow is highly effective in responding to infectious events, so that the demand for neutrophils almost never exceeds the capacity of the mitotic pool to supply them. In contrast, neutrophil consumption in patients with autoimmune neutropenia and hypersplenism can outstrip marrow production. Whether this reflects absence in such patients of the complete humoral stimulatory mechanisms that evolve in the infected host or the rate of destruction in these patients actually exceeds the rate of utilization in patients with infections is not known.

In summary, the causes of neutropenia are heterogeneous and best categorized in pathophysiologic terms (Fig. 140–3).

CLINICAL MANIFESTATIONS. Neutropenia can occur in a wide variety of systemic diseases (see Fig. 140–2), the manifestations of which may dominate the clinical picture. Many neutropenic

TABLE 140–1. DRUGS THAT CAUSE NEUTROPENIA

Antiarrhythmics
    Procainamide, propranolol, quinidine, tocainide
Antibiotics
    Chloramphenicol, penicillins, sulfonamides, para-aminosalicylic acid
        (PAS), rifampin, vancomycin, isoniazid, nitrofurantoin
Antimalarials
    Dapsone, quinine, pyrimethamine
Anticonvulsants
    Phenytoin, mephenytoin, trimethadione, ethosuximide, carbamazepine
Hypoglycemic agents
    Tolbutamide, chlorpropamide
Antihistamines
    Cimetidine, brompheniramine, tripelennamine
Antihypertensives
    Methyldopa, captopril
Anti-inflammatory agents
    Aminopyrine, phenylbutazone, gold salts, ibuprofen, indomethacin
Antithyroid agents
    Propylthiouracil, methimazole, thiouracil
Diuretics
    Acetazolamide, hydrochlorothiazide, chlorthalidone
Phenothiazines
    Chlorpromazine, promazine, prochlorperazine
Immunosuppressive agents
    Antimetabolites
Cytotoxic agents
    Alkylating agents, antimetabolites, anthracyclines, vinca alkaloids, cisplatin,
        hydroxyurea, actinomycin
Other agents
    Recombinant interferons, allopurinol, ethanol, levamisole, penicillamine,
        AZT, streptokinase

patients remain asymptomatic, most often those whose neutrophil count exceeds 1.0×10^9 per liter or those whose neutropenia is acute and self-limited in duration. When symptoms do occur, they generally result from recurrent, often severe, bacterial infections. This is not surprising in view of the pivotal importance of the neutrophil in the defense of the host against microorganisms (see Ch. 139).

The risk of bacterial infection increases slightly as the peripheral neutrophil count falls below 1.0×10^9 per liter but is greatly increased at levels below 0.5×10^9 per liter. The degree to which monocytosis compensates for neutropenia may modify the risk. I have personally followed a young patient with severe congenital neutropenia for more than 20 years, whose total leukocyte count is normal because of marked monocytosis. Because of the capacity of monocytes to "cover" for neutrophil deficiencies, this patient has had very few bacterial infections.

Lungs, genitourinary system, gut, oropharynx, and skin are the most frequent sources of infection in neutropenic patients. The infecting organisms are the "usual suspects" for the given anatomic site, with the caveat that in patients who have recurrent infections and require prolonged and recurrent antibacterial therapy, unusual (often hospital-acquired) organisms can colonize and subsequently cause infection. The antibiotic history of infected neutropenic patients is important to obtain. The usual signs and symptoms of infection are often diminished or absent in patients with neutropenia because the cell that mediates much of the inflammatory responses to infection is absent. Thus, neutropenic patients with severe bilateral bacterial pneumonia can present, initially, with minimal infiltrates demonstrable on chest radiograph and can have benign-looking nonpurulent sputum; patients with pyelonephritis may not exhibit pyuria; patients with bacterial pharyngitis may not have purulence in the oropharynx; and patients with severe bacterial infection of the skin may present only with erythroderma rather than furunculosis. In the neutropenic patient, infections that in an otherwise normal individual might have been well localized become quickly disseminated. Therefore, not only is the infected neutropenic patient a diagnostic problem but, in addition, because any given infection is more likely to be widespread at the time of diagnosis, these patients are often dangerously ill.

DIAGNOSIS. The diagnostic evaluation of neutropenia is influenced by its severity and the clinical setting in which it occurs. The assessment of patients with neutrophil counts of <0.5 to 1.0×10^9 per liter should obviously proceed briskly. The patient with fever, sepsis, or both in whom neutropenia is discovered for the first time presents a particularly difficult problem. In such patients it is impossible to determine immediately whether the neutropenia antedated sepsis, a situation with both prognostic and therapeutic implications, or whether the neutropenia is merely a short-lived response to the infection itself (Fig. 140–3). Examination of the peripheral blood smear and differential WBC count can be helpful in such cases. An increase in the fraction of circulating band neutrophil forms to levels above 20% suggests that marrow granulopoietic activity is responding appropriately (Fig. 140–4). It is then presumed

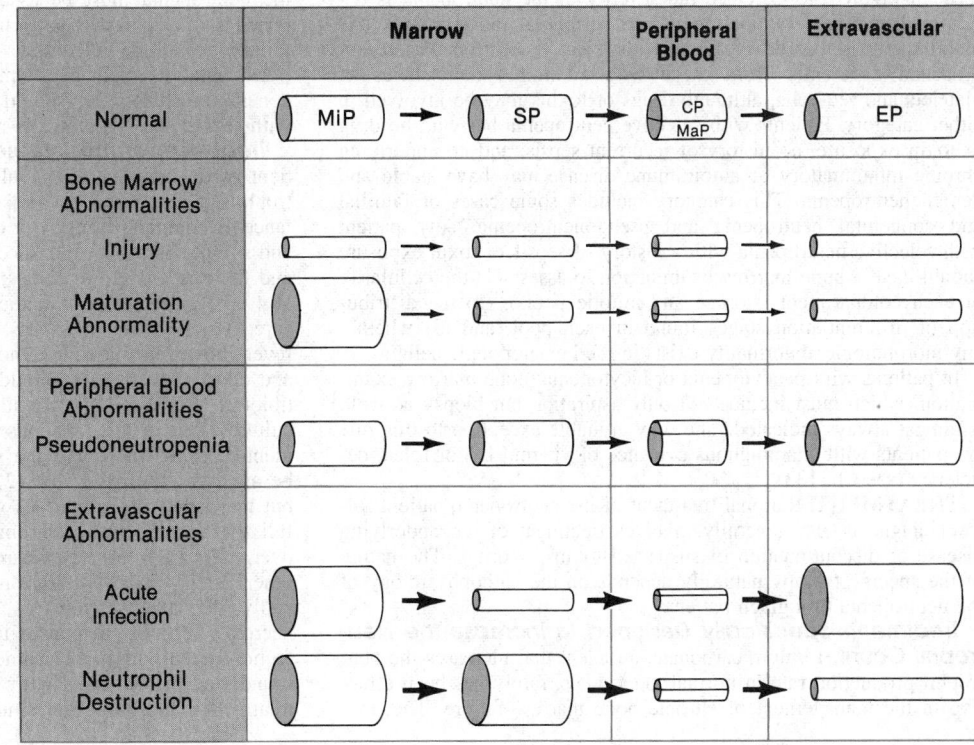

FIGURE 140–3. Pathophysiologic mechanisms of neutropenia. The size of a given compartment is represented by the size of the corresponding cylinder. The number of cells leaving a compartment for the next compartment can vary substantially, but flow between compartments is unidirectional. Notice that in every case the circulating neutrophil pool is small, but the size of the other pools is variable. Marrow injury causes a global decline in the size of all pools. A maturation abnormality, however, is characterized by an increase in the number of precursor cells that do not mature. Pseudoneutropenia is characterized by a movement of circulating neutrophils to the marginated pool. In severe infections, the acute demand for neutrophils in the infected extravascular site results in a transient loss of storage pool neutrophils before the hypercellular (but as yet immature) mitotic compartments can renew the storage pool. Finally, excessive destruction of neutrophils can result in neutropenia. MiP = mitotic pool; SP = storage pool; CP = circulating pool; MaP = marginated pool; EP = extravascular pool.

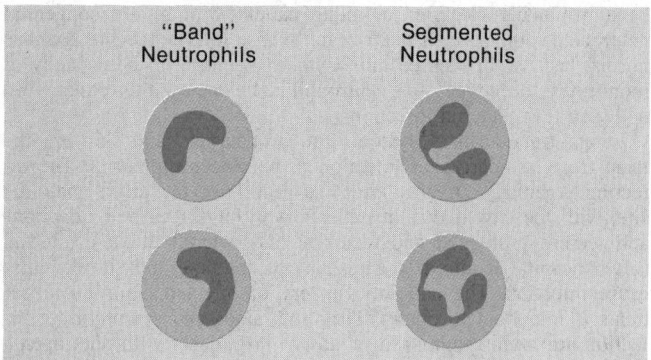

FIGURE 140–4. Band neutrophils are somewhat "younger" forms than segmented neutrophils. The nuclear lobes in a segmented form are separated by fine filaments absent in the band.

either that the marrow is recovering from injury or that the neutropenia is derived from a transient shift to the marginated pool or to the extravascular compartment.

The diagnostic evaluation of neutropenia must first address the question of the severity and then whether the patient has fever, sepsis, or both. The patient with sepsis and severe neutropenia should be treated promptly with intravenous antibiotics following appropriate cultures but without waiting for the results of those cultures. Once these important initial questions are answered, the remainder of the diagnostic evaluation can proceed (Fig. 140–5): (1) identifying any potential drugs and toxins to which the patient might have been exposed; (2) determining, if possible, the chronicity of the neutropenia; (3) ascertaining whether there have been recurrent infections; (4) identifying any underlying systemic disease that might be causative; and (5) examining the blood counts and blood morphology and bone marrow (the latter is usually indicated) to determine the most likely pathophysiologic explanation. The latter is important even if a specific, likely causative, underlying disease is promptly identified. Felty's syndrome, for example, is a well-recognized cause of neutropenia, but there are at least two separate pathophysiologic mechanisms in groups of these patients, one mediated by antineutrophil antibodies, the other by T lymphocyte–mediated bone marrow failure. Each mechanism has different therapeutic implications.

One approach to the neutropenic patient is shown in algorithmic form in Figure 140–5. Once the severity of the neutropenia is determined, careful examination of the peripheral blood counts and blood smear is in order. Patients with selective neutropenia are approached differently from those with additional deficiencies of platelets and red cells, although drugs or toxins may be involved in either category. Patients with selective neutropenia but with no drug or toxin exposure, no history of recurrent sepsis, and no underlying chronic inflammatory or autoimmune disease may have stable and benign neutropenia. This category includes some cases of familial and congenital neutropenia and pseudoneutropenia. Any patient with selective neutropenia with a history of sepsis or toxin exposure should have a bone marrow examination to assess (1) the cellularity of each compartment (storage and mitotic pools), (2) the distribution of differentiation stages found in each pool, and (3) whether any morphologic abnormality exists in the hematopoietic cells.

In patients with pancytopenia or bicytopenia, bone marrow examination, which must include not only aspiration but biopsy as well, is almost always indicated. The only arguable exception to this rule are patients with unambiguous evidence of vitamin B_{12} or folate deficiency (see Ch. 133).

TREATMENT. Rational treatment of the neutropenic patient follows diagnosis and generally involves treatment of the underlying disease or discontinuation of suspected toxins or drugs. The nature of the specific therapy naturally depends on the pathophysiology of the neutropenia in a given patient.

Treatments Specifically Designed to Increase the Neutrophil Count. Lithium carbonate, an agent that increases the neutrophil production rate in normal individuals, rarely has been effective in the management of chronic bone marrow failure. The dose

used in adults is 300 mg by mouth three times daily. In view of the frequency of toxicity, trials of therapy should be considered only as a last resort. No test to predict individual responsiveness has yet been developed.

Immunosuppressive therapy, including glucocorticoids or cyclosporin, almost always elicits a favorable response in patients with marrow failure mediated by cytotoxic T lymphocytes. *In vitro* clonogenic cultures of bone marrow cells in severely neutropenic patients can aid in the identification of patients likely to respond to such therapy. Some responses to immunosuppressive therapy have also occurred in patients whose neutropenia resulted from antineutrophil antibodies. Splenectomy is rarely helpful in the management of neutropenic patients, even those with Felty's syndrome. It is now reserved for patients with unambiguous hypersplenism in whom bone marrow function is normal.

Recombinant Human Granulopoietic Factors. Both GM-CSF and G-CSF are FDA-approved agents and are available to clinicians. In normal volunteers, GM-CSF and G-CSF reliably induce neutrophilic leukocytosis; GM-CSF also induces the appearance of eosinophils and monocytes. As a general rule, patients with drug-induced neutropenia (e.g., following cancer chemotherapy) recover more rapidly if they receive either GM-CSF or G-CSF, but apart from the setting of bone marrow transplantation, the role of these agents in clinical practice is still unclear. The widespread availability of recombinant human G-CSF and GM-CSF for clinical use has resulted in widespread inappropriate use. Although clear-cut indications exist for the use of G-CSF in the management of certain severe hereditary neutropenias, the role of these agents in the management of cancer and leukemia patients is not established, notwithstanding the hundreds of therapeutic trials published to date. Although in widespread use in this country to support bone marrow recovery in cancer patients following cytotoxic therapy, this cannot be considered routine at this time. Neither agent has been adequately tested as an auxiliary tool in the infected neutropenic patient, and this setting does not yet constitute an indication. Like all exciting new therapeutic agents, GM-CSF and G-CSF have peaked in popularity. Now new evidence is emerging that the use of these agents routinely in certain cancer patients may not be cost effective and that their use in certain settings of acute infection may actually result in excess morbidity.

Bone Marrow Transplantation. In severe aplastic anemia the role of bone marrow transplantation is well established (see Ch. 151). Other marrow failure states (e.g., myelodysplastic syndromes and congenital neutropenias) also respond to transplantation. Allogeneic transplantation is associated with high mortality; its use in patients with selective neutropenia is therefore uncertain. Before transplantation is seriously considered, the duration and severity of the neutropenia must be assessed; marrow failure must be established as the primary cause; and immunologically mediated marrow failure should be ruled out. If the patient has an identical twin, transplantation might be attempted with fewer constraints, but allogeneic transplantation should always be reserved for individuals with severe and symptomatic neutropenia caused by marrow failure.

Treatment of the Infected Neutropenic Patient. Each patient with neutropenia should understand the function of neutrophils, the consequences of neutrophil deficiency, and the importance of communicating with his or her physician the moment signs and symptoms of infection occur. If a neutropenic patient is afebrile and there is no sign of sepsis, the diagnostic workup should generally take place in the outpatient clinic to avoid unnecessary exposure to nosocomial infections. Patients with severe neutropenia and fever, however, should be hospitalized. Cultures of urine, blood, and other relevant sites should be obtained, but broad-spectrum antibiotics should be given without waiting for the results of these cultures. One of three responses is seen: (1) A causative organism is identified, in which case the spectrum of antimicrobial agents can be appropriately narrowed. (2) A candidate organism is not found, but the patient still improves with empiric therapy. In this setting a full course of broad-spectrum antibiotics should be given. Moreover, after a full course of parenteral antibiotics has been given, another 7 to 14 days of oral antibiotics should be considered, especially in patients with (a) invasive infections associated with necrosis, (b) slow responses to initial antibiotic therapy, or (c) infections recurrent in the same anatomic site. (3) No organism is found, and the clinical picture is not altered after 3 days of empiric treatment. This unsettling situation occurs with some regularity in

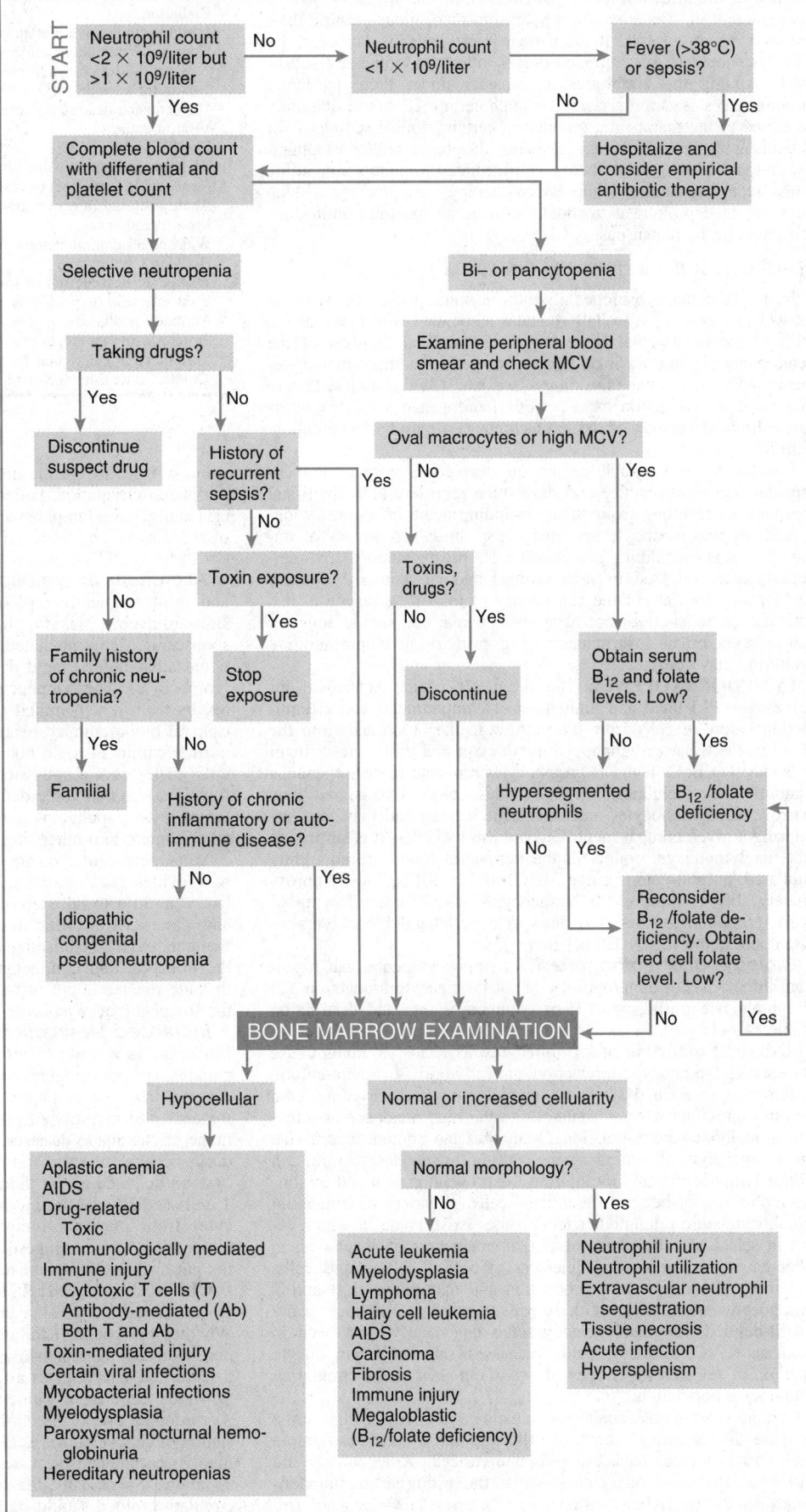

FIGURE 140–5. An algorithm for the evaluation of patients with neutropenia.

practice. The approach to a patient at this point depends on the seriousness of the infection. For a patient with localized disease who is not critically ill, it is sometimes helpful to discontinue empiric therapy and repeat cultures. If the patient is critically ill, however, antibiotics should be discontinued only if other antibiotics are substituted. Among the antibiotics to consider under these particular circumstances is amphotericin B. Amphotericin B should definitely be added to the therapeutic regimen in certain clinical settings—for patients with acute leukemia, diabetes, dysphagia and/or esophagitis, endophthalmitis, or defective cell-mediated immunity (including those receiving immunosuppressive therapy) and for those who have received prolonged treatment with broad-spectrum antibacterial agents in the recent past.

DEFICIENCIES OF OTHER CIRCULATING PHAGOCYTES

Monocytopenia, eosinopenia, and basophilopenia are seen in most of the bone marrow failure states associated with neutropenia. Isolated monocytopenia, however, is very unusual. In view of the heterogeneous and critical roles played by the monocyte-macrophage in normal physiology (see Ch. 139), complete failure of monocyte production for a period of more than 9 to 10 months (the estimated lifespan of tissue macrophages) may be incompatible with life.

Eosinopenia and basophilopenia are more common than monocytopenia in clinical practice and most often represent redistributional mechanisms resulting from stress, including acute infections, widespread neoplasms, and severe injury (e.g., burns). A variety of humoral factors, including glucocorticoids, prostaglandins, and epinephrine, are released in such settings and are known to induce eosinopenia. In view of the consistency of this stress response, if a patient with sepsis does not have eosinopenia, one should consider that adrenocortical insufficiency or a primary myeloproliferative syndrome may coexist.

LYMPHOCYTOPENIA. The life cycle of the neutrophil involves a well-defined and limited set of compartments and a unidirectional flow of cells from the marrow to the blood and from the blood to the tissues. Lymphocyte production and traffic are difficult to assess: (1) Both T and B lymphocytes replicate in heterogeneous anatomic sites, including the lymph nodes, spleen, tonsils, and bone marrow; (2) lymphocytes are capable of leaving and then later re-entering a given compartment. Given these variables, it is surprising that the lymphocyte counts in the peripheral blood are so tightly regulated; normal counts range from 2 to 4×10^9 per liter. Approximately 20% of these are B lymphocytes, and 70% are T lymphocytes. Lymphocytopenia is defined as a peripheral blood lymphocyte count below 1.5×10^9 per liter.

Etiology and Pathogenesis. Lymphocytopenia can result from three types of abnormalities: (1) of lymphocyte production, (2) of lymphocyte traffic, and (3) of lymphocyte loss and destruction (Table 140–2).

Reduced Production of Lymphocytes. The most common cause of reduced lymphocyte production in the world is protein-calorie malnutrition (see Ch. 194). The immunologic paresis resulting from malnutrition contributes substantially to the high incidence of infection in malnourished populations. Radiation and immunosuppressive agents, including alkylating agents and antithymocyte globulin, can induce lymphocytopenia by injuring the progenitor pool and inhibiting replication of better-differentiated cells. A variety of congenital lymphocytopenic immunodeficiency states exist, some of which result in selective deficiencies of B lymphocytes or of T cells or, in other cases, in combined deficiencies of both T cells and B cells. The mechanisms by which production and maturation of B and T lymphocytes are impaired in these patients are heterogeneous; many are ill-defined. Immunodeficiency states can clearly exist even in the absence of lymphocytopenia because of abnormal lymphocyte function or selective deficiency of one component of the circulating lymphocyte population.

Certain viruses are capable of inducing lymphocytopenia; some of these agents infect lymphoid cells and cause their destruction. Such viruses include measles, polio, and varicella-zoster viruses and HIV (human immunodeficiency virus, the acquired immunodeficiency syndrome [AIDS] virus) (see Ch. 361). HIV does not frequently cause lymphocytopenia but does infect the helper (CD4+) subset of T lymphocytes and destroys them, a process that results in

TABLE 140–2. CAUSES OF LYMPHOCYTOPENIA

Abnormalities of lymphocyte production
 Protein-calorie malnutrition
 Radiation
 Immunosuppressive therapeutic agents
 Congenital immunodeficiency states
  Wiskott-Aldrich syndrome
  Nezelof's syndrome
  Adenosine deaminase deficiency
 Viral infections
 Hodgkin's lymphoma
 Widespread granulomatous infection (mycobacterial, fungal)
Alterations in lymphocyte traffic
 Acute bacterial infection, trauma, stress, glucocorticoids
 Viral infection
 Widespread granulomatous infection
 Hodgkin's lymphoma
Lymphocyte destruction or loss
 Viral infection (e.g., HIV-1)
 Antibody-mediated lymphocyte destruction
 Protein-losing enteropathy
 Chronic right ventricular failure
 Thoracic duct drainage or rupture

a marked decline in the absolute numbers of helper T cells in the peripheral circulation. Patients with untreated Hodgkin's disease occasionally have lymphocytopenia, especially during the late stages of the disease and with the least favorable histologic subtypes (see Ch. 146).

Alterations in Lymphocytic Traffic. Alterations are common and most frequently represent transient responses to a variety of stressful events, including bacterial infections and trauma. These responses are likely mediated by high levels of endogenous glucocorticoids that induce rapid declines in circulating levels of B and T lymphocytes. The lymphocytopenic response to this type of steroid results from a self-limited shift of lymphocytes away from the peripheral blood compartment. Lymphocyte values generally return to normal within 24 to 48 hours. For this reason, the transient declines induced by endogenous steroid production are not associated with functional immunologic deficiency. Certain viruses can also bind to lymphocyte populations and cause their departure from the blood compartment into other sites.

More persistent lymphocytopenia has been described in patients with widespread granulomatous disease, a phenomenon that is likely multifactorial, deriving from both inhibition of production and alterations of traffic. Patients with these disorders are often difficult to treat. Establishing a cause-and-effect relationship between the infection and lymphocytopenia is difficult when one considers that the reverse might just as easily be true; consider, for example, the frequency of mycobacterial infection in patients with AIDS.

Increased Destruction of Lymphocytes. Lymphocytopenia can occur as a result of viral infection, as outlined above. In some patients lymphocytopenia results from antilymphocyte antibodies. As was the case in patients with immunologically mediated neutropenia, the majority of such individuals have underlying autoimmune or rheumatic diseases. Losses of viable lymphocytes can also occur because of structural defects in sites of high-density lymphocyte traffic, such as via thoracic duct fistulas. In such patients, both T cells and B cells decline in the peripheral blood. Loss of lymphocytes from intestinal lymphatics can occur in protein-losing enteropathies, severe congestive heart failure, or primary diseases of the gut or intestinal lymphatics (Table 140–2).

CLINICAL MANIFESTATIONS AND DIAGNOSIS. There are no specific clinical manifestations of lymphocytopenia *per se.* Whether the patient exhibits signs of immunologic deficiency depends on the pathophysiology of the disorder, the duration of the disease, the lymphocytes affected most significantly, and the degree to which cellular or humoral immunity is functionally perturbed. Accordingly, unless the clinical setting is clearly one in which transient lymphocytopenia is likely, the approach to diagnosis should involve comprehensive assessment of the integrity of the immune apparatus. Specifically, the subsets of lymphocytes remaining in the circulating blood should be identified and should at least include B cells, helper-inducer T cells, and cytotoxic-suppressor T cells. In addition, quantitative immunoglobulin levels should be measured in the serum and a series of skin tests performed to detect deficiencies of cell-mediated immunity.

TREATMENT. Because lymphocytopenia ordinarily represents a response to an underlying disease, primary attention must be paid to establishing the nature of that disease and instituting therapy for it. Patients whose lymphocytopenia is accompanied by hypogammaglobulinemia may benefit significantly from administration of immunoglobulin intravenously. The treatment of severe deficiencies of cell-mediated immunity remains experimental. Responses have been described with transplantation of allogeneic marrow, fetal liver, or thymic epithelial cells. Recent progress has been made in the therapy of adenosine deaminase deficiency (a cause of severe combined immunodeficiency) using adenosine deaminase conjugated to polyethylene glycol, and it is likely that this particular disease will be one of the early successes in the field of gene therapy.

Bagby GC, Segal GM: Growth factors and the control of hematopoiesis. In Hoffman R, Benz EJ, Shattil SJ, et al. (eds.): Hematology: Basic Principles and Practice. New York, Churchill Livingstone, 1994. *A comprehensive and up-to-date review of the growth factors known to govern white cell production, their biologic activity, and the biologic factors that control their production.*

Crawford J, Ozer H, Stoller R, et al.: Reduction by granulocyte colony-stimulating factor of fever and neutropenia induced by chemotherapy in patients with small-cell lung cancer. N Engl J Med 325:164, 1991. Nichols CR, Fox EP, Roth BJ, et al.: Incidence of neutropenic fever in patients treated with standard-dose combination chemotherapy for small-cell lung cancer and the cost impact of treatment with granulocyte colony-stimulating factor. J Clin Oncol 12:1245, 1994. *Hundreds of studies (e.g., Crawford et al.) have shown that treatment of patients with G-CSF or, in other studies GM-CSF, after they have received cytotoxic chemotherapy for malignancies, clearly causes an earlier-than-expected recovery of neutrophils. Such results are not sufficient to warrant widespread use of these factors in routine treatment of cancer patients. Caregivers must first know whether the use of GM-CSF or G-CSF in cancer patients (a) prolongs survival (so far they have not), (b) reduces actual infection rates (so far they do not), (c) is cost effective (Nichols et al. demonstrate that for at least one common malignancy, it is not), and (d) does not enhance the growth of the patient's cancer cells (not enough work on this has been done, but studies in animal models suggest that it should be studied with great care).*

Kaplan LD, Kahn JO, Crowe S, et al.: Clinical and virologic effects of recombinant human granulocyte-macrophage colony-stimulating factor in patients receiving chemotherapy for human immunodeficiency virus–associated non-Hodgkin's lymphoma: Results of a randomized trial. J Clin Oncol 9:929, 1991. *The bone marrow failure that complicates HIV-1 infection is a therapeutic problem. Even patients with blood counts reasonably close to normal are unusually intolerant of cytotoxic therapy and develop prolonged periods of post-therapy myelosuppression. Because myelosuppressive antiviral and anticancer chemotherapies are commonly required in AIDS patients, strategies for avoiding bone marrow toxicity have been sought recently, including the use of hematopoietic growth factors G-CSF and GM-CSF. Although these agents may be helpful in selected settings, they should be used with caution. Early in vitro work with hematopoietic growth factors, suggested that HIV-1 proviral gene expression could be enhanced by exposure of mononuclear phagocytes to cytokines that activate them (e.g., GM-CSF). The concern that such a phenomenon might occur during therapy of AIDS patients with GM-CSF has been realized, as revealed in the studies by Kaplan et al. and others. Combining GM-CSF with AZT (zidovudine) seems to prevent this undesirable effect.*

Louache F, Henri A, Bettaieb A, et al.: Role of human immunodeficiency virus replication in defective in vitro growth of hematopoietic progenitors. Blood 80:2991, 1992. *Bone marrow failure is a common complication of HIV infection, and a good number of laboratories are trying to determine the mechanisms by which it occurs because it complicates treatment substantially. Early proposals that HIV-1 infects purified progenitor cells have not been confirmed in studies that examined progeny of committed stem cells. Louache et al. provide evidence that infection of auxiliary cells (cells that produce growth factors and mitotic inhibitory factors for hematopoietic stem cells and progenitor cells) is a key factor in hematopoietic suppression by HIV-1.*

Shastri KA, Logue GL: Autoimmune neutropenia. Blood 81:1984, 1993. *Important new information on the nature of and diagnostic strategies for sorting different types of autoimmune neutropenias from one another is presented. Focusing on humoral more than cell-mediated immune mechanisms, the authors cover antineutrophil antibodies, hematopoietic inhibitory T cells (HIT cells), T-gamma lymphocytosis, antibody testing, and therapeutic options.*

140.2 Leukocytosis and Leukemoid Reactions

Circulating leukocytes consist of neutrophils, monocytes, eosinophils, basophils, and lymphocytes (T cells, B cells, and natural killer cells are all lymphocytes). Any one or all of these cell types can increase in peripheral blood to abnormal levels, depending on the stimulus. Each type of leukocyte is produced in the bone marrow (and in the case of lymphocytes, in lymph nodes, spleen, and thymus as well) in response to specific growth factors. The term *leukocytosis* describes a total leukocyte count $> 11.0 \times 10^9$

per liter. It is an important signal to examine the differential white blood cell (WBC) count and determine which of the WBC types is increased. Because the specifically elevated cell type is of greatest importance, however, one should understand that abnormal elevations of specific leukocyte types in the blood can occur without elevating the total leukocyte count. The terms *neutrophilia* (neutrophilic leukocytosis), *monocytosis, lymphocytosis, eosinophilia,* and *basophilia* suggest specific diagnostic considerations.

Leukocytosis is common in acutely ill patients. When the leukocyte count exceeds 25 to 30×10^9 per liter, it is termed a *leukemoid reaction.* Leukemoid reactions reflect a response of healthy bone marrow to molecular signals stimulated by infection, trauma, and similar stresses. Leukemoid reactions are not synonymous with leukoerythroblastosis, which indicates the presence of immature WBC and nucleated red cells in the peripheral blood irrespective of the total leukocyte count. Leukoerythroblastosis is less common than leukemoid reactions but often, especially in the adult patient, reflects serious marrow dysfunction (Table 140–3). Consequently, leukoerythroblastosis provides a strong indication to perform bone marrow aspiration and biopsy, unless the clinical setting is acute severe hemolytic anemia, sepsis in a patient with hyposplenism, or acute massive trauma (with multiple fractures).

NEUTROPHILIA

PATHOPHYSIOLOGY. There are three major anatomic sites of neutrophil traffic: the bone marrow, the peripheral blood, and the extravascular space (Fig. 140–6). Traffic moves unidirectionally from marrow to blood to extravascular space. The number of neutrophils within each site can be independently regulated. The number of neutrophil precursors in the marrow mitotic pool (MiP) is largely influenced by the granulopoietic growth factors: granulocyte-macrophage colony stimulating factor (GM-CSF) and granulocyte colony stimulating factor (G-CSF). These factors, the products of separate genes, not only function to stimulate the growth and differentiation of granulocyte and/or macrophage progenitor cells but also functionally activate neutrophils. The marrow storage pool is sufficient to provide the periphery with neutrophils for 5 days in the steady state, even if it were unsupported by the MiP. A variety of physiologic stresses can release neutrophils from the storage pool into the circulating pool (Fig. 140–6B). Also, peripheral neutrophils normally segregate into two equal pools—the circulating pool and the marginated pool. Neutrophilia can result rapidly from a shift of neutrophils from the marginated to the circulating pool—"demargination" (Fig. 140–6C). The response can be induced by injections of epinephrine. In patients with acute inflammatory illnesses, storage pool release and demargination usually occur together (Fig. 140–6D).

Neutrophilic leukocytosis is the most common type of leukocytosis in clinical practice. It evolves in response to the release of factors that govern its production and traffic. The factors themselves are produced by a complex network of cross-talking auxil-

TABLE 140–3. CAUSES OF LEUKOERYTHROBLASTOSIS

Normal marrow
  Severe acute hemolytic anemia
  Acute infection in hyposplenic patients
Abnormal marrow
  Multiple fractures
  Marrow infiltration
    Tuberculosis
    Fungal disease
    Fibrosis
    Malignant cells (carcinoma, sarcoma, lymphoma, myeloma, acute leukemia)
  Chronic myeloproliferative disorders
    Agnogenic myeloid metaplasia
    Chronic myelogenous leukemia
  Other disorders
    Osteopetrosis
    Gaucher's disease
    Amyloidosis
    Paget's disease of bone
    Severe tissue hypoxia

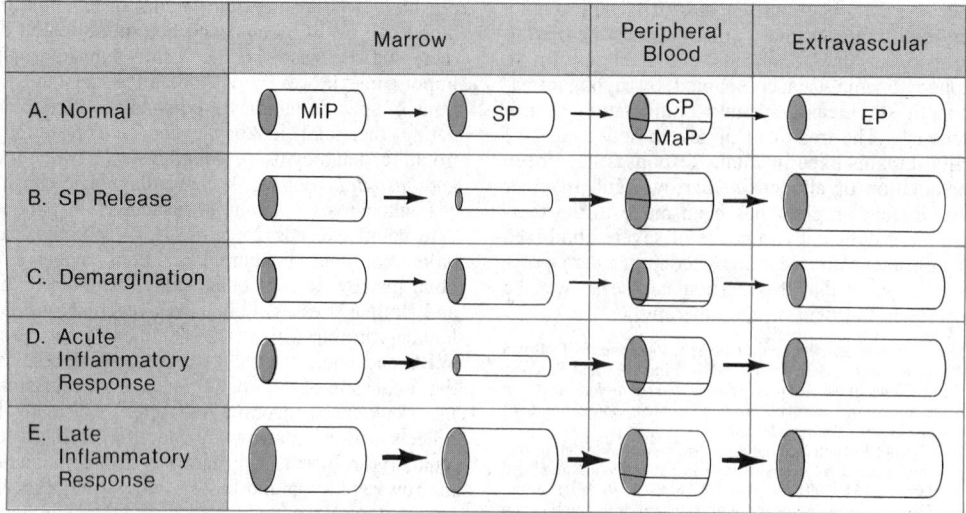

FIGURE 140–6. Pathophysiologic mechanisms of neutrophilia. In this figure the size of a given compartment is represented by the size of a given cylinder. The number of cells leaving a compartment for the next compartment is reflected by the size of the arrows between compartments. *A,* MiP = the mitotic pool of granulocyte precursor cells; SP = the granulocyte storage pool; CP = the circulating granulocyte pool; MaP = the marginated pool; EP = the extravascular pool. Notice that in every case the circulating neutrophil pool is large, but the size of the other pools is variable. *B,* A variety of stresses on the organism can result, perhaps through the action of glucocorticoid hormones, in the release of storage pool granulocytes. This occurs commonly as an acute response to acute infections. *C,* The circulating granulocyte pool can also increase in size by virtue of a shift of neutrophils from the marginated to the circulating pool. The demargination response can be regularly elicited by the administration of epinephrine and can also result from a variety of stresses, including acute infection. *D,* With most bacterial infections and other inflammatory processes, the acute demand for neutrophils in the infected extravascular sites results in the simultaneous release of storage pool neutrophils and demargination. *E,* Once the hematopoietic growth factor released in response to the inflammatory stimulus (see Fig. 140–7) has induced a few days of proliferation in the mitotic pool, the content of granulocytes in all pools increases, and delivery to the tissues becomes maximal.

iary cells in the bone marrow, including mononuclear phagocytes, microvascular endothelial cells, fibroblasts, and lymphocytes. These growth factor–producing cells respond to acute inflammatory events by augmenting production of the crucially important colony-stimulating factors (CSF's) (Fig. 140–7). The CSF's stimulate replication of granulopoietic progenitor cells, ultimately expanding the storage pool and increasing the circulating pool (see Fig. 140–6E). This new state persists until the inflammatory process is resolved.

CAUSES. Neutrophilia (neutrophil counts $> 7.5 \times 10^9$ per liter), a common clinical finding, usually reflects the inflammatory response to acute or subacute infections (Fig. 140–7; Table 140–4). Its presence should trigger a diagnostic search for an underlying cause. Such searches usually involve only a careful history and physical examination and a few inexpensive laboratory tests (the nature of which depends upon the findings on physical examination) because in most cases the site of infection is clinically apparent.

When neutrophilia occurs in the absence of evidence of acute inflammation or illness, three explanations should be considered: (1) Chemical effects; certain agents such as glucocorticoids, lithium chloride, or epinephrine commonly produce neutrophilia. (2) Malignant tumors; certain cancer cells may inappropriately express CSF genes, thereby increasing CSF blood levels. (When such cancers are effectively treated, the neutrophilia resolves.) (3) Chronic myeloproliferative disorders; chronic myelogenous leukemia, agnogenic myeloid metaplasia, essential thrombocytosis, and polycythemia rubra vera may result in substantial neutrophilia. Patients with these last-mentioned diseases can have few symptoms. When faced with an acute inflammatory illness, it is most prudent to await its resolution before seeking a myeloproliferative disorder.

DIAGNOSIS. Figure 140–8 provides an algorithm for the evaluation of patients with neutrophilia. Notice that the path leads quickly to bone marrow aspiration and biopsy as an essential strategy for evaluation of leukoerythroblastosis. In patients without leukoerythroblastosis, neutrophilic leukocytosis generally results from acute toxic, inflammatory, or traumatic stresses, and it is usually best to observe the course of neutrophilia to determine its degree of linkage with the underlying disease. If the underlying disease resolves and the neutrophilia does not, other, less common, explanations must be pursued.

Neutrophil Morphology. Neutrophil morphology can lead to early diagnosis (Fig. 140–8). Toxic granulation of neutrophils, the presence of Döhle bodies, and the presence of vacuoles in the neutrophil cytoplasm suggest that overt or subclinical inflammation, toxin exposure, trauma, or neoplasia exists. Because glucocorticoids

TABLE 140–4. COMMON CAUSES OF NEUTROPHILIA

I. Infections
Bacteria	Parasites
Viruses	Rickettsiae
Fungi	

II. Rheumatic and autoimmune disorders
Rheumatoid arthritis	Colitis
Vasculitis	Gout
Autoimmune hemolytic anemia	

III. Neoplastic disorders
Pancreatic, gastric, bronchogenic, and renal cell carcinoma; melanoma
Any cancer metastatic to bone marrow
Hodgkin's disease
Chronic myeloproliferative disorders (chronic granulocytic leukemia, agnogenic myeloid metaplasia, essential thrombocytosis, polycythemia vera)
Myelodysplastic disorders and acute myelomonocytic leukemia

IV. Chemicals
Mercury poisoning	Ethylene glycol
Venoms (reptiles, insects, jellyfish)	Histamine

V. Trauma
Thermal injury	Crush injuries
Hypothermia	Electric shock

VI. Endocrine and metabolic disorders
Ketoacidosis	Thyrotoxicosis
Lactic acidosis	

VII. Hematologic disorders (non-neoplastic)
Acute hemolytic anemias and transfusion reactions
Postsplenectomy
Recovery from marrow failure

VIII. Other disorders
Tissue necrosis	Exfoliative dermatitis
Pregnancy	Severe hypoxia
Eclampsia	

Drugs: corticosteroids, lithium chloride, and epinephrine

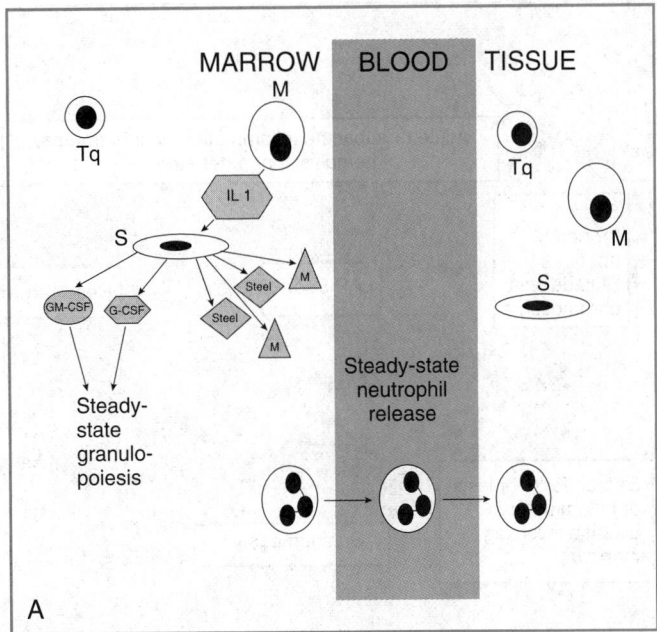

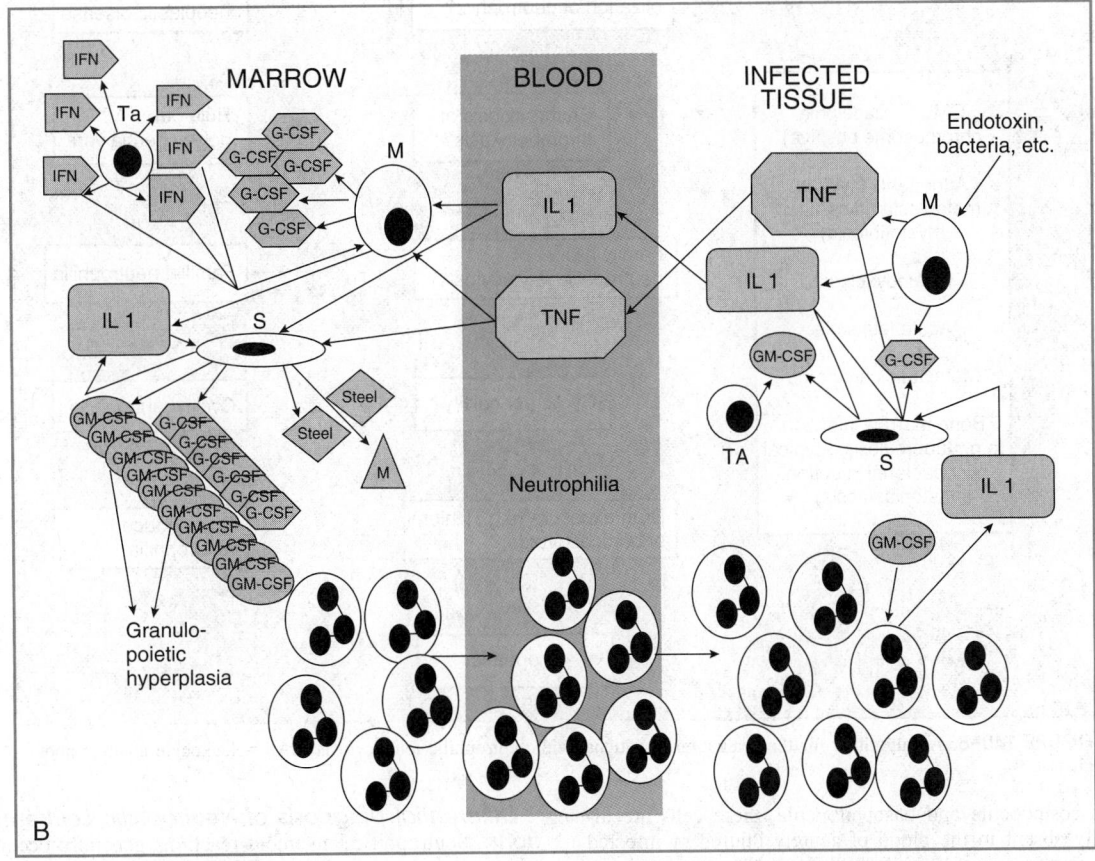

FIGURE 140–7. The likely mechanisms by which neutrophil production occurs in the steady state *(A)* and during inflammatory responses *(B)*. Virtually every mesenchymal cell can produce G-CSF and GM-CSF when induced to do so by inflammatory stimuli. Two key master switches in the inflammatory response are IL-1 and TNF α, both of which induce G-CSF and GM-CSF expression in a wide variety of stromal cells, including those in the bone marrow. These inductive cytokines also induce expression of adhesion molecules, IL-6, IL-11, and IL-8. *A,* In the steady state there is little detectable IL-1 or TNF in the tissues or in the circulation. Quiescent T cells (Tq), mononuclear phagocytes (M), and stromal cells (S) release little if any of these cytokines. In the marrow, these same cells exist but produce only a little, if any, GM-CSF, G-CSF, or IL-1 and release no TNF at all. *B,* To meet the needs of tissues that are infected, new neutrophils are supplied by a complex and interdependent intercellular network of interleukins, adhesion molecules, and growth factors. As above, growth factors and interleukins are shown as shaded figures. Auxiliary cells that participate in the release of these factors include M, S, and activated T cells (TA). Most inflammatory stimuli first influence mononuclear phagocytes, resulting in prompt release of IL-1 and TNF. These inductive factors stimulate the release of G-CSF and GM-CSF. As shown at the bottom right, GM-CSF induces the expression of IL-1 by neutrophils, thereby amplifying the inductive signal even more. The IL-1 and TNF from infected tissue are released into the circulation during periods of inflammation and ultimately influence the auxiliary cells of the bone marrow, shown on the left of the figure.

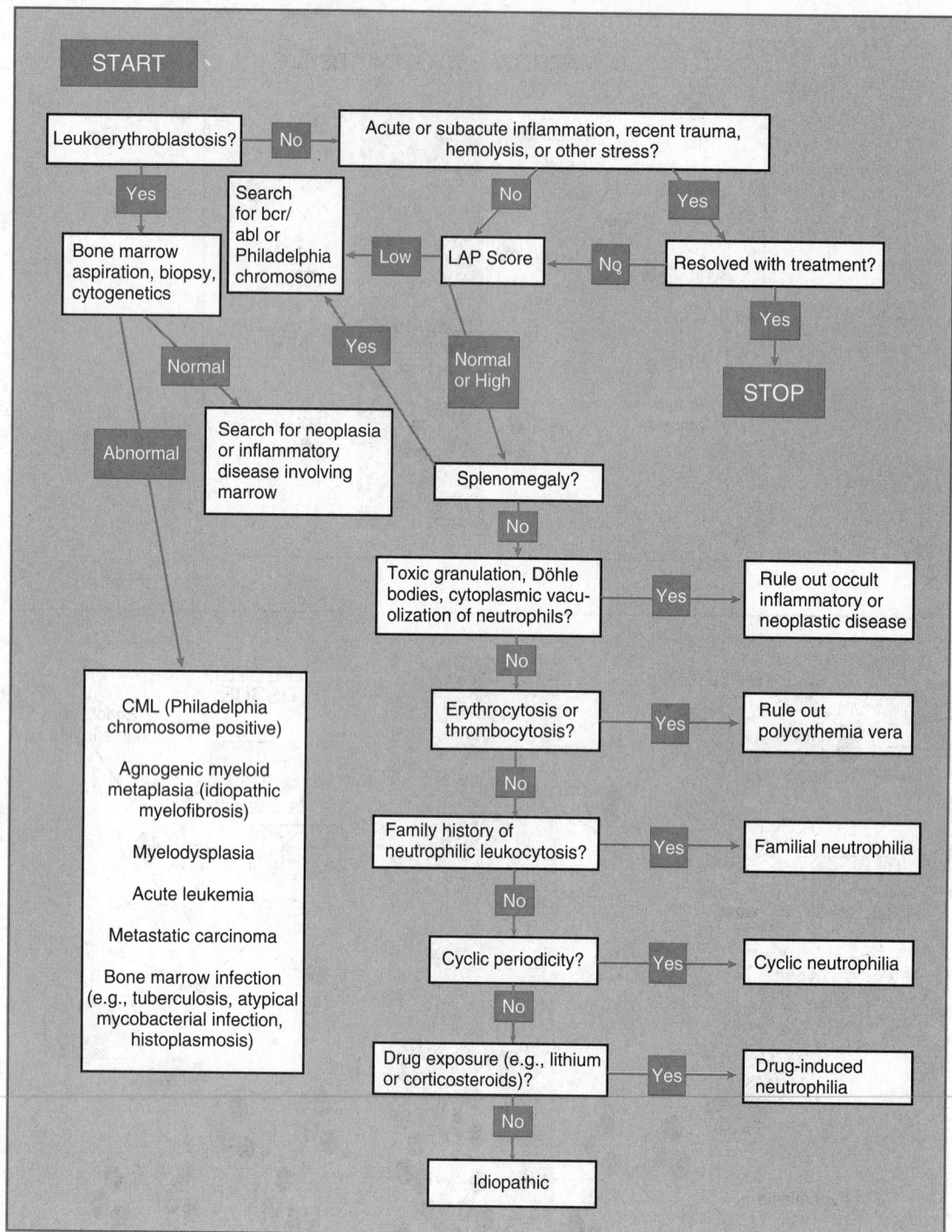

FIGURE 140–8. An algorithm for the evaluation of patients with neutrophilic leukocytosis. LAP = leukocyte alkaline phosphatase.

induce prompt eosinopenia and basophilopenia, these cells are almost universally absent in the blood of acutely injured or infected patients. Their presence should indicate that (1) the acutely ill patient may have concurrent adrenocortical insufficiency, (2) the neutrophilia derives from the inappropriate production of GM-CSF (e.g., by malignant cells), or (3) the neutrophilia is one manifestation of a hematopoietic neoplasm (a chronic myeloproliferative disorder, myelodysplastic syndrome, or certain of the acute nonlymphocytic leukemias).

Leukocyte Alkaline Phosphatase. Leukocyte alkaline phosphatase (LAP) is an enzyme found in neutrophils. When neutrophilia represents a reaction to an acute illness, the LAP levels usually increase substantially. In chronic myelogenous leukemia (CML), by contrast, the LAP score markedly decreases. Accordingly, a low LAP level should therefore lead to an evaluation designed to rule out CML (Table 140–5 and Fig. 140–8).

Differential Diagnosis of Neutrophilic Leukemoid Reactions. Neutrophilic leukemoid reactions generally occur in patients who are obviously systemically ill. When the neutrophil count exceeds 80×10^9 per liter or when the mildness of the systemic illness seems discordant with the extremely high level of neutrophils in the peripheral blood, the diagnosis most often considered is CML. A number of additional features distinguish leukemoid reactions from CML (Table 140–5). The diagnostic tests for CML are those designed to identify the classic balanced chromosomal rearrangement either morphologically (cytogenetic analysis) or by molecular methods (identification of the bcr/abl DNA, mRNA, or protein) (Table 140–5).

MONOCYTOSIS

Monocytosis is defined as absolute peripheral blood monocyte counts $>0.80 \times 10^9$ per liter in children and $>0.50 \times 10^9$ per liter

TABLE 140-5. DISTINCTIONS BETWEEN NEUTROPHILIC LEUKEMOID REACTIONS AND CHRONIC MYELOGENOUS LEUKEMIA (CML)

Finding/Result	Leukemoid Reaction	CML
Presence of fever or other manifestations of acute or subacute illness	Usual*	Infrequent†
Splenomegaly	Rare	Frequent
Natural course of neutrophilia	Resolution linked temporally with abatement of underlying disease	Progressive slow increase over time
Peripheral blood:		
Basophilia	Rare‡	Common
Leukocyte alkaline phosphatase	High	Low§
Philadelphia chromosome	Never	Frequent (85%)
Abnormal DNA: Rearrangement of breakpoint cluster region in DNA (chromosome 22)	Absent‖	Frequent (>85%)

* Regular exceptions to this rule are patients with leukemoid reactions associated with certain carcinomas (see Table 140-3).

† Patients with CML are not exempt from developing infections. Some patients with infectious processes may be found to have CML. The ideal time to evaluate them diagnostically is after the inflammatory process resolves.

‡ Patients with acute allergic reactions and patients with widespread parasitic diseases are frequently exceptions to this rule.

§ Leukocyte alkaline phosphatase scores are sometimes normal in CML patients after splenectomy.

‖ The Philadelphia chromosome forms when chromosome 22 breaks in a region called the breakpoint cluster region (bcr). Some CML patients have no Philadelphia chromosome on karyotypic analysis yet have bcr rearrangement on DNA analysis.

in adults. Monocytes present processed antigens to lymphocytes, mediate cellular cytotoxicity, release procoagulants, participate in bone remodeling and wound repair, dispose of damaged cells, and regulate immune and hematopoietic responses by producing interleukin-1 (IL-1), tumor necrosis factor (TNF) α, G-CSF, IL-6, and certain types of interferon-α. Two factors stimulate the growth and differentiation of mononuclear phagocytes: M-CSF and GM-CSF (Fig. 140-8). Stromal cells, including endothelial cells and fibroblasts, constitutively produce M-CSF and can be induced to release GM-CSF by inflammatory stimuli (see Fig. 140-7).

The mononuclear phagocyte is more sluggish than the neutrophil in moving toward and killing bacteria but is equally or more effective in killing obligate intracellular parasites such as fungi, yeast, and viruses. In addition, it participates substantially in all types of granulomatous inflammation. Monocytosis often occurs in patients with tuberculosis, syphilis, fungal infections, ulcerative and granulomatous colitis, and sarcoidosis (Table 140-6). Mild monocytosis is common in patients with Hodgkins's disease and a variety of cancers. High levels of monocytes in the blood are most often encountered in patients with hematopoietic malignancies, including

acute and chronic myelomonocytic leukemia, acute monocytic leukemia, and chronic myelogenous leukemia of the juvenile type.

EOSINOPHILIA

Eosinophilic leukocytosis (eosinophilia) exists when the eosinophil count in the peripheral blood exceeds 0.4×10^9 per liter. Eosinophils are produced by progenitor cells in the marrow, largely under the influence of IL-5, a protein that also stimulates the growth and differentiation of B lymphocytes. Eosinophils not only function as phagocytes but also play an essential role in modulating the potentially toxic effects of mast cell degranulation in hypersensitivity reactions. Because eosinophils have a unique capacity to release substances toxic to vascular endothelial cells, very high levels of eosinophils in the circulation can result in vascular, pulmonary, and cardiac injury. The eosinophilic syndromes and the causes of eosinophilia are described in Ch. 148.

LYMPHOCYTOSIS

Lymphocytosis is defined as any lymphocyte count in excess of 5.0×10^9 per liter. Atypical lymphocytosis is present when atypical lymphocytes account for more than 20% of the total peripheral blood lymphocyte population. The production and traffic of lymphocytes are clearly under tight control. A number of factors induce growth of T lymphocytes (IL-2, IL-3, IL-7), natural killer cells (IL-2, IL-12, IL-1), and B lymphocytes (IL-2, IL-10, IL-6, IL-5, IL-4, IL-7).

DIAGNOSIS. Mild to moderate lymphocytosis (lymphocyte counts $< 12 \times 10^9$ per liter) is most commonly caused by viral infections, including infectious mononucleosis and infectious hepatitis. Careful examination of the peripheral blood lymphocyte morphology can help distinguish between these two disorders. In infectious mononucleosis (see Ch. 341), many of the lymphocytes are large, with abundant cytoplasm and a "ballerina skirt"–like cytoplasmic border. These are the characteristic "atypical" lymphocytes that exceed 20% of the total lymphocyte population during the course of this disease. Interestingly, although the B lymphocyte is the target of the causative Epstein-Barr (EB) virus, the majority of the cells in the peripheral blood of patients with this disease are T lymphocytes. This proliferative response of T cells probably plays a major role in eradicating the potentially oncogenic EB.

Acute bacterial infections rarely cause lymphocytosis. One exception is pertussis (in children), in which profound lymphocytosis (up to 60×10^9 per liter) may occur (see Ch. 284). Table 140-7 lists a diversity of additional disorders associated with mild to moderate lymphocytosis. Perhaps with the exception of those with early chronic lymphocytic leukemia, most patients have overt signs of an underlying illness involving anatomic sites other than the lymphohematopoietic system. This rule also holds true for patients with substantial lymphocytosis (> 12 to 15×10^9 per liter), the differential diagnosis of which is limited (Table 140-7). Diagnosis depends upon establishing a tissue diagnosis to rule out malignant disease in patients who lack clear-cut evidence of a more benign disorder. Bone marrow aspiration and biopsy are required when (a) lympho-

TABLE 140-6. CAUSES OF MONOCYTOSIS

I. Infections

Tuberculosis	Syphilis
Brucellosis	Fungal infections
Bacterial endocarditis	Recovery from acute infections
Typhoid and paratyphoid fevers	Protozoal infections
Listeriosis	

II. Neoplastic disorders
Hodgkin's disease
Carcinoma (many)
Acute and chronic myelomonocytic leukemia, myelodysplastic syndromes, and chronic myelogenous leukemia of the juvenile type

III. Gastrointestinal disorders

Ulcerative colitis	Cirrhosis
Granulomatous colitis	

IV. Sarcoidosis
V. Drug reactions
VI. Recovery from marrow suppression
VII. Congenital neutropenia

TABLE 140-7. CAUSES OF LYMPHOCYTOSIS

I. High ($> 15 \times 10^9$ per liter)

Infectious mononucleosis	Chronic lymphocytic leukemia
Pertussis	Acute lymphocytic leukemia
Acute infectious lymphocytosis	

II. Moderate ($< 15 \times 10^9$ per liter)
Many viral infections

Infectious mononucleosis	Coxsackie
Measles	Adenovirus
Varicella	Mumps
Hepatitis	Cytomegalovirus

Other infectious diseases

Toxoplasmosis	Typhoid fever
Brucellosis	Syphilis (secondary)
Tuberculosis	

Neoplastic disorders
Carcinoma
Hodgkin's disease
Acute lymphocytic leukemia (early)
Chronic lymphocytic leukemia (early)
Other disorders (Graves' disease)

cytosis coexists with leukoerythroblastosis, (b) peripheral lymphocytes are immature (lymphoblasts), (c) the lymphocytosis persists without evidence of acute or subacute infection.

Immunophenotype ("lymphocyte markers") should be assessed using monoclonal antibodies to definitive integral membrane proteins. Such studies provide evidence for or against dominance of one lymphocyte type. Also, analyses of immunoglobulin light chain types can determine whether all circulating B lymphocytes are members of a single (therefore, likely neoplastic) clone.

Bagby GC, Segal GM: Growth factors and the control of hematopoiesis. In Hoffman R, Benz EJ, Shattil SJ, et al. (eds.): Hematology: Basic Principles and Practice. New York, Churchill Livingstone, 1994. An up-to-date review of the cellular and molecular regulation of granulopoiesis in response to inflammatory stimuli.

Bishop MR, Anderson JR, Jackson JD, et al.: High dose therapy and peripheral blood progenitor cell transplantation: Effects of recombinant human granulocyte-macrophage colony-stimulating factor on the autograft. Blood 83:610, 1994. This work reports that peripheral "stem cells" collected after the administration of GM-CSF and administered as the sole source of hematopoietic progenitors and stem cells are sufficient to permit bone marrow reconstitution after high-dose chemotherapy. This and other related works emphasize the important granulopoietic activity that each of these factors exhibits. That the expression of the endogenous genes that encode these proteins is activated by inflammatory stimuli clearly demonstrates their unambiguous importance in regulating white cell production.

Daley GQ, Van Etten RA, Baltimore D: Induction of chronic myelogenous leukemia in mice by the p210$^{bcr/abl}$ gene of the Philadelphia chromosome. Science 247:824, 1990. This work demonstrated the cause-and-effect relationship between the molecular defect and the pathogenesis of CML. More recent work in other laboratories is characterizing the signal-transducing proteins activated by the chimeric p210$^{bcr/abl}$ protein.

Peters WP, Rosner G, Ross M, et al.: Comparative effects of granulocyte-macrophage colony-stimulating factor (GM-CSF) and granulocyte colony-stimulating factor (G-CSF) on priming peripheral blood progenitor cells for use with autologous bone marrow after high-dose chemotherapy. Blood 81:1709, 1993. This paper focuses on two biologic activities of GM-CSF and G-CSF that make them valuable to transplanters and, potentially, to gene therapists: (1) They hasten granulopoietic recovery, and (2) they induce progenitor cells to circulate freely in the peripheral blood (so they can be harvested for engineering and transplantation by simply performing leukapheresis). The work demonstrates that the capacity of GM-CSF and G-CSF to induce the emergence of hematopoietic progenitor cells into the peripheral blood can be used to collect such cells for patients undergoing autologous bone marrow transplantation following high-dose chemotherapy. The use of "peripheral stem cells" collected under these conditions shortens the duration of neutropenia and, in the case of G-CSF, reduces overall costs of hospitalization.

141 PROLIFERATIVE DISORDERS OF THE HEMATOLOGIC SYSTEM

141.1 Erythrocytosis and Polycythemia Vera

Murray N. Silverstein and
Ayalew Tefferi

ERYTHROCYTOSIS

DEFINITIONS. The normal level of hemoglobin in adults ranges from 12 to 18 grams per deciliter and the normal hematocrit varies from 38 to 56%. In general, the concentration of hemoglobin is about 2 grams per deciliter less in females and 1 gram per deciliter less in African Americans. Higher concentrations are referred to as "erythrocytosis" and are classified as "absolute erythrocytosis" (accompanied by an increase in the red cell mass) or "apparent erythrocytosis" (not accompanied by an increase in red cell mass). The red cell mass is calculated by a radiodilution method, either directly by injecting radiolabeled autologous erythrocytes or indirectly by injecting radiolabeled albumin and measuring the whole blood volume first (red cell mass = whole blood volume × hematocrit).

When absolute erythrocytosis represents a clonal hematologic disorder associated with an increase in other myeloid cells, it is

known as "polycythemia vera." Nonclonal absolute erythrocytosis is called "secondary erythrocytosis."

When apparent erythrocytosis is associated with decreased plasma volume, it is categorized as "relative erythrocytosis." Note that apparent erythrocytosis is not always associated with decreased plasma volume and may result from an increased red cell mass-to-plasma volume ratio despite both measurements being within the normal range.

The distinction among the above-mentioned subclasses of erythrocytosis is clinically relevant (Table 141–1). For example, patients with polycythemia vera may have thrombohemorrhagic events and decreased cerebral blood flow unless the hematocrit is maintained (by phlebotomy or drug therapy) below 45%. Despite retrospective correlation of thrombotic events with either apparent or secondary erythrocytosis, the risk is probably smaller in nonclonal erythrocytosis. No convincing evidence exists that nonselective phlebotomy in such cases is beneficial. Therefore, the clinically relevant point during evaluation of erythrocytosis is whether the patient has polycythemia vera.

Currently, the evaluation of erythrocytosis begins with measurement of the red cell mass. This practice is influenced largely by the absolute requirement of increased red cell mass in the criteria devised by the Polycythemia Vera Study Group during initial treatment trials. What is often overlooked is that these criteria were not intended to be diagnostic and that they were used for purposes of accruing a uniform group of patients. For example, a patient with early disease or concomitant bleeding may not have an increased red cell mass. Furthermore, measurements of the blood volume are costly and not always accurate.

The current availability of reliable serum erythropoietin assays and appreciation of the pitfalls in blood volume measurements allow for an alternative and possibly cost-effective diagnostic evaluation of erythrocytosis. Erythrocyte production is regulated by erythropoietin, a glycoprotein hormone produced by the peritubular interstitial cells of the kidney in response to hypoxia. An autonomous proliferation of erythrocytes, as in polycythemia vera, is associated with low levels of erythropoietin, whereas secondary erythrocytosis is always accompanied by increased levels of the hormone. It should be noted that measurements of the red cell mass cannot distinguish between polycythemia vera and secondary erythrocytosis.

DIAGNOSIS. A diagnostic algorithm is given in Figure 141–1. Apparent erythrocytosis is unlikely when the hematocrit is greater than 58% in males and 52% in females. Therefore, under such conditions, measurements of the red cell mass are superfluous, and one should proceed directly to the measurement of serum levels of erythropoietin to distinguish polycythemia vera from secondary erythrocytosis. When the hematocrit is in the upper normal range (52 to 58% in males and 45 to 52% in females), polycythemia vera is unlikely in asymptomatic patients who do not have splenomegaly or

TABLE 141–1. CAUSES OF ERYTHROCYTOSIS

Absolute erythrocytosis—accompanied by increased red cell mass
  Clonal erythrocytosis—independent of erythropoietin
    Polycythemia vera
  Nonclonal erythrocytosis—erythropoietin-dependent
    Increased erythropoietin due to physiologic demand
      Central hypoxia
        High-altitude habitat
        Chronic lung disease (e.g., chronic obstructive pulmonary disease, pickwickian syndrome)
        Arteriovenous and intracardiac shunts
      Tissue hypoxia
        High oxygen-affinity hemoglobins
        Decreased 2,3-diphosphoglycerate
    Pathologic production of erythropoietin
      Tumors (liver, kidney, cerebellum)
      Renal disorders (cysts, renal transplant)
      Uterine fibroids
      Exogenous administration of erythropoietin
Apparent erythrocytosis—not accompanied by increased red cell mass
  Relative erythrocytosis—accompanied by decreased plasma volume
    Dehydration (diuretics)
    Smoking
    Hypertension
  Decreased ratio of red cell mass to plasma volume

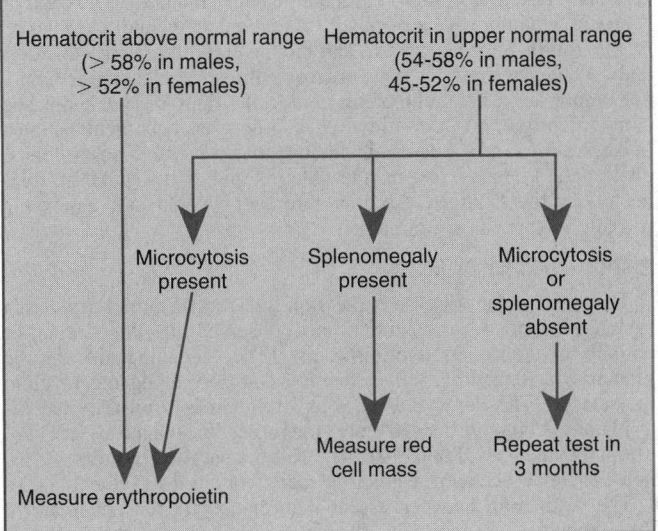

FIGURE 141–1. A diagnostic guideline to differentiate among causes of erythrocytosis. (From Tefferi A, Hoagland HC: Issues in the diagnosis and management of essential thombocytopenia. Mayo Clin Proc 69:651, 1994. By permission of Mayo Foundation for Medical Education and Research.)

microcytosis. These patients may represent the tail end of a normal Gaussian distribution, and repeating the blood cell count in 3 to 6 months is adequate.

It is appropriate, however, to investigate polycythemia vera when a hematocrit in the upper normal range is associated with splenomegaly or microcytosis (microcytosis is frequently found in polycythemia vera and is due to concomitant iron deficiency, which may prevent an obvious increase in the hematocrit). Splenomegaly increases plasma volume, and a true increase in red cell mass may be masked by an apparently normal hematocrit. This is the one situation for which measurement of the red cell mass is indicated and helpful. Microcytosis associated with a hematocrit in the upper normal range is suggestive of polycythemia vera. In this situation, measurement of the red cell mass may give a normal value; the diagnosis is supported by the demonstration of low serum levels of erythropoietin.

Increased serum levels of erythropoietin (more than 2 standard deviations from the normal mean value) indicate secondary erythrocytosis. In this respect, measurement of oxyhemoglobin percent saturation (to detect central hypoxia from cardiopulmonary disease), computed tomographic scans of the abdomen (to look for erythropoietin-producing tumors in the liver or the kidney), and determination of P_{50} (to diagnose high oxygen-affinity hemoglobin) are reasonable laboratory investigations. (P_{50} is the partial oxygen tension necessary to saturate 50% of the available hemoglobin and is determined from an oxygen-hemoglobin dissociation curve.)

POLYCYTHEMIA VERA

Polycythemia vera is a myeloproliferative disease characterized by the sustained persistence of an increased level of hemoglobin and an increased hematocrit. Its physiologic features are based on an increase in blood viscosity caused by the increase in red cell mass: The red cell mass dominates and defines the clinical syndrome. Polycythemia vera is an autonomous lesion that is not associated with or controlled by erythropoietin. It is a clonal hemopathy, and glucose-6-phosphate dehydrogenase heterozygotes with this disease have only one type of isoenzyme in the cells that arise from the bone marrow.

CLINICAL PRESENTATION AND LABORATORY DIAGNOSIS. The disease has a peak incidence at about age 60 and involves both genders equally. It affects Caucasians mostly, and its incidence is less in patients of African or Asian descent. Family prevalence is higher than expected, and increased incidence has been noted in persons exposed to radiation. With increasing use of laboratory screening tests, the diagnosis is being made in more and more asymptomatic patients. It is thought that some of the symptoms are related to hyperviscosity and decreased cerebral blood flow.

Table 141–2 lists the diagnostic criteria used by the Polycythemia Vera Study Group. The diagnosis is suggested when a patient has all three major criteria or the first two major criteria plus any two of the minor criteria as listed in Table 141–2. However, these criteria were formulated to accrue a uniform group of patients who had the disease and do not exclude the diagnosis in patients with early disease or concomitant iron deficiency. Recent studies have suggested the use of nonconventional criteria (serum level of erythropoietin and spontaneous erythroid colony formation from the peripheral blood) for conclusive diagnosis.

Important clinical and laboratory findings are listed in Table 141–3. Bone marrow examination reveals hypercellularity in more than 90% of patients with trilineage involvement. In addition, megakaryocytic clusters and reticulin fibrosis may be noted. As the disease progresses, more fibrosis is found in up to 20% of patients. Iron stores are low in more than 90% of the patients, and chromosome studies at presentation are abnormal in approximately 20%.

Spuriously abnormal laboratory findings include arterial hypoxia and hypoglycemia (*in vitro* consumption by increased cell count) and serum hyperkalemia (*in vitro* release of potassium from platelets). Immediate processing of laboratory studies and measurement of plasma levels of potassium are helpful for further investigation.

CLINICAL COURSE. More than 50% of the patients may develop thrombohemorrhagic complications, which are partly controlled with adequate treatment. In as many as 20% of patients, the disease may transform into postpolycythemia myeloid metaplasia, which is indistinguishable from agnogenic myeloid metaplasia. In 5 to 15% of patients, the disease evolves into acute myeloid leukemia. Overall median survival is greater than 10 years, which is better than the survival in agnogenic myeloid metaplasia but worse than the survival in essential thrombocythemia.

TREATMENT. The cornerstone of therapy for this disease is phlebotomy. The initial approach to all patients with polycythemia vera must be to decrease the red cell mass. We recommend drawing 500 ml of blood weekly and continuing that approach to maintain a hematocrit of 42% or less. Therapy with phlebotomy alone is associated with an increased risk of thrombosis, especially for patients older than 70 years, those with a history of thrombosis, and those requiring an increased frequency of phlebotomy.

Concurrent treatment with myelosuppressive agents decreases the risk of thrombotic complications. Chlorambucil and radiophosphorus are *not* recommended as myelosuppressive agents because they increase the risk of acute leukemia and other malignancies. A similar risk has not been found with the use of hydroxyurea. Accordingly, we favor the use of hydroxyurea in conjunction with phlebotomy among patients who are older than 70 years, have a history of thrombosis, frequently require phlebotomy, or concurrently have thrombocytosis greater than 600,000 per microliter. The initial dose of hydroxyurea usually is 500 mg 2 to 4 times per day. The hematocrit, platelet, and leukocyte counts are monitored carefully. The goal is to maintain the hematocrit below 42%, the platelet count below 500,000 per microliter, and the leukocyte count greater than 3000 per microliter. Hydroxyurea should be continued as long as there is a need for continued phlebotomy or persistence of thrombocytosis. During the advanced stages of the disease (spent phase), the hematocrit and platelet count may decrease to the normal range and specific therapy may not be needed. The risk of long-term hydroxyurea treatment has not been determined. Because of the con-

TABLE 141–2. THE POLYCYTHEMIA VERA STUDY GROUP DIAGNOSTIC CRITERIA FOR POLYCYTHEMIA VERA

Major Criteria	Minor Criteria

1 Increased red cell mass
  Males, ≥ 36 ml/kg
  Females, ≥ 32 ml/kg
	1 Platelets $> 400,000/\mu l$

	2 Leukocytes $> 12,000/\mu l$
2 Normal arterial oxygen saturation, $\geq 92\%$	3 Leukocyte alkaline phosphatase > 100 or Vitamin B$_{12}$ > 900 pg/ml
3 Splenomegaly	or
	Unbound B$_{12}$ binding capacity $> 2,200$ pg/ml

TABLE 141-3. PRESENTING CLINICAL AND LABORATORY FEATURES OF POLYCYTHEMIA VERA

Nonspecific symptoms of headache, dizziness, epigastric distress, fatigue, paresthesias	~ 30%
Generalized pruritus	~ 50%
Thrombohemorrhagic complications	~ 30%
Gastrointestinal tract hemorrhage	
Cerebrovascular accident, transient ischemic attack	
Angina, myocardial infarction	
Pulmonary embolus, deep venous thrombosis	
Arterial emboli	
Large vein thrombosis	
Budd-Chiari syndrome	
Palpable splenomegaly	~ 70%
Palpable hepatomegaly	~ 35%
Ruddy cyanosis	~ 70%
Increased blood pressure	~ 30%
Leukocytosis	~ 70%
Thrombocytosis	~ 50%
Hyperuricemia	~ 50%

cern about a leukemogenic potential, we do not recommend the use of hydroxyurea in younger patients with normal platelet counts.

Recently, interferon-α has been shown to have therapeutic activity in polycythemia vera. Because it is a relatively expensive drug with substantial side effects, it is not likely to replace current treatment modalities. The role of the new antiplatelet agent anagrelide, which is effective in treating essential thrombocythemia, has not been defined.

Birgegård G, Wide L: Serum erythropoietin in the diagnosis of polycythaemia and after phlebotomy treatment. Br J Haematol 81:603, 1992. *The authors evaluated serum erythropoietin (S-Epo) levels in 17 patients with secondary polycythemia, 14 patients with relative polycythemia, and 36 patients with polycythemia vera. They found increased S-Epo levels in all patients with secondary polycythemia, normal S-Epo levels in all but one patient with relative polycythemia, and low S-Epo levels in all but two patients with polycythemia vera.*

Pearson TC: Apparent polycythaemia. Blood Rev 5:205, 1991. *An authoritative review article on the classification of erythrocytosis, with emphasis on differentiation of apparent polycythemia from relative and polycythemia vera.*

Schwarcz TH, Hogan LA, Endean ED, et al.: Thromboembolic complications of polycythemia: Polycythemia vera versus smokers polycythemia. J Vasc Surg 17:518, 1993. *This study compares the incidence of thromboembolic events in patients with polycythemia vera with those with secondary polycythemia caused by tobacco use. Patients with polycythemia vera had a greater number of thromboembolic events and more peripheral arterial thromboemboli.*

Silver RT: A new treatment for polycythemia vera: Recombinant interferon alfa. Blood 76:664, 1990. *Initial demonstration of the therapeutic efficacy of recombinant interferon-α in polycythemia vera. The dose used was 3.0×10^6 U given subcutaneously three times a week. The usual interferon side effects were noted. Along with improved blood cell count, regression of spleen size was observed.*

Westwood N, Dudley JM, Sawyer B, et al.: Primary polycythaemia: Diagnosis by nonconventional positive criteria. Eur J Haematol 51:228, 1993. *The authors demonstrated the value of combined assessment of spontaneous peripheral blood erythroid colony formation, serum erythropoietic assay, platelet nucleotide ratio, platelet distribution width, and clinical evidence of ischemic vascular disease in making the diagnosis of polycythemia vera.*

141.2 CHRONIC MYELOPROLIFERATIVE DISEASES

Ayalew Tefferi and
Murray N. Silverstein

Chronic myeloid disorders represent clonal hematopoietic cell processes that affect the myeloid cell lineage (granulocytes, monocytes, erythrocytes, and platelets) and result in overproliferation of relatively mature cell elements with or without morphologic dysplasia. In the presence of dyshematopoiesis, the process is classified as a "myelodysplastic syndrome." Otherwise, it is classified as a "chronic myeloproliferative disorder."

The chronic myeloproliferative disorders are further subdivided on the basis of the predominantly proliferating myeloid cell type. Erythrocyte excess is classified as "polycythemia vera," platelet ex-

cess as "essential thrombocythemia," and granulocyte excess as "chronic granulocytic leukemia." "Agnogenic myeloid metaplasia" is the fourth subcategory of chronic myeloproliferative disorders and is characterized by bone marrow fibrosis and extramedullary hematopoiesis. The multipotent stem cell origin of the neoplastic clone in chronic myeloproliferative disorders has been demonstrated in several *in vitro* studies, including analyses of glucose-6-phosphate dehydrogenase isoenzyme patterns and X-linked DNA fragments. In this chapter, essential thrombocythemia and agnogenic myeloid metaplasia are discussed.

ESSENTIAL THROMBOCYTHEMIA

The predominant disease expression in essential thrombocythemia is thrombocytosis, a condition also observed in other acute or chronic myeloproliferative disorders. (The latter include chronic granulocytic leukemia, polycythemia vera, and agnogenic myeloid metaplasia.) The Polycythemia Vera Study Group arbitrarily has set a platelet count $\geq 6 \times 10^5$ per microliter to diagnose essential thrombocythemia (Table 141-4). This range of thrombocytosis, however, may occur in reaction to many conditions (Table 141-5).

The distinction between essential thrombocythemia and reactive thrombocytosis is clinically relevant because thrombohemorrhagic complications are more common in essential thrombocythemia than in reactive thrombocytosis. It is equally important to distinguish essential thrombocythemia from other chronic myeloproliferative disorders because of considerable differences in prognosis and management. For example, life expectancy may not be shortened by essential thrombocythemia, but it declines measurably in agnogenic myeloid metaplasia. Similarly, chronic granulocytic leukemia inevitably transforms into acute leukemia unless altered by allogeneic bone marrow transplantation.

The treatment of essential thrombocythemia is an evolving matter as to both therapeutic indications and the choice of new specific measures. Young or pregnant patients require special consideration. This chapter discusses our approach to essential thrombocythemia.

CLINICAL PRESENTATION. Most patients are asymptomatic when essential thrombocythemia is diagnosed, usually through incidental discovery of increased peripheral blood platelet count. Approximately one quarter, however, present with either thrombotic or hemorrhagic events. These include acute strokes, transient cerebral ischemic attacks, sagittal vein thromboses, epistaxis, ecchymoses, gastrointestinal tract hemorrhages, myocardial infarctions, angina, splanchnic vein thromboses (e.g., Budd-Chiari syndrome), deep vein thromboses, and digital microvascular ischemia. Additional, more frequent symptoms include vasomotor disturbances, vascular headaches, paresthesias, acrocyanosis, and erythromelalgia. The latter consists of distal extremity (palms and soles) pain, warmth, dysesthesias, and erythema, presumably due to microvascular obstruction by abnormal platelets. The condition responds well to aspirin therapy. Less than half of the patients with essential thrombocythemia have palpable splenomegaly when first diagnosed. Hepatomegaly and lymphadenopathy are rare.

DIAGNOSIS. The initial evaluation of thrombocytosis includes identifying concurrent conditions known to be associated with reactive thrombocytosis (Table 141-5), reviewing previous platelet counts, and abstracting historical data pertinent to thrombohemorrhagic events and vasomotor symptoms. In the absence of any obvious cause, persistent thrombocytosis likely represents essential thrombocythemia. The possibility, however, of chronic granulocytic leukemia presenting with isolated thrombocytosis and the (disputed)

TABLE 141-4. THE POLYCYTHEMIA VERA STUDY GROUP CRITERIA FOR THE DIAGNOSIS OF ESSENTIAL THROMBOCYTHEMIA

Platelet count $> 6 \times 10^5/\mu L$
Absence of conditions associated with reactive thrombocytosis
Documentation of normal iron stores
Normal red blood cell mass
No Philadelphia chromosome
Bone marrow collagen fibrosis must be absent or, in the absence of both splenomegaly and leukoerythroblastic picture, must be restricted to $< 1/3$ of the biopsy area

From Tefferi A, Hoagland HC: Issues in the diagnosis and management of essential thombocytopenia. Mayo Clin Proc 69:651, 1994. By permission of the Mayo Foundation for Medical Education and Research.

TABLE 141–5. CONDITIONS ASSOCIATED WITH REACTIVE THROMBOCYTOSIS

Infectious or inflammatory states—vasculitis, allergic reactions, etc.
Surgery and tissue damage—myocardial infarctions, pancreatitis, etc.
Malignancy—solid tumors, lymphoma
Iron deficiency anemia, hemolytic anemia, acute blood loss
Postsplenectomy state
Rebound effect after chemotherapy or immune thrombocytopenia
Renal disorders—renal failure, nephrotic syndrome

need to initiate specific therapy in essential thrombocythemia make further investigation mandatory.

The great majority of adult cases of thrombocytosis are reactive and do not require examination of the bone marrow. Practical factors commonly used to differentiate essential thrombocythemia from reactive thrombocytosis include the clinical assessment of spleen size and the degree and duration of thrombocytosis. Because less than half have palpable splenomegaly, immediate diagnosis occasionally remains uncertain. In general, examination of a peripheral blood smear is of limited value, although giant platelets and platelet aggregates are suggestive—but not diagnostic—of essential thrombocythemia. As a result, several laboratory variables have been investigated in an attempt to provide a positive diagnosis of essential thrombocythemia (Table 141–6). These are discussed below.

Tests of Platelet and Megakaryocyte Functions.
Only a minority of patients with essential thrombocythemia have laboratory evidence of functional platelet abnormalities. These include prolonged bleeding time, spontaneous platelet aggregation, decreased platelet aggregation in response to conventional platelet aggregants (including adrenaline), and abnormal intraplatelet and serum contents of β-thromboglobulin, 5-hydroxytryptamine, and platelet factor 4. The rarity of these findings makes them not applicable to most patients. Moreover, they have limited value in distinguishing essential thrombocythemia from reactive thrombocytosis. Also, the widespread use of nonsteroidal anti-inflammatory drugs makes it difficult to interpret the results.

A scoring system based on variables that include platelet distribution width, platelet nucleotide ratio, and unstimulated erythroid colony growth has a strong discriminatory value. Similarly, another recent study showed that spontaneous megakaryocyte or erythroid colony formation in vitro by progenitors from the bone marrow or blood (or both) occurred in 77% of patients with essential thrombocythemia and in none with reactive thrombocytosis. More importantly, patients with essential thrombocythemia who had spontaneous megakaryocyte growth underwent significantly more thrombotic events.

Bone Marrow Abnormality in the Diagnosis of Essential Thrombocythemia.
Bone marrow studies have revealed a specific, but not sensitive, association of decreased iron stores and increased reticulin content with essential thrombocythemia compared with reactive thrombocytosis. Megakaryocyte clusters occurred in all cases of essential thrombocythemia but also in 25% of cases of reactive thrombocytosis (see Table 141–6). Bone marrow cellularity and the presence or absence of platelet aggregates or megakaryocytic emperipolesis (a process in tissue culture by which one cell actively penetrates another, which nevertheless remains intact) did not have differential diagnostic usefulness. Definite clonal assignment is possible in women with the use of X-linked genetic probes. The usefulness of cytogenetic studies is limited by the low incidence of clonal abnormalities ($\approx 5\%$) in essential thrombocythemia.

Among the chronic myeloproliferative disorders, chronic granulocytic leukemia and polycythemia vera are easily identified by demonstrating the Philadelphia chromosome and increased red cell mass, respectively. Diagnostic difficulty occurs in distinguishing essential thrombocythemia from an early stage of agnogenic myeloid metaplasia (cellular phase of disease). Substantial or progressive collagen fibrosis, peripheral leukoerythroblastosis, or marked splenomegaly is most consistent with the diagnosis of agnogenic myeloid metaplasia. In the absence of these features, we favor the diagnosis of essential thrombocythemia, regardless of the degree of reticulin fibrosis. Authorities on the subject restrict the degree of allowable collagen fibrosis in essential thrombocythemia to less than one third of the cross-sectional area of the biopsy section (see Table 141–4).

Measurement of Acute-phase Reactants.
Plasma levels of interleukin-6 (IL-6) are elevated during the acute-phase response and in chronic conditions associated with infection, inflammation, or malignancy. Several studies have shown increased levels of IL-6 in reactive thrombocytosis compared with normal levels in clonal thrombocytosis, suggesting that IL-6 has a pathogenic rather than an associated role in reactive thrombocytosis. Similar increases have been found in C-reactive protein levels. Fibrinogen and the von Willebrand factor antigen are other acute-phase reactants whose plasma levels frequently are increased in reactive thrombocytosis. A plasma fibrinogen level greater than 500 mg per deciliter was found to be highly sensitive and relatively specific for reactive thrombocytosis. Intelligent interpretation of plasma C-reactive protein or fibrinogen levels may provide a rapid, inexpensive method of distinguishing essential thrombocythemia from reactive thrombocytosis.

MANAGEMENT. General Considerations. Essential thrombocythemia rarely transforms into acute leukemia or agnogenic myeloid metaplasia, and most patients have a normal life expectancy. Overall, however, at least one third of patients with essential thrombocythemia sooner or later undergo major thrombohemorrhagic complications. Such thrombotic events occur more frequently than hemorrhagic events and are often evident at presentation rather than during follow-up evaluation. Vasomotor symptoms develop in an even higher proportion of patients; these symptoms are easily controlled with nonsteroidal anti-inflammatory drugs.

The risk of thrombotic episodes relates directly to a history of previous thrombosis, inadequate control of thrombocytosis, the presence of cardiovascular risk factors, and the in vitro occurrence of spontaneous megakaryocyte colony formation. Some investigators consider advanced age a risk factor for thrombosis. However, neither the degree of thrombocytosis nor the in vitro or in vivo platelet function profile has been useful in predicting such events. The risk of hemorrhage may be increased when platelet levels are greater than 2×10^6 per microliter and is certainly related to the ingestion of nonsteroidal anti-inflammatory drugs. The mechanism for bleeding diathesis in extreme thrombocytosis may be related to the adsorption of large von Willebrand factor polymers by platelets.

Treatment Indications.
The ideal management of patients with essential thrombocythemia remains unsettled. Most authorities agree that treatment aimed at decreasing the level of platelets is indicated for patients with a history of thrombosis as well as those with cardiovascular risk factors. Less clear is whether to treat asymptomatic patients who lack such risk factors. The risk of major thrombohemorrhagic complications developing in asymptomatic patients of all ages may be as high as 20%. However, the benefit of specific therapy has not been established, and there is concern about the leukemogenic potential of the available therapeutic agents. Currently, however, no evidence supports the notion that therapy induces acute leukemia in essential thrombocythemia. Acute leukemia that develops from essential thrombocythemia is rare and has occurred even

TABLE 141–6. CLINICAL AND LABORATORY FEATURES HELPFUL IN DISTINGUISHING BETWEEN ESSENTIAL THROMBOCYTHEMIA AND REACTIVE THROMBOCYTOSIS

	Essential Thrombocythemia	Reactive Thrombocytosis
Chronic increase in platelets	+	−
Known causes of reactive thrombosis	−	+
Thrombosis or hemorrhage	+	−
Splenomegaly	+	−
Bone marrow reticulin fibrosis	+	−
Bone marrow megakaryocyte clusters	+	−
Acute-phase reactants* increased	−	+
Spontaneous colony formation†	+	−

* Including C-reactive protein and fibrinogen. † Erythroid or megakaryocyte colonies.

From Tefferi A, Hoagland HC: Issues in the diagnosis and management of essential thrombocytopenia. Mayo Clin Proc 69:651, 1994. By permission of Mayo Foundation for Medical Education and Research.

in the absence of specific therapy. Therefore, we currently recommend specific therapy (for platelet counts >600,000 per microliter) to all patients older than 50 years, especially those who have cardiovascular risk factors or a history of thrombosis. Treatment of younger patients and pregnant women is discussed below.

Choice of Therapeutic Agents.
When treatment is decided upon, the best initial drugs are hydroxyurea or anagrelide. Hydroxyurea is an oral agent that inhibits ribonucleotide reductase. Side effects include mild gastrointestinal complaints, reversible neutropenia in approximately 15% of patients, and mucocutaneous lesions (hyperpigmentation, maculopapular rash, skin and nail atrophy, violaceous papules, and ulcers) in up to 33%. The starting dose is 500 mg given orally twice a day. The goal is to keep platelets between 100,000 and 400,000 per microliter and leukocytes greater than 3000 per microliter.

Anagrelide is also an oral agent (not approved by the FDA yet and available under a research protocol only). Its mechanism of action may involve inhibition of megakaryocyte maturation. Its side effects include palpitations (forceful heartbeat and tachycardia), anemia, headache, fluid retention, nausea, diarrhea, and dizziness. Anagrelide rarely precipitates heart failure in elderly patients with heart disease. Accordingly, it is relatively contraindicated in that group. The starting dose is 0.5 mg given orally four times a day.

If treatment with hydroxyurea or anagrelide fails, interferon-α therapy may be considered (3 to 5 million units per square meter daily subcutaneously). Such treatment is effective, but its cost and toxicity prevent it from being used as initial therapy. We usually avoid the use of alkylating agents and radioactive phosphorus because of their established leukemogenic potential. Occasionally, however, the use of radioactive phosphorus is appropriate and effective in elderly patients as well as in those who are noncompliant or relatively inaccessible to follow-up treatment.

Management of Young Patients.
We recently updated our experience with essential thrombocythemia in young adults (age 12 to 40 years). In 56 patients followed for a median of 4.5 years, 5 had serious thrombotic episodes. None died of these complications, which did not appear to be influenced by the presence or absence of specific therapy. Similarly favorable outcomes in young persons have been noted by other investigators. One study reported that serious thrombohemorrhagic events occurred in 23% of the patients and were fatal in two patients. It may be helpful to note that none of the serious episodes was associated with platelet levels less than 5×10^5 per microliter.

On the basis of these data, it can be concluded that life-threatening complications can occur in less than one fourth of young patients with essential thrombocythemia. In symptomatic patients, maintaining the platelet level less than 5×10^5 per microliter may prevent recurrence of serious events. Until additional data are available, no strong recommendations can be made for or against specific therapy for asymptomatic young patients. We favor treatment for asymptomatic patients with cardiovascular risk factors and no treatment for asymptomatic women who are pregnant or of childbearing age.

Management of Pregnant Patients.
In a 15-year period, we have observed 34 pregnancies in 18 women with essential thrombocythemia. Of these pregnancies, 18 resulted in live births. Neither a history of disease complications, the presence or absence of specific therapy during pregnancy, nor prepregnancy platelet counts predicted miscarriages. Complications during the course of the pregnancy were rare, and all live deliveries were uncomplicated, despite no therapeutic interventions in 14 cases.

AGNOGENIC MYELOID METAPLASIA

Agnogenic myeloid metaplasia is unique among the chronic myeloproliferative disorders in that significant bone marrow fibrosis accompanies the clonal myeloproliferative process. Bone marrow fibroblasts are polyclonal in agnogenic myeloid metaplasia, whereas the hematopoietic cells are clonal, as evidenced by cytogenetic and glucose-6-phosphate dehydrogenase isoenzyme studies. Therefore, the bone marrow fibrosis is a reactive process that results from functional and kinetic stimulation of nonclonal fibroblasts by growth factors shed from clonal megakaryocytes.

Agnogenic myeloid metaplasia relates closely to other myeloproliferative diseases. By about 10 years after the diagnosis of poly-

cythemia vera, approximately 14% of patients develop a syndrome indistinguishable from agnogenic myeloid metaplasia. Agnogenic myeloid metaplasia may evolve into an acute nonlymphocytic leukemic state in 5 to 15% of patients.

PATHOGENESIS. The cause of the bone marrow fibrosis in agnogenic myeloid metaplasia is uncertain. Current data implicate transforming growth factor (TGF)-β as the major putative cytokine involved. TGF-β is a glycoprotein synthesized and secreted primarily by the monocyte-macrophage system and endothelial cells but also by megakaryocytes. TGF-β is capable of enhancing the production and secretion of extracellular matrix proteins, including collagen types I and III, from fibroblasts. Several other growth factors are also implicated in the stimulation of fibroblasts and include platelet-derived growth factor and epidermal growth factor.

Recent studies confirm the growth factor mediation of bone marrow fibrosis in agnogenic myeloid metaplasia. Higher levels of platelet-derived growth factor and TGF-β (but not of epidermal growth factor) have been reported in circulating platelets of patients with agnogenic myeloid metaplasia. Similarly, greater TGF-β activity and TGF-β mRNA expression were observed with megakaryoblasts than with other leukemic cell types. In vitro, anti–TGF-β antibodies decrease collagen synthesis mediated by megakaryoblast-conditioned media, and tumor necrosis factor-α and interferon-γ suppress the activation of type I collagen gene expression by TGF-β. In vivo, interferon-γ decreases intraplatelet levels of platelet-derived growth factor and TGF-β. These observations form the basis for anti–TGF-β and anti–platelet-derived growth factor therapeutic endeavors to reverse or arrest bone marrow fibrosis in agnogenic myeloid metaplasia.

CLINICAL FEATURES. Approximately 20% of patients with agnogenic myeloid metaplasia are asymptomatic when first seen, and, of this cohort, approximately 80% remain without symptoms for 5 years. Conversely, 80% of patients have symptoms, of whom 60% develop anemia, 24% suffer from the mechanical effects of the enlarged spleen, and 16% have abnormal bleeding. Those with anemia may have symptoms of weakness, fatigue, or palpitations. Painful splenomegaly results from the internal pressure of an increasingly enlarging spleen and is often associated with profound cachexia. Because of the marked turnover and proliferative nature of agnogenic myeloid metaplasia, hypermetabolism is a frequent feature of agnogenic myeloid metaplasia, causing weight loss, night sweats, and low-grade fever.

Bleeding may occur from a series of mechanisms. Platelet dysfunction may lead to purpura and ecchymoses. Acquired Factor V deficiency may precipitate serious bleeding. Thrombocytopenia or disseminated intravascular coagulopathy may develop during the clinical course of the disease. Occasionally, patients with agnogenic myeloid metaplasia develop symptoms due to extramedullary hematopoiesis (Table 141–7).

DIAGNOSIS. Diagnosis is based on (1) splenomegaly, (2) leukoerythroblastic blood picture, (3) the presence of teardrop poikilocytes in the peripheral blood, and (4) various degrees of bone marrow fibrosis. Differential diagnosis includes several marrow-invading diseases, including chronic granulocytic leukemia, infectious processes such as tuberculosis or histoplasmosis, and metastatic carcinoma.

LABORATORY FEATURES. Teardrop red blood cells and leukoerythroblastosis in a well-prepared blood smear strongly suggest agnogenic myeloid metaplasia. Teardrop red blood cells originate in the spleen and are a sign of extramedullary erythropoiesis. Leukoerythroblastosis reflects the presence of fibrosis in the marrow. Bone marrow aspirates tend to be hypocellular in 85%

TABLE 141–7. ORGAN INVOLVEMENT WITH EXTRAMEDULLARY HEMATOPOIESIS IN AGNOGENIC MYELOID METAPLASIA

Organ	Manifestation
Small intestine	Gastrointestinal tract hemorrhage
Spinal cord	Paralysis and paresthesias
Brain	Seizures
Lungs	Respiratory distress
Peritoneum	Ascites
Bladder	Hematuria

of patients, hypercellular in 5%, and normocellular in 10%. Bone marrow biopsy specimens may be hypercellular with reticulin fibrosis (cellular phase) or, in most cases, have substantial collagen fibrosis with or without osteosclerosis. Clonal cytogenetic abnormalities occur in one third of the patients and include 20q−, 13q−, and trisomy 21.

Anemia, with hemoglobin levels of 10 grams per deciliter or less, is observed in 50 to 60% of patients on initial examination. This is mostly due to ineffective erythropoiesis, but in about half of the patients, red blood cell survivorship is shortened. Thrombocytopenia may affect one third of the patients because of a decreasing megakaryocytic mass in the marrow and excessive destruction or sequestration of platelets by the enlarged spleen. Thrombocytopenia may also reflect "inapparent disseminated intravascular coagulopathy." Thus, patients may have a combination of thrombocytopenia, Factor V and VIII deficiency, and an increase of fibrin split products. Some of these patients remain stable with no clinical manifestations, but others can bleed excessively or even exsanguinate during a major surgical procedure. Isolated deficiencies of Factor V have been observed in patients with agnogenic myeloid metaplasia. Most patients with this disease have qualitative platelet defects, with no platelet aggregation occurring in response to either epinephrine or collagen. Leukopenia may occur in approximately 5 to 15% of patients. It is due to failing granulopoiesis in compromised bone marrow and to splenomegaly.

Serum levels of the N-terminal propeptides correlate with disease activity. Collagen types I and III are the major components of bone marrow fibrosis in agnogenic myeloid metaplasia. Initially, collagen is synthesized by fibroblasts as procollagen, a soluble precursor of collagen. Intracellular procollagen secreted into the bone matrix immediately cleaves the N- and C-terminal extensions, resulting in the release of these soluble propeptides into blood. Thus, the presence of increased concentrations suggests active collagen synthesis.

TREATMENT. Currently, no cure exists for patients with agnogenic myeloid metaplasia. Ongoing studies with antifibrosis agents, including penicillamine and suramin, have not been rewarding. A long-term study on the effects of colchicine in inhibiting fibrosis is under way. It has been observed recently that the new antiplatelet agent anagrelide may impede the development of fibrosis or reverse existing fibrosis in selected patients with agnogenic myeloid metaplasia. A large study is under way to test the consistency of this finding.

The management of agnogenic myeloid metaplasia is directed to symptoms. Androgens have been helpful in patients with normocytic normochromic anemia. The drug of choice is oxymetholone in doses of 50 mg three times daily. Because about 50% of patients have shortened red blood cell survival, the addition of prednisone, 30 mg daily, has been helpful. In patients with refractory hemolytic anemia (which may occur in up to 7% of patients), adrenal steroids might be helpful. If these measures fail, splenectomy is indicated.

The treatment of bleeding in agnogenic myeloid metaplasia varies. If it is caused by qualitative platelet defects, platelet transfusions may be helpful. In patients with thrombocytopenia, a trial of prednisone may be worthwhile. If adrenal steroids fail to treat thrombocytopenia, splenectomy may be indicated. Patients with Factor V deficiency should be given fresh frozen plasma.

Hydroxyurea taken orally should be considered for patients with painfully enlarged spleens. Radiation is not indicated because it usually is followed within 4 to 6 months by the spleen enlarging to more than its initial size.

The role of splenectomy has been fairly well defined in patients with agnogenic myeloid metaplasia. It is worthwhile for good surgical candidates in the following situations: (1) mechanically symptomatic splenomegaly, (2) refractory hemolytic anemia, (3) refractory thrombocytopenia, and (4) portal hypertension.

Before splenectomy is considered, it should be determined that the patient is not at risk because of impaired cardiac, pulmonary, hepatic, renal, or metabolic function. All patients should have full coagulation surveys. The preoperative preparation of patients who have only qualitative platelet disorders should include treatment with adrenal steroids and fresh platelet packs. For those who have all the features of apparent disseminated intravascular coagulopathy but are not bleeding, splenectomy is totally contraindicated. These patients may be reconsidered for splenectomy after the disseminated intravascular coagulopathy resolves. Patients with mechanically painful splenomegaly who are good candidates for splenectomy

have an impressive postoperative response. Approximately 50% of patients with refractory hemolytic anemia or refractory thrombocytopenia also improve measureably after splenectomy. Splenectomy also has been effective to relieve portal hypertension.

PROGNOSIS. The survival rate at 5 years of patients with agnogenic myeloid metaplasia is approximately 60%. The prognosis tends to be better for those who are asymptomatic, who are not anemic or thrombocytopenic, and who do not have enlarged livers. Hopefully, newer approaches to the control of the disease should lead to improved survival rates within the next decade.

Anagrelide Study Group: Anagrelide, a therapy for thrombocythemic states: Experience in 577 patients. Am J Med 92:69, 1992. *An original clinical study on the role of a new platelet-lowering agent anagrelide in chronic myeloproliferative disorders.*

Donehower RC: An overview of the clinical experience with hydroxyurea. Semin Oncol 19(3 suppl 9):11, 1992. *A comprehensive review of the clinical uses of hydroxyurea and associated side effects.*

Juvonen E, Ikkala E, Oksanen K, et al.: Megakaryocyte and erythroid colony formation in essential thrombocythaemia and reactive thrombocytosis: Diagnostic value and correlation to complications. Br J Haematol 83:192, 1993. *A study of in vitro megakaryocyte and erythroid colony formation in patients with essential thrombocythemia compared with those with reactive thrombocytosis.*

Martyré M-C: Platelet PDGF and TGF-β levels in myeloproliferative disorders. Leuk Lymphoma 6:1, 1991. *An excellent review of current knowledge about the pathogenesis of bone marrow fibrosis in agnogenic myeloid metaplasia.*

Middelhoff G, Boll I: A long-term clinical trial of interferon-alpha therapy in essential thrombocythemia. Ann Hematol 64:207, 1992. *Six patients with essential thrombocythemia were treated with recombinant interferon alpha 2b and followed for up to 4 years.*

Tefferi A, Barrett SM, Silverstein MN, Nagorney DM: Outcome of portal-systemic shunt surgery for portal hypertension associated with intrahepatic obstruction in patients with agnogenic myeloid metaplasia. Am J Hematol 46:325, 1994. *A long-term retrospective study describing the outcome of patients with agnogenic myeloid metaplasia who underwent portal-systemic shunt surgery for portal hypertension.*

Tefferi A, Ho TC, Ahmann GJ, et al.: Plasma interleukin-6 and C-reactive protein levels in reactive versus clonal thrombocytosis. Am J Med 97:374, 1994. *The authors demonstrated the use of plasma IL-6 or C-reactive protein levels in the differentiation of essential thrombocythemia from reactive thrombocytosis.*

Tefferi A, Silverstein MN, Plumhoff EA, et al.: Suramin toxicity and efficacy in agnogenic myeloid metaplasia. J Natl Cancer Inst 85:1520, 1993. *The authors investigated suramin as an antigrowth factor (i.e., antifibrosing agent) in the treatment of agnogenic myeloid metaplasia. In four treated patients, clinical benefit was not apparent, and accelerated splenomegaly was a notable complication.*

Visani G, Castelli U, Petti MC, et al.: Myelofibrosis with myeloid metaplasia: Clinical and haematological parameters predicting survival in a series of 133 patients. Br J Haematol 75:4, 1990. *A well-presented clinical study of 133 patients with agnogenic myeloid metaplasia.*

Watson KV, Key N: Vascular complications of essential thrombocythaemia: A link to cardiovascular risk factors. Br J Haematol 83:198, 1993. *The authors report on the association of increased arterial thromboembolic complications in patients with essential thrombocythemia suffering from cardiovascular risk factors.*

142 THE CHRONIC LEUKEMIAS

Michael J. Keating

CHRONIC MYELOGENOUS LEUKEMIA (Chronic Myeloid Leukemia, Chronic Myelocytic Leukemia, Chronic Granulocytic Leukemia)

DEFINITION. Chronic myelogenous leukemia (CML) is a disease characterized by overproduction of cells of the granulocytic, especially the neutrophilic, series and occasionally the monocytic series (see Color Plate 7F, right), leading to marked splenomegaly and very high white blood cell counts. Basophilia and thrombocytosis are common. A characteristic cytogenetic abnormality, the Philadelphia (Ph[1]) chromosome, is present in the bone marrow cells in more than 95% of cases. The granulocytes usually appear relatively normal, although many patients exhibit dysplastic changes, including Pelger-Huët anomalies. Neutrophil functions, such as phagocytosis and bactericidal activity, are largely preserved. Before effective treatment was available, patients survived, on the average, approximately 2 years after diagnosis.

ETIOLOGY. Usually no etiologic agent can be incriminated in CML. Exposure to ionizing radiation increases the risk of subsequent CML. Survivors of the atomic bomb explosions in Japan in 1945 have had an increased incidence of CML, with a peak occurring 5 to 12 years after exposure and seeming to be dose related

The relative risk has been falling since that time, but is still above the expected rate for Japan. Radiation treatment of ankylosing spondylitis and cervical cancer has increased the incidence of CML. No increase in the risk of CML has been demonstrated in individuals working in the nuclear industry. Radiologists working without adequate protection prior to 1940 were more likely to develop myeloid leukemia, but no such association has been found in recent studies. Benzene exposure increases the risk of acute myelogenous leukemia (AML) but not of CML. Patients with CML have an increased frequency of the Cw3 and Cw4 human leukocyte antigens (HLA's). Chronic myelogenous leukemia is not a frequent secondary leukemia following the treatment of other cancers with radiation and/or alkylating agents.

INCIDENCE. Chronic myelogenous leukemia constitutes one fifth of all cases of leukemia in the United States. CML is diagnosed in 1 or 2 persons per 100,000 per year, with a slight male preponderance. This incidence has not changed significantly in the past few decades. The incidence of CML increases with age; the median age at diagnosis is approximately 45 to 50 years. Ph^1-positive CML is uncommon in children and adolescents. Patients older than 60 years have a poorer prognosis. No familial association of CML has been noted.

MOLECULAR PATHOGENESIS. The striking feature in CML is the presence of Ph^1 chromosome in the bone marrow cells of more than 90% of patients with typical CML. The Ph^1 chromosome results from a balanced translocation of material between the long arms of chromosomes 9 and 22. As more chromosomal material is lost from chromosome 22 than is gained from chromosome 9, the Ph^1 chromosome is a shortened chromosome 22 containing approximately 60% of its normal complement of DNA. The break, which occurs at band q34 of the long arm of chromosome 9, allows translocation of the cellular oncogene *C-ABL* to a position on chromosome 22 called the breakpoint cluster region (bcr). The breakpoint in the bcr varies from patient to patient, but is identical in all cells of any one patient. *C-ABL* is a homologue of *V-ABL*, the Abelson virus that causes leukemia in mice (see Ch. 156). The apposition of these two genetic sequences produces a new hybrid gene *(BCR/ABL)*, which codes for a novel protein of molecular weight 210,000 kD (P210). The P210 protein, a tyrosine kinase, may play a role in triggering the uncontrolled proliferation of CML cells. The Ph^1 chromosome occurs in erythroid, myeloid, moncytic, and megakaryocytic cells, less commonly in B lymphocytes, rarely in T lymphocytes, but not in marrow fibroblasts. This extensive cellular distribution places the abnormality in CML close to the pluripotent stem cell. Studies of glucose-6-phosphate dehydrogenase (G6PD) isoenzymes support the finding of multilineage monoclonal proliferation, since a single isoenzyme is present in the aforementioned cells in some patients with CML. *C-sis,* the homologue of the simian sarcoma virus, is also translocated from chromosome 22 to chromosome 9 in CML but is distant from the breakpoint and not expressed in benign-phase CML. *C-sis* codes for a protein identical to platelet-derived growth factor (PDGF). Insertion of a retrovirus encoding P210 *(BCR/ABL)* into cells of mice has led to the development of a disease closely resembling CML in some of these animals, giving credence to the hypothesis that the *BCR/ABL* hybrid gene is sufficient to cause CML.

The fusion *BCR/ABL* gene and the P210 protein can be found in many cases of typical CML in which no cytogenetic abnormality occurs or in which changes other than typical t(9;22)(q34;q11) are identified. These patients have a survival rate and a response to therapy that are similar to those in Ph^1-positive patients. Patients with atypical CML who are Ph^1 and *BCR/ABL* negative have a different natural history than do patients who are either Ph^1 positive or Ph^1 negative with *BCR/ABL* positivity. They resemble more closely patients with myelodysplastic syndrome (MDS). Thus, three groups of patients with CML can be identified: (1) positive for Ph^1 and *BCR/ABL,* (2) Ph^1 negative and *BCR/ABL* positive, and (3) negative for Ph^1 and *BCR/ABL* (Table 142–1).

Although 100% of the metaphases on cytogenetic analysis usually show the presence of the Ph^1 chromosome, some normal stem cells must remain. Normal diploid cells appear on long-term bone marrow culture and following treatment with interferon, high-dose chemotherapy, and autologous bone marrow transplantation.

TABLE 142–1. CLASSIFICATION OF CHRONIC MYELOGENOUS LEUKEMIA (CML)

Disease	Ph^1 Present	*BCR/ABL* Rearrangement	Prognosis
Classic CML	Yes	Yes	Median, 4 yr
bcr+, Ph^{1-}	No	Most	Median, 4 yr
CMML/CMoL/bcr-CML	No	No	18–24 mo

bcr = Breakpoint cluster region; *BCR/ABL* = a hybrid gene (see text); CMML = chronic myelomonocytic leukemia; CMoL = chronic monocytic leukemia.

SYMPTOMS AND SIGNS. CML is diagnosed in many asymptomatic patients because of the use of hematologic studies in routine annual physical examinations or in evaluations of other illnesses. In these patients the white blood cell (WBC) count may be relatively low at the time of diagnosis. The WBC count correlates well with tumor mass as defined by spleen size. Patients with higher WBC counts and larger spleens have more symptoms. The symptomatology of CML, usually nonspecific, is secondary to anemia, spleen size, or an increased basal metabolic rate, but most patients are asymptomatic or only mildly symptomatic. Fatigue, weight loss, malaise, easy satiety, and a sense of left upper quadrant fullness are the major symptoms of CML. Rarely, bleeding (associated with a low platelet count and/or platelet dysfunction) or thrombosis (associated with thrombocytosis and/or marked leukocytosis) occurs. The serum uric acid level is commonly elevated at diagnosis, and acute gouty arthritis may follow treatment. An elevated blood histamine level (related to the basophil cell mass) can cause upper gastrointestinal ulceration and bleeding. Neutrophil function is usually normal or only modestly impaired, and neutrophil numbers are markedly increased; infections are therefore uncommon at the time of diagnosis. Headaches, bone pain, arthralgias, pain from splenic infarction, and fever are uncommon in the early stages of CML but become more common as the disease progresses. Priapism is occasionally noted, usually in patients with marked leukocytosis or thrombocytosis. Leukostatic symptoms, such as dyspnea, drowsiness, loss of coordination, or confusion, which are due to sludging in the pulmonary or cerebral vessels, are uncommon in the benign phase of CML despite WBC counts that may exceed 400,000 per microliter. These symptoms appear more frequently in later stages of the disease (i.e., in the accelerated or blast crisis phases, in which more premature cells predominate). All symptoms subside as the WBC count falls and the splenomegaly decreases as a result of effective treatment.

Splenomegaly, by far the most consistent physical sign in CML, occurs in more than 60% of cases. The spleen may extend to the pelvic brim and across the midline of the abdomen in some cases. Hepatomegaly is less common and is usually minor (1 to 3 cm below the right costal margin). Lymphadenopathy is very uncommon, as is infiltration of skin and other tissues. If present, these findings suggest Ph^1-negative CML or accelerated or blastic transformation of CML. Rarely, patients initially have a blast crisis; these patients can have any of the clinical manifestations of acute leukemia.

NATURAL HISTORY. More than 90% of patients present with CML in the benign phase, in which the disease behaves in a predictable fashion, with the symptoms, abnormal physical signs, and abnormal blood findings returning to normal following treatment. This satisfactory response is transient; all patients eventually develop a variety of changes in the behavior of the disease. Most frequently there is a "blast crisis," a clinical picture resembling that of acute leukemia. This change can be abrupt, but more frequently it is preceded by a period of progressively greater difficulty in maintaining the WBC count at a level of less than 20,000 per microliter and of other manifestations, such as increasing splenomegaly, hepatomegaly, and infiltration of nodes, skin, bones, or other tissues; the appearance of blast cells or basophils in the peripheral blood; development of anemia and/or thrombocytopenia; or fever, malaise, and weight loss. This last group of features, termed the accelerated phase of CML, demands reevaluation of the bone marrow, which, in the accelerated phase, shows dysplastic changes in the myeloid and other cell lineages and may show an increase in the percentage of blast cells (5 to 29%) and an increase in basophils. Aspiration of bone marrow may be difficult, especially in patients who have developed myelofibrosis subsequent to the CML. Chromosomal abnormalities, in addition to the Ph[1] chromosome, occur in both the accelerated and the blastic phases of CML. Blast crisis is diagnosed when 30% or more blast cells are present in the bone marrow and/or peripheral blood.

When the accelerated phase or blast crisis is suspected (i.e., 10 to 40% blasts in bone marrow), the patient should be further observed in 2 to 4 weeks, since the percentage of blasts in the blood and bone marrow can increase transiently after the treatment of CML is discontinued, especially if the patient had been treated with hydroxyurea or interferon. It is important to be cautious in classifying patients as having blast crisis or accelerated phase because of the adverse prognostic implications (Fig. 142–1). Criteria for the accelerated phase are the following: an increase in blast cells (>15%) or basophils (>20%) in the blood or bone marrow, thrombocytopenia (<100,000 per microliter), serious anemia (hemoglobin [Hb] <7 grams per deciliter); documented extramedullary leukemia, or development of clonal evolution (new chromosomal changes in addition to the Ph[1] chromosome).

The risk of developing accelerated phase or blast crisis in CML is relatively low in the first 2 years after diagnosis (~10% per year), but then increases and remains constant (15 to 20% per year) after that unless therapy such as bone marrow transplantation is used.

LABORATORY FINDINGS. All patients with untreated CML have an elevated WBC count ranging from 10,000 per microliter to more than 1,000,000 per microliter. The predominant cells are of the neutrophil series, with a left shift extending to blast cells (see Color Plate 7F, right). In addition, eosinophils and basophils are commonly increased in number. Monocytes may be slightly increased in some cases that overlap with chronic myelomonocytic leukemia (CMML). The bone marrow is hypercellular with marked myeloid hyperplasia and sometimes shows evidence of increased reticulin or collagen fibrosis. The myeloid-erythroid ratio is 15:1 to 20:1. About 15% of patients have 5% or more blast cells in the peripheral blood or bone marrow at diagnosis. T cells (both T helper and T suppressor), but not B cells, are increased in number in CML. A hemoglobin of less than 11 grams per deciliter is present in one third of patients. The red cells are usually normochromic and normocytic, but nucleated red cells are present in the blood of one quarter of the patients at diagnosis. Autoimmune hemolytic anemia and thrombocytopenia (<100,000 per microliter) are rare in CML, but thrombocytosis (>450,000 per microliter) occurs in almost half of the patients.

Biochemical abnormalities in CML include a markedly decreased leukocyte alkaline phosphatase (LAP) score in the neutrophils of 90% or more of patients, being completely absent in 5 to 10% of cases. A low LAP score also occurs in some patients with agnogenic myeloid metaplasia, which is sometimes difficult to differentiate from CML. The serum levels of transcobalamins I and III, cobalamin-binding glycoproteins produced by neutrophils, are elevated in accord with the increased neutrophils. This elevation leads to extremely high serum cobalamin values (e.g., vitamin B_{12} levels >10 times normal). Serum levels of lactate dehydrogenase, uric acid, and lysozyme are often increased. The lysozyme levels are modestly increased in CML compared with CMML, in which the

levels in blood and urine are often markedly increased. Kinetic studies show an increased neutrophil production rate related to a markedly expanded myeloid mass. The number of colony-forming cells in the blood in CML is increased, but the number in the bone marrow is in the normal range. Defective feedback control of WBC production is common in CML; some patients demonstrate a cyclic oscillation of the WBC count. The labeling index of myeloblasts in CML is lower than in normal bone marrow, and the generation time is prolonged, confirming the concept that CML is an accumulative rather than a proliferative disease. Neutrophils in CML survive intravascularly slightly longer than do normal granulocytes.

DIAGNOSIS. The diagnosis of typical CML is not difficult. The presence of unexplained myeloid leukocytosis with splenomegaly should lead to a leukocyte alkaline phosphatase (LAP) test on the peripheral blood neutrophils and bone marrow examination with a cytogenetic analysis. Marrow myeloid hyperplasia and hypercellularity further suggest the diagnosis. The ultimate test, however, remains the cytogenetic analysis; the presence of the Ph[1] chromosome in this clinical setting establishes the diagnosis. When the Ph[1] chromosome is not found in a patient with suspected CML, molecular evidence for the presence of the hybrid *BCR/ABL* gene should be sought, as 40 to 50% of Ph[1]-negative patients with CML have *BCR/ABL* rearrangement. The Ph[1] chromosome is usually present in 100% of metaphases, ordinarily as the sole abnormality. Ten to 15% of patients at initial presentation have an additional chromosomal change, such as loss of the Y chromosome, trisomy 8, an additional loss of material from 22q, or an atypical translocation. The patients who have atypical complex chromosomal changes, which may or may not involve chromosome 9 or 22 morphologically, demonstrate evidence of the hybrid *BCR/ABL* gene when molecular techniques are used.

Chronic myelogenous leukemia must be differentiated from leukemoid reactions, which usually produce WBC counts lower than 50,000 per microliter, toxic granulation vacuolation, Döhle bodies in the granulocytes, absence of basophilia, a normal or increased LAP level, and a clinical history and physical examination suggesting the origin of the leukemoid reaction. Corticosteroids can rarely cause extreme neutrophilia together with the left shift, but this response is self-limited and short in duration and thus seldom a cause of diagnostic difficulty.

Chronic myelogenous leukemia may be more difficult to differentiate from other myelodysplastic or myeloproliferative syndromes. Patients having agnogenic myeloid metaplasia with or without myelofibrosis have splenomegaly and often have neutrophilia and thrombocytosis. Polycythemia rubra vera with associated iron deficiency, which allows a normal hemoglobin level and hematocrit value, can manifest with an elevated neutrophil and platelet count. Such patients usually have a normal or increased LAP score and a WBC count less than 25,000 per microliter, and the Ph[1] chromosome is not present.

The greatest diagnostic difficulty lies with patients who have splenomegaly and leukocytosis but who do not have the Ph[1] chromosome. Many of these patients have the usual blood and marrow findings of Ph[1]-positive CML, and the *BCR/ABL* hybrid gene can be demonstrated despite a normal or atypical cytogenetic pattern. Patients who are Ph[1] negative and *BCR/ABL* negative are considered to have Ph[1]-negative CML or CMML (Table 142–1). The cytogenetic findings in patients with CMML are normal or involve an additional chromosome 8 or findings other than the Ph[1] chromosome. Patients with CMML have *ras* mutations in 50 to 60% of cases. Rarely, patients have myeloid hyperplasia, which involves almost exclusively the neutrophil, eosinophil, or basophilic cell lineage. These patients are described as having chronic neutrophilic, eosinophilic, or basophilic leukemia and do not have evidence of the Ph[1] chromosome or *BCR/ABL* gene. Isolated megakaryocytic hyperplasia can give rise to a syndrome called idiopathic thrombocythemia with marked thrombocytosis and splenomegaly. These conditions are considered to fall under the general category of myeloproliferative disorders and have a better prognosis than does CML.

EVOLUTION OF CML. Death occurs rarely during the chronic phase of CML, but over time the clinical behavior of the disease changes. One third of patients abruptly develop an acute transformation (blast crisis of CML); the other two thirds respond progressively less well in the control of the WBC count and spleen size

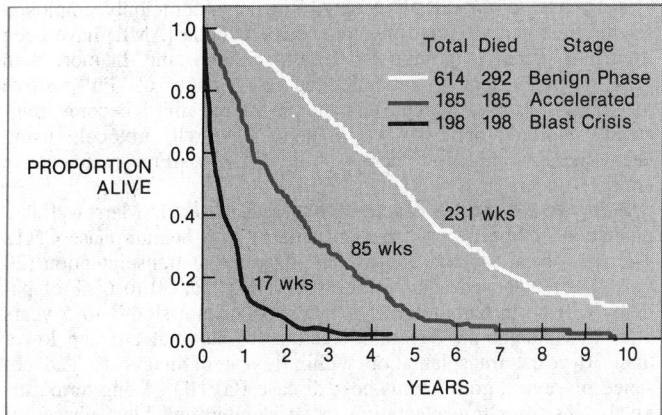

Total	Died	Stage
614	292	Benign Phase
185	185	Accelerated
198	198	Blast Crisis

FIGURE 142–1. Survival of M. D. Anderson Cancer Center patients with chronic myelogenous leukemia by phase of disease.

with conventional agents such as busulfan and hydroxyurea. This loss of control (accelerated phase) is often associated with an increased proportion of blasts, promyelocytes, and basophils in the peripheral blood and bone marrow and is often accompanied by anemia and thrombocytopenia. Some patients develop bone marrow failure in which anemia and thrombocytopenia are accompanied by increasing evidence of dysplastic changes in the marrow and myelofibrosis. The median survival after developing a blast crisis of CML is only 3 months (Fig. 142–1). The survival after development of the accelerated phase of CML is 12 to 18 months if the blood and bone marrow contain more than 30% blasts plus promyelocytes or more than 20% basophils or if the platelet count falls to less than 100,000 per microliter. Most patients with blast crisis or accelerated phase have additional chromosomal abnormalities (clonal evolution), such as duplication of the Ph^1 chromosome, trisomy of chromosome number 8, or development of an isochromosome number 17. Clonal evolution usually presages the accelerated phase or blast crisis of CML. The blast cells in blast crisis are usually myeloblasts, but less commonly erythroid, monocytoid, or megakaryoblastic transformations occur. In one quarter of cases, the blast cells are lymphoid in origin, as demonstrated by cytochemical stains (terminal deoxynucleotidyl transferase), immunophenotyping, and immunoglobulin heavy-chain rearrangement studies. In 10% of cases, the blast cells are completely undifferentiated. Some patients with acute leukemia and the Ph^1 chromosome abnormality presumably have had blast crises that occurred before the diagnosis of CML was made. These cases have the P210 protein and 8.5-kb fusion messenger RNA. Patients with acute lymphoblastic leukemia (ALL) with a Ph^1 usually have a P190 protein or a 7.0-kb fusion messenger RNA probably restricted to the lymphoid cells. Extramedullary blast crisis of CML can occur in the spleen, lymph nodes, skin, meninges, bone, and other sites. This initial extramedullary transformation is usually shortly followed by evidence of marrow involvement.

Chronic myelomonocytic leukemia and Ph^1- and *BCR/ABL*-negative CML appear to overlap clinically in some instances, and their clinical behavior, progress, and response to therapy resemble those of the MDS more than Ph^1-positive CML. A male preponderance is noted, splenomegaly is common (60 to 70%), and the WBC count, while elevated, is usually in the 25,000 to 100,000 per microliter range. Anemia and thrombocytopenia are more common than in Ph^1-positive CML, and eosinophilia and basophilia are less common. The median survival is 18 to 24 months, with patients dying of infection, bleeding, or transformation to acute leukemia.

TREATMENT. Immediate treatment of CML is not necessary unless the WBC count exceeds 200,000 per microliter or there is evidence of leukostasis (priapism, venous thrombosis, confusion, or dyspnea) or unless painful splenomegaly suggests splenic infarction. Hyperuricemia is common at the diagnosis of CML and should be treated with allopurinol, 100 mg three times a day, and adequate hydration while the WBC count is higher than 25,000 per microliter to prevent renal dysfunction. Acute gouty arthritis is rare.

PALLIATIVE TREATMENT. Chronic myelogenous leukemia has been treated traditionally with oral busulfan, which, if used prudently, gives smooth, sustained control of the WBC count, platelet count, and spleen size. Since overdosage with busulfan can cause prolonged myelosuppression, another active oral agent, hydroxyurea, has been increasingly used. Both agents have a high level of acceptance by the patient, and both control the manifestations of the disease in 90% of cases when first used, but over time they produce progressively shorter and less complete reductions in the WBC count and spleen size.

Busulfan is usually started at a dosage of 4 to 8 mg per day, depending on the WBC count and the patient's body size. Use of higher dosages of 12 to 16 mg per day should be restricted to patients with WBC counts greater than 200,000 per microliter. Leukapheresis can also be used on a short-term basis to decrease the leukocyte or platelet counts rapidly. When the initial WBC count halves, the starting dose should be decreased by 50%. The leukocyte count decreases exponentially and is closely correlated with reduction in spleen size. Since the WBC count continues to fall for 2 to 4 weeks after cessation of busulfan administration the drug should be discontinued when the WBC count reaches 20,000 to 25,000 per microliter to prevent severe pancytopenia from marrow

hypoplasia. The WBC count may not begin to rise again for several months or for more than a year, at which time a lower dose (2 to 4 mg per day) should be reinstituted. Few acute side effects are noted with busulfan, although premature menopause does occur in 20 to 40% of young women, and sterility is frequent in both men and women. Hyperpigmentation, weight loss, and fatigue, which can mimic Addison's disease, occur with prolonged use, and in a small number of patients pulmonary fibrosis develops. As the disease progresses, intervals between courses of busulfan shorten and the rate of rise in the WBC count at relapse increases.

Hydroxyurea is given at dosages of 1 to 4 grams per day, again according to the WBC count and body size. The WBC count falls in similar fashion to that induced by busulfan, but severe marrow hypoplasia is rare. The dosage of hydroxyurea is decreased as the leukocyte count decreases and can be discontinued when the WBC count is 5 to 10×10^3 per microliter. Some physicians prefer to treat patients with intermittent courses, whereas others maintain patients on 0.5 to 2 grams per day. The drug can be given as a single dose or fractionated throughout the day. While close monitoring of the blood count is necessary initially with hydroxyurea, the pattern of response is usually predictable with repeated courses. Side effects are uncommon, although rash, mucositis, and diarrhea can occur. The survival of patients treated with hydroxyurea is probably superior to that of those treated with busulfan. Busulfan exposure before allogeneic transplant is an adverse factor for survival. Splenic irradiation is not recommended for the treatment of CML.

CYTOGENETICALLY DIRECTED THERAPY. Busulfan and conventional-dose hydroxyurea rarely eliminate the Ph^1 chromosome from marrow cells. With high-dose hydroxyurea, however, diploid metaphases have been observed in several patients. A return to a normal chromosomal pattern would seem to be a reasonable therapeutic goal, and it might be anticipated that patients who achieve a normal karyotype may survive better than those who do not. Three therapeutic initiatives have been developed based on this concept: the use of interferons, intensive chemotherapy, and bone marrow transplantation.

Interferon Therapy. Both human leukocyte interferon and recombinant alpha-interferon (r-IFnα) have been demonstrated to produce hematologic and cytogenetic remissions in CML. Complete hematologic remissions are obtained in 75 to 80% of patients treated with r-IFnα, and 30 to 40% of the patients have complete or partial suppression in the Ph^1 chromosome. Gamma-interferon alone or combined with alpha-interferon does not have a significant therapeutic effect. Return of normal metaphases following the use of r-IFnα is associated with a longer survival than is seen in patients without a cytogenetic response. The dosage of r-IFnα is 2 to 5 million units per square meter per day, administered subcutaneously. The response rate is higher with the higher dose. The most common acute side effects—musculoskeletal discomfort, fever, and chills—subside in most patients but are often replaced by symptoms of fatigue, depression, lethargy, inattention, loss of weight, lack of libido, and mild alopecia. These toxicities are more common in patients over 60 years of age. Reactions at the injection site occur in approximately 5% of patients. Thrombocytopenia, anemia, arthritis, nephrotic syndrome, and seizures occur rarely. Loss of disease control, together with lack of side effects, may signal the development of neutralizing antibodies to interferon.

Aggressive Chemotherapy. Regimens commonly employed for the treatment of acute myelogenous leukemia (AML) have been used in an attempt to suppress the Ph^1 chromosome. In more than 50% of the treated patients, the percentage of Ph^1-positive metaphases is greatly reduced, and about one third become transiently diploid for 2 to 12 months. Research protocols using chemotherapy induction therapy followed by r-IFnα maintenance are now under way.

Allogeneic Bone Marrow Transplantation. Marrow transplantation has been performed in patients with benign-phase CML. The risk of early death due to complications of transplantation (20 to 30%) is balanced against the observation that 50 to 60% of patients will be in hematologic or cytogenetic remission 3 to 5 years after transplantation. Favorable factors for survival are age lower than 30 years, transplantation within 1 year of diagnosis, and absence of severe graft-versus-host disease (GVHD). Long-term survival rates after transplantation in accelerated and blast phases of CML are only approximately 10 to 15%. After syngeneic (identical twin) bone marrow transplantations, 84% of patients treated at the

Fred Hutchinson Cancer Center (Seattle, Washington) are alive and 75% continue in complete hematologic and cytogenetic remission. The possibility exists that many of these patients will be cured. Autologous marrow and peripheral blood stem cell support following ablative chemotherapy and radiation therapy is currently being evaluated. As only one third of all patients have a matched related donor, matched unrelated donor transplants are being investigated.

TREATMENT OF ACCELERATED CML AND BLAST CRISIS OF CML. Loss of control of CML with agents such as busulfan, hydroxyurea, or interferon is marked by development of increasing splenomegaly, leukocytosis, and thrombocytosis. Many of these patients develop additional cytogenetic abnormalities (clonal evolution). Some patients develop severe anemia and thrombocytopenia. Splenectomy occasionally corrects the thrombocytopenia. The bone marrow often develops increasing dysplasia of one or multiple cell lines, together with an increasing left shift (5 to 29% blast cells), eosinophilia, and basophilia. Change of therapy from busulfan to hydroxyurea or vice versa is successful for a short time (3 to 6 months) in 10 to 25% of patients. These patients are considered to have an accelerated phase of the disease. If the proportion of blast cells in bone marrow exceeds 30%, the patient is considered to be in blast crisis (acute transformation of CML) (see Color Plate 7G). The blast crisis or refractory accelerated phase of CML is usually treated with regimens designed for the treatment of acute leukemia. Treatment of myeloid, undifferentiated, or mixed-lineage blast crisis is usually unsatisfactory, with only 25 to 30% of patients achieving complete remission. Patients with a lymphoid blast crisis phenotype have a better chance (50 to 65%) of achieving complete remission on regimens utilizing vincristine, corticosteroids, asparaginase, and/or anthracyclines. The Ph[1] chromosome persists, and the duration of response is usually short (2 to 6 months), with no prospect of cure. Only 10 to 15% of patients with blast crisis survive for more than 1 year (Fig. 142–1). Allogeneic marrow transplantation should be offered to patients with blast crisis (with active disease or after remission is obtained) if a suitable donor is available, since few of these patients have survived more than 5 years. The mortality rate and relapse rate after allogenic transplantation for CML blast crisis are much higher than for CML in the benign phase. Patients who have an HLA-compatible sibling should have an allogeneic transplantation performed before the accelerated or blast phases of CML develop.

PROGNOSIS. The median survival in Ph[1]-positive CML was 3 to 4 years for patients treated in the 1970's, with a range of 1 to 20 years (Fig. 142–2). The median survival at the M. D. Anderson Cancer Center in Houston, Texas, for patients in whom diagnosis was made after 1980 is greater than 5 years. The risk of death is 5 to 8% per year for the first 24 months and increases to 15 to 20% per year for the next 2 years and 25% per year thereafter. No patients are projected to be cured with palliative use of busulfan and/or hydroxyurea. The influence of treatment with interferon, aggressive chemotherapy, and allogeneic transplantation on the improved survival of patients in whom diagnosis was made after 1980 is not certain at this time. Large spleen, increased liver size, elevated platelet counts, high marrow and blood blast and basophil percentages, advanced age, and clonal evolution are consistent adverse prognostic factors (Table 142–2) and have been combined into a simple staging system. This system identifies a high-risk group (30 to 40%) of patients with a median survival of only 2 years. The quality of life of patients in the benign phase is usually excellent.

TABLE 142–2. ADVERSE PROGNOSTIC FACTORS IN CHRONIC MYELOGENOUS LEUKEMIA (CML)

Older age
Large spleen
Large liver
Increase or decrease in platelets
High white count
Basophilia
Clonal evolution

From Kantarjian HM, Keating MJ, Smith TL, et al.: Proposal for a simple synthesis prognostic staging system in chronic myelogenous leukemia. Am J Med 88:1, 1990; with permission.

Ahuja H, Bar-Eli M, Arlin Z, et al.: The spectrum of molecular alterations in the evolution of chronic myelocytic leukemia. J Clin Invest 87:2042, 1991. *An overview of molecular events during the course of cases.*
Daley GQ, Van Etten RA, Baltimore D: Induction of chronic myelogenous leukemia in mice by the P210abl/bcr gene of the Philadelphia chromosome. Science 247:824, 1990. *Seminal report of role of BCR/ABL gene as causative factor in CML.*
Hehlmann R, Heimpel H, Hasford J, et al. and the German CML Study Group: Randomized comparison of busulfan and hydroxyurea in chronic myelogenous leukemia: prolongation of survival by hydroxyurea. Blood 83:398, 1993. *Demonstration of superior tolerance and survival of those receiving hydroxyurea compared with those given busulfan.*
Kantarjian HM, Dixon D, Keating MJ, et al.: Characteristics of accelerated disease in chronic myelogenous leukemia. Cancer 61:1441, 1988. *Quantitative analysis of impact on survival of various features of accelerated-phase CML.*
Kurzrock R, Gutterman JU, Talpaz M: The molecular genetics of Philadelphia chromosome-positive leukemias. N Engl J Med 319:990, 1988. *Detailed analysis of molecular genetic data in Ph[1] chromosome–positive acute and chronic leukemias.*
Strife A, Lambek C, Wisniewski D, et al.: Discordant maturation as the primary biological defect in chronic myelogenous leukemia. Cancer Res 48:1035, 1988. *Analysis of morphologic changes associated with various clinical stages of CML.*
Talpaz M, Kantarjian H, Kurzrock R, et al.: Interferon-alpha produces sustained cytogenic responses in chronic myelogenous leukemia. Ann Intern Med 114:532, 1991. *Long-term follow-up of interferon-induced cytogenetic responses.*
The Italian Cooperative Study Group on Chronic Myeloid Leukemia: Interferon α-2a compared with conventional chemotherapy for the treatment of chronic myeloid leukemia. N Engl J Med 330:820, 1994. *A comparative study demonstrating an unusual advantage for interferon over conventional therapy.*
Wagner JE, Zahurak M, Piantadosi S, et al.: Bone marrow transplantation of chronic myelogenous leukemia in chronic phase: evaluation of risks and benefits. J Clin Oncol 10:779, 1992. *A thoughtful discussion of transplantation in CML.*

HAIRY CELL LEUKEMIA

CLINICAL FEATURES. Hairy cell leukemia (HCL) is uncommon (1 to 2% of all leukemias). The median age at diagnosis is 50 years, with a 4:1 male preponderance. Patients have symptoms of fatigue due to anemia, fever, weight loss, and/or abdominal discomfort produced by splenomegaly. Sometimes the disease is diagnosed when patients have infection secondary to granulocytopenia or monocytopenia. The only consistent physical findings are slight to marked splenomegaly (75 to 80% of cases) caused by massive infiltration by hairy cells and slight to moderate hepatomegaly (33% of cases). Clinical lymphadenopathy is very uncommon, although retroperitoneal lymphadenopathy is noted on computed tomography (CT) in 20 to 25% of cases. More than two thirds of patients have anemia (< 10 grams per deciliter), neutropenia (< 1500 per microliter), thrombocytopenia (< 100,000 per microliter), and monocytopenia (< 100 per microliter). The WBC count is usually lower than 4000 per microliter at diagnosis, but marked thrombocytopenia is rare. The cytopenias are due to a combination of bone marrow production failure caused by leukemic infiltration and of hypersplenism. Marrow failure may be due in part to inhibitory factors (e.g., tumor necrosis factor) produced by the leukemic infiltrate, since the pancytopenia is often much more marked than would be anticipated from the degree of leukemic infiltration. During the course of the illness, patients often experience repeated infections

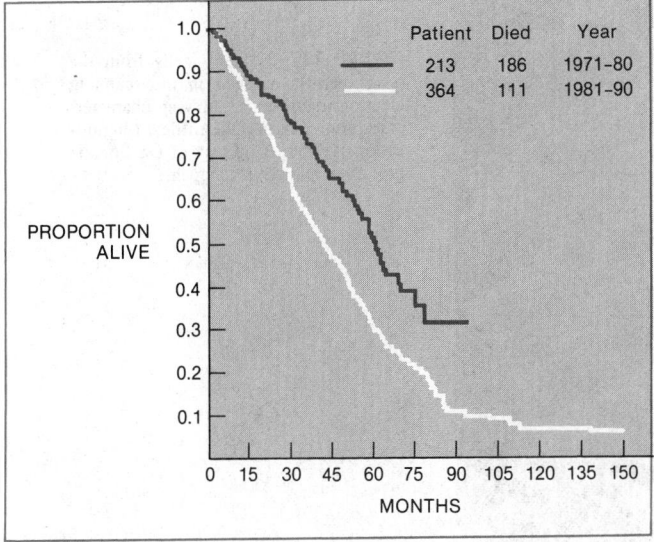

FIGURE 142–2. Survival of M. D. Anderson Cancer Center patients with benign-phase chronic myelogenous leukemia by year of diagnosis.

and more rarely a systemic vasculitis resembling polyarteritis nodosa or osteolytic bone lesions, usually affecting the upper femora. Although gram-positive or gram-negative infections occur as expected with neutropenia, patients with HCL have a predilection to develop tuberculosis, atypical mycobacterial infections, or fungal infections, perhaps related to the severe monocytopenia that is characteristic of this disorder. Pneumonia and septicemia are common causes of death in HCL.

DIAGNOSIS. In conjunction with the described clinical features, examination of the blood often suggests the diagnosis of HCL. In addition to the cytopenias described above, the peripheral blood film usually demonstrates relative or absolute lymphocytosis, composed of cells with cytoplasmic projections, giving rise to the name *hairy cell* leukemia (Fig. 142–3) (see Color Plate 7*J*, left). The cytoplasmic projections are best seen using phase contrast or electron microscopy. The hairy cells are 10 to 15 μm in diameter with pale blue cytoplasm and a nucleus with a loose chromatin structure and one or two indistinct nucleoli. Bone marrow aspiration is usually inadequate owing to increased reticulin, collagen, and fibrin deposition, and a bone marrow biopsy is necessary. The biopsy demonstrates increased cellularity with a diffuse or occasionally patchy infiltrate with hairy cells. The infiltrate is loose and spongy, with pale-staining cytoplasm surrounding bland, monotonous round or ovoid nuclei.

Hairy cells exhibit a strong acid phosphatase (isoenzyme 5) cytochemical reaction in 95% of cases, a reaction that is resistant to the inhibitory effect of tartaric acid (TRAP). Other lymphoproliferative diseases are rarely TRAP positive. Electron microscopy exquisitely demonstrates the microvillar projections. Often, ribosomal-lamellar complexes can be identified; these are characteristic, but not diagnostic, of HCL. The peroxidase stain is negative, and lysozyme activity is absent in hairy cells, differentiating the cells from monocytes.

The cell of origin of HCL is the B lymphocyte, as documented by the demonstration of heavy- and light-chain immunoglobulin gene rearrangements. Hairy cells express CD19 and CD20, FMC7, and CD22, but not CD21 or CD5. Cell-surface immunoglobulins can be immunoglobulin G (IgG) or immunoglobulin A (IgA), which are rare in chronic lymphocytic leukemia (CLL). The cells demonstrate a kappa or lambda light-chain phenotype excess. The cells are CD25 (TAC or low-affinity interleukin-2 [IL-2] receptor) positive and anti-HC2 positive, and they are positive for an early plasma cell antigen PCA-l, but not a late plasma cell antigen PCl. These findings suggest that hairy cells are late B lymphocytes or early plasma cells. High levels of soluble IL-2 receptors (>5 times normal) are present in the sera of almost all patients with HCL, with extremely high levels being noted in many cases. Some cases of HCL have a 14q+ cytogenetic abnormality with a breakpoint at 14q32 (the locus of the Ig heavy-chain gene). Hairy cells have a low proliferative index, with fewer than 1% being in the S phase of the cell cycle. Immune dysfunction is wide-ranging in HCL. Monocytopenia is universal, B and T lymphocytes are decreased in number; the CD4/CD8 ratio is often inverted; and skin test reactivity to recall antigens is impaired, as is antibody-dependent cellular cytotoxicity. Humoral immunity is relatively preserved with normal immunoglobulin levels. Markedly impaired ability of patients with HCL to produce alpha-interferon has been reported.

DIFFERENTIAL DIAGNOSIS. The differential diagnosis is most difficult between HCL and patients with lymphoma or chronic lymphocytic leukemia who have predominant splenomegaly and minimal lymphadenopathy. Some patients with a myelodysplastic or myeloproliferative syndrome have marked splenomegaly and pancytopenia with only a few atypical cells. Patients with other diseases, such as systemic lupus erythematosus and other autoimmune diseases, infiltrative splenomegaly, or tuberculosis, may have splenomegaly and cytopenia, but these diagnoses can usually be made by history, physical examination, and appropriate blood and bone marrow tests. Splenomegaly, cytopenia, and inaspirable marrow in a male should create a very high index of suspicion for HCL.

Other pathologic conditions to be differentiated from HCL requiring special tests are HCL variant, splenic lymphoma with villous

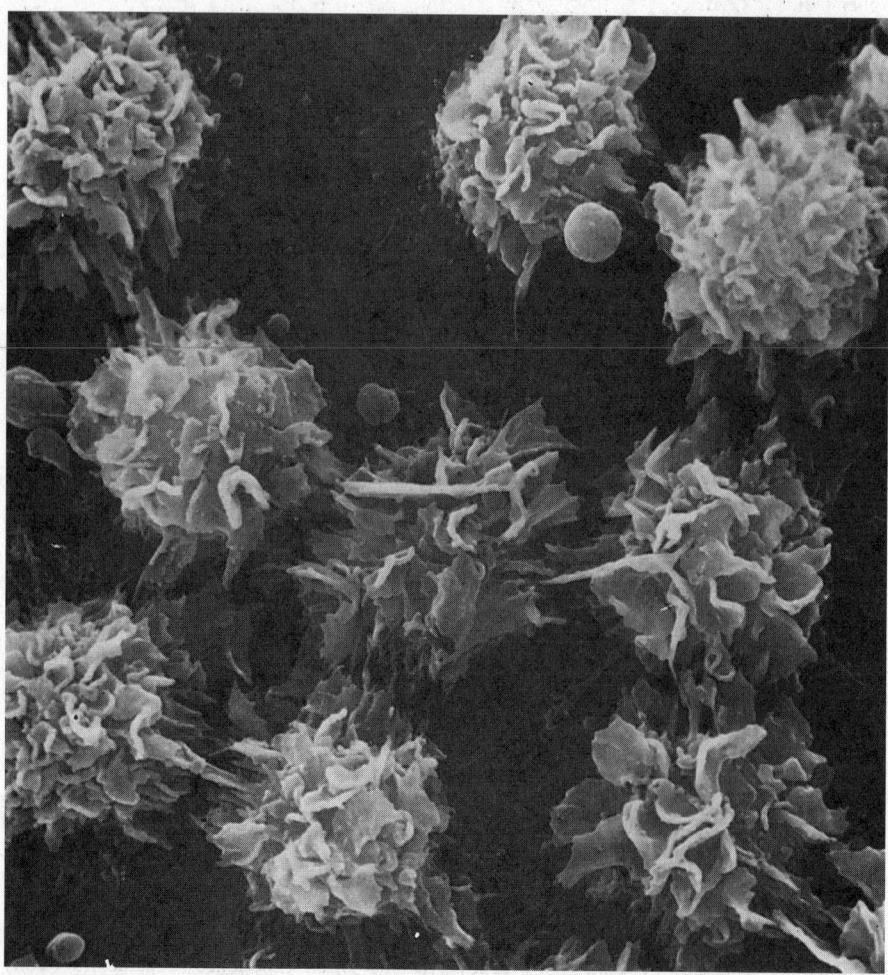

FIGURE 142–3. Hairy cells from the bone marrow as seen in the scanning electron microscope, showing characteristic prominent surface ruffles. Magnification ×8750. (Courtesy of Dr. Etienne deHarven and Nina Lampen.)

lymphocytes, B cell and T cell prolymphocytic leukemia, and CLL with splenomegaly and no lymphadenopathy. Splenectomy and lymph node biopsy are sometimes necessary to establish the diagnosis in difficult cases. Cases of HCL variant manifest with higher WBC counts are TRAP negative, have prominent nucleoli, and are only occasionally positive for antibodies against CD25. HCL variant responds poorly to interferon or deoxycoformycin, which are very effective agents in the management of typical HCL.

PROGNOSIS AND TREATMENT. A small proportion ($<5\%$) of patients with HCL do not require therapy. These patients have mild cytopenias, are not transfusion dependent, have no history of infections, and have a low level of marrow infiltration by hairy cells.

Splenectomy. Because splenomegaly can itself cause pancytopenia, splenectomy was used in the past as the first treatment of most patients with HCL when complications such as splenic infarction or abdominal discomfort occurred, when infections became frequent, or when anemia, neutropenia, or thrombocytopenia worsened. Splenectomy was temporarily effective in improving blood counts in two thirds of patients, with improvement usually noted within 1 to 4 weeks. Splenectomy was usually ineffective if the spleen was not palpable. Removal of the spleen does not decrease the infiltration of hairy cells in the marrow or reduce the incidence of infections. Usually within 2 years, pancytopenia recurs owing to progressive marrow infiltration. The median survival of most patients in whom splenectomy alone was utilized was 4 to 5 years. Splenectomy is now recommended mainly for patients with splenic infarcts or massive splenomegaly.

Interferon. Chemotherapy for HCL with alkylating agents, corticosteroids, androgens, and anthracyclines is not effective and, when used in the past, was associated not infrequently with prolonged myelosuppression and severe infections. Low-dose chlorambucil was better tolerated but seldom resulted in significant clinical improvement. The use of human leukocyte interferon (HuIFn), however, has revolutionized the present approach to therapy. The use of HuIFn or r-IFnα rapidly improves (1 to 3 months) granulocyte, platelet, and hemoglobin levels; reduces spleen size; and consistently decreases marrow infiltration. Peripheral blood counts return to normal in 80% of cases, and these patients achieve complete remission (no hairy cells in the marrow) or partial remission ($>50\%$ reduction in marrow HCL infiltration). The most commonly used dosage of IFn is 3×10^6 units given subcutaneously three times a week, although daily schedules for 6 months reduce the marrow HCL infiltration more effectively. Higher doses (3 to 5 $\times$ 10^6 units daily) increase the complete remission rate from 5 to 10% to 25%, with partial remission rate of 55 to 65% and a total failure rate of less than 5%. Most patients achieve partial remission by 6 months and complete remission by 12 to 18 months. Response to therapy is most satisfactory in patients who are less anemic and monocytopenic and who have lower marrow cellularity. Lack of response or loss of an initial response may result from the development of neutralizing antibodies to r-IFnα, especially if the antibody titer is high. When treatment is discontinued, most cases relapse within 1 to 2 years, but most will again respond to treatment. Relapse occurs more quickly in patients who achieve only partial remission than in those who respond completely. Treatment is usually reintroduced when patients become granulocytopenic. The presence of active, severe infection is not a contraindication to treatment with interferon. Indeed, the response to therapy provides patients with the best chance to recover from the infection.

Investigational Agents. Pentostatin (2-deoxycoformycin), an adenosine deaminase inhibitor, has marked activity in HCL. At the low dosages used to treat HCL (4 mg per square meter every 2 weeks), pentostatin produces complete remissions in 50 to 60% of patients and partial remissions in 40%. Higher dosages of pentostatin are associated with a high rate of infections, usually with opportunistic infections, since the agent is very immunosuppressive, decreasing both T cell number and function. The response rate of the higher dose regimen is 80 to 90%, with more than 60% of patients achieving a complete response. The response to treatment is more rapid than for interferon, occurring within 2 to 4 months following the initiation of therapy. Pentostatin is active in patients previously treated with interferon. Responses appear to be more durable than those seen in interferon-treated patients. Toxicity includes nausea and vomiting, infection, renal and hepatic dysfunction, conjunctivitis, and photosensitivity.

2-Chlorodeoxyadenosine (2-CDA), an adenosine analogue, has been reported to produce complete remissions in more than 90% of HCL patients with a single course of 0.1 mg per kilogram per day for 7 days by continuous intravenous infusion. Since the remissions appear to be very durable, 2-CDA promises to be the most effective agent developed to treat HCL. The drug is very well tolerated, with a low infection rate. *Granulocyte colony–stimulating factor (G-CSF)* has been reported to correct the granulocytopenia in HCL.

PROGNOSIS. The median survival of patients with HCL prior to interferon was 2 to 3 years. A return to normal leukocyte counts in HCL diminishes the risk of infection and is certain to improve the survival of patients with HCL. More than 90% of patients treated with interferon, 2-CDA, or pentostatin are projected to be alive at 5 years.

Bouroncle BA: Thirty-five years in the progress of hairy cell leukemia. Leuk Lymph 14(sl):1, 1994.
Quesada J: Hairy cell leukemia. *In* Freireich EJ, Kantarjian HM (eds.): Therapy of Hematopoietic Neoplasia. New York, Marcel Dekker, 1991, p 221. *A balanced analysis of the biology, clinical features, treatment, and prognosis of HCL.*
Robbins BA, Ellison DJ, Spinosa JC, et al.: Diagnostic application of two-color flow cytometry in 161 cases of hairy cell leukemia. Blood 82:1277, 1993.
Saven A, Piro LD: Treatment of hairy cell leukemia. Blood 79:1111, 1992.
Van Norman AS, Nagorney DM, Martin JK, et al.: Splenectomy for hairy cell leukemia. A clinical review of 63 patients. Cancer 57:644, 1986. *Describes features associated with response to splenectomy in HCL.*

CHRONIC LYMPHOCYTIC LEUKEMIA

Chronic lymphocytic leukemia (CLL) is a neoplasm characterized by accumulation of monoclonal lymphocytes, usually of B cell immunophenotype ($>95\%$ of cases), more rarely of T cell immunophenotype (see Color Plate 7I). The cells accumulate in the bone marrow, lymph nodes, liver, spleen, and occasionally other organs. CLL is the most common leukemia (one third of all cases) in the Western world and is twice as common as CML. The disease occurs rarely in those below the age of 30; most patients with CLL are over 60 years of age. Chronic lymphocytic leukemia increases in incidence exponentially with age; by age 80 the incidence rate is 20 cases per 100,000 persons per year. The male-female ratio is approximately 2:1. Asian countries such as Japan and China have an incidence of CLL only 10% of that in the United States and other Western countries. Intermediate incidence rates exist for persons of Hispanic origin.

ETIOLOGY. The cause of CLL is unknown. Ionizing radiation and viruses have not been associated with CLL. Familial clustering in CLL is more common than in other leukemias; first-degree relatives of patients have a twofold to fourfold higher risk than does the general population. Farmers have a higher incidence of CLL than do those in other occupations, raising the question of the possible etiologic role of herbicidal or pesticidal chemicals. No specific leukemogenic role of chemicals, including benzene, has been established for CLL.

PATHOGENESIS. Leukemia cells in CLL are usually remarkably homogeneous. The cells express low-intensity monoclonal surface immunoglobulin (SmIg, usually immunoglobulin M [IgM] $\pm$ immunoglobulin D [IgD]) of a single kappa or lambda light-chain phenotype. A number of patients with CLL have SmIg molecules that cross-react with IgM rheumatoid factor paraprotein. CLL cells are early B cells and have lost terminal deoxynucleotidyl transferase activity. The CLL cells express the pan B antigens CD19, CD20, and CD24 in almost all cases and CD21 (which includes the receptor for the Epstein-Barr virus and the C3D component of complement) and CD23 in more than 75% of cases. In fewer than 20% of cases is the C3B complement component receptor expressed. The vast majority of cells exhibit Ia antigen, have receptors for the Fc fragment of IgG, and spontaneously form rosettes with mouse erythrocytes. In 95% of cases, the CLL cells coexpress pan B cell antigens and CD5 (Leu 1, T1, and T101), a pan T cell antigen. Other T cell antigens and common acute lymphocytic leukemia antigen (CALLA) (CD10) are absent. CD25 (TAC, IL-2 receptor) antigen is positive in more than 20% of cells in 20% of cases.

Monoclonality of the B cells is demonstrated by marked preponderance of kappa or lambda light chains, by evidence of immunoglobulin gene rearrangement, by the presence of monoclonal serum Ig peaks in some cases, and by glucose-6-phosphate dehydrogenase isoenzyme studies.

CLL is an accumulative rather than a proliferative disease, since the CLL cells have a low proliferative index. Patients with higher WBC counts and more advanced stages have higher proliferative indices and shorter survivals. Most of the CLL cells in the blood and bone marrow are in the G_0 phase of the cell cycle, with only a small proportion of larger cells in the marrow and lymph nodes being in the other phases. The CLL cells have a longer lifespan in the blood than do normal B cells and have impaired egress from the blood. The CLL B cells have impaired responses to B cell mitogens and to B cell growth factors. The cells appear to be blocked in differentiation, with a high content of cytoplasmic IgM but a low surface IgM. Although most of the cells do not secrete immunoglobulins, in about 5% of cases a paraprotein of the same type as that on the surface of the CLL cells is present in the plasma or urine. The stimulatory effect of the CLL cells is low or absent in allogeneic or autologous mixed lymphocyte cultures. The CLL cells can be stimulated to differentiate into cells resembling hairy cells or plasma cells under the influence of phorbol esters, B cell mitogens, or growth factors.

T cell function is invariably abnormal in CLL. T cells are increased in number in the blood, bone marrow, and lymph nodes of patients with CLL, but they are polyclonal, and T cell receptor gene rearrangement is rare. The CD4/CD8 (T-helper/T-suppressor) ratio is often close to unity or is inverted owing to a relatively greater increase in the CD8-positive cells. The T cells have a blunted response to T cell mitogens in unseparated blood and decreased delayed hypersensitivity reactions to recall antigens. The T cell defects worsen as the disease progresses to a more advanced stage. Purified T cells have a normal response to T cell mitogens.

CLINICAL FEATURES. Most patients with CLL are asymptomatic, and the disease is diagnosed when absolute lymphocytosis is noted in the peripheral blood during evaluation for other illnesses or when the patient undergoes a routine physical examination. Symptoms such as fatigue, lethargy, loss of appetite, weight loss, or reduced exercise tolerance are nonspecific. These features are occasionally greater than can be explained by the degree of anemia or extent of tumor burden. Many patients have enlarged lymph nodes, usually cervical, noted by themselves or others. Fever and night sweats, or documented infections, are uncommon initial symptoms (<5%) but become more prominent as the disease progresses. Sinopulmonary infections are most common during the early phase of the disease, but as the disease progresses, the frequency of neutropenia, T cell deficiency, and hypogammaglobulinemia increases, resulting in gram-negative bacterial, fungal, and viral infections. Herpes zoster, herpes simplex, and cytomegalovirus infections usually occur later in the disease. An intriguing but unexplained common feature of CLL is an exuberant reaction to insect bites.

The major physical findings relate to infiltration of the reticuloendothelial system. Lymphadenopathy with discrete, rubbery, mobile lymph nodes is present in two thirds of patients at diagnosis. Later, as the lymph nodes enlarge, they become matted. Enlargement of the liver or spleen is less common at diagnosis (approximately 10% and 40% of cases, respectively). Less commonly, and usually late in the disease, clinically significant infiltration of skin, eyelids, heart, lungs, pleura, or gastrointestinal tract may occur. Organ failure due to infiltration with CLL is uncommon, with pulmonary symptoms being most likely to cause clinical problems. Infiltration of the central nervous system in CLL is rare, and central nervous system symptoms are more likely to be due to opportunistic infections, such as cryptococcosis or listeriosis. The extent of involvement varies from only a single node or node group to enlargement of virtually all nodes. Later in the disease, massive adenopathy may develop and cause luminal obstruction, such as obstructive jaundice, obstructive uropathy, dysphagia, or partial bowel obstruction. Unilateral or bilateral leg edema can occur owing to obstruction of the lymphatic and/or venous systems. Pleural effusions and ascites can also develop and are associated with a poor prognosis.

DIAGNOSTIC FEATURES. CLL is characterized by absolute lymphocytosis in the peripheral blood, a minimal level of more than 5000 per microliter, but more usually in the range of 40,000 to 150,000 per microliter. Extreme leukocytosis approaching 1×10^6 per microliter occurs only late in the disease, and hyperviscosity symptoms can occur if the WBC count is higher than 500,000/μl per microliter. If the lymphocyte count is 5000 to 15,000 per microliter, supportive evidence for clonality (kappa or lambda light-chain excess or immunoglobulin gene rearrangement) should be present before the diagnosis is made. Most physicians also document lymphocytosis in the bone marrow (>30% lymphocytes) and perform a bone marrow biopsy. Anemia (<11 grams per deciliter) is present in 15 to 20% of patients at diagnosis and thrombocytopenia (<100,000 per microliter) in 10%. Bone marrow replacement and hypersplenism contribute to the anemia and thrombocytopenia in most cases. The anemia is usually normochromic and normocytic, and the reticulocyte count is normal unless the patient has autoimmune hemolytic anemia, which usually results from the development of a warm-reacting IgG antibody. The diagnosis of autoimmune hemolytic anemia, which occurs in the course of 8 to 10% of cases, is confirmed by a positive direct Coombs test, reticulocytosis, a low serum haptoglobulin value, and an elevated unconjugated serum bilirubin level. In such patients, reactive erythroid hyperplasia as a response to the hemolysis may be masked in the bone marrow by the marked lymphocytic infiltration. Autoimmune thrombocytopenia can be diagnosed in some cases with a positive test for platelet antibodies. Cold agglutinin hemolysis occurs rarely in CLL. The antibodies causing the red cell and platelet destruction are not produced by the CLL cells, and the mechanism for the autoimmune diseases is not known. Pure red cell aplasia associated with T-suppressor cell activity is an additional reported cause of anemia in CLL.

The lymphocytes in CLL are indistinguishable on light or electron microscopy from normal small B lymphocytes. On bone marrow aspiration, the proportion of lymphocytes is greater than 30% and may extend up to 100% in patients with newly diagnosed CLL. The rest of the cells are normal myeloid and erythroid cells. Four patterns of lymphocyte infiltration on bone marrow biopsy occur and have prognostic value in CLL: (1) nodular (15%), (2) infiltrative (30%), (3) mixed nodular and infiltrative (30%), and (4) diffuse (35%). Most early-stage cases have patterns 1, 2, or 3; diffuse histology is most common in advanced-stage disease and becomes more prominent as the disease evolves. A diffuse histologic pattern confers a poor prognosis regardless of the stage of disease. Hypogammaglobulinemia is common in CLL and predisposes to infec-

TABLE 142–3. RAI AND BINET STAGING SYSTEMS IN CHRONIC LYMPHOCYTIC LEUKEMIA (CLL)

	Lymphocytosis	Lymphadenopathy	Hepatomegaly or Splenomegaly	Hemoglobin (grams/dl)	Platelets $\times 10^3/\mu l$
Rai stage					
0	+	−	−	≥ 11	≥ 100
I	+	+	−	≥ 11	≥ 100
II	+	±	+	≥ 11	≥ 100
III	+	±	±	< 11	≥ 100
IV	+	±	±	Any	< 100
Binet stage					
A	+	±	± (< 3 Lymphatic groups* positive)	≥ 10	≥ 100
B	+	±	± (≥ 3 Lymphatic groups* positive)	≥ 10	≥ 100
C	+	±	±	< 10 or	< 100

* (1) Cervical, axillary, and inguinal nodes; (2) liver; and (3) spleen; each group is considered one group whether unilateral or bilateral.

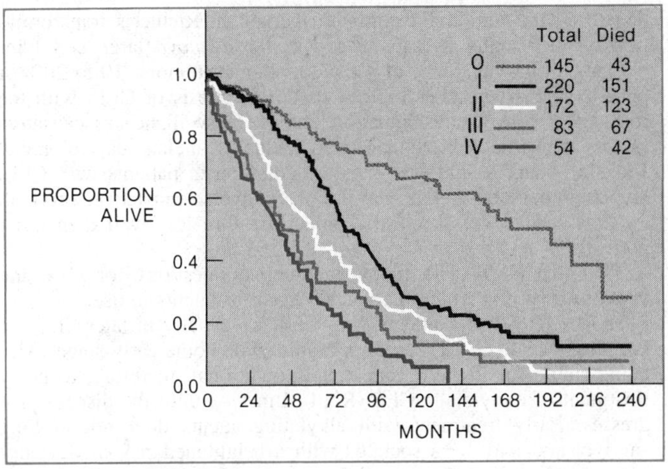

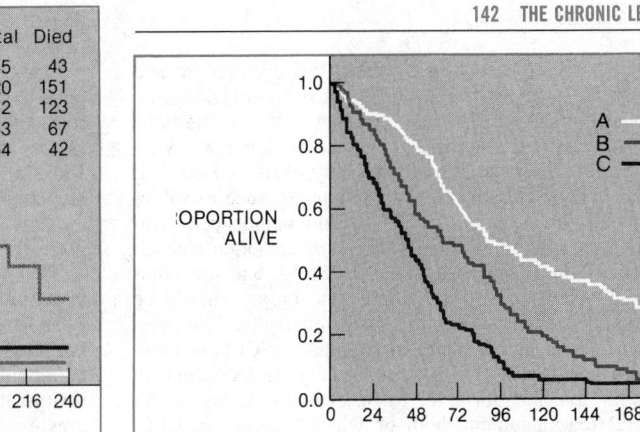

FIGURE 142–4. Survival of untreated patients with chronic lymphocytic leukemia by Rai stage.

FIGURE 142–5. Survival of untreated patients with chronic lymphocytic leukemia by Binet stage.

tions, especially with encapsulated microorganisms. Low levels of IgG, IgA, or IgM occur in 25% of newly diagnosed patients, are more common in advanced stages, and increase in frequency to 50 to 70% as the disease progresses.

Nonrandom cytogenetic abnormalities in CLL include trisomy 12 (40%), 14q+ abnormalities (25%), and abnormalities in the long arm of chromosomes 6 and 11. Single abnormalities are more common in early and recently diagnosed diseases, and additional changes develop with time (clonal evolution). The site of the breakpoint on chromosome 14 (q32) is close to the site of the Ig heavy-chain gene.

STAGING SYSTEMS. Two major staging systems are used. The Rai staging system (1975) defines five stages and is most frequently used in the United States, whereas the Binet system (1981) defines three stages and is most frequently used in Europe (Table 142–3). Both systems have the advantage of simplicity, low cost, and reproducibility and have been prospectively validated (Figs. 142–4 and 142–5). Within the stages, outcome is variable and other prognostic factors, such as the bone marrow histologic pattern, provide additional prognostic information. Patients with anemia and thrombocytopenia (Rai stages III and IV, Binet C) have, on the average, a poor prognosis; patients with lymphocytosis alone (Rai 0, some Binet A patients) have an excellent prognosis. The prognosis of the other patients is heterogeneous and, as might be expected, is worse in patients with a greater tumor burden. Rai stage II patients who have splenomegaly without lymphadenopathy (pure splenic form) have a better prognosis than do other stage II patients. While useful in the design and analysis of clinical trials, the staging systems are not particularly useful for individual patients because of the heterogeneity of outcome. A group of patients with a lymphocyte count of less than 30,000 per microliter, hemoglobin higher than 11 grams per deciliter, platelet count lower than 100,000 per

microliter, with fewer than three involved node areas, and lymphocyte doubling time of greater than 12 months has been described as having "smoldering" CLL, with a survival equal to that of an age- and sex-matched population.

Patients tend to progress through stages, with many patients developing more sites of involvement with time and eventually experiencing marrow failure, but anemia and thrombocytopenia can develop abruptly even without antibody-mediated destruction or increasing tumor burden.

DIFFERENTIAL DIAGNOSIS. Many diseases can cause lymphocytosis: pertussis, infectious lymphocytosis, cytomegalovirus and Epstein-Barr virus mononucleosis, tuberculosis, toxoplasmosis, chronic inflammatory disorders, and autoimmune syndromes. Although they may superficially resemble CLL, their clinical pictures seldom are confused with that of B cell CLL. Many of these patients are younger and have fever or other acute symptoms, or exhibit other clinical features, such as rash and joint symptoms, that are uncommon in CLL. The lymphocytosis (usually < 15,000 per microliter) is not sustained. If doubt persists, monoclonal antibodies will distinguish the monoclonal lymphocytosis in CLL from the polyclonal B cell proliferation in the other disorders. The more difficult differential diagnosis is from other lymphoproliferative disorders, such as prolymphocytic leukemia, HCL, the leukemic phase of mantle cell lymphoma, Waldenström's macroglobulinemia, and T cell CLL. While certain clinical features are more common in some of these disorders—for example, marked splenomegaly with minimal or no lymphadenopathy in prolymphocytic leukemia and HCL versus extensive lymphadenopathy with or without splenomegaly in CLL—none of these differential features is specific. The differential diagnosis therefore depends largely on histopathologic and more specifically immunophenotypic features (Table 142–4).

TABLE 142–4. DIFFERENTIAL DIAGNOSIS OF INDOLENT LYMPHOPROLIFERATIVE DISORDERS

Disease	Lymphadenopathy (%)	Splenomegaly (%)	Cell of Origin (B/T)	Positive Markers*			
				Smlg	*CD5*	*CD19, 20* (%)	*Other Positives*
CLL	75	50	B (20:1)	Weak	>90%	≥90	Mouse red blood cell (RBC) receptors
Prolymphocytic leukemia	33	95	B (4:1)	Bright	T cell PLL	75	FMC-7
Hairy cell leukemia	< 10	80	B(T rare)	Bright	—	>90	CD25, CD11C
Lymphoma (leukemic phase)	90	80	B(T rare)	Bright	Some	>90	CD10
Waldenström's macroglobulinemia	33	33	All B	Weak	Some	Many	CD38, PCA-1
Large granular lymphocytosis	10	10	All T	Absent	—	—	CD2, CD3, CD8

* CD5 —pan T cell, B CLL
CD19 —early pan B cell
CD20 —pan B cell
FMC-7—PLL and hairy cell
CD2 —pan T cell
CD3 —pan mature T cell

CD8 —T cell (suppressor-cytotoxic)
CD10 —early B cell
CD11C—hairy cells, activated T cell, NK cell
CD38 —activated B cell, thymocytes, plasma cells
PCA-1 —plasma cell
CD25 —low-affinity interleukin 2 (IL-2) receptor

Small lymphocytic lymphoma (SLL) shares histopathologic and immunophenotypic features with CLL, differing only in lacking absolute monoclonal lymphocytosis in the peripheral blood. The bone marrow in SLL may or may not have more than 30% lymphocytes. LFA-1 adhesion protein is much more commonly expressed on SLL cells than CLL cells. Occasionally, other lymphomas, such as follicular small cleaved cell lymphoma (FSCCL) and mantle cell lymphoma, manifest in a leukemic phase. These cells are often cleaved on light microscopy, have bright staining for SmIg, and are commonly FMC-7 and CD10 positive. Lymph node biopsy should be performed to identify these cases with greater precision. The presence of lymphoma cells in the blood in SLL and FSCCL is more common later in the disease. FSCLL can usually be identified by the presence of the translocation t(14;18) on cytogenic analysis and consequent BCL2 rearrangement, both of which are rare in CLL. The WBC count in Waldenström's macroglobulinemia at diagnosis is usually much lower than in CLL ($< 10,000$ per microliter), and many patients are leukopenic. The cells have a plasmacytoid appearance, CD38 and PCA-1 positivity, and more SmIg and cytoplasmic Ig. A monoclonal IgM plasma peak is present in almost all cases of Waldenström's macroglobulinemia but is rare in CLL. Prolymphocytic leukemia (PLL) is an uncommon disease (10% of the incidence of CLL), and its characteristics of massive splenomegaly, minimal lymphadenopathy, WBC count commonly $> 100,000$ per microliter, with 10 to 90% of the cells being prolymphocytes, distinguish this disease from typical B cell CLL. Prolymphocytes are larger cells than typical CLL lymphocytes; they have a distinct nucleolus and are often FMC-7 positive. The male-female ratio is 4:1, and the median age at diagnosis is 70 years. Survival is shorter than in CLL (median, 3 years), and response is poor to therapies usually applied in CLL. A monoclonal spike, usually IgG or IgA, is present in one third of cases. The immunoglobulin on the surface of the cells is usually IgG or IgA, not IgM ± IgD, as in CLL. A specific karyotypic abnormality, t(6;12) (q15;q13), has been reported in PLL. One fifth of the cases are of T cell phenotype. The predominant clinical manifestation in Sézary's syndrome (a CD4+ T cell malignant disorder related to mycosis fungoides) is chronic exfoliative erythroderma with a low number of circulating monoclonal T cells. The clinical and laboratory differential diagnosis from CLL is not difficult. Other T cell malignant disorders with peripheral blood involvement are adult T cell leukemia-lymphoma and large granular lymphocytosis (LGL). Adult T cell leukemia-lymphoma is associated with a retrovirus (human T cell leukemia-lymphoma virus [HTLV-1]) and is common in Japan and the Caribbean. It is frequently manifested by lytic bone lesions and hypercalcemia. In LGL the absolute lymphocyte count is usually low (< 5000 per microliter), with a CD2+, CD3+, and CD8+ (T-suppressor) phenotype (T-gamma cells). These patients often have splenomegaly, neutropenia, and rheumatoid arthritis–like symptomatology and serology. The lymphocytes have abundant cytoplasm with azurophilic granules. In most patients a benign course is noted, although repeated infections can occur.

PROGNOSTIC FACTORS. In addition to the impact of tumor burden and marrow function on prognosis, as reflected in the Rai and Binet staging systems, other adverse factors are as follows: (a) a diffuse pattern of lymphocytic infiltration observed on bone marrow biopsy; (b) an abnormal karyotype (e.g., trisomy 12 or multiple chromosomal abnormalities); (c) advanced age; (d) male sex; (e) elevated serum levels of thymidine kinase, β_2 microglobulin, uric acid, alkaline phosphatase, or lactate dehydrogenase; (f) rapid lymphocyte doubling time; and (g) an increased proportion of large or atypical lymphocytes in the peripheral blood. A poor response to therapy is an adverse factor in all phases of the disease. As the disease progresses, a worsening of stage and the development of prolymphocytic leukemia (10% of cases), large cell lymphoma, or myelomatous or acute lymphocytic leukemia (rare) are grave prognostic features. Multiple chromosomal abnormalities identify patients at risk of developing a large cell lymphomatous transformation (Richter's syndrome), which occurs in 5 to 10% of CLL patients as a terminal event. Richter's syndrome should be suspected whenever a single lymph node area or the spleen begins to enlarge in CLL or when unexplained clinical deterioration occurs. The transformation does not always share immunophenotypic or cytogenetic features with the original CLL clone and may be a coinci-

dental second tumor. Response to therapy in Richter's transformation is not usually as satisfactory as for *de novo* large cell lymphoma. A high incidence of second malignant tumors (10 to 20% of patients) either precedes or follows the diagnosis of CLL, with the roles of therapy versus impaired immune surveillance as causative factors being unclear. Skin cancer, including melanoma, colorectal and lung cancers, and sarcomas are common in patients with CLL. Hypogammaglobulinemia may have an adverse impact on survival. Patients who develop repeated infections fare less well than other patients.

TREATMENT. The major therapeutic questions for CLL are when to treat and which therapeutic agent or agents to use.

When to Treat. Patients with CLL are usually in later life, and the prognosis of the disease is variable (with some early-stage cases being stable for 5 to 20 years). It is traditional, therefore, to delay treatment of early-stage CLL (Rai 0, Binet A) until the disease progresses. Early treatment with alkylating agents does not prolong survival and may be associated with a heightened risk of developing second malignant tumors. Treatment of Rai stages III and IV (Binet stage C) patients is recommended at the time of diagnosis because of the poor survival of these patients (median, 2 years). Treatment of intermediate-stage disease (Rai stages I and II, Binet stage B) is recommended if symptomatic disease (fever, sweats, weight loss, severe fatigue), massive lymphadenopathy, or hepatosplenomegaly is present. Progressive organ and/or node enlargement and lymphocytosis ($> 100,000$ per microliter) are other common indications for treatment. Development of anemia, thrombocytopenia, or neutropenia associated with infections is usually an indication for systemic antileukemic therapy unless an autoimmune cause of the cytopenia (positive direct Coombs' test, antiplatelet or antineutrophil antibodies) is found. In the latter group of cases, the use of corticosteroids, such as prednisone, should be tried prior to the initiation of cytotoxic therapy. A doubling of blood lymphocytes in less than 12 months is an adverse prognostic factor and suggests that treatment is indicated.

Chemotherapy. Chlorambucil (less commonly, cyclophosphamide) is usually the first chemotherapeutic agent used. Corticosteroids are often used concurrently, but with no clearly demonstrated advantage in therapeutic response or survival. Chlorambucil regimens vary widely. In the chronic low-dosage daily regimen, 0.1 to 0.2 mg per kilogram per day of chlorambucil is continued for 3 to 6 weeks until the desired effect is obtained or until thrombocytopenia or neutropenia develops. The dosage is then adjusted for maintenance and is continued for 6 to 12 months. For intermittent high-dosage (pulse) schedules, chlorambucil (0.5 to 2 mg per kilogram) is given over 1 to 4 days every 4 weeks or given at half-dosage every 2 weeks. Neither dosage schedule for chlorambucil has been established as definitely superior. If prednisone is given concurrently with chlorambucil, the dosage is 60 to 100 mg per day in the pulse schedule. Continuous prednisone is not recommended in this elderly population, but can be given at a dosage of 40 to 60 mg per day for 4 weeks initially, tapering to 10 to 20 mg per day when combined with chlorambucil in the continuous-therapy schedule. Following therapy, the condition of many patients remains stable for months to years before disease progression indicates the need for further treatment. The endpoints for response to therapy have not been well defined, since treatment is usually strictly palliative. Most physicians try to achieve the disappearance of lymphadenopathy and splenomegaly and the return to a normal WBC count, but rarely normal bone marrow. Myelosuppression is the most common toxicity with chlorambucil, although occasionally rash, nausea, or pulmonary toxicity occurs.

The COP regimen (cyclophosphamide, 100 to 300 mg per square meter per day given orally on days 1 through 5; vincristine [Oncovin], 2 mg given intravenously on day 1; and prednisone, 100 mg administered orally on days 1 through 5) does not appear to have any advantage over chlorambucil. Indeed, vincristine has never been demonstrated to have activity in CLL. Sixty to 75% of patients obtain at least a partial clinical response with these alkylating agents, but a complete remission, including fewer than 30% lymphocytes in the bone marrow aspirate, is achieved in only 10 to 15% of the cases. Repeated rechallenge with the same drug combinations is usually associated with less satisfactory and shorter responses. Damage to DNA gives rise to concern regarding the role of alkylating agents as contributory factors to the high incidence of second malignant tumors in CLL. Two sets of recommen-

TABLE 142–5. DEFINITION OF REMISSION IN CLL: COMPARISON OF THE INTERNATIONAL WORKSHOP IN CLL (IWCLL) AND THE NATIONAL CANCER INSTITUTE WORKING GROUP (NCI-WG) CRITERIA

Criteria	Complete Remission (CR)		Partial Remission (PR)	
	IWCLL	*NCI-WG*	*IWCLL*	*NCI-WG*
Physical examination				
Nodes	None	None	Shift to a lower Binet stage, e.g., C → A or B, B → A	≥ 50% decrease
Liver/spleen	Not palpable	Not palpable		≥ 50% decrease
Symptoms	None	None		N/A
Peripheral blood				
Neutrophils	≥ 1500/μl	≥ 1500/μl		>1500/μl or ≥ 50% ↑ from baseline
Platelets	> 100,000/μl	> 100,000/μl		100,000/μl or > 50% ↑ from baseline
Hemoglobin	Not specified	> 11 grams/dl		> 11 grams/dl or > 50% ↑ from baseline
Lymphocytes	< 4000/μl	< 4000/μl		> 50% decrease
Bone marrow				
Lymphocytes	Normal aspirate and biopsy*	< 30%		N/A
		Normal*		N/A

* Nodules or focal aggregates of lymphocytes are comparable to CR.

dations address response and eligibility criteria in CLL studies (Table 142–5).

Regimens utilizing cyclophosphamide, doxorubicin (Adriamycin), and prednisone with vincristine (CHOP) or without vincristine (CAP) have produced response rates of 50 to 70% in previously untreated Binet stage C patients and are well tolerated in CLL despite the advanced age of most patients. The CAP regimen resulted in a complete remission rate of 45% in CLL, with a median survival of 7 years in the Binet C patients.

Corticosteroid Therapy. Corticosteroids, usually prednisone (60 to 100 mg per day), are indicated as treatment for Coombs-positive autoimmune hemolytic anemia and for some cases of immune-mediated thrombocytopenia in CLL. If there is no response in 3 to 4 weeks, the treatment has failed and the dose should then be tapered over 1 to 2 weeks. If a response is obtained, the dose is usually reduced by 25% each week over 4 weeks. Patients in whom corticosteroids fail often respond well to splenectomy and less well to intravenous high-dose immunoglobulin. Autoimmune hemolytic anemia and immune-mediated thrombocytopenia do not correlate closely with the activity of CLL.

Radiation Therapy. In CLL, radiation therapy is usually restricted to external irradiation of localized nodal masses or an enlarged spleen that has been refractory to chemotherapy. Repeated leukapheresis and extracorporeal irradiation of blood can decrease the tumor burden in CLL and occasionally increase hemoglobin and platelet levels but are not practical for long periods.

Experimental Therapies. Two adenosine analogues, fludarabine monophosphate and 2-CDA, and pentostatin (deoxycoformycin), an adenosine deaminase inhibitor, have exhibited therapeutic potential in CLL. Fludarabine monophosphate (25 to 30 mg per square meter per day for 5 days every 4 weeks) leads to complete remission in 70% of untreated patients and 35% of those previously treated with alkylating agents. The dose-limiting toxicity is myelosuppression. The course of therapy may be complicated by infections with organisms usually associated with immunodeficiency syndromes involving T lymphocytes (e.g., those caused by *Pneumocystis carinii*, herpesviruses). 2-CDA and deoxycoformycin have not been as widely studied in CLL.

Intravenous immunoglobulin (400 mg per kilogram every 3 to 4 weeks) significantly decreases the incidence of infections of minor to moderate severity in CLL patients with hypogammaglobulinemia, but the cost of this therapy is substantial. Although ineffective in patients with advanced-stage CLL, alpha-interferon may significantly decrease the lymphocyte count in 50 to 70% of early-stage cases as well as increase the absolute granulocyte count, improve the serum immunoglobulin level, and improve T-helper/T-suppressor ratios. Interleukin-2 has been administered sparingly to patients with refractory CLL, with no consistent improvement in disease pa-

rameters. Similarly, monoclonal antibodies directed against CLL cells have not as yet resulted in consistent benefit to patients.

PROGNOSIS IN CLL (Figs. 142–4 and 142–5). The median survival of patients with CLL is 4 to 5 years following initiation of treatment. As expected, patients with early-stage cases (Rai 0 to II) survive significantly longer, a median of 7 to 8 years. No current treatment strategy has demonstrated a survival advantage over conventional therapy with chlorambucil.

CLL tends to develop in elderly patients; death often occurs, therefore, from other intercurrent illnesses of this age group. Younger patients (< 60 years of age) almost all die as a result of CLL or one of its complications, especially infections. Gram-positive organisms usually cause nonfatal infections early in CLL, but most deaths due to infection are associated with gram-negative bacterial or fungal infections. Other opportunistic organisms such as *Mycobacterium tuberculosis*, herpesvirus, and *Pneumocystis carinii* may also contribute to death.

Bennett JM, Catovsky D, Daniel M-T, et al.: Proposals for the classification of chronic (mature) B and T lymphoid leukaemias. J Clin Pathol 42:567, 1989. *Classification of common and less common chronic leukemias using an integrated clinical, morphologic, and immunophenotypic approach.*

Cheson BD, Bennett JM, Rai KR, et al.: Guidelines for clinical protocols for chronic lymphocytic leukemia: Recommendations of the National Cancer Institute–Sponsored Working Group. Am J Hematol 29:152, 1988. *Standard guidelines for eligibility criteria, indications for treatment, and response criteria in B cell CLL.*

French Cooperative Group on Chronic Lymphocytic Leukemia: Effects of chlorambucil and therapeutic decision in initial forms of chronic lymphocytic leukemia (Stage A): Results of a randomized clinical trial on 612 patients. Blood 75:1414, 1990. *Randomized trial comparing outcome of early versus late treatment with chlorambucil in CLL. Disturbing data on second malignant tumors in early treatment group.*

Juliusson G, Oscier DG, Fitchett M, et al.: Prognostic subgroups in B-cell chronic lymphocytic leukemia defined by specific chromosomal abnormalities. N Engl J Med 323:720, 1990. *Major report on prognostic and biologic importance of cytogenetic abnormalities in CLL.*

Keating MJ, O'Brien S, Plunkett W, et al.: Fludarabine phosphate: A new active agent in hematologic malignancies. Semin Hematol 31:28, 1994. *A broad overview of the role of fludarabine in CLL and other diseases.*

Montserrat E, Rozman C: Chronic lymphocytic leukaemia: Prognosis and natural history. Bailliere's Clin Haematol 6:849, 1993. *A critical review of clinically relevant prognostic factors in CLL.*

Montserrat E, Vinolas N, Reverte JC, et al.: Natural history of chronic lymphocytic leukemia: On the progression and prognosis of early clinical stages. Nouv Rev Fr Hematol 30:359, 1988. *Illustrates features associated with risk of progression in early-stage CLL.*

O'Brien S, del Giglio A, Keating M: Advances in the biology and treatment of B-cell chronic lymphocytic leukemia. Blood 85:307, 1995. *A concise, advanced review.*

Rozman C, Montserrat E, Rodriguez-Fernandez JM, et al.: Bone marrow histologic pattern—The best single prognostic parameter in chronic lymphocytic leukemia: A multivariate analysis of 329 cases. Blood 64:642, 1984. *Bone marrow histologic pattern in CLL is shown to be a major prognostic factor for survival in all stages of disease.*

Saven A, Carrera CJ, Carson DA, et al.: 2-Chlorodeoxyadenosine treatment for refractory chronic lymphocytic leukemia. Leuk Lymph 5:133, 1991. *Large series of CLL patients treated with 2-CDA.*

143 THE ACUTE LEUKEMIAS
Frederick R. Appelbaum

DEFINITION

Normal hematopoiesis requires tightly regulated proliferation and differentiation of pluripotent hematopoietic stem cells to become mature peripheral blood cells. Acute leukemia is the result of a malignant event, or events, occurring in an early hematopoietic precursor. Instead of proliferating and differentiating normally, the affected cell gives rise to progeny that fail to differentiate and instead continue to proliferate in an uncontrolled fashion. As a result, immature myeloid cells (in acute myelogenous leukemia) or lymphoid cells (in acute lymphocytic leukemia), often called blasts, rapidly accumulate and progressively replace the bone marrow, leading to diminished production of normal red cells, white cells, and platelets. This loss of normal marrow function in turn gives rise to the common clinical complications of leukemia: anemia, infection, and bleeding. With time, the leukemic blasts pour out into the bloodstream and eventually occupy the lymph nodes, spleen, and other vital organs. If untreated, acute leukemia is rapidly fatal; most patients die within several months of diagnosis. With appropriate therapy, the natural history of acute leukemia can be markedly altered, and many patients can be cured.

ETIOLOGY

In most cases acute leukemia develops for no known reason, but sometimes a possible cause can be identified.

Radiation

Ionizing radiation is leukemogenic. Acute lymphocytic leukemia (ALL), acute myelogenous leukemia (AML), and chronic myelogenous leukemia (CML) are all increased in incidence in patients given radiation therapy for ankylosing spondylitis and in survivors of the atomic bomb blasts of Hiroshima and Nagasaki. The magnitude of the risk depends on the dose of radiation, its distribution in time, and the age of the individual. Greater risk results from higher dose radiation delivered over shorter periods to younger patients. In areas of high natural background radiation (often due to radon), chromosomal aberrations have been reported to be more frequent, but an increase in acute leukemia has not been consistently found. Recently concern has been raised about possible leukemogenic effects of extremely low frequency nonionizing electromagnetic fields emitted by electrical installations. If such an effect exists at all, the magnitude of the effect is small.

Oncogenic Viruses

The search for a viral cause of leukemia has been intensely pursued, but none has been found, except for two rare leukemias associated with retroviruses. Human T cell lymphotropic virus type I (HTLV-I), an enveloped, single-stranded RNA virus, is considered the causative agent of adult T cell leukemia (ATL). This distinct form of leukemia is found within geographic clusters in southwestern Japan, the Caribbean basin, and Africa. The virus can be spread vertically from mother to fetus or horizontally by sexual contact or through blood products. Although previously rare in the United States, HTLV-I seropositivity has been found with increasing frequency among patients undergoing frequent transfusions and among intravenous drug users. Screening of blood products for antibodies to HTLV-I is now a routine practice in blood banks in the United States. A second human retrovirus, genetically distinct from HTLV-I, termed HTLV-II, has been isolated from several patients with a syndrome resembling hairy cell leukemia. The etiologic link between HTLV-II and malignancy is uncertain.

Genetics and Congenital Factors

If leukemia develops before age 10 in a patient with an identical twin, the unaffected twin has a one in five chance of subsequently developing leukemia. In occasional families, multiple members have developed an identical form of leukemia. Several autosomal recessive disorders associated with chromosomal instability are prone to terminate in acute leukemia, including Bloom syndrome, Fanconi anemia, and ataxic telangiectasia. Other congenital disorders associated with an increased incidence of leukemia are Down syndrome and infantile X-linked agammaglobulinemia.

Chemicals

Heavy occupational exposure to benzene frequently results in marrow hypoplasia, which sometimes evolves into acute leukemia. Prior exposure to alkylating agents, such as chlorambucil, melphalan, and nitrogen mustard, is associated with an increased risk of AML. Increasing exposure to the agent and increased patient age accentuate the risk. Patients often have a myelodysplastic syndrome before developing secondary AML. Cytogenetic studies in these secondary leukemias frequently reveal abnormalities of chromosomes 5, 7, and 8. Prolonged exposure to epipodophyllotoxins (teniposide or etoposide) has been identified as a risk factor for the development of AML with monocytic morphology and abnormalities of the long arm of chromosome 11 (band q23).

INCIDENCE

The annual new case incidence of all leukemias is 8 to 10 per 100,000. This rate has remained static over the past three decades. The relative incidences for the four categories of leukemia are as follows: ALL, 11%; CLL, 29%; AML, 46%; and CML, 14%. The leukemias account for about 3% of all cancers in the United States. The impact of leukemia is heightened because of the young age of some patients. For example, ALL is the most common cancer and the second leading cause of death in children under 15 years of age. Acute lymphocytic leukemia has a maximal incidence between 2 and 10 years of age, with a second, more gradual rise in frequency in later life. The incidence of AML gradually increases with age, without an early peak. Approximately half of AML cases occur in patients under age 50.

PATHOPHYSIOLOGY

The precise molecular event or events that cause leukemic transformation are unknown; the end result, however, is relentless proliferation of immature hematopoietic cells that have lost their capacity to differentiate normally. The development of leukemia may be a multistep process, as demonstrated by the fact that in many cases acute leukemia develops in patients with a pre-existing myelodysplastic disorder. The disease is monoclonal, i.e., the final leukemic event occurs in a single cell. The level of differentiation at which malignancy becomes evident is variable. In some cases of AML, it appears that malignancy occurs in a very undifferentiated cell similar to the normal hematopoietic stem cell, in that red cell, platelet, and myeloid precursors are all products of the malignant clone. In other cases of AML, the malignant event may occur in a more differentiated cell, and only granulocyte and monocyte precursors develop from the malignant cell, while red cell and platelet precursors do not. In almost all cases of ALL, the myeloid lineage is not malignant, suggesting that in ALL, the malignant event occurs in a cell that is at least partially differentiated. Although the majority of leukemic cells are relatively undifferentiated, some mature circulating cells may be products of the malignant clone.

As the malignant clone expands, it does so at the expense of normal hematopoiesis. The mechanism of normal marrow suppression in leukemia is complex; in many patients with hypercellular marrows, pancytopenia is probably the result, at least in part, of physical replacement of normal marrow precursors by leukemic cells. Some patients with acute leukemia develop pancytopenia with a hypocellular marrow, however, suggesting that marrow failure is not simply due to physical replacement of the marrow space but also may be due to substances released by the malignant cells.

CLASSIFICATION

The acute leukemias can be classified in a variety of ways, including morphology, cytochemistry, cell-surface markers, cytoplasmic markers, cytogenetics, and oncogene expression. The most important distinction is between AML and ALL, since these two diseases differ considerably in their clinical behavior, prognosis, and response to therapy. Within the various subgroups of AML and ALL, there are also some important differences. A summary of the major subtypes of acute leukemia is provided in Table 143–1.

Morphology

Leukemic cells in AML typically are 12 to 20 μm in diameter, with discrete nuclear chromatin, multiple nucleoli, and cytoplasm that usually contains azurophilic granules. Auer rods, which are slender, fusiform cytoplasmic inclusions that stain red with Wright-Giemsa Stain, are virtually pathognomonic of AML. The French-American-British (FAB) collaborative group has subdivided AML into eight subtypes based on morphology and histochemistry (Table 143–1). M0, M1, M2, and M3 reflect increasing degrees of differentiation of myeloid leukemic cells. M4 and M5 leukemias have features of the monocytic lineage, M6 has features of the erythroid cell lineage, and M7 is acute megakaryocytic leukemia (see Color Plates 7K, 7L, and 8A).

The leukemic cells in ALL tend to be smaller than AML blasts and relatively devoid of granules. Acute lymphocytic leukemia can be divided, using FAB criteria, into L1, L2, and L3 subgroups. L1 blasts are uniform in size, with homogeneous nuclear chromatin, indistinct nucleoli, and scanty cytoplasm with few, if any, granules. L2 blasts are larger and more variable in size and may have nucleoli. L3 blasts are quite distinct, with prominent nucleoli and deeply basophilic cytoplasm with vacuoles (see Color Plates 8B and 8C).

Cell-Surface Markers

Monoclonal antibodies reactive with cell-surface antigens have been used to classify acute leukemias. Antibodies that react with antigens found on normal immature myeloid cells, including CD13, CD14, CD33, and CD34, also react with blast cells from most patients with AML. Exceptions are the M6 and M7 variants, which have antigens restricted to the red cell and platelet lineages, respectively. Myeloid leukemia blasts also express Ia antigens, but usually lack T cell, B cell, and other lymphoid antigens. In 10 to 20% of patients, however, AML blasts will express antigens usually restricted to B or T cell lineages. Expression of lymphoid antigens by AML cells does not change either the natural history or therapeutic response of these leukemias.

Acute lymphocytic leukemia can be divided into several forms based on cell-surface antigen expression. Approximately 60% of cases of ALL express the common ALL antigen, or CALLA, on the cell surface. CALLA (CD10) is a glycoprotein also found on occasional normal early lymphocytes and other nonhematopoietic tissues. Cases of CALLA-positive ALL are thought to represent a very early B cell differentiative state. About 20% of cases of CALLA-positive ALL have intracytoplasmic immunoglobulin and are termed pre-B cell ALL. B cell ALL is signified by the presence of immunoglobulin on the cell surface and accounts for fewer than 5% of cases of ALL. About 20% of cases of ALL are of the T cell phenotype, expressing antigens found on normal early T cells, such as CD5, CD3, or CD2. Approximately 15% of cases of ALL fail to express CALLA, B, or T cell markers and are termed null cell ALL. Leukemic cells in about 25% of patients with ALL also express myeloid antigens. The presence of such antigens defines a group of patients with a poorer prognosis.

Cytoplasmic Markers

Of the cytoplasmic markers identified, only one is commonly used clinically, deoxynucleotidyl transferase (TdT), a nuclear enzyme that is not found on normal mature myeloid or lymphoid cells. In more than 90% of cases of ALL, however, the lymphoblasts contain large amounts of the enzyme. Only 4% of cases of AML stain positively for TdT. Other cytoplasmic enzymes of occasional relevance include adenosine deaminase, which is increased in T cell ALL; 5'-nucleotidase, which is low in T cell ALL; and lysozyme, which is produced by monocytic leukemia cells.

Cytogenetics

In most cases of acute leukemia, there is a numerical or structural chromosomal abnormality within the leukemic cell population. The simplest chromosomal change is a gain or loss of a whole

TABLE 143–1. CLASSIFICATION OF ACUTE LEUKEMIAS

| Subtype | Morphology | Histochemistry | | | Monoclonal Reactivity | Cytogenetic Abnormalities |
		Myeloperoxidase	Nonspecific Esterase	PAS		
M0, Acute undifferentiated leukemia	Uniform, very undifferentiated	−	−	−	For subtypes M0–M5b, approximately 90% of cases will react with at least one of the following antimyeloid antibodies: Anti-CD13 Anti-CD14 Anti-CD33 Anti-CD34	Various
M1, Acute myeloid leukemia with minimal differentiation	Very undifferentiated, few azurophilic granules	+/−	+/−	−		Various
M2, Acute myeloid leukemia with differentiation	Granulated blasts predominate; Auer rods may be seen	+++	+/−	+		Various
M3, Acute promyelocytic leukemia	Hypergranular promyelocytes predominate	+++	+	+		t(15;17)
M4, Acute myelomonocytic leukemia M4E	Both monoblasts and myeloblasts present; like M4 but with eosinophils	++	+++	++		Various inv/del(16)
M5, Acute monocytic leukemia M5a M5b	Monoblasts predominate type a >80% monoblasts type b >20% promonocytes	+/−	+++	++		Various, including t(9,11)
M6, Acute erythroleukemia	Erythroblasts and megaloblastic red cell precursors seen	−	−	++	Antiglycophorin, antispectrin	Various
M7, Acute megakaryocytic leukemia	Undifferentiated blasts	−	+/−	+	Antiplatelet GpIIb/IIIa	Various
L1, Acute lymphoid leukemia Childhood variant	Small, uniform blasts, nucleoli indistinct	−	−	+++	65% react with anti-CD10 (anti-CALLA)	Various
L2, Acute lymphoid leukemia Adult variant	Larger, more irregular nucleoli present	−	−	++	20% react with anti-CD5, 3, or 2 (anti-T cell)	Various, including t(1;19)
L3, Burkitt-like acute lymphoid leukemia	Large with strongly basophilic cytoplasm and vacuoles	−	−	−	Antisurface immunoglobulin, anti-CD19, anti-CD20	t(8;14)

PAS = periodic acid–Schiff.

chromosome. Other common structural changes include translocations, which involve the exchange of material between two chromosomes; deletions, in which part of a chromosome is lost; or inversions, in which a single chromosome is broken in two places and the middle piece is inverted and rejoined. When patients with acute leukemia and a chromosomal abnormality are treated and there is complete remission of the disease, the chromosomal abnormality disappears, but it reappears when relapse occurs.

In more than 80% of cases of AML, a clonal chromosomal abnormality is found. The most frequent changes are a gain of chromosome 8 or loss of part or all of chromosome 7 or 5. These abnormalities are each seen in approximately 7 to 12% of cases of AML and are not associated with a particular subtype of AML, but are, in general, associated with a somewhat unfavorable prognosis. Other chromosomal abnormalities are associated with specific syndromes of AML. Acute promyelocytic leukemia virtually always has a translocation involving chromosomes 15 and 17 [t(15;17)]. Acute myelomonocytic (M4) leukemia with abnormal eosinophilia is associated with an inversion in chromosome 16. Patients with M2 AML with t(8;21) express CD56 on the surface of leukemic blasts, commonly have extramedullary disease, and have a relatively favorable outcome with chemotherapy.

Between 15 and 20% of adults with ALL have a Philadelphia (Ph) chromosome [t(9;22)]; the precise breakpoint of the translocation in ALL differs from that in CML. Other common changes in ALL are t(4;11), an abnormality seen mostly in neonatal ALL, t(8;14), an abnormality associated with the L3 variant of ALL, and t(1;19), a translocation common in pre–B cell ALL. The leukemic cells in about 20% of patients with ALL have a propensity to gain many chromosomes, often reaching an average of 50 to 60 chromosomes per cell. Patients with such hyperdiploid leukemias tend to respond well to chemotherapy.

Oncogenes

It is generally believed that the above-mentioned abnormalities in chromosomal structure are important in the development of leukemia, either by altering the expression of a normal gene (a proto-oncogene) necessary for cell growth and development or by causing the loss of inactivation of certain "tumor suppressor genes" (anti-oncogenes) (see Ch. 156). While the exact mechanisms by which abnormalities in chromosomal structure lead to leukemia are still uncertain, in some cases the normal genes involved have been identified. The t(15;17) associated with acute promyelocytic leukemia results in the fusion of a transcription factor (PML) on chromosome 15 with the alpha retinoic acid receptor gene (RARα) on chromosome 17. The *abl* proto-oncogene is affected in the t(9;22) translocation, while the *myc* proto-oncogene is altered with t(8;14). Approximately 25% of AML samples and 10% of ALL cases exhibit point mutations in the *N-ras* oncogene.

CLINICAL MANIFESTATIONS

The signs and symptoms of acute leukemia result from decreased normal marrow function and invasion of normal organs by leukemic blasts. *Anemia* is present at diagnosis in most patients, causing fatigue, pallor, and headache and, in predisposed patients, angina or heart failure. *Thrombocytopenia* is usually present, and approximately one third of patients have clinically evident bleeding at diagnosis, usually in the form of petechiae, ecchymoses, bleeding gums, epistaxis, or hemorrhage. Most patients with acute leukemia are significantly *granulocytopenic* at diagnosis. As a result, approximately one third of patients with AML, and slightly fewer patients with ALL, have significant or life-threatening infections at presentation, most of which are bacterial in origin.

In addition to suppressing normal marrow function, leukemic cells can infiltrate normal organs. The prevalence and degree of organ infiltration differ between ALL and AML. In general, ALL tends to infiltrate normal organs more often than AML. Enlargement of lymph nodes, liver, and spleen is common at diagnosis. Bone pain, thought to result from leukemic infiltration of the periosteum or expansion of the medullary cavity, is a common complaint, particularly in children with ALL, in many of whom the original diagnosis was juvenile rheumatoid arthritis. Leukemic cells may infiltrate the leptomeninges, causing leukemic meningitis. Signs of leukemic meningitis are headache and nausea. As the dis

ease progresses, central nervous system (CNS) palsies and seizures may develop. Although fewer than 5% of patients have CNS involvement at diagnosis, the CNS is a frequent site of relapse, particularly with ALL, and because of the so-called blood-brain barrier, the CNS requires special therapy, as will be discussed. Testicular involvement is also seen in ALL and is a frequent site of relapse. In AML, collections of leukemic blast cells, often referred to as chloromas or myeloblastomas, can occur in virtually any soft tissue, presenting as rubbery, fast-growing masses.

Certain clinical manifestations are unique to specific subtypes of leukemia. Patients with acute promyelocytic leukemia (M3) commonly have subclinical or clinically evident disseminated intravascular coagulation, caused by tissue thromboplastins present in the leukemic cells, which are released as the leukemic cells die. Acute monocytic or myelomonocytic leukemias are the forms of AML most likely to have extramedullary involvement. M6 leukemia often has a long prodromal phase. Patients with T cell ALL often have mediastinal masses.

LABORATORY MANIFESTATIONS

Abnormalities of peripheral blood counts are usually the initial laboratory evidence of acute leukemia. Anemia is present in most patients. Most are also at least mildly thrombocytopenic, and up to one quarter have severe thrombocytopenia (< 20,000 per micro­liter). Although most patients are granulocytopenic at diagnosis, the total peripheral white cell count is more variable, approximately 25% of patients having very high white cell counts (> 50,000 per microliter), approximately 50% having white cell counts between 5000 and 50,000, and 25% having a low white cell count (< 5000 per microliter). In most cases, blasts are present in the peripheral blood, although in some patients the percentage of blasts may be quite low, or blasts may be absent.

The diagnosis of acute leukemia is generally established by marrow aspiration and biopsy, usually from the posterior iliac crest. Marrow aspirates and biopsy specimens are usually hypercellular and contain 30 to 100% blast cells, which largely replace the normal marrow. Occasionally, in addition to the blast cell infiltrate, other findings are present, including marrow fibrosis (especially with M7 AML) or bone marrow necrosis.

Other laboratory abnormalities often seen are hyperuricemia, especially in ALL, and increased serum lactate dehydrogenase (LDH). Increased serum or urinary levels of muramidase, a hydrolytic enzyme present in the primary granules of primitive granulocytes and especially monocytes, are sometimes seen with M4 and M5 AML. Rarely, lactic acidosis may complicate acute leukemia, especially in patients with extreme hyperleukocytosis and L3 ALL.

DIFFERENTIAL DIAGNOSIS

The diagnosis of acute leukemia is usually straightforward, but occasionally can be more difficult. Leukemia and aplastic anemia can both manifest with peripheral pancytopenia, but the finding of hypoplastic marrow without blasts usually distinguishes aplastic anemia. Occasionally a patient may have hypocellular marrow and a clonal cytogenetic abnormality, which establishes the diagnosis of myelodysplasia or hypocellular leukemia. A number of processes other than leukemia can lead to the appearance of immature cells in the peripheral blood. Although other small round cell neoplasms can infiltrate the marrow and sometimes mimic leukemia, immunologic markers are effective in differentiating between the two. Leukemoid reactions to infections such as tuberculosis can result in the outpouring of large numbers of young myeloid cells, but virtually never does the percentage of blasts in marrow or peripheral blood reach 30% in a leukemoid reaction (see Ch. 140.2). Infectious mononucleosis and other viral illnesses can sometimes resemble ALL, particularly when large numbers of atypical lymphocytes are present in the peripheral blood and when the disease is accompanied by immune thrombocytopenia or hemolytic anemia.

TREATMENT

With the development of effective programs of combination chemotherapy and advances in marrow transplantation, many patients with acute leukemia can be cured. These therapeutic measures are complex and therefore are best carried out at centers with appropriate support services and experience in treating leukemia. Because leukemia is a rapidly progressive disease, specific antileukemic therapy should be started as soon after diagnosis as possible, usually within 48 hours. Before therapy is started, hemorrhage and infection should be brought under control, if possible. To prevent uric acid nephropathy, patients should be hydrated and given allopurinol, 100 to 200 mg orally, three times per day. The diagnosis of leukemia usually comes as a profound psychological shock to the patient and family. Therefore, in addition to stabilizing the patient hematologically and metabolically, it is worthwhile having at least one formalized conference in which the patient and the family are advised about the meaning of the diagnosis of leukemia and the consequences of therapy before treatment is initiated.

Management of Emergencies

Patients sometimes have treatable emergencies that require immediate attention before specific antileukemic therapy is begun. Severe bleeding usually results from thrombocytopenia, which can be reversed with platelet transfusions. Once thrombocytopenic bleeding is stopped, continued prophylactic transfusions of platelets to maintain the platelet count above 20,000 per microliter are warranted. Occasionally, patients also have evidence of disseminated intravascular coagulation (DIC), usually associated with the diagnosis of M3 AML. If active bleeding is due to DIC, the use of low doses of heparin (50 units per kilogram) given intravenously every 6 hours can often be of benefit. Whether heparin should be given prophylactically to patients with laboratory evidence of DIC but no active bleeding is an often debated, but unsettled, question. Patients with fever and granulocytopenia should have cultures, but infection should be assumed, and broad-spectrum antibiotics should be begun empirically. It is preferable to bring an infection under control before starting initial chemotherapy if the patient has an adequate granulocyte count. Patients often have infection and essentially no granulocytes, and delaying chemotherapy in such patients is unlikely to be of benefit. Patients with very high blast counts (>150,000 per microliter) may develop symptoms attributable to the effect of masses of these immature cells on blood flow. The leukostasis may evolve into vascular injury and local hemorrhage. If this situation occurs in the CNS, the outcome may be fatal. Leukapheresis, immediate whole-brain irradiation (600 cGy in one dose), and administration of hydroxyurea, 3 grams per square meter given orally for 2 or 3 days, can usually prevent this complication. Patients with very high white cell counts may also have uremia and anuria secondary to greatly increased serum uric acid levels, with subsequent intratubular crystallization. Rehydration, urine alkalinization with acetazolamide (500 mg per day), and prevention of uric acid production with allopurinol may lead to improved renal function. If patients do not respond and remain uremic, dialysis should be begun before institution of chemotherapy.

Treatment of ALL

After the patient's condition has been stabilized, antileukemic therapy should be started as soon as possible. Initial therapy for ALL can be divided into three phases: remission induction, postremission therapy, and CNS prophylaxis.

REMISSION INDUCTION. The initial goal of treatment is to induce complete remission, which is usually defined as the reduction of leukemic blasts to undetectable levels and restoration of normal marrow function. A number of different chemotherapeutic combinations can be used to induce remission; all include vincristine and prednisone, and most add L-asparaginase and/or daunorubicin, administered over 3 to 4 weeks. With such regimens, complete remission is achieved in 90% of children and 75% of adults. Since vincristine, prednisone, and L-asparaginase are relatively nontoxic to normal marrow precursors, the disease often enters complete remission after a relatively brief period of myelosuppression. Failure to achieve complete remission is usually due either to resistance of the leukemic cells to the drugs used or to progressive infection. These two complications occur with approximately equal frequency.

POSTREMISSION CHEMOTHERAPY. If no further therapy is given after induction of complete remission, virtually all cases relapse, most within several months. This fact demonstrates the need for further postremission therapy. Chemotherapy after complete remission can be given in a variety of combinations, dosages, and schedules. The term "consolidation chemotherapy" generally refers to short courses of further chemotherapy given at doses similar to those used for initial induction and thus requiring rehospitalization. Attempts are usually made to select drugs for consolidation that were not used in inducing the initial remission. In the case of ALL, such drugs include high-dose methotrexate, cyclophosphamide, and cytarabine, among others. "Maintenance" involves the administration of low-dose chemotherapy on a daily or weekly outpatient basis for long periods. The most commonly used maintenance regimens in ALL are daily 6-mercaptopurine and weekly or biweekly methotrexate. The optimal duration of maintenance chemotherapy is unknown, but maintenance is usually given for 2 to 3 years. Optimal chemotherapy for ALL requires both consolidation and maintenance chemotherapy.

CENTRAL NERVOUS SYSTEM PROPHYLAXIS. Most chemotherapeutic agents, when given intravenously or orally, do not penetrate the CNS well, making it a common site of relapse unless specific measures are taken. Effective regimens for CNS prophylaxis include the use of intrathecal methotrexate alone, intrathecal methotrexate combined with 2400 cGy to the cranium, or 2400 cGy to the craniospinal axis.

PROGNOSIS AFTER INITIAL CHEMOTHERAPY. A number of factors are predictive of outcome in ALL, the most consistent of which are age, white cell count at diagnosis, and expression of myeloid antigens by ALL blasts. With currently available treatment regimens, in 50 to 70% of children and 25 to 45% of adults in whom complete remission is achieved, remission remains complete for >5 years, and thus these patients are probably cured of their disease. In both children and adults, a low white cell count at diagnosis predicts a favorable outcome, while a high white cell count at diagnosis does the reverse. Patients with lymphoblasts that express myeloid antigens including CD13 or CD33 have both a lower initial complete remission rate and a shorter duration of remission than patients without such markers. Specific syndromes of ALL with a poor prognosis include the L3 variant of ALL or the presence of the Philadelphia chromosome or the t(4;11) chromosomal abnormality.

TREATMENT OF RELAPSED ALL. Most relapses occur within 2 years of diagnosis, and most occur in the marrow. Occasionally, relapse may first be found in an extramedullary site, such as the CNS or testes. Extramedullary relapse is usually followed shortly by systemic (marrow) relapse and so should be considered part of a systemic recurrence. With the use of chemotherapeutic regimens similar to those used for initial induction, 50 to 70% of cases achieve at least short-lived second remissions. A small percentage of cases in which first remission was longer than 2 years may be cured with salvage chemotherapy. If the CNS or testes were the initial site of the relapse, specific therapy to that site is also required along with systemic retreatment. Since the prognosis of relapsed leukemia treated with chemotherapy is so poor, marrow transplantation is now generally recommended in this setting.

MARROW TRANSPLANTATION (see Ch. 153). The use of high-dose chemoradiotherapy followed by marrow transplantation from a human leukocyte antigen (HLA)-identical sibling can cure 20 to 40% of patients with ALL in whom there is failure to achieve an initial remission or in whom there is relapse after an initial complete remission. The major limitations of transplantation are graft-versus-host disease, interstitial pneumonia, and disease recurrence. If an HLA-identical sibling is not available, alternative sources of marrow are from a partially matched family member; from an HLA-matched unrelated donor; or autologous marrow that has been removed during remission, treated in vitro to remove contaminating tumor cells, and then subsequently stored. The outcome of transplantation using either autologous marrow or alternative sources of marrow has not been as favorable as that using matched allogeneic family member donors.

Treatment of AML

REMISSION INDUCTION. Treatment with a combination of an anthracycline (daunomycin or idarubicin) and cytarabine leads to complete remission in 60 to 80% of patients with AML. Profound myelosuppression always follows when these agents are used at doses capable of achieving complete remission. Failure to achieve complete remission is usually due either to drug resistance or to fatal complications of myelosuppression.

POSTREMISSION THERAPY. Intensive consolidation chemotherapy using repeated courses of daunomycin and cytarabine at conventional doses, high-dose cytarabine, or other agents prolongs the average remission duration and improves the chances for long-term disease-free survival. Unlike the situation in ALL, low-dose maintenance therapy is of limited benefit after intensive consolidation treatment. In AML, leukemic recurrence occurs less often in the CNS, being seen in only approximately 10% of cases, most commonly in patients with M4 or M5 variants. There is no evidence that CNS prophylaxis improves overall disease-free survival in AML.

PROGNOSIS AFTER INITIAL CHEMOTHERAPY. Among those patients in whom complete remission is achieved, 15 to 30% remain alive in continuous complete remission for more than 5 years, suggesting probable cure. As with ALL, younger patients and those with a low white cell count at diagnosis have a more favorable outcome. Patients whose disease is characterized by certain chromosomal abnormalities, particularly t(8;21), t(15;17), and inv 16, do somewhat better, whereas those with 5q-, -7, 11q23, inv3, or t(6;9) do worse. Patients who have a long preleukemic phase before their condition evolves into acute leukemia and those whose leukemia is secondary to prior exposure to alkylating agents or radiation respond poorly to chemotherapy.

TREATMENT OF RECURRENT AML. Patients whose AML recurs after initial chemotherapy can achieve second remission in about 50% of cases following retreatment with daunomycin-cytarabine or high-dose cytarabine. Unfortunately these remissions tend to be short lived, and few patients in whom relapse occurs after first-line chemotherapy are cured by salvage chemotherapy.

THE TREATMENT OF ACUTE PROMYELOCYTIC LEUKEMIA (APL). Recent studies demonstrate that complete remissions can be induced in at least 80% of patients with APL using all-trans-retinoic acid (ATRA). Patients treated with ATRA usually have correction of coagulation disorders within several days, but up to 2 or 3 months of therapy may be required to achieve complete remission. ATRA works by inducing differentiation of leukemic cells. A unique toxicity of ATRA in the treatment of APL is the development of hyperleukocytosis accompanied by respiratory distress and pulmonary infiltrates. The syndrome responds to temporary discontinuation of ATRA and the addition of corticosteroids. If patients are treated for APL with ATRA alone, disease recurrence appears inevitable, suggesting that ATRA should be combined with, or followed by, other therapy.

BONE MARROW TRANSPLANTATION (see Ch. 151). For patients with AML in whom there is failure to achieve an initial remission or in whom there is relapse after chemotherapy, marrow transplantation from an HLA-identical sibling offers the best chance for cure. If carried out when patients have end-stage disease, approximately 15% of patients can be saved. If the procedure is applied earlier, the outcome with marrow transplantation improves, with approximately 30% of patients undergoing transplantation at first relapse or second remission being cured, and with cure rates of 50 to 60% if transplantation is carried out in the first remission. Several studies have prospectively compared the outcome of marrow transplantation with that of chemotherapy in patients with AML in first remission. The trend in all of these studies has been in favor of transplantation, although in not all the studies was there a statistically significant difference. Currently, transplantation is the treatment of choice for patients with AML who have suffered an initial relapse, and it should be strongly considered for most patients while in first remission. The major limitations to transplantation are graft-versus-host disease, interstitial pneumonia, and disease recurrence. Since the incidence of graft-versus-host disease increases with age, most centers limit transplantation to patients age 55 or less. Alternative sources of marrow include the use of partially matched family members, matched unrelated donors, and autologous transplantation. As with ALL, these alternative sources of marrow do not yield results as good as those obtained using a fully matched family member.

Supportive Care

Treatment of acute leukemia, especially AML, is accompanied by a number of complications, the two most serious and frequent being infection and bleeding. During the granulocytopenic period following induction and consolidation chemotherapy, most patients become febrile, and in approximately 50% of cases, a bacterial infection can be documented. The most commonly isolated organisms vary somewhat from medical center to medical center, but usually gram-positive organisms, such as *Staphylococcus epidermidis,* and gram-negative enteric organisms, such as *Pseudomonas aeruginosa, Escherichia coli,* and *Klebsiella aerobacter,* are the most commonly isolated bacteria. Even if no cause for fever is found, bacterial infection should be assumed, and in general, all patients with fever and neutropenia should begin receiving broad-spectrum antibiotics. Commonly used antibiotic combinations include a cephalosporin and a semisynthetic penicillin or a semisynthetic penicillin and an aminoglycoside. Once begun, antibiotics should be continued until patients recover their granulocyte count, even if the patients become afebrile first. If documented bacterial infections persist despite appropriate antibiotics, removal of indwelling catheters and granulocyte transfusions should be considered. It may be possible to reduce the incidence of bacterial infection through the use of selective gastrointestinal decontamination, using, for example, ciprofloxacin or a combination of trimethoprim-sulfamethoxazole plus colistin. The use of protective environments can also reduce the incidence of infection, but it is costly and has not been shown to influence overall survival.

Frequently, patients taking broad-spectrum antibiotics become afebrile for a time, only to develop a second fever. Such patients should be carefully reassessed with a high index of suspicion for fungal infection. Granulocytopenic patients who remain febrile for more than a week while taking broad-spectrum antibiotics should be treated empirically with amphotericin for presumed fungal infection.

In addition to being granulocytopenic, patients undergoing induction chemotherapy for leukemia have deficient cellular and humoral immunity, at least temporarily, and so are subject to those infections common in other immunodeficiency states, including *Pneumocystis carinii* infection and a variety of viral infections. *Pneumocystis carinii* infection can be prevented by prophylactic use of trimethoprim-sulfamethoxazole. Cytomegalovirus (CMV) infection can be prevented in the CMV-seronegative patient by the sole use of CMV-seronegative blood products. Herpes simplex can often complicate existing mucositis and can be treated successfully with acyclovir. Acyclovir is also useful for the treatment of disseminated varicella zoster.

The platelet count that signals a need for platelet transfusion has been the subject of recent debate. Traditionally, platelet transfusions from random donors were used to maintain platelet counts above 20,000 per microliter, but more recently it has been demonstrated that lowering this threshold to 10,000 is safe in patients with no active bleeding. In 30 to 50% of cases, patients eventually become alloimmunized and require the use of HLA-matched platelets. Occasionally, cells (presumably T cells) within the blood product can engraft in the immunosuppressed leukemic patient and cause a graft-versus-host reaction. Transfusion-induced graft-versus-host disease manifests with a rash, low-grade fever, elevated values in liver function tests, and falling blood counts. This syndrome can be prevented by irradiating all blood products with at least 1500 cGy before transfusion.

Appelbaum FR, Fisher LD, Thomas ED, et al.: Chemotherapy and marrow transplantation for adults with acute nonlymphocytic leukemia: A five-year follow-up. Blood 72:179, 1988. *Comparison of the outcome of marrow transplantation with that of continued chemotherapy for adults with AML.*

Baer MR, Bloomfield CD: Cytogenetics and oncogenes in leukemia. Curr Opin Oncol 4:24, 1992. *A thoughtful review.*

Bennett JM, Catovsky D, Daniel MT, et al.: Proposed revised criteria for the classification of acute myeloid leukemia. Ann Intern Med 103:626, 1985. *Update of the French-American-British (FAB) classification of acute leukemia.*

Champlin R, Gale RP: Acute myelogenous leukemia: Recent advances in therapy. Blood 69:1551, 1987. *Very good review of therapy for AML with excellent bibliography.*

Champlin R, Gale RP: Acute lymphoblastic leukemia: Recent advances in biology and therapy. Blood 73:2051, 1989. *Like above reference, but this time directed at ALL.*

Cheson BD, Cassileth PA, Head DR, et al.: Report of the National Cancer Institute–sponsored workshop on definitions of diagnosis and response in acute myeloid leukemia. J Clin Oncol 8:813, 1990. *A report of the recently adopted NCI definitions of diagnostic and response criteria for AML.*

Clarkson B, Ellis S, Little C, et al.: Acute lymphoblastic leukemia in adults. Semin Oncol 12:160, 1985. *Review of chemotherapy for adult ALL centering on Sloan-Kettering experience.*

Mayer RJ: Current chemotherapeutic treatment approaches to the management of previously untreated adults with de novo acute myelogenous leukemia. Semin Oncol 14:384, 1987. *Comprehensive, balanced review of chemotherapy for adult AML.*

Rowley JD: Recurring chromosome abnormalities in leukemia and lymphoma. Semin Hematol 27:122, 1990. *Updated review of chromosomal abnormalities seen in malignant hematologic diseases.*

Warrell RP, Frankel SR, Miller WH, et al.: Differentiation therapy of acute promyelocytic leukemia with tretinoin (all-trans-retinoic acid). N Engl J Med 324:1385, 1991. *Description of a new approach.*

144 INTRODUCTION TO NEOPLASMS OF THE IMMUNE SYSTEM

Carol S. Portlock

Neoplasms of the immune system are a heterogeneous group of tumors whose cells of origin may be the lymphocyte, the histiocyte, or other cell components of the immune system. Each neoplasm is thought to be a monoclonal expansion of malignant cells, although this has been conclusively demonstrated only for lymphocytic tumors. Characteristically, these neoplasms often retain many morphologic, functional, and migratory properties common to their normal cell counterparts.

With increasing understanding of the normal immune system, it has become possible to classify many malignant immune disorders according to their cell of origin. Monoclonal antibodies to cell-surface antigens permit the identification of B or T lymphocyte proliferations. By such immunophenotyping, malignant lymphocytic neoplasms can be related to stages of normal B or T lymphocyte development and maturation. Table 144–1 lists these diseases according to their normal cell lineage counterpart.

Establishing clonality of a B lymphocyte proliferation is usually accomplished by the demonstration of a single class of heavy- and/or light-chain cell-surface immunoglobulin. At the DNA level, clonality can be confirmed by the presence of a single immunoglobulin gene rearrangement. In precursor B lymphocyte neoplasms, which lack surface immunoglobulins, gene rearrangement studies are necessary to demonstrate clonality.

For T lymphocyte proliferations, clonality can be conclusively shown only by T lymphocyte receptor gene rearrangement. Studies of cell-surface antigens alone are not sufficient. Clonal lymphocyte proliferations are not always malignant, as exemplified by the chronic monoclonal T lymphocyte disorder of lymphomatoid papulosis.

Tumors of histiocytic lineage have not yet been shown to be monoclonal. These cells lack endogenous immunoglobulin but may acquire exogenous immunoglobulin on their cell surface. They may be rich in lysozyme or muramidase, and as phagocytic cells, they ingest latex particles or sensitized erythrocytes. The cell lineage of the Reed-Sternberg cell in Hodgkin's disease is uncertain. It shares *in vitro* characteristics with both histiocytes and lymphocytes. Recent molecular studies demonstrating immunoglobulin gene rearrangement and the presence of *bcl-2* oncogene suggest a B lymphocyte origin.

In addition to a specific immunotype and genotype, chromosomal abnormalities can be detected in the majority of immune system neoplasms. Among B lymphocyte lymphomas, these abnormalities most often include translocations involving chromosome 14 q 32 (the heavy-chain immunoglobulin gene locus) and the cellular oncogenes *c-myc* (chromosome 8), *bcl-1* (chromosome 11), or *bcl-2* (chromosome 18). The 14;18 translocation is associated with >75% of follicular lymphomas and up to one third of diffuse large cell lymphomas; t(11;14) with most diffuse small cleaved (centrocytic) lymphomas; and t(8;14) with Burkitt's lymphoma. Specific translocations of the T lymphocyte receptor gene loci appear to be involved in T-cell lymphocyte lymphomas. These include chromosome 14 q 11 (T lymphocyte receptor α- and δ-chain genes) or chromosomes 7q 34-36 or 7 p 15 (T lymphocyte receptor β- and γ-chain genes). The presumed oncogene translocation partners remain unidentified for most T-lymphocyte neoplasms. Other important genetic alterations that have recently been elucidated include p53 mutations in follicular lymphoma transformation and the presence of *bcl-6* oncogene rearrangement in up to one third of diffuse large cell lymphomas. No specific chromosomal changes have been identified thus far in Hodgkin's disease. Reed-Sternberg cells are difficult to isolate, are few in number, and possess complex hyperdiploid karyotypes. Another apparently specific marker is the presence of antibodies to the human retrovirus HTLV-I (human T cell leukemia/lymphoma virus) found in patients with adult T cell leukemia/lymphoma. These and other *in vitro* methods may provide additional information for defining prognostically important patient subsets.

Although each neoplasm of the immune system has a distinct clinicopathologic entity, these disorders tend to share some common clinical features. Systemic symptoms of fever, night sweats, and weight loss may be present and tend to correlate with advanced stage of disease. The neoplasm usually arises in one or more organs of the hematopoietic system (lymph nodes, spleen, liver, bone marrow), and if untreated or ineffectively treated, it tends to disseminate to all those organs, as well as to other sites. Bone marrow involvement with or without peripheral blood manifestation is common in certain disorders and may be the predominant feature. Meningeal infiltration often develops when aggressive neoplasms involve the bone marrow.

PATHOLOGY AND CLASSIFICATION

Neoplasms of B or T lymphocytic lineage are termed *non-Hodgkin's lymphomas*. The histopathologic classification of these tumors is complex and continually evolving as new entities are identified and the cellular/molecular biology is clarified. A well-accepted schema is that of the National Cancer Institute (NCI) Working Formulation (Table 144–2). Prognostic groups are termed low-, intermediate-, and high-grade lymphomas according to 5-year survival.

Many non-Hodgkin's lymphomas may exhibit two distinct histologic subtypes. Both the architecture and the cell type may change, usually evolving from a low-grade to an intermediate- or high-grade lymphoma. Rarely, two histologic subtypes may be present at diagnosis in the same lymph node (composite lymphoma). More often, two histologic subtypes may occupy two separate biopsy specimens; most frequently, one is seen at diagnosis and a second at relapse or autopsy. It is thought that such "transformation" represents

TABLE 144–1. LYMPHOMAS AS NEOPLASMS OF THE IMMUNE SYSTEM

Cell of Origin	Neoplasm
B cell	
Medullary B cell	Chronic lymphocytic leukemia, diffuse small lymphocytic lymphoma
Follicular B cell	Follicular lymphomas, diffuse mixed lymphoma, diffuse large cell lymphoma, Burkitt's lymphoma
Immunoblastic B cell	Diffuse immunoblastic lymphoma
T cell	
Thymic T cell	Lymphoblastic lymphoma
Mature T cell	Peripheral T-cell lymphomas, chronic lymphocytic leukemia (rare), HTLV-I-associated lymphoma, mycosis fungoides, Sézary's syndrome
Immunoblastic T cell	Diffuse immunoblastic lymphoma
Histiocytic	
Histiocyte	Malignant histiocytosis, true histiocytic lymphoma (rare)
Unknown	Hodgkin's disease

TABLE 144–2. CLASSIFICATIONS OF NON-HODGKIN'S LYMPHOMAS

NCI Working Formulation (1982)
Low-grade
Small lymphocytic (SLL)
Follicular, small cleaved cell (FSCL)
Follicular, mixed small cleaved and large cell (FML)
Intermediate-grade
Follicular, large cell (FLCL)
Diffuse, small cleaved cell (DSCL)
Diffuse, mixed small cleaved and large cell (DML)
Diffuse, large cell (cleaved and noncleaved) (DLCL)
High-grade
Large cell immunoblastic (IBL)
Lymphoblastic (convoluted and nonconvoluted) (LL)
Small noncleaved cell (Burkitt and non-Burkitt) (SNCL)

expansion of a more aggressive subclone. Its emergence may dramatically alter both therapy and prognosis.

In contrast to non-Hodgkin's lymphomas, the diagnostic malignant cells (Reed-Sternberg cells) of Hodgkin's disease appear similar in all four histologic subtypes of the neoplasm. Instead, distinguishing pathologic features include the number of Reed-Sternberg cells and the composition of normal background cells and stroma (see Ch. 146).

DIAGNOSIS AND STAGING

The diagnosis of a neoplasm of the immune system is based on pathologic classification of biopsy material. Such diagnoses require adequate tissue (preferably lymph node, so that both architecture and cell type may be assessed), proper handling, and expert hematopathologic interpretation. Special studies, such as imprints, immunotyping, gene rearrangement, karyotyping, deoxynucleotidyl transferase (TdT) determination, and electron microscopy, may provide additional information for classification. Because these latter studies require fresh tissue and special handling, it is important that the pathologist be involved *before* biopsy. Similarly, it is important that each case be evaluated jointly by a medical oncologist, radiation therapist, surgeon, and radiologist from the outset.

Once diagnosis becomes established, the extent of disease should be completely defined. Because each neoplasm has distinct clinicopathologic features, the choice of staging studies will be based on that information. All patients should have a complete history, particularly assessing the presence or absence of systemic symptoms, and physical examination. All nodal areas should be examined, including Waldeyer's ring and preauricular, epitrochlear, and popliteal lymph nodes. Epigastric or other abdominal masses may be found in addition to those in liver and spleen. The lungs, skin, breasts, testicles, and central nervous system should be carefully examined for extranodal involvement. All suspected patients require blood counts as well as liver and renal function tests. Computed tomography (CT) may be indicated if chest radiography is abnormal. Abdominal CT and lymphography are often complementary and not mutually exclusive. Gallium scanning may be useful but is not a diagnostic method. Liver and spleen scans are of minimal value. Studies of bone or gastrointestinal tract should be performed when symptoms indicate. However, with Waldeyer's ring involvement, associated upper gastrointestinal disease may be asymptomatic, and therefore it should be sought routinely. Bone marrow biopsy is often indicated, particularly if advanced clinical disease is present or the patient has a low-grade lymphoma. Cerebrospinal fluid cytology should be determined in all patients with intermediate- and high-grade lymphomas who have bone marrow involvement and in all patients with Burkitt's lymphoma, lymphoblastic lymphoma, or malignant histiocytosis.

Several different staging systems are applied to neoplasms of the immune system. Their purpose is to define disease extent, to assist in treatment strategies, to evaluate therapeutic results, and to determine prognosis. In Hodgkin's disease the utility of staging has been well demonstrated, so that appropriate care demands careful clinical and often pathologic staging. Staging laparotomy with splenectomy and biopsy of liver, lymph nodes, and bone marrow was developed for adequate intra-abdominal assessment of Hodgkin's disease (see Ch. 146). The Ann Arbor staging system for Hodgkin's disease has also been applied to non-Hodgkin's lymphomas (see Ch. 145). In this setting it has less value in determining therapy but remains an important predictor of prognosis. Modified staging systems are used in pediatric lymphomas, chronic lymphocytic leukemia, Burkitt's and lymphoblastic lymphomas, and mycosis fungoides. Intra-abdominal tissue assessment is rarely needed to determine treatment in non-Hodgkin's lymphomas. Nonetheless, careful clinical staging is imperative in all cases. Recently, an International Prognostic Index has been introduced for intermediate-grade non-Hodgkin's lymphomas. This schema uses the clinical factors of age, performance status, tumor bulk, and lactate dehydrogenase level in predicting outcome.

DIFFERENTIAL DIAGNOSIS

The differential diagnosis of neoplasms of the immune system consists of the evaluation of lymphadenopathy. Reactive processes, infections, other malignant tumors, and collagen vascular disorders all may cause enlarged lymph nodes, hepatosplenomegaly, or both. The location or locations of the lymph nodes, their size, shape, consistency, rapidity of onset, and other characteristics may aid in determining cause.

Regional lymph node hyperplasia may accompany acute or chronic infections of the extremities as well as vaccinations or insect bites. Diffuse lymphadenopathy may follow ingestion of phenytoin. Other diffuse reactive processes, such as acquired immunodeficiency syndrome (AIDS), angioimmunoblastic lymphadenopathy, and collagen vascular disorders, may be associated with an increased likelihood of developing lymphoma. Consequently, a single lymph node biopsy may not provide diagnosis, which is why we recommend pathologic consultation before biopsy.

Among infectious causes, viral illnesses predominate and often produce bizarre pathologic material. Infectious mononucleosis may produce features common to Hodgkin's disease. Cytomegalovirus, cat-scratch disease, toxoplasmosis, tuberculosis, syphilis, and sarcoidosis are other considerations. Other malignant neoplasms usually involve lymph nodes by regional spread. For example, cervical lymphadenopathy may be the first symptom of a malignancy involving the oropharynx or nasopharynx. Similarly, breast cancer may manifest with axillary adenopathy and a microscopic primary tumor.

In almost all instances, the only way to determine conclusively the cause of unexplained lymphadenopathy is by pathologic tissue examination. Low cervical and supraclavicular lymph nodes are more likely to yield diagnostic material than are axillary and inguinal nodes. When only intrathoracic or abdominal disease is present, bone marrow biopsy may provide diagnostic information and obviate surgery. Fine-needle aspiration is of lesser value in neoplasms of the immune system than in solid tumors because cell morphology and architecture are both important diagnostic parameters.

Knowles DM: Immunophenotypic and immunogenotypic approaches useful in distinguishing benign and malignant lymphoid proliferations. Semin Oncol 20:583, 1993. *An outstanding review of the complementary laboratory studies available in evaluating lymph node histology.*

Pangalis GA, VassilaKopoulos TP, Boussiotis VA, Fessas P: Clinical approach to lymphadenopathy. Semin Oncol 20:570, 1993. *An extensive review of causes and a mathematical algorithm for assessing need for biopsy.*

Simon R, Durrleman S, Hoppe RT, et al.: The non-Hodgkin's lymphoma pathologic classification project: Long-term follow-up of 1153 patients with non-Hodgkin's lymphomas. Ann Intern Med 109:939, 1988. *A median follow-up of 11 years, again demonstrating the clinical relevance of the Working Formulation.*

Straus SE, Cohen JI, Tosato G, Meier J: NIH conference: Epstein-Barr virus infections: Biology, pathogenesis, and management. Ann Intern Med 118:45, 1993. *A comprehensive review of EBV-associated lymphoproliferation and lymphomagenesis.*

145 NON-HODGKIN'S LYMPHOMAS

Carol S. Portlock

Non-Hodgkin's lymphomas are the single largest group of neoplasms of the immune system. Composed of more than 10 distinct disease entities, non-Hodgkin's lymphomas are best understood as a heterogeneous group whose common link is a characteristic monoclonal expansion of malignant B or T cells.

EPIDEMIOLOGY

Non-Hodgkin's lymphomas may appear at any age, although they are rarely diagnosed during the first year of life. They occur with increasing frequency throughout adulthood. The incidence is estimated to be approximately 43,000 cases per year in the United States (1993), with men affected more than women. Moreover, male predominance is most evident among young patients in association with the aggressive histologic subtypes of lymphoblastic and Burkitt's lymphomas.

Geographic clustering is characteristic of some non-Hodgkin's lymphomas: Burkitt's lymphoma in central Africa; adult T cell leukemia/lymphoma in southwestern Japan and the Caribbean; and small intestinal lymphoma with associated immunoglobulin disorders in the Middle East.

Preceding immune dysfunction has been associated with the development of aggressive non-Hodgkin's lymphomas. Congenital immunodeficiency states associated with lymphoma include severe combined immunodeficiency, ataxia-telangiectasia, Wiskott-Aldrich syndrome, X-linked lymphoproliferative syndrome, and common variable immunodeficiency (see Ch. 223). Transplant recipients, patients with autoimmune states, and patients with AIDS (acquired immunodeficiency syndrome) also have increased risk of developing lymphoma.

ETIOLOGY AND PATHOGENESIS

The etiology of non-Hodgkin's lymphomas is unclear. Perhaps the best studied lymphoma is Burkitt's, with which the Epstein-Barr virus (EBV) has been associated and for which specific chromosomal and oncogene translocations have been implicated in its pathogenesis.

Burkitt's lymphoma is the most common childhood malignant disorder in Uganda. The disease is found along a "lymphoma belt" lying approximately 10 degrees north and 10 degrees south of the African equator. The belt contains altitude, temperature, and rainfall restrictions that are similar to those of Papua, New Guinea, where Burkitt's lymphoma is also common. Holoendemic or hyperendemic malaria accompanies the geography of the lymphoma belt and originally suggested to Burkitt a mosquito-borne vector and/or associated host immune dysfunction.

Nonendemic Burkitt's lymphoma, a similar disease occurring rarely and sporadically in other areas of the world (less than one case per million annually in the United States), has also been reported to occur in time-space clusters. Nonendemic Burkitt's lymphomas may be associated with preceding immune dysfunction (e.g., organ transplantation and AIDS).

The EBV is present in almost 90% of African Burkitt's lymphoma but fewer than half of nonendemic cases. Whether the virus plays a causative role or is merely a passenger in Burkitt's lymphoma remains controversial. Typically, primary EBV infection precedes the development of Burkitt's lymphoma by at least 7 or more months. Ugandan children with high EBV capsid antigen titers have a 30-fold greater risk of developing Burkitt's lymphoma than do control subjects. Elevated EBV/VCA (viral capsid antigen) titers are associated with a favorable prognosis in both African and nonendemic tumors.

Adult T cell leukemia/lymphoma (ATL), a rare and recently discovered disorder, is associated with a unique human retrovirus, HTLV-I (human T cell leukemia/lymphoma virus). This disease is endemic to southwestern Japan, where 12 to 15% of normal persons have HTLV-I antibodies; it is also found in the Caribbean basin.

The specific chromosomal translocations seen in Burkitt's lymphoma have uniformly involved the c-myc oncogene on chromosome 8 and the immunoglobulin heavy- or light-chain genes on chromosomes 14, 2, or 22. These translocations—t(8;14), t(8;2), and t(8;22)—deregulate the myc gene and result in the constitutive production of a DNA binding protein that appears to control aspects of gene expression or DNA replication. The biologic correlate of this molecular event is the finding of spontaneous B cell lymphomas in transgenic mice carrying DNA sequences from the 8;14 translocation breakpoint. The bcl-2 gene product has been shown to block or delay apoptosis (active cell death), and its overexpression in follicular lymphomas appears to be the mechanism by which tumor cells accumulate.

In addition to the etiologic considerations of oncogenic viruses and oncogene transformation, other factors that have been associated with an increased incidence of lymphoma include ionizing radiation (whole-body dose greater than 100 cGy), hereditary predisposition, congenital or acquired immunodeficiency, and exposure to pesticides.

PATHOLOGY AND CLINICAL FEATURES

Many different pathologic classifications have been proposed for non-Hodgkin's lymphomas (see Ch. 144). The National Cancer Institute Working Formulation (1982) (see Table 145–2) is well accepted and clinically relevant. Pathologic interpretation of non-Hodgkin's lymphomas can be supplemented with a variety of complementary studies. Immunophenotyping may identify the cell of origin by demonstrating B cell monoclonal surface immunoglobulin, and B or T cell differentiation antigens. Clonality may also be ascertained by detecting the rearrangement of the B cell im-

munoglobulin genes or the T cell receptor gene loci. The karyotype may reveal a specific chromosomal translocation. The presence of antibody against HTLV-I suggests a T cell lymphoma, whereas human immunodeficiency virus (HIV) antibody suggests an aggressive B cell neoplasm (see Color Plate 8E).

Each disease entity of the Working Formulation has a distinct clinical presentation and prognosis, as noted below. Tables 145–1 and 145–2 list the pathologic appearance and some of the clinical characteristics of each category.

LOW GRADE (see Color Plate 8D, left). The low-grade lymphomas (small lymphocytic [SLL]; follicular, predominantly small cleaved cell [FSCL]; and follicular, mixed, small cleaved and large cell [FML]) share several clinical characteristics: (1) Each has a history of waxing and waning or of slowly progressive lymphadenopathy. (2) Affected nodes are rubbery, mobile, and rarely fixed and have no overlying skin infiltration; they may be bulky but are rarely painful. (3) Liver and spleen are frequently involved pathologically and may be enlarged; liver function tests are usually normal, although the alkaline phosphatase level may be mildly increased. (4) Bone marrow involvement is common; circulating lymphoma cells may be identified on smear or by cell-sorting techniques. (5) Blood counts are usually normal at diagnosis. Elevation of the white blood cell count with circulating cells, anemia with autoimmune hemolytic anemia, and cytopenias secondary to hypersplenism or bone marrow replacement are uncommon. (6) Other extranodal disease sites may include pleura, lung, skin, breast, and gastrointestinal tract. (7) Enlarged lymph nodes may cause lymphedema, ureteral obstruction, or epidural spinal cord compression. (8) Central nervous system (meningeal or parenchymal), renal, or testicular infiltration rarely occurs.

INTERMEDIATE GRADE AND HIGH GRADE. (see Color Plate 8D, right). As a group, the intermediate (follicular, predominantly large cell [FLCL]; diffuse, small cleaved cell [DSCL]; diffuse, mixed small and large cell [DML]; and diffuse, large cell [DLCL]) and high-grade lymphomas (large cell immunoblastic [IBL]; lymphoblastic [LBL]; and small noncleaved cell, including Burkitt's lymphoma and diffuse and undifferentiated lymphoma, non-Burkitt's type [SNCL]) have several general clinical features in common: (1) They appear abruptly with rapidly enlarging lymph node masses. (2) Lymph nodes may be rubbery and mobile but may also be hard and fixed with overlying skin infiltration. Masses may be warm, erythematous, and painful. (3) Bulky lymph node masses (> 10 cm) may invade the mediastinum, retroperitoneum, and/or mesentery. (4) Waldeyer's ring may be involved and is often associ-

TABLE 145–1. PATHOLOGIC CHARACTERISTICS OF NON-HODGKIN'S LYMPHOMAS

Subtype	Architectural Pattern	Malignant Lymphocyte Cytology	Immunophenotype/ Immunogenotype
SLL	Diffuse	Small round cells	B cell; rarely T cell
FSCL	Follicular	Small cleaved cells	B cell
FML	Follicular	Small cleaved cells admixed with large cells, cleaved or noncleaved	B cell
FLCL	Follicular	Large cells, cleaved or noncleaved	B cell
DSCL	Diffuse	Small cleaved cells	B cell; occasionally T cell
DML	Diffuse	Admixture of small and large cells, cleaved or noncleaved	B cell; T cell
DLCL	Diffuse	Large cells, cleaved or noncleaved	B cell; T cell
IBL	Diffuse	Large cells; plasmacytoid, clear, or polymorphic cell variants	B cell; T cell
LBL	Diffuse "starry sky"	Lymphoblasts, convoluted or nonconvoluted nuclei	Thymic T cell
SNCL	Diffuse "starry sky"	Noncleaved cells, round nuclei with prominent nucleoli	B cell

TABLE 145–2. CLINICAL CHARACTERISTICS OF NON-HODGKIN'S LYMPHOMAS

Subtype	% All Lymphomas	Median Age (yr)	Sex Ratio M:F	% PS I, II*	% PS III, IV*	% Bone Marrow Involvement
SLL	3.6	61	1.2:1	11	89	71
FSCL	22.5	54	1.3:1	18	82	51
FML	7.7	56	0.8:1	27	73	30
FLCL	3.8	55	1.8:1	27	73	34
DSCL	6.9	58	2:1	28	72	32
DML	6.7	58	1.1:1	45	55	14
DLCL	19.7	57	1:1	46	54	10
IBL	7.9	51	1.5:1	52	49	12
LBL	4.2	17	1.9:1	27	74	50
SNCL	0.5	30	2.6:1	34	66	14

* PS = pathologic stage (according to the Working Formulation, 1982).

ated with extranodal disease of the stomach or small bowel or both. (5) Hepatosplenomegaly may occur and be accompanied by abnormal liver function tests. Porta hepatis or even intrahepatic obstructive patterns may develop. (6) Extranodal involvement is common and can include stomach, small bowel, lung, skin, bone, and central nervous system (particularly meningeal disease in association with bone marrow involvement). Rarely ovarian, testicular, or renal disease may be present. (7) Bone marrow involvement and circulating cells are less commonly seen at diagnosis than in low-grade lymphomas. A leukemic picture may emerge, however, when progressive disease develops. (8) Lymph node masses may cause lymphedema, ureteral obstruction, vascular obstruction (superior vena cava syndrome, thrombophlebitis), and epidural cord compression.

MISCELLANEOUS. A miscellaneous category of the Working Formulation includes mycosis fungoides (see Color Plate 7J, right)—a rare helper T cell lymphoma of the skin; composite lymphoma—multiple histologic subtypes (e.g., FSCL and IBL) occurring simultaneously; and true histiocytic lymphoma.

Since the Formulation's publication in 1982, additional mature T cell lymphomas have been recognized. The peripheral T cell lymphomas are a diverse group of "postthymic" neoplasms, whose cell of origin is the differentiated T cell. Their morphology includes diffuse small cell, mixed cell, large cell, or immunoblastic lymphoma, as well as subgroups with histologic features of angioimmunoblastic lymphadenopathy, lymphomatoid granulomatosis, or Lennert's lymphoma. The most important subgroup is that of Ki-1 lymphoma, a diffuse large cell lymphoma often confused with Hodgkin's disease. If treated as a non-Hodgkin's lymphoma, this and other peripheral T cell lymphomas appear to have outcomes that parallel their B cell counterparts in the Working Formulation.

HTLV-I–associated adult T cell leukemia/lymphoma is characterized by geographic clustering, the presence of antibody to HTLV-I, and a rapidly fatal clinical course. Clinical features include abrupt onset of generalized lymphadenopathy, hepatosplenomegaly, skin infiltration, lytic bone disease, bone marrow involvement with circulating cells, and hypercalcemia. In spite of intensive chemotherapy, median survival is less than 1 year. Although clinically distinct, this rare T cell lymphoma is not easily distinguishable pathologically from other T cell lymphomas. Diffuse small cell, mixed cell, large cell, and undifferentiated cell types have all been described. Clinical suspicion and the presence of HTLV-I antibody are necessary to confirm the diagnosis.

DIAGNOSIS AND STAGING

The diagnosis of non-Hodgkin's lymphoma requires skilled interpretation of adequate tumor tissue, preferably from an involved lymph node, so as to assess tumor architecture as well as cell type. B cell and T cell typing studies may complement the pathologic interpretation but do not supplant it. The clinical history and ancillary studies, e.g., HTLV-I or HIV antibody, may also contribute. Once a diagnosis has been established, it is useful to determine the extent of disease through staging.

The Ann Arbor staging system used for Hodgkin's disease (see Ch. 146) is clinically helpful in the management of non-Hodgkin's lymphomas. It has several shortcomings, however, when applied to non-Hodgkin's lymphomas because it omits factors such as disease site, disease bulk, and extent of extranodal involvement. Also, the

presence of systemic symptoms plays a lesser role in influencing treatment planning and prognosis in non-Hodgkin's lymphoma. Nevertheless, thorough pretreatment staging is necessary in all patients. Table 145–3 lists noninvasive studies, which should be obtained in all patients.

On the basis of the above information, the clinical stage of the lymphoma can be determined. Because bone marrow involvement is so common, particularly in low-grade lymphoma, bilateral percutaneous bone marrow biopsies are often the simplest way to establish pathologic stage IV disease. Pathologic confirmation of other extranodal sites also may be appropriate, as when gastroscopic biopsy, pleural cytology, or skin biopsy is obtained. Laparotomy or thoracotomy is indicated only in patients with no other evident disease or when a gastrointestinal tumor is removed prior to treatment. Staging laparotomy as performed for Hodgkin's disease is rarely, if ever, indicated.

TREATMENT

In defining a treatment approach for patients with non-Hodgkin's lymphoma, it is necessary to consider such factors as histologic subtype, stage, sites of disease, tumor bulk, thoroughness of initial staging, general medical condition, and age, as well as the goals and effectiveness of therapy. In practical terms, non-Hodgkin's lymphomas can be considered in two broad categories: those that progress slowly and have an indolent natural history (the low-grade lymphomas) and those that present aggressively, progress rapidly, and, if unsuccessfully treated, are soon fatal (the intermediate- and high-grade lymphomas).

LOW-GRADE LYMPHOMAS. As outlined above, low-grade lymphomas infrequently present with truly localized disease (pathologic stage I or II). Only 11 to 27%, depending upon histologic subtype, are therefore eligible for regional treatment with radiation therapy. Although uncommon, such a presentation appears to be highly favorable, with more than 75% of patients remaining free of disease for 10 years or longer after irradiation alone (3500 to 4400 cGy to the region).

TABLE 145–3. NONINVASIVE STUDIES IN NON-HODGKIN'S LYMPHOMA

History with assessment of systemic symptoms, predisposing epidemiologic factors
Physical examination
Complete blood count and platelet count; Coombs' test if anemic
Liver and renal function tests
Serum immunoglobulins in low-grade lymphomas
Antibody for HTLV-I or HIV, if indicated
Chest radiograph, posteroanterior and lateral
Chest computed tomography, if indicated
Abdominal and pelvic computed tomography
 If unavailable, abdominal ultrasound study
 If normal, lymphography possibly indicated
Bone scan and bone radiographs if clinical involvement suspected
Upper gastrointestinal series, if clinical involvement suspected or if Waldeyer's ring involved
Gallium scan, optional in aggressive histologies
Cerebrospinal fluid cytology (in all patients with intermediate- or high-grade lymphomas and known bone marrow disease)

Many more patients appear to have clinically localized disease after noninvasive staging and bone marrow biopsy but have not undergone complete laparotomy staging. Under these circumstances, radiation therapy may still accomplish good local control. Many patients, however, have undetected microscopic disease outside the treatment portal that will slowly progress and lead to disease recurrence several years after initial therapy. Nevertheless, irradiation may still be a reasonable choice, because relapse may occur years later, and salvage treatment at relapse may be effective. Patients eligible for this approach are those with peripheral lymph node presentations (stages I and II) involving cervical, supraclavicular, axillary, or inguinal regions. Abdominal masses usually require whole-abdominal irradiation in which this approach may not be justified. Thoracic presentations are rare.

Most (74 to 89%) patients with low-grade lymphomas have advanced stage (III or IV) disease, making them ineligible for localized treatment approaches. Optimal management of such patients remains controversial. Single-agent or multiagent chemotherapy with or without irradiation induces complete disappearance of all known tumor (including bone marrow) in more than 80% of such patients. Unfortunately, median remission durations are usually limited to 2.5 to 5 years. "Complete" responders usually have persistent lymphoma cells in their peripheral blood and bone marrow that may be detected by molecular methods. The presence of such cells often correlates with subsequent relapse.

Autologous stem cell transplantation (ASCT) using cells collected from peripheral blood and/or bone marrow has been studied in both first and second remissions. It is unclear as of this writing whether such an intensive consolidation therapy prolongs survival, although it does appear to increase the duration of remission. Future research needs to address issues of stem cell product contamination, molecular definition of remission, acute/chronic toxicities, and expense.

In summary, a standard treatment regimen in advanced low-grade lymphoma has not been established. Daily single-agent cyclophosphamide; daily or pulse chlorambucil; or combinations of cyclophosphamide, vincristine, prednisone with or without procarbazine, or doxorubicin (Adriamycin) are reasonable choices, depending upon the clinical circumstances. Enrollment in a protocol regimen is encouraged whenever possible because an optimal treatment regimen has not been identified.

Another management approach in patients with advanced low-grade non-Hodgkin's lymphomas is to defer initial treatment, instituting therapy when disease progresses. This approach is based on the premise that treatment at diagnosis does not appear curative. Many patients have indolent, slowly progressive disease, and deferral does not appear to compromise therapeutic outcome. Approximately one half of all patients may be eligible for such an approach at diagnosis; the median treatment-free period correlates with histology: more than 8 years for SLL, 5 years for FSCL, and 10 months for FML.

Biologic therapies have also been investigated in low-grade lymphomas and appear to have some efficacy. These include monoclonal antibody therapy directed specifically against the malignant B cell immunoglobulin idiotype or against B cell differentiation antigens, vaccine therapy using the idiotype as immunogen, and interferon-α.

In up to half of patients, low-grade lymphomas may change with or without treatment from an indolent to an aggressive form by the eighth year following diagnosis. Most often the transformation manifests as rapidly growing disease in one or more sites, while the low-grade component remains stable or progresses slowly. Pathologic study reveals DLCL, IBL, or other aggressive subtypes, and clonal analyses are consistent with the low-grade histology. Most transformations represent the emergence of an aggressive subclone from the original indolent disease, but some cases appear to represent the emergence of a completely new second neoplasm that is a clonally distinct, aggressive lymphoma.

Histologic transformation has prognostic and therapeutic implications. Median survival is less than 1 year following its emergence, and intensive treatment programs are necessary to gain disease control. Some patients appear to have the aggressive component eradicated by such measures, often with persistence or later relapse of the indolent histology.

INTERMEDIATE-GRADE AND HIGH-GRADE LYMPHOMAS. Combination chemotherapy is the mainstay of curative treatment in aggressive non-Hodgkin's lymphomas. This is because the intent and realistic goal of treatment are always cure, and relapse must be avoided whenever possible.

The expectation of cure in the majority of patients with aggressive lymphomas, regardless of stage, is based on the following observations in advanced disease: (1) Tumors are rapidly proliferating and initially very sensitive to combination chemotherapy. (2) Survival curves in advanced disease are biphasic, revealing a rapid death rate during the first 2 years (composed of partially responding and nonresponding patients) and then a plateau of cured cases (composed of complete responders). (3) With intensifying drug regimens, the proportion of complete responders may be increased and, similarly, the proportion cured. (4) Increasing tumor bulk correlates with decreased complete response, the emergence of drug resistance, and poor survival. (5) The highest complete response rates to combination chemotherapy are achieved in patients with regional or disseminated nonbulky disease.

Commonly used agents in combination regimens include cyclophosphamide, doxorubicin, vincristine, prednisone, methotrexate, bleomycin, etoposide, and cytosine arabinoside. Representative regimens are listed in Table 145–4. Treatment should be initiated promptly after diagnosis and appropriate noninvasive staging; the regimen must be intensive (leading to at least moderate toxicity), administered in high and often escalating doses on a rigorous schedule, and attention must be paid to rapidity of response and any evidence of early drug resistance. After a defined treatment course, complete restaging is undertaken. With these guidelines, at least 60% of patients with advanced disease and more than 80% with localized disease achieve complete response. Most complete re-

TABLE 145–4. REPRESENTATIVE DRUG COMBINATIONS FOR INTERMEDIATE- AND HIGH-GRADE NON-HODGKIN'S LYMPHOMAS

MACOP-B		
Methotrexate	400 mg/m² IV	Weeks 2, 6, 10 with leucovorin
Adriamycin (doxorubicin)	50 mg/m² IV	Weeks 1, 3, 5, 7, 9, 11
Cyclophosphamide	350 mg/m² IV	Weeks 1, 3, 5, 7, 9, 11
Oncovin (vincristine)	1.4 mg/m² IV	Weeks 2, 4, 6, 8, 10, 12
Prednisone	75 mg PO	Daily, dose tapered over the last 15 days
Bleomycin	10 U/m² IV	Weeks 4, 8, 12
Co-trimoxazole	2 tab PO	Twice daily throughout
ProMACE-CytaBOM (21-day cycles)		
Prednisone	60 mg/m² PO	Days 1–14
Adriamycin (doxorubicin)	25 mg/m² IV	Days 1 and 8
Cyclophosphamide	650 mg/m² IV	Day 1
Etoposide (VP-16)	120 mg/m² IV	Day 1
Cytarabine	300 mg/m² IV	Day 8
Bleomycin	5 mg/m² IV	Day 8
Oncovin (vincristine)	1.4 mg/m² IV	Day 8
Methotrexate	120 mg/m² IV	Day 8 with leucovorin
Co-trimoxazole	2 tab PO	Twice daily throughout
m-BACOD (28-day cycles)		
Methotrexate	200 mg/m² IV	Days 8 and 15 with leucovorin
Bleomycin	4 mg/m² IV	Day 1
Adriamycin (doxorubicin)	45 mg/m² IV	Day 1
Cyclophosphamide	600 mg/m² IV	Day 1
Oncovin (vincristine)	1 mg/m² IV	Day 1
Dexamethasone	6 mg/m² PO	Days 1–5
CHOP (21- to 28-day cycles)		
Cyclophosphamide	750 mg/m² IV	Day 1
Hydroxydaunomycin/ Adriamycin (doxorubicin)	50 mg/m² IV	Day 1
Oncovin	1.4 mg/m² IV	Day 1
Prednisone	100 mg PO	Days 1–5

IV = intravenous; PO = by mouth.

sponses (>70%) are durable, and maintenance chemotherapy is unnecessary.

A recently completed prospective study of these four standard chemotherapy regimens (Table 145–4) has demonstrated no significant differences in complete remission rate, remission durability, or survival. The drug regimen CHOP has become the gold standard by which newer therapies are judged. Identification of prognostic factors that may influence outcome is of increasing importance. The recently introduced International Prognostic Index uses clinical factors of age, performance status, stage, tumor bulk, and LDH level. Biologic factors may also be incorporated into future prognostic models, such as the presence of bcl-2 or bcl-6 oncogenes in intermediate-grade lymphomas or p53 mutations in low-grade lymphomas.

Autologous stem cell transplantation (ASCT) is the mainstay of second remission therapy in intermediate- and high-grade lymphomas. Its role in poor risk or slowly responsive initial therapy regimens is currently under investigation. At this time, ASCT is not a standard consolidation approach in first remission therapy.

SPECIAL CONSIDERATIONS. *Histopathologic Subtype.* Lymphoblastic lymphoma and SNCL are often treated with modified intensive drug programs, and all patients require central nervous system prophylaxis.

Mediastinal Disease. Superior vena cava syndrome may be present and is effectively managed with chemotherapy and/or irradiation. Biopsy of undetermined mediastinal masses must pay close attention to problems of airway compression during anesthesia and avoid whenever possible low-dose irradiation or steroid therapy prior to the procedure.

Gastrointestinal Disease. Perforation and/or bleeding may be complications prior to or following treatment. To avoid this, surgical resection of the involved segment is often recommended, prior to therapy. Gastric lymphomas, however, may often be treated with combination chemotherapy and/or irradiation regimens without the need for surgical resection.

Central Nervous System. All patients with lymphoblastic lymphoma and SNCL, as well as those with other aggressive histologic types and bone marrow involvement, are at risk for meningeal disease. Cerebrospinal fluid cytology is determined before therapy, and meningeal prophylaxis is given.

Primary brain lymphoma, as often identified in immunodeficient patients, requires high-dose whole-brain irradiation with or without chemotherapy.

Tumor Masses Larger than 10 cm. Supplementary irradiation is sometimes administered concurrently with or following chemotherapy. Residual fibrosis may occasionally persist after therapy. Surgical resection of tumor masses has been shown to be of value only with intra-abdominal Burkitt's lymphoma.

Tumor Lysis Syndrome. Rapid tumor shrinkage with excess urate production should be anticipated in all patients and allopurinol administered. With bulky or disseminated tumor or both, rapid cell lysis may lead to hyperkalemia, hypocalcemia, hyperphosphatemia, hyperuricemia, and acute renal failure. Patients with SNCL and lymphoblastic lymphoma are most often affected.

AIDS-Associated Lymphomas. The presence of immunodeficiency, multiple infections, and extranodal disease may make standard chemotherapy regimens excessively toxic and unsuccessful in this group of patients (see Color Plate 8E).

PROGNOSIS

The Working Formulation identifies more than 10 distinct disease entities and groups them according to prognosis. The survival curves upon which these prognostic groups were initially based are no longer entirely valid because of improved treatment methods. Nevertheless, it is still important to recognize a low-grade category in which the lymphoma progresses slowly and has an indolent natural history, as well as intermediate- and high-grade categories in which the disease presents aggressively, progresses rapidly, and, if unsuccessfully treated, is soon fatal.

In Figure 145–1A are the overall survival curves of the original Working Formulation (based on 1975 data) according to prognostic category. The median survivals are approximately 6½ years for the low-grade, 2½ years for the intermediate-grade, and 1½ years for the high-grade categories. Figure 145–1B illustrates representative

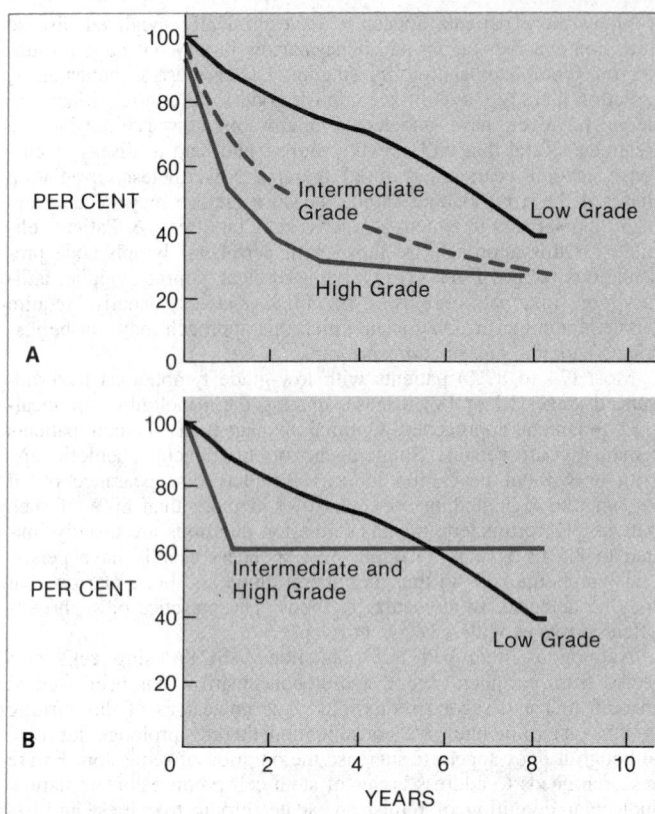

FIGURE 145–1. *A,* Actuarial survival according to histologic grade, based on 1975 data, as reported in the Working Formulation (1982). *B,* Hypothetical actuarial survival according to histologic grade, based on 1985 data (see text).

overall survival curves based on 1985 data, according to prognostic category. The median survival in the low-grade category is 6½ years, unchanged from the original Working Formulation, whereas the median survival for the intermediate- and high-grade categories has not yet been reached, and at least 60% of all patients remain alive and disease free at 5 years. Followed to 8 years, the curves overlap as patients in the low-grade category succumb to progressive lymphoma, while those in the intermediate- and high-grade categories continue to be disease free.

This, then, is the prognostic paradox of non-Hodgkin's lymphomas: Initially favorable, the low-grade histologic types become unfavorable with longer observation; and initially unfavorable intermediate- and high-grade histologic types become favorable because cure may be regularly achieved.

Armitage JO: Treatment of non-Hodgkin's lymphoma. N Engl J Med 328:1023, 1993. *A complete review of management approaches in non-Hodgkin's lymphomas.*

Fisher RI, Gaynor ER, Dahlberg S, et al.: Comparison of a standard regimen (CHOP) with three intensive chemotherapy regimens for advanced non-Hodgkin's lymphoma. N Engl J Med 328:1002, 1993. *A pivotal prospective study comparing four chemotherapy regimens for intermediate-grade non-Hodgkin's lymphomas.*

The International Non-Hodgkin's Lymphoma Prognostic Factors Project: A predictive model for aggressive non-Hodgkin's lymphoma. N Engl J Med 329:987, 1993. *A clinical prognostic factor index applied to intermediate-grade lymphomas.*

Knowles DM, Chamulak GA, Subar M, et al.: Lymphoid neoplasia associated with the acquired immunodeficiency syndrome (AIDS): The New York University Medical Center experience with 105 patients (1981–1986). Ann Intern Med 108:744, 1988. *A comprehensive study of the epidemiology, clinical features, and treatment outcome of 105 patients with AIDS-associated lymphomas.*

Magrath I: The pathogenesis of Burkitt's lymphoma. Adv Cancer Res 55:133, 1990. *A comprehensive review of the clinical, epidemiologic, and biologic features of Burkitt's lymphoma.*

The Non-Hodgkin's Lymphoma Pathologic Classification Project: National Cancer Institute sponsored study of classifications of non-Hodgkin's lymphomas: Summary and description of a working formulation for clinical usage. Cancer 49:2112, 1982. *The Working Formulation is presented in detail with pathologic and clinical analyses.*

Williams SF, Golomb HM (eds.): Non-Hodgkin's lymphoma. Semin Oncol 17:1, 1990. *A complete journal issue devoted to all aspects of non-Hodgkin's lymphomas: Pathology, basic science, clinical management, and complications of disease and therapy.*

146 HODGKIN'S DISEASE

Carol S. Portlock and
Joachim Yahalom

Hodgkin's disease, a distinct malignant disorder of the lymphatic system that primarily affects the lymph nodes, serves as a paradigm of the successful evolution of modern oncologic concepts. The management of Hodgkin's disease provides a multidisciplinary challenge, from an accurate diagnosis to a comprehensive staging evaluation and appropriate treatment recommendation. Particularly important is the collaboration between the medical and radiation oncologist because treatments often involve combined chemotherapy/irradiation strategies, and single-modality alternatives may affect future treatment options if relapse occurs. These complexities make the disease best treated by experienced multidisciplinary teams working in major medical centers.

EPIDEMIOLOGY AND ETIOLOGY

In the United States, approximately 7800 new cases of Hodgkin's disease are diagnosed annually. In contrast to the increasing incidence of non-Hodgkin's lymphoma, the annual incidence of Hodgkin's disease has remained stable over the past several decades. In developed western countries, the age-specific incidence of the disease is bimodal, with its greatest peak in the third decade of life and a second, smaller peak after age 50. The second peak is probably an artifact of histologic misclassification because recent studies have shown that many of the older-age cases originally diagnosed as Hodgkin's disease turned out to be non-Hodgkin's lymphomas. The age-specific incidence differs markedly in different countries. In Japan, where the overall incidence is low, no early peak exists. In some Third World countries the peak shifts into childhood. Hodgkin's disease is less common in African Americans, with a male to female ratio of 1.3 to 1.0.

Genetic factors appear to affect disease expression in Hodgkin's disease. Same-sex siblings have a 10 times greater risk of the disorder, and highly significant concordances of certain human leukocyte antigens (HLA) have been found among affected family members. Parent-child combinations have been more common than spouse pairing incidences, which possibly could reflect the influence of an infectious or environmental agent during childhood or early adolescence. Persons who grow up with few siblings, in single-family houses, who had early birth order and fewer playmates, show a higher risk of Hodgkin's disease. The incidence of clinical infectious mononucleosis is also associated with these factors; indeed, infectious mononucleosis becomes clinically detectable only after early childhood. Some believe that a viral infection at a certain age and host circumstances may induce a malignant transformation. For a short period, it was thought that Hodgkin's disease might be contagious because of reports of clustering, but that concern has been effectively dispelled.

In the past, because of the high incidence of tuberculosis in Hodgkin's disease, *Mycobacterium tuberculosis* was suspected to be the causative organism. More recently, the Epstein-Barr virus (EBV) has been implicated in epidemiologic and serologic studies. A small increase in incidence of Hodgkin's disease has been detected among patients with a history of infectious mononucleosis. More importantly, perhaps, the proportion of patients with Hodgkin's disease who possess high titers of antibody against the viral-capsid antigen of EBV was found to be larger than expected. Furthermore, enhanced activation of EBV was shown to precede the development of Hodgkin's disease. A variety of techniques have demonstrated that 50% or more of Hodgkin's biopsy specimens contain the EBV genome, that the EBV nucleic acid is localized to the Reed-Sternberg cell and its variants, and that the infected cells are monoclonal. These data suggest that EBV alone or with other carcinogens may contribute directly to the pathogenesis of Hodgkin's disease. Alternatively, it is possible that EBV is only a marker of a more fundamental disruption of the immune system of the host. Hodgkin's disease may represent a final common response to diverse pathologic processes such as viral infection, environmental or occupational exposures (e.g., woodworking), and a genetically determined host response.

PATHOLOGY

The diagnosis of Hodgkin's disease requires expert hematopathologic interpretation of a properly processed lymph node specimen. The Reed-Sternberg (R-S) cell is the diagnostic tumor cell that must be identified within the appropriate cellular milieu of lymphocytes, eosinophils, and histiocytes. Hodgkin's disease is unique pathologically because the tumor cells compose a minority of the cell population, whereas normal inflammatory cells are the major cell component. As a result, it sometimes may be difficult to identify the diagnostic R-S cells. Also, other lymphoproliferations may have cells that resemble R-S cells.

The R-S cell is characterized by its large size and classic binucleated structure with large eosinophilic nucleoli. R-S variants may have single nuclei, so-called popcorn cells and lacunar cells. The cellular origin of the R-S cell is uncertain. It has characteristics of both a macrophage and a lymphocyte, including the ability to phagocytose. Genetically the cell is hyperdiploid without recurring karyotypic abnormalities. As noted, the EBV genome has been identified in some specimens but is not consistently a feature. Two antigenic markers are thought to provide diagnostic information: CD-30 or Ber-H2 and CD-15 or Leu M-1. These reside on the R-S cells or their variants and not on the background inflammatory cells.

Hodgkin's disease has four histologic subtypes. Each is based upon the number and appearance of R-S cells as well as the background milieu. Lymphocyte-predominant Hodgkin's disease (LPHD) is a rare form of Hodgkin's disease in which few R-S cells may be identified. The cellular background consists primarily of lymphocytes in a diffuse or sometimes nodular pattern which may be mistaken for a low-grade non-Hodgkin's lymphoma. Unlike other histologic types of Hodgkin's disease, the lymphocytic infiltrate in LPHD is of B-cell polyclonal origin. This has led investigators to propose that LPHD is a non-Hodgkin's lymphoma unrelated to the other three histologic types of Hodgkin's disease. LPHD is more often clinically localized, usually effectively treated with irradiation alone, and may have late relapses (clinical features reminiscent of low-grade lymphoma).

Nodular sclerosing Hodgkin's disease (NSHD) is the most common subtype and typically affects young females with early-stage supradiaphragmatic presentations. The number of R-S cells is greater than in LPHD, and they may sometimes be found in clusters. The distinguishing feature is the presence of broad birefringent bands of collagen that divide the cellular process into macroscopic nodules. The tumors contain large numbers of T lymphocytes, eosinophils, neutrophils, and histiocytes. The so-called lacunar cell R-S variants often appear in the "cellular phase" of NSHD. Sclerosis is not a diagnostic feature limited to Hodgkin's disease. It may occur in non-Hodgkin's lymphomas as well, particularly those involving the mediastinum or retroperitoneum. The most difficult differential diagnosis pathologically is between NSHD and Ki-1 diffuse large cell lymphoma. Both entities may include sclerosis, large binucleated giant cells, and a T-cell lymphocytic infiltrate. Ki-1 lymphoma is a T-cell malignancy in which both the large and small cells are malignant. In such lymphomas, R-S–like cells are found that are CD30+ or Ber H-2–positive but CD15+ or Leu M-1–negative. Accurate pathologic diagnosis is critical because the two diseases often affect the same young, female population and present with large mediastinal masses, but treatment and prognosis may be decidedly different.

Mixed-cellularity Hodgkin's disease (MCHD) is the second most common histologic type. It is diagnosed more often in males, usually presents with generalized lymphadenopathy or with disease in extranodal sites, and produces associated systemic symptoms. R-S cells are frequently identified and bands of collagen are absent, although a fine reticular fibrosis may exist. The cellular background includes lymphocytes, eosinophils, neutrophils, and histiocytes.

Lymphocyte-depletion Hodgkin's disease (LDHD) is a rare disorder, particularly so because antigen marker studies have demonstrated that in the past many such cases were misdiagnosed as T-cell non-Hodgkin's lymphomas. R-S cells are numerous and may be pleomorphic, the cellular background is sparse, and diffuse fibrosis and necrosis may be present. This is the histologic subtype that may be associated with HIV infection and is most commonly diagnosed in elderly persons and in underdeveloped countries. By the time of diagnosis, affected patients usually have advanced-stage disease, extranodal involvement, an aggressive clinical course, and poor prognosis.

As a general rule, findings in extranodal tissues should not be used to diagnose Hodgkin's disease unless R-S cells are conclusively identified. Extranodal sites may contain noncaseating granulomas that are neither diagnostic of Hodgkin's nor connoters of active disease. Rather, granulomas appear to be a nonspecific finding in Hodgkin's disease which some experts believe may denote a favorable prognosis.

DIFFERENTIAL DIAGNOSIS

Hodgkin's disease is a lymph node–based malignancy and uniquely consists of lymphadenopathy in predictable clinical locations. More than 80% of patients present with lymphadenopathy above the diaphragm, often involving the anterior mediastinum; less than 10 to 20% present with lymphadenopathy limited to regions below the diaphragm. Therefore, the differential diagnosis is usually not that of generalized lymphadenopathy, but more commonly, that of regional lymphadenopathy in selected sites.

MEDIASTINAL PRESENTATIONS. Hodgkin's disease frequently affects the anterior mediastinum, and this may be the only site of involvement. In this location, the differential diagnosis is limited to neoplasms (Hodgkin's disease, aggressive non-Hodgkin's lymphomas, germ cell tumors, thymoma), infections (tuberculosis), and sarcoidosis. Hodgkin's disease is remarkably silent when it involves the mediastinal structures. Masses may reach a large size before patients complain of symptoms such as cough, wheeze, chest discomfort, or tightness. Unlike aggressive non-Hodgkin's lymphomas or other neoplasms, Hodgkin's disease rarely causes superior vena cava obstruction, phrenic nerve involvement with diaphragmatic paralysis, or laryngeal nerve compression and hoarseness. A common complaint of patients with large mediastinal masses due to Hodgkin's disease compressing the trachea is a cough or shortness of breath that intensifies when lying supine but is relieved by sitting upright.

REGIONAL LYMPH NODE PRESENTATIONS. Cervical, supraclavicular, axillary, or, uncommonly, inguinal lymphadenopathy may be the initial complaint. Lymph nodes that are unlikely to be involved with Hodgkin's disease at diagnosis include those in Waldeyer's tonsillar ring, as well as at preauricular, occipital, epitrochlear, posterior mediastinal, mesenteric, and popliteal sites. Involvement, if any, of these areas is more likely to occur in non-Hodgkin's lymphomas. In addition, retroperitoneal lymphadenopathy rarely occurs as the only site of Hodgkin's disease, but rather is accompanied by other supradiaphragmatic presentations and/or inguinal adenopathy. Many conditions can cause regional lymphadenopathy, including the following: infections with reactive lymphadenopathy (particularly frequent in the cervical and inguinal distributions); neoplasms (such as primary head and neck, lung or thyroid, breast, rectum); and autoimmune disorders. It is important to keep in mind that patients with lymphoma may develop superimposed regional reactive lymphadenopathy that may improve partially with a course of antibiotics. When residual lymphadenopathy persists, however, it deserves further investigation.

GENERALIZED LYMPH NODE PRESENTATIONS. Disseminated lymphadenopathy is infrequent in Hodgkin's disease. When present, it is usually associated with systemic symptoms and often extranodal involvement as well. This presentation is sufficiently uncommon that one must consider other causes of widespread lymphadenopathy: infections (viral, bacterial, fungal, mycobacterial), autoimmune disorders, HIV-associated lymphadenopathy, and non-Hodgkin's lymphomas.

EXTRANODAL INVOLVEMENT. Hodgkin's disease may affect extranodal tissues by direct invasion (contiguity), the so-called E-lesion, or by hematogenous dissemination, that is, stage IV disease. Isolated extranodal presentations (for example, cutaneous nodules or gastric involvement) without nodal involvement are generally absent and their presence usually denotes a non-Hodgkin's lymphoma except when associated with HIV disease. When extranodal involvement is suspected, one must also consider the possibility that the patient has an infection concurrent with regional Hodgkin's disease. Examples include patients who have bulky mediastinal involvement that produces tracheal or bronchial compression and an obstructive pneumonia as well.

Sites of extranodal involvement which suggest a diagnosis other than Hodgkin's disease include meninges, parenchymal brain involvement, nasal sinuses, lung lesions without mediastinal adenopathy, gastrointestinal tract invasion, ascites or mesenteric nodal disease, and genitourinary structures (kidney, bladder, testis, or ovary). All these areas are more commonly affected by a non-Hodgkin's lymphoma, other neoplasms, or infectious processes.

SYSTEMIC MANIFESTATIONS OF HODGKIN'S DISEASE. Occasionally patients come to attention because of systemic complaints or findings. These include chronic pruritus, which may be intense and produce destructive excoriation; systemic "B" symptoms of fever, night sweats, or weight loss; lymph node pain with alcohol consumption; an abnormal blood profile, such as leukocytosis with neutrophilia, eosinophilia, thrombocytosis; or rarely hypercalcemia, nephrotic syndrome, or pancytopenia with a fibrotic bone marrow and splenomegaly.

STAGING

The next step following the diagnosis of Hodgkin's disease is the staging process—the classification of the tumor according to its extent. Precise definition of the extent of nodal and extranodal involvement with Hodgkin's disease is made according to a standard staging classification system and is critical for selection of the proper treatment. Detailed documentation of the extent of disease also provides the baseline for evaluating the response to therapy and for monitoring potential relapse. Accurate delineation of disease sites is mandatory for the design of radiation therapy fields. The use of a standard staging system also allows comparison of the results of therapeutic interventions in different clinical trials.

The Ann Arbor staging classification has been the basis for treatment decisions for Hodgkin's disease patients since 1971. It was originally designed to distinguish patients who would benefit from extended-field radiation therapy from those who would require systemic chemotherapy. The staging system is an anatomic one and describes the sites of tumor in relation to the diaphragm. The anatomic regions for the staging of the disease are illustrated in Figure 146–1. The Ann Arbor staging classification has recently been revised at a meeting in Cotswolds, England. The most important contribution of the latter is the recognition of the importance of tumor bulk, adding a definition of bulky disease. The updated staging classification is detailed in Table 146–1.

The assignment of stage is based upon the number of sites of involvement, whether lymph nodes are involved on both sides of the diaphragm, whether this involvement is bulky (particularly in the mediastinum), whether there is contiguous extranodal involvement (E sites) or disseminated extranodal disease, and, additionally, whether typical systemic symptoms (B symptoms) are present. In defining a patient's stage, it is important to note how the information was obtained because this reflects on remaining uncertainties in the extent of disease evaluation. Clinical staging (CS) refers to information that has been obtained by initial biopsy, history and physical examination, and radiographic studies only. A pathologic stage (PS) is determined by more extensive surgical assessment of potentially involved sites, such as by surgical staging laparotomy and splenectomy. Table 146–2 outlines the staging evaluation.

HISTORY AND PHYSICAL EXAMINATION. The history should give special attention to the presence or absence of disease-associated symptoms, which may occur in up to one third of patients. These may include fever, night sweats, weight loss (B symptoms), pruritus, and, less commonly, pain in involved regions after ingestion of alcohol. In each anatomic stage, the presence of B symptoms is an adverse prognostic indicator that may affect the treatment choice. Unexplained fever should be significant (temperatures above 38° C) and recurrent during the previous month, night sweats should be drenching and recurrent, and unexplained weight loss is significant only if 10% of body weight is lost within the preceding 6 months. Although pruritus is no longer considered a B symptom, the presence of generalized itching is considered by many to be an adverse prognostic symptom. Certain combinations of B symptoms have been found to be more prognostically significant than others. For example, the combination of fever and weight loss has a more adverse prognosis than night sweats alone. B symp-

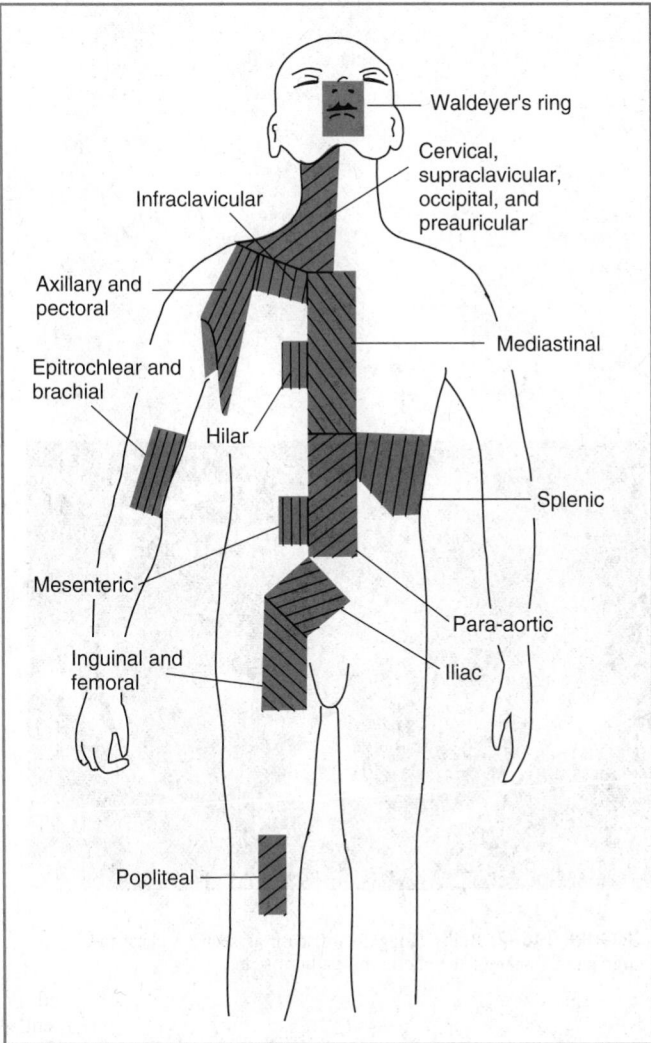

FIGURE 146–1. Anatomic definition of lymph node regions for staging of Hodgkin's disease. (From Kaplan HS, Rosenberg SA: The treatment of Hodgkin's disease. Med Clin North Am 50:1591, 1966.)

toms probably reflect end-product manifestation of cytokines produced by the tumor cells.

The physical examination should carefully determine the location and size of all palpable lymph nodes. An inspection of Waldeyer's ring, detection of splenomegaly or hepatomegaly, and evaluation of the cardiac and respiratory status are important.

LABORATORY STUDIES. The initial laboratory work should include a complete blood count with white cell differential and platelet count, an erythrocyte sedimentation rate (ESR), tests for liver and renal function, and assays for serum alkaline phosphatase and lactate dehydrogenase (LDH).

Mild to moderate anemia with normal indices of the type often found in patients with other malignancies or chronic disease may accompany Hodgkin's disease and does not necessarily indicate bone marrow involvement or hypersplenism. A moderate to marked leukemoid reaction and thrombocytosis are common, particularly in symptomatic patients, and usually disappear with treatment. Mild eosinophilia frequently exists, especially in patients with pruritus. Patients with advanced stage disease may show absolute lymphopenia (< 1000 cells per cubic millimeter), which usually denotes a poor prognostic sign. HIV-related Hodgkin's disease may present in this manner.

The ESR may provide helpful prognostic information. At some centers, treatment programs for patients with early-stage disease are influenced by the degree of ESR elevation. Changes in the ESR following therapy also may correlate with response and relapse. Other acute-phase reactants, such as serum copper, have been proposed as reliable nonspecific markers of disease activity but have shown no advantage over ESR.

TABLE 146–1. THE COTSWOLDS STAGING CLASSIFICATION FOR HODGKIN'S DISEASE

Stage I   Involvement of a single lymph node region or a lymphoid structure (e.g., spleen, thymus, Waldeyer's ring)

Stage II Involvement of two or more lymph node regions on the same side of the diaphragm (i.e., the mediastinum is a single site, hilar lymph nodes are lateralized). The number of anatomic sites should be indicated by a subscript (e.g., II_2).

Stage III Involvement of lymph node regions or structures on both sides of the diaphragm:
    III_1: With or without involvement of splenic, hilar, celiac, or portal nodes
    III_2: With involvement of para-aortic, iliac, or mesenteric nodes

Stage IV Involvement of extranodal site(s) beyond that designated E

Designations applicable to any disease stage
  A: No symptoms
  B: Fever, drenching sweats, weight loss
  X: Bulky disease:
    > 1/3 the width of the mediastinum
    > 10 cm maximal dimension of nodal mass
  E: Involvement of a single extranodal site, contiguous or proximal to a known nodal site
  CS: Clinical stage
  PS: Pathologic stage

Abnormalities of liver function studies should prompt further evaluation of that organ, with imaging and possible biopsy. An elevated alkaline phosphatase may be a nonspecific marker, but it also may indicate bone involvement that should be appropriately evaluated by a radionuclide bone scan and directed skeletal radiographs. An appreciably elevated LDH has been associated with a poor prognosis in some studies.

IMAGING STUDIES. Radiologic studies should include a chest radiograph and computed tomography (CT) scan of the chest, abdomen, and pelvis with intravenous contrast. In most patients a bipedal lymphogram and a gallium radionuclide scan provide important information and are highly recommended. Radionuclide bone scan, magnetic resonance imaging (MRI) of the chest or abdomen, and CT scan of the neck are contributory only under special circumstances.

The standard chest radiograph provides basic information regarding the extent of disease in the chest and offers a simple test for monitoring patients following treatment (Fig. 146–2). The thoracic CT scan details the status of intrathoracic lymph node groups, lung parenchyma, pericardium, pleura, and the chest wall. This additional information may alter the treatment recommendation in at least 10% of patients. The information obtained with chest CT also helps in the design of the radiation field and in assessing response.

TABLE 146–2. RECOMMENDED PROCEDURES IN STAGING HODGKIN'S DISEASE

1. Adequate surgical biopsy reviewed by an experienced pathologist
2. History and physical examination with particular attention to the presence and duration of B symptoms and pruritus
3. *Imaging studies*
  Plain chest radiograph
  CT scan of thorax
  CT scan of abdomen and pelvis
  Bipedal lymphography
  Gallium scan
4. *Hematologic studies*
  Complete blood count
  Erythrocyte sedimentation rate
  Bone marrow biopsy
5. *Biochemical studies*
  Liver function tests
  Renal function tests
  LDH, albumin, calcium
6. *Under special circumstances*
  Magnetic resonance imaging
  Technetium bone scan
  Percutaneous or laparoscopic liver biopsy
  Staging laparotomy

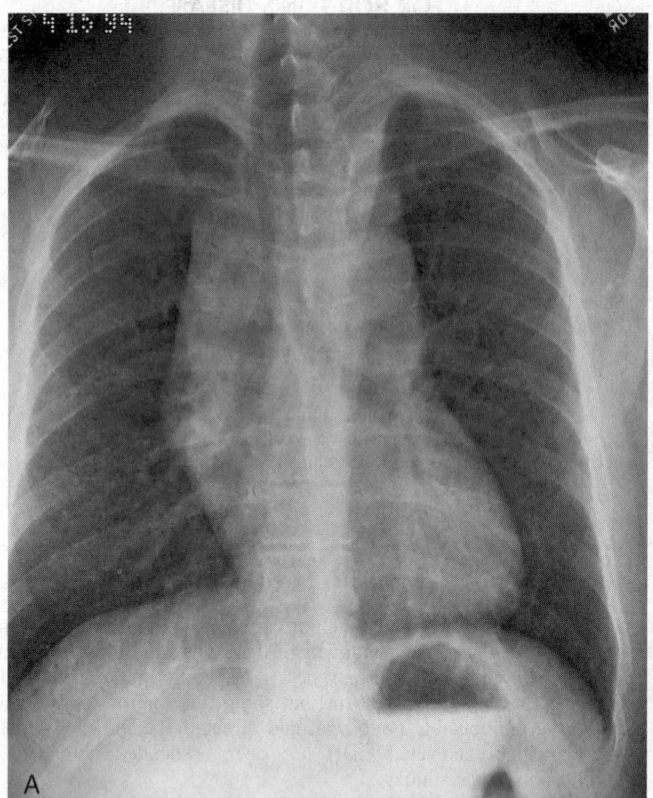

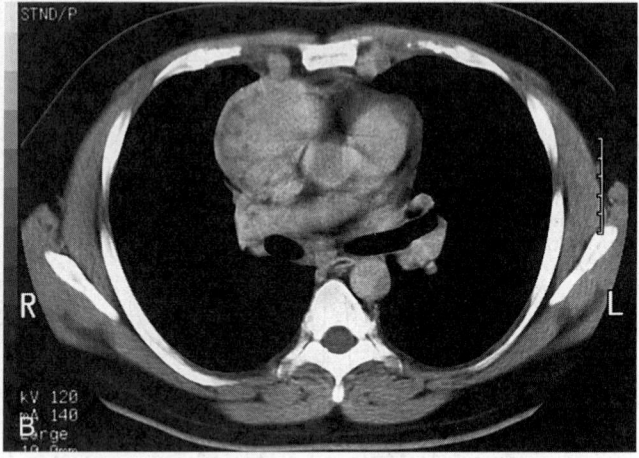

FIGURE 146–2. Bulky Hodgkin's disease as seen on chest radiograph, CT scan of the chest, and gallium scan.

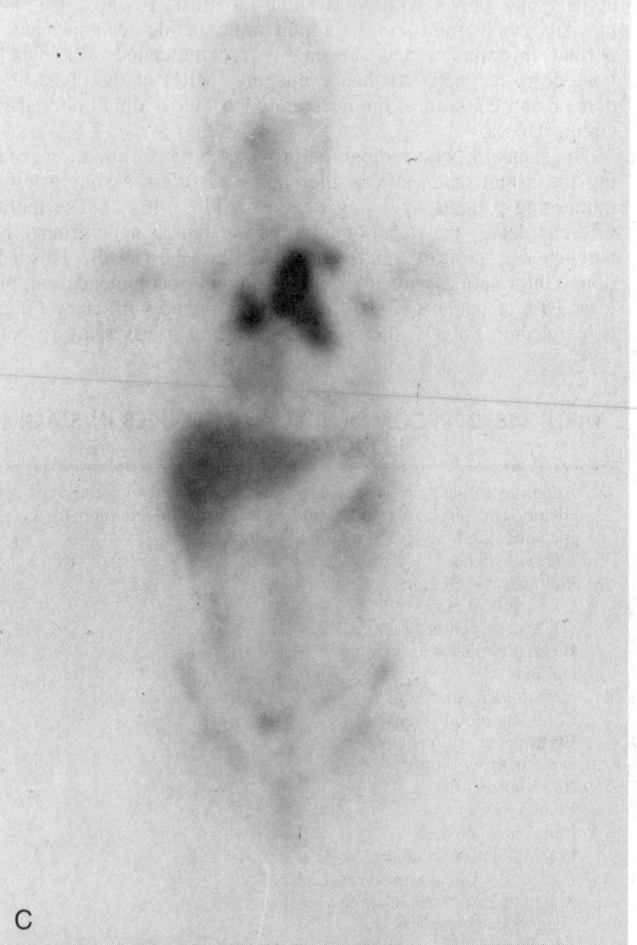

Because chest CT scans may remain abnormal long after completion of therapy, a gallium scan assists in the evaluation of pretreatment involvement and response to therapy. The gallium scan also may be a sensitive indicator of disease above the diaphragm, particularly when a dose of 10 mCi and a single photon emission CT (SPECT) technique are used. A negative gallium scan after completion of treatment supports the supposition that no active disease exists despite residual abnormality on the CT scan.

CT scans and bipedal lymphography provide the basic imaging studies for evaluation of the abdomen and pelvis. The lymphogram detects not only abnormal lymph node size but also abnormalities of internal lymph node architecture. The lymphogram is particularly accurate in evaluation of retroperitoneal and pelvic lymph nodes. In one large series, the overall accuracy of lymphography in identifying involved nodes was 92%. Lymphography also helps in designing radiation fields and assessing the response to therapy. The internal iliac, splenic hilar, porta hepatis, and mesenteric nodes are not opacified during lymphography and are best evaluated with a CT scan. Although the information from CT scan and lymphogram may be complementary, lymphograms are performed in only selected medical centers. As a result, CT scans have become the preferred study for the abdomen and pelvis in most institutions.

The current use of MR imaging is under study. MR imaging of the chest may help to differentiate residual fibrosis from active disease and to assess chest wall and pericardial invasion. So far MR imaging has been found to be of little advantage over CT scan in evaluating abdominal involvement. Radionuclide bone scans are appropriate for investigating the nature of bone pain or an elevated serum alkaline phosphatase. MR imaging may be a sensitive indicator of bone or bone marrow involvement.

BONE MARROW BIOPSY. Bone marrow involvement is relatively uncommon, but because of the impact of a positive biopsy on further staging and treatment, unilateral iliac crest bone marrow biopsy should be part of the staging process. Because the disease involves the marrow nonhomogeneously, single biopsies are not always adequate, and bilateral biopsies may be warranted in evaluating extent of disease in patients with widespread nodal disease or B symptoms.

STAGING LAPAROTOMY. Staging laparotomy is the most definitive method for detecting occult infradiaphragmatic Hodgkin's disease. A major problem with all imaging techniques for Hodgkin's disease is their inability to identify splenic involvement. In about one third of patients with normal-size spleens, Hodgkin's disease is found in the resected organ. Conversely, approximately half of patients found to have clinical or radiologic enlargement of the spleen do not have pathologic involvement of the removed organ. Staging laparotomy includes splenectomy and sampling of the splenic hilar, porta hepatis, para-aortic, and iliac nodes (with special attention given to areas that look suspicious on imaging studies). The procedure also samples the liver with a wedge and needle biopsy under direct vision and obtains open iliac crest bone marrow biopsy, if not performed previously. Areas of biopsy are marked with a clip, and an abdominal radiograph during or after laparotomy assists in verifying the removal of suspicious nodes shown by lymphography.

The complications of staging laparotomy include the nonspecific risks of general anesthesia and abdominal surgery. Reviews of laparotomy series report the risk of major postoperative complications to be 3 to 7%. Surgical mortality is rare (< 1%) and is absent from many large series. Because of occasional severe bacterial infections occurring after splenectomy, pneumococcal vaccine should be administered prior to staging laparotomy.

Laparotomy is not a routine staging procedure and should be considered only if the additional information may alter the choice of treatment. Thus, it is relevant only for patients who are potential candidates for radiation therapy alone. Although staging laparotomy remains the most precise way to determine the presence and extent of infradiaphragmatic Hodgkin's disease, it is currently used less frequently than in the past. This is because chemotherapy in many treatment plans has replaced localized radiation therapy. Furthermore, retrospective studies have provided data for determining the likelihood of infradiaphragmatic disease with different clinical presentations. Certain subgroups have < 10% risk of abdominal involvement. These include clinical stage I females, patients with involvement of the mediastinum alone, stage I males with lymphocyte-predominant histology, and young (< 27 years) females

with limited stage II disease. These patients may be treated with radiation therapy alone without a staging laparotomy.

TREATMENT

Over the last three decades, advances in radiation therapy and the development of effective combination chemotherapy have resulted in the cure of > 75% of all newly diagnosed patients with Hodgkin's disease. All patients, regardless of stage, can and should be treated with curative intent.

The stage of the disease is the most important determinant of treatment options and outcome. This makes precise definition of the extent of nodal and extranodal involvement during the staging critical for the selection of the proper treatment strategy. Hodgkin's disease is very sensitive to radiation and to many chemotherapy drugs; in most stages, more than one option provides effective treatment. Because most patients are expected to have a normal life expectancy, in designing new treatment programs particular attention must be paid to minimizing potential future toxicity. Any changes must be undertaken without compromising the excellent cure rates obtained by well-established therapies.

Effective treatment of Hodgkin's disease is complex, requiring the expertise of a multidisciplinary team consisting of a pathologist, diagnostic radiologist, and medical and radiation oncologists during staging of the disease and subsequent treatment. Because radiation plays an important role in the treatment, the use of a modern, high-quality radiation therapy facility staffed with an experienced team has been shown to bring about the best treatment results.

EARLY-STAGE DISEASE. The curative treatment of early stage Hodgkin's disease was established in the 1960's and 1970's using radiation alone, and this single modality remains the gold standard for the management of most patients with early-stage disease. In patients who were pathologically (laparotomy) staged and treated with primary irradiation alone, several large series reported a 15- to 20-year survival of nearly 90% and relapse-free survival rate of 75 to 80%. Most relapses (75%) occur within the first 3 years after completing therapy; late relapses are uncommon. It is important to note that more than half of the patients who relapse after radiation therapy alone are still curable with standard chemotherapy.

The standard approach in many United States centers has been to insist on a pathologic staging of the disease prior to recommending radiation therapy alone. This notion has been challenged by data from Canadian and European studies that show excellent overall survival results in patients selected for radiation therapy on the basis of clinical prognostic factors alone. Thus, treatment with radiation alone can be safely offered to clinically staged patients with favorable prognostic factors. With a clinical staging policy, however, more patients receive chemotherapy, either as initial or as salvage therapy.

An alternative treatment approach to early-stage disease is to use both radiation therapy and chemotherapy in selected patients. Combined-modality therapy reduces the relapse rate but in most studies does not change the overall survival rate while exposing all patients to the added toxicity of chemotherapy. New strategies that combine less intensive and less toxic chemotherapy regimens with radiation therapy to clinically involved sites are currently under evaluation. The preliminary data from several small studies are encouraging, but long-term results with these combined-modality programs are not yet available.

Early-stage patients with bulky mediastinal disease and significant B symptoms or clinically staged patients at high risk for subdiaphragmatic involvement (e.g., mixed cellularity or lymphocyte-depletion histology, age > 40) attain better relapse-free survival rates with combined-modality therapy than with radiation therapy alone. (Table 146–3 spells out the components of the acronym-designated chemotherapeutic regimens.)

Recently, two prospective randomized studies compared the efficacy of MOPP chemotherapy alone with radiation therapy alone in early-stage patients. Whereas a study from the National Cancer Institute (NCI) showed equivalent results for both modalities, other analyses found a significantly lower survival rate among patients treated with MOPP than among those treated with standard radiation therapy. Although other drug combinations such as ABVD may be more effective and less toxic than MOPP, they have not been

TABLE 146–3. COMBINATION CHEMOTHERAPY REGIMENS IN ADVANCED HODGKIN'S DISEASE

ABVD
Adriamycin (doxorubicin), 25 mg/m^2 IV
Bleomycin, 10 mg/m^2 IV
Vinblastine (Velban), 6 mg/m^2 IV
DTIC, 375 mg/m^2 IV
ABVD is repeated every 2 weeks; two treatments equal one cycle.

MOPP
Nitrogen mustard, 6 mg/m^2 IV days 1 and 8
Oncovin (vincristine) 1.4 mg/m^2 IV days 1 and 8
Procarbazine, 100 mg/m^2 PO days 1–14
Prednisone, 40 mg/m^2 PO days 1–14 (cycles 1 and 4 only)
MOPP is repeated every 28 days; each cycle is one 28-day course of therapy.

MOPP-ABVD
One 28-day cycle of MOPP with prednisone is alternated with one 28-day cycle of ABVD

MOPP-ABV hybrid
Nitrogen mustard, 6 mg/m^2 IV day 1
Oncovin (vincristine), 1.4 mg/m^2 IV day 1
Procarbazine, 100 mg/m^2 PO days 1–8
Prednisone, 40 mg/m^2 PO days 1–14
Adriamycin (doxorubicin), 35 mg/m^2 IV day 8
Bleomycin, 10 mg/m^2 IV day 8
Vinblastine, 6 mg/m^2 IV day 8
Pneumocystis carinii pneumonia prophylaxis is recommended with the hybrid regimen.

tested without irradiation in early-stage Hodgkin's disease and should not be used outside a controlled clinical trial.

RADIATION THERAPY. The cure of early-stage Hodgkin's disease with radiation alone became possible only after the recognition that all involved sites as well as adjacent nodal areas need to be treated with tumoricidal doses. Proper irradiation technique requires the use of linear accelerators that produce 6 to 10 megavolt photons. This degree of energy permits the exposure of large volumes to an adequate and homogeneous radiation dose with a modest degree of skin sparing. Treatment planning should be performed on a dedicated irradiation simulator that duplicates the features of the treatment unit. The plan itself is based on detailed imaging information that has been obtained during the staging process. The irradiation field is shaped to conform to the patient's anatomy and tumor configuration. Routine field verification (port films) is essential for controlling the proper delivery of treatment.

Successful therapy with radiation alone requires treatment of all clinically involved lymph nodes and all nodal and extranodal regions at risk for subclinical involvement. Certain standard large radiation therapy fields have been designed for the treatment of Hodgkin's disease. The fields are shaped to include multiple adjacent lymph node sites while accounting for normal tissue tolerance and the technical constraints of field size.

The classic irradiation fields are illustrated in Figure 146–3. The *mantle* irradiation field covers the lymph node areas above the diaphragm, including the submandibular, cervical, supraclavicular, infraclavicular, axillary, mediastinal, and hilar nodal areas. The *para-aortic* field includes the para-aortic lymph nodes from the diaphragm to the aortic bifurcation and the spleen or the splenic pedicle (after splenectomy). The *pelvic* field encompasses the iliac, inguinal, and femoral nodes. The *inverted-Y* field combines the para-aortic and pelvic fields. The term *total lymphoid irradiation* refers to treatment of all three fields. *Subtotal lymphoid irradiation* indicates treatment of the mantle and para-aortic fields only. To avoid excessive toxicity, the radiation fields are treated sequentially, the total dose is fractionated, and the irradiated volumes are carefully tailored with individualized divergent blocks. When patients require separate treatment to adjacent regions, the calculation of field separation is particularly important to avoid overlap at the spinal cord.

The dose required to eradicate Hodgkin's disease in demonstrably involved nodes is approximately 40 to 45 Gy (4000 to 4500 rad). A standard course of therapy with radiation alone includes treatment of the whole field to a total dose of 36 Gy (in 20 daily fractions of 1.8 Gy each, over a period of 4 weeks), with additional irradiation restricted to the clinically apparent disease sites of 4 to 9 Gy (1 Gy = 100 rad). A lower dose of radiation, in the range of 24 to 36 Gy, is used when irradiation is administered as adjuvant or consolidation treatment after chemotherapy. In such programs the radiation port may be limited to the clinically involved sites.

SIDE EFFECTS AND COMPLICATIONS OF RADIATION THERAPY. *Early Effects.* These depend on the irradiated volume, dose administered, and technique employed. They are also influenced by the extent and type of prior chemotherapy, if any, and by the patient's age.

The acute side effects of mantle field irradiation are usually mild and transient. They may include mouth dryness, change in taste, pharyngitis, nausea, dry cough, dermatitis, and fatigue. These side effects are managed symptomatically and subside gradually soon after the completion of radiation therapy. The main potential side effects of subdiaphragmatic irradiation are loss of appetite, nausea, and increase in bowel movements. These reactions are usually mild and can be minimized with standard antiemetic medications. Irradiation of more than one field, particularly after chemotherapy, can cause myelosuppression, and treatment delays may be required during therapy.

Six weeks to 3 months after completion of mantle therapy, approximately 15% of patients may develop Lhermitte's sign. Patients note an electric shock sensation radiating down the backs of both legs when the head is flexed. Lhermitte's sign may be secondary to transient demyelinization of the cervical spinal cord; it resolves spontaneously after a few months and is not associated with late or permanent cord damage. During the same period, radiation pneumonitis and/or acute pericarditis may occur in <5% of patients, more often in those who had extensive mediastinal disease. Both inflammatory processes have become rare with modern radiation techniques. Patients with Hodgkin's disease, regardless of treatment type, have a propensity to develop herpes zoster infection within 2 years after the onset of therapy. Usually the infection is confined to a single dermatome and is self-limited. If the cutaneous eruption is identified promptly, treatment with systemic acyclovir limits the duration and intensity of the infection.

Late Effects. Mantle field radiation therapy can induce subclinical hypothyroidism in about one third of patients. This is detected by elevation of the level of thyroid-stimulating hormone (TSH). Thyroid replacement with L-thyroxine is recommended, even for asymptomatic patients, to prevent the development of overt hypothyroidism and to decrease the risk of developing benign thyroid nodules. Irradiation of the pelvic field may have deleterious effects on fertility. In most patients this can be avoided by appropriate

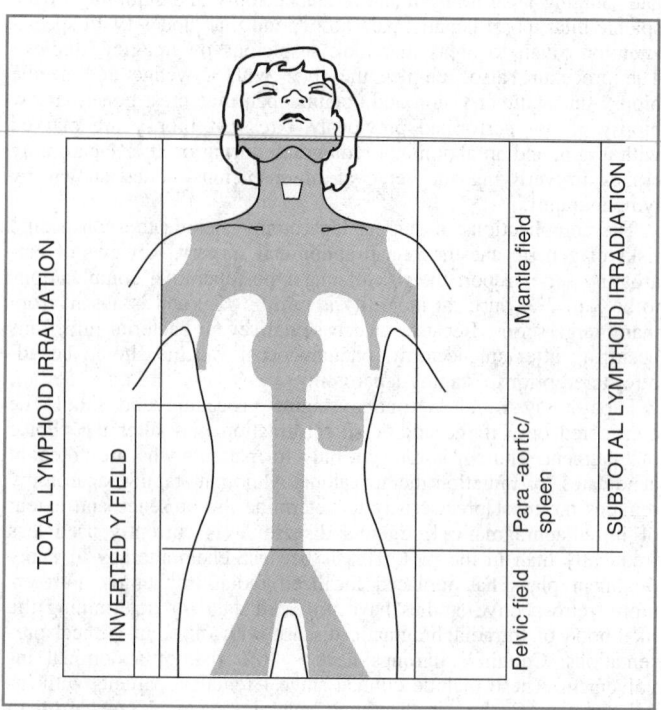

FIGURE 146–3. Standard radiation fields for Hodgkin's disease.

gonadal shielding. In females, the ovaries can be moved (oophoropexy) into a shielded area laterally or inferomedially near the uterine cervix. Irradiation of the mantle and para-aortic fields alone does not increase the risk of sterility.

Hodgkin's disease patients who were cured with radiation therapy and/or chemotherapy have an increased risk of developing secondary solid tumors and non-Hodgkin's lymphoma 10 or more years after treatment. Unlike MOPP and similar chemotherapy combinations, radiation therapy for Hodgkin's disease is not leukemogenic. The most frequent solid tumors reported after radiation therapy or chemotherapy for Hodgkin's disease are lung cancer, breast cancer, stomach cancer, and melanoma. Patients who are smokers should be strongly encouraged to eliminate the habit because the increase in lung cancer after irradiation or chemotherapy has been detected mostly in smokers. The increase in breast cancer risk is inversely related to the age at Hodgkin's disease treatment; in women irradiated after the age of 30 years, no increase in the risk of breast cancer has been found. Breast cancer is curable in its early stages, and early detection significantly improves survival. Breast examination should be part of the routine follow-up program for women cured of Hodgkin's disease, and routine mammography should begin about 8 years after treatment of Hodgkin's disease.

An increase in the risk of coronary artery disease has been reported for patients who have received mediastinal irradiation. To reduce this hazard, patients should be monitored and advised to avoid other established coronary disease risk factors such as smoking, hyperlipidemia, hypertension, and poor dietary and exercise habits. In children, high-dose irradiation affects bone and muscle growth and may result in deformities. Current programs for pediatric Hodgkin's disease are chemotherapy-based, and radiation therapy is limited to low doses.

ADVANCED-STAGE DISEASE. The mainstay of treatment in advanced Hodgkin's disease (stages IIIB and IV) is combination chemotherapy. Before embarking upon a therapeutic regimen, it is important to document carefully diagnosis, clinical or pathologic stage, and possible medical contraindications to systemic therapy. The possible side effects of the treatment plan should be outlined given the reasonable expectation of a curative outcome.

In selecting a combination chemotherapy regimen, it is important to evaluate the relative effectiveness, as well as potential acute and long-term side effects. Several combination chemotherapy regimens have been developed since their introduction in the 1960's and 1970's, but few studies have prospectively compared their efficacy. The most frequently used drug programs are listed in Table 146–3—MOPP, ABVD, MOPP-ABVD, and MOPP-ABV hybrid. MOPP and ABVD are considered non–cross-resistant drug regimens; alternating and hybrid regimens have been developed to take advantage of this characteristic. To date, none of these combination programs has been shown conclusively to be statistically superior in terms of remission rate, remission duration, or survival. In recently published, prospectively randomized studies, ABVD chemotherapy has been found to be at least as effective as MOPP and MOPP-ABVD; likewise, MOPP-ABV hybrid has been shown to be equivalent to MOPP-ABVD. Ongoing clinical trials will determine whether ABVD is also equivalent to MOPP-ABV hybrid.

Results of combination chemotherapy reveal a complete response rate of approximately 80%, a disease-free survival of 50 to 60%, and an overall survival of 40 to 50%. Adverse prognostic factors include the presence of systemic symptoms, tumor bulk, multiple extranodal sites, age >40 years, and male gender.

Strategies that increase the cure rate of advanced Hodgkin's disease include the following: The most important is to administer the planned drug regimen according to the dose and schedule of the empirically developed schema. Each drug was selected historically for its individual activity in Hodgkin's disease as well as for its relative lack of overlapping toxicity in the regimen. Retrospective analyses have demonstrated that the relative dose intensity (amount of drug per unit time) of the drug regimen correlates with treatment outcome. Another approach is to add regional irradiation as a consolidative local therapy after chemotherapy induction. This is routinely recommended when patients have bulky disease presentations (masses >10 cm) and often applied when residual masses remain following chemotherapy. Routine use of wide-field consolidative irradiation, either low dose or full dose, without these specific indications remains controversial, although retrospective studies and some prospective trials support this approach. Investigative strategies to

further increase the cure rate include the use of intensive combination chemotherapy with growth factor support and consolidative autologous stem cell transplantation in first clinical remission. These approaches have not yet proven to be superior to the standard drug regimens listed in Table 146–3.

When administering chemotherapy, one must pay attention to the rate of disease regression, remaining particularly alert to the rare situation in which response is sluggish (<50% tumor reduction in the first three cycles) or completely absent. In this setting one must seriously question the pathologic diagnosis (e.g., the disease may be a non-Hodgkin's lymphoma) or decide that the patient has primary refractory disease requiring a change in chemotherapy. In most patients, response is rapid, although a residual mass often persists at the completion of four to six cycles of chemotherapy. It is generally recommended to continue treatment for at least two cycles beyond a clinical complete remission. Measurement of response is accomplished by physical examination, chest radiography, CT scanning (when appropriate), and gallium scanning. If the response remains equivocal at the end of a chemotherapy regimen, it may be appropriate to evaluate the treatment effect with biopsy, particularly if there is residual gallium avidity.

TOXICITIES OF COMBINATION CHEMOTHERAPY. ABVD is a well-tolerated drug regimen whose major consistent toxicities include modest hair loss, fatigue, and myelosuppression (particularly neutropenia). Side effects in some patients include nausea and vomiting not completely controlled by the routine use of ondansetron or granisetron; bleomycin pulmonary toxicity (which must be monitored closely with diffusing capacity measures and drug discontinuance as soon as symptoms or a significant decrease in lung diffusion capacity is identified); vinblastine-associated peripheral or autonomic neuropathy; and symptomatic phlebitis. Rarely, patients may develop doxorubicin-induced cardiomyopathy or extravasation necrosis at injection sites.

In cancer centers, MOPP is used less frequently than ABVD because it is considered an equivalent drug program in terms of efficacy and has several less-acceptable side effects. These include greater myelosuppression (particularly thrombocytopenia); permanent infertility in most males and many older females; greater autonomic and peripheral neuropathy with vincristine; and, most importantly, the possible late toxicity of secondary myelodysplasia or acute myeloid leukemia in approximately 5% at 10 years. MOPP-ABV hybrid uses half the number of MOPP treatments and thereby reduces some of these risks. Nevertheless, one must still be concerned with permanent infertility and secondary blood dyscrasias. Secondary myelodysplasia or leukemia has been reported rarely after ABVD. However, an increased incidence of secondary solid tumors and non-Hodgkin's lymphoma has been detected in patients treated for Hodgkin's disease with any form of chemotherapy alone or with combined-modality therapy.

ABVD causes a transient azoospermia but not permanent infertility in men and only temporarily disrupts menstrual function in most women. Older women, however, may suffer permanent menopause or infertility. Because preservation of fertility is an important consideration in this young, potentially curable patient group, sperm banking should be recommended prior to chemotherapy. Many men have low sperm counts prior to any treatment as a result of chronic illness or general anesthesia. After ABVD or pelvic irradiation, counts generally recover within 1 to 2 years.

RELAPSED HODGKIN'S DISEASE. Hodgkin's disease may be cured even if the initial treatment fails. The choice of salvage approach depends on the history of prior treatments, considering the relapse sites as well as the patient's age and general medical condition.

For patients who relapse after radiation therapy, combination chemotherapy such as ABVD is the treatment of choice. If the relapse is regional and outside the prior irradiation field, involved or extended field irradiation may be added. The salvage rate in this group is excellent (10-year relapse-free survival of 50 to 60%). The most important prognostic factor following relapse after radiation therapy is the extent of disease at the time of relapse, emphasizing the importance of careful follow-up.

Standard-dose chemotherapy seldom salvages patients who fail to attain a complete response with chemotherapy or who relapse early after completion of combination chemotherapy (or combined modality therapy). High-dose chemotherapy accompanied by autologous stem cell transplantation (HD-ASCT) has become the preferred choice in this situation. A recent randomized study demonstrated the advantage of HD-ASCT over standard-dose salvage in refractory and relapsed patients. Results of transplantation are best in patients who have chemoresponsive disease at relapse, few prior therapies, and good performance status and lack bulky disease or bone/bone marrow involvement. Favorable patients have a curative potential of approximately 50 to 80% in most series. By contrast, only 10 to 30% of poor-risk patients remit and about 20% die of transplant complications. Carefully selected patients with a late first relapse (> 1 year after completion of standard-dose chemotherapy) may be salvaged with a second standard-dose combination chemotherapy, with or without involved field irradiation.

HD-ASCT is a cumbersome, toxic, and expensive process, making it important to identify proper candidates accurately. All should have histologic proof of active Hodgkin's disease at relapse because residual masses are common and may not represent active tumor. Consolidation HD-ASCT is not recommended in first remission. There is no standard reinduction chemotherapy at relapse, and it may include drugs used at initial therapy or new agents. The most commonly used HD-ASCT conditioning regimen is CBV (cyclophosphamide, BCNU, and VP-16). Other combinations also have demonstrated efficacy, and some programs also incorporate standard involved-field or intensive large-field radiation therapy. The autologous stem cell product may be provided from the patient's own bone marrow and/or peripheral blood with hematopoietic growth factor support.

SPECIAL CIRCUMSTANCES. *Pregnancy* may complicate the initial or relapse management of Hodgkin's disease. When the pregnancy is first diagnosed, it is important to clinically stage the patient by history and physical examination, single posteroanterior chest radiograph, ultrasonography, MRI or CT scan of the abdomen and pelvis, and bone marrow biopsy. In recommending medical management, one must keep in mind that Hodgkin's disease is often an indolent tumor and may be clinically silent or asymptomatic for many months. For that reason, it may be possible to monitor a patient and defer treatment during the pregnancy. If treatment is indicated, options include involved field irradiation with shielding of the pregnant uterus, single-agent chemotherapy such as vinblastine, or even combination chemotherapy. Treatment selection depends upon disease sites at risk, age and size of the developing fetus, tumor bulk, patient symptomatology, and predicted delivery date. Rarely it may be necessary to consider therapeutic abortion if the diagnosis of Hodgkin's disease in advanced symptomatic stage is made early in the pregnancy.

Pediatric Hodgkin's disease is unusual, and no large clinical trials exist that address all therapeutic questions. Special considerations surround the pediatric age group: bone growth, the asplenic state, and future infertility. To avoid these complications, most pediatric patients are treated without staging laparotomy to avoid splenectomy. Chemotherapy regimens use ABVD, MOPP-ABV, or its variants, and consolidative irradiation (when utilized) is administered in low dose and with attention to the treatment portals (encompassing the entire growing bone, rather than just a segment).

HIV-associated Hodgkin's disease is much less frequent than non-Hodgkin's lymphoma; the most important consideration is to establish an accurate diagnosis. The pathology of HIV-associated Hodgkin's disease has a sparse cellular background, a more pleomorphic histologic appearance, and an aggressive clinical course. Clinical staging often reveals more advanced disease than in non-HIV patients, and extranodal involvement is more frequent. It is important to distinguish between Hodgkin's disease and infectious causes of apparent extranodal involvement (such as pulmonary nodules) prior to determining a final treatment plan.

Staging laparotomy is generally not justified in HIV-affected patients. Primary irradiation, based on clinical stage, with or without adjuvant chemotherapy is appropriate for early-stage presentations; chemotherapy alone, with or without consolidative irradiation, is given in advanced disease. ABVD is a suitable combination regimen but may need to be modified to avoid bleomycin pulmonary toxicity. *Pneumocystis carinii* pneumonia prophylaxis should be instituted routinely. Zidovudine or other HIV antiviral treatment is generally not administered during chemotherapy. These patients

TABLE 146–4. RECOMMENDED FOLLOW-UP IN TREATED HODGKIN'S DISEASE

1. **End of therapy**
   Repeat all studies initially positive for baseline. If suspicious, consider biopsy.
2. **0 to 3 years following therapy**
   Visits: Every 3 to 4 months
   Imaging: Chest radiography each visit, unless CT chest obtained
        CT chest every 6 months × 2, then yearly
        CT abdomen and pelvis yearly
   Laboratory: With each visit: CBC, platelets, ESR
        Liver and renal function
        LDH
        Every 6 months: TSH
3. **3 to 5 years following therapy**
   Visits: Every 6 months
   Imaging: Chest radiography each visit, unless CT chest obtained
        CT chest, abdomen, pelvis yearly
   Laboratory: As in 2
4. **More than 5 years following therapy**
   Visits: Yearly
   Imaging: Chest radiography; CT only as indicated
   Laboratory: As in 2
5. **Other considerations, as indicated**
   Mammography
   Lipid profile
   Pulmonary function studies
   Echocardiography
   Hormone replacement if menopausal

should be approached whenever possible with curative intent. Primary Hodgkin's disease regimens are not so immunosuppressive as to be contraindicated except in unusual circumstances.

TREATMENT RECOMMENDATIONS

After an accurate histologic diagnosis and staging, the following general guidelines may be used in recommending therapy. For clinical stage I and IIA good-risk patients with a low likelihood of abdominal involvement, primary irradiation without staging laparotomy is appropriate. Combined-modality therapy (ABVD plus extended field irradiation) is a less acceptable alternative because it exposes patients to the toxicities of both modalities in a low-risk setting.

For clinical stage I and IIA or B, moderate-risk (see above) patients in whom the risk for abdominal involvement is > 10%, primary irradiation remains appropriate therapy but requires staging laparotomy to confirm pathologic stage I or II disease. Patients with pathologic stage III$_1$ A with minimal splenic involvement are also candidates for radiation therapy alone. An acceptable alternative in many patients is to use combined modality therapy (ABVD or MOPP-ABV hybrid plus extended-field irradiation).

For bulky early-stage presentations, clinical stage Ix or IIx disease, combined-modality therapy is essential. The choice of combination chemotherapy regimen is discussed above; usually this is ABVD or MOPP-ABV hybrid. Following successful induction of complete clinical remission, extended-field consolidation should be administered.

For clinical stage IIIA patients, combination chemotherapy (ABVD or MOPP-ABV hybrid) is usually used in conjunction with extended-field irradiation.

For advanced-stage disease (IIIB and IV), combination chemotherapy alone (ABVD or MOPP-ABV hybrid) or combined with involved- or extended-field irradiation is recommended.

Follow-up studies for successfully treated patients are listed in Table 146–4.

Bierman PJ, Armitage JO: Role of autotransplantation in Hodgkin's disease. Hematol/Oncol Clin North Am 3:591, 1993. *A comprehensive review of high-dose therapy with stem-cell transplant in Hodgkin's disease.*

Canellos GP, Anderson JR, Propert KJ et al.: Chemotherapy of advanced Hodgkin's disease with MOPP, ABVD, or MOPP alternating with ABVD. N Engl J Med 327:1478, 1992. *A prospective randomized trial demonstrating the value of doxorubicin-containing regimens.*

Glaser SL, Swartz WG: Time trends in Hodgkin's disease incidence: The role of diagnostic accuracy. Cancer 66:2196, 1990. *This analysis demonstrates a statistical decline in Hodgkin's disease incidence in older adults due to changes in pathologic diagnosis.*

Gospodarowicz MK, Sutcliffe SB, Clark RM: Analysis of supradiaphragmatic clinical stage I and II Hodgkin's disease treated with radiation alone. Int J Radiation Oncol Biol Phys 22:859, 1992. *The experience of using radiation alone to treat early-stage, pathologically staged patients.*

Leibenhaut M, Hoppe RT, Efron B et al.: Prognostic indicators of laparotomy findings in clinical stage I-II supradiaphragmatic Hodgkin's disease. J Clin Oncol 7:81, 1989. *An analysis of staging laparotomy information indicating that pathologic staging provides some subgroups with only minimal benefit.*

Lister TA, Crowther D, Sutcliffe SB et al.: Report of a committee convened to discuss the evaluation and staging of patients with Hodgkin's disease: The Cotswolds meeting. J Clin Oncol. 7:1630, 1989. *A clarification of the clinical and pathologic staging system for Hodgkin's disease, with practical examples.*

Mauch PM: Controversies in the management of early stage Hodgkin's disease. Blood 83:318, 1994. *A comprehensive review expanding upon staging treatment options and potential toxicities of therapy in early-stage Hodgkin's disease.*

Swerdlow AJ, Douglas AJ, Vaughan Hudson G, et al.: Risk of secondary primary cancers after Hodgkin's disease by type of treatment: Analysis of 2846 patients in the British National Lymphoma Investigation. Br Med J 304:1137, 1992. *One of the largest studies evaluating the risk of secondary malignancies after curative Hodgkin's disease therapy.*

Urba WT, Longo DL: Hodgkin's disease. N Engl J Med 326:678, 1992. *A comprehensive review of all clinical aspects, including chemotherapy in early-stage Hodgkin's disease.*

Young RC, Bookman MA, Longo DL: Late complications of Hodgkin's disease management. J Natl Cancer Inst Monogr 10:55, 1990. *An excellent overview of late treatment side effects (surgical staging, radiation therapy, and/or chemotherapy).*

147 LANGERHANS CELL (EOSINOPHILIC) GRANULOMATOSIS

Diane M. Komp

The term *Langerhans cell histiocytosis* (LCH) includes a group of proliferative disorders that affect children more commonly than adults. In all age groups, the diseases attack more males than females. Histiocytosis X was an earlier, now obsolete, classification for these granulomas that included, among other conditions, the syndromes of *Letterer-Siwe disease,* a frequently fatal disorder affecting the skin and multiple other organs of young children, and *Hand-Schüller-Christian disease,* a triad of calvarial bone defects, diabetes insipidus, and exophthalmos. Currently, LCH abnormalities are classified into *unifocal* and *multifocal eosinophilic granulomas;* they are not to be confused with the leukocytic eosinophilic syndromes discussed in Ch. 148. The multifocal forms are more common among children, sometimes taking on a malignant form. Unifocal eosinophilic adenomas arise at any age as solitary lesions in osseous structures and take a benign course. This section discusses both forms, primarily as they affect adults.

PATHOPHYSIOLOGY. The Langerhans cells originate from dendritic histiocytes that belong to the general class of bone marrow–generated phagocytes. The cell is characterized microscopically by cytoplasmic Birbeck granules. Langerhans' histiocytes normally reside primarily in the skin and to a lesser degree in other body organs, where they serve as accessory immune cells, being HLA-DR positive and expressing the CD1 antigen. Irritating stimuli such as smoking can induce relatively benign proliferation of Langerhans' cells in the lung. The factors that sometimes lead them, along with eosinophils and other marrow-engendered cells, to form enlarging nodular granulomas (eosinophilic granulomas) remain unknown, but a dysimmune response is suspected. Although LCH is characterized by pathologically bland cells that appear to be benign, lesional cells may exhibit clonality. A few reports suggest that LCH or subtypes of LCH occasionally may be malignant disorders, but this has not been well established.

PULMONARY INVOLVEMENT. Pure pulmonary histiocytosis, a rare disorder in children, represents an important clinical problem in adults, especially young males. Typically, multifocal LCH begins in the lung parenchyma and progresses to a stage of interstitial thickening that is represented radiographically by a reticulonodular pattern affecting predominantly mid- and basal areas of the lungs. As the proliferative-destructive process continues, a typical honeycomb pattern emerges that can predispose to restrictive lung disease, spontaneous pneumothorax., and, eventually, chronic cor pulmonale. Lung biopsy is diagnostic.

Cigarette smoking importantly contributes to pulmonary eosinophilic granulomatous disease. Electron microscopy or immunochemical methods can demonstrate typical Langerhans cells in the absence of granulomas in bronchoalveolar fluid after the inhalation of cigarette smoke. Stimulation of pulmonary LCH by smoking provides the only etiologic clue for any of the eosinophilic granulomatous disorders. The role of passive smoking in the onset of LCH in children and young adults is under epidemiologic investigation.

BONE LESIONS. Langerhans cell eosinophilic granulomas involving bone may be unifocal or multifocal. Unifocal granulomas affect males more than females and predominate in children. Solitary bone lesions in adults most often affect a rib but can involve the mandible, vertebral bodies, or pelvis. Some lesions remain asymptomatic, although local pain and swelling usually occur. Extensive and recurrent involvement of the mandible is particularly disturbing. Such lesions usually infiltrate the dental apices, eroding the lamina dura of surrounding teeth. Panoramic plain films have been the standard method for demonstration of these lesions, but newer computed tomography (CT) methods ("Dentascan") provide a more sensitive method for monitoring this anatomic area.

Vertebral granulomas can present a special problem of diagnosis and therapy among older persons, in whom LCH is uncommon. Direct removal is difficult because of the danger of vertebral collapse, but diagnosis usually is possible using CT-monitored stereotaxic needle aspiration. When lymphoma is a strong consideration, bone marrow aspiration and biopsy may be a safer first step. Spinal cord compression from extraosseous extension is unusual but should be considered strongly in patients who show leg weakness or sensory loss. Emergency corticosteroid and/or radiation therapy may be required in such instances; decompressive surgery seldom is necessary (see Ch. 441). In patients with pathognomonic radiographic lesions, immediate therapy may take precedence over pathologic documentation.

Radionuclide scans are used to determine whether one or more than one bone lesion exists and for follow-up searches for new disease. Bone scans alone, however, identify only a minority of lesions. Because the granulomas tend to be highly osteolytic with delayed repair, radioscintillation uptake identifies only 35% of lesions, with another 11% appearing as a cold spot. In non–weight bearing bones, open biopsy is the preferred diagnostic test. The insertion of bone chip fillings at the time of biopsy almost always heals the lesion. Inaccessible lesions are best treated by low-dose local supervoltage irradiation.

ENDOCRINE MANIFESTATIONS. Solitary basal skull eosinophilic granulomas rarely impair hypothalamic-pituitary function; most such associated neuroendocrine abnormalities accompany the multifocal forms of the disease. Characteristically, skull lesions involve the calvarium, sphenoid bones, sella turcica, and mandible. Lesions of the long bones of the upper extremity sometimes accompany the skull granulomas. Bone changes usually appear and progress for many years before endocrine symptoms arise. Often, permanent damage predates actual diagnosis. Complications of skull lesions include chronic otitis media, proptosis, and other deformities of the bone. Pituitary-hypothalamic damage by LCH most often produces temporary or permanent diabetes insipidus (DI); all persons developing unexplained DI deserve a careful search for LCH. Hypothalamic impairment in children can result in precocious puberty, infertility, or growth hormone deficiency. Accompanying granulomas may affect liver, spleen, lymph nodes, and skin. Gadolinium-enhanced magnetic resonance imaging is the most sensitive method to detect LCH in the pituitary-hypothalamic area. Transnasal biopsy can confirm the diagnosis of solitary granulomas occupying the region.

ASSOCIATION WITH MALIGNANCY. The presence of Langerhans' cells in pathologic material does not necessarily indicate a diagnosis of LCH. Especially in adults, Langerhans' cells may accompany true malignancies, particularly breast cancer and lymphoma. Nonmalignant LCH proliferation may precede or follow a diagnosis of leukemia or lymphoma.

TREATMENT. LCH occasionally undergoes spontaneous resolution. Such disappearances are particularly true of bony disease and complicate the analysis of clinical treatment trials. Milder chemotherapeutic agents such as vinblastine, 6-mercaptopurine, and methotrexate are used singly or in combination with corticosteroids. Recent evidence indicates that the morbidity of chronic disease may be avoided by the early use of VP 16 in multiorgan disease; some authorities have suggested, however, that VP 16 may induce non-lymphocytic leukemia. Corticosteroids play an important role in systemic treatment. Intralesional steroid injection is an important but little-known treatment for single bone lesions, particularly those of the mandible.

Earlier enthusiasm for immunotherapeutic agents has waned. Currently, cyclosporine is attracting attention as a potentially useful agent for aggressive, multinodular disease. To date, bone marrow transplantation cannot be recommended as an established method of treatment. Nevertheless, the results in a few treated patients with debilitating chronic multiosseous disease have been encouraging. In a handful of children who received liver transplants for life-threatening cirrhosis, active LCH in bones and skin improved when cyclosporine was used to prevent graft rejection.

Ben-Ezra JM, Koo CE: Langerhans' cells histiocytosis and malignancies of the M-PIRE system. Am J Clin Pathol 99:464, 1993. *Discusses the immunology of Langerhans cells.*

Bom LP: Langerhans Cell Histiocytosis. The Hague, CIP-Gegevens Koninklijke Bibliotheek, 1994.

Broadbent V, Gadner H, Komp DM, et al.: Histiocytosis syndromes in children. II. Approach to the clinical and laboratory evaluation of children with Langerhans cell histiocytosis. Med Pediatr Oncol 17:492, 1989.

Egeler RM, Neglia JP, Pucetti DM, et al.: Association of Langerhans cell histiocytosis with malignant neoplasms. Cancer 71:865, 1993. *A careful discussion addresses LCH as a primary or secondary response.*

Komp DM: Concepts in staging and clinical studies for treatment of Langerhans' cell histiocytosis. Semin Oncol 18:18, 1991. *A good review of therapy for these disorders.*

148 EOSINOPHILIC SYNDROMES
Peter F. Weller

Eosinophilia, often with heightened production of eosinophils as well as increased blood and tissue eosinophil accumulations, is associated with distinctive disease processes that include helminthic parasitic infections, allergic diseases, and a diversity of diseases of often ill-defined causes. Several eosinophil-related diseases are discussed in other chapters. This chapter provides an overview on eosinophils as a distinct class of leukocytes and considers the variety of diseases associated with eosinophilia.

STRUCTURE OF EOSINOPHILS. Eosinophils are distinguished from other leukocytes by their morphologies, constituents, products, and associations with specific diseases. Eosinophils are produced in the bone marrow. The cytokine interleukin 5, which specifically promotes the development and terminal differentiation of eosinophils, is principally responsible for increases in eosinophilopoiesis. Eosinophils normally dwell primarily in tissues, especially in tissues with an epithelial interface with the environment, including the respiratory, gastrointestinal, and lower genitourinary tracts. The lifespan of eosinophils, longer than that of neutrophils, may extend for weeks within tissues. Eosinophils usually possess bilobed nuclei and are morphologically characterized by their cytoplasmic granules. Specific granules, the most numerous of several types of cytoplasmic granules, have unique crystalloid cores and contain eosinophil-specific cationic proteins. These proteins bind acidic dyes such as eosin and are responsible both for the tinctorial properties and for many of the functional properties of eosinophils. The four eosinophil cationic proteins are major basic protein, eosinophil peroxidase, eosinophil cationic protein, and eosinophil-derived neurotoxin. Lysophospholipase, another predominant eosinophil protein, forms bipyramidal Charcot-Leyden crystals, often found in sputum, feces, and tissues as a hallmark of eosinophil-related diseases. In addition to their content of preformed granule proteins, eosinophils also elaborate newly synthesized lipid mediators, including the 5-lipoxygenase pathway–derived eicosanoid, leukotriene C_4, and platelet-activating factor.

FUNCTION OF EOSINOPHILS. Eosinophils serve several immunologic functions. They are capable of phagocytosing and killing bacteria and other small microbes. *In vivo*, however, eosinophils do not have a major role in host defense against such microbial pathogens and cannot constitute an effective defense against bacterial infections when neutrophil function is deficient. Rather, eosinophils primarily defend against large, nonphagocytosable organisms, most notably the multicellular, helminthic parasites, utilizing several mechanisms, including their cytotoxic cationic granule proteins. In allergic diseases, including asthma, eosinophils elaborate specific lipid mediators, leukotriene C_4 and platelet-activating factor. These can contract airway smooth muscle, promote mucus secretion, alter vascular permeability, and elicit eosinophil and neutrophil infiltration. Eosinophils also can stimulate mast cells and basophils to release allergic mediators. Some of the mechanisms beneficial in the eosinophils' role in host defense can prove detrimental to the host. Released eosinophil cationic proteins are toxic to host cells and may contribute to the pathogenesis of diseases in which heightened numbers of eosinophils are found within involved tissues. The effector functions of mature eosinophils can be stimulated by cytokines, including interleukin 5 and granulocyte-macrophage colony–stimulating factor. Additional immunologic functions, based on the eosinophil's capabilities to release cytokines and interact collaboratively with lymphocytes and other cells, are being defined. Such steps may add to our understanding of how eosinophils participate in normal mucosal immune responses and in eosinophil-related diseases.

Blood eosinophil numbers do not always reflect the extent of eosinophil involvement in disease-affected tissues. Eosinophils usually number less than 450 per microliter in the blood, and vary diurnally, being higher in the early morning and falling as endogenous glucocorticosteroid levels rise. Eosinopenia occurs with corticosteroid administration and also with active bacterial and viral infections. Some patients with sustained blood eosinophilia develop organ damage, especially cardiac damage, as found in the idiopathic hypereosinophilic syndrome. The genesis of sustained eosinophilia in some patients but not others is unclear. It suggests that some other activating events, as yet ill-defined, promote eosinophil-mediated tissue damage in the face of eosinophilia. Patients with sustained eosinophilia should be monitored for evidence of cardiac disease (see below).

DISEASE ASSOCIATED WITH EOSINOPHILIA (Table 148–1)

PARASITIC DISEASES. Eosinophilia is not elicited by infections with single-celled protozoan parasites (with the exception of the intestinal parasites *Isospora belli* and *Dientamoeba fragilis*), but rather by the multicellular helminthic parasites. The level of eosinophilia tends to parallel the magnitude and extent of tissue invasion, especially by larvae. Eosinophilia may be absent in established infections that are well contained within tissues or are solely intraluminal in the gastrointestinal tract (e.g., *Ascaris*, tapeworms). Even with helminthic diseases, superimposed bacterial infections (e.g., in disseminated strongyloidiasis) can suppress eosinophilia. In evaluating a patient with unexplained eosinophilia, geographic and dietary histories may indicate potential exposures to helminthic parasites. The stool should be examined for diagnostic ova and larvae, although with some infections more than the usual three examinations may be needed. In addition, for a number of the helminthic parasites that cause eosinophilia, diagnostic parasite stages never appear in feces. Hence, normal stool examinations do not necessarily exclude a helminthic cause for eosinophilia, and examination of appropriate blood or tissue biopsy specimens as guided by the clinical findings and exposure histories, may be needed. Specific tissue or blood-dwelling infections capable of causing eosinophilia include trichinosis, strongyloidiasis, filarial infections, and, in children, visceral larva migrans.

OTHER INFECTIOUS DISEASES. Two fungal diseases may be associated with eosinophilia: aspergillosis, but only in the form of allergic bronchopulmonary aspergillosis and not as invasive disease and coccidioidomycosis, following primary infection, especially in conjunction with erythema nodosum, and at times with progressive disseminated disease.

ALLERGIC DISEASES. These diseases, including allergic rhinitis and asthma, are discussed elsewhere (see Ch. 225 and 51). Hypersensitivity drug reactions can elicit eosinophilia, not necessarily accompanied by other manifestations, such as drug fever or or-

TABLE 148-1. DISEASES ASSOCIATED WITH EOSINOPHILIA

I. Infectious diseases
  A. Tissue-invasive helminth infection
    1. Principally outside North America
      a. Filariasis (especially in those from nonendemic regions)
      b. Schistosomiasis, acute and chronic
      c. Fascioliasis, acute
      d. Paragonimiasis
      e. Clonorchiasis
      f. Echinococcosis (often absent unless cyst fluid leakage)
    2. Indigenous to North America and other regions
      a. Trichinosis
      b. Toxocariasis (visceral larva migrans)
      c. Strongyloidiasis (may be suppressed with sepsis in hyperinfection syndrome)
      d. Ascariasis and hookworm disease (especially with early lung and tissue invasive stages)
  B. Other infections
    1. Coccidioidomycosis (acute and less commonly chronic)
    2. Bronchopulmonary aspergillosis
    3. Afebrile tuberculosis
    4. Convalescent phase of some infections, especially scarlet fever
    5. Chlamydial pneumonia of infancy
II. Allergic diseases
  A. Allergic rhinitis
  B. Asthma
  C. Atopic dermatitis
  D. Acute urticaria
  E. Hypersensitivity drug reactions
III. Myeloproliferative and neoplastic diseases
  A. Idiopathic hypereosinophilic syndrome
  B. Solid tumors, principally of mucin-secreting, epithelial cell origin, when metastatic to serosa or bone
  C. Lymphoid
    1. Lymphomas, especially T cell type and Hodgkin's disease
    2. Acute lymphoblastic leukemia, only uncommonly
    3. Occasionally with myeloma (heavy-chain disease)
  D. Myelogenous
    1. Eosinophilic leukemia—rare
    2. Chronic myelogenous leukemia
    3. Acute myelogenous leukemia, with some subtypes
  E. Other
    1. Angioimmunoblastic lymphadenopathy
    2. Histiocytosis with cutaneous involvement
    3. Angiolymphoid hyperplasia (Kimura's disease)

IV. Other cutaneous diseases
  A. Bullous pemphigoid
  B. Herpes gestationis
  C. Scabies
  D. Eosinophilic cellulitis (Well's disease)
  E. Episodic angioedema with eosinophilia
  F. Pruritic urticarial papules and plaques of pregnancy
V. Other pulmonary diseases
  A. Transient pulmonary eosinophilic infiltrates (Löffler's syndrome)
  B. Hypersensitivity pneumonitis
  C. Allergic bronchopulmonary aspergillosis
  D. Tropical pulmonary eosinophilia
  E. Eosinophilic pneumonia—acute and chronic
VI. Connective tissue diseases
  A. Vasculitis
    1. Allergic granulomatosis with angiitis (Churg-Strauss syndrome)
    2. Hypersensitivity vasculitis
  B. Rheumatoid arthritis (severe)
  C. Eosinophilic fasciitis
VII. Immunodeficiency diseases
  A. Hyper-IgE syndrome
  B. Wiskott-Aldrich syndrome
  C. Nezelof's syndrome with thymic dysplasia and increased IgE
  D. Selective IgA deficiency, when associated with increased IgE
  E. Graft-versus-host reactions
VIII. Gastrointestinal diseases
  A. Eosinophilic gastroenteritis
  B. Inflammatory bowel disease
IX. Occasional causes of eosinophilia
  A. Cholesterol embolization
  B. Long-term peritoneal dialysis
  C. Postirradiation
  D. Hypoadrenocorticosteroidism: Addison's disease, hypopituitarism
  E. Other localized disorders with occasional blood eosinophilia
    1. Eosinophilic lymphadenitis
    2. Eosinophilic cystitis
    3. Eosinophilic cholecystitis
    4. Eosinophilic meningitis
  F. Toxic: L-tryptophan, toxic oil syndrome (Spain)

gan dysfunction. When organ dysfunction develops, the drug must be stopped. Drug-induced interstitial nephritis (see Ch. 80) may be accompanied by blood eosinophilia, and eosinophils may be found in the urine.

MYELOPROLIFERATIVE DISEASES. The idiopathic hypereosinophilic syndrome is a leukoproliferative disease characterized by sustained overproduction of eosinophils. The three diagnostic criteria for this disorder are (1) eosinophilia in excess of 1500 per microliter of blood persisting for longer than 6 months, (2) lack of an identifiable parasitic, allergic, or other etiologic cause for eosinophilia; and (3) signs and symptoms of organ involvement. Not all patients with prolonged eosinophilia develop organ involvement, and many have benign courses. Moreover, the above diagnostic criteria are sufficiently broad to include eosinophilic disorders of other currently unrecognized etiologies, that may have more favorable courses. The presence of angioedema represents a good prognostic sign in hypereosinophilic patients. The finding may be related to the more recent identification of a distinct clinical syndrome of recurrent episodic angioedema with eosinophilia, not complicated by hypereosinophilic cardiac disease. The clinical signs and symptoms of the hypereosinophilic syndrome can be heterogeneous because of the diversity of potential organ involvement. One of the most serious and more frequent complications is cardiac disease due to endomyocardial thrombosis and fibrosis. Chordae tendineae may sustain progressive fibrotic damage, leading to mitral and tricuspid regurgitation and congestive heart failure from valvular incompetence and endomyocardial fibrosis. Echocardiography can facilitate detection and monitoring of these changes. Neurologic involvement can take three forms: embolic disease originating from the heart, diffuse encephalopathy, and peripheral neuropathy, especially mononeuritis multiplex. Other organ systems that can be in-

volved include the skin, liver, spleen, gastrointestinal tract, and lungs. For patients with prominent organ involvement and no therapy, mortality is about 75% after 3 years. Therapy is aimed at suppressing eosinophilia and is initiated with corticosteroids, which induce remission in about one third of patients. In those unresponsive to corticosteroids, hydroxyurea may be beneficial. For those unresponsive to or intolerant of hydroxyurea, vincristine or chlorambucil, alone or with lower doses of hydroxyurea, can control the disease. Cardiac involvement similar to that seen in the hypereosinophilic syndrome, which may require surgical valve replacement, may occur rarely with eosinophilias of other causes, including parasitic infections. A pathologically similar disease, Löffler's endocarditis and endomyocardial fibrosis, occurs in tropical regions, where antecedent parasite-elicited eosinophilias likely are responsible.

NEOPLASTIC DISEASES. Eosinophilic leukemia is uncommon. Eosinophilia may accompany chronic myelogenous leukemia (often with basophilia) and some subtypes of acute myelogenous leukemia but is uncommon with acute lymphoblastic leukemia. A minority of patients with Hodgkin's disease have elevated blood eosinophil levels, occasionally to high values. Increases in marrow and lymph node eosinophilia are more common. A small proportion of patients with carcinomas, especially those of mucin-producing epithelial cell origins, have associated blood eosinophilia. About a third of patients with angioimmunoblastic lymphadenopathy have eosinophilia. Eosinophilia may accompany mycosis fungoides, Sézary's syndrome, and lymphomatoid papulosis.

CUTANEOUS DISEASES. In addition to the neoplastic involvement of skin noted above, a number of cutaneous diseases can be associated with eosinophilia, including scabies, bullous pemphigoid, and two diseases associated with pregnancy, herpes gestationis and the syndrome of pruritic urticarial papules and plaques of pregnancy. In episodic angioedema with eosinophilia, recurrences are marked by blood eosinophilia; at times with significant weight gain from fluid retention; and less frequently by fever. The entity responds to corticosteroids.

PULMONARY EOSINOPHILIAS. These are discussed in Ch. 54 and 149.

GASTROINTESTINAL DISEASES. Eosinophilic gastroenteritis (see Ch. 98) and inflammatory bowel diseases (see Ch. 104) are considered elsewhere. Although eosinophils are present in the lesions of ulcerative colitis, on occasion increased blood eosinophilia can accompany both ulcerative colitis and Crohn's disease.

IMMUNE DISEASES. Of the various forms of vasculitis (see Ch. 243), only two are commonly associated with eosinophilia: hypersensitivity vasculitis and allergic granulomatous angiitis, the Churg-Strauss syndrome, in which asthma, eosinophilia, and pulmonary and neurologic involvement are frequent. Cholesterol embolization is at times associated with eosinophilia and hypocomplementemia, suggesting a secondarily elicited immunologic component. Some primary immunodeficiency syndromes are associated with eosinophilia, either commonly with the hyperimmunoglobulin E (IgE) syndrome, the Wiskott-Aldrich syndrome, and graft-versus-host disease or more selectively with Nezelof's syndrome and selective immunoglobulin A (IgA) deficiency when these are accompanied by increased levels of IgE. Eosinophilic fasciitis (see Ch. 456) and rheumatoid arthritis (see Ch. 237) are considered elsewhere. Eosinophilia may uncommonly accompany rheumatoid arthritis itself but is more commonly due to treatment medications.

OTHER DISEASES. Irritation of serosal surfaces can be associated with eosinophilia, e.g., Dressler's syndrome, eosinophilic pleural effusions, peritoneal and, at times, blood eosinophilia that develops during chronic peritoneal dialysis, and perhaps the eosinophilia that follows abdominal irradiation. Two notable apparently toxic diseases, the eosinophilia-myalgia syndrome due to contaminated L-tryptophan and the earlier toxic oil syndrome in Spain, were prominently associated with eosinophilia. Loss of normal adrenoglucocorticosteroid production in Addison's disease, adrenal hemorrhage, or hypopituitarism can cause modest eosinophilia (see Ch. 207).

Weller PF: Eosinophilia in travelers. Med Clin North Am 76:1413, 1992. *Considers the parasitic diseases associated with eosinophilia.*

Weller PF: The immunobiology of eosinophils. N Engl J Med 324:1110, 1991. *A brief review of the structure and immunologic functions of eosinophilic leukocytes.*

Weller PF, Bubley GJ: The idiopathic hypereosinophilic syndrome. Blood 83:2759, 1994. *Reviews the etiology, manifestations, differential diagnosis, therapy, and prognosis of the idiopathic hypereosinophilic syndrome.*

149 PLASMA CELL DISORDERS
Robert A. Kyle

The plasma cell disorders are a group of neoplastic or potentially neoplastic diseases associated with proliferation of a single clone of immunoglobulin-secreting plasma cells derived from the B cell series of immunocytes. This group of disorders has been referred to as monoclonal gammopathies, immunoglobulinopathies, paraproteinemias, and dysproteinemias.

The plasma cell disorders are characterized by the secretion of electrophoretically and immunologically homogeneous (monoclonal) proteins. Each monoclonal protein (M-protein, myeloma protein, or paraprotein) consists of two heavy (H) polypeptide chains of the same class and subclass and two light (L) polypeptide chains of the same type (see Fig. 221-2). The heavy polypeptide chains are designated by Greek letters: γ in immunoglobulin G (IgG), α in immunoglobulin A (IgA), μ in immunoglobulin M (IgM), δ in immunoglobulin D (IgD), and ϵ in immunoglobulin E (IgE). The subclasses of IgG are IgG1, IgG2, IgG3, and IgG4. There are two subclasses of IgA—IgA1 and IgA2. No subclasses of IgM, IgD, or IgE have been recognized. The light-chain types are kappa (κ) and lambda (λ). Both heavy chains and light chains have "constant" and "variable" regions with respect to amino acid sequence. Class specificity of each immunoglobulin is defined by a series of antigenic determinants on the constant regions of the heavy chains (γ, α, μ, δ, and ϵ) and the two major classes of light chains (κ and λ). The amino acid sequence in the variable regions of the immunoglobulin molecule corresponds to the active antigen-combining site of the antibody, whereas the constant regions convey other biologic properties (see Ch. 221).

RECOGNITION OF MONOCLONAL PROTEINS

Electrophoresis with cellulose acetate membrane is satisfactory for screening. High-resolution agarose gel electrophoresis is more sensitive for the detection of small monoclonal proteins. Immunoelectrophoresis or immunofixation with agarose gel or both should be used to confirm the presence of a monoclonal protein and to distinguish the immunoglobulin class and its light-chain type.

Analysis of Serum for Protein

Serum protein electrophoresis should be done when multiple myeloma, macroglobulinemia, or amyloidosis is suspected. Electrophoresis is also indicated with unexplained weakness or fatigue, anemia, back pain, osteoporosis, osteolytic lesions or spontaneous fracture, elevation of the erythrocyte sedimentation rate, hypercalcemia, Bence Jones proteinuria, renal insufficiency, immunoglobulin deficiency, or recurrent infections. It should also be performed in adults with sensorimotor peripheral neuropathy, carpal tunnel syndrome, refractory congestive heart failure, nephrotic syndrome, orthostatic hypotension, or malabsorption, because a spike or localized band is strongly suggestive of primary systemic amyloidosis (AL).

A monoclonal protein (M-protein) is usually seen as a narrow peak (like a church spire) in the densitometer tracing or as a dense, discrete band on the cellulose acetate membrane (Fig. 149-1A). Although the immunoglobulins (IgG, IgA, IgM, IgD, and IgE) compose the gamma component, they are also found in the β-γ or β region, and IgG may actually extend to the α_2-globulin area. Consequently, an IgG M-protein may range from the slow gamma (cathode) to the α_2-globulin region. In contrast, an excess of polyclonal immunoglobulins (having one or more heavy-chain types and both κ and λ light chains) produces a broad-based peak or broad band. It is usually limited to the γ region (Fig. 149-1B). It is important to differentiate between an M-protein and a polyclonal increase because the former is associated with a malignant process or a potentially neoplastic condition, whereas a polyclonal increase in immunoglobulins is associated with a reactive or inflammatory process. In 2 to 3 percent of sera with a monoclonal peak, there is an additional M-protein of a different immunoglobulin class. This condition is designated as a biclonal (double) gammopathy.

The presence of an M-protein is most suggestive of monoclonal gammopathy of undetermined significance (MGUS), multiple myeloma, primary amyloidosis, Waldenström's macroglobulinemia, or other lymphoproliferative disease. Rarely, other conditions may also simulate the presence of an M-protein in the serum, e.g., free hemoglobin-haptoglobin complexes resulting from hemolysis, large amounts of transferrin in patients with iron deficiency anemia, or the presence of fibrinogen. On the other hand, an M-protein may appear as a rather broad band on the cellulose acetate membrane or as a broad peak in the densitometer tracing, owing to the complexing of an M-protein with other plasma components or aggregates of IgG, polymers of IgA, or dimers of IgM.

An M-protein can be present when the total protein concentration, β and γ globulin levels, and quantitative immunoglobulin values are all within normal limits. A small M-protein may be concealed in the normal β or γ areas and may be overlooked. In addition, the presence of a monoclonal light chain (Bence Jones proteinemia) is rarely seen in the cellulose acetate tracing. In the heavy-chain diseases, the M-component is usually not apparent. Immunoelectrophoresis, a useful technique for identifying an M-protein, should be performed when a peak or band is seen in the cellulose acetate tracing or when multiple myeloma or related disorders are suspected (Fig. 149-2). Immunofixation, which is more sensitive, is useful when results of immunoelectrophoresis are equivocal or when one is searching for a small M-protein in primary amyloidosis, solitary plasmacytoma, or extramedullary plasmacytoma, or after successful treatment of multiple myeloma or macroglobulinemia.

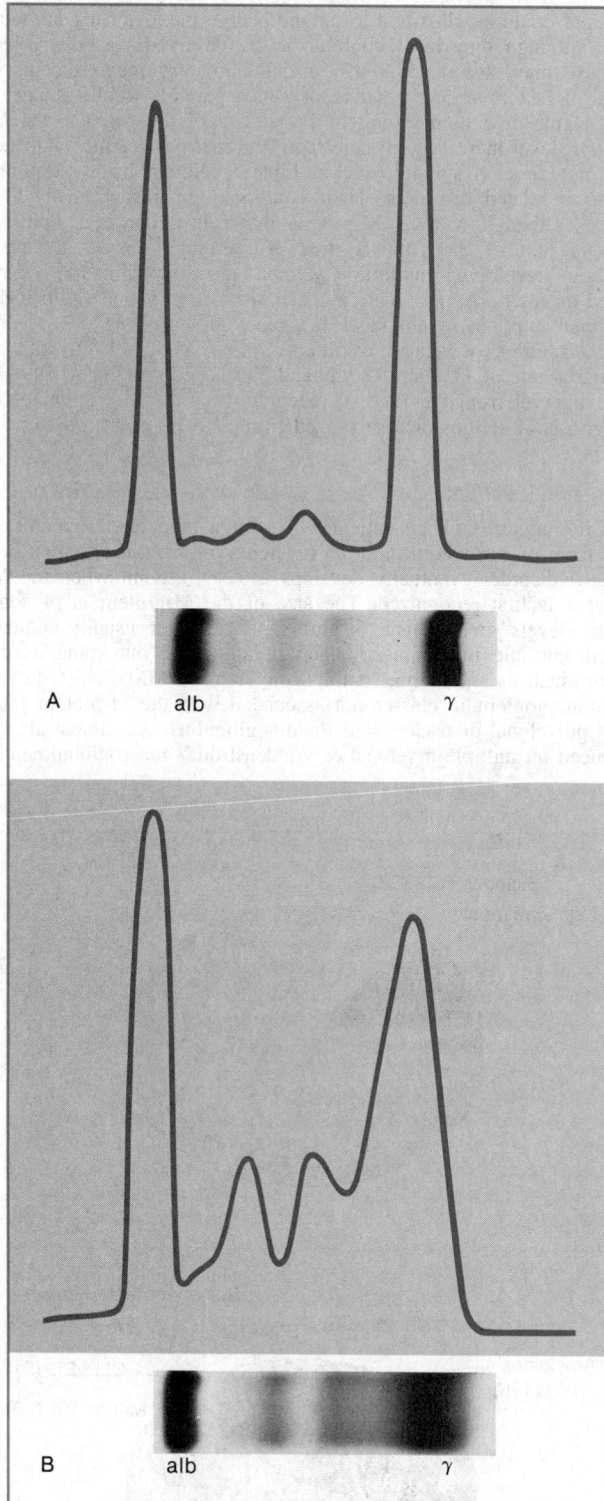

FIGURE 149–1. *A, top,* Monoclonal pattern of serum protein from densitometer tracing after electrophoresis on cellulose acetate (anode on left): tall, narrow-based peak of γ mobility. *Bottom,* Monoclonal pattern from electrophoresis of serum on cellulose acetate (anode on left): dense, localized band representing monoclonal protein in γ area. *B, top,* Polyclonal pattern of serum protein from densitometer tracing after electrophoresis on cellulose acetate (anode on left): broad-based peak of γ mobility. *Bottom,* Polyclonal pattern from electrophoresis of serum on cellulose acetate (anode on left): γ band is broad. *(A and B from Kyle RA, Garton JP: Laboratory monitoring of myeloma proteins. Semin Oncol 13:310, 1986.)*

Quantitation of Immunoglobulins

This procedure is more useful than immunoelectrophoresis or immunofixation for the detection of hypogammaglobulinemia. Quantitation can be performed by radial immunodiffusion, but this is tedious and subject to spurious abnormalities. Rate nephelometry is

the preferred method. The degree of turbidity produced by antigen-antibody interaction is measured by nephelometry in the near-ultraviolet region.

Serum Viscometry

Serum viscometry should be measured when the IgM monoclonal level is more than 3 grams per deciliter, when the IgA or IgG value is more than 4 grams per deciliter, or when the patient has oronasal bleeding, blurred vision, or other symptoms suggestive of a hyperviscosity syndrome.

Analysis of Urine

Dipstick tests are used in many laboratories to screen for protein, but unfortunately they are often insensitive to Bence Jones protein. Consequently, sulfosalicylic acid or Exton's reagent is best for the detection of protein.

Screening tests for Bence Jones proteins (monoclonal light chain in the urine) that utilize their unique thermal properties are not recommended because of their serious shortcomings. Immunoelectrophoresis or immunofixation of an adequately concentrated 24-hour urine specimen reliably detects Bence Jones protein. An M-protein appears as a dense, localized band on the cellulose acetate strip or a tall, narrow, homogeneous peak in the densitometer tracing, and its amount can be calculated on the basis of the size of the spike and the amount of total protein in the 24-hour specimen. It is not uncommon to have a negative reaction for protein and no obvious spike on electrophoresis and yet for immunoelectrophoresis or immunofixation of a concentrated urine specimen to show a monoclonal light chain. Immunoelectrophoresis or immunofixation should also be done on the urine of every adult older than 40 who develops a nephrotic syndrome of unknown cause. The presence of a monoclonal light chain in a nephrotic urine is strongly suggestive of primary amyloidosis. The differential diagnosis of an M-protein in the serum or urine is given in Table 149–1.

Kyle RA: The monoclonal gammopathies. Clin Chem 40:2154, 1994.
Kyle RA, Garton JP: Laboratory monitoring of myeloma proteins. Semin Oncol 13:310, 1986. *A guide for analysis of serum and urine for monoclonal proteins, with many illustrations of immunoelectrophoresis and immunofixation.*

MONOCLONAL GAMMOPATHY OF UNDETERMINED SIGNIFICANCE (MGUS)

The term "monoclonal gammopathy of undetermined significance" (MGUS) (benign monoclonal gammopathy) denotes the presence of an M-protein in persons without evidence of multiple myeloma, macroglobulinemia, amyloidosis, or other related diseases. The term "benign monoclonal gammopathy" is misleading because at diagnosis it is not known whether a process producing

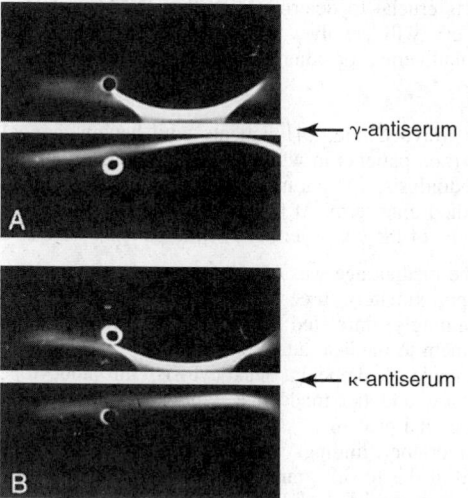

FIGURE 149–2. Immunoelectrophoretic pattern of serum. *A, top,* Antiserum to IgG (γ) shows a thickened arc. *B, top,* Antiserum to κ chains shows a thickened arc similar to the IgG arc. *A and B, bottom,* Antiserum to γ and to κ chains shows a faint normal arc. Patient's serum contains a monoclonal IgG κ protein. *(From Kyle RA, Greipp PR: 3. The laboratory investigation of monoclonal gammopathies. Mayo Clin Proc 53:719, 1978. By permission of Mayo Foundation for Medical Education and Research.)*

TABLE 149–1. CLASSIFICATION OF PLASMA CELL PROLIFERATIVE DISORDERS

I. Monoclonal gammopathies of undetermined significance (MGUS)
   A. Benign (IgG, IgA, IgD, IgM, and, rarely, free light chains)
   B. Associated neoplasms or other diseases not known to produce monoclonal proteins
   C. Biclonal gammopathies
   D. Idiopathic Bence Jones proteinuria
II. Malignant monoclonal gammopathies
   A. Multiple myeloma (IgG, IgA, IgD, IgE, and free light chains)
      1. Overt multiple myeloma
      2. Smoldering multiple myeloma
      3. Plasma cell leukemia
      4. Nonsecretory myeloma
      5. IgD myeloma
      6. Osteosclerotic myeloma (POEMS syndrome)
      7. Solitary plasmacytoma of bone
      8. Extramedullary plasmacytoma
   B. Waldenström's macroglobulinemia
      1. Other lymphoproliferative diseases
III. Heavy-chain diseases (HCD's)
   A. γ HCD
   B. α HCD
   C. μ HCD
IV. Cryoglobulinemia
V. Primary amyloidosis (AL)

From Kyle RA: Classification and diagnosis of monoclonal gammopathies. *In* Rose NR, Friedman H, Fahey JL (eds.): Manual of Clinical Laboratory Immunology. 3rd ed. Washington, DC, American Society for Microbiology, 1986, p 152.

an M-protein will remain stable and benign or will develop into symptomatic multiple myeloma, macroglobulinemia, amyloidosis, or a related disorder. MGUS is characterized by a serum M-protein concentration less than 3 grams per deciliter; fewer than 5% plasma cells in the bone marrow; no or only small amounts of M-protein in the urine; absence of lytic bone lesions, anemia, hypercalcemia, and renal insufficiency; and, most important, the stability of the presence of the M-protein and the failure of other abnormalities to develop.

Incidence

During 1992, 1026 patients with a serum M-protein were seen at the Mayo Clinic. The most frequent clinical diagnosis was MGUS (benign monoclonal gammopathy), occurring in more than half of patients (Fig. 149–3).

The prevalence of MGUS is 1% of patients older than 50 years and 3% of those older than 70 years. Because of this high prevalence, it is crucial to determine whether the M-protein will remain benign or will evolve to multiple myeloma, amyloidosis, macroglobulinemia, or other lymphoproliferative disease.

Prognosis

At the Mayo Clinic, 241 patients with benign monoclonal gammopathy (i.e., patients in whom multiple myeloma, macroglobulinemia, amyloidosis, lymphoma, or related diseases were excluded) were studied long term. At the time when the M-protein was recognized, some of the characteristics of the patients were as follows:

1. The median age was 64 years.
2. Approximately three fourths of the patients had other conditions seemingly unrelated to the monoclonal gammopathy that brought them to medical attention.
3. Anemia, leukopenia, leukocytosis, thrombocytopenia, renal insufficiency, and hypercalcemia, when present, were unrelated to the monoclonal protein.
4. Laboratory findings were as follows: The M-protein level ranged from 0.3 to 3.2 grams per deciliter (median, 1.7 grams per deciliter) and consisted of IgG (73%), IgA (11%), and IgM (14%), or was biclonal (2%); an M-protein was found in the urine in only 9 patients; bone marrow plasma cells ranged from 1 to 10% (median, 3.0%).

At the time of current follow-up (median, 22 years; range, 20 to 35 years), the 241 patients can be divided into four groups (Table 149–2). Approximately one fifth of the patients have remained sta-

ble and could be classified as having benign monoclonal gammopathy, although they must continue to be observed because serious disease may still develop. No initial laboratory measurements or clinical factors were predictive of which patients would remain in this stable or benign group. In 10 percent of the patients, the M-protein level increased to more than 3 grams per deciliter, but they did not develop symptomatic multiple myeloma, macroglobulinemia, or related disorders. Their condition remains clinically "benign," although with an M-protein that causes concern. Approximately half of the patients died of seemingly unrelated causes without developing multiple myeloma, macroglobulinemia, or related disorders. Approximately one fourth of the patients (24%) developed multiple myeloma (16%), macroglobulinemia (3%), amyloidosis (3%), or related disorders (2%) (Table 149–2), with an actuarial rate of 17% at 10 years and 33% at 20 years (Fig. 149–4). The interval from the time of recognition of the M-protein to the diagnosis of serious disease ranged from 2 to 29 years (median, 10 years).

Differentiation of MGUS from Multiple Myeloma and Macroglobulinemia

Differentiation of the patient with benign monoclonal gammopathy from one in whom multiple myeloma, macroglobulinemia, or a related disorder eventually develops is very difficult when the M-protein is first recognized. The size of the M-protein is of some help—levels greater than 3 grams per deciliter usually indicate overt multiple myeloma or macroglobulinemia, but some exceptions, such as smoldering multiple myeloma (SMM), exist. Levels of immunoglobulin classes not associated with the M-protein (normal polyclonal or background immunoglobulins) are almost always reduced in multiple myeloma or Waldenström's macroglobulinemia,

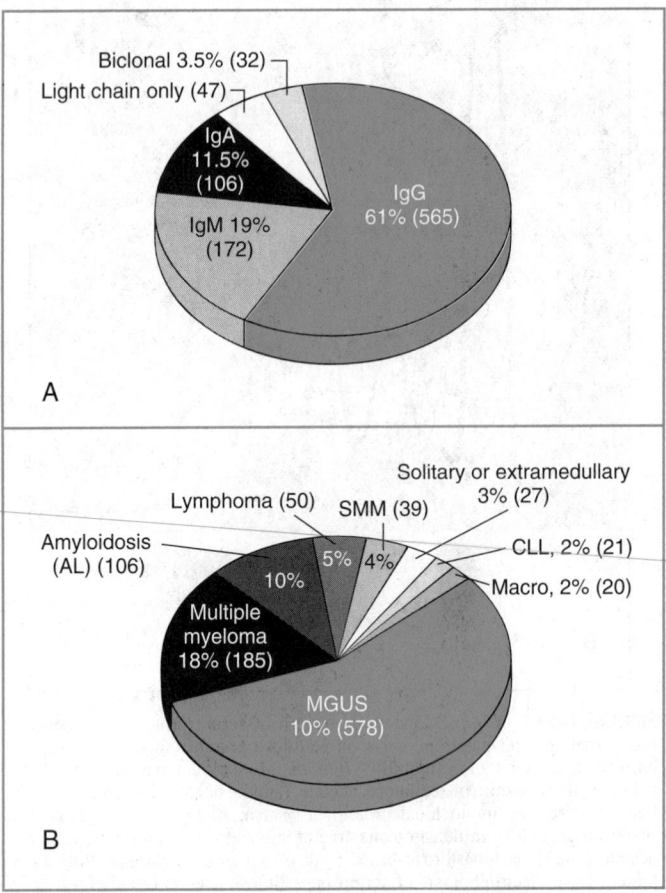

FIGURE 149–3. *A*, Distribution of monoclonal serum proteins in 922 patients seen at the Mayo Clinic during 1992. *B*, Diagnoses in 1026 cases of monoclonal gammopathy seen at the Mayo Clinic during 1992. CLL = chronic lymphocytic leukemia; Macro = macroglobulinemia; MGUS = monoclonal gammopathy of undetermined significance; SMM = smoldering multiple myeloma. (From Kyle RA: Multiple myeloma and other plasma cell disorders. *In* Hoffmann R, Benz EJ Jr, Shattil SJ, et al. [eds]: Hematology: Basic Principles and Practice. 2nd ed. New York, Churchill Livingstone, 1995, pp 1354–1374; with permission of the publisher.)

TABLE 149-2. COURSE IN A SERIES OF 241 PATIENTS WITH BENIGN MONOCLONAL GAMMOPATHY*

Group	Status	Percentage of Patients
1	No significant increase of serum or urine M-protein (benign)	19
2	Increase of M-protein to > 3 grams/dl	10
3	Died of unrelated cause	47
4	Developed myeloma (16%), macroglobulinemia (3%), amyloidosis (3%), or related diseases (2%)	24
Total		100

* During first 22 years (median) of follow-up.
Modified from Kyle RA: Monoclonal gammopathy of undetermined significance and smoldering multiple myeloma. Eur J Haematol 43 (Suppl 51):70, 1989; with permission of Munksgaard International Publishers.

but a reduction may also occur in benign monoclonal gammopathy. The association of a monoclonal light chain (Bence Jones protein-uria) with a serum monoclonal gammopathy suggests multiple myeloma or macroglobulinemia, but in many patients with small amounts of monoclonal light chain in the urine, the M-protein in the serum remains stable for many years. The presence of more than 10% plasma cells in the bone marrow suggests multiple myeloma, but some patients with more plasma cells have remained stable for long periods. The presence of osteolytic lesions strongly suggests multiple myeloma, but metastatic carcinoma may produce lytic lesions as well as plasmacytosis and may be associated with an unrelated monoclonal gammopathy.

Certain procedures show promise in differentiating the patient with MGUS or SMM from the patient with multiple myeloma. The plasma cell labeling index measures the synthesis of DNA, and when elevated it is good evidence that the patient has multiple myeloma or will soon have symptomatic disease. The use of a monoclonal antibody (BU-1) reactive with 5-bromo-2-deoxyuridine (BrdUrd) detects those cells synthesizing DNA, and the test can be performed in 4 to 5 hours. The presence of circulating plasma cells in the peripheral blood indicates active multiple myeloma.

In summary, no single technique reliably differentiates a patient with a benign monoclonal gammopathy from one who will subsequently have symptomatic multiple myeloma or other malignant disease. The M-protein level in the serum and urine should be serially measured, together with periodic re-evaluation of clinical and other laboratory features, to determine whether multiple myeloma or another related disorder is present.

If the serum M-protein is less than 2.0 grams per deciliter, electrophoresis should be repeated 6 months later, and if it is stable, it should be checked annually. If the serum M-protein is 2.0 grams per deciliter or more without evidence of myeloma or related disorders, electrophoresis should be repeated in 3 months, and if it is stable, the test should be repeated annually. If an M-protein is present in the urine, the patient should be followed more closely.

Association of Monoclonal Gammopathies with Other Diseases

Monoclonal gammopathy frequently exists without other abnormalities, but certain diseases are associated with it, as would be expected in an older population. The association of two diseases depends on the frequency with which each occurs independently. Furthermore, an association may be biased because of differences in a referral pattern or in other selected patient groups. Of the myriad associations that have been described, those listed below are the best established.

LYMPHOPROLIFERATIVE DISORDERS. An M-protein is found in 3 to 4% of patients with a diffuse lymphoproliferative process but in fewer than 1% of those with a nodular lymphoma. IgM monoclonal gammopathies are more common than IgG or IgA in lymphoproliferative diseases.

In a large series of patients in whom a serum IgM monoclonal gammopathy had been identified at the Mayo Clinic, more than half were originally considered to have MGUS (Table 149-3). During follow-up, 17% of patients with MGUS of the IgM class developed a malignant lymphoid disease, most frequently Waldenström's macroglobulinemia.

LEUKEMIA. M-proteins occur in the sera of some patients with chronic lymphocytic leukemia (Table 149-3), but with no recognizable effect on the clinical course. M-proteins have also been recognized in hairy cell, adult T cell, chronic myelogenous, acute promyelocytic, and acute myelomonocytic leukemias, but without a documented increased incidence over that in the normal population. M-proteins may also be found after liver, bone marrow, or kidney transplantation.

NEUROLOGIC DISORDERS. Approximately 5% of patients with sensorimotor peripheral neuropathy of unknown cause have an associated monoclonal gammopathy. In half of those with an IgM monoclonal gammopathy and peripheral neuropathy, the M-protein binds to myelin-associated glycoprotein (MAG). These patients have a slowly progressive sensorimotor neuropathy beginning in the distal extremities and extending proximally. Sensory involvement is more prominent than motor involvement. Cranial nerves and autonomic function are intact. The clinical and electrodiagnostic manifestations resemble those of chronic inflammatory demyelinating polyneuropathy. The relationship of the M-protein to the peripheral neuropathy is not clear.

DERMATOLOGIC DISEASES. Lichen myxedematosus (papular mucinosis, scleromyxedema) is characterized by papules, macules, and plaques infiltrating the skin and is associated with a cathodal IgG λ protein. Pyoderma gangrenosum and necrobiotic xanthogranuloma have also been associated with an M-protein.

Monoclonal Gammopathies with Antibody Activity

In some patients with MGUS, myeloma, or macroglobulinemia, the M-protein has exhibited unusual specificity to one of various antigens. Examples include actin, dextran, antistreptolysin O, antinuclear antibody, riboflavin, von Willebrand factor, thyroglobulin, insulin, double-stranded DNA, and apolipoprotein.

The binding of calcium by an M-protein may produce hypercalcemia without symptomatic or pathologic consequences. Affected patients should not be treated for hypercalcemia. M-proteins have also been found to bind to copper and to phosphate.

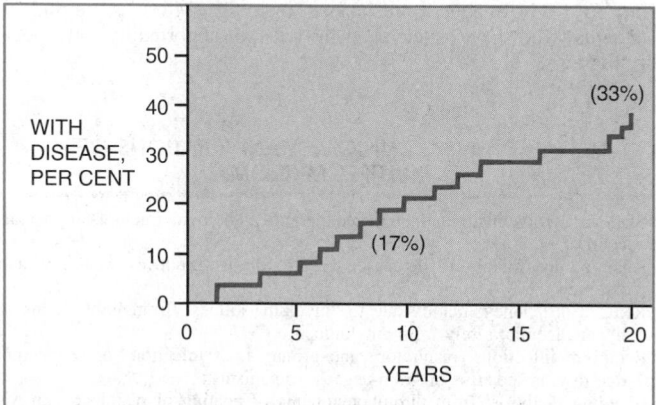

FIGURE 149-4. Incidence of multiple myeloma, macroglobulinemia, amyloidosis, or lymphoproliferative disease after recognition of monoclonal protein. (From Kyle RA, Lust JA: The monoclonal gammopathies [paraprotein]. Adv Clin Chem 28:145, 1990; with permission of Academic Press.)

TABLE 149-3. CLASSIFICATION OF IgM MONOCLONAL GAMMOPATHIES AMONG 430 PATIENTS

Classification	Percentage of Patients
Monoclonal gammopathy of undetermined significance	56
Waldenström's macroglobulinemia	17
Lymphoma	7
Chronic lymphocytic leukemia	5
Primary amyloidosis (AL)	1
Lymphoproliferative disease	14
Total	100

From Kyle RA, Garton JP: The spectrum of IgM monoclonal gammopathy in 430 cases. Mayo Clin Proc 62:719, 1987; with permission of the Mayo Foundation, Rochester, MN.

BICLONAL GAMMOPATHIES

Biclonal gammopathies occur in 2 to 3% of patients with monoclonal gammopathies. Biclonal gammopathy of undetermined significance accounts for about two thirds of patients. The remainder have multiple myeloma, macroglobulinemia, or other lymphoproliferative diseases. Triclonal gammopathies may also occur.

IDIOPATHIC BENCE JONES PROTEINURIA

Bence Jones proteinuria is a recognized feature of multiple myeloma, primary amyloidosis, Waldenström's macroglobulinemia, and other malignant lymphoproliferative disorders. A benign Bence Jones proteinuria may also occur. Patients have been documented to have a stable serum level of M-protein and Bence Jones proteinuria for more than 15 years without developing multiple myeloma or related disorders.

Kyle RA: "Benign" monoclonal gammopathy—after 20 to 35 years of follow-up. Mayo Clin Proc 68:26, 1993. *Of 241 patients with MGUS, 24% developed multiple myeloma, macroglobulinemia, amyloidosis, or related disorders.*
Kyle RA, Lust JA: Monoclonal gammopathies of undetermined significance. Semin Hematol 26:176, 1989. *Reviews the pathogenesis of monoclonal gammopathies as well as results of a long-term follow-up of benign monoclonal gammopathy. The association of monoclonal gammopathies with various diseases is emphasized.*

MULTIPLE MYELOMA

Multiple myeloma (myelomatosis, plasma cell myeloma, or Kahler's disease) is characterized by the neoplastic proliferation of a single clone of plasma cells engaged in the production of a monoclonal immunoglobulin. This clone of plasma cells proliferates in the bone marrow and frequently invades the adjacent bone, producing extensive skeletal destruction that results in bone pain and fractures. Anemia, hypercalcemia, and renal insufficiency are other important features.

Etiology and Epidemiology

The cause of multiple myeloma is unclear. Exposure to radiation, benzene and other organic solvents, herbicides, and insecticides may play a role. Multiple myeloma has been reported in familial clusters of two or more first-degree relatives and in identical twins.

Multiple myeloma accounts for 1% of all malignant disease and slightly more than 10% of hematologic malignancies in the United States. The annual incidence of multiple myeloma is 4 per 100,000. An apparent increased incidence in recent years is probably related to increased availability and use of medical facilities. Multiple myeloma occurs in all races and all geographic locations. Its incidence in blacks is almost twice that in whites. Multiple myeloma is slightly more common in men than in women. The median age of patients at the time of diagnosis is 61 years; only 2% of patients are younger than 40.

Biologic Aspects

Multiple myeloma is a B-cell malignancy with mature plasma cell morphology. In most cases, the plasma cells are CIg$^+$, CD38$^+$, and PCA-1$^+$, and only a minority express CD10, HLA-DR, and CD20. However, the nature of clonogenic cells in myeloma is still unknown. Circulating clonogenic pre-myeloma cells, by means of adhesion molecules, may home to the marrow, where they find an appropriate microenvironment (cytokine network) to differentiate and further expand. T cells play an important role. In patients with multiple myeloma, CD4 T cells are often reduced. Resting B cells enter into DNA synthesis stimulated by interleukin-4 (IL-4), proliferate with IL-5, and differentiate into plasma cells with IL-6. IL-6 is an important growth factor for myeloma cells. Elevated levels of IL-6 have been found in patients with progressive myeloma, in contrast to those with MGUS.

Increased expression of c-*myc*, H-*ras*, and bcl-2 has been found in myeloma. *Ras* mutations as well as point mutations of the tumor suppressor gene p53 have been seen. Thus, c-*myc*, H-*ras*, and p53 genes may be involved in the pathogenesis of myeloma.

Cytogenetic Abnormalities

Flow cytometry studies have shown aneuploidy in about 80% of patients, hyperdiploidy in 70%, and hypodiploidy in the remaining 10%. Chromosome abnormalities have been detected in about half of patients with multiple myeloma, but no specific abnormality has been demonstrated. Structural changes of chromosomes 1, 11, and 14, monosomies and trisomies, and translocations have been observed.

Clinical Manifestations

SYMPTOMS (Table 149–1). Bone pain, particularly in the back or chest and less often in the extremities, is present at the time of diagnosis in more than two thirds of patients. The pain is usually induced by movement and does not occur at night except with change of position. The patient's height may be reduced by several inches be-cause of vertebral collapse. Weakness and fatigue are common and often are associated with anemia. Fever is rare and, when present, is usually from an infection. The major symptoms may result from an acute infection, renal insufficiency, hypercalcemia, or amyloidosis.

PHYSICAL FINDINGS. Pallor is the most frequent physical finding. The liver is palpable in about 20% of patients and the spleen in 5%. Occasionally, extramedullary plasmacytomas may appear.

Laboratory Findings

A normocytic, normochromic anemia is present initially in two thirds of patients but eventually occurs in nearly every patient with multiple myeloma. The serum protein electrophoretic pattern (cellulose acetate) shows a peak or localized band in 80% of patients (see Fig. 149–1), hypogammaglobulinemia in almost 10%, and no apparent abnormality in the remainder. IgG M-protein is found in 53%, IgA in 20%, light chain only (Bence Jones proteinemia) in 17%, IgD in 2%, and biclonal gammopathy in 1%, and 7% have no serum M-protein at diagnosis.

Immunoelectrophoresis or immunofixation of the urine reveals an M-protein in approximately 75% of patients. The κ/λ ratio is 2:1. Ninety-eight percent of patients with multiple myeloma have an M-protein in the serum or urine at the time of diagnosis.

In the bone marrow of patients with multiple myeloma, plasma cells usually account for 10% or more of all nucleated cells, but they may range from less than 5% to almost 100% (Fig. 149–5). Bone marrow involvement may be focal rather than diffuse, requiring repeated bone marrow examinations for diagnosis. Identification of a monoclonal immunoglobulin in the cytoplasm of plasma cells by immunoperoxidase staining is helpful for differentiating monoclonal plasma cell proliferation in multiple myeloma from reactive plasmacytosis due to connective tissue disease, metastatic carcinoma, liver disease, and infections. The immunoperoxidase technique is also useful in recognizing neoplastic plasma cells that have atypical features.

Radiologic Findings

Conventional roentgenograms reveal abnormalities consisting of punched-out lytic lesions (Fig. 149–6), osteoporosis, or fractures in nearly 80% of patients. The vertebrae, skull, thoracic cage, pelvis, and proximal humeri and femora are the most frequent sites of involvement. Technetium-99m bone scanning is inferior to conventional roentgenography and should not be used. Computed tomography (CT) or magnetic resonance imaging (MRI) is helpful in patients who have skeletal pain but no abnormality on roentgenograms.

TABLE 149–4. CLINICAL MANIFESTATIONS OF MULTIPLE MYELOMA

Skeletal involvement: pain, reduced height, pathologic fractures, hypercalcemia
Anemia: due mainly to decreased erythropoiesis; produces weakness and fatigue
Renal insufficiency: mainly due to "myeloma kidney" from light chains or hypercalcemia; rarely from amyloidosis
Recurrent infections: respiratory and urinary tract infections or septicemia due to gram-positive or gram-negative organisms
Bleeding diathesis: from thrombocytopenia or coating of platelets with M-protein
Amyloidosis: develops in 10% to 15%
Extramedullary plasmacytomas: occurs late in the disease
Cryoglobulinemia type I: rarely symptomatic

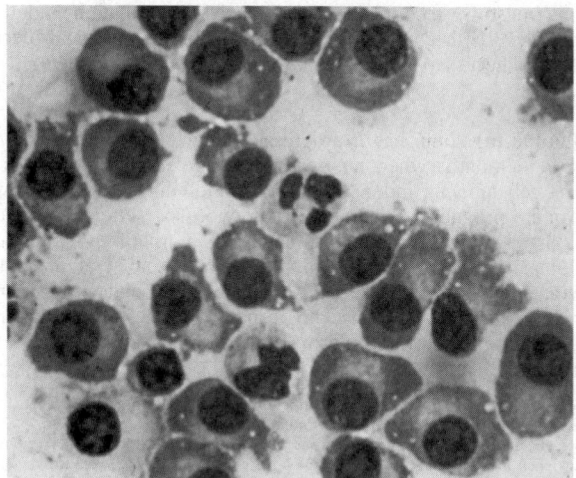

FIGURE 149–5. Bone marrow aspirate containing increased numbers of abnormal plasma cells.

Diagnostic Criteria

Minimal criteria for the diagnosis of multiple myeloma are a bone marrow containing more than 10% plasma cells or a plasmacytoma plus at least one of the following: (1) M-protein in the serum (usually greater than 3 grams per deciliter, (2) M-protein in the urine, and (3) lytic bone lesions. These findings must not be from metastatic carcinoma, connective tissue diseases, chronic infection, or lymphoma. Patients with multiple myeloma must be differentiated from those with MGUS and smoldering multiple myeloma.

Organ Involvement

RENAL. Bence Jones proteinuria detected by immunoelectrophoresis or immunofixation is present in 75%. The serum creatinine value is increased initially in almost half of patients and is ≥ 2 mg/dl in one fourth.

The two major causes of renal insufficiency are "myeloma kidney" and hypercalcemia. Myeloma kidney is characterized by the presence of large waxy laminated casts in the distal and collecting tubules. The casts are composed mainly of precipitated monoclonal light chains. The extent of cast formation correlates directly with the amount of free urinary light chain and with the severity of renal insufficiency. With dehydration, acute renal failure may occur.

Hypercalcemia, which is present in 25% of patients initially, is a major and treatable cause of renal insufficiency. Hyperuricemia may contribute to renal failure. Amyloidosis occurs in 10 to 15% of patients and may produce a nephrotic syndrome or renal insufficiency or both. Acquired Fanconi's syndrome, characterized by proximal tubular dysfunction, results in glycosuria, phosphaturia, and aminoaciduria (see Ch. 82). Deposition of monoclonal light chains in the renal glomerulus (light-chain deposition disease) may produce renal insufficiency and the nephrotic syndrome.

NEUROLOGIC. Radiculopathy, the single most frequent neurologic complication, is usually in the thoracic or lumbosacral area and results from compression of the nerve by the vertebral lesion or by the collapsed bone itself. Compression of the spinal cord occurs in up to 10% of patients. Peripheral neuropathy is uncommon in multiple myeloma and, when present, is usually caused by amyloidosis. Rarely, myeloma cells diffusely infiltrate the meninges. Intracranial plasmacytomas almost always represent extensions of myelomatous lesions of the skull.

Other Systemic Involvement

Hepatomegaly from plasma cell infiltration is uncommon. Ascites is rare. Plasmacytomas of the ribs are common and present either as expanding bone lesions or as soft tissue masses. The incidence of infections is increased in multiple myeloma. *Diplococcus pneumoniae* and *Staphylococcus aureus* organisms have been the most frequent pathogens, but gram-negative organisms now account for more than half of all infections. Propensity to infection results from impairment of antibody response, deficiency of normal immunoglobulins, and neutropenia. Bleeding from coating of the platelets by the M-protein may occur. Occasionally, a tendency to thrombosis is present.

Treatment

Not all patients who fulfill the minimal criteria for the diagnosis of multiple myeloma should be treated. The patient's symptoms, physical findings, and all laboratory data must be considered. If there are doubts about whether to begin chemotherapy, treatment should be withheld and the patient re-evaluated in 2 or 3 months.

Chemotherapy is the preferred initial therapy for overt symptomatic multiple myeloma. Palliative irradiation should be limited to patients with disabling pain from a well-defined focal process that has not responded to chemotherapy. In most cases, analgesics together with chemotherapy control the pain.

The major controversy in chemotherapy is whether melphalan and prednisone or a combination of alkylating agents should be used. The oral administration of melphalan (L-phenylalanine mustard, Alkeran) and prednisone, a standard form of therapy, produces objective response in 50 to 60% of patients. Melphalan may be given orally in a daily dose of 0.15 mg per kilogram for 7 days (8 to 10 mg per day), with 20 mg of prednisone given three times daily for the same period. Leukocyte and platelet levels should be determined at 3-week intervals, and the melphalan and prednisone therapy repeated in cycles every 6 weeks. The dose of melphalan should be adjusted until modest midcycle cytopenia occurs.

Many combinations of chemotherapeutic agents have been used. The best-known combination, the M2 protocol, includes melphalan, cyclophosphamide, carmustine (bischloroethylnitrosourea, or BCNU), vincristine, and prednisone. This regimen produces an objective response in 70 to 75% of patients, but the median survival is approximately 2.5 years, which is not significantly different from that produced by melphalan and prednisone. M2 and various other drug combinations have not clearly been shown to produce longer survival than does melphalan-prednisone.

Chemotherapy should be continued for at least 1 year, and if the patient is in plateau (stable serum and urine M-protein and no evidence of progression), treatment should be stopped. Continued chemotherapy may lead to the development of a myelodysplastic syndrome or acute leukemia. α_2-Interferon seems to prolong the duration of the plateau state but not survival. Patients should be followed closely, and the same chemotherapy should be reinstituted when relapse occurs.

Bone Marrow Transplantation

Allogeneic bone marrow transplantation has the advantage that the graft contains no tumor cells, and there may be a graft-versus-tumor effect. However, a significant early mortality rate of 20 to 25% is seen during the first 3 months, the risk of graft-versus-host disease is troublesome, and relapse of multiple myeloma is common. Furthermore, only 5 to 10% of patients with multiple

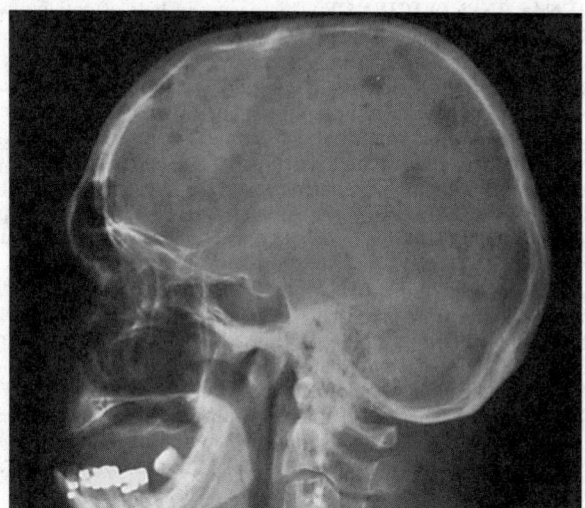

FIGURE 149–6. Skull roentgenogram showing multiple lytic lesions.

myeloma are eligible because of their age, renal function, and the lack of an HLA-matched sibling donor. Autologous peripheral blood stem cell or bone marrow transplantation is applicable for up to 50% of patients because the age limit is higher and a matched donor is unnecessary. However, it is difficult to eradicate multiple myeloma with our current preparative regimens, and the infused autologous peripheral stem cells or bone marrow may be contaminated by myeloma cells or their precursors.

It is essential to develop more sensitive techniques for detection of residual myeloma with the advent of more aggressive therapy. When the M-protein is not detected in the serum and urine with immunofixation and the bone marrow contains no identifiable myeloma cells, the patient still frequently relapses with myeloma of the same isotype that was present initially. Oligonucleotide primers to amplify regions of rearranged heavy-chain alleles with polymerase chain reaction in patients with multiple myeloma can detect 1 myeloma cell in 100,000 cells.

Treatment of Refractory Multiple Myeloma

Almost all patients with multiple myeloma who respond to chemotherapy eventually relapse. The highest response rates for patients with multiple myeloma resistant to alkylating agents have been with VAD (vincristine, Adriamycin [doxorubicin], and dexamethasone). Most of the activity of VAD is from dexamethasone. Intravenous methylprednisolone, 2 grams three times weekly for a minimum of 4 weeks, is helpful in patients with pancytopenia, and we find fewer side effects than from dexamethasone. If there is a response, methylprednisolone is reduced to once or twice weekly. VBAP—vincristine, carmustine (BCNU), and doxorubicin (Adriamycin) on day 1 and prednisone daily for 5 days every 3 to 4 weeks—benefits approximately 40% of patients. α_2-Interferon produces objective response in 10 to 20% of patients. Cyclophosphamide (600 mg/m^2 intravenously daily for 4 days) plus prednisone (100 mg daily for the same 4-day period) followed by granulocyte-colony–stimulating factor has been helpful in refractory patients with advanced disease. The use of agents such as verapamil, quinine, cyclosporine, and PSC-833 to reverse resistance to doxorubicin is a potentially important approach.

Management of Complications

HYPERCALCEMIA. Hypercalcemia, present in one fourth of patients at diagnosis, should be suspected in the presence of anorexia, nausea, vomiting, polyuria, polydipsia, increased constipation, weakness, confusion, or stupor. If it is untreated, renal insufficiency may develop. Hydration, preferably with isotonic saline plus prednisone (25 mg four times per day), relieves the hypercalcemia in most cases. The dosage of prednisone must be reduced and its use discontinued as soon as possible. If these measures fail, diphosphonates or gallium nitrate is beneficial. Patients with myeloma should be encouraged to be as active as possible because prolonged bed rest contributes to hypercalcemia. The manifestations and treatment of hypercalcemia are also discussed in Ch. 214.

RENAL INSUFFICIENCY. This occurs in half of patients with multiple myeloma and may develop insidiously or rapidly (acute renal failure). Hydration and prednisone are necessary if there is an accompanying hypercalcemia. Furosemide is helpful for maintaining a high urine flow rate (100 ml per hour). Hemodialysis is necessary in the event of symptomatic azotemia. Plasmapheresis may be helpful for regaining renal function, but patients with severe myeloma cast formation or other irreversible changes are unlikely to benefit from plasmapheresis. Allopurinol is necessary if hyperuricemia is present. For a more general discussion of renal insufficiency, see Ch. 76 and 77.

INFECTION. Prompt, appropriate therapy for bacterial infections is necessary. Prophylactic penicillin often benefits patients with recurrent gram-positive infections. Intravenously administered gamma globulin is helpful but expensive. Pneumococcal and influenza immunizations should be given to all patients.

SKELETAL LESIONS. Patients should be encouraged to be as active as possible but to avoid trauma. Fixation of fractures or impending fractures of long bones with an intramedullary rod and methyl methacrylate has produced good results.

MISCELLANEOUS COMPLICATIONS. Symptomatic hyperviscosity should be treated with plasmapheresis. Extradural plasma-

cytoma must be recognized and treated with radiation and dexamethasone. If the neurologic deficit increases, surgical decompression is necessary.

Prognosis

Multiple myeloma has a progressive course, with a median survival of 6 months when no treatment is given. The bone marrow plasma cell labeling index and β_2-microglobulin level are the most important prognostic factors in previously untreated multiple myeloma. Advanced age, plasmablastic morphology, circulating myeloma cells in the peripheral blood, increased myeloma colony growth, and increased levels of IL-6 are all associated with more aggressive disease. Patients who respond rapidly to chemotherapy and who have an elevated plasma cell labeling index have a shorter remission and survival.

Alexanian R, Dimopoulos M: The treatment of multiple myeloma. N Engl J Med 330:484, 1994. *A succinct review of multiple myeloma management.*
Barlogie B, Epstein J, Selvanayagam P, et al.: Plasma cell myeloma—new biological insights and advances in therapy. Blood 73:865, 1989. *This excellent review includes advances in the molecular biology and immunologic aspects of multiple myeloma.*
Gregory WM, Richards MA, Malpas JS: Combination chemotherapy versus melphalan and prednisolone in the treatment of multiple myeloma: an overview of published trials. J Clin Oncol 10:334, 1992. *A meta-analysis of 18 published trials comparing multiple and single alkylating agents, with no significant difference in overall duration of survival.*
Kyle RA: Monoclonal proteins and renal disease. Annu Rev Med 45:71, 1994. *Renal aspects of multiple myeloma, primary systemic amyloidosis, light-chain deposition disease, Waldenström's mcroglobulinemia, acquired Fanconi's syndrome, and cryoglobulinemia are reviewed.*
Kyle RA, Greipp PR: Plasma cell dyscrasias: Current status. CRC Crit Rev Oncol Hematol 8:93, 1988. *A comprehensive review of monoclonal gammopathies with more than 450 references.*

VARIANT FORMS OF MULTIPLE MYELOMA (see Table 149–1)

Smoldering Multiple Myeloma

The diagnosis of smoldering multiple myeloma (SMM) depends on the presence of an M-protein level greater than 3 grams per deciliter in the serum and greater than 10% plasma cells in the bone marrow, but no anemia, renal insufficiency, or skeletal lesions. Often a small amount of M-protein is found in the urine, and the concentration of normal immunoglobulins in the serum is decreased. The plasma cell labeling index is low. SMM should be recognized because patients must not be treated unless progression occurs. Biologically, patients with SMM have a benign monoclonal gammopathy (MGUS), but it is difficult to accept that diagnosis initially when the M-protein level is greater than 3 grams per deciliter and the bone marrow contains more than 10% plasma cells.

Plasma Cell Leukemia

Patients with plasma cell leukemia have greater than 20% plasma cells in the peripheral blood and an absolute plasma cell count of at least 2000 per microliter. Plasma cell leukemia is classified as primary when it is diagnosed in the leukemic phase (60%) or as secondary when there is leukemic transformation of a previously recognized multiple myeloma (40%). Patients with primary plasma cell leukemia are younger and have a greater incidence of hepatosplenomegaly and lymphadenopathy, a higher platelet count, fewer bone lesions, a smaller serum M-protein component, and a longer survival (median, 6.8 versus 1.3 months) than patients with secondary plasma cell leukemia. Treatment of plasma cell leukemia is unsatisfactory, but partial responses do occur with melphalan and prednisone or with a combination of alkylating agents. Secondary plasma cell leukemia rarely responds to chemotherapy because the patients have already received chemotherapy and are resistant.

Nonsecretory Myeloma

Patients with nonsecretory myeloma have no M-protein in either the serum or the urine and account for only 1% of those with myeloma. For certainty of diagnosis, an M-protein must be identified in the plasma cells by immunoperoxidase or immunofluorescence methods. More than a dozen patients in whom no M-protein could be found within the myeloma cell have been described.

IgD Myeloma

The M-protein is smaller than in IgG and IgA myelomas, and Bence Jones proteinuria of the λ type is more common. Amyloidosis and extramedullary plasmacytomas are more frequent with IgD myeloma. Survival is generally believed to be shorter than with other myeloma types, but IgD myeloma is often not diagnosed until later in its course.

Osteosclerotic Myeloma (POEMS Syndrome)

This syndrome is characterized by *p*olyneuropathy, *o*rganomegaly, *e*ndocrinopathy, *M*-protein, and *s*kin changes (POEMS). The major clinical features are a chronic inflammatory-demyelinating polyneuropathy with predominantly motor disability and sclerotic skeletal lesions. Except for the presence of papilledema, the cranial nerves are not involved. The autonomic nervous system is intact. Hepatomegaly occurs in almost one half of patients, but splenomegaly and lymphadenopathy occur in a minority. Hyperpigmentation and hypertrichosis are usually evident. Gynecomastia and atrophic testes as well as clubbing of the fingers and toes may be seen. In contrast to multiple myeloma, the hemoglobin level is usually normal or elevated, and thrombocytosis is common. The bone marrow usually contains fewer than 5% plasma cells, and hypercalcemia and renal insufficiency rarely occur. Most patients have a λ protein. Evidence of Castleman's disease may be found. Diagnosis is confirmed by the identification of monoclonal plasma cells obtained at biopsy of an osteosclerotic lesion.

If the lesions are in a limited area, radiation therapy will produce substantial improvement of the neuropathy in more than half of the patients. If the patient has widespread osteosclerotic lesions, chemotherapy with melphalan and prednisone may be helpful.

Solitary Plasmacytoma (Solitary Myeloma) of Bone

Diagnosis of this disease is based on histologic evidence of a tumor consisting of monoclonal plasma cells identical to those seen in multiple myeloma. In addition, complete skeletal roentgenograms must show no other lesions of myeloma, the bone marrow aspirate must contain no evidence of multiple myeloma, and immunoelectrophoresis or immunofixation of the serum and concentrated urine should show no M-protein. Exceptions to the last-mentioned criterion occur, but therapy for the solitary lesion usually results in the disappearance of the M-protein. Disease-free survival at 10 years ranges from 15 to 25%. Almost 50% of patients with solitary plasmacytoma are alive at 10 years. Treatment consists of radiation in the range of 40 to 50 Gy. The most uncertain criterion for diagnosis is the length of observation necessary before certainty that the disease will not become generalized.

Extramedullary Plasmacytoma

Extramedullary plasmacytoma is a plasma cell tumor that arises outside the bone marrow. The tumor is found in the upper respiratory tract in approximately 85% of cases, especially in the nasal cavity and sinuses, nasopharynx, and larynx. Extramedullary plasmacytomas may also occur in the gastrointestinal tract, central nervous system, urinary bladder, thyroid, breast, testes, parotid gland, and lymph nodes. The diagnosis is based on the finding of a plasma cell tumor in an extramedullary site and the absence of multiple myeloma on bone marrow examination, roentgenography, and appropriate studies of blood and urine. Treatment consists of tumoricidal irradiation. The plasmacytoma may occur locally, metastasize to regional nodes, or develop into multiple myeloma.

WALDENSTRÖM'S MACROGLOBULINEMIA (PRIMARY MACROGLOBULINEMIA)

Macroglobulinemia is the result of an uncontrolled proliferation of lymphocytes and plasma cells in which a large IgM M-protein is produced. The cause is unknown, but it does occur more frequently in certain families. The median age of patients at the time of diagnosis is 60 years, and about 60% are male.

Clinical Presentations

Weakness, fatigue, and bleeding (especially oozing from the oronasal area) are common presenting symptoms. Blurred or impaired vision, dyspnea, loss of weight, neurologic symptoms, recurrent infections, and congestive heart failure may occur. In contrast to multiple myeloma, lytic bone lesions, renal insufficiency, and amyloidosis are rare. Physical findings include pallor, hepatosplenomegaly, and lymphadenopathy. Retinal hemorrhages, exudates, and venous congestion with vascular segmentation ("sausage" formation) may occur. Sensorimotor peripheral neuropathy is common. Pulmonary involvement is manifested by diffuse pulmonary infiltrates and isolated masses. Pleural effusion may occur. Diarrhea and steatorrhea are uncommon.

Laboratory Evaluation

Almost all patients have moderate to severe normocytic, normochromic anemia. Coombs-positive hemolytic anemia is uncommon. The serum cholesterol value is often low. The serum electrophoretic pattern is characterized by a tall, narrow peak or dense band and is almost always of γ mobility. Seventy-five percent of the IgM proteins have a κ light chain. Low molecular weight IgM (7S) is present and may account for a significant part of the elevated IgM level. A monoclonal light chain is present in the urine of 80% of patients. The amount of urinary protein is usually modest.

The bone marrow aspirate is often hypocellular, but the biopsy is hypercellular and extensively infiltrated with lymphoid cells and plasma cells. The number of mast cells is frequently increased. Rouleaux formation is prominent, and the sedimentation rate is markedly increased unless gelation of the plasma occurs. About 10 percent of macroglobulins have cryoproperties.

Diagnosis

The combination of typical symptoms and physical findings, the presence of a large IgM M-protein (usually greater than 3 grams per deciliter), and lymphoid–plasma cell infiltration of the bone marrow provide the diagnosis. Multiple myeloma, chronic lymphocytic leukemia, and MGUS of the IgM type must be differentiated.

Treatment

Patients should not be treated unless they have anemia; constitutional symptoms such as weakness, fatigue, night sweats, or weight loss; hyperviscosity; or significant hepatosplenomegaly or lymphadenopathy. Chlorambucil (Leukeran) is usually given orally in a dosage of 6 to 8 mg per day and is reduced when the leukocyte or platelet value decreases. Patients should be treated until the disease has reached a plateau state; the treatment can be discontinued and the patients followed closely. Chemotherapy should be reinstituted when the disease relapses. Combinations of alkylating agents, such as the M2 protocol (vincristine, BCNU, melphalan, cyclophosphamide, and prednisone), may be beneficial. α_2-Interferon may be of some use. Eighty percent of previously untreated patients respond to fludarabine or 2-chlorodeoxyadenosine.

Transfusions of packed red blood cells should be given for symptomatic anemia. Spuriously low hemoglobin and hematocrit levels may occur because of the increased plasma volume from the large amount of M-protein. Consequently, transfusions should not be given solely on the basis of the hemoglobin or hematocrit value. Symptomatic hyperviscosity should be treated with plasmapheresis. The median survival in macroglobulinemia is 5 years.

Bladé J, Lust JA, Kyle RA: IgD multiple myeloma: presenting features, response to therapy, and survival in a series of 53 cases. J Clin Oncol 12:2398, 1994. *Review of 53 patients with IgD myeloma from a single institution.*

Dimopoulos MA, Alexanian R: Waldenström's macroglobulinemia. Blood 83:1452, 1994. *Covers features of the disease, complications, and therapy.*

Dimopoulos MA, Goldstein J, Fuller L, Delasalle K, Alexanian R: Curability of solitary bone plasmacytoma. J Clin Oncol 10:587, 1992. *Of 45 patients with solitary plasmacytoma of bone, 46% developed multiple myeloma; 53% were alive at 10 years.*

Frassica DA, Frassica FJ, Schray MF, et al: Solitary plasmacytoma of bone: Mayo Clinic experience. Int J Radiat Oncol Biol Phys 16:43, 1989. *In 46 cases of solitary plasmacytoma of bone, the presence of an M-protein did not significantly alter the survival or duration of disease-free survival.*

Kyle RA, Garton JP: The spectrum of IgM monoclonal gammopathy in 430 cases. Mayo Clin Proc 62:719, 1987. *This study of 430 patients with an IgM monoclonal protein emphasizes the variable clinical patterns of disease. Clinical and laboratory features are provided for 63 patients with Waldenström's macroglobulinemia.*

Kyle RA, Greipp PR: Smoldering multiple myeloma. N Engl J Med 302:1347, 1980. *Six patients fulfilled the criteria for the diagnosis of multiple myeloma, but their conditions behaved like a benign monoclonal gammopathy. The authors emphasize that such patients must be recognized and not treated.*

Noel P, Kyle RA: Plasma cell leukemia: an evaluation of response to therapy. Am J Med 83:1062, 1987. *This review of 43 patients with plasma cell leukemia differentiates primary and secondary plasma cell leukemia. Short survival is emphasized.*

Soesan M, Paccagnella A, Chiarion-Sileni V, et al: Extramedullary plasmacytoma: clinical behaviour and response to treatment. Ann Oncol 3:51, 1992. *The median survival of 22 patients with stage I extramedullary plasmacytoma was not reached after 163 months.*

Waldenström JG: POEMS: a multifactorial syndrome (editorial). Haematologica 77:197, 1992. *Describes the clinical and laboratory features of POEMS syndrome (osteosclerotic myeloma).*

HYPERVISCOSITY SYNDROME

Chronic nasal bleeding and oozing from the gums are frequent, but postsurgical or gastrointestinal bleeding may occur. Retinal hemorrhages are common, and papilledema may be seen. The patient occasionally complains of blurring or a loss of vision. Dizziness, headache, vertigo, nystagmus, decreased hearing, ataxia, paresthesias, diplopia, somnolence, and coma may occur. Hyperviscosity can precipitate or aggravate congestive heart failure. Most patients have symptoms when the relative viscosity is greater than 4 centipoises (cP), but the relationship between serum viscosity and clinical manifestations is not precise. Patients with symptomatic hyperviscosity should be treated with plasmapheresis. Plasma exchange of 3 to 4 liters should be performed daily until the patient is asymptomatic. The plasma should be replaced with albumin rather than plasma.

HEAVY-CHAIN DISEASES

The heavy-chain diseases (HCD's) are characterized by the presence of an M-protein consisting of a portion of the immunoglobulin heavy chain in the serum or urine or both. These heavy chains are devoid of light chains and represent a lymphoplasma cell proliferative process. There are three major types: γ HCD, α HCD, and μ HCD.

Gamma Heavy-Chain Disease (γ HCD)

The abnormal protein consists of a γ chain with significant deletions of amino acids, including the C_{H1} domain of the constant region.

The median age of patients is approximately 60 years, although the condition has been noted in persons younger than 20. Patients with γ HCD often present with a lymphoma-like illness, but the clinical findings are diverse and range from an aggressive lymphoproliferative process to an asymptomatic state. Hepatosplenomegaly and lymphadenopathy occur in about 60% of patients. Anemia is found in about 80% initially and in nearly all eventually. A few patients have had a Coombs-positive hemolytic anemia. The electrophoretic pattern often shows a broad-based band more suggestive of a polyclonal than an M-protein. The urinary protein value ranges from a trace to 20 grams daily, but it is usually less than 1 gram per 24 hours.

Increased numbers of lymphocytes, plasma cells, or plasmacytoid lymphocytes are seen in the bone marrow and lymph nodes. The histologic pattern varies, usually including generalized or localized lymphoma or myeloma, but in some cases there is no evidence of a lymphoplasmacytic proliferative process.

Treatment is indicated only for symptomatic patients. Many different drugs have been used, but the results have been inconsistent and generally disappointing. Therapy with cyclophosphamide, vincristine, and prednisone is a reasonable choice. If there is no response to this regimen, doxorubicin should be added.

The prognosis of γ HCD is variable and ranges from a rapidly progressive downhill course of a few weeks' duration to the asymptomatic presence of a stable monoclonal heavy chain in the serum or urine.

Alpha Heavy-Chain Disease (α HCD)

This most common HCD occurs in patients from the Mediterranean region or Middle East, usually in the second or third decade of life. About 60% are men. Most commonly, the gastrointestinal tract is involved, resulting in severe malabsorption with diarrhea, steatorrhea, and loss of weight. Plasma cell infiltration of the jejunal mucosa is the most frequent pathologic feature. Immunoproliferative small intestinal disease is restricted to patients with small intestinal lesions who have the same pathologic features as those of α-HCD, but these patients do not synthesize α heavy chains.

The serum protein electrophoretic pattern is normal in half the cases, and in the remainder an unimpressive broad band may appear in the α_2 or β regions. The diagnosis depends on the recognition of a monoclonal α heavy chain. The amount of α heavy chain in the urine is small, and Bence Jones proteinuria has never been reported.

Most often, α HCD is progressive and fatal, but response to melphalan or cyclophosphamide and prednisone may occur. Unexpectedly, antibiotics may also produce a remission.

Mu Heavy-Chain Disease (μ HCD)

This disease is characterized by the demonstration of a monoclonal μ chain fragment in the serum. The patient may present with

chronic lymphocytic leukemia or lymphoma, but it is likely that the clinical spectrum will broaden when more cases are recognized.

The serum protein electrophoretic pattern is usually normal except for hypogammaglobulinemia. Bence Jones proteinuria has been found in two thirds of cases. The course of μ HCD is variable, and survival ranges from a few months to many years. Treatment with corticosteroids and alkylating agents has produced some benefit.

Gertz MA, Kyle RA: Hyperviscosity syndrome: An analytic review. J Intensive Care Med (in press). *Comprehensively reviews the pathophysiology, clinical features, and treatment of hyperviscosity.*

Kyle RA, Greipp PR, Banks PM: The diverse picture of gamma heavy-chain disease: Report of seven cases and review of literature. Mayo Clin Proc 56:439, 1981. *This report of seven cases of γ HCD from a single institution includes a detailed literature review of 49 cases. The clinical picture is emphasized.*

Rambaud JC, Halphen M, Galian A, et al.: Immunoproliferative small intestinal disease (IPSID): Relationships with α-chain disease and "Mediterranean" lymphomas. Springer Semin Immunopathol 12:239, 1990. *Reviews immunoproliferative small intestinal disease and its relationship with α-chain disease.*

Wahner-Roedler DL, Kyle RA: μ-Heavy chain disease: Presentation as a benign monoclonal gammopathy. Am J Hematol 40:56, 1992. *A report of a case of μ-HCD that began as a benign monoclonal gammopathy but became an aggressive malignant lymphoproliferative process 3 years later. Reviews the 28 cases of μ-HCD in the literature.*

CRYOGLOBULINEMIA

Cryoglobulins are proteins that precipitate when cooled and dissolve when heated. They are designated as idiopathic or essential when they are not associated with any recognizable disease. Cryoglobulins are classified into three types: type I (monoclonal), type II (mixed), and type III (polyclonal).

Type I (monoclonal) cryoglobulinemia is most commonly of the IgM or IgG class, but IgA and Bence Jones cryoglobulins have been reported. Most patients, even with large amounts of type I cryoglobulin, are completely asymptomatic from this source. Others with monoclonal cryoglobulins in the range of 1 to 2 grams per deciliter may have pain, purpura, Raynaud's phenomenon, cyanosis, and even ulceration and sloughing of skin and subcutaneous tissue on exposure to the cold because their cryoglobulins precipitate at relatively high temperatures. Type I cryoglobulins are associated with macroglobulinemia, multiple myeloma, or MGUS.

Type II (mixed) cryoglobulinemia typically consists of an IgM M-protein and polyclonal IgG, although monoclonal IgG or monoclonal IgA may also be seen with polyclonal IgM. Serum protein electrophoresis usually shows a normal pattern or a diffuse, polyclonal hypergammaglobulinemic pattern. The quantity of mixed cryoglobulin is usually less than 0.2 gram per deciliter. Vasculitis, glomerulonephritis, lymphoproliferative disease, and chronic infectious processes are common. Purpura and polyarthralgias are frequently seen. Involvement of the joints is symmetric, but joint deformities rarely develop. Raynaud's phenomenon, necrosis of the skin, and neurologic involvement may be present. In almost 80% of renal biopsy specimens, glomerular damage can be identified. Nephrotic syndrome may result, but severe renal insufficiency is uncommon. Hepatic dysfunction and serologic evidence of infection with hepatitis C virus are common.

Early administration of corticosteroids is the most frequent therapy. Cyclophosphamide, chlorambucil, or azathioprine should be used if there is no response. Plasmapheresis has been effective in some instances. α_2-Interferon has been of benefit.

Type III (polyclonal) cryoglobulinemia is not associated with a monoclonal component. Type III cryoglobulins are found in many patients with infections or inflammatory diseases and are of no clinical significance.

Levey JM, Bjornsson B, Banner B, et al.: Mixed cryoglobulinemia in chronic hepatitis C infection: a clinicopathologic analysis of 10 cases and review of recent literature. Medicine 73:53, 1994. *A review of 10 cases of mixed cryoglobulinemia in hepatitis C patients. Presents clinical, serologic, and pathological data.*

Misiani R, Bellavita P, Fenili D, et al.: Interferon alfa-2a therapy in cryoglobulinemia associated with hepatitis C virus. N Engl J Med 330:751, 1994. *This prospective randomized study of 53 patients with HCV-associated type II cryoglobulinemia demonstrates the therapeutic efficacy of α_2-interferon.*

PRIMARY AMYLOIDOSIS (AL)

Amyloid, stained with Congo red, produces an apple-green birefringence under polarized light. It is a fibrous protein that consists of rigid, linear, nonbranching, aggregated fibrils of 7.5 to 10 nm width and of indefinite length. The type of amyloid cannot be differentiated by organ distribution or by electron microscopy. The amyloid fibrils in AL consist of the variable portion of a monoclonal light chain or, in some instances, the intact light chain

(Table 149–5). The light-chain class is more frequently λ than κ (2:1), with a predominance of the λ_{VI} subclass. Patients with AL may have aberrant de novo synthesis or abnormal proteolytic processing of light chains. Amyloid P-component (AP) is a glycoprotein found in all types of amyloid, but its function is unknown. The catabolism, or breakdown, of amyloid fibrils is an important but poorly understood factor in pathogenesis.

Clinical Features

The median age at diagnosis is 64 years, and only 1% of patients are younger than 40. Two thirds are male. Weakness or fatigue and loss of weight are the most frequent symptoms. Dyspnea, pedal edema, paresthesias, light-headedness, and syncope are frequently seen in patients with congestive heart failure or peripheral neuropathy. Hoarseness or change of voice as well as jaw claudication may occur.

The liver is palpable in one fourth of patients, but splenomegaly occurs in only 5%. Macroglossia is present in 10%. Purpura often involves the neck, face, and eyes. Ankle edema is common.

Almost one third of patients have a nephrotic syndrome. Carpal tunnel syndrome, congestive heart failure, peripheral neuropathy, and orthostatic hypotension are other major presenting syndromes (Fig. 149–7). The presence of one of these syndromes and an M-protein in the serum or urine is a strong indication of amyloidosis, for which appropriate biopsy specimens must be taken for diagnosis.

Laboratory Findings

Anemia is not a prominent feature, but, when present, it is usually due to renal insufficiency, multiple myeloma, or gastrointestinal bleeding. Thrombocytosis occurs in 10% of patients. Proteinuria is present initially in 80% and renal insufficiency in almost 50% of patients. Elevation of the serum alkaline phosphatase value is not uncommon. Hyperbilirubinemia is infrequent, but, when present, is an ominous sign. Hypoalbuminemia and elevation of the cholesterol and triglyceride values are common with the nephrotic syndrome. The Factor X level is decreased in fewer than 5% of patients and is rarely the cause of bleeding. The prothrombin time is increased in about 15% of patients, and the thrombin time is prolonged in 40%.

Immunoelectrophoresis or immunofixation reveals an M-protein in the serum and in the urine of more than 70% of patients. An M-protein is found in the serum or urine in 89% of patients at diagnosis.

Bone marrow plasma cells are usually only modestly increased. Less than one fifth of patients have more than 20% plasma cells in the marrow. Roentgenograms of the bones are normal unless the patient has multiple myeloma.

Organ System Involvement

CARDIAC AND CIRCULATORY. Congestive heart failure is present in approximately 20% of patients at diagnosis and develops during the course of the disease in an additional 5%. The electrocardiogram frequently shows either low voltage in the limb leads or features consistent with an anteroseptal infarction (loss of anterior forces). Atrial fibrillation, atrial or junctional tachycardia, ventricular premature complexes, and heart block are common electrocardiographic features.

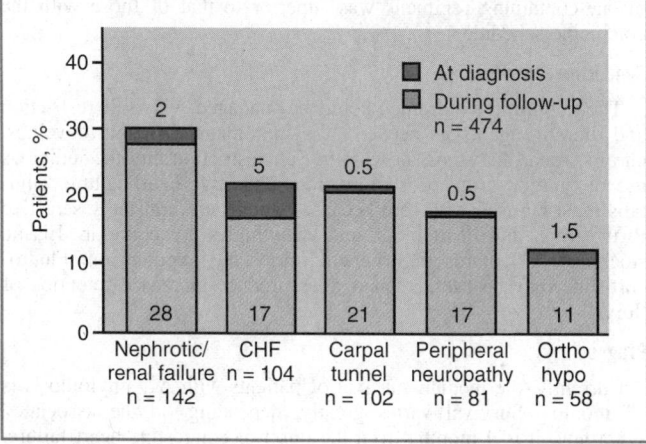

FIGURE 149–7. Syndromes seen at diagnosis and during follow-up of patients with primary amyloidosis (AL). Some patients had more than two syndromes at presentation. CHF = congestive heart failure; Ortho hypo-orthostatic hypotension. (From Kyle RA, Gertz MA: Primary systemic amyloidosis: Clinical and laboratory features in 474 cases. Semin Hematol 32:45, 1995.)

Echocardiography is valuable for evaluation of amyloid heart disease. Increased thickness of the ventricular wall and septum correlates with an increased incidence of congestive heart failure. Early cardiac amyloidosis is characterized by abnormal relaxation, whereas advanced involvement is characterized by restrictive hemodynamics. Intermittent claudication of the lower extremities, the upper extremities, or the jaw may be a prominent feature.

OTHER ORGANS. Nephrotic syndrome is present in more than one fourth of patients at the time of diagnosis. The degree of proteinuria does not correlate well with the extent of amyloid deposition in the kidney. Gross hematuria is rare. Other organ involvement includes the lungs and gastrointestinal tract, but it is asymptomatic in most instances. Sensorimotor peripheral neuropathy characterized by dysesthetic numbness involving the lower extremities occurs in one sixth of patients. Autonomic dysfunction may be a prominent feature and is usually manifested by orthostatic hypotension, diarrhea, or impotence. Amyloidosis can involve the periarticular structures and produce the shoulder pad syndrome. Rarely, osteolytic lesions from amyloid may occur. Pseudohypertrophy of skeletal muscles from amyloid deposition may be impressive. Petechiae, ecchymoses, papules, plaques, nodules, tumors, bullous lesions, thickening of the skin, and dystrophy of the nails may occur.

The diagnosis of amyloidosis depends on histologic proof. The initial diagnostic procedure should be abdominal fat aspiration, which is positive in 80% of patients. A bone marrow aspiration and biopsy should be done to determine the degree of plasmacytosis, and results are positive for amyloid in more than one half of patients. The abdominal fat or bone marrow biopsy results are positive in 90%. If subcutaneous fat and bone marrow biopsies are negative, a rectal biopsy should be done, including submucosa or kidney, liver, carpal tunnel tissue, sural nerve, or endomyocardium.

Specific antisera are helpful for identifying the type of systemic amyloidosis. Antiserum to AP reacts with all amyloid types and is useful in demonstrating the presence of amyloid.

Treatment

Therapy of AL amyloidosis is not satisfactory. In a prospective study of treatment with melphalan and prednisone compared with colchicine, no significant difference in survival was noted (25 and 18 months, respectively). When the survival of patients who received only one regimen was analyzed, or when survival was determined from the time of entry into the study to the time of death or progression of disease, significant differences favoring melphalan and prednisone therapy were evident.

In another prospective study, patients with AL were randomized to receive melphalan and prednisone, colchicine, or a combination of the three. Survival of those receiving the two melphalan-pred-

TABLE 149–5. CLINICAL CLASSIFICATION OF AMYLOIDOSIS

Amyloid Type	Classification	Major Protein Component
AL	Primary	κ or λ light chain
AA	Secondary	Protein A
AL	Localized	κ or λ light chain
ATTR	Familial	
	Neurologic	Transthyretin (prealbumin)
	Cardiopathic	Transthyretin (prealbumin)
	Nephropathic	
	Familial Mediterranean fever	Protein A
	Senile systemic amyloidosis	Transthyretin (prealbumin)
Aβ₂M	Long-term dialysis	β₂-Microglobulin

nisone-containing regimens was superior to that of those with the colchicine schedule.

Supportive Measures

The nephrotic syndrome should be managed with salt restriction and diuretic agents as needed. If symptomatic azotemia develops, chronic renal dialysis is necessary. Salt restriction and the judicious use of diuretic drugs are helpful for congestive heart failure. Digitalis must be used with care because patients are unusually sensitive to the drug, and heart block and arrhythmias are common. Elastic stockings or leotards may benefit orthostatic hypotension. Fludrocortisone may be useful, but it does produce increased retention of fluids.

Prognosis

Currently, the median survival of patients with AL amyloidosis is 13 months. Survival varies greatly, depending on the associated syndrome; it is 4 months from the onset of congestive heart failure. Patients with only peripheral neuropathy have a median survival of 2 years.

Buxbaum JN, Chuba JV, Hellman GC, et al.: Monoclonal immunoglobulin deposition disease: Light chain and light and heavy chain deposition diseases and their relation to light chain amyloidosis: clinical features, immunopathology, and molecular analysis. Ann Intern Med 112:455, 1990. *Emphasizes the presence of amyloidosis and light-chain deposition of monoclonal light chains.*

Kyle RA, Gertz MA: Systemic amyloidosis. CRC Crit Rev Oncol Hematol 10:49, 1990. *A comprehensive review of primary, secondary, localized, hereditary, senile, and endocrine amyloidoses with more than 550 references.*

Kyle RA, Gertz MA: Primary systemic amyloidosis: Clinical and laboratory features in 474 cases. Semin Hematol 32:45, 1995. *A review of the clinical and laboratory data on 474 primary amyloidosis patients seen at one institution from 1981–1992 within 30 days of diagnosis.*

Stone MJ: Amyloidosis: a final common pathway for protein deposition in tissues. Blood 75:531, 1990. *An excellent overview of systemic amyloidosis.*

150 DISEASES OF LYMPH NODES AND SPLEEN
Douglas V. Faller

PHYSIOLOGY AND FUNCTIONS OF THE LYMPH NODES

The lymph node is divided structurally into three primary areas: the cortex, paracortex, and medulla. The areas are physically and functionally interlaced and surrounded by a series of sinuses. The *cortex* is the outermost portion of the lymph node, located immediately beneath the subcapsular sinus, and is the major site of B cells (antibody-producing lymphocytes) in the node. *Afferent lymphatic* drainage, carrying antigens and microorganisms, flows into this space and into immediate contact with lymphocytes, antigen-presenting nonphagocytic cells (histiocytes), and phagocytic cells (macrophages) of the cortex. Such immune stimulation results in enlargement of *lymphoid follicles* in the cortex, producing *germinal centers,* sites of intense B-lymphocyte proliferation and antibody production. The *paracortex* lies between the cortex and medulla, and represents the primary localization of T lymphocytes. It additionally contains macrophages and histiocytes. The paracortex is also the site of lymphocyte trafficking, where recirculating T and B cells enter the lymphatics from the venous system. The *medulla* of the lymph node is made up of a tortuous network of endothelial cell–lined sinuses that coalesce at the hilus to form the *efferent lymphatic.* Antigens are effectively trapped during the slow percolation of lymphatic fluid through the node. In addition, the sinuses are decked with macrophages, which actively scavenge particulate matter and microorganisms. The lymph node medulla supports a transient phase of postantigenic B-cell development associated with a long-lived antigen-specific B-cell subset. Noradrenergic sympathetic and peptidergic fibers innervate both primary and secondary lymphoid organs, but their significance is unknown.

The lymph node functions as the major site where antigens interact with cells of the immune system. Macrophages and histiocytes, which are capable of taking up and presenting antigen, are placed in intimate contact with helper T cells and B cells to facilitate lymphocyte stimulation and production of antibody. Antigen can reach the node in two ways: It can flow in passively via the afferent lymphatics or it can be actively carried into the node by recirculating lymphocytes and macrophages.

Enlargement of lymph nodes *(lymphadenopathy)* can thus result from proliferation of resident lymphocytes following antigen exposure during infection. Hyperplasia of nonlymphoid cells in the nodes, including macrophages and circulating inflammatory cells, can result from inflammation or infection and also cause node enlargement. In either situation, the nodal architecture is preserved despite the cellular hyperplasia. Malignant proliferation of lymphocytes within the lymph node, as seen in lymphomas or leukemias, is easily distinguishable from benign hyperplasia because normal nodal structures are effaced. Lymph nodes also serve as effective traps for circulating tumor cells and provide fertile ground for their continued growth. Thus, malignant metastases are another cause of lymph node enlargement.

EVALUATION OF THE LYMPH NODES

NODAL GROUPS AND DRAINAGE PATTERNS. Because lymphatic flow is regionally distributed, an understanding of the relationship between the anatomic location of the superficial lymph node groups and the origin of afferent lymphatics that drain into them is critical for guiding the examination and making a differential diagnosis of the patient with lymphadenopathy. Several lymph node subgroups draining structures in the head and neck comprise the cervical nodes. The submental nodes, located under the chin, and the submandibular nodes, near the angles of the jaw, receive drainage from structures in the mouth and salivary glands. The jugular nodes, which lie along the anterior border of the sternocleidomastoid muscle; the supraclavicular nodes, found behind the midportion of the clavicle; and the suboccipital nodes, which lie in the posterior cervical triangle, receive lymphatics from many head and neck structures. In addition, the supraclavicular nodes also drain intrathoracic and intra-abdominal organ systems. Lymphatic flow from the eyes, ears, and scalp is directed toward the preauricular and postauricular node groups that lie in front of and behind the ear, respectively. The central and lateral axillary node groups, which are located in the chest wall and along the upper humerus, respectively, receive drainage from the upper extremity, chest wall, breast, and intrathoracic structures. Other node groups with similar drainage patterns include the subscapular nodes, lying anterior to the latissimus dorsi muscle; the pectoral nodes, lying under the edge of the pectoralis major muscle; and the infraclavicular nodes, lying under the distal clavicle. The epitrochlear nodes, located just above the medial humeral epicondyle, receive lymphatic flow from the forearm and hand. The inguinal nodes lie along the inguinal ligament and drain the lower extremity and genitalia. The external iliac and femoral nodes, found in the femoral triangle, have a similar drainage pattern but also receive afferents from pelvic structures.

The deep nodal systems of the thorax and abdomen, including the hilar, mediastinal, abdominal, retroperitoneal, and pelvic nodes, receive afferent lymphatic flow directly from organs of the thorax, abdomen, and pelvis. In addition, they receive secondary drainage from the superficial nodal groups. Discovery of enlargement of these deep nodal groups is usually the result of a directed diagnostic workup, or occasionally from surveillance roentgenography. The mass effect that sometimes results from enlargement of deep node groups, however, can result in distinctive symptoms, which should suggest a disease process producing internal adenopathy. Enlargement of thoracic nodes (hilar or mediastinal) can compress the trachea or mainstem bronchi (producing cough, dyspnea, or wheezing), the esophagus (resulting in dysphagia), the superior vena cava or subclavian vein (causing venous congestion in the face, neck, and arm), the phrenic nerve (causing paralysis of the diaphragm), or the recurrent laryngeal nerve (producing hoarseness). Because the abdomen and pelvis are less rigidly enclosed than the thorax, compression syndromes resulting from enlargement of deep node groups here are less common, but internal iliac or pelvic node enlargement can lead to venous or lymphatic congestion in the leg or external genitalia. Extremely large abdominal and pelvic nodes are occasionally detectable by deep palpation.

Lymph node enlargement is a common finding on physical examination. Certain lymph nodes are palpable under normal circumstances. Submandibular nodes less than 1 cm in diameter are common in children and young adults, and inguinal nodes 0.5 to 2 cm in diameter are frequently found in healthy adults. The first component of an efficient approach to lymphadenopathy is to evaluate its significance. Assessment of three factors permit an interpretation of the finding of lymphadenopathy and, in addition, begin to establish a differential diagnosis.

CLINICAL SETTING. The age of the patient is of major importance, with lymph node enlargement more often reflecting serious disease in adults. Lymphadenopathy in patients less than 30 years of age is due to benign (and usually infectious) causes in at least 80% of cases. In those more than 30 years of age, however, lymphadenopathy is due to a benign process only 40% of the time. Clinical features and the setting frequently guide and direct the workup. For example, coexistence of fever and signs of localized or systemic infection, especially in a younger patient, usually suggests an infectious cause. Alternatively, the presence of constitutional symptoms, such as weight loss, night sweats, or low-grade fevers, points to a malignant cause of localized adenopathy. The differential diagnosis of mediastinal adenopathy in a young patient from an endemic area must include histoplasmosis as well as lymphoma. Generalized lymphadenopathy in a homosexual, a hemophiliac, or an intravenous drug abuser suggests a human immunodeficiency virus (HIV)–related syndrome. HIV infection is both active and progressive in the lymphoid organs during the clinically latent period of HIV infection.

PHYSICAL CHARACTERISTICS. Palpation of lymph nodes is best performed with the fingertips, using a circular motion and gradually increasing pressure. Examination of enlarged lymph nodes reveals physical characteristics such as firmness, mobility, and tenderness, that help in narrowing the diagnostic choices. Because of rapid enlargement and stretching of the nodal capsule, lymphadenopathy due to infectious processes is often tender. Nodes enlarged by infection can be matted or asymmetric, and the overlying skin may be inflamed and tender. The nodes may be suppurative, especially when the infectious agent is a mycobacterium or a pyogenic bacterium like *Staphylococcus*. Metastatic tumor produces enlarged nodes that are firm, nontender, and frequently fixed to underlying tissue. Lymphomatous processes result in large, often symmetric lymph nodes that are firm, mobile, nontender, and rubbery.

LOCATION OF NODES. The anatomic patterns of regional lymphatic drainage to lymph node groups can provide valuable clues as to the cause of lymph node enlargement. Table 150–1 lists the most common causes of regional lymphadenopathy by location. Enlargement of certain node groups almost always indicates serious disease. Palpable supraclavicular or scalene nodes are always abnormal and frequently the result of lymphoma or metastases from breast, intrathoracic, or gastrointestinal malignancy. Virchow's node is an enlarged, firm left supraclavicular node due to metastatic gastrointestinal malignancy. Enlarged abdominal or retroperitoneal nodes are usually the result of a malignant process. Enlarged lymph nodes associated with a satellite mass and/or pleural or peritoneal effusions are often caused by malignancy. Although palpable inguinal nodes are common in healthy adults, progressive changes or association with femoral or external iliac adenopathy should raise the suspicion of an underlying malignancy.

DIAGNOSTIC APPROACH TO LYMPH NODE ENLARGEMENT

The workup of a patient with newly discovered palpable adenopathy is directed by the factors mentioned previously: the clinical setting, physical characteristics, and location of the nodes. When an infectious cause is strongly suspected, a 14-day period of observation, with or without antimicrobial therapy, is appropriate. It is imperative to record the location and characteristics of the adenopathy carefully, including pertinent negative findings in order to validate follow-up observations. If, however, nodes are fixed or firm, or any of the aforementioned findings associated with malignancy are discovered, the node should be biopsied immediately.

Biopsy can consist of surgical excision or percutaneous lymph node biopsy by fine-needle aspiration. Aspiration can establish the diagnosis in infectious processes or metastatic malignancies, but is less helpful in lymphoid malignancies, in which assessment of

TABLE 150–1. CAUSES OF LYMPH NODE ENLARGEMENT BY LOCATION

Cervical nodes
Infections of head, neck, sinuses, ears, eyes, scalp, pharynx
Mononucleosis syndromes (Epstein-Barr virus, cytomegalovirus, toxoplasmosis)
Rubella
Tuberculosis (often suppurative nodes)
Lymphoma (often unilateral)
Head and neck malignancy (often unilateral)

Scalene/supraclavicular nodes
Lung, retroperitoneal, or gastrointestinal malignancy (e.g., Virchow's node)
Lymphoma
Thoracic or retroperitoneal bacterial or fungal infections

Axillary nodes
Infections, bites, trauma to hands or arms
Cat-scratch disease
Lymphoma
Breast carcinoma
Brucellosis
Melanoma

Epitrochlear nodes
Infections of hand (unilateral)
Lymphoma (unilateral)
Sarcoidosis (bilateral)
Tularemia (often unilateral)
Secondary syphilis (bilateral)

Inguinal nodes
Infections of leg or foot
Lymphoma
Pelvic malignancy
Venereal diseases (lymphogranuloma venereum, syphilis)
Pasteurella pestis

Hilar nodes
Sarcoidosis
Tuberculosis
Systemic fungal infections
Lung carcinoma (unilateral)

Mediastinal nodes
Mononucleosis syndromes
Sarcoidosis
Tuberculosis
Histoplasmosis
Lung carcinoma
Lymphoma

Abdominal/retroperitoneal nodes
Mesenteric lymphadenitis (tuberculosis)
Lymphoma
Germ cell tumors/seminoma
Prostatic carcinoma and other malignancies

Generalized lymphadenopathy (more than two separate sites)
Infections (Epstein-Barr virus, cytomegalovirus, toxoplasmosis, tuberculosis, hepatitis, syphilis, HIV/AIDS, histoplasmosis)
Malignancy (lymphoma, chronic myelogenous leukemia, chronic lymphocytic leukemia, acute leukemias)
Drug reactions
Systemic lymphadenopathy syndromes

nodal architecture is often required for diagnosis. In addition to routine pathologic studies, analysis of the biopsied node may include (where appropriate) microbial cultures, antigenic typing of lymphocytes, chromosomal analysis, and molecular studies for gene rearrangements. Analysis of biopsied superficial lymph nodes in adults establishes the diagnosis in approximately 50% of cases. One fourth of those patients in whom a diagnosis cannot be established by biopsy go on to develop a disease, usually a lymphoma, within 1 year. Therefore, close follow-up of patients with nondiagnostic first biopsies is indicated, including repeat biopsies if adenopathy and symptoms persist, plus consultation with experienced hematopathologists.

Evaluation of deep lymph node groups for enlargement usually requires roentgenography or ultrasonography. Enlarged nodes deep in the axilla may be visualized by mammographic or xerographic techniques. Hilar and mediastinal nodes can be evaluated by standard chest radiographs or computed tomography (CT). Lymphangiography, formerly the standard for evaluation of pelvic, retroperitoneal, and abdominal nodes, has become obsolete.

DISEASE PROCESSES RESULTING IN LYMPHADENOPATHY

A number of mechanisms can enlarge the lymph nodes: (1) hyperplasia of benign lymphocytes in response to infection and/or antigenic stimulation; (2) proliferation of circulating inflammatory and phagocytic cells in response to infection; (3) proliferation and infiltration of phagocytic cells in the lipid storage disorders; (4) neoplastic proliferation of malignant lymphocytes or phagocytes; (5) infiltration by metastatic malignant cells. Involvement of regional lymph nodes by tumor cells is a prognostic index of survival and a biologic indicator of more distant metastatic disease. In most solid tumors in humans, removing the draining lymph nodes seems to have little impact on survival, although it may be important in local control of disease.

Table 150–2 lists the most common diseases associated with lymphadenopathy and the pathophysiologic mechanism responsible for nodal enlargement. In addition, there are a number of other uncommon diseases of unknown cause which primarily involve the lymph nodes or in which lymphadenopathy is prominent or even the cardinal manifestation of the disease.

Amyloidosis is a condition manifested by deposition of fibrillar material in various organs, including the lymph nodes (see Ch. 248). The disease states associated with this deposition may be inflammatory, neoplastic, or hereditary. If the function of internal organs is not compromised by the deposited amyloid, lymphadenopathy, which is characteristically firm and nontender and can be either diffuse or localized may be the first manifestation of the condition. Microscopic analysis of a biopsied node reveals the characteristic staining and ultrastructural properties of the amyloid material.

Sarcoidosis (see Ch. 61) is a granulomatous disease of young adults involving multiple organ systems, most commonly the lungs, skin, eyes, and nervous system. Bilateral symmetric hilar adenopathy, often associated with peritracheal adenopathy in an asymptomatic patient, is characteristic of the disease. Peripheral lymphadenopathy is modest or absent. The differential diagnosis of hilar adenopathy must include lymphoma, lung carcinoma, histoplasmosis, and tuberculosis, although the symmetry of the adenopathy and frequent lack of associated symptoms in sarcoidosis are distinctive.

Mucocutaneous lymph node syndrome (Kawasaki's syndrome) is a disease of children and occasionally young adults, manifested by a distinctive erythematous and desquamative exanthem, conjunctivitis, and fever. Asymmetric cervical adenopathy is found in 75% of patients.

Lymphomatoid granulomatosis (see Ch. 243) is an infiltration of blood vessel walls with atypical lymphoid and plasmacytoid cells that form granulomas. The vessels of the lung, skin, kidneys, and central nervous system are most often involved, and the intrathoracic lymph nodes are enlarged in 40% of cases. The invading lymphocytes are most likely premalignant T cells because as many as half of patients develop a T-cell lymphoma.

Angioimmunoblastic lymphadenopathy is characterized by a distinctive proliferation of immature and mature plasma cells in a setting of neovascularization. Hepatosplenomegaly and generalized lymphadenopathy are accompanied by a polyclonal hyperglobulinemia, hemolytic anemia, and systemic symptoms. Diagnosis can usually be established by lymph node biopsy, although the disease can be confused with the immunoblastic lymphadenopathy associated with drug reactions, especially phenytoin and allopurinol. One quarter to one half of patients with angioimmunoblastic lymphadenopathy develop a B-cell lymphoma (immunoblastic sarcoma).

HISTIOCYTIC DISORDERS

An array of diseases characterized by proliferation of normal or malignant histiocytes (antigen-presenting and antigen-processing mononuclear phagocytes) can express prominent lymphadenopathy. The benign proliferative disorders can be subdivided as to whether or not the proliferating cell is a Langerhans (or Langerhans-like) histiocyte. The Langerhans cell histiocytoses (once designated *histiocytosis X* (X for unknown etiology) (see Ch. 147) occur most often in children with three overlapping presentations. These include the following: (1) *eosinophilic granuloma* occurs in older children and adults and presents with solitary or multiple bony lesions; (2) *Hand-Schuller-Christian syndrome,* defined as the triad of lytic skull lesions, exophthalmos, and diabetes insipidus, usually affects young children; (3) *Letterer-Siwe* disease, a systemic histiocytosis disorder, occurs in infants and is manifested by fever, eczematoid rash, otitis, lymphadenopathy, hepatosplenomegaly, and other visceral involvement.

The non–Langerhans cell histiocytoses are also nonmalignant proliferative disorders and can all result in regional or generalized lymphadenopathy. *Familial erythrophagocytic lymphohistiocytosis* and *infection-associated hemophagocytic syndrome* are both characterized by constitutional symptoms, pancytopenia, hepatosplenomegaly, lymphadenopathy, and the distinctive pathologic finding of phagocytosed erythrocytes in bone marrow or lymph node specimens. *Sinus histiocytosis* frequently manifests with massive, painless cervical lymphadenopathy, fever, weight loss, leukocytosis, and, less often, generalized lymphadenopathy. *Malignant histiocytosis (histiocytic medullary reticulosis)* is a progressive proliferation of atypical (but not clearly malignant) histiocytes and immature monocytoid cells, producing severe constitutional symptoms, generalized lymphadenopathy in 50% of cases, hepatosplenomegaly, pancytopenia, and papulonodular skin lesions. Malignancies of histiocytes are rare. They include histiocytic sarcoma, true malignant histiocytosis, and monocytic leukemia, all of which produce prominent lymphadenopathy.

PHYSIOLOGY AND FUNCTIONS OF THE SPLEEN

The spleen, the largest lymphoid organ in the body, plays a major role in the cellular and humoral immune response to infection and inflammation. In addition, with its unique architecture and network of fixed phagocytic cells, the spleen acts as the primary filter for circulating senescent cells, antigens, and microorganisms in the blood. Unlike the lymph nodes, the spleen receives no direct lymphatic drainage. A spleen of average size (135 grams) receives a blood flow of 300 ml per minute. Splenic vessels from the hilus penetrate trabeculations formed by invaginations of the splenic capsule. The central arterioles, surrounded by sheaths of lymphoid tis-

TABLE 150–2. CAUSES OF LYMPHADENOPATHY

Infection (lymphoid and/or phagocytic hyperplasia)
Viral (herpes viruses [cytomegalovirus, Epstein-Barr virus, varicella zoster (V-Z)], rubella, HIV, hepatitis A, vaccinia)
Bacterial (streptococcal, staphylococcal, *Brucella,* tularemia, *Listeria,* cat-scratch disease, *Pasteurella pestis, Haemophilus ducreyi,* syphilis, leptospirosis)
Fungal (histoplasmosis, coccidioidomycosis)
Mycobacterial (tuberculosis, leprosy)
Chlamydial (trachoma, lymphogranuloma venereum)
Parasitic (toxoplasmosis, trypanosomiasis, filariasis)

Inflammation (lymphoid hyperplasia)
Rheumatoid arthritis, sarcoidosis, systemic lupus erythematosus, dermatomyositis, immune complex disease/serum sickness, angioimmunoblastic lymphadenopathy, drug reactions

Neoplasms
Hematologic (myeloproliferative or lymphoproliferative): lymphomas (including primary splenic lymphoma), Hodgkin's disease, acute or chronic myeloid and lymphoid leukemias, adult T-cell leukemia/lymphoma (caused by HTLV), malignant histiocytosis
Metastatic (infiltrative): tumors of breast, lung, kidney, prostate, head and neck, and gastrointestinal tract; melanoma, germ cell tumors, seminoma, neuroblastoma, sarcoma

Infiltration
Gaucher's disease, Niemann-Pick disease, amyloidosis

Endocrine (lymphoid hyperplasia)
Hyperthyroidism

Disease of unknown cause with prominent lymphadenopathy
Mucocutaneous lymph node syndrome
Lymphomatoid granulomatosis
Dermatopathic lymphadenitis
Histiocytic disorder (Letterer-Siwe disease, erythrophagocytic lymphohistiocytosis, sinus histiocytosis, histiocytic medullary reticulosis, malignant histiocytosis)
Giant follicular lymph node hyperplasia

sue, have branches (follicular arterioles) that take off at right angles, effectively skimming plasma and circulating antigens from the blood and delivering them directly to the splenic immune system. The terminal arterioles are open-ended and dump the remaining concentrated blood cells into the splenic cords. Some cells are shunted rapidly into the venous collection system, but many percolate slowly through the open splenic cords for several minutes before squeezing through 0.5- to 2.5-μm slits between the endothelial cells and the discontinuous basement membrane of the venous sinusoids in order to re-enter the splenic venous system. The cut surface of the spleen displays a prominent red pulp, dotted with islands of white pulp, which serve to compartmentalize its filtration and immunologic functions.

THE WHITE PULP. The white pulp consists of periarteriolar lymphatic sheaths, with a mantle of small lymphocytes (predominantly T lymphocytes) surrounding lymphoid germinal centers, which contain B cells and plasmablasts. Blood-borne antigens and pathogens are concentrated and contact immune responder cells in the white pulp. Circulating particulate antigens and opsonized microorganisms are rapidly phagocytosed by macrophages in both the white and the red pulp and are presented to the lymphocytes surrounding the germinal centers in the white pulp. Within 4 hours, such antigens can be detected within the germinal centers. Reactive plasmablasts secreting immunoglobulin M (IgM) appear, and the germinal centers enlarge within 24 hours. The spleen is therefore important in mounting a response to new immune challenges and serves as the major source of IgM production in the body. The marginal zone of the spleen surrounds these periarteriolar lymphatic sheaths of the white pulp with a dense reticulum in which the terminal arterioles end. This marginal zone blends into the red pulp.

THE RED PULP. The splenic cords (of Billroth) make up the red pulp. Erythrocytes slowly traverse these nonendothelialized cords and are subjected to metabolic conditions (including hypoxia, glucose deprivation, and low pH) that stress senescent or mildly damaged cells. Defective erythrocytes with abnormally stiff cytoplasm (as in the sickle cell hemoglobinopathies), deficient cellular membranes (as in the spherocytic hemolytic diseases), or excessive rigidity of membrane and cytoskeleton (as in the thalassemia syndromes) are culled from this delayed microcirculation by the avidly phagocytic macrophages, reticular cells, and littoral cells that line the cords. *Pitting* of inclusions from erythrocytes is also performed by the phagocytes as the red cells squeeze through narrow fenestrations into the venous sinuses. This pitting function removes Howell-Jolly bodies (nuclear remnants), Heinz bodies (denatured hemoglobin), and intraerythrocytic parasites, such as *Plasmodium* and *Bartonella.* New reticulocytes are *conditioned* in this environment, losing up to 30% of their cell membrane and any remaining mitochondria. Iron from ingested red blood cells is stored by the splenic phagocytes and released to the plasma for *reutilization of iron.* States of abnormal hemolysis engender a build-up of hemosiderin in these cells.

The spleen serves as a *reservoir* for platelets, sequestering in a freely exchangeable pool up to a third of the total platelet mass. In certain disease states, this reservoir function can be exaggerated. Acute entrapment of erythrocytes in the splenomegalic crisis of hemoglobin SC or SS disease *(splenic sequestration crisis)* or the blackwater crisis of falciparum malaria can induce profound shock. Although the spleen is a blood-forming organ until 5 months of gestation, *hematopoiesis* in the adult spleen occurs only as a result of pathologic, usually neoplastic, conditions. The spleen also contributes to the *regulation of blood volume* and the *catabolism of low-density lipoproteins.*

EVALUATION OF THE SPLEEN

The spleen lies against the posterior abdominal wall and the diaphragm. When the organ enlarges, its lower pole moves down, anteriorly, and to the right. It is best identified by detection of its movement during respiration. Except in the very young, a palpable spleen is nearly always significantly enlarged. Palpation and percussion are complementary but less sensitive than noninvasive imaging techniques. Imaging of the spleen and liver can be performed after injection of radiolabeled colloid. To visualize the spleen alone or to identify accessory spleens, heat-damaged or chemically damaged red blood cells tagged with ^{51}Cr or ^{99m}Tc are used. The same test can be used to monitor splenic function. CT of the abdomen (with or without contrast medium) is an excellent imaging modality for

demonstrating the size, shape, and position of the spleen, as well as for depicting intrasplenic pathologic features but has limited value in the diagnosis of splenic involvement by lymphoma. Ultrasonography complements the spleen scan and CT scan in diagnostic studies.

SPLENOMEGALY

Five general mechanisms may enlarge the spleen: (1) reactive proliferation of lymphoid cells; (2) infiltration by neoplastic cells or lipid-laden macrophages; (3) extramedullary hematopoiesis; (4) proliferation of phagocytic cells; and (5) vascular congestion. Diseases may cause splenomegaly by one or a combination of these mechanisms (Table 150–3). The causes of massive splenomegaly (> 3000 grams) are somewhat more limited (Table 150–4). The myelodysplastic disorders and lymphoid malignancies are the most common causes of chronic massive splenomegaly in nontropical countries. Splenomegaly can present as an isolated finding on physical examination, can exist in association with a systemic disorder, or can be discovered as a consequence of the secondary hematologic effects of splenic enlargement—the hypersplenism syndrome. Symptoms arising from splenomegaly may include pain from the stretched capsule of an acutely enlarged spleen or shock from atraumatic rupture of a tense capsule.

Evaluation of splenomegaly should include examination of the peripheral blood and frequently the bone marrow. A spleen scan is recommended to determine the size and shape of the spleen and to look for defects suggestive of tumors, cysts, or displacement by extrasplenic masses. In general, diagnostic tests are not performed on the spleen itself; they are oriented toward the diagnosis of disease states producing splenomegaly. Chest radiography or liver function tests may reveal the cause of the splenic enlargement. If lymphadenopathy is present, lymph node biopsy may yield a diagnosis. When systemic symptoms accompany splenomegaly but no lymphadenopathy is appreciated, a laparotomy with biopsies of liver, spleen, and lymph nodes is sometimes indicated. Such a study produces a diagnosis of lymphoma in one third of cases, congestive splenomegaly in one quarter, and an inflammatory state in one fifth.

INFECTION. Systemic infections are the most common causes of moderate and transient splenomegaly. Splenic enlargement is the rule in mononucleosis due to Epstein-Barr virus infection but is less frequent in the heterophile-negative mononucleosis syndromes associated with cytomegalovirus, adenovirus, or acquired toxoplasmosis. Splenomegaly can be massive in congenital toxoplasmosis or other

TABLE 150–3. CAUSES OF SPLENOMEGALY

Infection (lymphoid hyperplasia)
Viral, parasitic, bacterial, fungal

Inflammation (lymphoid hyperplasia)
Rheumatoid arthritis, sarcoidosis, systemic lupus erythematosus, renal dialysis, beryllium, serum sickness

Neoplasms (infiltration or myeloproliferative)
Leukemia, lymphoma (including HTLV-associated adult T-cell leukemia lymphoma, polycythemia vera, myeloid metaplasia, Hodgkin's disease, metastatic tumors, primary tumors)

Hemolytic disease (phagocytic hyperplasia)
Spherocytosis, thalassemia major, pyruvate kinase deficiency, paroxysmal nocturnal hemoglobinuria, hemoglobinopathies, immune cytopenias

Deficiency diseases
Iron deficiency, pernicious anemia

Infiltration
Gaucher's disease, Niemann-Pick disease, amyloidosis, extramedullary hematopoiesis

Splenic vein hypertension (vascular congestion)
Cirrhosis, splenic or portal vein thrombosis, hepatic schistosomiasis, congestive heart failure

Endocrine
Graves' disease, Hashimoto's thyroiditis

Hemophilia (subsequent to intensive therapy with clotting factor concentrate)

Other
Cysts, angioimmunoblastic lymphadenopathy, histiocytoses, hyperlipidemia

TABLE 150–4. CAUSES OF MASSIVE SPLENOMEGALY

Acute
    Malaria (falciparum) with splenic sequestration crisis
    Sickle cell anemia with splenic sequestration crisis

Chronic
    Myelodysplastic
        Chronic myelogenous leukemia
        Myeloid metaplasia/myelofibrosis
        Polycythemia vera (end-stage)
        Primary thrombocythemia
    Neoplastic
        Lymphoma
        Malignant reticuloendotheliosis
        Hodgkin's disease
        Hairy cell leukemia
        Chronic lymphocytic leukemia
    Hematologic
        Thalassemia major
        Sickle cell anemia (rarely)
    Inflammatory-infiltrative
        Gaucher's disease
        Sarcoid
        Felty's syndrome
    Infectious
        Malaria
        Kala-azar

infectious causes of the TORCH syndrome (toxoplasmosis, rubella, cytomegalovirus, and herpes simplex). A palpable spleen often accompanies viral hepatitis and influenza and less frequently in association with infectious lymphocytosis, pertussis, and roseola infantum. Bacterial infections causing splenomegaly include secondary syphilis, subacute bacterial endocarditis, and acute brucellosis. Hematogenous spread of tuberculosis or histoplasmosis can involve the spleen. Splenomegaly is common in tropical populations due to malaria, schistosomiasis, leishmaniasis (kala-azar), chronic worm infestation, and other disorders. Rickettsial infection can produce splenic enlargement, with a palpable organ being noted in up to 40% of patients with Rocky Mountain spotted fever. Between 30 and 80% of patients with the lymphadenopathy accompanying the HIV disease–related complex (ARC) have modest splenomegaly.

INFLAMMATION. Splenomegaly commonly accompanies systemic lupus erythematosus (20%), rheumatoid arthritis (5 to 10%), and Behçet's disease, often producing hypersplenic cytopenias. (Angio)immunoblastic lymphadenopathy, sometimes associated with anticonvulsant administration, is characterized by splenomegaly, autoimmune hemolytic anemia, and dysproteinemia. Regional ileitis is occasionally accompanied by a histiocytic infiltration of the spleen.

NEOPLASMS. The myelodysplastic disorders and acute and chronic leukemias commonly infiltrate the spleen, causing modest to massive enlargement. Splenic involvement is noted in 30 to 40% of adult non-Hodgkin's lymphoma at presentation. Primary malignant tumors of the spleen are rare and include lymphangiosarcomas, hemangiosarcomas, fibrosarcomas, and leiomyosarcomas. Occasionally (less than 1% of all lymphomas), non-Hodgkin's lymphoma may present with the spleen as the initial and only site of involvement (primary splenic lymphoma). Metastatic tumor is a rare cause of splenomegaly.

STORAGE DISEASES. Previously undiagnosed Gaucher's disease can cause asymptomatic splenomegaly. Niemann-Pick disease and the sea-blue histiocyte syndrome may also present in this way. Diagnosis can be made by bone marrow biopsy.

CHRONIC CONGESTIVE SPLENOMEGALY (BANTI'S SYNDROME). This complex is characterized by splenomegaly, hypersplenic pancytopenia, and gastrointestinal bleeding secondary to portal hypertension. The splenic vein hypertension is due to either intrahepatic disease (cirrhosis or schistosomiasis) or extrahepatic disease (such as portal or splenic vein thrombosis). Splenic vein thrombosis is most commonly caused by compression of the vein by tumor or fibrosis. Pregnancy, trauma, or intravascular coagulation can predispose to portal vein thrombosis. In these conditions, the spleen is enlarged and congested, with distended veins and venous sinuses. Periarteriolar hemorrhages, siderotic nodules, hyper-

plasia of the red pulp, and progressive fibrosis occur. Symptoms can range from vague gastrointestinal complaints to catastrophic bleeding from esophageal or gastric varices. Hematologic cytopenias may be severe but are rarely the major medical concern. Etiologic studies of congestive splenomegaly should include evaluation for alcoholism, liver function tests, liver-spleen scan, liver biopsy, and a search for varices. If no liver disease is found, venous obstruction should be considered and splenoportal venography performed. Splenic or hepatic vein thrombosis may be the initial manifestation of an occult myeloproliferative disease, particularly polycythemia vera.

HYPERSPLENISM

Hypersplenism describes an exaggeration of normal spleen function, with enhanced filtration and phagocytosis of the blood's cellular elements. The hyperplastic spleen can sequester as much as 90% of the total platelet pool or 45% of the red cell mass. Four criteria support the diagnosis of hypersplenism: (1) cytopenia of one or more hematologic cell lines; (2) compensatory reactive marrow hyperplasia; (3) splenomegaly; and (4) correction of abnormalities by splenectomy.

Although hypersplenism frequently accompanies splenic enlargement, splenomegaly due to infiltrative diseases (lymphoma, chronic leukemia, Gaucher's disease, amyloidosis) seldom produces the severe cytopenias of hypersplenism. On the other hand, enlargement of the spleen due to hypertrophy of the phagocytic elements (inflammatory diseases) or secondary to congestive splenomegaly with slowing of the cellular transit time through the organ frequently produces anemia, thrombocytopenia, or granulocytopenia of various degrees. The erythrostatic environment of hypersplenism especially threatens mildly abnormal red blood cells. Patients with well-compensated hereditary spherocytosis or elliptocytosis, for example, may experience acute, severe hemolysis from the transient splenic enlargement that accompanies mononucleosis. Similarly, the anemia of chronic liver disease may worsen as the increasing pressure in the portal system causes stasis and destruction of acanthocytes in the spleen. The harsh metabolic environment of the splenic cords is exaggerated in the enlarged and congested spleen. In addition, phagocytosis of red cells or platelets stimulates the reactive hyperplasia of splenic histiocytes, begetting more hypersplenism. This is the mechanism underlying *primary hypersplenism,* in which the spleen hypertrophies because of phagocytosis of defective red cells (hereditary spherocytosis), antibody-coated red cells (autoimmune hemolytic anemia), or antibody-coated platelets (autoimmune thrombocytopenia). Hypersplenism can be identified and quantified by demonstrating a decrease in the circulating half-life of labeled erythrocytes along with an increase in the spleen-liver uptake ratio.

INDICATIONS FOR SPLENECTOMY

Splenectomy may be indicated for either of two medical conditions: (1) to stage or control a basic disease process (Hodgkin's disease, hereditary spherocytosis, autoimmune cytopenias), or (2) to alleviate the consequences of hypersplenism secondary to other disease processes. The spleen also may have to be removed because of traumatic or, rarely, spontaneous rupture causing intra-abdominal hemorrhage.

THROMBOCYTOPENIA. *Chronic autoimmune thrombocytopenia* (ITP) refractory to corticosteroid therapy usually improves after splenectomy, with platelet counts rising to greater than 150,000 per cubic milliliter in 90% of patients on long-term follow-up. Those who do not respond completely often can be maintained on a lower corticosteroid dose. The thrombocytopenia accompanying *systemic lupus* responds only occasionally to splenectomy, whereas the thrombocytopenia that occasionally accompanies *discoid lupus* is due to a consumptive coagulopathy and splenectomy is not indicated. *Thrombotic thrombocytopenic purpura* has been treated in the past with splenectomy and corticosteroid therapy. Currently, however, preferred treatment includes plasmapheresis or plasma exchange, along with corticosteroids, platelet inhibitor drugs, and vincristine (see Ch. 152). Splenectomy is a safe and effective treatment in HIV-infected patients with severe symptomatic thrombocytopenic purpura resistant to medical therapy; durable, complete responses occur in 70%, and partial responses in 20%. The procedure also may induce sustained increases in peripheral absolute CD4 lymphocyte counts.

HEMOLYTIC ANEMIAS. *Autoimmune hemolytic anemia* caused by warm-reacting antibodies which does not resolve after 2 months of corticosteroid therapy may be treated by splenectomy. Two thirds of such patients have complete or partial remission but a high relapse rate. Splenectomy is a uniformly effective treatment for the anemia of *hereditary spherocytosis* (see Ch. 134). Surgery should be delayed until the age of 5 years, if possible, to decrease the risk of overwhelming sepsis. Other congenital hemolytic anemias do not respond consistently, and the decision to remove the spleen should be based on the severity of the anemia and lack of response to alternative treatments.

LEUKEMIAS. Splenectomy is routinely performed for symptomatic cytopenias or splenomegaly in *hairy cell leukemia* (leukemic reticuloendotheliosis). Improvement occurs in up to 85% of patients, but recurrence of cytopenia is common. Early splenectomy is no longer recommended, and the advent of 2'-deoxycoformycin, interferon-α, and 2'-chlorodeoxyadenosine therapy may relegate splenectomy to a secondary role for this disease (see Ch. 142). In the past, splenectomy was commonly carried out in patients with *chronic myelogenous leukemia* for relief of symptoms or prior to bone marrow transplantation. Any benefit is transient, however; survival is not affected and the operation in this setting carries a high mortality. Splenectomy can provide useful palliation in patients with *prolymphocytic leukemia* and *chronic lymphocytic leukemia* who have symptomatic splenomegaly or autoimmune hemolytic anemia and are refractory to chlorambucil, fludarabine, and 2'-chlorodeoxyadenosine. Splenectomy improves the hematologic status and the quality of life in patients with severe *agnogenic myeloid metaplasia* (see Ch. 141.2).

STORAGE DISEASES. Splenectomy can be performed in *Gaucher's disease* when splenomegaly produces mechanical or cytopenic problems. The spleen serves as a storage area for undigested cerebroside, so it is possible that splenectomy might accelerate the disease (see Ch. 174.2).

FELTY'S SYNDROME. Neutropenia of variable degrees and splenomegaly, occasionally accompanied by thrombocytopenia or anemia, occur in about 1% of patients with rheumatoid arthritis. The spleen appears to be both the source of the antibody coating the neutrophils and the means of their destruction. If the neutropenia is severe enough to cause frequent infections or skin ulcerations, splenectomy benefits 60 to 80% of patients.

THALASSEMIA MAJOR. In the setting of longstanding thalassemia, therapeutic splenectomy is often required as progressive splenomegaly results in increasing transfusion requirements.

RENAL DIALYSIS HYPERSPLENISM. Up to 10% of uremic patients undergoing long-term dialysis develop signs of hypersplenism. Splenectomy may decrease bleeding tendencies and transfusion requirements.

ALTERNATIVES TO SPLENECTOMY. Therapy with glucocorticoids inhibits phagocytosis and can provide a useful "chemical splenectomy" in short-term situations. Authorities may recommend partial splenectomy in children to reduce the risk of post-splenectomy complications. Partial or complete embolization of the spleen using percutaneous catheterization is a relatively safe, effective, and noninvasive approach when surgery is contraindicated. Splenic irradiation (100 to 500 cGy) can provide transient therapy for hypersplenism or splenomegaly due to infiltrative diseases.

POST-SPLENECTOMY SYNDROMES AND HYPOSPLENISM

HEMATOLOGIC SEQUELAE. The hyposplenic or post-splenectomy state often can be diagnosed from the peripheral blood smear (see Color Plate 6K). In the absence of splenic culling and pitting functions, nucleated red blood cells, Howell-Jolly and Heinz body inclusions, siderocytes, and acanthocytes enter the circulation. Reticulocytes are no longer conditioned, and their redundant cell membrane produces target cells.

A transient and modest increase in the leukocyte count occurs after splenectomy and lasts 1 to 2 weeks. The bulk of this *leukocytosis* is accounted for by an early *neutrophilia*. Later, *lymphocytosis* and *monocytosis* become more prominent.

Splenectomy routinely results in a prominent postoperative *thrombocytosis*, often producing platelet counts of 1 million or more per cubic millimeter for weeks to months thereafter. The elevation may persist indefinitely in 40% of patients. The risk of consequent thromboembolic phenomena after splenectomy is high only in the setting of myeloproliferative disease or paroxysmal nocturnal hemoglobinuria. Attempts should be made to decrease the platelet count with chemotherapy before surgery in such cases. Following surgery, therapy with anticoagulants and antiplatelet agents should be considered, especially if the patient is bedridden.

INFECTION. In the absence of the spleen or in the setting of functional hyposplenism, certain inadequacies of immune function can be demonstrated. IgM levels fall and complement-mediated opsonization declines. The latter is in part due to a fall in the levels of tuftsin and properdin, two spleen-produced opsonic proteins. The ability to phagocytose circulating antigens is compromised, as is cell-mediated immunity.

The risk of *overwhelming sepsis* following splenectomy or in functional hyposplenism is especially high in children, reaching as much as 16% per year in debilitated infants. The annual incidence falls to 4% by the age of 16 years, and seldom affects adults; in any event, mortality is extremely high. The causative organisms are encapsulated bacteria, predominantly pneumococci and less commonly meningococci or *Haemophilus influenzae*. These are poorly opsonized in the body, and the intact spleen, with its slow, tortuous blood flow past avid phagocytes, appears to be the primary site for clearance of these pathogens. Following splenectomy, infected children contract primarily a meningitis, which is less frequently fatal than the septicemia that may occur in splenectomized adults. All patients with decreased splenic function, whether due to functional hyposplenism or to splenectomy (traumatic or therapeutic), must be warned against the advent of any febrile illness. Prophylaxis with penicillin is recommended for all children with asplenia or splenic hypofunction (e.g., sickle cell anemia). Immunization with polyvalent vaccines to pneumococci, meningococci, and *H. influenzae* is advised for patients over 3 years. Serologic response to these vaccines may not be normal in the setting of hyposplenia or asplenia. The timing of vaccine administration (with respect to splenectomy) is not established, but vac-cination should precede splenectomy and any chemotherapy, if possible. Serious infections with unusual organisms like *Babesia* or *Bartonella* also occur in hyposplenic individuals. A concurrent viral infection may predispose hyposplenic patients to fulminant bacteremias.

FUNCTIONAL HYPOSPLENISM. Repeated symptomatic or silent infarction of the spleen in the course of veno-occlusive diseases such as sickle cell syndromes results in substantial or total loss of splenic tissue *(autosplenectomy)*. The spleen shrinks and becomes fibrotic. Reflecting the lost splenic filtration processes, circulating erythrocytes are found to contain mitochondrial remnants and inclusions of nuclear fragments (Howell-Jolly bodies) and denatured hemoglobin (Heinz bodies). Bizarrely shaped red cells, target cells, and large platelets appear. Hyposplenism can occur even with a large or normal-sized spleen if splenic tissue has been replaced by sarcoid granulomas, amyloid, or multiple myeloma, or if splenic phagocytes have been paralyzed by high-dose corticosteroid therapy. Other diseases linked with hyposplenism include ulcerative colitis, celiac disease, dermatitis herpetiformis, systemic lupus erythematosus, primary thrombocythemia, and Graves' disease. Such patients run the same risk of fulminant bacteremia as do those who have had their spleen surgically removed.

CONGENITAL ASPLENIA. This uncommon condition is associated with symmetric development of normally asymmetric organs or pairs of organs. Complex and multiple cardiovascular anomalies are the rule.

OTHER DISEASES OF THE SPLEEN

SPLENIC RUPTURE. Rupture of the capsule may be spontaneous in the setting of acute splenomegaly, precipitated by trauma, by overly zealous palpation of an enlarged spleen (secondary to mononucleosis, sepsis, or leukemia) or rarely by dissection of a pancreatic pseudocyst into the spleen. Rupture produces acute left upper quadrant pain, sometimes radiating to the left scapular region as well as abdominal guarding and rigidity, quickly progressing to hypovolemic shock. Often nonoperative management and the use of hemostatic agents, or splenorrhaphy, including gluing or wrapping of the ruptured capsule ("hair netting"), are attempted in place of splenectomy. After traumatic rupture of the spleen, especially in children, every effort should be made to preserve the spleen or to perform only a partial splenectomy.

perform only a partial splenectomy.

SPLENIC INFARCTION. Infarction usually occurs in the setting of splenic enlargement secondary to myeloproliferative disease or vascular occlusive phenomena (sickle hemoglobinopathies, including SS, Sβ-thalassemia, and SC diseases). Infarctions may be silent or produce severe left upper quadrant pain.

ARTERIAL ANEURYSMS. Splenic aneurysms are most common in women beyond middle age. They may be asymptomatic, cause left upper quadrant pain, or produce vague gastrointestinal complaints. Aneurysms of the spleen sometimes can be palpated; a bruit may be heard. Radiologic studies can reveal a calcified aneurysmal wall, and the diagnosis is made by sonography or angiography. Embolization of such aneurysms has been successful when surgery is contraindicated.

SPLENIC HEMANGIOMATOSIS. Diffuse cavernous hemangiomatosis of the spleen is rare, but the cavernous hemangioma is the most common benign tumor involving the spleen. The patient can present with splenic infarctions, splenomegaly, or thrombocytopenia secondary to platelet destruction within the hemangiomas. Alternatively, the finding of hemangiomatosis may be incidental. The diagnosis can usually be made by CT or sonography. *Littoral cell angioma* is an unusual splenic vascular tumor demonstrating histiocytic differentiation.

SPLENIC CYSTS AND BENIGN TUMORS. Echinococcal infection should be suspected in a patient with an appropriate travel history, single or multiple splenic cysts with calcified walls, and eosinophilia. Serologic studies may help in establishing the diagnosis. True splenic cysts (dermoids and mesenchymal inclusion cysts) are embryonic rests and can be diagnosed by CT, sonography, and angiography. *Inflammatory pseudotumors of the spleen* are benign lesions with infiltrating T cells and can be confused with malignant lymphoma. *Splenic hamartomas* are often mistaken for the nodular lesions of malignant lymphoma.

SPLENIC ABSCESS. Splenic abscesses usually follow a bout of septicemia and can be difficult to diagnose. The initial source of the organism is not consistent, but predisposing splenic abnormalities often exist. These include previous infarction (secondary to sickle cell disease or leukemia), trauma, and infection (malaria, typhoid, ameba, cysts). Some abscesses extend into the spleen from adjacent perforated abdominal organs (stomach, transverse colon, tail of pancreas). In most series, streptococci are the most common agents, followed by staphylococci and, with increasing frequency, by gram-negative organisms (*Salmonella,* Enterobacteriaceae, *Pseudomonas, Serratia, Bacteroides*) and anaerobes. Presenting symptoms include fever, chills, and left upper quadrant pain, often accompanied by tenderness, muscle spasm and subcutaneous edema over the spleen. Infection localized to the upper pole of the spleen can produce pleuritic pain and even left pleural effusion. An abscess in the lower pole may result in signs of peritoneal inflammation, including an audible friction rub. Splenic scan, sonography, and CT aid in diagnosis. The differential includes subphrenic abscess, pulmonary empyema, splenic infarction, perinephric abscess, neoplasms, and pancreatic pseudocyst. A combination of antibiotics and surgical intervention, usually splenectomy, is indicated. Single abscesses respond well, but multiple ones often are the result of generalized sepsis in a debilitated or immunocompromised patient and carry a high mortality.

Brigden ML: Overwhelming postsplenectomy infection still a problem. West J Med 157:461, 1992. *A review of the diagnosis of hyposplenism and asplenism in adults and their sequelae, with recommendations for prophylaxis.*

Chun CH, Raff MJ, Contreras L, et al.: Splenic abscess. Medicine 59:50, 1980. *Comprehensive review of this often fatal disease discussing cause, predisposing factors, diagnosis, and treatment.*

Coad JE, Matutes E, Catovsky D: Splenectomy in lymphoproliferative diseases: A report of 70 cases and review of the literature. Leuk Lymphoma 10:245, 1993. *Seventy percent of 70 patients had a complete hematologic response and 23% had a partial response. Improvements were more pronounced in B-cell than in T-cell disorders. A continuing role for splenectomy in symptomatic lymphoid malignancies is advocated.*

Freeman JL, Jari SZ, Roberts JL, et al.: CT of congenital and acquired abnormalities of the spleen. Radiographics 13:597, 1993. *Demonstrates the value and limitations of CT in the examination of patients with congenital and acquired abnormalities of the spleen.*

Heys SD, Eremin O: The relevance of tumor draining lymph nodes in cancer. Surg Gynecol Obstet 174:533, 1992. *Regional lymphatics may have an important role at the early stage of tumor development, but with progressive growth of tumor, the lymphatics are unlikely to be beneficial, both because of a failure of nodal antitu-*

mor defense mechanisms and because they may provide a preferred biologic environment for tumor cell proliferation and an anatomic route for dissemination to distant tissues and organs.

Hibberd PL, Rubin RH: Approach to immunization in the immunosuppressed host. Infect Dis Clin North Am 4:124, 1989. *A discussion of the roles of vaccines and adjunctive measures, such as antimicrobials and immunoglobulin, in the asplenic patient.*

Holdsworth RJ, Irving AD, Cuschieri A: Postsplenectomy sepsis and its mortality rate: Actual versus perceived risks. Br J Surg 78:1031, 1991. *A collective clinical review of the literature on post-splenectomy sepsis from 1952 to 1987, with detailed analysis of 5902 reports.*

Knecht H: Angioimmunoblastic lymphadenopathy: Ten years' experience and state of current knowledge. Semin Hematol 26:208, 1989. *A review of the idiopathic and drug-related forms of this disease and their natural histories.*

Lawrence DD, Carrasco CH, Fornage B, et al.: Percutaneous lymph node biopsy. Cardiovasc Intervent Radiol 14:55, 1991. *Reviews the advances in imaging modalities for detecting lymphadenopathy, and the use and limitations of fine-needle aspirations in the diagnostic workup of lymphadenopathy.*

Lucas CE: Splenic trauma. Choice of management. Ann Surg 213:98, 1991, with comment in 215:92, 1992. *A comprehensive review of current surgical and nonsurgical techniques aimed at preserving splenic function.*

Naouri A, Feghali B, Chabal J, et al.: Results of splenectomy for idiopathic thrombocytopenic purpura. Acta Haematol 89:200, 1993. *A review of 72 cases, demonstrating excellent responses and suggesting that factors associated with a good response to splenectomy included a high postoperative platelet count, preoperative corticosteroid dependence, and predominantly splenic sequestration.*

Pantaleo G, Graziosi C, Fauci AS: The role of lymphoid organs in the pathogenesis of HIV infection. Semin Immunol 5:157, 1993. *During the prolonged latency period of HIV infections, viremia is low and few infected cells circulate, but immune function deteriorates and CD4 lymphocyte levels fall. Active and progressive, but occult, HIV infection within the lymph nodes may explain the evolution to clinically apparent disease.*

Pochedly C, Sills RH, Schwartz AD (eds.): Disorders of the Spleen: Pathophysiology and Management. New York, Marcel Dekker, 1989. *Detailed description of splenic anatomy, physiology, and pathophysiology, with extensive discussion of the causes and sequelae of splenic hypofunction and hyperfunction.*

151 BONE MARROW TRANSPLANTATION
Joel Rappeport

DEFINITION

Bone marrow transplantation involves re-establishment of normal blood cell production through long-term engraftment of the pluripotential hematopoietic stem cell (a stem cell capable of both self-renewal and maturation to a variety of committed hematopoietic progenitors). The procedure is used to replace an absent, malignant, or genetically abnormal stem cell or to rescue a patient from myeloablative chemoradiation therapy. Several sources may serve as a reservoir of pluripotential stem cells, including bone marrow from a monozygotic twin (syngeneic transplant), a family member or unrelated donor with an identical human leukocyte antigen (HLA) type (allogeneic transplant) (see Ch. 229), autologous (self) bone marrow or peripheral blood, and more recently HLA-matched umbilical cord blood. Single HLA-mismatched donor bone marrow has also resulted in successful grafts. In more limited situations, T cell–depleted bone marrow from haploidentical (50% identical at the HLA locus) donors have also been successful. In many situations, a number of transplant sources may exist, and the relative merits of each source of marrow needs to be weighed for the particular situation. Donor and recipient erythrocyte ABO differences do not prohibit the use of a donor.

PRETRANSPLANTATION MEASURES

In virtually all situations a preparative regimen is necessary to immunosuppress the host, ablate abnormal hematopoiesis, or successfully treat an underlying malignant disease. Not all chemotherapeutic agents have similar properties. For example, cyclophosphamide is an excellent immunosuppressant with little effect on the hematopoietic stem cell, while busulfan primarily affects hematopoiesis. A variety of preparative regimens have been developed for different clinical situations. In autologous marrow and peripheral blood stem cell transplants, the marrow or peripheral blood is harvested and cryopreserved prior to administration of the preparative regimen. In some settings the autologous marrow is purged *ex vivo* (in the laboratory) of possible malignant cell contamination. The total marrow obtained from the donor in an allogeneic marrow transplant is usually $1-4 \times 10^8$ bone marrow cells per kilogram of recipient weight. This is obtained with multiple small-volume bone marrow aspirations from the iliac bone, and adequate numbers of cells for the average adult are usually obtained in approximately 600 ml. Following the preparative regimen, the bone marrow is infused intravenously. Hematopoiesis in the host becomes established within the milieu of the bone marrow stroma, with proliferation in the peripheral blood noted within 2 to 4 weeks. In the stable engrafted state, all cells are donor derived, including tissue macrophages. Peripheral blood counts normalize indefinitely.

POSTTRANSPLANT MANAGEMENT AND COMPLICATIONS

Bone marrow transplantation carries the risk of many complications, the frequency of which depend on the type performed as well as the patient's age and underlying medical condition. Short-term toxicity from the preparative regimen includes hepatic veno-occlusive disease, noninfectious interstitial pneumonia, mucositis, and cardiomyopathy. Long-term toxicity includes cataract formation, secondary malignant disease, and sterility. Children may undergo disturbances in growth and development. The incidence of graft rejection is related to the underlying disease and nature of the donor marrow.

The major complication associated with allogeneic transplantation is the *graft-versus-host disease (GVHD) reaction,* resulting from recognition by the engrafted donor T cell of a foreign recipient HLA antigen or a minor non-HLA transplant antigen. All allogeneic transplantations carry this risk. The primary target organs include the liver, gastrointestinal tract, and skin in both acute and chronic GVHD.

A number of prophylactic maneuvers may be undertaken to prevent GVHD. Prevention may include *ex vivo* marrow purging to deplete mature T cells, the putative initiator of the GVHD reaction. Prophylactic low-dose chemotherapeutic drugs, such as methotrexate, immunosuppressive agents such as corticosteroids, cyclosporine or antithymocyte globulin, or some combination of these agents may be administered for 6 to 12 months post-transplant. In most cases a state of immunologic tolerance develops after a period of months, allowing discontinuance of immunosuppression. Despite prophylactic treatment, acute GVHD occurs within a few weeks of engraftment in 30 to 60% of recipients of HLA-matched transplants. A greater incidence of severe GVHD is associated with marrow obtained from multiparous women, partially mismatched donors, and matched unrelated donors. Severe GVHD may be lethal, with patients dying from electrolyte imbalance, hepatic failure, or infection. Treatment of severe acute GVHD includes high-dose corticosteroids and/or antithymocyte globulin.

The chronic GVHD reaction appears a few months to a year following transplantation and shares many characteristics of autoimmune disorders, particularly scleroderma. Chronic GVHD may be associated with long-term disability as well as death from opportunistic infections. The disorder has been successfully treated with corticosteroids ± azathioprine or cyclosporine. The incidence of recurrent leukemia is less in patients with GHVD. This effect most commonly noted in acute lymphoblastic leukemia and chronic granulocytic leukemia has been designated the *graft-versus-leukemia (GVL) effect.*

Patients receiving marrow transplants have considerable risk of developing a wide range of infections. Immediate posttransplant risk consists of neutropenia–associated bacterial and fungal infections. Use of indwelling venous catheters has resulted in an increased incidence of gram-negative and gram-positive bacterial infections. After recovery from neutropenia the patient is susceptible to a variety of viral and fungal infections, including cytomegalovirus (CMV), herpes simplex, herpes zoster, and aspergillus. Interstitial pneumonia infections peak 2 to 4 months posttransplant, and if herpes zoster develops, it usually does so during the first 6 months. The risk of CMV pneumonia is increased in patients who have had prior CMV exposure or received transfusions or marrow from CMV-antibody–positive donors. Potential bone marrow recipients should be tested for the presence of the CMV antibody, and if negative should receive CMV-antibody–negative blood products. Many authorities recommend prophylactic administration of antiviral agents to persons at risk of reactivation of CMV infection. Late opportunistic infections result most often from the absence of immune function. Recapitulation of the newly engrafted

immune system reconstitutes the patient's immune system over a matter of months, the length of time depending on the type of marrow transplantation performed, as well as the presence or absence of GVHD. For most patients without chronic GVHD the immune system reconstitutes within 1 year following transplantation, and subsequently they have an appropriate response to immunizations. For patients with chronic GVHD the immunoincompetent state may persist for years. In situations in which the patient suffers from long-term immunodeficiency, gamma globulin replacement therapy may be beneficial.

CLINICAL APPLICATIONS

Aplastic Anemia

Acquired aplastic anemia (see Ch. 130) commonly results from loss of pluripotential stem cells. The preparative regimen for allogeneic transplantations consists entirely of immunosuppressive agents, most frequently high-dose cyclophosphamide. A major complication of marrow transplantation in aplastic anemia is graft rejection, which results from sensitization of the recipient to minor non-HLA transplantation antigens, exposure to which occurs primarily through transfusions. Therefore, at diagnosis a decision must be made whether or not the patient is a candidate for transplant as primary therapy. The patient and family should be immediately tissue typed, and if an appropriate transplant situation is identified, the patient should immediately be prepared for grafting. Judicious use of transfusions should be undertaken, with only clinically dictated transfusions administered. Sensitization may be decreased by transfusing filtered blood products. For the sensitized patient more intense immunosuppression may be required for transplantation. Complete recovery and survival in the young untransfused patient approaches 85%. Success in multiply transfused patients 30 years or older is in the range of 50% (Fig. 151–1). With an increased likelihood of the need for transplantation in older patients, an initial therapeutic approach may be a course of immunosuppression. However, the necessary transfusion support may ultimately result in a poorer transplant outcome. Hematopoietic reconstitution appears to be permanent, with patients having survived for more than 20 years.

Different preparative regimens are necessary for the patient whose aplastic anemia results from an underlying constitutional defect, such as Fanconi's anemia (Ch. 130). The aplastic anemia of these disorders may occur in young adulthood as well as in childhood, and a vigorous attempt should be made to rule out these scenarios. A number of successful transplantations have been performed in Fanconi's anemia utilizing umbilical cord blood as a source of stem cells. Patients with paroxysmal nocturnal hemoglo-

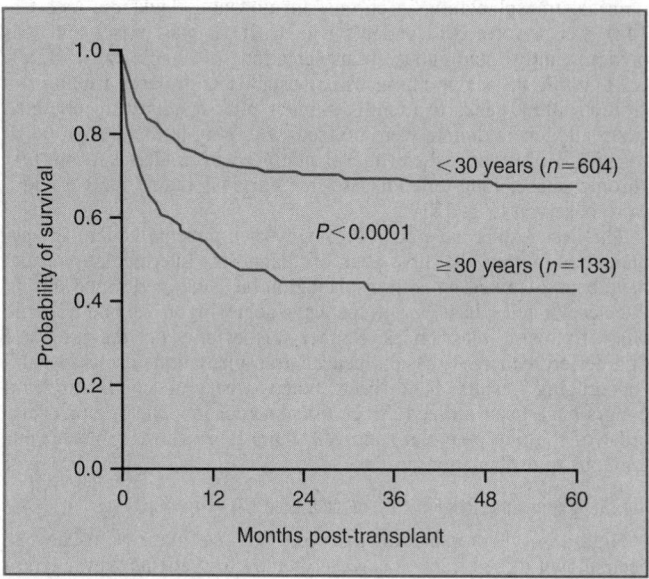

FIGURE 151–1. Probability of survival after HLA-identical sibling marrow transplants for severe aplastic anemia by patient age, 1985–1991. (From Bortin MM et al. and the International Bone Marrow Transplant Registry: 1993 Progress Report. Bone Marrow Transplant 12:97, 1993.)

binuria with or without aplasia have also been cured with allogeneic bone marrow transplantation.

Acute Nonlymphocytic Leukemia (see Ch. 143)

Some of the earliest successes in marrow transplantation occurred in patients with end-stage acute nonlymphocytic leukemia. Patients receiving allogeneic transplants in first remission currently have a prolonged disease-free survival of 45 to 60%. For patients electing to be initially managed with chemotherapy, success of transplants performed in second remission or "early" relapse are approximately 30 to 35%. This approach prevents exposing patients cured by chemotherapy to the vicissitudes of transplantation.

Whether to pursue transplantation in first-versus-subsequent remission should be determined individually with young patients with bad prognostic leukemic features undergoing transplant in first remission. Results of transplants performed later in the clinical course are poor, with a cure rate of approximately 10 to 15%. Experience of utilizing autologous chemotherapy–purged marrow has resulted in early outcomes similar to allogeneic transplants with a 2-year survival of 50% for patients in first remission. Patients with an underlying myelodysplastic syndrome should have an allogeneic rather than an autologous transplant, since the patient's pluripotential stem cell is qualitatively defective. Age-appropriate patients with myelodysplastic syndrome should be considered for transplantation prior to the evolution of leukemia. Matched unrelated registry donors for patients with acute nonlymphocytic leukemia have demonstrated approximately 40% long-term survival, although there is an increased incidence of both graft rejection and severe GVHD.

Acute Lymphoblastic Leukemia (ALL) (see Ch. 143)

Long-term disease-free survivals of approximately 30% have been noted in patients undergoing allogeneic transplantation who had had a previous relapse despite intensive initial chemotherapy. As sophisticated prognostic features were identified, patients with poor-prognosis ALL have undergone transplantation in first remission with success rates of 50 to 60%. Autologous transplantation has also been performed in lymphoblastic leukemia, with *ex vivo* marrow purging with monoclonal antibodies directed against specific leukemic antigens. Again, encouraging survival results of approximately 40 to 50% have been noted.

For those patients with a related allogeneic donor in second remission, particularly if relapse has occurred during maintenance chemotherapy, an allogeneic transplant should be pursued. If a family donor is not identified, the possibility of an autologous transplant should be pursued rather than seeking a matched unrelated donor.

Chronic Myelogenous Leukemia (CML)

Initial transplantation in chronic myelogenous leukemia (see Ch. 142) was performed in patients with CML in blast crises and was predominantly autologous transplantation of stable-phase CML cells. While the stable phase was re-established, relapse usually occurred within weeks to months. Similar poor results were obtained when allogeneic donors were utilized, with long-term survival of 10 to 15%. However, when transplantation was undertaken in first chronic phase, long-term disease-free survival rates of 50 to 60% were observed (Fig. 151–2).

The best results have been obtained when patients undergo transplantation within the first year of diagnosis. Intermediate results have been obtained when transplantation has been performed during the accelerated phase, or in patients achieving a second chronic phase following blast crises. Neither splenectomy nor the prior use of interferon therapy has influenced transplantation results. Again, encouraging results have been noted when matched unrelated donors have been utilized. Since this disorder involves a clonal disorder of the pluripotential stem cell, there is no current role for autologous transplantation.

Non-Hodgkin's and Hodgkin's Lymphoma (see Ch. 145 and 146)

High-dose chemoradiation followed by bone marrow rescue has been shown to be effective salvage therapy for patients with aggressive non-Hodgkin's lymphoma, with superior results being observed in chemosensitive disease compared with results in chemoresistant disease. It is currently unclear which source of pluripotential stem cell is preferable, autologous bone marrow, peripheral blood stem cells, or allogeneic bone marrow. Those patients with a secondary

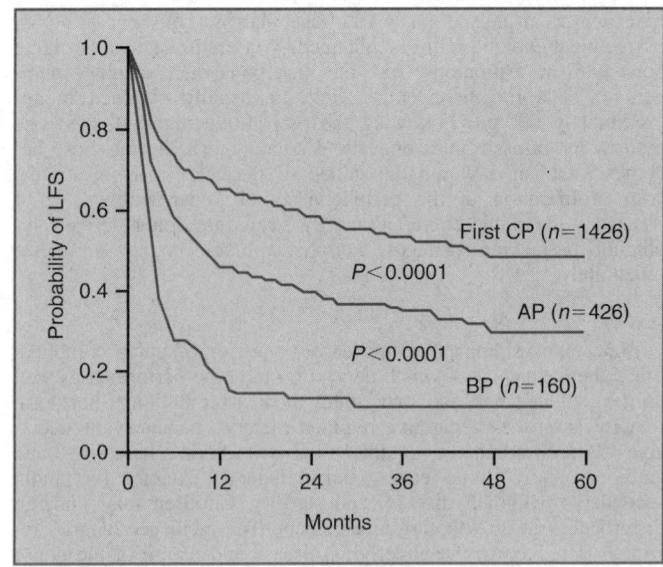

FIGURE 151–2. Probability of leukemia-free survival after HLA-identical sibling BMT for CML, 1985–1991. CP, chronic phase; AP, accelerated phase; BP, blast phase. (From Bortin MM et al. and the International Bone Marrow Transplant Registry, 1993 Progress Report. Bone Marrow Transplant 12:97, 1993.)

chemotherapy–induced hematopoietic disorder or an underlying immunologic abnormality should be offered an allogeneic transplant. Studies are under way to evaluate the role of marrow transplantation in patients with aggressive lymphoma and bad prognostic features in first complete remission. Sufficient evidence exists to suggest that appropriate candidates with low-grade non-Hodgkin's lymphoma should be considered for transplantation. Evaluation should be carried out in young patients with evidence of conversion to more aggressive lymphoma, as well as a short response to intensive chemotherapy. Patients with advanced Hodgkin's disease have also been effectively rescued.

OTHER APPLICATIONS

In addition to the diseases noted above, bone marrow transplantation has been successful in a number of other disorders, including breast cancer, multiple myeloma, germ cell cancers, neuroblastoma, and acute myelofibrosis. The precise role of marrow transplantation in these disorders is still under investigation. A large number of congenital hematopoietic disorders have been cured, including rare immunodeficiency and neutrophilic diseases, as well as more common hemoglobinopathies such as sickle cell anemia and thalassemia. Inborn errors of metabolism such as malignant osteopetrosis, Gaucher's disease, Hunter's syndrome, Hurler's syndrome, and adrenoleukodystrophy have all been successfully corrected with allogeneic bone marrow transplantation.

Sufficient advances have been made in prevention and treatment of the complications of bone marrow transplantation to consider the use of this therapeutic method as part of the management of a number of disorders. In virtually all disease states, success rates with marrow grafting are superior in early as opposed to late disease, and therefore the potential role of transplantation should be evaluated at the time of diagnosis rather than as a last desperate maneuver. The addition of matched unrelated donors as well as other sources of stem cells has increased the number of patients who may benefit from this therapeutic method.

Burakoff SJ, Deeg HJ, Ferrara J, Attkinson K (eds.): Graft-vs-Host Disease; Immunology, Pathophysiology and Treatment. New York, Marcel Dekker, 1990. *Superb and extensive multiple-author discussion of both the laboratory and clinical aspects of graft-versus-host disease. Can be used as clinical reference or for extensive review.*

Forman SJ, Blume KG, Thomas ED (eds.): Bone Marrow Transplantation. Boston, Blackwell Scientific Publications, 1994. *Most extensive multiple-author discussion of entire topic of bone marrow transplantation.*

Hansen JA, Choo SY, Geraghty DE, Mickelson E: The HLA system in clinical marrow transplantation. Hematol/Oncol Clin North Am 4:507, 1990. *Complete review of the HLA system, of value for both novice and expert.*

Kernan NA, Bartsch G, Ash RC, et al.: Analysis of 462 bone marrow transplantations from unrelated donors facilitated by the National Marrow Donor Program. N Engl J Med 328:593, 1993. *Large and recent report of the experience of transplantation utilizing matched unrelated donors.*

152 HEMORRHAGIC DISORDERS: ABNORMALITIES OF PLATELET AND VASCULAR FUNCTION

Marc Shuman

MECHANISMS OF HEMOSTASIS

NORMAL HEMOSTASIS. Normally, blood clots in response to vascular damage to form a local seal. The mechanisms involved can be divided into three categories: (1) vasoconstriction, (2) platelet adhesion and aggregation, and (3) fibrin formation and stabilization. All three processes are intimately related and are initiated simultaneously. Once the clot is formed and tissue repair has started, digestion of the clot (fibrinolysis) begins, eventually leading to vascular patency. Blood coagulation and fibrinolysis are largely described in Ch. 153.

The normal sequence of events leading to clotting is initiated by trauma to the vessel, which constricts reflexly to reduce blood flow (Fig. 152–1). With damage to the vascular endothelium, platelets adhere to the subendothelial matrix (Fig. 152–2). Tissue factor, a protein-phospholipid complex, is exposed in the vessel wall and activates clotting by binding Factor VII.

After the first platelets adhere to the injured vessel, platelet aggregation begins, initiated probably through multifactorial mechanisms (Fig. 152–2). Collagen fibers bind to platelet surface receptors that activate aggregation and stimulate secretion of intracellular granular contents, including adenosine diphosphate (ADP), prostaglandin G_2 (PGG_2), and thromboxane A_2. These secreted substances mediate and further amplify aggregation. Besides collagen, thrombin in minute concentrations ($\cong 1$ nM) aggregates platelets. Presumably, this is an additional stimulus to aggregation once the soluble clotting factors have been activated.

Platelets secrete serotonin and thromboxane A_2, which enhance vasoconstriction and expose surface sites that bind and accelerate the activation of Factors X and II (prothrombin) (Fig. 152–2). In addition to aggregating platelets, thrombin converts fibrinogen to fibrin, which becomes incorporated into the platelet plug. With crosslinking of fibrin strands by Factor XIIIa, a stable clot is formed.

Normally, activation of clotting and platelets is inhibited by an intact vascular endothelium and continuous blood flow (see Fig. 152–3*A*). Endothelium makes PGI_2, which inhibits platelet activation and is vasodilatory. Thrombomodulin, an integral membrane endothelial protein, serves as a receptor for thrombin, which in this way activates protein C, a potent inhibitor of coagulation (see Ch. 153). Endothelial cells also make tissue plasminogen activator, the primary activator of intravascular fibrinolysis. Platelets do not bind to the surface of normal endothelial cells. Vascular endothelium contains large amounts of heparan sulfate, a glycosaminoglycan, on its luminal surface. Antithrombin III binds with high affinity to heparan, thus providing a rapid and potent mechanism for inhibiting activated clotting factors. Clearly, the inner lining of blood vessels has a critical function in maintaining vascular patency by inhibiting activation of hemostasis.

PATHOLOGIC HEMOSTASIS. Platelet thrombi in the arterial system, called white thrombi, are composed primarily of fibrin and platelets. Red thrombi, found in the venous circulation, are composed of red blood cells trapped in the fibrin meshwork and usually contain few platelets. Clotting is activated pathologically in response to abnormalities in (1) the vessel wall, e.g., atherosclerosis; (2) platelets, e.g., myeloproliferative disorders; and (3) the coagulation system, e.g., antithrombin III deficiency. Anatomic and/or biochemical alterations of the vascular intima are by far the most frequent causes of pathologic thrombosis. A variety of pathologic alterations of the vessel wall modify endothelial function in a prothrombotic fashion (Fig. 152–3*B*). At one extreme, the endothelial lining may be physically disrupted, with exposure of circulating blood to extracellular matrix and tissue factor. Also, several substances may induce intact endothelium to promote thrombosis. Thus, interleukin-1, tumor necrosis factor, and endotoxin increase both endothelial plasminogen activator inhibitor-1, an inhibitor of fibrinolysis, and endothelial tissue factor. Moreover, endothelial cells express receptors for several of the coagulation factors, including Factors Va, IXa, and Xa, so that once coagulation is initiated, it can be amplified on the endothelial cell surface. It is not difficult to imagine how rupture of an atherosclerotic plaque results in pathologic initiation of clotting, terminating in vascular occlusion. Thrombosis is an important event in atherosclerotic vascular disease: (1) Platelet thrombi are found in the coronary circulation in fatal myocardial infarction, and (2) fibrinolytic therapy can restore blood flow early in coronary occlusion.

APPROACH TO THE PATIENT WITH A POSSIBLE BLEEDING DISORDER

When evaluating a putative bleeding disorder, useful information comes first from the patient. The history may suggest whether a bleeding diathesis is congenital or acquired and, if the latter, the most likely category into which it falls. Moreover, careful examination may reveal signs that indicate a platelet, vascular, or coagulation defect. Based on this information, one can focus the laboratory investigation on particular disorders of hemostasis (Table 152–1).

HISTORY. The following information should be obtained:

1. What is the duration of the bleeding tendency? Has it been present since birth? Was there excessive bleeding at the time of circumcision?

2. What are the frequency and duration of episodes? A history of intermittent episodes (bleeding on some occasions but not others) does not exclude the diagnosis of a hemorrhagic diathesis. Patients

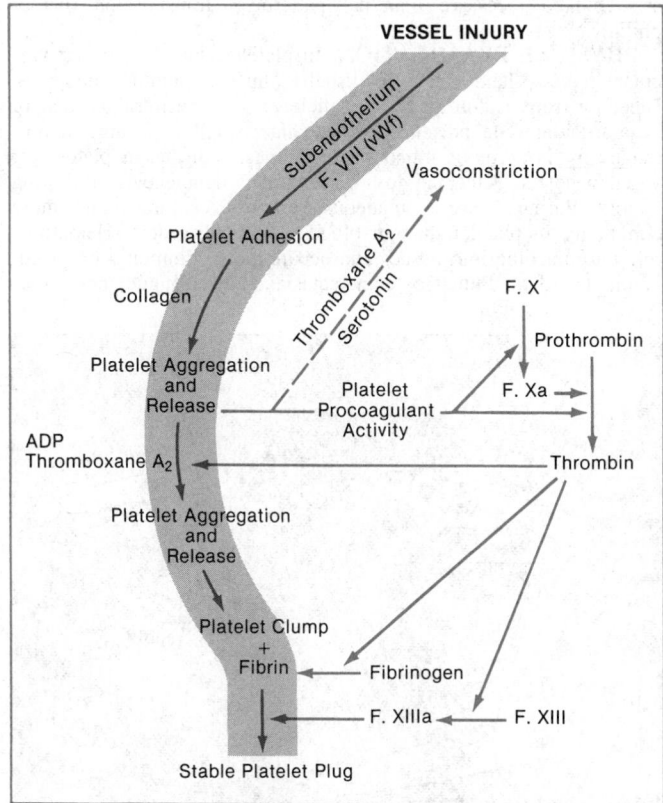

FIGURE 152–1. Schematic representation of platelet participation in hemostasis. Following vascular injury, platelets adhere to exposed subendothelial extracellular matrix. Under high shear conditions, von Willebrand factor (vWf) is required for adhesion. Collagen stimulates platelet secretion and aggregation. Secretion of adenosine diphosphate (ADP) and thromboxane A_2 further amplifies aggregation. Secretion of serotonin and thromboxane A_2 stimulates vasoconstriction. Factors IXa and VIIIa bind to specific platelet receptors, amplifying activation of Factor X. Factors Xa and Va bind to platelet receptors, amplifying thrombin formation. Thrombin aggregates platelets and converts Factor XIIIa and fibrinogen to fibrin. The end-product of these reactions is a crosslinked platelet-fibrin thrombus.

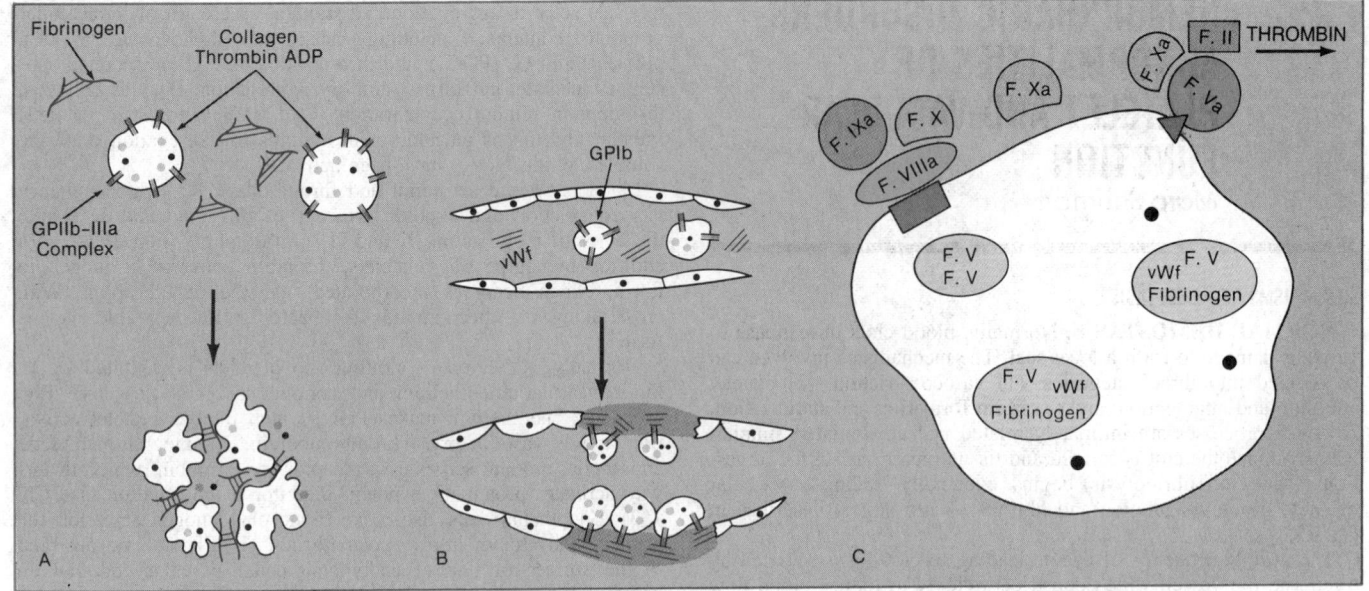

FIGURE 152–2. Platelet aggregation, adhesion, and enhancement of coagulation. *A,* Platelet aggregation. Several physiologic stimuli activate platelets, resulting in fibrinogen binding to specific receptors, GPIIb–IIIa. Binding of fibrinogen is followed by platelet aggregation. *B,* Platelet adhesion. Injury to the vascular endothelium results in exposure of extracellular matrix. Under high shear, von Willebrand factor (vWf) binds to the platelet receptor GPIb. The platelet-vWf complex then binds to the subendothelium. *C,* Amplification of thrombin formation by platelets. Coagulation Factors IXa, VIIIa, and X form a Ca^{2+}-dependent trimolecular complex on the platelet surface. Activation of Factor X is amplified several hundred thousand–fold. Coagulation Factors Xa, Va, and prothrombin form a Ca^{2+}-dependent trimolecular complex on platelets. Thrombin formation is amplified several hundred thousand–fold.

with mild von Willebrand disease or Factor XI deficiency may give this type of history.

3. What are the triggering events? Is hemorrhage spontaneous? Has excessive bleeding complicated surgery or dental work? Is menstrual bleeding excessive (menorrhagia)? Was bleeding abnormal at the time of childbirth?

4. What is the location of hemorrhage? Skin, joints, gastrointestinal or genitourinary tracts? In platelet disorders, epistaxis, cutaneous bleeding, and excessive vaginal bleeding are common. Joint hemorrhage is common in hemophilia but rare in platelet disorders.

5. What medication(s) is the patient taking? (Table 152–2)

6. What is the family history? Are only males affected? Is there an X-linked recessive maternal pattern of transmission (hemophilia)?

PHYSICAL EXAMINATION. In platelet abnormalities or vascular defects, hemorrhage is usually mucosal and/or cutaneous. Bleeding from a clotting factor deficiency is often intramuscular or intra-articular. The presence of petechiae, small (<3 mm) hemorrhages in the skin or mucous membranes, indicates a platelet or vascular defect. Petechiae do not accompany deficiencies of clotting factors. Purpura, larger cutaneous hemorrhages, are found more commonly in platelet than in blood clotting disorders. Hematoma refers to bleeding into tissues and occurs more commonly in coagulation disorders. Punctate telangiectasia on the tongue, nasal mu-

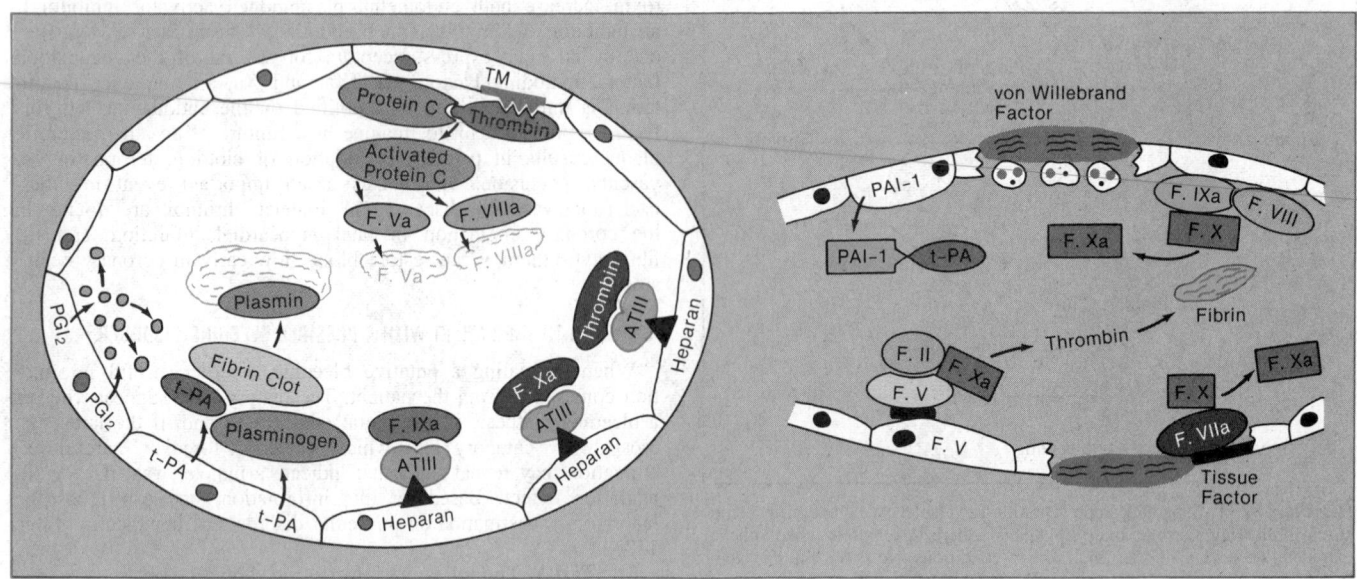

FIGURE 152–3. Regulation of coagulation by vascular endothelium. *Left,* Inhibition of activation of clotting by endothelium. Endothelial cells make substances that inhibit platelet secretion and aggregation and activate clotting factors. In addition, endothelium initiates degradation of the fibrin clot. *Right,* Activation of clotting by vascular endothelium. Injury to endothelium exposes tissue factor, which initiates the extrinsic pathway of clotting. Receptors for activation of Factor X and prothrombin amplify coagulation on the endothelial surface. Endothelium also secretes an inhibitor of clot lysis. PGI_2 = prostaglandin I_2; t-PA = tissue-plasminogen activator; PAI–1 = plasminogen activator inhibitor–1; TM = thrombomodulin; AT III = antithrombin III.

TABLE 152–1. DIFFERENTIAL DIAGNOSIS OF BLEEDING DISORDERS

| | Hereditary | | | |
	Hemophilia	Von Willebrand Disease	Qualitative Platelet Abnormalities	Blood Vessel Disorders
Genetics	X-Linked recessive	Autosomal dominant	Autosomal dominant Autosomal recessive	Autosomal dominant
Type of bleeding	Hemarthrosis Visceral CNS Soft tissues	Mucocutaneous	Mucocutaneous	Mucocutaneous Arterial rupture (connective tissue disorders)
Onset of bleeding	Delayed	Immediate	Immediate	Immediate
Physical examination	Joint deformities Hematomas Ecchymoses	Ecchymoses	Petechiae Ecchymoses	Ecchymoses Telangiectasia (HHT) Skin, joint, and eye abnormalities (connective tissue disorders)
Coagulation tests	aPTT: Abn	aPTT: Abn/N	N	N
Bleeding time	N	Abn	Abn	N/Abn

| | Acquired | | |
	Coagulation	Platelet	Blood Vessel Disorders
Type of bleeding	Visceral Soft tissues	Mucocutaneous	Mucocutaneous
Onset of bleeding	Delayed	Immediate	Immediate
Physical examination	Hematomas Ecchymoses	Petechiae Ecchymoses	Ecchymoses Perifollicular hemorrhage (scurvy)
Coagulation tests	PT: Abn/N aPTT: Abn/N	N	N
Bleeding time	N	Abn	N/Abn

CNS = central nervous system; HHT = hereditary hemorrhagic telangiectasia; N = normal; Abn = abnormal; aPTT = activated partial thromboplastin time; PT = prothrombin time.

cosa, lips, or fingertips reflects hereditary hemorrhagic telangiectasia. The history and physical examination alone may strongly indicate into which category a bleeding diathesis falls (see Table 152–1).

LABORATORY EVALUATION. Laboratory evaluation should be directed by the history and physical examination. For example, a strong family history of a mild bleeding disorder affecting both genders raises the possibility of von Willebrand disease. The finding of petechiae suggests a platelet or blood vessel disorder. When the history and physical examination fail to focus the investigation, the prothrombin time (PT), activated partial thromboplastin time (aPTT), and platelet count provide helpful initial screening tests. Figure 152–4 provides an algorithm for proceeding with further evaluation.

BLOOD PLATELETS

FORMATION AND KINETICS. Platelets are disc-shaped cells, 2 to 4 μm in diameter, normally found in the peripheral blood (150,000 to 300,000 per microliter). In Wright's-stained blood smears, they are identified by their blue-gray cytoplasm and red (lysosomal) granules and by lack of a nucleus (see Color Plate 5A). Their physiologic role in hemostasis has been described above (see Fig. 152–2).

Platelets are formed in the bone marrow from giant polyploid cells called megakaryocytes. Megakaryocytes mature by a series of nuclear replications within a common cytoplasm (endomitosis), leading to four- to six-lobed nuclei, and by elaboration of specific granules in the cytoplasm. Following maturation, the megakaryocyte cytoplasm becomes demarcated into platelet subunits, and the platelets are released into the circulation through the marrow sinusoids. Recently, the cDNA for a hematopoietic growth factor specific for megakaryocytes has been identified. It is anticipated that production of the recombinant protein will lead ultimately to therapy for patients with thrombocytopenia due to inadequate production of platelets.

Ordinarily, each megakaryocyte produces 1000 to 3000 platelets. Normally, 3 to 10 megakaryocytes are seen in bone marrow smears under low-power magnification, but none appears in peripheral blood. Platelets circulate for 9 to 10 days. Approximately one third reside in a splenic pool, which exchanges freely with the circulating pool. In diseases associated with platelet antibodies, the spleen is frequently the site of destruction. In addition, in disorders causing secondary splenic enlargement, thrombocytopenia may result from splenic sequestration (see Ch. 150). Conversely, following splenectomy, the platelet count may increase to 10^6 per microliter.

An estimate of platelet number in the peripheral blood film (normal, increased, decreased) is useful in detecting patients with abnormally low platelet counts. Normally, 3 to 10 platelets per high-power (oil immersion) field appear on peripheral smears. Platelets are counted directly by an automated particle counter.

PLATELET FUNCTION. Platelets contain three types of secretory granules: *lysosomes,* α-*granules,* and *dense bodies* (electron-dense organelles) (Fig. 152–5). α-Granules contain platelet-specific proteins: platelet factor 4; β-thromboglobulin; and several growth factors, including platelet-derived growth factor (PDGF), endothelial cell growth factor (PD-ECGF), and transforming growth factor-β (TGF-β). α-Granules also contain several hemostatic proteins, including fibrinogen, Factor V, and von Willebrand factor, which is synthesized by megakaryocytes. Dense bodies (δ granules) contain adenosine triphosphate (ATP), ADP, Ca^{2+}, and serotonin.

In hemostasis, platelets (1) release potent vasoconstrictors—thromboxane A_2 and serotonin—from their intracellular granules, (2) aggregate and form a plug at the site of vessel injury, and (3) provide a surface for the activation of soluble coagulation factors (see Fig. 152–2C).

At high shear rates, platelets require a plasma protein, von Willebrand factor, to adhere to subendothelial extracellular matrix (see Fig. 152–2). Platelets aggregate and secrete their granular contents in response to a variety of substances.

Platelets contain a membrane phospholipase C, which, upon stimulation by activating agents, hydrolyzes endogenous phosphatidylinositol to form a diglyceride. The diglyceride, in turn, is converted to arachidonic acid by a diglyceride lipase. Arachidonic acid acts as a substrate for prostaglandin synthetase and is subsequently converted to prostaglandins. The prostaglandin endoperoxide PGG_2 is required for ADP-induced aggregation and release; both PGG_2 and thromboxane A_2 are potent platelet-aggregating agents.

Activated platelets expose specific receptors that bind Factor Xa and Va and in this way increase their local concentration, thus accelerating prothrombin activation (see Fig. 152–2). Factor X is also activated by Factors IXa and VIII:AHF on the platelet surface.

Platelet dysfunction is a less common cause of bleeding than is thrombocytopenia.

PLATELET FUNCTION TESTS. *Bleeding Time.* The bleeding time measures the time required for bleeding to stop from a shallow incision, made under standardized conditions. It reflects the platelet and vascular components of coagulation and is normal with coagulation factor deficiencies (except von Willebrand disease). The bleeding time is prolonged when the platelet count falls below 90,000 per microliter or when a functional platelet abnormality ex-

TABLE 152-2. DRUGS THAT MAY ALTER HEMOSTASIS

I. Drugs reported to cause thrombocytopenia
A. Immune mechanism proposed*

Quinine/quinidine	Ranitidine
Sulfa compounds	Cimetidine
Ampicillin	Danazol
Penicillin	Procainamide
Thiazide diuretics	Carbamazepine
Furosemide	Acetaminophen
Chlorthalidone	Phenylbutazone
Phenytoin	p-Aminosalicylate
α-Methyldopa	Rifampin
Heparin	Acetazolamide
Digitalis derivatives	Anazoline
Aspirin	Arsenicals
Valproic acid	

B. Nonimmune mechanisms
(hemolytic-uremic syndrome)
Mitomycin C
Cisplatin
Cyclosporine
C. Mechanism undefined
Gold compounds
Indomethacin

II. Drugs that alter platelet function
A. Primary antiplatelet agents

Aspirin	Sulfinpyrazone
Dextran	Ticlopidine
Dipyridamole	

B. Drugs in which inhibition of platelet function is associated with prolongation of the bleeding time
Nonsteroidal anti-inflammatory agents
β-Lactam antibiotics
ε-Aminocaproic acid (> 24 grams/day)
Heparin
Plasminogen activators (streptokinase, urokinase, tissue plasminogen activator)

III. Drugs that affect coagulation factors
A. Induction of antibodies inhibiting function
Lupus anticoagulant†‡
Phenothiazines
Procainamide
Factor VIII antibodies
Penicillin
Factor V antibodies
Aminoglycosides
Factor XIII antibodies
Isoniazid
B. Inhibitors of synthesis of vitamin K–dependent clotting factors
(Factors II, VII, IX, X, proteins C and S)
Coumarin compounds
Moxalactam
C. Inhibitor of fibrinogen synthesis
L-Asparaginase‡

* List is limited to drugs for which there are multiple reports and there is *in vitro* or *in vivo* evidence for antiplatelet antibodies.
† Does not cause bleeding.
‡ May cause thrombosis.

ists. Von Willebrand disease prolongs the bleeding time; this is due not to a platelet defect but rather to the lack of a plasma factor important for normal platelet function (see Ch. 153). The bleeding time is the only test of platelet function that correlates with susceptibility to bleeding. Although patients with a prolonged bleeding time are at risk for increased bleeding with surgery, not all have abnormal bleeding.

Platelet Aggregometry. The response of platelets to a variety of aggregating agents can be quantitated in platelet-rich plasma or whole blood. The aggregometer measures temporal, semiquantitative, and qualitative parameters of *in vitro* aggregation. Agents typically used are ADP, collagen, and epinephrine. This technique is of greatest value in diagnosing congenital qualitative platelet disorders.

ABNORMALITIES IN PLATELET COUNT

Thrombocytopenia

Low platelet counts (thrombocytopenia) (Fig. 152–6) can be caused by disturbances in production, distribution, or destruction.

The consequences are entirely hemostatic. With normally functioning platelets, the following is expected:

1. Platelet count $\geq 100,000$ per microliter—patients have no abnormal bleeding even with major surgery.

2. Platelet count of 50,000 to 100,000 per microliter—patients may bleed longer than normal with severe trauma.

3. Platelet count of 20,000 to 50,000 per microliter—bleeding occurs with minor trauma, but spontaneous bleeding is unusual.

4. Platelet count < 20,000 per microliter—patients may have spontaneous bleeding.

5. Platelet count < 10,000 per microliter—patients are at high risk for severe bleeding.

DECREASED PRODUCTION OF PLATELETS

Hypoplasia of hematopoietic stem cells may cause thrombocytopenia (Table 152–3); most of these disorders are discussed in other chapters. They include decreased numbers of megakaryoblasts and replacement of the bone marrow by abnormal tissue. Examination of the bone marrow reveals decreased numbers of megakaryocytes and either an overall decrease in cellularity or an infiltration by abnormal cells.

Decreased production of platelets may also be due to abnormal maturation of megakaryocytes. Deficiency of either vitamin B_{12} or folate can cause thrombocytopenia owing to ineffective thrombocytopoiesis (see Ch. 133). Similarly, abnormal platelet production is common in hematopoietic dysplasias (see Ch. 130). In both disorders, megakaryocytes are usually increased. In hematopoietic dysplasia, megakaryocytes may be abnormal in appearance, such as micromegakaryocytes occasionally with a single-lobed nucleus.

INCREASED PERIPHERAL DESTRUCTION OF PLATELETS (Table 152–3)

IMMUNE DISORDERS. Three types of immunologic reactions cause premature destruction of platelets: (1) the development of autoantibodies against platelet-membrane antigens, (2) the binding of immune complexes to platelet Fc receptors, and (3) the lysis of platelets due to fixation of complement on their surface.

Idiopathic Thrombocytopenic Purpura (ITP). ITP is an autoimmune bleeding disorder characterized by the development of antibodies to one's own platelets, which are then destroyed by phagocytosis in the spleen and, to a lesser extent, the liver. Childhood ITP is usually acute and follows recovery from a viral infection. The incidence is equal in boys and girls. In adults, the onset is usually more gradual, without a preceding illness and with a chronic course. In a small percentage of adult cases, the disease has an acute onset. Ninety per cent of adults with ITP are under the age of 40, and the ratio of women to men is 3 to 4:1. Some patients' sera contain antibodies against platelet glycoproteins IIb and IIIa. Patients develop petechiae, ecchymoses, and epistaxis. Women may develop menorrhagia. Death due to hemorrhage amounts to about 5% in chronic ITP. Cerebral bleeding occurs in approximately 1% of cases.

The diagnosis of ITP depends on excluding underlying systemic disorders that result in increased peripheral destruction or decreased production of platelets. On physical examination, the spleen is not enlarged, although it may be in childhood ITP as a consequence of viral infection. In ITP, the hemoglobin is normal unless the patient has significant bleeding. Peripheral blood smears reveal normochromic, normocytic red blood cells. Similarly, the leukocyte count and differential are normal, although these values may reflect a preceding viral illness in children. Several assays for detecting antiplatelet antibodies on the platelet surface have been proposed. The value of these assays in diagnosing ITP is unclear. Most of the tests do not distinguish between autoantibodies and immune complexes that bind to the platelet Fc receptor. Furthermore, the assays do not differentiate between specific antiplatelet antibodies and nonspecifically absorbed immunoglobulin G (IgG). In most cases of ITP, the diagnosis is clear-cut, making it unnecessary to confirm the presence of antiplatelet antibodies. In complex cases, the antibody test may be helpful. The level of platelet-associated IgG does not correlate with the severity of thrombocytopenia. In >90% of cases of chronic ITP, the antibody is IgG.

If the general clinical evaluation and blood tests do not confirm the diagnosis of systemic disorders causing thrombocytopenia, the bone marrow should be examined. In ITP, the marrow is normal, al-

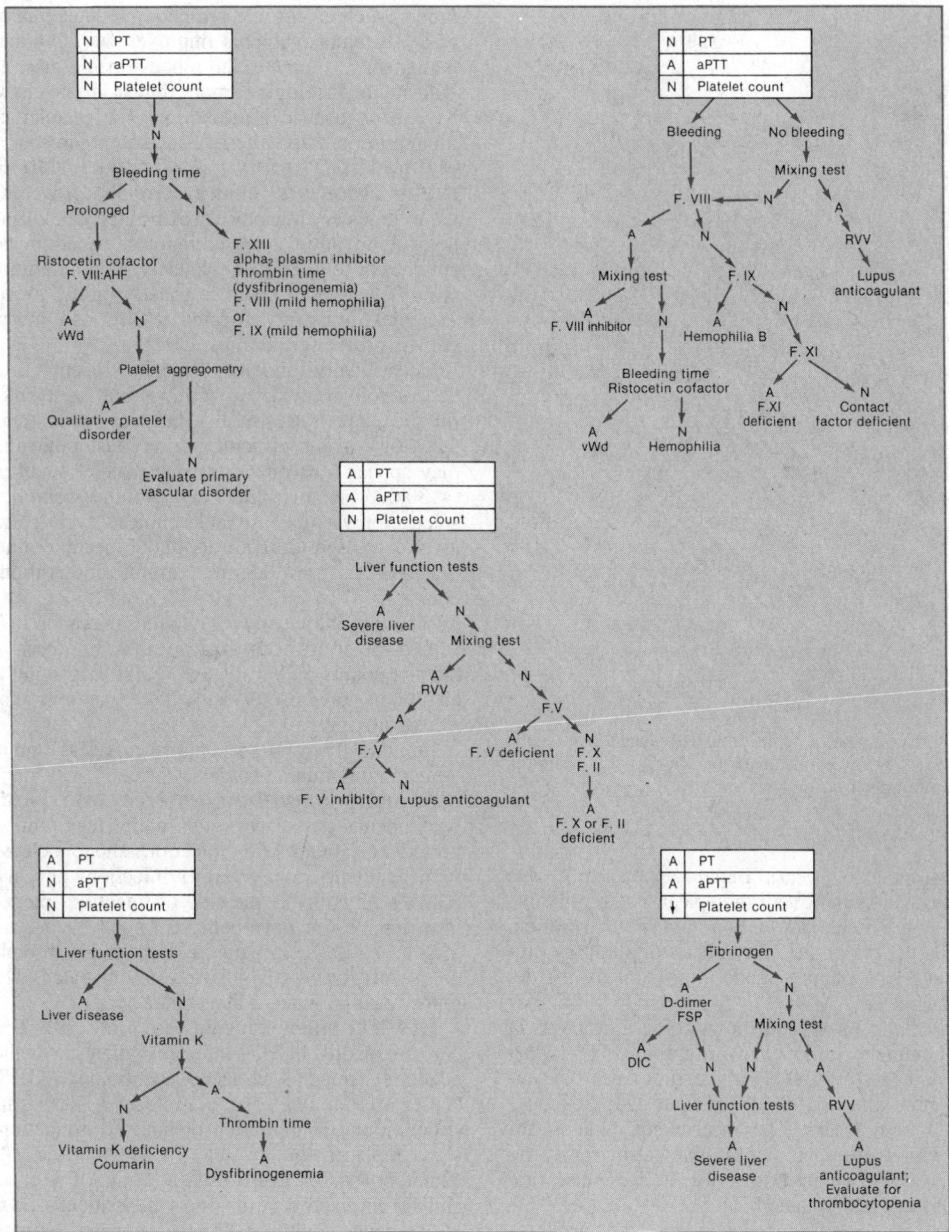

FIGURE 152–4. Algorithm for laboratory evaluation of bleeding disorders. vWd = von Willebrand disease; A = abnormal; N = normal; RVV = Russell viper venom test; FSP = fibrin split products; PT = prothrombin time; aPTT = activated partial thromboplastin time; AHF = antihemophilic factor; DIC = disseminated intravascular coagulation.

though megakaryocytes may be increased in number (see Color Plate 8J).

In children, ITP is self-limited. Approximately 70% recover within 4 to 6 weeks. In adults, indications for treatment depend on the severity of bleeding and the degree of thrombocytopenia. Asymptomatic patients with platelet counts >40,000 per microliter can be observed with periodic evaluation to determine the natural fluctuations of their disease. Patients with platelet counts <20,000 per microliter are usually symptomatic and require treatment. Patients with platelet counts >30,000 per microliter who have bleeding may have an acquired platelet function abnormality due to the antibody. Initially, bleeding associated with ITP is treated with prednisone or a similar corticosteroid at a dose of 1 to 2 mg per kilogram per day. Prednisone inhibits macrophage ingestion of antibody-coated platelets, in addition to suppressing antibody synthesis. Prednisone has also been shown to have a stabilizing effect on small blood vessels in thrombocytopenic animals. In 80 to 90% of patients, the platelet count rises to hemostatic levels within 2 to 3 weeks. Failure to respond to steroids is indicated by a platelet count <50,000 per microliter after 4 weeks of treatment. A subnormal platelet count after 6 weeks of treatment indicates steroid failure also. Once the platelet count has reached its apex and is stable, steroids should be tapered slowly. When the dose of prednisone is tapered, however, most patients (~90%) exhibit a relapse of thrombocytopenia. Thus, the primary benefit of prednisone is in the acute management of bleeding.

Another effective approach to managing patients who are actively bleeding or for whom major surgery is necessary is the use of intravenous γ globulin. Immunoglobulin G concentrates raise the platelet count within 3 to 5 days in most patients and is the most rapidly active agent. Unfortunately, the therapeutic effect is usually transient, because the platelet count falls to baseline levels over the next month. In a few instances, repeated infusions of γ globulin have led to sustained remissions after discontinuation of therapy. It is proposed that IgG works by blocking Fc receptors on macrophages, thereby inhibiting phagocytosis. The dosage is 1 gram per kilogram per day on 2 successive days. In 80% of patients, subsequent platelet counts rise above 50,000 per microliter. Owing to the lack of a sustained remission in most patients with severe thrombocytopenia treated with steroids or IgG, a more definitive approach is necessary. Splenectomy improves the platelet count in 70% of patients with ITP and induces sustained remission in approximately 60%, but no tests can predict reliably which patients will respond. The platelet count rises within a few days after

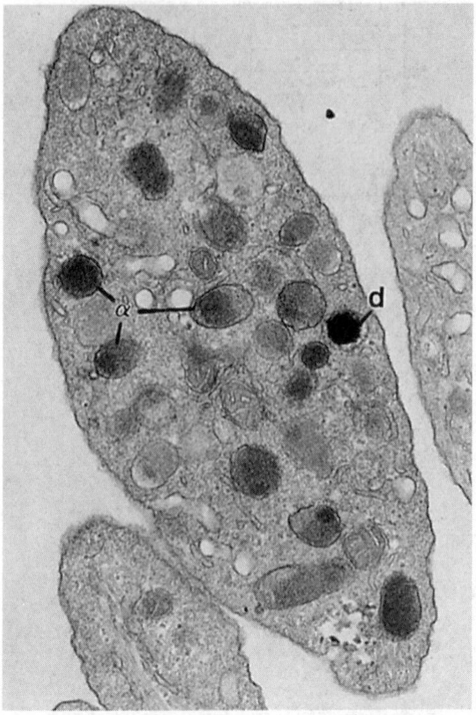

FIGURE 152–5. Electron micrograph of an unstimulated platelet. α = alpha granule; d = dense body ($\times$ 24,000). (Courtesy of Dr. Dorothy Bainton, University of California, San Francisco.)

splenectomy, or at most in 1 to 2 weeks. Benefit appears to be due to at least two mechanisms. As indicated, the spleen is the principal reticuloendothelial site of platelet destruction in ITP. In addition, the spleen appears to be the major site of synthesis of antibody production in ITP, with sufficient amounts made to account for the degree of thrombocytopenia seen.

A variety of other therapies have been shown to be efficacious in inducing partial or complete remissions in chronic ITP when splenectomy has failed. Danazol, 200 mg three times per day, induces a remission in approximately 40% of chronic ITP. Response is delayed and takes 4 to 6 weeks. The mechanism remains unknown. Intravenous vincristine and vinblastine also raise the platelet count in ITP, usually within 1 to 2 weeks. Responses are transient, and remissions are not sustained.

Immunosuppressive agents—cyclophosphamide and azathioprine—have also been used to induce remissions in chronic ITP. Because of the small numbers of patients reported, the relative efficacy of these two drugs is unclear. Success in improving the platelet count has been reported in 20 to 30% of cases. The potential benefit of these drugs must be weighed against the risks of toxicity, immunosuppression, suppression of hematopoiesis, and, in the case of cyclophosphamide, acute leukemia. Combination chemotherapy has also been used successfully to treat refreactory ITP. In one small series, 60% of patients remitted completely. Pulsed high-dose dexamethasone has also been reported to be effective therapy in patients with refractory ITP.

Management of ITP in pregnancy is complicated by the additional risk to the fetus of developing thrombocytopenia secondary to maternal antibodies. Intraventricular hemorrhage, gastrointestinal bleeding, and death have been reported in such newborns. Whether the mother had ITP prior to pregnancy is critical. When women first develop ITP during pregnancy, the risk of serious bleeding in the newborn is negligible. Conversely, neonates born to women with a history of ITP preceding pregnancy have a 20% risk of severe thrombocytopenia. In addition to treating the underlying ITP, cesarean delivery is recommended to decrease the risk of intracranial bleeding in these newborns.

Platelet Antibodies Associated with Systemic Disorders. Antibodies directed against platelets and causing thrombocytopenia occur in several types of disorders, in all of which bone marrow megakaryocytes are normal or increased in number.

Immune Thrombocytopenia Due to Cancer. Antibody-mediated destruction of platelets occurs in lymphoproliferative disorders, such as chronic lymphocytic leukemia and lymphoma. Generally, thrombocytopenia improves with treatment of the underlying malignancy. Immune thrombocytopenia has also been associated with nonhematologic tumors, but it is unclear whether or not these have been chance associations. The platelet count improves with immunosuppressive therapy such as prednisone.

Thrombocytopenia Associated with Systemic Autoimmune Disorders. Immune thrombocytopenia is common in systemic lupus erythematosus (SLE) (see Ch. 240). Whether this is due to specific antiplatelet antibodies, to antibodies against common antigens also found on platelets, or to immune complexes is unclear. The platelet count is usually mildly to moderately decreased. Treatment is usually directed at SLE, as other manifestations of the disease are present in most cases.

Occasionally, immune thrombocytopenia occurs in patients who have serologic evidence of lupus but fail to meet all of the criteria for the diagnosis of SLE. The decision to treat such patients with splenectomy is a difficult one, because other manifestations of SLE may appear subsequently. If the platelet count is severely decreased (< 30,000 per microliter) and no other complications of SLE exist, splenectomy is a reasonable choice. If the platelet count is moderately decreased (230,000 to 40,000 per microliter) and major bleeding problems are absent, careful observation may be the best course.

Monthly intravenous cyclophosphamide, 0.75 to 1.0 gram per square meter of body surface area, has been shown to normalize platelet counts within 2 to 18 weeks in patients with SLE who were also taking prednisone. Such therapy allows substantial reduction in steroid dosage.

Immune thrombocytopenia occurs less commonly in other systemic autoimmune disorders.

Immune Thrombocytopenia with Viral Illnesses. Thrombocytopenia associated with antiplatelet antibodies has been reported in patients with infectious mononucleosis, with human immunodeficiency virus (HIV) infection, and with cytomegalovirus (CMV) infection. In the case of infectious mononucleosis and CMV infection, thrombocytopenia is usually self-limiting, with recovery in 3 to 4 weeks. In patients with severe thrombocytopenia, a short course of glucocorticoids may be indicated. The nature of the immune reaction has not been characterized.

HIV Thrombocytopenia (see Ch. 369). Thrombocytopenia occurs frequently in HIV-infected patients, whether or not they have acquired immunodeficiency syndrome (AIDS). Frequently, the causes are multifactorial: (1) infection causing increased platelet destruction and/or inhibition of platelet production due to granulomatous replacement of the bone marrow, (2) suppression of hematopoiesis by drugs used to treat AIDS or associated infections, and (3) immune destruction of the patient's own platelets. Antibodies associated with platelets have been demonstrated in these patients, although the cause is unclear. Treatment with prednisone is hazardous owing to their immunocompromised status. Splenectomy has the disadvantage of further compromising the immune system. Zidovudine (AZT) treatment sometimes raises the platelet count with mild to moderate thrombocytopenia. For acute bleeding, intravenous globulin raises the platelet count within a few days.

Immune Thrombocytopenia Due to Drug-Induced Antibodies (see Table 152–2). More than 50 drugs have been reported to cause immune thrombocytopenia, but infrequently with conclusive confirmation. Quinine and quinidine often cause immune thrombocytopenia, and drug-dependent antibodies have been demonstrated. Sulfa compounds, including sulfisoxazole, sulfonamide, sulfamethoxypyridazine, and sulfamethazene, have also been demonstrated to cause immune thrombocytopenia. Multiple reports describe immune thrombocytopenia caused by hydrochlorothiazide, phenytoin, methyldopa, heparin, and digitalis derivatives. In most instances, the drug must be present to cause antibody binding and thrombocytopenia, and the platelet count returns to normal within a few days after discontinuation. Glucocorticoids do not accelerate recovery. Platelet antibody tests with and without the putative offending agent are useful in determining the cause of thrombocytopenia, but cannot be performed until the drug clears from the plasma. In addition, a drug metabolite, rather than the parent compound, may be responsible for antibody formation and binding to platelets. Unless the metabolite is specifically tested, a negative result will be obtained.

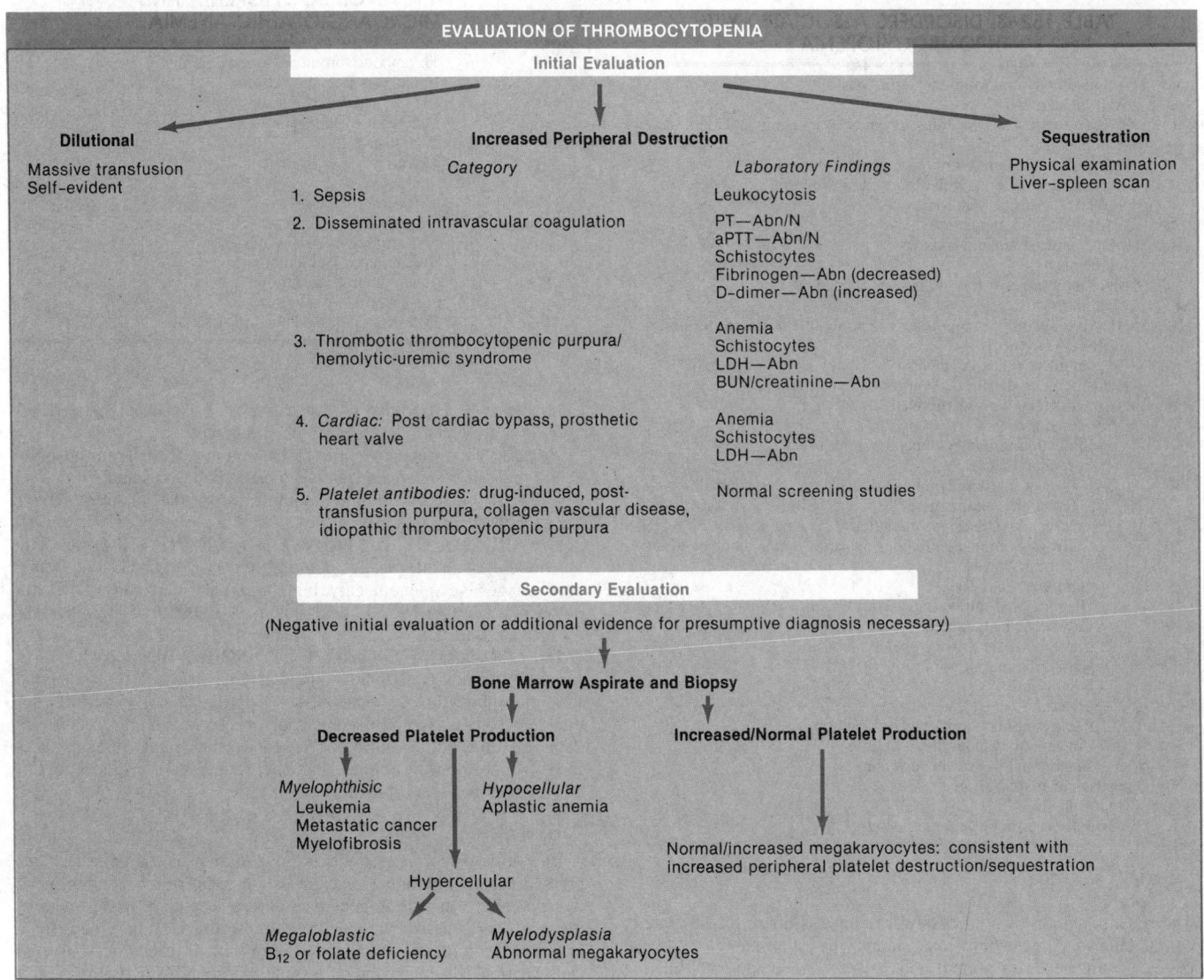

FIGURE 152–6. Evaluation of thrombocytopenia. Abn = abnormal; N = normal; PT = prothrombin time; aPTT = activated partial thromboplastin time; LDH = lactate dehydrogenase; BUN = blood urea nitrogen.

Heparin-Induced Thrombocytopenia. The incidence of thrombocytopenia associated with heparin therapy appears to be 3 to 5%, with a higher percentage of cases associated with bovine than with porcine preparations. The platelet count usually decreases gradually after the first few days of treatment and seldom induces bleeding. The count corrects rapidly after heparin is discontinued. Nevertheless, if the platelet count falls below 50,000 per microliter, heparin should be discontinued. Thrombocytopenia has been reported with the usual therapeutic doses as well as with the very low doses used for procedures such as hemodialysis.

NONIMMUNE DISORDERS ASSOCIATED WITH INCREASED CONSUMPTION OF PLATELETS. *Disseminated Intravascular Coagulation (DIC)* (see Ch. 153). In this syndrome coagulation is pathologically activated, resulting in thrombin formation and the subsequent removal of platelets from the circulation.

Thrombotic Thrombocytopenic Purpura (TTP). This is a rare disease of unknown etiology, characterized by severe thrombocytopenia, microangiopathic hemolytic anemia (>96% of patients), and neurologic abnormalities (>92% of patients). Fever and renal involvement—proteinuria, hematuria, azotemia, and casts—are present in 98% and 88% of patients, respectively. Renal abnormalities are usually mild; the creatinine rarely exceeds 3.0 mg per deciliter. Azotemia is usually reversible, concomitant with remission, in contrast to the hemolytic-uremic syndrome (see below). In the involved organs arterioles and capillaries become occluded by a hyaline material consisting principally of platelet thrombi plus fibrin deposits in the vessel wall. Virtually any organ may be involved. Symptoms frequently wax and wane, presumably owing to platelet aggregation

and disaggregation. Thus, patients may have evanescent headache, aphasia, or stupor one moment and be alert the next.

TTP must be considered when thrombocytopenia and anemia occur acutely with microangiopathic changes of red blood cells on the peripheral blood smear and the absence of evidence of other disorders (Tables 152–4 and 152–5) (see Color Plate 6*E*, right). Although findings in DIC are similar, patients with TTP have minimal changes in coagulation tests. Evans' syndrome, autoimmune hemolytic anemia and thrombocytopenia, is characterized by microspherocytes on peripheral smear, rather than by schistocytes, and by a positive Coombs test. Rarely, TTP has been reported to complicate SLE. More commonly, patients with SLE have immune thrombocytopenia and anemia of chronic disease or immune hemolytic anemia (see Ch. 240). TTP has also been reported in association with oral contraceptives and pregnancy. In most cases, the diagnosis of TTP is straightforward. When the diagnosis is uncertain, gum, skin, or bone marrow biopsy may be helpful, with positive results reported in 40 to 60% of cases. It is critical to establish the diagnosis and begin treatment rapidly, as delay can result in severe morbidity or mortality. Most untreated patients die within 3 months. Large-volume plasmapheresis, approximately two plasma volumes, with replacement infusion of normal plasma, is the treatment of choice for TTP, curing approximately 70% of patients. Infusion of large volumes of plasma without pheresis sometimes but not always induces remission, in which case concomitant plasmapheresis becomes imperative. Furthermore, because repeated courses of plasma infusion are usually necessary, the practical management of TTP is facilitated by plasmapheresis, which prevents excessive expansion of the blood volume and the risk of cardiovascular compromise.

TABLE 152–3. DISORDERS ASSOCIATED WITH THROMBOCYTOPENIA

I. **Hypoplasia of hematopoietic stem cells**
    Aplastic anemia
    Marrow damage from drugs, chemicals, ionizing radiation, alcohol, infection
    Congenital and hereditary thrombocytopenias
        Thrombocytopenia with absent radii syndrome
        Wiskott-Aldrich syndrome
        May-Hegglin anomaly
II. **Replacement of normal marrow**
    Leukemias
    Metastatic tumor (prostate, breast, lymphoma)
    Myelofibrosis
III. **Ineffective thrombocytopoiesis (normal or increased numbers of megakaryocytes)**
    Cobalamin or folate deficiency
    Hematopoietic dysplastic syndromes
IV. **Increased destruction of platelets**
    A. Immune disorders
        Idiopathic thrombocytopenic purpura (ITP)
        Secondary causes:
            Cancer: chronic lymphocytic leukemia, lymphoma, and so on
            Systemic autoimmune disorders: SLE, polyarteritis nodosa
            Infectious diseases: infectious mononucleosis, CMV, HIV
            Drugs: quinine/quinidine, heparin, sulfa compounds (see Table 152–1)
    B. Nonimmune disorders
        Disseminated intravascular coagulation
        Cavernous hemangioma
        Thrombotic thrombocytopenic purpura
        Hemolytic-uremic syndrome
        Sepsis
        Malaria
        Paroxysmal nocturnal hemoglobinuria
        Congenital cyanotic heart disease
        Acute renal transplant rejection
V. **Disorders of distribution**
    Hypersplenism
VI. **Dilutional: secondary to transfusion**

The best indication of a successful response is a rise in the platelet count. Plasmapheresis/infusion should be continued until the platelet count becomes normal and stable. Normalization of anemia and neurologic abnormalities usually follows. Approximately 10% of patients have a chronic, relapsing form of TTP. The plasma of patients with chronic TTP in remission contains abnormally large multimers of von Willebrand factor.

Hemolytic-Uremic Syndrome (HUS). Primarily a disorder of infants and young children, HUS rarely occurs in adults. Like TTP, HUS produces a microangiopathic hemolytic anemia, but thrombocytopenia is mild to moderate and neurologic abnormalities are absent. Unlike TTP, acute renal failure is a prominent feature in HUS, frequently requiring hemodialysis. Severe hypertension is a prominent feature. Children typically present with gastrointestinal signs and symptoms, abdominal pain, and diarrhea. HUS may occur in women who are in the postpartum period or who are taking oral

TABLE 152–4. DIFFERENTIAL DIAGNOSIS OF ANEMIA AND THROMBOCYTOPENIA

Diagnostic Study	Autoimmune Disorders (Evans' Syndrome, Collagen-Vascular Disease)	Disseminated Intravascular Coagulation	Thrombotic Thrombocytopenic Purpura/Hemolytic-Uremic Syndrome
Peripheral blood smear	Microspherocytes	Schistocytes (+)	Schistocytes (+++)
Reticulocyte count	Increased (+++)	N/Increased (+)	Increased (+++)
Coombs' test	Positive	Negative	Negative
Coagulation tests	N	Abn (+++)	N/Abn (+)

N = normal; Abn = abnormal.

TABLE 152–5. DISORDERS ASSOCIATED WITH THROMBOCYTOPENIA AND MICROANGIOPATHIC ANEMIA

Thrombotic thrombocytopenic purpura
Hemolytic-uremic syndrome
Disseminated intravascular coagulation
Malignant hypertension
Eclampsia
Vasculitis
    SLE
    Polyarteritis nodosa
Cavernous hemangioma
    (Kasabach-Merritt syndrome)
Disseminated carcinoma
Renal allograft rejection
Prosthetic heart valves
Malignant angioendotheliomatosis

---

contraceptives. HUS also has been reported in cancer patients receiving mitomycin C or cisplatin chemotherapy.

Sepsis. Gram-negative (more commonly than gram-positive) sepsis causes accelerated platelet destruction, presumably due to binding of bacterial immune complexes to the platelet. Severe thrombocytopenia may follow.

DISORDERS OF DISTRIBUTION OF PLATELETS. With splenic enlargement, platelet pooling increases (e.g., Gaucher's disease, congestive splenomegaly, lymphoma) and may cause thrombocytopenia (see Ch. 150). Platelet counts < 30,000 to 50,000 per microliter are unusual.

DILUTIONAL THROMBOCYTOPENIA. When packed erythrocytes or non-fresh whole blood is transfused to replace blood loss, thrombocytopenia may ensue. Approximately 35 to 40% of platelets remain after replacement of one blood volume; microvascular bleeding due to thrombocytopenia occurs rarely after replacement of one to two volumes. Platelets should be transfused only if thrombocytopenia and bleeding exist.

Thrombocytosis

Elevation of the platelet count above the normal range reflects increased production, either reactive or the result of a myeloproliferative disorder. Most thrombocytosis occurs secondary to an underlying disorder unassociated with complications. When due to a primary disorder of hematopoiesis, however, thrombocytosis can cause serious bleeding and/or thrombotic complications, making it important to determine its cause.

ESSENTIAL THROMBOCYTHEMIA. Essential thrombocythemia, a myeloproliferative disorder, is discussed in Ch. 141.2. Other myeloproliferative diseases, such as *agnogenic myeloid metaplasia* and *polycythemia vera,* also are associated with an elevated platelet count. The count may be elevated in chronic myelogenous leukemia but rarely results in complications.

REACTIVE THROMBOCYTOSIS. Elevated platelet counts occur secondarily in a number of unrelated disorders, but counts higher than 10^6 per microliter are unusual: *iron deficiency anemia; hemorrhage; splenectomy* (see Ch. 150); *inflammatory disorders, particularly inflammatory bowel disease; neoplasms (e.g., lung, gastrointestinal); leukemoid reaction* (see Ch. 140.2).

No convincing evidence exists that reactive thrombocytosis increases the risk of thrombosis. Therefore, it should not be treated. With successful treatment of the primary disease, the count returns to normal.

ABNORMALITIES IN PLATELET FUNCTION

Acquired Disorders of Platelet Function

DRUGS THAT INHIBIT PLATELET FUNCTION (see Table 152–2). *Nonsteroidal anti-inflammatory agents* inhibit platelet function by blocking platelet synthesis of prostaglandins. Aspirin (acetylsalicylic acid, or ASA) irreversibly acetylates prostaglandin synthetase and, as a result, impairs platelet function for its lifespan. One ASA tablet (300 mg) is sufficient to cause this effect. Fortunately, in normal people, this does not result in excessive bleeding, but in patients with von Willebrand disease or with severe coagulation factor deficiency (Factor VIII or IX), serious bleeding can result. For this reason, aspirin is contraindicated in these disorders.

High doses of the *β-lactam antibiotics,* such as penicillin and related compounds, induce an abnormality in platelet function that persists for 2 to 3 days after the drug is discontinued. The mechanism is unclear. The bleeding time is prolonged, and patients may have increased bleeding.

Renal Failure. Platelets function abnormally in patients with renal failure. The uremic metabolites responsible for this dysfunction are uncertain. Guanidinosuccinic acid and phenolic compounds that accumulate in uremia may inhibit platelet aggregation. Abnormal platelet adhesion and activation may occur in uremia as well as thrombocytopenia. The latter is usually mild and may be due to the underlying cause of renal disease.

Uremic bleeding is usually mucocutaneous and reflects abnormal platelet and/or vascular hemostatic functions. The bleeding time is commonly prolonged, but other causes of prolongation must be excluded (e.g., medication, congenital platelet disorders, and von Willebrand disease). Low hematocrits (< 24%) prolong the bleeding time in uremia. Transfusion of packed red blood cells to elevate the hematocrit above 26% improves the bleeding time. Tests of coagulation are normal.

When a uremic patient bleeds one must evaluate the possibility of a structural lesion or other hemostatic abnormalities. Platelet abnormalities are seldom the cause. When the hemostatic defect of renal failure is believed to be a significant contributing factor in bleeding, the patient should be dialyzed. Either peritoneal dialysis or hemodialysis usually can reverse the hemostatic defect. If the bleeding time remains prolonged and the patient is bleeding, other agents can be tried: low-dose estrogens, 1-deamino-8-D-arginine vasopressin (DDAVP), or cryoprecipitate. Their efficacy, however, has not been firmly established. All three raise the plasma levels of Factor VIII:AHF/vWf, but these patients usually remain in normal concentrations in uremia. Platelet transfusion usually has no benefit.

HEPATIC FAILURE (see Ch. 123). Platelet function is sometimes abnormal in liver disease, but why this is so and the extent to which it contributes to bleeding are unclear. The bleeding time may be prolonged in moderately severe liver disease when the platelet count is > 90,000 per microliter. DDAVP has been reported to improve the bleeding time in these circumstances. More commonly in hepatic failure, a bleeding diathesis is due to deficiencies of coagulation factors.

PARAPROTEINEMIAS (see Ch. 149). Abnormal platelet function occurs in a subset of patients with multiple myeloma or Waldenström's macroglobulinemia. The bleeding time is usually prolonged, and bleeding can be moderately severe. If the level of the paraprotein is lowered by plasmapheresis and/or chemotherapy, the bleeding time and bleeding improve, suggesting a direct effect of the paraprotein on platelet function. Paraproteins may impair platelet function by inhibiting platelet-fibrinogen interaction.

ACQUIRED STORAGE POOL DISEASE. Patients may develop mild platelet function abnormalities from loss of storage granules. Some of the disorders in which this has been reported include cardiopulmonary bypass surgery, hairy cell leukemia, and conditions with antiplatelet autoantibodies. Platelet dysfunction following bypass surgery is transient and not of clinical importance beyond the first 24 hours after surgery.

MYELOPROLIFERATIVE DISORDERS. Patients with essential thrombocythemia and, less commonly, agnogenic myeloid metaplasia may have abnormalities of platelet function. In essential thrombocythemia, abnormalities usually occur at platelet counts greater than 10^6 per microliter and may lead to abnormal bleeding, thrombosis, or both. Although the functional abnormalities are not specific, a prolonged bleeding time indicates that the patient is at risk for bleeding. Treatment of bleeding patients with thrombocytosis should be directed at lowering the platelet count as rapidly as possible.

Hereditary Disorders of Platelet Function

The bleeding history is similar among these rare diseases. Patients provide a lifelong history of easy bruising, epistaxis, and prolonged oozing after venipuncture, dental extractions, and other challenges to hemostasis.

GLANZMANN'S THROMBASTHENIA. This autosomal recessive bleeding disorder is characterized by a prolonged bleeding time and platelets that fail to aggregate normally when stimulated with ADP, epinephrine, collagen, or thrombin. In Glanzmann's thrombocytopenia, two membrane glycoproteins (GPIIb-IIIa) that normally serve as the receptor for fibrinogen in activated platelets are markedly deficient (see Fig. 152–2). Fibrinogen binding to platelets is required for platelet aggregation. The diagnosis is confirmed by demonstrating deficiency of platelet GPIIb-IIIa. The platelet count is always normal.

BERNARD-SOULIER SYNDROME. This autosomal recessive disorder is caused by a deficiency of a platelet membrane glycoprotein complex, GPIb-IX. As a result, "giant" platelets appear in the peripheral blood smear (see Color Plate 8K, left). Frequently, the platelet count is mildly decreased. In laboratory studies, platelets aggregate normally in response to ADP, collagen, or epinephrine but fail to aggregate in response to ristocetin. Physiologically, platelets fail to adhere normally to subendothelial connective tissue owing to defective binding of von Willebrand factor.

STORAGE POOL DISEASE (SPD). In this autosomal dominant disorder, platelet storage granules are decreased in number and/or content, presumably because of abnormal granule formation in megakaryocytes. The bleeding diathesis is mild and affects mostly women. With the deficiency in dense granules, platelets aggregate abnormally owing to inadequate secretion of ADP. Dense-granule SPD is also associated with several other congenital disorders, including oculocutaneous albinism in both the Hermansky-Pudlak and Chédiak-Higashi syndromes, the Wiskott-Aldrich syndrome, and a syndrome that includes thrombocytopenia and absent radii (TAR). Patients may also be deficient in α-granules, either in combination with dense granule deficiency or independently. The gray platelet syndrome refers to the latter situation, in which the absence of granule staining confers a gray color to the platelets. Mild thrombocytopenia may also be present in this disorder.

VON WILLEBRAND DISEASE. This disease, the most common congenital bleeding disorder, is discussed in Ch. 155.

PLATELET TRANSFUSIONS

INDICATIONS. When serious bleeding complicates thrombocytopenia, platelet transfusions are effective only when the cause is decreased production. Thrombocytopenia due to increased peripheral destruction or sequestration is usually refractory to platelet transfusion. Bleeding due to qualitative platelet disorders ordinarily responds to platelet transfusions except when secondary to uremia or hepatic failure or when an offending drug remains present in the circulation.

For patients with congenital platelet disorders, platelet transfusion must be given judiciously because repeated transfusions stimulate alloantibodies. Eventually, it may become impossible to raise the platelet count through transfusion. Accordingly, platelet transfusions should be reserved for serious bleeding or in preparation for surgery on patients with moderately severe platelet defects.

Platelet transfusions are indicated for patients who are bleeding actively and have either a platelet count below 50,000 per microliter or a qualitative platelet abnormality as manifested by a prolonged bleeding time. Platelet transfusions may also be indicated prophylactically before surgery or other invasive procedures. Prior to surgery, platelet counts should be above 50,000 per microliter in most cases, and above 90,000 per microliter for procedures such as neurosurgery or ophthalmologic surgery in which any abnormal bleeding may cause excessive morbidity. For invasive procedures, such as kidney or liver biopsies, a platelet count above 50,000 per microliter is probably sufficient, assuming normal platelet function.

CHRONIC THROMBOCYTOPENIA. In the absence of active bleeding, recommendations are based on the cause of thrombocytopenia. When thrombocytopenia is due to decreased production, the platelet count should be maintained above 10,000 to 20,000 per microliter. When accelerated destruction of platelets exists, transfusion is seldom effective. ITP patients frequently tolerate low platelet counts with little bleeding.

DOSAGE. For patients who require platelet transfusions chronically, platelets should be obtained from a single donor for each transfusion (generally six to seven units) to reduce the risk of forming multiple alloantibodies (see below). In a 70-kg patient, one unit of platelets usually raises the platelet count by approximately 10,000 per microliter. The count should be repeated 10 to 60 minutes after transfusion to assess the compatibility of the transfused platelets and to determine whether the desired count has been achieved. In actively bleeding patients, the platelet count should be maintained above 50,000 per microliter.

ALLOANTIBODIES AGAINST PLATELETS. In approximately 50 to 60% of patients who become refractory to random donor platelets, anti-HLA (human leukocyte antigen) antibodies appear to be responsible. The other presumed antigens have not yet been identified. In one rare form of alloimmunization, antibodies develop against the PL antigen, an epitope on platelet glycoprotein IIIa. The difference between PL^{A1} positive and negative (PL^{A2}) is a single amino acid. Ninety-eight per cent of the normal population have PL^{A1}-positive platelets.

When PL^{A1}-negative patients are transfused with PL^{A1}-positive blood, they may develop anti-PL^{A1} antibodies and *post-transfusion purpura* (PTP). Previous immunization is necessary, either by transfusion or by pregnancy. Why this syndrome is rare and selectively high in women despite the frequency of PL^{A1} negativity in the population is unknown. These patients not only rapidly clear transfused platelets from their circulation but also destroy their own platelets, becoming thrombocytopenic usually 5 to 10 days after transfusion. If patients with antibodies against the PL^{A1} antigen become severely thrombocytopenic, treatment with plasmapheresis or exchange transfusion is necessary, as bleeding from thrombocytopenia can be life-threatening.

Neonatal Alloimmune Thrombocytopenia. Thrombocytopenia due to maternal alloantibodies against fetal platelet antigens occurs in approximately 1 in 2000 to 4000 fetuses. Affected infants may have intracranial hemorrhages (estimated between 10 and 30%); in families with an affected infant, the risk of recurrence is at least 75%. PL^{A1} antibodies have been identified in most cases as being responsible for thrombocytopenia. Affected infants are treated by transfusion with washed maternal platelets. Women with a prior history of an affected infant should be delivered by cesarean section. Also, intravenous globulin given to pregnant mothers with a prior affected infant raises fetal platelet counts and reduces the rate of intracranial hemorrhage.

VASCULAR DISORDERS (Table 152–6)

Normal vascular function is necessary for effective hemostasis (see Fig. 152–1). Alteration in the integrity or structure of blood vessels can lead to a bleeding diathesis, the symptoms and signs of which are indistinguishable from those of a platelet disorder.

Congenital Vascular Disorders Associated with Bleeding

HEREDITARY HEMORRHAGIC TELANGIECTASIA (RENDU-OSLER-WEBER DISEASE). This disorder, the most common genetic cause of vascular bleeding, is inherited as an autosomal dominant trait. Its most frequent symptom is spontaneous epistaxis. More than half of the patients have epistaxis by age 20 and 90% by age 45. Telangiectasia occurs most frequently on the face in two thirds of patients, on the mouth in half, and on the cheeks, tongue, nose, and lower lip in approximately one third. In

TABLE 152–6. VASCULAR DISORDERS ASSOCIATED WITH BLEEDING

Congenital
  Hereditary hemorrhagic telangiectasia
  Cavernous hemangioma
  Connective tissue disorders
    Ehlers-Danlos syndrome
    Osteogenesis imperfecta
    Pseudoxanthoma elasticum
Acquired disorders affecting vascular hemostatic function
  Scurvy
  Immunoglobulin disorders
    Cryoglobulinemia
    Benign hyperglobulinemia
    Waldenström's macroglobulinemia
    Multiple myeloma
    Henoch-Schönlein purpura
  Glucocorticoid excess
    Cushing's syndrome
    Glucocorticoid therapy

about 40%, the hands and wrists are also involved. Beyond this cutaneous or mucosal involvement, the organ system affected most often is the gastrointestinal tract ($\sim 12\%$). Death from intestinal bleeding occurs in 12 to 15% of symptomatic patients. The liver, lungs, central nervous system, and urinary tract are involved in decreasing order of frequency. Pulmonary arteriovenous fistulas, present in approximately 5% of patients, are manifested by cyanoses, dyspnea, clubbing, and thoracic murmurs. Hemoptysis is unusual. Surgical resection is successful in managing this complication in most instances. Stroke may occur with central nervous system involvement, a complication that tends to affect younger patients (mean age, 33). Careful inspection of the nose and mouth usually reveals the diagnosis. In other cases, endoscopy or angiography may be necessary. Pathologic examination of involved tissue demonstrates dilated capillaries with loss of subendothelial structures.

Tests of platelet function and bleeding time are normal. There is no consistently effective therapy, but the prognosis is relatively good.

CAVERNOUS HEMANGIOMA (KASABACH-MERRITT SYNDROME). Congenital subcutaneous and visceral hemangiomas may be associated with thrombocytopenia and bleeding in infants and children. Bleeding occurs at the site of the lesions or systemically owing to thrombocytopenia. Platelets are activated within the hemangioma and subsequently removed from the circulation. In addition, mild DIC may occur with consumption of fibrinogen. Thrombocytopenia is more severe than coagulation abnormalities. Spontaneous regression of hemangiomas may occur over a period of years. In cases in which thrombocytopenia is severe and tumors are few, surgery and/or radiation therapy may be effective. Intentional thrombosis of hemangiomas by administration of inhibitors of fibrinolysis, with or without cryoprecipitate, has been successful in managing thrombocytopenia in a few cases.

DISORDERS OF CONNECTIVE TISSUE. Genetic abnormalities in structural glycoproteins such as collagen can result in vascular fragility caused by weakening of the vessel wall. Bleeding may be limited to increased bruising or may manifest as internal hemorrhaging. Ehlers-Danlos syndrome, osteogenesis imperfecta, and pseudoxanthoma elasticum, discussed elsewhere in this book, are examples of inherited disorders of connective tissue that may be associated with a bleeding diathesis on this basis.

Acquired Disorders of Blood Vessels Causing Bleeding

SCURVY. Severe vitamin C deficiency results in defective collagen formation in small blood vessels. Bleeding may occur in any tissue but is prominent in the lower extremities and is perifollicular in distribution. Other sites where bleeding is common include the gums, the subperiosteum in children, and the muscles.

PURPURA ASSOCIATED WITH IMMUNOGLOBULIN DISORDERS. *Cryoglobulinemia* (see Ch. 149). Patients with all three types of cryoglobulinemia have purpura as a complication of their disease. In type I, bleeding may be due to obstruction of blood flow in the microcirculation at cold temperatures by cryoprecipitates, resulting in increased vascular fragility. In type II and type III cryoglobulinemia, bleeding may be due to leukocytoclastic vasculitis associated with the immune complexes. Purpura occurs most commonly in the distal extremities.

Benign Hyperglobulinemia (Waldenström's Purpura). In this syndrome, patients have polyclonal hyperglobulinemia associated with purpura of the lower extremities. Leukocytoclastic involvement of the vessel wall may account for increased vascular fragility and bleeding. Commonly, the onset of purpura is preceded by a stinging sensation in areas of involvement. Although there is generally no evidence of systemic vasculitis, the disorder may evolve into Sjögren's syndrome or SLE.

Amyloidosis (see Ch. 248). Amyloid deposition in the skin and subcutaneous tissues alters the normal structural support for small blood vessels, resulting in increased vascular fragility (see Color Plate 8*I*, right). Purpura can occur at any site; for unclear reasons, periorbital hemorrhage is a characteristic finding.

Waldenström's Macroglobulinemia and Multiple Myeloma (see Ch. 149). Abnormalities in platelet function may occur with M proteins, as noted above. An additional contributing factor is hyperviscosity when it complicates these diseases. Slowing of blood flow and increased hydrostatic pressure may increase vascular fragility, leading to purpura.

Henoch-Schönlein Purpura. This childhood disorder is characterized by symmetric purpura and arthralgias of the lower extremities, abdominal pain, and melena. Rarely, adults are affected. Patients may give a history of a recent infectious illness. The disease has an acute onset with a maculopapular rash evolving into palpable purpura. Other complications include glomerulonephritis and hypertension (both of which are self-limiting) and intussusception. Involved tissues, including the skin, demonstrate vasculitis with immunoglobulin A (IgA) and complement deposition.

Henoch-Schönlein purpura usually remits spontaneously over a period of 1 to 2 months, although the course is often punctuated by flaring of symptoms and signs. Symptomatic improvement is obtained with glucocorticoids.

Miscellaneous Disorders

CUSHING'S SYNDROME. Cushing's disease or chronic administration of glucocorticoids results in increased bruising, particularly in the extremities. Abnormal bleeding probably results from alterations in the structure of the perivascular matrix, with loss of normal elasticity.

AUTOERYTHROCYTE SENSITIZATION (GARDNER-DIAMOND SYNDROME). This bizarre syndrome is characterized by the development of purpura at any site on the body, preceded by pain and burning. It occurs almost exclusively in women. Usually, affected women have a history of severe stress and emotional problems. Tests for abnormalities in hemostasis are all normal.

The diagnostic test is the development of large ecchymoses within 24 to 48 hours at the site of subcutaneous injection of a small amount ($\sim$ 0.1 ml) of the patient's own blood or erythrocytes. Injection should be at sites inaccessible to the patient, and a concurrent control injection should be administered. The primary differential diagnosis is factitious purpura.

PURPURA SIMPLEX. Purpura simplex denotes easy bruisability, commonly observed in young children and middle-aged women, affecting primarily the lower extremities. Laboratory evaluation, including the bleeding time, is normal, and no evidence exists of vascular abnormalities. Affected women do not experience excessive bleeding with surgery, nor do they suffer from internal bleeding.

Bennett JS, Shattil SJ: Congenital qualitative platelet disorders. *In* Williams WJ, Beutler E, Erslev AJ, et al. (eds.): Hematology. 4th ed. New York, McGraw-Hill, 1990, p 1407.

Berchtold P, McMillan R: Therapy of chronic idiopathic thrombocytopenic purpura in adults. Blood 74:2309, 1989. *Reviews current experience with therapeutic options in ITP as well as experimental approaches.*

Fresh-Frozen Plasma, Cryoprecipitate, and Platelets Administration Practice Guidelines Development Task Force of the College of American Pathologists: Practice parameter for the use of fresh-frozen plasma, cryoprecipitate, and platelets. JAMA 271:777, 1994. *Current guidelines for the transfusion of platelets as well as other blood products.*

George JN, Shattil SJ: Medical progress: The clinical importance of acquired abnormalities of platelet function. N Engl J Med 324:27, 1991. *An excellent recent review of this important topic.*

Kaplan BS, Trumpeter RS, Moake JL (eds.): Hemolytic Uremic Syndrome and Thrombotic Thrombocytopenic Purpura. New York, Marcel Dekker, 1992. *Comprehensive examination of both disorders.*

Mitus AJ, Schafer AI: Thrombocytosis and thrombocythemia. *In* Colman RW, Rao AK (eds.): Platelets in health and disease. Hematol Clin North Am 4:157, 1990. *Complete discussion of the pathophysiology of thrombocytosis and its complications in myeloproliferative disorders as well as its differentiation from secondary causes.*

Tomasulo PA, Petz LD: Platelet transfusion. *In* Petz LD, Swisher SN (eds.): Clinical Practice of Transfusion Medicine. 2nd ed. New York, Churchill Livingstone, 1989, p 427. *Excellent review of specific indications for platelet transfusion and management of alloimmunized patients.*

153 DISORDERS OF BLOOD COAGULATION
Deane F. Mosher

Normal hemostasis requires interactions among blood vessels, the formed elements of blood, especially platelets and monocytes, and blood coagulation proteins. The general biology of hemostasis and the approach to a patient suspected of having a hemorrhagic diathesis have been discussed in Ch. 152. In this chapter, attention is focused on hemorrhagic and thrombotic disorders that occur as a consequence of abnormalities of blood coagulation proteins.

OVERVIEW OF BLOOD COAGULATION MECHANISMS

Blood coagulation is initiated by substances in injured tissues and propagated by an interlocking network of zymogen-to-proteinase conversions. These reactions are both highly efficient and highly controlled to ensure that blood coagulation happens quickly and yet remains localized. Blood coagulation results in the formation of a protein scaffolding, the fibrin clot, that controls bleeding and serves as a nidus for subsequent cellular ingrowth and tissue repair. After several days, the fibrin clot is lysed and replaced by a more permanent scaffolding of connective tissue matrix molecules. Abnormalities that result in delay of clot formation or premature fibrinolysis are associated with a bleeding tendency (hemophilia). Abnormalities that result in inappropriate activation or localization of blood coagulation are associated with thrombosis (thrombophilia).

COAGULATION MOLECULES. Blood coagulation and fibrinolysis are initiated and modulated by molecules embedded in the external membrane of cells (tissue factor, thrombomodulin, urokinase receptor), deposited in extracellular matrix (heparan sulfate and dermatan sulfate proteoglycans), or secreted by vascular cells in a regulated manner (von Willebrand factor, plasminogen activators, and plasminogen activator inhibitors). These "extrinsic" molecules interact specifically with a host of plasma proteins "intrinsic" to flowing blood (Table 153–1).

Structural and functional similarities allow useful groupings of plasma proteins. Some are zymogens of serine proteinases and hence members of the serine proteinase family of proteins. Proteinases activated during blood coagulation are inhibited by specific serpins (*ser*ine *p*roteinase *in*hibitors). Among the serine proteinase family are five proteins (Factors II, VII, IX, and X and protein C) that are modified by vitamin K–dependent post-translational carboxylation of glutamic acid residues. A sixth plasma protein, protein S, is also modified by this reaction. The modification allows the six proteins to bind Ca^{2+} and phospholipids and thereby function efficiently in reactions on membrane surfaces. Factors V and VIII are homologous to one another and organize the vitamin K–dependent factors on membrane surfaces. Most of the proteins listed in Table 153–1, including fibrinogen and the vitamin K–dependent factors, are synthesized by hepatocytes. A number of the proteins, however, can be synthesized by other cell types such as megakaryocytes, monocyte-macrophages, and endothelial cells.

EXTRINSIC AND INTRINSIC PATHWAYS. Blood coagulation can be initiated by exposure of blood to tissue factor (the "extrinsic system") or by activation of "contact factors" of plasma (the "intrinsic system"). The two initiation pathways come together in a common pathway leading to generation of thrombin (activated Factor II), the master coagulation enzyme. As shown in Figure 153–1A, the concept of two initiation pathways and a common pathway is useful in understanding the two major classes of coagulation tests. One class, which includes the whole blood clotting time and the activated partial thromboplastin time (APTT), is based on activation of the "intrinsic pathway" by contact with glass or other negatively charged surfaces. The second class, represented by the prothrombin time (PT), involves addition of tissue factor to citrated plasma so that activation proceeds by the "extrinsic pathway."

The two initiation pathways are not clearly delineated *in vivo*. Activation of Factor IX, an "intrinsic factor," by Factor VII, an "extrinsic factor," is of obvious physiologic importance. Deficiency of Factors VII or IX or any of the proteins that follow Factor IX in the intrinsic and common pathways—Factors VIII, X, V, and II and fibrinogen—are associated with a bleeding tendency. In contrast, deficiency of any of three "contact factors"—Factor XII, prekallikrein, or high molecular weight kininogen (HMWK)—does not cause a bleeding problem. Deficiency of Factor XI, which links contact activation to Factor IX, is variably associated with a bleeding tendency.

TISSUE FACTOR AND THE EXTRINSIC PATHWAY. Factor VII circulates in a potentially active conformation but must combine with tissue factor to express this activity. Thus, tissue factor is the "match" that ignites the coagulation cascade (Fig. 153–1B). Sites rich in tissue factor include brain, adventitia of blood vessels, organ capsules, epidermis, and mucosal epithelium. Tissue factor is

TABLE 153-1. PROTEINS INVOLVED IN BLOOD COAGULATION AND FIBRINOLYSIS

Proteins	Synonym	Chromosomal Location	Size (Kilodaltons)*	Plasma Concentrations (mg/dl [μM])*	Kind of Protein	Function†
Fibrinogen	Factor I	4	340	300(9)	Structural protein	Gels to form clot
Factor II	Prothrombin	11	72	15(2)	Vitamin K–dependent zymogen of serine proteinase	Activates I, V, VIII, XIII, protein C, and platelets
Factor V	Proaccelerin	1	330	2(0.05)	Multifunctional binding protein	Supports X_a activation of II
Factor VII	Stable factor	13	50	0.05(0.01)	Vitamin K–dependent zymogen of serine protease	Activates IX and X
Factor VIII	Antihemophilic factor	X	330	0.01(0.0003)	Multifunctional binding protein	Supports IX_a activation of X
Factor IX	Christmas factor	X	56	0.5(0.1)	Vitamin K–dependent zymogen of serine proteinase	Activates X
Factor X	Stuart-Prower factor	13	56	1(0.2)	Vitamin K-dependent zymogen of serine proteinasse	Activates II
Factor XI	Plasma thromboplastin antecedent	4	160	0.5(0.03)	Zymogen of serine proteinase	Activates IX
Factor XII	Hageman factor	5	80	3(0.2)	Zymogen of serine proteinase	Activates XI and prekallikrein
Factor XIII	Fibrin-stabilizing factor	1(b) 6(a)	320	3(0.08)	Zymogen of transglutaminase	Crosslinks fibrin and other proteins
von Willebrand factor	Factor VIII–related antigen	12	800–20,000	2(0.05)	Multifunctional binding protein	Binds VIII, mediates platelet adhesion
Extrinsic pathway inhibitor	EPI, LACI	2	33	10(0.02)	Kunitz-type inhibitor	Inhibits VII/tissue factor in concert with X_a
Antithrombin III	Major antithrombin	1	60	20(2.5)	Serpin	Inhibits II_a, X_a, and other proteinases; cofactor for heparin
Protein C	—	2	62	0.4(0.06)	Vitamin K–dependent zymogen of serine proteiase	Inactivates V and VIII
Protein S	—	3	80	3(0.4)	Vitamin K–dependent protein	Cofactor for protein C_a, binds C4b-binding protein
Plasminogen	—	6	86	10(1.2)	Zymogen of serine proteinase	Lyses fibrin and other proteins
α_2-Antiplasmin	—	18	67	3(0.5)	Serpin	Inhibits plasmin
Prourokinase	—	10	54	tr	Zymogen of serine proteinase	Activates plasminogen
Tissue plasminogen activator	TPA	8	72	tr	Serine proteinase	Activates plasminogen
Plasminogen activator inhibitor-1	PAI-1	7	52	tr	Serpin	Inactivates TPA and urokinase
Plasminogen activator inhibitor-2	PAI-2	18	55	tr	Serpin	Inactivates TPA and urokinase

* For comparison, the size of albumin is 68 kilodaltons, and the plasma concentration of albumin is 3500 mg/dl (510 μM).
† For zymogens, the function after activation is given.
tr = trace.

not exposed to blood unless there is an anatomic disruption that allows blood access to the "hemostatic envelope" around blood vessels, organs, or the body itself.

In the presence of tissue factor, phospholipid, and Ca^{2+}, Factor VII can activate Factors IX and X. Activated Factor X then activates Factor II to thrombin, and thrombin cleaves fibrinogen to fibrin. The PT is the time to clot formation after addition of tissue factor, phospholipid, and Ca^{2+} to citrated platelet-poor plasma. When determined with an excess of tissue factor, the PT measures only factors of the extrinsic and common pathways and does not measure Factor VIII or IX. PT's of clinical specimens are often expressed as the International Normalized Ratio (INR), the ratio of the patient's PT and a normal PT, further normalized for source of tissue factor.

CONTROL OF FACTOR VII/TISSUE FACTOR BY EXTRINSIC PATHWAY INHIBITOR. Extrinsic pathway inhibitor (EPI) is a double-headed protease inhibitor of the Kunitz class. One head of EPI binds to activated Factor X_a, and its second head inhibits Factor VII in association with tissue factor. Therefore, EPI extinguishes the Factor VII/tissue factor "match" (Fig. 153–1B). Because activated Factor X is consumed in formation of the complex with EPI, the "fuse" that propagates blood coagulation, especially in areas of the body where tissue factor is low, begins with activated Factor IX, not Factor X (Fig. 153–1B).

CONTACT FACTORS AND THE INTRINSIC SYSTEM. Negatively charged surfaces, such as glass, sulfatide micelles, kaolin, and celite, bind Factor XII and HMWK. HMWK in turn binds prekallikrein and Factor XI. Binding to surfaces initiates a series of reciprocal cleavages of Factor XI and prekallikrein by activated Factor XII and of Factor XII by activated Factor XI and kallikrein. Activated Factor XI activates Factor IX in a reaction that requires Ca^{2+}. In the activated partial thromboplastin time (APTT), platelet-poor citrated plasma is allowed to incubate for 3 to 5 minutes with kaolin or ellagic acid to activate Factor XI optimally. Ca^{2+} and phospholipid are then added so that activated Factor XI can activate Factor IX, activated Factor IX can activate Factor X, and so on.

AMPLIFICATION OF ACTIVATION PATHWAYS. Activation of Factor X by activated Factor IX in the presence of Factor VIII and activation of Factor II by activated Factor X in the presence of Factor V are similar reactions that constitute the "fuse" that leads to the formation of thrombin (Fig. 153–1B). The two reactions require

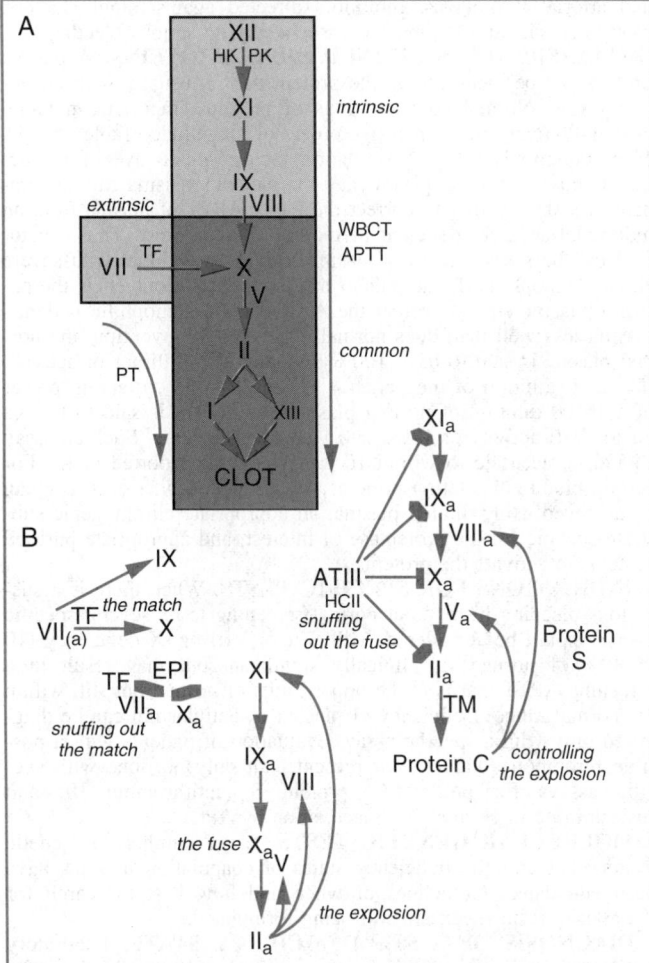

FIGURE 153–1. Diagrams of interactions among coagulation factors. Abbreviations: PT, prothrombin time; PK, prekallikrein; HK, high molecular weight kininogen; TF, tissue factor; TM, thrombomodulin; WBCT, whole blood clotting time; APTT, activated partial thromboplastin time; ATIII, antithrombin III; HCII, heparin cofactor II. Arrows indicate enzymic events. *A* is organized around the three important screening tests: the PT, WBCT, and APTT. *B* shows the steps of activation and control of clotting described in the text. The subscript "a" refers to factors that have been activated.

Ca^{2+} and phospholipid. The lipid requirement *in vivo* is satisfied by phospholipids on the surface of activated platelets, so-called platelet Factor 3 activity. Binding of Factors IX, X, and II to the phospholipid surface is defective if vitamin K–dependent gamma-carboxylation of glutamic acid residues does not occur during biosynthesis. Factors VIII and V serve to localize the IX/X and X/II reactions, respectively, on phospholipid surfaces. Factor V and Factor VIII are most effective after cleavage by thrombin (Fig. 153–1*B*). Thus, thrombin is generated initially at a sluggish rate, but once a small amount of thrombin is produced so that it can cleave Factor V and VIII to more active forms, subsequent thrombin generation is "explosively" rapid and efficient, consuming almost all of the Factor II in plasma. In addition, thrombin can activate Factor XI and thus cause activation of additional Factor IX molecules.

LOCALIZATION AND INHIBITION OF BLOOD COAGULATION. Activation of blood coagulation on a phospholipid surface *per se* localizes activation to the area of injury. Important additional localizing mechanisms include the protein C pathway to inactivate Factors V and VIII on the phospholipid surface and complexation of activated factors that diffuse away from the phospholipid surface by serpins (Fig. 153–1*B*).

The protein C pathway is initiated by binding of thrombin to thrombomodulin on the surface of endothelial cells. Thrombomodulin-bound thrombin activates protein C rather than acting upon fibrinogen or Factors V and VIII (Fig. 153–1*B*). Activated protein C (APC), in turn, inactivates Factors V and VIII. Activation of protein C by thrombin-thrombomodulin complex, therefore, is a powerful

anticoagulant event, just as the activation of Factors V and VIII by thrombin is a powerful procoagulant event. Efficient cleavage of Factors V and VIII by activated protein C is enhanced by the sixth vitamin K–dependent protein of plasma, protein S. A portion of circulating protein S is complexed to C4 binding protein (C4bp). Only the free form of protein S is active in the protein C pathway.

Two serpins in plasma, antithrombin III and heparin cofactor II, inhibit thrombin and other serine proteinases that are generated during blood coagulation. The rates at which both serpins combine with coagulation proteinases are accelerated many-fold by heparin and heparan sulfate–bearing proteoglycans in the vessel wall. The acceleration explains the anticoagulant action of heparin. The rate at which heparin cofactor II combines with thrombin is accelerated also by dermatan sulfate.

As described in more detail below, inherited deficiency of protein C, protein S, and antithrombin III and inherited resistance of Factor V to cleavage by APC have all been associated with a thrombotic diathesis.

STRUCTURE OF FIBRINOGEN AND FIBRIN. Fibrinogen and fibrin monomer are extended trinocular molecules made up of pairs of three polypeptide chains. The three chains run through half of the molecule, that is, through half of the central E nodule and the whole of one of the two peripheral D nodules. The chains adopt a coiled-spring structure between E and D nodules. The coiled-spring portion is susceptible to degradation by the principal fibrinolytic enzyme, plasmin, whereas the nodules resist degradation by plasmin. Thus, the products of complete lysis of fibrinogen by plasmin are one E nodule, two D nodules, and small fragments.

Thrombin cleavage releases negatively charged A and B fibrinopeptides to convert fibrinogen to a clottable derivative called fibrin monomer. Fibrin monomer assembles to form an infinite branching network of fibrils. At physiologic fibrin concentrations, this network constitutes a strong gel and immobilizes blood. Fibrinogen is usually completely converted to fibrin during blood coagulation. Thus, the concentration of fibrinogen antigen in serum is about 0.02 mg per deciliter (or 2 μg per milliliter), compared with 200 mg per deciliter in plasma.

The fibrin gel is modified by thrombin-activated Factor XIII. This enzyme, a transglutaminase, catalyzes covalent protein-protein crosslinking. Crosslinks are introduced between γ-chains of adjacent D domains, thus ligating the fibrin fibril end to end. Thus, the products of complete lysis of fibrin are an E nodule and crosslinked dimers of D nodules. Crosslinking of γ-chains renders the clot insoluble in protein denaturants such as 6M urea. The α-chains can ligate side to side among themselves or be crosslinked to α_2-antiplasmin. Both the "hardening" of the fibrin clot by crosslinking and the incorporation of other proteins into the clot are probably important. Deficiency of Factor XIII or α_2-antiplasmin is associated with a bleeding tendency, and some patients with Factor XIII deficiency suffer from poor wound healing.

FIBRINOLYSIS. Cleavage of plasminogen to the active proteinase, plasmin, is carried out by two plasminogen activators: tissue plasminogen activator (TPA) and urokinase. TPA is secreted as an active serine proteinase, whereas urokinase can be activated from a somewhat active precursor, prourokinase. TPA, plasminogen, and plasmin all bind to fibrin, and it is in a fibrin clot that TPA can activate plasminogen to plasmin most efficiently. Prourokinase works best when bound to urokinase receptors on the surface of cells.

Cells secrete specific inhibitors of TPA and urokinase, called plasminogen activator inhibitors 1 and 2, to regulate fibrinolysis in their local environment. Indeed, tightly controlled secretion of activator and inhibitor may allow a cell to localize plasminogen activation to volumes that are only nanometers across. Activator inhibitors are present in the circulation in low concentrations. Also in the circulation is α_2-antiplasmin, which inhibits plasmin in solution extremely rapidly and efficiently. Deficiency of plasminogen activator inhibitor 1 or, as described above, of α_2-antiplasmin is associated with a bleeding diathesis.

Epsilon-aminocaproic acid (EACA) and its cyclic analogue, tranexamic acid, bind to plasminogen and plasmin and inhibit binding of these molecules to fibrin. As a result, the molecules are good inhibitors of plasminogen activation.

Streptokinase, a bacterial protein, forms a complex with plasminogen and causes a conformational change that opens up the active site of plasminogen. The streptokinase-plasminogen complex can degrade fibrin and activate free plasminogen to plasmin. The complex is not inhibited by α_2-antiplasmin.

Drake TA, Morrissey JH, Edgington TS: Selective cellular expression of tissue factor in human tissues. Am J Pathol 134:1087, 1989. *Immunohistochemical localization of tissue factor defining the "hemostatic envelope."*
Hoffman R, Benz EJ Jr, Shattil SJ, et al. (eds.): Hematology: Basic Principles and Practice. 2nd ed. New York, Churchill Livingstone, 1995. *Comprehensive and systematic review of the hemostatic system with subsequent chapters on clinical disorders. Extensive references through 1994.*

APPROACH TO PATIENTS WITH COAGULATION DISORDERS

HISTORY AND PHYSICAL EXAMINATION. Three components are involved in effective hemostasis: the blood vessel, the platelets, and the network of soluble factors. Abnormal bleeding occurs with much greater frequency when two of the three components are compromised, as, for example, in a hemophilic patient who suffers trauma or takes aspirin or in a patient with peptic ulcer and thrombocytopenia. Disorders of platelets or blood vessels or blood coagulation factors in the extrinsic and common pathways often cause mucosal or superficial bleeding; deficiency of coagulation Factor VIII or IX results in a tendency to form soft tissue hematomas or to suffer from repeated hemarthroses. Thrombosis tends to occur when there is inflammation, abnormalities of the luminal surface of a large blood vessel, or stasis.

A personal history, family history, and physical examination are important parts of the evaluation of someone with a coagulation problem. In taking a history, it is not enough to simply ask: "Do you or your relatives bleed or clot abnormally?" One must also determine how the hemostatic system has been stressed: "Have you had any operations or tooth extractions? If so, did you bleed abnormally or require blood transfusions afterward? Are your menstrual periods heavy? Do you bruise easily? Do you take iron tablets? Have you ever had a limb immobilized?" And so on. A formal family tree indicating how many family members are at risk and which ones have symptoms or laboratory evidence of a coagulation disorder should be constructed.

LABORATORY SCREENING TESTS. When a bleeding disorder is suspected, a group of reproducible and fairly inexpensive laboratory tests should detect most clinically significant abnormalities of platelets, blood vessels, and the coagulation factor network:

1. A complete blood count and examination of the blood smear screen for abnormalities in bone marrow function or platelet number and morphologic changes in red cells caused by intravascular thrombosis or microangiopathy.

2. A quantitative platelet count provides more definitive information about platelet number.

3. The PT and APTT screen for abnormalities of the extrinsic and intrinsic coagulation pathways, respectively. Both tests are sensitive to abnormalities of the common pathway. The PT or APTT should be abnormally long if a single factor is below 20 to 40% of its normal concentration.

4. A template bleeding time screens for abnormalities of platelets, blood vessels, and von Willebrand factor.

5. The solubility of the fibrin clot in concentrated (6M) urea detects clinically significant deficiency of Factor XIII. The clot will not be covalently crosslinked and therefore will be soluble.

EVALUATION OF A PROLONGED PT OR APTT. The first step is to perform mixing experiments of normal plasma and the abnormal plasma to decide whether the abnormal plasma is deficient in a coagulation factor or contains an inhibitor of coagulation. If the screening test of the mixture is normal, the abnormal plasma likely is deficient in one or more factors, and specific factor assays should be done to identify the deficiency. Deficiency states causing a prolonged PT are all associated with increased risk of hemorrhage. Deficiency states causing a prolonged APTT, in contrast, may or may not be associated with a hemorrhagic diathesis, depending on which factor is missing. If the screening test of the mixture is abnormal, the abnormal plasma likely contains an inhibitor. Inhibitors may be of the so-called lupus type and directed against the phospholipid used in the assays or more rarely may be directed against a single coagulation factor. Lupus-type inhibitors rarely cause clinical bleeding. Indeed, as described below, some patients with lupus-type inhibitors suffer from repeated episodes of venous

and arterial thrombosis. Inhibitors directed against single factors, especially VIII and IX, may be associated with serious bleeding.

SPECIFIC TESTS OF INDIVIDUAL PROTEINS. A plasma protein can be measured as the protein *per se,* usually with an immunoassay. Normal concentrations of proteins important in blood coagulation vary more than five orders of magnitude (Table 153–1). More commonly, blood coagulation factors are assayed for functional activity. Normal plasma and the patient's plasma can be compared for their ability to correct the PT or APTT of plasma from an individual severely deficient in the factor of interest. Thus, Factor VIII can be measured using plasma from an individual with severe classic hemophilia. If the patient has Factor VIII deficiency, the patient's plasma should correct the APTT of the hemophilic patient's plasma less well than does normal plasma. By convention, the normal plasma is said to have 100% or 1 unit per milliliter of activity. If a 1:10 dilution of the patient's plasma has the correcting power of a 1:100 dilution of normal plasma, the patient is said to have a Factor VIII activity of 10%, or 0.1 unit per milliliter. Such an assay should be accurate to within 10 to 20% of the reported value. For certain blood coagulation proteins, assays with higher accuracy can be achieved using diluted plasma, an appropriate chromogenic substrate specific for the proteinase of interest, and appropriate purified proteins to activate the proteinase.

INDICATIONS FOR SPECIFIC TESTS. When there is a suspicious bleeding history but normal screening tests, several specific assays should be considered. Mild Factor VIII or IX deficiency (10 to 40% of normal) is clinically significant but may result in a screening APTT that is at the upper limits of normal but still within the normal range. Deficiency of plasma α_2-antiplasmin can be diagnosed only with a specific assay. Evaluation of patients with a possible thrombotic diathesis, at present, can only be done with specific assays for protein C, protein S, antithrombin III, and susceptibility of Factor V to inactivation by APC.

MOLECULAR GENETIC TESTS. Large numbers of genetic lesions that underlie deficiency states of coagulation proteins have been elucidated. Guidelines of when and how best to search for these lesions, however, are still being formulated.

DIAGNOSIS OF A 50% DEFICIENCY STATE. Laboratory studies of family members are often crucial to the evaluation of a patient, especially when the diagnosis centers on a heterozygous (50% of normals) deficiency. Because the normal level (i.e., the value in 99% of normal) of a coagulation factor is typically 70 to 140%, the level of the factor in individuals with heterozygous deficiency is typically 35 to 70% and the assay for the factor is accurate to within 5 to 10% of the reported value, the problem of distinguishing the 50% deficiency state from normal is a formidable one. If the apparent deficiency is found in other family members at risk, one can be much more confident that a true deficiency state exists. This problem is exemplified particularly by heterozygous deficiency states associated with thrombosis (i.e., deficiency of antithrombin III, protein C, or protein S). Workup of possible thrombophilia is further complicated by the possibility of dual deficiencies associated with more severe risk of thrombosis. The most important facet of the care of a patient with heterozygous deficiency is appropriate counseling. There should be general acceptance of the need for extensive family studies, including molecular genetic analyses, without prejudicing the insurability of newly identified affected individuals. To give an example, it would be much more efficient (and cost-effective) to identify a patient with antithrombin III deficiency as part of a family study and counsel that patient that he or she is at risk for thrombosis after surgery than to screen all patients prior to surgery with a specific assay for antithrombin III.

Coller BS, Schneiderman PI: Clinical evaluation of hemorrhagic disorders: Bleeding history and differential diagnosis of purpura. *In* Hoffman R, Benz EJ Jr, Shattil SJ, et al. (eds.): Hematology: Basic Principles and Practice. 2nd ed. New York, Churchill Livingstone, 1995, p. 1606. Santoro SA, Eby CS: Laboratory evaluation of hemostatic disorders. *In* Hoffman R, Benz EJ Jr, Shattil SJ, et al. (eds.): Hematology: Basic Principles and Practice. 2nd ed. New York, Churchill Livingstone, 1995, p. 1622. *Extensively referenced chapters on the clinical and laboratory evaluation of patients with congenital and acquired coagulation disorders.*

INHERITED DISORDERS OF BLOOD COAGULATION

The factors named with Roman numerals, with the exception of Factor XII, were identified as a consequence of patients presenting with bleeding disorders that were eventually recognized as unique and familial. Deficiency states associated with a familial tendency to thrombosis were identified as a more detailed understanding of the biochemistry of blood coagulation became available. Considerable information about the exact genetic defects that underlie inherited bleeding and thrombotic disorders has been generated. A bleeding or thrombotic diathesis may be due to a point mutation and hence a structural defect in the protein or to a mutation or deletion that causes lack of its synthesis. Deficiencies of Factors VIII and IX are inherited as X-linked traits, with bleeding occurring in the male hemizygotes. Von Willebrand disease can be an autosomal dominant or recessive disease. Deficiencies of all the other coagulation factors are transmitted as autosomal recessive traits, with clinically significant bleeding usually manifested only in patients with homozygous or compound heterozygous deficiency. In the case of protein deficiencies associated with familial tendency to thrombosis, heterozygotes with 50% of the normal level of the protein are at risk, and risk is influenced by other gene loci.

McKusick VA: Mendelian Inheritance in Man. 9th ed. Baltimore, The Johns Hopkins University Press, 1990. *Catalogs genetic defects.*

Hemophilia A (Factor VIII Deficiency)

CLINICAL MANIFESTATIONS. Hemophilia A is the most frequently encountered serious disorder of blood coagulation, occurring in 1 of 5000 male births. The degree of Factor VIII deficiency correlates well with the frequency of clinically significant bleeding. Furthermore, the degree of deficiency and bleeding severity tends to be similar in affected members of a given family. Hemophilia therefore can be classified as severe (< 1% normal activity), moderate (1 to 5% normal activity), or mild (5 to 25% normal activity).

Bleeding from the umbilical cord is rare at birth. Soft tissue hematomas may develop during early infancy. More difficulties begin when the child becomes physically active, and these continue throughout life. When bleeding follows trauma, it may be delayed because the primary hemostasis furnished by vessels and platelets is intact (see Ch. 152). Bleeding episodes can develop spontaneously without a history of trauma or other provoking causes. Such spontaneous bleeding may occur during periods of stress, such as before school examinations or following family dissension.

The bleeding of hemophilia can involve virtually any anatomic area. Repeated hemarthrosis of knees, elbows, or other joints is common and can result is progressive destruction of the joint. Hematomas often occur in muscles and soft tissues. Blood loss into thigh muscles or the retroperitoneum may be difficult to discern clinically and is frequently underestimated. If bleeding occurs on the pharynx or neck, airway obstruction can result. Severe bleeding may occur from peptic ulcerations. Partial intestinal obstruction may result from hemorrhage into the bowel wall. Mesenteric bleeding can lead to the development of bowel ischemia and necrosis. Hematuria can be painless or present as ureteral colic due to formation of clots that obstruct the ureter. Subdural hematomas and other central nervous system hemorrhages are uncommon but represent a major cause of death and disability.

Major or minor surgery, including dental extractions, can result in marked blood loss in a hemophilic patient. Even those patients with mild hemophilia, Factor VIII levels of 5 to 25% of normal, can be expected to develop clinically significant bleeding with surgery or trauma.

GENETICS. The majority of hemophilic patients give a positive family history with an X-linked inheritance pattern. In the remainder, the mutation of the Factor VIII gene may be new. A variety of nonsense and missense mutations, frameshifts, deletions, duplications, and insertions have been described, with each family having its own genetic defect. In addition, an inversion that arises from a particular vulnerability of the Factor VIII gene to homologous recombination appears to have occurred independently in 40 to 50% of families with severe disease.

DIAGNOSIS. A history of joint and soft tissue bleeding, a family history compatible with X-linked inheritance, and the presence of arthropathy on physical examination all point to the diagnosis of X-linked hemophilia. Factor IX deficiency (hemophilia B) must also be considered. Laboratory screening tests should show a normal PT and prolonged APTT. The abnormal APTT should be corrected by all deficient plasmas except those from individuals with known Factor VIII deficiency. In particular, the abnormal APTT should be corrected by plasma from a patient with Factor IX deficiency. If plasmas from patients with known deficiencies are not available, corrections can be attempted with normal plasma absorbed with barium salts (which remove Factor IX but not Factor

VIII) and serum (which contains Factor IX but not active Factor VIII). Absorbed plasma, but not serum, corrects the abnormal APTT of a patient with Factor VIII deficiency.

Because von Willebrand factor binds and stabilizes Factor VIII in the circulation, severe deficiency of von Willebrand factor is accompanied by severe deficiency of Factor VIII, and hemophilia A can be confused with von Willebrand disease. Unlike hemophilia, von Willebrand disease is inherited as an autosomal dominant trait, and the patient may present with a history of vascular-type bleeding. Upon screening, the bleeding time should be grossly prolonged in von Willebrand disease, whereas the bleeding time is usually at the upper limit of normal or only slightly prolonged in hemophilia. Further investigation should demonstrate deficiency or abnormality of von Willebrand factor and defective platelet aggregation mediated by the antibiotic ristocetin in von Willebrand disease but not in hemophilia. If the diagnosis remains in doubt, it may be helpful to perform laboratory tests on family members to determine the inheritance pattern of the deficiency.

TREATMENT. A major goal of patient, family, and physician is to have the patient lead as normal a life as possible. This entails some restrictions as a child and limitations on career choices. A hemophilic child should be reared in a protective environment until he understands the consequences of hemophilia and can take responsibility for his actions. Guided by the medical history, the degree of physical impairment, the severity of bleeding in affected family members, and the plasma level of Factor VIII, the patient should be advised to participate in activities commensurate with the severity of his disease. A very fine line can exist between physical exertions that preserve muscle tone and joint mobility and those that result in hemarthroses and hematomas. The physician should be alert for denial mechanisms sometimes constructed by patient and parents about the disease. With maturity, the patient usually is comfortable with the constraints imposed by his disease. He should be encouraged to develop his education and interests as fully as possible and counseled to adopt a career that does not expose him to undue hazards, is compatible with his physical capabilities, and allows him access to adequate health insurance coverage. Patient advocacy organizations can offer considerable support to the patient, his family, and his physician.

The patient must participate in a major way in his medical care. This has led to the widespread adoption of hemophilia treatment centers from which the patient can treat himself at home with the backup of a primary physician, a nurse coordinator, and a multidisciplinary team of a hematologist, orthopedic surgeon, infectious disease specialist, dentist, social worker, financial counselor, and others. It is reasonable to expect a patient to work or go to school full time, require a minimum of emergency room visits, and be hospitalized only for major trauma, medical illness, or elective surgery. The main cost of such a program is replacement therapy: A patient may consume many thousands of dollars in blood products each year. Home care programs, however, are cost-effective because bleeding episodes are treated when first symptomatic and do not proceed to the point where hospitalization is required for aggressive replacement therapy and pain management. About 50% of patients with hemophilia A have enough problems to make home care worthwhile.

Patients receiving long-term replacement therapy can be followed day to day by their primary care physician but need regular evaluation at 6- to 12-month intervals. The clinic visit should include a physical examination, with special attention paid to joints, an inhibitor screen, a chemistry panel including tests of liver function, and tests for antibodies to hepatitis viruses and HIV. Patients should carry identification to alert caregivers about their disease in an emergency.

REPLACEMENT THERAPY. Bleeding episodes are managed primarily by administration of concentrated Factor VIII in the form of cryoprecipitate or lyophilized purified protein. Cryoprecipitate is prepared by freezing individual bags of fresh plasma, each containing approximately 200 units of Factor VIII activity in 200 ml of plasma, at −20°C and then thawing at 4°C. Approximately 50% of the Factor VIII contained in the plasma remains as a precipitate, which is separated from the bulk of the plasma and stored frozen in individual bags containing approximately 100 units of Factor VIII activity in 20 to 40 ml of residual plasma. When needed, the appropriate number of bags is thawed at 37°C, and the contents are pooled and administered intravenously to the patient. Lyophilized Factor VIII concentrate is available in vials containing different amounts of Factor VIII activity (exact amounts stated on the labels). The concentrates are readily soluble upon addition of diluent and thus can be prepared and administered intravenously within 30 minutes.

The most important problem with replacement therapy is contaminating viruses. Each batch of Factor VIII concentrate is made from thousands of units of plasma. There is a high likelihood that recipients of untreated concentrates in the past are infected with hepatitis B, hepatitis C, and/or HIV. Patients should be vaccinated against hepatitis B at the time of diagnosis and are prime candidates for vaccines that may be developed in the future for non-A, non-B hepatitis viruses and HIV. The infectivity of concentrates can be minimized by additional purification steps and subjecting the concentrates to a treatment (e.g., heating or extraction with an organic solvent) that inactivates the viruses but preserves the activity of Factor VIII. Alternatively, Factor VIII is made by recombinant DNA techniques. These products are significantly more expensive than former concentrates. Several treatment strategies, therefore, have been developed that do not require exposure to blood products at all (e.g., use of desmopressin to raise transiently the level of Factor VIII and EACA to minimize mucosal bleeding).

The major advantage of cryoprecipitate was that it exposed the recipient to fewer donors and thus minimized the chance of blood-transmitted viral infection. Indeed, individuals have been supported from infancy to young adulthood with cryoprecipitate prepared from plasma donated sequentially by the same donor. The major disadvantages of cryoprecipitate are the inconvenience of thawing and pooling bags prior to administration and the need for the bags to stay frozen at −20°C until the time of administration. Major advantages of lyophilized concentrate are stability on storage and convenience of administration. Further, currently available concentrates have been processed to eliminate or inactivate HIV totally and possibly also hepatitis B and C and thus can be considered safer than cryoprecipitate.

Because of its large size, Factor VIII distributes mainly in the blood plasma. There is approximately 40 ml of plasma per kilogram of body weight, and a 70-kg patient with severe hemophilia A requires somewhat more than 2800 units of Factor VIII to raise the plasma level to 100% normal. As a rule of thumb, infusions of 15, 30, and 60 units per kilogram should raise the plasma level to 25%, 50%, and 100% of normal, respectively. The half-life of infused Factor VIII is 10 to 12 hours. Replacement therapy is ordinarily given three times a day when tight control of the level is needed and twice a day when deeper troughs in the level can be tolerated. Alternatively, a constant infusion of 1 to 2 units per kilogram per hour can be given after a loading dose.

Very early hemarthrosis can be self-managed with a single infusion to attain a peak Factor VIII level of 25 to 50% of normal. For more extensive hemorrhage, Factor VIII infusions usually are continued for 2 days after the cessation of symptoms or signs of bleeding. Muscle hematomas require a longer period of sustained Factor VIII levels, in the range of 40 to 60% of normal for 4 to 6 days. Major trauma or surgery requires that the Factor VIII level be maintained at more than 70% of normal until hemostasis is achieved and then in the range of 25 to 50% of normal for 10 to 14 days. When infusions are being given over several days, plasma Factor VIII levels should be measured after administration of the first dose to document that the desired level has been achieved and prior to subsequent scheduled administrations as needed to determine whether desired levels have been sustained and to adjust the dose. If a low Factor VIII persists despite replacement therapy, it may simply be that not enough Factor VIII is being given or that the patient has developed an inhibitor that neutralizes infused Factor VIII.

TREATMENT OF HEMARTHROSES. Joint bleeding is helped initially by immobilization of the affected limb and application of ice packs to diminish swelling and discomfort. Hemarthroses should not be aspirated unless such acute pain and tension are present that pressure necrosis is a major possibility or there is worry of infection. Aspiration should be performed only after giving replacement Factor VIII. When pain and swelling have subsided, the pa-

tient should begin rehabilitation to regain motion and strength in conjunction with prophylactic replacement therapy. Patients with joint disease may benefit from periodic assessment by an orthopedic surgeon. In properly selected patients, synovectomy and artificial joint replacement have been very successful in improving the usefulness of severe chronic joint deformity.

DENTAL CARE. The patient should be instructed about the importance of dental hygiene and should have frequent dental examinations. Bleeding in deep tissues of the oropharynx can be life threatening. Therefore, a local anesthetic by needle puncture should be given only after prophylactic Factor VIII concentrate. Extraction also requires prior administration of Factor VIII concentrate. For patients with mild or moderate hemophilia, it is likely that adequate levels of Factor VIII can be achieved with use of desmopressin, as described below for patients with von Willebrand disease. Administration of EACA or tranexamic acid by mouth, also described below, is useful in prevention of rebleeding after tooth extraction.

ANALGESICS. Bleeding can cause extraordinary pain. Injudicious use of narcotics can lead to addiction in hemophilic patients. Aspirin must be avoided by the hemophilic because it decreases platelet aggregation and accentuates bleeding. Acetaminophen and codeine are recommended as the first choices of analgesics. In selected cases, ibuprofen can be given for chronic joint pain. The likelihood that ibuprofen will cause increased bleeding can be assessed by a template bleeding time after the patient has been on the drug for several days. If the bleeding time is prolonged, the drug should be discontinued.

FACTOR VIII INHIBITORS. Up to 15% of hemophilic patients develop inhibitory antibodies to Factor VIII activity (Factor VIII inhibitor). The antibodies usually appear in childhood but should be of constant concern throughout the life of a hemophilic patient. The inhibitor need not be associated with any obvious change in the clinical severity of the disorder, and therefore specific testing for an inhibitor should be done before procedures that require replacement of Factor VIII. Treatment of patients with inhibitors is problematic. Much depends on the titer of the inhibitor, which is commonly expressed in Bethesda units: 1 Bethesda unit, by definition, inhibits 1 unit of Factor VIII, that is, the Factor VIII in 1 ml of normal plasma. If one calculates the amount of Factor VIII required to neutralize the inhibitor and achieve a 50% normal level of circulating Factor VIII in a 70-kg patient who has an inhibitor titer of 10 Bethesda units per milliliter, the amount (and cost) is immense:

$$10.5 \text{ units/ml} \times 40 \text{ ml/kg} \times 70 \text{ kg} = 29,400 \text{ units}$$

Several strategies are available, all expensive and none totally adequate. Because some inhibitors take up to several hours to complex with and inhibit Factor VIII, it may be possible to maintain Factor VIII levels at a therapeutic level by constant infusion. If the inhibitor is of modest titer (1 to 10 Bethesda units per milliliter), it may be possible to remove enough inhibitor by plasmapheresis to make therapy feasible with lower amounts of Factor VIII. A patient receiving Factor VIII concentrate may have an anamnestic immune response with an increase in the titer and avidity of his inhibitor. Therefore, everything possible should be done to achieve permanent hemostasis in the 4- to 6-day "golden period" during which replacement therapy is possible. Patients with high titers of rapidly acting inhibitor can be given porcine Factor VIII that is not neutralized by the antibodies or purified activated Factor VII that "bypasses" Factor VIII in the coagulation cascade.

CARRIER DETECTION. Women who have relatives with hemophilia frequently seek help to determine whether they may pass the disorder to their children. Only about 15% of the instances of hemophilia arise because of spontaneous mutation. Daughters of men with the disorder, mothers of more than one hemophilic son, and mothers who have a hemophilic son and another hemophilic male relative in their pedigree are obligate carriers of the hemophilic gene. A carrier woman has a 50% chance of producing a hemophilic male or a female carrier. Because of random clonal inactivation of the X chromosome, the carrier is a genetic mosaic with two populations of cells with an active normal X chromosome or active abnormal X chromosome (bearing the hemophilic gene). Therefore, a carrier should have about 50% of the normal level of Factor VIII activity. If the preponderance of cells has the active X chromosome with the hemophilic gene, the Factor VIII level can be less than 40% of normal and the woman may have clinical features of mild hemophilia. The opposite can occur as well. Determination of Factor VIII activity, therefore, is of limited usefulness in the identification of carrier women because low normal levels overlap with Factor VIII levels found in obligate heterozygotes. Preferably, the potential carrier and her family should be studied to identify the altered DNA sequence responsible for hemophilia or restriction fragment length polymorphisms that segregate with hemophilia. This information also can be used to diagnose hemophilia in fetuses in the first trimester, whereas assays of Factor VIII *per se* can be done only in the second trimester, when the fetal circulation is accessible for blood sampling by fetoscopy.

PROGNOSIS. The major long-term complications of moderate and severe hemophilia are (1) progressive joint deformity and crippling, (2) development of inhibitors to Factor VIII activity, (3) hepatitis and cirrhosis, and (4) AIDS. Despite the availability of replacement therapy, many hemophilics, for a variety of reasons, are treated inadequately or haphazardly and become severely crippled and, ultimately, chronic invalids. It has been shown that twice-weekly prophylactic infusions of Factor VIII from an early age eliminate arthropathy. Widespread prophylaxis, however, is not possible because of cost and a limit of Factor VIII worldwide. The latter three complications are seen more often in patients who receive frequent replacement therapy. A large proportion of patients who received significant quantities of blood products in the early and mid-1980's were infected with HIV. It is difficult to overemphasize the enormity of the physical and psychosocial hardship facing these patients and their infected spouses and children. The comprehensive treatment center and community resources such as the Hemophilia Foundation chapter are crucial in providing access to the latest treatment protocols and needed counseling and psychological support. The scourge of AIDS has negated the gains in life expectancy and freedom from disability that were achieved by the widespread availability of Factor VIII concentrates in the 1970's. Newer concentrates are much safer. The several hemophilic patients who have undergone liver transplantation for hepatic failure were cured of their hemophilia by Factor VIII produced by the transplanted organ. The challenge now is to introduce the normal Factor VIII gene stably into the patient's own cells. One hopes that future cohorts of hemophilic patients will enjoy both the benefits of replacement therapy and eventually cure through gene therapy.

Green D, McMichel DM: Hemophilia: Factor VIII deficiency. *In* Loscalzo J, Schafer AI (eds.): Thrombosis and Hemorrhage. Boston, Blackwell Scientific, 1994, p 683. Furie B, Limentani SA, Rosenfeld CG: A practical guide to the evaluation and treatment of hemophilia. Blood 84:3, 1994. Hoyer LW: Hemophilia A. N Engl J Med 330:38, 1994. *Three somber reviews of hemophilia A.*
Kaufman RJ, Antonarakis SE: Structure, biology and genetics of Factor VIII, *In* Hoffman R, Benz EJ Jr, Shattil SJ, et al. (eds.): Hematology: Basic Principles and Practice. 2nd ed. New York, Churchill Livingstone, 1995, p. 1633. *Reviews Factor VIII mutations causing hemophilia.*
Lakich D, Kazazian HH Jr, Antonarakis SE, et al.: Inversions disrupting the factor VIII gene are a common cause of severe hemophilia A. Nature Genetics 5:236, 1993. *This paper proposes a mechanism causing severe hemophilia A in approximately 45% of affected families. The mechanism is without precedent in other inherited diseases and appears to solve what was a deepening mystery.*

Von Willebrand Disease

CLINICAL MANIFESTATIONS. This disorder is due to a deficiency or abnormality of a plasma protein, von Willebrand factor, that binds and stabilizes Factor VIII in the circulation and also mediates adherence of platelets to sites of vascular injury. Thus, the clinical manifestations are a mix of the manifestations of hemophilia and a qualitative platelet disorder. Some patients have a severe hemorrhagic disorder, in which the level of Factor VIII is low enough and the bleeding problems severe enough that the disease must be differentiated from classic hemophilia. For others, an abnormality of von Willebrand factor is a laboratory curiosity. The severity of symptoms due to von Willebrand disease can vary even among afflicted family members, probably because there are a number of interacting genes and physiologic factors that control the synthesis and secretion of von Willebrand factor.

The principal bleeding problems are of the superficial type. In patients with severe disease, epistaxis and easy bruising are frequent complaints, especially early in life. Hematuria and gastrointestinal bleeding occur less frequently, and hemarthroses are quite rare. Postoperative bleeding is a major hazard. In patients with less severe disease, the hemorrhagic tendency usually becomes evident or troublesome only with trauma, surgery, or dental extractions. Women commonly experience excessive menses and postpartum bleeding. In all forms of the disease, the frequency and severity of bleeding tend to lessen with age.

DIAGNOSIS. Hallmarks of von Willebrand disease historically have been a low Factor VIII level, a long bleeding time, and autosomal inheritance. The latter two characteristics distinguish von Willebrand disease from hemophilia A. With the characterization of von Willebrand factor has come a broadening of the definition of von Willebrand disease so that the name now encompasses a heterogeneous group of defects of von Willebrand factor. These defects are described by a still-evolving classification system of numbers and letters. It has been estimated that up to 1% of people have a quantitative or qualitative abnormality of von Willebrand factor.

Classic (type 1) von Willebrand disease is due to a quantitative deficiency of von Willebrand factor and characterized by a prolonged bleeding time, prolonged APTT, and low level of Factor VIII. Confirmatory testing should reveal a low level of immunoreactive von Willebrand factor that parallels the level of Factor VIII and diminished or absent platelet aggregation when ristocetin is added to the patient's platelet-rich plasma. The analysis using ristocetin can be made more sensitive and quantitative by testing the ability of dilutions of the patient's plasma to support agglutination of washed platelets, the so-called ristocetin cofactor titer. Patients with severe disease can have less than 1% of normal von Willebrand factor in plasma and platelets. Their Factor VIII levels may be less than 5% of normal. Such patients may be heterozygous for a dominant negative mutation. More commonly, severe disease is a recessive disorder passed on by asymptomatic or minimally symptomatic parents. The recessive disease is sometimes called type 3.

Patients with variant (type 2) von Willebrand disease are suspected on the basis of bleeding problems, prolonged bleeding time, and abnormal ristocetin-induced platelet aggregation but normal or only slightly decreased levels of von Willebrand factor and Factor VIII. Such patients have qualitative abnormalities of von Willebrand factor. Electrophoretic analysis of the size distribution of von Willebrand factor multimers is key to further evaluation. This is done by probing separated plasma proteins with antibodies to von Willebrand factor after agarose gel electrophoresis. The normal pattern is a series of multimers ranging in size from 850,000 to 12,000,000 daltons. All sizes of multimers bind and stabilize Factor VIII, but only the large multimers adsorb to collagen and other components of the vessel wall and thus mediate attachment and spreading of platelets to the subendothelium of damaged vessels. In type 2A disease, the larger multimers are missing in both plasma and platelets, and von Willebrand factor function (e.g., ristocetin cofactor activity) is decreased more than von Willebrand factor antigen. In type 2M disease, ristocetin cofactor activity is decreased even though the multimer pattern is normal.

In type 2B disease, platelets in the patient's platelet-rich plasma are hypersensitive to aggregation by ristocetin, and the larger multimers are missing in plasma but not in platelets. It is thought that the largest multimers are missing from plasma because the multimers bind spontaneously to platelets. In principle, such a spontaneous interaction could be due to defects in the patient's von Willebrand factor or in the patient's platelets ("pseudo von Willebrand disease"), and indeed patients have been identified in whom the defect is in glycoprotein Ib that functions as one of the platelet cell surface receptors for von Willebrand factor (see Ch. 152).

Rare patients have von Willebrand factor that functions normally in platelet adhesion but cannot bind and stabilize Factor VIII, giving rise to type 2N von Willebrand disease, or so-called autosomal hemophilia. Platelet-dependent functions are normal.

Results of evaluations for mild type 1 von Willebrand disease can be ambiguous owing to absence of clear diagnostic criteria and the multitude of factors that influence the concentration of von Willebrand factor. Endothelial cells and megakaryocytes-platelets synthesize, store, and secrete von Willebrand factor. Secretion increases when endothelial cells are stimulated or injured. Therefore, the concentration of plasma von Willebrand factor is labile and can be increased by stimuli as innocuous as a vigorous Valsalva maneuver. Increases of 2- to 10-fold are common in ill patients. People with type O blood have lower concentrations than do people with types A and B. Hypothyroidism causes the concentration of von Willebrand factor to fall. Aging is associated with an increase in concentration. Thus, one must worry about both overdiagnosis and underdiagnosis of type 1 von Willebrand disease in someone with decreases in von Willebrand factor and Factor VIII to 50% of normal. Serial studies of von Willebrand factor levels over several months and studies of other family members can be helpful. Because symptoms in such patients are mild and tend to decrease with age, it may suffice to be honest with such patients about the ambiguities of the laboratory tests and counsel them to alert their physician about the possibility of von Willebrand disease in the event of trauma or major surgery.

GENETICS. Identification of mutations that result in the various qualitative (type 2) abnormalities of von Willebrand factor has revealed much about structure/function of the protein. Studies with type 1 von Willebrand disease have not been nearly so revealing. Data pooled from multiple families have demonstrated statistically significant linkage to the gene for von Willebrand factor. This information suggests, in a given family, that type 1 disease may be due to a defect in the von Willebrand factor gene, but a defect in another gene cannot be excluded. In other words, more than one molecular mechanism may be identified eventually as the basis for type 1 disease.

TREATMENT. Indications for therapy in von Willebrand disease include surgery, severe epistaxes, severe menorrhagia, and recurrent gastrointestinal bleeding. Therapy should be planned and modified based on quantitative estimates of plasma Factor VIII and consideration of the bleeding time.

Cryoprecipitate is equally rich in Factor VIII and von Willebrand factor, including the large multimers, and therefore corrects both the deficiency of Factor VIII and the long bleeding time of type 1 von Willebrand disease. Most Factor VIII concentrates are poor in von Willebrand factor and do not correct the bleeding time defect. Hence, replacement therapy in von Willebrand disease should be with cryoprecipitate or with Factor VIII concentrates of intermediate purity that have been documented to contain multimeric von Willebrand factor. Because the largest multimers of von Willebrand factor are cleared rapidly after infusion, the bleeding time is usually corrected only transiently. Infused von Willebrand factor allows the patient's own Factor VIII to circulate, and the Factor VIII level may remain elevated for considerably longer than would be predicted based on the amount of infused Factor VIII. Cryoprecipitate or concentrate should be given initially using the guidelines described above for Factor VIII replacement in hemophilia A. The infusion should be given immediately prior to maneuvers designed to achieve hemostasis. This practice ensures that the bleeding time as well as the Factor VIII level is maximally corrected. It is not practical to give cryoprecipitate often enough to keep the bleeding time corrected continuously or to quantify the correction with serial bleeding times. Therefore, once hemostasis is achieved, therapy should be directed toward keeping the level of Factor VIII in the appropriate therapeutic ranges as described above for hemophilia A. This probably requires less cryoprecipitate or concentrate than if one is treating a hemophilic.

Considerable attention has been devoted to the therapeutic potential of desmopressin (1-desamino-8-D-arginine vasopressin, DDAVP) in patients with mild hemophilia A and mild to moderately severe von Willebrand disease. Desmopressin causes release of von Willebrand factor and plasminogen activator from endothelial cells. Typically, a dose of 0.3 μg per kilogram of body weight in 50 ml saline given over 15 minutes causes several-fold increases of both Factor VIII and von Willebrand protein. The increases peak 15 to 30 minutes after infusion with a concomitant decrease in the bleeding time and may last for several hours. Desmopressin is also formulated as a nasal spray, 150 μg per nostril. The magnitude and duration of the response vary among individual patients, especially those with type 2A disease. Desmopressin is contraindicated in type 2B disease because appearance of the large multimers in the circulation can cause thrombocytopenia. To learn if the treatment is feasible in a given patient, one should quantify the response to a test dose of desmopressin at the time of diagnosis or 5 to 7 days prior to a planned procedure. Desmopressin is likely to produce a diminished response if used more than once every 24 hours. Restriction of fluid intake is necessary to reduce the possibility of hyponatremia.

EACA or tranexamic acid suppresses baseline and desmopressin-stimulated fibrinolysis. For oral surgical procedures, therefore, EACA or tranexamic acid is given orally in a dosage of 75 mg per kilogram every 6 hours or 20 mg per kilogram every 8 hours, respectively, beginning the evening before the procedure and finishing when all wounds are healed. It is controversial whether an antifibrinolytic agent should be given with major surgery.

MENSTRUATION AND PREGNANCY. Excessive menstrual blood loss can be managed with hormonal suppression. Levels of Factor VIII, von Willebrand factor, and ristocetin cofactor activity may become normal during pregnancy. Therefore, these tests, along with the bleeding time, should be repeated during the third trimester to plan for replacement therapy during delivery. Cryoprecipitate should be given if the Factor VIII level remains low. If the Factor VIII level is greater than 50%, but the bleeding time remains long, cryoprecipitate should be on call because postpartum blood loss is frequently severe enough to require replacement infusion.

COMPLICATIONS OF THERAPY. Chronic arthropathy is less common in von Willebrand disease than hemophilia A. The complications of replacement therapy for severe von Willebrand disease are the same as those described above for hemophilia A. Rarely, antibodies that inhibit the activity of von Willebrand protein develop. Patients receiving blood products should be vaccinated against hepatitis B and monitored for the acquisition of hepatitis viruses and HIV.

Sadler JE, Gralnick HR: Commentary: A new classification for von Willebrand disease. Blood 84:676, 1994. *Reference for simplified classification scheme used above.*
White GC, Montgomery RR: Clinical aspects of and therapy for von Willebrand disease. *In* Hoffman R, Benz EJ Jr, Shattil SJ, et al. (eds.): Hematology: Basic Principles and Practice. 2nd ed. New York, Churchill Livingstone, 1995, p. 1725.

Hemophilia B (Factor IX Deficiency)

CLINICAL MANIFESTATIONS. The incidence of Factor IX deficiency is about 1 in 30,000 male births. Factor IX deficiency is inherited as an X-linked disorder that presents with the historical and clinical features described above for Factor VIII deficiency. The severity of bleeding is usually similar within a family. Factor IX–deficient patients have fewer symptoms than do patients with Factor VIII deficiency; for example, patients with severe ($<1\%$ of normal) Factor IX deficiency have the symptoms of patients with moderate (1 to 5% of normal) Factor VIII deficiency. Nevertheless, Factor IX deficiency causes serious bleeding problems. Patients with severe disease can develop muscle hematomas, gastrointestinal hemorrhage, and bleeding into large joints with progression to crippling joint deformities. Because many are asymptomatic until their hemostatic system is stressed by surgery or trauma, patients with Factor IX deficiency can be more cavalier about their disease than patients with Factor VIII deficiency and may not seek medical attention until hemorrhage is far advanced.

DIAGNOSIS. This disorder is suspected with the finding of a prolonged APTT that can be corrected by normal serum but not by barium sulfate–adsorbed plasma. The inability of the patient's plasma to correct the prolonged APTT of plasma from a patient with known Factor IX deficiency establishes the diagnosis. A minority of patients with hemophilia B have an abnormal Factor IX that causes mild prolongation of a PT carried out with bovine tissue factor.

GENETICS. More than 300 mutations leading to hemophilia B have been identified. These include partial and total deletions, missense mutations, frameshifts, and premature stop codons and result in decreased or absent production of Factor IX or production of an abnormal molecule. Mutations in the promoter region (hemophilia B Leiden) cause poor expression of Factor IX that corrects partially after puberty.

TREATMENT. The care and long-term goals of therapy for the patient with Factor IX deficiency are similar to those described above for the patient with hemophilia A. Most patients need less care than if they had hemophilia A, but they require the same intensity of education and counseling.

REPLACEMENT THERAPY. Fresh-frozen plasma is used to treat mild to moderate bleeding, especially in those patients who have hemorrhagic episodes infrequently. Ordinarily, transfusion of 500 ml of plasma twice daily is sufficient to maintain a level of Factor IX activity 10 to 12% above baseline. EACA can be used as an adjunct to transfusions of plasma in patients with mucosal bleeding or dental work.

Patients with moderate to severe hemorrhage, such as large hemarthrosis or muscle hematomas, and patients being prepared for surgery can be treated with commercially prepared Factor IX concentrate, aiming for levels that are approximately two thirds as high as those described above for Factor VIII replacement therapy. Factor IX is smaller than Factor VIII and distributes in a volume 1.5- to 2-fold greater than the distribution volume of Factor VIII. Thus, proportionately more Factor IX than Factor VIII must be infused to achieve a similar response. As a rule of thumb, infusion of 50 units per kilogram should raise the plasma level of Factor IX to 50% of normal. Because of its longer half-life in the body, however, Factor IX needs to be given less often than Factor VIII in order to maintain a therapeutic level. The length of therapy depends on the severity of the hemorrhage and the patient's response. Therapy is generally continued for 2 days after bleeding and related symptoms have subsided.

COMPLICATIONS OF THERAPY. Two types of concentrates are available, highly purified Factor IX concentrates and prothrombin complex concentrates that are a mixture of the six vitamin K–dependent factors—Factors II, VII, IX, and X and proteins C and S. Recently improved viral inactivation methodology is thought to render these concentrates free of infectious HIV or hepatitis viruses. Nevertheless, patients should be immunized against hepatitis B. Prothrombin complex concentrates contain trace amounts of activated vitamin K–dependent factors and therefore are thrombogenic and carry a risk for thromboembolism, especially when used in high dosage in patients who have liver disease or are immobilized following surgery. EACA greatly enhances the risk of thromboembolism and should not be used as an adjunct to Factor IX replacement therapy. Indeed, some advocate low-dose heparin (5000 units every 12 hours) be given to surgical patients receiving prothrombin complex concentrates. Limited experience indicates that use of purified Factor IX concentrates is not associated with thromboembolic complications.

Antibody inhibitors to Factor IX develop in 5 to 10% of treated patients.

CARRIER DETECTION. The normal range for Factor IX is narrower than the normal range for Factor VIII, and therefore carrier testing based on coagulation assays is better for hemophilia B than for hemophilia A. Nevertheless, laboratory definition of the carrier state is still an exercise in probabilities and is best done with genetic markers. The Factor IX gene exhibits considerable polymorphism, and informative genetic markers are found in most families. It is still worthwhile to do Factor IX activity assays in potential carriers because women who are carriers may have Factor IX levels that are sufficiently low to cause mild bleeding, especially after trauma or surgery.

Limentani SA, Furie B: Biochemistry of factor IX and molecular biology of hemophilia B. *In* Hoffman R, Benz EJ Jr, Shattil SJ, et al. (eds.): Hematology: Basic Principles and Practice. 2nd ed. New York, Churchill Livingstone, 1995, p. 1664.
Roberts HR, Gray TF III: Clinical aspects of and therapy for hemophilia B. *In* Hoffman R, Benz EJ Jr, Shattil SJ, et al. (eds.): Hematology: Basic Principles and Practice. 2nd ed. New York, Churchill Livingstone, 1995, p. 1678.

Deficiencies of Contact Factors

Deficiencies of Factor XII, prekallikrein, or HMWK are clinically benign, and deficiency of Factor XI may sometimes be benign. Patients with these abnormalities, nevertheless, have APTT's that are as prolonged as patients with Factor VIII or IX deficiency. Therefore it is important to establish the correct diagnosis and counsel the patient whether he or she has a laboratory abnormality that carries a risk for bleeding.

DEFICIENCY OF FACTOR XII, PREKALLIKREIN, OR HMWK. These autosomal recessive disorders are almost always asymptomatic and are usually identified as an abnormality in a routine APTT. The APTT of a mixture of patient's plasma and normal plasma should be normal, that is, no demonstrable inhibitor. The plasma concentrations of Factors XI, IX, and VIII should be normal. The coagulation defect can be identified by the inability of the patient's plasma to correct the APTT of the appropriately deficient plasma.

FACTOR XI DEFICIENCY. Three separate gene defects that cause Factor XI deficiency are common in Ashkenazi Jews. The prevalence of autosomally recessive Factor XI deficiency in this population is 1 in 500 compared with 1 in 1 million in other populations. Types II and III are associated with an increased risk of bleeding problems when present in the homozygous or mixed heterozygous state. One of these mutations results in synthesis of a truncated molecule. The second is a missense mutation. The genetic heterogeneity helps explain why Factor XI deficiency is asymptomatic in some families and associated with bleeding in others. Severe (<20 to 30% normal) Factor XI deficiency causes the APTT to be prolonged. The PT, bleeding time, and specific assays for Factors VIII and IX should be normal. The diagnosis is established by a specific assay for Factor XI. Whether heterozygous individuals are also at risk for bleeding is controversial. Only a quantitative Factor XI assay defines the heterozygous 50% deficiency state.

Clinically significant bleeding usually occurs in association with trauma, surgery, or dental extractions. Hemorrhage seems more likely when tissues rich in fibrinolytic activity such as prostate are traumatized. Major bleeding into muscles or joints is rare. A decision to replace Factor XI should be made on the clinical assessment of ongoing bleeding, the baseline level of Factor XI, the genotype, and the personal and family history of bleeding. Patients with levels less than 20% normal or with a bleeding history should receive prophylaxis for surgery. Fresh-frozen plasma, 15 to 20 ml per kilogram followed by 3 to 6 ml per kilogram every 12 to 24 hours, should be given as treatment of bleeding or as prophylaxis for surgery. Only a few infusions may suffice, because Factor XI has a half-life of about 72 hours.

Seligsohn U, Griffin JH: Contact activation and factor XI. *In* Scriver CR, Beaudet AL, Sly WS, Valle D (eds.): Metabolic and Molecular Basis of Inherited Disease. New York, McGraw-Hill, 1995, pp. 3289–3311. *Detailed description on how to approach patients with Factor XI deficiency.*

Deficiencies of the Extrinsic and Common Factors

Deficiencies of Factors VII, X, V, and II are all associated with clinically significant bleeding. The hemorrhagic diathesis is not as predictable or severe as in hemophilia A or B, but replacement therapy probably will be required at some point in a patient's lifetime, especially to control bleeding from mucous membranes, after dental extractions, or during menses.

DEFICIENCY OF FACTOR VII. This is a rare autosomal recessive defect. Patients have a history of bleeding, usually beginning in infancy or early childhood. Bleeding, however, is frequently mild, even in patients with severe deficiency. Heterozygous relatives have no bleeding tendency. Mucous membrane bleeding, epistaxis, intramuscular hemorrhage, hemarthroses, and menorrhagia are the most common problems; gastrointestinal bleeding is less common, hematuria occurs only occasionally, and central nervous system bleeding is rare. Bleeding after dental extractions is predictable, and such extractions should be done with prophylactic replacement therapy. Clinical manifestations of bleeding can vary from mild to severe in the same patient. In fact, patients with impressive bleeding histories have undergone major surgery without accompanying hemorrhage. This phenomenon is unexplained and not consistent with the central role assigned to Factor VII in the physiologic initiation of blood coagulation. Also incongruent are observations of thromboembolism in Factor VII–deficient patients.

A diagnosis of Factor VII deficiency should be considered if the PT is prolonged but the APTT is normal. The coagulation time of the patient's plasma in response to Russell's viper venom, which directly activates Factor X, is normal. The diagnosis is established by the inability to correct the patient's PT with Factor VII–deficient plasma.

Bleeding is treated with plasma. The half-life of Factor VII is 2 to 6 hours, and therefore frequent treatment is needed during a bleeding episode. Levels of 15 to 20% of normal can be obtained with a loading dose of plasma of 10 to 20 ml per kilogram followed by 3 to 6 ml per kilogram every 12 hours and should suffice to stop bleeding or as prophylaxis for surgery. Commercially available prothrombin complex concentrate, which contains Factors VII, IX, X, and II, can be used if it is essential to avoid any possibility of intravascular volume overload; such concentrates carry the risk of thromboembolism. Menorrhagia may require treatment with oral contraceptive agents.

DEFICIENCY OF FACTOR X. This deficiency is also a rare autosomal recessive disorder. Clinical symptoms include epistaxis; occasional mucous membrane, joint, and muscle hemorrhages; and gastrointestinal bleeding. Women may have severe, life-threatening menses and postpartum hemorrhage. The diagnosis is suspected when both the PT and APTT are prolonged. The abnormal tests are corrected with normal serum but not with barium sulfate–adsorbed plasma. The clotting time of plasma in response to Russell's viper venom is usually prolonged, although an abnormal Factor X has been described which is activated normally by Russell's viper venom but not by the intrinsic or extrinsic systems of blood coagulation. The diagnosis is established by demonstration that the abnormal plasma does not correct Factor X–deficient plasma. Bleeding episodes are treated with plasma as described above for Factor VII deficiency; plasma needs to be given less often because the plasma half-life of Factor X is 24 to 48 hours.

DEFICIENCY OF FACTOR II (PROTHROMBIN DEFICIENCY). Like deficiency of Factors VII and X, Factor II deficiency (hypoprothrombinemia) is a rare recessive disorder. Bleeding ranges from mild to severe and generally occurs only if the Factor II activity level is below 20% of normal. Symptoms include umbilical bleeding at birth, epistaxis, menorrhagia, postpartum hemorrhage, and bleeding after trauma or minor surgical procedures. The diagnosis is suspected if the PT and APTT are prolonged and the thrombin time is normal. Neither serum nor barium sulfate–absorbed plasma corrects the abnormalities. A specific assay can be done based on the ability of the unknown to correct the PT of known Factor II–deficient plasma. Alternatively, a test can be done in which clotting of plasma is initiated with Taipan viper venom, a specific activator of Factor II. Bleeding is treated with infusions of fresh-frozen plasma as described above for Factor VII deficiency. Infusions are necessary only every 2 days because the half-life of Factor II is about 72 hours.

GLOBAL DEFICIENCY OF VITAMIN K–DEPENDENT FACTORS. These patients present as infants with bleeding, grossly prolonged PT and APTT, and low levels (<5% of normal) of Factors II, VII, IX, and X even though there is no evidence of liver disease, malabsorption, or ingestion of coumarin drugs. The levels of the vitamin K–dependent factors generally increase to 30 to 40% of normal when patients are given pharmacologic doses (10 mg per day) of vitamin K, and the patients do well with minimal symptoms. This syndrome is probably due to an abnormality of vitamin K metabolism, such as a dysfunctional vitamin K epoxide reductase.

DEFICIENCY OF FACTOR V. This disorder usually is inherited as an autosomal recessive trait. As with deficiencies of Factor VII, X, or II, symptoms are variable, and hemorrhage most often involves the mucous membranes of the nose and oral cavity. Hemarthroses are unusual. Menorrhagia may be so severe as to be life threatening. Some women with Factor V deficiency, however, have normal menses or only mild menorrhagia. Obstetric deliveries may occur with little or no bleeding, but postpartum hemorrhage is frequent and requires replacement therapy.

Both the APTT and PT are prolonged. The PT can be corrected by barium sulfate–adsorbed fresh plasma but not by serum. Definitive diagnosis is established if the patient's plasma does not correct the deficiency of a patient known to lack Factor V activity. For unknown reasons, the bleeding time is prolonged in about one third of Factor V–deficient patients.

Because Factor V is an extremely labile protein, treatment should be with plasma that is either fresh or was frozen while fresh and has not been stored for more than several months. The therapeutic goal should be a Factor V activity level greater than 25% of normal. Because Factor V is larger than the vitamin-K–dependent factors, it should be possible to achieve such a level with the doses of plasma described above for Factor VII deficiency. The plasma half-life of Factor V activity is 12 to 36 hours. Cryoprecipitate and Factor VIII concentrate are not enriched in Factor V. Surgery should be done under the "cover" of prophylactic replacement therapy.

Platelets contain 10 to 20% of the Factor V in blood, and therefore platelet concentrates are a good source of Factor V. Several patients have responded well to platelet transfusions after developing neutralizing antibodies to Factor V.

COMBINED DEFICIENCIES OF FACTORS V AND VIII. A number of patients have mild deficiencies of both Factors V and VIII inherited as an autosomal recessive trait. The basis of the syndrome is unknown but probably related to some post-translational modification of the two homologous proteins necessary for their function. Therapy should be directed toward replacement of both proteins.

Roberts HR, Eberst ME: Other coagulation factor deficiencies. *In* Loscalzo J, Schafer AI (eds.): Thrombosis and Hemorrhage. Boston, Blackwell Scientific, 1994, p 701.

DISORDERS OF FIBRINOGEN. These disorders fall into two categories: absent (afibrinogenemia) or a low (hypofibrinogenemia) content of plasma fibrinogen and abnormally functioning plasma fibrinogen (dysfibrinogenemia). Afibrinogenemia and hypofibrinogenemia are autosomally recessive traits. Dysfibrinogenemia can be autosomally dominant or recessive.

AFIBRINOGENEMIA. In patients with absence or low content of fibrinogen, the bleeding tendency may be noted at birth as a continued oozing from the umbilical stump. The intensity and frequency of bleeding after trauma or surgery vary from mild to severe. Death from intracranial hemorrhage may occur in infancy or early childhood. It is not understood why some patients have a minimal bleeding tendency whereas others are quite symptomatic. All assays that require formation of fibrin as an endpoint are abnormal. Plasma fibrinogen cannot be detected by immunologic or chemical (salting-out) methods. The bleeding time may be markedly prolonged. Bleeding episodes should be treated with cryoprecipitate, which contains 8-fold to 10-fold more fibrinogen than does an equivalent amount of plasma. Plasma fibrinogen concentrations greater than 100 mg per deciliter are generally adequate and can be achieved by administering 1 bag of cryoprecipitate for each 10 kg of body weight.

DYSFIBRINOGENEMIA. Dysfibrinogenemias are usually named after the cities in which they were discovered. The clinical features are quite variable. Most individuals are asymptomatic. Some have mild to moderate bleeding tendencies, usually manifest only after surgery or trauma. Wound dehiscence is a problem in some. Some have a tendency for thrombosis. The abnormal proteins have a fascinating array of defects. For instance, several of the abnormal fibrinogens are poor substrates for thrombin, so that the fibrinopeptides are released slowly. Other abnormal fibrinogens, once converted to fibrin monomer by thrombin, display impaired aggregation into a fibrin gel. The diagnosis of these disorders should be suspected when delayed or poorly formed fibrin endpoints are observed in PT, APTT, and thrombin time assays. The fibrinogen level, measured immunologically or chemically, is normal to low normal. The majority of patients do not require treatment. In instances of bleeding or before surgical procedures on a patient known to have a propensity to bleed, replacement therapy in the form of cryoprecipitate should be given to attain a plasma fibrinogen level of 100 to 150 mg per deciliter. Because the half-life of fibrinogen is 4 days, such infusions need to be given only every several days. There are no absolute guidelines for how long therapy must be continued, but infusions of cryoprecipitate should be administered for 2 days after bleeding stops.

DEFICIENCY OF FACTOR XIII. Bleeding symptoms in Factor XIII deficiency are in individuals with less than 1 to 2% of normal plasma Factor XIII activity. The symptomatic deficiency state is an autosomal recessive trait. The bleeding diathesis is commonly apparent at birth as umbilical stump hemorrhage and continues throughout life. Wounds ooze slowly for days and heal poorly with scar formation. Intracranial hemorrhage after inapparent or only minor trauma is common. Males tend to be sterile, and women with the disorder have a high incidence of fetal loss unless they receive replacement therapy during pregnancy. Thrombin formation or conversion of fibrinogen to fibrin is not impaired. Consequently, the PT and APTT are normal. Platelet function tests are also normal. The laboratory diagnosis consists of demonstrating that a fibrin clot, made by recalcification of the patient's plasma, dissolves overnight at room temperature in 6M urea or 1% monochloroacetic acid. Fibrin clots formed in the presence of greater than 1 to 2% of the normal concentration of Factor XIII remain intact indefinitely in these solvents.

Treatment consists of giving fresh-frozen plasma. Correction of the plasma concentration of Factor XIII to 5 to 10% of normal provides normal hemostasis. The half-life of Factor XIII is approximately 12 days, and thus prophylactic replacement therapy is feasible. Because central nervous system hemorrhage is a major risk, Factor XIII–deficient patients are commonly given 5 to 10 ml per kilogram of fresh-frozen plasma every 3 weeks. Extra plasma should be given in preparation for surgery or after head trauma. Development of inhibitory antibody to Factor XIII as a consequence of transfusion therapy is apparently rare.

DEFICIENCY OF α_2-ANTIPLASMIN. Congenital homozygous deficiency of α_2-antiplasmin is associated with a severe, hemophilia-like bleeding tendency. Heterozygous family members with plasma concentrations of the inhibitor 50% of normal have a mild bleeding tendency characterized by postoperative bleeding, excessive bleeding after tooth extraction, and easy bruising after trauma. Levels of α_2-antiplasmin can be quantified with an activity assay. Patients with severe homozygous deficiency have fewer bleeding episodes when treated chronically with tranexamic acid. Heterozygotes would probably also benefit from treatment with tranexamic acid or EACA when symptomatic or when their antiplasmin level is depleted by stresses such as major surgery.

DEFICIENCY OF PLASMINOGEN ACTIVATOR INHIBITOR-1. Congenital deficiency of this protein was recently shown to result in a bleeding tendency.

Fay WP, Shapiro AD, Shih JL, et al.: Brief report: Complete deficiency of plasminogen-activator inhibitor type 1 due to a frameshift mutation. N Engl J Med 327:1729, 1992.
Leebeek FWG, Stibbe J, Knot EAR, et al.: Mild haemostatic problems associated with congenital heterozygous alpha-2-antiplasmin deficiency. Thromb Haemost 59:96, 1988. *Update on hemorrhagic diathesis associated with 50% deficiency state.*
Lijnen HR, Collen D: Molecular and cellular basis of fibrinolysis. *In* Hoffman R, Benz EJ Jr, Shattil SJ, et al. (eds.): Hematology: Basic Principles and Practice. 2nd ed. New York, Churchill Livingstone, 1995, p. 1588.
Martinez J: Quantitative and qualitative disorders of fibrinogen. *In* Hoffman R, Benz EJ Jr, Shattil SJ, et al. (eds.): Hematology: Basic Principles and Practice. 2nd ed. New York, Churchill Livingstone, 1995, p. 1703.

Inherited Tendencies Toward Thrombosis

There has been considerable recent progress in the biochemical definition of hypercoagulability. Quantitative or functional deficiencies of four plasma proteins—protein C, protein S, antithrombin III, and Factor V—are known to be associated with a tendency toward thrombosis in affected families. Abnormalities of homocysteine metabolism have been shown to be associated with arterial thrombosis (see Ch. 180). Currently, ongoing "knock-outs" of genes for plasminogen and plasminogen activators in transgenic mice should provide insight into whether defects of any of these proteins are associated with thrombosis in humans.

APPROACH TO THE PATIENT WITH A SUSPECTED THROMBOTIC TENDENCY. The spectrum of syndromes associated with a thrombotic diathesis is only now being appreciated. In general, the following patients should be evaluated: those with family histories of thrombosis, those with thrombosis in unusual sites such as the portal vein or sagittal sinus, and those less than 40 years old. The evaluation should include a consideration of risk factors such as obesity, prolonged immobilization, and injury to or abnormalities of vessels. Secondary causes of hypercoagulability such as myeloproliferative syndrome, paroxysmal nocturnal hemoglobinuria, malignancy, and lupus anticoagulant should be excluded. It has been estimated that of patients with otherwise unexplained thrombosis, 1 to 2% have deficiency of antithrombin III, 2 to 5% have deficiency of protein C, 2 to 5% have deficiency of protein S, and 20 to 50% have abnormal Factor V that resists inactivation by APC. Evaluation of individuals with a possible inherited thrombotic diathesis should include an activity assay of antithrombin III (readily available), activity and immunologic assays of protein C and immunoassay of protein S (available in coagulation reference laboratories), and a screening assay for APC resistance (under development for widespread use). Evaluations of families should search for segregation of two traits in a single individual inasmuch as carriers of two gene defects have an increased risk for thrombosis compared with carriers of a single defect. Patients should be registered in anticipation that more informative tests will become available in the future.

DEFICIENCY OF PROTEIN C. Two syndromes of hereditary protein C deficiency have been described: (1) heterozygous deficiency, in which half-normal concentrations of protein C are associated with an increased risk of venous thromboembolism, and (2) homozygous deficiency, in which total lack (<1% of normal) of protein C is associated with neonatal purpura fulminans (ischemic necrosis of skin and digits) and massive venous thrombosis. Homozygous deficiency is invariably associated with severe problems. Not all individuals with heterozygous deficiency, however, have thrombosis. In families in which there is thrombosis, some family members with 50% levels are asymptomatic; that is, the phenotype displays autosomal dominance with incomplete penetrance. In some kindreds ascertained because of infants with homozygous defi-

ciency, obligate heterozygotes with deficiency do not seem at risk for thrombosis at all. This phenotypic heterogeneity is due partly to co-inheritance of the Factor V Leiden mutation as described below.

The diagnosis of protein C deficiency is usually based on decreased amounts of antigen in plasma. For patients on long-term therapy with warfarin, other vitamin K–dependent proteins, such as Factor X and II, are also measured with an immunoassay to correct for the 35 to 50% drop in the level of circulating vitamin K–dependent proteins caused by undercarboxylation. Dysfunctional protein C can be detected with activity assays.

Because not everyone with heterozygous protein C deficiency has thrombosis, long-term anticoagulation should be reserved for individuals who have had a thrombotic episode or have other risk factors. Asymptomatic family members should be counseled that they are at greater risk for thrombosis than normal and advised about the dangers of prolonged immobilization of limbs, obesity, and smoking. Protein C levels fall more quickly than the vitamin K–dependent procoagulant factors after a large "loading dose" of warfarin. When warfarin is started on a patient with heterozygous deficiency, therefore, the anticoagulant effect should be achieved at a leisurely pace by daily administration of the predicted maintenance dose. It is preferable to begin warfarin while the patient is being treated with heparin. However, one should be aware that heparin induces thrombocytopenia and thrombosis in some patients, especially those who have received it for more than 10 days.

Infants with homozygous protein C deficiency respond acutely to administration of plasma or prothrombin complex concentrate, which is rich in protein C. Oral anticoagulants can be used to decrease the frequency of thrombotic events.

DEFICIENCY OF PROTEIN S. Decreased levels of plasma protein S antigen or activity are associated with venous thrombosis. Correlation between antigen and anticoagulant activity is poor because a fraction of protein S in plasma is complexed with C4b-binding protein and only the fraction of protein S that is free has anticoagulant activity. The tendency toward thrombosis is inherited as an autosomal dominant trait with incomplete penetrance, and affected individuals tend to have levels of protein S which are 50% of normal; that is, they are heterozygous for the deficiency. The incidence of symptomatic heterozygous protein S deficiency is probably the same as the incidence of symptomatic protein C deficiency. Pending further information about this syndrome, it seems reasonable to approach and treat heterozygous protein S deficiency using the guidelines described above for heterozygous protein C deficiency.

DEFICIENCY OF ANTITHROMBIN III. The average concentration of the antithrombin III in deficient patients is approximately 50% of normal. The most frequent manifestation of thromboembolism is lower-extremity thrombophlebitis, often bilateral and recurrent and often with pulmonary embolism. Patients may develop venous insufficiency and chronic leg ulcers. Upper extremity thrombophlebitis and mesenteric vein thrombosis are less common. Rare patients may develop retinal or cerebral vein thrombosis, thrombosis of the renal vein or inferior vena cava, Budd-Chiari syndrome, priapism, or widespread clotting and defibrination syndrome. The cumulative incidences of thromboembolism are estimated to be 15% by age 19, 50% by age 29, and 85% in individuals over 40. Complete—that is, homozygous—lack of the antithrombin III has not been described. Patients homozygous for a dysfunctional antithrombin, however, have been reported.

Antithrombin III deficiency can be ascertained by an activity assay in which diluted plasma and heparin are mixed with a known concentration of thrombin and the amount of uninhibited thrombin is quantified with a chromogenic substrate. Ongoing thrombosis and heparin therapy both lower the concentration of plasma antithrombin III. Therefore, the diagnosis of antithrombin III deficiency is best made after the patient has recovered from a thrombotic event.

A patient with acute thrombosis should be treated with heparin. Because of depletion of antithrombin III, the level of antithrombin III may become so low that the patient is resistant to heparin. In this case, a source of antithrombin III should be infused, either in the form of fresh-frozen plasma or antithrombin III concentrate. The half-life of antithrombin III is 16 to 24 hours. Administration of warfarin should be started promptly, and the patient probably should receive warfarin indefinitely.

Prophylactic use of anticoagulants should be considered in view of the spontaneous and unpredictable occurrence of thromboembolism with the potential for a fatal outcome. At the very least, affected individuals should be counseled about the risks of the disorder. Pregnancies should be managed in high-risk clinics prepared to cope with the difficult questions of how, when, or whether anticoagulants should be administered during the pregnancy.

APC RESISTANCE. The most common of the described inherited predispositions to thrombosis is the recently characterized Leiden mutation of Factor V. This mutation renders Factor V resistant to inactivation by APC and accounts for most cases of APC resistance. APC resistance is ascertained by prolongation of an APTT done in the presence of APC. If the APTT is prolonged normally three- to four-fold when APC is added, the presence of 50% Factor V Leiden causes the prolongation to be only about two-fold. Homozygous Factor V Leiden is associated with a 1- to 1.5-fold prolongation. Diagnosis of the Leiden mutation can be made by polymerase chain reaction amplification of Factor V genes followed by restriction fragment analysis.

The prevalence of the Leiden allele in Northern European populations is approximately 2%. The prevalence of mutations causing protein C deficiency in the same population is approximately 0.4%. The likelihood of a history of thrombosis in individuals with heterozygous and homozygous Factor V Leiden has been estimated at 13% and 50%, respectively, compared with 0.5% in normals. When heterozygous protein C deficiency is present, the likelihood rises to 73% and 90%, respectively, in the Factor V Leiden heterozygotes and homozygotes, compared with 31% in protein C–deficient individuals with normal Factor V. Other genetic risk factors likely will be identified that interact with Factor V Leiden or protein C deficiency and account for thrombosis in individuals in whom the two risk factors do not segregate.

Long-term anticoagulation should be considered for APC-resistant individuals who have had a thrombotic episode or have other risk factors. Asymptomatic family members should be counseled that they are at greater risk for thrombosis than normal and advised about the dangers of surgery, pregnancy, and prolonged immobilization. These guidelines need to be reviewed and updated as more kindreds and populations are studied.

Bauer KA: Hypercoagulable states. In Hoffman R, Benz EJ Jr, Shattil SJ, et al. (eds.): Hematology: Basic Principles and Practice. 2nd ed. New York, Churchill Livingstone, 1995, p. 1781.
Dahlbäck B: Physiological anticoagulation. Resistance to activated Protein C and venous thromboembolism. J Clin Invest 94:923, 1994. *Perspective on APC resistance by the discoverer of the phenomenon.*
Koeleman BPC, Reitsma PH, Allaart CF, et al: Activated Protein C resistance as an additional risk factor for thrombosis in Protein C–deficient families. Blood 84:1031, 1994. *Addresses the question of whether APC resistance contributes to the familial clustering of thrombosis.*

ACQUIRED ABNORMALITIES OF BLOOD COAGULATION

In a number of clinical situations, the APTT and/or PT becomes prolonged: use of heparin, use of fibrinolytic agents, vitamin K deficiency secondary to malabsorption or dietary deficiency, severe liver disease, use of coumarin anticoagulants to lower the activity of vitamin K–dependent factors, and consumption coagulopathy associated with severe illness. Rarer causes of acquired deficiencies include selective urinary loss of a coagulation factor in nephrotic syndrome; selective adsorption of a coagulation factor, especially Factor X, to amyloid; and selective neutralization or depletion of a clotting factor due to development of an antibody to the factor.

Heparin

Heparin is used commonly for its anticoagulant properties in the prevention and therapy of thromboembolism and to keep blood fluid during extracorporeal circulation. By definition, 1 unit of heparin renders 1 ml of sheep blood incoagulable. The therapeutic concentration in humans (i.e., a patient with an APTT 1.5 to 2.5 times longer than normal) is 0.2 to 0.4 unit per milliliter. The concentration typically can be achieved and attained in an adult by a loading dose of 5,000 units and infusion of 30,000 units per 24 hours.

Bleeding is the most common complication of heparin therapy. This can be minimized by (1) administration of the drug by a loading dose followed by continuous infusion rather than by repeated boluses, (2) quantification of the anticoagulant effect at regular intervals by whole blood clotting times or APTT followed by adjustment of the dose, (3) selection of patients who do not have an occult bleeding site or underlying bleeding diathesis, and (4) prohibition of aspirin and intramuscular injections. Despite this, purpura, ecchymoses, hematomas, gastrointestinal hemorrhage, hematuria, retroperitoneal bleeding, or bleeding at sites of invasive procedures may occur. Heparin is cleared from the circulation within 2 to 4 hours. Therefore, if bleeding is minimal and can be controlled by local measures, discontinuing heparin may be all that is necessary. If bleeding is severe, the effects of heparin can be counteracted by giving 1 mg of protamine sulfate for each 100 units of heparin estimated to be in the patient's circulation.

After 7 to 10 days of heparin therapy, thrombocytopenia sometimes occurs, subsiding when heparin is discontinued. Mild thrombocytopenia is likely due to a direct effect of heparin on platelets. The incidence of thrombocytopenia is higher with heparin derived from bovine lung than that from porcine gut. In some patients, the thrombocytopenia can be severe and associated with venous and/or arterial thrombosis and disseminated intravascular coagulation (DIC). In these patients the thrombocytopenia is probably immunologically mediated. It is important to be alert for such a patient, because one's tendency is to treat the thrombosis by increasing the dose of heparin, only to make the situation worse. Heparin therefore should be discontinued if the platelet count drops precipitously. The best defense against platelet problems is prophylactic, that is, to initiate coumarin therapy early so that a stable anticoagulant effect is achieved during the first week of heparin therapy.

Low molecular weight heparin holds the promise of providing anticoagulant activity with more favorable pharmacokinetics and fewer bleeding problems. Heparin congeners (heparinoids) may be a therapeutic option in the future for patients with heparin-induced thrombocytopenia.

Several patients with neoplastic plasma cell disorders have presented with clinical bleeding due to a circulating heparin-like proteoglycan that requires antithrombin III for its function and can be neutralized by protamine sulfate.

Hirsh J: Heparin. N Engl J Med 324:1565, 1991.

Therapeutic Fibrinolysis (Thrombolysis)

Intravenous administration of streptokinase, urokinase, or TPA is accepted useful therapy for deep vein thrombosis, pulmonary embolism, acute myocardial infarction, and peripheral arterial thromboembolism. These agents re-establish patency of vessels more quickly than heparin. The dosage and method of administration of the agents are specific for the different conditions, and in some instances the agent is administered by selective catheterization of the involved vessel.

In the case of streptokinase or urokinase administered systemically, therapeutic effectiveness requires that systemic fibrinolysis be achieved—that the patients develop iatrogenic primary fibrinolysis. Prolongation of the thrombin time to twice normal is often taken as evidence that the desired effect has been achieved. Such patients also have decreased plasma fibrinogen, plasminogen, and α_2-antiplasmin. In the case of streptokinase administered locally or TPA administered systemically or locally, thrombi can be lysed with variable and sometimes minimal evidence of systemic fibrinolysis.

If the level of plasminogen falls to zero, the patient is relatively resistant to further infusion of fibrinolytic agents. At that point, or at the end of the planned infusion, there is hypercoagulability, and anticoagulation with heparin should be carried out.

The main complication of fibrinolytic therapy is hemorrhage, usually in the form of continuous slow oozing at sites of invasive procedures. If a pressure dressing does not control this bleeding, administration of the agent can be discontinued with the anticipation that fibrinolytic activity will subside within a few hours. Fresh-frozen plasma can be given if the bleeding is severe.

Bell WR: Fibrinolytic therapy: Indications and management. In Hoffman R, Benz EJ Jr, Shattil SJ, et al. (eds.): Hematology: Basic Principles and Practice. 2nd ed. New York, Churchill Livingstone, 1995, p. 1814.

Vitamin K Deficiency and Coumarin Anticoagulants

METABOLISM AND FUNCTION OF VITAMIN K. Vitamin K is required for post-translational gamma-carboxylation of specific glutamyl residues in Factors VII, IX, X, and II, proteins C and S, and certain other proteins (e.g., osteocalcin, which constitutes 1% of the protein in bone). In vitamin K–deficient states, immunologic testing shows that levels of the vitamin K–dependent plasma proteins are nearly normal; however, the functions to these proteins in reactions and assays (e.g., the PT) that require a phospholipid surface are severely impaired. As vitamin K deficiency develops, the activities of Factor VII and protein C decrease rapidly, followed by diminished activities of Factors IX, X, and II.

Body stores of vitamin K are limited. A normal diet containing green, leafy vegetables provides 300 to 500 μg of vitamin K, more than enough to meet the adult daily requirement of 1 μg per kilogram of body weight. In addition, vitamin K synthesized by normal gastrointestinal bacterial flora contributes to meeting the daily requirement. Vitamin K is a fat-soluble vitamin, and solubilization of fat must occur before vitamin K can be absorbed (see Ch. 103). Hence, vitamin K deficiency may occur in bile salt–deficient states, in all malabsorption disorders, or with an inadequate dietary intake combined with gastrointestinal sterilization by orally administered antibiotics. Vitamin K occurs naturally in two forms, vitamin K_1 (phylloquinone) and vitamin K_2 (menaquinone), both of which require lipid for absorption. A synthetic water-soluble form, vitamin K_3 (menadione), is commercially available. Despite its ready absorption from intestine, menadione must be converted to vitamin K_2 by the liver and therefore is not as rapidly effective as vitamin K_1 in promoting the gamma-carboxylation reaction.

VITAMIN K DEFICIENCY OF THE NEWBORN. At birth, vitamin K levels are low, and production of vitamin K by intestinal bacteria is insufficient to meet an infant's requirements for production of normally functioning coagulation factors. The vitamin K–deficient state lasts for 3 to 5 days and may be the reason why Israelites did not circumcise their babies until the eighth day (Leviticus 12:3). Cow's milk contains some vitamin K, but human milk contains essentially none (1 to 2 μg per liter). Unless vitamin K is given, the physiologic state of neonatal hypoprothrombinemia can lead to hemorrhagic disease of the newborn in the following high-risk groups: premature infants; breast-fed infants; infants of mothers who are receiving vitamin K antagonists, especially hydantoin anticonvulsants; and infants with malabsorption. If the PT is prolonged to an INR of 2.5 to 3.5, it is common to encounter bleeding from the umbilicus, ecchymoses and hematomas, hematuria, and, most importantly, intracranial hemorrhage. Prophylactic intramuscular administration of a 1-mg dose of vitamin K_1 at delivery virtually eliminates the risk of subsequent hemorrhage. Excessive administration (5 mg or more) of vitamin K_3 may cause hemolytic anemia and kernicterus in the newborn and should be avoided.

MALABSORPTION SYNDROMES. Malabsorptive states (see Ch. 103) with impaired absorption of fat, such as adult celiac disease, regional enteritis, use of cholestyramine or neomycin, or deficient intraluminal bile salts (obstruction of biliary ducts, cholestatic liver disease), are often associated with vitamin K deficiency. Similarly, various chronic diarrheas can cause vitamin K deficiency, presumably due to decreased transit time and a relative malabsorption of fats. The hallmark of vitamin K deficiency is a prolonged PT. If the INR is greater than 2.5, the patient is likely to have ecchymoses, gingival bleeding, hematomas, hematuria, and/or melena. Daily oral administration of vitamin K_1 in supraphysiologic doses (2 to 10 mg) prevents the deficiency and should be routine in patients with malabsorption of fat. The bleeding tendency, once developed, is easily corrected by giving 10 to 25 mg of vitamin K_1 intramuscularly. In cases in which the bleeding diathesis is so severe that intramuscular injections are contraindicated, 10 to 20 mg of vitamin K_1 may be infused intravenously. It should be infused slowly at a rate of 1 mg per minute because the vehicle in which the vitamin is dissolved can cause an adverse reaction. If this dose does not correct the PT, additional vitamin K is unlikely to have any effect.

DEBILITATED PATIENTS WHO MAY BE RECEIVING ANTIBIOTICS. Patients who are without oral intake for more than several days and on antibiotics should be given parenteral vitamin K_1 at a dose of 150 μg per day because they are likely to become vitamin K deficient. Patients with uremia or malignancy are at special risk and may become vitamin K deficient on the basis of poor oral intake alone.

Some third-generation cephalosporins have a hypoprothrombinemic effect greater than would be expected from elimination of bowel flora. It has been suggested that the N-methyl-thiotetrazole side chain shared by cefamandole, moxalactam, and cefoperazone is cleaved from the antibiotic and interferes with the action of vitamin K, especially in patients who are borderline deficient in vitamin K.

COUMARIN ANTICOAGULANTS. Warfarin and the other coumarin anticoagulants competitively inhibit the effects of vitamin K in the post-translational gamma-carboxylation of vitamin K–dependent plasma proteins. Coumarin anticoagulants are administered for prevention of recurrent thromboembolism in patients who have experienced deep vein thrombosis and pulmonary embolism or myocardial infarction. Patients should be reliable, able to be supervised, and without known potential foci of hemorrhage in the central nervous, gastrointestinal, or genitourinary systems.

The art of administration of warfarin involves balancing drug intake against vitamin K intake to prolong the PT into the therapeutic range. Results of PT's of patients on coumarin anticoagulants are best reported as the INR. The purpose of the INR is to standardize the PT so that results are consistent no matter what reagent, instrument, or laboratory is used. The INR is derived by the formula:

$$INR = (\text{patient's PT/normal PT})^{ISI}$$

The ISI (International Sensitivity Index) depends on the type of reagent and is derived in comparison to a World Health Organization standard with an ISI of 1.0. The more sensitive the reagent is to the effect of coumarin anticoagulation, the lower the ISI. The current trend is to change to more sensitive reagents. Thus, a sample with a therapeutic INR of 2.0 to 3.0 might clot in 18 seconds using a traditional reagent and 26 seconds using a more sensitive reagent, even though the control plasma using both reagents clots in 12 seconds. Someone experienced in adjusting coumarin doses according to the raw clotting time of the old test would make inappropriate decisions without the frame of reference provided by the INR.

An adult receiving a normal diet usually needs 5 to 10 mg of warfarin per day to achieve the desired INR. Upon initiation of therapy, the activities of the vitamin K–dependent proteins with the most rapid half-lives are lost first. Factor VII and protein C fall in the first 24 hours, followed by Factors IX, X, and II over the next 72 hours. Thus, a minimum of 3 to 4 days is required before a patient is therapeutically anticoagulated. The dose then can be altered to maintain the PT in the therapeutic range.

The syndrome of coumarin-induced skin necrosis recapitulates the syndrome of homozygous protein C deficiency. Upon initiation of warfarin therapy, the plasma concentration of protein C, which has a half-life of 6 hours, falls more quickly than the concentrations of Factors II, IX, and X, thus causing a hypercoagulable state. Therefore, therapy should be initiated with the predicted maintenance dose (rather than a "loading dose"), preferably while the patient is receiving heparin.

Once the INR is stabilized, it needs to be checked only every 3 to 4 weeks if the patient is on a stable diet and in usual health. The therapeutic dose of warfarin may change dramatically if the diet is changed or if changes are made in the intake of one of the many drugs that enhance or depress the effect of warfarin (Table 153–2). Patients should wear a bracelet or neck tag stating that they are receiving an oral anticoagulant. They should not take aspirin in any of its forms.

It is not uncommon for patients to experience slight gingival bleeding, purpura with minimal trauma, or trace hematuria while receiving anticoagulants in the therapeutic range. These symptoms become more marked when the patient is over-anticoagulated, and the patient is at risk for severe gastrointestinal or genitourinary hemorrhage, bleeding, or hematoma formation after trauma, and intracranial bleeding. If the INR is increased but increased bleeding is not a clinical problem, warfarin, which has a half-life of 35 hours, can be omitted until the desired INR is obtained. When over-anticoagulation results in clinically significant bleeding, the physician can give fresh-frozen plasma, 10 to 20 ml per kilogram, as a source of normal vitamin K–dependent proteins and/or give vitamin K, depending on the immediacy of the problem and whether continuation of warfarin is necessary. Inasmuch as volume overload should not be a problem in a bleeding patient, there is no role for prothrombin complex concentrate. Oral or intramuscular vitamin K_1, 5 to 25 mg, should correct the PT within 8 to 24 hours. Slow intravenous infusion of vitamin K_1, 20 to 40 mg, should correct the PT in 4 to 6 hours. Administration of more than 5 mg of vitamin K makes the

TABLE 153–2. DRUGS AND CONDITIONS THAT INFLUENCE RESPONSE TO WARFARIN

Increased Resistance to Warfarin

Hereditary warfarin resistance	Increased warfarin metabolism
Increase in dietary vitamin K	Barbiturates
Reduced drug absorption	Primidone
Malabsorption syndrome	Carbamazepine
Liquid paraffin laxatives	Ethchlorvynol
Cholestyramine resin	Glutethimide
Magnesium trisilicate	Meprobamate
	Griseofulvin
	Rifampin
	Nafcillin

Increased Sensitivity to Warfarin

Vitamin K deficiency	Synergism with warfarin
Malabsorption syndrome	Vitamin E
Wide-spectrum antibiotics	Anabolic steroids
Liquid paraffin	Danazol
Clofibrate	Blocking of warfarin metabolism
Displacement of albumin binding	Phenytoin sodium
Phenylbutazone	Chloramphenicol
Aspirin	Clofibrate
Indomethacin	Tricyclic antidepressants
Sulindac	Erythromycin
Mefenamic acid	Cimetidine
Tolmetin	Sulfamethoxazole-trimethoprim
Ibuprofen	Sulfinpyrazone
Naproxen	Unknown mechanism
Fenoprofen	Quinine
Phenytoin sodium	Quinidine
Oral hypoglycemic agents	Phenothiazine
Nalidixic acid	Disulfiram
Estrogen	Sulfisoxazole
Miconazole	Amiodarone

Adapted with permission from Peterson CE, Kwaan HC: Current concepts of warfarin therapy. Arch Intern Med 146:581, 1986. Copyright 1986, American Medical Association.

patient warfarin resistant and necessitates a round of re-anticoagulation. Therefore, the best strategy for the patient who needs continued anticoagulation is to give plasma and small doses (1 to 2 mg) of vitamin K while closely monitoring the INR and clinical state.

Patients occasionally present with bleeding complications after ingestion of a coumarin compound, either surreptitiously or as a suicide attempt. Patients who take coumarins surreptitiously are usually depressed and receive gain from medical attention. They may belong to a health profession. The coumarin compounds in rat poisons are much more powerful than warfarin and can cause extreme resistance to vitamin K for weeks and even months.

Coumarin anticoagulants should not be given from the sixth to the twelfth week of gestation owing to the high likelihood that characteristic facial and skeletal malformation, the so-called coumarin embryopathy, will be induced. Use of coumarin drugs in the second and third trimesters may be associated with an increased incidence of central nervous system malformations, presumed to be due to sporadic intracranial hemorrhages. If anticoagulation is needed during pregnancy, one approach is to switch to subcutaneous heparin between the sixth and twelfth week and after the thirty-eighth week.

Dalen JE, Hirsh J (eds): Third ACCP Consensus Conference on Antithrombotic Therapy. Chest 102:303S, 1992. *Situation-by-situation analyses of risk-benefits, cost-benefits, and rationale for recommended therapy. Has been reprinted for wide distribution.*
Furie B: Oral anticoagulant therapy. *In* Hoffman R, Benz EJ Jr, Shattil SJ, et al. (eds.): Hematology: Basic Principles and Practice. 2nd ed. New York, Churchill Livingstone, 1995, p. 1795.
Furie BC, Furie B: Vitamin K: Metabolism and disorders. *In* Hoffman R, Benz EJ Jr, Shattil SJ, et al. (eds.): Hematology: Basic Principles and Practice. 2nd ed. New York, Churchill Livingstone, 1995, p. 1737.

Liver Disease

The liver is the major site of synthesis of fibrinogen, plasminogen, the vitamin K–dependent proteins, antithrombin III, and most other plasma proteins. The mechanisms by which steady-state concentrations of these proteins in plasma are regulated are obscure. As part of the "acute-phase reaction" in response to interleukin-1, interleukin-6, and tumor necrosis factor, the synthesis of many of plasma proteins, especially fibrinogen, increases at the expense of albumin synthesis. The normal liver seems to have a considerable reserve for production of fibrinogen but seems to be working at nearly maximum capacity in the synthesis of vitamin K–dependent proteins.

Patients with liver diseases occasionally develop petechiae, ecchymoses, prolonged bleeding from venipunctures, and/or gastrointestinal hemorrhage. Clinically significant bleeding may occur with biopsies and surgery. The causes of these problems are diverse.

In patients with alcoholic liver disease, bleeding can be secondary to dietary vitamin K deficiency and responds promptly to oral vitamin K. With more advanced disease, patients may become vitamin K deficient on the basis of fat malabsorption as well as poor nutrition, and parenteral vitamin K must be given. The synthesis of vitamin K–dependent factors becomes impaired as hepatocytes are lost, rendering the patient resistant to parenteral vitamin K. A poor prognosis is associated with a prolonged PT (INR > 2.0) that does not become corrected with intravenous vitamin K. If the patient no longer responds to parenteral vitamin K, abnormal bleeding or correction of the PT prior to invasive procedures requires transfusions of fresh-frozen plasma. In fulminant hepatocellular disease, plasma fibrinogen levels can fall low enough to be considered the cause of bleeding; in such cases, both fresh-frozen plasma and cryoprecipitate should be given.

Acquired dysfibrinogenemia, manifested by abnormal fibrin polymerization, has been observed in a number of patients having hepatic disease such as alcoholic cirrhosis, postnecrotic cirrhosis of unknown cause, drug-induced hepatic failure, and hepatoma. The fibrinogen in these patients has an increased content of sialic acid. The clotting of these fibrinogens by thrombin is delayed in proportion to the increase of sialic acid. If the liver disease improves, the defect may disappear.

Patients with liver disease commonly have increased fibrinolysis because of an inability to maintain normal levels of α_2-antiplasmin and/or decreased hepatic clearance of plasminogen activators. Enhanced fibrinolysis, however, is rarely the primary cause of bleeding. Occasionally, chronic, smoldering DIC may develop so that the platelet count is decreased and levels of several coagulation factors fall because of consumption. These patients do not require therapy unless they exhibit clinically significant bleeding, in which case the approach should be the same as for patients with other causes of DIC (see below). Patients in whom Leveen peritoneovenous shunts have been placed and women with acute fatty liver of pregnancy and marked deficiency of antithrombin III (< 25% of normal) are at particular risk to develop DIC.

Efforts should be made to normalize the PT, fibrinogen concentration, and platelet count in patients with liver disease prior to surgery, biopsies, or other invasive procedures. Prothrombin complex concentrates are not recommended for prophylaxis in patients in whom the PT will not be corrected with parenteral vitamin K because such patients are likely to be deficient in plasma antithrombin III, to have decreased hepatic clearance of activated clotting factors, and therefore to be at risk for thromboembolism. Platelet concentrates should be given if the platelet count is less than 75,000 per microliter. If hypersplenism is the cause of the thrombocytopenia, however, it may be difficult to achieve a satisfactory platelet count.

Martinez J, Barsigian C: Coagulopathy of liver failure and vitamin K deficiency. *In* Loscalzo J, Schafer AI (eds.): Thrombosis and Hemorrhage. Boston, Blackwell Scientific, 1994, p. 945.

Renal Disease

Patients with uremia occasionally develop purpura, mucous membrane bleeding, gastrointestinal hemorrhage, and prolonged bleeding from venous and arterial needle puncture sites. Such patients usually have a long bleeding time. The pathogenesis of the bleeding tendency is complex. The platelet count may be low. More importantly, platelet function is abnormal owing to accumulation of a dialyzable substance in the circulation (see Ch. 152). Anemia contributes to platelet dysfunction *in vivo* because the stirring action of red cells causes a large increase in the diffusivity of platelets and allows platelets to be transported efficiently to areas where the vessel wall is injured. Erythropoietin therapy, therefore, normalizes the bleeding time. Daily infusion of cryoprecipitate has been useful in correcting the bleeding tendency in uremia. Although uncertain, the correction may be related to the high-molecular-weight von Willebrand factor multimers contained in cryoprecipitate. Desmopressin, which is effective in raising the plasma level of von Willebrand factor in patients with von Willebrand disease (see above), temporarily corrects the bleeding time in patients with uremia. Daily intravenous administration of conjugated estrogens may also correct the bleeding time over a period of days. Thus, a number of therapeutic maneuvers can be tried in a symptomatic uremic patient: dialysis to restore platelet function; transfusion to normalize red cell and platelet number; and administration of cryoprecipitate, desmopressin, or conjugated estrogen.

Coagulation factors, especially vitamin K–dependent factors and Factor V, tend to be at low concentration in chronic renal disease, although not to levels that should cause bleeding. Some of these deficiencies probably result from hepatic insufficiency or from vitamin K deficiency secondary to oral antibiotic therapy, malabsorption caused by uremic enteritis, and diminished dietary intake. Very low plasma Factor IX levels (10% of normal) have been observed in patients with severe nephrotic syndrome and preferential loss of Factor IX into the urine. Subclinical DIC occasionally occurs in chronic renal disease, as evidenced by elevated amounts of fibrin degradation products in serum and urine. It has been suggested that loss of antithrombin III in nephrotic syndrome may cause renal vein thrombosis. There are no clear guidelines as to when and how to treat such deficiencies. If the PT is long or the Factor IX level is low in a patient who is bleeding, fresh-frozen plasma is the replacement product of choice, although it may be difficult to give enough to someone who cannot compensate for the large volume.

Van Geet C, Hauglustaine D, Verresen L, et al.: Haemostatic effects of recombinant human erythropoietin in chronic hemodialysis patients. Thromb Haemost 61:117, 1989. *Documents favorable effect of erythropoietin on the bleeding time.*

Factor VIII Inhibitors

An endogenously produced anticoagulant, usually referred to as a circulating anticoagulant or a circulating inhibitor, is an antibody that interacts with a clotting factor in a manner that neutralizes the functional activity of the factor. Production of such an antibody is pathologic and often results in hemorrhage. Factor VIII inhibitors are commonly observed in hemophilia A (Factor VIII deficiency) but are rare in nonhemophilic patients. Conditions in which sporadic Factor VIII inhibitors occur include the postpartum state, diseases of immunologic dysfunction, and old age. The sporadic inhibitors induce a hemophilia-like state (i.e., a significant bleeding diathesis) but are unlike the inhibitors of hemophilic patients in several ways. They tend to be of low titer ($<$ 1 to 20 Bethesda units) and to bind Factor VIII weakly. Titers often drop when patients are treated with cyclophosphamide (Cytoxan), 1 gram intravenously, and prednisone, 80 mg per day to be tapered once an effect is seen. Such a therapeutic response is rare in patients with hemophilia and an inhibitor. Acute bleeding episodes can be managed with variable success by continuous infusion of Factor VIII concentrate or cryoprecipitate.

When a Factor VIII inhibitor is present, the PT is normal but the APTT is prolonged. If the patient's plasma is incubated for several hours with an equal quantity of normal plasma, the APTT of the mixture should be prolonged. The Factor VIII level in the patient's plasma and in the mixture of patient's plasma and normal plasma should be low no matter what dilutions are tested, whereas the Factor IX level should be normal. These characteristics distinguish Factor VIII inhibitors from the antiphospholipid inhibitors associated with lupus erythematosus (lupus-type inhibitors). A lupus-type inhibitor may cause prolongation of the PT, especially when the test is done with diluted thromboplastin; does not require an incubation period to express inhibitory activity in mixtures of patient's and normal plasma; and may interfere with the assays for both Factors VIII and IX when the patient's plasma is tested at a 1:10 dilution but not when the patient's plasma is tested at a 1:200 or 1:500 dilution. The implications of having a Factor VIII inhibitor versus a lupus-type inhibitor are very different, and the physician and laboratory must be sure that the correct diagnosis is made, even though no single test can make the distinction.

Lupus-type Inhibitors

Patients with systemic lupus erythematosus sometimes develop a circulating anticoagulant unrelated to the severity or duration of disease. A similar inhibitor is found in patients who do not have lupus. Patients who have the lupus-type inhibitor also may have anticardi-

olipin antibodies. The lupus-type inhibitor and the anticardiolipin are members of a cross-reacting family of antibodies that react with phospholipids bound to various plasma proteins. Only rarely, as when the inhibitor is associated with thrombocytopenia, platelet dysfunction, and/or acquired Factor II deficiency, is there clinically significant bleeding. Instead, patients with the lupus-type inhibitor are at increased risk to have recurrent thromboembolic events. Thrombosis can involve both veins and arteries. There is probably accelerated atherosclerosis. Women with the inhibitor have a greatly increased incidence of spontaneous abortion. Some patients have neurologic abnormalities that may be due to cerebral thrombosis or myelitis or both. In short, the problems associated with a lupus-type inhibitor can be devastating.

Inhibition of clotting tests is thought to be a consequence of binding of the inhibitor to the acidic phospholipids used in the PT and APTT. The prolongations of both assays can be impressive. Presumably, platelet membranes, rather than phospholipid micelles, provide the surface for activation of Factors X and II, thus accounting for the fact that clinically significant bleeding does not occur. The pathogenesis of the thrombotic diathesis associated with lupus-type inhibitors is unknown. A reasonable hypothesis is that affected individuals have antibodies that react in a noxious fashion with endothelial cells, for example, to bind to heparan sulfate proteoglycan, block prostacyclin production, or inhibit the cofactor activity of thrombomodulin in the protein C–protein S pathway.

The laboratory evaluation should ensure that blocking antibodies to Factor VIII or IX are not present and that the concentration of Factor II is not low. Without knowledge of the pathogenesis of the thromboembolism, no rational approach to treatment is possible. Anticoagulants should be tried but may not be effective. It also is reasonable to try immunosuppressive therapy or plasmapheresis. Administration of corticosteroids and low-dose aspirin during pregnancy had favorable laboratory and clinical effects in a group of women with the inhibitor and histories of spontaneous abortion.

Love PE, Santoro SA: Antiphospholipid antibodies: Anticardiolipin and the lupus anticoagulant in systemic lupus erythematosus (SLE) and non-SLE disorders. Ann Intern Med 112:682, 1990. Vianna JL, Khamashta MA, Ordi-Rosj, et al.: Comparison of the primary and secondary antiphospholipid syndrome: A European multicenter study of 114 patients. Am J Med 96:3, 1994. *Illustrate well the dilemmas of lupus-type inhibitors.*
Santoro SA: Antiphospholipid antibodies and thrombotic predisposition: Underlying pathogenetic mechanisms. Blood 83:2389, 1994. Roubey RAS: Autoantibodies to phospholipid-binding plasma proteins: A new view of lupus anticoagulants and other "antiphospholipid" autoantibodies. Blood 84:2854, 1994. *Review mechanisms and speculate on possible pathophysiologic insights offered by the recently popular paradigm that "antiphospholipid" autoantibodies are part of a linked set of autoantibodies directed against various phospholipid-binding plasma proteins.*

Miscellaneous Inhibitors of Clotting Factors

Antibody inhibitors to Factor V arise frequently as part of the immune response of post-surgery patients to bovine thrombin used as a hemostatic agent or as a component of fibrin glue. Such inhibitors usually are not associated with bleeding but can raise havoc with the laboratory control of anticoagulation. Acquired inhibitors to other clotting factors and to von Willebrand factor activity have developed in isolated patients. Such inhibitors, like inhibition of Factor VIII, may be associated with bleeding.

Myeloma or macroglobulinemia may give rise to defective fibrin polymerization as a result of interference by high concentrations of immunoglobulin. If overt bleeding occurs, plasmapheresis may restore adequate hemostasis by reducing plasma protein concentration.

Bäninger H, Hardegger T, Tobler A, et al.: Fibrin glue in surgery: Frequent development of inhibitors of bovine thrombin and human factor V. Br J Haematol 85:528, 1993. *Documents that these inhibitors are common, especially in patients with multiple operations.*

Sporadic Acquired Factor Deficiency

A number of patients with amyloidosis have Factor X deficiency because of its removal from the circulation through binding of zymogen Factor X to the amyloid deposits. Patients present with mild to severe bleeding, just like individuals with the inherited form of Factor X deficiency. Replacement therapy can be given with plasma or factor concentrates. However, the *in vivo* half-life of Factor X is shortened.

Occasionally, a patient is seen with isolated factor deficiency but no evidence of a neutralizing antibody; for example, when the patient's plasma is mixed 1:1 with normal plasma, the factor level in the mixture is 50%. Such a patient with Factor II deficiency was recently studied in depth and shown to have a non-neutralizing antibody to Factor II. Administration of corticosteroids was associated with a rise in Factor II activity and cessation of bleeding, but circulating Factor II was bound to antibody. These observations suggested that non-neutralizing antibodies to Factor II cause plasma Factor II deficiency because of rapid clearance of the antigen-antibody complexes, which is slowed by corticosteroids. Demonstration of non-neutralizing antibodies requires special techniques and takes some time. Therefore, in a patient who is bleeding seriously, one may need to begin corticosteroids, possibly supplemented with fresh-frozen plasma, before the diagnosis is established.

SYNDROMES OF DISSEMINATED INTRAVASCULAR COAGULATION (DIC)

In the following discussion, DIC is divided into four clinical syndromes: (1) compensated DIC, which may be associated with thrombosis but does not result in bleeding; (2) defibrination syndrome, in which the mechanisms that localize blood coagulation are overwhelmed by release of tissue factor, leading to massive utilization and depletion of fibrinogen and platelets and resultant thrombosis and/or bleeding; (3) primary fibrinolysis, in which the mechanisms that localize fibrinolysis are overwhelmed by release of plasminogen activators, leading to bleeding; and (4) microangiopathic thrombocytopenia, in which platelet microthrombi are widespread, leading to depletion of platelets, ischemic necrosis of tissues, and microangiopathic changes in red cells. The causes of DIC syndromes are many, and there is considerable overlap among syndromes. Patients with DIC often have multiple medical problems, including bone marrow failure, liver failure, renal failure, vitamin K deficiency, and the like, which may complicate the clinical and laboratory analysis of a given patient. Much of the controversy that surrounds DIC undoubtedly stems from attempts to lump diverse conditions and patients together. Despite its oversimplicity, the following scheme is useful because the treatments of the four syndromes are quite different. For many of the diseases associated with DIC, specific descriptions of the DIC and recommendations for treatment can be found under individual disease headings elsewhere in this textbook.

COMPENSATED DIC. Patients with serious underlying diseases (trauma, infection, malignancy) usually have increased production and consumption of platelets, fibrinogen, and other coagulation proteins. Patients with traumatized or inflamed tissues manifest the acute-phase reaction and a number of plasma α_1, α_2, and β globulins, including α_2-antiplasmin and fibrinogen, increase in concentration, whereas other plasma proteins, including transferrin and albumin, decrease in concentration. Areas of trauma or inflammation demonstrate ongoing coagulation and fibrinolysis. Under such conditions, unclottable fibrin degradation products can be detected by immunoassay in serum. However, the PT is normal, the platelet count is normal or only minimally decreased, and plasma fibrinogen concentration is elevated. There is speculation that low-grade DIC is associated with microemboli and microthrombi that contribute to the organ failure commonly found in patients with severe illnesses. At this point, however, the only indication to use heparin or other anticoagulants in such patients is as prophylaxis or treatment of thrombosis in large vessels. An outstanding example of the need for anticoagulation is the Trousseau syndrome of "migratory" venous thrombosis in patients with malignant disease (see Ch. 158.1). Warfarin therapy is often ineffective in such patients, and they must instead be started on a long-term regimen of heparin therapy.

DEFIBRINATION SYNDROME. The prototype of defibrination syndrome is the rapid onset of generalized bleeding that occurs when tissue factor is released into the circulation after massive brain trauma or during amniotic fluid embolization. Laboratory tests in such patients demonstrate gross depletion of platelets and fibrinogen, elevated fibrin degradation products, prolonged PT, and variable decreases in Factors V and VIII, Factor II, and the other vitamin K–dependent factors, antithrombin III, and plasminogen. Defibrination syndrome occurs most frequently with shock, sepsis, cancer, burns, and obstetric complications. Patients with sepsis, especially due to meningococci, may develop purpura fulminans and

the Waterhouse-Friderichsen syndrome (hemorrhagic necrosis of vital organs, including the adrenals). The patient's hemostatic system must be supported while the patient is resuscitated and the underlying cause is treated. Thus, the patient should receive platelet concentrates, cryoprecipitate as a source of fibrinogen, and fresh-frozen plasma as a source of other plasma proteins, especially the antithrombins. An appropriate mix is 10 bags of cryoprecipitate for every 2 to 3 units of plasma. One's goals should be a platelet count of more than 50,000 per microliter, a fibrinogen concentration greater than 100 mg per deciliter, an INR that is 1.5 or less, and a concentration of antithrombin III which is greater than 40% of normal. The role of heparin is controversial. It is my view that unless the patient improves quickly or active bleeding cannot be controlled, heparin should be infused in low doses (10 to 15 units per kilogram per hour after a loading dose of 30 to 40 units per kg) with the goal of dampening further defibrination as the patient's clotting components are replenished with cryoprecipitate and plasma. If the patient has overt thrombosis, the dose of heparin can be increased. The low dose of heparin should not cause lengthening of the PT or APTT or exacerbate the bleeding diathesis. Current studies may demonstrate a role for concentrates of protein C in patients with purpura fulminans associated with gross depletion of protein C. Patients who are severely ill and have defibrination syndrome are at high risk to become vitamin K deficient and therefore should receive parenteral vitamin K.

PRIMARY FIBRINOLYSIS. Primary fibrinolysis, in its pure form, results from massive release of plasminogen activator. Conditions associated with DIC that cause "primarily" fibrinolysis, if not primary fibrinolysis, include carcinoma of the prostate, acute promyelocytic leukemia, hemangiomas, and sustained release of plasminogen activator by endothelial cells produced by injection of venoms. A critical point is reached when enough plasmin is activated to deplete the circulation of α_2-antiplasmin. This allows plasmin to work unopposed on a variety of substrates in blood. Fibrinogen is lysed to fibrinogen degradation products. Because of the lack of fibrinogen and the inhibitory effect of degradation products on fibrin polymerization, the PT and thrombin time are prolonged. The platelet count, however, is appropriate for the state of the bone marrow, and antithrombin levels are normal. Ecchymoses, mucosal bleeding, and bleeding from needle puncture sites can be extensive. It is usually possible to give enough cryoprecipitate to keep plasma fibrinogen at a concentration greater than 100 mg per deciliter. There is, however, no concentrated source of α_2-antiplasmin. EACA, 1 gram per hour in an adult, may be effective in minimizing bleeding and should be given a therapeutic trial in a symptomatic patient if the activity of α_2-antiplasmin in plasma is less than 35 to 40% of normal. If there is a worry about induction of thrombosis with EACA, heparin in a low dose can be infused simultaneously, as described above.

MICROANGIOPATHIC THROMBOCYTOPENIA. The hallmarks of microangiopathic thrombocytopenia are a low platelet count and fragmented red cells on blood smear. Although the serum may contain fibrin degradation products, the PT is generally not elevated and the fibrinogen concentration is normal or increased. Microangiopathic thrombocytopenia can be seen in patients with sepsis, malignancy, immune complex disease, vasculitis, malignant hypertension, eclampsia, vascular malformations, and intravascular aspergillosis. The prototype conditions, however, are hemolytic uremic syndrome (HUS) and thrombotic thrombocytopenia purpura (TTP) (see Ch. 152). HUS involves mainly the vessels of the kidney, usually occurs in children, and ordinarily is self-limited. TTP involves many organs including the brain, ordinarily occurs in adults, and usually causes death unless aggressively treated. Acute neurologic symptoms are the most striking feature of full-blown TTP. The pathogenetic mechanism of HUS and TTP are obscure. It has been suggested that patients lack prostacyclin; have von Willebrand factor multimers that are extra large and cause spontaneous platelet aggregation; have autoantibodies that damage endothelial cells; or have a circulating substance, possibly of microbial origin, that causes spontaneous platelet aggregation and is neutralized by immunoglobulin present in normal plasma. The best documented cause is infection with *Shigella dysentariae* or *Escherichia coli,* such as 0157:H7, which encodes a Shiga-like exotoxin. There are intriguing instances in which HUS or TTP occurs in small clusters, is recurrent, or is familial. Underlying causes should be sought and treated specifically if found. Empiric treatment of HUS and TTP is infusion of fresh-frozen plasma and use of pharmacologic doses of glucocorticoids. The requirement for plasma is so great that plasma exchange is usually necessary. In other cases, occasional infusion of 1 to 2 units of plasma suffices. If extensive plasmapheresis fails, therapeutic options include use of drugs that inhibit platelet aggregation, splenectomy, and use of vincristine.

SNAKE BITES. Venoms from various snakes, especially the vipers and rattlesnakes, contain proteins that can, depending on the species, clot fibrinogen, activate Factor II, Factor X, protein C, or platelets, or cause release of plasminogen activator from endothelial cells. Fortunately, the clinical problems associated with the DIC syndromes from venoms are not as striking as the laboratory abnormalities displayed by the victims. Treatment in most instances can be conservative: administration of antivenoms, transfusion of platelets and/or plasma, and general supportive therapy. In some instances, hypofibrinogenemia and thrombocytopenia persist for weeks.

Moake JL: Thrombotic thrombocytopenic purpura and the hemolytic uremic syndrome. In Hoffman R, Benz EJ Jr, Shattil SJ, et al. (eds.): Hematology: Basic Principles and Practice. 2nd ed. New York, Churchill Livingstone, 1995, p. 1879. Wiliams EC, Mosher DF: Disseminated intravascular coagulation. In Hoffman R, Benz EJ Jr, Shattil SJ, et al. (eds.): Hematology: Basic Principles and Practice. 2nd ed. New York, Churchill Livingstone, 1995, p. 1758. *These two chapters give more detailed exposition of the subject.*

PART XIV

ONCOLOGY

154 INTRODUCTION
Joseph V. Simone

BACKGROUND

DEFINITIONS, INCIDENCE, AND MORTALITY. Cancer describes a class of diseases characterized by the uncontrolled growth of aberrant cells. Cancers kill by the destructive invasion of normal organs through direct extension and spread to distant sites via the blood, lymph, or serosal surfaces. The abnormal clinical behavior of cancer cells is often mirrored by biologic aberrations such as genetic mutations, chromosomal translocations, expression of fetal or other discordant ontologic characteristics, and the inappropriate secretion of hormones or enzymes. All cancers invade or metastasize, but each specific type has unique biologic and clinical features that must be appreciated for proper diagnosis, treatment, and study. About 1.2 million new cases of invasive cancer are diagnosed each year in the United States, and about 500,000 people die annually of the disease. Cancer is the second most deadly disease and is expected to surpass heart disease early in the twenty-first century to top that nefarious list. Over the past half century, the frequency of most cancers has been stable, but some dramatic changes have taken place (Fig. 154–1). Steady declines in stomach and uterine cancer have occurred, the latter undoubtedly due to routine cytologic screening for cervical cancer. The cause of the decline in stomach cancer is unknown. The most striking change has been the increases in lung cancer in both men and women, undoubtedly related to smoking. Other cancers with increasing mortality, particularly in the elderly, include melanoma, non-Hodgkin's lymphoma, and brain tumors. There have been speculations but little firm evidence to explain these changes. The overall mortality from cancer, particularly for those under age 65, has declined, primarily due to more effective therapy for cancers of fetal and hematopoietic origin that occur in the younger population. See Ch. 157 for more detailed treatment of cancer epidemiology.

ETIOLOGY AND PREVENTION. A broad array of agents can cause or directly contribute to a sequence of events or sensitize cells in such a way that cancer develops. The final common pathway in virtually every instance is a cellular genetic mutation that converts a well-behaved cellular citizen of the body into a destructive renegade that is unresponsive to the ordinary checks and balances of a normal community of cells. Promoters (oncogenes) and suppressors (like the retinoblastoma or *p53* gene) play a central role in many cases (see Ch. 156). Chemicals such as benzene and nitrosamines, physical agents such as gamma and ultraviolet radiation, and biologic agents such as the Epstein-Barr and hepatitis viruses contribute to carcinogenesis under certain circumstances. Evidence exists to link dietary factors to carcinogenesis; although not as clear as one would like, the evidence is strong enough to recommend diets low in fat and high in fiber. A sensible diet is based on grains, vegetables, and fruits, with smaller than the current average proportions of fat. Inherited susceptibilities are becoming more evident and probably play a key role in a significant number of cancers of the breast and colon. Down syndrome and the Li-Fraumeni syndrome are well-known harbingers of a substantial risk for developing cancer.

The single most important carcinogen in the United States and Europe is tobacco, because it causes or contributes to the development of about one-third of all cancers—primarily lung, esophageal, head and neck, and bladder. Less well appreciated is the contribution tobacco may make to causing breast, colon, and gastric cancer. Tobacco-related cancer is also important because it is preventable by the obvious, inexpensive, and 100% effective means of abstention. Although the total number of smokers in the United States has declined, through the skillful and irresponsible efforts of tobacco companies women smoke more than ever, adolescents continue to view smoking as socially chic, and the number of smokers in Asia and the third world countries is growing at an alarming rate. Cancer etiology and prevention are treated in more detail in Ch. 155.

EARLY DETECTION OF CANCER. When prevention of cancer is not possible because effective means are lacking, early detection is the next best strategy to reduce cancer mortality. The American Cancer Society (ACS) has recommended a series of cancer screening procedures for asymptomatic individuals (Table 154–1). Not all experts agree on the frequency or age ranges for employing such procedures, but the ACS recommendations are a well-considered and useful guide that, at the very least, indicates the cancers most amenable to clinically useful early detection by conventional techniques. An even more exciting development in this effort has been the emergence of genetic screening and counseling of families at high risk for developing cancer. Individuals at risk are identified largely by analysis of family pedigrees, and the increasing availability of the revolutionary tools of molecular biology can identify specific genetic mutations (see Ch. 156). As this is being written, the cloning of a mutated gene associated with a large minority of breast cancers appears imminent. It is certain that many such genes will be identified, focusing the cancer screening and early detection efforts more efficiently and productively on high-risk populations (see Ch. 155).

CANCER TUMOR GROWTH. While it is impossible to know the specific details of early *in vivo* tumor growth and the efficiency of tumor cell renewal of human cancer, clinical and laboratory observations have provided a reasonable conceptual framework. This framework should be used with caution, however, because it is certain that the intrinsic factors that control tumor growth and propagation are far more complex, episodic, and heterogeneous than we know, even within a single tumor mass. Furthermore, the stromal environment and neovascularization of tumors have become more central to our understanding of this process than heretofore. Nonetheless, the following description can be a useful reference point.

A tumor has reached the size of clinical detectability when it contains about 10^9 cells, weighing about 1 gram and occupying a volume of about 1 cc. A three-log increase to 10^{12} cells, 1 kg, and 1000 cc is often lethal. Below 10^9 cells, the tumor is usually undetectable, but it has already undergone at least 30 doublings, and only 10 further doublings will produce the 1 kg of tumor. This exercise illustrates how much has already occurred, with all the opportunities for the cancer to undergo advantageous mutation and metastasis, before clinical detection. Once the tumor has grown into the clinically evident range, it tends to grow progressively slower with increasing size. This deceleration of growth probably occurs because the tumor outgrows its blood supply, reaches anatomic boundaries, and responds to yet undiscovered feedback regulation from other members of the now larger and more heterogeneous mass of tumor cells. Thus cancers probably grow much like bacteria after inoculation into a favorable medium. The phases of bacterial growth describe a sigmoid curve (Fig. 154–2): an early lag phase of inapparent or slow growth followed by exponential growth. Growth then slows when new cell production and cell

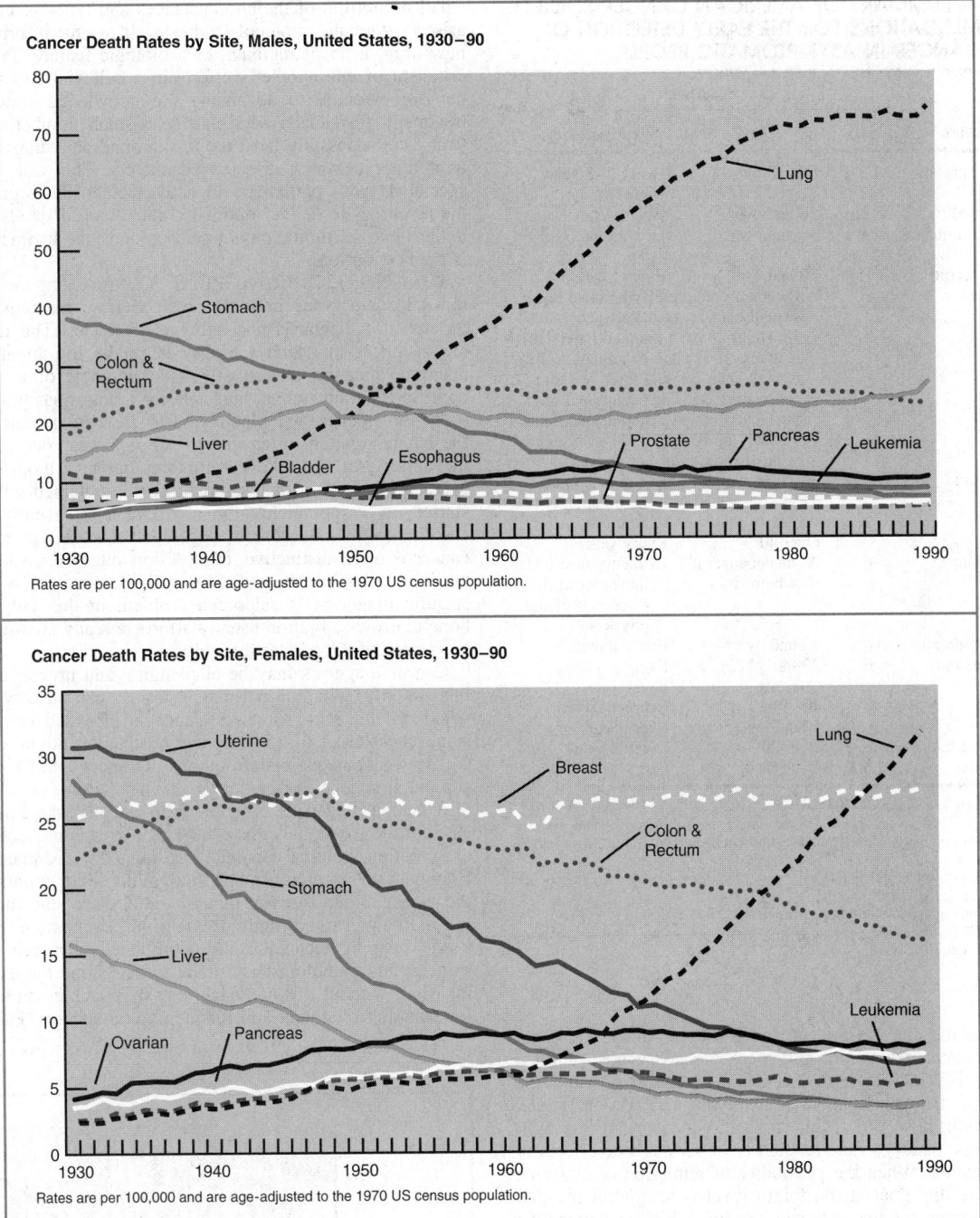

FIGURE 154–1. Cancer death rates in the United States. (From Cancer Facts and Figures—1994. Atlanta, American Cancer Society, 1994.)

death are nearly equal, with the latter phase in culture due to crowding and inadequate nutrients. Of course, in bacteria as well as cancers, the specific growth characteristics differ among types as well as within types that have developed subpopulations of mutant clones.

Most chemotherapy acts by damaging DNA, so it tends to be most effective in rapidly growing tumors such as acute leukemia, lymphomas, and testicular cancers. Also, after gross surgical removal, residual cancer cells may grow more rapidly and be more sensitive to subsequent ("adjuvant") chemotherapy. The sensitivity or resistance to chemotherapy or radiation, however, probably has as much or more to do with the specific biochemical and metabolic features of the cancer cell as with its growth characteristics (see Ch. 165).

MANAGEMENT OF THE PATIENT WITH CANCER

Oncology has been transformed over the past 40 years. From a diverse set of orphan diseases usually managed by surgeons alone and viewed with despair by most physicians, it has become a complex and exciting discipline that draws its strength from the essential partnership of specialists in medicine, surgery, pediatrics, pathology, radiation oncology, diagnostic imaging, psychiatry, and others. This remarkable evolution can be credited to therapeutic successes and biologic advances that could not be imagined in the early 1950's. At its best, oncology has pointed the way to an understanding of the biologic variability of cancer and the success that is possible with a coordinated multimodal approach to therapy.

GOALS. The oncologist—that is, anyone who seriously and expertly assumes responsibility for the management of patients with cancer—should have three sets of goals: therapeutic, human, and scientific. The initial therapeutic goal is to cure patients and return them to a normal place in society. This should be attempted in virtually all cancers, even when the likelihood of cure is small. It requires an attitude of reasonable hope and determination as well as a willingness to attempt difficult, dangerous, and sometimes daring approaches to fundamentally resistant diseases. If after a reasonable

TABLE 154–1. SUMMARY OF AMERICAN CANCER SOCIETY RECOMMENDATIONS FOR THE EARLY DETECTION OF CANCER IN ASYMPTOMATIC PEOPLE

Test or Procedure	Population		
	Sex	Age	Frequency
Sigmoidoscopy, preferably flexible	M & F	50 and over	Every 3–5 years
Fecal occult blood test	M & F	50 and over	Every year
Digital rectal examination	M & F	40 and over	Every year
Prostate examination*	M	50 and over	Every year
Papanicolaou test	F	All women who are or who have been sexually active, or have reached age 18, should have an annual Papanicolaou test and pelvic examination. After a woman has had three or more consecutive satisfactory normal annual examinations, the Papanicolaou test may be performed less frequently at the discretion of her physician.	
Pelvic examination	F	18–40	Every 1–3 years with Papanicolaou test
		Over 40	Every year
Endometrial tissue sample	F	At menopause, if at high risk†	At menopause and thereafter at the discretion of the physician
Breast self-examination	F	20 and over	Every month
Breast clinical examination	F	20–40	Every 3 years
		Over 40	Every year
Mammography‡	F	40–49	Every 1–2 years
		50 and over	Every year
Health counseling and cancer checkup§	M & F	Over 20	Every 3 years
	M & F	Over 40	Every year

From Cancer Facts and Figures—1994. Atlanta, American Cancer Society, 1994.

* Annual digital rectal examination and prostate-specific antigen should be performed on men 50 years and older. If either is abnormal, further evaluation should be considered.

† History of infertility, obesity, failure to ovulate, abnormal uterine bleeding, or unopposed estrogen or tamoxifen therapy.

‡ Screening mammography should begin by age 40.

§ To include examination for cancers of the thyroid, testicles, prostate, ovaries, lymph nodes, oral region, and skin.

attempt permanent cure is not possible, the physician must not abandon the patient but should aim for a secondary goal, a long, qualitatively satisfactory remission. If this is no longer possible, the tertiary level of therapeutic intent is to obtain a remission of any kind and duration; however, at this stage and later, one is less willing to expose the patient to the possibility of serious side effects or long hospitalization. When the possibility of remission of any type becomes remote, the goal at the fourth level is to control the disease and symptoms by the judicious use of palliative therapeutic measures.

The objective in the final stage is terminal care, which is always difficult because it requires the admission that specific therapy is no longer of any value. The only goal now is to provide comfort. Instead of blood transfusions, antibiotics, or chemotherapeutic agents, the physician must use pain medications, sedation, psychosocial support, and other comfort measures with the thought of returning the patient to the home or other appropriate setting and to the support of family.

The human goals in oncology are inextricably linked with the therapeutic and scientific goals. Physicians, nurses, and other health care providers wish to cure patients or improve their conditions so that they may fulfill their human destiny as well as possible. This requires sensitivity to the particular needs of the patient and family and an understanding of the social environment from which they came and to which they must return. The physician must help them maintain their dignity, understand their weaknesses, and refuse to allow any frustration, animosity, or excessive friendship to develop and threaten good judgment and the best interests of the patient.

The use of scientific methods in oncology is only in its adolescence, and definitive treatment has been established for only a small proportion of the circumstances and types of cancers that can arise. Systematic protocol studies yield useful information about a new drug, a novel regimen, or a biologic feature. Presentation and criticism of one another's efforts in a collegial and scientific manner are essential to advancing the knowledge about a particular treatment. Physicians who manage a small number of patients per year cannot possibly have the background and support necessary to treat these complex diseases adequately. This task is best left to specialists who participate in active scientific programs and have the resources to deliver optimal clinical care. It is also important to understand the limitations of science and that at times no treatment is the best option.

DIAGNOSTIC PRINCIPLES. The first diagnostic principle is that adequate tissue must be obtained from the tumor to establish the specific diagnosis and subtype of cancer. The rare exceptions are instances in which a biopsy might be life-threatening and the anatomic location is virtually pathognomonic of a specific histology. Some brain tumors and anterior mediastinal tumors that compress the trachea and blood vessels are two notable examples. In the latter situation, often due to a lymphoma, steroids may reduce the tumor size and relieve symptoms before a biopsy is attempted. More often, an adequate sample must be obtained before therapy is started unless complete surgical excision is definitively diagnostic and therapeutic. Because management of each type and subtype of cancer is often distinctive, every effort must be made to obtain appropriate samples, even if therapy is delayed for a short time. A specific diagnosis is seldom a problem in the leukemias because bone marrow aspiration usually affords a ready answer; the solid tumors present the greater difficulty.

Cancer diagnosis may be challenging and urgent; an understanding of some of its unusual manifestations can be very helpful. Elsewhere in this text, sound guidance is provided on paraneoplastic syndromes (see Ch. 158), endocrine manifestations of cancer (see Ch. 159), cutaneous manifestations of cancer (see Ch. 161), and oncologic emergencies (see Ch. 163).

A second diagnostic principle is to establish the extent of the disease. In the leukemias, this can be readily accomplished by physical examination, routine laboratory tests, chest roentgenography, and examination of cerebrospinal fluid. With solid tumors, determining the extent of the disease, that is, the *stage* of the tumor, often involves major surgery and an extensive examination that uses diagnostic imaging techniques. A coordinated approach involving the surgeon and pathologist is crucial to determine the extent of tumor invasion; without this approach, one may lack essential information for planning treatment and for judging its success. Failure to detect

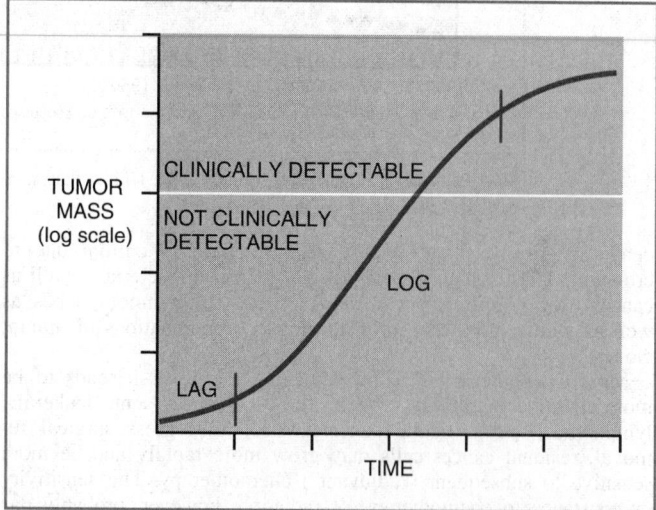

FIGURE 154–2. A schematic representation of the phases of growth of a cancer. After a period of inapparency (lag phase), growth tends to be logarithmic, followed by deceleration due to inadequate nutrients, competitive inhibition among cells, or a lack of neovascularization. (This resembles the growth of bacteria inoculated into a favorable medium.) The tumor has gone through many doublings before it becomes clinically apparent.

a tumor that has extended to regional lymph nodes can lead to undertreatment and a false impression that the local treatment, whether surgery or radiation therapy, was adequate. A simplified generic staging system is shown in Table 154–2. More detailed and specific staging systems have been developed for most cancers that take into account peculiar pathogenetic features, modes of spread, and potential curability. In addition, modern oncology demands an extensive biologic classification of leukemias and solid tumors, often requiring sophisticated scientific approaches not available a few years ago. This includes the use of monoclonal antibodies to determine the phenotype of lymphomas and leukemias, light and electron microscopy with special stains to determine the presence of glycogen, enzymes, or other substances that help to classify solid tumors, chromosomal analysis and modern molecular probes that identify unique characteristics of a disease and responsible oncogenes, suppressor genes, and familial genes (see Ch. 156 and 158).

THERAPEUTIC PRINCIPLES. The first step in treatment is to know the patient. All pertinent information—medical, developmental, and social—must be sought before treatment is planned. The second step is to know the tumor: its usual behavior, usual rate of growth, mode of spread, whether it is local or systemic, and any features that may provide prognostic or therapeutic leads. Third, one must know the available therapies: not only the therapeutic modalities such as chemotherapy, radiation therapy, and surgery but also the skills and limitations of colleagues. Finally, one must know oneself: one's skills, experience, objectivity, and limitations. All these factors shape decisions concerning the patient. Treating patients with cancer is not easy; one must be prepared for losses as well as gains while keeping overall progress and success in mind.

As indicated above, clarity of intent—whether curative, palliative, or supportive—will avoid the confusion of approach and method. Treatment protocols—either research or "standard of care" regimens—are important tools in this regard because they allow strategies to be planned should any momentary decisions be necessary. Protocols are also more likely to provide useful conclusions from a study or experience, because a scientific question or a uniform approach has been formulated and data have been collected in a systematic manner. A protocol is, however, only a road map. The planned therapy may require adjustment if complications develop after treatment has begun. Although many of these adjustments can be anticipated and specified in the protocol, not every circumstance can be foreseen. A protocol is also intended to provide practical information that will lead to improved treatment of subsequent patients.

THERAPEUTIC MODALITIES. There are four principal therapeutic modalities for cancer. *Surgery* is the oldest and most definitive when the tumor is localized under the most favorable anatomic circumstances. For example, for a small tumor localized in the breast, the interior of one kidney, or the peripheral edge of the liver, surgery is usually definitive, curative, and leaves no undue side effects. For many solid tumors, however, surgery alone is inadequate because of local or distant spread. Surgery is also crucial in establishing the extent of a tumor. Considerable surgical skill and experience are required to approach a tumor that may or may not be re-

sectable, achieve tumor-free margins, and obtain the necessary tissue without causing further dissemination.

Radiotherapy is most useful for localized tumors that cannot be resected at all or without serious morbidity and for tumors, such as Hodgkin's disease, that tend to spread to predictable contiguous sites. Therefore, a port of radiation can be enlarged beyond the known extent of the tumor and be quite effective. Unfortunately, radiotherapy can have serious side effects, especially in children who are growing and developing. Nonetheless, the skilled use of radiotherapy is an essential part of oncology; as with all modalities, its role changes depending on new knowledge about a particular tumor. The dosage of radiotherapy is based on an estimate of the dose absorbed by tumor, measured in equivalent units called "centigrays" (cGy) or "rads."

Chemotherapy was the first systemic treatment for any cancer. It most often consists of a combination of drugs, which is almost always more effective than the sequential use of single agents. Since tumors develop subpopulations of cells that differ in their sensitivity to antineoplastic drugs, combinations of agents destroy more cells more rapidly, thereby reducing the frequency of emergence of resistant clones. The mechanisms of action of common chemotherapeutic agents differ widely, although DNA damage is the common final pathway. Toxicity also differs among agents; myelosuppression and gastrointestinal disorders are the most common disturbances. Although toxicity is a concern, for many cancers the best therapeutic results depend on the intensity of the dosage; that is, effective agents given at higher doses over a shorter period are more efficacious than less intensive regimens. One must straddle the fine line between too much and too little.

Chemotherapy is used (1) as a definitive treatment, as in leukemia and some lymphomas; (2) as a principal form of treatment, as in testicular cancer and Ewing's sarcoma; or (3) as an adjuvant to another modality, such as amputation for osteosarcoma or surgical resection for breast or bowel cancer.

Biologic therapy for cancer includes, in addition to bone marrow transplantation, the newer uses of biologic response modifiers such as lymphokines or monoclonal antibodies and agents such as retinoic acid that may cause tumor cells to undergo differentiation and become harmless. These approaches, although still under development, show promise for the future.

The success of cancer therapy often depends on the skillful combination of two or more treatment modalities necessitating close cooperation of medical specialists. Failure to coordinate the effort may lead to the use of modalities in a useless or harmful sequence with an ineffective result.

Supportive care encompasses skilled general medical care. It includes management of infectious, metabolic, and cardiopulmonary disorders that frequently occur in patients undergoing aggressive treatment or surgical procedures. The judicious use of blood products is an essential part of supportive care, and infectious complications in the immunosuppressed patient must be anticipated. Because infections account for a large proportion of hospitalizations and deaths in patients with cancer, one cannot provide modern therapy without appropriate support from specialists in infectious diseases.

MEASURES OF SUCCESS. The measures of success in the treatment of patients with cancer are relatively simple, although not always precise. The first is survival without recurrence of tumor. Unfortunately, some malignancies recur many years after apparently successful control. An operative definition of cure, therefore, differs for each cancer. A patient who remains tumor-free for 2 years after completing therapy is probably cured if the tumor was neuroblastoma, lung cancer, acute myeloid leukemia, or lymphoblastic lymphoma. A much longer period would be needed to conclude a cure for breast cancer, Ewing's sarcoma, Hodgkin's disease, or acute lymphoblastic leukemia of childhood.

The second measure of success is resumption of a normal life pattern without sequelae from the disease or its treatment. The Karnofsky scale (Table 154–3) is a useful guide to measure "performance status." Unfortunately, late side effects, such as second malignancies, may occur 10 to 15 years after treatment is completed. A good estimate of success and failure is usually apparent in a few years, but long-term follow-up of patients is essential for definitive answers.

TABLE 154–2. SIMPLIFIED GENERIC CANCER STAGING SYSTEM

Stage 1	Localized. Usually confined to the organ of origin. Usually curable with locally effective measures such as surgery or irradiation.
Stage 2	Regional. Extends beyond organ of origin but remains nearby, in lymph nodes, for example. Often curable by local measures alone or in combination (surgery ± irradiation) or by a local modality with chemotherapy.
Stage 3	Extensive. Has extended beyond regional site of origin, crossing several tissue planes or extending more distantly via lymphatics or blood. Also may be confined to an organ or region, but be unresectable because of anatomic extent or location. This stage is used rather than stage 2 or stage 4 depending upon the usefulness of local and systemic treatment modalities and the likelihood of cure for that specific cancer.
Stage 4	Widely disseminated. Often involves the bone marrow or multiple distant organs. Rarely curable with current armamentarium.

TABLE 154–3. PERFORMANCE STATUS (KARNOFSKY SCALE)

Criteria of Performance Status (PS)

Able to carry on normal activity; no special care is needed	100	Normal; no complaints; no evidence of disease
	90	Able to carry on normal activity; minor signs or symptoms of disease
	80	Normal activity with effort; some signs or symptoms of disease
Unable to work; able to live at home and care for most personal needs; a varying amount of assistance is needed	70	Cares for self; unable to carry on normal activity or to do active work
	60	Requires occasional assistance but is able to care for most needs
	50	Requires considerable assistance and frequent medical care
Unable to care for self; requires equivalent of institutional or hospital care; disease may be progressing rapidly	40	Disabled; requires special care and assistance
	30	Severely disabled; hospitalization is indicated although death not imminent
	20	Very sick; hospitalization necessary; active supportive treatment is necessary
	10	Moribund, fatal processes progressing rapidly
	0	Dead

PATIENT-FAMILY-PHYSICIAN RELATIONSHIP. Patients with cancer and their families face an extremely difficult time. They need a physician who is hopeful, truthful, compassionate, understanding, accessible, informative, and knowledgeable. Although cancer patients understand that several physicians and other professionals will be involved in their care, they prefer and need one physician who can assume ultimate responsibility for their myriad needs.

Patients should be told of plans and procedures in language that is understandable and appropriate. Some idea of the nature of cancer can be provided by analogy. For example, one may compare leukemia to the overgrowth of a farmer's field (bone marrow) by weeds (leukemia cells) that prevent the growth and export of crops (normal blood cells). Because the weeds cannot be removed manually from the marrow, chemicals are used to destroy the weeds and allow the crops to grow.

Physicians and family often mistakenly believe that the patient is only concerned with the possibility of death. In fact, patients are often equally or more concerned with the immediate implications of disease, for example, separation from family, pain, disfigurement, lengthy hospitalization, financial ruin, or missed time at work or school. Sensitive caregivers will understand and try to address these issues. Some patients and families become very knowledgeable about the disease and in fact may know as much as or more than physicians about certain details; this should be viewed as an asset that can aid the physician in management. Physicians, nurses, and other caregivers may become emotionally attached to a patient or the family. This need not be avoided as long as the necessary professional relationship and sound medical judgment are sustained. The physician must realize that above all the patient and family want an expert physician, not a pal or buddy.

When the cancer becomes resistant to therapy and death is imminent, the patient and family need support more than ever to help them through the last days. The family must understand that no known effective therapy remains and that the goal of management must change from destroying cancer cells to providing comfort. Once this is decided, chemotherapy, transfusions, antibiotics, blood counts, and other laboratory tests are no longer necessary. The patient needs to be hospitalized only if proper supportive care or pain medication cannot be given at home. For pain that cannot be controlled by oral analgesics, parenteral morphine is the drug of choice and is most effective when given by continuous intravenous infu-

sion. The inadequate control of cancer pain in the United States is a national scandal. The demonstrably unwarranted fear of narcotic addiction, the rigid adherence to timed dosages irrespective of need, and the lack of knowledge and plain human sensitivity of doctors and nurses are widespread and indefensible. There is no reason for any cancer patient to suffer severe unremitting pain, a consequence of cancer more feared than death by most patients. Very effective narcotic regimens, including self-regulated intravenous drips, are both safe and readily available.

Patients themselves seldom ask the physician at this time whether they are going to die, probably because they already know or suspect the truth and do not want to confront the physician with an uncomfortable question. Should the question be asked, however, the patient probably knows the answer already; to deny this is worse than useless. Although guidelines can be provided for caring for patients during this difficult period, the medical staff must adopt an approach that is suitable to the particular patient and circumstances. Most of all, the patient needs palpable demonstration that the medical staff is readily available and willing to listen, to comfort, to provide any possible service, and simply to be there. Even patients who are at home should not be abandoned; telephone communication can provide welcome support to the family. Both hospice care and home visits by nurses can be a godsend to patients and their families.

155 CANCER PREVENTION
Gilbert S. Omenn

Cancers are diagnosed in 1.2 million people in the United States and claim over 500,000 lives each year, one fourth of all deaths. Fear of cancer, suffering from cancers and their treatment, and the limited benefit of treatments for most common cancers combine to make prevention an increasing priority in clinical medicine and in public health.

As Figure 155–1 shows, the leading cancer killer by far in both men and women is lung cancer, followed by cancers of the prostate, colon and rectum, and pancreas in men and by cancers of the breast, colon and rectum, ovary, and pancreas in women. Pancreatic and pulmonary cancers are particularly lethal.

The primary modalities for cancer prevention (see Table 155–1) involve behavior change, including smoking, alcohol, diet, and physical activity. Reduction of exposures to carcinogenic agents from all environmental sources comes next. Under intensive investigation are hormonal, nutritional, and pharmacologic interventions and genetic screening, counseling, and eventual treatments for those with testable inherited predispositions.

HEALTH-PROMOTING/CANCER-PREVENTING BEHAVIOR CHANGES

SMOKING CESSATION AND SMOKING PREVENTION. Diseases related to cigarette smoking represent a twentieth-century epidemic, now spreading globally. Smoking is the primary cause of cancers of the lung, larynx, oral cavity, and esophagus (approximately 10 to 20 times the risk compared with nonsmokers) and contributory to cancers of the pancreas, bladder, kidney, stomach, and cervix and to leukemia (about 2 times the risk). Smoking acts synergistically with chemical and radiation carcinogens in the lung and with alcohol in the esophagus and oral cavity. Former smokers, after a lag of up to 4 years, show a progressively lower relative risk compared with continuing smokers and even compared with the slowly rising rate as never-smokers age. However, the absolute risk of lung cancer probably never declines, in sharp contrast with coronary heart disease endpoints. Low-tar, low-nicotine, and filtered cigarettes have had little or no protective effect, because the smokers tend to inhale more deeply and more frequently.

Snuff dipping and smokeless tobacco have been promoted successfully to adolescents in recent years; their predisposition to cancer is similar to that of inhaled smoking. Leukoplakia, a white patch involving the oral mucosa epithelium, is a telltale premalignant lesion found in up to half of tobacco chewers, with a 5% risk

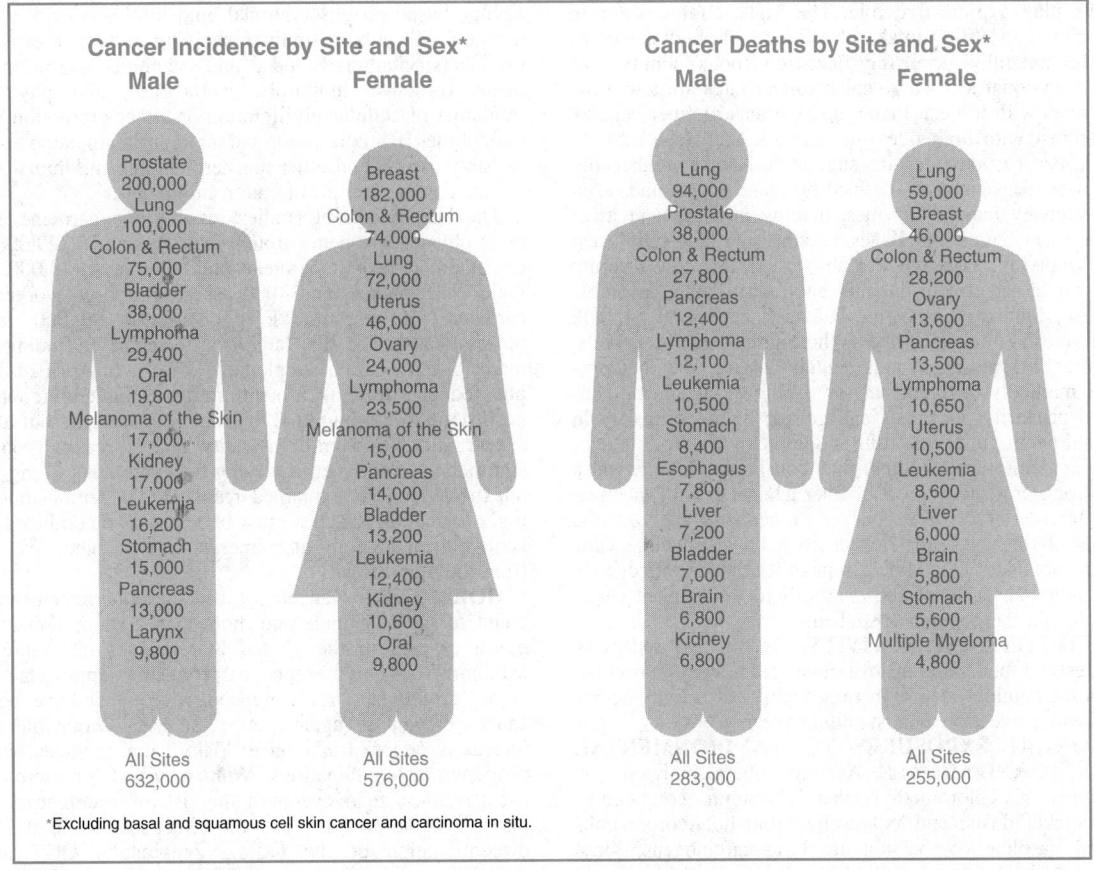

Cancer Incidence by Site and Sex*

Male	Female
Prostate 200,000	Breast 182,000
Lung 100,000	Colon & Rectum 74,000
Colon & Rectum 75,000	Lung 72,000
Bladder 38,000	Uterus 46,000
Lymphoma 29,400	Ovary 24,000
Oral 19,800	Lymphoma 23,500
Melanoma of the Skin 17,000	Melanoma of the Skin 15,000
Kidney 17,000	Pancreas 14,000
Leukemia 16,200	Bladder 13,200
Stomach 15,000	Leukemia 12,400
Pancreas 13,000	Kidney 10,600
Larynx 9,800	Oral 9,800
All Sites 632,000	All Sites 576,000

Cancer Deaths by Site and Sex*

Male	Female
Lung 94,000	Lung 59,000
Prostate 38,000	Breast 46,000
Colon & Rectum 27,800	Colon & Rectum 28,200
Pancreas 12,400	Ovary 13,600
Lymphoma 12,100	Pancreas 13,500
Leukemia 10,500	Lymphoma 10,650
Stomach 8,400	Uterus 10,500
Esophagus 7,800	Leukemia 8,600
Liver 7,200	Liver 6,000
Bladder 7,000	Brain 5,800
Brain 6,800	Stomach 5,600
Kidney 6,800	Multiple Myeloma 4,800
All Sites 283,000	All Sites 255,000

*Excluding basal and squamous cell skin cancer and carcinoma in situ.

FIGURE 155–1. Leading sites of cancer incidence and death—1994 estimates. (From Cancer Facts and Figures—1994. Atlanta, American Cancer Society, 1994.)

of epidermoid carcinoma. Finally, environmental tobacco smoke (ETS), or second-hand smoke, has been declared a definite human carcinogen by the Environmental Protection Agency; 6000 cases of lung cancer per year are attributed to ETS by the National Research Council.

A huge literature attests to the difficulty of helping smokers quit. About 5% "quit" by themselves (for at least a 6-month period) each year, but others relapse. Physicians play a key role in urging smokers to quit and in guiding them to self-help materials, classes, or pharmacologic quitting aids. Work-site, family, and community reinforcement is essential; increased taxes on tobacco products reinforce as well. Prevention of smoking, especially in young people, minorities, and women, can be enhanced by organized community and school programs as well as regulatory actions.

MODERATION OF ALCOHOL INTAKE. The National Cancer Institute *Dietary Guidelines* recommend that consumption of alcoholic beverages, if any, should be moderate. Alcohol intake is highly associated with cancers of the esophagus, oral cavity, pharynx, and larynx and, less strikingly, with liver, rectal, pancreatic, and breast cancer. It acts synergistically with cigarette smoking.

DIET. Guidelines for healthy diets strongly recommend decreases in fat and increases in fiber intake, most easily described as "five-a-day" fruits and vegetable portions. Such advice aims at preventing cancers, heart disease, and bowel disorders too.

The typical U.S. diet has 39% of calories from fat or about 150 grams per day. Dietary fat intake correlates positively with incidence and mortality rates for breast, prostate, and colon cancers. International, migrant, and time-trend data indicate that reduction in dietary fat to 20% of caloric intake would reduce breast cancer risk by two thirds. Unfortunately, most case-control (retrospective) and cohort (prospective) epidemiologic studies have found less striking correlations or none at all. Similar inconsistencies underlie positive associations of fat intake with colorectal and prostate cancers. Fat intake involves many variables, including percentage of calories, grams per day, saturated versus unsaturated fats and fatty acids, overweight, and duration of diet. Each type of cancer

possesses other confounding or interacting risk factors. Experimental studies in rodents show that dietary fat may exert tumor-enhancing or -promoting effects on the breast directly through changes in cell membranes or indirectly through neuroendocrine systems. In the colon, fat may influence bile acids, sterol substrates, and fecal microflora.

Clinical trials are essential to test hypothesized mechanisms and behavior change for cancer prevention. A feasibility study for the Women's Health Trial showed that women aged 45 to 69 can lower mean dietary fat intake to below 25% of energy requirements and maintain the diet and good health for 2 years. Reduction in dietary fat intake is a major component of the Women's Health Initiative, a massive trial aimed at reducing breast cancer, heart disease, and osteoporosis in postmenopausal women.

INCREASE IN DIETARY FIBER. The surgeon Dennis Burkitt deduced from widely varying country rates for colon cancer that

TABLE 155–1. PROPORTIONS OF CANCER DEATHS ATTRIBUTED TO VARIOUS RISK FACTORS

Factor or Class of Factor	Best Estimate	Range of Estimates
Tobacco	30	25–40
Alcohol	3	2–4
Diet	35	10–70
Food additives*	<1	−5–2
Reproductive/sexual behavior	7	1–13
Occupation	4	2–8
General pollution	2	1–5
Industrial products	<1	<1–2
Medicines/medical procedures	1	0.5–3
Geophysical factors†	3	2–4
Infections	10?	1–?

* Minus indicates potential benefits from antioxidants and other additives.
† UV and cosmic radiation included; perhaps 1% truly avoidable.
From Doll R, Peto R: The causes of cancer: Quantitative estimates of avoidable risks of cancer in the United States today. J Natl Cancer Inst 66:1193, 1981.

fiber-rich diets play a protective role. The highest rates occur in western countries with a high intake of refined carbohydrates compared with the naturally occurring fiber-rich foods common in African and Asian countries, where colon cancer rates are low. Low colon cancer rates with a mean intake of 31 grams of fiber per day in Finland contrast with high rates in Denmark and New York on 17 grams of fiber per day despite similar fat intakes. Fiber describes a heterogeneous category, defined by plant origins and resistance to digestion by human enzymes, making measurement awkward. Soluble fibers (gums, mucilages, pectins, and hemicelluloses) delay gastric emptying, slow glucose absorption, and lower serum cholesterol, with lesser effects on bulk and transit time. Insoluble fibers (cellulose, lignin, other hemicelluloses) increase fecal bulk and decrease intestinal transit time. Whole-grain breads, cereals, fruits, vegetables, legumes, and nuts contain lots of fiber but provide fibers of markedly different natures. Cellulose and hemicellulose are found primarily in cereals and grains; lignin, primarily in berry fruits; and pectin, in citrus fruits and apples.

Dozens of epidemiologic studies give consistent findings of a moderate-to-strong protective effect of fiber against colon cancer, as well as a protective effect of vegetables. When one analyzes the different forms of fiber or foods rich in fiber, however, more variable results are obtained. One should remember that no effect of a dietary component can be identified unless there is sufficient variation in intake within the population studied.

INCREASED PHYSICAL ACTIVITY. Overcoming sedentary or inactive lifestyles benefits cardiovascular, respiratory, muscular, cognitive, and metabolic systems. Increased physical activity seems to offer significant protection against colon cancer.

REDUCTION IN EXPOSURES TO ENVIRONMENTAL CARCINOGENIC CHEMICALS. Asbestos fibers, inorganic arsenic compounds, bis-chloromethyl ether, chromium compounds, mustard gas, nickel dusts, and polycyclic aromatic hydrocarbons from coal and gasoline combustion are lung carcinogens; vinyl chloride causes a distinctive angiosarcoma of the liver; some pesticides are associated with the development of non-Hodgkin's lymphoma; aromatic amine dyestuffs can cause bladder cancer; leather production and isopropyl alcohol manufacturing are associated with nasal cancers; and benzene can cause acute myelocytic leukemia. Tobacco smoke is the most prevalent chemical carcinogen, possibly followed by charbroiling of meats and fish.

PHYSICAL AGENTS. Ultraviolet radiation is the primary cause of skin cancers, including melanoma and lip cancer. Ionizing radiation (including radiotherapy) increases rates at essentially all exposed sites. Nonionizing radiation and electromagnetic fields have been suspected of increasing leukemia and brain cancer and possibly breast cancer rates, but the data are not consistent and the relationship is far from demonstrated.

DRUGS. Alkylating agents can cause leukemias; androgen anabolic steroids, liver cancer; chlornaphazine, bladder cancer; estrogens (possibly also "environmental estrogens"), cancers of the vagina and cervix (diethylstilbestrol), endometrium (postmenopausal estrogens), or liver and cervix (steroid contraceptives); azathioprine and cyclosporine immunosuppressants, non-Hodgkin's lymphoma; and phenacetin-containing analgesics, renal pelvic tumors.

INFECTIOUS AGENTS. Specific infectious agents can cause several cancers: primary hepatocellular cancer is associated, with hepatitis B and C (with distinctive mutations in gene *p53* and with synergistic effects of aflatoxins derived from *Aspergillus flavus* growth on crops); cervix, with certain human papillomaviruses; Burkitt's lymphoma and nasopharyngeal, with Epstein-Barr virus; Kaposi's sarcoma and non-Hodgkin's lymphoma, with HIV-1; T-cell leukemia, with HTLV-I; urinary bladder (*Schistosoma haematobium*) and cholangiocarcinoma of the liver (*Clonorchis sinensis*), with parasites; and gastric cancer, with *Helicobacter pylori*. Environmental or antibiotic control of these infections and/or vaccines to protect against exposure can be effective. Population-wide neonatal hepatitis B virus immunization is expected to reduce or eliminate the scourge of primary liver cancer in Taiwan.

CANCER PREVENTION INTERVENTIONS

CHEMOPREVENTION. Population trials of chemopreventives are currently under way worldwide. Because of their apparent antioxidant, tumor suppressor, and immunomodulatory actions, micronutrients (especially carotenoids and retinoids) have been prime agents, based on observational epidemiologic work as well as animal and cell culture findings showing protective effects. Other antioxidants (vitamins E and C and selenium), anticarcinogens in soybeans (protease inhibitors, isoflavones, and phytosterols), and inhibitors of cellular proliferation or tumor promotion are in phase I and phase II studies. For example, calcium supplementation and possibly aspirin and other nonsteroidal anti-inflammatory agents can reduce colonic cell proliferation in humans.

The largest current studies involve beta-carotene alone (22,000 male physicians), beta-carotene plus vitamin E (29,000 male smokers in Finland), beta-carotene plus vitamin A (14,000 male and female U.S. smokers and 4000 asbestos-exposed workers), and beta-carotene plus vitamin E plus aspirin (40,000 female health professionals). The first large trial to report its findings shocked the medical and vitamin supplement worlds. In April of 1994, the Alpha-Tocopherol/Beta-Carotene study in Finland reported not only no benefit from vitamin E or from beta-carotene but also 18% lung cancer and 8% overall mortality rate increases (both statistically significant) in the men receiving beta-carotene, 20 mg per day. This unexpected and unexplained result firmly demonstrates that seemingly logical approaches must be tested in randomized, clinical preventive trials before their merits are accepted. We await results from the other trials.

HORMONES. Cancers of the hormone-responsive tissues account for 20% of male and more than 40% of female newly diagnosed cancers in the United States. Thus chemoprevention with "antihormones" represents a promising approach. Progesterone is the prototype. Oral contraceptives (OC's) have become potent cancer prevention agents, once the early sequential OC's (which increased endometrial cancer risk) were replaced with estrogen-progesterone combinations. Women with 6 or more years of OC use have less than one-sixth the risk of endometrial cancer compared with never-users, and the effect lasts at least 15 years after discontinuation of the OC's. Combination OC's also suppress gonadotropin levels and ovulation, thereby decreasing the risk for epithelial ovarian cancers by about 40%, independent of parity. The breast is different: Progesterone increases the rate of cell division beyond that induced by estrogen. Combination therapy is now also preferred for postmenopausal hormone replacement therapy.

A strategy in premenopausal women for gaining the benefits of the OC's while actually reducing breast cancer (and cardiovascular) risk involves use of luteinizing hormone–releasing hormone (LHRH) antagonists, a "reversible bilateral oophorectomy," plus low-dose estrogen to overcome hypoestrogenic effects plus a quarterly progestogen. Antiestrogenic agents, such as tamoxifen, also are being subjected to multiple-endpoint trials.

Diethylstilbestrol and LHRH agonists are effective therapeutically against metastatic prostate cancer by reducing testosterone-mediated maintenance of prostate tissue. Inhibitors of 5-α-reductase may become useful in high-risk patients or even in primary prevention.

GENETIC SCREENING. Molecular studies in cancer reveal numerous oncogenes, tumor-suppressor genes, genes affecting cell division, cell cycle, and cell proliferation, and a host of other potential targets for cancer prevention. Known inherited cancer syndromes, such as retinoblastoma and polyposis coli, have specific mutations of general interest in carcinogenesis. If and when highly predisposing breast cancer gene(s) and cell-cycle/tumor-suppressor genes (such as the already discovered multiple-tumor-suppressor [MTS-1] p16 mutant) can be identified and converted into diagnostic tests, genetic screening and counseling programs are bound to increase. The discovery of other genetic mechanisms will bring new types of interventions as well.

American Cancer Society: Cancer Facts and Figures—1994. Atlanta, American Cancer Society, 1994. *Excellent annual update on cancer statistics and advances.*

DeVita VT Jr, Hellman S, Rosenberg SA (eds.): Cancer, Principles and Practice of Oncology. 4th ed. Philadelphia, JB Lippincott, 1993. *See Chapters 9 (Causes of Cancer) and 20 (Cancer Prevention).*

Doll R, Peto R: The causes of cancer: Quantitative estimates of avoidable risks of cancer in the United States today. J Natl Cancer Inst 66:1193, 1981. *Now-classic analysis of the preventable causes of cancer mortality.*

The Alpha-Tocopherol, Beta-Carotene Cancer Prevention Study Group: The effect of vitamin E and beta-carotene on the incidence of lung cancer and other cancers in male smokers. N Engl J Med 330:1029, 1994. *The first large-scale antioxidant chemoprevention trial reported unexpected and unexplained results.*

156 ONCOGENES AND SUPPRESSOR GENES: GENETIC CONTROL OF CANCER

Edison T. Liu

THE ONCOGENE THEORY AND HUMAN CANCERS

Oncogenes figure prominently in the study of human carcinogenesis, first as empiric associates of disease, second as genetic and biochemical explanations for cancer progression, and finally as targets for gene-directed therapeutics of the future. Equally important is the impact of oncogene investigations on how we conceptualize cancer. The older models favoring the influence of alien genes of viral origin were superseded by a new model that stressed the importance of mutations in resident genes. In this process, the genetics of cancer and the genetics of normal development and growth have merged, allowing for a more unified theory of cell proliferation and transformation.

THE MANY ROADS TO CANCER: ABERRATIONS OF SIGNALING PATHWAYS

Viral oncogenes were the first evidence that endogenous genes can directly cause cancer. Here, normal cellular genes (proto-oncogenes, designated by the c-prefix) are "captured" or transduced by the retrovirus and mutated through the error-prone replicative process of the retroviral life cycle. This results in a viral oncogene (v-*onc*) that is often structurally distinct from its normal cellular counterpart and is functionally arrested in a biochemically activated form. Extensions of these early investigations revealed that the oncogene precursors, the proto-oncogenes, act as biochemical switches in cellular command and control processes, specifically relaying signals from the outside of the cell to the nucleus. The progressive and controlled transfer of extracellular signals is bypassed when one of the relay members is rendered constitutively activated, resulting in a characteristic of a cancer cell: unmanaged growth.

Nature has provided ample evidence for oncogenic mutations in members of signaling pathways: the receptor tyrosine kinase, epidermal growth factor receptor (EGFR, homologous retroviral oncogene = v-*erbB*), when stimulated with one of its ligand, TGF-α (found to be overexpressed in some human cancers), interacts with *ras* (retroviral homologue = v-H-*ras,* or v-K-*ras*) through bridging proteins. *Ras,* in turn, is controlled by GTPase-activating proteins (GAPs, oncogenic homologue = NF1) and transmits signals through activation of *raf* (retroviral homologue, v-*raf*). Stimulation of the *ras/raf* pathway leads to augmented expression of the nuclear proteins *jun, fos,* and *myc* (retroviral homologues = v-*jun,* v-*fos,* v-*myc*). Thus, every relay node in this signal transduction pathway is a potential site for oncogenic conversion. The complexity of the transformation process is further augmented by the existence of multiple parallel signaling pathways that are promiscuous in their selection of biochemical partners. For example, the receptor tyrosine kinase HER-2 forms dimers either with itself or with related receptor tyrosine kinases, such as EGFR and HER-4; *ras* can be regulated by either *ras*-GAP or NF1; and stimulation of the *ras* pathway activates a number of mitogen-activated protein kinases (MAPKs).

THE MANY ROADS TO CANCER: BLOCK IN CELL DEATH

Until recently, the study of molecular oncogenesis has concentrated on these positive growth signals. However, kinetically, the accumulation of cancer cells can be accomplished by a decrease in cell loss as well as by an increase in cellular proliferation. Current evidence suggests that the abrogation of programmed cell death (apoptosis) may be an important concomitant to neoplastic transformation. The clearest example of an oncogene involved in the apoptotic process is *bcl*-2, found to be the important oncogene in patients with the t(14q;18q) translocation frequently detected in follicular lymphomas. *bcl*-2 blocks apoptosis when overexpressed or inappropriately expressed, and, in lymphomas, perturbations in

bcl-2 may be among the earliest oncogene abnormalities acting to prolong the lifespan of cells that are prone to accumulate genetic mutations. In experimental lymphomas, *bcl*-2 does not cause cancer directly, but subsequent mutations/rearrangements at other oncogenes, such as the c-*myc,* result in accelerated progression of the lymphoma, suggesting strong functional interaction between *bcl*-2 and *myc.* This *bcl*-2/*myc* interaction underscores another principle of oncogene action in that more than one cancer gene must be perturbed for a malignancy to emerge. This rule is well illustrated in the progression of colon cancer, in which four or five detectable oncogenic mutations must be present before overt cancer is observed.

THE MANY ROADS TO CANCER: RELEASE OF SUPPRESSION

Whereas proto-oncogenes are identified by a gain of function after mutational damage, another class of cancer genes—tumor suppressor genes—contribute to malignancy by a loss of function. To this end, well-known tumor suppressor genes such as the retinoblastoma gene (Rb-1) and p53 act as "brakes" to cellular proliferation, and each appears to function through distinct pathways. Rb-1 negatively regulates an important transcription factor, E2F, and the deletion of the Rb gene (as seen in congenital retinoblastoma) or sequestration of protein product (as seen in the presence of the adenovirus E1A protein, or the human papilloma viral protein, E7) releases the suppression of E2F. P53 enhances the expression of p21/CIP1, which is a potent suppressor of cell cycle regulatory kinase (CDK's). This suggests that loss of p53 and the associated loss of p21/CIP1 expression result in unmanaged progression through the cell cycle.

That both Rb and p53 are involved in the genesis of cancer is supported by the identification of germline mutations in patients with cancer predisposition syndromes such as congenital retinoblastoma (Rb), and the Li-Fraumeni multicancer syndrome (p53). As is the case with transforming oncogenes, the presence of a single abnormal tumor suppressor allele is alone insufficient for cancer to form; lesions at other genetic loci are necessary. For example, both Rb and p53 may need to be inactivated for some primary human cells to be rendered immortal, one of the first steps in transformation. In colon cancers, mutations in p53 frequently accompany several other genetic lesions, including those involved in cytoskeletal organization (APC), signal transduction *(ras),* and cellular adhesion (DCC) in order for an invasive cancer to emerge.

ONCOGENES AS MOLECULAR POINTS OF ORIGIN

Certain oncogenes are closely associated with specific malignancies, suggesting that they may be causative for that disease. Chronic myelogenous leukemia (CML) is characterized by a genetic rearrangement juxtaposing the beginning of the *bcr* gene on chromosome 22 with the *abl* proto-oncogene on chromosome 9. The resultant *bcr-abl* hybrid protein activates the tyrosine kinase activity of *abl* and, in animal models, has been shown to be the direct cause of the CML phenotype. Intriguingly, 10 to 25% of *de novo* acute lymphoblastic leukemias (ALL) also harbor the same t(9;22) translocation, but the rearrangement occurs at a slightly different genetic location. This generates a distinctly smaller hybrid *bcr-abl* oncoprotein with increased biochemical activity. Thus, not only does the *bcr-abl* induce a specific hematologic disease, CML, but minor alterations of the same aberrant protein result in a different clinical picture, ALL. Other examples exist of specific oncogene/cancer associations: the t(15;17) translocation seen exclusively in acute promyelocytic leukemia brings about the aberrant fusion of the retinoic acid receptor alpha (RARA) with another transcription factor, PML. This abnormal protein is seen in no other cancers. Rearrangements of the *bcl*-2 locus and translocations involving the *myc* proto-oncogene are found solely in lymphomas. In solid tumors, genetic perturbations of the *ret* oncogene have been identified only in thyroid cancers, and germline mutations in this receptor tyrosine kinase give rise to the heritable multiple endocrine neoplasia syndrome.

Less exclusive oncogene/cancer associations occur more frequently and are also helpful in mapping pathways of cancer progression. Overexpression or amplification of the HER-2 gene is seen in 20 to 30% of invasive breast cancers and is correlated with a worse outcome. The concordance observed in the HER-2 status between carcinomas *in situ,* invasive carcinomas, and their metastases from individual patients suggests that perturbations at the HER-2 locus occur early in breast tumorigenesis and mark a distinct progression pathway for the tumor. Similar findings have been observed in other cancers. p53 mutations are found in cervical carcinomas except in those induced by oncogenic papilloma viruses. *Ras* mutations are detected in 20 to 25% of *de novo* acute myelogenous leukemia but are very rare in chronic myelogenous leukemia (in either chronic or blast phase) or in acute promyelocytic leukemia, both being leukemic subgroups known to be induced by other oncogenes. The initiation by one gene may not only define a particular molecular progression pathway but may also predict some tumor characteristics as well. *Bcr-abl*–positive ALL's are associated with earlier relapse; HER-2 overexpression or amplification is found frequently in ductal breast carcinomas but rarely in lobular carcinomas; and N-*myc* amplification remains one of the most potent predictors of poorer survival in childhood neuroblastomas. Thus, oncogene mutations can be used not only in cancer diagnostics but also as useful markers of prognosis.

CONVERGENCE OF PATHWAYS: UNIFYING OBSERVATIONS

The many oncogenes involved in malignancies highlight the complexity of the cancer process. However, the dissection of the biochemical pathways used by these oncogenes is uncovering interactions that may begin to unify empiric observations of human tumor biology. One example is found in *ras. Ras* activity is downregulated by the GTPase-activating protein (or GAP), and oncogenic *ras* is resistant to the effects of GAP. The biochemistry therefore suggests that mutations abrogating GAP's negative effects on *ras* might promote cancer. Although abnormalities in *ras*-GAP have not been found, the gene associated with congenital neurofibromatosis, NF1, is structurally a GTPase-activating protein that functionally interacts with *ras.* Mutations in NF1, seen in neurofibromatosis, block its ability to downregulate *ras* activity. This biochemical interaction between *ras* and NF1 is manifested clinically in an unusual form of leukemia. Mutations in *ras* are the most common genetic abnormality in adult AML, and epidemiologic and molecular data support a role for *ras* in the induction of myeloid leukemias. Interestingly, children with neurofibromatosis have a higher rate of development of a rare myeloproliferative syndrome that often progresses to acute myelogenous leukemia. Thus, the biochemical pathway predicts the clinical convergence.

ONCOGENES AND CANCER THERAPY

A goal of oncogene research has been the potential targeting of oncogenes as specific therapies for cancer. This goal is now in reach because of a better understanding of their biochemistry and the growing awareness that activating some oncogenes may render cancer cells more sensitive to chemotherapy. Because activation of *ras* appears to be involved in a wide variety of cancers, *ras* has become an attractive target for gene-directed therapeutics. The transforming activity of *ras* requires that the oncoprotein be bound to the cell membrane through fatty acid modification at a four amino acid motif: CAAX (cysteine–aliphatic amino acid–aliphatic amino acid–any amino acid). Synthetic CAAX peptides effectively block *ras* transformation *in vitro,* but the excitement is in the fact that the growth of cancer cells not transformed by *ras* can also be inhibited by these CAAX peptides. The requirement, however, is that the activated pathway uses *ras* as an intermediary. Therefore, cells transformed by membrane-bound tyrosine kinases such as *src,* HER-2, and the EGFR are predicted to be inhibited by anti-*ras* approaches.

Recently, the stimulation of HER-2 and EGFR by antibodies against their respective extracellular domains has been found to augment sensitivity to alkylating agents, potentially by inhibiting DNA repair. In clinical trials, the adverse effects of HER-2 overexpression and amplification on the survival of women with node-positive breast cancer can be reversed by dose-intensive adjuvant therapy. Thus, the presence of oncogene abnormalities may be used to choose optimal therapy.

FROM MOLECULAR BIOLOGY TO PUBLIC HEALTH

In the past, oncogene sciences have centered on understanding molecular mechanisms and applications to clinical care. Recent advances have placed oncogenes more prominently in public health, and, in the process, have moved the field into the realm of cancer prevention. This fusion of disciplines has been necessitated by the identification of a growing number of cancer susceptibility genes and by the finding that oncogene mutations in some cases may represent "signatures" of carcinogen exposure. Data emerging from molecular epidemiologic investigations have identified predictable mutations in the p53 gene associated with aflatoxin exposure in hepatocellular carcinoma and with UV exposure in skin cancers. Cancer susceptibility genes for colon cancer (APC, MSH2, MLH1), for retinoblastoma (Rb), for the Li-Fraumeni syndrome (p53), for the multiple endocrine neoplasia syndrome (RET), and for neurofibromatosis (NF1) have already been cloned and can be used for direct screening of cancer susceptibility. The availability of these genetic tests raises some interesting, and, simultaneously, troubling questions: Who should be tested, and how young? What are the environmental factors modifying the genetic risk? Do all mutations in the susceptibility gene give the same cancer phenotype? What kind of screening or surveillance is optimal? What is the best timing for surgical prophylaxis? Is surgical prophylaxis efficacious? What safeguards to privacy can we provide our patients?

Perhaps the most intriguing of the susceptibility genes are those identified as causing the hereditary non-polyposis colorectal cancer (HNPCC). The prototype is the MSH2 gene localized on chromosome 2p, a DNA repair gene whose protein product is part of a complex that corrects DNA base mismatches. Here again, what we know molecularly and biochemically of MSH2 might predict the next clinical observations: that mutations in this gene involved in repairing damage after carcinogen exposure can induce colon cancer, but only in the presence of potentially identifiable mutagens. Because MSH2 is not a specific detoxification gene, the threshold for carcinogen effect in affected individuals may be lowered for all colonic carcinogens. Studies on MSH2, therefore, underscore the importance of gene-environment interactions in cancer induction and the potential of integrating molecular biology into cancer prevention interventions. For example, intensive colonoscopic screening and chemoprevention approaches can be targeted to these high-risk populations.

LESSONS LEARNED, FUTURE CHALLENGES

Our understanding of cancer genes has dramatically altered the conceptual landscape of basic biology. Its impact on clinical cancer care, however, is just beginning to be felt but will undoubtedly be equally profound. The promise of oncogene research is for more precise and effective therapy and for more rational prevention measures. Our arrival at this point has been due to discoveries arising from a basic research–clinical interface, a familiar paradigm that will undoubtedly lead to translation into novel therapies. The lesson learned is that groundbreaking ideas often come from unexpected corners: the secrets of human cancer from avian retroviruses and a major colon cancer gene from yeast genetics. The challenge in the future, however, will be to extend this process to the public health arena, where politics and ethics play a greater role in deciding what questions will be asked and how the solutions will be formulated.

ACKNOWLEDGMENTS: This review was written with the support of the NCI grant RO1-CA49240. Dr. Liu is a Scholar of the Leukemia Society.

Greenblatt MS, Bennett WP, Hollstein M, Harris CC: Mutations in the p53 tumor suppressor gene: clues to cancer etiology and molecular pathogenesis. Cancer Res 54:4855, 1994.

Liu ET, Weissman B: Oncogenes and Tumor Suppressor Genes. In Oncogenes and Tumor Suppressor Genes in Human Malignancies. Boston, Kluwer Academic Publishers, 1993, pp 1-14.

These references provide a general background on oncogenes and their role in human cancers.

Gibbs JB, Oliff A, Kohl NE: Farnesyltransferase inhibitors: *Ras* research yields a potential cancer therapeutic. Cell 77:175, 1994.

Muss HB, Thor AD, Berry DA, et al: c-*erbB*-2 expression and response to adjuvant therapy in women with node-positive early breast cancer. N Engl J Med 330:1260, 1994.

These references address the issue of oncogenes and cancer treatment.

Miki Y, Swensen J, Shattuck Eidens D, et al: A strong candidate for the breast and ovarian cancer susceptibility gene BRACA1. Science 266:66, 1994.

Ledger GA, Khosla S, Lindor NM, et al: Genetic testing in the diagnosis and management of multiple endocrine neoplasia type II. Ann Intern Med 122:118, 1995.

These references discuss the genetic basis of cancer susceptibility.

157 THE EPIDEMIOLOGY OF CANCER

William J. Blot

DESCRIPTIVE PATTERNS

THE GEOGRAPHY OF CANCER. Cancer affects all the world's populations, with about a threefold difference between areas with the highest and lowest age-adjusted rates. For certain cancers, the difference exceeds 100-fold (Table 157–1). Perhaps the most distinctive geographic patterns are seen for esophageal cancer. Pockets of exceptionally high mortality exist in areas of north central China, the Caspian littoral of Iran, and South Africa. In Linxian, China, for as yet unknown reasons, esophageal/gastric cardia cancer is the most common cause of death, causing over one third of all fatalities among adults. Clustering of elevated esophageal cancer rates also has been observed in parts of Europe and the United States, primarily due to heavy alcohol intake.

Geographic variation for other tumors is also noteworthy. Rates of oral cancer are highest in India and parts of south central Asia. Within the United States, elevated oral cancer mortality among females is found in the southern states, especially in rural areas. In both instances, the cause is the same—high use of smokeless tobacco. In southeastern China, nasopharyngeal cancer is the most common malignancy. It is also a leading cancer among Alaskan Aleuts and Eskimos and occurs more frequently among Chinese than white or black Americans. The primary cause of the cancer in southern China appears to be consumption of salted fish, especially during weaning and early childhood. The importance of early life events is also suggested by the up to threefold higher rates of nasopharyngeal cancer among Chinese-Americans born and raised in China than among those born and raised in the United States. Similar migrant effects are seen for stomach cancer. Japanese-Americans born in Japan, where rates of stomach cancer are among the highest in the world, have a two- to threefold higher incidence of this cancer than Japanese-Americans born in the United States. American-born Japanese in turn experience more than twice the incidence of

TABLE 157–1. INTERNATIONAL VARIATION IN AGE-ADJUSTED INCIDENCE RATES FOR SELECTED CANCERS

Cancer Site	High-Rate Areas*	Rate†	Baseline Rate‡
Oral cavity	France, India	35–45	1–2
Nasopharynx	China, Hong Kong	30	<1
Esophagus	China, Iran	100+	1–2
Stomach	Japan	80	5
Colon/rectum	U.S., Australia	50–60	6
Liver	China	30	1
Pancreas	U.S. blacks	15	1
Larynx	Brazil	20	2
Lung	U.S. blacks	100	6
Skin melanoma	Australia	30	<1
Breast	U.S.	90	20
Uterine cervix	Brazil, Colombia, India	40–80	4
Ovary	Norway, Pacific Islands	15–25	4
Prostate	U.S. blacks	90	2
Bladder	U.S. whites, Spain	25–30	2
Non-Hodgkin's lymphoma	Switzerland	10	1
Hodgkin's disease	Canada	5	<1
Multiple myeloma	U.S. blacks	10	<1
Leukemia	Canada	12	2–3
Total	U.S. blacks	**400**	**100**

* Country in which high-rate areas occur is listed. The high rates do not necessarily persist throughout the country.
† Approximate age-adjusted (world standard) incidence rate per year per 100,000 population among males (except for breast, cervix, and ovarian cancers). Data collection periods vary by area, but typically center around 1980.
‡ Approximate age-adjusted incidence rate in typical low-rate area.

TABLE 157–2. AGE-ADJUSTED CANCER INCIDENCE RATES* IN THE UNITED STATES, 1986–1990, BY SEX

Cancer Site	Males	Females
Oral and pharynx	16.5	6.2
Esophagus	6.4	1.9
Stomach	11.8	5.0
Small intestine	1.5	1.0
Colon/rectum	59.7	41.2
Gallbladder and biliary	2.2	2.3
Pancreas	10.6	8.0
Larynx	8.1	1.7
Lung	82.6	39.3
Bone	0.9	0.7
Soft tissue	2.5	1.7
Skin melanoma	12.8	9.5
Breast	0.9	108.4
Uterine cervix	—	8.7
Uterus, corpus	—	20.9
Ovary	—	14.3
Prostate	107.7	—
Testis	4.4	—
Bladder	29.4	7.5
Kidney and renal pelvis	11.8	5.9
Eye	0.8	0.5
Brain and nervous system	7.3	5.3
Thyroid	2.5	6.4
Hodgkin's disease	3.3	2.4
Non-Hodgkin's lymphomas	17.1	11.2
Multiple myeloma	5.2	3.6
Leukemia	13.1	7.6
Total	450.4	340.0

* Age-adjusted (1970 U.S. population) incidence rates per year per 100,000 population.

stomach cancer of white Americans. Such differences in rates imply the influence of environmental factors.

The most common cancers in western countries, those of the lung, large bowel, and breast, also vary geographically. Within the United States, the highest rates of lung cancer are now found in the South. In the 1980's lung cancer mortality in southern rural counties surpassed that in northern cities, reversing a longstanding pattern. These shifts follow changes in cigarette smoking, now more prevalent in the south than elsewhere in the country. In addition, certain southern port and coastal areas still maintain excess lung cancer rates among males as a legacy of occupational exposures to asbestos in shipyards during World War II, when shipbuilding was the largest manufacturing industry in the United States. Colon and breast cancer show a contrasting pattern, with high rates in the Northeast and low rates in the South, but the differentials are not large.

U.S. CANCER RATES AND TRENDS. It is estimated that in 1994 1 million Americans will develop and more than 500,000 will die of cancer. Table 157–2 presents age-adjusted incidence rates during 1986 to 1990 for 28 cancers. The data derive from areas of the country participating in the SEER program of cancer registries (covering approximately 10% of the population). Cancer, excluding basal and squamous cell skin cancers, was newly diagnosed in 450 of every 100,000 males and 340 of every 100,000 U.S. females each year during this period. The leading cancers among men are those of the prostate, lung, and colon/rectum, while among women the top three are breast, colon/rectum, and lung. If mortality rather than incidence data are considered, the order shifts. Among males, lung cancer is by far the leading cause of cancer death (74.9 deaths per year per 100,000), followed by colon/rectum (23.9 per 100,000) and prostate (25.0 per 100,000) cancer. Among females, death rates of lung cancer (29.5 per 100,000) now exceed rates for breast (27.4 per 100,000) and colon/rectum (16.3 per 100,000) cancer.

For nearly all cancers, the incidence rates are higher among men than women, the exceptions being gallbladder and thyroid cancers. For some cancers, explanations for the male excess are evident (e.g., higher tobacco and alcohol intake account for most of the higher rates of oral, esophageal, laryngeal, and lung cancer among males), but for others (e.g., stomach cancer, leukemia) the reasons are enigmatic.

Rates of most cancers, particularly those deriving from epithelial tissue, rise steadily with advancing age, often exponentially. Some cancers show a bimodal age distribution. Leukemia and nervous system tumors display an early childhood (age <5 years) peak; then rates decline before rising again in late middle age. Testis cancer occurs primarily between the ages of 20 and 40, while Hodgkin's disease incidence is highest at ages 20 to 30, declines somewhat, then rises again after age 50.

Racial differences in cancer occurrence are sometimes marked. Total cancer incidence during 1986 to 1990 was higher among black than white males by 20%, while rates were higher among white than black females by 5%. The black/white differences among males were particularly pronounced for esophageal, stomach, pancreas, and lung cancer, and multiple myeloma, with age-adjusted incidence from 50 to 300% higher among blacks than whites.

Mortality rates of several cancers have changed over the past decades (Fig. 157–1). Most notable has been the rise in lung cancer. Lung tumors were rarely diagnosed prior to the early 1900's, but incidence and mortality began a steady rise in the 1920's which has continued until today. The epidemic increase in lung cancer, almost entirely attributable to cigarette smoking, has almost ended. Mortality from lung cancer between the mid-1970's and mid-1980's declined by nearly 30% among white males below age 45, with smaller declines affecting white females and nonwhites of both sexes. As younger persons in the U.S. age and their more favorable lung cancer experience extends to older age groups, the overall rates of lung cancer should begin to decline. For white males, the total age-adjusted rates have already plateaued, but the leveling off and subsequent decrease in lung cancer rates among females will not take place until after the year 2000. Rates of stomach and cervical cancers, the leading tumors early in this century, have declined, the former for reasons not yet fully understood, the latter at least in part due to cytologic screening for cervical pathology. The decreases in these tumors are beginning to end, however, and rates of gastric cardia cancer are now rising.

Although not shown in Figure 157–1, there has been nearly a doubling in incidence of melanoma and · a 50% rise in non-Hodgkin's lymphomas among whites since the early 1970's. In addition, the excess among blacks for certain cancers has been increasing. This is occurring for lung, oral, laryngeal, and esophageal cancer. Rates of adenocarcinomas of the esophagus have been rising especially among whites. Reasons for the growing racial disparity are not entirely evident, although higher prevalences of cigarette smoking, heavy alcohol consumption, and nutritional disadvantages are suspect.

THE CAUSES OF CANCER

Cancer is believed to be largely preventable. The causes of most cancers of the oral cavity and pharynx, esophagus, liver, larynx, lung, and uterine cervix are now known. Risk factors also have been identified for other cancers, but the search continues to clarify the factors that account for the bulk of malignancies in the United States and around the world. Most current information on risk factors for cancer has come from case-control studies assessing various characteristics and exposures of patients with individual cancers and from cohort studies determining rates of cancer among groups exposed to particular agents suspected of carcinogenic potential. The leads for these epidemiologic investigations often have arisen from descriptive studies of cancer rates and statistics and from alert clinical observations.

The striking variation in cancer rates within and between countries, the differing rates among migrants from one place to another, and the often marked trends over time suggest that environmental factors induce most cancers, perhaps through interaction with host susceptibility traits. Factors known to be related to the risk of cancer in humans are summarized below.

TOBACCO. Cigarette smoking is the dominant cause of the leading cancer (i.e., lung cancer) in the United States and many other western nations. The association was first suspected by clinical observation that new lung cancer patients were often smokers and then confirmed in the 1950's by case-control and cohort studies in the United States and Great Britain. In the years since the first U.S. Surgeon General's report on smoking in 1964, additional evidence has documented that risks of lung cancer rise in proportion to both duration of smoking and amount smoked per day, with risks of lung cancer more than 20 times greater among long-term heavy smokers than among nonsmokers. Lifelong filter smokers have experienced a somewhat lesser risk than lifelong nonfilter smokers, but the greatest protection comes from smoking cessation. Risks 10 years after quitting are typically only one third or less those of continuing cigarette smokers. Smoking affects all the major types of lung cancers, although squamous and small cell carcinomas more than adenocarcinomas. Cigarette smoking also increases the risk of other cancers. It is a principal cause of cancers of the oral cavity and pharynx, esophagus, larynx, and renal pelvis; is a major contributor to cancers of the pancreas, bladder, and kidney; and is implicated to a moderate degree in cancers of the stomach and uterine cervix. Smokeless tobacco is the predominant cause of buccal mucosa cancers in some populations. In total, tobacco use is thought to account for nearly one third of all cancers in the United States and thus is the largest single preventable cause of cancer.

While the effects of smoking are far greater for smokers themselves, the consensus of evidence from nearly 30 worldwide epidemiologic studies in the past 15 years indicates that long-term exposure to environmental tobacco smoke also increases the risk of lung cancer among nonsmokers. The excess risk of lung cancer among nonsmoking women married to smokers has averaged about 30%. Because of tobacco's harmful effects, efforts to induce smokers to quit and to encourage nonsmokers, particularly adolescents, not to start smoking must be continued. Smoking prevalence among adult men in the United States has declined from a peak of nearly 60% in the 1950's to nearly 25% today. Further reductions are attainable and critical to the nation's public health.

ALCOHOL. Alcohol combines with tobacco to cause cancers of the oral cavity and pharynx, esophagus, and larynx. Alcoholic beverages also have been implicated in the etiology of liver, rectal, and breast cancers, although the latter associations remain to be verified. A large recent case-control study involving over 1100 oral and pharyngeal cancer patients in the United States found that cancer risk increased progressively with increasing intake of alcoholic beverages among nonsmokers as well as smokers. Smoking and drinking multiplied each other's effects so that the risk of oral cancer was increased over 35-fold among two-pack-a-day smokers who consumed more than four alcoholic drinks per day compared with abstainers of both products. Similar tobacco-alcohol interactions have been observed for esophageal and laryngeal cancer. Although not carcinogenic in animal models, ethanol seems likely to be the etiologic agent in humans, since all types of alcoholic beverages—beer, wine, dark and light spirits—have been linked with increased risk in epidemiologic studies.

OCCUPATIONAL HAZARDS. Occupational exposures have long been recognized as causes of cancer, beginning with the observation in the 1700's of scrotal cancer among chimney sweeps in London. Today at least 20 substances in the workplace have been associated with increased cancer risk (Table 157–3). About one-half have been implicated in lung cancer, occasionally in an interactive manner with cigarette smoking. Asbestos exposure accounts for the largest number of occupational cancers. Increased rates of lung cancer and mesothelioma have been found among asbestos miners and millers; factory workers handling asbestos textile and other products; shipyard, railroad, and construction workers; and employees working in other industries which manufacture or use this material. Smoking and asbestos interact to enhance lung cancer risk, so removing either agent significantly lowers the cancer burden.

Radon and its daughter products, another group of potent carcinogens, exist in high levels in underground mines throughout much of the world. Over 20-fold increases of lung cancer have been reported in some groups of radon-exposed miners, most of whom are also smokers, with the excesses most pronounced for small cell anaplastic carcinomas. Several chemicals, including inorganic arsenic, benzene, β-naphthylamine and other aromatic amines, bischloromethylether, mustard gas, certain nickel compounds, and polycyclic hydrocarbons also have induced cancer in exposed workers (Table 157–3). All except arsenic also are carcinogenic in animals, with the carcinogen often (but not always) inducing similar tumors in the animals as in humans.

Among all cancers, those of the nasal cavity and sinuses and the urinary bladder have the highest proportion related to occupational exposures. In a nationwide survey of all nasal adenocarcinomas in Sweden over a recent 19-year period, nearly 25% occurred among

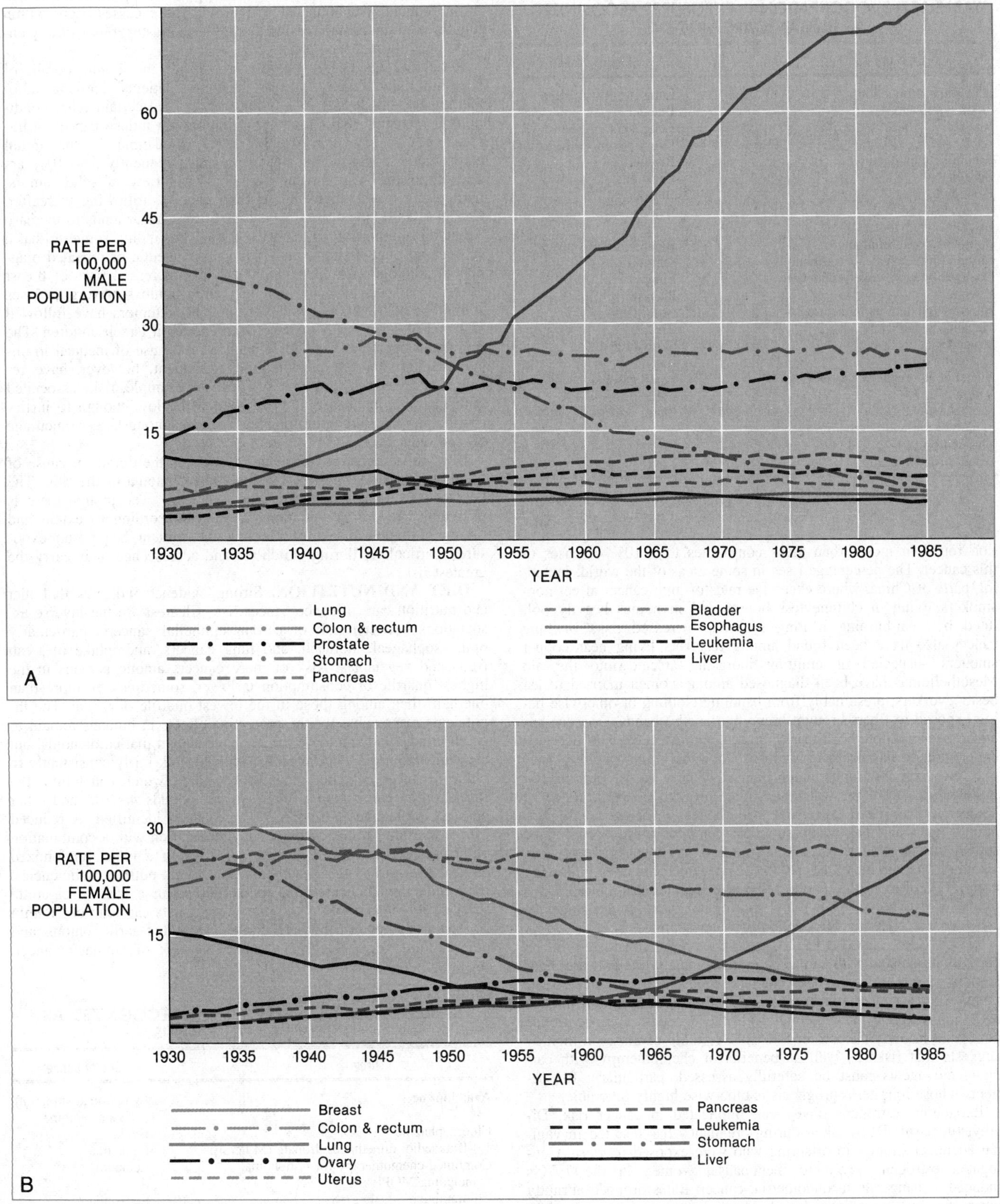

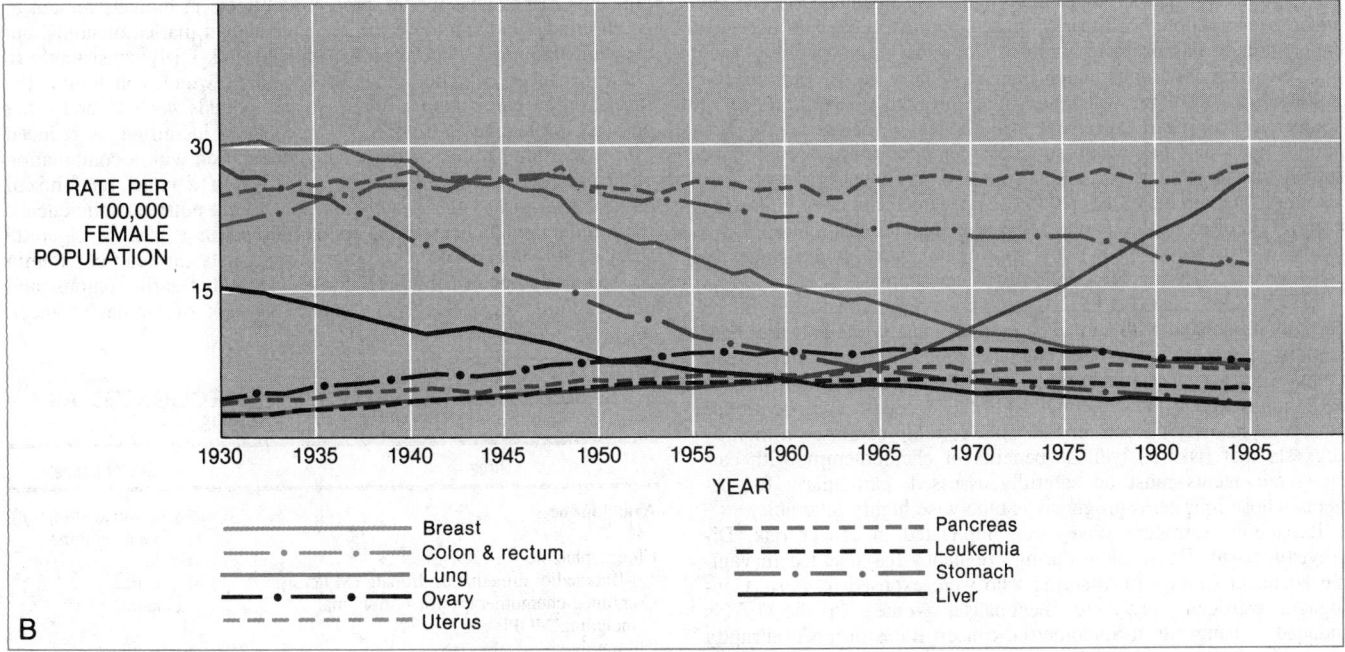

FIGURE 157-1. Trends during 1930–1985 in age-adjusted mortality rates for selected cancers in the United States. (From Boring CC, Squires TS, Tong T: Cancer statistics, 1991. Ca 41:19, 1991.)

furniture makers, possibly as a result of wood dust exposures. It has been estimated that among American men, up to 25% of all bladder cancers are occupationally related. The percentages for other tumors are less, and for all cancers combined, it is generally thought that fewer than 5% have been induced by workplace exposures.

ENVIRONMENTAL POLLUTION. Carcinogens have in some instances been identified in the air we breathe and the water we

drink. Quantifying the effects of air and water pollution has been extremely difficult, however, because of uncertainty over the amount and characteristics of exposures actually received by individuals. Prior to the discovery of the carcinogenic effects of cigarette smoking, air pollution, primarily from combustion products, was thought to be involved in the rise in lung cancer in the U.S. and other countries. It is now believed that the degree of air pollu-

TABLE 157–3. OCCUPATIONAL EXPOSURES RECOGNIZED AS HUMAN CARCINOGENS

Exposure	Site of Cancer
Aluminum production	Lung
4-Aminobiphenyl	Bladder
Arsenic	Lung, skin
Asbestos	Lung, pleura, peritoneum
Auramine manufacture	Bladder
Benzene	Leukemia
Benzidine	Bladder
β-Naphthylamine	Bladder
Bischloromethylether	Lung
Boot and shoe manufacture	Bladder, nasal sinuses
Chromium (hexavalent) compounds	Lung
Coal gasification, coke production	Lung
Erionite	Pleura
Isopropyl alcohol manufacture	Nasal sinuses
Magenta manufacture	Bladder
Mineral oils	Skin, other
Mustard gas	Lung
Nickel compounds	Lung, nasal sinuses
Radon	Lung
Soots, tars, and oils (polycyclic hydrocarbons)	Lung, skin
Vinyl chloride	Liver
Wood dusts (furniture)	Nasal sinuses

tion found in most urban areas contributes to <10% of cases of this cancer. The percentage rises in some areas of the world, including parts of China, where excessive rates of lung cancer affect nonsmokers living in chimneyless houses and in homes heavily polluted by coal-burning heating systems. Increased risks of lung cancer also have been found among residents living near copper smelters suspected of emitting inorganic arsenic into the air. Mesotheliomas have been diagnosed among women married to asbestos workers, presumably from handling clothing or otherwise being exposed to fibers brought home by their husbands. Concern has arisen over possible health risks from much lower levels of asbestos exposure that may occur in homes, schools, and other public places, but few such environmentally induced cancer cases seem likely. Pollutants in drinking water also have aroused concern. Rates of bladder cancer have correlated with levels of halogenated compounds in municipal water supplies; some of these agents have shown carcinogenicity in animal studies. Recent laboratory tests also indicate an increased risk of osteogenic sarcomas following high levels of exposure to fluoride in exposed animals, but epidemiologic investigations have found few or no unexpected changes in cancer rates following fluoridation of water supplies.

MEDICINAL AGENTS. Among chemicals considered to be causally associated with cancer in humans, nearly one-half are medications (Table 157–4). These include drugs used in cancer treatment, especially alkylating agents, which have been found to induce acute nonlymphocytic leukemias and other cancers. The occurrence of second primary cancers in 5 to 10% or more of those on therapy suggests that risks as well as benefits of chemotherapy with carcinogenic agents must be carefully assessed, particularly for patients whose long-term prognosis is otherwise highly favorable.

Exogenous estrogens have been implicated in cancer risk. Diethylstilbestrol (DES) taken during pregnancy has resulted in vaginal adenocarcinomas in offspring who were exposed *in utero*. Conjugated estrogens given to menopausal women in the 1970's induced a rising rate of endometrial cancer. Rates dropped abruptly when the drug was discontinued. The link to breast cancer is less clear, although several investigations have found an increased risk among women receiving long-term estrogen replacement therapy for menopausal symptoms. Extended use of oral contraceptives prior to first pregnancy also has been reported to increase subsequent risk of breast cancer, but the widespread introduction of oral contraceptives in the 1960's has not significantly influenced national rates of breast cancer in the United States. Combined (estrogen plus progestogen) oral contraceptives have been associated with a reduced risk of endometrial and ovarian cancer.

Certain immunosuppressive agents sharply increase risk of cancer. When given to renal transplant recipients, they increase the risk of subsequent lymphomas over 30-fold. The excesses occur within months of immunosuppressive therapy—the fastest onset of any environmentally induced cancer.

RADIATION. Follow-up of survivors of the atomic bombs of Hiroshima and Nagasaki and of groups of patients receiving radiotherapy for ankylosing spondylitis, cancer, and certain other conditions demonstrates that ionizing radiation can induce cancer in humans as it does in lower animals. Leukemia is the initial carcinogenic consequence, occurring most frequently 5 to 10 years after exposure, with increased risks of a variety of solid tumors, particularly breast, thyroid, and lung cancers, following thereafter. Cancer risk for some tumors such as breast cancer tends to increase linearly in proportion to radiation dose. The finding suggests that a similar risk may result from low-dose therapeutic or repeated diagnostic radiologic procedures. Significantly increased risks of breast cancer have been detected among atomic bomb survivors at doses somewhat below 50 rad, and head and neck tumors have followed <10 rad of scalp irradiation for tinea capitis in Israeli children. The findings suggest the need for prudence in the use of medical irradiation. Improvements in radiologic equipment, however, have resulted in lower radiation doses. Thus, for example, risks associated with mammography are now believed to be low enough to justify routine periodic screening for breast cancer among U.S. women age 50 and older.

Ultraviolet radiation from sun exposure is the dominant cause of basal and squamous cell carcinoma and melanoma of the skin. The key to prevention is reduced solar exposure, even though there is uncertainty regarding variations in effect according to extent and timing of exposure. For melanoma, intermittent heavy sun exposures, particularly during childhood and adolescence, may carry the greatest risk.

DIET AND NUTRITION. Strong evidence indicates that diet and nutrition can influence cancer risk. Clearest are the inverse associations between risk of certain epithelial cancers, particularly oral, esophageal, stomach, and lung cancers, and intake of fresh fruits and vegetables. Risk of these cancers among persons in the highest quartile of consumption is lower, sometimes by more than one-half, than among those in the lowest quartile of intake. The ingredients responsible for the protective effects in humans remain to be clarified. Epidemiologic studies have shown that carotenoids, but not animal sources of vitamin A (retinols), link fairly consistently to reduced cancer risk, but vitamins C and E, which can inhibit the formation of carcinogenic N-nitroso compounds *in vivo*, and other possibly protective nutrients also have been identified. A reduced cancer mortality followed daily supplementation with a combination of beta-carotene, vitamin E, and selenium in a large, randomized clinical trial in an area of China with chronic nutrient deficiencies. No similar benefit, however, was observed in a trial of cigarette smokers in Finland taking supplements of beta-carotene or vitamin E. Recent studies in China and Italy suggest that garlic, onions, and other allium vegetables may reduce the risk of stomach cancer.

TABLE 157–4. MEDICINAL AGENTS RECOGNIZED AS HUMAN CARCINOGENS

Drug	Site of Cancer
Azathioprine	Lymphoma, skin, soft tissue sarcoma
Chlornaphazine	Bladder
1,4-Butanediol dimethanesulfonate (Myleran)	Leukemia
Combined chemotherapy for lymphoma, including MOPP*	Leukemia
Chlorambucil	Leukemia
Cyclophosphamide	Leukemia, bladder
Estrogens—conjugated	Endometrium
Estrogens—synthetic (DES)	Vagina, cervix
Estrogens—steroid contraceptives	Benign liver tumors
Melphalan	Leukemia
Methoxsalen with ultraviolet A therapy (PUVA)	Skin
Phenacetin-containing analgesics	Renal pelvis
Treosulfan	Leukemia

* MOPP: procarbazine, nitrogen mustard, vincristine, and prednisone.

Some food contaminants, including aflatoxins sometimes found in moldy peanuts or grains, are strong animal carcinogens. Rates of liver cancer tend to be high in parts of Asia and Africa where aflatoxin contamination is common.

Dietary fat, particularly saturated fat, and calories have been implicated in the risk of colon and other cancers, although the etiologic nature of the associations is still not well established. Dietary fiber has been reported to reduce the risk of colon cancer, but its role vis-à-vis that of other constituents in vegetables, grains, and other fiber-rich foods is not clear. Despite these uncertainties, it has been estimated that a high percentage of colorectal cancers have a dietary etiology. Diet and breast cancer have been linked, in part because of the much higher rates of these cancers in western nations with high-fat, low-fiber diets, but the evidence is inconsistent. In total, some estimates suggest that one third or more of all cancers may be related to dietary and nutritional practices.

INFECTIOUS AGENTS. Several viral agents have been associated with human cancer, particularly cancers of the liver in endemic areas and of the uterine cervix worldwide. Hepatitis B virus (HBV) is the primary cause of hepatocellular carcinoma in China and other areas where infections are prevalent. Prospective follow-up studies show large increases in risk, with nearly all liver cancers arising among persons with prediagnosis HBV surface antigen positivity. The epidemiologic patterns of cervical cancer (with risks elevated among those with multiple sexual partners and/or early age at coitus) have long suggested a venereal component to etiology. Only recently have laboratory techniques enabled detection of human papillomavirus (HPV) as a likely etiologic agent in a high percentage of cases. Herpes simplex virus type 2 has been associated with cervical cancer, but its independent or interactive role with HPV remains to be clarified. The Epstein-Barr virus has been implicated in both nasopharyngeal cancer and Burkitt's lymphoma, while certain human retroviruses have been associated with adult T-cell leukemias in Japan and the Caribbean. The human immunodeficiency virus, the cause of AIDS, is associated not only with Kaposi's sarcomas but also with increased risk of lymphoma among survivors of AIDS.

GENETIC SUSCEPTIBILITY. A history of cancer in the family often increases cancer risk. The increases for common cancers such as those of the lung, colon, and breast are typically on the order of two- to threefold. Shared environmental factors may contribute to the familial clustering, but strong associations among subgroups with early age at onset of cancer or bilateral presentation of breast cancer indicate a genetic predisposition. The most marked genetic effects are seen for skin cancer, with tumors rarely appearing in persons inheriting darkly pigmented skin. A few cancers show mendelian inheritance patterns, including melanomas arising from familial dysplastic nevi and retinoblastomas. In addition, certain hereditary precancerous syndromes have been linked to increased cancer risk. Included are neurofibromatosis and other phacomatoses (associated with nervous system cancer), xeroderma pigmentosum and albinism (skin cancer), ataxia telangiectasia and certain other immunodeficiency syndromes (lymphoma, leukemia, and other cancers), Bloom's syndrome (lymphoma, leukemia, and other cancers), and Fanconi's anemia (leukemia). Investigations of families with unusually large numbers of members with the same or different cancers have provided insight into genetic patterns. In larger epidemiologic studies, increasing attention is being paid to systematic evaluations of genetic factors as reliable markers of host susceptibility become available. Lung cancer risk, for example, has recently been associated with the genetically controlled ability to metabolize the antihypertensive drug debrisoquine. Information on susceptibility factors will be crucial in understanding the mechanisms of carcinogenesis as well as delineating groups and individuals at high risk for targeted interventions.

International Agency for Research on Cancer: Overall Evaluations of Carcinogenicity: An updating of IARC Monographs Volumes 1 to 42. Monographs on the Evaluation of Carcinogenic Risks to Humans. Supplement 7. Lyon, World Health Organization, 1987. *A systematic review of epidemiologic and experimental evidence regarding carcinogenicity of over 150 substances.*

Miller RA, Ries LA, Hankey BF, et al. (eds.): Cancer Statistics Review 1973–1990. Bethesda, MD, US Department of Health and Human Services, NIH Publication No. 93-2789, 1993. *Up-to-date listing of cancer incidence, mortality, and survival rates in the United States.*

Schottenfeld D, Fraumeni JF Jr (eds.): Cancer Epidemiology and Prevention, 2nd ed. Oxford, Oxford University Press (in press). *A comprehensive review of cancer epidemiology, with individual chapters assessing cancers and causative agents, as well as basic concepts in cancer etiology and control.*

158 SYSTEMIC SECRETIONS OF CANCER CELLS AND THEIR EFFECTS

158.1 Paraneoplastic Syndromes

Kenneth R. Meehan and Marc S. Ernstoff

Paraneoplastic syndromes represent a constellation of signs and symptoms that result from distant effects by tumor on various body systems. These "remote" signs and symptoms may result from the production and release of ectopic hormones or growth factors, the development of autoimmunity or other as-yet-unknown factors. Many paraneoplastic syndromes are related to the excess production of hormones, creating a symptom complex indistinguishable from primary endocrine diseases. Successful treatment of these malignancies is associated with dramatic improvement in the paraneoplastic syndrome.

In general, paraneoplastic syndromes, except for cachexia, are rare. Recognition of a paraneoplastic syndrome alerts the clinician to a new diagnosis of cancer or the recurrence of a prior malignancy. The diagnosis of a paraneoplastic syndrome, such as dermatomyositis, or the discovery of specific autoantibodies in the serum may direct the patient's evaluation and treatment. Paraneoplastic syndromes may cause signs and symptoms that can be confused with the direct effects of the primary tumor or metastases, infection, toxicity of therapy, and comorbid illnesses. Thus, it is important that a correct diagnosis be made, allowing for the institution of appropriate cancer-directed treatment and symptomatic therapy.

The presentation, pathophysiology, diagnosis, and treatment of the more important paraneoplastic syndromes are described on a system basis (Table 158–1).

PARANEOPLASTIC NEUROLOGIC SYNDROMES

Although paraneoplastic involvement of the nervous system can result in debilitating disorders, they are often a diagnosis of exclusion. Some of the more common syndromes include myasthenia gravis, Eaton-Lambert syndrome, paraneoplastic cerebellar degeneration, and paraneoplastic eye syndromes.

MYASTHENIA GRAVIS (MG). *Presentation.* Although thymoma is the most common malignancy seen with MG, extrathoracic malignancies include leukemia, lymphomas, sarcomas, and tumors of the breast, lung, thyroid, skin, and gastrointestinal tract.

TABLE 158–1. PARANEOPLASTIC SYNDROMES

1. Endocrine	See Ch. 159
2. Neurologic	See Ch. 160
3. Dermatologic and arthritic	See Ch. 161
4. Renal	Glomerular abnormalities miscellaneous: amyloidosis, myeloma, kidney. See Ch. 79
5. Hematologic	Erythrocytosis, thrombocytosis, leukemoid reaction, anemia (chronic disease, aplastic anemia, microangiopathic hemolytic anemia), granulocytopenia and thrombocytopenia
6. Coagulation	Disseminated intravascular coagulation, superficial venous thromboembolus, marantic endocarditis and thrombotic microangiopathy
7. Miscellaneous	Hepatopathy, cancer-related cachexia

MG may present at any time during the course of a malignancy. Fifty percent or more of patients with MG possess gross or microscopic thymomas.

Pathophysiology. MG is an autoimmune disorder characterized by the production of antibodies directed against the acetylcholine receptor on the motor endplates within the synaptic junction. The deficiency of acetylcholine receptor results in episodic muscle weakness and fatigue, often involving muscles innervated by the cranial nerves, commonly resulting in ocular or bulbar manifestations. Patients often complain of progressive fatigue and blurred vision due to ptosis.

Diagnosis. The diagnosis of MG is based upon the clinical presentation of episodic muscle weakness, especially of the ocular and bulbar areas. A comprehensive physical examination should be performed, with attention to the breast, pelvis, and rectum. Although proximal muscle weakness can also be seen with Eaton-Lambert syndrome, sensation and deep tendon reflexes are preserved in MG. Clinical and laboratory tests that confirm the diagnosis of MG include improvement of muscle strength on physical examination with anticholinesterases such as edrophonium or neostigmine (Tensilon test), progressive decrease in amplitude of the muscle action potential upon repetitive electrical stimulation on electromyography (EMG) testing, and autoantibodies against the acetylcholine receptor. Radiographic evaluation of the mediastinum should be performed to evaluate the presence of a thymoma.

Treatment. Because MG is a syndrome caused by the deficiency of acetylcholine receptors, anticholinesterase inhibitors, such as pyridostigmine or neostigmine, maintain an elevated level of acetylcholine in the synaptic cleft and may improve symptoms. Thymectomy may benefit the majority of patients, although results vary widely. The prognosis after thymectomy may be based on the stage of the thymoma and not the presence of the associated syndrome of MG nor the duration of MG symptoms preoperatively. Other treatments include plasmapheresis, steroids, or cytotoxic drugs.

EATON-LAMBERT SYNDROME (ELS). *Presentation.* ELS is characterized by proximal muscle weakness in the legs, arms, and pelvic girdle, in association with reduced or absent deep tendon reflexes. Autonomic dysfunction is common (dry mouth, impotence, and peripheral paresthesias). Unlike MG, ELS generally spares the ocular and bulbar muscles. The onset of ELS may precede the diagnosis of cancer by up to 4 years.

Pathophysiology. Seventy percent of patients with ELS have an underlying malignancy, most commonly small cell carcinoma of the lung. A defective release of acetylcholine at the presynaptic nerve terminal, possibly due to autoantibodies to presynaptic voltage-gated calcium channels, results in a decreased amount of acetylcholine within the synaptic cleft.

Diagnosis. The diagnosis of ELS should be suspected in any patient presenting with proximal muscle weakness in association with autonomic dysfunction. The physical examination demonstrates minimal cranial nerve involvement and decrease or loss of deep tendon reflexes. An EMG reveals an increased muscle response to each stimulation secondary to accumulation of acetylcholine in the synaptic cleft. There is a poor response to the Tensilon test. The diminished deep tendon reflexes, minimal cranial nerve involvement, the results of EMG and the Tensilon test, as well as the absence of antiacetylcholine receptor antibody, distinguish ELS from MG.

Treatment. In malignancy-associated ELS, treatment should be directed at the primary cancer. Guanidine hydrochloride is a medication that may improve symptoms by increasing acetylcholine release. 4-Aminopyridine has been used but is associated with central nervous system (CNS) abnormalities including confusion and seizures. Plasmapheresis/plasma exchange and immune therapy (azathioprine, glucocorticoids) have also been used.

PARANEOPLASTIC CEREBELLAR DEGENERATION (PCD). *Presentation.* Although CNS paraneoplastic syndromes are rare, PCD is probably the most common. Patients present with progressive cerebellar dysfunction manifested as symmetric ataxia, dysarthria, and nystagmus. The onset of this syndrome generally precedes but may coincide with the diagnosis of various malignancies, including gynecologic tumors, breast cancer, bronchogenic cancer, and lymphoma.

Pathophysiology. PCD appears to be associated with autoantibodies specific to antigens on the surface of tumor cells and neuronal cells of the CNS (Purkinje cells or cerebellar cells), although their role in the pathogenesis of PCD is uncertain. These autoantibodies (anti-Yo with specificity to a Purkinje cell 62-kD antigen and anti-Hu with specificity to a cerebral cortex neuronal 35- to 40-kD antigen) may be found in serum or cerebrospinal fluid.

The clinical behavior of patients affected with PCD depends upon the presence or absence and type of autoantibody. For example, patients with the anti-Yo antibody are generally women who have a gynecologic malignancy, with the onset of CNS symptoms generally preceding the diagnosis of cancer. Patients with PCD without autoantibodies may be of either gender and harbor various malignancies, and CNS symptoms appear after the diagnosis of cancer.

Diagnosis. A diagnosis of PCD must be suspected in any patient who presents with signs and symptoms of progressive cerebellar deterioration occurring over a short period of time. Patients suspected of having PCD should have both serum and CSF evaluated for the presence of appropriate autoantibody.

Treatment. Pathologically, this disease involves a progressive loss of neurons in the CNS. As a result, any treatment benefit usually results in stabilization of neurologic deficits without improvement. After some patients are cured of their malignancy, the autoantibodies may persist in the serum, despite the lack of neurologic progression. Treatment options include treating the underlying malignancy, plasmapheresis, and immunosuppression with steroids, gamma globulin, and pulse cyclophosphamide.

PARANEOPLASTIC EYE SYNDROMES (PES). PES include opsoclonus-myoclonus (OM) and cancer-associated retinopathy (CAR), which are associated with an immune response to autoantigens. The symptoms of OM include diplopia, blurred vision, and oscillopsia, with physical finding of opsoclonus, myoclonus of the head, trunk and limbs, hyperreflexia, dysmetria, ataxia, and equivocal Babinski signs. The syndrome is associated with antineuronal antibodies (anti-Ri) which react with a 53- to 59-kD and a 68- to 76-kD antigen found in cerebral cortical neuronal nuclear extracts. OM can be seen with breast cancer and gynecologic malignancies. CAR presents with visual symptoms and rapidly progresses to bilateral, unexplained vision loss. Optic atrophy can be seen on the funduscopic examination. CAR has been associated with an autoantibody reactive to a 23-kD retinal antigen ("recoverin").

SKIN AND JOINT INVOLVEMENT

DERMATOMYOSITIS/POLYMYOSITIS (DM/PM). *Presentation.* Both DM and PM are idiopathic inflammatory myopathies characterized by proximal symmetrical muscle weakness, evidence of myositis on muscle biopsy, elevated serum muscle enzymes, and abnormal electromyographic changes. In addition, DM possesses characteristic skin changes. Although PM has been considered "dermatomyositis without the rash," this is probably incorrect and improperly assumes similar causes. The association of malignancy with DM/PM is controversial. The incidence ranges from 10 to 50% and increases with age.

Pathophysiology. Although DM/PM can exist in the absence of malignancy, the association of cancer with these disorders may result from an altered immune system. Recent data suggest that DM may be due to humorally mediated capillary necrosis. PM is thought to occur through T cell–mediated inflammation causing destruction of muscle fibers. Other possible causes of these syndromes include complement activation, infection, drugs, stress, and vaccines.

Diagnosis. The chief complaint at presentation is generally progressive proximal muscle weakness, and, in the case of DM, skin rash. The striated muscles of the esophagus can be involved, resulting in dysphagia. The characteristic skin changes of DM include a symmetrical rash surrounding the eyelids (heliotrope rash); plaques or papules over joints, especially the knuckles (Gottron's papules); and nail changes including cuticle hypertrophy or periungual telangiectasias.

The differential diagnosis of DM/PM includes MG, muscular dystrophy, endocrinopathies, and central or peripheral neurologic disease. Serum enzymes of muscle tissues (creatinine kinase or aldolase) are elevated, and electromyographic studies are confirmatory. A biopsy of the affected muscle group reveals perivascular and muscle fiber inflammatory infiltrates comprised of lymphocytes and macrophages. In addition to joints and skin involvement, other affected organ systems include lung, heart, gastrointestinal tract, and kidney.

The great majority of malignancies are found with a simple screening physical examination, routine blood tests, stool guaiac, urinalysis, chest radiography, and mammography in females.

Treatment. Whether the course of DM/PM is affected by treatment of the underlying disease is debated. The use of immunosuppressive agents may be useful. The development of DM/PM may herald the recurrence of a pre-existing malignancy.

SWEET'S SYNDROME (SS). ***Presentation.*** Sweet's syndrome, also known as acute febrile neutrophilic dermatosis, consists of fever, neutrophilia, and rash. The rash, made up of tender red or bluish firm papules or nodules, may coalesce to form irregular border plaques and may be asymmetrically located on the upper extremities. A biopsy reveals a diffuse infiltrate of mature neutrophils in the superficial dermis. Ten to 20% of patients with SS have an underlying malignancy, most commonly a hematologic malignancy such as acute leukemia and rarely cancers of the genitourinary tract, breast, and gastrointestinal tract. SS may precede, coincide with, or follow the diagnosis of a malignancy.

Pathophysiology. Skin lesions of SS, with its associated neutrophilia and fever, may represent a hypersensitivity reaction to an infection. Of note, the benign or idiopathic form of SS often follows a respiratory infection, and when associated with *Yersinia enterocolitica* SS improves with antibiotic therapy.

Although the cause of SS is unknown, nonspecific cytokine stimulation by granulocyte colony stimulating factor (G-CSF), granulocyte-macrophage colony stimulating factor (GM-CSF), interleukin (IL)-1, IL-4, and IL-8 can result in recruitment and proliferation of polymorphonuclear cells. Case reports have identified SS in patients receiving recombinant G-CSF. Circulating antibodies to neutrophilic cytoplasmic antigens have been detected in some patients, but their role is controversial. •

Diagnosis. Not all patients possess the classic triad of rash, temperature, and neutrophilia. Specific skin findings associated with malignancy-associated SS include bullous or ulcerated lesions and/or oral lesions. There are rare reports of kidney, lung, and liver involvement in this syndrome. SS may precede the diagnosis of malignancy by 1 year or herald the recurrence of a pre-existing malignancy. Owing to the high prevalence of leukemia, patients should undergo a thorough hematologic evaluation with continued follow-up. Associated laboratory and pathologic findings include elevated sedimentation rate, anemia, thrombocytopenia, and skin lesion revealing diffuse or perivascular neutrophil infiltration in the lower dermis.

Treatment. SS is generally a self-limited process if left untreated. The treatment of choice is steroids, often resulting in a complete remission within days. Treatment of the underlying disease or the administration of oral potassium iodide or colchicine has been successful.

ACANTHOSIS NIGRICANS (AN). ***Presentation.*** AN is a rare dermatologic syndrome characterized by symmetrical dark hyperpigmentation and thickening of the skin involving intertriginous areas of the body. Malignancy-associated AN has a sudden onset, spreads rapidly, and is generally associated with abdominal adenocarcinomas, most commonly of the gastrointestinal tract.

Pathophysiology. A possible role of insulin is suggested by the association of insulin resistance and AN. Transforming growth factor-α (TGF-α) and EGF have been implemented as causes of AN as well.

Diagnosis. Hyperpigmented skin lesions in the intertriginous areas are characteristic of AN. Oral lesions may be more common with malignancy-associated AN. A biopsy reveals hyperkeratosis, papillary hypertrophy, and increased melanin pigmentation in the stratum corneum.

Treatment. The malignancies associated with AN often behave aggressively. AN may or may not improve with the treatment of the underlying tumor. Topical steroids, retinoids, and podophyllin have been attempted with some success.

ERYTHEMA GYRATUM REPENS (EGR). ***Presentation.*** EGR involves serpiginous, whirled concentric erythematous bands that appear on the trunk and extremities of patients, most commonly those with lung and breast cancer. The lesions advance rapidly, sometimes centimeters daily, and may appear at any time during the clinical course.

Pathophysiology. Autoantibodies against skin antigens and immune complex deposition into the skin have been implicated as causes of EGR.

Diagnosis and Treatment. The clinical appearance is sufficient to make the diagnosis. Approximately half of the patients describe pruritus. Laboratory evaluation may demonstrate eosinophilia, and histologic features are often nonspecific. The differential diagnosis includes erythema chronicum migrans, lupus erythematosus, and psoriasis.

Treatment of the cancer with chemotherapy or irradiation has resulted in resolution of the skin lesions. Radiation therapy directed at the skin lesion and topical/systemic steroids have been used.

BAZEX'S SYNDROME (BS). Bazex's syndrome, or acrokeratosis paraneoplastica, is a syndrome associated with symmetrical distal erythematosquamous eruptions affecting the ears, nails, nose, fingers, palms, soles, toes, knees, elbows, cheeks, trunk, and scalp (descending order), and nail dystrophy. It is always associated with an underlying malignancy, most commonly squamous cell carcinomas of the upper aerodigestive tract. BS may precede overt malignancy by months or several years. The skin lesions disappear with successful treatment of the underlying cancer.

Two possible causes for this syndrome are growth factor production by the tumor and immunoglobulin deposition in the basal cell layer and basement membrane zone of the skin.

PARANEOPLASTIC PEMPHIGUS (PP). The term *paraneoplastic pemphigus* was first coined in 1990 by Anhalt and colleagues in a report of five patients presenting with painful mucosal ulcerations and polymorphous blistering skin eruptions on the trunk and extremities. PP has been associated with non-Hodgkin's lymphoma, chronic lymphocytic leukemia, thymomas, poorly differentiated spindle cell sarcomas, and extragonadal germ cell tumor. Histopathology of these lesions reveals vacuolization of epidermal basal cells, keratinocyte necrosis, acantholysis, and autoantibodies in the serum and perilesional epithelium. Autoantibodies have specificity to desmoplakin I and the 230-kD bullous pemphigoid antigen.

ERYTHRODERMA OR EXFOLIATIVE DERMATITIS (ED). The clinical signs of patients with erythroderma or exfoliative dermatitis include a generalized erythematous rash, usually sparing the palms and soles; minimal to severe exfoliation; dystrophic nails; alopecia; lower extremity edema; and hepatosplenomegaly. Associated symptoms include malaise, pruritus, and changes in body temperature.

Two forms exist. The nonparaneoplastic form of ED is characterized by direct malignant skin involvement (e.g., cutaneous T cell lymphoma and Sézary syndrome). The paraneoplastic form is associated with Hodgkin's disease, non-Hodgkin's lymphoma, leukemia, and myelodysplasia. The association of solid tumors with ED is less certain.

ACQUIRED ICHTHYOSIS (AI). AI is characterized by small whitish brown scales on the trunk and extensor surfaces of the legs and arms and is indistinguishable from the autosomal dominant ichthyosis vulgaris. The histopathologic characteristics include hyperkeratosis, parakeratosis, thinning of the granular layer, acanthosis, and a mild perivascular lymphohistiocytic infiltrate. Paraneoplastic AI is most commonly associated with Hodgkin's disease and can be seen in patients with lymphomas and leukemias as well as solid tumors (sarcomas, breast cancer, bronchogenic carcinoma, and cervical carcinoma).

PITYRIASIS ROTUNDA (PR). PR is characterized as round, slightly scaly, hyperpigmented lesions located on the trunk, buttocks, and thighs. Although it may be associated with a number of illnesses, including tuberculosis, dysentery, and malnutrition, it is also rarely seen in association with hepatocellular carcinoma, gastric carcinoma, squamous cell carcinomas of the upper aerodigestive tract, leukemia, and multiple myeloma.

TRIPE PALMS (TP) OR ACANTHOSIS NIGRICANS OF THE PALMS. In TP, the palms of the hands develop a velvety thickened appearance resembling the foregut of the cow (tripe). TP is commonly found in association with acanthosis nigricans or other cutaneous paraneoplastic syndromes. It has been most commonly associated with bronchogenic carcinoma and gastric carcinoma and less commonly with breast cancer, head and neck cancers, and genitourinary cancers. Elevated levels of growth hormone have been reported in some of the patients with malignancy-associated TP.

LESER-TRÉLAT (LT) SYNDROME. The eruptive appearance of multiple seborrheic keratoses is known as the sign of Leser-Trélat after the first description of the syndrome by Leser and Trélat in 1890. LT is seen predominantly in elderly patients and is associated with adenocarcinoma of the gastrointestinal tract as well as other internal malignancies and lympoproliferative disorders. Reports suggest that LT is related to the production of cytokines such as tumor-specific epidermal growth factor, insulin-like growth factor, and transforming growth factor-α.

PULMONARY OSTEOARTHROPATHY (POA)

Presentation. The clinical scenario of POA consists of symmetric clubbing of nails, active synovitis, and periosteal inflammation of the long bones. This syndrome is generally seen with lung carcinoma (non–small cell lung histologies) but has also been described with metastatic lung lesions, nonpulmonary malignancies, and a number of nonmalignant conditions.

Pathophysiology. The development of POA may be based upon two components: a neurogenic vascular component and a humorally mediated osteogenic element. A vagotomy partially reverses some symptoms, supporting the neurogenic vascular cause. Other possible causes include an immune-mediated response or release of growth factor(s) by the tumor.

Diagnosis. The classic triad of clubbing, synovitis, and periostitis may appear at different times in the clinical course. Although the joints of the lower extremities may be painful, red, and swollen, the physical examination may reveal that the "arthritis" is discomfort due to pain in the adjacent long bone, especially the distal radius/ulna and tibia/fibula. Plain radiographs may reveal the periosteal elevations. Bone scans appear to be more sensitive than plain radiographs and may confirm the diagnosis.

POA can be differentiated from metastatic bone disease or rheumatoid arthritis by the symmetrical bilateral finding and the absence of rheumatoid factor.

Treatment. The presence of POA does not alter the prognosis of a patient with a malignancy. Because POA is not life-threatening, treatment is often palliative. Arthritic symptoms may be treated with aspirin and/or nonsteroidal anti-inflammatory drugs. A vagotomy often results in analgesia within days to weeks. Atropine may also be helpful. Surgery of the primary malignancy may improve articular complaints, sometimes within hours. Chemotherapy or radiation therapy directed at the tumor may provide a gradual beneficial effect.

RENAL PARANEOPLASTIC SYNDROMES

Nephrotic syndrome in the setting of malignancy can be due to direct involvement of cancer in the kidney, renal vein thrombosis, or paraneoplastic syndrome. Paraneoplastic nephrotic syndrome (PNS) usually improves dramatically when the underlying malignancy is successfully treated. PNS is most commonly seen in association with Hodgkin's disease and is usually characterized by lipoid nephrosis (minimal glomerular nephrosis). Other glomerular lesions occurring in approximately 20% of PNS include membranous glomerulopathy, focal sclerosis, and membranoproliferative glomerulonephritis and may be associated with non-Hodgkin's lymphoma, colon cancer, bronchogenic carcinoma, and prostate cancer. Deposition of tumor-associated antigen-antibody complexes has been identified in membranous glomerulonephritis. It has been suggested that lipoid nephrosis may be caused by deficient T lymphocyte function.

PARANEOPLASTIC ENDOCRINE SYNDROMES

Two of the more common endocrine paraneoplastic syndromes are hypercalcemia and the syndrome of inappropriate secretion of antidiuretic hormone (SIADH).

HYPERCALCEMIA. Presentation. Paraneoplastic hypercalcemia (PHC) is characterized by the production of tumor-related molecules, which increase serum calcium levels by affecting calcium metabolism in the bones, kidneys, and gastrointestinal tract. Although any malignancy can be associated with this syndrome, the most common include breast cancer, renal cell carcinoma, squamous cell carcinomas (lung and upper aerodigestive tract), ovarian cancer, and multiple myeloma. Clinically occult cancer can cause this syndrome.

Pathophysiology. Parathyroid hormone–related peptide (PTHrP) plays a critical role in the development of PHC in many cancers. This peptide has been isolated and characterized. It shares 70% homology with the PTH molecule in the amino-terminal region, the binding site to receptors in the kidney and bone. PTHrP is produced in low amounts by nonmalignant tissues, including squamous epithelial cells and smooth and skeletal muscle cells and likely acts as a regulator of cell growth. PTHrP acts alone, synergistically, or additively with other humoral factors such as 1,25-dihydroxyvitamin D, IL-1, IL-6, tumor necrosis factor-α, TGF-α and β, leukemia inhibitory factor, GM-CSF, and prostaglandin E_2, resulting in hypercalcemia.

Diagnosis. Hypercalcemia from any cause can cause dysfunction of the heart (prolonged QT interval), gastrointestinal tract (nausea, vomiting, cachexia, and constipation), kidney (polyuria), and neuromuscular system (muscle weakness, fatigue, and coma). The onset of signs and symptoms depends upon the absolute level of the calcium and the rapidity with which this level was achieved. Laboratory data associated with PHC include a normal or low PTH level, a normal or low 1,25-dihydroxyvitamin D level, a mild metabolic alkalosis, and increased urinary cyclic AMP levels. In addition to the hypercalcemia, hypercalciuria, hypophosphatemia, and hyperphosphaturia, are present. PTH can be distinguished from PTHrP by carboxy- and amino-terminal PTH assays. Elevated PTHrP can occur in patients without a cancer and normal serum calcium levels.

Treatment. Because hypercalcemia can cause nausea and vomiting with polyuria, patients are generally dehydrated at presentation. Initial efforts should be directed at promoting euvolemia with normal saline hydration. Hydration improves glomerular filtration and promotes calcium excretion. Furosemide may be added once euvolemia has been achieved in an attempt to improve calcium excretion. Inhibition of bone resorption can be promoted with a number of agents, including bisphosphonates (etidronate, pamidronate), mithramycin, calcitonin, glucocorticoids, and gallium nitrite. The best therapy is treatment directed at the underlying disease. Nutritional supplements containing calcium need not be avoided because gastrointestinal absorption of calcium does not play a major role.

SYNDROME OF INAPPROPRIATE RELEASE OF ANTIDIURETIC HORMONE (SIADH). Presentation. Small cell carcinoma of the lung accounts for the majority of patients with inappropriate production of antidiuretic hormone (ADH) or vasopressin and can also be seen in other malignant and nonmalignant conditions (pulmonary and CNS processes). A number of commonly used medications in oncology, including narcotics, tricyclic antidepressants, and chemotherapy (vincristine, vinblastine, cyclophosphamide), have been associated with SIADH.

Pathophysiology. The body's fluid balance is governed by the sodium ion transfer under tight regulation of ADH. Inappropriate production of ADH results in hyponatremia, resulting in weakness, lethargy, fatigue, or coma.

Diagnosis. The patient with SIADH is generally euvolemic on physical examination and shows no signs of fluid overload or dehydration. Abnormal neurologic signs associated with hyponatremia may be present. Factitious hyponatremia should be considered and is due to elevated levels of triglycerides, protein, or glucose or excessive free water intake. The diagnosis of SIADH is made only in the setting of normal thyroid and adrenal function, and euvolemia by the observation of a low serum sodium, low serum osmolality, urine osmolality greater than serum osmolality, and an elevated urinary excretion of sodium.

Treatment. SIADH is best managed with treatment of the underlying tumor. Hyponatremia is initially treated by fluid restriction in an attempt to promote a gradual improvement in the patient's serum osmolality. Hypertonic saline (3%) can be used in life-threatening situations. Demeclocycline, a medication that creates nephrogenic diabetes insipidus, has also been used.

PARANEOPLASTIC HEMATOLOGIC DISORDERS

Paraneoplastic hematologic disorder can be quite diverse and includes clotting or bleeding abnormalities, erythrocytosis, leukemoid reaction, and thrombocytosis.

COAGULATION ABNORMALITIES. Presentation. The interaction of components of the coagulation cascade and tumor cells is intricate and complex, resulting in many effects, including thrombotic and hemorrhagic tendencies. Systemic activation of coagulation may result in disseminated intravascular coagulation (DIC), superficial venous thromboembolus (Trousseau syndrome), marantic endocarditis, or thrombotic microangiopathy. Although abnor-mal coagulation parameters are seen frequently in patients with malignancies, the relationship to signs and symptoms of coagula-tion abnormalities is often unrelated and the significance unknown.

Pathophysiology. Tumor cells may release procoagulant materials such as tissue factor–like substances, cytokines that activate Factor X, sialic acid portion of secreted mucin, or "thromboplastin-like" substances. Tumor-stimulated monocyte/macrophage may release procoagulant materials. Tumor cell–activated platelets result in adhesion and aggregation, thereby forming the nidus for clot formation as well as stimulating the intricate system of platelet–tumor cell interaction.

Diagnosis. Although mixed opinion exists with regard to the relationship of occult malignancy and thrombosis, about 10% of patients with a new thrombotic event are subsequently found to harbor cancer. Signs or symptoms suggestive of underlying malignancy and migratory or recurrent thrombophlebitis should precipitate a search for an occult cancer. It is important to rule out inherited clotting disorders, such as deficiencies of protein C, protein S, antithrombin III, dysfibrinogenemia, and plasminogen deficiency, which may appear in young patients (i.e., age 20 to 40) and can result in recurrent thrombosis in unusual locations.

Treatment. The initiation of anticoagulation therapy in any patient with cancer should take into consideration increased risk of hemorrhage due to a tumor invading blood vessels or the presence of CNS metastasis. Treatment is often initiated with heparin, followed by warfarin. Others advocate using aspirin and dipyridamole. The most effective therapy is directed at the underlying disease.

PARANEOPLASTIC LEUKEMOID REACTION (PLR). A leukemoid reaction is defined as a peripheral white blood cell count of greater than 20,000 cells per milliliter without evidence of either infection or leukemia. PLR should be differentiated from leukoerythroblastosis secondary to malignant involvement of the bone marrow. PLR is observed in a variety of solid tumors and can be associated with fever. G-CSF production has been observed in a number of different malignancies (malignant fibrous histiocytoma, nasopharyngeal carcinoma, transitional cell carcinoma of the urinary bladder) and is likely the cause of PLR. Clinically, the diagnosis of PLR is made by exclusion. The treatment for PLR involves therapy directed at the underlying malignancy.

CANCER-ASSOCIATED ERYTHROCYTOSIS (CAE) AND ANEMIA (CAA). CAE is most frequently seen in malignant and benign conditions of the kidney (renal cell carcinoma, Wilms' tumor, cystic kidney, and hydronephrosis). Other malignant and benign conditions associated with CAE include hepatoma, cerebellar hemangioblastoma, pheochromocytoma, sarcomas, and uterine fibroids. This paraneoplastic syndrome is most commonly associated with increased levels of endogenous erythropoietin but in some cases can be seen secondary to overproduction of androgens, prostaglandins, and other unidentified substances.

CAA is much more common in the setting of malignancy and may be secondary to chronic disease, red cell aplasia, bone marrow invasion, blood loss, chemotherapy, radiation therapy, nutritional deficiencies, and autoimmune and microangiopathic hemolysis. Pure red cell aplasia is most frequently associated with thymoma. Autoimmune hemolytic anemia is seen in association with B-cell lymphomas and rarely with solid tumors. Chemotherapy may directly affect the marrow or, in the case of cisplatin, cause a reduction of endogenous erythropoietin production. Treatment for chemotherapy-induced anemia with recombinant erythropoietin is successful in 30 to 40% of cases.

CANCER-ASSOCIATED THROMBOCYTOSIS (CAT). A true paraneoplastic CAT is seen in patients with Hodgkin's disease, non-Hodgkin's lymphoma, leukemias, and other solid malignancies and may be related to the overproduction of thrombopoietin(s).

MISCELLANEOUS PARANEOPLASTIC SYNDROMES

PARANEOPLASTIC HEPATOPATHY. *Introduction.* Paraneoplastic hepatopathy, also known as Stauffer syndrome, is characterized by hepatic dysfunction, fever, and weight loss and is most commonly seen in nonmetastatic renal cell carcinoma.

Pathophysiology. The cause of Stauffer syndrome is uncertain but likely involves an autoimmune process directed at hepatic cells or substances released by the tumor, resulting in elevated liver enzymes and hepatic dysfunction.

Diagnosis. Patients often present with fever and weight loss, in addition to hepatomegaly, elevated transaminases, and poor liver synthesizing ability (indicated by elevated prothrombin time). Hematologic abnormalities, such as thrombocytosis, may also exist. A liver biopsy may reveal Kupffer cell hyperplasia with fairly nonspecific inflammatory changes.

Treatment. In the presence of nonmetastatic hypernephroma, treatment directed at the primary lesion generally results in resolution of the syndrome. If signs or symptoms persist, an evaluation for metastatic disease should be initiated.

TUMOR-RELATED CACHEXIA. Most patients with cancer ultimately develop cachexia. Cachexia in the cancer patient is likely due to multiple factors, including change in taste and smell resulting in decreased caloric intake, loss of protein through effusions and hemorrhage, gastrointestinal obstruction, malabsorption, increased metabolic activity, and treatment-related nausea, vomiting, and appetite loss. Tumor-secreted factors like TNF-α, also known as cachexin, inhibit lipogenic enzymes, and contribute to the wasting syndrome. The resulting cachexia may be out of proportion to the size of the underlying malignancy.

Therapy is directed at the underlying malignancy and supplemental alimentation when appropriate (e.g., surgical candidates, patients with significant likelihood of response to treatment). High doses of the progestational hormone megestrol acetate have been shown to improve appetite in a significant percentage of cancer patients.

Davies RA, Darby M, Richards MA: Hypertrophic pulmonary osteoarthropathy in pulmonary metastatic disease. A case report and review of the literature. Clin Radiol 43:268, 1991.
Patel AH, Davila DG, Peters SG: Paraneoplastic syndromes associated with lung cancer. Mayo Clin Proc 68:278, 1993. *A review of the paraneoplastic syndromes associated with bronchogenic carcinoma and proposed mechanisms.*
Posner JB: Pathogenesis of central nervous system paraneoplastic syndromes. Rev Neurol 148:502, 1992. *Reviews pathogenesis of CNS paraneoplastic syndromes including hypothesis that these syndromes are immune disorders arising from an immune response to the underlying neoplasm.*
Prandoni P, Lensing AWA, Buller HR, et al: Deep-vein thrombosis and the incidence of subsequent symptomatic cancer. N Engl J Med 327:1128, 1992. *Presents a study of deep-vein thrombosis patients assessed for subsequent development of underlying malignancy.*
Sigurgeirsson B, Lindelof B, Edhag O, Allander E: Risk of cancer in patients with dermatomyositis or polymyositis. N Engl J Med 326:363, 1992. *Describes a population-based cohort study evaluating the association between malignancy and polymyositis or dermatomyositis.*
Singer FR: Pathogenesis of hypercalcemia of malignancy. Semin Oncol 18:4, 1991. *Reviews the causes of malignancy-associated hypercalcemia.*

158.2 Tumor Markers
Dennis L. Cooper

Serum tumor markers include a group of hormones, oncofetal proteins, enzymes, and tumor antigens that can be secreted into the bloodstream by malignant and, often, nonmalignant cellular types. Initially introduced as having potential as diagnostic screening agents, most of them have turned out to be useful in evaluating other aspects of cancer care. These include prognosticating, monitoring therapeutic effectiveness, and detecting evidence of tumor recurrence. This chapter reviews the uses and limitations of tumor markers and emphasizes their role in diagnosis and treatment. Discussion is limited to the use of tumor markers that have proven clinical value. Tissue tumor markers are important tools for the diagnostic pathologist but lie outside the scope of this section (Table 158–2).

COLORECTAL CARCINOMA (CEA)

SCREENING. Although an increase in serum carcinoembryonic antigen (CEA) was initially thought to indicate colorectal cancer, it turns out that CEA is a "broad-spectrum" tumor marker, being elevated in a variety of adenocarcinomas (lung, pancreas, breast, and stomach) as well as some head and neck squamous cancers and

TABLE 158-2. USE OF SERUM TUMOR MARKERS FOR SCREENING, PROGNOSIS, MONITORING RESPONSE TO THERAPY, AND DETECTING RECURRENCE

Tumor	Marker(s)	Utility of Markers			
		Screening	Prognosis	Monitoring	Recurrence
Colorectal	CEA	No	Yes	Yes	Yes
Ovary	CA 125	Possibly in high-risk groups in combination with pelvic exam, ultrasound	No	Yes	Yes
Testicle	HCG, AFP	No	In some studies, independent of stage	Yes	Yes
Prostate	PSA	Possibly in combination with DRE, TRAS	Yes	Yes	Yes
Breast	CA 15-3, CEA	No	No	Yes	Yes
Non-Hodgkin's lymphoma (aggressive)	LDH	—	Yes	No	Yes
Multiple myeloma	β₂-microglobulin	—	Yes	Yes	Yes
Hepatoma	AFP	Yes, in combination with ultrasound in high-risk patients*	No	Yes	Yes

CEA = carcinoembryonic antigen; HCG = human chorionic gonadotropin; AFP = alpha-fetoprotein; PSA = prostate-specific antigen; DRE = digital rectal examination; TRAS = transrectal ultrasonography.

* Screening studies have been positive in Asian patients with evidence of a previous hepatitis infection. Screening in European patients with non–hepatitis-related cirrhosis has not proved to be effective thus far (see text).

medullary cancer of the thyroid. Serum CEA is not increased in most early-stage (A–B₂) colorectal tumors and may be modestly increased in smokers and in association with a variety of benign conditions, including bronchitis, diverticulitis, peptic ulcer disease, fibrocystic breast disease, and a number of liver disorders. This lack of sensitivity and specificity makes CEA an inappropriate screening test for colorectal cancer as well as for adenocarcinomas of unknown origin. An increased CEA, in fact, does not help localize the tumor to either the colon or the gastrointestinal tract.

PROGNOSIS. The CEA level appears to provide independent prognostic information in patients with surgically staged colorectal cancers. Higher preoperative levels may correlate with a worse outcome because of undetected tumor. Also, recent data indicate that CEA is an adhesion molecule, suggesting that tumors expressing higher levels of CEA have an increased capacity for invasion and metastasis. Finding a high preoperative CEA, however, has limited value because treatment remains the same. Because recent data show a benefit for adjuvant chemotherapy in some patients with colon cancer, it is possible that a high CEA associated with lower stage lesions will identify patients who may benefit from such treatment. This has not been tested in randomized studies.

MONITORING. In patients undergoing therapy for metastatic colorectal cancer, a decline in CEA generally indicates a favorable response; in such circumstances the CEA can be used periodically to substitute for more expensive radiographic examinations. Conversely, a rising CEA may indicate tumor progression. Because salvage treatment is not available, such patients should have confirmation of disease progression before therapy is stopped. The CEA is most useful when serial measurements indicate a trend over a few months. Because therapy sometimes increases CEA as an early response, measurements should be continued as long as possible after treatment; individual results should not be overemphasized.

SURGICAL RE-EXPLORATION. A small percentage of patients with local-regional recurrence or single liver metastases from colon cancer can be cured with second resections. Although CEA elevations may precede radiographic or other clinical evidence of recurrence by several months, available information suggests that CEA determinations do not separate curable from incurable patients with colon cancer. For example, in one large study of adjuvant therapy in patients with resected stage B2 and C colon cancer, only 2.3% of patients who underwent routine postoperative monitoring of CEA had a potentially curative resection (disease-free for longer than one year). This represented 2.9% of patients with an elevated CEA and 1.9% of those with no elevation. Among a third group of patients who did not have CEA monitoring, 2% had a curative resection of recurrent tumor. The limitation of CEA monitoring is evident from these data.

OVARIAN CARCINOMA (CA 125)

SCREENING. CA 125 is a monoclonal antibody that recognizes an antigen secreted by ovarian and other cancers. Analogous to CEA in colon cancer, the serum CA 125 is neither sensitive nor specific for the diagnosis of ovarian cancer. Thus, the CA 125 may be normal in up to 50% of stage I (limited to one ovary) cancers and may be increased in patients with breast, lung, pancreas, and colorectal cancers. In addition, CA 125 elevations are not limited to patients with malignant disease; increased levels have been found in patients with endometriosis, pelvic inflammatory disease, benign ovarian cysts, the first trimester of pregnancy, menstruation, and liver disease. Ongoing studies are utilizing CA 125 in combination with pelvic examination and transvaginal ultrasonography to determine whether aggressive screening can reduce the mortality from ovarian cancer. Given known facts about the CA 125 antigen, a major concern in this kind of study is the number of women without ovarian cancer who may needlessly be subjected to laparotomy. Because the prevalence of ovarian cancer is low, it has been estimated that only 2.3% of unselected women with CEA elevations will be found to have ovarian cancer and nearly 98% will not. Even if CEA screening is limited to women with pelvic tumors, the positive predictive value (the percentage of patients with an abnormal value who have ovarian cancer) depends on the age of the patient. Benign pelvic masses in premenopausal women often elevate serum CA 125 levels; this means that only about 15 to 36% of their CA 125–associated pelvic masses will be ovarian cancer. The relationship increases among women older than 50 years. In that group, 80 to 90% of those with a pelvic mass and an elevated CA 125 have ovarian cancer, and the rate climbs to 98% if the CA 125 exceeds 65 U per milliliter. Patients in the last category are best referred to a gynecologic oncologist for a definitive initial laparotomy.

Although a high CA 125 in a postmenopausal woman with a pelvic mass indicates ovarian cancer, a normal CA 125 does not exclude the disease; one study found at laparotomy that 18 to 28% of women with pelvic masses and a normal CA 125 had ovarian cancer.

MONITORING THERAPY. Most patients with surgical-chemotherapy treatment for advanced ovarian cancer have a complete clinical remission, defined by a normal physical examination, CT scan, and CA 125 level. About half of those with clinical remission retain microscopic cancer deposits in the tumor bed, however, and even among those who are pathologically "clean," another half die of recurrence. CA 125 fails to identify the microscopic disease in these cases.

If the CA 125 fails to return to normal following chemotherapy, it indicates drug-resistant residual disease. Also, in patients with an initial response, a rising CA 125 may herald recurrence. Because second-line therapy is generally given for palliative intent, knowledge of asymptomatic residual disease has little benefit. Given the circumstances, the tumor markers contribute limited benefits.

BREAST CANCER (CA 15-3, CEA)

SCREENING. No present evidence indicates that the most commonly used tumor markers, CA 15-3 or CEA, have a useful role in screening patients for breast cancer. They are neither increased in most patients with early stage disease nor specific for patients with breast cancer.

MONITORING RESPONSE TO THERAPY. Rising levels of CA 15-3 or CEA in patients with breast cancer often provide the first sign of progressive or recurrent disease. In the absence of effective salvage treatment, however, such information is of limited value. Perhaps the most valuable use of tumor markers is in patients who are difficult to evaluate with radiographic examinations. For example, in patients with metastases limited to bone, bone scans may lag behind clinical improvement by many months. Similarly, in patients with abdominal carcinomatosis, serial tumor markers may accurately reflect tumor bulk and substitute for more expensive CT scans. In view of the increased (but unproved) use of high-dose chemotherapy and bone marrow rescue in patients with a 50% or greater response to conventional chemotherapy, the use of tumor markers may identify potential candidates for therapy who do not have otherwise measurable disease.

An important caveat to the use of tumor markers in patients receiving hormonal therapy is that some of them have a "flare" (worsening clinical disease and increase in tumor markers) weeks to months after beginning a course of hormonal therapy that may induce an excellent clinical response. Such patients should not have therapy terminated or changed prematurely.

PROSTATE CANCER (PSA)

SCREENING. PSA is secreted by prostate cells, reaching especially high levels in prostate cancer. Elevated serum acid phosphatase levels most often reflect extension-metastasis of prostate cancer outside the organ itself. Studies with large cohorts of asymptomatic men show that screening with PSA consistently detects approximately one third more cancers than digital rectal examination (DRE). Nevertheless, 20 to 30% of prostate cancers detected by transrectal ultrasonography (TRAS) and DRE are not associated with PSA elevations. To date, however, early detection by PSA has shown little or no effect on disease mortality. Accordingly, the American Cancer Society has recommended screening with DRE and PSA and reserving TRAS for patients with abnormalities on either examination. As Table 158–1 indicates, the PSA normally increases with age, and using an age-adjusted PSA increases the accuracy of the test. In patients on finasteride (Proscar) for benign prostatic hypertrophy, the clinician should divide the age-adjusted PSA range by half to define a new normal range. Patients with levels above this range or in whom the PSA does not fall by 50% after 1 year of finasteride should be evaluated for prostate cancer. Because approximately 30% of men over the age of 50 have evidence of microscopic organ-confined prostate cancer at autopsy, excessive application of PSA to diagnosis makes it possible that men with clinically "unimportant" prostate cancer will receive expensive, potentially morbid therapy. Although preliminary evidence shows that the tumors diagnosed after PSA screening are not microscopic, it seems reasonable to withhold aggressive screening in patients unlikely to live another 10 years. More general recommendations require the completion of ongoing studies.

ASSESSMENT OF THE ADEQUACY OF DEFINITIVE THERAPY. PSA determination is most usefully applied following radical prostatectomy for cancer. Because the antigen is organ specific, measurable levels of PSA 6 to 8 weeks after surgery indicate persistent disease. Chapter 209.2 discusses management in such instances.

In patients treated with radical radiation, the PSA generally falls to within the reference range within 1 year. Undetectable levels are not as common as after radical surgery and do not necessarily indicate residual disease. A PSA that does not fall within the reference range after 12 months usually indicates recurrent disease.

MONITORING THE RESPONSE OF HORMONAL ABLATION THERAPY. PSA remains an excellent tumor marker in pa-

tients receiving androgen ablation treatment even though the treatment independently lowers PSA values. This is important, as the progress of metastatic prostate cancer is not easily measured. The rate and depth of fall of PSA after androgen ablation correlate with the duration of response; it is rare for disease to progress in the absence of an increasing PSA.

TESTICULAR CANCER (HUMAN CHORIONIC GONADOTROPIN [HCG], ALPHA-FETOPROTEIN [AFP])

SCREENING. Normally, HCG is secreted by the placenta and AFP by the fetus. The presence of either protein in males or non-pregnant females is diagnostic of cancer. Neither protein offers value as a screening marker.

DIAGNOSIS. Although 15% of seminomatous tumors are associated with an increased HCG, high levels often are associated with a nonseminomatous tumor component. An increased level of AFP is diagnostic of the presence of nonseminomatous tumor. The importance of the distinction is that nonseminomatous tumors are treated with chemotherapy, and nonbulky seminomas confined to the abdomen are treated with radiation. Markedly elevated germ-cell markers accompanying poorly differentiated midline tumors (pineal, mediastinal, and retroperitoneal regions) are diagnostic of a testicular or extragonadal germ-cell tumor. Biopsy becomes unnecessary. Patients with lung, breast, gastrointestinal, and ovarian tumors may secrete low levels of HCG that are not diagnostic of a germ-cell tumor.

MONITORING RESPONSE TO THERAPY. Because either HCG or AFP is increased in 89% of patients with nonseminomatous tumors, they are useful in monitoring response after chemotherapy or for detecting subsequent recurrence. Generally, after chemotherapy, the HCG falls more predictably than the AFP, and the failure of the HCG to decrease by one or more logs on day 22 of therapy bodes a poor response. In view of the exquisite sensitivity of germ-cell tumors to therapy, tumor markers sometimes rise early after chemotherapy before a subsequent fall. Markers that do not subsequently return to normal indicate residual disease. Conversely, nearly one third of patients with normal markers and residual masses have residual disease.

HEPATOMA (AFP)

SCREENING. Screening with AFP and liver ultrasonography has been relatively successful and cost-effective in Asian countries because hepatoma is common and high-risk patients can be identified by hepatitis B and C serology tests. In Europe, where the prevalence of hepatoma is much lower and most screened patients have cirrhosis unrelated to hepatitis infection, AFP screening has not detected small and potentially resectable tumors. Prevalence and specificity importantly influence medical costs. Because of the lower prevalence of hepatoma and more expensive testing in the United States, estimated cost of detecting one hepatoma is as high as $270,000, compared with $8,000 in Japan.

MULTIPLE MYELOMA (β_2-MICROGLOBULIN [β_2-M])

PROGNOSIS. Multiple myeloma is a malignant lymphoproliferative disorder that is inevitably fatal in a period ranging from a few months to several years. Because of the extreme variability in disease aggressiveness and the absence of curative treatment, it is helpful to separate patients who require less aggressive or no treatment from those for whom experimental therapy would be appropriate as part of initial management. β_2-M, an HLA class I antigen, is a cell surface component of most nucleated cells. Secreted into the plasma in excessive amounts in multiple myeloma, β_2-M represents the most important, generally available prognostic factor in that disease. For example, in one study myeloma patients with a β_2-M level less than 6 μg per milliliter had a median survival of 36 months compared with 23 months in patients with a β_2-M greater than 6 μg per milliliter. If serum albumin level also was considered, median survival of younger patients (<60 yrs) with a serum albumin greater than 3.0 and a β_2-M less than 6 μg per milliliter lasted longer than 48 months, whereas older patients with both a low serum albumin and a high β_2-M survived an average of just over 1 year. Patients with either a low albumin or a high β_2-M, but not both, had an intermediate prognosis.

MONITORING. After treatment, the β_2-M level generally parallels the decline in the serum monoclonal protein; persistently elevated levels of β_2-M occasionally identify patients with brief responses. In patients with light chain disease or nonsecretory myeloma (and who do not have a measurable serum monoclonal protein), the β_2-M can be used to follow the response to treatment.

NON-HODGKIN'S LYMPHOMA (LACTIC DEHYDROGENASE [LDH])

PROGNOSIS. In patients with non-Hodgkin's lymphoma, it has become critically important to identify patients who are appropriate for more intensive treatment, including high-dose chemotherapy and autologous bone marrow transplant. A recent multi-institutional study has shown that age, performance status, clinical stage, and the pretreatment serum LDH can effectively separate patients with a good prognosis using current therapy from those who are unlikely to be cured. High pretreatment LDH has been consistently shown to be an adverse risk factor and presumably reflects the growth rate and tumor burden of the lymphoma. In contrast to the value of the pretreatment LDH, values obtained during therapy are less helpful. Also, the LDH value may increase in patients treated with granulocyte colony stimulating factors, presumably owing to increased progenitor cell turnover in the bone marrow.

TUMORS OF UNKNOWN ORIGIN

Approximately 5 to 10% of patients with cancer initially have tumors of unknown primary. In view of the lack of specificity of tumor markers for a specific tissue and the lack of effective therapy for most adenocarcinomas, tumor markers are not generally helpful in predicting the site of origin or in recommending therapy. An important exception is prostate cancer, in which a high serum PSA should result in an examination of the tumor specimen for expression of PSA.

Cannistra SA: Cancer of the ovary. N Engl J Med 329:1550, 1993.

Catalona WJ, Smith DS, Ratliff TL, et al.: Measurement of prostate-specific antigen in serum as a screening test for prostate cancer. N Engl J Med 324:1156, 1991.

Colombo M, de Franchis R, Del Ninno E, et al.: Hepatocellular carcinoma in Italian patients with cirrhosis. N Engl J Med 325:675, 1991.

Crawford ED, Schutz MJ, Clejan S, et al.: The effect of digital rectal examination on prostate-specific antigen levels. JAMA 267:2227, 1992.

Durand F, Buffet C, Pelletier G, et al.: Hepatocellular carcinoma [letter]. N Engl J Med 328:64, 1993.

Fisher RI, Gaynor ER, Dahlberg S, et al.: Comparison of a standard regimen (CHOP) with three intensive chemotherapy regimens for advanced non-Hodgkin's lymphoma. N Engl J Med 328:1002, 1993.

Fletcher RH: CEA monitoring after surgery for colorectal cancer. When is the evidence sufficient? [editorial]. JAMA 270:987, 1993.

Guess HA, Heyse JF, Gormley GJ, et al.: Effect of finasteride on serum PSA concentrations in men with benign prostatic hyperplasia. Results from the North American phase III clinical trial. Urol Clin North Am 20:627, 1993.

Miller JI, Ahmann FR, Drach GW, et al.: The clinical usefulness of serum prostate specific antigen after hormonal therapy of metastatic prostate cancer. J Urol 147:956, 1992.

Moertel CG, Fleming TR, Macdonald JS, et al.: An evaluation of the carcinoembryonic antigen (CEA) test for monitoring patients with resected colon cancer. JAMA 270:943, 1993.

Oesterling JE, Andrews PE, Suman VJ, et al.: Preoperative androgen deprivation therapy: Artificial lowering of serum prostate specific antigen without downstaging the tumor. J Urol 149:779, 1993.

Oesterling JE, Jacobsen SJ, Chute CG, et al.: Serum prostate-specific antigen in a community-based population of healthy men: Establishment of age-specific reference ranges. JAMA 270:860, 1993.

Okuda K: Advances in detection and treatment of liver cancer. Gann Monogr Cancer Res 38:3, 1991.

Ruckle HC, Klee GG, Oesterling JE: Prostate-specific antigen: Concepts for staging prostate cancer and monitoring response to therapy. Mayo Clin Proceed 69:69, 1994.

Shipp MA: A predictive model for aggressive non-Hodgkin's lymphoma. N Engl J Med 329:987, 1993.

Walsh PC: Using prostate-specific antigen to diagnose prostate cancer: Sailing in uncharted waters [editorial]. Ann Intern Med 119:948, 1993.

159 ENDOCRINE MANIFESTATIONS OF TUMORS: "ECTOPIC" HORMONE PRODUCTION

Stephen B. Baylin

The clinical manifestations of cancer arise not only through the consequences of the invasive properties of primary and metastatic lesions, but also through the hormonal activity of proteins and small peptides secreted by tumor cells. Even though the tumor-associated production of these protein products is common, the incidence of paraneoplastic syndromes is less frequent. This is because these hormones are made, in tumors, either in amounts too small to result in a biologic response or in forms that are biologically inactive. For a given cancer, the spectrum of hormones produced often appears "foreign" with respect to the tissue of origin for the neoplasm. Hence, the term "ectopic" has been applied to this cancer-associated activity. In reality, studies over the past decade have increasingly demonstrated that such basic aspects of normal tissue development as cell lineage relationships and steps in embryogenesis and in cell differentiation during renewal of adult tissues often provide logical explanations for patterns of hormone production by specific cancer types. Also, the rapid elucidation of molecular events regulating gene expression is bringing further understanding of cellular relationships underlying hormonal production patterns in cancer.

Before considering individual endocrine syndromes associated with tumors, it is helpful to broadly classify cancer-associated hormone production patterns according to biologic concepts thought to underlie this phenomenon (Table 159–1). Much of this activity can be associated with the small polypeptide hormones normally secreted by cells that constitute classic endocrine tissues. Common neuroendocrine characteristics of these cells have been recognized and encompassed in the eponym *a*mine *p*recursor *u*ptake *d*ecarboxylase, or "APUD" cells. Much of the "ectopic" hormone production by tumors involves the peptides from such cells, and the cancer most frequently represented—small cell lung carcinoma—has direct links to cells with APUD features. A common pattern of gene expression events in these cells during development may explain why APUD-associated tumors may often produce more than one small polypeptide hormone at a time.

A group of larger molecular weight glycoprotein hormones is more often produced by non-APUD-associated cancers (Table 159–1). Also, non-APUD tumors are more often associated with products of peptides which result in disorders of calcium homeostasis. The association of tumors and these gene expression events is much less well understood than that outlined above for APUD-cell tumors.

ECTOPIC ACTH PRODUCTION

Cushing's syndrome resulting from tumor cell production of ACTH is one of the first recognized and most common cancer-associated endocrine disorders. This disease is prototypical for the ectopic hormone syndromes associated with APUD cells and almost always occurs in tumors that arise from cells with endocrine features (Table 159–1). The cancer most commonly responsible for tumor-associated Cushing's syndrome is small cell lung carcinoma (SCLC), a common pulmonary neoplasm long recognized to have APUD features similar to those found in normal lung endocrine cells.

The expression of ACTH and related peptides by tumors, as was noted earlier for tumor-associated hormone production in general, is much more frequent than the actual occurrence of Cushing's syndrome. Thus, among all patients with SCLC, the incidence of clinical evidence of excess ACTH production is only 3 to 5%. The biosynthetic events underlying production of biologically active ACTH are complex and involve a series of post-translational steps that cleave biologically active ACTH and other peptides from the precursor gene product, pro-opiomelanocortin (POMC). Normal

TABLE 159-1. HORMONE-SECRETING TUMORS

	Hormones Secreted
Tumors most frequently secreting APUD hormones	
Small cell lung carcinoma	ACTH,* CRF,* ADH,* calcitonin, GRP, GRF
Carcinoid tumors (lung, pancreas, GI tract, thymus, ovary)	ACTH.* GRF
Islet cell tumors of pancreas	ACTH,* GRF
Medullary thyroid carcinoma	ACTH,* GRF, GRP, somatostatin
Pheochromocytoma	ACTH,* GRF
Neural tumors (ganglioneuroma)	ACTH,* VIP,* GRF
Melanoma	ACTH*
Prostate	ACTH*
Tumors most frequently secreting large glycoprotein hormones	
Non-small cell lung carcinomas	hCG*
Testicular carcinomas (embryonal components)	hCG*
Sarcomas	hCG*
Tumors most frequently causing hormonally mediated hypercalcemia	
Squamous cell carcinoma (lung, head, and neck)	PTH RP*
Renal carcinomas	PTH RP*
Bladder carcinomas	PTH RP*
Adenocarcinomas	PTH RP*
Lymphomas	PTH RP*

* Responsible for producing a clinical syndrome.
ACTH = adrenocorticotropic hormone
ADH = vasopressin
CRF = corticotropin-releasing factor
GRF = growth hormone–releasing factor
GRP = gastrin-releasing peptide
VIP = vasoactive intestinal polypeptide
hCG = human chorionic gonadotropin
PTH RP = parathyroid hormone–related peptide

pituitary cells contain all of the enzymes required for this processing. However, most cancer cells, even SCLC, cannot fully process the precursor POMC molecule even though they express, to variable levels, the POMC gene. In rare but well-documented situations, tumor-associated Cushing's syndrome can result from production of corticotropin-releasing factor (CRF) by cancer cells. The excess CRF then stimulates pituitary cells to release excess ACTH.

The symptoms of Cushing's syndrome in patients with cancer are much more varied and subtle than those in patients with pituitary-adrenal Cushing's disease (see Ch. 204.1). The virulent behavior of the cancer most frequently involved, SCLC, means that the patients do not have time to develop the full spectrum of symptoms associated with Cushing's disease. The most prominent manifestations are therefore those associated with the early metabolic consequences of excessive glucocorticoid production, including generalized weakness, carbohydrate intolerance, and mental changes, and problems secondary to mineralocorticoid excess, including edema, hypertension, and hypokalemic alkalosis. Hypokalemia, especially, is more prominent in patients with tumor-associated ACTH excess than in patients with pituitary Cushing's disease. These symptoms and/or electrolyte changes in patients with cancer, and especially those with SCLC, should alert the physician to the possibility of ectopic Cushing's syndrome.

The diagnostic questions in ectopic Cushing's syndrome relate to documenting the source of excess ACTH secretion. A first clue for a nonpituitary tumor-related source is the finding of an extraordinarily high plasma ACTH value, much in excess of those found in pituitary Cushing's disease. Urinary free cortisol levels are always elevated and, unlike in Cushing's disease (see Ch. 204.1), are usually *not* suppressible during a high-dose (8 mg per day) dexamethasone suppression test. Only in some patients with carcinoid tumors, and in the rare situation of tumors producing CRF, does this high-dose suppression test lower urinary cortisol in patients with "ectopic" Cushing's syndrome.

The treatment of tumor-associated Cushing's syndrome is often frustrating because of the aggressive nature of the cancers most frequently associated with this condition. An exception to this is carcinoid tumors, in which the clinical course is often protracted. The most efficacious therapy is primary eradication of the responsible neoplasm, either through chemotherapy or surgery. For SCLC, such complete tumor ablation is not usually possible. Alternatively, transient improvement may be obtained by using drugs, discussed in Ch. 204.1, which block steroid synthesis in the adrenal gland (such as metyrapone, aminoglutethimide, or ketoconazole).

CANCER-ASSOCIATED HYPERCALCEMIA

Hypercalcemia in patients with cancer is probably the most frequently seen paraneoplastic syndrome. In turn, cancer is the most commonly recognized cause of hypercalcemia in hospitalized patients. It is then imperative to rule out the presence of a tumor in any patient, especially one in the older age range, who has documented hypercalcemia.

The causes of tumor-associated hypercalcemia are varied. Direct effects of tumor metastases on bone resorption must always be considered, but it has become increasingly apparent that hormonal factors are more often involved. For many years, it was believed that parathyroid hormone (PTH), synthesized and secreted by tumor cells, was the etiologic agent. This hypothesis was based on detection of PTH immunoreactivity in sera of patients with tumors and hypercalcemia and presence of increased cyclic AMP levels in urine of such individuals.

However, during recent years, several groups have reported that a different small peptide, PTH-like peptide (PLP), which has partial homology to PTH only in the first 13 amino acids, is probably the humoral agent most frequently responsible for tumor-associated hypercalcemia. Interestingly, the gene for this hormone is normally ubiquitously expressed, and is not, as are other small polypeptide hormones, especially associated with normal cells having APUD endocrine features. Levels are especially high in normal keratinocytes, lactating mammary tissue, placenta, and other sites where the peptide appears to have a physiologic role. This distribution may explain why non-APUD tumors such as squamous cell, bladder, ovarian, and renal carcinomas have been most frequently associated to date with PLP secretion and hypercalcemia (Table 159–1).

Other humoral factors also play a variable role in producing hypercalcemia in patients with cancer. Growth factors, such as transforming growth factor (TGF-β), bone resorbing factors such as are found in hematologic malignancies, prostaglandins, and occasionally, active vitamin D metabolites have all been documented as tumor products that can cause hypercalcemia. It is apparent, then, that multiple factors can be simultaneously active to cause the hypercalcemia associated with tumors.

The diagnosis of tumor-associated hypercalcemia should be suspected in any patient with hypercalcemia. The suspicion is obviously highest for a patient with known cancer who develops or presents with this metabolic abnormality. The most important alternative and treatable cause for hypercalcemia is primary hyperparathyroidism (see Ch. 214). Features favoring this latter condition include a longstanding history of hypercalcemia and presence of subperiosteal bone resorption and renal stones. High circulating PTH levels with high urinary cyclic AMP levels are characteristic of patients with primary hyperparathyroidism. In contrast, patients with cancer and hypercalcemia have relatively low PTH levels in conjunction with high urine cyclic AMP.

The treatment for tumor-associated hypercalcemia can be difficult because the cancers most frequently associated are often extensive and aggressive at the time of diagnosis. Direct ablation of, or reduction in, tumor mass is the optimal treatment when feasible. When this is not possible, treatment of the hypercalcemia depends upon its severity and consequences for the patient. The simplest therapeutic approaches employ combinations of hydration and diuretics. For more refractory and severe hypercalcemia, drugs such as mithramycin or diphosphonates may have to be added to this regimen. These treatments for hypercalcemia are discussed in more detail in Ch. 214.

TUMOR PRODUCTION OF HUMAN CHORIONIC GONADOTROPIN

The production by tumors of chorionic gonadotropin (hCG), a large molecular weight glycoprotein, is another example of hormonal activity most associated with the non-APUD group of cancers (Table 159–1). As for other hormones, asymptomatic production of hCG is far more frequent than the situation in which enough biologically active hCG is produced to cause symptoms in the patient. hCG is composed of α and β subunits, which are often discordantly produced by neoplasms. Production of the α subunit is particularly common, and elevated circulating levels of this peptide are often found in patients with multiple types of cancer. Production of intact hCG is common in tumors of trophoblastic origin (i.e., choriocarcinomas, testicular embryonal carcinomas, and seminomas), the normal source for hCG, and less often seen in cancers of the lung, pancreas, and other types.

The infrequent symptoms associated with tumor-associated secretion of hCG include precocious puberty in children and gynecomastia in adult males, usually associated with advanced tumors such as lung carcinoma. The treatment for these syndromes, especially in adults, is usually ineffective given the advanced nature of the tumors.

HYPOGLYCEMIA AND TUMORS

A long-recognized syndrome, most often associated with mesenchymal tumors (retroperitoneal fibrosarcomas, hemangiopericytomas and leiomyosarcomas, adrenocortical carcinomas, and hepatomas), is hormonally induced hypoglycemia. This metabolic disorder, first thought to be secondary to excess insulin produced by tumor cells, has subsequently been linked to production of insulinlike factors or so-called nonsuppressible insulin-like activity. Recently, the association of one such factor, insulin-like growth factor II (IGF-II), with tumor-related hypoglycemia has been strengthened by the demonstration of IGF-II mRNA and peptide in mesenchymal tumors associated with hypoglycemia. However, the physiologic role of IGF-II remains uncertain because serum IGF-II levels in patients with these tumors have not been found to be uniformly elevated. The interpretation of these studies is made difficult by the presence of serum-binding proteins, and further studies are needed to establish convincingly the role of IGF-II in tumor hypoglycemia.

HYPONATREMIA, INAPPROPRIATE ANTIDIURETIC HORMONE SYNDROME (SIADH), AND CANCER

An important metabolic abnormality occurring in patients with cancer is hyponatremia. The classic syndrome is associated with the presence of hyponatremia, increased urine osmolality, increased urine sodium (> 20 mEq per liter), and decreased serum osmolality (< 275 mOsm per liter). A series of investigators over the years, using first biologic assays and later immunoassays, has established that these electrolyte imbalances result from production and secretion by tumor cells of a polypeptide hormone, vasopressin, or antidiuretic hormone (ADH). As for other "ectopic" hormone syndromes associated with small polypeptide hormones, inappropriate secretion of ADH is most often associated with, but not restricted to, the APUD tumor, SCLC (Table 159–1). Such tumors most frequently have the cellular features necessary to synthesize a 20,000-dalton glycosylated prohormone, provasopressin, and to process this peptide to the smaller biologically active ADH molecule.

Recognition of SIADH is important because the symptoms of hyponatremia, such as lethargy and mental changes, can present severe problems for patients with cancer. Also, the hyponatremia can be successfully managed by fluid restriction, careful administration of saline solutions, and/or treatment with drugs such as demeclocycline.

OTHER TUMOR-ASSOCIATED HORMONE SYNDROMES

Although the syndromes discussed above constitute the majority of cancer-related endocrine diseases, there are other less frequent tumor-associated hormonal states that are important for the clinician to recognize.

ONCOGENIC OSTEOMALACIA

A syndrome associated with bone pain and muscle weakness, together with the radiologic features of osteomalacia, can occur in patients with mesenchymal tumors such as benign osteoblastomas, giant cell osteosarcomas, hemangiomas, and occasionally epithelial tumors such as prostate and SCLC. Biochemical studies show hypophosphatemia and subnormal 1,25-dihydroxyvitamin D levels. The pathophysiology of this disorder is unclear but appears to involve a hormonally mediated and severe renal phosphate loss as the primary event. The tumor origin of the inciting factor is inferred from the observations that the syndrome can remit dramatically with irradiation of the neoplasm. When primary treatment of the tumor is not feasible, treatment with phosphorus replacement and vitamin D can provide substantial improvement of symptoms and hypophosphatemia.

POLYCYTHEMIA

Tumors such as hepatomas, hemangiomas, and renal carcinomas can cause polycythemia. Recently, such tumors have been shown to produce erythropoietin mRNA, and patients with this syndrome have been found to have elevated erythropoietin levels in their serum by immunoassay. In general, no treatment is required. However, intermittent phlebotomy is occasionally required to alleviate symptoms.

TROPHOBLASTIC HYPERTHYROIDISM

The thyrotropic activity inherent to the choriogonadotropin (hCG) molecule can occasionally account for appearance of a small goiter and mild hyperthyroidism in patients with choriocarcinomas or hydatidiform moles. Occasionally, the hyperthyroidism can be severe enough to require treatment with antithyroid drugs.

HYPERTENSION

Renin-secreting tumors must be considered in the differential diagnosis of hypertension and hypokalemia. Most commonly, these tumors arise in the juxtaglomerular cells, the normal source of renin. Extrarenal renin-secreting tumors are rare and include pancreatic, ovarian, and pulmonary tumors. In general, hypertension subsides upon removal of the tumors. However, extrarenal renin-secreting tumors are usually aggressive and quite advanced at the time of presentation. In these situations, angiotensin-converting enzyme inhibitors such as captopril may be required for treatment of hypertension.

ACROMEGALY

The production of growth hormone or, more rarely, growth hormone–releasing factor (GRF), has been documented in nonpituitary tumors such as carcinoids, pancreatic islet cell neoplasms, pulmonary carcinomas, and gastric, ovarian, and breast carcinomas. Uncommonly, this can produce the full manifestations of acromegaly. For production of GRF (Table 159–1), the associated tumors generally arise from endocrine cells. The treatment of tumor-associated acromegaly is, when feasible, removal of the causative neoplasm.

OTHER HORMONES PRODUCED BY TUMORS

A number of other hormones, often in the small polypeptide hormone category (some are shown in Table 159–1), may be found in tumor tissue and/or secreted by the tumor. Examples include calcitonin, somatostatin, and GRP in endocrine tumors. These hormones have not been associated with clinical syndromes in patients with these diseases but in some instances may be useful tumor markers to follow in monitoring disease course.

Ball, DW, de Bustros, AC, Baylin, SB: Endocrine manifestations of cancer. *In* Moore WT, Eastman R (eds.): Diagnostic Endocrinology, 2nd ed. St. Louis, Mosby, 1995.

Odell WD, Appleton WS: Humoral manifestations of cancer. *In* Wilson, JD, Foster, DF (eds.): Textbook of Endocrinology, 8th ed. Philadelphia, WB Saunders, 1992.

Ectopic ACTH Production

Shepherd FA, Laskey J, Evans WK, et al.: Cushing's syndrome associated with ectopic corticotropin production and small-cell lung cancer. J Clin Oncol 10:21, 1992. *Extensive review of complications associated with ectopic ACTH in lung cancer patients.*

White A, Clark AJL: The cellular and molecular basis of the ectopic ACTH syndrome. Clin Endocrinol 39:131, 1993. *Possible defects in glucocorticoid feedback suppression of ACTH production by tumors.*

Hypercalcemia and Cancer

Mundy GR: Mechanisms of osteolytic bone destruction. Bone 12, Suppl. 1:S1, 1991.

Seymour JF, Gagel RF: Calcitriol: the major humoral mediator of hypercalcemia in Hodgkin's disease and non-Hodgkin's lymphoma. Blood 82:1383, 1993. *An excellent review of the role of vitamin D in tumoral hypercalcemia.*

Wysolmerski JJ, Broadus AE: Hypercalcemia of malignancy: The central role of parathyroid hormone-related protein. Ann Rev Med 45:189, 1994. *A good overall review of the biology and clinical aspects of the humorally-mediated hypercalcemia syndrome.*

Hypoglycemia and Cancer

Daughaday WH, Kapadia M: Significance of abnormal serum binding of insulin-like growth factor II in the development of hypoglycemia in patients with non-islet cell tumors. Proc Natl Acad Sci USA 86:6778,1989. *Questions regarding the role of IGF-II in tumoral hyperglycemia are addressed.*

Gorden P, Hendricks CM, Kahn CR, et al.: Hypoglycemia associated with nonislet-cell tumor and insulin-like growth factors: A study of the tumor types. N Engl J Med 305:1452, 1981. *This paper reviews the tumor types associated with hormonally mediated hypoglycemia.*

Vasopressin and Cancer

Moses AM, Scheinman SJ: Ectopic secretion of neurohypophyseal peptides in patients with malignancy. Endocrinol Clin N Am 20:489, 1991. *A recent review of abnormal vasopressin secretion in cancer patients.*

Osteomalacia and Cancer

Nuovo MA, Dorfman HD, Sun C-C, Chalew SA: Tumor-induced osteomalacia and rickets. Am J Surg Pathol 13:588, 1989. *This is a good overall review.*

Polycythemia and Cancer

DaSilva J-L, Lacombe C, Bruneval P, et al.: Tumor cells are the site of erythropoietin synthesis in human renal cancers associated with polycythemia. Blood 75:577, 1990. *This paper documents erythropoietin production from tumor cells.*

Trophoblastic Hyperthyroidism

Wilber JF, Spinella P: Identification of immunoreactive thyrotropin-releasing hormone in human neoplasia. J Clin Endocrinol Metab 59:432, 1984. *Describes the syndrome and the role of hCG.*

Hypertension and Cancer

Atlas SA, Hesson TE, Sealey JE, et al.: Characterization of inactive renin ("prorenin") from renin-secreting tumors of non-renal origin. J Clin Invest 73:437, 1984.

Ruddy MC, Atlas SA, Salerno FG: Hypertension associated with a renin-secreting adenocarcinoma of the pancreas. N Engl J Med 307:993, 1982.

Acromegaly and Cancer

Asa SI, Kovacs K, Thorner MO, et al.: Immunohistological localization of growth hormone-releasing hormone in human tumors. J Clin Endocrinol Metab 60:423, 1985.

Melmed, S: Extrapituitary acromegaly. Endocrinol Clin N Am 20:507, 1991.

160 NONMETASTATIC EFFECTS OF CANCER ON THE NERVOUS SYSTEM

Jerome B. Posner

When patients with cancer develop nervous system dysfunction, metastasis is usually the cause. Cancer also can exert deleterious effects on the nervous system by mechanisms other than metastasis. Recognition of these nonmetastatic neurologic complications can prevent inappropriate and perhaps harmful therapy directed at a nonexistent metastasis. Sometimes nervous system symptoms precede the discovery of the cancer and can, if correctly interpreted, lead the physician to the diagnosis of an otherwise occult neoplasm.

An almost bewildering variety of neurologic disorders has been

TABLE 160–1. NONMETASTATIC EFFECTS OF CANCER ON THE NERVOUS SYSTEM

Paraneoplastic syndromes or remote effects of cancer (see Table 160–2)
Side effects of therapy
  Chemotherapy
  Radiation therapy (see Table 160–3)
Metabolic and nutritional abnormalities
  Destruction of vital organs (e.g., liver)
  Elaboration of hormonal substances by tumor
  Competition between tumor and brain for essential substrates (e.g., glucose)
  Malnutrition
Infections (usually associated with lymphomas)
  Parasites (e.g., toxoplasmosis)
  Fungi (e.g., cryptococcosis, aspergillosis, mucormycosis)
  Bacteria (e.g., *Listeria monocytogenes*)
  Viruses (e.g., herpes zoster)
Vascular disease
  Intracranial hemorrhage
  Cerebral infarction

ascribed to effects of systemic cancer (Table 160–1). Most patients with nervous system dysfunction not caused by metastases are eventually found to be suffering from infection, vascular or metabolic disorders, or neurotoxicity of chemotherapy. This chapter discusses two other types of nervous system damage related to cancer not described elsewhere in this book: paraneoplastic syndromes (Table 160–2) and radiation injury.

PARANEOPLASTIC SYNDROMES

Paraneoplastic syndromes, also called "remote effects of cancer on the nervous system," refer to neurologic dysfunction caused by cancer but not ascribable to such well-defined secondary effects of cancer as infection, coagulation abnormalities, metabolic disorders, or side effects of therapy (see Table 160–1). Similar clinical disorders occur in the absence of cancer, and thus, in any given patient, the cancer must be found to be certain that the neurologic disorder is paraneoplastic. Excluding patients with mild

TABLE 160–2. PARANEOPLASTIC SYNDROMES AFFECTING THE NERVOUS SYSTEM

Brain and cranial nerves
  Dementia–limbic encephalitis
  Retinal degeneration
  Optic neuritis
  Opsoclonus-myoclonus
  Subacute cerebellar degeneration
  Brain stem encephalitis
Spinal cord
  Subacute motor neuropathy
  Necrotizing myelopathy
  Myelitis
  Motor neuron disease?
Dorsal root ganglia
  Subacute sensory neuronopathy
Peripheral nerve
  Subacute or chronic sensorimotor peripheral neuropathy
  Acute polyradiculoneuropathy (Guillain-Barré syndrome)
  Remitting and relapsing peripheral neuropathy
  Mononeuropathies
  Mononeuritis multiplex
  Brachial neuritis
  Autonomic neuropathy
  Peripheral neuropathy associated with paraproteinemia
  Neuromyotomia, stiff-man syndrome
Neuromuscular junction and muscle
  Lambert-Eaton myasthenic syndrome
  Myasthenia gravis
  Dermatomyositis, polymyositis
  Acute necrotizing myopathy
  Carcinoid myopathies
  Myotonia
  Cachectic myopathy
  "Neuromyopathy"

peripheral neuropathy or myopathy possibly associated with cachexia, remote effects of cancer affect less than 1% of patients with cancer. Lung cancer accounts for more than 50% of cases; the incidence is greatest among patients with ovarian and small cell lung cancer and Hodgkin's disease. Because of its rarity, the diagnosis of paraneoplastic syndrome should never be accepted until a thorough evaluation has excluded metastatic or other nonmetastatic causes of neurologic dysfunction. In particular, infiltration of nerve roots by tumor in the leptomeninges may mimic paraneoplastic peripheral neuropathy.

Increasing evidence suggests that the etiology of most or all remote effects is autoimmune. Patients with the Lambert-Eaton myasthenic syndrome (see below) harbor an IgG antibody that reacts with voltage-gated calcium channels on the presynaptic neuromuscular junction. Complexing of these channels by the antibody prevents normal release of acetylcholine, which, in turn, causes the clinical symptoms of the disorder. About two-thirds of patients with the Lambert-Eaton myasthenic syndrome have, or will shortly develop, evidence of small cell lung cancer. The tumors possess a protein antigen homologous with or identical to the calcium channels in the neuromuscular junction against which the antibody response is presumed to be directed. Removal of IgG from the serum of a patient with Lambert-Eaton myasthenic syndrome ameliorates the neuromuscular symptoms, and injection of that IgG into experimental animals reproduces the neurologic disorder. High titers of antibodies against other onconeural antigens (antigens shared between tumor and nervous system) are found in several other paraneoplastic syndromes (see below), suggesting a mechanism similar to that in the Lambert-Eaton syndrome. However, paraneoplastic syndromes may be a heterogeneous group of disorders in which other etiologies, such as opportunistic viral infections, competition between tumor and the nervous system for essential metabolites, and secretion by tumor of neurotoxins, also may play a role.

Paraneoplastic syndromes are usually classified by the anatomic site of neurologic disability (Table 160–2). However, it is common for more than one anatomic site to be involved (e.g., Lambert-Eaton syndrome and cerebellar degeneration; dementia and myelopathy; limbic encephalitis and sensory neuronopathy). When more than one symptom is present, the disorder can be called "paraneoplastic encephalomyelitis" or "paraneoplastic encephalomyeloneuritis." Some of the more characteristic paraneoplastic syndromes are described below.

Brain and Cranial Nerves

CEREBRUM. Loss of recent memory (limbic encephalitis) and affective alterations, either anxiety or depression, are the usual findings. Seizures are prominent in some patients; others have a fluctuating confusional state. When other abnormal neurologic signs are present, they usually point to the brain stem, cerebellum, or peripheral nerves (encephalomyelitis). The cerebrospinal fluid (CSF) usually contains 10 to 40 lymphocytes per cubic milliliter, with a slight elevation of the protein concentration. Computed tomography (CT) and magnetic resonance imaging (MRI) are usually normal, but in some patients, abnormalities can be found in the medial temporal areas. Antibodies reacting with neuronal nuclei can be found in patients with limbic encephalitis associated with small cell lung cancer.

Pathologically, there are two main groups: In some patients, no significant pathologic changes are found in the cerebrum despite clinical dementia. Other patients demonstrate widespread cerebral neuronal loss, gliosis, and perivascular collections of lymphocytes, particularly in the medial temporal lobes (limbic encephalitis) or the thalamus. In those patients who have antineuronal antibodies in blood and CSF, the same antibodies also can be identified in the brain. The differential diagnosis includes brain or leptomeningeal metastases; fungal, parasitic, or viral infections (including multifocal leukoencephalopathy); and metabolic encephalopathy. Appropriate imaging, CSF examination, and other laboratory tests usually identify these disorders. The rapid onset of dementia in middle age accompanied by cerebellar, brain stem, or peripheral nerve dysfunction, but no other focal cerebral signs, suggests paraneoplastic dementia as a remote effect of cancer. Degenerative dementias such as Alzheimer's disease usually are slower in onset and have a more protracted course. However, paraneoplastic dementia may be confused with Creutzfeldt-Jakob disease. There is no specific treatment for paraneoplastic dementias, but they occasionally improve spontaneously on successful therapy of the cancer.

CEREBELLUM. Cerebellar symptoms usually evolve over weeks, with bilateral and symmetric ataxia of gait, arms, and legs. Severe dysarthria is usually present; vertigo and diplopia are common, but nystagmus may be absent. Some patients have neurologic signs pointing to disease outside the cerebellum (e.g., extensor plantar responses, diminished or exaggerated tendon reflexes, dementia). Early in the disorder there is a cerebrospinal fluid pleocytosis, and an elevated IgG content is common. In about one half of patients the neurologic findings precede discovery of the cancer, but the clinical picture is so characteristic that cancer should be suspected. Cerebellar atrophy may be seen on MR scan. In a subset of patients with gynecologic cancers (ovarian, uterine, fallopian tube, breast), an antibody (anti-Yo) reacting exclusively with cerebellar Purkinje cells and with the underlying tumor allows a definitive diagnosis to be made before the tumor is discovered. Other antibodies may be present in some other patients with nongynecologic tumors. The role of the antibody in the pathogenesis of the disease is unknown.

Pathologic changes consist of loss of cerebellar Purkinje cells with or without lymphocytic cuffing of blood vessels in the deep nuclei. Cerebellar dysfunction is also caused by cerebellar or leptomeningeal metastases and by *Listeria* meningitis or progressive multifocal leukoencephalopathy. These disorders can easily be identified by MRI and CSF examination. In alcohol-nutritional cerebellar degeneration, truncal and lower extremity ataxia is prominent, but nystagmus, dysarthria, and upper extremity ataxia are mild or absent. Sporadic or familial cerebellar degenerative disorders are much slower in onset. Cerebellar dysfunction associated with viral infections (varicella, infectious mononucleosis) or with chemotherapy (5-fluorouracil, cytosine arabinoside) may mimic paraneoplastic cerebellar degeneration. Paraneoplastic cerebellar degeneration usually runs a subacute course and then stabilizes or occasionally improves with successful treatment of the tumor.

Cranial Nerves

Two rare but striking paraneoplastic syndromes affect the eyes. The first is characterized by rapid onset of blindness associated with retinal degeneration, usually of photoreceptors. In some such patients, antibodies that react with cells in the retina can be identified in the serum, suggesting that the disorder is an immune one. Optic neuritis, which does not differ clinically in any way from the idiopathic disorder, also has been described in some patients with underlying neoplasms. Opsoclonus (saccadic conjugate involuntary movement of the eyes), also called "saccadomania," is often a paraneoplastic disorder. About 50% of infants and children with opsoclonus have underlying neuroblastoma. In adults, about 20% of patients with opsoclonus probably have an underlying cancer, usually breast or lung cancer. The disorder in adults may be associated with an antibody (anti-Ri) different from that found in encephalomyelitis associated with small cell lung cancer (see below). Except when the autoantibody is present, there is no way of clinically distinguishing paraneoplastic opsoclonus from opsoclonus caused by metabolic or structural abnormalities of the brain stem or cerebellum.

Spinal Cord

Two distinct myelopathies complicate cancer: *Subacute motor neuronopathy* affects anterior horn cells, usually in patients with Hodgkin's disease or other lymphomas. The course is subacute, with progressive painless asymmetrical lower motor neuron weakness of legs and arms. Some patients complain of sensory symptoms, but sensory loss is mild or absent despite profound weakness. The major pathologic finding is degeneration of anterior horn cells. Sometimes there is inflammation in the anterior horns and demyelination in the white matter of the spinal cord. The clinical course is different from most remote effects in that many patients improve spontaneously, independently of the course of the underlying lymphoma. The etiology is unknown, but a similar disorder in mice harboring lymphomas appears to be caused by a retrovirus. Typical amyotrophic lateral sclerosis is rarely paraneoplastic.

In *subacute necrotic myelopathy,* both gray and white matter are affected equally. Clinically, there is rapidly ascending sensory and motor loss, usually to midthoracic levels, the patient becoming paraplegic and incontinent within hours or days. The neurologic symptoms often precede the discovery of the neoplasm, and the illness is clinically and pathologically indistinguishable from idiopathic subacute necrotic myelopathy. Because epidural or intramedullary spinal metastases and arteriovenous spinal cord anomalies may present similar clinical signs, an MRI scan is essential.

Peripheral Nerves and Dorsal Root Ganglia

Four clinical peripheral nerve disorders occur in association with cancer. Characteristic of carcinoma is *subacute sensory neuronopathy* marked by loss of sensation with relative preservation of motor power. The illness usually precedes the appearance of the carcinoma and progresses over a few months, leaving the patient with moderate or severe disability. CSF pleocytosis and increased IgG content are common. Pathologically, there is destruction of posterior root ganglia with perivascular lymphocytic cuffing and wallerian degeneration of sensory nerves. Many of the patients have inflammatory and degenerative changes in brain and spinal cord as well (encephalomyelitis). The disorder, when associated with small cell carcinoma, is characterized by serum antibodies (anti-Hu) reacting against neuronal nuclei and small cell lung cancer cells. There is no treatment.

More common than sensory neuronopathy is a *distal sensorimotor polyneuropathy,* characterized by motor weakness, sensory loss, and absence of distal reflexes in the extremities. The illness is pathologically characterized by either segmental demyelination or wallerian degeneration (or both) of sensory and motor peripheral nerves. Pathologically and clinically, the sensorimotor neuropathy is indistinguishable from polyneuropathies not associated with cancer. Indeed, some have suggested that late or terminal polyneuropathy may be due to nutritional deprivation associated with cancer. Its etiology, however, is not clear, and it does not respond to treatment with vitamins or other nutritional supplements.

A *polyneuritis* clinically and pathologically indistinguishable from acute postinfectious polyneuropathy (Guillain-Barré syndrome) also complicates cancers, particularly Hodgkin's disease. A few patients with *neuropathy limited to the autonomic nervous system* have been reported.

Neuromuscular Junction and Muscles

NEUROMUSCULAR JUNCTION. *Myasthenia gravis* is associated with thymomas but usually not other systemic tumors. The *Lambert-Eaton myasthenic syndrome* is characterized by weakness and fatigability of proximal muscles, particularly of the pelvic girdle and thighs. The cranial nerves and respiratory muscles are usually spared. Patients often complain of dryness of the mouth, impotence, pain in the thighs, and peripheral paresthesias. Proximal muscles are weak, but strength increases over several seconds of sustained contraction. The deep tendon reflexes are diminished or absent. The diagnosis is made by electromyographic studies in which repeated nerve stimulations at rates above 10 per second cause a progressive *increase* in the size of the muscle action potential (the opposite of myasthenia gravis). About two-thirds of patients with this syndrome either have or will develop cancer, usually small cell carcinoma of the lung. Plasmapheresis and immunosuppressant drugs usually relieve symptoms, as may successful treatment of the neoplasm. The illness responds poorly to anticholinesterase drugs but does respond to 3,4-diaminopyridine in doses up to 100 mg per day.

MUSCLE. Typical *dermatomyositis* or *polymyositis* may occur as a remote effect of cancer. Fewer than 10% of patients with this disorder have cancer, but the figure is higher in older patients. The clinical picture of polymyositis associated with cancer (i.e., subacute development of weakness, particularly involving proximal muscles and sometimes bulbar muscles) is indistinguishable from dermatomyositis or polymyositis not associated with cancer. Pathologically, there may be two groups: one with the typical inflammatory lesions of polymyositis and one with little inflammation but severe muscle necrosis. The latter group may suffer an explosive clinical course. The patients respond less well to corticosteroid therapy than do those with dermatomyositis unaccompanied by cancer, although substantial improvement with steroid treatment does occur in some. Intravenous immunoglobulin may help.

Muscle Weakness. Some patients with cancer complain of *weakness* and *fatigability* that seem worse than can be accounted for by their cancer alone. Cachexia and weight loss alone do not usually cause measurable muscle weakness. The weakness is usually proximal and produces particular difficulty climbing stairs or getting out of low chairs. Ankle reflexes may be diminished or absent. Further neurologic evaluation does not yield findings diagnostic of one of the remote effects of cancer described above. Brain and colleagues have labeled this entity "neuromyopathy" because its exact anatomic locus is unclear, but others have suggested that it is a nonspecific accompaniment of cachexia and systemic illness. Specific (type II) muscle fiber atrophy develops early in patients with systemic cancer. The cause and treatment of the weakness are unknown.

Bunn PA Jr, Ridgway EC: Paraneoplastic syndromes. *In* DeVita VT Jr, Hellman S, Rosenberg SA (eds.), Cancer Principles and Practice of Oncology. 4th ed. Philadelphia, JB Lippincott, 1993, pp 2026–2071. *A description of both neurologic and nonneurologic paraneoplastic syndromes.*

Posner JB: Neurologic Complications of Cancer. Philadelphia, FA Davis, 1995. *A comprehensive monograph with chapters on metastatic and nonmetastatic complications of cancer including paraneoplastic syndromes.*

Vecht ChJ: Paraneoplastic syndromes. *In* Twijnstra A, Keyser A, Ongerboer de Visser BW (eds.), Neuro-Oncology: Primary Tumors and Neurological Complications of Cancer. Amsterdam, Elsevier, 1993, pp 385–418. *The title is self-evident; a clinical description.*

NERVOUS SYSTEM INJURY FROM THERAPEUTIC RADIATION

Adverse effects of ionizing radiation on the nervous system (Table 160–3) are related to the total dose of radiation, the size of each fraction, the total duration over which the dose is received, and the volume of nervous system tissue irradiated. Other factors, such as underlying nervous system disease (e.g., brain tumor, cerebral edema), previous surgery, concomitant use of chemotherapeutic agents, and individual susceptibility make it impossible to define precisely a safe dose of radiation therapy for a given individual. However, guidelines allow the radiation therapist to calculate generally safe nervous system doses. Adverse effects may involve any portion of the central or peripheral nervous system and may occur acutely or be delayed weeks to years following irradiation.

CLINICAL MANIFESTATIONS. *Acute encephalopathy* may follow large radiation doses to the brains of patients with increased intracranial pressure, particularly in the absence of corticosteroid prophylaxis. Immediately following treatment, susceptible patients develop headache, nausea and vomiting, somnolence, fever, and occasionally worsening of neurologic signs, rarely culminating in cerebral herniation and death. Acute encephalopathy usually follows the first radiation fraction and becomes progressively less severe with each ensuing fraction. This disorder is believed to result from increased intracranial pressure or brain edema from radiation-in-

TABLE 160–3. RADIATION INJURY TO THE NERVOUS SYSTEM

Time After RT	Organ Affected	Clinical Findings
Primary injury		
Immediate (minutes to hours)	Brain	Acute encephalopathy
Early delayed (6 to 16 weeks)	Brain	Somnolence, focal signs
	Spinal cord	Lhermitte's sign
Late delayed (months to years)	Brain	Dementia, focal signs
	Spinal cord	Transverse myelopathy
	Peripheral nerves	Paralysis, sensory loss
Secondary injury (years)	Several	Brain, cranial and/or peripheral nerve sheath tumors
	Arteries (atherosclerosis)	Cerebral infarction
	Endocrine organs	Metabolic encephalopathy

duced alteration of the blood-brain barrier. It responds to corticosteroids. Acute worsening of neurologic symptoms does not occur after spinal cord irradiation.

Early delayed reactions appear 6 to 16 weeks after therapy and persist for days to months. A transient, diffuse encephalopathy commonly follows prophylactic irradiation of the brain for leukemia in children and for small cell lung cancer in adults. The disorder is characterized by somnolence, often associated with headache, nausea, vomiting, and sometimes fever. The electroencephalogram may be slow, but there are no focal signs. Whole-brain irradiation for brain tumor sometimes causes lethargy and worsening of focal neurologic signs, simulating progression of the brain tumor. CT and MRI scans also may suggest worsening. Both disorders usually respond to steroids but resolve spontaneously even if untreated. Rarely, a brain stem disorder characterized by diplopia, ataxia, dysarthria, and dysphagia, and associated with foci of demyelination resembling acute multiple sclerosis, follows irradiation to the brain stem. *Early delayed myelopathy* follows radiation therapy to the neck or upper thorax and is characterized by Lhermitte's sign (an electric shock–like sensation radiating into various parts of the body when the neck is flexed). The symptoms resolve spontaneously. Early delayed radiation syndromes are believed to result from demyelination, possibly due to radiation-induced damage to oligodendroglia.

Late delayed radiation injury appears after months to years and may affect any part of the nervous system. In the brain, there are two clinical syndromes. The first follows whole-brain irradiation either prophylactically or in some patients with primary and metastatic brain tumors. The disorder is characterized by dementia without focal signs. There is cerebral atrophy on CT or MRI scan; pathologic changes are nonspecific, and there is no treatment. The second disorder affects patients who receive either focal brain irradiation during therapy of extracranial neoplasms or whole-brain irradiation for intracranial neoplasms. Neurologic signs suggest a tumor and include headache, focal or generalized seizures, and hemiparesis. MRI or CT scans reveal a hypodense mass, sometimes with contrast enhancement. Neuropathologic features include coagulative necrosis of white matter, telangiectasia, fibrinoid necrosis of blood vessels with thrombus formation, glial proliferation, and bizarre multinucleated astrocytes. The clinical and imaging findings cannot be distinguished from those of brain tumor, and the diagnosis can be made only by biopsy. Positron emission tomography, using radiolabeled glucose, generally shows decreased metabolism in areas of radiation damage, whereas most tumors show increased metabolism. Corticosteroids sometimes ameliorate symptoms. Improvement in symptoms may be sustained even after corticosteroid withdrawal, but if symptoms recur, the treatment of the disorder, if focal, is surgical removal.

Late delayed myelopathy is characterized by progressive paralysis, sensory changes, and sometimes pain. A Brown-Séquard syndrome (weakness and loss of proprioception in the extremities of one side with loss of pain and temperature sensation on the other) is often present at onset. Patients occasionally respond transiently to steroids, and the disorder may stop progressing, but generally patients become paraplegic or quadriplegic. Pathologic changes include necrosis of the spinal cord. *Late delayed neuropathy* may affect any cranial or peripheral nerve. Common disorders are blindness from optic neuropathy and paralysis of an upper extremity from brachial plexopathy after therapy for lung or breast cancer. The pathogenesis is probably fibrosis and ischemia of the plexus. There is no treatment.

Radiation-induced tumors, including meningiomas, sarcomas, or, less commonly, gliomas, may appear years to decades after cranial irradiation and may follow low-dose irradiation. Malignant or atypical nerve sheath tumors may follow irradiation of the brachial, cervical, and lumbar plexuses. The central nervous system may also be damaged when radiation alters extraneural structures. Radiation therapy accelerates *atherosclerosis,* and cerebral infarction associated with carotid artery occlusion in the neck may occur many years after neck irradiation. *Endocrine* (pituitary, thyroid, parathyroid) dysfunction from radiation may be associated with neurologic signs. Hypothyroidism often presents as a neurologic disorder, and hyperthyroidism or hyperparathyroidism from radiation may also cause an encephalopathy.

Delattre JY, Posner JB: Neurologic complications of chemotherapy and radiation therapy. *In* Aminoff MJ (ed.), Neurology and General Medicine. New York, Churchill-Livingstone, 1995. *Describes neurologic complications of most currently used chemotherapeutic agents and of therapeutic irradiation.*

Gutin P, Leibel S, Sheline G (eds.): Radiation Injury to the Nervous System. New York, Raven Press, 1991. *A comprehensive description of all the nervous system side effects of therapeutic irradiation.*

161 CUTANEOUS MANIFESTATIONS OF INTERNAL MALIGNANCY

Frank Parker

Cutaneous changes associated with internal malignant disease are diverse. Some skin alterations are clear indicators of underlying malignant disease. Others, less specific, arise in either the presence or absence of malignancy but occur with sufficient frequency to arouse suspicion and require a search for underlying carcinoma or lymphoma. These various skin findings may precede any signs associated with the internal malignant disease; they are therefore of crucial importance in early identification and cure of internal neoplasms.

Skin manifestations of internal malignant disease can be classified into two major groups: (1) those in which malignant cells can be found in the skin on biopsy (specific skin lesions) and (2) those in which malignant cells cannot be identified on a skin biopsy (nonspecific skin lesions). The specific lesions are diagnostic of the internal malignant disease, whereas the nonspecific skin alterations may or may not be associated with an internal neoplasm. Some of the nonspecific skin changes are clear indicators of underlying tumor; others merely arouse concern.

SPECIFIC SKIN LESIONS ASSOCIATED WITH INTERNAL MALIGNANT DISEASE

Carcinomas, leukemia, lymphoma, plasma cell dyscrasias, and sarcomas can all affect the skin specifically in clinically identifiable patterns. A biopsy of a suspicious skin lesion is helpful because the tissue of origin (primary underlying neoplasm) can often be identified.

Skin Metastases (Table 161–1 and Color Plate 16A)

Metastases to the skin are comparatively rare (approximately 1 to 5% of internal malignancies), but when present are readily diagnosed by biopsy. Cutaneous metastases usually appear as flesh-colored to red-purple or brownish solitary papules or nodules, stony-hard to the touch, and often innocent in appearance. There is no relationship between site of origin and size, color, and consistency of the metastatic deposit. Lung cancer in men and breast cancer in women most commonly involve the skin; other sources include malignant tumors of the gastrointestinal tract, kidney, ovary, uterus, and urinary bladder and oral cavity carcinomas.

Clinical patterns of metastatic spread to skin depend on several factors such as the organ of origin and whether tumor is disseminated by lymphatics or blood. In general, those neoplasms that spread via lymphatics, such as breast and oral cavity carcinoma, localize in the skin late in the clinical course. Tumors that often embolize through venous channels, such as those arising in the lung, kidney, and ovary, can appear early in the skin and thus may be the first indication of the internal malignant disease.

Certain areas of the skin are predisposed to metastases, localizing near the site of the primary cancer (Table 161–1). Thus, abdominal wall metastases, especially around the umbilicus (Sister Mary Joseph's nodules), arise from neoplasms of the stomach, kidney, and ovary. The lower abdominal wall and external genitalia metastases arise from cancers of the genitourinary systems; face and neck skin metastases, from carcinomas of the oropharynx; and the scalp is a common site for metastases from breast, lung, and the genitourinary system.

TABLE 161–1. INTERNAL MALIGNANCIES METASTATIC TO SKIN: CLINICAL FEATURES AND AREAS OF DISTRIBUTION

Primary Internal Malignancy	Cutaneous Clinical Features	Areas of Distribution
Breast	Papules, nodules—rock hard En cuirasse—scirrhous form Erysipeloides—cellulitis form Alopecia neoplastica	Chest wall Trunk Scalp
Lung	Papules, nodules Scirrhous—morpheic form Erysipeloides—cellulitis form Alopecia neoplastica	Chest wall Scalp Face
Kidney	Angiomatous, pulsatile nodules Scirrhous—en cuirasse form Alopecia neoplastica	Abdominal wall, trunk Scalp Face External genitalia
Stomach, bowel, pancreas	Nodules Scirrhous—en cuirasse form Cellulitis—erysipeloides	Anterior abdomen Periumbilical
Ovary, uterus	Nodules Cellulitis—erysipeloides form	Umbilicus, abdomen
Oral cavity	Nodules	Face and neck
Thyroid	Pulsatile angiomatous nodules	Anywhere

Some patterns of metastatic disease are characteristic. For example, metastases to the scalp simulate wens or turban (pilar) tumors that may ulcerate. More distinctive is "alopecia neoplastica"—that is, areas of scarring alopecia in the scalp with induration and atrophy that simulate alopecia areata. Metastases from the breast and, less commonly, from the stomach, prostate, lung, uterus, and pancreas can produce dramatic changes in the chest wall: carcinoma en cuirasse. This scirrhous form of cutaneous metastatic spread produces extensive fibrosis of the dermis as a result of lymphatic involvement and obstruction by the cancer cells so that large areas of the chest are girdled by a thick, rigid encasement on which pink to flesh-colored papules and nodules evolve to form morphea-like plaques. The distinctive skin lesion of inflammatory carcinoma, or "carcinoma erysipeloides," is usually caused by breast cancer (less frequently by malignant tumors of the uterus, lung, and gastrointestinal tract) and simulates cellulitis over the ipsilateral chest wall anteriorly. Renal cell carcinoma and medullary and anaplastic forms of thyroid cancer, which are highly vascularized tumors, may simulate hemangiomatous nodules that pulsate on palpation when deposited in the skin. *Inflammatory oncotaxis* is a term describing the attraction of cancer cells to an area of tissue trauma resulting presumably because trauma (surgery and radiation) causes inflammation and capillary disruption, thus predisposing cancer cells to settle in these areas. For example, cutaneous metastases from colon, kidney, and cervix have been known to localize in abdominal wall surgical incisions.

Prognosis among patients with cutaneous metastases is poor, as they imply metastases elsewhere internally. If a cutaneous metastatic lesion is discovered years after the primary cancer is diagnosed, a second internal cancer should be ruled out because only 10% of internal cancers (mostly breast carcinoma) spread to the skin after 5 years' time. Clearly any skin nodule or papule of obscure origin and uncertain diagnosis should undergo biopsy, especially if there are reasons to suspect malignancy.

Lymphomas

Specific cutaneous involvement (neoplastic cellular proliferation in the skin) is seen less frequently in the lymphoma-leukemia group of neoplasms than in carcinomas. Rather, cutaneous manifestations are more often nonspecific (i.e., pruritus, petechiae, purpura, infections) in patients with leukemias and lymphomas, occurring in 25 to 40% of such patients (see below, Nonspecific Skin Lesions Associated with Internal Malignant Disease). The specific skin lesions that are seen are similar in patients with lymphoma and leukemia, regardless of the various types of these neoplasms. Thus, skin lesions in all forms of lymphomas and leukemias appear as red, blue, and violaceous asymptomatic macules, nodules, and plaques that may ulcerate. Particularly suggestive are thickened, beefy-red arcuate lesions as well as poikilodermatous plaques (hyperpigmentation and hypopigmentation with telangiectasis throughout the thickened patches).

CUTANEOUS T-CELL LYMPHOMAS (Table 161–2). These lymphomas are lymphoproliferative disorders of helper T lymphocytes with an affinity for skin (epidermotropism) in which atypical lymphocytes accumulate in clusters in the epidermis to form so-called Pautrier's abscesses. They represent at least three types of lymphoma: mycosis fungoides, Sézary syndrome, and adult T-cell lymphoma, each of which presents with variable clinical characteristics and biologic behavior.

Mycosis fungoides (see Color Plate 16B) usually follows a prolonged course, beginning with nonspecific skin lesions (so-called premycotic stage) that, after a variable number of years, evolve into histologically specific skin lesions (cutaneous patches, plaques—the mycotic stage) and then into ulcerative nodules and tumors (tumor stage).

Extracutaneous disseminated disease involves first lymph nodes and then, in advanced stages, liver and spleen and other internal organs. Less commonly the disease may begin with cutaneous nodules and tumors without evolving from patches and plaques. Several types of clinical lesions (patches, plaques, and tumors) may coexist in any one patient. The premycotic stage (biopsy of lesions is nonspecific) can persist from a few months to more than 40 years, the morphology of the skin lesions resembling a number of banal dermatoses: psoriasis or eczema or poikilodermatous telangiectatic, stippled pigmented patches. In the plaque stage the premycotic lesions become infiltrated, although indurated, red-purple plaques also arise from previously uninvolved skin. The lesions usually are oval to round, but they may also be arciform or annular or assume a horseshoe shape, or the entire integument may be infiltrated, producing a thickened, red hide (erythroderma). In the final stage, tumors develop from preexisting plaques, erythroderma, or previously

TABLE 161–2. CUTANEOUS T-CELL LYMPHOMAS

Lymphoma	Skin Lesions	Other Features
Mycosis fungoides	Erythematous patches, plaques, tumors, erythroderma	Late involvement of lymph nodes, internal organs
Sézary syndrome	Erythroderma with ectropion and leonine facies; often spares body folds	Sézary cells in blood with high WBC, hepatosplenomegaly, lymphadenopathy
Adult T-cell lymphoma	Erythroderma, papules, nodules	HTLV 1 virus antibodies, hepatosplenomegaly, osteolytic bone lesions, hypercalcemia
T immunoblastic lymphoma	Plaques, tumors	Arise from pre-existing mycosis fungoides or Sézary syndrome
Chronic lymphoblastic leukemia, T-cell type	Erythroderma, plaques, nodules	Prolonged course
T lymphoblastic lymphoma	Tumors of skin	Rapidly fatal with bone marrow and mediastinal involvement

uninvolved skin. Tumors may be a few centimeters to 10 cm in size and often ulcerate. It is difficult to diagnose mycosis fungoides in the premycotic stage; it requires multiple skin biopsies over extended periods. However, the detection of rearranged T-cell receptor genes can be readily demonstrated in skin lesions of mycosis fungoides, and this may prove to be a sensitive and practical method for the early diagnosis of T-cell neoplasms (including mycosis fungoides, human T-cell lymphomas, and chronic lymphocytic leukemia). Clonal rearrangements for the β T-cell receptor genes are also found in lymph nodes removed from patients with mycosis fungoides and considered histologically to contain only benign lymphadenopathy.

The *Sézary syndrome* (see Color Plate 16C), the leukemic variant of mycosis fungoides, consists of generalized exfoliative dermatitis with edema, redness, and thickening of the skin associated with ectropion, leonine facies, keratoderma of the palms and soles, hepatosplenomegaly, and lymphadenopathy as well as with large numbers of atypical T lymphocytes in the circulation. The latter, so-called Sézary cells, represent T cells with highly convoluted nuclei identical to the cells infiltrating the skin in mycosis fungoides. The immediate source of the circulating Sézary cells appears to be the skin, as the bone marrow is rarely involved. In many patients mycosis fungoides pursues a chronic course, and the patients die of unrelated causes; some experience rapid progression to cutaneous tumors and ulcerative lesions and disseminated disease (visceral involvement is frequently dif-fuse and resembles leukemic infiltrates). Sézary syndrome has a particularly poor prognosis. Staphylococcal or *Pseudomonas* septicemia is the most common terminal event, accounting for half of the deaths.

Adult T-cell lymphoma, which is associated with a retrovirus, human T-cell lymphoma virus (HTLV), occurs mainly in blacks in the United States. Cutaneous findings are prominent in 70% of patients and may be the presenting feature. Flesh-colored papules, nodules, and tumors as well as generalized erythroderma may be present. The papules are diffusely disseminated over the trunk and coalesce to form plaques. Patients also display peripheral and mediastinal lymphadenopathy, and hepatosplenomegaly is found in half of the patients. A unique feature of this lymphoma is trabecular and bone marrow involvement with multiple "punched-out" osteolytic lesions in the axial skeleton and long bones associated with extreme hypercalcemia.

Several other forms of T-cell lymphomas occur with skin involvement and are outlined in Table 161–2.

NON-HODGKIN'S LYMPHOMAS AND CUTANEOUS B-CELL LYMPHOMAS (see Ch. 145). Red, blue, or violaceous skin lesions occur in all forms of non-Hodgkin's lymphoma. They appear as papules, nodules, and plaques with occasional large, ulcerated tumors that evolve in the skin after lymph node involvement. Skin involvement can be seen as the initial presentation, or it may occur late in the course of the disease. It appears to have no impact on prognosis.

HODGKIN'S DISEASE (see Ch. 146). The skin is not commonly involved in a specific way, but when it is, the erythematous papules, nodules, and plaques that often ulcerate are indistinguishable from the skin lesions found in non-Hodgkin's lymphoma. The site of predilection is the thoracic wall, spread being via retrograde lymphatic drainage pathways from massively enlarged axillary and cervical lymph nodes. Specific cutaneous involvement is seen in those patients with extensive and highly aggressive Hodgkin's disease.

Leukemias

Leukemia cutis usually develops months after the diagnosis of leukemia (55% of patients) or at the time of diagnosis (38%), but it can occasionally precede systemic disease and be the first sign of the underlying condition. Red to violaceous papules, nodules, and thickened plaques are the usual forms that leukemic infiltrates take, but rarely erythroderma is found. When chronic myelogenous leukemia (CML) enters the blast phase, greenish tumors may develop in the skin, forming chloromas or granulocytic sarcomas (see Ch. 142). Skin lesions in acute leukemias and chronic lymphocytic leukemia (CLL) are found on the face and extremities, whereas those associated with CML are more commonly seen on the trunk. In monocytic leukemia, widespread leukemia skin infiltrates occur,

and oral mucosal involvement (gingival hyperplasia) is commonplace. In general, the histology of leukemic cells in skin for various forms of leukemia mimics that seen in the blood and bone marrow, but it is difficult to diagnose the type of leukemia from skin biopsies.

Plasma Cell Dyscrasias

Specific skin manifestations of multiple myeloma, extramedullary plasmacytoma, and Waldenström's macroglobulinemia consist of lymphoplasmacytoid cell infiltrates or deposition of monoclonal paraprotein immunoglobulins (see Ch. 149). Bluish red and flesh-colored nonulcerated nodules and plaques on the trunk are observed in 4% of patients with multiple myeloma, representing in most instances extensions from underlying medullary plasma cell proliferation.

Cutaneous Histiocytic Malignant Tumors

Malignant tumors of histiocytes may be solitary or present as disseminated disease. *Malignant histiocytosis* (histiocytic medullary reticulosis), a systemic, progressive proliferation of atypical histiocytes, produces wasting, fever, lymphadenopathy, hepatosplenomegaly, pancytopenia, and skin lesions. Children and adults are affected, and skin lesions are an integral part of the disease, especially in children (up to 90% have cutaneous changes). The reddish purple papulonodular and ulcerative plaques occur over the trunk and face early in the clinical course. Malignant histiocytosis is fatal in adults but somewhat less aggressive in children.

Angioblastic Lymphadenopathy

Immunologically mediated, this often fatal disorder is characterized by proliferation of plasmacytoid immunoblasts and plasma cells. Fever, malaise, weight loss, hepatosplenomegaly, and generalized lymphadenopathy are accompanied in 40% of cases by generalized, maculopapular, purpuric, and, at times, exfoliative erythroderma. Biopsy findings of involved lymph nodes are diagnostic (proliferation of plasma cells, arborizing vessels, and deposition of amorphous material), while skin biopsy reveals a lymphohistiocytic vasculitis composed of plasma and immunoblast-like cells.

Neuroblastoma

Neuroblastoma, a poorly differentiated tumor derived from primordial neural crest cells, arises within the sympathetic ganglion (cervical, thoracic, and pelvic tumors) and adrenal glands of children. It frequently metastasizes to bone, lymph nodes, liver, and skin. Bluish nodules appear over a wide area (causing these children to be called blueberry-muffin children). A helpful clinical sign occurs after rubbing these lesions: They blanch with a halo of surrounding erythema, probably related to the release of catechols contained in the cells of the tumors. Even though patients with neuroblastoma are not hypertensive, 85% have increased urinary catecholamine metabolites.

Kaposi's Sarcoma (see Color Plates 12D and 16D)

Kaposi's sarcoma, a multifocal, vascular malignant tumor, can occur in four major clinical settings: African Kaposi's, classic Kaposi's in elderly Jewish or Mediterranean males, Kaposi's secondary to immunodeficiency conditions, and Kaposi's sarcoma occurring as a complication of acquired immunodeficiency syndrome (AIDS). In each instance the skin lesions are identical histologically and clinically; they present as purplish brown macules, plaques, papules, or nodules. The distribution and course of these sarcomatous lesions, however, vary according to the clinical setting (Table 161–3). Thus, classic Kaposi's sarcoma occurs in elderly males of Mediterranean background as purplish macules that may progress to infiltrative plaques and nodules on the distal extremities, following an indolent course. The Kaposi's sarcoma occurring in young homosexuals and others with AIDS is characterized by widely distributed, red-brown macules, papules, and nodules over the upper body and progresses in a fulminant course. The Kaposi's lesions in AIDS often follow skin cleavage lines and frequently involve the oropharyngeal mucosa, appearing as purple hemorrhagic plaques. The importance of the immune status in the evolution of Kaposi's sarcoma is dramatically illustrated in renal transplant patients who are immunosuppressed. Kaposi's sarcoma develops after 9 to 16 months following transplantation and initiation of immunosuppressive drugs. Rapidly progressive, widespread, red to purple papules en-

TABLE 161-3. KAPOSI'S SARCOMA: COMPARISON OF VARIOUS FORMS

	Classic Form	African Form	Immunologic Deficiency State	AIDS Associated
Age	40–70 years	Middle age	Any age	20–50 years
Gender	M:F, 10–15:1	—	M or F	Mostly males
Social characteristics	Mediterranean or Jewish ancestry	Blacks in equatorial Africa	Patients taking immuno-suppressive drugs—renal transplant, etc.	Homosexuals, drug addicts, hemophiliacs
Occurrence	0.2% cancers in USA	10% of all malignant tumors in Africa	400% greater incidence than population at large	Increasing; 35% of AIDS patients
Clinical appearance of skin lesion	Multiple purple-brown macules, papules, plaques, nodules	Nodules, exophytic lesions, infiltrative, burrowing plaques	Papules, nodules	Multiple purple-brown macules, papules, nodules; follow cleavage lines of skin
Cutaneous location	Lower legs most often, occasionally arms	Extremities	Trunk, neck—widespread lesions	Widespread—upper body, face, neck
Mucosal involvement	Rare	Rare	—	Common
Node and systemic involvement	Rare—occasionally nodes, GI tract, liver in 10% of patients	Uncommon	—	Frequent; 75% with visceral involvement; 5% visceral lesions only
Course and prognosis	Indolent course, 15% mortality within 10 years	Indolent course	Good; may regress if immunosuppressive drugs can be stopped	Fulminant condition, poor prognosis
Response to therapy	Excellent	—	Good	Poor

sue, but they may regress when immunosuppressive therapy is withdrawn.

NONSPECIFIC SKIN LESIONS ASSOCIATED WITH INTERNAL MALIGNANT DISEASE (Table 161-4)

Malignant cells cannot be identified in the skin in a wide variety of cutaneous manifestations of internal malignant disease. The pathogenesis of these disparate skin reactions is obscure. Often the only evidence that malignancy and cutaneous changes are related is the observation that following removal of the tumor or treatment of the neoplasm the skin change subsides or disappears and may subsequently exacerbate if the neoplasm recurs. Skin manifestations may coincide with, antedate, or follow the clinical diagnosis of internal malignant disease.

Although nonspecific manifestations are often highly suggestive of underlying malignant disease, they are more frequently seen with other nonmalignant conditions. When these skin changes are observed, therefore, an internal neoplasm is only one of several possibilities in the differential diagnosis.

Nonspecific skin manifestations can be considered under two major headings: (1) skin changes common to many skin diseases, including internal malignancy; and (2) syndromes and entities commonly associated with internal neoplasia.

Skin Changes Common to Many Skin Conditions, Including Internal Malignancy

Pruritus, unassociated with detectable abnormalities of the skin except for secondary lesions such as excoriations or prurigo-like papules, may be an important manifestation of various internal malignant diseases, including Hodgkin's disease, lymphocytic leukemia, carcinoid, polycythemia vera (in which pruritus often occurs after exposure to heat), and, less commonly, carcinoma. The itching may be mild or severe, localized or generalized, intermittent or constant. In Hodgkin's disease, itching is usually continuous and may be localized to the feet and lower part of the body, only later to become generalized. Up to 30% of patients with Hodgkin's disease may itch. Pruritus of leukemia has a greater tendency to be generalized and may evolve into generalized erythroderma. Carcinomas of the gastrointestinal tract, lung, ovary, and prostate may also be associated with itching, which may precede recognition of these cancers by a year. Although dry skin (xerosis) is the most common cause of pruritus, other systemic causes of this bothersome symptom should be sought in addition to malignant disease, including drug reactions, cholestatic liver disease, uremia, diabetes, and thyroid disease.

Erythroderma, or exfoliative dermatitis, is a cutaneous reaction pattern with various causes. In 10% of patients, total-body cutaneous redness, edema, scaling, and lichenification are associated with malignancy. In clinical practice the usual cause of exfoliative dermatitis is either a drug reaction or a generalized exacerbation of a pre-existing dermatosis such as atopic dermatitis, psoriasis, or contact dermatitis. When it is due to malignant disease, erythroderma is most pathognomonic of Hodgkin's disease, less frequently seen in lymphocytic leukemia, or rarely associated with underlying carcinoma. Erythroderma may be the first sign of Hodgkin's disease or leukemia. Skin biopsies do not reveal lymphomatous or leukemic infiltrates, although the patients clinically look similar to those with Sézary's syndrome (in which skin biopsies display diagnostic Sézary cells).

Figurate erythemas are red, gyrate, serpiginous, and annular bands that take on a pattern reminiscent of a wood grain and have been given descriptive names such as erythema gyratum repens and erythema annular centrifugum. These lesions are occasionally associated with neoplasia, especially breast and lung cancer.

Urticaria-like lesions, flesh-colored to red pruritic papules, nodules, and plaques, at times accompany leukemia, so-called

TABLE 161-4. NONSPECIFIC SKIN LESIONS ASSOCIATED WITH INTERNAL MALIGNANCIES

I. Skin lesions common to many skin conditions, including internal malignancy
II. Syndromes and entities commonly associated with internal malignancy
  A. Nongenetic syndromes
    1. High incidence of association with internal malignancy
      Paget's disease
      Stewart-Treves syndrome
      Acanthosis nigricans
      Dermatomyositis
      Leser-Trélat syndrome
      Glucagonoma syndrome
      Bazex syndrome
      Pulmonary osteoarthropathy
      Carcinoid syndrome
      Lymphomatoid papulosis
    2. Low incidence of association with malignancy
      Sweet's syndrome
      Amyloid
      Urticaria pigmentosa and mastocytosis syndrome
      Bowen's disease
  B. Genetic syndromes
    1. High incidence of association with malignancy
      Torre's syndrome
      Gardner's syndrome
      Cowden's syndrome
      Multiple endocrine neoplasia IIB
      Ataxia-telangiectasia
    2. Low incidence of association with malignancy
      Neurofibroma
      Peutz-Jeghers syndrome
      Basal cell carcinoma nevus syndrome
      Bloom's syndrome

leukemids. They may precede the development of leukemia by many months, and biopsy of the lesions does not show malignant cells. Treatment and control of leukemia often result in clearing.

Acquired hypertrichosis lanuginosa (malignant down), the sudden onset of excessive growth of fine, long, unpigmented fetal hair (lanugo) over the face, trunk, and limbs, has been associated with breast, uterine, pancreatic, pulmonary, and gastrointestinal carcinomas as well as lymphomas.

Herpes zoster is increased in incidence in patients with Hodgkin's disease and chronic lymphocytic leukemia as well as with a variety of neoplasms that are being managed with chemotherapy. This is evidence of the important role that impaired cellular immunity plays in activating viral replication. The painful, unilateral, grouped, clear, and often hemorrhagic umbilicated vesicles in a dermatomal distribution are readily recognized (see Ch. 336).

A number of miscellaneous dermatoses have occasionally been associated with internal malignant disease, but it is not entirely clear whether these associations are real or fortuitous. Table 161–5 lists some of these.

Syndromes and Entities Associated with Internal Neoplasia

A number of unique cutaneous syndromes, both genetic and nongenetic, are associated with internal neoplasms with sufficient frequency to alert the clinician to look for these potentially curable neoplasms early in their evolution. In some instances there is a high incidence of associated neoplasms, whereas in others this association is less clear.

NONGENETIC SYNDROMES AND ENTITIES ASSOCIATED WITH INTERNAL MALIGNANT DISEASE

HIGH INCIDENCE OF CUTANEOUS LESIONS ASSOCIATED WITH MALIGNANCY. *Paget's disease* of the breast is invariably found with an underlying intraductal mammary carcinoma. Erythematous scaling or weeping, sharply marginated patches on the nipple and areola of one breast should alert the clinician to examine the breast carefully. A breast mass may not be palpable or may not be definitely found with mammography, but in virtually every case an underlying carcinoma is present. Paget's disease can also occur in the anogenital region (extramammary Paget's disease). In this disorder, eczematous, pruritic, crusted, lichenified, well-demarcated patches may involve the lower abdominal wall, inguinal regions, genitalia, or perianal area. In up to 50% of such patients, an underlying carcinoma of the rectum, prostate, urethra, other parts of the genitourinary tract, or apocrine gland is found. Biopsies taken from mammary and extramammary Paget's disease show the same diagnostic features, namely, large, round cells with clear cytoplasm in the epidermis (Paget's cells).

Stewart-Treves syndrome is the occasional occurrence of lymphoangiosarcoma as a complication of chronic lymphedema of the arm after radical mastectomy for carcinoma of the breast. Angiomatous, livid, or dusky red blebs and nodules exuding fluid may evolve from 2 to 20 years following mastectomy and the onset of the lymphedema. Angiosarcoma has also developed in congenital lymphedema as well as in lymphedema of the legs following surgery for cervical cancer.

TABLE 161–5. DERMATOSES ASSOCIATED WITH INTERNAL MALIGNANT DISEASE

Dermatosis	Associated Cancer
Bullous lesions: pemphigoid, pemphigus, dermatitis herpetiformis	Rectal, breast, larynx, lymphoma
Tylosis: palmar hyperkeratosis	Esophagus
Acquired ichthyosis	GI leiomyosarcoma, lymphoma, multiple myeloma, lung, breast
Palmar fasciitis and polyarthritis: palmar fascial thickening with erythema, swelling of palms and dorsum of hands	Ovary

Acanthosis nigricans (see Color Plate 16G) presents as soft, velvety, verrucous, brown hyperpigmentation of the body folds, especially those of the neck, axillae, and groin. When it occurs in patients over the age of 40 years, it is often a sign of an underlying malignant tumor, usually adenocarcinoma (most often stomach, gastrointestinal tract, and uterus; less commonly, ovary, prostate, breast, and lung) and rarely lymphoma. Acanthosis nigricans involving the tongue and oral mucosa is highly suggestive of underlying malignancy. Acanthosis nigricans may appear before the malignant neoplasm 20% of the time. Regression of the skin sign following therapy for the tumor and reappearance with reactivation of the tumor have been observed, suggesting that the underlying tumor secretes an unidentified substance that is responsible for the verrucoid skin lesions. Acanthosis nigricans is more commonly found in individuals under 40 years of age, and then it is not usually associated with malignancy but rather with obesity or a variety of endocrinopathies (Cushing's disease, acromegaly, polycystic ovaries, hypothyroidism and hyperthyroidism, insulin-resistant diabetes). It also occurs on a familial basis. Special concern must be given to nonobese adults who have recently developed the verrucous areas in body folds. In 80 to 90% of all instances the cancer arises in the stomach.

Dermatomyositis (see Color Plate 16H) developing in individuals over 40 years of age also calls for a careful search for underlying carcinoma (see Ch. 247). Although there is disagreement whether the incidence of internal malignant disease is increased in dermatomyositis, numerous cases have been reported with this association. Not uncommonly the dermatomyositis resolves upon removal of the carcinoma, but the syndrome recurs if the tumor reappears. In some instances the dermatomyositis precedes the cancer by several years. The search for neoplasm should be continued, therefore, even if the initial evaluation fails to find it, especially with (1) failure of the dermatomyositis to respond to conventional therapy (i.e., after systemic steroids), (2) a history of previous malignant disease, or (3) presence of atypical symptoms of the dermatomyositis. Malignant tumors of the breast and lung are those most commonly associated with dermatomyositis. Dermatomyositis is recognized by proximal muscle pain and weakness and a characteristic dermatitis that includes heliotrope rash (edematous, dusky, violaceous discoloration of the eyelids) along with a brilliant violaceous, erythematous telangiectatic scaling rash over the cheeks, forehead, V of the neck, elbows, and knees. Gottron's papules, slightly elevated red to violaceous papules or small plaques over the knuckles, are also an important finding in dermatomyositis.

The *Leser-Trélet sign,* the sudden appearance and growth of multiple seborrheic keratoses, occurs with underlying cancer in the elderly. This sign has been the subject of controversy because seborrheic keratoses of the same histologic type are common in the elderly. Nevertheless, several case reports have described new and enlarging keratoses in association with cancer of the lung, adenocarcinoma of the bowel, mycosis fungoides, and Sézary's syndrome and, in some of these patients, the keratoses regressed when the malignant tumor was treated.

Lymphomatoid papulosis is a disease of cutaneous lymphoid infiltration characterized clinically by involuting and recurring purplish-red papules, plaques, and nodules. Ten to 20% of patients develop a lymphoma (cutaneous T-cell lymphoma, K_1 large cell lymphoma, Hodgkin's disease). Pathologically the skin lesions appear in one of two forms: Type A lesions contain large anaplastic-appearing tumor cells, whereas Type B lesions have cerebriform mononuclear cells and epidermotropism similar to or indistinguishable from those of mycosis fungoides. The lesions may wax and wane; some patients do not develop underlying lymphoma. Unfortunately, no single clinical or pathologic characteristic distinguishes lymphomatoid papulosis from lymphoma. At onset, however, the presence of skin lesions >3 cm in diameter, persistence without spontaneous regression, and the presence of lymphadenopathy all indicate that the condition is malignant. Lymph node biopsy will help to diagnose lymphoma. Later in the disease course, rapidly growing lesions that fail to regress spontaneously or become resistant to therapy (such as PUVA) usually signal transformation to lymphoma.

Necrolytic migratory erythema, associated with α-cell tumors of the pancreas and elevated glucagon levels, evolves as gradually enlarging erythematous patches with central, superficial blister formation progressing to central crusting and healing. Annular and figurate lesions result, with exudative, erosive, and crusting areas most pronounced in the perineum, groin, and perioral areas. Painful glossitis may be another prominent sign of the glucagonoma syndrome. The skin rash and stomatitis often resolve within a week after the tumor is removed. The pathogenesis of the skin and mucous membrane lesions is unclear. The glucagonoma syndrome is discussed more completely in Ch. 206. Similar skin lesions may be seen in association with severe zinc deficiency.

Bazex syndrome, or acrokeratosis paraneoplastica, is a unique cutaneous marker of carcinomas of the upper respiratory tract, especially seen with squamous cell carcinomas of the oral, pharyngeal, laryngeal, esophageal, and bronchial areas, primarily in males. When the tumor is asymptomatic, red to violaceous, scaling, psoriasis-like patches are found confined to the bridge of the nose, fingers, toes, and margins of the ear helices. The nail folds are often red, scaling, and tender with grooving of the nails and onycholysis. Later the eruption on the acral areas becomes more extensive, spreading from the fingers to the palms and soles, which, in turn, become red and scaling and form a honeycomb-like thickening. The fingers and toes become violaceous and bulbous, and the rash evolves on the nose. In the last stage, if the tumor has not been treated and has progressed, new scaling lesions resembling psoriasis spread over the face, trunk, knees, arms, and scalp. Nail dystrophy (ridged, brittle, crumbling nails) is extensive.

Clubbing of the fingers is a well-known manifestation of bronchogenic carcinoma, mesothelioma, metastatic carcinoma to the thorax (from the colon, larynx, breast, or ovary) and occasionally Hodgkin's disease. *Hypertrophic pulmonary osteoarthropathy* is the term used when clubbing is accompanied by subperiosteal new bone formation along the shafts of the long bones of the extremities and digits. Joints of the ankle, knees, wrists, and hand may be painful and swollen. In some patients cutaneous thickening of the forearms and legs produces cylindric enlargement of the limbs, and the facial features become coarse with deep facial furrows simulating acromegaly. At times, deep confluent skin wrinkles evolve over the forehead and scalp, a condition termed *pachydermoperiostosis* when the skin changes accompany acromegaloid features.

Carcinoid, malignant tumor of the chromaffin cells of the gastrointestinal tract and, less frequently, the bronchus, may be associated with intermittent scarlet to violet red flushing of the head, neck, and upper part of the trunk. Eventually the erythema becomes permanent, and telangiectasis and tortuous veins evolve in the flushed areas. This syndrome and its cutaneous manifestations are described more fully in Ch. 210.2.

LOW INCIDENCE OF CUTANEOUS LESIONS ASSOCIATED WITH MALIGNANCY. *Amyloid deposits* in the skin may occur without obvious cause (cutaneous amyloidosis) as part of an inherited syndrome or secondary to plasma cell dyscrasias—either primary systemic amyloidosis or multiple myeloma. In the case of plasma cell dyscrasias, shiny, translucent, waxy, firm purpuric papules and plaques occur on the mucocutaneous junctions of the eyes, nose, and mouth along with macroglossia. Occasionally, infiltrated papules are not apparent, and only purpuric lesions evolve around the eyes ("raccoon eyes").

Urticaria pigmentosa consists of skin lesions that appear as numerous red-brown macules and papules on the trunk and extremities. Light stroking of the skin lesions causes urtication with edema and a red flare due to the release of histamine from the mast cells infiltrating the skin (Darier's sign). These skin lesions are sometimes associated with systemic mastocytosis (see Ch. 231) or, more rarely, with mast cell leukemia or myeloproliferative disorders (myelofibrosis, myeloid metaplasia, polycythemia, and granulocytic leukemia) with extensive infiltration of mature mast cells in the marrow and mast cells or basophils in the peripheral blood.

Bowen's disease of the skin consists of multiple superficial squamous cell cancers occurring in non-sun-exposed areas of the body, particularly in individuals with a history of long-term ingestion or exposure to arsenicals (drinking of well water, exposure to insecticides or industrial arsenicals). Bowen's skin lesions appear as discrete, red, scaling, flat to slightly raised patches that mimic eczematous or psoriatic patches. These skin lesions should be removed to prevent progression to invasive squamous cell carcinoma. The relationship of these lesions to internal malignancy is controversial, but a careful search for cancers of the larynx, lung, esophagus, liver, and bladder is warranted.

Sweet's syndrome may be the harbinger of underlying myelogenous or lymphoblastic leukemia, hairy cell leukemia, lymphomas and solid carcinomas (breast, stomach, lung, colon) in 25% of cases. The unique syndrome consists of painful, raised erythematous plaques on the face, trunk, and extremities; often the surfaces of the plaques have vesicles or sterile pustules. Intermittent fever occurs in 80% of patients along with polyarteritis, leukocytosis, and elevated sedimentation rate. Skin biopsy shows bandlike infiltration in the upper dermis with neutrophils. Identical pathology is seen with or without underlying internal malignancy, so a careful search must be made for hemoproliferative diseases or solid tumors. Frequent reassessments are advisable because Sweet's syndrome can occur very early in the evolution of the underlying malignancies.

GENETIC SYNDROMES ASSOCIATED WITH INTERNAL MALIGNANT DISEASE

HIGH INCIDENCE OF ASSOCIATION WITH INTERNAL MALIGNANCY. *Gardner's syndrome* consists of multiple epidermoid and sebaceous cysts of the face and scalp, fibrous tissue tumors of the skin (desmoid tumors, fibromas and fibrosarcomas), osteomas of the membranous bones of the face and head, and polyps of the colon and rectum (see Ch. 106). No patients with this syndrome live beyond the seventh decade without developing adenocarcinoma of the bowel.

Cowden's disease, a condition in which there are numerous hamartomas of the skin, mucous membranes, and internal organs, is associated with malignant neoplasms of the breast and thyroid in a high percentage of patients. The hamartomas present on the skin as keratotic, warty papules and nodules on the central area of the face and on the hands and arms. Papular, cobblestone lesions may appear on the gingiva, palate, tongue, and larynx.

Torre's syndrome, another autosomal dominant condition, consists of multiple sebaceous gland tumors, sebaceous adenomas, sebaceous hyperplasia, and basal cell cancers with sebaceous differentiation. It is associated with cancers of the colon, duodenum, ampulla of Vater, uterus, and genitourinary tract. The skin tumors in this condition are yellowish or red papules and nodules.

Multiple Endocrine Neoplasia Type IIB (see Ch. 210.1). Medullary carcinoma of the thyroid and pheochromocytoma are found in association with a marfanoid habitus and multiple whitish to pink papular mucosal neuromas studding the lips, tip of the tongue, and, less often, the buccal mucosa, gingivae, palate, and pharynx. Neuromas also develop on the conjunctivae and corneas, and thickened corneal nerves may be found with slit-lamp examination.

Ataxia-telangiectasia, an autosomal recessive disorder associated with lymphomas, is recognized by telangiectasias over the ears, eyelids, nose, butterfly area of the face, and conjunctivae in association with progressive cerebellar ataxia, profound immunologic deficiency, and sinopulmonary infections (see Ch. 223). Hodgkin's disease, non-Hodgkin's lymphoma, or leukemia develops in 10% of patients, with other malignant neoplasms such as ovarian dysgerminomas, gliomas, cerebellar medulloblastomas, and gastric adenocarcinomas occurring less frequently. Persons with *Wiskott-Aldrich syndrome* also display a propensity to malignant lymphomas (79%) or leukemias (13%) by the age of 10 years, probably related to widespread immunologic abnormalities of both the humoral and cell-mediated systems found in this condition. The skin changes are similar to atopic dermatitis (and are associated with petechiae due to thrombocytopenia).

LOW INCIDENCE OF ASSOCIATION WITH INTERNAL MALIGNANCY. Some dominant inherited conditions are associated with internal malignancy, but the relationship is not frequently found. Thus, patients with *neurofibromatosis* have café-au-lait spots, axillary freckles, and multiple neurofibromas. They are prone to develop pheochromocytomas (10% of patients by the age of 60 years), acoustic neuromas, and neurofibrosarcomas.

Patients with the *Peutz-Jeghers syndrome* have numerous brown-black macules on the lips, perioral regions, hands, and feet in association with hamartomatous polyps of the small bowel, stomach, and, less commonly, colon (see Ch. 106). Malignancy occasionally develops in the polyps. *Nevoid basal cell carcinoma syndrome* is occasionally associated with the development of medulloblastoma or fibrosarcoma of the jaw.

Bloom's syndrome (telangiectatic redness of the skin in photoexposed areas and stunted growth) and the *Chédiak-Higashi syndrome* (light coloration of skin and hair) are autosomal recessive conditions associated with a propensity to develop leukemias and lymphomas.

Callen JP (ed.): Dermatological Signs of Internal Disease, 2nd ed., Philadelphia, WB Saunders, 1995. *Has chapters on the cutaneous signs of internal malignancy, metastatic disease to the skin, leukemias, and lymphomas, all written by experts. Most pictures are black and white; bibliography is limited.*

Fett DL, Gibson LE, Su WPD: Sweet's syndrome: Systemic signs and symptoms and associated disorders. Mayo Clin Proc 70:234, 1995. *Reviews the experience with this subcutaneous marker of malignancy in 48 patients encountered over 12 years.*

Kurzrock E, Cohen PR, Markowitz A: Clinical manifestations of vasculitis in patients with solid tumors. A case report and review of the literature. Arch Intern Med 154:334, 1994. *A comprehensive review of the clinical manifestations of cutaneous vasculitis in patients with solid tumors.*

Politi Y, Ophir J, Brenner S: Cutaneous paraneoplastic syndromes. Acta Derm Venereol 73:161, 1993. *An up-to-date review with tables, figures, and a good bibliography.*

Poole S, Fenske NA: Cutaneous markers of internal malignancy. I. Malignant involvement of the skin and the genodermatoses. J Am Acad Dermatol 28:1, 1993. Poole S, Fenske NA: Cutaneous markers of internal malignancy. II. Paraneoplastic dermatoses and environmental carcinogens. J Am Acad Dermatol 28:147, 1993. *A comprehensive review of cutaneous signs of internal malignancy both metastatic and paraneoplastic; multiple colored pictures and an extensive bibliography.*

162 PRINCIPLES OF CANCER THERAPY

Sydney E. Salmon and Joseph R. Bertino

Over the past few decades the development of effective anticancer drugs has progressively integrated medical management with surgery and radiation therapy in the multimodal treatment of cancer. The development of new cytotoxic and endocrine agents and the introduction of biologic therapy based on recombinant synthesis of interferons and cytokines have expanded such medical management, as has the treatment of the complications of cancer. Furthermore, the internist also must be familiar with palliative aspects of cancer care, including management of pain (see Ch. 17) and treatment of life-threatening complications (see Ch. 163).

Although current systemic therapy can cure few forms of metastatic cancer, it is now increasingly effective as a component of multimodal management of apparently localized cancers known to have a high frequency of occult micrometastatic spread. This approach is predicated on the availability of specific systemic agents with antitumor activity in advanced cancers of the same histopathology. Not all patients are candidates for attempts at cancer therapy because of limitations in available drugs or comorbidity from other medical problems associated with increasing age. To a significant extent, cancer is a disease of the elderly, and treatment for many types of cancer in patients over the age of 65 remains difficult owing to reduced host tolerance to the toxicities of many cancer chemotherapeutic agents. Patients and families must be fully informed about the nature of planned treatment, whether curative or palliative in intent. Inasmuch as prognosis for individual patients is currently based on statistical estimates, the physician must evaluate each patient individually in relation to relevant prognostic factors in attempting to establish prognosis and develop a treatment plan.

DEVELOPMENT OF A TREATMENT PLAN

The major clinical features of cancer to be considered in developing a treatment plan include (1) specific histologic diagnosis of the neoplasm, (2) tumor burden and extent of specific organ involvement (stage), and (3) biologic characteristics and other prognostic factors relevant to the specific type of cancer.

DIAGNOSIS. Accurate histologic diagnosis and staging critically influence treatment selection. Increasingly, immunohistochemical analysis helps in subtyping lymphomas and distinguishing among various morphologically "undifferentiated" neoplasms. Undifferentiated or poorly differentiated tumors can be proven with

immunohistochemistry to be lymphoma, melanoma, germ cell neoplasm, sarcoma, and so on. Tumors of diverse histogenesis can have markedly different prognosis and treatment. Electron microscopy sometimes can help by identifying specific morphologic features such as melanosomes (in melanoma) or desmosomes (in carcinomas) that permit more specific classification. Other distinctive biologic markers include immunohistochemistry, hormone receptor expression, serum or urinary tumor markers (e.g., β-hCG, α-fetoprotein, carcinoembryonic antigen, CA-125, myeloma proteins, urinary 5-hydroxyindole acetic acid), karyotype, or molecular analysis. Increasingly, molecular biologic methods for DNA analysis are also playing a role in diagnosis by identifying characteristic gene rearrangements (e.g., Southern blots), gene deletions, or oncogene expression. Cellular proto-oncogene amplification and expression have been linked to the pathogenesis of various neoplasms (Table 162–1). Recently, genes have also been identified that regulate the cell cycle and provide "checkpoints" when damage to DNA occurs. Thus, in the presence of the tumor suppressor gene p53, cells damaged by drugs or x-rays undergo "apoptosis," or cell death. A large percentage of tumor cells have abnormal p53 function (loss or mutation) and continue to divide and generate further genetic abnormalities (translocations, rearrangements) even when exposed to DNA damage. Another important tumor suppressor gene is the retinoblastoma gene (Rb). Cells homozygous for this deletion become malignant, as this protein is important for cell cycle regulation. Determination of the status of these two gene products is becoming increasingly important in assessing tumor biology and prognosis.

In the leukemias and lymphomas, such information can prove important for selecting appropriate treatment approaches. For example, the approach to treatment of T-cell or B-cell lymphomas differs as a function of cell lineage, and this often cannot be identified with standard histologic approaches. Accordingly, it is important that the surgeon provide fresh tissue to the pathologist. Many specialized tests cannot be performed on tumor tissue that has been fixed. These specialized studies can in some instances provide evidence for a treatable or curable form of cancer that otherwise might go unrecognized.

STAGING. Assessment of the body burden and spread of cancer by clinical means (staging) is important in developing the treatment plan. Most staging systems assess the size of the primary tumor and define regional lymph node involvement, as well as the presence or absence of distant metastatic disease. It is important to distinguish between clinical and pathologic staging and to recognize that pathologic staging employing surgical biopsy is generally more accurate. Increasingly, staging can be accomplished by using noninvasive imaging procedures such as chest radiography and magnetic resonance (MR) imaging or computed tomography (CT) scanning. In the diagnostic workup of specific forms of cancer, such as breast or prostate cancer, bone scans can be useful to evaluate advanced disease but have minimal use in early localized disease unless the patient has skeletal symptoms. For multiple myeloma, bone scans are of less use than skeletal radiographs. The temptation to use a variety of redundant and expensive tests such as CT, MR, and ultrasonography to examine the same site should be avoided. It is important to focus on the benefit-to-risk ratio of invasive procedures such as staging laparotomy. The patient's age, performance status, concomitant medical problems, and histologic diagnosis all must be considered and the procedure carried out only if it may influence the treatment plan. For patients who present with life-threatening local complications of cancer (e.g., spinal cord compression, upper airway obstruction, the superior vena cava syndrome, or obstructive

TABLE 162–1. PROTO-ONCOGENE EXPRESSION OF IMPORTANCE IN PATHOGENESIS OF HUMAN NEOPLASMS

Neoplasm	Oncogene
Burkitt's lymphoma	c-myc
Follicular lymphoma	bcl-2
Chronic myelogenous leukemia	c-abl
Breast cancer	HER-2/neu
Ovarian cancer	HER-2/neu
Neuroblastoma	n-myc

jaundice), it is usually necessary first to treat the local complication. Even in these cases, a pathologic diagnosis should be established if at all possible before treatment is started.

OVERALL ASSESSMENT. Once diagnosis and staging have been performed, the information must be integrated into an optimal treatment plan. For patients with apparently localized cancers, multidisciplinary input is important, as a combined-modality approach may be indicated. The biologic characteristics of the specific cancer must be considered. For many tumor types, histopathologic features such as grade of tumor cell differentiation are important, with a less differentiated or undifferentiated phenotype indicating a more aggressive neoplasm. For some sites, other biologic factors are of greater value than histologic grade. For example, in breast cancer, the presence or absence of estrogen or progesterone receptors and the DNA-index and ploidy status as determined by flow cytometry provide useful information in developing a treatment plan. Some patients with a minimal tumor burden (e.g., stage I) of currently incurable B-cell neoplasms (e.g., chronic lymphocytic leukemia [CLL] and multiple myeloma) are best watched expectantly rather than treated. By contrast, almost all patients with diffuse large cell (intermediate or high grade) lymphoma should be treated aggressively with curative intent irrespective of stage unless they are very elderly and have other major medical problems.

In any given patient, it is important to decide whether curative therapy is available or not, and if so, whether the patient's age and overall medical condition permit a curative approach. If cure is not an option, one must consider whether palliation with prolongation of survival (and relief of symptoms) can be achieved. For old and infirm patients a palliative approach may be preferable—particularly if there is significant morbidity associated with the treatment approach under consideration. On the other hand, some forms of cancer therapy are very effective and well tolerated even with advanced age (e.g., use of tamoxifen in adjuvant therapy of postmenopausal breast cancer or of chlorambucil for CLL). For many tumor types it is important to examine results of recent prospective clinical trials relevant to the patient's diagnosis and clinical setting and, if possible, to enter patients on clinical trials.

THERAPEUTIC MODALITIES

Three primary therapeutic approaches dominate the treatment of cancer: surgery, radiation therapy, and medical therapy.

Surgery

Cancer surgery is most useful to establish a tissue diagnosis, to excise the primary tumor with clear surgical margins free of tumor, and to determine the extent of cancer with staging procedures (Table 162–2). Surgery is a simple and safe means to remove solid tumors when the tumor is confined to a specific anatomic site of origin. However, in the case of some solid tumors, most patients already have metastatic disease at the time of presentation. In evaluating major surgery for an individual patient it is important to assess the operative risk-to-benefit ratio for the procedure in light of the patient's general health status, the extent of the tumor, and the likelihood that it can be completely removed. Additionally, the technical complexity of the surgical procedure, the type of anesthesia needed, and the experience of the personnel must also be considered.

With advances in both radiation and chemotherapy, the need for radical surgery has diminished. However, it remains a major primary approach to curative cancer therapy. For testicular cancer,

TABLE 162–2. APPLICATIONS OF SURGERY IN THE TREATMENT OF CANCER

1. Definitive treatment for primary cancer as a single modality
2. Use in combination with radiation and/or chemotherapy
3. Debulking residual disease (e.g., ovarian cancer) after resection of the primary
4. Resection of metastatic disease with curative intent (testicular cancer, pulmonary metastases in sarcoma, liver metastasis in colorectal cancer)
5. Determining the extent of cancer, including regional node involvement (pathologic staging)
6. Treatment of emergency complications (e.g., obstructed viscus)
7. Palliation of symptoms and signs of locally invasive or metastatic cancer
8. Reconstruction and rehabilitation

even in the presence of limited metastatic disease, regional lymphadenectomy following radical orchiectomy can be curative and eliminate the need for chemotherapy in some patients who have metastases only to retroperitoneal lymph nodes. For many other sites, surgical resection of regional lymph nodes is carried out for diagnostic rather than therapeutic purposes. For example, in breast cancer, the presence or absence of axillary lymph node involvement is the single most important factor in evaluating the likelihood of distant recurrence, and this information is currently not obtainable by nonsurgical means. Similarly, surgical staging of nodal involvement in colorectal cancer plays an important role in deciding on whether adjuvant systemic chemotherapy is indicated.

Initial cancer therapy often requires a multimodal approach to maximize the chance of cure while simultaneously reducing the extent of surgery required. Multimodal approaches require close communication among the involved physicians prior to surgery. Early communication is improved by obtaining histopathologic diagnosis by needle biopsy or local excision of the primary cancer before more extensive therapy. Two examples are of note in this regard: (1) the management of osteogenic sarcoma with limb salvage surgery, irradiation, and adjuvant chemotherapy and (2) the management of early breast cancer with lumpectomy, axillary staging followed by primary irradiation, and adjuvant systemic administration of cytotoxic or endocrine agents. In both instances, the combined approach yields a better cosmetic and functional outcome. With advances in breast conservation surgery, screening mammography is now more widely used because a diagnosis of breast cancer is no longer tantamount to a subsequent mastectomy. The result is an increased ability to establish a diagnosis of breast cancer when the tumor is less extensive and when likelihood of cure is greater. Improved plastic surgical techniques have also made breast reconstruction possible for women who either require or prefer mastectomy.

In addition to its use in diagnosis, staging, and primary therapy, cancer surgery also plays an important role in the management of some patients with more extensive cancer. In ovarian cancer, when the gynecologic oncologist "debulks" peritoneal and omental spread to the status of minimal residual disease, patients become better candidates for systemic chemotherapy and have a better survival. Additionally, early resection of pulmonary metastases of soft tissue sarcomas, and of solitary brain metastases in melanoma, colon, or breast cancer, may provide marked palliation and improved survival, albeit with only occasional cures.

Radiation Therapy

Radiation therapy has made major strides in instrumentation, physics, radiobiology, treatment planning, and applications to curative and palliative cancer therapy. In general, the term "radiation" refers to ionizing radiation that is either electromagnetic or particulate (e.g., γ rays). Compared with surgery, radiation therapy has distinct advantages in the locoregional treatment of cancer. Radiation causes less acute morbidity and can be curative for some specific sites while preserving organ or tissue structure and function. An example is the use of radiation for the curative treatment of early-stage laryngeal cancer wherein vocal function can be preserved.

The basic unit of ionizing irradiation is the gray (Gy), which has superseded the rad (1 Gy = 100 rads). By interaction with molecular oxygen, radiation induces the formation of superoxide, hydrogen peroxide, or hydroxyl radicals that damage or break cellular DNA, the critical target for radiation-induced cell death. Both single- and double-strand breaks of the DNA helix can be induced, with the latter constituting lethal damage. Single-strand breaks, if not repaired by the cell, can also result in cell death. High linear energy transfer (LET) radiation can induce direct damage to the molecular structure of DNA.

Radiation has limitations in treatment of bulky tumors. Large tumors frequently have poorly perfused, hypoxic zones in which radiation often fails to induce needed reactive intermediaries. Various forms of irradiation are used for differing therapeutic objectives. For example, electron beam irradiation deposits most of its energy in the skin and soft tissues and can be useful for superficial therapy in skin neoplasms such as mycosis fungoides. Low-energy (kilovoltage) x-rays expend most of their effects on the overlying tissues above a deep-seated tumor and therefore cause considerable normal tissue damage. By contrast, higher energy x-rays (megavoltage) or γ-irradiation from a cobalt-60 source spare the skin, deposit their energy at greater depth, and provide a better approach to treating deep-seated neoplasms. Use of radioactive implants also can be useful in some settings (e.g., cervical cancer). The use of multiple irradiation fields reduces the dose to normal tissue while increasing the dose to the tumor. The use of fractionated doses or radiation causes less cumulative damage to normal tissues than to the tumor, as the normal tissues are often able to repair sublethal damage more quickly. Additionally, as a tumor shrinks with therapy, its oxygenation can improve and render it more radiosensitive. The selection of treatment is based on the relative radiosensitivity of the tumor and of the normal organs and tissues within the radiation field (Table 162–3).

The combined use of multiple fields, fractionated irradiation, and megavoltage radiation equipment is optimized by detailed treatment planning individualized to the patient's tumor. Although the major uses of radiation therapy involve local irradiation of sites of tumor involvement, total body irradiation is a valuable part of a preparative regimen together with high-dose chemotherapy for allogeneic or autologous bone marrow transplantation for leukemia or lymphoma (see Ch. 151).

Radiation therapy has important palliative applications. One of these is for bone pain due to metastatic involvement of the skeleton. Irradiation can also cause sufficient cytoreduction of tumor in bone to permit healing of osteolytic lesions and thereby prevent pathologic fractures of weight-bearing bones. Other examples include tumor shrinkage to relieve postobstructive infection in lung cancer and to suppress bronchial or gastric bleeding secondary to cancer.

Although modern radiation therapy with megavoltage equipment has proved to be extremely useful, even higher energy radiation approaches are currently in development. These include the use of higher LET sources of irradiation (e.g., neutrons, charged particles, heavy ions), which may also provide selective advantages for specific tumor sites and reduce the need for oxygenation of tumor tissue. Additionally, several classes of compounds are under study as radiosensitizers to enhance the cytotoxic effects of radiation on tumor cells. One class is the halopyrimidines, including bromodeoxyuridine, fluorouracil, and fluorodeoxyuridine, which sensitize DNA to strand breakage by radiation. A second class includes the nitroimidazoles (structural analogues of metronidazole [Flagyl]), which can enhance radiation damage to hypoxic cells by accepting free electrons and forming free radicals with oxygen. Several sulfhydryl compounds are also under investigation as potential radioprotective agents. Such compounds would need to exhibit selective uptake in normal cells in order to increase the therapeutic index of radiation for tumor cells, and this approach also remains experimental.

Although the term "radiation" normally refers to ionizing irradiation, several other forms of radiation are also used in cancer treatment. These include hyperthermia and photodynamic therapy, both of which are still undergoing development. Some tumors show thermal sensitivity to temperatures in the range of 41 to 43°C and may be more sensitive than surrounding normal tissues. Hyperthermia

TABLE 162–3. TOLERANCE OF NORMAL TISSUES TO IRRADIATION

Tissue	Toxic Effect	Limiting Dose (Gy)*
Bone marrow	Aplasia	2.5
Lung	Pneumonitis, fibrosis	15.0
Kidney	Nephrosclerosis	20.0
Liver	Hepatitis	25.0
Spinal cord	Infarction, necrosis	45.0
Intestine	Ulceration, fibrosis	45.0
Heart	Pericarditis, myocarditis	45.0
Brain	Infarction, necrosis	50.0
Skin	Dermatitis, sclerosis	55.0

* Radiation in 2.0-Gy fractions to the whole organ for 5 days weekly produces a 5% incidence of the listed toxicities at the limiting doses listed.

TABLE 162–4. RESPONSIVENESS OF CANCER TO CHEMOTHERAPY

Cure (>30%) of advanced disease
  Choriocarcinoma
  Acute lymphocytic leukemia (childhood)
  Malignant lymphoma (Hodgkin's disease, diffuse high-grade or intermediate-grade non-Hodgkin's lymphoma)
  Hairy cell leukemia
  Testicular cancer
  Childhood solid tumors (embryonal rhabdomyosarcoma, Ewing's sarcoma, Wilms' tumor)
  Acute myelocytic leukemia
  Acute lymphocytic leukemia (adult)
  Promyelocytic leukemia
Significant palliation, some cures of advanced disease (5–30%)
  Ovarian cancer
  Bladder cancer
  Small cell lung cancer
  Gastric cancer
Palliation, probably increases survival
  Breast cancer
  Multiple myeloma
  Head and neck cancer
Adjuvant treatment leading to increased cure
  Breast cancer
  Colon cancer
  Osteogenic sarcoma
  Early-stage large cell lymphoma

appears to work best on bulky tumors with poor blood supply in which the tumor cells are in an acidic environment. A variety of approaches can induce local or regional hyperthermia (e.g., ultrasonography, microwaves, regional perfusion) and may enhance the effects of ionizing irradiation or chemotherapy on local tumors.

Photodynamic therapy (PDT) is another form of nonionizing radiation therapy. PDT involves the preliminary systemic administration of a photosensitizing compound such as a hematoporphyrin derivative (e.g., dihematoporphyrin ether, Photofrin II). Such hematoporphyrins are concentrated in the vicinity of local tumors and can be activated with local exposure to visible red light (usually 630 nm), with a resulting preferential toxicity to cancer cells. The intense light used for PDT can be delivered via a fiberoptic probe which can be used for various internal sites as well as on the skin. The mechanism of action of PDT is poorly understood but may involve vascular damage or a direct toxic effect on tumor cells. Side effects of photodynamic therapy include hypersensitivity to light (skin and eyes). Locally, PDT induces transient sunburn and hyperpigmentation as well as local tumor necrosis. Tumor sites amenable to PDT include skin recurrences of breast cancer (e.g., chest wall) and malignant lesions in the endobronchus, peritoneal cavity, and bladder. Photodynamic therapy has not been approved by the Food and Drug Administration in the United States and remains investigational.

Medical Therapy

Curative therapy has been developed for a series of relatively uncommon neoplasms, and useful palliative therapy has been developed for some common forms of cancer (Table 162–4). With rare exceptions, effective therapy has utilized combinations of anticancer drugs. Increasingly, anticancer drugs are used in concert with surgery and/or irradiation.

Ideally, anticancer drugs should eradicate cancer without harming normal tissues; however, this goal has not been achieved, and most useful drugs have significant side effects. The introduction of anticancer drugs for clinical use has largely been predicted from animal tumor models. Perhaps because the initial murine models were for acute leukemia, many of the developed drugs are general antiproliferative agents. Accordingly, they are more effective against rapidly proliferating tumors than against some of the more slowly growing solid tumors and are more toxic to rapidly growing tumors than to normal host tissues. Nevertheless, such generally antiproliferative agents can have important toxic side effects on normal tissues that divide rapidly such as bone marrow, gastrointestinal mucosa, and skin.

CELL KINETICS AND RESPONSE TO CHEMOTHERAPY. A number of related factors, including total tumor burden, cell kinetics, and intrinsic sensitivity, influence the response to anticancer drugs. In both animal models and human tumors, growth occurs in accord with gompertzian kinetics. Initially growth occurs rapidly, and most tumor cells traverse the complete cell cycle. As the tumor burden grows larger, the rate of tumor cell doubling progressively slows (Fig. 162–1), and the fraction of cells traversing the cell cycle decreases as more and more cells remain "hung up" in a G_0 phase. Whereas the population doubling time may be in the range of 1 to 2 days at the subclinical phase (with less than 1 gram of tumor), by the time the tumor burden has reached 1 kg or more, the tumor cell population doubling time may be 3 to 6 months. A significant problem in the treatment of high tumor burden metastatic solid tumors is that the tumor exhibits a significant degree of heterogeneity; subpopulations of cells exhibit differing biologic, kinetic, antigenic, and drug-sensitivity profiles.

Several important features related to cell kinetics and tumor burden are important with respect to drug dose, scheduling, and response to chemotherapy. Anticancer drugs can be classified as either cell cycle specific (CCS) or cell cycle nonspecific (CCNS) (Table 162–5). CCNS agents have greater effects on cycling than on noncycling cells but nonetheless can exert anticancer effects on noncycling cells, whereas CCS agents do not. Endocrine agents are also in a sense cycle-active, as they block the transition of tumor cells from G_1 to the S phase of the cell cycle. However, certain endocrine agents (e.g., tamoxifen, progestins) are considered to suppress growth rather than kill tumor cells. Endocrine agents are therefore often given for many years, whereas cytotoxic agents are usually given over a time course measured in months.

An important concept in cancer chemotherapy is that cellular killing with cytotoxic agents follows first-order kinetics, with a given dose of drug killing only a fraction of the tumor cells. This "fractional kill hypothesis" is particularly relevant to CCNS agents and predicts that the greater the dose of drug administered, the greater the "log kill" of tumor cells which will occur.

TABLE 162–5. RELATIONSHIP OF TUMOR CELL CYCLE TO ACTIVITY OF MAJOR CLASSES OF CYTOTOXIC ANTICANCER DRUGS

Cell Cycle–Specific (CCS) Agents	Cell Cycle–Nonspecific (CCNS) Agents
Antimetabolites (cytarabine, fluorouracil, methotrexate, mercaptopurine, hydroxyurea)	Alkylating agents (busulfan, cyclophosphamide, mechlorethamine, melphalan, thiotepa, chlorambucil)
Bleomycin	Antibiotics (dactinomycin, daunorubicin, doxorubicin, mitomycin)
Plant alkaloids (vincristine, vinblastine, etoposide, taxol)	Platinum compounds (cisplatin, carboplatin)
	Nitrosoureas (BCNU, CCNU)
	Dacarbazine
	Mitoxantrone
	L-Asparaginase

The concept of combination chemotherapy was developed to take advantage of the fact that many anticancer agents have differing mechanisms of action and side effects. This concept was based on the hypothesis that giving drugs with differing mechanisms of action may achieve synergistic antitumor effects while simultaneously retarding the rate of development of drug resistance. Additionally, by careful selection of drugs in a combination to include those with known single-agent activity against the tumor and different normal tissue toxicities, the side effects would be "spread" across different tissues and organs. The validity of this concept has been borne out clinically. Optimal results for most tumor types sensitive to chemotherapy have been achieved with drug combinations, often employing CCNS and CCS agents possessing different mechanisms of action. For example, cisplatin has demonstrated clear-cut synergy with etoposide in testicular cancer and small cell lung cancer and with fluorouracil in both head and neck and esophageal cancer. The major potential toxicity for cisplatin is renal, whereas myelosuppression is the major side effect for both etoposide and fluorouracil.

New drugs entering clinical trials are normally first tested in patients with a large tumor burden of metastatic cancer who have relapsed from known effective chemotherapy regimens. Although this approach is ethically most acceptable, it nonetheless represents a significant obstacle to new drug development, as these patients have a lower probability of response to a new drug than those with a lower tumor burden or those who have not been previously treated. The presence of the blood-brain barrier has been a major obstacle to the development of chemotherapy for primary or metastatic tumors in the brain. At present brain tumors are treated chiefly with surgery and radiation therapy.

DRUG RESISTANCE. For many of the drug-responsive tumor types listed in Table 162–3, major cytoreduction occurs with initial chemotherapy. Some months to years thereafter, however, tumor regrowth occurs and continues even though the same drugs are reinstituted. This observation usually reflects the acquisition of drug resistance by the tumor to the specific drugs. Most drug resistance is considered to result from the high spontaneous mutation rate of cancer cells, which leads to the development of heterogeneous subpopulations, some of which exhibit resistance to various drugs. Perhaps the most important form of multidrug resistance (MDR) is mediated by a cell membrane glycoprotein (the P-glycoprotein), which is thought to function as an energy-dependent efflux pump that actively extrudes a variety of cytotoxic agents from the cell (Fig. 162–2).

Drugs pumped out of the cancer cell by the P-glycoprotein include natural products such as plant alkaloids (vincas, podophyllotoxins), antibiotics (dactinomycin, doxorubicin, daunorubicin) and some synthetic agents (e.g., melphalan, mitoxantrone). The P-glycoprotein is normally expressed in tissues such as the gut and the kidney, perhaps to deal with toxic products in the environment. Cancer cells with mutations to "switch on" the expression of the gene responsible for encoding the P-glycoprotein show resistance to a wide variety of useful anticancer drugs. Techniques such as immunohistochemistry, Western blots, and Northern blots can be used to detect the presence of P-glycoprotein in tumor tissues. Clinical studies suggest that patients whose tumors express P-glycoprotein have a

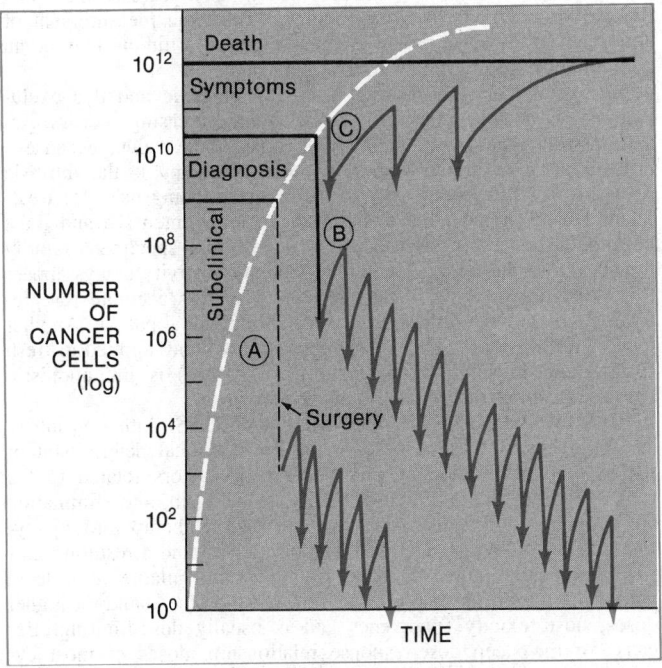

FIGURE 162–1. The relationship of tumor growth and tumor burden to treatment strategies and outcome with systemic chemotherapy. Human tumors grow in accord with the "Gompertz curve" (*dashed line*), with a decreasing doubling time as tumor burden increases. Treatment interventions relate to tumor type and extent of disease. *A,* Surgery followed by pulse courses of adjuvant chemotherapy. *B,* Systemic chemotherapy for stage III Hodgkin's disease. *C,* Palliative chemotherapy for advanced non–small cell cancer. In *A,* combined modality has curative potential with the addition of chemotherapy after surgery. Cure is also possible in *B* with prolonged administration of combination chemotherapy. In *C,* the patient's tumor burden is too great and potency of the drugs for this specific form of cancer is inadequate because of development of drug resistance. (Modified from Salmon SE, Sartorelli AC: Cancer chemotherapy. In Katzung BG [ed.]: Basic and Clinical Pharmacology, 4th ed. Norwalk, CT, Appleton and Lange, 1989, p 685.)

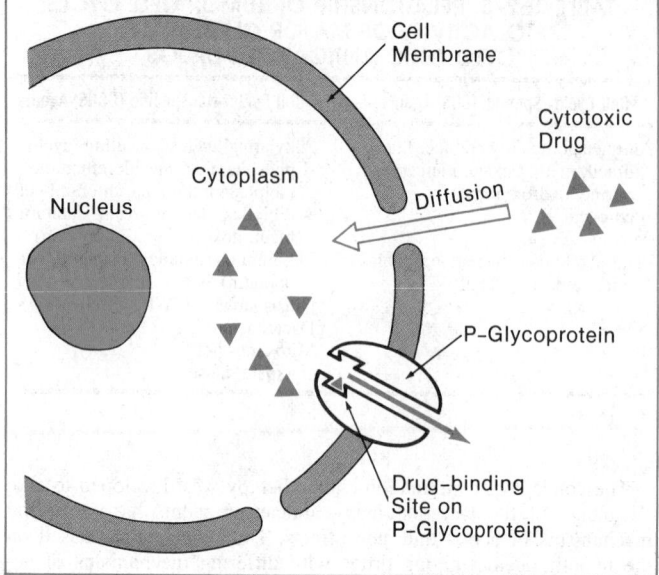

FIGURE 162–2. Model of cancer cell expressing P-glycoprotein. This transmembrane protein is believed to function as an energy-dependent efflux pump or drug transporter. It has acceptor sites to which various natural product anticancer drugs bind, after which they are pumped out of the cell. Chemosensitizers such as verapamil also bind to the drug acceptor sites on P-glycoprotein and can competitively inhibit its function.

poor prognosis. Culture studies performed on biopsy specimens *in vitro* have documented that P-glycoprotein-positive tumors usually exhibit resistance to doxorubicin. Tumor types such as sarcoma, neuroblastoma, malignant lymphoma, and myeloma are usually P-glycoprotein-negative at the time of diagnosis but are frequently positive for P-glycoprotein when the patient relapses from chemotherapy. A series of noncytotoxic drugs has been identified which reverse drug resistance mediated by P-glycoprotein (e.g., verapamil, cyclosporine). In drug-resistant patients with malignant lymphoma and multiple myeloma, high doses of verapamil given simultaneously with vincristine and doxorubicin can reverse resistance to these agents, with some patients regaining remission. Although verapamil is not an ideal chemosensitizer (owing to its cardiovascular side effects), other potential chemosensitizers (cyclosporine analogues, cyclosporine, nontoxic verapamil analogues) are now being tested in an effort to identify more effective and less toxic chemosensitizers. In the long run, such chemosensitizers may find their major use to prevent development of MDR expression. Other mechanisms of multidrug resistance have also been identified; these include an increase in a protein called MRP, and mutations in topoisomerase II, the target for the anthracycline drugs, and etoposide.

An example of a more drug-specific mechanism of resistance has been identified for the antimetabolite methotrexate (MTX). MTX and its polyglutamated metabolites inhibit the function of the enzyme dihydrofolate reductase (DHFR). The normal function of DHFR in nucleic acid synthesis is to reduce inactive dihydrofolate to its active tetrahydrofolate form, which serves as a one-carbon donor for the synthesis of purine nucleotides and thymidylate. Some tumor cells that acquire MTX resistance have been found to have an increased number of DNA gene copies encoding for DHFR. This form of multiple gene reduplication is called gene amplification. The amplified DHFR genes in MTX-resistant cells produce a markedly increased number of copies of the DHFR enzyme, far exceeding the amount of MTX that can be delivered to the cell, and thereby allow tumor cell DNA synthesis and proliferation to continue. Gene amplification in mammalian cells has been observed only in tumor cells, but the phenomenon is not unique to MTX resistance.

PREDICTIVE TESTING *IN VITRO*. Many approaches have been developed to assess the probability of a patient's relapsing after primary therapy or responding to a given type or class of en-

docrine or cytotoxic agent. The goal of such efforts is to identify which patients might benefit from planned treatment. The "S-phase" fraction of the tumor cell population undergoing DNA synthesis as well as DNA ploidy can be determined by flow cytometry. For several tumor types, patients with a high percentage of tumor cells in DNA synthesis and/or hyperdiploidy have a high likelihood of relapsing early after local primary cancer therapy. Taken with other prognostic characteristics, such flow cytometry assays may aid in identifying patients who should receive adjuvant chemotherapy. This approach is currently being applied in patients with stage I breast cancer in an effort to decide which patients are at higher risk for recurrence.

The results of S-phase and DNA ploidy analysis are often provided by diagnostic laboratories on breast cancer specimens, along with the findings from estrogen and progesterone receptor testing. Estrogen and progesterone receptor assays in breast cancer are used primarily to identify patients likely to respond to endocrine agents in either the adjuvant or recurrent cancer setting. The sex steroid hormone receptors are located in the cell nucleus and must bind the hormone and translocate it to cellular DNA to exert endocrine action via gene activation or suppression. Additionally, in the absence of adjuvant therapy, tumors that are estrogen or progesterone receptor-positive take longer times to recur and have a better overall prognosis than tumors that are receptor negative. Recent studies of another tumor cell constituent, the HER-2/neu oncogene, can be of prognostic value. Amplification of the number of copies of the HER-2/neu gene or increased expression of the gene product by RNA or protein analysis appears to predict a poor prognosis in both breast and ovarian cancer. The protein product of HER-2/neu is expressed on the surface of tumor cells and structurally appears to be a hormone receptor analogous to the epidermal growth factor (EGF) receptor. Abnormalities in expression of p53, the tumor suppressor gene, have been associated with a worse prognosis when present in a wide variety of solid tumors. Recent studies indicate that the lack of wild type p53 protects cells from chemotherapy-induced apoptosis. Lack of the retinoblastoma protein may also decrease the sensitivity of tumor cells to antimetabolites. Thus, the measurement of abnormalities of these tumor suppressor genes in tumors may be an additional prognostic factor in treatment outcome.

For specific anticancer drug testing, clonogenic and dye exclusion assays *in vitro* have been applied with increasing success. Assays of this type are potentially of considerable value, because a critical factor regarding response to chemotherapy is the intrinsic sensitivity of the specific tumor to the agents being used for treatment. However, available techniques are labor intensive and must be applied to freshly biopsied and viable tumor specimens rapidly transferred to the testing laboratory. Chemosensitivity assays appear to predict drug resistance but are somewhat less accurate for predicting which drugs will be useful for an individual patient. Another type of testing for drug resistance that is now being applied to fresh frozen (and in some instances to fixed tissues) is immunohistochemical testing for P-glycoprotein expression.

PHARMACOKINETIC CONSIDERATIONS. Although intrinsic drug sensitivity appears to be the most critical determinant of response to chemotherapy, pharmacokinetic factors related to the route of administration, bioavailability, metabolism, and elimination are probably of greater importance in cancer therapy. Many cytotoxic agents have a steep dose-response curve and a resulting narrow therapeutic index. Thus at too low an available dose level within the tumor, no response is seen. On the other hand, at higher doses, host toxicity supervenes and is usually dose-limiting. Because of the steep dose-response relationship, doses of most cytotoxic agents are calculated in relation to body surface area, a more accurate approach than dose calculations based on body weight. Patients usually prefer the oral route of drug administration, but marked variations in bioavailability among oral formulations plus inconsistent patient compliance tend to rule it out. For example, with the alkylating agent melphalan, more than a 10-fold variation in plasma levels has been documented after standard dosing. Unfortunately, plasma assays are not routinely available for most anticancer drugs, and the only semiquantitative indicator of bioavailability of cytotoxic agents is the occurrence of myelosuppression after drug administration. For patients presenting with hypercalcemia or other dire complications of myeloma, oral melphalan therefore seems undesirable, as such patients need good drug bioavailability immediately. Similar difficulties are faced with oral administration of fluorouracil, methotrexate, and 6-mercaptopurine. Bioavailability is good after oral administration of agents such as tamoxifen and cyclophosphamide.

The intravenous route of drug administration is preferable for most cytotoxic anticancer drugs, as it assures producing adequate plasma levels while minimizing compliance problems. For some agents, continuous intravenous drug administration for 4 days or longer provides better results and less toxicity than do bolus or short-duration infusions. This is because tumor response for many agents can be related to the "area under the plasma disappearance curve (AUC)" for the drug, whereas toxicity generally relates more directly to peak plasma concentrations than to the AUC. With the advent of vascular access devices such as subcutaneous ports, external catheters, and infusion pumps, outpatient continuous infusion chemotherapy can now be used for stable drugs such as fluorinated pyrimidines, anthracyclines, and vinca alkaloids. Subcutaneous administration can be used effectively with drugs such as cytarabine, interferon-α, and erythropoietin. Subcutaneous dosing provides more sustained plasma levels than can be obtained with intravenous administration. Depot intramuscular formulations are available for a variety of endocrine agents used in treatment of breast or prostate cancer.

Regional administration of chemotherapy can be used effectively for several tumor sites. One is metastatic colon cancer limited to the liver. Hepatic artery catheterization for arterial infusion of 5-fluorodeoxyuridine or 5-fluorouracil can be used effectively by connection of the catheter to an external pump or to an implantable perfusion pump. In either instance, arterial infusions are often administered for 14 days followed by a similar rest period. A relatively high objective response rate of metastatic colon cancer in the liver can be obtained by this means, but this route is ineffective for metastases outside the liver. Hepatic artery chemotherapy is expensive and associated with complications, including arterial thrombosis, biliary sclerosis, and chemical hepatitis. Nonetheless, it can induce sustained remissions for a year or more in selected patients. Regional infusion or isolated perfusion has been used with melanomas or sarcomas of the lower extremity. With in-transit melanoma metastases of the lower extremity, melphalan or cisplatin has been administered in this fashion with or without regional hyperthermia.

Intracavitary drug administration with instillation of a biologic agent such as BCG (bacille Calmette-Guérin) or interferon or a variety of cytotoxic agents (e.g., thiotepa, doxorubicin, mitomycin, cisplatin) is used to treat superficial bladder cancer. Intraperitoneal drug administration has also gained increasing popularity and appears to show particular promise for patients with peritoneal carcinomatosis. It can induce remissions of established metastatic disease. In ovarian cancer intraperitoneal chemotherapy is being studied as a follow-up to cytoreductive surgery. Diffusion of intraperitoneally administered drugs is limited to a few millimeters of tumor tissue. Accordingly, intraperitoneal chemotherapy is seldom warranted in patients with bulky tumor masses. For optimal distribution, the drug is usually diluted in 2 liters of parenteral fluid for injection. Preferred drugs for intraperitoneal administration are those that tend to be largely limited to the peritoneal cavity and have good properties for tumor penetration. Mitoxantrone, fluorodioxyuridine, and cisplatin have these favorable characteristics and can be quite useful. With each of these drugs, the intraperitoneal concentration can be 1000-fold higher than measured in the systemic circulation. Other agents sometimes used in intraperitoneal administration include thiotepa, fluorouracil, and methotrexate. Intraperitoneal drug administration can be performed at repeated intervals with relative ease if a surgically implanted Tenkoff catheter is connected to a subcutaneous port. Mild to moderate chemical peritonitis and the development of peritoneal adhesions are common complications of intraperitoneal chemotherapy and limit repeated use.

The intrathecal route can be used to deliver therapy to the meninges. Both methotrexate and cytarabine can be given by this route to prevent meningeal leukemia and treat central nervous system leukemia or lymphoma. Intrathecal methotrexate has been used effectively for acute lymphoblastic leukemia as an adjuvant to initial systemic chemotherapy and has reduced the frequency of central nervous system relapse in patients in complete peripheral remission.

EVALUATION OF RESPONSE. Objective measurement of tumor shrinkage with medical or radiation therapy has prognostic im-

portance. Reduction of symptoms alone does not indicate a response. Cure or significant prolongation of survival occurs in patients who achieve complete response (disappearance of all evidence of cancer). Whenever possible, confirmation of response should be obtained pathologically through the use of restaging procedures. Many patients achieve only a partial response, defined as a reduction of tumor burden by 50% or more. Patients achieving partial responses generally have palliation of symptoms and usually have a prolonged period without tumor growth. Modest improvements in survival accompany some partial responses.

Tumor markers in the blood or urine can be useful in monitoring response to therapy (Table 162-6). Patients with testicular germ cell tumors and gestational choriocarcinoma cannot be considered potentially cured unless the titer of marker substance falls below the limit of detection. Tumor marker studies are also useful in judging responses in ovarian cancer, prostatic carcinoma, colon cancer, multiple myeloma, neuroblastoma, and the carcinoid syndrome.

Response to adjuvant chemotherapy cannot be evaluated by these methods, as insufficient tumor usually remains to employ physical or imaging studies or tumor markers. However, in the neoadjuvant setting wherein chemotherapy is used prior to local surgery, the response to chemotherapy provides an *in vivo* sensitivity test to determine whether the employed agents can provide adjuvant therapy after surgery. This approach has been used effectively in osteosarcoma even though calcified bone tumors do not shrink with therapy. This is because neovascularization, as detected by pre- and post-therapy angiography, regresses with effective chemotherapy. Furthermore, pathologic findings at the time of surgical resection after neoadjuvant chemotherapy can be important. In general, cure of osteosarcoma is achieved in patients whose tumors exhibit at least 90% necrosis.

CYTOTOXIC ANTICANCER DRUGS. Safe and effective use of cytotoxic cancer chemotherapy requires considerable understanding of the pharmacology and toxicology of these drugs. This section provides a brief synopsis of some of the more important agents. The drug doses cited are for single-agent chemotherapy. When drugs are used in combinations, lower doses may be required for some agents. Therefore, it is generally wise to use effective and well-established combination protocols with known side-effect profiles rather than improvising combinations. The development of new combinations of standard drugs is best done in the research setting.

Alkylating Agents (Table 162-7). The major clinically useful alkylating agents kill cells by binding to and crosslinking DNA via a bis(chloroethyl)amine, ethylenimine, or nitrosourea moiety. Although these agents likely kill cells by alkylating DNA (primarily at the N7 position of guanine), they also react chemically with sulfhydryl, amino, hydroxyl, and phosphate groups of all cellular nucleophilic (electron-rich) sites. Alkylating agents differ in the severity of early and late side effects. The major acute side effects are gastrointestinal (nausea and vomiting) and hematologic (myelosuppression). Most alkylating agents have strong vesicant action and can cause local tissue injury when infiltrated into the skin.

All alkylating agents can potentially induce ovarian or testicular failure as well as acute leukemia. Agents such as melphalan and chlorambucil appear to be more leukemogenic than cyclophosphamide, whereas busulfan and the nitrosoureas cause more persis-

TABLE 162-6. APPLICATIONS OF TUMOR MARKERS TO CANCER DIAGNOSIS AND THERAPY

Tumor Type	Marker*	Applications
Choriocarcinoma	hCG	Diagnosis, response
Testicular cancer	hCG, AFP	Diagnosis, response
Hepatoma	AFP	Diagnosis
Prostate cancer	PSA	Diagnosis, response
Multiple myeloma	M-proteins	Diagnosis, response
Carcinoid	5-HIAA	Diagnosis, response
Neuroblastoma	VMA	Diagnosis, response
Colon cancer	CEA	Response
Ovarian cancer	CA-125	Response

* hCG = human chorionic gonadotropin; AFP = α-fetoprotein; PSA = prostatic specific antigen; M-proteins = monoclonal immunoglobulins; 5-HIAA = 5-hydroxyindoleacetic acid; VMA = vanillylmandelic acid; CEA = carcinoembryonic antigen.

TABLE 162-7. ALKYLATING ANTICANCER DRUGS

Drug	Major Indications
Nitrogen mustard	Hodgkin's disease
Melphalan	Multiple myeloma
Chlorambucil	Chronic lymphocytic leukemia
Busulfan	Chronic myelocytic leukemia
Cyclophosphamide	Lymphoma, breast cancer, bladder cancer
Ifosfamide	Soft tissue sarcomas
Nitrosoureas (carmustine, lomustine)	Brain tumors, lymphoma
Procarbazine	Hodgkin's disease
Dacarbazine	Melanoma, Hodgkin's disease

tent damage to hemopoietic stem cells and more prolonged myelo-suppression.

Cyclophosphamide (Cytoxan) and Ifosfamide (Ifex). Cyclophosphamide is the most widely used alkylating agent and is effective in the treatment of both hematologic malignancies and solid tumors. It does not have significant vesicant effects, as it is a prodrug and must be biotransformed in the liver, which breaks down cyclophosphamide to the active metabolite phosphoramide mustard plus acrolein. Cyclophosphamide is available in both intravenous and oral formulations and is well absorbed by the oral route. A commonly used single-agent dosage schedule for intravenous cyclophosphamide is 1.0 gram per square meter every 3 weeks. Cyclophosphamide produces a less severe pattern of myelosuppressive toxicity than other alkylating agents. Cyclophosphamide can cause severe neutropenia but usually of relatively short duration. Thrombocytopenia is less severe than with other alkylators, a useful feature. Other toxicities of cyclophosphamide include alopecia and immunosuppression. When high doses are used (e.g., for bone marrow transplantation), cyclophosphamide can also cause myocardial necrosis or inappropriate renal water retention. Although cyclophosphamide can cause acute nonlymphocytic leukemia and pulmonary fibrosis, these toxicities are more common with other alkylating agents. Both cyclophosphamide and a related analogue ifosfamide (Ifex) can cause hemorrhagic cystitis. Bladder toxicity can be blocked by administration of the uroprotective agent mesna (Mesnex), which is concentrated in the urine and neutralizes active moieties causing bladder toxicity. Mesna is particularly valuable with ifosfamide, which otherwise routinely causes bladder toxicity. Ifosfamide causes somewhat less hematologic toxicity than other alkylating agents and at present is used mostly for second-line therapy (e.g., for therapy of testicular cancer, lymphoma, or metastatic sarcomas).

Chlorambucil (Leukeran). Chlorambucil has antitumor activity similar to that of cyclophosphamide and is also well absorbed after oral administration. It is used primarily in the treatment of chronic lymphocytic leukemia, low-grade lymphomas, macroglobulinemia, and polycythemia vera. Chlorambucil does not cause hemorrhagic cystitis or alopecia, and gastrointestinal side effects are mild. However, it is myelosuppressive. Acute nonlymphocytic leukemia has been reported in patients treated with chlorambucil for polycythemia vera or other disorders.

Melphalan (Alkeran). Melphalan is L-phenylalanine mustard and gains access to cells through an amino acid transport system. Melphalan is commonly given orally in a dosage of 10 mg per square meter per day for 4 days every 3 to 4 weeks. It is essential to follow serial CBC's closely, as some patients do not absorb the drug and the only clue to this is the absence of myelosuppression. If myelosuppression does not occur, melphalan dosage should be increased in subsequent courses until moderate myelosuppression is induced. Melphalan is commonly used in the treatment of multiple myeloma and ovarian cancer and occasionally for other tumor types. The drug induces acute nonlymphocytic leukemia in some patients treated for myeloma or ovarian cancer.

Busulfan (Myleran). Busulfan is a methane-sulfonate-based alkylating agent that has specificity for myeloid neoplasms and appears to have less antitumor activity in other forms of cancer. It is available only for oral administration and is used primarily for treatment of chronic myeloid leukemia (CML). Busulfan can pro-

duce protracted myelosuppression, and hematologic recovery should be complete before the next course is administered. Myleran can cause pulmonary fibrosis, hyperpigmentation, weakness, and wasting. Adrenal function remains normal.

Nitrosoureas. Carmustine (BCNU) and lomustine (CCNU) are rapidly biotransformed via nonenzymatic hydrolysis to release moieties with alkylating and carbamoylating activities. Carmustine is available for intravenous use and lomustine for oral administration. The major toxicity of nitrosoureas at standard dosage levels is on hematopoietic stem cells, and delayed, prolonged myelosuppression can result. At high dosage (e.g., in preparative regimens for bone marrow transplantation) nitrosoureas can induce a chemical hepatitis or pneumonitis. Prolonged use with total doses greater than 1500 mg per square meter can also result in pulmonary fibrosis or renal failure. Because of their high lipid solubility and ability to cross the blood-brain barrier, the nitrosoureas have some activity against primary brain tumors. The nitrosoureas also are useful in the management of Hodgkin's disease and multiple myeloma and as part of combined-modality therapy for cancers of the anal canal.

Platinum Compounds. Cisplatin and carboplatin are platinum-coordination compounds with broad-spectrum antitumor activity and synergistic interactions with a variety of other cytotoxic agents, including alkylating agents, antimetabolites, and natural products. Although their mechanism of action is not completely understood, they act similarly to alkylating agents in terms of their ability to bind to the N7 position of guanine and crosslink DNA. However, crosslinking with adenine and cytosine also occurs, as does binding to RNA and protein.

Cisplatin and carboplatin differ in their toxicity profiles. Both drugs are administered intravenously. Cisplatin is commonly given in a dose of 100 mg per square meter every 3 weeks, whereas the dose of carboplatin is in the range of 450 mg per square meter at similar intervals, although larger doses may be tolerated. After intravenous infusion, the major acute toxicity for both cisplatin and carboplatin is nausea and vomiting, worse with cisplatin. Satisfactory suppression of the gastrointestinal side effects of platinum compounds requires potent antiemetic agents, often in combination. Cisplatin has the additional potentials of renal toxicity and a progressive neuropathy following large cumulative doses of drug. The nephropathy can be largely prevented if the patient is well hydrated with simultaneous saline infusions and diuretics are given with cisplatin. Myelosuppression is minimal with cisplatin but is dose-limiting with carboplatin. Although carboplatin is less toxic than cisplatin, its efficacy is equivalent for some, but not all tumors. The lack of myelosuppression favors cisplatin for use in some drug combinations with myelosuppressive agents.

Antimetabolites (Table 162-8). The antimetabolites are structural analogues of normal biochemical compounds, most of which are involved in DNA or RNA synthesis and generally function as CCS agents. Antimetabolites are classed in relation to their mechanisms of action.

Pyrimidine Antagonists. *Cytarabine (Cytosine Arabinoside, Cytosar-U, Ara-C).* Cytarabine is an S-phase–specific agent that is particularly useful in acute nonlymphocytic leukemia and to a lesser extent in other hematologic malignancies. Its active form, ara-CTP, competitively inhibits DNA polymerase, blocking DNA synthesis. Ara-C also blocks chain elongation and ligation of fragments into newly synthesized DNA. Ara-C is given intravenously and crosses

TABLE 162-8. ANTIMETABOLITE ANTICANCER DRUGS

Drug	Major Indications
Folic acid antagonists (methotrexate)	Acute lymphocytic leukemia, choriocarcinoma, breast cancer, bladder cancer, head and neck cancer
5-Fluorouracil	Gastrointestinal cancer, breast cancer
5-Fluorodeoxyuridine	Regional therapy (intra-arterial or intraperitoneal) for colon cancer metastasis
Cytosine arabinoside	Acute leukemia
6-Mercaptopurine, 6-thioguanine	Acute leukemia
Fludarabine	Chronic lymphocytic leukemia
2-Chlorodeoxyadenosine	Hairy cell leukemia
Deoxycoformycin	Hairy cell leukemia, T-cell lymphoma
Hydroxyurea	Chronic myelocytic leukemia

the blood-brain barrier. It is administered either by continuous infusion or in bolus doses by the intravenous or subcutaneous route for 5 to 7 days. In an alternative schedule which exceeds the manufacturer's recommended maximum, high-dose ara-C is administered in doses of 1 to 3 grams every 12 hours for 3 to 5 days and causes higher response rates. The duration of intracellular retention of ara-CTP appears to predict ara-C antileukemic effects, with best results in patients who have the longest ara-CTP retention times. Both standard and high-dose ara-C can produce severe myelosuppression. With the high-dose regimen, chemical conjunctivitis is common and can be ameliorated with steroid ophthalmic drops. With rare exception, in order to achieve complete remissions in acute leukemia, ara-C must be administered with sufficient intensity to drive the bone marrow to severe hypocellularity and destroy the leukemic blast population. Thereafter the marrow is repopulated by residual normal progenitors that were suppressed by the leukemia. Ara-C is generally used in combination with daunorubicin in the treatment of acute nonlymphocytic leukemia but also acts synergistically with other drugs including cisplatin. Cytarabine can also be given intrathecally in doses of 75 to 100 mg as treatment for leukemic or carcinomatous meningitis.

Fluorouracil (5-FU) and Floxuridine (5-FUDR). 5-FU is an important anticancer agent used to treat a variety of solid tumors, including cancers of the head and neck, esophagus, breast, and colon. It acts synergistically with a variety of agents, including platinum compounds and radiation therapy. Recent studies indicate that "pulse" or bolus injections of 5-FU are cytotoxic as a result of incorporation into RNA, whereas continuous infusions of this drug (2 or more days) kill cells by inhibiting DNA synthesis and producing "thymineless death." 5-FU is usually given intravenously by bolus or infusion schedules but can also be used in intra-arterial, intracavitary, and topical therapy. An optimal schedule for 5-FU administration is a 5-day continuous infusion at a dose rate of 1.0 gram per square meter per day. This schedule causes some gastrointestinal toxicity but only a mild degree of myelosuppression. Full doses of cisplatin can be administered additionally, providing an active treatment program in the neoadjuvant chemotherapy of head and neck and esophageal cancer. 5-FU administered on a weekly intravenous bolus schedule produces greater hematologic toxicity and mucositis than lower total doses. Less common toxicities observed with 5-FU include a neurologic syndrome associated with ataxia, chemical conjunctivitis, and a syndrome including chest pain and cardiac enzyme elevation consistent with myocardial ischemia. The bioavailability of 5-FU after oral administration is erratic, and the drug is metabolized mostly during its first pass through the liver.

Both the gastrointestinal toxicity and the antitumor activity of 5-FU can be enhanced by administration of leucovorin, which increases the binding of fluorodeoxyuridine phosphate to thymidylate synthetase. This combination appears to increase the antitumor activity of 5-FU in breast and colon cancer. Interferon-α and levamisole also appear to enhance 5-FU activity in colorectal cancer. Levamisole potentiation has been observed only in the adjuvant setting. Both 5-FU and 5-FUDR can be given by hepatic artery infusion to treat patients with colorectal carcinoma with metastases confined to the liver. With the use of a surgically placed vascular access catheter, outpatient hepatic artery infusions can be administered using either an internal or portable external pump. A limitation is that either 5-FU or 5-FUDR can induce a chemical hepatitis and biliary sclerosis with jaundice. Hepatic dysfunction can be most readily detected by obtaining liver chemistries on day 14 when 5-FU is to be discontinued. Recent studies indicate that the response rate and duration of remission are increased by the addition of leucovorin (folinic acid) or dexamethasone to 5-FUDR.

Purine Antagonists. *6-Mercaptopurine and 6-Thioguanine.* In contrast to 6-MP, some 6-TG metabolites are incorporated into both DNA and RNA. 6-TG has some uses in acute nonlymphocytic leukemia in combination with cytarabine, whereas 6-MP is used primarily in acute lymphoblastic leukemia, particularly in childhood. Absorption of 6-MP is variable, but plasma monitoring can identify poor absorbers who have a high likelihood of developing recurrent leukemia, presumably because of inadequate bioavailability of 6-MP. The 6-MP analogue azathioprine is a useful immunosuppressive agent. Because both 6-MP and azathioprine are catabolized by xanthine oxidase, patients must have their thiopurine doses reduced to 25% of their standard doses if they are also receiving the xanthine oxidase inhibitor allopurinol. 6-TG is not catabolized

by xanthine oxidase, and dose correction is not required for allopurinol.

Fludarabine (Fludara, 5-Fluoroadenosine Monophosphate). Fludarabine is an analogue of adenine which appears to inhibit DNA polymerase and ribonucleotide reductase. Fludarabine is the single most active agent available in the treatment of chronic lymphocytic leukemia and also exhibits some antitumor activity in other indolent lymphomas and macroglobulinemia. Fludarabine is often given intravenously in a dose of 25 mg per square meter per day over 30 minutes for 5 days every 4 weeks. The major toxicity is myelosuppression. Higher doses administered in early trials in patients with acute nonlymphocytic leukemia occasionally produced cortical blindness. In the lower-dosage schedule used in chronic lymphocytic leukemia and other lymphoid neoplasms, side effects are usually mild and reversible.

Additional purine antagonists are deoxycoformycin (DCF) and 2-chlorodeoxyadenosine (2-CDA). Both DCF and 2-CDA are extremely active agents in the treatment of hairy cell leukemia and can produce prolonged remissions after a single course of treatment. Both agents also exhibit some antitumor activity in other lymphoid neoplasms (e.g., CLL).

Folic Acid Antagonists. Methotrexate is a structural analogue of folic acid and is currently the only FDA-approved member of this group. Clinical trials of new antifolates are targeting not only dihydrofolate reductase (e.g., trimetrexate) but also other folate-requiring enzymes such as thymidylate synthase (e.g., Tomudex). Methotrexate can be administered orally, intramuscularly, or intravenously and is useful primarily as a component of chemotherapy combinations for various types of cancer, including acute lymphoblastic leukemia, small cell lung cancer, bladder cancer, head and neck cancer, and breast cancer. When used in high dosage with leucovorin rescue, it exerts antitumor activity in osteogenic sarcoma. Intracellular formation of polyglutamated forms of MTX is important to the action of MTX, as the polyglutamated forms have equivalent ability to inhibit dihydrofolate reductase action but have a longer intracellular retention time than MTX. The polyglutamates also inhibit other folate-dependent enzymes, including thymidylate synthase. Given satisfactory renal function and adequate hydration, MTX is excreted unchanged in the urine within 12 hours of administration.

Major toxicities of MTX are to rapidly dividing tissues, including the bone marrow, and affect gastrointestinal mucosa, and to a lesser extent skin. At high dosages or in patients with impaired renal function, MTX also can induce renal toxicity. The toxic effects on the rapidly dividing tissues can be circumvented by administering the reduced folate leucovorin (folinic acid) within 36 hours after MTX administration. Leucovorin rescue also can be used when MTX is intentionally administered in higher than manufacturer's recommended maximum dose (e.g., 1500 mg per square meter or more). When high-dose MTX is administered, leucovorin must be administered in dosage of 15 to 50 mg per square meter every 6 hours for 48 hours, with the duration of rescue contingent on the serum MTX level. Increased leucovorin dosage and longer periods of rescue are needed in patients with impaired renal function. The high-dose MTX/leucovorin rescue regimen therefore requires good renal function.

NATURAL PRODUCT ANTICANCER DRUGS (Table 162–9). The two main classes of natural antitumor products are plant alkaloids and antibiotics. Resistance to the natural products discussed below (with the exception of bleomycin) can be mediated by the P-glycoprotein multidrug resistance mechanism.

Plant Alkaloids. **Vincristine and Vinblastine.** The vinca alkaloids were isolated from the common periwinkle (*Vinca rosacea*). The major vincas in clinical use, vincristine (Oncovin) and vinblastine (Velban), precipitate tubulin and disrupt cellular microtubules. Whereas the primary toxicity of vinblastine is hemopoietic, vincristine's major toxicity affects peripheral nerves, resulting in sensorimotor and autonomic neuropathies. Common symptoms are paresthesias ("pins and needles sensation") in the digits and progressive muscular weakness with areflexia, particularly in the lower extremities. Foot drop can develop, as can occasional cranial, bladder, or bowel neuropathies. The neurotoxicity subsides slowly after the drug is discontinued, with improvement requiring months, especially if motor function is impaired. The lack of bone marrow tox-

TABLE 162–9. NATURAL PRODUCT ANTICANCER DRUGS

Drugs	Major Indications
Plant alkaloids	
Vincristine	Lymphoid malignancies
Vinblastine	Hodgkin's disease, testicular cancer
Podophyllotoxins	
Etoposide (VP-16)	Small cell lung cancer, lymphoma
Tenoposide (VM-26)	Acute lymphocytic leukemia
Taxol	Ovarian cancer, breast cancer
CPT-11	Colon cancer
Antibiotics	
Anthracyclines	
Doxorubicin	Lymphoma, breast cancer, sarcomas
Daunorubicin	Acute leukemia
Idarubicin	Acute leukemia
Mitoxantrone (synthetic)	Acute leukemia, lymphoma
Mitomycin	Gastrointestinal malignancies
Actinomycin D	Choriocarcinoma, Wilms' tumor or Ewing's sarcoma, rhabdomyosarcoma
Bleomycin	Lymphoma, head and neck cancer
Miscellaneous agents	
Hexamethylmelamine	Ovarian cancer
Asparaginase	Acute lymphocytic leukemia

icity of vincristine has made it useful for combination chemotherapy regimens. The vincas have vesicant effects and can be administered only intravenously. Both provide antitumor activity in leukemias and lymphomas as well as in selected solid tumors, including small cell lung cancer and breast cancer. Vincristine is used in various drug combinations, including MOPP, CHOP, MACOP-B, and M-BACOD used in the treatment of lymphomas and VMCP and VAD used in the treatment of multiple myeloma. Vinblastine's greatest use has been in its incorporation into the PVB regimen for the treatment of nonseminomatous testicular cancers, and in the ABVD regimen to treat Hodgkin's disease. Vinblastine is also used in combination with cisplatin in non–small cell lung cancer and with mitomycin in metastatic breast cancer.

Podophyllotoxins. Etoposide (VP-16, VePesid), a semisynthetic glucoside, is produced from extracts of the root of the mayapple or mandrake (*Podophyllum peltatum*). A closely related analogue, teniposide (VM-26), has not been approved in the United States by the FDA. Mechanistically, podophyllotoxins are thought to act as inhibitors of nuclear topoisomerase II, leading to DNA strand breaks. Additional effects include inhibition of nucleoside transport and mitochondrial electron transport. Etoposide is highly lipid soluble and water insoluble and requires a special formulation for intravenous administration. An oral formulation is also available. Good tissue distribution is achieved in all sites other than the brain. A commonly used schedule administers etoposide intravenously for 3 days at a dosage of 150 to 200 mg per square meter per day. Etoposide is excreted primarily in the urine and to a lesser extent in the bile. Its dosage should be reduced by half in patients with impaired renal function. The main side effect is myelosuppression, although gastrointestinal toxicity and alopecia also can occur. Etoposide is used primarily to treat metastatic testicular cancer in combination with cisplatin and bleomycin. The combination substitutes etoposide for vinblastine, yielding a less toxic but equally effective regimen. Etoposide also, exerts potent effects against small cell lung cancer, lymphomas, and monocytic leukemia.

Taxol. Taxol is a newly approved anticancer agent derived from the bark of the western yew tree (*Taxus brevifolia*). Taxol stabilizes cellular microtubules, thereby preventing cell division. It is water insoluble and formulated for intravenous administration. The major toxicities are myelosuppressive and gastrointestinal. Taxol has confirmed activity in the treatment of refractory ovarian, breast, and esophageal cancer and is being tested in other tumor types as well.

ANTITUMOR ANTIBIOTICS. *Doxorubicin, Daunorubicin, and Idarubicin.* These anthracycline antibiotics were isolated from a variant of *Streptomyces peucetius* and are extremely useful in cancer chemotherapy. Daunorubicin (daunomycin) was the first agent in this class and is active in the treatment of acute leukemia. Its congener, doxorubicin (Adriamycin), has a broader spectrum of antitumor activity, including both hematologic malig-

nancies and a variety of solid tumors such as carcinoma of the breast and thyroid, lymphoma, and myeloma, as well as osteogenic and soft tissue sarcomas. Daunorubicin is frequently used in combination with cytarabine in the treatment of acute leukemia, whereas doxorubicin is incorporated into regimens for solid tumors along with cyclophosphamide, fluorouracil, etoposide, vincristine, or cisplatin. Mechanistically, the anthracyclines intercalate with high affinity into DNA and inhibit the action of topoisomerase II, resulting in DNA strand breaks. Anthracycline cardiac toxicity may also be related in part to the generation of free radicals. Both doxorubicin and daunorubicin must be administered intravenously by either bolus injection or prolonged infusion. Extravasation can lead to severe tissue injury. Immediate topical application of 1.5 ml of 99% dimethylsulfoxide (DMSO)* has been reported to prevent subsequent ulceration. For prolonged anthracycline infusions, use of a vascular access catheter is advisable. Ulceration and necrosis following anthracycline extravasation usually require surgical debridement of the damaged tissues plus skin grafting.

The most common acute toxicities of the anthracyclines include alopecia, nausea, vomiting, mucositis, and myelosuppression. A dose-dependent, delayed, and potentially irreversible cardiomyopathy with reduced cardiac contractility can develop in patients who receive large cumulative doses of doxorubicin or daunorubicin. Acute cardiac arrhythmias are uncommon. Various drugs have been tried in as yet unsuccessful efforts to block cardiac-related free radical generation.

Periodic monitoring for cardiac effects of anthracyclines is normally initiated when a patient has received a total doxorubicin dose of 350 to 400 mg per square meter. Endomyocardial biopsy can also be used. Cardiac toxicity is uncommon with cumulative bolus doses of doxorubicin of less than 550 mg per square meter, above which the incidence rises progressively. Elderly patients and others with risk factors for cardiac disease (e.g., hypertension) are at somewhat higher risk for anthracycline cardiomyopathy. Anthracyclines are not recommended for patients who have major pre-existing heart disease. When doxorubicin is administered by continuous infusion (e.g., for 4 to 5 days), there is less cardiotoxicity, and a significantly larger cumulative dose in the range of 1000 mg per square meter can usually be administered. However, regular cardiac monitoring is required, and doxorubicin should be discontinued if the left ventricular ejection fraction falls below 50%. Idarubicin is another anthracycline recently approved for use in the treatment of acute myelocytic leukemia. In controlled studies, idarubicin in combination with cytosine arabinoside induced higher remission rates than daunorubicin and cytosine arabinoside.

Bleomycin. Bleomycin (Blenoxane) comprises 11 closely related glycopeptide moieties produced by *Streptomyces verticillus*. The major components are bleomycins A2 and B2. Bleomycin action involves its binding to DNA and generation of superoxide and other reactive oxygen species, including hydroxyl radicals. DNA fragmentation appears to result from the oxidation of a DNA-bleomycin-Fe^{2+} complex. Bleomycin's antitumor activity is schedule-dependent, and it is a CCS agent. It can be administered by subcutaneous, intramuscular, and intravenous routes. Bleomycin is in synergy with vinblastine or etoposide and with cisplatin. Its major uses are in carcinoma of the testis as well as squamous cell carcinomas of the head and neck, cervix, skin, penis, and rectum. It is also used in combination regimens for treatment of lymphomas.

Bleomycin has minimal myelosuppressive effects and is useful in combination with drugs that cause leukopenia. Acute toxicities include anaphylactoid reactions and fever associated with hypotension and dehydration. Patients who have not received bleomycin previously should receive a test dose (e.g., 1 to 2 mg) to discover such adverse reactions. Individual therapeutic doses of bleomycin are usually in the range of 5 to 10 units per square meter.

The most serious chronic reaction to bleomycin is pulmonary fibrosis related to the cumulative dose of drug and manifested by cough, dyspnea, and bilateral basilar infiltrates on chest radiography. It is possible to screen for earlier pulmonary abnormalities such as a decline in the diffusion capacity, which is usually detectable at total doses of bleomycin above 250 units. If the pulmonary diffusion capacity falls abnormally, bleomycin should be discontinued. The incidence of pulmonary fibrosis rises at total

---

* Although commercially available, DMSO has not been approved for use by the United States Food and Drug Administration.

doses above 450 units and is higher in patients with pre-existing pulmonary disease, after lung irradiation, and in the elderly. No effective agents can reverse this toxicity, although steroids may be of some use. Other reactions to bleomycin include skin toxicity with blistering, desquamation, hyperkeratosis of the palms, and hyperpigmentation of creases.

Mitomycin. Mitomycin (Mutamycin, Mitocin-C, Mitomycin C) is isolated from *Streptomyces caespitosus.* Its structure includes quinone, carbamate, and aziridine groups, which may contribute to its antitumor activity. Mitomycin functions as a CCNS alkylating agent after it has been activated in various tissues by the cytochrome P-450 system. Thereafter it can alkylate DNA to form intrastrand and interstrand crosslinks resulting in cell death. Mitomycin has "bioreductive" properties, with increased cytotoxic effects on poorly oxygenated tumor cells in solid tumors. Mitomycin's clinical spectrum of antitumor activity includes breast, lung, gastrointestinal, genitourinary, and gynecologic cancers. Mitomycin has been incorporated into a variety of cytotoxic drug combinations for systemic administration, often as second-line therapy for patients who relapse from initial chemotherapy. It is usually administered intravenously but can be used for intravesical therapy of superficial bladder cancer. Its normal intravenous dosage range is 10 to 15 mg per square meter.

The major toxicity of mitomycin is myelosuppression, usually appearing 4 to 6 weeks after injection. Mitomycin has a cumulative effect on bone marrow stem cells, which can lead to protracted marrow hypoplasia for 3 to 6 months after discontinuing the drug. Nausea and vomiting and anorexia often occur at the time of administration but can usually be managed effectively with antiemetic agents. Occasionally, mitomycin can induce interstitial pneumonitis, nephrotoxicity, or hemolytic-uremic syndrome.

Actinomycin D. Actinomycin D (dactinomycin, Cosmegen) is the first effective antitumor antibiotic isolated from *Streptomyces.* It binds to the DNA helix by intercalation between adjacent guanine-cytosine base pairs and inhibits DNA-dependent RNA synthesis. This leads to cessation of most protein synthesis in sensitive cells. The drug is administered intravenously, and its major toxicity is myelosuppression, usually appearing 7 to 10 days after injection. Actinomycin D also causes significant gastrointestinal toxicity with abdominal cramps and diarrhea as well as mucositis. The drug also can cause a radiation "recall" reaction wherein cutaneous erythema redevelops at a site of prior irradiation. Actinomycin D's principal use is in pediatric oncology in combination chemotherapy for the treatment of Wilms' tumor, Ewing's sarcoma, and embryonal rhabdomyosarcoma. It has some utility in adults in third-line therapy of germ cell tumors of the testis or ovary, gestational choriocarcinoma, and soft tissue sarcomas.

MISCELLANEOUS ANTICANCER AGENTS. Procarbazine. Procarbazine (Matulane) is an orally administered methylhydrazine derivative that has antitumor activity in Hodgkin's disease (as part of MOPP combination chemotherapy) and some use also in non-Hodgkin's lymphomas, lung cancer, and brain tumors. Procarbazine is usually given in a dose of 100 mg per square meter per day for 10 to 14 days in each chemotherapy cycle. Procarbazine is activated metabolically to provide a methyldiazonium ion that binds to nucleic acids and proteins as well as phospholipids and inhibits macromolecular synthesis. Its mechanism of cytotoxicity is thought to involve DNA strand scission, possibly via generation of H_2O_2. Procarbazine's principal toxicities are nausea, vomiting, and myelosuppression. One of procarbazine's metabolites is a monoamine oxidase (MAO) inhibitor that can cause toxicity when the patient is taking other MAO inhibitors. Patients taking procarbazine are potentially subject to hypertension if they ingest tyramine-rich foods such as ripe cheese, wine, and bananas. Disulfiram-like reactions are also seen, with sweating and headache after alcohol ingestion. Other infrequent reactions include hemolytic anemia and pulmonary reactions. Procarbazine is also known to be leukemogenic, carcinogenic, and mutagenic and is considered to play a significant role in the late leukemias and other second malignancies in patients with Hodgkin's disease. Procarbazine also produces azoospermia and anovulation. Because alternative combinations lacking procarbazine can be used in the treatment of Hodgkin's disease, e.g., ABVD, the benefits versus risks of using this agent must be carefully considered.

Dacarbazine. Dacarbazine (DTIC, dimethylimidazole carboxamide) is activated by oxidative N-demethylation. A methyl carbo-

nium ion metabolite is thought to be the cytotoxic intermediate with alkylating activity. Dacarbazine is administered intravenously either in a single-day infusion schedule of 750 mg per square meter or in fractionated bolus doses over 5 days or more. DTIC causes severe nausea and vomiting, and potent antiemetic agents are required. Myelosuppression is relatively mild. Dacarbazine is used in combination chemotherapy for Hodgkin's disease (ABVD), for soft tissue sarcomas in combination with doxorubicin and other agents, and in single-agent chemotherapy for metastatic melanoma.

Hexamethylmelamine (HMM). This agent is available only in an oral formulation because of its sparing solubility. Oral bioavailability of HMM is quite variable, however, and nausea and vomiting can be dose-limiting. The gastrointestinal distress increases with daily use, limiting the length of treatment courses (at doses of up to 12 mg per kilogram per day) to 2 to 3 weeks. Mild myelosuppression occurs. Additionally, HMM can induce both central and peripheral neurotoxicities, including altered mood, hallucinations, and peripheral neuropathy. HMM is thought to act as an alkylating agent, possibly via the enzymatic hydroxylation of its demethyl metabolites to cytotoxic methylol compounds. HMM exhibits antitumor activity in alkylating agent–resistant ovarian cancer and to a lesser extent in several other neoplasms (lung, breast cancer, lymphomas).

Hydroxyurea (Hydrea, HU). Hydroxyurea acts as an inhibitor of ribonucleotide reductase, resulting in intracellular depletion of deoxynucleoside triphosphates and inhibition of DNA synthesis. It is available for clinical use in oral formulation. HU's major toxicity is to the bone marrow, and it causes transient dose-related myelosuppression. At high dosage, a megaloblastic anemia can develop, which is nonresponsive to vitamin B_{12} or folic acid. Gastrointestinal side effects of nausea and vomiting are also common with high-dose therapy. HU is used primarily to treat chronic myeloid leukemia, but it also has some use in head and neck cancer and metastatic melanoma, and as a radiosensitizer.

Mitoxantrone (Novantrone). Mitoxantrone is an anthracenedione with a structure that appears analogous to that of the anthracyclines. It has been approved by the FDA as a second-line agent for treatment of acute leukemia in relapse but is also useful in the treatment of breast cancer and lymphoma. Mitoxantrone binds to DNA and causes strand breaks and inhibits DNA and RNA synthesis. In terms of cellular response by tumor cells, there is not complete cross-reactivity between mitoxantrone and the anthracyclines. Mitoxantrone dosage for acute leukemia is higher than for solid tumors. Comparative studies in patients with advanced breast cancer suggest that it is less active and toxic than doxorubicin. Its major acute toxicity is myelosuppression. Gastrointestinal side effects, including nausea, vomiting, and mucositis as well as alopecia, are less severe than with the anthracyclines. Mitoxantrone can cause some cardiac toxicities, usually manifest by development of arrhythmia at the time of injection, and can exacerbate pre-existing anthracycline-induced cardiomyopathy. It can be used intraperitoneally in patients with ovarian cancer, as most of the drug remains in the peritoneal cavity. This reduces systemic toxicity but it can induce chemical peritonitis and adhesions.

Asparaginase (Crasnitin, Elspar). L-Asparaginase is a bacterial enzyme isolated from *Escherichia coli* or *Erwinia carotovora.* Its major use is to treat lymphoblastic leukemias and some lymphomas with a deficiency in asparagine synthetase and cellular dependence on exogenous asparagine. L-Asparagine is a nonessential amino acid, and most normal cells can synthesize their required asparagine. Therapeutically, L-asparaginase depletes the plasma of asparagine by catalyzing it to aspartic acid and ammonia. Most patients develop fever and chills as well as nausea and vomiting after administration, but these symptoms can usually be reduced or prevented by premedication with antiemetics and anti-inflammatory agents. Asparaginase toxicity can produce abnormal liver function tests (SGOT, alkaline phosphatase, and bilirubin) as well as hypoalbuminemia and reductions in plasma levels of clotting factors and insulin. Other occasional toxicities include pancreatitis and central nervous system abnormalities, which can lead to confusion or coma. Repeated use of asparaginase leads to the development of antibodies that can inhibit its activity and accelerate its clearance as well as induce hypersensitivity reactions. Patients developing hypersensitivity after asparaginase administration may exhibit hypotension, laryngeal edema, bronchospasm, and urticaria. Switching to an asparaginase derived from a different bacterial species can bypass neutralizing antibodies in hypersensitive patients. The lack of myelosuppressive or gastrointestinal toxicity has facilitated incorporation of L-asparaginase into drug combinations for the treatment of acute lymphocytic leukemia.

Management of Toxicity

Most cytotoxic drugs are also toxic for host cells, and treatment schedules must take this into account.

DOSE ADJUSTMENTS FOR BONE MARROW TOXICITY. Myelosuppressive agents often must be downwardly adjusted to avoid serious or life-threatening side effects such as granulocytopenic fever and thrombocytopenic bleeding. For most drugs, empiric schedules have been developed for drug administration with single agents or combinations of myelosuppressive drugs normally given every 3 to 4 weeks. The interval between treatments provides time for hematopoietic recovery of normal myeloid progenitors in the bone marrow and avoids cumulative myelosuppression. It is essential to check the patient's WBC, differential, and platelet count immediately prior to each course of myelosuppressive chemotherapy. During the first few cycles of chemotherapy, and at intervals thereafter, it is useful to check counts between treatment courses, particularly in order to determine the nadir of absolute granulocyte count (AGC). Falls of AGC below 1000 per microliter, increase the risk of infection; AGC's below 500 represent a potentially fatal risk. As hematopoietic recovery can occur rapidly after the nadir, the AGC immediately prior to the next course can be normal even though the nadir count may have been very low. For some drug combinations with low but brief AGC nadirs, prophylactic anti-infective agents (e.g., sulfamethoxazole-trimethoprim) that will bracket the AGC nadir can protect against infection secondary to neutropenia. In general, if the AGC immediately prior to the next course of chemotherapy is less than 2000 per microliter, the dose of myelosuppressive drugs should be reduced by 50%. With an AGC of less than 1500 per microliter, dosage should be reduced by 75%. If less than 1000, the drug should be withheld until hematologic recovery occurs. An additional approach to problems of myelosuppression involves the use of bone marrow growth factors as discussed below under "Biological Agents."

DOSE ADJUSTMENTS FOR IMPAIRED HEPATIC OR RENAL FUNCTION. It is important to make downward dosage adjustments for specific drugs when altered hepatic or renal function plays a major role. The metabolism of doxorubicin depends upon good hepatobiliary function. Patients with a serum bilirubin of greater than 3.0 mg per deciliter should have their doxorubicin dose reduced by at least 50% until drug tolerance is established.

Cisplatin, methotrexate, etoposide, hydroxyurea, and bleomycin all clear predominantly via renal excretion. Doses of these agents should be decreased approximately in proportion to the decline in renal function as determined by creatinine clearance and reflected by the serum creatinine.

Endocrine Agents

Cancer cells often exhibit susceptibility to hormonal control mechanisms that regulate growth of the normal organ or tissue from which the neoplasm arose. Endocrine therapy appears generally to work through cytostatic rather than cytotoxic mechanisms and usually requires long-term suppression. Endocrine therapy includes the use of both hormones and "antihormones," which are either antagonists or partial agonists for a given endocrine mechanism. Inasmuch as the effects of hormones are receptor mediated, evaluation of receptors capable of binding hormones has played an important role in assessing both tumor types and individual patients for possible endocrine therapy. Dose schedules and applications of some major endocrine agents are summarized in Table 162–10.

STEROID HORMONES AND ANTIHORMONES. Cancers arising from endocrine organs and the immune system are susceptible to the effects of steroid hormones, steroid hormone antagonists, and hormone deprivation. The sex steroids and their antagonists

TABLE 162–10. HORMONALLY ACTIVE AGENTS IN CANCER TREATMENT

Representative Agents	Dose (oral unless specified)	Toxicity A = Acute D = Delayed	Uses
Glucocorticoids			
Prednisone	20–100 mg/day or 50 mg qod (single dose)	A: Fluid retention, hyperglycemia, euphoria, depression, hypokalemia	Leukemia Lymphoma Myeloma Breast cancer Brain metastases
Dexamethasone	4–16 mg/day or 40 mg/day for 4-day pulses every 2–4 weeks	D: Osteoporosis, immunosuppression, gastrointestinal ulcers, cushingoid appearance, cataracts	
Estrogen			
Diethylstilbestrol	5 mg tid (breast) 1–3 mg qd (prostate)	A: Nausea, vomiting, fluid retention, hypercalcemia (flare reaction with bone metastases), uterine bleeding D: Feminization, accelerated coronary artery disease	Breast cancer Prostate cancer
Antiestrogen			
Tamoxifen	20 mg qd	A: Occasional nausea, fluid retention, hot flashes D: Retinal degeneration	Breast cancer
Aromatase inhibitor			
Aminoglutethimide (plus hydrocortisone 20 mg bid)	250 mg bid (breast) 250 mg qid (prostate)	A: Dizziness D: Rash (transient)	Breast cancer Prostate cancer
Progestins			
Megestrol acetate	40 mg qid	A: Increased appetite (megestrol), fluid retention	Breast cancer Endometrial cancer
Hydroxyprogesterone	1 gm IM biw	D: Weight gain, thromboembolism	Renal cancer
Androgens			
Fluoxymesterone	10–20 mg qd	A: Cholestatic jaundice (with oral drug)	Breast cancer
Testosterone	600 mg IM q 4–6 wks	D: Virilization	
Antiandrogen			
Flutamide	250 mg tid	D: Gynecomastia	Prostate cancer
Gonadotropin-releasing hormone agonists (depot formulations)			
Leuprolide acetate	7.5 mg SQ monthly	A: Transient flare of symptoms	Prostate cancer
Goserelin acetate	3.6 mg SQ monthly		Breast cancer (?)

represent major agents for the treatment of common cancers arising from the breast, prostate gland, and uterus. The role of endocrine ablation procedures (hypophysectomy, adrenalectomy, oophorectomy, orchiectomy) has diminished as systemic agents have been identified which can replace surgical procedures. Nonetheless, oophorectomy and orchiectomy are still useful in the treatment of endocrine-sensitive cancers of the breast and prostate, respectively.

Estrogens and Antiestrogens. Pharmacologic doses of estrogen have therapeutic effects in cancers of the prostate and the breast. Estrogen therapy remains a mainstay in the treatment of metastatic prostate cancer. Orchiectomy is equally efficacious and lacks feminizing side effects. No evidence suggests an additive effect of the two.

For breast cancer, the antiestrogen tamoxifen (Nolvadex) is better tolerated than high-dose estrogen therapy. Tamoxifen improves survival of postmenopausal women with estrogen and/or progesterone receptor-positive breast cancer in both the adjuvant and metastatic settings. Recent but still controversial studies also suggest that tamoxifen may be a useful adjuvant for hormone receptor-negative cancers in postmenopausal women. In general, cytotoxic chemotherapy rather than endocrine therapy is recommended for women with hormone-receptor-negative breast cancer. Tamoxifen is available only in 10 mg tablets for oral administration, with a manufacturer's recommended dose of 10 mg twice daily. The schedule lacks a good scientific rationale because with chronic therapy, tamoxifen and its active metabolite dihydroxytamoxifen achieve a steady state with a large deep tissue reservoir. Accordingly, use of a single dose of 20 mg should be an acceptable alternative schedule with fewer problems with compliance. Serious or life-threatening toxicities of tamoxifen (thromboembolic disease, retinitis) are rare. Common side effects include hot flashes and weight gain, sometimes due to fluid retention. Mild nausea also may occur. In premenopausal women with hormone receptor-positive neoplasms and overt metastatic disease, both oophorectomy and antiestrogen therapy can be useful. However, cytotoxic chemotherapy remains indicated, as it appears to have curative potential. The role of ovarian ablation or antiestrogen therapy added to chemotherapy in the adjuvant setting remains to be defined. Tamoxifen has been reported as occasionally having palliative effects in other neoplasms such as ovarian or endometrial cancer.

Androgens and Antiandrogens. Androgen therapy is contraindicated in prostate cancer because it stimulates growth. Virilizing androgens such as testosterone propionate, fluoxymesterone (Halotestin), and testosterone enanthate (Delatestryl) have all been used beneficially in the treatment of metastatic breast cancer with hormone receptor-positive disease. However, androgen therapy has largely been replaced with antiestrogen therapy because the antiestrogen does not cause hirsutism, deepening of the voice, or changes in libido. Additionally, the oral halogenated androgens (e.g., fluoxymesterone) also can cause cholestatic jaundice. The antiandrogen flutamide (Eulexin) is a useful agent in the treatment of prostate cancer in combination with one of the gonadotropin-releasing hormone agonists (Lupron, Zoladex), and these combinations function as a "medical orchiectomy."

Progestins. Progestins are useful in palliative management of metastatic breast or endometrial cancer and can cause tumor regression in endocrine-sensitive disease. No evidence suggests their utility in the adjuvant setting in either of these neoplasms. Occasional patients with prostate cancer also appear to benefit from progestational therapy. The most commonly used progestins include megestrol acetate (Megace), medroxyprogesterone (Provera), and hydroxyprogesterone caproate (Delalutin). Megestrol acetate is useful for second-line endocrine therapy for patients with metastatic breast cancer who initially respond to tamoxifen. In patients who experience disturbing side effects from tamoxifen (e.g., severe hot flashes), megestrol acetate may represent a reasonable alternative. In addition to its antitumor effects, megestrol acetate improves appetite in some patients with cancer-induced cachexia.

Glucocorticoids. Adrenal steroid hormones of the glucocorticoid class (e.g., prednisone, methylprednisolone, dexamethasone) are useful in treating lymphoid malignancies and may also potentiate the effects of cytotoxic agents in these tumor types as well as in breast cancer and perhaps other neoplasms. The glucocorticoids play an important role in treating complications of cancer (hypercalcemia, cerebral edema). Glucocorticoids are lympholytic and nonmyelosuppressive and have been incorporated into combination chemotherapy for acute and chronic lymphocytic leukemia, malignant lymphoma, and multiple myeloma. Glucocorticoids appear to induce cell death in some lymphoid malignancies by apoptosis.

AROMATASE INHIBITORS. Aminoglutethimide (Cytodren) inhibits the first step in adrenal steroid synthesis. Additionally, and probably more importantly, aminoglutethimide also inhibits the extra-adrenal conversion of the adrenal androgen androstenedione to estrone by the enzyme aromatase. Aromatase is found in body fat and some other tissues and explains the presence of the weak estrogen estrone in the plasma of postmenopausal women. Aminoglutethimide is useful in the palliative treatment of recurrent breast cancer in hormone receptor-positive patients. Used in combination with hydrocortisone, it suppresses endogenous steroid hormone synthesis (including androstenedione) as well as ACTH production and slows the catabolism of aminoglutethimide. Aminoglutethimide is commonly administered in a dose of 250 mg twice daily along with 20 mg of hydrocortisone. Somewhat higher doses have been employed for second-line endocrine therapy for metastatic prostate cancer. Patients receiving aminoglutethimide and hydrocortisone should be cautioned against abrupt cessation of therapy to avoid symptoms of adrenal insufficiency.

GONADOTROPIN-RELEASING HORMONE (GnRH, LHRH) AGONISTS. Several synthetic analogues of natural GnRH (LHRH) are now clinically available. Both leuprolide acetate (Lupron) and goserelin acetate (Zoladex) are available in long-acting parenteral-depot formulations. These analogues function more potently than natural GnRH agonists and also have an unusual effect on the pituitary, consisting of initial stimulation followed by long-term inhibition of the release of FSH and LH. This initial increase in gonadotropins can cause a transient increase in symptoms in patients with bone metastases. The inhibition of release of the gonadotropin reduces testicular androgen synthesis in men and ovarian estrogen production in women. Accordingly, GnRH offers an alternative to surgical orchiectomy in patients with prostate cancer and avoids the gynecomastia, nausea, vomiting, edema, and thromboembolic disease that estrogens may induce. The effectiveness of GnRH agonists is enhanced by administration in combination with an antiandrogen (flutamide), and the combination has been reported to be more effective than a GnRH agonist alone in patients with stage D metastatic prostate cancer. Impotence results from this form of "medical orchiectomy," as it does from surgical orchiectomy, but the effects of medical therapy are potentially reversible if treatment is discontinued. Medical orchiectomy is more expensive but acceptable to patients who decline surgical orchiectomy. GnRH agonists now show promise in combination with antiestrogens as endocrine therapy for premenopausal women with hormone receptor–positive breast cancer. The GnRH agonists are abortifacients in animals and should not be given to women who are or may become pregnant.

BIOLOGIC THERAPY

A new form of cancer therapy, still early in its evolution, is the use of recombinant cytokines, growth factors, and monoclonal antibodies for the treatment of cancer (Table 162–11). The term "biologic therapy" describes this heterogeneous group of agents that either are normal mammalian mediators or achieve antitumor effects through endogenous host defense mechanisms. The biologic agents have also been termed "biologic response modifiers" (BRM's). Both the cellular and humoral limbs of immunity can be exploited in cancer therapy. The cellular defenses include several classes of cytotoxic lymphocytes (natural killer [NK] cells), lymphokine-activated killer (LAK) cells, tumor infiltrating lymphoma (TIL), and cytotoxic T lymphocytes (CTL), as well as antibody-dependent cytotoxic cells (ADCC). The nonspecific cells of the reticuloendothelial system including activated macrophages also may be important. Humoral agents with antitumor activities include cytokines such as interferons and interleukins as well as specific antibodies. Most of these humoral agents interact with specific immune effector cells in coordinated and synergistic fashion. The general availability of cytokines and growth factors has been facilitated by the development of recombinant DNA technology. Antibodies are highly specific and generally interact directly with their tumor targets when they are directed against cell surface constituents. Some humoral agents including the tumor necrosis factors α and β have demonstrated po-

TABLE 162–11. BIOLOGIC THERAPY OF CANCER: APPROACHES AND AGENTS

Approach	Agents
Active immunotherapy	
Nonspecific	Adjuvants: BCG, levamisole
	Cytokines: Interferons
	Interleukin-2
Specific	Tumor cell vaccines
Passive serotherapy	
Antibodies	Polyclonal or monoclonal antibodies (alone or conjugated with drugs, radionuclides, or toxins)
Adoptive cellular therapy	Lymphokine-activated killer cells
	Tumor-infiltrating lymphocytes
Immunomodulators	Levamisole, thymic hormones
Bone marrow growth factors (see Table 162–13)	G-CSF, GM-CSF, M-CSF, IL-3, EPO
Growth factor antagonists	Suramin
	Antibodies to growth factor receptors (e.g., EGF, HER-2/neu, IL-2 receptors)
Antiangiogenesis agents	

tent local antitumor properties in preclinical models but have yet to be shown to be clinically useful.

Vaccines based on specific bacterial agents or extracts from bacteria can nonspecifically activate the host immune system. Using BCG, this approach has been applied successfully to intravesical therapy of in situ cancer of the urinary bladder. Specific cancer-associated antigen vaccines have been under active investigation for many years, so far without success.

INTERFERONS. The interferons (IFN's) are a family of antiviral proteins that differ in their cellular origin and polypeptide structure as well as in their clinical applications. The three major molecular species are IFN-α, -β, and -γ. IFN-α and -β mediate their action by binding to the same cell surface receptor, whereas a second cell surface receptor mediates the action of IFN-γ. IFN-α is the major species for use in the treatment of hematologic malignancies and solid tumors. Whether IFN-β or -γ will have sufficient advantage over IFN-α in any specific cancer indication to gain regulatory approval is uncertain.

Interferon-α. Recombinant IFN-α (IFN-α_2, Intron-A, Roferon) is a polypeptide cytokine with antiviral properties which is useful for single-agent treatment of selected hematologic malignancies and solid tumors. The precise mechanism of action of IFN is still poorly understood, but it is known to activate the transcription of a number of cellular genes. Additionally, IFN action inhibits the synthesis of a number of proteins in sensitive tumor target cells including ornithine decarboxylase, a rate-limiting enzyme in polyamine metabolism. Although IFN-α also has antiviral and immunoregulatory properties that alter the biologic function of many cell types involved in humoral and cellular immunity, it is unclear whether these functions influence its antitumor properties above and beyond its direct receptor-mediated effects on sensitive tumor cells. The antitumor properties of IFN-α also appear to be schedule-dependent with a cytostatic mode of action. Most remissions induced by IFN are only partial.

IFN-α can be administered parenterally by intravenous, intramuscular, subcutaneous, and intracavitary routes. Its preferred route is by subcutaneous administration, which provides the longest duration of action. The dosage schedules are quite variable, with higher dosages required for some tumor types. Hairy cell leukemia (HCL) is the tumor most sensitive to IFN-α. Usual dosages are in the range of 3 million IU administered subcutaneously three times weekly. At these low levels, IFN usually causes only mild side effects such as fever and chills with the first few doses. For Kaposi's sarcoma, far more aggressive and toxic IFN schedules are required and can cause anorexia, weight loss, failure in concentration, and profound weakness. High-dose IFN can also induce occasional cardiac arrhythmias, nausea, vomiting, leukopenia, myalgias, proteinuria, and hepatic dysfunction ("transaminitis"). Thus, optimal biologic and antitumor effects of IFN-α appear to be more related to tumor type and biologic response modification than to dose alone. Elderly patients appear to develop more marked side effects at all

dosage schedules. Some of the major current uses and dosage levels for IFN-α are summarized in Table 162–12.

IFN-α is also useful in the treatment of chronic myeloid leukemia, multiple myeloma, some of the low-grade non-Hodgkin's lymphomas, and in some examples of metastatic melanoma or renal cell carcinoma. In myeloma, IFN-α appears to lengthen remissions induced by chemotherapy. Patients receiving recombinant IFN-α for HCL, CML, or renal cancer have developed neutralizing antibodies to the recombinant product when the disease progresses again after an IFN-induced remission. A limited number of patients with neutralizing antibodies have been successfully retreated by switching to nonrecombinant IFN-α. IFN-α has recently been incorporated into combination therapy with various cytotoxic and endocrine agents. At present, use of IFN-α in combination with 5-FU is being explored in the treatment of metastatic colorectal cancer and in combination with *cis*-retinoic acid to treat renal and cervical cancers. Although the clinical indications for IFN therapy continue to grow gradually, it has lacked the type of broad-spectrum anticancer effects that were initially envisioned.

INTERLEUKIN-2 (IL-2, PROLEUKIN). IL-2 is an immunomodulatory cytokine that acts on T-cell progenitors to produce LAK cells. Recombinant IL-2 has been approved for therapeutic use in renal cancer. Direct intravenous infusion induces LAK cells in the patient. Additionally, after leukapheresis to obtain circulating lymphocytes from the patient, these can then be exposed to IL-2 in tissue culture to activate lymphoid progenitors into LAK cells, which are then reinfused into the patient. There is now general agreement that either IL-2 or IL-2/LAK can induce tumor regression in 10 to 20% of patients with renal carcinoma, melanoma, lymphoma, or other neoplasms.

Whereas the infusion of LAK cells causes relatively few side effects, IL-2 induces considerable toxicity. Patients receiving high-dose IL-2 must be in an intensive care unit with close management of blood pressure, fluids, and electrolytes. The high-dose regimens are suitable only for younger patients without other significant disease or impairment of cardiac, pulmonary, hepatic, or renal function. Common side effects of high-dose IL-2/LAK are probably due to lymphoid infiltrates in major organs and an induced capillary leak syndrome. Shortly after initiation of high-dose IL-2 therapy, tachycardia develops, and a significant drop in arterial blood pressure occurs. As IL-2 administration continues, compensatory fluid retention occurs in association with weight gain, oliguria, and azotemia. Vasopressors are often needed. Even at lower doses that can be used in a conventional hospital or outpatient setting (e.g., 3 million IU per square meter daily by intravenous infusion for 2 weeks), hypotension and fluid retention are not uncommon.

Pulmonary metastases appear to be somewhat more sensitive to IL-2 or IL-2/LAK therapy than are other tumors. With the adoptive immunotherapy approach using IL-2/LAK, a small percentage of patients treated at the National Cancer Institute who had undergone prior removal of the primary tumor achieved complete remission with all evidence of metastatic disease disappearing for prolonged periods of time. Some controversy nonetheless remains as to whether the use of high-dose IL-2/LAK has any advantage over administration of IL-2 alone at a lower and better-tolerated dosage level.

LEVAMISOLE (ERGAMISOLE). Levamisole is an anthelmintic agent possessing immunopotentiating properties. Levamisole has been reported to enhance various tests of cell-mediated immunity in patients with Hodgkin's disease but has not been shown to have a therapeutic effect. When combined with 5-FU, however, levamisole has been reported to enhance adjuvant chemotherapy of patients with Duke's C colon cancer. The combined use with surgery reduces the recurrence rate by two thirds; the mechanism remains unknown. In patients with overt metastatic colon cancer, the combination of 5-FU and levamisole does not appear to be any more useful than 5-FU alone.

ANTITUMOR ANTIBODY THERAPY. At the present time, antibody-based therapy for cancer remains investigational and has not been approved by the FDA.

Antibody therapy has shown some encouraging results in malignant B-cell lymphoma (both Hodgkin's disease and non-Hodgkin's lymphomas as well as chronic lymphocytic leukemia) and perhaps in acute myelocytic leukemia. Objective tumor regressions have been observed after administration of unconjugated, radionuclide-conjugated, and toxin-conjugated antibodies directed at lymphoma cells. One pilot observation used murine anti-idiotypic antibodies to

TABLE 162–12. SOME CURRENT USES OF INTERFERON-α IN CLINICAL ONCOLOGY

Tumor Type	Dose (mU)	Response Rate (%)
Hairy cell leukemia	3/day or 3 times weekly	75–90
Chronic myeloid leukemia	5/m²/day	50–80
Multiple myeloma	3/m²/day or 3 times weekly	20–30*
Cutaneous T-cell lymphoma	10/day or 3 times weekly	45
Follicular (B-cell) lymphoma	5/day or 3 times weekly	30–50*
Kaposi's sarcoma	10/m²/day or 3 times weekly	30
Metastatic melanoma	5–10/m² 3 times weekly	10–20
Renal cell carcinoma	5–10/m² 3 times weekly	10–30
Carcinoid syndrome	5/m² 3 times weekly	20–30†

* Also being used for remission maintenance therapy.
† Reduction in symptoms and 5-HIAA excretion.

the cell surface Ig on neoplastic B cells and achieved at least one prolonged complete remission. Development of anti-idiotypic antibodies, however, requires preparing a specific antibody for each patient. Recent efforts in lymphoma have been focused on employing antibodies that recognize "shared idiotypes" or other lymphoid-associated antigens as targets for antibodies. For other tumor types, results with antibody-based therapy have been disappointing.

GROWTH FACTOR ANTAGONISTS. The use of antagonists to polypeptide growth factors is an extension of neuroendocrine therapy but represents a form of biologic therapy as well. One growth factor antagonist that has recently been recognized to have anticancer properties is suramin, which has been used since the 1920's for the treatment of African sleeping sickness. Suramin is a polysulfonated naphthylurea that binds tightly to heparin-binding growth factors such as fibroblast growth factor (FGF), platelet-derived growth factor (PDGF), and insulin-like growth factor (IGF-1). Exclusion of growth factors from their receptors can result in "programmed cell death." Suramin actively treats prostate cancer, presumably by blocking the action of FGF and other growth factors. Suramin also inhibits the function of a variety of enzymes and other proteins, so its precise mechanism of antitumor action remains to be defined. Suramin's multiple actions also account for a broad range of toxicities, which can be severe or irreversible. One of these is adrenal insufficiency, which requires long-term adrenal steroid replacement. Frequent plasma monitoring of suramin concentrations is essential, because there is the potential for serious neuropathy when suramin concentrations exceed 300 μg per milliliter. The use of suramin in cancer therapy is currently investigational. Suramin represents the first member of a new class of investigational agents for cancer therapy. Another approach to growth factor receptor blockade involves use of monoclonal antibodies to epidermal growth factor (EGF) receptor and the IL-2 receptor.

BONE MARROW GROWTH FACTORS. A new approach to supportive care for bone marrow failure associated with cancer and for maintaining adequate hematopoietic function between courses of myelosuppressive chemotherapy is to administer bone marrow growth factors to stimulate an increased rate of production of myeloid progenitors. The bone marrow growth factors are glycoproteins that function in overlapping and hierarchic manner on bone marrow progenitors and not only result in cell proliferation but also activate differentiation and cell trafficking. The factors currently in clinical trials in cancer patients are summarized in Table 162–13.

TABLE 162–13. RECOMBINANT BONE MARROW GROWTH FACTORS OF POTENTIAL IMPORTANCE IN SUPPORTIVE CARE OF CANCER PATIENTS

Growth Factor*	Effects
G-CSF	Stimulates granulocyte production
GM-CSF	Stimulates granulocyte, macrophage, and eosinophil production
M-CSF	Stimulates macrophage production and activation
IL-3	Stimulates granulocyte, macrophage, and platelet production
EPO	Stimulates production of RBC's

* G-CSF = granulocyte colony stimulating factor; GM-CSF = granulocyte macrophage colony stimulating factor; M-CSF = macrophage colony stimulating factor; IL-3 = interleukin-3; EPO = erythropoietin.

The major factors also potently stimulate the proliferation of myeloid precursors. Several of these recombinant proteins, including granulocyte colony stimulating factor (G-CSF), granulocyte macrophage colony stimulating factor (GM-CSF), and erythropoietin (Epogen, EPO) (see Table 162–6), are widely used in cancer treatment. Both IL-3 and macrophage colony stimulating factor (M-CSF) are at an earlier stage of development and their role in supportive care is currently uncertain. Clinical trials using subcutaneously administered G-CSF or GM-CSF have shown that either can shorten the duration of granulocytopenia, the frequency of infectious complications, and the duration of hospitalization after chemotherapy combinations that normally require inpatient administration. With bone marrow transplantation (wherein high-dose chemotherapy and/or total body radiation is employed) both myelosuppressive and nonmyelosuppressive side effects can be diminished with the use of G-CSF or GM-CSF. Preliminary evidence suggests that IL-3 (multi-CSF) can stimulate platelet and red blood cell as well as granulocyte production.

In preclinical studies, IL-3 also appears to act synergistically with GM-CSF to produce more complete and rapid recovery of circulating granulocytes and platelets. The major toxicities of the growth factors that stimulate white cell production include fever, myalgias, and occasional skin rashes. Pericarditis has been reported with high-dose GM-CSF or G-CSF. Recombinant EPO is already in general clinical use for the anemia of renal failure. Preliminary studies also suggest that when used in pharmacologic doses, EPO can restore normal red blood cell counts in some patients with multiple myeloma and perhaps in some other hematologic malignancies as well. EPO also has promise for reducing the degree of anemia induced by cytotoxic chemotherapy.

Chabner BA, Collins JM: Cancer Chemotherapy: Principles and Practice. Philadelphia, JB Lippincott Company, 1990. *An excellent reference on cancer chemotherapy, including detailed discussion of the pharmacology of anticancer drugs.*
DeVita VT, Hellman S, Rosenberg SA: Cancer: Principles and Practice of Oncology, 3rd ed. Philadelphia, JB Lippincott Company, 1989. *A standard reference.*
Holland JF, Frei E III, Bast RC Jr, et al.: Cancer Medicine, 3rd ed. Philadelphia, Lea & Febiger, 1993. *A comprehensive textbook covering clinical, diagnostic, and therapeutic approaches for all major forms of cancer. Major modalities of treatment as well as drug combination schedules are delineated in detail in relation to relevant tumor types.*

163 ONCOLOGIC EMERGENCIES
Stephen M. Hahn

The care of patients with cancer is characterized by the management of chronic illnesses. Acute oncologic emergencies require rapid evaluation and institution of therapy. Several types of cancer are now routinely cured and in others treatment brings an increase in quality of life and survival time. Therefore, the early recognition and treatment of oncologic emergencies have an important role in the medical management of cancer patients.

FEVER AND NEUTROPENIA. The most common oncologic emergency consists of fever (temperature greater than 38°C) and neutropenia (absolute neutrophil count less than 1000 per cubic millimeter). Neutropenic cancer patients have an increased risk of systemic infection and the rapid development of the septic syndrome. Emergent empiric antibiotic therapy is crucial.

Infection risk increases once the neutrophil count drops below 1000 per cubic millimeter. Disruptions of other host defenses also predispose to infection. Paramount among these is breakdown of the gastrointestinal barrier with mucositis. Additional factors include the presence of indwelling catheters, invasive procedures, and abnormal cellular and humoral immunity.

The febrile, neutropenic patient usually presents with few signs or symptoms other than fever. Localized infection may be present but not clinically apparent. The absence of an adequate number of leukocytes may make the detection of an active infection difficult. A careful history and physical examination focusing on common sites of infection must be performed. The oral cavity should be inspected for evidence of mucositis as well as lesions suggestive of anaerobic, viral (especially herpes simplex), and fungal (especially *Candida* species) infection. Examination of soft tissue and skin, especially at catheter sites, may show early cellulitis or septic phlebitis. A perirectal abscess should be sought by careful palpation of the anorectal area for induration, fluctuance, or tenderness.

Cultures should be performed on all patients before antibiotic therapy is begun and should be sent routinely for isolation of bacteria and fungi. Blood cultures are obtained both from the port of an indwelling central catheter and from peripheral veins. If an indwelling catheter is suspected to be the source of infection, removal of the catheter may not always be required but must be considered. If the catheter is removed, the tip should be sent for Gram stain and culture. Sputum examination by Gram stain and culture is usually not helpful but is obtained if sputum is produced. Gram stain and bacterial, fungal, and viral cultures should be sent on all oral, skin, and soft tissue lesions. Biopsies of cutaneous lesions may be especially helpful in the diagnosis of systemic viral and fungal infections and can be safely performed in the neutropenic patient. Chest radiography, urinalysis with microscopy, and evaluation of ascites and pleural fluid should be performed. Although meningitis is not typically encountered in febrile neutropenic cancer patients, a lumbar puncture should be performed when suggestive clinical signs or symptoms exist.

Indwelling urinary tract catheters and unnecessary intravenous catheters are to be avoided. Strict handwashing by all hospital personnel is required. Aggressive prophylactic or therapeutic mouth care (suggested regimen: nystatin suspension, benadryl/antacid/lidocaine mixture, and 5% sodium bicarbonate solution, alternating each every 2 hours, administered as swish and spit) provides relief of symptoms and may improve the patient's course.

Once evaluated and hospitalized, the patient should be started without delay on broad-spectrum antibiotics that include coverage for *Pseudomonas* species and other gram-negative organisms. Based upon the isolate patterns at an individual institution and clinical suspicions regarding the source of the fever, coverage for gram-positive organisms may be necessary. Suggested regimens are (1) a third-generation cephalosporin (ceftazidime, 1 to 2 grams every 8 hours intravenously) or (2) a semisynthetic penicillin (piperacillin or mezlocillin, 3 to 4 grams every 4 hours intravenously) plus an aminoglycoside (gentamicin or tobramycin, 2 mg per kilogram loading dose followed by one to three divided doses daily, depending upon renal function). If a specific organism is suspected, appropriate antibiotics should be added to the initial regimen. For example, if infection of an indwelling catheter is likely, additional gram-positive coverage with vancomycin (500 mg every 6 hours intravenously) should be added for *Staphylococcus aureus* and *S. epidermidis*. Rotation of the antibiotic dose among the ports of a multilumen catheter is recommended. We recommend anaerobic coverage with clindamycin (300 mg intravenously every 6 hours) for patients with mucositis, periodontal infections, or perianal infections. Newer oral antifungal agents such as fluconazole should be given to patients who present with suspected thrush or esophagitis. These agents do not replace amphotericin B in the treatment of documented or suspected invasive fungal infections. Fluconazole prophylaxis to prevent invasive mycotic infections is now under active study.

If fever persists after the initiation of antibiotics, cultures and diagnostic studies should be repeated and broader coverage added to the patient's regimen. Patients with prolonged neutropenia who are receiving broad-spectrum antibiotics are at high risk for fungal infection. Early institution of antifungal therapy may be life saving. If after 5 to 7 days, the patient remains febrile, empiric antifungal therapy with amphotericin B should be started (0.5 to 1.0 mg per kilogram per day intravenously). In general, if neutropenic patients remain febrile despite broad-spectrum therapy, one should consider the following diagnostic possibilities: a second bacterial isolate, abscess, anaerobic infection, gram-positive bacteria, atypical organisms, fungi, viruses, and drug fever.

One can identify an infection in approximately 50% of patients with fever and neutropenia. If a causative organism or a specific infection is discovered, specific therapy should be initiated; however, broad-spectrum antibiotics should not be discontinued because there is a 40% chance of developing infection with a second isolate when antibiotic therapy is narrowed. Patients with documented infections require treatment for a full course (usually a 2-week course of antibiotic therapy). If the patient is afebrile and no specific infection has been identified, antibiotics may be discontinued when the absolute neutrophil count exceeds 1000 per cubic millimeter. Antibiotics should be continued in the patient who remains neutropenic even if he becomes afebrile. Otherwise, clinical deterioration or the return of fever occurs in a significant proportion of these patients.

The introduction of recombinant hematopoietic cytokines such as granulocyte colony stimulating factor (G-CSF) and granulocyte-macrophage colony stimulating factor (GM-CSF) has improved the treatment of neutropenia in cancer patients. These cytokines may be administered prophylactically (24 hours after the last dose of cytotoxic chemotherapy) or therapeutically (when the patient develops fever and/or neutropenia). In most clinical settings, the hematopoietic cytokines should not be given immediately prior to or concurrently with cytotoxic chemotherapy because the increased cycling of the hematopoietic progenitors produced by these agents may increase myelotoxicity. The prophylactic use of cytokines reduces the duration of neutropenia induced by chemotherapy. Some studies also report that the use of cytokines decreases the number of febrile neutropenic episodes, the duration of hospitalization, and the number of infections. The therapeutic use of cytokines is theoretically attractive, but their full value awaits the final results of randomized trials. The preliminary results of one randomized trial do suggest a modest decrease in the duration of neutropenia and days of hospitalization. Clinical judgment with regard to the severity of the patient's illness and the expected duration of neutropenia determines whether therapeutic administration of cytokines is indicated. G-CSF is administered initially as a subcutaneous injection (5 μg per kilogram). Higher doses (10 μg per kilogram) may be necessary in some patients. The drug is well tolerated by most patients. GM-CSF is initially administered subcutaneously in doses of 1 to 6 μg per kilogram per day. Subsequent bone pain, fever, allergic reactions, and lethargy have been reported.

At one time, white cell transfusions were thought to benefit patients with gram-negative infection and prolonged neutropenia. Such transfusions are not now recommended because their benefit is questionable and the risks, such as alloimmunization, pulmonary toxicity, and infections, are significant. Prophylaxis with absorbable or nonabsorbable antibiotics is controversial and not routinely recommended. *Clostridium difficile* infection and vitamin K deficiency may occur in the setting of prolonged broad-spectrum antibiotic use.

SPINAL CORD COMPRESSION. Back or neck pain due to cancer can be a harbinger of neurologic disaster and merits immediate, careful evaluation. The pain of intraspinal lesions is worsened by straining, sneezing, coughing, movement, and recumbency. Complaints may precede the diagnosis by days to months, but once neurologic signs exist, progression is usually rapid. Typically, midline back pain progresses to radicular pain followed by weakness, sensory loss, paralysis, and/or loss of sphincter control at or below the level of the lesion. Early recognition is important, as ambulatory ability and maintenance of bowel and bladder control at the time when therapy is begun correlates highly with the ultimate functional outcome. Fewer than 15% of patients with paraplegia or loss of sphincter tone due to metastatic or primary spinal cancer regain function. The location of such lesions correlates with the volume and number of involved vertebral bodies (thoracic > lumbar > cervical).

The physical examination determines the pace of evaluation and treatment (Fig. 163–1). Patients who show signs of spinal compres-

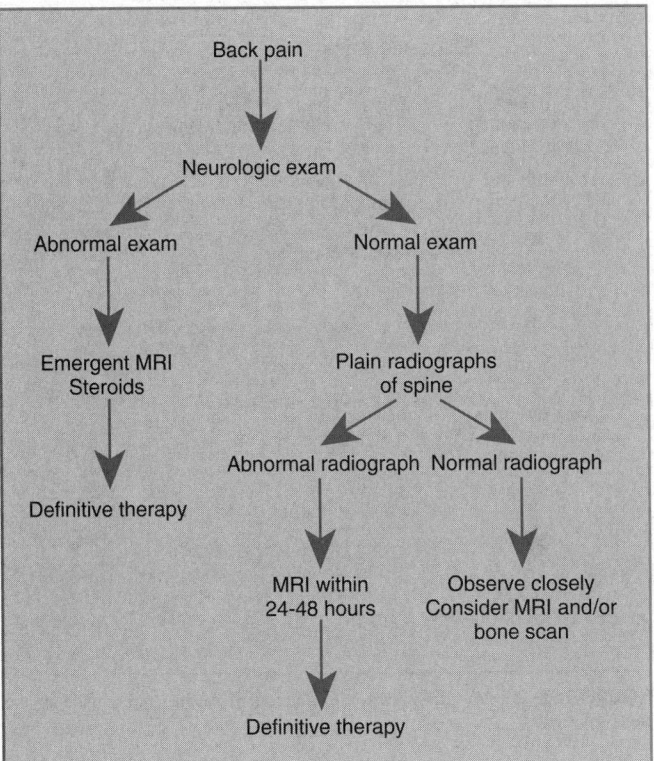

FIGURE 163–1. Flow diagram for evaluation of spinal cord compression in the cancer patient.

sion require immediate treatment with dexamethasone (10 mg intravenously plus 4 to 6 mg every 6 hours) followed by emergent evaluation. Patients with no neurologic findings but plain film evidence of spine metastases similarly carry a high risk of epidural metastases and deserve to be evaluated emergently. Patients with no neurologic findings and no plain film abnormalities may be expeditiously evaluated as outpatients. Two thirds of patients with spinal cord compression have plain film spine radiographs showing erosion or loss of pedicles, partial or complete collapse of vertebral bodies, or a paraspinous mass. When neurologic abnormalities exist, however, one should proceed directly to magnetic resonance (MR) imaging with gadolinium enhancement, which has replaced myelography as the diagnostic test of first choice. MR scans are noninvasive and delineate intramedullary, extramedullary, intradural, and extradural lesions. MR images also demonstrate encroachment on the cord through the spinal foramina. Furthermore, MR imaging avoids the 14% risk of neurologic deterioration that myelography causes in patients with complete obstruction. Although MR imaging of the suspected site of compression is usually performed emergently, we recommend an MR scan of the entire spine. This is especially important in patients with malignancies that produce multiple bone metastases (lung, breast, prostate) and may have other noncontiguous areas of epidural disease. Complete spine MR imaging also is imperative for patients scheduled to receive radiation therapy because of the need to include other sites of disease in the radiation portals. Metrizamide myelography is another diagnostic option in the patient with spinal cord compression and should still be considered the diagnostic gold standard. If after a lumbar injection, a myelographic block is identified, a C1-2 puncture should be performed to visualize fully the extent of the block, as well as to define other rostral lesions (15%). A computed tomography (CT) scan focused on the spinal block is often useful to further delineate the lesion.

Palliative radiation therapy is the treatment of choice in patients who have slowly evolving neurologic symptoms, incomplete block, cauda equina involvement, or widely metastatic disease. Treatment may be initiated with high-dose fractions, followed by lower dose fractions. Steroids can be reduced judiciously as radiation therapy proceeds. Surgery in spinal cord compression is recommended if a tissue diagnosis is needed, if neurologic dysfunction progresses despite radiation treatment, if spinal cord compression recurs in an area of previous radiation therapy, and if spinal instability arises from vertebral body collapse or bony protrusion into the spinal cord. Simple laminectomy is not usually effective and may lead to spinal instability. The surgical procedure is dictated by tumor location and surgical experience and expertise. Radiation therapy should be used postoperatively. Chemotherapy for chemosensitive malignancies is used in addition to radiation or surgery.

INTRACRANIAL METASTASES. Complaints of headache, altered mental status, and seizures in cancer patients may signal intracranial metastases. These processes are amenable to treatment and, if left untreated, can be fatal. The differential diagnosis of altered mental status, seizures, and headache in a cancer patient include iatrogenic causes (chemotherapy agents, narcotic analgesics, hypnotics, and antiemetics), metabolic disorders (hypercalcemia, hyponatremia, hypoglycemia, hypomagnesemia, hyperviscosity, hepatic encephalopathy), paraneoplastic syndromes (subacute cerebral degeneration, dementia, limbic encephalitis, optic neuritis, angioendotheliosis, progressive multifocal leukoencephalopathy), strokes (coagulation abnormalities, thrombocytopenia, Trousseau's syndrome), sepsis, and intracranial metastases. Careful history, physical examination, and laboratory evaluation are primary and should guide decisions as to further workup. In acutely ill cancer patients, cranial CT should be done to define the presence and characteristics of the intracerebral lesion. MR imaging is more sensitive in defining metastatic lesions and differentiating between vascular and malignant lesions and should be considered if there is a need to clarify CT scan findings. If no mass lesion is demonstrable, leptomeningeal carcinomatosis as the cause of neurologic signs and symptoms is sought by examination of spinal fluid.

Neurologically deteriorating patients who show signs of impending intracerebral herniation should be intubated and hyperventilated to maintain the P_{CO_2} between 25 and 30 mm Hg. Mannitol, up to 1.5 grams per kilogram, should be administered immediately and repeated, if necessary, every 6 hours. If signs of increased intracranial pressure exist with or without impending herniation, high-dose intravenous dexamethasone (16 mg every 6 hours) should be administered to lessen cerebral edema. Status epilepticus requires immediate-acting drugs such as benzodiazepines and close attention to respiratory status. Seizures, other than status epilepticus, caused by intracranial metastasis are managed by phenytoin, oral loading dose 15 mg per kilogram followed by 300 mg per day. Drug levels should be monitored. This is particularly important, because accompanying dexamethasone therapy can accelerate the metabolism of phenytoin. Other than in those who have had seizures, the routine use of phenytoin in patients is not recommended.

Radiation therapy for intracranial metastasis is usually palliative. A total dose of 30 Gy delivered over 10 to 15 fractions decreases motor deficits in approximately 33% of paralyzed patients and reduces or stops headaches in about half. For patients with controlled or no systemic disease and a solitary intracranial metastasis in a site not amenable to surgery, radiation at higher doses (40 to 50 Gy) to the site of disease is justified. By and large, a surgically accessible solitary lesion in patients with controlled systemic disease merits removal.

SUPERIOR VENA CAVA SYNDROME: Superior vena cava (SVC) syndrome is caused by extrinsic compression (90%) or, less likely, fibrosis, thrombosis, or invasion of the SVC. Signs and symptoms can be subtle and evolve slowly over a 2- to 5-week period. A spectrum of signs can be associated with the SVC syndrome, including cyanosis, edema, venous engorgement of the head, neck, arms, chest, and upper abdomen, varying degrees of airway obstruction, pleural and pericardial effusions, and tracheal edema. Nonpitting edema of the neck (Stokes' collar) can also be found. Symptoms, which frequently worsen when the patient lies down or leans forward, may include fullness or stuffiness in the ears or nose, eye disturbances, facial swelling, shortness of breath, cough, chest pain, voice changes (hoarseness), dysphagia, headache, stupor, seizures, and syncope. Back pain may herald simultaneous spinal cord compression by a contiguously extending tumor. Upper extremity venography complements either CT scan or MRI in defining the level of SVC obstruction.

In the past, malignancy-associated SVC syndrome was considered an oncologic emergency that merited immediate radiation treatment to avoid death from respiratory arrest or intracranial hemorrhage. Immediate therapy is indicated for impending airway obstruction (stridor) or increased intracranial pressure (stupor, seizure), particularly in a thrombocytopenic patient. Given the many benign causes of SVC syndrome and the frequency of chemosensitive malignancies such as small cell lung cancer and lymphomas, its cause should be determined while judiciously managing the patient. Sputum cytology, bone marrow, lymph node biopsy, thoracentesis, bronchoscopy, and thoracotomy may confirm the diagnosis.

Once a neoplastic cause of SVC syndrome has been established, appropriate treatment should be initiated. In most cases, radiation therapy remains the primary treatment, employing doses of 1.5 to 4.0 Gy per day to a total dose of 30 to 50 Gy. About 85% of patients improve within 3 weeks, but symptoms usually recur. If small cell lung cancer, testicular cancer, or lymphoma causes SVC obstruction, one should deliver chemotherapy through a lower extremity vein. Corticosteroids may improve cerebral or laryngeal edema. The role of anticoagulation remains undefined. The increasing use of subclavian catheters to deliver chemotherapy has raised the frequency of SVC thromboses. Fibrinolytic therapy should be considered in patients who have recently developed SVC syndrome and are not at high risk of dangerous bleeding. After successful fibrinolysis, heparinization and subsequent warfarin therapy should be instituted to prevent recurrent SVC syndrome and to maintain the indwelling catheter.

CARDIAC TAMPONADE. Cardiac tamponade in a cancer patient may have a noncancerous cause, may be the first manifestation of malignancy, or may signify disease progression. Prompt diagnosis is necessary because tamponade is life threatening and successful treatment improves survival. Either primary tumors of the pericardium (mesothelioma, sarcoma, and teratoma) or, more frequently, metastatic disease from breast, lung, leukemia, lymphoma, melanoma, or epidemic or nonepidemic Kaposi's sarcoma can cause tamponade. When fluid pressure within the pericardial sac equals right atrial and ventricular diastolic pressure, cardiac tamponade occurs. As intrapericardial pressure increases, heart rate, myocardial contractility, and systemic resistance increase. If intrapericardial pressure increases rapidly, between 150 and 250 ml of fluid (normal volume <50 ml) may cause tamponade; if fluid accumulates slowly, however, greater than 1 liter may be accommodated without producing decompensation. Symptoms are nonspecific and include shortness of breath, chest pain, cough, hoarseness, nausea, abdominal pain, hiccups, and anxiety. Signs associated with rapid effusion are a falling systolic pressure, elevated jugular venous pressure, a small, quiet heart (Beck's triad), and a narrowed arterial pulse pressure. Pulsus paradoxus is a classic, but not constant, sign of tamponade. The chest radiograph may show an enlarged globular (water bottle) heart and possibly pleural effusions. The pathognomonic finding on electrocardiogram of electrical alternans is rare; decreased voltage is frequent. Two-dimensional echocardiography is the noninvasive, preferred diagnostic study and provides both anatomic and physiologic information. Right heart catheterization establishes the diagnosis and allows monitoring during therapeutic maneuvers (Fig. 163–2).

Pericardiocentesis is lifesaving: it provides fluid for diagnosis and, with insertion of a pigtail catheter, permits one to measure the rate of fluid reaccumulation and to instill drugs for treatment. Fluid can be serous, serosanguineous, or frankly hemorrhagic. In the case of hemorrhagic fluid, the absence of clot and a hematocrit lower than systemic levels weigh against the fluid resulting from puncture of the myocardium. Fluid should be sent for cultures and cytology. Once a malignancy has been established, three treatments are available: radiation, chemotherapy, and surgery. Radiation therapy up to 40 Gy is highly successful (approaching 100%) in treating effusion caused by leukemias or lymphomas. Systemic chemotherapy, however, is most often considered the treatment of choice for leukemic and lymphomatous pericardial effusions. A lower success rate accompanies therapy for effusions due to melanoma, lung, and breast carcinoma. Surgical approaches to effusion include pericardiectomy, pleuropericardial window, and subxiphoid pericardiotomy. Pericardiectomy is effective for malignant pericardial effusions but carries more morbidity than either a window or subxiphoid pericardiotomy. A pleuropericardial window has a low complication rate (<5%) and a relatively low recurrence rate. Subxiphoid pericardiotomy, unlike the window procedure, requires local anesthesia

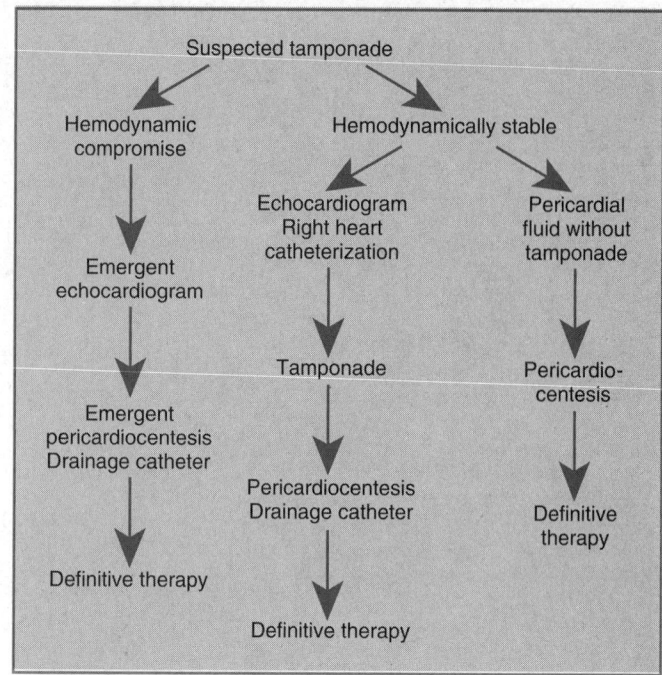

FIGURE 163–2. Flow diagram for evaluation of cardiac tamponade in the cancer patient.

and has virtually no complication or recurrence rate; however, it carries an increased incidence of tumor cell dissemination. Drug instillation into the pericardial sac has been tried with various chemotherapeutic agents (thiotepa, methotrexate, nitrogen mustard), radioisotopes, and tetracycline. Tetracycline is highly effective in obliterating the pericardial space and eliminating fluid recurrence. However, there can be a period of transient fevers, arrhythmias, and chest pain after treatment.

HEMOPTYSIS. The most common causes of hemoptysis (tuberculosis, fungal infections, lung abscess, bronchiectasis, bronchial adenoma) are not neoplastic; however, malignancies, especially of bronchogenic origin, are most common among older patients. Hemoptysis associated with respiratory compromise should be considered an emergency.

Minor hemoptysis often presages massive hemoptysis. Therefore, while the cause of hemoptysis is pursued, observation, oxygen, and prevention of aspiration are prudent. Patients with massive hemoptysis should be admitted to an intensive care unit. Correction of coagulopathy and thrombocytopenia, repletion of blood volume, and determination of the site and cause of bleeding are undertaken simultaneously. Bronchoscopy is the diagnostic procedure of choice to determine the site and cause of bleeding and to provide direct therapeutic intervention. Surgical resection, if the patient can tolerate the procedure and if the site can be localized, represents the intervention of choice. Radiation therapy can be delivered to sites of hemoptysis and is effective in up to 80% of patients. Other, less ideal treatment options include neodymium yttrium-aluminum-garnet (Nd:YAG) laser–induced coagulation, endobronchial tamponade with a venous catheter, bronchial artery catheterization with embolization, and ice lavage. Nd:YAG laser is usually restricted to lesions causing nonmassive hemoptysis; endobronchial tamponade should not be used for right upper lobe hemorrhages; embolization can result in spinal cord damage.

AIRWAY OBSTRUCTION. Airway obstruction by an intrinsic or extrinsic malignancy is an emergency, and management depends on the tempo of narrowing, its location, previous treatment, and the type of tumor. Steroids should be given to lessen edema and, in the case of lymphomas, begin treatment. Obstruction at or above the larynx and high tracheal region should first be relieved by tracheostomy with subsequent radiation therapy or surgery performed in a nonemergency setting. More distal obstructions can be treated with surgery or radiation therapy (external and/or brachytherapy). Nd:YAG laser has been useful in treating high-grade, incomplete, centrally obstructing airway lesions. The technique is quick and safe and provides immediate relief. Restrictions to its use include lobar or segmental level lesions, extraluminal compression, total luminal obstruction, upper lobe lesions, and tracheoesophageal fistula. The use of visible light lasers and fiberoptics with photosensitizers (photodynamic therapy, PDT) also may relieve obstructed airway lesions. In this case, the lesion can be totally obstructing the airway and because cylindrical light-emitting fibers are used, complete removal of tumor may be possible. Furthermore, PDT can be repeated. Repeat bronchoscopy 2 to 3 days following endobronchial PDT should be performed to remove necrotic tissue and evaluate the status of treatment.

HYPERCALCEMIA. Hypercalcemia occurs in approximately 10% of all cancer patients. Lung, particularly squamous cell, and breast cancers account for 40 to 60% of all cases. Hypercalcemia frequently accompanies bone metastases but may occur in their absence.

Malignancy-associated hypercalcemia is often caused by tumors that secrete a parathyroid-related protein, which results in increased bone and renal tubular calcium reabsorption. Assays for this protein are now available. Likewise, osteolytic metastases can act directly on bone to cause calcium resorption or can secrete factors that result in bone resorption or activation of osteoclasts. Calcium homeostasis is tightly regulated between 9 and 10 mg per deciliter. Approximately 45% of calcium is ionized (non–protein bound) and total calcium levels must be corrected for changes in serum albumin concentration. Many laboratories are now reporting ionized calcium levels. Laboratory values usually show an elevated serum calcium, commonly above 12 mg per deciliter.

The clinical manifestations may be manifold and nonspecific and depend in part on the general metabolic condition and associated illnesses of the patient, as well as the degree and rapidity of calcium elevation. Symptoms include polyuria, nocturia, polydipsia, anorexia, nausea, vomiting, abdominal pain, fatigue, lethargy, confusion, psychosis, agitation, stupor, obtundation, and coma. The electrocardiogram may show a narrowed QT interval.

For patients who are symptomatic or have serum calcium levels above 13 mg per deciliter, treatment should be immediate and aggressive. Because of the reversible defects of renal tubular absorption and subsequent fluid loss coupled with decreased oral intake, affected patients are invariably volume depleted. Volume repletion with normal saline at a rate of 200 to 300 ml per hour results in calciuresis. Once rehydration is accomplished, urinary output should be maintained at 200 to 300 ml per hour. Saline-induced calciuresis can be augmented by furosemide. Electrolytes, including magnesium should be checked frequently and, when necessary, repleted. Calcitonin (4 IU per kilogram every 12 hours increased to 8 IU per kilogram every 8 hours) can lower the serum calcium by 2 to 3 mg per deciliter within a few hours. Unfortunately, the effects of natriuresis and calcitonin are short lived. Once the patient is initially stabilized, the optimal treatment becomes therapy for the underlying malignancy. Steroids can be effective in reducing hypercalcemia in multiple myeloma, lymphoma, and occasionally breast cancer. For the chronic management of hypercalcemia, several agents are available. The bisphosphonates bind to hydroxyapatite crystals and inhibit their dissolution. Two bisphosphonates, etidronate and pamidronate, are now available for use in the United States. Etidronate is initially given intravenously (7.5 mg per kilogram per day) for 3 days. This is usually followed by oral etidronate, 20 mg per kilogram per day if a response to intravenous drug is observed. Pamidronate is administered in a single dose of 60 to 90 mg by slow intravenous infusion over 24 hours. Bisphosphonates reduce serum calcium levels to the normal range in at least 60% of patients. Gallium nitrate is also available for the treatment of hypercalcemia. Gallium is usually administered as a continuous infusion (200 mg per square meter per day) for 5 days; toxicities include nephrotoxicity and acute optic neuritis. Finally, intravenous mithramycin (10 to 25 μg per kilogram over a period of 4 to 6 hours) may be given every 48 hours for up to three doses. The response to mithramycin may last up to 3 weeks. After the initial course, mithramycin may be administered up to twice weekly to maintain normocalcemia. The use of mithramycin to treat hypercalcemia has declined because of concern over toxicities, which include hypotension, hepatic and renal dysfunction, and bone marrow suppression, especially thrombocytopenia. Patients treated with any of these agents should be observed closely for the development of hypocalcemia.

TUMOR LYSIS SYNDROME. Tumor lysis syndrome is a metabolic emergency that can be anticipated and prevented. Rapid tumor lysis is usually encountered upon initiation of chemotherapy for rapidly proliferating malignancies such as high-grade lymphomas or acute leukemias. Rarely it has been reported to occur in solid tumors. The syndrome can occur within 48 hours after arterial embolization of large tumors within the liver. Tumor lysis syndrome causes rapid and severe metabolic changes, including hyperkalemia, hyperuricemia, hyperphosphatemia, and hypocalcemia. Hyperuricemia or hyperphosphatemia can cause renal failure secondary to uric acid or calcium phosphate crystallization in the tubules. Hypocalcemia caused by precipitation of calcium phosphate and lowered calcitriol levels can result in neuromuscular irritability, tetany, and obtundation. Hyperkalemia can be sufficiently severe to cause cardiac arrhythmias and sudden death.

Treatment begins with identification of the patient at risk and prevention of the metabolic and end-organ changes. Patients likely to develop rapid tumor lysis associated with chemotherapy should be hospitalized for initial treatment and to circumvent the syndrome. Volume status, electrolytes, blood urea nitrogen, creatinine, uric acid, phosphorus, and calcium serum levels are obtained before beginning chemotherapy. If patients present with evidence of tumor lysis syndrome prior to chemotherapy, every effort should be made to correct the metabolic abnormalities before starting the drugs. It is not always possible to postpone chemotherapy, however, and in such a setting, hemodialysis may be necessary. Hyperkalemia must be treated aggressively with sodium polystyrene sulfonate (kayexalate) or, if electrocardiographic changes are noted, calcium chloride, insulin, dextrose, and sodium bicarbonate. The next treatment priority is to avoid uric acid precipitation in the renal tubules. This is done by alkalinizing the urine with one quarter normal sodium chloride containing two ampules (100 mEq) of sodium bicarbonate and maintaining a urinary output between 100 to 200 ml per hour. Additional bicarbonate is titrated to maintain urine pH between 7 and 8. Loop diuretics (furosemide) may be necessary to maintain urine flow. Acetazolamide (250 mg by mouth once or twice daily) may be administered in the first days to further hasten urine alkalinization. Allopurinol should be administered prior to chemotherapy (500 mg per square meter on day one and 300 mg by mouth on subsequent days) because it decreases uric acid production by inhibiting xanthine oxidase. Theoretically, calcium phosphate crystal formation can be increased by alkalinization of the urine (pH > 8). Practical considerations, however, dictate that excretion of uric acid is of primary importance, and high-volume urinary output, even when alkaline, dilutes calcium phosphate in the urine and lessens the danger of phosphate crystalluria. Hypocalcemia occasionally requires therapy with intravenous calcium. Rarely, calcitriol replacement is necessary to obviate persistent hypocalcemia caused by low calcitriol levels. Hemodialysis is initiated when volume status, urinary output, acid/base status, and electrolyte changes signal its necessity.

HEMORRHAGIC CYSTITIS. Patients who have received or are receiving cyclophosphamide or ifosfamide may develop a life-threatening hemorrhagic cystitis, caused by metabolites (chlorethylazeridine, chloroacetic acid, and acrolein) of either chemotherapy agent. The metabolites are excreted by the kidney, producing high concentrations in the bladder. The bladder grossly appears hyperemic and edematous, with areas of punctate hemorrhage; mucosal erosions and sloughing are common. The best management entails prevention by maintaining a high urinary output to decrease the concentration of metabolites achieved in bladder and by correcting any coagulation defect. Systemic use of sodium 2-mercaptoethanesulfonate (mesna) prevents mucosal irritation by detoxifying the metabolites within the bladder. Once hemorrhagic cystitis occurs, conservative management with care to ensure excellent urinary output is often adequate. Blood product replacement may be necessary. The use of urethral catheters to remove metabolites and rest the bladder is controversial because catheters can provoke spasm and may prevent passage of clots. If conservative management is not effective, the bladder may be irrigated by N-acetylcysteine. If that fails, irrigation with 1.0 to 2.0% formalin solution frequently (85%) stops bleeding after one treatment. To avoid ureteral reflux of formalin, the formalin-containing irrigation bag should not be elevated more than 15 cm above the pubis. Other agents that may be efficacious include the intravesicular administration of 1.0% alum or prostaglandin E_2 and F_2. If conservative measures fail to control hemorrhage, diversion of hypogastric arteries with ureteral diversion and cystectomy may be necessary.

HEMATOLOGIC EMERGENCIES. Thrombocytopenia is common in patients undergoing chemotherapy. When the platelet count drops to 20,000 per cubic millimeter or less, platelets should be administered prophylactically. Uremia, fever, and drugs also may alter platelet function and number and may affect the decision to transfuse platelets prophylactically. If the platelet count is less than 50,000 per cubic millimeter, platelets should be transfused for active bleeding, before surgery, or before an invasive procedure. When the patient is symptomatic or has a hemoglobin less than 8.0 grams per deciliter, red blood cells should also be administered, but platelet infusion should underpin treatment.

Leukostasis may result when white blood cell counts exceed 100,000 per cubic millimeter. An oncologic emergency is defined not by the degree of leukocytosis but by its associated symptoms. The problem most often accompanies chronic or acute myelogenous leukemia. The ensuing clinical dysfunction results from the lack of deformability of white blood cell blasts, with subsequent plugging of small vessels. The leukostasis syndrome affects the central nervous system, causing stupor, dizziness, visual problems, ataxia, coma, intracranial hemorrhage, and sudden death, as well as the lungs, producing pulmonary infiltrates and hypoxia proceeding to pulmonary failure with a scenario similar to adult respiratory distress syndrome. Because extreme leukocytosis results in hyperviscosity, diuresis and volume depletion should be avoided. The goal of treatment is to reduce the white blood cell count by leukapheresis (decrease white blood count by 20 to 60% over 3 to 4 hours), followed immediately by effective therapy of the underlying leukemia. Because of the potential of leukemic cell lysis, measures should be instituted to prevent tumor lysis syndrome.

Bilezikian JP: Drug therapy: Management of acute hypercalcemia. N Engl J Med 326:1196, 1992. *An excellent review of the causes, pathophysiology, and treatment of acute hypercalcemia.*

Byrne TN: Current concepts: Spinal cord compression from epidural metastases. N Engl J Med 327:614, 1992. *A comprehensive review of clinical and pathologic aspects of spinal cord compression. Included is a practical guide to the evaluation and treatment of patients with suspected epidural tumor.*

Nieto AF, Doty DB: Superior vena cava obstruction: Clinical syndrome, etiology, and treatment. Curr Prob Cancer 10:443, 1986. *Classic review of the topic of superior vena cava syndrome.*

Pizzo PA: Drug therapy: Management of fever in patients with cancer and treatment-induced neutropenia. N Engl J Med 328:1323, 1993. *A practical and well-referenced review of the most recent developments in the approach to the patient with fever and neutropenia.*

164 APPROACH TO THE PATIENT WITH METASTATIC CANCER, PRIMARY SITE UNKNOWN

Daniel C. Ihde

DEFINITION. For a malignant neoplastic disease first to manifest itself by the appearance of visceral or nodal metastases, without any clue to the location of the primary cancer on initial assessment, is not uncommon. Patients presenting in this fashion are said to have metastatic cancer, primary site unknown (MCPSU). Other terms employed to denote this clinical entity include cancer (or carcinoma) of unknown primary site and metastases of unknown origin. This syndrome has been heterogeneously defined both clinically and, as discussed later, pathologically. There is no consensus regarding the extent of evaluation required before the conclusion is reached that the site of primary cancer cannot be readily ascertained, but most authorities agree that complete history and physical examination, blood count and chemistry screening panel, tests of urine and stool for occult blood, chest radiograph, and routine histologic evaluation of the diagnostic pathologic specimen should be performed.

ETIOLOGY. The syndrome of MCPSU by definition results from occult but metastatic primary cancer, the etiology of which varies markedly, depending upon the organ of origin of the malignant process. Interestingly, in a minority of patients the underlying primary site is not apparent even at autopsy. In 302 patients with MCPSU who eventually had postmortem examination, the primary site of cancer was identified in 27% during life and in an additional 57% at autopsy, with a residual 16% in whom even autopsy did not disclose the primary neoplasm. If autopsy is not performed, the fraction of patients in whom the origin of cancer is not discovered is as high as 70 to 80%.

INCIDENCE. Since there is no standard definition of the MCPSU syndrome, its incidence can only be estimated. Various authorities suggest that 2 to 12% of all cancer patients present in this fashion, with the higher estimates generally based on case series from tertiary care centers. Since the number of persons with malignant neoplasms in the United States is approximately 1,000,000 per year, it is likely that the MCPSU syndrome is diagnosed in as many as 50,000 to 60,000 patients annually.

PATHOGENESIS AND PATHOLOGY. The primary pathogenesis of the MCPSU syndrome is the sequence of events that led to the formation and dissemination of the primary cancer. This of course differs greatly depending upon the causative primary neoplasm. Why the primary cancer is not discovered by routine diagnostic evaluation is a question of major interest. The most common explanation is that the tumor is simply too small to be detected by physical examination and imaging studies. Other possibilities include prior surgical excision of the primary, as can occasionally be established in malignant melanoma presenting as MCPSU; hemorrhagic infarction with resultant necrosis and scarring, as is thought to occur in some testicular choriocarcinomas; and spontaneous regression, perhaps mediated by immunologic mechanisms.

Since pathologic confirmation of malignant neoplasm must be obtained and a search for the primary cancer by routine evaluation must be unrewarding before a tentative diagnosis of MCPSU is made, further scrutiny of the pathologic specimen assumes critical importance in the subsequent approach to the patient. Discussion between clinician and pathologist should always occur and may reveal that available pathologic material is inadequate for a more specific diagnosis because of suboptimal amount of preparation. This is more often the case with pathologically undifferentiated neoplasms or when the diagnosis of malignancy rests solely on cytologic material obtained by fine-needle aspiration, which provides little information on tissue architecture and is often insufficient for the detailed immunohistochemical or electron microscopic studies that can help elucidate the primary site or type of malignant neoplasm. If the pathologist believes examination of more tissue could be beneficial, careful communication among pathologist, clinician, and surgeon is essential to ensure that repeat biopsy yields sufficient, properly processed material.

Once an adequate pathologic specimen is available, routine light microscopic examination reveals adenocarcinoma in approximately 40% of MCPSU patients, undifferentiated carcinoma or malignant neoplasm in 40%, squamous carcinoma in 10 to 15%, and, in fewer than 5% each, melanoma, neuroblastoma, or other types of cancer. The pathologist must determine that the presumed metastasis is not the primary site of cancer. Carcinoma occurring in a setting of adjacent epithelial dysplasia suggests a primary neoplasm, whereas types of cells not normally present in the biopsy site, such as epithelial acinar structures in lymph nodes, confirm that the tumor is metastatic. Light microscopic examination can sometimes reveal structural features that suggest the origin of the cancer. For example, papillary adenocarcinoma most often arises in the thyroid, ovary, or lung, and signet ring adenocarcinoma in the gastrointestinal tract. Rosetting malignant cells are characteristic of neuroblastoma and psammoma bodies of thyroid or ovarian carcinoma.

More specialized studies are especially helpful in evaluating undifferentiated carcinomas or malignant neoplasms, which can prove to be poorly differentiated squamous cell carcinoma or adenocarcinoma, lymphoma, amelanotic melanoma, germ cell carcinoma, or undifferentiated sarcoma, and can also identify the organ of origin of some carcinomas. Immunohistochemical techniques are now more widely utilized than electron microscopy. Analysis with panels of monoclonal or polyclonal antibodies can suggest specific diagnoses, such as lymphoma with leukocyte common antigen positivity, melanoma or sarcoma with neuroectodermal S-100 antigen positivity, carcinoma with cytokeratin or epithelial membrane antigen positivity, prostatic carcinoma with prostate-specific antigen (PSA) positivity, thyroid carcinoma with thyroglobulin positivity, and germ cell carcinoma with reactivity to antibodies against human chorionic gonadotropin (hCG) or α-fetoprotein (AFP). However, it is not firmly established that the clinical behavior and response to therapy of malignant neoplasms, particularly undifferentiated neoplasms, diagnosed solely by immunohistochemical means are identical to the behavior and response of corresponding neoplasms diagnosed by light microscopy.

Electron microscopic findings may likewise be of value, particularly in undifferentiated neoplasms. Ultrastructural demonstration of microvilli is characteristic of adenocarcinoma, desmosomes of squamous carcinoma, premelanosomes or melanosomes of malignant melanoma, and cytoplasmic dense-core granules of neuroendocrine carcinomas such as small cell lung cancer.

Differing degrees of certainty which individual pathologists require to make a more specific diagnosis and differing numbers and types of specialized pathologic studies employed before the diagnosis of MCPSU is made account for the second major source of heterogeneity in patients reported to have the MCPSU syndrome.

CLINICAL MANIFESTATIONS. The first clinical manifestation and site of initial pathologic diagnosis of cancer in patients with MCPSU most often occurs in the lung or pleural space, liver, bone, or lymph nodes. Other sites include cancer in the peritoneal space and pelvis, brain, epidural space, and skin. The distribution of metastases is clearly different in patients with MCPSU and those with an obvious primary site. For example, bone metastases are not common in overt pancreatic cancer but are frequent in pancreatic cancer presenting as MCPSU. Liver and lung metastases are uncommon in overt prostatic cancer but occur much more frequently in prostatic cancer with a clinically undetected primary site.

The most common eventually detected primary sites of cancer in MCPSU patients are the pancreas, lung, colon, and hepatobiliary structures. In MCPSU cases presenting above the diaphragm, the lung is the most common primary cancer site that is later discovered, while for infradiaphragmatic presentations, the pancreas is the most frequently documented primary site.

The distribution of eventually proven sites of cancer origin in patients with MCPSU is somewhat different from that of various cancers in the general population. Germ cell, adrenal, hepatobiliary, pancreatic, and renal cancers are relatively overrepresented among patients with the MCPSU syndrome, whereas malignant tumors of breast, uterus and uterine cervix, lung, and prostate are relatively underrepresented. Cancers in the latter group are more readily diagnosed by simple means such as physical examination and chest radiograph than are malignant neoplasms in the former group.

STAGING EVALUATION. The oncologic staging evaluation, or determination of the extent of tumor dissemination, is somewhat atypical in patients with MCPSU. With the presence of metastatic cancer already proven, considerable effort is often expended in attempting to document the site of the primary tumor. However, this is frequently inappropriate, since most MCPSU patients prove to have advanced carcinoma refractory to therapy, and performing extensive testing to locate the primary tumor site could occupy a considerable fraction of the patient's life expectancy with only minimal prospects of affecting the ultimate outcome.

Identifying the primary tumor site benefits the patient in only three circumstances: (1) Tumor confined to a single peripheral lymph node region may be potentially completely eradicated, making control of the primary cancer in the area drained by affected nodes the dominant determinant of survival. An example is occult primary squamous carcinoma of the head and neck region occurring in cervical lymph nodes. (2) Documenting that the primary tumor arises in an organ for cancers of which effective systemic treatment is available, such as breast cancer, strongly supports the administration of such therapy. (3) Localizing a primary tumor producing or about to produce disabling symptoms may allow institution of palliative therapy.

Identification of additional asymptomatic visceral metastatic sites of tumor is of no value in a patient with known visceral metastases. However, in patients whose MCPSU arises in a single peripheral lymph node region, discovery of visceral or distant nodal metastases may avert unnecessarily radical locoregional therapy.

There is universal agreement that radiographic barium studies of the upper gastrointestinal tract and colon and intravenous pyelogra-

phy are of no value in the absence of symptoms or signs suggestive of an occult primary cancer in the region being imaged, since false-positive studies occur more frequently than the uncommon true-positive result. Computed tomography (CT) of the abdomen and chest probably has a higher yield, but in most cases detects only an untreatable primary cancer, especially pancreatic and non–small cell lung cancer. In all patients with MCPSU, any imaging studies suggested by the comprehensive evaluation of the pathologic specimen that might support the diagnosis of a treatable malignant neoplasm, such as prostatic ultrasonography in an adenocarcinoma reacting with antibodies to PSA, or CT to detect retroperitoneal lymphadenopathy in an undifferentiated neoplasm reacting with antibodies to leukocyte common antigen, should be performed. Imaging studies for evaluation of symptoms are always appropriate, since detection of a primary or metastatic tumor that requires palliative treatment, such as intestinal bypass for impending obstruction, may result.

Serum biochemical studies that may help diagnose a treatable neoplasm, such as hCG and AFP (germ cell carcinoma) and PSA and prostatic acid phosphatase (prostatic cancer), should be obtained in the appropriate clinical and pathologic setting. However, only markedly elevated values of these biomarkers are specific for germ cell (or hepatocellular in the case of AFP) carcinoma and prostatic cancer, respectively, since other cancers and benign conditions, such as liver disease and prostatic hypertrophy, are associated with more modest elevations. Moderate elevations do, however, support further evaluation for the specific treatable neoplasm in question. Estrogen receptor determinations can be performed on an appropriately prepared tumor biopsy, but only markedly elevated values strongly support the diagnosis of hormonally responsive breast or endometrial cancer, as many types of carcinoma can exhibit modestly elevated receptor protein levels.

The remainder of the staging evaluation in patients with MCPSU should be closely tailored to the specific clinical presentation. It is most useful to segregate patients into two groups, those with known tumor confined to lymph nodes and those with tumor in visceral site(s) with or without node involvement.

MCPSU Confined to Lymph Nodes. Malignant melanoma and lymphoma can occur as isolated lymphadenopathy in any node-bearing region, and, if neither is excluded by pathologic evaluation, a primary cutaneous melanoma (along with pathologic review of previously excised skin lesions) or other sites of adenopathy (and possibly evidence of bone marrow involvement), respectively, should be sought. Likely sites of origin of other primary cancers vary markedly by nodal area.

In patients with middle and upper cervical adenopathy in whom biopsy reveals squamous or poorly differentiated carcinoma, complete endoscopic examination with blind biopsies and CT to identify areas of submucosal thickening may disclose a primary cancer of the upper aerodigestive tract. Patients with supraclavicular adenopathy more often prove to have adenocarcinoma, which is likely to originate in the lung, breast, or (only in the left fossa) the gastrointestinal tract.

Adenocarcinoma occurring as isolated axillary adenopathy most likely originates in the breast in the female, with lung cancer another possibility in both sexes. Careful breast examination and mammography are always performed in this setting. With other pathologic diagnoses, lung and skin of the upper extremity should be considered as possible primary sites. Isolated inguinal malignant adenopathy may be either squamous cell carcinoma or adenocarcinoma, and the primary cancer often originates in the genitalia, skin of the lower extremity, and anorectal structures, which should be carefully examined. A fraction of MCPSU patients with poorly differentiated tumor confined to the mediastinal or retroperitoneal nodes prove to have germ cell carcinoma, and testicular examination and ultrasonography are appropriate.

MCPSU in Visceral Sites. Approximately 85% of MCPSU patients have visceral metastases, and no reproducibly effective systemic therapy is currently available for the great majority. The clinician should focus on identifying neoplasms for which effective systemic treatment exists, specifically chemotherapy-responsive breast and ovarian cancer, pulmonary and extrapulmonary small cell carcinoma, germ cell carcinoma, and lymphoma; hormone-responsive prostatic, breast, and endometrial carcinoma; and papillary carcinoma of the thyroid, which is responsive to radioactive iodine administration. Unfortunately, no more than 10% of MCPSU patients with visceral metastases are found to have one of these neoplasms.

In women, pelvic examination should be performed and mammography obtained if pathologic evaluation does not exclude breast cancer. Any suspicion of gynecologic neoplasm should lead to abdominal and pelvic CT or pelvic ultrasonography. Some women with malignant ascites revealing adenocarcinoma on cytologic examination and no evidence of metastases outside the peritoneal cavity have tumors with clinical behavior similar to that of ovarian carcinoma and may be candidates for exploratory laparotomy. The thyroid gland should be carefully palpated in both sexes.

In men, prostatic examination and perhaps ultrasonography should be performed, and blind prostatic biopsy may be appropriate if suspicion of prostate cancer is high. The possibility of an overlooked subareolar mass due to male breast cancer should not be forgotten. In younger men with predominant midline nodal presentations and minimal visceral tumor, especially confined to the lung, historical evidence of rapid tumor growth or response to previous therapy suggestive of the incompletely characterized syndrome of "poorly differentiated carcinoma of unknown primary site" should be sought, and testicular examination and ultrasonography performed.

TREATMENT. *MCPSU Confined to Lymph Nodes.* Patients who, after the staging evaluation outlined above, have all known tumor confined to a single lymph-node–bearing region should be approached aggressively, as a fraction of them will attain 5-year survival and even cure. Those with melanoma should undergo radical lymphadenectomy, with the expectation of 5-year survival of 15 to 35%, depending upon the number and volume of nodal metastases, an outcome similar to stage III melanoma managed with excision of the primary skin lesion and radical lymphadenectomy. If malignant lymphoma is the suspected diagnosis, combination chemotherapy appropriate for lymphoma followed by local irradiation is a reasonable approach.

Squamous and undifferentiated carcinoma in middle to upper cervical nodes is most often managed with radical neck dissection and irradiation, although irradiation alone may be sufficient for low-volume disease. The radiation field often includes the nasopharynx, oropharynx, and laryngopharynx to treat possible primary tumor sites. Five-year survival of 25 to 50% can be anticipated, depending upon tumor volume. The outlook for patients with adenocarcinoma and supraclavicular node metastases is much more grim, with only occasional patients living 5 years after irradiation.

Isolated axillary adenopathy in women with biopsy-proven adenocarcinoma is often treated as breast cancer. Axillary node dissection and modified radical mastectomy are usually advocated in this setting and yield 5-year survival rates of 30 to 70%, results at least as good as in overt stage II breast cancer. Only half of mastectomy specimens reveal a primary tumor. More recently, similar survival has been reported in patients treated only with axillary dissection or excision, often in conjunction with breast irradiation. Since a fraction of patients clearly have breast cancer, systemic adjuvant therapy appropriate for stage II breast cancer, either chemotherapy or tamoxifen depending upon the individual patient, should be considered. Men and women with squamous or undifferentiated carcinoma confined to axillary nodes should have evaluation for node dissection, since approximately 20% will live 5 years after surgery. Although physical examination usually reveals the primary cancer in patients with malignancy in inguinal nodes, surgical extirpation or irradiation alone yields 5-year survival of approximately 25% in patients without a documented primary site.

If MCPSU of undifferentiated pathology is confined to mediastinal or retroperitoneal nodes, a trial of aggressive combination chemotherapy, especially in younger patients, may be appropriate, since these nodal regions are common areas in which extragonadal germ cell tumors and lymphomas arise.

MCPSU in Visceral Sites. Palliative or supportive care is often the major focus of management in MCPSU patients with visceral metastases, since most have widely disseminated cancer for which no effective systemic treatment is available. Occasionally, surgical resection of metastases may be beneficial, as in the case of a solitary brain metastasis or an obstructing intestinal lesion. Palliative irradiation, to brain or bone metastases, for example, is often effective. Chemotherapy or in some instances hormonal therapy or

radioactive iodine, which are the only maneuvers that address the problem of distant metastatic disease, can be administered with realistic expectation of success in only a few subgroups of patients.

If either detailed review of the pathologic material or the staging evaluation raises reasonable suspicion of one of the primary cancers discussed above that might be expected to respond to systemic treatment, a trial of appropriate therapy should be initiated, provided that a favorable risk-benefit ratio is thought to exist in the individual patient.

Two other clinical settings also merit strong consideration of chemotherapy. In women with isolated malignant ascites, laparotomy with maximum feasible resection of tumor masses, provided they are confined to the peritoneal cavity, may be appropriate. Whether or not a primary ovarian tumor is identified, a recent study reports a relatively indolent clinical course in these patients, with some complete responses to chemotherapy regimens utilized in ovarian cancer.

The syndrome of poorly differentiated carcinoma of unknown primary site is not well defined, but a fraction of patients with some or all of the characteristics enumerated above have complete remissions, some durable, with cisplatin-containing chemotherapy regimens utilized for testicular cancer. Regrettably, such success has not always been observed. Originally these cases were thought to represent germ cell carcinomas in which a definitive pathologic diagnosis could not be rendered, but in one series of patients in whom more than one fourth completely responded to chemotherapy, even detailed retrospective pathologic review suggested that no more than 5% of patients had initially unrecognized germ cell tumors. Thus the pathogenesis of this syndrome remains obscure, and until therapeutic results are obtained after the prospective application of strict diagnostic criteria, utilized to select a group of patients who are then uniformly treated, the proportion that derives substantial benefit from chemotherapy will remain uncertain.

For the remaining patients with visceral MCPSU, there is no evidence that any treatment improves survival. Close observation with palliation of symptoms as they arise is an appropriate management strategy. Chemotherapy regimens for which responses in the MCPSU syndrome have been reported or investigational treatments may be given to fully ambulatory patients who understand the limitations of therapy but still desire it.

PROGNOSIS. The prognosis of MCPSU in most patients is poor. Median and 5-year survival in several large series of consecutive patients accrued in single institutions is approximately 5 to 10 months and 3 to 7%, respectively. The most important prognostic features, as in most other cancers, are sites and volume of tumor involvement, ambulatory status, and degree of weight loss. Five-year survival is reported to be 25 to 50% for patients whose tumor is confined to peripheral lymph nodes and less than 3% for all other patients.

Abbruzzese JL, Abbruzzese MC, Hess KR, et al.:Unknown primary carcinoma: Natural history and prognostic factors in 657 consecutive patients. J Clin Oncol 12:1272, 1994. *A recent large institutional series of consecutive MCPSU patients, with detailed information on prognostic factors.*

Greco FA, Vaughn WK, Hainsworth JD: Advanced poorly differentiated carcinoma of unknown primary site: Recognition of a treatable syndrome. Ann Intern Med 104:547, 1986. *Initial detailed description of clinical characteristics and prognostic features of a subgroup of MCPSU patients surprisingly responsive to combination chemotherapy.*

Haskell CM, Cochran AJ, Barsky SH, et al.: Metastasis of unknown origin. Curr Probl Cancer 12:1, 1988. *Comprehensive and critical review of MCPSU syndrome.*

165 MOLECULAR MECHANISMS OF DRUG RESISTANCE

Michael W. DeGregorio and
Edith A. Perez

The development of drug resistance to antineoplastic agents represents a major reason for treatment failures in hematologic and oncologic malignancies. The mechanism(s) underlying drug resistance in cancer can be broadly attributed to many cellular adaptations. In fact, many mechanisms responsible for causing drug resistance in cancer are also thought to be responsible for detoxification of normal tissues. Therefore, unique molecular mechanisms responsible for drug resistance are difficult to discern from normal cellular defenses. However, some forms of drug resistance in cancer are known to be associated with the overexpression of certain tumor suppressor and/or regulatory gene(s).

Classic Multidrug Resistance

The term *multidrug resistance* (MDR) denotes the ability of malignant cells to withstand exposure to lethal doses of several structurally and functionally unrelated antineoplastic agents (Table 165–1). MDR can be inherent in a particular neoplastic clone or may arise as the result of a spontaneous somatic mutation. According to current theories of tumor growth, such mutations could occur during one of every 10^6 cell divisions. Thus, multidrug-resistant cells are very likely to be found in a typical tumor mass that measures 1 cm^3 and contains 10^9 cells. Several mechanisms of drug resistance have been identified in human cancer cells. These include overexpression of P-glycoprotein ("classic MDR"), alteration in quantity or quality of topoisomerase II, and overexpression or mutation of genes that control cell cycle kinetics and modulate programmed cell death (apoptosis).

A variety of normal tissues constitutively express P-glycoprotein. These include epithelial cells of the kidney, colon, small intestine, pancreas, bile canaliculi, and adrenal glands; endothelial cells in the brain and testis; and placental trophoblasts. The location of P-glycoprotein on the luminal surfaces of these organs is consistent with its role as a transporter protein, perhaps functioning to protect normal cells from natural toxins.

Among chemotherapeutic agents, substrates for P-glycoprotein include the anthracyclines, epipodophyllotoxins, vinca alkaloids, taxanes, mitomycin C, and actinomycin D. P-glycoprotein functions as an energy-dependent efflux pump that reduces the intracellular concentration of certain antineoplastic agents by actively extruding them across the cell membrane. Although these agents are structurally and functionally disparate classes of chemotherapeutic agents, they are all lipophilic compounds derived from natural products. In general, resistance to one of the agents of the MDR phenotype implies cross-resistance to the other classes of drugs.

Innately resistant tumors arising from tissues that normally express the *mdr*1 gene are inherently multidrug resistant. Significant *mdr*1 gene expression has also been found in some untreated leukemias, lymphomas, and non–small cell lung cancers with neuroendocrine features. More commonly, elevated *mdr*1 RNA levels are seen in malignancies that have recurred after successful initial treatment with antineoplastic agents. Numerous studies have documented the emergence of the MDR phenotype in relapsed cancers of the breast and ovary, neuroblastoma, leukemias, and lymphomas, the apparent result of negative selection of clones that express P-glycoprotein. Clinical studies have found *mdr*1 gene expression and P-glycoprotein positivity to be adverse prognostic factors in leukemia, breast cancer, neuroblastoma, and childhood soft tissue sarcoma.

TABLE 165–1. CLASSES OF DRUGS AFFECTED BY THE MDR PHENOTYPE

Drug Class	Cellular Target
Anthracyclines	Topoisomerase II
Doxorubicin	(intercalation)
Daunorubicin	
Mitoxantrone	
Epipodophyllotoxins	Topoisomerase II
VP-16 (etoposide)	
VM-26 (teniposide)	
Vinca alkaloids	Microtubules
Vincristine	
Vinblastine	
Taxanes	Microtubles
Taxol (Paclitaxel)	
Taxotere	
Antibiotics	DNA intercalator
Actinomycin D	Alkylator
Mitomycin C	
Mithramycin	

.Another form of MDR involves alterations in topoisomerase II and confers resistance to cytotoxic agents that target this enzyme. Topoisomerases are nuclear enzymes that modulate the topologic structure of DNA by inducing transient DNA breaks. When this type of MDR develops, resistance to epipodophyllotoxins and anthracyclines but not vinca alkaloids is observed. P-glycoprotein is not detectable, and changes in intracellular accumulation of drug are not seen. Drug resistance is associated with quantitative or qualitative abnormalities of topoisomerase II that lead to decreased enzyme activity. Decrements in topoisomerase activity can result from spontaneous mutations, down-regulation of transcription, or altered phosphorylation patterns of topoisomerase II. The normal down-regulation of topoisomerase II in quiescent cells may explain their relative resistance to inhibitors of topoisomerase II.

A more recently emerging field in MDR involves the use of recombinant biologic molecules in the treatment of cancer. Primarily these molecules are of the class known as cytokines. These molecules were originally identified as messenger or signaling molecules between cells of the immune system. Because of the ability of these molecules to recruit or stimulate the immune system, some have been rapidly moved to the clinical arena. Included in this group are the interferons, interleukins, and colony stimulating factors. With increasing knowledge and experience of the biologic effects of the cytokines, it is now appreciated that a phenomenon of multiple cytokine resistance ("mcr") exists, and by the use of cytokines as drugs, this is a form of MDR.

However, as more cytokines have been identified, a very complex picture has emerged which shows multiple biologic effects from a single cytokine, depending on the dose, cell type treated, or assay system used. In cancer research, an important focus has been on cytokines that affect negative growth regulation. The classic example of this type of cytokine is transforming growth factor-β (TGF-β). More recently, interleukin 6 (IL-6) has been studied for its growth inhibitory effects. Both TGF-β and IL-6 can inhibit the growth of certain epithelial and hematopoietic cells.

Recent studies suggest that changes in cell cycle kinetics, particularly in pathways that lead to apoptosis, may be important in the development of MDR. Apoptosis (also called programmed cell death) is an active form of cellular suicide that is energy-dependent, requires protein synthesis, and usually culminates in the activation of endogenous endonucleases that degrade the cell's DNA. Apoptosis may represent a common final pathway for cell death caused by a variety of antineoplastic agents.

Apoptosis and Therapeutic Resistance

The energy-dependent biologic process of apoptosis has now been linked to the responses of cancers to radiation, chemotherapy (both cytotoxic and DNA-damaging), immunoantibody therapy, and cytokine treatment. Indeed, MDR can result from the failure of cells to carry out this process. The tumor suppressor gene product p53 is required in many cases for apoptosis. As this gene is the one found most frequently mutated in all types of human cancers and presumably inactivated, any cell carrying the mutation is resistant to that type of apoptosis. A p53-independent pathway for apoptosis has also been identified, but this process may be restricted to only certain cell types. A better understanding of the p53-independent pathway will likely yield new targets for overcoming MDR at a basic level.

The p53-dependent apoptotic pathway is responsible for mediating the cytotoxicity of 5-fluorouracil, etoposide, and doxorubicin. Thus, patients harboring mutations in the p53 gene in their tumors would likely be resistant to those drugs even in the absence of *mdr*1 overexpression. The p53 tumor suppressor protein itself has been linked to the human *mdr*1 gene. The p53 protein is a DNA-binding protein that activates transcription of some genes and represses transcription of others. For example, the normal or wild-type p53 protein can repress transcription of the *mdr*1 and IL 6 genes. A mutant form of p53 is inefficient at repression of expression of IL 6 and actually results in stimulation of expression of the *mdr*1 gene. In clinical studies of both B-cell chronic lymphocytic leukemia (B-CLL) and acute myelogenous leukemia (AML), the presence of p53 mutations in patients was not associated with overexpression of the *mdr*1 gene. However, in that B-CLL study, the p53 mutations were associated with increased drug resistance.

APPROACHES TO OVERCOMING DRUG RESISTANCE.

The circumvention of MDR has been an active area of oncologic research. Several classes of pharmacologic agents are capable of reversing the MDR phenotype in preclinical studies (Table 165-2). However, because of unacceptable toxicities, only a few of these have been used effectively in humans. Although verapamil and cyclosporine showed early promise as chemosensitizing agents in the treatment of some hematologic malignancies, the results of many clinical trials have been disappointing. In studies using high-dose verapamil, for example, nearly all patients developed heart block or hypotension before optimal MDR-reversing concentrations of the drug could be achieved. Furthermore, even if ideal levels of a chemosensitizing agent could be achieved *in vivo,* it is likely that cancer cells are simultaneously protected by other mechanisms of MDR. It is probably overly simplistic to think that P-glycoprotein alone holds the key to the problem of MDR.

With a rapidly expanding understanding of the cell cycle, new strategies to interrupt cell proliferation and promote cell death are being pursued. The *bcl-2* and p53 genes offer just two of many potential targets in the molecular therapy of cancer. Early clinical trials have begun using p53 antisense oligonucleotides in patients with leukemia in the hope of counteracting the effects of mutant p53. *Bcl-2* and *bcr/abl* (in chronic myelogenous leukemia) are also being targeted by antisense therapy as a means to remove malignant cells that contaminate autologous bone marrow grafts. Other approaches aim to induce apoptosis directly by initiating the chain of events that leads to autodigestion of nuclear DNA and cell death.

Chin K-V, Pastan I, Gottesman MM: Function and regulation of the human multidrug resistance gene. Adv Cancer Res 60:157, 1993. *A current comprehensive review of the clinical ramifications of MDR.*

Kastan MB, Onyekwere O, Sidransky D, et al.: Participation of p53 protein in the cellular response to DNA damage. Cancer Res 51:6304, 1991. *A significant scientific article associating a tumor suppressor gene with cellular response, potentially representing a new therapeutic target.*

RESISTANCE TO ALKYLATING AGENTS

The alkylating agents are a diverse series of chemical compounds that react strongly with various negatively charged, electron-rich nucleophilic substances. A variety of chemical groups (sulfhydryl, carboxylic, imidazole, phosphate, and amino) serve as targets in biologic systems. The cellular effects of alkylating agents are probably mostly related to the alkylation of components of DNA; the N^7 position of guanine is particularly susceptible, although other sites may be alkylated as well. These reactions may lead to the formation of DNA interstrand or intrastrand crosslinks and the formation of DNA-protein links, as well as modulation of oncogene expression and activity. Because these effects may interfere with DNA replication, transcription, and translation, alkylating agents have played a central role as chemotherapy agents for the treatment of cancer.

The alkylating agents in clinical use fall into five chemical classes: (1) the nitrogen mustards (chlorambucil, cyclophosphamide, ifosfamide, mechlorethamine, and melphalan); (2) the ethylenamines (thiotepa, hexamethylmelamine); (3) the alkyl sulfonates (busulfan); (4) the nitrosoureas (carmustine, lomustine, semustine, streptozotocin); and (5) the triazines (dacarbazine). Another group of agents, the platinum derivatives cisplatin and its analogue carboplatin, are also classified as alkylating agents.

TABLE 165–2. CLASSES OF CHEMOSENSITIZING AGENTS AND THEIR DOSE-LIMITING TOXICITIES

Drug	Class/Function	Dose-limiting Toxicity
Verapamil	Ca²⁺ channel blocker	Cardiovascular
Diltiazem	Ca²⁺ channel blocker	(hypotension, heart block)
Quinine	Cinchona alkaloid	Gastrointestinal
Quinidine	Antiarrhythmic	Neurologic
Amiodarone	Antiarrhythmic	
Trifluoperazine	Calmodulin inhibitor	Neurologic
Cyclosporin A	Immunosuppressant	Renal, biliary
Tamoxifen	Triparanol analogue	Neurologic
Toremifene	Triparanol analogue	Neurologic

TABLE 165–3. MECHANISMS OF ALKYLATING RESISTANCE

Drug	Resistance Mechanism
Nitrogen mustard	Transport reduction
	Glutathione transferase increase
	DNA repair increase
Melphalan	Transport reduction
	Glutathione increase
Nitrosoureas	DNA repair increase
Cyclophosphamide	Aldehyde dehydrogenase increase
Cisplatin	Transport reduction
	Detoxification associated with thiol-containing compounds
	DNA repair increase
	Modulation of oncogene expression
	Modulation of signal transduction

Intrinsic and acquired resistance to the alkylating agents is unfortunately a common and complex clinical problem in cancer. A wide range of metabolic or structural properties of cells may lead to drug resistance; its molecular basis is one of the most important and actively studied problems in clinical oncology. Several recent studies indicate different mechanisms of resistance to the same alkylating agent in different cell lines and differing mechanisms for the different alkylating agents. Resistance to alkylating agents and platinum compounds is associated with decreased drug accumulation, increased drug inactivation, and increased repair of drug-induced DNA damage (Table 165-3).

The mechanism(s) by which alkylating agents and cisplatin enter the cell is the subject of intense study. Impaired cisplatin accumulation is one of the earliest changes detectable in some human cancer cell lines selected *in vivo* and probably contributes to clinical resistance. Detoxification or inactivation of electrophilic alkylating agents and platinum compounds has also been associated with their reactions with thiol-containing compounds, such as glutathione (GSH) and metallothionein. GSH is the predominant nonprotein thiol compound in mammalian cells and has been shown to play a role in cellular homeostasis, metabolism, transport, and drug detoxification. In its chemically reduced form, GSH can inactivate peroxides and free radicals or bind to positively charged electrophilic molecules, such as the active groups of alkylating agents, rendering them less toxic and potentially leading to drug resistance. These reactions are catalyzed by nonenzymatic mechanisms and by the enzymes glutathione peroxidase and glutathione S-transferase (GST). Although the clinical importance of GSH and GST in alkylating drug resistance is still somewhat controversial, preclinical data have prompted clinical trials utilizing GST or GSH synthesis inhibitors.

The second type of a detoxification mechanism associated with thiol-containing compounds is through metallothioneins. These are the most prominent cellular protein sulfhydryl–containing cysteine residues and are believed to play a role in heavy metal regulation and detoxification. Increased levels of metallothioneins have also been associated with resistance to cisplatin and alkylating agents in some preclinical models.

Repair Mechanisms

An increased ability to repair alkylating damage appears to contribute to the drug resistant phenotype as well. Cisplatin toxicity is thought to be mediated primarily by the formation of lethal intrastrand DNA crosslinks, and several reports suggest that increased DNA repair is indeed associated with resistance to this compound. For example, unscheduled DNA synthesis, which is thought to be indicative of DNA repair, is relatively increased in response to cisplatin treatment in cisplatin-resistant ovarian cancer cells compared with drug-sensitive parental cells.

For the cell to repair cisplatin-DNA complexes, a source of deoxynucleotides is required. The deoxythymidine monophosphate (dTMP) synthase cycle is the sole source of *de novo* thymidine, and the incorporation of thymidine is rate limiting in DNA synthesis. Increased levels of dTMP synthase and thymidine kinase have been associated with cisplatin resistance. Therefore, modulators of intracellular folate metabolism are expected to play a role in cisplatin resistance. Recent studies have indeed documented modulation of cisplatin resistance by the methotrexate analogue edatrexate.

Another example of alkylating drug resistance with an increased capacity to repair DNA is the reported increased levels of O^6-alkyl-guanine DNA alkyltransferase, an enzyme that removes adducts from the O^6 position of the base guanine in cell lines resistant to alkylating agents.

Oncogenes and Alkylating Resistance

Some oncogenes, most notably c-*fos* and c-H-*ras,* appear to be involved in alkylator drug resistance. The c-*fos* nuclear oncogene has been proposed to play an important role in resistance to cis-platin. The c-*fos* oncogene is one of a group of immediate-early genes activated in response to a variety of stimuli, including growth factors and chemotherapy agents. It has previously been shown that cisplatin-resistant human carcinoma cells contain elevated mRNA for c-*fos*. This has been supported by clinical data demonstrating c-*fos* gene amplification in tumor samples isolated from patients resistant to cisplatin-based combination chemotherapy.

The postulated mechanisms of c-*fos* action in cisplatin resistance may involve DNA synthesis and repair processes, including dTMP synthase and DNA polymerase. This is consistent with the DNA-binding and transcriptional activation functions of the *fos* protein in its interaction with other genes. Interestingly, the aforementioned enzymes comprise a multienzyme complex, and *fos* may act to regulate expression of the entire complex. The fact that cisplatin administration results in a cascade of events, beginning with activation of c-*fos* and leading to induction of dTMP synthase and DNA polymerase, is highly suggestive of this explanation. Even though the precise mechanism by which repair of cisplatin-induced DNA damage occurs is not known, any repair pathway ultimately requires polymerases, ligases, and deoxynucleotides.

The H-*ras* oncogene has also been implicated in resistance to cis-platin. The biochemical mechanisms by which *ras* may be implicated in drug resistance are unclear, but the location of the *ras* protein on the inner surface of the cell membrane suggests that it might function by affecting drug transport. It is also possible that the association with resistance may be through modulation of signal transduction pathways, as *ras* modulation has been shown to affect protein kinase C and to act upstream of *fos* in signal transduction.

Berger NA: Alkylating agents. *In* DeVita VT, Hellman S, Rosenberg SA (eds.): Cancer: Principles and Practice of Oncology. Philadelphia, JB Lippincott, 1993, p. 400. *A comprehensive review of the alkylating agents used in the treatment of cancer.*

Colvin M: Alkylating agents and platinum antitumor compounds. *In* Holland JF, Frei E III, Bast RC, et al. (eds.): Cancer Medicine. Philadelphia, Lea & Febiger, 1993, p 733. *An additional review of the alkylating agents, with emphasis on the platinum compounds.*

Hamilton TC, Ozols RF, Dabrow MB: Multidrug resistance to alkylating agents and platinum compounds: State of our knowledge. Oncology 4:101, 1990. *A review regarding the mechanisms of alkylating cross-resistance.*

METHOTREXATE RESISTANCE

Consideration of the mechanism of action and metabolism of methotrexate (MTX) serves as the basis for understanding mechanisms of resistance. Following uptake by the folate transport system, the antimetabolite MTX can bind avidly to and inhibit its primary enzyme target, dihydrofolate reductase (DHFR). Then, in the presence of adequate thymidylate synthase activity, inhibition of DHFR results in depletion of the reduced folate pools essential for thymidylate and *de novo* purine synthesis. The cytotoxicity of MTX is significantly influenced by intracellular metabolism involving polyglutamation, in a manner similar to physiologic folates. MTX polyglutamates bind more effectively to DHFR and are preferentially retained by the cells. Additionally, these polyglutamyl derivatives can inhibit other folate-dependent enzymes, including thymidylate synthase and 5-aminoimidazole carboxamide ribotide (AICAR) transformylase enzymes (involved in thymidylate and *de novo* purine synthesis, respectively). Therefore, resistance to MTX can result from a number of alternative mechanisms in the complex pathway of drug transport, reduced polyglutamation leading to decreased drug retention, as well as reduced inhibition of enzymes as described above and either elevated levels of DHFR or reduced affinity of DHFR for MTX. Whereas all of these mechanisms have been described in examples of experimental resistance of cultured cells to MTX, increased DHFR levels secondary to gene amplification is the only mechanism identified to date that has been associated with clinical MTX resistance.

Bertino JR, Romanini A: Folate antagonists. *In* Holland JF, Frei E III, Bast RC, et al. (eds.): Cancer Medicine. Philadelphia, Lea & Febiger, 1993, p 698. *A general review of methotrexate: clinical uses and mechanisms of resistance.*

TAMOXIFEN RESISTANCE

Tamoxifen (TAM) prolongs both the disease-free and overall survival of postmenopausal women following primary surgery, and induces tumor regression in about 50% of women with advanced estrogen receptor–positive (ER+), metastatic breast cancer. Although approximately 50% of ER+ tumors respond to TAM, only 60% of patients with metastatic breast cancer have hormone-dependent, ER+ tumors. Therefore, only 30% of all breast cancer patients actually benefit from TAM therapy. In addition, the majority of patients who initially respond to therapy may eventually develop acquired TAM resistance following prolonged administration. Unfortunately, the cellular and molecular mechanisms underlying the development of acquired resistance to the antiestrogens are still poorly understood. The rest of this chapter reviews the mechanism of action, the multiple mechanisms associated with acquired TAM resistance, and potential clinical strategies to overcome this resistance.

Mechanism of Action

The mechanism(s) by which TAM inhibits tumor cell growth was at one time believed to be solely mediated through interaction with estrogen receptors. Binding of TAM to the estrogen receptors is believed to form a complex that is then bound to specific chromatin sites, thus blocking the expression of estrogen-induced genes. The resulting blockade is believed to inhibit cell growth (cytostatic). This cytostatic effect on cell growth is fully reversible with estrogen administration.

Several studies have now shown that cellular inhibition by TAM may involve much more than a simple competitive antagonism of estrogen receptors. Modulation of breast cancer cell growth by the differential stimulation or inhibition of growth factor production from cells may also play a role in antiestrogen action. Recent evidence suggests that estrogens may stimulate cell growth by inducing cells to synthesize growth factors and/or receptors. TAM, on the other hand, may act by decreasing the production of growth factors while at the same time stimulating the production of growth-inhibitory factors.

At least one pathway may involve the stimulation of growth inhibition–transforming growth factor (TGF-β) production by TAM. TGF-β has both growth-inhibitory and stimulatory effects but is selective in its actions. In stromal cells or fibroblasts, it stimulates cell growth. However, in most types of tumor cells, including breast tumors, it is a highly potent growth inhibitor. Although the exact mechanism of TGF-β growth-inhibitory effects is poorly understood, it does appear to inhibit tumor cell growth independently of the estrogen receptor. The association between a number of other growth factors and control over breast cancer cell growth has also been examined, including TGF-α, epidermal growth factor (EGF), and insulin-like growth factors (IGF-I and IGF-II). However, the exact role of each of these growth factors in the induction of cell growth by estrogen and the inhibition of cell growth by TAM remains to be elucidated.

The antiestrogenic activity of TAM appears to depend on both the species studied and the target tissue examined. In rats and humans, tamoxifen has similar biologic activity. In both species TAM has partial estrogen agonist effects on uterine tissues but is considered primarily an estrogen antagonist on breast tissue. TAM's estrogenic effects have been noted in postmenopausal patients on gonadotropins, plasma proteins, and vaginal epithelium. Whether the difference in antiestrogenic action is related to species-specific or tissue-specific metabolism or is the result of altered signal interpretation by the cell following interaction of the antiestrogen with the estrogen receptor is unknown.

Potential Mechanisms of Tamoxifen Resistance

A variety of mechanisms have been implicated in the development of acquired resistance to TAM. The absence or loss of estrogen receptors could explain the development of hormonal independence or TAM resistance, particularly since ER− tumors rarely respond to TAM. However, clinical studies suggest that resistance to TAM is not always caused by selection of a hormone-independent and/or ER− clone of tumor cells. Maintenance of ER and/or progesterone receptor levels and responses to secondary hormonal therapies are typically seen in patients with acquired TAM-resistant tumors.

A number of recent clinical reports also suggest that TAM can have growth-stimulatory effects on tumors in some patients. Following initial response to TAM in premenopausal patients, patients developing therapeutic failure frequently respond to ovariectomy when TAM is discontinued at the time of tumor progression. In contrast, ovariectomy appears to be ineffective in patients if TAM is continued after castration. These clinical observations suggest that TAM stimulates the growth of tumor cells by some unknown mechanism. Additional data show that patients with tumor progression on TAM therapy can have a tumor response from the mere discontinuation of TAM.

ESTROGEN RECEPTOR VARIANTS. Protein structure modifications leading to altered affinity of the ER for TAM is a plausible resistance mechanism. Site-specific mutations, including nonsense or frameshift mutations in the structural gene coding for the ER, may result in various types of functionally abnormal receptors. These mutations may render the ER entirely nonfunctional; thus the tumor would appear clinically as if it were ER −. Alternatively, if mutations result in amino acid substitutions in important domains of the receptor, the result may be the generation of ER species that are functionally active but exhibit altered specificities for estrogens and antiestrogens.

It is postulated that tumors with ER variant cell populations may escape the normal growth dependence of estrogens, and subclones may be selected by TAM treatment. Thus the selection of TAM-resistant ER variants may be clinically significant in regard to TAM resistance.

GROWTH FACTORS AND TAMOXIFEN. Recent studies have demonstrated that TAM may act independently of the ER altogether and that its effects are the result of the counterbalance between TAM-induced growth-inhibitory and growth-stimulatory factors secreted by breast cancer cells and their adjacent cells. A number of growth factors have been identified which are associated with estrogen's modulating effects on the cell cycle. These primarily involve polypeptide growth factors, which regulate the progression of the cell through the cell cycle.

Several autocrine growth factors have been identified which regulate the growth of breast cancer cells. TGF-α–like growth factors are believed to be associated with the stimulation of cell cycle growth, whereas TGF-β is a polypeptide that inhibits cell growth. Estrogens are believed to inhibit TGF-β production, whereas TAM is believed to stimulate its production. TAM appears to stimulate the production of TGF-β from stromal and breast cancer cells, as mentioned earlier. It has been suggested that TAM-induced TGF-β production from either ER + cells or stromal cells may act to inhibit cell growth of ER − cells. TAM resistance may therefore occur once the stromal cells can no longer produce TGF-β.

Interestingly, apoptosis is now known to be associated with the growth inhibitory effects of the antiestrogens. The TGF-β1 gene is one of the hallmarks of induced apoptosis. When resistance develops to the antiestrogens, apoptosis may be inhibited by turning off the production of TGF-β. Furthermore, TAM switches from a growth-inhibitory agent to an agent that stimulates growth in both preclinical and clinical settings, which may be regulated by TGF-β or other growth factors.

Decreased Cellular Accumulation

A decrease in cellular drug concentration is one mechanism by which cells become resistant to TAM. Although no similar efflux pump has been identified in TAM resistance, compared with MDR, several recent studies suggest some overlapping factors between the two forms of resistance. An increase in P-glycoprotein has been noted following estradiol treatment in a preclinical rat mammary adenocarcinoma model. Although little other evidence has been published on the interaction between MDR and antiestrogen resistance, further studies may help to determine the link between these forms of resistance. Interestingly, the more impressive correlation between these forms of resistance is that both appear to share the common characteristic of a drug accumulation defect. The reduced cellular levels of drug in MDR have been well documented and appear to be directly correlated with overexpression of the P-glycoprotein pump. However, not until recently did preclinical and clinical studies show that reduced TAM accumulation is also apparent in breast cancers that are resistant to TAM.

Other Factors Contributing to Antiestrogen Failure

A variety of factors may contribute to therapeutic failure of TAM which are not related to cellular or molecular resistance. These include patient noncompliance, weight gain, the ingestion of foods high in phytoestrogens such as soy products, and drug interactions. Cellular or molecular resistance is therefore considered the primary contributing factor for patients who develop resistance to TAM.

Circumvention

The information from a variety of recent studies suggests that TAM resistance is complex and may involve multiple mechanisms. Genetic mutations, whether already present in cancerous cells or induced by TAM, most likely underlie the phenotypic changes noted in resistant cells. These changes may be manifested by altered receptor number or affinity of the ER, increased production of TGF-α or decreased production of TGF-β, increased binding of drug to antiestrogen binding sites, altered signal interpretation by the cell, decreased cellular accumulation of drug, or altered metabolism of drug.

Pure steroidal antiestrogens, such as a 7-alkylamine derivative of 17-estradiol, have been studied in TAM resistance. These agents are specifically designed to decrease the partial agonist activity associated with TAM. Although prolonged use of these agents may be associated with a number of side effects, including atherosclerosis and osteoporosis, they may nevertheless be effective in the treatment of TAM-resistant patients.

Research involving growth stimulation and/or inhibition of breast cancer cells by growth factors has led to much of the well-supported knowledge on TAM resistance and will likely provide much further information on the mechanisms involved. If TAM resistance does correlate with the loss of TGF-β production, synthesis and administration of growth factors that inhibit cell proliferation should be explored.

Other potential methods of circumvention have also been suggested, including intermittent pulse therapy, which is based on the belief that continuous exposure of cells to drug may select for hormone-independent resistant cells, and gene therapy, which may become plausible once the genetic basis of breast cancer and resistance is better understood.

Johnston SRD, Dowsett M, Smith IE: Towards a molecular basis for tamoxifen resistance in breast cancer. Ann Oncol 3:503, 1992. *A review of the potential molecular mechanisms of resistance to tamoxifen.*

Legha SS: Tamoxifen in the treatment of breast cancer. Ann Intern Med 109:219, 1988. *A useful review of the clinical utility of tamoxifen in breast cancer.*

Wiebe VJ, Osborne CK, Fuqua S, et al.: Tamoxifen resistance in breast cancer. Crit Rev Oncol Hematol 14:173, 1993. *A comprehensive review of proposed and known mechanisms of tamoxifen resistance.*

166 TREATMENT OF NEOPLASTIC DISEASE DURING PREGNANCY
Valerie J. Wiebe

The incidence of cancer spontaneously arising during pregnancy is reported to be low (0.07 to 0.1%). However, this incidence may be on the rise. The decision by many women to delay pregnancy until later in their reproductive years is expected to increase the incidence of neoplasms diagnosed during pregnancy. Therefore, many clinicians may be confronted more frequently with the management of neoplasms during pregnancy. Few situations are faced by the patient and her physician which involve so many ethical and moral dilemmas. Although termination of pregnancy is not medically indicated for most neoplasms diagnosed during pregnancy, treatment involving radiation and chemotherapy pose obvious risks to the fetus. Unfortunately, few therapeutic guidelines exist in regard to the therapeutic management of neoplasms arising during pregnancy. This is primarily due to the fact that large prospective studies cannot be performed in pregnant patients. Therefore, most information relies on data from limited case reports. This chapter summarizes some of the information available in the literature concerning the management of neoplasms during pregnancy. However, it must be kept in mind that therapy should be tailored to the individual patient and that much more needs to be learned concerning the treatment of neoplasms during pregnancy.

BREAST CANCER

EPIDEMIOLOGY AND NATURAL HISTORY. The incidence of breast cancer in association with pregnancy is reported to be between 0.03 and 3.8% (Table 166–1). The diagnosis of breast cancer during pregnancy may account for as much as 2 to 5% of all patients diagnosed with the disease. Breast and cervical cancers are reported to account for more than half of all malignancies occurring during pregnancy. The high incidence of these neoplasms in pregnancy is probably related to the fact that they are frequently seen in women of childbearing age.

DIAGNOSIS. The majority of patients with breast cancer during pregnancy present with a painless lump that may be easily overlooked. Unfortunately, the diagnosis of breast cancer is often delayed in pregnant patients by as much as 2 to 7 months. This is primarily due to the assumption that changes occurring within the breasts are related to normal physiologic changes associated with pregnancy. Breast tenderness and engorgement may complicate routine physical examination. Owing to the delay in diagnosis of breast cancer in the pregnant patient, there is often a higher rate of nodal metastasis and a poorer overall survival of patients. Although early diagnosis is key in determining the prognosis of this disease and is a factor that can be controlled by the physician, any breast lump occurring during pregnancy should be closely evaluated.

Because of the difficulty in detecting breast cancer during pregnancy, some investigators recommend that mammographic screening be performed during the initial prenatal examination in all women over the age of 25. However, others report that mammographic screening is of limited value in the pregnant patient. False-negative mammograms have been reported in up to 75% of pregnant patients who were found to have breast cancer on subsequent biopsy. Increased water density of the breast and normal tissue changes associated with pregnancy are believed to make mammograms difficult to interpret. Therefore, this procedure may be unreliable during pregnancy and is not considered worth the added risk of fetal exposure to radiation. Fine-needle aspiration may also be of limited benefit because cellular hyperplasia occurs normally in breast tissue during pregnancy. Excisional biopsy may therefore be the diagnostic procedure of choice because it poses little risk to the mother and fetus and is perhaps the most accurate method of establishing a definitive diagnosis of breast cancer in the pregnant patient.

The use of diagnostic radiographs in pregnancy is recommended only when documentation of metastasis will result in a change in therapeutic recommendations. Because most diagnostic radiographs to the chest and pelvis are below the level of radiation (0.008 to 0.04 rad) associated with significant risk to the fetus, they are considered relatively safe in pregnancy. However, proper precautions should be taken to reduce fetal radiation exposure, including the use of abdominal shielding and careful calculation of the radiation dose received by the fetus.

The use of hormone receptor assays, including estrogen receptors (ER's) and progesterone receptors (PR's), are also of limited value in pregnancy. Most studies suggest that the majority (>75%) of breast cancers in pregnant patients are both ER- and PR-negative. However, these results are difficult to interpret because high levels

TABLE 166–1. ESTIMATED INCIDENCE OF VARIOUS TYPES OF CANCER ASSOCIATED WITH PREGNANCY

Cancer	Estimated Incidence per 1000 Pregnancies
Breast	0.3–38.0
Cervical	0.45–0.81
Colorectal	0.01–0.02
Leukemia	0.01
Lymphoma	0.01–1.00
Melanoma	0.3–2.8
Ovarian	0.02–0.06
Thyroid	?

of circulating estrogen and progesterone during pregnancy may significantly alter hormone receptor levels. Furthermore, assays that measure only unbound receptors may not be an accurate assessment of receptor number if concentrations of hormone are high and most receptors are in the bound form.

MANAGEMENT. Historically, therapeutic abortion was recommended in patients developing breast cancer during pregnancy. High circulating levels of estrogen during pregnancy were believed to further stimulate the growth of hormonally sensitive breast tumors. However, most evidence now suggests that the majority of breast cancers arising during pregnancy are ER-negative (hormone-independent). Surgical oophorectomy has also been shown to be ineffective in pregnant patients with breast cancer. Furthermore, retrospective studies evaluating the efficacy of therapeutic abortion in patients developing breast cancer during pregnancy suggest that therapeutic abortion does not exert any beneficial effects on the course of breast cancer. Because termination of pregnancy does not appear to improve the survival rate of breast cancer patients, it should be considered only in patients who do not desire to continue their pregnancies.

For those patients choosing to bring their pregnancies to term, surgical management of breast cancer is the treatment of choice, particularly when the procedure is considered curative. Surgery spares the fetus from the significant risk of fetal anomalies induced by radiation and/or chemotherapy. Furthermore, in early-stage breast cancer, local-regional control of the disease is often achieved by primary surgery alone. Although breast-sparing surgical procedures are commonly used in the nonpregnant population, these procedures are less of an option for pregnant patients because they are used in combination with radiation therapy, which poses a substantial risk to the fetus.

Unfortunately, many women who develop breast cancer during their childbearing years are likely to have ER-negative, lymph node–positive breast cancer. In this subset of patients, surgery alone may not be curative. In the nonpregnant population, studies have indicated that adjuvant chemotherapy is effective in the treatment of premenopausal patients with breast cancer regardless of nodal status. The use of adjuvant chemotherapy in nonpregnant patients may improve survival by as much as 20 to 30%. Although adjuvant chemotherapy is effective in ER-negative, lymph node–positive patients, it is effective only if treatment is not delayed.

Typically, CMF (cyclophosphamide, methotrexate, and 5-fluorouracil) is the chemotherapeutic regimen of choice in nonpregnant patients. However, the use of folate antagonists such as methotrexate should be avoided during pregnancy because they are highly teratogenic. Folate antagonists are associated with the "aminopterin syndrome." The syndrome involves multiple congenital anomalies, including cranial dysostosis, and is commonly seen in infants exposed to folic acid antagonists during the first trimester. In patients who require chemotherapy during the first trimester, a doxorubicin-containing regimen such as CAF (cyclophosphamide, doxorubicin, and 5-fluorouracil) or one that contains only cyclophosphamide may be used. In the second or third trimesters, CMF may be considered if necessary. In patients diagnosed late in pregnancy or those with greatly advanced disease at the time of diagnosis, for whom chemotherapy will not significantly alter the course of the disease, chemotherapy may be delayed until after delivery.

Little is known about the use of hormonal therapy, such as tamoxifen, during pregnancy. Theoretically, because oophorectomy has not proven effective in the treatment of breast cancer during pregnancy and most patients have ER-negative breast cancer, antiestrogen therapy would be expected to be of limited value. Moreover, the risk of teratogenic effects from antiestrogens on the developing fetus far outweighs the limited benefits of therapy that is merely cytostatic in nature and not considered curative.

CERVICAL CANCER

EPIDEMIOLOGY AND NATURAL HISTORY. Cervical cancer is currently the most frequently diagnosed type of invasive cancer associated with pregnancy. The incidence of cervical cancer in association with pregnancy is between 1 in 1240 and 1 in 2200 pregnancies. This accounts for approximately 1 in 34 cases of cervical cancer diagnosed. The incidence of cervical cancer does not appear to be altered in pregnancy. Although the incidence of cervical cancer has been substantially reduced by the routine use of Pap smears, cervical neoplasia is still the most common gynecologic neoplasm to occur during pregnancy. The clinical course and symptoms of cervical cancer in pregnant patients do not significantly differ from those of nonpregnant patients. Approximately 70 to 95% of all cases diagnosed during pregnancy are squamous cell carcinoma. Adenocarcinoma accounts for the remaining cases.

DIAGNOSIS. The majority of cervical cancers (93%) are diagnosed late in pregnancy. Only a minority of patients (6.3%) are diagnosed with stage I disease early in pregnancy. This suggests that delayed diagnosis of cervical cancer during pregnancy is a significant problem. Delayed diagnosis may stem from the fact that patients present with symptoms that may easily be passed off as normal problems associated with pregnancy, including vaginal bleeding or spotting. Sanguinopurulent discharge may also occur. With more advanced disease, the pregnant patient may have symptoms of weight loss, pelvic pain, and lower-extremity edema.

The overall characteristics of carcinoma of the cervix during pregnancy do not differ significantly from those in the nonpregnant population (Table 166–2). The cytologic and histologic findings associated with the precancerous state in adenocarcinoma are difficult to define and often require conization to make a reliable diagnosis. Adenocarcinoma *in situ* is even more difficult to diagnose. In fact, patients presenting with early invasive adenocarcinoma often present with a history of negative Pap smears within a year of diagnosis. In pregnancy, the diagnosis of adenocarcinoma is further complicated by the fact that lesions are typically found high in the endocervical canal or deep within the endocervical crypts. Routine Pap smears in these cases are not diagnostic, although most clinicians prefer to avoid the use of more invasive procedures during pregnancy. Therefore, the avoidance of invasive biopsy procedures during pregnancy may lead to a delay in the diagnosis of cervical cancer.

In order to detect early-stage cervical cancer during pregnancy, it is recommended that patients undergo Pap smear screening during either their preconceptional or initial prenatal visit. Repeat Pap smears should be performed at each trimester if the patient has been treated for cervical dysplasia within the last 2 years. If cervical dysplasia is detected on Pap smear, a detailed examination should be performed. This includes repeat cytologic analysis, colposcopy, aimed biopsy, and in some cases conoid excision of the cervix uteri. Colposcopy should be used to follow up any abnormal cervical cytologic specimens. Although this procedure is inadequate in 20% of unselected nonpregnant patients, it is reported to have a greater accuracy during pregnancy.

In patients with highly abnormal cytology not explained by colposcopic examination or with colposcopic evidence of invasive disease that cannot be proven with a simple punch biopsy, cervical conization may be performed as a diagnostic procedure. However, this procedure carries a high degree of risk to both the fetus and mother and therefore should be avoided during pregnancy unless absolutely necessary, particularly during the first trimester. This procedure has been associated with significant morbidity in pregnancy, including profuse cervical hemorrhage. A high incidence of incomplete resection of precancerous lesions in pregnant patients has also been reported. Therefore, conization should be performed during pregnancy only in order to determine if frank invasive disease is present so that therapy may be initiated during pregnancy.

MANAGEMENT. *Cervical Dysplasia and in Situ Cervical Cancers.* The management of cervical cancer during pregnancy depends on the trimester of pregnancy and the stage of the disease at diagnosis. If cervical dysplasia or carcinoma *in situ* arises during pregnancy, careful observation until delivery may be all that is necessary. For patients with Pap smears showing classes III, IV, and V, repeat cytologic examination should be performed as well as colposcopy. In patients with incompletely visualized transformation zones and no evidence of invasive disease, colposcopic procedures may be repeated in 2 to 3 weeks before carrying out more invasive procedures. If patients do not show pathology on repeat examination, then pregnancy should be continued and a detailed examination should be performed following delivery (after regression of gestational changes). Some investigators suggest that a minimum of 10 weeks after delivery is necessary for regression of gestational changes, whereas others suggest that 6 to 8 weeks is sufficient.

If pathology is retained on repeat cytologic examination and/or colposcopy, then aimed biopsy should be performed (Fig. 166–1). If no pathology is detected on biopsy, then the pregnancy should continue and a detailed examination should be performed after delivery. If dysplasia is noted on biopsy, the pregnancy should continue and treatment should be instituted after delivery. In patients who chose to continue their pregnancy, it is recommended that dysplastic lesions be coloscoped at least every 3 months during pregnancy. This is primarily to monitor disease progression and avoid the chance of unmonitored progression to invasive disease. Once the presence of invasive disease is ruled out by colposcopic examination and biopsy, there is no pressing indication to treat cervical dysplasia during the pregnancy regardless of the degree of disease. If dysplasia occurs in the first trimester, therapeutic abortion may be considered for some patients. Re-evaluation and treatment may then be performed after regression of gestational changes.

If the initial biopsy shows cancer *in situ*, pregnancy should be preserved and treatment instituted after delivery. Typically *in situ* cervical cancer has been shown to be slow growing. In fact, its rate of growth has been reported to be much slower than the gestational period. If patients present with cancer *in situ* during the first trimester, interuption of pregnancy may be considered in some patients. In this case, the patient should be re-evaluated and treated after termination. If cancer *in situ* is detected during the second and third trimesters of pregnancy, pregnancy should be preserved and cytologic examination repeated. Repeat evaluation with conization of the cervix should be performed after delivery.

Invasive Cervical Cancer. The treatment of invasive cervical cancer during pregnancy depends on the characteristics of the tumor and the stage of gestation at diagnosis. With early-stage disease, a modest tumor volume, and early pregnancy (< 20 weeks' gestation), a laparotomy with the fetus *in situ* may be performed. It is also recommended that a pelvic lymphadenectomy be performed initially and if no gross nodal metastases are present, a potentially curative radical hysterectomy should be performed. Treatment using this surgical procedure has resulted in survival rates similar to those noted in nonpregnant patients treated surgically or with radiation.

For patients presenting in the second trimester (> 20 weeks' gestation) with early-stage disease (stage I or IIB) and a large tumor (> 5 cm), the timing of treatment depends on the stage of fetal maturity. Fetal survival increases significantly after 27 weeks' gestation. Therefore, the decision to institute therapy depends on how far the patient is from that time point. A delay of a few weeks may be reasonable, but a month delay may be excessive in some patients. However, in patients who present in the second trimester with a modest tumor volume (< 5 cm), a delay in treatment until after early delivery may be reasonable. In this case, tumor volume should be monitored carefully to avoid undetected rapid enlargement.

TABLE 166–2. CHARACTERISTICS OF CERVICAL CARCINOMA IN PREGNANT AND NONPREGNANT PATIENTS

	Nonpregnant Patients (%) (N = 386)	Pregnant Patients (%) (N = 37)
Tumor localization		
Endocervical	73.3	78.4
External os	2.3	2.7
Portio	24.4	18.9
Tumor growth		
Endophytic	58.5	51.4
Exo-endophytic	25.9	43.2
Exophytic	15.5	5.4
Tumor grade		
Poor	27.8	16.2
Moderate	54.5	67.6
Well	17.7	16.2
Tumor invasion		
Absent	49.1	45.0
Lymph vessels	43.9	40.0
Blood vessels	7.0	15.0

Modified from Baltzer J, et al.: Carcinoma of the cervix and pregnancy. Int J Gynecol Obstet 31:317, 1990.

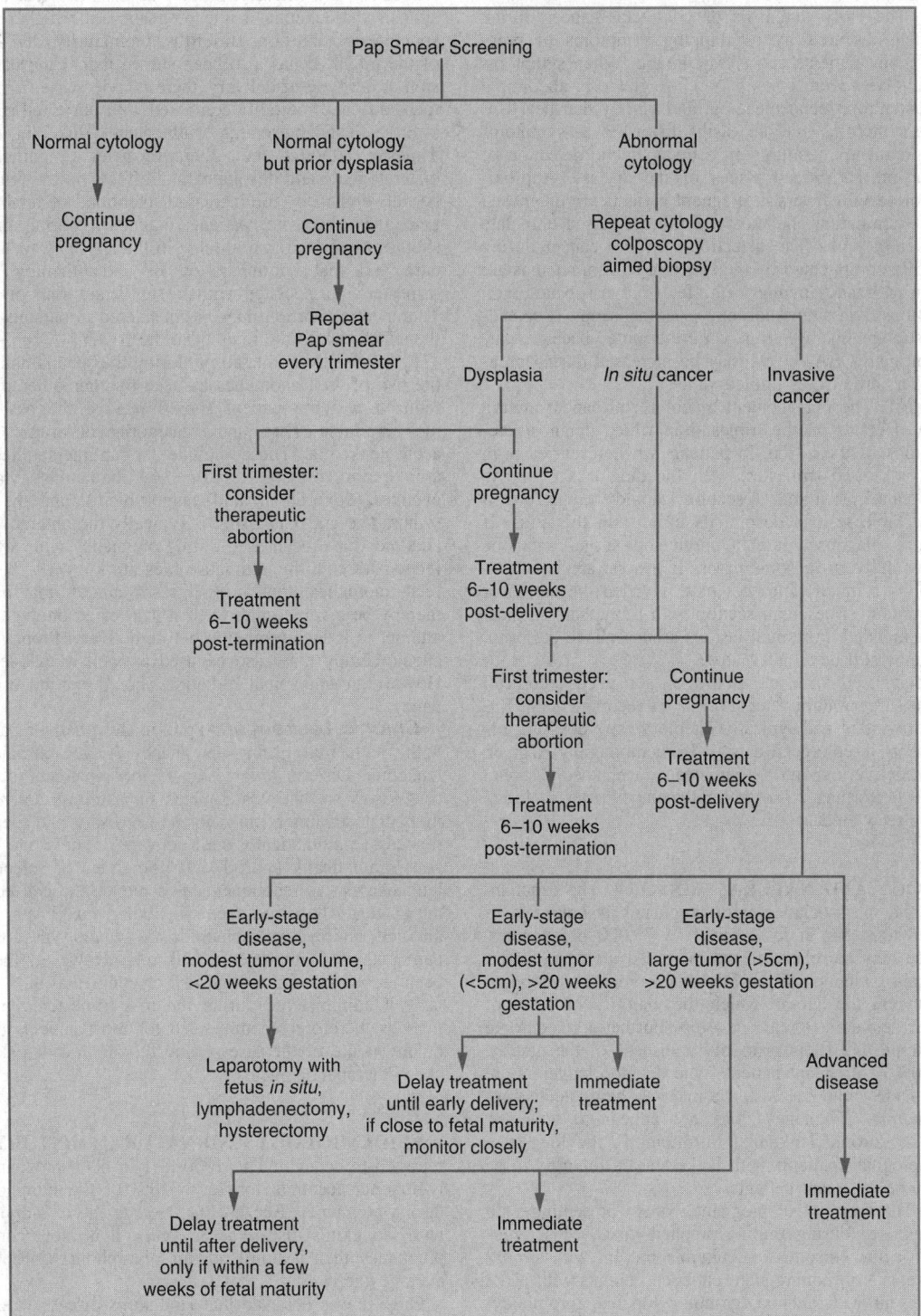

FIGURE 166–1. Diagnosis and management of cervical cancer during pregnancy.

Advanced Disease. For patients in their first trimester who present with advanced disease and who are not candidates for radical hysterectomy, immediate lymph node evaluation followed by external beam therapy is recommended. Spontaneous abortion results near the conclusion of external beam therapy. Uterine curettage should then be performed following spontaneous abortion to decrease the chance of incomplete termination and subsequent sepsis.

In the second trimester, spontaneous abortion induced by radiation therapy may not be an effective method of abortion. Therefore, for those patients requesting or requiring therapeutic abortion, a therapeutic abortion should be performed near the conclusion of planned external beam therapy. For patients wishing to continue with their pregnancy, a cesarean section and lymphadenectomy without hysterectomy may be performed if the chance for fetal sur-

vival is good. In patients presenting with disease extending to both pelvic side walls, maternal survival is considered remote and in this case a delay in therapy to await fetal maturity is reasonable.

COLORECTAL CANCER

EPIDEMIOLOGY AND NATURAL HISTORY. The incidence of colorectal cancer in association with pregnancy is low, between 1 in 50,000 and 1 in 100,000 pregnancies. The low incidence of colorectal cancer is probably related to the fact that colorectal cancer is found in < 5% of patients 40 or younger. The distribution of colorectal cancer does not appear to vary from that found in nonpregnant patients. Most cases of colorectal cancer have been reported to occur below the peritoneal reflection. Approximately 57% arise in the rectum, 20% in the sigmoid, and the remaining 23% throughout the colon.

DIAGNOSIS. The early diagnosis of colorectal cancer during pregnancy is often obscured by overlapping symptoms of pregnancy. Typically many patients are asymptomatic. When symptoms do occur, they involve severe constipation, weight loss, abdominal pain, anorexia, distention, rectal bleeding, and bloody diarrhea. Unfortunately, these symptoms may be easily dismissed as symptoms associated with pregnancy, resulting in a delay in the detection of colorectal cancer until advanced stages of the disease. Approximately 75% of colorectal cancers in pregnant patients are diagnosed by digital rectal examination and most are not diagnosed until late in pregnancy or early labor. The detection of colon cancer during pregnancy is further complicated by the fact that barium enemas are contraindicated in pregnancy owing to the fetal risk associated with this procedure. Biopsy via sigmoidoscopy or colonoscopy is considered the diagnostic method of choice. Furthermore, because carcinoembryonic antigen (CEA) levels may be increased during pregnancy, these markers are also of limited value.

MANAGEMENT. The management of colorectal cancer arising during pregnancy depends on the trimester in which diagnosis occurs and the location of the lesion. In patients who present early in pregnancy (first or second trimester) with the diagnosis of early-stage colorectal cancer, surgical resection should be performed promptly on resectable lesions despite its effects on the fetus. If colorectal cancer is diagnosed late in pregnancy, surgery may be delayed until after delivery in some cases. If lesions are large and lie below the pelvic brim or if tumors have invaded the uterus or adjacent pelvic structures, cesarean section with immediate surgical resection is recommended. For small lesions arising above the brim, vaginal delivery may still be an alternative.

For patients diagnosed with metastatic or advanced colorectal cancer, a delay in surgery until after delivery is recommended. Radiation should be avoided and typically chemotherapy does not offer sufficient benefits in colorectal cancer. If chemotherapy is given during pregnancy, delivery should be induced or a planned cesarean section should be performed close to fetal maturity after maternal blood counts have recovered.

LEUKEMIA

EPIDEMIOLOGY AND NATURAL HISTORY. The exact incidence of leukemia in association with pregnancy is unknown. It has been reported to occur in less than 1 in 75,000 pregnancies. The low incidence may be related to the increased incidence of infertility in leukemia patients and the fact that women of reproductive years are beyond the age in which the majority of cases of acute lymphocytic leukemia (ALL) develop. Furthermore, chronic lymphocytic leukemia (CLL) is primarily a disease of the elderly. Approximately 50% of pregnant patients who develop leukemia are reported to have acute leukemia, with the majority being acute non-lymphocytic leukemia. Pregnancy does not appear to alter the course of acute or chronic leukemia. Furthermore, the long-term survival rates of pregnant patients with leukemia are reported to be similar to those in nonpregnant patients.

DIAGNOSIS. The majority of pregnant women presenting with leukemia are diagnosed during routine prenatal visits. Most pregnant patients with acute episodes of leukemia present with similar symptoms to those seen in nonpregnant patients. Patients with acute leukemia may present with anemia, granulocytopenia, thrombocytopenia, splenomegaly, bone pain, bleeding, and infectious episodes.

Few patients are diagnosed with chronic leukemia during pregnancy. Because chronic lymphocytic leukemia (CLL) is found primarily in the older population, the majority (90%) of cases diagnosed in association with pregnancy are chronic myelocytic leukemia (CML). The diagnosis of chronic leukemia during pregnancy does not differ from that of the nonpregnant patient. Symptoms typically include fatigue, malaise, weight loss, night sweats, and low grade fevers. Patients may also present with splenomegaly and leukocytosis.

MANAGEMENT. *Acute Leukemia.* Treatment decisions for patients presenting with acute leukemia during pregnancy should be based on a number of factors, including the stage of gestation, health of the mother and fetus, mother's prognosis, potential for future pregnancies after treatment, and carcinogenic and teratogenic potential of the drugs. For leukemia patients who desire to bring their pregnancies to term, the consequences to the fetus of maternal leukemia appear directly related to the health of the mother during pregnancy and delivery. Studies have shown that the earlier the diagnosis of leukemia in the pregnancy, the higher the incidence of spontaneous abortion, stillbirths, prematurity, and low birth weight of the infant. It has also been shown that if the patient is in remission at the time of delivery, there is a decrease in maternal and fetal morbidity and mortality compared with untreated patients.

In patients presenting with acute leukemia during the first trimester, although chemotherapy carries a significantly higher risk of teratogenic and developmental effects on the fetus, the risks may be outweighed by the increased likelihood of fetal survival to a viable age. Therefore, patients diagnosed during the first trimester should be advised that a delay in therapy may reduce the chance of cure and that administration of chemotherapy during the first trimester is associated with a significant risk of fetal anomalies. Therapeutic abortion may be considered in patients unable to accept the added risk to the fetus from therapy.

If the disease is diagnosed during the second and third trimesters, the risk of fetal anomalies induced by chemotherapy is significantly reduced and the patient should receive the best treatment regimen available. Three main categories of drugs are used to treat acute leukemia. These include the antimetabolites (methotrexate, aminopterin, 6-mercaptopurine, 6-thioguanine, cytarabine), anthracyclines (doxorubicin and daunorubicin), and the vinca alkaloids (vincristine and vinblastine). Typically the anthracyclines and vinca alkaloids have been used during pregnancy with few deleterious effects. Although the antimetabolites are known to be associated with fetal anomalies, most investigators suggest that induction chemotherapy be given similar to treatment of a nonpregnant patient in an attempt to induce remission before delivery. Prophylactic intrathecal chemotherapy may also be used as well as whole-brain radiation. However, craniospinal radiation should not be used during pregnancy.

Chronic Leukemia. Approximately half of patients diagnosed with leukemia during pregnancy have chronic myelogenous leukemia. Disease progression in these patients is considered relatively slow so that most patients survive until delivery. In this case, immediate treatment may not be necessary and the disease may be treated symptomatically until delivery. If the white blood cell count rises dramatically ($> 250 \times 10^9$ per liter) or splenomegaly occurs, leukapheresis is recommended to reduce the cell count and size of the spleen. Alkylating agents including melphalan, busulfan, chlorambucil, and cyclophosphamide are typically used to treat nonpregnant patients with chronic leukemia. However, these agents have been associated with a high risk of congenital birth defects, particularly if administered during the first trimester. Symptomatic treatment is therefore recommended for most patients owing to the indolent nature of the disease and the significant risk to the fetus of chemotherapeutic agents.

LYMPHOMA

EPIDEMIOLOGY AND NATURAL HISTORY. Lymphoma is reported to occur in 1 in 1000 to 1 in 6000 pregnancies. Hodgkin's lymphoma accounts for 25 to 40% of the lymphomas that occur during pregnancy. Because the average age of individuals diagnosed with Hodgkin's disease is 32 years, it is more commonly seen in pregnancy than is non-Hodgkin's lymphoma (NHL), for which the average age is 42.

Once it was believed that Hodgkin's disease was exacerbated by pregnancy. However, most studies have now concluded that the survival rates of pregnant and nonpregnant patients with Hodgkin's lymphoma are not significantly different. Furthermore, Hodgkin's lymphoma does not appear to adversely effect pregnancy because most women go on to deliver normal, healthy infants.

Although the effects of pregnancy on Hodgkin's lymphoma appear minimal, the effects of pregnancy on NHL remain controversial. Many investigators now believe that when NHL occurs in association with pregnancy, it typically has a more aggressive histology and results in disseminated disease. Furthermore, in patients presenting with Burkitt's lymphoma during pregnancy, tumors appear to be unusually aggressive. Patients with Burkitt's lymphoma may present with rapidly progressive disease that may involve the ovaries or breast. When the disease involves breast tissue, it is associated with a particularly poor prognosis. The underlying mechanism for the altered biology of NHL and Burkitt's lymphoma in pregnancy is unclear at this time.

DIAGNOSIS. The diagnosis of lymphoma during pregnancy is generally based on the finding of lymphadenopathy because the majority of pregnant patients are typically asymptomatic at the time of diagnosis. Approximately 80% of patients present with superficial adenopathy. The most common form is cervical adenopathy. Some patients may have symptoms including fever, night sweats, weight loss, and pruritus. In these cases, it has been suggested that a more aggressive form of the disease is present.

The diagnosis of lymphoma during pregnancy must often rely heavily on an accurate history (including onset and course of adenopathy), physical examination, blood tests, bilateral bone marrow biopsies, and chest radiography with abdominal shielding. Although diagnostic chest radiography does pose a radiation risk to the fetus, in general the millirad doses of radiation associated with diagnostic procedures such as chest radiography are considered safe, provided that proper abdominal shielding is instituted. The use of tomograms and isotope studies are contraindicated in pregnancy owing to the significant risk to the fetus.

The staging of lymphoma during pregnancy is complicated by the relative contraindication to the use of many diagnostic procedures during pregnancy. Staging often includes the use of lymphangiograms. This procedure exposes the fetus to a significant amount of radiation. However, it has been suggested that a single-image abdominal film taken 24 hours after injection of contrast is relatively safe to the fetus if administered in the second and third trimesters. Using this technique, the fetus should be subjected to less than 1 rad of radiation. This procedure is believed to provide the most information and the least amount of fetal exposure.

The pathologic staging of Hodgkin's disease involves the use of staging laparotomy and splenectomy. However, most investigators agree that it should not be routinely performed in pregnant patients. In fact, even in nonpregnant patients, staging laparotomy may not be required unless the results will influence the form of therapy the patient is to receive. For patients with NHL, clinical staging of disseminated disease can be performed in most cases without the use of staging laparotomy.

MANAGEMENT OF HODGKIN'S DISEASE IN EARLY PREGNANCY. Although the opinion is controversial, many investigators agree that if a patient presents with Hodgkin's lymphoma in early pregnancy (up to 20 weeks), therapeutic abortion should be recommended. Furthermore, therapeutic abortion has been recommended in patients who have been exposed to chemotherapy or radiation (> 10 rad) either at the time of conception, during weeks 8 to 12 of gestation, or in those patients who will require radiation or chemotherapy at those times. Therapeutic abortion should also be considered in patients with infradiaphragmatic disease requiring pelvic irradiation, systemic symptoms, visceral disease, aggressive disease, and bulky mediastinal disease. Furthermore, therapeutic abortion should be considered in patients unwilling to accept the added risk to the fetus from chemotherapy or radiation. For patients with localized disease treatable with modified-field supradiaphragmatic radiation that exposes the fetus to less than 10 rad, therapeutic abortion may not be indicated. In these cases, the patients may be treated with modified-field/modified-dose irradiation and full staging and therapy instituted after delivery.

If patients choose to continue their pregnancies, chemotherapy may be delayed until after the first trimester. However, the patient should be closely monitored for disease progression. If disease progression occurs, therapy should be promptly initiated. In most cases, a short delay in therapy does not affect the patient's prognosis. However, if subdiaphragmatic disease is present, treatment should not be delayed.

The treatment of choice for patients with either localized or advanced disease is chemotherapy. Although chemotherapy may be teratogenic, it is considered safer than radiation during pregnancy and may also be more efficacious. Single-agent vinblastine and limited supradiaphragmatic radiation with abdominal shielding may be used in patients requiring treatment in the first trimester. Once the patient is in the second and third trimesters, vinblastine alone may be continued or supradiaphragmatic irradiation may be considered if supradiaphragmatic disease is life threatening.

MANAGEMENT OF HODGKIN'S DISEASE IN LATE PREGNANCY. In patients presenting after 20 weeks of gestation with localized disease, most investigators suggest that treatment be delayed until after delivery. If disease progression threatens the mother or infant, then therapy should be instituted. In patients with

localized supradiaphragmatic disease, localized irradiation with dose and field modification or chemotherapy may be given. However, definitive treatment should be delayed until after delivery with complete staging.

In patients presenting with subdiaphragmatic or advanced Hodgkin's disease in late pregnancy (> 20 weeks), a delay in therapy until after delivery may not be possible. For patients who require more than localized irradiation, chemotherapy is generally recommended. Single-agent vinblastine may be used to control disease progression in some patients until delivery. However, in many patients, single-agent chemotherapy may not be sufficient to slow disease progression and in these cases combination chemotherapy should be administered. It is recommended that first-line combination chemotherapy be instituted in these patients in order to provide the maximum cure rates.

If combination chemotherapy is required, curative regimens such as MOPP (mechlorethamine hydrochloride, vincristine, procarbazine, and prednisone) or ABVD (doxorubicin, bleomycin, vinblastine, and dacarbazine) can be given during the second or third trimester. Few data are available on the safety of these regimens in pregnant patients. However, the ABVD regimen may be somewhat safer than MOPP because mechlorethamine and procarbazine have been associated with a significant risk of fetal malformations.

Non-Hodgkin's Lymphoma (NHL)

The management of NHL during pregnancy depends on the grade of the disease diagnosed as well as the gestational age at the time of diagnosis. For low-grade NHL, treatment may be delayed until after delivery. Unfortunately, many patients diagnosed during pregnancy are found to have intermediate- or high-grade disease and may die of the disease prior to delivery. Any delay in therapy in these patients may reduce the chance of cure from initial therapy. Furthermore, salvage therapy is typically not considered curative in this disease. The use of aggressive chemotherapy in advanced NHL has improved the survival rate of pregnant patients and permitted successful delivery in some patients. However, most patients with NHL who have gone on to deliver live infants have had localized disease or disease that was diagnosed late in pregnancy.

MANAGEMENT OF NON-HODGKIN'S LYMPHOMA IN EARLY PREGNANCY. For patients presenting during early pregnancy (< 20 weeks) with favorable histology (limited stages I, II or advanced), therapy may be delayed until after the first trimester or until after delivery. If disease progression is noted, localized involved field irradiation plus abdominal shielding or chemotherapy may be used. Fetal exposure should be limited to < 10 rad.

For most patients presenting in early pregnancy with unfavorable histology (stage IA, contiguous IIA), therapeutic abortion is recommended. Therapeutic abortion is also recommended for patients who present with progressive disease (stages II, III, IVA, or IVB), lymphoblastic lymphoma, Burkitt's lymphoma, or bulky abdominal disease during the first trimester. It has also been recommended for patients who will be exposed to chemotherapy or radiation (> 10 rad) in the first trimester, as well as for patients who are unwilling to accept the risk to the fetus from potentially teratogenic therapy.

In patients with unfavorable histology (stage IA, contiguous IIA) who refuse therapeutic abortion, therapy may be delayed until the second trimester. Chemotherapy or involved field irradiation can then be given. For patients with more advanced disease, Burkitt's lymphoma, or bulky disease, combination chemotherapy is typically required. Treatment can be delayed until after the first trimester in some patients. However, for patients with lymphoblastic lymphoma or Burkitt's lymphoma, any delay in therapy significantly affects the mother's prognosis.

MANAGEMENT OF NON-HODGKIN'S LYMPHOMA IN LATE PREGNANCY. The management of non-Hodgkin's lymphoma in late pregnancy (> 20 weeks) typically involves observation until delivery. Early delivery may be considered in order to initiate therapy. If the patient demonstrates disease progression and early delivery is not feasible, then treatment should be initiated. Involved field irradiation using an acceptable fetal dose or combination chemotherapy can be instituted.

Combination chemotherapy regimens including COP-BLEO (cyclophosphamide, vincristine, prednisone, and bleomycin), AVTEP (doxorubicin, vincristine, teniposide, cyclophosphamide, and prednisone), BLEO with IT-MTX (bleomycin and intrathecal methotrexate), and CHOP (cyclophosphamide, doxorubicin, vincristine, and prednisolone) can be given. These regimens have been administered during the second and third trimesters of pregnancy.

MELANOMA

EPIDEMIOLOGY AND NATURAL HISTORY. Malignant melanoma is reported to occur in as many as 2.8 per 1000 deliveries and comprises about 8% of all cancers arising during pregnancy. Approximately 90% of malignant melanomas in association with pregnancy are cutaneous in origin, and many arise from a pre-existing nevus. Other sites of origin include the eye, vagina, upper respiratory tract, and anorectum. It has been speculated that pregnancy alters the natural history of malignant melanoma. However, many recent studies have not supported this notion.

Malignant melanoma is noted to have a higher rate of metastasis to the placenta and fetus than other forms of cancer associated with pregnancy. However, the incidence of this is extremely rare. Only 16 cases have been reported, and of these only 4 infant deaths were directly attributed to the transplacental metastasis of malignant melanoma.

DIAGNOSIS. The diagnosis of malignant melanoma during pregnancy is similar to that in the nonpregnant patient (Table 166-3). Because most malignant melanomas arise from existing nevi, careful skin examination and excisional biopsy should be performed on any suspicious nevi. The morphologic characteristics of malignant melanoma include asymmetry, irregular borders, variation in color, horizontal or vertical growth, ulceration, bleeding, and satellite lesions.

TABLE 166-3. CHARACTERISTICS OF MELANOMA IN PREGNANT AND NONPREGNANT PATIENTS

Characteristic	Pregnant Patients (N = 100)	Nonpregnant Patients (N = 86)
Stage at diagnosis		
1	88%	92%
2	10%	6%
3	2%	2%
Primary site		
Trunk	40%	52%
Extremity	50%	30%
Head and neck	6%	13%
Other	4%	5%
Histology		
Lentigo maligna	0%	2%
Superficial spreading	69%	63%
Nodular	18%	23%
Other	13%	12%
Clark level		
I	2%	1%
II	9%	10%
III	49%	50%
IV	26%	27%
V	7%	4%
Unknown	7%	8%
Median thickness	1.30 mm	1.20 mm
Number of ulcerations	25%	24%
Site of first metastasis		
Nodes	71%	61%
Local skin	13%	18%
Lung	6%	12%
Liver	2%	6%
CNS	2%	3%
Other	6%	0%
Later metastases		
Nodes	39%	26%
Local skin	11%	10%
Distant metastases	27%	26%
Mean follow-up	6 years	7.7 years
Recurrence rate	48%	38%
Death rate	25%	23%

Modified from Slingluff CL, et al.: Malignant melanoma arising during pregnancy: A study of 100 patients. Ann Surg 211:552, 1990.

MANAGEMENT. Malignant melanoma arising during pregnancy is best managed surgically. Cure rates as high as 95% have been reported following surgery depending on a number of variables, including the size and depth of the tumor, nodal involvement, and anatomic site. Excisional biopsy with a narrow margin should be performed on any suspicious nevi. Wider excision can then be performed following microscopic confirmation of disease. Excisions approximately twice the diameter of the lesion should be used for small lesions (< 1.5 mm). This is reported to result in recurrence rates of less than 2.5%. Wider excisions are recommended for larger lesions.

Management of Metastatic Disease. Prophylactic lymphadenectomy is typically not recommended during pregnancy if regional lymph nodes are not palpable. However, some investigators suggest that there is a shortened time to lymph node metastasis in pregnant patients and that lymph node basins should be examined carefully on a regular basis because of an increased risk of nodal metastasis. If nodal metastasis is present, then regional lymphadenectomy should be performed. For patients who have isolated hematogenous metastasis, surgical management may be used which results in clinical remission of variable lengths.

Typically, chemotherapy does not offer sufficient benefit to the mother to warrant the risk to the fetus. Single-agent therapy such as dacarbazine (DTIC) has been given. Various other combination regimens have been used including BOLD (bleomycin, vincristine, lomustine, and dacarbazine). While most of these agents have the potential to cause teratogenic effects in the fetus as well as neutropenia and infection, it is best to delay the use of chemotherapy if possible until after delivery.

Despite several reports in the literature of melanoma tumor regression following delivery, at this time there is insufficient evidence supporting the role of therapeutic abortion in order to induce regression of the maternal tumor. To date, malignant melanoma has shown little sensitivity to endocrine manipulation, including the use of estrogens, antiestrogens and androgens, suggesting that the elevated levels of hormones circulating during pregnancy have little overall effect on the growth of malignant melanoma. Furthermore, biopsies of tissues have failed to demonstrate either ER's or PR's during pregnancy, lending support to the notion that tumors are hormone insensitive.

OVARIAN CANCER

EPIDEMIOLOGY AND NATURAL HISTORY. Although rare, ovarian cancer is the second most common gynecologic cancer to occur during pregnancy. The incidence of ovarian cancer in association with pregnancy is reported to be between 1 in 17,000 and 1 in 47,000 pregnancies. The distribution of ovarian tumors in pregnant patients is very different from that seen in nonpregnant patients and typically consists of tumors of low grade and stage. In general, these tumors are associated with a favorable maternal outcome. Most cases are diagnosed in stage I disease before extraovarian dissemination occurs. Approximately two thirds of ovarian cancers arising during pregnancy are of the epithelial type. Germ cell and stromal cell tumors make up the remaining cases. Dysgerminomas are the most common germ cell tumor diagnosed. The mortality rate following a diagnosis of germ cell cancer has been reported to be as high as 93% by 2 years after diagnosis.

DIAGNOSIS. Most ovarian neoplasms diagnosed during pregnancy are asymptomatic. The majority are detected by physical examination during the first prenatal visit. However, the diagnosis of ovarian tumors occurring during pregnancy is frequently missed even when very large tumors are present. Ultrasound scanning may help in the early detection of ovarian masses in some pregnant patients. Patients may present with acute symptoms, including abdominal pain and increasing abdominal girth. This is typically associated with adnexal torsion or rupture and frequently occurs during weeks 8 to 16 of gestation.

The definitive diagnosis of ovarian cancer may be delayed until the second trimester when surgery becomes less of a risk to the fetus. Owing to the high risk of inducing spontaneous abortion during the first trimester following surgery, most physicians suggest that surgical exploration of asymptomatic ovarian masses be delayed until the second trimester unless the mass is very large (> 6 cm). Surgical exploration should also be performed on all solid masses and any cystic mass greater than 5 cm which persists into the second trimester.

MANAGEMENT. Management of an adnexal mass diagnosed during pregnancy depends on the gestational age of the fetus and the size and other characteristics of the mass. In patients who present with masses that are unilateral, unilocular, mobile and < 6 cm during the first trimester, observation until delivery may be all that is necessary. Patients presenting with asymptomatic mobile unilateral adnexal masses in the first trimester of pregnancy without any ascites should be electively explored in the second trimester. For larger masses (> 6 cm) and those that are solid, bilateral, or persist after 14 weeks' gestation, laparotomy is recommended.

For patients who present with an ovarian mass during the latter half of pregnancy (> 20 weeks), the decision to perform surgery is less clear. The risk of premature delivery is greater at this point. In most cases, if there is no evidence of extraovarian disease, surgery can be delayed until after fetal maturity. A short delay in treatment of a few weeks to a month may not significantly affect maternal prognosis but may have a major impact on fetal survival. If the patient becomes symptomatic, emergency laparotomy should be performed. During the second trimester, a midline upper abdominal incision can be used for surgical exploration of ovarian masses. Using this technique, the ovaries can be isolated without extensive manipulation of the uterus. If the mass appears malignant, the incision can be extended inferiorly to allow for staging, and exploration of the abdomen for metastatic disease can be performed.

Because the majority of patients diagnosed with ovarian cancer during pregnancy are early stage and low grade, therapeutic abortion is usually not indicated. Most patients can be treated using conservative surgical management. Surgery alone (salpingo-oophorectomy) may be curative for ovarian cancers in stage IA or IIB, regardless of whether it is of germ cell or epithelial origin. If patients present during the first two trimesters with epithelial tumors that are of high stage and grade, therapeutic abortion is recommended. Some investigators recommend that a total hysterectomy, bilateral salpingo-oophorectomy with omentectomy, and sacrifice of the fetus be performed.

For patients with advanced disease who refuse therapeutic abortion and cannot be surgically managed, chemotherapy should be considered. Administration should be delayed until after the first trimester if possible. Standard chemotherapeutic regimens for nonpregnant patients with epithelial ovarian carcinomas involve the use of cisplatin and cyclophosphamide. The use of alkylating agents such as cyclophosphamide has been associated with an increased risk of teratogenic effects when used in the first trimester. However, the use of cyclophosphamide and cisplatin in the second and third trimesters has not demonstrated a significant risk to the fetus from the limited data available.

The management of nonpregnant patients with germ cell tumors typically involves surgical resection, followed by combination chemotherapy. Because germ cell tumors are generally aggressive in nature, they are considered almost uniformly fatal without the use of chemotherapy. Therefore, patients diagnosed with malignant germ cell tumors should begin chemotherapy soon after recovery from exploratory surgery. Regimens incorporating vincristine, actinomycin D, and cyclophosphamide are effective against germ cell tumors. More recently, regimens such as PVB (cisplatin, vinblastine, and bleomycin) have been used with somewhat increased efficacy. Cure rates as high as 85% have been reported in nonpregnant patients with stage I disease treated with this regimen. Few data are available on the use of the PVB regimen in pregnancy. However, as single agents these drugs have been used successfully in pregnant patients.

THYROID CANCER

EPIDEMIOLOGY AND NATURAL HISTORY. The incidence of thyroid cancer arising during pregnancy is unknown. However, because the peak incidence of epithelial cancer of the thyroid in the nonpregnant population is in the early 30's, it is a disease of women in their childbearing years. The most frequent histologic type of thyroid cancer diagnosed is papillary, followed by follicular, then anaplastic. Medullary cancer is much less frequent (5%) and appears to be associated with multiple endocrine neoplasms.

DIAGNOSIS. The diagnosis of thyroid cancer during pregnancy often relies heavily on physical examination because many patients do not present with symptoms of hypothyroidism or hyperthyroidism. Patients are often diagnosed by palpation of nodules in the first or third trimester. When evaluating the thyroid, it must be kept

in mind that the gland undergoes a number of physiologic changes during pregnancy. The thyroid increases to approximately twice its size during pregnancy. This is a result of follicular cell hyperplasia and abundant colloid formation. However, hypertrophy generally does not significantly hinder physical palpation of thyroid nodules. Thyroid function also changes during pregnancy: Serum thyroxine levels become elevated, but there is a corresponding decrease in T_3 resin uptake, resulting in a normal free serum thyroxine.

Ultrasonography may be used to aid in the characterization of thyroid nodules as well as to guide needles for fine-needle biopsy. Fine-needle aspiration may be used for definitive diagnosis. In pregnant patients it is reported to be approximately 80% accurate. Although some biopsies clearly demonstrate thyroid carcinoma, other carcinomas are less apparent and may appear only as cellular, reactive needle aspirates. Radioisotope scanning and radioactive iodine are both contraindicated in pregnancy owing to fetal uptake of radioisotope.

MANAGEMENT. Thyroid cancer in the pregnant patient is best managed surgically. If diagnosed in early pregnancy, a subtotal thyroidectomy may be used to treat thyroid cancers of the papillary, follicular, and mixed papillary-follicular types. Subtotal thyroidectomy reduces the risk of hypoparathyroidism, which can be a major problem in the pregnant patient. If possible, surgery should be delayed until after the first trimester to avoid potential risks to the fetus. If patients present during the first trimester, thyroid suppression with exogenous thyroxine may be used to slow the growth of the tumor until surgery can be performed in the second or third trimester. If nodules continue to enlarge during thyroid suppression, surgical resection should be performed in a timely fashion.

If papillary, follicular, and mixed papillary-follicular thyroid cancers are diagnosed in late pregnancy, surgery may be delayed until fetal lung maturity, at which time early delivery can be induced or a caesarean section performed. Thyroid suppression may also be used until surgery can be performed. Because the majority of thyroid cancers diagnosed during pregnancy are of the papillary, follicular, and mixed papillary-follicular types and are of low stage and grade, these cancers are typically considered indolent in nature and a short delay in surgery may not significantly affect maternal prognosis. However, if medullary or anaplastic thyroid cancer is diagnosed, the disease is much more aggressive and surgery should not be delayed. In this case total thyroidectomy should be performed. Because the prognosis following a diagnosis of anaplastic thyroid cancer is considered extremely poor, the goal of treatment is to prolong the life of the mother for as long as possible and potentially until an early delivery can be performed.

The use of radiation therapy during pregnancy is typically contraindicated. However, it may be used to treat lesions of the upper airway. In this case, abdominal shielding and calculation of the fetal dose should be performed. In general, chemotherapy does not offer sufficient benefits in thyroid cancer to outweigh the risks to the fetus.

MISCELLANEOUS NEOPLASMS

EPIDEMIOLOGY. A variety of other neoplasms have been diagnosed in association with pregnancy. Neoplasms of the pituitary gland are fairly common in women of childbearing age, and have been diagnosed in association with pregnancy. Typically most pituitary tumors are prolactin-secreting pituitary adenomas. The diagnosis of pheochromocytoma during pregnancy is rare, but at least 200 cases have been reported. Other malignancies in association with pregnancy are less frequent (< 100 cases). These include parathyroid adenoma, sarcoma, Cushing's syndrome, meningioma, renal cell carcinoma, hepatic cancer, adrenal cancer, insulinoma, and stomach and pancreatic cancers in decreasing order of occurrence.

DIAGNOSIS AND MANAGEMENT. *Pituitary tumors* are often asymptomatic and may go undetected until they become enlarged. Because the pituitary gland significantly enlarges during pregnancy, many undiagnosed tumors may become symptomatic. Patients may present with headache or visual changes. If patients develop symptoms during pregnancy, visual field testing and computed tomography may be used for diagnosis. Although prolactin-secreting adenomas have been reported in pregnancy, one of the primary symptoms associated with this tumor type is infertility.

Management of pituitary tumors during pregnancy involves the use of bromocriptine therapy. In patients diagnosed with macroadenoma before becoming pregnant, surgery or radiation may be given before conception, or bromocriptine may be administered throughout pregnancy. Although bromocriptine therapy has been used during pregnancy with few harmful effects, it is generally recommended to discontinue therapy after conception in patients with microadenoma. Patients should be monitored closely for signs of headache or visual changes.

The diagnosis of *pheochromocytoma* is much less common in the pregnant patient. Patients typically present with symptoms similar to those in nonpregnant patients, including paroxysmal or sustained hypertension, tachycardia, sweating, and headache. Many patients do not present with symptoms until puerperium, at which time they may present with preeclampsia, sudden antepartum shock, and hyperpyrexia. Magnetic resonance imaging may be safely used to localize pheochromocytomas during pregnancy.

If pheochromcytomas are diagnosed early in pregnancy, it is recommended that patients be treated with α-adrenergic blockade and surgical resection of the tumor. A short-acting α-blocker such as phentolamine should be given. Therapeutic abortion is also indicated because the mortality rate of the fetus with or without therapy is high (40 to 67%). Patients presenting in late pregnancy should begin α-adrenergic blockade at least 3 days before a planned cesarean section. An α-blocker that is considered safe for the fetus, such as phenoxybenzamine, should be instituted in this case.

DRUG KINETICS DURING PREGNANCY

A number of physiologic changes take place in the pregnant patient that may have significant effects on the pharmacology of antineoplastic agents. An increase in plasma volume by almost 50% is noted in pregnancy. The amniotic fluid may also act as a third space for some water-soluble drugs. These factors may alter the volume of distribution for some drugs, which may result in a dilutional effect. An increased volume of distribution may result in lower peak concentrations and/or a longer half-life of some agents unless there is a corresponding increase in excretion or elimination of the drug. Although there is an overall increase in plasma proteins, there is a decrease in plasma albumin concentrations, which may lead to a decrease in the unbound active fraction of drugs bound to these proteins.

Gastrointestinal function is also changed, slowing the absorption of some orally administered drugs and potentially altering the amounts absorbed. There is an increase in the enterohepatic circulation of drugs, resulting in an increased bioavailability (F) of drugs that undergo enterohepatic circulation. Changes in renal and hepatic function during pregnancy may also alter the elimination of drugs. Renal excretion of drugs is typically enhanced because of increases in the glomerular filtration rate and creatinine clearance. Hepatic clearance of drugs may be either increased or decreased. Increased drug clearance may reduce the area under the concentration $\times$ time curve (AUC) of some agents, which may significantly influence their efficacy.

When chemotherapeutic agents are administered during pregnancy, the altered physiology of the patient and its effects on the pharmacokinetics of agents must be evaluated (Table 166–4). In general, these physiologic changes may not affect the pharmacokinetics of agents until the latter part of pregnancy. However, chemotherapeutics are often administered in the second or third trimester owing to the increased fetal risk in the first trimester. The pharmacokinetics (volume of distribution, peak drug concentrations, half-life of administration, area under the concentration curve, clearance) of some antineoplastics may therefore be significantly altered in pregnant patients.

ADVERSE EFFECTS OF CHEMOTHERAPEUTICS ON THE FETUS

Following *in utero* exposure to chemotherapeutics, fetal death, miscarriage, premature birth, low birth weight, teratogenesis, organ toxicity, hematopoietic depression, and hormonal alterations have all been reported. Delayed effects may also occur, and because most patients are lost to follow-up, their exact incidence may never be known (Table 166–5). Although the risk of these toxicities is considered significantly high following the use of some antineoplastics such as aminopterin, not all agents present such an extreme risk to the fetus. The risk of fetal toxicities following antineoplastic use depends largely on the timing of antineoplastic exposure with respect to gestational age, the total amount of drug exposed to the fetus, and the drug's mechanism of action.

During the first trimester, when cells are rapidly dividing, the fetus is highly sensitive to antineoplastics. Most investigators believe that exposure of the fetus to antineoplastics at this time presents a significant risk to the fetus (Table 166–6). Although the use of antineoplastics during the first trimester has been associated with a 7.5 to 25% incidence of malformations, the incidence is probably overestimated because radiation therapy, which is a known teratogenic agent, may have contributed to the overall incidence of malformations in some cases. When patients receiving either radiation therapy or folate antagonists are excluded from analysis, the incidence of fetal malformations following single-agent chemotherapy approaches 6%. Furthermore, the overall incidence of fetal malformations occurring in normal patients without the use of chemotherapy is estimated to be 3%, and the incidence of minor malformations may be as high as 9%.

In the first trimester it is best to avoid the use of antineoplastics altogether. However, because not all agents are associated with the same degree of fetal risk, withholding therapy in a patient who has advanced cancer may not be justified. When chemotherapy must be used, both the vinca alkaloids (vincristine, vinblastine) and antibiotics (doxorubicin and daunoubicin) appear to be somewhat less teratogenic than other agents used in first trimester pregnancy. In the second and third trimester, single-agent antineoplastics or combination chemotherapy has been given successfully with few reported adverse effects on the fetus. However, careful fetal monitoring evaluating intrauterine growth and fetal stress should be performed routinely because intrauterine growth retardation, low birth weight, and premature birth may still occur. When combination chemotherapy is given, each agent should be selected carefully because drugs may interact together or with radiation to produce synergistic teratogenic effects.

The timing of delivery with respect to the administration of the

TABLE 166–4. PHARMACOKINETIC FACTORS THAT MAY BE ALTERED DURING PREGNANCY AND MECHANISMS OF CIRCUMVENTION

Pharmacokinetic Factor	Effect	Comments
Volume of distribution (V_d)	Increased	Avoid drugs that may accumulate in third spaces, such as methotrexate.
Half-life ($t_{1/2}$)	Increased or decreased	Measure drug concentrations. Assume extended half-life of some drugs and allow sufficient time after administration of drugs to permit recovery of blood counts prior to delivery.
Concentration $\times$ time (AUC)	Increased or decreased	Be aware that altered AUC's may result in altered efficacy and toxicity of some drugs. Reduced AUC's may account for poor therapeutic responses in some patients. Alternatively, increased AUC's may improve drug efficacy at the risk of increased maternal and fetal toxicity.
Bioavailability (F)	Increased or decreased	Avoid giving orally administered drugs.
Enterohepatic circulation	Increased or decreased	Avoid giving orally administered drugs or those known to undergo extensive enterohepatic circulation.
Protein binding	Increased or decreased	Avoid administration of other agents that are highly protein bound concurrently with antineoplastic agents.
Renal clearance	Increased	For drugs that undergo extensive renal clearance, serum concentrations should be measured if feasible and subsequent doses adjusted if necessary.
Hepatic clearance	Increased or decreased	Measure serum concentrations if feasible and adjust doses if necessary.

TABLE 166–5. COMMON TOXICITIES IN INFANTS EXPOSED *IN UTERO* TO ANTINEOPLASTICS

Toxicities Noted at Birth	Potential Long-term Complications
Bone marrow toxicities	Carcinogenesis
Low birth weight	Mental retardation
Organ toxicities	Mutation
Premature birth	Physical retardation
Spontaneous abortion	Second-generation teratogenesis
Teratogenesis	Sterility

antineoplastic agents may also dictate the amount of fetal toxicity experienced following delivery. The physician should pay close attention to the timing of blood count nadirs for each antineoplastic used and attempt to deliver the infant at a time when both maternal and fetal blood counts have recovered. Delayed nadirs may indicate delayed elimination of drug and the need for more time to recover from chemotherapy before the next dose or a planned cesarean section. Because elimination of drug from the fetus also depends on the maternal system, delivery when blood counts remain low may not only predispose the mother to bleeding problems and infection but may also increase the fetal risk of toxicity from drugs that may not be easily eliminated by the immature infant liver and kidneys.

Fetal exposure to the antineoplastic agent may be the most important factor in determining risk to the fetus. Fetal exposure involves many factors, including physiochemical properties of the antineoplastic agent, dose and schedule of the drug, and pharmacokinetics of the drug in both the maternal and fetal systems. Increased fetal exposure to cytotoxic drugs may be the result of large total doses of drug, prolonged infusions of drug, intraperitoneal administration of antineoplastics, or delayed elimination of drug from the maternal system (such as third spacing with methotrexate). The amniotic fluid may itself act as a third compartment or sink, in which the slow release of drug over time may increase the exposure time of the fetus to drug. This may be particularly true if high-dose methotrexate is administered to the pregnant patient. In this case, methotrexate levels should be carefully monitored and calcium leucovorin rescue considered.

The blood-placental barrier is easily penetrated by most agents, although drug diffusion across the placenta depends on the molecular weight, degree of protein binding, lipophilicity, and degree of drug ionization. Agents that easily penetrate the blood-placental barrier are generally low in molecular weight, have low plasma protein binding, are lipophilic, and remain in the unionized state. Typically, drug is detected in fetal tissues or blood samples following administration to the mother, in the form of parent compound or metabolites. This suggests that many antineoplastics do penetrate the maternal/fetal placental barrier. However, exposure of the fetus to antineoplastics does not necessarily result in teratogenesis or fetal toxicity. For instance, doxorubicin has been detected in a variety of fetal tissues but has not been directly associated with significant teratogenic or toxicologic effects on the fetus, although long-term follow-up is not available in most cases.

The incidence and degree of fetal anomalies produced are also related to the mechanism of action of the individual drug. Drugs that interfere with the biosynthesis of DNA, RNA, and proteins appear to be particularly teratogenic. These include folic acid antagonists (methotrexate, aminopterin), purine antagonists (6-mercaptopurine, 6-thioguanine), and pyrimidine antagonists (5-fluorouracil, FUdR, ftorafur, ara-C, 5-azacitidine, 6-azauridine, hydroxyurea, guanazole). Alkalating agents including nitrogen mustard, busulfan, and cyclophosphamide are also considered highly teratogenic. Agents that have been used with relative safety include the plant alkaloids and antibiotics.

Although the teratogenic effects are perhaps the most obvious concern surrounding the use of antineoplastics during pregnancy, a number of other toxicities may follow *in utero* exposure to these agents. Although some are only mild side effects, others are severe and can result in the death of the infant following delivery (Table 166–7).

EFFECTS OF RADIATION ON THE FETUS

The effects of radiation on the developing fetus are well known. In humans, radiation exposure during pregnancy can result in em-

bryonic death, congenital malformations, or intrauterine growth retardation. Small doses of radiation received from diagnostic procedures (1 to 2 rad) have been associated with an increased risk of childhood malignancies, particularly leukemia. The extent and type of effect on the fetus depend on the dose administered, dose rate, field size, energy of the radiation, and gestational age of the fetus. Irradiation consisting of small doses (< 5 rad or 0.05 Gy) does not appear to be associated with an increased incidence of spontaneous abortions, growth retardation, or congenital malformations. Typically, most diagnostic procedures are in the dose range below 0.01 Gy. Radiation exposure to the fetus following diagnostic procedures to the extremities, shoulders, cervical spine, skull, chest roentgenogram, and pelvis are estimated below 100 mrad. Procedures including cholecystography, intravenous pyelography, upper gastrointestinal series, barium enema, and radiography to the lumbar spine, abdomen, and hips are below 1000 mrad. However, procedures such as lymphangiography and computed tomography to the abdomen are associated with a much higher radiation dose to the fetus (> 0.05 Gy) and should be avoided during pregnancy.

Exposure to Therapeutic Levels of Radiation in Early Pregnancy

Exposure of the fetus to higher doses of radiation, as would be required for many therapeutic protocols, has been associated with severe toxic effects to the fetus. Fifty per cent of infants exposed to doses of 2.5 Gy between the third and tenth week of gestation have been reported to develop mental retardation, microcephaly, cataracts, retinal degeneration, low birth weight, and skeletal and genital abnormalities. The effects of radiation on the fetus are directly related to the gestational age (Table 166–8). The minimal lethal dose of radiation increases with the age of the fetus. On day one after con-

TABLE 166–6. FETAL MALFORMATIONS FOLLOWING USE OF ANTINEOPLASTIC AGENTS DURING THE FIRST TRIMESTER OF PREGNANCY

Drug Used	No. of Patients Exposed to Drug	No. of Fetal Malformations
Alkylating agents		
Busulfan	22	2
Chlorambucil	5	1
Cyclophosphamide	7	3
Mechlorethamine HCl	6	0
Nitrogen mustard	6	0
Thiotepa	0	0
Triethylene melamine	4	0
	50	6 (12%)
Antimetabolites		
Aminopterin	52	10
Azathioprine	35	0
Azoserine	1	0
Cytarabine	1	1
5-Fluorouracil	1	1
6-Mercaptopurine	20	0
Methotrexate	3	3
	113	15 (13%)
Antibiotics		
Daunorubicin	1	0
Doxorubicin	3	0
	4	0 (0%)
Plant alkaloids		
Vinblastine	14	1
	14	1 (7%)
Miscellaneous		
Amsacrine	1	1
Cisplatin	1	0
Colchicine	10	0
Dactinomycin	0	0
Procarbazine	1	1
Urethane	3	1
	16	3 (19%)
Overall incidence	197	25 (13.0%)
Overall incidence in previous reports		(7.5–25%)
Estimated overall incidence of all malformations in normal patients without chemotherapy		3%
Estimated incidence of minor malformations in normal patients without chemotherapy		9%

TABLE 166–7. TOXICITIES OCCURRING IN INFANTS FOLLOWING *IN UTERO* EXPOSURE TO SPECIFIC ANTINEOPLASTIC AGENTS

Toxicity in Infant	Gestational Age at Exposure	Drugs Used
Spontaneous abortion	NS	Busulfan*
Premature	NS	Busulfan, 6-MP*
Anemia, neutropenia	8 wks–delivery	Busulfan
Slowed growth	Conception–delivery	Busulfan
Diarrhea	2nd, 3rd trimester	DN, VCR, PDN, L-ASP, 6-MP, MTX
Severe bone marrow hypoplasia	2nd, 3rd trimester	DN, PDN, VCR, MTX, L-Asp, CY
Severe bone marrow hypoplasia	2nd, 3rd trimester	MTX, VCR, DN, L-ASP, CY, PDN, 6-MP*
Leukopenia	2nd, 3rd trimester	DX, VCR, PDN, L-ASP, CY, 6-MP, MTX
Pancytopenia, septicemia, death	1st–3rd trimester	CY, Ara-C, PDN, 6-MP, VCR, MTX
Chromosomal rings and gaps	2nd, 3rd trimester	CY, Ara-C, DN, VCR, PDN, L-ASP, MTX, 6-MP*
Premature	2nd, 3rd trimester	CY, DX, Bleo, VCR, Dactinomycin
Gastroenteritis, death	2nd, 3rd trimester	Ara-C, VCR, PDN, 6-MP, MTX
Premature, iris adhered to cornea	2nd, 3rd trimester	Ara-C, DN, 6-TG
Perinatal seizures, pneumothorax	2nd, 3rd trimester	Ara-C, DN
Fetal death following chemotherapy	2nd trimester	Ara-C, 6-TG
Respiratory distress	2nd, 3rd trimester	Ara-C, DX, 6-TG, PDN, VCR
Thrombocytopenia	3rd trimester	Ara-C, 6-TG, DN
Polycythemia, hyperbilirubinemia	Conception–delivery	MTX, 6-MP, VCR, PDN, DX, Ara-C
Cushingoid	3rd trimester	MTX, VCR, 6-MP, PDN

NS = Not stated.
* = Radiation also received.
Abbreviations: Ara-C = cytabarine; L-ASP = L-asparaginase; Bleo = bleomycin; CY = cyclophosphamide; DN = daunorubicin, DX = doxorubicin; 6-MP = 6-mercaptopurine; MTX = methotrexate; PDN = prednisone; 6-TG = 6-thioguanine; VCR = vincristine

ception the approximate minimal lethal dose is 0.1 Gy, whereas the minimal lethal dose in a fetus > 12 weeks of age is approximately 1 Gy. In the early blastocyst stage the effects are considered all or none, because any surviving embryo generally does not experience any teratogenic effects. However, during early organogenesis the developing embryo is very sensitive to the lethal, teratogenic, and growth-retarding effects of irradiation. In humans, the period during which the embryo is highly sensitive to multiple system malformations is the ninth to the eleventh weeks of gestation.

During the first trimester no dose of radiation can be considered safe. For patients exposed at any time during pregnancy to doses of < 0.05 Gy, there is little increased risk of abortion, growth retardation, and congenital malformations. However, above this dose the risk substantially increases with exposures of 0.1 to 0.15 Gy. With doses greater than 2.5 Gy given during organogenesis, malformations are noted in the majority of fetuses exposed, and for doses exceeding 3.0 Gy spontaneous abortion usually occurs. In general, it is now thought that following doses of radiation in the range of 0.5 Gy there is a very strong possibility of fetal damage. It has also been recommended that therapeutic abortion be considered in patients receiving radiation doses of greater than 0.1 Gy during the first trimester.

Exposure to Therapeutic Levels of Radiation in the Second and Third Trimesters

During the second and third trimesters of pregnancy, the chance of lethal effects and congenital abnormalities in the fetus from radiation diminishes over time. Although exposure of the fetus to radiation may not result in severe deformities at this time, it can still result in permanent cell depletion in organs or tissues exposed to radiation. Although most fetal organ systems become less susceptible to radiation damage beyond the first trimester, the central nervous, ocular, and hematopoietic systems continue to be vulnerable to the effects of radiation throughout pregnancy. Radiation exposure during weeks 12 to 20 of gestation has been associated with mental retardation, stunted growth, and microcephaly. Exposure to radiation after week 20 of gestation appears to avoid most gross malformations but has resulted in epilation, dermal erythema, and hematologic depression.

Abdominal shielding can be used during pregnancy to limit fetal exposure to radiation. Although abdominal shielding during supradiaphragmatic radiation does significantly reduce fetal exposure, there remains a significant risk of fetal exposure from internal scatter of radiation. Furthermore, because the size of the uterus may significantly differ between pregnant patients, which changes the distance between the fetus and the radiation field, a radiation dose or procedure considered safe for one patient may not be for another.

BREAST-FEEDING

Little is known about the short- and long-term effects of breast-feeding on the infant and/or mother following a diagnosis of neoplastic disease in pregnancy. In the case of breast cancer, breast-feeding would not be recommended if surgery is to take place following delivery because hormonal changes may complicate

TABLE 166–8. SUMMARY OF MALFORMATIONS IN 26 INFANTS EXPOSED TO RADIATION *IN UTERO*

Gestational Age (wks)	Rads Received	No. of Patients	Infant Outcome (Incidence)
2–4	15	1	No abnormalities (1/1)
3–6	16–37	5	Undersized (5/5) microphthalmus (4/5), microcephaly (4/5), mental retardation (4/5), other abnormalities (4/5), retinal degeneration (2/5), cataracts (1/5), acute death (1/5), delayed death (1/5)
5–7	35–39	2	Undersized (2/2), mental retardation (2/2), microphthalmus (2/2), microcephaly (2/2), cataracts (1/2), retinal degeneration (1/2)
6–8	2–44	5	Undersized (5/5), microcephaly (5/5), microphthalmus (4/5), mental retardation (3/5), acute death (2/5), skeletal abnormalities (2/5), other abnormalities (2/5), genital abnormalities (1/5), cataracts (1/5), degeneration of retina (1/5)
8–11	1–29	3	Undersized (3/3), microcephaly (3/3), microphthalmus (3/3), mental retardation (3/3), degeneration of retina (2/5), genital abnormalities (1/5), other abnormalities (1/5)
10–12	19	1	Undersized (1/1), mental retardation (1/1), microcephaly (1/1), delayed death (1/1), other abnormalities (1/1)
10–14	43	1	Undersized (1/1), microcephaly (1/1), mental retardation (1/1)
12–16	28–32	2	Undersized (2/2), microcephaly (2/2), mental retardation (2/2)
16–18	34–41	2	Mild microcephaly (2/2), mental retardation (1/2), mild mental retardation (1/2), undersized (1/2)
16–20	30	1	Mild mental retardation (1/1), mildly undersized (1/1)
19–25	18–40	3	No abnormalities (3/3)

Modified from Dekban AS: Abnormalities in children exposed to x-irradiation during various stages of gestation: Tentative timetable of radiation injury to the human fetus. J Nucl Med 9:471, 1968.

surgery. However, little evidence suggests that breast-feeding should not be permitted in other cases unless the patient has had or requires chemotherapy. In this situation breast-feeding is contraindicated because many drugs are known to penetrate into breast milk, and the effects of low doses of antineoplastics in infants are unknown. At least one incidence of cyclophosphamide-induced neutropenia and thrombocytopenia in a breast-fed infant has been reported. Other agents have also been reported to penetrate breast milk in significant concentration, including doxorubicin, cisplatin, methotrexate, and hydroxyurea.

Allen H, Nisker J (eds.): Cancer in Pregnancy—Therapeutic Guidelines. Mount Kisco, NY, Futura, 1986. *Detailed review of the therapeutic management of cancer during pregnancy.*

Caligiuri MA, Mayer RJ: Pregnancy and leukemia. Semin Oncol 16:388, 1989. *This article, written by two authorities in leukemia, summarizes treatments and outcomes of pregnant patients with leukemia.*

Colbourn DS, Nathanson L, Belilos E: Pregnancy and malignant melanoma. Semin Oncol 16:377, 1989. *An excellent review of melanoma during pregnancy; stresses the natural history of the disease and the effects of pregnancy on melanoma.*

Doll DC, Ringenberg QS, Yarbro JW: Antineoplastic agents and pregnancy. Semin Oncol 16:337, 1989. *Summarizes the literature on the use of chemotherapy during pregnancy, including pharmacology, pharmacokinetics and effects of fetal exposure to antineoplastics.*

Doll DC, Ringenberg QS, Yarbro JW: Management of cancer during pregnancy. Arch Intern Med 148:2058, 1988. *Reviews the pharmacology of antineoplastics in pregnancy, adverse effects on the fetus, and management recommendations.*

Galenberg MM, Loprinzi CI: Breast cancer and pregnancy. Semin Oncol 16:369, 1989. *Excellent summary of the incidence, diagnosis, prognosis, and treatment of breast cancer during pregnancy.*

Jacob JH, Stringer CA: Diagnosis and management of cancer during pregnancy. Semin Perinatol 14:79, 1990. *Reviews the therapeutic management of a variety of cancers developing during pregnancy.*

Jolles CJ: Gynecologic cancer associated with pregnancy. Semin Oncol 16:417, 1989. *Details the management of gynecologic cancers during pregnancy.*

Ringenberg S, Doll DC: Endocrine tumors and miscellaneous cancers in pregnancy. Semin Oncol 16:445, 1989. *Discusses diagnosis and management of the more rare types of cancers occurring during pregnancy.*

Ward FT, Weiss RB: Lymphoma and pregnancy. Semin Oncol 16:397, 1989. *Therapeutic guidelines for treatment of lymphoma during pregnancy.*

167   THE FUTURE OF ONCOLOGY
Donald M. Miller

The past 20 years has been one of the most exciting periods in the history of biology and medicine, particularly for the field of oncology. A steady stream of important discoveries during this period has produced a dramatic improvement in our understanding of malignant transformation and tumor progression. Indeed, much of our current knowledge about the physiologic regulation of cell growth has come from observations made in malignant cells. Identification of the genes responsible for the abnormal growth regulation of tumor cells has elucidated many of the normal growth control pathways.

Until recently, little of this new information has been translated into treatments for patients with cancer. However, during the past 5 years, the concept of "translational research" has been developed to describe research that uses basic molecular insights to find new treatments for clinical problems. Clinical trials are more commonly incorporating molecular markers and intermediate endpoints based on the molecular biology of malignancy. Clinically, many exciting advances during the past decade have been in the field of immunotherapy. The development of effective cancer vaccines and the use of recombinant cytokines and growth factors have assumed important roles in the practice of oncology.

It is likely that the immediate future of oncology will include the successful application of modern molecular biology to the development of novel antiproliferative therapies for cancer. Just as the cancer cell has provided a window through which to view the normal growth regulatory processes, cancer patients are likely to provide a window through which we will begin to modulate gene expression in a therapeutically useful manner.

The major discoveries of the past two decades in the field of cancer biology have centered on characterization of the molecular processes of malignant transformation (see Ch. 156). Major advances have surrounded discovery of oncogenes and tumor suppres-

sor genes, elucidation of signal transduction pathways, development of molecular epidemiology, and understanding of metastasis at the molecular level. Over 100 genes have been classified as oncogenes based on their participation in the abnormal growth characteristics of tumor cells. It has become clear that each of these genes also participates in signal transduction "cascades" that control growth and differentiation of normal cells. The characterization of the mechanisms by which oncogenes induce malignant transformation has provided ideal targets for novel antiproliferative therapies. In addition, this new information has allowed us to understand carcinogenesis on the molecular level. This has led to new and more accurate measures of carcinogenesis.

The discovery of *tumor suppressor genes*—genes that are frequently deleted or inactivated in malignant cells—has stimulated attempts to use their antiproliferative functions therapeutically (see Ch. 156). An improved understanding of signal transduction pathways has allowed the initial characterization of inhibitors of enzymes involved in these pathways. It has become clear that a relatively large number of signaling pathways exist, each with multiple members. In addition, there is now substantial evidence of "crosstalk" (cross-signaling) between different pathways. Likewise, the improved understanding of the molecular basis of metastasis has allowed the initial development of agents that inhibit this process. Although considerable effort has been expended to understand the metastatic process at the molecular level, many questions remain. Clinical trials of metastasis inhibitors are currently under way. Each discovery in these areas has provided new targets for the development of novel effective therapies. Improved understanding of the interplay between the external environment and individual genetic makeup in the development of cancer has stimulated the search for agents with the potential to prevent malignant transformation, leading to successful clinical trials of chemoprevention.

Each new insight into the pathophysiology of malignant transformation has provided new targets for therapy. The opportunity to develop new agents with rational targets has produced collaborations between academic scientists and the pharmaceutical and biotechnology industry with the goal of developing better treatments based on the molecular biology of cancer. Many of the new approaches have come from serendipitous observations, such as the development of retinoids as chemopreventive agents based on their ability to differentiate leukemic cells. In other instances, such as the successful use of antibodies targeted to Her2/*neu* in breast cancer, development of these therapies has been more traditional.

IMPROVED UNDERSTANDING OF CANCER BIOLOGY

Many of the discoveries of cancer biology that have occurred during the past 20 years have been unexpected. Although the genetic basis of cancer has been accepted for the past 50 years, the concepts of human oncogenes and tumor suppressor genes are relatively recent. While it is clear that at least two genetic events are required to induce malignant transformation, we know very little about the specific requirements for sequential molecular events in the induction of many malignancies. Additionally, we know very little about how the environment and genetic influences interact to modulate the risk of malignant transformation during the early events in malignant transformation.

The identification of tumor suppressor genes and the development of positional cloning have allowed the discovery and characterization of a series of tumor-specific genes. Family studies have been crucial in this work. The retinoblastoma gene was the first tumor suppressor gene to be identified, although its presence was predicted by genetic studies that predated its cloning by almost 30 years. The detailed characterization of families with inherited retinoblastoma and a comparison with sporadic patients made it clear that both inherited and sporadic retinoblastomas are caused by the same genes. This observation, subsequently confirmed when the gene was cloned and sequenced, has established an important principle.

These studies have shown that the study of high-risk populations can provide important clues about the genes involved in the much more common sporadic tumors. This is demonstrated by the fact that the penetration of tumors such as hereditary retinoblastoma and polyposis coli is 90%, while the incidence of cancer in individuals with carcinogen exposure such as diethylstilbestrol (DES) exposure is only 0.1% per year. This means that if there are very small increments in risk for specific populations, they will be very hard to detect. On the other hand, the identification of inherited genes that may participate in malignant transformation with a much higher penetrance may allow the identification of individuals at high risk.

The discovery and characterization the genes responsible for cell cycle control has increased our understanding of the complexity of growth regulation. It is clear that the cyclins and the cyclin-dependent kinase (CDK) enzymes interact with transcriptional regulatory proteins in a number of ways. In addition, the recent discovery of CDK inhibitors suggests that both positive and negative regulatory mechanisms exist which control the effect of these proteins. The loss of the tight regulation of cell cycle control by malignant cells allows them to avoid the requirement for growth factors in order to divide. Obviously, the loss of the genes encoding the inhibitory proteins can result in increased cell cycling, producing an abnormal growth pattern and malignant transformation. On the other hand, abnormal expression of these genes may be one mechanism by which to induce apoptosis, or programmed cell death (see later discussion).

It has become clear that mammalian cells have a complicated system of checks and balances to guard against uncontrolled cell growth. One mechanism is the progressive shortening of the ends of chromosomes, or telomeres, that accompanies normal cell division and may contribute to cellular aging. Recent reports have appeared of a dramatic correlation between malignant transformation and the expression of telomerase, an enzyme that prevents the shortening of telomeres. As shown in Figure 167–1, telomerase may represent one of the factors that select between aging and malignancy. The number of cell divisions correlates well with the initial length of the telomeres, and progressive loss of telomeres is observed in culture. Thus 50 to 200 nucleotides are lost with each cell division and some 4000 nucleotides are lost by the time of senescence. This provides a partial explanation for the mechanism by which, in many

malignant cells, the aging process has been arrested. This has been shown to relate to the decreased intracellular activity of telomerase. This enzyme, which normally "shortens" the telomere, appears to play a role in the limited number of cell cycles that can occur. The characterization of this enzyme's role as a factor in the continued cellular division of malignant cells suggests that it will provide an important target for new chemotherapy agents.

The increased understanding of how cells die could play an important role in the development of new anticancer therapy. It has become clear that the regulation of cell death is just as complex as the regulation of cell growth. Most, if not all, animal cells self-destruct by activation of an intrinsic cell suicide program accompanied by a set of characteristic morphologic and biochemical changes known as *apoptosis,* or programmed cell death. During apoptosis, the nucleus and the cytoplasm condense and the dying cell fragments into apoptotic bodies, which are ingested and absorbed by macrophages or normal neighboring cells. The initiation of apoptosis is tightly regulated by numerous intracellular and extracellular signals capable of inducing cell death.

Recent evidence suggests that cells from a variety of human malignancies have a decreased ability to undergo apoptosis in response to at least some physiologic stimuli. In tumor cell lines, overexpression of the Bcl-2 gene specifically prevents cells from undergoing apoptosis in response to a number of signals. On the other hand, mere overexpression of Bcl-2 is not enough to prevent apoptosis. Bax is a protein that binds to Bcl-2 and inactivates its life-giving functions. Korsmeyer and coworkers have suggested that the Bcl-2/Bax protein pair constitute a "rheostat of cell death," with the ratio of Bcl-2 to Bax determining whether a cell that receives a death signal will accept or ignore it (Fig. 167–2).

It is now clear that Bcl-2 is only one of a family of genes that can control the apoptotic threshold. The discovery of Bcl-x, a Bcl-2-like protein, suggests that other proteins may exist which control the ability of cancer cells to undergo cell death. This possibility has been substantiated by studies with *C. elegans,* which contains at least 14 genes that participate in the apoptosis pathway. An in-

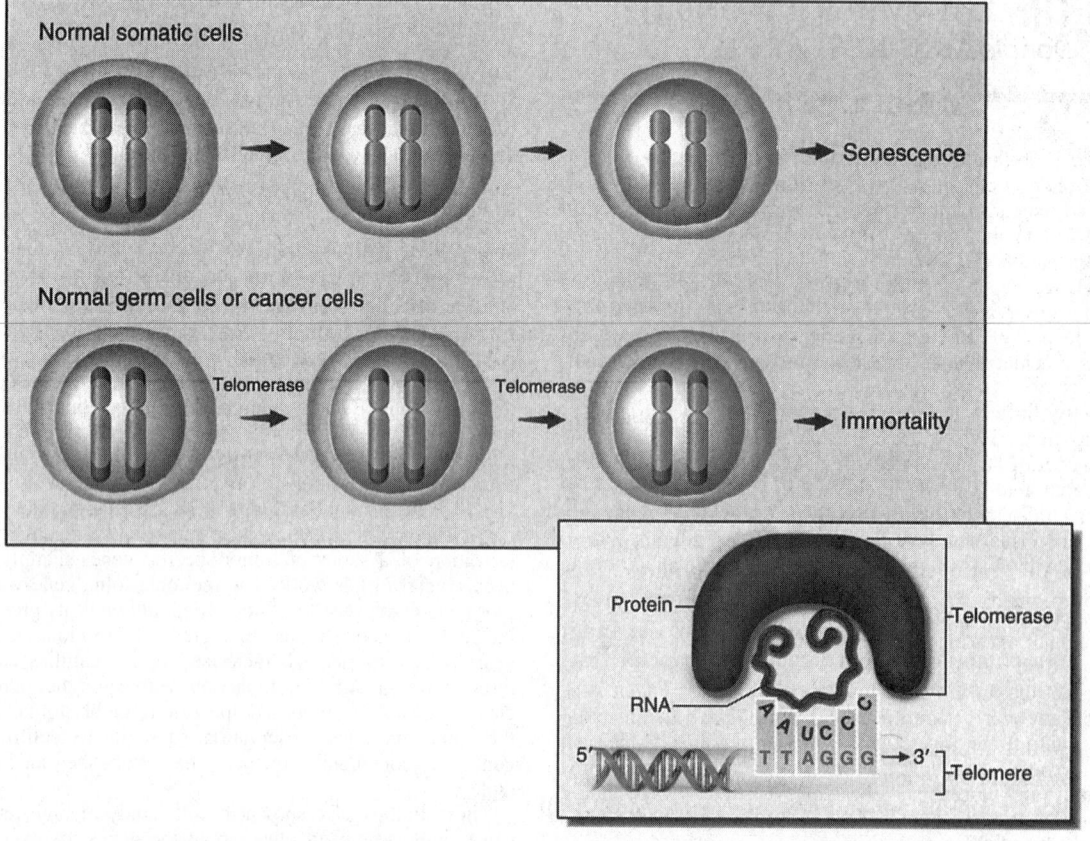

FIGURE 167–1. Role of telomeres in aging and cancer. In this model, the progressive loss of telomeres (red tips of chromosomes) is associated with the senescence of normal somatic cells. The maintenance of normal telomere length is associated with the immortality of normal germ cells and cancer cells. (From Haber DA: Clinical implications of basic research: Telomeres, cancer and immortality. N Engl J Med 332:955, 1995. Copyright by the Massachusetts Medical Society.)

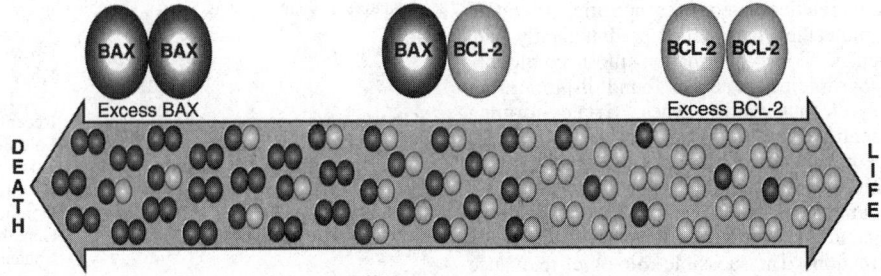

FIGURE 167–2. Interaction of Bcl-2/Bax controls cell death. The ratio of the two proteins called Bcl-2 and Bax, which bind to themselves or each other, determines whether cultured lymphocytes live or die. (From Barinaga M: Cell Suicide: By ICE, not fire. Science 263:754, 1994. Copyright 1994 by the American Association for the Advancement of Science.)

creased understanding of the signaling mechanisms of apoptosis will also improve our potential abilities to modify the process. The Fas ligand (FasL) is a cell surface molecule that binds to its receptor, Fas, and induces apoptosis of Fas-bearing cells. This mechanism appears to play an important role in death of T cells. Other genes such as the ICE gene (interferon-1B–converting enzyme) may modify apoptosis-inducing signals.

Improved understanding of cell death may have immediate implications for cancer treatment. Although it has been generally accepted that chemotherapy drugs are effective because they are selectively toxic to malignant cells, evidence accumulates that these agents, in many instances, induce apoptosis. This implies that factors that increase the tendency to apoptosis may dramatically improve the efficacy of specific chemotherapeutic agents. Likewise, because apoptosis requires a genetic program, mutations of the genes involved in this pathway could cause drug-resistant tumors. For example, cells that are "p53 deficient" are much less sensitive to treatment with γ irradiation or Adriamycin than are identical cells containing normal p53.

The identification by a number of investigative groups of a series of DNA mismatch repair enzymes inactivated in cancer cells has provided an important opportunity to improve our understanding of the genetic instability of malignant cells. In fact, mismatch repair deficiency appears to be important in a number of inherited human tumors. In Lynch's syndrome, for example, 90% of the tumors appear to have a defect in one of several mismatch repair enzymes, while in sporadic colon tumors, 12 to 15% have a mismatch repair defect. Sporadic breast, lung, and prostate tumors have an incidence that is commonly 5 to 10% but in some cases may be up to 50%.

Most cancer patients die of metastatic disease rather than of their primary tumor. It is quite likely that during the next 10 years the molecular mechanism of metastasis will be much more clearly understood. Metastasis is a multistep process involving the expression of many cellular genes. The selection process that determines which cells will successfully traverse the circulatory impediments and establish viable metastases is not clear. Interruption of specific steps of this process has been successful in animal models, but no viable clinical interventions to prevent metastasis exist at this time. A more complete understanding of the molecular basis of this process will allow development of novel approaches to prevent the metastasis of common tumors in a clinical setting. The ability to inhibit expression of specific genes and the development of receptor ligands that prevent the adherence of tumor cells to basement membrane are possible directions for development of antimetastatic drugs.

Despite the burgeoning amount of information about the genetic basis of cancer, little is known about the *epigenetic* aspects of malignant transformation. Why, for instance, do cells containing an activating mutation of a specific oncogene become malignant in some tissues but not others? Why are some tumors chemosensitive and others, such as colon carcinoma and renal cell carcinoma, not? Why can we cure testicular cancer but not prostatic? Why do individuals who have inherited an abnormality of a specific tumor suppressor gene have a marked increase in their risk of certain tumors but not others? As an example, individuals who have inherited an abnormal BRCA1 gene may have an 85% risk of developing breast or ovarian carcinoma but a normal risk of other tumor types. The answers to these questions will probably affect development of new therapies over the next decade or so.

A number of techniques have allowed the rapid characterization of tumor-related genes and their mechanisms of action. The devel-

opment of polymerase chain reaction (PCR), which has revolutionized molecular biology, is rapidly being applied in clinical settings. This technique allows the detection of very rare cells containing a specific translocation (such as residual leukemic cells following bone marrow transplantation). In addition, this technique is now being used to detect small numbers of circulating cells in patients with solid tumors. The development of transgenic mice has allowed the study of the effects of overexpression or mutation of specific genes. More importantly, the development of animals containing activated human oncogenes will allow the characterization of complementary genes that interact in the production of human tumors. A logical extension of transgenic technology has been the development of animals in which both copies of a single gene are inactivated. These "knockout" mice provide important information about the normal functions of genes that have been inactivated. In addition, the development of immunodeficient murine model systems, such as nude mice and severe combined immunodeficiency (SCID) mice, has allowed the growth of human tumors in animals. These model systems will become crucial with the development of "gene-specific" therapies that will require "human" target DNA sequences.

DEVELOPMENT OF NEW TREATMENTS BASED ON CANCER MOLECULAR BIOLOGY

ANTIGENE THERAPY. The identification of oncogenes and the improved understanding of normal growth regulation have provided excellent targets for the design of novel antiproliferative therapeutic approaches. Gene expression inhibition represents an attractive approach to rational design of chemotherapeutic agents. Early attempts to inhibit expression of oncogenes have centered on the use of antisense oligonucleotides. Similar approaches for using triplex-forming oligonucleotides and ribozymes are being developed. Whereas each of these modalities has unique advantages and disadvantages, their promise may lie in an ability to inhibit expression of single genes.

Antisense inhibition of gene expression uses a complementary oligonucleotide to bind to the mRNA of a specific target gene and to inhibit its expression. This may occur either by inhibition of transcriptional activity or by stimulation of RNAse H activity resulting in selective digestion of the mRNA. There has been considerable *in vitro* documentation of the inhibitory activity of either antisense oligonucleotides or vectors expressing antisense transcripts. Clinical trials of antisense oligonucleotides have demonstrated that these molecules are relatively nontoxic. Although oligonucleotides have a limited oral bioavailability, they are well absorbed from all sites and have a relatively long half-life (48 hours). They are primarily excreted via urine with no known end-organ toxicity. Modified oligonucleotide backbones are resistant to circulating endonucleases and may be crucial to the clinical use of these molecules. The biotechnology industry has successfully synthesized new classes of oligonucleotides are currently being tested in humans within the next year. Animal studies have demonstrated very good antitumor effects in selected model systems and clinical trials are under way. Early evidence suggests that the simultaneous inhibition of two or more genes involved in the abnormal growth patterns of leukemic or tumor cells may have markedly synergistic growth inhibitory effects.

Another approach that attempts to inhibit expression of specific genes involved in the malignant process is the use of *triplex-forming oligonucleotides*. Triple-stranded DNA is formed by the binding of a third strand in an antiparallel manner in the major groove (Fig.

167–3). This interaction is relatively sequence specific, providing the opportunity to create molecules that interact predominantly with a single genomic sequence. Triplex formation most commonly occurs in polypurine/polypyrimidine sequences found disproportionately in the promoters of eukaryotic genes. Triplex-forming sequences have been identified in the promoters of the c-*myc*, Ha-*ras*, Ki-*ras*, EGF receptor, *neu*, and interleukin-2 (IL-2) receptor genes. Triplex-forming oligonucleotides have been shown to inhibit expression of a number of human genes. These sequences may have important regulatory functions, expressed through intramolecular triplex formation. The possible biologic relevance of these sequences is further suggested by the presence of physiologic triplex-binding proteins and the binding of antitriplex antibodies to intact cellular chromatin. Triplex-forming oligonucleotides may provide a sequence-specific means of inhibiting expression of single genes, although this approach is further from actual clinical application.

A third approach to "antigene therapy" is the use of *ribozymes*. Ribozymes are catalytic RNA molecules that can be targeted to specific mRNA sequences. Anti-HIV (human immunodeficiency virus) ribozymes have been shown to have antiviral effects in infected tissue culture cells and are currently being tested in patients with acquired immunodeficiency syndrome (AIDS). Likewise, ribozymes targeted to the translocated BCR/Abl transcript of Philadelphia chromosome–positive (Ph+) CML cells have been shown to have dramatic antiproliferative effects. The use of these catalytic RNA molecules has considerable promise as a gene therapy modality. However, it is likely that several means to inhibition of a single gene or multiple genes will be necessary for the successful application of the antigene approach.

Several major problems exist with the current applications of oligonucleotide therapy, including the lack of means of successful delivery of adequate oligonucleotide concentrations to the target cell nucleus, the need to identify possible toxic effects, the need to synthesize stable oliognucleotides modified to allow cost-effective administration of therapeutic doses to patients, and the possible development of resistance to these agents. However, the ability to inhibit expression of single genes remains an attractive approach to cancer therapy.

THERAPY TARGETED TO GENE PRODUCTS. The development of new agents targeted to the products of genes that participate in malignant transformation has several advantages: (1) These compounds may be small molecules that act as enzyme inhibitors. (2) Improved recombinant DNA technology may allow development of genetically engineered inhibitors, such as dominant negative mutants of signal transduction enzymes (mutants that are inactive but

that compete for substrates). (3) Traditional approaches to new drugs have concentrated on enzyme inhibitors and/or growth factors. This means that the infrastructure for the development of this type of agent is in place and will allow more rapid synthesizing of these drugs.

As shown in Table 167–1, there are many potential targets for this type of therapy. Growth factor inhibitors provide an excellent target for therapy because they are localized to the membrane of malignant cells. In clinical trial the use of antibodies to the Her2/*neu* receptor on breast cancer cells has demonstrated inhibition of growth of tumors overexpressing this gene. Other approaches include the development of mutant growth factors that bind to target growth factor receptors as inactive ligands. The development of soluble forms of growth factor receptors and dominant negative growth factor receptors has shown promise *in vitro*. Suramin is a new agent being tested in prostate cancer that appears to exert its antiproliferative effect in part through specific binding to growth factor receptors.

There are a number of approaches to the inhibition of signal transduction mutants. Because these gene products generally are en-

TABLE 167–1. NEW TARGETS FOR CANCER THERAPY

Inhibitors of Gene Products

Growth factors	Growth factor–specific antibodies
	Dominant negative analogues
	Small molecule ligands
Growth factor receptors	Receptor specific antibodies
	Soluble receptors
Signal transduction proteins	Farsenylation inhibitors
	Substrate analogues
	Dominant negative proteins
Tumor suppressor genes	Gene replacement
	Enhanced expression
Nuclear oncogenes	Double-stranded decoy sequences

Inhibitors of Gene Expression

mRNA	Antisense oligonucleotides
	Ribozymes
Transcription machinery	Triplex-forming oligonucleotides
	Transcription factor decoys
	DNA-binding drugs

Treatments That Use Genetic Programs

Apoptosis pathway	Induction of apoptosis
Differentiation pathway	Differentiating agents
Immune response	Cancer vaccines

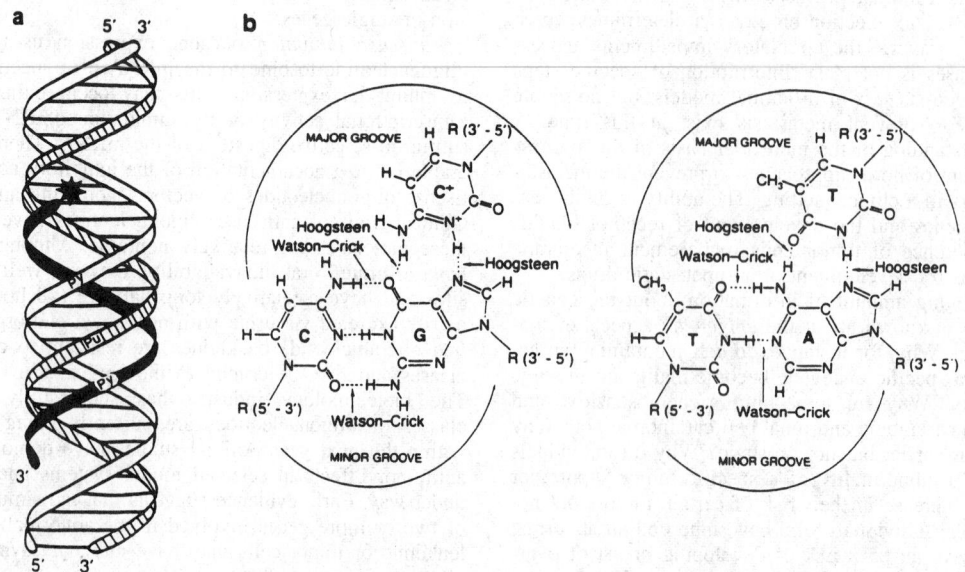

FIGURE 167–3. Structure of triplex DNA. *A,* Ribbon model of intermolecular triplex DNA. *B,* Watson-Crick and Hoogsteen hydrogen bonding of triplex bases. (From Helene C, Toulme J-J: Specific regulation of gene expression by antisense, sense, and antigene nucleic acids. Biochem Biophys Acta 1049:99, 1990.)

zymes, it is possible to develop competitive inhibitors. This has been done for the *ras* proteins with agents that are currently in clinical trials. Likewise, the inhibition of necessary modifications of these proteins may be an effective means to interfere with growth. Farsenylation inhibitors prevent farsenylation of the *ras* proteins, a necessary step in their activation. Agents that downregulate specific signal transduction pathways will probably be effective antiproliferative agents in cells using these pathways to stimulate growth in an abnormal manner.

One major difficulty with the development of therapeutic modalities based on our understanding of the molecular biology of cancer has been the identification of molecules that specifically interact with proteins or polynucleotides. The development and use of "combinatorial libraries" promise to allow empirical identification of peptides or oligonucleotides that interact specifically with target sequences. Effective combinatorial libraries could revolutionize the drug discovery process. In this approach, multiple randomly generated peptides or oligonucleotides are bound to the target protein or DNA sequence of choice. The molecules that bind, even at relatively low affinity, are purified, and the binding cycle is repeated several times, each time resulting in the further enrichment of the binding species. This allows the purification of binding agents that might not be predicted otherwise.

CANCER GENE THERAPY (see Ch. 25)

The rapid evolution of gene therapy as a viable alternative for cancer therapy has resulted in a number of approaches currently being tested in clinical trials. Indeed, cancer is an ideal disease in which to test this type of therapy. Cancer patients often have limited life expectancy, in many cases there are no effective treatments available, and in general the genetic defect of malignant cells can be defined. For these reasons, cancer gene therapy trials have made up the majority of gene therapy trials approved by the National Institutes of Health (NIH) Recombinant Advisory Committee (RAC).

IMMUNOPOTENTIATION. Because current delivery systems do not allow the reliable transfection of every cell in a human tumor, most of the current clinical trials have chosen approaches relying on immunologic therapies. Initial studies at the National Cancer Institute used tumor-invasive lymphocytes (TIL) as delivery cells for the tumor necrosis factor (TNF) gene; results have shown that this approach causes the delivery and expression of this gene in human tumors. As is often the case, the choice of approach has often been dictated by the problems associated with delivery systems. The vectors currently in use include retroviruses, adenovirus vectors, and adeno-associated viral vectors. In addition, a number of groups have begun testing the use of liposomes and viral/DNA/polylysine complexes as delivery vehicles.

The most popular and widely investigated modality of cancer gene therapy has been immunopotentiation. This reflects the fact that, for immunopotentiation, delivery of genetic material to every cell is not required. Several laboratories have shown that tumor cells transfected with cytokine genes, including IL-2, GM-CSF, and interferon, stimulate an immune response when they are reinjected into the parent tumor. The mechanism of this stimulation is most likely related to the continued secretion of recombinant cytokine by these cells. Another area of immunopotentiation is the development of recombinant vaccines. Tumor-associated antigens have been characterized for a number of tumors, including breast cancer, colon cancer, and melanoma. In the case of melanoma, for example, five distinct tumor antigens have been identified and their interactions with immune T cells characterized. The sequencing of these genes has allowed development of expression vectors that can be effectively utilized as vaccines against their parent tumors. Although it is too early to determine the efficacy of these immunopotentiation methods, they are likely to be more effective in adjuvant settings.

GENE REPLACEMENT. Perhaps the most logical approach to cancer gene therapy is the replacement of tumor suppressor genes that have been lost or those inactivated by mutation. Because it is possible in many cases to identify the genes involved in malignant transformation, it seems relatively straightforward to replace defective tumor suppressor genes. However, the major drawback of this approach is that it is theoretically necessary to replace the defective gene in every cell in order to eradicate the tumor. On the other hand, as more effective vectors and delivery systems are developed, it may soon be possible to use tumor suppressor gene products as

gene therapy reagents. In fact, it may be possible to suppress cell growth by overexpression of tumor suppressor genes that are not actually involved in the pathophysiologic mutation of a given tumor.

GENETIC CHEMOTHERAPY. Another attractive approach to cancer gene therapy is "genetic chemotherapy." This has been widely used to sensitize malignant cells to inactive prodrugs. For example, the transfection of tumor cells with the herpes simplex thymidine kinase (HStk) gene makes them markedly sensitive to ganciclovir, which is activated by the HSV thymidine kinase to its toxic product but not altered by the mammalian enzymes. Animal studies have shown that expression of HStk in a minority of cells is adequate to eradicate a much larger proportion of malignant cells. This potentiation of effect, known as the "bystander effect," is poorly understood but promises to play an important role in future gene therapy trials. Likewise the characterization of tissue-specific promoters has allowed the development of gene therapy vectors that express toxin genes selectively in tumor cells. For example, the tyrosinase promoter that is functional only in melanoma cells can be used to drive the tissue-specific expression of genes that would be quite cytotoxic if expressed in normal tissue.

There are many problems with cancer gene therapy in its current state which will continue to delay the development of curative therapies. The primary problem at this time is how to deliver genetic material to target cells. However, other issues, including the cost of this type of treatment, issues of patient safety, and regulatory difficulties, are also daunting problems. It appears likely that continued advancement of vector technology and close collaboration among molecular biologists, virologists, and clinical investigators will stimulate the rapid development of new approaches.

CANCER PREVENTION (see Ch. 155)

Prevention of cancer in the aging United States population is an extremely important area. Effective education is a critical element of cancer prevention. It appears that information about high-risk behaviors should be targeted to children and adolescents. This education has been quite effective in alerting the public about the dangers of smoking, smokeless tobacco, sun exposure, and imprudent diet (see Ch. 9). Important aspects of effective cancer prevention include avoiding carcinogen exposure, maintaining a healthy lifestyle, and being aware of the means of early cancer detection. The development of effective chemoprevention agents is also crucial. Identifying high-risk populations such as individuals who have smoked heavily for many years and are at increased risk of lung cancer or individuals at high risk for head and neck cancer has allowed the testing of specific chemopreventive drugs. The initial trials of these agents have provided convincing evidence that, at least in the case of head and neck cancer, intensive chemoprevention measures can be quite effective.

An important aspect of cancer prevention is nutritional modification. There is considerable public interest about the potential role of diet in cancer causation. It has been reasonably estimated that as many as 30% of tumors in the United States are related to dietary habits. Population studies have shown that ethnic groups consuming diets high in fat or low in fiber have an increased cancer risk. However, direct links in individual patients have been difficult to prove, because the relative risk may be only slightly increased and the dietary habits of local populations as well as family units vary greatly. An example of a significant decrease in the incidence of a specific tumor presumed to be caused by dietary changes has been the dramatic decrease in gastric carcinoma in this country during the past 50 years (from an incidence of 38 in 100,000 to 5 in 100,000 in U.S. men). This decrease is apparently related to improved food preservation and decreased usage of nitrates in food processing. Epidemiologic research into the role of specific nutritional elements is a high priority at present. It is likely that our understanding of the role of nutrition in cancer causation will improve considerably over the next several decades.

The identification of cancer susceptibility genes has allowed recognition of certain individuals with high risk of cancer. These individuals should be followed closely to detect and treat tumors at an early stage. However, the characterization of specific inherited mutations will predict only a very small proportion of individuals who will actually develop malignancy. The vast majority of human tumors are sporadic, with mutations that may be similar to or different from those causing the inherited tumors.

TUMOR MARKERS AND SUSCEPTIBILITY GENES (see also Ch. 158.2)

The study of families with an increased risk of cancer has led to the discovery of a series of "tumor susceptibility" genes. These genes represent several classes of genes including tumor suppressor genes, mismatch repair genes, transcription factor genes, and several genes that have been incompletely characterized. In many ways, colon cancer has provided a paradigm for the understanding of sequential molecular changes that participate in malignant transformation *in vivo*. Through the use of tumor families and positional cloning, researchers have extensively characterized a set of genetic events eventually leading to the development of colon cancer. The genetic changes accompanying the progression from normal colonic mucosa to frank carcinoma are shown in Figure 167-4. Sequential changes in the structure or level of expression of these genes appear to accumulate over time. It is likely that at least three genetic abnormalities are required for the evolution of frank malignancy.

It is interesting to consider the advantages inherent in the study of malignant disease of the colon. First, there are a number of familial syndromes in which the risk of eventual malignancy is quite high. Second, the colonic mucosae can be observed directly via the colonoscope, so that malignancy can be detected quite early. Finally and most importantly, the multistage development of colonic tumors from small adenomas to larger adenomas and then to frank tumors provides a series of steps that can be analyzed sequentially. These characteristics have been partly responsible for the development of a stepwise model for colon cancer. It is likely that this type of tumor evolution will be observed in other tumors as well.

Breast cancer (see Ch. 208.5) has also been, because of its frequency in U.S. women, an area of intense research. The announcement in late 1994 of the cloning of BRCA1—the gene responsible for inherited predisposition to breast and ovarian cancer—was the exciting climax to a race that started 4 years earlier. Inherited breast cancer represents approximately 10% of all breast cancer in the U.S.; BRCA1 is involved in half of these cases. The decreased expression of BRCA1 in invasive breast cancers and the loss of normal alleles of BRCA1 in breast and ovarian cancer suggest that BRCA1 is a tumor suppressor gene. The detailed characterization of mutations in families with inherited breast cancer has been somewhat disappointing for those investigators who had hoped to develop a straightforward test for mutation. Of the first 38 mutations characterized, 27 were seen once, 8 were seen twice, and 3 were seen more often. Most of the mutations are frameshift or nonsense mutations leading to premature termination of the protein and conferring high risk. Interestingly, clinical factors such as age at cancer onset or development of ovarian cancer as well as breast cancer do not appear to be related to the specific mutation inherited by individual patients. This suggests that genotype/phenotype interactions may be much more important than previously recognized. It is clear that, to the individual with two family members with ovarian cancer, total risk of malignancy is 20 to 30%.

Other genes also play a role in inherited breast cancer. BRCA2, a gene located on chromosome 13q12, appears to be a less common culprit in inherited breast cancer; there is apparently at least one additional BRCA gene. The role of the BRCA genes in sporadic breast cancer is unclear; however, it is likely that these genes participate in the development of certain sporadic tumors. The interaction between these genes and the risk factors for breast cancer remains unclear. It is likely that other oncogenes—in particular the *ras* oncogene family—may interact with these genes to cause inherited cancer.

The identification of BRCA1 has crystallized many of the controversies surrounding the possible utility of cancer genes as markers of risk of malignancy. The identification of multiple mutations has

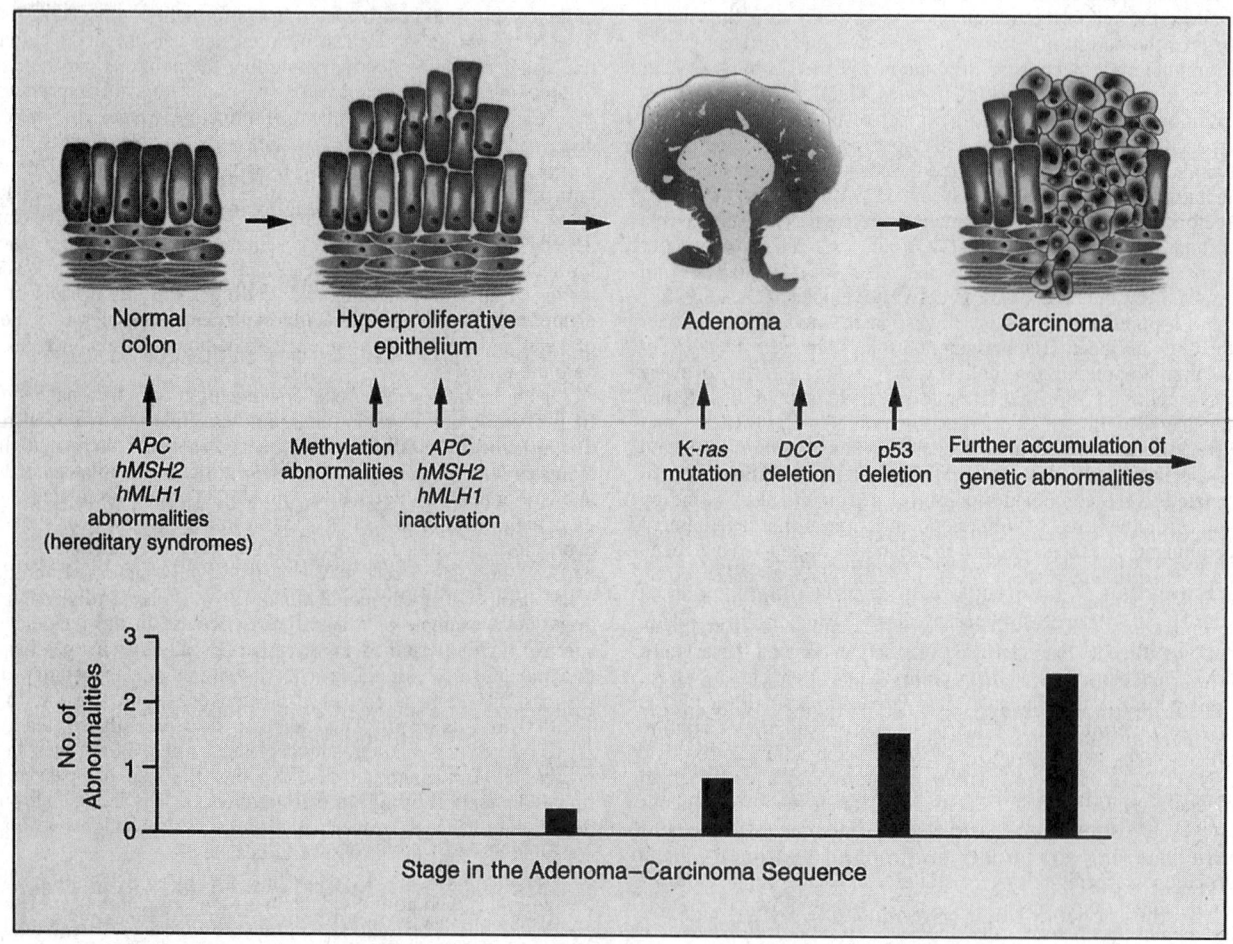

FIGURE 167–4. Sequential genetic events responsible for colon cancer. The molecular changes may vary in their order of occurrence; the most common sequence is shown. (From Toribara NW, Sleisenger MH: Current concepts: screening for colorectal carcinoma. N Engl J Med 332:861, 1995. Copyright by the Massachusetts Medical Society.)

raised the question of why all women with BRCA1 do not get breast cancer. The answers to this question may include such variables as chance, different mutations, preventive surgery, environmental differences, or other genes. Parity seems to decrease the risk; each birth decreases risk by 15%. In addition, other genes such as H-*ras* may play a role in modulating risk of cancer. However, the characterization of BRCA1 has also raised a number of additional questions. For example: What will we advise women with BRCA1 mutations? Should testing be freely available?

Genetic counseling is a crucial aspect of genetic testing for cancer. Indeed, the personnel requirements for a complete testing facility include clinical geneticists, genetic counselors, psychologists, oncologists, persons to perform screening, and surgeons. There is considerable potential for harm with genetic testing whether the result is negative or positive. If the test is negative, the possible detrimental effects include survivor guilt, family discord, and concern about testing error. Likewise, if the test is positive, there may be resultant confusion, loss of job and insurance, social stigma, anxiety, depression, and considerable additional cost of medical surveillance and care. However, there are also many positive effects of genetic testing. If the test is negative, the benefits include the fact that the cancer risk is lowered, allowing effective career and family planning. If the test is positive, the advantages include increased medical survival with early detection and treatment, the opportunity to avoid carcinogens and to pursue prenatal testing for potentially affected pregnancies, empowerment to make informed medical decisions, and the opportunity to participate in chemoprevention clinical trials. A number of genes are related with a strong predisposition for malignancy. This list, which currently includes between 10 and 15 genes, is likely to grow rapidly. These genes have been characterized by family studies and positional cloning and are also involved with sporadic tumors of the same types. Although the identification of genes that confer an extremely high risk of cancer provides important clues to human tumors, only the minority of human tumors are caused by single genes; the vast majority are polygenic.

One of the most important developments in understanding the genetics of cancer has been the ability to characterize small sequence differences directly in DNA. In the context of a group of individuals, these differences are known as *polymorphisms*. They may occur either in coding or noncoding regions of the genome. The ability to characterize thousands of these polymorphisms has made it possible to perform family studies to track genes involved in familial tumors. These polymorphisms provide markers for the loss of specific chromosomal segments during the evolution of a tumor. They have been crucial in the identification of genes important in the development of common tumors, such as colon cancer, as well as less common tumors, such as Wilms' tumor.

The issue of genetic testing is emphasized by the frequency of commonly inherited cancer risk genes. It is estimated, for example, that the incidence of BRCA1 mutations in the United States is 1 million. Individuals with the mutation have an 80% risk of developing breast or ovarian cancer during their lifetime. Likewise the incidence of familial colon cancer (FCC) predisposition is estimated to be 1 million. These individuals also have an 80% risk.

Another development that promises to make the identification of cancer causing genes more straightforward is the ability to more easily characterize loss of heterozygosity. It is now possible using PCR techniques to determine which sequences within a specific tumor have lost heterozygosity and are therefore candidate tumor suppressor genes. This may allow for detection of novel genes without the need for detailed family studies or positional cloning. Several other techniques, including fluorescent *in situ* hybridization (FISH), chromosomal painting, and PCR analysis of gene rearrangement have greatly enhanced characterization of the genetic abnormalities of specific tumors.

An important aspect of the earlier diagnosis of malignancy is the discovery of improved cancer markers. For example, the use of the prostatic specific antigen (PSA) has allowed early diagnosis in many men with prostatic carcinoma. Unfortunately, this has not translated into a high rate of cure for these individuals. There is considerable debate among oncologists and urologists about the appropriate use of this test as a screening device. It is hoped that identifying markers to distinguish those tumors with more rapid progression will allow the distinction of subpopulations of patients with prostatic carcinoma who should be treated more aggressively.

It is likely that the remarkable progress of the past several decades will result in more effective means of preventing malignant transformation and metastasis. Cancer prevention will take on new importance as we learn more about the molecular basis of agents that reduce cancer risk. We have passed through a period of remarkable expansion of our understanding of basic cancer biology that has pointed the way to new therapeutic approaches. While it is interesting to speculate on the new directions, it is almost impossible to imagine where the "molecular revolution" will take us during the next decade. The next two decades should see advances in the clinical arena to match those made in the laboratory during the past two decades.

Fishel R, Lescoe MK, Rao MRS, et al.: The human mutator gene homolog MSH2 and its association with hereditary nonpolyposis colon cancer. Cell 75:1027, 1993; Toribara NW, Sleisenger MH: Current concepts: screening for colorectal carcinoma; N Engl J Med 332:861, 1995. *The first article describes the techniques used to characterize the genetic abnormalities in a group of patients with the hereditary nonpolyposis colon cancer syndrome; the review article is an excellent summary of the sequential changes that occur in the development of colon cancer.*

Karp JE, Broder S: Molecular foundations of cancer: New targets for intervention. Nature Med 1:309, 1995. *Conceptual and practical advances in molecular medicine are changing our understanding of cancer pathogenesis. In time this should provide the opportunity to alter the natural history of many cancers.*

Levitzki A, Gazit A: Tyrosine kinase inhibition: An approach to drug development. Science 267:1782, 1995. *An excellent discussion of many chemotherapy targets and how the pharmaceutical industry is developing agents to inhibit specific enzymes.*

Miki Y, Swenson J, Skolnick MH, et al.: A strong candidate for the breast and ovarian cancer susceptibility gene BRCA1. Science 266:66, 1994; JAMA 273:535, 1995. *These are the classic articles describing the discovery of BRCA1 and characterization of its mutations.*

Oltvai ZN, Korsmeyer SJ: Checkpoints of dueling dimers foil death wishes. Cell 79:189, 1994. *An excellent discussion of the factors that regulate apoptosis and its role in the development of malignancy.*

PART XV

METABOLIC DISEASES

168 APPROACH TO THE PATIENT WITH METABOLIC DISEASE
Louis J. Elsas II

In this chapter we approach the principles of screening, diagnosing, and treating inherited metabolic diseases, many of which are detailed in subsequent chapters. In Ch. 24, inborn errors of metabolism are defined in terms of the function and location of proteins and the pathophysiologic consequences to the human organism when they are impaired. Here we invoke the predictive power of a genetic approach in identifying and preventing irreversible damage from an inborn error of metabolism. The goal is to diagnose the disorder and intervene to prevent damage by a return to metabolic homeostasis before disease is irreversible. Genetic screening is used to accomplish this objective. Once the disorder is detected, if its pathophysiology is understood, intervention can restore metabolic homeostasis and prevent progressive disease.

Genetic screening is a process by which a small population of high-risk individuals is selected from a much larger group. From the smaller population, a diagnosis, preferably presymptomatic, is made. Screening is performed in at least five categories of heritable risk, age, or reproductive condition.

Nonselected screening at a population base is performed to identify the homozygously affected individual and to prevent death, mental retardation, and other irreversible clinical manifestations. Certain principles are used to determine which diseases would be ethically, legally, and socially acceptable for such a public health activity (Table 168–1) (see Ch. 2). At present this type of screening is limited to the newborn owing to this population's accessibility, the rapidity of progression, and the lifelong burden of disease processes. Disorders currently being screened for in various combinations include phenylketonuria, maple syrup urine disease, galactosemia, homocystinuria, tyrosinemia, sickle cell disease, congenital adrenal hyperplasia, biotinidase deficiency, hypothyroidism, and cystic fibrosis.

Selective screening of newborns, children, and adults is performed to identify inherited disorders that may not be preventable. The objectives are to provide amelioratory treatment; determine the genetic component of the disorder; provide genetic counseling to patients, parents, and relatives; provide new information about the disorder's pathophysiology; and develop prevalence data. The laboratory diagnostic methods used in selective screening are different from those used in nonselective mass screening, and clinical judgment is the primary criterion for entry into this type of genetic screening. The preventive aspects of genetic screening of the symptomatic patient are important, particularly in disorders in which the onset of irreversible manifestations requires time for full expression. Given a specific diagnosis, genetic counseling may alter reproductive or life-planning behavior. Examples of heritable disorders amenable to selective screening are peroxisomal disorders, Wilson's disease, cystinuria, familial hypercholesterolemia, various organic acidemias, mucopolysaccharidosis and other lysosomal disorders, cystinosis, Duchenne's muscular dystrophy, disorders of mitochondrial function, and disorders of connective tissue.

Selective and nonselective genetic screening in pregnant women is achieved by fetal sonography, chorionic villus biopsy, or amniocentesis coupled with biochemical, chromosomal, or molecular analyses of cultured fetal cells. Maternal blood is a useful screening source for the fetal disorders Down syndrome and spina bifida. If maternal blood concentrations of α-fetoprotein, chorionic gonadotropin, or estriol vary above or below mean values of normal at a specific age of gestation, further fetal studies by sonography and amniocentesis are indicated. Considerable research is in progress to isolate fetal cells from maternal blood to avoid invasion of the amniotic cavity in prenatal screening.

Screening selected populations at risk for environmental hazards is generally applied to the adult population. Pharmacogenetic disorders fall into this category and include screening plasma pseudocholinesterase concentrations preoperatively to detect *pseudocholinesterase deficiency* and prevent death from succinyldicholine, and determining α-antitrypsin genotypes in individuals exposed to dust to prevent occupation-related, early-onset emphysema from α_1-antitrypsin deficiency.

Screening for asymptomatic heterozygotes in a "high-risk" population is another preventive approach to inborn errors of metabolism. The objective is to provide genetic counseling and reproductive alternatives in high-risk mating. An example is screening for *Tay-Sachs disease* carriers in the Ashkenazi Jewish population (see Ch. 24). Implementing newborn screening for sickle cell hemoglobin detects not only the homozygously affected infant, but also the SA heterozygote. The data from either genotype could be used to develop pedigrees and provide genetic counseling to at-risk family members.

THERAPY OF INHERITED DISEASE

Because the metabolic diseases considered in this section have in common that they are inherited and caused by single genes of large effect, a general approach to their treatment is appropriate. These approaches are outlined in Table 168–2. The level at which therapy is rendered depends on the level of understanding of the pathophysiologic mechanisms producing disease and the interventional methods available. Thus genetic counseling is used for diseases whose mechanisms are not yet understood, whereas engineered enzyme is replaced in *Gaucher disease, type I* by recurrent intravenous infusion.

Genetic counseling is a unique and fundamental aspect of management in inherited metabolic diseases. Patients and relatives usually ask the following questions: Why did this disease occur? Will this disease happen in me or my children? Can it be cured or prevented? Genetic counseling tries to answer these questions through complex processes involving several elements (see Ch. 29). One cannot overemphasize the importance of an accurate diagnosis before entering into formal genetic counseling.

TABLE 168–1. PRINCIPLES FOR NONSELECTIVE GENETIC SCREENING

The disorder should produce a high burden to the affected individual yet be preventable.

Methods for screening, retrieval, diagnosis, and management must be practical and available to the target population as a whole.

Inheritance and pathogenesis of the disease should be understood and genetic counseling available.

Benefit-to-cost ratio of the program should be greater than 1.

Patients' rights should be protected (voluntariness, informed consent, confidentiality).

Sensitivity and specificity should be high for the methods used.

TABLE 168–2. GENETIC APPROACHES TO THERAPY OF INHERITED DISEASE

Genetic Counseling: Prospective therapy
  Diagnosis, risk assessment, informational transfer, support for resource allocation
Reproductive Alternatives: Contraception, abstinence, artificial insemination, *in vitro* fertilization, risk-taking with or without prenatal monitoring

Environmental Engineering
  Avoiding offending agent
  Supplemental physical, speech, developmental therapy
  Nutritional management
    Limit toxic precursor
    Provide deficient product
    Detoxify through alternate metabolic route
    Provide feedback inhibitor
    Provide supraphysiologic amounts of vitamin precursor
    Induce protein (enzyme) production

Protein and Enzyme Replacement
  Infuse protected pure enzyme
  Provide clotting factors and peptide hormones
  Transplantation (prospective)
    Organ transplant
    Bone marrow transplant

Genetic Engineering
  Somatic gene therapy
    Random insertion
    Homologous recombination (site specific)
  Germ line therapy

Surgical intervention may be a useful adjunct for treating heritable disorders. For example, stabilizing hypoplastic cervical vertebrae may prevent quadriparesis or death in a variety of *chondrodysplasias* and *mucopolysaccharidoses,* accompanied by hypoplasia of the odontoid process. In *Marfan syndrome,* careful monitoring of aortic root diameter with surgical removal and prosthesis may prevent a lethal aortic dissection. Similarly, evaluation of polyps and early colectomy may prevent disseminated adenocarcinoma in families with the autosomal dominant forms of *familial polyposis coli.* Preventing heritable cancer by early surgical excision is therapeutic for thyroid carcinoma in *medullary thyroid carcinoma, Wilms' tumors,* and neurofibromas of *von Recklinghausen's disease.* Other examples of the benefit of preventive surgery for inborn errors include splenectomy for hemolytic anemias associated with spherocytosis and pyloroplasty in pyloric stenosis.

Environmental engineering is the most commonly used approach to preventing disease in patients affected by inherited metabolic disease. The environment (nutritional intake, exposure to toxins, sun, stress, climatic variation, and drug therapy) may produce a disease state in individuals who have inherited single genes or polygenic susceptibility to the environmental stress. Pharmacogenetic disorders exemplify the simple treatment of *avoidance* once the genetic susceptibility is identified. Health then can be viewed as a continual adaptation between the individual and the environment. Environmental engineering is a form of genetic therapy in which individual genetic susceptibility is identified and the environment is altered to provide optimal health for that individual's unique genetic constitution. The frequency of diseases caused by genetic susceptibility to the environment varies from rare to 100%. All humans develop *scurvy* unless ascorbate is provided in the diet because we are all homozygously deficient for the ability to convert glucuronic acid to glucuronolactone and ascorbate. Humans and primates lost this anabolic pathway during evolution. By contrast, humans readily synthesize tetrahydrobiopterin (BH_4), a cofactor in many hydroxylase reactions including phenylalanine hydroxylase. There are rare diseases (about 1 in 500,000) of increased blood phenylalanine and severe progressive neurodegeneration in which biopterin (BH_2) is not synthesized. BH_2 replacement may treat defects in biosynthesis and exemplifies a group of metabolic disorders known as *vitamin-dependency disorders.*

Nutritional management involves correcting the metabolic block and returning the patient to homeostasis through diet manipulation and drug therapy. Many of the diseases listed in this section are amenable to this approach and use the pathophysiologic mechanisms listed in Table 24–2. For example, in disorders of the urea cycle, protein intake is limited to reduce ammonia accumulation. Arginine is supplemented to provide deficient product of the blocked reaction and alternate pathways are induced for nitrogen excretion. The latter therapy is made possible by a ubiquitous enzyme *N*-glycine-acylase, which forms adducts with benzoic acid and glycine to produce hippuric acid that is excreted, thus ridding the body of one nitrogen molecule. *Orotic aciduria* is caused by mutations in the bifunctional enzyme orotate phosphoribosyl transferase-orotidine-5'-monophosphate decarboxylase. The disease process, which includes severe anemia and immune deficiency, is caused by deficient end-product, uridine, and is treated by replacing 100 to 200 mg per kilogram per day of uridine (orally). Feedback inhibition is important in treating *congenital adrenal hypertrophy* with replacement doses of hydrocortisone to prevent virilization from testosterone overproduction. Glucose decreases overproduction of the precursors δ-aminolevulinic acid and porphobilinogen in *acute intermittent porphyria* caused by porphobilinogen deaminase deficiency. Using supraphysiologic amounts of a specific vitamin is important if it is the precursor for coenzyme in a genetically impaired holoenzyme. There are many vitamin-dependent metabolic disorders such as pyridoxine (vitamin B_6)–dependent *homocystinuria,* and vitamin C–dependent *Ehlers-Danlos syndrome type VI.* In vitamin B_6–dependent homocystinuria mutant cystathionine synthase is stabilized to biologic degradation when saturated with pyridoxal phosphate. Others include vitamin B_{12}-dependent methylmalonic aciduria, thiamine-dependent maple syrup urine disease, and biotin-dependent propionic aciduria. Some blocked metabolic reactions can be augmented by inducing transcription of their gene. For example, phenobarbital and several other drugs induce hepatic UDP–glucuronyl transferase gene expression and reduce the accumulation of unconjugated bilirubin in *Gilbert syndrome.*

If the specific protein or enzyme has been purified and engineered to function in its specified organ or subcellular organelle, it can be used to treat an inherited metabolic disease. One good example is glucocerebrosidase, which has been purified in large quantities from placenta and biochemically engineered to contain the mannose recognition site for cellular uptake into lysosomal compartments. It has been used successfully to prevent and reverse the pancytopenia and bone disease of *type I Gaucher disease* (see Ch. 174.2). Many proteins are now made through recombinant techniques to treat metabolic disease and bypass the risks of AIDS and hepatitis attendant on using human-derived biologicals. These include Factor VIII for *hemophilia type A,* and growth hormone for *growth hormone deficiency.* Several other engineered proteins used to treat inherited metabolic disease include 1-deamino-8-D-arginine vasopressin to treat *X-linked recessive diabetes insipidus,* and recombinant $α_1$-antitrypsin made stable by inactivating methionine 385 in the treatment of $α_1$-antitrypsin deficiency. Some enzymes such as adenosine deaminase have been modified with polyethylene glycol to reduce immunogenicity and prolong biological half-life in the blood. It is used to treat *severe combined immunodeficiency (SCID).*

For metabolic disorders that are lethal and have no other available therapy, organ transplantation may be life-saving. Transplantation with histocompatible organs has become clinically important due to advances in immunology which not only allow for better tissue typing but also enable chronic immunosuppression with such drugs as cyclosporine, azathioprine, and prednisone to prevent rejection.

Several principles are required for successful treatment of an inherited metabolic disorder by organ transplant: (1) The normal enzyme, protein, or function must be provided by the transplanted organ. (2) Usually the affected organ must be removed. (3) The host must be immunologically tolerant to the gene product being introduced in addition to the transplanted organ itself. These principles are particularly relevant when displacement bone marrow transplantation is used. In the latter, normal donor stem cells differentiate and provide their enzymes to the recipient's reticuloendothelial system. Diseases associated with accumulation of products in the central nervous system are not yet ameliorated by bone marrow transplantation, although accumulation in bone, liver, and spleen is reduced. One group of metabolic diseases uses stem cell bone marrow transplantation to prevent leukemia caused by syndromes that include defective DNA repair, such as *Fanconi's anemia, Bloom syndrome,* and *ataxia-telangiectasia.* Organ transplantation of liver or kidney can reverse growth and developmental delay in type I glycogen storage disease, cystinosis, acute intermittent porphyria, type I tyrosinemia, Fabry's disease, oxalosis, and non-neuronotrophic lysosomal storage diseases. Lung transplantation has been successful in cystic fibrosis and α_1-antitrypsin deficiency, and prophylactic aortic transplantation has prevented aortic dissection in Marfan syndrome.

In the past decade somatic cell gene therapy to treat patients afflicted with genetic disease has entered the arena of clinical research. Numerous laboratories throughout the world are actively designing strategies by which exogenous DNA can be incorporated in the genomic DNA of patients to provide a missing gene function. It is not overly optimistic to assume that some form of *gene therapy* for a number of inherited metabolic diseases will be routinely available by the end of the century (see Ch. 25).

Desnick RJ: Treatment of Genetic Diseases. New York, Churchill Livingstone, 1991. *A multiauthored review of various approaches to metabolic disease therapy.*

Elsas LJ: Newborn screening. *In* Rudolph AM (ed.): Pediatrics. 20th ed. New York, Appleton-Century-Crofts, 1994. *Approaches to genetic screening.*

Elsas LJ, Acosta PB: Nutrition support of inherited metabolic disease. *In* Shils ME, Olson JA, Shike M (eds.): Modern Nutrition in Health and Disease. 8th ed, Philadelphia, Lea & Febiger, 1993. *Complete discussion of how to manage metabolic disease by diet.*

Disorders of Carbohydrate Metabolism

169 GALACTOSEMIA
Stanton Segal

The galactosemias are toxicity syndromes exhibited by patients with an inherited inability to metabolize the sugar galactose, a constituent of the disaccharide lactose found in milk and milk products. There are three disorders, each resulting from a deficiency of one of the enzymes that catalyze the normal conversion of galactose to glucose. Uridyltransferase deficiency is the most prevalent and is commonly referred to as classic galactosemia (Table 169–1). For all three disorders, the elevations of the level of galactose and its metabolites in blood, urine, and tissues can be diminished and acute neonatal clinical manifestations alleviated by omitting dietary galactose.

ETIOLOGY. Galactokinase, galactose-1-phosphate (P) uridyltransferase, and uridine diphosphate-4-epimerase deficiencies are all autosomal recessive genetic disorders. The individual human genes have been located on chromosomes 17, 9, and 1, respectively. The tissues of obligate heterozygotes contain about 50% of the normal enzyme activity, whereas homozygotes exhibit absence or very little activity of enzymes. Immunoelectrophoretic analysis has shown that patients with transferase deficiency produce a protein similar to the normal, but with severely reduced or no enzyme activity. Sequence analysis of the cloned uridyltransferase gene reveals several mutations responsible for single amino acid substitutions. The most common is the replacement of an arginine for glutamine at amino acid 188 near the active site of the enzyme, which results in a protein with no catalytic activity. More than 70% of Caucasian patients are either homozygous or heterozygous for this mutation.

TABLE 169–1. GALACTOSEMIA ENZYME DEFICIENCIES

Enzyme Defect	Accumulated Metabolite(s)	Effects
Galactokinase	Galactose	Cataracts early in life; no multiple organ involvement
Galactose-1-P uridyltransferase	Galactose Galactose-1-P	Syndrome of nutritional failure, liver disease, abnormal renal tubule function, cataracts, mental retardation, ovarian abnormalities
Uridine diphosphate-4-epimerase	Galactose Galactose-1-P UDP galactose	Resembles transferase deficiency, but may occur in a benign form

PREVALENCE. Uridyltransferase deficiency has a prevalence of 1 per 40,000 births and a carrier rate of about 1% in the United States population. A gene known as the Duarte variant is allelic to the normal transferase and codes for a protein that is electrophoretically different and enzymatically less active. The gene frequency of the Duarte variant is about 0.05%, and homozygotes for the Duarte variant have about 50% of normal transferase activity in their red blood cells (RBC's). With widespread neonatal screening, a number of babies have been detected with low red cell transferase activity who are compound heterozygotes with one gene for defective transferase and another for the Duarte variant. Such infants have only 10 to 25% of red cell enzyme activity but rarely have impaired galactose utilization that requires treatment.

Galactokinase deficiency is quite rare, having a prevalence of 1 in 500,000 to 1 in 1 million births. Epimerase deficiency is also rare. The benign type has mainly been described in Swiss and Japanese populations, whereas only a few cases of symptomatic epimerase deficiency have been detected.

PATHOGENESIS. Galactose is converted to glucose by a unique series of three enzyme reactions (Fig. 169–1). Normally this pathway functions efficiently. Galactose rapidly disappears from blood after intravenous infusion, even faster than a comparable amount of glucose. In normal individuals liver extraction of galactose results in a rise in the level of blood glucose.

In each of the three forms of galactosemia, diminished enzyme activity produces an accumulation of the substrates proximal to the metabolic block (Fig. 169–1). When galactose is increased, alternative pathways form large amounts of otherwise trace metabolites. In one reaction galactose is reduced to form the sugar alcohol galactitol, whereas in another galactose is oxidized to galactonic acid. These metabolites accumulate in tissues and are excreted in considerable amounts in the urine.

Identification of accumulated metabolites and the elucidation of alternative pathways have provided insights into the relationship of biochemical toxicity and clinical manifestations of the disorders. Cataract formation appears to be due to the galactitol formed by lens aldose reductase. Galactitol, which cannot be further metabolized, accumulates in the lens and produces osmotic changes with inhibition of fluid, lens swelling, and protein precipitation. The exact biochemical alterations in other target organs affected by transferase deficiency have not been defined. No specific structural alterations of the brain are associated with mental retardation in cases of transferase deficiency, although white matter changes have been seen on magnetic resonance imaging and cerebellar atrophy noted on computed tomography scans. Liver dysfunction may be accompanied by altered architecture of liver characterized by pseudoacinar formation of hepatic cells.

There are several possibilities for the pathogenesis of the long-term complications of mental retardation, speech abnormalities, ataxia, and hypogonadism in women affected with transferase-deficient galactosemia despite strictly eliminating galactose from the diet. (1) There is *in utero* damage. Elevated levels of galactitol are

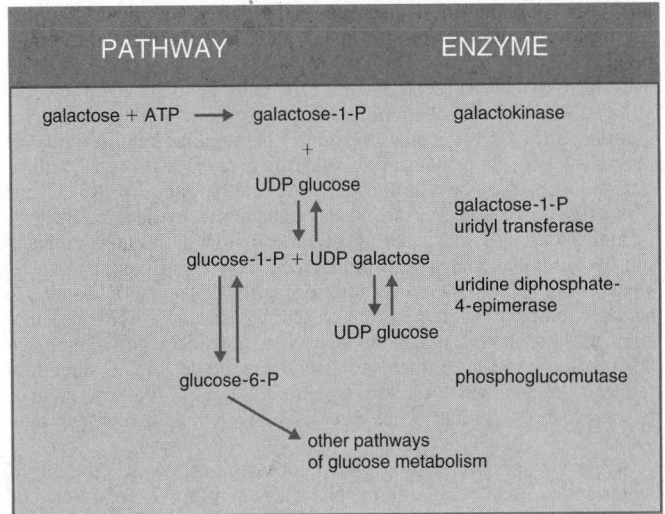

FIGURE 169–1. Normal enzymatic pathway that converts galactose to glucose.

found in affected fetuses and galactose-1-P is increased in cord RBC's. Indeed, cataractous change can be found in the embryonal and fetal lens, and the ovaries of females with hypergonadotropic gonadism may be small, fibrotic, or streaked, consistent with a developmental abnormality. (2) There is continuous self-intoxication, a concept based on the constantly elevated red cell galactose-1-P and urinary galactitol in patients on galactose-restricted diets. This could occur from galactose liberated by the turnover of complex carbohydrates or from galactose-1-P resulting from pyrophosphorylatic cleavage of UDP galactose derived from UDP glucose. (3) There may be depletion of essential metabolites. Tissue inositol levels are low in the galactose toxic state and a decrease in red cell UDP galactose levels has been reported in some patients. (4) There may be hidden sources of galactose in the diet even when extreme care has been taken to eliminate known sources. Tomatoes and watermelon are now known to be rich in free galactose.

CLINICAL MANIFESTATIONS. Cataracts are the principal finding in patients with galactokinase deficiency, who otherwise are healthy. The cataracts are usually discovered in infants and children examined for other medical reasons. Pseudotumor cerebri has been described in some galactokinase-deficient patients as well as those with transferase deficiency. Cataracts have been observed in some heterozygous carriers, and patients younger than 40 with cataracts frequently have lower than normal red cell galactokinase levels.

Uridyltransferase deficiency usually manifests itself shortly after birth or within the first few weeks of life with growth failure, vomiting, diarrhea, hepatomegaly, ascites, jaundice, hemolytic anemia, hypoglycemia, proteinuria, and a renal Fanconi's syndrome. Cataracts may not be easily observed with an ophthalmoscope in young infants but are found on slit-lamp examination. Infants with this disease may die in the first few days of life from overwhelming *Escherichia coli* sepsis before other manifestations are evident. Without eliminating galactose from the diet, severely affected infants die of inanition and liver failure. Occasionally, because of vomiting, the infant's formula is changed to one that is galactose-free, with subsequent cessation of the toxicity syndrome. Later in childhood these patients with undetectable red cell transferase activity have severe mental retardation and cataracts after milk is reintroduced into the diet.

Black patients with transferase deficiency may have a milder toxicity syndrome and in some cases have no symptoms. This has been called the Negro variant. Such patients have been found to metabolize some galactose because of the presence of 10% of normal transferase activity in liver and intestinal mucosa. A toxicity syndrome resembling transferase deficiency can occur in some cases of epimerase deficiency.

DIAGNOSIS. Suspect galactokinase deficiency in any infant or child with cataracts, and confirm the diagnosis by assaying RBC or cultured fibroblast galactokinase. A presumptive diagnosis is possible by detecting reducing sugar in urine that is glucose oxidase negative (galactose) or by chromatographic analysis for galactitol in the urine. These urinary findings also obtain in transferase defi-

ciency, whose definitive diagnosis requires assaying RBC transferase activity. Because severely affected babies may be given blood transfusions before a diagnosis of galactosemia is considered, red cell transferase assay should be delayed until transfused blood has been replaced by the infant's own cells. However, an assay of transferase of parents' red cells with 50% of normal activity found in both may be helpful in making presumptive diagnosis in such infants or in those who may have died before specimens for assay were obtained.

Besides the quantitative assay of RBC transferase, starch gel electrophoresis or isoelectric focusing to determine isoenzyme banding may be useful in distinguishing the carrier for classic galactosemia, the homozygous Duarte variant whose RBC enzyme activity is comparable to that of carriers for the classic disease, and mixed Duarte-classic galactosemia carriers who have 10 to 25% of normal activity.

In the differential diagnosis, hereditary fructose intolerance with hepatomegaly, liver dysfunction, hypoglycemia, renal Fanconi's syndrome, and nonglucose reducing substance in the urine should be considered. Lactosuria, a common finding in a variety of gastrointestinal disorders, also causes a positive test result for reducing substance. However, many laboratories use glucose oxidase–based tests for determining blood and urinary sugar, and in such instances, galactosemia and galactosuria would go undetected. The greatest confusion in differential diagnosis is the distinction between transferase deficiency and primary liver disease. Because the liver is the major organ metabolizing galactose, any disruption of hepatocellular function may result in galactosemia and galactosuria. Red cell transferase assay should make the distinction. Patients with clinical findings resembling classic transferase deficiency galactosemia who have normal red cell transferase activity should also be tested for red cell epimerase activity.

Many cases are currently diagnosed as a result of neonatal screening. More than 40 U.S. states and several foreign countries test all newborns by analyzing heel-stick blood spots on filter paper. All positive test results require confirmation by quantitative assay of the individual enzymes and isoelectric focusing analysis. Such screening has resulted in delineation of the benign form of epimerase deficiency in which galactose-1-phosphate appears to accumulate only in RBC's. Subsequent studies have indicated that the epimerase in such cases is unstable because of increased requirement for cofactor NAD, which can be supplied by other cells but not by RBC's.

TREATMENT. A galactose-free diet is the cornerstone of treatment. Eliminating galactose early in classic galactosemia may cause cataracts to regress, liver dysfunction and renal tubule abnormalities to disappear, and early growth and development to be normal. Besides banning milk and all milk products, care should be taken to eliminate foods in which milk is used in cooking and baking or lactose has been added. Attention should be paid to fruits and vegetables (watermelon and tomatoes). There is no indication that the ability to metabolize galactose increases with age, so dietary restrictions should not be relaxed in older children. Despite cessation of postnatal galactose toxicity with an early-instituted lactose-free diet, there are later manifestations of slow mental development, speech abnormalities called verbal dyspraxia, ataxia, and ovarian failure with hypogonadotropic hypogonadism in affected females.

PROGNOSIS. Dietary galactose restriction does not ensure a normal outcome. Despite excellent treatment from birth, many patients with transferase deficiency have below-average mental development with learning defects, diminished attention span, and visual perceptual difficulties. More than 60% have speech abnormalities and 80% of affected females have hypergonadotropic hypogonadism. The outcome does not differ in patients without neonatal symptoms treated at birth from those recognized within the first several weeks of life on the basis of the acute galactose toxicity syndrome due to ingesting galactose-containing feeds. Untreated infants, however, may not survive. Older patients may develop an ataxic neurologic syndrome while on galactose-restricted diets.

PREVENTION. Prenatal diagnosis can be performed by assaying transferase of a chorionic villus biopsy or cultured amniotic cells or by determining galactitol in amniotic fluid. Galactose restriction during pregnancy in which the fetus is at risk has not altered the prognosis.

Elsas LJ, Fridovich-Kiel JL, Leslie N: Galactosemia: A molecular approach to the enigma. Int Pediatr 8:101, 1993. *Presents the structure of the human uridyltransferase gene and the frequency of mutations, demonstrating the high incidence of the arginine substitution for glutamine at position 188 (Q188R) in the amino acid sequence.*

Segal S, Berry G: Disorders of galactose metabolism. *In* Scriver CH, Beaudet AL, Sly WS, et al. (eds.): The Metabolic and Molecular Bases of Inherited Disease. 7th ed, New York, McGraw-Hill, 1995. *A monograph and molecular bases on all aspects of galactose metabolism, galactosemia, and the pathophysiology of galactose intoxication.*

170 GLYCOGEN STORAGE DISEASES

Harry L. Greene

Glycogen is the storage form of glucose and is present in varying amounts in virtually all cells, although the liver is the primary organ for storage and subsequent release of glucose into the circulation. Glycogen is synthesized from glucose and glucose hydrolyzed and released from glycogen; this highly regulated process helps maintain normal blood glucose concentrations during fasting. At least eight enzymes involved in glycogen synthesis and the hydrolysis to glucose are utilized in this control.

Glycogen storage diseases are characterized by an abnormal tissue concentration (>70 mg per gram of liver or >15 mg per gram of muscle) and/or an abnormal structure of the glycogen molecule. During the past 40 years, patients who have deficient activity in virtually every enzyme important in the normal synthesis or degradation of glycogen have been identified. With the exception of phosphorylase kinase deficiency, all are inherited in an autosomal recessive manner. Although the enzyme deficiency may vary among patients, the clinical expression of the disease can usually be traced to either the liver or the muscle.

HEPATIC FORMS OF GLYCOGENESIS

The various hepatic enzymatic deficiencies are expressed primarily as hypoglycemia and hepatomegaly, and three defects (branching enzyme, glycogen synthetase, and debranching enzyme) result in the accumulation of abnormally structured glycogen and may cause progressive hepatic cirrhosis and associated splenomegaly. Conversely, the accumulation of normally structured glycogen, as seen with deficiency of phosphorylase, phosphorylase b kinase, acid alpha-glucosidase, or glucose-6-phosphatase, is usually not associated with hepatic fibrosis and splenomegaly. Figure 170–1 summarizes the general location of enzymatic defects resulting in the hepatic forms of glycogenesis. With the exception of lysosomal acid glucosidase deficiency, hypoglycemia is a common presenting feature. Clinical and biochemical expressions of the various types of glycogen storage diseases are summarized in Table 170–1, and the more commonly diagnosed types are discussed below.

GLUCOSE-6-PHOSPHATASE DEFICIENCY (TYPE I GLYCOGEN STORAGE DISEASE). This disorder has been subcategorized into types a, b, or c, with type a the most common; but all types have similar clinical features. As noted in Figure 170–1, all other enzymatic defects directly affect the formation or degradation of glycogen, with the exception of glucose-6-phosphatase. Similarly, the clinical expression of this defect is distinctly different from that of the other forms of glycogenosis. For example, fasting-induced hypoglycemia may be extreme, and lactic acidosis, hyperlipidemia, and hyperuricemia may be unique to patients with type I. The mechanism for the striking abnormalities in lipid and purine metabolism as well as carbohydrate metabolism results primarily from overproduction of substrate in response to a decline in blood glucose, as indicated in Figure 170–1. The documented reversal of these abnormalities by treatment that maintains the blood glucose level between 80 and 90 mg per deciliter supports the postulate that these changes are the result of hormonal responses to the hypoglycemia. Therapeutic intervention has been evaluated more extensively in patients with this defect than any other. As a result, it

has been possible to devise reasonably effective dietary control for these patients that results in favorable development into adulthood.

Late Complications. As more patients have survived and developed into active, functioning adults, two subsequent, unexpected complications have become apparent: (1) single or multiple hepatic adenomas and (2) progressive glomerulosclerosis with renal failure. Adenomas usually develop in patients between ages 16 and 22, and it is unusual for a patient not to have adenomas by age 25. Because adenomas tend to subsequently become malignant, annual monitoring by ultrasonography is recommended. Any rapidly expanding lesion should be considered potentially malignant and should undergo surgical biopsy because serum α-fetoprotein measurements have been an unreliable marker for malignant transformation. There has been some indication that the adenomas could be prevented or reduced in younger children by more stringent dietary control; however, this hypothesis has not been substantiated in older individuals.

The development of progressive glomerulosclerosis, proteinuria, hypertension, and renal failure has been a recent observation and usually occurs in older patients (>18 years) who are less well managed and exhibit recurrent hypoglycemic episodes, chronic hypertriglyceridemia, and lactic acidosis. The mechanism causing the renal lesion is not defined, although some improvement in proteinuria has been seen following treatment with angiotensin-converting enzyme inhibitors.

DEBRANCHING ENZYME DEFICIENCY (TYPE III GLYCOGEN STORAGE DISEASE). This disease most often affects only the liver but may affect muscle as well. When muscles are involved, the serum creatine phosphokinase (CPK) level is elevated, and patients are usually classified as having type IIIb disease. Some patients may not show elevated CPK levels during early life, and so evaluation during later childhood or adolescence should be performed. Hypoglycemia with fasting is less severe (usually 40 to 50 mg per deciliter) than in patients with type I, although hepatic enlargement may be substantially greater. Serum aspartate aminotransferase (AST) and alanine aminotransaminase (ALT) concentrations are commonly above 500 units per milliliter. Correspondingly, hepatic fibrosis of varying degrees is usually present during childhood and may be progressive. At least two adult patients (ages 43 and 55) presenting with "cryptogenic cirrhosis" and bleeding esophageal varices have been diagnosed as having debrancher enzyme deficiency.

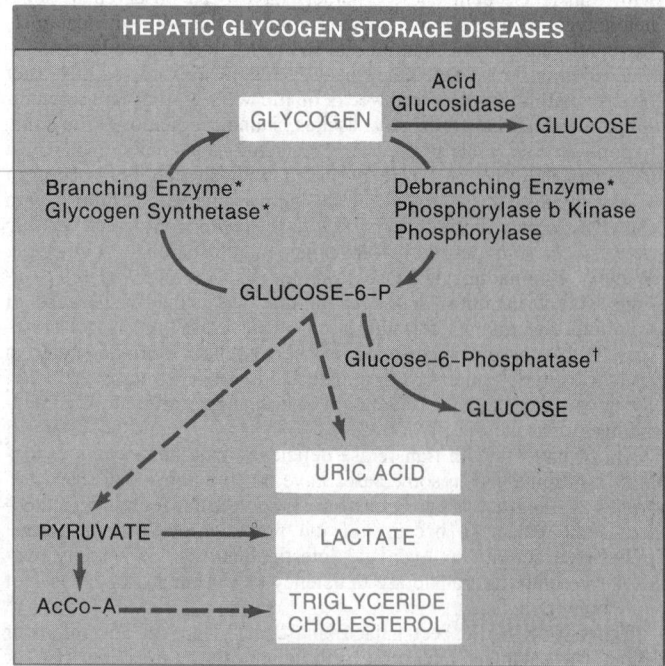

FIGURE 170–1. Mechanism for abnormalities in lipid, purine, and carbohydrate metabolism in type I (glucose-6-phosphatase deficiency) glycogen storage disease. * = associated with hepatic cirrhosis. † = associated with elevated serum uric acid, lactate, and lipid levels and with hepatic adenoma.

TABLE 170–1. CLASSIFICATION OF GLYCOGEN STORAGE DISEASES

Type	Enzyme Affected	Primary Organ Involved	Manifestations
O	Glycogen synthetase	Liver	Hypoglycemia, hyperketonia, FFT, early death
Ia	Glucose-6-phosphatase	Liver	Enlarged liver and kidney growth failure, fasting hypoglycemia, acidosis, thrombocyte dysfunction
Ib	Microsomal membrane G-6-P translocase	Liver	As in Ia; in addition, recurrent neutropenia, bacterial infections
Ic	Microsomal membrane P-transporter	Liver	As in Ia
II	Lysosomal acid glucosidase	Skeletal and cardiac muscle	*Infantile form:* early-onset, progressive muscle hypotonia, cardiac failure, death before 2 years *Juvenile form:* late-onset myopathy and variable cardiac involvement *Adult form:* limb-girdle muscular dystrophy-like feature
III	Amylo-1,6-glucosidase (debrancher enzyme)	Liver, skeletal muscle, heart	Fasting hypoglycemia, hepatomegaly in infancy; some have myopathic features, rarely clinical cardiac features
IV	Amylo-1,4-1,6-transglucosidase (brancher enzyme)	Liver, muscle	Hepatosplenomegaly, cirrhosis; may have late-onset myopathy
V	Muscle phosphorylase	Skeletal muscle	Exercise-induced muscular pain, cramps, and progressive weakness, sometimes with myoglobinuria; symptoms usually begin during adolescence or early adulthood
VI	Liver phosphorylase	Liver	Hepatomegaly, mild hypoglycemia, good prognosis
VII	Phosphofructokinase	Muscle, red blood cells	As in V; in addition, mild hemolytic anemia
Formerly VIb, VIII, or IX	Phosphorylase b kinase	Liver, leukocytes, (?) muscle	As in VI; X-linked inheritance
X	Cyclic AMP-dependent kinase	Liver, muscle	Hepatomegaly, mild hypoglycemia

Treating these patients has not been advocated because the natural course of the disease has been thought to be benign. However, because growth retardation and cirrhosis may be serious complications, several patients have been treated with frequent feedings and raw cornstarch to maintain blood glucose levels between 75 and 100 mg per deciliter. Treated patients often show a significant reduction in serum transaminase levels and improvements in growth, and they may demonstrate improved muscle strength, although serum CPK activities remain elevated.

Clinical and laboratory features of the other, more unusual forms of hepatic glycogenesis are presented in Table 170–1.

MUSCULAR FORMS OF GLYCOGEN STORAGE

ACID ALPHA-GLUCOSIDASE DEFICIENCY (POMPE'S DISEASE, TYPE II GLYCOGEN STORAGE DISEASE). In this condition, virtually all tissues have an increased glycogen content. However, presenting clinical manifestations of the illness are cardiac enlargement, myocardial failure, and generalized muscle hypotonia without muscle wasting. The classic infantile form manifests during the first months of life, and few survive past the first year. The juvenile variant presents in later infancy or early childhood and progresses more slowly, with death in the second or third decade. The adult type manifests as a slowly developing adult-onset myopathy. In each case, the diagnosis is dependent on finding deficient activity of acid α-1, 4-glucosidase in muscle specimens or cultured fibroblasts. No treatment, including bone marrow transplantation and systemic enzyme infusion, has proved to be of long-term benefit to these patients.

MYOPHOSPHORYLASE DEFICIENCY (TYPE V GLYCOGEN STORAGE DISEASE, MCARDLE'S DISEASE). Most of these patients are asymptomatic during early childhood and escape diagnosis until the second or third decade of life. A history of muscle pain and cramps after exercise, signs of myoglobinuria, and painful cramping on an ischemic exercise test are characteristic. The diagnosis is suggested by an elevation in serum muscle CPK isoenzyme activity and by failure to elevate the serum lactate level with exercise. The diagnosis is established by documenting elevated muscle glycogen in the sarcolemmal regions and reduced muscle phosphorylase activity. Glucose or fructose ingestion prior to exercise is said to reduce the symptoms.

MUSCLE PHOSPHOFRUCTOKINASE DEFICIENCY (MUSCLE PHOSPHOGLYCERATE MUTASE DEFICIENCY, LACTATE DEHYDROGENASE [LDH-M] SUBUNIT DEFICIENCY, TYPE VII GLYCOGEN STORAGE DISEASE). These muscle glycogenoses are rare and clinically similar to myophosphorylase deficiency. Patients with phosphofructokinase deficiency may also show a mild hemolytic anemia. Diagnosis depends on muscle enzyme analysis. Treatment is aimed at avoiding strenuous exercise.

DIAGNOSIS AND PRENATAL DIAGNOSIS OF GLYCOGEN STORAGE DISEASE

Diagnostic enzyme analysis on hepatic or muscle tissue for most types of glycogen storage diseases is currently funded at Duke Medical Center, Division of Genetics. Prenatal diagnosis of three types of glycogen storage diseases (types II, III, and IV) is also possible and is performed on cultured amniotic cells in this laboratory.

Chen YT, Cornblath M, Sidbury JB: Cornstarch therapy in type I glycogen storage disease. N Engl J Med 310:171, 1984. *The usefulness of dietary raw cornstarch to maintain blood glucose concentrations is demonstrated.*

Ding JH, deBarsy T, Brown B, et al.: Immunoblot analyses of glycogen debranching enzyme in different subtypes of glycogen storage disease type III. J Pediatr 116:95, 1990. *Provides newer insights into the molecular basis of type III glycogenoses.*

Ghishan FK, Greene HL: Inborn errors of metabolism that lead to permanent liver injury. *In* Zakim D, Boyer TD (eds.): Hepatology: A Textbook of Liver Disease. 2nd ed. Philadelphia, WB Saunders, 1990. *An extensively referenced review that focuses on the altered metabolism, treatment, and outcome of the hepatic forms of glycogenesis.*

Hers HG, Van Hoof F, deBarsy T: The glycogen storage diseases. *In* Scriver CR, Brandet AL, Sly WS, Valle D (eds.): The Metabolic Basis of Inherited Disease, 6th ed. New York, McGraw-Hill, 1989. *This extensively referenced article provides information on the clinical and biochemical aspects of the glycogen storage diseases.*

Parker PH, Ballew M, Greene HL: Nutritional management of glycogen storage disease. Annu Rev Nutr 13:83, 1993. *Combines the biochemical abnormalities of the glycogenoses and associated research findings with a practical guide to dietary management of children and adults.*

171 FRUCTOSE INTOLERANCE
Harry L. Greene

Fructose, a normal dietary constituent of fruits, vegetables, honey, and the disaccharide sucrose (table sugar), is present at a level of 50 to 100 grams per day in the average Western diet. At this level of intake, it is rapidly absorbed in the proximal small intestine by a specific transport mechanism and is extracted on the first pass from the portal vein. Because fructose malabsorption has been described in some individuals, the relative tolerance of dietary fructose in normal children was evaluated by feeding 31 children 2 grams of fructose per kilogram of body weight. Four children developed gastrointestinal symptoms and 71% developed abnormal breath hydrogen excretion, suggesting that a significant increase in dietary fructose can result in malabsorption in some individuals.

Initial metabolism of fructose primarily involves three enzymes: fructokinase, aldolase B, and triokinase (Fig. 171–1), although hexokinase phosphorylates some of the fructose. Five enzymatic defects involving fructose metabolism have been identified: (1) fructokinase deficiency, (2) aldolase A deficiency, (3) aldolase B deficiency, (4) fructose-1, 6-diphosphatase deficiency, and (5) D-glycerate kinase deficiency. The enzymatic defects in fructose metabolism are illustrated in Figure 171–1, and each of the defects is discussed below.

FRUCTOKINASE DEFICIENCY (Essential Fructosuria)

Fructokinase deficiency is a rare (about 1 in 130,000 births), asymptomatic, autosomal-recessive condition caused by deficient activity of fructokinase, the first enzyme in fructose utilization. Because no pathologic condition results from this defect, the primary concern relates to the fact that fructose is a reducing sugar. Thus, a positive reaction with urinary Clinitest tablets may result in the erroneous suggestion of diabetes unless glucose oxidase is determined with a dipstick. The precise nature of the enzymatic defect is not known because the gene for fructokinase has not yet been identified.

ALDOLASE DEFICIENCY

Three aldolases (A, B, and C) are responsible for the conversion of fructose-1, 6-diphosphate into glyceraldehyde-3-phosphate and dihydroxyacetone phosphase. Embryonic tissue produces aldolase A; adult liver, kidney, and intestine expresses aldolase B; and nervous tissue expresses aldolase C. Although all three aldolases are tetramers of identical 40-kDa subunits, each is coded for different genes on different chromosomes: aldolase A on chromosome 16,16q22-q24, aldolase B on chromosome 9,9q13-q32, and aldolase C on chromosome 17,17 cen-q 21.

ALDOLASE A DEFICIENCY. Aldolase A deficiency may be detrimental because of its pivotal role in glycolysis. This is apparently of special relevance to the developing embryo, which ex-

presses only aldolase A. Only a few patients with this deficit have been described, and not all symptoms are expressed to the same degree. Potential symptoms include mental retardation, short stature, hemolytic anemia, and abnormal facial appearance. Because aldolase B becomes normal at birth, patients do not show fructosuria; thus, restricting dietary fructose is of no benefit.

ALDOLASE B DEFICIENCY (HEREDITARY FRUCTOSE INTOLERANCE, HFI). Aldolase B deficiency (prevalence about 1 in 20,000 births) is a potentially life-threatening autosomal-recessive disorder than can be effectively treated by eliminating dietary fructose. This disorder is due to deficiency of fructose-1-phosphate aldolase (aldolase B). Aldolase B is normally present in large amounts in the liver, intestine, and renal cortex; thus, excessive fructose intake by patients with HFI adversely affects each of these organs.

Symptoms do not become manifested until the patient ingests fructose or fructose-containing foods. Because lactose is the carbohydrate source in mammalian milk, infants do not develop symptoms until the introduction of dietary fruits or other fructose-containing foods or medication, i.e., fruits, fruit juices, medicinal syrups, sucrose-containing infant formulas, and so forth. The primary presentation is vomiting and other features hypoglycemia within 20 to 30 minutes after fructose ingestion. These acute manifestations may not be apparent following lower chronic intakes, for example with fructose-containing infant formulas. In these instances, failure to thrive, hepatomegaly, and cirrhosis may represent the dominant presenting features. Concomitant laboratory findings include an acute decrease in serum glucose and phosphate concentrations and an elevated uric acid concentration. With continued exposure to fructose, hyperbilirubinemia, lactic acidosis, hepatosplenomegaly, and liver failure develop in conjunction with renal tubular dysfunction (bicarbonaturia, aminoaciduria, phosphaturia). At this stage, liver biopsy shows fatty infiltration of hepatocytes with cellular necrosis and mild bile duct proliferation with fibrosis. If exposure to fructose continues, progressive fibrosis, cirrhosis, and death from liver failure follow. The brain may also show diminished neurons.

The diagnosis is suggested by the presence of urinary reducing sugar detectable by Clinitest tablets and not by urinary dipstick,

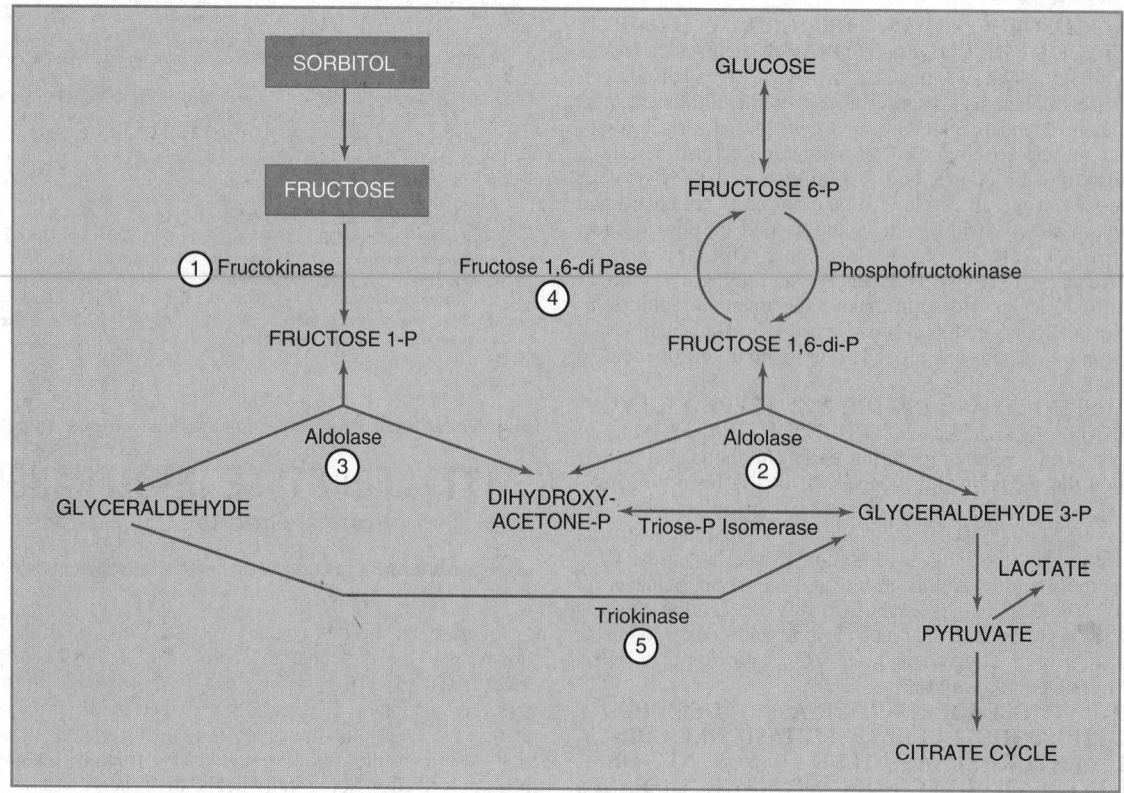

FIGURE 171–1. The major pathway for fructose metabolism in the liver, showing the five defects discussed in the text. Aldolase deficiency consists primarily of defects in aldolase B(③). Aldolase A deficiency(②) is extremely rare and is expressed primarily during embryogenesis.

which measures glucose oxidase. Because similar clinical features may be present with galactosemia or tyrosinemia, diagnosis can be confirmed by measuring fructose-1-phosphate aldolase activity in liver or intestinal biopsy specimens. An intravenous fructose tolerance test (0.2 to 0.3 gram per kilogram in adults or 3 grams per square meter in children) after restriction of dietary fructose for several weeks has been used to confirm the illness, but this procedure may cause hypoglycemia. Patients should be monitored closely to prevent complications during fructose tolerance tests. Fructose loading cannot detect heterozygotes; for this purpose, ^{31}P magnetic resonance spectroscopy applied to fructose metabolism is necessary.

Five mutations have been identified in the aldolase B gene: two large deletions of 1.65 and 1.4 kb and three small deletions of 7 and 4 bp. In addition, six point mutations have been identified: (1) a single G → C mutation changing alanine to proline at position 149 of the protein subunit; (2) a change of alanine to aspartate at position 174; (3) a change of asparagine to lysine at position 334; (4) a change of alanine to valine at position 337; (5) a stop codon at position 288, the consequence of a deletion of cytosine of the leucine codon; and (6) a stop codon at position 297, shortening the carboxy terminus by 67 residues.

In spite of recurrent bouts of hypoglycemia and substantial liver disease, restriction of dietary fructose usually results in almost complete recovery during a 3- to 5-week period, and affected adults have normal intelligence. Older children and adults are protected from large dietary intakes of fructose by an aversion to sweets, although small amounts taken chronically may result in isolated, often reversible, somatic growth retardation.

FRUCTOSE-1, 6-DIPHOSPHATASE (FDPase) DEFICIENCY

This rare disorder was first described in 1970. Patients usually present before age 6 months with fasting-induced lactic acidosis, hypoglycemia, and hepatomegaly. The reaction to glycerol is similar to that from fructose ingestion but is less severe than that of patients with HFI. The condition is due to a defect of hepatic fructose-1, 6-diphosphatase, a gluconeogenic enzyme (Fig. 171–1). Thus, when hepatic glycogen stores are depleted, fasting hypoglycemia develops. During fasting, urinary organic acids are similar to those of tyrosinemia type I but with an absence of succinyl acetate. In addition, starvation leads to increased excretion of glycerol.

The human gene for FDPase has not been isolated, so prenatal diagnosis is unlikely. The enzyme is a tetramer for identical 36 kD. The diagnosis is suspected when, after about 12 to 16 hours of fasting, the blood sugar concentration falls and is not restored when glucagon is administered, and acidosis (lactate) is present. Loading tests with fructose or glycerol may be dangerous because they lead to hypoglycemia and lactic acidosis. Diagnosis is confirmed by measuring the enzyme in hepatic biopsy material. Treatment consists of avoiding fasting and restricting dietary fructose and glycerol.

D-GLYCERATE KINASE DEFICIENCY (D-GLYCERIC ACIDURIA)

This is a rare (10 patients described), clinically variable disorder resulting in either no symptoms, metabolic acidosis and failure to thrive, or profound psychomotor retardation and seizures. The variable phenotypic expression has not been fully explained on the basis of the enzymatic defect, but all patients who show a substantial increase in D-glycerate excretion after fructose ingestion should avoid dietary fructose.

Baker L, Winegrad AI: Fasting hypoglycemia and metabolic acidosis associated with deficiency of hepatic fructose-1, 6-diphosphatase activity. Lancet 2:13, 1970. *The first description of a patient with deficient fructose-1, 6-diphosphatase activity.*

Ghishan FK, Greene HL: Inborn errors of metabolism that lead to permanent liver injury. *In* Zakim D, Boyer TD (eds.): Hepatology: A Textbook of Liver Disease. 2nd ed. Philadelphia, WB Saunders, 1990. *An extensively referenced review that focuses on the altered metabolism, treatment, and outcome of fructose intolerance.*

Hommes FA: Inborn errors of fructose metabolism. Am J Clin Nutr 58(Suppl):788, 1993. *A recent correlation between the genotype and phenotype of the five various defects in fructose metabolism.*

Odievre M, Gentil C, Gautier M, et al.: Hereditary fructose intolerance in childhood. Am J Dis Child 132:605, 1978. *This article is an excellent presentation of the clinical, hepatic, and biochemical changes that can be expected in children with HFI.*

Schulte MJ, Lenz W: Fatal sorbitol infusion in a patient with fructose-sorbitol intolerance. Lancet 2:188, 1977. *This paper illustrates the need to restrict sorbitol as well as fructose in patients with HFI.*

172 PRIMARY HYPEROXALURIA
Richard E. Hillman

Primary hyperoxaluria refers to two different peroxisomal enzyme deficiencies that are characterized by massive synthesis and urinary excretion of oxalic acid. Oxalate is also deposited in the heart, the eye, the skin, and other organs, leading to a variety of clinical pictures. Particularly in type I disease, the clinical manifestations present early in childhood with nephrolithiasis or nephrocalinosis and lead to renal failure within the first decade of life. However, the ready availability of oxalate assays in the last few years has led to the description of milder cases, mostly type II, which are either asymptomatic or present only with water deprivation. Both types are inherited as autosomal recessive traits and must be distinguished from secondary hyperoxalurias due to increased absorption of oxalate by the gut. These secondary causes include inflammatory bowel disease and fat malabsorption, which may tie up calcium and convert insoluble calcium oxalate to more absorbable salts. Although most adult patients with calcium oxalate nephrolithiasis excrete normal amounts of oxalate, it is now clear that hyperoxaluria must be considered in the differential diagnosis.

Primary hyperoxaluria type I (glycolic aciduria) is caused by a defect in the peroxisomal enzyme alanine:glyoxylate aminotransferase. This enzyme normally converts glycolic acid to the amino acid glycine. In its absence, glycolic acid leaves the peroxisome and is converted to oxalic acid by lactic dehydrogenase (LDH). Both glycolic and oxalic acids are excreted in large amounts, usually > 60 mg per 1.73 meters^2 per 24 hours. In most cases, this concentration exceeds the solubility of oxalic acid. This enzyme has been cloned, and multiple defects have been demonstrated.

Primary hyperoxaluria type II (glyceric aciduria) is due to one of two defects. Until recently it was believed that the defect lay in the enzyme D-glyceric dehydrogenase. This enzyme leads to the accumulation of hydroxypyruvic acid, which is reduced in the cytoplasm to L-glyceric acid. It had been unclear why this defect caused hyperoxaluria. Recently, it was suggested that this enzyme may be the same as glyoxalate reductase, which leads to accumulation of glyoxalate and production of oxalate by LDH. Type II is a much milder disease in most cases than type I. Asymptomatic cases or cases with only a single attack of oxaluria have been reported. Two recent cases only became symptomatic following severe water deprivation, one while sailing, one while running in hot weather.

Some patients with type I disease respond to large doses of pyridoxine (20 to 200 mg per day). This vitamin is the cofactor for the enzyme. It appears to act by stabilizing the remaining activity and is effective only in patients with some enzyme, in general the milder cases. Dilute urine should be maintained by high fluid intake, and some reports suggest that diuretics may help. Attempts to form more soluble salts of oxalate, particularly with magnesium, have met with some success. The only "cure" for this disease has been a combined renal and liver transplant. Renal transplants alone have failed due to the accumulation of oxalate from other organs. Type II patients are very variable. Pyridoxine has no effect. Other measures that maintain a dilute urine seem to be enough in the milder cases.

Danpure CJ, Purdue PE, Fryer P, et al.: Enzymological and mutational analysis of a complex primary hyperoxaluria type I phenotype. Am J Hum Genet 53:417, 1993. *The latest data on type I enzyme deficiencies, including variability.*

Hillman RE: Primary hyperoxalurias. *In* Scriver CR, Beaudet AL, Sly WS, et al. (eds.): The Metabolic Basis of Inherited Disease. 6th ed. New York, McGraw-Hill, 1989, p 933. *A general review of the biochemistry of primary oxalosis and related secondary disorders.*

Seageant LE, de Groot GW, Dilling LA, et al.: Primary oxaluria type 2 (L-glyceric aciduria): A rare cause of nephrolithiasis in children. J Pediatr 118:912, 1991. *A review of clinical information on type II disease.*

Disorders of Lipid Metabolism

173 THE HYPERLIPOPROTEINEMIAS

Joseph L. Witztum and Daniel Steinberg

Hyperlipidemia, abnormal elevation of plasma cholesterol and/or triglyceride levels, is one of the most common clinical problems that confront the physician in daily practice. Much attention has been focused on these disorders because there is a strong association of hyperlipidemia—especially hypercholesterolemia—with development of atherosclerosis, and of hypertriglyceridemia with pancreatitis. Hyperlipidemia may occur because of a primary genetic disorder or as a result of environmental influences secondary to other medical conditions, or any combination of these factors. Because lipids are transported in plasma as components of lipoprotein complexes, understanding lipoprotein physiology is necessary for informed diagnosis and therapeutic planning.

PHYSIOLOGY OF LIPOPROTEIN TRANSPORT

Lipoproteins are complex macromolecules that transport nonpolar lipids through the aqueous environment of plasma. The more nonpolar lipids—triglycerides and cholesteryl esters—are carried almost exclusively in the central core of the spherical lipoprotein particles. The more polar lipids (such as phospholipids and free cholesterol), together with amphipathic apolipoproteins, form a surface monolayer that serves to "solubilize" the particles and allows them to remain in stable solution in the aqueous plasma.

Each lipoprotein particle contains on its surface one or more apolipoproteins that have a variety of functional and structural roles. Some apolipoproteins provide structural stability to the lipoprotein, serve as ligands for cellular lipoprotein receptors that help determine the metabolic fate of individual particles and act as cofactors for plasma enzymes involved in plasma lipid and lipoprotein metabolism. Other apolipoproteins play several roles, e.g., apolipoprotein B (apo B) is the major structural apolipoprotein of the triglyceride-rich lipoproteins secreted by the liver (very low-density lipoproteins [VLDL]), but it also serves as the ligand for binding of low-density lipoproteins (LDL) (formed from VLDL) to cellular LDL receptors. Table 173–1 lists major apoproteins, lipoproteins on which they reside, and known or postulated functions.

The most widely used classification of lipoproteins is based on their different densities, which determine their behavior during preparative equilibrium ultracentrifugation. The fact that lipoprotein particles exist as relatively discrete species when separated this way led to the currently used density classification system outlined in Table 173–2. A second classification system originally proposed many years ago assigns priority to the apoprotein content of the lipoproteins. For example, in the high-density lipoprotein (HDL) density class there are lipoprotein particles that contain mainly apo A-I and others that contain both apo A-I and apo A-II; these are designated LpA-I and LpA-I, A-II, respectively. Current research suggests that it is primarily LpA-I that confers the antiatherogenic properties of HDL. Thus, in the future, full evaluation may include this type of analysis, but for now more research is needed to determine its clinical value.

An older classification system of the lipoproteins, based on their electrophoretic patterns (lipoprotein pattern typing), while important historically for the development of our understanding of lipid transport disorders, is not used commonly today. However, for the sake of completeness, the electrophoretic mobility of each lipoprotein class is also given in Table 173–1.

SYNTHESIS AND TRANSPORT OF ENDOGENOUS LIPIDS. The endogenous lipid transport system can be divided into two major classes: the apo B-100 lipoprotein system (VLDL, IDL [intermediate-density lipoprotein], and LDL) and the apo A-I lipoprotein system (HDL).

Metabolism of Very Low-Density Lipoproteins (VLDL). Between meals, free fatty acids are mobilized from the adipose tissue and serve as a major source for hepatic triglyceride synthesis. Lipogenesis, the synthesis of fatty acids *de novo* from carbohydrate or protein, also can occur in the liver. Fatty acids can either enter mitochondria (where beta oxidation occurs) or they can undergo esterification to form triglycerides in the cytosol. Control of triglyceride synthesis is a complex process that appears to be regulated in part by changes in insulin and glucagon that occur with feeding. Glucagon enhances fatty acid oxidation, whereas insulin prevents it. In addition, insulin may induce lipogenic enzymes in the liver. Triglycerides, together with cholesterol synthesized *de novo* in the liver or delivered to the liver by chylomicron remnants, are packaged together with apo B and phospholipids and form a nascent VLDL (Fig. 173–1). Plasma VLDL also contain other apolipoproteins, including the C apoproteins, and apo E. Apo B is found as a full-length protein termed apo B-100 (or apo B), which is made by the liver, or as a shortened form termed apo B-48, which is made in humans only by the intestine. Apo B is an obligatory component for nascent VLDL assembly and secretion from the hepatocyte; other apoproteins are added to VLDL after their entry into plasma. The size of the VLDL particle released depends on the availability of triglycerides in the liver. Very large triglyceride-rich VLDL are secreted when excess hepatic triglyceride synthesis is occurring, as in obesity, non–insulin dependent diabetes, and excess alcohol consumption. In contrast, small VLDL are secreted when availability of triglyceride, but not cholesterol, is decreased. Each VLDL particle contains one molecule of apo B, yet under ordinary circumstances the rate of apo B synthesis is not rate limiting for VLDL secretion. Although enhanced triglyceride synthesis can lead to enhanced triglyceride output, the *number* of VLDL particles released is not necessarily increased. Instead, *larger* individual VLDL particles containing more triglyceride are released. Understanding the processes regulating VLDL assembly and release by the hepatocytes is necessary to understand the etiology of clinically important disorders, such as familial combined hyperlipidemia (FCH) or hyperapobetalipoproteinemia, which are characterized by increased rates of secretion of VLDL particles from the liver. Other lipoprotein disorders (familial hypertriglyceridemia) are caused by hepatic secretion of a normal number of VLDL particles but ones that are enriched with triglycerides. The half-life of VLDL is about 1 hour or less.

TABLE 173–1. APOLIPOPROTEIN CHARACTERISTICS

Apoprotein	Lipoproteins	Function
Apo B-100	VLDL, IDL, LDL	Secretion of VLDL from liver. Structural protein of VLDL, IDL, and LDL. Ligand for the LDL receptor
Apo B-48	Chylomicrons, remnants	Secretion of chylomicrons from intestine
Apo E	Chylomicrons, VLDL, IDL, HDL	Ligand for binding of IDL and remnants to LDL receptor and LRP
Apo A-I	HDL, Chylomicrons	Structural protein of HDL Activator of LCAT
Apo A-II	HDL, Chylomicrons	Unknown
Apo C-II	Chylomicrons, VLDL, IDL, HDL	Activator of LPL
Apo C-III	Chylomicrons, VLDL, IDL, HDL	Inhibitor of LPL (*in vitro*)

TABLE 173–2. CHARACTERISTICS OF MAJOR LIPOPROTEIN CLASSES

Lipoprotein Class	Density (gm/ml)	Diameter (nm)	Major Lipid	Electrophoretic Mobility
Chylomicron and remnants	<< 1.006	5000–800	Dietary triglycerides	Remains at origin
VLDL	< 1.006	800–300	Endogenous triglycerides	Pre-β
IDL	1.006–1.019	350–250	Cholesteryl esters, triglycerides	Slow pre-β
LDL	1.019–1.063	250–180	Cholesteryl esters	β
HDL	1.063–1.210	50–120	Cholesteryl esters, phospholipids	α
Lp(a)	1.055–1.085	300	Cholesteryl esters	Slow pre-β

The primary function of lipoprotein particles is to transport lipids from one site to another. Triglyceride-rich lipoproteins serve to transport endogenously synthesized triglyceride to adipose tissue for storage in the fed state or to muscle for utilization in the fasting state. The enzyme that catalyzes peripheral triglyceride uptake is lipoprotein lipase (LPL). This enzyme is synthesized in adipose tissue and skeletal muscle cells, secreted, and transported across the capillary endothelial cell, where it binds to glycoproteins on the endothelial luminal surface. When VLDL bind to LPL, the LPL is activated by apo C-II present on the surface of the VLDL particle. This leads to triglyceride hydrolysis and release of fatty acids, which are then transported into the fat (or muscle) cell where they are re-esterified with glycerol and stored as intracellular triglyceride. The vast majority of triglyceride in adipose tissue is acquired by this mechanism because essentially no lipogenesis occurs *de novo* from glucose in human adipose tissue. The activity of LPL in adipose tissue is increased in the fed state, effectively providing for triglyceride storage. Insulin is required to maintain adequate LPL levels in adipose tissue. It appears to do so by maintaining synthesis and release, but it does not acutely affect changes in LPL levels. This is in contrast to "hormone-sensitive lipase" (HSL), an enzyme that hydrolyzes intracellular triglycerides, releasing fatty acids to plasma for uptake by the liver. HSL is acutely inhibited by insulin, while glucagon increases its activity. Thus, following a meal, high insulin levels serve to promote storage of fatty acids in the adipocyte as triglyceride, while in the fasting state hydrolysis is promoted, providing fatty acids for uptake by muscle and liver.

As noted above, the action of LPL requires the cofactor, apo C-II. Shortly after VLDL enters into plasma, apo C-II is transferred to VLDL from a reservoir on circulating HDL. After hydrolysis of triglyceride in VLDL, the apo C-II is released and presumably picked up again by HDL. The importance of apo C-II is demonstrated by individuals with genetic deficiency of C-II, which leads to impaired LPL activity and massive hypertriglyceridemia. Other apolipoproteins, such as C-III, are also transferred between VLDL and HDL. *In vitro*, apo C-III can inhibit LPL-mediated hydrolysis, but its physiologic role *in vivo* is still unclear.

Hydrolysis of triglycerides in VLDL profoundly alters the structure of the VLDL with collapse of the core. The excess surface components, including cholesterol, phospholipids, and the non-apoB apoproteins, are transferred to HDL. The triglyceride-depleted VLDL, with its associated loss of other lipids and apoproteins, now becomes an IDL, cholesterol-enriched and containing only apo B and apo E. Under normal conditions this particle is rapidly removed from plasma by the liver through a complex interaction with several hepatic receptors, including the LDL receptor, which recognizes apo B and apo E, and with another receptor, termed the remnant receptor, which is specific for apoprotein E. This latter receptor is thought to be the LDL-receptor–related protein (LRP). While the majority of IDL particles are normally removed from plasma by

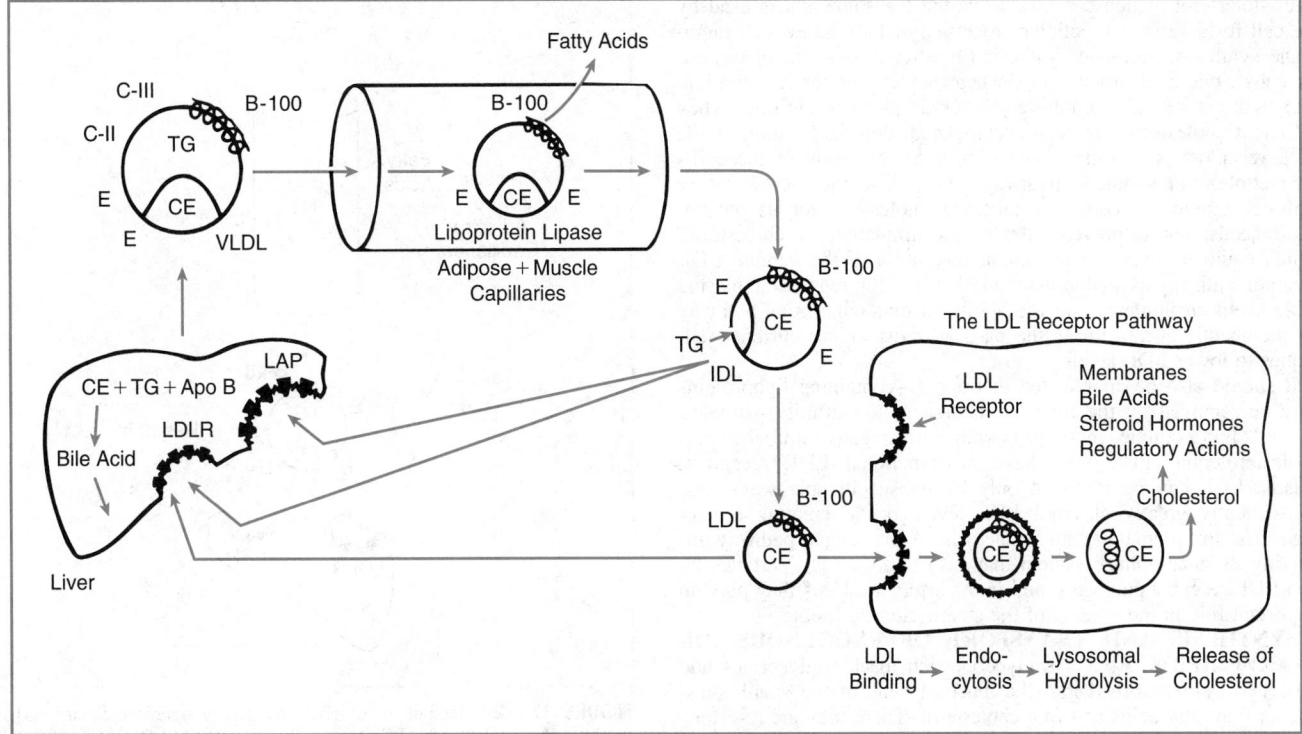

FIGURE 173–1. Simplified scheme of metabolism of apo B-containing lipoproteins. In the liver, triglyceride *(TG)*, cholesteryl esters *(CE)*, and apolipoprotein B-100 *(B-100)* are packaged and released into plasma as very low-density lipoproteins *(VLDL)*. In capillary beds, lipoprotein lipase hydrolyzes TG to release free fatty acids. The TG-depleted particle is termed an intermediate-density lipoprotein *(IDL)*. The particle is further metabolized to CE-rich low-density lipoprotein *(LDL)*. A major fraction of IDL particles is removed from plasma by hepatic receptors, both by LDL receptors *(LDLR)* and LDL receptor-related protein *(LRP)*. A portion of IDL is converted to LDL, which is then removed from plasma by LDLR on liver and peripheral cells. Uptake of LDL via the LDLR pathway leads to regulation of cholesterol synthesis and LDLR synthesis as explained in text. (Modified from Witztum, JL: Current approaches to drug therapy for the hypercholesterolemic patient. Circulation 80:1101, 1989. By permission of the American Heart Association, Inc.).

this process in other species, in humans a significant fraction is converted into LDL. By the time the cholesterol-rich LDL has been formed, most of the triglyceride has been removed and apo B is now the sole apoprotein remaining from the original VLDL particle. Under normal circumstances, most of the cholesterol found in plasma is present in the form of LDL particles, and only minute amounts of IDL are present.

Apo E, which acts as a ligand for both the LDL receptor and the LRP, appears to be crucial for both the direct removal of IDL and conversion of IDL particles to LDL. Patients who either lack apo E or are homozygous for apo E isoforms (E_2) that bind less efficiently to these receptors may have excess plasma accumulation of IDL particles (and chylomicron remnants) and are both hypercholesterolemic and hypertriglyceridemic, a condition known as dysbetalipoproteinemia.

Metabolism of LDL. Each LDL particle is derived from VLDL via IDL and contains one copy of apo B. All other apolipoproteins have now been removed, together with much of the phospholipid and triglyceride and some of the cholesterol. Although only a small percentage of VLDL particles ultimately end up as LDL, the bulk of plasma cholesterol is accounted for by LDL particles because of the relatively slow rate of clearance of LDL from plasma (half-life of 2 to 3 days). Because LDL particles contain only apo B, their efficient clearance can occur only by way of the LDL receptor pathway. In normal humans, approximately 75% of LDL particles are cleared by the LDL receptor pathway and approximately two thirds of LDL particles are removed by the liver. Nobel prize winners Brown and Goldstein elucidated the LDL receptor pathway, one of the major achievements of modern medical science. The rate of LDL removal via this pathway is the primary determinant of LDL levels. The LDL receptor, which binds apo B with high affinity and leads to internalization of the LDL particle via the LDL receptor pathway, is found on virtually every mammalian cell. As shown in the right side of Figure 173–1, the LDL particle binds to the receptor on the surface of the cell, and subsequently the receptor and the bound LDL particle are internalized. LDL is then delivered to the lysosome, but the receptor recycles to the surface of the cell. Within the lysosome, the protein component, apo B, is degraded to amino acids or oligopeptides. The cholesteryl ester is hydrolyzed to free cholesterol, which can now leave the lysosome and is used by the cell for a variety of cellular processes, including new cell membrane synthesis, hormone synthesis (in adrenal, ovarian, or testicular cells), bile acid production (in hepatocytes), or for re-esterification to be stored as a cholesteryl-ester droplet. In addition, when sufficient cholesterol has been accumulated, down-regulation of the LDL receptors is accomplished, as well as inhibition of the cell's own cholesterol synthetic pathway. Thus, this efficient regulatory pathway provides a cell with sufficient cholesterol for its physiologic needs, but it prevents the overaccumulation of cholesterol, which could be toxic. In particular, regulation of the *hepatic* LDL receptor pathway is a dominant mechanism for regulating plasma LDL levels in humans, and the ability to manipulate this pathway by therapeutic agents forms the basis of most of our current techniques to lower LDL levels.

It should also be appreciated that apo B–containing lipoproteins may be removed by the liver by inefficient, low-affinity pathways as well. For example, in subjects with homozygous familial hypercholesterolemia (FH), who have no functional LDL receptors, plasma LDL can be removed only by nonspecific pathways, and consequently greatly elevated LDL levels occur, creating a very high risk for premature atherosclerosis. A scavenger pathway involving the macrophage system may also remove LDL particles by non-LDL receptor pathways, and in the artery wall this may play an important role in the genesis of the atherosclerotic lesion.

SYNTHESIS AND TRANSPORT OF EXOGENOUS (DIETARY) LIPIDS. After a triglyceride-rich meal, triglycerides and cholesterol are absorbed into the mucosal cells of the small intestine as free fatty acids and free cholesterol. There they are re-esterified to triglyceride and cholesterol esters and incorporated into the core of a nascent lipoprotein, the chylomicron. The surface coat of the chylomicron is composed of phospholipid and apoproteins A-I, A-II, and A-IV. Apo B-48 is a crucial component of chylomicrons and is a product of the same gene that codes for apoprotein B-100. Apo B-48 is so named because it is identical to the first 48% (the

amino terminal portion) of apo B-100. In humans, the intact, full-length apo B-100 is made only in the liver, while apo B-48 is made only in the intestine. Apo B-48 appears to be required for the small intestine to produce chylomicrons, as individuals with abetalipoproteinemia, who are incapable of secreting apo B from intestinal (or hepatic) cells, cannot assemble chylomicron particles. Apo B-48 is transcribed from the apo B-100 gene, but the mRNA is first edited by a cytosine-to-uracil change creating a stop-codon. The domain of intact apo B-100 that binds to the LDL receptor is contained in the carboxy terminal end. Because apo B-48 lacks this domain it is unable to bind to LDL receptors. Thus, once the chylomicron has been secreted by the intestine, apo B-48 functions primarily as a structural component.

Triglycerides constitute >90% by weight of the chylomicron particle, and consequently the density of this lipoprotein is the lowest of any in plasma. When plasma is left overnight in the refrigerator, if chylomicrons are present, they will float to the top and appear as a layer of "cream" on top, which is the basis for the chylomicron test. In normal individuals, this test is always negative after an 8- to 12-hour fast, as chylomicrons have a short half-life in plasma. The presence of a positive chylomicron test in a 12-hour fasting sample is abnormal and indicative of marked delay in chylomicron clearance.

Chylomicrons are delivered to the plasma via the thoracic duct (Fig. 173–2). While in the lymph and after entering plasma, chylomicrons acquire apo C-II, C-III, and apo E by transfer. After having acquired sufficient apo C-II, which is absolutely required for LPL activity, the chylomicron can interact with LPL in a manner

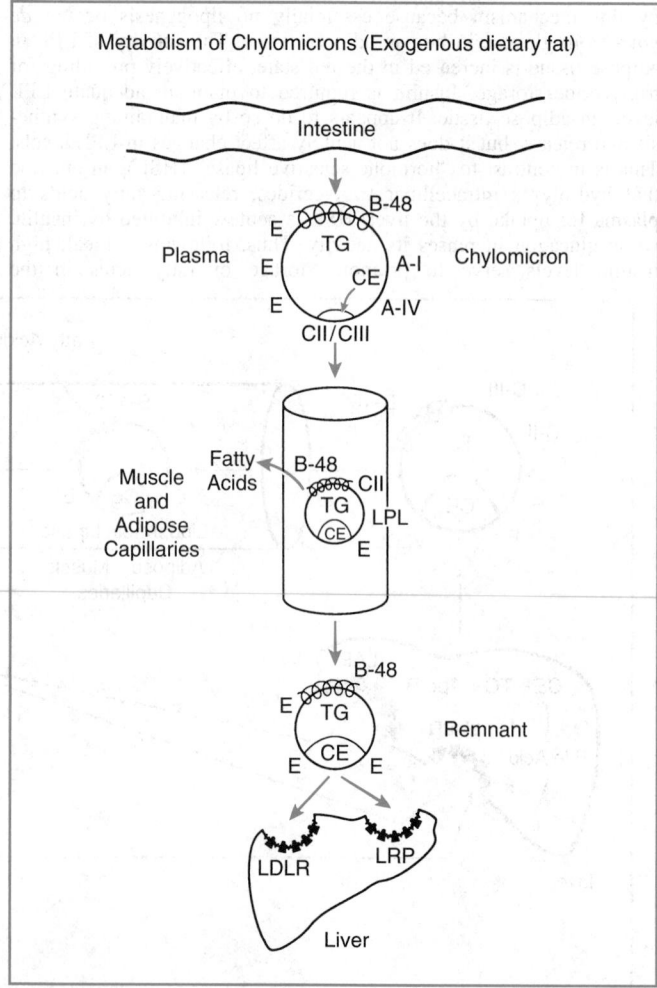

FIGURE 173–2. Metabolism of chylomicrons (exogenous dietary fat). In the intestine, triglyceride (TG) and small amounts of cholesteryl esters (CE) are packaged with apo B-48, apo A-I, and apo A-IV and released into lymph. The chylomicron particle acquires apo E and apo C-II/C-III in lymph and plasma. In capillary beds, TG is hydrolyzed by lipoprotein lipase (LPL). The remnant particle is then removed primarily by liver, mediated by binding to LRP and LDLR as well as to surface proteoglycans. Chylomicron remnants are not a source of LDL.

analogous to that of VLDL. After sufficient triglyceride hydrolysis has occurred, the remaining chylomicron particle, now termed a remnant, has a markedly reduced core volume and its excess surface components, including apoproteins such as C-II, C-III, and some of the apo E, are transferred to HDL as described for VLDL. The remnant particle is still relatively cholesterol-ester–rich. In part, this cholesterol comes from dietary sources, but a significant amount is also transferred into the particle from HDL mediated by cholesterol ester transfer protein (CETP). In addition, because it is still a relatively large particle, it contains many copies of apo E on its surface, and it is believed that this represents the ligand that leads to rapid interaction with remnant receptors in the liver and efficient removal from the circulation. The exact pathway for uptake of chylomicron remnants by the liver is still being investigated but probably includes the LRP, the LDL receptor itself, as well as cell-surface glycosaminoglycans that can also bind apo E. Apo E is central to the process of remnant removal, just as it is for IDL uptake. Individuals who either lack apo E or synthesize only apo E isoforms that bind poorly to receptors can accumulate chylomicron remnants in plasma.

HDL-CONTAINING LIPOPROTEINS. When chylomicrons and VLDL are hydrolyzed by LPL to release fatty acids for peripheral use, their surface coat of unesterified cholesterol, phospholipid, and various apoproteins forms excess surface material that must be disposed of. HDL play a principal role in this by acting as an acceptor or "sink" for this excess surface material (Fig. 173–3). Nascent HDL particles are synthesized by the liver and the intestine and are composed primarily of phospholipid and two major structural proteins, apoproteins A-I and A-II. HDL accepts the phospholipid (mainly lecithin) and unesterified cholesterol from the excess surface of triglyceride-rich lipoproteins as they are catabolized. An enzyme associated with HDL—lecithin-cholesterol acyl transferase (LCAT)—removes a fatty acid from lecithin and transfers it to cholesterol, producing cholesteryl ester and lysolecithin. The esterified cholesterol moves into the core of the HDL particle, making it possible to accept another free cholesterol molecule onto the surface of the HDL particle. In turn, the cholesteryl esters are then transported back to the liver (reverse cholesterol transport) either directly or by transfer to other lipoproteins, such as VLDL, IDL, or LDL via CETP. The uptake of these cholesteryl-ester–enriched lipoproteins by the liver results in net removal from plasma of cholesteryl esters. This HDL/LCAT/CETP system plays a pivotal role in removing excess cellular cholesterol, facilitating its transfer back to the liver for excretion. The removal of excess cholesterol from arterial wall cells by such a mechanism could play a crucial role in mini-

mizing cholesterol accumulation in the artery wall and thus inhibiting atherogenesis (see Ch. 40). Thus, HDL may be viewed as playing a vital role in transporting excess cholesterol from extrahepatic tissues back to the liver where it is excreted in the bile. In addition to its role in reverse cholesterol transport, HDL may also serve as the reservoir for apoproteins such as C-II, C-III, and E as they shuttle back and forth from triglyceride-rich lipoproteins while being catabolized.

BILE ACID PRODUCTION (see Ch. 126). Nearly all cells of the body have the capacity to synthesize cholesterol *de novo,* but none has the ability to degrade it completely. However, hepatocytes have the capacity to convert cholesterol into bile acids, which can then be secreted into the bile along with free cholesterol and phospholipids. Nearly 95% of secreted bile acids are reabsorbed in the distal ileum and enter the enterohepatic circulation, i.e., they are taken up by the liver and recycled. Cholesterol delivered to the liver in the form of chylomicrons or other lipoproteins could be recycled and secreted as VLDL or converted to bile acids for secretion into the bile.

DISORDERS OF LIPOPROTEIN METABOLISM

Disorders of lipoprotein metabolism can lead to hypercholesterolemia or hypertriglyceridemia or both. While these disorders appear to be common in the general population, the molecular events responsible for them are only currently being elucidated. For purposes of organization the hyperlipoproteinemias are grouped into disorders leading primarily to hypercholesterolemia (due to elevations of LDL levels) or to hypertriglyceridemia (due to elevations of VLDL or chylomicrons) or to combined elevations of both triglycerides and cholesterol. Several monogenic disorders have been defined that lead to each type of hyperlipidemia, but for many cases the etiology is likely to be polygenic. These disorders affect plasma lipoprotein levels by overproduction of lipoproteins and/or decreased clearance.

Hyperlipoproteinemia Resulting Primarily in Hypercholesterolemia

FAMILIAL HYPERCHOLESTEROLEMIA AND FAMILIAL DEFECTIVE APOLIPOPROTEIN B. *Familial hypercholesterolemia* (FH) is a common autosomal dominant disorder due to absence of or defective LDL receptors resulting in decreased capacity to remove plasma LDL. Familial defective apolipoprotein B is an autosomal dominant disorder in which the ligand binding region of apo B is defective, also leading to delayed plasma LDL clearance. In both disorders LDL cholesterol levels are strikingly increased, frequently associated with characteristic xanthomas in the Achilles tendons, the patellar tendons, the extensor tendons of the hands, and by the presence of xanthelasma. It is frequently associated with early coronary artery disease (CAD). In heterozygous FH, estimated to be present in 1 in 500 individuals, there is one abnormal allele for the LDL receptor. The abnormal allele may produce no receptors or produce abnormal LDL receptors that are largely nonfunctional. In the heterozygote a 50% decrease exists in hepatic LDL receptor number, a corresponding decrease in LDL catabolism, and an approximately twofold to threefold increase in plasma LDL levels. In the rare homozygous FH patient (only 1 in 1,000,000 people) almost no functional LDL receptors are found, and plasma LDL levels may be increased sixfold to tenfold. In this situation, LDL can be removed from plasma only by low-affinity pathways. In familial defective apolipoprotein B, the ligand-binding domain of apo B is defective because of a missense mutation at amino acid 3500. This mutation leads to impaired binding of LDL to the LDL receptor and clinical consequences similar to those seen in FH. It is likely that other mutations in apo B affecting its ability to bind to the LDL receptor also occur.

These disorders are characterized by greatly elevated concentrations of LDL cholesterol. If untreated, patients with FH have premature CAD, as well as other clinical manifestations of atherosclerosis (see Ch. 41). Peripheral vascular disease and cerebral vascular disease are also increased, although not as much as CAD. Tendon xanthomas are seen only in FH and in patients with familial defective apo B. Bilateral, irregular, firm and nodular thickenings in the Achilles tendons or extensor tendons of the hands or knees are usually present and can be so large as to interfere with normal functions, such as wearing shoes. Xanthelasma typically occurs in this

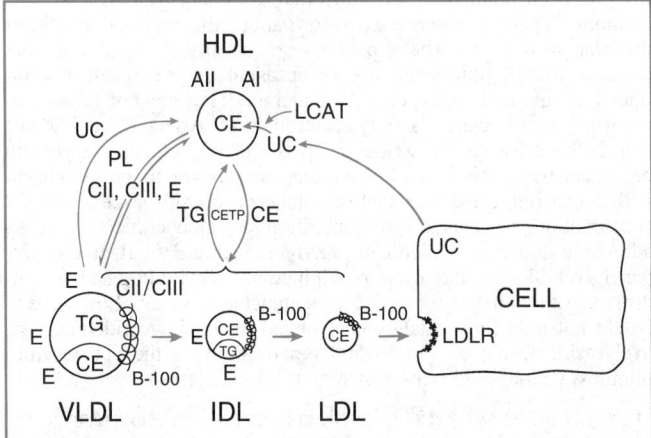

FIGURE 173–3. Interactions of high-density lipoproteins *(HDL)* and apo B-containing lipoproteins. HDL has particles containing apo A-I and particles containing apo A-I, A-II. Nascent HDL, made primarily by liver and intestine, accepts unesterified cholesterol *(UC)* from VLDL and from membranes of cells. The enzyme lecithin-cholesterol-acyltransferase *(LCAT),* which is associated with HDL, esterifies the cholesterol to form cholesteryl esters *(CE),* which then form the core of the HDL. The enzyme cholesterol ester transfer protein *(CETP)* transfers CE from HDL into apo B-containing lipoproteins in exchange for TG. HDL also serves as a "sink" for apoproteins C-II/C-III and E, which shuttle back and forth from the HDL to VLDL and IDL.

setting, and corneal arcus is frequently seen as well, although this latter is seen in other lipoprotein disorders and can be seen in elderly, normolipidemic patients as well.

Plasma cholesterol levels in heterozygous FH exceed the upper 1% of levels seen in the general population and are generally in the range of 300 to 500 mg per deciliter. In rare patients, homozygous for FH, plasma cholesterol levels can exceed 800 to 1000 mg per deciliter. Triglyceride levels are usually normal, but in 10% of subjects may be mildly elevated. Patients with defective remnant removal or with marked chylomicronemia may also have markedly elevated cholesterol levels, but they will have very high triglyceride levels as well. In addition, their plasma will appear turbid or creamy, in contrast to plasma in FH patients, which is always clear.

Because myocardial infarction can occur in men with heterozygous FH when they are in their early 40's, these subjects deserve vigorous therapy to lower LDL levels and to decrease other risk factors as well. Women with FH also have an accelerated risk for CAD, although the absolute risk is less than that of men and the CAD occurs at a later age. For both men and women the risk of atherosclerosis is greatly accelerated by the presence of other risk factors such as smoking, hypertension, diabetes, low HDL cholesterol levels, and high Lp(a) levels. A diet low in saturated fat and cholesterol should be initiated in all affected individuals with this disorder, although frequently only modest reductions in LDL levels occur. Effective therapy can be achieved using a bile acid-binding resin, frequently combined with high-dose nicotinic acid (niacin) given with meals. HMG-CoA reductase inhibitors, a class of compounds termed *statins,* are increasingly being used as first-line therapy as they effectively lower LDL cholesterol levels by 20 to 40% and infrequently have side effects. When these statins are combined with a bile acid–binding resin, decreases of LDL levels by 50 to 60% can frequently be achieved. In some individuals, triple therapy with a statin, a bile acid-binding resin, and niacin may be necessary to normalize LDL levels. Unfortunately, subjects homozygous for FH will usually not respond to these measures, which work in large part by increasing the LDL receptor activity. For such individuals heroic measures are required, such as repeated plasmapheresis or a more specialized procedure, termed LDL apheresis, in which apo B-containing lipoproteins are removed from blood as it passes extracorporeally through a column that binds apo B. In selected individuals, liver transplantation has been used. In the future it is hoped that gene therapy may lead to correction of the primary genetic defect.

POLYGENIC HYPERCHOLESTEROLEMIA. Irrespective of one's definition of hypercholesterolemia, it is clear that a large number of individuals in the general population have elevated LDL-cholesterol levels (see Table 173–4). If one uses the conventional definition that the top 5% of the general population have hypercholesterolemia, then on average only 1 of 25 of such hypercholesterolemic individuals will have FH, and only 2 will have familial combined hyperlipidemia (FCH) (described below). The large majority have hypercholesterolemia due to a complex interaction of multiple genetic factors and environmental factors, i.e., polygenic hypercholesterolemia. The cause of the hypercholesterolemia is unknown, but it is likely due to the convergence of several subtle alterations that affect regulation of LDL levels. Differences may exist in dietary responsiveness to cholesterol and saturated fat, differences in regulation of cholesterol and/or bile acid biosynthesis, and/or differences in regulation of LDL receptor activity and in the secretion and intravascular catabolism of apo B-containing lipoproteins.

FAMILIAL HYPERALPHALIPOPROTEINEMIA. Occasionally, patients are seen who have mildly elevated total cholesterol levels due to elevated HDL cholesterol. They usually have normal levels of LDL and VLDL. In these individuals the elevated HDL cholesterol level is genetic, and in some families it is inherited as an autosomal dominant trait. In other families the etiology appears to be polygenic. High levels of HDL can also be seen with chronic alcoholism, in response to estrogen administration, and after exposure to chlorinated hydrocarbon pesticides. In some families a genetic deficiency of CETP is associated with strikingly elevated HDL cholesterol levels, especially in Japanese populations. Individuals with hyperalphalipoproteinemia do not have any unusual clinical features, and they have been reported to have slightly increased longevity due to a decreased incidence of CAD.

Hyperlipoproteinemias Resulting Primarily in Hypertriglyceridemia

LIPOPROTEIN LIPASE DEFICIENCY AND APO C-II DEFICIENCY. LPL deficiency is a rare autosomal recessive trait that is characterized by the absence of active LPL in all tissues, leading to massive hypertriglyceridemia from birth and the clinical consequences of eruptive xanthoma and episodes of pancreatitis. This same clinical syndrome may also occur with deficiency of apo C-II, an obligatory activator of LPL, though clinical manifestations tend to occur later in life.

In infants and young children with LPL deficiency, the hypertriglyceridemia results primarily from chylomicron accumulation, while impairment of VLDL triglyceride removal becomes more important in later life. Homozygosity for LPL deficiency or for apo C-II deficiency is necessary for this disorder to occur. Heterozygosity for LPL deficiency may lead to moderate hypertriglyceridemia and may be one factor in the etiology of FCH. Infants with homozygous LPL deficiency have massive hypertriglyceridemia and grossly lipemic serum. They frequently fail to thrive and have severe abdominal pain and pancreatitis as a consequence of their marked hyperchylomicronemia. Eruptive xanthomas can occur on the extensor surfaces, notably on the elbows, knees, back, and buttocks but can occur elsewhere, and when seen are pathognomonic for chylomicronemia. Hepatomegaly is frequent, as is splenomegaly, which occurs because of the accumulation of lipid-laden foam cells. LPL activity can be measured by assaying plasma after injection of heparin, which releases LPL into plasma. Apo C-II levels can be assayed by immunoassay. The clinical manifestations will rapidly disappear with elimination of fat from the diet, which leads to elimination of the chylomicronemia. With effective fat restriction, plasma triglyceride levels can usually be maintained between 500 and 800 mg per deciliter or lower, and at this level, episodes of eruptive xanthoma, abdominal pain, and pancreatitis can usually be avoided. Substances that increase endogenous VLDL output, such as alcohol and glucocorticoids, must be avoided. With effective attention to diet, individuals can grow and easily reach adulthood without difficulty. There is no indication that any increased risk for atherosclerosis exists in this disorder.

FAMILIAL HYPERTRIGLYCERIDEMIA. Individuals with this condition have marked hypertriglyceridemia, normal to low LDL levels, and marked decreases in HDL cholesterol levels. When studied in detail, the number of VLDL particles is relatively normal, but they are triglyceride enriched. LPL-related triglyceride removal and remnant removal appears to be normal. HDL particle number is also relatively normal, but the triglyceride content in the HDL, which is normally very low, is considerably increased at the expense of cholesterol. The underlying defect in this disorder is postulated to be enhanced hepatic triglyceride synthesis. This disorder has been defined as an autosomal dominant trait that is quite common. There is some controversy about the association of this disorder with CAD. These patients are usually detected only because of routine lipid screening, or occasionally as a result of complications of marked hypertriglyceridemia. They do not have xanthomas unless there is chylomicronemia. Affected individuals usually have hypertriglyceridemia in adulthood, and they appear to be unusually sensitive to factors that are known to be associated with hypertriglyceridemia such as diabetes, obesity, excess alcohol consumption, or use of estrogen, diuretics, glucocorticoids, or β-adrenergic blockers, which can greatly exaggerate the degree of hypertriglyceridemia and even precipitate the chylomicronemia syndrome. Although the reasoning is somewhat circular, most experts would not treat individuals with isolated hypertriglyceridemia, e.g., triglyceride levels of 250 to 500 per deciliter, if they come from families without evidence of increased atherosclerosis.

Hyperlipoproteinemias Resulting in Mixed or Combined Hyperlipidemia

DYSBETALIPOPROTEINEMIA. Dysbetalipoproteinemia, also known as broad-beta or type III hyperlipoproteinemia, is a condition in which there is abnormal accumulation of cholesterol-rich IDL-type particles, commonly termed β-VLDL. This disorder is due to interaction of (1) an autosomal recessive defect in apo E that leads to abnormal remnant catabolism and (2) an independent aggravating environmental factor (e.g., obesity, diabetes, pregnancy) or genetic factor (FCH) leading to overproduction of apo B-containing lipoproteins. The combination of these two factors leads to accumulation of IDL-like particles (resulting from impaired VLDL catabolism) and remnants (resulting from impaired chylomicron metabolism) that lead to xanthomas, peripheral vascular disease, and CAD.

There are three major alleles for apo E, differing from each other by a single amino acid substitution at one or two sites. These are termed E_2, E_3, and E_4. An individual can be homozygous for any of these alleles, or heterozygous for any combination. The apo E encoded by the E_2 allele has sharply reduced ability to bind to lipoprotein receptors. Individuals homozygous for this allele (i.e., E_2/E_2 homozygotes), who compose about 2% of the population, have a relative defect in IDL and remnant catabolism. This can lead to relative accumulation in plasma of cholesteryl-ester–rich IDL and chylomicron remnant particles (β-VLDL) and corresponding decrease in LDL levels because of defective conversion of VLDL to LDL (see Fig. 173–1). Yet, in the absence of aggravating factors, total plasma cholesterol levels are actually low in such individuals and triglyceride levels are normal. However, in an estimated 1 of 100 individuals with E_2/E_2 homozygosity, there is also an associated condition leading to overproduction of VLDL. This combination results in the absolute accumulation of β-VLDL particles, which are atherogenic when present in excess. This is expressed as marked hypertriglyceridemia and hypercholesterolemia. Normally, VLDL particles have "pre-β" mobility on agarose gel electrophoresis, but the VLDL remnants in dysbetalipoproteinemia are much closer to LDL in composition and therefore have "β" mobility ("β-VLDL"). Hence, the designation *dysbetalipoproteinemia*. Because individuals who are homozygous for the E_2 allele will have low levels of such qualitatively abnormal VLDL present in plasma even when total lipids are normal (or even low), some experts use the term dysbetalipoproteinemia to refer to the condition of homozygosity for E_2, while the term type III hyperlipoproteinemia or broad-beta syndrome is reserved for those individuals with associated hyperlipidemia. The type III hyperlipoproteinemia phenotype can also be caused by total absence of apo E, which has been observed in rare families.

If VLDL is not overproduced, there are no clinical manifestations. However, when overproduction of VLDL occurs, marked hyperlipidemia appears, and this disorder may present as premature clinical atherosclerosis with peripheral vascular disease and/or CAD. The presence of hypothyroidism has been noted frequently in individuals with clinical symptoms. These patients frequently have highly characteristic planar xanthomas in the creases of the palms as well as tuberous or tuberoeruptive xanthomas on the elbows or knees that are virtually diagnostic for this disorder. Occasionally these manifestations can be seen with obstructive liver disease. Although the apo E abnormality is present from birth, it is unusual to see hyperlipidemia in a male younger than age 30 and in a female before menopause. The presence of hypertriglyceridemia accompanied by unusual degrees of hypercholesterolemia when associated with palmar or tuberous xanthomas is highly suggestive of this disorder. Liver disease and hypothyroidism need to be excluded. Electrophoresis of a VLDL fraction of plasma will reveal particles of beta mobility, rather than the typical pre-β mobility. The E_2 isoforms can be identified by isoelectric focusing in specialty laboratories, and genotyping is also available. The concentration of LDL is typically low even in hyperlipidemic patients, and a normal or elevated LDL level should make one consider an alternative diagnosis. HDL levels are normal or slightly decreased, depending on the degree of hypertriglyceridemia.

In many E_2/E_2 adults with clinical manifestations of hyperlipidemia, there is associated obesity, and weight reduction is of primary importance. In postmenopausal women, low-dose estrogen replacement frequently normalizes the abnormal lipoprotein profile and corrects the hyperlipidemia. All patients should be checked for mild degrees of hypothyroidism using sensitive TSH assays; if hypothyroidism is present, treatment may frequently completely normalize the lipoprotein profile. Gemfibrozil is frequently effective in decreasing lipid levels in these individuals; high-dose nicotinic acid may also be useful. Use of an HMG-CoA reductase inhibitor has been found to be quite successful in reducing the hypercholesterolemia and, when combined with low-dose gemfibrozil, has frequently normalized triglyceride levels in severe cases.

FAMILIAL COMBINED HYPERLIPIDEMIA. Among patients with myocardial infarction, a significant number have an apparently dominantly inherited pattern of hyperlipoproteinemia that is expressed by a variable lipoprotein phenotype. Thus, individuals may have increased levels of VLDL, or LDL, or both lipoproteins.

Some first-degree relatives have elevated VLDL levels, some have elevated LDL, and some have both. This entity appears to be monogenic and inherited in an autosomal dominant manner and has been termed familial combined hyperlipidemia (FCH) or familial multiple lipoprotein-type hyperlipidemia. The lipoprotein phenotype is not stable over time. A person can have VLDL elevations noted on one visit but marked increases in LDL, or both VLDL and LDL, at another visit. While there remains much uncertainty about classification of this disorder, all clinicians seeing patients with premature CAD recognize the frequency of this pattern. A characteristic of this disorder is increased accumulation of small LDL particles, which are cholesterol depleted. Thus, patients may have a relatively normal "LDL cholesterol" level, yet the number of LDL particles is increased and therefore the LDL-apo B level is increased. Some investigators have termed this condition familial hyper*apo*betalipoproteinemia. Most evidence suggests that the underlying defect is increased hepatic secretion of VLDL. These VLDL appear to be smaller than normal, with less triglyceride per particle. Undoubtedly this disorder represents several different genetic traits interacting with the basic defect–overproduction of VDL. For example, overproduction of VLDL may become manifested primarily as elevations in VLDL if a relative or absolute defect in VLDL catabolism occurs in addition, as for example, with relative deficiency in LPL activity. Recently, a number of cases of heterozygous LPL deficiency have been found in association with this phenotype. Conversely, in the face of appropriate VLDL and IDL catabolism, LDL may accumulate because of the increased rate of generation of LDL and/or functional disturbances in LDL catabolic mechanisms. These individuals also typically have low levels of HDL with decreases in both HDL cholesterol and apo A-I.

This phenotype is associated with a clinical constellation that includes mild abdominal obesity, insulin resistance, mild hypertension, elevated VLDL levels, the presence of an excess number of small dense LDL, and decreased HDL. This syndrome has been referred to as the insulin-resistance syndrome or syndrome X (see Ch. 205). This disorder is more typically seen in men and is associated with a strikingly high rate of premature CAD. The effect of other risk factors appears to be greatly exaggerated in these individuals, and a history of smoking is frequently found in those with early CAD. Patients do not have any characteristic xanthomas, and the diagnosis is made by a characteristic family history that is unusually positive for early CAD, by documentation of the variable lipoprotein phenotype, and, if possible, by lipoprotein phenotyping of first-degree relatives. Women may also be affected by this phenotype, although the clinical manifestations of CAD appear to be expressed later in life. Because this disorder is associated with a high risk of premature CAD, vigorous efforts should be made to lower lipoprotein levels of affected individuals. Nicotinic acid may be quite efficacious in some individuals in lowering VLDL and raising HDL levels. Other regimens include the use of an HMG-CoA reductase inhibitor alone or in combination with gemfibrozil. The use of gemfibrozil alone to lower VLDL levels will often be highly effective but is almost always associated with significant rises in LDL.

OTHER FORMS OF HYPERTRIGLYCERIDEMIA. Mild hypertriglyceridemia is one of the most commonly encountered hyperlipidemias. Although many patients with hypertriglyceridemia will fit into one of the categories noted above, there are many other patients with triglyceride levels of 400 to 2000 mg per deciliter who do not seem to fall into any of those categories. They may have a family history of hypertriglyceridemia and/or quite commonly have one of the secondary forms of hypertriglyceridemia, such as that due to excess alcohol use or diabetes mellitus. Frequently, treating the underlying cause will ameliorate the hypertriglyceridemia, but often a milder form remains, probably indicative of an underlying as yet undefined genetic defect.

ACQUIRED DISORDERS OF LIPOPROTEIN METABOLISM

Many medical conditions are associated with mild or even severe hyperlipidemia in the absence of underlying genetic hyperlipoproteinemia. With underlying genetic hyperlipidemia, acquired disorders can lead to greatly exaggerated effects on lipoprotein levels. Table 173–3 lists disorders commonly associated with changes in lipoprotein levels.

TABLE 173-3. ACQUIRED DISORDERS OF LIPOPROTEIN METABOLISM

Hypercholesterolemia
Nephrotic syndrome
Hypothyroidism
Dysgammaglobulinemia
Acute intermittent porphyria
Obstructive liver disease

Combined Hyperlipidemia
Nephrotic syndrome
Hypothyroidism
Glucocorticoid excess/Cushing's disease
Diuretics
Uncontrolled diabetes

Hypertriglyceridemia
Diabetes mellitus
Uremia
Sepsis
Obesity
Systemic lupus erythematosus
Dysgammaglobulinemia
Glycogen storage disease, type I
Lipodystrophy
Drugs
  Alcohol
  Estrogens
  β-Adrenergic blocking agents
  Isotretinoin (13-*cis*-retinoic acid)

DIABETES MELLITUS (see Ch. 205). Persons with untreated insulin-dependent diabetes, as well as uncontrolled non–insulin-dependent diabetes, frequently have hypertriglyceridemia, low HDL levels, and associated small dense LDL particles. These individuals appear to have low adipose tissue or muscle LPL activity that leads to relative impairment in VLDL clearance. Although LDL levels are not absolutely elevated in these individuals as a rule, for the degree of hypertriglyceridemia, the LDL levels are higher than expected. In part, this may be due to nonenzymatic glycosylation of the LDL particle caused by hyperglycemia as well as by down-regulation of LDL receptors because of insulin lack.

CHRONIC UREMIA AND DIALYSIS (see Ch. 78.1). Many individuals with chronic uremia have elevated VLDL levels with associated hypertriglyceridemia and low HDL cholesterol levels. This condition persists even after initiation of maintenance hemodialysis or peritoneal dialysis. These lipoprotein abnormalities are related to defects in LPL-mediated triglyceride removal and/or associated overproduction.

ALCOHOL AND OTHER DRUGS. Among the many associated factors that cause mild degrees of hypertriglyceridemia, alcohol consumption is probably the most common; it increases triglyceride levels in most individuals. This occurs because both fatty acid synthesis and VLDL output are stimulated, and LPL activity is inhibited. In individuals with normal baseline VLDL levels this is not usually a problem, but in those in whom there is excess VLDL secretion or some other additional basis for impairment in VLDL clearance, marked hypertriglyceridemia ensues with alcohol use. Diuretic agents and β-adrenergic blocking agents are also frequently associated with mild increases in triglyceride levels in patients with no underlying abnormality in lipoprotein metabolism but with quite marked increases in those with underlying hypertriglyceridemia. In individuals with genetic hypertriglyceridemia or FCH, estrogen use may also lead to marked increases in VLDL levels. Hypertriglyceridemia occurs in 25% of people given isotretinoin (13-*cis*-retinoic acid) for cystic acne.

HYPOTHYROIDISM (see Ch. 203). Thyroid hormone is crucial in many steps of lipoprotein metabolism. LDL receptor activity is particularly sensitive to thyroxine levels, and in hypothyroidism LDL levels are elevated because of down-regulation of LDL receptor number. In addition, LPL activity is low, leading to elevated VLDL levels and even, rarely, chylomicronemia, especially in subjects with dysbetalipoproteinemia.

NEPHROTIC SYNDROME (see Ch. 79). With massive proteinuria and with hypoalbuminemia, a compensatory increase occurs in overall hepatic protein synthesis, and in particular there is

marked increase in VLDL output. An associated defect in VLDL catabolism is also seen, in part due to depressed LPL activity.

HYPERLIPOPROTEINEMIA AND ATHEROSCLEROSIS

The etiology of atherosclerosis is multifactorial; a more general discussion of its pathogenesis can be found in Ch. 40. However, the cause-and-effect relationship between hypercholesterolemia and atherosclerosis has been proved in a large number of animal model studies and by large randomized, double-blind clinical intervention trials. Reducing plasma LDL cholesterol levels sharply reduces the risk of subsequent clinical CAD in both patients with pre-existing CAD and in patients free of CAD at the beginning of the study. In studies extending over 5 to 7 years, morbidity and mortality from new coronary events have been reduced by as much as 20 to 40%. A statistically significant decrease in *total* mortality was also seen in two large studies, the Coronary Drug Project (in the group of men treated with nicotinic acid) and in a recent Scandinavian trial using an HMG-CoA reductase inhibitor to lower plasma cholesterol levels. Angiographic studies have documented that intensive cholesterol-lowering regimens slow progression of coronary lesions: In some cases there has even been significant regression of lesions. Plasma triglyceride levels also correlate very significantly with risk of CAD, but the interpretation of this correlation is less clear, as elevation of triglyceride levels is frequently associated with other factors that may be more immediately relevant to the increase in CAD risk. The atherogenicity of individual lipoprotein classes is discussed below.

CHYLOMICRONS AND VLDL. Almost no evidence exists that chylomicrons are proatherogenic, and they are probably too large to penetrate into the artery. VLDL may also be too large, but CAD risk correlates with hypertriglyceridemia almost as well as it does with hypercholesterolemia in the fasting state and most of the triglycerides in plasma are carried in VLDL. This correlation may be explained by the frequent association of hypertriglyceridemia with obesity, low HDL levels, small, dense LDL, and diabetes mellitus. More likely is the possibility that the catabolic products of VLDL, the IDL, are atherogenic. Indeed, in hyperlipidemic patients with dysbetalipoproteinemia, the lipoprotein that accumulates is a type of IDL—so-called β-VLDL. Such patients are at increased risk of atherosclerosis and its complications. Moreover, the lipoprotein class that accumulates in experimental animals fed a high-fat, high-cholesterol diet is predominantly the same sort of β-VLDL.

LDL. There is no doubt about the atherogenicity of LDL. Patients with FH have strikingly premature atherosclerosis. However, in addition to greatly increased LDL, they also have some increase in IDL. Yet patients with a mutation of apo B that reduces its affinity for the LDL receptor accumulate *only* LDL, and their risk of premature CAD at any given plasma cholesterol level appears to be just as great as that of patients with LDL receptor deficiency. Increasing evidence suggests that oxidative modification of LDL within the artery is important, if not obligatory, for mediating the atherogenicity of LDL. Much evidence has been obtained that oxidized LDL is formed in the artery wall. Products of oxidized LDL may contribute to atherogenesis by many mechanisms, including attracting monocytes to the lesion and facilitating their conversion into macrophages. In turn, macrophages express scavenger receptors that take up oxidized LDL, leading to foam cells and the fatty streak lesion. In addition, products of oxidized LDL are toxic, producing endothelial damage and initiation of thrombosis. Treatment with antioxidants has been shown to slow the progress of atherosclerosis in several animal models, but similar data are not yet available in humans.

HDL. A wealth of epidemiologic evidence establishes that a high level of plasma HDL is associated with a lower risk of CHD. Until recently it was not certain whether the protective effect of a high HDL level was referable to a direct effect of the HDL or whether it represented a "marker" for some other factor. Studies in transgenic mice have now shown that increasing HDL reduces the susceptibility of these mice to atherosclerosis. It is widely believed that HDL protects against atherosclerosis by facilitating reverse cholesterol transport, i.e., the ability of HDL to accept excess cholesterol from tissues and return it to the liver, either directly or via other lipoproteins, but this has not been explicitly proved.

Lp(a). An increased risk for CAD has been found in many populations in association with increased levels of Lp(a), in particular when elevated levels of LDL are also present. However, Lp(a) appears to be an independent risk factor. Lp(a) is an LDL particle to which an additional large protein, termed apo (a), is attached via a disulfide bond. There are many different allelic forms of apo (a) protein, varying widely in molecular size and determined in large part by genetic factors. Apo (a) has high homology to plasminogen, but lacks the catalytically active site. Speculation has centered on the possibility that it interferes with plasminogen binding to its receptors and thus inhibits plasmin formation and thrombolysis. Alternatively, Lp(a) may have increased binding to the extracellular matrix of the artery, leading to greater deposition of the associated LDL. To date, no effective therapy has been found to lower elevated Lp(a) levels.

PRACTICAL MANAGEMENT OF HYPERLIPIDEMIA

TREATMENT OF HYPERCHOLESTEROLEMIA. Irrespective of the cause of elevated LDL levels, patients are usually managed similarly. In almost all cases, lowering LDL levels is achieved first by dietary intervention and then, if necessary, by adding drug therapy. Because the LDL receptor plays such an important role in regulating plasma LDL levels, therapy is aimed at achieving maximal expression of hepatic LDL receptor activity. Dietary cholesterol and saturated fat both lead to suppression of hepatic LDL receptor activity, and therefore reduction of these dietary components leads to up-regulation of hepatic LDL receptors and lowered plasma cholesterol levels. Individuals heterozygous for FH are more restricted in their response, and generally even stringent diets lower their LDL levels by no more than 5 to 10% below baseline levels. However, all individuals should be instructed in these diets, because some are unusually responsive.

Regulation of hepatic LDL receptor activity also appears to underlie mechanisms by which many commonly used hyperlipidemic drugs affect plasma cholesterol levels. As shown in Figure 173–4, the hepatocyte is the primary site of cholesterol synthesis. The cholesterol made by this cell is either excreted into plasma in the form of VLDL or is converted into bile acids, which are released into the intestine in response to meals. Normally, >95% of bile acids are reabsorbed and transported to the liver via the enterohepatic circulation and recycled through the liver up to six to seven times per day. Bile acid–binding resins work by binding bile acids in the intestine and promoting their subsequent loss in the stool. This prevents reabsorption and results in depletion of hepatic bile acid pools. In response, the hepatocyte actually increases cholesterol (and triglyceride) synthesis, as well as compensatory bile acid synthesis to replete the depleted bile acid pool. Despite this enhanced cholesterol synthesis, it is not sufficient to compensate for depletion of some crucial intracellular sterol pool, and the hepatocyte responds by also increasing LDL receptor expression. In turn, this directly removes LDL particles (or their precursors) from circulation. In this way, a nonsystemic agent leads to enhanced removal of plasma LDL particles and lowered plasma cholesterol levels. Very likely the soluble dietary fibers, such as oat bran, also lower plasma cholesterol by binding bile acids in a similar manner. For many individuals, this degree of plasma cholesterol lowering is sufficient.

However, in others the enhanced cholesterol (and triglyceride) synthesis leads to enhanced VLDL synthesis and release, and in effect, negates in part the cholesterol-lowering effect. In fact, many patients develop a transient or even permanent increase of plasma triglycerides (VLDL) in response to bile sequestrant therapy, even as LDL levels are lowered. This enhanced production of VLDL leads to generation of more LDL, which offsets in part the enhanced LDL removal, leading to suboptimal lowering of LDL levels. For this reason, a second agent, in combination with a bile sequestrant, is frequently used and leads to synergistic lowering of LDL levels. For example, nicotinic acid, which effectively inhibits release of lipoproteins from the liver, is quite effective when combined with a bile acid–binding resin. Even more effective is the use of an HMG-CoA reductase inhibitor. This class of drugs, which have been termed statins, directly inhibits cholesterol biosynthesis and as a result not only inhibits the production of new lipoproteins but also, by apparently depleting still further specific hepatic sterol pools, leads to maximal expression of hepatic LDL receptor activity (see Fig. 173–4). This effect is greatly enhanced when used in combination with a bile acid–binding resin and can lower LDL levels by >50%. If these two drugs are combined with nicotinic acid as a third agent, LDL levels can be lowered by as much as 70% or more.

WHOM TO TREAT. The definition of hypercholesterolemia has been undergoing marked changes in recent years as it has become clear that "ideal" or "optimal" cholesterol levels are quite different from "normal" levels, which have been arbitrarily defined as values below the 90th or 95th percentile of the bell-shaped curve of the general population. The expert panel of the National Cholesterol Education Program (NCEP) has recommended specific desirable blood cholesterol levels for the population as a whole (Table 173–4). Many experts have argued that any plasma cholesterol level above 160 to 180 mg per deciliter is above *ideal* values, such as those found in the Japanese, for example, who have a low incidence of CAD. Unfortunately the vast majority of people in the United States have plasma cholesterol levels that are far above this ideal. For this reason, there is an intensive ongoing effort to educate the general public as to appropriate dietary guidelines to lower plasma cholesterol levels.

It should be appreciated that these cutoff points are appropriate for the population as a whole, but assessment of appropriate cholesterol levels for any given patient must take into account the presence of other risk factors. Although many individuals with very high plasma cholesterol levels clearly are at increased risk for CAD (see Ch. 41), most patients who develop CAD actually have total and LDL cholesterol levels that would place them in the borderline or, not infrequently, even below the borderline category. Thus, individuals with hypertension, smoking history, obesity, or diabetes are clearly at increased risk at any given plasma cholesterol level. Individuals with low levels of HDL (i.e., <35 mg per deciliter) are also at significantly increased risk. A strong family history of heart disease is highly predictive of those individuals who are at increased risk. Finally, for patients who have existing CAD and, in particular, for those who have already undergone coronary artery bypass graft or other types of intervention, the cholesterol levels listed above are probably still too high. Achievement of ideal plasma cholesterol levels (i.e., 160 mg per deciliter) is probably more appropriate. Studies in experimental animals and data from clinical trials show that the greater the reduction in plasma cholesterol levels, the greater the clinical benefit achieved.

The NCEP has devised a protocol for screening and management of blood cholesterol in the general population. It is recommended that plasma total cholesterol levels should be measured in all adults over age 20 at least once every 5 years. HDL cholesterol should be measured at the same time whenever possible. These measurements may be made in the nonfasting state. In individuals free of CAD,

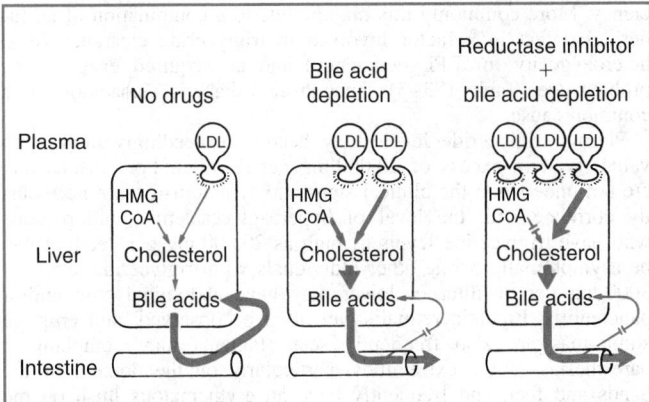

FIGURE 173–4. Mechanisms by which a bile acid–binding resin and an HMG CoA-reductase inhibitor lower plasma LDL levels (From Brown MS, Goldstein JL: A receptor-mediated pathway for cholesterol homeostasis. Science 232:34, 1986. Copyright 1986 by the American Association for the Advancement of Science.)

TABLE 173–4. BLOOD CHOLESTEROL LEVELS

(mg per dl)	Desirable	Borderline	High
Total blood cholesterol	<200	200–239 (borderline high)	>240
LDL	<130	130–159	>160

total cholesterol levels are classified into desirable, borderline, and high levels. It should be appreciated that the cutoff point that defines high blood cholesterol, 240 mg per deciliter, is a value that represents the top 20th percentile of the U.S. adult population and corresponds to a value at which risk for CHD rises more steeply. Similarly, an HDL-cholesterol level < 35 mg per deciliter is defined as low and represents an independent risk factor. For individuals with desirable blood cholesterol levels (< 200 mg per deciliter) the level of HDL cholesterol determines the appropriate follow-up. Those with HDL cholesterol levels > 35 mg per deciliter are advised about dietary modification, physical activity, and other risk-reduction activities and to have repeat determinations of total and HDL cholesterol levels in 5 years. Those with HDL cholesterol levels < 35 and/or those who have two or more risk factors should have a formal lipoprotein analysis in the fasting state. These risk factors include man > 45 years, woman > 55 years or premature menopause not taking estrogen, a positive family history of premature CAD, history of smoking, hypertension, diabetes, obesity, and an HDL cholesterol level below 35 mg per deciliter. The lipoprotein analysis includes measurement of fasting levels of total cholesterol, total triglyceride, and HDL cholesterol. From these values, LDL cholesterol is calculated as follows:

$$LDL\ cholesterol = Total\ cholesterol - HDL\ cholesterol - (triglycerides/5).$$

Further classification is based on LDL values: LDL cholesterol levels < 130 mg per deciliter are defined as desirable; those 130 to 159 mg per deciliter as borderline high-risk; and those >160 mg per deciliter as high-risk LDL cholesterol levels. Patients with desirable LDL cholesterol levels can be provided education about general dietary habits and risk factor modification. Patients with borderline elevated levels and with fewer than two risk factors can similarly be given dietary instruction with re-evaluation annually. Patients with borderline LDL elevations and two or more risk factors should undergo thorough evaluation, receive dietary therapy, and be considered for drug therapy if they fail to respond. Finally, individuals with high-risk LDL cholesterol levels, > 160 mg per deciliter, should have a thorough evaluation to rule out any secondary causes and the presence of a familial lipoprotein disorder and then should begin dietary therapy. Presently the American Heart Association step I or step II diets, which restrict dietary saturated fat and cholesterol, should be prescribed to all individuals with greater than desirable cholesterol levels. This diet is safe for a wide spectrum of individuals, from those as young as age 2 years to the elderly, and usually works best when followed by the whole family.

The NCEP guidelines suggest that all patients with existing CAD have a formal lipoprotein analysis. If LDL cholesterol levels are < 100 mg per deciliter, patients should receive individual instruction on diet and risk-factor reduction. If LDL cholesterol levels are > 100 mg per deciliter, patients should be instructed on an appropriate diet and be considered for drug therapy. The therapeutic goal for treatment of hypercholesterolemia is listed in Table 173–5. The decision to initiate drug therapy for elevated LDL cholesterol levels should be considered in most patients only after the individual has been on a diet for 3 to 6 months. In general, a young or middle-aged adult who has been on such a diet, yet continues to have LDL cholesterol levels > 190 mg per deciliter is a candidate for drug therapy even in the absence of other risk factors. Individuals with existing CAD or those who have high LDL cholesterol levels of 160 to 190 mg per deciliter and other risk factors are also candidates for drug therapy, including an HMG-CoA reductase inhibitor, bile acid–binding resins, and nicotinic acid.

The statin class of drugs, which are being used increasingly as primary therapy, lower LDL levels by 25 to 35%. Combinations of a statin and a bile acid–binding resin are also highly efficacious, and LDL lowering of > 50% can frequently be achieved. They have now been in use for more than 10 years with practically no serious side effects. A myositis-like picture has been rarely associated with their use, particularly when combined with nicotinic acid, gemfibrozil, or rarely, with erythromycin. This appears as muscle pain and is associated with increases in muscle creatine kinase (creatine phosphokinase; [CPK]). Rarely, frank rhabdomyolysis has occurred. This side effect has been seen particularly in transplant patients treated with cyclosporine. Abnormalities in liver function tests oc-

TABLE 173–5. THERAPEUTIC GOAL FOR TREATMENT OF HYPERCHOLESTEROLEMIA

Therapeutic Goal LDL cholesterol (mg per dl)	Patient Categories
< 130	Moderate risk for CAD
	Patients with no family history of CAD and no other CAD risk factors
	Young adults with familial hypercholesterolemia
	Adults with familial hypercholesterolemia and no other risk factors
< 100	High risk for CAD
	With family history of CAD or two or more CAD risk factors
	Adult familial hypercholesterolemia patients with family history of CAD or one or more risk factors
	Individual with existing CAD
	Individual after CABG
	Individual with low HDL cholesterol and family history of CAD

LDL = low-density lipoprotein; HDL = high-density lipoprotein; CAD = coronary artery disease; CABG = coronary artery bypass graft surgery.

cur occasionally, but frequently when this occurs there is associated excess alcohol use. CPK levels should be measured prior to the start of statin therapy to obtain baseline levels, at bimonthly intervals during initial use of therapy, and semiannually after that.

TREATMENT OF MILD HYPERTRIGLYCERIDEMIA. The NCEP guidelines do not directly address the issue of hypertriglyceridemia. As noted above, the link between triglycerides and CAD is complex and may be explained by associations between high triglyceride and low HDL levels and atherogenic forms of LDL. Patients with milder degrees of hypertriglyceridemia should be treated initially with nonpharmacologic therapy. This should include weight reduction in overweight patients, increased physical activity, and low-fat diets. Alcohol should be restricted. Gemfibrozil lowers VLDL levels, but frequently there is an associated rise in LDL levels. Niacin has been used to both decrease VLDL and increase HDL. Many experts now use a statin as initial therapy for treating patients with familial combined hyperlipidemia. VLDL levels are lowered, HDL increases, and there is no increase in LDL. In some patients the combined use of gemfibrozil and a statin has been useful, but this combination may increase slightly the risk of myositis.

RECOGNITION AND TREATMENT OF MARKED HYPERTRIGLYCERIDEMIA: THE CHYLOMICRONEMIA SYNDROME. Marked chylomicronemia with plasma triglyceride levels >1000 mg per deciliter is associated with a combination of signs and symptoms that has been termed the *chylomicronemia syndrome*. Prompt and effective therapy is indicated to prevent severe medical complications, including pancreatitis. This syndrome occurs whenever there is excess accumulation of chylomicrons. Rarely this occurs as a result of homozygous LPL deficiency, or apo C-II deficiency. More commonly this may be due to a combination of an inherited defect in a factor involved in triglyceride clearance (e.g., heterozygosity for LPL deficiency) and an acquired exacerbating problem (see Table 173–3). Uncontrolled diabetic ketoacidosis is a common cause.

Plasma triglyceride levels may become exceedingly high, with values well in excess of 20,000 mg per deciliter. For reasons that are not understood the clinical signs and symptoms do not necessarily correlate with the level of hypertriglyceridemia, and patients who have triglyceride levels as high as 20,000 mg per deciliter can be asymptomatic, while other individuals with triglyceride levels of 3000 mg per deciliter or lower may have abdominal pain and/or pancreatitis. Lipemia retinalis can often be observed, and eruptive xanthomas are also frequently seen. Patients may complain of paresthesias of the extremities, particularly on the dorsum of the hands and feet, and frequently have an erythematous flush on the face and chest. With marked hyperchylomicronemia, impairment of recent memory has been noted. Patients also may complain of symmetric arthralgia, although physical findings or joint involvement is not found. In diabetics, this syndrome may be associated with marked insulin resistance, marked hyperglycemia, and frequently diabetic ketoacidosis. Because of the marked hyperchylomicrone-mia, an increased proportion of the total blood volume is occupied by fat, and many routine laboratory tests will be invalid because fat is sampled as well as the water space. For example, hyponatremia is frequently seen in samples from hyperchylomicronemic subjects, but this is a "pseudo hyponatremia" that occurs because of inclusion of lipid in the aliquot of blood sampled, and lipid does not contain sodium. Simple removal of chylomicrons from plasma by a brief centrifugation step before laboratory tests can eliminate such artifacts. Frequently a false-negative test for amylase occurs in lipemic plasma, apparently due to an inhibitor of amylase activity.

The diagnosis is made by the presence of chylomicrons in fasting plasma, which will always appear milky. Plasma will usually appear turbid when plasma triglycerides are > 350 mg per deciliter, because of the excess accumulation of VLDL, and will appear grossly lipemic when triglycerides are > 1000 mg per deciliter. With extreme degrees of hypertriglyceridemia the whole blood takes on the appearance of cream of tomato soup, and plasma allowed to sit in a refrigerator overnight will develop a thick layer of chylomicrons on top. Since the major cause of hyperchylomicronemia is accumulation of dietary-induced fat, the treatment is absolute elimination of fat from the diet until triglyceride levels have fallen to a safe level. With associated pancreatitis, patients usually receive nothing orally, and in this setting plasma triglyceride levels will usually fall by 50% every 2 to 3 days. When refeeding begins, fat (of all kinds) must be totally avoided initially and then replaced very gradually.

RARE DISORDERS OF LIPOPROTEIN METABOLISM

There are a number of inherited disorders of lipoprotein metabolism that are rare but that have taught us a great deal about lipoprotein function. Patients with *hypobetalipoproteinemia* have mutations in one or both apo B alleles that lead to truncated apo B proteins. Because of defective synthesis and/or enhanced intravascular catabolism, there are markedly reduced levels of apo B–containing lipoproteins in plasma. Heterozygotes may have LDL cholesterol levels of ≤ 50 mg per deciliter, and rare compound heterozygotes may have LDL cholesterol levels of ≤ 5 mg per deciliter. Usually these patients are asymptomatic and long lived. Patients with the rare autosomal recessive disorder of *abetalipoproteinemia* have total inability to release apo B-48 from intestinal cells or apo B-100 from liver. They have a normal apo B gene, but lack a lipid transfer protein required for assembly of lipoproteins. Because they cannot make chylomicrons, they malabsorb fat and fat-soluble vitamins. They manifest ataxia, neuropathy, and retinitis pigmentosa and are responsive to high doses of vitamin E. Patients with *Tangier disease* have virtually no HDL in plasma, apparently because of abnormally rapid removal of HDL from plasma. This leads to generation of abnormal chylomicron remnants, which are stored as cholesteryl esters in phagocytic cells. Patients typically have enlarged, orange tonsils and develop corneal opacities and polyneuropathy. Premature atherosclerosis does not seem to occur. No therapy is indicated.

Patients with mutations in *cholesterol ester transfer protein* (CETP) have also recently been described, particularly in Japanese populations, and this is associated with cholesteryl ester enrichment of HDL and greatly elevated HDL cholesterol values, frequently > 100 mg per deciliter. Although not proven, it is generally believed that this mutation is associated with protection from CAD. In contrast, in patients with deficiency of *lecithin cholesterol acyltransferase* (LCAT), unesterified cholesterol accumulates in plasma and tissues, and patients may develop premature CAD. In addition, they have corneal opacities, hemolytic anemia, and early renal failure. Therapy consists of renal transplantation and fat-restricted diets. Two rare disorders leading to accumulation of abnormal sterols have also been described. Patients with *cerebrotendinous xanthomatosis* have defective bile acid synthesis with associated oversynthesis and accumulation of cholestanol and cholesterol in brain, tendons, and other tissues. They can have neurologic symptoms (including cerebellar ataxia and dementia), tendon xanthomas, atherosclerosis, and cataracts. Finally, patients may have large tendon xanthomas due to abnormal accumulation of plant sterols, chiefly β-sitosterol. Normally, plant sterols are not absorbed, but in patients with *sitosterolemia* there is unexplained intestinal absorption and accumulation of β-sitosterol in plasma and tendons. Treatment consists of diets low in plant sterols and cholesterol and the use of cholestyramine to promote gastrointestinal loss.

Breslow J: Familial disorders of high-density lipoprotein metabolism. *In* Scriver CR, Baudet AL, Sly WS, Valle D (eds.): The Metabolic and Molecular Basis of Inherited Disease. New York, McGraw-Hill, 1995, p. 2031. *Comprehensive overview of HDL metabolism.*
Brown MS, Goldstein JL: A receptor-mediated pathway for cholesterol homeostasis. Science 232:34, 1986. *Classic citation describing the LDL receptor pathway—this was the lecture delivered on the occasion of receipt of the Nobel Prize.*
Brunzell JD: Familial lipoprotein lipase deficiency and other causes of the chylomicronemia syndrome. *In* Scriver CR, Baudet AL, Sly WS, Valle D (eds.): The Metabolic and Molecular Basis of Inherited Disease. New York, McGraw-Hill, 1995, p. 1913. *Comprehensive description of disorders leading to accumulation of chylomicrons.*
Goldstein JL, Hobbs HH, Brown MS: Familial hypercholesterolemia. *In* Scriver CR, Baudet AL, Sly WS, Valle D (eds.): The Metabolic and Molecular Basis of Inherited Disease. New York, McGraw-Hill, 1995, p. 1981. *Comprehensive description of pathogenesis and clinical description of this important cause of hypercholesterolemia.*
Havel RJ, Kane JP: Introduction: Structure and metabolism of plasma lipoproteins. *In* Scriver CR, Baudet AL, Sly WS, Valle D (eds.): The Metabolic and Molecular Basis of Inherited Disease. New York, McGraw-Hill, 1995, p. 1841. *Excellent overview of lipoprotein metabolism.*
Kane JP, Havel RJ: Disorders of the biogenesis and secretion of lipoproteins containing the B-apolipoproteins. *In* Scriver CR, Baudet AL, Sly WS, Valle D (eds.): The Metabolic and Molecular Basis of Inherited Disease. New York, McGraw-Hill, 1995, p. 1853. *Comprehensive and current concepts of metabolism of apo B-containing lipoproteins.*
Mahley RW, Rall SC: Type III hyperlipoproteinemia (dysbetalipoproteinemia): The role of apolipoprotein E in normal and abnormal lipoprotein metabolism. *In* Scriver CR, Baudet AL, Sly WS, Valle D (eds.): The Metabolic and Molecular Basis of Inherited Disease. New York, McGraw-Hill, 1995, p. 1953. *Most comprehensive and up-to-date discussion of role of apo E in lipoprotein metabolism.*
Steinberg D, Olefsky JM: Hypercholesterolemia and Atherosclerosis: Pathogenesis and Prevention. New York, Churchill Livingstone, 1987. *Easy-to-read book covering both basic research and clinical aspects of lipoprotein metabolism and their relationship to atherosclerosis.*
Witztum JL, Steinberg D: The role of oxidized LDL in atherogenesis. J Clin Invest 88:1785, 1991. *Overview of hypothesis that oxidation of lipoproteins contributes to their atherogenicity.*

174 LYSOSOMAL STORAGE DISEASES

Margaret M. McGovern and Robert J. Desnick

The lysosomal storage diseases are a family of more than 30 disorders resulting from different defects in lysosomal function. Although most of these disorders are caused by the deficiency of a specific hydrolytic enzyme, others are due to impaired receptors or deficiencies of crucial cofactors or protective proteins. Prevalent among these disorders are Fabry's disease, Gaucher's disease, and Niemann-Pick disease, lipid storage diseases that result from mutations in specific genes that encode lipid-degrading enzymes. The respective enzymatic defects lead to the storage in lysosomes of specific lipids and their metabolites. All three of these disorders have later-onset forms that can present in adult life. In addition, Gaucher's disease and Niemann-Pick disease have severe, fatal infantile forms that are described briefly.

FABRY'S DISEASE

DEFINITION. Fabry's disease is an X-linked inborn error of glycosphingolipid metabolism characterized by angiokeratomas (telangiectatic skin lesions), hypohidrosis, corneal and lenticular opacities, acroparesthesias, and vascular disease of the kidney, heart, and/or brain. The disease has an estimated incidence of 1 in 40,000 males.

ETIOLOGY AND PATHOGENESIS. Fabry's disease is an X-linked recessive trait that is manifested in affected hemizygous males. Atypical hemizygous males with residual α-galactosidase A activity may be asymptomatic or have late-onset, mild disease manifestations primarily limited to the heart. Heterozygous females are usually asymptomatic or exhibit mild manifestations. The disease results from the deficient activity of a lysosomal hydrolase (Table 174–1). The course of the disease is more severe in affected males with blood group B or AB, since the blood group B substance also

TABLE 174–1. BIOCHEMICAL AND PHENOTYPIC CHARACTERISTICS OF LYSOSOMAL STORAGE DISEASES

	Deficiency	Accumulation	Accumulation Site	Resultant Complications
Fabry's	α-Galactosidase A	Primarily globotriaosylceramide	Lysosomes of vascular endothelial and smooth muscle cells	Ischemia, infarction
Gaucher's				
Type 1	Acid β-glucosidase	Primarily glucosylceramide	Macrophage-monocyte system	Infiltration of bone marrow, progressive hepatospleno-megaly, skeletal complications
Type 2	Acid β-glucosidase	Primarily glucosylceramide	Macrophage-monocyte system; CNS	Infiltration of bone marrow, progressive hepatospleno-megaly, skeletal complications, neurodegeneration
Type 3	Acid β-glucosidase	Primarily glucosylceramide	Macrophage-monocyte system; CNS	Progressive neurodegeneration
Niemann-Pick				
Type A	Acid sphingomyelinase	Sphingomyelin	Monocyte-macrophage system; CNS	Hepatosplenomegaly, no neurologic disease
Type B	Acid sphingomyelinase	Sphingomyelin	Monocyte-macrophage system	Progressive hepatosplenomegaly, infiltrative lung disease

accumulates as it is normally degraded by α-galactosidase A. The molecular basis of Fabry's disease has been identified for a number of patients (Table 174–2).

PATHOLOGY. Fabry's disease is characterized by marked deposition of globotriaosylceramide and related glycosphingolipids with terminal α-galactosyl moieties primarily in the plasma and in the lysosomes of endothelial, perithelial, and smooth muscle cells of blood vessels. These glycosphingolipid deposits also are prominent in epithelial cells of the cornea, in glomeruli and tubules of the kidney, in muscle fibers of the heart, and in ganglion cells of the dorsal roots and autonomic nervous system. The skin lesions are telangiectases. Capillaries, venules, and arterioles show pathologic lipid storage, and there is marked dilatation of the capillaries of the dermal papillae just below the epidermis. The larger lesions are usually located in the upper dermis, where they may produce elevation, flattening, or hypertrophy of the epithelium, with keratosis—hence the term angiokeratoma. Ultrastructurally the glycosphingolipid inclusions in lysosomes have a concentrically arranged lamellar or myelin-like structure.

CLINICAL MANIFESTATIONS. The angiokeratomas usually occur in childhood, which may lead to early diagnosis. They increase in size and number with age and range from barely visible to several millimeters in diameter. The lesions are punctate, dark red to blue-black, and flat or slightly raised. They do not blanch with pressure, and the larger ones may show slight hyperkeratosis. Characteristically the lesions are most dense between the umbilicus and knees, in the "bathing trunk area," but may occur anywhere, including the oral mucosa. The hips, thighs, buttocks, umbilicus, lower abdomen, scrotum, and glans penis are common sites, and there is a tendency toward bilateral symmetry. Variants without skin lesions have been described. Sweating is usually decreased or absent. Corneal opacities and characteristic lenticular lesions, observed in slit-lamp examination, are present in affected males as well as in about 70% of asymptomatic heterozygotes. Conjunctival and retinal vascular tortuosity are common and result from the systemic vascular involvement.

Pain is the most debilitating symptom in childhood and adolescence. Fabry crises, lasting from minutes to several days, consist of agonizing, burning pain in the hands and feet and proximal extremities and are usually associated with exercise, fatigue, and/or fever. These painful acroparesthesias usually become less frequent in the third and fourth decades of life, although in some men they may become more frequent and severe. Attacks of abdominal or flank pain may simulate appendicitis or renal colic.

With increasing age, the major morbid symptoms result from the progressive involvement of the vascular system. Early in the course of the disease, casts, red cells, and lipid inclusions with characteristic birefringent "Maltese crosses" appear in the urinary sediment. Proteinuria, isothenuria, and gradual deterioration of renal function and development of azotemia occur in the second to fourth decades of life. Cardiovascular findings may include hypertension, left ventricular hypertrophy, anginal chest pain, myocardial ischemia or infarction, and congestive heart failure. Mitral insufficiency is the most common valvular lesion. Abnormal electrocardiographic and echocardiographic findings are common. Cerebrovascular manifestations result primarily from multifocal small vessel involvement. Other features may include chronic bronchitis and dyspnea, lymphedema of the legs without hypoproteinemia, episodic diarrhea, osteoporosis, retarded growth, and delayed puberty. Death most often results from uremia or vascular disease of the heart or brain. Prior to hemodialysis or renal transplantation, the mean age at death for affected men was 41 years. Atypical male variants with residual α-galactosidase A activity who are asymptomatic or mildly affected have been described, and more recently, several patients with late-onset isolated cardiac or cardiopulmonary disease have been reported. These patients do not have the early classic manifestations. These "cardiac variants" have cardiomegaly, usually involving the left ventricular wall and interventricular septum, and electrocardiographic abnormalities consistent with cardiomyopathy. Others have had hypertrophic cardiomyopathy and/or myocardial infarctions.

DIAGNOSIS. The diagnosis in classically affected males is most readily made from the history of painful acroparesthesias, hypo-

TABLE 174–2. MOLECULAR GENETICS OF FABRY'S, GAUCHER'S, AND NIEMANN-PICK DISEASES

	Chromosome Assignment	Molecular Characteristics	Comments
Fabry's	Xq22	cDNA, entire genomic sequences, >50 mutant alleles known	Many mutations responsible for disease include amino acid substitutions, gene rearrangements, mRNA splicing defects
Gaucher's	1q21	cDNA, functional and pseudogenomic sequences, >35 mutant alleles known	4 mutations (N370S, L444P, 84insG, IVS2^{+1}) account for 90–95% of mutant alleles in Ashkenazi Jewish patients
Niemann-Pick			
Types A and B	11p15.1 to p15.4	cDNA, entire genomic sequence, >30 mutant alleles known	3 mutations account for >90% of mutant alleles in Ashkenazi Jewish patients with type A disease
Type C	Chromosome 18	—	Specific gene and nature of cholesterol defect unknown

cDNA = complimentary DNA; mRNA = messenger RNA.

hidrosis, the presence of characteristic skin lesions, and the observation of the characteristic corneal opacities and lenticular lesions. The disorder is often misdiagnosed as rheumatic fever, erythromelalgia, or neurosis. The skin lesions must be differentiated from the benign angiokeratomas of the scrotum (Fordyce's disease) or from angiokeratoma circumscriptum. Angiokeratomas identical to those of Fabry's disease have been reported in fucosidosis, aspartylglycosaminuria, late-onset GM$_1$ gangliosidosis, galactosialidosis, α-N-acetylgalactosaminidase deficiency, and sialidosis. The diagnosis of the mild cardiac variants should be considered in individuals with left ventricular hypertrophy and/or cardiomyopathy. The diagnosis of classic and variant cases is confirmed biochemically by markedly decreased α-galactosidase A activity in plasma, isolated leukocytes, or cultured fibroblasts or lymphoblasts.

Heterozygous females may have corneal opacities, isolated skin lesions, and intermediate activities of α-galactosidase A in plasma or cell sources. Rare female heterozygotes may have manifestations as severe as those in affected males. However, in asymptomatic at-risk females in families affected by Fabry's disease, optimal diagnosis should be by direct analysis of their family's specific mutation. Prenatal detection of affected males can be accomplished by demonstrating deficient α-galactosidase A activity or by detecting the family's specific gene mutation in chorionic villi obtained in the first trimester of pregnancy or in cultured amniocytes obtained by amniocentesis in the second trimester.

TREATMENT. Phenytoin and carbamazepine have been shown to decrease the frequency and severity of the chronic acroparesthesias and the periodic crises of excruciating pain. Otherwise, treatment of the disease complications is supportive and nonspecific. Renal transplantation and long-term hemodialysis have become life-saving procedures. Replacement therapy using partially purified human enzyme has proved to be biochemically effective in pilot trials; however, sufficient enzyme has not been available to evaluate the clinical effectiveness of long-term replacement therapy. The recent availability of the cDNA encoding human α-galactosidase A should permit the future expression of sufficient quantities of recombinantly produced, active enzyme for further trials of enzyme replacement therapy and future trials of gene therapy.

Desnick RJ, Ioannou YA, Eng CM: Fabry disease: α-Galactosidase deficiency and Schindler disease: α-N-acetylgalactosaminidase deficiency. *In* Scriver CR, Beaudet AL, Sly WS, Valle D (eds.): The Metabolic and Molecular Bases of Inherited Disease, 7th ed. New York, McGraw-Hill, 1995. *Definitive chapter describing clinical, pathologic, biochemical, and molecular manifestations of Fabry's disease with more than 400 references.*

Eng CM, Desnick RJ: Molecular basis of Fabry disease: Mutations and polymorphisms in the human α-galactosidase A gene. Hum Mutation 3:103, 1994. *Description of mutations in classic and variant cases.*

GAUCHER'S DISEASE

DEFINITION. Gaucher's disease is a lipid storage disease characterized by deposition of glucocerebroside in cells of the macrophage-monocyte system. There are three clinical subtypes delineated by the absence or presence and progression of neurologic involvement: Type 1 or the adult, non-neuronopathic form; type 2, the infantile or acute neuronopathic form; and type 3, the juvenile or Norrbotten form. All three subtypes are inherited as autosomal recessive traits. Type 1 disease is the most common lysosomal storage disease and the most prevalent genetic disorder among Ashkenazi Jewish individuals, with an incidence of about 1 in 1000 and a carrier frequency of about 1 in 16 to 18.

ETIOLOGY AND PATHOGENESIS. All three subtypes of Gaucher's disease result from deficient activity of a lysosomal hydrolase (Table 174–1). The molecular basis of Gaucher's disease has been identified for 90 to 95% of Ashkenazi Jewish patients (Table 174–2). Genotype/phenotype correlations have been noted for the different subtypes and may provide the molecular basis for the remarkable clinical variation in type 1 Gaucher's disease. Presumably the amount of residual enzymatic activity determines disease subtype and severity. For example, type 1 patients homozygous for the milder N370S mutation tend to have a later onset and milder course than patients with one N370S allele and another mutant allele. However, the wide variability in clinical presentation among Gaucher's disease patients cannot be fully explained by the underlying acid β-glucosidase mutations. The lesions causing the severe type 2 (infantile) disease express little, if any, enzymatic activity *in vitro*.

PATHOLOGY. The pathologic hallmark is the presence of the Gaucher cell in the macrophage-monocyte system, particularly in the bone marrow. These cells, which are 20 to 100 μm in diameter, have a characteristic wrinkled-paper appearance resulting from intracytoplasmic substrate deposition. These cells stain strongly positive with periodic acid–Schiff, and their presence in bone marrow and/or other tissues suggests the diagnosis (Fig. 174–1). The accumulated glycolipid, glucosylceramide, is derived primarily from the phagocytosis and degradation of senescent leukocytes and to a lesser extent erythrocyte membranes. Glycolipid storage results in organomegaly and pulmonary infiltration. Neuronal cell loss in patients with types 2 and 3 disease presumably results from accumulation of the cytotoxic glycolipid, glucosphingosine, in the brain due to the severe deficiency of acid β-glucosidase activity. Glucosylceramide accumulation in the bone marrow, liver, spleen, lungs, and kidney leads to pancytopenia, massive hepatosplenomegaly, diffuse infiltrative pulmonary disease, and nephropathy or glomerulonephritis. The progressive infiltration of Gaucher cells in the bone marrow causes thinning of the cortex, pathologic fractures, bone pain, bony infarcts, and osteopenia. Central nervous system (CNS) involvement occurs only in patients with types 2 and 3 disease.

CLINICAL MANIFESTATIONS. There is a broad spectrum of clinical expression among patients with type 1 disease, in part due to a combination of different mutant alleles. Onset of clinical manifestations occurs from early childhood to late adulthood with most seen by adolescence. At presentation, patients may have easy bruisability due to thrombocytopenia, chronic fatigue secondary to anemia, hepatomegaly with or without elevated liver function tests, splenomegaly, and bone pain or pathologic fractures. Occasional patients have pulmonary involvement. Patients whose disease is diagnosed in the first 5 years of life are frequently non-Jewish and typically have a more malignant disease course. Patients with milder disease are discovered later in life during evaluations for hemato-

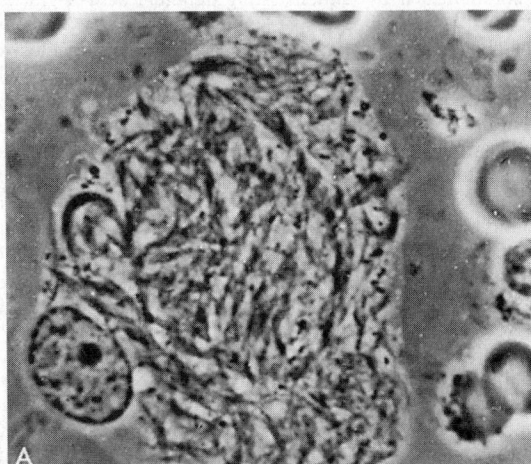
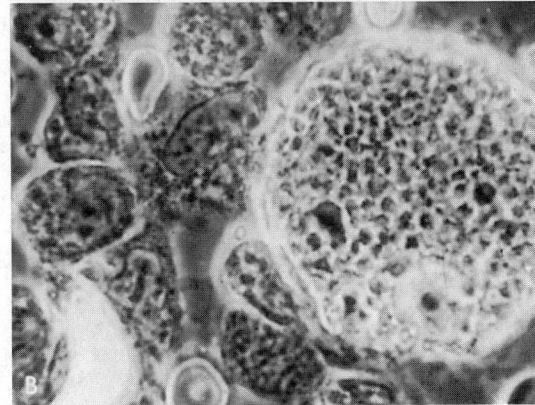

FIGURE 174–1. Typical Gaucher cell *(A)* and a foam cell seen in Niemann-Pick disease *(B)*. Both are viewed under phase microscopy in unstained smears of aspirated bone marrow. Magnification can be estimated from adjacent red cells.

logic or skeletal problems or are found to have splenomegaly on routine examinations. In symptomatic patients, splenomegaly is progressive and can become massive. Clinically apparent bony involvement, which occurs in >20% of patients, can present as bone pain or pathologic fractures. Most patients have radiologic evidence of skeletal involvement, including an Erlenmeyer flask deformity of the distal femur, which is an early skeletal change. In patients with symptomatic bone disease, lytic lesions can develop in the long bones, ribs, and pelvis, and osteosclerosis may be evident at an early age. Bone crises with severe pain and swelling can occur. Bleeding secondary to thrombocytopenia may manifest as epistaxis and bruising and is frequently overlooked until other symptoms become apparent. Children with massive splenomegaly are short of stature because of energy expenditure required by the enlarged organ.

Type 2 disease, which is rare and panethnic in distribution, is characterized by a rapid neurodegenerative course with extensive visceral involvement and death within the first 2 years of life. The disease occurs in infancy with increased tone, strabismus, and organomegaly. Failure to thrive and stridor due to laryngospasm are typical. The progressive psychomotor degeneration leads to death, usually due to respiratory compromise.

Type 3 disease is noted in infancy or childhood. In addition to the organomegaly and bony involvement, neurologic involvement is present. There is a high frequency of type 3 disease in Sweden (1 in 50,000), which has been traced to a common founder in the 17th century. Type 3 has been further classified as type 3a and 3b based on the extent of neurologic involvement and whether there is progressive myotonia and dementia (type 3a) or isolated supranuclear gaze palsy (type 3b).

DIAGNOSIS. Gaucher's disease should be considered in the differential diagnosis of patients with unexplained organomegaly, easy bruisability, and/or bone pain. Bone marrow examination usually reveals the presence of Gaucher cells; however, all suspect diagnoses should be confirmed by demonstrating deficient acid β-glucosidase activity in isolated leukocytes or cultured fibroblasts. For possible genotype/phenotype correlations, the specific acid β-glucosidase mutation may be determined, particularly inAshkenazi Jewish patients. Carrier identification can be achieved by enzymatic assay confirmed with DNA testing in most Jewish families. Testing should be offered to all family members, but it should be kept in mind that heterogeneity even among members of the same kindred can be so great that cases may be diagnosed in asymptomatic affected individuals during such testing. Prenatal diagnosis is available by determining enzymatic activity or specific mutations in chorionic villi or cultured amniotic fluid cells.

TREATMENT. In the past, management of patients with type 1 disease was primarily symptomatic, including blood transfusions for anemia, partial or total splenectomy for severe mechanical cardiopulmonary compromise or hypersplenism, analgesics for bone pain, and orthopedic procedures for joint replacement. A small number of patients also have undergone bone marrow transplantation, which, if successful, is curative. However, a matched donor is required, and there are significant morbidity and mortality due to the procedure. There is no effective treatment for the neurologic involvement in types 2 and 3 disease. More recently, the safety and efficacy of enzyme replacement with purified placental or recombinant acid β-glucosidase has been demonstrated in type 1 disease. Clinical trials have demonstrated that most extraskeletal symptoms are reversed by initial debulking doses of enzyme (30 to 60 IU per kilogram) administered by intravenous infusion every other week. The effectiveness of enzyme replacement in reversing and preventing bony manifestations is still under study; however, early data indicate that it may be efficacious. Efforts are also under way to develop gene therapy for type 1 disease.

Beutler E, Grabowski G: Gaucher disease. *In* Scriver CR, Beaudet AL, Sly WS, Valle D (eds.): The Metabolic and Molecular Bases of Inherited Disease, 7th ed. New York, McGraw-Hill, 1995. *Comprehensive review of the clinical, biochemical, and molecular features of Gaucher's disease.*

Pastores GM, Sibille AR, Grabowski GA: Enzyme therapy in Gaucher disease type 1: Dosage efficacy and adverse events in 33 patients treated for 6 to 24 months. Blood 82:408, 1991. *Description of initial experience with enzyme replacement therapy.*

DEFINITION. The four major subtypes of Niemann-Pick disease (NPD) are characterized by accumulation of sphingomyelin and cholesterol in lysosomes of cells of the macrophage-monocyte system. Type A disease is a fatal disorder of infancy, whereas type B disease is a non-neuronopathic form in which most affected individuals live into adulthood and suffer primarily from hepatic and pulmonary involvement. Types C and D disease are neurodegenerative disorders with onset in early or late childhood. All four subtypes are inherited as autosomal recessive traits and display variable clinical features.

ETIOLOGY AND PATHOGENESIS. Types A and B NPD result from deficient activity of a lysosomal hydrolase (Table 174–1). In Types C and D NPD the genetic defect(s) involve the defective transport of cholesterol from the lysosome to the cytosol. The gene encoding the defect in type C disease has been localized (Table 174–2), but the specific gene and nature of the cholesterol transport defect remain unknown.

PATHOLOGY. The pathologic hallmark in types A and B NPD is the histochemically characteristic lipid-laden foam cell, often referred to as the Niemann-Pick cell. These cells, which can be readily distinguished from Gaucher cells by their histologic and histochemical characteristics, are not pathognomic for NPD, since histologically similar cells are found in patients with Wolman's disease, cholesterol ester storage disease, lipoprotein lipase deficiency, and in some patients with GM_1 gangliosidosis, type 2. Sphingomyelin is the major lipid that accumulates in the cells and tissues of patients with types A and B NPD. In most normal tissues, sphingomyelin constitutes 5 to 20% of the total cellular phospholipid content; however, in patients with types A and B NPD the sphingomyelin levels may be elevated up to 50-fold, constituting about 70% of the total phospholipid fraction. Lysosomal sphingomyelin accumulation in brain, liver, kidney, and lungs has been documented with organs from patients with types A and B NPD which contain about the same amount of sphingomyelin, with the notable exception that patients with type B NPD have little or no lipid storage in their CNS. In general, patients with type A disease have less than 5% of normal acid sphingomyelinase activity when determined in cultured fibroblasts and/or lymphocytes, whereas cells from type B patients typically have 10 to 20% of normal activity that presumably prevents development of the neurologic symptoms.

CLINICAL MANIFESTATIONS. The clinical presentation and course of type A NPD is relatively uniform and is characterized by normal appearance at birth, although the newborn period is sometimes complicated by prolonged jaundice. Hepatosplenomegaly, moderate lymphadenopathy, and psychomotor retardation are evident by 6 months of life and are followed by rapid neurodegeneration. The loss of motor function and deterioration of intellectual capabilities are progressive. In later stages, spasticity and rigidity are evident with affected infants experiencing complete loss of contact with their environment.

In contrast to the stereotyped type A phenotype, the clinical presentation and course in patients with type B disease are more variable. Most cases are diagnosed in infancy or childhood when enlargement of the liver and/or spleen is detected during a routine physical examination. At diagnosis, type B patients also have evidence of mild pulmonary involvement, usually detected as a diffuse reticular or finely nodular infiltration on chest roentenogram. In most patients, hepatosplenomegaly is particularly prominent in childhood, but with increasing linear growth the abdominal protuberance decreases and becomes less conspicuous. In mildly affected patients the splenomegaly may not be noted until adulthood, and there may be minimal disease manifestations. In most patients with type B disease, decreased pulmonary diffusion due to alveolar infiltration becomes evident in childhood and progresses with age. Severely affected individuals may experience significant pulmonary compromise by age 15 to 20. Such patients have low PO_2 values and dyspnea on exertion. Life-threatening bronchopneumonia may occur and cor pulmonale has been described. Severely affected patients also may have liver involvement leading to life-threatening cirrhosis, portal hypertension, and ascites. Clinically significant pancytopenia due to secondary hypersplenism may necessitate partial or total splenectomy. Typically, patients with type B disease do not have neurologic involvement and are intellectually intact.

Patients with type C disease often have prolonged neonatal jaundice, appear normal for 1 to 2 years, and then experience a slowly progressive and variable neurodegenerative course. Their hepatosplenomegaly is less severe than in patients with types A or B disease, and they may survive into adulthood. Patients with type D NPD develop neurologic symptoms later in childhood and have a slower neurodegenerative course than patients with type C. Most patients with type D disease share a common ancestry traceable to the Acadians from Yarmouth County, Nova Scotia. It appears that these patients also have an abnormality in cholesterol metabolism and that the defect may be allelic with that causing type C disease.

DIAGNOSIS. Type A disease is diagnosed in the patient's first year of life with failure to thrive, organomegaly, and severe psychomotor retardation. In type B NPD, splenomegaly is usually noted early in childhood; however, in very mild cases, the enlargement may be subtle and detection may be delayed until adolescence or adulthood. The presence of the characteristic Niemann-Pick cells in the bone marrow supports the diagnosis. However, patients with types C and D disease also have extensive infiltration of these cells in the bone marrow. Thus, all suspect cases should be evaluated enzymatically to confirm the clinical diagnosis by measuring the sphingomyelinase activity level in peripheral leukocytes, cultured fibroblasts, and/or lymphoblasts. Patients with type A and B disease will have markedly decreased levels of enzymatic activity (1 to 10% of normal), whereas patients with types C and D disease may have slightly decreased sphingomyelinase activity (50 to 75% of normal), and patients with Gaucher's disease and other storage disorders presenting with hepatosplenomegaly and/or neurologic involvement will have normal or near-normal levels. Types C and D disease can be biochemically documented by demonstrating the cholesterol transport defect in cultured fibroblasts. The enzymatic

identification of type A and B carriers is problematic. However, in families in which the specific molecular lesion has been identified, family members can be accurately tested for heterozygote status by DNA analysis. Heterozygote identification for types C and D disease is unavailable. Prenatal diagnosis of types A and B disease may be reliably made by measuring acid sphingomyelinase activity in cultured amniocytes or chorionic villi. In families in which the specific molecular lesions are known, the prenatal diagnosis can be made by DNA analysis of the fetal cells.

TREATMENT. At present there is no specific treatment available for any of the NPD subtypes. Orthotopic liver transplantation in an infant with type A disease and amniotic cell transplantation in several patients with type B disease have been attempted with little or no success. Bone marrow transplantation in a type B patient was successful in reducing the spleen and liver volumes, the sphingomyelin content of the liver, the number of Niemann-Pick cells in the marrow, and the radiologic infiltration of the lungs. However, no long-term information is available as this patient died 3 months after transplantation. To date, lung transplantation has not been performed in any severely compromised patient with type B disease. Future prospects for treatment of type B disease include enzyme replacement and gene therapy. Treatment of types A, C, and D disease are presently precluded by the severe neurologic involvement.

Schuchman EH, Desnick RJ: Types A and B Niemann-Pick Disease. *In* Scriver CR, Beaudet AL, Sly WS, Valle D (eds.): The Metabolic and Molecular Bases of Inherited Disease, 7th ed. New York, McGraw-Hill, 1994. *The most up-to-date description of the clinical, metabolic, and molecular nature of Niemann-Pick types A and B.*

Inborn Errors of Amino Acid Metabolism

175 HYPERAMINOACIDURIA
(With a Classification of the Inborn and Developmental Errors of Amino Acid Metabolism)
Charles R. Scriver

Study of inborn errors has improved our knowledge of amino acid metabolism, as well as the diagnosis and treatment of associated diseases. The inborn errors of renal amino acid transport affect either a carrier or a metabolic process coupled to the transcellular flux that achieves normal reabsorption.

L-Aminoaciduria, representing less than 2 to 3% of the total urinary nitrogen, is a normal phenomenon. More than 95% of the filtered amino acid load is reabsorbed by the proximal portion of the renal tubule; the remainder is excreted in the urine. Efficiency of renal tubular transport of an amino acid is related to its chemical and steric structure, the amount in the glomerular filtrate, and the gender, age, and physiologic state of the subject. Abnormal aminoaciduria (hyperaminoaciduria) is a result of acquired or hereditary disturbances of cellular metabolism or transport. Table 175–1

shows the known hyperaminoacidurias. (The table includes several disorders of amino acid metabolism that do not show hyperaminoaciduria but affect organic acid and fatty acid derivatives; they can be detected in urine by gas chromatography.)

The hyperaminoacidurias are explained by several mechanisms acting on net reabsorption in the proximal tubule (Fig. 175–1):

1. *Saturation:* The concentration of amino acid in filtrate approaches or exceeds the capacity of the tubular system to reabsorb it (overflow or prerenal aminoaciduria).

2. *Competition:* One amino acid at elevated concentration competes with another sharing the same transporter ("combined" aminoaciduria).

3. *Modification of transporter:* The amino acid is not transported efficiently because its carrier is altered (renal aminoaciduria).

4. *Inhibition of substrate transfer:* The coupling of energy to the transporter is altered, and flux is impaired (renal aminoaciduria).

Renal transporters show preferences for either single free amino acids or specific groups of them. The transport systems identified in Table 175–1 (group III) were revealed through loss of function in the variant (mutant or developmental) state. Oligopeptides are transported on carriers different from those used by free amino acids.

Scriver CR, Beaudet A, Sly W, Valle D (eds.): The Metabolic and Molecular Bases of Inherited Disease. 7th ed. New York, McGraw-Hill, 1995. *The mendelian disorders of amino acid metabolism (catabolism or transport) are described, chapter by chapter, in detail.*

Scriver CR, Tenenhouse HS: Mendelian phenotypes as "probes" of renal transport systems for amino acids and phosphate. *In* Windhager E (ed.): Handbook of Physiology: Renal Physiology. New York, Oxford University Press, Section 8, Vol. II, pp. 1977–2016, 1992. *A review of the inborn errors of renal amino acid transport and associated transport systems.*

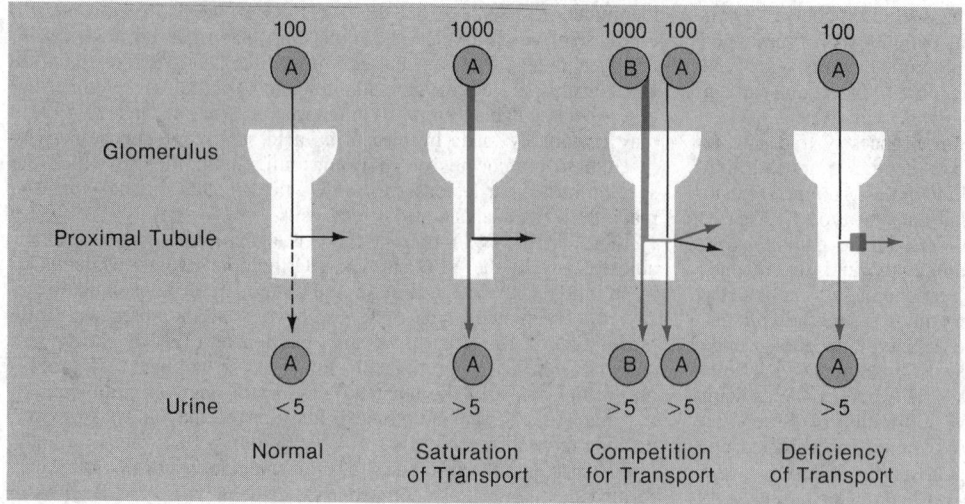

FIGURE 175–1. Mechanism of hyperaminoaciduria. *Panel 1:* Normal reabsorption reclaims >95% of filtered amino acid molecules. Hyperaminoaciduria can occur if *(Panel 2)* filtered load increases (10× increase shown) and transport mechanism is saturated, if *(Panel 3)* amino acid (B) (in excess) competes with another (A) on a shared carrier, or if *(Panel 4)* carrier itself or coupling of energy to carrier is impaired.

TABLE 175–1. HEREDITARY AND ACQUIRED AMINOACIDOPATHIES

The aminoacidurias presented in this table are divided into acquired and inherited types. Disturbances related to perinatal adaptive phenomena of multifactorial origin are included. The classification recognizes physiologic factors affecting amino acid distribution between plasma and urine, and whether the disorder primarily affects catabolism or membrane transport of the amino acid(s).

Thus the disorders are grouped according to mechanism and preferred fluid for detection. The data refer to those conditions associated with perturbation of the normal content of ninhydrin-reactive metabolites in plasma or urine; some exceptions have been made to include ninhydrin-negative metabolites where it is relevant.

GROUP IA

The primary defect is in catabolism. There is a low renal clearance of amino acid but a hyperaminoaciduria by saturation of transepithelial transport. Detection in the plasma is preferable unless otherwise indicated, but using urine for screening (or diagnosis) is not precluded; assignment to this group implies primarily that diagnosis (or screening) of the condition is feasible by virtue of significant metabolite accumulation in blood (or plasma).

Amino Acid Affected:
↓ = decreased; ↑ = increased. Source of enzyme number is *Enzyme Commission.* IP = apparent inheritance pattern; AR = autosomal recessive; AD = autosomal dominant; (AR) = probably autosomal recessive; XL = X-linked. *Remarks:* CNS = central nervous system; CoA = coenzyme A; CSF = cerebrospinal fluid.

Condition or Disease	Amino Acid Affected	Enzyme Affected (Synonym) In Group A	IP	Remarks
*Common Perinatal (Adaptive) Traits**				
Neonatal hyperphenylalaninemia	Phenylalanine	? Phenylalanine 4-mono-oxygenase (phenylalanine-hydroxylating system) [1.14.16.1]	—	Benign; may respond to folic acid; often occurs with tyrosinemia
Neonatal tyrosinemia	Tyrosine	4-Hydroxyphenylpyruvate dioxygenase (p-hydroxyphenyl pyruvic acid hydroxylase) [1.13.11.27]	—	Benign; responds to ascorbic acid and reduced protein intake
Hypermethioninemia	Methionine	Methionine adenosyltransferase (ATP:L-methionine S-adenosyltransferase) [2.5.1.6]; hepatic isoenzyme	—	Benign; usually found with high protein intake
Hyperhistidinemia	Histidine	? L-Histidine ammonia-lyase [4.3.1.3]	—	Benign; related to high protein intake
Inherited Traits				
Hyperphenylalaninemia				
Classic phenylketonuria	Phenylalanine	Phenylalanine 4-mono-oxygenase (L-phenylalanine, tetrahydropteridine:oxygen oxidoreductase [4-hydroxylating]) [1.14.16.1]	AR	Plasma phenylalanine >1 mM; causes mental retardation when untreated; L-phenylalanine tolerance in diet is 250–500 mg/day
"Mild" phenylketonuria	Phenylalanine	Same	AR	Plasma phenylalanine >1 mM; similar to entry above, but dietary tolerance for L-phenylalanine is >500 mg/day
Transient "hyperphenylalaninemia"	Phenylalanine	Pterin-4α-carbinolamine hydratase	AR	Plasma phenylalanine elevated; change in status to that of next entry or normal, several months (or years) after birth
Non-PKU hyperphenylalaninemia	Phenylalanine	Phenylalanine 4-mono-oxygenase	AR	Plasma phenylalanine <1 mM on normal diet; less effect on IQ
Dihydropteridine reductase deficiency	Phenylalanine	Dihydropteridine reductase [1.6.99.7]	AR	Deficient tetrahydrobiopterin cofactor recycling also impairs biosynthesis of L-dopa and 5-hydroxytryptamine (5-HT) in CNS; low-phenylalanine diet does not correct this

TABLE 175–1. HEREDITARY AND ACQUIRED AMINOACIDOPATHIES *Continued*

Condition or Disease	Amino Acid Affected	Enzyme Affected (Synonym) In Group A	IP	Remarks
		Inherited Traits (Continued)		
Biopterin synthesis defects	Phenylalanine	GTP-cyclohydrolase [3.5.4.16] or 6-pyruvoyltetrahydropterin synthase [4.6.1.10] in pathway for tetrahydrobiopterin synthesis	AR	Deficient cofactor synthesis; see preceding entry for effect
Hypertyrosinemia				
Tyrosinosis (Medes)	Tyrosine	? Tyrosine aminotransferase (L-tyrosine:α-ketoglutarate aminotransferase) [2.6.1.5]	(AR)	One case known; myasthenia gravis probably incidental finding
Hypertyrosinemia I	Tyrosine (and methionine in acute stage)	Fumarylacetoacetate hydrolase [3.7.1.2]	AR	Hepatic cirrhosis and renal tubular failure; usually fatal in absence of effective treatment
Hypertyrosinemia II	Tyrosine	Soluble (cytosol) tyrosine aminotransferase [2.6.1.5]	AR	Can be associated with developmental retardation; Richner-Hanhart syndrome in most patients
Hawkinsinuria	Tyrosine	4-Hydroxyphenylpyruvate dioxygenase [1.13.11.27]	AD	Disease signs are variable and include failure to thrive; reflect formation of epoxides and adducts of glutathione
Hyperhistidinemia†				
Classic form	Histidine (alanine high in some cases)	L-Histidine ammonia-lyase [4.3.1.3]; liver, epidermis	AR	Harmless condition in majority
Branched-chain hyperaminoacidemia‡	Leucine, isoleucine, valine, alloisoleucine	Branched-chain α-keto acid lipoate oxidoreductase (probably decarboxylase component) [1.2.4.3(4)]	AR	Clinical variants from: postnatal collapse and mental retardation in survivors (diet therapy can be effective); to intermittent symptoms (development may be otherwise normal); to unremittent (milder than classic form).
Maple syrup urine disease (classic)				
Thiamine-responsive form	Same	Same	AR	Mild form; responsive to thiamine (vitamin B_1)
Multiple dehydrogenase form; E_3 deficiency	Same (plus pyruvate and α-ketoglutarate)	Dihydrolipoamide dehydrogenase [1.8.1.4]	AR	Congenital lactic acidosis plus branched-chain amino-keto acid disorder
Hypervalinemia	Valine	Branched-chain amino-acid aminotransferase (valine aminotransferase) [2.6.1.66]	AR	Retarded development and vomiting; responds to diet
Hyperlysinemia and related disorders				
Hyperlysinemia	Lysine (and saccharopine); (secondary pipecolic acidemia)	Deficient "α-aminoadipic semialdehyde synthase" (bifunctional enzyme with lysine-ketoglutarate reductase [1.5.1.8] + saccharopine reductase [1.5.1.9] activities)	AR	Probably benign
Saccharopinuria variant	Saccharopine (and lysine)	Only saccharopine reductase activity of bifunctional enzyme is deficient	AR	Same as above
α-Aminoadipic aciduria	α-Aminoadipic acid	? Mitochondrial α-aminoadipate amino transferase [2.6.1.39]	(AR)	Variable clinical features
α-Ketoadipic aciduria	α-Aminoadipic and α-ketoadipic acids	? α-Ketoadipic decarboxylase	(AR)	Mental retardation
2-Hydroxyglutaric aciduria	Hyperlysinemia (in some patients)	? Glutaryl CoA dehydrogenase [1.3.99.7]	AR	Progressive ataxia, mental retardation, leukoencephalopathy, cerebellar atrophy
Pipecolic acidemia (primary form)	Pipecolic acid	L-Pipecolate dehydrogenase (pipecolate oxidase) [1.5.99.3]		A peroxisomal disease with hepatomegaly and mental retardation (variant of Zellweger syndrome and adrenoleukodystrophy)
Hypermethioninemia	Methionine	Hepatic ATP: L-methionine S-adenosyltransferase [2.5.1.6]	AR	Variable associations, probably benign
Homocyst(e)inemia/uria				
Classic form	Methionine high; homocyst(e)ine high	Cystathionine β-synthase [L-serine hydrolase (adding homocysteine)] [4.2.1.22]	AR	Risk factor for occlusive vascular disease in heterozygotes. Homozygotes have dislocated optic lens and osteoporosis and may have impaired mental development
Tetrahydrofolate-deficient form	Methionine low; homocyst(e)ine high	5,10-Methylene tetrahydrofolate reductase [1.7.99.5]		Variable manifestations: developmental delay to severe psychomotor retardation. Heterozygotes for thermolabile variant putatively at elevated risk for coronary artery disease

Table continued on following page

TABLE 175–1. HEREDITARY AND ACQUIRED AMINOACIDOPATHIES *Continued*

Condition or Disease	Amino Acid Affected	Enzyme Affected (Synonym) *In Group A*	IP	Remarks
Inherited Traits (Continued)				
Homocyst(e)inuria (with methylmalonic aciduria)	Homocyst(e)ine (high), methionine (low): methylmalonate (high)	Defective cobalamin coenzyme biosynthesis	AR	Defective remethylation of homocysteine and impaired methylmalonyl-CoA mutase (MMA mutase) activity; developmental delay
		Defective cobalamin transport (lysosomal)	(AR)	
Cystathioninuria†	Cystathionine	Cystathionine γ-lyase [4.4.1.1]	AR	Probably benign trait; vitamin B_6 corrects biochemical trait in most patients
Hyperglycinemia				
Ketotic form	Glycine and other glucogenic amino acids	Propionyl-CoA carboxylase [6.4.1.3]	AR	Ketosis, neutropenia, mental retardation; often fatal
Ibid.	Ibid.	Methylmalonyl-CoA mutase [5.4.99.2]	AR	Symptoms are those of methylmalonic aciduria with acidosis (some mutase-affected patients are responsive to vitamin B_{12})
Ibid.	Ibid.	Acetyl-CoA acyltransferase (β-ketothiolase) [2.3.1.16] deficiency¶	AR	Signs are those of α-methyl-β-hydroxybutyric aciduria (with or without tiglic aciduria) and acidosis
Nonketotic form	Glycine	Glycine cleavage reaction (CO_2, NH_3, and hydroxymethyltetrahydrofolate formed) [2.1.2.10] P, H, T, & L proteins in complex; P is deficient in 80% of cases	AR	Severe CNS depression; high CSF: plasma glycine ratio. Benzoate and dextromethorphan (NMDA blocker) for therapy
Sarcosinemia				
Sarcosinemia (classic form)†	Sarcosine	Sarcosine oxidase (sarcosine:oxygen oxidoreductase [demethylating]) [1.5.3.1]	AR	Benign trait
"Sarcosinemia" (glutaric aciduria, type II)	Sarcosine (glutaric acid and multiple fatty acids)	Electron transfer flavoprotein (affecting multiple aryl-CoA dehydrogenases) [1.3.99.2–3]	AR	Postnatal lethargy, vomiting, coma, and acidosis; odor; multiple abnormalities of fatty acid oxidation
Hyperprolinemia				
Type I	Proline	L-Proline dehydrogenase (oxidase) [1.5.99.8]	AR	Benign trait
Type II	Proline	1-Pyrroline dehydrogenase (Δ¹-nicotinamide-pyrroline-5-carboxylate: adenine dinucleotide [NAD⁺] oxidoreductase) [1.5.1.12]	AR	Δ¹-pyrroline-5-carboxylate and 3-hydroxy-1-pyrroline-5-carboxylate excreted in urine. Proline concentration higher in type II than type I; seizures
Hyperhydroxyprolinemia	Hydroxyproline	4-Hydroxy-L-proline dehydrogenase (oxidase) [1.1.1.104]	AR	Benign trait
Hydroxylysinemia	Free hydroxylysine	? Hydroxylysine kinase [2.7.1.81]	(AR)	Mental retardation
Tryptophanemia	Tryptophan (with indoleketonuria)	? Formamidase [3.5.1.9]	(AR)	Variable, probably benign
Hyperammonemia Carbamoyl phosphate synthetase (CPS) deficiency	Glycine, glutamine	Carbamate kinase (ATP carbamate phosphotransferase) [2.7.2.2]	AR	Ammonia intoxication, protein intolerance, hepatomegaly, vomiting
Ornithine transcarbamoylase (OTC) deficiency	Glutamine	Ornithine carbamoyltransferase (carbamoylphosphate:L-ornithine carbamoyltransferase) [2.1.3.3]	XL	Same as above
Citrullinemia	Citrulline	Argininosuccinate synthetase (L-citrulline:L-aspartate ligase (adenosine monophosphate [AMP]-forming)) [6.3.4.5]	AR	Same as above
Argininosuccinicaciduria†	Argininosuccinic acid	Argininosuccinate lyase (L-argininosuccinate arginine-lyase) [4.3.2.1]	AR	Same as above; also has trichorrhexis nodosa
Hyperargininemia	Arginine	Argininase (L-arginine amidinohydrolase) [3.5.3.1]	AR	Deterioration of CNS function and IQ in childhood; hyperammonemia (inconstant) aggravated by protein
Hyperornithinemia	Ornithine	Unknown (mitochondrial ornithine transport system?)	AR	Associated with hyperammonemia and homocitrullinemia (HHH syndrome)
Hyperornithinemia (without hyperammonemia)	Ornithine	L-Ornithine; 2-oxoacid aminotransferase [2.6.1.13]	AR	Associated with gyrate atrophy of choroid and retina but no hyperammonemia

TABLE 175–1. HEREDITARY AND ACQUIRED AMINOACIDOPATHIES *Continued*

Condition or Disease	Amino Acid Affected	Enzyme Affected (Synonym) *In Group A*	IP	Remarks
Inherited Traits (Continued)				
Hyperalaninemia	Alanine	Pyruvate dehydrogenase (lipoate) (pyruvate dehydrogenase) [1.2.4.1] deficiency, pyruvate carboxylase [6.4.1.1] deficiency, and other defects	AR	Lactic acidosis, various other manifestations
Aspartylglucosaminuria	Glycoasparagine	Aspartylglucosylaminase (2-acetamido-1[β¹-L-aspartamidol]-1,2-dideoxyglucose amidohydrolase) [3.5.1.26]	AR	Lysosomal disease; mental retardation
Glutathionemia†	Glutathione or related peptides	γ-Glutamyltransferase (γ-glutamyltranspeptidase) [2.3.2.2]	AR	Mental retardation?
Hyperthreoninemia	Threonine	Unknown	(AR)	Seizures
Other Conditions That May Affect Amino Acids in Plasma				
Protein-calorie malnutrition	Tryptophan/leucine/isoleucine/valine ↓; tyrosine/glycine/proline ↑	—	—	Severity of change related to severity of malnutrition
Prolonged fasting	Alanine ↓; threonine, glycine ↑	—	—	Early fasting does not show same pattern
Obesity	Leucine/isoleucine/valine/phenylalanine/tyrosine ↑; glycine ↓	—	—	Reflects insulin insensitivity
Hepatitis	Methionine/tyrosine ↑	—	—	Reflects severity of liver disease

* These conditions have been detected by screening methods applied in the newborn period of life. They should not be misdiagnosed as permanent disorders of amino acid metabolism also identifiable by screening.

† Urine screening is as efficient as, or even more reliable than, blood screening in these conditions.

‡ A number of disorders of branched-chain amino acid catabolism cause accumulation of substances that are ninhydrin negative. These compounds can usually be detected by gas-liquid chromatographic methods (see Goodman SI: Am J Hum Genet 32:781, 1980).

§ Partial activity; >2% of normal.

¶ Hyperglycemia observed only in some patients with this enzyme deficiency.

GROUP IB

The primary defect is in catabolism. There is a high renal clearance of amino acid and a hyperaminoaciduria by saturation of transepithelial transport. Detection in the urine is preferable.

Source of enzyme number is *Enzyme Commission*. IP = apparent inheritance pattern; AR = autosomal recessive; (AR) = probably autosomal recessive; AD = autosomal dominant.

Condition or Disease	Substance Affected (Synonym)	Enzyme Affected (Synonym) [Enzyme Commission No.]	IP	Remarks
Hypophosphatasia	Phosphoethanolamine	Deficiency of alkaline phosphatase (tissue nonspecific (liver, body, kidney) isoenzyme) [3.1.3.1]	AR	"Rickets" unresponsive to vitamin D; craniosynostosis; hypercalcemia, elevated pyridoxal phosphate (blood marker)
Pseudohypophosphatasia	Phosphoethanolamine	Same as above; activity present but altered	AR	Same as above
β-Aminoisobutyricaciduria	β-Aminoisobutyric acid	Hepatic R-β-aminoisobutyrate-pyruvate transaminase [2.6.1.40]	AD/AR	Benign metabolic polymorphic trait

Condition or Disease	Substance Affected (Synonym)	Enzyme Affected (Synonym) *In Group A*	IP	Remarks
4-Hydroxybutyricaciduria (γ-aminobutyrate pathway)	γ-OH butyrate	Succinic semialdehyde dehydrogenase [1.2.1.24]	AR	Mental retardation, hypotonia; detectable by gas chromatographic analysis of urine, plasma, CSF
Hyper-β-alaninemia	β-Alanine	? β-Alanine-pyruvate aminotransferase (β-alanine transaminase) [2.6.1.18]		Seizures; somnolence; mental retardation
Carnosinemia	Carnosine	Serum aminoacyl-histidine dipeptidase (carnosinase) [3.4.13.3]	AR	Benign (most cases)
Pyroglutamic aciduria*	L-Pyroglutamic acid (5-oxo-L-proline; pyrrolidone-2-carboxylic acid)	Glutathione synthetase [6.3.2.3]	AR	L-Pyroglutamic acid formed via modified γ-glutamyl cycle. Associated metabolic acidosis

GROUP II

There is a primary defect in catabolism and a secondary defect in transport. Hyperaminoaciduria is of combined origin–saturation and competition.

Detection is possible in both plasma and urine.

Disease	Amino Acids Affected in Plasma	Amino Acids Present in Urine	Remarks
Hyperprolinemia, types I and II	Proline	Proline, + hydroxyproline and glycine	See entries in group 1A; competition occurs on iminoglycine transport system (see group III)
Hyper-β-alaninemia	β-Alanine	β-Alanine, + β-aminoisobutyric acid and taurine	See entry in Hyper-β-alaninemia in group IB; competition occurs on β-amino transport system

Table continued on following page

TABLE 175–1. HEREDITARY AND ACQUIRED AMINOACIDOPATHIES *Continued*

Disease	Amino Acids		Remarks
	Affected in Plasma	*Present in Urine*	
Hyperlysinemia	Lysine	Lysine, + ornithine and arginine	See entries in group IA; competition occurs on "dibasic" transport system (see group III)
Hyperargininemia	Arginine	Ornithine and lysine and sometimes generalized hyperaminoaciduria	See entry in group IA; competition occurs on "dibasic" transport system (see group III); pathogenesis of generalized aminoaciduria unknown

* Urine screening is as efficient as, or even more reliable than, blood screening in these conditions.

GROUP III

The primary defect is in the renal membrane transport site. There is a high renal clearance of amino acid, and detection is possible only in the urine. *Activity Affected:* Presumed gene product activity affected by mutant gene. IP = apparent inheritance pattern; AD = autosomal dominant; (AD) = probably autosomal dominant; AR = autosomal recessive; (AR) = probably autosomal recessive; XL = X-linked. *Remarks:* PTH = parathyroid hormone.

Trait	Substance Affected	Activity Affected	Other Tissues Affected	IP	Remarks
Common Perinatal (Adaptive) Trait					
Neonatal iminoglycinuria	Proline, hydroxyproline, glycine	Specific proline and specific glycine transport (probably)	—	—	Benign adaptive trait; prolinuria subsides at ~100 days, glycinuria at ~200 days after full-term birth
Neonatal cystine-lysinuria	Cystine and dibasic amino acids (lysine, ornithine, and arginine)	Specific dibasic transport system	—	—	Reflects heterozygosity for cystinuria (see below) plus ontogeny
Inherited Hyperaminoacidurias					
Selective					
Hyperdibasic aminoaciduria type 2 (Lysinuric-protein intolerance)	Lysine, ornithine, arginine ("dibasic" group)	Shared "dibasic" amino acid transport system in basolateral membrane	Intestine (basolateral membrane, efflux defect); fibroblasts (plasma membrane; efflux defect on y$^+$ system)	AR	Associated with protein intolerance, failure to thrive, hyperammonemia
Hyperdibasic aminoaciduria type I	Lysine, ornithine, arginine	Shared "dibasic" amino acid transport system (brush-border membrane)	Intestine	AR	Associated with mental retardation in one reported patient; heterozygotes have hyperdibasic aminoaciduria
Isolated hyperlysinuria	Lysine	Lysine-specific system (brush border)	Intestine	AR	One proband reported
Classic cystinuria	Lysine, ornithine, arginine, and cystine	Shared system in brush border membrane	Intestine	AR	"Negative" reabsorption of affected amino acid can occur; three alleles (? same locus), each causing different phenotypes: in type I carrier (vs. types II and III) no excess of amino acids in urine ("silent"); in type III patient, intestinal transport intact (or partial defect)
Hypercystinuria	Cyst(e)ine	Specific system for cyst(e)ine	?	(AR)	One pedigree only
Iminoglycinuria	Proline; hydroxyproline; glycine	Shared system for imino acids, glycine (and sarcosine)	Intestine	AR	Benign; 4 alleles (? same locus); I and II are silent carriers; III and IV are hyperglycinuric carriers; I associated with intestinal defect; IV with K$_m$ mutant
Hartnup disorder	Neutral amino acids (excluding imino acids, glycine, cyst(e)ine, and β-amino acids)	Shared system for large neutral amino acid group (luminal membrane)	Intestine	AR	Usually benign; 3 alleles (? same locus); II, intestine affected; II, intestine normal; III, kidney normal; carrier "silent" in all
Hyperhistidinuria	Histidine	Specific system for histidine	Intestine	AR	Associated with mental retardation in siblings
Hyperdicarboxylic aminoaciduria (glutamate-aspartate transport defect)	Glutamic acid, aspartic acid	Shared dicarboxylic amino acid transport system (brush border membrane)	Intestine ±	AR	Benign
Idiopathic (primary genetic) Fanconi's syndrome	Generalized effect on all solutes and water	? Mitochondrial defect disrupted ATP energized ion pump (basolateral membrane); impaired sodium-coupled transporter (apical membrane)	Secondary to renal phenotype	AR (and AD)	Adult-onset and infantile-childhood forms are differentiated

TABLE 175–1. HEREDITARY AND ACQUIRED AMINOACIDOPATHIES *Continued*

Trait	Substance Affected	Activity Affected	Other Tissues Affected	IP	Remarks
Inherited Hyperaminoacidurias (Continued)					
Secondary genetic forms of renal Fanconi's syndrome					
Cystinosis; type I, type II	Same as above (secondary response)	Cystine storage (lysosomal defect), with secondary damage to tubule and glomerulus (later)	Organ damage from cystine storage (thyroid, retina, CNS)	AR*	Several alleles; infantile (type I) and adolescent (type II) forms have differing rates for onset of nephropathy; "adult" form (type III) has no nephropathy
Hereditary fructose intolerance	Same as above, + fructose	Fructose-1-phosphate aldolase (fructose biphosphate aldolase) (with secondary effects on cellular ATP)	Secondary to renal phenotype (hepatic cirrhosis)	AR	Nephropathy dependent on intact PTH-cAMP axis in kidney; responds to fructose withdrawal
Galactosemia	Same as above, + galactose	Galactose-1-phosphate uridyltransferase (with secondary effects on cellular ATP)	Secondary to renal phenotype (cataracts, CNS effects)	AR	Fanconi's syndrome responds to galactose withdrawal; "galactosemia" due to galactokinase deficiency does *not* have Fanconi's syndrome
Hereditary tyrosinemia	Same as above, + tyrosine metabolites	Fumarylacetoacetate hydrolase	Secondary to renal phenotype (hepatic cirrhosis)	AR	Fanconi's syndrome responds to tyrosine restriction
Wilson's disease	Same as above, with proximal and distal renal tubular acidosis	WND protein, in P-type ATPase family of cation transporters	Hepatolenticular degeneration	AR	Fanconi's syndrome responds to depletion of copper burden
Lowe's oculocerebrorenal syndrome	Generalized dysfunction with defective urinary NH_3 production	? In OCRL-1 protein (strong homology with inositol polyphosphate-5-phosphatase)	An oculo-cerebro-intestinal-renal syndrome	XL†	Treatment does not improve mental retardation or the cataracts and hydrophthalmia
Vitamin D dependency (pseudodeficiency rickets)	Generalized defect (secondary response)	Type I: 25-Hydroxyvitamin D-1-α-hydroxylase Type II: defective binding of hormone	Impaired receptor synthesis or ligand binding affects intestinal absorption of calcium and initiates PTH response	AR	Nephropathy dependent on PTH excess and hypocalcemia (phenocopy occurs in vitamin D deficiency)

* For each type.
† Recessive.

Data from Benson PF, Fensom AH: Genetic Biochemical Disorders. Oxford Monographs on the Medical Genetics No. 12. Oxford, Oxford University Press, 1985. *A "handbook," leaner than* The Metabolic and Molecular Bases of Inherited Disease *(the standard "encyclopedia"), that covers, in short essays, nearly all entries in Table 175–1.* Scriver CT, Tenenhouse HS: Mendelian phenotypes as "probes" of renal transport systems for amino acids and phosphate. Handbook of Physiology (Renal Section, 1987). *A review of the amino acid transport systems (in kidney and other tissues) delineated by mutations in humans and of their relative importance in metabolic homeostasis.* Wellner D, Meister A: A survey of inborn errors of amino acid metabolism and transport in man. Annu Rev Biochem 50:911, 1981. *A crisp review of events in a field that now moves more slowly than it once did.*

176 THE HYPERPHENYLALANINEMIAS AND ALKAPTONURIA

Charles R. Scriver

A widely accepted medical model of disease attributes manifestations (signs and symptoms) to a deviant underlying process (pathogenesis) that has its origins in both proximate and ultimate causes. According to this model, phenylketonuria, the best known form of hyperphenylalaninemia, is no longer a disease, although it continues to be a risk factor, because its principal manifestations (mental retardation, pigment dilution, mousy odor, neurotransmitter deficiency) occur only in rare cases escaping early diagnosis. This satisfactory turn of events came about because pathogenesis from hyperphenylalaninemia (the risk factor) is offset by treatment. Genetic forms of hyperphenylalaninemia are described here; they are all autosomal recessive disorders. About 0.01% of live births are affected. Physicians for adult-age patients must be aware of maternal hyperphenylalaninemia (see below).

PHENYLALANINE METABOLISM. Phenylalanine is an essential amino acid. The normal concentration in plasma is < 125 μmole per liter (1 μmole = 165 μg). The balance between intake and utilization is largely controlled by a hydroxylation reaction (Fig. 176–1A). Impaired hydroxylation is the chief explanation for hyperphenylalaninemia. The reaction requires the apoenzyme *phenylalanine hydroxylase,* molecular oxygen, and *tetrahydrobiopterin* cofactor; the last-named is consumed in stoichiometric amounts to form tyrosine, the reaction product. The catalytic property of phenylalanine hydroxylase requires both moment-to-moment regeneration of tetrahydrobiopterin from dihydrobiopterin, a byproduct of the hydroxylating reaction, and long-term renewal of the tetrahydrobiopterin pool by synthesis from precursors. The former is achieved by the enzyme *dihydropteridine reductase,* the latter by a *synthesis pathway* in which several enzymes act in sequence (Fig. 176–1B). Accordingly, there are several ways to impair phenylalanine hydroxylation. Failure to recognize the biologic heterogeneity of hyperphenylalaninemia may lead to erroneous counseling and ineffective (or unnecessary) treatment; all of its forms require special management of women during the reproductive years.

DISORDERS OF PHENYLALANINE HYDROXYLASE INTEGRITY. The phenylalanine hydroxylase enzyme is multimeric and homopolymeric. The polypeptide is encoded by a gene on chromosome 12, region q24.1, which is expressed only in liver in humans. Mutations at this locus cause either phenylketonuria (with plasma phenylalanine values >1 mM on a normal diet) or nonphenylketonuric hyperphenylalaninemia (values <1 mM, but >0.125 mM). Phenylketonuria is typically associated with mental retardation in the untreated patient; the other form is not. The incidence of the phenylketonuric form (about 1 per 10,000 births) varies widely by population.

The hydroxylation reaction accounts for about three quarters of the moment-by-moment outflow of phenylalanine; incorporation into protein is the other important route (Fig. 176–1A). If there is deficient hydroxylating activity, and dietary intake is not curtailed, phenylalanine accumulates in body fluids. Overflow into the alternative pathways generates excessive amounts of metabolites derived from phenylalanine, such as the pyruvic (causing phenylketonuria), lactic, and acetic acid derivatives (Fig. 176–1A). Overburden of phenylalanine and its by-products impairs brain development in ways still not fully understood.

Phenylketonuria was first described as a clinical entity in 1934 by Asjborn Fölling, who surmised that the disorder was autosomal recessive and an inborn error of metabolism. In the following three decades, phenylketonuria was seen as a paradigm for the biochemical basis of mental disease, of disease that could be prevented by deliberately restoring normal metabolism, and of chemical individuality that could be used as the basis for a screening test and early diagnosis. Newborn screening for hyperphenylalaninemia is now one of the most widely applied "genetic" tests. The incidence of the risk factor has not changed, but the frequency of the associated disease is now trivial in screened populations. The practical issues for physicians are interpretation of a positive screening test result, accuracy of the test, and maternal hyperphenylalaninemia (all discussed below).

TETRAHYDROBIOPTERIN-DEFICIENT FORMS OF HYPERPHENYLALANINEMIA. Not every case of persistent hyperphenylalaninemia is explained by a primary hydroxylase deficiency. Tetrahydrobiopterin insufficiency impairs function of three hydroxylases (for phenylalanine, tryptophan, and tyrosine) and synthesis of their products, notably 5-hydroxytryptophan (the precursor of serotonin) and L-dopa (the precursor of catecholamines) (Fig. 176–1B). The products function as neurotransmitters in the brain, and a deficiency of them gives rise to central nervous system disease (including retarded psychomotor development, basal ganglion dysfunction, and unstable body temperature). Regeneration of tetrahydrobiopterin is necessary to maintain catalytic function of the three hydroxylases. *Deficient activity of quininoid dihydropteridine reductase* (gene on chromosome 4, region p15.3) or of *4α-carbinolamine dehydratase* (gene on chromosome 10q22) impairs recycling of dihydrobiopterin. *Deficient activity of guanosine triphosphate cyclohydrolase 1 or 6-pyruvoyl tetrahydropterin synthase* (gene on chromosome 11q22.3-q23.4) impairs synthesis of tetrahydrobiopterin.

SCREENING AND DIAGNOSIS. Screening newborn infants for hyperphenylalaninemia is public policy. Capillary blood collected on filter paper from heel puncture is analyzed by the bacterial inhibition (Guthrie) assay, fluorimetric analysis, or other quantitative methods. Blood phenylalanine values >2 mg per deciliter ($125\mu M$) on the first day of life or thereafter are considered abnormal and require further investigation. The screening test is not infallible, and false-negative results do occur, some for biologic reasons. Urine screening for "phenylketones" is not reliable.

Every infant with persistent hyperphenylalaninemia is investigated to rule out disorders of tetrahydrobiopterin homeostasis. Urine pterin metabolites or blood cofactor levels are measured under special conditions; there are distinctive urine profiles as well as low blood levels in the disorders of tetrahydrobiopterin synthesis. The tests are done at established centers and require experienced interpretation. Measures of phenylalanine hydroxylase require liver biopsy and are seldom done. Dihydropteridine reductase can be measured in blood spots, fibroblasts, and amniocytes, the cyclohydrolase in phytohemagglutinin-stimulated leukocytes, and the synthase in erythrocytes.

After excluding disorders of tetrahydrobiopterin metabolism, hyperphenylalaninemia is classified as follows. About one half of cases with primary phenylalanine hydroxylase deficiency have "phenylketonuria," a generic term for severe hyperphenylalaninemia (>1 mM), low phenylalanine tolerance (<500 mg per day), and high risk of mental retardation in the absence of treatment. The remainder have nonphenylketonuric hyperphenylalaninemia with lower blood phenylalanine values (<1 mM), higher tolerance for dietary phenylalanine (>500 mg per day), and no elevated risk for mental retardation if not treated. There is a correlation between level of hepatic hydroxylase activity and clinical form; in broad terms, activity is $<1\%$ of normal in phenylketonuria and $>1\%$ of normal in nonphenylketonuric hyperphenylalaninemia.

DNA analysis identifies mutations at the hydroxylase (Fig. 176–2) and other cloned loci. Interpretation of phenotype by mutation analysis is clinically relevant. Prenatal diagnosis by analysis of

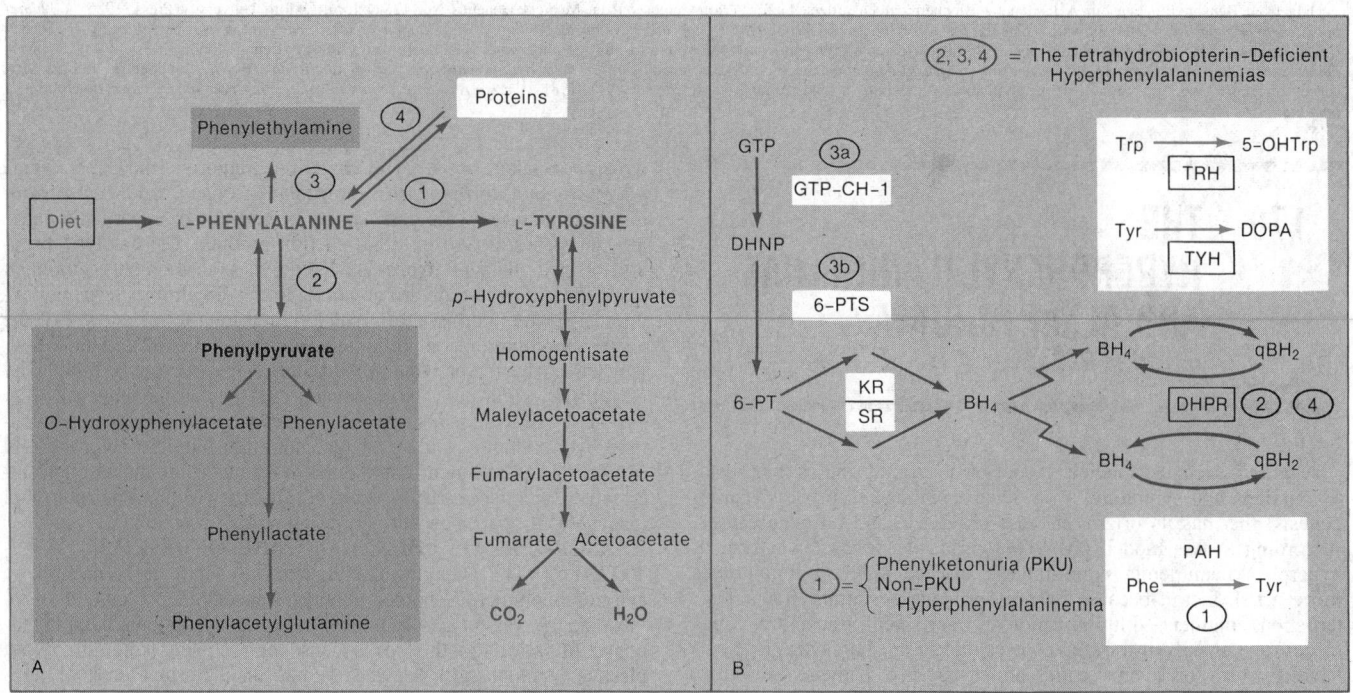

FIGURE 176–1. *A,* Intake of phenylalanine (an essential amino acid supplied only by diet) and its disposal by hydroxylation (1) (representing three quarters of normal runout), transamination (2), decarboxylation (3), and incorporation into proteins (4) (representing under a quarter of runout). *B,* Interrelations between phenylalanine hydroxylase (PAH), dihydropteridine reductase (DHPR), and the tetrahydrobiopterin (BH$_4$) biosynthesis pathway serving aromatic amino acid hydroxylation reactions. Mutations at the relevant chromosomal loci impair the hydroxylation reactions with effects on PAH activity only (1); DHPR activity (2); GTP-cyclohydrolase 1 (GTP-CH-1) activity (3a); 6-pyruvoyltetrahydropterin synthase activity (6-PTS) (3b); and 4α-carbinolamine dehydratase (4). Disorders 2, 3a, 3b, and 4 can impair function of three hydroxylases: PAH, tyrosine hydroxylase (TYH), and tryptophan hydroxylase (TRH). GTP = guanosine triphosphate; DHNP = dihydroneopterin triphosphate; 6-PT = 6-pyruvoyltetrahydropterin; KR = 2'-ketotetrahydropterin reductase; SR = sepiapterin reductase; qBH$_2$ = quinonoid dihydrobiopterin.

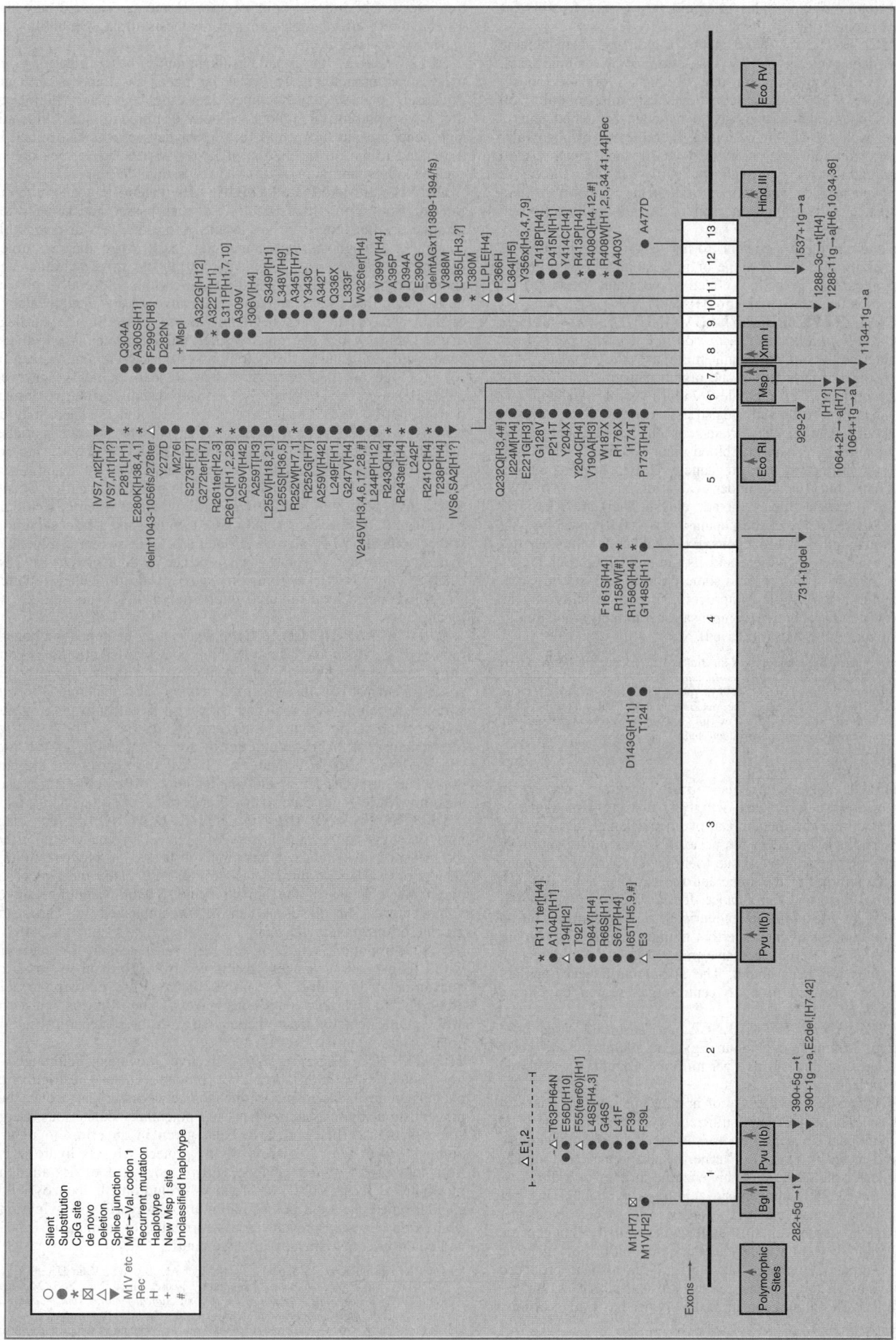

FIGURE 176–2. Diagram of the phenylalanine hydroxylase (PAH) gene (≈ 90 kb, chromosome 12q24.1), showing exons (*vertical bars*), polymorphic restriction sites (*arrows*), and regions of some associated with phenylketonuria. The code (e.g., MIV) indicates normal residue, position in the PAH polypeptide, and replacement residue. Several mutations involve hypermutable CpG dinucleotides; some are "recurrent." Over 200 mutations were known before this edition went to press.

DNA in chorionic villus samples or amniocytes is now feasible for most (≈ 85%) couples at risk.

TREATMENT. The main treatment for primary phenylalanine hydroxylase deficiency is dietary restriction of the amino acid. There are several semisynthetic diet products ("orphan foods") for this purpose. Phenylketonuric patients can tolerate only 250 to 500 mg of phenylalanine per day to maintain the blood phenylalanine level well below 1 mM. Intake, blood levels of phenylalanine, and growth rate are monitored at frequent intervals to avoid undertreatment or overtreatment. *Treatment into adult life is now recommended to maintain normal neuropsychologic function.* Well-treated patients have normal or near-normal intellectual development.

The tetrahydrobiopterin-deficient forms require continuous replacement therapy of cofactor alone or in combination with neurotransmitter precursors. Whether effective postnatal treatment of these disorders is feasible remains to be seen.

MATERNAL HYPERPHENYLALANINEMIA. *This problem is relevant to all practitioners who counsel women about pregnancy.* Intrauterine hyperphenylalaninemia places the fetus at risk of microcephaly, mental retardation, and organ malformations (notably cardiac). Accordingly, all females with hyperphenylalaninemia should be identified, followed (registries exist for this purpose), counseled about risk when they attain reproductive age, and treated with diet to maintain near-normal blood phenylalanine levels before conception and throughout the pregnancy. This treatment prevents harm to the fetus, but it is still under evaluation.

GENETICS. Mutant alleles (at all relevant loci) are recessive. Their aggregate frequency in the population is ≈ 0.01, meaning that 2% of the population is heterozygous. Explanations for the high frequency of this "rare" phenotype and its genes include founder effects and genetic drift (observed in some populations), selective advantage in the heterozygote (unproved), hypermutability at the locus (observed), reproductive compensation (unlikely), and multiple loci involved in the trait (observed).

Levy HL: Maternal phenylketonuria. Prog Clin Biol 281:227, 1988. *A good discussion of a major problem (maternal hyperphenylalaninemia).*

Scriver CR, Kaufman S, Woo SLC: The hyperphenylalaninemias. *In* Scriver CR, Beaudet AL, Sly WS, et al. (eds.): The Metabolic and Molecular Bases of Inherited Disease. 7th ed. New York, McGraw-Hill, 1995. *A reference covering all major issues concerning the hyperphenylalaninemias.*

ALKAPTONURIA*

DEFINITION. Alkaptonuria is a rare hereditary disease in which homogentisic acid oxidase activity is missing. Homogentisic acid produced during the metabolism of phenylalanine and tyrosine accumulates and is excreted in the urine. It causes pigmentation of cartilage and other connective tissue (ochronosis) and in later years a degenerative arthritis of the spine and the larger peripheral joints. The disease has historical significance, for it was chiefly on the basis of study of families with alkaptonuria that Sir Archibald Garrod developed the concept of inborn errors of metabolism. The disease is inherited as an autosomal recessive trait. No method of detection of heterozygotes has been found. The alkaptonuria gene (symbol AKU) has been mapped to a 16 centimorgan region on human chromosome 3q2.

INCIDENCE AND PREVALENCE. At least 600 cases have been reported, including one in an Egyptian mummy 3500 years old. A prevalence of three to five per million individuals was found in Northern Ireland.

PATHOGENESIS. The activity of homogentisic acid oxidase in the normal adult human liver is sufficient to metabolize over 1600 grams of homogentisic acid per day. Normally, no homogentisic acid can be detected in plasma or urine. In alkaptonuric individuals there is no detectable activity of this enzyme in liver or kidney tissue. Plasma levels of homogentisic acid rise to about 3 mg per deciliter, and the urinary excretion ranges from 4 to 8 grams per day. Mammalian tissue contains an enzyme called homogentisic acid polyphenoloxidase that catalyzes the oxidation of homogentisic acid to an ochronotic pigment, but pigment can also be produced nonenzymatically in the presence of oxygen and alkali, as, for example, in urine. The homogentisic acid polymer has a high affinity

for cartilage and connective tissue macromolecules. The stained tissue is fragile and eventually may break down, leading to degenerative intervertebral disc or joint disease. Homogentisic acid may also have a direct effect upon collagen synthesis through inhibition of lysyl hydroxylase.

PATHOLOGY. In an adult alkaptonuric patient, cartilage in many areas, particularly the costal, laryngeal, and tracheal cartilage, is densely pigmented, sometimes appearing coal-black. Pigmentation is also present throughout the body in fibrous tissue, fibrocartilage, tendons, and ligaments. To a lesser degree, it is also found in the endocardium, in the intima of larger vessels, in various organs such as kidney and lung, and in the epidermis.

CLINICAL MANIFESTATIONS. Homogentisic acid is present in urine from birth. Urine is colorless when passed but darker when alkaline or after long exposure to air. Before the days of disposable diapers, the diagnosis was sometimes made when diapers turned brown in alkaline soaps. Pigment may appear in perspiration and stain clothing in the axillary and genital regions. Generally, the earliest change that can be detected externally is a slight pigmentation of the sclerae or the ears, beginning at age 20 to 30. The cartilage of the ears may be slate blue or gray and feel irregular and thickened. Sometimes dusky discolorations of underlying tendons can be seen through the skin over the hands. In many patients, however, pigment is scarcely evident. The arthritis usually produces limitation of motion of the hips, knee joints, or shoulders. There may be periods of acute inflammation, and later there is usually rather marked limitation of motion and ankylosis in the lumbosacral region. The arthritic complications are often severe and painful and may lead to extensive crippling. In addition, alkaptonuric patients appear to have a high incidence of cardiovascular disease, including generalized arteriosclerosis and chronic mitral and aortic valvulitis, with calcification of valves and annulus. At least one degenerated pigmented aortic valve has been replaced with a prosthesis. Myocardial infarction is a common cause of death. Other reported complications include ruptured intervertebral discs, prostatitis, and renal stones.

RADIOGRAPHIC CHANGES. These may be almost pathognomonic of alkaptonuria. The vertebral bodies of the lumbar spine show degeneration of the intervertebral discs with narrowing of the space and dense calcification of remaining disc material. There is variable fusion of vertebral bodies, but little osteophyte formation and minimal calcification of intervertebral ligaments. The degenerative changes of ochronotic arthritis are most severe in the hip, shoulder, and knee, and there may be calcific deposits in the tendons. The sacroiliac joints and smaller joints of the extremities usually show little or no abnormality. Ear cartilage may be calcified.

DIAGNOSIS AND DIFFERENTIAL DIAGNOSIS. The diagnosis is suggested by the history of pigmentary changes of urine, the presence of nonglucose reducing substance, the pigmentation of sclerae or cartilage, arthritic episodes, and especially the typical radiographic changes of the lumbar spine. Specific identification of homogentisic acid in urine can be accomplished by chromatographic or enzymatic assays.

The ochronotic changes of skin and cartilage may be confused with pigmentary changes resulting from prolonged use of quinacrine hydrochloride (Atabrine) or from use of carbolic acid dressings for chronic cutaneous ulcers. The arthritis must be differentiated chiefly from rheumatoid arthritis, osteoarthritis, and gout.

TREATMENT. There is no effective treatment although a low protein diet for life would be prudent. Dietary restriction of phenylalanine and tyrosine of the degree necessary to reduce homogentisic aciduria is impractical and potentially deleterious. Large amounts of ascorbic acid have been given in an effort to reduce pigment formation. Ascorbic acid protects lysyl hydroxylase from inhibition by homogentisic acid *in vitro.* It does not alter the metabolic defect. NTBC (2-(2-nitro-4-trifluoromethylbenzoyl)-1,3-cyclohexanedione), the potent inhibitor of p-hydroxyphenylpyruvic acid oxidase, would prevent excess formation of homogentisic acid and could be a new therapy in alkaptonuria.

La Du BN: Alkaptonuria. *In* Scriver CR, Beaudet AL, Sly WS, Valle D (eds.): The Metabolic and Molecular Bases of Inherited Disease. 7th ed. New York, McGraw-Hill, 1995. *A detailed discussion of the history, clinical features, and biochemical derangements of alkaptonuria and ochronosis.*

Pollak M, Chou Y-H W, Cerda JJ, et al.: Homozygosity mapping of the gene for alkaptonuria to chromosome 3q2. Nature Genetics 5:201, 1993. *A significant step in the history of this classic disease.*

---

*James B. Wyngaarden, M.D., wrote this section for the 19th edition. His text is used here with minor revisions; there is some new material.

177 THE HYPERPROLINEMIAS AND HYDROXYPROLINEMIA

James M. Phang

There are three autosomal recessive genetic disorders in the degradative pathways for proline and hydroxyproline. Although these rare disorders are generally benign, the resulting metabolic abnormalities, at least for one, is associated with neurologic manifestations in childhood.

The α-nitrogen of the imino acids proline and hydroxyproline is incorporated within a pyrrolidine ring. This feature confers structural and functional properties to proteins. Owing to the ring structure, the metabolism of proline, including biosynthesis from glutamate and ornithine and degradation back to glutamate, is catalyzed by a specific set of enzymes. Both synthetic and degradative pathways share Δ^1-pyrroline-5-carboxylate as an intermediate. The cycling of proline may mediate the transfer of reducing-oxidizing potential to regulate metabolic pathways. Preformed hydroxyproline is not incorporated into proteins. Instead, hydroxyproline is formed from peptide-linked proline primarily in collagen.

HYPERPROLINEMIAS. The two genetic disorders in proline metabolism are characterized by hyperprolinemia and iminoglycinuria, but they are due to different enzyme deficiencies; type II hyperprolinemia can be diagnosed directly. This disorder is due to a deficiency of Δ^1-pyrroline-5-carboxylate dehydrogenase, which catalyzes the second step in the degradative pathway for proline (Fig. 177–1); the deficiency in enzyme activity can be determined in extracts of circulating leukocytes or cultured fibroblasts. Hyperprolinemia in type II is more marked than in type I, but the distinguishing feature of type II is the accumulation of Δ^1-pyrroline-5-carboxylate in plasma and its excretion in urine. The hyperprolinemia in type I is due to a deficiency of the first enzyme in the pathway, proline oxidase. Although plasma proline is generally lower than in type II, the diagnosis of type I is one of exclusion, i.e., hyperprolinemia unaccompanied by Δ^1-pyrroline-5-carboxylate in urine or plasma.

Clinical manifestations have been described with the hyperprolinemias, but the association may be due to chance because in most cases hyperprolinemia was identified fortuitously in patients presenting with clinical abnormalities (biased ascertainment). This is true especially for type I hyperprolinemia: Renal disease and mental retardation found in some pedigrees were shown to segregate independently of hyperprolinemia. For type II hyperprolinemia, however, clinical associations untainted by biased ascertainment have been identified. Screening of a large pedigree in Ireland identified 14 new cases confirmed by elevated plasma Δ^1-pyrroline-5-carboxylate and undetectable enzyme activity in leukocytes. Nine of these 14 new subjects had a history of recurrent childhood febrile seizures requiring hospitalization and treatment with anticonvulsants. Thus, the association of type II hyperprolinemia with a predisposition to seizures appears convincing. Adults in this pedigree were fertile and otherwise normal. Although the mechanism for this association remains unclear, the recent cloning of a high-affinity proline transporter in rat brain suggests that proline or its metabolites may have a neuromodulatory function.

HYDROXYPROLINEMIA. Hydroxyprolinemia with hydroxyprolinuria, but without hyperprolinemia or hyperprolinuria, has been described in members of several families. Although the degradation of hydroxyproline parallels that of proline, the pathway enzymes are distinct except that the second degradation step is catalyzed by a common enzyme that dehydrogenates both Δ^1-pyrroline-5-carboxylate (see above) and 3-OH-Δ^1-pyrroline-5-carboxylate. The first step in the degradation, however, is catalyzed by distinct oxidases. The absence of urinary Δ^1-pyrroline-5-carboxylate or its hydroxylated congener leads to the conclusion that this autosomal recessive disorder is due to a deficiency of hydroxyproline oxidase. In this disorder there are no clinical manifestations related to abnormalities in collagen metabolism or central nervous system function, and therapy is not indicated.

Flynn MP, Martin MC, Moore PT, et al.: Type II hyperprolinaemia in a pedigree of Irish travellers (nomads). Arch Dis Child 64:1699, 1989.
Fremeau RT Jr, Caron MG, Blakely RD: Molecular cloning and expression of a high affinity L-proline transporter expressed in putative glutamatergic pathways of rat brain. Neuron 8:915, 1992.
Phang JM, Scriver CR: Disorders of proline and hydroxyproline metabolism. *In* Scriver CR, Beaudet AL, Sly WS, et al. (eds.): The Metabolic Basis of Inherited Disease. 6th ed. New York; McGraw-Hill, 1989, p 577.

178 DISEASES OF THE UREA CYCLE

Stephen D. Cederbaum

Ammonia is a highly toxic metabolic product, which, when present at levels no more than two times the upper limits of normal (10 to 25 μM), may cause symptoms. The urea cycle is a five-step metabolic pathway in which two ammonia molecules and one bicarbonate molecule are converted to the relatively easily excreted and nontoxic urea. It is the only major pathway to remove waste nitrogen derived from ingested protein or from normal or augmented protein turnover in the body. The urea cycle occurs predominantly or possibly exclusively in the liver.

In children, the vast majority of cases of hyperammonemia are the result of inborn errors of metabolism, primarily of the urea cycle. In adults, a larger proportion are due to liver failure and less frequently to toxic ingestion. Nevertheless, with the wider availability of blood ammonia tests, the increased recognition of urea cycle disorders, and more successful treatment modalities, the inherited disorders of ammonia metabolism are being recognized with greater frequency in adolescents and adults with acute or intermittent organic brain syndrome. Hyperammonemia appears to be better tolerated in infants and young children, in part because the cranium is more compliant. Ammonia levels that leave minimal residual damage in infants may be deadly in adults. Ammonia itself appears to be the metabolite toxic to the central nervous system; however, there is some speculation that the accumulation of glutamine, a compound in equilibrium with ammonia, may be involved as well. The primary toxic effect appears to be the uptake of fluid into as-

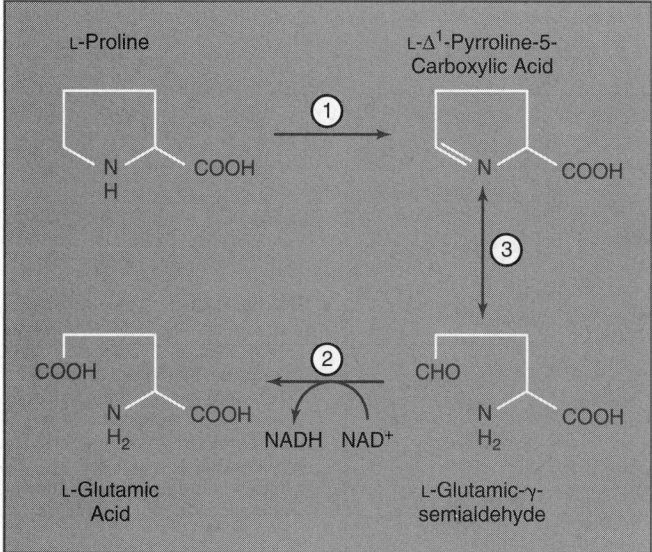

FIGURE 177–1. Schematic of the degradative pathway for proline. Reaction 1 is catalyzed by proline oxidase (EC number unassigned); reaction 2 is catalyzed by Δ^1-pyrroline-5-carboxylic acid dehydrogenase (EC 1.5.1.12) and reaction 3 is spontaneous. Type I hyperprolinemia is due to blockade at reaction 1 (deficiency of proline oxidase), and type II hyperprolinemia is due to blockade at reaction 2 (deficiency of Δ^1-pyrroline-5-carboxylic acid dehydrogenase).

trocytes causing cerebral edema. Death is caused acutely by herniation of the brain through the foramen magnum with consequent cerebral ischemia, but survivors may have various degrees of brain damage.

The urea cycle is shown in Figure 178–1. The five enzymes generally associated with it are carbamoylphosphate synthetase 1 (CPS-1) and ornithine transcarbamoylase (OTC), found in the mitochondrion; and argininosuccinate synthetase (ASAS), argininosuccinate lyase (ASAL), and arginase 1 (ARG-1) found in the cytoplasm. N-Acetylglutamate synthetase catalyzes the synthesis of N-acetylglutamate, which activates CPS-1 and modulates urea cycle function, and the ornithine transporter recycles ornithine to the mitochondrion. Deficiency of these latter enzymes has been associated with symptomatic hyperammonia, the former only in infants.

The normal urea cycle can increase its ureagenic capacity greatly in response to ammonia challenge. The genes for all five enzymes have been cloned and are available for defining mutations, prenatal diagnosis, and population studies.

Disorders of the urea cycle are estimated to occur in 1 in 25,000 births. It is probable that 2 to 4% of the population is heterozygous for a urea cycle defect, although only women who are carriers of ornithine transcarbamoylase deficiency are known to be prone to disease. It is unclear whether patients receiving intensive chemotherapy for leukemia, in whom hyperammonemia occurs rarely, or patients receiving valproate anticonvulsant therapy, in whom it occurs more mildly, are heterozygotes for one or another of these enzyme deficiencies.

Complete deficiency of any of the first four enzymes in the cycle usually leads to severe hyperammonemia in the first 2 to 4 days of life. The patients have irritability, lethargy, and poor feeding that progress rapidly to stupor, seizures, coma, respirator dependence, and death. The plasma ammonia level often exceeds 1000 μM, and urea levels are extremely low. Episodic hyperammonemia occurs in association with periods of endogenous protein catabolism and severely affects patients, such as those with severe OTC deficiency; they almost certainly die or suffer severe neurologic impairment during one of these episodes. Patients with partial deficiency of urea cycle enzymes or those who avoid hyperammonemia in the neonatal period may present at any time later in life, from infancy to adulthood. Older patients have irritability, vomiting, and disorientation, which may progress (as in the infants) to stupor, seizures, coma, and death. These episodes are often precipitated by severe infection, excessive protein intake, parturition, or rarely by menstruation, or they may have no apparent cause.

Some general genetic characteristics of defects in the urea cycle are presented in Table 178–1.

TABLE 178–1. GENETIC CHARACTERISTICS OF DISORDERS OF THE UREA CYCLE

Enzyme Defect	Inheritance Pattern	Heterozygote Detection	Heterozygote Symptoms	Prenatal Diagnosis*
Carbamoyl phosphate synthetase	AR†	No‡	No	Yes
Ornithine transcarbamoylase	X-linked	Yes, in most instances*	Yes	Yes
Argininosuccinate synthetase	AR	No‡	No	Yes
Argininosuccinate lyase	AR	Yes	No	Yes
Arginase I	AR	Yes	No	Yes

* With varying degrees of ease.
† AR = Autosomal recessive.
‡ Heterozygotes for all disorders can be detected, if the specific base change in the gene has been ascertained. This is not practical at this time outside of the research laboratory.

ENZYME DEFICIENCIES

DEFICIENCY OF CARBAMOYL PHOSPHATE SYNTHETASE. This, the first enzyme in the urea cycle, constitutes up to 25% of the mitochondrial matrix protein in liver, and ordinarily all of the carbamyl phosphate synthesized from ammonium and bicarbonate by CPS-1 is used to produce urea. Orotic acid and pyrimidine are products of carbamoylphosphate as well, which is synthesized by a second, independently regulated cytoplasmic enzyme. Patients with both the neonatal and later-onset forms have been described. Diagnosis may be inferred from hyperammonemia, low to absent levels of citrulline in the plasma amino acid profile, and normal or elevated bicarbonate levels. During acute hyperammonemia there is usually a generalized hyperaminoacidemia with particular prominence of glutamine. Liver transplantation alone offers definitive treatment. Restricting dietary protein, supplementing essential amino acids and citrulline, hospitalizing for "catabolic crises," hemodialysis or peritoneal dialysis, and administering phenylacetate (or phenylbutyrate) and benzoate to divert ammonia to phenylacetylglutamine and benzoylglycine (hippurate) are used to control symptoms and treat crises (Fig. 178–2). Patients with this and other urea cycle defects are prone to develop severe hyperammonemia with valproate anticonvulsant therapy.

DEFICIENCY OF ORNITHINE TRANSCARBAMOYLASE. This mitochondrial enzyme catalyzes the reaction of carbamyl phosphate with ornithine to form citrulline, which is then transported out of the mitochondrion for further metabolism. The acute form of this X-linked enzyme deficiency usually occurs in males. Uncommonly

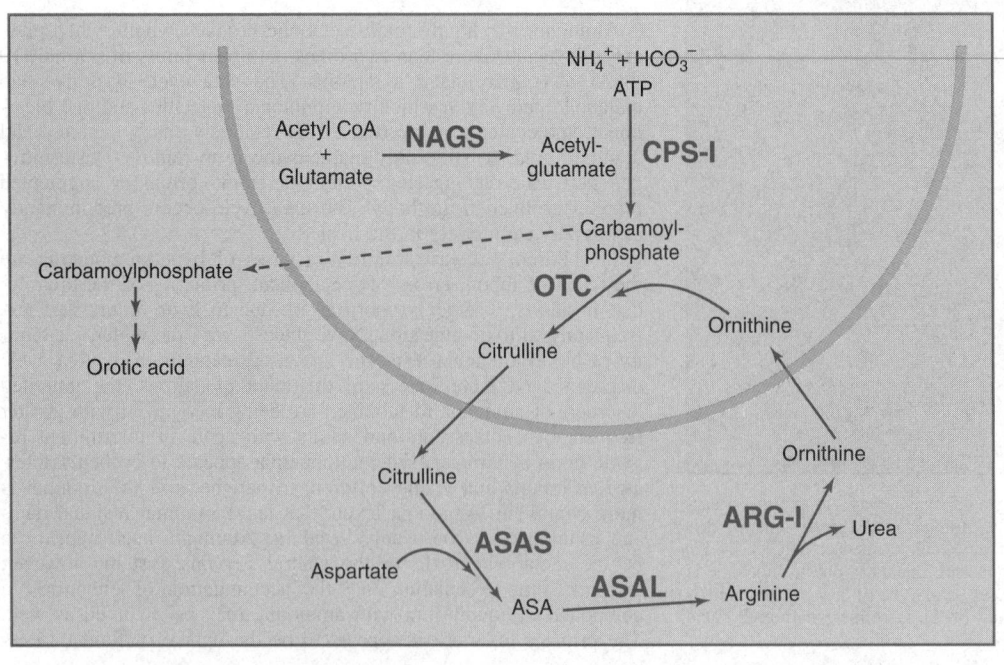

FIGURE 178–1. Abbreviated pathway for the urea cycle. NAGS = N-acetylglutamate synthetase; CPS-1 = carbamoylphosphate synthetase 1; OTC = ornithine transcarbamoylase; ASAS = argininosuccinate synthetase; ASAL = argininosuccinate lyase; ARG-1 = arginase 1. Enzymes within the bold line function within the mitochondrial matrix.

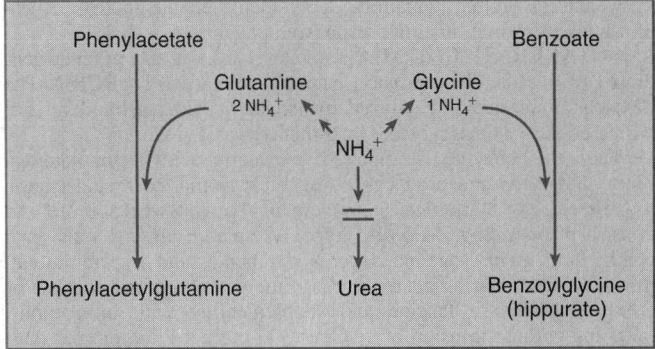

FIGURE 178–2. Mechanisms of ammonia diversion from the urea cycle with administration of sodium phenylacetate and sodium benzoate.

a newborn female may be severely affected, thought to be due to random X-chromosome inactivation. Female carriers of this codominant trait usually escape obvious symptoms, but those who have them usually present later in life or at parturition with hyperammonemic crises, some of which may be severe enough to be fatal. A smaller number of males with partial enzyme deficiency may present later as well. Patients with this "later-onset" form of the disease may suffer from severe and otherwise inexplicable protein intolerance. The amino and organic acid profiles resemble those of CPS-1 deficiency. OTC deficiency is distinguished by extraordinarily high levels of orotic acid in the urine, formed when the excess carbamoyl phosphate accumulating in the mitochondrion leaks into the cytoplasm and is channelled into the pyrimidine biosynthetic pathway (see Fig. 178–1). Orotic acid levels may be normal when ammonia has been controlled. Because of this typical clinical biochemical picture, liver biopsy to confirm enzymes is less frequently undertaken than in CPS-1 deficiency. An allopurinol challenge may be necessary to detect carrier females, a test with <100% accuracy. The treatment is identical to that described for CPS-1 deficiency.

DEFICIENCY OF ARGININOSUCCINATE SYNTHETASE (CITRULLINEMIA). This cytoplasmic enzyme condenses the citrulline synthesized by OTC with aspartate to form argininosuccinate in a reaction that introduces the second ammonia nitrogen for excretion as urea. ASAS deficiency leads to hyperammonemia, greatly increased blood citrulline levels, and excretion of excessive amounts of citrulline and orotic acid in the urine. Here, too, neonatal, later-onset, or symptomless deficiency of the enzyme has been reported. Genetic heterogeneity at the ASAS locus has been demonstrated by residual enzyme activity or by study of the gene and its mRNA.

Treatment is similar to that for CPS-1 and OTC deficiencies except that arginine is supplemented instead of citrulline. Citrulline excretion is more complete than that of ammonia, and managing this condition is somewhat easier.

DEFICIENCY OF ARGININOSUCCINATE LYASE (ARGININOSUCCINIC ACIDURIA). ASA is cleaved into two smaller product molecules, arginine and fumarate, in a reaction catalyzed by ASA lyase. This enzyme deficiency results in massive accumulation and excretion of ASA. Variable onset or lack of symptoms characterizes this enzyme deficiency as well. ASA is actively secreted by the renal tubules and its synthesis can be stimulated by stoichiometric amounts of arginine as a source of ornithine to drive the urea cycle. By this means, ammonia levels are rapidly reduced and can be controlled more reliably than in any other urea cycle disorder.

DEFICIENCY OF ARGINASE 1 (HYPERARGININEMIA). Arginase, the final enzyme in the urea cycle, catalyzes the hydrolysis of arginine to urea and ornithine, the latter returned to the mitochondrion to participate in another cycle of ammonia detoxification (see Fig. 178–1). Clinical symptoms of hyperargininemia, the rarest of the urea cycle defects, are of later onset, are more gradual and relentless in progression, and are less frequently or seriously punctuated by apparent episodes of acute hyperammonemia and organic brain syndrome. Rather typically, normal patients begin to develop gait abnormalities and spasticity at age 2 to 3, and cortical and pyramidal tract dysfunction progresses slowly. More than 80% of the reported patients are still alive, some at age 30 or older. The di-

agnosis is often suspected when arginine levels are found to be elevated in blood or urine. Excess arginine excretion in urine along with secondary cystinuria pattern is more variable and less reliable as a screening method. Hyperammonemia is usually seen only during acute catabolic episodes.

Although most patients have been moderately to severely retarded at detection, treatment by limiting protein and diverting ammonia reverses many of the most severe manifestations of the disease, and presymptomatic treatment has allowed two patients to reach the age of 20 or older without apparent clinical manifestations.

FUTURE TREATMENT

Urea cycle defects, originally considered a pediatric problem, are moving into the realm of internal medicine. Internists must cast aside the lactulose used for hyperammonemia of liver failure and gastrointestinal bleeding in favor of diversion therapy and hemodialysis. Soon liver replacement, the artificial liver, and gene therapy will be more widely used. As breakthroughs in gene technology allow us to dissect the pathobiology of the acute catabolic process, efforts to control this process rather than control its consequences will become increasingly important.

Bachmann C: Urea cycle disorders. *In* Fernandes J, Saudubray J-M, Tada K (eds.): Inborn Metabolic Diseases. New York, Springer-Verlag, 1990, p 211. *A practical clinical chapter on urea cycle disorders reflecting a transatlantic perspective.*

Brusilow SW, Horwich AL: Urea cycle enzymes. *In* Scriver CR, Beaudet AL, Sly WS, Valle, D (eds.): The Metabolic and Molecular Bases of Inherited Disease. 7th ed. New York, McGraw-Hill, 1995. *The definitive clinical and molecular discussion of these inborn errors.*

Elsas III LJ, Acosta PB: Nutritional support of inherited metabolic diseases. *In* Shils ME, Olson JA, Shike M (eds.): Modern Nutrition in Health and Disease. 8th ed. Malvern, PA, Lea & Febiger, 1994, p 1147. *A practical guide to the nutritional aspects of treating this and other metabolic disorders.*

179 BRANCHED-CHAIN AMINOACIDURIAS

Louis J. Elsas

Leucine, isoleucine, and valine are essential amino acids that share branching, aliphatic chains.

MAPLE SYRUP URINE DISEASE (MSUD). This disorder, also called branched-chain α-ketoaciduria, derives its name from the burnt-sugar smell of affected infants. MSUD is caused by impaired branched chain α-ketoacid dehydrogenase, which catalyzes decarboxylation of the α-ketoacid derivatives of all three of these amino acids. Isovaleric acidemia affects only the next step of leucine catabolism and is caused by defects in isovaleryl CoA dehydrogenase. Both disorders conform to autosomal recessive patterns of inheritance. The affected homozygote exhibits impaired activity in the branched-chain α-ketoacid dehydrogenase (BCKD) multienzyme complex. This enzyme catalyzes oxidative decarboxylation and transacylation of α-ketoisocaproate, α-keto-β-methylvalerate, and α-ketoisovalerate, which are derived from deamination of leucine, isoleucine, and valine, respectively. The blocked reaction is

$$\text{Branched chain} - \overset{\overset{\displaystyle O}{\|}}{C} - COOH + CoASH + NAD^+ \longrightarrow$$

$$\text{Branched chain} - \overset{\overset{\displaystyle O}{\|}}{C} - CoA + CO_2 + NADH + H^+$$

If impaired, branched chain α-ketoacids and amino acids accumulate throughout the body and produce neurotoxicity by poorly defined mechanisms.

The disease is caused by mutations in one of six genes, which code for the six different proteins that make up the branched chain α-ketoacid dehydrogenase multienzyme complex. A wide range of mutations is defined, along with the consequent severity of impaired enzyme and clinical manifestations (Table 179–1).

TABLE 179–1. GENES, PROTEINS, AND MUTATIONS IN THE HUMAN BRANCHED-CHAIN α-KETOACID DEHYDROGENASE COMPLEX

Name (Function)	Chromosome Locus	Gene Size (kb)	Mature Protein (kd)	Mutation
E1α (decarboxylase)	19q13.1-q13.2	55	47	Y393N (Mennonite missense mutation)
E1β (stabilizes decarboxylase)	6p21-p22	100	37	11bp deletion (frameshift with premature STOP)
E2 (acyltransferase)	1p31	68	52	E163STOP
				F215C (exonic and intronic insertions, deletions, and transitions)
E3 (dehydrogenase)	7	?	55	Affects other substrate-specific dehydrogenases (α-ketoglutarate and pyruvate)
E1α kinase (inactivates)	?	?	43	?
E1α phosphatase (activates)	?	?	?	?

These proteins are encoded in the nuclear genome. Once translated in the cytosol, they are guided to the mitochondria by amino terminal leader sequences, transmigrate through outer and inner membrane, and assemble in the mitochondrial matrix. The six proteins are (1) a dimeric E1 or branched-chain α-ketoacid decarboxylases (E1α and E1β); (2) a branched-chain dihydrolipoamide acyltransferase (E2); (3) lipoamide oxidoreductase (E3); (4) E1 α kinase; and (5) E1 α phosphatase.

Several cofactors are involved in the overall reaction, including thiamin pyrophosphate, lipoamide covalently bound to E2, coenzyme A, and nicotinamide adenine dinucleotide. Many patients respond to pharmacologic excesses of thiamine supplement (8 mg per kilogram per day). The presumed mechanism is that by saturating binding sites for thiamine pyrophosphate on E1α, the multienzyme complex is stabilized to biologic degradation.

Diagnosis. In typical MSUD, feeding difficulties and apnea develop in a newborn who was normal at birth. Convulsions and decorticate rigidity may develop, and, before newborn screening, affected infants died or were severely damaged. With newborn screening, retrieval, diagnosis, and diet intervention before age 2 weeks, these children not only survive but have reached adulthood and can reproduce.

In surveyed populations the frequency of MSUD varies from 1 in 760 (in Mennonites) to an average United States figure of 1 in 200,000 newborns. Atypical cases with less severe clinical manifestations may be missed in newborn screening and appear with intermittent ataxia in later childhood or early adulthood. The diagnosis should be suspected clinically by the patient's intermittent symptoms related to protein ingestion and sweet smell to the earwax. A positive dinitrophenylhydrazine reaction is seen in urine, and the diagnosis is confirmed by the abnormal excesses of branched-chain amino acids and ketoacids in blood and urine. The enzyme defect is demonstrable in leukocytes and fibroblasts, and prenatal monitoring has been accomplished both biochemically and through DNA analysis.

Treatment. Treatment is aimed at limiting intake of branched-chain amino acids to prevent accumulation of neurotoxic branched-chain α-ketoacids. However, these essential amino acids must be ingested in large enough quantities to enable new protein synthesis and normal growth. Commercial formulas are available to accomplish this goal. In infancy and early childhood, anabolism is encouraged by providing excess calories and maintaining total protein intake at the recommended daily allowance. Treatment is monitored clinically by growth and development and biochemically by analyzing plasma amino acid concentrations. Because leucine residues are more frequent than isoleucine and valine in natural proteins, care must be given not to overrestrict isoleucine and valine while attempting to lower blood concentrations of leucine by restricting dietary natural protein. Thiamine supplements enable increased protein intake in some thiamine-responsive patients.

ISOVALERIC ACIDEMIA. Isovaleryl CoA is the product generated from α-ketoisocaproate (leucine's derivative) by BCKD. The next catabolic step is catalyzed by isovaleryl CoA dehydrogenase, which coverts isovaleryl CoA to β-methylcrotonyl CoA.

When this enzyme is impaired, isovaleric acid accumulates in blood and urine and produces a foul odor similar to rancid cheese or sweaty feet. Symptoms are severe in the first week of life and consist of vomiting, acidosis, hypoglycemia, tremors, coma, and death. Leukopenia, anemia, thrombocytopenia, and hyperammonemia may occur during acute attacks. Emergency therapy consists of eliminating dietary leucine and supplementing with intravenous, oral, and colonic infusion of glycine (300 mg per kilogram per day) to provide an alternate excretory pathway for the nontoxic adduct, isovaleryl glycine. Carnitine (100 mg per kilogram) may provide nontoxic adducts of isovaleryl carnitine. Both adducts are excreted in the urine. As patients mature, they have less frequent attacks and are developmentally normal. "Attacks" are caused by excess leucine ingestion, starvation, infections, or other causes of catabolism. Chronic intermittent forms of this disorder have not been differentiated from acute infantile forms at the biochemical or molecular level of enzyme or gene analysis and may result from epigenetic phenomena.

Diagnosis. The diagnosis is suspected from the clinical presentation and associated odor and is established by demonstrating excess isovaleric acid and its adducts in the urine by gas-liquid chromatography. The gene has been cloned and sequenced and some mutations have been defined.

Treatment. Chronic therapy includes reduced intake of leucine. Unlike MSUD, valine and isoleucine are normally catabolized and are required as essential nutrients in normal amounts in the diet. Supplements of glycine (90 to 100 mg per kilogram per day) and carnitine (10 mg per kilogram per day) are used as part of chronic dietary management. Outcome is excellent in both infantile and later-onset forms of isovaleric acidemia diseases if the acute, irreversible effects of the neonatal disease are prevented.

Danner DJ, Elsas LJ: Disorders of branched chain amino and keto acid metabolism. In Scriver CR, Beaudet A, Sly W, Valle D (eds.): The Metabolic and Molecular Bases of Inherited Disease. 7th ed. New York, McGraw-Hill, 1995. *Sophisticated discussion of clinical, biochemical, and pathophysiologic characteristics of these diseases (268 references).*

Elsas LJ, Acosta PB: Nutrition support of inherited metabolic disease. In Shils ME, Olson JE, Shike M (eds.): Modern Nutrition in Health and Disease. 8th ed. Malvern, PA, Lea & Febiger, 1994, p 1147. *A complete approach to dietary therapy of these diseases.*

180 HOMOCYSTINURIA

Bruce A. Barshop

Homocystinuria *per se* refers to abnormal urinary excretion of the disulfide form of homocysteine, and excessive blood homocysteine or homocystine, that is, homocyst(e)inemia, is a sign of a small number of specific metabolic disorders. Cardinal signs of the homocyst(e)inemia sequence include ocular lens dislocation, mental retardation, skeletal abnormalities, and thromboembolic complications. Cystathionine β-synthase deficiency is the most common cause. Rarer causes are disorders of homocysteine remethylation due to methylenetetrahydrofolate reductase deficiency or a variety of disorders of vitamin B_{12} distribution or metabolism to the active methylcobalamin cofactor for methionine synthase. Homocystinuria may also arise pharmacologically, as with triacetyl-azauridine, possibly related to pyridoxine depletion.

BIOCHEMISTRY

Homocysteine is a nonprotein amino acid that is the transmethylation product of methionine (Fig. 180–1). Homocysteine may be remethylated to methionine or may participate in a transulfuration sequence. The proportion of remethylation to transulfuration is regulated in humans, varying with availability of methionine and cysteine.

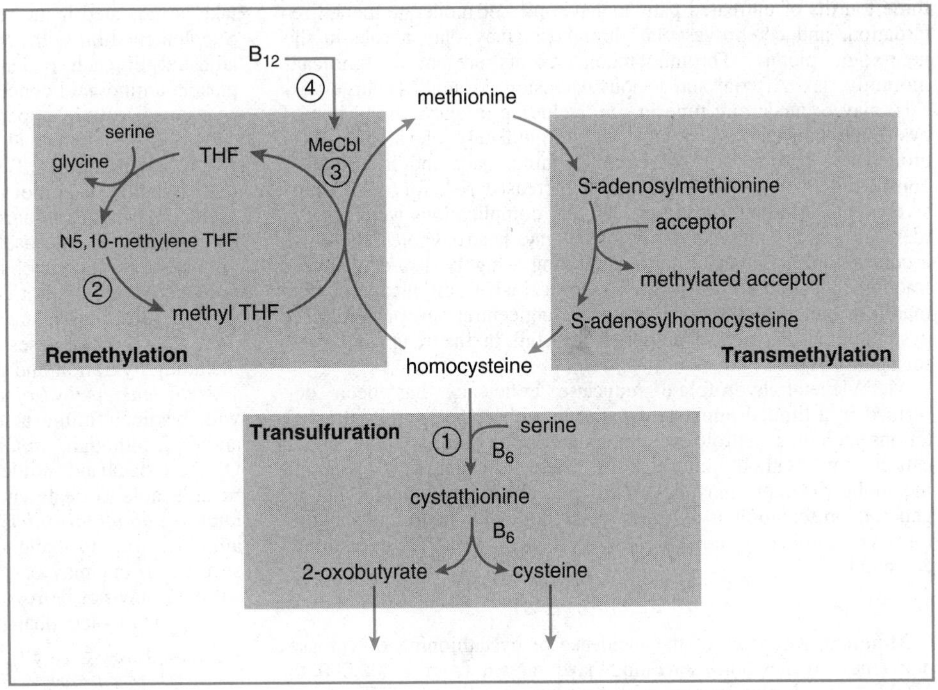

FIGURE 180-1. Pathways of homocysteine metabolism. The systems of transmethylation, remethylation, and transulfuration are marked. Steps discussed are numbered: (1) cystathionine β-synthase; (2) methylenetetrahydrofolate reductase; (3) methionine synthase; (4) systems of cobalamin absorption, distribution, and reduction: THF = tetrahydrofolate; MeCbl = methylcobalamin; B_{12} = cyanocobalamin/hydroxocobalamin; B_6 = pyridoxine.

Deficiency of cystathionine β-synthase results from a range of structural enzyme mutations, with heterogeneity in severity, most notably with respect to responsiveness of the biochemical abnormalities to pyridoxine. Approximately half of reported patients are pyridoxine responsive, and in these patients the course is generally less severe. While there is intrafamilial as well as interfamilial variability in clinical expression, there is complete concordance at the extremes of pyridoxine unresponsiveness or absence of immunoreactive material. Defects in homocysteine remethylation arise from deficiency of methylenetetrahydrofolate reductase or disorders of cobalamin metabolism, due to either impaired cellular accumulation in both adenosylcobalamin and methylcobalamin (Cbl C and D defects), defective cobalamin reduction on methionine synthase (Cbl E and G), or decreased lysosomal cobalamin entry or efflux (transcobalamin II deficiency or Cbl F, respectively). All of these inborn conditions are inherited in an autosomal recessive manner.

Cystathionine β-synthase maps to chromosome 21q22, a region associated with the Down syndrome phenotype. Transcobalamin II maps to chromosome 22q11-q13.1, and the remaining disorders are not mapped.

CLINICAL FEATURES

Cystathionine β-synthase deficiency is pleiotropic, with effects in eye, skeleton, and central nervous and vascular systems (Table 180-1). Nontraumatic dislocation of the ocular lens can be a presenting finding. Almost all untreated patients develop some abnormality of the skeletal system. Eye and skeletal system changes resemble those in Marfan syndrome, which is due to a defect in the fibrillin gene. Fibrillin, present in high concentration in the zonular fibers and the matrix of the periosteum and perichondrium, is extremely rich in cysteine; fibrillin structure may be affected either by cysteine limitation or homocysteinylation. Between one third and

TABLE 180-1. HOMOCYSTINURIA

Class	Cause	Biochemical Features			System	Clinical Features Signs
		hcys	met	MMA		
Homocysteine transulfuration defect	Cystathionine β-synthase deficiency	↑	↑	—	Ocular	Ectopia lentis, myopia, glaucoma, optic atrophy, retinal detachment
					Skeletal	Elongated and thinned bones, arachnodactyly, genu valgum, pectus malformation, scoliosis
					Vascular	Thromboembolic events (arterial or venous)
					Neurologic	Mental retardation often in untreated cases Cerebrovascular thromboses, seizures Psychiatric disorders, personality disorder
Homocysteine remethylation defect	Methylenetetrahydrofolate reductase deficiency	↑	↓	—	Ocular	Ectopia lentis
					Vascular	Thromboses
					Neurologic	Variable—psychiatric to severe neurologic
	Cobalamin metabolic defects B_{12} uptake/distribution Transcobalamin II deficiency Cbl F (lysosomal B_{12} efflux defect)	—/↑	—/↓	+/−	Hematologic Pansystemic	Pancytopenia, macrocytosis Methylmalonic acidemia, ketoacidosis
	B_{12} reduction/synthesis of adenosyl-cobalamin and methylcobalamin Cbl C, Cbl D	—/↑	—/↓	+	Pansystemic Hematologic Neurologic	Methylmalonic acidemia, ketoacidosis Pancytopenia Mental retardation
	B_{12} reduction/fixation of methyl-cobalamin to methionine synthetase Cbl E, Cbl G	↑	—/↓	—	Vascular	Vaso-occlusive phenomena

Hcys = homocyst(e)inemia/homocystinuria; met = elevated plasma methionine; MMA = methylmalonic acidemia

three fourths of untreated patients have mild or moderate mental retardation, and cerebrovascular thrombosis may play a role in the neurologic picture. Thromboembolic events present a significant mortality risk. Arterial and venous occlusion, in small or large vessels, may occur at any time in life, including infancy. Blood homocyst(e)ine concentrations may be intermediately elevated in heterozygotes, particularly after a methionine load, and it has been considered that heterozygotes are at increased risk for vaso-occlusive events. Although increased vascular complications were not evident in a large outcome survey of obligate heterozygotes, there are a considerable number of studies showing a highly disproportionate fraction of patients with various vaso-occlusive complications who manifest either blood homocyst(e)ine concentrations or fibroblast cystathionine β-synthase activities that fall in the range observed for heterozygotes.

Methylenetetrahydrofolate reductase deficiency has been described in a limited number of patients, with a spectrum of presentations including neurologic symptoms, thromboses, and lens dislocation, but without conspicuous skeletal changes. Cobalamin metabolic disorders may have clinical features in common, but in general, presentation is in early childhood with neurologic symptoms, megaloblastic anemia, and in some cases, methylmalonic acidemia.

PREVALENCE

Minimum estimates of the incidence of cystathionine β-synthase deficiency by newborn screening have ranged from $1:300,000$ to $1:60,000$ live births, varying with population and method. Estimates for incidence have been in the range of $1:40,000$ in Europe, corresponding to a carrier frequency of about 1%. The incidence of homocysteine remethylation defects appears to be $<1:800,000$.

DIAGNOSIS

Urine metabolic screening generally reveals a positive reaction with cyanide-nitroprusside, but this is neither specific nor particularly sensitive. Quantitative amino acid analysis is superior. Urine, which normally has no measurable homocysteine or homocystine, may have up to 700 μmol homocysteine per day in affected individuals. Diagnosis also requires measuring plasma amino acids, since artifactual homocystinuria (e.g., bacterial contamination of cystathioninuric urine) can be excluded, and since various causes of homocystinuria may be distinguished (Table 180–1). In cystathionine β-synthase deficiency, methionine (normally below 30 μM) may be up to 2000 μM in the plasma, whereas in methylenetetrahydrofolate reductase deficiency or cobalamin metabolic defects that affect methionine synthase, the concentrations of methionine are decreased or normal. In urinary organic acid analysis, the presence of methylmalonic acid (and associated propionate metabolites) in addition to homocystinuria and/or homocysteinemia is characteristic of the defects of cobalamin metabolism. Anemia and macrocytosis are characteristic of the cobalamin metabolism defects, but not of uncomplicated cystathionine β-synthase or methylenetetrahydrofolate reductase deficiency. Associated immunodeficiency is also unique to the cobalamin metabolic defects among these disorders. Methionine loads have been used diagnostically. An oral bolus of methionine (typically 100 mg per kilogram) can distinguish heterozygotes and homozygotes on the basis of peak blood homocysteine concentration at around 4 hours, but overlap with the normal range is considerable for heterozygotes. Assay of cultured cells or biopsy tissue may confirm the diagnosis. Cystathionine β-synthase deficiency can be assayed in liver biopsy specimens, lymphocyte preparations, or fibroblasts; heterozygotes can be distinguished, but there is considerable overlap with normal values. Methylenetetrahydrofolate reductase can be assayed in fibroblasts or liver biopsy specimens, and the cobalamin defects can be distinguished by complementation or uptake studies in cultured fibroblasts.

TREATMENT

In *cystathionine β-synthase deficiency* it is important to determine initially whether a patient is responsive to pyridoxine. Doses of 100 to 500 mg or greater are given per day, and levels of plasma and urinary amino acids should be followed over the course of a few weeks. Folic acid repletion should precede the trial of pyridox-

ine. If the patient responds, pyridoxine supplementation should be continued indefinitely. Dietary management with low methionine intake is indicated if the response to pyridoxine is less than complete. Supplementation with cysteine may be beneficial. The diet must be adjusted in each patient individually so as to approach normal plasma amino acid concentrations. The incidence of certain progressive complications appears to be reduced with dietary therapy, and certainly the intellectual outcome is improved with early institution of dietary treatment. Betaine (N,N,N-trimethylglycine) allows for remethylation of homocysteine by an alternate pathway and may be useful in pyridoxine-unresponsive patients. Dipyridamole and low-dose aspirin may be useful adjuvants, and avoiding agents that can promote thromboembolism, such as oral contraceptives, is probably prudent. Surgery is not contraindicated, but requires special caution; surgical procedures are without thromboembolic complication in more than 95% of cases in which appropriate precautions are taken, including hydration and possibly perioperative pyridoxine treatment.

Methylenetetrahydrofolate reductase deficiency can be treated with betaine, folinic acid, methionine, and additional vitamins B$_6$ and B$_{12}$, although, *uniformly,* results have been less than complete. On the other hand, milder variants may occur in adulthood and may be amenable to treatment aimed at decreasing homocysteine. *Cobalamin metabolic disorders* may be treated with large amounts of vitamin B$_{12}$ (up to 1 mg daily). The response may be dramatically successful, but may be incomplete, and neurologic damage already suffered may not be reversible. Hydroxocobalamin may be more effective than cyanocobalamin.

Mudd SH, Skovby F, Levy HL, et al.: The natural history of homocystinuria due to cystathionine β-synthase deficiency. Am J Hum Genet 37:1, 1985. *The course of the untreated disease is defined in this international questionnaire study covering more than 600 patients, and some effects of treatment are analyzed statistically.*
Pyeritz RE: Homocystinuria. *In* Beighton P (ed.): McKusick's Heritable Disorders of Connective Tissue. St. Louis, CV Mosby, 1993, pp 137–178. *Complete discussion of clinical and metabolic features of homocystinuria with insights into possible effects on fibrillin structure.*

181 DISORDERS OF PURINE AND PYRIMIDINE METABOLISM

Beverly S. Mitchell and
Michael S. Hershfield

PURINE ENZYME DEFICIENCIES AND DISORDERS OF IMMUNE FUNCTION

ADENOSINE DEAMINASE DEFICIENCY. Adenosine deaminase (ADA) deficiency in its usual severe form causes the syndrome of severe combined immunodeficiency disease (SCID) with absence of both T- and B-lymphocyte function. Less complete ADA deficiency is associated with T-cell dysfunction and more variable loss of B-cell function. It is now recognized that ADA deficiency can result in slowly progressive immune dysfunction presenting in adolescents or adults. ADA deficiency accounts for approximately 20% of all SCID's and for one third to one half of those with autosomal recessive inheritance. Several hundred families with ADA deficiency have been identified to date. The frequency of ADA deficiency has been estimated at 1 in 200,000 to 1 in 1 million births.

Etiology and Pathogenesis. The gene for ADA is located on chromosome 20q. More than 25 single base changes within the coding region, as well as several deletions and splicing mutations leading to loss of enzymatic activity, have been identified. The majority of affected individuals are compound heterozygotes for two different molecular defects. A so-called partial deficiency of ADA activity resulting from mutations that cause a less severe loss of enzymatic activity in the absence of clinical manifestations has been identified in population screening programs.

ADA catalyzes the irreversible deamination of adenosine to inosine, and of 2'-deoxyadenosine to 2'-deoxyinosine (Fig. 181–1). In the absence of ADA activity, increased plasma levels of both adenosine and 2'-deoxyadenosine in the range of 0.5 to 10 μM occur; high levels of 2'-deoxyadenosine, but not adenosine, are excreted in

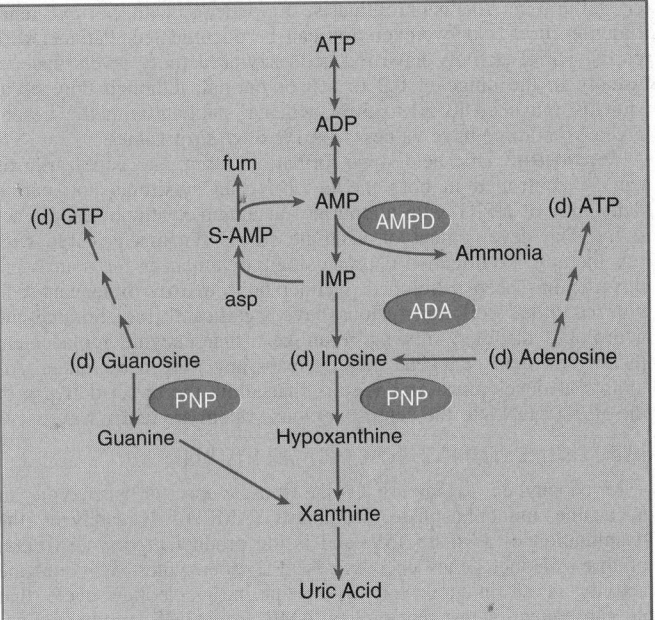

FIGURE 181–1. Schema of purine metabolism demonstrating metabolic reactions catalyzed by adenosine deaminase (ADA), purine nucleoside phosphorylase (PNP), and AMP deaminase (AMPD). asp = aspartate; fum = fumarate.

the urine. The pathogenesis of this disorder and its selectivity for cells of the immune system are not completely understood. The major pathogenic mechanism involves the accumulation of 2′-deoxy ATP derived from 2′-deoxyadenosine in lymphocyte progenitors and the toxicity of this metabolite for lymphoid cells. Deoxy ATP pool expansion inhibits ribonucleotide reductase, thus inhibiting DNA replication. In addition, 2′-deoxyadenosine inactivates the enzyme S-adenosylhomocysteine hydrolase, which may result in the accumulation of S-adenosylhomocysteine, an inhibitor of trans-methylation reactions mediated by S-adenosylmethionine.

Clinical Manifestations. ADA deficiency is most frequently diagnosed in children with signs of immunodeficiency manifested by lymphopenia, failure to thrive, and recurrent infections with both ordinary pathogens and opportunistic organisms. *Pneumocystis carinii* infections and candidiasis are commonly observed, as well as cytomegalovirus, varicella, and other viral pneumonias and infections. Vaccination with live organisms may be fatal, and an increased incidence of B-cell lymphomas has been reported. Although the diagnosis has most commonly been made in very young children, there is increasing recognition of less severe forms of ADA deficiency presenting over the first two decades of life with milder forms of immunodeficiency. Chronic respiratory infections may lead to pulmonary insufficiency in older individuals. Physical findings are unremarkable with the exception of an absence of lymph nodes and tonsillar tissue and the presence in some affected infants of very prominent costochondral junctions. Neurologic abnormalities have been reported in occasional cases, as have autoimmune abnormalities such as hypothyroidism, hemolytic anemia, and immune thrombocytopenic purpura. Chest radiography reveals the absence of a thymus and peripheral blood examination usually demonstrates an absolute lymphopenia of <500 per microliter with a marked reduction in mature T cells and a more variable decrease in B cells associated with hypogammaglobulinemia and lack of specific antibody response to immunization. *In vitro* tests of lymphocyte function, including proliferative responses to mitogens and antigen, are abnormal.

Diagnosis. The disorder should be looked for in individuals with recurrent infections associated with unexplained lymphopenia. The diagnosis is made by measuring ADA activity in the hemolysates of untransfused patients. Determining the degree of elevation of 2′-deoxy ATP and the reduction of S-adenosylhomocysteine hydrolase activity in erythrocytes is useful to gauge the severity of ADA deficiency. In kindreds in which the mutations in

the ADA gene have been identified because of a previously affected sibling, the diagnosis can be made at the molecular level by amplifying specific regions of the gene using the polymerase chain reaction (PCR) and DNA sequencing. Prenatal diagnosis can be accomplished by ADA activity assay of cultured amniotic or chorionic villus cells, as well as by DNA analysis when the mutations are known.

Treatment. Specific antibiotic treatment for infections is essential. In addition, patients should receive prophylaxis for *Pneumocystis carinii* and fungal infections and should not receive live virus vaccines or unirradiated blood products. Most patients are also treated with intravenous immunoglobulin. Once the diagnosis is established, the patient is a candidate for either bone marrow transplantation from an HLA-identical or haploidentical donor or enzyme replacement therapy with polyethylene glycol (PEG)–conjugated bovine ADA. The long-term survival with engraftment for second siblings (who are less ill at diagnosis) with HLA-identical transplants is >90%, and this remains the treatment of choice if a donor is available. Haploidentical transplants with T-cell–depleted marrow have been less successful, with the probability of long-term survival ranging from 28 to 67%. Enzyme replacement with PEG-conjugated ADA (PEG-ADA), which maintains high levels of ADA activity in plasma, is uniformly effective in correcting metabolic abnormalities caused by ADA deficiency. Improving lymphocyte counts and function by restoring the thymus has occurred within weeks to a few months of intramuscular treatment with PEG-ADA given once or twice weekly. Although lymphocyte counts do not return to normal, the majority of patients have a major reduction in infectious episodes and have resumed growth and normal activities. Experimental somatic cell gene therapy (see Ch. 25) has been used in several patients who have been treated concomitantly with PEG-ADA. Retroviral vector–mediated transduction of ADA cDNA into the patients' interleukin-2–activated peripheral blood T cells has increased ADA activity that has persisted for several months. This disorder has been considered a prime target for gene therapy directed at lymphohematopoietic stem cells derived from bone marrow, and umbilical cord blood in prenatally diagnosed patients and clinical trials using this approach are in progress.

PURINE NUCLEOSIDE PHOSPHORYLASE DEFICIENCY. Purine nucleoside phosphorylase (PNP) catalyzes the reversible phosphorolysis of the nucleosides inosine and 2′-deoxyinosine to the base hypoxanthine and guanosine and 2′-deoxyguanosine to guanine (Fig. 181–1). Deficiency of PNP has been reported in approximately 30 families, and mutations in the PNP gene located on chromosome 14q have been identified in several individuals. Lack of PNP activity is associated primarily with T-cell depletion and cellular immune dysfunction, although either B-cell dysfunction or B-cell hyperactivity associated with autoimmune disorders also occurs in about one third of patients. Neurologic abnormalities including spasticity, ataxia, behavioral abnormalities, hypertonia, and hypotonia have been seen in >50% of affected individuals. Patients generally present in childhood with recurrent infections associated with markedly reduced lymphocyte counts with specific loss of T cells and are found to lack a thymus gland. Absence or marked reduction of PNP activity in erythrocytes is diagnostic. Supportive laboratory tests consist of a marked decrease in uric acid due to the inability to convert PNP substrates to hypoxanthine and guanine. Serum and urinary levels of all four nucleoside substrates of PNP are increased. The metabolite of 2′-deoxyguanosine, 2′-deoxy GTP, is found in erythrocytes and is thought to be causally associated with the T-cell depletion because it accumulates in T-cell precursors leading to a block in DNA replication. Treating this disorder with either red cell transfusions or with infusions of deoxycytidine aimed at restoring DNA replication has not resulted in any consistent therapeutic response. The efficacy of bone marrow transplantation to date remains poor. PEG-conjugated PNP and gene therapy remain developmental, and the small number of affected patients makes clinical research on this disorder difficult.

LESCH-NYHAN SYNDROME

The Lesch-Nyhan syndrome is an X-linked disorder caused by absence or severe deficiency of the enzyme hypoxanthine-guanine phosphoribosyltransferase (HPRT). It is manifested as a devastating neurologic disorder consisting of compulsive self-mutilation, choreoathetosis, spasticity, and often mental retardation. The syndrome occurs with a frequency of 1 in 100,000 births and is associated with a marked overproduction of purines, resulting in hyperuricemia and gout (see Ch. 251). Partial deficiency of the enzyme also causes hyperuricemia, but without severe neurologic deficits, and accounts for < 1% of patients with gout.

Etiology and Pathogenesis. The molecular basis of HPRT deficiency has been studied in detail, and a large number of point mutations, splicing defects, and deletions have been identified. HPRT catalyzes the reaction whereby the purine bases hypoxanthine and guanine are condensed with ribose-5-PO_4 derived from PP-ribose-P to form the corresponding nucleotides, inosine and guanosine monophosphate, thus salvaging the purine bases for nucleotide metabolism. In the absence of HPRT activity, hypoxanthine and guanine can be catabolized only through xanthine to uric acid, causing hyperuricemia and markedly increased uric aciduria. In addition, an increase in the intracellular concentration of PP-ribose-P and reduced formation of inosine monophosphate (IMP) and guanosine monophosphate (GMP) leads to a marked increase in the overall rate of de novo synthesis of purine nucleotides, further increasing the generation of uric acid. The clinical sequelae of hyperuricemia and increased uric acid excretion are the juvenile onset of uric acid stone formation and gouty arthritis. The pathogenesis of the neurologic defects is not well understood but could involve guanine nucleotide deficiency as a result of decreased guanine salvage in neurons that depend on the salvage pathway for purine nucleotide synthesis. Positron emission tomography has demonstrated a selective decrease in glucose metabolism in the caudate nucleus, but anatomic studies of the brains of affected individuals have not revealed any structural lesions.

Clinical Manifestations. The Lesch-Nyhan syndrome is manifested in affected males during the first year of life by an initial delay in motor development, followed by extrapyramidal signs leading to choreoathetosis and, at approximately age 1, by pyramidal tract involvement with hyperreflexia, clonus, and scissoring of the legs. Compulsive self-destructive behavior appears sometime between early childhood and adolescence and constitutes a behavior pattern unique to this disorder. Affected individuals bite their fingers, lips, and buccal mucosa, necessitating restraints and in some cases edentulation. Repeated attempts at self-injury, such as placing extremities in dangerous areas and self-inflicted head trauma, are common. Mental and growth retardation also occur in the majority of cases. Uric acid crystalluria may be noted as orange crystals in the diaper during the first weeks of life and, if untreated, may lead to nephrolithiasis, obstructive uropathy, and azotemia. Hyperuricemia is usually present and may attain levels of 18 mg per deciliter. Gout may develop later in the course of the disease, but generally not before puberty. Death usually occurs in the second or third decade from infection or renal failure.

Patients with partial deficiency of HPRT develop uric acid crystalluria and renal calculi in childhood, and gouty arthritis often occurs before age 20. Neurologic manifestations, including mental retardation, mild spastic quadriplegia, dysarthria, cerebellar ataxia, and seizures, are noted in 20% of patients, but self-mutilation does not develop. Patients with partial HPRT deficiency may seek medical attention due to passing a renal calculus or an attack of gouty arthritis. Life expectancy is normal.

Diagnosis. The clinical diagnosis of the Lesch-Nyhan syndrome is strongly suggested by the self-mutilation and characteristic choreoathetosis; mental retardation of other origins is very rarely accompanied by the induction of self-injury, especially in the presence of intact sensation. The presence of hyperuricemia supports the diagnosis. The definitive diagnosis is made by demonstrating a lack of HPRT enzymatic activity in red cells or other tissues. The molecular defect has been established in many patients. Female carriers cannot be definitively identified by HPRT activity assay of peripheral blood cells but may be detected using cultured skin fibroblasts or by DNA analysis if the nature of the mutation in an affected male relative has been defined.

Partial deficiency of HPRT is manifested by the early onset of gouty arthritis in male patients or by the early onset of uric acid

crystalluria and/or nephrolithiasis. In patients with normal renal function, uric acid overexcretion can be documented. Patients with partial HPRT activity have red cell enzyme activity levels that are usually in the range of 0.2 to 5% of normal, although they occasionally range up to 30 to 50%, whereas patients with the Lesch-Nyhan syndrome have values < 0.01% of control values.

Treatment. Uric acid stone formation, tophi, and gouty arthritis can be controlled in both the Lesch-Nyhan syndrome and partial deficiency of HPRT with allopurinol to inhibit xanthine oxidase activity. The development of xanthine stones remains possible with this therapy. No effective pharmacologic treatment of the neurologic disorder has been developed. Neither bone marrow transplantation nor red blood cell transfusions have significantly ameliorated the neurologic disorder, making it unlikely that enzyme replacement therapy or stem cell gene therapy plays any role in treatment. Attempts at developing viral vectors that allow the direct delivery of the HPRT cDNA to the central nervous system are under way.

MYOADENYLATE DEAMINASE DEFICIENCY AND MYOPATHY

Myoadenylate deaminase is the muscle-specific isoenzyme of adenosine monophosphate deaminase (AMPD). It catalyzes the deamination of AMP to IMP and is the product of one (AMPD1) of three distinct genes encoding AMPD isoenzymes. This enzyme activity is an integral part of the purine nucleotide cycle that in subsequent steps regenerates AMP from IMP, producing fumarate (Fig. 181–1), and appears to play a major role in energy production in skeletal tissue. Deficiency of AMPD1 has been documented in 2% of all muscle biopsies submitted for histologic examination. Inherited deficiency of myoadenylate deaminase is associated with exercise-related cramps and myalgias. An acquired deficiency of AMPD1 is associated with a number of primary muscle disorders.

ETIOLOGY AND PATHOGENESIS. The AMPD1 gene is located on chromosome 1 and is expressed predominantly in skeletal muscle, whereas AMPD2 and 3 are expressed in other tissues. The normal expression of AMPD1 is associated with an alternatively spliced 12 bp second exon of the gene, so that 0.6 to 2% of the mRNA in human skeletal muscle lacks exon 2 and encodes a protein of four fewer amino acids. A single nonsense mutation within this second exon has been identified at frequencies ranging from 0.13 to 0.19 in the general population and is associated in its homozygous form with a marked reduction in AMPD1 protein. To date, no other mutations have been identified as causing this enzyme deficiency state. Acquired AMPD1 deficiency is associated with decreased AMPD1 mRNA levels that may be due to a regulatory defect in gene expression in a variety of muscle disorders.

AMPD1 protein has been shown to bind to myosin heavy chain in skeletal muscle. During contraction, the activity of AMPD1 increases markedly. Operation of the next two steps in the purine nucleotide cycle regenerates AMP and produces fumarate, an intermediate in the citric acid cycle, as a by-product. Patients deficient in AMPD1 do not generate IMP, NH3, or fumarate in skeletal muscle during exercise.

CLINICAL MANIFESTATIONS. Individuals with the inherited form of AMPD deficiency may develop fatigue, cramps, or myalgias following vigorous exercise; myoglobinuria has been reported occasionally. The majority of these patients have presented between childhood and early adulthood. The disorder has been documented in > 200 individuals. With the high frequency of the nonsense mutation in the general population, it is apparent that a large number of homozygous mutant individuals must exist who do not have clinical symptoms severe enough to warrant medical evaluation. It has been postulated that the low level of normal alternative splicing that eliminates the exon containing the nonsense codon results in production of a protein product with some enzymatic activity in many homozygous individuals. Acquired deficiency of AMPD1 is found in a number of muscle diseases, including neurogenic disorders, divergent myopathies, and collagen vascular disorders. The clinical symptoms of these individuals are dictated by the primary muscle disease. Whether the clinical heterogeneity of this disorder relates to the expression of the spliced variant of the enzyme and/or to the expression of other AMPD's in muscle tissue or indeed whether the enzyme deficiency state is causally associated with symptoms is under investigation.

DIAGNOSIS. Individuals with AMPD1 deficiency do not produce NH$_3$ on ischemic exercise of the forearm and may have an elevated CPK in 50% of cases. Histochemical stains and enzyme activity determinations demonstrate an absence of AMPD1 enzyme in muscle biopsies. The genetic abnormality may be detected by an altered restriction enzyme digestion site in genomic DNA.

TREATMENT. No treatment has been demonstrated to be highly effective. Oral ribose has been administered in an attempt to enhance the synthesis of purine nucleotides with variable subjective improvement.

2,8-DIHYDROXYADENINE RENAL STONES

Deficiency of the enzyme adenine phosphoribosyltransferase (APRT) leads to an accumulation of its substrate—adenine—which in turn is oxidized, although inefficiently, by xanthine oxidase to 2,8-dihydroxyadenine. Because of the insolubility of this product, patients with the autosomal recessive form of this disorder are predisposed to develop radiolucent renal calculi composed of 2,8-dihydroxyadenine. Renal stones may develop within the first months of life or present as late as the fifth decade, although many APRT-deficient individuals never develop stones. The diagnosis may be made by analyzing the stones with ultraviolet, infrared, or mass spectrometry or x-ray crystallography. Definitive diagnosis requires demonstrating the absence of APRT activity in erythrocyte lysates. No other biochemical or clinical abnormalities have been reported in individuals homozygous for this enzyme deficiency; heterozygous individuals have no clinical abnormalities. Mutations at the APRT locus are particularly common in individuals of Japanese ancestry, and investigation of the molecular basis of this defect reveals a single base mutation at codon 136 in 68% of the defective alleles, with two other mutations accounting for 28% of defects. Analysis of both germline and somatic cell mutations in non-Japanese subjects has revealed clustering of the mutations at the intron 4 splice donor site and at codon 87. Thus, the molecular basis of this disorder appears to result from relatively few mutations. Therapy for individuals with 2,8-dihydroxyadenine calculi consists of restricting dietary purines, high fluid intake, and treatment with allopurinol to prevent the oxidation of adenine by xanthine oxidase.

XANTHINURIA

Classic xanthinuria results from deficiency of the enzyme xanthine oxidase. As a consequence, xanthine and hypoxanthine produced by the catabolism of purines cannot be oxidized to uric acid, resulting in very low serum urate and urinary uric acid excretion values. Serum oxypurine (xanthine and hypoxanthine) concentrations and urinary oxypurine excretion are increased. This disorder has been identified in >60 individuals, with approximately one third of these developing radiolucent renal calculi composed of xanthine. Crystalline deposits of xanthine and hypoxanthine in muscle have been described in a few individuals with muscle cramps following exercise and may also be associated with polyarthritis. The diagnosis is strongly suggested by the presence of low serum and urinary uric acid levels in conjunction with elevated serum and urinary oxypurine concentrations. Deficiency of xanthine oxidase activity can be confirmed by direct enzymatic assay. Therapy for xanthine calculi consists primarily of increasing fluid intake.

A combination of xanthine oxidase deficiency and sulfite oxidase deficiency may also result in xanthinuria and has been attributed to an absence of the molybdenum cofactor for catalytic activity required for both enzymes to be active. The few reported patients with this disorder have presented in infancy with a severe neurologic disorder characterized by seizures, nystagmus, enophthalmos, ocular lens dislocation, and Brushfield spots characteristic of sulfite oxidase deficiency.

DISORDERS OF PYRIMIDINE METABOLISM

Hereditary orotic aciduria is a rare genetic disorder of pyrimidine metabolism that is characterized by megaloblastic anemia, leukopenia, retarded growth and development, and high levels of urinary orotic acid excretion, frequently associated with crystal or stone formation. The disorder is inherited as an autosomal recessive defect and results from deficiency of activity of the bifunctional enzyme uridine monophosphate (UMP) synthase that in two steps catalyzes the conversion of orotic acid to UMP. This enzyme is, therefore, essential for the *de novo* synthesis of pyrimidine nucleotides. The gene encoding this enzyme has been localized to the long arm of chromosome 3 and two point mutations in the cDNA encoding the enzyme have been described that result in loss of its activity and the clinical syndrome. Administering uridine (2 to 4 grams per day) has been demonstrated to ameliorate the clinical sequelae of this enzymatic defect because uridine can be directly phosphorylated to UMP.

Pyrimidine 5′-nucleotidase deficiency is an autosomal recessive disorder that results in hereditary hemolytic anemia associated with prominent basophilic stippling of red blood cells. Erythrocytes contain high levels of cytidine and uridine monophosphates that are substrates for the enzyme, as well as a number of pyrimidine conjugates, including cytidine diphosphate (CDP)-choline and CDP-ethanolamine and uridine diphosphate-glucose. Acquired pyrimidine 5′-nucleotidase activity is found associated with lead toxicity and also with the induction of basophilic stippling due to undegraded ribosomal nucleoprotein and with accumulation of pyrimidine nucleotides. Diagnosis of the hereditary disorder is made by measuring erythrocyte pyrimidine 5′-nucleotidase enzymatic activity or by demonstrating elevated pyrimidine nucleotides by UV absorption spectra in red cell lysates.

Dihydropyrimidine dehydrogenase deficiency is a rare autosomal recessive disorder characterized by deficiency of the enzymatic activity responsible for degrading the pyrimidine bases uracil and thymidine. High excretion levels of these metabolites are found in the urine and may be detected when screening for organic aciduria. Although no clinical symptoms have been associated with this defect, administering fluoropyrimidines (5-fluorouracil; 5-fluorodeoxyuridine) to enzyme-deficient patients with malignancy can result in severe and prolonged drug-related toxicity.

Diasio RB, Beavers TL, Carpenter JT: Familial deficiency of dihydropyrimidine dehydrogenase: Biochemical basis for familial pyrimidinemia and severe 5-fluorouracil-induced toxicity. J Clin Invest 81:47, 1988. *This study documents the lack of dihydropyrimidine dehydrogenase activity as a causal factor in 5-FU toxicity.*

Hershfield MS, Mitchell BS: Immunodeficiency diseases caused by adenosine deaminase deficiency and purine nucleoside phosphorylase deficiency. In Scriver CR, Beaudet AL, Sly WS, Valle D (eds.): The Molecular and Metabolic Bases of Inherited Disease. 7th ed. New York, McGraw-Hill, 1995. *Highly detailed discussion of clinical, metabolic, and molecular aspects of ADA and PNP deficiency states.*

Kamatani N, Hakoda M, Otsuka S, et al.: Only three mutations account for almost all defective alleles causing adenine phosphoribosyltransferase deficiency in Japanese patients. J Clin Invest 90:130, 1992. *Analyzes 141 defective APRT alleles from 71 Japanese families to document that the number of mutations underlying the defect in the Japanese population is limited.*

Markert ML: Purine nucleoside phosphorylase deficiency. Immun Def Rev 3:45, 1991. *An excellent, comprehensive clinical review of patients with PNP deficiency.*

Sabina RL, Holmes EW: Myoadenylate deaminase deficiency. In Scriver CR, Beaudet AL, Sly WS, Valle D (eds.): The Molecular and Metabolic Bases of Inherited Disease. 7th ed. New York, McGraw-Hill, 1995. *In-depth description of the clinical and biochemical abnormalities associated with myoadenylate deficiency states.*

Sculley DG, Dawson PA, Emmerson BT, et al.: A review of the molecular basis of hypoxanthine-guanine phosphoribosyltransferase (HPRT) deficiency. Hum Genet 90:195, 1992. *A general review of the Lesch-Nyhan syndrome, HPRT gene structure, and HPRT mutations.*

Webster D, Becroft DMO, Suttle DP: Hereditary orotic aciduria and other deficiencies of pyrimidine metabolism. In Scriver CR, Beaudet AL, Sly WS, Valle D (eds.): The Molecular and Metabolic Bases of Inherited Disease. 7th ed. New York, McGraw-Hill, 1995. *An excellent review describing the clinical syndrome and the biochemistry of the enzyme deficiency state in great detail.*

Inherited Disorders of Connective Tissue

182 THE MUCOPOLYSACCHARIDOSES

Hans C. Andersson and Emmanuel Shapira

The mucopolysaccharidoses (MPS's) are a heterogeneous group of inherited lysosomal storage disorders. The common feature of these disorders is intracellular storage and urinary excretion of glycosaminoglycans (GAG's), previously termed acidic mucopolysaccharides. The GAG's result from proteolytic cleavage of large macromolecules—the proteoglycans. They are highly glycosylated and sulfated molecules that are normally degraded in a stepwise manner in the lysosome by specific enzymes that either cleave terminal sulfate or glycosyl groups or acetylate the GAG to facilitate further degradation. The MPS's result from the deficient activity of one of these lysosomal enzymes. This deficiency arrests further degradation of GAG's and leads to their storage in various tissues. The storage causes progressive disruption of cellular function and leads to physical deformation of various tissues.

The group of MPS disorders demonstrates two principles of human genetics—heterogeneity and variability. Heterogeneity refers to the observation that mutations in different enzymes located at different loci can lead to clinically indistinguishable phenotypes. This phenomenon is exemplified by the four types of MPS III (Sanfilippo). Within each type of MPS, a considerable clinical variability exists as to the age of onset, the rate of progression, and the extent to which various organs are involved. Typically, they manifest within a spectrum of severity from early, severe childhood forms to milder, late childhood or adolescent forms. This clinical variability can sometimes be explained by the biochemical and molecular observation of particular mutations with varying degrees of residual enzyme activity. Many of the genes coding for enzymes involved in the MPS diseases have been cloned, making possible mutation analysis in individual patients. The more severely affected patients have a mutation resulting in the complete absence of detectable enzyme protein in their tissues, whereas mildly affected patients have point mutations leading to an amino acid substitution with detectable enzyme protein but with markedly decreased residual activity. Other factors in addition to the specific gene mutation may also be involved in modifying the patient's clinical presentation.

CLINICAL FEATURES

Most patients with MPS diseases appear normal at birth and gradually develop pathologic findings in the first 2 years of life. The various MPS's share multiple organ system involvement, organomegaly, dysostosis multiplex, and facial coarsening. Dysostosis multiplex refers to the collective bony abnormalities, including thickened calvarium, J-shaped sella, anterior vertebral hypoplasia leading to kyphoscoliosis, impaired long bone growth with irregular metaphyses, poorly formed pelvis, and oar-shaped ribs that invariably lead to short stature. MPS I, II, III, and VII are usually also characterized by central nervous system (CNS) storage, resulting in progressive mental retardation. MPS IV (Morquio) spares the CNS but has unusually severe skeletal abnormalities, including odontoid hypoplasia that may become life-threatening. In many of the MPS's, sensorineural and conductive hearing loss and vision defects (corneal and retinal) may also contribute to poor intellectual development. Cardiac disease from GAG stored in valve leaflets, endocardium, myocardium, and coronary arteries is a common feature in middle childhood and is often the cause of death.

The MPS's are inherited as autosomal recessive disorders, with the exception of MPS II, which has an X-linked mode of inheritance. The incidence of each of the various MPS's is relatively rare, in the range of 1 in 40,000 to 1 in 100,000 live births. Table 182–1 summarizes some of the distinguishing clinical and biochemical features of the MPS's.

DIAGNOSIS

Whenever the diagnosis of MPS is suspected, a urine-screening test for GAG's should be performed. The most commonly used screening test is the toluidine blue spot test; it is relatively sensitive but has a significant false-positive rate owing to reactivity with chondroitin sulfate, which is a normal finding in the urine. In some MPS III and IV patients, the spot test can be falsely negative. In patients with a positive spot test and those suspected of being falsely negative, the various GAG's in the urine should be identified by either thin-layer chromatography or electrophoresis. Based on the clinical presentation and the pattern of urinary GAG's, the diagnosis should be established by demonstration of the specific enzyme deficiency in leukocytes, fibroblasts, or other tissues (Table 182–1). Mutation analysis is available for most MPS disorders, and a genotype-phenotype correlation has been established for some mutations.

MANAGEMENT AND TREATMENT

SUPPORTIVE CARE. In managing families with an MPS-affected member, proper counseling is one of the most important and difficult tasks (see Ch. 29). The basic explanation of the pathophysiology of the disease, emphasizing that nothing that the parents did or did not do led to the disorder, can alleviate the guilt and anger that parents of newly diagnosed MPS patients experience. The risk for other unaffected family members should be provided, including the option of prenatal diagnosis in future pregnancies in all family members with an increased risk for having affected offspring.

Treatment for patients with MPS is mainly symptomatic because treatments for the primary defect are few and variably effective. Supportive treatment should be aimed at the following complications:

1. Orthopedic: Because of the generalized and progressive nature of the skeletal involvement, a conservative orthopedic approach is most appropriate, minimizing surgical treatment. Surgical intervention is critical in patients with spinal cord compression and atlantoaxial instability. Orthopedic shoes and ankle braces can be used to maintain mobility in the early stages of the disease. In some patients, elongating the Achilles tendon may be helpful. Surgery is advised for carpal tunnel syndrome when progressive median nerve compression is documented.

2. Cardiorespiratory: Early alveolar involvement is relatively common in some of the MPS's. Small airway obstruction by accumulated storage material, thickened mucosal secretions, hypertrophy of tonsils/adenoids, and the associated macroglossia all contribute to the respiratory problems. Sleep apnea should be considered and treated in the early stages of the disease, whereas tracheostomy might be considered in the very advanced stages of the disorder. Managing a tracheostomy can be difficult owing to tenacious secretions. Cardiac insufficiency may be palliated by medical therapy, but valvular dysfunction is more difficult to correct, especially because these are very high-risk anesthesia patients.

3. Hernias: Inguinal and umbilical hernias are relatively common and often require surgical correction.

4. Neurologic: Only the relatively rare complication of hydrocephalus can be treated by ventriculoperitoneal shunting. Anticipatory diagnostic studies should attempt to ascertain those patients at risk for atlantoaxial dislocation.

5. Anesthesia: Patients with MPS should be considered at high risk whenever general anesthesia is considered. This is due to the associated respiratory complications, temporomandibular ankylosis, and atlantoaxial instability. General anesthesia should be restricted to mandatory surgical procedures that cannot be performed under local anesthesia.

TABLE 182-1. THE MUCOPOLYSACCHARIDOSES

MPS Type	Eponym	Enzyme Deficiency	Urinary GAG	Clinical Presentation
I				
I-H	Hurler	α-L-Iduronidase	DS HS	Onset < 2 yrs, early corneal clouding and organomegaly, coarse facies, MR; later onset of cardiorespiratory failure
I-S	Scheie	α-L-Iduronidase	DS	Later onset (> 5 yrs), similar to I-H but with normal intellect, milder skeletal involvement, and slower progression
II	Hunter	Iduronate sulfatase	DS HS	Onset < 4 yrs, early skeletal involvement, organomegaly, but no corneal clouding; X-linked inheritance, MR usually severe; mild form with normal intelligence and slower progression
III	Sanfilippo			Same for all types (A–D)
IIIA		Heparan-N-sulfatase	HS	Onset > 2 yrs, rapidly progressive neurologic/intellectual regression; late mild visceral and skeletal involvement
IIIB		α-N-Acetylglucosaminidase		
IIIC		N-Acetyl-CoA : α-glucosaminide acetyltransferase		
IIID		N-Acetylglucosamine-6-sulfatase		
IV	Morquio			
IVA		N-Acetyl-galactosamine-6-sulfatase	KS	Onset < 4 yrs, mainly skeletal involvement, rapidly progressive kyphoscoliosis, short stature, odontoid hypoplasia, late corneal clouding, and normal intellect
IVB		β-Galactosidase	KS	Same as IVA, but may develop MR
VI	Maroteaux-Lamy	Arylsulfatase B	DS	Onset < 4 yrs, phenotype as in MPS I-H, but with normal intellect; rare adult form with slower progression
VII	Sly	β-Glucuronidase	HS DS ChS	Variable age of onset, MR and skeletal involvement; few patients present as hydrops fetalis

DS = dermatan sulfate; HS = heparan sulfate; KS = keratan sulfate; ChS = chondroitin sulfate; MR = mental retardation.

6. Dental care: Dental care is a relatively common problem in patients with MPS's owing to the decreased mouth opening, gingival hypertrophy, and poor dental hygiene in patients with mental retardation. Awareness of the need for continuous dental care should be maintained.

ENZYME AND GENE THERAPY. Attempts to treat patients with MPS types I and II by high-volume plasma transfusions were made nearly 25 years ago. The amount of enzyme that could be provided with the maximal plasma transfusion led to some decreased urinary excretion of the GAG's but no meaningful phenotypic improvement. Attempts to purify large quantities of enzymes from human tissues (placental) or by genetic engineering are currently under way in several laboratories. Thus far, the amount of purified enzyme required for clinical trials is not available for MPS therapy (see Ch. 25). The additional problem of targeting enzyme to the affected tissue, especially the brain, must still be overcome.

Enzyme replacement by bone marrow transplantation has been attempted in a limited number of patients. Some of the patients with MPS VI who have received a bone marrow transplant had significant clinical improvement with complete or nearly complete arrest of the progressive disorder. Bone marrow transplantation did not prevent the severe skeletal deformities in MPS IV nor the severe neurologic regression in patients with MPS III. The clinical indications for bone marrow transplantation in patients with MPS I-H and MPS II are not established owing to the lack of consistent improvement in the neurologic sequelae. As this transplantation can only arrest the progression but not reverse the symptoms, attempts were made to provide this treatment to patients within the early stages of the disease. It is not clear whether the few patients who appeared to benefit from bone marrow transplantation had mutations with residual activity and therefore had better outcomes. The correlation of genotype with phenotype that is becoming available might enable a conclusive answer to this question. A national collaborative study is being done to evaluate the possible role of bone marrow transplantation in patients with certain MPS's.

Gene therapy (see Ch. 25) for MPS's by providing the normal gene carried by one vector or another to the desirable tissue remains a desirable goal for the future. Major hurdles that need to be overcome include choosing vector, establishing stable incorporation of the normal gene, and targeting the gene to the affected tissue.

Gieselmann V: Lysosomal storage diseases. Biochem Biophys Acta 1270:1, 1995. *An excellent review of the molecular understanding of lysosomal enzymes and their mutations, with an emphasis on genotype-phenotype correlation.*
Neufeld EF, Muenzer J: The mucopolysaccharide storage diseases. *In* Scriver CR, Beaudet AL, Sly WS, Valle D (eds.): The Metabolic and Molecular Bases of Inherited Disease. 7th ed. New York, McGraw-Hill, 1995. *The most comprehensive review of MPS's available in the definitive reference text for metabolic diseases. This discussion of basic science and clinical issues related to lysosomal storage diseases offers a biochemical understanding of these diseases.*
Whitley CB: The mucopolysaccharidoses. *In* Beighton P (ed.): McKusick's Heritable Disorders of Connective Tissue. 5th ed. St. Louis, Mosby-Year Book, 1993. *An extremely readable clinical summary of MPS's with many illustrative graphs and clinical photographs. Gives the nongeneticist a concise overview of the MPS's.*

183 THE MARFAN SYNDROME
Peter H. Byers

DEFINITION. The Marfan syndrome is a dominantly inherited connective tissue disorder characterized by musculoskeletal abnormalities (arachnodactyly, tall stature, scoliosis, pectus deformities, and ligamentous laxity), cardiovascular abnormalities (mitral valve prolapse [MVP] and regurgitation, aortic valve insufficiency, and aortic dilatation, aneurysm, and dissection), lens dislocation, and myopia.

ETIOLOGY AND PATHOGENESIS. The Marfan syndrome results from mutations in the gene (FIBN1) that encodes fibrillin I, located on chromosome 15q21. Fibrillin is a 350-kDa glycoprotein that contains 43 repeats of a calcium binding EGF-precursor–like motif and other cysteine-rich motifs. This protein is ubiquitously distributed in the extracellular matrix and is a major constituent of microfibrils of elastic tissue and of the zonular fibrils of the lens. Many different mutations in the gene have now been identified and have been shown to interfere with the synthesis, secretion, or accumulation in the extracellular matrix of the normal protein. Genetic linkage studies suggest that most, if not all, individuals with typical Marfan syndrome have mutations in the FIBN1 gene.

PREVALENCE. The Marfan syndrome affects about 1 in 15,000 individuals without racial or ethnic predilection. About 60 to 70% of affected individuals have an affected parent; the remainder have new mutations.

PATHOLOGY. The mitral and aortic valves are characterized by "myxomatous degeneration" or the appearance of large pools of nonfibrous material that separates the normal cells of the valves. The valves may be thickened. In the absence of dissection, metachromatic material accumulates in the aortic media and the normal elastic laminae are disrupted. Aortic dissection characteristically begins in the ascending aorta and may proceed in both directions. Death frequently results from cardiac tamponade due to hemopericardium, coronary occlusion, occlusion of the arteries to the brain, or loss of perfusion of multiple abdominal organs.

CLINICAL MANIFESTATIONS. The Marfan syndrome is highly variable in its clinical manifestations, and affected members within the same family may differ in the manner in which they express the mutation. The differences between families may be explained, in part, by different mutations in the FIBN1 gene. The diagnosis of the Marfan syndrome requires that criteria in two or more major areas be met (family history, cardiac, musculoskeletal, or ocular findings) with a family history, and an additional criterion if there is a new mutation. The diagnosis can be made occasionally in newborns because of lens dislocation, MVP, scoliosis, and tall stature with arachnodactyly; in addition, there is a particularly severe newborn variant of the condition. More commonly, diagnosis is made during childhood or adolescence because of tall stature, MVP, lens dislocation, and arachnodactyly. Aortic root diameter is generally within the normal range during childhood, although it tends to be in the upper range. Scoliosis may progress rapidly during the adolescent growth spurt. More than half the individuals with the Marfan syndrome have lens subluxation, usually in the superior direction. Lens subluxation is generally not progressive after adolescence but if the position of the lens interferes with vision, replacing it with an artificial lens is often beneficial. Cataracts and glaucoma are occasional complications of ectopia lentis.

The major life-threatening complication of the Marfan syndrome is aortic dissection and rupture, and most deaths result from cardiovascular disease when the aorta is untreated. The risk of dissection is correlated with aortic diameter. Commonly aortic diameters do not exceed the normal adult range (20 to 37 mm) until the third decade and then enlarge slowly, although the rate varies with individuals. Aortic dissection in the Marfan syndrome is occasionally asymptomatic, but usually there is prolonged, severe substernal chest pain of a tearing or searing quality, often with radiation into the neck, back, and arms. It is often accompanied by diaphoresis, hypotension, and shock. Blood pressure in the two arms may differ. Rarely, pregnancy is complicated by aortic dissection.

DIFFERENTIAL DIAGNOSIS. *Isolated ectopia lentis,* a dominantly inherited disorder, also results from mutation in the FIBN1 gene but is not accompanied by significant aortic dilatation or dissection. *Congenital contractural arachnodactyly (CCA)* is a dominantly inherited disorder characterized by arachnodactyly, joint contractures, small cup-shaped ears, pectus deformity, mild scoliosis, and MVP, but lens dislocation is absent and aortic dilatation is not a complication. CCA has been linked to the FIBN2 gene on chromosome 5. *Homocystinuria* (see Ch. 180) is characterized by autosomal recessive inheritance, tight joints, peripheral vascular disease, thrombosis of arterial vessels, lens dislocation, osteoporosis, and, in some, mild mental retardation. The diagnosis is confirmed by detecting excessive homocysteine in the urine. Because of MVP, tall stature, and some of the skeletal features, the *mitral valve prolapse syndrome* is commonly mistaken for the Marfan syndrome. The disorder is dominantly inherited but quite variable; the absence of lens dislocation and lack of aortic root dilation distinguish the MVP syndrome from the Marfan syndrome. Individuals with the *Stickler syndrome* may have a marfanoid habitus, degenerative arthritis of multiple joints, cleft palate, and vitreal degeneration. In most families, the condition results from mutations in the COL2A1 gene that encodes the chains of type II collagen. The marfanoid habitus may be found in some people with sickle cell disease, the Klinefelter syndrome (the 47,XXY karyotype), and multiple endocrine adenomatosis type IIB (see Ch. 210.1).

TREATMENT AND CARE. The major objective of treating people with the Marfan syndrome is to prevent or treat aneurysm and dissection. Because aortic dissection is the principal cause of death, efforts to slow the rate of increase of aortic diameter hold promise to delay major complications. Recent studies suggest that aortic enlargement may slow in some people treated with β-blockers. It is not clear if some physical or molecular features identify those who respond. Blood pressure should always be maintained in the normal range. Advances in surgical technique have made replacing aneurysmal portions of the aorta a routine treatment that increases life expectancy. Replacement should be considered when aortic root diameter reaches approximately 55 to 60 mm and before

decompensation of the left ventricle from aortic valvular insufficiency. Yearly echocardiographic examination permits a sound basis for following aortic enlargement. A family history of aortic dissection at smaller diameters may be considered in timing the replacement. Either a human cadaver homograft that includes the aortic valve or a composite graft that contains a prosthetic valve is now used. Replacing the proximal aorta leaves the remainder of the vessel at risk, and follow-up by imaging of the remaining vessel is important in planning further surgery. Routine care consists of yearly echocardiography with referral to the cardiac surgeon when the aortic diameter reaches 50 to 55 mm, regular ophthalmologic evaluation, and continuing follow-up by a physician familiar with the syndrome.

There may be an increased risk for the mother with Marfan syndrome during pregnancy if the aortic diameter is greater than normal. There is a 50% risk of transmitting the gene for Marfan syndrome with each pregnancy, and molecular diagnosis of affected status of the fetus may be available in some families. Genetic counseling is important to determine if others are affected and to provide detailed information about the condition (see Ch. 29).

Dietz HC, Cutting GR, Pyeritz RE, et al.: Marfan syndrome caused by a recurrent de novo missense mutation in the fibrillin gene. Nature 352:337, 1991. *The demonstration that mutations in fibrillin produce the Marfan syndrome.*
Pyeritz RE: The Marfan syndrome. *In* Royce PM, Steinmann B (eds.): Connective Tissue and Its Heritable Disorders: Molecular, Genetic, and Medical Aspects. New York, Wiley-Liss, 1993, p 437. *The most recent, comprehensive review of the Marfan syndrome in all its aspects.*
Shores J, Berger KR, Murphy EA, et al.: Progression of aortic dilation and the benefit of long-term β-adrenergic blockade in Marfan's syndrome. N Engl J Med 330:1335, 1994. *The only published controlled trial of treatment with β blocker.*

184 EHLERS-DANLOS SYNDROME
Peter H. Byers

DEFINITION. Ehlers-Danlos syndrome (EDS) is a group of more than 10 inherited connective tissue disorders characterized by abnormalities of the skin, ligaments, and internal organs. The clinical manifestations include skin fragility, abnormal scar formation, excessive bruising, joint laxity, and, in one variety, rupture of viscera and arteries (Table 184–1).

ETIOLOGY. Some forms of EDS result from defects in the synthesis and processing of types I and III collagens, the major proteins of skin, ligaments, tendons, blood vessels, and viscera. The known defects include mutations affecting the structure, synthesis, processing, or stability of type III collagen (EDS type IV); deficient hydroxylation of lysyl residues in type I and type III collagen (EDS type VI); defective conversion of type I procollagen to collagen (EDS type VII); defective collagen cross-linking and abnormal cellular utilization of copper (EDS type IX); and a functional defect in fibronectin (EDS type X). The molecular bases of EDS types I, II, III, V, and VIII are not known.

PREVALENCE. The prevalence of EDS is estimated at about 1 in 5000 births. EDS type III, benign familial hypermobility, accounts for most patients identified as having EDS; some forms are uncommon (EDS types IV, VI, VII, and VIII); others have been found in only a few families (EDS types IX and X). There is no racial or ethnic predisposition for any of the common types of EDS.

PATHOLOGY AND PATHOGENESIS. Dermal collagen fibrils in patients with EDS types I, II, III, and VI are larger than normal and irregular in outline when viewed by electron microscopy. In EDS type IV, skin is thin and collagen fibril diameter is frequently smaller than normal. Arterial wall thickness is usually less than normal, and tensile strength is diminished. Fibroblastic cells in dermis frequently have marked dilatation of the rough endoplasmic reticulum as a result of defective secretion of type III procollagen. There are no specific pathologic features of the other types of EDS.

CLINICAL MANIFESTATIONS. The clinical manifestations of each type of EDS are different (Table 184–1); it is important to identify patients with EDS type IV because of the grave consequences of the disease and to identify those with EDS types V, VI, and IX because of the risk of recurrence in their families.

EDS types I and II are characterized by marked joint laxity; soft, velvety, and hyperextensible skin; easy bruising; and "cigarette-paper" scars in areas of trauma. They differ in severity. Prematurity is common in EDS type I but rare in EDS type II. The major complications of both are recurrent joint dislocations, skin fragility, and early-onset osteoarthritis. The manifestations of joint laxity are more severe in childhood and decrease following puberty. At present the diagnosis depends on recognizing the appropriate clinical findings; electron microscopic studies of dermis may be confirmatory but are not specific. Patients with EDS type III are commonly seen by rheumatologists because of the joint discomfort and early onset of degenerative joint disease.

EDS type IV, the most severe form, results from dominant mutations in the genes of type III collagen. The diagnosis is confirmed by finding decreased amounts of type III collagen in skin, by identifying a defect in the structure, synthesis, or secretion of type III procollagen by cultured dermal fibroblasts, or by identifying a defect in gene structure. In the newborn period some infants already have bruising, but most affected infants are difficult to identify. By adolescence the veins are readily visible on the trunk and extremities, and bruising is common. Vascular or bowel rupture is rare during childhood. Arterial fragility may manifest as sudden death, stroke, shock from retroperitoneal or intra-abdominal bleeding, or compartmental syndromes, depending on the site of vessel rupture. Prompt surgical intervention may be lifesaving, although tissue friability may make repairs difficult. Pregnancy may be complicated by arterial or uterine rupture, either of which is often fatal. Recurrent abdominal pain may result from repeated mural hemorrhage in the small intestine. Sigmoid rupture is common. Survival beyond the fifth decade is rare.

EDS type VI is an autosomal recessive disorder characterized by a marfanoid habitus, skin and joint findings similar to those in EDS type II, ocular fragility, and scoliosis. The diagnosis is made by finding decreased amounts of hydroxylysine in skin and confirmed by low levels of lysyl hydroxylase measured in cultured dermal fibroblasts. Mutations have been identified in lysyl hydroxylase. Late complications may include vascular rupture, as well as blindness from retinal detachment or globe rupture.

EDS type VII is often detected in the newborn period, because of bilateral congenital hip dislocation and marked joint laxity. The hips are often difficult to stabilize, and recurrent dislocation may continue at the hips and other joints. When suspected clinically the diagnosis can be confirmed in some patients by identifying intermediates in the conversion of type I procollagen to collagen in skin and confirming the defect in cultured dermal fibroblasts. The most common defect recognized is an abnormal structure of the proα2(I) chain caused by exon 6 skipping in the COL1A2 gene. Similar mutations in the COL1A1 gene produce a somewhat more severe phenotype. Both these disorders result from loss of the cleavage site for the N-terminal procollagen proteinase. A recessively inherited deficiency of the proteinase itself results in the clinical picture of dermatosparaxis (EDS type VIIC), a very rare disorder characterized by extreme joint laxity and skin fragility and laxity.

EDS type VIII is characterized by the combination of noninflammatory gingival loss (often leading to loss of teeth) and the cutaneous and joint signs of the EDS type II phenotype.

EDS type IX is noted in childhood with skin hyperextensibility and laxity, drooping facies, and minor skeletal anomalies. Evidence of bladder dysfunction may be present by age 6, and diverticula of the bladder and hydronephrosis may occur. Mild chronic diarrhea, orthostatic hypotension, short upper arms with limited pronation and supination, and the occipital inferior horns become apparent during adolescence. Intelligence is usually in the normal range; inheritance is X-linked recessive. The diagnosis is made by the low serum copper and ceruloplasmin levels and confirmed by low lysyl oxidase levels in cultured dermal fibroblasts. The disease is allelic to Menkes' syndrome, a defect of copper metabolism. Maintaining normal urinary drainage is important to prevent renal failure, and continuing bladder drainage may be essential to prevent rupture. There is some variation in severity among families.

DIFFERENTIAL DIAGNOSIS. The differential diagnosis is generally limited to the varieties of EDS, although some individuals with the Marfan syndrome have marked joint laxity and others with forms of osteogenesis imperfecta have joint laxity and easy bruising. Patients with EDS type IV and EDS types I and II are often investigated for a bleeding diathesis before the correct diagnosis is made. Because of joint instability and laxity many patients with EDS types I, II, III, VI, and VII are investigated for developmental delay before it is recognized that they have a form of EDS.

TREATMENT. The gaping skin wounds that occur in some forms of EDS should be approximated carefully, and the removable sutures should be left in place for twice the usual time. Recurrent dislocations can often be repaired surgically, although further recurrence is more common than in unaffected individuals. Arterial rupture in patients with EDS type IV needs to be treated surgically unless bleeding is controlled by compartmental limitation (e.g., some

TABLE 184–1. CLINICAL FEATURES, MODE OF INHERITANCE, AND BIOCHEMICAL DISORDERS OF THE EHLERS-DANLOS SYNDROME

Type	Clinical Features	Inheritance	Molecular Defect
I: Gravis	Soft, velvety, hyperextensible skin; easy bruising; "cigarette paper" scars; hypermobile joints; varicose veins; prematurity	AD	Not known
II: Mitis	Similar to EDS type I but less severe	AD (AR, rare)	Not known COL1A2 null alleles
III: Familial hypermobility	Soft skin, no scarring, marked large and small joint hypermobility	AD	Not known
IV: Arterial	Thin, translucent skin with visible veins; marked bruising; skin and joints have normal extensibility; arterial, bowel, and uterine rupture	AD	Mutations in the COL3A1 gene that alter type III collagen synthesis, secretion, and structure
V: X-linked	Similar to EDS type II	XLR	Not known
VI: Ocular	Soft, velvety, hyperextensible skin; hypermobile joints; scoliosis; ocular fragility and keratoconus	AR	Lysyl hydroxylase deficiency due to mutations in the LOH gene
VII: A and B: Arthrochalasis multiplex congenita	Congenital hip dislocation; joint hypermobility; soft skin with normal scarring	AD	A: COL1A1 exon 6 skipping mutation that deletes N-proteinase cleavage site B: COL1A2 exon 6 skipping mutation that deletes N-proteinase cleavage site
C: Dermatosparaxis	Very soft, fragile, bruisable skin; marked joint hypermobility	AR	Procollagen N-proteinase deficiency
VIII: Periodontal	Generalized periodontitis; skin similar to EDS type II	AD	Not known
IX: X-linked cutis laxa; occipital horn syndrome	Soft, extensible, lax skin; bladder diverticula and rupture; short arms, limited pronation and supination; broad clavicles, occipital horns	XLR	Abnormal intracellular copper utilization with defect in lysyl oxidase; allelic to Menkes' syndrome
X: Fibronectin defect	Similar to EDS type II	AR	Defect in fibronectin

AD = Autosomal dominant; AR = Autosomal recessive; XLR = X-linked recessive.

retroperitoneal bleeding). The repair of affected arteries is often difficult because of extreme friability. If colon rupture recurs, the colon can be excised to prevent further episodes. Rupture of the small bowel is very rare. Some patients with EDS type VI respond to ascorbic acid (1 to 4 grams per day) with some symptomatic improvement and increased excretion of hydroxylysine in the urine. There is no metabolic treatment for other forms of EDS, and management is largely symptomatic.

PROGNOSIS. The prognosis in EDS depends on the specific type with which the patient is affected. Life expectancy is considerably shortened in EDS type IV because of organ and vessel rupture and may be decreased in EDS type VI; in all others, life expectancy is normal. With the exception of EDS type VI, no specific therapy is available that affects the natural history of the condition.

Prevention by prenatal diagnosis is feasible for some types of EDS. Heterozygosity for the EDS type VI mutation has been recognized by examination of amniotic fluid cells in a family at risk for recurrence. The structural mutations in EDS type VII and in EDS type IV should be recognizable by studies of collagens synthesized by chorionic villus cells in culture or by analysis of the specific mutation. Analysis of copper uptake and distribution by amniotic fluid cells should facilitate prenatal diagnosis of EDS type IX. All families should have access to genetic counseling once a proband is identified.

McKusick VA: Heritable Disorders of Connective Tissue. 4th ed. St Louis, CV Mosby, 1972, p 292. *Although the classification is not up to date, the richness of clinical detail is unsurpassed. A delight to read because of the many case histories and the personal touch.*

Steinmann B, Royce PM, Superti-Furga A: The Ehlers-Danlos syndrome. *In* Royce PM, Steinmann B (eds.): Connective Tissue and Its Heritable Disorders: Molecular, Genetic, and Medical Aspects. New York, Wiley-Liss, 1992, p 351. *The most comprehensive recent review of the clinical, biochemical, and molecular genetic aspects of EDS.*

185 OSTEOGENESIS IMPERFECTA

Peter H. Byers

DEFINITION. Osteogenesis imperfecta (OI) is a heterogeneous group of disorders characterized by bone fragility and associated connective tissue involvement. The clinical picture depends on the nature of the mutation and ranges from a form that is lethal in the perinatal period to a mild phenotype in which stature is normal and bone fractures are only slightly more common than usual.

ETIOLOGY AND PATHOGENESIS. In virtually all instances, OI results from mutations in one of the two genes, COL1A1 and COL1A2, that encode the proα1(I) and proα2(I) of type I collagen,

respectively. Type I collagen is the major structural protein of bone and of many other connective tissues (tendon, skin, sclera, ligament). The protein contains three chains—two α1(I) chains and a single α2(I) chain in a triple helix—that require glycine in every third position of each chain. OI phenotypes result from mutations that substitute for virtually any of the third position glycine residues, splice junction mutations, and short genomic deletions or duplications. The severity of the OI reflects the nature of the mutation, the location, and the gene in which the mutation occurred and the effect of the mutations on the protein. OI type I, the mildest form, results from synthesis of about half the normal amount of type I collagen, whereas the other forms (Table 185–1) result from mutations that alter the protein's structure. These mutations alter the ability of the molecules to be secreted, to form extracellular fibrils, and to be mineralized. The deficit of normal collagen in bone leads to fracture and deformity, the extent of which depends on the nature of the protein abnormality.

PREVALENCE. The incidence of OI is thought to be approximately 1 in 15,000 to 20,000 births. The mild dominant form, OI type I, is most prevalent. The incidence of the lethal perinatal form is approximately 1 in 50,000 to 60,000.

CLINICAL MANIFESTATIONS (Table 185–1).

OI Type I. Fracture rate is highest during childhood, decreases at puberty, and may increase in the postmenopausal period for women. Adult-onset hearing loss is common.

OI Type II. Affected infants have very marked bone deformity and diminished mineralization of bone. Death is usually the consequence of pulmonary insufficiency due to a very small thorax.

OI Type III. This form is characterized by marked short stature, progressive limb deformity, scoliosis, and thin bones that are susceptible to fracture. People with this form of OI frequently use a wheelchair for most of their activities and may be among the shortest adults an internist encounters, with some less than 3 feet tall. Progressive pulmonary and cardiac insufficiency may decrease life span. Basilar impression, compression of the brain stem due to settling of the skull on the vertebral column, may lead to neurologic impairment, tussive headache, neurologic compromise, sleep apnea, and death. Life expectancy is shortened, although some individuals with this form of OI live an average span.

OI Type IV. Severity is between OI type III and OI type I. Stature is decreased but generally above 4 feet for males.

DIFFERENTIAL DIAGNOSIS. In the perinatal period, OI needs to be distinguished from forms of *hypophosphatasia* and *severe chondrodysplasia (e.g., spondyloepiphyseal dysplasia, achondrogenesis, and hypochondrogenesis), and Menkes' syndrome.* Radiographs and serum levels of alkaline phosphatase and of copper distinguish among these conditions. During early childhood, *nonaccidental trauma* may be confused with OI in some children; the characteristic radiographic features of trauma may be helpful in the diagnosis. During adolescence, *idiopathic juvenile osteoporosis* may be confused with OI, and biochemical studies of cultured dermal fibroblasts may help to distinguish the two. Other forms of brittle bone disorders, including sclerosing bone disease such as *pykno-*

TABLE 185–1. OSTEOGENESIS IMPERFECTA

Type	Clinical Features	Inheritance	Biochemical and Genetic Abnormalities
I	Normal stature, little or no deformity; blue sclerae; hearing loss in 50%; dentinogenesis imperfecta is rare and may distinguish a subset	AD	*Common:* "Nonfunctional" COL1A1 allele
II	Lethal in the perinatal period; minimal calvarial mineralization; beaded ribs; compressed femurs; marked long-bone deformity; platyspondyly	AD (new)	*Common:* Substitutions for glycyl residues in the triple-helical domains of both chains of type I collagen *Rare:* Rearrangement in the COL1A1 and COL1A2 genes; exon deletions in triple-helical domain of COL1A1 and COL1A2
		AR (rare)	Small deletion in COL1A2 on the background of null allele
III	Progressively deforming bones, usually with moderate deformity at birth; sclerae variable in hue, often lighten with age; dentinogenesis common; hearing loss common; stature very short	AD AR (uncommon)	Point mutations in the COL1A1 and COL1A2 gene Frame-shift (4 bp deletion) in COL1A2 that prevents incorporation of chains into molecules
IV	Normal sclerae; mild to moderate bone deformity and variable short stature; dentinogenesis is common and hearing loss occurs in some	AD	Point mutations in COL1A1 and COL1A2 gene; exon skipping mutations in COL1A2

AD = autosomal dominant; AR = autosomal recessive.

dysostosis and *osteopetrosis* are rarely confused with OI. In adult life, OI may be thought to be *osteoporosis*.

TREATMENT AND CARE. Currently no medical therapies have been demonstrated to alter growth or decrease fracture rate in any form of OI. As a consequence, treatment is largely mechanical and directed toward preservation of function and, especially for those who depend on wheelchairs for mobility, ensuring independence in adult life. The mainstays of care are active physical therapy and habilitation and appropriate orthopedic intervention. Recurrent fracture of long bones may lead to periods of inactivity which, in turn, may decrease bone mineralization and predispose to further fracture. Placing intramedullary rods in the bones of the legs can short-circuit this cycle and lead to ambulation in some who fracture readily. Monitoring hearing, particularly in the adult, is important, and awareness of the symptoms of basilar impression in people with OI type III and OI type IV may reduce complications if intervention is necessary.

Prenatal diagnosis by ultrasonography is available for OI type II (14 to 16 weeks' gestation) and OI type III (15 to 19 weeks' gestation). Biochemical studies of chorionic villus cells can identify a fetus that synthesizes abnormal type I collagen molecules (OI types II, III, and IV), if the abnormality is known from study of an affected individual. In appropriate families, linked DNA markers can identify the affected allele and can be used for presymptomatic and prenatal diagnosis.

Byers PH: Osteogenesis imperfecta. *In* Royce PM, Steinmann B (eds.): Connective Tissue and Its Heritable Disorders: Molecular, Genetic, and Medical Aspects. New York, Wiley-Liss, 1993, p 317. *A detailed review of biochemical, molecular, genetic, and clinical abnormalities in OI.*

186 PSEUDOXANTHOMA ELASTICUM

Jouni Uitto

Pseudoxanthoma elasticum (PXE) (synonyms: Grönblad-Strandberg syndrome, systemic elastorrhexis) is a generalized progressive connective tissue disorder primarily affecting the elastic fibers. Clinically, PXE manifests as characteristic cutaneous lesions, ocular changes, and widespread vascular abnormalities. The relative severity of these changes results in a variety of clinical pictures. The on-

set of the disease may be in early childhood, and in most cases the cutaneous changes are evident before age 30. The exact incidence of PXE is not known, although estimates are about 1 in 160,000 persons. The male-female ratio is probably 1:1.

CLINICAL MANIFESTATIONS. *Skin.* The primary cutaneous lesions are relatively small (1 to 3 mm) yellowish papules that give the affected area a pebbly, "plucked chicken skin" appearance. The primary lesions tend to coalesce into larger plaques, and the skin of the involved areas becomes thickened and leathery (Fig. 186–1). Gradually, the affected skin becomes redundant, lax, and inelastic. The predilection sites are the face, neck, axillary folds, lower abdomen, and thighs. The nasolabial folds and chin creases may be strikingly accentuated. Yellowish lesions similar to those noted on the skin can also be seen on the mucous membranes.

Eye. The ocular changes are characterized by angioid streaks, i.e., grayish or brownish-red, poorly defined streaks radiating across the fundus of the eye. Their development usually starts later than that of the cutaneous lesions, often during the third or fourth decade. The ocular changes are commonly bilateral and include hemorrhages and exudates in Bruch's membrane, an elastin-rich structure located between the retina and the choroid. The degenerative changes of the eye frequently lead to impaired vision, and complete blindness, although rare, is one of the major complications of PXE. Angioid streaks may be present without noticeable cutaneous changes, but other accompanying observations, such as vascular changes, may lead to correct diagnosis of PXE. Angioid streaks can also be associated with other diseases—for example, Paget's disease of bone, sickle cell anemia, tumoral calcinosis, lead poisoning, and idiopathic thrombocytopenia.

Vascular Manifestations. The early manifestations of arterial involvement include hypertension, weak peripheral pulses, and, occasionally, intermittent claudication. The most devastating complications develop as a result of coronary occlusion or cerebral hemorrhage; the most frequent complication is recurrent bleeding from the gastrointestinal tract. A common site of the gastrointestinal bleeding is the gastric mucosa, where the elastic fibers of the arteries are particularly affected. Bleeding from the urinary tract can also occur.

INHERITANCE. Most cases of PXE are inherited as an autosomal recessive disease. However, autosomal dominant inheritance has been documented in some families, although delayed onset, incomplete expression, and lack of carrier detection complicate the genetic analysis. In addition to the inherited forms, several cases with cutaneous findings consistent with PXE but without family history and without vascular or ocular involvement have been re-

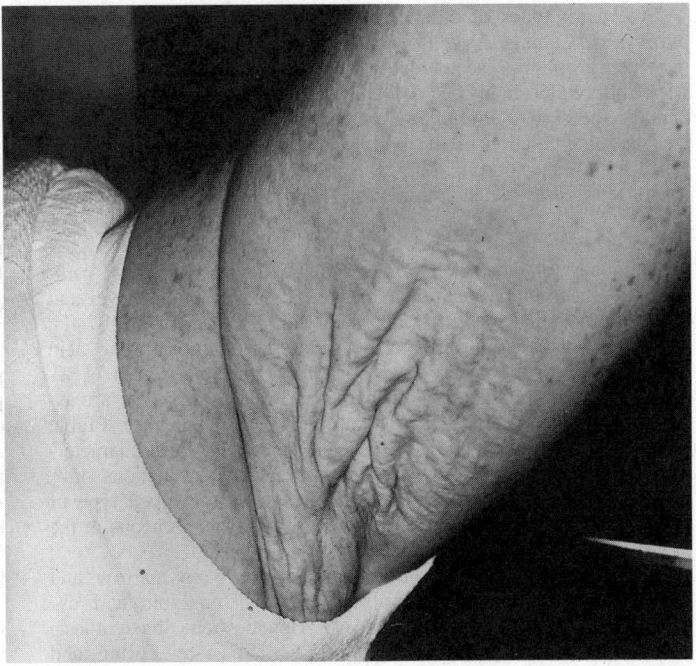

FIGURE 186–1. Typical cutaneous manifestations of pseudoxanthoma elasticum. The lesion demonstrates redundant and inelastic skin in the axillary fold.

ported. Periumbilical perforating PXE appears to be a distinct acquired form of the disease.

PATHOLOGY. Histopathologic examination of the involved skin demonstrates an accumulation of structures in the middle or lower dermis that stain positively with stains specific for elastic fibers, e.g., Verhoeff's stain. In contrast to the elastic fibers in normal skin, the elastic material in PXE appears irregularly clumped and fragmented. The accumulation of elastic fibers has also been quantitated by computerized morphometric analyses and by assay of desmosine, an elastin-specific crosslink compound. Characteristically, the fragmented elastic fibers contain calcium that appears bluish on routine hematoxylin-eosin stain and that can be demonstrated by calcium-specific stains. Electron microscopy of affected skin demonstrates that the amorphous elastin component has been replaced by bundles of granular material with staining properties different from those of normal elastin. Also, foci containing calcium hydroxyapatite crystals can be detected in the elastic fibers. These morphologic findings thus provide evidence for derangement in the organization of the elastic structures in PXE. Biochemical proof of the exact molecular defect in the structure or metabolism of elastin is, however, lacking, and it is unclear whether the calcification of elastic fibers is a primary or secondary event.

THERAPY. No specific treatment is available, and the primary prevention entails genetic counseling (see Ch. 29). Although treatment with vitamin E, vitamin C, or a low-calcium diet has been advocated in isolated case reports, there is no clinical proof of their efficacy. In selected cases, plastic surgery may be helpful to improve the skin's cosmetic appearance.

Christiano AM, Uitto J: Molecular pathology of the elastic fibers. J Invest Dermatol 103:53S, 1994. *A review of the molecular defects of elastin in heritable connective tissue diseases, including PXE.*
Lebwohl M, et al.: Classification of pseudoxanthoma elasticum. J Am Acad Dermatol 30:103, 1994. *Report of a consensus conference on PXE.*
Neldner KH: Pseudoxanthoma elasticum. Clin Dermatol 6:1, 1988. *Extremely useful clinical account of PXE, based on the author's data on 100 patients followed over a 10-year period.*
Neldner KH, Martinez-Hernandez A: Localized acquired cutaneous pseudoxanthoma elasticum. J Am Acad Dermatol 1:523, 1979. *Clinical description of a distinct acquired form of pseudoxanthoma elasticum.*

Disorders of Porphyrins and Metals

187 THE PORPHYRIAS
Karl E. Anderson

Porphyrias are due to deficiencies of specific enzymes of the heme biosynthetic pathway and, when clinically expressed, are associated with striking accumulations of heme pathway intermediates. These conditions are more prevalent, and more often manifested, in adults than are most well-characterized metabolic diseases, and are likely to be encountered by physicians in many disciplines. The three most common porphyrias differ considerably from each other and are managed very differently. Most porphyrias are inherited, but other factors are important in determining their severity.

Two major types of clinical manifestations are characteristic of porphyrias. *Cutaneous photosensitivity* occurs in types of porphyria in which porphyrins accumulate. Porphyrins are activated by long-wave ultraviolet light (UV-B) and generate oxygen radicals that damage the skin. *Neurologic effects* occur in porphyrias characterized by accumulation of the porphyrin precursors δ-aminolevulinic acid (ALA) and porphobilinogen (PBG). (Standard abbreviations for these diseases are shown in Table 187–1.)

THE HEME BIOSYNTHETIC PATHWAY AND THE PORPHYRIAS

The genes for most of the eight enzymes of this important pathway have been cloned and characterized at the molecular level and their chromosomal locations identified (Fig. 187–1; Table 187–1). Mutations of the erythroid-specific form of δ-aminolevulinic acid synthase, the first enzyme, have been found in some cases of X-linked sideroblastic anemia. Porphyrias and related disorders are associated with deficiencies of the other seven enzymes (Table 187–1). Mutations in genes for these enzymes have been characterized in detail in five types of porphyria. Different mutations have generally been found in unrelated families with any given type of porphyria. Thus these diseases are probably all heterogeneous at the molecular level.

Heme is synthesized in largest amounts in bone marrow and liver, where it is used primarily to make hemoglobin and cytochrome P-450 enzymes, respectively. Hepatic heme biosynthesis is regulated primarily by ALA synthase, which is rate-limiting, and under sensitive feedback control by cellular free heme content. Hepatic ALA synthase is induced by many of the same drugs and steroids that induce P-450 enzymes. Additional pathway enzymes and cellular uptake of iron are important in regulating heme synthesis in erythroid cells.

Most heme pathway intermediates are conserved and excreted only in small amounts. ALA and PBG are normally excreted in much larger amounts than porphyrins. Porphyrinogens (hexahydroporphyrins) undergo auto-oxidation outside cells and are excreted primarily as porphyrins. ALA, PBG, and porphyrinogens are colorless and nonfluorescent. Porphyrins are reddish and fluoresce when exposed to long-wave UV light. ALA, PBG, uroporphyrin, and hepta-, hexa-, and pentacarboxyl porphyrins are excreted mostly in urine, coproporphyrin (a tetracarboxyl porphyrin) in urine and bile, and harderoporphyrin (a tricarboxyl porphyrin) and protoporphyrin (a dicarboxyl porphyrin) in bile and feces.

CLASSIFICATION

Traditionally, porphyrias have been divided into erythropoietic and hepatic types, based on whether the excess production of intermediates takes place primarily in bone marrow or liver (Table 187–1). Some porphyrias have both erythroid and hepatic features. Porphyrias with neurovisceral symptoms are also termed "acute porphyrias." They share many clinical features and are similarly managed. Several "cutaneous porphyrias" manifest similar skin lesions but differ considerably in their treatment and prognosis. The cutaneous features of erythropoietic protoporphyria (EPP) are distinct. Now that these disorders are better characterized, they are best classified in terms of their specific enzyme deficiencies.

THE MOST COMMON PORPHYRIAS

It is important to appreciate that the three most common types of porphyria, which are likely to be encountered periodically by any physician, differ markedly from each other with regard to major clinical manifestations, exacerbating factors, tests important for diagnosis, and effective therapies (Table 187–2). Because their features are so distinct, a feature learned about one of these porphyrias will not apply to the others. On the other hand, these three conditions are prototypic: They share some important features with the other less common porphyrias. This should be evident from the brief descriptions of each of the porphyrias that follow.

ALA DEHYDRATASE DEFICIENT–PORPHYRIA (ADP). In this very rare autosomal recessive disorder, ALA dehydratase is markedly reduced (1 to 2% of normal). Symptoms resemble acute

TABLE 187-1. ENZYMES OF THE HEME BIOSYNTHETIC PATHWAY AND CLASSIFICATION AND INHERITANCE OF DISEASES ASSOCIATED WITH THEIR DEFICIENCIES*

Enzyme	Chromosomal Location	Disease	Inheritance	Classifications of Porphyrias			
				Hepatic	*Erythropoietic*	*Acute*	*Cutaneous*
ALA synthase							
Erythroid	Xp11.21	Sideroblastic anemia	X-linked recessive				
Nonerythroid	3p21	None known					
ALA dehydratase	9q34	δ-Aminolevulinic acid dehydratase–deficient porphyria (ADP)	Autosomal recessive	?X		X	
Porphobilinogen deaminase†	11q24.1 -> q24.2	Acute intermittent porphyria (AIP)	Autosomal dominant	X		X	
Uroporphyrinogen III cosynthase	10q25.2 -> q26.3	Congenital erythropoietic porphyria (CEP)	Autosomal recessive		X		X
Uroporphyrinogen decarboxylase	1p34	Porphyria cutanea tarda (PCT)‡	Autosomal dominant	X			X
		Hepatoerythropoietic porphyria (HEP)	Autosomal recessive	X	X		X
Coproporphyrinogen oxidase	9	Hereditary coproporphyria (HCP)	Autosomal dominant	X		X	X
Protoporphyrinogen oxidase	?14	Variegate porphyria (VP)	Autosomal dominant	X		X	X
Ferrochelatase	18q21.3 or 22	Erythropoietic protoporphyria (EPP)	Autosomal dominant		X		X

* The most precise classification is according to the specific enzyme deficiencies. Other classifications based on the major tissue site of overproduction of heme pathway intermediates (hepatic versus erythropoietic) or the type of major symptoms (acute neurovisceral versus cutaneous) are useful but not precise or mutually exclusive.
† This enzyme is also known as hydroxymethylbilane synthase and formerly as uroporphyrinogen I synthase.
‡ PCT is primarily acquired. Inherited deficiency of uroporphyrinogen decarboxylase is partially responsible for familial (type II) PCT.

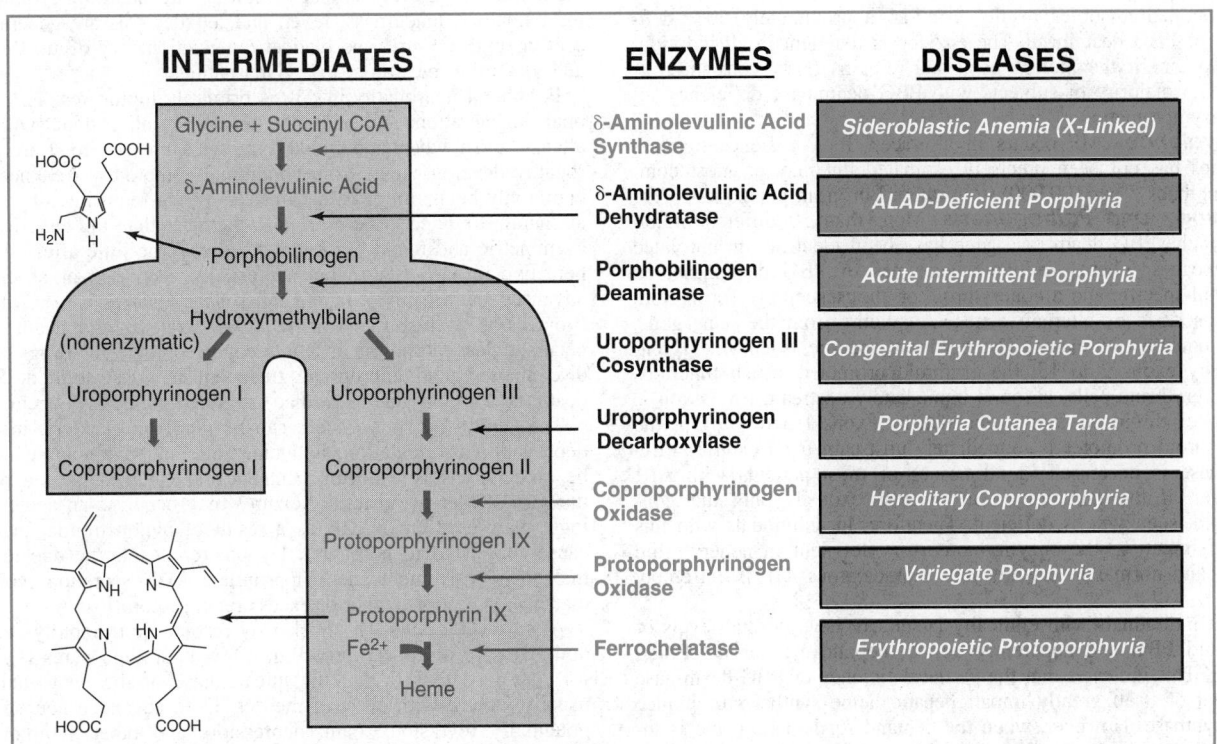

FIGURE 187-1. Intermediates and enzymes of the heme biosynthetic pathway and the major diseases of porphyrin metabolism that have been associated with deficiencies of specific enzymes. The initial and last three enzymes (in red) are mitochondrial and the other four (in black) are cytosolic. Heme is synthesized from glycine and succinyl CoA. Intermediates in the pathway include δ-aminolevulinic acid (an amino acid), porphobilinogen (a pyrrole), and hydroxymethylbilane (a linear tetrapyrrole). Uroporphyrinogen III cosynthase catalyzes closure of hydroxymethylbilane, with inversion of one of the pyrroles, to form a porphyrin macrocycle, uroporphyrinogen III. (Nonenzymatic closure occurs without inversion of this pyrrole, forming uroporphyrinogen I, which is not metabolized beyond coproporphyrinogen I.) The next two enzymes result in decarboxylation of six of the eight side chains of uroporphyrinogen III, with sequential formation of 7-, 6-, and 5-carboxylate porphyrinogens, coproporphyrinogen III, 3-carboxylate porphyrinogen, and protoporphyrinogen IX. The final two enzymes catalyze oxidation of protoporphyrinogen IX to protoporphyrin IX and insertion of ferrous iron into the porphyrin macrocycle to form heme (iron protoporphyrin IX). With the exception of protoporphyrin IX, all porphyrin intermediates are in their reduced forms (hexahydroporphyrins or porphyrinogens). Chemical structures of two intermediates are shown.

TABLE 187–2. THREE MOST COMMON HUMAN PORPHYRIAS AND THEIR MAJOR DISTINGUISHING FEATURES

	Presenting Symptoms	Exacerbating Factors	Most Important Screening Tests	Treatment
Acute intermittent porphyria (AIP)	Neurovisceral (acute)	Drugs (mostly P-450 inducers); progesterone; dietary restriction	Urinary porphobilinogen	Heme; glucose
Porphyria cutanea tarda (PCT)	Blistering skin lesions (chronic)	Iron; alcohol; estrogens; hepatitis C virus; halogenated hydrocarbons	Plasma (or urine) porphyrins	Phlebotomy; low-dose chloroquine
Erythropoietic protoporphyria (EPP)	Painful skin and swelling (mostly acute)		Plasma (or erythrocyte) porphyrins	β-Carotene

intermittent porphyria (AIP) but may begin in childhood. Hemolysis is sometimes present. Urinary ALA and coproporphyrin III and erythrocyte zinc protoporphyrin are increased. In this and other disorders in which ALA accumulates, coproporphyrin III may originate from excess ALA that is metabolized to coproporphyrinogen III in tissues other than the tissue of origin of the excess ALA.

Several other conditions are associated with ALA dehydratase deficiency and increased ALA. *Lead poisoning* and *hereditary tyrosinemia* can present with symptoms (abdominal pain, ileus, and motor neuropathy) that are strikingly similar to those of the acute porphyrias. Lead concentrates in erythroid cells and also inhibits ferrochelatase, leading to excess erythrocyte zinc protoporphyrin. Urinary coproporphyrin excretion is also increased. Deficient erythrocyte ALA dehydratase in lead poisoning can be restored to normal with dithiothreitol *in vitro*. In hereditary tyrosinemia, a deficiency of fumarylacetoacetase leads to accumulation of succinylacetone (2,3-dioxoheptanoic acid). This structural analogue of ALA is a potent inhibitor of ALA dehydratase. Other heavy metals or styrene exposure can also inhibit ALA dehydratase.

ACUTE INTERMITTENT PORPHYRIA (AIP). This autosomal dominant disorder results from an approximately 50% deficiency of PBG deaminase. The enzyme is deficient in all individuals who inherit the mutant gene and remains fairly constant over time. The majority of subjects with PBG deaminase deficiency remain asymptomatic.

Prevalence. AIP occurs in all races. Its prevalence in most countries has not been precisely estimated but may be most common (perhaps 5 per 100,000) in northern European populations.

Etiology and Pathogenesis. More than 50 different mutations of the PBG deaminase gene have been identified in unrelated AIP lineages. There are two isoenzymes of PBG deaminase, an erythroid-specific and a nonerythroid or "housekeeping" form. Both are transcribed by alternative mRNA splicing from the same gene, which contains 15 exons. The erythroid-specific isoenzyme is encoded by exons 2 to 15; the erythroid promoter, which functions only in erythroid cells, is found immediately upstream from exon 2. The nonerythroid enzyme is encoded by exons 1 and 3 to 15; the nonerythroid promoter is immediately upstream from exon 1. PBG deaminase is decreased in all tissues of most patients with AIP. However, if the mutation is in or near exon 1, only the nonerythroid isoenzyme is deficient. Therefore, in individuals with this type of mutation, the enzyme activity is deficient in nonerythroid tissues and normal in erythrocytes. Homozygous AIP is extremely rare.

Most individuals with clinically latent AIP have normal levels of ALA and PBG and apparently normal hepatic cytochrome P-450 content. This indicates that the partial deficiency of PBG deaminase does not of itself greatly impair hepatic heme synthesis or induce ALA synthase. However, when the demand for hepatic heme is increased by drugs, hormones, or nutritional factors, the deficient enzyme can become limiting for heme synthesis, induction of hepatic ALA synthase is accentuated, and ALA and PBG accumulate in liver and increase in plasma and urine. Excess porphyrins originate nonenzymatically from PBG or enzymatically from ALA transported to tissues other than the liver.

Most drugs that are harmful in AIP induce hepatic ALA synthase and cytochrome P-450 enzymes. Sulfonamide antibiotics are not inducers and may inhibit PBG deaminase. Reduced caloric and carbohydrate intakes enhance induction of ALA synthase in animals and in AIP can increase ALA and PBG and precipitate symptoms. Administering carbohydrate can reduce hepatic ALA synthase and P-450 enzymes.

The mechanism of neural damage in AIP is unknown. Porphyrias and related disorders associated with increased ALA have similar neurologic manifestations. ALA is structurally analogous to γ-aminobutyric acid (GABA) and can interact with GABA receptors. However, ALA and other products of the heme pathway have not been convincingly shown to be neurotoxic. The suggestion that heme deficiency may occur in nervous tissue in these disorders is also unproven.

Clinical Manifestations. Symptoms rarely occur before puberty and seldom if ever recur throughout adult life. Characteristically, attacks last for several days or longer, often require hospitalization, and are followed by complete recovery. Abdominal pain is the most common symptom; it is usually steady and poorly localized but may be cramping. Tachycardia, hypertension, restlessness, fine tremors, and excess sweating may be due to sympathetic overactivity. Other manifestations include nausea; vomiting; constipation; pain in the limbs, head, neck, or chest; muscle weakness; and sensory loss. Ileus, with distention and decreased bowel sounds, is common. However, increased bowel sounds and diarrhea may be seen. Because the abdominal symptoms are neurologic rather than inflammatory, tenderness, fever, and leukocytosis are generally absent or mild. Dysuria and bladder dysfunction may occur. Recurrent attacks tend to be similar in a given patient.

Peripheral neuropathy in AIP is primarily motor, results from axonal degeneration, and does not develop in all patients with acute attacks, even when abdominal symptoms are severe. Rarely, neuropathy develops apart from abdominal symptoms. Weakness most commonly begins in proximal muscles (often requiring a careful examination to detect), more often in the arms than the legs. It can be asymmetric and focal. Tendon reflexes may be little affected or hyperactive in early stages but are usually decreased or absent with advanced neuropathy. Cranial and sensory nerves can be affected. Progression to respiratory and bulbar paralysis and death seldom occurs unless porphyria is not recognized, harmful drugs are not discontinued, and appropriate treatment is not instituted. Sudden death, presumably due to cardiac arrhythmia, may also occur.

The central nervous system can be involved. Anxiety, insomnia, depression, disorientation, hallucinations, and paranoia, which can be especially severe during acute attacks, may suggest a primary mental disorder or hysteria. Seizures may occur as an acute neurologic manifestation of AIP, as a result of hyponatremia, or due to causes unrelated to porphyria. Hyponatremia may be due to hypothalamic involvement and inappropriate ADH secretion; vomiting, diarrhea, and poor intake; or excess renal sodium loss.

After several days, an attack may resolve quite rapidly, with abdominal pain disappearing within a few hours and paresis within a few days. Attacks during the luteal phase of the menstrual cycle usually resolve with onset of menses. Even advanced neuropathy is potentially reversible. Pain, depression, and other symptoms are sometimes chronic.

Chronic hepatic abnormalities are common in AIP, and there is an increased risk of hepatocellular carcinoma (apparently not associated with hepatitis B or C). AIP may predispose to chronic hypertension and be associated with impaired renal function. The mechanisms of these associations are unknown.

Precipitating Factors. Recognition of precipitating factors is important for management. Endogenous steroid hormones are probably most important. This is indicated by rarity of symptoms and excess ALA and PBG before puberty, more frequent clinical expression in women, premenstrual attacks in some women, and exacerbations after use of sex steroid preparations. Some patients manifest increased proportions of 5β-H steroid metabolites that are potent inducers of hepatic ALA synthase. Recurrent cyclic attacks are troublesome in some women and occur when progesterone levels are highest; progesterone and its metabolites are potent inducers of ALA synthase, whereas estrogens are not. Pregnancy is usually well tolerated despite high progesterone levels. Some women are more prone to attacks during pregnancy, possibly due in part to hyperemesis gravidarum and reduced caloric intake.

Drugs remain important as causes of AIP attacks. The major drugs known to be harmful or safe in the acute porphyrias are listed in Table 187–3. Barbiturates and sulfonamides are most notorious. Benzodiazepines are much less hazardous. Published information is insufficient to allow most drugs to be classified as definitely harmful or safe. Advice can be sought from a center with experience in porphyria with regard to unpublished information.

Reduced caloric intake, usually instituted in an effort to lose weight, is a common cause of attacks. Attacks are also provoked by intercurrent infections, major surgery, and other conditions. Attacks are almost always due to two or more factors acting in an additive fashion. Probably for this reason (a) drugs may produce attacks in adults but are rarely reported to do so in children with PBG deaminase deficiency; (b) anticonvulsants do not produce attacks in some PBG deaminase–deficient subjects; and (c) barbiturate anesthetics more frequently exacerbate porphyria if symptoms were present prior to anesthetic exposure.

Diagnosis and Differential Diagnosis. AIP and other acute porphyrias are uncommon, their symptoms are nonspecific, and physical findings are minimal. Therefore, a high index of suspicion is necessary for diagnosis. The diagnosis is established by demonstrating a marked increase in urinary PBG, using a quantitative method (see later discussion of laboratory methods). During an acute attack, PBG excretion generally is in the range of 50 to 200 mg per day (reference range 0 to 4 mg per day), and ALA excretion 20 to 100 mg per day (reference range 0 to 7 mg per day). Such increases virtually assure a diagnosis of AIP, variegate porphyria (VP), or hereditary coproporphyria (HCP). ALA and PBG excretion generally decrease with clinical improvement. Such decreases are particularly dramatic (but transient) after heme therapy. After an attack of AIP it is distinctly unusual for ALA and PBG to decrease to persistently normal levels, except after prolonged periods of latency. In HCP and VP, excretion of ALA and PBG may decrease to normal levels more readily. Fecal porphyrins are usually normal or minimally increased, which distinguishes AIP from HCP and VP. Urinary uroporphyrin and coproporphyrin and erythrocyte protoporphyrin may be increased, but these are not specific findings.

Decreased PBG deaminase (most conveniently measured in erythrocytes) confirms the diagnosis of AIP. However, as already noted, some mutations of the PBG deaminase gene reduce only the nonerythroid enzyme. Furthermore, erythrocyte PBG deaminase has a wide normal range (up to threefold) that somewhat overlaps the AIP range and is increased by inapparent concurrent conditions that stimulate erythropoiesis. The enzyme is not reduced in HCP and VP, which is also important to consider when acute porphyria is suspected. For these reasons, measurement of erythrocyte PBG deaminase is not useful in acutely ill patients. On the other hand, its measurement is highly useful to analyze pedigrees of known AIP patients, if it is established that the propositus has a low value. In screening family members, urinary PBG should also be measured. Diagnosis of AIP *in utero* is possible but is seldom indicated in view of the favorable outlook for most PBG deaminase–deficient subjects.

No single laboratory test fully excludes AIP, HCP, and VP. However, a normal result of a quantitative test for urinary PBG virtually excludes these disorders as a cause of current symptoms. Attempting to provoke increases in ALA and PBG for diagnostic purposes by glycine loading or administering phenobarbital may be dangerous and is not definitive.

Treatment. Acute attacks usually require hospitalization for treatment of severe pain, nausea, and vomiting and for administration of intravenous glucose and heme. Hospitalization also facilitates observation for neurologic complications, electrolyte imbalances, and nutritional status and investigation of precipitating factors. Symptomatic therapy includes narcotic analgesics, which are usually required for abdominal pain, and small to moderate doses of a phenothiazine for nausea, vomiting, anxiety, and restlessness. Chloral hydrate can be used for insomnia. Diazepam in low doses is probably safe if a minor tranquilizer is required. Bladder distention may require catheterization. After recovery, continued treatment with a phenothiazine is seldom indicated.

Heme therapy and carbohydrate loading are specific therapies because they repress hepatic ALA synthase and overproduction of ALA and PBG. Heme therapy is most effective in this regard and should be initiated early, but only after the diagnosis of a porphyric attack is confirmed by a marked increase in urinary PBG. Diagnosis is more difficult after heme therapy, which can at least transiently normalize ALA and PBG.

The standard regimen for heme therapy is 3 mg heme per kilogram of body weight, infused intravenously once daily for 4 days. A longer course of treatment is seldom necessary if treatment is started early. Efficacy is reduced and recovery is less rapid when treatment is delayed and neuronal damage is more advanced. It is not effective for chronic symptoms of AIP. A lyophilized hematin (hydroxy-heme) preparation is available in the United States. The manufacturer recommends reconstitution with sterile water. However, the product is unstable and degradation products adhere to endothelial cells, platelets, and coagulation factors, causing a transient anticoagulant effect and phlebitis at the site of infusion. Reconstitution with human albumin enhances the stability of hematin and prevents these side effects. Heme arginate, which is available in Europe and South Africa, is much more stable than hematin and also does not have these side effects. It is an investigational drug in the United States.

Carbohydrate loading may suffice for mild attacks and can be given orally as sucrose, glucose polymers, or carbohydrate-rich foods. If oral intake is poorly tolerated or is contraindicated by distention and ileus, glucose administered intravenously (at least 300 grams daily) is usually indicated. A central venous line facilitates more complete parenteral nutritional support and avoids excess fluid volumes. Parenteral nutritional support may be indicated in some patients who require heme therapy.

Treatment of seizures is problematic because virtually all antiseizure drugs (except bromides) can exacerbate AIP. β-Adrenergic blocking agents may control tachycardia and hypertension in acute attacks of porphyria but may be hazardous in patients with hypovolemia, in whom increased catecholamine secretion may be an im-

TABLE 187–3. DRUGS CONSIDERED UNSAFE AND SAFE IN AIP, HCP, AND VP

Unsafe	Safe
Barbiturates*	Narcotic analgesics
Sulfonamide antibiotics*	Aspirin
Meprobamate*	Acetaminophen
Carisoprodol*	Phenothiazines
Glutethimide*	Penicillin and derivatives
Methyprylon	Streptomycin
Ethchlorvynol*	Glucocorticoids
Phenytoin*	Bromides
Mephenytoin	Insulin
Succinimides (ethosuximide, methsuximide)	Atropine
Carbamazepine*	Cimetidine
Clonazepam	Ranitidine*·†
Primidone*	?Estrogens*·‡
Valproic acid*	
Pyrazolones (aminopyrine, antipyrine)	
Griseofulvin*	
Ergots	
Metoclopramide*	
Rifampin*	
Pyrazinamide*	
Diclofenac*	
Progesterone and synthetic progestins*	
Danazol*	
Alcohol	

* Porphyria is listed as a contraindication, warning, precaution, or adverse effect in US labeling for these drugs.

† Although porphyria is listed as a precaution in US labeling for this drug, it is regarded as safe by other sources.

‡ There is little evidence that estrogens alone are harmful in acute porphyrias. They have been implicated as harmful based mostly on experience with estrogen-progestin combinations and because they can exacerbate PCT.

portant compensatory mechanism. Numerous other therapies have been tried in this disease but have not been consistently useful.

Prognosis. In the past 20 years, attacks of porphyria have rarely been fatal. If acute attacks are treated appropriately, inciting factors removed, and precautions taken to prevent further attacks, the outlook for patients with AIP is usually excellent. Recurrent attacks of porphyria occur in some patients and can be disabling but do not occur throughout adult life. The great majority of relatives with PBG deaminase deficiency never develop symptoms, especially if they have normal urinary porphyrin precursors. Although such individuals are less sensitive to inducing drugs than are patients with prior porphyric symptoms, they should follow the same precautions as AIP patients. Latent AIP should never be construed as a health risk that limits availability of health insurance.

Prevention. Some specific measures are helpful in preventing clinical expression of AIP. (1) Family members should be screened to detect latent cases. (2) Harmful drugs should be avoided. (3) "Crash diets" for weight reduction and even brief periods of starvation (e.g., during postoperative periods or intercurrent illnesses) should be avoided. Diet regimens for obesity should provide for gradual weight loss during periods of clinical remission of porphyria. (4) Investigational approaches for preventing frequent attacks include use of gonadotropin-releasing hormone analogues (for women with frequent cyclic attacks) or periodic heme infusions. Oophorectomy is not an acceptable option for preventing cyclic attacks.

CONGENITAL ERYTHROPOIETIC PORPHYRIA (CEP).
This autosomal recessive disorder is due to a deficiency of uroporphyrinogen III cosynthase. Less than 200 cases have been reported. CEP occurs in several animal species (including all fox squirrels).

Etiology and Pathogenesis. At least six different mutations of the uroporphyrinogen III cosynthase gene have been identified in CEP. Most patients have unrelated parents and have inherited a different mutation from each parent. Severity of the disease is variable and relates to the degree of enzyme deficiency caused by the particular mutations. Intramedullary hemolysis and shortened survival of circulating erythrocytes are caused by porphyrins produced and accumulated in bone marrow erythroid cells that are actively synthesizing hemoglobin. Even in the most severe cases there is some residual cosynthase activity, and heme production is actually increased in response to hemolysis. Increased heme production occurs at the expense of a considerable accumulation of hydroxymethylbilane (the substrate of the deficient enzyme), which is converted nonenzymatically to uroporphyrinogen I. Excretion of type III porphyrin isomers is also increased. Splenomegaly can contribute to anemia and cause leukopenia and thrombocytopenia. Sunlight, other sources of UV light, and minor trauma to friable skin are other determinants of clinical expression. Drugs, steroids, and nutrition have little influence.

Clinical Manifestations. In most cases, reddish urine and severe cutaneous photosensitivity are noted in early infancy. Recently, patients with very severe cases have presented as nonimmune hydrops, received intrauterine transfusions, and soon after birth developed marked photosensitivity when phototherapy was initiated for neonatal jaundice. In at least five cases symptoms began in adult life. Cutaneous features resemble those in porphyria cutanea tarda (PCT) but are usually more severe. Lesions on sun-exposed skin include bullae and vesicles, which are prone to rupture and become infected, hypopigmented or hyperpigmented areas, and hypertrichosis. Loss of digits and facial features and corneal scarring can be severe. Porphyrins are deposited in the teeth (producing a reddish-brown color termed *erythrodontia*) and in bone. Bone demineralization can be substantial. There are no neurologic manifestations. Hemolysis and splenomegaly are almost always present. Life expectancy is often shortened by infections or hematologic complications.

Diagnosis and Differential Diagnosis. Porphyrin excretion and porphyrin levels in red cells and plasma are generally much greater than in other forms of porphyria. Porphyrins in urine are primarily uroporphyrin and coproporphyrin, and in feces mostly coproporphyrin. ALA and PBG are normal. In most cases uroporphyrin I predominates in erythrocytes. A predominance of protoporphyrin in red cells has been described in some cases and is characteristic of bovine CEP. Stimulating erythropoiesis increases

uroporphyrin and coproporphyrin in erythrocytes in this condition. CEP is readily distinguished from EPP clinically but may resemble HEP and homozygous cases of AIP, VP, and HCP.

Treatment. Protection of the skin from sunlight and minor trauma and prompt treatment of secondary bacterial infections help prevent scarring and mutilation. Blood transfusions sufficient to suppress erythropoiesis may be the most effective treatment. Improvement may occur after splenectomy. Oral charcoal may be helpful by increasing fecal excretion of porphyrins.

Prevention. In affected families heterozygotes with intermediate deficiencies of the cosynthase can be detected, and CEP can be diagnosed *in utero*. Therefore, there are options for preventing genetic transmission.

PORPHYRIA CUTANEA TARDA (PCT).
This, the most common and readily treated form of porphyria, is caused by a deficiency of uroporphyrinogen decarboxylase in the liver. It is most common in men but has become more frequent in women, associated with alcohol and estrogen use.

Etiology and Pathogenesis. PCT is fundamentally an acquired disorder, although in some cases an inherited deficiency of uroporphyrinogen decarboxylase is a predisposing factor. Currently, PCT is classified into three types. In the "sporadic" form (type I), which constitutes the majority of cases, the enzyme is deficient in liver but not in erythrocytes and other tissues, and there are no mutations at the uroporphyrinogen decarboxylase locus. Moreover, the amount of hepatic uroporphyrinogen decarboxylase protein, as measured immunochemically, is normal, suggesting that an acquired process has inactivated the enzyme. With treatment and remission of the disease, the enzyme activity gradually increases to normal. Familial (type II) PCT is distinguished from type I by an approximately 50% deficiency of the decarboxylase in nonhepatic tissues, such as erythrocytes, and mutations in the uroporphyrinogen decarboxylase gene. The mutant alleles do not express detectable enzyme protein. The inherited autosomal dominant trait is not associated with overt disease unless the product of the normal allele is inactivated by the same acquired factors that are important in type I PCT. In type III PCT, the enzyme is deficient in liver but not other tissues, as in type I. However, unlike type I, more than one family member is affected. All three types are clinically similar and difficult to distinguish, and they respond to the same therapies.

Examples of *toxic porphyria* have resembled PCT. Most notably, an extensive outbreak of porphyria occurred in eastern Turkey in the late 1950's after seed wheat containing the fungicide hexachlorobenzene was used for food. Di- and trichlorophenols and 2,3,7,8-tetrachlorodibenzo-*p*-dioxin (TCDD, dioxin) have been implicated in smaller outbreaks and single cases in humans. When administered to animals, these chemicals decrease uroporphyrinogen decarboxylase (only in liver) and induce a pattern of excess porphyrins resembling PCT. There is seldom a history of exposure to such chemicals in sporadic (type I) PCT.

A notable feature of PCT is massive accumulation of porphyrins in liver, which may develop over many months. This precedes the appearance of excess porphyrins in plasma and urine. Hepatic ALA synthase may be little increased because amounts of porphyrins produced in PCT are small relative to rates of hepatic heme formation. By contrast, during attacks of the acute porphyrias much larger amounts of intermediates are excreted (as porphyrin precursors) and ALA synthase is substantially induced. Worsening of PCT by factors (other than alcohol) that induce heme synthesis is seldom reported.

The pattern of porphyrins that accumulate in PCT is complex and characteristic. The enzyme-catalyzed decarboxylation of uroporphyrinogen occurs in four sequential steps. Therefore, when the enzyme is markedly deficient, uroporphyrin and the hepta-, hexa-, and pentacarboxyl porphyrins (type I and III isomers, and derived from the corresponding porphyrinogens) accumulate. In addition, pentacarboxyl porphyrinogen can be metabolized by coproporphyrinogen oxidase to a series of tetracarboxyl porphyrins termed isocoproporphyrins. These are excreted primarily in bile and feces and are diagnostic of uroporphyrinogen decarboxylase deficiency.

Acquired factors may contribute to inactivation of hepatic uroporphyrinogen decarboxylase as follows: (1) A normal or increased amount of hepatic iron seems essential in this disease. One or more mechanisms may be involved. Ferrous iron may directly inhibit the enzyme. Iron may catalyze the formation of free radicals that damage the enzyme protein or oxidize its porphyrinogen substrates to porphyrins. (2) Cytochrome P-450 enzymes may also be involved in the oxidation of porphyrinogen substrates. (3) Alcohol intake may promote iron absorption, stimulate hepatic heme and porphyrin synthesis, or generate free radicals that damage the decarboxylase. (4) Estrogens, but apparently not other steroids, can exacerbate PCT, perhaps by an unknown oxidative mechanism. (5) The strong association with chronic hepatitis C virus infection suggests that hepatocellular damage induced by this virus, which appears to be accentuated by iron, can involve specific cellular proteins including uroporphyrinogen decarboxylase.

Clinical Manifestations. Most PCT patients have a history of moderate or heavy alcohol intake. The disease may develop in men treated with estrogens for prostate cancer and women taking oral contraceptives or replacement estrogens. Cutaneous photosensitivity is the major clinical feature. Vesicles and bullae develop on the face, dorsa of the hands and feet, forearms, and legs. Sun-exposed skin becomes friable, and minor trauma may precede the formation of bullae or cause denudation of the skin. Small white plaques ("milia") may precede or follow vesicle formation. Involved skin tends to heal slowly. Hypertrichosis and hyperpigmentation sometimes present even in the absence of vesicles. Thickening, scarring, and calcification of affected skin ("pseudoscleroderma") may be striking. Neurologic effects are not observed.

Liver histopathology is usually not diagnostic of alcoholic liver disease. Cirrhosis and hepatocellular carcinomas are most common in older patients and at autopsy. In many locations as many as 80% of PCT patients are chronically infected with hepatitis C virus. This strong association may explain much of the chronic liver damage and many of the hepatocellular carcinomas that have been observed in PCT. The disease is also associated with systemic lupus erythematosus and the acquired immunodeficiency syndrome (AIDS).

PCT sometimes occurs in patients with advanced renal disease. Skin lesions may be more severe and plasma porphyrin levels much higher in this setting because urinary excretion of porphyrins is not possible, and they are poorly dialyzed.

Very rarely, hepatic tumors themselves contain and presumably produce excess porphyrins. Some of these cases have resembled PCT.

Diagnosis and Differential Diagnosis. Skin lesions in PCT, VP, and HCP are indistinguishable clinically and histologically. It is important to differentiate these conditions by laboratory testing before starting therapy. A predominance of uroporphyrin and 7-carboxylate porphyrin in urine and increased isocoproporphyrin in feces are diagnostic of PCT. In PCT, urinary ALA may be slightly increased; PBG is normal. Total fecal porphyrins are usually less increased in PCT than in other types of porphyria with photosensitivity. Plasma porphyrins are always increased in patients with skin lesions due to any type of porphyria; the fluorescence spectrum of plasma can distinguish VP and EPP from PCT (see below).

Treatment. A course of phlebotomies is the preferred treatment and almost always produces a remission. Patients are also advised to discontinue alcohol, estrogens, iron supplements, or other contributing factors. Because iron stores in PCT are seldom markedly increased and may be normal, removal of only 5 to 6 units of blood at 1- to 2-week intervals is usually sufficient. Plasma (or serum) ferritin and porphyrin levels should be followed. Ferritin decreases before porphyrins. Phlebotomies should be stopped when the ferritin is near the lower limit of normal. Further iron depletion is of no additional benefit and may cause anemia and associated symptoms. Remission may be prolonged even if the ferritin level later returns to normal. In some cases relapses occur and respond to another course of phlebotomies. Deferoxamine, an iron chelator, may be effective in PCT but is much less efficient.

A course of low-dose chloroquine (e.g., 125 mg twice weekly for several months or as needed) or hydroxychloroquine is usually effective when repeated phlebotomies are contraindicated. The mechanism of their effects in PCT is not established. One hypothesis is that chloroquine forms complexes with porphyrins and promotes their removal from the liver. Chloroquine given in usual doses to PCT patients can cause marked increases in photosensitivity and porphyrin levels in plasma and urine, and nausea, malaise, fever, and hepatocellular damage. Although these adverse effects are generally transient and are followed by complete remission, it is prudent to avoid them by using a low-dose regimen.

Therapy is more difficult when PCT occurs with advanced renal disease because phlebotomy is usually contraindicated by anemia

(usually due to erythropoietin deficiency). Recent studies indicate that genetic recombinant erythropoietin can mobilize excess iron, support phlebotomy, and lead to remission of PCT in these patients.

HEPATOERYTHROPOIETIC PORPHYRIA (HEP). This rare, recently recognized autosomal recessive disease is clinically similar to CEP but is distinguished by excess isocoproporphyrin in feces and urine and decreased uroporphyrinogen decarboxylase activity in erythrocytes (and other tissues). The mutations in the uroporphyrinogen decarboxylase gene found in this disease are associated with some residual enzyme activity, unlike those in familial PCT. Therefore, strictly speaking, HEP is not the homozygous form of familial PCT. Increased erythrocyte protoporphyrin probably reflects an earlier accumulation of uroporphyrinogen in erythroblasts, which after completion of hemoglobin synthesis is metabolized to protoporphyrin. A similar explanation can account for increased erythrocyte protoporphyrin in other homozygous forms of porphyria.

HEREDITARY COPROPORPHYRIA (HCP) AND VARIEGATE PORPHYRIA (VP). These autosomal dominant acute hepatic porphyrias are clinically similar to AIP but are much less common in most countries. However, VP is quite prevalent in South Africa, where most cases have been traced to a couple who immigrated from Holland in the late 1600's. Unlike AIP, these disorders can cause cutaneous photosensitivity.

Etiology and Pathogenesis. HCP and VP are due to approximately 50% deficiencies of coproporphyrinogen oxidase and protoporphyrinogen oxidase, respectively. As in AIP, ALA and PBG are increased during acute attacks. This reflects induction of hepatic ALA synthase by factors such as endogenous steroids, drugs, and nutritional alterations, and the fact that PBG deaminase activity is almost as low as ALA synthase even in normal liver. When coproporphyrinogen III accumulates in HCP and coproporphyrinogen III and protoporphyrinogen IX in VP, they are auto-oxidized to the corresponding porphyrins. Coproporphyrinogen III may accumulate in VP because there is a functional association between coproporphyrinogen oxidase and the deficient protoporphyrinogen oxidase in mitochondria. Furthermore, coproporphyrinogen is more readily lost from the liver than are other porphyrinogens, and its loss increases further when heme synthesis is stimulated. In one form of HCP, termed *harderoporphyria,* a structurally altered coproporphyrinogen oxidase with reduced substrate affinity results in accumulation of harderoporphyrin as well as coproporphyrin. A few homozygous cases of HCP and VP have been described.

Clinical Manifestations. Drugs, steroids, and nutritional factors that are detrimental in AIP also exacerbate HCP and VP. Neurologic manifestations are identical to those in AIP. Skin manifestations are similar to those of PCT and usually occur apart from the neurovisceral symptoms. Impaired biliary excretion by concurrent liver diseases or drugs such as contraceptive steroids can cause porphyrin retention and worsen photosensitivity.

Diagnosis and Differential Diagnosis. Urinary ALA, PBG, and uroporphyrin are increased during acute attacks. When symptoms resolve, these normalize more readily than in AIP. Urinary coproporphyrin is markedly increased in both HCP and VP. A marked, isolated increase in fecal coproporphyrin is distinctive for HCP. Fecal coproporphyrin and protoporphyrin are about equally increased in VP. The fluorescence spectrum of plasma porphyrins (at neutral pH) is characteristic and very useful for rapidly distinguishing VP from the other porphyrias. This test is probably the most sensitive method for detecting VP, including latent cases, at least in adults.

Treatment and Prognosis. Acute attacks of VP are treated as in AIP. Striking decreases in attacks and deaths from VP in South Africa are attributed to identifying latent cases, avoiding harmful drugs, and providing better treatment during acute attacks. Measures that protect the skin from sunlight are helpful for photosensitivity. Phlebotomies and chloroquine are not effective. Cholestyramine may decrease photosensitivity occurring with liver dysfunction.

ERYTHROPOIETIC PROTOPORPHYRIA (EPP). This is an autosomal dominant condition due to a deficiency of ferrochelatase.

Etiology and Pathogenesis. At least 10 different point mutations in the ferrochelatase gene have been identified in various EPP families. Ferrochelatase is deficient in all tissues in EPP but becomes rate-limiting for protoporphyrin metabolism primarily in bone marrow. Some obligate carriers have little or no increase in red cell protoporphyrin. Increases in plasma and fecal protoporphyrin are also variable. This marked variation in clinical expression is evident within individual kindreds and is not well explained.

Individuals with clinically expressed EPP accumulate excess protoporphyrin in erythroid cells, plasma, bile, and feces. Bone marrow reticulocytes are the primary source of the excess protoporphyrin. Circulating erythrocytes and the liver contribute smaller amounts. Protoporphyrin in erythrocytes in EPP is not complexed with zinc and compared with zinc protoporphyrin (found in lead poisoning, iron deficiency, and homozygous forms of porphyria) diffuses more readily into plasma. Zinc protoporphyrin dissociates less readily from hemoglobin binding sites and persists in the red cell as long as it circulates. Disposition of the excess protoporphyrin in EPP depends on hepatic uptake, biliary excretion, and degree of enterohepatic circulation. These processes are impaired by liver damage.

Clinical Manifestations. Cutaneous manifestations usually begin in childhood and are distinctly different from those of other porphyrias. Burning, itching, erythema, and swelling can occur within minutes of sun exposure. Diffuse edema of sun-exposed areas may resemble angioneurotic edema. Other characteristic skin changes include lichenification, leathery pseudovesicles, labial grooving, and nail changes. Scarring is rarely severe or deforming. Vesicles, pigment changes, friability, and hirsutism are unusual. There is no fluorescence of the teeth and no neuropathic manifestations. Drugs that exacerbate hepatic porphyrias are not known to worsen EPP, although they are generally avoided as a precaution.

Hemolysis is uncommon or very mild in uncomplicated cases. Erythropoiesis and iron metabolism are generally normal. Mild anemia with hypochromia and microcytosis is noted in some cases and is unexplained. Patients with EPP may develop gallstones containing protoporphyrin.

Liver function is usually normal in EPP. A minority of patients with EPP develop liver disease, which can progress rapidly to death from liver failure. Excess protoporphyrin itself may have cholestatic effects and damage hepatocytes. Intercurrent factors such as viral hepatitis, alcohol, iron deficiency, fasting, and oral contraceptive steroids have played a role in some patients.

Diagnosis and Differential Diagnosis. Protoporphyrin is increased in bone marrow, erythrocytes, plasma, bile, and feces of EPP patients. Urinary porphyrins and porphyrin precursors are normal. Hepatic complications of EPP are often preceded by increasing levels of erythrocyte and plasma protoporphyrin, abnormal liver function tests, marked deposition of protoporphyrin in liver cells and bile canaliculi, and increased photosensitivity.

Treatment and Prognosis. β-Carotene was developed primarily for treating EPP. Its clinical benefits have been substantiated in large series of patients. No side effects other than a mild and dose-related skin discoloration due to carotenemia have been noted. Its mechanism of action may involve quenching of singlet oxygen or free radicals. Cholestyramine may reduce protoporphyrin levels by interrupting its enterohepatic circulation. Iron deficiency, caloric restriction, and drugs or hormone preparations that impair hepatic excretory function should be avoided.

Hepatic complications may resolve spontaneously if a reversible cause of liver dysfunction, such as viral hepatitis or alcohol, is contributing. Transfusions or heme therapy may suppress erythroid and hepatic protoporphyrin production. Splenectomy, correction of iron deficiency, and use of cholestyramine or activated charcoal may be beneficial. Liver transplantation is sometimes required.

DUAL PORPHYRIA. This term refers to patients with porphyria and deficiencies of more than one enzyme of the heme biosynthetic pathway. Examples include double heterozygotes with both VP and familial PCT, deficiencies of both porphobilinogen deaminase and uroporphyrinogen decarboxylase (with symptoms of AIP, PCT, or both), and deficiencies of both coproporphyrinogen oxidase and uroporphyrinogen III cosynthase.

LABORATORY DIAGNOSIS OF PORPHYRIAS

Appropriate laboratory testing for these disorders is both specific and sensitive. An array of tests for porphyria is available, but some are subject to overuse and misinterpretation. Porphyrias can be readily detected and misdiagnoses avoided by relying primarily on

TABLE 187–4. FIRST-LINE LABORATORY TESTS FOR SCREENING FOR PORPHYRIAS AND SECOND-LINE TESTS FOR FURTHER EVALUATION WHEN INITIAL TESTING IS POSITIVE

	Symptoms Suggesting Porphyria	
Testing	*Acute Neurovisceral Symptoms*	*Cutaneous Photosensitivity*
First-line	Urinary ALA and PBG (quantitative; random urine)	Total plasma porphyrins†
Second-line	Urinary ALA, PBG, and total porphyrins* (quantitative; 24-hour urine)	Erythrocyte porphyrins
		Urinary ALA, PBG, and total porphyrins* (quantitative, 24-hour urine)
	Total fecal porphyrins*	
	Erythrocyte PBG deaminase	
	Total plasma porphyrins†	Total fecal porphyrins*

* Urinary and fecal porphyrins are fractionated only if the total is increased.
† The preferred method is by direct fluorescent spectrophotometry.
Abbreviations: ALA = δ-aminolevulinic acid; PBG = porphobilinogen.

a few first-line tests. The preferred approach for screening, as outlined in Table 187–4, is to rely on measurement of *urinary porphyrin precursors (ALA and PBG)* in patients with neurovisceral symptoms and a fluorometric measurement of *total plasma porphyrins* when it is suspected that skin photosensitivity may be due to porphyria.

In acutely ill patients, it is important to identify or exclude acute porphyria promptly. Urinary PBG is always markedly increased during acute attacks of AIP, HCP, and VP. A normal level effectively excludes these disorders as a cause of current symptoms. Because PBG is so strikingly increased during an attack, quantitation on a spot sample is highly informative. Assays for PBG use Ehrlich's aldehyde (*p*-dimethylaminobenzaldehyde), which forms reddish-purple chromogens with PBG, urobilinogen, and other substances in urine. Qualitative methods (e.g., Watson-Schwartz and Hoesch tests) are still widely used to screen for increased PBG. They are subject to misinterpretation and false-positive readings, do not quantitate PBG, and are less sensitive and only slightly more rapid than quantitative methods, which separate PBG from interfering substances by ion-exchange chromatography. If a qualitative test for PBG is used for screening, positive samples should be retested by a quantitative method. Urinary ALA and coproporphyrin, but not PBG, are increased in ADP.

Total plasma porphyrins are always increased in patients with active skin lesions. Normal plasma porphyrin levels exclude porphyria as a cause of cutaneous symptoms if the measurement is carried out by a simple and direct fluorometric method. Plasma porphyrins in VP are mostly covalently bound to plasma porphyrins and may not be detected by other methods.

The interpretation of urine, fecal, and erythrocyte porphyrin levels is often problematic, for the following reasons: (1) In contrast to plasma porphyrins, these measurements do not individually detect all cutaneous porphyrias. (2) Urine and erythrocyte porphyrins can be increased in many conditions other than porphyria, whereas an increased plasma porphyrin concentration is much more specific for porphyria. (3) Fecal porphyrin determinations are semiquantitative and subject to interference by diet and other factors.

More extensive testing is required if an initial screening test for porphyria is positive or may also be necessary initially if subclinical porphyria is suspected. Laboratory testing of relatives is not appropriate until test results have firmly established a diagnosis of porphyria in the propositus. Results of testing the propositus guide the choice of tests for relatives. Consultation with a physician and laboratory with experience in testing for porphyrias is done in these situations. Incorrect diagnoses of porphyria are not uncommon in patients with symptoms due to other diseases. Therefore, the laboratory data that were the basis for an original diagnosis of porphyria should remain available for future reference.

Anderson KE: The porphyrias. *In* Zakim D, Boyer T (eds.): Hepatology. Philadelphia, WB Saunders, in press. *One of several recent and detailed reviews on the genetic, biochemical, and clinical aspects of the porphyrias.*
Bonkovsky HL, Healey BS, Lourie AN, et al.: Intravenous heme-albumin in acute intermittent porphyria: Evidence for repletion of hepatic hemoproteins and regulatory heme pools. Am J Gastroenterol 86:1050, 1991. *This article describes a*

method for reconstituting and stabilizing lyophilized hematin with human albumin to prevent phlebitis and other side effects.

Herrero C, Vicente A, Bruguera M, et al.: Is hepatitis C virus infection a trigger of porphyria cutanea tarda? Lancet 341:788, 1993. Discussion of the recently described strong association of PCT with hepatitis C infection.

Kauppinen R, Mustajoki P: Prognosis of acute porphyria: Occurrence of acute attacks, precipitating factors, and associated diseases. Medicine 71:1, 1992. A recent review of clinical aspects of the acute porphyrias, emphasizing new developments.

Long C, Smyth SJ, Woolf J, et al.: Detection of latent variegate porphyria by fluorescence emission spectroscopy of plasma. Br J Dermatol 129:9, 1993. Measurement of total plasma porphyrins is an underutilized laboratory method that is useful for diagnosis, differential diagnosis, and assessing treatment of cutaneous porphyrias. This article demonstrates its usefulness in detecting latent as well as overt VP.

Mustajoki P, Nordmann Y: Early administration of heme arginate for acute porphyric attacks. Arch Intern Med 153:2004, 1993. A large series of patients treated with intravenous heme, emphasizing the importance of early treatment.

Ratnaike S, Blake D, Campbell D, et al.: Plasma ferritin levels as a guide to the treatment of porphyria cutanea tarda by venesection. Australas J Dermatol 29:3, 1988. Experience showing that plasma ferritin and total porphyrins are the best predictors of response of PCT during treatment by phlebotomy.

Verstraeten L, Van Regemorter N, Pardou A, et al.: Biochemical diagnosis of a fatal case of Gunther's disease in a newborn with hydrops-fetalis. Eur J Clin Chem Clin Biochem 31:121, 1993. A case report describing recent developments in molecular and clinical aspects of CEP, and presentation of severe disease in utero.

188 WILSON'S DISEASE

Andrew Deiss

DEFINITION. Wilson's disease (hepatolenticular degeneration) is a hereditary disorder characterized by the accumulation of copper in the body, especially in the liver, brain, kidneys, and corneas. The excess copper leads to tissue injury and ultimately, if effective treatment is not instituted, to death.

ETIOLOGY AND PREVALENCE. Wilson's disease is inherited as an autosomal recessive trait. The gene has been mapped to chromosome 13q14.3. It probably codes for a copper-transporting ATPase. The prevalence of the disease is approximately 30 per million.

PATHOGENESIS. Normally, loss of copper from the body occurs primarily through the bile. Much of biliary copper is secreted in a poorly absorbable form and thus is lost in the feces. Copper balance is normally maintained by this mechanism. In Wilson's disease biliary excretion of copper is impaired, and as a consequence total body copper is progressively increased. The specific nature of the metabolic abnormality that causes this defect is not known.

Positive copper balance begins in infancy in Wilson's disease and continues thereafter unless appropriate therapy is given. However, the distribution of copper changes as the disease progresses. Liver copper is actually greater in presymptomatic homozygotes than in symptomatic ones. Thus not only does net deposition of liver copper cease, but also a portion of previously deposited copper is lost from the liver and deposited elsewhere. This copper redistribution probably takes place when liver injury occurs. If this injury occurs abruptly in many hepatocytes, liver disease may be clinically manifested, and a large amount of copper may be released over a short period, creating the potential for acute erythrocyte injury and hemolytic anemia as well. However, if hepatocyte injury is more gradual, acute liver disease does not occur and the patient remains asymptomatic as the important site of copper deposition shifts to the brain. With the latter course, most patients later develop neurologic or psychiatric symptoms, usually with clinically inapparent cirrhosis.

The serum concentration of the copper-containing protein ceruloplasmin is low in 95% of patients with Wilson's disease. The hypoceruloplasminemia is probably due in part to a decrease in ceruloplasmin gene transcription.

PATHOLOGY. The diagnosis cannot be made on the basis of histologic sections of the liver. Fatty change and glycogen-filled nuclei are present early, followed later by piecemeal necrosis, lymphocytic infiltration, erosion of limiting plates, parenchymal collapse, and fibrosis. Ultimately, these abnormalities evolve into postnecrotic cirrhosis. Stains for copper are unreliable, being negative most frequently during the early stages of the disease, when diagnostic help is most needed.

In the brain, abnormal astrocytes and neuronal necrosis are widely distributed, and there is atrophy or cavitation of the basal ganglia and occasionally the cerebral cortex.

CLINICAL MANIFESTATIONS. Wilson's disease is a disorder of young persons. Although the disease may occur at any time from the age of 5 into the sixth decade, two thirds of patients seek medical attention between the ages of 8 and 20. The physician should suspect the disorder in young people with signs of chronic or recurrent hepatic dysfunction or with characteristic neurologic abnormalities.

The hepatic symptoms are quite diverse. Commonly, a brief illness characterized by malaise, anorexia, jaundice, and increased aminotransferases is mistaken for viral hepatitis. Similar episodes may recur at intervals of months or years, or a latent period may occur during which the patient is asymptomatic until neurologic symptoms begin. If clinically overt hepatocyte injury persists over a longer period, a syndrome resembling chronic active hepatitis results. Occasionally, liver injury occurs precipitously. The need for prompt diagnosis is urgent because without rapid institution of appropriate treatment, death is likely in these patients. More commonly, however, hepatocyte injury is gradual and is not accompanied by symptoms of liver disease; nevertheless, cirrhosis develops ultimately in all patients. This liver injury may not be recognized until neurologic disease is evaluated.

Episodes of hemolytic anemia occur when massive release of copper from the liver takes place. Thus hemolysis is usually accompanied by overt liver disease; it occurs regularly in patients with fulminant hepatic failure. Hemolysis usually lasts only a short period and disappears spontaneously.

Neurologic disease may begin with a variety of motor symptoms, including involuntary movement, such as tremor or chorea, or decreased movement. The tremor is primarily proximal, often characterized by a "wing-beating" rhythmic oscillating tremor of the upper extremities that may eventually extend to the trunk. Dystonic signs include slowness of movement or speech, unsteady gait, dystonic posturing, and dystonic facies in which the upper lip is drawn tightly over the teeth. Frequently, loss of coordination of fine movements, such as those required for handwriting, is the earliest neurologic sign. As the disease progresses, patients may develop combinations of these abnormalities. Dysarthria, rigidity, drooling, and titubation are late features. Seizures are infrequent and sensory abnormalities absent. The Kayser-Fleischer (K-F) ring, described below, is definitively diagnostic in the neurologic variety and nearly so in the hepatic form of the disease.

Psychological symptoms of Wilson's disease are prominent and consist of early development of intellectual deterioration, personality changes, and unstable behavior. Children begin to fail at school, and young adults may show difficulty in performing jobs once considered routine. Schizophreniform symptoms and other forms of bizarre behavior may appear, but the mental status examination always shows signs of organic dementia. Effectively removing excess copper often improves but usually fails to eliminate these symptoms completely.

K-F rings are golden brown or greenish rings or arcs in Descemet's membrane at the limbus of the cornea. They are composed of copper-containing granules and develop primarily after redistribution of liver copper. They may be visible with the unaided eye, but slit-lamp examination should always be obtained. K-F rings are present in all or nearly all patients in the neurologic or psychiatric stage of the disease but are not present in about one third of those with hepatic symptoms.

Rare symptoms ascribable to Wilson's disease include cholelithiasis, sunflower cataracts, arthropathy, renal calculi, heart disease, and Fanconi's syndrome.

DIAGNOSIS. The classic diagnostic features are K-F rings, low serum ceruloplasmin concentration (< 20 mg per deciliter), and increased amounts of liver and urinary copper (> 250 μg per gram of dry weight and > 100 μg per 24 hours, respectively). Computed tomography or preferably magnetic resonance scans may show atrophy or cavitation even in patients with no neurologic abnormalities, but they may be entirely normal. The role of genetic diagnosis is not established, but it is likely to be complicated by the reported great allelic heterogeneity.

The classic diagnostic signs are present in nearly all patients with fully evolved neurologic Wilson's disease but only in about two thirds of those presenting with liver disease. In these patients, K-F rings often have not yet formed, and the serum ceruloplasmin concentration may be difficult to interpret. Even in Wilson's disease, serum ceruloplasmin increases during inflammation, estrogen administration, and pregnancy and may decrease during liver failure. Measurement of the copper content of the liver should resolve the problem. Hepatic copper is often greater than normal (50 μg per gram of dry weight) in a variety of chronic liver diseases, but it seldom reaches the concentration seen in most patients with Wilson's disease (>250 μg per gram of dry weight). In a patient with a disease clinically suggestive of Wilson's disease, hepatic copper of this magnitude is essentially diagnostic. If the diagnosis is still in doubt, incorporation of radioactive copper into ceruloplasmin can be measured; incorporation is negligible in Wilson's disease, normal in other liver disease, even with copper loading, and intermediate in 75% of heterozygotes, but there is much overlap between groups. All measurements of copper metabolism should be entrusted only to laboratories experienced with their determination, and the normal values of that laboratory should be used. In patients with fulminant hepatic failure, it has been proposed that the ratios of alkaline phosphatase (IU per liter) to total bilirubin (mg per deciliter) and of AST (IU per liter) to ALT (IU per liter) of <2.0 and >4.0, respectively, identify patients with Wilson's disease, but the specificity has been questioned.

In primary biliary cirrhosis and chronic cholestasis, diseases with acquired abnormalities of copper excretion, liver copper may be greatly increased and K-F rings occur rarely. The age, symptoms, and laboratory abnormalities of patients with these diseases help distinguish them from those with Wilson's disease.

Early during the hemolytic anemia the urinary copper excretion is very great. The Coombs test result is negative. When hemolysis and acute liver disease occur concurrently in a young person, Wilson's disease is the most probable cause.

Examination of all siblings of patients with Wilson's disease is mandatory to identify presymptomatic homozygotes. K-F rings are usually absent. Serum ceruloplasmin concentration is reduced in 95% of homozygotes and 20% of heterozygotes. If it is low, liver copper content should be measured. Hepatic copper is slightly increased in most heterozygotes. If the copper is >250 μg per gram of dry weight, Wilson's disease is present, and it should be treated as in symptomatic patients. Heterozygotes never become symptomatic and should not be treated. Some homozygotes are missed by this evaluation, so continued follow-up is necessary.

TREATMENT. Without effective lifetime therapy, Wilson's disease is inevitably fatal. If treatment is begun early enough, symptomatic recovery usually is complete, and a life of normal length and quality can be expected. If treatment is begun too late, death may not be prevented, or recovery will be only partial.

Effective therapy depends on establishing negative copper balance, thereby preventing deposition of more copper and mobilizing for excretion excess copper already deposited. Three agents are available that seem to be equally efficacious.

D-Penicillamine remains the drug of choice, at least until there is substantially more experience with the other agents. The usual dosage is 1 gram per day, given in divided doses 1 hour before meals and at bedtime. Pyridoxine, 25 mg per day, is also given. Response typically is quite slow, occurring over months, but it may occur more rapidly. A year or more is often required to obtain maximum improvement. At least 10% of patients experience a worsening of neurologic symptoms during the first month or two of treatment, and this phenomenon should not suggest that the diagnosis is in error. Compliance and the effectiveness of therapy must be monitored at 1- to 2-month intervals for the first year and twice yearly thereafter; monitoring consists of measurements of urinary copper, serum ceruloplasmin, and serum nonceruloplasmin copper (total serum copper minus ceruloplasmin copper). Nonceruloplasmin copper should decrease early and ceruloplasmin more gradually if treatment is adequate. Urinary copper levels increase at once to 1 to 5 mg per 24 hours during the first few months and then gradually decline as the excess of copper decreases.

Toxic effects are frequent. Rash, fever, adenopathy, neutropenia, or thrombocytopenia often occurs during the first 2 weeks of treatment. In such circumstances, penicillamine should be discontinued; when the symptoms have cleared, prednisone should be begun at a dose of 40 mg per day and penicillamine resumed at 250 mg per day and gradually increased to full dose over a period of a few weeks. The steroids can then be tapered and stopped. Side effects that occur later after penicillamine is begun include proteinuria, nephrotic syndrome, systemic lupus erythematosus, Goodpasture's syndrome, and a variety of chronic skin diseases. These side effects can often be reversed by temporarily stopping penicillamine and resuming it after the symptoms have abated, sometimes adding steroids. Treatment should never be suspended for more than a few months.

If penicillamine toxicity is not manageable, either trientine (250 mg 1 hour before meals and at bedtime) or zinc (50 mg of elemental zinc 1 hour before meals, preferably as the acetate) is an effective alternative. Experience is not extensive with either, but side effects have been minimal.

Some patients, especially those with fulminant hepatic failure, are so severely ill that the benefits of medical treatment cannot occur rapidly enough to prevent death. In these patients, liver transplantation, if successful, is curative.

Brewer GJ, Yazbasiyan-Gurkan V: Wilson disease. Medicine 71:139, 1992. *A good review, with emphasis on zinc treatment, by the authors who developed it.*
Cartwright GE: Diagnosis of treatable Wilson's disease. N Engl J Med 298:1347, 1978. *An excellent description of the protean and often confusing clinical presentations of Wilson's disease and a few illustrations of what happens when the diagnosis is missed.*
Scheinberg IH, Sternlieb I: Wilson's Disease. Philadelphia, WB Saunders, 1984. *The authoritative monograph based on the authors' extensive experience with all aspects of Wilson's disease.*
Walshe JM: Diagnosis and treatment of presymptomatic Wilson's disease. Lancet 2:435, 1988. *Criteria for identifying asymptomatic homozygotes in families of patients with Wilson's disease. Liver biopsies should be obtained for confirmation as the author recommends, and therefore more frequently than he has actually done.*

189 IRON OVERLOAD
(Hemochromatosis)
Virgil F. Fairbanks and William P. Baldus

DEFINITION. Hemochromatosis is a state of total body iron overload due to increased iron absorption that results in parenchymal tissue damage. In persons of European descent, the disorder arises most often as the genetic disorder known as *hereditary* or *primary hemochromatosis. Secondary hemochromatosis* occurs in a variety of chronic anemias caused by ineffective erythropoiesis, the most common being homozygous β-thalassemia; multiple transfusions; and less frequent conditions listed in Table 189–1.

PREVALENCE, GENETICS, AND ETIOLOGY. Hereditary hemochromatosis, transmitted by an autosomal recessive gene, is the most common single gene disorder of people of Caucasian descent. Approximately 3 to 5 persons per 1000 are homozygous for the disease in the United States, Canada, France, Sweden, the

TABLE 189–1. DISORDERS ASSOCIATED WITH IRON OVERLOAD

Hereditary hemochromatosis
Chronic anemias
  Thalassemia major
  Sideroblastic anemia
    Hereditary sideroblastic anemia
    Refractory anemia with ringed sideroblasts
  Congenital dyserythropoietic anemia
Exogenous iron overload
  Transfusion-dependent anemia
  Chronic oral iron ingestion (in absence of iron deficiency)
African (Bantu) hemochromatosis
Porphyria cutanea tarda
Portacaval shunt
Juvenile hemochromatosis
Neonatal hemochromatosis
Congenital transferrinemia

United Kingdom, Australia, New Zealand, and South Africa. Heterozygotes are approximately 10% of the Caucasian population of these countries. Northern Portugal has the highest incidence, with an estimated 24% of the population being heterozygous and 2% homozygous. African-Americans have a lower prevalence of homozygous hemochromatosis, but it is thought to be about 0.3 to 0.5 per thousand. Hemochromatosis is rare in Asians. The paradoxical occurrence of clinical hemochromatosis in successive generations of kindreds carrying a recessive gene is best explained by homozygotes marrying heterozygotes. Statistically, this must occur in 10% of matings, reflecting the high heterozygote frequency in Caucasians.

The hemochromatosis gene is in linkage disequilibrium with the HLA-A and HLA-B genes. Seventy percent of persons with hemochromatosis have HLA-A3 antigens, compared with 28% in the general population. They also exhibit increased frequencies of HLA-B7 and B14 antigens. In the course of numerous generations, the effect of normal meiotic recombination should be to render the HLA allele frequencies in hemochromatosis similar to those of the general population. The most likely explanation for the high frequencies of certain HLA alleles is that the mutation is relatively recent, although it occurred and became widely prevalent before Europeans colonized North America, Australia, New Zealand, and South Africa.

Hereditary hemochromatosis is due to a mutation in a gene on the short arm of chromosome 6. The exact site of the mutation remains unknown. The gene product also remains unknown. Preliminary laboratory studies show that in persons with hereditary hemochromatosis there is increase in a membrane iron-binding protein that is normally present on the surface of intestinal mucosal cells and hepatocytes.

Normal adult men absorb approximately 1 mg of iron daily from the intestinal tract in order to balance iron loss. Normal women, during the reproductive years, absorb approximately 2 mg of iron each day, the greater need reflecting menstrual iron loss. Persons homozygous for hereditary hemochromatosis absorb from their intestinal tracts only a few milligrams of iron each day in excess of need. Clinical signs and symptoms, when they appear, reflect an iron accumulation of 15 to 40 grams. Manifestations can begin even before age 20. Not all homozygotes develop overt disease, however, because clinical manifestations also depend on cofactors of age, gender, iron content of the diet, alcohol, and other unknown factors. Women, for example, regularly lose iron during menses and childbirth. Therefore, despite an equal frequency of homozygosity, they express the disease one-tenth as often as do men. Ethanol abuse or hepatitis accelerates liver and pancreatic disease in hereditary hemochromatosis. Either ethanol abuse or hepatitis may increase serum iron concentration due to marked ferritinemia that results from hepatocyte injury. Alcohol abuse occurs in as many as one third of patients with hemochromatosis. The frequency of serum antibodies to hepatitis C also is higher than in the normal population.

METABOLIC AND TISSUE EFFECTS. Iron accumulates over decades, as ferritin and hemosiderin, in nearly all cells of the body. Tissue damage that leads to morbidity occurs in liver, thyroid, hypothalamus, heart, pancreas, gonads, and joints. This leads to cirrhosis of the liver, hypothyroidism, hypothalamic hypogonadotropic hypogonadism, cardiomyopathy, diabetes mellitus, arthralgias, and deforming arthritis. There is pigment deposition in skin, principally melanin. Cardiac deposition of ferritin and hemosiderin causes cardiac arrhythmias and impaired contractility of cardiac muscle.

The liver is a target organ because iron absorbed from the intestinal tract enters the portal circulation and passes through the liver before it enters any other organ. Iron that exceeds the binding capacity of transferrin is deposited in the liver. In hereditary hemochromatosis, excess iron is deposited initially as hemosiderin granules in hepatocytes, in a periportal pattern, i.e., the heaviest deposition is at the periphery of the lobule. Marked deposition of hemosiderin also occurs in the epithelial cells of the biliary canaliculi. As iron overloading progresses, hemosiderin deposition occurs in Kupffer cells. Signs of hepatocellular injury are also first apparent and most pronounced in the periphery of the lobule. These changes consist of cytoplasmic ballooning and fatty change. As the disease progresses, filaments of fibrous tissue begin to traverse the lobule and periportal fibrosis occurs. The other changes of severe cirrhosis follow. Similar histologic changes occur in the pancreas, heart, and other organs.

In secondary hemochromatosis, as in that which may follow numerous transfusions for chronic anemia, hemosiderin deposition is initially more marked in the Kupffer cells. Ultimately, however, the histologic pattern becomes indistinguishable from that of hereditary hemochromatosis. Furthermore, other histologic changes may be indistinguishable between late-stage hemochromatosis and alcoholic cirrhosis, except for the marked hemosiderosis in the former.

CLINICAL MANIFESTATIONS. Although many people with hemochromatosis are asymptomatic, all are at risk for developing severe dysfunction of the heart, liver, pancreas, pituitary, gonads, or joints, as well as for fatal peritonitis or sepsis.

Clinical manifestations are more common in men older than 20 and in postmenopausal women. Rare cases may involve adolescent children and young women. Table 189–2 lists the potential symptoms, signs, and laboratory abnormalities of hemochromatosis. The most common symptoms are fatigue, that may be overwhelming; arthralgias; abdominal discomfort; impotence; amenorrhea; and palpitations. Cardiac arrhythmia is a common presenting sign and may be either atrial or ventricular. Suntan-like hyperpigmentation of the skin can affect both exposed and nonexposed areas as well as scars. In advanced cases, the skin may be slate gray. Hepatosplenomegaly, ascites, pleural effusion, or arthritis may develop early or late. The arthritis may affect any joint but most commonly involves the second and third metacarpophalangeal joints, knees, and hips. The affected joints may be deformed, with or without inflammatory signs. Signs of hypothyroidism and testicular atrophy often appear. There may be loss of hair on body and extremities. Mild abdominal pain is common. Infrequently, there may be an abrupt onset of abdominal pain followed by prostration, shock, and death. In some cases of fatal acute peritonitis or septicemia, *Yersinia enterocolitica* or *Vibrio vulnificus* have been incriminated.

Hemochromatosis, because of its associated asthenia and cardiac, hypogonadal, or multiple-organ pathology, may bring patients initially to seek the attention of general physicians, cardiologists, pediatricians, urologists, endocrinologists, neurologists, or psychiatrists. Its features should be understood by all physicians because concentrating on a particular organ system—like one of the six blind men of Hindustan describing an elephant—may preclude early diagnosis and preventive treatment, which crucially influence prognosis.

LABORATORY ABNORMALITIES AND DIAGNOSIS. The most useful laboratory test to ascertain hemochromatosis is measuring serum iron concentration, total iron-binding capacity, and transferrin saturation. These should be done together. The transferrin saturation is calculated from $100 \times$ serum iron concentration divided by total iron-binding capacity. Characteristically, the transferrin saturation is $>60\%$ and may approach 100% in hemochromatosis, whereas normally it is 20 to 50%. Other conditions may

TABLE 189–2. CLINICAL AND LABORATORY MANIFESTATIONS OF HEMOCHROMATOSIS

Symptoms	Signs	Laboratory Abnormalities
None (common)	Alopecia	Increased serum iron concentration
Fatigue	Hyperpigmentation	
Weakness	Tender, swollen joints	Serum transferrin saturation $>60\%$
Arthralgia	Cardiac arrhythmia	
Abdominal pain	Cardiomegaly	Increased serum ALT or AST transaminases
Impotence	Hepatomegaly	
Amenorrhea	Splenomegaly	Increased blood glucose
Dyspnea	Pleural effusion	Abnormal glucose tolerance
Abdominal swelling	Ascites	Low serum testosterone
Weight loss	"Spider" telangiectasia	Low serum estrogen and progesterone
	Signs of hypothyroidism	Low FSH and LH
	Testicular atrophy	Low serum T_4, high TSH
		Azoospermia
		Thrombocytopenia
		Macrocytosis
		Electrocardiographic abnormalities
		Echocardiographic abnormalities
		Roentgenographic and imaging abnormalities

also elevate serum iron concentration and transferrin saturation, particularly the recent ingestion of medicinal iron, iron-fortified vitamin preparations, or oral contraceptives (Table 189–3). Therefore, if the transferrin saturation is elevated, the test should be repeated after eliminating such confounding variables. If it is still elevated, serum ferritin assay should be performed. When iron overload is marked, as in advanced hemochromatosis, the serum ferritin concentration commonly exceeds 500 μg per liter and may be >5000 μg per liter. However, because serum ferritin is an acute phase reactant, elevated values may result from chronic disease, such as inflammation (as in rheumatoid arthritis), or from malignancies. Liver injury from hepatitis or alcohol abuse also elevates the serum ferritin concentration. Elevated concentration of serum ferritin may be observed in Gaucher's disease. Therefore, elevated values of serum ferritin concentration must be interpreted in the context of the presence or absence of these other conditions.

Among other frequent laboratory abnormalities are elevated blood glucose concentration, abnormal glucose tolerance test results, elevated serum AST or ALT activity, low serum thyroxine, elevated serum thyroid-stimulating hormone, low serum values for pituitary gonadotropins, and thrombocytopenia (reflecting liver disease). Hemoglobin concentration, hematocrit, erythrocyte count, erythrocyte indices, leukocyte count, and differential are usually normal, although chronic liver disease may be reflected in macrocytosis. Bone marrow examination with iron stain variably shows increase in hemosiderin; hence, it is not reliable for diagnosis of iron overload.

Roentgenographic examinations of affected joints show soft tissue swelling, narrowing of joint spaces, irregular articular surfaces, osteoporosis, and subcapsular cysts. There may be chondrocalcinosis or calcification of periarticular ligaments. Synovial fluid often contains calcium pyrophosphate and apatite crystals. Distinction from either degenerative arthritis or rheumatoid arthritis may be difficult.

Electrocardiography may reveal atrial or ventricular arrhythmia, low QRS amplitude, and repolarization abnormalities of ST segment and T waves. Echocardiography and cinecardiography may

TABLE 189–3. PHENOMENA KNOWN TO AFFECT SERUM IRON CONCENTRATION, TOTAL IRON-BINDING CAPACITY, AND TRANSFERRIN SATURATION

Phenomenon	Effect
Menstrual cycle	Premenstrually, elevated values (SI increased by 10–30%); at menstruation, low values (SI decreased by 10–30%)
Pregnancy	May elevate SI due to increased progesterone; may lower SI due to Fe deficiency
Ingestion of iron (including iron-fortified vitamins)	High values (SI may rise by 300+ μg/dL and transferrin saturation to 75%)
Iron contamination of Vacutainer tube or other glassware (phenomenon may be rare, sporadic, very difficult to prove)	High values (SI 200–300 μg/dL, transferrin saturation of 75–100%)
Iron dextran injection	Very high values (SI may be >500 μg/dL, transferrin saturation 100%, probably from circulating iron dextran; effect may persist for several weeks)
Hepatitis (including steatohepatitis)	Very high values (SI may exceed 1000 μg/dL due to hyperferritinemia from hepatocyte injury)
Acute inflammation (respiratory infection), abscess, immunization, myocardial infarction	Low or normal SI; normal or low Tsat
Chronic inflammation or malignancy	Low or normal SI; normal or low Tsat
Iron deficiency	Low or normal SI; increased TIBC; low or normal Tsat
Iron overload (hemochromatosis)	High SI, high Tsat

Abbreviations: SI = serum iron; TIBC = total iron binding capacity; Tsat = transferrin saturation (in %).

show dilated, or, less commonly, restrictive cardiomyopathy. There may be radiographic evidence of pulmonary vascular congestion or pleural effusion.

Definitive diagnosis usually requires liver biopsy. This also permits evaluation of the severity of liver injury and thus the prognosis. In addition to hematoxylin and eosin stain, the biopsy specimen should be stained for iron by Perls' Prussian blue method. In the absence of iron overload, the stainable iron is 0 to 1+. In heterozygotes or those with alcoholic cirrhosis, it may be 1 to 2+; in those with homozygous hemochromatosis, it is usually 3 to 4+. These semiquantitative estimates from iron stain correlate with quantitative measurements of hepatic iron concentration. The hepatic iron concentration can be measured in the liver biopsy specimen. Normal hepatic iron concentrations are <40 (men) and <33 (women) μmol per gram of tissue (dry weight). In alcoholic cirrhosis and in heterozygotes for hemochromatosis, the hepatic iron concentration is <100 μmol per gram of tissue. In homozygous hemochromatosis, the hepatic iron concentration usually exceeds 200 μmol per gram of tissue. A useful index is obtained by dividing the hepatic iron concentration in μmol per gram by the patient's age in years. This "hepatic iron index" is usually >1.9 in homozygous hemochromatosis.

Imaging methods, such as computed tomography or magnetic resonance imaging, have led to the correct diagnosis of hemochromatosis in many instances. However, compared with conventional laboratory methods, imaging procedures are both too insensitive and too expensive to be used in the screening of patients for hemochromatosis.

HLA typing has almost no role in diagnosis of hemochromatosis. Of persons whose leukocytes have the HLA-A3 antigen, only about 1 in 90 are found to have hemochromatosis. Such persons are more likely to be normal or to have alcoholic cirrhosis than hereditary hemochromatosis. As a screening test, HLA typing would yield unacceptably high frequencies of both false-positive and false-negative results. It may be used, however, to help identify affected siblings of a known patient. When so used, it does not matter what the HLA type is: Within a sibship, anyone whose HLA genotype is identical with that of a sibling who has proven disease is also presumed to have homozygous hemochromatosis.

Physicians must examine other members of a sibship for hemochromatosis because within any hemochromatosis sibship, on average 25% of sibs are homozygous for hemochromatosis. Measuring transferrin saturation and serum ferritin concentration is sufficient to identify other affected sibs.

TREATMENT. The treatment of hemochromatosis is repeated phlebotomy, the most efficient, least inconvenient, and least expensive way to remove excess iron from the body. Chelating therapy or dietary manipulation has no place in treating hereditary hemochromatosis. Because iron stores may be 25 to 40 grams of iron, and each half-liter of blood removed contains approximately 200 mg of iron, phlebotomies can be sustained at the rate of one to two times per week for 1 to 3 years or longer before the iron stores become depleted. Patients should be advised that they may need to have 50 to 100 or more phlebotomies before their iron stores are reduced to normal. This is usually done at the rate of one to two phlebotomies per week until the venous hemoglobin concentration or hematocrit begins to decline and does not return to normal (Fig. 189–1). Then, serum ferritin assay determines whether additional phlebotomies are required. The objective is to lower the serum ferritin concentration to <20 μg per liter before reducing the rate of phlebotomy. After that, most patients require four to six phlebotomies annually to keep the serum ferritin concentration in the normal range. Because the transferrin saturation is often high irrespective of the state of iron stores, the measurement of serum iron, total iron-binding capacity, and transferrin saturation is less reliable for determining when additional phlebotomies are needed.

People with hemochromatosis should abstain from handling or eating uncooked shellfish or marine fish because they are susceptible to fatal septicemia from the marine bacterium *V. vulnificus* (see Ch. 109). No other dietary restrictions should be imposed. However, complete abstinence from use of alcohol must be observed.

In addition to measures directed toward removing iron from the body, treating cardiac dysfunction may require cardiac glycosides or diuretics, diabetes may require insulin, hypothyroidism requires thyroid replacement, impotence may be relieved with androgens, and

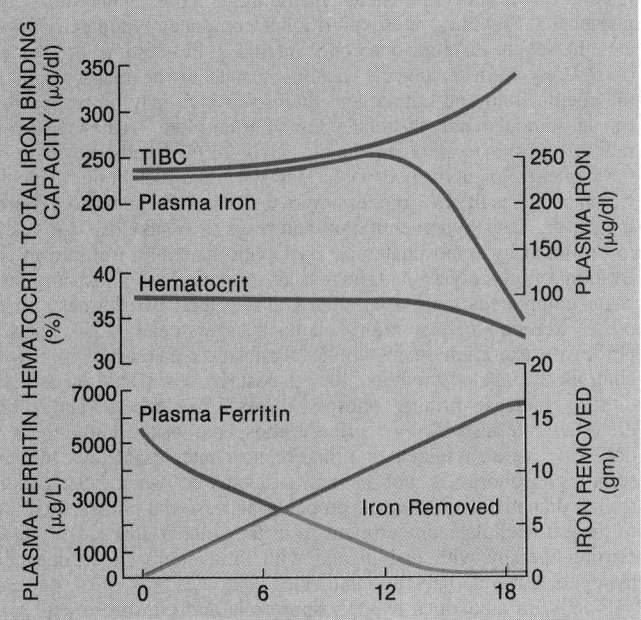

FIGURE 189–1. Serial changes in the hematocrit, plasma iron concentration, total iron-binding capacity, and plasma ferritin concentration in a subject with idiopathic hemochromatosis on repeated venesection therapy. Plasma iron = serum iron, plasma ferritin = serum ferritin. (N.B.: Plasma from EDTA-anticoagulated specimen will have spuriously low plasma iron due to chelation of iron by EDTA. Therefore, *only serum specimens are tested.*) (From Bothwell TH, Charlton RW, Cook JD, et al.: Idiopathic haemochromatosis. *In* Iron Metabolism in Man. Oxford, Blackwell Scientific, 1979.)

painful joints may require salicylates or nonsteroidal anti-inflammatory agents. In advanced cases, liver transplant may be required. Early diagnosis and vigorous treatment should prevent the need for these drastic and costly measures that have high morbidity and uncertain outcomes.

PROGNOSIS. Historically, the median survival was about 2 years from diagnosis. A greatly improved prognosis results from early diagnosis and treatment. When the diagnosis precedes onset of signs and symptoms, and in the absence of hepatic cirrhosis or diabetes, survival is the same as for the age- and gender-matched cohort of the general population. When cirrhosis or diabetes is already present at the time of diagnosis, the outlook is poorer. Cirrhosis rarely disappears as a result of phlebotomy therapy. Patients may die of hepatic or cardiac failure or may exsanguinate from ruptured esophageal varices. They are at risk of death from infections, such as peritonitis. Patients with cirrhosis have a 30% probability of developing hepatocellular carcinoma, even after iron stores are depleted by phlebotomy. Diabetes is not improved by removing iron, although it may not progress as rapidly. Arthritis is not improved by iron removal and, unfortunately, may first appear after adequate removal of excess iron. However, cardiac dysfunction is often substantially improved. Impotence requires continued androgen therapy. Azoospermia is not alleviated. Amenorrhea may rarely be alleviated. Osteoporosis that follows premature menopause requires estrogen therapy. The risk of sudden death from sepsis or peritonitis is diminished.

It is tragic whenever this easily diagnosed and easily treated disorder is permitted to evolve unrecognized and untreated. Patients for whom the diagnosis is not made in a timely manner may develop cirrhosis, severe cardiac dysfunction, or both. A few dozen such patients, who could not otherwise be salvaged, have had liver or heart transplantation or both. Such procedures may be warranted, although extremely costly and attended by long-term morbidity even when successful. The long-term survival of patients who have had these transplants is still unknown, although a few have survived as long as 5 years following liver transplant.

Balan V, Baldus WP, Fairbanks VF, et al.: Screening for hemochromatosis. A cost-effectiveness study based on 12,258 patients. Gastroenterology, 107:453, 1994.

Edwards CQ, Kushner JP: Screening for hemochromatosis. N Engl J Med 328:1616, 1993. *These two references extensively analyze all considerations in screening for hemochromatosis, follow-up tests, and examinations. A reasonable cost estimate of screening and the potential for salvaging years of life is approximately $2000 per year of life saved per person who is homozygous for hereditary hemochromatosis. Even when morbidity and productivity loss that attend hemochromatosis are not considered, cost-benefit relationship is favorable.*

Fargion S, Mandelli C, Piperno A, et al.: Survival and prognostic factors in 212 Italian patients with genetic hemochromatosis. Hepatology 15:655, 1992. *Patients adequately treated by phlebotomy before developing cirrhosis had normal survival; for cirrhotic patients, median survival was 8 years. Hepatocellular cancer occurred in 17% of cirrhotic patients and was the most common cause of death. Other prognostic variables are considered.*

Summers KM, Halliday JW, Powell LW: Identification of homozygous hemochromatosis subjects by measurement of hepatic iron index. Hepatology 12:20, 1990. *The hepatic iron index, obtained by dividing hepatic iron concentration, in μmol per gram by patient's age, provides the best criterion for identifying homozygotes with iron overload.*

190 PHOSPHORUS DEFICIENCY AND HYPOPHOSPHATEMIA
Wadi N. Suki

Phosphorus is an integral constituent of all body tissues. It is a component of hydroxyapatite, the main crystalline structure of bone, and of the phospholipids in all cell membranes. It is a component of nucleotides and furnishes the backbone of DNA. It is also a component of the second messengers, cyclic adenosine monophosphate (cAMP) and cyclic guanosine monophosphate (cGMP). It combines with a number of proteins, under the influence of various kinases, to activate their enzyme activity. As a component of 2,3-diphosphoglycerate (2,3-DPG), it facilitates the release to tissues of oxygen from oxyhemoglobin. In ATP and creatine phosphate, it serves as an energy store, and when excreted in the urine, it serves as an important buffer to facilitate excretion of urinary acid. When all the functions of phosphate are taken into consideration, it becomes evident why severe deficiency of this anion can lead to disordered function of a large number of systems.

NORMAL PHOSPHORUS METABOLISM. More than 700 grams (22 moles) of phosphorus are present in an average-sized adult: 80% of the total phosphorus is present in bone, 10% is present in skeletal muscle. In muscle cells and in other cells, phosphate in the form of phospholipids, phosphoproteins, and phosphosugars represents the major intracellular anion and is present in a concentration of approximately 100 mmol per liter of cell water.

In the extracellular fluid, phosphorus is present in a concentration of 4.0 to 7.0 mg per 100 ml in children and 2.7 to 4.5 mg per 100 ml in adults. Phosphate in blood is mostly free (only 10% is protein bound) and is present in two ionic forms, dibasic (HPO_4^-) and monobasic ($H_2PO_4^-$), the relative amounts of which vary with the blood pH, being present in a ratio of 4:1 at pH 7.4. Therefore, phosphate concentration in blood should be considered in terms of millimoles (0.9 to 1.5 mmol per liter in adults and 1.4 to 2.2 mmol per liter in children) rather than milliequivalents (which would vary with blood pH).

Depending on the composition of the diet, the average adult in the United States consumes 800 to 1500 mg of phosphorus daily, derived primarily from dairy products and meat. Most of the ingested phosphorus is absorbed, and, except in growing children, most is excreted in the urine. Urinary excretion depends on glomerular filtration and tubular reabsorption, with only 12% of the filtered load being excreted in the urine. Intestinal absorption of phosphate is augmented by the active metabolites of vitamin D, whereas tubular absorption is inhibited by parathyroid hormone acting through its second-messenger cAMP.

HYPOPHOSPHATEMIA. Moderate or severe hypophosphatemia is seen in approximately 2% of hospitalized patients.

Etiology. (Table 190–1). Hypophosphatemia may result from a shift into cells, in which case body phosphorus stores are normal.

TABLE 190–1. CLASSIFICATION OF HYPOPHOSPHATEMIA

Transient hypophosphatemia with normal body stores
  Ingestion of carbohydrates
  Respiratory alkalosis
Sustained hypophosphatemia with reduced body stores
  Moderate hypophosphatemia
    Depressed tubular absorption
      Hyperparathyroidism
      Expanded ECF volume
      Alkali administration
      Glucocorticoids
      Magnesium depletion
      Fanconi's syndrome
      Familial hypophosphatemic rickets
    Reduced intestinal absorption
      Reduced intake
      Malabsorption
      Vitamin D deficiency
      Phosphate-binding antacids
    Extracorporeal losses—dialysis
  Severe hypophosphatemia
    Prolonged use of phosphate-binding antacids
    Parenteral alimentation
    Nutritional recovery syndrome
    Recovery phase of severe burns
    Severe respiratory alkalosis
    Poorly controlled diabetes mellitus
    Alcoholism and alcohol withdrawal

On the other hand, hypophosphatemia may be associated with depleted total body stores, resulting from poor dietary intake, reduced gastrointestinal absorption, or increased renal losses.

Hypophosphatemia may be sustained or may be transient, as seen after ingestion of carbohydrates due to the phosphorylation of sugars before they enter the body cells, or in respiratory alkalosis, wherein alkalinization of the cytosol activates intracellular glycolysis and increases the formation of phosphorylated sugars.

Moderate Hypophosphatemia. In addition to carbohydrate administration and respiratory alkalosis, which cause transient hypophosphatemia, a number of other disorders can result in moderate hypophosphatemia (serum phosphorus 1 to 2.5 mg per deciliter). These disorders may be classified into those that increase renal losses of phosphate, decrease intestinal absorption of phosphate, or increase extracorporeal loss of phosphate such as in hemodialysis against a phosphate-free dialysate. Renal losses of phosphate are increased when tubular absorption is depressed, as seen in hyperparathyroidism (see Ch. 214), in expansion of the extracellular fluid volume, in administration of alkali or glucocorticoids, in hypomagnesemia and magnesium depletion, and in renal tubular defects such as Fanconi's syndrome (see Ch. 82) or familial hypophosphatemic rickets (see Ch. 213).

Reduced intestinal absorption may be caused by drastically reduced intake, malabsorption, vitamin D deficiency, and the use of phosphate-binding antacids. Moderate hypophosphatemia causes only osteomalacia.

Severe Hypophosphatemia (serum phosphorus < 1 mg per deciliter). This causes serious systemic manifestations that demand prompt attention and correction. The most common causes of this disorder are prolonged use of phosphate-binding antacids, hyperalimentation, nutritional recovery syndrome and recovery from severe burns, severe respiratory alkalosis, poorly controlled diabetes mellitus, and alcoholism and alcohol withdrawal syndrome. Phosphate-binding compounds, such as aluminum and magnesium oxides, bind phosphate in the intestinal lumen and impair its absorption. The excessive use of these compounds by patients with peptic ulcer disease or by patients with chronic renal failure who are treated with these compounds to prevent the development of hyperphosphatemia, results in phosphate depletion. Enteral and parenteral alimentation, if not accompanied by phosphate, can also result in phosphate depletion. Phosphate excretion in the urine is increased by administering glucose and amino acids. Furthermore, glucose and amino acids entering into cells and their incorporation into intracellular compounds consume phosphate and deplete body stores. Overzealous refeeding of severely malnourished subjects also may

result in multiple deficiencies including thiamine, potassium, and phosphate. Providing these nutritional components generally obviates the severe disorder once encountered in this setting. In the case of severely burned subjects, healing results in the reabsorption of the edema fluid and consequent diuresis, which may be responsible for substantial renal phosphate loss. Furthermore, as new tissue is rebuilt, phosphate is taken up by newly formed cells, aggravating the depletion of body phosphate stores. Unlike metabolic alkalosis, which may result in a modest drop in the serum phosphorus, prolonged vigorous hyperventilation and respiratory alkalosis can result in profound hypophosphatemia. Hypophosphatemia results from activation of glycolysis and increased formation of phosphorylated sugar compounds caused by raised intracellular pH. Urinary phosphate excretion in respiratory alkalosis is extremely low, whereas phosphate excretion in metabolic alkalosis is increased. In poorly controlled diabetes mellitus, the glucosuria and resulting osmotic diuresis increase urinary phosphate loss. Acetoacetate and β-hydroxybutyrate also increase urinary phosphate loss. Finally, the acidosis *per se* also increases urinary phosphate loss. However, the serum phosphorus is not generally depressed when poorly controlled diabetics first present, probably because the phosphate shifts to the extracellular compartment from the cellular space. Only after starting therapy with insulin and with intravenous fluids does the hypophosphatemia become manifested.

Finally, in alcoholics hypophosphatemia and phosphate depletion are caused by multiple factors: the phosphaturic effect of ethanol, the phosphaturia resulting from magnesium depletion, poor dietary intake, and ketoacidosis. Other contributing factors can be vomiting, diarrhea, and the use of phosphate-binding antacids.

MANIFESTATIONS (Table 190–2). Severe hypophosphatemia alters cell membrane composition and function, depletes intracellular phosphorylated compounds, such as ATP and 2,3-DPG, and increases intracellular calcium. This constellation of disorders results in disturbed function of multiple body systems.

MANAGEMENT (Table 190–3). When total body phosphorus stores are normal, phosphate supplementation is unnecessary. When body phosphate stores are reduced, urinary losses need to be mini-

TABLE 190–2. MANIFESTATIONS OF HYPOPHOSPHATEMIA

Symptoms and Signs	Comments
Central nervous system	
Symptoms and signs of metabolic encephalopathy	Irritability, malaise, ataxia, seizures, coma
Neuromuscular	
Generalized muscle weakness or paralysis	Ventilatory insufficiency, respiratory failure
Rhabdomyolysis	Increased creatine kinase; large muscle tenderness; may mask underlying hypophosphatemia
Cardiac muscle dysfunction	Congestive cardiomyopathy
Hematologic	
Altered red cell function	Depleted 2,3-DPG shifts oxyhemoglobin dissociation curve to the left and impairs tissue oxygen delivery. Depleted ATP, increases intracellular calcium causing hemolysis
Impaired leukocyte function	Impaired leukotaxis, phagocytosis, and bactericidal activity, susceptibility to infection
Impaired platelet aggregation	Bleeding tendency from lips and oral mucosa
Bone	
Bone resorption, osteomalacia, increased 1α-hydroxylation of vitamin D	Increased calcium absorption, mild increase of serum calcium, depressed PTH secretion, and marked renal hypercalciuria
Renal	
Impaired tubular function	Increased urine calcium and magnesium, renal glucosuria, decreased ammoniagenesis and metabolic acidosis
Liver	
Transient hyperbilirubinemia	
Metabolism	
Hypoglycemia	

TABLE 190–3. MANAGEMENT OF HYPOPHOSPHATEMIA

	Treatment	Dose
Normal body phosphorus stores		
Transient hydrophosphatemia	Treat underlying disorder	No phosphate replacement
Reduced body phosphorus stores		
Moderate hypophosphatemia	Minimize urinary losses, reduce sodium diuresis, enhance gastrointestinal absorption, discontinue phosphate binders	
	If patient capable of oral intake:	
	High-phosphate foods	e.g., skimmed cow's milk (contains 1 mg P/ml)
	Oral supplements:	
	Sodium salt	Phospho-Soda 750 mg P per 5 ml
	Potassium salt (potassium not contraindicated/desirable)	Neutra-Phos 250 mg P/capsule with 7 mEq of K; Neutra-Phos K; 250 mg P/capsule with 14 mEq of K; K Phos 150 mg P/tablet with 3.65 mEq K; or K-Phos Neutral 250 mg P with 2 mEq K
Severe hypophosphatemia		
Patient incapable of oral/enteral intake, or with organ manifestations of P depletion	Parenteral P	P 2.5–5 mg/kg body weight (0.08–0.16 mmol/kg) infused over 6 hrs, repeated every 6 hrs until serum P is 2.0–2.5 mg/dl
Hypocalcemic patient, renal failure		Lower dose than above

mized, gastrointestinal absorption needs to be enhanced, and phosphate supplements may be necessary. To replete body phosphorus stores, 1000 to 2000 mg of phosphorus may need to be supplemented daily for up to 2 weeks. Whenever phosphate replacement is given, the serum calcium, magnesium, phosphorus, and electrolytes should be monitored closely. The complications of administering phosphate include diarrhea (after oral administration), hypocalcemia, metastatic calcification, hypotension, hyperkalemia and/or hypernatremia, and metabolic acidosis.

Stoff JS: Phosphate homeostasis and hypophosphatemia. Am J Med 72:489, 1982. *A concise review of the physiology of hypophosphatemia, its manifestations, and treatment.*

191 DISORDERS OF MAGNESIUM METABOLISM

Allen C. Alfrey

Magnesium is the second most common intracellular cation, with only three other cations—potassium, calcium, and sodium—occurring with greater abundance in the body. It plays a crucial role in storing and using energy, as all enzymatic reactions involving ATP frequently require magnesium. Because magnesium is also an essential element for plants, being a constituent of chlorophyll, it is present in virtually all food sources. Despite this wide distribution, the average dietary intake of magnesium is about 25 mEq per day, which only marginally meets recommended daily requirements for this element. Fractional absorption of magnesium varies from 80% on a magnesium-restricted diet to < 10% when large oral loads of magnesium are consumed. Renal magnesium reabsorption occurs in multiple nephron segments, and a tubular maximum (TM) mechanism can be described for the whole kidney. The normal tubular reabsorption for magnesium is very close to the TM_{Mg} glomerular filtration rate (GFR). Therefore, small changes in the serum magnesium are accompanied by rather rapid increases or decreases in urinary magnesium excretion. This intrinsic TM phenomenon, which is not directly controlled hormonally, allows the kidney to be the major determinant of plasma magnesium levels.

MAGNESIUM DEPLETION

The prevalence of hypomagnesemia in a general hospital setting has been estimated to range from 6.9 to 12%, being as high as 20% in patients in an ICU. Clinical findings of severe hypomagnesemia are confined mainly to the neuromuscular system and consist of muscle fasciculations and tremors, positive Chvostek's and Trousseau's signs, overt tetany, weakness, anorexia, apathy, and rarely seizures. The biochemical findings of symptomatic hypomagnesemia are serum magnesium levels usually < 1 mEq per liter associated with hypokalemia and hypocalcemia.

MECHANISMS. Magnesium depletion can result from either gastrointestinal or renal causes (Table 191–1). When serum magnesium falls only slightly, and if the kidneys respond normally, urine magnesium excretion falls to < 12 mg (1 mEq) per day. Therefore, urine magnesium is low if magnesium depletion results from gastrointestinal causes; however, it is in the normal range (120 to 160 mg per day) if depletion results from a renal leak.

Magnesium depletion has been found in 35% of patients with steatorrheic states. Fecal magnesium content correlates with the amount of stool fat, suggesting that magnesium malabsorption is a result of magnesium forming an insoluble complex with fat in the gastrointestinal tract. Any severe diarrheal state such as ulcerative colitis, amebic colitis, and intestinal resection can also deplete magnesium. Another gastrointestinal cause of magnesium depletion is an isolated defect in magnesium absorption that usually occurs in infants.

Renal magnesium wasting (Table 191–1) can result from either an intrinsic disorder of the renal tubule or from extrinsic or reversible factors. The three major intrinsic causes of renal magnesium wasting are familial or sporadic renal magnesium wasting, Bartter's syndrome, and drug nephrotoxicity. Familial or sporadic renal magnesium wasting can severely deplete magnesium.

TABLE 191–1. CAUSES OF HYPOMAGNESEMIA

Gastrointestinal
   Steatorrheic states
   Severe diarrhea
   Familial magnesium malabsorption
Renal
   Intrinsic
      Familial or sporadic renal magnesium wasting
      Bartter's syndrome
      Nephrotoxic agents
   Extrinsic (intrarenal)
      Volume expansion
      Hypercalciuria
      Diabetic ketoacidosis
      Diuretics
Miscellaneous
   Alcoholism
   Thyrotoxicosis
   Burns
   Parathyroidectomy
   Lactation

Although hypomagnesemia is common in Bartter's syndrome, it rarely, if ever, is severe enough to cause symptoms. Drugs that most commonly cause this complication are the aminoglycosides, cyclosporine, and cis-diamminodichloride platinum (cis-DDP). Cis-DDP commonly causes renal magnesium wasting that can persist for months after the drug has been discontinued. A number of extrinsic or intrarenal factors, including virtually all diuretics, volume expansion, diabetic ketoacidosis, and hypercalciuria, can cause mild to moderate renal magnesium wasting. There are several miscellaneous causes of magnesium depletion, including alcoholism, thyrotoxicosis, pancreatitis, lactation, parathyroidectomy, and burns. Alcoholism is the most important. Magnesium depletion in this condition results from a number of causes, including poor dietary intake and some enhanced renal excretion of this cation. Hypomagnesemia, which correlates with the severity of the hyperthyroid state, is a result of redistribution rather than deficiency of this element. Hypomagnesemia can also result from redistribution following parathyroidectomy, which results from magnesium being incorporated into bone, along with calcium salts, during the rapid healing that follows parathyroid surgery.

EFFECT OF MAGNESIUM ON CALCIUM METABOLISM. Magnesium depletion is the most common cause of hypocalcemia in a general hospital population. Parathyroid hormone (PTH) levels have been shown to be either low or inappropriately normal when the patient has hypomagnesemia-induced hypocalcemia. This is a problem of release rather than synthesis of PTH in that PTH levels rapidly increase within minutes of giving magnesium replacement. Besides affecting PTH secretion, with more severe magnesium depletion there is also bone resistance to PTH, as manifested by a lack of calcemic response.

INTERRELATIONSHIP BETWEEN MAGNESIUM AND POTASSIUM. Approximately 40% of hypomagnesemic patients have coexisting hypokalemia. In muscle and myocardium, when either intracellular magnesium or potassium falls, there is a corresponding decrease in the other cation. Conversely in primary potassium depletion there is intracellular muscle magnesium depletion without hypomagnesemia. The interrelationship between intracellular potassium and magnesium is further demonstrated by the fact that repletion of potassium frequently cannot be accomplished without concomitantly administering magnesium. The term "refractory potassium repletion states" has been used to describe this condition. Intracellular depletion of magnesium has been suggested as responsible for causing a variety of cardiovascular alterations, including increased sensitivity to digitalis toxicity, cardiac arrhythmias such as premature ventricular contractions, and torsades de pointes. However, it is unclear whether these cardiovascular alterations are a direct result of magnesium depletion or a consequence of the associated intracellular potassium depletion.

DIAGNOSIS AND MANAGEMENT OF MAGNESIUM DEPLETION. Magnesium depletion is usually readily diagnosed by measuring the serum magnesium level. Mild asymptomatic magnesium depletion requires no treatment if the patient is able to eat a normal diet. Patients with symptomatic hypomagnesemia usually require parenteral magnesium replacement. As a rule, the magnesium deficit can be roughly calculated by assuming that the space of distribution is the extracellular volume. Because half the administered magnesium is excreted in the urine, replacement is approximately twice the calculated deficit. Although an occasional patient may require intravenous replacement, the intramuscular route is safer and the preferred method of administering magnesium. Suggested magnesium replacement for hypomagnesemic states is given in Table 191-2. It has been suggested that intravenous magnesium should be routinely given to patients with acute myocardial infarction to replace depleted intracellular magnesium, partially based on the finding of reduced muscle magnesium and potassium levels, especially in patients on diuretics. This has been suggested to enhance tissue potassium repletion, decrease death rates, and reduce the number of episodes of arrhythmias in this patient population. The evidence is good that magnesium replacement can enhance intracellular potassium replacement and under certain conditions is necessary for potassium repletion. However, there is continuing controversy about what if any other benefit magnesium therapy affords patients with acute myocardial infarction.

TABLE 191-2. MANAGEMENT OF HYPOMAGNESEMIA

Severe hypomagnesemia (serum Mg < 1 mEq/L)
Intramuscular replacement
  4 ml of 50% $MgSO_4 \cdot 7(H_2O)$ (magnesium sulfate heptahydrate), 16.3 mEq (196 mg/Mg) IM every 4 hours for the first 24 hours.
  Subsequent replacement as required for persistent hypomagnesemia should be 2 ml 50% $MgSO_4 \cdot 7(H_2O)$ IM every 6 hours.
Intravenous replacement
  Initially 12 ml of 50% $MgSO_4 \cdot 7(H_2O)$ (49 mEq Mg) in 1000-ml solution in 5% dextrose infused over 3 hours.
  Additional 2 liters containing 12 ml of 50% $MgSO_4 \cdot 7(H_2O)$ administered over the remainder of the first 24-hour period.
  Over the next 3 to 4 days, 49 mEq Mg per day may be given intravenously.
Symptomatic hypomagnesemia (tetany or seizures)
  4 ml (16.3 mEq) of a 50% $MgSO_4 \cdot 7(H_2O)$ solution diluted to 100 ml and infused over a 10-minute period.
Chronic oral replacement therapy (steatorrheic states and renal magnesium wasting)
  Magnesium oxide (550 mg Mg/gram), 250 to 500 mg four times daily as tolerated without developing diarrhea.

HYPERMAGNESEMIA

Mild hypermagnesemia is seen in hypothyroidism, adrenal insufficiency, and advanced renal failure. The majority of cases of symptomatic hypermagnesemia have resulted from administering large oral loads of magnesium, in the form of laxatives or antacids, to patients with advanced renal insufficiency. In patients with normal renal function, life-threatening hypermagnesemia has been described in only a few unusual circumstances. Several fatalities in children have resulted from accidentally ingesting Epsom salts (magnesium sulfate). Normal subjects receiving 800 to 1600 mEq of magnesium sulfate per rectum have been found to have serum magnesium levels of 6 to 16 mEq per liter. Administering hypertonic magnesium solutions poses an additional risk of producing magnesium intoxication in patients with normal renal function. With hypertonic magnesium solutions, i.e., 50% $MgSO_4$, fluid moves from the extracellular space into the gastrointestinal tract. This decreases effective blood volume and reduces renal perfusion, which compromises the ability to excrete the magnesium absorbed from the large gastrointestinal load. This combination of increased absorption and decreased ability to excrete magnesium can cause life-threatening hypermagnesemia.

SYMPTOMS. Usually no symptoms are noted until the serum magnesium is >4 mEq per liter, at which time deep tendon reflexes may be slightly depressed. When serum magnesium increases to 10 to 15 mEq per liter, deep tendon reflexes are absent and the patient may also develop a flaccid quadriplegia. Other symptoms include lethargy, nausea, dilated pupils, respiratory depression, hypotension, bradycardia, and rarely complete heart block and cardiac arrest.

TREATMENT OF ACUTE HYPERMAGNESEMIA. Severe hypermagnesemia requires emergency management because patients can die of respiratory failure or cardiac arrest. Calcium is a direct antagonist to magnesium, and as little as 5 to 10 mEq of calcium administered intravenously can readily reverse these potentially lethal complications. This should be followed by methods to reduce the serum magnesium concentration. In patients with reasonable renal function, the combination of furosemide and 0.5N saline to replace urine volume and maintain diuresis can augment magnesium excretion. The most effective way of reducing plasma magnesium levels is hemodialysis using a magnesium-free dialysate.

Millane TA, Ward DE, Camm AJ: Electrophysiology, pacing and arrhythmia. Clin Cardiol 15:103, 1992. *An excellent, well-referenced review on the interrelationship between magnesium and potassium and cardiac arrhythmias.*

Rude RK: Magnesium metabolism and deficiency. Endocrinol Metab Clin North Am 22:377, 1993. *A recent review with 142 articles referenced.*

Whang R, Whang DD, Ryan MP: Refractory potassium repletion. A consequence of magnesium deficiency. Arch Intern Med 152:40, 1992. *Emphasizes the need for combined replacement with potassium and magnesium in certain conditions.*

Woods KL, Fletcher S, Roffe C, et al.: Intravenous magnesium sulphate in suspected acute myocardial infarction: Results of the second Leicester intravenous magnesium intervention trial (LIMIT-2). Lancet 1:1553, 1992. *A double-blind study supporting the benefits of magnesium replacement in acute myocardial infarction.*

192 NUTRITION'S INTERFACE WITH HEALTH AND DISEASE

192.1 Introduction
Douglas C. Heimburger

OLD AND NEW PARADIGMS

Nutrition science has been characterized by two major phases in the twentieth century. During the first, nutrition scientists discovered, characterized, and synthesized the various vitamins and described their deficiency syndromes in detail. The dietary requirements for these nutrients were determined and have been periodically updated by the National Academy of Sciences as the *Recommended Dietary Allowances* (RDA's, Table 192–1). These are estimated with a margin of error designed to prevent classic deficiencies in practically all persons and do not represent minimum requirements. For nutrients for which too little information exists to estimate recommended intakes, the Academy has published *Estimated Safe and Adequate Daily Dietary Intakes* (Table 192–2).

The second phase of modern nutrition science has focused on the relationships of diet and nutritional status to the diseases that plague western societies, such as coronary heart disease, cancer, and the other leading causes of death. Particularly during the last decade, this has led to expansion of the perspectives of nutrition scientists and the evolution of a new paradigm for understanding nutrition, which is contrasted with the older paradigm in Table 192–3. It is likely that this development will produce exciting changes in the way nutrition and health are understood during the next decade. Specifics of the new paradigm are detailed in Ch. 192.2.

NUTRITION'S INFLUENCE ON MORTALITY AND MORBIDITY

The causal connections between diet and chronic disease are difficult to tease out of the complex network of other risk factors, including social and behavioral variables, so a wide variety of studies must be relied on to establish them with reasonable certainty. The first links between diet and disease are often derived from epidemiologic studies, but these are unable to infer causal relationships and may be confounded by variables that have not been examined. Epidemiologic studies are also challenged by the difficulty of accurately assessing the diets of free-living individuals. Animal and *in vitro* studies can overcome some of these drawbacks, but may be confounded by experimental conditions that differ from those encountered by humans. A large number of prospective, randomized human intervention trials have been undertaken to test the effects of dietary change on the risk for disease. However, even these will not always be conclusive because of pitfalls associated with selecting study populations and isolating individual dietary factors.

Nevertheless, taken together, epidemiologic, animal, *in vitro*, and intervention studies are proving that human dietary habits contribute importantly to the pathogenesis of most of the major causes of death in developed countries. The 10 leading causes of death in the United States are listed in Table 9–4. Table 192–4 lists those causes as well as several other morbid conditions that have well-established dietary links.

Nutritional influences on the most common cause of death in the United States, coronary heart disease (CHD), have been the subject of a great deal of productive research. The overall US mortality rate from CHD peaked in the 1960's and, in a trend that surprised medical science, has declined steadily ever since. While the causes of the decline are not firmly established, it is apparent that changes in lifestyle, including diet, are probably more responsible than is high-tech care of patients with established CHD. Elevated plasma low-density lipoprotein cholesterol (LDL-C) levels are a major risk factor for CHD and peripheral atherosclerosis correlating strongly with dietary saturated fat intake and less strongly with cholesterol intake. Both of these in the United States derive largely from foods of animal origin such as meats, dairy products, and eggs. Attempts to produce less atherogenic substitutes for some of these foods have not always proven beneficial. For instance, hydrogenation of vegetable oils to create margarine and shortening results in the formation of *trans* fatty acids that affect serum cholesterol levels in a manner similar to the saturated fatty acids found in butter and lard. LDL-C levels can be lowered modestly by increasing the intake of soluble fibers from legumes, fruits, and vegetables. LDL must be oxidized before it induces injury to arterial wall epithelial cells; adequate dietary levels of the antioxidant vitamins C and E, and β-carotene, have been shown to inhibit LDL oxidation.

Epidemiologic evidence suggests that fish consumption may reduce CHD risk, perhaps through the action of ω-3 fatty acids. Evidence also indicates that moderate consumption of alcohol, especially wine, is associated with decreased risk for CHD, possibly through increasing high-density lipoprotein cholesterol (HDL-C) levels or preventing oxidation of LDL. Circulating levels of the amino acid homocysteine, which are asymptomatically elevated in 20 to 25% of Americans, have been strongly correlated with risk for CHD. Homocysteine levels can be reduced by increasing the intake of folic acid (mainly from legumes and vegetables) and decreasing the intake of methionine (principally from animal protein). A conservative estimate suggests that moderate dietary modification by the US population, consisting mainly of replacing saturated fats with complex carbohydrates, fiber, monounsaturated fats, and fish, should lead to a 10% reduction in serum cholesterol levels and a 20% reduction in CHD mortality compared to 1987 levels.

Nutrients, non-nutritive dietary constituents, and nutritional status can influence the risk for cancer in a variety of ways. Nutrition interacts with each step of carcinogenesis (carcinogen activation and tumor initiation, promotion, and progression). Humans are exposed to countless potential carcinogens, but to many anticarcinogens as well, each day through dietary and other means. Excess caloric intake may favor the generation of free radicals and reduce the body's ability to detoxify carcinogens. By contrast, antioxidant nutrients scavenge free radicals and other (pre)carcinogens, inhibiting their activation and/or their ability to initiate mutations. Folic acid may improve a cell's ability to preserve or repair its DNA, either preventing or reversing the tendency to mutation. Obesity, excess dietary fat intake, and excess alcohol appear to promote tumor growth.

Much evidence indicates that the number one cancer killer, lung cancer, is strongly influenced by diet. While the most important causal factor is cigarette smoking, the consumption of fruits and vegetables and of one of their major micronutrient constituents, β-carotene, associates inversely with lung cancer risk in both smokers and nonsmokers. This is also true of plasma levels of β-carotene. It is probable that other nutrients in fruits and vegetables, such as folic acid, as well as non-nutritive components, are partly responsi-

TABLE 192–1. FOOD AND NUTRITION BOARD, NATIONAL ACADEMY OF SCIENCES—NATIONAL RESEARCH COUNCIL RECOMMENDED DIETARY ALLOWANCES,[a] REVISED 1989

Designed for the maintenance of good nutrition of practically all healthy people in the United States

Category	Age (years) or Condition	Weight[b] (kg)	Weight[b] (lb)	Height[b] (cm)	Height[b] (in)	Protein (g)	Fat-Soluble Vitamins Vitamin A (μg RE)[c]	Vitamin D (μg)[d]	Vitamin E (mg α-TE)[e]	Vitamin K (μg)	Water-Soluble Vitamins Vitamin C (mg)	Thiamine (mg)	Riboflavin (mg)	Niacin (mg NE)[f]	Vitamin B6 (mg)	Folate (μg)	Vitamin B12 (μg)	Minerals Calcium (mg)	Phosphorus (mg)	Magnesium (mg)	Iron (mg)	Zinc (mg)	Iodine (μg)	Selenium (μg)
Infants	0.0–0.5	6	13	60	24	13	375	7.5	3	5	30	0.3	0.4	5	0.3	25	0.3	400	300	40	6	5	40	10
	0.5–1.0	9	20	71	28	14	375	10	4	10	35	0.4	0.5	6	0.6	35	0.5	600	500	60	10	5	50	15
Children	1–3	13	29	90	35	16	400	10	6	15	40	0.7	0.8	9	1.0	50	0.7	800	800	80	10	10	70	20
	4–7	20	44	112	44	24	500	10	7	20	45	0.9	1.1	12	1.1	75	1.0	800	800	120	10	10	90	20
	7–10	28	62	132	52	28	700	10	7	30	45	1.0	1.2	13	1.4	100	1.4	800	800	170	10	10	120	30
Males	11–14	45	99	157	62	45	1,000	10	10	45	50	1.3	1.5	17	1.7	150	2.0	1,200	1,200	270	12	15	150	40
	15–18	66	145	176	69	59	1,000	10	10	65	60	1.5	1.8	20	2.0	200	2.0	1,200	1,200	400	12	15	150	50
	19–24	72	160	177	70	58	1,000	10	10	70	60	1.5	1.7	19	2.0	200	2.0	1,200	1,200	350	10	15	150	70
	25–50	79	174	176	70	63	1,000	5	10	80	60	1.5	1.7	19	2.0	200	2.0	800	800	350	10	15	150	70
	51+	77	170	173	68	63	1,000	5	10	80	60	1.2	1.4	15	2.0	200	2.0	800	800	350	10	15	150	70
Females	11–14	46	101	157	62	46	800	10	8	45	50	1.1	1.3	15	1.4	150	2.0	1,200	1,200	280	15	12	150	45
	15–18	55	120	163	64	44	800	10	8	55	60	1.1	1.3	15	1.5	180	2.0	1,200	1,200	300	15	12	150	50
	19–24	58	128	164	65	46	800	10	8	60	60	1.1	1.3	15	1.6	180	2.0	1,200	1,200	280	15	12	150	55
	25–50	63	138	163	64	50	800	5	8	65	60	1.1	1.3	15	1.6	180	2.0	800	800	280	15	12	150	55
	51+	65	143	160	63	50	800	5	8	65	60	1.0	1.2	13	1.6	180	2.0	800	800	280	10	12	150	55
Pregnant						60	800	10	10	65	70	1.5	1.6	17	2.2	400	2.2	1,200	1,200	320	30	15	175	65
Lactating	1st 6 months					65	1,300	10	12	65	95	1.6	1.8	20	2.1	280	2.6	1,200	1,200	355	15	19	200	75
	2nd 6 months					62	1,200	10	11	65	90	1.6	1.7	20	2.1	260	2.6	1,200	1,200	340	15	16	200	75

[a] The allowances, expressed as average daily intakes over time, are intended to provide for individual variations among most normal persons as they live in the United States under usual environmental stresses. Diets should be based on a variety of common foods in order to provide other nutrients for which human requirements have been less well defined.

[b] Weights and heights of Reference Adults are actual medians for the designated age, as reported by NHANES II. The use of these figures does not imply that the height-to-weight ratios are ideal.

[c] Retinol equivalents. 1 retinol equivalent = 1 μg retinol or 6 μg β-carotene.

[d] As cholecalciferol: 10 μg cholecalciferol = 400 IU of vitamin D.

[e] α-Tocopherol equivalents; 1 mg D-α-tocopherol = 1 α-TE.

[f] 1 NE (niacin equivalent) is equal to 1 mg of niacin or 60 mg of dietary tryptophan.

TABLE 192-2. ESTIMATED SAFE AND ADEQUATE DAILY DIETARY INTAKES OF SELECTED VITAMINS AND MINERALS[a]

Category	Age (years)	Vitamins			Trace Elements[b]			
		Biotin (μg)	Pantothenic Acid (mg)	Copper (mg)	Manganese (mg)	Fluoride (mg)	Chromium (μg)	Molybdenum (μg)
Infants	0–0.5	10	2	0.4–0.6	0.3–0.6	0.1–0.5	10–40	15–30
	0.5–1	15	3	0.6–0.7	0.6–1.0	0.2–1.0	20–60	20–40
Children and	1–3	20	3	0.7–1.0	1.0–1.5	0.5–1.5	20–80	25–50
adolescents	4–6	25	3–4	1.0–1.5	1.5–2.0	1.0–2.5	30–120	30–75
	7–10	30	4–5	1.0–2.0	2.0–3.0	1.5–2.5	50–200	50–150
	11 +	30–100	4–7	1.5–2.5	2.0–5.0	1.5–2.5	50–200	75–250
Adults		30–100	4–7	1.5–3.0	2.0–5.0	1.5–4.0	50–200	75–250

[a] Because there is less information on which to base allowances, these figures are not given in Table 192–1 and are provided here in the form of ranges of recommended intakes.

[b] Since the toxic levels for many trace elements may be only several times usual intakes, the upper levels for the trace elements given in this table should not be habitually exceeded.

From the National Research Council: Recommended Dietary Allowances, 10th ed. Washington, DC, National Academy Press, 1989.

ble for the protective effects. This argues against relying on antioxidant supplements to reduce disease risk. It is noteworthy that the plasma levels of antioxidant nutrients (β-carotene and vitamins C and E) and folic acid are lower in smokers than nonsmokers and intermediate in persons passively exposed to smoke. Probably caused in large part by oxidants in cigarette smoke, this is an example of an interaction between nutritional factors and environmental exposures that explains more of the variation in cancer incidence than does either factor alone.

The second largest cause of cancer deaths in women, breast cancer, associates positively with dietary fat intake and obesity, especially when the latter affects predominantly the abdomen. Because of the inconsistencies between ecologic and cohort studies noted earlier, however, it is unclear whether dietary fat per se, total calorie intake, or other factors are responsible for the associations. Epidemiologic evidence suggests that alcohol intake may also be a risk factor for this disease. Colorectal cancer is the second highest cause of cancer mortality in men and the third in women. Its risk correlates positively with dietary fat intake in both ecologic and cohort studies and inversely with intake of dietary fiber, calcium, and folic acid. Other malignant diseases for which dietary fat intake appears to increase risk include prostate and ovarian cancers.

The interaction of all these influences is powerful enough to indicate that diet contributes to about 35% of cancer deaths in western countries. Even though the independent influences of potentially protective nutrients such as carotenoids, vitamins C and E, folic acid, and fiber are not known because they are all present in vegetables and fruits, the evidence that a liberal intake of fruits and vegetables reduces cancer risk is overwhelming, supported by 128 of 156 epidemiologic studies reviewed in 1992.

Hypertension is a major risk factor for stroke, CHD, congestive heart failure, peripheral vascular disease, and renal disease. It often associates with obesity, especially abdominal obesity, and weight reduction in obese hypertensives usually leads to improvements in blood pressure. Sodium restriction also usually reduces blood pressure levels. In addition to these well-known effects, blood pressure levels have correlated inversely with the intake of potassium, calcium, and magnesium and are sometimes reduced when these nutrients are supplemented. Because alcohol intake elevates blood pressures, its use should be minimized in hypertensive patients.

Type II diabetes mellitus is strongly associated with obesity (see Ch. 205). This is especially true for abdominal obesity and less so for peripheral obesity. Sugar consumption does not lead to diabetes except to the extent that it may promote weight gain. Past recommendations to restrict total carbohydrate intake in diabetics have been abandoned, so that 55 to 60% of a diabetic's energy intake should come from carbohydrate, preferably unrefined carbohydrates that include fiber. Because higher fat diets tend to promote both obesity and CHD, for which diabetics are at high risk, dietary fat intake should be kept low. Alcohol can cause hypoglycemia, hyperglycemia, and increased triglyceride levels in diabetics, and its use should be minimized. In both diabetics and nondiabetics, excess alcohol intake is responsible for many deaths, particularly from accidents and liver disease, and is a factor in some suicidal deaths.

Osteoporosis is influenced by several dietary factors. Inadequate calcium intake during adolescence may result in suboptimal peak bone mass in early adulthood, and during later life it may lead to more rapid bone loss, thereby increasing the risk for osteoporosis. Other nutrients that influence bone mass have received much less attention. Sodium, phosphorus, and protein, all of which are consumed by Americans in greater quantities than required, may promote excess bone loss. Vitamin D and magnesium assist in maintaining optimal bone mass.

The causes and health effects of obesity, one of the most prevalent nutritional disorders in the United States, are reviewed in Ch. 196. Low dietary fiber intake causes constipation, and although not conclusively established, it is thought to be a cause of intestinal diverticular disease. Inadequate maternal folic acid intake has been conclusively proven to be a major risk factor for congenital neural tube defects such as spina bifida and myelomeningocele.

TRANSLATING EVIDENCE INTO DIETARY CHANGE

Thus there is strong evidence that dietary habits can influence the incidence and severity of many potentially incapacitating or lethal diseases in the United States. No justification exists for the belief that modification of the "usual" American diet is unnecessary or futile. The only questions are whether it is feasible and what is re-

TABLE 192-3. OLD AND NEW PARADIGMS IN NUTRITION

Old Paradigm	New Paradigm
Major nutritional problems = classic deficiency syndromes	Major nutritional problems = chronic diseases
Micronutrients (vitamins, minerals, trace elements) function primarily as cofactors in biochemical reactions	Micronutrients also function as antioxidants, regulators of genes and cell-cell communications, hormones, and pharmacologic agents
Nutrient needs (Recommended Dietary Allowances) determined by amounts required to prevent classic deficiency syndromes	Nutrient needs (not yet distilled into consensus recommendations) determined by amounts required to provide optimal function and health and prevent chronic disease; amounts are affected by individual's genetic makeup and environmental exposures
Micronutrient deficiencies are global, affecting whole body	Micronutrient deficiencies may be localized, and affect the functions of specific tissues
General effects of nutrients	Specific effects of nutrient subtypes, e.g., individual fatty acids, amino acids, and particular forms of micronutrients
All benefits of food are derived from nutrients; many can be obtained from supplements	Many non-nutritive components of foods, e.g., fiber, pigments, protease inhibitors, flavonoids, and others have important effects; even if some become available through supplements, many undetected ones may exist in foods

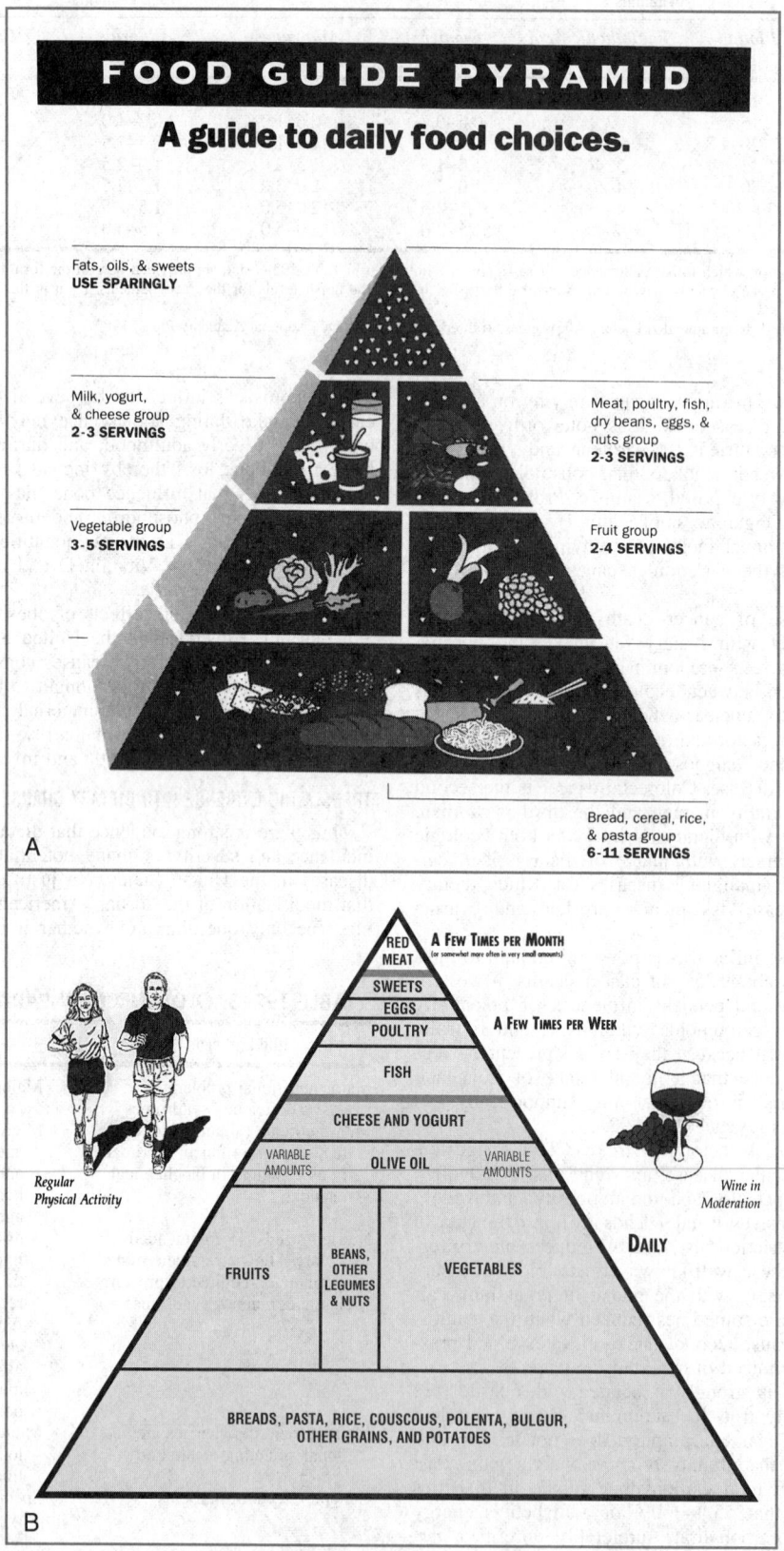

FIGURE 192.1–1. *A*, USDA/DHHS Food Guide Pyramid. *B*, Traditional healthy Mediterranean diet pyramid. (*A*, From USDA/DDHS. *B*, Copyright 1994, Oldways Preservation & Exchange Trust and The President and Fellows of Harvard College. Used by permission.)

TABLE 192–4. DIETARY INFLUENCES ON MAJOR CAUSES OF DEATH AND MORBIDITY IN UNITED STATES

	Possible Beneficial Influences	Possible Deleterious Influences
Cause of Death		
Coronary heart disease	Complex carbohydrates, particular fatty acids (e.g., mono-unsaturated, polyunsaturated, and ω-3 fatty acids from fish), soluble fiber, antioxidants (vitamins E, C; β-carotene, selenium), folic acid, moderate alcohol	Saturated fat, cholesterol; excess calories, sodium, animal protein; abdominal distribution of body fat
Cancer	Fruits and vegetables (for β-carotene, vitamins A, C, D, E, folic acid, calcium, selenium, phytochemicals), fiber	Excess calories, fat, alcohol, red meat, salt- and nitrite-preserved meats, possibly grilled meats; abdominal distribution of body fat
Stroke	Potassium, calcium, ω-3 fatty acids	Sodium, alcohol (as with hypertension)
Accidents		Alcohol
Diabetes mellitus	Fiber	Excess calories, fat, alcohol; abdominal distribution of body fat
Suicide		Alcohol
Chronic liver disease		Alcohol
Atherosclerosis (peripheral)	Particular fatty acids (e.g., monounsaturated and ω-3 fatty acids), soluble fiber, antioxidant vitamins	Saturated fat, cholesterol
Cause of Morbidity		
Obesity		Excess calories and fat
Hypertension	Potassium, calcium, ω-3 fatty acids	Sodium, alcohol, excess calories; abdominal distribution of body fat
Osteoporosis	Calcium, vitamin D	Sodium, phosphorus, protein
Diverticular disease, constipation		Fiber
Neural tube defects	Folic acid	

quired to effect change. Various health agencies and the US government have used public education, particularly the publication of dietary goals, as their primary means. The US Departments of Agriculture (USDA) and Health and Human Services (USDHHS) developed the food guide pyramid to replace the traditional basic four food groups in educating the public (Fig. 192–1A). It indicates that a healthy diet should be founded on ample servings of the complex carbohydrates present in breads, cereals, rice, and pasta. Vegetables and fruits should be a prominent component as well. Foods of animal origin, such as meat, eggs, and dairy products, should form a less central part of the diet, and fats, oils, and sweets should be used sparingly.

Even these recommendations do not typify an ideal diet based on the available evidence, but reflect a consensus on what can be realistically expected of the American public. A potentially more "ideal" pyramid, based on observations of low rates of chronic disease and high adult life expectancies in the Mediterranean region in 1960, has been promulgated by the Department of Nutrition at Harvard University (Fig. 192–1B). In this pyramid, sources of monounsaturated fatty acids, such as olive oil and nuts, are given a more prominent place in the diet, as are beans and other legumes. Fish and poultry are preferable over red meat. Moderate consumption of wine (normally with meals) is recommended as optional, unless it would put the individual or others at risk.

Beginning in May 1994, the US Food and Drug Administration and USDA initiated a major public education effort by requiring substantial changes in the listing of nutrient contents and health claims on food labels. Issues that were previously left to the discretion of food manufacturers, such as the serving sizes and particular nutrients listed, are now stipulated. Labels must delineate total calories and percentage of calories from fat, amounts of total fat, saturated fat, cholesterol, sodium, total carbohydrates, dietary fiber, sugars, protein, vitamins A and C, calcium, and iron. Labels also must indicate how a food's contents of these nutrients conform to recommended intakes, based on a reference 2000 calorie diet. Definitions for "low," "high," "light," "reduced," "free," and "healthy" have been standardized (Table 192–5). Further, only the particular health claims listed in Table 192–6 are permitted on food labels. As further evidence accumulates on the relationships between diet and disease, the approved claims will undoubtedly be revised.

For more details on the rationale for and methods of implementing the recommended dietary changes, please see Ch. 9.2. Physicians can importantly influence their patients' health by encouraging them to optimize their dietary habits and providing them with instructional materials and assistance from dietitians that can help them make needed changes.

National Academy of Sciences; Diet and Health: Washington, DC, 1989. *Comprehensive and easily readable analysis of the scientific evidence on the role of diet in the etiology and prevention of chronic disease in the United States, prepared by a committee of experts.*

Shils ME, Olson JA, Shike M (eds.): Modern Nutrition in Health and Disease, 8th ed. Malvern, PA, Lea & Febiger, 1994. *Comprehensive and detailed source for information on all aspects of human nutrition.*

US DHHS. Washington, DC, DHHS, 1989. Promoting Health/Preventing Disease: Year 2000 Objectives for the Nation. *Health promotion/disease prevention priorities and goals for the nation in nutrition and other areas.*

TABLE 192–5. DEFINITIONS OF TERMS USED ON FOOD LABELS

Low fat	≤ 3 grams per serving
Low saturated fat	≤ 1 gram per serving, ≤15% of calories
Low calorie	≤ 40 calories per serving
High	≥ 20% of desired daily value per serving
Light	Half the fat or one-third the calories of the regular product
Reduced	≤ 75% of content of regular product
Free	None, or insignificant amount (e.g., < 1 gram fat or < ½ gram sugar per serving)
Healthy	Low total and saturated fat, sodium, and cholesterol; ≥ 10% daily value for vitamin A, vitamin C, iron, calcium, protein, or fiber

From USDHHS, FDA, USDA,

TABLE 192–6. PERMISSIBLE HEALTH CLAIMS FOR FOOD LABELS

Calcium	May lower risk for osteoporosis
Fat	May increase risk for cancer
Saturated fat and cholesterol	Increase risk for coronary heart disease
Fiber-containing grain products, fruits, and vegetables	May reduce risk for coronary heart disease and cancer
Sodium	May increase risk for high blood pressure
Folic acid supplementation	Reduces risk for neural tube defects

From USDHHS, FDA, USDA.

192.2 Consequences of Altered Micronutrient Status

Joel B. Mason

Micronutrients are a highly diverse array of dietary components necessary to sustain health. The physiologic roles of micronutrients are as varied as their composition: Some are used in enzymes as either coenzymes or prosthetic groups; others, as biochemical substrates or hormones; and in some instances, the functions are not well defined. Under normal circumstances, the average daily dietary intake for each micronutrient required to sustain normal physiologic operations is measured in milligram or smaller quantities. This quantification distinguishes micronutrients from macronutrients, the latter category encompassing carbohydrates, fats, and proteins, as well as the macrominerals calcium, magnesium, and phosphorus.

For homeostasis to proceed properly, most dietary nutrients must be ingested in quantities that are neither too small nor too great. Disorders may arise when this "physiologic window" is either not met or is exceeded. The size of the window varies for each micronutrient and should be kept in mind, particularly in present-day circumstances when the administration of large quantities of certain micronutrients is being increasingly explored for possible therapeutic implications. Many factors determine the dietary requirement for a particular micronutrient, only one of which is the amount needed to sustain those physiologic functions for which it is used (Table 192–7). The *US Recommended Daily Allowances* (RDAs) provides dietary guidelines that indicate how much of each nutrient is "adequate to meet the known nutrient needs of practically all healthy persons"; the RDAs are listed in Table 192–1. Adequate intake, which is the amount necessary to prevent a deficiency state, is not necessarily synonymous with optimal intake, an issue this chapter discusses in more detail.

SALIENT FEATURES OF VITAMINS AND TRACE ELEMENTS: TRADITIONAL PERSPECTIVES

VITAMINS (Table 192–8). Vitamins have long been categorized as either fat soluble (A,D,E,K) or water soluble (all the others). This remains a physiologically meaningful manner of categorization. None of the fat-soluble vitamins appears to serve as a coenzyme. Their absorption is primarily through a micellar route, and pathophysiologic conditions associated with fat malabsorption frequently are associated with selective deficiencies of the fat-soluble vitamins. In contrast, most water-soluble vitamins function as coenzymes. Furthermore, the water-soluble vitamins are not absorbed through the lipophilic phase in the intestine.

TRACE ELEMENTS (Table 192–9). Fifteen trace elements have been identified as essential for health in animal studies: iron, zinc, copper, chromium, selenium, iodine, fluorine, manganese, molybdenum, cobalt, nickel, tin, silicon, vanadium, and arsenic. Nevertheless, only for the first 10 of these is there compelling evidence of essentialness in humans. Cobalt seems to be essential solely as a component of vitamin B_{12}; an isolated deficiency state has never been described. Deficiency syndromes for several of the other essential trace elements were not recognized until recently because of their exceedingly small requirements and their ubiquitous nature in foodstuffs. Only under exceptional circumstances, such as long-term dependence on total parenteral nutrition (TPN) that lacked the elements (a situation that has since been corrected), have some of the deficiency syndromes been observed.

The biochemical functions of trace elements have not been as well characterized as those for the vitamins, but most of their functions appear to be as components of prosthetic groups or as cofactors for a number of enzymes. Determination of essential trace element status is problematic except for iron, selenium, and iodine. The vanishingly low concentrations of these elements in bodily fluids and tissues, the fact that blood levels frequently do not correlate well with levels in the target tissues, and the fact that functional tests cannot be devised until biochemical functions are better understood, preclude an accurate and convenient laboratory method of assessment for most of the trace elements.

CONDITIONS THAT INCREASE THE REQUIRED DIETARY INTAKE FOR VITAMINS AND MINERALS

Many physiologic, pathophysiologic, and pharmacologic factors increase the dietary requirements for micronutrients (Table 192–7), and these factors when compounded enhance the risk of developing a deficiency state.

PHYSIOLOGIC FACTORS. Stages of the life cycle have an important impact on the requirements of certain nutrients. Phases of rapid growth and development, such as in utero development, infancy, adolescence, and pregnancy, are associated with remarkable increases in the utilization of certain micronutrients on a per-kilogram basis. Requirements for most micronutrients increase in pregnancy; those for iron and folate are particularly increased, because of the rapid proliferation of placental and fetal tissues. Periods of lactation are similarly associated with remarkable increases in requirements. A lactating woman experiences disproportionately large increases in her requirements for zinc and vitamins A, E, and C, in addition to the needs for pregnancy, to meet the metabolic demands incurred by milk production.

Infancy carries with it particular vulnerabilities to specific micronutrient inadequacies: Healthy infants in the United States are typically supplemented with vitamin K at birth and with iron and vitamin D during the course of the first year because of their particular susceptibility to deficiencies of these nutrients.

The ability to maintain adequate iron status from menarche through menopause is compromised in women by the additional losses incurred by menstruation, pregnancy, and lactation. As a result, the highest rate of iron deficiency affects women of childbearing age.

Specific dietary recommendations for the elderly have not yet been formally adopted, but these will inevitably appear because aging also affects the requirements for certain micronutrients. Vitamin B_{12} status, for instance, declines significantly with aging because of the high prevalence of atrophic gastritis and its associated impairment in protein-bound B_{12} absorption. The average decline is big enough to put a measurable proportion of the elderly population at risk of clinically important B_{12} deficiency and thus warrants an increase in B_{12} intake in this age group. Elderly persons, particularly those institutionalized for a long time, are also susceptible to vitamin D deficiency; increased intake is therefore indicated. The causes include diminished cutaneous synthesis of vitamin D by senile skin and decreased sun exposure, as well as in many instances to smaller dietary intakes.

PATHOPHYSIOLOGIC AND PHARMACOLOGIC FACTORS. Intestinal malabsorptive and maldigestive states predispose to multiple micronutrient deficiencies. Both fat-soluble and water-soluble micronutrients are absorbed predominantly in the proximal small intestine, the only exception being vitamin B_{12}. Diffuse mucosal diseases, therefore, that affect the proximal portion of the gastrointestinal tract are very likely to result in deficiencies. Even in the absence of mucosal disease of the proximal small intestine, however, extensive ileal disease, small bowel bacterial overgrowth, and chronic cholestasia can each interfere with the maintenance of adequate intraluminal conjugated bile acid concentrations and thereby impair absorption of fat-soluble vitamins. Maldigestion is usually the result of chronic pancreatitis. Untreated, it frequently

TABLE 192–7. FACTORS THAT DETERMINE THE DIETARY REQUIREMENT FOR A MICRONUTRIENT

Physiologic Factors
1. *Bioavailability:* the proportion of an ingested micronutrient that can be assimilated and utilized for physiologic purposes
2. Quantity required to fulfill physiologic roles
3. Extent to which the body can reutilize the micronutrient
4. Distribution of nutrient in the body: storage compartments, etc.
5. Influence of gender
6. Stage of life cycle: intrauterine development, childhood, adulthood, elder adulthood, pregnancy, lactation

Pathophysiologic and Pharmacologic Factors
1. Inborn errors of metabolism that variously affect assimilation, utilization, or excretion of micronutrients
2. Acquired disease states that alter the amounts required to sustain homeostasis (e.g., malabsorption, maldigestion, states that increase utilization)
3. Lifestyle habits, e.g., smoking, ethanol consumption
4. Drugs: may alter bioavailability and/or utilization

TABLE 192–8. VITAMINS AND THEIR FUNCTIONS

	Fat-Soluble Vitamins			
	Biochemistry and Physiology	Deficiency	Toxicity	Assessment of Status
Vitamin A	A subset of the retinoid compounds with biologic activity qualitatively similar to retinol. Carotenoids are structurally related to retinoids. Some carotenoids, most notably β-carotene, are metabolized into compounds with vitamin A activity and are considered to be provitamin A compounds. Vitamin A is an integral component of rhodopsin and iodopsins, light-sensitive proteins in retinal rod and cone cells.	Follicular hyperkeratosis and night blindness are early indicators. Conjunctival xerosis, degeneration of the cornea (keratomalacia), and de-differentiation of rapidly proliferating epithelia indicate more severe deficiency. Bitot spots (focal areas of the conjunctiva or cornea with foamy appearance) are an indication of xerosis. Blindness, due to corneal destruction and retinal dysfunction, ensues if left uncorrected. Increased susceptibility to infection also a consequence.	> 500,000 IU may cause acute toxicity: intracranial hypertension, skin exfoliation and hepatocellular necrosis. Chronic toxicity may occur with habitual daily intake of > 33,000 IU: alopecia, ataxia, dermatitis, cheilitis, pseudotumor cerebri, hepatocellular necrosis, and hyperlipidemia. Daily ingestion of > 25,000 IU during early pregnancy can be teratogenic. Excessive intake of most carotenoids causes a benign, yellowish discoloration of the skin. Large doses of canthaxanthin, a carotenoid, can induce retinopathy.	Retinol concentration in the plasma as well as vitamin A concentrations in the milk and tears are reasonably accurate measures. Toxicity best assessed by elevated levels of retinyl esters in plasma. A quantitative measure of dark adaptation for night vision or an electroretinogram are useful functional tests.
Vitamin D	A group of sterol compounds whose parent structure is cholecalciferol (vitamin D_3). Cholecalciferol is formed in the skin from 7-dehydrocholesterol by exposure to UV-B radiation. A plant sterol, ergocalciferol, can be similarly converted into vitamin D_2, and has similar vitamin D activity. Maintains intracellular and extracellular concentrations of calcium and phosphate by enhancing intestinal absorption of the two ions and, in conjunction with parathormone, promoting their mobilization from bone mineral.	Deficiency results in rickets in childhood and osteomalacia in adults. Expansion of the epiphyseal growth plates and replacement of normal bone with unmineralized bone matrix are the cardinal features. Deformity of bone and pathologic fractures occur. Serum concentrations of calcium and phosphate may decline.	Excess amounts result in abnormally high serum concentrations of calcium and phosphate: metastatic calcifications, renal damage, and altered mentation may ensue.	The serum concentration of the major circulating metabolite, 25-hydroxy vitamin D, indicates systemic status except in chronic renal failure, in which the impairment of renal 1-hydroxylation results in disassociation of the monohydroxy and dihydroxy vitamin concentrations. Measuring the serum concentration of 1,25-dihydroxy vitamin D is then necessary.
Vitamin E	A group of at least 8 naturally occurring compounds that share a spectrum of biologic activities. Some are tocopherols and some tocotrienols. The most biologically active of the vitameric forms is α-tocopherol. Acts as an antioxidant and free radical scavenger in lipophilic environments, most notably in cell membranes. Acts in conjunction with other antioxidants such as selenium.	Deficiency due to dietary inadequacy rare in developed countries. Usually affects premature infants, individuals with fat malabsorption, and persons with abetalipoproteinemia. Red blood cell fragility can produce hemolytic anemia. Neuronal degeneration produces peripheral neuropathies, ophthalmoplegia, and destruction of posterior columns of spinal cord. Neurologic disease frequently irreversible if deficiency is not corrected early enough. May contribute to hemolytic anemia and retrolental fibroplasia in premature infants.	Depressed levels of vitamin K-dependent procoagulants and potentiation of oral anticoagulants has been reported, as has impaired leukocyte function. Doses of 800 IU/d may increase the incidence of hemorrhagic stroke.	Plasma or serum concentration of α-tocopherol is most commonly used. Additional accuracy is obtained by expressing this value per mg of total plasma lipid. Red blood cell peroxide hemolysis test is not entirely specific, but is a useful functional measure of antioxidant potential of cell membranes.
Vitamin K	A family of naphthoquinone compounds with similar biologic activity. Phylloquinone (vitamin K_1) is derived from plants; a variety of menaquinones (vitamin K_2) are derived from bacterial sources. Serves as an essential cofactor in the posttranslational α- or gamma-carboxylation of glutamic acid residues in many proteins. These proteins include several circulating procoagulants and anticoagulants as well as proteins in the bone matrix and renal epithelium.	Deficiency syndrome uncommon except in (1) breast-fed newborns, in whom it may cause "hemorrhagic disease of the newborn"; (2) adults with fat malabsorption or who are taking drugs that interfere with vitamin K metabolism (e.g., coumarin, phenytoin, broad-spectrum antibiotics); and (3) individuals taking large doses of vitamin E and anticoagulant drugs. Excessive hemorrhage is usual manifestation.	Rapid intravenous infusion of K_1 has been associated with dyspnea, flushing and cardiovascular collapse, probably related to dispersing agents in the solution. Supplementation may interfere with coumarin-based anticoagulation. Pregnant women taking large amounts of the provitamin menadione may deliver infants with hemolytic anemia, hyperbilirubinemia and kernicterus.	The prothrombin time is typically used as a measure of functional K status; it is neither sensitive nor specific for vitamin K deficiency. Determination of undercarboxylated prothrombin in the plasma is more accurate but less widely available.

Table continued on following page

causes malabsorption and deficiencies of fat-soluble vitamins. Vitamin B_{12} malabsorption often can be demonstrated in this setting, a result of inadequate R-protein digestion, but clinical B_{12} deficiency is rarely reported in patients with pancreatitis.

A myriad of rare inborn errors of metabolism has been described that impair an individual's ability to assimilate, utilize, or retain a particular vitamin or mineral. Such defects are usually partial and can often be overcome, at least in part, by administering doses of the nutrient that are several degrees of magnitude greater than is usually required. Suspicion for such defects should be entertained if: (1) a known defect exists in the family, (2) a deficiency syndrome arises at birth or during infancy, and (3) the deficiency syndrome is present despite adequate dietary intake and the absence of any disease that would impair the ability to assimilate the nutrient.

The long-term administration of many drugs may adversely affect micronutrient status and may either induce an overt deficiency syn-

TABLE 192–8. VITAMINS AND THEIR FUNCTIONS *(Continued)*

Water-Soluble Vitamins

	Biochemistry and Physiology	Deficiency	Toxicity	Assessment of Status
Thiamine (vitamin B₁)	A water-soluble compound containing substituted pyrimidine and thiazole rings and a hydroxyethyl side chain. The coenzyme form is thiamine pyrophosphate (TPP). Serves as a coenzyme in many -keto acid decarboxylation and transketolation reactions. Inadequate thiamine availability leads to impairments of above reactions, resulting in inadequate ATP synthesis and abnormal carbohydrate metabolism. May have an additional role in neuronal conduction independent of above mentioned actions.	Classic deficiency syndrome ("beriberi") described in Asian populations consuming polished rice diet. Alcoholism and chronic renal dialysis are also common precipitants. High carbohydrate intake increases need for B₁. Deficiency produces various combinations of peripheral neuropathy, cardiovascular and cerebral dysfunction. Cardiovascular involvement ("wet beriberi") includes congestive heart failure and low peripheral vascular resistance. See Ch. 406 for neurologic changes. Deficiency syndrome responds to parenteral thiamine, but is at least partially irreversible after a certain stage.	Excess intake is largely excreted in the urine although parenteral doses of >400 mg/d are reported to cause lethargy, ataxia, and reduced tone of the gastrointestinal tract.	The most effective measure of B₁ status is the erythrocyte transketolase activity coefficient, which measures enzyme activity before and after addition of exogenous TPP: Red cells from a deficient individual express a substantial increase in enzyme activity with addition of TPP. Thiamine concentrations in the blood or urine are also used.
Riboflavin (vitamin B₂)	A compound consisting of a substituted isoalloxazine ring with a ribitol side chain. Serves as a coenzyme for diverse biochemical reactions. The primary coenzymatic forms are flavin mononucleotide (FMN) and flavin adenine dinucleotide (FAD). Riboflavin holoenzymes participate in oxidation-reduction reactions in myriad metabolic pathways.	Deficiency is usually found in conjunction with deficiencies of other B vitamins. Isolated deficiency of riboflavin produces hyperemia and edema of nasopharyngeal mucosa, cheilosis, angular stomatitis, glossitis, seborrheic dermatitis and a normochromic, normocytic anemia.	Toxicity not reported in humans.	The most common assessment is determining the activity coefficient of glutathione reductase in red blood cells (the test is invalid for individuals with glucose-6-phosphate dehydrogenase deficiency). Measurements of blood and urine concentrations are less desirable methods.
Niacin (vitamin B₃)	Refers to nicotinic acid and the corresponding amide, nicotinamide. The active coenzymatic forms are composed of nicotinamide affixed to adenine dinucleotide, forming NAD or NADP. Over 200 apoenzymes use these coenzymes as electron acceptors or hydrogen donors. The essential amino acid, tryptophan, is utilized as a precursor of niacin; 60 mg of dietary tryptophan yields approximately 1 mg of niacin. Dietary requirements depend partly on tryptophan content of diet.	*Pellagra* is the classic deficiency syndrome and often affects populations where corn is the major source of energy. Still endemic in parts of China, Africa, and India. Diarrhea, dementia (or associated symptoms of anxiety or insomnia) and pigmented dermatitis that develops in sun-exposed areas are typical. Glossitis, stomatitis, vaginitis, vertigo, and burning dysesthesias are early signs. Seen also in carcinoid syndrome, which diverts tryptophan to other synthetic pathways.	Human toxicity known largely through studies examining hypolipidemic effects. Includes vasomotor phenomenon (flushing), hyperglycemia, parenchymal liver damage, and hyperuricemia.	Assessment is problematic: Blood levels of vitamin not reliable. Measurement of urinary excretion of the niacin metabolites, N-methylnicotinamide and 2-pyridone are thought to be the most effective means of assessment at present.
Vitamin B₆	Refers to several derivatives of pyridine, including pyridoxine (PN), pyridoxal (PL), and pyridoxamine (PM). The coenzymatic forms are pyridoxal-5-phosphate (PLP) and pyridoxamine-5-phosphate (PMP). As a coenzyme, B₆ is involved in many transamination reactions (and thereby in gluconeogenesis), in the synthesis of niacin from tryptophan, of several neurotransmitters, and of ∂-aminolevulinic acid (and therefore in heme synthesis).	Deficiency usually seen in conjunction with other water-soluble vitamin deficiencies. Stomatitis, angular cheilosis, glossitis, irritability, depression and confusion occur in moderate to severe depletion; normochromic, normocytic anemia has been reported in severe deficiency. Abnormal EEG's and, in infants, convulsions have been observed. Some sideroblastic anemias respond to B₆ administration. Isoniazid, cycloserine, penicillamine, ethanol, and theophylline can inhibit B₆ metabolism.	Chronic use with doses exceeding 200 mg/d (in adults) may cause peripheral neuropathies and photosensitivity.	Many laboratory methods of assessment exist. The plasma or erythrocyte PLP levels are most common. Urinary excretion of xanthurenic acid after an oral tryptophan load or activity indices of RBC alanine or aspartic acid transaminases (ALT and AST, respectively) all are functional measures of B₆-dependent enzyme activity.

drome or predispose to one. The manner in which drug-nutrient interactions occur varies; some of the more common mechanisms are outlined in Table 192–10. Some drugs exert their therapeutic effects by specifically inhibiting the actions of a micronutrient. Examples include coumarin, which inhibits gamma-carboxylation re-actions mediated by vitamin K, and methotrexate, which binds tightly to dihydrofolate reductase, thereby inhibiting folate metabolism.

Tobacco smoking alters the metabolism of several micronutrients, including folate, β-carotene, and vitamins C and E. In large surveys, diminished plasma levels of folate and ascorbic acid have been observed in long-time smokers. Smoking is also associated with diminished levels of folate in cells of the oral mucosa, diminished ascorbic acid levels in leukocytes, and decreased concentrations of vitamin E in lung alveolar fluid.

NEW FRONTIERS IN MARGINAL DEFICIENCY STATES

REDEFINING THE CONCEPT OF NUTRIENT DEFICIENCY. An important evolution in the understanding of micronutrient requirements has occurred over the past century: As nutritional science has expanded its appreciation for additional

TABLE 192–8. VITAMINS AND THEIR FUNCTIONS *(Continued)*

Water-Soluble Vitamins

	Biochemistry and Physiology	Deficiency	Toxicity	Assessment of Status
Folate	A group of over 35 related pterin compounds. The fully oxidized form, folic acid, is not found in nature but is the pharmacologic form of the vitamin. All folate functions relate to their ability to transfer one-carbon groups. The step is essential in the *de novo* synthesis of nucleotides, in the metabolism of several amino acids, and is an integral component for the regeneration of the "universal" methyl donor, S-adenosylmethionine. Inhibition of bacterial and cancer cell folate metabolism is the basis for the sulfonamide antibiotics and chemotherapeutic agents such as methotrexate and 5-fluorouracil.	Women of childbearing age are the most likely individuals to develop deficiency. The "classical" deficiency syndrome is megaloblastic anemia. The hemopoietic cells in the bone marrow develop megaloblastic features, reflecting ineffective DNA synthesis. The peripheral blood smear demonstrates macroovalocytes and polymorphonuclear leukocytes with an average of more than 3.5 nuclear lobes. Megaloblastic changes in the oral and gastrointestinal epithelia often occur, producing glossitis and diarrhea, respectively. Sulfasalazine and phenytoin inhibit absorption and predispose to deficiency.	Doses >400 $\mu g/d$ may partially correct the anemia of B_{12} deficiency and mask (and perhaps exacerbate) the associated neuropathy. Doses >400 μg also reported to lower seizure threshold in individuals prone to seizures. Rarely parenteral administration is reported to cause allergic phenomena, but are probably due to dispersion agents.	Serum folate measures short-term folate balance, whereas RBC folate better reflects tissue status. Serum homocysteine rises early in deficiency but is nonspecific since B_{12} deficiency or renal insufficiency also may cause elevations.
Vitamin C (ascorbic and dehydroascorbic acid)	Ascorbic acid readily oxidizes to dehydroascorbic acid. Since the latter can be reduced *in vivo*, it possesses vitamin C activity. Total vitamin C is therefore measured as the sum of ascorbic and dehydroascorbic acid concentrations. Because of its reductant properties, it serves primarily as a biologic antioxidant and free radical scavenger in aqueous environments. The biosyntheses of collagen, carnitine, bile acids, and norepinephrine, as well as proper functioning of the hepatic mixed-function oxygenase system, all depend on these properties. Vitamin C in foodstuffs increases the intestinal absorption of non-heme iron.	Overt deficiency is uncommonly observed in developed countries. The classic deficiency syndrome is *scurvy*, characterized by fatigue, depression, and widespread abnormalities in connective tissues such as inflamed gingivae, petechiae, perifollicular hemorrhages, impaired wound healing, coiled hairs, hyperkeratosis, bleeding into body cavities. In infants, defects in ossification and bone growth may occur. Tobacco smoking lowers plasma and leukocyte vitamin C levels.	Quantities exceeding 500 mg/d (in adults) sometimes cause nausea and diarrhea. Acidification of the urine with supplementation, and the potential for enhanced oxalate synthesis, have raised concerns regarding nephrolithiasis, but this has yet to be demonstrated. Supplementation may interfere with laboratory tests based on redox potential (e.g., fecal occult blood testing, serum cholesterol and glucose). Withdrawal from chronic ingestion of high doses of vitamin C supplements should occur gradually over a month since accommodation does occur, raising a concern of "rebound scurvy."	Plasma ascorbic acid concentration reflects recent dietary intake whereas leukocyte levels more closely reflect tissue stores. Women's plasma levels are approximately 20% higher than men's for any given dietary intake.
Vitamin B_{12}	A group of closely related cobalamin compounds composed of a corrin ring (with a cobalt atom in its center) connected to a ribonucleotide via an aminopropanol bridge. Microorganisms are the ultimate source of all naturally occurring B_{12}. The two active coenzyme forms are desoxyadenosylcobalamin and methylcobalamin. Both are needed for the synthesis of succinyl CoA, which is essential in lipid and carbohydrate metabolism, as well as the synthesis of methionine. The latter reaction is essential for amino acid metabolism, for purine and pyrimidine synthesis, for many methylation reactions, and for the intracellular retention of folates.	Dietary inadequacy rarely causes deficiency except in strict vegetarians. Most deficiencies reflect loss of intestinal absorption: this may result from pernicious anemia, pancreatic insufficiency, atrophic gastritis, small bowel bacterial overgrowth, or ileal disease. Megaloblastic anemia and megaloblastic changes in other epithelia (see Folate) are the result of sustained depletion. Details of the hematologic (see Ch. 133) and neurologic (see Ch. 406) complications are described elsewhere. Hematologic and neurologic complication may occur independently.	A few allergic reactions have been reported to crystalline B_{12} preparations and are probably due to impurities, not the vitamin.	Serum, or plasma, concentrations are generally accurate. Subtle deficiency with neurologic complications, as described in the Deficiency column, can best be confirmed by measuring the concentration of serum methylmalonic acid, which is a sensitive indicator of cellular deficiency.
Biotin	A bi-cyclic compound consisting of a ureido ring fused to a substituted tetrahydrothiophene ring. Most dietary biotin is linked to lysine, a compound called biotinyl lysine, or biocytin. The lysine must be hydrolyzed by an intestinal enzyme called biotinidase before intestinal absorption occurs. Acts primarily as a co-enzyme for several carboxylases; each holoenzyme catalyzes an ATP-dependent CO_2 transfer. The carboxylases are critical enzymes in carbohydrate and lipid metabolism.	Isolated deficiency is rare. Deficiency in humans has been produced experimentally, by prolonged diets lacking the vitamin, and by ingestion of large quantities of raw egg white, which contains avidin, a protein which binds biotin with extremely high affinity. Alterations in mental status, myalgias, hyperesthesias, and anorexia occur. Later, a seborrheic dermatitis and alopecia develop. Biotin deficiency is usually accompanied by lactic acidosis and organic aciduria.	Toxicity has not been reported in humans with doses as high as 60 mg/d in children.	Plasma and urine concentrations of biotin are diminished in the deficient state. Elevated urine concentrations of methyl citrate, 3-methylcrotonylglycine and 3-hydroxyisovalerate are observed in deficiency.

Table continued on following page

TABLE 192–8. VITAMINS AND THEIR FUNCTIONS *(Continued)*

Water-Soluble Vitamins

	Biochemistry and Physiology	Deficiency	Toxicity	Assessment of Status
Pantothenic acid	Consists of pantoic acid linked to β-alanine through an amide bond. Pantothenate serves as an essential precursor of coenzyme A(CoA). CoA is essential for the synthesis and β-oxidation of fatty acids, and the synthesis of cholesterol, steroid hormones, vitamins A and D, and other isoprenoid derivatives. CoA is also involved in the synthesis of several amino acids and ∂-aminolevulinic acid, a precursor for the corrin ring of vitamin B_{12}, the porphyrin ring of heme, and of cytochromes. CoA is also necessary for the acetylation and fatty acid acylation of a variety of proteins.	Usually seen in conjunction with other water-soluble vitamin deficiencies. Experimental, isolated deficiency in humans produces fatigue, abdominal pain and vomiting, insomnia, and paresthesias of the extremities.	Doses exceeding 10 g/d may induce diarrhea.	Whole blood and urine concentrations of pantothenate are indicators of status; serum levels are not accurate.

TABLE 192–9. NUTRITIONAL TRACE ELEMENTS AND THEIR CLINICAL IMPLICATIONS

Trace Elements

	Biochemistry and Physiology	Deficiency	Toxicity	Assessment of Status
Chromium	Dietary chromium consists of both inorganic and organic forms. Its primary function in humans is to potentiate insulin action. It accomplishes this as a circulating dinicotino-glutathione complex called glucose tolerance factor. It thereby impacts on carbohydrate, fat, and protein metabolism.	Deficiency in humans described only in long-term TPN patients receiving insufficient chromium. Hyperglycemia, or impaired glucose intolerance, is uniformly observed. Elevated plasma free fatty acid concentrations, neuropathy, encephalopathy, and abnormalities in nitrogen metabolism are also reported. Whether supplemental chromium may improve glucose tolerance in mildly glucose intolerant but otherwise healthy individuals remains controversial.	Toxicity after oral ingestion is uncommon and seems confined to gastric irritation. Airborne exposure may cause contact dermatitis, eczema, skin ulcers, and bronchogenic carcinoma.	Plasma or serum concentration of chromium is a crude indicator of chromium status; it appears to be meaningful when the value is markedly above or below the normal range.
Copper	Copper is absorbed by a specific intestinal transport mechanism. It is carried to the liver where it is bound to ceruloplasmin, which circulates systemically and delivers copper to target tissues in the body. Excretion of copper is largely through bile into feces. Absorptive and excretory processes vary with the levels of dietary copper, providing a means of copper homeostasis. Copper serves as a component of many enzymes, including amine oxidases, ferroxidases, cytochrome c oxidase, dopamine β-hydroxylase, superoxide dismutase, and tyrosinase.	Dietary deficiency is rare; it has been observed in premature and low birth weight infants fed exclusively a cow's milk diet and in individuals receiving long-term TPN lacking copper. The clinical manifestations include depigmentation of skin and hair, neurologic disturbances, leukopenia, hypochromic microcytic anemia, and skeletal abnormalities. The anemia arises from impaired utilization of iron and is therefore a conditioned form of iron deficiency anemia. The deficiency syndrome, except for the anemia and leukopenia, is also observed in Mencke's disease, a rare inherited condition associated with impaired copper utilization.	Acute copper toxicity has been described after excessive oral intake and with absorption of copper salts applied to burned skin. Milder manifestations include nausea, vomiting, epigastric pain and diarrhea; coma and hepatic necrosis may ensue in severe cases. Toxicity may be seen with doses as low as 70 µg/kg/d. Chronic toxicity is also described. Wilson's disease is a rare, inherited disease associated with abnormally low ceruloplasmin levels and accumulation of copper in the liver and brain, eventually leading to damage to these two organs (see Ch. 188).	Practical methods for detecting marginal deficiency are not available. Marked deficiency is reliably detected by diminished serum copper and ceruloplasmin concentrations as well as low erythrocyte superoxide dismutase activity.
Fluorine	Known more commonly by its ionic form, fluoride. It is incorporated into the crystalline structure of bone, thereby altering its physical characteristics.	An intake of < 0.1 mg/d in infants, and < 0.5 in children is associated with a decreased incidence of dental caries. Optimal intake in adults is between 1.5 and 4 mg/d.	Acute ingestion of > 30 mg/kg body weight fluoride is likely to cause death. Excessive chronic intake (> 0.1 mg/kg/d) leads to mottling of the teeth (dental fluorosis), calcification of tendons and ligaments, exostoses, and may increase the brittleness of bones.	Estimates of intake or clinical assessment are used since no good laboratory test exists.

TABLE 192–9. NUTRITIONAL TRACE ELEMENTS AND THEIR CLINICAL IMPLICATIONS *(Continued)*

Trace Elements			
Biochemistry and Physiology	Deficiency	Toxicity	Assessment of Status
Iodine: Readily absorbed from the diet, concentrated in the thyroid, and integrated into the thyroid hormones, thyroxine (T_4), and triiodothyronine (T_3). The hormones circulate largely bound to thyroxine-binding globulin. They modulate resting energy expenditure and, in the developing human, growth and development.	In the absence of supplementation, populations relying primarily on food from soils with low iodine content have endemic iodine deficiency. Maternal iodine deficiency leads to fetal deficiency, which produces spontaneous abortions, stillbirths, hypothyroidism, cretinism, and dwarfism. Permanent cognitive deficits may also be induced by iodine deficiency during infancy and childhood. In the adult, compensatory hypertrophy of the thyroid (goiter) occurs along with varying degrees of hypothyroidism.	Large doses (> 2 mg/d in adults) may induce hypothyroidism by blocking thyroid hormone synthesis. Supplementation with > 100 μg per day to an individual who was formerly deficient occasionally induces hyperthyroidism.	Iodine status of a population can be estimated by the prevalence of goiter. Urinary excretion of iodine is an effective laboratory means of assessment. The TSH (thyroid-stimulating hormone) level in the blood is an indirect, and therefore not an entirely specific, means of assessment.
Iron: Participates in redox reactions in a number of metalloproteins such as hemoglobin, myoglobin, and the cytochrome enzymes. Primary storage form is ferritin Intestinal absorption is 15–20%. for "heme" iron and 1–8% for the iron contained in vegetables. Absorption of the latter form is enhanced by the ascorbic acid in foodstuffs, by poultry, fish, or beef and by an iron-deficient state; it is decreased by phytate and tannins.	The most common micronutrient deficiency in the world. Women of childbearing age constitute the highest risk group because of menstrual blood losses, pregnancy, and lactation. The classic deficiency syndrome is hypochromic, microcytic anemia. Glossitis and koilonychia (spoon nails) are also observed. Easy fatigability often develops as an early symptom. In children, mild deficiency insufficient to cause anemia is associated with behavioral disturbances and poor school performance.	Iron overload occurs when habitual dietary intake is extremely high, intestinal absorption is excessive, or repeated parenteral administration occurs. Excessive iron stores usually accumulate in reticuloendothelial tissues and cause little damage (hemosiderosis). If overload continues, iron eventually begins to accumulate in tissues such as the liver, pancreas, heart, and synovium; the result is hemochromatosis (see Ch. 189). Hereditary hemochromatosis arises as a result of homozygosity of a common, recessive trait. Excessive intestinal absorption of iron is observed in homozygotes.	Negative iron balance initially leads to depletion of iron stores in the bone marrow and an associated decrease in serum ferritin. As the severity of deficiency proceeds, serum iron (SI) decreases and total iron-binding capacity (TIBC) increases. An iron saturation ($=$ SI/TIBC) of $< 16\%$ suggests iron deficiency (see Ch. 132).
Manganese: A component of several metalloenzymes. Most manganese is in mitochondria, where it is a component of manganese superoxide dismutase.	Manganese deficiency in the human has not been conclusively demonstrated. It is said to cause hypocholesterolemia, weight loss, hair and nail changes, dermatitis, and impaired synthesis of vitamin K-dependent proteins.	Toxicity by oral ingestion unknown in humans. Toxic inhalation causes hallucinations, other alterations in mentation, and extrapyramidal movement disorders.	Until the deficiency syndrome is better defined, an appropriate measure of status will be difficult to develop.
Molybdenum: A cofactor in several enzymes, most prominently xanthine oxidase and sulfite oxidase.	A probable case of human deficiency is described secondary to parenteral administration of sulfite. This resulted in hyperoxypurinemia, hypouricemia, and low sulfate excretion.	Toxicity not well described in the human although it may interfere with copper metabolism at high doses.	Laboratory means of assessment not meaningful until deficiency syndrome is better defined.

Table continued on following page

physiologic functions of micronutrients, an ever increasing need to redefine the concept of deficiency has ensued. The original means by which the necessary intake of these nutrients was defined was typically based on a disease entity that occurred as a result of a flagrant deficiency of the nutrient, the so-called classic deficiency syndrome. In retrospect, this was naive, since it is now evident that most, if not all, micronutrients serve important functions in a wide variety of distinct biochemical systems. As the science of nutrition has come to appreciate this diversity in function, new deficiency syndromes are being defined.

Nevertheless, the redefinition of micronutrient deficiencies and the re-examination of recommended daily intakes have proven difficult for several reasons. In some instances there continues to be less than definitive evidence for the role of a particular micronutrient in a new function that has been proposed. Furthermore, even if a novel biochemical or physiologic role is well demonstrated for a nutrient, an appropriate question is whether optimization of such function translates into optimization of health. For example, providing supplemental vitamin E to elderly individuals who are vitamin E replete enhances T lymphocyte responsiveness to mitogens. Nevertheless, it is unclear whether this diminishes infection rates among the elderly. Another difficult problem pertains

to the use of micronutrients in supraphysiologic quantities, i.e., intakes that greatly exceed all conventional concepts of what is necessary for health. When taken in large quantities, some micronutrients affect physiologic functions beneficially (e.g., gram quantities of niacin to reduce low density lipoprotein [LDL] cholesterol). Such physiologic effects are not observed at more conventional levels of intake and are therefore usually considered to be "pharmacologic" effects of the nutrient. Nevertheless, if the dietary requirement of a nutrient is strictly defined as the minimal dose necessary for the maintenance of optimal health, as has been suggested, then supraphysiologic doses may have to be considered as the dietary requirement in such instances. Thus, the determination of "optimal" nutrient intake depends considerably on which physiologic effect is sought. Furthermore, if only a segment of the population will benefit from supraphysiologic quantities of a nutrient, should dietary guidelines for the entirety be established according to this effect?

Determining an adequate level of intake implies the existence of a means of measuring nutrient status. In seeking such indices, the diversity of function often makes it difficult to decide the most germane measurement. Tobacco smoking, for example, appears to diminish vitamin E levels in alveolar fluid but not in the serum. The

TABLE 192–9. NUTRITIONAL TRACE ELEMENTS AND THEIR CLINICAL IMPLICATIONS (Continued)

Trace Elements

	Biochemistry and Physiology	Deficiency	Toxicity	Assessment of Status
Selenium	Selenium is a component of several enzymes, most notably glutathione peroxidase and superoxide dismutase. These enzymes appear to prevent oxidative and free radical damage of various cell structures. Evidence suggests that the antioxidant protection conveyed by selenium operates in conjunction with vitamin E, since deficiency of one seems to enhance damage induced by a deficiency of the other. Selenium also participates in the enzymatic conversion of thyroxine to its more active metabolite, tri-iodothyronine.	Deficiency is rare in North America except in individuals receiving long-term total parenteral nutrition (TPN) lacking selenium. Such individuals have myalgias and/or cardiomyopathies. Populations in some regions of the world, most notably some parts of China, have marginal intake of selenium. In these regions, *Keshan's disease*, a condition characterized by cardiomyopathy, is endemic. The disease can be prevented (but not treated) by selenium supplementation.	Toxicity is associated with nausea, diarrhea, alterations in mental status, peripheral neuropathy, loss of hair and nails; such symptoms were observed in adults who inadvertently consumed between 27 and 2400 mg.	Erythrocyte glutathione peroxidase activity and plasma, or whole blood, selenium concentrations are moderately accurate indicators of status.
Zinc	Intestinal absorption occurs by a specific process that is enhanced by pregnancy and corticosteroids and diminished by coingestion of phytates, phosphates, iron, copper, lead, or calcium. Diminished intake of zinc leads to increased efficiency of absorption and decreased fecal excretion, providing a means of zinc homeostasis. Zinc is a component of over 100 enzymes; among these are DNA polymerase, RNA polymerase and tRNA synthetase.	Mild deficiency causes growth retardation in children. More severe deficiency is associated with growth arrest, teratogenicity, hypogonadism and infertility, dysgeusia, poor wound healing, diarrhea, a dermatitis on the extremities and around orifices, glossitis, alopecia, corneal clouding, loss of dark adaptation and behavioral changes. Impaired cellular immunity is observed. Excessive loss of gastrointestinal secretions through chronic diarrhea, fistulas, etc., may precipitate deficiency. *Acrodermatitis enteropathica* is a rare, recessively inherited disease in which intestinal absorption of zinc is impaired.	Acute zinc toxicity can usually be induced by ingestion of > 200 mg of zinc in a single day (in adults). It is manifested by epigastric pain, nausea, vomiting, and diarrhea. Hyperpnea, diaphoresis, and weakness may follow inhalation of zinc fumes. Copper and zinc compete for intestinal absorption: chronic ingestion of > 25 mg/d of zinc may lead to copper deficiency. Chronic ingestion of >150 mg/d has been reported to cause gastric erosions, low HDL cholesterol levels, and impaired cellular immunity.	There are no accurate indicators of zinc status available for routine clinical use. Plasma, erythrocyte, and hair zinc concentrations are frequently misleading. Acute illness, in particular, is known to diminish plasma zinc levels, in part by inducing a shift of zinc out of the plasma compartment and into the liver. Functional tests that determine dark adaptation, taste acuity, and rate of wound healing lack specificity.

concepts of "localized" nutrient deficiencies and tissue-specific requirements add a level of complexity to the determination of nutrient status.

The following examples illustrate how advances in nutritional science are prompting the redefinition of micronutrient requirements.

Folate. Guidelines regarding the necessary intake of folate were based, until recently, on the prevention of megaloblastic anemia. Measurements of serum and erythrocyte folate concentrations have been the most common means of assessing status; maintaining such levels within accepted normative ranges provides good assurance that folate status is adequate to prevent anemia.

It has become increasingly evident, however, that low folate levels that are insufficiently severe to cause anemia may still disturb normal biochemical and physiologic homeostasis. This is evidenced in part by an increase in serum homocysteine, an amino acid that is normally metabolized by a folate-dependent pathway. Some nutritional surveys identify elevated serum homocysteine levels in certain individuals whose habitual intake of folate is at or just above the US RDA (see Table 192–1), as well as in those whose serum folate levels are marginally above the conventional thresholds of deficiency. This elevation reflects less than optimal disposal of homocysteine, which is now believed to enhance the development of occlusive vascular disease. Vitamins B_6 and B_{12} are also important components of the biochemical pathways by which the body disposes of homocysteine, although their responsibility for hyperhomocysteinemia in the population is less evident.

The ingestion of folate in quantities considerably above the present recommended allowances appears to have other health benefits. Women taking folate supplements at the time of conception have a significantly lower risk of delivering a baby with a neural tube defect compared to women who do not take folate supplements but whose dietary intake or serum folate levels fall within

conventionally accepted ranges. A more controversial observation is the inverse relationship that exists between the ingestion of folate and the incidence of epithelial neoplasia of the uterine cervix, the colorectum, and the bronchopulmonary tree; the inverse relationship is observed even when folate status (or dietary intake) falls within the range of conventionally accepted norms.

These observations suggest that the ingestion of folate in quantities above what is presently regarded as adequate may contribute to the optimization of health. Substantial increases in the suggested intake of any micronutrient must be tempered, however, by the consideration of toxicity: with folate, this is primarily related to its ability to mask B_{12} deficiency when taken in doses exceeding 400 μg per day.

TABLE 192–10. EXAMPLES OF DRUG-MEDIATED EFFECTS ON MICRONUTRIENT STATUS

Drug(s)	Nutrient	Mechanism of Interaction
Dextroamphetamine, fenfluramine, levodopa	Potentially all micronutrients	Induce anorexia
Cholestyramine	Vitamin D, folate	Adsorbs nutrient, decreases absorption
Omeprazole	Vitamin B_{12}	Induces modest bacterial overgrowth; decreases gastric acid, impairing absorption
Sulfasalazine, methotrexate	Folate	Impair absorption and/or inhibit folate-dependent enzymes
Isoniazid	Pyridoxine	Impairs utilization of B_6
Nonsteroidal anti-inflammatory agents	Iron	Gastrointestinal blood loss
Penicillamine	Zinc	Increases renal excretion

Antioxidant and Free-Radical Scavenging Vitamins/ Provitamins. Vitamins A, C, and E, as well as many of the carotenoids, are effective antioxidants. In addition, vitamins C and E and some of the carotenoids can scavenge free radicals when taken in adequate quantities. Such properties have long been appreciated, but it is only recently that oxidation and free radical damage have been thought to play important roles in common degenerative illnesses such as atherosclerosis, cancer, cataracts, retinal degeneration, and neurodegenerative disorders.

Growing evidence indicates that LDL can undergo oxidation in vivo and that LDL thus transformed is particularly atherogenic. Prevention of LDL oxidation, at least in animal models, retards the process of atherogenesis. Supplementation in human subjects with severalfold the RDA of vitamin E, and perhaps some of the other antioxidant micronutrients, is an effective means of preventing LDL oxidation. Such intervention, however, remains unproved as a way to confer beneficial effects on human atherogenesis. Some evidence suggests that large doses of β-carotene may protect against the recurrence of coronary heart disease. If so, it is not yet clear whether this possible effect is mediated through the prevention of LDL oxidation.

Many epidemiologic studies indicate that the occurrence of cancers of the oral cavity, lung, esophagus, stomach, and perhaps colorectum is inversely related to dietary intake of fresh vegetables and fruits. Careful dissection of dietary data suggests that β-carotene and vitamin E content are the most protective components of these foodstuffs. High doses of vitamin A and some of its synthetic analogues (e.g., 13-cis-retinoic acid) can effectively reduce the recurrence of head and neck cancers, although hepatic toxicity is sometimes a limiting factor. Similarly, when taken in large doses, these agents as well as β-carotene or vitamin E have been shown to promote the regression of oral leukoplakia, a premalignant lesion. Daily supplementation with one to three times the US RDA of β-carotene, selenium, and vitamin E has been found to reduce the incidence of gastric adenocarcinoma in a disease-prevalent region of China. Contrarily, an intervention trial in Finland showed, if anything, an increase in lung cancer in smokers with daily supplementation of β-carotene. Further investigation is necessary to define any circumstances under which antioxidant nutrients can effectively prevent cancer.

Epidemiologic associations also suggest an inverse relationship between lens cataracts, macular degeneration, and the intake of vitamins C, E, and β-carotene. Considerable experimental evidence indicates that photo-oxidation can contribute to both of these common degenerative conditions of the eye. In animal models these degenerative processes have been retarded by supraphysiologic supplementation with vitamin C or E. Individuals who ingest vitamin C in excess of the US RDA have a lower incidence of cataract than those ingesting the RDA, suggesting a preventive role for larger than conventionally recommended doses of these nutrients. Nevertheless, insufficient prospective data exist at the present time to conclude that antioxidants specifically prevent cataracts and macular degeneration.

Vitamin B₁₂ and Neuropsychiatric Disease. Plasma B_{12} concentrations are considered to be an accurate indication of B_{12} status. The normal range for a healthy population has typically been considered 150 to 900 pg per milliliter; values above 150 or 200 pg per milliliter were felt to exclude B_{12} deficiency as a cause of neurologic or psychiatric syndromes. Some observations, still controversial, suggest that 7 to 10% of individuals who have plasma B_{12} values between 150 and 400 pg per milliliter may develop neuropsychiatric complications of B_{12} deficiency in the absence of megaloblastic anemia. Such persons can be identified by an elevated level of methylmalonic acid in the blood that decreases to normal after parenteral B_{12} administration. An elevation in serum methylmalonic acid is both a sensitive and specific indication of cellular B_{12} deficiency. Awareness of this phenomenon is particularly important, since it is now clear that atrophic gastritis, an asymptomatic condition that affects approximately 30% of the elderly population, frequently produces a modest decrease in B_{12} absorption.

Table 192–11 lists several examples of biochemical functions of vitamins that have only recently been identified. As nutritional science proceeds with defining the clinical significance of each of these new roles, and determines what quantities of each vitamin are necessary to optimize such functions, redefinition of the desirable range of vitamin status may well occur.

TABLE 192–11. NEWLY IDENTIFIED ROLES FOR VITAMINS

Vitamin or Provitamin	Classic Role(s)	New Role(s)
β-Carotene	Provitamin A	Antioxidant, free radical scavenger, cell-cell gap junction modulation
Niacin	NAD/NADP coenzyme	Reduction of LDL, and elevation of HDL, cholesterol
Folate	Hemopoietic factor	Diminishes homocysteinemia, incidence of neural tube defects
Vitamin A	Transduction of visual input in retina	Induction and maintenance of epithelial differentiation, maintenance of cell-mediated immunity, morphogenetic signal in embryogenesis
Vitamin D	Regulator of calcium, phosphate metabolism	Modulates epithelial proliferation and promotes differentiation
Vitamin B₆	Coenzyme for transamination	Modulation of steroid activity
Vitamin C	Hydroxylation coenzyme	Antioxidant

Sauberlich H, Machlin L (eds.): Beyond Deficiency: New Views on the Function and Health Effects of Vitamins. Ann NY Acad Sci 1992, vol. 669. *Excellent collection of discussions pertaining to new perspectives on functions of vitamins and how these perspectives impact on the definition of deficiency.*

Shils M, Olson J, Shike M (eds.): Modern Nutrition in Health and Disease, 8th ed. Malvern, Pa, Lea & Febiger, 1994, vol. 1. *Comprehensive, up-to-date reviews of biochemistry, physiology, and nutrition of each micronutrient.*

193 NUTRITIONAL ASSESSMENT
Bruce R. Bistrian

Nutritional assessment in clinical medicine has three primary goals: to identify the presence and type of malnutrition, to define health-threatening obesity, and to devise suitable diets as prophylaxis against disease later in life. The focus of this chapter is on the diagnosis of protein energy malnutrition (PEM) because of its wide prevalence and major impact on disease outcome. Other deficiency diseases are of much less relevance, since most occur in conjunction with PEM or with specific disease states such as thiamine deficiency with alcoholic liver disease, or fat-soluble vitamin deficiency with malabsorptive states. The classic deficiency diseases, either primary or secondary, are considered elsewhere in this volume. The widespread availability of parenteral and enteral therapeutic measures over the past decade that can provide adequate feeding regimens in virtually any disease condition make a rudimentary knowledge of the pathophysiology of PEM and its nutritional assessment essential for all primary care practitioners. (See Ch. 194.)

CLINICAL NUTRITIONAL ASSESSMENT

The clinical assessment of protein nutritional status is based principally on clinical history, simple anthropometry, and measurements of the levels of several secretory proteins. Although detailed dietary assessment can at times be helpful, in most circumstances physicians can safely limit their diet questions to whether patients have been following a prescribed diet and how much alcohol they drink. In ambulatory patients the ability to maintain usual and adequate weight generally indicates that serious micronutrient deficiency is not likely due to dietary inadequacy. Isolated vitamin deficiencies in the absence of weight loss or symptoms are rare, except perhaps for folate and B_{12}. Although nutritional anemias do exist, the role of dietary deficiency in folic acid or vitamin B_{12}-related anemias is minimal in the absence of underlying disease or weight loss. Only iron deficiency is a reasonable cause as a dietary anemia. By contrast, full dietary assessment and diet prescriptions are likely to help conditions such as fat malabsorption accompanied by weight loss, cramps, or diarrhea. Such evaluations are most effectively carried out by dietitians. Thus, detailed nutritional assessment of PEM with secondary assessment of vitamin and mineral deficiencies usually is needed only when PEM or a specific disorder known to interfere with nutrient metabolism, such as celiac disease, pernicious anemia, or nutrient-drug interactions, coexists. Even then the assessment should emphasize the likely deficiencies. For fat malabsorption, one should check levels of the fat-soluble vitamins, A, D, E, and K as well as important divalent and trivalent cations (Ca^{tt}, Zn^{tt}, Mg^{tt}, Fe^{ttt}). When ileal resection has occurred, serum B_{12} levels should be measured. Weight loss due to short gut syndrome should prompt assessment of the fat-soluble vitamins, folic acid, vitamin B_{12}, calcium, magnesium, zinc, and iron. Measurements of body water status (BUN, creatinine, serum sodium) and acid-base balance (CO_2 combining power, chloride, potassium, urine, and arterial pH) should be obtained if the diarrhea is profuse.

Clinically obvious marasmus and hypoalbuminemic malnutrition affect 25 to 50% of patients hospitalized for acute care. Many of these patients can benefit from nutritional support and require a thorough clinical nutritional assessment, including dietary history, physical examination, and laboratory tests that serve to confirm clinical impressions. The history should list information about the timing and amount of weight loss, medical illnesses, medications, gastrointestinal symptoms (abdominal pain, diarrhea, dysphagia), diet habits (eating fewer than two meals a day, alcohol consumption, dental status), social habits (eats alone, needs assistance in self-care), economic status (enough money for food), and mental status, particularly the presence of depressive symptoms. A special focus should be reserved for the elderly in whom PEM due to these last factors is more common.

WEIGHT LOSS

A recent unintended weight loss of 10 pounds should prompt efforts to diagnose the underlying disorder or social circumstance. Weight loss alone does not distinguish the composition of tissue loss, which can range from 25 to 30% lean tissue in semistarvation to 50% lean tissue loss following starvation plus injury. Therefore, unintentional weight loss of more than 10 pounds indicates a need for thorough nutritional assessment. Weight loss in excess of 10% of usual weight should be considered to represent PEM that will impair physiologic function, particularly muscle strength and endurance. Weight loss in excess of 20% should be considered severe PEM that will substantially impair most organ systems. If major elective surgery is planned, such individuals would likely benefit from adequate feeding preoperatively. If palliative or curative radiotherapy or systemic chemotherapy is planned, adequate feeding during therapy by use of supplemental formulas, tube feeding, or parenteral nutrition (in that order) is indicated. However, if the weight loss represents end-stage systemic illness (e.g., cancer, end-stage liver disease, AIDS) for which no primary therapy is planned or effective, invasive nutritional support is rarely indicated.

PHYSICAL EXAMINATION

Although the patient's external appearance and a check of his or her skin, eyes, mouth, hair, and nails often provide a clue to the presence of nutritional abnormalities (Table 193–1), the physical findings of deficiency syndromes of vitamins, essential fatty acids, and trace metals are relatively insensitive and nonspecific. With respect to PEM, only the marasmic form of semistarvation is evident at examination. Loss of subcutaneous fat and skeletal muscle is manifested by sunken temples, thin extremities, wasting of the muscles of the hand, and rarely edema. While kwashiorkor in children is characterized by severe edema, and a pot-belly appearance due to hepatomegaly and ascites, one rarely encounters these clinical signs in hypoalbuminemic malnutrition.

The most useful element in the physical examination is body weight, which is expressed as a relative value to evaluate the patient in relation to the healthy population. Weight and height are easily obtained and there are established standards for comparison (Table 193–2). Although newer standards are available, they reflect the increasing prevalence of obesity in the U.S. population. Use of the 1959 standards allows the same tables to be used to diagnose significant PEM (less than 85% desirable weight, which approximates the 5th percentile) and significant obesity defined as incurring excessive mortality risk (greater than 130% desirable weight). Although severe PEM will often occur at levels greater than 85% desirable weight, this generally will be detected by percent weight loss or upper arm anthropometry. Height can be measured in the reclining patient by using a tape measure, and in certain situations patient history may be relied upon. The major confounding variable that limits the value of weight and height as an index of PEM is the tendency for water retention with disease, and thus weight gain may not reflect an increase in lean body mass or protein content. Fluid retention is particularly a problem with hypoalbuminemic malnutrition because of the effects of aldosterone, antidiuretic hormone, and insulin stimulated by the stress response to cause sodium and fluid retention. Fluid retention, however, is not common on presentation to the physician's office or initially to the hospital except in diseases such as cardiac failure, end-stage liver disease, and severe renal disease.

TABLE 193–1. DESIRABLE WEIGHT IN POUNDS IN RELATION TO HEIGHT FOR ADULT MEN AND WOMEN, 25 YEARS OR OLDER*

Men Medium Frame				Women Medium Frame			
Height Ft.	In.	Range	Midpoint	Height Ft.	In.	Range	Midpoint
				4	8	93–104	98.5
				4	9	95–107	101
				4	10	98–110	104
				4	11	101–113	107
				5	0	104–116	110
5	1	113–124	118.5	5	1	107–119	113
5	2	116–128	122	5	2	110–123	116.5
5	3	119–131	125	5	3	113–127	120
5	4	122–134	128	5	4	117–132	124.5
5	5	125–138	131.5	5	5	121–136	128.5
5	6	129–142	135.5	5	6	125–140	132.5
5	7	133–147	140	5	7	129–144	136.5
5	8	137–151	144	5	8	133–148	140.5
5	9	141–155	148	5	9	137–152	144.5
5	10	145–160	153	5	10	141–156	148.5
5	11	149–165	157				
6	0	153–170	161.5				
6	1	157–175	166				
6	2	162–180	171				
6	3	167–185	176				

Adapted from the Metropolitan Life Insurance Company Statistical Bulletin 40:1, 1959.
* Corrected to nude weights and heights by assuming 1-inch heel for men, 2-inch heel for women, and indoor clothing weight of 5 and 3 pounds for men and women, respectively.

TABLE 193–2. CLINICAL SIGNS AND SYMPTOMS OF NUTRITIONAL INADEQUACY IN ADULT PATIENTS

	Clinical Sign or Symptom	Nutrient
General	Wasted, skinny	Calorie
	Loss of appetite	Protein-energy
Skin	Psoriasiform rash, eczematous scaling	Zinc, vitamin A, EFA
	Pallor	Folate, iron, vitamin B_{12}, copper
	Follicular hyperkeratosis	Vitamin A, vitamin C
	Perifollicular petechiae	Vitamin C
	Flaking dermatitis	Protein-energy, niacin, riboflavin, zinc
	Bruising	Vitamin C, vitamin K
	Pigmentation changes	Niacin, protein-energy
	Scrotal dermatosis	Riboflavin
	Thickening and dryness of skin	Linoleic acid
Head	Temporal muscle wasting	Protein-energy
Hair	Sparse and thin, dyspigmentation	Protein
	Easy to pull out	Protein
	Corkscrew hairs	Vitamin C
Eyes	History of night blindness (also impaired visual recovery after glare)	Vitamin A, zinc
	Photophobia, blurring, conjunctival inflammation	Riboflavin, vitamin A
	Corneal vascularization	Riboflavin
	Xerosis, Bitot spots, keratomalacia	Vitamin A
Mouth	Glossitis	Riboflavin, niacin, folic acid, vitamin B_{12}, pyridoxine
	Bleeding gums	Vitamin C, riboflavin
	Cheilosis	Riboflavin, pyridoxine, niacin
	Angular stomatitis	Riboflavin, pyridoxine, niacin
	Hypogeusia	Zinc
	Tongue fissuring	Niacin
	Tongue atrophy	Riboflavin, niacin, iron
	Nasolabial seborrhea	Pyridoxine
Neck	Goiter	Iodine
	Parotid enlargement	Protein
Thorax	Thoracic rosary	Vitamin D
Abdomen	Diarrhea	Niacin, folate, vitamin B_{12}
	Distention	Protein-energy
	Hepatomegaly	Protein-energy
Extremities	Edema	Protein, thiamine
	Softening of bone	Vitamin D, calcium, phosphorus
	Bone tenderness	Vitamin D
	Bone ache, joint pain	Vitamin C
	Muscle wasting and weakness	Protein, calorie, vitamin D, selenium, sodium chloride
	Muscle tenderness, muscle pain	Thiamine
Nails	Spooning	Iron
	Transverse lines	Protein
Neurologic	Tetany	Calcium, magnesium
	Paresthesias	Thiamine, vitamin B_{12}
	Loss of reflexes, wrist drop, foot drop	Thiamine
	Loss of vibratory and position sense	Vitamin B_{12}
	Ataxia	Vitamin B_{12}
	Dementia, disorientation	Niacin
Blood	Anemia	Vitamin B_{12}, folate, iron, pyridoxine
	Hemolysis	Phosphorus, vitamin E

Modified from Russel RM: Nutritional assessment. *In* Wyngaarten JB, Smith LH Jr, Bennett JC: Cecil Textbook of Medicine, 19th ed. Philadelphia, 1992, WB Saunders, pp 1151–1155.

The body mass index (BMI), which is the weight in kilograms divided by the height in meters squared, has recently gained favor as a nutritional measure because of two valuable attributes. The measure is relatively independent of height, and the same standards apply to males and females. Normal nutrition is defined as a BMI of 18 to 25 with significant obesity defined as a BMI > 28. Evidence from less developed countries suggests the BMI is better correlated with outcome than weight/height.

UPPER ARM ANTHROPOMETRY

Approximately 50% of body fat is subcutaneous. The use of skinfold calipers to define the triceps skinfold is the most practical technique to estimate body fat. Standards for skinfold measurements are available from the Health and Nutrition Examination Survey (HANES I and II), which were derived from a probability sample of the U.S. population. Generally less than the 5th percentile is used to define abnormality (Table 193–3). The principal value of the triceps skinfold (TSF) is to determine the arm muscle circumference (AMC) or arm muscle area.

$$AMC(cm) = Arm\ Circumference - \frac{(\pi)\ (TSF\ in\ mm)}{10}$$

The arm muscle circumference is a specific measure of PEM if the 5th or 10th percentile is chosen as the cutoff point and is particularly valuable in edematous states or in amputees in whom weights are inaccurate or insensitive. The triceps skinfold and arm muscle circumference measurements are most useful in initial defining of marasmic-type malnutrition or the mixed disorder. Nearly all dietitians are skilled in upper arm anthropometry.

SERUM PROTEINS

Despite many concerns, the serum albumin level remains the traditional standard for nutritional assessment by virtue of its extensive history and its continued use to separate the two principal forms of PEM. Hypoalbuminemia is a strong predictor of risk for morbidity and mortality in both hospitalized and ambulatory patients. In almost all cases, except perhaps for hereditary analbuminemia, excessive loss due to nephrosis, and occasionally in protein-losing enteropathy, hypoalbuminemia identifies the injury response and thus the presence of an illness with the accompanying effects of anorexia and depression of immune function. Given the half-life for albumin of 18 to 20 days and the fractional replacement rate of about 10% per day, the return of serum albumin to normal takes about 2 weeks of feeding when the stress response remits. Levels of other proteins such as transferrin, prealbumin, and

TABLE 193–3. 5TH, 10TH, AND 50TH PERCENTILE FOR TRICEPS SKINFOLD (TSF) AND MID UPPER ARM MUSCLE CIRCUMFERENCE (MUAMC) OF AMERICAN MEN AND WOMEN FROM THE NHANES I SURVEY

Age Group	MUAMC (cm) Percentile			TSF (mm) Percentile		
	5TH	10TH	50TH	5TH	10TH	50TH
Male						
18–24	23.8	24.8	27.9	4.5	6.0	11.0
18–24	23.5	24.4	27.2	4.0	5.0	9.5
25–34	24.2	25.3	28.0	4.5	5.5	12.0
35–44	25.0	25.6	28.7	5.0	6.0	12.0
45–54	26.0	26.9	28.1	5.0	6.0	11.0
55–64	22.8	26.4	27.9	5.0	6.0	11.0
65–74	22.5	23.7	26.9	4.5	5.5	11.0
Female						
18–24	13.4	19.0	21.8	11.0	13.0	22.0
18–24	17.7	18.5	20.6	9.4	11.0	18.0
25–34	18.3	18.9	21.4	10.5	12.0	21.0
35–44	18.5	19.2	22.0	12.0	14.0	23.0
45–54	18.8	19.5	22.2	13.0	15.0	25.0
55–64	18.6	19.5	22.6	11.0	14.0	25.0
65–74	18.6	19.5	22.5	11.5	14.0	23.0

From Bishop CW, Bowen PE, Ritchey SJ: Norms for nutritional assessment of American adults by upper arm anthropometry. Am J. Clin. Nutr. 34:2530, 1981.

retinol-binding protein with respective half-lives of 7 days, 2 days, and ½ day also fall acutely with injury and respond more quickly when stress remits. However, serum transferrin also varies with iron status, and prealbumin and retinol-binding protein vary with dietary carbohydrate and renal function. As a result, these proteins do not identify the presence and severity of the stress response any better than albumin.

NUTRITIONAL THERAPY AND ITS ASSESSMENT

The same indices that are used in the baseline nutritional assessment can be used to assess response to therapy, provided certain points are kept in mind. In the stressed, hospitalized patient receiving nutrition, day-to-day weight changes generally reflect shifts in fluid balance rather than energy balance. In the ambulatory setting, weight increases or decreases are most likely to reflect changes in protein nutritional status and body fat, because the underlying illness is usually less severe. Even the most sensitive research methods for assessing changes in lean body mass, however, do not offer major improvements in diagnosis in the more seriously ill. Techniques that measure total body water such as isotope dilution and underwater weighing, from which lean tissue is extrapolated, fail to account for the distortion in hydration of lean tissue with illness. Surrogate measures of total body protein to estimate lean tissues such as total body potassium measurement do not adjust for differing potassium/nitrogen ratios with disease. A newer method, multi-frequency body impedance, does show promise as a simple, accurate, noninvasive method that may allow distinction between intracellular and extracellular water, with the former used to estimate lean tissue.

In the unstressed patient with marasmus, appropriate protein and calorie intake should cause a positive nitrogen balance of 2 to 6 grams per day (60 to 180 grams lean tissue) and slow weight gain depending on the positive energy balance. For instance, a 300 kilocalorie excess of intake over expenditure would provide approximately 120 grams of lean tissue (100 kilocalorie equivalent) plus 200 kilocalories (22 grams) as fat for a total of 140 grams or about ⅓ pound of weight per day. Weight gains in excess of this probably reflect sodium and water retention due to the insulin stimulated by dietary carbohydrate. Such overhydration can be improved by reducing salt and limiting fluid intake. In patients with hypoalbuminemic malnutrition who are no longer stressed, a similar nutritional regimen will lead to a comparable gain of tissue, but weight change may vary as edema becomes mobilized, with normalization in serum albumin in 2 to 4 weeks. In stressed patients with hypoalbuminemic malnutrition, appropriate nutritional support will often not restore lean tissue but will improve other important functions such as wound healing and immune competence. Both the stress response and the limited activity level reduce the efficiency of skeletal muscle repletion, which represents 30% of body weight and 75% of actively metabolizing lean tissue. Functional testing of muscle strength and endurance such as hand dynamometry may prove useful as assessment tools in the future. Similarly, any reduction of other physiologic function or impairment in performing the usual activities of daily living will accentuate PEM.

Although caloric expenditure can now be reliably and easily measured with portable indirect calorimeters, estimated energy expenditures are sufficient in most clinical situations. The three components of total energy expenditure (TEE) are basal energy expenditure (about 55 to 65% of TEE), thermal effect of feeding (about 10% of TEE), and activity energy expenditure (the remainder). An energy intake of 30 to 35 kilocalories per kilogram of body weight will maintain most sedentary ambulatory patients, with adjustments upward or downward in 200- to 300-kilocalorie increments as prompted by biweekly changes in weight. Although young, severely burned or traumatized patients may require 35 to 40 kilocalories per kilogram in the acute phase to meet TEE, most postoperative patients who require invasive nutritional support for mechanical or infectious complications need no more than 30 kilocalories per kilogram because of their older age and reduced activity energy expenditure. Overfeeding should be avoided in such patients.

Daley BJ, Bistrian BR: Nutritional assessment. *In* Zaloga G (ed.): Nutrition in Critical Care. St Louis, CV Mosby, 1993, pp 9–33. *Discusses etiologic factors in development of protein-caloric malnutrition (PCM) and nutritional assessment methods.*

Functional tests of PCM and indirect calorimetry are adjunctive measures of nutritional status.

Hill G: Body composition research: Implications for the practice of clinical nutrition. JPEN 16:197, 1992. *Superb presentation of clinical nutritional assessment in critically ill patients evaluated in terms of functional indices, protein kinetic studies, and basic body composition techniques of* in vivo *neutron activation analysis and labeled water.*

McMahon MM, Bistrian BR: Anthropometric assessment of nutritional status in hospitalized patients. *In* Himes JH (ed.): Anthropometric Assessment of Nutritional Status. New York, Wiley-Liss, 1991, pp 365–381. *Discusses in detail the value of upper arm anthropometry and creatinine excretion in nutritional assessment.*

194 PROTEIN-ENERGY MALNUTRITION

Robert B. Baron

Protein-energy malnutrition (PEM) occurs when inadequate protein and/or calories are ingested to meet an individual's nutritional requirements. PEM may be primary, as a result of inadequate food intake, or secondary, as a result of illness. In developing nations, PEM is most often primary and affects predominantly infants and children. It is the most important nutritional disorder and one of the developing world's most important health problems. In industrialized nations, PEM is most often secondary to other diseases and affects both children and adults. In North America and Europe, 28 to 80% of hospitalized patients have been reported to have secondary PEM. This chapter emphasizes clinical features of secondary PEM as seen in industrialized nations.

Pathogenesis

Secondary PEM is caused by decreased intake of calories and protein, increased nutrient losses, or increased nutrient requirements (Table 194–1). It can develop slowly owing to chronic illness or chronic semistarvation or rapidly owing to acute illness.

In uncomplicated starvation and semistarvation, metabolism adapts to reduce the breakdown of lean body mass. Fat and fat-derived fuels gradually replace glucose as the major energy source. During the initial phase of a complete fast, glucose requirements for the brain, bone marrow, renal medulla, and peripheral nerves are provided by glycogen. Glycogen stores, however, last for only 12 to 24 hours. As glucose levels decline, insulin levels also decline and glucagon levels increase. Amino acids, particularly alanine, are released by muscle. Hepatic gluconeogenesis from amino acids provides glucose for the central nervous system and other glycolytic tissues. The changes in insulin and glucagon also favor lipolysis. Mobilized fatty acids provide the fuel for the remaining tissues. By the second week of a complete fast, fatty acids are less completely oxidized and more of them form ketone bodies. Ketones become the primary energy source for the brain and reduce the need for glucose. The muscles catabolize less protein and release less alanine, thus conserving their protein content.

TABLE 194–1. CAUSES OF PROTEIN-ENERGY MALNUTRITION IN HOSPITALIZED PATIENTS

Decreased Oral Intake	
Anorexia	Poverty
Nausea	Old age
Dysphagia	Social isolation
Pain	Substance abuse
Gastrointestinal obstruction	Depression
Poor dentition	
Increased Nutrient Losses	
Malabsorption	Nephrosis
Diarrhea	Fistula drainage
Bleeding	Protein-losing enteropathy
Glycosuria	
Increased Nutrient Requirements	
Fever	Trauma
Infection	Burns
Neoplasms	Medications
Surgery	

Adaptation also decreases the body's total energy requirement, by as much as 40% in severe chronic undernutrition. Absolute requirements decrease as body weight diminishes owing to a decrease in body mass. More importantly, however, energy requirements also decrease per unit of body mass. Both ingested food and circulating endogenous substrates are utilized more efficiently. More endogenous amino acids, for example, are utilized for protein synthesis than for oxidation. In addition, virtually all of the body's biochemical and physiologic processes are curtailed. Less energy is expended for the sodium-potassium pump, protein turnover, temperature regulation, the inflammatory response, and the function of most body organs during chronic undernutrition.

During a severe acute illness, hormonal and inflammatory responses prevent this adaptation to starvation and result in changes in protein and energy metabolism that can rapidly lead to PEM (Table 194–2). Circulating levels of the catecholamines, glucocorticoids, glucagon, and growth hormone are all increased. Although necessary to mediate the body's response to physical stress, these hormonal and inflammatory changes result in marked increases in energy expenditure, nitrogen loss, gluconeogenesis, and the failure of ketoadaptation. In this manner, changes in body composition, including depletion of protein and fat stores, may occur rapidly. Several other compounds mediate the systemic response to inflammation, including cytokines such as tumor necrosis factor, interleukin (IL)-1, IL-2, IL-6, interferon-γ, and lipid mediators such as platelet-activating factor, thromboxane A_2, leukotriene B_4 and prostaglandin E_2. Complex interconnections relate hormones, cytokines, and lipid mediators and are only partially understood. Rather than a simple cascade, mediators may respond variably to different stimuli; some with overlapping effects may be initiated simultaneously, whereas others may be interconnected by amplification and feedback loops.

The resting metabolic expenditure (RME) may increase significantly during the response to illness. In burns involving greater than 40% of the body surface area, for example, the RME may double. In other critical illnesses such as trauma or sepsis, the RME typically increases by 20 to 50%. Nitrogen losses also typically increase by 20 to 100%. During the response to illness, skeletal muscles release amino acids at an accelerated rate. These can then be metabolized for energy or shifted to the liver or other visceral organs, where their need for protein synthesis is more immediate. During prolonged illness and continued energy and protein deficiency, however, depletion of visceral protein also occurs and can lead to functional impairment of body organs.

Physiologic Consequences

Virtually every organ and organ system of the body can undergo marked morphologic and functional changes during protein-energy malnutrition.

BODY WEIGHT. The most obvious manifestation of chronic PEM is loss of body weight. Most patients can tolerate a loss of 5% to 10% without significant consequences, but losses greater than 40% below ideal weight are almost always fatal. Both adipose tissue and the lean body mass are depleted, but losses of adipose tissue are greater. Extracellular water remains nearly constant, resulting in its relative increase. In severe PEM, the body's visceral organs also decrease in size. In experimental animals, for example, a 7-day fast results in a 40% decrease in liver mass, 28% decrease in the gastrointestinal tract, 20% decrease in the kidneys, and 17% decrease in cardiac mass. During acute PEM caused by critical illness, changes in body weight and adipose stores may be less marked despite changes in organ morphology and function. Many patients may actually gain weight owing to retention of sodium and body water.

HEART. Severe PEM results in both quantitative and qualitative changes in the heart. In the "Minnesota Experiment," in which 32 male volunteers were semistarved for 6 months, a 24% decrease in body weight was associated with an 18% decrease in cardiac stroke volume and a 38% decrease in cardiac index. Animal studies have demonstrated similar findings, as well as decreases in left ventricular contractility and compliance, decreased myocardial glycogen, myofibrillar atrophy, and interstitial edema. These changes are reversed with nutritional repletion.

LUNG. The lung parenchyma is minimally affected during PEM, but marked changes in pulmonary function can occur as a result of the loss of mass and strength of the muscles of breathing. In the Minnesota Experiment, vital capacity, tidal volume, and minute volume declined by 8%, 19%, and 30%, respectively, after 24 weeks of semistarvation. The ventilatory response to hypoxia is also decreased during semistarvation, but the clinical significance of this is unclear.

GASTROINTESTINAL TRACT. During severe PEM, gastric motility slows and gastric acid secretion decreases. The most significant effects of PEM on the luminal gastrointestinal tract affect the small intestine. Total small bowel mass decreases, primarily owing to mucosal atrophy and loss of villi. Lymphocytic infiltration of surface epithelial cells can occur, and epithelial cell renewal slows down. Both disaccharidase enzyme activity and the rate of absorption of amino acids decline. Although pancreatic endocrine activity is spared, exocrine insufficiency can accompany severe PEM. Similar changes in the gastrointestinal tract are observed in individuals fed exclusively with parenteral nutrition, suggesting that stimulation of the gut by intraluminal nutrients is necessary for normal structure and function.

LIVER. In typical secondary PEM, liver mass decreases but its histology remains normal. Fat, protein, and glycogen are depleted, but the number of hepatocytes is preserved. In contrast, children with severe, primary protein deficiency resulting in kwashiorkor have enlarged livers with fatty infiltration and excess glycogen. In both instances, serum levels of albumin and other serum transport proteins commonly go down owing to diminished hepatic synthesis.

KIDNEY. Renal mass decreases during PEM, but histology remains normal. Renal function is well preserved except for an impaired concentrating ability due to a lowering of the medullary osmotic gradient.

ENDOCRINE. The endocrine response to PEM is complex and affected by the extent of concurrent illnesses, as discussed above. Serum thyroxine typically falls to the lower limits of normal or slightly below. Peripheral conversion of thyroxine (T_4) to triiodothyronine (T_3) is commonly decreased, favoring the conversion to reverse triiodothyronine. Serum TSH and the TSH response to TRH remain unaltered. Gonadal hormones are also affected. In men, testosterone levels are decreased and LH and FSH levels are appropriately increased. In women, gonadotropin release is depressed despite low levels of circulating estrogens.

IMMUNOLOGIC FUNCTION. Severe PEM importantly affects the immune system. Virtually all components of the immune system are adversely affected in rough proportion to the degree of nutritional impairment. Peripheral blood lymphocyte counts commonly decline to values often < 1200 per cubic millimeter. Both the percentage of T cells and T-cell functions are depressed. Skin tests for delayed hypersensitivity reactions often become nonreactive, and lymphocyte responses, weaken to phytohemagglutinin and poke weed mitogens.

Humoral immunity is affected in a more variable fashion. Specific antibody responses are depressed in some instances and preserved in others. For example, antibody production following administration of poliovirus, tetanus, diphtheria, measles, and pneumococcal polysaccharide antigens remains normal, whereas impaired responses follow the administration of yellow fever and

TABLE 194–2. PHYSIOLOGIC COMPARISON OF UNCOMPLICATED STARVATION AND SEVERE CATABOLIC ILLNESS

Physiologic Characteristics	Uncomplicated Starvation	Catabolic Illness
Catecholamines	Decreased	Increased
Glucagon	Decreased	Increased
Cortisol	Decreased	Increased
Insulin	Decreased	Increased
Cytokines	Variable	Increased
Metabolic rate	Decreased	Increased
Proteolysis	Decreased	Increased
Gluconeogenesis	Decreased	Increased
Nitrogen excretion	Decreased	Increased
Fatty acid utilization	Increased	Increased
Adaptation to starvation	Present	Absent

Adapted from Weinsier RD, Heimburger DC, Butterworth CE: Handbook of Clinical Nutrition. 2nd ed. St. Louis, CV Mosby, 1989.

influenza A vaccines. In some instances, the affinities and binding capacity of antibodies are reduced.

Slight neutropenia may occur during PEM but the usual concurrent bacterial infections cause leukocytosis. Neutrophils are normal morphologically, but some measures of neutrophil function, including chemotaxis and bacterial killing, are abnormal. Phagocytosis is usually normal.

Levels of individual complement components, other than C4, and total serum hemolytic complement activity are commonly decreased. Other nonspecific host defense mechanisms, including interferon production, opsonization, and plasma lysozyme production, may also be adversely affected by protein-calorie undernutrition. Acute phase reactants such as C-reactive proteins, α_2-macroglobulin, α_1-antitrypsin, and haptoglobin tend to be elevated. Changes in the body's anatomic barriers to infection, including atrophy of the skin and gastrointestinal mucosa, may contribute to an increased risk of infection.

It is not possible to define the exact mechanisms of enhanced susceptibility to infections observed with PEM. Each of the abnormalities of the immune response probably contributes in part. Micronutrient deficiencies may occur concurrently with PEM and can also cause significant abnormalities in the immune response.

WOUND HEALING. Almost all aspects of wound healing are adversely affected in patients with severe PEM. Neovascularization, fibroblast proliferation, collagen synthesis, and wound remodeling are delayed. Local factors, such as edema associated with hypoalbuminemia and micronutrient deficiencies, may contribute to poor wound healing in undernourished patients. In mild PEM, however, wound healing is relatively well-preserved despite negative nitrogen balance. Even during complete starvation, endogenous substrates can be effectively utilized for collagen synthesis during the early phases of wound healing.

Clinical Manifestations

The diverse clinical manifestations of PEM range from mild growth retardation and weight loss to several distinct clinical syndromes. This diversity reflects differences in the relative degree of protein and energy deficiency, the cause of the deficiency, the severity and duration of the deficiency, the age of the patient, and the association of other illnesses or nutritional deficiencies. In children in the developing world with severe PEM, for example, the classic syndromes of kwashiorkor (predominant protein deficiency) and marasmus (predominant energy deficiency) may develop. Marasmic kwashiorkor and intermediate syndrome may be seen when protein deficiency develops in combination with chronic energy deficiency.

KWASHIORKOR. Children with severe kwashiorkor commonly have a decreased blood pressure, bradycardia, and hypothermia. Body weight is usually low but may be normal owing to edema and anasarca. Affected children are characteristically apathetic, lethargic, and anorectic. They may move about little, or not at all. Their skins develop a "flaky paint" dermatitis with dry, hyperpigmented, hyperkeratotic lesions over the face, extremities, and perineum. The hair is typically sparse, dry, and brittle and may be reddish or yellowish. The abdomen is distended owing to hepatomegaly and ascites. The extremities are commonly wasted and edematous. Clinical signs of concurrent micronutrient deficiency may also be present (see Ch. 192.2).

The serum albumin typically falls below 2.8 grams per deciliter with a lymphocyte count less than 1200 cells per cubic millimeter. A mild anemia is common; it is usually normochromic and normocytic unless other deficiencies coexist. The serum transferrin usually declines but may be normal or slightly elevated if iron deficiency coexists. Other serum transport proteins, including prealbumin and retinol-binding protein, decrease. Serum glucose and lipids likewise go down. Serum levels of liver enzymes most often remain normal and may be low. Blood urea nitrogen and urinary urea nitrogen are low. Fluid and electrolyte disorders are common, particularly hypokalemia, hypophosphatemia, and a hyperchloremic metabolic acidosis.

MARASMUS. Children with marasmus have less characteristic manifestations. Although their pulse, blood pressure, and body temperature may be low, they tend to be less apathetic and lethargic and to have a good appetite. Growth is retarded and the weight low. Muscle wasting is obvious, as is loss of body fat. Such children look emaciated, but have no edema. The skin is dry and loose with decreased turgor. The dermatitis of kwashiorkor is usually absent. The hair is thin, dry, and dull. The abdomen is thin without signs of hepatomegaly or edema. Typically, there are fewer laboratory abnormalities than in children with kwashiorkor. Serum albumin and other transport proteins are often normal. A mild anemia is common. Any of the other laboratory abnormalities of kwashiorkor may exist but usually are absent.

SECONDARY PROTEIN-ENERGY MALNUTRITION. The clinical manifestations of secondary PEM also vary considerably, in large part reflecting the associated illness that has caused the malnutrition, the nutritional status of the patient prior to the illness, and the rate at which it develops (Table 194–3). Marasmus-like secondary PEM typically results from chronic indolent diseases such as chronic obstructive pulmonary disease or cancer. Most patients experience a gradual wasting process that begins with weight loss and proceeds through stages of mild, moderate, and severe cachexia. In its most severe form, virtually all body fat stores disappear and muscle mass wastes away, most noticeably in the temporal and interosseous muscles. Laboratory studies may be relatively unremarkable. Serum albumin, for example, may be normal or slightly decreased, rarely decreasing to < 2.8 grams per deciliter.

In contrast, kwashiorkor-like secondary PEM occurs primarily in association with acute life-threatening illnesses such as trauma, burns, and sepsis. Owing to the rapidity of onset, subcutaneous fat and muscle mass reflect the patient's baseline nutritional status and are typically normal or, if the patient is obese, increased. Serum proteins, however, typically decline with serum albumin < 2.8 grams per deciliter. Dependent edema, ascites, and anasarca may be present and the hair may be easily pluckable. As with primary PEM, combinations of marasmus-like secondary PEM and kwashiorkor-like secondary PEM can occur simultaneously, typically in patients with indolent chronic diseases who develop a superimposed acute illness.

Diagnosis

The absence of distinct clinical manifestations can make the diagnosis of PEM difficult. A high index of suspicion based on the patient's risk factors for malnutrition, the overall clinical setting, and close observation is often necessary.

BODY WEIGHT. The most sensitive diagnostic measure is a documented history of weight loss, quantified as a percent of origi-

TABLE 194–3. COMPARISON OF SEVERE MARASMUS-LIKE AND KWASHIORKOR-LIKE SECONDARY PROTEIN-ENERGY MALNUTRITION

Syndrome	Clinical Setting	Time Course	Clinical Features	Laboratory Findings	Prognosis
Marasmus-like PEM	Chronic illness	Months	History of weight loss Muscle wasting Absent subcutaneous fat	Normal or mildly reduced serum proteins	Variable; depends on underlying disease
Kwashiorkor-like PEM	Acute, catabolic illness	Weeks	Normal fat and muscle Edema Easily pluckable hair	Serum albumin < 2.8 g/dl	Poor

Adapted from Weinsier RL, Heimburger DC, Butterworth CE: Handbook of Clinical Nutrition. 2nd ed. St. Louis, CV Mosby, 1989.

nal body weight. Weight changes, however, may be obscured by edema. Some patients, particularly those with a severe acute illness such as sepsis, burns, or multiple trauma, can develop severe protein depletion rapidly without undergoing much weight loss. Nevertheless, most authors consider a 10% loss of body weight occurring during an acute illness to be clinically significant.

LABORATORY TESTS. Each of the clinical abnormalities affecting patients with severe PEM can be used as a diagnostic test to detect undernutrition. Most valuable are the serum albumin, other serum transport proteins such as transferrin, prealbumin, and retinol-binding protein, anergy to skin test antigens, total lymphocyte count, blood urea nitrogen, urinary excretion of creatinine, and anthropometric measures of body composition such as skinfold thickness and mid-arm muscle circumference. Each of these tests when abnormal has been shown to predict poor clinical outcomes in patients in a variety of clinical settings. It remains unclear whether the poor outcomes predicted by excessive weight loss or by abnormalities in these tests reflect the consequences of PEM or the severity of the underlying illness.

CLINICAL ASSESSMENT. A thorough, nutritionally focused history and physical examination can predict outcomes as well as can any of the above tests and indices. The history should examine recent reduction in dietary intake, changes in body weight, gastrointestinal symptoms, the underlying illness, and the patient's functional status. The physical examination should emphasize loss of subcutaneous fat, muscle wasting, volume status, and signs of micronutrient deficiencies (see Ch. 192.2). The initial clinical assessment is often equivocal; that is, the presence of clinically meaningful undernutrition is uncertain. In such cases, serial evaluations of the clinical examination, body weight, and laboratory parameters, as well as close observation of the patient's nutrient intake as a function of estimated requirements, are necessary to make the diagnosis of PEM.

Treatment

The goals of treatment of PEM are to provide adequate energy, protein, and micronutrients to restore body composition to normal and treat the underlying process that caused the deficiency.

STRATEGY. Treatment should proceed in two stages. In severe PEM, the first priority should be to correct fluid and electrolyte abnormalities and treat acute medical problems, especially infections. Although any combination of electrolyte and acid-base abnormalities can occur, most common are hypokalemia, hypocalcemia, hypophosphatemia, hypomagnesemia, and a hyperchloremic metabolic acidosis.

In the second phase one must provide adequate nutritional substrate to begin repletion. Nutrients should be provided gradually to prevent complications of overfeeding. In most adult patients no more than 0.8 gram of protein per kilogram and 30 Kcal per kilogram of actual body weight should be provided per day. As the patient's condition stabilizes, protein and energy intake can be increased to 35 to 40 Kcal per kilogram and 1.0 to 1.5 grams of protein per kilogram per day. Adequate micronutrients must be simultaneously provided. Patients with severe, life-threatening PEM should be fed even more cautiously.

ROUTE OF THERAPY. Nutrients can be provided either enterally or parenterally. Patients whose gastrointestinal tract is functioning and who can protect their airway should be fed enterally, either by mouth, feeding tube, or tube enterostomy. Patients with contraindications to enteral feeding can be given required nutrients parenterally via either peripheral or central veins (see Ch. 198). An algorithm for selecting the most appropriate method of nutritional support is shown in Figure 194–1.

REHABILITATION. Treating patients with PEM requires more than the provision of nutrients. Physical therapy and other measures to improve functional status are effective adjuncts to nutrition. Physical therapy may result in greater repletion of muscle mass and smaller adipose tissue stores than nutritional repletion without muscle contraction.

The most important non-nutritional factor in treatment is the resolution of the disease or social process that caused the PEM. In most instances, if the underlying process cannot be effectively treated, little benefit is derived from treating the patient's nutritional deficiencies. In particular, patients with terminal illnesses who become progressively malnourished as they near death will obtain little benefit from aggressive nutritional treatment. In these instances,

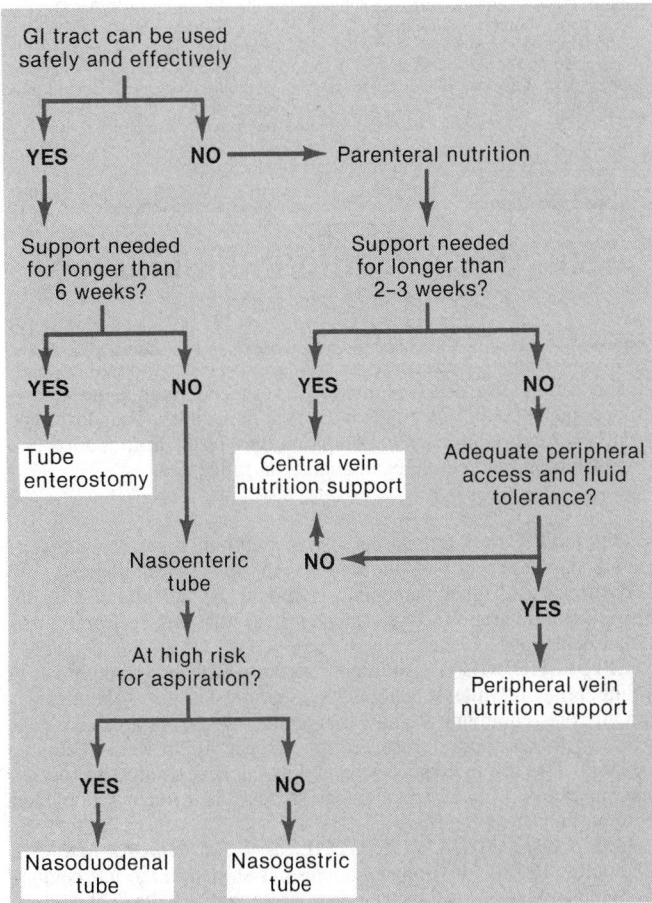

FIGURE 194–1. Decision tree concerning method of nutritional support.

such therapy can be withheld using the same criteria as for other life-sustaining treatments.

Prevention

In industrialized societies protein-calorie undernutrition is best prevented by the early identification of high-risk patients during admission to the hospital. Each such patient should be screened for predisposing risk factors (see Table 194–1). Patients at risk should receive more formal assessment of their nutritional status. Those identified early in the course of their illness, while PEM is still mild, can often be treated with noninvasive nutritional support, preventing the consequences of PEM and the complications of nutritional support. Patients who require prolonged hospitalization, including those in chronic care facilities, should be regularly re-evaluated for the development of new evidence of PEM.

The prevention of primary PEM in the developing world is much more complex and difficult. Poverty and underdevelopment are the primary causes of undernutrition in those areas. Although the direct transfer of food during periods of famine can be lifesaving, the development of agricultural techniques, food distribution systems, and other public health improvements is more important for the long-term prevention of PEM. The identification and early treatment of individual cases of protein-calorie undernutrition among children are also of great importance. Programs that monitor growth and development, that provide nutritional information and supplements to pregnant and lactating women, infants, and children, and that provide family planning and prenatal care are important measures. It is particularly important to abolish programs that distribute infant formulas and discourage traditional breast feeding practices.

Detsky AS, Smalley PS, Chang J: Is this patient malnourished? JAMA 271:54, 1994. *A systemic clinical approach for identifying patients with PEM.*

Hardin TC: Cytokine mediators of malnutrition: Clinical implications. Nutrition Clin Pract 8:55, 1993. *Practical review of current data suggesting that cytokines are important mediators of the metabolic changes associated with critical illness.*

Torun B, Chew F: Protein energy malnutrition. *In* Shils ME, Olson JA, Shike M (eds.): Modern Nutrition in Health and Disease. 8th ed. Malvern, PA, Lea & Febiger, 1994. *Comprehensive review of PEM with emphasis on prevention, pathophysiology, diagnosis, and treatment.*

Wilmore DW: Catabolic illness: Strategies for enhancing recovery. N Engl J Med 325:695, 1991. *Excellent discussion of the metabolic and nutritional events of critical illness and potential strategies for modifying them.*

195 THE EATING DISORDERS
Douglas A. Drossman

The eating disorders—anorexia nervosa and bulimia nervosa—attract much public attention and scientific inquiry. Diagnosis and treatment require an understanding that they result from a combination of biologic, psychological, and social influences.

ANOREXIA NERVOSA

DEFINITION. Anorexia nervosa is a chronic disorder characterized behaviorally by self-induced weight loss, psychologically by body-image and other perceptual disturbances, and biologically by physiologic alterations (e.g., amenorrhea) that result from nutritional depletion.

EPIDEMIOLOGY. Anorexia nervosa afflicts predominantly young, affluent white females (95%). The incidence may be increasing. In one community study the number of new cases per year over a 10-year period rose from 0.55 per 100,000 to 3.26 per 100,000. The disorder is associated with higher social class, occurring in up to 1 in 250 adolescent students in private school and with an incidence of 1%.

ETIOLOGY AND PATHOGENESIS. *Sociocultural Factors.* The cultural ideal for women's bodies has shifted in the last century from that of plumpness (formerly representing wealth, abundance, maternalism, and fertility) to a slimmer female image (representing independence, assertiveness, and success). Thinner women predominate on prime-time television and among beauty pageant contestants and high-fashion models. Social pressures from peers, particularly during adolescence, seem to influence young women and girls to engage in anorectic behaviors. These factors are probably not sufficient for the disorder to develop, but may create the proper environment for its expression in the predisposed individual. Recent studies also report an association of childhood sexual abuse history among patients with anorexia nervosa.

Psychological Factors. It is believed that anorectics have an incompletely developed personal identity and struggle to maintain a sense of control over their environment. Psychiatric interviews suggest that the patient develops within a family that values outward appearance, proper behavior, and achievement more than self-actualization. In response to parental expectations, the pre-anorectic child learns to be hard working, eager to please, and attentive to family needs. In turn, the parents support and indulge in the behaviors of their model child ("best little girl in the world"). Therefore, these actions are mutually reinforced, leading to interdependence among the family members (enmeshment). However, the high standards within the family are rarely achieved by the child, who obsessively struggles for parental approval.

It follows that "negative" childhood behaviors (e.g., assertiveness, rebellion) are not permitted. These behaviors are believed necessary for the development of individual identity. As a result, the pre-anorectic child comes to rely on externally imposed ideal values to maintain self-esteem, but at the expense of self-actualization and a sense of autonomy.

It is not surprising that a distressing period for the pre-anorectic child occurs during or soon after puberty, when physical, social, and psychological events (menarche, growth spurt, school, and adolescent peer pressure) encourage separation from the family and individuation. Over 80% of anorectic patients develop the disorder within 7 years of menarche. The compounded life events at this time are experienced with feelings of helplessness and ineffectiveness. The decision to diet, while not fully understood, may be a desperate attempt for control of one's body, at least, in a distressing new environment.

Biologic Factors. There is increased risk of anorexia nervosa among siblings (6%), with a four- to five-fold difference in concordance rates for monozygotic twins, suggesting a predisposing role for genetic factors. Also, there are more perinatal complications reported among anorexia nervosa patients. The higher birth weight and the increased prevalence of obesity preceding the onset of illness suggest that premorbid obesity is an influencing factor. Abnormalities in satiety, temperature regulation, and endocrine function suggest that a hypothalamic abnormality exists, although no specific lesion has been identified. It is more likely that the hypothalamus serves a modulating role. In the predisposed individual, the biologic and psychosocial events around the time of adolescence may produce neurotransmitter, endocrine, or immune changes via the hypothalamus, leading to the physiologic and behavioral changes characteristic of the disorder.

CLINICAL MANIFESTATIONS. There are no characteristic pathologic or physiologic findings, and no consistent psychiatric diagnosis is found. The consistency of the medical and behavioral features, however, argues for classifying the disorder as a clinical entity.

Psychological and Behavioral Features. Pursuit of Thinness. Patients are not truly anorectic, but struggle against hunger to achieve an unrealistic degree of weight loss. Interestingly, they are preoccupied with food and exhibit bizarre food preferences or elaborately prepare food for others. For most anorectics, weight loss is accomplished through dietary restriction and exercise (restrictor subgroup), although up to 50% will also self-induce vomiting or take purgatives (bulimic subgroup).

Perceptual Disturbances. Anorectics overestimate their body width, insisting they are too fat despite profound weight loss. Their assessment of the body habitus of others is not affected. Anorectics may also exhibit abnormalities in the perception of enteroceptive stimuli. They distort hunger awareness, deny fatigue, and fail to recognize emotional states such as anger and depression.

Sense of Ineffectiveness. Patients feel as though they are controlled by their environment and seem unable to function separately from family or other relationships. They gauge their responses to the expectations of others.

Cognitive Deficits. Patients may exhibit deficits in conceptual thought and abstract reasoning. They may be unable to view situations in anything but extremes, and they interpret events in a rigid and highly personalized form.

Medical Features. Most of the physical, metabolic, and endocrine abnormalities of anorexia nervosa are also seen in starvation secondary to the other conditions. The severity of the findings correlates with the nutritional state.

Physical Signs. Patients may have severe loss of subcutaneous fat and exhibit bony prominences. Core temperature, blood pressure, and pulse are decreased. Examination of the skin may reveal acrocyanosis, downy hair (lanugo), and yellow discoloration (hypercarotenemia). Elevated serum carotene and vitamin A levels are due either to excess intake of dietary carotenoids or to an acquired defect in the utilization or metabolism of these compounds. Secondary sexual features remain absent when anorexia develops before puberty.

Endocrine Abnormalities. *Gonadal.* The endocrine hallmark is gonadal dysfunction. Females develop amenorrhea, have decreased follicle-stimulating (FSH) and luteinizing hormone (LH), and do not exhibit secretory bursts of LH throughout the day in response to endogenous luteinizing hormone releasing factor (LH-RF). Normal menses usually recur with weight gain, when body fat content reaches 22%. Male anorectics lose libido and are infertile.

Thyroid. Clinical features, such as decreased vital signs, dry skin, constipation, cold intolerance, and a delayed ankle jerk, suggest hypothyroidism. T_3 levels tend to be low, with a corresponding increase in reverse T_3, the relatively inactive isomer of T_3. Under the stress of malnutrition, the liver preferentially deiodinates T_4 to rT_3. The clinical findings of mild hypothyroidism may arise from decreased availability of the more active T_3 isomer, which preferentially binds to the thyroid receptor. Free thyroxine, total T_4 levels, and the TSH response to TRH are normal. Clinically significant hypothyroidism does not occur, and treatment with exogenous thyroid is not indicated.

Adrenal. Anorectic patients usually have normal or slightly elevated plasma cortisol levels with decreased urinary excretion of 17-hydroxycorticosteroids. This is due to a decrease in the metabolic clearance of cortisol from plasma with an increase in cortisol-binding capacity. The 24-hour cortisol production rate and basal ACTH secretion are normal. The response to ACTH stimulation may be increased, and the response to metyrapone stimulation is normal. Decreased libido and delayed virilization in males may reflect a shift of androgen metabolism from the 5α-reductase enzyme system (yielding testosterone and its congeners) to the 5β-reductase system, producing the weaker androgen etiocholanolone.

Growth Hormone. Human growth hormone (hGH) levels are normal or slightly elevated. Concurrently there is a decrease in somatomedin levels. This growth-promoting peptide is produced by the liver and other tissues under the influence of hGH. Somatomedin mediates the anabolic effects of hGH but not its lipolytic effects. Thus, anorectic patients and other malnourished individuals maintain their adipose tissue breakdown (increased hGH) without growth effects.

Cardiovascular Abnormalities. Cardiovascular function deteriorates with decreased cardiac O_2 consumption, left ventricular wall thickness, cardiac chamber size, and blood pressure. These are adaptive responses to malnutrition and decreased catecholamine levels. Electrocardiographic changes include bradycardia, decreased QRS amplitude, prolonged QT interval, nonspecific ST segment changes, and U waves. Patients may also develop arrhythmias (tachycardia, sinus arrest, and ectopic atrial, junctional, or ventricular rhythms) due either to the primary disorder or to metabolic disturbances secondary to purgation. Sudden death has been reported among severely emaciated patients.

Hematologic Findings. Leukopenia and decreased white cell function, anemia, thrombocytopenia, and hypocomplementemia may occur. Anorectic patients do not seem to have a greater susceptibility to infection, however.

Gastrointestinal Findings. Changes in gastrointestinal function from malnutrition underlie the common complaints of early satiety, bloating, belching, vomiting, and constipation. Generally, transit times throughout the gastrointestinal tract are increased, so constipation and delayed gastric emptying are common. Pancreatic fibrosis and jejunal dilatation may occur. Malabsorptive diarrhea and acute gastric dilatation may develop with rapid refeeding.

DIAGNOSIS. Social and cultural factors promote and maintain anorectic behaviors, making medical diagnosis difficult. Within some population groups (e.g., high-fashion models, ballerinas) low body weight is an economic necessity, and the associated anorectic behaviors are accepted. The use of criteria such as those proposed by the American Psychiatric Association (Table 195–1) is recommended for clinical diagnosis. The diagnosis is confirmed by identifying the described behavioral features and by excluding any treatable medical disorders.

The differential diagnosis in this young population includes primary endocrine disorders (panhypopituitarism, Addison's disease, hyperthyroidism, diabetes mellitus), gastrointestinal disease (Crohn's disease, celiac sprue), chronic infection (tuberculosis), neoplastic disorders (lymphoma), AIDS, and, rarely, CNS disorders (hypothalamic tumor, vascular malformation).

All patients should receive a nutritional assessment to determine the severity of the malnutrition and to establish a baseline for follow-up. Height and weight are usually sufficient. Other nutritional measures (serum transferrin, albumin, measurement of triceps skin fold thickness, skin test reactivity to *Candida* antigen) should be obtained in patients with marked weight loss to gauge the approach to nutritional treatment.

TREATMENT. There are two goals in the treatment of patients with anorexia nervosa: nutritional restitution with alleviation of medical complications, and modification of the psychological and environmental factors that promote anorectic behavior. No single treatment is superior, and a multidisciplinary approach involving medical, psychiatric/psychological, and nutritional (dietitians, pharmacists) personnel is needed.

General Medical Care. The medical physician performs the initial clinical assessment, is responsible for the medical and nutritional care of the patient, and provides psychological support. The general approach should include (1) fostering a sense of autonomy in the patient by encouraging her to take personal responsibility in the treatment plan, (2) remaining objective, consistent, and honest to maintain the patient's trust, (3) involving the family as part of the treatment program, (4) serving as liaison and patient advocate with the various consultants and counselors.

Nutritional Care. With mild degrees of weight loss (e.g., weight 80% of ideal or better), nutritional and psychological counseling is sufficient. The physician's role includes personal support, education about adolescent body development and its relationship to diet, and scheduling of periodic visits to observe for clinical deterioration. With moderate malnutrition (weight 65 to 80% of ideal) nutritional supplements may be necessary, but hospitalization usually is not required. Oral replacement with a palatable, nutritionally complete formulation (e.g., Ensure Plus) may help, with the goal being intake of 250 to 500 calories above daily energy requirement. In some cases, cisapride, metoclopramide, or bethanechol may be used to improve gastric emptying and the patient's tolerance of larger meals. With severe malnutrition (weight less than 65% of ideal), hospitalization is usually required. Oral replacement may be attempted, but if the patient is unable or unwilling to comply, tube feeding into the duodenum may be necessary. The patient can receive 400 to 600 calories above daily caloric need, with the goal being no more than 1 to 2 kg weight gain per week.

Severely malnourished patients who tolerate feeding tubes poorly or refuse to eat, must be nourished parenterally. The peripheral venous route is preferred, since central hyperalimentation is more expensive and is associated with a greater frequency of complications. If a central venous route is chosen, it should be supervised by an experienced hyperalimentation team. Caloric delivery should begin with one half of the daily requirement, progressing to full requirement by day three or four. Electrolytes, serum chemistry, and hepatic and renal function must be monitored.

The goal of enteral or parenteral supplementation is to *slowly* get the patient to a body weight out of the range of medical risk. Rapid refeeding produces excess water stores and edema, secondary metabolic disturbances, and possibly cardiac failure. Continued nutritional intervention beyond achieving a "dry weight" of 80% of ideal is not recommended because it is psychologically invasive and minimizes the patient's involvement in the treatment. Supplements interfere with appetite and with attempts to re-establish normal eating patterns.

Pharmacotherapy. No pharmacologic agent is of proven value. Chlorpromazine, amitriptyline, lithium carbonate, and cyproheptadine have been reported effective in small, short-term inpatient treatment trials. Their use should be ancillary to the long-term nutritional and behavioral approaches.

Psychotherapy. Psychotherapy is used to help the patient modify the aberrant eating behavior and to improve psychosocial function. Behavior modification is an effective means of achieving short-term weight gain. Family therapy offers the best potential for long-term benefit, since treatment is directed toward modifying the family interactions that maintain the anorectic behavior. Insight therapy may occasionally help the motivated patient.

TABLE 195–1. DIAGNOSTIC CRITERIA FOR ANOREXIA NERVOSA*

A. Refusal to maintain body weight over a minimal normal weight for age and height (e.g., weight loss leading to maintenance of body weight 15% below that expected) or failure to make expected weight gain during period of growth, leading to body weight 15% below that expected.

B. Intense fear of gaining weight or becoming fat, even though underweight.

C. Disturbance in the way in which one's body weight, size, or shape is experienced (e.g., claiming to "feel fat" even when emaciated or belief that one area of the body is "too fat" even when obviously underweight).

D. In females, absence of at least three consecutive menstrual cycles when otherwise expected to occur (primary or secondary amenorrhea; a woman is considered to have amenorrhea if her periods occur only following hormone [e.g., estrogen] administration).

* Used by permission from the American Psychiatric Association Diagnostic and Statistical Manual of Mental Disorders (DSM-IIIR), 4th ed. Washington, D.C., American Psychiatric Association, 1987.

PROGNOSIS. The short-term prognosis is generally favorable; over 75% of patients will attain a body weight above 75% of ideal. Menses will resume in at least half; however, less than one third of patients will resume normal eating patterns. The long-term prognosis varies, and relapses requiring hospitalization occur in about half of the patients. The mortality rate among hospitalized patients averages 6%, with the main causes of death being inanition and severe electrolyte disturbances; suicide occurs in 1%. A poorer prognosis is associated with a late age of onset, self-induced vomiting or laxative abuse, long duration of illness, male sex, and the presence of associated psychiatric disturbance. A better prognosis is associated with the patient's ability to achieve a degree of social integration (e.g., with parent, spouse, and friends). Whatever the immediate outcome, anorexia nervosa is a lifelong behavioral disorder with periodic exacerbations requiring medical, psychological, and nutritional intervention.

BULIMIA NERVOSA

DEFINITION. Bulimia, derived from the Greek meaning "ox-eating," is a behavioral disorder characterized by episodes of overeating (binging), usually followed by acts to "undo" the threatened weight gain with self-induced vomiting, cathartic or diuretic abuse (purging), fasting, or excessive physical activity. Bulimia nervosa particularly describes patients who binge *and* purge. Compared to anorectics, bulimics have normal body weight and tend to have less distortion of body image. Bulimics are more aware that their behavior, although secretive, is aberrant, and they may therefore be more accepting of treatment.

EPIDEMIOLOGY. Binge eating, at least once, occurs in half of the population, and weekly binge eating is reported by up to 15%. Self-induced vomiting or laxative/diuretic abuse associated with binge eating occurs in up to 20% of college students, and 4% report this type of behavior at least weekly. Bulimia is almost exclusively diagnosed in young (< 30 years) women (> 95%). Most bulimics carry on their activity secretly; less than one third discuss their behavior with physicians. In one survey only 2.5% were under medical care.

ETIOLOGY AND PATHOGENESIS. Affected persons commonly report obesity during childhood or adolescence, and the onset of bulimia in association with a conscious decision to diet. At some point they lose control of their compulsion to eat large amounts of "forbidden foods" and binge. Self-induced vomiting is discovered as a convenient method of re-establishing weight control. Thus, a binge-purge cycle becomes established.

As with anorexia nervosa, societal influences seem to play a prominent role in the desire not to be fat. The ancient Romans ate lavishly and then induced vomiting at feasts. Socialites who must attend many dinner parties sometimes induce vomiting. Bulimics report coming from families that emphasize hearty eating and use food to celebrate happy times and to console during sad times: Eating takes on greater meaning than simply to achieve nutritional benefit, and this may help to explain the emotional and behavioral investment present in food and eating.

These behaviors appear to have biochemical correlates. Neurotransmitters, including serotonin (5-HT), dopamine, norepinephrine, opioids, and cholecystokinin (CCK), modulate hunger and regulation of food intake. All have been implicated as contributing to clinical expression of this disorder. For example, 5-HT has a satiety-promoting effect, and reduced brain levels in animals lead to carbohydrate binges similar to those affecting bulimics. Bulimic women, compared to normal persons, have blunted meal-induced secretion of CCK, and this correlates with satiety.

These and other data suggest that the behavioral features of bulimia may relate to dysregulation of CNS neurotransmitter systems. This would support the association of this disorder with its psychological features and with the potential therapeutic role for psychopharmacologic agents.

CLINICAL MANIFESTATIONS. *Psychological and Behavioral Features.* The characteristic behavioral feature is the binge-purge cycle: an eating compulsion associated with failure to achieve or to respond to normal satiety. The episodes occur secretly and are often associated with feelings of frustration, loneliness, or the sight of tempting foods. Binges are usually planned, and the preparation is associated with anxiety and excitement. The binge is usually terminated when feelings of guilt or physical discomfort such as nausea, abdominal pain, or headache occur. At this point patients self-induce vomiting and/or take cathartics or laxatives. Bulimics generally look healthy, and their behaviors go unnoticed by friends and family. They are more outgoing than their anorectic counterparts. Some patients may exhibit impulsive or antisocial behaviors such as drug abuse, kleptomania, and sexual promiscuity. The patient who seeks help does so because of feelings of guilt, anxiety, or depression, or when he or she is no longer able to continue the habit and still function in daily activities.

Medical Features. The medical findings of bulimia derive from the vomiting and laxative abuse. The physical examination may reveal parotid or salivary gland swelling due to vomiting, bruising of the knuckles from their rubbing against the upper incisors during the induction of vomiting ("Russell's" sign), pharyngitis and dental erosions from reflux of gastric acid, or conjunctival hemorrhages from retching.

Frequent vomiting may be complicated by esophagitis, Mallory-Weiss tears, or aspiration pneumonitis. Hypokalemic hypochloremic metabolic alkalosis due to loss of H^+, Cl^-, and K^+ is the most common metabolic complication, and this may lead to cardiac arrhythmias or renal injury. Secondary metabolic disturbances may produce weakness, tetany, and seizures. Emetics such as ipecac may produce cardiac conduction defects and arrhythmias. The use of stimulant laxatives can produce a "cathartic colon" with degeneration of Auerbach's plexus.

Most bulimic patients are clinically depressed by the time they request medical help, and 5% sooner or later attempt suicide. A large proportion of bulimic patients have first-degree relatives with major affective disorders.

DIAGNOSIS. The diagnosis is based on recognition of the binge eating pattern and the exclusion of other medical diseases that might explain the behavior. The differential diagnosis, which is limited in this young population group, would include schizophrenia, use of oral contraceptives, seizures, and rare neurologic disorders. The latter may include *Klüver-Bucy syndrome,* a disorder of bilateral temporal lobe damage associated with indiscriminate sexual behavior, hyperphagia, and pica, and *Kleine-Levin syndrome,* a sleep disorder associated with hypersomnia and overeating.

TREATMENT. The goal of treatment is to help the patient overcome the urge to overeat. Bulimic patients recognize their behaviors as maladaptive. Compared to anorectics, they are more aware of associated psychological difficulties and are more willing to work with physicians and counselors in a treatment plan.

The currently most favored psychotherapeutic approach consists of cognitive-behavioral treatment in which the patient identifies the abnormal behaviors and then uses behavioral techniques to extinguish them, thereby accomplishing greater self-control. The treatment is safe and probably effective.

Antidepressants have been reported to be successful in decreasing the binge activity and in increasing the patient's sense of well-being. They appear effective regardless of whether symptoms of clinical depression exist. One recent study also indicates that combined treatment using cognitive-behavior and antidepressant therapy is superior to antidepressant treatment alone.

Agras WS, Rossiter EM, Arnow B, et al.: Pharmacologic and cognitive-behavioral treatment for bulimia nervosa: A controlled comparison. Am J Psychiatry 149:82, 1992. *Well-controlled study shows that both cognitive-behavioral and antidepressant treatment can be helpful for bulimia nervosa. Cognitive-behavioral therapy more effective in preventing relapse; combined treatment approach may have additional advantages.*

Bemporad JR, Beresin E, Ratey JJ, et al.: A psychoanalytic study of eating disorders: I. A developmental profile of 67 index cases. J Am Acad Psychoanal 20:509, 1992. *Supports idea that clinical expression of the disorder results from disturbances in early relationships leading to impaired feelings of security and interpersonal difficulties.*

Drossman DA: Approach to unexplained weight loss and the eating disorders. *In* Yamada T (ed.): Textbook of Gastroenterology, 2nd ed. Philadelphia, JB Lippincott, 1994. *Comprehensively reviews epidemiology, pathophysiology, medical and psychosocial characteristics, diagnosis, and treatment of major eating disorders.*

Freund KM, Graham SM, Lesky LG, Moskowitz MA: Detection of bulimia in a primary care setting. J Gen Intern Med 8:236, 1993. *Offers simple questions that can be used to identify patients with bulimia.*

Kennedy SH, Garfinkel PE: Advances in diagnosis and treatment of anorexia nervosa and bulimia nervosa. Can J Psychiatry 37:309, 1992. *Reviews treatment approach and outcome of patients having anorexia nervosa and bulimia nervosa.*

196 OBESITY

F. Xavier Pi-Sunyer

Obesity is a frustrating condition for patient and physician alike. Its underlying cause is rarely clear, and its treatment is fraught with difficulty and failure. Management of obesity therefore requires much understanding and persistence.

About 34 million adult Americans (26% of those aged 20 to 75 years) are overweight, 12.4 million severely so. The percentage of adult women who are overweight (27.1%) is somewhat greater than that of men (24.2%).

DEFINITION

Visual inspection of a patient can give a subjective but fairly accurate estimate of the degree of obesity. More objective measures are height-weight tables, weight-related indices, and other anthropometric measurements.

The three most commonly used indices are (1) tables of average weights by height and age; (2) tables of desirable weights for height associated with lowest mortalities in insured populations; and (3) indices derived from height and weight, of which the body mass index is the most useful.

TABLES OF AVERAGE WEIGHTS. National Health and Nutrition Examination Surveys (NHANES) are periodically conducted on a representative United States population and then compiled in percentile tables as weights for height for gender. These cross-sectional data can be used for defining obesity, with a commonly made arbitrary decision that a weight above the 85th percentile for a young adult population is "overweight" for everyone. This comparison to a reference population makes no statement as to health risk involved at any weight level. The biggest problem is finding an appropriate reference population, particularly for minorities.

IDEAL WEIGHT TABLES. The Metropolitan Life Insurance Company Tables of Heights and Weights indicate the weight at which longevity is greatest, based on those insured. The 1983 tables were derived from the pooled data of 25 insurance companies in the United States and Canada, including about 4.2 million policies issued between 1950 and 1971. People with major diseases were screened out. The tables show weights based on lowest mortality for men and women at ages 25 to 59 by height and body frame.

The Metropolitan tables have been criticized as being inaccurate because (1) insured subjects do not represent a random sample of the population; (2) insured subjects are screened for illness and so are healthier than average; (3) no actual body frame measurements were taken when data were gathered so that the division into three frame categories (small, medium, and large) was a *post hoc* manipulation of the data; (4) about 20% of the subjects used in the tables reported their heights and weights but were not actually measured (the bias being that women tend to under-report their weight and men to over-report their height); (5) the tables do not distinguish between obesity and overweight.

BODY MASS INDEX (BMI). A third way to classify overweight is by computing the BMI:

$$BMI = kg/(ht \text{ in meters})^2$$
$$\text{or } BMI = lb/(ht \text{ in inches})^2 \times 703.1$$

This simple measurement correlates well with other estimates of fatness, although some very muscular individuals may be classified as obese when they are not. It is also a somewhat more accurate index of fatness for males than for females.

The mean BMI (weighted for the height distribution of the US population) taken from the mid-point of the medium frame of the 1983 Metropolitan tables is 22.4 kg per square meter for men and 22.5 kg per square meter for women. Patients can be divided for degree of obesity as shown in Figure 196–1. Health risks increase as BMI increases above 25.

Aging is a fattening process, so that a young and old person of comparable body weight are not comparably obese (Fig. 196–2). This has led to controversy concerning whether it is the total weight of an individual that should stay constant from 25 years to 70 years or the fat-free mass, that is, the working cellular mass of

the body plus the skeleton. The average weight data from the US population show a gradually increasing weight with age, more pronounced and sustained for women than for men (Fig. 196–3).

Whereas many studies suggest that an increase from one's weight at 25 years old may increase mortality, a number have suggested that for the lowest mortality, the pattern of body weight should be leanness in the twenties followed by a very moderate weight gain as one gets older. The minimal mortality points in relation to BMI for each age-gender grouping have been calculated. The regression lines, computed separately for men and women, are presented in Figure 196–4. Clearly, age strongly affects the BMI associated with the lowest mortality in this study. Also, the regression lines for men and women are nearly the same. The "best" BMI gradually increases with age in both genders, with no consistent difference between men and women. As a result, a single set of weight goal tables (Table 196–1) can be constructed which are applicable for both men and women. The goals, which are somewhat more liberal for certain age groups than are the Metropolitan tables, are given by decade of age, with generally higher allowable weights as persons get older. Until the issue is further clarified, these goals seem to be reasonable for a physician to utilize in counseling patients in preventive medicine. Two caveats must be added. First, these tables have been derived from and are applicable primarily to white men and women in the United States. Second, the tables have been derived from populations without known risk factors. Patients with significant risk factors such as coronary artery disease, hypertension, and diabetes mellitus are better counseled on stricter tables, such as the Metropolitan Life Tables of 1983 (see Ch. 193).

OTHER METHODS. Over half of the fat in the body is deposited under the skin. Its thickness can be measured at various sites using standard skin calipers. It is not difficult to become adept in the use of the calipers, and a running record of a patient's estimated body fat can be easily kept. The most useful and accurate tables are based on the measurement of four skinfold thicknesses—biceps, triceps, subscapular, and suprailiac. For such tables, see the *British Journal of Nutrition* 2:77, 1974.

Other methods of defining obesity are more difficult and expensive and therefore are used mostly for research purposes: (1) Total body water can be measured by dilution with tritiated or deuterated water. Water is then assumed to be a fixed proportion of fat-free

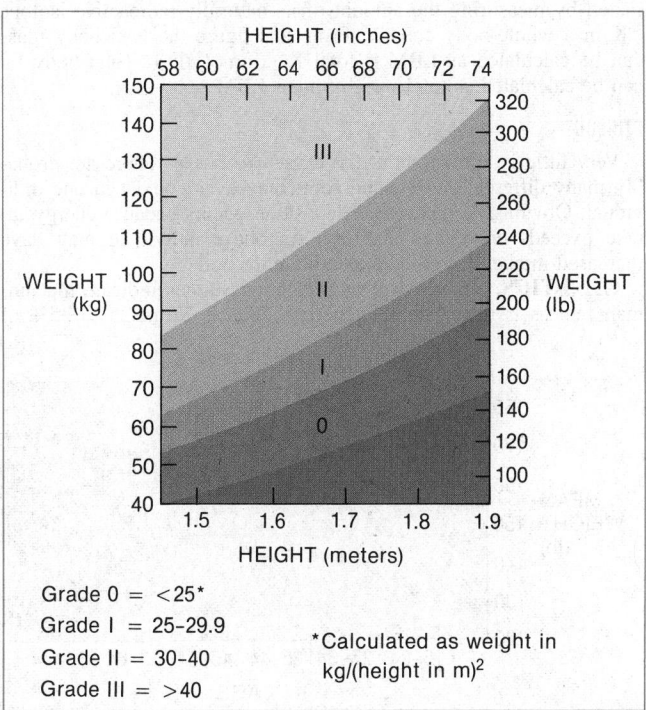

FIGURE 196–1. Grades of obesity as defined by body mass index. (From Garrow JS: Obesity and Related Diseases. New York, Churchill Livingstone, 1988.)

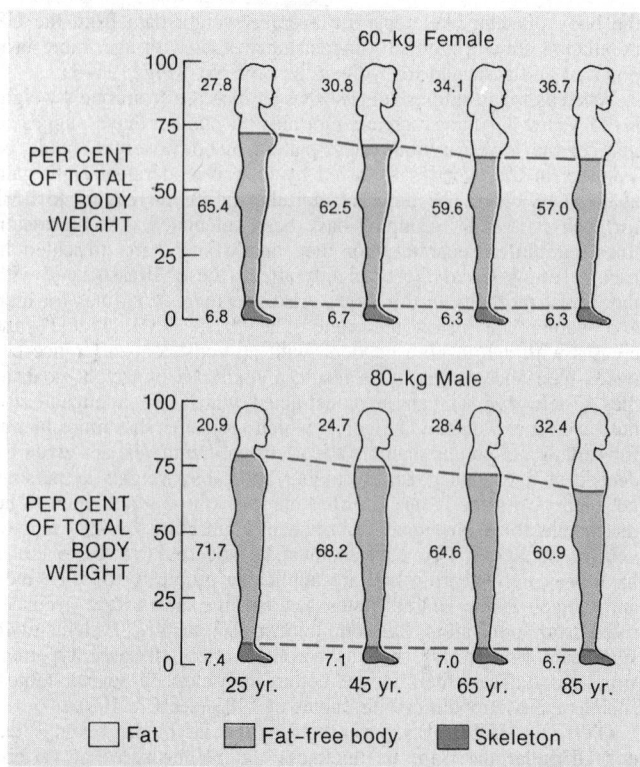

FIGURE 196-2. Body composition change with aging of representative normal adults. (Adapted from Moore FD, Olesen KH, McMurrey JE, et al.: The Body Cell Mass and Its Supporting Environment. Philadelphia, WB Saunders, 1963.)

mass (FFM = water mass/0.73), and FFM is subtracted from total body weight to obtain total body fat. (2) Body density can be measured by underwater weighing (with accurate correction for lung and abdominal air) and the amount of fat-free mass and body fat can be calculated. (3) The amount of body potassium can be estimated by measuring the amount of its naturally radioactive isotope ^{40}K in a whole-body counter. From this figure the lean body mass can be calculated as LBM = total K^+ (mmol)/68.1. Total body fat can be calculated as total weight minus LBM.

ETIOLOGY

Very little is known about the cause of obesity. There are probably many different causes, and some may even coexist in one individual. Obviously excess lipid deposition occurs because energy intake exceeds energy expenditure. An obese individual may have increased intake, decreased expenditure, or both.

GENETICS. Recent twin and adoption studies indicate that human fatness is under strong genetic influence. From 25 to 35% of

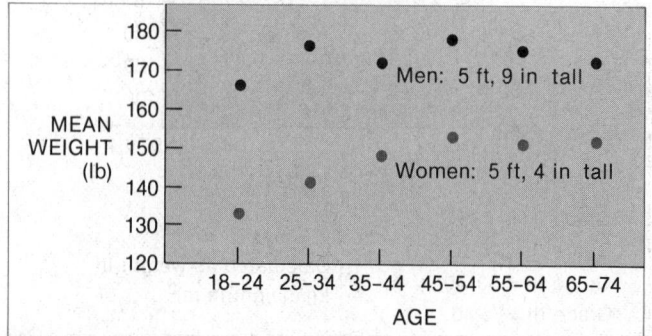

FIGURE 196-3. Weight change with aging for men and women. (Adapted from National Center for Health Statistics: Weight by height and age for adults 18–74 years, United States, 1971–1974. DHEW Publication No. [PHS] 79-1656, Series 11, No. 208, 1979.)

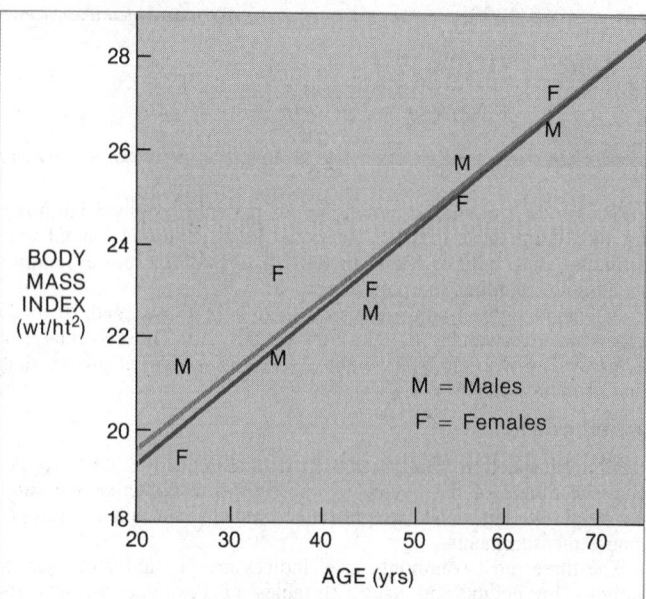

FIGURE 196-4. The effect of age on the body mass index (BMI) associated with lowest mortality. Minimal mortality points were computed for each age-gender group. The regression lines were computed separately for men *(dark red line)* and for women *(light red line)*. Note that there is a strong effect of age on the BMI associated with lowest mortality and that the regression lines for men and women are nearly identical. (From The Build Study, 1979. Adapted by Andres R: *In* Andres R, Bierman EL, Hazzard WR, Blass JP [eds.]: Principles of Geriatric Medicine. Copyright © 1990 by McGraw-Hill, Inc. Used by permission of McGraw-Hill Book Company.)

the variance in skinfold thickness, body mass index, and relative weight has been attributed to genetic factors. The studies that have shown this degree of variance describe the genetic influences found in persons living under particular environmental conditions, namely those of Western society. Because the environment in which heritable characteristics are expressed affects the expression, these variance ranges may not apply to all societies. Not only is there a strong genetic component to fatness, but there is also a similarly strong genetic component to regional fat distribution. Thus, a person's genotype is an important determinant of how adaptation to excess energy intake occurs. Environment is also clearly important, and the interrelation of genetics to particular environments needs to be further investigated.

A number of rare genetic diseases are associated with obesity, but through unknown mechanisms: the Prader-Willi syndrome, the Laurence-Moon-Biedl syndrome, the Alstrom syndrome, the Cohen syndrome, the Carpenter syndrome, and Blount's disease. The reader is referred to textbooks on genetic disorders for further descriptions of these entities.

ENERGY INTAKE. Hyperphagia is the striking cause of obesity in a number of animal models (both genetic and brain-lesioned). The cause of human obesity is much less straightforward. Obesity has been regarded as an eating disorder for centuries, but the presumed abnormality has been difficult to document. Measuring food intake in a free-living environment is subject to large errors. Most studies have suggested that obese persons do overeat (at least in their weight-gaining phases). Many reports describe individuals who categorically deny overeating but lose weight when brought into a metabolic ward and placed on a calculated weight-maintaining diet for their height and age.

Possibly obese persons are unduly attracted by the hedonic aspects of food, or they have impaired feedback signals registering satiety, or they have insensitive brain receptor centers for the feedback signals. It has also been suggested that feeding behavior is learned and that satiety is a conditioned response. Maladaptive conditioning is said to occur in obese persons. None of these theories has been scientifically validated.

ENERGY EXPENDITURE. *Resting Metabolic Expenditure.* Obese individuals may gain weight because they are "thrifty"; i.e., less ingested nutrient is spent as heat and thus more is available for storage. Impaired thermogenesis exists in certain animal

TABLE 196-1. AGE-SPECIFIC WEIGHT-FOR-HEIGHT TABLES*
(GERONTOLOGY RESEARCH CENTER)

Height (ft–in)	Weight Range (lbs) for Men and Women by Age (Years)†				
	25	35	45	55	65
4–10	84–111	92–119	99–127	107–135	115–142
4–11	87–115	95–123	103–131	111–139	119–147
5–0	90–119	98–127	106–135	114–143	123–152
5–1	93–123	101–131	110–140	118–148	127–157
5–2	96–127	105–136	113–144	122–153	131–163
5–3	99–131	108–140	117–149	126–158	135–168
5–4	102–135	112–145	121–154	130–163	140–173
5–5	106–140	115–149	125–159	134–168	144–179
5–6	109–144	119–154	129–164	138–174	148–184
5–7	112–148	122–159	133–169	143–179	153–190
5–8	116–153	126–163	137–174	147–184	158–196
5–9	119–157	130–168	141–179	151–190	162–201
5–10	122–162	134–173	145–184	156–195	167–207
5–11	126–167	137–178	149–190	160–201	172–213
6–0	129–171	141–183	153–195	165–207	177–219
6–1	133–176	145–188	157–200	169–213	182–225
6–2	137–181	149–194	162–206	174–219	187–232
6–3	141–186	153–199	166–212	179–225	192–238
6–4	144–191	157–205	171–218	184–231	197–244

* Values in this table are for height without shoes and weight without clothes. To convert inches to centimeters, multiply by 2.54; to convert pounds to kilograms, multiply by 0.455.

† Data from Andres R: Gerontology Research Center, National Institute of Aging, Baltimore, MD.

models of obesity. Although it has been more difficult to document in humans, recent studies in both adults and infants have reported that a low rate of energy expenditure may predispose to obesity.

Thermogenesis can be divided into three components—resting metabolic rate (RMR), thermic effect of food (TEF), and thermic effect of exercise or activity (TEE).

RMR is the energy expended in the postabsorptive state to drive basic life-supporting processes under thermoneutral conditions. RMR, expressed as total amount of energy spent per unit time, is higher in obese persons than in lean ones. RMR can be well correlated with total weight but can be better correlated with lean body mass (LBM). This explains why men have higher RMR's than women and why RMR's decrease with age.

Obese individuals have a higher LBM than those who are lean because they require an extra amount of sustaining cell mass to maintain the extra fat. When RMR is expressed as kilocalories per kilogram of LBM, obese persons have values equivalent to the lean. It is only when RMR is expressed as kilocalories per kilogram of body weight that they have values below those who are lean. This is because per unit of weight they have a relatively lower amount of metabolizing cell mass and a larger amount of stored fat, which is relatively inert in energy utilization. In terms of basal or resting energetics, therefore, the obese once they are obese do not have impaired RMR's and are not more "efficient" than lean persons.

The RMR varies as much as ± 15% from individual to individual, even when they are matched for age, gender, and surface area. If a difference in metabolic rate between individuals can be as great as one third, it is clear that at a given caloric intake one individual may gain weight and another may lose it. Energy balance depends on matching intake to expenditure. It is not surprising that different individuals maintain weight on widely differing caloric intakes.

Expenditure in Activity. The obese expend more energy during physical activity because an obese person is moving a greater load through space, whether walking, running, or climbing stairs. This is true, although less so, even when body weight is supported, as in cycle ergometer exercise, because of the higher cost of moving the larger leg mass. Thus, more kilowatts of energy are expended.

Studies of obese persons show most of them to be less active, both in engaging in physical activities and in moving about once engaged. The amount of energy expended over 24 hours in physical activity varies considerably from individual to individual, however, and it is difficult to generalize.

Expenditure After Food. Food is an important thermogenic stimulant because it generates heat as it is metabolized. Because of this, a fed person has a higher metabolic rate than a fasting one. This elevation of postcibal metabolic rate above basal has been called the thermic effect of food (TEF). With a mixed diet, about 10% of the metabolizable energy ingested is lost as heat.

Obese persons may have equivalent or somewhat depressed TEF responses compared with lean persons. The impaired response appears to be related to insulin resistance, which leads to a slower glucose disposal. The impaired utilization of glucose by the cells of the body slows down heat production. This impaired thermogenic effect can be normalized by giving insulin, so that a thermic response equivalent to that of insulin-sensitive persons occurs. Therefore, it seems likely that a thermogenic defect relating to carbohydrate disposal is found in obese patients who are insulin resistant and not found in those who are equivalently obese but insulin sensitive. Thus, there is evidence for an overall somewhat diminished thermic effect of food in obese compared with lean individuals. However, even insulin-resistant obese persons with a decreased TEF have a total energy expenditure greater than do lean persons for the 3- to 4-hour period after the meal, because the slight decrease in TEF is less than the inherent elevation in their RMR.

In summary, although hypometabolism may predispose to obesity in some cases, RMR is higher once obesity is present. Thermogenic responses to ordinary stimuli (food, stress, cold) are small *per se,* and differences between lean and obese persons are small to nonexistent. The net result is that 24-hour energy expenditure in the typical obese person is greater than that of the typical sedentary lean person.

Expenditure After Overfeeding. Small rodents can waste rather than store much of excess ingested calories. This seems to be mediated through the sympathetic nervous system, which activates and causes hypertrophy of brown adipose tissue (BAT), a tissue that is specialized to generate heat. A deficient ability to burn off excess calories in this fashion has been documented in a number of genetically obese rodents. Little evidence suggests that humans have an adequate amount of brown fat to mount a similar excess of heat production.

In lean humans, significant overfeeding (of the order of 2000 extra calories per day) for about 10 days or more may lead to energy wastage. In the few studies of overfeeding done in obese volunteers, no evidence of similar energy wastage was found, but few long-term studies are available.

Do obese people lack a protective mechanism, i.e., heat dissipation, that lean people possess if they overeat? There is not much convincing experimental evidence to date, although it is a tempting hypothesis that needs to be further investigated.

PATHOPHYSIOLOGY

FAT CELLS. Fat cells (adipocytes) form a reservoir of energy that expands or contracts according to the energy balance of the organism. Fat cells develop from precursor preadipocytes to accommodate excess nutrient calories. Adipocytes gradually increase in volume to about 1 μg of mass, at which point little further enlargement seems to be possible. With continuing positive energy balance, new adipocytes form from precursor cells and the total cell number increases. Adipocytes can increase in number in an unlimited fashion, so that fat mass can reach huge dimensions through hyperplasia.

Once fat cells are formed, it is difficult to dedifferentiate them. This has been termed the "ratchet effect," because a ratchet turns in only one direction. Even though weight may be lost, fat cell numbers remain fixed. As a result, fat cell size reverts toward normal and with sustained weight loss may actually go below normal.

What the stimulus is for the differentiation of preadipocytes into adipocytes is unknown. Adipose tissue lipoprotein lipase (LPL) may be involved. LPL acts to break down triglyceride to glycerophosphate and free fatty acids (FFA). Whereas LPL activity seems to rise with weight loss and is thought to be important in the accelerated weight regain of many patients, it seems to drop after the maintenance of weight loss for a time, suggesting that its elevation in the obese patient may be secondary rather than primary.

REGIONAL DISTRIBUTION OF ADIPOSE TISSUE. Fat mass is distributed differently in men and women. The android, or male, pattern is characterized by fat distributed predominantly in the upper body above the waist, whereas the gynecoid, or female, pattern shows fat predominantly in the lower body, that is, lower abdomen, buttocks, hips, and thighs. Upper body fat has a significantly worse prognosis for morbidity and mortality than does lower body fat. Evidence suggests that the intra-abdominal or visceral component of fat rather than the subcutaneous abdominal component is responsible. The regional distribution can be measured in a variety of ways. The easiest, most common, and very useful way is by measuring body circumference at the waist and at the hips and calculating a waist:hip ratio. A ratio of greater than 0.85 in women and greater than 1.0 in men can be considered abnormally high.

Fat cells from the upper body seem to be functionally different from fat cells in the lower body. They are more sensitive to catecholamines and insulin. It is likely that the greater lipolytic and lipogenic potential of the upper body cells is related to an underlying difference in sex-hormone response of the two tissues. Thus, testosterone and estrogen influences may be important and may act differently on upper and lower body fat cells.

Abdominal or android fatness carries a greater risk for hypertension, cardiovascular disease, hyperinsulinemia, diabetes mellitus, gallbladder disease, stroke, and cancer of the breast and endometrium. It also carries a greater risk of overall mortality. Because more men than women have the android distribution, they are more at risk for most of these conditions. Also, women who deposit their excess fat in a more android manner have a greater risk than women whose fat distribution is more gynecoid. Upper body fat deposition tends to occur primarily by hypertrophy of the existing cells, whereas lower body fat deposition is by differentiation of new fat cells, i.e., hyperplasia. Reducing a normal number of enlarged fat cells to normal size is easier than reducing large numbers of the cells in the lower body hyperplastic depot to normal or below normal size. This may explain the weight loss difficulties of many women with lower body obesity.

Thus, three components of body fat are associated with health risk: percent body fat, subcutaneous truncal or abdominal fat, and visceral fat in the abdominal cavity. While partly correlated with each other, they do show independence of expression.

SET POINT. The concept of a "set point" of body weight suggests that each person has a control system that "sets" how much weight, or alternatively how much fat, he or she should have. How the control system is regulated, that is, where the feedback signals from "weight" or "fat" originate and how they might be transmitted (humoral, neural, both?) to the hypothalamic feeding and satiety areas are totally unknown.

This set-point theory suggests that people possess a given weight because they are "set" there. That is, one's set point is the weight one normally maintains. Although this is circular thinking, set-point theory has been used to suggest that weight loss programs are misguided and that the effort to lose weight is inevitably fraught with failure because set point will bring individuals up to their pre-weightloss weight.

The set-point theory has been used to suggest that exercise and some drugs lower set point and most palatable foods raise it. Once these statements have been made, however, no closer understanding of the regulation of body weight and of food intake has been attained. Certainly, if there is a "set point," it is a very movable one that seems to change easily under the influence of a number of environmental conditions.

CLINICAL MANIFESTATIONS

INSULIN RESISTANCE. Obesity induces an insulin-resistant state in man, one that is associated with both basal and stimulated hyperinsulinemia. This results from a change in β-cell insulin release rather than in the threshold to glucose stimulation. The enlarged fat cell is less sensitive to the antilipolytic and lipogenic actions of insulin. Although a decreased number of insulin receptors contributes to the insulin resistance, the resistance is generally much greater than would be predicted from the magnitude of this decrease. A "postreceptor" defect therefore occurs as well. This defect in glucose utilization occurs also in other insulin-sensitive tissues, particularly muscle. The liver is also less responsive to insulin. As the insulin resistance becomes more profound, glucose uptake in peripheral tissues is impaired and hepatic glucose output increases.

DIABETES MELLITUS. In a certain number of obese individuals, diabetes mellitus occurs, as the non–insulin-dependent (NIDDM) type (see Ch. 205). The prevalence of diabetes is approximately three times higher in overweight than in nonoverweight persons. In the United States about 85% of patients with NIDDM are obese. Clinically manifest diabetes develops only with the appropriate genetic legacy, but obesity, by enhancing insulin resistance, increases the demand on the pancreatic islets and tends to unmask and exacerbate an underlying genetic propensity.

HYPERTENSION. The prevalence of hypertension (blood pressure greater than 140/90 mm Hg) is approximately three times higher for the obese than for the nonobese. In the Framingham Study, high blood pressure developed 10 times more often in persons who were 20% or more overweight than in those of normal weight.

The mechanism by which obesity contributes to high blood pressure is not clear. Hyperinsulinemia leading to increased tubular reabsorption of sodium may be a factor; increased sympathetic tone may be another. Whatever the mechanism, weight loss from dieting leads to a fall in arterial pressure, even when salt intake is not restricted.

CARDIOVASCULAR DISEASE. In obesity, increased blood volume, stroke volume, left ventricular end-diastolic volume, and filling pressure result in a high cardiac output. This can lead to predominantly left ventricular hypertrophy and dilatation. Hypertension also contributes to left ventricular hypertrophy. Thus, obese hypertensive patients are at greater risk for congestive heart failure and sudden death.

BLOOD LIPIDS. Obese people seem to have an adverse pattern of plasma lipoproteins. This is manifested particularly by a low concentration of high density lipoprotein (HDL) cholesterol. LDL cholesterol may be elevated. Hypertriglyceridemia is more prevalent in obese persons, possibly because the insulin resistance and hyperinsulinemia of obesity lead to increased hepatic production of triglycerides. The hypertriglyceridemia generally improves with weight loss, but if a true genetic lipoprotein disorder coexists, more intensive therapy specific for the lipoprotein abnormality may be required (see Ch. 173).

RESPIRATORY PROBLEMS. Severe obesity can lead to chronic hypoxia with cyanosis and hypercapnia. Associated with this are an increased demand for ventilation, an increased breathing workload, respiratory muscle inefficiency, and decreased functional reserve capacity and expiratory reserve volume. Peripheral lung units can close, resulting in a ventilation-perfusion mismatch.

The end-stage associated with severe obesity is the pickwickian syndrome, in which hypoventilation is so marked that hypoxia leads to long periods of somnolence. In these patients, pulmonary hypertension occurs and cardiac failure may supervene.

SLEEP APNEA. Sleep apnea is common in severely obese patients (see Ch. 65). The relationship between obesity and sleep apnea is unclear because the most obese individuals are not necessarily the most severely affected. Apnea can be obstructive or central in nature; both forms are more prevalent in obese persons. In obese persons the upper airways may be obstructed by the large local accumulation of fat tissue, often in combination with micrognathia and enlarged tonsils and adenoids. The obstruction leads to hypoventilation and hypoxia, which somehow trigger apneic episodes that then worsen the hypoxia and hypercapnia. Affected patients benefit from weight loss and sometimes from surgical removal of some of the obstructive tissues. Central apnea is characterized by a cessation of ventilatory drive from brain centers, so that diaphragmatic excursions stop for periods of 10 to 30 seconds. The reason obese persons are prone to this condition is unknown. Pharmacotherapy sometimes helps. Daytime somnolence is common in obese patients with apnea, partly from hypoxia and partly from the continual disturbance of sleep at night, because they tend to awaken after each apneic episode.

VENOUS CIRCULATORY DISEASE. Severely obese individuals often have varicose veins and venous stasis. Congestive heart failure may add to dependent edema, with the further complications of trophic changes of the skin and an increased propensity for thrombophlebitis and thromboembolism. Pulmonary embolism is much more common in the obese than in those of normal weight (see Ch. 59).

CANCER. Endometrial cancer is two to three times more common in obese than in lean women. Risk of breast cancer increases with increasing BMI in postmenopausal women. It has been speculated that this increased risk is due to the stimulatory effect of increased levels of estrogen in the postmenopausal period. Obese women also have a higher incidence of cancer of the gallbladder and of the biliary system. Obese men have a higher mortality from cancer of the colon, rectum, and prostate for reasons that are unknown.

GASTROINTESTINAL DISEASE. Cholesterol gallstones are more prevalent in obesity. The pathogenetic sequence is presumed to be that of greater cholesterol production in the increased body fat depots, greater biliary excretion of cholesterol, and a resulting supersaturation of the cholesterol in bile. The gallstones can lead to cholecystitis (see Ch. 126) and the need for cholecystectomy. The obese carry a greater risk for complications and mortality from such abdominal surgery.

Many obese patients have fatty livers with modest abnormalities of liver function tests, but hepatic diseases in general are not more common in obese than in lean persons.

ARTHRITIS. As the severity of obesity increases, joint symptoms related to osteoarthritis become common. Excess stress is particularly placed on joints of the lower extremities and the lower back.

Body weight and serum uric acid level often correlate. With obesity, urate clearance is decreased and urate production increased. Because hypertension and diabetes mellitus also correlate with elevated uric acid levels, the relationship between hyperuricemia and obesity is multifactorial.

SKIN. Skin problems are common in obesity, particularly intertrigo in redundant folds of skin. Fungal and yeast infections of skin are common. Acanthosis nigricans occurs in a minority of morbidly obese patients. These patients can manifest a syndrome that includes severe insulin resistance.

PSYCHOLOGICAL MANIFESTATIONS

The psychological toll of severe obesity is large. Poor self-image and impaired social relationships are common. Obese individuals are often discriminated against in educational and professional settings, engendering anxiety, anger, and self-doubt. There is no evidence, however, of any particular neurotic or psychotic character in obese individuals. The depression and anxiety seem to be situational rather than endogenous; they often improve if the obesity can be ameliorated.

MORTALITY

Obesity is associated with increased mortality. The effect of obesity on cardiovascular mortality generally occurs through linkage with other risk factors such as hypertension, diabetes, and dyslipidemia. Obesity, however, can also make independent contribution to mortality. In the Framingham Study, for every 10% rise in relative weight, systolic blood pressure rose 6.5 mm Hg, plasma cholesterol 12 mg per deciliter, and fasting blood glucose 2 mg per deciliter. The causes of increased mortality for those 20% or more overweight include coronary heart disease, stroke, diabetes, digestive diseases, and cancer (Table 196–2). The risk of mortality is higher for those with upper body obesity than those with lower body obesity. A number of prospective studies have now described this, particularly as it relates to cardiovascular disease risk.

OBESITY AND THE ENDOCRINE SYSTEM

Although obesity has often been described as an "endocrine" disease, <1% of obese patients have any measurable endocrine dysfunction. Hypothalamic, pituitary, thyroid, adrenal, ovarian, and possibly pancreatic endocrine syndromes have been related to obesity.

HYPOTHALAMIC DISEASE. In this type of obesity, the appetite systems or tracts located in the hypothalamus are affected. Bilateral damage in the ventromedial hypothalamus produces hyperphagic obesity in the rat; conversely, bilateral damage in the extreme lateral portion of the hypothalamus causes aphagia. Rather than a single balance of a "feeding center" and a "satiety center," however, it is now clear that diffuse excitatory and inhibitory neuronal systems controlling feeding course through the limbic system and the whole brain. Following trauma, inflammation, or a tumor (particularly craniopharyngioma) involving the hypothalamus, a few patients develop hyperphagic obesity, most of them after surgery for hypothalamic tumors. The diagnosis is usually based on history, physical findings, and brain imaging studies.

PITUITARY AND ADRENAL DYSFUNCTION. Cushing's disease is the most common form of pituitary dysfunction leading to obesity (see Ch. 207). ACTH is excessively produced, which leads to excess production of cortisol by the adrenal cortex. Cushing's syndrome can also have a variety of other causes, including exogenous glucocorticoids, primary disorders of the adrenal, and paraneoplastic syndromes of excess ACTH production. The hypercortisolism causes adipocytes located primarily at the center of the body to expand, while those at the extremities do so much less. With this central obesity comes hypertension and diabetes.

THYROID DISEASE. Obesity is often ascribed to "hypometabolism" caused by underactivity of the thyroid gland, but this is in fact seldom true. Severe hypothyroidism can lead to some increased fat, but most of the excess weight is actually edema, which is lost with the institution of thyroid hormone replacement.

POLYCYSTIC OVARIAN SYNDROME. Mild hirsutism, irregular menses or amenorrhea, and obesity have been linked in the "polycystic ovarian syndrome." In this disorder the ovaries have atretic follicles, the patient is anovulatory, and menstrual disturbance (long-term amenorrhea to oligomenorrhea) is the rule. The ovaries overproduce androgens. Although hirsutism is common, virilization is not. The relation of obesity to the polycystic ovarian syndrome is not clear, but the two conditions often coexist.

ENDOCRINE CONSEQUENCES OF OBESITY. One of the pathophysiologic consequences of obesity may be certain endocrine abnormalities. The sex-hormone abnormalities associated with obesity are different in males and females. Whereas mildly obese men have no detectable abnormalities, severely obese men have mild hypogonadotropic hypogonadism, with less than two thirds the normal mean plasma levels of total testosterone, free testosterone, and follicle-stimulating hormone. Gonadotropic hormones are suppressed by elevated plasma estrogens derived from increased aromatization of adrenal steroids in the excessive body fat. Obesity may be associated with increased metabolic clearance rates of testosterone, caused partly by decreased sex hormone-binding globulin (SHBG). Spermatogenesis, libido, and potency, however, are normal.

Estrogens are not elevated in obese premenopausal women, probably because the amount of estrone conversion by the adipose tissue is small in comparison with regular ovarian estradiol production. Estrogens are elevated, however, in postmenopausal obese women, most likely owing to increased peripheral conversion of the prehormone androstenedione to estrone. This may be a partial explanation as to why there is less osteoporosis in obese women.

There are differences in the androgen-estrogen environment in persons with upper (UBO) and lower (LBO) body obesity. This is more clearly defined in women. Women with UBO have higher androgen production rates and higher concentrations of testosterone and estradiol levels than those with LBO. They also have decreased levels of SHBG, so that free testosterone concentrations are higher. Women with LBO have increased estrone from peripheral aromatization of circulating androgens.

In obesity, insulin resistance develops and hyperinsulinemia results. Whether impaired glucose tolerance or frank diabetes ensues depends on the degree of insulin resistance and the underlying genetic make-up of the individual. Triiodothyronine (T_3) may be elevated to high normal in conditions of high caloric intake with adequate carbohydrate, while thyroxine levels and TSH levels are normal. Slightly low blood cortisol levels may be present in obe-

TABLE 196–2. PATTERN OF EXCESS MORTALITY VARIATION WITH EXCESS WEIGHT (MEN AGES 15–34 YRS AT ENTRY)

Weight Relative to Average Weight (Percent)	Mortality Ratio
105–115	110
115–125	127
125–135	134
135–145	141
145–155	211
155–165	227

Adapted from Society of Actuaries and Association of Life Insurance Medical Directors of America: *Build Study 1979*. Chicago, Society of Actuaries, March 1980, p 82.

sity, probably because of enhanced turnover rates of cortisol. The circadian rhythm of cortisol secretion is usually normal in obesity. Urinary free cortisol levels are normal if related to the lean body mass or urinary creatinine. Also, obese patients usually suppress normally with dexamethasone (see Ch. 207).

Pseudotumor cerebri (benign intracranial hypertension) occurs most commonly in obese young women. No intracranial pathology has been found, although headache, blurred vision, and papilledema occur. Why obesity affects so many of these patients is unclear.

Hypothalamic control of prolactin and growth hormone is often defective in obesity, with poor responses to insulin hypoglycemia. These abnormalities generally revert to normal with weight loss, but not always. Whether these pituitary abnormalities reflect altered hypothalamic control due to obesity or abet the obesity in some way is unclear.

TREATMENT

Obesity is very difficult to treat, because the primary emphasis must be on active patient self-control rather than on passive drug therapy. The responsibility of the physician is to be as supportive and helpful as possible. The three approaches to weight control are diet, exercise, and drugs.

DIET. A truly motivated individual will generally stay on a diet for a long time, initially for weight loss and then for weight maintenance. Crash diets for a few days or weeks are ineffective. Because of the long-term requirement for a diet, it must be tailored to a person's tastes and habits.

The diet must be nutritionally adequate. It is not possible to calculate a diet under 1100 calories that contains adequate amounts of vitamins and minerals. If the diet is lower in calories than this, vitamin and mineral supplements are necessary. The goal of weight loss is to lose as much fat as possible while losing as little lean body mass as possible. A mixed, balanced diet is a sensible approach to long-term weight reduction. A diet that contains at least 0.8 to 1.2 grams of protein per kilogram of desirable body weight will minimize nitrogen losses. The protein should be of high quality, so that essential amino acids can be utilized to maintain lean body mass.

A useful strategy to induce and maintain weight reduction is to educate the obese patient appropriately with regard to the caloric content of foods. Particularly important is to emphasize the high caloric density of some foods, especially those high in fat. An attempt should be made to get the fat content of the diet below 30% of total calories. The lower the fat content, the lower the caloric content of the diet is likely to be. Foods high in fiber should be used liberally because of their low caloric density. Refined sugars should be reduced because these provide calories without any useful vitamins or minerals.

Very Low Calorie Diets.
Very low calorie diets (VLCD) severely limit daily intake to 300 to 700 calories. Some diets are strictly limited to protein and have been called protein-supplemented modified fasts (PSMF). Others allow both protein and carbohydrate. The concept of protein-supplemented fasting arose because the regimen improves nitrogen balance over fasting programs. There is little evidence, however, that at equicaloric levels protein alone is better than protein with carbohydrate. The extra weight lost early in the diet when protein alone is given is that of water. With this water diuresis there is electrolyte loss as well. The calories can be given either in liquid formula form or as natural foods. High-quality protein must be given. It is also imperative that adequate supplements of vitamins and minerals be taken. These very severe diets have been given for extensive periods of time, but it is unwise to allow them to last longer than 16 weeks. The heavier the patient, the safer the diet seems to be. The lighter the patient, the more LBM is lost per unit of weight loss, so that more caution, more liberal calories, and a shorter time period of dieting should be followed. These diets, especially those relying on liquid formulas, have been popular because of their relative ease and because, since they are so hypocaloric, the weight loss is more rapid. However, they can have serious side effects.

Side effects of these severe diets include orthostatic hypotension (secondary to both sodium loss and impaired norepinephrine secretion), fatigue, cold intolerance, dry skin, hair loss, and menstrual irregularities. Cholelithiasis, cholecystitis, and rarely pancreatitis occur. Unfortunately, most individuals rapidly regain weight after being on these crash programs, perhaps in large measure because the very low caloric content and the liquid form of the diet do not educate the patient to make the adjustments in lifestyle and eating behavior necessary to maintain the weight loss.

Behavior Modification.
Psychoanalysis and psychotherapy have not been very helpful in weight control. An extended change in eating behavior requires a great change in lifestyle, however, so behavior modification programs have proliferated. Behavior therapy is a fundamental departure from the traditional "dietary" training of the past, in which a list of foods, the allowable quantities, and specific menus were supplied. In behavior modification the patient is first made aware of what and how much he or she eats as a background for changing that behavior. Many persons eat quite unconsciously, with little thought of how much they eat and with little or no knowledge of its caloric content. Initially, in the education process, careful food intake diaries are kept. Patients record not only what and how much was eaten, but where, with whom, how, their feelings, and their degree of hunger. These diaries are analyzed, and nutrient densities of foods are discussed. New modes of eating are suggested, including not eating between meals, eating always at table, eating only three times per day, watching the portions of food eaten, not doing other activities while eating, and eating slowly with concentration. Behavior modification also strives at stimulus control and environmental management. The aim is to break learned associations between environmental cues and food intake. Particular situations that trigger eating are avoided or controlled. Behavior modification therapy is usually done in groups, with continued dialogue between the trained group leader (psychologist, nutritionist, physician), the other group members, and the patient.

EXERCISE. Obesity is a consequence of greater energy intake than energy expenditure. To lose weight, the imbalance must be tipped the other way, with expenditure becoming greater than intake. This is done not only by hypocaloric dieting, but also by increasing activity. Obese persons tend to be inactive; it is therefore important to increase caloric utilization. Patients should be taught the approximate number of calories being expended over basal level in individual activities. Most are surprised at how much exercise it takes to expend just a few calories (Table 196–3).

Moderate exercise only transiently increases the metabolic rate. The calories expended are the calories of work done. In the obese, moderate exercise does not actually lower food intake, but intake does not increase to keep pace with the extra expenditure, as it does in lean persons. This is helpful in inducing weight loss.

DRUG THERAPY. Drugs in weight control have been used as short-term adjunctive therapy to diet and exercise. Over the long term the use of drugs has been disappointing, owing to small effects on weight loss or adverse side effects. In general, drugs affect appetite modestly. Anorectic drugs act centrally through brain catecholamine, dopaminergic, or serotoninergic pathways. For example, amphetamine and its derivatives seem to produce anorexia through stimulating the central hypothalamic neurochemical pathways in which norepinephrine and/or dopamine is the principal neurotransmitter.

Amphetamine not only decreases appetite; it also elevates mood and increases arousal, probably mediated through making norepinephrine and dopamine more abundant at synapses. In contrast, fenfluramine is thought to increase brain serotonin. Mazindol probably works through a dopaminergic mechanism. It therefore appears that increasing the activity of norepinephrine, dopamine, and/or serotonin at certain central nervous system sites can lead to anorexia and weight loss.

All of the drugs mentioned have a greater effect on appetite control than do placebos. Problems arise, however, from abuse potential and side effects. Amphetamine has clearly addictive properties. Amphetamine and phenmetrazine may have disturbing side effects, such as sleep disturbances, agitation, and psychosis. Irritability and insomnia have been reported with diethylpropion, mazindol, and phentermine. Fenfluramine may cause depression, sedation, and diarrhea. Contraindications include severe hypertension, coronary artery disease, glaucoma, and a history of drug abuse.

These drugs are generally prescribed for short periods of time, in an effort to help patients over difficult weight "plateaus" or crisis periods. Some experts suggest that certain of the drugs lower "set point" of weight and should be given chronically. This is not generally accepted practice.

TABLE 196–3. APPROXIMATE ENERGY EXPENDITURE IN SELECTED ACTIVITIES FOR PEOPLE OF DIFFERENT WEIGHTS (CALORIES PER 30 MINUTES)*

Activity	Weight (Pounds)					
	110	130	150	170	190	210
Aerobic dancing						
"walking pace"	99	114	132	150	168	186
"jogging pace"	159	186	213	243	270	300
"running pace"	204	240	276	315	351	387
Basketball	207	243	282	318	357	396
Canoeing—leisure	66	78	90	102	114	126
Canoeing—racing	156	183	210	237	267	294
Carpentry	78	93	105	120	135	147
Cycling—5.5 mph	96	114	132	147	165	183
Cycling—9.4 mph	150	177	204	231	258	285
Dancing—ballroom	78	90	105	117	132	144
Dancing—disco	156	183	210	237	267	294
Gardening	150	177	204	231	258	285
Golf	129	150	174	195	219	243
Judo	294	345	399	450	504	558
Lying or sitting down	33	39	45	51	57	63
Mopping floor	96	105	120	138	153	171
Running						
11.5 minutes per mile	204	240	276	315	351	387
9 minutes per mile	291	342	393	447	498	552
7 minutes per mile	366	417	468	522	573	624
5.5 minutes per mile	435	513	591	669	747	828
Skiing, cross-country	216	252	291	330	369	408
Standing quietly	39	45	51	57	66	72
Swimming						
backstroke	255	300	345	390	435	486
crawl	192	228	261	297	330	366
Table tennis	102	120	138	156	174	195
Tennis	165	192	222	252	282	312
Walking						
3 mph	102	114	126	138	153	165
4 mph	120	141	162	186	207	228

* Adapted from The High Energy Factor, by Bernard Gutin. Copyright © 1983 by Bernard Gutin and Gail Kessler. Reprinted by permission of Random House, Inc.

GOALS. Very often patients, and sometimes physicians, have unrealistic goals of what can be accomplished. One pound of fat is equivalent to 4000 kilocalories. With a deficit of 400 kilocalories per day, losing one pound takes 10 days. The more accurate the knowledge of daily energy expenditure and energy intake is, the closer a physician can predict the rate of weight loss. This may prevent unrealistic goals and disappointment by both patient and therapist. The initial goal for weight loss should be modest, with an effort made to lose 10 to 15% of weight rather than to strive for an "ideal" or "normal" weight. With even this amount of loss, detectable improvement can occur in co-morbid conditions. If such weight loss can be maintained for a period of months, a further effort can be attempted.

SURGERY. Certain patients have severe obesity (greater than 100% over desirable weight), have tried weight control programs without success, and often have complications such as sleep apnea, heart failure, phlebitis, and arthritis. Their life expectancy is much lower than normal. These patients may be candidates for surgery because nonoperative management rarely leads to permanent weight reduction.

Surgery for obesity should be considered experimental, as there is no one accepted procedure and all carry significant risks and complications. Because of the severe side effects of previously done intestinal surgery, gastric surgical procedures have become popular. A small fundic pouch or reservoir is created so that individuals are severely limited in the amount of food that they can eat. The distal stoma created for the pouch has variably been designed to empty into the rest of the stomach or into a loop of jejunum, with the rest of the stomach and duodenum becoming a blind loop. Alternatively, in vertical banded gastroplasty, as opposed to horizontal banding, only a small tubular reservoir remains for food entering from the esophagus. Side effects include gastric distress, vomiting, and electrolyte disturbances. Also, some patients do not lose much weight, because many eat "around" the small reservoir with frequent servings of liquid or semisolid foods. A mean weight loss of two thirds of excess weight has been reported, but failure is not uncommon. Dilatation of the gastric pouch, stomal dilation, stomal obstruction, and gastric dehiscence can occur as complications.

Surgery is still unsatisfactory and experimental, but it may be advisable in some cases. Because life-long follow-up and vitamin and mineral supplementation are necessary, a responsible and cooperative patient and an experienced surgeon are a requisite duo.

WEIGHT REGAIN

The most difficult problem in the treatment of obesity is the maintenance of a reduced body weight. The ability to maintain weight loss may depend on the severity of obesity and the amount of hypercellularity of the adipocytes in a given individual.

A person who is modestly overweight with enlarged adipocytes but little proliferation of extra adipocytes can more easily maintain weight loss. The adipocyte hyperplasia of greater obesity is likely to create a much greater problem in maintenance of weight loss. The degree of filling of adipocytes is very likely a regulated factor in energy balance. Obese persons with adipocyte hyperplasia begin to decrease the mass of each adipocyte as they lose weight. If the adipocyte mass drops below a normal lower level of about 0.5 μg per cell, individuals seem to have greater difficulty in maintaining weight reduction. Adipocyte mass seems to be a regulated factor with a feedback effect on energy intake, so that the reduced obese seem to experience strong food intake cues that they have trouble resisting.

Lipogenic enzyme activities increase when a hypocaloric diet is liberalized as a patient goes from a weight-loss to a weight-maintenance period. This is consequent to an increase in caloric intake rather than being primarily caused by the reduction in weight. Reduced obese individuals have been reported to require about 25% fewer calories per square meter of surface area to maintain their body weight than do either normal persons or obese individuals who have not dieted and lost weight. This is because, as obese persons reduce, the energy expended in general activity decreases owing to the smaller mass they carry. Their RMR is appropriate to the new lean body mass, but their thermic effect of activity drops unless they can greatly increase their activity pattern over the previous one. Therefore, exercise is very important in the weight maintenance phase.

PREVENTION

The propensity toward obesity is partially inherited, but a large component is also environmental. Obesity leads to an increased morbidity and mortality from a number of diseases, especially for those who are under 45 years old. Being overweight in early adult life is more dangerous than it is at older ages.

It is incumbent on physicians to make their patients aware of these risks and try to keep patients at a body mass index of grade 0 to grade 1 (see Fig. 196–1). This is particularly true for those patients who already have, or have a family history of, the diseases that are precipitated and abetted by obesity.

Atkinson R, Dietz W, Foreyt J, et al. (NIH Task Force on Obesity): Very low calorie diets. JAMA 270:967, 1993. *A review of very low and low calorie diets, their risks and benefits.*

Bjorntorp P: The associations between obesity, adipose tissue distribution and disease. Acta Med Scand (Suppl)723:121, 1988. *A review of the impact of upper body obesity on morbidity and mortality.*

Bouchard C: Genetic factors in obesity. Med Clin North Am 73:67, 1989. *The role of biologic inheritance in human body fat variation is reviewed.*

Danford D, Fletcher SW (eds.): Methods for voluntary weight loss and control. Ann Intern Med 119:641, 1993. *Report of an NIH Consensus Conference. A very useful summary of the papers detailing the present knowledge of weight loss and weight maintenance strategies, including benefits and risks.*

Garrison RJ, Castelli WP: Weight and 30 year mortality of men in the Framingham Study. Ann Intern Med 103:1006, 1985. *A report of the degree of obesity and mortality in a prospective study of men.*

Lew EA, Garfinkel L: Variations in mortality by weight among 750,000 men and women. J Chron Dis 32:563, 1979. *A description of the mortality experience of men and women in a long-term prospective study by the American Cancer Society, documenting that individuals 30 to 40% heavier than average had a mortality rate 50% higher than those of average weight. Mortality comparisons as a function of weight for all common diseases are included.*

Manson JE, Colditz GA, Stampfer MJ, et al.: A prospective study of obesity and risk of coronary heart disease in women. N Engl J Med 322:882, 1990. *A prospective study in women, specifically targeted to coronary heart disease but also following all-cause mortality.*

Pi-Sunyer FX: Health implications of obesity. Am J Clin Nutr 53:1595S, 1991. *A review of the clinical side effects of obesity.*

Ravussin E, Lillioja MB, Knowler WC, et al.: Reduced rate of energy expenditure as a risk factor for body-weight gain. N Engl J Med 318(8):467, 1988. *A report of hypometabolism as a predisposing cause of obesity.*

Segal KR, Pi-Sunyer FX: Exercise, resting metabolic rate, and thermogenesis. Diabetes/Metab Rev 2:19, 1986. *A review of the differences in thermogenic response to food and to exercise in lean and obese persons.*

Stunkard AJ, Sorensen TIA, Harris C, et al.: An adoption study of human obesity. N Engl J Med 314:193, 1986. *A study of the contributions of genetic factors and the family environment to human fatness, concluding that genetic influences have an important role in determining human fatness in adults.*

197 ENTERAL NUTRITION
John L. Rombeau

Enteral nutrition is the provision of liquid formula diets into the gastrointestinal (GI) tract. When compared with total parenteral nutrition (TPN), enteral nutrition measurably increases intestinal mucosal growth and function and is less costly. Because of these acknowledged benefits, enteral nutrition is being used with increasing frequency in medical patients. It is therefore incumbent upon physicians to be familiar with the rationale, indications, administration, and prevention of complications of enteral nutrition.

RATIONALE FOR PROVISION OF ENTERAL NUTRIENTS

EFFECTS ON INTESTINAL GROWTH AND FUNCTION. The most important stimulus for gut growth and function is the presence of nutrients within the GI tract. Enteral nutrients mediate such effects both directly and indirectly. The presence of nutrients within the intestinal lumen directly increases epithelial desquamation and enhances mucosal cell renewal. In the absence of luminal stimuli or intestinal nutrients, the small and large bowel atrophy, not only in the absorptive cells and brush-border enzymes, but in the mucus-secreting cells and the gut-associated lymphoid tissue. These are important protective components of the intestinal barrier against bacteria, endotoxins, and other antigenic macromolecules and may provide a rationale for using small volumes (e.g., 10 ml per hour) of continuous enteral feeding in critically ill patients even if they cannot tolerate larger volumes and must be fed parenterally as well.

Enteral nutrients mediate many of their indirect enterotrophic effects by stimulating gut hormones such as gastrin, neurotensin, bombesin, and enteroglucagon. Gastrin exerts trophic effects on the stomach, duodenum, and possibly the colon. Enteral nutrients given to animal models increase production of additional enterotrophic hormones. Furthermore, because of reduced manufacturing costs of its nutrient components, enteral feeding is less costly than TPN and may be more cost-effective than hand-feeding disabled or debilitated patients.

INDICATIONS

General indications for enteral nutrition include the following: (1) the presence of protein-energy malnutrition (see Ch. 194), (2) a GI tract that can safely tolerate the agents, and (3) anticipated inadequate oral intake for at least 7 days. Safe usage of the GI tract is possible in the absence of obstruction, severe intractable diarrhea, or massive bleeding. The anticipated duration of inadequate oral intake is based solely upon the clinical judgment of the primary physician. Table 197–1 indicates examples of specific medical indications for enteral nutrition. Figure 197–1 gives an algorithm for determining the method of feeding.

DIETARY FORMULAS

Commercial enteral formulas have proliferated rapidly. Table 197–2 outlines the nutrient composition of some of these agents, including polymeric-balanced diets, modified formulas, and modular supplements.

POLYMERIC-BALANCED FORMULAS. Polymeric formulas are "complete" balanced, isotonic diets containing 100% of the

Recommended Daily Allowance (RDA) for substrates, vitamins, and minerals when prescribed in recommended amounts. These formulas are palatable and are the first choice for oral supplementation or tube feeding when digestion and absorption are reasonably normal. The nitrogen source consists of an intact or partially hydrolyzed natural protein (e.g., soy, egg, lactoalbumin), requiring the patient's ability to digest protein, in addition to carbohydrate and fat. The caloric density of these formulas is usually 1 kcal per milliliter, but it can be as high as 1.5 to 2 kcal per milliliter. Calorie-dense formulas are reasonable choices for patients who have unusually high caloric requirements, can tolerate only limited feeding volumes, or require fluid restriction. Most importantly, polymeric-balanced formulas are less expensive than the other formulas. Their major disadvantage is a fixed nutrient composition.

MODIFIED FORMULAS. Conventional modified diets are also "complete" diets. Composed primarily of predigested or "elemental" nutrients, they require minimal digestion and are almost completely absorbed. Although the protein source can be crystalline amino acids, some pancreatic function is required to digest carbohydrates (oligosaccharides and disaccharides) and fats (up to 30% of which are provided as medium-chain triglycerides). In addition, absorption of glucose, sodium, amino acids, fat, vitamins, and trace elements requires intact mucosal transport systems.

Unlike the polymeric-balanced diets, modified diets are hyperosmolar, unpalatable, and relatively expensive, costing between 3 and 10 times as much per calorie as polymeric-balanced formulas. They may produce osmotic diarrhea if administered too rapidly and require flavoring supplements for oral use. Modified diets may be indicated in conditions of digestive or absorptive insufficiency, in which polymeric diets are not well tolerated. Examples of such limiting conditions include chronic pancreatitis, short bowel syndrome, and prolonged ileus.

Disease-Specific. Certain modified formulas are designed for patients with specific nutritional needs. Formulas that contain only essential amino acids as the protein source are designed for patients with renal failure. Formulas that have a protein source high in branched-chain amino acids (BCAA) and low in aromatic amino acids have been formulated for patients with hepatic encephalopathy, severe trauma, and sepsis. Formulas that are high in fat content ($\sim 55\%$ of calories) and low in carbohydrate content ($\sim 28\%$ of calories) have been recommended for patients with respiratory insufficiency because their oxidation produces less carbon dioxide. The high fat content of these formulas may produce diarrhea in critically ill patients. Little objective evidence justifies the use of any of these expensive, disease-specific formulas; their use should be restricted to patients with specific nutrient needs who cannot tolerate polymeric and conventional modified diets.

MODULAR SUPPLEMENTS. Modular supplements, which consist of single or multiple nutrients, can be added to existing "fixed-ratio" diets without affecting the quality or quantity of other nutrients. They are designed for patients for whom standard fixed-ratio formulas are suboptimal. Commercially available modules include carbohydrate, fat, protein, mineral, electrolyte, and vitamin formulations.

ENTERAL NUTRITION ADMINISTRATION

ACCESS. Selection of the access site for delivery of enteral nutrients is based upon the anticipated duration of forced feeding and the potential risk of aspiration. Ideally, enteral nutrition is given by the oral route in alert patients with intact gag reflexes who require nutritional supplementation only with meals. For patients who cannot tolerate oral nutrition, other access techniques include nasogastric tube, nasoenteric tube, and tube enterostomy.

Nasogastric or nasoenteric tubes are ideal for patients who require short-term (less than 4 weeks) enteral nutrition. To use these

TABLE 197–1. INDICATIONS FOR THE USE OF ENTERAL NUTRITION IN THE ADULT MEDICAL PATIENT

Protein-energy malnutrition with anticipated significantly decreased oral intake for at least 7 days
Anticipated significantly decreased oral intake for 10 days
Severe dysphagia
Massive small bowel resection (used in combination with TPN)
Low output (< 500 ml per day) enterocutaneous fistula

TABLE 197–2. COMMONLY USED COMMERCIAL ENTERAL FEEDING FORMULAS*

Category	1.0 kcal/ml	1.5 kcal/ml	2.0 kcal/ml
Polymeric Balanced			
≤16% protein	Ensure, Resource, Isocal, Osmolite, Nutren 1.0	Nutren 1.5, Ensure Plus, Resource Plus, Sustacal HC	Nutren 2.0, Deliver, Magnacal
17–20% protein	Osmolite HN, Isocal HN, Ensure HN, Ultracal, Jevity	Ensure Plus HN	TwoCal HN
≥20% protein	Sustacal, Replete, Promote	TraumaCal	
Modified-conventional			
≤16% protein	Peptamen, Reabilan, Vivonex Plus, Criticare HN		
17–20% protein	Vital HN, Reabilan HN, AlitraQ		
Modified-disease			
Specific (% protein)†			
Critical Care	Impact (22%)	Perative (20%)	
Glucose Intolerance	Glucerna (17%)		
Hepatic	Travasorb Hepatic (11%), Hepatic-Aid (15%)		
Malabsorption		Lipisorb (17%)	
Renal		Travasorb Renal (7%)	Nepro (14%), Suplena (6%), Amin-Aid (4%)
Pulmonary		Pulmocare (17%), NutriVent (18%)	
Modular supplements			
Protein	Propac, Casec, ProMod, Nutrisource		
Carbohydrate	Moducal, Polycose, Sumacal, Nutrisource		
Fat	Microlipid, MCT Oil, Nutrisource		

* This table includes only a partial listing of commercial products.

† Manufacturers market these products as disease specific. The author's use of this designation is intended neither to endorse the manufacturers' claims of special efficacy in the diseases specified nor to deny that some of the polymeric-balanced or modified-conventional formulas might be appropriate, or even superior, in these conditions.

access routes safely, patients must have intact gag reflexes and competent lower esophageal sphincters. Ideal candidates are those with poor oral intake such as occurs with cancer of the head and neck and the lung. The stomach is the preferred site of delivery, but the nasoenteric tube should be advanced into the jejunum in patients with gastroparesis and a high risk of aspiration.

Permanent access through tube enterostomies is the preferred route of delivery for long-term enteral nutrition (more than 4 weeks). Tube enterostomies are inserted either endoscopically, laparoscopically, or operatively into the pharynx, stomach, and jejunum.

The percutaneous endoscopic approach (PEG) is the preferred method for gastrostomy placement. It has the advantage of decreased procedure time, local anesthesia, absence of an incision, and avoidance of ileus. The speed, simplicity, low cost, and low complication rate of PEG have resulted in its replacement of surgical gastrostomy in most hospitals. Surgical gastrostomy for feeding is indicated for patients unable to tolerate PEG, or in individuals undergoing concomitant GI surgery.

Jejunostomy is indicated for patients who need long-term enteral nutrition and have chronic aspiration, gastric outlet obstruction, stomach or duodenal cancer, or have had a gastrectomy.

DELIVERY. Formulas are delivered intermittently or continuously. Intermittent feeding is preferred for delivery into the stomach because it is more physiologic and "frees" the patient from the feeding equipment. Feedings of polymeric diets in a volume of 240 to 400 ml every 4 hours are well tolerated. The disadvantages of intermittent feedings consist of an initial requirement for nursing supervision, such as monitoring for gastric residuals, and a higher risk of aspiration if delayed gastric emptying exists. Slow administration of small volumes into the stomach (25 to 40 ml per hour) is well tolerated and avoids the abdominal discomfort often caused by the increased rate and volume of intermittent feedings.

Continuous feeding, administered by infusion pump over 18 to 24 hours, requires less nursing supervision and results in smaller residual volumes as well as a lower risk of aspiration than intermittent feeding. When feeding into the duodenum or jejunum, continuous feeding is required to avoid distention of the bowel, fluid and electrolyte shifts, and diarrhea, all of which can occur with intermittent feeding. Feedings into the small bowel usually employ isotonic polymeric solutions, initially at a rate of 30 ml per hour. The rate is increased approximately 25 ml per hour per day until the desired volume is achieved to meet the patient's nutrient requirements. Infusions should be initiated at very low rates (10 ml per hour) in critically ill patients. Disadvantages of continuous feeding include

the expense of the volumetric infusion pump and the limitation it places on the ambulatory patient.

MONITORING. Patients receiving enteral feedings require the same careful monitoring as do those who receive parenteral nutrition. This is especially true in critically ill ones. Routine monitoring is best accomplished by following a protocol that ensures complete and detailed surveillance, reducing the possibility of error in formula choice and nutrient administration, and assessing progress toward nutritional goals (Table 197–3).

Special attention must be paid to the GI tolerance to the formula. The patient's condition should be evaluated daily for diarrhea, constipation, nausea, cramping, vomiting, and abdominal distention. One must give close attention to the patient's metabolic status and fluid and electrolyte balance. In many instances, potential complications can be avoided by simple maneuvers such as changing the infusion rate, caloric density, or formulation.

Periodic nutritional assessment is required to evaluate the adequacy of the nutritional support. Nitrogen balance, body weight change, and serum protein status should be monitored and the nutrient prescription amended when indicated. Because of frequent disruptions in feeding attempts, it is not uncommon for hospitalized patients to receive as little as 70% of the enteral calories ordered on a daily basis. These considerations may make it necessary to increase the infusion rate or to supplement infusions with parenteral feeding until satisfactory enteral intake is achieved.

COMPLICATIONS

Clinically significant complications of enteral feeding, although few, should be promptly recognized and treated aggressively. As noted, a standardized monitoring protocol helps to prevent and detect possible problems. Complications of enteral feeding are grouped into four major categories: gastrointestinal, metabolic, infectious, and mechanical.

GASTROINTESTINAL. Diarrhea, defined as stool weight (or volume) of more than 200 grams (or milliliters) per 24 hours, the most common complication of enteral nutrition, occurs in 10 to 20% of patients. Its possible causes are listed in Table 197–4. Tube feeding–related factors that have been suggested to predispose to diarrhea but not documented by controlled studies, include formula hyperosmolality, lactose in the presence of relative lactase deficiency, and bacterial contamination of the enteral products and delivery systems. Although contamination has not been documented as a cause for diarrhea, formula containers and administration tubing should be changed daily to avoid this complication. High-fat formulas may cause diarrhea when patients suffer from fat

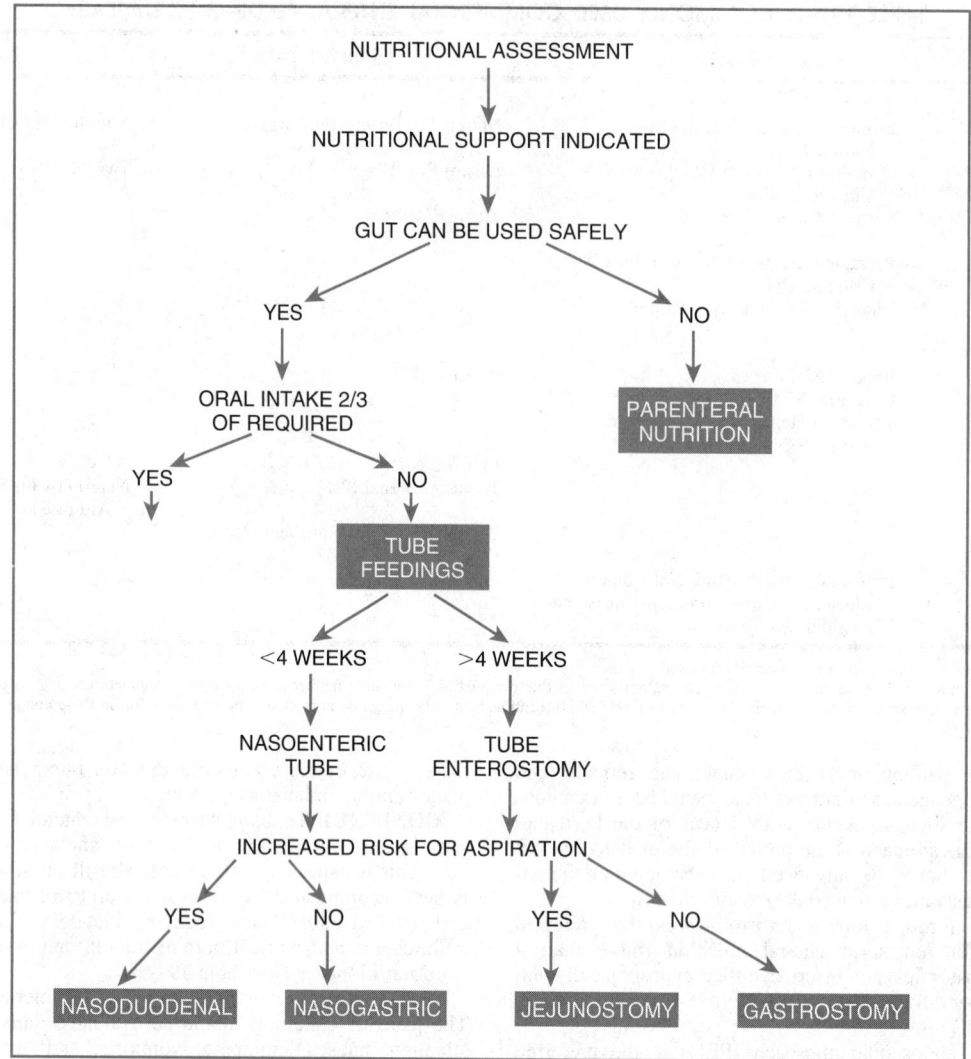

FIGURE 197–1. Decision approach for type and route of nutritional support.

malabsorption (as with pancreatic exocrine insufficiency, biliary obstruction, ileectomy, or ileitis). Enterally administered medications, including antibiotics, hyperosmolar drug solutions such as sorbitol-containing elixirs, and magnesium-containing antacids, can cause diarrhea. Many elixir medications contain substantial amounts

(up to 65%) of sorbitol, although the agent is listed in alphabetical order in the drug information insert only as an "inactive" ingredient. For this reason, all elixir medications must be considered potential causes for diarrhea in tube-fed patients, and it is often prudent to discontinue them or change them to tablet or intravenous forms to determine their responsibility.

Treatment of diarrhea is directed at the underlying cause; however, several therapeutic options are available when there is no clearly identifiable cause. Decreasing the feeding flow rate may alleviate diarrhea by allowing time for intestinal mucosal adaptation to occur when the GI tract has not been used for extended periods (i.e., in starvation and TPN-induced intestinal atrophy). The flow rate is then slowly increased over several days. Parenteral feeding may be necessary to meet full nutrient requirements during this in-

TABLE 197–3. STANDARD ORDER FORM FOR PATIENTS RECEIVING ENTERAL NUTRITION

Obtain abdominal radiograph to confirm tube location before feeding.

Elevate head of bed 30 degrees when feeding into the stomach.

Record name, volume, and strength of formula, and duration and rate (ml/hr) of feeding.

Do not allow formula to hang for more than 8 hours.

Check gastric residual every 4 hours in patients receiving gastric feedings. Withhold feedings for 4 hours if residual is 50% greater than ordered volume. Notify physician if two consecutive measurements detect excessive residual.

Weigh patient on Monday, Wednesday, and Friday. Record weight on graph.

Record input and output daily. Every 8 hours, chart volume of formula administered separately from water or other oral intake.

Change administration tubing and cleanse feeding bag daily.

Irrigate feeding tube with 20 ml of water at the completion of each intermittent feeding, when tube is disconnected, after the delivery of crushed medications, or if feeding is stopped for any reason.

When patient is ingesting oral nutrients, request calorie counts daily for 5 days, then weekly thereafter.

Obtain complete blood count with red blood cell indices, SMA 12, serum iron, and serum magnesium every Monday.

Obtain SMA 6 every Thursday.

Collect urine for 24 hours, starting at 8 A.M., and analyze for urea nitrogen and creatinine each week.

TABLE 197–4. CAUSES OF DIARRHEA IN TUBE-FED PATIENTS

Common Causes Unrelated to Tube Feeding
  Elixir medications containing sorbitol
  Magnesium-containing antacids
  Antibiotic-induced sterile gut
  Pseudomembranous colitis
Possible Causes Related to Tube Feeding
  Inadequate fiber to form stool bulk
  High fat content of formula (in presence of fat malabsorption syndrome)
  Bacterial contamination of enteral products and delivery systems (causal association with diarrhea not documented)
  Rapid advancement of rate (after GI tract is unused for prolonged periods)
Unlikely Causes Related to Tube Feeding
  Formula hyperosmolality (proven not to be a cause for diarrhea)
  Lactose (absent from nearly all enteral feeding formulas)

terval. Nonspecific treatment with antidiarrheal agents can also be tried cautiously. Supplementation of formulas with pectin may help solidify the stool and slow transit time in patients not receiving broad-spectrum antibiotics. The fiber contained in some commercial formulas (usually soy polysaccharide) has not been shown to reduce the incidence of diarrhea.

METABOLIC. Metabolic complications include abnormalities of fluid and electrolyte balance, hyperglycemia, trace element deficiencies, vitamin K deficiency, and abnormalities in protein tolerance.

Overhydration occurs in 20 to 25% of patients receiving enteral nutrition. Cardiac failure and renal insufficiency aggravate the problem and complicate its management. Slowing of the infusion rate or substitution of a 1.5 to 2 kcal per milliliter formula usually provides adequate treatment, and diuretics are rarely necessary for acute control. Although uncommon, hypertonic dehydration also can occur in patients fed calorie-dense formulas, especially when they cannot communicate their thirst.

Hyperglycemia occurs in 10 to 30% of tube-fed patients. High-caloric enteral diets may unmask adult-onset diabetes mellitus. Hyperglycemia is corrected by decreasing the formula flow rate or administering insulin or implementing both of these measures. Because hyperglycemia can cause osmotic diuresis, the patient's fluid status must be carefully monitored.

Abnormalities of most electrolytes and trace elements have been reported. Routine screening of these substances permits early detection before clinical manifestations are apparent. This is especially important in patients with renal, cardiac, or hepatic insufficiency.

INFECTIOUS. The most common infectious complication of enteral nutrition is aspiration pneumonia, which is potentially fatal. Its incidence varies from 1 to 44%, depending on how it is defined. Aspiration can occur subtly, without witnessed episodes of vomiting, and it should be suspected with new onset of tachycardia, tachypnea, fever, hypoxemia, or chest radiographic changes. Patients fed nasogastrically appear to have a higher likelihood of aspiration than patients fed by gastrostomy or jejunostomy. Those with an endotracheal tube or a tracheostomy have an especially high risk. Feeding beyond the pylorus probably lowers the incidence of aspiration, although no conclusive evidence supports this premise.

Preventive measures include elevating the head of the bed to 30 degrees, periodic measuring of gastric residuals, and inflating endotracheal tube cuffs. Correct techniques to insert the soft feeding tubes and careful observation of the tube's position may prevent potentially lethal bronchopleural complications. A chest radiograph should be obtained prior to initiating feeding in every patient with a newly inserted nasogastric or nasoenteric tube. Methods for detecting the "silent" aspiration of enteral formulas in intubated patients include checking tracheal aspirates for the presence of glucose with the use of oxidant reagent strips or placing methylene blue dye in the formula, as a potential marker in tracheal aspirates.

MECHANICAL. Mechanical complications associated with enteral nutrition generally relate to the tube itself or to its anatomic position. Nasoenteric tubes can cause nasopharyngeal erosions and discomfort, sinusitis, otitis media, gagging, esophagitis, esophageal reflux, tracheoesophageal fistulas, and rupture of esophageal varices. Feeding tubes can become knotted or clogged. Gastrostomy or jejunostomy tubes can cause mechanical obstruction of the pylorus or small bowel. Additional complications of percutaneous tubes include leakage around the tube, dislodgment to an intraperitoneal position, and occlusion, especially of small-bore needle-catheter jejunostomies.

Guenther PA, Settle RG, Perlmutter S, et al.: Tube feeding–related diarrhea in acutely ill patients. J Parenter Enter Nutr 15:277, 1991. *Review of the causes and potential treatments for diarrhea in patients receiving enteral nutrition.*

Moore FA, Feliciano DV, Andrassy RJ, et al.: Early enteral feeding, compared with parenteral, reduces postoperative septic complications: The results of a meta-analysis. Ann Surg 216:172, 1992. *Review of published clinical trials of enteral nutrition versus TPN. Significant increases in infectious complications were noted in patients receiving TPN.*

Rombeau JL, Caldwell MD (eds.): Clinical Nutrition: Enteral and Tube Feeding, 2nd ed. Philadelphia, W.B. Saunders, 1990. *Detailed and extensively illustrated text includes scientific principles and practical clinical aspects of enteral nutrition.*

The Veterans Affairs Total Parenteral Nutrition Cooperative Study Group: Perioperative total parenteral nutrition in surgical patients. N Engl J Med 325:525, 1991. *Largest published prospective, controlled, clinical trial of TPN. Significant increases in infectious complications were noted in patients receiving TPN.*

198 PARENTERAL NUTRITION
M. Molly McMahon

It was first appreciated in 1968 that patients could receive all of their nutritional requirements intravenously. This advance was a landmark for the field of nutrition and clinical medicine. While parenteral nutrition can be essential, or even lifesaving, its substantial cost and potential for complications necessitate that it be used judiciously.

DEFINITION. The term *parenteral nutrition* (PN) should be used in place of intravenous hyperalimentation. The latter was coined at a time when provision of an excess of calories was believed to be beneficial; it is now accepted that overfeeding should be avoided. PN provides amino acids (nitrogen), dextrose (carbohydrate), fat, electrolytes, minerals, trace elements, vitamins, and water by central vein (central parenteral nutrition, CPN) or by peripheral vein (peripheral parenteral nutrition, PPN). The enteral route should always be selected for the provision of nutrition in malnourished patients with a functional gastrointestinal tract because the bowel atrophies when nutrients are provided exclusively by vein.

NUTRITIONAL CONTENT

PROTEIN. An essential component of PN is nitrogen. All currently manufactured PN solutions use crystalline amino acids as the source of nitrogen for protein synthesis. Each gram of protein provides 4.0 kilocalories. The protein solutions are available with or without added electrolytes and minerals. For the well-nourished healthy subject without stress, the recommended dietary allowance of protein is 0.8 gram per kilogram per day provided that total caloric intake is adequate. Protein is a metabolic fuel although its structural functions are as important as its fuel functions. At steady-state, amino acid oxidation equals protein intake. Therefore, caloric requirements should be estimated as total calories rather than as nonprotein calories.

Protein breakdown and synthesis are dynamic processes. During severe stress, protein catabolism exceeds protein synthesis, resulting in a net loss of body protein. Body protein stores are minimal, and because all amino acids exist as structural protein, net protein loss results in a loss of tissue function. The increase in proteolysis is caused by the actions of hormones and cytokines. Additional protein losses may occur with specific disease states. Diminished protein synthesis results from bed rest and decreased food intake. Most hospitalized patients receiving PN should receive between 1.0 and 1.5 grams of protein per kilogram of body weight per day. Stressed patients should receive the higher end of the protein range. For most patients, provision of greater amounts of protein does not provide benefit, and the excess protein results in ureagenesis. The provision of nutrition support to critically ill, immobilized patients can decrease but not prevent the loss of body protein.

Modified amino acid solutions have been formulated for use in specific disease states. For example, the use of branched-chain enriched amino acid solutions (providing up to 50% of the amino acids as leucine, isoleucine, and valine) has been suggested for patients with hepatic encephalopathy. These patients have decreased plasma levels of branched-chain amino acids and increased levels of the aromatic amino acids. Branched-chain amino acids are uniquely oxidized in skeletal muscle and adipose tissue rather than the liver. Several studies indicate that patients prone to encephalopathy can be given more protein using branched-chain enriched solutions (compared with standard solution) without worsening the encephalopathy. The clinical effectiveness of formulas with high levels of branched-chain amino acids is controversial, however, as few prospective randomized trials have compared results of this treatment with standard therapy. Once the encephalopathy resolves, the less costly standard amino acid solution should be used. Patients with liver disease without encephalopathy can also tolerate the less costly standard amino acid solutions. Insufficient data support the use of branched-chain amino acid solutions in patients with renal failure or severe stress.

Another example of a modified amino acid formulation is a more concentrated (15%) amino acid base solution. Use of this product enables higher caloric and protein provision in less volume for patients with excess total body water and salt. Again, the disadvantages of this product are its expense and the lack of prospective, randomized trials confirming efficacy. PN supplementation with the amino acid glutamine is undergoing investigation. Currently, glutamine is not present in commercially available PN solutions in the United States, because it has a shorter shelf life than the more commonly used amino acids and has been considered a nonessential amino acid. During critical illness, however, glutamine appears to be a conditionally essential amino acid for the intestinal tract. For patients undergoing bone marrow transplantation, use of glutamine-supplemented PN (compared with standard amino acid solution) improved clinical outcome with fewer infections and shortened hospital stay. Additional prospective randomized trials of these modified formulas are needed.

CARBOHYDRATE. Parenteral carbohydrate is provided in the form of dextrose. Solutions of dextrose in concentrations of 10 to 70% are mixed with the appropriate amount of amino acids to obtain the desired solution. The dextrose is hydrated, and each gram of dextrose monohydrate provides 3.4 kilocalories. Body carbohydrate stores are limited. The minimum daily glucose requirement is the amount necessary to meet brain glucose needs (100 to 150 grams per day). In healthy subjects, dextrose infusion suppresses hepatic glucose release (decrease in need for protein-derived gluconeogenic precursors) and stimulates glucose oxidation (decrease in requirement for amino acid oxidation as an energy source). In addition, dextrose infusion stimulates insulin, which is a strong inhibitor of protein breakdown. The beneficial effects of dextrose as a substrate in PN are attributed to the provision of calories with a nitrogen-sparing effect.

INTRAVENOUS FAT EMULSION. Currently available intravenous fat emulsions consist of 10% (1.1 kcal per milliliter) or 20% (2.0 kcal per milliliter) emulsions of long-chain fatty acids derived from safflower and/or soybean oil, egg yolk phospholipid, and an emulsifying agent (glycerin) to render it isotonic. Parenteral fat is calorically dense, isotonic, protein sparing, and can prevent essential fatty acid deficiency. In addition, provision of a portion of calories as fat allows lower rates of dextrose infusion and results in less hyperglycemia and hyperinsulinemia, as well as a lower incidence of abnormalities in liver function tests. The fat can be administered intravenously either by piggyback infusion or as a 3-in-1 admixture of fat, dextrose, and protein in one container. The fat emulsion is hydrolyzed by lipoprotein lipase to free fatty acids and glycerol. When fatty acids are oxidized for fuel, the respiratory quotient and therefore carbon dioxide production rates are lower than those observed if carbohydrate or protein is oxidized; this may be advantageous in certain clinical situations (e.g., severe pulmonary disease).

Adverse effects, including hypoxemia, hepatic dysfunction, and impaired immune function due to uptake of fat by the reticuloendothelial system, have been reported with intravenous fat administration. However, all of the effects have been demonstrated at the higher infusion rates achieved during 8- to 12-hour infusions rather than during 24-hour infusions. At very high infusion rates, enzymatic removal systems for free fatty acids become saturated, a step that can lead to hypertriglyceridemia. No data suggest that intravenous administration of long-chain triglyceride emulsions at rates of 30 to 50 mg per kilogram per hour (for 70-kg patient, approximately 50 to 85 grams per day) to normolipemic patients results in any adverse effects. Thus, continuous lipid infusion is preferable to discontinuous lipid infusion. If the plasma triglyceride concentration exceeds 400 mg per deciliter, the lipid infusion rate should be reduced or the infusion discontinued. The optimal percentage of calories that should be infused as fat is not known. Essential fatty acid deficiency can be prevented if approximately 5% of total calories is given as fat, and provision of 30% of total calories as fat is generally recommended for stressed patients receiving PN. The role of lipid extends beyond that of energy substrate alone, as substitution of different lipid sources has been reported to beneficially modify the host's response to illness. There is active investigation to determine the optimal type (e.g., medium-chain triglycerides, short-chain triglycerides, structured triglycerides, omega-3 fatty acids) and quantity of fat to be provided in PN solutions.

ELECTROLYTES, MINERALS, TRACE ELEMENTS, AND MULTIVITAMINS. Electrolytes and minerals required for health are sodium, potassium, chloride, calcium, phosphorus, magnesium, and sulfur. The electrolytes are supplied as salts, e.g., calcium gluconate, magnesium sulfate, potassium chloride, sodium chloride, and potassium phosphate. Most sodium and potassium cations are added to the PN solution as chloride or acetate salts after the phosphate requirement is met. Acetate is further metabolized by the liver to bicarbonate, providing an alkaline buffer.

The composition of intravenous multivitamin products has been formulated according to the guidelines of the American Medical Association Nutrition Advisory Group. One adult and one pediatric multivitamin formulation are commercially available. The adult formulation provides the daily maintenance for three fat-soluble and nine water-soluble vitamins (Table 198–1). For patients requiring short-term nutrition, vitamin K often is not routinely added to PN solutions. Accordingly, the prothrombin time should be monitored to determine whether vitamin K supplementation is needed. The daily multivitamin dose may be increased for patients with suspected or documented vitamin deficiencies. Serious consequences can result if standard replacement amounts for vitamins are not provided. During a recent nationwide shortage of intravenous multivitamin preparations, three patients receiving thiamine-deficient PN died with refractory lactic acidosis and a clinical course suggestive of beriberi. Autopsy of the brain of two of these patients revealed lesions diagnostic of acute thiamine deficiency.

Trace elements are available commercially as combination products or as single-item injections; 1 ml of the multiple trace element injection contains zinc, copper, manganese, and chromium in amounts that are suggested for medically stable adult patients (Table 198–2). This amount may be adjusted as needed for individual patients. Since iron, iodine, and selenium are not routinely added to PN solutions for patients requiring short-term nutrition support, monitoring of levels and supplementation of these elements may be required for patients receiving long-term PN.

INDICATIONS FOR NUTRITION SUPPORT

MALNUTRITION. Protein catabolism (with eventual depletion of body protein leading to protein-calorie malnutrition) can be a consequence of starvation, severe illness, or a combination. Malnutrition is difficult to define and inevitably arbitrary. It reflects the timing and extent of recent (previous 3- to 6-month interval) unintentional weight loss; the presence or absence of clinical markers of stress; and the anticipated time that the patient will be unable to meet nutritional requirements orally that determine the need for nutritional support. Nutritional support should be provided promptly for severely stressed patients because the metabolic response to illness affects the malnourished individual more seriously than the nourished person. Studies that have demonstrated a beneficial influence of nutritional support on clinical outcome have provided nutrition for a minimum of 1 week. Currently there is no evidence that suggests that nutrition support of briefer duration is beneficial. Additional research is needed to develop clinical markers for malnutrition and identify patients who will benefit from nutrition support.

DELIVERY OF PN

INDICATIONS. Once it has been determined that nutritional support should be initiated, the route for nutrient delivery should be selected. Parenteral nutrition should be used whenever nutrition

TABLE 198–1. STANDARD ADULT MULTIVITAMIN INJECTION

Vitamin	Amount per Dose per Day
A (retinol)	3300 IU
D (ergocalciferol)	200 IU
E (dl-alpha tocopheryl acetate)	10 IU
C (ascorbic acid)	100 mg
B_1 (thiamine)	3 mg
B_2 (riboflavin)	3.6 mg
B_6 (pyridoxine)	4 mg
B_{12} (cyanocobalamin)	5 µg
Folic acid	400 µg
Niacinamide	40 mg
Dexpanthenol	15 mg
Biotin	60 µg

TABLE 198–2. STANDARD ADULT TRACE ELEMENT INJECTION

Trace Element	Amount / Dose / Day
Zinc	4 mg
Copper	1 mg
Manganese	500 μg
Chromium	10 μg

support is indicated in a patient with a nonfunctioning gastrointestinal tract. In particular, PN should be considered for malnourished patients who have persistent bowel obstruction, gastrointestinal motility disorders (other than isolated gastroparesis), malabsorption, short bowel syndrome with insufficient intestinal adaptation to maintain nutritional status using the enteral route, prolonged postoperative ileus, hypotension, severe pancreatitis, and in patients in whom a feeding tube cannot be placed in the desired location. PN can be added supplementally for patients who tolerate tube feeding at a low rate but not at a rate sufficient to meet caloric requirements. While it is difficult to establish absolute criteria for the use of PN, the American Society for Parenteral and Enteral Nutrition has published guidelines for the general use of PN as well as recommendations for its use in selected disease states. Once the decision has been made that PN is indicated, the clinician is faced with the challenge of selecting CPN or PPN as the preferred form of nutrition.

CENTRAL VS. PERIPHERAL PN: INDICATIONS, ADVANTAGES, AND LIMITATIONS.

Peripheral parenteral nutrition (PPN) should be considered in medically stable patients requiring short-term (e.g., 7 to 10 days) parenteral support, because it avoids the risks of central venous catheterization. Central parenteral nutrition (CPN) is necessary to provide adequate nutrition to patients who are moderately or severely stressed or who are anticipated to require longer use of parenteral support. It is not possible to administer by PPN the high osmolarity solutions used in CPN because a high incidence of infiltration and phlebitis follows administration of such solutions via peripheral veins. For this reason the osmolarity of PPN solutions should not exceed 1000 mOsm per liter. The addition of isotonic lipid to dextrose and amino acids is believed to enhance vein tolerance to PPN solutions. There are limitations to the use of PPN. The cost is similar to that of CPN solutions. Further, critically ill patients will often not tolerate the high volume rates required to meet nutrition needs.

Parenteral nutrition is an essential form of nutrition for malnourished patients with nonfunctioning gastrointestinal tracts. An understanding of the indications for use, appreciation of the significant cost and potential complications, and the ability to design a nutrition program and monitoring plan are important to effective use of this therapy. Future prospective randomized trials are needed to establish outcome data in appropriate patient groups. Evidence that the use of alternate fuel sources may beneficially modify the body's response to illness is stimulating research that may expand the role of nutritional support.

Vascular Access. Selection of the site for catheter insertion should be individualized for each patient. Cannulation of a high-flow central vessel permits infusion of hyperosmolar nutrient solutions that are not tolerated by smaller low-flow peripheral veins. In general, the preferred site of central catheter insertion is the subclavian vein, both for patient comfort and ease of management. Central vein cannulation for PN should never be considered an emergency procedure. Coagulation studies should be checked prior to catheterization, and patients should be adequately hydrated. Sterile technique during catheter insertion is mandatory. While placement of double- or triple-lumen catheters is appropriate in patients who require multiple infusions or hemodynamic monitoring in addition to PN, medically stable patients should receive nutrition via a single-lumen catheter. Prior to initiation of CPN, a chest radiograph should be obtained to confirm catheter tip location in the distal superior vena cava.

The peripherally inserted central (PIC) catheter, which has long been used successfully in children, may also be used effectively in selected adult patients. These radiopaque catheters, inserted in the basilic or cephalic vein via the antecubital fossa and advanced to the distal superior vena cava for infusion of CPN, provide reliable venous access for medically stable patients requiring from 1 week to as much as 6 months of CPN. Early reports noted a high incidence of phlebitis with PIC catheter use, but more recent reports have had more favorable results. The use of PIC catheters preserves existing peripheral vasculature, eliminates many of the risks associated with central venous catheter insertion, and is time and cost efficient.

ESTIMATION OF DAILY CALORIC REQUIREMENTS.

The daily caloric requirement of patients can be estimated by use of a formula, such as the Harris-Benedict equation, or measured by indirect calorimetry (Table 198–3). For many years it was believed that patients requiring nutritional support had elevated caloric requirements, especially when stressed by surgery, trauma, or sepsis. Over the last decade, however, numerous studies have shown that the majority of hospitalized patients have surprisingly normal energy expenditure, usually between 100% and 120% of predicted caloric expenditure. Overfeeding is poorly tolerated by stressed patients. Excess calories can increase oxygen consumption, carbon dioxide production, minute ventilation, and the work of breathing, which can fatigue patients with impaired lung function. Overfeeding also can cause hyperglycemia, which may adversely affect leukocyte and complement function. Finally, excessive calories can cause abnormal liver test results. To design a specific PN program, the clinician should first determine the appropriate volume for the individual patient, then estimate the caloric requirement, and finally estimate the protein and fat requirements (approximately one third of total calories), providing the remaining calories as carbohydrate.

TABLE 198–3. GUIDELINES FOR ESTIMATING DAILY CALORIC, PROTEIN, AND LIPID REQUIREMENTS OF HOSPITALIZED PATIENTS

Requirements	Moderately to severely stressed patient in intensive care unit*	Mildly to moderately stressed patient in hospital ward*
Calories†	Basal Harris-Benedict	Basal Harris-Benedict to Harris-Benedict plus 20%
Protein‡	1.5 g/kg body weight	1.0–1.5 g/kg of body weight
Lipid	30% of total calories during 24	30% of total calories during 24

Modified from McMahon M, Farnell M, Murray M: Nutritional support of critically ill patients. Mayo Clin Proc 68:911–920, 1993.

Harris-Benedict equation
  Females: 655 + (9.6 × weight, kg) + (1.7 × height, cm) − (4.7 × age, yr)
  Males: 66 + (13.7 × weight, kg) + (5.0 × height, cm) − (6.8 × age, yr).

* If patient weight ≥ 120% of ideal body weight, basal Harris-Benedict estimate of caloric needs (based on current weight) and 1.5 grams of protein per kilogram (based on ideal weight) are adequate. Ideal body weight can be estimated by the following method: females, 45.4 kg for 1.5 meters and 2.3 kg for additional 2.5 cm; males, 48.1 kg for 1.5 meters and 2.7 kg per additional 2.5 cm.

† An indirect calorimetric measurement of daily caloric needs is particularly helpful in the following groups of patients: severely stressed patients (e.g., following closed-head injury, multiple trauma, severe burn), volume-overloaded patients in whom the "dry weight" estimate is uncertain, nutritionally supported patients in whom weaning from mechanical ventilation is difficult, morbidly obese patients, or severely malnourished patients.

‡ Assumes normal or near-normal hepatic and renal function.

MONITORING PN. After initiation of PN, one must carefully monitor the patient's vital signs and laboratory values. The presence of fever should always be explained in a patient with a central catheter. Hemodynamic data, fluid balance, creatinine, urea, and sodium should be reviewed to help determine the appropriate PN volume. Daily weight should be interpreted in light of the fluid balance; weight increases exceeding 0.25 kg over a 24-hour period usually reflect fluid gain. Biochemical monitoring should include a complete blood count, electrolytes, glucose, creatinine, urea nitrogen, amino transferase, bilirubin, alkaline phosphatase, phosphorus, calcium, and albumin. Plasma magnesium, zinc, and copper levels should be measured in patients with impaired absorption or increased gastrointestinal (zinc, copper) or renal (magnesium) output. The calcium, magnesium, and zinc values should be interpreted with knowledge of the albumin level, as they are albumin-bound. For patients receiving fat emulsion, triglyceride levels should be checked prior to and following initiation of PN. The extent and frequency of biochemical monitoring following initiation of PN should be individualized; at a minimum, plasma glucose, electrolytes, and phosphorus levels should be checked until stable. During short-term hospitalization, a serum glucose goal range of 100 to 200 mg per deciliter is appropriate. If glucose values exceed 180 to 200 mg per deciliter, regular insulin may be added to the PN admixture. Initiation of a subcutaneous regular insulin algorithm or a variable intravenous insulin infusion should be considered if glycemic control is not adequate using PN insulin alone.

PN should not constitute the sole treatment for acute abnormalities in volume or electrolyte disturbances, but it is an effective vehicle to replace chronic losses. Knowledge of the volume of gastrointestinal and renal losses allows estimation of electrolyte and mineral losses and appropriate PN supplementation. A daily review of the medication profile is important in an attempt to anticipate and manage metabolic changes (e.g., amphotericin: hypokalemia, hypomagnesemia, renal tubular acidosis; corticosteroids: hyperglycemia, hypokalemia; insulin: hypokalemia, hypophosphatemia, hypomagnesemia; diuretics: hypokalemia, hypomagnesemia, metabolic alkalosis; propofol: this anesthetic agent is in a 10% fat emulsion, and its administration may temporarily eliminate or decrease the requirement for additional fat. The acetate and chloride content of the PN admixture should be adjusted for acid-base disturbances. The acetate and chloride balance should be based on the blood gases (arterial or venous), electrolytes, and the source and volume of gastrointestinal or renal losses. The acetate content may be increased and the chloride content decreased in metabolic acidosis; the converse is true for metabolic alkalosis. Although the extent of the daily examination must be individualized, the catheter site, heart, and lungs should always be examined, and the possible development of peripheral edema assessed. Use of a clinical monitoring record that combines information about the PN composition with biochemical data facilitates prompt recognition of metabolic abnormalities. The daily goal is to determine whether the PN program (volume or composition) needs modification in light of the patient's current condition. Once the gastrointestinal tract regains function, the enteral route should always be used for nutrition. Although sudden discontinuation of PN has been reported to precipitate hypoglycemia, these results occurred when excessive calories were received which could lead to exaggerated insulin responses. In the absence of overfeeding, a 50% decrease in the PN infusion rate for 1 hour prior to discontinuation appears safe and should not cause hypoglycemia.

Volume-Restricted PN. Patients with excess total body water and salt following major surgery or illness are often those most in need of nutrition support. The ability to concentrate CPN solutions may allow earlier and more adequate nutrition support. By use of concentrated commercial solutions of 10% amino acids and 70% dextrose, 1 liter can, for example, provide 70 grams of protein and 200 grams of dextrose (960 total calories). Fat should be added when a larger volume can be tolerated. To further restrict volume the PN admixture may be used as a vehicle for drugs with a stable dose requirement, provided therapeutic efficacy has been documented for continuous drug infusion. Medications commonly added to the PN admixture include histamine receptor antagonists and insulin.

COMPLICATIONS

The complications associated with PN can be categorized into catheter related (mechanical, infectious, and thrombotic), metabolic, and gastrointestinal. Studies have demonstrated that the use of organized interdisciplinary nutrition support teams reduces complications.

Pneumothorax, the most common mechanical complication, is most often related to improper central vein cannulation technique. Anatomic factors (such as cachexia, barrel chest deformity, kyphosis, and morbid obesity) can increase the risk even with satisfactory technique. An important predictor of complications associated with central catheter insertion is the physician's experience in catheter insertion.

Catheter malposition is generally not serious if recognized early. Misdirection most often involves a subclavian catheter traveling up the ipsilateral internal jugular vein. The catheter usually can be repositioned, employing either the catheter guide wire technique or fluoroscopic manipulation. Other uncommon complications related to catheter placement include air embolism, subclavian or internal carotid artery puncture, hemothorax, hemomediastinum, catheter embolism, thoracic duct injury, and brachial plexus injury.

Bacteremia and fungemia are serious complications, and the catheter should always be evaluated as a potential source of infection. Most catheter-related septicemias begin with focal infections of the catheter wound; organisms from the patient's own cutaneous flora invade the intracutaneous tract when the catheter is inserted and thereafter. Hub contamination may also cause catheter-related septicemia. In addition, hematogenous seeding of the fibrin sheath on the catheter tip can occur during an episode of bacteremia or fungemia. Sterile technique and the use of effective antiseptics during catheter insertion are the most important measures to prevent catheter sepsis.

The two types of infection that occur most are catheter infection and catheter-related septicemia. Quantitative cultures of the external surface of the catheter differentiate infection from contamination more reliably than the broth-culture method. Infection is diagnosed when the culture of the catheter grows >15 colony-forming units. Catheter-related septicemia is diagnosed by semiquantitative catheter cultures and blood cultures that are positive for the same species. The most common organisms that cause catheter-related sepsis are coagulase-negative staphylococci, *Staphylococcus aureus,* and yeast. In selected circumstances (unexplained fever or leukocytosis), replacement of the catheter by guide wire exchange technique is appropriate. Catheters should always be removed immediately if patients appear septic. Blood (peripheral and central) and catheter cultures should always be obtained; if applicable, the catheter site should also be cultured. New types of catheters and cuffs are being developed to reduce the risk of device-related infection.

While subclinical venous thrombosis commonly occurs in patients receiving CPN, clinically important thrombosis is uncommon during short-term nutrition use. The incidence, however, is higher in patients receiving long-term PN. The diagnosis should always be considered when a patient develops swelling in the arm and neck ipsilateral to the catheter and develops swollen veins in the neck. The use of very low doses of heparin (5000 to 6000 U in PN per day) or warfarin (approximately 1 mg per day) can reduce the incidence of central vein thrombosis without causing adverse hemorrhagic effects and should be considered for patients requiring long-term PN.

Profound metabolic consequences can result from several causes, including providing parenteral calories in excess of needs, the exclusive use of dextrose as the caloric source, or either an excess or deficiency of nutrients. Serious and life-threatening complications have been recognized since the advent of PN therapy. The risks increase when chronically malnourished patients are too rapidly refed, principally as a result of fluid and electrolyte abnormalities. Sudden refeeding results in an acute increase in plasma insulin concentration, which can affect salt and water balance and electrolyte homeostasis. Hyperinsulinemia promotes renal tubular reabsorption of sodium, which can expand extracellular fluid and provoke cardiac decompensation in extremely malnourished patients with decreased left ventricular mass. Hyperinsulinemia also can cause a decrease in the plasma concentrations of potassium, phosphorus, and magnesium. Hyperinsulinemia promotes the passage of potassium from the extracellular space into the intracellular space and results in hypokalemia. Glucose- and insulin-stimulated glycolysis enhance cellular uptake and use of phosphorus for the phosphorylation of glycolytic intermediates and for adenosine triphosphate synthesis. Hyperinsulinemia can increase tissue uptake of magnesium, resulting in hypomagnesemia. The adverse sequelae resulting from hypokalemia, hypophosphatemia, and hypomagnesemia are discussed in Chs. 75.3, 190, 191. Patients receiving long-term PN suffer an increased risk of developing metabolic bone disease.

Hepatic abnormalities are the most common gastrointestinal complications associated with PN. The spectrum reflects not only a complication of the therapy itself, but also relates to the patient's underlying medical status and use of medication. In adults, PN-related hepatic abnormalities are common and are generally benign and temporary. Some patients requiring long-term PN, however, have persisting abnormalities in liver function tests associated with fibrotic and/or cholestatic damage. Complications may be biochemical (elevation of serum aminotransferase, alkaline phosphatase, or bilirubin) or histologic (steatosis, portal triaditis). Transaminase elevations generally occur early in therapy (1 to 2 weeks after initiation of PN) and often resolve without change in the PN program. Bilirubin and alkaline phosphatase elevations usually appear slightly later (2 to 3 weeks into therapy). While the etiology of PN-related hepatic abnormalities has not been clearly elucidated, many factors have been proposed, including the PN solution (excessive dextrose or total calories, or fat-free PN), nutritional deficiencies (carnitine, taurine, essential fatty acid deficiency), and cholestasis. Biliary complications associated with PN include acalculous cholecystitis, gallbladder sludge, and cholelithiasis. Sludge, the most common of these, occurs when the gastrointestinal tract is not used.

Abnormalities of the liver function test should not automatically lead to stopping or altering the PN solution, since abnormal liver function tests may not represent true liver dysfunction. Other causes of abnormal hepatic function, such as extrahepatic obstruction, medications, or infection, should be excluded. The nutrition program should be reviewed to be certain that the caloric intake is not excessive and that a mixed-fuel system (i.e., dextrose, protein, and fat) is being infused.

ASPEN: Guidelines for the use of parenteral and enteral nutrition in adult and pediatric patients. JPEN 17S:1SA, 1993. *Provides concise guidelines (and recent references) for the use of PN.*

Driscoll DF, Baptista RJ, Mitrano FP, et al.: Parenteral nutrient admixtures as drug vehicles: Theory and practice in the critical care setting. Ann Pharmacother 25:276, 1991. *Important resource for pharmaceutical information regarding PN admixtures.*

McMahon M, Farnell MB, Murray MJ: Nutritional support of critically ill patients. Mayo Clin Proc 68:911, 1993. *Discusses metabolic response to illness, hormonal and cytokine effects on nutritional assessment, and design of nutritional programs for hospitalized patients.*

Rose BD: Clinical Physiology of Acid-Base and Electrolyte Disorders. New York, McGraw-Hill, 1989. *Superb resource on electrolyte and acid-base metabolism.*

Solomon S, Kirby DF: The refeeding syndrome: A review. JPEN 14:90, 1990. *Discusses pathophysiology of the refeeding syndrome.*

Subcommittee on the Tenth Edition of the RDA's: Recommended Dietary Allowances. National Academy Press, 1989. *A valuable and concise resource on clinical deficiencies and recommended allowances for macronutrients, vitamins, minerals, trace elements, and electrolytes.*

PART XVII

ENDOCRINE AND REPRODUCTIVE DISEASES

---

199 PRINCIPLES OF ENDOCRINOLOGY

Gordon N. Gill

Communication is essential for all life processes. Accurate sensing of the environment and appropriate coordinated responses depend on the nervous and endocrine systems, which are tightly interwoven. Nervous system functions are mediated by hormones and the endocrine system is centrally controlled by the nervous system. Communication between cells is necessary for development from a single fertilized egg to a mature adult, for an orderly reproductive cycle, and for homeostatic adjustments to a constantly changing environment. Hormones, distinct chemical messengers, transmit information from one cell to another to coordinate homeostatic adaptations, growth, development, and reproduction. *Hormones,* a word derived from Greek meaning "excite" or "set in motion," bind with high affinity and specificity to receptors, which are allosteric proteins. Receptor proteins have two essential functional characteristics: a recognition site, which binds hormones with high specificity and affinity, and an activity site, which transduces the information received into a biochemical message. Allosteric receptor proteins adopt various conformational states; binding of the hormone ligand results in the active conformation. The initial event in hormone action is thus a bimolecular reaction dependent on the concentration of hormone, the concentration of receptor, and the affinity of receptor for hormone.

$$\text{[Hormone]} + \underset{\text{Inactive}}{\text{[Receptor]}} \underset{k_{-1}}{\overset{k_1}{\rightleftharpoons}} \underset{\text{Active}}{\text{[Hormone-Receptor]}}$$

Factors that control the concentration of both hormone and receptor determine biologic responses of cells, of organs, and of the whole organism.

Classic endocrinology dealt with the glands that produce hormones and the concentration of hormone to which cells expressing receptors are exposed. Biosynthesis, secretion, transport of hormone to target cells, and metabolic inactivation determine the effective hormone concentration. Diseases of endocrine glands that impair hormone production result in deficiency states, whereas diseases that cause excessive production result in hormone excess states. Expression of receptor is equally important in forming the active hormone-receptor complex. Genetic and acquired diseases that impair receptors result in deficiency states even though hormone concentrations are compensatorily increased. Increased receptor expression results in an excess state, an event that occurs with growth factor receptors in malignant transformation.

Hormones are produced not only by the glands of internal secretion but by a variety of cells throughout the body. Neurohormones, produced in the hypothalamus, are also produced in cells throughout the nervous system to modulate neuronal function. Gastrointestinal hormones are produced within the nervous system. Hormones that regulate production and maturation of cells of the hematopoietic and immune systems are made in cells of these lineages and in endothelial and mesenchymal cells. Growth-promoting and -inhibiting hormones (growth factors and growth inhibitors) are produced by macrophages and mesenchymal cells. Many of these signaling molecules do not travel long distances through the blood to reach target cells as do classic hormones (endocrine) but act on target cells in the vicinity of the producer cell (paracrine) or even on the producer cell itself (autocrine). During development, cell surface hormones may act on the cell surface receptor of a neighbor cell as a cell-cell communication system. Regardless of signaling distance, the same principles of hormone-receptor interactions operate.

HOW HORMONES WORK

Two classes of hormones operate via two types of receptors (Fig. 199–1). Peptide hormones are synthesized as parts of larger protein molecules and processed as secretory proteins. They act via receptors located in the cell membrane with the recognition/binding site exposed on the cell surface and the activity domain facing the inside of the cell. Activated cell surface receptors use a variety of strategies to transduce signal information, often activating second messengers, which amplify and distribute the molecular information. Many peptide hormones ultimately signal via regulation of protein phosphorylation. In this most common process through which proteins are covalently modified, a phosphate group is do-

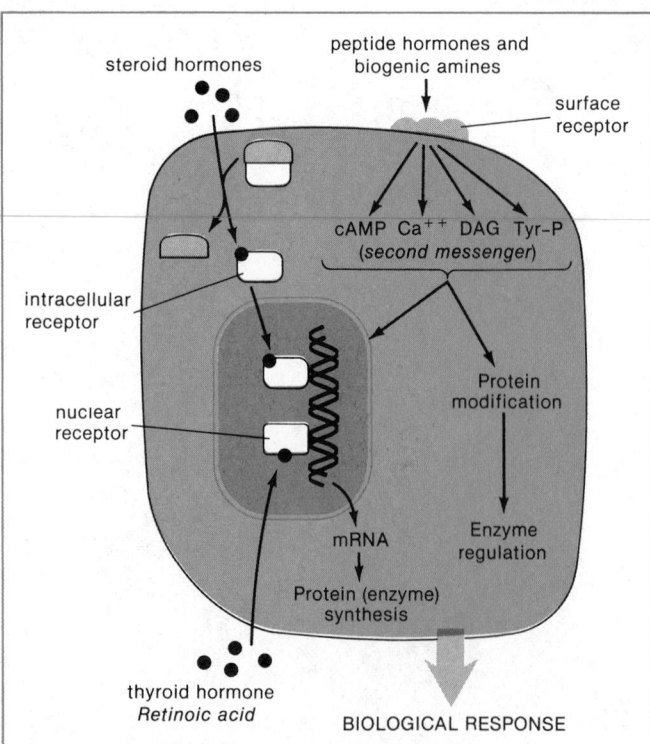

FIGURE 199–1. Mechanisms by which peptide and steroid hormones signal.

nated to the protein by adenosine triphosphate. This allows peptide hormones to change rapidly the conformation and thus the function of existing cell enzymes. It also allows somewhat slower changes in gene transcription to regulate the concentration of enzyme proteins. Biogenic amines function like peptide hormones.

Steroid hormones are synthesized from precursor cholesterol. Thyroid hormone, retinoic acid (vitamin A), and vitamin D are synthesized via separate pathways but act through the same family of receptors and mechanisms as do steroid hormones. This group of hormones acts via structurally related receptors that bind to DNA recognition sites to regulate transcription of target genes. They change the concentration of cell proteins, primarily enzymes, and thus the metabolic activity underlying the physiologic response.

Peptide Hormones Act Via Cell Surface Receptors

HORMONE BINDING AND SIGNAL TRANSDUCTION. Peptide hormone receptors have one of three general structures (Fig. 199–2): (1) a seven-membrane spanning structure in which the recognition site is formed by exterior sequences between membrane-spanning helices and the activity site is formed by interhelical regions inside the cell, (2) a single membrane-spanning helical structure separating the recognition domain from the cytoplasmic domain, which contains an intrinsic enzyme activity, and (3) a single membrane-spanning helix that separates the recognition domain from an intracellular domain that couples to second messenger systems, as do the seven-membrane spanning receptors. The protein coupled may be an intracellular tyrosine kinase or other enzyme.

Hormone ligands and receptors bind with high affinities (equilibrium dissociation constants [K_D] of nanomolar to picomolar), thus providing the specificity necessary for cells to decode the information provided by the low concentration of hormone present among the many other circulating and extracellular proteins. The conformational change resulting from peptide hormone binding activates receptors to signal from the cell surface. Removal of receptors from the cell surface results in down-regulation and attenuation of response. Binding affinities and dose-response curves for the initial event in cell signaling are the same. Biologic responses consequent to these initial events occur via a series of amplifications, each with its own affinity. The result is a dose-response curve for biologic activities which is more sensitive than that for binding and activation of the initial response. Full biologic responses may thus occur at a low concentration of hormone, resulting in occupancy of only 10% or less of receptors. This provides high sensitivity to small changes in hormone concentration. It also provides significant reserve. Hormone-induced down-regulation may remove 90% of receptors from the cell surface. This renders the cell refractory to the initial hormone concentration, but if the need is great enough, hormone concentrations can increase 10-fold and fully activate the residual 10%

of receptors to give full biologic responses. Such a response system provides high initial sensitivity, buffering via down-regulation against excessive hormone responses, but reserve that can operate when the signal strength is strong enough.

Receptors are mobile in the plane of the membrane. Ligand binding not only transduces signals but also induces down-regulation by removing receptors from the cell surface. Ligand binding may induce sequestration of receptors and their retention inside the cell via interactions with cell proteins, as occurs with rhodopsin and adrenergic receptors. Ligand binding may induce endocytosis via clathrin-coated pits with ultimate degradation via lysosomal enzymes, as occurs with insulin and epidermal growth factor receptors. The concentration of cell surface receptors is regulated by interaction with hormone ligand and by other signals that regulate its synthesis and affinity. The concentration of receptors determines the cells' responsiveness. Antagonists occupy receptors but in general do not induce desensitization. When antagonists are removed, receptor concentrations are high and cells are very responsive to hormone exposure. Effects on receptor concentration are seen clinically as up-regulation (e.g., as excessive adrenergic responses when β blockers are rapidly withdrawn) and as down-regulation (e.g., insulin resistance in type II diabetes). Regulation of receptor synthesis is an important mechanism by which one hormone regulates responsiveness to another to coordinate biologic effects.

A class of cell surface receptors serves a nutrient delivery rather than an informational function. These molecules include the low density lipoprotein (LDL) receptor, the transferrin receptor, and the asialoglycoprotein receptor. LDL and transferrin receptors, which are clustered in coated pits, internalize, deliver LDL (cholesterol) and iron to the cell interior, and then recycle to the cell surface. Such receptors do not down-regulate but undergo repeated rounds of recycling to provide the cell with essential nutrients.

INTRACELLULAR SECOND MESSENGERS. *Cyclic AMP and Cyclic GMP.* The concept of second messengers was established by Earl Sutherland, who discovered cAMP, an intracellular allosteric effector that mediates the action of many peptide hormones. Hormone receptors are coupled to catalytic adenylate cyclase via guanosine nucleotide binding (G) proteins, the β-adrenergic receptor being a paradigm for this signaling pathway (Fig. 199–3). This receptor belongs to the seven-membrane spanning class. On ligand binding, the receptor interacts with a G protein trimer consisting of α, β, and γ subunits. Because G proteins bind GDP with higher affinity than GTP, guanine nucleotide exchange is triggered by proteins that facilitate exchange of GTP for GDP; activity is reversed by hydrolysis of GTP to GDP. Binding of hormones to receptors that operate through the cAMP second messen-

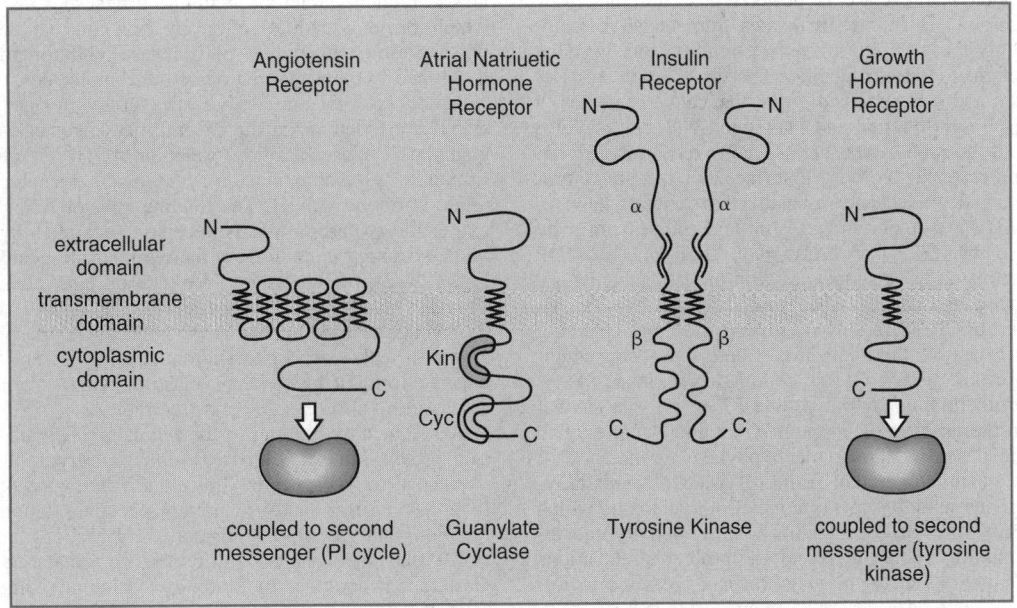

FIGURE 199–2. Structures of peptide hormone receptors.

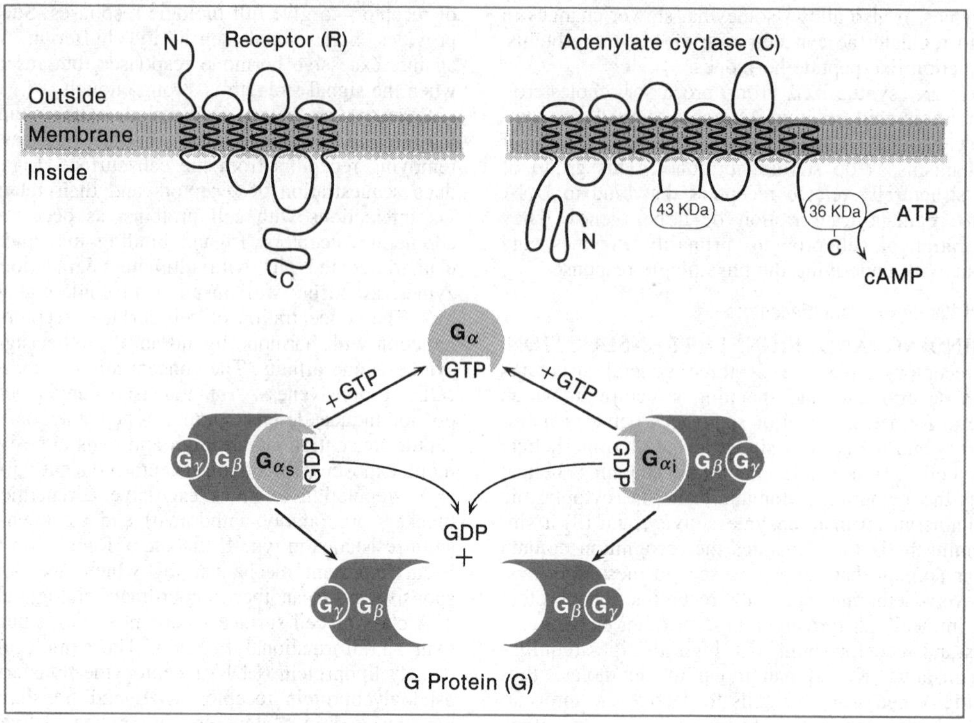

FIGURE 199–3. Hormone-regulated adenylate cyclase.

ger system results in a conformational change causing receptors to bind to G proteins. Ligand-activated receptors facilitate exchange of GTP for GDP so that the activated $G_\alpha s$ (stimulating α GTP binding subunit) dissociates from the β and γ subunits. The [ligand · hormone receptor] · [$G_\alpha s$ · GTP] complex activates adenylate cyclase to catalyze formation of cAMP from ATP. Each hormone ligand induces formation of multiple cAMP molecules via this mechanism. Inhibitory G proteins operate in a similar manner to decrease cAMP formation. In both cases ligand-activated receptors act to exchange GTP for GDP, analogous to proteins that catalyze this process to regulate protein synthesis.

Adenylate cyclase is a large complex molecule with a 12-membrane spanning structure. The two large cytoplasmic domains have internal sequence similarities and are related to sequences in guanylate cyclase. Eight adenylate cyclases have been identified, and their channel-like structure suggests that they may function as transporters in addition to catalyzing formation of cAMP.

Activation of adenylate cyclase is buffered and terminated by several mechanisms: (1) Hormone dissociates from receptor. Binding of G_α · GTP to the receptor decreases affinity for hormone about one order of magnitude to facilitate this dissociation. (2) Receptors desensitize and are removed from the cell surface by a process involving phosphorylation and interaction with cell proteins termed *arrestins*. If hormone exposure is short, receptors are dephosphorylated and reappear on the cell surface; if exposure is prolonged, receptors are degraded and resensitization requires new receptor synthesis. (3) Most importantly, G_α proteins possess intrinsic GTPase activity so that GTP is hydrolyzed to GDP and, on GDP binding, G_α is inactivated and reassociates with the β/γ subunits.

There are many consequences when this mechanism of signal transduction is perturbed. Mutations in seven-membrane spanning receptors may inactivate so that signaling is defective; some mutations, such as those observed in thyroid-stimulating hormone (TSH) receptors in hyperfunctioning thyroid nodules, may activate so that receptors signal in the absence of hormone. Continuous exposure to hormone results in desensitization or tachyphylaxis. Deficiency of G protein, which occurs in certain forms of pseudohypoparathyroidism, results in insensitivity to hormone. Cholera toxin, which activates ADP ribosylation of $G_\alpha s$, inhibits GTPase activity and interferes with reversibility so that profound and prolonged elevations in cAMP occur. Mutations in G_α proteins that are predicted to impair GTPase activity have been described in endocrine tumors.

cAMP, an intracellular allosteric effector, binds to the regulatory subunit of cAMP-dependent protein kinase. A-kinase is a tetrameric protein consisting of two regulatory and two catalytic subunits. Binding of cAMP dissociates the inhibitory regulatory subunits as a dimer from the two catalytic subunits. The latter then catalyze the transfer of the γ phosphate of ATP to serine and threonine residues in proteins. This covalent modification by phosphorylation causes an allosteric conformational change in the substrate protein which results in a change in its activity. The hormonal signal is transduced into an alteration in enzyme activity and thus in cell function. Phosphorylation of cytoplasmic proteins results in alterations such as glycolysis; the activated catalytic kinase subunit also migrates to the nucleus to phosphorylate and activate transcription factors such as the cAMP response element binding protein (CREB).

cAMP actions are reversed by hydrolysis of cAMP by phosphodiesterase to 5′ AMP, and protein phosphorylation is reversed by the action of phosphatases. Phosphodiesterases are regulated and are a frequent target of inhibitor drugs such as methylxanthines, which prolong cAMP action by blocking its degradation. Phosphatases are regulated by phosphatase-inhibitor proteins, which are fine tuned by phosphorylation of these molecules.

A conceptually similar but structurally distinct system provides signal transduction via the second messenger cGMP. Two forms of guanylate cyclase catalyze formation of cGMP from GTP. The best-characterized mammalian enzyme is the receptor for atrial natriuretic hormone (ANH). The binding site for ANH is located on the extracellular portion of its receptor separated by a single membrane-spanning domain from the cytoplasmic guanylate cyclase (see Fig. 199–2). In contrast to adenylate cyclase, receptor and catalytic activities reside in the same molecule. Activity is regulated primarily by ligand binding but also depends on phosphorylation of the enzyme, with dephosphorylation causing desensitization. A cytoplasmic form of guanylate cyclase contains a heme moiety and is activated by nitrous oxide and free radicals.

cGMP acts by binding to the regulatory domain of cGMP-dependent protein kinase. G-kinase, a dimeric enzyme that is evolutionarily related to A-kinase, is allosterically activated on cGMP binding. Like A-kinase, it catalyzes protein phosphorylation to alter enzyme function and physiologic responses. Reactions are terminated by cGMP phosphodiesterase and protein phosphatases. cGMP phosphodiesterase is activated by binding of calcium · calmodulin, a mechanism providing biochemical communication between two signaling systems.

Calcium and Diacylglycerol. Hormone receptors that activate the phosphatidylinositol (PI) cycle transmit information to the interior of the cell via two second messengers: calcium (Ca^{2+}) and diacylglycerol (DAG) (Fig. 199–4). The cycle of PI metabolism consists of synthesis of this phospholipid, its breakdown, and its resynthesis. PI is composed of a 3-carbon glycerol backbone with long-chain fatty acids esterified at carbons 1 and 2 and an inositol ring esterified via a phosphoester bond at carbon 3. Distinct kinase enzymes catalyze phosphorylation of the inositol ring at positions 3, 4, and 5. Quantitatively the principal phosphorylations occur sequentially at positions 4 and then 5. The principal function of activated hormone receptors is to stimulate phosphoinositidase (phospholipase C), which releases the phosphorylated inositol to generate inositol trisphosphate (IP_3, inositol 1,4,5 P_3) and DAG (the glycerol backbone with fatty acids attached at carbons 1 and 2). IP_3 increases the concentration of cytoplasmic [Ca^{2+}]. It mobilizes stored intracellular Ca^{2+} by binding to specific receptors on intracellular membranes and by facilitating opening of calcium channels. The concentration of basal cytoplasmic Ca^{2+} is at least 1000-fold less than that in storage sites and outside the cell. The release from intracellular stores or entry of Ca^{2+} into the cell rapidly increases cytoplasmic [Ca^{2+}].

Ca^{2+} plays a regulatory role in muscle contraction, in neuromuscular transmission, and in hormone signaling. Ca^{2+} binds to calmodulin and alters its conformation, causing the $Ca^{2+}\cdot$ calmodulin complex to bind to a variety of enzymes to regulate their activities. $Ca^{2+}\cdot$ calmodulin regulates protein kinases, including myosin light chain kinase involved in smooth muscle contraction, phosphorylase kinase involved in breakdown of glycogen, and calmodulin-dependent protein kinase important in synaptic transmission. $Ca^{2+}\cdot$ calmodulin regulates cyclic nucleotide phosphodiesterase and adenylate and guanylate cyclases to influence cAMP and cGMP concentrations, and it is involved in microtubule assembly and disassembly. $Ca^{2+}\cdot$ calmodulin is thus able to bind to a variety of other proteins and to alter their activity in response to information provided by the cytoplasmic Ca^{2+} concentration.

DAG acts as a second messenger by binding to protein kinase C to activate this important regulatory enzyme. Protein kinase C also requires Ca^{2+} for activation, so both second messengers of this pathway cooperate to increase the activity of this enzyme. Tumor promoters, such as active phorbol esters, are DAG analogues and act via protein kinase C.

The components of this second messenger system are diverse and complex. There are multiple isoenzyme forms of protein kinase C and of phosphoinositidase. Although one isoenzyme form of phosphoinositidase is activated via receptor-coupled G proteins, another is activated by binding to receptor tyrosine kinases and undergoing tyrosine phosphorylation. Additional kinases phosphorylate alternate positions on the inositol ring; PI 3-kinase is activated by certain tyrosine kinases to yield unique PI metabolites with functions distinct from Ca^{2+} mobilization. Sphingosine, a component of glycosphingolipid metabolism, inhibits protein kinase C, which provides dual regulation of this protein. Specific phosphatases remove the phosphate groups from the inositol ring to terminate its activity; lithium blocks the activity of one of these phosphatases to enhance accumulation of the biologically active inositol phosphates. Like other information pathways, this one is diffused to generate coordinated cellular responses and is buffered and ultimately turned off when the signal strength decreases.

Protein Tyrosine Kinases. A group of peptide hormone receptors contains intrinsic protein tyrosine kinase activity. Ligand binding to the extracellular domain results in an allosteric change that is transmitted across the single membrane-spanning segment to activate the cytoplasmic kinase domain (see Fig. 199–2). In a second structural motif a transmembrane receptor is coupled to a distinct cytoplasmic tyrosine kinase subunit. The lymphocyte receptor CD4 and cellular p56[lck] belong to this second class.

Within the cell the great majority of protein-bound phosphate is attached to serine and threonine residues, with only a small fraction being attached to tyrosine. Numerous kinases, however, covalently modify tyrosine residues in proteins as a central regulatory function in cell proliferation, developmental processes, and differentiated function. The extracellular ligand-binding domains of receptors of this class contain cysteine-rich regions that create the binding sites either as monomers (epidermal growth factor [EGF] receptor) or as dimers (insulin receptor) or contain immunoglobulin-like structures (platelet-derived growth factor [PDGF] and fibroblast growth factor [FGF] receptors). The cytoplasmic protein tyrosine kinase domains are highly homologous, containing ATP and substrate-binding sites, but different receptors recognize distinct substrates to give specific biologic responses. For example, insulin stimulates glucose uptake while EGF stimulates cell proliferation. The tyrosine kinases contain variable domains on both sides of the tyrosine kinase core as well as inserts within the kinase domain

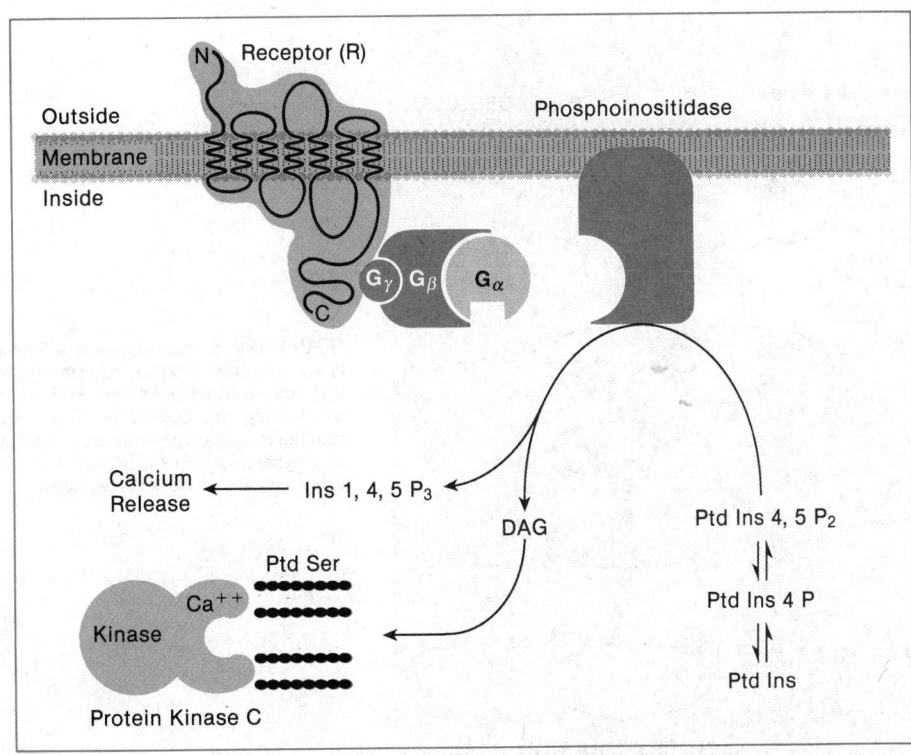

FIGURE 199–4. The phosphatidylinositol signaling pathway.

which provide regulatory sites that modulate ligand-activated tyrosine kinase activity.

Information received by a cell surface tyrosine kinase receptor is transmitted via a signal transduction pathway that begins with direct physical coupling of two proteins and proceeds via the GTP-binding protein *ras* (Fig. 199–5). In response to ligand binding, receptor tyrosine kinases either self-phosphorylate or phosphorylate a linker substrate. Proteins that contain a 100 amino acid domain homologous to a region in *src*, SH2, bind tightly to these sites of tyrosine phosphorylation. The growth factor receptor binding protein 2 *(Grb2)* is a molecular coupler containing an SH2 domain that plugs into a tyrosine phosphorylation site. *Shc* is another molecule coupler frequently used. *Grb2* also contains two SH3 domains that act as a receptacle for proline-rich domains of the guanine nucleotide exchange protein *SOS*. These high-affinity protein-to-protein interactions bring *SOS* to the cell membrane, where *ras* is present in its inactive GDP-bound form. Activated GTP-bound *ras* then couples to a serine/threonine protein kinase cascade involving first *raf*-1, then MEK and MAP (mitogen-activated protein) kinases. Information is thus relayed, expanded, and diffused to ultimately control gene expression and cell division. Operative mechanisms for this, as for other hormone-signaling pathways, include ligand or protein-protein interactions, activated GTP-bound G proteins, and protein phosphorylation. Receptor tyrosine kinases also couple to additional signaling pathways via SH2 domains in other proteins and via tyrosine phosphorylation of these proteins including phospholipase C-γ, a transcription control protein STAT 91, and PI 3-kinase.

Increased tyrosine kinase activity is reversed by four principal mechanisms: (1) ligand-induced endocytosis and down-regulation of surface receptors, (2) tyrosine phosphatases, which specifically remove phosphate from tyrosine residues, (3) reversal of the kinase reaction to transfer the phosphate from tyrosine residues in protein to ADP, and (4) hydrolysis of *ras*-bound GTP to GDP.

Regulation and reversibility of ligand-activated tyrosine kinases are important. Mutations involving these proteins occur frequently in cells transformed from normal to cancerous patterns of growth. Mutations may bypass regulatory features so that the kinases are constitutively active. The kinases may be overexpressed, most frequently owing to gene amplification but also owing to enhanced transcription, or the ligand may be constitutively expressed to activate receptors continuously. Mutant *ras* proteins may be constitutively active owing to decreased GTPase activity or to a defect in a protein that stimulates the GTPase activity of *ras*. Any of these changes converts a normal regulatory protein into an oncoprotein, one capable of causing neoplastic transformation.

Steroid Hormones Act Via Nuclear Receptors

THE SUPERFAMILY OF STEROID HORMONE RECEPTORS. All steroid hormone receptors share structural similarities indicative of a common ancestral molecule. The most conserved structural feature is the DNA-binding domain that contains zinc "fingers" (Fig. 199–6). The diagnostic spacing of cysteine residues creates a structure coordinated to a Zn^{2+} atom and an α helix that binds to the major groove of DNA. Because the energy of protein-DNA interaction depends on the area of contact, most proteins bind DNA as complexes. Steroid hormone receptors of the glucocorticoid receptor subfamily bind to DNA as homodimers; receptors of the thyroid hormone receptor subfamily may bind as homodimers but more commonly bind as heterodimers with a common partner, the retinoid X receptor (RXR).

The DNA recognition element consists of two half-sites of six base pairs, each half binding one monomer surface of the dimeric receptor protein. The half-sites are arranged as direct, inverted, or everted repeats. Receptors of the glucocorticoid receptor subfamily most often bind to palindromic sites, whereas receptors of the thyroid hormone receptor subfamily most often bind to sites made up of directly repeated DNA sequences. Small variations in the DNA-binding domain and in the DNA recognition element provide specificity for hormone action. One important determinant for receptor binding and activity is the spacing between the two half-sites for dimeric receptor binding. The spacing rules for DNA recognition elements that are arranged as direct repeats (DR) indicate that a spacing of 1 (DR + 1) directs RXR homodimer binding and 9-*cis*-retinoic acid responses, DR + 3 directs vitamin D receptor · RXR binding and vitamin D responses, DR + 4 directs thyroid hormone receptor · RXR binding and thyroid hormone responses, and DR + 5 directs retinoic acid receptor · RXR binding and all-*trans*-retinoic acid responses. RXR binds to the upstream half and the hormone-specific receptor binds to the downstream half of these DNA response elements to mediate hormone-dependent changes in transcription. Spacing between half-sites is crucial for binding homodimeric receptors of the glucocorticoid receptor class, but the

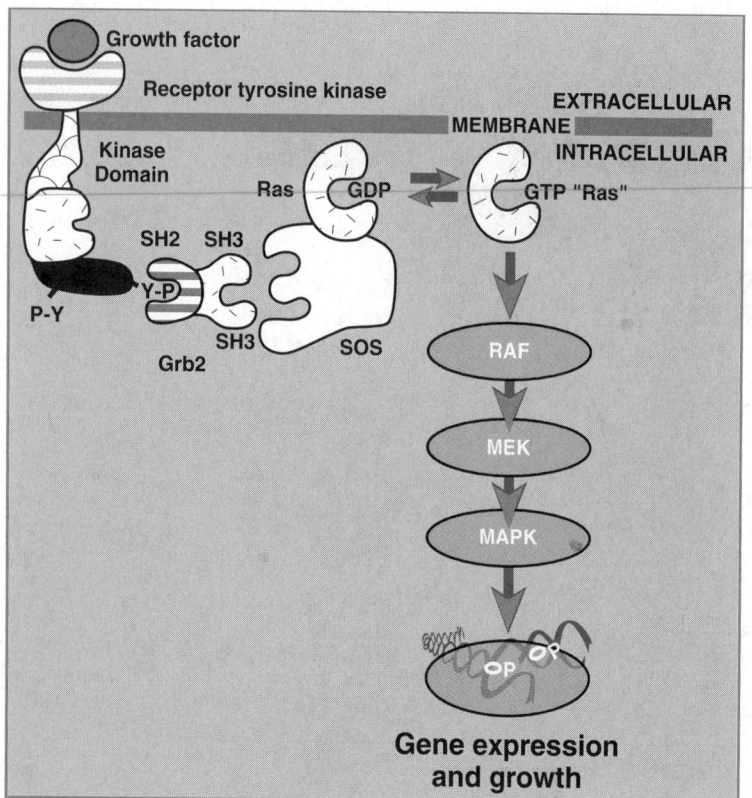

FIGURE 199–5. Information transfer through a receptor tyrosine kinase pathway. Sites of receptor tyrosine self-phosphorylation, Y-P, are recognized by the SH2 domain of the linker *Grb2*, which brings the guanine nucleotide exchange factor *SOS* to the membrane where *ras* is located. Activated GTP-bound *ras* initiates signaling by contacting *raf*, a serine/threonine kinase, to initiate a cascade of kinase activations.

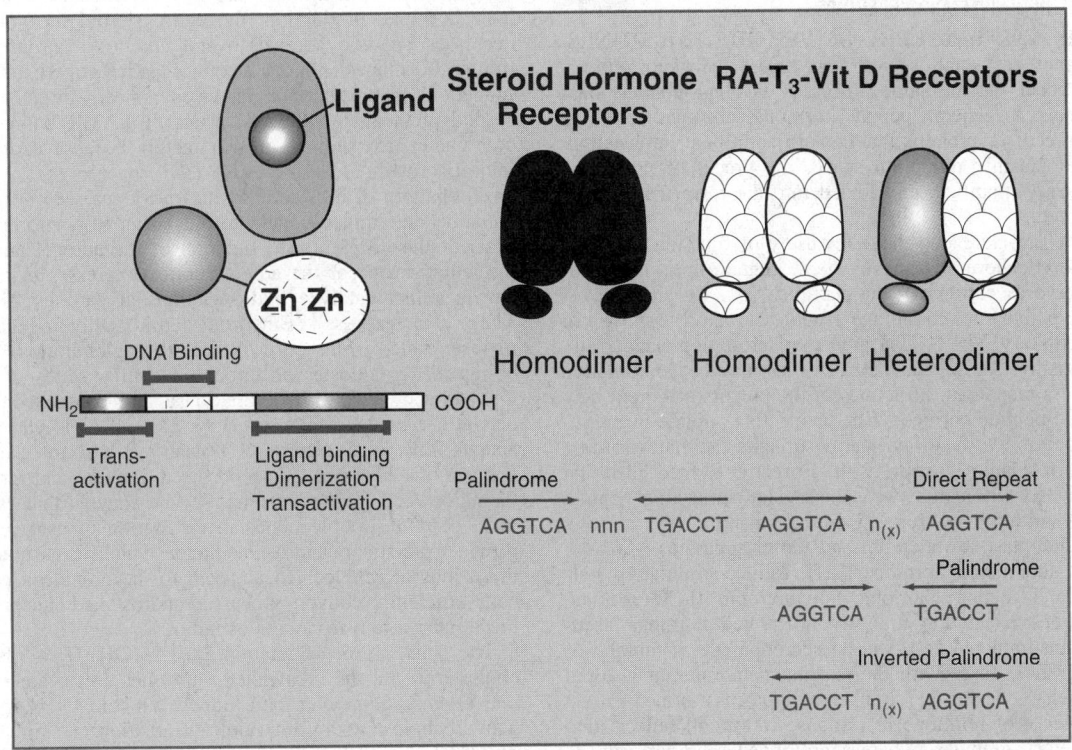

FIGURE 199–6. Structural features of steroid hormone receptors. *Left,* The DNA-binding domain, which consists of two zinc finger structures, is flanked by N′ terminal activation sequences and by C′ terminal ligand binding, dimerization, and activation sequences. *Right,* Glucocorticoid receptor family members bind as homodimers to palindromes. Thyroid hormone receptor family members bind primarily as heterodimers with retinoid X receptor to direct repeat motifs separated by varying numbers of base pairs.

sequence of the half-site provides an essential discriminant. Specificity is quantitative, not absolute. For example, progesterone receptors bind to glucocorticoid response elements, and retinoic acid receptors bind to thyroid hormone receptor DNA response elements. Specificity is sufficient for generating hormone-specific responses but may permit overlapping functions as in ligand-activated progesterone receptor induction of glucocorticoid-regulated genes.

Hormone binding activates the biologic function of the receptor. Cortisol receptors exist in inactive complexes with other proteins; cortisol binding induces an allosteric change that facilitates dissociation, allowing the ligand-bound receptor to bind to DNA. Thyroid hormone and retinoic acid receptors exist bound to DNA rather than complexed to protein; hormone binding results in an allosteric change that activates the receptor, so it interacts with other components of the transcription machinery.

The steroid hormone receptor family is a large one that includes subfamilies of receptors: at least four for retinoic acid, two for thyroid hormone, several for 1,25(OH)$_2$ vitamin D and for fatty acids or metabolites causing perixosome proliferation, and a group of "orphans" whose ligands remain to be identified. The general structural motif is an important one, which, in evolution, has diverged to specify responses to many hormonal signals and to control expression of numerous genes.

REGULATION OF GENE TRANSCRIPTION. Hormone-activated receptor proteins bound to their DNA response element targets act as *cis*-active enhancers. They act from various positions relative to the start of transcription and in various combinations with other regulatory proteins to control the rate of initiation of gene transcription. Gene promoters lie upstream of the site where eukaryotic RNA polymerase II initiates transcription of messenger RNA. The best characterized promoter contains a TATA box that binds a protein, transcription factor II D (TF II-D), which directs accurate transcription by RNA polymerase II ~ 30 base pairs downstream. Seven proteins (TATA-associated factors or TAF's) associate with TF II-D in a specific complex that provides a molecular surface for interaction with the transcription-regulatory proteins, which are bound elsewhere to DNA. Other promoter motifs include a basal initiator and GC-rich regions in which multiple transcription start sites exist. Gene expression is induced by increasing the rate

of transcription. The gene must contain a DNA response/binding element for the receptor to generate a response; multiple binding sites give greater enhancement. The DNA-binding elements position the steroid hormone receptors so that other regions of the protein can interact with proteins in the transcription initiation complex. Adaptor proteins may connect the proteins bound at enhancer sites to the proteins of the basal transcription complex bound at the promoter.

Hormone-activated receptors can also repress transcription. Negative feedback loops operate through this process. Activated cortisol receptors repress transcription of the gene encoding the ACTH precursor; activated thyroid hormone receptors inhibit transcription of both α- and β-TSH subunit genes. The principle of ligand-activated receptors binding to specific DNA target sequences in the regulated gene is the same as that required for inductive responses. The receptor may inhibit transcription by displacing positive enhancers, by blocking RNA polymerase engagement, or by silencing transcription through interactions with the core transcriptional machinery, analogous to protein-protein interactions that enhance transcription.

Many other proteins regulate initiation of transcription, both as inducers and as inhibitors. These bind to DNA via specific sequences, as do steroid receptors, or they may interact with proteins which do. These proteins may be modified in response to hormonal signals initiated at the cell surface. Such alterations account for the changes in gene transcription due to hormones acting via surface receptors. Two general and cooperative mechanisms exist: phosphorylation and translocation of transcription factors from cytoplasm to nucleus. Genes regulated by cAMP contain DNA sequences that specify binding of a specific nuclear transcription regulator (CREB). CREB, which undergoes changes in activity upon phosphorylation, is a required final mediator of gene induction by peptide hormones that act at the cell surface to activate adenylate cyclase and cAMP-dependent protein kinase. STAT-91 and related proteins are phosphorylated on tyrosine residues and, when phosphorylated, enter the nucleus to activate transcription of specific genes. This chain of effects alters transcription of mRNA's and cell protein concentrations to dictate changes in cell function and organ physiology.

BIOSYNTHESIS OF HORMONES AND RECEPTORS

SYNTHESIS AND DELIVERY OF PEPTIDE HORMONES.
Peptide hormones are small secretory proteins; their biosynthesis and secretion occur via the same processes as other nonhormonal secretory proteins. In general, peptide hormones are synthesized as part of larger precursor proteins that contain additional information. Within the endoplasmic reticulum space, the precursor protein is cleaved, covalently modified, and folded into the form that will be ultimately secreted.

The precursor structure may have a variety of functions. Precursors for antidiuretic hormone and oxytocin contain specific neurophysins that serve as carriers of the peptides from the site of synthesis in the hypothalamus to storage granules in axon terminals in the posterior pituitary. The ACTH precursor, pro-opiomelanocortin, contains information for several peptides that may be coordinately involved in stress responses. Structures in the precursor protein may serve to fold the peptide correctly. The connecting peptide in the insulin precursor between the β and the α subunits facilitates folding for formation of mature insulin with correctly formed disulfide bonds between and within the two chains. The connecting peptide is then excised and removed from mature α-β insulin.

Within the endoplasmic reticulum and Golgi apparatus, glycosylation of TSH, luteinizing hormone (LH), follicle-stimulating hormone (FSH), and human chorionic gonadotropin (hCG) occurs. Secretory granules containing highly concentrated hormone accumulate in the unstimulated cell. During secretion the membrane of the secretory granule fuses with the plasma membrane, and stored hormone is discharged into the circulation, a process termed *exocytosis*. Rapid release of hormone in response to stimuli reflects discharge of secretory granules, whereas prolonged secretion reflects release of newly synthesized hormone.

Peptide hormones may also be derived from precursors with receptor-like structures or from circulating forms. EGF and transforming growth factor-α (TGF-α) are made as a part of the surface domain of a transmembrane protein with a receptor-like structure. These are released by proteolysis, although they may act on adjacent cells without processing to provide cell-to-cell communication. Renin, an enzyme released from juxtaglomerular cells, acts on angiotensinogen secreted from liver. Active angiotensin is synthesized by progressive proteolysis of a precursor outside of cells: renin to yield angiotensin I and angiotensin-converting enzyme to yield angiotensin II.

Secreted peptide hormones have a short half-life of about 3 to 7 minutes in the circulation. Glycoprotein hormones have longer half-lives of 1 to 4 hours. The short circulating half-life and peptide degradation by gastric acid and intestinal enzymes have precluded oral use of this class of hormones. Several attempts to prolong half-lives have met with partial success: Complexing with Zn^{2+} and protamine creates a slowly absorbed and longer-acting form of injectable insulin; removing the amino group from the N' terminal amino acid and substituting a D-arginine creates a longer-acting ADH, which can be absorbed from nasal mucous membranes. At present direct use of peptide hormones is limited to injectable forms. Prolonged action results in receptor desensitization, so recapitulation of normal cyclic secretion typical of endogenous production presents a second difficulty. Use of GnRH must be both by parental routes and pulsatile in nature to induce ovulation and successful pregnancy.

SYNTHESIS AND TRANSPORT OF STEROID HORMONES.
Steroid hormones are derived from cholesterol provided by *de novo* cellular synthesis from acetate or by uptake of circulating cholesterol made in the liver and delivered to cells via low density lipoprotein (LDL) particles. Synthesized steroid hormones are not stored, so secretory rates directly reflect production rates. In adrenal and gonadal tissues the rate-limiting step for increased steroid hormone biosynthesis is transfer of substrate cholesterol to the side chain cleavage enzyme located in the inner mitochondrial membrane. Cleavage of the side chain of cholesterol is catalyzed by a cytochrome P-450 enzyme that resembles other steroid hydroxylases. These enzymes progressively modify the cholesterol nucleus by the sequential addition of hydroxyl groups to specific sites. The rate-limiting step is stimulated in target cells by ACTH, LH, and FSH to result in rapid increases in steroid hormone biosynthesis. The trophic stimulatory hormones also maintain the structure of the target glands and induce each of the enzymes involved in hormone biosynthesis. With hypophysectomy or feedback inhibition of pituitary hormone production, the entire steroid biosynthetic pathway decreases and the adrenal, ovary, and testis atrophy. Addition of trophic hormones induces enzymes and regrowth of target glands. Induction of biosynthetic enzymes appears directly mediated via second messenger pathways, primarily cAMP, but growth requires coordinate provision of growth factors because cAMP, in general, inhibits growth.

The pattern of biosynthetic enzymes expressed during cell differentiation determines which steroid hormone is produced and is the basis of the differentiated function of the adrenal and gonads. The fascicularis zone of the adrenal cortex expresses cytochrome P-450 enzymes that catalyze hydroxylations at carbons 21, 17, and 11. They also express 3β-hydroxysteroid dehydrogenase, $\Delta^{4,5}$ isomerase, which forms cortisol. The zona glomerulosa of the adrenal cortex makes aldosterone through a similar series of reactions, but the pathway lacks 17α-hydroxylase and contains an activity that acts at carbon 18. The testis lacks 21- and 11β-hydroxylases, so reactants flow to testosterone. Ovarian synthesis of estradiol requires cooperation between adjacent theca interna and granulosa cells. Granulosa cells express aromatase, the enzyme that catalyzes placement of three double bonds in the A ring of estrogens but cannot provide precursor androstenedione, which is synthesized in the theca interna cell located adjacent to the granulosa cell. Granulosa cells efficiently convert precursor androstenedione provided by the theca interna to estrone and estradiol.

The active form of vitamin D, 1,25(OH)$_2$D, is also made from cholesterol, but the biosynthetic enzymes are located in three separate organs: skin, liver, and kidney. Vitamin D$_3$ is formed from 7-dehydrocholesterol by ultraviolet irradiation of skin. D$_3$ is then hydroxylated at carbon 25 in the liver to yield 25(OH)D. This is converted by 1α-hydroxylase to 1,25(OH)$_2$D in proximal tubule cells of the kidney. In this unique endocrine system, the major site for regulation is the final 1α-hydroxylation in renal proximal tubule cells, a step controlled by parathyroid hormone and phosphate.

In contrast to peptide hormones, steroid hormones have longer circulating half-lives and may be active when administered orally. Following secretion into the circulation, steroid hormones are bound to transport glycoproteins made in the liver. The transport proteins, which have a binding but not an activity site, provide a reservoir of hormone, protected from metabolism and renal clearance, which can be released to cells. Three transport proteins have been characterized: corticosteroid-binding globulin (CBG), which binds cortisol and progesterone, sex steroid hormone–binding globulin (SHBG), which binds testosterone with greater affinity than estradiol, and vitamin D–binding protein, which binds precursor 25(OH)D with greater affinity than 1,25(OH)$_2$D. Thyroid-binding globulin (TBG) binds L-thyroxine to provide its uniquely long half-life of 7 days. Estrogens induce and androgens inhibit synthesis of these transport proteins. Albumin provides a large carrier system that weakly binds hormones.

Free steroid hormone, which is in equilibrium with that bound to transport protein, enters cells to bind intracellular receptors and generate biologic responses. The free fraction is also the active one in feedback regulation, so it is the concentration of free hormone that is altered in homeostatic responses. The free fraction is very small compared with the bound fraction, but total hormone concentrations from both fractions are measured in most clinical assays. Conditions such as pregnancy, which alter binding protein concentrations, alter total measured hormone but not the biologically relevant free hormone concentration. In special clinical situations measurement of binding protein concentration and of free hormone may be required for accurate assessment.

Steroid hormones are metabolized principally in the liver to inactive water-soluble metabolites. Cortisol is inactivated by reduction of the double bond in the A ring and conjugation to glucuronide or sulfate at carbon 3 to make it water-soluble for renal excretion. However, not all peripheral metabolic alterations are inactivating. 5α-Reductase converts testosterone to 5α-dihydrotestosterone, which is the biologically active species in male reproductive tract and skin. Androstenedione produced in ovary and adrenal can be converted to testosterone in peripheral tissues. Significant quantities of estradiol are produced by conversion of circulating precursors.

Like their hormonal ligands, receptor synthesis is highly regulated to control cellular responses and sensitivity to hormones. Receptor synthesis is increased in response to environmental or developmental need or is repressed in negative feedback loops and during stages of development. Receptor concentration is as important as hormone concentration in determining cell responses. Regulation of receptor synthesis is therefore central to providing coordinated and appropriate endocrine responses.

INTEGRATION OF ENDOCRINE RESPONSES

FEEDBACK LOOPS. Multiple hormones cooperate to coordinate development, reproduction, and homeostasis. When a hormone has elicited an appropriate response, the signal must be terminated. In addition to the buffering that occurs in target cells, feedback control is the principal mechanism through which this occurs (Fig. 199–7). Feedback loops are especially important for communication between organs that are spatially separated. The hormonal products of peripheral endocrine glands such as thyroid, adrenal cortex, ovary, and testis exert negative feedback control over the synthesis and secretion of the stimulatory pituitary hormone. Feedback, which occurs at the level of the pituitary cell and in the hypothalamus, operates via control of several essential steps. The neurohormone thyrotropin-releasing hormone (TRH) stimulates thyrotropes of the anterior pituitary to synthesize and secrete TSH, which in turn increases synthesis and secretion of thyroid hormone. Increased production of thyroid hormone induces appropriate metabolic responses in target organs; it also inhibits production of TSH to return the system to baseline. The prohormone L-thyroxine (T_4) is converted in the pituitary thyrotrope to active T_3, and T_3 binds to nuclear T_3 receptors to inhibit transcription of both α and β TSH subunit genes. T_3-bound receptors also decrease synthesis of TRH receptors, rendering cells less responsive to stimulatory TRH. In addition, T_3 inhibits hypothalamic production of TRH. Conversely, when thyroid hormone concentrations are low, feedback inhibition is relieved and TRH stimulates increased production of TSH, which increases production of T_4 and thus re-establishes homeostasis. Feedback principles provide an exquisitely sensitive system for making appropriate changes and then returning to the homeostatic set point.

Feedback operates not only via steroid and thyroid hormones but also through peptides and ions. Pituitary FSH production is feedback regulated by the ovarian steroid hormone estrogen and by the ovarian peptide hormone inhibin. Parathyroid hormone (PTH) regulates serum Ca^{2+} concentrations; with hypocalcemia PTH increases and re-establishes normocalcemia. The increase in serum $[Ca^{2+}]$ feedback inhibits PTH synthesis and secretion to re-establish serum PTH concentrations appropriate to normocalcemia. With mutations in the $[Ca^{2+}]$ receptor on parathyroid cell membranes, feedback sensing is impaired and excessive PTH is made.

RECRUITMENT OF COORDINATE RESPONSES. Physiologic responses result from many different cell types and organs acting in concert. The necessary coordination is provided both by a hormone acting at multiple sites and by each hormone eliciting multiple responses, which sum to give the overall effect. Integrated responses require that one hormone regulate the synthesis or action of another; the nervous system is integrated into the overall response. Paradigms of such coordinated responses include stress, fasting, and reproduction.

A major stress, such as trauma with pain and hypovolemia, initiates a central nervous system response that includes synthesis and secretion of corticotropin-releasing hormone (CRH) and antidiuretic hormone. CRH is the major stimulus to increase pituitary secretion of ACTH, which increases adrenal cortisol production. Cortisol maintains not only blood glucose but also vascular responsiveness to epinephrine and norepinephrine. It limits excessive inflammatory responses to prevent further volume loss and tissue damage. CRH acts, in the central nervous system, to stimulate the peripheral sympathetic nervous system. Increased sympathetic nervous system activity mediates adaptive cardiovascular responses, including increased blood pressure and pulse rate. It also induces appropriate

FIGURE 199–7. Forward regulation and negative feedback.

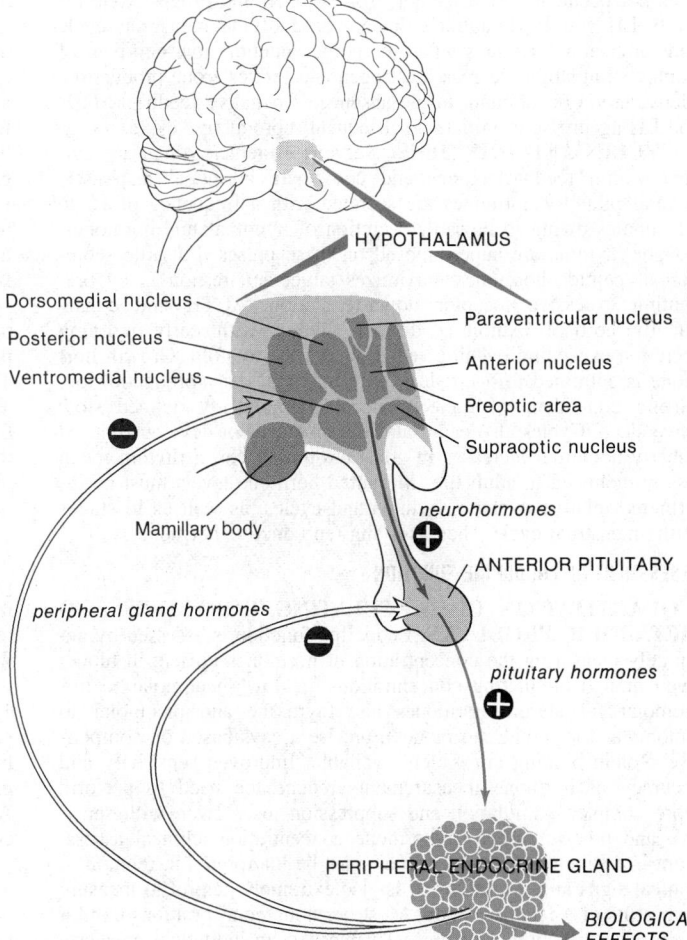

behavioral responses. ADH increases permeability of the collecting duct of the distal nephron to conserve water and intravascular volume. It facilitates CRH-stimulated ACTH secretion. With hypovolemia the renin-angiotensin-aldosterone system is also activated to enhance vasoconstriction and to conserve sodium and intravascular volume. These responses of the hypothalamus, pituitary, and adrenal cortex together facilitate survival from stresses.

With fasting, blood glucose concentrations are maintained for 12 to 24 hours by glucagon- and epinephrine-mediated release of glucose from glycogen stores. With more prolonged fasting cortisol-stimulated gluconeogenesis is the major mechanism that sustains blood glucose. Insulin secretion is suppressed. Metabolic demands are decreased by inhibition of 5'-deiodinase to decrease conversion of T_4 to active T_3 in peripheral tissues. Growth-promoting hormones, such as insulin-like growth factor I, are also suppressed under conditions of substrate lack. With starvation, gonadotropin secretion decreases and reproductive capacity is diminished.

Female reproductive cycles result from coordinated signaling by hypothalamic, pituitary, and ovarian hormones. Pulsatile secretion of gonadotropin-releasing hormone stimulates pituitary production of LH and FSH. During the follicular phase of the menstrual cycle these peptide hormones regulate ovarian secretion of estrogen and direct maturation of follicles, one of which increases 1000-fold in diameter and becomes dominant for ovulation. FSH induces LH receptors in ovarian granulosa cells, and both LH and FSH induce aromatase as part of the mechanism that enhances estrogen production. LH and FSH increase during the follicular phase and, with follicle development, estrogen secretion rises. Positive feedback effects of estrogen result in the mid-cycle surge of LH and FSH, which induces ovulation. The remaining granulosa and theca cells reorganize to form the corpus luteum, which produces progesterone as well as estrogen. Concentrations of these hormones negatively inhibit FSH and LH production and induce additional uterine changes necessary for implantation. Ovarian inhibin also inhibits FSH production. If fertilization and implantation occur, the corpus luteum is regulated by hCG until placental steroidogenesis is established. If fertilization does not occur, negative feedback of estrogen and progesterone inhibits LH and FSH, and the luteal phase of the menstrual cycle ends after about 10 days when the corpus luteum, now deprived of trophic stimulation, decreases estrogen and progesterone production. Menstruation occurs and, in the absence of negative feedback, FSH and LH again rise to initiate a subsequent reproductive cycle.

CYCLES AND RHYTHMS. Nervous system rhythms are evident within feedback loops and coordinate hormonal responses. Several pituitary hormones are secreted with a frequency of 15 to 60 minutes owing to pulsatile secretion of hypothalamic hormones. Longer rhythms are superimposed on these pulses. Pulsatile secretion of peptide hormones maximizes target cell responses by preventing excessive receptor down-regulation. ACTH and consequently cortisol exhibit a diurnal rhythm with early morning secretion exceeding evening secretion at least twofold. Growth hormone is entrained to deep sleep with maximal daily production occurring coincident with electroencephalographically defined slow wave sleep. Cycles also occur at different stages of development. At puberty nocturnal increases in gonadotropins occur, a rhythm much less pronounced in adult life. Measured hormone levels must be interpreted relative to these rhythms and cycles, as well as to stages of the menstrual cycle when assaying reproductive hormones.

ASSESSMENT OF ENDOCRINE FUNCTION

QUANTITATION OF CIRCULATING HORMONES AND METABOLIC PRODUCTS. Endocrine function is assessed by accurately measuring the concentration of hormones present in blood. Even though circulating concentrations are low (nanomolar to micromolar for steroid hormones and thyroxine and picomolar to nanomolar for peptide hormones), precise assays based on competitive protein binding are widely available. Improved sensitivity and accuracy of hormone measurements reduce the need to perform more complex stimulation and suppression tests. Even with sensitive and precise assays of hormone concentration, clinical assessment is essential. Measured values must be interpreted in relation to clinical signs and symptoms. It is also extremely helpful to measure both arms of a feedback loop. Most hormone concentrations exhibit a gaussian distribution of normal values, so an individual measurement at either end of the normal range may be normal or abnormal

for that individual. Coincident measurement of TSH and T_4, LH and testosterone, ACTH and cortisol, PTH and Ca^{2+} gives greater information than either alone. A T_4 at the lower end of the normal range with an elevated TSH indicates thyroid gland failure, whereas the same T_4 with a normal TSH likely indicates a euthyroid state. An elevated cortisol with suppressed ACTH indicates autonomous production of cortisol by an adrenal tumor. Cycles and rhythms of hormone secretion must also be considered. Evening cortisol concentrations are half or less of peak morning values. Coincident measurement of ACTH clarifies whether a low cortisol represents diurnal rhythm or adrenal insufficiency; an elevated ACTH when cortisol is low suggests adrenal insufficiency. Measurement of gonadotropins, estradiol, and progesterone must be related to normal values for follicular and luteal phases of the menstrual cycle.

Steroid and thyroid hormones are bound to carrier proteins. In pregnancy, in which estrogen increases hepatic production of carrier proteins, total cortisol and T_4 values are elevated but ACTH and TSH are normal. On occasion, however, it is necessary to measure the free, active hormone concentration. Because the free fraction is very small relative to the total amount, careful separation of bound from free fractions without the use of organic solvents is necessary, and very sensitive detection systems are required. Assays for free T_4 and for ionized Ca^{2+} are available for specialized clinical circumstances. One can assess the amount of binding globulin directly, or indirectly measure unoccupied binding sites (T_3 resin uptake test).

Measurement of urinary excretion of some hormones provides an integrated value for daily production rates. Measurement of urinary free cortisol is particularly useful because cortisol-binding globulin, which binds 1 cortisol molecule per molecule of protein, is approximately saturated at the peak morning cortisol concentration. Free unbound cortisol that exceeds binding capacity is filtered at the glomerulus, so an elevated 24-hour urine free cortisol provides an accurate assessment in cortisol excess syndromes.

Measurement of metabolic effects is an essential component of endocrine evaluation. Insulin function is assessed by measuring plasma and urine glucose concentrations, PTH by measuring serum $[Ca^{2+}]$, aldosterone by measuring serum $[K^+]$, and ADH by measuring serum and urine osmolalities.

STIMULATION AND SUPPRESSION TESTS. Measurement of both arms of a feedback loop provides sufficient laboratory information in most endocrine deficiency or excess states. Additional diagnostic information can be gained, however, by perturbing the feedback system through administration of hormones. For stimulation tests a hormone is administered and the ability of the target gland to respond is assessed by measuring its product. This provides an estimate of the ability of the target gland to synthesize hormone, of its trophic maintenance, and its exposure to feedback inhibition. Baseline measurements are made before hormone administration and at the established normal time of peak target gland response. Ranges of normal responses have been established for comparison. Examples include TRH stimulation tests, in which levels of pituitary-produced TSH are measured. In hypopituitarism, serum TSH fails to rise in response to a standard intravenous injection of TRH. In primary hypothyroidism, in which feedback inhibition by thyroid hormone is small, TSH rises excessively, whereas in hyperthyroidism excessive feedback inhibition results in minimal or no increases in TSH. For ACTH stimulation tests, $ACTH_{1-24}$ is administered as an intravenous injection to assess the ability of the adrenal cortex to produce cortisol. A low baseline cortisol that fails to rise indicates adrenal insufficiency. Interpretation requires integration of clinical information because failure to respond to ACTH may also occur when the adrenal cortex has been suppressed owing to treatment with synthetic glucocorticoids. A variation of stimulation tests involves interruption of the feedback loop by metabolic inhibitors of hormone biosynthesis. Metyrapone, an inhibitor of 11β-hydroxylase, decreases serum cortisol, relieving feedback suppression of ACTH production. The resulting increase in ACTH can be measured directly, or ACTH-stimulated 11-desoxycortisol, the precursor of cortisol, can be measured as an indicator of increased ACTH. The metyrapone test provides an assessment of pituitary corticotrope function and reserve. Stimulation tests are most useful in suspected endocrine deficiency states.

Suppression tests, which measure the ability of administered hormone to provide feedback inhibition, are most useful in evaluating hormone excesses. Dexamethasone, a potent synthetic glucocorticoid, is administered to inhibit ACTH production. Because dexamethasone is not detected in cortisol assays, more easily measured cortisol rather than ACTH can be used as an endpoint. In Cushing's syndrome, the source of cortisol excess can be deduced using dexamethasone suppression. Pituitary tumors that produce excess ACTH frequently retain susceptibility to feedback inhibition. These tumors are resistant to doses of dexamethasone that suppress normal corticotrope ACTH production but are inhibited by higher doses of dexamethasone. In contrast, adrenal gland tumors and tumors that ectopically produce ACTH are resistant to even high doses of dexamethasone.

ANATOMIC ASSESSMENT. Imaging of endocrine glands is important, especially when considering surgical therapy. The high sensitivity and precision of computed tomography and nuclear magnetic resonance imaging allow detection of even small endocrine tumors such as pituitary, parathyroid, and adrenal adenomas. Sonographic techniques are also useful for imaging the thyroid gland, ovaries, testes, and pancreas. Radionuclide imaging may also be useful. Radioactive isotopes of iodine (^{123}I, ^{131}I) or compounds that are concentrated by the thyroid gland similar to iodine, such ^{99}Tc, are used to determine anatomy and imply function of the thyroid gland.

Measurement of hormone concentrations in venous effluent of glands may be useful in specialized circumstances to localize the source of abnormal production. Measurement of ACTH in petrosal sinus blood may be useful in localizing pituitary tumors, of PTH in neck and chest veins in localizing unusually located parathyroid adenomas, and of insulin in mesenteric venous drainage in localizing pancreatic insulinomas.

Cytologic and immunocytochemical techniques are important. Fine-needle aspiration of thyroid nodules with cytologic examinations analogous to those used in Papanicolaou smears has become the procedure of choice to distinguish benign and malignant thyroid nodules. Staining of surgical tissues with antihormone antibodies provides proof of hormone production and a guide to future therapy.

Receptors are not routinely measured but can be quantitated using immunologic techniques. Recombinant DNA technologies can be used to define inherited defects in receptors. When oncogenes are identified in specific endocrine neoplasms, these can be measured and mutations identified using DNA hybridization techniques. Autoimmune endocrine diseases can be documented by quantitating antibodies directed against specific organs (thyroid-stimulating immunoglobulin, anti-islet cell antibodies, antiadrenal antibodies).

ABERRATIONS IN DISEASE

DEFICIENCY STATES. The most prevalent endocrine disorders result from hormone deficiencies. A variety of disease states impair or destroy endocrine glands: defects in organ development, genetic defects in biosynthetic enzymes, immune-mediated destruction, neoplasia, infections, hemorrhage, nutritional deficits, and vascular insufficiency. Endocrine gland failure may be acute with rapid development of symptoms or chronic with slower development of symptoms but more pronounced physical changes. Defects in a gland such as the thyroid may result in a multisystem disorder due to failure to produce a single hormone, whereas defects in the hypothalamus or pituitary may result in a multisystem disorder, including thyroid deficiency, due to failure to produce many hormones. Multiple endocrine gland deficiencies may also result from autoimmune-mediated mechanisms in the polyglandular autoimmune deficiency syndromes. Because hormones participate in coordinated responses, secondary changes in other endocrine responses often result from deficiency of a single hormone.

Deficiency states also result from defects in hormone receptors and in signaling mechanisms. Defects may be inherited or acquired. Genetic abnormalities in androgen receptors result in unresponsiveness to androgens and an XY male with a female phenotype; defects in vitamin D receptors result in vitamin D–resistant rickets; defects in thyroid hormone receptors result in the resistance to thyroid hormone of Refetoff's syndrome; defects in growth hormone receptors result in ateliotic dwarfism of Laron's syndrome. Acquired receptor defects most often result from immunologic mechanisms where antibodies bind to receptors, blocking ligand access.

Postreceptor defects may occur. A defect in $G_{\alpha}s$ results in pseudohypoparathyroidism, in which unresponsiveness to PTH occurs. Such patients fail to respond normally to other hormones whose receptors couple to adenylate cyclase (TSH, glucagon, LH). Type II diabetes mellitus, which is inherited, is characterized by in-

sulin resistance. The molecular defect has not yet been characterized, but understanding this pathophysiology underlies therapeutic approaches directed at reducing resistance to and augmenting secretion of insulin. Because receptor and postreceptor defects are characterized by hormone resistance, feedback does not occur and producer glands enlarge and circulating hormone concentrations are high despite clinical evidence for deficiency.

EXCESS STATES. Excessive production of hormone and clinical evidence of such excess implies failure of normal feedback mechanisms. This occurs most commonly with neoplasia and with autoimmunity, in which antireceptor antibodies act as hormone agonists. Tumors of endocrine glands characteristically produce excessive amounts of the hormone made by the cell of origin but are no longer subject to normal feedback controls. Some tumors, such as pituitary adenomas that produce ACTH, retain feedback but require higher concentrations of cortisol to suppress ACTH. Prolactinomas retain dopamine suppression, and both their function and growth can be inhibited by dopamine agonists. Tumors arising in peripheral endocrine glands that are under pituitary trophic hormone regulation are autonomous because they are not normally subject to negative feedback. More undifferentiated tumors may also be insensitive to feedback regulation.

Hormones may be produced in excess by tumors arising from cells that do not normally produce the hormone. Ectopic production of peptide hormones is common in a variety of neoplasms, and symptoms due to the hormone excess may contribute significantly to morbidity. Because steroid hormones are made via a multienzyme pathway, excesses of these hormones occur only with tumors arising in the producer gland or with excessive production of the trophic peptide hormone. Cortisol excess may result from adrenocortical tumors or from excessive stimulation by ACTH produced by pituitary or ectopic neoplasms.

The most prevalent disease due to agonistic antibodies is Graves' disease, in which antibodies are produced that activate the TSH receptor. Because many hormones are available as therapeutic agents, some patients take excessive amounts and present with an endocrine excess syndrome.

GENETIC DETERMINANTS OF DISEASE. Many endocrine diseases result from genetic mutations. Genetic defects in biosynthetic enzymes may result in deficiency states: Hypothyroidism may result from thyroid peroxidase or deiodinase enzyme defects; adrenal insufficiency may result from 21-hydroxylase deficiency or a defect in other steroid biosynthetic enzymes; a form of male hypogonadism may result from 5α-reductase deficiency. Receptor defects are thought to be uncommon, but methods to define these have only recently become available. Type II diabetes, the most common endocrine abnormality, is inherited but its molecular basis is not yet known. Autoimmune endocrine disease also has a genetic basis involving an inherited defect in immune surveillance. Multiple endocrine neoplasia syndromes are due to activating mutations in the *ret* tyrosine kinase receptor so that cell growth and function are constitutively stimulated without ligand.

In the future, methods using nucleic acid probes can be used to make precise diagnoses in disease states and to provide predictive information before overt disease develops. Because genetic defects are present in all DNA, peripheral blood cells or skin fibroblasts provide a ready source of material for assay. Acquired mutations can be assessed by assay of material obtained by biopsy.

Darnell J, Lodish H, Baltimore D (eds.): Cell to cell signaling: Hormones and receptors. *In* Molecular Cell Biology. New York, WH Freeman, 1990. *Good overview of principles of mechanisms of hormone signaling.*

Egan SE, Weinberg RA: The pathway to signal achievement. Nature 365:781, 1993. *Overview of the central mitogenic pathway important for normal growth, which is often deranged in cancer.*

Fantl WJ, Johnson DE, Williams LT: Signalling by receptor tyrosine kinases. Annu Rev Biochem 65:453, 1993. *Review of structure and signaling by an essential class of peptide hormone receptors.*

Goodrich JA, Tjian R: TBP/TAF complexes: Selectivity factors for eukaryotic transcription. Curr Opin Cell Biol 6:403, 1994. *A thoughtful discussion of the way by which regulatory proteins contact the transcriptional machinery.*

Lazar MA: Thyroid hormone receptors: Multiple forms, multiple possibilities. Endocrinol Rev 14:184, 1993. *Review with primary references of how thyroid hormone and related receptors work.*

Mulligan LM, Kwok JBJ, Healey CS, et al.: Germ-line mutations of the RET proto-oncogene in multiple endocrine neoplasia type 2A. Nature 363:458, 1993. *First demonstration of an inherited mutation that activates a receptor, resulting in neoplasia.*

Tang W-J, Gilman AG: Adenylyl cyclases. Cell 70:869, 1992. *Minireview of the prototypic signal-transducing molecule.*

200 ENDORPHINS/OPIOID PEPTIDES, PROSTAGLANDINS, AND NATRIURETIC HORMONES

200.1 The Endorphin Family of Opioid Peptides: Biochemistry, Anatomy, and Physiology

Stanley J. Watson

Many central and peripheral nervous system structures contain cells that secrete endogenous neuropeptides capable of mimicking opiate alkaloids, such as morphine and heroin. These peptides have a common pentapeptide sequence at their amino terminus [Tyr-Gly-Gly-Phe-Met (or-Leu)], which is important for their opiate activity. Such *endogenous opioid peptides* carry the generic name of endorphins and are divided into three main families: (1) *Pro-Opio-Melano-Cortin* (or POMC), (2) *Pro-Enkephalin*, and (3) *Pro-Dynorphin/Neo-Endorphin* (Fig. 200–1). POMC produces one opiate peptide, β-endorphin, and several nonopioid products, e.g., ACTH and α-, β-, and γ-melanocyte-stimulating hormones (MSH). In contrast, pro-enkephalin has seven repeated opioid sequences, and pro-dynorphin has three.

The structural pharmacology of the opiate alkaloids includes active and inactive stereoisomers of both opiate agonists and antagonists. Radiolabeling of the active alkaloids in the 1970's made it possible to identify opiate receptors in brain. A search for their natural ligands followed, and more than 20 active peptide fragments were extracted. Among these are β-endorphin, met- and leu-enkephalin, and dynorphin. Gene and mRNA information has radi-

cally improved our knowledge of the sequences of the endorphins within their precursors and provided better understanding of their relationships with their nonopiate fragments.

Members of all endorphin families are widely distributed in brain, heart, lung, adrenal, ovary, pituitary, testes, and gut. POMC is found in the corticotrophs of the anterior lobe of the pituitary, in the arcuate nucleus in the base of the hypothalamus, and in the nucleus tractus solitarius in the brain stem. POMC fibers project through limbic, autonomic, and pain systems. The dynorphin system is more widespread both within the brain and in the periphery and also resides in testes, ovary, gut wall, adrenal cortex, and LH and FSH cells of anterior pituitary. In brain the dynorphin system is linked to sympathetic tone, pain systems, motor systems, endocrine control, limbic system, and cortical functions. The enkephalin system, even more widespread than dynorphin and POMC, is found with the catecholamine cells of the adrenal medulla. It also resides in heart, lung, gut wall, sympathetic ganglia, pituitary, and many brain fiber systems. Although enkephalin cells are widely distributed in brain, few linking circuits have as yet been identified. The most obvious systems involved by enkephalins are motor, pain, endocrine, autonomic, limbic (reward), cortex, and hippocampus.

Several different endocrine and neural tissues process endorphin peptides. The most obvious example is found with POMC in the pituitary of the rat. In the anterior lobe the corticotrophs produce, among other peptides, the stress hormone ACTH (1-39). In contrast, in the intermediate lobe (found in most species, but in humans present only in pregnant women and fetuses) that same molecule is further processed to make α-melanocyte-stimulating hormone [or N-acetyl ACTH 1-13 amide and ACTH (18-39)]. Similar tissue-specific processing patterns are found for other POMC peptides, such as β-endorphin, as well as for pro-dynorphin– and pro-enkephalin–produced peptides. For example, pro-enkephalin in adrenal is cleaved into larger fragments, whereas in brain it is actively processed to much smaller peptides. In the last 5 years many of the enzymes capable of participating in the cleavage and amidation of peptide precursors and their products have been cloned and studied.

Several principles have emerged about the above processing. A given precursor can give rise to one set of products in one tissue and a different set in another tissue. General processing differences reflect the chosen cleavage site, indicated by the presence of a dibasic peptide bond (e.g., lysine-argenine). In a second type of processing variant, other chemical moieties are added to a given site in a peptide sequence, e.g., amidation, acetylation, sulfation, or phos-

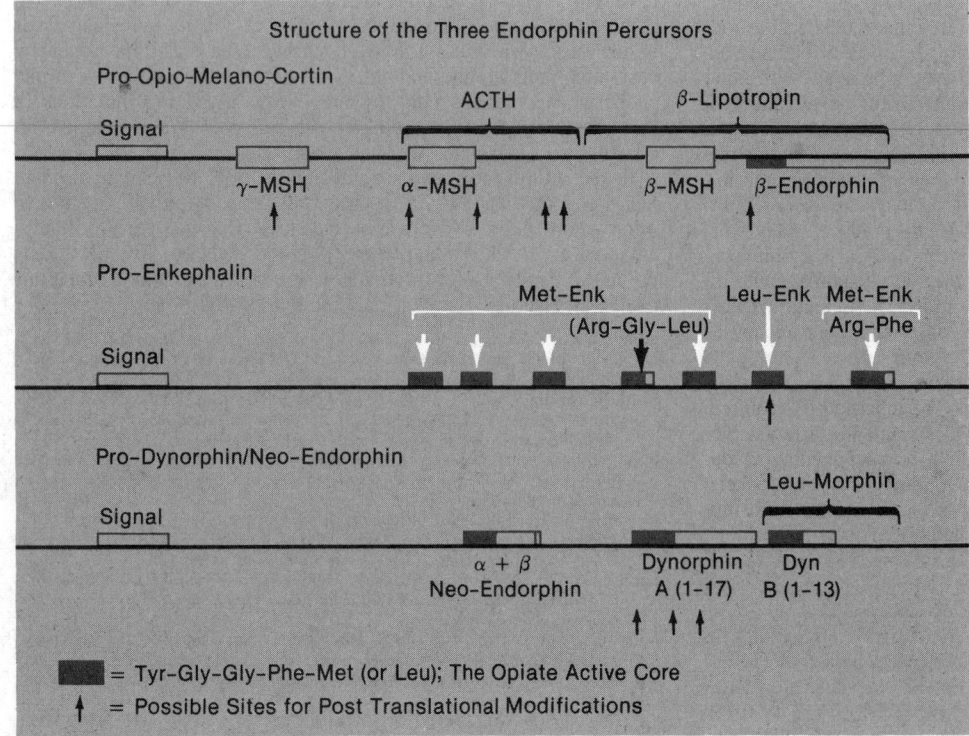

FIGURE 200–1. Simplified schematic of the precursors for all three endorphin families. Note the many peptides produced from each precursor, their similar size, and in the case of pro-enkephalin and pro-dynorphin, the multiple copies of opioid peptides produced by each.

phorylation. Both types of processing choices can alter the nature and potency of these molecules. For example, the addition of an acetyl group to the amino terminal tyrosine of β-endorphin decreases its opiate activity by more than 1000-fold. Thus, two of the largest problems in peptidergic systems, especially in brain, lie in understanding the precursor-processing pathways and the final structure of the peptides produced by each precursor in tissues of interest. Figure 200–1 provides a simplified version of the information.

Peptidergic cells have a range of control over the materials they secrete. To add further complexity, several peptides arise from each of the three endorphin precursors, and nonopioid peptides can be co-produced and co-secreted along with the endorphins (e.g., ACTH and β-endorphin from anterior lobe).

Three main opiate receptor subclasses, each with a different distribution pattern in brain, gut, pituitary, adrenal, and reproductive tissues, have been described (μ, κ, δ).

The μ receptor is very sensitive to morphine; the δ receptor seems to prefer enkephalin-like peptides; the κ receptor was characterized by the action of dynorphin-like peptides. All three opiate receptors have now been cloned, expressed, and localized and are under structural analysis. They are all members of the seven transmembrane G protein-linked receptor class. The selectivity of the receptors is not absolute. For example, dynorphin, while κ preferring, is also a potent μ agonist, and enkephalins, while δ preferring, can interact with the μ site. There is not a one-to-one anatomic link between κ receptors and dynorphin-producing cells and fibers; nor is there one for the δ receptor and pro-enkephalin systems. Rather, one tends to see two or even three opiate receptor subtypes associated with the terminal systems of the peptidergic neurons. Possibly the processing choices of a cell, by altering the peptide products, can alter the receptor preference of the materials secreted. If so, the cell may modulate its products to act on different receptor subtypes at the synapse. Such a system would be extremely flexible in modulating synaptic transmission.

With a multiplicity of peptides and receptors occupying a variety of tissues, it is clear that endorphins do not have a single physiologic role. Furthermore, multiple active transmitters and modulators may exist in the same cell. A particularly clear example of "co-transmission" can be found with the pro-dynorphin peptides in the hypothalamus. Pro-dynorphin peptides (and mRNA) are found in the same cells that produce vasopressin. Consistent with this finding, arginine vasopressin (AVP) and dynorphin are co-released from the posterior pituitary with the same stimuli. It is hypothesized that dynorphin provides local feedback inhibition on further AVP secretion. Other examples of co-transmission among the endorphins include enkephalin and catecholamines in the adrenal medulla, enkephalin and catecholamines in the sympathetic nervous system, and dynorphin and LH/FSH in the anterior pituitary.

Table 200–1 summarizes the main physiologic changes observed with the endorphins. The endorphins have been classically associated with modulation of stress and pain. The neuronal and endocrine systems involved in these responses are the hypothalamic-pituitary-adrenal system and the limbic system. In fact, each major component of the stress-response system contains endorphins. For example, the hippocampus, a main site of corticosteroid feedback, contains enkephalin and dynorphin neurons; the hypothalamus contains all three opioid families; the anterior pituitary contains POMC and enkephalin; the adrenal medulla produces enkephalin; and the adrenal cortex, dynorphin. A similar pattern accompanies pain-modulatory systems in the spinal cord, periaqueductal central gray, thalamus, and the limbic system.

Table 200–1 outlines several patterns effected by the endorphins: (1) These peptides are implicated in a wide variety of physiologic events. (2) Many of these events correlate with their anatomic locus. For example, all three endorphins are found in the nucleus tractus solitarius and are implicated in cardiovascular regulation; gut motility is controlled from the brain and gut opiatergic loci; respiration is regulated partially by the parabrachial nucleus, an area with both opiate peptides and receptors; and motor integration actively involves the nigrostriatal system, rich in opioid anatomy. (3) The functions associated with the endorphins are basic, homeostatic, limbic, "core" activities; they express affective or "drive"-related activities, rather than cognitive ones. (4) There are a few "unexpected" physiologic links, such as appetite modulation, drinking, and thermoregulation.

Coming years undoubtedly will see consolidation and organization of the great wealth of biologic data on these important systems.

TABLE 200–1. PROPOSED FUNCTIONS AND KNOWN ANATOMIC LOCALIZATIONS OF THE ENDOGENOUS OPIOID SYSTEMS

Function	Anatomic Localization
Appetite modulation and eating behavior	Limbic system, including hypothalamus and amygdala
Cardiovascular regulation	NTS, parabrachial nucleus
Drinking and water balance	Subfornical organ, magnocellular hypothalamic-pituitary system
Endocrine responses	Hypothalamic-pituitary-peripheral axis
Stimulatory effects on Growth hormone Melanocyte-stimulating hormone Prolactin	Hypothalamus and anterior lobe
Inhibitory effects on Follicle-stimulating hormone Luteinizing hormone Thyroid-stimulating hormone	Hypothalamus and anterior lobe
Inhibition of release of vasopressin and oxytocin	Hypothalamus and posterior lobe
Gastrointestinal motility	NTS, area postrema, and GI nervous plexuses
Pain inhibition	Thalamus, periaqueductal gray, substantia gelatinosa, NTS, spinal cord
Respiration	Parabrachial nucleus, NTS
Response to stress	Hypothalamic-pituitary-adrenal axis
Sensory-motor integration	Nigrostriatal system, globus pallidus, inferior and superior colliculi
Thermoregulation	Hypothalamus

NTS = Nucleus tractus solitarius.

One of the main foci will be a clearer view of the physiology-peptide-receptor interface; the other will be increased understanding of the genetic regulation of these systems. With the increasing clarity will come improved appreciation of the regulation of a whole series of crucial basic brain functions.

Akil H, Bronstein D, Mansour A: Overview of the endogenous opioid systems. In Rodgers RJ, Cooper SJ (eds.): Endorphins, Opiates and Behavioral Processes. Chichester, John Wiley and Sons Limited, 1988, pp 1–23. General overview of biochemistry, anatomy, and physiology of endorphins.

Fowler CJ, Fraser GL: μ-, δ-, κ-opioid receptors and their subtypes. A critical review with emphasis on radioligand binding experiments. Neurochem Int 24:401, 1994.

Herbert E, Seasholtz A, Comb M, et al.: Study of the regulation of expression of neuropeptide genes by gene transfer methods. In Psychopharmacology: The Third Generation of Progress. New York, Raven Press, 1987, pp 373–384. Summary of the gene structure and promoter elements of several peptide genes.

Mansour A, Watson SJ: Anatomical distribution of opioid receptors in mammalians: An overview. In Herz A (ed): Opioids I. Handbook of Experimental Pharmacology. Vol. 104/I. New York, Springer-Verlag, 1993, pp 79–105. Comprehensive overview of opioid peptide producing and ligand binding structure in brain.

Mansour A, Fox CA, Akil H, Watson SJ: Opioid receptor mRNA expression in the rat CNS: Anatomical and functional implications. Trends Neurosc 18:22, 1995.

Pasternak GW: Review: Pharmacological mechanisms of opioid analgesics. Clin Neuropsychopharmacol 16:1, 1993.

Reisine T, Bell GI: Molecular Biology of Opioid Receptors. Trends Neurosc 16:56, 1993. Overview of structure and pharmacology of all three opioid receptors.

200.2 Prostaglandins and Related Compounds

Garret A. FitzGerald

Arachidonic acid, derived from dietary sources, is transported in plasma in both esterified and nonesterified forms, primarily bound to lipoproteins and albumin, respectively. The relative importance of these two sources for cellular delivery is poorly understood. Esterified arachidonic acid in low density lipoproteins is taken up by cells by a process dependent on the low density lipoprotein receptor. The fatty acid is compartmentalized in the phospholipid domain

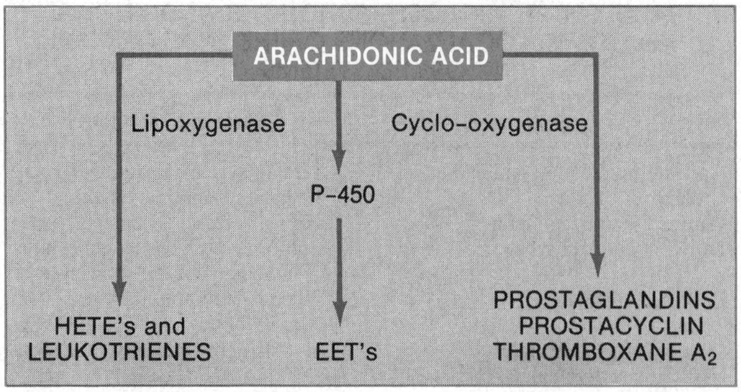

ARACHIDONIC ACID

Lipoxygenase   Cyclo-oxygenase

P-450

HETE's and   EET's   PROSTAGLANDINS
LEUKOTRIENES   PROSTACYCLIN
                                       THROMBOXANE A_2

FIGURE 200–2. Major pathways of metabolism of arachidonic acid.

of cell membranes. This localization appears relevant to the availability of arachidonate for release. A cytosolic phospholipase (PL) A_2 with high affinity for arachidonic acid is thought to be central to this process. Phosphorylation by mitogen-activated kinase and protein kinase C permits its calcium-dependent translocation to the cell membrane. Other PL's may also participate in arachidonate release. Subsequent oxygenation by either cyclo-oxygenase or lipoxygenase gives rise to biologically active compounds. A third pathway of metabolism via cytochrome P450 also exists (Fig. 200–2).

All cells can release arachidonic acid, but the predominant enzymatic products that are formed are highly cell specific. Because

they are derived from a polyunsaturated eicosanoic (C_{20}) fatty acid, these compounds—thromboxane A_2, the prostaglandins (PG's), epoxygenases, leukotrienes, and lipoxins—are collectively known as eicosanoids. Because of their diverse biologic properties and rapid metabolism to inactive products, the eicosanoids have been implicated as local mediators of receptor-dependent events in a range of physiologic processes and in diverse human diseases, including bronchial asthma, inflammation, and unstable coronary disease. Arachidonic acid itself and its metabolites may also function as intracellular second messengers, particularly in the modulation of ion channels, ras activity, and perhaps gene expression.

THE CYCLO-OXYGENASE PATHWAY (Fig. 200–3)

The biotransformation of arachidonic acid into thromboxane (Tx)A_2, prostacyclin (PGI$_2$), PGE$_2$, PGF$_{2\alpha}$, and PGD$_2$ is catalyzed by a common enzyme, the fatty acid cyclo-oxygenase (COX). The product of the COX reaction is an unstable endoperoxide, PGG. A second oxygen molecule is then introduced at C_{15}; this results in the 15-hydroperoxy endoperoxide PGH, and liberates a free radical. There are two COX genes; a constitutive form (COX-1), which is expressed ubiquitously and has recently been crystalized. Although COX-1 is inducible in certain constrained circumstances (e.g., by certain cytokines in bone marrow-derived mast cells or by male sex hormones in ram seminal vesicle), COX-2, which is expressed in a more limited repertoire of cells, is induced by cytokines, tumor promoters, growth factors, and gonadotropins. Consequently, it is presumed to be the COX of predominant importance in the generation of prostaglandins in inflammation and, perhaps, cancer.

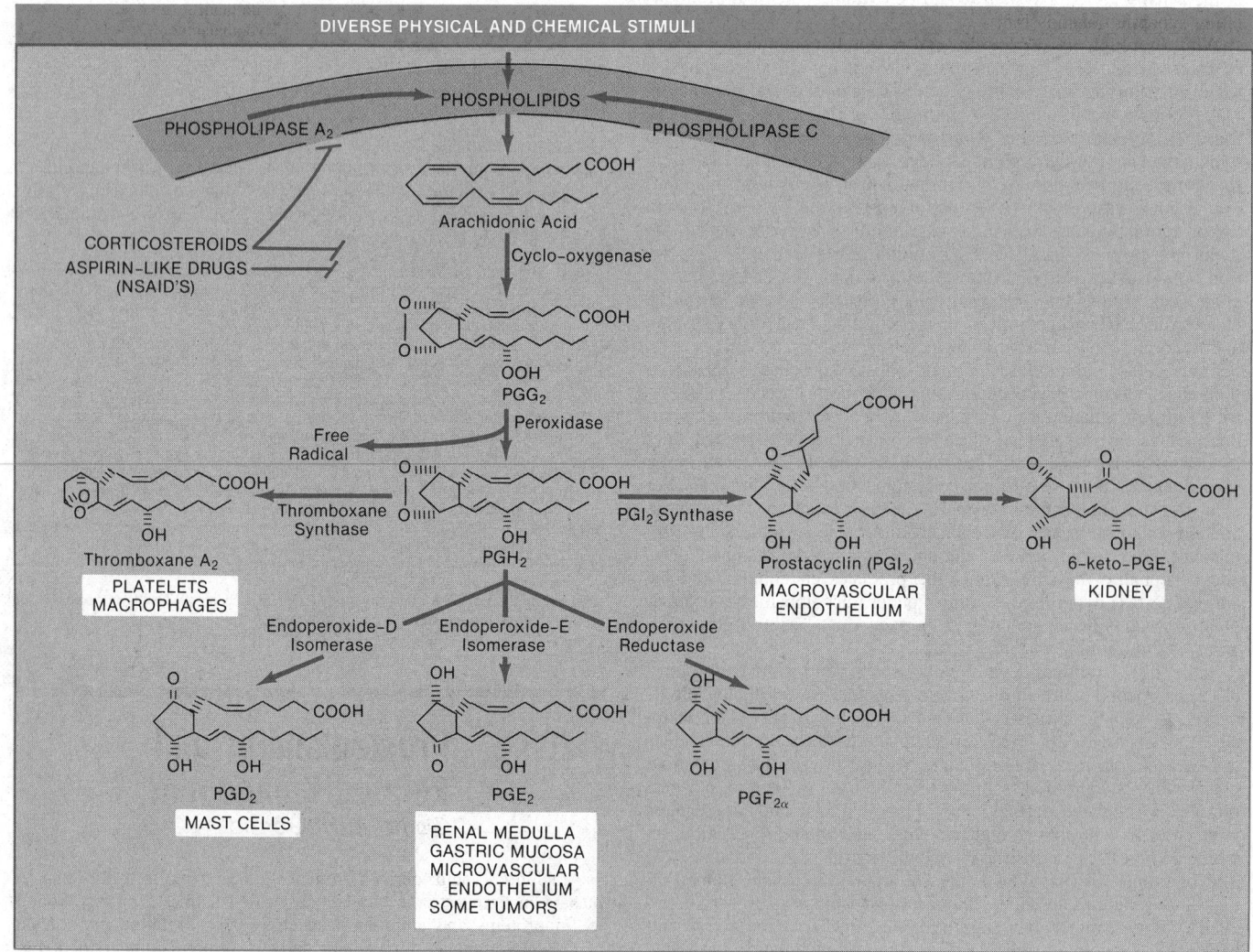

FIGURE 200–3. Metabolism of arachidonic acid by fatty acid cyclo-oxygenase. The major tissues of origin of the eicosanoids are shown.

PGH is metabolized by cell-specific enzymes to form either the "classic" prostaglandins of the D, E, and F series, PGI_2, or TxA_2. Arachidonic acid contains four double bonds ($\Delta^{5,8,11,14}$). It is apparent from the sequence of biosynthesis (Fig. 200–3) that two double bonds remain in its (bisenoic) COX products. This is denoted by the subscript 2, as in TxA_2 and PGE_2. Analogous metabolism of other fatty acid substrates gives rise to monoenoic or trienoic prostaglandins and thromboxanes (Fig. 200–4). For example, metabolites of eicosatrienoic acid ($C_{20:3}$n-6) contain only one (Δ^{13}) double bond. Eicosapentaenoic acid (EPA) ($C_{20:5}$n-3), which is prevalent in certain fish and aquatic mammals, is transformed by COX to metabolites with three ($\Delta^{5,13,17}$) double bonds, such as PGI_3 and TxA_3. Structurally, prostaglandins of the D, E, and F series possess a cyclopentane ring and differ only in their substituent groups. The F series prostaglandins are referred to as $PGF_{1\alpha}$, $PGF_{2\alpha}$, and $PGF_{3\alpha}$.

THROMBOXANE A_2. TxA_2, the predominant COX product formed by platelets, stimulates aggregation of these cells and constricts vascular and bronchial smooth muscle. These biologic properties are shared by the PG endoperoxides. A single thromboxane (Tx) receptor gene encodes a member of the G protein–coupled receptor superfamily. Distinct placental and endothelial isoforms have been cloned. Tissue-specific splice variants may differ in their preferential linkage to intracellular effector molecules and in aspects of their desensitization. Although the Tx receptor is phosphorylated, the molecular events that underlie eicosanoid receptor desensitization are poorly understood. Expression of the receptor appears to be transcriptionally regulated by certain growth factors and male sex steroids. Recently, a mutation in the first intracellular loop of the Tx receptor has been linked to a bleeding disorder characterized by a selective defect in the aggregability of platelets *ex vivo* by Tx agonists.

PROSTACYCLIN. Prostacyclin (PGI_2), the predominant COX product of arachidonic acid formed by vascular endothelium and also by subendothelium, both inhibits the aggregation of platelets by all recognized agonists and disaggregates previously aggregated platelets. PGI_2 inhibits the adherence of platelets and neutrophils to foreign surfaces and damaged endothelium and dilates both bronchial and vascular smooth muscle. A PGI receptor has recently been cloned and exhibits about 30 to 40% homology with other eicosanoid receptors. Another potentially important property of PGI_2 is the modulation of cholesterol efflux from arterial walls. Nanomolar quantities of PGI_2 stimulate the activity of both the lysosomal and cytoplasmic cholesterol ester hydrolases when added experimentally to vascular smooth muscle cells but have no effect on the microsomal acyl-CoA cholesterol acyl transferase (ACAT), which re-esterifies free cholesterol. Both PGI and TxA synthase en-

zymes have been cloned. Although the sequence homology between them is less than 40%, they are both P450 enzymes.

PGI_2 biosynthesis is increased in several human diseases in which evidence of platelet activation is present, including severe peripheral arterial disease and unstable coronary disease. Although this implies a homeostatic role for this eicosanoid, its biologic importance remains ill defined in the absence of pharmacologic antagonists. Recently, local vascular delivery of the COX-1 gene has been reported to limit platelet-dependent vascular occlusive events in a canine model, perhaps by enhancing vascular PGI formation.

PROSTAGLANDIN D_2. Prostaglandin D_2, the principal COX product of the mast cell, is released, together with histamine and other mediators, by IgE-dependent and other stimuli. Infusion of PGD_2 in humans results in nasal stuffiness, systemic hypotension, and flushing. PGD_2 is increased in bronchoalveolar lavage fluid following antigen challenge in atopic individuals, suggesting that it may contribute to the bronchomotor response in allergic asthma. PGD_2 is a minor product of the platelet COX. Both PGD_2 and its 9α, 11β-PGF metabolite inhibit platelet aggregation by stimulating adenylate cyclase, thereby increasing intraplatelet cyclic AMP. In experimental animals, central administration of PGD_2 induces sleep, an event that is countered by infusion of PGE_2. Two forms of the PGD synthase exist—one in brain, which has been cloned, and the other in blood cells. The former is highly expressed in rat leptomeninges and choroid plexus, where it may increase PGD levels in the CSF. Elevated CSF levels of PGD have been reported in patients with African sleeping sickness. Selective knock-out of the PGD synthases and/or the recently cloned PGD receptor may clarify the role of this eicosanoid in sleep regulation and immune function.

PROSTAGLANDIN E_2. The formation of PGE_2 from PGH_2 is catalyzed by a PGE_2 isomerase that is present in renal medulla, gastric mucosa, and platelets. PGE_2 rather than PGI_2 may be the predominant prostaglandin formed by microvascular endothelium. In the kidney, PGE_2 can act both as a vasodilator and as an inhibitor of tubular sodium absorption. It helps maintain renal blood flow, together with PGI, during activation of the renin-angiotensin and sympathoadrenal systems. Three E prostaglandin receptor genes (EP_1, EP_2, and EP_3) have been cloned. Analogous to the Tx receptor, tissue-specific carboxyl terminal splice variants of the EP receptor couple with differing preference for discrete effector pathways in expression systems.

PGE_2 is the predominant COX product of arachidonic acid formed in gastric mucosa. It participates in the regulation of gastric blood flow and limits the effects of diverse physical and chemical

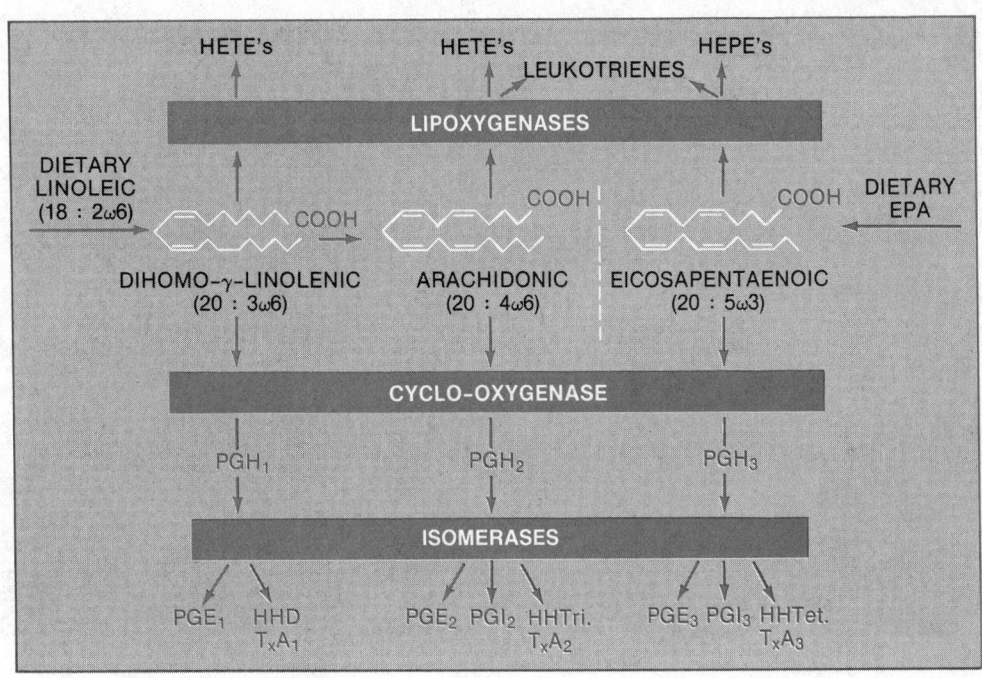

FIGURE 200–4. Analogous formation of mono-, bis-, and trienoic prostaglandins. (Reproduced with permission from FitzGerald GA, Price P, Knapp HR: Biochemical and functional effects of dietary substrate modification in man. *In* Simopoulos AP, Kifer RR, Martin RE [eds.]: Health Effects of Polyunsaturated Fatty Acids in Seafoods. Orlando, FL, Academic Press, 1986, pp 61–80.)

insults to the gastric mucosa. This "cytoprotective" property is shared by PGI_2, but the mechanism by which this protection occurs is unknown. Other biologic properties of PGE_2 include relaxation of bronchial smooth muscle, contraction of uterine smooth muscle (19-hydroxylated E prostaglandins are the major arachidonic acid products in human semen), and modulation of lymphocyte function. PGE_2 modulates neurotransmission via presynaptic receptors on adrenergic neurons in vitro and appears to be important in the sleep/wakefulness cycle.

In a minority of patients with solid tumors, PGE_2 production by the tumor causes hypercalcemia via stimulation of osteoclast activity (see Ch. 159). In such cases, suppression of PGE_2 biosynthesis lowers the level of serum calcium. When metastases to bone occur, however, local mechanisms for hypercalcemia supervene.

PROSTAGLANDIN $F_{2\alpha}$. $PGF_{2\alpha}$, formed from PGH_2 by the action of an endoperoxide reductase, contracts bronchial and uterine smooth muscle and vasoconstricts some uterine beds. Although increases in $PGF_{2\alpha}$ metabolites have been described during dysmenorrhea and allergen-evoked bronchospasm, a unique site for formation of this prostaglandin and its role in pathophysiology remain to be determined. High concentrations of $PEF_{2\alpha}$ and Tx receptor mRNA are found in myometrium.

THE LIPOXYGENASE PATHWAY (Fig. 200–5)

Arachidonic acid is also widely subject to lipoxygenation reactions (Fig. 200–5). In neutrophils, insertion of an oxygen molecule adjacent to one of the double bonds yields the hydroperoxy derivative, 5-hydroperoxyeicosatetraenoic acid (5-HPETE). This can undergo further metabolism to either a 5-hydroxyeicosatetraenoic acid (5-HETE) or to an unstable 5,6-epoxide intermediate, leukotriene (LT)A_4. This compound can be hydrolyzed to 5,12-dihydroxyeicosatetraenoic acids, one of which is LTB_4. The subscript 4 refers to the number of double bonds. Thus, analogous to the nomenclature for COX products, substitution of eicosapentaenoic acid for arachidonic acid as a substrate would result in formation of LTB_5. The site of the initial lipoxygenation reaction tends to vary with cell type. Thus, 12-HETE is formed predominantly in platelets, 5-HETE by polymorphonuclear leukocytes, and 5-HETE, 11-HETE, and 15-HETE by endothelial cells as measured in culture.

The 5-lipoxygenase (5-LO) of human neutrophils, a cytosolic enzyme, is translocated to the membrane for metabolism of arachidonic acid. It requires an 18K protein, termed the five lipoxygenase activating protein (FLAP), to achieve full activation. Analogous activating proteins do not appear necessary for expression of 12- and 15-lipoxygenase activity. The primary structures of two distinct 12-lipoxygenases have been reported. One, in porcine leukocytes, is immunologically identical to that in porcine brain and human tracheal cells. It is closely related to the 15-lipoxygenase. The human platelet 12-lipoxygenase is a distinct gene product. The role of 12-HETE in platelets is unknown. Platelet 12-lipoxygenase is translocated from the cytosol to the membrane in a calcium-dependent manner, and 12-HETE inhibits the mobilization of a glycoprotein IIb/IIIa complex in tumor cell lines. This complex is analogous to that which serves as a receptor for adhesive macromolecules, such as fibrinogen, in activated platelets. 12-Lipoxygenase products regulate potassium channel flux in Aplysia. Formation of 15-HETE is reportedly increased in atherosclerotic blood vessels, and in situ hybridization studies suggest that expression of the enzyme is increased and co-localized with oxidized low density lipoproteins in human atherosclerotic plaques.

LTA_4 is conjugated enzymatically with glutathione to yield LTC_4. This compound is metabolized to LTD_4 and LTE_4 by successive elimination of a γ-glutamyl residue and glycine. The cysteinyl-containing leukotrienes are powerful bronchoconstrictors and vasoconstrictors. These compounds also dilate microvessels, increase vascular permeability, and stimulate mucus secretion. LTC_4 causes pulmonary bronchoconstriction, an effect that is partially blocked by COX inhibitors. This implies that LTC_4 may mediate this effect via the release of a bronchoconstrictor prostaglandin, such as thromboxane A_2. LTC_4 may cooperate with luteinizing hormone-releasing hormone (LHRH) in the control of LH release by cells of the anterior pituitary, judged by in vitro studies.

LTB_4 stimulates adhesion, migration, aggregation, enzyme release, and generation of superoxide by polymorphonuclear leukocytes. These biologic properties strongly suggest a role for lipoxygenase products in both inflammation and antigen-evoked bronchoconstriction.

Embryonic stem cell knock-out of the 5-LO gene results in a normal phenotype. However, the lethal effects of intravenous injection of platelet-activating factor and the local inflammatory response to topical application of arachidonic acid are modified by gene disruption. It is likely that imminent information from the inactivation and/or overexpression of other enzymes and receptors will clarify further the biologic role of eicosanoids.

DiHETE's can be formed via transcellular metabolism, at least in vitro. Examples include 12,20-DiHETE formed by a mixed suspen-

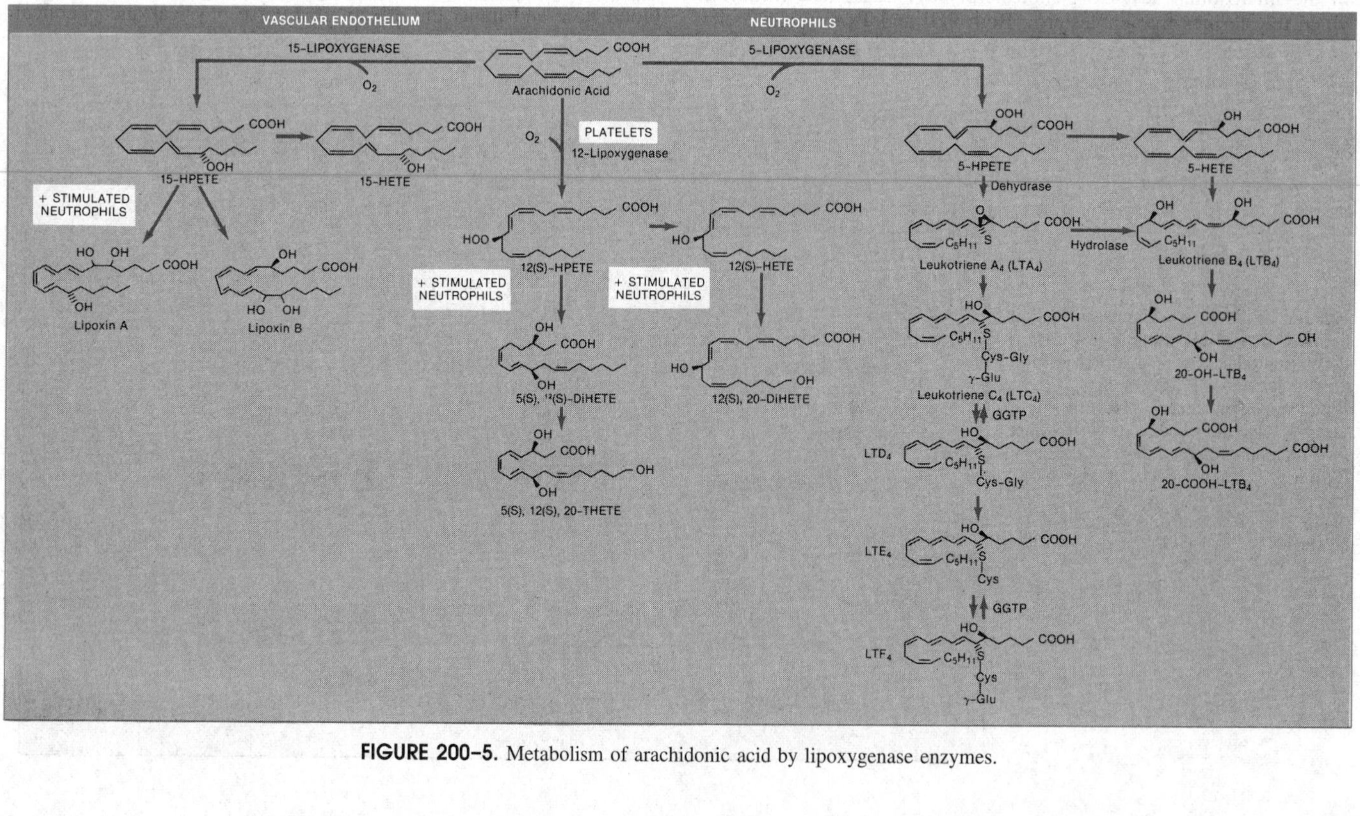

FIGURE 200–5. Metabolism of arachidonic acid by lipoxygenase enzymes.

sion of platelets and polymorphonuclear leukocytes. Leukocytes can utilize erythrocyte LTA_4 to generate LTB_4 and endothelial cells can utilize platelet-derived PGH_2 to generate PGI_2.

Stimulated human leukocytes can convert 15-HPETE to products termed lipoxins (LX) containing a characteristic tetraenoic structure (Fig. 200–5). The two major products are identified as LXA and LXB. LXA is a potent stimulus to superoxide generation by neutrophils and contracts pulmonary tissue. Both LXA and LXB inhibit natural killer cell cytotoxicity *in vitro*, by a mechanism distinct from that of PGE_2, which decreases the binding between target and effector cells. Another series of compounds with potent biologic properties *in vitro* are the hepoxilins, formed by an intramolecular rearrangement of 12-HETE. Glutathione conjugates of hepoxilin A_3 cause hyperpolarization of rat brain neurons at nanomolar concentrations.

THE EPOXYGENASE PATHWAY (Fig. 200–6)

In addition to metabolism by COX and lipoxygenase enzymes, arachidonic acid is subject to ω and ω-1 oxidation by cytochrome P450 enzymes in microsomal preparations. A specific P450 enzyme with high affinity for arachidonic acid has been cloned. This results in the formation of 19-OH and 19-oxo-eicosatetraenoic acid (by ω-1-oxidation) and 20-OH-eicosatetraenoic and eicosatetraene-1,20-dioic acids (by ω oxidation). In addition, a series of epoxides 14(15)-epoxy-, 11(12)-epoxy-, 8(9)-epoxy-, and 5(6)-epoxy-eicosatrienoic acids (EET's) can be formed by this enzyme from arachidonic acid. These compounds can then be further transformed to vicinyl diols by epoxide hydrolases. One such compound, 11,12-dihydroxyeicosatrienoic acid, inhibits the Na^+-K^+-ATPase enzyme in vascular smooth muscle. 5(6)-EET inhibits sodium absorption and potassium secretion by the rabbit cortical collecting duct, and synthetic 5(6)-EET stimulates the release of LH and somatostatin by pituitary cells in culture. Interestingly, 8,9-EET and 14,15-EET stereospecifically inhibit human platelet COX. By contrast, all EET's studied inhibit platelet aggregation *in vitro* by a nonspecific mechanism, independent of an effect on Tx formation. EET's weakly inhibit monocyte and platelet adherence to endothelial cells. Finally, 5(6)-EET is metabolized to epoxides of PGG_1, PGH_1, and PGE_1 and to the 5S, 6S and 5R, 6R isomers of 5-hydroxy-PGI_1. The biosynthesis of EET's has recently been confirmed *in vivo*. Urinary excretion of their vicinyl diols (DHET's) is increased in normal pregnancy, and further increments, particularly of 14(15)-

DHET, are observed in patients with pregnancy-induced hypertension. 5(6)-EET biosynthesis is increased in syndromes of salt and water retention.

THE ISOPROSTANES. Free radicals may catalyze the formation of prostaglandin and leukotriene isomers from arachidonic acid in the sn-2 position of phospholipids. These isoprostanes are potentially susceptible to cleavage by PLA's and may function as either intracellular mediators of oxidant stress and/or as autacoids. Indeed, two such compounds, 8-epi $PGF_{2\alpha}$ and 8-epi PGE are vasoconstrictors—an effect prevented by Tx receptor antagonists. Isoprostane excretion in urine is elevated in clinical conditions putatively associated with oxidant stress, such as reperfusion, certain poisonings, and in apparently healthy cigarette smokers, perhaps due to neutrophil activation.

PHARMACOLOGIC AND DIETARY REGULATION OF BIOSYNTHESIS

With the exception of P450-derived metabolites, and the isoprostanes, none of the oxygenated products of arachidonic acid have the potential for storage in significant quantities for subsequent release by cells. Release is equivalent to biosynthesis. Arachidonate release may occur by several mechanisms. Phosphatidylinositol (PI) may be hydrolyzed by a PI-specific PLC, yielding diacylglycerol (DAG) and inositol phosphate. DAG is then further hydrolyzed, yielding free arachidonic acid and other fatty acids. Alternatively, phosphatidylcholine (PC) may be hydrolyzed by phospholipase A_2(PLA_2), yielding arachidonic acid from the sn-2 position. PLA_2 may also liberate arachidonic acid from phosphatidylethanolamine. Selectivity of phospholipid compartmentalization and phospholipase action permits some HETE's and EET's to modulate second messenger formation. Thus, 15-HETE incubated with endothelial cells is selectively incorporated into PI, and agonist-evoked activation of PLC results in release of a 1-stearoyl-2(15-HETE)-DAG. 15-HETE enrichment of lipidic second messengers modifies β-adrenergic receptor sensitivity in cardiomyocytes. PLD-catalyzed formation of a modified phosphatidic acid has also been demonstrated.

CORTICOSTEROIDS. The effects of steroids on eicosanoid biosynthesis are complex. It is thought that they induce formation of a phospholipase-inhibitory protein, variously named lipocortin, macrocortin, lipomodulin, and renomodulin (see Fig. 200–3). It is

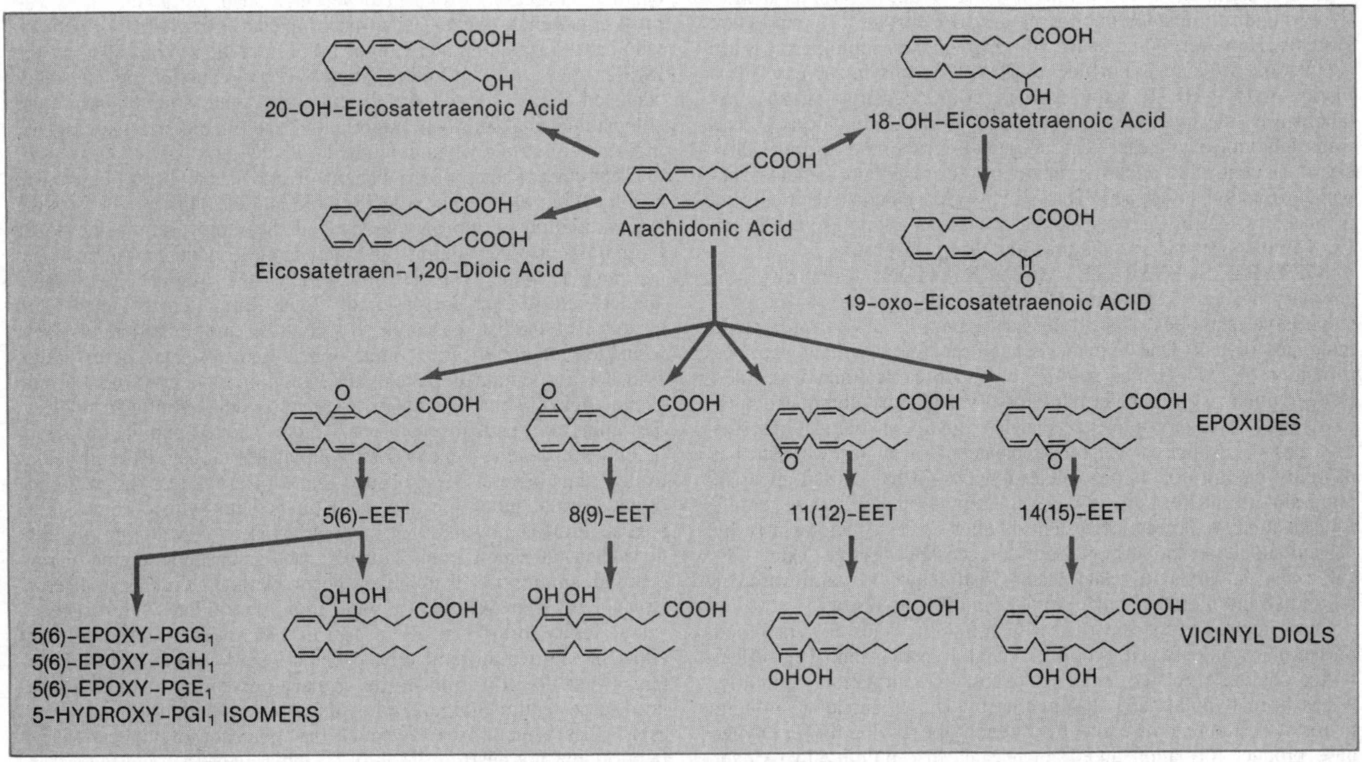

FIGURE 200–6. Metabolism of arachidonic acid by cytochrome P450.

hypothesized that initially steroids bind to specific cytosolic receptors and that the complex is then transferred to the nucleus where steroids regulate the expression of genes and subsequently the synthesis of a PLA$_2$-inhibitory protein (see Ch. 199). The lipocortin family is derived from a monomeric 40K protein, phosphorylation of which by protein kinases results in its activation as an inhibitor. Interestingly, there is a striking sequence homology between this protein and the 40K protein that is phosphorylated following the binding of epidermal growth factor to its receptor. The amino acid sequence of one member of the family, lipocortin III, is identical to that of inositol 1,2-cyclic phosphate 2 phosphohydrolase. Such a role for lipocortin has been disputed, however, especially as lipocortins bind nonspecifically to phospholipids.

More recently, steroids have been shown to down regulate induction of COX-2 and several PLA's. Regulation of other inducible enzymes, such as nitric oxide synthase, is also of likely relevance to the anti-inflammatory properties of these compounds.

COX INHIBITORS. Nonsteroidal anti-inflammatory drugs (NSAID's) prevent the formation of prostaglandins by inhibiting COX. This group of drugs includes aspirin, salicylates, indomethacin, ibuprofen, piroxicam, fenoprofen, paracetamol, phenylbutazone, oxyphenbutazone, bolmetin, sulfinpyrazone, and sulindac. Paracetamol (acetaminophen) is a considerably less potent inhibitor than the other compounds, except perhaps in the brain. Aspirin is also unlike the other compounds in that it acetylates a serine residue at position 529, close to the active site of the platelet PGG/H synthase, and inhibits the enzyme irreversibly. This accounts for the unique effects of aspirin on the platelet COX-1. Whereas other cells have the capacity for de novo protein synthesis, the anucleate platelet does not; thus inhibition of TxA$_2$ formation by aspirin persists for the lifetime of the platelet. By contrast, the effects of aspirin on eicosanoid formation by other cells (e.g., prostacyclin biosynthesis by vascular endothelium), which expresses both COX-1 and COX-2 are not so prolonged owing to their capacity to generate new enzymes. The irreversible actions of aspirin on platelet COX also account for the cumulative inhibition of platelet TxA$_2$ formation by the repeated administration of low dosages of aspirin (20 to 40 mg per day; a regular aspirin tablet contains 325 mg). This results in partial inhibition of platelet COX after single-dose administration. Even though low doses of aspirin tend to depress PGI$_2$ formation, its effect is more pronounced on platelet TxA$_2$ biosynthesis during long-term therapy. The serine target for aspirin acetylation is conserved in COX-2, and aspirin is a relatively nondiscriminant inhibitor of the two enzymes in expression systems. However, coincident with prostaglandin inhibition, aspirin acetylation of COX-2, but not of COX-1, results in increased formation of 15-R-HETE. Aspirin is subject to extensive first-pass metabolism by the liver, and its deacylated product, salicylic acid, is a weak inhibitor of platelet COX. Reduction in the rate of drug delivery in a controlled-release preparation permits more efficient hepatic extraction of aspirin. This still permits cumulative inhibition of platelet COX in the presystemic circulation, while protecting the COX in the systemic vasculature from aspirin exposure.

DIETARY SUBSTRATE MODIFICATION. Mortality from coronary heart disease seems to be lower in populations who consume large quantities of n-3 fatty acids, such as EPA, from aquatic mammals or fish. One hypothesis has been that a shift toward the formation of TxA$_3$ (which is less biologically active than TxA$_2$) and PGI$_3$ (which is a platelet-inhibitory, vasodilator compound like PGI$_2$) may favorably influence platelet-vessel wall interactions (see Fig. 200–4). Although fish oil supplementation of the western diet has only modest effects on platelet function, it has caused apparent regression of atherosclerosis in several animal models. However, efforts to modify the rate of restenosis after coronary angioplasty by fish oil supplementation have been unsuccessful in large-scale clinical trials. Attempts to relate dietary fish intake to cardiovascular morbidity and mortality have provided conflicting results.

Supplementation of the diet with n-3 fatty acids lowers blood pressure in patients with mild essential hypertension. This effect is not obviously related to altered eicosanoid formation. Similarly, it has been hypothesized that marine oils might modulate inflammatory or immune diseases by altering the profile of lipoxygenase product formation and/or increasing susceptibility to oxidant injury.

LIPOXYGENASE INHIBITORS AND ANTAGONISTS. Recent clinical studies have demonstrated the efficacy of 5-LO inhibitors and sulfidopeptide receptor antagonists in asthma. They appear to be additive to the effects of β-adrenoreceptor agonists.

FUNCTIONS OF ARACHIDONIC ACID METABOLITES *IN VIVO*

The evidence implicating arachidonate metabolites in mechanisms of some human diseases includes measurements of their biosynthesis and the effects of drugs that prevent their formation or antagonize their actions. Because of the evanescence of the primary compounds, estimates of in vivo synthesis have largely been based upon measurement of long-lived but biologically inactive metabolites. Quantitative assays for the major urinary metabolites of primary prostaglandins, PGI$_2$ and TxA$_2$, have been useful in identifying potential targets for drugs designed to modulate their actions. Similar methodology is now available to explore lipoxygenase and epoxygenase product formation in vivo. The capacity of tissues to generate arachidonic acid metabolites greatly exceeds the actual production rates in vivo. Thus, artifacts related to sample collection (for example, platelet activation ex vivo during blood sampling, catheter-induced vascular trauma, or formation of free radical-catalyzed derivatives during sample storage) can seriously confound attempts to measure these compounds in the bloodstream. Measurement of metabolite excretion in urine has been favored as a noninvasive, albeit indirect, approach. The most specific and sensitive method for measurement of eicosanoid metabolites is gas chromatography-mass spectrometry, which has been used to validate radioimmunoassays and enzyme immunoassays for selected compounds.

THE CARDIOVASCULAR SYSTEM. TxA$_2$ is one of many platelet agonists generated in vivo. While aspirin inhibits Tx-dependent aggregation, other agonists, such as thrombin and high doses of collagen, can induce aggregation in vitro despite the presence of aspirin. In view of these properties, it is superficially surprising that aspirin has been shown to influence clinical outcome in a variety of trials in cardiovascular disease, presumably because of its effects on TxA$_2$ formation. This may reflect the importance of TxA$_2$ as an amplifying signal for other platelet agonists.

Aspirin reduces significantly the incidence of stroke in patients suffering transient ischemic attacks or with nonvalvular atrial fibrillation. It also reduces the incidence of thrombotic occlusion following coronary artery bypass graft implantations and the incidence of myocardial infarction and death in patients with unstable coronary disease. The drug reduces the risk of a combined endpoint of myocardial infarction, stroke, and vascular death by about 25%. The most convincing evidence that aspirin reduces mortality in patients who have suffered an acute myocardial infarction is provided by the ISIS-2 study of >17,000 patients. The reduction in mortality achieved by aspirin and the thrombolytic agent streptokinase were comparable and additive. Importantly, aspirin did not increase the incidence of stroke when combined with streptokinase.

Clear-cut evidence of the benefit of aspirin has been obtained in smaller trials of patients with unstable angina. This may reflect the early initiation of aspirin therapy and the more prominent role of thrombosis in determining outcome in these patients. Angioscopic and angiographic evidence of thrombosis is present in unstable angina, and phasic increases of TxA$_2$ formation coincide with episodes of cardiac ischemia. By contrast, the alteration of TxA$_2$ formation after myocardial infarction is transient, and there is little evidence of sustained platelet activation in patients with chronic stable angina. Thus, if entry to the trial is delayed after a myocardial infarction, patients represent a more "dilute" population potentially susceptible to benefit from antiplatelet therapy. Recently, controlled trials have also established that aspirin reduces the incidence of myocardial infarction and death in patients with chronic stable angina. Presumably, they are at greater risk of developing platelet-dependent unstable coronary events, such as unstable angina or myocardial infarction, then their peers without coronary disease. Nonetheless, they represent a population more dilute with respect to susceptibility to the benefits of aspirin than patients presenting with either of the two aforementioned conditions. Exploration of the potential benefits of aspirin in the primary prevention of cardiovascular disease requires larger studies than those reported to date. Thus, aspirin has been shown to reduce the incidence of myocardial infarction, but not death, in healthy US physicians. A trend toward increased hemorrhagic stroke in the aspirin group did not attain statistical significance. Although aspirin has been used in combination with dipyridamole in many of these studies, there is little evidence that this latter drug contributes to the antithrombotic efficacy of aspirin in humans. The lowest dose of aspirin that has been shown to be effective in unstable angina has been 75 mg per day.

THE RESPIRATORY SYSTEM. Although TxA_2 as well as LT biosynthesis is increased coincident with the bronchoconstrictor response to inhaled allergen, experiments with aspirin and throboxane antagonists suggest that its functional importance is marginal. A minority of asthmatics, perhaps 10%, exhibit bronchoconstrictive, hypersensitivity reactions to aspirin. This appears to reflect a role for prostaglandins, TxA_2, or leukotrienes, as these attacks are provoked by a range of structurally distinct inhibitors of COX but rarely by salicylate, which resembles aspirin but is a weak inhibitor of that enzyme. No evidence currently supports an allergic basis for this condition. Drug-induced reactions in such patients may be quite severe and often feature profuse rhinorrhea and flushing in addition to bronchospasm. Whether such attacks are mediated by differential inhibition of bronchoconstrictor versus bronchodilator prostaglandins, by a shunting of the arachidonate substrate toward lipoxygenation and the formation of bronchoconstrictor leukotrienes, or by reduced formation of a prostaglandin that normally inhibits release of other mediators of bronchoconstriction is unknown.

Aspirin may also trigger a hypersensitivity response in which alterations in blood pressure, flushing, tachycardia, and diarrhea predominate over bronchospasm. Some of these patients have systemic mastocytosis (see Ch. 231).

THE GASTROINTESTINAL SYSTEM. Both PGI_2 and PGE_2 are cytoprotective of gastric mucosa *in vitro* and are thought to contribute to the regulation of mucosal blood flow. The dose-related gastrointestinal side effects of NSAID's are thought to reflect increased susceptibility to local injury (e.g., H^+ backdiffusion) due to inhibition of these prostaglandins. Interestingly, COX-1 but not COX-2 appears to be expressed in the normal gastrointestinal (GI) tract. Thus, recently developed highly selective COX-2 inhibitors may provide a potent anti-inflammatory effect devoid of GI side effects. An alternative approach has been to combine dimethyl PGE analogues as an adjunct to NSAID therapy. The watery diarrhea associated with multiple endocrine neoplasia often responds to treatment with prostaglandin inhibitors. Excessive formation of LTB_4 has been demonstrated in colonic mucosa and rectal dialysates obtained from patients with inflammatory bowel disease.

Recent epidemiologic data have suggested the possibility that aspirin intake may be inversely associated with the incidence of colon cancer. Controlled trials suggest that a preferential COX-1 inhibitor, sulindac, may cause regression of familial polyposis coli. Although preliminary reports suggest expression of COX-2 in such lesions and in colonic cancers, the clinical potential of COX inhibitors in these disorders remains to be explored.

RENIN RELEASE AND RENAL FUNCTION. Although sympathoadrenal activity is the principal regulator of renin release, it appears to be via a COX metabolite of arachidonic acid. PGI_2 is the most potent of the prostaglandins as a renin secretagogue. Inhibition of COX by NSAID's has implications for the diagnostic application of renin measurements. The associated reduction in aldosterone production may be deleterious for patients with hyperkalemia.

Metabolites of arachidonic acid contribute little to the regulation of renal blood flow under physiologic circumstances. Under conditions of increased vasoconstrictor tone, however, preservation of renal blood flow becomes increasingly dependent upon the generation of vasodilator prostaglandins. This is particularly so in patients with chronic glomerulonephritis, Bartter's syndrome, the nephropathy of systemic lupus erythematosus, congestive heart failure, or combined hepatic and renal dysfunction. It has been proposed that the decline in renal function in such patients following administration of NSAID's is less likely to occur with sulindac as a result of retroconversion of the sulfide to the sulfone. It is important to determine if elaboration of vasodilator prostaglandins in these circumstances is dependent on induction of COX-2. Physiologic stress has been shown to induce spatially selective expression of COX-2 in the central nervous system. Should this mechanism operate in the renal vasculature, it would have serious implications for the clinical development of selective inhibitors of COX-2.

The kidney possesses the capacity to generate TxA_2 in addition to vasodilator prostaglandins. Renal biosynthesis of TxA_2 is in-

creased in some patients with severe nephropathy in association with systemic lupus erythematosus, and infusion of a PGH_2-TxA_2 receptor antagonist improves indices of renal function in such patients. Increased TxA_2 biosynthesis by the kidney has been demonstrated in animal models in response to ureteric obstruction, renal vein thrombosis, and development of hypertension following partial renal ablation and coincident with the development of cyclosporine-induced nephrotoxicity. Increased TxA_2 formation during renal allograft rejection has been reported in humans; however, it is unknown whether this is an epiphenomenon or of primary importance in the rejection process. 16,16-Dimethyl PGE_2 delays renal allograft rejection in man, although the mechanism is unknown.

PGE_2 is the major product formed from arachidonic acid in the renal medulla, where it appears to inhibit sodium reabsorption in the distal tubule. EP receptor subtypes are spatially segregated within the kidney as determined by *in situ* hybridization. The consequent sodium retention caused by administration of a COX inhibitor persists only for a day or two, after which sodium balance is reversed despite continued treatment. Prostaglandins may also influence free water clearance. Indomethacin diminishes the excessive water elimination in nephrogenic and lithium-induced diabetes insipidus. Interestingly, disruption of the COX-2 gene results in marked polydipsia and polyuria in surviving animals.

Although P450-catalyzed metabolism of arachidonate occurs in renal tissue and several of the compounds influence tubular ion flux, glomerular filtration rate, and vascular tone, their precise role in renal physiology and pathology remains to be established.

THE REPRODUCTIVE SYSTEM. Both PGE_2 and $PGF_{2\alpha}$ are potent stimulants of myometrial contraction. Both they and their methylated analogues have been utilized as abortifacients and in the induction of labor, usually as an adjunct to low amniotomy. COX inhibitors are currently being evaluated in the treatment of premature labor. A potential hazard of this approach has been premature closure of the ductus arteriosus, although the incidence of the complication is unknown. Closure of a persistent ductus arteriosus can be achieved with indomethacin in the neonatal period. This implies that a COX metabolite contributes to ductal patency. Infusion of PGE_1 has been used to maintain an open ductus in infants with pulmonary atresia until corrective surgery is performed.

Biosynthesis of the prostaglandins increases during pregnancy, particularly during labor. This may reflect induction of COX-2, which is regulated by gonadotropic hormones. Efforts to create COX-2 knock-outs (many of the homozygotes were lethal) have emphasized the likely importance of this enzyme in developmental biology. COX-2 inhibitors may have potential as "morning after" birth control pills. In the case of PGI_2, biosynthesis is increased markedly from as early as the first trimester. Interestingly, this increment is less pronounced in patients with pregnancy-induced hypertension (PIH). Indeed, diminished PGI_2 biosynthesis is apparent prior to the rise in blood pressure. Studies of TxA_2 biosynthesis indicate that platelet activation is present in normal pregnancy and is further increased in patients with severe PIH. TxA_2 is a potent vasoconstrictor in the placental bed and may contribute to the depressed placental blood flow that is a hallmark of PIH. Multicenter trials have been performed to determine if aspirin will reduce the incidence of PIH in women at risk of developing the disease. They have yielded equivocal results. It has been difficult to document a teratogenic risk from maternal consumption of aspirin in the first trimester.

FEVER AND INFLAMMATION. COX inhibitors share antipyretic, analgesic, and anti-inflammatory actions. Paracetamol differs from the other compounds in being an efficient antipyretic despite weak anti-inflammatory properties in the periphery. The prostaglandins that mediate fever are unknown. Vasodilator prostaglandins seem to act in concert with other mediators to augment the inflammatory response. Among these may be the leukotrienes, which enhance capillary permeability and function as chemoattractants and leukocyte activators. Cross-overs of COX and LO knock-out mice may elucidate the interactive role of these families of eicosanoids in inflammatory disease.

Chen X-S, Sheller JR, Johnson EN, Funk CD: Role of leukotrienes revealed by targeted disruption of the 5-lipoxygenase gene. Nature 372:179, 1994. *The first embryonic stem cell knock-out of a gene encoding an eicosanoid-related protein.*

Lecomte M, Laneuville O, Ji C, et al.: Acetylation of human prostaglandin endoperoxide synthase-2 (cyclooxygenase-2) by aspirin. J Biol Chem 269:13207, 1994. *Inhibition of prostaglandin formation by the inducible COX.*

Morrow JD, Hill KE, Burk RF, et al.: A series of prostaglandin F₂-like compounds are produced *in vivo* in humans by a non-cyclooxygenase, free radical-catalyzed mechanism. Proc Natl Acad Sci 87:9383, 1990. *The first description of isoprostanes in human plasma and urine.*

Namba T, Sugimoto Y, Negishi M, et al.: Alternative splicing of C-terminal tail of prostaglandin E receptor subtype EP3 determines G-protein specificity. Nature 365:166, 1993. *Differential linkage of receptor splice variants to intracellular signals.*

Patrono C: Aspirin as an antiplatelet drug. N Engl J Med 330:1287, 1994. *A comprehensive review of the prototypic prostaglandin inhibitor.*

Picot D, Loll PJ, Garavito RM: The x-ray crystal structure of the membrane protein prostaglandin H₂ synthase-1. Nature 367:243, 1994. *The first crystal structure of an eicosanoid-related protein.*

Samuelsson B: Leukotrienes: Mediators of immediate hypersensitivity and inflammation. Science 220:568, 1983. *A review that concentrates on the biosynthesis and metabolism of these compounds and their role in inflammation.*

200.3 Natriuretic Hormones

Dennis A. Ausiello

In the last decade, considerable interest has focused on endogenous factors that play a role in the regulation of water and electrolyte balance. The isolation and cloning of the cardiac-derived atrial natriuretic peptide (ANP) has led to a rapid definition of its biosynthesis, storage, release response, and action. Although there are still some uncertainties, a picture of its role in physiology and pathophysiology and as a possible therapeutic agent has been developed. A second compound (or compounds), called natriuretic hormone (NH), whose presumed structure and function are distinct from those of ANP, has not yet been completely characterized. Therefore, its physiology, pathophysiology, and therapeutic potential are still unclear.

NATRIURETIC HORMONE (NH)

Experimental observations led to the concept of the existence of an endogenous regulator of mammalian Na⁺-K⁺-ATPase (the Na⁺ pump) more than 25 years ago. At that time intravascular expansion with saline in dogs produced a brisk natriuresis with no change in renal perfusion pressure, glomerular filtration rate, or mineralocorticoid activity. The natriuretic effects of extracellular fluid volume expansion in one animal also occurred in a second animal cross-circulated with the blood of the first. The presumption was that the natriuresis was due to a circulating substance that exerted its effects directly on the renal tubular Na⁺ reabsorptive process without affecting renal hemodynamics. Further experiments confirmed that active extracts from plasma, urine, and tissue sources that were natriuretic *in vivo* had a direct effect on transepithelial sodium transport. These substances have digitalis-like characteristics, although there was no reason to assume a structural identity between the postulated endogenous Na⁺-K⁺-ATPase inhibitor and the cardiac glycosides. Digitalis is a potent inhibitor of Na⁺-K⁺-ATPase and causes both natriuresis and an increase in vascular resistance, although these are not its major pharmacologic effects. Using the digoxin radioimmunoassay, digitalis-like immunoactivity has been found in the urine and plasma of sodium-loaded normal human subjects and in uremic and hypertensive subjects. Whether NH and digitalis-like compounds are the same endogenous Na⁺-K⁺-ATPase inhibitors remains to be defined.

BIOLOGIC ACTIVITIES. The biologic effects that have been claimed for the putative NH include (a) natriuresis *in vivo*, (b) inhibition of sodium transport *in vitro*, (c) Na⁺-K⁺-ATPase inhibition, (d) positive cardiac inotropism, and (e) increased vascular reactivity.

BIOCHEMICAL CHARACTERIZATION. Recently, the chemical structure of the endogenous Na⁺-K⁺-ATPase inhibitor from hypothalamus was chemically characterized as an isomer of the plant-derived cardiac glycoside, ouabain. This mammalian molecule inhibits active sodium transport in renal tubular cells and has positive inotropic and vasoconstrictive properties consistent with the NH/hypertension hypothesis.

SITE OF ORIGIN. The site of origin of the NH also remains uncertain, but the brain has been favored because the natriuretic effects of extracellular fluid volume expansion appear to depend on an intact central nervous system. An ouabain-like compound has been isolated from human cerebrospinal fluid. The hypothalamus represents an enriched source of an endogenous inhibitor of Na⁺-K⁺-ATPase, if not the site of its production.

NH AND THE PATHOPHYSIOLOGY OF ESSENTIAL HYPERTENSION. NH may play a role in normal volume regulation and in the pathophysiology of hypertension and secondary edema states. NH may have an extrarenal action leading to enhanced vascular reactivity. The hypothesis proposed is that in hereditary forms of hypertension, there is a persistent tendency toward renal retention of sodium. This may be due to increased Na⁺-K⁺ cotransport or Na⁺-H⁺ exchange in the proximal tubule, occurring as a manifestation of a generalized genetic defect in Na⁺-Na⁺ (Na⁺-Li⁺) countertransport. This defect exists in the erythrocytes of some patients with essential hypertension and in their first-degree normotensive relatives. The renal sodium retention leads to a transient increase in extracellular fluid volume, which serves as a stimulus for the release of a Na⁺-K⁺-ATPase inhibitor. The sodium pump inhibitor acts on the renal tubule to promote sodium excretion, thus restoring extracellular fluid volume to normal levels. It has similar inhibitory effects on Na⁺-K⁺-ATPase in vascular smooth muscle cells, resulting in a tonic increase in vascular tone, increased total peripheral resistance, and hypertension. It is assumed that Na⁺-K⁺-ATPase inhibition in vascular smooth muscle results in an increase in cytosolic free calcium concentration, which must occur to produce the arterial vasoconstriction. How this occurs is unclear. One of the hypotheses is that altered Na⁺-Ca²⁺ exchange resulting from partial sodium-pump inhibition may account for an increase in intracellular free Ca²⁺ concentration. At this time, this hypothesis remains attractive but unproven.

ATRIAL NATRIURETIC PEPTIDE (ANP)

ANP, a peptide hormone, is secreted primarily by the cardiac atria and produces natriuresis, diuresis, smooth muscle relaxation, and inhibition of renin and aldosterone secretion. Its major sites of action include the cardiovascular, renal, and endocrine systems. Although the exact mechanisms triggering the release of ANP are not clear, stretching of the atria appears to be the principal stimulus.

It has been known for several decades that membrane-bound secretory granules exist in the cardiac atria. In 1981 in a pioneering report, DeBold and his colleagues observed that bolus injection of crude extracts of rat atria, but not ventricles, produced a rapid, massive, and short-lasting diuresis and natriuresis and a modest kaliuresis. This suggested the existence of a natriuretic hormone in the atrial granules. Subsequently, this unique hormonal system has been thoroughly studied. The amino acid sequence of the active circulating peptide and its prehormone forms have been defined together with their gene structure, target tissue receptors, and signal transduction pathways.

STRUCTURE, BIOSYNTHESIS, AND SECRETION. The atrium first produces a pre-pro ANP (151 amino acids), the final 126 amino acids of which is pro ANP. The pro ANP, the principal storage form of the hormone in the atrial granules, is the immediate precursor of the biologically active 28 amino acid ANP, the predominant circulatory peptide. Circulatory ANP has a cysteine-cysteine disulfide crosslink that is essential for its activity.

The human gene for pre-pro ANP is located on the short arm of chromosome 1. Transcription of the pre-pro ANP gene proceeds at a high rate in the cardiac atria, estimated to be 1 to 3% of all mRNA in the atrial cardiocytes. ANP gene expression is transcriptionally regulated by dexamethasone and thyroid hormone. ANP is also expressed at very low levels in other tissues, such as brain, anterior pituitary, adrenal medulla, lung, kidney, thyroid, and submandibular gland. The major site of ANP synthesis is the monocytes of the right cardiac atrium, with lesser production in the left atrium. Pro ANP is cleaved by a specific atrial protease, probably at the time of exocytotic fusion of atrial granules with the plasma membrane and possibly even soon after secretion from the myocyte, resulting in ANP as the predominant form entering the coronary sinus blood.

STIMULI FOR RELEASE. Atrial stretch, measured as atrial transmural pressure, is the principal stimulus for ANP secretion into the circulation. Atrial pressure is also correlated with release of ANP. During infusion of isotonic saline in humans, plasma ANP increases in parallel with the increase of right atrial pressure. This results from rapid conversion of pro ANP to ANP and/or release of ANP. With cardiovascular or pulmonary disease, a significant correlation exists between circulating ANP levels and the right and left atrial pressures.

Mineralocorticoids, as well as glucocorticoids administered in high doses, increase mRNA encoding for pre-pro ANP and circulating ANP levels, indicating an increase in ANP production and release. In addition, adrenalectomized rats do not respond to increased atrial pressure with increased atrial and circulating ANP levels in the absence of glucocorticoid or mineralocorticoid replacement. Thus these hormones may play a permissive role in the volume response mediating ANP release as well as inducing ANP secretion directly.

BIOLOGIC AND PLASMA HALF-LIFE. A sensitive radioimmunoassay, generally specific for the mid to C-terminal peptides of ANP, will detect levels of 1 to 10 pg of the peptide in plasma. In subjects on varied sodium diets, the plasma ANP levels range from 10 to 40 pg per milliliter.

After release from the atrium or after intravenous administration, ANP is rapidly cleared with a plasma half-life between 2 and 4 minutes in humans. Biologic activity of ANP critically depends on the intact ring structure and carboxy-terminal residues. The rank order of tissue degradative potency appears to be kidney > liver > lung > plasma > heart.

ANP RECEPTORS. ANP receptors are localized on the cell surface of target tissues, including most notably adrenal, kidney, and the vasculature. They are also found, to a lesser extent, in the central nervous system, hepatocytes, colonic smooth muscle, and lung. In kidney, ANP binding sites are most prevalent in large vessels, glomeruli, and the renal medulla. In the adrenal, ANP binding is limited primarily to the zona glomerulosa.

Molecular cloning has defined three ANP receptors. The first is the ANP-C (or ANP-R2) clearance receptor, which is not coupled to cGMP production, the signal transduction pathway involved in ANP action. Clearance receptors do not mediate any known physiologic effect. The receptors for ANP in the kidney and vascular smooth muscle are predominantly clearance receptors. Their abundance accounts for the short half-life of circulatory ANP. It seems probable that the atrial peptide system has a novel receptor-mediated sequestration and clearance mechanism that is responsible, at least in part, for maintaining plasma levels of the hormone. The other ANP receptors are two structurally similar plasma membrane receptors, ANP-R1 and ANP-R3, the biologically active receptor forms. ANP binding to the extracellular domain of R1 or R3 activates the cytoplasmic domain of the receptor, which is a guanylate cyclase responsible for the generation of the second messenger, cGMP.

CELLULAR ACTION. The most apparent action of ANP is to increase intracellular cGMP concentration. ANP is a unique peptide hormone in its use of cGMP as a second messenger, which mediates most of the physiologic actions of the hormone. ANP also influences intracellular calcium homeostasis, which may be responsible for some of its biologic effects.

The physiologic responses to ANP include (1) relaxation of vascular and other smooth muscles, (2) increase in glomerular filtration rate and inhibition of tubular water and sodium transport in the kidney, and (3) inhibition of hormone secretion (Fig. 200-7).

KIDNEY ACTION. The kidney is the primary target organ for ANP. ANP causes natriuresis and diuresis by a concerted action at several nephron segments. The primary sites of action of ANP are the glomerulus, the renal vasculature, and the inner medullary collecting duct, although other nephron segments may be involved in the response to ANP. ANP can increase glomerular filtration rate by raising the glomerular hydraulic pressure gradient from capillary lumen to Bowman's space through differential effects on afferent and efferent arteriole tone. By relaxing glomerular mesangial cells, ANP also increases the glomerular ultrafiltration coefficient, Kf. The combined effects result in an increased filtration pressure and thus an increased filtration fraction, with a higher load of salt and water being delivered to the tubules for excretion.

The increased quantity of sodium filtered is not completely reabsorbed. There is an increased delivery of sodium to the distal tubule and collecting duct, where ANP reduces sodium reabsorption and vasopressin-induced water reabsorption, leading to a profound natriuresis. In addition, redistribution of blood flow from the cortex to inner medulla, which dilutes the papillary interstitium, results in an increase in sodium and water excretion.

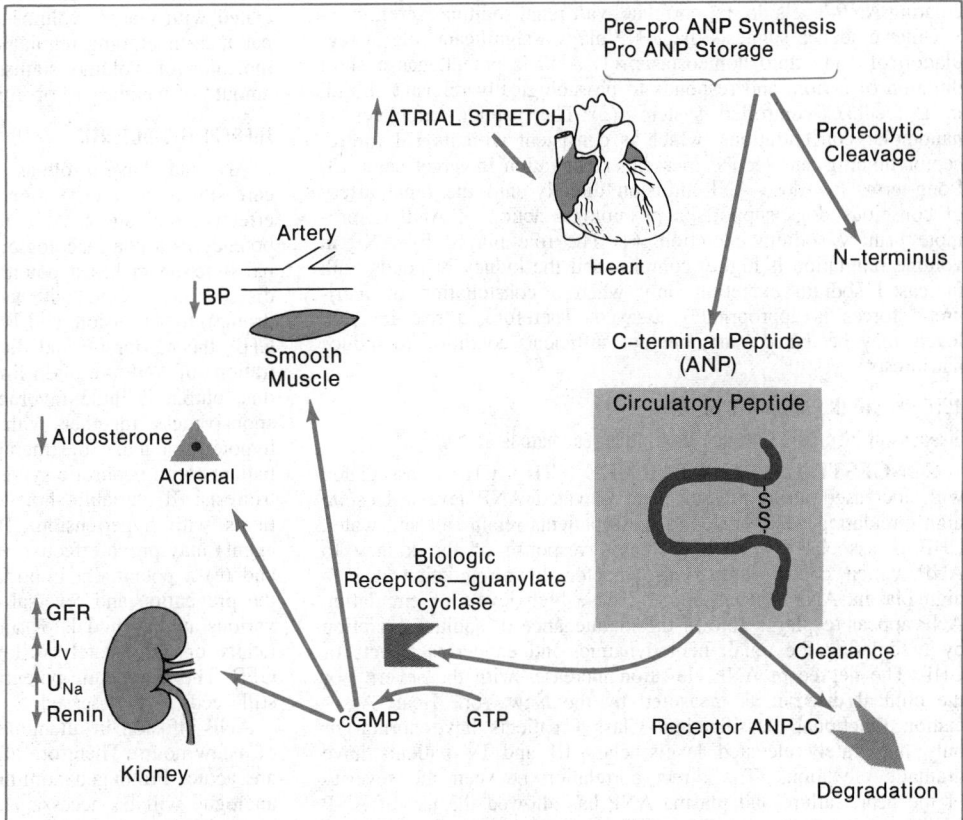

FIGURE 200-7. Major target organs and actions of atrial natriuretic peptide (ANP).

CARDIOVASCULAR ACTION. ANP directly relaxes arterial vascular smooth muscle through the action of its second messenger, cGMP. This ANP-induced vasorelaxation occurs independent of the presence of endothelium. ANP most effectively relaxes large-caliber arteries, such as the aorta and renal and iliac arteries. The more peripheral vascular segments of the arterial tree are less sensitive to the hormone. ANP causes vasorelaxation of aorta constricted with norepinephrine or angiotensin II, compatible with its role as one of the most potent vasodilators known and as a functional antagonist of a variety of vasoconstrictors.

ANP at pharmacologic concentrations reduces mean arterial pressure in man by reducing peripheral vascular resistance and decreasing intravascular volume. This is followed by a decrease in cardiac output attributed to (1) a shift of volume from the intravascular to extravascular space, probably due to alteration in capillary permeability or an increase in resistance to venous return at the site of postcapillary circulation. Hemoconcentration, secondary to a decreased plasma volume, may occur in humans in response to ANP. (2) Preload reduction due to relaxation of venous smooth muscle, leading to an augmentation of venous capacitance and a reduction of venous return.

ENDOCRINE ACTION. ANP modulates renin-angiotensin-aldosterone secretion. Administration of ANP causes a prompt decline in circulatory renin and aldosterone levels. ANP blocks both basal and agonist-stimulated (angiotensin II, ACTH, K$^+$) secretion of aldosterone in isolated adrenal zona glomerulosa cells. This appears to be a direct action of ANP on these cells. In addition, ANP decreases the biosynthesis and release of vasopressin. The decrease in vasopressin may potentiate a decrease in vascular tone and augment the diuresis and natriuresis induced by ANP.

SIGNIFICANCE OF ANP IN BODY FLUID HOMEOSTASIS

It is not yet possible to describe definitively the physiologic relevance of ANP. Some evidence suggests that ANP exerts a trivial influence on the normal regulation of body fluid homeostasis: (1) Infusion of ANP into conscious animals and normal human subjects results in plasma concentrations slightly above the physiologic range but produces only a slowly developing and relatively modest natriuresis. (2) Ingestion of food containing salt does not increase plasma ANP, yet a natriuresis routinely occurs postprandially. (3) In a number of common physiologic and experimental conditions, circulating ANP levels do not correlate with renal sodium excretion.

Other evidence suggests that ANP plays a significant role in regulation of body fluid homeostasis: (1) ANP is potent, has a short duration of action, and responds to physiologically relevant stimuli in a feedback-controlled system. (2) The peptide circulates at nanomolar concentrations, which is consistent with its Kd for receptor binding and second messenger activation in target cells. (3) Long-term, low-dose ANP infusion directly into the renal artery of conscious dogs supports a physiologic action of ANP to promote urinary sodium excretion. (4) The role played by ANP in volume regulation is highly complex and the kidney responds with increased sodium excretion only when a constellation of natriuretic forces is appropriately assayed. Therefore, a rise in ANP levels may be a necessary, but not sufficient, condition to induce natriuresis.

ROLE OF ANP IN PATHOPHYSIOLOGY
Diseases of Disordered Volume Regulation (Edematous States)

CONGESTIVE HEART FAILURE (CHF). CHF is associated with increased atrial pressure and elevated ANP levels. Despite high circulating ANP, however, these patients retain salt and water. CHF is associated with a decreased response of the kidney to ANP, which could result from receptor down-regulation due to high plasma ANP concentrations. These high levels of circulating ANP appear to play a role in the maintenance of sodium excretion by modulating the renal, hemodynamic, and endocrine effects of CHF. The degree of ANP elevation increases with the severity of the clinical disease, as measured by the New York Heart Association functional classification. Class I patients have normal or only moderately elevated levels; class III and IV patients have dramatic elevations. The direct correlation between the severity of the heart failure and plasma ANP has allowed the use of ANP levels to serve as a marker for CHF in adults and children, including those with congenital heart disease. ANP levels correlate directly with right atrial pressure, pulmonary capillary wedge pressure, and pulmonary artery pressure and inversely with cardiac output and cardiac index.

CIRRHOSIS. Progressive cirrhosis of the liver is accompanied by renal sodium and water retention with the development of ascites and edema. This state is usually accompanied by elevated plasma ANP levels, consistent with the "overflow" theory of ascites formation. As in CHF, raised ANP plasma concentrations in the presence of total body volume expansion implies a "refractory" or "reset" response to ANP. This hyporesponsiveness to ANP in cirrhosis is supported by the observation that ANP levels can be stimulated to increase further by water immersion, peritoneovenous shunting, and acute volume expansion with a resultant natriuresis in some patients. It is probable that a complex balance between ANP and antinatriuretic factors is responsible for renal sodium retention in early and late cirrhosis. In the former, hepatic venous outflow obstruction results in renal salt retention and intravascular volume expansion (overflow hypothesis). This in turn leads to an elevation in ANP levels counterbalanced by antinatriuretic factors such that the net effect is ascites formation. In late cirrhosis, with loss of intravascular volume into the peritoneal compartment (underfill hypothesis), there is a reduced stimulus for ANP secretion such that ANP plasma levels no longer offset antinatriuretic processes.

NEPHROTIC SYNDROME. Why edema forms in the nephrotic syndrome is not completely understood. Traditionally it has been suggested that renal sodium and water retention is a consequence of the lower plasma oncotic pressure from hypoalbuminemia and the resultant reduction in plasma volume. Consistent with this hypothesis, nephrotic syndrome is found to be associated with normal or diminished circulatory levels of ANP that can be stimulated to rise after intravascular volume expansion. Head-out water immersion conducted on patients with nephrotic syndrome demonstrated that ANP levels increased, but renal salt and water excretion was blunted. There thus appears to be an impaired renal response to ANP in the nephrotic syndrome.

ESSENTIAL HYPERTENSION. Patients with essential hypertension have a wide range of plasma ANP concentrations, suggesting that the contribution of ANP may vary in the heterogeneous population of patients with this disease. This finding precludes the use of ANP levels to differentiate among the various causes of hypertension.

RENAL DISEASE. Progressive renal disease is frequently associated with plasma volume expansion and elevated ANP levels. In patients undergoing regular dialysis, ANP levels can be used as an indicator of volume status. Decreased levels correlate with the amount of weight loss of fluid removal in dialysis patients.

THERAPEUTIC POTENTIAL

ANP may have a role as a therapeutic agent, especially in critical care situations. Intervention, in general, is limited by a lack of an effective oral agent. ANP must be administered intravenously. Its potency as a pharmacologic agent in altering cardiovascular and renal function makes it potentially attractive in treating patients with diseases associated with edema (CHF, cirrhosis, nephrotic syndrome), hypertension, and ischemic renal injury: (a) In patients with CHF, the natriuretic and diuretic effects of pharmacologic concentrations of ANP are often limited, but the effect on augmenting cardiac output is quite favorable; (b) in cirrhosis, the renal hyporesponsiveness together with a relatively increased sensitivity to hypotension make the therapeutic use of ANP problematic; (c) in patients with nephrotic syndrome, ANP infusion may result in a natriuresis; (d) variable short-term benefits have been reported in patients with hypertension. The use of low-dose ANP with other agents may prove effective if a satisfactory oral agent is developed; and (e) a potentially important therapeutic action of ANP may be the prevention and reversal of acute renal failure (see Ch. 76). In various animal models of acute renal failure, ANP given prophylactically or immediately following the hemodynamic insult restores GFR. The therapeutic potential of ANP in human acute renal failure still needs to be assessed.

ANP infusion in all human studies has not exceeded a duration of a few hours. Therefore all reported responses to ANP in humans are acute. Prolonged administration of ANP with a nonparenteral analogue will be necessary to evaluate its therapeutic potential in chronic human diseases.

Blaine EH: Atrial natriuretic factor plays a significant role in body fluid homeostasis. Hypertension 15:2, 1990. *Debate on the role ANP plays in body fluid homeostasis.*

Brenner BM, Ballermann BY, Gunning ME, et al.: Diverse biological actions of atrial natriuretic peptide. Physiol Rev 70:665, 1990. *Comprehensive review of the current understanding of the structure of ANP, its synthesis, secretion, cellular and target organ action, and its role in various pathophysiologic states.*

Floras JS: Sympathoinhibitory effects of atrial natriuretic factor in normal humans. Circulation 81:1860, 1990. *Integrative cardiovascular responses to ANP in normal humans.*

Goetz KL: Evidence that atriopeptin is not a physiological regulator of sodium excretion. Hypertension 15:9, 1990. *Debate on the role ANP plays in body fluid homeostasis.*

Haupert GT: Structure and biological activity of the Na^+-K^+-ATPase inhibitor isolated from bovine hypothalamus: Difference from ouabain. In Bamberg, E, Schoner, W (eds.): The Sodium Pump. New York; Steinkopff Darmstadt Springer, 1994, pp 732–742. *Review of current knowledge of the hypothalamic ouabain-like factor.*

ACKNOWLEDGMENT: I would like to thank Eliezer Holtzman for his invaluable help in preparing this chapter.

201 NEUROENDOCRINOLOGY

201.1 The Neuroendocrine System

Mark E. Molitch

NEUROENDOCRINE REGULATION

Neuroendocrinology refers to the general area of endocrinology in which the nervous system interacts with the endocrine system, serving to link aspects of cognitive and noncognitive neural activity with metabolic and hormonal homeostatic activity. Neural cells that can secrete hormones, i.e., *neurosecretory* cells, serve as the final common pathway linking the brain with the endocrine system. The *neurohypophyseal* neurons originate from the paraventricular and supraoptic nuclei, traverse the hypothalamic-pituitary stalk, and release vasopressin and oxytocin from nerve endings in the posterior pituitary. The *hypophysiotropic* neurons, localized in specific hypothalamic nuclei, project their axons to the median eminence to secrete their peptide and bioamine release and inhibiting hormones into the proximal end of the hypothalamic-pituitary portal vessels (Fig. 201–1). Neurons from other nuclei within the hypothalamus and other parts of the brain influence pituitary hormone secretion by interacting with these specific neurons. The median eminence receives its blood supply from the superior hypophyseal artery, which arborizes into a rich capillary bed. The capillary loops extend into the median eminence and coalesce to form the long portal veins that traverse the pituitary stalk and end in the pituitary. The capillary walls are "fenestrated," allowing entry of peptides secreted by the axon terminals. At the pituitary end of the stalk, the portal vessels again branch to form an extensive capillary plexus.

The neuroendocrine system operates through a series of feedback loops that control pituitary and target organ hormone levels precisely. Target organ hormones feed back at both the hypothalamic and pituitary levels to complete the loop, and efferent controller factors from the hypothalamus include both stimulatory and inhibitory substances. The feedback loops can be perturbed, resulting in temporary or prolonged alterations of set points by such factors as length of day (circadian periodicity), stress, nutritional status, and systemic illness. The suprachiasmatic nuclei, located just above the optic chiasm, are important in regulating circadian rhythms of the body.

HYPOPHYSIOTROPIC HORMONES

The regulation of pituitary hormones by hypophysiotropic hormones is quite complex, in part because of the multiplicity of substances present in the hypothalamus that can affect pituitary hormone secretion and in part because of the redundancy and overlapping nature of the feedback loops. In addition, some hypophysiotropic hormones exert effects on more than one pituitary

hormone (Fig. 201–2). Some of the hypophysiotropic hormones are also found elsewhere in the body, particularly the gastrointestinal tract and placenta, in which they may have significant physiologic functions. All of the hypophysiotropic hormones are also present in extrahypothalamic brain and function as neurotransmitters. Several hormones can occur in the same hypothalamic nucleus. In each instance, the action of the hypophysiotropic hormone is mediated first by binding to specific receptors and then by alteration of intracellular transduction mechanisms.

THYROTROPIN-RELEASING HORMONE (TRH). TRH is a tripeptide whose secretion is stimulated by norepinephrine and dopamine and inhibited by serotonin. The primary neuroendocrine functions of TRH are to stimulate the synthesis and release of thyroid-stimulating hormone (TSH) and prolactin (PRL). It has been estimated that a single molecule of TRH, through its TSH-releasing effect, induces the release of > 100,000 molecules of thyroxine from the thyroid. In hypothyroidism, TRH synthesis and binding to the pituitary are increased, resulting in increased basal and TRH-stimulated TSH and PRL levels. Correction of the hypothyroidism with thyroid hormones decreases the elevated TSH and PRL levels. Conversely, in hyperthyroidism, basal and TRH-stimulated TSH levels are markedly suppressed; basal PRL levels are not low, but the PRL response to TRH is markedly blunted and returns to normal with correction of the hyperthyroidism. The feedback effects of

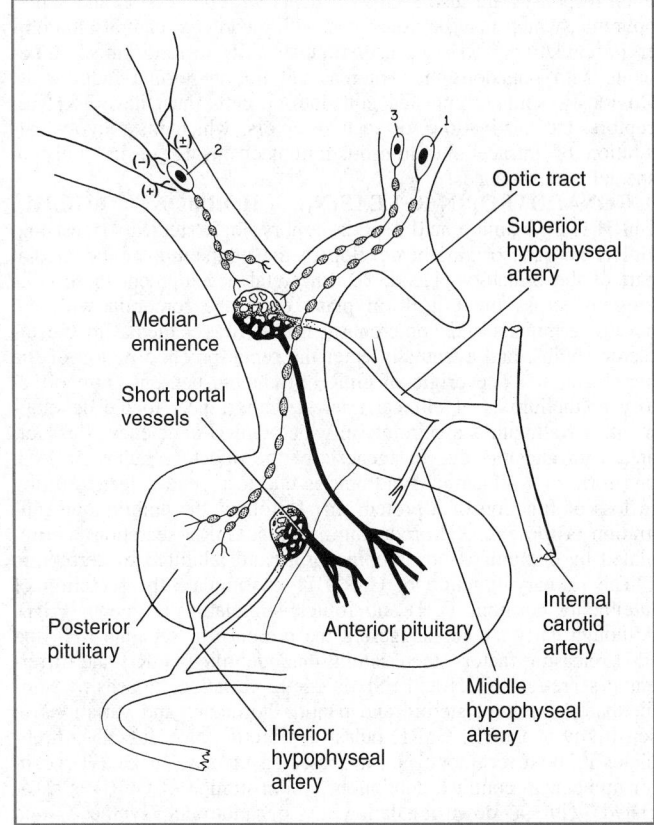

FIGURE 201–1. Neuroendocrine organization of the hypothalamus and pituitary gland. The posterior pituitary is fed by the inferior hypophyseal artery and the hypothalamus by the superior hypophyseal artery, both branches of the internal carotid artery. Most of the blood supply to the anterior pituitary is venous by way of the long portal vessels, which connect the portal capillary beds in the median eminence to the venous sinusoids in the anterior pituitary. Hypophysiotropic neurons (2) terminate in the median eminence on portal capillaries. These neurons of the tuberoinfundibular system secrete hypothalamic hormones into the portal veins for conveyance to the anterior pituitary gland. Multiple inputs to such neurons can be stimulatory, inhibitory, or neuromodulatory. Neuron 1 represents a peptidergic neuron originating in the magnocellular nuclei and projecting directly to the posterior pituitary by way of the hypothalamic-neurohypophyseal tract. Neuron 3 represents a vasopressinergic neuron projecting to the median eminence. (Modified from Lechan RM: Neuroendocrinology of pituitary hormone regulation. Endocrinol Metab Clinic North Am 16:475, 1987.)

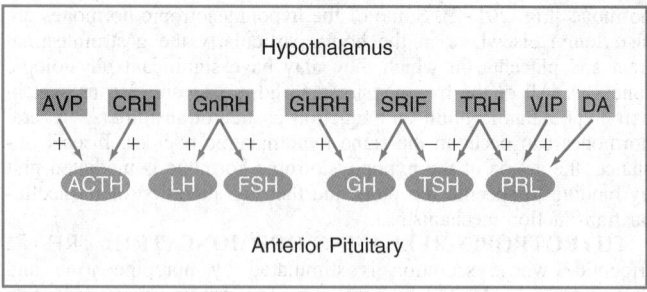

FIGURE 201–2. Interrelationships between hypothalamic and pituitary hormones. (+) indicates stimulatory effect and (−) indicates inhibitory effect. (See text for abbreviations.)

thyroid hormones, therefore, while occurring primarily at the pituitary, also occur at the hypothalamus.

Although TRH is the major regulator of TSH synthesis and secretion, the role of TRH as a physiologic PRL-releasing factor remains questionable. TRH can also stimulate growth hormone (GH) secretion in acromegaly, and in several states in which there is decreased insulin-like growth factor-1 (IGF-1) feedback on GH secretion, such as cirrhosis, renal insufficiency, anorexia nervosa, poorly controlled insulin-dependent diabetes mellitus, and malnutrition. Such responses are also seen in patients with depression and schizophrenia, which may be associated with disordered central bioaminergic regulation. TRH can also stimulate FSH secretion in some patients with gonadotroph adenomas but not in normal individuals. Obviously, somatotroph and gonadotroph cells must have TRH receptors, but "activation" of such receptors, which may involve alteration of intracellular transduction mechanisms, occurs only in special circumstances.

GONADOTROPIN-RELEASING HORMONE (GnRH). GnRH is a 10-amino acid peptide. Embryologic studies suggest that GnRH neurons originally develop in the epithelium of the medial part of the olfactory placode. During fetal development these cells migrate across the cribriform plate, enter the forebrain with the nervus terminalis and vomeronasal nerves, travel medial to the olfactory bulbs, and eventually enter the septal-preoptic region of the hypothalamus. The origin of GnRH-producing neurons from olfactory epithelium is of clinical interest with respect to the development of Kallmann's syndrome, in which GnRH deficiency is associated with anosmia due to agenesis of the olfactory bulbs. At least one form of Kallmann's syndrome is due to a gene defect resulting in loss of function of a protein that facilitates the embryologic migration of these GnRH-producing neurons. GnRH secretion is stimulated by dopamine and norepinephrine and inhibited by serotonin.

The primary function of GnRH is to stimulate the secretion of luteinizing hormone (LH) and follicle-stimulating hormone (FSH). Although early studies suggested the presence of separate LH- and FSH-releasing factors, there is only one identified GnRH and differential secretion of LH and FSH is due to variations in sensitivity of feedback effects of steroid and peptide hormones and variations in sensitivity to GnRH. GnRH pulsatile secretion also directly up-regulates its own receptors; i.e., it causes an increase in GnRH receptor number. In contrast, continuous administration of GnRH is associated with a down-regulation of gonadotropin synthesis and secretion due to decreased receptor numbers as well as postreceptor mechanisms.

In women, positive and negative steroid hormone feedback regulation of the hypothalamic-pituitary-gonadal axis occurs at both the pituitary and hypothalamic levels, the hypothalamic effects being the alteration of GnRH pulse amplitude and frequency and the pituitary effects being the modulation of the gonadotropin response to GnRH. In the follicular phase of the menstrual cycle estrogen feeds back negatively on gonadotropin secretion. At mid-cycle, estrogen feedback becomes positive and rising estrogen levels from the developing follicle stimulate the ovulatory surge of LH and FSH. Following ovulation, the feedback again becomes negative, and the estrogen and progesterone produced by the corpus luteum result in decreasing levels of LH and FSH. In the male, testosterone decreases GnRH pulsatile secretion with resultant decreased go-

nadotropin pulse amplitude and frequency as well as the gonadotropin response to exogenous GnRH.

The negative feedback effects of inhibin, a peptide produced by testicular Sertoli cells and ovarian granulosa cells, are predominantly on FSH at the pituitary. Inhibin causes a dose-related decrease in the sensitivity of gonadotrophs to GnRH, but there may also be a hypothalamic site of action. The related ovarian protein, activin, stimulates FSH synthesis and release from the pituitary. Another gonadal peptide, follistatin, also inhibits the oophorectomy- and GnRH-induced rises in FSH selectively, primarily by binding to activin. These ovarian peptides are also found in the pituitary and therefore may have additional local effects on gonadotropin secretion.

The hormone levels and feedback loops mentioned are primarily those of mature adults. In children, gonadotropin and gonadal steroid levels are very low. At puberty, negative feedback of steroid hormones decreases and gonadotropin and steroid levels gradually rise. During this pubertal development, in females the variation in negative and positive estrogen feedback develops, eventually resulting in the ovulatory menstrual cycle. At menopause, ovarian estrogen production ceases, gonadotropin levels rise markedly, and the symptoms associated with estrogen deficiency develop. In men, aging sometimes produces a decrease in testosterone production with a modest rise in gonadotropins, but there is no clinical syndrome similar to menopause.

GnRH has been successfully administered in a pulsatile manner to individuals with hypogonadotropic hypogonadism due to GnRH deficiency, resulting in restoration of normal sexual function and fertility. Long-acting GnRH agonists have been used to down-regulate GnRH receptors and gonadotropin secretion in a variety of conditions, including precocious puberty, prostate cancer, breast cancer, uterine fibroids, and endometriosis. Direct GnRH antagonists that competitively compete for the GnRH receptor are being explored for similar conditions.

SOMATOSTATIN. Somatostatin (also known as somatotropin release-inhibiting factor [SRIF]) is a tetradecapeptide; a 28-amino acid precursor also has GH inhibitory properties. Somatostatin blocks the rise in GH that occurs with all stimuli in a dose-dependent manner. The interaction of somatostatin and growth hormone–releasing hormone (GHRH) on GH secretion is complex. GH secretory episodes are associated with increased GHRH secretion often accompanied by low somatostatin levels; the basal or trough GH levels are associated with low GHRH levels and more elevated somatostatin levels. Somatostatin also inhibits basal and stimulated TSH secretion. However, dose-response studies in humans using somatostatin infusions have shown that GH is about 10-fold more sensitive to inhibition by somatostatin than is TSH. This suggests that the physiologic role of somatostatin in inhibiting TSH secretion is limited.

Somatostatin is also present in the D cells of the pancreatic islets and the gut mucosa as well as the myenteric neural plexus. Via paracrine and endocrine actions it suppresses the secretion of insulin, glucagon, cholecystokinin, gastrin, secretin, vasoactive intestinal polypeptide (VIP), and other gastrointestinal hormones, as well as such functions as gastric acid secretion, gastric emptying, gallbladder contraction, and splanchnic blood flow. Recently, analogues of somatostatin have been found to be effective in the treatment of acromegaly, carcinoid tumors, VIP-secreting tumors, TSH-secreting pituitary tumors, islet-cell tumors, and diarrhea of a number of causes.

CORTICOTROPIN-RELEASING HORMONE (CRH). CRH releases ACTH, β-endorphin, β-lipotropin, melanocyte-stimulating hormone (MSH), and other peptides generated from pro-opiomelanocortin (POMC) in equimolar amounts. CRH mediates 75% of the ACTH response to stress, and the remaining 25% is due to vasopressin. CRH and vasopressin have synergistic effects on ACTH release. In fact, CRH and vasopressin coexist in about half of the CRH-containing paraventricular neurons and even in the same neurosecretory granules. CRH and vasopressin are not always released coordinately, however, and stress has been shown to selectively activate the vasopressin-containing subset of CRH neurons.

Cortisol feeds back to decrease ACTH secretion at both the hypothalamic and pituitary levels. ACTH and β-endorphin also feed back negatively to decrease CRH release by the hypothalamus. Morphine suppresses the ACTH response to CRH in humans, acting presumably through opioid μ receptors. Central bioamines and peptides also influence CRH secretion. Acetylcholine, dopamine, norepinephrine, and epinephrine stimulate and GABA inhibits hypothalamic CRH secretion. Norepinephrine and epinephrine also stimulate pituitary ACTH secretion directly and are additive to the stimulatory effect of CRH.

Monokines released by inflammatory tissue, such as interleukin-1 and tumor necrosis factor-α stimulate the synthesis and release of CRH and vasopressin from the hypothalamus and the release of ACTH by the pituitary. The consequent increase of cortisol then reduces the intensity of the inflammatory response and release of these monokines, completing the feedback loop. Thus, this neuroendocrine-immune loop serves to modulate the inflammatory response.

Both ovine and human CRH have been given to humans in a variety of experimental paradigms, although CRH has not yet been approved by the U.S. Food and Drug Administration for commercial use. These preparations have been found to be of some use in stimulating ACTH secretion during petrosal sinus sampling in the differential diagnosis of Cushing's disease versus ectopic ACTH syndrome.

GROWTH HORMONE–RELEASING HORMONE (GHRH). GHRH dose-dependently stimulates GH secretion, and in some individuals GHRH is capable of eliciting a small increase in PRL as well. With repetitive administration every 3 hours, GHRH can cause the release of sufficient GH in children with GHRH deficiency to result in an increase in IGF-I levels and an acceleration of growth. Both IGF-I and GH itself feed back negatively on GH secretion, mediated by both a decrease in GHRH and an increase in somatostatin. This feedback effect of IGF-I is clinically relevant, as documented by the high circulating GH levels that occur in IGF-I–deficient states, such as renal insufficiency and cirrhosis. In children with mutations of the GH receptor resulting in their not being responsive to GH (GH insensitivity syndrome, also known as Laron-type dwarfism), IGF-I levels are very low and GH levels are correspondingly elevated. α_2-Adrenergic receptors and serotonin activate GHRH and GH secretion, but γ-aminobutyric acid (GABA) is inhibitory to GHRH secretion.

PROLACTIN-INHIBITORY FACTOR (PIF). The inhibitory component of hypothalamic regulation of PRL secretion predominates over the stimulatory component. Dopamine (DA) is the predominant, physiologic PIF, and the concentration of DA found in the pituitary stalk plasma is sufficient to decrease PRL levels. It is likely that in most physiologic circumstances that cause a PRL rise, such as lactation, there is a simultaneous fall in DA along with a rise in a PRL-releasing factor (PRF), such as vasoactive intestinal peptide (VIP). Blockade of endogenous DA receptors by a variety of drugs, such as the neuroleptics, causes a rise in PRL. Lesions that interrupt the basal hypothalamic neuronal pathways carrying dopamine to the median eminence or that interrupt portal blood flow result in decreased dopamine reaching the pituitary and hyperprolactinemia.

PROLACTIN-RELEASING FACTOR (PRF). A number of hypothalamic peptides other than TRH have also been shown to have PRF activity. VIP stimulates PRL synthesis and release at concentrations found in hypothalamic-pituitary portal blood. Within the VIP precursor is another similarly sized peptide known as peptide histidine methionine (PHM), which also has PRF activity. Complicating the role of VIP as a PRF is the finding that VIP is also synthesized by anterior pituitary tissue. The precise roles of VIP versus PHM and hypothalamic VIP versus pituitary VIP still are not clear.

ENDOGENOUS OPIOID PEPTIDES. The endogenous opioid peptides have only a minor role in neuroendocrine regulation. There are three major opioid peptide receptors and three major groups of opioid peptides, but the correspondence is not one for one. The μ receptor mediates most of the endocrine effects and analgesia; morphine is its prototypic agonist and naloxone is its prototypic antagonist; the primary peptide ligand for the μ receptor is β-endorphin. The δ receptor mediates behavioral, analgesic, and some endocrine effects and has as its primary peptide ligands met- and leu-enkephalins, which are derived from proenkephalin A. The κ receptor mediates sedation and ataxia and binds primarily dynorphin and the neoendorphins, which are derived from proenkephalin B (prodynorphin). All neuronal perikarya containing POMC-derived peptides are located in the arcuate nucleus, from which β-endorphin- and α-MSH–containing fibers project to the median eminence,

other parts of the hypothalamus, and other areas of the brain. Anterior pituitary β-endorphin is secreted with ACTH with CRH and vasopressin stimulation.

Various opioid peptides are linked to a number of bodily functions, including stress, mental illness, narcotic tolerance and dependence, eating, drinking, gastrointestinal function, learning, memory, reward, cardiovascular responses, respiration, thermoregulation, seizures, brain electrical activity, locomotor activity, pregnancy, and neuroimmune activity. The anterior pituitary itself is poor in opioid receptors, but the hypothalamus is quite rich. It has been suggested that the effects of opioid peptides on anterior pituitary hormone secretion occur via modulation of hypothalamic bioamines and hypophysiotropic factors. In general, endogenous opioids have an inhibitory influence on gonadotropin secretion through action on GnRH secretion, probably by inhibition of noradrenergic neuronal input. Opioids feed back negatively on ACTH and β-endorphin secretion and naloxone can increase basal and stimulated ACTH levels. Endogenous opioids have minimal effects on GH, PRL, and TSH secretion.

CNS RHYTHMS AND NEUROENDOCRINE FUNCTION

Pituitary hormones are secreted in a pulsatile fashion with a number of rhythms superimposed. The pulse amplitude of a pituitary hormone reflects the amount of releasing hormone as well as factors that may alter sensitivity to that releasing hormone. Thus, the amplitude can be altered by inhibitory factors (e.g., GHRH versus somatostatin), nutritional factors, feedback effects of target organ hormones, and prior stimulation that depletes a readily releasable pool of hormone. The frequency is generally governed by the frequency of release of the hypophysiotropic factor, regulated by the hypothalamic pulse generator system.

The pituitary has an intrinsic rhythm of small amplitude with a frequency of every 2 to 10 minutes. Superimposed upon this intrinsic rhythm is that from the pulsatile release of hypophysiotropic releasing factors, with or without the withdrawal of a corresponding inhibitory factor. Rhythms that are shorter than a day are referred to as *ultradian* rhythms. The next layer of rhythmicity is the *circadian* rhythm, i.e., rhythms with approximately 24-hour periodicity. These rhythms are usually synchronized with the 24-hour period by a periodic environmental cue, such as the dark-light cycle. The suprachiasmatic nucleus functions as a circadian pacemaker and receives light-induced electrical impulses from the retina via the retinohypothalamic tract, finally transmitting those impulses to the pineal, where they are converted to hormonal signals. Signals for a rhythm with a periodicity longer than 24 hours, i.e., an *infradian* rhythm, include the gravitational influence of the moon, giving rise to the menstrual cycle.

A number of factors may influence circadian and infradian rhythms. One of the most important is the sleep-wake cycle. GH, TSH, PRL, ACTH, and pubertal LH secretion are all entrained more to the sleep-wake cycle than the dark-light cycle. Each has an increase and maximal level that occur following sleep onset. The profound diurnal variation of cortisol and ACTH is often used as an index of "normality" of the system. Loss of this diurnal rhythm occurs with disordered regulation by CRH, which may be due to endogenous depression or excessive alcohol intake, as well as autonomous secretion of ACTH in Cushing's disease. Loss of diurnal rhythm of cortisol has been used as a diagnostic test for Cushing's syndrome.

Interesting changes occur in gonadotropin secretion as the child passes through puberty into adulthood. Early in puberty the amplitude of pulses increases during sleep at night, especially for LH, but in adulthood this nocturnal rise is lost. In patients with anorexia nervosa, the pattern of gonadotropin secretion often reverts to this pubertal pattern, only to lose this pattern again with weight gain. This suggests that body composition may in some way affect the regulation of the pulsatile secretion of the gonadotropins. In fact, the percentage of body composition that is fat has been proposed as being important in the timing of the onset of puberty.

Endocrine rhythms appear to reflect a rather primitive organizing influence that helps the animal to adapt to the environment. The circadian synchronization with the light-dark cycle and sleep and the infradian synchronization with seasonal changes are present very early phylogenetically. However, because humans are able to alter the light-dark cycles, they are less tied to environmental changes. This has led to new, modern problems with these rhythms such as jet-lag, which involves the rapid resynchronization of the rhythms with several hour time-zone displacements. Because not all rhythms resynchronize at the same rates, some of the disorientation and other symptoms associated with jet-lag may be due to abnormal phase relationships of various body rhythms to each other and to the dark-light cycle.

Frohman LA, Downs TR, Chomczynski P: Regulation of growth hormone secretion. Front Neuroendocrinol 14:344, 1992. *A thorough, molecularly oriented review of the regulation of GH secretion.*

Lechan RM: Neuroendocrinology of pituitary hormone regulation. Endocrinol Metab Clinic North Am 16:475, 1987. *An excellent discussion of the anatomic features of neuroendocrine regulation. MRI scans and accompanying diagrams clarify hypothalamic structural anatomy.*

Orth DN: Corticotropin-releasing hormone in humans. Endocr Rev 13:164, 1992. *A thorough review of CRH: its tissue distribution, blood levels, responses to its administration in normals and patients, its diagnostic use, and its secretion ectopically.*

Reichlin S: Neuroendocrine-immune interactions. N Engl J Med 329:1246, 1993. *A critical review of the various interactions between the endocrine and the immune systems, including possible psychological influences. It asks more questions than it answers in this exciting new field.*

Schwanzel-Fukuda M, Jorgenson KL, Bergen HT, et al.: Biology of normal luteinizing hormone–releasing hormone neurons during and after their migration from olfactory placode. Endocrine Rev 13:623, 1992. *Reviews the fascinating unfolding story regarding the migration of GnRH neurons from the olfactory placode to the hypothalamus. Defects in this migration result in Kallman's syndrome.*

Van Cauter E: Diurnal and ultradian rhythms in human endocrine function: A minireview. Horm Res 34:45, 1990. *Reviews the physiology and clinical relevance of the rhythms characterizing hormone secretion.*

NEUROENDOCRINE DISEASE

DISEASES OF THE HYPOTHALAMUS. Diseases may affect the hypothalamus by being localized to the hypothalamus, by being part of more generalized central nervous system (CNS) disease, such as neurosarcoidosis, or by indirect means, such as by causing hydrocephalus (Table 201–1). Furthermore, hormonal changes may occur in a variety of psychiatric disorders, mediated by functional alterations in hypothalamic regulation.

The axons projecting to the median eminence that contain the various hypophysiotropic factors are concentrated in the basal portion of the hypothalamus. Thus, lesions located within this final common pathway might be expected to cause significant decreases in the secretion for some or all of the pituitary hormones except PRL, which may increase because of the elimination of the tonic inhibition by dopamine. Diabetes insipidus may also occur. Other functions of the hypothalamus are more diffusely located, such as the regulation of temperature, food intake, and blood pressure.

Symptoms due to hypothalamic dysfunction are related to size of the lesion and consequently to the area of the hypothalamus involved, as well as to the rapidity of increase in lesion size. Slowly growing lesions tend to cause problems of hormone dysregulation rather than dramatic symptoms. Large, slowly growing lesions can cause more acute problems, however, when a slight increment in growth eliminates remaining vestiges of vasopressin or ACTH secretion or completely occludes the aqueduct of Sylvius, causing hydrocephalus.

The best way of discerning lesions affecting the hypothalamus is by magnetic resonance imaging (MRI) with gadolinium enhancement, although computed tomographic (CT) scanning with intravenous contrast is also quite good. Formal visual field testing may discern impingement of the optic nerves and chiasm by hypothalamic lesions, including the suprasellar extension of pituitary tumors. Detailed testing of hypothalamic-pituitary function may reveal evidence of functional hypothalamic disruption with great sensitivity.

Congenital Embryopathic Disorders. The most common embryopathic disorders to affect the hypothalamus are the midline cleft syndromes, which cause varying degrees of defects of midline structures, especially the optic and olfactory tracts, the septum pellucidum, the corpus callosum, the anterior commissure, the hypothalamus, and the pituitary. The clinical presentation of patients with midline cleft defects varies in severity from cyclopia to cleft lip and from isolated hypothalamic hormone defects to panhypopituitarism. The combination of absent septum pellucidum associated with optic nerve hypoplasia is referred to as *septo-optic dysplasia* and is associated with abnormalities of hypothalamic and other di-

TABLE 201–1. ETIOLOGY OF HYPOTHALAMIC DISEASE

Neonates

Intraventricular hemorrhage
Meningitis: bacterial
Tumors: glioma, hemangioma
Trauma
Hydrocephalus, hydranencephaly, kernicterus

1 Month–2 Years

Tumors: glioma, especially optic glioma, histiocytosis X, hemangiomas
Hydrocephalus, meningitis
"Familial" disorders: Laurence-Moon-Bardet-Biedl, Prader-Labhart-Willi

2–10 Years

Tumors: craniopharyngioma, glioma, dysgerminoma, hamartoma, histiocytosis X, leukemia, ganglioneuroma, ependymoma, medulloblastoma
Meningitis: bacterial, tuberculous
Encephalitis: viral and demyelinating, various viral encephalitides and exanthematous demyelinating encephalitides, disseminated encephalomyelitis
"Familial" disorders: diabetes insipidus, etc.
Damage from nasopharyngeal radiation therapy

10–25 Years

Tumors: craniopharyngioma, pituitary tumors, glioma, hamartoma, dysgerminoma, histiocytosis X, leukemia, dermoid, lipoma, neuroblastoma
Trauma
Subarachnoid hemorrhage, vascular aneurysm, arteriovenous malformation
Inflammatory diseases: meningitis, encephalitis, sarcoidosis, tuberculosis
Disease associated with midline brain defects: agenesis of corpus callosum
Chronic hydrocephalus or increased intracranial pressure

25–50 Years

Nutritional: Wernicke's disease
Tumors: glioma, lymphoma, meningioma, craniopharyngioma, pituitary tumors, angioma, plasmacytoma, colloid cysts, ependymoma, sarcoma, histiocytosis X
Inflammatory: sarcoidosis, tuberculosis, viral encephalitis
Subarachnoid hemorrhage, vascular aneurysms, arteriovenous malformation
Damage from pituitary radiation therapy

50 Years and Older

Nutritional: Wernicke's disease
Tumors: sarcoma, glioblastoma, lymphoma, meningioma, colloid cysts, ependymoma, pituitary tumors
Vascular: infarct, subarachnoid hemorrhage, pituitary apoplexy
Infectious: encephalitis, sarcoidosis, meningitis

Adapted from Plum F, Van Uitert R: Non-endocrine diseases of the hypothalamus. *In* Reichlin S, Baldessarini RJ, Martin JB (eds.): The Hypothalamus. New York, Raven Press, 1978, p 415.

encephalic structures. Some patients with septo-optic dysplasia and hypothalamic hypopituitarism have sexual precocity, presumably due to lack of inhibitory influences from other parts of the hypothalamus and intact GnRH-producing structures. Children with very mild midline cleft defects consisting of cleft lip or palate or both have been found to have a markedly increased risk of having GH and other pituitary hormone deficiencies. A recent evaluation with MR scanning of patients with "idiopathic" GH deficiency showed absence of the infundibulum in 43%.

Kallmann's syndrome is an autosomal dominant condition characterized by anosmia or hyposmia and hypogonadotropic hypogonadism. It is due to a gene defect resulting in loss of function of a protein that facilitates the embryologic migration of GnRH-producing neurons. The pituitary is usually intact, and treatment with pulsatile GnRH therapy or gonadotropins results in spermatogenesis and normal gonadal function. In some patients, other neurologic abnormalities may be present, including cerebellar ataxia, nerve deafness, color blindness, cleft lip and palate, mental retardation, and disordered thirst.

Tumors. The most common tumors affecting the hypothalamus are *pituitary adenomas* that have significant suprasellar extension. These tumors can cause varying degrees of hypopituitarism, diabetes insipidus, and hyperprolactinemia by either compressing the normal pituitary or, more commonly, affecting the pituitary stalk and mediobasal hypothalamus. Evidence that hypopituitarism is from pituitary compression includes a low serum PRL level and a lack of TSH response to TRH; pituitary function in such cases usually does not improve after treatment. In patients with normal or elevated PRL levels, pituitary function often returns following therapy.

Craniopharyngiomas are the next most common tumors affecting the hypothalamus. Microscopically, craniopharyngiomas consist of cysts alternating with stratified squamous epithelium. The cyst fluid is usually thick and dark and the material is often calcified. They arise from remnants of Rathke's pouch. A closely related, less common lesion is *Rathke's cleft cyst,* which develops from the space between the anterior and rudimentary intermediate lobes. Rathke's cleft cysts are lined with cuboidal as opposed to squamous epithelium, and the cyst fluid is usually white and mucoid. Craniopharyngiomas sometimes recur postoperatively whereas Rathke's cleft cysts rarely recur. Craniopharyngiomas most commonly present during childhood, but they also may occur in adults and even the elderly. These tumors present because of mass effects, including headache, vomiting, visual disturbance, seizures, hypopituitarism, and polyuria. Some patients present with galactorrhea, amenorrhea, and hyperprolactinemia, suggestive of a prolactinoma. Careful endocrine testing reveals varying degrees of hypopituitarism in 50 to 75% and modest hyperprolactinemia in 25 to 50%. Surgical extirpation of craniopharyngiomas commonly causes a worsening of pituitary function, often resulting in complete panhypopituitarism and diabetes insipidus because of stalk section. Irradiation may also be helpful, especially in children.

Suprasellar dysgerminomas arise from primitive germ cells that have migrated to the CNS during fetal life and structurally are identical to germ cell tumors of the gonads. They most commonly occur in children, where they cause decreased growth because of hypopituitarism, diabetes insipidus, and visual problems. Hyperprolactinemia occurs in >50%, and 10% have precocious puberty due to the production of chorionic gonadotropin by the tumor. As opposed to craniopharyngiomas, these tumors are very radiosensitive, and radiation therapy is the preferred treatment.

A hypothalamic *hamartoma* is a nodule of growth of hypothalamic neurons attached by a pedicle to the hypothalamus between the tuber cinereum and the mammillary bodies and extending into the basal cistern. Asymptomatic hamartomas may be present in up to 20% of random autopsies; rarely, these lesions may enlarge, causing disruption of hypothalamic function because of compression of adjacent tissue. A variant of the hamartoma consisting of similar tissue within the anterior pituitary but without a neural attachment to the hypothalamus is called a choristoma or gangliocytoma. These neuronal tumors are of particular endocrine interest because they can produce hypophysiotropic hormones. A number of cases associated with precocious puberty have been reported in which the hamartomas produce GnRH. Successful treatment has been reported with surgery and with the administration of a long-acting GnRH analogue, which suppresses gonadotropin secretion but does not affect the tumor itself. Medical therapy with the GnRH analogue may be the best choice, as surgery can be noncurative or even fatal, if the hamartoma does not cause other problems from mass effects. Some gangliocytomas have been reported which produce GHRH and acromegaly and CRH and Cushing's syndrome.

Other tumors and space-occupying lesions occurring in the suprasellar area include arachnoid cysts, meningiomas, gliomas, astrocytomas, chordomas, infundibulomas, cholesteatomas, neurofibromas, lipomas, and metastatic cancer (particularly breast and lung). Any such lesion may present with varying degrees of hypopituitarism, diabetes insipidus, and hyperprolactinemia, and surgical therapy often worsens the hormonal deficit.

Inflammatory Disorders. CNS involvement in *sarcoidosis* occurs in 1 to 5% of patients, as determined on clinical grounds, and in up to 16% of cases at autopsy. Isolated CNS sarcoidosis is quite uncommon, however. When sarcoidosis does involve the CNS, the hypothalamus is involved in 10 to 20%. Sarcoid granulomas can involve the hypothalamic stalk or pituitary and may be infiltrative or present as a mass lesion. The most common endocrine findings are varying degrees of hypopituitarism, diabetes insipidus, and hyperprolactinemia. Obesity due to hypothalamic involvement by sarcoidosis has also been reported. In patients with isolated CNS sarcoidosis, the diagnosis may be extremely difficult. Examination of the CSF usually shows elevated protein levels, low glucose levels, a pleocytosis, and variable elevations of angiotensin-converting enzyme. However, biopsy is often necessary. Although corticosteroid therapy has been reported to at least partially reverse the thirst dis-

orders, anterior pituitary hormone deficits usually do not respond. *Langerhans cell histiocytosis* or eosinophilic granulomatous infiltration of the hypothalamus may cause diabetes insipidus, varying degrees of hypopituitarism, and hyperprolactinemia. It is the most common cause of diabetes insipidus in children. Usually this infiltration appears as a thickening of the pituitary stalk, but it may also appear as a mass lesion of the hypothalamus or the pituitary. Osteolytic lesions may be present in the jaw or mastoid and radiographs of the jaw are a worthwhile part of the diagnostic evaluation of an unknown suprasellar mass or diabetes insipidus for this reason. Therapy consists of local surgery, focal irradiation, or chemotherapy with alkylating agents and high-dose corticosteroids.

Vascular Disease. An enlarging aneurysm may present as a mass lesion of the hypothalamic-pituitary area and may cause hypopituitarism and visual field defects. Obviously, the distinction must be made before surgery. Tumors and aneurysms may also coexist, and careful radiologic evaluation with MRI is necessary to discern this. Hypothalamic disease due to vascular infarction is extremely rare.

Trauma. Head trauma can cause defects ranging from isolated ACTH deficiency to panhypopituitarism with diabetes insipidus. Within the first 72 hours of trauma, GH, LH, ACTH, TSH, and PRL levels may actually be elevated in blood, perhaps due to acute release. These levels subsequently fall, and patients either return to normal or develop hypopituitarism. In patients dying of head injury, anterior pituitary infarction has been found in 16% of cases, posterior pituitary hemorrhages in 34%, and hypothalamic hemorrhages or infarction in 42% of cases. The paraventricular and supraoptic nuclei and median eminence are particularly involved with microhemorrhages, resulting in the high frequency of panhypopituitarism with diabetes insipidus. With frontal injuries, the brain travels backward but the pituitary cannot move, resulting in the pituitary stalk becoming avulsed, with interruption of the portal vessels. Most patients with head injury are hyperprolactinemic, confirming clinically that the hypothalamus and/or stalk is the primary site of injury.

Irradiation. Whole brain irradiation for intracranial neoplasms frequently results in hypothalamic dysfunction, as evidenced by endocrine abnormalities and behavioral changes. The most common endocrine abnormality is hyperprolactinemia, but hypopituitarism can also occur. When the radiation therapy is targeted to the hypothalamic area, as in patients with tumors in that area or nasopharyngeal carcinomas, hypopituitarism occurs even more frequently. The frequencies of loss of pituitary function are so high that all patients who have had their pituitary and hypothalamic areas irradiated must be followed closely to detect these deficits when they occur.

EFFECTS OF HYPOTHALAMIC DISEASE ON PITUITARY FUNCTION. Hypothalamic disease can cause both pituitary hyperfunction and hypofunction in varying degrees of severity. Although severe disease can cause absolute deficiencies of the various hormones, milder disease may cause a subtle alteration of feedback loops and timing such that, for example, the integration of signals necessary for menstrual cycling is lost, resulting in "hypothalamic" amenorrhea. Furthermore, the hypothalamic defects may be interrelated, so that the rather common finding of hyperprolactinemia occurring with hypothalamic dysfunction causes a hypogonadotropic hypogonadism that is reversible when the elevated PRL levels are brought down to normal. In many cases no structural lesion can be found on MRI, and a functional defect due to altered neurotransmitter regulation is invoked.

Growth Hormone. Loss of normal GH secretion is the most common hormonal defect occurring with structural hypothalamic disease. Congenital idiopathic GH deficiency (IGHD) is a heterogeneous disorder consisting of hypothalamic and pituitary defects. The diagnosis is usually made between 1 and 3 years of age because of impaired growth. Between 5 and 30% of IGHD subjects have an affected relative, and thus their defect is thought to have a genetic basis; some have been associated with a deletion of the GH gene. In about three-quarters of cases there is a normal GH response to exogenous GHRH, suggesting that the defect is likely disordered hypothalamic regulation. Children with IGHD should be treated with biosynthetic GH, although experimental studies suggest that GHRH treatment is also often successful. Other hormonal defects that may be present also must be treated simultaneously, although therapy with gonadal steroids should be delayed to prevent epiphyseal closure before the final desired height is achieved. A reversible form of IGHD due to inadequate parental care and affection is referred to as the *emotional deprivation syndrome* or *psychosocial dwarfism.* Restoration of a proper social environment for such a child results in prompt normalization of GH secretion and growth. It has been hypothesized that the disordered GH regulation is due to a psychogenic alteration of the neurotransmitter balance necessary for normal GHRH and somatostatin secretion.

Gonadotropins. **Hypothalamic Hypogonadism.** The primary defect in this group of disorders involves secretion of GnRH, with resultant impairment in pituitary gonadotropin secretion and gonadal function. The disorders causing these conditions may be primary, i.e., congenital defects, or acquired. Depending upon the time of onset, they present either as delayed puberty, interruption of pubertal progression, or loss of adult gonadal function. The lesions causing these disorders may cause loss of other hormones or may be isolated to GnRH. Loss of gonadotropin secretion as the result of hypothalamic structural damage is the second most common defect after GH deficiency. However, a substantial portion of these defects is due to hyperprolactinemia and is reversible with correction of the hyperprolactinemia.

Lesions presenting prepubertally result in the failure of onset of puberty or incomplete progression of puberty if the defect is partial. If the disorder is limited to GnRH and the gonadotropins, prior growth and development are normal. However, the growth spurt occurring at puberty is lost. The most common congenital lesion causing prepubertal GnRH deficiency is Kallmann's syndrome, comprising 50% of males and 37% of females presenting with isolated gonadotropin deficiency. In patients with idiopathic GnRH deficiency, the GnRH gene appears to be normal. However, indirect measures of functional GnRH secretion show that there may be disorders of pulse amplitude and/or frequency. When hyperprolactinemia occurs before puberty, it can prevent the onset of puberty and must always be looked for in this setting.

The ideal therapy for patients with GnRH deficiency is the replacement of GnRH via subcutaneous administration every 2 hours using a portable pump. This causes a rapid rise in the LH and FSH responses to the GnRH and a rise in testosterone to normal, as well as development of normal spermatogenesis. Similar studies in women result in ovulatory cycles in 80%. In men, comparable results can be obtained with exogenous gonadotropins given three times per week. Replacement with testosterone alone causes adequate androgenization but does not result in an increase in testicular size or in spermatogenesis.

Loss of formerly normal GnRH secretion in adults may be due to structural hypothalamic damage such as a tumor, a functional change unassociated with a detectable lesion, or hyperprolactinemia. Structural disease must be excluded in such patients by CT or MR scanning. Most but not all functional hypogonadotropic hypogonadism occurs in women, the most common causes being weight loss, excessive exercise, or psychogenic stress. In some the exercise results in a loss of body fat not detected with total body weight measures and it is unclear whether the hypogonadism is directly due to the loss of body fat or to the exercise *per se*. Studies of pulsatile gonadotropin secretion in such patients reveal absent pulses. Usually there is a normal gonadotropin response to injected GnRH. Regain of weight and stopping of the exercise result in resumption of normal gonadal function. Hyperprolactinemia occurring postpubertally can also decrease GnRH and the pulsatile secretion of LH and FSH, resulting in anovulation with oligo/amenorrhea in women and impotence and infertility in men.

Therapy should be directed at the underlying process, if possible. Efforts at weight gain and restricting exercise should be made when appropriate. In idiopathic, functional hypogonadotropic amenorrhea there are two goals: (1) restoration of a normal estrogen status to promote well-being and to prevent osteoporosis and (2) facilitation of ovulation for fertility. The former can generally be achieved with cyclic estrogen and progesterone, whereas the latter may require clomiphene, GnRH, or gonadotropin therapy.

Hypothalamic Hypergonadism (Precocious Puberty). Precocious puberty is defined as the onset of puberty before the ages of 8 in girls and 9 in boys. "Pseudo"-precocious puberty is that due to peripheral (gonadal or adrenal) causes. Central, "true," or GnRH-dependent precocious puberty is characterized by hormonal changes

similar to those that occur at the time of normal puberty, i.e., an increase in the pulsatile release of LH, an increase in the gonadotropin response to GnRH, and an increase in gonadal steroid secretion. GnRH-dependent precocious puberty therefore represents a premature activation of this GnRH pulse generator by a variety of lesions, or it may also be idiopathic. Less than one-quarter of cases of central precocious puberty occur in boys, but they tend to have more serious underlying disease. In boys with central, GnRH-dependent precocious puberty, hypothalamic hamartomas account for 38% of cases, other CNS lesions represent 31%, familial disease accounts for 23%, and idiopathic disease accounts for only 8%. The picture is quite different in girls, however, as hypothalamic hamartomas account for only 15% of cases, other CNS lesions represent 14%, the McCune-Albright syndrome (polyostotic fibrous dysplasia) accounts for 6%, and fully 65% are idiopathic. Dysgerminomas in the suprasellar or pineal region can produce hCG, which acts like LH in its stimulation of gonadal function. Usually such tumors cause increased sex steroid formation but fail to cause ovulation.

Therapy of central GnRH-dependent precocious puberty consists of surgical removal of the tumor or medical therapy with a long-acting GnRH analogue. The latter can suppress gonadotropin and sex steroid hormone levels and cause a stabilization or even regression of secondary sex characteristics and a slowing of growth and bone maturation in most cases. When therapy is discontinued at the normal time of puberty, sex steroid levels increase, secondary sexual characteristics again develop, growth increases, and regular menses develop spontaneously. For those patients who do not respond to the GnRH analogues, treatment with medroxyprogesterone acetate or testolactone, an aromatase inhibitor, is indicated.

Prolactin. **Hypothalamic Hyperprolactinemia.** Structural or infiltrative lesions of the hypothalamus, such as those discussed above, can decrease the amount of dopamine reaching the lactotrophs, causing modest hyperprolactinemia. PRL elevations due to such lesions rarely exceed 150 ng per milliliter and usually are less than 100 ng per milliliter. Similar elevations are also seen in patients with an empty sella. Because their therapy is quite different, it is very important to differentiate nonsecreting pituitary adenomas with extensive suprasellar extension causing PRL elevations in this range from PRL-secreting adenomas which, when of such a large size, usually cause PRL elevations 5 to 50 times higher. A number of medications can cause hyperprolactinemia, primarily by interfering with central catecholamines, dopamine in particular (Table 201–2).

Therapy is generally directed at the underlying cause. The hyperprolactinemia itself may impair gonadal function so that efforts may also be made to lower PRL levels with bromocriptine or other dopamine agonists. PRL levels usually fall quite readily in such pa-

TABLE 201–2. CAUSES OF HYPERPROLACTINEMIA

Pituitary Disease	Neurogenic	Medications
Prolactinomas	Chest wall lesions	Phenothiazines
Acromegaly	Spinal cord lesions	Haloperidol
"Empty sella syndrome"	Breast stimulation	Monoamine-oxidase
Lymphocytic hypophysitis		inhibitors
Cushing's disease		Tricyclic antidepressants
Pituitary stalk section		Reserpine
		Methyldopa
		Metoclopramide
		Amoxepin
		Cocaine
		Verapamil

Hypothalamic Disease	Other
Craniopharyngiomas	Pregnancy
Meningiomas	Hypothyroidism
Dysgerminomas	Chronic renal failure
Nonsecreting pituitary adenomas	Cirrhosis
	Pseudocyesis
Other tumors	Adrenal insufficiency
Sarcoidosis	Idiopathic
Eosinophilic granuloma	
Neuraxis irradiation	
Vascular	

Modified from Molitch ME: Management of prolactinomas. Annu Rev Med 40:225, 1989.

tients. Restoration of gonadal function is not automatic, however, as the primary hypothalamic lesion may also directly impair release of GnRH. In that circumstance both bromocriptine and sex steroid replacement may be necessary. When psychotropic medications that cause the hyperprolactinemia cannot be stopped, dopamine agonists may be used but may exacerbate the psychosis. In such cases and others in which fertility is not an issue, treatment with cyclic estrogen/progestin replacement can be carried out safely.

Idiopathic Hyperprolactinemia. Idiopathic hyperprolactinemia is a diagnosis of exclusion. PRL levels in this condition are usually < 100 ng per milliliter. In such cases, small pituitary or hypothalamic tumors could exist that are beyond the resolution of current imaging techniques, but when such patients are followed for many years, it is very uncommon for tumors to later be visualized. Idiopathic hyperprolactinemia can cause amenorrhea, galactorrhea, impotence, infertility, and loss of libido, just as occurs with hyperprolactinemia of other causes, and therefore may need to be treated. Premature osteoporosis related to the estrogen deficiency may also occur. The only possible treatment is bromocriptine or another dopamine agonist, and these are successful in >90% of cases. Alternatively, cyclic estrogen/progesterone replacement may be given, but fertility will not be restored.

TSH. *Hypothalamic hypothyroidism,* also referred to as tertiary hypothyroidism, is due to a central lesion that impairs the secretion of TRH, usually along with loss of other hormones. It occurs considerably less commonly than hypothalamic GH and gonadotropin deficiency. TSH levels in this syndrome generally are normal or even slightly elevated, and the response to TRH is delayed, peaking at 60 to 120 minutes rather than at 20 to 30 minutes. TSH in these patients is biologically less active than normal and binds to the TSH receptor less well owing to altered glycosylation as a result of the TRH deficiency. Treatment is with L-thyroxine.

ACTH. *Hypothalamic ACTH deficiency* due to hypothalamic lesions is uncommon. It may occur with loss of other hormones but may also appear as an isolated deficiency. In the absence of CNS lesions or a history of trauma, most cases of isolated ACTH deficiency appear to be a pituitary autoimmune disorder. However, in patients with hypothalamic disease as the cause, basal ACTH levels are low and the ACTH response to injected CRH may be prolonged and exaggerated, much as is the TSH response to TRH. The best test remains the comparison of the ACTH responses to hypoglycemia, which is clearly mediated by the hypothalamus, and to CRH. The ACTH response is low in response to hypoglycemia but increased and delayed in response to CRH in most patients with hypothalamic CRH deficiency. Treatment is with glucocorticoids, and mineralocorticoids are not needed.

Vasopressin (see Ch. 75). Diabetes insipidus can develop as a result of destructive lesions in the supraoptic and paraventricular nuclei or in the mediobasal hypothalamus in the path of the neural fibers containing vasopressin that are passing on to the posterior pituitary. Irritative lesions can trigger the release of vasopressin in an unregulated fashion, resulting in the syndrome of inappropriate ADH (vasopressin) secretion (SIADH).

EFFECTS OF HYPOTHALAMIC DISEASE ON OTHER NEUROMETABOLIC FUNCTIONS. A number of functions that affect the internal milieu, in addition to anterior and posterior pituitary function, are regulated, at least in part, by the hypothalamus, including temperature control, behavior, consciousness, memory, sleep, food intake, and carbohydrate metabolism.

Alterations in Food Intake. Body weight is kept relatively constant in nonobese individuals through an integration of a number of factors relating to the intake of nutrients and the output of energy, which are affected by hormonal, environmental, and genetic factors. As with the regulation of hormone secretion, the regulation of food intake can be conceptually regarded as an adjustment of food intake and energy expenditure around "set-points," which may be different for body weight, total body fat, and lean body mass. A number of areas of the hypothalamus are involved in the regulation of energy balance.

Hypothalamic Obesity. Destruction of the mediobasal hypothalamus sometimes inhibits satiety and may result in hyperphagia and hypothalamic obesity. The hyperphagia is due to destruction of noradrenergic fibers originating in the paraventricular nucleus that pass through the mediobasal hypothalamus. Because of their location, such lesions usually also produce hypopituitarism and diabetes insipidus. There are a number of rare syndromes in which obesity is a

major part for which a hypothalamic cause has been postulated. Prader-Willi is the most common of these syndromes, occurring in 1 in 25,000 births. It is characterized by hypotonia, obesity, short stature, mental deficiency, hypogonadism, and small hands and feet. About half have a chromosome 15 deletion. In the few cases studied at autopsy, no discernible hypothalamic lesions were detected. In the other syndromes (Laurence-Moon-Biedl-Bardet, Altrom-Hallgren), no specific hypothalamic lesions have been found.

Hypothalamic Anorexia. Lesions of the lateral hypothalamus, which destroy nigrostriatal dopaminergic fibers that pass through this area, produce hypophagia along with an increase in peripheral norepinephrine turnover and metabolic rate. This syndrome is very rare, probably owing to the requirement of bilateral lesions. The hormonal changes that occur in anorexia nervosa appear to be all secondary to the weight loss, and there is no evidence for a primary hypothalamic disorder in this syndrome.

Hyperglycemia. Hypothalamic activation as part of the generalized response to stress can cause a release of GH, PRL, and ACTH, which serve as counterregulatory hormones with respect to insulin. Of more importance in the acute response to stress, this hypothalamic response results in sympathetic activation with release of catecholamines that inhibit insulin secretion and stimulate glycogenolysis. In rare circumstances of acute hypothalamic injury from trauma, stroke, or infection, severe hyperglycemia can occur which is similar to the hyperglycemia seen in animals when the floor of the fourth ventricle is pricked with a needle, a phenomenon referred to as "piqûre" diabetes by Claude Bernard.

Temperature Regulation. The anterior hypothalamus and preoptic area contain temperature-sensitive neurons that respond to internal temperature changes by initiating certain thermoregulatory responses necessary to maintain a constant temperature. Measures that dissipate heat include cutaneous vasodilation, sweating, panting, and behavioral changes that result in attempts to alter the environment. Measures that increase body heat include increasing metabolic heat production, shivering, cutaneous vasoconstriction, and similar behavioral changes. In humans, much of the increase in metabolic heat production occurs via sympathetic activation. The thermosensitive neurons are affected by endogenous pyrogens and drugs that alter thermoregulation as well as input from thermoreceptors in the skin and spinal cord.

Rare patients have been reported with anterior hypothalamic lesions that caused sustained hypothermia due to failure of heat generation by shivering and vasoconstriction but who had intact heat dissipation or downward resetting of the temperature set point. Paroxysmal hypothermia lasting for minutes to days due to the sudden onset of sweating, vasodilation, and a fall in core temperature has been reported in a number of patients in association with demonstrated lesions such as tumors and agenesis of the corpus callosum. Some of these patients had evidence of other hypothalamic dysfunction, including diabetes insipidus, hypogonadism, and precocious puberty.

Fever as a manifestation of hypothalamic disease is uncommon but has been reported in relation to trauma or bleeding into the region of the anterior hypothalamus. Such fevers rarely persist more than two weeks. Paroxysmal hyperthermia due to hypothalamic dysfunction also occurs. Some cases of paroxysmal hypothermia and hyperthermia respond to anticonvulsant medications, suggesting that the neuronal discharge causing the temperature changes is seizure-like.

Poikilothermia results from the inability to dissipate or generate heat to keep the body temperature constant in the face of varying ambient temperatures. This condition results from bilateral lesions in the posterior hypothalamus and rostral mesencephalon, which are the areas responsible for the final integration of thermoregulatory neural efferents. Patients with this condition do not feel discomfort with temperature changes and are unaware of having a problem. Depending upon the ambient temperature, they may present with life-threatening hypothermia or hyperthermia. Poikilothermia is normally present in infants and frequently occurs in elderly individuals.

Abrahams JJ, Trefelner E, Boulware SD: Idiopathic growth hormone deficiency: MR findings in 35 patients. AJNR 12:155, 1991. *In this series of children with idiopathic GH deficiency, a high proportion were found to have structural abnormalities of the pituitary stalk, making these disorders of midline embryologic development. As imaging techniques improve, more and more "idiopathic" disorders may be found to have structural causes.*

Chapelon C, Ziza JM, Piette JC, et al.: Neurosarcoidosis: Signs, course and treatment in 35 confirmed cases. Medicine 69:261, 1990. *Features of neurosarcoidosis are reviewed and the hypothalamic dysfunction that may occur is described.*

Constine LS, Woolf PD, Cann D, et al.: Hypothalamic-pituitary dysfunction after radiation for brain tumors. N Engl J Med 328:87, 1993. *In this series of 32 patients, more than two thirds had some hormonal dysfunction 2 to 13 years following cranial irradiation. Studies like this point out the need for endocrine evaluation of all patients undergoing cranial irradiation.*

Loes DJ, Barloon TJ, Yuh WTC, et al.: MR anatomy and pathology of the hypothalamus. AJR 156:579, 1991. *This article shows what can be achieved with modern imaging techniques. Hypothalamic anatomy and pathology are shown with great clarity.*

Molitch ME: Pathologic hyperprolactinemia. Endocrinol Metab Clin North Am 21:877, 1992. *Covers current knowledge of regulation of prolactin secretion, various causes of hyperprolactinemia, and therapies available.*

Stein DT: New developments in the diagnosis and treatment of sexual precocity. Am J Med Sci 303:53, 1992. *This review carefully delineates the pathophysiology of sexual precocity, diagnostic maneuvers necessary to establish a precise diagnosis, and various treatment modalities.*

201.2 The Pineal Gland

Alfred J. Lewy

The mammalian pineal is located in the "center" of the brain (above the quadrigeminal plate, just behind the posterior commissure) but is actually outside of the blood-brain barrier. Postganglionic neurons from the superior cervical ganglia release norepinephrine that stimulates β_1-adrenergic receptors on the pinealocytes (Fig. 201–3). This results in the synthesis and release into the CSF and venous circulation of melatonin, the principal putative hormone of the pineal gland. The (paired) suprachiasmatic nuclei are the source of an approximately 24-hour rhythm in melatonin production that persists in conditions of constant darkness or blindness. Photic input, conveyed to the suprachiasmatic nuclei (SCN) via the retino-

hypothalamic tracts, synchronizes (entrains) the SCN and its output circadian rhythms to the 24-hour light-dark cycle. Between the SCN and the cell bodies of the preganglionic sympathetic neurons in the spinal cord, there are synapses in the paraventricular nuclei.

Melatonin production by the human pineal is decreased by β-blockers and α_2 agonists and is increased by certain tricyclic antidepressants that block reuptake of norepinephrine. Melatonin production is also increased by extreme physical exercise, norepinephrine, and psoralen. In general, diet and activity have no effect. Increased melatonin in manic states and decreased melatonin in depression probably occur but most likely represent epiphenomena following changes in adrenergic activity.

FUNCTION OF MELATONIN

The function of melatonin in humans remains elusive. In some fish and reptiles melatonin coalesces melanin-containing melanosomes and in this way causes blanching, but this effect has been lost in most animals. Melatonin may possibly have this effect on the mammalian retinal pigmented epithelium. The association of pineal tumors with disorders of puberty is most likely explained by compression of the hypothalamus, since no melatonin-secreting tumor has yet been found. Furthermore, it now appears that the main effect of melatonin on the reproductive system lies in its ability to communicate the time of the year to animals that are seasonal breeders. In such animals it can have either anti- or progonadal activity depending on whether the species is a spring or fall breeder, respectively. Reproductive and endocrine effects of exogenous melatonin administration, not to mention endogenous melatonin secretion, have not been well documented in humans, with the possible exception that melatonin at certain doses can increase prolactin levels in humans.

CHRONOBIOLOGY OF MELATONIN

Melatonin is produced only during nighttime darkness in both diurnal and nocturnal animals with an approximately 12-hour "on" phase and 12-hour "off" phase. Many blind people with a complete absence of light perception have free-running endogenous circadian rhythms. When these individuals' melatonin rhythms are out of phase with their sleep-wake cycles (which have remained more or less synchronized to clock time), they are prone to develop nocturnal insomnia and daytime sleepiness. A pattern of insomnia that recurs every few weeks is almost pathognomonic for free-running circadian rhythms in totally blind individuals.

Although darkness does not induce melatonin production, in sighted people exposure to sufficiently bright light during the night immediately suppresses melatonin production. Two models have been proposed to explain how the nightly melatonin profile is shaped. In the *two-pacemaker model*, it is hypothesized that separate endogenous pacemakers control the onset and offset of melatonin production, cued primarily to dusk and dawn, respectively. In the *"clock-gate" model*, the suppressant effect of light (unique to melatonin) participates in the shortening of the duration of nighttime melatonin production during long photoperiods. Both models attempt to explain the shorter duration of melatonin secretion during the briefer summer nights compared to the longer winter nights.

The changing duration of nighttime melatonin secretion during the calendar year seems to be responsible for the reproductive effects of the light-dark cycle in seasonal breeders. Seasonal rhythms have not been well documented in humans, but it is clear that humans have most, if not all, of the circadian rhythms found in other higher animals. Whereas seasonal rhythms respond to the duration of the photoperiod or scotoperiod, circadian rhythms respond to the 24-hour light-dark cycle. In animals, the light-dark cycle's phase-shifting effects on circadian rhythms can be described by a phase response curve (PRC). This appears to be the case in humans as well. The PRC can be explained as follows: Delay responses (shifts to a later time) result when exposure to light occurs during the first part of the night; advance responses (shifts to an earlier time) result when exposure occurs during the latter part of the night. These phase shifts are greatest in magnitude in the middle of the night and are least during the middle of the day.

Although the suppressant effect of light is unique to melatonin, phase-shifting by light affects the endogenous circadian pacemaker (SCN) and all of its driven rhythms. In fact, the timing of the SCN's circadian rhythms is best measured by the circulating levels of melatonin. In some species injections of exogenous melatonin

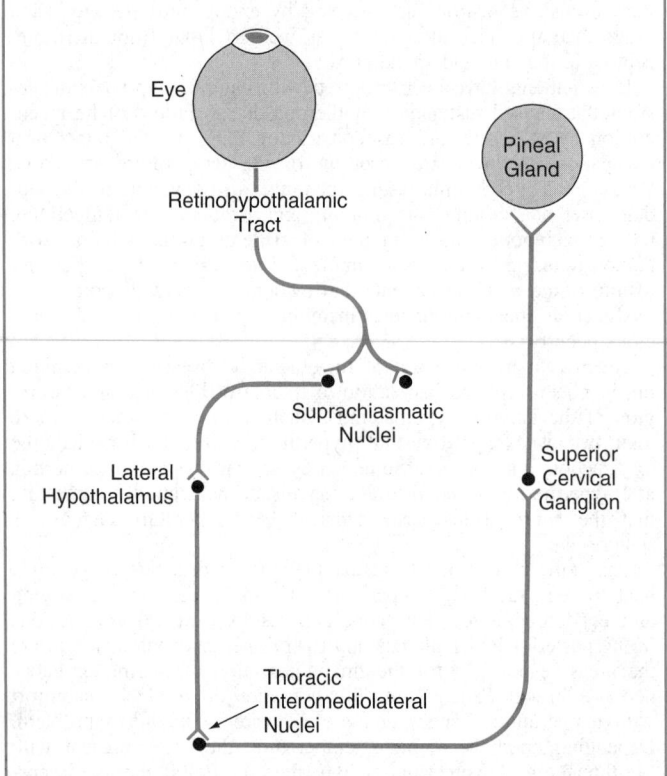

FIGURE 201–3. Schematic diagram for the neuroanatomic regulation of the timing of mammalian melatonin production (see text). (Adapted by permission of the publisher from "Biochemistry and regulation of mammalian melatonin production" by AJ Lewy, in The Pineal Gland, edited by RM Relkin, pp 77–128. Copyright 1983 by Elsevier Science Publishing Co., Inc.)

Eye

Retinohypothalamic Tract

Pineal Gland

Suprachiasmatic Nuclei

Lateral Hypothalamus

Superior Cervical Ganglion

Thoracic Interomediolateral Nuclei

are capable of causing phase shifts and/or entrainment. In lizards, a PRC for melatonin has been described that is about 12 hours out of phase with the PRC for light; that is, the melatonin PRC resembles a dark-pulse PRC. In humans, exogenous melatonin appears to have circadian phase-shifting effects, which can be described by a PRC that resembles a dark-pulse PRC. Thus, melatonin—which is produced only during the night—may be the chemical messenger of darkness. Therefore, human melatonin production may normally have a role, however small, in the entrainment of the SCN's circadian rhythms. Not being seasonal breeders, perhaps humans have retained the suppressant effect of light in order to use endogenous melatonin to more effectively augment entrainment and phase-shifting effects of the light-dark cycle. The melatonin PRC may also provide the rationale for precise scheduling of exogenous melatonin administration for therapeutic purposes, such as to treat chronobiologic sleep and mood disorders and to facilitate adaptation to shift work and air travel.

PINEAL TUMORS

Three main types of tumors that usually arise in the pineal are (1) pineoblastomas or pineocytomas, the term used depending on the degree of differentiation of this tumor of the pineal parenchyma; (2) germ cell tumors, including germinomas and embryonal carcinomas; and (3) glial tumors. Symptomatic enlargement of pineal by cysts has also been reported, but these are almost always asymptomatic. Destruction of pineal tissue can reduce or even ablate melatonin production, but pineocytomas have rarely been associated with increased circulating levels of melatonin. Melatonin production decreases with age, but this does not seem to be related to pineal calcification. By occluding the cerebral aqueduct, pineal tumors can produce symptoms associated with increased intracranial pressure, sometimes necessitating a shunt. Through pressure on the quadrigeminal plate, pineal tumors can produce Parinaud's syndrome, which includes paresis of upward conjugate gaze. Some germinomas and embryonal carcinomas secrete human chorionic gonadotropin, which has been implicated in cases of delayed onset of puberty. Treatment modalities include surgical extirpation, radiation, and chemotherapy, depending on tumor type and location and the absence or degree of metastases.

Lewy AJ, Sack RL, Singer CM, et al.: Winter depression and the phase shift hypothesis for bright light's therapeutic effects: History, theory and experimental evidence. J Biol Rhythms 3:121, 1988.
Lewy AJ, Wehr TA, Goodwin FK, et al.: Light suppresses melatonin secretion in humans. Science 210:1267, 1980.
Lewy AJ, Ahmed S, Jackson JML, Sack RL: Melatonin shifts circadian rhythms according to a phase-response curve. Chronobiol Int 9:380, 1995.
Neuwelt EA (ed.): Diagnosis and Treatment of Pineal Region Tumors. Baltimore, Williams & Wilkins, 1984.

202 THE PITUITARY

202.1 Anterior Pituitary

J. Larry Jameson

ANATOMY AND EMBRYOLOGY

The pituitary is a relatively small gland located in the sella turcica at the base of the brain. It has a bilobed shape and weighs about 0.6 gram (range 0.4 to 0.9 gram), being somewhat larger in women than in men. The pituitary is divided into anterior and posterior lobes, with the anterior lobe comprising about 80% of the gland. The posterior pituitary, or neurohypophysis, consists of the pituitary stalk as well as the posterior lobe (see Ch. 202.2). Superiorly, the pituitary is covered by the diaphragma sellae, a reflection of the dura mater that forms the roof of the sella and is attached to the clinoid processes. The diaphragma sellae has a central opening that is penetrated by the pituitary stalk and its blood vessels. Importantly, the optic chiasm, formed by the union of the optic nerves, is positioned directly above the pituitary gland and below the third ventricle. The exact position of the chiasm is variable, and the de-

gree to which it is tethered may affect the pattern of visual field changes experienced by patients with pituitary tumors that expand into the suprasellar region. The lateral boundaries of the sella are formed by the cavernous sinuses, which contain the internal carotid artery and branches of cranial nerves III, IV, V, and VI.

The blood supply to the pituitary gland is derived from the superior and inferior hypophyseal arteries, which are connected by a portal system of small vessels and capillaries. Specialized vascular structures, referred to as gomitoli, are located in the median eminence of the hypothalamus and consist of short terminal arterioles draining into portal veins that course down the pituitary stalk to join the sinusoidal capillaries of the anterior lobe. Hypothalamic hormones enter fenestrations in the perigomitolar capillaries to flow from the hypothalamus to the anterior pituitary. Venous drainage from the anterior lobe enters the posterior pituitary capillary bed before draining into the cavernous sinus.

The six major pituitary cell types include somatotropes (growth hormone [GH]–producing), lactotropes (prolactin [Prl]–producing), corticotropes (adrenocorticotropic hormone [ACTH]–producing), thyrotropes (thyroid-stimulating hormone [TSH]–producing), gonadotropes (follicle-stimulating hormone [FSH]– and luteinizing hormone [LH]–producing), and folliculostellate cells, which do not produce the classic pituitary hormones but may have paracrine functions. The biochemical characteristics of the major anterior pituitary hormones are summarized in Table 202–1.

The pituitary is formed early in embryonic life from the fusion of Rathke's pouch (which gives rise to the anterior pituitary) and a portion of the ventral diencephalon (which gives rise to the posterior pituitary). Rathke's pouch is an ectodermal evagination in the roof of the primitive oropharynx. The ontogeny of hormone production during anterior pituitary development has been characterized in detail. The pituitary anlage expresses the glycoprotein hormone α gene even as the progenitor cells are arising from Rathke's pouch. Subsequently, proopiomelanocortin-producing cells can be seen in the hypothalamus and in the pituitary. An evanescent group of TSH-producing cells appear but then fade away, to be followed later by a distinct population of TSH cells in a different location in the pituitary. After gonadotropes develop, GH- and Prl-producing cells appear and later form distinct populations of somatotropes and lactotropes. The transcription factor, Pit-1, a member of the Pou-Homeo domain family, is produced in somatotropes, lactotropes, and thyrotropes. Mutations in Pit-1 prevent the development of these cells and cause hormone deficiencies. This lineage relationship probably accounts for the observation that some GH-producing tumors also secrete Prl and about one third of TSH-producing tumors cosecrete GH.

Anterior pituitary hormone production is largely established by the ninth week of gestation, and the anatomic and biosynthetic mechanisms that comprise an active hypothalamic-pituitary system are functional by 12 to 17 weeks of gestation. In anencephaly, all anterior pituitary cell types, with the exception of corticotropes, are capable of hormone synthesis and secretion, indicating that the embryonic pituitary develops relatively normally in the absence of hypothalamic stimulation.

Somatotropes, which constitute 40 to 50% of anterior pituitary cells, are located predominantly in the lateral aspects of the anterior pituitary. Lactotropes comprise 15 to 25% of cells and are scattered throughout the anterior pituitary. Corticotropes constitute 10 to 20% of anterior pituitary cells and are located mainly in the central region of the anterior pituitary. Gonadotropes, which account for about 10% of pituitary cells, produce both FSH and LH, although a small fraction of gonadotropes appear to selectively secrete only one of the hormones. Only 5% of pituitary cells are thyrotropes. The folliculostellate cells have long, irregular processes that extend between the hormone-producing cells. They do not contain secretory granules but have been shown to produce growth factors such as basic fibroblast growth factor, vascular endothelial growth factor, and follistatin, among others.

Horvath E, Kovacs K: Morphology of adenohypophyseal cells and pituitary tumors. In Imura H (ed.): The Pituitary Gland, 2nd ed. New York, Raven Press, 1994, p. 29. A definitive summary of pituitary pathology.
Voss JW, Rosenfeld MG: Anterior pituitary development: Short tales from dwarf mice. Cell 70:527, 1992. A review of a remarkable series of studies that define pituitary cell lineages.

TABLE 202-1. FEATURES OF THE MAJOR ANTERIOR PITUITARY HORMONES

Hormone	Amino Acids	MW	Serum Half-life	Cell Type	Target Gland
Growth hormone (GH)	191	22 kD	20 min	Somatotrope	Multiple
Prolactin (Prl)	198	23 kD	20 min	Lactotrope	Breast
Adrenocorticotropic hormone (ACTH)	39	4.5 kD	8 min	Corticotrope	Adrenal
Thyroid-stimulating hormone (TSH)	α-subunit, 92 aa	14 kD	50 min	Thyrotrope	Thyroid
	β-subunit, 118 aa	17 kD			
Luteinizing hormone (LH)	α-subunit, 92 aa	14 kD	50 min	Gonadotrope	Gonad
	β-subunit, 121 aa	18 kD			
Follicle-stimulating hormone (FSH)	α-subunit, 92 aa	14 kD	220 min	Gonadotrope	Gonad
	β-subunit, 111 aa	18 kD			

The amino acid lengths are based upon the cloned cDNA's and the molecular weights (MW) include the contributions of the carbohydrates in the case of the glycoprotein hormones (TSH, LH, FSH). The serum half-lives assume single-compartment monexponential decay.

RADIOLOGY OF THE PITUITARY

Currently, radiologic imaging of the pituitary gland primarily involves computed tomography (CT) and magnetic resonance imaging (MRI). CT scans are performed using high-resolution (1.5-mm), contrast-enhanced procedures with direct coronal sections. Although CT provides excellent resolution, problems include artifacts from metallic objects and dental fillings, and some patients have difficulty assuming the position required for coronal sections. Pituitary tumors typically enhance with contrast on CT, and cystic components are hypodense.

Overall, MRI is the technique of choice for evaluating the sellar region. MRI scans provide multiplanar imaging and excellent resolution of the pituitary and surrounding cerebrovascular fluid (CSF), vascular, and central nervous system structures. There is less radiation exposure with MRI than with CT, allowing repeated imaging as required for evaluation and follow-up. However, bone structures are not well-defined by MRI. The normal anterior pituitary appears isointense with brain white matter, whereas the posterior pituitary exhibits high signal intensity. The optic chiasm can be readily identified superior to the pituitary gland because it is surrounded by hypodense structures. MRI scans detect pituitary microadenomas in nearly all patients with surgically proven tumors. Pituitary adenomas typically appear hypointense on T1-weighted images and show less gadolinium contrast enhancement than surrounding normal tissue. Focal hypodense areas are also seen in about a quarter of normal individuals, which may correspond to cysts or small adenomas that have been described in autopsy series, emphasizing the importance of endocrine evaluation in making the diagnosis of pituitary tumors.

Elster AD: Modern imaging of the pituitary. Radiology 187:1, 1993. *A review focused on MRI of the sellar region.*
Tindall GT: Disorders of the Pituitary. St. Louis, CV Mosby, 1986. *This book reviews multiple pituitary disorders and has particularly good chapters on anatomy, radiology, and transsphenoidal surgery.*

REGULATION OF THE PITUITARY AXIS

The concept of positive and negative feedback control represents a fundamental tenet of endocrinology. The pituitary gland integrates the influences of an array of positive and negative signals to modulate hormone secretion within a narrow range (Table 202-2). The major hypothalamic–pituitary–target gland axes include TRH–TSH–thyroid hormone, CRH–ACTH–cortisol axis, GnRH–LH/FSH–gonads, and GRF–GH–IGF-1. Prolactin is the only major pituitary hormone that is not subject to feedback inhibition by hormones produced in target tissues. However, it is controlled by positive and negative input from the hypothalamus.

The principles of feedback regulation are well-illustrated by the hypothalamic–pituitary–thyroid axis (see Fig. 203–1). Hypothalamic TRH stimulates TSH secretion from the pituitary. TSH increases thyroid hormone secretion, which in turn suppresses hypothalamic TRH as well as pituitary TSH. A typical regulatory loop therefore has both positive (TRH,TSH) and negative (T_4,T_3) components, allowing a high degree of control of hormone levels. In this case, the pituitary gland integrates positive TRH signals and the negative effects of thyroid hormone. The concept of feedback regulation is important not only for understanding pituitary physiology, but because it provides the basis for analyzing pituitary gland function using stimulation and suppression tests.

Feedback regulatory systems are superimposed upon hormonal rhythms that are used for adaptation to the environment. Seasonal changes, the daily occurrence of the light-dark cycles, and stress are but a few of many environmental events that have major impacts on the secretion of pituitary hormones. Some hormonal pathways, such as ACTH secretion, are entrained to the light-dark cycle, causing characteristic peaks of ACTH and cortisol production in the early morning, with a nadir in the late afternoon and evening. The secretion of other hormones, such as GH, is altered by sleep, stress, and meals. The early pubertal surges of LH occur at night and usually in association with sleep. The menstrual cycle provides an example of a pituitary rhythm that occurs on a much longer time scale (approximately 28 days). The pattern of the menstrual cycle is coupled to cycles of follicular development in the ovary. As follicular development progresses, levels of gonadal steroids and inhibin feed back upon the hypothalamus and pituitary to modulate LH and FSH secretion.

Because many hormones are released in a pulsatile manner and in a rhythmic fashion, it is important to be aware of these characteristics of secretion when attempting to relate serum measurements to normal values. Although it is possible to characterize pulsatile patterns of hormone secretion using frequent blood sampling (every 10 min) over several hours, this is not practical in a clinical setting. Alternative approaches include stimulation and suppression tests or the use of "integrated" measurements of hormone production, such as 24-hour urine free cortisol as an index of ACTH secretion or IGF-1 as a biologic marker of GH action.

Crowley WF Jr, Filicori M, Spratt DI, et al.: The physiology of gonadotropin-releasing hormone (GnRH) secretion in men and women. Recent Prog Horm Res 41:473, 1985. *Summary of neuroendocrine control of reproduction with emphasis on the importance of pulsatile secretion.*

HYPOPITUITARISM

Hypopituitarism implies diminished production of one or more anterior pituitary hormones. Although the recognition of complete or panhypopituitarism is usually straightforward, the detection of partial or selective hormone deficiencies is more challenging. Pituitary hormone deficiencies can be caused by loss of hypothalamic stimulation (tertiary hormone deficiency) or by direct loss of pituitary function (secondary hormone deficiency). The distinction between hypothalamic and pituitary causes of hypopituitarism is important for establishing the correct diagnosis and for applying and

TABLE 202-2. FACTORS THAT REGULATE PITUITARY HORMONE SECRETION

Hormone	Releasing Factors	Inhibiting Factors
Growth hormone (GH)	GRF	SMS, IGF-1
Prolactin (Prl)	TRH, VIP, E_2	Dopamine
Adrenocorticotropic hormone (ACTH)	CRH, vasopressin	Cortisol
Thyroid-stimulating hormone (TSH)	TRH	T_4, T_3, SMS, dopamine
Luteinizing hormone (LH)	GnRH	E_2, testosterone
Follicle-stimulating hormone (FSH)	GnRH, activin	Inhibin, E_2, testosterone

GRF, growth hormone–releasing factor; SMS, somatostatin; IGF-1, insulin-like growth factor-1; TRH, thyrotropin-releasing hormone; VIP, vasoactive intestinal peptide; E_2, estradiol; CRH, corticotropin-releasing hormone; T_4, thyroxine; T_3, triiodothyronine. The gonadal steroids, E_2 and testosterone, exert much of their inhibitory effects on gonadotropin secretion at the hypothalamic level.

interpreting the relevant diagnostic endocrine tests. With improved procedures for testing the hypothalamic-pituitary axis, it is apparent that hypothalamic causes of hypopituitarism are more common than previously appreciated (see Ch. 201.1). When hypopituitarism is accompanied by diabetes insipidus, one should particularly consider hypothalamic causes of pituitary dysfunction.

CAUSES OF HYPOPITUITARISM. A variety of congenital causes of hypopituitarism have been described (Table 202–3). Sporadic and familial forms of panhypopituitarism occur, but the underlying genetic or developmental defects have not been elucidated. Congenital combined deficiencies of GH, Prl, and TSH are caused by mutations in the gene encoding Pit-1, a pituitary-specific transcription factor that is involved in the development of somatotrope, lactotrope, and thyrotrope cell lineages. Different types of Pit-1 mutations are inherited in an autosomal dominant or recessive pattern. Congenital GH deficiency can be caused by a heterogeneous group of mutations in the GH gene. These include large deletions of the GH gene that are inherited in an autosomal recessive manner and involve genetic recombination between related DNA sequences in the duplicated GH gene cluster. Point mutations have also been described in the GH gene, and some of these can be inherited in an autosomal dominant manner, apparently because the mutant hormone impairs GH biosynthesis and normal function of the somatotrope cell. Mutations have also been described in the LH-β, FSH-β, and TSH-β genes that cause autosomal recessive forms of selective hormone deficiencies.

Neoplastic lesions, particularly pituitary adenomas, are the most common cause of acquired hypopituitarism. Pituitary adenomas cause hypopituitarism in several different manners. In some cases, there is direct destruction or compression of the normal pituitary. Compression of the pituitary stalk can impair blood supply to the pituitary as well as decrease input from hypothalamic hormones. Hemorrhage into tumors can lead to pituitary infarction. When tested carefully, most patients with macroadenomas have partial deficiencies of one or more pituitary hormones, most often involving GH and gonadotropins. A mild degree of hyperprolactinemia is characteristic of disorders that cause stalk compression, and hyperprolactinemia further impairs gonadotropin secretion. A variety of other neoplasms that occur near the sella, such as craniopharyngiomas, can also cause hypopituitarism (Table 202–3).

Pituitary apoplexy is usually caused by hemorrhage into a tumor with associated infarction. In the absence of a tumor, predispositions to apoplexy include trauma, pregnancy, anticoagulation, sickle cell anemia, and diabetes mellitus. Pituitary infarction in the peripartum period is referred to as Sheehan's syndrome and is usually associated with significant hemorrhage and hypovolemia. It is often heralded by the inability to lactate, amenorrhea, and symptoms of adrenal insufficiency. Sheehan's syndrome is now infrequent owing to improvements in obstetrical care.

Radiation causes hypopituitarism primarily because of its effects on hypothalamic function, although high-dose radiation (e.g., proton beam) can also cause direct pituitary damage. The sellar region is subjected to radiation in the treatment of pituitary adenomas, craniopharyngiomas, clivus chordomas, optic gliomas, meningiomas, dysgerminomas, and other neoplasms. Importantly, the effects of radiation can be delayed as much as several years, and patients at high risk should be evaluated at yearly intervals for radiation-induced hypopituitarism. Although GH and gonadotropin deficiencies develop first in most patients, ACTH or TSH deficiencies occasionally occur first, emphasizing the need to evaluate each of the major axes.

Empty sella syndrome can occur as a primary or an acquired condition. It is caused by defects in the diaphragma sellae which allow herniation of the arachnoid membrane into the hypophyseal fossa. In longstanding cases, sellar enlargement occurs, probably because of persistent transduction of intracranial pressure. With appropriate imaging studies, the pituitary gland can be seen as a flattened rim of tissue along the floor of the sella. Primary empty sella occurs most commonly in women and may be associated with features of benign intracranial hypertension. Pituitary function in patients with primary empty sella syndrome is usually normal, although 15% have mild hyperprolactinemia, probably because of stretching of the pituitary stalk. Acquired forms may occur as a result of surgery, radiation, or pituitary infarction (usually of an adenoma).

DIAGNOSIS AND TREATMENT. The diagnosis of hypopituitarism rests upon the stimulation tests summarized in Table 202–4. The therapy of hypopituitarism depends upon the nature and severity of the hormone deficiencies as well as the desired clinical endpoint. The goal is to replace hormones in a physiologic manner, with efforts to avoid the consequences of overreplacement. In patients with acquired forms of hypopituitarism (e.g., pituitary tumors, radiation treatment), it is not uncommon to encounter a mixture of partial hormone deficiencies. It is generally prudent to provide hormone replacement if partial deficiency is suspected, as patients may experience symptoms over a number of years before an unequivocal diagnosis of hormone deficiency is made. Examples of hormonal replacement paradigms are provided in Table 202–5.

TABLE 202–3. HYPOTHALAMIC AND PITUITARY CAUSES OF HYPOPITUITARISM

Congenital
  Panhypopituitarism, pituitary aplasia
  Combined deficiency of GH, Prl, TSH
  Kallmann syndrome (selective GnRH deficiency with anosmia)
  Isolated GHRH, CRH, TRH deficiencies
  Isolated deficiencies of GH, Prl, ACTH, LH, FSH, or TSH
Neoplastic
  Pituitary adenomas
  Craniopharyngioma
  Metastatic tumors
  Teratomas, dysgerminomas, chordomas, gliomas, meningiomas
  Leukemia/lymphoma
  Hypothalamic hamartoma
  Third ventricular cysts, Rathke's pouch and other cysts
Inflammatory/infiltrative
  Sarcoidosis
  Tuberculosis, syphilis, eosinophilic granulomas, other granulomatous diseases
  Autoimmune lymphocytic hypophysitis
  Histiocytosis X, Hand-Schuller-Christian disease
Vascular
  Neonatal intraventricular hemorrhage
  Pituitary apoplexy
  Sheehan syndrome (postpartum necrosis)
  Internal carotid aneurysm
  Diabetic necrosis
  Sickle cell anemia
  Vasculitis
  Subarachnoid hemorrhage
  Trauma associated with stalk section or necrosis
Metabolic/neurogenic
  Anorexia nervosa
  Hemochromatosis
  Amyloidosis
  Critical illness
  Psychosocial dwarfism
Iatrogenic
  Radiation
  Post-surgical

Phillips JA, Cogan JD: Genetic basis of endocrine disease. 6. Molecular basis of familial human growth hormone deficiency. J Clin Endocrinol Metab 78:11, 1994. *Overview of the heterogeneous types of growth hormone gene mutations.*
Radovick S, Nations M, Du Y, et al.: A mutation in the POU-homeodomain of Pit-1 responsible for combined pituitary hormone deficiency. Science 257:1115, 1992. *One of several reports of Pit-1 mutations in humans.*
Vance ML: Hypopituitarism. N Engl J Med 330:1651, 1994. *A review of causes, diagnosis, and management of hypopituitarism.*
Wakai S, Fukushima T, Teramoto A, et al.: Pituitary apoplexy: Its incidence and clinical significance. J Neurosurg 55:187, 1981. *A summary of clinical features associated with 93 cases of pituitary apoplexy occurring in a series of 563 patients.*

PITUITARY TUMORS

CLASSIFICATION. Pituitary tumors are classified according to the hormones that they produce. The approximate prevalence of the different types of pituitary adenomas is summarized in Table 202–6. Histologically, pituitary tumors are also classified according to their tinctoral staining characteristics (acidophilic, eosinophilic, chromophobe adenomas), but these analyses correlate only loosely with type of hormone produced. In recent years, immunohistochemical studies, using antibodies specific for each of the major pituitary hormones, have been used to define tumor phenotype. Electron microscopy can provide additional ultrastructural information but is

TABLE 202-4. TESTS OF PITUITARY INSUFFICIENCY

Hormone	Test	Interpretation
Growth hormone	*Insulin tolerance test:* Regular insulin (0.05–0.15U/kg) is given IV and blood is drawn at −30, 0, 30, 45, 60, and 90 min for measurement of glucose and GH.	If hypoglycemia occurs (glucose <40 mg/dL), GH should increase >10 µg/L. Careful supervision is required during testing.
	L-Dopa test: 10 mg/kg PO with GH measurements at 0, 30, 60, and 120 min.	Normal response is GH >7 µg/L.
	L-Arginine test: 0.5 gm/kg IV over 30 min with GH measurements at 0, 30, 60, and 120 min.	Normal response is GH >7 µg/L.
Prolactin	*TRH test:* 200–500 µg IV with measurements of TSH and Prl at 0, 20, and 60 min.	Normal prolactin is >2 µg/L and >200% increase after TRH
ACTH	*Insulin tolerance test:* Regular insulin (0.05–0.15 U/kg) is given IV and blood is drawn at −30, 0, 30, 45, 60, and 90 min for measurement of glucose and cortisol.	If hypoglycemia occurs (glucose <40 mg/dL), cortisol should increase by >7 µg/dL or to >20 µg/dL. Careful supervision is required during testing.
	CRH test: 1 µg/kg ovine CRH IV at 8 AM with blood samples drawn at 0, 15, 30, 60, 90, 120 min for measurement of ACTH and cortisol.	In most normals, the basal ACTH increases 2- to 4-fold and reaches a peak (20–100 pg/mL). ACTH responses may be delayed in cases of hypothalamic dysfunction. Cortiso levels usually reach 20–25 µg/dL.
	Metyrapone test: Metyrapone (30 mg/kg) at midnight with measurements of plasma 11-deoxycortisol and cortisol at 8 AM. ACTH can also be measured. A 3-day test is also available.	A normal response is 11-deoxycortisol >7.5 µg/dL or ACTH >75 pg/mL. Plasma cortisol should fall below 4 µg/dL to ensure an adequate response.
	ACTH stimulation test: ACTH 1-24 (cosyntropin), 0.25 mg IM or IV. Cortisol and aldosterone are measured at 0, 30, and 60 min. A 3-day ACTH stimulation test consists of 0.25 mg ACTH 1-24 given IV over 8 h each day.	A normal response is cortisol >18 µg/dL and aldosterone response of >4 ng/dL above baseline. In suspected hypothalamic-pituitary deficiency, 3-day ACTH test should result in 17-OH steroids of >25 mg/24h.
TSH	*Basal thyroid function tests:* T$_4$, T$_3$, THBI, TSH.	Low free thyroid hormone levels in the setting of TSH levels that are not appropriately increased.
	TRH test: 200–500 µg IV with measurements of TSH and Prl at 0, 20, and 60 min.	TSH should increase by >5 mU/L unless thyroid hormone levels are increased.
LH, FSH	*Basal levels of LH, FSH, testosterone, estrogen*	Basal LH and FSH should be increased in postmenopausal women. Low testosterone levels in conjunction with low or low-normal LH and FSH are consistent with gonadotropin deficiency.
	GnRH test: GnRH (100 µg) IV with measurements of serum LH and FSH at 0, 30, 60 min.	In most normals, LH should increase by 10 IU/L and FSH by 2 IU/L. Normal responses are variable and repeated stimulation may be required.
	Clomiphene test: Clomiphene citrate (100 mg) is given orally for 5 days. Serum LH and FSH are measured on days 0, 5, 7, 10, and 13.	A 50% increase should occur in LH and FSH, usually by day 5.
Multiple hormones	*Combined anterior pituitary test:* GHRH (1 µg/kg), CRH (1 µg/kg), GnRH (100 µg), TRH (200 µg) are given sequentially IV. Blood samples are drawn at −30, 15, 30, 60, 90, and 120 min for measurements of GH, ACTH, LH, FSH, and TSH.	Combined or individual releasing hormone responses must be evaluated in the context of basal hormone values and may not be diagnostic.

TABLE 202-5. HORMONAL REPLACEMENT THERAPY IN HYPOPITUITARISM

Pituitary Axis	Hormonal Replacements
Growth hormone	In children, GH (0.06–0.1 mg/kg) SC 3×/week or daily.
Prolactin	None
ACTH-cortisol	Prednisone (5 mg PO qAM; 2.5 mg PO qPM) or cortisone acetate (25 mg PO qAM; 12.5 mg PO qPM) or hydrocortisone (20 mg PO qAM; 10 mg PO qPM). Fluorohydrocortisone (0.05–0.1 mg PO qd) is rarely required for secondary adrenal insufficiency.
TSH-thyroid	L-Thyroxine (0.1–0.15 mg) PO qd
Gonadotropins-gonads	Pulsatile GnRH (via pump) can be used for GnRH-deficient subjects, or FSH and LH (or hCG) can be used to induce ovulation in women. hCG alone, or FSH and LH can be used to induce spermatogenesis in men. In men, testosterone enanthate (100–200 mg) IM q1–3 weeks or testosterone cyclopentylpropionate (100–250 mg) IM q1–3 weeks. In women, conjugated estrogens (0.625–1.25 mg) or mestranol (35 µg) PO days 1–25 each month cycled with medroxyprogesterone acetate (5–10 mg) PO qd days 15–25 each month. Low-dose contraceptive pills may also be used.
Posterior pituitary	Desmopressin (DDAVP), 0.05–0.2 ml (5–20 µg) intranasally once or twice daily, or 1/10th this dose can be given SC.

Replacement therapy is dictated by the types of hormone deficiencies and by the clinical circumstances. In each case, the recommended preparations and doses are representative but need to be adjusted for individual patients. Other hormonal preparations are also available.

not used routinely. Tumor grade is not particularly useful for predicting invasiveness, and pituitary adenomas are rarely malignant. Radiologic or clinical evidence of tumor size, impingement, or invasion of local structures surrounding the sella, or evidence of metastasis (usually within the CNS) can provide more practical indices of the biologic behavior of the tumor.

THEORIES OF PITUITARY TUMORIGENESIS. A long-standing controversy exists concerning the clonality of pituitary tumors. Monoclonal tumors arise from a single progenitor cell, presumably because of a somatic mutation to create an oncogene or to inactivate a tumor suppressor gene. Polyclonal tumors, on the other hand, reflect hyperplasia caused by exogenous stimulation of a group of cells by a growth factor or hypothalamic-releasing hormone. Using recombinant DNA techniques to track X-chromosome inactivation as an index of cell lineage, it has been shown that the vast majority of pituitary tumors are monoclonal in origin. This finding does not exclude a role for hormonal stimulation as a predisposing factor for somatic mutations, and the hormonal environment may also affect the rate of tumor growth (e.g., Nelson's syndrome).

Supporting the concept that somatic mutations lead to pituitary tumorigenesis, a subset (35 to 40%) of somatotrope adenomas has mutations in two different amino acids (Arg 201 and Gln 227) which result in activation of the Gsα subunit. Either mutation prevents GTP hydrolysis, causing the Gsα subunit to stimulate adenylyl cyclase in a constitutive manner. The elevated intracellular cAMP levels lead to increased cell growth as well as GH production. Mutations in other oncogenes, such as *ras*, Rb, and p53, are uncommon in pituitary tumors. Thus, the nature of the somatic defects in most pituitary tumors remains unknown.

Two types of inherited predispositions to pituitary tumors are recognized. Patients with McCune-Albright syndrome occasionally de-

TABLE 202–6. PREVALENCE OF DIFFERENT TYPES OF PITUITARY ADENOMAS

Type of Pituitary Adenoma	Disorder	Hormone Produced	Prevalence (%)*
Somatotrope	Acromegaly/gigantism	GH	10–15
Lactotrope (prolactinoma)	Hypogonadism, mass effects	Prolactin	25–40
Corticotrope	Cushing's disease	ACTH	10–15
Gonadotrope	Mass effects, hypopituitarism	FSH and/or LH	10–15
α-subunit	Mass effects, hypopituitarism	Free α-subunit	5
Thyrotrope	Hyperthyroidism	TSH	<3
Nonfunctioning/null cell	Mass effects, hypopituitarism	None	10–25

* The prevalence rates represent ranges described in several different large series. Mixed tumors (e.g., GH and prolactin) and plurihormonal adenomas are not shown. Prolactinomas were underestimated in most recent pathologic series because they are largely managed medically. Most glycoprotein hormone–producing pituitary tumors were classified as nonfunctioning adenomas until the application of immunohistochemical studies.

velop pituitary adenomas as well as characteristic abnormalities in other tissues, particularly the ovary, bone, and thyroid. Interestingly, McCune-Albright syndrome is also caused by mutations in the Gsα subunit. However, the somatic mutations in McCune-Albright syndrome occur early during development, rather than only in the pituitary gland, so that multiple tissues are affected. In multiple endocrine neoplasia type 1 (MEN-1), the predisposition to pituitary tumors is inherited in an autosomal dominant manner and occurs in conjunction with tumors of the parathyroid and pancreas. The MEN-1 gene has been localized on the long arm of chromosome 11 (11q13). Individuals with MEN-1 are thought to inherit one mutant allele, with tumorigenesis occurring after a "second hit" mutates or deletes the normal MEN-1 gene. Deletions of portions of chromosome 11 have also been described in sporadic pituitary tumors. Deletions of other chromosomal regions (loss of heterozygosity) suggest that several different tumor suppressor genes may play a role in the development of pituitary tumors.

Alexander JM, Biller BM, Bikkal H, et al.: Clinically nonfunctioning pituitary tumors are monoclonal in origin. J Clin Invest 86:336, 1990. *One of several studies using X-chromosome inactivation to demonstrate that pituitary tumors are monoclonal in origin.*

Landis CA, Masters SB, Spada A, et al.: GTPase inhibiting mutations activate the alpha chain of Gs and stimulate adenylyl cyclase in human pituitary tumours. Nature 340:692, 1989. *A classic study showing that mutations in the Gsα subunit cause constitutive activation of adenylyl cyclase, leading to somatotrope neoplasia.*

MASS EFFECTS OF PITUITARY ADENOMAS.

Many of the clinical manifestations of pituitary adenomas are related to the hypersecretion of hormones. However, the mass effects of the enlarging tumor can also lead to specific signs and symptoms. Particularly in the case of nonfunctioning tumors or those that produce gonadotropins, the primary clinical manifestations are related to effects of the tumor on surrounding structures.

Headaches are common in patients with macroadenomas and appear to be caused by expansion of the diaphragma sellae or by invasion of bone. Headaches may be retro-orbital or referred to the top of the skull, but the location is variable. Severe headache associated with nausea, vomiting, and altered consciousness can also be caused by infarction of a pituitary adenoma. In severe cases, pituitary apoplexy can occur and may require urgent surgical decompression.

The effects of pituitary tumors on the visual fields are well-explained by the relationship of the optic chiasm to the sella turcica. Expansion of macroadenomas into the suprasellar region exerts pressure on the optic chiasm, usually in the central region where nerves emanating from the inferior and medial part of the retina (superior temporal visual fields) cross. Consequently, bitemporal hemianopsia is the most common visual field abnormality associated with pituitary adenomas. However, the exact pattern of visual field loss is variable and is affected by the location and flexibility of the chiasm as well as the direction and extent of tumor growth. Large tumors may grow asymmetrically and invade the cavernous sinus or surround an optic nerve, leading to other patterns of visual field changes or loss of visual acuity. It is essential for all patients with pituitary tumors to undergo high-resolution radiologic imaging to evaluate the size and location of the tumor. Formal visual field testing by an ophthalmologist is required to detect subtle visual field changes and should be performed in all patients with suprasellar extension. Longstanding visual field changes may not be reversed by surgical decompression, but dramatic improvements can occur if visual loss is recent.

The normal pituitary is often compressed into a thin rim of tissue by large pituitary adenomas. Hypopituitarism probably results more from compression of the hypothalamic-pituitary stalk than from direct replacement or pressure on the normal pituitary. GH deficiency and hypogonadotropic hypogonadism are particularly common. Slightly elevated prolactin levels (generally < 100 ng per milliliter) occur in cases of stalk compression because of diminished inhibition by dopamine. It is important not to mistake such tumors for prolactinomas, as they will not decrease in size in response to medical therapy with bromocriptine. Preoperative hypopituitarism caused by a large pituitary mass is reversible in up to half of patients after surgical decompression. Diabetes insipidus (vasopressin deficiency) is rarely caused by pituitary tumors and should raise the suspicion of a craniopharyngioma or other disorders likely to cause hypothalamic dysfunction.

Arafah BM: Reversible hypopituitarism in patients with large nonfunctioning pituitary adenomas. J Clin Endocrinol Metab 62:1173, 1986. *This study of 26 patients with macroadenomas illustrates how pituitary tumors can cause hypopituitarism by compression of the pituitary stalk.*

THERAPY OF PITUITARY ADENOMAS. Surgical Treatment.

Except for prolactinomas, surgery is the primary mode of therapy for most pituitary tumors that warrant intervention. Indications for surgery include reduction in hormone levels and decompression to relieve mass effects or to prevent further tumor expansion. Currently, the transsphenoidal route is used almost exclusively for decompression or extirpation of pituitary tumors. Because of substantially greater morbidity, transfrontal craniotomy is reserved for patients with tumors that require extensive exploration of the suprasellar region and surrounding structures, including invasion into the third ventricle. The transsphenoidal approach usually involves a sublabial incision, allowing ready access to the sphenoid sinus, which leads to the floor of the sella. After the sella is entered, the tumor is identified and resected in fragments under microscopy. Decompression of the sellar contents can allow tumor in the suprasellar region to drop into the surgical field to allow further resection. In experienced hands, transsphenoidal surgery is effective and complications are uncommon (<5% complication rate), but include CSF leak, hemorrhage, optic nerve injury, hypopituitarism, and sinusitis. Transient diabetes insipidus occurs in about 5% of patients following surgery but rarely persists long-term. Mortality rates are <1%.

Surgical cure rates are largely a function of the size and location of the pituitary mass. When stringent hormonal criteria are used to assess surgical success rates, <30% of macroadenomas are cured by transsphenoidal surgery, although considerable improvements in hormone levels or mass effects can be achieved. On the other hand, hormone hypersecretion by microadenomas (<1 cm in size) can be corrected completely in up to 80 to 90% of patients, although the cure rates vary considerably at different institutions.

Radiation Therapy.

Radiation therapy has been used as a primary mode of treatment of pituitary adenomas and as adjunctive therapy following surgery or in combination with medical therapy. Radiation therapy is typically administered over 4 to 5 weeks at a dose of 45 Gy using ^{60}Co or a linear accelerator. Proton beam therapy has also been used and delivers very high doses of radiation within a localized region, but it is limited to intrasellar lesions and is not widely available. Because response rates are slow (several years) and complete remission is rarely achieved, primary radiation therapy is generally reserved for patients who cannot or choose not to undergo surgery. Radiation therapy is more commonly used as adjunctive therapy following incomplete transsphenoidal resection. The decision regarding adjunctive radiation therapy involves a number of issues, including hormone levels, amount and location of residual tumor, rate of tumor growth, and degree of invasiveness. Because the time to recurrence for most macroadenomas is 5 to 10 years, it is often reasonable to follow patients with imaging techniques, reserving radiation therapy for those with evidence of recurrence. Complications of radiation therapy are dose-related but can also be idiosyncratic. Partial or complete hypopituitarism occurs in 50 to 70% of patients and is primarily due to hypothalamic injury. Less common complications include optic nerve damage, brain necrosis, vascular damage, and predisposition to sarcomas.

Medical Therapy. The emergence of medical therapies for pituitary tumors has dramatically impacted patient management. Dopamine agonists, which include the ergot derivatives (bromocriptine, lisuride, pergolide) and a D_2 selective agonist (CV205-502), have a primary role in the management of prolactinomas. They induce a rapid fall in prolactin levels and, importantly, decrease tumor size. Dopamine agonists are also used in the management of acromegaly, although the GH responses and effects on tumor size are generally much less pronounced than in prolactinomas. Somatostatin analogues, such as octreotide, act to suppress the secretion of a number of hormones, including GH and TSH. Octreotide has been used to treat acromegaly and TSH-producing tumors. Longacting GnRH agonists and antagonists have been studied in gonadotropin-producing tumors. Unlike the situation in normal individuals, the long-acting agonists do not cause desensitization and suppression of gonadotropins in most pituitary tumors. GnRH antagonists are more effective, reducing FSH in the majority of patients examined, but these agents have little effect on tumor growth. Medical therapy of Cushing's disease is primarily directed toward inhibition of steroid biosynthesis. Therapeutic drugs include ketoconazole, metyrapone, aminoglutethimide, and o′,p′, DDD (mitotane). Because of substantial side effects and because patients with Cushing's disease tend to respond to these drugs by producing more ACTH, medical therapy is used primarily as an adjunctive treatment or to reduce cortisol levels preoperatively.

Halberg FE, Sheline GE: Radiotherapy of pituitary tumors. Endocrinol Metab Clin 16:667, 1987. *A good summary of the use of radiation therapy in multimodality management of pituitary tumors.*
Klibanski A, Zervas NT: Diagnosis and management of hormone-secreting pituitary adenomas. N Engl J Med 324:8221, 1991. *A concise review of the diagnosis and managment of pituitary adenomas.*

GROWTH HORMONE

The pituitary gland contains a large amount of stored GH (5 to 10 mg), a 191 amino acid, single-chain protein that contains two intramolecular disulfide bonds (see Table 202–1). The GH gene is located on chromosome 17 and is part of a five-member gene cluster that includes a GH variant gene, two placental lactogen (hPL) genes that are also referred to as chorionic somatomammotropin (hCS) genes, and an hPL pseudogene that is not expressed. Highly repetitive sequences within the gene cluster appear to account for the propensity for recombination and deletions of the GH gene, causing one form of GH deficiency.

The predominant circulating form of GH is a 22-kD protein. However, a splicing variant creates a 20-kD form that constitutes about 10 to 15% of circulating GH and appears to be biologically active. GH also forms high molecular weight oligomers and is complexed in the circulation to two different binding proteins. The high-affinity binding protein has been identified as a circulating form of the extracellular domain of the GH receptor. In addition to greatly reducing the clearance of GH, this binding protein may also modulate GH action.

GH production is controlled by a complex interplay of hypothalamic stimulatory and inhibitory peptides, neurotransmitters, growth factors, sex steroids, and nutritional conditions. The most important regulators of GH are the hypothalamic factors; GH-releasing factor (GRF), which is stimulatory; and somatostatin, which is inhibitory. GH increases the production of IGF-1 (also known as somatomedin C), which in turn inhibits GH production. GRF acts by a G protein–coupled receptor that is structurally related to receptors in the VIP, glucagon, and secretin family. GRF stimulates cAMP, activates phospholipase C, and causes an increase in intracellular calcium. GRF causes somatotrope hyperplasia and stimulates GH biosynthesis and secretion. The Gsα subunit, which is coupled to the GRF receptor, is one of the targets for activating mutations that lead to somatotrope adenomas. Somatostatin binds to receptors that inhibit

adenylate cyclase and thereby lower cAMP levels. As a result, GRF and somatostatin act antagonistically at the level of signal transduction. When both hormones are added concomitantly, somatostatin appears to act dominantly and GH secretion is inhibited.

IGF-1 also inhibits GH secretion and acts at both the pituitary and hypothalamic levels. In addition to reflecting GH action (primarily at the liver), serum IGF-1 is also sensitive to nutritional and metabolic changes. In starvation and anorexia nervosa, IGF-1 levels are low, resulting in increased levels of GH. In obesity, GH levels are low and GRF responses are blunted. Stress, exercise, and a variety of neurogenic stimuli also increase GH secretion. Estrogens stimulate GH secretion, but its effects are less pronounced than for prolactin.

Large bursts of GH secretion characteristically occur at night in association with slow-wave sleep. GH levels tend to be greatest during puberty and decline gradually in adulthood. The amplitude of GH pulses is greater in women than in men, likely reflecting the effects of estrogens. Spontaneous GH pulses can reach 50 ng per milliliter and are cleared rapidly with a half-life of about 20 minutes. Consequently, random GH levels can be very low or high. In addition, GH responses to GRF are highly variable even within an individual, probably reflecting variations in endogenous somatostatin tone.

GH acts through a single transmembrane receptor that is structurally related to prolactin and cytokine receptors (e.g., erythropoietin and colony-stimulating factors). This group of receptors associates with adaptor tyrosine kinases, one of which is referred to as JAK2 (Janus associated kinase 2). After GH stimulation, JAK2 is phosphorylated and initiates a signaling cascade. The GH molecule has two distinguishable receptor-binding domains that allow it to contact two separate receptor molecules to induce receptor dimerization. Mutations in the GH receptor cause GH resistance and severe growth retardation, a condition referred to as Laron-type dwarfism. GH levels are elevated and IGF-1 levels are low, reflecting the inability of the mutant receptor to transduce the GH signal.

Many of the growth and metabolic effects of GH are transmitted indirectly through the actions of IGF-1. GH stimulates IGF-1 production in most tissues, where it then exerts autocrine or paracrine effects. Circulating IGF-1 is derived predominantly from the liver and is a useful marker of GH action because it has a longer half-life and integrates the effects of GH pulses. Although IGF-1 levels are used in the diagnosis of acromegaly and to assess the integrity of the GH axis, it must be remembered that factors other than GH (e.g., malnutrition) can alter IGF-1 levels. IGF-1 acts via widely distributed receptors that are structurally related to insulin receptors. In addition to its growth-promoting and anabolic effects, IGF-1 also stimulates mitogenesis in many tissues.

GH has its major effects on linear growth but also influences a variety of metabolic pathways. Some of these effects are mediated by GH directly, whereas others are conferred by IGF-1. Although the relative roles of GH and IGF-1 are debated, their actions are cooperative in many cases. The effects of GH on linear growth appear to be mediated largely by IGF-1, which has been used to stimulate growth in patients with GH insensitivity syndrome. Linear growth in the fetus and neonate is not GH-dependent, as illustrated by the fact that GH-deficient babies have normal birth lengths. In contrast, normal postnatal linear growth requires GH, as illustrated by the clinical manifestations of GH deficiency. GH and IGF-1 act together to markedly accelerate linear growth, particularly at the time of puberty when sex steroids enhance GH and IGF-1 levels.

GH also induces lipolysis and stimulates anabolic activity, including amino acid uptake and protein synthesis. As a result, it reduces body fat, increases lean body mass, and leads to positive nitrogen balance. These properties of GH are most striking in GH-deficient children who have undergone replacement. GH opposes many of the actions of insulin and can be considered diabetogenic. In diabetics, nocturnal GH secretion accounts in part for the dawn phenomenon in which there is a decrease in glucose utilization, causing a tendency towards hyperglycemia.

GROWTH HORMONE DEFICIENCY (see also Ch. 201.1). Causes of GH deficiency include hypothalamic disorders, GH gene mutations, combined pituitary hormone deficiencies, radiation, and psychosocial dwarfism (see Table 202–3). The clinical manifestations of GH deficiency depend upon the time of onset and the severity of hormone deficiency. Children with complete GH deficiency have slow linear growth rates (approximately 3 cm per year), and they rapidly fall below normal on standardized growth charts. GH-deficient children have normal skeletal proportions, and many have a pudgy, youthful appearance because of decreased lipolysis. Particularly in the setting of cortisol deficiency, there is a predisposition to hypoglycemia.

Basal GH does not provide a reliable measure of GH reserve, whereas low IGF-1 levels are consistent with GH deficiency. GH deficiency is most frequently assessed using insulin-induced hypoglycemia, which activates CNS pathways, leading to stimulation of both GH and ACTH secretion (see Table 202–4). The insulin tolerance test requires careful monitoring for symptoms of severe hypoglycemia, such as confusion or depressed consciousness. This test should be avoided in patients with seizure disorders or coronary artery disease. Insulin doses (approximately 0.1 U per kilogram) may need to be decreased if glucocorticoid deficiency is suspected, or increased in conditions of insulin resistance (e.g., obesity). Alternatives to the insulin tolerance test for evaluation of GH include stimulation by L-dopa or arginine. Stimulation tests with GRF have not been well-standardized and appear to show substantial variation even within an individual, perhaps because of changing somatostatin tone.

In children with well-documented GH deficiency, GH replacement is effective and is essential to increase final adult height. In a typical regimen, recombinant GH (0.06 to 0.1 mg per kilogram) is given three times a week or daily as subcutaneous injections. The efficacy of GH treatment depends upon when it is initiated as well as replacement of other hormone deficiencies, if they coexist. In the setting of multiple hormone deficiencies, replacement of thyroid hormone and cortisol is necessary for effective GH action. On the other hand, sex steroids (estrogen in particular) lead to epiphyseal closure and limit linear growth. Consequently, GH is more effective before puberty; if exogenous sex steroids are given, low doses should be used. For unclear reasons, the effects of GH appear to wane after about 1 year of treatment. The potential role of GH replacement in adults is debated. Short-term studies show that it can increase lean body mass and improve the sense of well-being in adults with documented GH deficiency, but safety data for long-term GH administration are still lacking.

GROWTH HORMONE EXCESS: ACROMEGALY AND GIGANTISM. *Etiology and Pathogenesis.* GH-producing pituitary tumors involve the neoplastic proliferation of somatotrope cells and account for about 10 to 15% of pituitary tumors (see Table 202–6). GH-producing tumors are frequently mixed tumors that secrete more than one hormone. Prolactin is produced in the majority of somatotrope adenomas when evaluated by immunohistochemistry, and elevated serum levels of prolactin occur in about 25% of cases. A subset of these tumors are categorized morphologically as mammosomatotrope adenomas. Cosecretion of prolactin may predict a greater likelihood of response to treatment with bromocriptine. GH-producing tumors can also cosecrete glycoprotein hormones, most frequently the common α-subunit (approximately 10 to 30%), or rarely, TSH.

Considerable progress has been made concerning the cause of GH-producing pituitary tumors. Ectopic production of GRF (usually carcinoid or pancreatic islets) is a well-documented but rare (< 1%) cause of acromegaly which can result in somatotrope hyperplasia. Gsα mutations occur in 35 to 40% of somatotrope adenomas. Molecular defects in the remaining 60 to 65% of somatotrope adenomas remain to be identified.

Clinical Features. GH-secreting tumors cause acromegaly in adults and gigantism in children in whom GH excess occurs before epiphyseal closure. The annual incidence of acromegaly has been estimated at about 3 per million. It affects men and women with equal frequency and is most often recognized when patients are in their 30's or 40's, usually after a decade of GH excess. The clinical features of acromegaly are summarized in Table 202–7. The most striking features of acromegaly usually involve the face, hands, and feet. The diagnosis is often suspected because of changes in facial appearance, including enlargement of the lower jaw (prognathism), the nose and lips, and the sinuses (causing frontal bossing) (Fig. 202–1). Oral cavity changes, including malocclusion, increased spacing between the teeth, and enlargement of the tongue, may lead to recognition of the disorder by dentists. A hollow, resonant voice is caused by changes in the vocal cords and the soft tissues of the hypopharynx. Sleep apnea can occur in patients with soft tissue obstruction of the pharynx. Few acromegalics wear rings because they

TABLE 202–7. CLINICAL FEATURES OF ACROMEGALY

Musculoskeletal
Acral enlargement of hands and feet
Prognathism
Frontal bossing
Arthritis/arthralgias
Carpal tunnel syndrome
Muscle weakness
Cutaneous
Increased skin folds (e.g., forehead)
Increased soft tissue thickness
Skin tags
Oily skin
Increased sweating
Acanthosis nigricans
Oral/dental (adjectival, as at)
Malocclusion
Increased spacing between teeth
Enlargement of tongue
Enlargement of lips
Reproductive
Decreased libido/impotence
Oligomenorrhea
Galactorrhea in women
Neuropsychiatric
Headaches
Visual field defects
Somnolence
Metabolic
Glucose intolerance or diabetes mellitus
Hypercalciuria
Hyperphosphatemia
Cardiopulmonary
Hypertension
Cardiac enlargement
Sleep apnea
Other
Goiter
Colonic polyps
Deep, resonant voice
Sinusitis
Generalized visceromegaly

have long since outgrown them, and they usually have a history of progressive increase in shoe size and width. In addition to bony enlargement, there is a marked increase in the soft tissue of the hands and feet. A moist, doughy, enveloping handshake is characteristic of acromegaly. Heel pad thickness (which can be assessed radiographically) correlates well with IGF-1 levels and other clinical features of the disease. Arthralgias (hands, feet, hips, knees) are common (approximately 75%) and are caused by cartilage and synovial overgrowth. Some degree of carpal tunnel syndrome is seen in about half of patients. Skin changes include increased skinfolds, particularly over the brow and forehead. The skin is usually oily owing to increased sebaceous activity and sweating. Skin tags are common, and the incidence of colonic polyps is increased. Galactorrhea may be seen in women and reproductive dysfunction occurs in both women and men. Headaches, visual field defects, and other neurologic symptoms depend upon the location and extent of tumor growth.

Acromegaly causes as much as a two- to three-fold increase in mortality. Most of the increased mortality can be attributed to cardiovascular and cerebrovascular diseases and may be related in part to the increased prevalence of hypertension (25 to 35%) and diabetes mellitus (10 to 25%) in acromegaly. There is evidence for cardiac hypertrophy in the majority of acromegalics, and symptomatic heart disease, consisting of coronary ischemia and/or congestive heart failure, occurs in 15 to 20% of patients. Sleep apnea may predispose patients to cardiac dysrhythmias. There is an increased risk of premalignant polyps and colon cancer in acromegaly, and screening with colonoscopy is generally recommended. The disfigurement, metabolic complications, and increased mortality associated with acromegaly emphasize the importance of early diagnosis and implementation of appropriate therapy to lower the GH levels into the normal range.

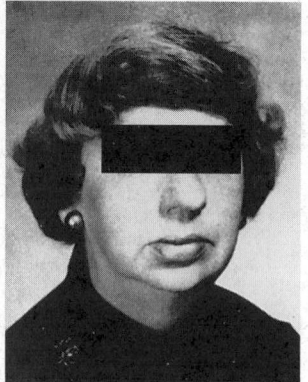

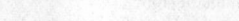

1977   1981

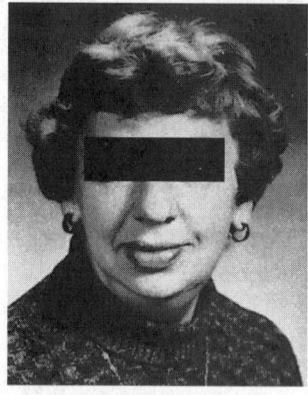   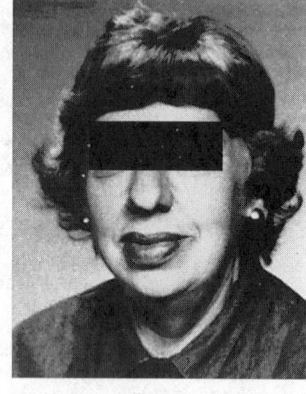

1983   1988

FIGURE 202–1. Clinical features of acromegaly. Serial photographs of a 64-year-old woman with acromegaly. Over an 11-year period, there is a progressive worsening of facial features, including enlargement of the nose and lips and development of prognathism. She also experienced hypertension, arthropathy, and enlargement of the hands. (Courtesy of Dr. Mark E. Molitch. Reprinted with permission from Molitch ME: Clinical manifestations of acromegaly. Endocrinol Metab Clin North Am 21:597,1992.)

Diagnosis. Because GH is secreted in a pulsatile manner and because the amplitude of GH pulses can be large (> 50 ng per milliliter), random GH levels are not very useful in making the diagnosis of acromegaly. IGF-1 levels provide an integrated index of GH production and provide a better screening test for acromegaly. IGF-1 levels are normally elevated during puberty and pregnancy and are suppressed during starvation. Otherwise, they correlate well with 24-hour GH production rates and with disease activity. The most reliable test for acromegaly is the glucose tolerance test (Table 202–8). In acromegaly, increased glucose levels fail to suppress GH below 2 ng per milliliter or cause a paradoxical increase in GH. More than half of patients with acromegaly exhibit a paradoxical stimulation of GH in response to TRH. Cosecretion of prolactin should be evaluated, and the common α-subunit of the glycoprotein hormones may provide an additional marker of tumor activity. After the diagnosis of acromegaly, radiologic studies, preferably using MRI, should be used to evaluate the extent of tumor growth. Unlike Cushing's disease and prolactinomas, the majority of patients with acromegaly have macroadenomas. In the absence of an apparent pituitary tumor, the possibility of ectopic GRF secretion causing somatotrope cell hyperplasia should be considered.

Therapy. The goals of therapy in acromegaly are to reverse or prevent tumor mass effects and to reduce the long-term morbidity and mortality that result from excess GH production. Correction of the disorder prevents further physical disfigurement and can result in substantial resolution of soft tissue changes and improvements in metabolic derangements. Although reductions in GH levels are associated with improvements in symptoms, the ultimate goal is to achieve normal GH and IGF-1 levels and to prevent tumor recurrence without incurring hypopituitarism.

Transsphenoidal surgery results in GH levels < 5 ng per milliliter in about 60% of patients with microadenomas. Not all of these patients are cured of their tumor when assessed by more stringent criteria, such as GH suppression below 2 ng per milliliter during an oral glucose tolerance test. Patients with macroadenomas are rarely cured by surgery (< 30%) but usually have reductions in GH levels.

Medical therapies for acromegaly include the somatostatin analogue octreotide and dopamine agonists such as bromocriptine. Responsiveness to both of these agents depends upon the presence and density of receptors on tumor cells. Octreotide reduces GH and IGF-1 levels in most patients and reduces tumor size in about half. Octreotide is useful as adjunctive therapy in patients who are not cured by surgery and/or radiation. There are also reports that preoperative treatment with octreotide can reduce tumor size and alter tumor consistency, thereby facilitating transsphenoidal resection. Although octreotide has a much longer half-life than somatostatin, it must be given in doses of 100 to 200 μg every 8 hours by subcutaneous injection to maintain GH suppression. Side effects include diarrhea and increased risk of cholelithiasis. Although bromocriptine was used extensively in early studies of medical therapy of acromegaly, it is less effective than octreotide in most patients and can require relatively high doses (up to 30 mg per day). However, some patients respond to bromocriptine but not octreotide, and it is also possible to combine the treatments.

Radiation is not recommended as primary therapy for acromegaly because of the length of time (5 to 10 years) required for reductions in GH levels and the high incidence of hypopituitarism. Adjunctive radiation therapy may be required for patients with macroadenomas when GH levels or mass effects persist after transsphenoidal surgery and medical therapy.

Ezzat S, Snyder PJ, Young WF, et al.: Octreotide treatment of acromegaly. A randomized, multicenter study. Ann Intern Med 117:711, 1992. *This large study shows that octreotide effectively decreases GH and IGF-1 concentrations in 53% and 68% of patients, respectively.*
Fahlbusch R, Honegger J, Buchfelder M: Surgical management of acromegaly. Endocrinol Metab Clin North Am 21:669, 1992. *Role of surgery in acromegaly.*
Melmed S: Acromegaly. N Engl J Med 322:966, 1990. *A review of the diagnosis and clinical management of acromegaly.*

PROLACTIN

Prolactin and GH are derived from a common ancestral gene, accounting for the similarities in structures and some overlap in functional properties. The prolactin gene is located on chromosome 6 and encodes a 198 amino acid protein (23-kD) that is produced in the lactotrope cells. Prolactin contains three intramolecular disulfide bonds, and high molecular variants are reported which may represent dimers or protein aggregates. Although the larger molecular weight forms of prolactin react in radioimmunoassays, they have diminished biologic potency. Prolactin is glycosylated to a small extent, but the role of the sugar chains is unclear. Estrogen stimulates lactotrope proliferation, and their number is consequently greater in women than in men and during pregnancy (approximately 70% of pituitary cells).

Prolactin secretion is controlled by tonic inhibition by dopamine, which acts through D_2-type receptors on lactotropes. Prolactin biosynthesis and secretion are stimulated by the hypothalamic peptides TRH and VIP. Hypothyroidism causes increased TRH output and can result in hyperprolactinemia. VIP, which acts via receptors that increase cAMP, may be responsible for prolactin increases associated with suckling. VIP is also found in the pituitary, where it may act as an autocrine or paracrine regulator of prolactin production. On balance, dopamine inhibition is the dominant influence for prolactin secretion. Prolactin is the one pituitary hormone that increases after pituitary stalk section. A variety of pharmacologic agents can stimulate prolactin secretion, in many cases by impairing dopamine secretion or action (Table 202–9).

Prolactin secretion is pulsatile and increases with sleep, stress, chest wall stimulation, and pregnancy. Prolactin levels are usually less than 15 to 20 ng per milliliter in women and 10 to 15 ng per milliliter in men. The primary function of prolactin is to induce and sustain lactation. However, prolactin binds to specific receptors that are located in several tissues, including breast, gonads, lymphoid cells, and liver. There are several different forms of prolactin receptors, which, like the GH receptor, are members of a cytokine family of receptors. During pregnancy, prolactin levels increase, and, in conjunction with other hormones (estrogens, progesterone, thyroid hormone, cortisol, and insulin), breast epithelium is stimu-

TABLE 202–8. SELECTED TESTS OF EXCESS PITUITARY FUNCTION

Hormone	Test	Interpretation
Growth hormone	*Basal IGF-1*	Elevated IGF-1 levels are consistent with acromegaly when interpreted in the context of age and nutritional status.
	Oral glucose suppression test: After 75-gm glucose load, GH is measured at −30, 0, 30, 60, 90, 120 min.	GH should be suppressed to <2 µg/L in normals. GH may paradoxically increase in acromegaly.
	TRH test: TRH (200 µg) is given IV with serum GH measurements at 0, 20, 60 min.	GH is not stimulated by TRH in most normals. A GH increase of 10 µg/L or >50% of baseline is consistent with acromegaly but can also occur in other disorders. The test is most useful for evaluating surgical cure.
Prolactin	*Basal prolactin levels*	Elevated prolactin (>200 µg/L) is consistent with a prolactinoma. When prolactin levels are between 20 and 100 µg/L, other causes of hyperprolactinemia should be considered.
ACTH	*Measurement of 24-hour urine free cortisol*	Elevated urine free cortisol is suggestive of Cushing's syndrome, but has several other causes as well.
	Overnight dexamethasone suppression test: Dexamethasone (1 mg) PO at midnight followed by 8 AM plasma cortisol.	AM cortisol should be suppressed to <5 µg/dL in normals. Normal dexamethasone suppression excludes Cushing's syndrome. Several other disorders can cause failure to suppress normally.
	Low-dose dexamethasone suppression test: Dexamethasone (0.5 mg) q6h for 8 doses with basal and end-of-treatment measurements that may include 24-hour urine collections for free cortisol or 17-hydroxysteroids and AM plasma cortisol and ACTH.	17-OH steroids should be suppressed to <4 mg/24h; urine free cortisol should be <20 µg/24h; serum cortisol should be suppressed to <6 µg/dl. Failure to suppress cortisol production is consistent with the diagnosis of Cushing's syndrome.
	High-dose dexamethasone suppression test: Dexamethasone (2 mg) q6h for 8 doses with basal and end-of-treatment measurements that may include 24-hour urine collections for free cortisol or 17-hydroxysteroids and AM plasma cortisol and ACTH.	The high-dose test is intended to distinguish Cushing's disease (pituitary adenoma), ectopic ACTH production, and adrenal adenoma. 50% suppression of 17-OH steroids or 90% suppression of urine free cortisol production is suggestive of Cushing's disease. Less than 50% suppression suggests ectopic ACTH or adrenal adenoma. Low ACTH levels are consistent with adrenal adenoma.
	CRH test: Ovine CRH (1 µg/kg) is administered IV, and ACTH and cortisol are drawn at −15, 0, 15, 30, 60, 90, and 120 min.	In Cushing's disease, there is usually a 50% increase in ACTH and 20% increase in cortisol. Adrenal adenoma is associated with suppressed ACTH. Ectopic ACTH is associated with high basal ACTH and cortisol levels that are not affected by CRH.
	Petrosal sinus ACTH sampling: The inferior petrosal sinus is catheterized, ideally bilaterally, and plasma ACTH is compared with simultaneous peripheral samples. The sampling can be done in conjunction with CRH stimulation.	In Cushing's disease, the ratio of ACTH in the petrosal sinus/periphery is at least 2. In ectopic ACTH, the ratio of petrosal sinus/peripheral level is <1.5.
TSH	*Basal thyroid function tests*	An inappropriately normal or elevated TSH in the setting of increased free thyroid hormone levels is consistent with a TSH-producing tumor or other causes of inappropriate TSH secretion.
	Free α-subunit level	Elevated free α-subunit levels associated with inappropriately elevated TSH are suggestive of a TSH-producing tumor.
FSH, LH	*Basal FSH, LH, testosterone*	Increased LH and testosterone levels in males are consistent with LH-secreting tumors. Elevated FSH and low-normal testosterone are suggestive of an FSH producing tumor if primary gonadal failure is not present. In females, assessment of excess hormone secretion is difficult because of changes during the menstrual cycle and at menopause.
	TRH test: TRH (200 µg) is given IV with measurements of serum FSH, LH, FSH β, and LH β subunits at 0, 20, 60 min.	Stimulation of LH, FSH, or their free β-subunits is suggestive of a gonadotropin-producing adenoma.

lated to proliferate and milk synthesis is induced. High levels of estrogen and progesterone inhibit lactation during pregnancy. The rapid decline in these steroids in the postpartum period permits lactation to occur. Neural pathways leading to the secretion of oxytocin provide the "let-down" reflex that induces lactation in response to suckling. Early in the postpartum period, prolactin secretion is stimulated by suckling, but this response becomes damped with time. Prolactin also suppresses gonadotropins, probably by a direct action on GnRH-secreting neurons. As a result, breastfeeding can suppress ovulation. The role of prolactin in other tissues is not well understood. High levels of prolactin are present in amniotic fluid, and it is produced in the decidual layer of the placenta.

PROLACTIN DEFICIENCY. Prolactin deficiency is rare and occurs primarily in the setting of combined hormone deficiencies. Prolactin levels at or below the limits of detection of radioimmunoassays and failure of prolactin to rise after TRH stimulation are consistent with the diagnosis. The only recognized consequence of prolactin deficiency is the absence of postpartum lactation. No effects on breast development or other tissues have been described in prolactin deficiency.

HYPERPROLACTINEMIA. *Etiology and Pathogenesis.* Hyperprolactinemia can occur as a consequence of pharmacologic alterations in the pathways that control prolactin secretion or of physiologic or metabolic effects on prolactin production and clearance or as a neoplastic condition (Table 202–9). Prolactinomas are neoplastic growths of lactotrope cells and are the most common type of pituitary adenoma (approximately 25 to 40%). Theories concerning the causes of prolactinomas have centered on hormonal stimuli that influence lactotrope growth and prolactin secretion. Estrogen is a potent stimulus for lactotrope proliferation. In rats, chronic estrogen exposure induces lactotrope hyperplasia and prolactinomas, but no clear association exists between estrogens (e.g., oral contraceptive use) and the incidence of prolactinomas in humans. It is possible that estrogen stimulates the growth of pre-existing prolactinomas, and this may account for the fact that some tumors appear to increase in size during pregnancy. Diminished dopamine tone results in increased prolactin but has not been

TABLE 202-9. DIFFERENTIAL DIAGNOSIS OF HYPERPROLACTINEMIA

Hypothalamic-pituitary disease
  Prolactinomas
  Acromegaly (somatomammotrope tumors)
  Pituitary tumors causing stalk compression
  Craniopharyngiomas and other hypothalamic neoplasms
  Metastatic tumors
  Infiltrative and inflammatory disorders
  Post-irradiation
  Empty sella syndrome
Drugs
  Dopamine antagonists (e.g., phenothiazines, butyrophenones, pimozide, domperidone, sulpiride, metoclopramide)
  Tricyclic antidepressants (e.g., imipramine, amitriptyline)
  Monoamine antihypertensives (e.g., methyldopa, reserpine)
  Verapamil
  Estrogens
  Opiates
  H_2 blockers (e.g., cimetidine)
Physiologic/metabolic
  Pregnancy
  Hypothyroidism
  Pseudocyesis
  Renal failure
  Cirrhosis
  Spinal cord lesions
  Chest wall or nipple stimulation
  Exercise, stress, sleep, sexual intercourse
Idiopathic

shown to cause prolactinomas. Prolactin secretory dynamics are generally restored to normal upon resection of prolactinomas, suggesting that an underlying hypothalamic abnormality is not present. Analyses of tumor DNA from a relatively small number of prolactinomas are consistent with a monoclonal origin, but molecular defects in prolactinomas have not been readily identified. Mutations in the *ras* oncogenes have been found in case reports but are not found in most prolactinomas.

Microprolactinomas constitute the great majority of tumors in premenopausal women. In contrast, macroadenomas are more commonly seen in men and postmenopausal women. The predominance of smaller tumors in premenopausal women may be accounted for by a bias of ascertainment, as elevated prolactin levels in this group lead to clinical manifestations (amenorrhea, galactorrhea, or infertility). Subclinical prolactinomas likely exist in men and many older women, as about 10% of individuals have prolactin-positive microadenomas in autopsy series.

Clinical Features. Hyperprolactinemia causes galactorrhea and oligomenorrhea in premenopausal women. Estrogen facilitates prolactin-induced galactorrhea, explaining why it is less common in postmenopausal women or in women with prolonged hypogonadism. Amenorrhea is primarily a consequence of prolactin suppression of GnRH, although prolactin may also have inhibitory effects at the level of the pituitary and the gonad. Amenorrhea is associated with infertility, and prolactin levels should be a routine part of the hormonal evaluation of infertility. Estrogen deficiency can cause decreased libido, vaginal dryness, and dyspareunia. Long-standing estrogen deficiency also leads to osteopenia in some women. A subset of patients have hirsutism and can exhibit elevations of adrenal androgens. Oral contraceptives may mask prolactin-induced oligomenorrhea that becomes apparent upon their discontinuation. In postmenopausal women, prolactinomas are often identified because of mass effects rather than because of their hormonal effects.

In men, hyperprolactinemia causes hypogonadism with suppressed LH and FSH levels and low testosterone levels. Hypogonadism causes diminished libido, impotence, and rarely gynecomastia or galactorrhea. Diminished libido may also reflect suppression of GnRH, as testosterone replacement is not as effective as suppression of hyperprolactinemia. Hyperprolactinemia is found in up to 5% of men being evaluated for sexual dysfunction.

Diagnosis. The four primary causes of hyperprolactinemia must be distinguished if the correct therapy is to be instituted: (1) physi-

ologic hyperprolactinemia; (2) pharmacologic hyperprolactinemia; (3) hypothalamic or pituitary stalk compression; and (4) prolactinoma (Table 202-9). With the exception of pregnancy and renal failure, physiologic causes of increased prolactin (e.g., transient pulses) result in minor elevations in prolactin (usually < 50 ng per milliliter) which may not be present upon repeat testing. Primary hypothyroidism should also be excluded as a cause of mild hyperprolactinemia. A careful drug history should be obtained in all patients with hyperprolactinemia because of the large number of agents that can stimulate prolactin secretion. Psychotropic medications, in particular, can increase prolactin either by reducing dopamine production or by blocking its action. In most cases, the degree of hyperprolactinemia caused by drugs is less than 100 ng per milliliter. A variety of suprasellar and parasellar mass lesions cause hyperprolactinemia (generally between 20 and 100 ng per milliliter) because of compression of the hypothalamus or pituitary stalk. Unless evidence is very good for physiologic or drug-induced hyperprolactinemia, patients with mild hyperprolactinemia should be evaluated with CT or MRI scans to distinguish between microprolactinomas and other large mass lesions that cause stalk compression. To a first approximation, prolactin levels correlate with tumor size. When no pituitary lesions are seen by radiographic studies and physiologic and pharmacologic causes of hyperprolactinemia cannot be identified, the diagnosis of idiopathic hyperprolactinemia is made. Idiopathic hyperprolactinemia may represent small microprolactinomas or altered hypothalamic regulation of prolactin secretion. Whether such patients should be treated depends upon the clinical effects of hyperprolactinemia. Like patients with microprolactinomas, few of these patients develop large tumors.

Therapy. The natural history of prolactinomas has been evaluated in several series. Although large prolactinomas clearly must evolve from smaller lesions, it is uncommon for microprolactinomas to progress to macroadenomas. When patients with microadenomas are followed without treatment over 3 to 5 years, prolactin levels decrease in 10 to 20% and increase in < 10% of patients. Decreased prolactin may occur because of spontaneous tumor infarction. Because of the slow rate of growth, it is reasonable to monitor patients with microprolactinomas without treatment unless the hyperprolactinemia is causing symptoms that warrant therapy.

When hyperprolactinemia causes hypogonadism, osteopenia, or infertility, a dopamine agonist such as bromocriptine is the therapy of choice. Dopamine agonists normalize prolactin levels and correct amenorrhea-galactorrhea in the majority of patients. They also reduce tumor size. Bromocriptine is usually started as a half tablet (1.25 mg) given at bedtime with a snack to avoid side effects (nausea, dizziness, somnolence, and nasal stuffiness). After adaptation to the drug, the dose can be increased gradually over several weeks. A typical final dose is 2.5 mg, two or three times a day with meals, but up to 30 mg per day may be required. The lowest effective dose should be used after achieving adequate suppression of prolactin levels. Unless spontaneous infarction of the tumor occurs, it is uncommon to be able to stop bromocriptine without recurrence of hyperprolactinemia. Some patients who cannot tolerate the side effects of bromocriptine may be able to take other dopamine agonists (e.g., pergolide). In some cases, prolactinomas appear resistant to bromocriptine, but it is important to ensure compliance and to be certain that the underlying lesion is a prolactinoma and not some other cause of hyperprolactinemia. In cases unresponsive to dopamine agonists, transsphenoidal surgery is the treatment of choice. Although initial remission rates (60 to 90%) for transsphenoidal surgery of microprolactinomas are good, long-term recurrence is seen in up to 50% of patients. Radiation therapy is not recommended for microprolactinomas because responses are slow and often incomplete and there is a high incidence of hypopituitarism.

Bromocriptine therapy for infertility or when there is a possibility of pregnancy deserves special consideration. Bromocriptine can induce ovulation in 80 to 90% of patients with hyperprolactinemia. Although bromocriptine has not been associated with congenital malformations or complications during pregnancy, most physicians and patients prefer to avoid its use during pregnancy if possible. A form of barrier contraception is usually recommended until two to three regular menstrual cycles have occurred. Subsequently, pregnancy can be confirmed if a menstrual period is missed, allowing discontinuation of bromocriptine. Less than 2% of patients with microadenomas but 15% of patients with macroadenomas develop symptoms of tumor enlargement (headaches, visual field defects) during pregnancy. If symptoms develop, radiologic studies should be performed. If there is evidence of visual field compromise or tumor growth, bromocriptine therapy should be restarted. Prolactin levels are not very useful because they are normally increased in pregnancy, and prolactin production by an enlarging tumor may not increase substantially. Because problems of tumor growth occur most often in patients with macroadenomas, consideration should be given to the option of transsphenoidal decompression before pregnancy in women with large tumors, as long as fertility can be preserved.

Macroprolactinomas also respond well to dopamine agonists. However, because the tumors are larger and produce greater amounts of prolactin, a longer period of treatment may be required for reduction of prolactin levels. Reversal of hypogonadism can require 3 to 6 months. Visual field defects are a very sensitive index of tumor size, and improvements can be seen in about 90% of patients. A significant reduction in tumor size (approximately 50%) is seen in about half of patients assessed by radiologic studies. Thus, it is reasonable to use bromocriptine as a first-line therapy even in patients with visual field defects as long as visual acuity is not threatened by rapid progression or recent tumor hemorrhage. Bromocriptine doses should be advanced (up to 20 to 30 mg per day) until prolactin levels reach the normal range or a plateau. After prolonged treatment, it is usually possible to reduce the dose of bromocriptine. However, discontinuation of bromocriptine is not recommended for macroadenomas because rapid regrowth of the tumor can occur. Surgery results in remission of macroprolactinomas in < 40% of patients and should be reserved for those who do not respond to dopamine agonists. Radiation therapy can be used as an adjunctive measure in patients with large, aggressive tumors that are inadequately controlled by treatment with dopamine agonists and surgical decompression.

Klibanski A, Biller BM, Rosenthal DI, et al.: Effects of prolactin and estrogen deficiency in amenorrheic bone loss. J Clin Endocrinol Metab 67:124, 1988. *This study suggests that estrogen deficiency and amenorrhea associated with hyperprolactinemia reflect a greater risk of developing osteopenia.*

Molitch ME: Management of prolactinomas. Annu Rev Med 40:225, 1989. *A concise and practical summary of the management of prolactinomas.*

Molitch ME: Pregnancy and the hyperprolactinemic woman. N Engl J Med 312:1364, 1985. *A balanced and well-referenced review of issues pertaining to hyperprolactinemia and pregnancy.*

Schlechte J, Dolan K, Sherman B, et al.: The natural history of untreated hyperprolactinemia: A prospective analysis. J Clin Endocrinol Metab 68:412, 1989. *A long-term prospective study of the natural history of hyperprolactinemia in 30 women.*

ACTH (see also Ch. 204)

ACTH is a 39 amino acid peptide that is derived from a precursor polypeptide, pro-opiomelanocortin (POMC). In the anterior pituitary, POMC (241 aa) encodes several peptides, including an aminoterminal peptide, joining peptide, ACTH, and β-lipotropin. The functional roles of the POMC-encoded peptides other than ACTH have not been fully defined. β-lipotropin, in addition to ACTH, may stimulate melanocytes and contribute to hyperpigmentation in conditions of POMC stimulation. β-lipotropin can be processed further to yield γ-lipotropin and β-endorphin. The biologically active portion of ACTH resides within the first 18 of its 39 amino acids. However, because a synthetic peptide (cosyntropin) that includes the first 24 amino acids has a longer half-life, it is used clinically to assess adrenocortical function.

The half-life of ACTH is relatively short (< 10 min), and pulses of ACTH secretion are discrete. Levels of precursor peptides, such as β-LPH, do not always parallel those of ACTH because of their slower clearance rates. β-LPH, but not ACTH, is also elevated in renal failure. In neoplastic conditions, particularly ectopic production of ACTH, the levels of precursor peptides or their processed products may be elevated. The POMC gene can also be expressed from alternate transcription start sites, giving rise to aberrant POMC transcripts in ectopic tumors.

The primary effect of ACTH is to stimulate the adrenal gland to produce cortisol. It also stimulates secretion of adrenal androgens and mineralocorticoids, although production of mineralocorticoids is controlled primarily through non–ACTH-dependent mechanisms (see Ch. 204). Consequently, mineralocorticoid function is preserved in ACTH deficiency, in contrast to primary adrenal insufficiency, which is characterized by loss of glucocorticoid and mineralocorticoid function.

ACTH binds to a high-affinity receptor that is a member of the seven-transmembrane class of receptors that are coupled to G pro-

teins. ACTH acts as a trophic hormone and stimulates the immediate secretion of cortisol and other adrenal steroids. Long-term stimulation by ACTH causes adrenal hyperplasia and enlargement. On the other hand, ACTH deficiency leads to adrenal atrophy, and several days of ACTH stimulation are required before steroid synthesis returns to normal.

The secretion of ACTH is regulated by the hypothalamic-pituitary-adrenal (HPA) axis. Hypothalamic corticotropin-releasing hormone (CRH) is the most important stimulator of ACTH secretion. CRH is a 41 amino acid peptide that is produced in the paraventricular nucleus of the hypothalamus and in other sites in the nervous system and peripheral tissues (see Ch. 201.1). The CRH receptor is structurally related to the calcitonin/VIP/GRF subfamily of seven-membrane spanning, G protein–coupled receptors. CRH stimulates cAMP production and increases POMC gene transcription as well as ACTH secretion. Chronic stimulation by CRH also causes corticotrope cell hyperplasia, which can be seen in cases of ectopic CRH production.

Arginine vasopressin (AVP) weakly stimulates ACTH when given alone, but it acts synergistically when administered with CRH. Several other hypothalamic factors (angiotensin II, VIP, gastrin-releasing peptide, catecholamines) also enhance ACTH secretion, either by stimulating CRH or by acting at the level of the pituitary gland.

ACTH secretion is inhibited by glucocorticoids, which act at both the hypothalamic and pituitary levels. Cortisol inhibits POMC gene transcription by binding to glucocorticoid receptors that interact with negative glucocorticoid response elements (nGREs) in the POMC promoter. Cortisol also inhibits ACTH secretion and blunts the ACTH response to CRH. Consequently, ACTH responses to CRH stimulation tests depend upon ambient concentrations of cortisol and are most robust at night when cortisol levels are low. Cortisol inhibits CRH production and may also act at higher CNS levels. After prolonged glucocorticoid suppression of the HPA axis, the amount of endogenous CRH secretion appears to be rate-limiting and can require several months to recover.

Plasma ACTH is secreted in discrete pulses (10 to 80 pg per milliliter) that occur about once an hour. Because of the marked variation in ACTH levels, random measurements are of little value, and most clinical tests are therefore based upon cortisol or its metabolites, which tend to integrate the effects of ACTH. ACTH secretion exhibits a marked diurnal rhythm, being greatest at night several hours after the initiation of sleep. Cortisol levels are greatest in the early morning and reach a nadir in the late afternoon and evening. Patients with Cushing's disease lose or exhibit a blunted diurnal rhythm of ACTH secretion. ACTH secretion can be stimulated by a variety of different forms of stress, including psychological stimuli such as fright, anticipation of athletic competition, or surgery. Depression is associated with activation of the HPA axis and impairs dexamethasone suppressibility. Hypoglycemia induces ACTH secretion, probably through a central mechanism. The resulting increase in cortisol secretion represents one of several counterregulatory mechanisms that increase glucose production. Insulin-induced hypoglycemia provides a mechanism for testing the integrity of the HPA axis (see Table 202–4). Serious trauma and infection activate an array of cytokines that stimulate CRH and ACTH secretion. Because cortisol levels are often increased up to 10-fold in these circumstances, similar adjustments in cortisol replacement doses may be required in seriously ill patients with adrenal insufficiency.

ACTH DEFICIENCY: SECONDARY HYPOCORTISOLISM. Secondary hypocortisolism causes symptoms of glucocorticoid deficiency, including nausea, vomiting, weakness, fatigue, fever, and hypotension. In addition to reduced levels of cortisol, laboratory tests can detect hyponatremia, hypoglycemia, and eosinophilia. Depending upon its cause, the severity of cortisol deficiency in secondary adrenal insufficiency is often not as marked as in primary adrenal insufficiency. In addition, mineralocorticoid function is preserved in secondary adrenal deficiency. Consequently, the clinical manifestations of volume depletion are less pronounced and hyperkalemia is not a feature of ACTH deficiency. Because ACTH levels are low in secondary adrenal insufficiency, hyperpigmentation is not seen as in primary adrenal insufficiency. In women, reduced adrenal androgens can decrease libido and cause loss of axillary and pubic hair.

The most common cause of ACTH deficiency is treatment with exogenous glucocorticoids, which cause suppression of the HPA axis. Sudden withdrawal of glucocorticoids or an increased requirement induced by the superimposition of severe illness can elicit symptoms of glucocorticoid deficiency. Congenital forms of ACTH deficiency are rare and usually occur in combination with the loss of other pituitary hormones.

ACTH reserve is most often evaluated using CRH or the insulin tolerance test. Caution should be exercised before inducing hypoglycemia in patients with suspected adrenal insufficiency. Insulin-induced hypoglycemia stimulates central responses to neuroglycopenia and mimics some, but not all, stresses that activate ACTH secretion. CRH testing (ovine CRH, 1 μg per kilogram IV) is also useful for distinguishing hypothalamic and pituitary causes of ACTH deficiency, as it still induces an ACTH response in patients with hypothalamic dysfunction and blunted responses to hypoglycemia. The metyrapone test provides an alternative to the insulin tolerance test. Metyrapone inhibits cortisol production, resulting in stimulation of ACTH secretion and an increase in precursor adrenal steroids (e.g., 11-deoxycortisol). Patients should be monitored closely for evidence of adrenal insufficiency. The "short" and "long" ACTH stimulation tests have largely been replaced by more direct measurements of ACTH but can be used to demonstrate improvement in cortisol secretion with repeated infusions of ACTH. Incomplete or normal cortisol responses to the initial ACTH infusion do not exclude ACTH deficiency, as the adrenal may remain ACTH-responsive if ACTH deficiency is recent or incomplete.

ACTH deficiency is treated by replacement with glucocorticoids (see Table 202–5). Doses need to be individualized and are based largely on clinical criteria in which symptoms of glucocorticoid deficiency are balanced against features of glucocorticoid excess. Patients should wear MedicAlert tags and be instructed in the warning signs of cortisol deficiency, including nausea, vomiting, abdominal pain, low-grade fever, fatigue, and postural dizziness. Stress doses of steroids should be used during times of illness. Mineralocorticoid replacement is not usually required in patients with ACTH deficiency.

CUSHING'S DISEASE (see also Ch. 204). *Etiology and Pathogenesis.* Cushing's *disease* results from a pituitary neoplasm that causes excess production of ACTH. It is to be distinguished from a variety of other causes of Cushing's *syndrome* (glucocorticoid excess), which include adrenal causes of cortisol excess, ectopic production of ACTH, and physiologic states that result in overproduction of cortisol. Cushing's disease accounts for about 60 to 70% of cases of Cushing's syndrome. Approximately 10 to 15% of pituitary tumors secrete ACTH. For unknown reasons, Cushing's disease occurs about eight times more often in women than in men.

The cause of Cushing's disease has been the subject of a longstanding controversy. The observations that CRH stimulates corticotrope hyperplasia and that some patients with Cushing's disease have corticotrope hyperplasia when the pituitary is subjected to pathologic evaluation support the idea of a hypothalamic cause of Cushing's disease. This concept has been used to explain the frequent recurrence of Cushing's disease after apparent cure following transsphenoidal surgery. On the other hand, most ACTH-producing pituitary neoplasms, like other pituitary tumors, are monoclonal in origin. A primary defect in corticotrope cells is also supported by several clinical observations. First, most patients who undergo successful removal of a corticotrope adenoma exhibit suppression of the HPA axis after surgery, suggesting that CRH is low rather than high. Second, many patients with Cushing's disease respond to exogenous CRH, suggesting that endogenous CRH levels are not high. On balance, the great majority of cases of Cushing's disease likely arise from a primary defect at the level of the pituitary, with rare cases being caused by a hypothalamic disorder.

In contrast to other pituitary tumors, the great majority (80 to 90%) of ACTH-secreting tumors are microadenomas at the time of diagnosis. The clinical features of cortisol excess may allow detection of corticotrope adenomas before they have grown to a larger size. High levels of cortisol may also restrain tumor growth. ACTH-secreting macroadenomas tend to be locally invasive.

Clinical Features. The clinical features of Cushing's disease are caused by the effects of excess glucocorticoids and by the hypersecretion of ACTH and other POMC peptide products. The severity of the features of Cushing's disease varies greatly and ap-

pears to reflect not only the level of free cortisol, but also the duration of the disease and perhaps the sensitivity to glucocorticoid action. In florid cases of Cushing's disease (Fig. 202–2), the constellation of symptoms and physical features is readily recognized. However, early in the disease or in mild cases, it can be extremely challenging to distinguish the clinical features of Cushing's disease from similar traits that are seen in the normal population. Clinical suspicion is of paramount importance because it establishes the first screening test before embarking upon laboratory studies. On the

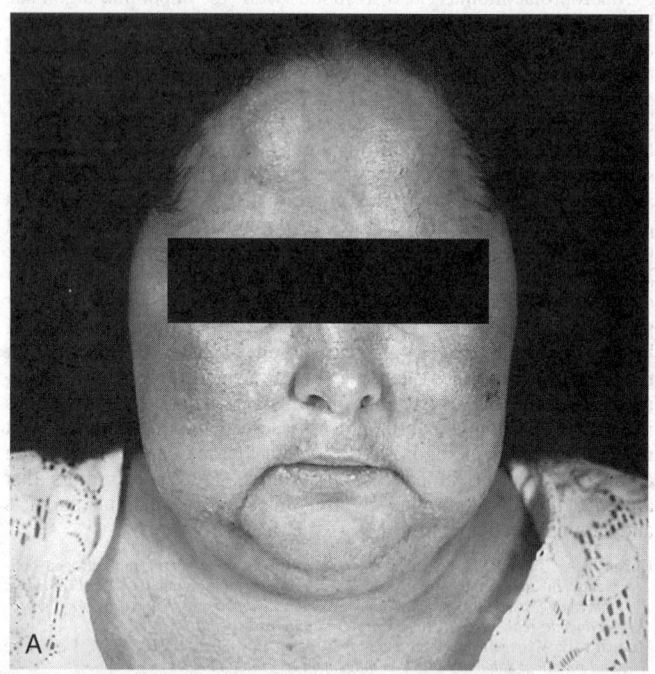

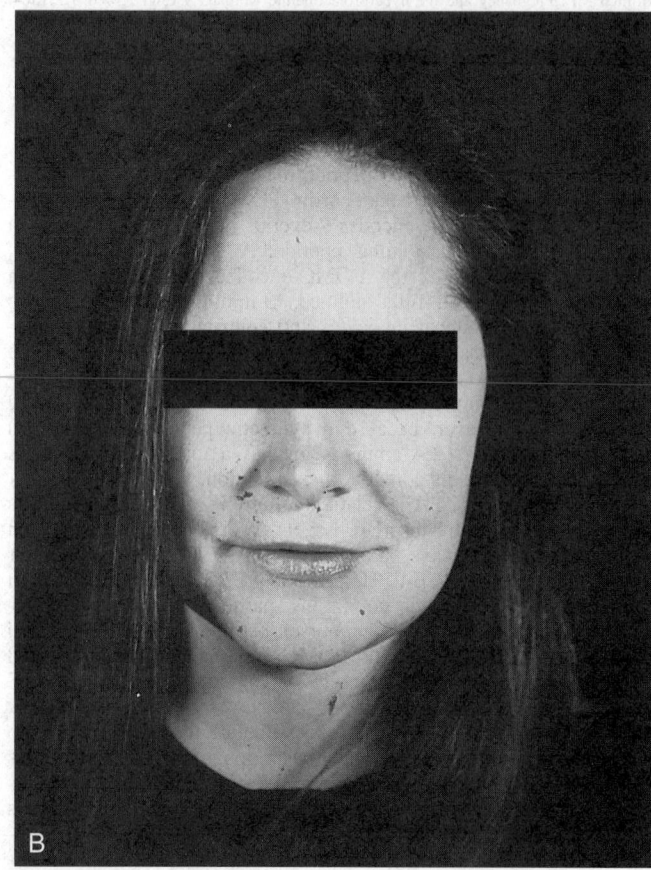

FIGURE 202–2. Clinical features of Cushing's disease. A 25-year-old woman with severe Cushing's disease. *A,* Facial features of Cushing's syndrome, including plethora, moon facies, and hirsutism, are evident. *B,* Dramatic resolution of the manifestations of cortisol excess after successful transsphenoidal surgery. (Courtesy of Dr. Beverly M. K. Biller.)

TABLE 202–10. CLINICAL FEATURES OF CUSHING'S DISEASE

General
Obesity (centripetal distribution)
"Moon facies" and mild proptosis
Increased supraclavicular fat and "buffalo hump"
Hypertension
Skin
Hyperpigmentation
Facial plethora
Hirsutism
Violaceous striae and thin skin
Capillary fragility and easy bruising
Acne
Edema
Musculoskeletal
Muscle weakness (proximal)
Osteoporosis and back pain
Reproductive
Decreased libido
Oligomenorrhea
Neuropsychiatric
Depression
Irritability and emotional lability
Psychosis
Metabolic
Hypokalemia and alkalosis
Hypercalciuria and renal stones
Glucose intolerance or diabetes mellitus
Impaired wound healing
Impaired resistance to infection
Granulocytosis and lymphopenia
Tumor mass effects
Headache
Visual field loss
Hypopituitarism

other hand, one must be discriminating and not formally evaluate everyone with obesity, hypertension, and glucose intolerance. Of the many features listed in Table 202–10, some are relatively specific for Cushing's disease. For example, the centripetal distribution of fat with the characteristic "buffalo hump," "moon facies," and deposition in the supraclavicular area, with minimal fat in the extremities, is much more specific than generalized obesity. Striae that are wide (>1 cm) and purple in color reflect steroid-induced thinning of the dermis and can be distinguished from the more common "stretch marks." Numerous spontaneous ecchymoses also occur because of thinning of the skin and capillary fragility. Proximal muscle weakness represents another relatively specific manifestation of glucocorticoid excess. Osteopenia and hypokalemia, when present, provide objective evidence consistent with ACTH excess. Hypokalemia results from the effects of ACTH on mineralocorticoid production and from the ability of high levels of cortisol to saturate 11β-dehydrogenase, an enzyme in the kidney that inactivates cortisol. As a result, cortisol can "spill over" and act on mineralocorticoid receptors in the distal tubule. The hyperpigmentation associated with Cushing's disease is not as striking as that in Addison's disease or ectopic ACTH syndrome, but in association with other findings, it should raise the suspicion of Cushing's disease and helps to distinguish it from adrenal causes of hypercortisolemia. Hirsutism and acne are caused by the increased production of adrenal androgens and are more prominent in Cushing's disease than in hypercortisolism caused by adrenal adenomas, in which glucocorticoids tend to be the predominant product. Oligomenorrhea probably has several causes, including androgen effects on the reproductive axis and glucocorticoid inhibition of GnRH, which may

also account for diminished libido. Hypertension and glucose intolerance are caused by glucocorticoid excess. Immune suppression, opportunistic infections, and impaired wound healing can lead to considerable morbidity. Neuropsychiatric symptoms, including depression, can be prominent effects of Cushing's disease. Suicide occurs with increased frequency in untreated Cushing's disease.

Diagnosis. The screening tests and differential diagnosis of Cushing's syndrome represent one of the greatest diagnostic challenges in endocrinology (see Ch. 204). In most cases, the complete evaluation of Cushing's syndrome can take place in the outpatient setting. The first step is to determine whether a patient truly has cortisol excess. After confirmation of Cushing's syndrome, one must distinguish among (1) adrenal causes of cortisol excess, (2) pituitary causes of ACTH excess (Cushing's disease), and (3) ectopic sources of ACTH (Table 202–11).

In screening for hypercortisolism, random cortisol levels are not useful because of diurnal variation of the hormone. The overnight dexamethasone test is the most widely used screening test (see Table 202–8). A normal dexamethasone test essentially excludes Cushing's syndrome. It should be noted, however, that abnormal overnight dexamethasone suppression can be seen in up to 30% of hospitalized patients and in many patients with depression. An elevated 24-hour urine free cortisol (UFC) provides an alternative or additional screening test for hypercortisolism. Often, two sequential specimens are collected because of day-to-day variations in hormone production. The sensitivity and specificity of UFC measurements are greater than those of the overnight dexamethasone suppression test, particularly in hospitalized patients.

After demonstrating that cortisol excess is present, the next step is to determine the source of excess ACTH or cortisol. The classic approach is to perform a low-dose, followed by a high-dose dexamethasone suppression test (see Tables 202–8 and 202–11). The low-dose dexamethasone test excludes or confirms the presence of Cushing's syndrome. On the second day of the test, normal individuals suppress plasma cortisol to <5 μg per deciliter and reduce the 17-hydroxysteroids to <2.5 mg per 24 hours or UFC to <20 μg per 24 hours. All forms of Cushing's syndrome fail to suppress according to these criteria.

The high-dose dexamethasone test is one of several means to distinguish ACTH-independent and ACTH-dependent causes of Cushing's syndrome and to discriminate between pituitary and ectopic causes of ACTH-dependent Cushing's syndrome (Table 202–11). Because adrenal sources of cortisol excess are autonomous and ACTH-independent, plasma and urinary cortisol levels are not affected by dexamethasone suppression, even at high doses. In addition, plasma ACTH levels are low in adrenal causes of Cushing's syndrome because the hypothalamic-pituitary axis is suppressed. Pituitary and ectopic causes of Cushing's syndrome are both ACTH-dependent but respond differently to high-dose dexamethasone. Pituitary adenomas have an altered set point for glucocorticoid inhibition but retain a partial ability to respond to high-dose dexamethasone. The exact criteria for dexamethasone suppression in the high-dose test are debated. In most cases of ACTH-producing pituitary adenomas, 17-hydroxysteroids are suppressed to <50% of baseline, and UFC is suppressed below 90% of baseline during the high-dose dexamethasone test.

The ectopic ACTH syndrome should be suspected in patients with known malignancies, particularly oat cell carcinoma, bronchial, thymic, or gastrointestinal carcinoids, islet cell tumors, medullary carcinoma of the thyroid, and others. Plasma ACTH levels are often very high (>200 pg per milliliter) and can be associated with hyperpigmentation. Clinical features of Cushing's syn-

TABLE 202–11. TESTS USED IN THE DIFFERENTIAL DIAGNOSIS OF CUSHING'S SYNDROME

Etiology	Overnight Dex test	Plasma ACTH	Low-dose Dex	High-dose Dex	CRH stimulation of ACTH	Petrosal/Peripheral ACTH Ratio
Normal	Suppression	Normal	Suppression		Normal	
Pituitary	No suppression	Normal or high	No suppression	Suppression	Normal or increased	>2
Ectopic	No suppression	High or normal	No suppression	No suppression	No response	<1.5
Adrenal	No suppression	Low	No suppression	No suppression	No response	<1.5

Classic responses are indicated. Certain cases of ectopic ACTH production are suppressed by high-dose dexamethasone (Dex) or are stimulated by CRH. In these cases, petrosal sinus sampling is the most reliable method for distinguishing pituitary and ectopic sources of ACTH.

drome may be altered by the rapid onset of extreme hypercortisolemia. Pronounced weakness, fluid retention, glucose intolerance, and poor skin integrity are often seen and can exacerbate problems associated with underlying tumors. Hypokalemia is more common than in other forms of Cushing's syndrome.

Ectopic ACTH syndrome is readily recognized in its classic form. However, a subset of tumors, particularly carcinoids, exhibit dexamethasone suppression similar to that seen with pituitary adenomas. When suspected, carcinoids can sometimes be detected by CT or MRI, but many are too small to be seen even with these techniques. Because of these exceptions to the high-dose dexamethasone test, a variety of procedures have been devised in an attempt to further distinguish ectopic and pituitary-dependent sources of ACTH. The metyrapone test takes advantage of the fact that inhibition of 11β-hydroxylase blocks cortisol production. As a result, negative feedback is reduced and pituitary-dependent sources of ACTH typically exhibit an increase in ACTH, which stimulates the production of precursor adrenal steroids (e.g., 11-deoxycortisol) (see Table 202–4). Although most ectopic causes of ACTH exhibit a blunted response to the decreased cortisol levels, the subset of ectopic tumors that respond atypically to dexamethasone are most likely to give a positive response in the metyrapone test.

In recent years, inferior petrosal sinus sampling has been used to distinguish pituitary and ectopic sources of ACTH when the source of ACTH is not obvious based upon the clinical circumstances or imaging studies. This test requires an experienced radiologist for safe and effective catheterization of the petrosal sinus (which drains the pituitary venous effluent). Blood samples are taken simultaneously from the left and right petrosal sinuses and from the periphery. In the case of ACTH-producing pituitary adenomas, there is a gradient in ACTH levels between the central and peripheral blood specimens. Administration of CRH stimulates ACTH and tends to enhance the gradient. A gradient of 2:1 (central:peripheral) on either the left or the right is consistent with a pituitary source of ACTH. After clinical or biochemical studies suggest the presence of a pituitary adenoma, pituitary imaging should be performed using CT or MRI. Most ACTH-secreting pituitary adenomas are small, and scans are normal in more than half of patients.

Therapy. The efficacy of transsphenoidal surgery for Cushing's disease is greatly aided by making the correct diagnosis preoperatively. In experienced hands, surgical cures of ACTH-producing microadenomas occur in about 75 to 95% of patients undergoing a first operation. As with other pituitary tumors, complete remissions with macroadenomas are much less common. In the event of surgical remission or cure, postoperative hypocortisolism is common because of suppression of the hypothalamic-pituitary axis. After coverage for steroid withdrawal in the postoperative period, cortisol replacement should be minimized to allow recovery of the HPA axis.

If transsphenoidal surgery is unsuccessful, reoperation may be indicated and can result in remission in up to 50% of patients. If transsphenoidal surgery cannot be performed or has failed, alternative forms of therapy should be used to prevent the long-term consequences of hypercortisolism. Pituitary irradiation is usually the second line of treatment for Cushing's disease. It is more efficacious in children and younger patients, but it has a slow therapeutic response, often requiring concomitant medical therapy. Bilateral adrenalectomy represents another alternative for patients with severe hypercortisolism following transsphenoidal surgery. It rapidly and effectively lowers cortisol levels but is associated with relatively high morbidity and mortality (as high as 5%) because of the associated metabolic and immune system alterations caused by hypercortisolism. After adrenalectomy, patients must be maintained on glucocorticoids and mineralocorticoids and are at risk for the development of Nelson's syndrome.

Medical therapy of Cushing's disease has its primary role in preparation for surgery or for control of hypercortisolism during the interval when radiation therapy is taking effect. Because most pituitary adenomas are responsive to changes in cortisol levels, they have a tendency to "escape" from adrenal blockade by producing higher levels of ACTH. Medical therapies include ketoconazole, metyrapone, aminoglutethimide, and mitotane (o,p'-DDD). Whether the glucocorticoid receptor antagonist RU486 has a role in the management of Cushing's syndrome remains to be established.

NELSON'S SYNDROME. Nelson's syndrome was initially described as the appearance of a pituitary adenoma after bilateral adrenalectomy. In addition to an enlarging pituitary mass, the syndrome is characterized by very high ACTH levels and hyperpigmentation. It is caused by a pre-existing ACTH-producing tumor that grows in the absence of feedback inhibition by high levels of glucocorticoids. The incidence of clinically significant Nelson's syndrome after adrenalectomy for Cushing's disease varies from 10 to 50% in different series. Patients with Cushing's disease who have undergone adrenalectomy should be followed with imaging studies and plasma ACTH levels, as tumors that cause Nelson's syndrome can be very aggressive. When there is evidence of mass effects or rapid growth, transsphenoidal surgery should be performed. Postoperative radiation therapy may provide additional benefit, although it appears to be less efficacious than in other ACTH-producing adenomas.

Kaye TB, Crapo L: The Cushing syndrome: An update on diagnostic tests. Ann Intern Med 112:434, 1990. *A critical review of the advantages and shortcomings of various tests used in the differential diagnosis of Cushing's syndrome.*
Mampalam TJ, Tyrrell JB, Wilson CB: Transsphenoidal microsurgery for Cushing disease. A report of 216 cases. Ann Intern Med 109:487, 1988. *A representative study of surgical results from a center with extensive experience.*
Oldfield EH, Doppman JL, Nieman LK, et al.: Petrosal sinus sampling with and without corticotropin-releasing hormone for the differential diagnosis of Cushing's syndrome. N Engl J Med 325:897, 1991. *This classic study shows that simultaneous bilateral sampling of plasma from the inferior petrosal sinuses, with the adjunctive use of CRH, distinguishes patients with Cushing's disease from those with ectopic adrenocorticotropin secretion.*
Schteingart DE: Cushing's syndrome. Endocrinol Metab Clin North Am 18:311, 1989. *This review emphasizes the therapeutic options for Cushing's disease.*

GONADOTROPINS (FSH AND LH)

The pituitary glycoprotein hormones include FSH, LH, and TSH. Chorionic gonadotropin (CG), which is structurally very similar to LH, is made in the placenta. Each of the glycoprotein hormones has a specific β-subunit that forms a noncovalent dimer with the common α-subunit. The α- and individual β-subunits are encoded by separate genes. The β-subunit genes are evolutionarily related and share a common gene structure as well as nucleotide and amino acid sequence homology. Similarities in the structures of the β-subunits account for their ability to form noncovalent dimers with the common α-subunit. The α- and β-subunits each undergo glycosylation, which is important for correct hormone folding, intracellular transport, and secretion. Glycosylation is also required for biologic activity, presumably because of effects on the tertiary structure of the hormones.

The half-life of LH (approximately 50 min) is shorter than that of FSH (approximately 220 min), accounting for the more rapid secretory dynamics of LH, even though both hormones are secreted together. Differences in FSH and LH sequences between the conserved cysteines provide distinct "determinant loops" that allow the hormones to bind to specific receptors. Receptor contacts are made by both the α- and β-subunits. The receptors for FSH and LH are also structurally related and are members of the G protein–coupled seven-transmembrane family. After binding to their receptors, LH and FSH stimulate cAMP production, phosphotidylinositol turnover, and mobilization of calcium.

The gonadotropins are involved in sexual differentiation, sex steroid production, and gametogenesis. The regulation and physiologic roles of gonadotropins are quite different in males and females. In males, receptors for FSH are located on Sertoli cells and seminiferous tubules, whereas LH receptors are located on Leydig cells in the testis. LH stimulates androgen production by the Leydig cells. FSH is involved primarily in sperm maturation in the seminiferous tubules. Thus, FSH and LH act together to induce spermatogenesis (see Ch. 209).

In females, ovarian FSH receptors are located on granulosa cells, where they induce enzymes involved in estrogen biosynthesis. LH receptors are located predominantly on thecal cells in the ovary and stimulate the production of ovarian androgens and steroid precursors that are transported to granulosa cells for aromatization to estrogens. The pattern of FSH and LH secretion during the menstrual cycle results in follicular recruitment and maturation (largely FSH-mediated), followed by ovulation (largely LH-mediated) and steroid production by the corpus luteum.

Gonadotropin secretion is regulated primarily by the hypothalamic decapeptide gonadotropin-releasing hormone (GnRH). The receptor for GnRH is a member of the G protein–coupled seven-transmembrane family of receptors. GnRH stimulates an immediate release of intracellular calcium, followed by a second phase of extracellular calcium influx. GnRH also activates phosphotidylinositol turnover, resulting in production of diacylglycerol (DAG) and inositol triphosphate (IP_3), which act together to stimulate the protein kinase C pathway. The gonadotrope cell is exquisitely sensitive to the pattern of GnRH stimulation. Continuous rather than pulsatile exposure to GnRH causes gonadotrope desensitization and suppression of LH and FSH. Gonadotrope sensitivity to GnRH is modulated by sex steroids and probably other hypothalamic peptides such as neuropeptide Y (NPY). Increased GnRH secretion in combination with a higher density of GnRH receptors and rising estradiol concentrations accounts in part for the dramatic release of gonadotropins that induces ovulation.

The hypothalamic-pituitary-gonadal (HPG) axis is activated during fetal development. However, during the first 2 years of life, LH and FSH levels fall and remain suppressed until puberty. The physiologic basis for gonadotropin suppression during early childhood is not well-understood but involves tonic inhibition of the GnRH pulse generator by the CNS, as the pituitary gland is still responsive to exogenous GnRH. Most theories hold that the onset of puberty reflects disinhibition of the pulse generator. Puberty occurs between ages 8 and 13 in girls and between ages 9 and 14 in boys. In the peripubertal period, sleep-associated bursts of LH secretion can first be detected at night. Subsequently, a gradual increase occurs in LH pulse frequency and amplitude, such that LH pulses are detected during the day and night.

In women, the pattern of GnRH pulse frequency varies across the menstrual cycle. The combination of GnRH stimulation with ovarian feedback regulation results in a complex orchestration of positive and negative hormonal signals that converge at the gonadotrope to regulate LH and FSH secretion. The typical 28-day menstrual cycle is divided into follicular and luteal phases that are separated by ovulation on day 14. Unlike chronic exposure to low concentrations of estrogens, which exert negative feedback regulation and inhibit GnRH, the increasing concentration of estrogen prior to the LH surge exerts positive feedback regulation that results in increased GnRH pulse frequency. Increased GnRH, in combination with increased gonadotrope sensitivity to GnRH, results in the LH/FSH surge. During the luteal phase, the gonadotropin pulse frequency is reduced. In addition to feedback regulation by steroids, ovarian peptides such as inhibin also play a role in control of the reproductive axis. Inhibin causes selective suppression of FSH without affecting LH secretion. A homodimer of inhibin β-subunits, referred to as activin, has opposite actions and selectively stimulates FSH. Circulating inhibin provides one of the negative feedback inputs that lead to FSH suppression as the follicle develops.

The perimenopause is characterized by a gradual cessation of ovarian function. After several years of menstrual cycles that are sometimes anovulatory or irregular, menses cease, thereby defining the menopause. Although there is considerable variation, menopause usually occurs at about age 50. At this point, ovarian follicles have been depleted, and the production of sex steroids changes such that there is minimal production of estrogen and progesterone, but ovarian androgens continue to be made, primarily by stromal cells. The chronic decline in estrogen and progesterone causes loss of feedback inhibition and a marked increase in LH and FSH levels.

In males, the regulation of the HPG axis is relatively constant. After early puberty, LH and FSH pulses occur about once an hour during the night and day. It is notable that there is considerable variation in LH pulse frequency among normal individuals. Because each pulse of LH stimulates testosterone secretion, one also observes pulses of testosterone following LH, although these pulses are muted somewhat by the presence of serum-binding proteins that delay clearance. Nevertheless, testosterone levels can drop below the "normal" range in individuals with slow LH pulse frequencies. Testosterone inhibits the hypothalamic-pituitary axis, although its actions are thought to be mediated, in part, by aromatization to estrogens. Much of the inhibition by gonadal steroids occurs at the hypothalamic level, but there is also evidence for weak inhibition of the gonadotrope at the level of the pituitary gland. The HPG axis in men, unlike that in women, remains intact with aging. However, a gradual decline in testosterone levels is associated with an increase in LH and FSH with aging.

HYPOGONADOTROPIC HYPOGONADISM. Clinical features of hypogonadotropic hypogonadism in women are due primar-

ily to estrogen deficiency and include breast atrophy, vaginal dryness, and diminished libido. Hot flushes are uncommon, in contrast to postmenopausal estrogen deficiency. In premenopausal women, normal menstrual cycles provide evidence for an intact HPG axis. LH and FSH levels should be increased in postmenopausal women. Hypogonadism in men causes decreased libido and sexual function. In men, low testosterone without elevation of LH and FSH is consistent with impaired hypothalamic-pituitary reserve. Because of the variability in circulating testosterone and gonadotropins, it is often necessary to evaluate these hormones on several occasions and at different times of the day. GnRH stimulation can distinguish hypothalamic and pituitary deficiency but may require multiple injections to prime the pituitary, if GnRH deficiency is longstanding.

In premenopausal women, preparations of estrogen and progestins should be used for hormonal replacement and to allow cyclical growth of the endometrium. Pulsatile GnRH (for GnRH-deficient subjects) or gonadotropins can be given to induce ovulation and fertility when desired. Testosterone can be replaced in men using intramuscular injections that are given at 2- to 4-week intervals. Doses and the intervals between injections should be adjusted on an individual basis, using libido and testosterone levels before the next injection as a guide. Oral preparations of androgens should be avoided because of hepatotoxicity. Transdermal preparations are also available, but there is less experience with their long-term acceptance and efficacy. Induction of spermatogenesis requires pulsatile GnRH (for GnRH-deficient subjects) or injections of gonadotropins.

A congenital form of hypogonadotropic hypogonadism is caused by deficiency of GnRH, which in turn causes deficiencies of LH and FSH. When associated with anosmia (absent sense of smell), the condition is referred to as Kallmann's syndrome. A gene defect that causes Kallmann's syndrome has been defined. The so-called KAL gene is located on the tip of the short arm of the X-chromosome and encodes a protein that is proposed to play a critical role in migration of the GnRH-producing neurons during development. Pulsatile GnRH has been used to induce puberty and fertility in both males and females with Kallmann's syndrome.

Secondary hypogonadotropic hypogonadism is relatively common. In most cases it is reversible and is caused by weight loss, anorexia nervosa, stress, heavy exercise, or severe illness. Reversible forms of secondary hypogonadotropic hypogonadism are caused by GnRH deficiency and are more common in women than men. The condition is ideally treated by correcting the underlying cause. Many women have a discrete threshold for weight or exercise level that causes loss of menstrual periods. When it is not possible to correct the underlying abnormality, hormonal replacement can be used in women for protection against osteopenia and to cycle the endometrium.

A variety of pathologic conditions can cause secondary hypogonadotropic hypogonadism, often in association with deficiencies of other pituitary hormones (see Table 202–3). These include hypothalamic lesions or CNS radiation therapy. Pituitary tumors can suppress gonadotropins because of stalk compression and disruption of pulsatile GnRH input as well as by direct destruction of normal pituitary tissue. Hyperprolactinemia can suppress GnRH and lead to reduced gonadotropin levels. In contrast to the aforementioned causes of hypogonadotropic hypogonadism, which result from GnRH deficiency, primary deficiencies of LH and FSH are uncommon. An acquired form of isolated gonadotrope deficiency is rarely encountered and may have an autoimmune basis. Mutations in the LH-β or FSH-β genes have been described in case reports and cause selective loss of individual gonadotropins.

FSH- AND LH-PRODUCING TUMORS. *Etiology and Pathogenesis.* Although most early series suggested that gonadotropin-producing adenomas were relatively uncommon, recent studies using sensitive techniques to characterize tumor phenotype show a prevalence (10 to 15%) that is similar to that of corticotrope or somatotrope adenomas (see Table 202–6). The majority (70 to 80%) of pituitary tumors classified previously as nonfunctioning adenomas can be shown to produce low levels of intact glycoprotein hormones or their uncombined α- or β-subunits. Biosynthetic defects in the tumor cells account for relatively inefficient hormone secretion as well as the propensity to produce uncombined subunits.

FSH is produced more commonly than LH. Elevated levels of free α-subunits are seen more often than increased free β-subunits.

Clinical Features. Gonadotropin-producing tumors are somewhat more common in men than women and increase in prevalence with age. FSH- and LH-producing tumors do not usually cause a characteristic hormone excess syndrome. The tumors are typically large macroadenomas and present as clinically nonfunctioning tumors with symptoms and signs related to local mass effects. Visual field loss due to suprasellar extension and compression of the optic chiasm is found in > 70% of patients. Many of these tumors are detected incidentally by CT and MRI scans performed for unrelated indications. Symptoms of hypopituitarism, including hypogonadism with loss of libido, are also common. Men with predominantly FSH-secreting tumors can paradoxically present with hypogonadal features that are related to low levels of testosterone. These patients must be distinguished from those with primary hypogonadism who have testicular dysfunction. Tumors that primarily secrete LH are rare but can cause increased testosterone levels. Premenopausal women with gonadotropin-producing tumors may experience menstrual irregularity or secondary hypogonadism. Postmenopausal women often show reduced gonadotropin levels because the mass effects of the gonadotropin-producing tumors cause stalk compression, impairing GnRH stimulation of gonadotropins from both normal and pituitary tumor cells.

Diagnosis. Because of the absence of a clinical syndrome in most patients, the preoperative diagnosis of gonadotropin-producing pituitary tumors has relied on imaging studies and laboratory tests. Unfortunately, the laboratory diagnosis of gonadotropin-producing tumors is less than satisfactory. First, the tumors synthesize gonadotropins inefficiently, and hormone levels are usually not markedly elevated. Second, because the secretion of gonadotropins is pulsatile, random LH and FSH values are difficult to interpret. Furthermore, gonadotropin levels vary widely and are normally elevated in postmenopausal women. GnRH stimulation tests also do not clearly distinguish patients with gonadotropin-producing tumors from normals, and suppression tests have not proven useful. However, paradoxical responses to TRH have helped to identify gonadotropin-secreting tumors. In contrast to its effect in normals, TRH stimulates secretion of intact gonadotropins or the uncombined FSH and LH β-subunits in most patients with gonadotropin tumors. Once identified, the uncombined α- or β-subunits can serve as tumor markers and can be useful for monitoring responses to therapy.

Men with proven gonadotropin-producing tumors typically have high-normal or elevated FSH levels but low levels of testosterone. Elevated prolactin levels are commonly seen and are caused by tumor mass effects. It is important to distinguish this group from patients with true prolactinomas. As noted above, many women, including those in the postmenopausal group, have paradoxically low gonadotropin levels. Thus, the absence of elevated gonadotropins does not exclude the diagnosis of a gonadotropin-producing tumor.

The postoperative diagnosis of gonadotropin-producing tumors can be made based upon immunohistochemical analyses or using more sophisticated studies of gonadotropin gene expression. These types of analyses confirm that the great majority of clinically nonfunctioning tumors are composed of gonadotropin-producing cell types.

Treatment. Because the major symptoms of the gonadotropin-producing tumors are due to extrasellar extension and local mass effects, the main aim of treatment is reduction in the size of the tumor. Complete or partial reversal of visual field defects and hypopituitarism can be accomplished by surgery unless these have been longstanding. However, transsphenoidal surgery is rarely curative of this group of macroadenomas. Patients with significant residual tumor may benefit from radiation therapy, although there are no large series in which patients have been randomly allocated to treatment groups. Because most tumors are slow growing, one approach is to monitor tumor recurrence using visual fields and CT or MRI. If tumor markers such as free α- or β-subunit levels are available, they can be used alone or in conjunction with TRH testing to monitor tumor function. When follow-up studies show rapid tumor growth, repeat surgery and/or radiation therapy is indicated.

There has been great interest in medical therapies that might be useful as adjuncts to surgery or even as primary therapies in pa-

tients not requiring immediate decompression. The success of bromocriptine and somatostatin analogues in treating hormone oversecretion and tumor mass in prolactinomas and acromegaly has not been seen in most patients with gonadotropin-producing tumors, although exceptions have been described in selected patients. The efficacy of long-acting GnRH agonists or antagonists, which suppress LH and FSH in normal individuals, has also been examined. The GnRH agonists stimulate gonadotropin secretion from tumors without apparent desensitization and have not been useful. GnRH antagonists have been shown to suppress FSH levels in small series of patients, but it is not clear whether these agents will be useful for reducing tumor size, and this treatment remains experimental.

Daneshdoost L, Pavlou SN, Molitch ME, et al.: Inhibition of follicle-stimulating hormone secretion from gonadotroph adenomas by repetitive administration of a gonadotropin-releasing hormone antagonist. J Clin Endocrinol Metab 71:92, 1990. *Repetitive administration of Nal-Glu GnRH antagonist decreased FSH secretion by gonadotroph adenomas in four of five patients.*

Jameson JL, Klibanski A, Black PM, et al.: Glycoprotein hormone genes are expressed in clinically nonfunctioning pituitary adenomas. J Clin Invest 80:1472, 1987. *This study used measurements of mRNA expression to demonstrate that most clinically nonfunctioning pituitary tumors are derived from gonadotrope cells.*

Snyder PJ: Gonadotroph adenomas of the pituitary. Endocrinol Rev 6:552, 1985. *A good summary of the diagnosis and management of FSH- and LH-producing tumors.*

THYROID-STIMULATING HORMONE

Like the other glycoprotein hormones, TSH is a heterodimer composed of the common α-subunit and the unique TSH β-subunit. Both subunits are glycosylated, and the composition of carbohydrates is thought to alter the biologic activity of the hormone. TSH is produced in thyrotrope cells, which account for about 5% of pituitary cell types. TSH is measured by highly sensitive immunoradiometric assays that use antisera directed toward the TSH β-subunit. Normal levels of TSH range from 0.5 to 5.0 μU per milliliter. The detection limit for current TSH assays is < 0.01 μU per milliliter, allowing measurement of suppressed TSH levels in hyperthyroidism.

TSH controls thyroid hormone (T_4 and T_3) synthesis and secretion from the thyroid gland. TSH receptors are members of the G protein–coupled seven-transmembrane family and are structurally related to LH and FSH receptors. TSH stimulates cAMP production, acts as a trophic hormone, and stimulates hormone biosynthesis in the thyroid. TSH secretion from the pituitary gland is regulated by the hypothalamic-pituitary-thyroid (HPT) axis. Hypothalamic thyrotropin-releasing hormone (TRH) is a tripeptide that stimulates TSH synthesis and secretion. TRH, acting through its G protein–coupled receptor, elicits phosphoinositol turnover and induces release of intracellular calcium followed by an influx of extracellular calcium. TSH secretion appears to be modulated by alterations in calcium flux, whereas biosynthesis may be controlled by activation of other pathways, such as protein kinase C. A variety of other hypothalamic hormones, including somatostatin and dopamine, can inhibit TSH secretion, but their role in normal physiology has not been clearly elucidated.

Thyroid hormones have an inhibitory effect on the production of TRH and TSH and comprise a powerful negative feedback loop in the HPT axis. The direct effects of thyroid hormone at the level of the pituitary gland are well-illustrated by TSH responses to TRH stimulation tests. In hypothyroidism, TSH responses to exogenous TRH are exaggerated. In hyperthyroidism, TSH responses to TRH are blunted or flat, indicating that the inhibitory effects of thyroid hormone override the stimulatory effects of TRH. Thyroid hormones act via nuclear receptors that function at the transcriptional level to suppress expression of the TRH gene as well as the α- and β-subunit genes of TSH. In hypothyroidism, expression of the TSH α and β genes is stimulated and hormone production is markedly enhanced.

TSH secretion is pulsatile, but the amplitude of the pulses is relatively small and does not create the difficulties that are encountered with measurements of other pituitary hormones. TSH levels are elevated in infants in the immediate postpartum period. Thereafter, thyroid function tests remain remarkably constant throughout life. There is a diurnal rhythm of TSH secretion with a small increase at night. Because of the integrated nature of the HPT axis, thyroid function tests are best interpreted when concentrations of TSH, free T_4, and free T_3 levels are known. Except in conditions of secondary hypothyroidism or TSH-secreting pituitary tumors, TSH levels provide an excellent screening test for thyroid dysfunction. In primary hypothyroidism, TSH levels are elevated, as TSH increases logarithmically in response to falling thyroid hormone levels (see Ch. 203). In hyperthyroidism, TSH is suppressed to levels below or near the detection limits of most sensitive assays.

CENTRAL HYPOTHYROIDISM. Central forms of hypothyroidism include secondary hypothyroidism, which is caused by TSH deficiency, and tertiary hypothyroidism, which is caused by TRH deficiency. Two different types of congenital TSH deficiency are caused by genetic mutations. One type involves the TSH β gene, in which several different types of have been described. The other involves mutations in Pit-1, which cause combined deficiencies of GH, Prl, and TSH. Central forms of hypothyroidism are often associated with other pituitary hormone deficiencies and usually there is no goiter because of low TSH levels. Suspicion of central hypothyroidism should prompt measurements of T_4, T_3, and TSH as well as other pituitary hormones. When TSH deficiency is documented, thyroid hormone is replaced using daily doses of L-thyroxine (0.05 to 0.15 mg per day). Because TSH cannot be used as an endpoint, one monitors serum levels of free T_4 and T_3.

Tests for TSH deficiency are best performed by analyzing free thyroxine levels in combination with TSH. Low free T_4 without elevated TSH is consistent with central hypothyroidism. Free T_4 measurements should be used rather than total T_4 to avoid confusion caused by TBG deficiency (which is suggested by high T_3 resin uptake tests). In some patients with hypothalamic disease, the TSH level is partially elevated in the presence of low free T_4, but the bioactivity of the TSH is reduced. Central forms of hypothyroidism must be distinguished from the sick-euthyroid condition (see Ch. 203). Laboratory tests in the sick-euthyroid syndrome progress through several phases but can include prolonged periods when both TSH and free thyroid hormone levels are low. It can be very difficult in these patients to unequivocally exclude central hypothyroidism. In addition to the clinical setting in which thyroid function tests are measured, the presence of normal thyroid function tests prior to the illness and the absence of known hypothalamic or pituitary disease make true central hypothyroidism unlikely. Increased levels of reverse T_3 are suggestive of sick-euthyroidism, and free T_4 and T_3 may be in the normal or low normal range in sick-euthyroid patients.

TSH-SECRETING TUMORS. *Etiology and Pathogenesis.* TSH-secreting tumors are rare and account for between 1 and 3% of pituitary tumors. Like gonadotropin-producing tumors, a subset of tumors classified as clinically nonfunctioning can be shown to produce TSH, often at subclinical levels. However, because TSH overproduction can cause hyperthyroidism, TSH-secreting tumors are more readily detected than FSH- and LH-producing tumors. As many as 30% of TSH-producing tumors are plurihormonal. Growth hormone and prolactin are co-secreted most often, perhaps reflecting a common cellular lineage for thyrotropes, somatotropes, and lactotropes. Longstanding severe hypothyroidism can cause thyrotrope hyperplasia and pituitary enlargement. However, these hyperplastic masses regress upon thyroid hormone replacement. Most true TSH-producing tumors are relatively autonomous and respond weakly, if at all, to TRH stimulation or thyroid hormone suppression.

Clinical Features. TSH-secreting tumors are usually macroadenomas by the time a diagnosis has been made. Consequently, many patients exhibit mass effects of the tumor as well as hyperthyroidism. The clinical features of TSH-secreting tumors resemble those of Graves' disease except that features of autoimmunity such as ophthalmopathy are absent. Circulating levels of T_4 and T_3 range widely but can be elevated as much as two- to threefold. Diffuse goiter is present in the majority of patients with TSH-producing tumors, and the 24-hour uptake of radioiodine is elevated.

Diagnosis. Because feedback inhibition of TSH is impaired in TSH-producing tumors, TSH levels are inappropriately elevated in the presence of high levels of T_4 and T_3. TSH levels produced by tumors range from the low-normal range to as high as 500 μU per milliliter, but most are minimally elevated. Using ultrasensitive TSH assays, it is now possible to detect nonsuppressed TSH levels without the need for TRH testing. Free α-subunit measurements can be very helpful in confirming the diagnosis of a TSH-secreting tumor. Most TSH-producing tumors ($>80\%$) secrete excess free α-subunit. Thus, the diagnosis of a TSH-secreting tumor can usually be made by demonstrating that a hyperthyroid patient has a detectable serum TSH associated with excess secretion of the free α-

subunit and/or GH. The finding of a mass lesion on CT or MRI scan confirms the diagnosis. Several other causes of inappropriate TSH secretion should be considered, including resistance to thyroid hormone and familial dysalbuminemic hyperthyroxinemia and other disorders that alter serum thyroid hormone binding proteins.

Treatment. The goals are to treat the underlying TSH-secreting tumor and to correct the hyperthyroidism. Transsphenoidal surgery alone is rarely curative because of the large size of most tumors, but it can alleviate mass effects and lower TSH levels. As with other large pituitary tumors, adjunctive radiation therapy may be required to control tumor growth. Somatostatin analogues (e.g., octreotide) have been used as adjunctive medical therapy and decrease TSH and α-subunit levels in about 80% patients with TSH-secreting tumors, but consistent effects on tumor growth have not been demonstrated. Hyperthyroidism caused by TSH-secreting tumors can also be treated using antithyroid drugs or radioiodine.

Comi RJ, Gesundheit N, Murray L, et al.: Response of thyrotropin-secreting pituitary adenomas to a long-acting somatostatin analogue. N Engl J Med 317:12, 1987. *This study of five patients with TSH-secreting tumors shows that the somatostatin analogue SMS 201-995 can reduce hypersecretion of TSH.*

NULL CELL PITUITARY TUMORS. Null cell adenomas, or clinically nonfunctioning tumors, are variably defined depending upon the criteria used to analyze tumor cell phenotype. As noted above, the majority of clinically nonfunctioning adenomas can be shown to produce low levels of the free α-subunit, FSH, and, to a lesser degree, LH when analyzed by immunocytochemistry or for mRNA expression. A smaller fraction can be shown to produce low levels of other pituitary hormones, particularly ACTH or GH, that escaped detection by routine endocrine testing. Even with detailed analyses of hormone production, a subset (10 to 20%) of nonfunctioning adenomas do not appear to produce one of the major pituitary hormones.

The clinical features and management of null cell tumors are similar to those for gonadotropin-producing tumors. The major signs and symptoms result from tumor mass effects that cause visual field defects, headache and other neurologic symptoms, and hypopituitarism. Transsphenoidal surgery is the primary mode of treatment, with a goal of debulking the tumor to relieve mass effects. Because there are no serum tumor markers, patients must be followed by CT or MRI scans in conjunction with visual field tests.

202.2 Posterior Pituitary
Alan G. Robinson

ANATOMY AND HORMONE SYNTHESIS. The hormones of the posterior pituitary, vasopressin and oxytocin, are synthesized in specialized neurons, the magnocellular neurons, that are noted for their large size. In the hypothalamus the magnocellular neurons are clustered in the paired paraventricular nuclei and the paired supraoptic nuclei (Fig. 202–3). Vasopressin and oxytocin are also synthesized in parvicellular (small cell) neurons of the paraventricular nuclei, and vasopressin (but not oxytocin) is synthesized in the suprachiasmatic nucleus. Transcription of vasopressin and oxytocin mRNA and translation of vasopressin and oxytocin prohormone occur entirely in the cell bodies of hormone-specific neurons. The preprohormones are cleaved from the signal peptide in the endoplasmic reticulum, and the prohormones, pro-pressophysin and pro-oxyphysin, are packaged with processing enzymes into neurosecretory granules. In the magnocellular neurons the neurosecretory granules are transported via microtubules down the long axons that form the supraopticohypophyseal tract to terminate in axon terminals in the posterior pituitary. During transport the processing enzymes cleave pro-pressophysin to vasopressin (8 a.a.), vasopressin neurophysin (95 a.a.), and vasopressin glycopeptide (39 a.a.) (Fig. 202–4). Pro-oxyphysin is similarly cleaved to oxytocin and oxytocin neurophysin, but not glycopeptide. Within the neurosecretory granules, neurophysins form neurophysin/hormone complexes that stabilize the hormones. Crystallography demonstrates that tetramers of neurophysin form specific binding sites for five molecules of

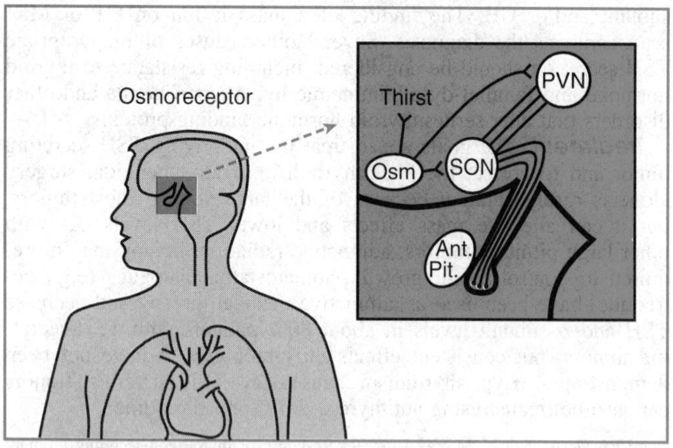

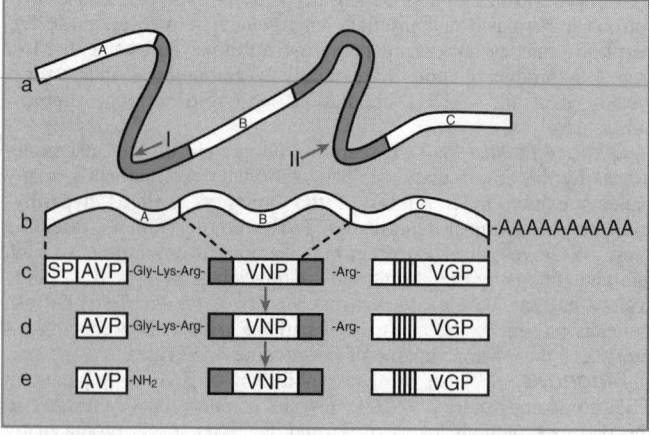

FIGURE 202–3. Sagittal view of the head demonstrating the position of the neurohypophysis. The magnocellular neurons are clustered in two paraventricular nuclei (PVN) and two supraoptic nuclei (SON). Only one nucleus of each pair is illustrated. The supraoptic nuclei are located lateral to the edge of the optic chiasm, while the paraventricular nuclei are central in the wall of the third ventricle. The osmostat and thirst center are located in the hypothalamus anterior to the third ventricle. The axons of the four nuclei combine to form the supraopticohypophyseal tract as they course through the pituitary stalk to their storage terminals in the posterior pituitary. (From Buonocore CM, Robinson AG: Diagnosis and management of diabetes insipidus during medical emergencies. Endocrinol Metab Clin North Am 22:411, 1993.)

hormone. Stimulatory (e.g., cholinergic and angiotensin) neurotransmitter terminals and inhibitory (e.g., γ-aminobutyric acid [GABA], noradrenergic, atrial natriuretic peptide [ANP]) neurotransmitter terminals control release of vasopressin by the activity of contacts on the cell body. Physiologic release of vasopressin and oxytocin into the general circulation is at the level of the posterior pituitary where, in response to an action potential, intracellular calcium is increased to cause the neurosecretory granules to fuse with the axon membrane to release (via exocytosis into the pericapillary) the entire contents of the granule. Once released, there is no further association of vasopressin with neurophysin, and each of the peptide products can be independently detected in the general circulation. Factors that stimulate the release of vasopressin also stimulate synthesis; however, whereas release is instantaneous, synthesis requires a longer time. This may explain the physiologic advantage of the large store of hormone in the posterior pituitary. In most species sufficient hormone is stored in the posterior pituitary to support maximum antidiuresis for several days and baseline levels of antidiuresis for weeks without synthesis of new hormone.

The axons of the parvicellular neurons of the paraventricular nuclei terminate in the median eminence of the basal hypothalamus where, similar to other hypothalamic releasing factors, the hormones are secreted into the portal capillary system and serve as regulators of secretion of adrenocorticotropic hormone (ACTH). Yet other axons secrete hormone into the cerebrospinal fluid of the third ventricle, where the function is unknown.

SECRETION. *Vasopressin and Regulation of Osmolality.* The primary physiologic action of vasopressin is its function as a water-retaining hormone. The central sensing system (osmostat) for control of release of vasopressin is located in a small area of the hypothalamus just anterior to the third ventricle (Fig. 202–3). The osmostat controls release of vasopressin to cause water retention and acts also in stimulation of thirst to cause water repletion. Osmotic regulation of vasopressin release and osmotic regulation of thirst are usually tightly coupled, but experimental lesions and some pathologic situations in humans demonstrate that the regulation can be independent. The primary extracellular osmolyte to which the osmoreceptor responds is sodium. Glucose and urea under normal physiologic conditions readily traverse neuron membranes and do not affect the release of vasopressin. Although the osmolality among normal subjects is between 278 and 294 mOsm per kilogram of water, for each person extracellular fluid osmolality is maintained in a narrow range. An increase in plasma osmolality as little as 1% will stimulate the osmoreceptors to cause release of vaso-

pressin. Basal levels of vasopressin are 0.5 to 2 pg per milliliter, which will maintain urine osmolality above plasma osmolality and urine volume at less than 2 liters per day. With increases in plasma osmolality, there is a linear increase in plasma vasopressin and a linear increase in urine osmolality as illustrated in Figure 202–5. At plasma osmolality of about 294 mOsm per kilogram of water, urine osmolality is maximally concentrated at about 1200 mOsm per kilogram. Thus the entire physiologic range of urine osmolality is accomplished by changes in plasma vasopressin of 0.5 to 5 pg per milliliter.

Water must be not just conserved but consumed as well, in order to replace obligate insensible water loss and obligate urine output. In animals, drinking behavior increases linearly with increases in osmolality similar to the release of vasopressin. In humans, thirst has been less well studied than vasopressin secretion, but it is thought that thirst is not stimulated until a somewhat higher osmolality than the threshold for release of vasopressin. Most humans get sufficient water from catabolism of food or fluids taken daily so that marked thirst is almost never sensed.

Vasopressin acts on V_2, antidiuretic, receptors in the kidney to cause water retention by stimulating cyclic AMP production in the luminal cell membranes of the collecting duct. This opens channels for water transport from the collecting duct to the hypertonic medullary interstitium, and maximum concentration of the final urine is isotonic with the inner medulla of the kidney (see Ch. 74). While the increase in urine osmolality is linear with increases in plasma vasopressin, the changes in urine volume are geometric. This is illustrated in Figure 202–5. Urine volume is maintained at less than 4 liters per day until plasma vasopressin is nearly absent; when maximum urine osmolality decreases to less than 50 mOsm per kilogram, urine volume increases rapidly to 18 to 20 liters per day.

Vasopressin and Pressure and Volume Regulation. In contrast to the osmoregulatory system, volume regulation is anatomically diffuse. High-pressure (baro) receptors are located in the aorta and carotid sinus, and low-pressure volume receptors are located in the left atrium. Stimuli for pressure and volume receptors pass via the glossopharyngeal, ninth, and vagal, tenth, cranial nerves to the brain stem and through the nucleus tractus solitarius to finally converge on the magnocellular neurons, where the predominant action is inhibitory. Decreases in blood pressure or vascular volume stimulate vasopressin release, whereas maneuvers that increase volume or left atrial pressure (e.g., negative pressure breathing) decrease secretion of vasopressin. The release of vasopressin in response to changes in volume or pressure is less sensitive than the release in response to osmoreceptors, and reduction of 10 to 15% in blood volume or pressure is needed to stimulate re-

FIGURE 202–4. Synthesis of vasopressin is via: *a,* three exons *(A,B,C)* with intervening intronic sequences. *b,* The introns are cut out to form mature cytoplasmic RNA. *c,* The preprohormone is synthesized, and signal peptide is cleaved in the endoplasmic reticulum. *d,* The intact precursor is packaged into neurosecretory granules. *e,* The prohormone is subsequently cleaved to the final products: vasopressin, vasopressin neurophysin, and vasopressin glycopeptide. The colored regions of vasopressin precursor are hormone specific. (From Robinson AG, Fitzsimmons MD: Diabetes insipidus. Advances in Endocrinology and Metabolism. Chicago, Mosby-Yearbook, Inc., 1994.)

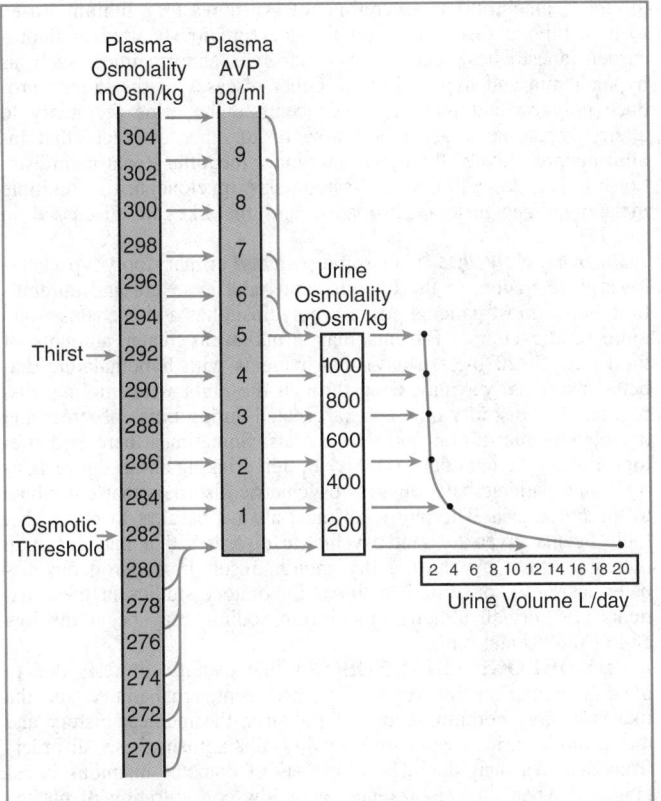

FIGURE 202–5. Idealized schematic of the normal physiologic relationships among plasma osmolality, plasma vasopressin, urine osmolality, and urine volume. The entire physiologic range of urine osmolality occurs with 0 to 5 pg per milliliter of vasopressin. Increases of plasma osmolality above approximately 294 result in increases in plasma vasopressin, but no further concentration of the urine, which is limited by the concentration of the renal inner medulla. Decreases in plasma osmolality below approximately 282 cause no further decrease in vasopressin or increase in urine volume. Note that urine volume is plotted as a horizontal scale to emphasize the geometric relationship between urine volume and urine osmolality. (Adapted from Robinson AG: Disorders of antidiuretic hormone secretion. Clin Endocrinol Metab 14:55, 1985.)

lease of vasopressin. However, once vasopressin is stimulated the increase in response to baroreceptors is logarithmic, and levels of vasopressin achieved are markedly above those achieved by osmotic stimulation. Other nonosmotic stimuli such as nausea and intestinal traction probably act through similar neural pathways to release vasopressin. The effector of the pressor component is the V_1 receptor located on vascular smooth muscle. For V_1 receptors the mechanism of action of vasopressin is to increase intracellular calcium rather than to stimulate adenylate cyclase. In intact animals, pressor activity of vasopressin is weak because of compensatory vasodilatory systems that tend to modulate the action. An action of vasopressin to regulate blood pressure is prominent only when other endocrine systems are deficient (e.g., in autonomic neuropathy).

Interaction of Osmotic and Volume Regulation. In physiologic regulation of water balance, osmotic regulation and volume regulation are usually synergistic. Dehydration causes an increase in osmolality and a decrease in volume, both of which stimulate release of vasopressin. Similarly, excess administration of fluid causes both expansion of volume and decrease in osmolality to inhibit vasopressin secretion. In pathologic situations there may be hyponatremia with inadequate volume, as with diuretic use, or a sense of inadequate volume, as with cardiac failure or cirrhosis. In these situations, volume regulation is predominant and vasopressin levels are high. ANP, described in detail in Ch. 200.3, may affect the osmotic release and action of vasopressin. With volume expansion, ANP is released from atrial myocytes and acts at the kidney to induce natriuresis. ANP is also synthesized in the hypothalamus where it may act to decrease vasopressin secretion.

Physiology of Oxytocin. Oxytocin has similar concentrations in the posterior pituitary of men and women, but a physiologic function for oxytocin has been described only in women. Stimulation of the nipple during suckling causes release of oxytocin to induce myocontraction of ductile smooth muscle in the breast to eject milk. At parturition the uterus becomes increasingly sensitive to oxytocin, and pulses of oxytocin enhance uterine tone at term and delivery. The greatest release of oxytocin occurs with delivery of the infant, probably secondary to stretching of the vaginal wall. Oxytocin may be more important for its effect of inducing uterine contraction that inhibits blood loss after delivery than for its role in initiating parturition. In animal studies, administration of oxytocin to males increases sperm transport, but this has not been documented in humans.

There are no defined syndromes of increased or decreased secretion of oxytocin. Women with diabetes insipidus secondary to traumatic damage of the magnocellular neurons and presumed absence of oxytocin may have normal pregnancy and delivery and breastfeed their infants. Excessive administration of oxytocin to induce labor can stimulate V_2 receptors of the kidney and cause abnormal water retention and hyponatremia.

DIABETES INSIPIDUS

DEFINITION. Diabetes insipidus is the excretion of a large volume of hypotonic, insipid (tasteless) urine, usually accompanied by excessive polydipsia. There are three pathophysiologic mechanisms in the differential diagnosis of diabetes insipidus: (1) *Hypothalamic diabetes insipidus* is the inability to secrete (and usually to synthesize) vasopressin in response to increased osmolality. There is no concentration of the dilute filtrate in the renal collecting duct, and a large volume of urine is excreted. This produces an increase in serum osmolality with stimulation of thirst and secondary polydipsia. Levels of vasopressin in plasma are unmeasurable or low. (2) *Nephrogenic diabetes insipidus* is a disorder in which the otherwise normal kidney is unable to respond to vasopressin. As in hypothalamic diabetes insipidus, the dilute filtrate entering the collecting duct is excreted as a large volume of hypotonic urine. There is a rise in serum osmolality that stimulates thirst and produces polydipsia. Unlike hypothalamic diabetes insipidus, however, measured levels of vasopressin in plasma will be high. (3) *Primary polydipsia* is a primary disorder of thirst stimulation. Ingested water produces a mild decrease in serum osmolality that turns off secretion of vasopressin. In the absence of vasopressin action on the kidney, there is lack of concentration of urine and excretion of a large volume. Measured vasopressin in plasma is low. While the pathophysiologic mechanisms for the three disorders are distinct, patients in each category usually have polyuria, polydipsia, and normal serum sodium. This is because the normal thirst mechanism is sufficiently sensitive to maintain fluid balance in the first two disorders, and the kidney is normally sufficiently responsive to excrete the water load in the third.

CLINICAL PRESENTATION. *Hypothalamic Diabetes Insipidus.* The sudden appearance of hypotonic polyuria after transcranial surgery in the area of the hypothalamus or after head trauma with basal skull fracture and hypothalamic damage obviously suggests the diagnosis of hypothalamic diabetes insipidus. In these situations if the patient is unconscious and unable to recognize thirst, hypernatremia is a common accompaniment. However, even in patients with more insidious progression of a specific disease or in patients with idiopathic hypothalamic diabetes insipidus, the onset of polyuria is often relatively abrupt, occurring over a few days. The presenting problem is the volume of urine and polydipsia, not the decrease in urine osmolality. Most patients do not complain of polyuria until urine volume exceeds 4 liters per day, and, as illustrated in Figure 202–5, urine volume is exponentially related to urine osmolality and plasma vasopressin. Thus, urine volume does not exceed 4 liters per day until the ability to concentrate the urine is severely limited and plasma vasopressin is nearly absent. This same relationship has been observed in dogs with experimental lesions of the hypothalamus. In such dogs there is little increase in urine volume until only 10% of the vasopressin cells remain, and then loss of the remaining 10% produces rapid and marked increase in urine volume to 10 to 15 times normal. Urine volume seldom exceeds the amount of dilute fluid delivered to the collecting duct (about 18 liters in humans), and in many cases is less because patients voluntarily restrict fluid intake, causing some mild volume contraction and increased proximal tubular reabsorption of fluid. Patients often express a preference for cold liquids, which are probably more effective in assuaging thirst. Both thirst and urine output persist through the night. In patients with partial diabetes insipidus there is some ability to secrete vasopressin, but this secretion is markedly attenuated at normal levels of plasma osmolality. Therefore, these patients have symptoms and urine volume only moderately different from patients with complete diabetes insipidus. As most patients with hypothalamic diabetes insipidus have sufficient thirst to drink fluid to match urine output, there are few laboratory abnormalities at the time of presentation. Serum sodium may be in the high normal range, while blood urea nitrogen (BUN) and uric acid may be low secondary to large urine volume.

A variant of hypothalamic diabetes insipidus is the syndrome of absent osmostat with intact volume receptors. This syndrome is referred to as essential hypernatremia because the patients have increased sodium and absence of thirst. Physiologic maneuvers demonstrate that when the patients are euvolemic, an increase in plasma osmolality produces neither secretion of vasopressin nor sensation of thirst. However, vasopressin is synthesized by the hypothalamus and stored in the posterior pituitary because stimulation of baroreceptors results in prompt secretion of vasopressin, and the kidney is responsive because vasopressin release by volume receptor stimulation causes urinary concentration. Because patients lack thirst, they are chronically dehydrated with increased serum sodium. The amount of urine output depends on the degree of dehydration-induced secretion of vasopressin. Given sufficient fluid replacement to return extracellular volume to normal, patients become markedly polyuric and manifest the underlying diabetes insipidus.

Rarely, hypothalamic diabetes insipidus occurs as an autosomal dominant pattern of inherited disease. In reported families, the disorders are due to single nucleotide substitution or deletion in the vasopressin gene. Interestingly, in an animal model of hereditary diabetes insipidus (the Brattleboro rat), which is also due to a single nucleotide deletion, the diabetes insipidus is autosomal recessive. Diabetes insipidus is expressed only in the homozygote rat because both alleles of the gene are expressed, and 50% expression of vasopressin is adequate to allow normal water balance. In the human disorder, diabetes insipidus is not present at birth, which suggests normal synthesis of vasopressin. But, by an as-yet-undetermined mechanism, the abnormal vasopressin translation product synthesized by the mutant allele causes destruction of vasopressinergic neurons. Cell death produces diabetes insipidus later in childhood or early in adult years.

Diabetes insipidus with onset during pregnancy may be due to rapid catabolism of vasopressin. The placenta produces a cystine-aminopeptidase (oxytocinase or vasopressinase) that enzymatically destroys vasopressin and thus increases the metabolic clearance rate of vasopressin. Polyuria most often becomes manifest in patients who have some underlying decreased ability to secrete vasopressin or to respond to vasopressin action, e.g., partial hypothalamic diabetes insipidus or compensated nephrogenic diabetes insipidus. Treatment may be required only during the pregnancy, and the patient may return to her previous baseline function without need for therapy when the pregnancy ends. In some patients, hypothalamic diabetes insipidus due to any cause first becomes symptomatic during pregnancy and then persists with the usual course.

Myxedema and adrenal insufficiency both impair the ability to excrete free water by renal mechanisms. The simultaneous occurrence of either of these diseases with diabetes insipidus (as may occur with a tumor of the hypothalamus or pituitary) may decrease the large urine output of diabetes insipidus. Replacement treatment for the anterior pituitary deficiency, especially glucocortocoids, may cause sudden and massive excretion of dilute urine. Similarly, the onset of either hypothyroidism or adrenal insufficiency during the course of diabetes insipidus may decrease the need for vasopressin replacement and even cause hyponatremia.

Nephrogenic Diabetes Insipidus. The gene for the V_2 receptor has been localized to the Xq 28 region of the X chromosome. In familial nephrogenic diabetes insipidus, symptoms are noted only in patients homozygous for the disorder, and affected males have excessive polyuria and dehydration from birth.

Nephrogenic diabetes insipidus may also be acquired during treatment with certain drugs such as demeclocycline (which is used

to treat inappropriate secretion of vasopressin), lithium (used to treat bipolar disorders), and fluoride (previously used in fluorocarbon anesthetics) and from electrolyte abnormalities such as hypokalemia and hypercalcemia. Other diseases of the kidney produce polyuria and inability to concentrate the urine secondary to altered renal medullary blood flow or to other disorders that inhibit maintenance of the hypertonic inner medulla. Renal manifestations of sickle cell disease, sarcoidosis, pyelonephritis, multiple melanoma, analgesic nephropathy, and the like are discussed in Ch. 77.

Primary Polydipsia. In some patients, primary polydypsia follows acute trauma to the hypothalamus and is severe and unremitting, but in most patients primary polydipsia has a slower onset and more erratic course. Patients may drink even greater amounts of fluid (e.g., >20 liters a day) than patients with hypothalamic diabetes insipidus, yet may sleep through the night with minimal disruption. The disorder may be exacerbated during times of stress and not bothersome during normal intervals. Sometimes there is a lifelong history of habitual excessive water drinking in an entire family. Some patients have obvious psychiatric disorders that contribute to the polydipsia. The physician must always be alert to pharmacologic agents given to treat psychiatric disorders that may result in increased thirst by causing dry mouth, result in nephrogenic diabetes insipidus, or stimulate thirst. Laboratory studies in these patients are normal, although the serum sodium may be at the low end of the normal range.

PHYSIOLOGIC DIAGNOSIS. While osmotic diuresis due to hyperglycemia, an intravenous contrast agent, renal injury, and the like is a more common cause of polyuria, the medical history and the isotonic urine osmolality readily distinguish these disorders from diabetes insipidus. The diagnosis of diabetes insipidus is established when there is absence of or low concentration of plasma vasopressin and inappropriately low urine osmolality in the presence of elevated serum osmolality due to increased serum sodium. These criteria may be met at presentation, especially in acute diabetes insipidus occurring after trauma or after surgery in which there has not been adequate fluid replacement. In a patient with hypernatremia and hypotonic urine osmolality with normal renal function, diabetes insipidus is diagnosed. One need only administer a vasopressin agonist and document a renal response with decreased urine volume and increased urine osmolality to confirm the diagnosis of hypothalamic diabetes insipidus. Sometimes in the postoperative state there is water diuresis secondary to water retention during the surgical procedure. Vasopressin is normally secreted in response to surgical stress, and intravenously administered fluid may be retained. During recovery, when vasopressin levels fall, there is diuresis of the retained fluid. If further fluid is administered to match the urine output, persistent polyuria might be mistaken for diabetes insipidus. In this situation the physician should decrease the rate of fluid administered and observe the urine output and the serum sodium. If the serum sodium rises above the normal range and the urine is still hypotonic, the response to a vasopressin agonist will document the diagnosis of diabetes insipidus.

Most outpatients will have polyuria, polydipsia, and normal sodium. In these patients it is necessary to perform a test to increase serum osmolality and to measure urinary response. The best described and easiest to administer is the dehydration test and subsequent response to vasopressin (Fig. 202–6). The test should be carried out under controlled observation in the hospital or an appropriately equipped outpatient area. The timing of test administration depends on the symptoms of the patient. If the patient has marked polyuria during the night, it is best to begin the test during the day because the patient readily may become dehydrated. If the patient has only two or three episodes of nocturia per night, it may be best to begin the test in the evening so the major part of the dehydration takes place when the patient is asleep. In either case, the patient is weighed at the beginning of the test and the volume and osmolality (usually determined by freezing point depression) of all excreted urine are measured. The patient is weighed after output of each liter of urine. When two consecutive urine samples have osmolality differing by no more than 10% and the patient has lost 2% of body weight, a blood sample is obtained for measurement of serum osmolality, sodium, and plasma vasopressin. The patient is then given 2 μg of desmopressin intravenously or intramuscularly (or 5 units of aqueous vasopressin). Patients with normal levels of vasopressin have $<5\%$ increase in urine osmolality in response to the administered desmopressin. Patients with complete hypothalamic diabetes

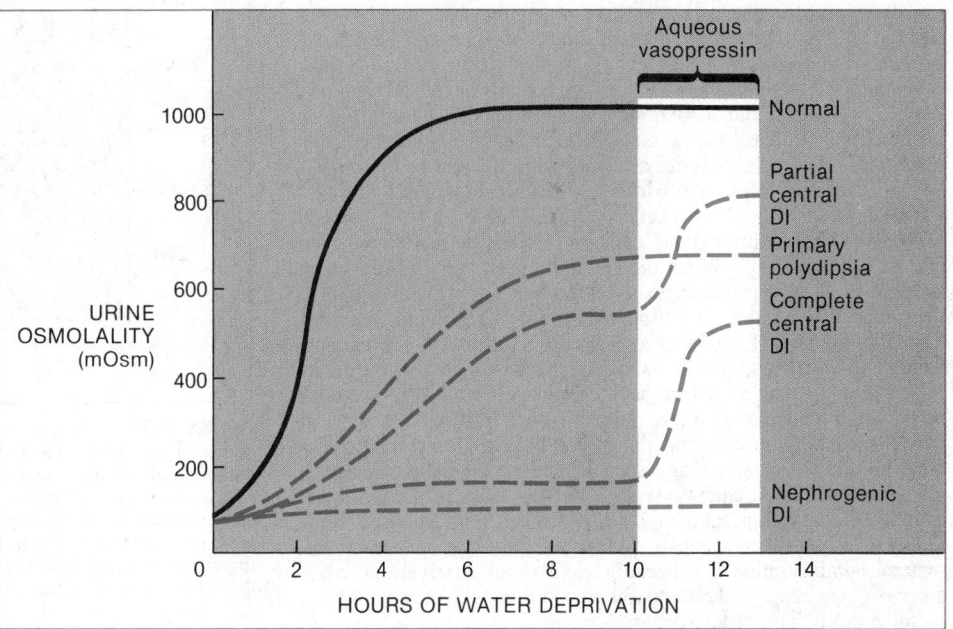

FIGURE 202–6. Responses to the dehydration test described by Miller et al., Annals of Internal Medicine (1970), to differentiate various types of diabetes insipidus and primary polydipsia. The response to dehydration shows a plateau, and the subsequent change in urine osmolality in response to administered vasopressin is illustrated. See discussion in text. *DI* = diabetes insipidus. (From Dennis VW: Investigations of renal function. *In* Wyngaarden JB, Smith LH, Jr, Bennett JC [eds.]: Cecil's Textbook of Medicine, 19th ed. Philadelphia, WB Saunders, 1992, p 495.)

insipidus have minimal concentration of the urine with dehydration and marked increase in urine osmolality in response to administered desmopressin (usually greater than 50%).

In patients with nephrogenic diabetes insipidus there usually is no urine concentration in response to administered vasopressin, although in some cases of acquired nephrogenic diabetes insipidus some urinary concentration may result. Nephrogenic diabetes insipidus is unequivocally distinguished from hypothalamic diabetes insipidus by measure of vasopressin in plasma by radioimmunoassay. Vasopressin levels are usually elevated in nephrogenic diabetes insipidus.

In patients with partial hypothalamic diabetes insipidus and patients with primary polydipsia, the urine is somewhat concentrated in response to dehydration, but it cannot be expected to be concentrated to the maximum of a normal person because the large urine volume, regardless of cause, washes out the medullary osmotic gradient that determines the maximum urine concentration. When vasopressin is administered, patients with partial hypothalamic diabetes insipidus have a further increase (usually greater than 10%) in urine osmolality, whereas patients with primary polydipsia have no further increase. There is controversy about the reliability of distinguishing these last two disorders. Some patients with primary polydipsia may not become sufficiently dehydrated with the test to secrete maximum vasopressin and hence will have an increase in urine osmolality in response to administered desmopressin. Alternatively, some patients with partial diabetes insipidus may become sufficiently dehydrated so there is maximal concentration of urine during the test and no further response to administered desmopressin. When plasma vasopressin assays become sufficiently sensitive, reliable, and available, plasma vasopressin levels at the end of dehydration may better distinguish these two disorders. In the meantime, it is important to have adequate follow-up of patients with partial diabetes insipidus to ensure that during treatment with vasopressin a good therapeutic response is obtained, as would be expected, and that hyponatremia does not occur, as might be expected if the patient had primary polydipsia.

ETIOLOGIC DIAGNOSIS. The dehydration test will confirm that absence of vasopressin is responsible for the polyuria, but the cause of the lack of vasopressin must then be determined. As noted above, vasopressin is synthesized in paired paraventricular nuclei high on the walls of the third ventricle and paired supraoptic nuclei lateral to and above the optic chiasm (see Fig. 202–3). As diabetes insipidus is symptomatic only when 80 to 90% of the vasopressin cells are destroyed, a lesion must be quite large or strategically located where the paths from the four nuclear groups converge into the pituitary stalk just above the diaphragma sellae. Such lesions can be recognized by nuclear magnetic resonance (NMR) scans of the brain. In about 80% of normal subjects, NMR shows a high intense signal (bright spot) in the posterior pituitary on T_1-weighted

images. Commonly in diabetes insipidus, there is loss of the hyperintense signal of the posterior pituitary, which is thought to be due to depletion of stored hormone. It is not known exactly what component of the hormone precursor store is responsible for the hyperintense signal.

Tumors that cause diabetes insipidus are most often benign primary intracranial tumors such as craniopharyngioma, ependymoma (suprasellar germinoma), or pinealoma that arises in the third ventricle. Primary tumors of the anterior pituitary cause diabetes insipidus only when there is suprasellar extension. Metastasis to the hypothalamus from lung, breast, melanoma, and the like may lodge in the portal capillaries of the median eminence and destroy the supraopticohypophyseal tract to cause diabetes insipidus. Granulomatous diseases, such as Langerhans' cell histiocytosis, sarcoidosis, or tuberculosis, may destroy vasopressin cells in the hypothalamus. Leukemic infiltrates of the hypothalamus may cause diabetes insipidus. In diseases with peripheral manifestations the diagnosis is usually suspected on the basis of general medical findings. Idiopathic diabetes insipidus is probably an autoimmune disease, and other autoimmune diseases are recognized in affected patients. When CNS disease is suspected but not diagnosed by NMR or general physical examination, cerebrospinal fluid obtained by lumbar puncture may be helpful in identifying tumor cells or tumor markers. Widening of the posterior pituitary stalk is observed on NMR with a variety of infiltrative diseases of the neurohypophysis, including idiopathic diabetes insipidus, Langherans' cell histiocytosis, suprasellar germinoma, sarcoidosis, tuberculosis, and metastatic disease. An NMR study with a widened pituitary stalk and absence of the hyperintense signal of the posterior pituitary on T_1 is especially suggestive of a granulomatous or inflammatory disease and should prompt the search for evidence of granulomatous disease elsewhere in the body.

Rarely, if patients with diabetes insipidus are unable to drink or are given a hypertonic solution, they develop severe acute hypernatremia. Osmotic equilibrium with intracellular water of neurons and glia produces shrinking of the brain. The brain is in a closed vault (skull), and when the brain shrinks there is engorgement of vasculature of the CNS. Rupture of vessels may produce subarachnoid hemorrhage, gross intracerebral hemorrhage, or intracerebral petechial hemorrhages producing permanent brain damage. If, however, the hypernatremia persists over a longer time, accommodation of the neurons occurs by production of "idiogenic osmoles," which decreases the amount of brain neuron shrinkage. These events, which also occur in nonketotic hyperosmolar coma, will affect treatment recommendations.

TREATMENT. Water diuresis is the primary manifestation of diabetes insipidus and water replacement in adequate quantities avoids metabolic complications. The aim of therapy is to reduce the amount of polyuria and polydipsia to a tolerable level while avoiding overtreatment that might produce water retention and hyponatremia. The best therapeutic agent is the vasopressin agonist desmopressin. Desmopressin is different from vasopressin in that the terminal amino group of cystine has been removed to prolong the duration of action and a D-arginine is substituted for L-arginine in position 8 to decrease the pressor effect. In therapeutic dosage, this agent acts on V_2, antidiuretic, receptors with minimal action on V_1, pressor, receptors. Desmopressin is available for intranasal administration in a spray bottle that delivers a fixed dose of 10 μg in 100 μl or in a bottle with a rhinal catheter that can deliver from 25 to 200 μl (2.5 to 20 μg). When therapy is initiated, it is best to begin at night to allow the patient to sleep through the night and then to determine the duration of action by quantifying polyuria the next day. The duration of action of a single dose varies between patients from 6 to 24 hours, but in most patients a dosage can be determined that gives a good therapeutic response on an every-12-hour schedule. If patients are never polyuric on a 12-hour schedule, it may be advisable to delay administration of a dose once or twice a week to allow diuresis of any accumulated water. Desmopressin is also available for parenteral use in 2 ml vials of 4 μg per milliliter; 5 to 10% of an intranasal quantity administered intravenously, intramuscularly, or subcutaneously gives an equivalent response. Parenteral administration is especially useful postoperatively or when a patient is unable to take the nasal preparation.

Some orally administered pharmacologic agents are also useful in treating diabetes insipidus. Chlorpropamide in doses of 100 to 500 mg daily enhances the effect of vasopressin at the renal tubule and is especially useful in patients with partial hypothalamic diabetes insipidus. Maximum antidiuresis is achieved after 4 days of administration. Carbamazepine (Tegretol) in doses of 200 to 600 mg per day causes release of vasopressin. Clofibrate also stimulates the release of endogenous vasopressin in doses of 500 mg every 6 hours. Thiazide diuretics cause sodium depletion and volume contraction and decrease urine volume by increasing proximal tubular reabsorption of glomerular filtrate. Ibuprofen blocks the normal inhibitory action of prostaglandin E on vasopressin action on the kidney. While ibuprofen is not a primary treatment, it may alter the antidiuretic response of other agents. For each of these pharmacologic agents the prescribing physician should be careful of potential toxicity and side effects.

Some situations require special attention in therapy. If the patient has been chronically hypernatremic and the brain has had time to adapt with production of idiogenic osmoles as described above, therapy should not be overly zealous. Too rapid lowering of osmolality in the extracellular fluid will produce a shift of water into the brain and cause cerebral edema. In this situation, desmopressin can be administered, but the amount of water should be regulated to decrease osmolality by no more than about 1 mEq every 2 hours. Postoperatively or after head trauma, diabetes insipidus may be transient (see prognosis below), and long-term maintenance therapy cannot be reliably established. Pregnant patients with diabetes insipidus can be treated with desmopressin, which has a normal duration of action because it is not destroyed by vasopressinase. It has the additional advantage of having very little action on the oxytocin receptors of the uterus. However, during pregnancy normal plasma osmolality decreases by 10 mOsm per kilogram because of changes in serum sodium. Patients with diabetes insipidus treated during pregnancy require sufficient desmopressin to maintain serum sodium at this lower level.

COURSE AND PROGNOSIS. The prognosis of properly treated diabetes insipidus is excellent. Historical complications of bladder hypertrophy and hydroureter secondary to voluntarily decreasing urine frequency are largely unseen with modern therapy. When the diabetes insipidus is secondary to a recognized disease process, it is that disease that determines the ultimate prognosis. There are some specific clinical situations in which the course is different and characteristic. Postoperative or post-traumatic diabetes insipidus is often due to rupture of the pituitary stalk and can follow a course referred to as "triphasic" (Fig. 202–7). The first phase is diabetes insipidus due to axon shock and lack of release of vasopressin. This lasts for 5 to 10 days. This is followed by a second phase of antidiuresis, which is thought to be produced by uncontrolled release of vasopressin from the large storage pool in the axon terminals of the posterior pituitary. This store is sufficient to

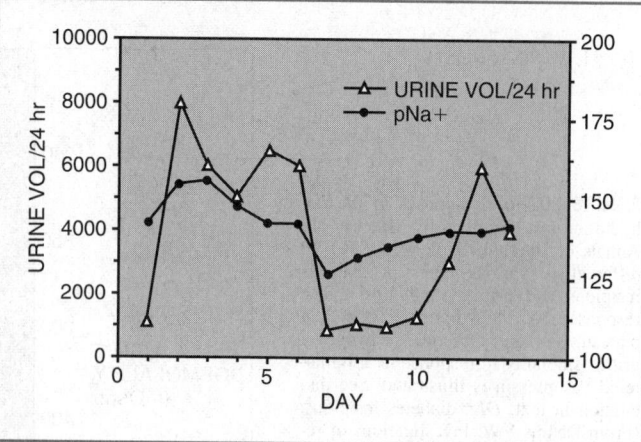

FIGURE 202–7. Triphasic response to trauma of the pituitary stalk. Urine output *(open triangles)* and serum Na+ *(solid dots)* are illustrated. Note the onset of diabetes insipidus immediately after the head trauma and lasting for 6 days. On days 7 through 10 there was a marked decrease in diuresis (with elevated urine osmolality) typical of the second phase with inappropriate release of vasopressin. During this time the patient actually became hyponatremic and required fluid restriction to treat the hyponatremia. After day 10 there was return of diabetes insipidus.

produce constant antidiuresis for an additional 5 to 10 days. The possibility of this course developing is one reason for closely following desmopressin therapy in the postoperative or post-traumatic patient. Continued administration of desmopressin and especially continued forcing of fluids either orally or parenterally will produce profound hyponatremia during the second phase. Hyponatremia is often heralded by nausea or vomiting, and severe hyponatremia may cause cerebral edema and serious neurologic sequelae. Thus, fluids may need to be restricted during this period, as they are in therapy of inappropriate secretion of antidiuretic hormone. The third or final phase is the return of diabetes insipidus after the pool of stored vasopressin has been exhausted. This may be permanent or transient. Eventually there may be return of sufficient vasopressin function to allow a lessening in intensity or discontinuation of treatment. This usually occurs within the first year of diabetes insipidus, but has occurred as long as 10 years after the initiating event. Potential return of function is another reason for occasionally withholding therapy during long-term treatment. Interestingly, the second phase of excess vasopressin and hyponatremia has been reported without preceding or subsequent diabetes insipidus. This is reported as postoperative syndrome of inappropriate secretion of antidiuretic hormone. It is probably due to trauma to only some vasopressin axons. There are sufficient functioning vasopressin neurons to prevent the diabetes insipidus of the first and third phase, but sufficient leakage of vasopressin to cause the second phase. It is only the setting and timing that identify this as an isolated second phase of the triphasic response.

Diabetes insipidus should not be considered idiopathic until after 4 years of follow-up. Over this interval, annual CT or NMR scans are indicated to test for the appearance of a tumor or infiltrative process that may not have been detected at the initial examination.

SYNDROME OF INAPPROPRIATE SECRETION OF ANTIDIURETIC HORMONE

Excess secretion of vasopressin can be caused by abnormal secretion from the posterior pituitary or by ectopic synthesis and secretion of vasopressin by a tumor. The excess vasopressin causes water retention, volume expansion, and natriuresis producing hyponatremia. This disorder is discussed in Ch. 75.

Holtzman EJ, Harris HW, Kolakowski LF, et al.: A molecular defect in the vasopressin V2-receptor gene causing nephrogenic diabetes insipidus. N Engl J Med 328:1534, 1993. *Molecular cause of hereditary nephrogenic diabetes insipidus.*

Ito M, Oiso Y, Murase T, et al.: Possible involvement of inefficient cleavage of preprovasopressin by signal peptidase as a cause for familial central diabetes insipidus. J Clin Invest 91:2565, 1993. *Identity of a genetic defect producing familial central diabetes insipidus.*

Iwasaki Y, Oiso Y, Kondo K, et al.: Aggravation of subclinical diabetes insipidus during pregnancy. N Engl J Med 324:522, 1991. *Compensated partial hypothalamic diabetes insipidus and compensated nephrogenic diabetes insipidus may both become symptomatic during pregnancy.*

Maghnie M, Villa A, Arico M, et al.: Correlation between magnetic resonance imaging of posterior pituitary and neurohypophyseal function in children with diabetes insipidus. J Clin Endocrinol Metab 74:795, 1992. *Describes characteristic hyperintense signal of posterior pituitary on T_1-weighted images with MRI and describes thickened pituitary stalk that may be seen in diabetes insipidus.*

Merendino JJ, Spiegel AM, Crawford JD, et al.: A mutation in the vasopressin V2-receptor gene in a kindred with X-linked nephrogenic diabetes insipidus. N Engl J Med 328:1538, 1993. *Molecular cause of hereditary nephrogenic diabetes insipidus.*

Miller M, Dalakos T, Moses AM, et al.: Recognition of partial defects in antidiuretic hormone secretion. Ann Intern Med 73:721, 1970. *Guide to performing and interpreting dehydration test, which is the "standard" for differential diagnosis of diabetes insipidus.*

Reeves WB, Andreoli TE: The posterior pituitary and water metabolism. *In* Wilson JD, Foster DW (eds.): Williams Textbook of Endocrinology, 8th ed. Philadelphia, WB Saunders, 1992, pp 311–356. *Extensively referenced chapter with detailed description of anatomy of neurohypophysis and physiology of vasopressin and oxytocin.*

Robinson AG, Verbalis JG: Diabetes insipidus. *In* Bardin CW (ed.): Current Therapy in Endocrinology and Metabolism, 5th ed. St. Louis, C.V. Mosby, 1994, pp 1–6. *Concise guide to various acute and chronic treatments of diabetes insipidus.*

203 THE THYROID

Wolfgang H. Dillmann

Anatomy and Physiology

The thyroid, the largest endocrine gland in the body, weighs about 20 grams, the right lobe usually being larger than the left. Adult size is reached at age 15. The two lateral lobes lie anterior to the thyroid cartilage and are connected by a small isthmus located just below the cricoid cartilage. The lobes have a pointed superior pole and a rounded inferior pole with a thickness of about 2 cm, a length of 4 to 5 cm, and a width of 2 to 3 cm. The lobes are divided by fibrous septae into pseudolobes composed of spherical structures called follicles. A dense capillary network surrounds the follicles, which are richly innervated by sympathetic and parasympathetic nerve endings. The follicles consist of a single layer of epithelial cells surrounding a lumen filled with a proteinaceous colloid material consisting of over 75% thyroglobulin. Thyroglobulin is formed by the epithelial thyroid cells, which both synthesize and store the hormone.

A feedback loop involving the hypothalamus, pituitary, and thyroid gland regulates the glandular secretion of thyroid hormone (Fig. 203–1). The hypothalamus generates thyroid-releasing hormone (TRH) to energize pituitary thyroid-stimulating hormone (TSH). TSH, in turn, stimulates thyroid hormonal output, which feeds back on both hypothalamus and pituitary to complete the regulatory circle.

Thyroid Hormone Formation

Thyroxine (T_4) is the major secretory product of the thyroid, with a daily production rate of 80 to 100 μg. T_4 is produced only by the thyroid gland. In contrast, only 20% of the daily production rate of triiodothyronine (T_3) is derived from thyroid secretion and 80% from peripheral T_4 conversion (Fig. 203–2). The daily production rate of T_3 is 30 to 40 μg. Normal thyroid hormone formation requires normal levels of TSH and an adequate but not excessive supply of iodine. Optimal iodine intake is about 150 to 300 μg per day. In some mountainous areas of the world, daily iodine supplies can be as low as 20 to 30 μg. The United States population, however, has a high iodine intake, with a daily supply of 600 to 700 μg, much of which derives from food additives such as iodized salt and flour. Iodine is reduced to iodide (I^-) in the gastrointestinal tract and readily absorbed. Iodide is removed from the bloodstream by uptake and concentration in the thyroid gland and excretion in the urine. Under normal conditions, the kidney clears iodide from plasma at about 30 ml per minute, whereas thyroid clearance is 8 ml per minute, so that only 25% of intake enters the thyroid under normal conditions. Excess iodine intake levels the percentage of uptake; reduced intake raises it. Thyroid uptake of iodide varies from 5 to 30%. Other organs such as the salivary glands, mammary glands, gastric mucosa, and choroid plexus also can take up iodine but cannot form thyroid hormone. The ability of the thyroid to actively accumulate iodine through an iodide transporter localized in the cell membrane leads to a 20 to 40:1 concentration gradient of cell to plasma. The iodide in the thyroid cells is rapidly oxidized and enzymatically incorporated via thyroid peroxidase into tyrosine molecules of thyroglobulin by a process called organification. Thyroid peroxidase requires activation by H_2O_2. A flavoprotein enzyme, presumably an NAPDH cytochrome C reductase, generates H_2O_2, but the precise identity of the H_2O_2-generating system is uncertain. Antithyroid medications such as propylthiouracil (PTU) and methimazole inhibit thyroid peroxidase, thereby decreasing thyroid hormone formation. Thyroid hormone formation occurs on thyroglobulin, a 660-kD glycoprotein, with 25% of its tyrosine residues accessible to iodination. The monoiodinated tyrosine (MIT) and the deiodinated tyrosine (DIT) are coupled by the thyroid peroxidase enzyme to form T_4 by linking two DIT's or, for T_3 formation, linking one MIT and one DIT molecule. Thyroglobulin contains only 3 or 4 T_4 and 0.2 to 0.3 T_3 residues. The organification and coupling reactions on thyroglobulin occur at the luminal border of the thyrocyte, which then exocytoses and stores it as colloid. Thyroid hormone secretion starts with endocytosis of a colloid droplet by the luminal cell membrane of the thyrocyte. The colloid droplet then combines with lysosomes to form phagolysosomes with thyroglobulin proteolysis and release of T_4 and T_3 at the basal border into the capillaries. Iodotyrosine and especially MIT and DIT, which are liberated from thyroglobulin, are deiodinated by a specific deiodinase. Iodide thus liberated mixes with iodide entering from the blood and is reused for organification. Decreased levels of this deiodinase rarely may cause goiter and hypothyroidism.

REGULATION OF THYROID HORMONE SYNTHESIS

Thyroid hormone synthesis is influenced by intrathyroidal factors, primarily the amount of iodide in the thyroid cell; by extrathyroidal factors, especially peptide hormones, which can occupy the TSH receptor especially under normal conditions; and by the thyroid-stimulating immunoglobulin (TSI) in Graves' disease. Under conditions of very low iodine intake, T_3 preferentially is formed instead of T_4. Iodide excess in the thyroid leads to a short-term inhibition of thyroid hormone formation. After about 48 hours, however, the iodide transporter system decreases and thyroid hormone formation returns to normal in spite of elevated circulating iodide levels. Excess iodide also inhibits thyroid hormone release. Increased iodination of thyroglobulin increases its resistance to proteolytic degradation, thereby freeing less T_4 and T_3. Paradoxically, excess iodide can also increase thyroid hormone formation, especially in abnormal

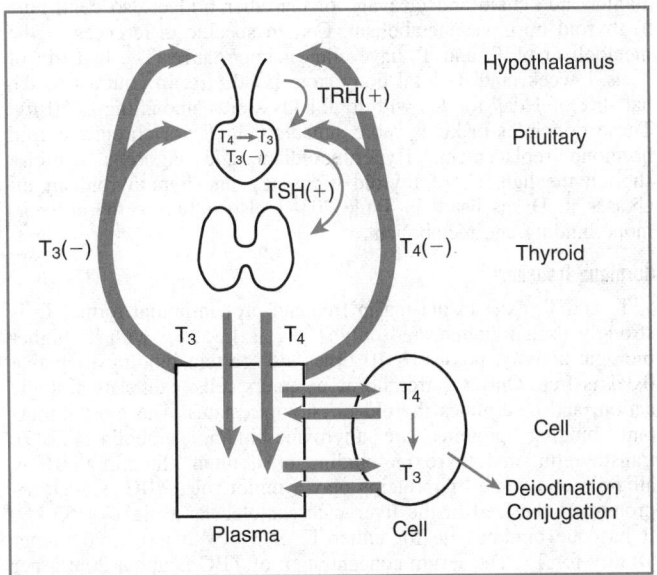

FIGURE 203–1. Hypothalamic-pituitary-thyroid interrelationship. TRH exerts a positive stimulatory effect on TSH secretion, which stimulates thyroid hormone formation. T_4 is the primary thyroid secretory product which is converted in the cells of specific organs, such as kidney and liver, to T_3. T_3 is the most biologically active thyroid hormone and is inactivated by further deiodination or conjugation and biliary excretion.

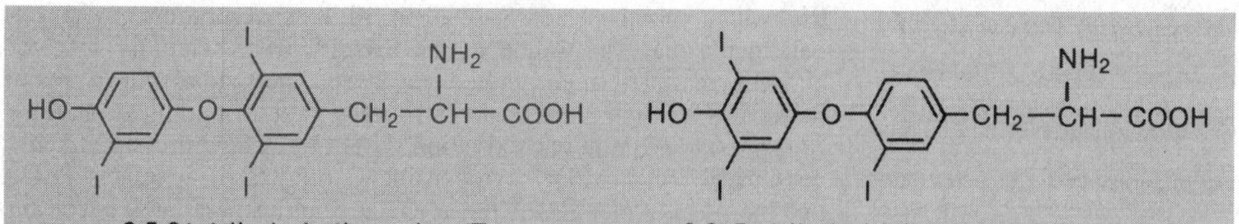

FIGURE 203–2. Structure of the thyroid hormones.

3,5,3′–triiodo L-thyronine (T_3)   3,3′,5′–triiodo L-thyronine (reverse T_3)

thyroid glands. For these reasons, iodine should not be used to treat thyroid diseases except under special conditions. In addition to iodide, TSH influences thyroid function by stimulating all steps of thyroid hormone formation. TSH binding to TSH receptors stimulates cAMP formation and subsequently protein kinase A activity. Such binding also stimulates the phospholipase C–based signaling system and the *ras* proto-oncogene kinase pathway. In addition to the marked influences that are exerted on thyroid hormone formation by iodide and TSH, IGF-1, EGF, prostaglandins, and cytokines such as interleukins and catecholamines modify thyroid function.

EXTRATHYROIDAL HORMONE PRODUCTION AND TURNOVER

Most T_3 is produced by extrathyroidal 5′ deiodination of T_4, which allows for alteration in T_3 production independent of changes in thyroid function. Because T_3 is three to four times as biologically active as T_4, extrathyroidal regulation of T_3 levels has important consequences reflected by the nonthyroidal illness syndrome discussed below. The conversion of T_4 to T_3 is performed by two forms of 5′ deiodinases. Type I 5′ deiodinase contains the rarely used amino acid selenocysteine and is most active in liver and kidney. The activity of Type I 5′ deiodinase declines with hypothyroidism and is inhibited by propylthiouracil and glucocorticoids. Type II 5′ deiodinase is active in the central nervous system (CNS), pituitary, brown adipose tissue, and placenta. It resists inhibition by PTU and increases with hypothyroidism, resulting in near-normal CNS T_3 levels. A third deiodinase, termed 5 deiodinase or Type III 5 deiodinase, removes the inner ring iodide to form the biologically inactive reverse T_3 from T_4 and metabolizes T_3 to diiodothyronine (T_2). The thyroid hormone derivatives, including reverse T_3 and the di- and monothyronine compounds, have no currently recognized biologic importance.

In addition to deiodination, by which 80% of T_4 is metabolized, thyroid hormones are metabolized by transfer of glucoronyl and sulfate residues to the phenolic hydroxyl group of thyroid hormone and by biliary excretion. Deamination and decarboxylation of the alanine side chain and cleavage of the ether bridge also contribute to thyroid hormone metabolism. Certain specific differences in the metabolism of T_4 and T_3 have clinical importance. The half-life of T_4 is 1 week, and its total body store is 800 μg, in contrast to the half-life of 1 day for T_3, with total body stores amounting to 50 μg. These principles make T_4 more suitable than T_3 for chronic thyroid hormone replacement. Hyperthyroidism and vigorous exercise shorten the half-life of thyroid hormones, and hypothyroidism increases it. Drugs listed in Table 203–1 also influence thyroid hormone binding and metabolism.

Hormone Transport

T_4 and T_3 exist in plasma in free and protein-bound forms. T_4 is strongly protein-bound, and only 0.03% is free. T_3, with its higher biologic activity, possesses 10 times less protein binding such that 0.3% is free. Only the free hormone enters cells, exerts its biologic action, and determines thyroid physiologic status. The most important binding proteins are thyroxine-binding globulin (TBG), transthyretin, and thyroxine-binding prealbumin albumin (TBPA); albumin and some lipoproteins play a minor role. TBG is a glycoprotein synthesized in the liver with a molecular weight of 55 kD. It has one binding site for either T_4 or T_3, with a 10-fold higher affinity for T_4. The serum concentration of TBG is about 20 mg per liter to allow for binding of 20 μg of T_4 per deciliter. Transthyretin has two binding sites for T_4, but with an affinity 100-fold lower than that of TBG. T_3 binds weakly to transthyretin. The total binding capacity of transthyretin for T_4 is very large at 200 μg of T_4 per deciliter. Albumin has one binding site for T_4 or T_3, with a 50-fold lower affinity compared to TBG. In normal plasma, the T_4-binding distribution is 80% of T_4 binding to TBG, 15% to transthyretin, and

5% to albumin and lipoproteins. For T_3, the distribution is 90% bound to TBG and the rest to albumin and lipoproteins, with little binding to transthyretin. Table 203–1 lists conditions leading to alterations in TBG. Changes in total T_4 or T_3 resulting from such alterations may be confused with conditions leading to thyroid hormone excess or deficiency due to hyperthyroidism or hypothyroidism. Elevated or decreased total T_4 or T_3 levels caused by abnormalities in binding proteins are always accompanied by normal free T_4 and free T_3 concentrations and a euthyroid state. Elevated levels of TBG as they occur, for example, in pregnant patients or patients with acute hepatitis lead to increased levels of total T_4 and T_3. Because more T_4 is bound, less T_4 is able to enter the tissue to be metabolized and inhibit TSH secretion. Slightly higher TSH levels result in increased thyroid hormone formation and a new steady state accompanied by normal free thyroid hormone concentrations. Specific drugs also can lower thyroid hormone concentrations without lowering thyroid hormone–binding proteins (Table 203–1). For example, salicylic acid or phenytoin competes with thyroid hormone for binding to TBG. The effects of phenytoin are more complex in that they reduce both total serum T_4 levels and slightly lower free T_4 concentrations. TSH concentrations remain normal under such circumstances, and the patients are not hypothyroid. In contrast to alterations in binding proteins, increases or decreases in thyroid hormone production lead to abnormalities in both total and free hormone concentrations.

THYROID HORMONE ACTION

Most thyroid hormone effects are mediated by the binding of T_3 to nuclear thyroid hormone receptor proteins. T_3 has a 10-fold higher affinity for this nuclear receptor than T_4, accounting for the higher biologic activity of T_3. T_3 nuclear receptors belong to the c erbA proto-oncogene family and are encoded by the genes c erbA α and c erbA β. Each gene has several splice variants, only some of which bind T_3. The T_3 nuclear receptor is a T_3-activated transcription factor that binds to specific nucleotide sequences located upstream or downstream of the transcription start site of T_3-responsive genes. Many T_3-responsive genes show an increase in transcription upon T_3 binding to the nuclear T_3 receptor protein. This leads to increased formation of specific mRNA's and proteins such as those coding for growth hormone, malic enzyme, myosin heavy chain α and the calcium pump of the sarcoplasmic reticulum. T_3 suppresses transcription of other genes such as the gene coding for the TSH-α and TSH-β subunits. In this scenario, specific mutations of the c erbA β receptor lead to the generalized thyroid hor-

TABLE 203–1. FACTORS INFLUENCING THYROID HORMONE BINDING TO TBG

Increased TBG concentration
  Congenital abnormality
  Hyperestrogenic state
    Pregnancy, estrogen therapy
  Disease related
    Hepatitis, biliary cirrhosis, acute intermittent porphyria
  Drugs
    Tamoxifen, perphenazine, clofibrate
Decreased TBG concentration
  Congenital abnormality
  Drugs
    Glucocorticoids (large doses), androgenic steroids, asparaginase
  Severe systemic illness
    Nephrotic syndrome, chronic liver disease, protein malnutrition
Drugs interfering with binding to normal TBG
  Salicylates, diazepam, phenytoin, furosemide, high levels of free fatty
    acids

mone resistant syndrome: The mutant $T_3\beta$ receptor interferes with the action of normal T_3 receptor proteins. In addition to its effects on transcription, T_3 influences the half-life of mRNA and proteins and affects the translation of mRNA, a step that may lead to rapid changes in ion transport.

Braverman LE, Utiger RD (eds.): Werner and Ingbar's The Thyroid, 6th ed., Philadelphia, JB Lippincott, 1991. *A basic text.*

Lazar MA: Thyroid hormone receptors: Multiple forms, multiple possibilities. Endocrinol Rev 14:184, 1993.

Refetoff S, Weiss RE, Usala SJ: The syndromes of resistance to thyroid hormone. Endocrinol Rev 14:348, 1993.

Vassart G, Dumont JE: The thyrotropin receptor and the regulation of thyrocyte function and growth. Endocrinol Rev 13:596, 1992. *The titles of the above articles are self-explanatory.*

EVALUATION OF PATIENTS WITH THYROID DISEASE

The evaluation of patients with thyroid disease includes a physical examination of the thyroid, laboratory tests for thyroid function and, when indicated, specific other procedures including ultrasonography, radioactive iodine uptake and scan, and fine-needle aspiration.

Physical Examination

Palpation of the thyroid gland is an important part of the general physical examination, and abnormalities in size, consistency, and contour of the gland are a common finding. For example, 6% of women have thyroid nodules. An enlargement of the thyroid, however, may be a first clue for Graves' disease; or a firm thyroid nodule can represent thyroid cancer. Examination of the thyroid begins by having the patient swallow while observing the contour of the neck from the side. Thyroid enlargements and irregularities, like a nodule, moving up from the substernal area can be identified. Palpation of the thyroid can be performed by standing behind the patient and using the fingers of both hands to identify the isthmus lying just below the cricoid cartilage. Moving laterally, the second, third, and fourth fingers can palpate both thyroid lobes. By exerting gentle pressure during swallowing, the surface of the thyroid moving past the fingers reveals enlargement or the presence of thyroid nodules. A thyroid examination should always include palpation of lateral and submandibular lymph nodes. The size of thyroid nodules can be recorded by measuring their two largest diameters.

Measurement of Thyroid Hormone Values

Techniques employed for measurement of T_4, free T_4, T_3, and TSH by radioimmunoassays or enzyme-coupled immunoassays are rapidly changing. The newer assays provide for increased assay sensitivity. Radioimmunoassays are progressively being replaced by enzyme-linked immunoabsorption assays, and new chemoluminescent compounds are available for supersensitive TSH assays. Serum thyroid hormone concentrations for T_4, free T_4, T_3, and TSH in normals and patients with thyroid disease are given in Table 203–2. These measurements accurately define thyroid function in most persons, making more specialized tests rarely needed.

TOTAL AND FREE T_4. Total T_4 values (4.5 to 12.5 μg per deciliter) are altered by changes in thyroid function or changes in the concentration affinities of thyroid hormone–binding proteins. Determination of free T_4 levels (non–protein-bound) corrects for these abnormalities. Current laboratory capacities involve quantitation of non–protein-bound T_4 by a two-step fluorometric enzyme immunoassay or by equilibrium dialysis. Normal values range from 0.9 to 2 ng per deciliter. Some of these assays occasionally falsely identify too high free T_4 values in patients with dysalbuminic hyperthyroxemia, but non–protein-bound T_4 measurement by the two-step immunoassay approach gives a good approximation of free T_4. This free T_4 index is constructed by multiplying the total T_4 by an estimated protein binding (usually the T_3 uptake test). The T_4 index does not adequately reflect the thyroid status in patients with the nonthyroidal illness syndrome, as discussed below.

Measurement of total T_3 levels by enzyme-coupled immunoassays has a normal range of 80 to 220 ng per deciliter and is also influenced by alterations in binding proteins, but to a lesser extent. The total T_3 assay should not be confused with the T_3 uptake or T_3 resin test, which is used to calculate the free thyroxine index.

SERUM REVERSE T_3. Reverse T_3 (rT_3) (normal range 20 to 40 ng per deciliter) should be determined only in special situations. Its level is elevated (40 to 120 ng per deciliter) in patients with various systemic illnesses, leading to the nonthyroidal illness syndrome (NTI). Because of decreased T_4, free T_4, and T_3 levels in some of these patients, its determination can help to distinguish NTI from hypothyroidism. In hypothyroid patients, reverse T_3 levels are decreased.

The levels of the thyroxine hormone–binding proteins, TBG, transthyretin, and albumin, can be directly measured by immunoassays. During pregnancy and with estrogen treatment, TBG levels are elevated 2- to 3-fold owing to a decreased metabolic clearance of TBG molecules which have an increase in glycosylation. An albumin variant with increased affinity for T_4 exists in the familial dysalbuminic syndrome and leads to elevated T_4 levels with normal T_3 values and uptake. A transthyretin variant with similar effects on T_4 binding has also been described. Table 203–3 lists causes of increased T_4 levels.

SERUM THYROGLOBULIN. Thyroglobulin is produced only by thyroid tissue. Normal persons have low but detectable thyroglobulin levels. Total surgical removal of thyroid tissue for cancer should result in undetectable thyroglobulin levels. Determination of thyroglobulin levels by immunoassays has its most useful application following thyroid cancer surgery. The upper normal limit of thyroglobulin is 20 to 25 ng per deciliter, and levels above that range may indicate a return of thyroid cancer. Thyroglobulin levels also increase when patients become hypothyroid, as occurs, for example, in preparation for radioactive iodine scanning and treatment. Determination of thyroglobulin levels at that time is strongly recommended. Normal thyroglobulin levels do not completely exclude the return of thyroid cancer because in about 10% of patients with thyroid cancer, thyroglobulin is normal in spite of the return of thyroid cancer. Intake of thyroid hormones leads to a decrease of thyroid tissue and thus lowers thyroglobulin levels. Patients with thyrotoxicosis factitia have, therefore, low thyroglobulin levels, in contrast to patients with thyroiditis. In both of these conditions, radioactive iodine uptake is low and thyroglobulin levels can help distinguish between these two conditions. In the presence of antithyroglobulin antibodies, accurate determination of thyroglobulin by immunoassays is not possible.

THYROID-STIMULATING HORMONE. Serum TSH levels correlate inversely with active thyroid hormone concentrations and represent the best single index to the presence of primary hyperthyroidism or primary hypothyroidism. In hypothyroidism with low thyroid hormone concentrations, TSH levels rise above the upper normal limit of 6 μU per milliliter. In hyperthyroidism with elevated thyroid hormone levels, TSH levels fall below the lower normal limit of 0.3 μU per milliliter. TSH levels as currently measured fall below the lower limit of normal in patients with hyperthyroidism, whatever the cause. Suppressed TSH levels also can accompany other conditions, including pituitary or hypothalamic disease; nonthyroidal illness; treatment with dopamine, glucocorticoids, and other drugs; and psychiatric illness or recent recovery from hyperthyroidism. In secondary hypothyroidism due to pituitary failure (<5% of all hypothyroidism), the formation and secretion of thyroid hormone is low but TSH levels fail to rise. Similarly, in hypothalamic disease leading to decreased TRH formation, TSH levels are not elevated in spite of decreased T_4 and T_3 concentrations. Elevated TSH levels rarely occur in the absence of hypothyroidism. TSH-producing pituitary tumors rarely cause hyperthyroidism. In the generalized thyroid hormone resistance syndrome, however, TSH levels are inappropriately elevated in proportion to the markedly elevated T_4 and T_3 levels. In hypothyroidism, markedly elevated TSH levels decline only slowly after thyroxine therapy achieves normal T_4 and T_3 concentrations. Hypothyroidism leads to an increase in the number of TSH-producing thyrotrophs, which de-

TABLE 203-2. SERUM THYROID HORMONE VALUES IN NORMAL PERSONS AND PATIENTS WITH THYROID DISEASE

	Normal	Hyperthyroid	Hypothyroid
T_4 μg/dl	4.5–12.5	>12.5	<4.5
free T_4 (ng/dl)	0.9–2	>2	<0.9
T_3 (ng/dl)	80–220	>220	<80
TSH (μU/ml)	0.3–6	<0.3	>6

TABLE 203-3. CAUSES OF INCREASED SERUM TOTAL T₄ CONCENTRATION

Thyroid State Condition	T₄	Free T₄	T₃	TSH	Comments
Hyperthyroid state	H	H	H or N	L	High T₄ combined with hypermetabolic state and hyperthyroidism
Euthyroid state					
Binding abnormalities					
TBG levels increased	H	N	H	N	Autosomal dominant
T₄ binding to albumin increased (familial dysalbuminemic hyperthyroxinemia)	H	N,H*	N	N	*Same "free T₄" methods lead to erroneous results
T₄ binding by transthyretin increased (familial)	H	N	N	N	
T₄ antibodies present	H	N,H	N,L,*H*	N	*Method based, anti-T₃ antibody may also be present
Drug effects					
Inhibitors of 5' deiodinase					
Oral cholecystographic contrast agents (ipodate, iopanoate)	H	H	L	H	Inhibition of T₃ formation
Amiodarone	H	H	L	L,N	
Propranolol	H	N	L,N	N,H	Only with large doses
Heparin	H	N,H	N	N	Temporary after IV doses
T₄ administration	H	H	N	L	Mild hyperthyroxinemia in patients on T₄ replacement
Various disorders					
Nonthyroidal illness syndrome	H,N	N,L	L	N,L,H	See text for detail
Hyperemesis gravidarum	H	H,N	N	L	During early part of pregnancy; remits
Acute psychiatric illness	H,N	H,N	N	L	During acute phase; remits without treatment
Extrathyroidal deiodinase defect	H	H	N	N	A few case reports but not completely documented
Thyroid hormone resistance syndrome (pituitary and generalized)	H	H	H	H	In generalized resistance syndrome, hypothyroid features can be present, especially related to CNS development. If only pituitary resistance, thyrotoxic symptoms

H = high; N = normal; L = low.
Sequence indicates frequency of occurrence, e.g., free T₄ = HN—more frequently free T₄ is high, but normal levels can also be encountered.

cline only slowly after euthyroidism returns. Accordingly, 4 to 6 weeks should be allowed before increasing replacement doses of thyroxine above average on the basis of TSH levels. Severe long-standing hypothyroidism can lead to pituitary enlargement, mimicking pituitary tumors. The availability of sensitive TSH levels allows adequate assessment of pituitary reserves under such circumstances and makes TRH tests less useful.

ANTITHYROID ANTIBODIES. Antibody formation can occur against the thyroid peroxidase enzyme, thyroglobulin, and the TSH receptors T₄ and T₃. These antibodies can be present in serum. The most frequently occurring is the antimicrosomal antibody for which the thyroid peroxidase enzyme is the antigen. In Hashimoto's disease, elevated antibodies occur in >80% of patients with no specific therapeutic requirements resulting from high antiperoxidase antibody titers. Antithyroglobulin antibodies are positive in 60% of Hashimoto's disease. Occurrence of antithyroglobulin antibodies precludes using thyroglobulin levels to follow patients after thyroid cancer surgery or radioactive iodine treatment. Different types of TSH receptor antibodies occur, some of which stimulate thyroid hormone formation, whereas others only stimulate DNA synthesis or block TSH action. The TSI is a TSH receptor antibody that stimulates thyroid hormone formation and accompanies >90% of cases of Graves' disease. The TSI is related to, but not the same as, the long-acting thyroid-stimulating antibody (LATS), a previously used assay. In patients in whom the diagnosis of Graves' disease cannot be made clinically, determination of the TSI may be helpful, but routine TSI determination is not recommended. Persistent high levels of TSI in patients with Graves' disease on long-term antithyroid medication suggests but does not guarantee that stopping the antithyroid medication will not be followed by continuous euthyroidism. Anti-TSH antibodies can cross the placenta and produce neonatal Graves' disease or hypothyroidism. Circulating antibodies to T₄ and T₃ can interfere with the accurate determination of these hormones.

Evaluation of the Thyroid by Radioisotope Tests

RADIOACTIVE IODINE (RAI) UPTAKE. The epithelial cells of the thyroid actively transport iodide (I⁻) and molecules of similar charge and configuration such as $^{99m}TcO^-_4$ pertechnetate and ^{201}Th. Only iodide is permanently retained in the thyroid cell by organification. Two separate tests use radioactive iodine: total radioactive uptake and thyroid scanning. Both are contraindicated during pregnancy. The radioactive iodine uptake only roughly indicates thyroid function. The 24-hour uptake ranges widely from 5 to 20%, and this, along with the marked decreased uptake in the presence of increased amounts of bodily cold iodine, makes it an unreliable indicator of thyroid function. Patients with subacute thyroiditis have a markedly reduced or absent uptake, whereas patients with active Graves' disease have a normal or increased uptake. Accordingly, the radioactive iodine uptake may be useful in diagnosing subacute thyroiditis. Its routine use for the diagnosis of Graves' disease is not recommended.

THYROID SCAN. Thyroid scans give graphic representations of the distribution of radioactive iodine in the gland. They are useful in identifying whether thyroid nodules show decreased ("cold") or increased ("hot") accumulation of radioactive iodine compared with normal paranodular tissue. Uptake also identifies thyroid tissue outside the gland. The isotopes ^{123}I, ^{131}I, and ^{99m}Tc can be used. ^{123}I is preferred because it provides a much smaller radiation dose to the thyroid than ^{131}I. With a ^{99m}Tc scan, good quality images can be obtained about 30 minutes after administration. Some thyroid nodules have a normal iodine transporter but lose the ability to organify iodine. Such nodules (about 10%) are not cold on ^{99m}Tc scans, a significant disadvantage of the technique. The ^{131}I isotope is sometimes preferred for identifying thyroid cancer metastases because it has a higher energy gamma ray and better penetrates the tissue. Scans in some patients fail to colocalize palpable nodules adjacent to areas of increased or decreased radioactive iodine retention. Such nodules may be autonomously either hot or cold. Because thyroid cancers exists in <1% of hot nodules compared with 20% of cold ones, the radioactive iodine uptake of thyroid nodules can be useful. In special cases, a suppression scan may be useful. After placing the patient on 150 to 200 μg of T_4 per day for 4 to 6 weeks, one repeats the thyroid scan. Thyroid hormone and TSH values should be normal before thyroxine is started. Autonomous nodules continue to show an increased iodine uptake (hot), whereas other nodules lose their radioactive iodine retention, becoming cold. Cold nodules need to be further evaluated with fine-needle aspiration, but this is not required for hot ones.

THYROID ULTRASONOGRAPHY. Ultrasonography gives a high-resolution image of the thyroid and can identify nodules 1 to 3 mm in diameter. Such small nodules are, however, not clinically relevant. Ultrasonography can distinguish solid from cystic lesions and determine changes in the size of the nodule in response to thyroid hormone suppression therapy. Ultrasound-guided fine-needle aspiration helps in obtaining cytologic material from nodules that are difficult to identify by palpation. Ultrasonography cannot distinguish between benign and malignant thyroid nodules, nor can the technique identify substernal extensions of the thyroid or spread of metastatic disease to this region. For the latter purpose, magnetic resonance imaging (MRI) or computed tomography (CT) can be useful.

Fine-Needle Aspiration of Thyroid Nodules

Aspiration of thyroid nodules with a fine needle (22 to 27 gauge) to obtain material for cytologic examination provides good diagnostic accuracy with minimal side effects. Bleeding into the aspirated nodule is the only unwanted effect and usually has no clinical consequence. Results obtained with this procedure are listed in Table 203–4. Seeding of malignant cells along the needle track does not present a clinical problem with fine-needle aspiration. An experienced cytopathologist is crucial for the successful use of this procedure. Since the advent and wide use of fine-needle aspiration, surgical removal of benign nodules has substantially decreased.

Bayer MF: Effective laboratory evaluation of thyroid status. Med Clin North Am 75:1, 1991. *Provides a succinct guide to modern testing.*
Nicoloff JT, Spencer CA: The use and misuse of sensitive thyrotropin assays. J Clin Endocrinol Metab 71:493, 1990. *A valuable paper on the do's and don'ts of the subject.*
Stocklig JR: Serum thyrotropin and thyroid hormone measurements and assessment of thyroid hormone transport. *In* Braverman LF, Utiger RD (eds.): The Thyroid, 6th ed. Philadelphia, JB Lippincott, 1991, p. 463. *Comprehensively discusses the subject.*

NONTHYROIDAL ILLNESS SYNDROME (NTI)

Severe systemic illness, physical trauma, and psychiatric disturbances can substantially alter thyroid hormone levels in patients without intrinsic thyroid disease. Various terms have been used for this condition, including the nonthyroidal illness syndrome, sick euthyroid syndrome, and low T_3 syndrome. The severity of the illness correlates roughly with the extent of thyroid hormone changes. A decreased serum T_3 concentration is the critical component of the syndrome. The frequent alterations of thyroid hormone levels in severe illness probably make NTI a more common cause of abnormal thyroid hormone values than intrinsic thyroid disease. NTI represents one end of a spectrum of endocrine responses to severe illness which include increases in ACTH and cortisol levels. Increases in cytokines, especially tumor necrosis factor and interleukins-1 and -6, also occur. The consequences, if any, of NTI for total body metabolism and the functional status of specific organs are unclear and therapy is not recommended. Diagnosing the simultaneous occur-

rence of hypothyroidism or hyperthyroidism in patients with NTI is a difficult diagnostic challenge. Different variants of NTI occur.

LOW T_3, NORMAL T_4 VARIANT. A marked decrease in serum total T_3 and free T_3 concentrations accompanied by normal serum T_4 and TSH levels is the most frequently encountered combination of thyroid hormone values in NTI. A rough correlation exists between the severity of the systemic illness and the decrease in T_3 levels. Decreased T_3 levels are most likely caused by an impairment of extrathyroidal T_4 to T_3 conversion. The decline is accompanied by an increase in rT_3 levels. Diminished 5′ deiodinase activity accounts for this reciprocal change, with T_3 no longer being formed from T_4 and reverse T_3 not being metabolized to rT_2. The decrease in T_3 levels may decrease protein turnover and exert a sparing effect on body proteins, but the overall impact on metabolic and organ function is unclear. Because of normal T_4 and TSH levels, this variant of NTI can be clearly distinguished from hypothyroidism.

LOW T_3, LOW T_4 VARIANT. In addition to low T_3 levels, T_4 levels also decline in patients with more severe illness. Several changes contribute: (1) decreases in thyroxine-binding proteins (TBG and transthyretin); (2) displacement of thyroxine from proteins by fatty acids; and (3) decreased thyroid hormone production because of lowered TSH levels. The degree of lowered T_4 levels correlates with disease severity: Mortality increases in patients with T_4 levels below 4 μg per deciliter and approaches 80% in patients with T_4 levels below 2 μg per deciliter. T_4 administration does not influence outcome, and the low levels reflect the severity of the underlying illness but appear not to contribute directly to mortality. In addition to low T_3 and T_4 levels, T_4 indexes are low but dialysis-measured free T_4 levels remain normal or only minimally lowered. TSH levels are low but may be slightly elevated during recovery from severe illness. TSH levels above 20 μU per milliliter are not compatible with NTI and point to hypothyroidism.

Unusual Variants of Nonthyroidal Illness

Elevated T_4 levels with initially normal T_3 levels that subsequently decline occur with liver disease, especially acute hepatitis. Increased synthesis and release of TBG most likely accounts for the increased T_4 levels. A delayed fall in T_3 levels can affect patients with AIDS, indicating a poor prognosis; rT_3 levels are not elevated. In psychiatric illness, especially manic depressive disease, elevated T_4 levels occur during the initial disease phase, T_3 levels are normal, and TSH results vary. Elderly patients frequently show low T_3 levels; possible causes include chronic illness, medication intake, or an adjustment to increasing age. T_3 levels remain normal in selected healthy elderly individuals.

Diagnostic Considerations

The diagnosis of hypothyroidism or hyperthyroidism in severely ill patients with nonthyroidal illness can be difficult. Signs indicating the prior existence of thyroid disease such as a goiter, a thyroidectomy surgical scar, exophthalmos, or pretibial myxedema should be sought. Organ manifestations such as marked bradycardia for hypothyroidism or tachycardia and fine tremor for hyperthyroidism may provide important clues, especially if no other reason for these signs can be identified. As described above, NTI-induced alterations in thyroid function tests suppress the standard indices of hypothyroidism or hyperthyroidism, but certain guidelines can help. A TSH level above 20 μU per milliliter in an NTI patient makes a diagnosis of hypothyroidism highly likely, and thyroxine therapy is indicated. Similarly, TSH levels below 0.03 μU per milliliter and only moderately elevated T_3 and T_4 levels make hyperthyroidism likely. As systemic illness improves, T_3 and T_4 levels rise further and hyperthyroidism becomes evident. If Graves' disease causes the hyperthyroidism, a TSI determination can be helpful. The preferred treatment for such hyperthyroidism is by medical therapy using PTU or methimazole.

THYROTOXICOSIS

Thyrotoxicosis occurs when tissues are exposed to excess amounts of thyroid hormone, resulting in specific metabolic changes and pathophysiologic alterations in organ function. A distinction can be made between thyrotoxicosis and hyperthyroidism. Hyperthyroidism denotes increased formation and release of thyroid hormone from the thyroid gland, whereas thyrotoxicosis describes

TABLE 203–4. RESULTS OBTAINED BY FINE-NEEDLE ASPIRATION OF THYROID NODULES

	Percent of Patients
Adequate tissue obtained	90
Benign tumor	74
Malignant tumor	4
Suspicious or indeterminate	12
Correct diagnosis	<90
False negative	4
False positive	1

One fifth of these nodules are malignant after surgery by final pathology.

the clinical syndrome that results. Excess intake of exogenous thyroid hormone would lead to thyrotoxicosis but by the definition given above, such a patient would not be hyperthyroid. The terms, however, are frequently used interchangeably. Table 203–5 lists causes for thyrotoxicosis. The major ones are (1) increased occupancy of TSH receptors by TSI, TSH, or human chorionic gonadotropin (hCG); (2) autonomous overproduction of thyroid hormone by thyroid nodules; (3) increased release of thyroid hormone during specific phases of thyroiditis; (4) excessive thyroid hormone intake or ectopic thyroid hormone formation. The most frequent cause of thyrotoxicosis is Graves' disease, accounting for 60 to 90% of cases and occurring among women with a frequency of 1.9%. Men experience one tenth of the occurrence in women. Other causes in decreasing order of frequency include toxic thyroid nodules, thyroiditis, factitious thyrotoxicosis, iodine-induced thyrotoxicosis, and hCG- and TSH-induced hyperthyroidism.

Graves' Disease

Graves' disease, also termed Basedow's or Parry's disease, carries the hallmarks of excess formation and secretion of thyroid hormone and diffuse goiter. Additional characteristics include exophthalmos, dermopathy (especially pretibial myxedema), and rarely thyroid acropachy. These supplementary manifestations seldom appear together and often run a divergent time course.

ETIOLOGY AND PATHOGENESIS. Graves' disease is most likely an autoimmune disorder with B lymphocytes producing immunoglobulins, some of which bind to and activate the TSH receptor, stimulating excess thyroid growth and hormone secretion. For these antibodies the TSH receptor appears to represent the antigenic site, and they act like TSH and are termed thyroid-stimulating immunoglobulins (TSI). Other antibodies occur in Graves' and other autoimmune diseases such as Hashimoto's disease. These antibodies bind to the TSH receptor but stimulate only thyroid growth without increasing thyroid hormone secretion. Some antibodies bind to the TSH receptor but block TSH action and lead to thyroid atrophy. A diversity of TSH antibodies occurs in autoimmune thyroid diseases, generating a spectrum of illnesses with Graves' disease and hyperthyroidism at one end and Hashimoto's disease and thyroid atrophy leading to hypothyroidism at the other. The role that specific antibodies play in causing the ophthalmopathy that occurs in 20 to 40% of patients with Graves' disease is less clear. Specific antibodies directed against non-TSH retro-orbital antigens localized on retro-orbital fibroblasts and muscle cells as well as antibodies directed at TSH-like antigens have been described. Retro-orbital fibroblasts appear to express a TSH receptor–like protein. Anti-TSH antibodies occur at a low frequency in Hashimoto's disease and in euthyroid relatives of patients with Graves' disease. The simultaneous occurrence of blocking TSH antibodies may prevent hyperthyroidism in such patients.

The precise sequence of events leading to TSH receptor antibody production and factors that initiate antibody formation have not been clearly identified. A genetically mediated antigen-specific defect in T lymphocyte suppressor function has been proposed. Such a defect in immune surveillance would allow T helper cell clones, which mistake part of the TSH receptor as a foreign antigen, to arise and persist. Such clones would then stimulate B cells to produce anti-TSH receptor antibodies. Alternatively, thyroid cells stimulated by specific cytokines produced in response to a viral infection may express on their cell surface Class II molecules of specific HLA-DR types which present fragments of the TSH receptor to T lymphocytes; these then would stimulate B lymphocytes to produce TSH receptor antibodies. The two mechanisms are not mutually exclusive and both could contribute to TSH receptor–directed antibody formation. The autoimmune response may be promoted by poorly defined factors including the following: (1) iodide excess; for example, the incidence of Graves' disease increases after iodine supplementation in deficient areas; (2) viral or bacterial infection; for example, outbreaks of Graves' disease can follow *Yersinia enterocolitica* infection; (3) glucocorticoid withdrawal or stress; the stress induction has been questioned and may relate to a worsening of symptoms by the combined occurrence of hyperthyroidism and physical or emotional stress which brings the patients to medical attention; (4) parturition: A state of relative immune tolerance develops during pregnancy and reverses after delivery; (5) lithium therapy; this may modify immune responses.

PATHOLOGY. The thyroid gland in Graves' disease enlarges diffusely and contains increased vascularity. The parenchyma exhibits hypertrophy and hyperplasia, with follicular cells showing increased height, surrounding a lumen containing a decreased amount of colloid. Infiltration by lymphocytes indicates the autoimmune nature of the disease. These cells probably generate a considerable amount of TSH receptor antibody. Iodide administration increases the colloid accumulation and decreases vascularity, making the gland firmer. A gland that increases in size in patients receiving antithyroid medication indicates either excess medication, inducing hypothyroidism, or too low a dose, providing inadequate receptor blockade and continued thyroid hormone formation and growth. Severe thyrotoxicosis can lead to muscle atrophy with muscle fiber degeneration, cardiac hypertrophy, focal hepatic necrosis with lymphocyte infiltration, a decrease in bone density, and hair loss. In patients with Graves' disease ophthalmopathy, an increase in retro-orbital contents leads to protrusion of the globe. The retro-orbital tissues show marked infiltration by lymphocytes, mast cells, and plasma cells along with increased amounts of mucopolysaccharide, especially hyaluronic acid. Extraocular muscles show edema, round cell infiltration, and mucopolysaccharide deposition eventually resulting in muscle fibrosis. In patients with pretibial myxedema, the skin shows prominent lymphocyte infiltration and mucopolysaccharide deposition.

CLINICAL FEATURES. Excess thyroid hormone action due to any of the causes listed in Table 203–5 can lead to an increased metabolic rate and changes in the function of several organs. In addition, patients with Graves' disease have specific clinical manifestations resulting from the underlying autoimmune process. The thyrotoxicosis and autoimmune-related manifestations can show independent variations in intensity and time course, causing diagnostic difficulties.

Features of Thyrotoxicosis. Table 203–6 lists common signs and symptoms of thyrotoxicosis. The typical patient with Graves' disease is a woman in her mid-20's to 30's experiencing recent onset of nervousness, difficulty in controlling emotions, and a state of agitated tiredness made worse by sleep disturbances. She speaks rapidly and cannot sit still. Problems of recent onset in interaction with others at home or at work are frequently reported. Questioning brings out feelings of intolerance with excess sweating, palpitations, muscle weakness, frequent bowel movements, and weight loss in spite of good appetite. Sometimes weight gain ensues because the increased appetite and caloric intake exceed the enhanced caloric consumption. Oligomenorrhea and amenorrhea occur in premenopausal women. On physical examination, the skin is warm and moist and has a fine velvety texture. The hair is fine and when combed, sheds substantial amounts, leading to thinning of the hair. Onycholysis with separation of the nail from the fingertip is fre-

TABLE 203–5. CAUSES OF THYROTOXICOSIS

Dependent on increased thyroid hormone production
    Dependent on increased occupancy of the TSH receptor by:
        Thyroid-stimulating immunoglobulin (TSI)
            Graves' disease
            Hashitoxicosis
        Human chorionic gonadotropin (hCG)
            Hydatiform mole
            Choriocarcinoma
        Thyroid-stimulating hormone (TSH)
            TSH-producing pituitary tumor
    Autonomous overproduction of thyroid hormone (independent of TSH)
        Toxic adenoma (TSH receptor mutant)
        Toxic multinodular goiter
        Follicular cancer (rare)
    Jodbasedow effect (excess iodine-induced hyperthyroidism)
Independent of increased thyroid hormone production
    Increased thyroid hormone release
        Subacute granulomatous thyroiditis (painful)
        Subacute lymphocytic thyroiditis (painless)
    Nonthyroidal source of thyroid hormone
        Thyrotoxicosis factitia
        "Hamburger" thyrotoxicosis
        Ectopic production by:
            Ovarian teratoma (struma ovarii)
            Metastasis of follicular cancer

TABLE 203–6. TISSUE-SPECIFIC SIGNS AND SYMPTOMS OF THYROTOXICOSIS

Tissue	Symptoms and Signs
Central nervous system	Nervousness and emotional lability Fine tremor of hands
Cardiovascular	Palpitations, tachycardia, atrial fibrillation, increased difference between systolic and diastolic blood pressure
Gastrointestinal (GI)	Hyperdefecation, GI hypermotility, diarrhea
Muscle	Proximal muscle weakness, muscle atrophy, hyperreflexia
Skin	Warm moist smooth skin, onycholysis, fine hair, hair loss, excessive perspiration
Metabolic	Heat intolerance, weight loss usually with increased appetite
Thyroid	Enlargement or nodule(s)

quent. Gynecomastia can occur in men because of increased estrogen production. Fine tremor is noted on the stretched-out hands, and tendon reflexes become hyperactive. The eye signs of thyrotoxicosis are most likely mediated by an increased sympathetic tone and include a widened distance between the upper and lower lid, lid lag on upward gaze, and frequent blinking. These signs do not indicate Graves' ophthalmopathy and are not accompanied by protrusion of the eyes. Cardiovascular manifestations can be marked, characterized by sinus tachycardia, a widened pulse pressure, and an often elevated systolic blood pressure. True hypertension is not frequent in hyperthyroidism but does occur in hypothyroidism. The heart beat is vigorous with a hyperactive pericardium. On auscultation the first sound is increased and a third sound and frequently a systolic murmur are audible. A harsh to-and-fro sound can be audible and is most likely caused by the pleural and pericardial surfaces rubbing each other. Cardiac arrhythmia, especially atrial fibrillation, can contribute to the development of heart failure. Muscle atrophy and weakness develop, and hypokalemic periodic paralysis has a measurable incidence in males of Asian extraction. Bone turnover can be increased, leading to hypercalcemia of as much as 12 mg per deciliter. Unusual blood-detected abnormalities ($<10\%$ of patients) include elevated alkaline phosphatase levels, increased direct bilirubin, mild anemia, and moderate neutropenia. Renal tubular acidosis can occur, and immune complex nephritis has been reported.

In older patients, the manifestations of thyrotoxicosis can be considerably modified. Affected patients frequently appear apathetic rather than nervous. Cardiovascular signs, general muscle weakness, and marked weight loss are more prominent. Cardiac arrhythmias that are refractory to conventional treatment, unexplained heart failure, or the recent onset or marked worsening of pre-existing angina pectoris should lead to a determination of thyroid hormone values.

Features Specific for Graves' Disease. Autoimmune processes mediate the enlargement of the thyroid gland, infiltrative ophthalmopathy, dermopathy, and acropachy, thereby distinguishing Graves' disease from other causes of thyrotoxicosis. Palpation most frequently reveals diffuse and symmetric thyroid enlargement (two to six times normal). Thyroid nodules can occur and should be biopsied because, although unusual, thyroid cancer can coincide with Graves' disease. Auscultation of the thyroid frequently reveals a thyroid bruit, reflecting the increased blood supply. In a small number of patients, the thyroid remains of normal size. A hallmark finding of Graves' disease is infiltrative ophthalmopathy. Clinically detectable eye disease occurs in 20 to 40% of patients with Graves' disease, but severe ophthalmopathy requiring aggressive treatment affects only about 5%. Affected persons complain of easy tearing, photophobia, a feeling of sand in the eyes, diplopia, and decreased visual acuity. Ophthalmopathy affects the anterior soft tissue structures of the eye and with progressive severity involves more posterior structures as well. Periorbital edema and chemosis occur early and result from impaired drainage of the orbital veins. The swollen and fibrotic muscles cause lid retraction and restrict ocular movement, leading to diplopia. Upward gaze is most frequently impaired; with limitations of lateral gaze occurring less frequently. Tissue edema and accumulation of hydroscopic hyaluronic acid lead to engorgement of extraocular muscles and swelling of retro-orbital connective tissue, pushing the globe forward and resulting in prop-

tosis and further restriction of eye movement. Proptosis and lid retraction prevent complete closure of the eyes, resulting in exposure keratitis and corneal ulceration. Adequate care to prevent drying and infection of the cornea is important. Compression of the optic nerve at the posterior apex by enlarged muscles may lead to blurring and impaired visual acuity, visual field defects, impairment of color vision, and papilledema. Optic nerve compression can occur in the absence of proptosis. Graves' ophthalmopathy that is clinically apparent in only one eye occurs in 5 to 14% of patients. Sensitive imaging techniques like CT, however, show that most of these patients have bilateral orbital disease. Most patients with Graves' ophthalmopathy are hyperthyroid, but dissociation can occur, with ophthalmopathy appearing in patients of euthyroid or hypothyroid status. More unusual manifestations include coexisting myasthenia gravis with Graves' disease. Other cases may include diffuse lymphadenopathy and splenomegaly. Rarely, other autoimmune disorders occur in patients with Graves' disease.

DIAGNOSIS AND DIFFERENTIAL DIAGNOSIS. In patients with severe Graves' disease showing typical signs of thyrotoxicosis and autoimmune-mediated manifestations such as ophthalmopathy, the diagnosis is not difficult (Table 203–6). Gauging the degree of thyroid hormone overproduction guides subsequent therapy. Measurement of free T_4, T_3, and TSH levels constitutes a sufficient laboratory workup. In all patients with Graves' disease, T_3 levels are markedly elevated, and in most such patients free T_4 levels are elevated as well. In some patients, however, the marked stimulation of TSH receptors leads to higher hormone production rates of T_3 so that serum T_3 levels rise markedly while T_4 levels remain normal. This combination of laboratory values is termed T_3 toxicosis and is most frequently found during the initial phases or a relapse of Graves' disease. TSH levels are undetectable and serve to exclude TSH-producing tumors or thyroid hormone resistance as causes for the elevated thyroid hormone levels. In typical Graves' disease, radioactive iodine–based tests and a determination of the TSI are unnecessary. The clinical diagnosis becomes more difficult in patients with milder disease, in older patients manifesting apathetic thyrotoxicosis, and in patients with coexisting illnesses. Determination of free T_4, T_3, and TSH levels adequately establish the degree of thyrotoxicosis in patients with mild disease and older patients with an apathetic picture. Undetectable TSH levels using an ultrasensitive TSH assay are especially helpful in establishing that the body contains an excess amount of thyroid hormone. Intercurrent illness modifies thyroid hormone values by lowering T_3 levels and in some patients T_4 levels. Elevated reverse T_3 levels further implicate an intercurrent illness as a modifier of thyroid hormone values. Obtaining TSI values can be helpful in these patients because their elevation confirms the diagnosis of Graves' disease. Palpation of the thyroid revealing a nodule, a somewhat painful thyroid, or no palpable thyroid tissue is unusual and requires additional diagnostic procedures. A radioactive iodine scan is especially helpful in identifying a cold thyroid nodule surrounded by high uptake in surrounding tissue, a combination compatible with Graves' disease with a cold nodule requiring biopsy. Alternatively, the nodule may be hot, with surrounding areas showing decreased or absent uptake, which makes it more likely that the patient has a toxic adenoma. Very low uptake in patients who experience pain on palpation of the thyroid area indicates thyroiditis. In patients with no palpable thyroid tissue and absent thyroid uptake, ectopic production of thyroid hormone or factitious intake should be suspected. Thyroglobulin levels are very low in such patients.

Discrepancies between the degree of thyrotoxicosis and the extent of autoimmune abnormalities can complicate the diagnosis of Graves' disease. Some patients can exhibit marked bilateral or unilateral ophthalmopathy with minimal or no signs of thyrotoxicosis. In such instances, T_4 and T_3 levels are in the upper normal range and TSH levels are in the low normal or decreased range. The condition has been termed euthyroid ophthalmopathy or euthyroid Graves' disease. Thyrotoxicosis is mimicked by few clinical syndromes, and thyroid hormone values are normal in most of these. Pheochromocytomas can lead to heat intolerance, profuse sweating, palpitations, tachycardia, elevated glucose levels, and a state of anxiety. Anxiety states by themselves also lead to irritability, tremor, weakness, tachycardia, and weight loss. Thyroid hormone values are normal in these conditions.

TREATMENT OF GRAVES' DISEASE. The ophthalmopathy and dermopathy of Graves' disease require separate therapeutic approaches. The therapy of thyrotoxicosis is aimed at decreasing thyroid hormone formation and secretion. Three different therapeutic approaches are used: (1) antithyroid drugs that inhibit the thyroid peroxidase enzyme involved in thyroid hormone formation, (2) radioactive iodine, and (3) surgery. Both of the latter treatments decrease the amount of functional thyroid tissue. The most frequently used treatment modalities are antithyroid drugs or radioactive iodine, and the choice between them depends on the phase and severity of the disease, the specific situation of the patient, and the preference and experience of the physician. Spontaneously occurring increases and decreases of the underlying autoimmune abnormality lead to cycles of worsening and improvement of the thyrotoxic symptoms, making variable the natural history of Graves' disease. Consequently, life-long follow-up is recommended. About 10 to 20% of patients with Graves' disease remit spontaneously, and about half become hypothyroid after 20 to 30 years in the absence of therapy, most likely due to continued autoimmune destruction of the thyroid. Not treating patients and awaiting a spontaneous remission is not recommended. Therapy directed against the autoimmune process is currently not available.

TREATMENT OF THYROTOXICOSIS. *Antithyroid Drug Therapy.* Amelioration of thyrotoxic symptoms by decreasing thyroid hormone formation and release is the initial task in severe thyrotoxicosis. The thionamide derivatives, propylthiouracil (PTU) and methimazole (MMI), are the preferred initial treatment options in Graves' disease in the absence of contraindications. Radioactive iodine can lead to increased release of thyroid hormone and, infrequently, worsen the thyrotoxic symptoms to the point of inducing thyroid storm. Thyroid surgery is contraindicated in severely hyperthyroid patients. PTU and MMI, as well as carbimazole, which is used in Great Britain and is metabolized to methimazole, interfere with organification and iodotyrosine coupling by inhibiting the peroxidase enzyme. Both compounds may exert a mild immunosuppressive effect; a decrease in the level of TSI occurs after the drugs are started. This could be due to a mild immunosuppressive effect but also could result from decreased thyroid hormone secretion. Both drugs are rapidly absorbed from the gastrointestinal tract and concentrated in the thyroid. PTU inhibits peripheral conversion of T_4 to T_3, contributing 10 to 20% to the decrease in T_3 levels. This effect does not occur with MMI. MMI, however, is at least 10 times more potent than PTU and has a longer intrathyroidal residence time. MMI administered once a day is effective, whereas PTU must be given every 6 to 8 hours to exert its full effect. Both PTU and MMI cross the placenta; given in high doses they can interfere with fetal thyroid function. The choice between PTU and MMI and particular dosing schemes vary considerably between different centers. PTU is most useful for patients with severe thyrotoxicosis; those with moderate thyrotoxicosis are started on MMI, which comes in 5- and 10-mg tablets. Starting doses of 20 to 30 mg once daily are used. Improvement of thyrotoxic symptoms, in general, takes 2 to 3 weeks and can lag behind the normalization of thyroid hormone values. Euthyroidism can be achieved in 4 to 6 weeks. Thyroid hormone values are checked 4 weeks after the start of therapy and if no decrease in values occurs in spite of compliance, the dose may be increased to 30 to 40 mg a day. Once thyroid hormone levels normalize, the dose is decreased. A decrease in dose which is accompanied by an increase in free T_4 or T_3 levels and symptoms suggesting disease reactivation requires maintenance at higher dose levels for a longer time. Most patients can be maintained on low doses of 2.5 to 5 mg of MMI for 12 to 24 months.

A few patients with severe hyperthyroidism are started on PTU (100 to 150 mg every 8 hours). The choice is based on the faster decrease in T_3 levels with PTU than MMI. In some patients, higher doses of 200 to 300 mg every 6 hours are required. PTU comes in 50-mg tablets and, when taken in doses of two or three tablets three times a day, can lead to compliance problems. With improvement, the physician can progressively lower PTU doses and switch to once-a-day MMI. Most patients are then maintained on the lower MMI dose (2.5 to 5 mg per day) for 12 to 24 months. It appears that longer duration of antithyroid therapy bodes well for patients staying euthyroid after the medication is stopped. Most relapses oc-

cur within the first 3 to 6 months after discontinuation of antithyroid therapy. In young adults, a second course of antithyroid drug therapy can be tried, but the chance of permanent remission declines.

Undesired occurrences during PTU and MMI therapy include an increase in thyroid size, which may result from overtreatment, shown by low T_4 levels and elevated TSH levels, or undertreatment and reactivation of disease. Unfavorable indicators of disease activity are a requirement for higher PTU and MMI doses and T_3 levels that increase excessively compared with T_4 levels. Favorable prognostic signs are continued normalization of thyroid hormone levels, especially a normal T_4 to T_3 ratio in spite of using lower PTU and MMI doses, and decreasing thyroid size and TSI levels. Routine monitoring of TSI is not recommended. A recent report suggests a different treatment protocol. Patients are treated initially with MMI until euthyroid. Subsequently a combination of MMI (10 to 20 mg) plus thyroxine (0.1 mg T_4 per day) is used for another 12 to 24 months, at which time all signs of active Graves' disease have disappeared. MMI is discontinued and the patient is continued on 0.1 mg T_4 for 1 more year. Long-term remissions have been reported to occur in >90% of patients treated with this regimen. Before such a protocol is adopted for routine use, however, confirmation of results in patients of a different ethnic background and iodine exposure should be obtained.

Table 203–7 lists side effects of thionamide compounds. These occur most frequently during the initial 3 to 6 months after the therapy is started. The most frequent complications are allergic in nature, and skin rashes occur in 2 to 3% of patients. The major toxic reaction is agranulocytosis, which develops suddenly and occurs in 0.2 to 0.5% of patients. Routine monitoring of leukocyte counts is not recommended, but a leukocyte count should be obtained before starting therapy. Patients need to be instructed to discontinue their medication and contact their physician when a fever occurs or infections develop, especially in the oropharynx. A white blood count below 0.5×10^9 per liter indicates agranulocytosis and requires both discontinuation of antithyroid drugs and administration of broad-spectrum antibiotics as well as supportive therapy. Other treatment modalities such as radioactive iodine should be chosen for further treatment.

Radioactive Iodine (RAI). RAI therapy (^{131}I) is used most frequently to treat hyperthyroidism in adults in the United States, in contrast to Europe and Japan, where antithyroid medication is the preferred approach. In either event, antithyroid drugs are the preferred initial therapy for thyrotoxicosis. RAI therapy is preferred for older patients with moderate hyperthyroidism and thyroid enlargement, for patients with a prior allergic or toxic reaction to the antithyroid medication, and when frequent medication intake cannot be guaranteed. ^{131}I is also used after a course of antithyroid medication has failed to induce a long-term euthyroid state. RAI treatment is contraindicated during pregnancy; the fetal thyroid becomes able to accumulate iodine at 10 to 12 weeks of gestation. RAI can induce a thyroiditis with glandular swelling leading to potential air-

TABLE 203–7. SIDE EFFECTS OF ANTITHYROID DRUGS

Severe
Agranulocytosis (0.2–0.5%)
Only rare cases reported
    Hepatitis (can result in hepatic failure)
    Cholestatic jaundice
    Thrombocytopenia
    Hypoprothrombinemia
    Aplastic anemia
    Lupus-like syndrome with vasculitis
    Hypoglycemia (insulin antibodies)

Less severe
Most frequent (1–5%)
    Rash
    Urticaria
    Arthralgia
    Decreased leukocyte level (drop in white cell counts by $2-3 \times 10^3$)
    Fever
Less frequent
    Arthritis
    Diarrhea
    Decreased sense of taste

way obstruction in patients with large retrosternal goiters. A very low RAI uptake caused by excessive iodine exposure also precludes ^{131}I use.

Before ^{131}I administration, antithyroid drugs should be stopped for 3 or 4 days. Different dosing methods have been proposed for ^{131}I application. One approach is to aim at delivering 80 μCi ^{131}I per gram of thyroid tissue. The 80 μCi is then multiplied by the estimated weight of the gland and corrected for ^{131}I uptake. This delivers 6000 to 8000 rad to the thyroid and most frequently requires doses of 5 to 10 mCi. In patients with low uptake, large glands, and severe thyrotoxicosis leading to rapid intrathyroidal iodine turnover, larger doses often are chosen. Improvement in thyrotoxicosis occurs after 4 to 5 weeks, and 40 to 70% of patients regain normal thyroid functions within 6 to 8 weeks. Almost 80% of patients are cured with one dose. The remaining need a second dose, which should not be undertaken before 6 months have elapsed. After giving radioactive iodine, antithyroid drugs can be added at day 5 to reach a euthyroid state more quickly. In addition, β-sympathetic blockade is used to relieve associated symptoms. RAI can induce a painful thyroiditis and lead to acute thyroid hormone release and worsening of thyrotoxicosis. Severe thyroiditis can be treated with anti-inflammatory agents such as aspirin; rarely glucocorticoids are required. RAI treatment–induced worsening of Graves' ophthalmopathy has been reported in some studies but not in others. Administration of glucocorticoids concurrently with RAI treatment may be beneficial, but such treatment is not well enough established to be recommended for routine use. Steroids, however, may be useful for patients with prominent eye disease in whom RAI therapy is the approach of choice. No increase of thyroid cancer, other malignancies, or malformations in subsequent pregnancies have been documented after RAI therapy. It is recommended, however, that pregnancy not occur for 6 to 12 months after RAI treatment. Hypothyroidism is a consequence of RAI treatment. More than 50% of patients become hypothyroid during the first year after therapy, with an additional 2 to 3% during each subsequent year. Unless otherwise treated, transient hypothyroidism occurs 2 to 3 months after radioactive iodine treatment, with subsequent spontaneous normalization of thyroid hormone values. Patients should be informed of this risk and be followed after the acute phase of treatment every 4 to 6 months and subsequently at least once a year.

Surgical Therapy. Surgical removal of a large part of the thyroid (subtotal thyroidectomy) is indicated in patients with large obstructing glands or glands containing nodules that are identified as malignant or equivocal on fine-needle aspiration. Pregnant women with severe hyperthyroidism, which is difficult to control with antithyroid drugs, can be treated with thyroidectomy during the second trimester. In addition, young patients who are difficult to control on antithyroid drugs, patients with toxic reactions to antithyroid drugs, and patients who are not candidates for antithyroid drugs and refuse radioactive iodine are treated by surgery. Nevertheless, patients must be euthyroid before surgery is undertaken. This is achieved by using PTU or MMI for approximately 6 weeks. In patients on PTU or MMI, a saturated solution of potassium iodide (1 drop 3 times a day) can be administered daily for 10 days prior to surgery to reduce the vascularity of the gland. Subtotal thyroidectomy should be performed by an experienced thyroid surgeon. Complications including hypoparathyroidism, recurrent laryngeal nerve paralysis, and hemorrhage should occur in less than 1 to 2% of patients. In addition, transient hypocalcemia, wound infection, and keloid formation leading to unsightly scars may occur. Hypothyroidism occurs to a somewhat lower extent than after RAI, but its frequency may be underestimated. Recurrent hyperthyroidism occurs in about 10% of patients.

ALTERNATIVE AND SUPPORTIVE THERAPIES. In a small number of patients with Graves' disease, the conventional therapies listed above cannot be used. In some, toxic reactions preclude the use of antithyroid drugs and ^{131}I cannot be employed because a very low uptake occurs due to excess iodine exposure or because of pregnancy. Also, some patients may present a high surgical risk because of underlying medical problems. In such cases, the oral cholecystographic agent iopanoic acid or sodium iopodate (Oragrafin), administered at 1 gram per day, inhibits T_4 to T_3 conversion and leads to rapid lowering of T_3 levels. In addition, because of release of iodine from the compound, T_4 levels fall. These compounds should be used for only 2 to 3 months because escape from their antithyroid effect occurs. The perchlorate ion (ClO_4^-) of

$KClO_4$ is a competitive inhibitor of thyroidal iodide transport. In doses limited to 1 gram per day, serious toxic effects such as anaplastic anemia and gastric ulcers can be avoided. The compound is especially effective in iodine-induced hyperthyroidism (Jodbasedow) as occurs, for example, in patients treated with the antiarrhythmic compound amiodarone. Potassium perchlorate should be used for only a short duration and with careful supervision. The isolated use of iodine to treat thyrotoxicosis is ill advised because its inhibitory effects on thyroid hormone secretion often fail. Iodine should be used only in patients who are on antithyroid medication and are prepared for thyroid surgery or in the treatment of thyroid storm (see below).

β-Adrenergic blocking agents such as propranolol, 60 to 120 mg per day in three or four divided doses, help to provide relief of symptoms such as tachycardia, tremor, anxiety, and heat intolerance. The rationale for their use is based on an increased sensitivity of the β-sympathetic system in thyrotoxicosis and on a small inhibitory effect of T_4 to T_3 conversion. Patients with a history of asthma or congestive heart failure should not receive propranolol because it constricts bronchial smooth muscle and has a negative inotropic effect. Propranolol should not be used as a sole agent to treat hyperthyroidism because it neither directly inhibits thyroid hormone action nor induces a euthyroid state. Multivitamin supplementation is advisable in patients with severe thyrotoxicosis, especially if nutrition is not well balanced and adequate.

TREATMENT OF OPHTHALMOPATHY AND DERMOPATHY. Clinically apparent ophthalmopathy affects 20 to 40% of patients with Graves' disease, but severe symptoms occur in only a minority. For most patients with mild eye signs, only general supportive measures are needed. These include elevation of the head at night and wearing of tinted glasses to protect the eyes from sunlight and foreign bodies. Application of 1% methylcellulose drops to the eyes and taking a diuretic to decrease periorbital swelling provide further relief. Patients with more severe ophthalmopathy should be managed in close consultation between an endocrinologist and an ophthalmologist. Severe inflammatory reactions are treated with 60 to 100 mg of prednisone in divided doses for 2 to 4 weeks, with subsequent tapering of the dose over 8 to 12 weeks. Combinations of prednisone and cyclosporine have also been used. External x-ray therapy to the retro-orbital area may be helpful but is less well established as desirable therapy. The total dose is 20 Gy (2000 rad) given in 10 fractions over 2 to 3 weeks. Signs of optic nerve compression such as papillary edema, decreased color vision, and decreased visual acuity require surgical decompression, for which a transantral approach is frequently favored. After the active inflammatory process subsides, corrective surgical procedures may be beneficial. Retro-orbital muscle surgery may correct for eyeball misalignment and double vision. Eyelid surgery aimed at protecting the cornea, relieving discomfort, and cosmetic improvement should be the last surgical step.

Other Causes of Thyrotoxicosis

TOXIC ADENOMA AND TOXIC MULTINODULAR GOITER. Increased formation and secretion of T_3 and T_4 can occur in a single nodule or in multiple thyroid nodules. The latter condition is also termed Plummer's disease. Single nodules need to be larger than 2 to 3 cm in diameter to engender hyperthyroidism. Histologically, these nodules are follicular adenomas. Frequently a large nodule is palpable on one side of the thyroid, with atrophy of the other side. In contrast, patients with toxic multinodular goiter may undergo general nodular enlargement. Such persons frequently are older and have had a goiter for a long time before autonomous overproduction of thyroid hormone ensues. The thyrotoxicosis can be precipitated by excess iodine intake (Jodbasedow effect) and appears to occur particularly frequently in autonomous thyroid tissue, which functions independently of TSH stimulation. On physical examination, multinodular goiters range from small to large with possible substernal extension. Laboratory values show suppressed TSH levels and marked elevation of T_3 levels, with T_4 levels showing a lesser increase. Antibodies against the TSH receptor (TSI) and thyroid peroxidase (anti-TPO) are absent, in contrast to patients with Graves' disease. On RAI scan two patterns can be distinguished. Some patients show an irregular and patchy distribution of increased RAI uptake. In others, one or more distinct hot nodules occur with marked, localized increased RAI accumulation and no uptake between the hot nodules. Both patterns are compatible with toxic goiter. Clinically affected patients may be difficult to diagnose because the disease affects elderly patients, who tend to present with apathetic hyperthyroidism. As noted earlier, typical thyrotoxic signs can be minimal in such patients, who often show apathy, lethargy, a depressed mood, weight loss, and cardiac abnormalities.

RAI is the treatment of choice for most patients with one toxic adenoma or multinodular toxic goiter. Severely thyrotoxic patients may need a course of antithyroid medication several weeks before they receive RAI to forestall acute worsening and decompensation after ^{131}I administration. The ^{131}I dose is 150 μCi per gram of tissue, twice that used for Graves' disease. Permanent hypothyroidism infrequently develops because remaining thyroid tissue resumes thyroid hormone secretion after ablation of toxic adenomas. Surgery can remove isolated adenomas, especially in younger patients.

RARE CAUSES. Thyrotoxicosis can be caused by TSH-producing pituitary tumors as well as by excess formation of hCG by hydatiform moles or choriocarcinoma. Surgical therapy is appropriate for both pituitary tumors and moles. Choriocarcinoma is treated by appropriate chemotherapy, and persistent thyrotoxicosis may require antithyroid drugs. Ectopic production of thyroid hormone by ovarian teratoma leads to mild thyrotoxicosis. Body scans detect RAI uptake in the location of the ovaries. Surgical removal is corrective. Follicular carcinoma of the thyroid with functioning metastases rarely leads to hyperthyroidism. Therapy is discussed in the section on thyroid cancer. Subacute or chronic thyroiditis can release high amounts of T_4 and T_3 and induce hyperthyroidism lasting for several weeks or months. RAI uptake is very low in such lesions. *Thyrotoxicosis factitia* results from inadvertent or planned ingestion of large amounts of thyroid hormone. It most frequently accompanies efforts at weight loss or occurs in patients with psychiatric problems. Many of these patients have easy access to thyroid hormone because they took it in the past, have relatives or acquaintances who are taking thyroid hormone, or are medical personnel. Ingestion of ground meat products prepared from neck trim containing thyroid tissue has also been reported (hamburger thyrotoxicosis). Patients with thyrotoxic symptoms, suppressed TSH levels, increased T_4 and T_3 levels, low RAI uptake, and suppressed thyroglobulin levels meet the diagnostic criteria for thyrotoxicosis factitia. Patients taking T_3 preparations have elevated T_3 levels but suppressed T_4 levels. Stopping thyroid hormone intake usually suffices. Additive β-sympathetic blockade or agents like ipodate to inhibit T_4 to T_3 conversion are rarely needed.

The term *Jodbasedow effect,* as noted before, designates iodine-induced hyperthyroidism. It occurs most frequently in patients with toxic nodular goiter exposed to excess amounts of iodine but has also been reported in Graves' disease. Problems with the autoregulation of thyroid hormone formation usually exist before iodine exposure; however, some patients have been reported who exhibited completely normal thyroid function after iodine was withheld. The Jodbasedow effect typically occurs in iodine-deficient areas after iodine supplementation is provided. Exposure to iodinated radiographic contrast media and iodinated drugs presents a frequent triggering event for the Jodbasedow effect in the United States. The antiarrhythmic agent amiodarone, which contains 37% iodine, can induce the Jodbasedow effect. The developing hyperthyroidism can worsen arrhythmias and lead to difficult management problems. In milder cases, antithyroid drugs like MMI are used. Potassium perchlorate prevents further iodine uptake and inhibits thyroid hormone formation. The usual dose is 200 mg four times a day.

Special Therapeutic Problems

THYROID STORM. Thyroid storm or thyrotoxic crisis is a life-threatening form of decompensated hyperthyroidism. Thyroid storm occurs most frequently in patients with severe thyrotoxicosis who develop an intercurrent severe illness such as an infection or sepsis or undergo a major surgical procedure. The distinction between severe thyrotoxicosis with an additional intercurrent illness and thyroid storm cannot be clearly drawn. Patients with severe thyrotoxicosis developing an intercurrent illness should be aggressively treated by the approach outlined in Table 203–8 because the illness can quickly decompensate into thyrotoxic crisis. Thyrotoxic crisis

TABLE 203–8. MANAGEMENT OF THYROID STORM

Inhibition of thyroid hormone formation and secretion
  PTU, 400 mg q8h PO or by nasogastric tube
  Sodium iodide, 1 gram IV in 24 hours, or saturated solution of KI, 5 drops q8h
Sympathetic blockade
  Propranolol, 20–40 mg q4-6h, or 1 mg IV slowly (repeat doses until heart rate slows); not indicated in patients with asthma or congestive heart failure that is not rate-related
Glucocorticoid therapy
  Hydrocortisone, 50–100 mg IV q6h
Supportive therapy
  Intravenous fluids (depending on indication: glucose, electrolytes, multivitamins)
  Temperature control (cooling blankets, acetaminophen; avoid salicylates)
  O$_2$ if required
  Digitalis for congestive failure and to slow ventricular response; pentobarbital for sedation
  Treatment of precipitating event (e.g., infection)

requires no acute increase in thyroid hormone values, and it cannot be identified by laboratory tests. An acute increase in tissue availability of free thyroid hormones caused by a decrease in plasma-binding proteins may cause it, but equally likely are coincident increases in cytokines such as TNF-α and IL-6. Clinical signs compatible with thyrotoxic crisis are fever in excess of the temperature elevation expected from the intercurrent illness, with temperatures of 41°C (105°F) and even higher. In addition, marked tachycardia, extreme restlessness, agitation, and tremor occur. Patients may deteriorate mentally and become delirious, psychotic, obtunded, and even comatose. Hypotension with congestive heart failure and signs of an acute abdomen can develop. Table 203–8 outlines therapy, which includes high doses of antithyroid medication and iodine after starting antithyroid drugs. Cortisol turnover increases markedly, inducing enhanced formation of 11-keto compounds (cortisone), which are less metabolically active. Administration of 300 mg of hydrocortisone in divided doses is therefore indicated. Propranolol provides effective sympathetic blockade that has a favorable effect on rapid heart rate and induced cardiac failure. The compound, however, has a negative inotropic effect and should be used cautiously in patients with congestive heart failure. A history of asthma attacks precludes the use of β-sympathetic blockers. Treatment of precipitating events and supportive therapy must be started immediately.

THYROTOXICOSIS AND PREGNANCY. The most frequent cause of thyrotoxicosis during pregnancy is Graves' disease, but hyperthyroidism can result from toxic multinodular goiter and more rarely an excess of hCG production by hydatiform moles or choriocarcinoma. Hyperthyroidism may be difficult to recognize because pregnancy itself can lead to a hyperdynamic cardiovascular state and heat intolerance. Total T_4 and T_3 levels are increased owing to elevated thyroid hormone–binding protein levels, but T_4 values above 15 μg per deciliter strongly suggest hyperthyroidism. Hyperemesis gravidarum leads to elevated T_4 levels (hyperthyroxinemia), with normal T_3 values. In addition to medical problems of the mother resulting from severe thyrotoxicosis, slight increases in neonatal mortality rate and low birth weight in newborns have been reported. Antithyroid drugs are the initial therapy of choice. RAI is contraindicated, and the patient needs to be euthyroid before surgery can be considered. Because PTU inhibits T_4 to T_3 conversion, crosses the placenta less readily, and is concentrated to a lower extent in mothers milk than MMI, PTU is preferred over MMI in pregnant patients. Isolated cases of aplastica cutis induced by MMI have been reported. At high doses, PTU can induce fetal hypothyroidism and goiter because it crosses the placenta. In contrast, thyroid hormone minimally crosses the placenta. PTU doses are therefore limited to 200 to 300 mg per day; the addition of thyroxine confers no advantage. PTU administered in this way during pregnancy is relatively safe and does not negatively affect either fetal development or the outcome of pregnancy. If adequate control of hyperthyroidism is not possible, subtotal thyroidectomy should be considered, which is best performed during the second trimester. Long-term treatment with propranolol is not recommended because low birth weight can result. In addition, postnatal bradycardia and poor responses to hypoxia have been noted in newborns of mothers treated with propranolol. During the postpartum period, the mother risks developing new Graves' disease, a recurrence of previously quiescent Graves' disease, or postpartum thyroiditis. A state of relative immunosuppression during pregnancy which disappears with delivery has been implicated. Newborns delivered by mothers with Graves' disease can have a state of transient hyperthyroidism due to placental passage of TSI or less frequently long-term Graves' disease because of a genetic propensity. Mild neonatal thyrotoxicosis requires no therapy because the disease is self-limiting. In severe and more long-term thyrotoxicosis, PTU at doses of 10 to 25 mg every 8 hours is given. Nursing mothers with thyrotoxicosis can safely receive PTU in doses of 200 to 300 mg per day; these doses do not lead to levels in the milk that impair a newborn's thyroid function. MMI is concentrated in the milk at higher levels and should not be used.

Cardiac Disease

Thyrotoxicosis in patients with pre-existing cardiac disease can worsen symptoms and induce cardiac decompensation. Rarely, however, does severe hyperthyroidism induce cardiac symptoms in patients without underlying cardiac disease. Nevertheless, angina pectoris or high output failure has been reported after resumption of a euthyroid state in patients with severe thyrotoxicosis without prior evidence of cardiac disease. An increased association exists between Graves' disease and mitral valve prolapse. Most patients with cardiac problems due to hyperthyroidism are elderly, and many have toxic multinodular goiter. It is important to restore a euthyroid state promptly in these patients. This is best achieved by adequate doses of PTU (300 to 600 mg per day). Atrial fibrillation occurs in 10 to 15%; signs of congestive heart failure may be due to the rapid ventricular response and the absence of atrial contraction. Prompt slowing of the ventricular heart rate with digitalis and inducing β-sympathetic blockade with propranolol or atenolol are important. Digitalis must be prescribed with care because thyrotoxic patients are somewhat digitalis resistant, and a narrow margin separates therapeutic and toxic doses. Similarly, β-sympathetic blockers with negative inotropic effects should be used with caution in patients with congestive heart failure. The presence of atrial fibrillation usually requires anticoagulant therapy with aspirin or warfarin sodium. Increased vitamin K metabolism, however, may require lower warfarin doses. Spontaneous reversion from atrial fibrillation to regular sinus rhythm occurs frequently as successfully treated patients achieve a euthyroid state. If sinus rhythm has not returned after a euthyroid period of 4 months, cardioversion should be considered. Angina pectoris can worsen sufficiently in hyperthyroid patients that preinfarction angina becomes a concern. In markedly hyperthyroid patients, interventional procedures such as coronary angioplasty or bypass surgery should not be undertaken without prior treatment with antithyroid drugs because of the danger of thyrotoxic crisis. Calcium channel blockers like diltiazem are useful in patients with contraindications to propranolol. Angiographic procedures using iodinated contrast agents can markedly worsen the thyrotoxicosis because of the induction of the Jodbasedow effect, which especially endangers patients with toxic multinodular goiter. The antiarrhythmic compound amiodarone also can induce the Jodbasedow effect, as described above.

Becks GP, Burrow GN: Thyroid disease and pregnancy. Med Clin North Am 75:121, 1991. *A useful article for physicians caring for pregnant women.*
Burch AB, Wartofsky L: Graves' ophthalmopathy: Current concepts regarding pathogenesis and management. Endocrine Rev 14:747; 1993. *A thorough exploration of this difficult clinical problem.*
Gavin LA: Thyroid crisis. Med Clin North Am 75:179; 1991. *Provides a clinically detailed consideration of the problem.*
McDougall R: Graves' disease. Med Clin North Am 75:79, 1991. *A longer review of the subject.*

HYPOTHYROIDISM

Hypothyroidism is the clinical syndrome that results from decreased secretion of thyroid hormone from the thyroid gland. It most frequently reflects a disease of the gland itself (primary hypothyroidism) but can also be caused by pituitary disease (secondary hypothyroidism) or hypothalamic disease (tertiary hypothyroidism). Hypothyroidism leads to a slowing of metabolic processes and in its most severe form to the accumulation of mucopolysaccharides in the skin, causing a nonpitting edema termed myxedema. The term *myxedema* is reserved by some for a severe form of hypothyroidism, whereas others use the terms interchangeably. The term *cretinism* is reserved for hypothyroidism dating from birth and leading to abnormalities of intellectual and physical development. The generalized thyroid hormone resistance syndrome (GTRS) results from an abnormality in the amino acid sequence of the β form of the nuclear thyroid hormone receptor, leading to decreased T_3 binding. Impairment of thyroid hormone effects in GTRS is partly overcome by increased thyroid hormone levels, thereby preventing significant hypothyroid symptoms in most patients. The condition is rare.

INCIDENCE, ETIOLOGY, AND PATHOGENESIS. The incidence of hypothyroidism varies somewhat with the geographic area. In areas of adequate iodine supply, like the United States, 0.8 to 1.0% of the population are hypothyroid. In iodine-deficient areas of the world, the incidence is 10- to 20-fold higher. Neonatal hypothyroidism occurs with a frequency of 0.02% in the Caucasian population, whereas among African Americans it falls to 0.003%. Table 203–9 lists the causes of hypothyroidism.

Primary hypothyroidism accounts for about 90 to 95% of all cases, the remainder being of pituitary or hypothalamic origin. Most patients with primary hypothyroidism develop thyroid hormone deficiency during adulthood. Only a minority of patients have congenital hypothyroidism resulting from defects in enzymes required for thyroid hormone synthesis, thyroid agenesis, dysgenesis, or ectopic thyroid tissue. Temporary congenital hypothyroidism can be induced by maternal iodine or antithyroid drug administration. Primary hypothyroidism can be of a thyroprivic form, with markedly reduced or absent thyroid tissue, or a goitrous form, with an enlarged thyroid. The most frequent cause of hypothyroidism in adults is autoimmune disease, with goitrous or thyroprivic Hashimoto's disease being the prime example. In autoimmune-based hypothyroidism, antibodies are directed against thyroperoxidase, thyroglobulin, and the TSH receptor. Antithyroglobulin and antiperoxidase antibodies probably serve only as markers of autoimmunity, but anti-TSH antibodies cause disease. TSH receptor antibodies can block TSH action and thus contribute to decreased thyroid hormone formation. In addition to antithyroid antibodies, antibodies can be directed against the proteins of other endocrine organs such as the pancreas, adrenals, parathyroids, and gonads. Affected patients suffer from polyglandular endocrine deficiency states (see Ch. 210.1). A strong family history can be identified in most of these conditions.

Thyroid autoimmune disease also has an increased association with nonendocrine abnormalities such as pernicious anemia, lupus

TABLE 203–9. CAUSES OF HYPOTHYROIDISM

Primary hypothyroidism
Insufficient amount of thyroid tissue
  Destruction of tissue by autoimmune process
    Hashimoto's thyroiditis (atrophic and goitrous forms)
    Graves' disease—end-stage
  Destruction of tissue by iatrogenic procedures
    ^{131}I therapy
    Surgical thyroidectomy
    External radiation
  Destruction of tissue by infiltrative processes
    Amyloidosis, lymphoma, scleroderma
Defects of thyroid hormone biosynthesis
  Congenital enzyme defects
  Congenital mutations in TSH receptor
  Iodine deficiency or excess
  Drug-induced: thionamides, lithium, sulfonamides, interleukins, tumor necrosis factor, and others
Secondary hypothyroidism
Pituitary
  Panhypopituitarism, e.g., neoplasm, radiation, surgery, Sheehan's syndrome
  Isolated TSH deficiency
Hypothalamic
  Congenital
  Infection
  Infiltration (sarcoidosis, granulomas)
Transient hypothyroidism
Silent and subacute thyroiditis
Thyroxine withdrawal
Generalized resistance to thyroid hormone

erythematosus, rheumatoid arthritis, Sjögren's syndrome, chronic hepatitis, and myasthenia gravis. Thyroprivic hypothyroidism due to iatrogenic destruction of thyroid tissue by RAI, external beam radiation, or surgery is second only to autoimmune disease in causing hypothyroidism in the United States. Worldwide, hypothyroidism due to iodine deficiencies and goitrogens predominates. Goitrous hypothyroidism develops because TSH hypersecretion results in excessive thyroid growth. Iodine excess also can lead to goitrous hypothyroidism through iodine-induced inhibition of thyroid hormone formation (Wolff-Chaikoff effect). This occurs especially in patients with underlying thyroid disease. The thyroid is unable to reduce iodide uptake in spite of increased iodide stores, and the inability to escape from the Wolff-Chaikoff effect leads to goitrous hypothyroidism.

Secondary hypothyroidism is due to destruction of pituitary thyrotrophs by pituitary or adjacent tumors or by necrosis, as in Sheehan's syndrome. Mutations in the TSH β-subunit can lead to biologically inactive TSH, resulting in secondary hypothyroidism. In addition, mutations in the TSH receptor leading to hypothyroidism are described. Hypothalamic hypothyroidism is due to decreased TRH secretion, resulting in diminished TSH synthesis. TSH produced in the absence of a TRH stimulus does not show normal glycosylation and has decreased biologic activity. In addition to permanent hypothyroidism, transient hypothyroidism affects patients with subacute or painless thyroiditis, including the postpartum variety. Withdrawal of long-time thyroid hormone replacement leads to several weeks of hypothyroidism until the pituitary thyrotroph population is replenished and normal thyroid-pituitary feedback resumes.

Pathologic changes in hypothyroidism depend on the cause. In patients with thyroprivic hypothyroidism, the thyroid atrophies and is replaced by fatty and fibrous tissue. By contrast, in iodine deficiency–induced goitrous hypothyroidism, the gland appears hyperplastic with tall columnar epithelium. Extrathyroidal pathology is more uniform and independent of the cause of hypothyroidism. It is characterized by increased accumulation of glycosaminoglycans in interstitial tissue, giving the skin a waxy appearance. Glycosaminoglycan accumulation occurs because of decreased removal of the substance. With severe longstanding hypothyroidism, increased capillary permeability leads to proteinaceous fluid accumulation which may involve the pericardium.

CLINICAL MANIFESTATIONS. The different causes of hypothyroidism lead to similar symptoms, the most common of which are listed in Table 203–10. The slow and progressive onset in most patients can make clinical diagnosis difficult. This is especially true in elderly patients exhibiting changes like dry skin, reduced body and scalp hair, and memory difficulties, all of which could be due to the aging process in the absence of hypothyroidism. Typical complaints in hypothyroid patients include increased tiredness and sleep requirement with a depressed mood, feeling cold, gaining weight on the same diet, constipation, increased forgetfulness and increased time needed to fulfill a task, and decreased exercise tolerance associated with muscle cramps on strenuous exercises. Affected patients relate these complaints in a low-pitched, hoarse voice with a slow speech pattern. Frequently the changes are only fully appreciated by the patient after thyroid hormone replacement

and return to a euthyroid state. The facial appearance is frequently dull and apathetic with puffiness around the eyes and loss of lateral eyebrows. The skin takes on a yellow complexion due to carotene accumulation and becomes cold, dry, and rough with nonpitting edema (myxedema). The thyroid may be normal, enlarged, or absent, depending on the cause of hypothyroidism. Cardiovascular changes can include bradycardia and an enlarged cardiac silhouette primarily due to pericardial effusion. Hypertension occurs in 10% of hypothyroid patients and resolves after thyroid hormone replacement. Because of the increased occurrence of hypercholesterolemia and hypertension, hypothyroid patients have more coronary artery disease. Angina pectoris sometimes develops only after starting thyroid hormone replacement. Anemias of different causes accompany hypothyroidism and can contribute to angina symptoms. Iron deficiency anemia results from decreased iron absorption. Absorption of folic acid is decreased. Pernicious anemia results from gastric mucosa atrophy with antibodies directed against the gastric mucosa. The decreased oxygen consumption in the hypothyroid state leads to diminished erythropoietin production, resulting in a mild anemia that can be thought of as an adaptive state. Pulmonary function is characterized by shallow and slow breathing and a decreased respiratory response to hypercapnia and hypoxia. Patients are very sensitive to sedatives that can depress the respiratory drive and lead to CO_2 retention and coma. Gastrointestinal motility decreases markedly and can lead to paralytic ileus and the megacolon of myxedema. The kidneys not only have an impaired ability to excrete a free water load, but an inappropriate ADH syndrome (SIADH) can develop and intensify hyponatremia. Because of physical resistance in associated tissues, slow Achilles tendon reflexes are a hallmark of hypothyroidism. Similarly, severe hypothyroidism can lead to cerebellar ataxia and peripheral neuropathy. Endocrine and metabolic abnormalities include hyperprolactinemia leading to galactorrhea, heavy menstrual bleeding, menorrhagia, hypoglycemia, and SIADH. Longstanding and severe hypothyroidism can induce marked thyrotroph hyperplasia, resulting rarely in increased pituitary size and sella enlargement suggesting a pituitary tumor. Hypothyroidism in newborns needs to be treated immediately with thyroxine replacement; otherwise severe retardation of mental development, short stature, and deaf mutism can develop.

DIAGNOSIS. Figure 203–3 gives an approach to the diagnosis of hypothyroidism. An elevated TSH combined with a below-normal free T_4 is diagnostic of primary hypothyroidism. T_3 levels are not useful in the diagnosis of hypothyroidism because they are frequently normal in mild hypothyroidism and are markedly lowered by the NTI syndrome. In pituitary or hypothalamic hypothyroidism, the TSH level is normal or decreased, and only below-normal T_4 or free T_4 levels are diagnostic. With third-generation sensitive TSH assays, the TRH stimulation test provides little additional information. Using the TRH stimulation test, an absent response of TSH indicates secondary hypothyroidism, whereas a partial or delayed TSH response indicates partial pituitary deficiency or hypothalamic disease. Patients with pituitary hypothyroidism frequently show other signs of pituitary deficiency, including low FSH and LH lev-

TABLE 203–10. TISSUE-SPECIFIC SIGNS AND SYMPTOMS OF HYPOTHYROIDISM

Tissue	Signs and Symptoms
Central nervous system	Forgetfulness, stoic appearance, myxedematous dementia, cerebellar ataxia
Cardiovascular	Bradycardia, pericardial effusion, hypertension
Respiratory	Depressed ventilatory drive, pleural effusion, sleep apnea
Gastrointestinal	Constipation, hypomotility
Muscle	Delayed tendon reflexes, muscle stiffness and cramps, increased muscle volume, weakness
Skin	Dry, rough, hyperkeratosis; nonpitting puffiness due to mucopolysaccharide deposits
Metabolic	Basal metabolic rate decreased, cold intolerance, decreased T_4 and drug turnover, weight gain

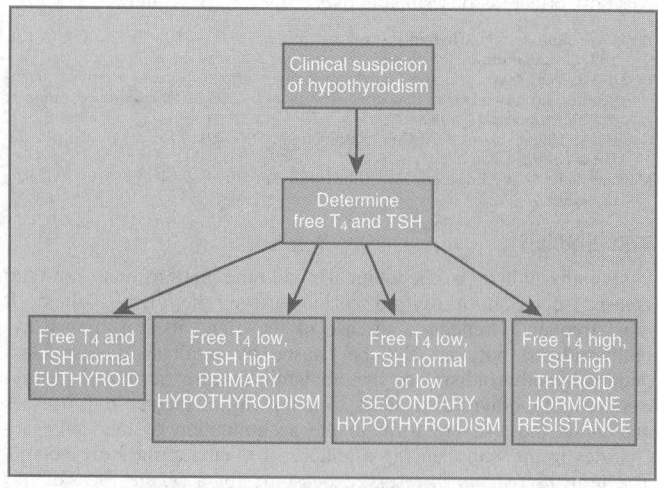

FIGURE 203–3. Diagnostic approach to hypothyroidism.

els in the face of low sex hormone levels. It is especially important to identify deficient ACTH secretion and resulting secondary adrenal insufficiency. When present, thyroid hormone replacement cannot be started before initiating cortisol replacement. Low TSH levels can also be found in patients who recently became hypothyroid after a prolonged period of hyperthyroidism which led to a decrease in the pituitary thyrotroph population. Other laboratory manifestations of hypothyroidism include elevated cholesterol, CPK, LDH, and aspartate transaminase levels.

The presence of antithyroid antibodies is compatible with Hashimoto's disease and presents a risk factor for developing hypothyroidism. During early phases of hypothyroidism, T_4 and free T_4 lie just below the lower normal range. T_3 is normal and TSH is barely elevated. This condition has been termed subclinical hypothyroidism, or the failing gland syndrome. Patients show minimal or no signs of hypothyroidism because a normal T_3 level maintains their metabolic status. Many such patients later develop clinical hypothyroidism with a further increase in TSH levels and a decrease in T_4 and free T_4 levels. In patients with Hashimoto's disease or after RAI treatment of Graves' disease, this pattern occurs frequently. Transient hypothyroidism frequently occurs in postpartum patients, with subacute thyroiditis, or after RAI treatment for Graves' disease. Changes in TSH levels lag behind alterations in T_4 and T_3 levels; careful follow-up is required to determine if permanent hypothyroidism ensues.

DIFFERENTIAL DIAGNOSIS. Fully developed hypothyroidism presents a distinct clinical picture with few imitations. Patients with renal disease resulting in a nephrotic syndrome and hypoalbuminemia can develop a puffy face, peripheral edema, a pale downy skin, anemia, and hypercholesterolemia. Goiter and thyroid nodules occur with increased frequency in patients with renal disease. Lowering of TBG levels leads to a decrease in total T_4 values. In contrast to hypothyroidism, however, free T_4 is not decreased and TSH is not increased. In children, Down syndrome can mimic hypothyroidism. Differential diagnosis is further complicated by an increased incidence of Hashimoto's thyroiditis and resultant hypothyroidism in patients with Down syndrome, but thyroid hormone values are normal in Down's patients without thyroid disease.

TREATMENT. Hypothyroidism is preferentially treated with levothyroxine (T_4), with doses ranging from 0.05 to 0.2 mg per day and an average replacement dose of 1.6 μg per kilogram per day. T_3 is formed from T_4 by intracellular conversion so that both T_4 and T_3 exist in the body. Synthetic T_4 has a long shelf life and uniform potency. Eighty percent is absorbed, and once a day intake leads to stable T_4, T_3, and TSH levels. Accordingly, thyroxine represents the preferred thyroid hormone preparation for chronic replacement. Patients should be informed that replacement probably is needed for the rest of their lives and that periodic evaluation is required. In young healthy adults without coronary artery disease, a starting dose of 75 to 100 μg per day can be used and then adjusted after 2- to 3-week intervals to reach the final replacement level. In elderly patients and those with coronary artery disease, the initial dose should be 12.5 to 25 μg per day and increased by 25 to 50 μg every 4 to 6 weeks to allow a slow increase in metabolic rates, avoiding a mismatch between coronary blood supply and metabolic demand. The aim is to achieve a euthyroid status with TSH, T_4, and T_3 levels in the normal range. Because in the complete absence of functioning thyroid tissue all T_3 is formed from the thyroxine medication and the 20% of thyroidal contribution to T_3 levels is missing, T_3 levels are frequently in the mid-normal range and T_4 levels are in the upper range of normal. A slight increase in T_4 levels occurs 2 to 6 hours after thyroxine intake so that blood for thyroid hormone determination should be drawn 20 to 24 hours later. The average replacement dose for thyroxine varies with age and to a lesser degree with the cause of hypothyroidism and the level of physical activity. Children (5 to 10 years), for example, require average replacement doses of 3 to 4 μg per kilogram. Required replacement doses in elderly persons, by contrast, are 20 to 30% lower (1.4 μg per kilogram per day) than those needed in middle-aged adults. Patients with malabsorption or those taking aluminum preparations (antacids), cholestyramine, lovastatin, ferrous sulfate, and rifampin need higher replacement doses. During pregnancy, especially in the third trimester, thyroxine replacement needs increase by 30 to 50%. After delivery, thyroxine replacement is decreased to standard levels.

The ease of approach, virtual absence of side effects, and observance of a revitalized patient make thyroxine treatment of hypothyroid patients a satisfying therapeutic experience. Thyroxine and T_3 levels normalize within 2 to 3 weeks. TSH levels lag behind for 3 to 4 weeks or more because of the increased number of thyrotrophs in the pituitary after longstanding hypothyroidism. Clinical improvement begins 2 to 3 weeks after therapy, but complete resumption of a euthyroid state can take several months.

Patients receiving chronic T_4 replacement should be evaluated by physical examination and free T_4, T_3, and TSH determination once or twice a year. The TSH level is a good indicator of adequate replacement. In patients with primary hypothyroidism, TSH levels below the normal range indicate overreplacement and levels above the upper normal range indicate underreplacement. Chronic overreplacement with thyroxine can increase bone turnover, which is a special concern in women; however, no evidence currently exists for an increased bone fracture rate. Chronic T_4 overreplacement also can lead to cardiovascular abnormalities, especially arrhythmias and cardiac hypertrophy. The treatment of subclinical hypothyroidism is controversial. Enlargement of the thyroid gland, elevated cholesterol levels—especially with LDL:HDL ratios above 3, or signs of decreased exercise tolerance and mild congestive heart failure warrant treatment.

In addition to thyroxine, triiodothyronine (T_3), combinations of T_4 and T_3, desiccated thyroid, and thyroxine plus iodine in one tablet are available. Only the use of T_3 is recommended in special situations. T_3 is useful for short-term treatment of patients with thyroid cancer after thyroid surgery and before RAI administration, because of its short half-life of 1 day versus the half-life of T_4 of 7 days (see section on thyroid cancer). Parenteral T_3 can be used to treat myxedema coma. In patients with the rare condition of 5' deiodinase deficiency, T_3 preparations are also useful. Other thyroid preparations have no advantage over thyroxine and are not recommended.

Special Clinical Conditions

ANGINA PECTORIS, CARDIAC SURGERY, AND THYROID HORMONE REPLACEMENT. Coronary artery disease occurs with increased frequency in hypothyroid patients. The complaint of angina pectoris most often arises with thyroid hormone replacement, which increases cardiac demand and O_2 consumption. Adequate thyroid hormone replacement is strongly recommended in these patients because in addition to the general benefit of a euthyroid state, cholesterol levels may decrease and blood pressure may normalize. Frequently, worsening of the angina precludes adequate thyroid hormone replacement. Treatment with β-sympathetic blockers such as propranolol (20 to 40 mg three times a day) can sometimes ameliorate the problem but may lead to significant bradycardia. Also, β-blockade fails to solve the basic dilemma between inadequate thyroid hormone replacement and angina production. In such patients with persistent mild to moderate hypothyroidism, percutaneous coronary transluminal angioplasty or coronary bypass surgery can be undertaken. Several studies have shown no deleterious consequences of a mild to moderate hypothyroid state on clinical outcome.

TREATMENT OF MYXEDEMA COMA. Patients with severe myxedema, either spontaneously or suffering from cold exposure, intake of analgesics or sedatives, or infection, may become progressively obtunded and lapse into coma. Myxedema coma is rare but presents a life-threatening emergency with a 20 to 50% mortality which is best treated in an intensive care unit. Treatment should be instituted immediately and if T_4 and TSH levels cannot be readily obtained, therapy may be started on clinical suspicion. Increasing obtundation and elevated P_{CO_2} levels especially indicate the need for thyroid hormone administration. Assessment of adrenal function should also be undertaken because giving hydrocortisone can disturb pituitary-adrenal feedback and make subsequent diagnosis difficult. Vigorous thyroid hormone replacement is required. Thyroxine can be given as a single 300 μg T_4 bolus followed by daily 50 to 100 μg intravenous T_4 maintenance doses. A T_3 replacement schedule using 10 μg T_3 intravenously every 4 hours until the patient greatly improves and oral therapy can be resumed has recently been advocated. T_3 administration offers the potential advantage that no conversion of T_4 to T_3 is required, a step that may be impaired in severely ill patients. The treatment of myxedema coma is outlined in Table 203-11.

Arlot S, Debussche X, Lalau JD, et al.: Myxedema coma: Response of thyroid hormone with oral and intravenous high-dose L-thyroxine treatment. Intensive Care Med 17:16, 1991.

Becker C: Hypothyroidism and atherosclerotic heart disease: Pathogenesis, medical management, and the role of coronary artery bypass surgery. Endocrinol Rev 6:432, 1985.

Fisher DA: Management of congenital hypothyroidism. Clinical Rev 19. J Clin Endocrinol Metab 72:523, 1991.

Mandel SJ, Larsen PR, Seeley EW, Brent GA: Increased need for thyroxine during pregnancy in women with primary hypothyroidism. N Engl J Med 323:91, 1990.

Mitchell JM: Thyroid disease in the emergency department. Thyroid function tests and hypothyroidism and myxedema coma. Emerg Med Clin North Am 7:885, 1989.

Roti E, Minelli R, Gardini E, et al.: The use and misuse of thyroid hormone. Endocrinol Rev 14:401, 1993.

THYROIDITIS

Thyroiditis includes infectious and autoimmune inflammatory diseases of the thyroid. Thyroiditis is divided into acute (suppurative), subacute painful (granulomatous), subacute painless (lymphocytic), chronic lymphocytic (Hashimoto's), and chronic fibrous (Riedel's) thyroiditis. Postpartum thyroiditis is classified as a variant of subacute painless lymphocytic thyroiditis.

Acute (Suppurative) Thyroiditis

Acute suppurative thyroiditis consists of a rare infection of the gland by bacteria, fungi, *Pneumocystis carinii*, or other organisms. Symptoms include tender swelling, sometimes with fluctuation and an erythematous skin overlying the area. Fever with leukocytosis frequently occurs. Identification of the microbial agent may require fine-needle aspiration of the lesion. Appropriate antibiotics and sometimes drainage of the abscess are required. Long-term sequelae are rare, but when a large part of the thyroid gland is involved, hypothyroidism may occur.

Subacute Painful (Granulomatous) Thyroiditis

INCIDENCE, ETIOLOGY, AND PATHOLOGY. Subacute painful thyroiditis, also termed de Quervain's thyroiditis, giant cell thyroiditis, subacute nonsuppurative thyroiditis, or granulomatous thyroiditis, is the most frequent cause of severe thyroid pain and tenderness. Subacute painful thyroiditis is not rare, resulting in 5% of all medical consultations for thyroid disease. It is most common in women 40 to 50 years old and shows an association with HLA-B35. The disease frequently follows a viral infection, and elevated titers to mumps, adeno-, entro-, echo-, influenza, coxsackie-, measles and other viruses have been found. Increased thyroid antibody titers (antimicrosomal, antithyroglobulin, anti-TSH receptor) occur in 10 to 20% of patients during the subacute phase and disappear as the disease fades. Such antibodies are polyclonal and most likely arise secondary to thyroid damage caused by viral infection. The thyroid is enlarged and edematous with destruction of follicular architecture and the presence of histocytes that coalesce into giant cells.

MANIFESTATIONS, DIAGNOSIS, AND TREATMENT. The disease frequently follows by 1 to 3 weeks the occurrence of viral pharyngitis, mumps, measles, or other viral syndromes. Severe pain develops over the thyroid area, radiates to the ear, and is enhanced by swallowing. A feeling of general malaise with muscle aches, pain, anorexia, and fever is present. On palpation, the thyroid is very tender and may be generally enlarged but can contain unilat-

eral painful areas. Cervical lymphadenopathy rarely occurs. Characteristic laboratory findings are an elevated sedimentation rate, often above 100 mm per hour Westergren, and a markedly decreased RAI uptake ($<2\%$ at 24 hours). The level of free T_4 and TSH depend on the phase of the disease, with high T_4 levels occurring during the early stage owing to follicle disruption and hormone release. At later stages, transient hypothyroidism may follow, with elevated TSH levels. Rarely, permanent hypothyroidism ensues. Thyroglobulin levels are elevated during the acute phase.

Subacute thyroiditis is an inflammatory, self-limiting disorder that at most requires symptomatic therapy. In mild cases, no therapy or analgesics such as aspirin (2 to 3 grams per day) are sufficient. Prednisone, 40 to 60 mg daily, can suppress more severe symptoms and bring relief. Within 8 to 10 days symptoms markedly decrease, and the dose can be tapered and completely stopped after 4 weeks. Sometimes symptoms flare up again and the prednisone taper needs to be reversed. In some patients, more than one attack may occur, leading to an increased risk of permanent hypothyroidism. During the initial phase, the patient may be thyrotoxic and need treatment with β-sympathetic blocking agents such as propranolol. Rarely hepatitis develops, requiring careful follow-up.

Subacute Painless (Lymphocytic) Thyroiditis with Transient Hyperthyroidism

INCIDENCE, ETIOLOGY, AND PATHOLOGY. Subacute painless thyroiditis with transient hyperthyroidism is also called subacute lymphocytic thyroiditis with spontaneously revolving hyperthyroidism and silent thyroiditis. The hallmark of the disorder is a self-limiting episode of thyrotoxicosis and a histologic picture of lymphocytic infiltration which differs from the changes found in Hashimoto's disease. Both postpartum thyroiditis and the sporadic disease occurring in the general population are forms of subacute lymphocytic thyroiditis. The incidence of sporadic subacute painless thyroiditis shows some geographic variability, with the sporadic form occurring more frequently in previously iodine-deficient areas which are now iodine replete, like the Great Lakes area of the United States, where the disease may account for 5 to 15% of all thyroiditis. Postpartum thyroiditis occurs in 2 to 6% of all pregnant women in the United States. The incidence is even higher in Sweden and Japan, reaching 7 to 12%. Eighty percent of cases of the sporadic form affect women between the ages of 30 and 40 years. The disease is most likely autoimmune in origin and independent of a preceding viral illness. Subacute lymphatic thyroiditis is distinguished from chronic lymphocytic thyroiditis (Hashimoto's disease) by a self-limiting course and a lower extent of lymphocyte infiltration with the absence of germinal centers.

MANIFESTATIONS, DIAGNOSIS, AND TREATMENT. Typical are an abrupt onset with signs of thyrotoxicosis such as nervousness, heat intolerance, tachycardia, and weight loss. A small, firm, but painless goiter is noted in about half the patients. Some may present in a hypothyroid state after the initial hyperthyroid phase was unnoticed. Postpartum thyroiditis usually occurs 3 to 6 months after delivery, with an initial transient hyperthyroid phase followed by hypothyroidism. The latter lasts 1 to 3 months, and most patients make a spontaneous recovery. During the initial hyperthyroid phase, which can last 2 to 4 months, T_4 and T_3 are elevated, with relatively higher T_4 levels due to thyroid hormone release from damaged follicles. Thyroid antibodies, especially antiperoxidase, are frequently positive but at low titers. Sedimentation rate is normal or only slightly elevated, in contrast to the marked elevation occurring in subacute painful thyroiditis. The RAI uptake is suppressed. Signs of Graves' disease, such as ophthalmopathy and pretibial myxedema, are absent, and the level of TSI, which is the hallmark of Graves' disease, is normal. Thyroid biopsy shows a typical histologic picture with abundant lymphocyte infiltration, but the procedure is not required for routine diagnosis. Treatment aims at sympathetic blockade using, for example, propranolol to alleviate symptoms during the thyrotoxic phase. Glucocorticoids are not needed. Prolonged hypothyroid episodes may be treated with thyroxine replacement, but with subsequent tapering of the dose and final withdrawal because most patients regain euthyroid status. Increased incidences of goiter and persistent hypothyroidism have been noted in patients who continue to show antiperoxidase antibodies. Similarly, the recurrence of postpartum thyroiditis has been noted in some patients with continued presence of antiperoxidase antibodies after the initial phase of the disease.

TABLE 203-11. TREATMENT OF MYXEDEMA COMA

Thyroid hormone administration
300 μg T_4 over 5-10 minutes initially, followed by 100 μg T_4 IV q24h until oral T_4 therapy can be started
Alternatively, 10 μg T_3 IV q4h until oral T_4 therapy can be started
Glucocorticoid administration
Hydrocortisone, 100 mg IV bolus followed by 25 mg q6h by IV drip
Cover to conserve heat
Intravenous fluids, electrolytes, and glucose to correct electrolyte abnormalities and hypoglycemia
Tracheal intubation and mechanical ventilation as required
Treat precipitating conditions (infection)
Avoid sedatives, narcotics, and overhydration

Chronic lymphocytic thyroiditis is the most prevalent form of thyroid autoimmune disease, affecting about 3 to 4% of the population in the United States. It is three times more common in women and most frequently diagnosed between the third and fifth decade of life. A genetic propensity for the disease is demonstrated by an increased familial incidence and an association with major histocompatibility antigens such as HLA-B8. The goitrous variant of Hashimoto's thyroiditis occurs more frequently in patients positive for HLA-DR5, whereas the atrophic variant is associated with HLA-DR3. The presence of antiperoxidase and antithyroglobulin antibodies indicates the autoimmune nature of the disease. Very high levels of thyroid antibodies distinguish Hashimoto's thyroiditis from other forms. In addition, anti-TSH receptor antibodies can occur which are frequently of the blocking variety, impairing TSH action. Rarely, TSI's are present, leading to hyperthyroidism and the combined occurrence of Graves' disease and Hashimoto's disease called Hashitoxicosis. Thyroid pathology is dominated by heavy lymphocyte infiltration destroying the normal follicular architecture. Lymph follicles and germinal centers can be identified. The presence of copious lymphocytes is a hallmark of the disease that distinguishes it from other forms of autoimmune thyroiditis. Differential diagnosis between the abundant lymphocyte infiltrates of Hashimoto's disease and the occurrence of a primary thyroid lymphoma is sometimes difficult. Thyroid lymphomas occur with an increased frequency in Hashimoto's disease but overall are rare. Also, the pathology of the thyroid gland in Hashimoto's disease is characterized by extensive fibrosis throughout the gland. Different manifestations of Hashimoto's disease can be distinguished. The occurrence of a goitrous versus an atrophic variant may be explained by the prevailing autoimmune antibodies. For example, in patients with atrophic thyroiditis, high titers of TSH receptor–blocking antibodies are found. In other patients with Hashimoto's disease, a goiter and features of Graves' disease occur which results from the TSI presence.

CLINICAL MANIFESTATIONS AND DIAGNOSIS.

In Hashimoto's thyroiditis, thyroid enlargement is the most frequent manifestation, with 75% of patients having a euthyroid goiter; the remainder have the atrophic variety and may not have a palpable gland. Hypothyroidism occurs as an initial manifestation in 20% of patients. Hyperthyroidism occurs in < 5% of patients and can be either self-limiting or longstanding, representing Hashitoxicosis. The principal abnormalities in the immune system discussed for Graves' disease also apply to Hashimoto's disease. The prevalence of specific forms of TSH receptor antibodies with a predominance of the TSI in Graves' disease versus the occurrence of TSH receptor–blocking antibodies in Hashimoto's disease distinguishes the two autoimmune diseases. In addition, lymphocyte infiltration is much more destructive to the architecture of the normal gland than in Graves' disease. Other autoimmune diseases occur with increased frequency in Hashimoto's patients, including autoimmune diseases of the endocrine system with adrenal, parathyroid, pituitary, and gonad destruction and damage to β cells of the pancreas. Furthermore, an association occurs with pernicious anemia, Sjögren's syndrome, lupus erythematosus, and idiopathic thrombocytopenic purpura. Graves' disease can occur in conjunction with the same illnesses.

On physical examination, a painless symmetrically enlarged thyroid gland is noted which feels firm and rubbery with an irregular surface. The gland can reach a size and firmness that leads to pressure symptoms, impairing swallowing and resulting in inlet obstruction with tracheal compression. Sometimes only one firm lobe or a single firm thyroid nodule may be palpable, representing the only remnant, with other parts of the gland destroyed by the autoimmune process. On laboratory examination, 90% of patients have positive antiperoxidase antibodies and 50% have antithyroglobulin antibodies. T_4 and TSH levels can be normal. In patients with the hypothyroid form, TSH levels are elevated and T_4 and free T_4 levels are decreased. RAI scans are not required for routine workup and are not diagnostic. They can show normal, increased, or decreased overall uptake with local patchy areas of increased and decreased iodine accumulation. Fine-needle aspiration is not routinely used but can be helpful in differentiating a firm nodule as a thyroid remnant in Hashimoto's disease versus a benign thyroid adenoma or thyroid cancer. The incidence of thyroid cancer is not increased in Hashimoto's disease except for the increased occurrence of lymphomas, a rare event.

TREATMENT. The autoimmune abnormality underlying Hashimoto's disease is currently not amenable to therapy. Therapy is directed at achieving a euthyroid state and dealing with mechanical problems resulting from the goiter. Thyroxine replacement is initiated when T_4 levels are low and TSH levels are high. In some patients, only the TSH is slightly elevated and the T_4 is low-normal, with signs of hypothyroidism being absent. These patients can be treated with thyroxine replacement to forestall further thyroid gland enlargement and future clinical hypothyroidism. In some patients, thyroxine therapy cannot decrease the goiter size and obstructive symptoms may require surgery for relief. During the early phases of Hashimoto's disease, transient hyperthyroidism can occur and requires only symptomatic treatment with sympathetic β-blockers. Hyperthyroidism developing in well-established Hashimoto's disease is treated like Graves' disease, with antithyroid medication as the treatment of choice.

Fibrous Thyroiditis (Riedel's Thyroiditis)

In fibrous thyroiditis, thyroid tissue is replaced by dense, chronically inflamed fibrous tissue. The thyroid is rock hard on palpation, a finding that can be compatible with thyroid cancer. Thyroid aspiration can clarify the diagnosis. Tracheal obstruction can occur and may require surgery. Sclerosing mediastinitis, retroperitoneal fibrosis, sclerosis of the biliary tract, and pseudotumors of the orbit have been described in such patients. When hypothyroidism exists, thyroxine replacement is required.

Rapoport B: Pathophysiology of Hashimoto's thyroiditis and hypothyroidism. Ann Rev Med 42:91, 1991. *A thorough review of the subject.*
Singer PA: Thyroiditis. Acute, subacute, and chronic. Med Clin North Am 75:61, 1991. *Provides a thorough discussion of the condition.*

NONTOXIC DIFFUSE AND NODULAR GOITER

The term *nontoxic* or *simple goiter* indicates an increase in the mass of the thyroid gland resulting from excessive replication of benign thyroid epithelial cells. In patients with nontoxic goiter, thyroid hormone levels are usually normal. The increase in thyroid size is a slow process evolving over many years, starting with a diffuse initial enlargement, which frequently becomes multinodular with time. Nontoxic goiter is the most common thyroid disease in America, affecting about 5% of the population. Its incidence increases with age and affects women three to five times more frequently than men. Goiters have been classified according to the epidemiologic pattern in which they occur as endemic or sporadic goiters. Thyroid enlargement occurring in > 10% of a population is termed *endemic goiter* and is presumed to result from environmental factors, such as iodine deficiency or the presence of goitrogens in the food chain which inhibit thyroid hormone formation. *Sporadic goiter* indicates thyroid enlargement in a small fraction of the population. The cause of sporadic goiter varies, with thyroid growth most frequently stimulated by extrathyroidal growth factors. TSH is the most frequent stimulator. The observation that goiters also occur in patients with adequate thyroid hormone levels and normal or low TSH levels indicates either that the sensitivity of thyroid cells to TSH can increase markedly or that other factors drive thyroid cell growth. Stimulatory effects of IGF-1 and EGF on thyroid cell growth have been reported. In addition, TSH receptor-directed antibodies that have only a growth-stimulating effect have been described. Different thyroid cells also have a varying propensity to grow and enter the mitotic cycle independent of stimulation by growth factors. Specific thyroid cells and their descendants that possess an increased noncancerous propensity to divide and grow can form new thyroid follicles. These different factors that contribute to goiter formation explain why not all goiters shrink or stop growing on thyroxine supplementation and resultant TSH suppression.

The pathology of the goitrous thyroid varies, depending on the stage and cause of the goiter. Initially, hypertrophic follicles with hypervascularity are prevalent throughout the gland. With increasing duration follicle size varies. Some follicles become involuted whereas others enlarge with colloid accumulation. Fibrotic areas sometimes separate hypertrophic from atrophic and involuted areas. This mixed pattern of follicle activity is reflected in RAI scans with patchy areas of increased and decreased uptake.

MANIFESTATIONS. Patients with nontoxic simple goiter can be asymptomatic or present with symptoms due to mechanical pressure exerted by the enlarged thyroid gland. Structures exposed to pressure are the trachea, esophagus, recurrent laryngeal nerve, and large cervical veins. Substernal goiters are most frequently responsible for tracheal pressure symptoms leading to deviation, narrowing, and chondromalacia. The trachea must be narrowed to 20 to 30% of its normal diameter to produce respiratory symptoms, especially inspiratory stridor. Pull and pressure on the laryngeal nerve leading to hoarseness can occur with benign goiters but should raise the suspicion of malignancy. The presence of a substernal goiter is made evident when patients raise both arms above the head, which pulls the goiter upward into the thoracic inlet. The resultant impediment of jugular venous return leads to a livid suffusion of the face and discomfort for the patient (Pemberton's sign). An acute painful enlargement of an area of the thyroid frequently reflects sudden bleeding into a thyroid nodule; symptoms improve as resorption of the hemorrhage occurs. In a slow and progressively developing dominant nodule, thyroid cancer must be excluded by cytologic examination of a fine-needle aspirate.

Congenital goiter in endemic areas results most frequently from insufficient thyroid hormone formation due to iodine deficiency or the presence of goitrogens and resultant TSH stimulation of the gland. Sporadic congenital goiter is often due to biosynthetic abnormalities in thyroid hormone formation resulting from defects in (1) iodide transport into the thyroid, (2) deficient peroxidase activity, (3) deficient iodotyrosine coupling, (4) formation of abnormal thyroglobulin, (5) impaired thyroglobulin proteolysis, or (6) deiodinases being deficient or absent and not allowing for intrathyroidal iodide conservation. These defects are rare and account for 10% of all congenital hypothyroidism. If these patients are left untreated, goiter and cretinism can result. In other patients, nontoxic goiter with mild hypothyroidism develops. The combination of congenital hypothyroidism and eighth nerve deafness has been termed Pendred's syndrome.

DIAGNOSTIC PROCEDURES. The most sensitive index to evaluate thyroid status in patients with goiter is the TSH level. TSH can be elevated in the face of normal or low-normal T_4 levels and mid-normal T_3 values. Most such patients benefit from thyroxine replacement, with TSH decreasing into the normal range and removing the thyroid growth stimulus. The thyroid status of patients with nontoxic goiter needs to be evaluated once or twice a year because some thyroid nodules develop autonomy over time, and toxic adenomas with resulting thyrotoxicosis can develop. In addition, ingestion of excess iodine can induce thyrotoxicosis due to the Jodbasedow effect. With progressive involution of the goiter, TSH values increase progressively and hypothyroidism develops. The presence of pressure symptoms requires evaluation for substernal extension of the thyroid gland which is best performed by CT scan or MRI. In the absence of such imaging, radiography reveals tracheal deviation, and pulmonary function tests can document inspiratory impairment. In patients with endemic goiter, especially due to iodine deficiency, laboratory values show a low T_4, normal T_3, and elevated TSH level stimulating the thyroid gland for further compensatory growth. The amount of iodine intake can be documented by determining iodide excretion in the urine which is correspondingly low in iodine-deficiency regions.

TREATMENT. The aim of therapy is to decrease the size of the thyroid, relieve pressure-induced symptoms, and achieve a euthyroid state. The approach to the patient with a goiter is outlined in Figure 203–4. In patients with sporadic goiter and elevated TSH levels, a clear rationale for thyroxine therapy is given. Thyroxine is started at 100 μg per day with subsequent dose adjustments to bring TSH into the low-normal but not the undetectable range. In patients with large, nontoxic diffuse goiters and normal T_4 and TSH levels, the same approach is chosen. The efficiency of this approach is indicated by a 20% decrease in thyroid volume after 1 year of treatment. In patients showing a response to therapy, treatment may be indefinite.

Treatment of multinodular goiter, especially in older patients, provides a more difficult problem. The TSH level must be determined, and if it is suppressed or in the low-normal range, thyroxine therapy should not be started. Thyroxine therapy also can be guided by results of an RAI scan and the suppression test, as described above. Identification of autonomous areas excludes thyroxine therapy. In patients with multinodular goiter without autonomous areas

and high-normal or elevated TSH levels, a trial of thyroxine therapy can be undertaken. In older patients, the initial dose of thyroxine should not be higher than 50 μg, and dose increases should be staggered at 25-μg steps at 4- to 6-week intervals. The results of thyroxine suppression therapy in patients with longstanding multinodular goiter are frequently disappointing, with little or no decrease in goiter size. Because thyroid tissue between nodules can decrease considerably, however, the nodules may appear more prominent. If no discernible decrease in size of multinodular goiter occurs after 6 to 12 months, thyroxine therapy should be stopped. In such patients, symptoms of temporary hypothyroidism can occur 1 month after stopping the medication and last for an additional month.

Endemic goiter is best treated by iodine supplementation, providing approximately 200 μg of iodine per day, or by the removal of identifiable goitrogens. Iodine supplementation can induce thyrotoxicosis due to the Jodbasedow effect. Surgical therapy of a goiter should be undertaken only if significant obstructive symptoms occur and goiter size cannot be reduced by thyroxine therapy. After partial thyroidectomy, thyroxine at 1.6 μg per kilogram per day should be supplied to prevent regenerative hyperplasia. RAI therapy for large goiters has been tried with modest success. ^{131}I can induce a thyroiditis and thyroid swelling, leading to an acute increase in obstructive symptoms, and should therefore be performed only in carefully observed patients.

Greenspan FS: The problem of the nodular goiter. Med Clin North Am 75:195, 1991. *Provides a detailed analysis of the problem.*
Studer H, Peter JH, Gerber H: Natural heterogeneity of thyroid cells: The basis for understanding thyroid function and nodular goiter growth. Endocrinol Rev 10:125, 1989. *An excellent explanatory treatise.*

BENIGN AND MALIGNANT THYROID NODULES

A thyroid nodule is a single palpable abnormality in the thyroid gland which can be a benign adenoma or thyroid cancer. Thyroid nodules are frequent and occur in about 5% of the population. In contrast, thyroid cancer is much less frequent, and among 100 patients with thyroid nodules only 4 have thyroid cancer. Distinguishing between benign and malignant lesions is an important task that is best accomplished by sampling cells from the lesions by fine-needle aspiration. This distinction is required to perform selective surgery.

Solitary Thyroid Nodules

INCIDENCE, ETIOLOGY, AND PATHOLOGY. Thyroid nodules must be at least 1 cm in diameter to be palpable. Such clinically detectable nodules occur in 6% of women and about 1.5% of men. The prevalence rises to 40 to 50% if smaller nodules are included which are discovered by autopsy or high-resolution ultrasonography. Ultrasound studies also reveal that abnormalities which appear as single nodules on palpation often represent conglomerates of multiple nodules. A solitary thyroid nodule identified on palpation is, therefore, a rather nonspecific finding. The most common benign lesion forming a single thyroid nodule is a thyroid adenoma. Most likely such adenomas result from clones of follicular cells which progress more quickly through the cell cycle but show benign growth characteristics. An adenoma is defined as a solitary encapsulated nodule composed of follicular cells arranged in an architecture that differs from that of the adjacent gland. The definition distinguishes adenomas from adenomatous nodules, which represent the early stage of a multinodular goiter. Adenomatous nodules lack a well-defined capsule or an architecture similar to the surrounding gland; clinically, adenomatous nodules and thyroid adenomas have a similar appearance. Adenomas vary in size, cell architecture, and appearance of follicular cells. Cell architecture nearly always follows a follicular pattern, with papillary adenomas being very rare. Follicular adenomas are classified into microfollicular or macrofollicular lesions and an embryonal variant containing almost no collagen. Hürthle cell adenomas are made up of follicular cells containing a large amount of mitochondria and have an eosinophilic staining pattern. No clear correlation between functional behavior or a propensity for malignant degeneration has been established for these different types of adenomas, and they are not precursors of thyroid cancer. Because adenomas are often hypercellular and contain mitotic figures, differentiation of a benign follicular adenoma from a follicular carcinoma on cytologic material obtained by aspiration is frequently not possible. Capsular invasion and vessel infil-

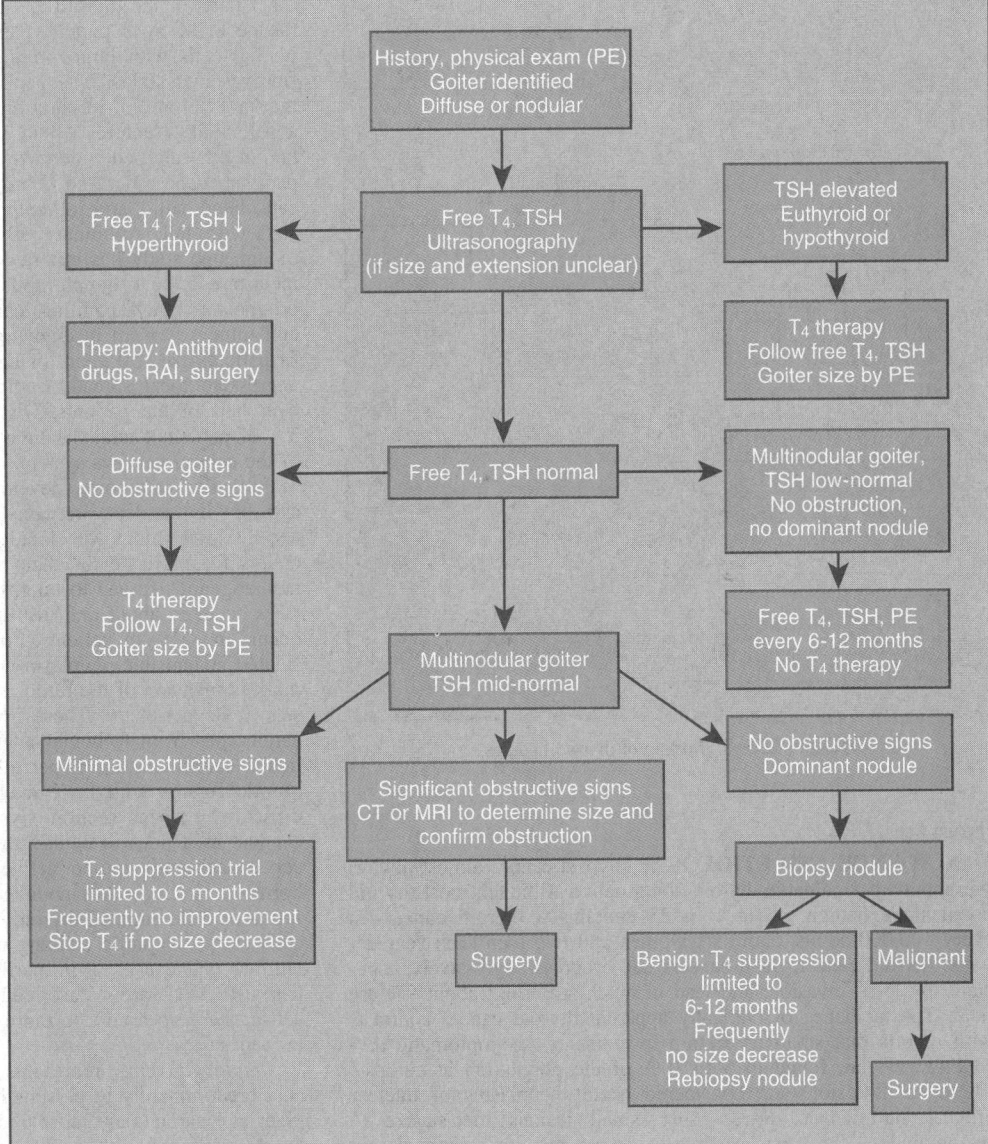

FIGURE 203–4. Evaluation and management of patients with nontoxic diffuse and nodular goiter and undetermined thyroid status.

tration are hallmarks of a malignant lesion, and these can be assessed only by histologic examination of the entire nodule. Frequently nodules outgrow their blood supply and undergo cystic degeneration. Ultimate pathologic evaluation of follicular neoplasms identifies benign adenomas in 85% and carcinomas in 15%.

MANIFESTATIONS, DIAGNOSIS, AND TREATMENT. Most thyroid nodules are discovered on routine physical examination. A systematic approach to thyroid nodules is outlined in Figure 203–5. Only rarely do solitary nodules become large enough or extend below the sternum to cause pressure symptoms. Bleeding into a nodule can lead to acute pain and enlargement. Most patients with thyroid nodules are euthyroid because 85 to 90% of the adenomas concentrate iodine very poorly and do not actively form thyroid hormone. The evaluation of a thyroid nodule includes a history, especially inquiries about the occurrence of specific risk factors such as radiation to the head and neck area. Examination reveals the presence of the nodule and should evaluate lymph nodes in the head and neck area as well as the clinical thyroid status of the patient. Blood determinations of free T_4 and TSH should be obtained to confirm the thyroid status. Fine-needle aspiration of the thyroid nodule to provide material for evaluation by a cytopathologist provides the most accurate assessment. Results to be expected from fine-needle aspiration are listed in Table 203–4. Identification of a nodule as a papillary carcinoma requires thyroid surgery. If a suspicious result is obtained and cannot distinguish between a follicular adenoma and a carcinoma, an RAI scan can be performed: 85 to 90% of thyroid nodules are nonfunctional or "cold" and 20% of such nodules contain a malignancy. Identification of a nodule with a

suspicious cytologic result as nonfunctional on RAI scan should result in surgical removal. About 10 to 15% of thyroid nodules are functional or "hot"; the incidence of thyroid cancer is <1% in such lesions. A recent report indicates that a mutant TSH receptor, which always stimulates thyroid hormone formation even when it is not occupied by TSH, is expressed in functional adenomas. If such patients are euthyroid, they can be followed with careful evaluation of thyroid size and functional status. Sooner or later 25% of these patients become hyperthyroid. Nodules in such patients are surgically removed after the patient is made euthyroid by treatment with PTU or MMI. In older patients or in patients with a high surgical risk, such nodules can be ablated with RAI.

In about 75% of patients, a thyroid nodule aspirate indicates a benign thyroid nodule. Most such patients have few or no pressure symptoms. In patients with a normal TSH level, thyroxine should be given, starting at 100 μg per day but choosing lower doses in elderly patients and those having cardiovascular symptoms, as discussed above. Approximately a one-fifth reduction in the size of these nodules occurs in a majority of patients within 6 to 12 months. If no response to thyroxine occurs, the medication can be stopped. The size of the nodule should then be followed carefully, and a growing nodule should be reaspirated at 1- to 2-year intervals. Rapid growth of a nodule, especially in a patient on thyroxine, requires reaspiration. Increase in nodule size can be due to the accumulation of fluid in a cystic lesion. Although the cyst can be aspirated, fluid frequently reaccumulates and the nodule progressively enlarges. Benign enlarging nodules can be removed surgically.

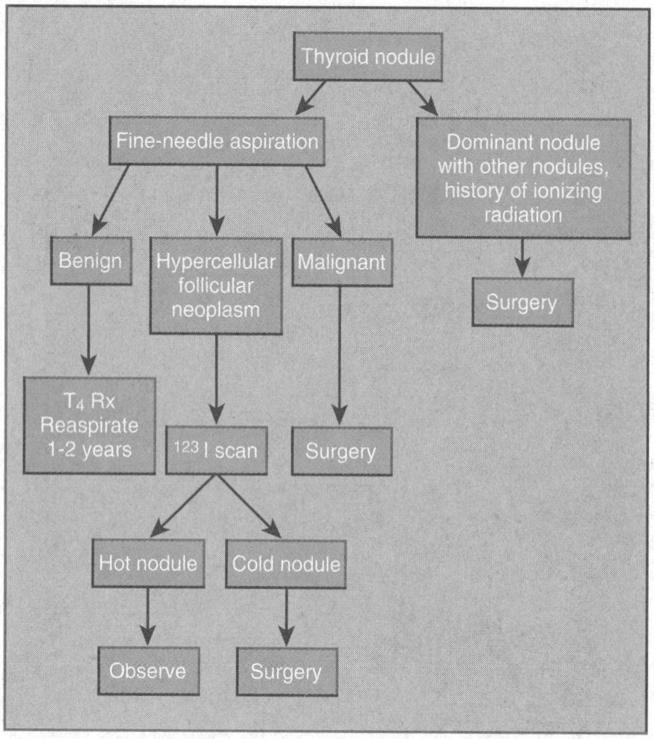

FIGURE 203–5. Workup of thyroid nodules.

Thyroid Cancer

INCIDENCE AND ETIOLOGY. Thyroid cancer almost always presents with a palpable thyroid abnormality. Although most thyroid nodules are benign, about 1 in 25 contains a thyroid cancer. In every 100,000 adults, about six women and two men each year develop thyroid cancer. Such cancers can progress aggressively, especially by local invasion, and lead to much suffering; about 9% are fatal. The incidence of clinically apparent thyroid cancer contrasts with reports that small (< 10 mm in diameter), asymptomatic thyroid cancers are found in 5 to 10% of the population at autopsy. These small lesions are considered occult neoplasms of unclear clinical significance. Rarely such small lesions metastasize to lymph nodes. The cause of thyroid cancer remains unknown, but activation of kinase genes *ret* and *trk* have been reported. In follicular cancer, mutations of the *ras* kinase gene occur in papillary cancer. Anaplastic cancer shows inactivating mutations of the p53 repressor gene. Despite these beginnings, however, a conclusive relationship between specific gene alterations and particular forms of thyroid cancer has not been established. Certain risk factors for thyroid cancer can be identified. Radiation to the head and neck area, especially during early childhood, leads to a 30-fold increase in thyroid cancer with radiation doses up to 1500 rad. Higher radiation doses of 5000 rad or more, as they are delivered to the thyroid by ^{131}I therapy for Graves' disease, do not lead to an increased incidence of thyroid cancer. Other risk factors are primarily genetic and include familial forms of papillary cancer, Gardner's and Cowden's syndrome for papillary cancer, and the multiple endocrine neoplasia (MEA) type II syndrome for medullary cancer. Most thyroid cancers are of follicular epithelial cell origin; chronic TSH stimulation appears to play a permissive but not causative role in differentiated papillary and follicular thyroid cancers. Papillary cancer is the least aggressive malignancy and represents about 70% of all thyroid cancer, with follicular cancers representing 15%. The rest are made up of medullary cancer, anaplastic cancer, lymphomas, and other rare tumors. Metastases to the thyroid occur primarily from malignant melanomas and cancers of breast, lung, and kidney.

PATHOLOGY. Papillary cancer is the most common thyroid cancer in the United States, being two to three times more common in women and relatively more common in young patients. The absolute incidence is higher in the fourth to seventh decades. Papillary cancers occur most frequently in parts of the world where iodine

supply is adequate. Papillary cancers generally are not encapsulated, and they grow slowly by infiltrative local spread, initially affecting other parts of the thyroid and extending to regional lymph nodes in the neck. Microscopically, papillary cancer is characterized by epithelial cells with large, irregular, frequently clear nuclei covering fibrovascular stalks. The papillae, which give the tumor its name, may not be present in parts of the tumor, and some parts may have a follicular structure. About half of papillary carcinomas contain laminated, calcified spherules called psammoma bodies. Variants of papillary cancer with good prognosis include the micropapillary encapsulated, solid, and follicular variants. A poor prognosis is associated with tall, columnar cells and diffuse sclerosis variants. Although one study has reported a higher mortality with lymph node metastases, local lymph node invasion is not necessarily a bad prognostic sign in papillary cancer because it occurs even with occult tumors < 1 cm in diameter, which have a favorable prognosis. In patients past 50 years of age, papillary cancers undergo a more aggressive local spread, leading to death from local invasions in over half of the patients. Distant metastases are uncommon (2 to 3% of patients), with the lung more frequently involved than bone or the central nervous system.

Follicular carcinoma develops more frequently with increasing age, but its incidence remains only one fifth that of papillary cancer. Despite this lower incidence, however, follicular cancer accounts for more deaths than papillary cancer because of its early hematogenous spread to lung, bone, brain, and liver. Distant metastases occur in about one fifth of patients. Lymph node involvement occurs in < 1% of patients. Follicular cancer presents as an encapsulated, expansile neoplasm with a microfollicular pattern. Its hallmark is invasion of the tumor capsule and extension into blood vessels at its periphery. These invasive features distinguish follicular carcinomas from follicular adenomas. Aspirates obtained from follicular carcinomas are hypercellular, containing cells with numerous mitotic figures with large nuclei. The diagnosis, however, can be difficult on frozen section. Cyst formation occurs in follicular cancer just as it does in benign thyroid nodules. Rarely follicular cancer concentrates iodine actively and generates sufficient thyroid hormone to create hot nodules leading to thyrotoxicosis. In some forms of differentiated thyroid cancer, epithelial cells called Hürthle cells show oxyphilic staining and contain numerous mitochondria. Hürthle cell cancer is primarily a variant of follicular cancer but has also been rarely described with a papillary structure. Hürthle cell cancer appears to be more aggressive than papillary or follicular cancer.

Anaplastic cancer represents about 5% of thyroid cancer and occurs predominantly in persons older than 70 years. The spindle and giant cell variants are most frequent, and the rare small cell variant can be confused with lymphomas or medullary cancer. Almost one third of anaplastic cancers arise in pre-existing differentiated cancers. The prognosis is dismal, with a mean survival of 7 to 12 months. Death most commonly results from aggressive local invasion causing progressive tracheal obstruction or massive hemorrhage. Distant metastases occur, but the local spread is so rapid that metastatic foci have little clinical importance.

Medullary carcinoma is a malignant tumor of calcitonin-secreting C cells which accounts for 2 to 3% of all thyroid cancer. The tumor produces calcitonin, calcitonin-related peptide, chromogranin A, ACTH, prostaglandins, and carcinoembryonic antigen. Densely packed cells form solid masses separated by hyalinized tumor stroma. Amyloid deposits occur frequently. Several variants of the tumor have been described, with the sporadically occurring form accounting for 80% and genetic or familial variants making up the remainder. The familial variants can be subdivided into those occurring with multiple endocrine neoplasia (MEN)2a, MEN2b, and a familial non-MEN variant. In MEN2a the medullary cancer occurs together with pheochromocytomas and parathyroid adenomas; in MEN2b pheochromocytomas and ganglioneuromas occur. In the familial form, the tumor is multicentric in origin and C cell hyperplasia precedes cancer development. The tumor metastasizes via the lymphatic route and the bloodstream. The peak incidence of the sporadic form is in the sixth and seventh decades. At the time of diagnosis, lymphatic spread has frequently developed. Medullary carcinoma is quite aggressive and less than half its carriers survive for 10 years.

Thyroid lymphoma most frequently consists of the diffuse B-cell variant and occurs most frequently in patients with Hashimoto's disease. Such lymphomas present as rapidly growing masses replacing thyroid tissue and extending through the capsule into adjacent soft tissue. Secondary involvement of the thyroid by malignant lymphoma arising elsewhere occurs in about one fifth of patients with advanced generalized lymphoma.

MANIFESTATIONS, DIAGNOSIS, AND TREATMENT. Thyroid nodules are frequent, but only about 1 in 20 contains a thyroid cancer. Figure 203–5 outlines the approach to such lesions. The task is to identify the cancerous lesion in order to perform selective surgery. Specific features in the patient's history and symptoms and signs can point to the occurrence of cancer but are not conclusive. Thyroid cancer is more likely in a nodule developing in a child or a patient over age 60, especially males. A single hard nodule showing rapid, painless growth is more likely to be a cancerous lesion. A history of radiation to the head and neck area during childhood, a family history of thyroid cancer, Gardner's syndrome, Cowden's syndrome, and MEN2 syndrome all represent strong risk factors. A single hard nodule noted on palpation which is fixed to surrounding tissue and the identification of firm, poorly mobile lateral lymph nodes may indicate cancer spread.

Laboratory tests offer little in the diagnosis of thyroid cancer. In most patients with thyroid nodules, thyroid hormone values are normal. Elevated thyroid hormone levels indicate a follicular carcinoma markedly overproducing thyroid hormone. In the rare patients with medullary cancer, calcitonin-related peptides and calcitonin levels are elevated. The evaluation of patients with MEN2 is discussed in Ch. 210. Fine-needle aspiration of thyroid nodules and examination of the obtained material by a cytopathologist provide the highest diagnostic yield. The procedure is easy to perform and, aside from occasional bleeding in the thyroid nodule, is without serious risk. Results obtained by fine-needle aspiration are listed in Table 203–4. When a trained cytopathologist is not available, the evaluation needs to be modified. A ^{123}I scan is performed to determine if the thyroid nodule is cold. Because 20% of cold nodules coming to attention in a referral center contain thyroid cancer, such nodules are surgically removed. Thyroid ultrasonography can provide further detail, especially related to the presence of fluid and cystic lesions. Most fluid accumulation in thyroid nodules represents cystic degeneration of thyroid nodules, and the incidence of cancer in such lesions is not markedly different from that in solid nodules.

Thyroid surgery should be performed by an experienced thyroid surgeon. Some diversity of opinion exists related to the extent of the operation. For example, some thyroid surgeons treat a 1.5- to 2.0-cm papillary cancer only with a lobectomy, whereas others prefer a near-total thyroidectomy. The author prefers the removal of such lesions by near-total thyroidectomy. In the hands of an experienced surgeon, complications from permanent hypoparathyroidism (2%) or vocal cord paralysis (2%) are no greater for a near-total thyroidectomy than for a lobectomy. A near-total thyroidectomy has the advantage that only small remnants of thyroid tissue remain which can be ablated with RAI. Because normal thyroid tissue accumulates RAI much more avidly than any thyroid cancer, it is not possible to treat thyroid cancer successfully by ^{131}I therapy in the presence of a large amount of normal thyroid tissue. In addition, after near-total thyroidectomy the patient can be followed with thyroglobulin levels. Increases in the level of thyroglobulin indicate a return of thyroid cancer.

^{131}I ablation is used in patients who undergo near-total thyroidectomy, especially if the primary lesion is a papillary cancer >2 cm in diameter or a follicular cancer. The regimen goes as follows: One day after surgery, patients are started on triiodothyronine (Cytomel 25 μg every day or twice a day) and maintained on this dose of T_3 for 4 to 6 weeks. T_3 has a half-life of 1 day and the patient becomes hypothyroid much more quickly than with thyroxine treatment. When medication is stopped at the end of the 4- to 6-week healing period, the patient becomes markedly hypothyroid, documented by an elevated TSH level. After the TSH has attained levels of at least 40 μU per milliliter, a scanning dose of 3 mCi of ^{123}I is administered. If a small remnant of thyroid tissue is left in the bed of the thyroid, an ablative dose of 29 mCi of ^{131}I is administered. Identification of a larger amount of thyroid tissue or lymph node metastases leads to the administration of a higher dose of ^{131}I, ranging from 75 to 125 mCi according to the amount of remaining tissue. Seven to 10 days after treatment, a second RAI scan can be performed. This post-treatment scan identifies areas of ^{131}I uptake that were not detected by the initial lower dose diagnostic scan. In the future, administration of human recombinant TSH will induce high TSH levels and stimulate ^{131}I uptake. This step will eliminate the need to achieve hypothyroidism before RAI is administered.

When patients become hypothyroid for RAI scanning, it is important to obtain a thyroglobulin level: Elevated levels indicate that a sizable mass of thyroid tissue was left after surgery. Patients who had considerable thyroid tissue left or tumor spread to lymph nodes should be rescanned 6 months after the initial scan to ensure that the initial RAI treatment ablated all thyroid tissue. Patients who had only a small amount of tissue left can be rescanned within 1 year. Patients whose thyroglobulin levels remain normal should be rescanned 3 years after surgery. If no evidence of RAI accumulation occurs, no subsequent rescanning is necessary and patients can be followed with thyroglobulin values. In about 10% of patients, thyroid cancer can dedifferentiate, resulting in a discrepancy between a positive RAI scan and undetectable thyroglobulin levels. Similarly, patients with elevated thyroglobulin level and minimal or absent RAI uptake on scans have been identified. Such individuals need to be followed carefully and may require additional RAI treatment because the elevated thyroglobulin level can indicate the presence of thyroid cancer. The best initial treatment of patients with near-total thyroidectomy for papillary cancer consists of giving sufficient thyroxine to suppress TSH into the low-normal range combined with RAI therapy. This regimen markedly decreases the late recurrence of papillary cancer. Follicular carcinoma is more aggressive and should be treated more vigorously than papillary cancer. Medullary cancer does not respond to RAI therapy and must be treated with surgery plus external radiation and chemotherapy, especially if bone metastases occur. Anaplastic cancer has a poor prognosis; attempts to increase survival time by treatment with chemotherapy and external radiation therapy have been unsuccessful, although palliative external radiation can especially alleviate obstruction.

Clark OH, Duh Q-Y: Thyroid cancer. Med Clin North Am 75:211, 1991.
Mazzaferri EL: Papillary thyroid carcinoma: Factors influencing prognosis and current therapy. Semin Oncol 14:315, 1987.
Ridgeway EC: Clinician's evaluation of a solitary thyroid nodule. J Clin Endocrinol Metab 74:231, 1992.
Robbins J, Merino MJ, Boice JD Jr, et al.: Thyroid cancer: a lethal endocrine neoplasm. Ann Intern Med 115:133, 1991.

204 THE ADRENAL GLAND

204.1 Adrenal Cortex

D. Lynn Loriaux

The two adrenal glands lie either on top of or next to each kidney (Fig. 204–1). Each gland, between 6 and 8 grams in weight, is composed of a cortex and medulla. The cortex makes steroid hormones, and the medulla, in essence a sympathetic ganglion, makes catecholamines. The cortex includes three histologic zones in the adult: zona glomerulosa, zona fasciculata, and zona reticularis (Fig. 204–2). Each zone can be thought of as an independent organ. The outermost zona glomerulosa produces aldosterone, the primary mineralocorticoid in humans. The zona fasciculata produces primarily cortisol, the primary glucocorticoid in humans, and the zona reticularis produces the "adrenal androgens." The adrenal androgens are, in fact, androgen and estrogen precursors, the parent compound being dehydroepiandrosterone (DHA) and its sulfate conjugate. The biologic actions of these steroid hormones are effected via intracellular receptors, cytoplasmic or nuclear in location, that regulate gene transcription upon binding with the appropriate ligand. DHA has no known receptor. The distribution of these receptors defines the responsive tissues for each hormone. Aldosterone regulates sodium balance, acting primarily on the distal tubule of the nephron. Cortisol maintains physiologic integrity in ways that re-

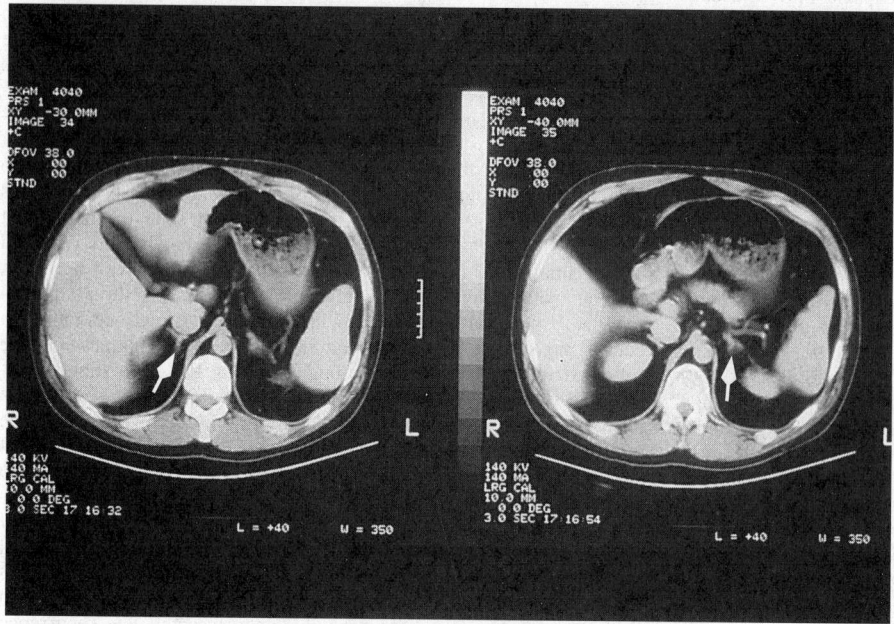

FIGURE 204-1. MRI of abdomen showing the position and relative size of the normal adrenal glands.

main poorly understood, and its receptors are found in virtually every cell in the body. DHA has no identifiable biologic action. The synthesis and secretion of each of these hormones are regulated, in the main, by a separate "feedback" system. The major trophic hormone for aldosterone secretion is renin, for cortisol adrenocorticotropic hormone (ACTH), and for DHA cortical androgen–stimulating hormone (CASH), which is not yet fully characterized. Thus,

in the case of the zona glomerulosa and the zona fasciculata, the functional status of each can be assessed by measuring two hormones: aldosterone and plasma renin, and cortisol and ACTH, respectively.

The adrenal medulla, in essence a sympathetic ganglion, produces catecholamines in response to neural input. Disorders of the adrenal medulla are discussed in Ch. 204.2.

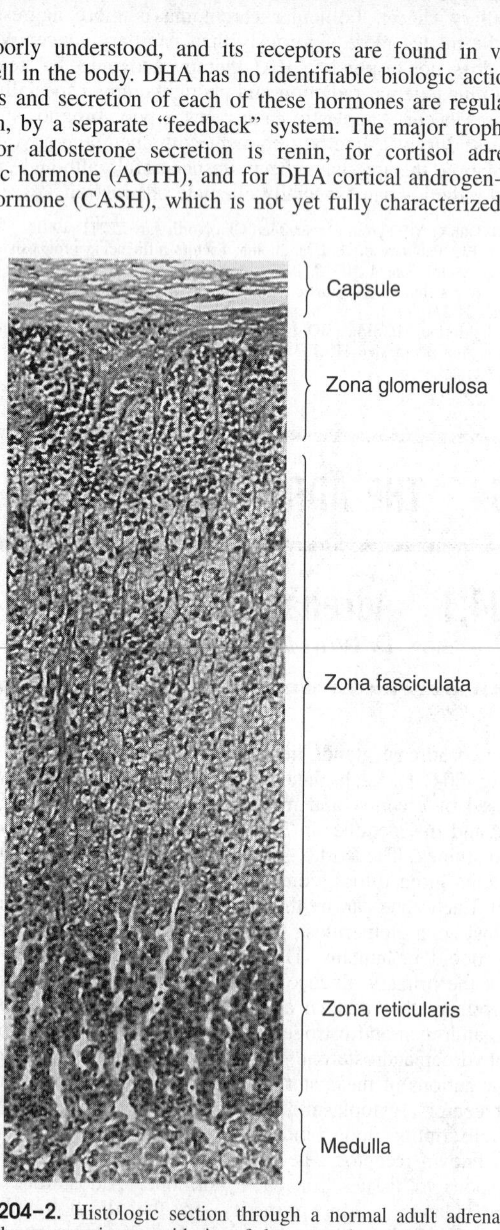

DISORDERS OF ADRENOCORTICAL FUNCTION

Disorders of adrenocortical function can be thought of as disorders of overproduction or underproduction of the four classes of steroid hormones produced by the adrenal gland: cortisol, aldosterone, androgen, and estrogen. In addition, "mixed" disorders, the congenital adrenal hyperplasias, are characterized by a clinical picture of combined hormone excess and deficiency. These disorders are considered separately.

The diagnosis of disorders of adrenocortical function, like that of other endocrine syndromes, requires a compatible clinical picture with biochemical confirmation of the associated underlying abnormality. In years past, the tests used in the diagnosis of adrenal disease were both confusing and many. Fortunately, the last several years have brought order and simplification to the process.

Tests of Adrenocortical Function

THE PORTER-SILBER CHROMOGENS. The 3-carbon side chain of cortisol reacts with meta-dinitrobenzene to form a colored adduct with an absorption maximum at 410 μm. Other adrenal steroids having this configuration in the side chain include cortisone, 11-deoxycortisol, tetrahydrocortisone, tetrahydro-11-deoxycortisol, and tetrahydrocortisol (Fig. 204–3). This reaction, called the Porter-Silber chromogen reaction, was the basis of the first test to provide some measure of cortisol production. It is still in widespread use. Because urinary metabolites are, for the most part, conjugated to glucuronic acid and sulfuric acid, the measurement of Porter-Silber chromogens first involves an acid hydrolysis to cleave these conjugates. This is followed by a lipid extraction with a solvent such as dichloromethane. The Porter-Silber reaction is performed on the steroids in the lipid extract. The absorption maximum is quantitated spectrophotometrically. The normal range for Porter-Silber excretion is 2 to 12 mg per day. The excretion of these steroids is markedly affected by body size, and the normal range is considerably narrowed by normalizing the measurement against urinary creatinine excretion. With this correction, the normal range is the same for all ages, 4.5 ± 1(SD) mg per gram of creatinine per day. The normal range includes the extinction point for the assay, which means that values below the normal range cannot be measured reliably with this assay.

URINE FREE CORTISOL. Urine free cortisol is that fraction of urinary cortisol that is neither conjugated to glucuronic or sul-

Capsule

Zona glomerulosa

Zona fasciculata

Zona reticularis

Medulla

FIGURE 204-2. Histologic section through a normal adult adrenal gland showing the progression, outside in, of the zona glomerulosa, zona fasciculata, and zona reticularis.

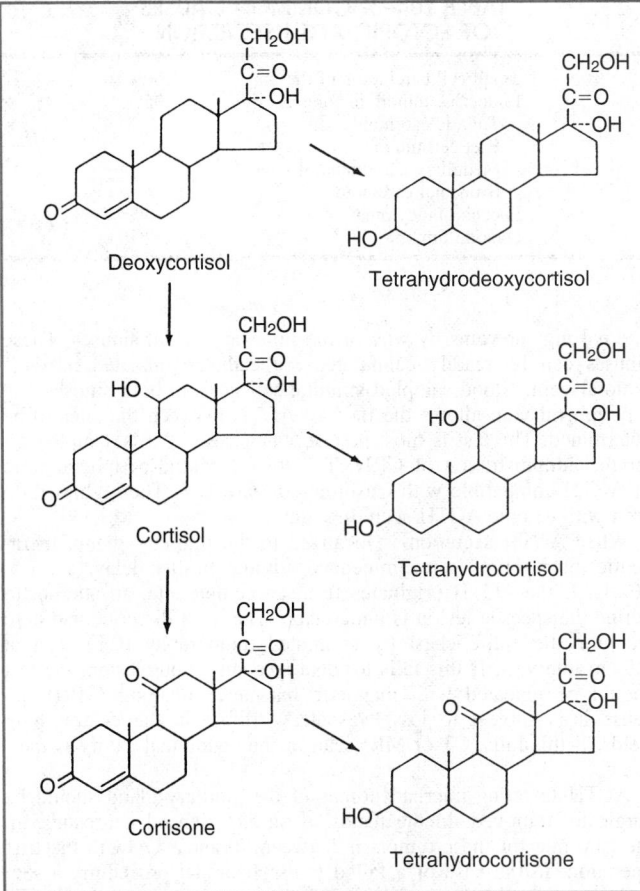

FIGURE 204–3. The family of steroids known as the Porter-Silber chromogens, commonly referred to as the 17-hydroxysteroids.

furic acid nor bound to a protein. Accordingly it is filtered by the renal glomerulus and can be extracted directly from urine with a lipid solvent. The detection limit of this assay also lies in the normal range of cortisol excretion and, hence, is not a reliable test for adrenal insufficiency.

PLASMA CORTISOL. Intuitively, the measurement of circulating plasma cortisol should provide the most direct assessment of adrenal cortisol secretion. The secretion of cortisol is pulsatile, with a steady frequency of about one pulse per hour in adults. The amplitude of these pulses, however, varies markedly, with 8 to 10 high-amplitude pulses clustering in the early morning hours. This pattern creates a diurnal secretory rhythm in plasma cortisol concentration. Cortisol circulates predominantly bound to a glycosylated 59-kD α_2-globulin, cortisol-binding globulin (transcortin [CBG]). This binding protects circulating cortisol from hepatic clearance and gives cortisol a relatively long plasma half-life of 60 to 80 minutes. Normal plasma cortisol concentrations range between 5 and 20 μg per deciliter. At some time each day, normal subjects have plasma cortisol concentrations that cannot be differentiated from zero. These biologic complexities make hazardous the interpretation of isolated plasma cortisol determinations. If cortisol is measured at frequent intervals (30 minutes) over a 24-hour period and the values are averaged, the mean plasma cortisol concentration amounts to 7.5 ± 1 μg per deci-liter. To work within this narrow confidence interval, however, requires the measurement of a large number of plasma cortisol concentrations, which is prohibitive except in extraordinary circumstances.

PLASMA ACTH CONCENTRATION. The development of the two-site immunoradiometric assay (IRMA) for ACTH simplified considerably the differential diagnosis of adrenal disease. The normal range of plasma ACTH extends up to 100 pg per milliliter.

Three provocative tests of adrenal function are in common use. The *ACTH stimulation test* is the most reliable screening test for adrenal hypofunction. It is also the standard method by which suspected enzymatic deficiencies in adrenal steroidogenesis are examined. The test is performed by administering 250 μg of synthetic ACTH (Cortrosyn) intravenously and measuring the serum steroids of interest 45 and 60 minutes later. The normal adrenal gland pro-

duces plasma cortisol concentrations > 20 μg per deciliter in response to this challenge. *Corticotropin-releasing hormone (CRH),* the 41-amino acid hypothalamic secretagogue for ACTH, is a useful test for separating ACTH-dependent from ACTH-independent hypercortisolism and is an essential component of the inferior petrosal sinus sampling procedure (IPSS) for localizing the site of ACTH secretion (see Ch. 204.2). The test is performed by infusing CRH, 1 μg per kilogram, intravenously over 1 minute and measuring the ACTH response between 3 and 30 minutes thereafter.

The *dexamethasone suppression test* is widely used to screen for adrenal hyperfunction. The test has so many false-positive and false-negative results (sensitivity and specificity of about 0.8), however, that it is superseded by the tests mentioned above. The test retains some value in the differential diagnosis of mineralocorticoid excess. Many iterations of this test are available, the simplest being 0.5 mg dexamethasone administered by mouth every 6 hours for 2 days.

Plasma and urine aldosterone and plasma renin activity are important tests to evaluate states of apparent mineralocorticoid excess and deficiency.

The differential diagnosis of congenital adrenal hyperplasia requires the measurement of specific steroid biosynthetic intermediates that accumulate proximal to the responsible enzymic deficiencies in the steroid biosynthetic cascade. The most commonly measured are 17-hydroxyprogesterone (21-hydroxylase deficiency) and 11-deoxycortisol (11-hydroxylase deficiency). These steroids are most reliably measured in the context of an ACTH stimulation test, as described above.

Adrenal Hyperfunction

There are four syndromes of adrenal hyperfunction: Cushing's syndrome, hypokalemic metabolic alkalosis, masculinization, and feminization. These result from the excessive secretion of cortisol, mineralocorticoid, androgen, and estrogen, respectively. These disorders can occur in isolation or, more commonly, in combination with one or more of the others.

GLUCOCORTICOID EXCESS—CUSHING'S SYNDROME.
Diagnosis. Cushing's syndrome is caused by glucocorticoid excess. The "classic" syndrome is defined clinically: weight gain, plethora, striae, hypertension, and proximal muscle weakness (Table 204–1). The weight gain is predominantly truncal, with increased fat deposited in a yokelike pattern around the neck, leading to the well-known dorsocervical fat pad (buffalo hump) and filling in of the supraclavicular fossae. Plethora is evident as a ruddy complexion. The striae of Cushing's syndrome are characteristically violaceous in appearance and occur in thin skin. Proximal muscle weakness is best assessed by testing the ability of the patient to rise unassisted from a squatting position. The biochemical diagnosis depends on the demonstration of an elevated plasma concentration of "bioactive" cortisol, which is best reflected in the excretion of urine free cortisol. If the clinical picture is "strong," urine free cortisol concentrations above the normal range are adequate for the diagno-

TABLE 204–1. CLINICAL FEATURES OF GLUCOCORTICOID EXCESS

	Frequency (%)
Weight gain	90
"Moon facies"	75
Hypertension	75
Violaceous striae	65
Hirsutism	65
Glucose intolerance	65
Proximal muscle weakness	60
Plethora	60
Menstrual dysfunction	60
Acne	40
Easy bruising	40
Osteopenia	40
Dependent edema	40
Hyperpigmentation	20
Hypokalemic metabolic alkalosis	15

sis. If the clinical picture is "weak," urine free cortisol excretion must be above the levels found in "physiologic" causes of adrenal activation, such as stress and depression. This level is generally taken to be 250 μg per day. This approach to the diagnosis of Cushing's syndrome occasionally identifies patients with an "atypical" picture. At one extreme are patients with minimal clinical manifestations of Cushing's syndrome but very high levels of free cortisol excretion. This constellation of findings is characteristic of Cushing's syndrome associated with systemic malignancy, typically a small cell carcinoma of the lung. The clinical picture is dominated by the "cachexia" of malignancy, and the typical "anabolic" features of Cushing's syndrome such as weight gain and dorsocervical fat distribution fail to develop. At the other extreme are patients with well-established clinical signs of Cushing's syndrome but without sufficient urine free cortisol excretion to confirm the diagnosis. This situation is usually the result of iatrogenic or surreptitious exogenous glucocorticoid administration. A careful history and review of systems usually reveal the source of the glucocorticoid. In the rare cases of surreptitious glucocorticoid abuse, measurement of the commonly prescribed synthetic glucocorticoids in randomly obtained serum samples is necessary for the diagnosis. Rarely, naturally occurring Cushing's syndrome can be cyclic or even intermittent. In this case, repeated measures of urine free cortisol at frequent intervals of 3 to 5 days are necessary to establish the diagnosis.

Differential Diagnosis and Treatment. The causes of Cushing's syndrome are shown in Table 204–2. They can be conveniently divided into ACTH-dependent and ACTH-independent causes. This differentiation is made on the basis of the plasma ACTH concentration following the administration of CRH. Values >10 pg per milliliter indicate ACTH-dependent disease; values <10 pg per milliliter indicate ACTH-independent disease.

The causes of ACTH-dependent Cushing's syndrome include *Cushing's disease* caused by an ACTH-secreting pituitary tumor and the *ectopic secretion of ACTH* from a neoplasm not of pituitary origin. Cushing's disease is the most common cause of Cushing's syndrome, accounting for 70 to 80% of all noniatrogenic cases (see Ch. 202.1). The ectopic secretion of ACTH by a nonpituitary neoplasm accounts for about 10% of cases. The common causes of ectopic ACTH secretion are listed in Table 204–3. More than 90% of these tumors are found in the chest. The most common cause is small cell cancer of the lung. Other neoplasms include bronchial carcinoid tumors, medullary cancer of the thyroid, islet cell tumors of the pancreas, and pheochromocytoma.

There are two forms of the ectopic ACTH syndrome. In the first, Cushing's syndrome occurs as classically described by Harvey Cushing. It can be thought of as the *anabolic form* of ectopic ACTH secretion because it is associated with weight gain and the characteristic central obesity of the disorder. It is usually caused by slow-growing benign tumors such as bronchial carcinoid tumors. The second form, *the catabolic form,* has none of the anabolic features associated with "classic" Cushing's syndrome. Weight loss, hypertension, edema, and hypokalemia dominate the clinical picture. This form of the disease is commonly associated with advanced and widely metastatic tumors that impair caloric intake and prevent weight gain and the development of central obesity.

Differentiating the two ACTH-dependent forms of Cushing's syndrome from each other depends on localizing the source of the ACTH secretion. The most effective method of doing this is by sampling inferior petrosal sinus blood for the measurement of ACTH levels (IPSS). Pituitary venous blood drains into the cavernous sinuses on either side of the sella turcica and thence into the

TABLE 204–2. CAUSES OF CUSHING'S SYNDROME

ACTH-dependent causes
  ACTH-secreting pituitary tumor (Cushing's disease)
  Nonpituitary ACTH-secreting neoplasm (ectopic ACTH syndrome)
ACTH-independent causes
  Adrenal adenoma
  Adrenal carcinoma
  Micronodular adrenal disease
  Factitious or surreptitious glucocorticoid administration

TABLE 204–3. COMMON CAUSES OF ECTOPIC ACTH SECRETION

Small cell carcinoma of the lung	50%
Endocrine tumors of foregut origin	35%
Thymic carcinoid	
Islet cell tumor	
Medullary carcinoma, thyroid	
Bronchial carcinoid	
Pheochromocytoma	5%
Ovarian tumors	2%

internal jugular veins by way of the inferior petrosal sinuses. These sinuses can be readily cannulated via catheters inserted into the femoral vein. Blood sampled simultaneously from both sinuses and a peripheral vein allows the ratio of ACTH between the sites to be determined. The test is most precise when the blood is sampled after the administration of CRH. The lowest central-peripheral ratio of ACTH compatible with Cushing's disease is 3. The highest ratio seen with ectopic ACTH-secreting tumors is 1.8.

When ACTH secretion is localized to the pituitary gland, therapeutic intervention is recommended without further delay (see Ch. 202.1). If the ACTH originates from an ectopic site, an attempt to define the specific lesion is undertaken. The most direct course is to examine the entire chest by computed tomography (CT) scan at 0.5-cm intervals. If this fails to identify a suspicious lesion, the test should be repeated with magnetic resonance imaging (MRI) because it is subject to less "vascular" artifact in the central lung fields. If this fails, CT or MRI scan of the abdominal cavity is indicated.

ACTH-secreting microadenomas of the pituitary gland should be surgically removed. In the hands of an experienced neurosurgeon, the cure rate for these tumors is between 90 and 95% with the first operation. In the case of a failed transsphenoidal procedure, a second procedure is successful in 50% of cases. The recurrence rate appears to be <5%. Ectopic tumors should be removed if found. If the tumor cannot be found or is found to be widely metastatic, adrenal blockade with ketoconazole, up to 1200 mg by mouth in divided doses, is an effective treatment for the associated glucocorticoid excess. Ultimately, if the process appears to be headed to a protracted course, bilateral adrenalectomy via flank incision or laparoscopy is a useful adjunct to management.

The causes of ACTH-independent Cushing's syndrome, if iatrogenic and factitious disease are excluded, are adrenal in origin: adrenal adenoma, adrenal cancer, and micronodular adrenal dysplasia. They account for 10 to 20% of naturally occurring cases of Cushing's syndrome. Adrenal adenomas are the most common, accounting for about 15% of cases of Cushing's syndrome. The tumors are typically unilateral, are <4 cm in diameter, and produce only a single steroid hormone, in this case, cortisol. Adrenal cancers are rare, having an incidence of 1 in 600,000 per year. They are generally unilateral and large at the time of discovery, usually >6 cm in diameter. Adrenal cancers typically produce more than one steroid hormone, the most common combinations being glucocorticoid and mineralocorticoid, or glucocorticoid and androgen. The differentiation of an adenoma from a carcinoma is made clinically; histologic examination of the tissue is of little value. The most important indicators of malignancy are size at the time of diagnosis, the number of steroid hormones clinically apparent, and any evidence of spread at the time of surgical intervention. Micronodular adrenal dysplasia is characterized by normal or small adrenal glands that show scattered 1- to 3-mm hyperplastic nodules separated by atrophic adrenal cortex. This disease can be sporadic or part of a larger syndrome, Carney's complex, in which the adrenal disease is associated with pigmented lentigines, atrial myxoma, and germ cell tumors (see references).

The differential diagnosis of ACTH-independent Cushing's syndrome depends almost exclusively on the findings produced by CT or MRI scan. Small unilateral lesions with no evidence of metastasis should be removed by a unilateral flank excision or by a laparoscopic procedure. Large lesions should be removed via a transabdominal approach so that the abdominal organs can be carefully examined and the liver biopsied at the time of operation. The treatment for micronodular adrenal dysplasia is bilateral adrenalectomy.

Metastases should be surgically excised until no longer feasible. The only known chemotherapy effective against this cancer is *ortho, para'*-DDD (OP'DDD). It is given orally to tolerance, usually a dose between 6 and 10 grams per day. Side effects are neuropsychiatric and gastrointestinal, with somnolence, ataxia, reduced attention span, nausea, and diarrhea predominating. One-fourth of patients have an objective remission, and the remissions average 7 months in duration. No-one has been cured of metastatic adrenocortical carcinoma.

MINERALOCORTICOID EXCESS. *Diagnosis.* There are no reliable symptoms of mineralocorticoid excess. Signs include arterial hypertension and dependent edema. Laboratory findings are more specific. The mineralocorticoid effect on the distal nephron is sodium retention at the expense of potassium and hydrogen excretion. Excess mineralocorticoid produces an expanded vascular volume in association with hypokalemia and metabolic alkalosis. Mineralocorticoid excess can be renin-angiotensin–independent or –dependent. Aldosterone-secreting tumors are examples of renin-angiotensin–independent disease. In renin-angiotensin–dependent disease, the mineralocorticoid is produced in response to the renin-angiotensin trophic signal. This is commonly encountered in states of contracted arterial volume such as congestive heart failure or cirrhosis with ascites. The two forms of mineralocorticoid excess can be differentiated on the basis of the plasma renin activity. If resting plasma renin activity is high, the mineralocorticoid excess is renin-angiotensin–dependent. If plasma renin activity is low and cannot be stimulated by 4 hours of upright posture, the mineralocorticoid excess is renin-angiotensin–independent.

***Renin-Angiotensin–Independent Mineralocorticoid Excess.* Differential Diagnosis and Treatment.** Table 204–4 lists the causes of renin-angiotensin–independent mineralocorticoid excess. Aldosterone is the offending mineralocorticoid in most but not all of these disorders. The first task is to differentiate cases caused by aldosterone excess from those caused by another mineralocorticoid. Urine and plasma aldosterone measurements provide the answers for this differentiation. If the aldosterone concentration is normal or above, aldosterone is the causative agent. If the aldosterone concentration is below the normal range or undetectable, the disorder is caused by a mineralocorticoid other than aldosterone.

There are two common causes of aldosterone-mediated renin-angiotensin–independent mineralocorticoid excess: aldosterone-producing adenoma and bilateral hyperplasia of aldosterone-secreting cells. Dexamethasone-suppressible hyperaldosteronism is a rare cause of aldosterone-mediated renin-angiotensin–independent mineralocorticoid excess. It can be excluded by finding normal or high levels of circulating aldosterone after 2 days of giving dexamethasone, 2 mg per day by mouth in divided doses. The remaining causes of renin-angiotensin–independent aldosterone excess must be separated from one another to guide the appropriate therapeutic intervention. Aldosterone-secreting adenomas respond well to surgical removal, whereas bilateral hyperplasia does not. The most direct approach to this differentiation is to measure cortisol-aldosterone ratios in adrenal venous blood sampled simultaneously from both glands following the administration of ACTH. The diagnostic accuracy of this test approaches 100%. Aldosterone-secreting adenomas are characterized by high levels of aldosterone from one side and none from the other, the secretion from the nonaffected side being suppressed by the volume-expanded state. Bilateral hyperplasia is characterized by comparable aldosterone levels from each gland, making cortisol-aldosterone ratios in effluent adrenal blood roughly equal on the two sides.

Unilateral adrenal adenomas should be surgically excised. In the hands of an experienced surgeon, the cure rate is very high. Bilateral hyperplasia does not respond well to surgery and is best treated with spironolactone to dampen the metabolic sequelae of mineralocorticoid excess and with antihypertensive medications if spironolactone inadequately controls blood pressure.

The causes of non–aldosterone-mediated renin-angiotensin–independent mineralocorticoid excess are rare (Table 204–5). The first task is to exclude adrenocortical carcinoma. This is best done by imaging the adrenal glands with CT or MRI scan. Failure to find adrenal asymmetry with a dominant mass, usually > 4 cm in diameter, essentially excludes the diagnosis. Symmetrically enlarged adrenal glands of moderate degree suggest congenital adrenal hyperplasia. The two congenital adrenal hyperplasias that lead to hypertension are 11-hydroxylase deficiency and 17-hydroxylase deficiency. The first can be diagnosed by measuring the circulating concentration of 11-deoxycortisol. Normally, this steroid does not circulate in plasma. 17-Hydroxylase deficiency is best diagnosed by a unique clinical picture (hypertension, pubertal delay, and genital ambiguity) coupled with an inappropriately elevated plasma progesterone concentration.

The enzyme 11β-hydroxysteroid dehydrogenase (HSD) catalyzes the conversion of cortisol to cortisone. Cortisol interacts with the mineralocorticoid receptor as an agonist; cortisone does not. Because the circulating concentrations of cortisol are 1000 times those of aldosterone, cortisol can have considerable mineralocorticoid activity in humans. This is prevented by the action of 11β-HSD, which converts cortisol to its inactive metabolite, cortisone. If the activity of this enzyme is impaired, cortisol assumes the role of aldosterone. Because cortisol secretion is not regulated by the renin-angiotensin system, a state of mineralocorticoid excess at normal plasma cortisol concentrations results. The appropriate treatment is to suppress cortisol secretion with an exogenous glucocorticoid having little or no mineralocorticoid activity, such as dexamethasone or prednisone.

The active ingredient in licorice, glycyrrhizic acid, is a competitive inhibitor of 11β-HSD. Thus, licorice intoxication can cause hypertension by the same mechanism as spontaneously occurring 11β-HSD deficiency. Licorice intoxication usually can be excluded by history. The most common source of licorice in the United States is chewing tobacco.

All causes of non–aldosterone-mediated renin-angiotensin–independent mineralocorticoid excess except for malignancy should "respond" to adrenal suppression with dexamethasone, 2 mg per day. If this fails, especially in the presence of an adrenal mass, adrenal malignancy is suggested. When adrenal suppression is successful, hydrocortisone, 12 to 15 mg per square meter per day, should be used for long-term treatment.

Adrenal Hypofunction

GLUCOCORTICOID DEFICIENCY (Table 204–6). ***Diagnosis.*** A broad spectrum of signs and symptoms can herald the presence of glucocorticoid deficiency. At one extreme is the *"chronic syndrome,"* characterized by symptoms of malaise, anorexia, and orthostatic hypotension. Occasionally, vague abdominal pain can occur. Signs include weight loss, hypotension with an orthostatic component, and, in certain cases, a melanin-based hyperpigmentation of the skin. The routine laboratory picture reveals a normochromic normocytic anemia, relative lymphocytosis often with

TABLE 204–4. COMMON CAUSES OF RENIN-ANGIOTENSIN–INDEPENDENT MINERALOCORTICOID EXCESS

Aldosterone-secreting adenoma
Adrenal cancer
Congenital adrenal hyperplasia
    11-hydroxylase deficiency
    17-hydroxylase deficiency
11β-hydroxysteroid dehydrogenase deficiency
Licorice intoxication
Glucocorticoid-suppressible hyperaldosteronism

TABLE 204–5. COMMON CAUSES OF RENIN-ANGIOTENSIN–DEPENDENT MINERALOCORTICOID EXCESS

Vomiting
Diuretics
Edematous disorders
    Congestive heart failure
    Hepatic cirrhosis
    Nephrotic syndrome
Renal ischemia
Bartter's syndrome
Renin-secreting tumors

TABLE 204-6. CAUSES OF GLUCOCORTICOID DEFICIENCY

ACTH-independent causes
    Tuberculosis
    Autoimmune (idiopathic)
    Other rare causes
        Fungal infection
        Adrenal hemorrhage
        Metastases
        Sarcoidosis
        Amyloidosis
        Adrenoleukodystrophy
        Adrenomyeloneuropathy
        HIV infection
        Congenital adrenal hyperplasia
        Medications (ketoconazole, OP'DDD)
ACTH-dependent causes
    Hypothalamic-pituitary-adrenal suppression
        Exogenous
            Glucocorticoid
            ACTH
        Endogenous—cure of Cushing's syndrome
    Hypothalamic-pituitary lesions
        Neoplasm
            Primary pituitary tumor
            Metastatic tumor
        Craniopharyngioma
        Infection
            Tuberculosis
            Actinomycosis
            Nocardiosis
    Sarcoid
    Head trauma
    Isolated ACTH deficiency

an unexplained eosinophilia, mild prerenal azotemia, and hyponatremia. If aldosterone secretion is impaired by the process, hyperkalemia also can be observed. At the other extreme is the *"acute syndrome,"* characterized by rapidly evolving agitation, confusion, fever, and abdominal pain, all associated with arterial hypotension. As the hypotension evolves into shock, it is relatively unresponsive to volume replacement and pressor agents, imitating the hemodynamic characteristics of "pump" failure in association with increased vascular volume. The laboratory findings are the same as those found in the chronic syndrome. Untreated, the acute syndrome quickly leads to coma and death. When first seen, the symptoms and signs of most patients with adrenal insufficiency lie somewhere on the continuum between these two extremes.

The diagnosis of glucocorticoid deficiency is confirmed by the inability of the adrenal glands to respond normally to an ACTH challenge. Synthetic ACTH, 250 μg, is administered intravenously, and plasma cortisol is determined 45 and 60 minutes later. The normal adrenal gland produces plasma cortisol concentrations of 20 μg per deciliter or more. Any value < 20 μg per deciliter implies a degree of adrenal compromise. Because the differential diagnosis of adrenal insufficiency relies on the plasma concentration of ACTH, it is prudent to draw a blood sample for ACTH prior to the administration of ACTH and to "hold" the sample in the laboratory pending the results of the plasma cortisol determination.

Differential Diagnosis and Treatment. The first task in the differential diagnosis of glucocorticoid deficiency is to define whether or not the process is ACTH-dependent. ACTH-dependent glucocorticoid deficiency implies disordered function of the hypothalamus and/or pituitary gland leading to ACTH deficiency, whereas ACTH-independent glucocorticoid deficiency is caused by disordered adrenal function, such as destruction of the gland by an infectious process like tuberculosis. This distinction is best made on the basis of plasma ACTH concentration measured at the time of glucocorticoid deficiency (i.e., before treatment with glucocorticoid has been initiated). ACTH concentrations in or below the normal range imply an ACTH-dependent process. ACTH concentrations above the normal range imply an ACTH-independent process.

Glucocorticoid Deficiency Related to Adrenal Suppression. The most common cause of ACTH-dependent glucocorticoid deficiency is hypothalamic-pituitary-adrenal "suppression" by exoge-

nously administered glucocorticoids, either iatrogenic or factitious. Whether or not a patient develops adrenal suppression as a result of exogenous glucocorticoid administration depends upon three variables: the dose of the glucocorticoid administered, the duration of administration, and the schedule of administration. It is unusual to develop clinically manifest adrenal suppression with doses of glucocorticoid equal to or less than the daily replacement dose of the preparation employed—20 mg per day of hydrocortisone, 5 mg per day of prednisone or prednisolone, and 0.5 mg per day of dexamethasone. Given doses that exceed these limits, it is unusual to develop clinically manifest glucocorticoid deficiency if the duration of administration is < 3 weeks. Finally, the dosage schedule can affect the rapidity with which the final state of adrenal suppression is reached. Glucocorticoids given as a single dose first thing in the morning are the least suppressive; glucocorticoids given in divided doses throughout the day are the most suppressive. Thus, at one extreme are patients given decreasing doses of prednisone for 14 days to treat an acute inflammatory process such as poison ivy. Signs and symptoms of glucocorticoid deficiency following cessation of the medication are extremely unlikely. At the other extreme are patients treated with large doses of glucocorticoids given in divided doses for long periods of time for the treatment of disorders such as chronic obstructive pulmonary disease. These patients develop many of the stigmata of Cushing's syndrome and manifest signs and symptoms of glucocorticoid deficiency within 48 hours if the glucocorticoid is stopped for any reason. The clinical manifestations of this deficiency can range from the "chronic" syndrome at one extreme to the "acute" syndrome at the other.

Glucocorticoid Deficiency Due to Hypothalamic-Pituitary Disease. Destructive lesions of the hypothalamus and pituitary gland are a rare cause of ACTH-dependent glucocorticoid deficiency. Although it is uncommon, diagnosis is imperative because early therapeutic intervention can prevent many of the serious sequelae of these tumors, including blindness. Examples include pituitary tumor, metastatic tumors to the region, sarcoid, amyloid, craniopharyngioma, and Rathke's pouch cyst. Pituitary infections such as actinomycosis and nocardiosis and vascular accidents such as Sheehan's syndrome also can lead to adrenal insufficiency. The most direct approach to the diagnosis of these lesions is imaging with CT scan using contrast enhancement or with MRI following gadolinium administration. A rare cause of ACTH-dependent glucocorticoid deficiency is *autoimmune lymphocytic hypophysitis.*

The treatment of chronic ACTH-dependent glucocorticoid insufficiency consists of replacing the missing hormone. Glucocorticoid should be replaced in the form of hydrocortisone, the naturally occurring glucocorticoid in humans, at a rate of 12 to 15 mg per square meter per day. Cortisol is secreted in bursts, between 7 and 10 per day, clustering in the morning hours. To reproduce this pattern with replacement steroid is impossible with currently available methods. Empirically, however, it has been found that patients do as well with a single morning dose of cortisol as with divided doses, and compliance is simplified with this regimen. Clinical measures best monitor the adequacy of replacement: Anorexia, weight loss, and hyponatremia suggest underreplacement; weight gain, plethora, and supraclavicular fat deposition suggest overreplacement. The current standard of practice is to increase cortisol dose in the context of "stress," actual or anticipated. The dose of cortisol is doubled for the duration of the stress and returned to replacement levels immediately upon cessation of the stress. Typical stresses include febrile illness; nausea and vomiting; trauma such as lacerations, contusions, and fractures; and surgical procedures, including dental extraction. Acute glucocorticoid deficiency is treated with large doses of cortisol given intravenously, 100 mg every 6 hours, coupled with emergency support of blood pressure plus volume expansion and pressors when indicated.

Primary Adrenal Insufficiency. The most common cause of primary adrenal insufficiency worldwide is tuberculosis. Tuberculosis causes adrenal insufficiency by destroying the adrenal cortex and replacing it with caseating granulomas. The most common cause of adrenal insufficiency in the industrialized west is an autoimmune process, usually as part of the polyglandular deficiency syndrome. In this disorder, an autoimmune "adrenalitis" leads to destruction of the adrenal cortex. This disease has two forms, types I and II. The relative features of the two forms are detailed in Table 204–7. Type I is a disease of childhood with a mean age of onset of 12 years.

TABLE 204–7. POLYENDOCRINE DEFICIENCY SYNDROMES

	Type I	Type II
Age of onset	12 yrs	24 yrs
Adrenal insufficiency	+	+
Diabetes mellitus	–	+
Autoimmune thyroid disease	–	+
Hypoparathyroidism	+	–
Mucocutaneous candidiasis	+	–
Hypogonadism	+	+/–
Chronic active hepatitis	+	–
Pernicious anemia	+	–
Vitiligo	+	+

Type II begins at an average age of 24 years. The dominant features of type I disease are adrenal insufficiency, hypoparathyroidism, and mucocutaneous candidiasis. The dominant features of type II disease are adrenal insufficiency, autoimmune thyroid disease, and insulin-dependent diabetes mellitus. Other important differences include the patterns of inheritance. Type I is transmitted as an autosomal recessive trait, occurring across sibships, whereas type II has a "dominant" pattern of inheritance, appearing in multiple generations of an affected family. Also, type I disease has no HLA association, whereas type II is associated with the DR3/DR4 haplotypes. Both disorders appear to be mediated by an autoimmune process. For example, circulating antibodies to one or more endocrine organs are found in most patients, and defects in T lymphocyte function such as a decrease in "suppressor" activity are described.

All of the clinically important fungi except *Monilia* can cause adrenal destruction. The most common cause is histoplasmosis, which is due to an organism particularly prominent in the Ohio and Tennessee valleys and along the Piedmont Plateau of the Middle Atlantic states. South American blastomycosis is the next most common fungal cause of adrenal insufficiency, followed by North American blastomycosis, coccidioidomycosis, and cryptococcosis. The pathophysiology of fungal adrenalitis is much like that of tuberculosis—destruction leading to adrenal enlargement with caseating granuloma formation. If healing occurs, the adrenal glands can shrink in size, sometimes resuming a relatively normal volume. The healing process is often accompanied by calcification.

The advent of CT scan has revealed adrenal hemorrhage as a more frequent cause of adrenal insufficiency than had been recognized previously. The usual setting is a stressed individual receiving long-term anticoagulation for the prevention of pulmonary or cardiac emboli or other thrombotic phenomena. Typically, affected patients complain of back pain followed, in a few days, by the onset of the first signs and symptoms of adrenal insufficiency.

Metastases to the adrenal gland are common, with a frequency as high as 70% in patients with disseminated breast or lung cancer. Adrenal insufficiency as a result of metastases, however, is uncommon, although moderate abnormalities in adrenal function often can be detected in patients with bilateral adrenal metastases. Tumors commonly associated with adrenal insufficiency are cancers of the breast, lung, stomach, and colon; melanoma; and some lymphomas.

The syndrome of acquired immunodeficiency (AIDS) can be associated with adrenal insufficiency in its late stages. Cytomegalovirus infection of the adrenal glands commonly accompanies this condition, as does infection with *Mycobacterium avium-intracellulare* and the various fungi that can colonize and destroy the adrenal glands. The plasma cortisol response to ACTH administration is abnormal in 10 to 15% of patients with AIDS and its advanced complications.

Adrenoleukodystrophy is an inborn abnormality of long-chain fatty acids causing adrenal insufficiency in association with several neurologically impaired phenotypes. Newborn adrenoleukodystrophy is transmitted as an autosomal recessive trait. Adrenoleukodystrophy, also known as brown Schilder's disease (brown being an adjective describing the hyperpigmentation of the skin) or sudanophilic leukodystrophy, is transmitted as an X-linked disease of children characterized by rapidly progressive central demyelination eventuating in seizures, dementia, cortical blindness, coma, and death. Death usually occurs before puberty is complete. X-linked

adrenomyeloneuropathy is a disease of young adults characterized by a slowly progressive mixed upper and lower motor and sensory neuropathy leading to an ascending spastic paraparesis. Signs and symptoms of spinocerebellar degeneration appear in some cases. Both forms of the disease are associated with progressive failure of all steroid-secreting cells, leading to adrenal and gonadal failure. The metabolic marker for these diseases is an elevated circulating level of very long chain fatty acids (VLCFA's), C-26 and greater in length. The cause of this abnormality seems to be an abnormal peroxisomal transporter protein that prevents the appropriate metabolism of the VLCFA's. Several treatments have been tried, but only autologous bone marrow transplantation appears to be successful.

Other rare causes of primary adrenal insufficiency include amyloidosis, congenital unresponsiveness to ACTH, congenital adrenal hypoplasia, and familial glucocorticoid insufficiency.

The treatment of ACTH-independent glucocorticoid deficiency is the same as that outlined for ACTH-dependent glucocorticoid deficiency except that the addition of a mineralocorticoid is usually required. This is because adrenal cortical destruction impairs both cortisol and aldosterone secretion. The available orally active mineralocorticoid is fludrocortisone acetate (Florinef). It is equipotent with aldosterone. The secretion rate of aldosterone in salt-replete humans is about 100 μg per day. Thus, fludrocortisone, 100 μg per day, is the appropriate replacement dose. The drug has a wide therapeutic window, and no specific monitoring for treatment effect other than an occasional plasma potassium concentration is necessary.

MINERALOCORTICOID DEFICIENCY. *Diagnosis.* The major clinical manifestations of mineralocorticoid deficiency are hyponatremia, hyperkalemia, and mild metabolic acidosis. These can lead to profound muscle weakness and cardiac arrhythmias. Combined glucocorticoid and mineralocorticoid deficiency is a common cause of this picture and should first be excluded with an ACTH stimulation test. If that test is normal, the diagnosis of isolated hypoaldosteronism depends upon the demonstration of an inappropriately low circulating aldosterone level. The causes of isolated hypoaldosteronism are listed in Table 204–8.

Differential Diagnosis and Treatment. Selective hypoaldosteronism was, until recently, believed to be rare. Recent studies, however, show that it accounts for as many as 10% of cases of unexplained hyperkalemia. The causes of hypoaldosteronism can be divided into renin-angiotensin–dependent (hyporeninemic) and renin-angiotensin–independent (hyper-reninemic) causes. The differentiation is made on the basis of the plasma renin activity. The usual test is a measurement of plasma renin activity following 4 hours of upright posture. Levels in the normal or low range identify cases that are renin-angiotensin–dependent, whereas high levels identify cases that are renin-angiotensin–independent.

Renin deficiency, overall, is the most common cause of selective aldosterone deficiency. It is usually found in elderly subjects with mild, nonoliguric renal disease. Many such patients have insulin-dependent diabetes, and diabetic nephropathy is thought to be an important contributing abnormality. Other causes of renin-angiotensin–dependent hypoaldosteronism include autonomic dysfunction associated with prolonged bed rest and, rarely, treatment with prostaglandin synthesis inhibitors such as indomethacin.

TABLE 204–8. CAUSES OF ISOLATED HYPOALDOSTERONISM

Renin-angiotensin–dependent
  Hyporeninemic hypoaldosteronism
  Autonomic neuropathy
  Prostaglandin synthesis inhibitors
Renin-angiotensin–independent
  Inhibition of aldosterone synthesis
    Heparin
    Cyclosporine
    Calcium channel blockers
  Following resection of an aldosterone-secreting adenoma
  18-hydroxylase deficiency
  Aldosterone resistance (pseudohypoaldosteronism)

The causes of renin-angiotensin–independent hypoaldosteronism include all causes of ACTH-independent adrenal insufficiency listed in Table 204–6. In this setting, selective hypoaldosteronism can result if treatment is confined to glucocorticoid replacement. The other causes of this disorder center on alterations in the synthesis and secretion of aldosterone. These include long-term heparin administration and the "salt-wasting" forms of congenital adrenal hyperplasia (21-hydroxylase deficiency, 3β-hydroxysteroid dehydrogenase deficiency, and 17-hydroxylase deficiency). Again, treating these disorders with glucocorticoid alone is a common cause of selective hypoaldosteronism. Finally, any defect in the conversion of corticosterone to aldosterone, such as 18-hydroxylase deficiency, leads to selective hypoaldosteronism.

Treating selective hypoaldosteronism of any cause is straightforward. Aldosterone deficiency does not produce clinical symptoms unless the subject is "salt deprived." This is unlikely to occur at levels of salt intake greater than 10 mEq per kilogram per day. For adults, this equals about 4 grams of sodium chloride per day, which is routinely ingested in the average American diet. Thus, a simple way to treat selective hypoaldosteronism is to ensure adequate dietary salt intake which, in the United States, is not a problem in young and otherwise healthy subjects. This approach, however, fails in patients with "fetish" diets or those who cannot maintain an adequate oral intake of salt for any reason. Important in this regard are the dietary restrictions that frequently accompany old age and those often imposed upon infants and toddlers. In these cases, it is advisable to supply exogenous mineralocorticoid. Fludrocortisone is the only available preparation of orally active mineralocorticoid. It is equipotent with aldosterone and is given in doses that approximate the daily production rate of aldosterone in the salt-replete individual, 100 μg per day. The preparation can be given as a single daily dose with the morning meal. The drug's therapeutic window is wide, so overtreatment is unlikely. Thus, an occasional serum potassium concentration measurement is adequate to monitor efficacy of treatment.

Disorders of Combined Insufficiency and Excess

THE CONGENITAL ADRENAL HYPERPLASIAS. Defects in the synthesis of cortisol lead to compensatory stimulation of adrenal steroidogenesis to maintain normal plasma cortisol concentrations. This inevitably leads to an accumulation of the steroid biosynthetic intermediate immediately before the enzymatic defect in the biosynthetic cascade. Clinically, the result is expressed as glucocorticoid deficiency (which can be so mild as to be inapparent or so severe as to be life threatening) in association with mineralocorticoid excess or deficiency and androgen excess or deficiency. These disorders are usually classified as "salt-wasting," "hypertensive," "virilizing," or "feminizing," depending upon the combination of hormone excess and deficiency. They are presented in detail in Ch. 207. Only the attenuated or "nonclassic" form of 21-hydroxylase deficiency is presented here.

21-Hydroxylase deficiency is one of the most prevalent autosomal recessive disorders, with a heterozygote frequency that may be as high as one in five. Although congenital in nature, the disorder usually makes its first appearance with the onset of puberty. Hirsutism, oligomenorrhea, and cystic acne are the most common clinical manifestations. The disorder is identical in presentation to idiopathic hirsutism–polycystic ovarian disease and cannot be differentiated from this disorder without specifically examining adrenal steroidogenesis looking for the 21-hydroxylase block. This is best done in the context of an ACTH stimulation test performed in the usual way, with measurements of 17-hydroxyprogesterone made at 45 and 60 minutes after administration of the ACTH. Normal subjects do not exceed 17-hydroxyprogesterone levels of 350 ng per deciliter, but patients with the disorder attain plasma levels > 1500 ng per deciliter. The incidence of this disorder in young hirsute patients varies between 1 and 30%, depending on ethnic background, averaging about 5% for the population as a whole.

As with the other congenital adrenal hyperplasias, treatment consists of exogenous glucocorticoid replacement to circumvent the deficiency in cortisol biosynthesis. The usual approach is to administer cortisol (Cortef), 12 to 15 mg per square meter per day as a single morning dose. Care should be taken that the adrenal gland is not completely suppressed by the replacement regimen chosen. This

can be assessed by an ACTH stimulation test 3 to 6 months following the initiation of treatment.

DISORDERS OF TISSUE RESPONSIVENESS: THE STEROID RESISTANCE SYNDROMES

Two disorders of end-organ resistance are relevant to a discussion of disorders of adrenal function: glucocorticoid resistance and mineralocorticoid resistance.

Glucocorticoid resistance is rare; only 17 separate probands have been described to date. The disease is characterized by markedly elevated indices of cortisol production (increased urine free cortisol excretion) in the absence of any of the clinical stigmata of Cushing's syndrome. Occasionally, signs and symptoms of mineralocorticoid and androgen excess are responsible for bringing the patient to medical attention. Like the situation in congenital adrenal hyperplasia, androgens and mineralocorticoids are elevated in this syndrome as a by-product of the increased adrenal steroidogenesis necessary to produce enough cortisol to maintain life. The cause of the disease, which has not been proved in all cases, is a defect in the ligand-binding domain of the glucocorticoid receptor. The disease is transmitted as an autosomal recessive trait, with heterozygote subjects sometimes manifesting attenuated forms of the disorder.

The diagnosis is suggested by finding elevated rates of urine free cortisol excretion in a subject with none of the stigmata of Cushing's syndrome. The diagnosis is confirmed by demonstrating abnormal binding characteristics of the glucocorticoid receptor, usually in mononuclear leukocytes. Treatment should be reserved for persons manifesting signs and symptoms of androgen or mineralocorticoid excess and consists of the exogenous administration of a synthetic glucocorticoid, usually dexamethasone, in doses sufficient to bring the urine free cortisol excretion into the normal range. This is usually accompanied by remission of the associated steroid excess syndromes.

Mineralocorticoid resistance is characterized by elevated levels of aldosterone and increased plasma renin activity in association with signs and symptoms of mineralocorticoid deficiency. The disorder is generally referred to as pseudohypoaldosteronism. It is commonly divided into two subtypes, but only type 1 appears to fulfill the usual criteria for receptor-mediated end-organ resistance.

Type 1 pseudohypoaldosteronism is a rare inherited disorder presenting with salt loss and failure to thrive in infancy, most commonly between 5 and 7 days of age. The cause appears to be an abnormal mineralocorticoid receptor, with decreased binding affinity and decreased receptor number both described. Hyponatremia, hyperkalemia, and metabolic acidosis in association with elevated plasma and urine aldosterone and an elevated plasma renin activity make the diagnosis. The treatment is to replace dietary salt at a rate of 10 to 40 mEq per kilogram per day.

Aubourg P, Blanche S, Jambaque' I: Reversal of early neurologic and neuroradiologic manifestations of X-linked adrenoleukodystrophy by bone marrow transplantation. N Engl J Med 322:1860, 1990. *Describes a successful outcome from a previously always progressive and often fatal disease.*

Carney JA, Young WF: Primary pigmented nodular adrenocortical disease and its associated conditions. Endocrinologist 2:6, 1992. *Describes an associated complex of abnormalities.*

Donovan DS, Dluhy RG: AIDS and its effect on the adrenal gland. Endocrinologist 1:227, 1991. *The title says it all in this informative review.*

Friedman RB, Oldfield EH, Nieman LK: Repeat transsphenoidal surgery for Cushing's disease. J Neurosurg 71:520, 1989. *Describes the surgical approach when transnasal hypophysectomy fails to remove the tumor.*

Gill JR: Primary hyperaldosteronism: Strategies for diagnosis and treatment. Endocrinologist 1:365, 1991. *The title is self-explanatory.*

Javier E, Reardon GE, Malchoff CD: Glucocorticoid resistance and its clinical presentations. Endocrinologist 1:141, 1991. *A helpful discussion of a rare disorder.*

Miller J, Crapo L: The biochemical analysis of hypercortisolism. Endocrinologist 4:7, 1994. *Brings order and simplification to the subject.*

Muir A, Maclaren NK: Autoimmune diseases of the adrenal glands, parathyroid glands, gonads, and hypothalamic-pituitary axis. Endocrinol Metab Clin North Am 20:619, 1991. *A detailed coverage of the mechanisms and treatment of the autoimmune syndrome.*

Schteingart DE: Treating adrenal cancer. Endocrinologist 2:149, 1992. *Describes treatment and outcome in greater detail.*

Speiser PW, DuPont B, Rubenstein P: High frequency of non-classical steroid 21-hydroxylase deficiency. Am J Hum Genet 37:650, 1985. *Discusses the adult form of the syndrome.*

Urbanic RC: Cushing's disease—18 years' experience. Medicine 60:14, 1981.

Veldhuis JD, Melby JC: Isolated aldosterone deficiency in man: Acquired and inborn errors in the biosynthesis of action of aldosterone. Endocrinol Rev 2:495, 1986. *A clearly stated description of the problem.*

204.2 ADRENAL MEDULLA

Daniel T. O'Connor

The catecholamines (norepinephrine, epinephrine, and dopamine) serve as neurotransmitters and circulating hormones. Catecholamines acquire their name by the catechol (3,4-dihydroxyphenyl) modification of their aromatic (phenyl) rings. *Norepinephrine* is the amine neurotransmitter released from terminals of postganglionic axons of the sympathetic nervous system, as well as from central nervous system noradrenergic axons. Adrenal medullary chromaffin cells store both epinephrine and norepinephrine in catecholamine secretory vesicles.

Chromaffin cells derive embryologically from neuroectoderm. Precursor cells differentiate in the center of the adrenal gland in response to cortisol; the precursors then differentiate into sympathetic neurons in response to nerve growth factor. A few such cells also migrate to form paraganglia, collections of chromaffin cells on both sides of the aorta. The largest such periaortic cluster, often found near the level of the inferior mesenteric artery, is referred to as the organ of Zuckerkandl. Both chromaffin cells and postganglionic sympathetic axons are part of the effector limb of the sympathetic branch of the autonomic nervous system and are innervated by thoracolumbar preganglionic axons emerging from the spinal cord.

Catecholamines are released from the adrenal medulla into the circulation through the adrenal vein. Norepinephrine from sympathetic neurons is released presynaptically and acts as a cell-to-cell neurotransmitter. Circulating plasma norepinephrine influences blood pressure and heart rate under only the most extreme circumstances of sympathetic activation. Relatively selective adrenal catecholamine release occurs during syncope and insulin-evoked hypoglycemia, whereas active, dynamic exercise selectively stimulates sympathetic neuronal norepinephrine release.

CATECHOLAMINE BIOSYNTHESIS AND METABOLISM

Catecholamine biosynthesis starts with the essential dietary amino acid phenylalanine, which is converted to tyrosine by phenylalanine hydroxlase. Tyrosine is hydroxylated to dihydroxyphenylalanine (DOPA) by the action of tyrosine hydroxylase (TH), the rate-limiting enzymatic step in catecholamine biosynthesis. DOPA decarboxylase then converts DOPA to dopamine, which is carried by the vesicular monoamine transporter (VMT) from cytosol into the catecholamine storage vesicle, where dopamine-β-hydroxylase (DβH) converts it to norepinephrine. In sympathetic axons and in 15 to 20% of chromaffin cells, norepinephrine is the final catecholamine product. In 80 to 85% of chromaffin cells a further enzymatic step occurs: phenylethanolamine-*N*-methyltransferase (PNMT), a cytosolic enzyme, catalyzes the *N*-methylation of norepinephrine to epinephrine.

Catecholamines in noradrenergic axons and chromaffin cells are sequestered from the cytosol in membrane-limited organelles: catecholamine storage vesicles (or chromaffin granules, in chromaffin cells). Chromaffin granule cores contain not only catecholamines but also soluble proteins such as DβH and chromogranin A.

The process of catecholamine discharge from chromaffin cells and sympathetic axons is *exocytosis*, wherein all soluble components of the granule are co-released and ultimately make their way to the circulation.

Neuronal uptake ("reuptake") is the major route of norepinephrine removal from synaptic clefts (Fig. 204–4). Characteristics of this process are its location at the presynaptic axonal membrane, high-affinity, stereoselectivity, saturability, dependence on extracellular sodium, and specific pharmacologic inhibition by agents such as tricyclic antidepressants (e.g., desipramine) and cocaine. After neuronal uptake, cytosolic catecholamines can be either retransported into storage vesicles or deaminated by the enzyme monoamine oxidase (MAO), yielding the catecholamine metabolite dihydroxymandelic acid (DHMA). The enzyme catecholamine-O-methyltransferase (COMT), which acts on both catecholamines and DHMA, is present mainly in the cytosol of liver and kidney cells. COMT adds a methyl group to one of the hydroxyl oxygens on the catecholamines' dihydroxyphenyl rings, yielding either metanephrine (or methoxyepinephrine; from epinephrine), normetanephrine (or methoxynorepinephrine; from norepinephrine), or methoxytyramine (from dopamine). The metanephrines can then be deaminated by MAO to yield vanillylmandelic acid (VMA), while deamination of methoxytyramine by MAO yields homovanillic acid (HVA). DHMA is also a substrate for COMT, yielding VMA. Thus, complete enzymatic degradation of catecholamines to VMA (from epinephrine or norepinephrine) or HVA (from dopamine) involves the sequential action of two enzymes (MAO and COMT), either of which may initiate the process. In the bloodstream, catecholamines have a very short half-life, 1 to 2 minutes. They are cleared from the circulation largely by neuronal uptake but are also subject to direct renal excretion or sulfoconjugation of a ring hydroxyl group.

CATECHOLAMINE ACTION

Catecholamine receptors are specific for ligands and are classified as subtypes of the α ($\alpha_{1a,b,c}$, $\alpha_{2a,b,c}$) and β ($\beta_{1,2,3}$) classes. The hemodynamic effects of circulating norepinephrine require extreme concentrations. Whereas plasma norepinephrine may vary normally over a range of 200 to 1000 pg per milliliter during physiologic stimulation of sympathetic neuronal activity, far higher concentrations of infused norepinephrine (in excess of 1000 to 2000 pg per milliliter) are required to substantially affect blood pressure or heart rate. At β receptors, norepinephrine is a strong agonist at β_1 (cardiac, inotropic, and chronotropic) sites, although a relatively weak agonist at β_2 (vascular, vasodilatory) sites. At α receptors, norepinephrine is an effective agonist at both α_1 (vascular, vasoconstrictive) and α_2 (neuronal and vascular) sites. Infused norepinephrine acutely raises both systolic and diastolic blood pressure by actions on both β_1 and α adrenergic receptors, with vasoconstriction accompanied by reflex bradycardia. The hemodynamic effects of circulating epinephrine (50 to 500 pg per milliliter) differ from those

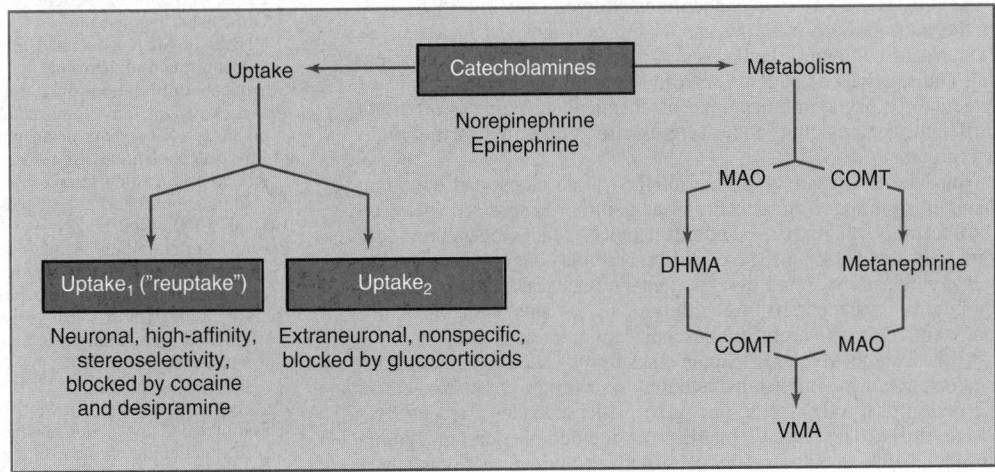

FIGURE 204–4. Catecholamine disposition and metabolism. MAO = monoamine oxidase; COMT = catechol-O-methyltransferase; VMA = vanillylmandelic acid; DHMA = dihydroxymandelic acid.

of norepinephrine. At β receptors, epinephrine is an agonist at both β_1 and β_2 sites. It is also a more potent agonist than norepinephrine at both α_1 and α_2 sites. During acute infusion, it increases systolic blood pressure, heart rate, and cardiac output, with a fall in diastolic blood pressure and systemic resistance, the latter effects resulting from actions at β_2 adrenergic receptors.

With chronic excess of circulating catecholamines, the hemodynamic profile may change substantially, in part as a consequence of desensitization of catecholamine target organs, resulting from adaptive changes in both receptor and postreceptor responses.

PHEOCHROMOCYTOMA

Pheochromocytoma is a chromaffin cell neoplasm that typically causes symptoms and signs of episodic catecholamine release, including paroxysmal hypertension. The tumor is an unusual cause of hypertension, accounting for at most 0.1 to 0.2% of cases of high blood pressure. In population-based cancer studies, its frequency was about two cases per million population. The diagnosis of pheochromocytoma is typically made in young to middle-aged adults, most commonly in the fourth or fifth decade of life; about 10% of diagnoses are made in children (usually male). Autopsy series indicate that the incidence of pheochromocytoma increases progressively with age. In adults, there is no gender difference in incidence.

About 90% of pheochromocytomas exist as solitary, unilateral, encapsulated adrenal medullary tumors. About 10% are bilateral, more commonly among several members of a family in which 40 to 70% may have bilateral tumors. The tumors are vascular, and large ones often contain internal hemorrhagic or cystic areas. Reported sizes have ranged from < 1 gram to several kilograms; the average is about 40 grams. About 10% of tumors are extra-adrenal (paragangliomas), and 90% of these are intra-abdominal, most commonly arising from chromaffin cells near the aortic bifurcation in the organ of Zuckerkandl or near the kidney. Other sites include the paravertebral sympathetic ganglia, the urinary bladder, other autonomic ganglia (celiac, superior or inferior mesenteric), the thorax (including the posterior mediastinum, the heart, and paracardiac regions), and the neck (in sympathetic ganglia, carotid body, cranial nerves, or glomus jugulare). Bilateral and extra-adrenal tumors are more common in children. Histologically, oval groups of cells, in clusters or "nests," stain for chromogranin A; a less frequently used stain identifies neuron-specific enolase. Less than 10% of the tumors are malignant; malignancy occurs more frequently in extra-adrenal tumors and is evidenced by local invasion or distant metastases but cannot be judged reliably from histologic appearance. Local invasion commonly involves adjacent vascular structures, such as the inferior vena cava. Distant metastatic sites include bone, lung, lymph nodes, and liver. Bilateral adrenal medullary hyperplasia has been reported in gene carriers from kindreds with multiple endocrine neoplasia type 2 (MEN-2). This hyperplasia may be a precursor of pheochromocytoma.

The "rule of 10's" is useful to recall approximate frequencies of pheochromocytoma that vary from the usual: 10% bilateral, 10% extra-adrenal, 10% extra-abdominal, 10% malignant, 10% familial, 10% pediatric, and 10% without blood pressure elevation.

ETIOLOGY. *Familial* pheochromocytomas constitute 5 to 10% of the total and are more frequently bilateral and extra-adrenal, although less commonly malignant. A careful family history is essential, and relatives of patients with the familial syndromes should be screened for pheochromocytoma; biochemical screening is often not sufficient, and imaging studies are also recommended in this high-risk group.

Von Hippel-Lindau syndrome (VHLS) is an autosomal dominant disorder resulting from mutations at a tumor-suppressor locus on chromosome 3p25-p26. Its manifestations include pheochromocytoma (in about 14% of gene carriers), retinal angioma, cerebellar hemangioblastoma, renal cysts and carcinoma, pancreatic cysts, and epididymal cystadenoma. Accordingly, all patients with pheochromocytoma deserve careful funduscopic examination.

MEN-2A and MEN-2B (Sipple's syndrome) are autosomal dominant disorders arising from mutations on chromosome 10q11.2 in the region of the *RET* proto-oncogene, which encodes a receptor tyrosine kinase. The features of MEN-2A include pheochromocytoma (in about 40% of gene carriers), medullary thyroid carcinoma, and primary hyperparathyroidism (adenoma or hyperplasia). Because of this syndrome, it is wise to screen all pheochromocytoma patients for medullary thyroid carcinoma with serum calcitonin. MEN-2B features include pheochromocytoma, medullary thyroid carcinoma, multiple mucosal neuromas (of lips, tongue, buccal mucosa, eyelids, conjunctivae, corneas, and gastrointestinal tract), and marfanoid body habitus (but without lens or aortic abnormalities).

Hereditary neurofibromatosis (von Recklinghausen's disease), an autosomal dominant disorder resulting from mutations at the NF1 (neurofibromin) locus on chromosome 17q11.2, presents with neurofibromas and café-au-lait spots; about 1% of neurofibromatosis patients have pheochromocytoma. Familial pheochromocytoma may also occur in isolation; whether such families represent disease processes etiologically distinct from VHLS or MEN is not clear.

In the 90 to 95% of pheochromocytomas which are *sporadic,* the cause of the neoplastic process remains obscure, although loss of heterozygosity on chromosomes 1p, 3p, 17p, and 22q suggests somatic cell deletion mutation of one autosomal allele at as-yet-uncharacterized tumor suppressor loci.

DIAGNOSIS. Because pheochromocytoma is a potentially curable form of hypertension, the diagnosis is worth considering in each new case of hypertension. However, because hypertension is so commonly encountered in clinical practice (~ 20 to 25% of the adult population), and pheochromocytoma is so distinctly unusual (~ 0.1 to 0.2% of patients with hypertension), laboratory evaluation should be selective and guided by the degree of clinical suspicion, based on criteria outlined below (Table 204–9).

Symptoms and Signs. Paroxysmal symptoms (such as the triad of episodic palpitations, diaphoresis, and headache) are the classic features of pheochromocytoma. These paroxysmal "attacks" characteristically begin abruptly, may last for minutes to hours, and subside gradually, with a frequency varying from many times daily to one or more per week (most commonly) or even every few months. Less common symptoms include apprehension or anxiety, tremulousness, pain in the chest or abdomen, weakness, or weight loss. In some series, > 90% of patients have experienced paroxysmal symptoms of one or more of the classic triad. Autopsy series indicate that as many as 50 to 75% of pheochromocytomas may be undiagnosed during life, suggesting that many pheochromocytomas do not give rise to these classic symptomatic features. Patients over the age of 60 years with pheochromocytoma are especially likely to report minor or no symptoms.

Other features in the history may suggest pheochromocytoma. Affected patients may report an increase in blood pressure after re-

TABLE 204–9. DIAGNOSTIC APPROACH TO PHEOCHROMOCYTOMA

Clinical clues or "tipoffs"
  History
    Paroxysmal symptoms (classic triad is headache, diaphoresis, palpitations)
    History of extraordinarily labile or refractory hypertension
    Family history of pheochromocytoma, von Hippel-Lindau syndrome (VHLS), or multiple endocrine neoplasia (MEN)
    Incidental adrenal abnormality on abdominal imaging test (rarely)
  Physical examination
    Labile, refractory hypertension
    Orthostatic hypotension
    VHLS- or MEN-associated findings (retinal angiomas, thyroid enlargement, mucosal neuromas)
Biochemical confirmation (only after clue or tipoff; begin with urinary tests)
  Urinary catecholamines and metabolites (24-hour sample, or 2-hour sample after a paroxysm; metanephrines, the first screening test)
  Plasma catecholamines (if urinary values are equivocal; take care to obtain a basal, resting sample)
  Clonidine suppression test (if plasma catecholamines are in the equivocal 1000–2000 pg/ml range)
  Plasma chromogranin A (storage vesicle protein released with catecholamines; also elevated by renal failure)
Anatomic localization (only after biochemical confirmation)
  By morphology (most sensitive, less specific)
    Computed tomography (the imaging test most frequently obtained)
    Magnetic resonance imaging (may have advantages for extra-adrenal tumors)
  By function (most specific, less sensitive)
    Radiolabeled metaiodobenzylguanidine (MIBG) scanning (accumulates in functioning chromaffin tissue)

ceiving certain antihypertensive drugs, especially β-adrenergic antagonists and guanethidine, or they may experience a remarkable fall in blood pressure after receiving α_1-adrenergic antagonists such as prazosin. Hypertension in such patients is relatively refractory to medical management. A history of extreme blood pressure lability during intubation, surgery, or induction of general anesthesia also suggests possible pheochromocytoma. A family history of pheochromocytoma, VHLS, or MEN should prompt an evaluation for pheochromocytoma. Paroxysmal symptoms on micturition or bladder distention or painless, gross hematuria may suggest pheochromocytoma of the bladder; the diagnosis is confirmed by cystoscopy.

Hypertension (usually severe and refractory to antihypertensive medications) is the cardinal sign of pheochromocytoma, although it is nonspecific and may be insensitive. In about half of patients, hypertension is sustained, with intermittent blood pressure surges in half or more of these; in about 40%, hypertension is paroxysmal, with relatively normal blood pressure between surges. Hypertensive surges may be precipitated by abdominal manipulation, but generally no antecedent is noted. The heart rate is usually elevated during blood pressure surges but may decline as a result of physiologic reflex bradycardia. Orthostatic hypotension is variably observed. As many as 15 to 20% of patients may have cholesterol gallstones.

Laboratory Diagnosis. Because hypertension is so common and pheochromocytoma so rare, further biochemical evaluation for pheochromocytoma in hypertensives should be selective and focused on subjects who display some relevant clue to pheochromocytoma on history, physical examination, or screening laboratory evaluation. If interpretation of urinary measurements is not clearcut, evaluation should proceed to plasma measurements, which require more careful sampling technique. The number and diversity of biochemical tests obtained should parallel the clinical index of suspicion. If suspicion is low, a single screening test may suffice, usually 24-hour urinary metanephrine excretion. If suspicion is high, multiple tests, both urine and plasma, are in order. Because anatomic or imaging studies may detect nonspecific adrenal abnormalities in up to 2% of the population, such studies should not be undertaken unless biochemical tests are positive.

Routine Tests. Results of routine screening tests obtained for other purposes (such as general health maintenance) may provide tipoffs. Hyperglycemia is common, and about half of pheochromocytoma patients manifest carbohydrate intolerance; frank diabetes requiring insulin is unusual. Lactic acidosis occurs rarely, even without shock. Serum lactic dehydrogenase activity may be elevated from adrenal isoenzyme 3. Rarely, pheochromocytoma may be an incidental finding on computed tomographic or magnetic resonance imaging of the abdomen undertaken for other indications.

Urine Tests. Widely available tests measure urinary free (unconjugated) catecholamines and catecholamine metabolites: the metanephrines and VMA. A 24-hour urine sample is collected, and creatinine is measured in the same sample as an index of adequacy and completeness of collection. Of the available tests, increased urinary metanephrines have the highest diagnostic sensitivity and specificity for pheochromocytoma. The urinary excretions of metanephrines and VMA remain normal until the very end stage of renal disease, so elevated levels validly diagnose pheochromocytoma.

Artifactual false-positive assay results have been greatly minimized in recent years with the introduction of more specific assay methods based on separation of catecholamines and metabolites in urine by high-pressure liquid chromatography. False-positive increases in free catecholamines may result from exogenous sources, such as catecholamines (which may be administered surreptitiously), α-methyldopa (but VMA excretion is characteristically normal), L-DOPA, labetalol, sympathomimetic amines (which release endogenous catecholamines from their stores), and fluorescent drugs such as tetracycline. Misleading elevations of endogenous catecholamines may occur as a consequence of the sympathoadrenal responses to shock, hypoglycemia, physical exertion, increased intracranial pressure, or withdrawal of central α_2 agonists such as clonidine. False-positive metanephrine elevations may result from excessive catecholamines (exogenous or endogenous) or the use of monoamine oxidase inhibitors or propranolol (which interferes with the spectrophotometric assay). False-positive VMA elevations may occur after ingesting carbidopa (a peripheral DOPA decarboxylase inhibitor) or monoamine oxidase inhibitors.

Blood Tests. Biochemical tests on blood samples offer the advantage of patient convenience but the disadvantage that even minor physical or mental stress can result in false-positive elevations. Plasma catecholamines are best sampled from a supine, resting patient in whom an indwelling antecubital venous cannula has been in place for at least 15 minutes. Plasma assay methods provide generally reliable results, with usual normal resting norepinephrine of 200 to 400 pg per milliliter and normal resting epinephrine of 20 to 60 pg per milliliter. Most patients with pheochromocytoma have markedly elevated (>2000 pg per milliliter) resting plasma catecholamines (norepinephrine plus epinephrine); plasma concentrations elevated beyond this point strongly suggest pheochromocytoma. The upper limit of normal (norepinephrine plus epinephrine) is <1000 pg per milliliter. Values between 1000 and 2000 pg per milliliter are equivocal and may represent either pheochromocytoma or sympathoadrenal activation by physical or mental stress. In these subjects the clonidine suppression test discussed below is of particular value.

False-positive plasma catecholamine elevations may result from the same factors that produce false-positive urinary elevations but are a more severe problem because measurements are made at only one time point. These factors include physical stress, such as trauma, surgery, upright posture, acute venipuncture, hypoglycemia, hypovolemia, hypotension, cold, sodium depletion, or mental stress, such as anxiety or pain. Drugs that increase plasma catecholamines include sympathomimetic amines which release catecholamines from their stores, cocaine which blocks catecholamine reuptake, and abrupt clonidine withdrawal. Illnesses known to elevate plasma catecholamines include both acute (e.g., myocardial infarction, diabetic ketoacidosis, or sepsis) and chronic conditions (e.g., congestive heart failure, anemia, respiratory failure, or hypothyroidism). Factors that diminish plasma catecholamines include drugs (clonidine, reserpine, and α-methylparatyrosine), autonomic neuropathy, and congenital deficiency of DβH activity.

As with urine biochemical tests, plasma catecholamine sampling during a paroxysmal attack of hypertension is of value. A finding of normal plasma catecholamines when blood pressure is elevated is quite a useful negative result. Because only extreme elevations of plasma norepinephrine perturb blood pressure, the finding of normal plasma catecholamines while blood pressure is elevated argues strongly against pheochromocytoma as the cause.

Other components of the catecholamine storage vesicle core are released into the bloodstream by pheochromocytomas. The plasma concentration of chromogranin A is elevated in patients with pheochromocytoma, with a diagnostic sensitivity of 83% and specificity of 96%. It is not substantially elevated by acute venipuncture, nor is it affected by drugs used in treatment or diagnosis of pheochromocytoma. Because chromogranin A is released by a variety of neuroendocrine secretory vesicles, its plasma concentration is also elevated in other neuroendocrine neoplasias. Chromogranin A values are also elevated in renal insufficiency because of retained immunoreactive fragments of the protein.

Pharmacologic Diagnostic Tests: Suppressive and Provocative. Pharmacologic tests for pheochromocytoma are generally not necessary because the diagnosis can usually be confirmed by urine and plasma biochemical measurements at rest or during spontaneous blood pressure surges.

The *clonidine suppression test* is of value if plasma catecholamine elevations in a patient with suspected pheochromocytoma are equivocal (that is, from 1000 to 2000 pg per milliliter). The rationale for the test is that pheochromocytoma chromaffin cells, ulike normal adrenal medullary chromaffin cells, are not innervated; hence, catecholamine release from pheochromocytoma chromaffin cells is autonomous and not susceptible to manipulation by drugs that decrease efferent sympathetic outflow, such as the central α_2 agonist clonidine. Blood is obtained for plasma catecholamines before and 3 hours after a single oral dose of 0.3 mg clonidine. In a subject without pheochromocytoma, plasma norepinephrine should fall to <500 pg per milliliter after clonidine. A positive test (failure of catecholamines to decline after clonidine) is sensitive but may not be entirely specific for pheochromocytoma. Although cat-cholamines do not fall after clonidine in pheochromocytoma, the blood pressure fall is comparable to that seen in essential hypertensives. To prevent inordinate falls in blood pressure during the test, prior volume depletion should be avoided; the test is most safely done in subjects whose diastolic blood pressure prior to clonidine is ≥ 100 mm Hg. Because beta blockers such as propranolol diminish circulating norepinephrine clearance (and hence plasma norepinephrine responses to clonidine), they should be discontinued 48 hours prior to and during the test. The test remains valid during α blockade.

Catecholamine provocative tests (such as the glucagon test) are used in only a few centers because of the potential hazard posed by inordinate catecholamine release.

Anatomic Localization. Tumor location must be known in order to plan the proper surgical route. Ninety-five per cent of pheochromocytomas are in the abdomen, and the great majority of these can be visualized by one of three modalities: computed tomographic (CT) scan, magnetic resonance imaging (MRI), or metaiodobenzylguanidine (MIBG) scintigraphy. CT and MRI are highly sensitive, although nonspecific, because they visualize any mass lesion, not just pheochromocytomas. MIBG scanning is highly specific for chromaffin tissue, although somewhat less sensitive than CT or MRI.

MIBG, a radiolabeled analogue of guanethidine, is transported into chromaffin cells by the reuptake cell membrane catecholamine carrier. Because it accumulates in chromaffin cells, an MIBG abnormality is extraordinarily specific (about 98%) for pheochromocytoma, although somewhat less sensitive (85 to 90%). MIBG imaging is especially useful for metastatic, recurrent, or extraadrenal tumors. Abdominal ultrasonography is a safe imaging tool but is less sensitive than CT or MRI. Plain abdominal radiographs, intravenous urograms (pyelograms), air insufflation retroperitoneal pneumography, arteriography, and venography are no longer done to localize pheochromocytoma. Indeed, arteriography or venography of the tumor may trigger hypertensive crises.

Differential Diagnosis. Because many conditions can mimic the diagnostic features of pheochromocytoma, as many as 90% of patients who present with some feature of the tumor turn out not to have one after diagnostic testing. Examples include certain drugs, such as surreptitiously self-administered epinephrine or isoproterenol. Abrupt withdrawal from clonidine can provoke a sympathoadrenal discharge with "rebound" blood pressure elevation. Subjects treated with monoamine oxidase inhibitors for depression may develop hypertensive crises if they inadvertently ingest foods rich in tyramine.

Disease states causing or simulating catecholamine excess and hypertension include thyrotoxicosis, acute intracranial disturbances such as subarachnoid hemorrhage or posterior fossa masses, hypertensive crisis of paraplegia which can be initiated by visceral manipulation or bladder distention, and hypoglycemia especially in the presence of β blockade. Damage to carotid sinus baroreceptors by surgery or tumor may result in baroreflex failure, with episodic blood pressure and plasma catecholamine surges; clonidine is the drug of choice. Episodic surges in plasma dopamine have been described in some patients with episodic blood pressure elevation but without pheochromocytoma; the mechanism has not been established.

PATHOPHYSIOLOGY AND COMPLICATIONS. Although circulating catecholamine excess is the ultimate cause of hypertension in pheochromocytoma, the correlation of blood pressure with plasma catecholamines is modest. Desensitization to catecholamine effects may contribute to underdiagnosis of the tumor in the elderly. Pheochromocytomas also release a number of potentially vasoactive substances in addition to catecholamines, which may modify blood pressure. Hemodynamic studies suggest that elevations in systemic vascular resistance rather than cardiac output account for the blood pressure rise.

Acute norepinephrine infusion leads to plasma volume contraction, and a past mainstay of pheochromocytoma management has been an effort to re-expand plasma volume, either spontaneously after therapeutic α blockade, or with preoperative saline infusion. However, recent careful measurements of plasma volume indicate that, on average, it is not as contracted as once believed. Orthostatic hypotension is variably observed in pheochromocytoma. It cannot be clearly attributed to plasma volume contraction and likely reflects catecholamine desensitization, the effects of vasodilator peptides and catecholamines, and dysautonomia.

The major catecholamine secreted by most pheochromocytomas is norepinephrine. Small intra-adrenal tumors (especially early in the course of MEN-2) may secrete predominantly epinephrine. Pure epinephrine secretion by pheochromocytomas is rare.

Cardiomyopathy (myocarditis) occurs in a minority of pheochromocytoma patients, presumably as a consequence of catecholamine excess. This process is generally reversible after tumor removal, and congestive heart failure responds to preoperative α-adrenergic blockade. In most patients, however, the degree of myocardial left ventricular hypertrophy on cardiac ultrasonography is no different from that seen in essential hypertension.

MANAGEMENT. Preoperative Preparation and Drug Treatment. Once pheochromocytoma has been diagnosed, the patient is prepared for surgery with adrenergic blockade for a period of 1 to 4 weeks. During α blockade, any catecholamine-induced plasma volume contraction is allowed to correct itself. α Blockade is usually accomplished with oral phenoxybenzamine, an irreversible, noncompetitive antagonist that acts predominantly at α_1 receptors. The drug is begun at 5 mg twice daily, and the dose is adjusted gradually upward by increments of 10 mg every 1 to 4 days to a maximum of 50 to 100 mg twice daily. The usual dose range required is 30 to 80 mg per day. Treatment goals are to normalize blood pressure (≤ 160/≤ 90 mm Hg), prevent paroxysmal hypertension, and abolish tachyarrhythmias (ventricular extrasystoles < 1 to 5 per minute), without inducing intolerable orthostatic hypotension (i.e., orthostatic falls of > 85/> 45 mm Hg). Side effects of adequate phenoxybenzamine dosage include orthostatic hypotension, tachycardia, nasal congestion, dry mouth, diplopia, and ejaculatory dysfunction. In patients intolerant of phenoxybenzamine, one can use the α_1-selective antagonist prazosin, in a dose range of 0.5 to 16 mg per day, given orally two to four times daily.

If blood pressure or tachyarrhythmias including sinus tachycardia are not fully controlled by α blockade, β blockade is instituted with oral propranolol, 10 to 40 mg four times daily. β blockade must not be undertaken before α blockade has been instituted; after blockade of vasodilatory vascular β_2-adrenergic receptors, catecholamines' continued access to vasoconstrictive α_1 receptors may induce unopposed vasoconstriction and exacerbation of hypertension. β Blockade may be especially useful for predominant epinephrine-secreting tumors. Metoprolol or labetalol are alternatives to propranolol. In subjects with contraindications to β blockade, lidocaine or amiodarone can be used for tachyarrhythmias.

If combined management with α- plus β-adrenergic antagonists is not fully effective, the tyrosine hydroxylase inhibitor α-methylparatyrosine is added, at an oral dose of 0.25 to 1.0 gram four times daily. Its use may be complicated by sedation, fatigue, anxiety, diarrhea, or extrapyramidal reactions.

For acute management of severe hypertensive crises, intravenous nitroprusside is effective. Intravenous nonselective α_1/α_2 blockade with phentolamine (1 mg bolus, then by continuous infusion) is also useful. Calcium channel blockade with sublingual nifedipine (10 mg broken under the tongue) has also been used.

Avoid opiates (narcotic analgesics), narcotic antagonists (such as naloxone), histamine, ACTH, saralasin, glucagon, or indirect sympathomimetic amines (such as phenylpropanolamine or tyramine). All of these agents may provoke hypertensive surges by releasing catecholamines from the tumor. Drugs that block catecholamine reuptake, such as tricyclic antidepressants (e.g., desipramine), cocaine, or guanethidine, may worsen hypertension. β-Adrenergic antagonists, by blocking vasodilatory vascular β_2 receptors, may cause unopposed α-mediated vasoconstriction by circulating catecholamines, resulting in severe hypertension, unless α blockade is first instituted. Dopaminergic antagonists (such as metoclopramide or sulpiride) may result in hypertension. All should be avoided.

Operative and Perioperative Management. Autopsy series of pheochromocytoma indicate that even clinically unsuspected cases can be lethal. At least 90% of pheochromocytomas are benign, and surgical resection provides a cure, although up to 25% of patients may retain some lesser degree of hypertension. Residual tumor may be diagnosed by urinary catecholamine measurement 1 to 2 weeks postoperatively. The operative mortality of pheochromocytoma resection should not exceed 2 to 3%. In malignant pheochromocytoma, the individual course is highly variable, but long-term 50% survival is < 5 years.

Several surgical approaches are feasible, depending on the particular pheochromocytoma presentation; the experience of the surgeon is crucial. The entire adrenal gland harboring a pheochromocytoma is usually excised. Anesthetic management is guided by selection of agents that do not cause catecholamine release or potentiate catecholamines' dysrhythmic effects. Intravenous glucose replacement (5% dextrose in water or saline) should be given to prevent hypoglycemia, a frequent occurrence after tumor removal. Times at which hypertensive surges are likely to occur include anesthetic induction, intubation, tumor palpation, and ligation of tumor veins. If intraoperative hypotension occurs, the initial treatment should be saline infusion to expand intravascular volume. Only after plasma volume expansion to euvolemia is norepinephrine infusion appropriate.

For intraoperative blood pressure surges, intravenous nitroprusside is often employed. Alternatively, α blockade can be accomplished with intravenous phentolamine (an α_1 and α_2 antagonist), starting with a 1-mg dose and proceeding to infusion. The calcium channel antagonist nicardipine has also been used.

In the postoperative period, several problems occur with some frequency:

1. Hypotension. Most commonly this results from hypovolemia and responds to saline infusion; several liters may be required, often with the guidance of central pressure measurements. After volume repletion, norepinephrine can be infused if needed.

2. Hypertension. Plasma catecholamines remain elevated for several days after complete pheochromocytoma resection. Even 2 weeks postoperatively, up to one fourth of patients still have hypertension. At this time, the differential diagnosis includes residual unresected tumor, essential hypertension, or hypertension secondary to renal damage caused by prior hypertension. A urine collection for catecholamines, obtained at least 1 to 2 weeks after tumor resection, will clarify matters.

3. Hypoglycemia. After correction of catecholamine excess, insulin release may be increased and end-organ responsiveness to insulin augmented, resulting in hypoglycemia. Hypoglycemia may masquerade as refractory hypotension. Infusion of glucose (5% dextrose in water or saline) during the intraoperative and immediate postoperative period is useful.

MALIGNANT PHEOCHROMOCYTOMA. Although most pheochromocytomas are well-encapsulated, localized growths, approximately 5 to 10% are malignant. Malignancy is diagnosed by the biologic behavior of the tumor, in the form of adjacent tissue invasion or distant metastatic spread. Extra-adrenal tumors are more likely to metastasize than are primary adrenal ones. Catecholamine biosynthesis tends to be especially deranged in malignant tumors, with secretion of substantial amounts of DOPA and dopamine (metabolized to HVA, which can be detected in the urine). Increased plasma DOPA in pheochromocytoma suggests malignancy.

In patients with malignant pheochromocytoma, α- and β-adrenergic blockade with phenoxybenzamine and propranolol remain the mainstay of management of symptoms and signs of catecholamine excess. If catecholamine effects are not controlled, the tyrosine hydroxylase inhibitor α-methylparatyrosine can be effective, from 0.25 to 1.0 gram four times daily.

Metastases tend to be slow growing, and the natural history of malignant pheochromocytoma is variable; the 5-year survival is < 50%. Common sites of metastasis are the retroperitoneum, skeleton (bone), lymph nodes, and liver. Periodic surgical debulking may help to control symptoms. The response to chemotherapy has been generally disappointing, but the combination of vincristine, cyclophosphamide, and dacarbazine shows promise in many patients. Skeletal metastases show some response to irradiation, although the neoplasm is not particularly susceptible to radiation therapy. High-dose (300 mCi) radiation therapy with intravenous ^{125}I-MIBG remains experimental but is of value in some patients.

CATECHOLAMINE DEFICIENCY DISEASE STATES

Loss of even both adrenal glands seldom produces a catecholamine deficiency state. In diabetics receiving insulin, the usual counterregulatory response to hypoglycemia involves the actions of epinephrine and glucagon to trigger hepatic glycogenolysis. In diabetics who also have autonomic neuropathy, deficient epinephrine release during hypoglycemia, coupled with deficient glucagon responses, may result in impairment of the usual counterregulatory response to hypoglycemia, prolonging its duration.

Several individuals have been described with an apparent congenital deficiency of DβH; such individuals have greatly diminished or undetectable norepinephrine and epinephrine in blood, urine, and cerebrospinal fluid. Presenting features of this lifelong syndrome include severe orthostatic hypotension, ptosis, nasal stuffiness, hyperextensible joints, and retrograde ejaculation. The diagnosis is made in patients with severe orthostatic hypotension, a plasma norepinephrine/dopamine ratio of < 1, and undetectable plasma DβH activity. During sympathoadrenal activation in these subjects, increments in efferent sympathetic nerve traffic occur, but sympathetic axons release the precursor dopamine instead of norepinephrine, perhaps compounding the hypotension.

THE INCIDENTAL ADRENAL MASS (OR "INCIDENTALOMA")

Up to 2% of all abdominal CT scans, as well as 9% of autopsies, incidentally discover minimal adrenal gland abnormalities. Rarely do these lesions require further attention.

Occasionally the appearance of an adrenal mass on CT or MRI is sufficiently characteristic for a firm diagnosis; an example is adrenal myelolipoma, a benign accumulation of bone marrow elements in an otherwise normally functioning adrenal, with a characteristic fat-density image on CT or MRI. Myelolipoma requires no treatment.

If an adrenal mass is > 4 to 6 cm in span, its chance of malignancy (especially adrenocortical carcinoma) increases, and such masses should be resected unless they have a clearly benign appearance (such as myelolipoma) on CT or MRI. In smaller lesions, adrenal carcinoma is unlikely unless other signs or symptoms of adrenocortical hormone excess are apparent. Incidental masses < 4 to 6 cm in span are followed by periodic CT scanning. In subjects with known metastatic carcinoma, adrenal abnormalities are likely to be adrenal metastases. In subjects with recent major abdominal trauma, adrenal abnormalities likely represent hemorrhage and should resolve with time.

Because not all pheochromocytomas manifest hypertension at all times, all patients with incidental adrenal masses should be screened for pheochromocytoma with a 24-hour urine collection for catecholamine metabolites.

Virtually all patients with aldosterone-producing adrenal adenoma have hypertension and hypokalemia. If blood pressure and serum potassium are normal on a diet of > 200 mEq sodium per day and < 100 mEq potassium per day (confirmed by 24-hour urine), no further evaluation is needed.

Cushing's disease is likely only if other signs or symptoms are suggestive. The diagnosis is made by giving 1 mg of oral dexamethasone at 11 P.M. and sampling serum cortisol the next morning at 8 A.M.

Cryer PE: Pheochromocytoma. West J Med 156:399, 1992. *A comprehensive review contrasting the diagnostic value of plasma versus urinary catecholamines.*

Grossman E, Goldstein DS, Hoffman A, et al.: Glucagon and clonidine testing in the diagnosis of pheochromocytoma. Hypertension 17:733, 1991. *A large series evaluating the sensitivity and specificity of these provocation and suppression tests of catecholamine release.*

Hsiao RJ, Parmer RJ, Takiyyuddin MA, et al.: Chromogranin A storage and secretion: Sensitivity and specificity for the diagnosis of pheochromocytoma. Medicine 70:33, 1991. *The chromaffin storage vesicle protein chromogranin A, co-released by exocytosis with catecholamines, is a sensitive and specific plasma marker of pheochromocytoma in hypertension patients.*

Jovenich JJ: Anesthesia in adrenal surgery. Urol Clin North Am 16:583, 1989. *Practical suggestions on anesthetics to use or avoid.*

Kailasam MT, O'Connor DT, Parmer RJ: The regulation and role of catecholamines in hypertension and pheochromocytoma. Curr Opinion Endocrinol Diabetes 1:135, 1994. *A review emphasizing recent diagnostic developments.*

Malone MJ, Libertino JA, Tsapatsaris NP, et al.: Preoperative and surgical management of pheochromocytoma. Urol Clin North Am 16:567, 1989. *Rationale for selection from several possible surgical approaches.*

Neumann HPH, Berger DP, Sigmund G, et al.: Pheochromocytomas, multiple endocrine neoplasia type 2, and von Hippel-Lindau disease. N Engl J Med 329:1531, 1993. *This large series highlights the importance and yield of screening patients with pheochromocytoma for familial syndromes.*

Ross NS, Aron DC: Hormonal evaluation of the patient with an incidentally discovered adrenal mass. N Engl J Med 323:1401, 1991. *A sensible approach to this increasingly frequent and vexing clinical problem.*

205 DIABETES MELLITUS
Robert S. Sherwin

OVERVIEW

Diabetes mellitus is a chronic disorder characterized by impaired metabolism of glucose and other energy-yielding fuels, as well as the late development of vascular and neuropathic complications. Diabetes mellitus consists of a group of disorders involving distinct pathogenic mechanisms with hyperglycemia as the common denominator. Regardless of cause, the disease is associated with insulin deficiency, which may be total, partial, or relative when viewed in the context of coexisting insulin resistance. Lack of insulin plays a primary role in the metabolic derangements linked to diabetes, and hyperglycemia, in turn, plays a key role in the complications of the disease.

In the United States diabetes mellitus is the fourth most common reason for patient contact with a physician and is a major cause of premature disability and mortality. It is the leading cause of blindness among working-age people, of end-stage renal disease, and of nontraumatic limb amputations. It increases the risk of cardiac, cerebral, and peripheral vascular disease two- to seven-fold and is a major cause of neonatal morbidity and mortality. On the bright side, recent data indicate that most of the debilitating complications of the disease can be prevented or delayed by prospective treatment of hyperglycemia and cardiovascular risk factors.

CLASSIFICATION

Diabetes mellitus can be divided into three subclasses (Table 205–1): (1) type I, or insulin-dependent diabetes mellitus; (2) type II, or non–insulin-dependent diabetes mellitus; and (3) secondary diabetes linked to another identifiable condition or syndrome. In addition, two conditions—impaired glucose tolerance and gestational diabetes—significantly increase the later risk of developing diabetes mellitus and may, in some instances, be part of its natural history.

TYPE I DIABETES MELLITUS. Patients with this disorder have little or no insulin secretory capacity and depend on exogenous insulin to prevent metabolic decompensation (e.g., ketoacidosis) and death. Commonly in previously healthy nonobese children or young adults diabetes appears abruptly over days or weeks, whereas in older age groups it may have a more gradual onset. At the time of initial presentation the patient appears ill, has marked symptoms (e.g., polyuria, polydipsia, polyphagia, and weight loss), and may demonstrate ketoacidosis. Type I diabetes is believed to

TABLE 205–1. CLASSIFICATION OF DIABETES

I. Clinical Diabetes
1. Type I or insulin-dependent diabetes (IDDM). Formerly called juvenile-onset diabetes.
2. Type II or non–insulin-dependent diabetes (NIDDM). Formerly called maturity- or adult-onset diabetes.
   A. Obese (~80–85%)
   B. Nonobese (~15–20%)
   C. Maturity-onset diabetes of the young (MODY)
3. Secondary diabetes
   A. Pancreatic disease (e.g., chronic pancreatitis, hemochromatosis, cystic fibrosis, pancreatic carcinoma)
   B. Endocrine disease (e.g., acromegaly, Cushing's syndrome, glucagonoma, polycystic ovary syndrome, pheochromocytoma)
   C. Drugs (e.g., thiazide diuretics, glucocorticoids, beta-adrenergic blockers, pentamidine, oral contraceptives, phenytoin)
   D. Genetic syndromes (e.g., Turner's syndrome, myotonic dystrophy, Huntington's disease, lipodystrophy, ataxia-telangiectasia)
   E. Insulin receptor abnormalities (due to defective insulin receptors or to antibodies directed toward the insulin receptor)
   F. Malnutrition-related diabetes

II. Risk Categories
1. Impaired glucose tolerance
2. Gestational diabetes

have a long asymptomatic preclinical stage, often lasting years, during which pancreatic beta cells are gradually destroyed by an autoimmune attack (Fig. 205–1). An acute illness may speed the transition from the preclinical to the clinical stage. Initially insulin therapy is essential to restore metabolism toward normal. A "honeymoon period" may follow, lasting weeks or months, during which time smaller doses of insulin are required due to partial recovery of beta cell function and reversal of insulin resistance caused by acute illness. Thereafter, insulin secretory capacity is gradually lost. This syndrome accounts for about 10% of diabetes in the United States.

TYPE II DIABETES MELLITUS. This is, by far, the most common form of the disease, comprising 85 to 90% of the diabetic population and taking heterogeneous forms. Affected patients retain some endogenous insulin secretory capacity, but insulin levels are low relative to the magnitude of insulin resistance and ambient glucose levels. They do not depend on insulin for immediate survival and rarely develop ketosis, except under conditions of great physical stress. Nevertheless, they may require insulin therapy to control hyperglycemia. Type II diabetes characteristically appears after the age of 40 years, has a high rate of genetic penetrance unrelated to HLA genes, and is associated with obesity. The clinical presentation is much more insidious. The classic symptoms of diabetes may be mild and tolerated for a long time before the patient seeks medical attention. Moreover, if hyperglycemia is asymptomatic, the disease may become evident only after complications develop.

SECONDARY DIABETES. A variety of diabetic syndromes can be attributed to a specific disease, drug, or condition. These include (1) pancreatic disease, (2) endocrine disease, (3) drugs, (4) genetic syndromes, (5) insulin receptor abnormalities, and (6) malnutrition. Severe illness (e.g., burns, trauma, sepsis) may provoke hyperglycemia due to hypersecretion of insulin antagonistic hormones. Although on some occasions this may reflect underlying diabetes, the metabolic disturbance is often self-limited and should not be classified as diabetes until the precipitating illness has resolved.

Most diabetes mellitus can be classified on clinical grounds. A small subgroup of patients differ and display features common to both type I and II diabetes. They are commonly nonobese and have diminished insulin secretion that is not sufficient to make them ketosis prone. Many initially respond to oral agents, but, with time, require insulin. Some may have a slowly evolving form of type I diabetes. Others defy easy categorization.

IMPAIRED GLUCOSE TOLERANCE. The term applies to the finding of glucose levels that are higher than normal but lower than those diagnostic of diabetes mellitus. Impaired glucose tolerance produces neither the symptoms nor the serious complications associated with diabetes. About 25%, however, eventually go on to develop typical type II diabetes.

GESTATIONAL DIABETES. The term categorizes increased glucose levels that are first detected during pregnancy. It excludes known diabetes preexisting conception. Gestational diabetes occurs in about 2% of pregnancies and usually appears in the second or third trimester at the time when pregnancy-associated insulin antagonistic hormones peak. After delivery, glucose tolerance usually reverts to normal. Nevertheless, within 5 to 10 years 30 to 40% develop type II diabetes. Occasionally, pregnancy may precipitate type I diabetes. Although gestational diabetes generally causes only mild, asymptomatic hyperglycemia, rigorous treatment, often with insulin, is required to protect against fetal morbidity and mortality.

DIAGNOSIS

The diagnosis is usually straightforward when diabetes presents with classic symptoms, and a random plasma glucose measurement that is 200 mg per deciliter or greater. Further diagnostic testing is unwarranted and delays treatment. Although glycosuria strongly suggests diabetes, urine testing should never be used exclusively because some persons have a low renal threshold for glucose. If diabetes is suspected but not confirmed by a random glucose determination, the screening test of choice is an overnight fasting plasma glucose level; it varies less from day to day and is more resistant to factors that nonspecifically alter glucose metabolism. Diagnosis is established if glucose equals or exceeds 140 mg per deciliter on at least two separate occasions. Fasting glucose levels <115 mg per deciliter generally do not warrant further testing; values between 115 mg and 140 mg per deciliter, although not diagnostic, should arouse suspicion. Because such individuals may show postprandial

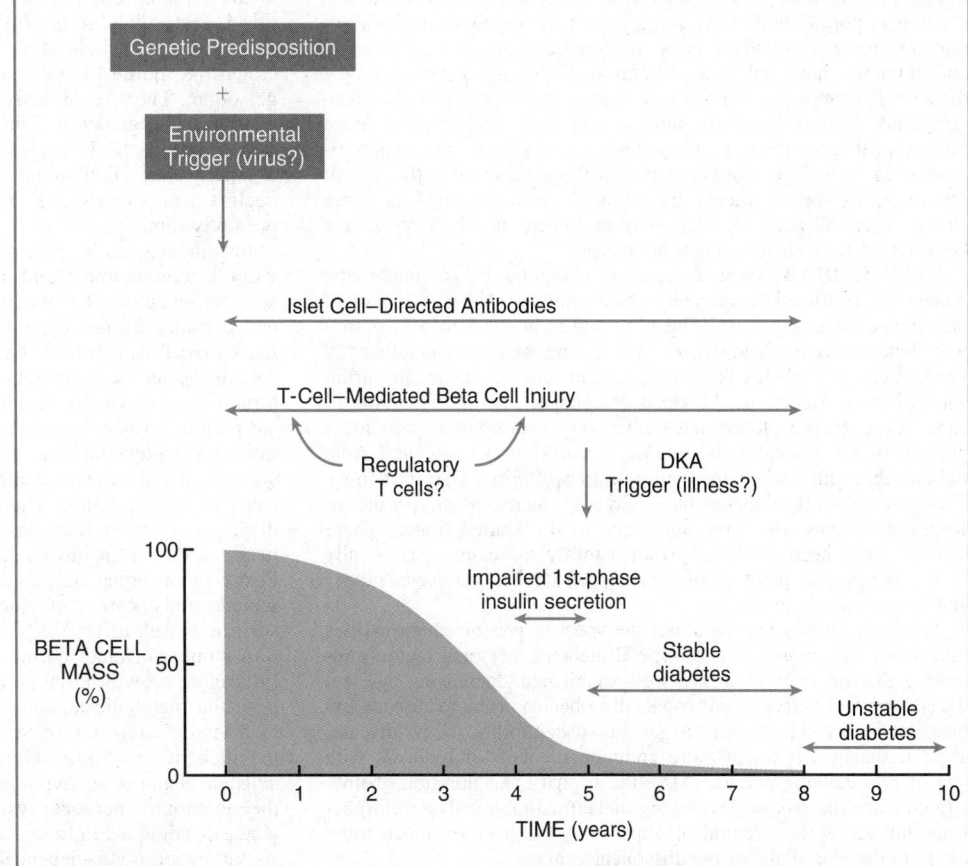

FIGURE 205-1. A summary of the sequence of events that lead to beta cell loss and ultimately to the clinical appearance of type I diabetes.

hyperglycemia, some experts recommend further testing using the oral glucose tolerance test (OGTT). The OGTT has the advantage of detecting diabetes at its earliest stage, when treatment is most effective. The disadvantage is that the test may lead to overdiagnosis unless the clinician recognizes its pitfalls. Common factors that nonspecifically impair glucose tolerance include (1) carbohydrate restriction (< 150 grams for 3 days), (2) bed rest (days) or severe inactivity (weeks), (3) medical or surgical stress, (4) drugs (e.g., thiazides, beta-blockers, glucocorticoids, or phenytoin), and (5) smoking during the test or anxiety from needle sticks.

The clinician has several choices when faced with a fasting glucose in the indeterminate range (115 to 140 mg per deciliter). Although the OGTT is the "gold standard" for diagnosing diabetes when fasting glucose is below 140 mg per deciliter and has proved useful as a research tool, its value in the clinical setting is questionable because of its high variability. When the OGTT is employed, some individuals neither meet the diagnostic criteria for diabetes (i.e., a 2-hour OGTT level >200 mg per deciliter) nor show a normal glucose profile. They are classified as having impaired glucose tolerance (IGT) if (a) fasting glucose is less than 140 mg per deciliter, (b) the 2-hour OGTT level is between 140 and 200 mg per deciliter, and (c) an intervening glucose is 200 mg per deciliter or greater. Because no diagnostic markers distinguish those individuals (about 25%) who will become diabetic, they should be tested annually using a fasting glucose measurement. It is also prudent to prescribe the same lifestyle changes suggested to overt diabetic patients, because IGT (like diabetes mellitus) is associated with a higher risk of premature cardiovascular disease.

Because many patients with type II diabetes have the disease years before symptoms are appreciated, it is important to screen (using a fasting glucose measurement) high-risk individuals (Table 205-2). Because mild glucose elevations may have adverse effects on the fetus, a more aggressive approach is recommended for pregnant women. Pregnant women should receive a screening 50-gram OGTT between 24 and 28 weeks of gestation. If fasting glucose is 105 mg per deciliter or the 1-hour OGTT value is > 150 mg per deciliter, an extended 100-gram OGTT should be performed. Gesta-

tional diabetes is diagnosed if two values equal or exceed the upper limits of normal: fasting, 105 mg per deciliter; 1 hour, 190 mg per deciliter; 2 hour, 165 mg per deciliter; and 3 hour, 145 mg per deciliter.

PREVALENCE/EPIDEMIOLOGY

TYPE I DIABETES. Prevalence rates for type I diabetes are relatively accurate because patients invariably become symptomatic. Estimates for the United States are about 0.30%. Type I diabetes is more prevalent in Finland, Scandinavia, Scotland, and Sardinia, less prevalent in Southern Europe and the Mid-East, and rare in Asian countries such as Japan. The annual incidence in Northern Europe appears to have risen in the last half century, implying the introduction of an unidentified environmental factor. Prevalence rates are strikingly different among different ethnic groups living in the same geographic environment. Caucasian children living in Allegheny County, Pennsylvania, or in Colorado are about 50 to 70% more likely to develop type I diabetes than nonwhites living in the same area, observations most likely explained by genetic differences in susceptibility.

The recognition that type I diabetes has a protracted preclinical phase has placed some epidemiologic characteristics of the disease in a new light. Its increased incidence in the winter months and its association with specific viral epidemics may be explained by the superimposition of illness-provoked insulin resistance in a patient with marginal beta cell function. Similarly, its common appearance

TABLE 205-2. CANDIDATES FOR DIABETES SCREENING

1. Presence of suggestive symptoms
2. Obesity (especially if centrally distributed)
3. Positive family history
4. Women with a morbid obstetric history or with large babies
5. Recurrent skin or genital infections
6. High-risk populations (African-Americans, Latinos, Native Americans)
7. The elderly (> 60 years)
8. Presence of other risk factors for atherosclerosis

during puberty may also be attributed to the appearance of insulin resistance; normal puberty is accompanied by impaired insulin-stimulated glucose metabolism. New methods for tracking islet-directed autoimmunity have led to a reappraisal of the age at which type I diabetes first appears. Although the age-specific incidence rises progressively from infancy to puberty and then declines, incidence rates appear to continue at a low level for many decades. Approximately 25 to 30% of patients develop the disease after the age of 20 years. In these patients the clinical syndrome evolves more slowly, islet cell antibody titers may be lower, and HLA types may be different from their younger counterparts.

TYPE II DIABETES. Systematic screening for asymptomatic diabetes is restricted to relatively small groups, making estimates of prevalence rates imprecise. The U.S. rate is about 3 to 5%, with a prevalence amounting to 10 to 15% among persons older than 50 years. Type II diabetes is more common and occurs at an earlier age in Native Americans, Mexican descendants, and African-Americans. Type II prevalence rates also vary worldwide, showing a propensity for Asiatic Indians, Polynesian/Micronesians, and Australian Aborigines when they migrate to westernized surroundings. Similarly, type II diabetes has markedly increased in people of Japanese descent who have emigrated to the United States. These changes have been attributed to an inability to adapt metabolically to the behavioral patterns of westernization, i.e., reduced activity and higher caloric intake.

Although little is known about the specific genetic abnormalities associated with most forms of type II diabetes, personal factors promoting disease expression are well-established. Increasing age, reduced physical activity, and especially obesity promote disease expression in individuals with a genetic susceptibility to the disease. Type II diabetes is much more common in obese individuals with one or two diabetic parents. Also, the severity and duration of obesity enhance the risk of developing diabetes. Individuals with higher waist-hip ratios (i.e., central or upper-body obesity) are much more likely to develop diabetes in subsequent years.

MALNUTRITION-RELATED DIABETES. This is a disorder of tropical underdeveloped countries occurring in nutritionally deprived adolescents or young adults and characterized by diminished insulin secretion and hyperglycemia, usually without ketosis. It has been divided on clinical grounds into two subclasses, fibrocalculous and protein-deficient pancreatic diabetes, but it is uncertain that these subclasses represent distinct disease entities. Patients with the fibrocalculous form are underweight and have recurrent attacks of abdominal pain in association with pancreatic duct stones and fibrosis. Exocrine pancreatic insufficiency is common. The disease may be linked to the consumption of cassava root, which contains toxic cyanogenic glycosides. The protein-deficient form is characterized by more pronounced wasting, without pancreatic calcifications and fibrosis or abdominal pain. The reduced beta cell function may be secondary to nutritional deficiency.

PATHOPHYSIOLOGY

INSULIN SECRETION AND ACTION. Insulin is initially synthesized in the pancreatic beta cells as a large single-chain polypeptide, proinsulin, which is cleaved, resulting in removal of a connecting strand (C-peptide) and the appearance of the smaller, double-chain insulin molecule (51 amino acid residues). Insulin and the C-peptide remnant are packaged in membrane-bounded storage granules; stimulation of insulin secretion results in the discharge of equimolar amounts of insulin and C-peptide and a small amount of unconverted proinsulin into the portal circulation. Because, unlike insulin, C-peptide escapes hepatic metabolism, its concentration provides a more precise marker of endogenous insulin secretion. The concentration of glucose is the key regulator of insulin secretion. For glucose to activate secretion, it must first be transported by a protein (GLUT 2) into the beta cell, phosphorylated by the enzyme glucokinase, and metabolized. The immediate triggering process is poorly understood but likely involves the activation of signal transduction pathways, closure of ATP-sensitive potassium channels, and the entry of calcium into the beta cell. Normally, when blood glucose rises even slightly above the fasting level of 75 to 100 mg per deciliter, beta cells secrete insulin, initially from preformed stored insulin and later from the synthesis of new insulin. The route of glucose entry as well as its concentration determines

the magnitude of the response. Higher insulin levels are produced when glucose is given orally than when given intravenously owing to the simultaneous release of gut peptides (e.g., glucagon-like peptide I, gastric inhibitory polypeptide, cholecystokinin). Other insulin secretagogues include amino acids and vagal stimulation. Once secreted into portal blood, insulin encounters the liver as its first target organ. The liver effectively removes approximately 50% of the insulin and degrades it. The consequence of this uptake is that the portal vein insulin is always at least two- to four-fold higher than in the peripheral circulation. Conversely, when blood glucose levels decline even slightly (e.g., to 70 mg per deciliter), insulin secretion promptly diminishes.

Insulin acts on responsive tissues by first passing through the vascular compartment and, upon reaching its target, binding to its specific receptor. The insulin receptor is a heterodimer with two α and β chains formed by disulfide bridges. The α subunit resides on the extracellular surface and is the site of insulin binding. The β subunit spans the membrane and can be phosphorylated on serine, threonine, and tyrosine residues on the cytoplasmic face. The intrinsic protein tyrosine kinase activity of the β subunit is essential for insulin receptor function. Rapid receptor autophosphorylation and tyrosine phosphorylation of cellular substrates are essential early steps in insulin action. Thereafter, a series of phosphorylation and dephosphorylation reactions are triggered that ultimately produce insulin's effects in insulin-sensitive tissues (liver, muscle, and fat). Postreceptor signal transduction pathways leading to insulin action include translocation of glucose transporters (GLUT 4) to the cell surface as well as activation of MAP and PI3-kinases.

A number of other hormones, termed counterregulatory hormones (glucagon, growth hormone [GH], catecholamines, and cortisol) oppose the metabolic actions of insulin. Among these, glucagon and to a lesser extent GH have important roles in the development of the diabetic syndrome. Glucagon is secreted by pancreatic alpha cells in response to hypoglycemia, amino acids, and activation of the autonomic nervous system. Its major effect is on the liver, where it stimulates glycogenolysis, gluconeogenesis, and ketogenesis via cyclic AMP–dependent mechanisms. It is normally inhibited by hyperglycemia but is absolutely or relatively increased in both type I and type II diabetes despite the presence of hyperglycemia. GH secretion by the anterior pituitary is also inappropriately increased in type I diabetes owing, at least in part, to an attempt to overcome a defect in insulin-like growth factor-1 generation caused by insulin deficiency. The major metabolic actions of GH are on peripheral tissues, where it acts to promote lipolysis and inhibit glucose consumption. In type I diabetic patients with reduced portal vein insulin levels, GH is also capable of stimulating hepatic glucose production.

METABOLIC EFFECTS OF INSULIN. Insulin's pivotal role in diabetes is best appreciated by first examining the extent to which it participates in fuel homeostasis in healthy subjects.

Fasted State. After an overnight fast, low basal levels of insulin diminish glucose uptake in peripheral insulin-sensitive tissues (muscle and fat). Most glucose uptake occurs in non–insulin-sensitive tissues, primarily the brain, which, because of its inability to use free fatty acids (FFA), is critically dependent on glucose for oxidative metabolism. Maintenance of stable blood glucose levels is achieved by release of glucose by the liver at rates (7 to 10 grams per hour) matching those of consuming tissues. The hepatic processes involved consist of glycogenolysis and gluconeogenesis, with gluconeogenesis contributing 25 to 60% and glycogenolysis contributing the remainder. Both play a significant role, and both depend on the balance of insulin and glucagon in the portal circulation. Reduced insulin levels decrease glycogen synthesis, allowing glucagon's effect on glycogenolysis to prevail. Glucagon also stimulates gluconeogenesis, whereas the lowered insulin promotes peripheral mobilization of glucose precursors (amino acids, lactate, pyruvate, glycerol) and fuels (FFA) for gluconeogenesis.

Fed State. Ingestion of a large glucose load triggers multiple homeostatic mechanisms that minimize glucose excursions and restore normoglycemia. These include (1) suppression of hepatic glucose production, (2) stimulation of hepatic glucose uptake, and (3) acceleration of glucose uptake by peripheral tissues, predominantly muscle. Each depends on insulin. In the liver, the increase in portal insulin rapidly suppresses glucose production, limiting glucose entry into the circulation at a time when it is flooded by exogenous glucose. In addition, about 30% of ingested glucose is deposited in the liver. The net effect is substantial hepatic retention of glucose as glycogen. The uptake of glucose by peripheral tissues is mediated predominantly by insulin and to a more limited extent by the mass effect of hyperglycemia itself. Insulin-stimulated glucose transport across the plasmalemma of both adipose and muscle tissue is attributable to the recruitment of glucose-transporting proteins (i.e., GLUT 4) from a cytosolic compartment to the plasma membrane. In muscle, glucose may be used for glycogen synthesis or undergo oxidative or nonoxidative metabolism. In adipose tissue, glucose is utilized for the formation of alpha-glycerophosphate, which is necessary for esterification of FFA to form triglycerides. Intracellular metabolic processes are also facilitated by the action of insulin. Insulin promotes glycogen formation by stimulating glycogen synthase and glucose oxidation by activating pyruvate dehydrogenase and decreasing lipolysis (FFA compete with glucose for oxidative metabolism).

Ingestion of large quantities of glucose is not representative of conditions during ingestion of ordinary meals. If the quantity of carbohydrate consumed and the resultant insulin response are small, glucose homeostasis is maintained largely by a reduction in hepatic glucose production rather than an increase in glucose uptake. This is because glucose production is much more sensitive than glucose uptake to the effects of small changes in insulin secretion. The rise in insulin that accompanies consumption of mixed meals also facilitates protein and fat storage. Because muscle is in negative nitrogen balance in the fasting state, repletion of muscle nitrogen depends on a net uptake of amino acids in response to protein feeding. In muscle, insulin acts to promote positive nitrogen balance by inhibiting the breakdown of protein and stimulating the synthesis of new proteins. Similarly, in adipose tissue insulin accelerates triglyceride uptake by stimulating lipoprotein lipase, while simultaneously inhibiting hormone-sensitive lipase that catalyzes the hydrolysis of stored triglycerides.

Metabolic Defects in Diabetes. In type II diabetes, fasting hyperglycemia is accompanied by an inappropriate increase in hepatic glucose production that is generally proportionate to the blood glucose elevation. In type I diabetes, portal insulin deficiency is invariably present and thus hepatic glucose production is consistently elevated. In addition, insulin deficiency leads to hypersecretion of glucagon and GH, which further accentuate glucose overproduction. Because basal glucose uptake occurs largely in non–insulin-sensitive tissues, total body glucose uptake tends to be increased owing to the mass action of hyperglycemia. This underscores the crucial role the liver plays in determining the fasting glucose level in diabetes. The increase in glucose production in both types of diabetes is due to an acceleration of gluconeogenesis. The loss of the restraining effect of insulin leads to a relative increase in portal glucagon and, in turn, an increase in the uptake and conversion of glycogenic substrates to glucose within the liver. In the extreme situation of total insulin lack, an excessive release of a variety of counterregulatory hormones causes gluconeogenesis to increase further and blocks compensatory increases in glucose disposal. The clinical correlate is profound hyperglycemia (Fig. 205–2). Fasting levels of FFA are also frequently elevated owing to accelerated mobilization of fat stores. In type II diabetes, FFA elevations occur in the presence of normal or increased insulin, suggesting resistance to insulin's inhibitory effect on lipolysis. Although FFA are not directly converted to glucose, they promote hyperglycemia by providing the liver with factors to support gluconeogenesis and by interfering with glucose consumption in muscle. Endogenous insulin secretion in type II diabetes provides sufficient levels of insulin in portal blood to suppress conversion of FFA to ketones in the liver. In type I diabetes, however, mobilized FFA are more readily converted to ketone bodies. The combined effects of insulin deficiency and the presence of glucagon suppress fat synthesis in liver. This reduces intrahepatic malonyl CoA, which together with carnitine stimulates the activity of hepatic acylcarnitine transferase I, facilitating the transfer of long chain fatty acids into mitochondria, where they are broken down via beta-oxidation and converted to ketone bodies. In addition, hypoinsulinemia, by decreasing ketone turnover, enhances the magnitude of the ketosis for any given level of ketone production. During diabetic ketoacidosis, ketone levels dramatically increase because of the concomitant release of counterregulatory hormones. The rise in glucagon accelerates hepatic ketogenesis, whereas elevations of catecholamines, GH, and cortisol act in concert to increase lipolysis and, in turn, the delivery of FFA to

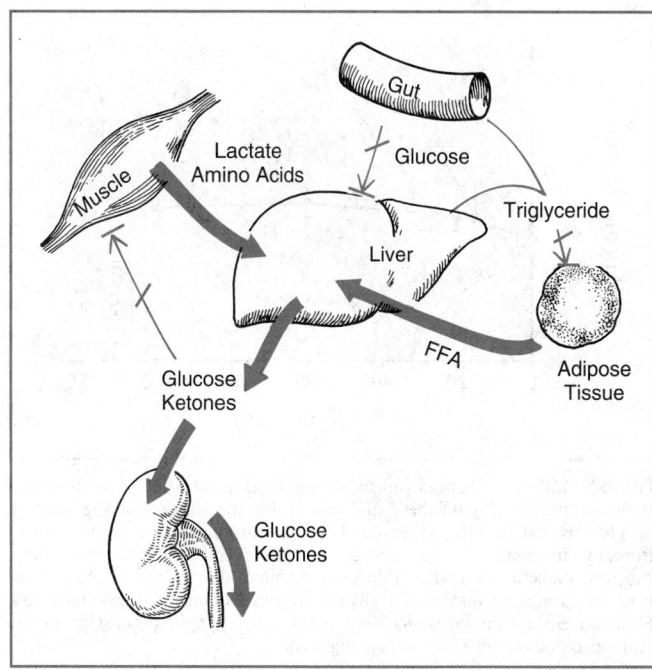

FIGURE 205–2. The effects of severe insulin deficiency on body fuel metabolism. Lack of insulin leads to mobilization of substrates for gluconeogenesis and ketogenesis from muscle and adipose tissue, accelerated production of glucose and ketones by the liver, and impaired removal of endogenously produced and exogenous fuels by insulin-responsive tissues. The net result is severe hyperglycemia and hyperketonemia that overwhelm renal removal mechanisms.

the liver (Fig. 205–2). The increase in substrate delivery may become so pronounced that it saturates the oxidative pathway, leading to a fatty liver and hypertriglyceridemia.

Diabetes is characterized by marked postprandial hyperglycemia after carbohydrate ingestion. In type II diabetes, the combined effects of delayed insulin secretion and hepatic insulin resistance impair the suppression of hepatic glucose production. Hyperglycemia ensues, even though insulin levels may rise to levels above those seen in nondiabetic individuals (insulin secretion remains deficient relative to the prevailing glucose level), because insulin resistance reduces the capacity of muscle to remove glucose and store it as glycogen. The normal increase in glucose-6-phosphate in muscle after insulin is markedly attenuated in diabetes, implying that the block in glycogen synthesis precedes glucose-6-phosphate formation and is mediated at either the level of glucose transport or its conversion to glucose-6-phosphate (by hexokinase) (Fig. 205–3). These defects are more pronounced in patients with severe hyperglycemia, in whom insulin secretion is further reduced. Type I patients show the most marked and prolonged elevations in blood glucose after ingestion of carbohydrate. These individuals have low portal vein insulin levels, which are not reversed by conventional subcutaneous insulin therapy. Consequently, the liver fails to reduce its glucose production or to appropriately take up glucose. In addition, glucose uptake by peripheral tissues is impaired by the lack of insulin and the development of insulin resistance secondary to chronic insulin deprivation. The net result is a gross defect in glucose disposal that is only partially compensated for by renal glycosuria. The insulin-deficient patient may exhibit defects in the disposal of ingested protein and fat as well. In the absence of a rise in insulin, meal ingestion may cause hyperaminoacidemia due to a failure to stimulate the net uptake of amino acids in muscle and hypertriglyceridemia due to reduced activity of lipoprotein lipase. Thus, type I diabetes may be viewed as a disorder of protein and fat tolerance as well as glucose tolerance.

PATHOGENESIS

Type I diabetes produces profound beta cell failure with secondary insulin resistance, whereas type II diabetes causes less severe insulin deficiency and a more severe impairment of insulin ac-

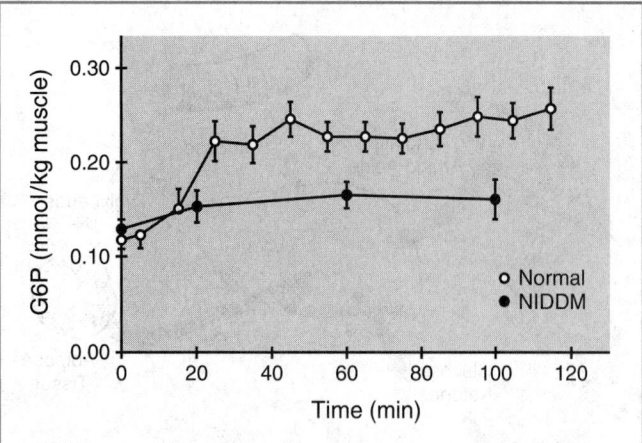

FIGURE 205–3. Changes in the concentration of glucose-6-phosphate (G6P) in muscle of nondiabetic and type II diabetic subjects during infusion of glucose and insulin as measured by nuclear magnetic resonance spectroscopy. In contrast to the increase in muscle G6P levels in nondiabetic subjects, diabetics exhibited little or no change, despite comparable elevations in circulating insulin and glucose. (From Rothman DI, Shulman RG, Shulman GI: J Clin Invest 89:1069, 1992, by copyright permission of the American Society for Clinical Investigation.)

tion. Given the similarity in the overall picture, it is not surprising that both forms of diabetes share many pathophysiologic features. However, despite the apparent phenotypic similarity, the underlying pathogenetic mechanisms leading to type I and type II diabetes are strikingly different.

TYPE I DIABETES. Type I diabetes results from an interplay of genetic, environmental, and autoimmune factors that selectively destroy insulin-producing beta cells. The role of genetic factors is underscored by data in identical twins showing concordance rates of 30 to 50%, rates much higher than those for nonidentical twins or siblings. It has been assumed that because concordance rates are not 100%, environmental factors must be important for disease expression. Even identical twins, however, do not have identical T cell receptor or immunoglobulin genes, and thus for autoimmune diseases, such as type I diabetes, total concordance would not be expected. Although all the genes linked to the disease have not been identified and are undoubtedly multiple, the HLA genes on the short arm of chromosome 6 play a dominant role. In nonaffected siblings, the risk of developing diabetes is 15 to 20% if they are HLA-identical, 5 to 10% if they share one HLA gene, and < 1% if they are HLA nonidentical. Specific HLA haplotypes are linked to type I diabetes: 90 to 95% express DR3 and/or DR4 class II HLA molecules, compared with an incidence of 50 to 60% in the general population; 60% of patients express both alleles, a rate more than 10-fold that of the general population. Another class II allele, HLA-DR2, has a negative association with disease. Specific class II DQ haplotypes even more strongly correlate with disease susceptibility in Caucasians. Susceptibility is associated with polymorphisms of the allele encoding the beta chain of the DQ class II HLA molecule. The presence of aspartic acid at position 57 protects against disease, whereas substitution of a neutral amino acid at this position is associated with a much higher frequency. Other polymorphisms, such as a substitution of arginine at position 52 of the DQ alpha chain, may confer additional risk. It is likely, however, that no single class II gene accounts for HLA-associated susceptibility to disease and that significant genetic heterogeneity exists. The association of the disease with specific class II HLA genes implies the involvement of CD4 T cells in the autoimmunity process, because these molecules are critical for the presentation of antigenic peptides to CD4 T cells and for the selection of the T-cell repertoire.

Although environmental factors such as diet (e.g., milk protein in newborns) and toxins have been proposed as initiating factors, most attention has focused on viruses. Epidemics of mumps, coxsackievirus, and congenital rubella have been associated with an increased frequency of type I diabetes. In one instance, a coxsackievirus B4 was isolated from the pancreas of a child who died of diabetic ketoacidosis, and inoculation of the virus into mice caused

disease, fulfilling Koch's postulates. Viruses that produce acute, lytic infection, however, are probably responsible for only an occasional case. Instead, if viruses are involved, it is more likely that they trigger an autoimmune response. It has been postulated that if a virus contains an epitope that resembles a beta cell protein, infection with the virus could abrogate self-tolerance, triggering autoimmunity. Interestingly, sequence homology has been identified between coxsackievirus B and glutamic acid decarboxylase (GAD), an important autoantigen in type I diabetes.

About 80% of new-onset patients with type I diabetes have islet cell antibodies (ICA). A variety of antibodies with specificity against beta cell constituents have been identified, including insulin and GAD. The idea that type I diabetes is a chronic autoimmune disease with an acute presentation has come from evidence that ICA are present in approximately 3% of asymptomatic first-degree relatives of patients, and these individuals have a high risk of developing type 1 diabetes, often many years later. ICA-negative relatives rarely develop the disease. These antibodies, however, appear to be markers for rather than the cause of beta cell injury. Beta cell destruction is more likely mediated by a variety of cytokines released by T cells and macrophages that are toxic to beta cells or by the direct actions of cytolytic T cells. Patients dying soon after disease onset have a monocytic cellular infiltration restricted to islets, termed insulitis. The infiltrate is composed of CD8 and CD4 T cells, macrophages, and B cells. As the disease progresses, the islets become completely devoid of beta cells and inflammatory infiltrate, leaving intact alpha, delta, and pancreatic polypeptide cells, illustrating the exquisite specificity of the attack. At the time of clinical diagnosis, about 5 to 10% of the beta cell mass remains (see Fig. 205–1).

The damaged beta cells of newly diabetic patients overexpress antigen-presenting class I HLA molecules, which would promote increased susceptibility to attack by cytotoxic CD8 T cells. A role for CD8 T cells is supported by studies involving pancreatic transplantation in identical twins. Monozygotic twins with diabetes who received kidney and pancreas grafts from their nondiabetic, genetically identical sibling required little or no immunosuppression for graft acceptance. Nevertheless, the islets were soon selectively invaded with mononuclear cells, predominantly CD8 T cells, leading to the recurrence of diabetes. Thus, decades after the original onset of disease, the immune system still had the ability to selectively destroy beta cells. Evidence implicating T cells also derives from clinical trials using immunosuppressive drugs. Drugs such as cyclosporine slow or prevent progression of recent-onset diabetes, but immunosuppression must be administrated continuously to maintain the effect. Supporting data for a primary role for T cells derives from animal models that spontaneously develop diabetes. NOD mice develop insulitis and islet autoantibodies at about 4 weeks of age and ultimately progress to diabetes after 12 to 24 weeks. A variety of treatments designed to deplete T cells prevent diabetes. Most importantly, adoptive transfer of T cells isolated from acutely diabetic mice donors into irradiated NOD mice rapidly produces diabetes. Both CD4 and CD8 T cells are required for transfer of disease, suggesting that both are necessary for disease expression. The specific antigens recognized by these diabetogenic T cells remain uncertain. A potential role for GAD is suggested by data showing that if NOD mice are made tolerant to GAD early in life, they fail to develop insulitis and diabetes. The chronic smoldering nature of the disease suggests the presence of regulatory or protective influences. In keeping with this, T cells that protect the islet from immune attack have been isolated from the islets of NOD mice. Such findings suggest that the rate of appearance and clinical expression of disease may be modulated by the balance between diabetogenic and protective populations of T cells.

TYPE II DIABETES. Hyperglycemia in type II diabetes results from an undefined genetic defect(s) (concordance rates in identical twins are nearly 100%), the expression of which is modified by environmental factors. Inasmuch as hyperglycemia itself impairs insulin secretion and action, a phenomenon termed "glucose toxicity" (Fig. 205–4), by the time full-blown hyperglycemia has become manifest, virtually all patients exhibit both insulin resistance and defective insulin secretion. The sequence makes it impossible to determine which one started the vicious cycle leading to the disease.

Insulin Secretion. Fasting insulin levels in type II diabetes are generally normal or increased. Yet, they are relatively low if one takes into account the coexisting presence of hyperglycemia. As hyperglycemia becomes more severe, basal insulin fails to increase or

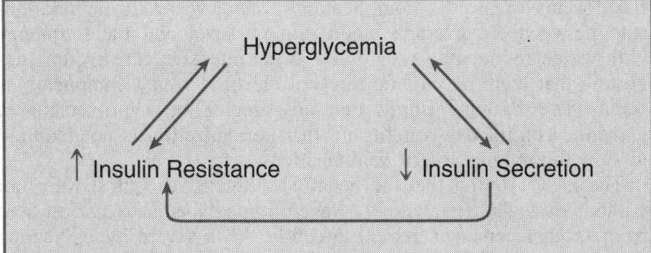

FIGURE 205–4. Elevations of circulating glucose initiate a vicious cycle in which hyperglycemia begets more severe hyperglycemia.

declines further. The insulin secretory defect usually correlates with the severity of fasting hyperglycemia and is more evident following carbohydrate ingestion. In its mildest form, the beta cell defect involves only the initial (or "first phase") secretory phase; the more delayed insulin response remains intact. When viewed in the context of simultaneous insulin resistance, however, a "normal" response is actually inadequate to maintain glucose tolerance. In these subjects, the beta cell defect is specific for glucose; i.e., it is spared from affecting other secretagogues (e.g., amino acids). Insulin deficiency is thus less pronounced during ingestion of mixed meals. Patients with more severe fasting hyperglycemia (>200 mg per deciliter), lose the capacity to respond to increases in circulating glucose. These observations suggest that a specific abnormality in recognition of glucose by the beta cell occurs in the earliest stages of type II diabetes and that this defect worsens as the disease progresses. Although the cause of beta cell failure is unknown, some French families with maturity-onset diabetes of the young (MODY) share a mutation in the gene encoding glucokinase, the key enzyme responsible for the phosphorylation of glucose within the beta cell and liver. A variety of glucokinase mutations have been identified in different families, each capable of interfering with transduction of the glucose signal to the beta cell. Because other families have no detectable glucokinase gene mutations, MODY appears to be a heterogeneous disorder much like more common type II diabetes, which is rarely associated with glucokinase gene mutations. Studies in rodents suggest that the loss of glucose-stimulated insulin secretion is associated with decreased expression of GLUT 2, the beta cell glucose transporter. This defect appears to be a secondary consequence of the diabetic state. Loss of GLUT 2 during the transition to the diabetic state could accelerate further loss in glucose-stimulated insulin secretion. Pathology studies of patients with longstanding type II diabetes have demonstrated amyloid-like deposits, within islets composed of islet amyloid polypeptide (IAPP) or "amylin," a peptide synthesized in the beta cell and cosecreted with insulin. Chronic hypersecretion of IAPP accompanying hyperinsulinemia may lead to precipitation of the peptide which, over time, might contribute to impaired beta cell function.

Insulin Resistance. With few exceptions (e.g., some African-American patients), type II diabetes is characterized by marked impairment in insulin action. The insulin dose-response curve for augmenting glucose uptake in peripheral tissues is shifted to the right (decreased sensitivity) and the maximal response is reduced, particularly with more severe hyperglycemia. Other insulin-stimulated processes, such as inhibition of hepatic glucose production and lipolysis, also show reduced sensitivity to insulin. The mechanisms responsible for insulin resistance remain poorly understood. Early studies focused on defects in insulin binding to its receptor. Mutations in insulin receptors result in the syndrome called Leprechaunism, characterized by severe growth retardation and insulin resistance. Two other rare syndromes of extreme insulin resistance have been identified, characterized by either a profound deficiency of insulin receptors (most often affecting young females with acanthosis nigricans, polycystic ovaries, and hirsutism) or the presence of anti–insulin receptor antibodies (associated with acanthosis nigricans and other autoimmune phenomena).

Although insulin receptors may be reduced in some type II diabetic patients, defects in more distal or "postreceptor" events appear to play the predominant role in insulin resistance. Abnormalities have been reported in β-subunit tyrosine kinase activity, protein tyrosine phosphatase, and the insulin-sensitive glucose transporter (GLUT 4) in adipose (but not muscle) tissue from patients with

type II diabetes. Whether the defects uncovered are primary or secondary to the disturbance in glucose metabolism is uncertain. Possibly, a variety of genetic abnormalities in the cellular transduction of the insulin signal may produce an identical clinical phenotype. No evidence suggests that the mechanisms of insulin resistance in nonobese patients differ from those of their obese diabetic counterparts, but the coexistence of obesity accentuates the severity of the resistant state. In particular, upper body or abdominal versus lower body or peripheral obesity is associated with insulin resistance and diabetes. It is now believed that intra-abdominal visceral fat (detected by CT or MRI) may be the real culprit. Abdominal fat cells have a higher lipolytic rate and are more resistant to insulin than fat derived from peripheral deposits. Cortisol hypersecretion and/or hereditary factors influence distribution of body fat, the latter contributing an additional genetic influence on expression of the disease.

What Is the Primary Defect? It remains uncertain whether insulin resistance or defective insulin secretion is the primary event leading to type II diabetes. Because it is difficult to resolve this issue once overt diabetes has developed, attention has focused on high-risk nondiabetic subjects. Studies in populations with high prevalence rates, such as Pima Indians and Mexican Americans, have found that insulin resistance is the initial predisposing defect. Similar results have been reported in nondiabetic first-degree relatives of type II diabetic patients and in healthy prediabetic offspring of two diabetic parents. Interestingly, hyperinsulinemia has been detected in prediabetic subjects one to two decades before the onset of diabetes, suggesting that the development of the diabetic syndrome is exceedingly slow. Although these studies support the view that insulin resistance generally antedates insulin deficiency, its presence was insufficient to produce overt diabetes. The finding implies that for diabetes to become manifest, the additional factor of impaired insulin secretion is required (Fig. 205–5). It is unclear whether the appearance of a secretory defect is a secondary phenomenon (e.g., due to beta cell exhaustion) or the result of a second independent defect that becomes evident only upon chronic beta cell stimulation (e.g., a subtle genetic defect in beta cell signal transduction). This sequence of events, although common, does not occur in all patients. The demonstration of functional glucokinase gene mutations in some MODY patients clearly indicates that primary beta cell defects are capable of producing an identical phenotype. Furthermore, a significant number of African-Americans with type II diabetes exhibit little or no insulin resistance, and diminished glucose-stimulated insulin secretion has been reported to be a feature of the subgroup of women with gestational diabetes who later develop type II diabetes. Thus, it is unlikely that a single pathogenetic mechanism is responsible for type II diabetes.

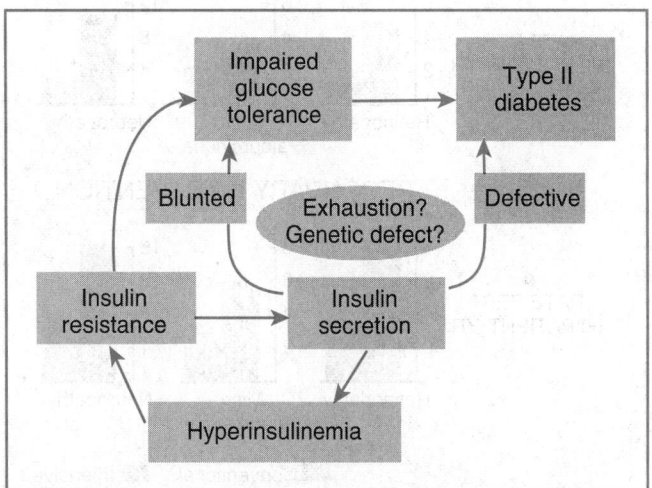

FIGURE 205–5. A proposed sequence of events leading to the development of type II diabetes: insulin resistance resulting from genetic influences, central obesity, inactivity, or a combination of these factors leads over time to a progressive loss of the beta cell's capacity to compensate for this defect.

RELATIONSHIP BETWEEN DIABETES CONTROL AND ITS COMPLICATIONS

Whether the vascular and neuropathic complications of diabetes can be prevented or delayed by improved glycemic control has been debated for more than a half century. To answer the question, the National Institutes of Health initiated the Diabetes Control and Complications Trial (DCCT) to determine if intensive insulin therapy can prevent diabetic complications and/or retard the progression of mild retinopathy. The 9-year trial involved 29 medical centers in North America and included 1441 type I patients aged 13 to 39 years who agreed to be assigned randomly to either intensive insulin therapy or conventional care. Intensive care consisted of three or more insulin injections per day or an insulin pump, self-monitoring of blood glucose at least four times per day, and frequent contact with a diabetes health care team. Conventional care consisted of one or more commonly two injections of insulin mixtures per day, less frequent monitoring, standard education, and less frequent visits. The target goals of therapy were markedly different. The intensive care group sought premeal blood levels of 70 to 120 mg per deciliter, postprandial blood levels of < 180 mg per deciliter, and a glycohemoglobin as close to normal as possible. In the conventional care group, the goal was clinical well-being. Patients were divided into two groups of comparable size: (1) a primary prevention group with diabetes for 1 to 5 years and no detectable complications, and (2) a secondary intervention group with diabetes for 1 to 15 years who had mild nonproliferative retinopathy. Remarkably, nearly 99% of the patients completed the trial.

The DCCT achieved a clear separation of glucose levels between the groups over the entire study period. Glycohemoglobin and mean glucose levels in the intensive care group were 1.5 to 2.0% and 60 to 80 mg per deciliter lower than those receiving conventional care. Although there was considerable variability among individual patients, most of the intensive care group failed to achieve normal glucose levels (glycohemoglobin averaged 1.1% above normal, or a glucose level of about 155 mg per deciliter). Despite this, intensive care reduced the development of retinopathy by 76% in the primary prevention group and the progression of retinopathy by 54% in the secondary intervention group (Fig. 205–6). The latter effect became apparent only after 4 years. In addition, intensive care reduced the risk of developing microalbuminuria by 39%, frank proteinuria by 54%, and clinical neuropathy by 60% compared with conventional care. The incidence of major cardiovascular events also tended to be lower, but the number of events was insufficient to provide statistical proof. At the least, intensive therapy did not seem to pose a

risk for macrovascular complications. There was a linear relationship between the average blood glucose level and the frequency with which retinopathy progressed in the intensive care group, suggesting that there may be no threshold level at which complications occur. The findings imply that any degree of improvement in glycemic control has benefit and that normalization is not required to slow the progression of complications.

The DCCT found that the benefits of intensive control were not without risk. The frequency of severe hypoglycemia requiring help from another person increased threefold. Also, severe hypoglycemia often occurred without classic warning symptoms (often while the patient was asleep). This is in keeping with data showing suppression of adrenergic responses to hypoglycemia in subjects treated with intensive insulin regimens. Weight gain was more common. These changes indicate that in some patients the risks of intensive therapy may outweigh the benefits. Included are patients with recurrent severe hypoglycemia and hypoglycemic unawareness, patients in whom the dangers of hypoglycemia are greater because of other coexisting medical conditions or their occupation, patients with far-advanced complications, young children, the elderly, and patients who are unable or unwilling to participate in their management (e.g., self-monitoring of blood glucose). Such individuals are likely to benefit from less aggressive therapy designed to lower glucose levels without provoking hypoglycemia. It is noteworthy that despite a higher rate of hypoglycemia, intensive care did not have any detectable effect on cognitive functioning.

What conclusions can be drawn from the DCCT? The primary message is that "control matters." In type I diabetic patients who are willing and able to participate actively in their management, the goal should be the best level of glycemic control possible without placing them at undue risk. It is crucial that there be in place a health care team that is able to provide the resources, guidance, and support required to achieve treatment goals. Although the DCCT did not involve type II patients, it is likely that the results of the DCCT apply to them as well. However, a larger subgroup of type II patients are not ideal candidates for tight control when viewed in the context of its potential risks. This is particularly true in elderly patients with coexisting cardiovascular disease. The DCCT suggests there are benefits to be gained in nearly all patients from lowering glucose from levels > 200 to levels in the 150 mg per deciliter range; for most type II patients this is achievable with diet, oral agents, or less complicated insulin regimens than are required in type I patients. The greatest challenge to the DCCT results relates to how they can be effectively applied to clinical practice, a formidable task. The study group was highly motivated and more compliant than the average patient with diabetes. Management was supervised by an experienced health care team that was able to devote more time to patients than is possible in most practices. Also, the immediate costs of intensive treatment are greater, although the long-term cost savings of having healthier, more productive patients is obvious. An important lesson from the DCCT experience was that successful treatment was largely accomplished by the efforts of the patients themselves as well as nonphysicians, principally nurse educators and dietitians. Thus, it may be more practical to use physician-directed health care teams to translate the findings of the DCCT.

TREATMENT

Treatment of diabetes mellitus involves changes in lifestyle and pharmacological intervention with insulin or oral glucose-lowering drugs. In type I diabetes, the primary focus is to replace insulin secretion; lifestyle changes are required to facilitate insulin therapy and optimize health. For most patients with type II diabetes, changes in lifestyle are the cornerstone of treatment. Pharmacologic intervention represents a secondary treatment strategy for individuals unable to adopt lifestyle changes. Although therapeutic strategies for the two forms of diabetes differ, the short-term and long-term goals of treatment are identical (Table 205–3).

Type I Diabetes

INSULIN PREPARATIONS AND PHARMACOKINETICS. A variety of highly purified insulin preparations are commercially available that differ mainly in their time of onset and duration of action (Table 205–4). Nearly all contain 100 units per milliliter (U-100), although a more concentrated regular insulin with a more prolonged action (500 units per milliliter or U-500) can be obtained for

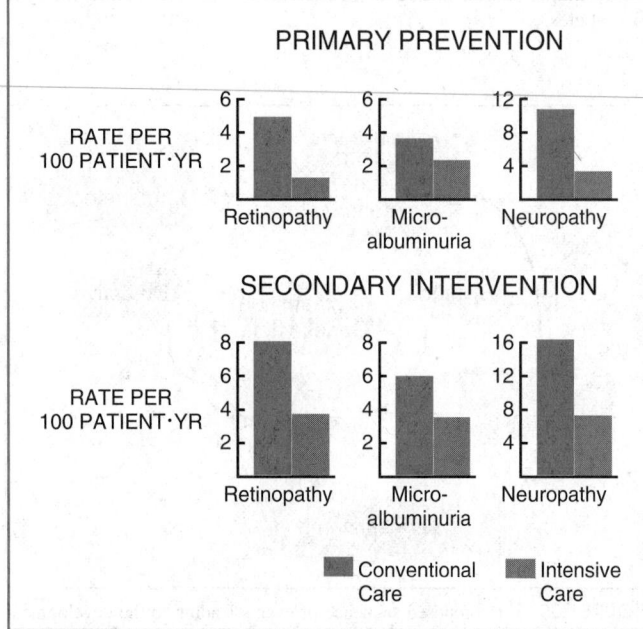

FIGURE 205–6. A summary of the results of the Diabetes Control and Complications Trial (DCCT).

TABLE 205–3. TREATMENT GOALS

I. *Short Term*
   A. Restore metabolic control to as close to normal as possible
   B. Improve sense of well-being
II. *Long Term:* Minimize risk of diabetic complications
   A. Accelerated atherosclerosis
   B. Microangiopathy (retinopathy, nephropathy)
   C. Neuropathy

resistant patients. Pure insulin preparations result in fewer problems related to insulin antigenicity, such as insulin allergy, insulin resistance, and lipoatrophy. Human insulin is the principal form of insulin sold in North America and other industrialized countries. Although animal (beef, pork, and beef/pork combination) insulins are still sold, they will be less available in the years to come. Human insulins are slightly less antigenic than porcine and much less antigenic than bovine insulin. Because they generate lower titers of insulin antibodies, human insulins act more rapidly after injection, and their effects tend to persist for a shorter time. This allows for better synchrony between insulin peaks and meal absorption after injection of rapid-acting insulin with meals but may produce earlier peaks of intermediate-acting insulin that cause hypoglycemia during sleep and/or fail to sustain effects for a full 24-hour period, thereby necessitating twice-daily injections. Human insulin is most useful in patients who are initiating insulin therapy and do not already have antibodies or who have the potential to require insulin intermittently (e.g., type II diabetics during an illness) because intermittent insulin use increases its antigenic potential. There is little clinical benefit in introducing human insulin to patients who are well controlled using animal preparations.

After subcutaneous injection regular insulin begins to act in about 30 minutes and therefore should be given 20 to 30 minutes before a meal. Because it acts quickly, it is most effective in blunting elevations in glucose following meals and in allowing for rapid adjustments in insulin dosage based on measurements of blood glucose by the patient. This is especially helpful in managing glucose elevations that occur during illness or with consumption of large meals. Because rapid-acting insulins afford much greater flexibility, they have assumed a greater role in intensive treatment regimens. Other insulin preparations are modified to delay their absorption from injection sites so as to prolong their action. Either protamine is added, yielding intermediate-acting NPH insulin, or the size of the zinc-insulin crystal is enlarged by adjusting the preparation process. The latter yields Lente (intermediate-acting) and Ultralente (long-acting) insulin. The intermediate-acting insulins (NPH and Lente) have a similar time course of action. They offer the compromise of some degree of coverage for meals coinciding with their peak actions and provision of basal levels of insulin when given twice per day. Longer-acting insulins (Ultralente), because they have less evident "peaks," offer some advantages for basal insulin replacement. Human Ultralente has a shorter duration of action and generally requires twice-daily dosing. Among individuals, the time course of a given preparation is highly variable, owing in part to differences in circulating insulin antibodies. Even in the same patient, a preparation may produce variable responses. This phenomenon is partially explained by the fact that insulin absorption depends on the site of injection. Absorption is faster when insulin is injected into the abdomen than into an extremity, and is faster in an upper than in a lower limb. Moreover, absorption is accelerated if it is injected into an extremity that is subsequently involved in exercise or if the injection site is massaged or warmed. The depth of injection is also a critical variable. Absorption is much faster if insulin is injected intramuscularly rather than subcutaneously, and intramuscular injection in thin individuals often may occur. These confounding factors lead to variations in blood glucose responses and frustration for the patient. Furthermore, insulin preparations are predominantly in hexameric form, which delays its absorption from subcutaneous injection sites because of the slow dissociation of hexamers into monomers. This factor has led to using recombinant DNA technology to construct monomeric insulin analogues that are more rapidly absorbed from subcutaneous tissues. Although the clinical utility of monomeric insulins is not established, the use of genetic engineering to design novel insulins is a promising development.

INSULIN REGIMENS. During the first few years of type I diabetes some degree of beta cell function typically persists, allowing many patients to achieve glycemic control with less intensive effort. Because intermediate-acting insulins generally are not sustained over a 24-hour period and because insulin requirements tend to increase early in the morning, most patients should be started on two daily injections of a mixture of intermediate-acting and rapid-acting human insulin before breakfast and dinner. Although Lente insulin has a theoretical advantage over NPH insulin because it does not contain a foreign protein (protamine), this appears to have negligible c ical significance. There is some advantage to using NPH when insulin mixtures are used. If regular insulin is mixed with NPH, it retains its pharmacokinetic characteristics, whereas if it is mixed with Lente, the excess zinc may cause regular insulin to precipitate out of solution, delaying its absorption. Initially, the doses of intermediate-acting insulin are adjusted to optimize predinner and fasting glucose levels. Once this is accomplished, the doses of rapid-acting insulin are varied so as to optimize prelunch and bedtime glucose values. Patients should inject in the same region but different locations at the same time each day, i.e., in the abdomen in the morning to optimize insulin delivery and in the leg or buttock at night to slow absorption. Some patients may experience a brief "honeymoon" period during which there is partial recovery of beta cell function and a need to reduce insulin doses. This should not be used as a signal to reduce efforts aimed at glycemic control; optimized insulin therapy may help preserve beta cell function.

Several years after the onset of type I diabetes, residual insulin secretion typically stops and twice-daily insulin injections no longer suffice. Optimal glycemic control requires that insulin delivery be directed toward more closely simulating the normal pattern of insulin secretion, namely continuous "basal" insulin secretion throughout the day and night and brief increases in insulin levels coinciding with ingestion of meals. The major problem with regimens relying on twice-daily injections is that the glucose-lowering effect of predinner intermediate-acting insulin is greatest at the time when requirements are lowest (i.e., 2:00 to 3:00 A.M.), whereas when requirements are increasing early in the morning (i.e. 5:00 to 8:00 A.M.) insulin levels decline. The result is a tendency to nocturnal hypoglycemia and/or fasting hyperglycemia.

It has become evident that successful management must begin with control of fasting glucose levels. Failure to do so leads to perpetuation of hyperglycemia for the remainder of the day or attempts at corrective measures with supplemental insulin that miss the mark. The therapeutic obstacle imposed by fasting hyperglycemia is best appreciated in the context of its pathogenesis, namely, glucose overproduction. Once hepatic gluconeogenesis has been activated in the morning, it is not readily suppressed by subcutaneous injections of insulin and hyperglycemia persists after breakfast. The key factors responsible for fasting hyperglycemia are inadequate overnight delivery of insulin and sleep-associated GH release. The "dawn phenomenon" is most pronounced in patients with type I diabetes because of their inability to compensate by raising endogenous insulin secretion. The magnitude of the dawn phenomenon can be attenuated by designing insulin regimens to ensure that the effects of exogenous insulin do not peak in the middle of the night and become dissipated by morning. Several approaches can deal with the problem (Fig. 205–7). The simplest is to use three injections, i.e., mixtures of intermediate- and short-acting insulin before breakfast, short-acting insulin before dinner, and intermediate-acting insulin at bedtime. The primary disadvantage of this approach is that meal schedules must be fixed rather rigidly. Alternative multidose regi-

TABLE 205–4. INSULIN PREPARATIONS: TIME-COURSE OF ACTION

Class	Preparation	Onset of Effect	Peak Effect	Duration of Action
Rapid-acting	Regular	30 min	2–4 hr	5–8 hr
Intermediate-acting	NPH or Lente	1–2 hr	6–10 hr	16–24 hr
Long-acting	Ultralente			
	Human	4–6 hr	8–20 hr	24–28 hr
	Bovine	4–6 hr	14–24 hr	28–36 hr

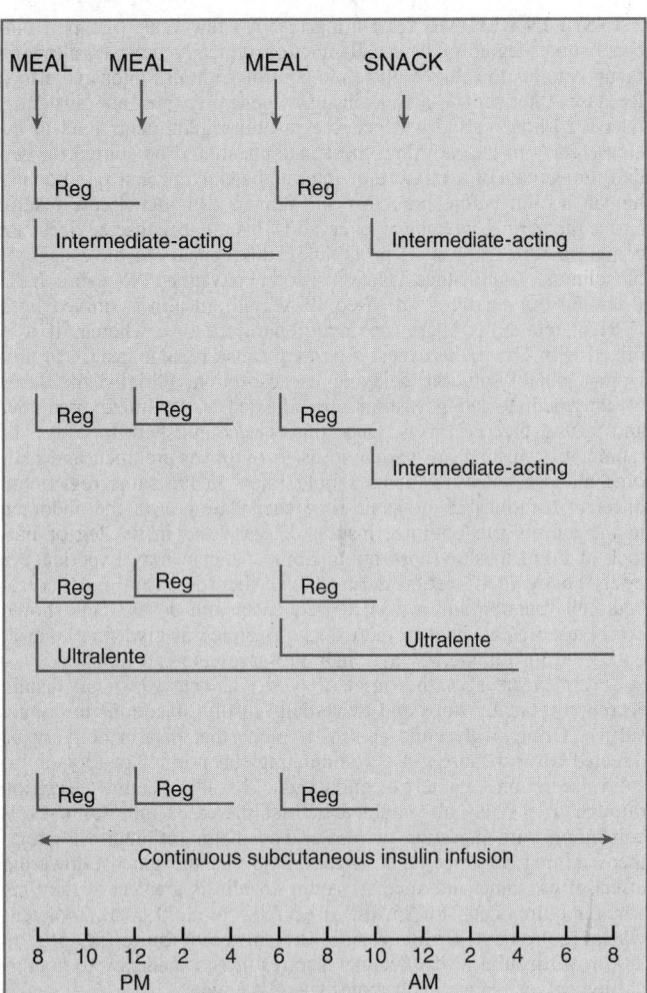

FIGURE 205–7. Several intensive insulin regimens commonly used in the treatment of diabetes. Each is designed to provide a continuous supply of insulin around the clock and to make extra insulin available at the time of meals, thereby simulating more closely the normal physiologic pattern of insulin secretion.

mens include (1) Ultralente (twice daily if human insulin is used) to replace basal insulin secretion and short-acting insulin before each meal, or (2) short-acting insulin before each meal and intermediate-acting insulin at bedtime. Pen injectors containing cartridges filled with insulin make multidose insulin regimens more convenient.

An alternative that provides greater flexibility in insulin dosing while minimizing variations in absorption is continuous subcutaneous insulin infusion (CSII). This method administers rapid-acting insulin around the clock using a battery-powered, externally worn, computer-controlled infusion pump. The pump delivers basal rates continuously and can be programmed to vary the flow rate automatically for set time periods, such as reducing the flow rate at 1:00 to 4:00 A.M. and then increasing it to compensate for increased insulin requirements early in the morning (i.e., 5:00 to 8:00 A.M.). Boluses determined by self-monitoring of blood glucose are given before meals by manually activating the pump. Most pumps contain a syringe filled with insulin attached to an infusion set consisting of a catheter and a 27-gauge needle which is inserted subcutaneously, preferably in the abdomen, to optimize absorption. Unfortunately, the approach has problems that limit its use. The most obvious disadvantage is wearing the pump itself. Because CSII uses short-acting insulin, any interruption in the flow (most commonly due to insulin precipitation within the catheter) leads to rapid deterioration in control. Local infections at the catheter site occasionally occur. Also, maintenance of the pump and appropriate infusion rates requires effort and sophistication. The intensive treatment regimens

described above are not for everyone. In patients appropriate for such care, however, intensive insulin therapy should be encouraged. An absolute indication for intensive therapy is pregnancy. In order to eliminate the excess neonatal morbidity and mortality which, in the past, were associated with diabetic pregnancy requires maintaining glycemic control. Ideally, intensive insulin therapy should be instituted prior to conception to minimize the higher risk of fetal anomalies. After conception, blood glucose targets are more stringently applied than at other times, with the aim to restore glucose levels to those found in nondiabetic pregnant individuals.

LIFESTYLE CHANGES. The management of diet and exercise contributes importantly to the care of patients with type I diabetes (Table 205–5). The patient must be advised of the need for a careful balance between calorie intake and energy expenditure (exercise), while taking into account the availability of injected insulin. The introduction of intensive insulin regimens has permitted more flexibility in meal planning by allowing more latitude in varying the size, content, and timing of meals. This offers the opportunity for a more normal lifestyle, minimizing compliance problems and optimizing patient acceptance. Meals should be nutritionally sound and provide sufficient calories to meet the energy needs of growing children, active young adults, or pregnancy. The 1800-kcal diet commonly used in type II patients is grossly insufficient in such active individuals. Furthermore, diets should be specifically aimed at minimizing long-term cardiovascular risk. Because type I patients depend on exogenous insulin, management is facilitated by using a meal plan designed to match the time course of the insulin dosage regimen selected. Patients should learn a system that allows for consistent nutrient (especially carbohydrate) intake each day (such as the Exchange System developed by the American Diabetes Association) to allow the appropriate substitution of foods within the meal plan and learn to compensate for departures from the meal plan by adjusting insulin doses or for periods of increased activity by consumption of extra food. Efforts should be made to avoid long delays between meals; frequent small snacks may be needed at times of peak insulin action to avoid hypoglycemia. Most patients, regardless of their regimen, require a bedtime snack to reduce the risk of nocturnal hypoglycemia. The potential for weight gain requires special emphasis on portion control and appropriate (but not excessive) food intake for treatment of hypoglycemia.

Regular exercise is important to promote well-being and reduce vascular complications. Little evidence suggests, however, that exercise substantially improves glycemic control in type I diabetes, even though it reduces overall insulin requirements by enhancing insulin sensitivity. Exercise may rapidly reduce blood glucose levels, particularly when it coincides with the time of the peak action of an insulin injection or if it accelerates insulin absorption from its injection site. Exercise also produces a marked increase in glucose uptake by muscle. Blood glucose levels nevertheless remain stable in normal subjects because insulin levels fall, promoting increases in hepatic glucose production that match the rate of glucose consumption. In the diabetic receiving insulin exogenously, this "finely

---

TABLE 205–5. LIFESTYLE MODIFICATIONS FOR THE PATIENT WITH DIABETES

I. Diet prescription
 1. Weight reduction (when appropriate)
 2. Carbohydrates: 45–60% (depending on severity of diabetes and triglyceride levels)
 3. Restriction of saturated fat (to < 10% of calories)
 4. Increased monounsaturated fat (depending on the need to limit carbohydrate)
 5. Decreased cholesterol intake to < 300 mg per day
 6. Sodium restriction in patients prone to hypertension

II. *Exercise prescription**
 1. *Type:* Aerobic strongly preferred. Avoid heavy lifting, straining, and Valsalva maneuvers that raise blood pressure.
 2. *Intensity:* Increase pulse rate to at least 120–140, depending on the age and cardiovascular state of the patient.
 3. *Frequency:* 3–4 days per week
 4. *Duration:* 20–30 minutes preceded and followed by stretching and flexibility exercises for 5–10 minutes.

* Limitations are imposed by pre-existing coronary or peripheral vascular disease, proliferative retinopathy, peripheral or autonomic neuropathy, and poor glycemic control.

tuned" homeostatic mechanism is disturbed. The continued presence of exogenous insulin further accelerates glucose uptake and, more importantly, blocks the compensatory increase in glucose production, so that circulating glucose falls. Because the magnitude of the fall is not easily titrated, hypoglycemia may be a complication. The tendency to overeat when hypoglycemic symptoms occur may lead to a rebound increase in blood glucose to hyperglycemic levels. Thus, if the patient is unable to adjust diet and insulin, intermittent exercise may intensify glucose fluctuations rather than improve glycemic control.

Type II Diabetes

In most type II diabetic patients, diet and exercise are the key or the only therapeutic intervention required to restore metabolic control (Table 205–5). They are especially effective in obese, sedentary persons who constitute the majority type II diabetic patients. For the obese patient, modest weight reduction (e.g., 5 kg), irrespective of starting weight, leads to a rapid decline in blood glucose levels. The dramatic impact of weight loss is mediated by changes in insulin-responsive tissues as well as the beta cell: Insulin resistance diminishes, glucose production declines, and the resulting fall in glucose leads to improved glucose-stimulated insulin secretion. The effect of weight loss is not restricted to glucose; lipoprotein profiles and blood pressure also improve. In general, *it matters little how weight loss is achieved* provided that adequate nutrition is maintained. In sedentary diabetic patients daily caloric requirements for weight maintenance are as low as 25 to 30 kcal per kg body weight per day. In such individuals the classic 1800-kcal diet commonly prescribed is generally ineffective. It is sensible to begin with a nutritionally sound, individually tailored restrictive diet aimed at producing a caloric deficit of about 500 kcal per day. Because a caloric deficit of 3500 kcal is required to lose 1 pound of body fat, weight loss can be expected to be approximately 1 pound per week. For some very obese patients with a history of failed weight loss attempts, very low calorie diets (600 to 800 kcal per day) can be useful when done under medical supervision. Regardless of the method used, most patients are unable to maintain a diet for an extended period of time, and if they are successful, most regain the lost weight. Although the reasons for the failure of most diet programs are unclear, confounding factors may make weight loss more difficult in type II diabetes. The normal decrease in basal metabolic rate during weight loss is accentuated in diabetic patients because the metabolic improvement produced by weight loss reverses the accelerated gluconeogenesis and futile cycling of substrates commonly seen in poorly controlled diabetes, both of which waste energy. Moreover, dieting reduces glycosuria, lessening urinary caloric loss. Success is best achieved by a combination of a supportive environment that emphasizes long-term goals (short-term weight changes mean little in the big picture), regular exercise to increase energy expenditure, behavior modification, and, most importantly, the patient's commitment.

Even when weight loss is not successful, the meal plan can remain a valuable tool to reduce the risk of cardiovascular disease in the patient with diabetes. This is best achieved by reducing saturated fat and in turn raising the carbohydrate content of the diet. Although it was originally thought that carbohydrate intake should be restricted, it is now appreciated that a diet high in carbohydrate (50 to 60%) can improve insulin action and glycemic control. This is particularly true in patients with mild hyperglycemia. In patients with more severe fasting hyperglycemia or with triglyceride elevations that may be aggravated by high-carbohydrate diets, a moderate carbohydrate intake (45 to 50% of total calories) may be preferable. It has been assumed that carbohydrate intake should be focused on complex carbohydrates (starches) and that simple sugars should be limited. Little evidence supports this assumption; simple sugars raise glucose levels to about the same extent as complex carbohydrates when they are consumed by diabetic patients. Thus, the total amount of carbohydrate in the diet rather than the source of carbohydrate should be the primary consideration. The optimal source of carbohydrate may be foods containing water-soluble fiber (e.g., oats, gums, legumes, fruit pectin). Such fiber blunts the meal-induced rise in blood glucose by delaying gastric emptying and, in turn, the rate of meal absorption. A mild lowering of triglycerides and LDL-cholesterol may occur as well. It is commonly believed that sucrose leads to excessive glycemic excursions and therefore must be omitted. This may not be the case, especially when modest

amounts of sucrose are eaten within the context of mixed meals. Glucose excursions are not significantly different when equivalent amounts of sucrose and complex carbohydrates are added to meals. This may be because other foods (e.g., protein and fat) act to delay the absorption and promote insulin secretion. Thus, it is unnecessary to forbid the use of foods containing sucrose, provided it is done in moderation. Such restrictions can lead to poor adherence to the meal plan.

A key component of the diabetic meal plan is to reduce or change the composition of dietary fat. The typical diet of Western countries, high in saturated or animal fat, appears to contribute to the development of atherosclerosis in patients with diabetes. Although substituting monounsaturated fatty acids (MUFA) rather than carbohydrates for saturated fat in the diet has been advocated to reduce LDL-cholesterol without raising triglycerides, the approach is difficult to achieve as the major sources of MUFA are olive, canola, and peanut oils.

Regular exercise is a useful adjunct in the therapy of diabetes (Table 205–5). It can improve insulin action and facilitate weight loss, but its major advantage is to lower cardiovascular risk. Experiments in monkeys fed atherogenic diets and retrospective population studies strongly suggest that regular exercise attenuates coronary artery disease. This is thought to apply to diabetic patients as well. In support of this view, regular exercise produces a fall in VLDL-triglyceride and a rise in HDL-cholesterol and fibrinolytic activity in type II diabetes. Limitations may be imposed by pre-existing coronary or peripheral vascular disease, proliferative retinopathy, peripheral or autonomic neuropathy, and poor control.

Pharmacologic Intervention

The temptation to use pharmacologic agents should be restrained in type II diabetes, particularly in obese patients. However, the clinician must also resist the temptation to stop at diet and exercise, if they are sufficient only to eliminate symptoms.

ORAL GLUCOSE-LOWERING AGENTS. Oral glucose-lowering agents are generally effective in patients in whom diet and exercise fail to achieve treatment goals. Oral agents tend to be favored as first-line therapy if hyperglycemia is mild, the patient is older, and obesity is pronounced. The response cannot be predicted with certainty based on clinical characteristics, and few circumstances contraindicate their use (e.g., severe insulin deficiency, allergy, pregnancy). Patients presenting with severe hyperglycemia generally require insulin to lower glucose levels in the initial phases of treatment. Once glucose levels have stabilized and the "toxic" effects of severe hyperglycemia on beta cell function and insulin action have been minimized, many such patients become responsive to oral agents.

Sulfonylurea drugs were the only class of oral agents available in the United States before 1995. Initially they enhance insulin secretion by virtue of their ability to bind to potassium channels on the surface of the beta cell, thereby facilitating cellular depolarization. The reduction in glucose that follows is accompanied by a decline in insulin levels toward baseline. Insulin resistance commonly diminishes, mainly due to partial reversal of postreceptor defects that are produced either by extrapancreatic effects of the drug or improved glycemic control *per se*. The clinical benefits of sulfonylureas are due to their combined effect on insulin secretion and action. The importance of the former is underscored by the fact that sulfonylureas are totally ineffective in type I diabetes. Although the sulfonylureas differ in relative potency, effective dosage, duration of action, metabolism, and side effects, from a clinical standpoint these differences have marginal practical significance (Table 205–6). Each drug has similar hypoglycemic effects when used in maximal doses. *Tolbutamide* has the shortest duration of action and is metabolized by the liver and therefore has advantages in elderly patients with impaired renal function who are more vulnerable to hypoglycemia. Because it usually must be taken two or three times a day, it tends to be less effective because of problems with compliance. *Chlorpropamide* is the longest-acting sulfonylurea and therefore requires only once per day dosing. It is partially metabolized in the liver, but it and its active metabolites are removed by the kidney. These properties enhance the risk of hypoglycemia in the patient who omits meals or has renal insufficiency. Chlorpropamide can cause significant hyponatremia by virtue of its capacity to pro-

TABLE 205-6. CHARACTERISTICS OF GLUCOSE-LOWERING AGENTS

Generic Name	Daily Dosage Range (mg)	Duration of Action (hr)
Tolbutamide	500–3000	6–12
Chlorpropamide	100–500	60
Tolazamide	100–1000	12–24
Glipizide	2.5–40	12–24
Glyburide	1.25–20	16–24
Micronized glyburide	0.75–12	12–24
Metformin	850–2550	8–12

mote the action of antidiuretic hormone. This effect is more common in elderly patients, especially when they are taking diuretics. Thus, chlorpropamide has the greatest potential for serious side effects. *Sulfonylureas* with an intermediate duration of action offer a reasonable compromise, although they still have a risk of producing severe hypoglycemia. These drugs may be given once per day, although twice-daily dosing may be required in patients with more severe hyperglycemia. After choosing an oral agent, treatment is initiated using low doses and then increasing dosage every 1 to 2 weeks until treatment goals or maximally effective doses are reached. Most patients (about 75%) initially respond with a lowering of glucose levels. It is not uncommon to see slippage after years of therapy owing to failure to sustain enthusiasm for diet and exercise, to progression of beta cell failure, to superimposition of other medical problems or drugs, or to drug tolerance. The deteriorating glycemic control begets even poorer control owing to the phenomenon of glucotoxicity (see Fig. 205–4). Secondary drug failure occurs at a rate of 5 to 10% per year. Early signs of secondary drug failure should provoke renewed attempts to enforce diet as well as an increase in drug dosage. Persistent hyperglycemia despite maximal drug doses signals the need to switch to insulin therapy or to add metformin; rarely is it helpful to switch to another oral agent.

Recently, the biguanide metformin became available in the United States as an alternative oral glucose-lowering agent. (The drug has been used for many years in Canada and Europe.) Unlike sulfonylureas, this drug acts mainly by reducing hepatic gluconeogenesis and diminishing intestinal glucose absoption. As a result, insulin levels fall, a potential advantage if the theory implicating hyperinsulinemia in the development of atherosclerosis proves correct. Because metformin tends to induce mild weight loss, it may be particularly suitable for obese patients either as monotherapy or as an additive drug when sulfonylureas are ineffective alone. The drug does not produce hypoglycemia when used as monotherapy; however, it can rarely produce lactic acidosis (approximately 0.03 cases per 1000 patient years) and should therefore not be given to patients with renal insufficiency, liver disease, or a history of hypoxemia or alcohol abuse. The major side effects are gastrointestinal, particularly anorexia and nausea, which may contribute to its effect on weight loss. Metformin has a relatively short half-life (it is eliminated exclusively by the kidney), generally necessitating administration as two or three divided doses given with meals.

INSULIN THERAPY. Insulin is most commonly used as first-line therapy for nonobese, younger, or severely hyperglycemic patients and is temporally required during severe stress (e.g., injury, infection, surgery) or in pregnancy. Insulin should not be used as first-line therapy in poorly compliant patients who are unwilling to self-monitor glucose levels or for patients possessing a high risk of hypoglycemia. In patients with severe obesity, profound insulin resistance often necessitates the use of large doses of insulin, which sometimes interferes with efforts to restrict caloric intake to achieve weight loss. In newly diagnosed patients or those with relatively mild fasting hyperglycemia who continue to maintain endogenous insulin secretory capacity, relatively small doses of insulin (e.g., 0.3 to 0.4 unit per kilogram of body weight per day) given once or twice a day may be sufficient to achieve target goals. Such patients retain some degree of meal-stimulated endogenous insulin secretion and therefore may require less rapid-acting insulin. Although it is common practice to administer a single dose of intermediate-acting insulin in the morning, frequently its glucose-lowering effect does not extend over a full 24-hour period. Because a key element of successful insulin treatment is to diminish accelerated rates of morning glucose production, it is generally more effective to split the dose, administering sufficient amounts of intermediate-acting insulin in the evening (before dinner or preferably at bedtime) to optimize control of the fasting glucose level. Alternatively, a single small dose of intermediate-acting insulin given at bedtime to control fasting hyperglycemia may be effective throughout the remainder of the day in patients who have retained the capacity to secrete insulin with meals. This approach has the advantage of greater simplicity and may be combined with oral glucose lowering agents during the day to facilitate endogenous insulin release with meals.

In practice, most insulin-treated patients are obese, have more severe hyperglycemia, and have already failed oral therapy. These patients are more insulin deficient and insulin resistant. As a result, they often require multiple-dose regimens involving insulin mixtures to control hyperglycemia. As in type I patients, it is best to distribute their insulin as evenly as possible throughout the day. The complexity of the regimen must be individualized based on the total clinical context of the patient's disease, the level of diabetes education and ability to perform self-care, and most importantly on the patient's motivation. Although some specialists have advocated combinations of insulin and oral hypoglycemic drugs in patients requiring large doses of insulin, combination therapy is no more effective than insulin alone in controlling blood glucose. However, less insulin may be required.

Monitoring

SELF-MONITORING OF BLOOD GLUCOSE (SMBG). SMBG has revolutionized diabetes management. It actively involves patients in the treatment process, allows more rapid treatment adjustments, and reinforces diet therapy. SMBG provides the patient with the tools necessary for crucial self-management. SMBG is especially useful in the care of patients receiving insulin or oral glucose-lowering agents during periods of stress and of patients susceptible to hypoglycemia. Urine glucose testing is unreliable and should be used only in patients who cannot or refuse to apply SMBG or in whom the treatment goal is only prevention of symptomatic hyperglycemia.

The newer glucose meters are small, portable, and accurate, give a digital readout, and have computerized memory to facilitate record keeping. These factors make them, for most patients, preferable to visual estimates from test strips. Blood sampling is facilitated and made less painful by automated spring-operated lancet devices. SMBG is of value only if the patient performs tests on a regular basis, can accurately measure glucose levels, and can make use of the results. The patient must become familiar with what a normal glucose value is, what the glucose targets are, and how they may vary with changes in diet, activity, and insulin absorption. Day-to-day adjustments in short-acting insulin, based on premeal values and a "sliding scale," can be readily accomplished by most patients. The patient also needs to examine the effects of longer-acting insulins and make small adjustments if glucose levels (e.g., prebreakfast and predinner values) are not within the target range. At a minimum, patients need to be able to adjust to repetitive patterns of hypoglycemia or hyperglycemia as well as to periods of illness ("sick days"). In the latter circumstance, urine testing for ketones should be done as well.

The success of insulin therapy depends on the frequency with which the patient monitors. Patients with type I diabetes should be encouraged to monitor before each meal and at bedtime. Periodic checks 90 to 120 minutes after meals help to control postprandial hyperglycemia, and patients may occasionally need to monitor blood levels in the middle of the night (e.g., 3 AM) to avoid nocturnal hypoglycemia. Type II patients who are treated with insulin should conduct SMBG daily, before breakfast and dinner and at bedtime. Here the aim is to reduce the risk of hypoglycemia. Those taking oral agents may benefit from less frequent testing (e.g., before breakfast or dinner, every 2 or 3 days), depending on their metabolic status. Type II patients on diet therapy should, at the very least, learn SMBG to prevent metabolic decompensation. They may benefit from monitoring glucose levels periodically so that they can better appreciate how individual foods or deviations from the meal plan adversely affect their glycemic control.

GLYCOHEMOGLOBIN. Glycohemoglobin (or glycated hemoglobin) assays have emerged as the "gold standard" by which glycemic control is measured. The test does not rely on the patient's ability to monitor or accurately record blood glucose levels, and it is not influenced by acute changes in blood glucose or by the interval since the last meal. Glycohemoglobin is formed when glucose reacts nonenzymatically with the hemoglobin A molecule and is composed of several fractions, the major one being hemoglobin A_{1c} (HbA_{1c}). Total glycohemoglobin (HbA_1) and HbA_{1c} (expressed as the percentage of total hemoglobin) vary in proportion to the average level of glucose over the lifespan of the red blood cell (RBC), thereby providing an index of glycemic control during the preceding 6 to 12 weeks. Several assay methods have been developed that vary in their precision, yield different ranges for nondiabetic values, and lack common standardization procedures. Clinicians must therefore become familiar with the assays used in their own laboratory and use that specific assay when evaluating changes in glycemic control in individual patients. Although the ambient glucose level is the dominant factor influencing glycohemoglobin, other factors may confound interpretation of the test. For example, any condition that increases RBC turnover (e.g., pregnancy or hemolytic anemia) spuriously lowers glycohemoglobin, regardless of the assay employed. Some assays yield spuriously low values in patients with hemoglobinopathies such as sickle cell disease or trait and hemoglobin C or D, or spuriously high values when hemoglobin F is increased (e.g., thalassemia, myeloproliferative disorders) or large doses of aspirin are consumed. Thus, for unexpected high or low values, factors that alter the specific test used should be excluded, including hemoglobin variants. In most cases, however, discrepancies between SMBG and glycohemoglobin results reflect problems with the former rather than the latter. Although glycohemoglobin provides the most accurate estimate of overall glycemic control, it is less valuable in determining what specific changes in therapy are indicated. Blood glucose measurements are essential to adjust the components of the insulin regimen appropriately.

MANAGEMENT PLAN/TREATMENT GOALS. A management plan should take into consideration the life patterns, age, work and school schedules, psychosocial needs, educational level, and motivation of the individual patient. The plan should include medications, recommendations for lifestyle changes, a meal plan, monitoring instructions (including "sick day" management), and hypoglycemia prevention and treatment strategies. Each component of the plan must be understood and agreed upon by the patient. Active patient participation in problem solving as well as ongoing, continued support from the health care team are critical for successful management. At each visit the management plan should be reviewed and an assessment made of the patient's progress in achieving target goals. If the goals are not met, the causes need to be identified and the plan modified accordingly. The history and physical examination should focus on early signs and symptoms of retinal, vascular, neurologic, and foot complications and reinforcement of the diet and exercise prescription. A complete ophthalmologic examination and a timed urine collection for albumin should be obtained annually in most patients.

The formulation of target glycemic goals must take into account the results of the DCCT, the patient's capacity to implement the treatment plan, the risk for hypoglycemia, and other factors that would alter the risk-benefit ratio. The risk-benefit ratio for intensive pharmacologic therapy may be less favorable for patients with type II than type I diabetes. However, in those patients considered appropriate for more intensive management, the glycemic targets should be much the same, regardless of the form of diabetes. Table 205–7 presents target glycemic guidelines for nonpregnant diabetic patients and targets for other factors that increase the potential for diabetic complications.

Pancreas/Islet Transplantation

Intensive insulin treatment rarely, if ever, restores glucose homeostasis to levels achieved in nondiabetic individuals. The search for more effective methods of treatment thus remains a long-term goal of diabetes research. Efforts have focused on transplantation of insulin-producing tissue, resulting in substantial improvement in the outcome of such pancreas transplant surgery in recent years. In major centers, most patients emerge from the perioperative period with a functioning graft, and, once insulin independence is established, the majority stabilize for many years. Unfortunately, because of the need for long-term immunosuppression, pancreas transplantation is, at present, an option for only a select group of patients, mainly for

TABLE 205–7. THERAPEUTIC TARGETS FOR NONPREGNANT DIABETIC PATIENTS

Parameters	Normal	Goal	Signals Possible Intervention*
Premeal glucose (mg/dl)	< 115	80–120	< 80 or > 140
Bedtime glucose (mg/dl)	< 115	100–140	< 100 or > 160
HbA_{1c}† (%)	< 6	< 7	> 8
LDL-cholesterol (mg/dl)	< 130	< 130	> 130
HDL-cholesterol (mg/dl)	> 35	> 35	< 35
Fasting triglycerides (mg/dl)	< 150	< 150	> 250–300
Blood pressure (mm Hg)	< 140/90	< 130/85	> 130/85

* Targets may vary depending on assessment of risk-benefit ratio.
† Targets need to be adjusted for local laboratory differences in assay method and nondiabetic reference ranges.

type I diabetes requiring immunosuppression for renal allografts. In such individuals successful pancreas transplantation may be more effective in preventing nephropathy in the grafted kidney. The application of islet transplantation to humans with diabetes has proved exceedingly difficult, largely because of difficulty in obtaining sufficient numbers of viable human islets. Thus far, only a few patients have become insulin independent. Interestingly, islet transplantation has been much more successful in patients with chronic pancreatitis who have undergone total pancreatectomy followed by intraportal injections of their own islets. The implication is that the use of immunosuppressive drugs and/or chronic low-grade rejection of the foreign islet grafts accounts for the high incidence of failure reported with early attempts. If correct, the future of islet transplantation therapy may depend more on the manipulation of the islet or the immune system to prevent rejection than on technical surgical advances.

COMPLICATIONS

Acute Metabolic Complications

HYPERGLYCEMIC STATES. Metabolic decompensation in diabetes manifests as severe hyperglycemia with or without ketoacidosis. Although diabetic ketoacidosis (DKA) generally is seen in type I patients and nonketotic hyperosmolar syndrome generally is seen in type II patients, exceptions are common. In both conditions mortality increases with age and is usually due to an associated catastrophic illness (e.g., myocardial infarction, cerebrovascular accident, sepsis) or acute complications (e.g., aspiration, arrhythmias, or cerebral edema). Thus, treatment does not simply depend on insulin to reverse the metabolic abnormalities that dominate the picture; it also depends on detection and treatment of precipitating illnesses as well as prompt attention to fluid and electrolyte disturbances.

DIABETIC KETOACIDOSIS. DKA may herald the onset of type I diabetes, but it most often (> 80%) occurs in established diabetic patients as a result of an intercurrent illness (e.g., infection), an inappropriate reduction in insulin dosage, or missed injections (especially in adolescents). A common scenario is the patient who fails to increase insulin therapy and consume extra fluids during illness. Prevention requires education in "sick day" management and assessment of urine ketones whenever blood glucose monitoring shows severe hyperglycemia or physical illness is noted.

The two cardinal biochemical features of DKA—hyperglycemia and hyperketonemia—are caused by the combined effects of severe insulin deficiency and excessive secretion of counterregulatory hormones that interact synergistically to magnify the effects of insulin lack. These changes mobilize the delivery of substrates from muscle (amino acids, lactate, pyruvate) and adipose tissue (FFA, glycerol) to the liver, where they are actively converted to glucose (via gluconeogenesis) or ketone bodies (beta-hydroxybutyrate, acetoacetate) and ultimately released into the circulation at rates that greatly exceed the capacity of tissues to utilize them. The net result is hyperglycemia (greater than 300 mg per deciliter), acidosis (pH < 7.35), and an osmotic diuresis leading to marked dehydration. Typically, the history indicates deterioration over days with symptoms of increasing hyperglycemia. Other features may include abdominal pain, anorexia, and nausea. The pain is normally periumbilical and constant in nature and can mimic that pain associated with surgical emergencies. Reduced motility of the gastrointestinal tract, or a paralytic ileus in severe cases, may further contribute to the diagnostic confusion. Vomiting is a threatening symptom, as it precludes oral replacement of the excessive fluid loss caused by the osmotic diuresis; severe volume depletion follows quickly. Physical findings are mainly secondary to dehydration and acidosis and include dry skin and mucous membranes, reduced jugular venous pressure, tachycardia, orthostatic hypotension, depressed mental function, and deep and rapid (termed Kussmaul) respirations. Ketosis is recognizable by a sweet, sickly smell on the patient's breath.

The diagnosis is usually straightforward and should be made promptly. The clinical picture and the presence of severe hyperglycemia should alert the clinician to test for serum ketones, and if possible, to measure arterial pH. The severity of hyperglycemia can vary from 250 to 300 mg per deciliter to > 1000 mg per deciliter, serum bicarbonate is depressed, and there is an increase in the anion gap (the difference between the serum sodium and the sum of the chloride and bicarbonate concentrations) that is generally proportional to the decrease in serum bicarbonate. There may be superimposed hyperchloremia if the patient maintains adequate glomerular filtration rate (GFR) and is able to exchange ketoacid anions for chloride in the kidney. The depression of arterial pH depends on the degree of respiratory compensation; in mild cases pH ranges from 7.20 to 7.35 and in severe cases it may be as low as 6.8 to 6.9. Usually the severity of the clinical presentation depends more on the magnitude of the acidosis than of the hyperglycemia. Occasionally a degree of superimposed metabolic alkalosis (e.g., caused by vomiting or diuretic use) may obscure the true severity of ketoacidosis. An increase in the anion gap out of proportion to the level of bicarbonate should suggest this possibility. Because quantitative measurements of beta-hydroxybutyrate and acetoacetate are not readily available, rapid diagnosis requires qualitative assessment of serum ketones using dilutions of serum and reagent strips (Ketostix) or tablets (acetest). These methods depend on a nitroprusside reaction with acetoacetate. Acetone, however, reacts weakly with nitroprusside and beta-hydroxybutyrate reacts not at all, making the test sometimes misleadingly low. Because of the presence of intracellular acidosis, beta-hydroxybutyrate levels are often much higher than acetoacetate, and the frequent presence of concomitant lactic acidosis farther reduces acetoacetate. Conversely, once insulin therapy begins, the nitroprusside reaction often remains "positive" and gives the false impression of sustained ketosis for many hours or days because some beta-hydroxybutyrate is converted to acetoacetate, and nonacidic acetone is cleared slowly from the body. Other laboratory abnormalities in DKA include reduced serum sodium (due to hyperosmolarity and the shift of water from the intravascular to the extravascular space), prerenal azotemia, and hyperamylasemia, which is usually of nonpancreatic origin but can lead to the erroneous diagnosis of pancreatitis. Normal, elevated, or reduced concentrations of potassium, phosphate, and magnesium may exist at the time of presentation of DKA. Nevertheless, large deficits of these electrolytes invariably accompany the osmotic diuresis and become apparent during the course of treatment. Mortality rates for DKA vary between 5 and 10%. For the most part, death occurs in elderly patients (> 65 years) in whom DKA is initiated or complicated by a serious underlying illness. DKA also remains a major cause of death in children with type I diabetes, especially if complicated by the development of cerebral edema.

NONKETOTIC HYPEROSMOLAR SYNDROME. Nonketotic hyperosmolar syndrome is characterized by severe hyperosmolarity (greater than 320 mOsm per liter), hyperglycemia (greater than 600 mg per deciliter), and dehydration. The major reason such severe hyperglycemia occurs is that patients cannot drink enough fluid to keep pace with the osmotic diuresis caused by hyperglycemia. This results in impaired renal function that reduces glucose loss via the kidney, leading to remarkable elevations in blood glucose. The history is usually of an insidious onset with a deterioration over weeks. Patients are often elderly with either mild or un-

diagnosed type II diabetes. They may be on medications that contribute to the diuresis as well as the impairment in insulin secretion (e.g., thiazide diuretics), or they may be demented or institutionalized and unable to recognize thirst or have access to fluids. Unlike DKA, severe acidosis and ketosis are absent. However, some type II patients with depressed endogenous insulin secretion may be unable to suppress ketone production in the face of elevations in counterregulatory hormones produced by physical illness. Because they have higher portal vein insulin concentrations than type I diabetic patients, ketone production by the liver and in turn the severity of the acidosis are usually mild. The level of consciousness generally correlates with the severity and duration of hyperosmolarity. Only about 10% of patients present in coma, and an equal number show no signs of mental obtundation. A variety of often reversible neurologic abnormalities may exist, including grand mal or focal seizures (about 10% of cases), extensor plantar reflexes, aphasia, hemisensory or motor deficits, delirium, and exacerbation of a preexisting organic mental syndrome. Clinical signs show profound dehydration; gastrointestinal symptoms are less frequent than in DKA. The laboratory picture is dominated by the effects of uncontrolled diabetes and dehydration; renal function is invariably impaired, hemoglobin is elevated, liver function tests may be abnormal owing to fatty liver, and hypertriglyceridemia may lead to a falsely low serum sodium ("pseudohyponatremia"). Although the severe hyperosmolarity would be expected to lower serum sodium as well, it is not uncommon to see "normal" or even elevated levels due to the severe dehydration. The severity of the hyperosmolar state can be measured directly or estimated according to a formula that excludes urea because it is freely diffusible throughout the body and therefore has little influence on the osmotic pressure gradient:

Effective osmolarity (in mOsm/L)
$$= 2[Na^+ + K^+ \,(mEqL)] + \frac{\text{plasma glucose (mg/dl)}}{18}$$

A value greater than 320 mOsm per liter reflects hyperosmolarity and greater than 350 mOsm per liter indicates a severe hyperosmolar state. Recent data suggest that mortality is approximately 10 to 20%. Poor outcome is related to age as well as elevated BUN and sodium concentrations. The syndrome may be complicated by thromboembolic events, aspiration, and rhabdomyolysis. Surprisingly, acute renal failure and cerebral edema are relatively uncommon.

MANAGEMENT. The goals of therapy for both DKA and nonketotic hyperosmolar syndrome are to reverse the metabolic disturbance and replace fluid and electrolyte deficits. This requires the prompt delivery of water, electrolytes, and insulin, as well as attention to potential complications that might arise during therapy and treatment of underlying precipitating events.

In the initial stages of therapy, the primary consideration is to restore vascular volume and correct hypoperfusion. At this time a massive total body deficit of water (5 to 12 liters) and sodium (about 5 to 10 mEq per kilogram) requires prompt attention (deficits usually are more profound in nonketotic hyperosmolar syndrome). Although water loss is greater than sodium, it is usually preferable initially to replace fluid deficits with isotonic normal saline (0.9% NaCl solution) so as to restore intravascular volume as quickly as possible. Fluid replacement regimens vary, but it is common to administer 1 liter of normal saline in the first 30 to 60 minutes followed by another liter over the next hour. Therefore, the regimen (normal or half-normal saline) and the rate of infusion (commonly 0.5 liter per hour) should be adjusted over the next 6 hours (and thereafter) based on the response to fluid replacement and the clinical status of the patient (e.g., underlying cardiovascular disease or oliguria). In general, normal saline and hypotonic solutions are alternated for DKA. For nonketotic hyperosmolar syndrome or older patients with DKA, hypotonic solutions are more commonly used. In the latter circumstance, normal saline generally provides more sodium and chloride than the patient needs and may result in hypernatremia; in DKA hypotonic solutions may accelerate the shift of water into the intracellular space and in turn contribute to the development of cerebral edema that may be seen in young patients. During the course of treatment, once blood glucose falls to 250 to 300 mg per deciliter, glucose should be added to the solution to avoid eventual hypoglycemia and to minimize the risk of cerebral edema.

Although insulin resistance is present in both DKA and nonketotic hyperosmolar syndrome, large supraphysiologic doses of insulin are not necessary and are more likely to provoke hypokalemia, hypophosphatemia, and delayed hypoglycemia. A typical insulin replacement regimen is to give an intravenous bolus of 0.1 U per kilogram of rapid-acting (regular) insulin followed by 0.1 U per kilogram per hour thereafter. Intravenous administration is the most predictable way of delivering insulin to target tissues, particularly in the severely hypovolemic patient with reduced peripheral blood flow. If this is not possible, the intramuscular site is preferred to the subcutaneous site because the latter predisposes to unpredictable absorption. It is ideal if blood glucose falls at a steady and predictable rate (about 100 mg per deciliter per hour), so it is important to monitor blood glucose closely after starting insulin to check that the rate of fall is appropriate. Blood glucose should not fall too rapidly, especially in young children, as a rapid fall may be associated with cerebral edema. A steady fall in blood glucose also means that the time at which glucose is added to the regimen may be predicted in advance. When reviewing the progress of treatment, it is important to consider a failure in insulin delivery if blood glucose fails to drop. In some this is due to severe insulin resistance and necessitates an increase in the insulin dose. Because the primary mechanism for lowering plasma glucose in the early stages of treatment is disposal of glucose via the urine rather than by insulin-stimulated glucose consumption, the problem may reflect inadequate replacement of intravascular volume and restoration of GFR or the development of renal failure.

Potassium replacement needs close attention because both hyperkalemia and hypokalemia are associated with cardiac arrhythmia. At the time of presentation, patients have a severe total body deficit of potassium (about 5 mEq per kilogram), yet serum potassium levels may be low, normal, or high (especially if acidosis or renal failure exists). Once one starts intravenous fluid and insulin, serum potassium falls quickly because of an insulin-mediated shift of potassium into the intracellular space. In addition, fluid replacement causes extracellular dilution of potassium and increases potassium removal because of improved renal perfusion. This trend can be countered by potassium replacement based on serum levels. A low potassium requires prompt treatment with 30 to 40 mEq per hour, whereas a normal serum potassium signals the need to ensure an adequate urine output before starting therapy at approximately 20 mEq per hour. In patients who may have lost potassium for other reasons such as diuretic use or gastrointestinal loss, one should anticipate the need for greater potassium supplementation. Patients with circulatory collapse or compromised renal function may not be able to tolerate a potassium load. Electrocardiograms may provide a more direct assessment of intracellular potassium and are recommended. Flat or inverted T waves suggest a low and peaked T waves a high intracellular potassium. The intracellular potassium deficit in renal tubular cells further promotes potassium loss by the kidneys, and this abnormality does not correct immediately. As a result, excess potassium loss may continue for days or weeks.

In most patients with DKA, acidosis disappears with standard therapeutic measures. Artificial correction with alkali (bicarbonate) is unnecessary. Insulin suppresses lipolysis, reducing FFA flux to the liver and ketogenesis. The remaining ketoacids are oxidized, leading to the regeneration of bicarbonate. In severe acidosis, bicarbonate is indicated. The hyperventilatory drive of severe acidosis is uncomfortable, and severe acidosis has a negative inotropic effect and causes vasodilation. However, bicarbonate must be used with caution because it may provoke hypokalemia, which in the context of a falling serum potassium may precipitate a cardiac arrhythmia. In addition, by causing a sudden left shift of the dissociation curve for oxyhemoglobin, bicarbonate may impair oxygen delivery to tissues. At the time of presentation, the dissociation curve for oxyhemoglobin is approximately in the normal position, as the expected right shift caused by acidosis is offset by a left shift due to reduced red cell 2,3-diphosphoglycerate. Sudden correction of acidosis moves the curve to the left, as red cell 2,3-diphosphoglycerate levels recover only slowly during the course of therapy. If alkali is given, small amounts should be slowly administered (44 mEq every 1 to 2 hours) when there is evidence of severe acidosis (pH < 7.0 to 7.1). Therapy should be discontinued when pH rises to about 7.1. Although substantial phosphate depletion occurs with both DKA and nonketotic hyperosmolar syndrome, the prophylactic use of phosphate in DKA has failed to show any significant benefit. Hypocalcemic tetany may complicate phosphate therapy unless magnesium supplements are provided. Because the longer prodro-mal period associated with nonketotic hyperosmolar syndrome may lead to more severe phosphate losses, they may need to be replaced as potassium phosphate together with magnesium.

The patient's fluid and cardiovascular status must be carefully monitored throughout treatment. When there is severe hypovolemia or renal dysfunction, central venous pressure monitoring is indicated. The presence of cardiac dysfunction or adult respiratory distress syndrome, both recognized complications in severe cases, calls for measuring pulmonary wedge pressure. Urinary catheterization is essential in unconscious or oliguric patients, and gastric decompression may be required to minimize the risk of aspiration. As in any intensive care situation, an accurate record of fluid input and output and key laboratory measurements (every 1 to 2 hours), such as plasma glucose, arterial pH, and electrolytes, allow an ongoing review of progress. Even more important is the need to search for a possible coexisting illness; serious medical illness may easily be overlooked for several hours during the early phases of therapy. In children, monitoring of mental status is crucial because of their risk of cerebral edema. Leukocytosis often accompanies DKA or nonketotic hyperosmolar syndrome and should not be taken as a rationale for antibiotic prophylaxis.

ALCOHOLIC KETOACIDOSIS. This syndrome may be confused with DKA, particularly when hyperglycemia is present. It typically is seen in people who have consumed large amounts of alcohol and then abstain from food or drink for an extended period. Commonly, the patient is anorectic and has nausea and vomiting, prolonging the period of starvation. The syndrome is characterized by severe ketoacidosis and dehydration. Hyperglycemia is inconsistent; it may exist in association with underlying diabetes (or pancreatitis) or be mildly present in nondiabetic subjects. The stress of the illness, volume depletion, activation of the sympathetic nervous system following alcohol withdrawal, prolonged starvation, or probably a combination of these factors results in a fall in insulin and a rise in glucagon levels. The combination markedly accelerates ketogenesis. Hyperglycemia is probably limited because hepatic metabolism of alcohol leads to an increase in the NADH/NAD ratio, which inhibits gluconeogenesis despite insulin deficiency. Alcoholic ketoacidosis is rapidly reversed by intravenous administration of fluids and glucose; insulin is rarely needed, except in diabetic persons.

HYPOGLYCEMIA. Severe hypoglycemia is the most frequent complication in type I diabetes. It symptomatically affects 10 to 25% of these patients at least once a year. The condition can vary widely, from requiring just the help of another person to being severe enough to require emergency medical assistance. The frequency of less disabling hypoglycemia is even higher. From a practical standpoint, data showing that near-normoglycemia prevents the long-term vascular complications of diabetes has resulted in a much greater frequency of severe hypoglycemia in insulin-treated patients and renewed interest in its physiology and prevention. The less common event of hypoglycemia induced by oral glucose-lowering agents should not be overlooked. This tends to occur in elderly diabetics with impaired renal function and is generally associated with the longer-acting sulfonylureas. The management is no different from the treatment of insulin-induced hypoglycemia, but because of the long-acting nature of oral agents hypoglycemia may recur for 24 to 48 hours after drug withdrawal. Prolonged and severe hypoglycemia can cause irreversible brain damage; it has been less clear what, if any, neurologic damage is caused by milder episodes of hypoglycemia. Some studies have shown that EEG abnormalities are more prevalent in young children who have a history of recurrent hypoglycemia. The DCCT, on the other hand, reported no evidence of neuropsychological impairment after an average of 7 years of intensified treatment, even in patients with recurrent severe hypoglycemic episodes. Nevertheless, hypoglycemia may provoke seizures, accidental injury, and a catecholamine response that can induce arrhythmias or cardiac ischemia in patients with underlying cardiac disease. Hypoglycemia is thought to account for 3 to 4% of deaths in insulin-treated diabetic patients. It also has far-reaching social implications. At a personal level, it can become the patient's greatest fear and lead the patient and clinician to aim deliberately for less than optimal glycemic control.

In normal persons, hypoglycemia provokes a response that returns blood glucose to normal. This involves three defense mechanisms: (1) insulin dissipation, (2) counterregulatory hormone secretion and action, and (3) a subjective awareness of hypoglycemia, resulting in ingestion of carbohydrate. The brain cannot synthesize or store more than a few minutes' supply of glucose and, in the short term, is wholly dependent on a constant supply of glucose. If glucose efflux from the circulation exceeds exogenous and endogenous influx, hypoglycemia results. Spontaneous recovery of blood glucose involves a complex response that includes activation of hepatic glucose production and, to a lesser extent, diminution of peripheral glucose uptake. These changes are triggered when plasma glucose begins to approach the hypoglycemic range (60 to 70 mg per deciliter). The rise in glucose production is initiated by the release of glucagon as well as epinephrine in conjunction with a fall in endogenous insulin release and, at the outset, probably reflects mainly the stimulation of hepatic glycogenolysis. When hypoglycemia is sustained, other hormones such as GH and cortisol help to ensure the continued glucose production via gluconeogenesis. Multiple factors contribute to the diminution in glucose uptake, including epinephrine's inhibitory effect on insulin-stimulated glucose uptake, insulin disappearance, elevations of free fatty acids and hypoglycemia *per se*.

Type I diabetic patients are much more prone to hypoglycemia for several reasons. Insulin enters the circulation from a nonphysiologic source (e.g., a subcutaneous depot) that is unaffected by regulatory responses to a falling blood glucose. In addition, these patients for unclear reasons have attenuated or absent glucagon secretion during hypoglycemia, although glucagon responses to other stimuli persist. Most patients develop defective glucagon responses after 2 to 5 years, about the time they become totally insulin-dependent. Consequently, they must rely heavily on their ability to release epinephrine. Unfortunately, nearly half of type I patients with disease for over 10 years also undergo a stimulus-specific diminution of their epinephrine response to hypoglycemia that increases its risk. The ability of type I patients to recognize hypoglycemia and take corrective action may be impaired as well, further adding to the risk. Symptoms result from changes in autonomic activity and brain function. Autonomic symptoms, including sweating, tremor, and palpitations, are often the earliest subjective warning of hypoglycemia. Symptoms and signs of glucose deficiency in the central nervous system, termed neuroglycopenia, may be nonspecific. (e.g., fatigue or weakness) or more clearly neurologic (e.g., double vision, oral paresthesias, slurring of speech, apraxia, and behavioral disturbances). The irritability and confusion that occur during hypoglycemia may prevent a patient's awareness of their cause. Some diabetic patients lose their normal autonomic warning symptoms of hypoglycemia and may recognize the condition only when somatic neurologic function becomes impaired. The loss of awareness of symptoms is more likely to be found in patients with long disease duration and is associated with an absent or impaired sympathoadrenal response. The duration of diabetes, however, is not the only factor responsible for impaired adrenergic and symptomatic responses to hypoglycemia. Similar phenomena may also occur when patients are switched to intensive insulin regimens, which at least partly may explain the increased frequency of severe hypoglycemia reported in the DCCT. Recent studies indicate that the introduction of intensified treatment regimens may lower the glucose level that triggers epinephrine release and adrenergic symptoms (Fig. 205–8). The major cause for this phenomenon is the increased appearance of iatrogenic hypoglycemia during intensified insulin therapy because brief periods of hypoglycemia suppress counterregulatory hormone responses and symptoms during subsequent hypoglycemia for several days. Defective glucose counterregulation induced by intensive insulin regimens appears to be reversible by scrupulous avoidance of hypoglycemia and a readjustment of treatment goals, underscoring the need to prevent hypoglycemia by improving self-management skills.

Pathogenesis of Chronic Diabetic Complications

The pathogenesis of the microvascular and neuropathic complications of diabetes remains poorly understood. Proteins are readily glycosylated *in vivo* in direct proportion to prevailing levels of glucose. The relative nonspecificity of the process is underscored by the fact that nonenzymatic glycosylation involves not only hemoglobin but also serum and membrane proteins, low density lipoproteins (LDL), peripheral nerve protein (tubulin), and structural pro-

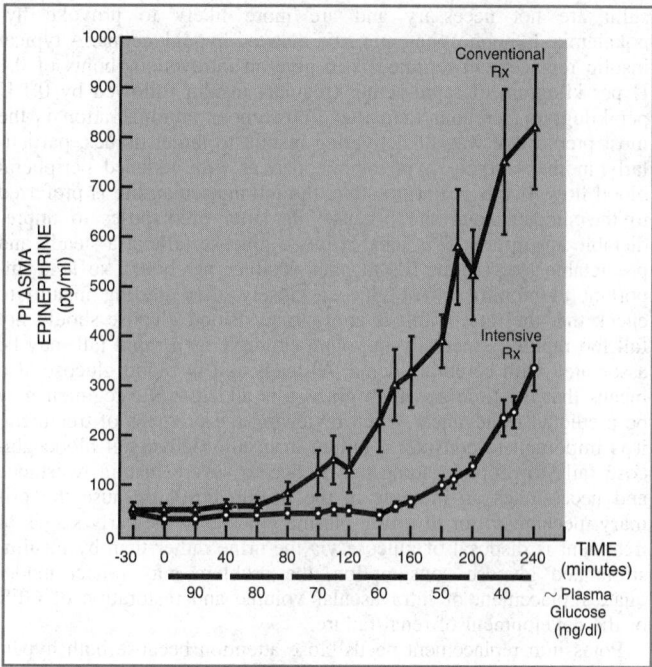

FIGURE 205–8. Plasma epinephrine levels during a stepwise reduction in plasma glucose levels from 90 to 40 mg per deciliter over 4 hours in patients with type I diabetes before *(triangles)* and after several months of intensive insulin treatment *(circles)*. (Adapted from Amiel SA, Sherwin RS, Simonson DC, Tamborlane WV: Diabetes 37:901, 1988.)

teins. This has led to the idea that hyperglycemia induces widespread modifications of cellular and structural proteins that contribute to long-term complications. Available data suggest that advanced glycosylation end products (AGE's) have adverse functional consequences. AGE's are generated by the nonezymatic glycosylation of long-lived proteins (e.g., collagen, laminin) that are further modified by the Maillard reaction, resulting in accumulation of proteins with glucose-derived cross-links in a variety of tissues, including the kidneys and blood vessels. In experimental diabetic animals, inhibition of AGE formation not only reduces tissue deposition of AGE's but also inhibits the expansion of glomerular volume and urinary protein excretion in the absence of changes in circulating glucose levels. These observations suggest that at least some complications may be amenable to agents that do not depend on reversing hyperglycemia. Another potential biochemical mechanism through which hyperglycemia could impair cell function involves the polyol pathway through which nonphosphorylated glucose is reduced to sorbitol by aldose reductase and sorbitol is converted to fructose by sorbitol dehydrogenase. Polyol pathway activity is regulated by the intracellular concentration of free glucose and therefore varies according to glucose levels in insulin-independent tissues. It has been postulated that accumulated sorbitol might exert osmotic effects that could lead to cell injury or to depletion of myoinositol. Beneficial effects of aldose reductase inhibitors and myoinositol therapy, however, have not been convincingly shown in patients.

Hemodynamic changes in the microcirculation may also contribute to microangiopathy. In the kidney, GFR is increased out of proportion to plasma flow owing to an elevation in the transglomerular pressure gradient. It has been postulated that the raised glomerular pressures contribute to renal disease based on the observation that single-nephron hyperfiltration after partial renal ablation in the nondiabetic rat causes proteinuria and progressive glomerular damage in the remnant kidney. Similarly, the hemodynamic alterations of diabetes may cause transglomerular passage of proteins and AGE's; with time their accumulation in the mesangium could trigger proliferation of mesangial cells and matrix production, eventually leading to glomerulosclerosis. Less affected glomeruli would develop compensatory hyperfiltration but ultimately succumb, as does the remnant kidney. Clinical studies support this view. Unilateral renal artery stenosis diminishes diabetic pathologic lesions in the affected kidney, and angiotensin-converting enzyme inhibitors, which reduce intraglomerular pressure, slow progression of diabetic nephropathy. The diabetes-associated increase in microcirculatory hydrostatic pressure also may contribute to the generalized capillary leakage of macromolecules in diabetic patients.

The above theories would predict the benefits of optimal glycemic control reported by the DCCT in patients with few or no complications. Whether similar benefits can be expected once severe damage has occurred is less clear. Extensive glycosylation of proteins with slow turnover rates would not be readily affected by correction of hyperglycemia. Moreover, the hemodynamic theory for nephropathy predicts that once glomerular injury causes compensatory hyperfiltration, progressive injury would continue in the remaining glomeruli, regardless of the metabolic state.

Diabetic Retinopathy

Diabetes is the leading cause of blindness in persons aged 30 to 65 years. Blindness occurs 20 times more frequently in diabetic patients than others and is most often seen after the disease has been manifest for at least 15 years. Approximately 10 to 15% of type I diabetic patients become legally blind (visual acuity of 20/200 or worse in the better eye), whereas in type II diabetic patients the risk is less than half that value. The primary cause of visual loss is retinopathy.

The earliest retinopathic changes are classified as nonproliferative. The first sign is microaneurysms (small red dots 20 to 200 μm), which typically arise in areas of capillary occlusion. Microaneurysms develop after about 3 to 5 years of diabetes and are seen in most conventionally treated patients who have had diabetes for 10 years. Subsequently, retinal blot hemorrhages (round with blurred edges) and hard exudates (variable size, sharply defined and yellow) appear due, respectively, to extravasation of blood and lipoproteins. Infarctions of the nerve fiber layer, called "cotton wool spots" or "soft exudates," may be observed as white or gray rounded swellings. These lesions generally do not affect visual acuity. Advanced nonproliferative lesions occur if retinal ischemia becomes more severe, including intraretinal microvascular abnormalities (IRMA), dilated capillaries that are very permeable, and venous irregularities. They compose the "preproliferative phase" of retinopathy, which predicts a high risk for proliferative retinopathy within 1 to 2 years. Proliferative retinopathy is characterized by the growth of fine tufts of new blood vessels and fibrous tissue from the inner retinal surface or optic nerve head. The vessels and fibrous tissue begin on the retinal surface and later grow into the vitreous, leading to retinal detachments and hemorrhages, the most important contributors to blindness. Occasionally, new vessels may invade the anterior chamber angle, leading to intractable glaucoma, severe pain, and blindness. Some patients without proliferative changes may also develop severe visual loss due to vascular leakage (macular edema) and/or vascular occlusion in the area of the macula. Macular edema may be suggested by the presence of large deposits of hard exudates surrounding the macular area but is often undetectable by direct ophthalmoscopy. Maculopathy is more common in type II diabetes and represents an important cause of decreased visual acuity in this group. Visual loss in diabetes is further complicated by high prevalence rates of cataracts and open angle glaucoma. Diabetic patients commonly report changes in vision resulting from osmotic swelling of the lens due to hyperglycemia. These changes are reversed by improved glycemic control and must be distinguished from more serious ocular pathology.

The eye provides a unique window through which to follow the appearance and progression of retinopathy. Regardless of the type of diabetes, the severity of retinopathy increases with increasing duration of the disease. The one exception is early childhood diabetes; before puberty retinopathy (as well as other complications) is less common regardless of disease duration. Prevalence rates of both nonproliferative and proliferative retinopathy are higher in type I than in type II diabetes. In conventionally treated type I diabetes, patients rarely, if ever, exhibit retinopathy when first diagnosed. Thereafter, the frequency of retinopathy rises to 20 to 25% at 5 years, 50 to 70% at 10 years, and >95% after 15 years. Proliferative retinopathy is rare within the first 10 years of type I diabetes, but increases to 50% after 20 years. It is less common in type II diabetes, appearing in about 10 to 15% of patients after 20 years. Retinopathy affects about 15 to 20% of type II diabetic patients at the time of disease detection, implying that the disease had previously been undetected.

Although retinopathy may be triggered by hyperglycemia, eventually retinal vascular perfusion diminishes, and this is believed to accelerate the process. New vessels generally appear in areas of nonperfusion. Ischemia may provoke local production of insulin-like growth factor I, a stimulator of retinal angioneogenesis in animals and other growth factors. Epidemiologic studies show a higher prevalence of retinopathy and macular edema in patients with hypertension; nephropathy and pregnancy also appear to accelerate retinopathy. At present, medical therapy is restricted to optimization of glycemic control, which delays and slows progression of nonproliferative retinopathy. Little evidence suggests that improving glycemic control benefits the more advanced stages of retinopathy. In addition, it makes sense to treat hypertension aggressively. Surgical therapy using retinal photocoagulation is the treatment of choice when progressive retinopathy threatens vision. Its value was established by the prospective Diabetic Retinopathy Study involving patients with proliferative retinopathy. The risk of severe visual loss in treated eyes was less than half of that in untreated eyes. The study also defined the advantage of panretinal photocoagulation for proliferative lesions (e.g., involving the disc, associated with hemorrhage), which posed the highest risk for visual loss. The more recent Early Treatment Diabetic Retinopathy Study involved patients at an earlier stage and showed an even more striking reduction in the risk of visual loss after laser therapy. It established the benefit of photocoagulation for all patients with new vessels, regardless of severity, and for macular edema. The trial found that interventions at the nonproliferative stage had no detectable value. In more advanced proliferative retinopathy, vitrectomy may be required to remove vitreous hemorrhage or to cut extensive fibrous bands causing retinal detachments. In such cases, surgery may restore vision although vitrectomy has risks, including retinal detachment, cataract formation, and glaucoma.

The above considerations make it imperative for physicians to identify prospectively patients at risk. Nonspecialists, including house officers, internists, and diabetologists, have difficulty in diagnosing proliferative retinopathy; in one study they correctly diagnosed proliferative retinopathy in less than half the cases! Accordingly, diabetic patients should be advised to have annual ophthalmologic examinations. In type I diabetes ophthalmologic visits should begin within 5 years, whereas type II diabetic patients should be seen from disease onset.

Diabetic Nephropathy

End-stage renal disease (ESRD) from diabetic nephropathy is a major cause of death, particularly in type I diabetes, in which it affects 30 to 35% of patients. Although it is less frequent (about 15 to 20%) in the type II diabetic population, this more common form of the disease still constitutes the majority of diabetic patients seeking therapy for ESRD. Overall, diabetes is the leading cause and accounts for one third of the ESRD cases in the United States.

The natural history of diabetic nephropathy has been well characterized in type I diabetes (Fig. 205–9); much less data are available in type II. Soon after diagnosis, GFR is commonly increased, associated with renal hypertrophy and an increase in glomerular volume and capillary surface area. Hyperfiltration appears to depend on hyperglycemia and is reversed by intensive treatment. After several years glomerulosclerosis appears, characterized by thickening of the glomerular capillary basement membrane and the expansion of collagen matrix material within the mesangial region, as well as arteriolosclerosis. In the early years of this histologic evolution, renal function is not impaired and on routine urinalysis test strips show no evidence of proteinuria. Although most patients continue to develop mesangial and capillary wall change as the duration of diabetes increases, only a minority develop sufficiently extensive glomerulosclerosis to cause ESRD. Renal biopsy specimens from these individuals generally show more pronounced expansion of mesangial volume and diffuse deposits of mesangial matrix that presumably encroach on glomerular filtering capacity. Accordingly, routine tests of renal function (e.g., serum creatinine and urinalysis) remain normal during a long "silent" period as glomerular compromise gradually progresses.

In patients destined to develop ESRD, gross proteinuria (greater than 0.3 gram of albumin per day) begins approximately 15 years after the diagnosis of diabetes. At this time, renal function remains

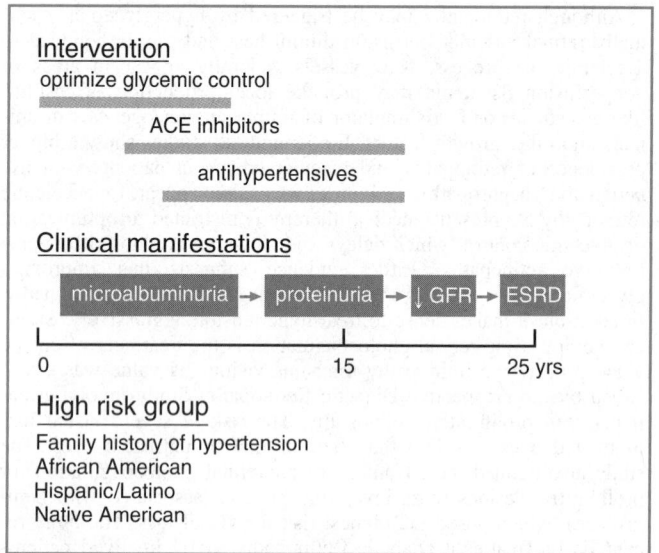

FIGURE 205–9. The natural history of diabetic nephropathy and the time sequence of various medical interventions.

normal, but hypertension is often present. After a variable period of time, however, (about 3 years), GFR diminishes, as reflected by an increase in serum creatinine. The appearance of massive proteinuria and the nephrotic syndrome is common in this context and often heralds progression to renal insufficiency. Once serum creatinine rises (reflecting a 40 to 50% decline in GFR), most patients develop ESRD within 10 years. The course is highly variable, however, particularly in type II diabetes, in which moderate proteinuria may persist for many years without substantive deterioration in renal function. A simple but useful method of following progression of renal failure is to plot the reciprocal of the serum creatinine as a function of time. This allows better assessment of therapeutic interventions and the time when dialysis will be necessary.

Several potential complications accentuate renal dysfunction in diabetes. Azotemic patients are at higher risk to develop acute renal failure after injection of contrast for diagnostic studies. When such tests are necessary, special attention should be given to ensure adequate hydration before and immediately after the procedure. Other types of renal disease are also more prevalent in diabetes. Asymptomatic bacteriuria and pyelonephritis are about twice as common, especially in women. This is due to multiple factors, including autonomic bladder dysfunction, impaired perfusion, and glycosuria, which enhances bacterial growth. Papillary necrosis is associated with diabetes in over half the cases, and renal artery stenosis is more common in patients with diabetes. Particularly in patients receiving ACE inhibitors, hyperkalemia may develop. A variety of other factors contribute to this, including insulin deficiency, metabolic acidosis, reduced GFR, tubulointerstitial disease, and the syndrome of hyporeninemic hypoaldosteronism commonly seen in older patients with impaired renal function.

A genetic predisposition to hypertension and persistent elevations of GFR predict an increased risk of nephropathy. Erythrocyte sodium-lithium countertransport, a marker of essential hypertension that is increased in some type I patients with nephropathy, may provide the link between a family history of hypertension and nephropathy. The risk of nephropathy is three- to six-fold higher in African-Americans, Latinos, and Native Americans with type II diabetes, a frequency similar to that seen in type I diabetes (Fig. 205–9). Although type I patients destined to develop nephropathy may have no signs on routine testing, they pass through a stage during which they excrete small amounts of albumin (or microalbuminuria) detectable only by sensitive assay techniques (40 to 300 mg per day). The appearance of hypertension increases the likelihood that microalbuminuria will progress to nephropathy. In patients with type II diabetes, progression of microalbuminuria to clinical proteinuria is slower and may reflect severe generalized vascular disease rather than nephropathy. The importance of detect-

ing microalbuminuria is underscored by evidence that its progression to nephropathy can be prevented or delayed by optimized glycemic control, angiotensin-converting enzyme (ACE) inhibitors, and hypertension control. Albumin excretion rates should be confirmed at least once before intervening because transient microalbuminuria can be induced by nonspecific factors such as severe hyperglycemia or heavy exercise.

Treatment of nephropathy varies depending on the stage of disease (Fig. 205–9). Early in the course of diabetes (no microalbuminuria), primary efforts should focus on optimizing glycemic control, especially in higher-risk patients. Other measures should include aggressive treatment of coexisting hypertension as well as routine screening for asymptomatic urinary tract infections and bladder dysfunction. We recommend strict glycemic control for patients with microalbuminuria. ACE inhibitors appear to have special value, with benefits such as retarding proteinuria, that are independent of their blood pressure–lowering effects. Once clinical nephropathy becomes evident, aggressive efforts at glycemic control have marginal value; reducing hypertension and intraglomerular pressure remain the only proven means of slowing progression. In addition to ACE inhibitors alone or in combination with other antihypertensives, calcium channel blockers have potential value, although their long-term benefits have not been formally tested. Dietary protein restriction (i.e., 0.8 gram per kilogram of body weight) may add limited benefit once GFR becomes subnormal. As ESRD approaches, long-term treatment plans should proceed much as they would in nondiabetic uremic patients, but therapy should be instituted earlier. Diabetic patients tolerate uremia poorly: retinopathy and neuropathy deteriorate more rapidly, hypertension becomes more difficult to control, glycemic excursions increase, and protein wasting is aggravated. Generalized atherosclerosis accelerates, leading to significant morbidity during dialysis or following transplantation. The decision between transplantation and dialysis should be individualized. Renal transplantation represents the treatment of choice for most young patients, especially if one can find a matched living-related donor. Survival rates for recipients of cadaver grafts remain high and are only about 10% less than for nondiabetic graft recipients. Cardiovascular disease provides the major cause of morbidity and mortality following transplantation. Accordingly, transplant candidates should be evaluated prospectively and treated for vascular insufficiency. Most older type II patients are offered dialysis. The preference between continuous ambulatory peritoneal dialysis and hemodialysis varies among centers. However, many diabetic patients have problems caused by the rapid shifts in blood volume that accompany hemodialysis. Although survival rates are considerably worse for dialysis than transplantation, this difference largely reflects the fact that the patients are older and have more severe underlying disease. Mortality is substantially higher in diabetic than nondiabetic patients receiving dialysis owing to the more rapid development of vascular insufficiency.

Diabetic Neuropathy

Symptomatic, potentially disabling neuropathy affects nearly 50% of diabetic patients. It may be symmetrical or focal and often involves the autonomic nervous system as well. The prevalence of symmetrical neuropathy is similar in type I and II diabetes, whereas focal neuropathy is more common in older type II patients. Because it is a heterogeneous collection of clinical syndromes, multiple pathogenetic factors are likely involved. Hyperglycemia figures prominently; however, other factors may also be important, especially ischemia. The chronic, more insidious neuropathic disorders may be mediated by a "metabolic" process, whereas the more acute, often self-limiting neuropathies may have a vascular cause. Nerve growth factor is diminished in nerves of patients with neuropathy, perhaps limiting regenerative capacity. Autonomic nerve bundles and ganglia from type I diabetic patients with autonomic neuropathy show monocytic infiltration, and their sera may contain complement-fixing antibodies to sympathetic ganglia, suggesting that autoimmune mechanisms contribute to this complication. Because the mechanisms producing such a heterogeneous clinical picture are poorly understood, neuropathy is classified according to areas affected (Table 205–8). Currently, therapy is limited to improving glycemic control. This is effective mainly before clinical symptoms have developed. The usefulness of aldose reductase inhibitors has been difficult to establish, perhaps because more advanced cases were studied.

TABLE 205–8. CLASSIFICATION OF DIABETIC NEUROPATHY

Polyneuropathies	Mononeuropathies
Distal symmetrical	Isolated nerve lesions
Chronic sensorimotor	Peripheral
Acute sensory	Cranial
Proximal motor	Radiculopathy
Autonomic	

DISTAL SENSORIMOTOR NEUROPATHY. This syndrome, characterized by axonal loss, is the most common presentation of diabetic neuropathy. The process involves all somatic nerves but has a distinct predilection for distal sites, i.e., the distal sensorimotor nerves of the feet and hands. Patients complain of numbness and tingling in the extremities, especially the feet. Symptoms characteristically worsen at night, and function usually declines relentlessly with time. In early cases, the neuropathy can be asymptomatic and may be discovered only during a clinical examination. Sometimes, distal neuropathy first expresses its presence via complications, such as foot ulceration or spreading cellulitis from a traumatic cut (see below). Bedside clinical testing typically demonstrates a symmetrical loss of sensation distally, with variable loss of distal reflexes (e.g., ankle) and muscle wasting of the intrinsic muscles of the hands and feet. Damage usually affects sensory more than motor fibers and usually encompasses both small (pain and temperature) and large (position and touch) sensory fibers. In less obvious cases, subtler deficits may be detected by testing thermal discrimination, vibration sense thresholds, and nerve conduction. Because the clinical picture is not distinguishable from other forms of distal neuropathy (e.g., alcohol, heavy metals, uremia, amyloidosis), the diagnosis is one of exclusion.

ACUTE SENSORY NEUROPATHY. This less common form of neuropathy is symptomatically distressing but usually self limiting. It may develop after a period of altered metabolic control, such as an episode of DKA. It is characterized by severe pain, hyperesthesias, and a worsening of pain at night. The hyperesthesia can be so severe that even contact with bedclothes brings on distressing pain. Some cases are associated with weight loss and depression. Pathologic studies show a loss of small sensory fibers. Occasionally, small fiber injury is selective, leaving vibratory and position sense and motor function intact.

PROXIMAL MOTOR NEUROPATHY. This syndrome, also known as diabetic amyotrophy or femoral neuropathy, affects males more than females and tends to occur in elderly type II patients. It is characterized by wasting and weakness of the major proximal muscle groups of the pelvis and may be accompanied by sensory defects, often with a femoral nerve distribution. The anterolateral muscles of the calf are less often involved. Occasionally there is extension plantar response. There is some overlap with the clinical features of acute sensory neuropathy in that most such patients have suffered recent severe weight loss and many are depressed. Nerve biopsies show ischemic changes in keeping with a vascular cause. This form of neuropathy has a good prognosis; most cases resolve within 12 months.

MONONEUROPATHIES. The mononeuropathies are a collection of isolated lesions affecting cranial or peripheral nerves. They usually have a sudden onset and occur most often asymmetrically. The oculomotor, trochlear, and abducens nerves mark the most common sites for a cranial nerve lesion, with lesions of the oculomotor nerve characteristically sparing the pupillary reflex. The median, radial, and lateral popliteal nerves are the most common sites of peripheral nerve lesions. The cause of such lesions is unknown, but the sudden onset suggests a vascular component. Nerve entrapment may contribute to peripheral nerve lesions. Painful radiculopathies may also occur in the distribution of one or a number of spinal roots, presenting as an asymmetric lesion in a well-defined dermatome(s) that may be confused with herpetic neuralgia or occasionally with abdominal or cardiac disease. The mononeuropathies and radiculopathies are symptomatically distressing, but all tend to resolve with time.

AUTONOMIC NEUROPATHY. Symptomatic, autonomic diabetic neuropathy produces a wide range of problems and carries a poor prognosis. It usually accompanies other chronic complications of diabetes and through disturbed regulation of local blood flow may play a role in their pathogenesis. Neuropathic lesions may result in abnormalities of the cardiovascular system, skin, gastrointestinal tract, bladder, and sexual function. In recent years a battery of tests of cardiac autonomic function based on reduced changes in the RR interval of the ECG following a Valsava maneuver or standing have proved useful diagnostically. The most disabling cardiovascular effect is orthostatic hypotension, caused by an impaired sympathetic vasoconstrictor response and possibly impaired cardiac reflexes. Medications that cause volume depletion or vasodilation may worsen the hypotension. More commonly, cardiac denervation results in a rapid heart rate and an impaired rate response to stress. Patients with cardiovascular autonomic neuropathy are more likely to have silent myocardial ischaemia or infarction, an abnormal prolongation of the QT interval, and defective heart rate and blood pressure responses to exercise, each of which is potentially capable of precipitating an acute cardiac event. Autonomic sudomotor dysfunction is characterized by distal anhidrosis, compensatory truncal and facial sweating, heat intolerance, and on occasion, gustatory sweating. Heat stroke and hyperthermia are the most serious risk, especially when vascular disease is present. It may also facilitate foot infections by creating breaks in the skin. Altered gastrointestinal function is frequent. The most common symptom is constipation, but diarrhea is often the most distressing. Diarrhea may have a variety of causes, including hypermotility due to impaired sympathetic inhibition, hypomotility leading to bacterial overgrowth, pancreatic insufficiency, or a spruelike syndrome. The problem may be compounded by fecal incontinence due to the loss of sphincter control and intensification of diarrhea during sleep. Gastroparesis may lead to complaints such as bloating and early satiety after meals, or nausea and vomiting. This is a problem for patients on insulin, in whom unpredictable food absorption may adversely affect glycemic control and exacerbate hypoglycemia. Bladder dysfunction caused by neuropathy leads to infrequent urination, incomplete bladder emptying, dribbling, and overflow incontinence. Bladder residual volumes may exceed 150 ml, predisposing to urinary tract infection. Psychologically, the most disturbing complication of autonomic neuropathy is impaired sexual function consisting of male impotence and retrograde ejaculation. The prevalence may be as high as 50% in males and 25% in females at some point in the disease. One must exclude psychogenic or other organic causes of impotence due to medications, alcohol, or vascular insufficiently which may be correctable.

TREATMENT. In the absence of specific ways to reverse established neuropathy, pain control is the highest priority. Some patients respond to standard analgesic therapies, and tricyclic antidepressants have shown some efficacy in prospective randomized trials. Intravenous lidocaine or the analogue oral mexiletine may be of benefit when pain is severe. Occasionally, opiates are the only option. Autonomic neuropathy causes specific problems for which more therapeutic interventions are available. Stocking supports, 9α-fluorohydrocortisone, pindolol (a β blocker with partial agonist properties), and clonidine have all been used with mixed success for orthostatic hypotension. Metoclopramide and cisapride can stimulate gastric emptying in cases of gastroparesis. Erythromycin also stimulates gastric emptying and may be helpful. These patients should avoid high-fiber diets, which interfere with treatment. Diarrhea may respond to broad-spectrum antibiotics, clonidine, or agents such as diphenoxylate or Imodium, and bladder emptying may be enhanced by drugs such as bethanechol. The treatment of impotence in males includes vacuum erection aids, intracorporeal papaverine or phentolamine injections, and penile prosthetic implants.

Diabetic Foot

The "diabetic foot" results from a complex interplay of factors. The syndrome is characterized by plantar ulcers that heal slowly and follow apparently insignificant trauma. In severe cases gangrene may be a complication and amputation the outcome. Diabetes accounts for about one half of nontraumatic limb amputations. To varying degrees, the diabetic foot is characterized by chronic sensorimotor neuropathy, autonomic neuropathy, and poor peripheral circulation; visual loss may also contribute to the difficulties with self-care. Sensorimotor neuropathy results in a loss of normal sensation, preventing detection of traumatic events. Accordingly, sharp objects left in the sole of the shoe or ill-fitting shoes may erode the skin surface without signalling pain. Neuropathy also produces abnormal motor function of the intrinsic muscles of the foot and abnormal proprioception, thereby altering weight distribution on the sole. Unnatural weight bearing on the metatarsal heads and clawing of the metatarsophalangeal joints result. Also callous formation occurs at these sites which may erode the softer underlying tissues. In severe cases the abnormal distribution of weight endured by the foot can result in repeated painless fractures and displacement of normal joint surfaces producing the so-called Charcot joint. Impaired peripheral circulation often coexists. Atheromatous plaques in the descending aorta, major vessels of the leg, or distal sites compromise flow. Diminished cardiac output due to cardiovascular disease and/or disturbed autoregulatory mechanisms of the microcirculation may contribute to impaired peripheral blood flow. Characteristically the diabetic foot, in the absence of severe atheromatous disease, appears well perfused with a skin surface that is normally warm and dry. This is thought to be due to increased skin blood flow and reduced sweating, both features of impaired autonomic regulation. Treatment of the diabetic foot is aimed primarily at prevention. This involves education (Table 205–9) and regular checking of the state of the feet of patients at risk during routine visits and by foot care specialists. Proper preventive foot care can reduce the rate of amputations by 50%. In cases of deformed feet, orthotics to minimize abnormal weight bearing or orthopedically fitted shoes may be required. It is essential that ulcers be treated early with antibiotics, dead tissue debridement, and appropriate dressings. Cast immobilization made for the foot may be a useful adjunct to the treatment of foot ulcers by redistributing weight away from an ulcerated area. Surgical removal or débridement is required for nonviable tissues such as gangrenous toes or deep soft tissue infections with evidence of gas gangrene. In extensive cases, foot or even leg amputation may be necessary; a compromised peripheral circulation makes this outcome more likely. If poor circulation is a dominant feature, one must attempt to improve distal flow by surgery or angioplasty.

Atherosclerosis and Hypertension

Atherosclerosis involving the arteries of the heart, lower extremities, and brain is the major cause of death from diabetes. The atherosclerotic process is indistinguishable from that affecting the nondiabetic population but begins earlier and is more severe. The predilection to atherosclerosis is uniformly observed over the entire spectrum of diabetes—from difficult-to-control insulin-dependent patients to patients with mild hyperglycemia not requiring insulin. For unclear reasons, the disparity between diabetic and normal subjects is more pronounced in women.

Accelerated atherosclerosis in diabetes is an independent risk factor not solely attributable to an increased frequency of the other recognized factors, e.g., hypertension or dyslipidemia. Whereas microvascular and neuropathic complications develop more commonly in individuals showing the highest glucose levels, this is not true for atherosclerotic complications. Other abnormalities induced by diabetes could be responsible such as small dense atherogenic LDL, oxidized or glycated LDL, increased platelet aggregation, hyperviscosity, endothelial cell dysfunction, decreased fibrinolysis, and increased clotting factors and fibrinogen. Clinical studies indirectly support the concept that hyperinsulinemia *per se* may contribute to macrovascular disease in diabetes, perhaps because of its stimulatory effects on smooth muscle proliferation. Both type II and type I diabetic patients (because they receive insulin via the systemic route) commonly have elevated insulin levels in the systemic circulation, despite the presence of hyperglycemia.

Diabetes may be accompanied by other risk factors for atherosclerosis that markedly increase the incidence of macrovascular complications. The prevalence of hypertension is increased at least twofold in patients with type II diabetes, owing in part to the clustering of both disorders in patients with obesity and insulin resistance. Hypertension is not associated with type I diabetes in the absence of renal disease but develops in most patients with nephropathy. Although LDL-cholesterol levels are not higher in diabetes, dyslipidemia characterized by elevated triglycerides, decreased HDL cholesterol, and smaller, denser LDL cholesterol commonly develops in type II diabetic patients and in poorly controlled type I diabetes. The major cardiovascular risk factors—hypertension, hypercholesterolemia, and smoking—synergize with diabetes to promote atherosclerosis. As a result, the risk of myocardial infarction is two- to three-fold greater in diabetes, but increases to about eight-fold in the presence of hypertension, and to about 20-fold if hypercholesterolemia coexists. Smoking enhances the risk even further. The diagnosis of diabetes should prompt a careful search for other risk factors for atherosclerotic vascular disease and initiate aggressive preventive measures.

Because hypertension accelerates not only atherosclerosis but also nephropathy and probably retinopathy, it is important to treat even minimal elevations of blood pressure that in nondiabetics might be dismissed. The normal nocturnal fall in blood pressure may be lost in diabetic patients, leading to more sustained hypertension throughout the day. Initially, nonpharmacologic measures such as weight loss, exercise training, and sodium restriction should be tried. If blood pressure is not lowered *below* 130/85 mm Hg, drug therapy is indicated. Among the various therapeutic options, ACE inhibitors offer special advantages, especially when there is concomitant renal disease. Unlike thiazide diuretics and β-adrenergic blockers, they do not adversely effect glycemic and lipid control. Their use should, however, be restricted in patients with hyperkalemia. Calcium channel blockers, α-adrenergic blockers, and vasodilators have no adverse metabolic effects and therefore are good alternatives. The selection of drugs should be individualized, taking into consideration other coexisting medical problems. Diuretics may be helpful as adjuncts if there is a volume component to the hypertension. If thiazides are used, they should be given in small doses to minimize their adverse metabolic effects. β blockers should be avoided in patients who are at risk for hypoglycemia.

Elevations of LDL cholesterol must also be treated. Because women with diabetes have a cardiovascular risk similar to that of men, all diabetic patients should be viewed as "high risk," regardless of gender. The goals should be an LDL-cholesterol below 130 mg per deciliter, and lower if there is already evidence of vascular disease (e.g., below 100 mg per deciliter). The first step lies in reinforcement of diet and optimization of glycemic control. If this fails, bile acid sequestrants or HMG CoA reductase inhibitors are recommended. Nicotinic acid is less useful because it increases insulin resistance and hyperglycemia. More commonly, diabetes is associated with elevations of VLDL-triglyceride and reductions of HDL-cholesterol. These variables often respond to weight reduction, diet modification, regular exercise, and other measures aimed at improving glycemic control. Only if this fails should drug therapy (e.g., fibric acid derivatives) be considered. Unfortunately, drug treatment is more effective in lowering triglycerides than raising HDL-cholesterol. Low-dose aspirin therapy reduces cardiovascular events in diabetic patients similarly to its effect in nondiabetic individuals. Large vessel disease in diabetics is as well treated surgically as it is in nondiabetic illness. Similarly, neither the frequency of multiple coronary vessel disease nor the outcome of coronary vascular surgery differs between diabetic and nondiabetic persons.

The association of diabetes with premature atherosclerosis may only represent the "tip of the iceberg." Impaired insulin-stimulated glucose metabolism commonly affects seemingly healthy people living in industrialized western countries but is generally counterbalanced by increased insulin secretion. Although this state of chronic hyperinsulinemia may successfully defend against the de-

TABLE 205–9. FOOT CARE PRESCRIPTION FOR HIGH-RISK PATIENTS (E.G., NEUROPATHY AND/OR VASCULAR INSUFFICIENCY)

Never walk barefooted
Do not apply hot water or heating pads to feet
Inspect feet daily (use mirror for plantar surfaces)
Keep feet clean, dry between toes
Lubricate dry skin using a nongreasy lotion or cream to avoid cracking
Wear properly fitting soft shoes
Break in new shoes slowly
Use second pair of shoes at night (larger size for edema)
Cut toenails straight across
Visit foot care specialist regularly
Stop smoking

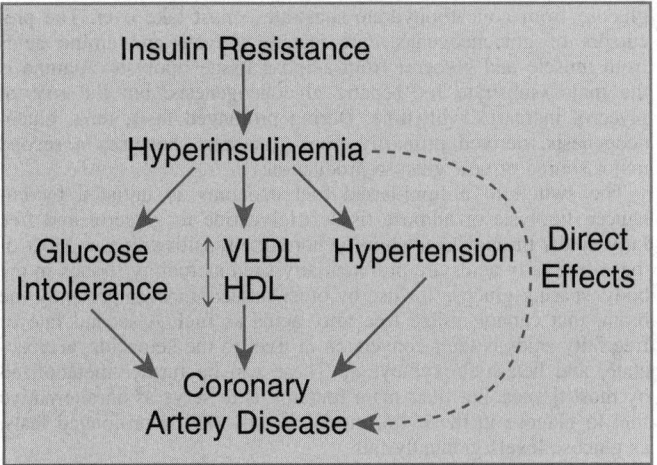

FIGURE 205-10. Syndrome X, a hypothesis based on the premise that insulin resistance accounts for the clustering of cardiovascular risk factors within a given individual.

velopment of diabetes, Reaven suggests that the price paid may be substantial (Fig. 205-10). According to his hypothesis, compensatory hyperinsulinemia has adverse effects on other systems affected by insulin such as sympathetic nervous system activity, renal sodium reabsorption, hepatic triglyceride synthesis, and arterial smooth muscle proliferation. Healthy, nonobese nondiabetic individuals with hyperinsulinemia have higher blood pressures, glucose, and triglyceride levels and lower HDL cholesterol concentrations than do subjects with normal insulin levels. The term syndrome X has been coined to describe this phenomenon, namely the clustering within the same persons of hyperinsulinemia, mild glucose intolerance, dyslipidemia, and hypertension, each of which is a risk factor for atherosclerosis. Several prospective population studies have found that the presence of hyperinsulinemia is closely related to the subsequent appearance of cardiovascular disease. Although statistical associations of this sort do not prove causality, they strongly suggest that insulin resistance has a potential role in the pathogenesis of atherosclerosis. If true, it further underscores the importance of lifestyle changes that improve insulin action in the treatment of type II diabetes and suggests that the same approach could benefit insulin-resistant patients with more subtle metabolic abnormalities (syndrome X). These data should not be a signal to lower therapeutic insulin doses, because the long-term adverse effects of hyperglycemia in diabetics are likely to be much greater than those caused by hyperinsulinemia. Instead, these observations suggest the

potential value of distributing smaller doses of insulin more evenly throughout the day to increase biologic effectiveness of the insulin regimen.

SUMMARY

The long-term goals of diabetes care consist of minimizing vascular and neurologic complications and maintaining a sense of well-being. These are best attained by early detection and treatment. Considering the wide array of potential problems and their multifactorial nature, diabetes care must be comprehensive in nature rather than limited to glycemic control. Attention should be devoted to risk factors that compound the adverse effect of diabetes on atherogenesis, the principal cause of mortality from the disease. Because the complications of diabetes develop slowly and are not readily reversible, it is crucial for the clinician to take a prospective approach, as is summarized in Figure 205-11.

American Diabetes Association: Position Statement: Standards of medical care for patients with diabetes mellitus. Diabetes Care 17:616, 1994. *An up-to-date summary of current standards of care for the management of diabetic patients, including the goals of treatment.*

Bouchard C, Despres J-P, Mauriege P: Genetic and nongenetic determinants of regional fat distribution. Endocrinol Rev 14:72, 1993. *This review summarizes the metabolic and clinical implications of variations in body fat distribution as well as the genetic and nongenetic factors influencing body fat topography.*

Brownlee M: Glycation products and the pathogenesis of diabetic complications. Diabetes Care 15:1835, 1992. *A short review of the process by which glucose modifies macromolecules and how these changes might lead to diabetic complications and be prevented.*

Castano L, Eisenbarth GS: Type I diabetes: A chronic autoimmune disease of man, mouse, and rat. Annu Rev Immunol 8:647, 1990. *A review of the evidence supporting the role of autoimmune mechanisms in the pathogenesis of type I diabetes.*

Consensus statement: Detection and management of lipid disorders in diabetes. Diabetes Care 16 (Suppl 2):106, 1993. *A summary of a consensus conference organized by the American Diabetes Association to develop strategies to better define and reduce the risk of vascular disease associated with diabetes.*

Cryer PE: Iatrogenic hypoglycemia as a cause of hypoglycemia-associated autonomic failure in IDDM. Diabetes 41:255, 1992. *A short review of the various clinical syndromes that lead to an increased risk of hypoglycemia in patients with type I diabetes.*

Davis MD: Diabetic retinopathy: A clinical overview. Diabetes Care 15:1844, 1992. *A review article that presents a description of the natural history of diabetic retinopathy and analyzes the results of clinical trials assessing treatment.*

Deckert A, Grenfell A: Epidemiology and natural history of diabetic nephropathy. In Pickup J, Williams G (eds.): Textbook of Diabetes. Oxford, Blackwell Scientific, 1992, p. 651. *A review of the natural history of diabetic renal disease and the factors influencing its development.*

DeFronzo RA, Bonodonna RC, Ferrannini E: Pathogenesis of NIDDM: A balanced overview. Diabetes Care 15:318, 1992. *A comprehensive review article dealing with the pathophysiology of type II diabetes and pathogenetic factors leading to its development.*

Diabetes Control and Complications Trial Research Group: The effect of intensive treatment of diabetes on the development and progression of long-term complications of insulin-dependent diabetes mellitus. N Engl J Med 329:927, 1993. *The report summarizes the results of the landmark multicenter prospective trial that evaluated the impact of intensive insulin therapy on its long-term complications.*

Fajans SS: Classification and diagnosis of diabetes. In Rifkin H, Porte D Jr (eds.): Diabetes Mellitus: Theory and Practice. New York, Elsevier, 1990, p 346. *Summarizes the classification of the various forms of diabetes and the diagnostic criteria used to detect disease.*

Greene DA, Sima AAF, Albert JW, Pfeifer MA: Diabetic neuropathy. In Rifkin H, Porte D Jr (eds.): Diabetes Mellitus: Theory and Practice. New York, Elsevier, 1990, p 710. *A general review of the pathogenesis and the management of diabetic neuropathy.*

Groop LC: Sulfonylureas in NIDDM. Diabetes Care 15:737, 1992. *A comprehensive review of the actions, pharmacokinetics, and clinical use of sulfonylurea drugs.*

Kreisberg RA: Diabetic ketoacidosis. In Rifkin H, Porte D Jr (eds.): Ellenberg and Rifkin's Diabetes Mellitus, 4th ed. New York, Elsevier, 1990, p 591. *A thorough and current review of the pathogenesis and treatment of this disorder.*

Lasker RD: The Diabetes Control and Complications Trial: Implications for policy and practice. N Engl J Med 329:1035, 1993. *This editorial discusses the health care implications of the DCCT results.*

Lewis EJ, Hunsicker LG, Bain RP, Rohde RD: The effect of angiotensin-converting enzyme inhibition on diabetic nephropathy. N Engl J Med 329:1456, 1993. *A report of a well-designed multicenter trial to examine the use of angiotensin-converting enzyme inhibitors in slowing the progression of diabetic nephropathy.*

Physician's Guide to Insulin Dependent (Type I) Diabetes: Diagnosis and Treatment, 2nd ed. Alexandria, VA, American Diabetes Association, 1994. *A monograph that provides a detailed review of the diagnosis and treatment of type I diabetes.*

Physician's Guide to Non–Insulin-Dependent (Type II) Diabetes: Diagnosis and Treatment, 3rd ed. Alexandria, VA, American Diabetes Association, 1994. *A monograph that reviews the diagnosis, pathogenesis, and treatment of type II diabetes.*

Reaven GM: Role of insulin resistance in human disease. Diabetes 37:1495, 1988. *A detailed review of the evidence linking insulin resistance with a variety of risk factors associated with atherosclerosis.*

Trucco M: To be or not to be Asp 57, that is the question. Diabetes Care 15:705, 1992. *A short review of the role of HLA genes in the pathogenesis of type I diabetes.*

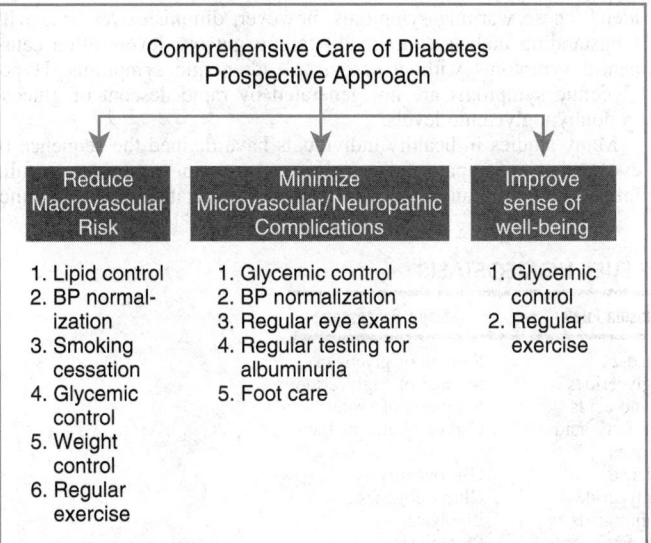

FIGURE 205-11. The key elements of a comprehensive management plan for patients with diabetes.

206 HYPOGLYCEMIA/PANCREATIC ISLET CELL DISORDERS
Jeffrey S. Flier

206.1 Hypoglycemia

In spite of food intake being intermittent and the unavoidability of periodic fasting, normal human plasma glucose concentrations remain within narrow limits. An abnormally low plasma glucose concentration, or hypoglycemia, may result from a variety of clinical disorders. Because glucose is the primary fuel of the brain, and the brain cannot synthesize glucose, transport it against a concentration gradient, or substitute alternative fuels in the short term, the consequences of hypoglycemia for brain function may be severe, including death. As a result, numerous and redundant adaptive mechanisms have evolved to prevent hypoglycemia. When these fail or become overwhelmed, the clinical syndrome of hypoglycemia results.

FUEL HOMEOSTASIS

Hypoglycemia is best viewed within the framework of disordered fuel homeostasis. Highly regulated changes in the rates of glucose production and use, coordinated with changes in the metabolism of muscle and fat, maintain glucose concentrations within narrow limits (usually between 70 and 150 mg per deciliter) despite intermittent and variable food intake. This is best seen as occurring in two contrasting physiologic conditions—the fed and fasted states (Table 206–1).

After food ingestion, circulating insulin levels rise, stimulated by increased plasma glucose and potentiated by meal-induced enteric hormones (incretins). Insulin is the dominant hormone of this anabolic postprandial period, and counterregulatory hormones are suppressed. Insulin shuts off hepatic glucose production, promotes the utilization of glucose as opposed to fat as an energy substrate, and directs storage of ingested nutrients such as glycogen, fat, and protein. In contrast, within 4 to 6 hours of food ingestion, metabolism switches to a fasted or catabolic phase characterized by falling insulin levels and rising levels of four counterregulatory hormones—glucagon, epinephrine, growth hormone, and cortisol. These hormonal changes result in critical changes in fuel metabolism: a switch from glucose use to production to maintain glucose levels sufficient for normal brain function and the change from a carbohydrate- to a lipid-based fuel economy for most other tissues of the body.

Hepatic glucose production derives initially from preformed glycogen, but the capacity of hepatic glycogen to sustain plasma glucose levels is limited to 8 to 12 hours, or even less after periods of exercise or illness. Thus, for more sustained fasting, including the normal overnight fast, gluconeogenesis, the generation of new glucose from noncarbohydrate substrates, must take over. The precursors of gluconeogenesis are lactate/pyruvate and amino acids from muscle and glycerol from adipose tissue lipolysis. Alanine is the major substrate for hepatic gluconeogenesis, but the role of glycerol increases with time. During prolonged fasts, renal gluconeogenesis, derived primarily from glutamine, becomes a second major source of new glucose production.

The switch to a lipid-based fuel economy is initiated by enhanced lipolysis of adipose tissue triglyceride to glycerol and free fatty acids, through activation of hormone-sensitive lipase. Most of these free fatty acids are preferentially used as fuel by tissues in the body, sparing glucose for use by other tissues, most importantly the brain, that cannot utilize free fatty acids as fuel. A second fate of free fatty acids is their conversion in liver to the ketoacids, acetoacetate, and beta-hydroxybutyrate. These can be further metabolized by most tissues, but their main function is to serve as an alternative fuel to glucose in the brain, most critically during prolonged fasts, as glucose levels gradually fall.

The defense against hypoglycemia requires both a fall in insulin levels and a rise in the four counterregulatory hormones. The fall in insulin levels is dominant, since if insulin fails to fall, hypoglycemia may result despite maximal counterregulatory response. A rising level of glucagon, by increasing hepatic glucose production, is the primary defender of the plasma glucose level under most circumstances. Epinephrine plays a secondary role, both by increasing glucose production and limiting its use, but may be critical under circumstances in which glucagon is deficient, as often occurs during the course of diabetes mellitus. Permissive levels of cortisol and growth hormone contribute to the defense against hypoglycemia by antagonizing insulin action. They also promote gluconeogenesis by enhancing provision of substrate and inducing the enzymes responsible for hepatic gluconeogenesis.

SIGNS AND SYMPTOMS OF HYPOGLYCEMIA

Hypoglycemia produces two distinct categories of symptoms (Table 206–2). The first results from secretion of the adrenal hormone, epinephrine; this provides a potential warning of hypoglycemia while simultaneously contributing to glucose counterregulation. Adrenergic symptoms include pallor, sweating, tachycardia, tremor, anxiety, and hunger. The second consists of central nervous system (CNS) symptoms of "neuroglycopenia," including headache, dizziness, altered mentation, visual disturbance, motor dysfunction, confusion, erratic behavior, convulsions, and loss of consciousness. Hypoglycemic patients often report a stereotyped subset of these symptoms with repeated episodes. No feature of these neuroglycopenic symptoms suggests their being caused by hypoglycemia as opposed to the many other structural or metabolic etiologic factors. This accounts for the common delay in considering hypoglycemia as a cause of altered mental status in other than insulin-treated diabetics. When glucose drops rapidly to hypoglycemic levels, as in response to exogenous insulin, adrenergic symptoms are usually evident. These warning symptoms, however, diminish over time with longstanding diabetes. Gradually falling glucose levels often cause neural symptoms without associated adrenergic symptoms. Hypoglycemic symptoms are not generated by rapid descent of glucose to nonhypoglycemic levels.

Many studies in healthy individuals have defined the sequence of events that accompany falling glucose levels in response to insulin infusions. Subtle and clinically inapparent alterations in CNS func-

TABLE 206–1. PHASES OF FUEL HOMEOSTASIS

Phase	Hormonal Determinants	Plasma Fuels	Major Processes
Fed (anabolic)	Rising insulin Falling glucagon	Glucose Triglycerides Amino acids Free fatty acids Ketones	Storage of glycogen Storage of triglyceride Synthesis of protein Carbohydrates as fuels
Fasted (catabolic)	Falling insulin Rising glucagon	Glucose Triglycerides Amino acids Free fatty acids Ketones	Glycogenolysis Gluconeogenesis Lipolysis Proteolysis Ketogenesis Lipid fuel economy

TABLE 206-2. SYMPTOMS OF HYPOGLYCEMIA

Adrenergic
  Sweating
  Tremor
  Anxiety
  Palpitations
  Weakness
  Hunger
Neuroglycopenic
  Headache
  Dizziness
  Altered mentation
  Visual disturbance
  Motor disturbance
  Convulsions
  Unconsciousness

tion may be detected in response to decrements in plasma glucose of only 15 mg per deciliter below that of an overnight fast. In one study, glucagon and epinephrine release appeared at 53 mg per deciliter, growth hormone at 52 mg per deciliter, and cortisol at 43 mg per deciliter. Neuroglycopenic symptoms generally develop when the plasma glucose level falls below 45 mg per deciliter, and major dysfunction is expected below 20 mg per deciliter. These figures are only guidelines, however, since considerable variability may be seen, some of which is predictable. Counterregulation typically occurs in diabetics with chronic hyperglycemia. These diabetics may have symptoms at higher glucose levels, and individuals with frequent hypoglycemia, including tightly controlled diabetics, have a lowered threshold for symptoms; they remain completely unaware of hypoglycemia prior to the onset of major CNS dysfunction. These adaptations may reflect changes in the system for transporting glucose into the CNS.

CAUSES OF HYPOGLYCEMIA

When the possible causes of hypoglycemia are being addressed (Table 206–3), the most important clinical distinction is to separate hypoglycemia induced by eating (reactive) and hypoglycemia occurring in the fasting state. The former is diagnosed excessively and rarely indicates a serious underlying disorder, while the latter demands a thorough search for a specific cause. Reactive hypoglycemia is not associated with hypoglycemia during a fast, but patients with true fasting hypoglycemia may experience the problem within 6 hours after ingesting food.

TYPES OF HYPOGLYCEMIA

POSTPRANDIAL HYPOGLYCEMIA. The most serious form of reactive hypoglycemia is alimentary hypoglycemia. Affected persons most often have had gastrectomy, but may also have had gastrojejunostomy, pyloroplasty, or vagotomy. Typically such patients develop adrenergic or neuroglycopenic symptoms of hypoglycemia from 30 to 120 minutes after a meal, and the blood sugar fall may be sufficient to produce seizures or coma. The pathogenesis is thought to involve rapid absorption of glucose, stimulating brisk insulin release, and, ultimately, inappropriately elevated insulin levels. The possible involvement of gut-derived incretins in causing the insulin hypersecretion has been suggested. Early diabetes is frequently cited as a condition that predisposes to reactive hypoglycemia, but the association appears to be exceedingly rare or nonexistent. Hypoglycemia may develop after ingestion of fructose or galactose in individuals with fructose intolerance or galactosemia.

Idiopathic reactive hypoglycemia includes two syndromes. The first is true idiopathic reactive hypoglycemia and is quite rare. Affected persons repeatedly exhibit symptoms of hypoglycemic-induced adrenergic excess following meals. Ingestion of carbohydrate relieves the symptoms as glucose levels rise. No specific mechanism for this disorder has been defined, and the hypoglycemia virtually never causes serious neuroglycopenia. A far more common situation involves patients with what has been called the idiopathic postprandial syndrome or pseudohypoglycemia. These individuals report symptoms suggesting either adrenergic discharge or mild neuroglycopenia in the 2 to 5 hours after meals but have normal accompanying glucose levels. Substantial confusion

has arisen from performance of oral glucose tolerance tests that were interpreted as demonstrating hypoglycemia, often defined as values below 60 mg per deciliter. Tests performed on control groups without symptoms demonstrate similar glucose values, suggesting that the "low" glucose levels are unrelated to the symptoms. It is no longer recommended that oral glucose tolerance tests be performed when evaluating postprandial "hypoglycemia." Instead, persistent symptoms in the postprandial state should be evaluated by measuring glucose levels during episodes as they occur during the course of a normal day. Patients with pseudohypoglycemia often remain convinced that they suffer from hypoglycemia even after such studies have proven normal. The popular press has proposed many remedies and unusual diets to deal with pseudohypoglycemia, but scientific explanations for the symptoms are lacking.

FASTING HYPOGLYCEMIA. Fasting hypoglycemia results from a mismatch between the rates of glucose production and glucose utilization. This can be due to impaired glucose production or to combinations of decreased production and increased utilization. Isolated increases in utilization with appropriate glucose production are not known to exist. The causes of isolated failure of hepatic glucose production can be divided into several categories based on pathogenetic mechanisms. These include defects in hormones that promote gluconeogenesis; defects in one or more of the enzymes critical to gluconeogenesis; severe generalized liver disease; deficiency of gluconeogenic substrates; and certain drugs. Overutilization of glucose may be caused by endogenous or exogenous insulin or insulin-like factors, by certain large metabolically active tumors, and by specific metabolic disorders that impair the availability of fat as a substrate for energy production. One clinical clue regarding the role of underproduction versus overutilization of glucose is the rate of glucose infusion needed to prevent hypoglycemia. Since the rate of glucose production during a fast approximates 2 mg per kilogram per minute, whereas the maximal rate of glucose utilization under the action of insulin is 12 mg per kilogram per minute,

TABLE 206-3. CLINICAL CLASSIFICATION OF HYPOGLYCEMIAS

I. Postabsorptive (fasting) hypoglycemia
  A. Drugs
    1. Insulin, sulfonylureas, ethanol
    2. Pentamidine, quinine, salicylates, propranolol
    3. Others
  B. Critical organ failure
    1. Liver disease
    2. Renal failure
    3. Cardiac failure
    4. Sepsis
    5. Inanition
  C. Hormone deficiencies
    1. Hypopituitarism
    2. Adrenal insufficiency
    3. Glucagon and epinephrine deficiency (esp. in diabetes)
  D. Non-beta cell tumors
  E. Endogenous hyperinsulinism
    1. Insulinoma
  F. Autoimmune
    1. Autoantibodies to insulin
    2. Autoantibodies to insulin receptor
  G. Factitious
    1. Insulin
    2. Sulfonylureas
  H. Hypoglycemia of infancy and childhood
    1. Ketotic hypoglycemia
    2. Enzyme deficiencies in pathways of glycogenolysis and gluconeogenesis
    3. Defects in amino acid, fatty acid, and ketoacid metabolism
II. Postprandial (reactive) hypoglycemias
  A. Alimentary hypoglycemia
  B. Idiopathic reactive hypoglycemia
  C. Deficiencies of enzymes of carbohydrate metabolism
    1. Galactosemia
    2. Hereditary fructose intolerance
  D. (Pseudohypoglycemia)

glucose requirements substantially above 10 grams per hour strongly suggest that overutilization must exist.

DRUG-INDUCED HYPOGLYCEMIA. When use of insulin and sulfonylureas in patients with diabetes is included, drugs are the most common cause of hypoglycemia. Drug-induced hypoglycemia is more likely to occur at the extremes of age, in the acutely or chronically undernourished, and in the presence of renal or hepatic dysfunction. Alcohol predictably inhibits hepatic gluconeogenesis. Ethanol oxidation generates reduced nicotinamide adenine dinucleotide (NADH) and increases the ratio of NADH to nicotinamide adenine dinucleotide (NAD). This inhibits gluconeogenesis at multiple steps, including the transformation of pyruvate to oxaloacetate, which is further transformed into phosphoenolpyruvate via the rate-limiting enzyme of gluconeogenesis, phosphoenolpyruvate carboxykinase. Even quite modest amounts of alcohol will induce hypoglycemia under conditions in which gluconeogenesis is driving hepatic glucose production, for example, when starvation has depleted hepatic glycogen. The CNS consequences of hypoglycemia may mimic intoxication, and alcoholic hypoglycemia can have serious consequences if not identified promptly. Salicylates may cause hypoglycemia, especially in children, by an uncertain mechanism. Propranolol may contribute to fasting hypoglycemia by reducing the glycogenolytic response to epinephrine and, in diabetics, by blunting the awareness of hypoglycemia due to epinephrine release. Pentamidine exerts a toxic effect on pancreatic beta cells to release insulin acutely and cause hypoglycemia; chronic effects can cause diabetes. Quinine treatment of malaria has been described as causing hypoglycemia secondary to drug-induced insulin release. Many other drugs have been associated with hypoglycemia as a rare event.

INSULINOMA. Insulinoma is a rare disorder that occurs in approximately one per 250,000 individuals. The median age of onset is about 50 years, except for those who develop it in the context of multiple endocrine neoplasia type I (MEN I), in which it occurs in the mid 20's. Such tumors are uncommon below the age of 20 years, and very uncommon below the age of 5 years. Most insulinomas are small, benign, and single. Tumors are multiple in 7% and malignant in about 5%. Eight percent of patients with insulinoma have MEN I, and these are much more likely to be multiple. These tumors will occasionally secrete other hormones, including gastrin, ACTH, glucagon, somatostatin, and 5-hydroxindoles. Nesidioblastosis is a rare condition affecting neonates in which pancreatic duct epithelium gives rise to endocrine cells that are distinct from true islets. The condition is more common than insulinomas in producing hyperinsulinism and hypoglycemia in this age group; its occurrence in adults is very rare.

Clinical Picture. Patients with insulinoma have varying combinations of neuroglycopenic and autonomic symptoms that tend to occur five or more hours after a meal, as after an overnight fast. The symptoms and extent of hypoglycemia are affected by exercise, diet, ingestion of ethanol, or religious fasts. Rarely, symptoms may occur only in the 2 to 4 hours after a meal rather than during fasting. Common symptoms include diplopia, blurred vision, palpitations, weakness, and confusion or bizarre behavior. Some patients will have a refractory seizure disorder in the absence of other symptoms. In such instances, insulinoma may be overlooked for prolonged periods. As many as 20% of patients may be mistakenly viewed as suffering from neurologic or psychiatric disorders. Many patients remain unaware that eating prevents attacks.

Diagnosis. The diagnosis of insulinoma is based on the presence of *Whipple's triad* (appropriate symptoms in association with hypoglycemia and relief of symptoms after elevation of the blood glucose level) together with inappropriately elevated plasma insulin and C-peptide levels in the absence of sulfonylurea in the plasma. The diagnosis is most straightforward when insulin, C-peptide, and sulfonylurea determinations are obtained concurrently during an episode of hypoglycemia. It is often useful to retain a separate aliquot of plasma for subsequent measurement of proinsulin, cortisol, anti-insulin, or receptor antibodies in the event that the diagnosis is unclear after measurement of insulin and C-peptide.

If the history suggests hypoglycemia but neither symptoms nor hypoglycemia can be identified at the initial evaluation, supervised fasting is usually the next step. The goal is to determine whether hypoglycemia develops and, if so, whether it is accompanied by endogenous hyperinsulinism. While extended overnight fasts may be useful in initial outpatient evaluation, the gold standard for safe and thorough evaluation is an inpatient fast of up to 72 hours. Plasma glucose, insulin, C-peptide, and cortisol should be measured every 6 hours, with the frequency of testing influenced by the patient's history and the obtained glucose values. The patient should be tested repeatedly for cognitive function. The diagnosis of hypoglycemia during a fast is complicated by the fact that normal individuals may have quite low levels of glucose during a 72-hour fast in the absence of symptoms. Although the mean minimal levels of glucose in one study were 62 mg per deciliter and 52 mg per deciliter in men and women, respectively, values as low as 22 mg per deciliter have been recorded in asymptomatic normal women. It is therefore essential to continue the fast to the point at which symptoms occur, or to 72 hours. In one large series, Whipple's triad was demonstrated within 12 hours of the last meal in 29% of patients, within 24 hours in 71%, within 36 hours in 79%, within 48 hours in 92%, and within 72 hours in 98%. At the time of symptoms, plasma glucose concentration was below 46 mg per deciliter in all patients. Rarely, exercise at the end of a fast will provoke hypoglycemia that is otherwise not demonstrable. Given the results in normal persons, the clinician should be wary of diagnosing hypoglycemia in the absence of symptoms that are relieved by food ingestion. Interpretation of insulin levels during a fast may also be a source of confusion and must be evaluated in the light of simultaneous glucose values. Insulin levels are of no value if simultaneous glucose values are normal or elevated; any measurable insulin level in the presence of hypoglycemia less than 45 mg per deciliter must be viewed as suspicious.

Some centers aim to avoid the use of the prolonged fast in diagnosing insulinoma. Several provocative tests rely on the tendency of insulinomas to release insulin excessively in response to specific secretagogues, including tolbutamide and glucagon, but these are not in wide use. The C-peptide suppression test is based on the fact that after exogenous insulin–induced hypoglycemia, patients with insulinoma have impaired suppression of endogenous insulin and C-peptide. These results are influenced by age and obesity. Proinsulin levels, both absolute and as a fraction of total immunoreactive insulin, are elevated in most patients with insulinoma.

Once insulinoma has been confirmed biochemically, the tumor should be localized before surgery. Preoperative and intraoperative ultrasonography has replaced celiac angiography and CT in many centers as the method of choice, with intraoperative sonograms approaching 90% sensitivity. If a tumor cannot be localized, a skilled surgeon may identify a tumor intraoperatively, and failing that, distal pancreatectomy may be successful, because tumors are evenly distributed through the pancreas, and ectopic insulinomas are exceedingly rare. Malignant insulinoma metastasizes to regional lymph nodes and liver but rarely produces distant metastases. Persistent hypoglycemia in patients with malignant insulinomas, in patients whose tumors could not be found at exploration, or in patients refusing surgery is best treated with diazoxide, which inhibits insulin release. Phenytoin, propranolol, and verapamil have been reported to be useful in some cases. A long-acting analogue of somatostatin, octreotide, reduces hyperinsulinemia and symptoms in many but not all patients with insulinoma. A chemotherapeutic regimen reported to have some benefit in malignant insulinoma consists of streptozotocin plus fluorouracil or chlorzotocin. Although the prognosis is generally poor, a few patients with metastatic insulinomas survive in relatively good health for long periods.

FACTITIOUS AND AUTOIMMUNE HYPOGLYCEMIA. Hypoglycemia induced by the surreptitious administration of insulin or sulfonylureas is probably more common than insulinoma. As a result, the coexistence of hypoglycemia and inappropriate insulin levels does not establish the diagnosis of insulinoma (Table 206–4). Most often, factitious hypoglycemia occurs in medical personnel or in family members of patients with diabetes. Insulin has been used for suicide, homicide, and child abuse. The best means to distinguish insulinoma from surreptitious insulin administration is to measure C-peptide along with insulin during hypoglycemia. C-peptide is released on an equimolar basis with endogenous insulin into the portal vein, and its level is elevated parallel to insulin in insulinoma. Exogenous insulin suppresses insulin secretion in normal

TABLE 206–4. DIFFERENTIAL DIAGNOSIS OF INSULINOMA AND FACTITIOUS HYPOGLYCEMIA

Test	Insulinoma	Exogenous Insulin	Sulfonylureas
Plasma glucose	Low	Low	Low
Plasma insulin	Inappropriately high	Inappropriately high (possibly very)	Inappropriately high
C-peptide	Increased	Not increased or low	Increased
Proinsulin	Increased	Not increased or low	Increased
Insulin antibodies	Absent	May be present	Absent
Sulfonylurea levels	Absent	Absent	Present

individuals, and C-peptide levels are similarly suppressed. Antibodies to insulin, if present in persons not known to have received insulin therapy, can also indicate surreptitious insulin use. Both insulin and C-peptide levels are increased as a consequence of sulfonylurea administration; this can be diagnosed only by identifying the drug in plasma or urine.

Hypoglycemia can be the result of autoimmune disease, due either to the occurrence of spontaneous autoantibodies against insulin or the insulin receptor. Both syndromes commonly occur in the context of other autoimmune features. The mechanism for hypoglycemia caused by anti-insulin autoantibodies has never been clearly defined, but is probably a consequence of erratic release of insulin bound to antibodies in the circulation. Hypoglycemia may be severe, may accompany either fasting or the postprandial state, and is typically self-limited. Autoantibodies to the insulin receptor most often cause insulin-resistant diabetes and the skin condition acanthosis nigricans. Such antibodies can act as insulin-like agonists after binding to the insulin receptor, thereby causing hypoglycemia. Patients with hypoglycemia due to anti-insulin receptor autoantibodies may have pure fasting hypoglycemia, they may develop fasting hypoglycemia after a previous phase of insulin-resistant diabetes, or they may have the otherwise very unusual combination of fasting hypoglycemia together with postprandial hyperglycemia. Such patients typically do not have acanthosis nigricans as a clue to diagnosis, and the diagnosis may be suggested by the presence of one or more findings suggestive of autoimmunity. During hypoglycemia caused by such insulin-mimetic antibodies, C-peptide levels are suppressed. Insulin levels may be suppressed, normal, or slightly elevated because of the ability of receptor autoantibodies to reduce clearance of the hormone. Glucocorticoids may be effective therapy, either by inducing cellular resistance to the agonist properties of the antireceptor antibodies or in some cases by lowering the antibody titer.

NON–BETA CELL TUMOR HYPOGLYCEMIA. Hypoglycemia may occur in a variety of extrapancreatic tumors of mesenchymal or epithelial origin, and some malignant hematologic diseases can result in systemic hypoglycemia. Sarcomas and fibromas are the most common, but renal, adrenal, and gastrointestinal cancers and hepatomas may have a similar effect, along with several other rare associations. The mesenchymal tumors are typically large tumors that arise in the retroperitoneum or thorax. Characteristic of these hypoglycemias is the suppression of plasma insulin levels. In some cases, very large tumors appear capable of inducing hypoglycemia through massive utilization of glucose that exceeds the capacity for hepatic compensation. In other cases, a humoral mediator apart from insulin has been sought; very high levels of insulin-like growth factor-II (IGF-II) mRNA have been identified in several such tumors. IGF-II bears homology to both insulin and IGF-I and may produce hypoglycemia through receptors for either or both of these ligands. IGF-II may also suppress growth hormone levels, and this additional consequence of IGF-II expression may contribute to hypoglycemia.

HYPOGLYCEMIA IN HEPATIC, RENAL, AND ENDOCRINE DISORDERS AND MISCELLANEOUS CONDITIONS. Although the liver has substantial reserve capacity, hypoglycemia may accompany fulminant hepatic failure and sometimes occurs for unclear reasons in association with less severe hepatic dysfunction due to viral hepatitis; cirrhosis; and hepatic congestion caused by severe right-sided heart failure. The hypoglycemia that sometimes accompanies renal failure is often multifactorial and may be due to reduced clearance of hypoglycemic drugs, reduced food intake, and reduced gluconeogenesis, possibly secondary to deficient gluconeogenic substrates. Most patients with hypopituitarism and adrenal insufficiency do not develop hypoglycemia, although this can occur, especially during fasts. Hypoglycemia is a common development in children below 6 years of age with hypopituitarism. Isolated deficiencies of glucagon and epinephrine are not known to cause hypoglycemia.

Children are susceptible to hypoglycemia because of a number of inherited or acquired abnormalities affecting the enzymes that regulate fuel metabolism. These include defects that affect the rate of glycogen breakdown, such as glucose-6-phosphatase deficiency; glycogen synthesis as in the glycogen storage diseases; and gluconeogenesis, as with deficiency of fructose-1,6-diphosphatase. Ketotic hypoglycemia of childhood may be due to substrate limitation, and alanine turnover is reduced. Hypoglycemia may also result from defects in the ability to utilize fatty acids or ketones, in which case the tissues become dependent on glucose for fuel, and the liver cannot meet the demand. Defects in the pathway of fatty acid oxidation or ketone formation can cause this result, as can systemic deficiency of carnitine, a molecule necessary for the transport of fatty acids into mitochondria, the site of their oxidation.

Hypoglycemia accompanies starvation and may occur in anorexia nervosa as well as in persons following unusual faddist diets. It may also accompany any state of extreme inanition or cachexia, during sepsis, or after prolonged, severe exercise, especially in the physically untrained.

THE APPROACH TO THE PATIENT WITH HYPOGLYCEMIA (Fig. 206–1)

Hypoglycemia may be suspected on the basis of symptoms that are nonspecific or identified through a blood test in a patient otherwise not suspected of being hypoglycemic. In the latter situation, the possibility of artifactual hypoglycemia, due to utilization of glucose by erythrocytes or leukemic leukocytes in the test tube, must be considered, as must the possibility that the patient has adapted to longstanding or mild hypoglycemia by nutritional or other modifications.

In the initial phase of consideration of hypoglycemia, several major questions must be addressed. These include the distinction between fasting and reactive hypoglycemia and the relationship between hypoglycemia and any symptoms or signs. This requires a careful history from both patient and family members including detailed evaluation of medication use, and an effort to obtain specimens for assay during any spontaneous episodes if possible before administration of food or intravenous glucose, should that be necessary. If hypoglycemia is suspected, 10 to 20 ml of blood should be drawn beyond that needed for glucose determination. Additional analyses, including insulin, C-peptide, cortisol, sulfonylurea level, and others can be determined on the basis of clues generated from the history and physical examination. If hypoglycemia is noted in a patient who is ill or if history and physical examination point to specific syndromes known to be associated with hypoglycemia, the subsequent evaluation should be led by this information and may be quite limited. If hypoglycemia is documented without a clear indication of its relationship to fasting or symptoms and the patient is generally healthy, fasting hypoglycemia and its provocation of symptoms should be documented. Once fasting hypoglycemia is demonstrated, insulinoma should be distinguished from hypoglycemia due to ingestion/administration of insulin or sulfonylureas or, less commonly, from hormone deficiency or inapparent solid tumor.

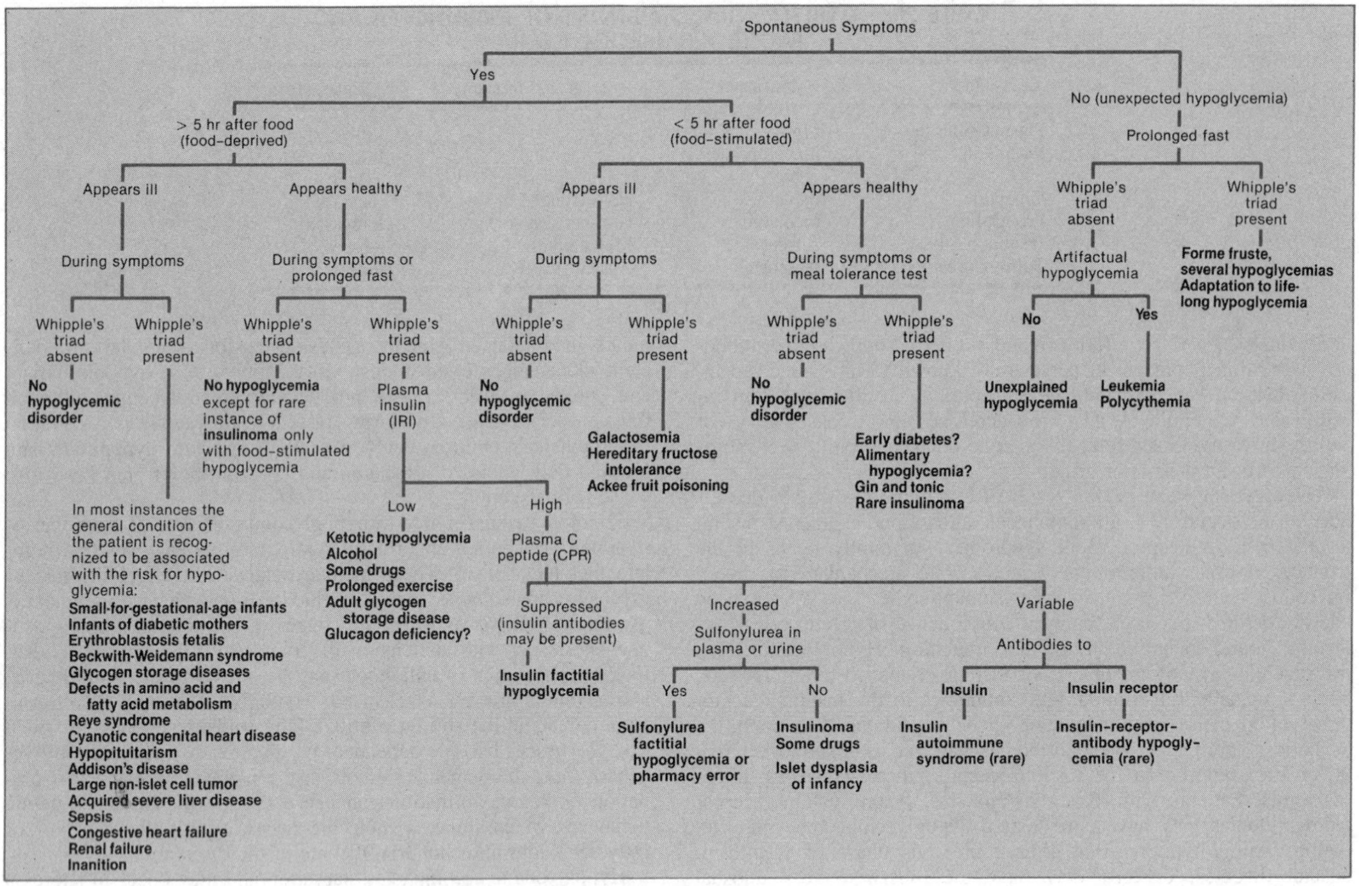

Spontaneous Symptoms

Yes — No (unexpected hypoglycemia)

Yes branch:

> 5 hr after food (food-deprived) — < 5 hr after food (food-stimulated)

No branch: Prolonged fast

> 5 hr after food (food-deprived)

Appears ill — Appears healthy

Appears ill: During symptoms
- Whipple's triad absent → **No hypoglycemic disorder**
- Whipple's triad present → In most instances the general condition of the patient is recognized to be associated with the risk for hypoglycemia:
  Small-for-gestational-age infants
  Infants of diabetic mothers
  Erythroblastosis fetalis
  Beckwith-Weidemann syndrome
  Glycogen storage diseases
  Defects in amino acid and fatty acid metabolism
  Reye syndrome
  Cyanotic congenital heart disease
  Hypopituitarism
  Addison's disease
  Large non-islet cell tumor
  Acquired severe liver disease
  Sepsis
  Congestive heart failure
  Renal failure
  Inanition

Appears healthy: During symptoms or prolonged fast
- Whipple's triad absent → **No hypoglycemia** except for rare instance of **insulinoma** only with food-stimulated hypoglycemia
- Whipple's triad present → Plasma insulin (IRI)
  - Low → **Ketotic hypoglycemia**, **Alcohol**, **Some drugs**, **Prolonged exercise**, **Adult glycogen storage disease**, **Glucagon deficiency?**
  - High → Plasma C peptide (CPR)
    - Suppressed (insulin antibodies may be present) → **Insulin factitial hypoglycemia**
    - Increased → Sulfonylurea in plasma or urine
      - Yes → **Sulfonylurea factitial hypoglycemia or pharmacy error**
      - No → **Insulinoma**, **Some drugs**, **Islet dysplasia of infancy**
    - Variable → Antibodies to
      - Insulin → **Insulin autoimmune syndrome (rare)**
      - Insulin receptor → **Insulin-receptor-antibody hypoglycemia (rare)**

< 5 hr after food (food-stimulated)

Appears ill — Appears healthy

Appears ill: During symptoms
- Whipple's triad absent → **No hypoglycemic disorder**
- Whipple's triad present → **Galactosemia**, **Hereditary fructose intolerance**, **Ackee fruit poisoning**

Appears healthy: During symptoms or meal tolerance test
- Whipple's triad absent → **No hypoglycemic disorder**
- Whipple's triad present → **Early diabetes?**, **Alimentary hypoglycemia?**, **Gin and tonic**, **Rare insulinoma**

No (unexpected hypoglycemia) — Prolonged fast

- Whipple's triad absent → Artifactual hypoglycemia
  - No → **Unexplained hypoglycemia**
  - Yes → **Leukemia Polycythemia**
- Whipple's triad present → **Forme fruste, several hypoglycemias Adaptation to life-long hypoglycemia**

FIGURE 206-1. Evaluation of hypoglycemic disorders.

Cryer PE: Glucose counterregulation: Prevention and correction of hypoglycemia in humans. Am J Physiol 264:E149, 1993. *Review of the physiologic response to hypoglycemia.*

Davis SN, Cherrington AD: The hormonal and metabolic responses to prolonged hypoglycemia. J Lab Clin Med 121:21, 1993.

De Feo et al.: Modest decrements in plasma glucose concentration cause early impairment in cognitive function and later activation of glucose counterregulation in the absence of hypoglycemic symptoms in normal man. J Clin Invest 82:436, 1988. *Evidence for subtle defects in cognitive function when glucose levels fall modestly below the fasting level.*

Grunberger G, et al.: Factitious hypoglycemia due to surreptitious administration of insulin: Diagnosis, treatment and long-term follow-up. Ann Intern Med 108:252, 1988. *An approach to this vexing disorder.*

Lowe WL, Roberts CT, JR, Leroith D, et al.: Insulin-like growth factor-II in nonislet cell tumors associated with hypoglycemia: Increased levels of messenger ribonucleic acid. J Clin Endocrinol Metab 69:1153, 1989. *Nonislet cell tumors associated with hypoglycemia were found to produce large amounts of IGF-II mRNA.*

Moertel CG, et al.: Streptozocin-doxorubicin, streptozocin-fluorouracil, or chlorozotocin in the treatment of advanced islet-cell carcinoma. N Engl J Med 326:519, 1992. *Comparative regimens for treatment of islet cell carcinoma.*

Palardy J, Havrankova, Lepage R, et al.: Blood glucose measurements during symptomatic episodes in patients with suspected postprandial hypoglycemia. N Engl J Med 321:1421, 1989. *Importance of measuring glucose during occurrence of spontaneous symptoms of hypoglycemia clearly demonstrated by data in this paper. When self-collected capillary blood specimens on filter paper were analyzed for glucose, only 5% had values less than 2.8 mM/L (50 mg/dl).*

Pandit MK, et al.: Drug-induced disorders of glucose tolerance. Ann Intern Med 118:529, 1993.

Service FJ: Hypoglycemias. J Clin Endocrinol Metab 76:269, 1993. *Excellent clinical review.*

Zeiger MA, et al.: Use of intraoperative ultrasonography to localize islet cell tumors. World J Surg 17:448, 1993. *Efficacy of this technique in identifying small insulinomas.*

the core of the islet. They are surrounded by a rim of glucagon-secreting A cells and pancreatic peptide-secreting PP cells. D cells containing somatostatin are found primarily between the A and B cells. Several other peptides, such as gastrin and vasoactive intestinal polypeptide (VIP), have less clear cells of origin and may be expressed only in perinatal islets under normal circumstances.

ISLET CELL TUMORS

Tumors can arise from any of the hormone-producing cells of the islets of Langerhans. Patients with islet cell tumors may seek medical attention as a result of distinct syndromes caused by hormone hypersecretion or because of the consequences of growth of either the primary tumor or its metastases. Nearly all benign islet cell tumors and more than 80% of carcinomas secrete clinically significant amounts of hormone; some secrete multiple hormones. Clinical presentation usually reflects the dominance of one hormone. The tumor is named after the hormone responsible for the clinical syndrome, or in asymptomatic patients, the hormone found in highest concentration in the circulation or in the tumor.

DIAGNOSIS. Islet cell tumors are generally slow growing and are compatible with prolonged survival. Nonfunctioning tumors are typically found during evaluation of symptoms or signs due to the pancreatic mass, and the diagnosis is made histologically. Alternatively, patients may have a characteristic clinical syndrome, which stimulates the measurement of circulating tumor products. Further evaluation often requires provocative or suppressive tests, evaluation to identify physiologic consequences of hormone oversecretion, and exclusion of alternative causes for elevated levels of the hormone.

Once biochemical criteria for a hormone-secreting tumor are satisfied, imaging studies are used to assess the site and extent of the tumor and the possibility of surgical cure. The combination of endoscopic and intraoperative ultrasonography plus computed tomography (CT) has proven the most sensitive approach, largely displacing angiography in most centers. Selective venous sampling has been applied with limited success. Preliminary indications suggest that external scanning after administration of a radiolabeled ana-

206.2 Islet Cell Tumors

The islets of Langerhans are nests of endocrine cells dispersed throughout the exocrine pancreas. Each islet may be viewed as a miniature organ in which four distinct cell types, each producing a single hormone, are organized in a specific manner. The insulin-producing B cells comprise 60% of islet cells and are located in

logue of somatostatin can identify islet cell tumors based on their expression of somatostatin receptors.

PATHOLOGY. Benign and malignant islet tumors cannot be readily distinguished on the basis of histologic appearance. The diagnosis of carcinoma requires the identification of metastases.

ASSOCIATED SYNDROMES. Pancreatic islet cell tumors may occur as part of the multiple endocrine neoplasia (MEN) syndrome. The islet cell tumors most commonly present in MEN I are gastrinomas and insulinomas. Compared with sporadic tumors, pancreatic tumors in MEN I are more likely to be multiple and malignant. The diagnosis of the MEN I syndrome should be considered when hypercalcemia is present in a patient with an islet cell tumor, as more than 90% of patients in whom MEN I is diagnosed have hyperthyroidism.

THERAPY. The initial aim of treatment is curative resection of the tumor. If this proves impossible, tumor syndromes may be attenuated either by diminishing hormone secretion or by blocking their untoward physiologic effects. Residual tumors can be palliated with chemotherapy or surgical debulking. Octreotide, a long-acting 8-amino acid analogue of somatostatin, reduces hormone production and has proven to be a mainstay in the treatment of symptoms due to hormone-secreting islet cell tumors. Unfortunately, gradual loss of efficacy of this agent often develops, presumably in association with advancing tumor burden.

TYPES OF TUMORS

INSULINOMA. Insulinoma is the most common islet cell tumor. This subject is discussed in Ch. 206.1.

GASTRINOMA. The second most common islet cell tumor is the gastrinoma, associated with the Zollinger-Ellison syndrome, in which recurrent gastric ulcers are produced as a result of hypersecretion of gastric acid. This is discussed in Ch. 99.6.

VIPOMA. VIP is a 28-amino acid peptide that has considerable homology with members of the secretin family. It was purified as a vasodilating activity from normal intestine in 1970 and was shown to have widespread distribution in the central and peripheral nervous systems. Although purified from this source, it is apparently not expressed in the endocrine cells of the normal gastrointestinal tract, where it plays the role of a local neurotransmitter, modulating ion and water transport as well as vascular tone.

Several years earlier, Verner and Morrison described the association of severe watery diarrhea with a non–insulin-producing islet cell tumor. The disorder subsequently was identified with VIP-producing tumors and circulating VIP, and it was shown that VIP infusion would produce secretory diarrhea, hypokalemia, and metabolic acidosis. Accordingly, the term *VIPoma* has superseded other designations, including Verner-Morrison syndrome, watery diarrhea hypokalemia achlorhydria (WDHA), and pancreatic cholera. These tumors may produce other peptides that can contribute to the features of this disorder. These include peptide histidine methionine (PHM), which is derived from a common precursor with VIP and has similar actions on intestinal secretion, as well as neurotensin and somatostatin.

Clinical Features and Diagnosis. The diagnosis of VIPoma is suggested by watery diarrhea that exceeds 3 liters per day in 80% of patients and hypokalemic acidosis due to major losses of potassium and bicarbonate in the stool. The volume depletion and hypokalemia can cause profound weakness, flaccid paralysis, and hypokalemic nephropathy, and may be fatal. Diabetes or glucose intolerance is common, due either to a glucagon-like effect of VIP or to an effect of hypokalemia to inhibit insulin secretion. Half of the patients may develop hypercalcemia, which may be due to coexpression of parathyroid hormone-related peptide by the tumor, rather than parathyroid adenomas; VIPomas rarely associate with the MEN syndrome.

Diagnosis requires demonstration of elevated levels of VIP in plasma. The sample should be carefully prepared with protease inhibitors, as the VIP molecule is highly unstable and may be degraded if such precautions are not carried out. Mild elevations of VIP below the range seen in VIPomas sometimes occur in diarrheal states associated with short bowel syndrome and inflammatory bowel disease. Secretory diarrhea may be seen in three other endocrine tumors (gastrinoma, carcinoid, and somatostatinoma), but peak volume of diarrhea rarely exceeds 3 liters per day in these disorders. The diarrhea in gastrinoma is caused by hypersecretion of

gastric acid and is reversed by treatments that reverse acid hypersecretion, whereas VIPomas are associated with hypochlorhydria or achlorhydria.

Pathology. Among patients with the VIPoma syndrome, 80% have islet cell tumors, of which approximately half are malignant, with hepatic metastases at the time of presentation. Pancreatic VIPomas are often large, up to 7 cm in diameter, and may be identified by immunocytochemistry using antibodies to the prepro-VIP molecule. Association with MEN I syndrome is rare. VIPoma may also be associated with neuroblastoma, ganglioneuroma, pheochromocytoma, and small cell tumors of the lung.

Treatment. The optimal treatment is surgical extirpation of the primary tumor. Localization of the tumor and identification of any metastases can be carried out with CT. In the occasional case in which localization of a biochemically identified tumor is impossible, including efforts at intraoperative ultrasonography, a blind distal pancreatectomy can be performed. Surgery may also be indicated to treat local effects or to remove a large primary tumor in the presence of metastases, although this is controversial.

Medical treatment includes support with fluid and electrolyte repletion, as well as an effort to limit the secretory diarrhea. Glucocorticoids may reduce diarrhea without affecting levels of VIP, and transient responses to clonidine, indomethacin, and a variety of other agents have been described. A major advance in the medical treatment of VIPomas has been the introduction of octreotide, which both reduces tumor output of VIP and reduces intestinal chloride secretion in response to VIP. Symptoms are ameliorated in most patients, although gradually increasing doses may be required, sometimes ending in loss of clinical response. In patients with inoperable tumors, chemotherapy with regimens combining streptozotocin and fluorouracil or streptozotocin and doxorubicin has induced partial remissions with lowered levels of VIP and reduction of symptoms. Hepatic embolization has also been used to reduce VIP production by hepatic metastases.

GLUCAGONOMA. Glucagon, a 29-amino acid peptide produced in the A cells located in the periphery of the islets of Langerhans, plays a key role in the regulation of hepatic glucose production. The glucagon gene is also expressed in the small intestine, where processing of preproglucagon yields the glucagon precursor enteroglucagon, as well as the glucagon-like peptides 1 and 2. These may function as "incretins," enhancing glucose-induced insulin secretion. Patients with glucagonoma typically have large forms of glucagon and glucagon-like peptide in the circulation, in addition to native glucagon.

Clinical Features and Diagnosis. Patients with glucagonomas most commonly present between the ages of 40 and 70 years. The disorder is most often brought to attention by a characteristic necrolytic, erythematous rash, which affects more than 80% of the patients and is usually a major source of disability. Located most often on the face, intertriginous areas, and extremities, the rash is initially erythematous and scaly, tends to become raised and bullous and then crusty, and heals as a hyperpigmented and indurated lesion. The rash may become superinfected, and glossitis, stomatitis, angular cheilitis, nail dystrophy, and thinning of the hair may also be seen. The etiology of the rash is linked to hyperglucagonemia and associated amino acid deficiency, although a role for zinc deficiency has been suggested based on similarities to the rash seen in zinc deficiency (acrodermatitis enteropathica) and a claimed response of some patients to treatment with zinc.

Mild, asymptomatic diabetes mellitus accompanies glucagonomas. The condition is evident only as an abnormal glucose tolerance test; ketoacidosis does not occur, presumably because of adequate insulin to suppress lipolysis. Other common clinical features are weight loss, anemia, psychological depression, and thromboembolic disease, as well as nonspecific abdominal complaints.

The diagnosis of glucagonoma requires finding elevated levels of glucagon in the plasma, and exclusion of other conditions associated with elevated, although typically much lower, levels of glucagon, such as uncontrolled diabetes mellitus, chronic renal failure, cirrhosis, sepsis, stress, or fasting. Normal circulating glucagon levels lie between 50 and 150 pg per milliliter. Most patients with glucagonoma have levels above 1000 pg per milliliter, often much higher. Patients usually seek attention for evaluation of the skin rash or thromboembolic disease; routine consideration of the diagnosis of glucagonoma in the patient with new-onset diabetes is not warranted in their absence.

Pathology. Glucagonoma is most often caused by single, large (3 to 5 cm) pancreatic tumors located in the body and tail of the organ. Although these tumors are typically slow growing, by the time of diagnosis as many as three quarters will have metastasized, most often to regional lymph nodes and liver, occasionally to distant sites. The syndrome accompanies MEN I.

Treatment. After localization of the tumor and assessment of metastatic disease, most often with CT, surgical cure can be achieved in approximately one third of patients. Surgery may also be indicated to relieve local effects or in an effort to reduce the tumor burden. Octreotide usually reduces glucagon levels and improves symptoms. The rash often resolves after several days of octreotide treatment or after successful surgery. Zinc supplementation and amino acid infusions also have been reported to diminish the severity of the rash. Arterial embolization or chemotherapy with combinations of streptozotocin, fluorouracil, doxorubicin, and dacarbazine may reduce hormone production from the tumor and induce partial remission. Tumor burden may gradually increase over a period of 2 to 10 years despite these treatments, and the clinical course may be complicated by production of additional hormones, such as gastrin.

SOMATOSTATINOMA. Somatostatin, an inhibitor of growth hormone secretion, is widely distributed in the nervous system and the gut. It acts as a neurotransmitter in the nervous system, as a paracrine regulator within endocrine glands, and as a hormone in the hypophyseal-portal system. Somatostatin inhibits the secretion of many hormones, including insulin, glucagon, growth hormone, prolactin, gastrin, and secretin, and in addition inhibits gastric acid and enzymes as well as pancreatic exocrine secretion. Somatostatin is produced by the D cells of the islets, which account for approximately 10% of islet cells.

Clinical Features and Diagnosis. Somatostatinoma may occur with a complex of symptoms, including mild diabetes mellitus, cholelithiasis, and diarrhea with steatorrhea. These result from the action of somatostatin to inhibit insulin release, gallbladder motility, and pancreatic enzyme and bicarbonate secretion. Patients may also develop weight loss, hypochlorhydria, anemia, and flushing. The diagnosis can be difficult, as somatostatinoma is very rare, its symptoms are nonspecific and often mild, and its associations (such as diabetes and cholelithiasis) occur much more often in its absence. As a result, at the time of diagnosis two thirds of patients have hepatic metastases. Some patients with documented somatostatinoma may lack any features of the syndrome, and in these cases the disorder is found incidentally or during the evaluation of jaundice or weight loss. Somatostatinomas have been documented to produce other hormones, including insulin, glucagon, adrenocorticotropic hormone (ACTH), calcitonin, gastrin, VIP, and prostaglandins. Somatostatin-producing tumors may also arise in the duodenum, where they are more typically small, well circumscribed, and amenable to resection. Duodenal somatostatinomas may be associated with neurofibromatosis, but are not associated with high circulating levels of somatostatin or the associated syndrome.

Pathology. Most somatostatinomas arise in the pancreas, where they are typically single, large, and metastatic at the time of diagnosis. Most other cases arise in the duodenum or jejunum. Secretion of somatostatin by other tumors, including pheochromocytomas and medullary carcinoma of the thyroid, has been reported.

Treatment. The treatment of pancreatic somatostatinomas resembles the treatment of other islet cell tumors, including surgery if possible, and palliation with hepatic embolization or chemotherapy. There is little evidence for utility of octreotide.

OTHER HORMONES PRODUCED BY ISLET CELL TUMORS. Pancreatic islet cell tumors that produce ACTH account for nearly 10% of cases of Cushing's syndrome due to ectopic ACTH production. However, in patients with islet cell tumors in the context of MEN I, the Cushing phenotype is more often a consequence of a pituitary adenoma. Some islet cell tumors have also been shown to produce corticotropin-releasing hormone, but Cushing's syndrome in a patient with islet cell tumor has yet to result from this mechanism. Acromegaly has been reported in patients with islet cell tumors secreting growth hormone-releasing factor, as has hypercalcemia due to secretion of parathyroid hormone-related pep-

tide. Many endocrine tumors of the pancreas and gut produce pancreatic polypeptide (PP) as a second hormone, and PP therefore can serve as a useful marker for islet cell tumors. PP is a 36-amino acid peptide from a family that includes neuropeptide Y and peptide YY. PP comprises 10% of islet cells, and although it is evolutionarily conserved, is released in response to food, and has biologic effects when given to experimental animals or humans, its precise physiologic role has not been defined. Most patients with PP-secreting tumors are asymptomatic.

NONFUNCTIONING ISLET CELL TUMORS. Approximately 10% of islet cell tumors have no identified syndrome of hormone excess. Some of these express peptides such as PP, and others undoubtedly express genes encoding presently unknown peptides. These tumors frequently reach a large size at the time of diagnosis and present symptoms such as malaise, abdominal pain, and jaundice. A mass can often be palpated, and at least half have hepatic metastases at first evaluation. Surgery cures approximately 20%, and chemotherapy with streptozotocin with or without fluorouracil provides objective palliation in approximately half of the remaining. Although 5-year survival is approximately 40%, many patients with metastatic disease enjoy a substantially longer survival.

Gorden P, Comi RJ, Maton PN, Go VL: Somatostatin and somatostatin analogue (SMS 201–995) in treatment of hormone secreting tumors of the pituitary and gastrointestinal tract and non-neoplastic diseases of the gut. Ann Intern Med 110:35, 1989. *Thorough review of somatostatin analogue as therapy.*

Kvols LK, Brown ML, O'Connor MK, et al.: Evaluation of a radiolabeled somatostatin analog (I-123 octreotide) in the detection and localization of carcinoid and islet cell tumors. Radiology 187:129, 1993. *Technique evaluated in 28 patients. Previously undetected lesions were found in four.*

Moertel CG, Lepkopoulo M, Lipsitz S, et al.: Streptozotocin-doxorubicin, streptozotocin-fluorouracil or chlorozocin in the treatment of advanced islet cell carcinoma. N Engl J Med 326:519, 1992. *Comparison of chemotherapeutic regimens.*

Rosch T, Lightdale CJ, Botet JF, et al.: Localization of pancreatic islet cell tumors by endoscopic ultrasonography. N Engl J Med 326:1721, 1992. *Describes advantages of the technique.*

Vinik AI, Moattari AR: Treatment of endocrine tumors of the pancreas. Endocrin Metab Clin North Am 18:483, 1989. *Comprehensive review with 186 references.*

207 DISORDERS OF SEXUAL DIFFERENTIATION

Maria I. New and Nathalie Josso

Gonads, genital ducts, and external genitalia become sexually dimorphic during fetal life, depending upon the presence or absence of genetic and endocrine factors, all of which actively impose maleness. Female differentiation requires no specific stimulus, occurring constitutively in the absence of male-determining factors. The asymmetric mechanism of sex differentiation has an important bearing upon the pathogenesis of intersex disorders: Male pseudohermaphroditism, defined as incomplete virilization of a 46,XY male, results from defects in the synthesis, metabolism, or action of one or several masculinizing factors. In contrast, female pseudohermaphroditism results from inappropriate exposure of female anlagen to masculinizing agents.

ANATOMY OF NORMAL SEX DIFFERENTIATION

MALE SEX DIFFERENTIATION. *Testicular Differentiation.* The gonadal primordium is represented by the gonadal ridge, which is progressively colonized by extraembryonic primordial germ cells. The first recognizable event of testicular differentiation, at 7 weeks' gestation, is the development of primordial Sertoli cells, which aggregate to form seminiferous tubules and produce anti-müllerian hormone (AMH). Leydig cells differentiate at 8 weeks of gestation and increase until 12 to 14 weeks, when they begin to degenerate. At birth, very few remain in the interstitial tissue; the Leydig cell population reappears at puberty.

Somatic Sex Differentiation. After gonadal differentiation, the internal reproductive tract consists of two pairs of ducts: the wolffian ducts and the müllerian ducts. In males, müllerian duct regression begins at 8 weeks and is more or less complete at 10 to 12 weeks. The wolffian ducts develop into the vasa deferentia, epididymides, and seminal vesicles. Prostatic buds develop around the opening of the ducts at 10 to 11 weeks of age while fusion of outgrowths of the urogenital sinus forms the prostatic utricle, the male equivalent of the vagina (Fig. 207–1). At 10 weeks, the genital tubercle elongates and the urethral folds fuse over the urethral groove, leading to formation of the penile urethra, while the genital swellings move posteriorly and fuse, forming the scrotum. Male anatomic development is completed by 90 days of gestation, but penile growth occurs only between 20 weeks and term, at a time when, paradoxically, serum testosterone levels are declining.

FEMALE DIFFERENTIATION. *Ovarian Differentiation.* Slower than the testis to differentiate initially, the fetal ovary eventually reaches a more advanced stage of maturation. At 12 to 13 weeks, some oogonia, located in the deepest layer of the cortex, have entered meiotic prophase. By 7 months' gestation, all germ cells have entered or completed meiotic prophase. Fetal granulosa cells produce estrogen at the same developmental stage at which fetal testes produce testosterone, but ovarian production of AMH can be demonstrated only after birth.

Somatic Sex Differentiation. Female fetal sex differentiation is characterized by degeneration of the wolffian ducts at 10 weeks, while the müllerian ducts develop into fallopian tubes, uterus, and upper vagina. The vagina differentiates at the level of the müllerian tubercle, between the openings of the wolffian ducts where the prostatic utricle forms in males. Whereas in males the prostatic utricle opens just beneath the neck of the bladder, in females, the lower end of the vagina slides down the posterior wall of the urethra to acquire a separate opening on the body surface (Fig. 207–1). Feminization of the external genitalia begins by the formation of the dorsal commissure, between the genital swellings, which in the fe-

male do not migrate posteriorly or fuse, and give rise to the labia majora. Because the genital folds do not fuse, they become the labia minora, and the genital tubercle becomes the clitoris. In the female, all these steps are constitutive and occur in the absence of hormonal stimulation.

MECHANISMS OF GONADAL SEX DETERMINATION: THE SRY GENE. Sex determination in mammals is governed primarily by gene(s) lying on the Y chromosome; the number of accompanying X chromosomes is irrelevant. The X and Y chromosomes each contain pseudoautosomal regions of approximately 2.6×10^6 base pairs, which enter into homologous recombination between the sex chromosomes at meiosis, ensuring their correct segregation. Loci on the Y chromosome proximal to the pseudoautosomal boundary normally are not involved in an exchange with the X chromosome and exhibit patrilineal inheritance. It is essential to the chromosomal basis of sex determination that the testis-determining gene be located in the nonrecombining, Y-specific region. The testis-determining gene (SRY), which is located on the short arm of the human Y chromosome, is conserved and Y-specific among a wide range of mammals and encodes a testis-specific transcript. Mutations of the SRY gene have been reported in sex-reversed XY individuals. Conversely, translocation of SRY leads to maleness in XX subjects, but these are sterile because XX germ cells do not survive in a testicular environment.

Although fetal ovarian development is constitutive, female germ cells survive only in the presence of two X chromosomes; 45,X individuals experience early loss of germ cells, leading to fibrous degeneration of the ovaries usually associated with Turner syndrome. Recently, it has been found that male to female sex reversal occurs in individuals with duplications of the short arm of the X chromosome, suggesting that there also may be a gene for femaleness. This locus has been termed DSS for dosage-sensitive sex reversal and has been localized to a 1.6×10^5 base pair region of the short arm of the X chromosome.

MECHANISM OF SOMATIC SEX DIFFERENTIATION. Sex differentiation of the reproductive tract is mediated by two discrete hormones produced by the fetal testis: AMH and testosterone (Fig. 207–2). In the absence of both, female differentiation proceeds unimpeded.

AMH, which is synthesized by immature Sertoli cells and by postnatal granulosa cells, is responsible for müllerian regression. The gene, located on chromosome 19, is a member of the transforming growth factor-β (TGF-β) superfamily and acts via a serine threonine kinase receptor located on chromosome 12.

Androgens are responsible for maintenance of the wolffian ducts and virilization of the urogenital sinus and external genitalia. Testosterone production by the fetal testis is detectable at 9 weeks in the human fetus, increases to a peak at 15 to 18 weeks, then falls sharply, so that serum concentrations of testosterone overlap in males and females in late pregnancy. In adult Leydig cells, the capacity to respond to sustained gonadotropin stimulation by increased androgen production is curtailed by the development of a refractory state, due to receptor down-regulation, which does not occur in the fetus. When human chorionic gonadotropin (hCG) declines in the third trimester, the hypothalamic-pituitary axis gains control over testicular functional activity.

Testosterone is the major steroid released by fetal testes in the bloodstream, and it enters cells by passive diffusion or pinocytosis. A local source of androgen is important for wolffian duct development, which does not occur if testosterone is supplied only via the peripheral circulation, as in female pseudohermaphroditism due to adrenal hyperplasia. Testosterone is converted intracellularly to dihydrotestosterone (DHT) by the enzyme 5α-reductase (Fig. 207–3). Two distinct isoforms of 5α-reductase have been cloned: Type 1 is present in very low levels in the prostate and the sebaceous glands; type 2 is present in high levels in the prostate and in the area of the external genitalia. DHT binds to the androgen receptor with greater affinity and stability than does testosterone. Therefore, in tissues equipped with 5α-reductase at the time of sex differentiation, such as the prostate, urogenital sinus, and external genitalia, DHT is the active androgen. However, at high concentrations, testosterone interacts with the androgen receptor similarly to DHT. The gene coding for the androgen receptor is located on the X chromosome.

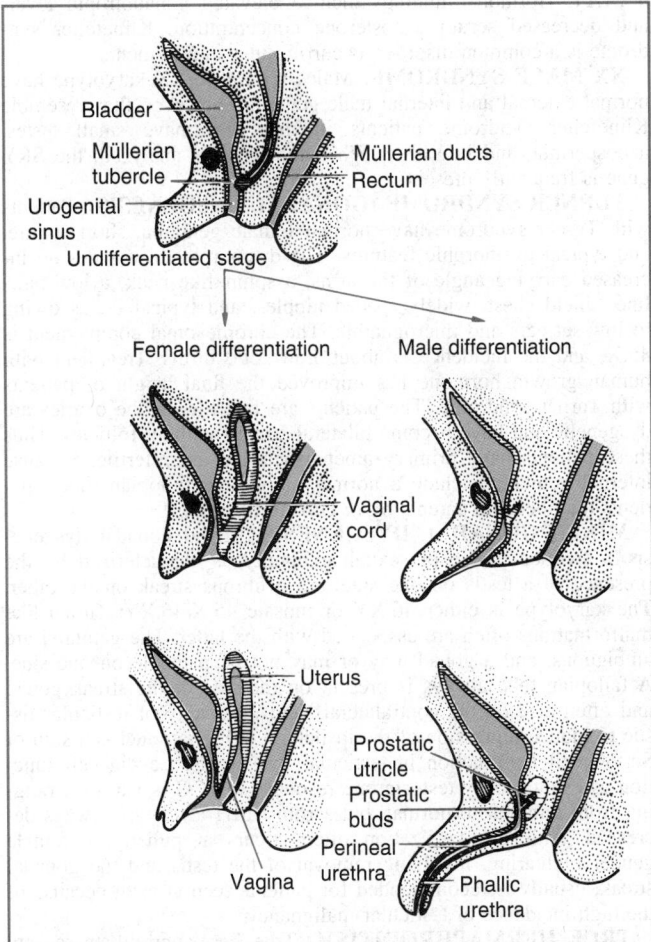

FIGURE 207–1. Differentiation of the urogenital sinus. (From Josso N: Physiology of sex differentiation: A guide to the understanding and management of the intersex child. *In* Josso N [ed.]: The Intersex Child. Basel, Karger, 1981, p 1.)

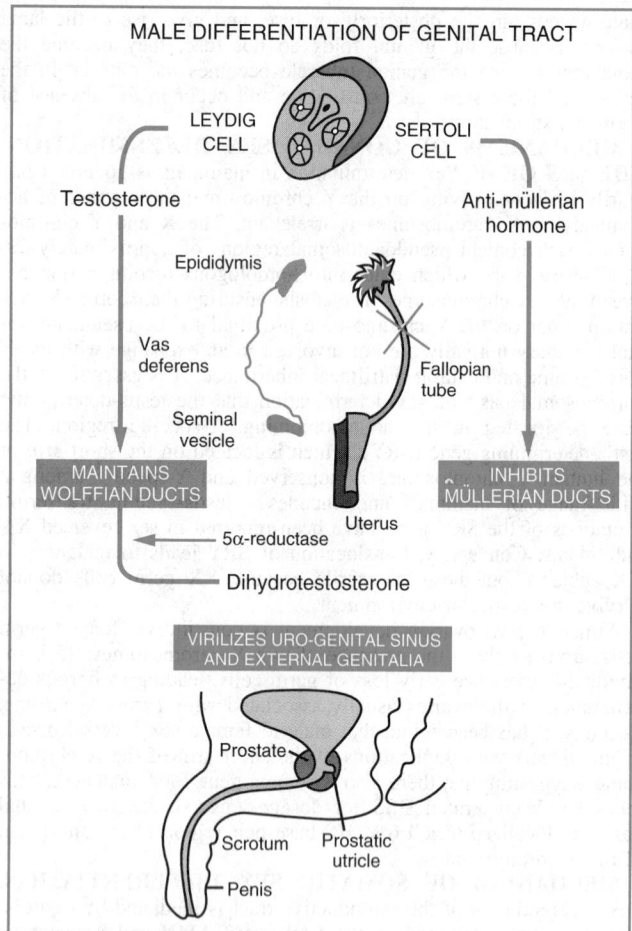

MALE DIFFERENTIATION OF GENITAL TRACT

FIGURE 207–2. Hormones involved in male differentiation of the reproductive tract. Testosterone, synthesized by Leydig cells, maintains the wolffian ducts and virilizes the urogenital sinus and external genitalia after reduction to dihydrotestosterone. Antimüllerian hormone, produced by fetal Sertoli cells, inhibits the development of the müllerian ducts, which would otherwise develop into uterus and tubes. (From Josso N: Physiology of sex differentiation: A guide to the understanding and management of the intersex child. *In* Josso N [ed.]: The Intersex Child. Basel, Karger, 1981, p 1.)

CLASSIFICATION OF INTERSEX STATES

Normal sex differentiation occurs at various levels (Fig. 207–4): Genetic sex is established at fertilization by the nature of the sex chromosome donated by the spermatozoon. The presence or absence of the SRY gene primarily determines gonadal sex, and the presence or absence of fetal testes determines somatic sex through the secretion of testosterone. Gender identity is established early in life by the sex of rearing but can exceptionally be disrupted at puberty by hormonal factors.

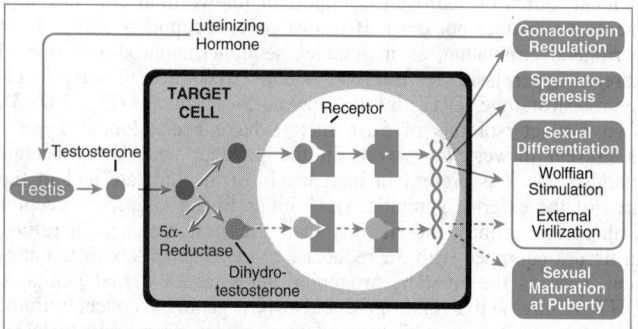

FIGURE 207–3. General scheme of androgen action. (From Wilson JD: Syndromes of androgen resistance. Biol Reprod 46:168, 1992.)

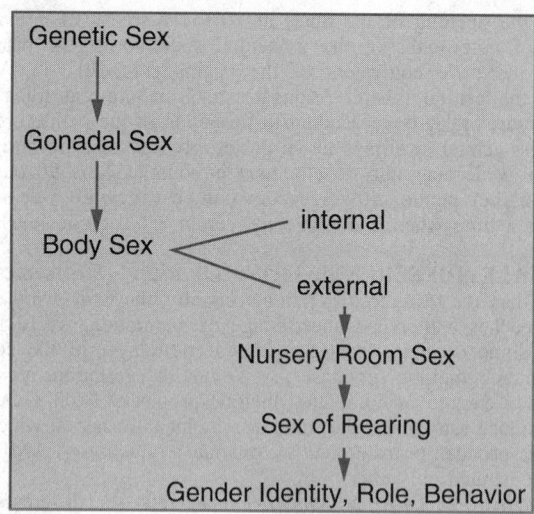

FIGURE 207–4. Stages of sex differentiation. Genetic sex specified at fertilization determines gonadal sex, which in turn determines somatic and legal sex. Gender identity usually is determined by the sex of rearing. (From New MI, Levine LS: Congenital adrenal hyperplasia. *In* Harris H, Hirschhorn K [eds.]: Advances in Human Genetics. New York, Plenum Press, 1973, p 251.)

DISORDERS OF CHROMOSOMAL SEX

KLINEFELTER SYNDROME. In this condition, males have normal development of the penis and scrotum, but the testes are small and firm. At adolescence, gynecomastia is frequent and infertility is common owing to azoospermia. The usual karyotype is 47,XXY. Hormonal findings include elevated gonadotropin levels and decreased serum testosterone concentration. Klinefelter syndrome is a common disorder, occurring in 1 in 500 men.

XX MALE SYNDROME. Males with a 46,XX karyotype have normal external and internal male genitalia; however, they resemble Klinefelter syndrome patients in that they have small testes, azoospermia, and infertility. When the DNA is analyzed, the SRY gene is frequently present.

TURNER SYNDROME (GONADAL DYSGENESIS). Patients with Turner syndrome have normal female genitalia, short stature, and typical dysmorphic features. The dysmorphism includes an increased carrying angle of the arms, a sphinxlike neck, a low hairline, shield chest, widely spaced nipples, and typical facies owing to low-set ears and micrognathia. The chromosomal complement is 45,X, and the incidence is about 1 in 2500 births. Treatment with human growth hormone has improved the final height of patients with Turner syndrome. The patients are infertile, as the ovaries are dysgenetic and have become bilateral streaks without follicles. Thus these patients have primary amenorrhea and are infertile. Because internal genitalia include a normal uterus and fallopian tubes, patients may become parents by *in vitro* fertilization.

MIXED GONADAL DYSGENESIS. Mixed gonadal dysgenesis, a frequent cause of sexual ambiguity, is characterized by the presence of a testis on one side and a fibrous streak on the other. The karyotype is either 46,XY or mosaic 45,X/46,XY; Turner-like malformations often are associated with the latter. The genitalia are ambiguous, and a gonad may or may not be palpable on one side. A fallopian tube always is present on the side of the streak gonad and often also on the contralateral side; incapacity of testicular tissue to induce regression of the ipsilateral müllerian duct is a sign of Sertoli cell malfunction in testicular dysgenesis. Leydig cell function as evaluated by testosterone response to hCG is variable, ranging from minimal to normal, but serum AMH levels are always decreased. Although virilization often occurs at puberty, a female gender of rearing, involving removal of the testis and the gonadal streak, usually is recommended for patients seen at birth because of the high incidence of testicular malignancy.

TRUE HERMAPHRODITISM. True hermaphroditism, a rare and usually sporadic disorder, is defined as coexistence of seminiferous tubules and ovarian follicles in the same subject. Most patients have an ovotestis with either an ovary or a testis on the opposite side; a testis is usually in the scrotum, an ovotestis more seldom. Histologically, ovarian tissue is more or less normal, whereas testicular tubules are markedly dysgenetic and may harbor gonadoblastomas or seminomas.

The genitalia are usually ambiguous; rare cases of completely masculine or feminine genitalia have been reported. The anatomy of the internal reproductive tract depends on the nature of the gonads. A uterus is present in approximately 90% of cases. Testosterone response to hCG is variable, and AMH levels are usually low. Most patients experience breast development, ovulation, and even menstruation at puberty; pregnancy and successful childbirth are possible if selective removal of testicular tissue is feasible. Unless gender has already been assigned, male orientation should be restricted to patients with no uterus and descended testicular tissue, because testicular tissue is usually dysgenetic and prone to malignant degeneration. The majority of true hermaphrodites have no Y chromosome: 68% have a 46,XX karyotype, 12% are 46,XY, and the remainder are mosaics. To resolve the discrepancy between the presence of testicular tissue and the lack of a Y chromosome, the DNA of 46,XX true hermaphrodites has been examined with probes for SRY. True hermaphrodites usually lack SRY, suggesting that the condition, at least in familial cases, is due to constitutive activation of a gene normally triggered by SRY.

DISORDERS OF GONADAL SEX

PURE GONADAL DYSGENESIS, TESTICULAR REGRESSION SYNDROME. Patients with pure gonadal dysgenesis have a normal female phenotype, including uterus and tubes, but have fibrous streaks instead of gonads; they are free of Turner-like malformations and develop to normal height. Familial cases have been described, with either a 46,XX or a 46,XY karyotype; in the latter, mutations of the SRY gene have been identified. Other 46,XY patients with absent gonads present with various degrees of sexual ambiguity and no müllerian derivatives. The implication that some testicular tissue was functional at least up to 10 weeks and subsequently regressed has led to the name "fetal testicular regression syndrome." Testicular regression may occur in late pregnancy or even postnatally; these fully virilized males present only with bilateral cryptorchidism. This condition also is known as *anorchia*.

TESTICULAR DYSGENESIS. Testicular dysgenesis is characterized by seminiferous tubule degeneration and invasion by connective tissue arranged in whorls as in a streak gonad. Germ cells are rare or absent; the gonad is often maldescended and prone to malignant degeneration. The clinical picture, as in true hermaphroditism, combines defects of AMH- and testosterone-dependent steps of sex differentiation, depending on the extent and timing of testicular degeneration. The incidence of gonadal tumors may reach 30%, making castration and subsequent hormonal replacement the safest therapeutic option.

DYSGENETIC MALE PSEUDOHERMAPHRODITISM. Patients with dysgenetic male pseudohermaphroditism have bilaterally differentiated dysgenetic testes. Their external genitalia are ambiguous and müllerian derivatives are always present. The clinical, endocrine, and cytogenetic picture is similar to that of mixed gonadal dysgenesis.

NONDYSGENETIC MALE PSEUDOHERMAPHRODITISM. Patients with bilateral nondysgenetic testes fail to masculinize because of biochemical alteration of the synthesis or action of a single testicular hormone. This is in contrast to subjects with true hermaphroditism or testicular dysgenesis, characterized by defects of testosterone- and AMH-dependent steps of sex differentiation. Defects of testosterone-mediated steps of sex differentiation are the most frequent and are characterized, in 46,XY subjects, by a variable degree of penile development and hypospadias. Usually, a single perineoscrotal opening leads into a urogenital sinus; the blind vaginal pouch opens into the posterior wall of the urethra, usually at the junction of the vertical and horizontal segments of the urethra. Extreme situations occur more rarely. Sometimes, the vagina and urethra have separate perineal orifices as in a normal female, or, in deeply virilized patients, the vaginal orifice opens beneath the bladder neck, differing only by size from the prostatic utricle of a normal male. Müllerian derivatives, the uterus and upper segment of the vagina, are always regressed. Serum levels of AMH are normal or elevated. Insufficient production of active androgens or androgen end-organ resistance may be involved. However, a large number of cases cannot be classified. "Idiopathic" male pseudohermaphroditism can be considered to be a malformation masquerad-

ing as a testosterone defect. Association of genital ambiguity with other developmental defects frequently is observed, sometimes as one of the several components of a recognized syndrome such as Smith-Lemli-Opitz; the WAGR syndrome, including Wilms tumor, aniridia, gonadal abnormalities, and mental retardation; or the hand-foot-genital syndrome.

DISORDERS OF PHENOTYPIC SEX

FEMALE PSEUDOHERMAPHRODITISM. Female pseudohermaphroditism, defined as the sexual ambiguity of a 46,XX fetus with two normal ovaries, is the most frequent type of intersex. Rarely, the female fetus is masculinized owing to transplacental transfer of androgens from an ovarian or adrenocortical tumor in the mother or from exogenous steroids. Most female pseudohermaphrodites have been exposed to endogenous androgens prenatally owing to congenital adrenal hyperplasia (CAH).

Virilization due to androgen excess is limited to the androgen-responsive external genitalia (the lower vagina, genital folds and swellings, and phallus). Masculinization ranges from minimal clitoromegaly and a mild degree of posterior labial fusion to formation of a urogenital sinus with the orifice located distally along the urethral groove, ending in extreme cases at the tip of the phallus. Because there is no testicular tissue, testosterone is not produced locally to support development of wolffian duct structures, nor is AMH produced; therefore the fallopian tubes, uterus, and upper vagina are normal. Thus, with proper medical treatment and vaginal reconstruction, there is capacity for normal childbearing.

CAH should be suspected in sexually ambiguous newborns with a uterus but no palpable gonadal tissue. Such patients should be karyotyped and have endocrine evaluation done immediately because of the life-threatening salt loss found in many cases of CAH.

CONGENITAL ADRENAL HYPERPLASIA. CAH is a family of monogenic autosomal recessive disorders of steroidogenesis in which enzymatic defects result in impaired synthesis of cortisol by the adrenal cortex (Table 207–1). Subsequent adrenocorticotropic hormone (ACTH) oversecretion via the negative feedback system stimulates the adrenal to become hyperplastic. As a result, both precursor steroids proximal to the enzyme block and hormonal products of unimpeded pathways are overproduced. In some forms, diversion of precursor steroids into androgen pathways results in excessive levels of potent androgens and virilization of the female fetus. In other forms, sex steroids are underproduced in both the adrenal and the testes, leading to ambiguous genitalia in genetic males. Abnormal secretion of mineralocorticoids in some cases results in disturbances in the regulation of electrolytes, plasma volume, and blood pressure.

STEROID 21-HYDROXYLASE DEFICIENCY. *Classic 21-Hydroxylase Deficiency.* Steroid 21-hydroxylase deficiency is the most common enzymatic defect causing CAH. Classic 21-hydroxylase deficiency occurs in about 1 in 14,000 live births, but the incidence may vary by population and geographic area (Fig. 207–5). The classic disorder has two forms: salt wasting and simple virilizing (non–salt wasting); both result in sexual ambiguity in the newborn genetic female. In the salt-wasting form, which occurs in about three fourths of cases, adrenal production of aldosterone and of cortisol is inadequate. Salt-wasting crises are associated with hyponatremia, hyperkalemia, and hypovolemia, with metabolic acidosis, loss of vascular tone, and, in some cases, shock and death. Crises usually arise between 7 days and 2 weeks of life, after discharge from the hospital. Thus, the affected first-born male who has normal genitalia is particularly at risk for a salt-wasting crisis at home. Ambiguous genitalia in the female usually prompt diagnostic procedures, placing females at lower risk. Salt wasting should be carefully ruled out even in newborns with mild genital ambiguity. Unlike salt wasters, simple virilizers can synthesize sufficient amounts of aldosterone for salt retention.

Nonclassic 21-Hydroxylase Deficiency. Nonclassic 21-hydroxylase deficiency, a genetic variant of the classic form, is associated with a milder enzyme defect and does not cause prenatal virilization in the genetic female. However, signs of androgen excess may appear postnatally in both sexes. Nonclassic 21-hydroxylase deficiency occurs in 1 in 100 births in the general population and with a higher frequency in specific ethnic groups, making this the most frequent autosomal recessive disease in humans.

TABLE 207–1. THE FORMS OF CONGENITAL ADRENAL HYPERPLASIA: CLINICAL AND HORMONAL ASPECTS

Deficiency	Genital Ambiguity	Postnatal Virilization	Salt Metabolism	Renin	Steroid Pattern	
					Increased	*Decreased*
21-hydroxylase				High		
A. Classic salt wasting	F	Yes	Salt wasting		17-OHP; Δ^4-A	aldo; cortisol
Simple virilizing	F	Yes	Normal		17-OHP; Δ^4-A	cortisol
B. Nonclassic (symptomatic and asymptomatic)	No	Yes	Normal		17-OHP; Δ^4-A	—
11β-hydroxylase				Low		
A. Classic	F	Yes	Salt retention		DOC; compound S	cortisol $\pm$ aldo
B. Nonclassic	No	Yes	Normal		Compound S $\pm$ DOC	
3β-hydroxysteroid dehydrogenase				High		
A. Classic	M/F	Yes	Salt wasting		17-OH-pregnenolone; DHEA	aldo; cortisol; T
B. Nonclassic	No	Yes	Normal		17-OH-pregnenolone; DHEA	—
17α-hydroxylase	M	No	Salt retention	Low	DOC; compound B	cortisol; T
17,20-lyase	M	No	Normal		None	DHEA; T; Δ^4-A
Cholesterol desmolase	M	No	Salt wasting	High	None	All

17-OHP = 17-hydroxyprogesterone; Δ^4-A = Δ^4-androstenedione; aldo = aldosterone; DOC = deoxycorticosterone; compound S = 11-deoxycortisol; DHEA = dehydroepiandrosterone; T = testosterone; B = corticosterone.

Clinical Presentation. In 21-hydroxylase deficiency, 17α-hydroxyprogesterone (17-OHP) and progesterone are overproduced and are converted to the androgens dehydroepiandrosterone (DHEA), Δ^4-androstenedione (AD), and testosterone, which cause virilization. Postnatally, in untreated classic and nonclassic children, growth accelerates in the early years but the epiphyses close prematurely, resulting in a tall child but a short adult. Even when treated, most patients do not reach the height potential indicated by family height. Pubertal development under hypothalamic-pituitary control may be suppressed by excess adrenal androgens, and fertility potential may not be achieved until proper treatment is instituted to suppress ACTH and adrenal androgen secretion. Without treatment, males may evidence pseudopuberty marked by phallic growth, small testes, and precocious growth of pubic, axillary, and body hair. Male internal and external genital development is normal. Untreated females may suffer from excessive androgenic symptoms such as cystic acne, secondary amenorrhea/oligomenorrhea, or polycystic ovarian syndrome (Fig. 207–6).

Molecular Genetics. The gene encoding 21-hydroxylase is located on the short arm of chromosome 6 within the human major histocompatibility complex. The gene locus for the 21-hydroxylase enzyme, termed CYP21, has a closely neighboring homologue, the pseudogene CYP21P, which is not expressed. Two forms of mutations observed are gene deletions, which result from chromosomal misalignment as well as unequal crossing over during meiosis, and gene conversions, which apparently involve the transfer of short sequences resident on the pseudogene to the active gene.

Diagnosis and Treatment. Screening of newborns for elevated serum 17-OHP identifies males and females with classic 21-

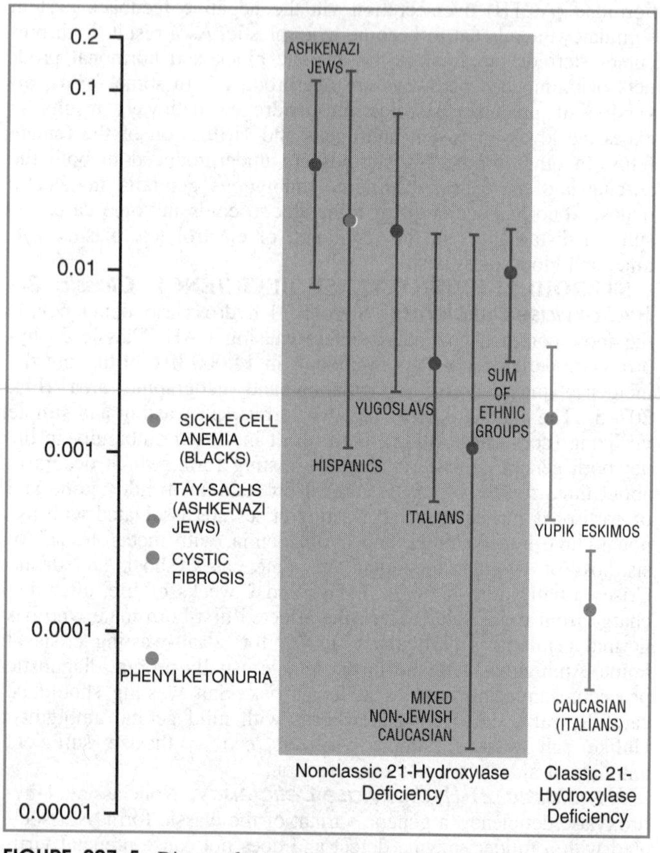

FIGURE 207–5. Disease frequencies of classic 21-hydroxylase deficiency (in two populations), nonclassic 21-hydroxylase deficiency (in five ethnic groups), and four other relatively common autosomal recessive disorders compared. (From Speiser PW, Dupont B, Rubinstein P, et al.: High frequency of nonclassical steroid 21-hydroxylase deficiency. Am J Hum Genet 37:650, 1985.)

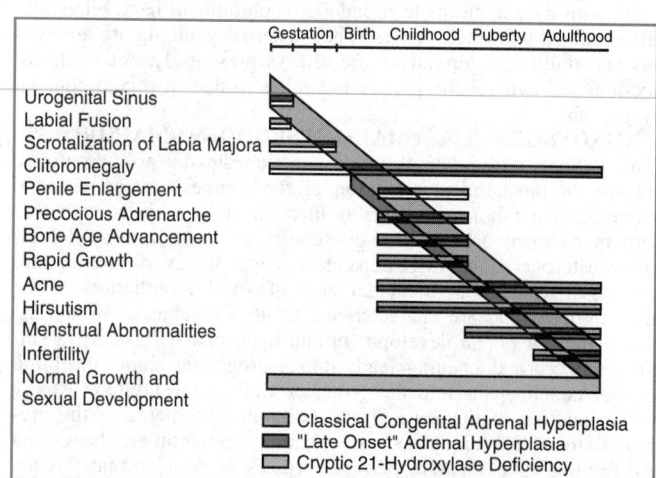

FIGURE 207–6. Clinical spectrum of HLA-linked steroid 21-hydroxylase deficiency. Clinical presentation in 21-hydroxylase deficiency ranges from prenatal virilization with labial fusion to precocious adrenarche, to pubertal or postpubertal virilization. During their lifetime, patients may change from symptomatic to asymptomatic with 21-hydroxylase deficiency. (From New MI, Dupont B, Grumbach K, et al.: The adrenal hyperplasias. *In* Stanbury JB, Wyngaarden JB, et al. [eds.]: The Metabolic Basis of Inherited Disease. 5th ed. New York, McGraw-Hill, 1983, p 973.)

hydroxylase deficiency irrespective of genital phenotype. In the United States, newborns currently are screened in 15 states. In suspected cases, the chromosomal or genetic sex should be determined by buccal smear for Barr bodies, karyotyping, fluorescent Y, or SRY analysis. Elevated 17-OHP, which may be several hundred times normal, confirms the enzyme defect. Routine screening does not detect the nonclassic form of 21-hydroxylase deficiency. In the nonclassic form, 17-OHP levels may be elevated in early morning readings but normal in midmorning and afternoon. Thus, the deficiency is best diagnosed with an ACTH stimulation test (an intravenous bolus injection of 0.25 mg synthetic ACTH and assay for serum 17-OHP at 0 and 60 minutes). The coordinates of the baseline and the ACTH-stimulated 17-OHP concentrations aggregate on a regression line into three diagnostic groups. Classic cases fall into the highest group on the regression line, nonclassic cases aggregate lower than classic cases, and an overlap of heterozygote carriers and unaffected cases appears in the lowest group (Fig. 207–7).

The female with classic 21-hydroxylase deficiency should almost always be assigned to the female gender, as she has the potential for normal sexual and reproductive function. In classically affected untreated females, surgical correction of genital ambiguity is required. Recent experience indicates that early one-stage vaginal and perineal reconstruction, which avoids a second-stage surgical procedure and decreases delayed vaginal stenosis, is effective in correcting the ambiguity.

Postnatal management involves lifelong hormonal replacement. It is necessary to monitor 17-OHP serum concentration (or daily urinary excretion of pregnanetriol) as well as plasma renin activity in the classic salt-wasting form. Hydrocortisone generally is given in infancy and childhood in a dose range of 10 to 25 mg per square

meter per day in order to maintain the serum 17-OHP concentration between 500 and 1000 ng per deciliter. Attempts to bring the 17-OHP concentration to normal results in cushingoid features and retarded growth. In adolescence and adulthood, hydrocortisone may be replaced with dexamethasone or prednisone. Mineralocorticoid (9α-fluorohydrocortisone) administration and added salt to the diet are necessary in patients with salt-wasting disease and may improve hormonal control in simple virilizers. Treatment of nonclassic 21-hydroxylase deficiency with dexamethasone in low doses (0.25 mg at bedtime) is usually effective in reversing symptoms of androgen excess, including reduced fertility.

Prenatal Management. Prenatal diagnosis is best performed with a direct molecular genetic approach but can also be achieved by assessment of 17-OHP or AD in amniotic fluid. Diagnosis by DNA testing requires sampling of chorion frondosum obtained by chorionic villus sampling or amniotic fluid cells obtained by amniocentesis. Chorionic villus sampling performed in the eighth to tenth week of gestation allows diagnosis earlier than amniocentesis performed in the second trimester. Direct examination of the CYP21 gene locus is carried out by Southern blotting for identification of gene deletions (10 to 35% of cases) and with allele-specific oligonucleotide probes for point mutations. Together, these two tests routinely identify about 90% of all mutations.

The recommended prenatal treatment of 21-hydroxylase deficiency is oral dexamethasone, 20 μg per kilogram per day (prepregnancy weight) divided in three equal doses and administered to the mother starting before the ninth week of gestation (Fig. 207–8). Therapy should continue to term if the fetus is found to be an af-

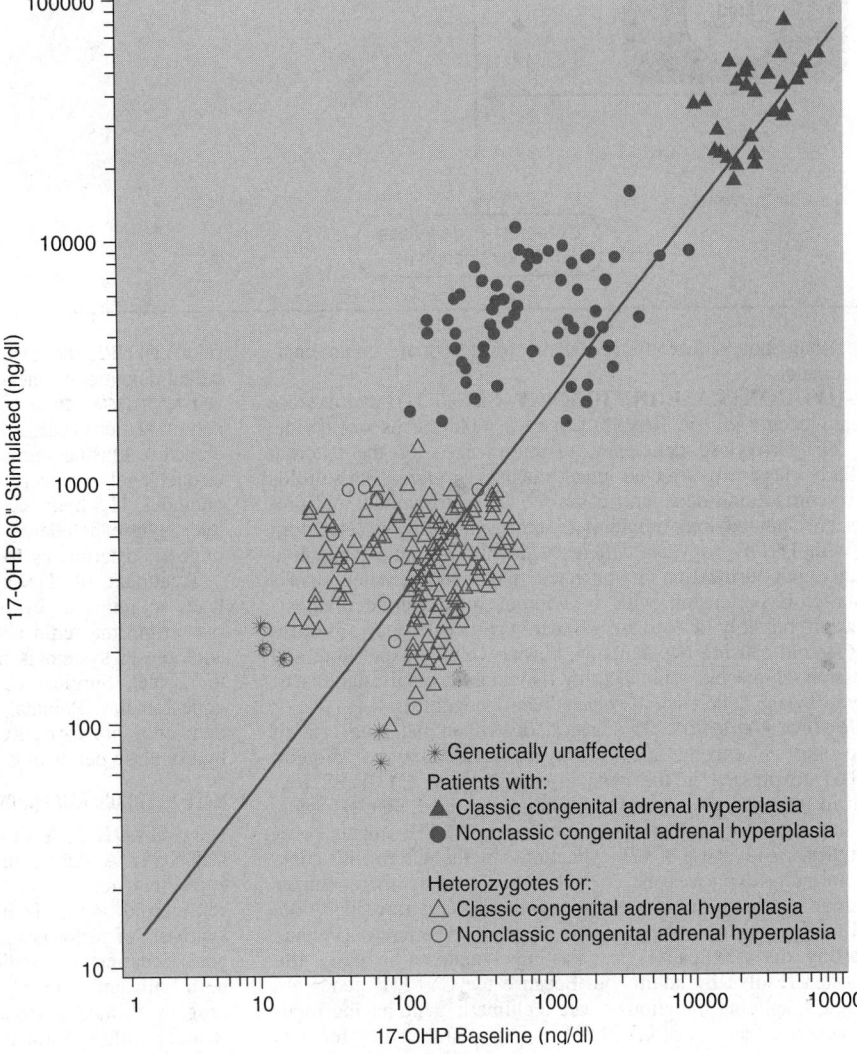

17-OHP NOMOGRAM FOR THE DIAGNOSIS OF STEROID 21–HYDROXYLASE DEFICIENCY
60 MINUTE CORTROSYN STIMULATION TEST

FIGURE 207–7. Nomogram relating baseline to ACTH-stimulated serum concentrations of 17-hydroxyprogesterone (17-OHP). The scales are logarithmic. A regression line for all data points is shown. The data for this nomogram were collected between 1982 and 1991 at the Department of Pediatrics, The New York Hospital–Cornell Medical Center, New York, New York.

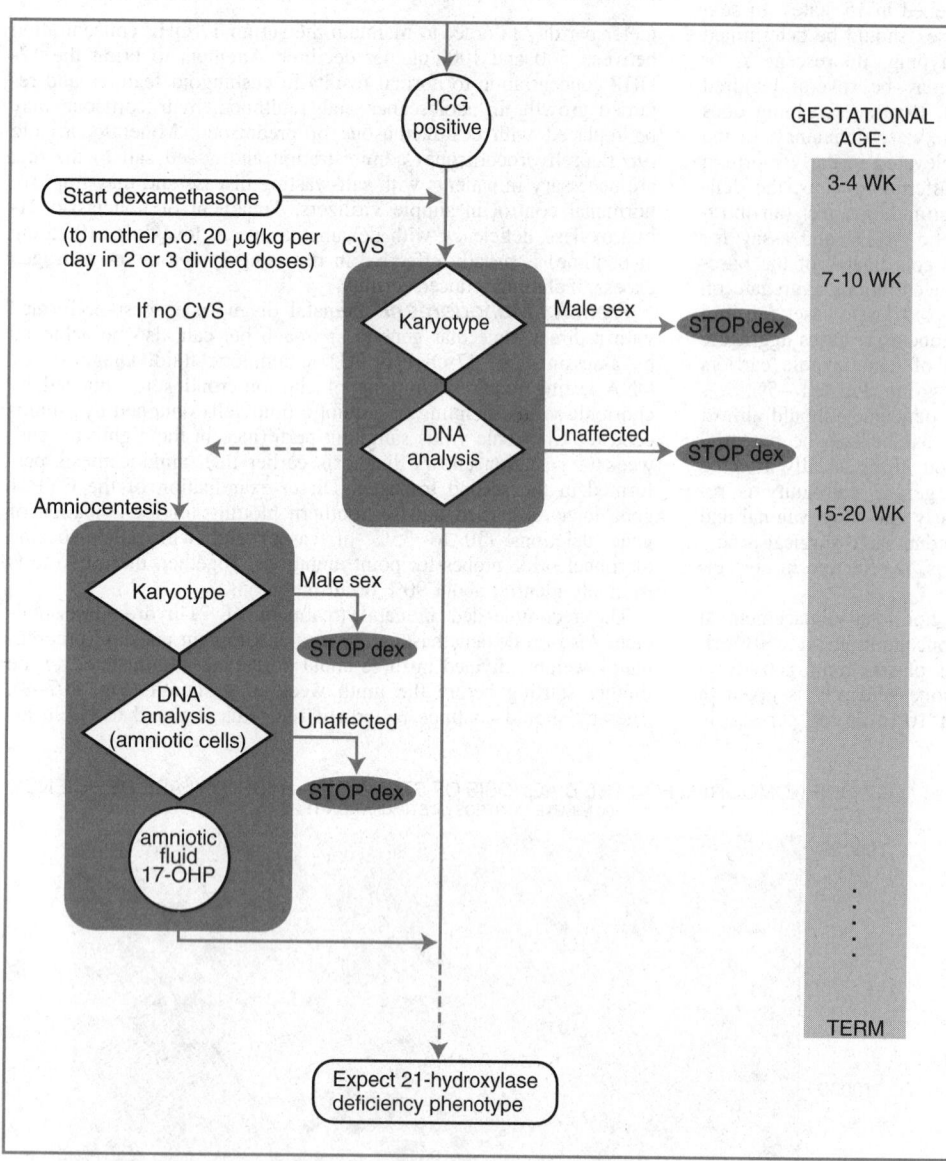

FIGURE 207–8. Algorithm depicting prenatal management of pregnancy in families at risk for a fetus affected with 21-hydroxylase deficiency. (From Speiser PW, Laforgia N, Kato K, et al.: First trimester prenatal treatment and molecular genetic diagnosis of congenital adrenal hyperplasia [21-hydroxylase deficiency]. J Clin Endocrinol Metab 70:838–848, 1990. © The Endocrine Society.)

fected female but is discontinued if the fetus is male or an unaffected female.

11β-HYDROXYLASE DEFICIENCY. Steroid 11β-hydroxylase deficiency occurs in 1 in 100,000 to 1 in 200,000 births worldwide. As in 21-hydroxylase deficiency, masculinization of the external genitalia in classically affected females occurs *in utero*. The steroids 11-deoxycortisol and deoxycorticosterone are oversecreted, and precursors are shunted into uninhibited androgen pathways. Newborn males with 11β-hydroxylase deficiency do not present with genital ambiguity, but virilization in untreated males and females ensues postnatally. Hypertension with or without hypokalemic alkalosis may occur, possibly due to excess deoxycorticosterone, a salt-retaining steroid causing hypokalemia; plasma volume expansion; and suppression of plasma renin activity. Nonclassic manifestations of 11β-hydroxylase deficiency also have been recognized.

Molecular Genetics. Two genes located on the long arm of chromosome 8 encode the 11β-hydroxylase enzyme protein: CYP11B1 (expressed in the zona fasciculata) and CYP11B2 (expressed in the zona glomerulosa). Mutations in the CYP11B1 gene, which has regulatory sequences responsive to ACTH, impair cortisol synthesis and cause CAH. Mutations in the CYP11B2 gene, which normally expresses the enzyme aldosterone synthase, impair aldosterone synthesis but not cortisol synthesis. This rare condition, termed corticosterone methyloxidase type II deficiency (Persian salt-wasting disease), causes salt-wasting symptoms in early life which often resolve by adulthood. Because the CYP11B genes are homologues, splicing mutations create a chimeric gene having regulatory sequence features of CYP11B1 and structural coding features

of CYP11B2; the result is a rare form of low-renin hypertension called dexamethasone-suppressible hyperaldosteronism.

Diagnosis and Treatment. In 11β-hydroxylase deficiency, serum 11-deoxycortisol (compound S) and deoxycorticosterone are elevated. Plasma renin activity is suppressed and/or plasma aldosterone levels are very low. In the genetic female with ambiguous genitalia, 11β-hydroxylase deficiency can be distinguished from 21-hydroxylase deficiency by elevated levels of compound S and deoxycorticosterone as well as suppressed plasma renin activity.

Treatment of 11β-hydroxylase deficiency with glucocorticoids leads to reduced levels of deoxycorticosterone with natriuresis, a rise in plasma renin activity, and normotension. Because the renin-angiotensin system is no longer suppressed, aldosterone levels rise to normal. Surgical correction may be necessary in untreated genetic females. Prenatal diagnosis and treatment of 11β-hydroxylase deficiency are carried out with the same protocol as in steroid 21-hydroxylase deficiency.

MALE PSEUDOHERMAPHRODITISM

3β-HYDROXYSTEROID DEHYDROGENASE DEFICIENCY. A defect in 3β-hydroxysteroid dehydrogenase, an enzyme that acts early in the pathway of cortisol synthesis, impairs sex steroid synthesis in both the adrenal and the gonads. As the synthesis of testosterone is impaired in 3β-hydroxysteroid dehydrogenase deficiency, males are incompletely masculinized and are born with ambiguous genitalia. In the genetic female fetus, Δ⁴ androgens formed peripherally from the excess secretion of DHEA produce mild clitoral enlargement. In the case of a severe enzyme block in either gender, salt wasting owing to aldosterone deficiency may develop.

A gene for the peripheral form of 3β-hydroxysteroid dehydrogenase (type I) and a gene for the adrenal-gonadal form of 3β-hydroxysteroid dehydrogenase (type II) have been identified and mapped to chromosome 1. Mutations in the type II gene have been described only in the classic form of the disorder.

Steroid 3β-hydroxysteroid dehydrogenase deficiency is diagnosed by a high ratio of Δ^5 to Δ^4 steroids. Elevated levels of pregnenolone, 17-hydroxypregnenolone, and DHEA are evident in serum; urinary Δ^5 metabolites pregnanetriol and 16-pregnanetriol are elevated. Steroid values in the newborn period may not be informative, as Δ^5 steroids are normally high during this time in unaffected persons. Glucocorticoid administration, with the addition of a mineralocorticoid to correct salt wasting, is effective.

Some women exhibiting clinically significant signs of androgen excess show a pattern of elevated Δ^5 to Δ^4 steroids; this may represent an underlying mild (nonclassic) 3β-hydroxysteroid dehydrogenase defect. No mutation has been identified to date in the nonclassic form. The nonclassic defect is diagnosed by 60-minute ACTH testing. Treatment consists of oral dexamethasone administration in small doses (0.25 mg at bedtime).

17α-HYDROXYLASE/17,20-LYASE DEFICIENCY.

Combined 17α-hydroxylase/17,20-lyase deficiency, a rare form of CAH, impairs the synthesis of cortisol and sex steroids. Males at birth may present with ambiguous genitalia or be mistakenly assigned to the female gender. Wolffian duct formation is incomplete owing to deficient androgen production, whereas normal AMH secretion by Sertoli cells inhibits formation of the uterus and fallopian tubes. Genetic females appear normal at birth and throughout childhood but may present with primary amenorrhea at puberty. Plasma gonadotropins are elevated in both sexes. Hypertension with hypokalemia due to excess deoxycorticosterone may develop and present clinically in childhood or may be found incidental to failure of puberty. The structural gene for P450c17 is located on chromosome 10.

The deficiency is diagnosed by high serum deoxycorticosterone and extremely high corticosterone (B) levels. Aldosterone levels are low owing to suppressed renin and hypokalemia from excess deoxycorticosterone. Before puberty, 17α-hydroxylase/17,20-lyase deficiency is treated with glucocorticoids. Sex steroids appropriate to the gender of rearing are given at pubertal age to induce the development of secondary sex characteristics. In genetic males raised as females, gonadectomy and vaginal reconstruction are required.

Isolated 17,20-lyase deficiency also can occur, in which the 17-hydroxylase function of the enzyme is intact and allows the synthesis of cortisol, but C_{19} steroid production is deficient.

CHOLESTEROL DESMOLASE DEFICIENCY.

Cholesterol desmolase deficiency (lipoid adrenal hyperplasia or Prader's syndrome), an extremely rare condition, involves a block in the conversion of cholesterol to pregnenolone. Affected males and females have a female external genital phenotype. Biochemical findings include profound deficiencies of all steroids, low plasma volume, hyperkalemia, and hyponatremia. Neonatal mortality is high from total adrenal insufficiency, but some patients maintained on hormonal replacement can survive to adulthood. The gene for the cholesterol desmolase enzyme has been cloned and mapped to chromosome 15.

LEYDIG CELL APLASIA.

Leydig cell aplasia or hypoplasia is a rare syndrome characterized by high basal luteinizing hormone (LH), normal follicle-stimulating hormone, and low testosterone, which does not respond to hCG stimulation. Adrenal steroidogenesis is normal, suggesting that the defect may reside at the level of the LH receptor.

5α-REDUCTASE DEFICIENCY.

Deficiency of 5α-reductase is a rare autosomal recessive disorder (Table 207–2). The membrane-bound enzyme 5α-reductase type 2 is responsible for the conversion of testosterone to DHT. A defect in 5α-reductase causes selective impairment of DHT-dependent steps of male sex differentiation. In patients with 5α-reductase deficiency, plasma testosterone levels are normal to elevated, whereas DHT levels are low. LH levels are normal or slightly elevated. Most patients have severe perineoscrotal hypospadias, and there may be a blind vaginal pouch opening into the urogenital sinus or the urethra. As the wolffian ducts are maintained by testosterone, patients have normal vasa deferentia, seminal vesicles, and epididymides. DHT-mediated virilization of the urogenital sinus and the external genitalia is impaired, and the prostate is small or absent. Patients have a female habitus without breast development but lack female internal genital structures. At puberty, testosterone-dependent masculinization occurs to a variable degree; affected males develop rugation and hyperpigmentation of the scrotum, growth of the phallus, an increase in muscle mass, and deepening of the voice. Some may have testicular descent (Fig. 207–9A). Gender change from female to male in untreated affected subjects has been documented.

Patients diagnosed with 5α-reductase deficiency in infancy and early childhood are best reared as males once hypospadias, ventral contraction and bowing of the penis (chordee), and cryptorchidism are surgically corrected. Because DHT is not available for general use, adults are usually treated by high doses of testosterone esters. In the absence of 5α-reduction, 19-nortestosterone is active and can be given by injection in an esterified form.

5α-Reductase isoform 2 is the major isoenzyme expressed in genital tissues, and a deletion in the type 2 gene has been found in affected subjects. Eighteen different mutations have been identified in 25 families, and approximately 40% of affected individuals are compound heterozygotes.

ABNORMALITIES OF THE TESTOSTERONE RECEPTOR: ANDROGEN INSENSITIVITY.

Masculinization of the reproductive tract depends upon androgen binding to the androgen receptor protein. Mutations of the X-linked gene coding for the androgen receptor in subjects hemizygous for the mutated gene therefore lead to androgen insensitivity, known in its complete form as testicular feminization syndrome (see Table 207–2). Androgen insensitivity is one of the most frequent forms of male pseudoher-

TABLE 207–2. DISORDERS OF SEXUAL DIFFERENTIATION IN MALES

Disorder	Defective Protein	Gene Localization	Phenotype				Endocrinology	
			Müllerian Ducts	Wolffian Ducts	External Genitalia	Other	Testosterone	AMH
Defects in enzymes involved in testosterone synthesis or metabolism	Side chain cleavage	15q23–24	Absent	Present	Ambiguous		Low	Normal
	17α-hydroxylase	10	Absent	Present	Female	Hypertension	Low	Normal
	3β-HSD type 2	1p13	Absent	Present	Ambiguous	Salt loss	Low	High*
	17β-HSD type 3	9q22	Absent	Present	Female		Low	Normal
	5α-reductase type 2	2p23	Absent	Present	Ambiguous		High	Normal
Androgen insensitivity A. CAIS	Androgen receptor	Xq11–12	Absent	Absent	Female		Normal	High*
B. PAIS	Androgen receptor	Xq11–12	Absent	Present	Ambiguous		Normal	High*
Persistent müllerian duct syndrome	AMH	19p13	Present	Present	Male		Normal	Low
	AMH receptor	12q13	Present	Present	Male		Normal	Normal

* In the neonatal and pubertal period; normal at other times.
AMH = anti-müllerian hormone; 3β-HSD = 3β-hydroxysteroid dehydrogenase; 17β-HSD = 17β-hydroxysteroid dehydrogenase; CAIS = complete androgen insensitivity; PAIS = partial androgen insensitivity.

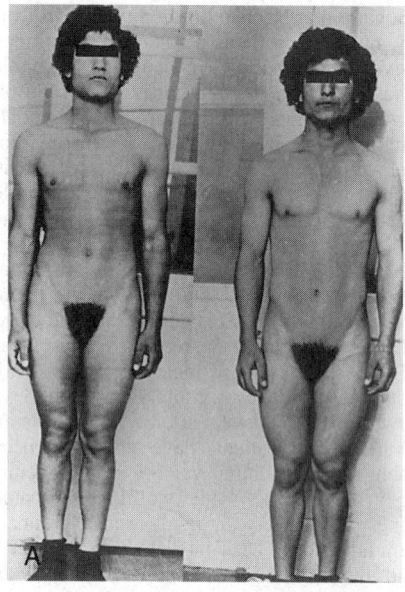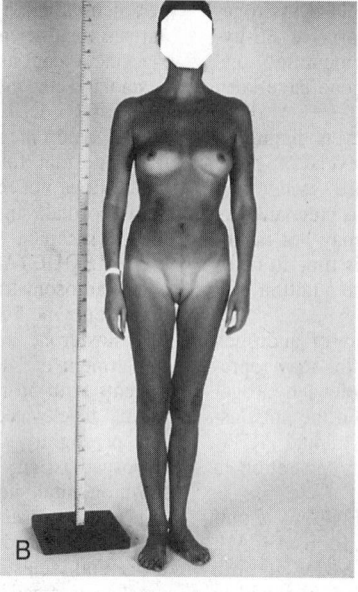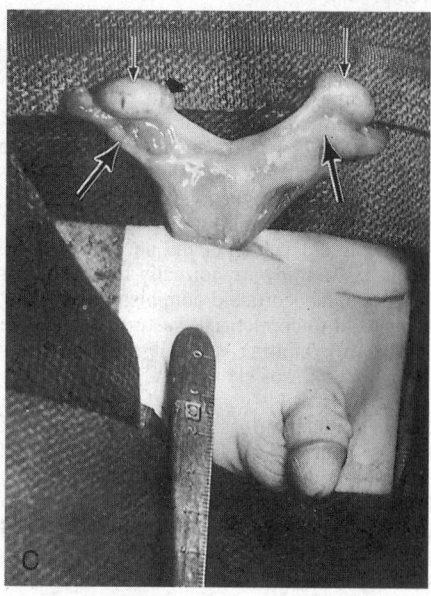

FIGURE 207–9. *A,* Pubertal virilization in brothers with 5α-reductase deficiency. (From Savage MO, Preece MA, Jeffcoate SL, et al.: Familial male pseudohermaphroditism due to deficiency of 5α-reductase. Clin Endocrinol 12:397, 1980.) *B,* Picture of patient with complete androgen insensitivity. *C,* A case of persistent müllerian duct syndrome; operative field. Above the normal, infantile, male genitalia are the contents of the right hernia sac. This consists of the testes *(small arrow)* and fallopian tubes *(large arrow)* which are separated by the uterus. A portion of an epididymis *(arrowhead)* caps the right testis. The vas deferens was palpable posteriorly on both sides. (From Harbison MD, Magid MLS, Josso N, et al.: Anti-Müllerian hormone in three intersex conditions. Ann Genet 34:226, 1991.)

maphroditism; estimates of incidence vary from 1 in 20,000 to 64,000 male births. It causes a spectrum of phenotypic abnormalities.

Clinical Features. Subjects affected by the complete form of androgen insensitivity have a normal female phenotype. They are rarely discovered before puberty unless masses are palpated in the groin or labia and discovered to be testes at surgical exploration. The vagina is usually shallow and ends blindly. Internal genital structures usually are absent, although some cases with residual müllerian derivatives have been described. The testes may be located in the abdomen or in the labia majora and do not undergo spermatogenesis. Testosterone and LH levels are elevated owing to a defective feedback regulation caused by androgen resistance at the level of the hypothalamus. Testicular estrogen production usually is increased; coupled with androgen insensitivity, this results in an unopposed estrogen effect and is the most likely explanation for breast development at puberty. Pubic and axillary hair is scant or absent (Fig. 207–9*B*).

Partial androgen insensitivity, also termed Reifenstein syndrome, presents with a variable degree of genital ambiguity, and both virilization and breast development occur at puberty (see Table 207–2). Partial androgen insensitivity also is consistent with a male phenotype with gynecomastia and infertility as the sole manifestations.

Molecular Genetics and Prenatal Diagnosis. The androgen receptor gene is located on the X chromosome, between Xq13 and Xp11, consistent with the sex-linked recessive mode of inheritance observed in affected families. *De novo* cases are not uncommon, contributing to the negative family history exhibited by approximately one third of complete androgen insensitivity sufferers.

At the cellular level, androgen insensitivity usually can be recognized by studying the affinity of cultured genital skin fibroblasts for DHT, but mutations can affect DNA binding and other aspects of receptor function. Prenatal diagnosis of androgen receptor defects is possible using chorionic villus tissue biopsy and DNA analysis.

Management. Management depends on the severity of the androgen receptor defect. Patients with complete androgen insensitivity should be raised as girls, and the testes should be removed to avoid malignant degeneration, which occurs in 1 to 2% of cases. The optimal time for castration is controversial. Some physicians prefer to delay it until after adolescence, to allow spontaneous feminization to occur. Estrogen treatment is then required to preserve breast development. Management of patients with partial androgen insensitivity is less straightforward because the diagnosis cannot always be confirmed by molecular studies in the neonatal period.

When the phallus is very small and other causes of male pseudohermaphroditism have been excluded, female gender assignment is the best option. Patients with partial androgen insensitivity who are raised as girls should have their testes removed early to avoid unwanted virilization.

PERSISTENT MÜLLERIAN DUCT SYNDROME. Male pseudohermaphroditism due to an isolated defect of AMH synthesis or action is a rare autosomal recessive disorder, characterized by the presence of uterus and tubes, tightly linked to the testes in otherwise normally virilized males. When these are held in the pelvis by the round ligament, they prevent the testes from descending and lead to bilateral cryptorchidism (Fig. 207–9*C*). In most cases, however, müllerian derivatives are mobile and are dragged into the inguinal canal and scrotum by the descending testis, resulting in an apparent inguinoscrotal hernia with contralateral cryptorchidism. The condition usually is discovered only at operation.

A dozen different mutations of the gene coding for AMH have been described in patients with low or undetectable serum concentrations of the hormone. End-organ insensitivities, perhaps due to mutations of the AMH receptor gene, are probably involved in subjects with normal serum levels of AMH. Treatment should aim at preserving fertility through early correction of cryptorchidism, paying great attention to the integrity of the vas deferens, which often is incorporated in the wall of the uterus and cervix.

CONCLUSIONS AND GENERAL MANAGEMENT

Sexual ambiguity, at least in the newborn, should be treated as a pediatric emergency. It may threaten the life of the patient if, as in most cases, the intersex condition is due to CAH and is associated with salt loss. Even if this is not the case, it is important to assign gender as early as possible. Gender identity is established very early in life, certainly by the time speech is established. Gender confusion owing to indeterminant or wrong assignment of gender may lead to severe emotional disorders later in life.

Three diagnostic clues are helpful: gonadal location, presence of a uterus, and karyotype. If no gonads are palpable in a 46,XX chromatin-positive baby, CAH should be suspected before the possibility of true hermaphroditism or idiopathic female pseudohermaphroditism is entertained. In patients with at least one palpable gonad, if a uterus can be visualized by ultrasonography, the most likely diagnosis is testicular dysgenesis in 46,XY subjects and true hermaphroditism or XX maleness in 46,XX subjects. If there are no müllerian derivatives, male pseudohermaphroditism due to testosterone defects or malformations should be considered. It is prudent to wait a few days to assign the gender until common causes of sexual ambiguity are investigated. However, once gender is assigned, the physician should proceed with certainty in counseling parents on the sex of rearing, thus avoiding confusion of gender.

Donahoe PK, Powell DM, Lee MM: Clinical management of intersex abnormalities. Curr Probl Surg 28:519, 1991. *A compendium of surgical approaches in the reconstruction of genital abnormalities.*

George FW, Wilson JD: Sex determination and differentiation. *In* Knobil E, Neill JD (eds.): The Physiology of Reproduction. 2nd ed. New York, Raven Press, 1994, p 3. *An up-to-date overview of the physiology of sex determination.*

Josso N, Cate RL, Picard JY, et al.: Anti-Müllerian hormone, the Jost factor. Rec Progr Hormone Res 48:1, 1993. *An update on AMH.*

McPhaul MJ, Marcelli M, Zoppi S, et al.: Genetic basis of endocrine disease: The spectrum of mutations in the androgen receptor gene that causes androgen resistance. J Clin Endocrinol Metab 76:17, 1993. *A study of the relationship between phenotype and genotype in androgen insensitivity.*

New MI: Congenital adrenal hyperplasia. *In* DeGroot L (ed.): Endocrinology. 3rd ed. Philadelphia, WB Saunders, 1994. *A comprehensive chapter on the various forms of congenital adrenal hyperplasia.*

New MI, White PC, Speiser PW, et al.: Congenital adrenal hyperplasia. *In* Emery AEH, Rimoin DL: Principles and Practice of Medical Genetics. 3rd ed. New York, Churchill Livingstone, 1995. *An overview of the molecular genetics of congenital adrenal hyperplasia.*

Polin RA, Fox WW (eds.): Fetal and Neonatal Physiology, vol 2. Philadelphia, WB Saunders, 1992. *Section XXVIII of this book comprises six chapters on the ovary and testis. Notable is the chapter "Germ Cells and the Indifferent Gonad" by Jirasek.*

Wachtel S (ed.): Molecular Genetics of Sex Determination. New York, Academic Press, 1994. *Articles on the basic biology of sex determination as well as human genetics of sex determination and clinical aspects of syndromes of abnormal sex differentiation.*

Wilson JD, Griffin JE, Russell DW: Steroid 5 alpha-reductase-2 deficiency. Endocr Rev 14:577, 1993. *A study of the molecular genetics of 5α-reductase deficiency.*

208 ENDOCRINOLOGIC DISEASES UNIQUE TO WOMEN

208.1 The Ovaries
Robert W. Rebar

The ovaries episodically release female gametes (oocytes or eggs) and secrete sex steroid hormones, principally androstenedione, estradiol, and progesterone. Oocytes are released only during the adult reproductive years, when sex steroid secretion is also greatest, but the ovaries are physiologically active throughout life.

Sex steroids affect the growth, differentiation, and function of a variety of tissues and organs throughout the body; therefore, abnormalities of the ovaries and of sex steroid secretion should be recognized by all physicians. A rational approach to the diagnosis and treatment of reproductive disorders in women requires an understanding of the functions of the ovaries and of their most important unit, the follicle, throughout life.

EMBRYOLOGY AND ANATOMY OF THE OVARIES

EMBRYOGENESIS AND DIFFERENTIATION (see also Ch. 207). Prior to 6 to 7 weeks of fetal age the gonads are paired, undifferentiated gonadal ridges overlying the mesonephros. By the sixth week of gestation, the primordial germ cells have migrated from their site of origin in the yolk sac to the gonadal ridges. Beginning during the sixth to eighth weeks the ovaries rapidly differentiate, and the number of germ cells, now called oogonia, increases by mitosis to 6 to 7 million. The germ cells next undergo meiosis such that all germ cells (now called oocytes) are arrested in meiotic prophase by the seventh month of gestation. From midgestation onward the number of germ cells progressively decreases until the menopause, by which time virtually no oocytes remain (Fig. 208–1). The germ cells are eliminated from ovaries by *ovulation* and by *atresia* (degeneration), which accounts for the elimination of 99.9% of all germ cells. The development of the ovaries is described in greater detail in Ch. 207.

THE ADULT OVARY. The adult ovary consists of two principal parts: a central medulla surrounded by the predominant outer cortex

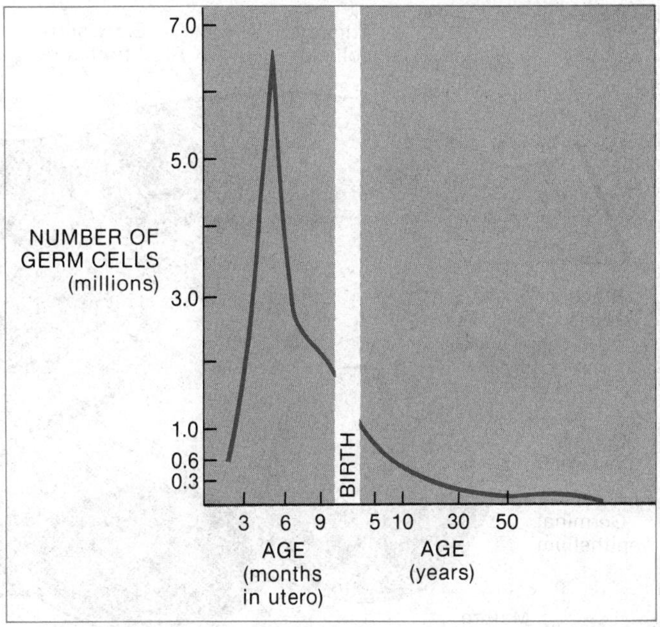

FIGURE 208–1. The number of oocytes present in both ovaries at different ages. (Adapted from Baker TG: *In* Austin CR, Short RJ [eds.]: Reproduction in Mammals. I. Germ Cells and Fertilization. London, Cambridge University Press, 1972, pp 14–45. Reproduced from Rebar RW: Semin Reproduct Endocrinol 1:169–176, 1983.)

(Fig. 208–2). The entire ovary is limited by a single cell layer termed the germinal epithelium. The medulla contains the blood vessels and nerves as well as nests of steroid-secreting hilus or ovarian Leydig cells. The cortex contains the *follicle complexes,* composed of the *oocyte, granulosa cells,* and *theca cells.* Characteristic changes occur in each component during follicle growth and differentiation. Interactions among the follicular components give rise to the gamete (ovum) and to sex steroid hormones necessary for establishing and maintaining early pregnancy following fertilization of the ovum.

Follicles can be divided into two major classes, nongrowing and growing. The nongrowing or *primordial* follicles comprise 90 to 95% of the ovarian follicles throughout the reproductive life of the female. The ability of a woman to menstruate and reproduce depends totally upon the pool of primordial follicles. Each primordial follicle contains a small oocyte arrested in meiotic prophase, surrounded by a layer of squamous cells from which granulosa cells originate. These cells are bounded by the basal lamina, which is selectively permeable to solutes in plasma. This complex is surrounded in turn by stroma, which consists of supporting connective tissue cells, contractile cells, and steroid-secreting thecal interstitial cells. Primordial follicles are recruited sequentially to become growing follicles, which then pass through primary, secondary, and tertiary (or graafian) phases. Atresia may occur in any phase.

Erickson GF, Schreiber JR: Morphology and physiology of the ovary. *In* Becker KL, (eds.): Principles and Practice of Endocrinology and Metabolism. Philadelphia, JB Lippincott, 1990, p 776. *A treatise on follicular growth and development.*

OVARIAN FUNCTION IN CHILDHOOD AND PUBERTY

PHYSICAL CHANGES AT PUBERTY. Puberty extends from the earliest signs of sexual maturation until the attainment of physical, mental, and emotional maturity. Pubertal changes in girls result directly or indirectly from maturation of the hypothalamic-pituitary-ovarian unit. Hormonally, human puberty is characterized by a resetting of the negative gonadal steroid feedback loop, the establishment of new circadian and ultradian (frequent) gonadotropin rhythms, and the acquisition in the female of a positive estrogen feedback loop controlling the menstrual cycle as interdependent expressions of the gonadotropins and ovarian steroids. In girls, pubertal development generally occurs between 8 and 14 years of age. The age of onset and the rate of progress through puberty are vari-

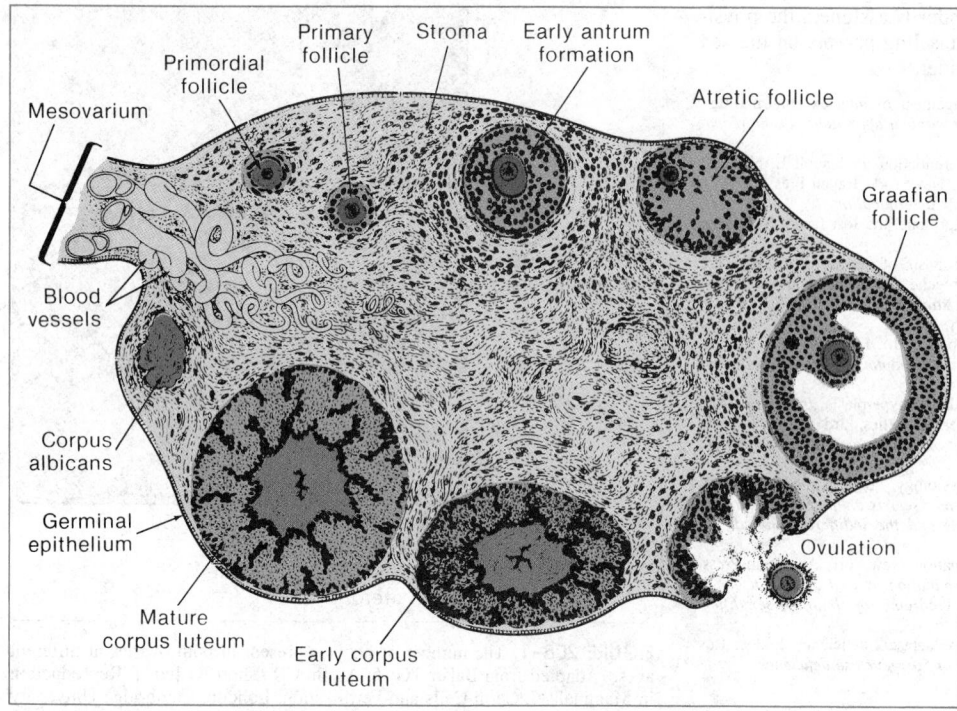

FIGURE 208–2. Diagrammatic illustration of the microscopic anatomy of the ovary. Changes in the components of the follicular complex occurring during atresia and ovulation are shown, progressing clockwise, from a primordial follicle *(upper left)* to a corpus albicans *(lower left)*. (Adapted from Ross GT, Schreiber JR: *In* Yen SSC, Jaffe RB [eds.]: Reproductive Endocrinology—Physiology, Pathophysiology and Clinical Management, 2nd ed. Philadelphia, WB Saunders, 1986, p 115.)

able and depend upon genetic, socioeconomic, nutritional, physical, and psychological factors.

Physical changes occur in an orderly sequence over a definite time frame during puberty (Fig. 208–3). Breast budding in girls is usually the first pubertal change, followed shortly by the appearance of pubic hair, with menarche occurring late in pubertal development. The time from breast budding (median age of onset 9.8 years) to menarche approximates 2 years. Breast development results from increasing ovarian estrogen production and pubic and axillary hair from increasing ovarian androgen production. Estrogens are required for growth of pubic hair as well.

The ovarian sex steroids join with growth hormone and adrenal androgens to produce the adolescent growth spurt. Peak growth velocity is achieved relatively early with little growth observed following menarche. Lean body mass, skeletal mass, and body fat are equal in prepubertal boys and girls, but by maturity women have twice as much body fat and less lean body mass and skeletal mass as men, as a result of differences in sex steroid secretion beginning at puberty. Estrogens are necessary for normal formation, mineralization, and maturation of bones. Well-established standards exist for determining radiographically, typically by examining radiographs of the bones of the wrist, whether bone age is appropriate

for chronologic age. Estrogen deficiencies retard and excesses advance bone age in relation to chronologic age.

HORMONAL CHANGES. The ovaries function even in early childhood. The low levels of luteinizing hormone (LH) and follicle-stimulating hormone (FSH), which are normally present, increase if the ovaries are removed prior to puberty, just as they do later in life, indicating exquisite sensitivity of the hypothalamic-pituitary unit to extremely low circulating sex steroid levels. As puberty nears there is a progressive decrease in sensitivity of the hypothalamic-pituitary unit to sex steroids, leading to increased secretion of pituitary gonadotropins, stimulation of sex steroid output, and the

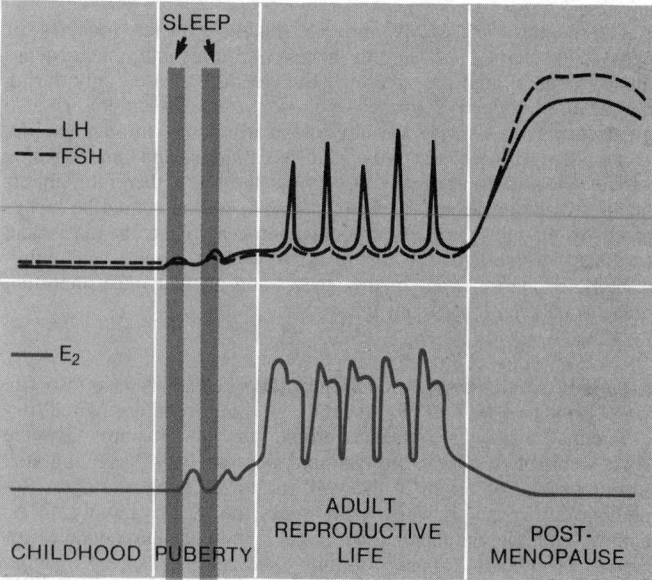

FIGURE 208–4. The changing patterns of LH, FSH, and estradiol (E_2) concentrations in peripheral blood throughout the life of a woman. The elevated levels of LH and FSH present in the first several weeks of life are not shown, nor is the fact that both LH and FSH are secreted in a pulsatile fashion. The pubertal period has been expanded to illustrate the sleep-associated increases in LH and FSH followed by morning increases in E_2 that are observed during puberty. (Reprinted with permission from *Endocrine and Metabolism Continuing Education Quality Control Program,* 1982. Copyright American Association for Clinical Chemistry, Inc.)

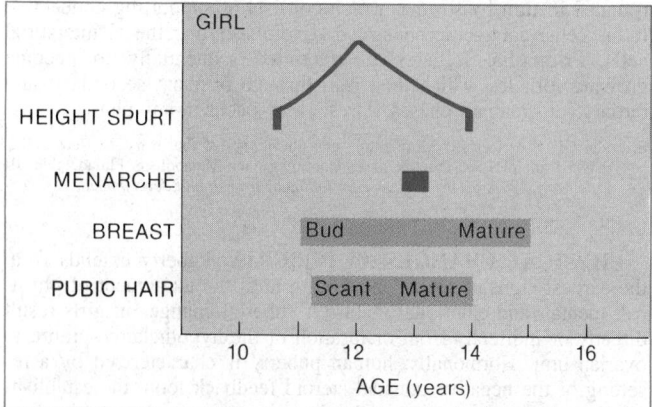

FIGURE 208–3. Temporal sequence of events for the "average" girl during puberty. (Reproduced from Rebar RW: *In* Yen SSC, Jaffe RB [eds.]: Reproductive Endocrinology—Physiology, Pathophysiology and Clinical Management, 3rd ed. Philadelphia, WB Saunders, 1991, p 830.)

development of secondary sex characteristics. Increased secretion of both LH and FSH initially occurs at night with sleep and is associated with increased estradiol secretion the following morning (Fig. 208–4). As is true for most hormones, both LH and FSH are secreted in an episodic or pulsatile rather than a continuous fashion. It is possible that the sleep-entrained pulsatile secretion of gonadotropins commences in response to increased pulsatile secretion of gonadotropin-releasing hormone (GnRH). Later in puberty, secretion of LH and FSH is increased, relative to childhood, throughout the 24-hour period, except during the early follicular phase when nighttime increases still occur. Basal levels of estradiol, the major estrogen secreted by the ovaries, increase throughout puberty. A "critical body mass" may be required for positive estrogen feedback and ovulation. During the first 2 years after menarche, up to 90% of menstrual cycles may be anovulatory because of a delay in the synchronization of the hypothalamic-pituitary-ovarian axis.

ABERRATIONS IN PUBERTAL DEVELOPMENT

DEFINITION. Abnormalities of pubertal development can be divided into four major categories (Table 208–1):

1. *Precocious puberty* represents any pubertal changes before the age of 8 years. The precocious development is *isosexual* when the development is common to the phenotypic sex of the individual and *heterosexual* when the development is characteristic of the opposite sex. *True* or *central precocious puberty* is due to premature maturation of the hypothalamic-pituitary axis. In the absence of increased hypothalamic-pituitary activity, *precocious pseudopuberty* (also known as precocious puberty of peripheral origin) exists.

2. *Delayed (or interrupted) puberty* is defined as the absence of any secondary sex characteristics by the age of 13 years or of menarche by age 16 or by passage of 5 or more years from breast budding to menarche.

3. *Asynchronous pubertal development* occurs when there is deviation from the normal pattern of pubertal development.

4. *Heterosexual pubertal development* is development occurring at the appropriate time, but with some features characteristic of the opposite sex.

PRECOCIOUS PUBERTY. *Differential Diagnosis.* The temporal sequence in which the signs and symptoms of sex steroid hormone excess appear is most important. *Incomplete isosexual precocious puberty* indicates premature development of only a single pubertal feature. If breast budding occurs prior to the age of 8 years in the absence of any other development, the diagnosis may be *premature thelarche*. Premature thelarche is believed due to transient increases in estrogen secretion or increased breast sensitivity to the small quantities of circulating estrogens present prior to puberty. If pubic and/or axillary hair develops alone and persists, *premature pubarche* and *adrenarche* must be considered. These abnormalities are associated with slight increases in adrenal androgen secretion, but not with clitoromegaly or other signs of virilization. These syndromes require no treatment, and affected girls typically begin true puberty at the usual age.

When precocious development is isosexual, the purpose of evaluation is to determine if the cause is central (true precocious puberty) or not. Careful questioning of the patient and her parents may indicate inadvertent ingestion or absorption of sex steroids (ia-

TABLE 208–1. ABERRATIONS OF PUBERTAL DEVELOPMENT

I. Precocious development (before age 8)
  A. Isosexual precocity
    1. Incomplete sexual precocity
      a. Premature thelarche
      b. Premature pubarche
      c. Premature adrenarche
    2. True (central) precocious puberty
      a. Idiopathic (constitutional)
      b. Due to CNS lesions
      c. Primary hypothyroidism
      d. Silver-Russell syndrome
    3. Precocious pseudopuberty (of peripheral origin)
      a. Ovarian neoplasms
      b. Adrenal neoplasms
      c. Iatrogenic (estrogen-containing preparations)
      d. hCG-secreting neoplasms distinct from CNS and ovarian tumors
      e. McCune-Albright syndrome
  B. Heterosexual precocity
    1. Ovarian neoplasms
    2. Adrenal neoplasms
    3. Congenital adrenal hyperplasia
    4. Other rare disorders of sexual differentiation

II. Delayed pubertal development
(no development by age 13; absence of menarche by age 16; passage of 5 years or more from breast budding without menarche)
  A. Anatomic abnormalities
    1. Müllerian agenesis or dysgenesis (Rokitansky-Küster-Hauser syndrome)
    2. Distal genital tract obstruction
      a. Transverse vaginal septum
      b. Imperforate hymen
      c. Vaginal agenesis
  B. Hypergonadotropic hypogonadism (FSH > 30–40 mIU per milliliter)
    1. Gonadal dysgenesis
      a. With stigmata of Turner's syndrome
      b. Pure (46,XX or 46,XY)
      c. Mixed
    2. Ovarian failure with normal ovarian development
      a. Autoimmune disorders
      b. Gonadotropin receptor and/or postreceptor defects (?resistant ovary or Savage syndrome)
      c. Enzymatic defects (17α-hydroxylase deficiency, galactosemia)

      d. Physical causes
        i. Irradiation
        ii. Chemotherapeutic agents
        iii. Viral agents
      e. Idiopathic
  C. Hypogonatotropic or normogonadotropic hypogonadism (LH and FSH < 10 mIU per milliliter or LH and FSH 6–25 mIU per milliliter with at least one being > 10 mIU per milliliter)
    1. Isolated gonadotropin deficiency
      a. In association with midline defects (Kallmann's syndrome)
      b. Independent of associated disorders
    2. Neoplasms of the hypothalamic-pituitary axis
      a. Craniopharyngiomas
      b. Pituitary tumors
      c. Others
    3. Infiltrative processes (Langerhans-type histiocytosis)
    4. Idiopathic hypopituitarism
    5. "Hypothalamic" forms of amenorrhea
      a. Psychogenic
      b. Exercise associated
      c. Associated with malnutrition
      d. Anorexia nervosa
    6. Miscellaneous disorders
      a. Prader-Labhardt-Willi syndrome
      b. Lawrence-Moon-Bardet-Biedl syndrome
      c. Primary hypothyroidism
    7. Constitutional delayed puberty

III. Asynchronous pubertal development
  A. Incomplete forms of androgen insensitivity
  B. Complete forms of androgen insensitivity

IV. Heterosexual pubertal development
  A. Polycystic ovary syndrome
  B. Congenital adrenal hyperplasia (female pseudohermaphroditism)
    1. 21-Hydroxylase deficiency
    2. 11β-Hydroxylase deficiency
    3. 3β-ol-Hydroxysteroid dehydrogenase deficiency
  C. Male pseudohermaphroditism due to 5α-reductase deficiency
  D. Male pseudohermaphroditism due to partial androgen insensitivity
  E. Mixed gonadal dysgenesis
  F. Androgen-producing neoplasms
    1. Ovarian
    2. Adrenal
  G. Cushing's syndrome

trogenic or factitious). About 10% of individuals with true precocious puberty have one of several organic brain diseases, including neoplasms, tuberous sclerosis, neurofibromatosis, encephalitis, meningitis, and hydrocephalus. The seriousness of intracranial lesions mandates that girls with precocious puberty have radiographic evaluation of the central nervous system, most effectively by magnetic resonance imaging (MRI). In almost 90% of girls with true precocious puberty, however, no cause is identified (idiopathic or constitutional).

The physical examination may also provide critical information about the cause of the precocious development. Cutaneous café-au-lait spots, facial asymmetry, polyostotic fibrous dysplasia and other skeletal abnormalities, cranial nerve deficits, and multiple ovarian follicular cysts suggest *McCune-Albright syndrome* in a girl with precocious puberty. It is now known that various clones of cells in the endocrine glands of girls with this disorder function autonomously with respect to cyclic AMP (cAMP) production as a consequence of a mutation within exon 8 of the G protein α subunit. This same mutation probably accounts for the bone lesions and café-au-lait hyperpigmentation. Precocious development associated with short stature, congenital bodily asymmetry, a triangular facies, and clinodactyly suggests the *Silver-Russell syndrome*. Characteristic signs and symptoms may suggest the coexistence of primary hypothyroidism and precocious puberty, especially if galactorrhea is also present. In these patients, thyroid hormone replacement therapy halts progression of pubertal development until the expected age of puberty. (Enigmatically, primary hypothyroidism may also lead to delayed pubertal development. Thyroid hormone replacement permits the onset of puberty.)

Abdominal and rectal examination may reveal a mass, suggesting an adrenal or ovarian tumor. Because palpable ovarian cysts may develop rarely prior to ovulation in true precocious puberty, the presence of a mass need not confirm the diagnosis of precocious pseudopuberty.

When vaginal bleeding is the only sign of development, the diagnosis of sexual precocity should be suspect. Common causes of bleeding in this age group include irritation from a vaginal infection or foreign body, sexual assault, prolapse of the urethral meatus, and ingestion of estrogen-containing medications (most commonly oral contraceptive preparations). A vaginal or cervical neoplasm is also a rare possibility. Thus, vaginal bleeding dictates the need for vaginal examination, often best performed under anesthesia, before further evaluation is undertaken.

Heterosexual precocity in an apparent prepubertal female is almost always due to congenital adrenal hyperplasia or to an androgen-secreting adrenal or ovarian neoplasm. Only very rarely must another disorder of sexual differentiation be considered (see Ch. 207). It is important to examine the external genitalia carefully because congenital adrenal hyperplasia is usually associated with some degree of sexual ambiguity.

Excessive androgens produced endogenously by abnormal fetal adrenal glands *in utero* or diffusing across the placenta to the fetus from the mother can virilize the external genitalia and result in female pseudohermaphroditism. The extent of virilization varies from an enlarged clitoris only to sexual ambiguity sufficient to make gender assignment difficult.

Excessive maternal androgen secretion, typically from an ovarian or adrenal neoplasm, can lead to virilization of a female fetus. This occurs very rarely, because of the great capacity of the placenta to aromatize naturally occurring androgens to estrogens. Virilization of a female fetus is much more likely to occur if a pregnant woman has ingested a synthetic steroid preparation with androgenic properties because available synthetic compounds generally cannot be aromatized.

Excessive androgen secretion beginning *in utero* is usually associated with defective cortisol synthesis. As a consequence, ACTH secretion is increased, resulting in congenital adrenal hyperplasia and excessive androgen secretion. The three different enzyme defects in the steroidogenic pathway that can lead to virilization of the female fetus are described in Ch. 207. 21-Hydroxylase deficiency is the most common form of congenital adrenal hyperplasia, accounting for the disorder in more than 90% of affected individuals. The defect may vary from partial to complete deficiency of the enzyme.

Diagnostic Tests. **Measurement of Peptide and Steroid Hormones.** Increased levels of immunoreactive human chorionic gonadotropin (hCG) may suggest an hCG-secreting neoplasm, most commonly an ovarian teratoma or dysgerminoma. In such cases, the hCG, which is antigenically and biologically similar to LH, stimulates ovarian steroid secretion and pseudopubertal development. Because even specific LH immunoassays show some cross-reactivity with hCG, values for serum LH may be elevated in individuals with hCG-secreting tumors. Immunoreactive hCG is always elevated in the presence of such tumors. Levels and ratios of FSH and LH typical of pubertal as opposed to prepubertal girls help in diagnosing true precocious puberty. Timed urine collections rather than blood samples can be used to measure gonadotropin secretion if necessary. The use of exogenous GnRH to stimulate endogenous LH and FSH secretion can be useful in differentiating gonadotropin-dependent from gonadotropin-independent precocious puberty. Excessively high circulating levels of estrogen suggest an estrogen-producing neoplasm. High levels of serum testosterone suggest an ovarian source of excess androgen in girls with heterosexual development, whereas increased levels of dehydroepiandrosterone (DHEA) or its sulfate (DHEA-S) (the principal precursors of 17-ketosteroids) suggest an adrenal source. High levels of serum 17-hydroxyprogesterone imply congenital adrenal hyperplasia (CAH) secondary to 21-hydroxylase deficiency, whereas high levels of serum 11-deoxycortisol imply an 11β-hydroxylase deficiency. In CAH these hormone levels should decrease promptly following oral administration of suppressive doses of dexamethasone. Suppression in response to exogenous corticoids occurs much less consistently in individuals with adrenal cortical adenomas and carcinomas and rarely in those with ovarian androgen-secreting neoplasms (see Ch. 204.1, 207).

Additional Studies. Ultrasonic scanning of the adrenals and ovaries and computed tomography (CT) of the adrenals may be indicated to confirm clinical suspicions. In girls with ovarian or adrenal neoplasms the tumor can almost always be localized radiographically. Catheterization of the ovarian and adrenal veins and measurements of the effluent steroids from each gland should be pursued only when CT, ultrasonography, or MRI fails to identify what is suspected to be a neoplasm. Although plain skull films are of use in screening for pituitary and parapituitary tumors, CT or MRI of the skull is indicated in the presence of definite neurologic deficits or if true precocious puberty is suspected. Radiographic estimation of bone age is indicated in all cases and serves as a useful tool to follow the results of treatment.

Treatment. Treatment for precocious puberty should be initiated promptly so that: (1) The patient's ultimate height is not compromised as a result of sex steroid–induced premature epiphyseal closure. (2) Emotional disturbances in the patient and her parents are prevented or attenuated.

GnRH analogues are now the preferred therapy for suppressing gonadotropin secretion and also may prevent early bone maturation. The analogues are not effective in children with McCune-Albright syndrome, and ketoconazole or testolactone has been only marginally successful. Medroxyprogesterone acetate (100 to 200 mg intramuscularly every 2 to 4 weeks) also may be used to suppress gonadotropin secretion. Medroxyprogesterone acetate, however, does not always prevent premature epiphyseal closure and the resultant short stature.

Individuals with CNS or steroid-secreting neoplasms must undergo therapy appropriate for the particular lesion. Girls with congenital adrenal hyperplasia are appropriately managed with glucocorticoids (plus mineralocorticoids when indicated) as outlined in Ch. 207.

DELAYED PUBERTY. Typically girls with delayed puberty present at the age of 16 years or later because of primary amenorrhea, but younger girls may present because of failure to initiate pubertal development. Because of the anxiety generated by delayed puberty, some evaluation is always indicated regardless of the age of the patient.

When pubertal development progresses normally but menstruation does not begin, an abnormality in the genital tract should be considered. Congenital malformations of the müllerian ducts are uncommon, occurring in 0.02% of all women. Most do not cause amenorrhea, and many do not impair reproduction. The anomalies associated with amenorrhea vary in severity from an imperforate hymen to complete aplasia of all müllerian duct derivatives with vaginal atresia. Although aplasia generally involves all of the müllerian duct derivatives, defects may involve only a single part of the distal genital tract.

A müllerian duct anomaly is suggested by (1) normal levels of serum gonadotropins and steroids, (2) an abnormal outflow tract, (3) a history of cyclic abdominal pain with or without a palpable mass, and (4) normal development of secondary sex characteristics. Normal ovarian function still induces endometrial growth and shedding after menarche if the uterus is normal. In the absence of a normal outflow tract, however, the menstrual effluent is retained and may or may not be able to escape into the abdominal cavity. Free in the abdominal cavity, the effluent may cause endometriosis. Constrained to the uterine cavity, the effluent causes hematometra and a large abdominal mass. In the absence of a mass or cyclic pain, a karyotype is indicated in girls with evidence of an abnormal genital tract to rule out any of several disorders of sexual differentiation (see Ch. 207). Such disorders, however, almost never occur together with completely normal pubertal development. In girls with a normal karyotype and a genital tract anomaly, examination under anesthesia and diagnostic laparoscopy should be undertaken to delineate the extent of the defect. When the abnormality consists of an imperforate hymen or transverse vaginal septum only, surgical restoration can be accomplished relatively simply. Attempts to provide an outflow tract for the uterus should not be undertaken if there is no cervix because of the high risk of recurrent pelvic infection. Even with a functional cervix, the creation of an outflow tract that will permit successful pregnancy is unlikely. A functional vagina can be created surgically or by the daily use of ever-larger dilators. To prevent shrinkage and scarring, surgery should be deferred until the patient is willing to use dilators postoperatively on a daily basis or she is about to become sexually active.

Other causes of delayed puberty and primary amenorrhea are the same as those that may cause amenorrhea in older women (see below). When no apparent cause for delayed development is found, constitutional delayed puberty must be entertained as a diagnosis of exclusion. A strong family history of delayed maturation adds support to this presumption. Small doses of estrogen may be administered to induce some pubertal development but may obscure a pathologic cause for the delay and may compromise linear growth and ultimate height.

ASYNCHRONOUS PUBERTAL DEVELOPMENT. Asynchronous pubertal development is characteristic of male pseudohermaphroditism due to androgen insensitivity, especially complete testicular feminization. This syndrome of androgen insensitivity is inherited either as an X-linked recessive or as a sex-limited autosomal dominant trait. Despite the presence of intra-abdominal or inguinal testes, there is complete failure of virilization. Affected individuals develop breasts (but only to Tanner stage 3) and a typical female habitus with unambiguous female external genitalia but with absence of internal female structures, generally having only a foreshortened blind-ending vagina. Little or no pubic and axillary hair develops. The karyotype is obviously 46,XY in these individuals. Circulating testosterone levels are equivalent to or higher than those found in normal men, and LH levels are elevated while FSH levels are normal compared to those in menstruating women. This syndrome is further discussed in Ch. 207.

HETEROSEXUAL PUBERTAL DEVELOPMENT. *Polycystic ovary (PCO) syndrome,* by far the most common cause of heterosexual pubertal development, is associated with the development of some secondary sex features characteristic of males at the normal age of puberty. Feminization occurs in affected girls, and they develop normal breasts and a typical female habitus, but masculinization also occurs. (In contrast, girls with congenital adrenal hyperplasia generally show little if any female development at puberty.) A heterogeneous syndrome, PCO syndrome most typically begins at or near puberty with hirsutism and irregular menses from the time of menarche. Menarche may be delayed as well, so that young women may present with primary amenorrhea. Basal LH levels tend to be somewhat elevated in perhaps 80% of cases, and circulating levels of all androgens are elevated moderately.

Congenital adrenal hyperplasia is generally diagnosed prior to puberty, and heterosexual precocious pseudopuberty is typical. However, if the defect is mild and changes to the external genitalia are minimal, masculinization may occur at the expected age of puberty. This attenuated or nonclassic form of 21-hydroxylase deficiency seems to occur in families with a strong family history of

hirsutism. Affected girls generally have some defeminization with flattening of the breasts, severe hirsutism, relatively short stature, and obesity.

Mixed gonadal dysgenesis designates asymmetric gonadal development, with a germ cell tumor or a testis on one side and an undifferentiated streak, rudimentary gonad, or no gonad on the other. The extent of genital virilization prior to puberty is variable in this rare disorder. The vast majority are reared as girls, in whom virilization occurs at puberty; some may note breast development as well. Affected individuals generally have a mosaic karyotype, with 45,X/46,XY being most common. Short stature and other stigmata associated with a 45,X karyotype in Turner's syndrome are less common in patients with tumors than in patients with testes. Gonadectomy is indicated in all individuals with a Y chromosome to eliminate the increased neoplastic potential of such dysgenetic gonads and in all patients in whom virilization occurs at puberty to remove the source of androgen. Estrogen replacement therapy is warranted following gonadectomy. Other causes of male pseudohermaphroditism associated with heterosexual pubertal development are described in Ch. 207.

An androgen-producing neoplasm or Cushing's syndrome may occur rarely during the pubertal years and lead to heterosexual development.

Marshall WA, Tanner JM: Variations in the pattern of pubertal changes in girls. Arch Dis Child 44:291, 1969. *A classic paper that is required reading for all serious students.*
Simpson JL, Rebar RW: Normal and abnormal sexual differentiation and development. *In* Becker KL, et al. (eds.): Principles and Practice of Endocrinology and Metabolism. Philadelphia, JB Lippincott, 1990, p 710. *A detailed discussion of the disorders of sexual differentiation organized similarly to the discussion in this chapter.*
Styne DM, Grumbach MM: Puberty in the male and female. Its physiology and disorders. *In* Yen SSC, Jaffe RB (eds.): Reproductive Endocrinology, 3rd ed. Philadelphia, WB Saunders, 1991, p 511. *A detailed and excellently referenced discussion of normal and abnormal pubertal development.*

THE NORMAL MENSTRUAL CYCLE

CHARACTERISTICS OF THE MENSTRUAL CYCLE. Between menarche at approximately age 12 years and the menopause at about age 51 years, the reproductive organs of normal women undergo a series of closely coordinated changes at approximately monthly intervals that together comprise the normal menstrual cycle. The menstrual cycle is the expression of the coordinated interactions of the hypothalamic-pituitary-ovarian axis, with associated changes in the target tissues (endometrium, cervix, vagina) of the reproductive tract.

A menstrual cycle begins with the first day of genital bleeding (day 1; menses) and ends just prior to the next menstrual period. The median menstrual cycle length is 28 days, but normal ovulatory menstrual cycles may range from about 21 to 40 days in length. Menstrual cycles vary most greatly in length in the years immediately following menarche and in the years immediately preceding menopause, largely because of an increased incidence of anovulatory cycles. Irregularities in menstrual cycle length also may be caused by abrupt changes in diet, exercise, or environment; serious emotional disturbances; and following parturition or abortion. The menstrual cycle can be divided into three distinct phases: *follicular, ovulatory,* and *luteal.*

The Follicular or Preovulatory Phase. Variable in length, the follicular phase begins with the first day of menstrual bleeding and extends to the day prior to the preovulatory LH surge. A rise in serum FSH begins in the late luteal phase of the previous menstrual cycle, continues into the early follicular phase, and initiates growth and development of a group of follicles (Fig. 208–5). The preovulatory follicle destined for ovulation is selected from this cohort in a manner that is not yet understood. Circulating LH levels rise slowly throughout the follicular phase, but FSH levels fall after the early follicular phase increase. Approximately 7 to 8 days before the preovulatory LH surge, estradiol (E_2) and estrone (E_1) begin to increase, generally reaching a maximum on the day before or the day of the LH surge. The divergence in LH and FSH levels may be related to the follicular secretion of *inhibin* (folliculostatin), a hormone that specifically inhibits the release of FSH. Several days before the LH surge, plasma androgens (androstenedione and testosterone) and some progestins (17α-hydroxyprogesterone and 20α-dihydroprogesterone) begin to increase. They peak on the day

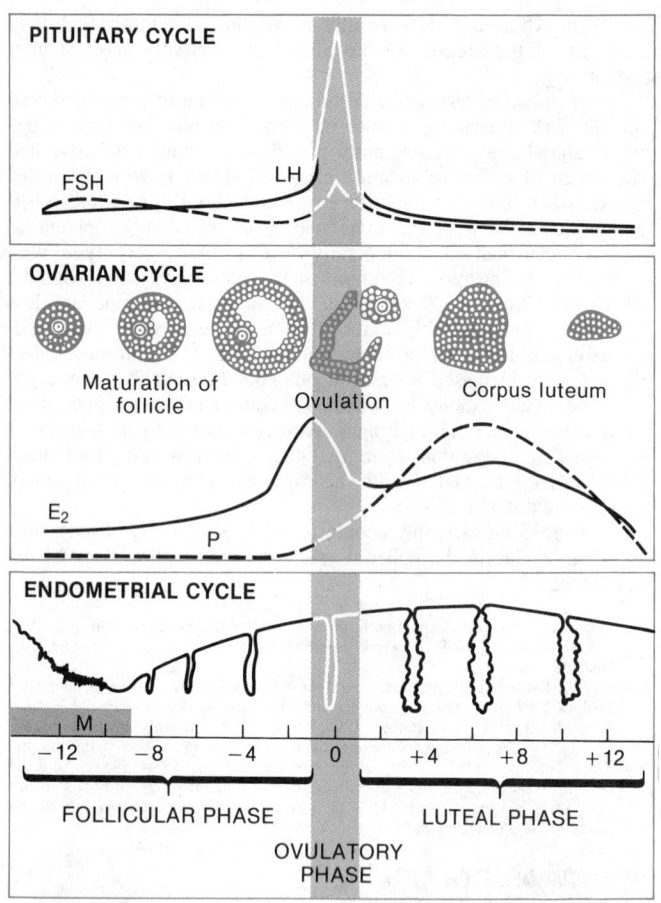

PITUITARY CYCLE

FSH

LH

OVARIAN CYCLE

Maturation of
follicle

Ovulation

Corpus luteum

E_2

P

ENDOMETRIAL CYCLE

M

−12   −8   −4   0   +4   +8   +12

FOLLICULAR PHASE   LUTEAL PHASE

OVULATORY
PHASE

FIGURE 208–5. The idealized cyclic changes observed in gonadotropins, estradiol (E_2), progesterone (P), and uterine endometrium during the normal menstrual cycle. The data are centered on the day of the LH surge (day 0). Days of menstrual bleeding are indicated by M. (Reprinted with permission from *Endocrine and Metabolism Continuing Education Quality Control Program*, 1982. Copyright American Association for Clinical Chemistry, Inc.)

of the LH surge. Progesterone itself does not increase until just prior to the onset of the LH surge.

The Ovulatory Phase. During this phase the ovum is released from the mature graafian follicle about 32 to 34 hours after the onset of the preovulatory surge of LH by the pituitary gland. The ovulatory phase extends from 1 day prior to the LH surge to 1 day following the LH surge. Some women experience brief (a few minutes to few hours in length), dull, unilateral pelvic pain near the time of ovulation, termed *mittelschmerz*. The association of this pain to ovulation is unknown, but it may be due to leakage of follicular fluid into the abdominal cavity at ovulation. *Mittelschmerz* may occur before or after actual ovulation or not at all in ovulatory women. During the ovulatory phase a rapid rise in plasma LH results in response to positive estrogen feedback, leading to final maturation of the follicle and to ovulation. As peak LH levels are reached, E_2 levels drop, but progesterone levels continue to increase.

The Luteal or Postovulatory Phase. The more constant half of the menstrual cycle, the luteal phase, is approximately 14 days in length and ends with the onset of menses. This phase represents the functional lifespan of the corpus luteum ("yellow body") of the ovary, which supports the released ovum by secreting progesterone. In the luteal phase, progesterone secretion increases to peak 6 to 8 days after the LH surge. Parallel but smaller increases in 17α-hydroxyprogesterone, E_2, and E_1 levels also occur. Progesterone levels decrease toward menses unless the ovum is fertilized and pregnancy results. The finding of serum progesterone levels greater than 10 ng per milliliter 1 week prior to menses is probably diagnostic of normal ovulation. Progestins increase basal morning body temperature so that a "thermogenic shift" of more than 0.3° C occurring after a nadir is a presumptive sign of ovulation and proges-

terone secretion. Unfortunately, taking basal temperatures on a daily basis is tedious, subject to error, and not very reliable.

CYCLIC CHANGES IN TARGET ORGANS. *Endometrium.* During the menstrual cycle the endometrium undergoes remarkable histologic and cytologic changes, which culminate with menstrual bleeding when the corpus luteum ceases to secrete progesterone. The *basal layer of the endometrium,* which is not lost during menses, then regenerates the *superficial layer* of compact epithelial cells lining the uterine cavity and an *intermediate layer of spongiosa,* both of which are shed at each menstruation. Endometrial glands in these layers proliferate under the influence of estrogen in the follicular phase so that the mucosa thickens. In the luteal phase, under the influence of progesterone, the glands become coiled and secretory, with increased vascularity and edema of the stroma. As both E_2 and progesterone decline in the late luteal phase, the stroma becomes increasingly edematous, endometrial and blood vessel necrosis occurs, and endometrial bleeding ensues. Local release of prostaglandins may initiate vasospasm and ischemic necrosis in the endometrium as well as the uterine contractions accompanying menstrual flow. Thus prostaglandin synthetase inhibitors can relieve dysmenorrhea (menstrual cramping). Fibrinolytic activity in the endometrium also peaks at the time of menstruation, accounting for the noncoagulability of menstrual blood. Because the histologic changes during the menstrual cycle are so characteristic, endometrial biopsies are used to date the stage of the cycle and to assess the tissue response to gonadal steroids.

Cervix and Cervical Mucus. During the follicular phase, cervical vascularity, congestion, and edema increase progressively under the influence of estrogen. The external cervical os opens to a diameter of 3 mm at ovulation and then decreases to 1 mm. Cervical mucus increases in quantity (10- to 30-fold) and in elasticity. "Palm leaf" arborization (ferning) becomes prominent just prior to ovulation (if cervical mucus is allowed to dry on a glass slide and is examined microscopically). Under the influence of progesterone during the luteal phase, cervical mucus thickens, becomes less watery, and loses its elasticity and ability to fern. The characteristics of cervical mucus are useful clinically to evaluate the stage of the cycle and the amount of estrogen present.

Vagina. When ovarian estrogen secretion is low, as in the early follicular phase, vaginal epithelium is pale and thin. In the follicular phase under the influence of estrogens the epithelium thickens, and the number of mature cornified epithelial cells increases. During the luteal phase, progesterone causes a decrease in the percentage of cornified cells and an increase in the number of precornified intermediate cells and polymorphonuclear leukocytes. There is also increased cellular debris and clumping of shed desquamated cells. Histologic changes in the vaginal epithelium and in the cervical mucus are the most sensitive indicators of estrogen status in the body. However, the reliability of vaginal smears depends upon the absence of infection or exogenously administered steroid hormones that have antiestrogenic effects. Steroid hormones also facilitate progression of spermatozoa toward the ovaries and of ova toward the uterine cavity through effects on the fallopian tubes.

Ovary. A small primordial follicle with a diameter of 50 μm transforms and grows into a mature graafian follicle 1 to 2 cm in diameter in two distinct phases: (1) The oocyte and follicle grow to form a *primary follicle,* apparently independent of gonadotropin control. The oocyte increases tenfold in diameter (from 15 to 150 μm) and becomes surrounded by a zona pellucida, a translucent "shell" of glycoproteins. In addition, the single layer of cells surrounding the oocyte becomes cuboidal and takes on the characteristics of granulosa cells. (2) In a second phase completely dependent upon gonadotropin and steroid hormones, the follicular unit develops into a *mature graafian follicle,* which is capable of being released in response to the midcycle surge of LH and FSH. Under the influence of FSH, granulosa cells acquire specific receptors for FSH, undergo mitosis, multiply to form secondary follicles consisting of several granulosa cell layers, and also acquire the ability to aromatize androgens to estrogens. Simultaneously, thecal interstitial cells begin to develop around the basement membrane surrounding the granulosa cells, develop specific cell membrane receptors for LH, and synthesize and secrete androgens, primarily Δ^4-androstenedione and testosterone, in response to LH. The androgens can diffuse across the basement lamina where they are aromatized to estrogens. The rising E_2 in the follicular phase then feeds back on the hypothalamic-pituitary unit via the systemic circulation (Fig. 208–6).

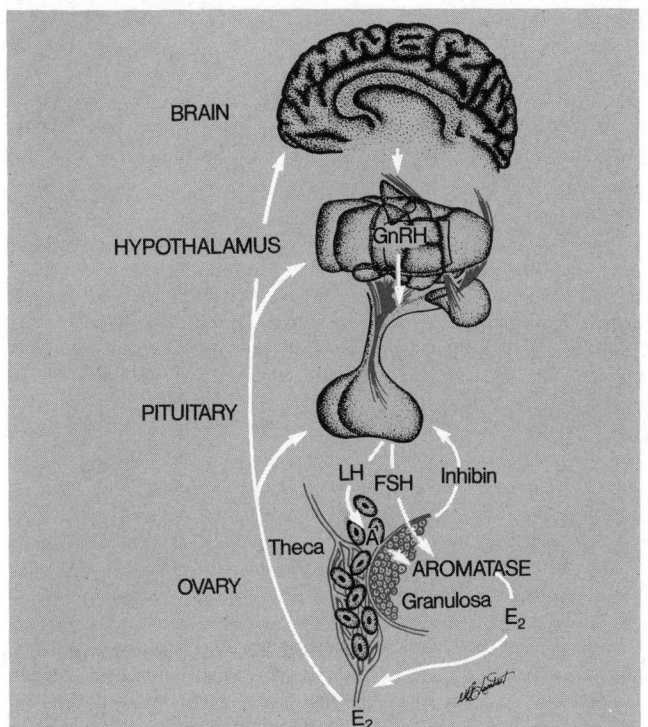

FIGURE 208-6. The hypothalamic-pituitary-ovarian axis in the regulation of follicular maturation and steroidogenesis. A = androgens; E_2 = estradiol. (Modified from *Endocrine and Metabolism Continuing Education Quality Control Program,* 1982. Copyright American Association for Clinical Chemistry, Inc.)

The so-called *two-cell theory* holds that both granulosa and theca cells are required for estrogen biosynthesis and maturation of the follicle.

A tertiary graafian follicle that contains an antrum or fluid-filled cavity increases from 200 μm to 1 to 2 cm in diameter, primarily because of accumulation of follicular fluid, again under the direct control of FSH. In tertiary follicles, FSH induces the appearance of specific LH receptors on granulosa cell membranes. These LH receptors are responsible for the stimulation of progesterone secretion prior to ovulation (luteinization) and for continued production of progesterone in the luteal phase.

Approximately 2 weeks are required for the presumptive preovulatory follicle to complete its growth and expel a mature oocyte. The oocyte is inhibited from resuming meiotic maturation by granulosa cell–oocyte interaction and an oocyte maturation inhibitor (OMI) until following the LH-FSH surge. Within 36 hours of the onset of the surge, the oocyte completes the first meiotic division (reduction to 22 + X chromosomes) and a first polar body is extruded. The second meiotic division is completed only if the oocyte is fertilized by a spermatozoon. During the LH-FSH surge the preovulatory follicle bulges above the surface of the ovary. A stigma or avascular area develops on the follicle surface. Under the influence of local prostaglandins, plasminogen activator, and other hormones, a cluster of granulosa cells surrounding the oocyte and the oocyte itself (together known as the cumulus oophorus) are extruded.

The corpus luteum is formed from the granulosa and theca cells of the former preovulatory follicle following ovulation and secretes progesterone and E_2 for approximately 14 days. It then degenerates unless fertilization occurs. The lifespan of the corpus luteum may depend in part upon prostaglandins and prolactin as well as upon progestin. If fertilization occurs, hCG, which is similar to LH, is secreted by the developing blastocyst and helps to support the corpus luteum until the fetoplacental unit can support itself. Pregnancy tests in common use have been developed utilizing antibodies to the specific β subunit of hCG and have little if any cross-reactivity with LH.

OVARIAN STEROIDOGENESIS. The ovaries and the developing follicles synthesize sex steroid hormones (estrogens, androgens, and progestins), which play important roles in feedback regu-

lation of the menstrual cycle and in preparing the uterus to accept a fertilized ovum via two separate pathways: (1) the so-called Δ^5 pathway, in which 17α-hydroxypregnenolone and DHEA with double bonds between carbons 5 and 6 are intermediates, and (2) the Δ^4 pathway, in which pregnenolone is converted to progesterone and in which 17α-hydroxyprogesterone and androstenedione with double bonds between carbons 4 and 5 are the alternative intermediates (Fig. 208–7).

Although cholesterol as substrate for steroid synthesis is obtained normally from circulating low-density lipoproteins (LDL's), it can be synthesized *de novo* from two-carbon fragments (acetate). Different structures and cells within the ovary synthesize different steroids, in part because of stimulation by the gonadotropins. Gonadotropin binding to its receptor activates adenylate cyclase and stimulates cAMP production. The cAMP in turn activates protein kinases that catalyze phosphorylation of proteins to mediate the cellular effects of each gonadotropin (see Ch. 199). LH also increases phosphatidylinositides within the ovary. LH acts primarily to regulate the first step in steroid hormone biosynthesis, that is, the conversion of cholesterol to pregnenolone. FSH acts to aromatize androgens to estrogens. Thus, LH acts to enhance substrate flow and the synthesis of androgens and/or progesterone. In the absence of LH, FSH action is reduced because of diminished substrate for aromatization.

Androgens, primarily androstenedione and testosterone, are secreted by interstitial and theca cells and serve as the substrate for the granulosa cell aromatase enzyme for synthesis of estrogens. Androstenedione, the major ovarian androgen, can also be converted to testosterone and estrogens in peripheral tissues. When ovarian androgen synthesis is excessive, as in ovarian androgen-producing tumors, or when conversion of androgen to estrogen in the ovary is reduced, as in PCO syndrome, hirsutism and even virilism can result. Testosterone, the most biologically potent androgen, is bound tightly to sex hormone–binding globulin (SHBG; also known as testosterone-estradiol–binding globulin, TeBG) so that only about 1% of circulating testosterone is biologically free and active. Secretion rates and circulating concentrations in normal adult premenopausal women are given in Table 208–2.

Estrogens are produced predominantly in ovarian follicles by granulosa cell aromatization of the A ring of theca cell androgens. Naturally occurring estrogens are 18-carbon steroids, which by definition stimulate proliferation of the endometrium and bind to specific, saturable cytosolic receptors. The amount of estrogen secretion depends on the phase of the menstrual cycle (Table 208–2). In the early follicular phase the secretion rates of E_2 and E_1 are almost equal (60 to 170 μg per day). As the dominant follicle is selected, E_2 secretion increases to as much as 800 μg per day, with almost all the E_2 synthesized by the dominant follicle. The corpus luteum also produces significant quantities of E_2 (250 μg per day). In the late follicular and luteal phases, E_1 secretion is about one-fourth that of estradiol. The dominant follicle and corpus luteum synthesize about 95% of circulating E_2; E_1 is of little significance in the ovulating woman. In the postmenopausal years, however, E_1 becomes the predominant estrogen in the absence of functioning follicles. E_1 is synthesized by peripheral conversion of adrenal androgens, especially androstenedione. As much estrogen is synthesized during the 9 months of pregnancy as would be synthesized during 100 years of normal menstrual cycles.

Progesterone synthesis is low in the follicular phase, but increases to 10 to 40 mg per day during the luteal phase (Table 208–2). Should pregnancy occur, progesterone production increases to as much as 300 mg per day at term. Why the corpus luteum atrophies at about 14 days is not known, but it may be due to the effects of intraovarian estrogen and/or prostaglandins. However, LH stimulation is required for progesterone production by the corpus luteum. Progesterone induces secretory changes in the endometrium in preparation for implantation of the fertilized ovum.

INTRAOVARIAN CONTROL OF FOLLICULAR DEVELOPMENT. Although the secretion of E_2 by granulosa cells is critical for the occurrence of normal menstrual cycles, any role for E_2 within the ovary in regulating follicular development in women is now questioned. Nuclear estrogen and progesterone receptors do not appear in the granulosa cells of the dominant follicle in women until just prior to the LH surge, and androgen receptors cannot be

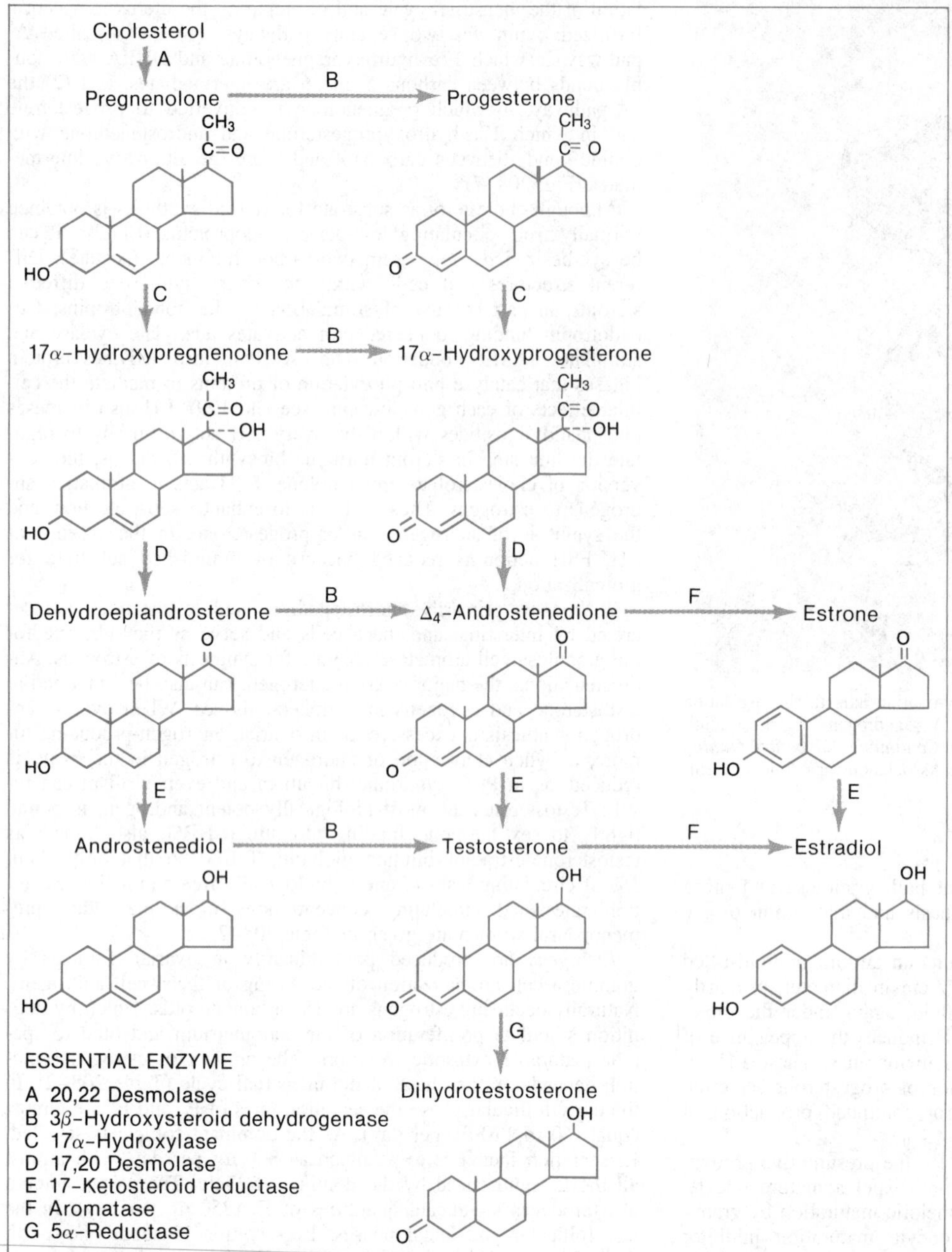

FIGURE 208–7. Steps in ovarian biosynthesis of steroid hormones. (Modified from data of Ross GT: *In* Rudolph AM [ed.]: Pediatrics 16:1726, 1977. Copyright American Academy of Pediatrics 1977.)

identified in either granulosa or theca cells until the secondary stage of development. Because steroids act by binding to these receptors, it appears that steroids are not essential for follicular development. Consistent with this conclusion is the surprising observation that normal follicular growth and development and successful fertilization *in vitro* can be accomplished with use of exogenous gonadotropins in women with 17α-hydroxylase deficiency, who have no ability to synthesize androgens and estrogens (Fig. 208–7).

Several peptides secreted by granulosa cells appear to play critical roles in intraovarian regulation of follicular development, whereas steroids are important for neuroendocrine feedback regulation and preparation of the endometrium to receive the fertilized oocyte. Although the physiologic roles of these peptides remain to be defined precisely, inhibin, insulin-like growth factors (IGF) I and II and their binding proteins, and perhaps other growth factors as well appear to have modulatory effects on follicular development. At present this is an evolving area of knowledge with potential implications for developing new strategies to induce ovulation in anovulatory women.

NEUROENDOCRINE REGULATION OF THE OVARIES.

Neurons containing various peptide hormones that can release or inhibit secretion of the gonadotropins are found in the hypothalamus

(see Ch. 201). Specifically, cells containing GnRH occur in the area including the arcuate nucleus and median eminence and the preoptic area. Axons from these neurons run in the tuberoinfundibular tract and terminate on capillaries within the median eminence; this allows for delivery of their products through the portal vascular system to the anterior pituitary gland. It appears that classic neurotransmitters, including norepinephrine, dopamine, and serotonin, as well as neuromodulators, such as endogenous opiates and prostaglandins, influence secretion of GnRH by the hypothalamus. In addition, estrogens and androgens bind to cells in the hypothalamus and the anterior pituitary, and progestins bind to cells in the hypothalamus to influence hypothalamic-pituitary regulation of ovarian function.

GnRH is secreted in a pulsatile fashion (perhaps because of an inherent oscillator within the arcuate nucleus) and is responsible for pulsatile release of gonadotropins. Pulsatile gonadotropin release in turn appears to account for the pulsatile secretion of sex steroids from the ovaries. The ovarian sex steroids then feed back on the hypothalamic-pituitary unit to modulate both the frequency and amplitude of the gonadotropin pulse (see Fig. 208–6). Thus, gonadotropin pulses vary throughout the menstrual cycle. Pulses occur at approximately 60- to 90-minute intervals in the

TABLE 208-2. CONCENTRATIONS, METABOLIC CLEARANCE RATES, PRODUCTION RATES, AND OVARIAN SECRETION RATES OF SEX STEROID HORMONES IN BLOOD

Steroid	Plasma MCR (liters/day)	Binding	Phase of Menstrual Cycle or Stage of Life	Plasma Concentration (ng/dl)	Plasma Production Rate (μg/day)	Ovarian Secretion Rate (μg/day)
Androstenedione	2000	Albumin	Premenopausal	40–240	3200	800–1600
			Postmenopausal	30–120	1600	
Testosterone	700	TeBG, albumin	Premenopausal	19–70	260	
			Postmenopausal	15–70	150	
Estradiol	1350	TeBG, albumin	Early follicular	2.5–6	70–200	60–170
			Late follicular	20–40	445–945	400–800
			Midluteal	15–25	270	250
			Postmenopausal	< 1.0–2.5		
Estrone	2200	Albumin	Early follicular	2–6	70–200	60–170
			Late follicular	10–20	300–600	250–500
			Midluteal	10–15	240	160
			Postmenopausal	1.5–5.0	55	
Progesterone	2200	CBG, albumin	Follicular	3–10	700–2500	1500
			Luteal	10–25	3000–30,000	24,000

CBG = Cortisol-binding globulin; MCR = metabolic clearance rate; TeBG = testosterone-estradiol–binding globulin.

follicular phase and at intervals of >180 minutes in the luteal phase.

Gonadal steroids can exert both negative and positive feedback effects on gonadotropin secretion. Among ovarian steroids, 17β-estradiol is the most potent inhibitor of gonadotropin secretion, acting on both the hypothalamus and the pituitary. For women to ovulate, E_2 must also elicit a positive feedback effect on gonadotropin release. The feedback effects are both time and dose dependent. In the normal menstrual cycle the positive feedback action of E_2 leading to the LH surge is preceded by a period when lower E_2 levels are present with their negative feedback effects.

It appears that the ovary is the "clock" for the timing of ovulation, with the hypothalamus stimulating pulsatile release of the gonadotropins. The follicle complex and corpus luteum develop in response to gonadotropin stimulation. For appropriate ovarian regulation of reproductive function in women, three biologic characteristics are necessary: (1) an appropriate balance and sequence of negative and positive feedback actions; (2) differential feedback effects on the release of LH and FSH; (3) local intraovarian controls on follicular growth and maturation, separate from but interrelated to the effects of gonadotropins on the ovaries.

Erickson GF, Schreiber JR: Morphology and physiology of the ovary. *In* Becker KL (eds.): Principles and Practice of Endocrinology and Metabolism. Philadelphia, JB Lippincott, 1990, p 776. *A detailed discussion of ovarian function.*

Richardson GS: Steroidogenesis. *In* Sciarra JJ (ed.): Gynecology and Obstetrics. Vol. 5. Philadelphia, Harper and Row, 1986 (rev. ed.), p 1. *A detailed summary of the steroidogenic pathway.*

Speroff L, Glass RH, Kase NG: Regulation of the menstrual cycle. *In* Clinical Gynecologic Endocrinology and Infertility, 5th ed. Baltimore, Williams & Wilkins, 1994, p 183. *A detailed and up-to-date summary of what is currently known about the human menstrual cycle.*

ABNORMALITIES OF THE REPRODUCTIVE YEARS

DYSMENORRHEA AND ENDOMETRIOSIS. Dysmenorrhea, perhaps the most common of all gynecologic disorders, affects about 50% of postpubertal women. Dysmenorrhea can be classified as primary or secondary.

Primary dysmenorrhea occurs only in ovulatory cycles. Prostaglandins that are released from the endometrium just prior to and during menstruation cause contraction of uterine smooth muscle and produce dysmenorrhea by initiating painful, exaggerated uterine contractions and myometrial ischemia. Associated systemic symptoms include nausea, diarrhea, headache, and emotional changes. Primary dysmenorrhea is much more common than is secondary dysmenorrhea.

In *secondary dysmenorrhea* there is a pathologic cause for the dysmenorrhea. Endometriosis, the ectopic occurrence of endometrial tissue generally within the abdominal cavity, is the most common cause in severe cases. Other possible causes include pelvic inflammatory disease, congenital abnormalities such as atresia of a portion of the distal genital tract and cystic duplication of the paramesonephric ducts, and cervical stenosis.

Prostaglandin synthetase inhibitors such as naproxen, ibuprofen, mefenamic acid, and indomethacin are the mainstays of treatment. If the dysmenorrhea is still severe, addition of an oral contraceptive preparation to inhibit ovulation and limit prostaglandin release is generally effective. In cases in which the pelvic pain still remains intractable, additional evaluation is warranted. If thorough evaluation of the gastrointestinal and urinary tracts fails to reveal a definitive cause, examination under anesthesia and diagnostic laparoscopy may be indicated.

If endometriosis is diagnosed at laparoscopy, treatment varies, depending on the severity of the disease and the goals of the patient regarding fertility. It may be possible to fulgurate implants or lyse adhesions through the laparoscope. In general, endometriosis should be treated medically, with additional surgery deferred until infertility (if present) becomes manifest. Medical therapy can consist of continuous suppression with GnRH analogues, progestins, oral contraceptive agents, or danazol for 3 to 6 months. GnRH analogues are rapidly becoming the most frequent form of medical suppressive therapy. After a course of therapy, use of oral contraceptive agents probably should be continued until fertility is desired. Conservative surgical resection of endometriotic tissue should almost always be deferred until it is established as the cause of infertility. Surgery may be required, however, for continuing severe pain, severe endometriosis, or large ovarian cysts containing endometriosis (endometriomas). If symptoms continue despite adequate treatment or if psychological overlay is suspected, psychiatric evaluation may be indicated. Medical causes of dysmenorrhea, however, should be eliminated first.

PREMENSTRUAL SYNDROME. Premenstrual syndrome (PMS), also known as premenstrual tension (PMT), is a complex of physical and/or emotional symptoms that occur repetitively in a cyclic fashion before menstruation and that diminish or disappear with menstruation. Typically these cyclic symptoms are sufficiently severe to interfere with some aspects of life. Women with established psychiatric disturbances probably should not be included among those with PMS. More than 150 different symptoms are now thought to vary with the menstrual cycle (Table 208–3). Estimates of the prevalence of PMS range from 25 to 100%. For most women the syndrome is merely annoying; it is likely that PMS causes serious difficulties for no more than 5 to 10%. The diagnosis is best established by requiring patients to keep prospective daily records of symptoms over a 2- to 3-month period. Fewer than 50% of women complaining of PMS are found to have the syndrome when such records are examined.

Most women seek help for PMS in their 30's after 10 or more years of symptoms. Many report that their symptoms began at menarche; approximately half state that symptoms followed childbirth. Severity and duration of symptoms are often reported to increase following each successive pregnancy, and to become more severe with advancing age. Women with severe longstanding PMS almost always describe associated psychological reactions, including social difficulties, such as marital discord, difficulty relating to their children, difficulty maintaining friendships, and withdrawal from social activities.

The cause of PMS is unknown and patients should be informed that no one therapy has been effective in all women. Women with mild premenstrual symptoms often benefit from simple changes in

TABLE 208-3. COMMON SYMPTOMS OF CYCLIC PREMENSTRUAL SYNDROME

Somatic Symptoms

Abdominal bloating	Constipation or diarrhea
Acne	Headache
Alcohol intolerance	Peripheral edema
Breast engorgement and tenderness	Weight gain
Clumsiness	

Emotional and Mental Symptoms

Anxiety	Insomnia
Change in libido	Irritability
Depression	Lethargy
Fatigue	Mood swings
Food cravings (especially salt and sugar)	Panic attacks
	Paranoia
Hostility	Violence toward self and others
Inability to concentrate	Withdrawal from others
Increased appetite	

lifestyle, including addition of mild aerobic exercise each day; reduction in intake of xanthine-containing beverages, salt, and refined sugar in the day, particularly in the luteal phase; stress reduction; and adequate rest. Women with more severe PMS may benefit from treating predominant complaints symptomatically. Thus bromocriptine* (generally 2.5 mg twice a day) or danazol (100 to 400 mg daily in two divided doses) may be given continuously for relief of mastalgia, with the understanding that both may have unpleasant side effects. Prostaglandin synthetase inhibitors may help reduce dysmenorrhea and may benefit headaches. Mild sedatives and tranquilizers may help reduce insomnia and anxiety. Low doses of fluoxetine (20 mg) either administered daily or for the last 2 weeks of each menstrual cycle have been reported to reduce the emotional symptoms associated with PMS. Mild diuretics (especially spironolactone at doses up to 100 mg each morning) may benefit cyclic edema if such can be confirmed.

Because PMS requires the occurrence of cyclic ovulation, oophorectomy is occasionally considered for patients with particularly intractable symptomatology. However, oophorectomy may create new problems related to estrogen deficiency for women with PMS treated in this permanent fashion. Several recent trials employing a GnRH agonist together with exogenous steroids (so-called add-back therapy) have been described as reducing PMS. Whether such therapy can be utilized long-term remains to be determined.

Natural progesterone, particularly in the form of vaginal suppositories given at doses of up to 800 mg per day, has been used but results of double-blind placebo-controlled trials have provided no evidence of efficacy. Likewise, the use of large quantities of multiple vitamins or of oil of evening primrose, containing the essential fatty acid γ-linolenic acid, a precursor of prostaglandins, is unsubstantiated.

Keye WR Jr (ed.): The Premenstrual Syndrome. Philadelphia, WB Saunders, 1988. *A simple multiauthored text detailing what is known about this disorder.*
Stillman R: Endometriosis. *In* Becker KL (ed.): Principles and Practice of Endocrinology and Metabolism. Philadelphia, JB Lippincott, 1990. *A succinct summary of this enigmatic disorder.*

ABNORMAL UTERINE BLEEDING. *Differential Diagnosis.* The causes of abnormal uterine bleeding in the reproductive years include complications from the use of oral contraceptive preparations; complications of pregnancy (especially threatened, incomplete, or missed abortion and ectopic pregnancy); coagulation disorders (most commonly idiopathic thrombocytopenic purpura and von Willebrand's disease); and pelvic disease such as intrauterine polyps, leiomyomas, and tumors of the vagina and cervix. Clearcell adenocarcinoma of the vagina or cervix may occur in women exposed to diethylstilbestrol (DES) during fetal life as a result of maternal ingestion. Affected women also may have congenital abnormalities of the upper vagina, cervix, and uterus. Because a history of DES exposure is not always obtained and because this malignant tumor may be fatal, clinical suspicion should remain high.

---

* This use is not listed in the manufacturer's directive.

Women with a history of DES exposure should be reassured, however, that the incidence of malignancy is extremely low. Trauma (coital or otherwise), foreign bodies, systemic illnesses including various endocrinopathies (such as diabetes mellitus, hypothyroidism and hyperthyroidism, Cushing's syndrome, and Addison's disease), leukemia, and renal disease may also be associated with abnormal bleeding as the presenting manifestation.

Dysfunctional uterine bleeding (DUB), abnormal uterine bleeding with no demonstrable organic genital or extragenital cause (75% of cases), is most frequently associated with anovulation. Postmenarchal bleeding in adolescents secondary to immaturity of the hypothalamic-pituitary-ovarian axis accounts for about 20% of all cases, and premenopausal bleeding consequent to incipient ovarian failure constitutes more than half of the cases. Most anovulatory bleeding is due to either estrogen withdrawal or estrogen breakthrough bleeding. In anovulatory women, estrogen stimulates the endometrium unopposed by progesterone. As a consequence, the endometrium proliferates, becomes thicker, and may shed irregularly, especially if estrogen levels drop. Anovulatory bleeding tends to occur at less frequent intervals, while organic lesions tend to cause bleeding more frequently than cyclic menses.

Evaluation and Treatment. All cases of abnormal bleeding should be evaluated, including obtaining a thorough history with special emphasis on the amount and duration of blood loss. Prospective charting of the days on which bleeding occurs may be required to evaluate the bleeding pattern. Complications of pregnancy or a bleeding diathesis must always be ruled out.

The physical examination (including the Papanicolaou smear) is normal in dysfunctional bleeding except for signs of anemia in the more severe cases. Laboratory tests should include a complete blood count, platelet count, coagulation studies, thyroid function tests, and fasting blood glucose. DUB must be a diagnosis of exclusion. Management of DUB depends upon the age of the patient and the extent of the bleeding. A sample of the endometrium should be obtained by biopsy or by dilatation and curettage from all women over age 35 and from those at increased risk of developing endometrial carcinoma because of prolonged anovulatory bleeding.

Even profuse bleeding in anovulatory women can almost always be successfully treated by administering one combination oral contraceptive pill every 6 hours for 5 to 7 days. Bleeding should cease within 24 hours, but patients should be warned to expect heavy bleeding 2 to 4 days after stopping therapy. If anemia and signs of acute blood loss are profound, blood transfusion may be necessary. If the bleeding continues despite therapy, curettage can be carried out. Recurrence can be prevented by giving the patient combination oral contraceptive agents cyclically for 3 or more months. If spontaneous cyclic menses do not resume and pregnancy is not desired, the patient can be treated with cyclic progestin (medroxyprogesterone acetate 5 to 10 mg for 10 to 14 days each month) or oral contraceptive agents. If pregnancy is desired, ovulation can be induced, as discussed subsequently.

Acute episodes of anovulatory bleeding also can be treated with conjugated estrogens administered intravenously (25 mg every 4 hours for up to three doses) until bleeding ceases. Progestin therapy (medroxyprogesterone acetate 5 to 10 mg orally for 10 days) should be started simultaneously. Withdrawal bleeding will occur after cessation of therapy, and the patient can then be treated with oral contraceptive agents for at least three cycles.

For individuals with anovulatory bleeding without an episode of profuse bleeding, treatment with cyclic oral contraceptive agents or progestin can be provided unless pregnancy is desired, in which case ovulation must be induced.

Speroff L, Glass RH, Kase NG: Dysfunctional uterine bleeding. *In* Clinical Gynecologic Endocrinology and Infertility, 5th ed. Baltimore, Williams & Wilkins, 1994, p 531. *A detailed and logical approach to the treatment of abnormal uterine bleeding.*

AMENORRHEA. *Definition and Etiology.* Amenorrhea is the absence of menstruation for 3 or more months in women with past menses (*secondary amenorrhea*) or the absence of menarche by the age of 16 years regardless of the absence or presence of secondary sex characteristics (*primary amenorrhea*). If an intact genital outflow tract exists and there is no primary disease of the uterus, amenorrhea is a sign of failure of the hypothalamic-pituitary-ovarian axis to produce cyclically the hormones necessary for menses. Amenorrhea is a sign of any of several disorders involving different organ systems. Amenorrhea is physiologic in the prepubertal girl, during pregnancy and early in lactation, and after the menopause. At any other time it is pathologic and demands evaluation. Use of the term *post-pill amenorrhea* to refer to failure to resume menses within 3 months of discontinuing oral contraceptives is inappropriate. Women so affected should be evaluated in the same manner as for any woman with amenorrhea. Similarly, individuals with menses occurring at infrequent intervals of greater than 40 days or having fewer than 9 menses per year, termed oligomenorrhea, should be evaluated identically to women with amenorrhea.

Clinical Evaluation. In patients with amenorrhea even subtle hormonal abnormalities may be manifested by obvious signs and symptoms. Breast development indicates exposure to estrogens, and the presence of pubic and axillary hair indicates androgenic stimulation.

Patients should be questioned especially closely for evidence of psychological disturbances, dietary and exercise habits, lifestyle, environmental stresses, a family history of genetic anomalies, and abnormal growth and development. Patients should also be asked about and examined for the presence of any signs of hyperandrogenism, including hirsutism, temporal balding, deepening of the voice, increased muscle mass, clitoromegaly, and increased libido, as well as for any signs of defeminization, including decreasing breast size and vaginal atrophy. Any history of galactorrhea, the nonpuerperal secretion of milk from the breasts, should be determined (see Ch. 208.4). A history of symptoms related to thyroid and adrenal dysfunction should also be sought.

The physical examination should focus on evaluating (1) body dimensions and habitus, (2) the extent and distribution of body hair, (3) breast development and secretions, and (4) the genitalia.

In normal adult women the arm span is similar to the height, whereas in hypogonadal women the span is generally more than 5 cm greater than the height. The general appearance of the patient should be evaluated to determine if the habitus is that of an adult female. The distribution and quantity of body hair should be considered in view of the family history. The extent of any hirsutism should be recorded, preferably by photographs. Other signs of virilization should be sought carefully. Breast development should be graded according to the method of Tanner (Table 208–4). Breast secretion should be sought by applying pressure to the breasts while the patient is seated. Any secretion should be examined microscopically for the presence of perfectly round fat globules of varying size, which are always present in milk and indicate galactorrhea. Finally, the female genitalia should be examined carefully because they are such sensitive indicators of hormonal milieu. The Tanner stage of pubic hair development should be noted (Table 208–4). Because the sensitivity of the genitalia to androgens decreases onward from early in fetal development, the extent of any virilization is important. Fusion of the labia and enlargement of the clitoris with or without formation of a penile urethra are observed in women exposed to androgens during the first 3 months of fetal development (see Ch. 207). Significant clitoromegaly in the absence of other signs of sexual ambiguity and in the presence of other signs of virilization requires marked androgenic stimulation and strongly implicates an androgen-secreting neoplasm in the absence

of a history of ingestion of exogenous steroids. The development of the labia minora in postpubertal women indicates the influence of estrogens. Overt anomalies of the distal genital tract and especially any evidence of obstruction to the escape of menstrual blood should be sought in the remainder of the pelvic examination. The vaginal mucosa and the cervical mucus are exquisitely sensitive to estrogen. Under the influence of estrogen the vaginal mucosa changes during sexual maturation from a tissue with a shiny, bright red appearance with sparse, thin secretions to a dull, gray-pink rugated surface with copious, thick secretions.

The history and physical examination quickly differentiate among several causes of amenorrhea, regardless of the age of the patient (Table 208–5). The various disorders of sexual differentiation and the other peripheral causes are often apparent on inspection. Distal genital tract obstruction should be identified at the time of pelvic examination even if the specific abnormality is not obvious. The physical stigmata of Turner's syndrome, discussed subsequently, generally make the diagnosis simple. Any sexual ambiguity indicates the need for chromosomal analysis and the measurement of 17α-hydroxyprogesterone to rule out congenital adrenal hyperplasia. Pregnancy and gestational trophoblastic disease may be suspected and confirmed by measuring circulating concentrations of hCG. The possibility of intrauterine synechiae or adhesions (Asherman's syndrome) must be considered in individuals developing amenorrhea following curettage or endometritis. Tuberculous endometritis, especially in younger women, may also lead to this disorder. Without hormonal measurements it may be impossible to distinguish among individuals with chronic anovulation, in whom hypothalamic-pituitary-ovarian function is insufficiently coordinated to produce cyclic ovulation, and those with ovarian failure, in whom in most cases the ovaries are devoid of oocytes. Still, it is generally possible to form some strong clinical impressions about the cause of the amenorrhea. It can be noted if the patient has absence of, incomplete, or complete development of secondary sex characteristics. The presence of excess body hair or galactorrhea may provide clinical evidence of the pathogenesis of the amenorrhea. Signs and symptoms of adrenal or thyroid dysfunction may be important as well.

The administration of a progestin has been advocated to assess the level of endogenous estrogen. This test is of limited value, however, because almost half the young women with premature ovarian failure experience withdrawal bleeding in response to progestin.

To ascertain if the outflow tract is intact, an orally active estrogen, such as 2.5 mg conjugated estrogen daily for 21 days, with 5 to 10 mg of oral medroxyprogesterone acetate for the last 5 to 10 days, may be administered. Withdrawal bleeding should occur if the endometrium is normal. Still, hysterosalpingography and hysteroscopy may be required to diagnose Asherman's syndrome because some patients do continue to have some withdrawal bleeding.

Laboratory Evaluation. Basal levels of FSH, prolactin, and TSH should be measured in all amenorrheic and oligomenorrheic women to confirm the clinical impression (Fig. 208–8).

TABLE 208–4. CRITERIA FOR DISTINGUISHING TANNER STAGES 1 TO 5 DURING PUBERTAL MATURATION

Tanner Stage	Breast	Pubic Hair
1 (Prepubertal)	No palpable glandular tissue or pigmentation of areola; elevation of areola only	No pubic hair; short, fine vellous hair only
2	Glandular tissue palpable with elevation of breast and areola together as a small mound; areolar diameter increased	Sparse, long, pigmented terminal hair chiefly along the labia majora
3	Further enlargement without separation of breast and areola; although more darkly pigmented, areola still pale and immature; nipple generally at or above midplane of breast tissue when individual is seated upright	Dark, coarse, curly hair, extending sparsely over mons
4	Secondary mound of areola and papilla above breast	Adult-type hair, abundant but limited to mons and labia
5 (Adult)	Recession of areola to contour of breast; development of Montgomery's glands and ducts on areola; further pigmentation of areola; nipple generally below midplane of breast tissue when individual is seated upright; maturation independent of breast size	Adult-type hair in quantity and distribution; spread to inner aspects of the thighs in most racial groups

Data from Ross GT: Disorders of the ovary and female reproductive tract. *In* Wilson JD, Foster DW (eds.): Textbook of Endocrinology, 7th ed. Philadelphia, WB Saunders, 1985, p 206; Speroff L, Glass RH, Kase N: Clinical Gynecologic Endocrinology and Infertility, 3rd ed. Baltimore, Williams & Wilkins, 1983, p 377; and Kustin J, Rebar RW: Menstrual disorders in the adolescent age group. Primary Care 14:139, 1987.

TABLE 208-5. CAUSES OF AMENORRHEA

Disorders of sexual differentiation
  Distal genital tract obstruction (müllerian agenesis and dysgenesis)
  Gonadal dysgenesis
  Ambiguity of external genitalia (male and female pseudohermaphroditism)
Other peripheral causes
  Pregnancy
  Gestational trophoblastic disease
  Amenorrhea traumatica (Asherman's syndrome)
Chronic anovulation or ovarian failure
  Degree of sexual development
  Galactorrhea
  Evidence of androgen excess
  Evidence suggestive of adrenal or thyroid dysfunction

Increased TSH levels with or without increased levels of prolactin imply primary hypothyroidism, and further evaluation for this disorder is indicated (see Ch. 203). Although hypothyroidism commonly results in anovulation, amenorrhea occurs in only some hypothyroid women. Menorrhagia and oligomenorrhea may occur as well. The very sensitive immunoassays for TSH permit identification of women with hyperthyroidism as well because TSH levels are suppressed in those individuals.

If the prolactin concentration is increased (typically >20 to 30 ng per milliliter) and the TSH level is normal (generally <5 μU per milliliter), measurement of the prolactin concentration in the basal state should be repeated before more extensive evaluation is undertaken. This is the case because prolactin levels are increased by nonspecific stressful stimuli, sleep, and food ingestion. Prolactin levels may be elevated in as many as one third of women with amenorrhea. Evaluation of galactorrhea and hyperprolactinemia is detailed in Ch. 208.4.

Increased FSH levels (generally >30 to 40 milli International Units [mIU] per milliliter) imply ovarian failure and require further evaluation. Chromosomal evaluation is indicated in all individuals with elevated FSH levels who are under the age of 30 years at the time the amenorrhea begins.

If prolactin and TSH concentrations are within normal ranges and FSH levels are low or normal, the measurement of total testosterone levels may be helpful whether or not there is any evidence of hirsutism or virilization. Hyperandrogenic women need not be hirsute because some have relative insensitivity of the hair follicles to androgens. Mildly increased levels of testosterone (and perhaps DHEA-S as well) suggest PCO syndrome. However, total circulating androgen levels are rarely not elevated because of the alter-

ations in metabolic clearance rate and SHBG that are present in PCO syndrome. Circulating levels of LH and FSH may aid in differentiating PCO syndrome from hypothalamic-pituitary dysfunction. LH levels are frequently elevated in PCO syndrome such that the ratio of LH to FSH is increased; however, LH levels may be identical to those observed in normal women in the follicular phase. In contrast, levels of LH and FSH are normal or slightly reduced in hypothalamic-pituitary dysfunction. There is some overlap between women with "PCO-like" disorders and those with hypothalamic-pituitary dysfunction. Radiographic assessment of the sella turcica is indicated in all amenorrheic women in whom both LH and FSH levels are very low (both < 10 mIU per milliliter) to exclude a pituitary or parapituitary neoplasm. Other pituitary functions should be evaluated in any individual with significantly impaired LH and FSH secretion, as detailed subsequently. Both total testosterone and DHEA-S levels should be measured in hirsute or virilized women. Testosterone levels of >200 ng per deciliter should lead to investigation for an androgen-producing neoplasm, most likely of ovarian origin. DHEA-S levels >7.0 μg per milliliter should lead to evaluation for an adrenal neoplasm, and DHEA-S levels between 5.0 and 7.0 μg per milliliter should lead to evaluation for "adult-onset" congenital adrenal hyperplasia (see Ch. 207).

Hypergonadotropic Amenorrhea (Presumptive Ovarian Failure, Primary Hypogonadism)

Differential Diagnosis. Gonadal failure may begin at any time during embryonic or postnatal development and may result from many causes (Table 208-6). Normally the ovaries fail at menopause when virtually no functioning follicles remain. However, premature loss of oocytes prior to age 40 may occur and lead to premature ovarian failure, possibly from abnormalities in the recruitment and selection of oocytes. Because FSH is the principal regulator of folliculogenesis, most causes of premature ovarian failure may somehow involve FSH secretion or action. Circulating gonadotropin levels increase whenever ovarian failure occurs because of decreased negative estrogen feedback to the hypothalamic-pituitary unit.

Genetic Abnormalities. Several pathologic conditions with dysgenetic gonads have elevated gonadotropin levels and amenorrhea. The term *gonadal dysgenesis* refers to individuals with undifferentiated streak gonads without any association with either extragonadal stigmata or sex chromosomal aberrations. Because individuals with gonadal dysgenesis have the normal complement of oocytes at 20 weeks of fetal age but virtually none by birth, this disorder is a form of premature ovarian failure.

Turner's syndrome describes patients with streak gonads composed of fibrous stroma and four cardinal features: (1) a female phenotype, (2) sexual infantilism, (3) short stature, and (4) several physical abnormalities, sometimes including a webbed neck, lowset ears, multiple pigmented nevi, double eyelashes, micrognathia, epicanthal folds, shieldlike chest with microthelia, short fourth

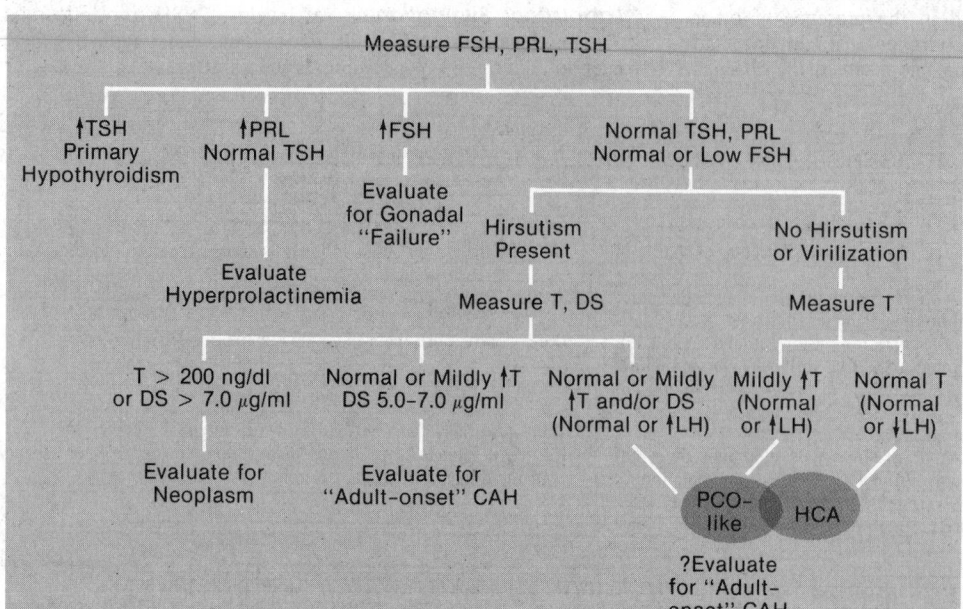

FIGURE 208-8. Biochemical evaluation of amenorrhea. This schema must be considered as an adjunct to the clinical evaluation of the patient. See text for details. **Abbreviations:** FSH = follicle-stimulating hormone; PRL = prolactin; TSH = thyroid-stimulating hormone; T = testosterone; DS = dehydroepiandrosterone sulfate; LH = luteinizing hormone; PCO-like = polycystic ovarian–like; HCA = hypothalamic chronic anovulation; CAH = congenital adrenal hyperplasia.

TABLE 208–6. CLASSIFICATION OF HYPERGONADOTROPIC AMENORRHEA (FSH > 40 mIU per milliliter)

I. Menopause
II. Genetic abnormalities
   A. Genetically reduced cell endowment
   B. Accelerated atresia
   C. Gonadal dysgenesis
      1. With stigmata of Turner's syndrome (45,X)
      2. Pure (46,XX or 46,XY)
      3. Mixed
   D. Trisomy X with or without chromosomal mosaicism
   E. In association with myotonia dystrophica
III. Physical causes
   A. Gonadal irradiation
   B. Chemotherapeutic (especially alkylating) agents
   C. Viral agents
   D. Surgical extirpation
IV. Autoimmune disorders
   A. Polyglandular, involving ovarian failure and any combination of thyroiditis, hypoadrenalism, hypoparathyroidism, diabetes mellitus, myasthenia gravis, vitiligo, mucocutaneous candidiasis, and pernicious anemia
   B. Isolated ovarian failure
V. Enzymatic defects
   A. 17α-Hydroxylase deficiency
   B. Galactosemia
VI. Defective gonadotropin secretion and/or action
   A. Resistant ovary or Savage syndrome
   B. Secretion of biologically inactive forms
   C. α or β subunit defects
VII. Congenital thymic aplasia
VIII. Circulating gonadotropin antibodies
IX. Idiopathic premature ovarian failure

metacarpals, an increased carrying angle of the arms, and certain renal and cardiovascular defects (most commonly coarctation of the aorta and aortic stenosis). The diagnosis can sometimes be made at birth because of unexplained lymphedema of the hands and feet. The syndrome is associated with an abnormality of sex chromosome number, morphology, or both. Most commonly the second sex chromosome is absent (45,X). This is the single most common chromosomal disorder in humans, but more than 95% of such fetuses are aborted so that the incidence in newborns is approximately 1 in 3000 to 5000. Chromosomal breakage and mosaicism occur frequently as well. In mosaic individuals with a normal 46,XX cell line, sufficient follicles may persist postnatally to initiate pubertal changes and to cause ovulation so that pregnancy is possible.

Pure gonadal dysgenesis is the term given to phenotypically female individuals with streak gonads who are of normal stature and have none of the physical stigmata associated with Turner's syndrome. Such individuals have either a 46,XX or 46,XY karyotype. The 46,XX defect may be inherited as an autosomal recessive, with 10% having associated nerve deafness. The 46,XY defect may be inherited as an X-linked recessive, with clitoromegaly occurring in 10 to 15% and gonadal tumors developing in 25% if the gonads are not removed.

Trisomy X (46,XXX karyotype) is also associated with premature menopause, while many such individuals actually have normal reproductive lives. Premature menopause can also occur in mosaic individuals with cell lines with excess X chromosomes. When gonadal abnormalities occur in women with excess X chromosomes, they seem to occur after ovarian differentiation so that some ovarian function is possible. Only later in life do such women develop secondary amenorrhea and premature ovarian failure.

Other Causes. *Physical, Chemical, and Infectious Causes.* Irradiation and chemotherapeutic agents, especially alkylating agents, utilized to treat various malignant diseases also may cause premature ovarian failure. Ovulation and cyclic menses return in some of these patients even after prolonged intervals of hypergonadotropic amenorrhea associated with signs and symptoms of profound hypoestrogenism. Rarely, mumps affects the ovaries and causes ovarian failure.

Autoimmune Disorders. Premature ovarian failure may occur in conjunction with a variety of autoimmune disorders. The most well-known syndrome involves hypoadrenalism, hypoparathyroidism,

and mucocutaneous candidiasis together with ovarian failure (see Ch. 210). Thyroiditis is the most commonly associated abnormality. Antibodies to the FSH receptor have been identified in a very few cases. These associations make it mandatory to rule out other potentially life-threatening endocrinopathies in young women with hypergonadotropic amenorrhea.

Enzymatic Defects. In girls with the rare syndrome of 17α-hydroxylase deficiency who survive until the expected age of puberty, sexual infantilism and primary amenorrhea occur together with elevated levels of gonadotropins. Increased synthesis of desoxycorticosterone leads to hypertension with hypokalemic alkalosis; serum progesterone levels are elevated as well. As with other causes of congenital adrenal hyperplasia, the hypertension is controlled by replacement therapy with glucocorticoids (see Ch. 207). Women with galactosemia also develop ovarian failure early in life, even when a galactose-restricted diet is introduced early in infancy (see Ch. 169).

Defective Gonadotropin Secretion and/or Action. The resistant ovary (Savage) syndrome occurs in young amenorrheic women who have (1) elevated peripheral gonadotropin concentrations, (2) normal (although immature) follicles present on ovarian biopsy, (3) a 46,XX karyotype with no evidence of mosaicism, (4) fully developed secondary sex characteristics, and (5) ovarian resistance to stimulation with human menopausal or pituitary gonadotropins. There seems to be some block to gonadotropin action within the ovary in this syndrome.

Therapeutic Considerations. Women with hypergonadotropic amenorrhea and ovarian failure should be treated identically whether or not they have signs of hypoestrogenism or desire pregnancy. Ovarian biopsy is not indicated to document the existence of follicles because only a small portion of each ovary can be sampled and because pregnancies have resulted in patients who had biopsies devoid of follicles. Estrogen replacement is warranted to prevent the accelerated bone loss known to occur in affected women (see Ch. 217). The estrogen should be given sequentially with a progestin to prevent endometrial hyperplasia. Young women with ovarian failure may require twice as much estrogen as postmenopausal women for relief of signs and symptoms of hypoestrogenism.

Women with hypergonadotropic amenorrhea are rarely able to become pregnant. Pregnancy is more likely to occur with estrogen replacement therapy than with any other therapy. It is not clear why pregnancy may rarely occur in such women. Even with estrogen replacement the pregnancy rate is less than 10%. The most successful treatment of young women with hypergonadotropic amenorrhea involves hormone replacement to mimic the normal menstrual cycle and embryo transfer utilizing donor oocytes. Pregnancy rates are higher than in other women undergoing *in vitro* fertilization and typically exceed 30% per cycle.

Differential Diagnosis and Treatment of Chronic Anovulation. Chronic anovulation, the most frequent form of amenorrhea encountered in women of reproductive age, implies that functional ovarian follicles remain and that cyclic ovulation can be induced or reinitiated with appropriate therapy (Table 208–7). Appropriate management requires that the cause of the anovulation be determined. The pathophysiologic bases for several forms of anovulation are unknown, but the anovulation can be interrupted transiently by nonspecific induction of ovulation in the majority of affected women. It is important to recognize that anovulation can result in either amenorrhea or irregular (generally less frequent) menses.

Hypothalamic Chronic Anovulation (HCA). HCA represents a heterogeneous group of disorders with similar manifestations. Emotional and physical stress, exercise, diet, weight loss, body composition, malnutrition, environment, and other unrecognized factors may contribute in varying proportions to the anovulation. Abrupt cessation of menses in women under 30 years of age who have no anatomic abnormalities of the hypothalamic-pituitary-ovarian axis and no other endocrine disturbances suggests a diagnosis of HCA. Affected individuals tend to be bright, educated, and engaged in intellectual occupations and may well give a history of psychosexual problems and socioenvironmental trauma. HCA is characterized by low to normal levels of gonadotropins and relative hypoestrogenism. Rarely, however, do affected women present with signs and symptoms of estrogen deficiency. Psychological counseling and/or a change in lifestyle, especially for those women engaged in strenu-

TABLE 208–7. CAUSES OF CHRONIC ANOVULATION

I. **Chronic anovulation of hypothalamic-pituitary origin**
  A. Hypothalamic chronic anovulation
    1. Psychogenic
    2. Exercise associated
    3. Associated with diet, weight loss, and/or malnutrition
    4. Anorexia nervosa and bulimia
    5. Pseudocyesis
  B. Forms of isolated gonadotropin deficiency (including Kallmann's syndrome)
  C. Due to hypothalamic-pituitary damage
    1. Pituitary and parapituitary tumors
    2. Empty-sella syndrome
    3. Following surgery
    4. Following irradiation
    5. Following trauma
    6. Following infection
    7. Following infarction
  D. Idiopathic hypopituitarism
  E. Hypothalamic-pituitary dysfunction or failure with hyperprolactinemia (multiple causes)
  F. Due to systemic diseases

II. **Chronic anovulation due to inappropriate feedback** (i.e., polycystic ovary syndrome)
  A. Excessive extraglandular estrogen production (i.e., obesity)
  B. Abnormal buffering involving sex hormone–binding globulin (including liver disease)
  C. Functional androgen excess (adrenal or ovarian)
  D. Neoplasms producing androgens or estrogens
  E. Neoplasms producing chorionic gonadotropin

III. **Chronic anovulation due to other endocrine and metabolic disorders**
  A. Adrenal hyperfunction
    1. Cushing's syndrome
    2. Congenital adrenal hyperplasia (female pseudohermaphroditism)
  B. Thyroid dysfunction
    1. Hyperthyroidism
    2. Hypothyroidism
  C. Prolactin and/or growth hormone excess
    1. Hypothalamic dysfunction
    2. Pituitary dysfunction (microadenomas and macroadenomas)
    3. Drug induced
  D. Malnutrition

Modified from Rebar RW: Chronic anovulation. *In* Serra GB (ed.): The Ovary. New York, Raven Press, 1983, p 217.

ous exercise programs, may be effective in inducing cyclic ovulation and menses. For women desiring pregnancy, ovulation can also be induced with clomiphene citrate (50 to 100 mg per day for 5 days beginning on the fifth day of withdrawal bleeding). Treatment with human menopausal gonadotropin and human chorionic gonadotropin (hMG-hCG) or with GnRH administered in a pulsatile fashion may be effective in women who do not ovulate in response to clomiphene. Most physicians advocate the use of exogenous steroids to prevent osteoporosis. A regimen can be used consisting of oral conjugated estrogens (0.625 to 1.25 mg), ethinyl estradiol (20 μg), or micronized estradiol-17β (1 to 2 mg) or transdermal estradiol-17β (0.05 to 0.10 mg) daily, with oral medroxyprogesterone acetate (5 to 10 mg) added for the first 12 to 14 days of each month. Sexually active women can be given oral contraceptive agents as an alternative. If steroid therapy is administered, patients must be informed that the amenorrhea probably will be present when therapy is discontinued. Other physicians believe only periodic observation is indicated, with barrier methods of contraception recommended for fertility control. Adequate ingestion of calcium should be ensured regardless of therapy. Contraception is needed for sexually active women with HCA, because the functional defect is mild in these disorders and may resolve spontaneously at any time, with ovulation occurring prior to any episode of menstruation.

Individuals with amenorrhea and significant weight loss should be examined for the possibility of *anorexia nervosa* (see Ch. 195). This disorder may be the most severe form of functional HCA, or it may be a distinct entity.

Kallmann's syndrome (isolated gonadotropin deficiency or familial hypogonadotropic hypogonadism) is a familial disorder consist-

ing of gonadotropin deficiency, anosmia or hyposmia, and color blindness in men or, more rarely, in women. Other midline defects such as cleft lip and palate can occur in the affected individual or in family members. The trait is transmitted as an X-linked recessive or a male-limited autosomal dominant trait, but genetic heterogeneity may occur. Partial or complete agenesis of the olfactory bulb is present on autopsy, accounting for use of the term *olfactogenital dysplasia*. The disorder affects only gonadotropin secretion, and all other pituitary hormones are secreted normally. Isolated gonadotropin deficiency in the absence of anosmia occurs as well. Sexual infantilism with a eunuchoid habitus is the clinical hallmark of this disorder, but moderate breast development may occur. Circulating LH and FSH levels are quite low, but almost always detectable. Ovulation induction requires use of hMG-hCG or pulsatile GnRH. Estrogen replacement therapy is indicated in these women until such time as pregnancy is desired. It may not be possible to distinguish between partial isolated gonadotropin deficiency and functional HCA in all cases.

Hypopituitarism may be obvious upon cursory inspection or sufficiently subtle to require endocrine testing (see Ch. 202.1). The clinical presentation depends on the age of onset, the cause, and the nutritional status of the individual. Failure of development of secondary sex characteristics or for development to progress once puberty is initiated must always raise the question of hypopituitarism. Ovulation can be induced successfully with exogenous gonadotropins when pregnancy is desired and after the hypopituitarism is treated appropriately. Replacement therapy with estrogen is indicated to prevent signs and symptoms of estrogen deficiency.

Galactorrhea associated with hyperprolactinemia, whatever the cause, almost always occurs together with amenorrhea caused by hypothalamic-pituitary dysfunction or failure. Many conditions can cause excess prolactin secretion (see Ch. 208.4). It is unclear if all individuals with chronic anovulation associated with hyperprolactinemia and no other cause have pituitary microadenomas, even in the absence of identifiable radiographic changes of the sella turcica. Hirsutism may be observed occasionally in association with amenorrhea-galactorrhea and hyperprolactinemia. Elevated levels of the adrenal androgens DHEA and DHEA-S may be observed and may account for the PCO-type ovaries present in some hyperprolactinemic women.

The hypothalamic-pituitary unit also may fail to function normally in a number of stressful, debilitating, systemic illnesses that interfere with somatic growth and development. Chronic renal failure, liver disease, and diabetes mellitus are the most prominent examples.

Chronic Anovulation Due to Inappropriate Feedback. PCO syndrome, which causes anovulation because of inappropriate feedback signals to the hypothalamic-pituitary unit, is a heterogeneous disorder in which there is considerable clinical and biochemical variability among affected individuals. Although patients usually present with amenorrhea, hirsutism, and obesity, affected women may instead complain of irregular and profuse uterine bleeding, may not have hirsutism, and may be of normal weight. Excess androgen from any source or increased extraglandular conversion of androgens to estrogens can lead to the typical findings of PCO syndrome. Included are such diverse disorders as Cushing's syndrome, mild congenital adrenal hyperplasia, virilizing tumors of adrenal or ovarian origin, hyperthyroidism and hypothyroidism, obesity, and primary PCO syndrome with no other recognizable cause. In the primary syndrome the irregular menses, mild obesity, and hirsutism begin during puberty and typically become more severe with time. Obesity alone can lead to a PCO-like syndrome, with the degree of obesity required to cause anovulation varying widely from individual to individual. All such patients are well estrogenized regardless of whether they present with primary or secondary amenorrhea or dysfunctional bleeding. As noted, LH concentrations tend to be elevated, with relatively low and constant FSH levels, but both may be in the normal range compared with levels in women in the follicular phase of the menstrual cycle. Levels of most circulating androgens, especially testosterone, tend to be mildly elevated. The cause of PCO syndrome is unknown, but current evidence suggests that the hypothalamic-pituitary unit is intact and that a functional derangement, perhaps involving insulin-like growth factors such as insulin-like (IGF-I) within the ovary, results in abnormal gonadotropin secretion.

The aim of the diagnostic evaluation is to rule out any causes (such as neoplasms) that require definitive therapy. Hirsutism should be evaluated as detailed in Ch. 208.3. PCO syndrome itself is a benign disorder. Patients generally require therapy for hirsutism, for induction of ovulation if pregnancy is desired, and for prevention of estrogen-induced endometrial hyperplasia and cancer. No ideal therapy exists, but rather the therapeutic approach must be individualized to the needs of each patient.

In the anovulatory woman not desiring pregnancy who is not hirsute, therapy with intermittent progestin administration (such as medroxyprogesterone acetate 5 to 10 mg orally for 10 to 14 days each month) or oral contraceptives can be provided to reduce the increased risk of endometrial carcinoma that is present in such a woman with unopposed estrogen. All women utilizing intermittent progestin administration should be cautioned about the need for effective contraception if they are sexually active, because these agents do not inhibit ovulation when administered intermittently.

The approach to the hirsute anovulatory woman not desiring pregnancy is detailed in Ch. 208.3. Oral contraceptive agents are the first line of therapy for such women with mild hirsutism and offer protection from endometrial hyperplasia.

In women with PCO syndrome desiring pregnancy, clomiphene citrate is the first approach to inducing ovulation because of its simplicity and high success rate. Approximately 75 to 80% conceive with such therapy. Other possible methods of inducing ovulation include use of hMG-hCG, purified FSH, pulsatile GnRH, wedge resection of the ovaries at laparotomy, and laser or cautery destruction of follicles at laparoscopy. Surgical treatment is warranted only rarely and only in women in whom all other methods fail, in whom there is a question of an ovarian tumor because of ovarian size or circulating androgen levels, and in whom fertility is not an issue (because of the risk of pelvic adhesions from the surgery leading to infertility).

A particularly severely affected subset of women present with marked obesity, anovulation, mild glucose intolerance and high levels of circulating insulin with insulin resistance, acanthosis nigricans, hyperuricemia, and severe hirsutism with markedly elevated circulating androgen levels. These women have *hyperthecosis of the ovaries* in which the androgen-producing cells in the stromal, hilar, and thecal components of the ovaries are increased greatly in number. Although considered a separate entity by some clinicians, hyperthecosis probably should be viewed as a part of the spectrum of disorders constituting PCO syndrome.

Chronic Anovulation Due to Other Endocrine and Metabolic Disorders.
Adrenal hyperfunction appears to cause chronic anovulation by inducing a PCO-like syndrome secondary to increased adrenal androgen secretion, but other possible mechanisms also exist.

Both hyperthyroidism and hypothyroidism are associated with a variety of menstrual disturbances, including dysfunctional uterine bleeding and amenorrhea as a result of alterations in the metabolism of androgens and estrogens. These metabolic changes in turn result in inappropriate steroid feedback and chronic anovulation.

Rebar RW: Premature ovarian failure. *In* Lobo RA (ed.): Treatment of the Postmenopausal Woman. Basic and Clinical Aspects. New York, Raven Press, 1994, p 25. *A detailed discussion of the diagnosis and treatment of premature ovarian failure.*

Yen SSC, Jaffe RB (eds.): Reproductive Endocrinology, 3rd ed. Philadelphia, WB Saunders, 1991. *Detailed chapters describe practical evaluation of hormonal status and chronic anovulation caused by peripheral endocrine disorders as well as by CNS-hypothalamic-pituitary dysfunction.*

DISORDERS OF FOLLICULOGENESIS.
Recognized disorders of folliculogenesis cannot be identified before ovulation begins. They are believed to reflect abnormalities in follicular development.

Luteinized Unruptured Follicle (LUF) Syndrome.
The LUF syndrome describes development of a dominant follicle without its subsequent disruption and release of the ovum. The abnormality can be diagnosed by ultrasonography or by the absence of evidence of ovulation when the ovary is viewed at laparoscopy. The disorder is believed to occur infrequently and sporadically and is probably not a significant cause of infertility. Menstrual cycles in which no ovum is released are characterized by presumptive evidence of ovulation, including biphasic basal body temperatures, secretory endometrium, a normal LH surge, and normal progesterone production in the luteal phase. In fact, although the syndrome is believed to occur, data to substantiate its existence are only circumstantial (although strongly suggestive) at present.

Luteal Phase Dysfunction.
Progesterone secretion in the luteal phase may be reduced in duration (termed luteal phase insufficiency) or in amount (termed luteal phase inadequacy). More rarely the endometrium may be unable to respond to secreted progesterone because of the absence of progesterone receptors. These disorders are believed to represent causes for infertility (because of inability of fertilized ova to implant) in approximately 5% of infertile couples. Abnormalities of the follicular phase, especially in the frequency of gonadotropin pulses, may account for most luteal phase defects. Luteal phase defects also may occur sporadically in normally ovulating women approximately once each year.

Luteal phase dysfunction may be associated with several clinical entities, including mild or intermittent hyperprolactinemia (of any cause), strenuous physical exercise, inadequately treated 21-hydroxylase deficiency, and habitual abortion. Luteal dysfunction occurs more commonly at the extremes of reproductive life and in the first menstrual cycles following full-term delivery, abortion, or discontinuation of oral contraceptives. It also may occur during ovulatory cycles induced with clomiphene citrate or hMG-hCG.

The diagnosis of luteal phase dysfunction can be made either by endometrial biopsy or by serial progesterone determinations. Endometrial biopsies obtained from the uterine fundus in the late luteal phases of two different cycles must be at least 2 days out of phase from the expected date of bleeding, as judged from the subsequent menstrual cycle, for the diagnosis to be made. The absolute concentration that progesterone must achieve and the length of time progesterone must be increased in the luteal phase to exclude luteal dysfunction are unclear. Luteal dysfunction is extremely rare in women with menstrual cycles greater than 25 days in length in whom a single random progesterone determination is greater than 15 ng per milliliter.

Treatment of luteal dysfunction is controversial. Any underlying defect should be treated. If subsequent luteal function depends on prior follicular development, modification of follicular development with either clomiphene citrate (25 to 100 mg daily by mouth for 5 days beginning on cycle day 3 to 5) or FSH (75 to 300 IU intramuscularly for 3 to 5 days beginning on cycle day 3 to 5) is reasonable. hCG (2500 to 5000 IU intramuscularly at 2- to 3-day intervals beginning with the shift in basal body temperature) or progesterone (12.5 mg intramuscularly in oil daily or 25 mg twice a day as rectal or vaginal suppositories) can be utilized as well. Bromocriptine may correct the abnormality in individuals with hyperprolactinemia. Synthetic progestational agents should not be used to treat luteal phase defects because of their possible (although unproven) association with congenital anomalies. Furthermore, the synthetic progestins produce an abnormal endometrium. None of these agents has been shown to increase the pregnancy rate.

Soules MR: Luteal phase deficiency: A subtle abnormality of ovulation. *In* Keye WR Jr, Chang RJ, Rebar RW, Soules MR (eds.): Infertility: Evaluation and Treatment. Philadelphia, WB Saunders, 1995. *A complete consideration of the etiology, diagnosis, and treatment of luteal phase abnormalities.*

INFERTILITY.
Infertility may be defined as involuntary inability to conceive. *Sterility* is total inability to reproduce. In either case the situation may or may not be correctable, especially for each particular couple. Failure to reproduce thwarts a basic human instinct and causes anger, guilt, and depression. More than 10% of couples in the United States seek medical assistance for infertility.

The requirements for pregnancy to occur are several:

1. The male must produce adequate numbers of normal, motile spermatozoa.
2. The male must be capable of ejaculating the sperm through a patent ductal system.
3. The sperm must be able to traverse an unobstructed female reproductive tract.
4. The female must ovulate and release an ovum.
5. The sperm must be able to fertilize the ovum.
6. The fertilized ovum must be capable of developing and implanting in appropriately prepared endometrium.

Infertility is too frequently viewed primarily as a problem of the female. In fact, in approximately 40% of cases, infertility is caused by the male (Table 208–8). In perhaps one third of couples more than one cause contributes to the infertility.

TABLE 208-8. CAUSES OF INFERTILITY AND THEIR APPROXIMATE INCIDENCE (%)

I. **Male factors (40%)**
  A. Decreased production of spermatozoa
   1. Variocele
   2. Testicular failure
   3. Endocrine disorders
   4. Cryptorchidism
   5. Stress, smoking, caffeine, nicotine, recreational drugs
  B. Ductal obstruction
   1. Epididymal (postinfection)
   2. Congenital absence of vas deferens
   3. Ejaculatory duct (postinfection)
   4. Postvasectomy
  C. Inability to deliver sperm into vagina
   1. Ejaculatory disturbances
   2. Hypospadias
   3. Sexual problems (i.e., impotence), medical or psychological
  D. Abnormal semen
   1. Infection
   2. Abnormal volume
   3. Abnormal viscosity
  E. Immunologic factors
   1. Sperm-immobilizing antibodies
   2. Sperm-agglutinating antibodies
II. **Female factors**
  A. Fallopian tube pathology (20 to 30%)
   1. Pelvic inflammatory disease or puerperal infection
   2. Congenital anomalies
   3. Endometriosis
   4. Secondary to past peritonitis of nongenital origin
  B. Amenorrhea and anovulation (15%)
  C. Minor ovulatory disturbances (<5%?)
  D. Cervical and uterine factors (10%)
   1. Leiomyomas and polyps
   2. Uterine anomalies
   3. Intrauterine synechiae (Asherman's syndrome)
   4. Destroyed endocervical glands (postsurgery or postinfection)
  E. Vaginal factors (<5%)
   1. Congenital absence of vagina
   2. Imperforate hymen
   3. Vaginismus
   4. Vaginitis
  F. Immunologic factors (<5%)
   1. Sperm-immobilizing antibodies
   2. Sperm-agglutinating antibodies
  G. Nutritional and metabolic factors (5%)
   1. Thyroid disorders
   2. Diabetes mellitus
   3. Severe nutritional disturbances
III. **Idiopathic or unexplained (<10%)**

Peak age of fertility in the female is 25 years. For nulliparous women of this age the average time during which unprotected intercourse occurs until conception is 5.3 months. For parous women the average duration of intercourse until conception is 2.7 months. The reproductive performance of couples is influenced by the ages of the female and male partners, the frequency of intercourse, and the length of time the couple has been attempting to conceive. There is a decline in both female and male reproductive performance after age 25.

Couples who complain of infertility merit evaluation regardless of the length of infertility. If the couple believes there is a problem, it is the physician's responsibility to reassure them by appropriate evaluation and subsequent explanation of all findings and the prognosis.

The evaluation begins with a detailed history obtained from both partners and physical examinations of both individuals. The couple should be seen together for the first visit. Each couple should be questioned together and separately because separate interviews may uncover information that would not be imparted in the presence of the partner.

Initial evaluation for infertility generally includes (1) assessment of semen, (2) documentation of ovulation by basal body temperature, serum progesterone determination approximately 6 to 8 days before menses, or endometrial biopsy less than 3 days before onset of menses, and (3) evaluation of the female genital tract by hysterosalpingography. Basal serum levels of prolactin and thyroid hormones should be measured. Diagnostic laparoscopy with tubal dye instillation should be performed if results of all previous tests are normal because 30 to 50% of women are found to have endometriosis or tubal disease on surgical evaluation. Treatment must be predicated on the findings of the infertility evaluation.

Glass RH: Infertility. *In* Yen SSC, Jaffe RB (eds.): Reproductive Endocrinology, 3rd ed. Philadelphia, WB Saunders, 1991, p 689. *A summary of the approach to the infertile couple.*

SEXUAL FUNCTION AND DYSFUNCTION. Although sexual responses begin following puberty, they can continue for the duration of a woman's life. Sexual responses generally are divided into four phases: excitement, plateau, orgasm, and resolution.

With sexual arousal and excitement, vasocongestion and muscular tension increase progressively, primarily in the genitals, manifested by vaginal lubrication in the female. The lubrication is due to formation of a transudate in the vagina. Sexual excitement is initiated by any of a variety of psychogenic or somatogenic sexual stimuli and must be reinforced to result in orgasm. With continued stimulation, the excitement phase increases in intensity into a plateau phase during which a high state of sexual interest is maintained. The plateau phase may be short or long, and it is from this phase that an individual can shift to orgasm. The orgasmic phase tends to be brief and is characterized by rapid release from the developed vasocongestion and muscular tension. The orgasmic release is also known as the climax because peak psychological and physical intensity is achieved and there is an attendant feeling of satisfaction. Copious secretions and transudate may flow during orgasm in women. Although women may resolve toward sleep following orgasm, many remain responsive to sexual stimulation and may return to plateau and subsequent orgasm.

Characteristic genital and extragenital responses occur during these phases. Estrogens magnify the sexual responses, but responses may occur in estrogen-deficient women. For women these changes occur in the breasts and in the pudendal region and are variable from one response cycle to another. For some women, excitement proceeds quickly through plateau to orgasm, and orgasm is explosive and accompanied by vocalization and involuntary contractions of the pelvic skeletal muscles. For other women, the responses are slow in building, controlled in amplitude, and long lasting. For a few women orgasm never occurs; for many it is intermittently absent.

The somatic sensate focus enabling orgasmic release is variable and may include stimulation of the breast, vagina, or clitoris. The psychological aspect of coitus may involve concentration on the current partner or act or fantasies about other times and persons. Although orgasms may vary in physiologic intensity, what is important is psychological satisfaction. Satisfaction for both men and women may be had without orgasm.

Women may seek consultation because of disturbances in normal sexual arousal or orgasm. Such sexual dysfunction may be due to either organic or functional disturbances.

A variety of diseases affecting neurologic function, including diabetes mellitus and multiple sclerosis, may prevent sexual arousal. So, too, may local pelvic disorders, such as endometriosis and vaginitis, which cause dyspareunia and lead to sexual avoidance. Estrogen deficiency causing vaginal atrophy and dyspareunia is a relatively common cause of sexual dysfunction. Debilitating systemic diseases such as malignant disease may also affect sexual function indirectly.

In most cases the cause of sexual dysfunction is psychological. For instance, vaginismus involves involuntary contractions of the muscles surrounding the introitus and leads to dyspareunia. It is a conditioned response engendered by a previous imagined or real traumatic sexual experience. Feelings of guilt, caused by incest or rape as examples; of inadequacy, caused by hysterectomy or mastectomy; or of depression or anxiety may lead to failure to be aroused. Failure to achieve orgasm may be viewed as a dysfunction if the woman is frustrated or dissatisfied.

Treatment of sexual dysfunction is best accomplished by eliminating functional causes and providing the patient, often together with her partner, with appropriate psychological counseling. Behavioral modification is effective in treating many women with psychological sexual dysfunction.

Kaplan HS: The Evaluation of Sexual Disorders: Psychological and Medical Aspects. New York, Brunner-Mazel, 1983. *A good general text detailing sexual disorders.*

Kaplan HS: The Illustrated Manual of Sex Therapy, 2nd ed. New York, Brunner-Mazel, 1987. *A simple text graphically detailing the therapeutic techniques first introduced by Masters and Johnson.*

Kolodny RC, Masters WH, Johnson VE: Textbook of Sexual Medicine. Boston, Little, Brown and Company, 1979. *A widely used text detailing sexual problems and their therapy.*

Masters W, Johnson V: Human Sexual Response. Boston, Little, Brown and Company, 1966. *The classic work detailing human sexual response. Required reading for all individuals seriously interested in this field.*

Nadelson CC, Marcotte DB (eds.): Treatment Interventions in Human Sexuality. New York, Plenum Press, 1983. *A multiauthored text that considers sexual problems in detail.*

HORMONAL THERAPY DURING THE REPRODUCTIVE YEARS

INDUCTION OF OVULATION. Induction of ovulation should never be attempted until serious disorders precluding pregnancy are ruled out or treated. Furthermore, ovulation induction should be utilized only in women with chronic anovulation, because women with ovarian failure are unresponsive to any form of ovulation induction. In general, the use of pharmaceutical agents does not improve the quality of an ovum, and thus the chance of pregnancy is not improved in women who ovulate regularly.

Clomiphene citrate is the agent that usually induces ovulation most easily. Clomiphene should be utilized in individuals without hyperprolactinemia who have the ability to release LH and FSH. A typical course of clomiphene therapy is begun on the fifth day following either spontaneous or induced uterine bleeding. The initial dosage is 50 mg daily for 5 days. Clomiphene appears to act as an anti-estrogen and stimulates gonadotropin secretion by the pituitary gland to initiate follicular development. If ovulation is not achieved in the very first cycle of treatment, the daily dosage is increased to 100 mg. If ovulation is still not achieved, dosage is increased in a stepwise fashion by 50-mg increments to a maximum of 200 to 250 mg daily for 5 days. The highest dose should be continued for 3 to 6 months before the patient is regarded as a clomiphene failure. The quantity of drug and the length of time that it can be used, as suggested here, are greater than those recommended by the manufacturers, but conform with published series.

The ovulatory surge of LH may occur 5 to 12 days (average, 7 days) after the completion of the last day of clomiphene treatment in each course. Couples are advised to have intercourse every other day during this time interval. Ovulation can be documented by monitoring changes in basal body temperature or preferably by measuring serum progesterone approximately 14 days after the last clomiphene tablet is taken. In addition, menses should occur about 3 weeks after the last day of therapy. Withdrawal bleeding with progestin can be induced if the patient fails to bleed within 4 weeks of therapy and if a serum hCG level documents that the patient is not pregnant. Testing the urine for an LH surge with any of several commercially available tests may also be useful in timing ovulation.

Some clinicians give 5,000 to 10,000 IU of hCG intramuscularly 7 days after the last day of clomiphene therapy to trigger ovulation, but this approach has not been established to increase effectiveness. The administration of hCG, however, does serve to time ovulation and may be helpful in selected couples. Ovulation can be expected to occur approximately 36 hours after hCG administration.

Of appropriately selected patients, 75 to 80% will ovulate and 40 to 50% can be expected to become pregnant. About 15% of pregnancies can be expected with each ovulatory cycle. The multiple pregnancy rate is about 8%, with almost all being twins. The incidence of congenital anomalies is not increased.

Side effects of clomiphene are uncommon and rarely serious. The most serious ones include vasomotor flushes (10%), abdominal discomfort (5%), breast tenderness (2%), nausea and vomiting (2%), visual symptoms (1.5%), and headache (1%). Ovarian enlargement may occur but is rare (5%). Concern has recently been raised about the potential for clomiphene to increase the risk of epithelial ovarian cancer. The evidence is insufficient to change current practices but suggests that clomiphene be administered prudently and for only a limited number of cycles.

The addition of dexamethasone, 0.5 mg orally at bedtime to blunt the nighttime secretion of ACTH, may be useful in hyperandrogenic women with an adrenal component who fail to ovulate in response to clomiphene. Other individuals failing to respond to clomiphene typically require hMG-hCG or perhaps pulsatile GnRH to induce ovulation.

Bromocriptine, a dopamine agonist, is effective in inducing ovulation in hyperprolactinemic women (see Ch. 208.4). The drug should be stopped once pregnancy is confirmed. Ovulatory menses and pregnancy are achieved in about 80% of patients with galactorrhea and hyperprolactinemia. The majority of women with prolactin-secreting pituitary tumors remain asymptomatic during pregnancy. It is extremely rare for a patient with either a microadenoma or a macroadenoma to develop a problem related to the tumor that affects either the mother or the fetus during pregnancy. Monitoring during pregnancy need consist only of questioning the patient about the development of visual symptoms and headaches. Formal assessment of visual fields and CT or MRI should be carried out in any patient developing suspicious symptoms. Symptoms generally abate with institution of bromocriptine therapy. No adverse effects of bromocriptine on fetuses or pregnancies have been reported.

hMG, a purified preparation of gonadotropins extracted from the urine of postmenopausal women, must be administered intramuscularly. Each vial contains 75 units of FSH and 75 units of LH. Purified FSH has become available for use recently. Biochemically engineered preparations of both products will become available in the future. hMG is administered at doses of two to four vials for 5 to 12 days to achieve follicular development as monitored by ultrasonography and serum or urinary E_2 concentrations. hCG, 5,000 to 10,000 IU, is administered as a single intramuscular dose when follicular maturation is apparent. The hCG should be withheld if more than three follicles mature together. GnRH analogues are now being utilized to suppress endogenous follicular activity before initiating therapy with hMG and continued until hCG is given in older women and those with poor responses to hMG alone. Use of the analogues necessitates administration of larger quantities of hMG. Success rates, however, seem to be somewhat improved with this combined therapy.

Because of the expense and the complication rate, thorough evaluation should be carried out to exclude other causes of infertility before hMG-hCG is used. Ovulation can be induced in almost 100% of patients, but pregnancy occurs in only 50 to 70%. There is no increased risk of congenital anomalies with hMG-hCG. Concerns have been raised that hMG may increase the risk of ovarian epithelial cancer, but the data are too tenuous to require any change in current practice.

The rate of multiple pregnancies with hMG-hCG may approach 30%, with 5% being triplets or more. Ovarian hyperstimulation is the major side effect and may be life threatening. The ovaries enlarge remarkably in this treatment-induced syndrome, and multiple follicle cysts, stromal edema, and multiple corpora lutea are present. There is a shift of fluid from the intravascular space into the abdominal cavity with resultant hypovolemia and hemoconcentration. The cause of the ascites is unknown. Treatment is conservative, with monitoring of fluid and electrolyte status. Pelvic examinations should not be performed for fear of rupturing the ovaries. The hyperstimulation generally resolves slowly over about 7 days.

GnRH, administered intravenously or less effectively subcutaneously at doses of 5 to 20 μg every 60 to 120 minutes, also can be used to induce ovulation in women with an intact pituitary gland. It is most effective in individuals with hypothalamic chronic anovulation. hCG can be administered to support the corpus luteum after ovulation at a dose of 1500 IU intramuscularly every 3 days for three to four doses. The advantage of GnRH rests in the fact that hyperstimulation is extremely unlikely. However, reported pregnancy rates have been no greater than those achieved with hMG-hCG. Furthermore, some patients do not tolerate wearing the infusion pump that must be utilized.

Speroff L, Glass RH, Kase NG: Induction of ovulation. *In* Clinical Gynecologic Endocrinology and Infertility, 5th ed. Baltimore, Williams & Wilkins, 1994, p 897. *A detailed and practical survey of how to induce ovulation.*

STEROIDAL CONTRACEPTION. *Physiologic Actions and Metabolic Effects.* Oral contraceptive pills are the most widely used contraceptives worldwide, with more than 50 million users. Combination (estrogen-progestin) and progestin-only preparations are available. The estrogen may be either mestranol or ethinyl estradiol, while the progestin is usually one of eight derivatives of 19-nor-testosterone: norethindrone, norethindrone acetate, norethynodrel, ethynodiol diacetate, norgestrel, levonorgestrel, desogestrel, and norgestimate. Combination products containing one of the last two progestins were recently approved for use in the United States.

The low-dose combination pills currently in use (containing 30 to 35 μg of estrogen with reduced amounts of progestin) were developed to reduce the biochemical changes produced by contraceptive steroids, but the majority of studies were conducted with the older high-dose preparations. It is known that virtually all biochemical changes are dose related.

Combination oral contraceptives inhibit the midcycle gonadotropin surge by inhibiting GnRH release from the hypothalamus. Cervical mucus becomes thick, viscid, and scanty in amount, thus retarding sperm penetration. Fallopian tube motility and secretion are altered as well, and the endometrial glands produce less glycogen. Efficacy is substantiated by a failure rate of 0.1% during the first year of combination oral contraceptive use.

Oral contraceptives decrease maturation of the vaginal epithelium and somehow render the vagina more susceptible to candidiasis. The endometrium becomes atrophic with variable degrees of decidual change, leading to diminished menstrual flow. Follicular development is arrested with low estrogen and progesterone secretion. Both circulating LH and FSH levels are reduced and constant.

The general metabolic effects of oral contraceptives resemble those of pregnancy. Glucose tolerance is impaired, with an increase in plasma insulin levels. The "mini-pill" containing progestin only in low dosage may cause no changes in glucose metabolism. Levels of circulating triglycerides and of very low density lipoproteins (VLDL's) are often increased, almost entirely because of the estrogenic component (see Ch. 173). Only slight changes accompany the low-dose combination preparations. The new progestins desogestrel and norgestimate are less androgenic than the earlier agents and stimulate lipid formation less than did the earlier ones. Only very high estrogenic formulations will increase mean serum cholesterol levels. Because of a direct effect of estrogens on the endoplasmic reticulum in the liver, α_2 globulins, including angiotensinogen, and β globulins are increased, while serum albumin levels are decreased somewhat. A number of blood coagulation factors and carrier proteins (including thyroid-binding globulin, transferrin, ceruloplasmin, SHBG, and corticosteroid-binding globulin) are also increased.

Interactions with Other Drugs. Oral contraceptive steroids interact with several other drugs, leading to reduced effectiveness of the contraceptives or of the other drug. Such interactions occur because of altered drug absorption or metabolism. The majority of these interactions occur only with long-term use of the pharmacologic agent. By inducing hepatic microsomal enzymes, long-term administration of antibiotics may reduce the contraceptive efficacy of the steroids. The short-term use of antibiotics is probably of little concern. Anticonvulsants also sharply reduce the efficacy of contraceptive steroids, as do antacids, which may decrease the absorption of steroids. Conversely, contraceptive steroids oppose the therapeutic effects of anticoagulants, antidiabetic agents, and certain antihypertensive agents, such as guanethidine and α-methyldopa, because of their metabolic effects. Because of the impaired elimination of certain drugs, such as phenothiazines, oral contraceptive users may require lower doses.

Complications, Side Effects, and Benefits. Although the complications and side effects of combination oral contraceptives have been widely reported, the low-dose formulations currently available have minimized the side effects compared with the older, high-dose preparations without sacrificing contraceptive efficacy or reducing the substantial health benefits associated with oral contraceptive use.

The use of oral contraceptives increases the risk of *thromboembolism,* possibly as much as 4- to 13-fold with the doses of estrogens used in early preparations. The estrogen content of oral contraceptives appears to be correlated roughly with the risk of venous thromboembolic disease. Lower dosages of estrogen than were used initially in oral contraceptive preparations may not significantly increase the risk of any cardiovascular complications. Advanced maternal age and smoking seem to be the major risk factors for thromboembolic phenomena in users of oral contraceptives. In the absence of smoking and in women under the age of 45 years who do not suffer from obesity, hypertension, diabetes mellitus, or inherited lipoprotein abnormalities, there is little, if any, increased risk for cardiovascular disease, including myocardial infarction, with use of low-dose combination oral contraceptives. Some clinicians believe that these preparations may be used safely in normal women until the menopause.

In the absence of smoking and hypertension, most recent epidemiologic studies indicate that the use of low-dose oral contraceptives approximately doubles the risk of fatal and nonfatal stroke in young women, compared with a fourfold risk associated with the earlier use of preparations containing larger amounts of estrogens. Some but not all women with migraine headaches may note increasingly frequent headaches with oral contraceptive use. Although anecdotes indicate otherwise, epidemiologic studies do not confirm that women with migraine headaches have a greater risk of stroke.

Women using oral contraceptives are more likely to become hypertensive, especially if over the age of 35 years. Smoking may contribute to the incidence of hypertension. Increases in blood pressure are generally reversible shortly after oral contraceptives are discontinued. Failure of the blood pressure to return to normal when oral contraceptives are discontinued suggests underlying disease.

Contraceptive steroids do not appear to be teratogenic. Derivatives of 19-nor-testosterone can virilize female fetuses when administered in large doses to women early in pregnancy, but the doses required are far in excess of those contained in oral contraceptives.

Use of oral contraceptives reduces the risk of benign breast neoplasia, including fibrocystic disease and fibroadenoma. Because benign breast disease is a significant risk factor for the subsequent development of breast cancer, oral contraceptives may afford protection against breast cancer in this manner. Indeed, the incidence of breast cancer does not seem to be increased by use of oral contraceptives. Furthermore, oral contraceptives reduce the risk of developing endometrial carcinoma by about half and of developing ovarian carcinoma by about 40%. In the cases of both endometrial and ovarian cancers, the protection is related to duration of use and persists for at least 10 years after stopping oral contraceptives.

Use of combined oral contraceptives may result in an increased risk for the development of *hepatocellular adenoma,* and this risk may increase with increased duration of contraceptive use. Rarely in patients with such adenomas the liver may rupture, and death may even occur because of hemorrhage. There is no evidence of any increased risk of developing liver cancer.

The relationships of oral contraceptive use to cervical carcinoma, pituitary tumors, and melanoma are unclear. Most studies show positive relationships between cervical dysplasia and oral contraceptive use. Cervical dysplasia is increased in women with first coitus at an early age and those who have multiple sexual partners. Current evidence suggests that the increased incidence of cervical dysplasia is not related to the oral contraceptive but to these behavioral characteristics. There is some evidence that the incidence of prolactinomas may be increasing in women, but the use of contraceptive steroids has not been shown to increase this risk.

So-called *post-pill amenorrhea* is sometimes regarded as a side effect of oral contraceptive use. The return to ovulation following discontinuation of contraceptive use is variable but occurs within 4 to 8 weeks in most patients. Approximately 1 in 500 patients have amenorrhea for 6 months or longer, with 15% of these having associated galactorrhea. This prolonged amenorrhea is probably caused by underlying disorders unrelated to oral contraceptive use. In normal women subsequent fertility is unimpaired.

Nausea and vomiting occur occasionally when use begins but generally abate with continued use. Mastalgia and increased breast size may occur but also tend to subside in several cycles. Chloasma (hyperpigmentation of the face) is a leading cause of pill discontinuation. Acne is usually improved, but occasionally may be exacerbated. Dizziness, headaches, visual disturbances, depression, and increased or decreased libido have been reported. Easy bruisability due to increased capillary fragility and edema also may occur.

Other therapeutic benefits exist with oral contraceptive use as well. The risk of pelvic inflammatory disease appears reduced by half. Decreased menstrual blood loss results in a lower incidence of iron deficiency anemia. Acne frequently improves and dysmenorrhea decreases in the majority of patients. Symptomatic relief of endometriosis occurs in some patients. The risk of functional ovarian cysts is decreased, as are the incidences of ectopic pregnancies and uterine fibroids. Women with PCO syndrome treated with oral contraceptives are afforded protection from endometrial carcinoma. Oral contraceptives have been linked to prevention of postmenopausal osteoporosis. Oral contraceptives may possibly afford protection against development of rheumatoid arthritis as well.

Absolute contraindications to the use of oral contraceptives include thrombophlebitis, thromboembolic disorders, cardiovascular disease, or a history of these conditions; markedly impaired liver function; known or suspected estrogen-dependent neoplasia; undiagnosed abnormal genital bleeding; known or suspected pregnancy; and congenital hyperlipidemia. Oral contraceptives generally should be administered with caution to smokers, women who are obese, and those with varicose veins. If headaches develop or become more frequent with pill use, oral contraceptives should be discontinued. Because of a possible increase in postsurgical thromboembolic complications in women using oral contraceptives, use of oral contraceptives should be discontinued 2 weeks prior to major surgery and begun again 2 weeks postoperatively.

Low-dose combination oral contraceptive pills offer superb protection for sexually active women not desiring pregnancy. For most such individuals the benefits of the low-dose preparations clearly outweigh the adverse effects, but possible side effects and complications must be considered in treating individual patients.

Two long-acting, implantable or injectable contraceptive steroid preparations are now approved for use in the United States. Levonorgestrel (Norplant) and depo-medroxyprogesterone (Depo-Provera) are extremely effective, contain no estrogen, and affect fertility by suppressing pituitary gonadotropin secretion. They also thicken cervical mucus and cause endometrial atrophy and irregular uterine bleeding.

Henzl MR: Contraceptive hormones and their clinical use. *In* Yen SSC, Jaffe RB (eds.): Reproductive Endocrinology, 3rd ed. Philadelphia, WB Saunders Company, 1991, p 807. *A detailed discussion of steroidal contraception.*
Speroff L, Darney P: A Clinical Guide for Contraception. Baltimore, Williams & Wilkins, 1992. *A monograph devoted to a consideration of contraceptive choices.*

THE MENOPAUSE AND POSTMENOPAUSAL YEARS

DEFINITIONS AND EPIDEMIOLOGY. The *menopause* is the final menstrual period denoting the cessation of cyclic ovarian function as manifested by cyclic menstruation. The *climacteric* is the physiologic period during which regression of ovarian function occurs. Its onset generally is signaled by alterations in the menstrual cycle or vasomotor symptomatology. Menopause occurs at a mean age of approximately 51 years. Today's average woman in the Western world can expect to live one third of her life in the postmenopausal phase.

SYMPTOMATOLOGY AND SIGNS. Most signs and symptoms associated with the postmenopausal years result from decreased circulating estrogen. Common symptoms include hot flushes, paresthesias, palpitations, cold hands and feet, headaches, vertigo, irritability, anxiety, nervousness, depression, fatigue, weight gain, insomnia, night sweats, forgetfulness, and inability to concentrate.

Vasomotor instability is perhaps the most common complaint. Over 75% of women experience hot flushes with decreasing estrogen levels, and these may persist for years. In a typical hot flush, the skin, especially of the head and neck, becomes red and warm for a few seconds to 2 minutes with cold chills thereafter. Accompanying physiologic changes include a rise in skin temperature, peripheral vasodilatation, increased heart rate, decreased skin resistance, and concomitant LH pulses. The mechanism for hot flushes is unknown but must involve thermoregulatory centers in the hypothalamus.

Any increase in bleeding or resumption of bleeding after 6 months of amenorrhea demands examination and sampling of the endometrium to exclude carcinoma. Women note relocation of fat deposits, with increased fat in the lower abdomen, hips, and breasts. The genital skin becomes thin and pale, with a decrease in the size of the labia minora, clitoris, uterus, and ovaries, and the women often complain of dyspareunia. Decreased elastic tissue of skin is noted, and osteoporosis may occur in about 25% of postmenopausal women (see Ch. 217).

Menopausal signs and symptoms may begin long before menses have ceased. Symptoms may be difficult to diagnose in women with previous hysterectomies. Following bilateral oophorectomy young women develop identical signs and symptoms.

ENDOCRINOLOGIC CHANGES. During the menopausal transition regular menstrual cycles may continue up to the menopause. The cycles may become shorter, due to shortened follicular phases, with increased FSH, normal LH, and decreased E_2 and progesterone levels compared with normal ovulatory cycles. Variable cycles also may occur prior to the menopause, with some being ovulatory and others being anovulatory. Waning ovarian follicular activity with decreasing E_2 production must be central to these changes, and yet some follicles have been found on occasion in ovaries of postmenopausal women.

In postmenopausal women, circulating FSH and LH concentrations are greatly increased. Estrogen levels are decreased markedly, but androgen levels are decreased only slightly. The postmenopausal ovaries continue to secrete substantial amounts of androgen (androstenedione and testosterone), which together with adrenal androgens are converted to estrogens by extraglandular conversion in the periphery. The peripheral conversion of androgens accounts for most circulating estrogen in postmenopausal women.

CLINICAL MANAGEMENT. Treatment of postmenopausal women must be individualized and based on a personal dialogue with each patient. Exogenous estrogen replacement stops or diminishes hot flushes, reverses atrophic genital changes, decreases osteoporotic fractures (see Ch. 217), and may decrease the incidence of atherosclerotic coronary artery disease.

Estrogen replacement therapy is absolutely contraindicated in postmenopausal women with estrogen-dependent tumors of the breast, uterus, or kidney; acute liver disease; cerebrovascular disease; active deep-vein thrombosis and embolism; malignant melanoma (?); and undiagnosed genital bleeding. Replacement therapy must be considered carefully and other therapy may require modification in women with estrogen-associated hypertension, diabetes mellitus, cholecystitis and cholelithiasis, pancreatitis, congestive heart failure, past endometriosis, and neuro-ophthalmologic vascular disease. Individual exceptions to even the absolute contraindications exist.

Many treatment regimens are currently being utilized. Estrogen should be administered together with a progestin in a cyclic fashion to women with a uterus to prevent an increased risk of endometrial hyperplasia and carcinoma. Oral estrone sulfate (0.625 to 1.25 mg), micronized estradiol-17β (1 mg), or transdermal estradiol (0.05 mg) may be given daily. To this should be added a progestin such as medroxyprogesterone acetate (5 to 10 mg orally for 12 to 14 days each month, beginning on the first day of the month). Menstrual bleeding occurs in more than half of the women. As a consequence, continuous daily administration of a combination of an estrogen and a progestin has been advocated. The ratios of estrogen to progestin utilized are empiric. Unfortunately, irregular breakthrough bleeding occurs frequently in the first several months of therapy, even though the majority of women eventually become amenorrheic. Although continuous combined therapy is an option, it cannot be advocated strongly until more data accumulate regarding its safety and efficacy. Similar dosages of estrogen alone may be administered continuously to women who have undergone hysterectomy, particularly because progestins may impact negatively on several beneficial metabolic effects of estrogen. Younger women may require twice as much estrogen as older women to alleviate symptoms.

Even the continuous combined replacement therapy differs from oral contraceptive preparations in that the doses of estrogen and progestin are lower. Moreover, the estrogens utilized in replacement therapy have fewer metabolic effects than do the synthetic estrogens used in oral contraceptives. There is no evidence that postmenopausal estrogen administration increases the risk of thromboembolic phenomena.

Before beginning estrogen replacement therapy, patients should have a complete history and physical examination. A pretreatment mammogram is indicated because estrogens stimulate glandular tissue and may make diagnosis of breast masses more difficult. Periodic Papanicolaou smears should be obtained, and patients should undergo endometrial biopsy for any breakthrough bleeding and perhaps at intervals of 1 to 2 years while receiving estrogen replacement therapy. Some clinicians believe endometrial biopsies are not needed so long as there is no abnormal bleeding and withdrawal bleeding does not begin until at least 11 days after beginning progestin.

Side effects of therapy are common and may require modifications of therapy. Breast tenderness occurs frequently if too much estrogen is given. The dose of progestin should be reduced in the woman who complains of depression and/or bloating.

Medroxyprogesterone acetate (20 to 40 mg) or megestrol acetate (40 to 80 mg) orally each day may be utilized to treat hot flushes in women who cannot or will not take estrogens. Clonidine skin patches programmed to deliver 0.1 mg per day may also reduce the intensity and frequency of hot flushes in individuals who cannot take estrogens. Postural hypotension, however, is a common side effect with this therapy. Vaginal lubricants may be used for symptomatic treatment of dyspareunia in such individuals.

EFFECTS OF ESTROGEN ON LIPIDS AND CARCINOMA. Unlike with the use of oral contraceptives in younger women, estrogen replacement in postmenopausal women does not raise blood pressure. This may be true because some estrogens, particularly the synthetic ones used in oral contraceptives, increase hepatic synthesis of renin substrate (angiotensinogen). In standard doses, the naturally occurring estrogens E_2 and E_1 do not increase renin substrate.

Estrogen administration tends to lower total cholesterol levels, with the degree of reduction varying with the dose and potency of the estrogen. Furthermore, estrogen decreases the LDL-cholesterol and increases the HDL-cholesterol fraction. Thus the net effect of estrogen administration is to shift the HDL-LDL ratio to one associated with a decreased risk of cardiovascular disease. Overall, the risk of cardiovascular disease appears reduced by half in postmenopausal users of estrogen, but this reduced risk has not yet been confirmed by prospective studies. Estrogen administration to postmenopausal women may increase plasma triglycerides slightly, but these increases are generally of no significance except in some individuals with genetic disorders of triglyceride metabolism in whom marked elevations may occur.

Progestins, especially those derived from 19-nor-testosterone (such as norethindrone and norgestrel), oppose the effects of estrogens on plasma lipid and lipoprotein fractions. Even orally administered medroxyprogesterone, which is relatively neutral when given alone, appears to reduce the favorable changes induced by estrogens when given in combination with estrogen.

Estrogens exert their cardiovascular effects in many ways. They appear to retard the oxidation of LDL and thereby may decrease the atherogenicity of LDL. Estrogens also suppress the uptake of LDL by blood vessel walls, inhibiting the development of endothelial atheroma. Estrogens cause vasodilation of coronary vessels. These vasodilatory effects may be mediated by estrogen-induced alterations in prostaglandin metabolism and by increasing the levels of prostacyclin (a vasodilator) and decreasing the levels of thromboxane (a vasoconstrictor). Estrogen receptors exist in the endothelial cells of the vascular system, and binding to these receptors may stimulate the release of nitric oxide, a potent endogenous vasodilator. A positive inotropic effect of estrogen on cardiac function also has been observed.

Estrogen-containing oral contraceptive preparations have not been linked conclusively to increased risks of endometrial or breast cancer. However, as noted, estrogen given alone to postmenopausal women greatly increases the risk of endometrial cancer over that in women never given estrogen. The risk of endometrial carcinoma is reduced markedly, if not abolished, by the cyclic addition of a progestin. Whether estrogen per therapy increases the risk of breast cancer is not clear. If so, the effect is approximately 25% with prolonged use of estrogen. Because the likelihood of death from cardiovascular disease is far greater than that from breast cancer, it appears that the benefits of estrogen replacement therapy outweigh the risks in most postmenopausal women.

Lobo R (ed.): Treatment of the Postmenopausal Woman. Basic and Clinical Aspects. New York, Raven Press, 1993. *A review by leading authorities on the physiologic changes and therapeutic approaches to the menopause.*

OVARIAN TUMORS

Ovarian tumors may cause ovarian dysfunction, either by secreting hormones or by stimulating adjacent non-neoplastic stromal cells. Only perhaps 5% of ovarian tumors, however, show functional activity. Most nonfunctional tumors are asymptomatic until late in their evolution; more than three fourths are diagnosed only in advanced stages. In contrast, women with functioning neoplasms commonly present with altered sexual development or reproductive abnormalities, and thus diagnosis is made much earlier. Ovarian tumors may occur in all age groups but are less common in younger women, especially before puberty.

Ovarian tumors generally are classified as (1) common epithelial tumors derived from coelomic epithelial cells; (2) sex cord stromal tumors composed of granulosa cells, theca cells, Sertoli-Leydig cells, or their progenitors; (3) lipid or lipoid cell tumors; (4) germ cell tumors, including teratomas, dysgerminomas, and choriocarcinomas; (5) gonadoblastomas; (6) soft tissue tumors not specific to the ovary; and (7) secondary metastatic tumors. Each of these major classes of tumors includes several different histologic types. Sex cord stromal tumors are most apt to be functioning.

Ovarian neoplasms must be distinguished from tumor-like conditions of the ovary, which include luteomas of pregnancy (nodular theca-lutein hyperplasia) that may result in virilization of the mother but regress spontaneously post partum; hyperplasia of ovarian stroma (hyperthecosis), frequently associated with severe hirsutism; functional follicle and corpus luteum cysts; germinal inclusion cysts lined by surface epithelium; simple cysts; paraovarian

TABLE 208–9. CLINICAL FEATURES OF HORMONE-PRODUCING OVARIAN TUMORS

Tumor	Hormones Produced*	Incidence				Size Range in cm (per cent Palpable)	Miscellaneous
		Age in Years		Malignancy	Bilaterality		
		Peak	Range				
Androblastoma (arrhenoblastoma)	*Androgens,* estrogens	20–40	4–69	20%	Rare	<5–>25 (85)	Most common virilizing ovarian neoplasm
Dysgerminoma	Androgens, *chorionic gonadotropin*	10–30	6–76	100%	15%	3–50 (60)	May be "mixed" with other tumors originating from germ cells
Gonadoblastoma	*Androgens,* estrogens	10–30	6–38	50%	40%	<1–>30 (?)	Usually occur in genetic males with female external genitalia
Granulosa-theca cell	*Estrogens,* androgens, progestogens	30–70	<1–92	5–20%	10–15%	<1–>30 (80–90)	Most common functioning ovarian neoplasm
Hilar cell	*Androgens,* estrogens	45–75	4–86	Rare	Rare	1–9 (50)	Hypertension in 50%, diabetes in 50%
Lipoid cell (adrenal-like)	*Androgens,* estrogens	20–50	6–78	20%	Rare	0.5–30	Diabetes associated with lesion in 50%
Teratomas, benign	Serotonin, thyroxine	10–40	<1–78	Rare	10%	2–45 (90)	Carcinoid syndrome only in patients with large carcinoid tumors
Teratomas, malignant	Chorionic gonadotropin	6–15	6–42	100%	Rare	>5 (100)	Not all secrete chorionic gonadotropin

Modified from data of Rose GI, Vande Wiele RL: *In* Williams RH (ed.): Textbook of Endocrinology, 5th ed. Philadelphia, WB Saunders, 1974, p 368.
* When more than one hormone is secreted, the major one is *italicized.*

cysts; inflammatory lesions; and endometrial cysts or endometriomas.

Ovarian neoplasms are diagnosed most commonly at the time of routine pelvic examination. Even most functioning neoplasms are palpable; those that are not may be identified by ultrasonography. As an ovarian tumor grows, it distends the abdomen, leading to pressure on the bladder or rectum and a sensation of pelvic fullness and discomfort. Ascites may develop if the neoplasm is malignant or sometimes when it is not (Meigs' syndrome). Abdominal and pelvic pain may occur with torsion, hemorrhage, or rupture of the tumor.

Functioning ovarian tumors can produce other clinical manifestations as well (Table 208–9). Some tumors are associated with clinical manifestations of decreased hormone production. Intervals of amenorrhea caused by steroid suppression of gonadotropins may alternate with excessive vaginal bleeding produced by steroid stimulation of the endometrium during the reproductive years. In some young girls, steroid-secreting ovarian tumors may cause pseudopubertal development. In postmenopausal women, increased estrogens, secreted by the tumor itself or from peripheral aromatization of androgens secreted by the tumor, may stimulate the endometrium and result in bleeding.

Any pelvic mass identified on examination must be investigated. What constitutes such a "mass" and what evaluation is indicated depend on the age of the individual. Adnexal masses < 5 cm in diameter may well be due to normal follicular development in women of reproductive age and may resolve with observation over 2 to 8 weeks. Even simple cystic masses > 5 cm in diameter, as documented by ultrasound examination, may resolve over a few weeks. Those that do not resolve require surgical removal. Any palpable, complex adnexal mass in a postmenopausal woman, in whom the ovaries normally atrophy and cannot be detected during examination, should be removed. Ultrasonography also may identify small simple cysts in postmenopausal women. Most regress spontaneously.

Yeh I-T, Zaloudek C, Kurman RJ: Functioning tumors and tumor-like conditions of the ovary. *In* Becker KL (ed.): Principles and Practice of Endocrinology and Metabolism. Philadelphia, JB Lippincott, 1990, p 848. *An excellent discussion of the clinical manifestations of ovarian tumors for any physician who undertakes the medical care of women.*

208.2 Ovarian Carcinoma
Howard W. Jones, III

Ovarian carcinoma is the most deadly of the gynecologic malignancies. The age-specific incidence gradually rises, reaching a peak at about age 70, at which time it is 55 per 100,000 among white women. The rate is somewhat lower among black women. The cause of ovarian cancer is unknown; except for some relatively rare familial groups, it has not been possible to identify any clinically useful high-risk groups for increased surveillance. The lifetime risk of ovarian cancer for women in the United States is about 1.4%, but women with one first-degree relative appear to have an increased risk of 3 to 5%. Rare familial groups with a high incidence of ovarian, breast, and colon cancer have been described. Multiple pregnancies and the use of oral contraceptives may be protective because of decreased ovulation and hormonal influences.

PATHOLOGY

Four types of ovarian tumors require separate consideration because of their clinical characteristics and prognoses: (1) The common *epithelial tumors* of the ovary include the serous, mucinous, endometrioid, clear cell, and otherwise unspecified adenocarcinomas. These tumors account for almost 90% of ovarian cancers and are most commonly found in postmenopausal women. (2) *Germ cell tumors*, which arise from the totipotent oocytes, are usually benign ("dermoid cysts"). They often occur in young women and are almost always unilateral. When malignant (e.g., dysgerminoma, teratoma), they are highly aggressive but respond very well to combination chemotherapy. (3) *Stromal tumors* are generally low grade, and because they arise from the granulosa, theca, and Sertoli-Leydig cells of the ovary, they may be hormonally functional. They are usually unilateral and may occur in any age group, but most typically in the fourth and fifth decades. Surgical excision alone may be all the therapy required, but combination chemotherapy is effective for metastatic or recurrent disease. (4) Malignancies of other sites that are metastatic to the ovary must always be considered in the evaluation of patients with a pelvic mass. In some cases a pelvic mass is the first indication of a primary gastrointestinal or endometrial carcinoma. Breast cancer also commonly metastasizes to the ovary.

DIAGNOSIS
Clinical Presentation

Early ovarian cancer is usually asymptomatic. Occasionally, ovarian enlargement is found on routine examination and cancer may be discovered incidentally at the time of abdominal or pelvic surgery for other indications. In most cases, however, widespread intra-abdominal metastases are present by the time the diagnosis is made. Symptoms of abdominal swelling, bloating, and pelvic fullness or pressure are common. It is not unusual for the patient to have had vague abdominal complaints or nonspecific gastrointestinal symptoms. Ascites or a palpable abdominopelvic mass may be found on examination. The presence of an irregular mass in the pelvis or cul-de-sac nodularity accompanied by ascites is often diagnostic. Some patients develop malignant pleural effusions and present with shortness of breath.

SCREENING TESTS. Screening tests for ovarian cancer are still controversial. Transvaginal ultrasonography, although quite effective for diagnosing ovarian cysts and tumors, is nonspecific and its use for screening results in surgical exploration of a large number of women with benign ovarian cysts. Even when a cancer is diagnosed by ultrasound screening in an asymptomatic patient, there is still no evidence that survival is improved. Serum levels of the tumor-associated antigen CA-125 above 35 U per milliliter are highly correlated with ovarian cancer in postmenopausal women. Unfortunately, many ovarian tumors do not cause elevated levels of CA-125, whereas endometriosis, pelvic inflammatory disease, and some benign ovarian tumors may do so. The relative rarity of ovarian cancer, combined with the nonspecific nature of currently available tests, makes ovarian cancer screening unsatisfactory.

DIFFERENTIAL DIAGNOSIS. A pelvic mass can be caused by either a benign or a malignant tumor of the ovary as well as by inflammatory conditions, physiologic cysts, and malignancies of other pelvic organs and structures. Initially, a careful history and physical examination are most helpful in suggesting possible primary sites. Pelvic ultrasonography may allow the dimensions and character of the mass to be determined. Smooth-walled, unilocular ovarian cysts are almost always benign, whereas malignancies are most commonly described as echogenically "complex," with both cystic and solid components. The possibility of ectopic pregnancy must always be considered, and a pregnancy test is therefore normally the first laboratory study done in women in the reproductive age group. A careful contraceptive history is important because functional ovarian cysts, including both follicle cysts and corpus luteum cysts, are common in ovulating women. Inflammatory masses and endometriosis can be confused with ovarian cancer and can cause an elevated CA-125 in addition to a complex adnexal mass. In the older age group, diverticular abscesses and carcinoma of the colon must be considered within the differential diagnosis.

Once a complete history and physical examination have been done and the size and character of the mass have been confirmed by ultrasonography, several additional studies may be helpful. A barium enema or colonoscopy is almost always indicated prior to surgery to rule out a primary lesion or secondary involvement of the colon. An abdominal and pelvic computerized tomography scan can identify evidence of upper abdominal metastases or ureteral obstruction.

Additional studies (e.g., brain scans, bone scans) should generally be reserved for patients whose symptoms or physical findings suggest involvement of the areas to be studied.

TREATMENT
Surgery

In almost all cases of suspected ovarian carcinoma, an exploratory laparotomy is the ultimate diagnostic procedure. If the diagnosis is sustained, tumor debulking, including total abdominal hysterectomy and bilateral salpingo-oophorectomy, if possible, should be done. At this point a definitive diagnosis can be made and the extent of the disease accurately staged (Table 208–10). Aggressive tumor debulking, even when all cancer cannot be removed, improves the length and quality of survival. If possible, this initial surgery should be done by a gynecologic oncologist whose special training and experience should provide the optimal surgical and postoperative management.

The goal of the initial operation for ovarian cancer is twofold. First, all tumor should be removed if possible to provide the greatest possibility of cure. In approximately two thirds of patients, however, widespread intra-abdominal metastases prevent complete surgical debulking. The second goal of surgery is accurate staging (Table 208–10). In addition to the stage of disease, the volume of residual tumor following initial surgery, the histologic type and grade of the tumor, and the age of the patient have important prognostic significance. Women with minimal residual disease and well-differentiated tumors have the most favorable outcome. Those under age 50 and those with tumors exhibiting mucinous and endometrioid histology also seem to do better.

Careful staging evaluation with peritoneal cytology and multiple biopsies of the upper abdomen (the omentum, diaphragm, and retroperitoneal nodes) is especially important in early-stage disease because microscopic metastases often escape clinical detection. Accurate staging guides the most appropriate postoperative management. Patients with Stage Ia well-differentiated epithelial ovarian cancers do not need additional therapy.

In patients with advanced disease, aggressive surgical debulking includes bowel resection or colostomy in as many as 25% of patients. Whether such extensive surgical resection actually improves 5- and 10-year survival rates is still controversial. It is agreed,

TABLE 208–10. DEFINITIONS OF THE STAGES IN PRIMARY CARCINOMA OF THE OVARY*

Stage I	Growth limited to the ovaries.
Stage Ia	Growth limited to one ovary; no ascites. No tumor on the external surface; capsule intact.
Stage Ib	Growth limited to both ovaries; no ascites. No tumor on the external surfaces; capsules intact.
Stage Ic	Tumor either Stage Ia or Ib, but with tumor on surface of one or both ovaries; or with capsule ruptured; or with ascites present containing malignant cells or with positive peritoneal washings.
Stage II	Growth involving one or both ovaries with pelvic extension.
Stage IIa	Extension and/or metastases to the uterus and/or tubes.
Stage IIb	Extension to other pelvic tissues.
Stage IIc	Tumor either Stage IIa or IIb, but with tumor on surface of one or both ovaries; or with capsule(s) ruptured; or with ascites present containing malignant cells or with positive peritoneal washings.
Stage III	Tumor involving one or both ovaries with peritoneal implants outside the pelvis and/or positive retroperitoneal or inguinal nodes. Superficial liver metastases equal Stage III. Tumor is limited to the true pelvis but with histologically proven malignant extension to small bowel or omentum.
Stage IIIa	Tumor grossly limited to the true pelvis with negative nodes but with histologically confirmed microscopic seeding of abdominal peritoneal surfaces.
Stage IIIb	Tumor involving one or both ovaries with histologically confirmed implants of abdominal peritoneal surfaces, none exceeding 2 cm in diameter. Nodes are negative.
Stage IIIc	Abdominal implants greater than 2 cm in diameter and/or positive retroperitoneal or inguinal nodes.
Stage IV	Growth involving one or both ovaries with distant metastases. If pleural effusion is present, there must be positive cytology to allot a case to Stage IV. Parenchymal liver metastases equals Stage IV.

* Nomenclature of the International Federation of Gynecology and Obstetrics (FIGO). Staging is based on findings at clinical examination and surgical exploration.

however, that optimal tumor debulking (<1 cm residual) results in prolongation of good-quality survival. This is where the skills and experienced judgment of the gynecologic oncologist are most important.

Chemotherapy

Most patients with ovarian cancer require postoperative chemotherapy. Cisplatin or carboplatin, which has fewer renal and neurologic side effects, is the cornerstone of most regimens. They are usually given in combination with other agents, such as cyclophosphamide, doxorubicin, hexamethylmelamine, or etoposide. Taxol has also been shown to be effective and is being used as second line and sometimes as primary therapy. Most patients are treated with intermittent intravenous therapy at 4-week intervals for six monthly cycles, but some centers use intraperitoneal chemotherapy instead. Response rates of 60 to 80% are generally seen, but only about 30% of the treatment group experiences a complete response. Some debilitated patients are still treated with a single alkylating agent, such as oral melphalan, but this therapy is probably not as effective as cisplatin alone or in combination with other cytotoxic drugs. Carboplatin is almost as well tolerated as oral melphalan.

Radiation Therapy

Postoperative external radiation therapy to the whole abdomen is probably as effective as chemotherapy for patients with minimal residual tumor. The toxicity of such therapy, especially that of gastrointestinal obstruction, has usually been greater than that associated with chemotherapy.

Intraperitoneal radioactive colloidal chronic phosphate is also used to treat some women with Stage I or II disease with no gross residual tumor. Only patients with very early disease are good candidates for this therapy, which requires a complete and uniform intraperitoneal distribution of the radioactive suspension.

"Second-look" Surgery

A planned re-exploration in order to evaluate the extent of disease following a course of therapy and to resect any residual malignancy has been called "second-look" surgery. This approach allows an excellent research evaluation of the effect of the primary therapy, but it has not proven to be of significant clinical benefit to patients with ovarian cancer. Measurements of tumor-associated antigens, such as CA-125, used in conjunction with periodic physical examinations and selected radiographic studies, have been helpful in monitoring the disease status of treated patients. Until more effective salvage therapy is available, second-look surgery in the asymptomatic patient with a normal physical examination is probably not indicated.

Treatment of Recurrent, Metastatic Disease

The overall survival of patients treated for ovarian cancer is only 30 to 40%; many women develop progressive disease despite appropriate primary therapy. Salvage chemotherapy protocols for recurrent disease lead to only a 10% response rate, which is usually partial and short term. Widespread intra-abdominal metastases with bowel obstruction are frequent, but reoperation with resection, bypass, or enterostomy may provide significant palliation. Pleural effusion may require thoracentesis and pleural sclerosis. With the relative effectiveness of current primary chemotherapy, patients may survive to develop late metastases to the liver, brain, and meninges. Localized radiation has been helpful in some of these patients.

PROGNOSIS

The long-term survival rate of patients treated for epithelial ovarian cancer is still disappointing (Table 208–11). Almost 60% of patients have Stage III or IV disease at the time of diagnosis. Although the majority of women with advanced disease live 2 years with a reasonable quality of life, recurrent cancer eventually becomes symptomatic in most, and by 5 years only about 15% still survive. The results are much better for patients diagnosed at an earlier stage. Almost three fourths of women with Stage I ovarian cancer survive 5 years.

TABLE 208-11. CARCINOMA OF THE OVARY: DISTRIBUTION BY STAGE AND 3- AND 5-YEAR SURVIVAL IN THE DIFFERENT STAGES*

Stage	Patients Treated		3-Year Survival (%)	5-Year Survival (%)
	Number	(%)		
I	2230	26.1	79.8	72.8
II	1313	15.4	60.5	46.3
III	3339	39.1	27.1	18.6
IV	1391	16.3	10.1	4.8
Unstaged	268	3.1	31.7	21.6
TOTAL	8541	100.0	43.4	34.9

* Data from Carcinoma of the ovary. In Pettersson F (ed.): Annual Report on the Results of Treatment in Gynecological Cancer, Vol. 22. Stockholm, Panorama Press AB, 1994. The "Annual Report" is published at regular intervals by the International Federation for Gynecology and Obstetrics and contains vast quantities of statistics generated from institutions which submit their treatment results from throughout the world.

Baker VV: Molecular biology and genetics of epithelial ovarian cancer. Obstet Gynecol Clin North Am 21:25, 1994. *A good update on the rapidly expanding knowledge of the molecular genetics of ovarian cancer.*

Herbst AL: The epidemiology of ovarian carcinoma and the current status of tumor markers to detect disease. Am J Obstet Gynecol 170:1099, 1994. *An excellent review of epidemiology and screening for ovarian cancer. Part of a mini-symposium.*

Hoskins WJ: Surgical staging and cytoreductive surgery of epithelial ovarian cancer. Cancer 71:1534, 1993. *This paper discusses the importance and controversies related to staging and aggressive debulking of ovarian cancer.*

Ozols RF: Treatment of ovarian cancer: Current status. Semin Oncol 21:1, 1994. *A complete review on the therapy of ovarian cancer.*

Soper JT: Management of early-stage epithelial ovarian cancer. Clin Obstet Gynecol 37:423, 1994. *The indications for chemotherapy and radiation and the results that can be expected are reviewed.*

Thigpen JT, Bertelsen K, Eisenhauer EA, et al.: Long-term follow-up of patients with advanced ovarian carcinoma treated with chemotherapy. Ann Oncol 4(54):35, 1993. *The authors report 5- to 10-year follow-up in a series of patients treated with platin-based combination chemotherapy.*

208.3 Hirsutism
Roger S. Rittmaster

DEFINITION. ***Normal Hair Growth.*** Most body hair can be classified as vellus or terminal. Vellus hairs are fine and unpigmented, such as those that cover the face of children. Terminal hairs, pigmented and coarser, may be sex hormone–dependent (such as those over the chin and abdomen of men) or sex hormone–independent (such as eyebrows and eyelashes) (Fig. 208–9). Androgens convert vellus hair to terminal hair in sex hormone–dependent areas.

Hirsutism. Hirsutism is the presence of excess hair in women. This is usually an androgen-dependent process. Twenty-five to 35% of young women have terminal hair over the lower abdomen, around the nipples, or over the upper lip. Most women gradually develop more androgen-dependent body hair with age. Nevertheless, "normal" patterns of female hair growth are unacceptable to many women. At the other extreme, severe hirsutism may rarely be the earliest sign of masculinizing diseases. More often, however, severe hirsutism reflects only increased androgen production in women with no serious underlying disorder.

ETIOLOGY. Hirsutism may be divided into androgen-dependent and androgen-independent causes. Androgen-dependent hirsutism is restricted to areas where men typically become hirsute and often begins with adolescence. In women, androgens arise from the ovaries, the adrenal glands, or exogenous sources such as anabolic steroids (Table 208–12). Often, no definite abnormality exists; the hirsutism simply results from modestly increased androgen production and/or increased skin sensitivity to androgens.

Androgen-independent hirsutism is caused by drugs (cyclosporine, glucocorticoids, minoxidil, diazoxide, and possibly phenytoin) or starvation (anorexia nervosa); it may be associated with the skin lesions of porphyria; or it may be an inherited condition. Androgen-independent hirsutism is characterized by long, fine hairs occurring over much of the body, including such areas as the forehead and flanks. Androgens may exacerbate androgen-independent hirsutism, giving rise to a clinically confusing presentation. The pathophysiology of androgen-independent hirsutism is unknown.

PATHOPHYSIOLOGY OF ANDROGEN-DEPENDENT HIRSUTISM. To be active in skin, testosterone, the major circulating androgen, must first be converted to dihydrotestosterone by the enzyme 5α-reductase. Hirsute women have elevated skin 5α-reductase compared with nonhirsute women. Nevertheless, increased 5α-reductase alone is usually insufficient to induce hirsutism.

Hirsute women as a group also have increased androgen production from the adrenal glands, the ovaries, or both. Either testosterone itself is secreted, or androgen precursors such as androstenedione are secreted, which are then converted in the liver or skin to active androgens. Most hirsute women do not have an underlying disease, but simply fall at one end of the spectrum of androgen production and skin 5α-reductase activity.

The ovarian and adrenal causes of hirsutism listed in Table 208–12 lead to increased androgen production. Virilizing tumors secrete androgens directly. The pituitary adenomas in Cushing's disease release ACTH, which stimulates the adrenals to secrete both cortisol and androgens (see Ch. 204.1). The virilizing forms of congenital adrenal hyperplasia involve enzyme defects that impair cortisol synthesis, leading to increased ACTH secretion (see Ch. 204.1). The enzyme block causes shunting of cortisol precursors to androgens. The most common form, 21-hydroxylase deficiency, leads to an overproduction of 17-hydroxyprogesterone. Whereas severe forms of 21-hydroxylase deficiency cause ambiguous genitalia in female infants, milder forms may lead only to hirsutism and/or irregular menses. This "attenuated" form of 21-hydroxylase deficiency is present in about 1% of hirsute women.

In the polycystic ovarian syndrome, both the ovaries and adrenals secrete excess androgens, although the majority of the androgens are usually of ovarian origin (see Ch. 208.1).

CLINICAL MANIFESTATIONS. Androgen-induced hirsutism of benign origin usually begins in adolescence and becomes gradually worse with time. Family history is often positive. The hirsutism may vary from mild to severe. Usually hair growth begins over the lower abdomen, on the breasts, and over the upper lip. Widespread hirsutism over the upper back, upper abdomen, and upper chest implies severe hyperandrogenism. Some women may have only facial hair or other unusual patterns of hirsutism, probably due to local variation in skin 5α-reductase activity.

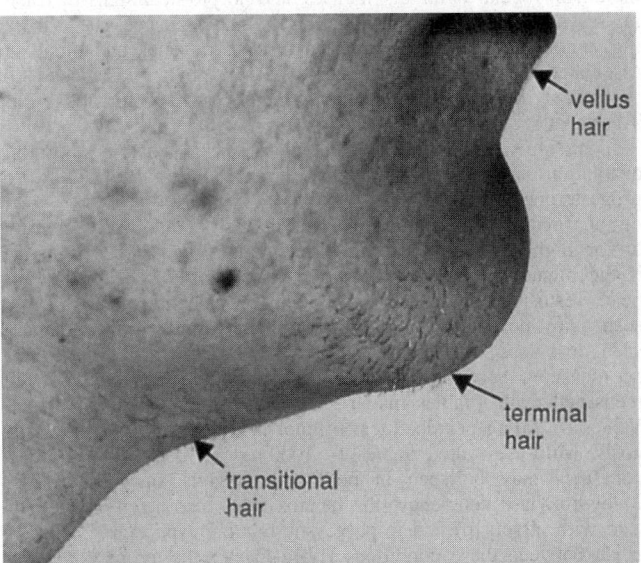

FIGURE 208-9. Facial hair growth in a hirsute woman. Vellus hair is fine, unpigmented hair. Terminal hair is coarse and pigmented. Transitional hair is intermediate between vellus and terminal. This woman also has mild acne, another androgen-dependent process. (Reprinted with permission from Rittmaster RS: Hirsutism. Med Clin North Am 14:2686, 1987.)

TABLE 208-12. CAUSES OF ANDROGEN-DEPENDENT HIRSUTISM

Ovarian causes
  Severe insulin resistance
  Virilizing ovarian tumors
Adrenal causes
  Congenital adrenal hyperplasia
    21-Hydroxylase deficiency
    3β-Hydroxysteroid dehydrogenase deficiency
    11-Hydroxylase deficiency
  Cushing's disease
  Ectopic ACTH-producing tumors
  Virilizing adrenal tumors
Combined ovarian and adrenal causes
  Polycystic ovary syndrome
  "Idiopathic" hirsutism
Exogenous androgens
  "Anabolic" steroids
  Danazol
  Postmenopausal hormone replacement formulations containing androgens

Severe, rapidly progressive hirsutism, beginning in childhood or beyond adolescence, suggests an androgen-secreting tumor. Such tumors can cause signs of virilization: deepening of the voice, excess muscle development, and marked clitoral enlargement. Signs of virilization, however, simply imply severe hyperandrogenism and can occasionally be seen with all causes of hirsutism. Androgen-secreting tumors are rare, and most severely hirsute women have either polycystic ovarian syndrome or hirsutism alone.

Attenuated congenital adrenal hyperplasia is clinically indistinguishable from simple hirsutism or polycystic ovarian syndrome, and the diagnosis must be made biochemically. Cushing's disease may be suspected when the patient presents with central obesity, hypertension, diabetes, and/or thinning of the skin (see Ch. 204.1).

DIAGNOSIS. The diagnostic evaluation of hirsutism is directed at ruling out a significant underlying cause. Important historical points include a drug history (including use of oral contraceptives), age of onset and rate of progression of hirsutism, presence of thinning of scalp hair or deepening of the voice, menstrual history, history of obesity, and family history of hirsutism. The physical examination should include an assessment of the quality and distribution of hair growth, signs of virilization or Cushing's syndrome, and presence of abdominal or pelvic masses.

Laboratory Evaluation. In women with androgen-dependent hirsutism, regular ovulatory menses, and no physical signs of Cushing's syndrome, hormonal evaluation is usually unnecessary. Virilizing tumors have not been reported in such patients, and hirsutism associated with attenuated congenital adrenal hyperplasia need not be treated differently from other benign forms of hirsutism (see Treatment section).

In hirsute women with irregular menses, a reasonable laboratory evaluation includes measurement of serum testosterone, 17-hydroxyprogesterone, prolactin, LH, and FSH. A testosterone level < 170 ng per deciliter (6 nmol per liter) makes an androgen-secreting tumor highly unlikely, although re-evaluation may be necessary if the hirsutism continues to progress or signs of virilization appear. Testosterone levels above 170 ng per deciliter may also be seen with polycystic ovarian syndrome. To rule out attenuated 21-hydroxylase deficiency, serum 17-hydroxyprogesterone should be measured between 7 and 9 A.M. during the first week of the menstrual cycle (values may be elevated during the luteal phase). Values < 200 ng per deciliter (6 nmol per liter) rule out this diagnosis. Mildly elevated values (< 1000 ng per deciliter) (30 nmol per liter) may be seen in both heterozygous and homozygous 21-hydroxylase deficiency (the heterozygous disorder is not associated with hirsutism) and in polycystic ovarian syndrome. To distinguish between these conditions, 17-hydroxyprogesterone should be measured 30 to 60 minutes after the intravenous administration of 250 μg synthetic ACTH. Levels are > 1500 ng per deciliter (45 nmol per liter) in homozygous 21-hydroxylase deficiency. Other forms of attenuated congenital adrenal hyperplasia are too rare to justify routine hormonal screening. Serum prolactin, LH, and FSH are used to evaluate the possibility that a prolactinoma, ovarian fail-

ure, or polycystic ovarian syndrome is contributing to the irregular menses. These tests are not directly relevant to the evaluation of hirsutism itself. Measurement of dehydroepiandrosterone sulfate (DHEAS) as an index of adrenal androgen production is generally unhelpful.

TREATMENT. Hirsutism is a cosmetic problem that may have severe psychosocial consequences. Because it is not a disease in itself, the benefits and risks of any therapy should be carefully weighed and the treatment individualized.

Mechanical Hair Removal. For mild hirsutism, bleaching and mechanical hair removal are adequate and safe. Shaving is the easiest method of temporarily removing visible hair. Although shaving does not increase hair growth rates, it may leave a stubble and is unacceptable to many women. Plucking and waxing may control mild hirsutism, but they also do not resolve the problem and may lead to scarring. Electrolysis can provide a safe, effective alternative for localized mild to moderate hirsutism and is a useful adjunct to medical therapy in more severe cases. Electrolysis is expensive, however, and long-term treatment may be necessary.

Drug Treatment. Successful medical therapy results in a gradual return of terminal hair to finer, less pigmented vellus hair. Younger women with mild hirsutism of brief duration respond best to medical therapy. More severe hair growth can be prevented, and resolution of the hirsutism is possible. Nevertheless, drug treatment is not a cure, and lifelong therapy may be necessary to prevent recurrence. Generally, 6 months is needed to judge the efficacy of a given therapy, although improvement may continue indefinitely. No drug is approved by the Food and Drug Administration for treatment of hirsutism.

Antiandrogens. Antiandrogens (spironolactone, cyproterone acetate, flutamide) block the androgen receptor and are the drug treatment of choice for hirsutism. They are effective in reducing hair growth in at least 70% of women, and hirsutism stabilizes in the remaining ones. Spironolactone is usually given in a starting dose of 50 mg twice daily. The most common side effect is increased frequency of menses, which can be controlled by combining spironolactone with an oral contraceptive. Spironolactone should not be given to women with renal insufficiency. Cyproterone acetate, a potent antiandrogen and progestin, is often given as 25 to 50 mg daily for the first 10 days of a birth control pill cycle. Although widely used in Europe and Canada, it is not available in the United States. Flutamide is given as 125 to 250 mg twice daily. Both flutamide and cyproterone acetate can cause a drug-induced hepatitis, and all antiandrogens should be avoided in pregnant women. Flutamide is more expensive than other antiandrogens.

5α-Reductase Inhibitors. This is a new class of drugs that blocks the formation of dihydrotestosterone. Finasteride, the only such inhibitor available at the time of publication, is approved for treatment of benign prostatic hyperplasia. Early studies suggest that it effectively treats hirsutism, but more experience is needed. It would be expected to cause ambiguous genitalia in the male offspring of women taking the drug during pregnancy.

Ovarian Suppression. Although oral contraceptives are often used to control menstrual cycles in women given antiandrogens, they are usually ineffective for treating hirsutism when used alone (although they may prevent the hirsutism from becoming worse). Birth control pills differ in the androgenicity of the progestational component, but this difference has never been shown to have clinical significance in the treatment of hirsutism. Gonadotropin-releasing hormone analogues suppress the ovary by suppressing LH and FSH secretion. They are effective in treating hirsutism associated with polycystic ovarian syndrome but are expensive and lead to menopausal symptoms unless estrogens are given concurrently.

Glucocorticoids. Glucocorticoids suppress adrenal cortisol and androgen secretion. They are frequently ineffective in low doses, and higher doses can cause Cushing's syndrome. They also can cause a drug-induced hirsutism in some women and cannot be recommended as a routine treatment. Although glucocorticoids have traditionally been used to treat congenital adrenal hyperplasia, antiandrogens are more effective in treating the hirsutism associated with this disorder.

PROGNOSIS. Untreated, hirsutism usually becomes gradually worse with time, and most therapies need to be continued indefinitely. However, worsening hirsutism is easily prevented with antiandrogen therapy, and most women experience a satisfactory improvement with the judicious use of mechanical and medical therapies.

Dunaif A, Givens J, Merriam G, Haseltine F (eds.): Polycystic Ovary Syndrome (Current Issues in Endocrinology and Metabolism). Cambridge, MA, Blackwell Scientific Publications, 1992. *A collection of excellent reviews on polycystic ovary syndrome.*

Jeffcoate W: The treatment of women with hirsutism. Clin Endocrinol 39:143, 1993. *A somewhat different approach (from mine) to the evaluation and treatment of hirsutism.*

Rittmaster RS: Hyperandrogenism. *In* Copeland LJ (ed.): Textbook of Gynecology. Philadelphia, WB Saunders, 1993, p 414. *A detailed review of the pathophysiology, evaluation, and treatment of hyperandrogenism.*

Rittmaster RS: Treating hirsutism. Endocrinologist 3:211, 1993. *An overview of recent advances in the evaluation and treatment of hirsutism.*

208.4 Nonmalignant Diseases of the Breast

Douglas J. Marchant

Approximately one in every four women in the United States requires medical attention for breast symptomatology. More than half of all women have some degree of fibrocystic changes during their lifetime, and most have histologic changes that could be described as "fibrocystic disease." It is recommended, however, that the term *fibrocystic disease* be abandoned and the term *fibrocystic change* or *condition* be substituted because it is more descriptive of the clinical entity.

The physician should be knowledgeable about these common benign conditions and provide treatment or referral when indicated. This chapter discusses growth and development of the breasts, puberty, pregnancy and lactation, and the common benign conditions for which consultation is requested. Diagnostic studies, including examination of the breast, aspiration, and indications for surgical biopsy and referral, are emphasized. Gynecomastia, the main nonmalignant abnormality of the male breast, is described in Ch. 209.1.

GROWTH AND DEVELOPMENT OF THE BREAST

The functional units of the breast are of ectodermal origin. The epithelial ridge that eventually forms the breast tissue, recognizable by the thirty-fifth day of embryonic life, undergoes a series of alterations to form the lactiferous ducts and alveolae. At 15 weeks, mesenchymal cells differentiate into the smooth muscle of the nipple and the areola. The breast unit is complete at birth, as demonstrated by the occasional appearance of "witch's milk" caused by high levels of maternal hormones. During the third trimester of pregnancy, placental hormones in the fetal circulation stimulate further development of the functional units. This colostral secretion declines within 3 to 4 weeks, the breast tissue involutes, and no additional differentiation occurs until puberty.

Development of the mature breast begins with the onset of puberty and continues for several years. Estrogen levels increase, and the areolae become enlarged and pigmented. Adipose tissue is deposited to form and shape the breast and to provide a steroidogenic milieu for the conversion of hormones directly in the breast. In addition to estrogen and progesterone, insulin, cortisol, thyroxin, growth hormone, and prolactin are required for complete functional development.

The mature breast consists of the functional units—the alveolae, lactiferous ducts, and their supporting tissues. The alveolae are inconspicuous in the nonpregnant, nonlactating breast. The much larger ducts lie embedded in a stromal network consisting of fibrous tissue, fat, blood vessels, and lymphatics.

ABNORMALITIES OF GROWTH AND DEVELOPMENT

A number of congenital anomalies may be referred to the clinician for evaluation and treatment. The most frequently observed is the accessory nipple, or polythelia. This tissue, which may be mistaken for a pigmented nevus, lies along the milk line extending from the axilla to the groin. Rarely, functioning breast tissue is found along this milk line. Most commonly this ectopic breast tissue is located in the axilla, where it may enlarge and become quite painful during pregnancy and lactation.

Patients may be referred for failure of breast development, premature development, and breast hypertrophy. Normal sexual development and puberty are discussed in Ch. 208.1. Complete absence of the breast is rare and usually is associated with defects in the chest wall and muscles. Premature development is usually associated with the appearance of a mass beneath the nipple-areola complex. Other manifestations of sexual maturation are absent and hormonal studies are normal. A vaginal smear reveals little or no estrogen effect, consistent with the prepubertal state. No treatment is required; in particular to be avoided is surgical removal of the mass in the mistaken belief that it represents a tumor. If this area is removed, breast tissue will not develop on the affected side. Asymmetric breast development is common and requires no further treatment. Breast hypertrophy, on the other hand, is often uncomfortable and disturbing both to the patient and to the parents. These patients require considerable counseling because if reduction mammoplasty is recommended too early, a repeat operation will be necessary. A reduction mammoplasty, if required, should be performed only after completion of breast development, which may take several years.

THE BREAST DURING PREGNANCY AND THE PUERPERIUM

With the completion of breast development during and following puberty, the breasts are quiescent until pregnancy. During pregnancy the breast grows and develops due to lobular alveolar growth, the formation of secretory cells, and changes in the supporting tissues. Insulin responsiveness also is acquired during pregnancy. Further growth requires estrogen, progesterone, prolactin, and human placental lactogen. During pregnancy, serum prolactin increases from a nonpregnant level of approximately 10 ng to 200 ng per milliliter or more at term. Human placental lactogen reaches serum concentrations of approximately 6000 ng per milliliter at term. Lactation is suppressed by estrogen and progesterone, which inhibit prolactin action at the receptor level. With the rapid drop in estrogen and progesterone levels following delivery, this inhibition is removed and milk production begins. A decrease in the prolactin-inhibiting factor (PIF) by suckling increases prolactin and further promotes lactation. In the final event oxytocin is released and acts on the myoepithelial cells to contract the duct system for the delivery of the milk. By the end of the third or fourth month, suckling is the only stimulus required for continued lactation. If breast-feeding does not occur, prolactin rapidly returns to nonpregnant levels.

Mastitis occasionally complicates lactation, usually following the first pregnancy. There is a localized area of inflammation and tenderness and slight elevation of temperature. Treatment includes continuation of breast-feeding and the use of appropriate antibiotics. Because the most common organism is *Staphylococcus aureus,* penicillin or one of its derivatives is the treatment of choice. If the patient does not respond and if the tenderness and fever persist, a breast abscess should be suspected, for which the treatment is adequate drainage under general anesthesia in an operating room setting. Antibiotics should be continued in full therapeutic doses for 7 to 10 days following adequate drainage. The breast rapidly returns to normal and the cosmetic result is excellent.

The discovery of a dominant mass during pregnancy or lactation requires careful consideration. Early in pregnancy, a dominant mass is easily distinguished from fibrocystic changes. Often the patient gives a history of a mass first discovered many years before and followed in the belief that it represented a benign fibroadenoma. With rare exception, the cause of all dominant masses discovered during pregnancy or the puerperium should be resolved. This requires an open biopsy using a local anesthesia. Biopsy can be safely performed during lactation. The patient is requested to empty the breast early on the day of the operation. The mass is removed with careful approximation of the breast tissues and a pressure dressing temporarily applied. This can be removed later in the day and often the patient can breast-feed on the operated side.

FIBROCYSTIC CHANGES

Fibrocystic changes, which represent an exaggerated physiologic response to a changing hormonal environment, include painful lumpy breasts (mastodynia, mastalgia), a dominant mass, and nipple discharge.

The peak incidence of fibrocystic changes occurs between the ages of 30 and 50. Breast tenderness often occurs premenstrually, which suggests that progesterone may play an important role in the development and symptomatology of these changes. In the resting breast there is minimal epithelial proliferation in the proliferative phase of the menstrual cycle and maximal proliferation in the secretory phase, a pattern quite different from that of the endometrium. Whether this dissimilarity between breast and endometrial epithelium reflects receptor content or some more indirect effect on proliferation is unclear. Estrogen is a mitogen for the endometrium but not for the breast, and the idea, derived largely from endometrial studies, that progestins are protective for the breast is difficult to sustain. The relative contributions of estrogen and progesterone to the origin of benign breast conditions require further investigation.

Most, if not all, women experience these fibrocystic changes, and to label this condition a "disease" is inappropriate. Physical examination usually reveals irregular thickening, particularly in the upper outer quadrants. The changes associated with this process and its symptomatology constitute one of the most difficult challenges in the office practice of the physician.

MASTODYNIA (MASTALGIA)

Breast pain is common; it may occur in as many as 50% of women. Usually the cause is unclear, and relief of symptoms often is proportional to the time that the physician spends with the patient. The discomfort generally is classified as (1) cyclic mastalgia or mastodynia occurring immediately prior to the menses; (2) fibrocystic changes, including duct ectasia and sclerosing adenosis; or (3) referred pain such as costochondritis.

Almost all women complain of occasional breast discomfort for the first few days preceding the onset of menses, and most do not seek medical attention. It is the discomfort occurring at other times during the menstrual cycle, or throughout the cycle, that brings the patient to the physician.

Perimenopausal patients not infrequently note breast discomfort. The cause is unknown. Postmenopausal patients should be carefully evaluated for referred pain. They often perceive the discomfort to be in the breast when in reality it is related to the pectoral muscles, the chest wall, or even the cardiovascular system. Trauma is not an infrequent cause of breast discomfort. The usual presentation is a tender erythematous or ecchymotic area. In some cases open biopsy must be performed to rule out carcinoma.

NIPPLE DISCHARGE

Nipple discharge may be physiologic or pathologic, provoked or spontaneous. In most cases the patient can be immediately reassured that cancer is unlikely because 10% or fewer of breast cancers present with nipple discharge. A careful and detailed history is essential. Is the discharge produced only at the time of breast self-examination when the nipple is squeezed? Does it occur only with sexual stimulation? What type of physical exercise does the patient do? Does she wear a sport brassiere? Does she take any medication? Has she ever been pregnant? What is the menstrual history? Most patients can describe the character of the discharge, although not necessarily in a reliable fashion. For example, many patients complain of bloody nipple discharge, but when the secretions are examined on a gauze or by cytology, the color is blackish green and no blood cells are found.

Three types of discharge deserve further comment: galactorrhea, serosanguinous or bloody discharge, and discharge from the postmenopausal breast.

GALACTORRHEA. Galactorrhea is the spontaneous secretion of a milky discharge not immediately associated with a pregnancy. Usually it is persistent and occasionally it is voluminous. Elevated prolactin levels may be associated with galactorrhea. Physiologic causes of hyperprolactinemia include breast stimulation, coitus, eating, exercise, pregnancy, sleep, and stress. Hyperprolactinemia may also be due to pathologic factors, including brain and pituitary disorders, encephalitis, and pituitary microadenomas or macroadenomas. In addition, a number of pharmacologic agents may produce hyperprolactinemia, as noted in Table 208–13.

Prolactin is secreted in a sleep-related circadian rhythm with maximal release between 3:00 A.M. and 5:00 A.M. Serum samples, therefore, should be obtained in a fasting state between 8:00 A.M. and 12:00 noon. Prolactin levels do not change during the menstrual cycle. A serum level of prolactin of >20 ng per milliliter

TABLE 208–13. CAUSES OF NONPUERPERAL GALACTORRHEA

I. **Central origin**
  A. Organic
    1. Suprahypophyseal lesions
      a. Hypothalamic disorders–infiltrative processes (histiocytosis, metatastic diseases); masses (craniopharyngioma, meningioma); infarction; embolism
      b. Pituitary stalk lesions–section; impingement by tumors (all types with suprasellar extension); vascular insult
    2. Hypophyseal tumors
      a. Prolactin secreting* (solitary; part of multiple endocrine adenomatosis syndrome mixed with GH, TSH, ACTH)
  B. Functional
    1. Drug related
      a. Psychotropic (butyrophenones, phenothiazines)*
      b. Antihypertensive (reserpine, α-methyldopa)
      c. Cannabinoids (morphine, heroin)
      d. Contraceptives
      e. Antigastroplegics (metoclopramide)*
    2. Unclassified (idiopathic, stress, empty sella syndrome)

II. **Peripheral origin**
  A. Due to pituitary prolactin
    1. Due to primary failure of target endocrine gland
      a. Hypothyroidism
      b. Addison's disease
    2. Due to excess estrogen formation from target endocrine glands
      a. Feminizing adrenal carcinoma
      b. Polycystic ovarian syndrome
    3. Due to decreased metabolic clearance of PRL
      a. Renal failure
      b. Liver failure
      c. Hypothyroidism
    4. Due to local breast conditions
      a. Mechanical stimulation or suckling
      b. Thoracic and/or breast trauma, burn
      c. Inflammation, i.e., mastitis, herpes zoster
  B. Due to ectopic prolactin production
    1. Renal neoplasia
    2. Bronchogenic neoplasia

* Most common causes of highest serum PRL levels.

may be abnormal and should be further evaluated. Other diagnostic studies include microscopic evaluation of the breast discharge, which may reveal refractile fat globules, confirming the diagnosis. A thorough history should be taken to rule out physiologic or pharmacologic causes, and the menstrual history should focus on amenorrhea, oligomenorrhea, infertility, or a short luteal phase.

Prolactinomas, or prolactin-secreting pituitary adenomas, are common causes for hyperprolactinemia in women. Prolactinomas may be microadenomas (<1 cm in diameter) or macroadenomas (>1 cm). The diagnosis usually is made by computed tomography (CT) scan using contrast media. Modern CT or magnetic resonance imaging has replaced older methods of diagnosing pituitary tumors, such as the cone view tomogram or plain skull film.

SEROUS OR BLOODY BREAST DISCHARGE. This type of nipple discharge must be investigated. Usually it is caused by a benign intraductal papilloma, but carcinoma occurs in 10 to 15% of these patients. Often it is difficult to demonstrate the exact quadrant of the breast from which the discharge appears at the nipple. A microscopic examination of the fluid may identify red blood cells, confirming the clinical impression and the need for open biopsy.

POSTMENOPAUSAL NIPPLE DISCHARGE. Any nipple discharge that occurs during the postmenopausal period must be viewed as suggestive of carcinoma of the breast. Careful examination of the breast may reveal a mass or other findings consistent with carcinoma, which must be followed up, as described in Ch. 208.5.

DETECTION AND DIAGNOSIS

HISTORY. The diagnostic evaluation begins with a careful history, noting the age of the patient, the date of the last menstrual period, family history of breast disease, use of medication, the date of birth of the first child, and any surgery related to previous breast disease. Inquiry should be made concerning the use of oral contraceptives, including the type of medication and for how long it has been taken. If the patient has received estrogen replacement therapy, the type of medication and the length of time that the medication has been used should be noted. Pelvic surgery, including oophorectomy and a history of pelvic malignancy, particularly ovarian carcinoma and endometrial carcinoma, should be recorded. Did the patient notice the symptom casually or by employing deliberate breast self-examination, or was it first noted by another health care provider? Does the patient wear a brassiere? What type of medication has the patient used to provide relief? Are there any emotional factors that should be considered? The history should be recorded with particular emphasis on the data of onset of the symptom, the exact location in the breast, and, finally, the disposition.

PHYSICAL EXAMINATION. For careful evaluation the breasts are first examined in the sitting or standing position. Contour, symmetry, and skin changes are noted. The vascular pattern is observed and the condition of the areola and nipple recorded. These changes may be exaggerated by asking the patient to elevate the arm or to place her hands on the hips, thus contracting the pectoralis major muscles and exaggerating any small change noted on routine observation. While the patient is in this position, the axilla is palpated, being careful to support the arm with the opposite hand. This relaxes the pectoralis muscle and permits careful evaluation of the axilla. While the patient is in the sitting or standing position, the supraclavicular area should be checked for a cervical rib or other unexpected finding. Examination of the neck may reveal thyroid enlargement.

Following these maneuvers, the patient is placed in the supine position. The breast is palpated in a systematic manner with the flat of the hand. The use of pHisoHex or talcum powder permits the identification of even minor alterations. Approximately 80% of American women discover their own lesions, often while taking a shower. The use of this so-called wet technique permits the identification of very subtle changes in breast texture. Following the careful evaluation of all quadrants, the areola and nipple should be carefully examined and the nipple gently squeezed. Any discharge is evaluated for location, consistency, and color.

The patient often presents with a chief complaint of a lump. This may or may not be confirmed by careful examination. The usual finding is a vague thickening, particularly in the upper outer quadrant.

The physician must carefully evaluate the chief complaint and then, on the basis of a thorough examination, decide whether the findings represent a dominant mass or an exaggeration of normal breast tissue associated with fibrocystic changes. In the obese patient with very large breasts, it is unlikely that any but the most obvious lesion will be discovered by routine examination. The large breast, therefore, is an indication for mammography to augment what in most cases is an inadequate physical examination.

Once a lesion has been characterized as a mass, a lump, or a dominant mass and has been measured or drawn, its cause must be established. There are no obviously benign lesions. The only exception is a mass in the teenager for whom elective treatment of an obvious fibroadenoma may be recommended.

CYST ASPIRATION

A mass may be cystic, solid, benign, or malignant. Attempts should be made to aspirate the mass with a fine (23 or 24 gauge) needle. Local anesthesia is not required. The mass is immobilized with the fingers, the needle inserted, and the fluid withdrawn. If the fluid is clear or cloudy and no residual mass is palpated immediately following the aspiration, it is sufficient to arrange a follow-up examination in 1 month with reassurance and monthly self-examination of the breast. If the mass remains immediately following the aspiration, if the fluid is bloody, or if there is a residual mass on the first follow-up visit, open biopsy is mandatory. If the mass is solid, open biopsy is recommended except for a teenager, for whom excision biopsy can be performed on an elective basis.

Cytologic evaluation of nipple discharge or cyst fluid is seldom rewarding. On the other hand, it is probably advisable to examine spontaneous nipple discharge microscopically, particularly if it is unilateral and serosanguinous or bloody. A positive cytologic examination of cyst fluid in the absence of other indications for biopsy is exceedingly rare. Cytology is not, therefore, recommended as a routine examination.

FINE-NEEDLE ASPIRATION (FNA)

The accurate use of FNA requires an understanding of the techniques involved and a cytopathologist capable of interpreting the smear. A standard disposable syringe can be used with a 23- to 25-gauge needle. Local anesthesia is helpful because several "passes" may be required to obtain an adequate sample of "tissue juice" for appropriate evaluation. The material should not enter the syringe and should be placed directly on the slide and fixed with an appropriate spray. The technique is most useful for the obvious dominant mass. FNA is useful only if positive; a negative finding is unreliable. Some radiologists prefer that a mammogram be performed prior to FNA because the procedure may distort the anatomy of the breast.

OTHER DIAGNOSTIC STUDIES

Ultrasonography is useful to confirm the presence or absence of macrocysts, particularly when these lesions are discovered by mammography and are nonpalpable. The procedure should not be performed on a routine basis because it is unsuitable for screening and is an extra expense to the patient. It is much simpler to immediately attempt aspiration with a fine-gauge needle. Thermography and diaphonography are experimental procedures and should not be employed, except with evaluative protocols.

Mammography may be used as a screening examination in the asymptomatic patient or to confirm the findings noted on physical examination. The accuracy of mammography depends upon a number of factors, including the size and density of the breast and the location of the lesion. False-negative results, which occur even in the best institutions, may reach 10% and in some centers approach 25%. The presence of a dominant mass and a negative mammogram clearly do not preclude the recommendation for referral and an open biopsy.

BREAST BIOPSY

Certain features of the breast biopsy are important when discussing such a recommendation with the patient. In the past, open biopsy was performed solely as a diagnostic procedure to determine the presence or absence of cancer. Currently, the biopsy often becomes part of conservative treatment, and therefore it must be executed by surgeons familiar with contemporary treatment for breast cancer (see Ch. 208.5). It is essential that the biopsy be performed in an operating room setting with trained personnel familiar with the biopsy technique and the use of local anesthesia.

MANAGEMENT OF BENIGN BREAST DISORDERS

The medical management of benign breast conditions often challenges even the most well-informed physician. For patients with mild fibrocystic changes and minimal symptomatology, reassurance only is indicated. Occasionally, a well-fitting brassiere, salt restriction, and a mild analgesic to control discomfort are all that is required.

For patients with greater discomfort, a detailed history is often the key to appropriate diagnosis and therapy. Mammography may be helpful in ruling out significant breast pathology and in reassuring the patient. Treatment strategy often depends upon the "complaint threshold of the patient and the safety threshold of the physician." In the absence of highly effective specific therapy, a number of treatment regimens have been proposed: the topical use of progestational agents, tamoxifen, bromocriptine, various vitamin formulations, and primrose oil. For most patients treatment is directed toward a reasonable and rational explanation rather than any specific medication.

Danazol is effective, but for most patients the cost and the side effects are prohibitive. Moderate doses of danazol decrease follicular maturation and increase anovulatory periods. Danazol has intrinsic androgenic activity and also decreases sex hormone–binding globulin, which increases free testosterone levels. Estradiol secretion is reduced because of the lack of follicular maturation. For some patients who have been incapacitated by breast discomfort and nodularity, a short course of danazol (400 to 600 mg daily for 6 months) may provide symptomatic relief and a marked change in the physical examination. The use of danazol should be restricted to those patients who have failed more conservative measures to control their symptomatology.

The treatment of patients with galactorrhea varies according to its cause and the patient's desires. For patients with a pituitary microadenoma, bromocriptine, 5 mg daily, is usually effective. Unfortunately, if bromocriptine is discontinued, hyperprolactinemia usually returns, leading to galactorrhea and amenorrhea. Therapy therefore must be continued indefinitely.

The objectives for therapy of prolactinomas are to normalize the prolactin levels and menstrual function, to preserve function of the anterior pituitary, and to reduce the tumor mass. Patients with macroadenomas or with extrasellar extension of the tumor should be treated first with bromocriptine, followed by surgery when maximal reduction of the tumor size has been obtained. Surgery should be performed without discontinuing bromocriptine because the adenoma may rapidly regrow.

Women with no evidence of pituitary adenoma but with unacceptable rates of galactorrhea may benefit from bromocriptine even if the serum prolactin level is normal. If galactorrhea is not symptomatic in such patients, however, treatment is not necessary. It is appropriate to refer most of these patients for further endocrine evaluation and to a reproductive endocrinologist if fertility is desired.

Occasional patients present with nonlactational mastitis, i.e., periodic drainage of purulent material from the nipple-areola complex in spite of previous attempts at drainage. In this condition, known as squamous metaplasia, it is not clear whether infection occurs initially followed by squamous metaplasia and intermittent discharge or whether squamous metaplasia occurs first followed by infection. The treatment, however, is complete excision of the involved duct system. Antibiotics are seldom helpful.

The most common benign neoplasm of the breast is the fibroadenoma, usually first presenting in the teenager but occasionally discovered on routine examination during the early reproductive years. Most of these lesions should be removed. In the occasional young patient with more than one mass, it is appropriate to use ultrasonography to document the actual number of lesions. Most surgeons prefer to remove the palpable lesion, usually as day surgery under local anesthesia, a procedure that is easy to do when the lesion is small. Patients who have discovered these lesions almost invariably request removal. The role of the primary care physician is to document the finding and then arrange for appropriate referral.

The diagnosis and treatment of nonmalignant diseases of the breast constitute one of the most difficult challenges facing the primary care physician. The symptomatology is extremely subjective, and conclusions based even upon the most careful examination are subject to error.

Even specific complaints, such as nipple discharge, require considerable judgment when recommending treatment or referral. No lesion is obviously benign. Because 80% of women with breast cancer have no identifiable risk factors, careful breast examination must be included as part of every physical examination.

Brookshaw JD: Danazol treatment of benign breast disease: A survey of U.S.A. multi center studies. Postgrad Med J 55:52, 1979. *Danazol has been approved by the FDA for the treatment of fibrocystic changes. It is costly, however, and there are a number of side effects. This article describes the results of a multicenter study in the United States.*

Feig SA: Decreased breast cancer mortality through mammographic screening: Results of clinical trials. State Art Radiol 167:659, 1988. *Although mammography screening can lead to a remarkable improvement in breast cancer survival, the degree to which any program achieves potential gain depends upon the technical quality of the study, the interpretive expertise of the radiologist, the screening facility, and the number of projections.*

Hindle WH: Fine needle aspiration. *In* Hindle WH (ed.): Breast Disease for Gynecologists, Norwalk, CT, Appleton and Lange, 1990, p 67. *This chapter covers the history and evolution of the fine-needle aspiration technique, including recommendations and contraindications for its use.*

Kleinberg DL, Noel GH, Frantz AG: Galactorrhea: A study of 235 cases including 48 with pituitary tumors. N Engl J Med 296:589, 1977. *This classic article is perhaps the most comprehensive report on the clinical entities associated with galactorrhea.*

Leis HP Jr: Management of nipple discharge. World J Surg 13:736, 1989. *This report of a series of over 8000 breast operations discusses the incidence of breast cancer in patients presenting with nipple discharge and the management of significant discharges.*

Love SM, Gelman SR, Silen W: Fibrocystic disease of the breast, a non disease. N Engl J Med 307:1010, 1983. *This article traces the history of fibrocystic "disease." Because most, if not all, women have these changes, the condition should not be called a disease. In most cases there is no relationship between fibrocystic changes and the later development of breast cancer.*

Yen SSC: Prolactin in human reproduction. *In* Yen SSC, Jaffe RB (eds.): Reproductive Endocrinology. Philadelphia, WB Saunders, 1986, p 237. *This chapter describes abnormalities in prolactin secretion and the treatment of the clinical sequelae.*

208.5 Breast Cancer

Brian J. Lewis and Robert M. Conry

EPIDEMIOLOGY AND PATHOGENESIS

In 1994, 182,000 new cases of female breast cancer and 1000 new cases of male breast cancer were projected for the United States. In terms of annual mortality, 46,000 women and 300 men die of breast cancer. These figures and the one in eight lifetime risk that a woman in the United States has for developing breast cancer make this disease a significant health problem.

The cause of breast cancer is unknown, but several factors correlate with its occurrence: age, family history, ethnic influences, and hormonal effects.

AGE. Only about 15% of cases of breast cancer occur before age 40. The age-adjusted incidence steadily increases thereafter, with two thirds of cases occurring in postmenopausal women.

FAMILY HISTORY. Daughters or sisters of breast cancer patients have a two- to threefold greater risk of developing breast cancer than do women without an affected first-degree relative. More specifically, this relative risk can range from 1.4 if only one first-degree relative is affected after age 60 to 4 to 6 if two first-degree relatives are affected. Unlike patients in the general population, women with the highest relative risk among those with a positive family history have a greater tendency to have their disease before age 40. Careful counseling, screening, and tracking of high-risk patients are essential. Increased monitoring should be performed on patients with prior definitive treatment for breast cancer because they have a 10 to 15% lifetime chance of developing a second primary breast cancer.

GENETICS. Five to 10% of breast cancer patients have inherited mutations leading to the disease. Two genes, BRCA1 and BRCA2, have recently been identified which together may account for most of these mutations (see Ch. 158.2). BRCA1, residing on the long arm of chromosome 17, is associated with female breast and ovarian carcinoma. BRCA2, residing on the long arm of chromosome 13, is associated with male and female breast cancer but not ovarian carcinoma. Mutations in either BRCA1 or BRCA2 are estimated to exist in 1% of all women and result in an extremely high risk of breast cancer, exceeding 50% before age 50 years and reaching 80% by age 65 years. Thus, as an inherited trait, breast cancer is among the most common genetic diseases in the world. BRCA1 and BRCA2 appear to be tumor suppressor genes, and their contribution to sporadic, nonhereditary forms of breast cancer remains uncertain. Diagnostic tests for mutations within these genes could be available within 2 years, raising numerous ethical, clinical, and psychological issues.

ETHNIC INFLUENCES. Ninety percent of breast cancer patients lack a positive family history. Although ethnic background has a role, it is necessary to control for the influences of allied cultural and nongenetic factors. Asian women have a much lower risk of breast cancer than women in Western countries, perhaps related to a later age of menarche. However, that these differences are not solely due to genetics has been suggested by studies of migrants. Japanese women immigrating to the United States were found to have an incidence of breast cancer almost equal to Caucasians in the same area.

HORMONAL EFFECTS. Estrogens have an impact on the development of breast cancer. Early menarche, late menopause, and late or no pregnancy correlate with a higher risk (relative risk of 1.3, 1.5 and 1.9, respectively). Conversely, premature loss of ovarian function, late menarche, early menopause, and early or more numerous pregnancies correlate with a decreased risk. The chance for developing breast cancer is increased in men with Klinefelter's syndrome or with other disturbances of estrogen metabolism.

Multiple trials examining the relationship between oral contraceptive use and the risk of developing breast cancer have yielded variable results. However, the data suggest that if oral contraceptives increase the overall risk of breast cancer, the magnitude of the increase is small and seen primarily among long-term users. Use of postmenopausal estrogen replacement therapy may be associated with a small increase in the relative risk of breast cancer in the range of 1.5 to 2.0 for moderate-dose conjugated estrogen therapy

TABLE 208–14. RISK FACTORS FOR BREAST CANCER IN WOMEN WITH PROLIFERATIVE BREAST DISEASE

Diagnosis	Relative Risk of Breast Cancer (95% Confidence Interval)
Nonproliferative lesions	1.0
Proliferative disease without atypical hyperplasia	1.9 (1.2 to 2.9)
Atypical hyperplasia	5.3 (3.1 to 8.8)
Atypical hyperplasia + family history of breast cancer	11.0 (5.5 to 24)

Data from DuPont WD, Page DL: Risk factors for breast cancer in women with proliferative breast disease. N Engl J Med 312:146, 1985.

over a 10- to 20-year period. Few data are available regarding the effects of long-term, low-dose therapy currently used for treatment and prevention of osteoporosis.

Historically, there has been a linkage between fibrocystic disease of the breast and an increased risk for breast cancer. A host of terms has been lumped under "fibrocystic disease" (i.e., macrocysts, microcysts, adenosis, apocrine change, fibrosis, fibroadenoma, and ductal hyperplasia). We now know that the majority of women (70%) who have a biopsy for benign disease are not at increased risk for cancer, but the presence of atypical hyperplasia and a family history of breast cancer greatly increase the probability of developing breast carcinoma (Table 208–14).

OTHER RISK FACTORS. Other risk factors include ionizing radiation and possibly diet. Surprisingly, consumption of even moderate amounts of alcohol is associated with an appreciable increase in risk. However, whether alcohol itself is responsible or whether it is associated with another responsible factor remains uncertain. Repeated chest fluoroscopy for tuberculosis, therapeutic radiation of mastitis, and exposure of Japanese women to the atomic bomb blast have been linked to increased rates of breast cancer. Animal models and geographic-ethnic differences in incidence suggest that dietary factors, in particular fat (increased in the Western diet), may contribute to the development of breast cancer.

DIAGNOSIS

Clinical Presentation

Breast cancer is usually noted as a painless lump and discovered incidentally by the patient, by routine physical examination, or by mammography. Pain and tenderness are nonspecific findings and herald cancer < 10% of the time. Physical findings suggestive of a malignancy include a hard, irregular mass and skin dimpling or nipple retraction. Nonbloody nipple discharges are rarely associated with cancer. Bloody discharges correlate with intraductal papillomas in about 30% of cases and with invasive cancer in about one third of cases.

Pertinent history includes a family history of breast cancer on the maternal side, especially in first-degree relatives, prior breast biopsies, whether the lump is new or old, and whether it fluctuates in size, consistency, and tenderness with the menstrual cycle. Such cycling is more suggestive of a benign process but by no means rules out cancer. Physical examination should include careful inspection and palpation of both breasts and assessment of the axillary, supraclavicular, and infraclavicular node areas.

Evaluating a Breast Mass

A suspicious breast mass requires systematic evaluation and follow-up. A negative mammogram or needle aspiration does not ensure that a mass is benign, and if it remains of concern, it must be excised. To avoid distortion of breast anatomy, a mammogram should precede any biopsy procedure. Breast imaging rules out contralateral lesions and multiple foci in the ipsilateral breast, and it is sometimes redone after biopsy to confirm that the area of interest was in fact removed.

Formerly, diagnosis and treatment were a one-step procedure. A woman with a suspicious lesion had an excision under general anesthesia with frozen section analysis of the tumor. If cancer was found, mastectomy immediately followed, and the woman awoke to confront both the diagnosis of cancer and the loss of her breast. A two-step procedure is now used. Fine-needle aspiration cytology or excisional biopsy under local anesthesia allows an outpatient diag-

nosis. If cancer is found, the patient and surgeon can then review treatment options.

Screening and Detection

Early detection of a tumor improves the chances for successful treatment. Efforts to screen for and detect early breast cancer have centered on self-examination, physician examination, and techniques for imaging the breast.

Self-examination is simple, without cost, and free of risk. It has been shown to result in earlier detection of tumors in several studies but has not been shown to reduce mortality. It is a reasonable practice to recommend for adult women, although its incremental benefit over that of mammography is uncertain. Any mass that is new and persists for more than a few weeks, is rapidly enlarging, or changes from a previously stable lump requires a physician's examination.

Examination by a physician as a screening tool is more costly and is applied less frequently than self-examination. Discovery of an unsuspected mass during a periodic examination by a physician leads to detection of tumors at an earlier stage than in patients who do not have periodic breast examinations. The American Cancer Society recommends that every woman over the age of 40 have a routine breast examination annually.

Breast imaging techniques include thermography, sonography, and radiographic mammography. Thermography has yet to prove sufficiently sensitive for widespread use. Sonography can help distinguish cystic from solid lesions initially found on radiography. Radiographic mammography is a well-studied and standardized methodology. Annual mammography lowers the mortality from breast cancer in screened populations by about 25% compared with unscreened control groups. It detects smaller lesions with fewer nodal metastases. Current technology allows a lower dose of radiation per examination. Table 208–15 shows guidelines for screening.

Breast cancer incidence rose gradually over the first half of the century and turned more sharply upward in the 1960's, concomitant with and possibly as a result of increased attention to education and screening. The mortality (deaths per 100,000), however, has remained constant. It may be that tumors are being found earlier and treated more readily, because more of the tumors found are smaller. Alternatively, a proportion of the early asymptomatic (subclinical) cancers being discovered may have a lower malignant potential than tumors that grow faster and more rapidly become clinically apparent. Thus, screening may appear more efficacious than it really is because some of the patients discovered to have an "early" cancer may represent a subpopulation with indolent disease who would not otherwise have had clinical expression of the tumor. Nonetheless, there has been a definite reduction in mortality from breast cancer in women who are screened with mammography.

TUMOR BIOLOGY

Breast cancer is more than just a local process; local control of tumor is necessary but not by itself sufficient to address the threat of distant metastases. Breast cancer is also a chronic illness with a potential for recurrence up to 40 years after removal of the primary tumor. Although one can extirpate apparent disease in the breast and in the axillary nodes in the majority of cases, at least 50 to 80% of women found to have tumor in the axillary nodes and 30% of those without axillary node metastases eventually have metastatic disease.

STAGING. The system for clinically staging breast cancer reflects the anatomic extent of tumor (Table 208–16). It allows consistent and comparable description and reporting of cases. The

TABLE 208–15. GUIDELINES FOR MAMMOGRAPHIC SCREENING OF ASYMPTOMATIC WOMEN

1. Mammography every 1 to 2 years for women aged 50 or older
2. Mammography annually for women at any age with a personal history of breast cancer
3. Mammography annually for women aged 40 and over who have a family history of breast cancer or who are otherwise at increased risk. The effectiveness of mammography in women aged 40 to 50 without increased risk is unproven.

TABLE 208–16. STAGING OF CARCINOMA OF THE BREAST

Stage I   Tumor ≤2 cm without skin or chest wall involvement and without regional lymph node metastases

Stage II   Tumor >2 cm without nodal metastases; tumor ≤5 cm with metastasis to moveable ipsilateral axillary nodes

Stage III   Tumor >5 cm with regional lymph node metastases; skin involvement or chest wall attachment; any size tumor with metastases to fixed ipsilateral axillary nodes or ipsilateral internal mammary nodes

Stage IV   Distant metastases

stages correlate with survival and are important in planning treatment, but they do not totally predict the clinical behavior of the tumor. A more complete classification scheme would ideally measure the balance between the inherent virulence of the cancer and the intrinsic antitumor defenses of the host. The combination of the presence and extent of metastases to the axillary nodes is the single most important prognostic factor for patients with breast cancer. Patients treated with radical mastectomy alone have 10-year survival rates of 70% with negative nodes, 50% with one to three positive axillary nodes, and only 20% with four or more positive axillary nodes. In addition to tumor size and nodal status, hormone receptor content and nuclear grade reproducibly correlate with prognosis. The infrequent histologic subtypes of papillary, colloid (mucinous), and tubular carcinoma are associated with a more favorable outcome. Other variables such as the percentage of cells in S-phase, oncogene expression, epidermal growth factor receptors, cathepsin-D, and stress response (heat shock) proteins may also predict who will have metastatic disease (Table 208–17), but the independent contribution of any of these factors remains to be established.

METHOD OF SPREAD. Breast cancer spreads directly to the bloodstream as well as to the draining lymphatics. Tumor emboli can traverse the lymph nodes and enter the venous system; and tumor cells can presumably reach lymph nodes by way of the bloodstream. In addition, upon discovery, a breast cancer mass usually contains 10^9 or more cells. Given what is known of doubling times, the cell number at diagnosis implies that the cancer may have been growing for a number of years. It seems logical that there will be shedding of the tumor cells into the venous and lymphatic circulation throughout the life of the tumor, especially early, when tumor growth rate is highest.

Accordingly, it is likely that many more patients with breast cancer have micrometastases than we see with clinical recurrence. Negative axillary nodes may not mean that the tumor was never present in the lymphatic system but rather that it had been there and was unable to flourish. Positive lymph nodes do correlate with subsequent metastases and poor survival. This could reflect simple anatomic spread of cancer past the last "line of defense" imposed by the lymph nodes (Halsted). More probably it implies that because the tumor persisted in the nodes, however it arrived there, it may also persist and grow in other organs.

CELL ORIGIN. Most breast tumors derive from mammary epithelium. Eighty percent of these are infiltrating ductal carcinomas. Less common are infiltrating lobular carcinoma, medullary carcinoma, comedocarcinoma, and tubular, papillary, and colloid carcinoma. Lobular and comedocarcinoma can be bilateral and require increased surveillance of the unaffected breast. Lobular carcinoma in situ poses a special problem. Although it is not an invasive lesion, it is associated with a 1% annual risk for the development of an invasive lesion in either breast. Some surgeons have therefore advocated prophylactic mastectomy. A more conservative approach is to do a "mirror image" biopsy of the contralateral breast to rule out invasive tumor and then to track the patient closely with periodic examinations and prompt biopsy of any suspicious lesions. Ductal carcinoma in situ carries a higher risk for evolving into invasive cancer and requires surgery. Inflammatory breast cancer represents a highly virulent pathologic variant. Clinically, the patient has a red, swollen, warm breast with a characteristic peau d'orange appearance. Microscopically, this is associated with involvement of dermal lymphatics by tumor. It has proven difficult to achieve long-term survival in patients with this diagnosis with local treatment, but the addition of systemic therapy has improved results somewhat.

HORMONE RECEPTOR PROTEINS. Estrogen and progesterone receptor proteins (ERP and PRP) are present in normal mammary epithelium and in a proportion of breast cancers. After binding to the steroid, the activated hormone-receptor complex interacts with specific sites on DNA, and this results in the initiation of steroid-specific protein synthesis. One product of estrogen stimulation is PRP, and the presence of PRP signifies functionally intact ERP. A tumor is considered ERP-positive when it contains more than 10 femtomoles of receptor per milligram of protein, as measured using a radioligand binding assay. Monoclonal antibodies against ERP are now available and permit microscopic visualization and enumeration of ERP-positive tumor cells.

ERP is found more frequently and in higher titer in tumors from postmenopausal patients (≥60% versus 30 to 40% positive in premenopausal women). ERP-positive tumors tend to be less virulent and are more likely to respond to hormonal therapy (see below). Tumors that contain both ERP and PRP have the greatest likelihood of regressing after an endocrine maneuver, and the probability of a response increases directly with the titer of the RP. Given the therapeutic and prognostic implications of hormone receptor levels, it is mandatory that all primary breast cancers be submitted for receptor analysis at the time of removal. There is an 80% concordance between the hormone receptor profile of a primary tumor and its metastases, in the absence of intervening hormone treatment. Breast cancers are heterogeneous in the sense that in RP-positive specimens, the majority but not necessarily all of the cells contain RP. When metastatic disease becomes refractory to hormonal therapy after initially responding, the progression reflects the outgrowth of hormone-independent cells that are usually RP-negative.

PRIMARY MANAGEMENT OF BREAST CANCER

Stage I and Stage II Disease

Since Halsted's time, almost three generations ago, the view of breast cancer as a local or regional process made radical mastectomy or one of its variants the standard approach to the management of resectable tumor confined to the breast and the axillary lymph nodes. Patients often received postoperative radiation therapy to the chest wall and the draining lymph node areas. These treatments have produced a local control rate of 95%, but variations in locoregional therapy have not differed significantly in their impact upon distant recurrence or overall survival. Furthermore, more extensive surgery or surgery followed by radiation increases the risk of arm edema.

These approaches entered general use without the testing of alternative approaches, but recently local tumor excision with breast irradiation has been gaining a wider acceptance. Older, largely uncontrolled studies seemed to indicate similar outcomes either with tumor excision and breast irradiation or with traditional mastectomy. Although one cannot refer to the decades of observation on local tumor control and side effects that exist for standard surgical approaches, multiple, controlled trials have recently shown that the techniques are equivalent in terms of tumor recurrence and overall survival.

Public interest in alternatives to mastectomy has increased, and patients are more informed and expect their physicians to provide a comprehensive overview of treatment possibilities, especially ones that would spare them the disfigurement and distress imposed by mastectomy. Likewise, the growing application of plastic surgery

TABLE 208–17. PROGNOSTIC FACTORS IN BREAST CANCER

Factor	Influence on Risk of Metastases
Tumor size	Risk increases with size
Nodal status	Risk increases with presence and number of nodal metastases
Hormone receptor status	Risk increased if receptors not present
Nuclear grade	Risk increased with high grade
Favorable histology	Risk decreases with favorable subtypes
Percent S-phase	Risk increases with percent S-phase
Oncogene expression	Risk appears to increase with increased oncogene expression
Cathepsin-D levels	Risk appears to increase with levels
Epidermal growth factor receptor levels	Risk appears to increase with levels
Stress response protein levels	Risk appears to increase with levels

for breast reconstruction after mastectomy has lessened the emotional trauma of the operation.

Breast conservation is appropriate therapy for Stage I or Stage II disease. Table 208–18 lists the requirements for its use. Mammography is essential to exclude patients with multifocal disease or with diffuse microcalcifications. (Even if the latter prove benign on biopsy, they will interfere with the subsequent mammographic follow-up used to screen for recurrent cancer.) An adequate surgical resection of the tumor with negative resection margins is essential and is facilitated by inking the margins of the specimen and orienting it for the pathologist. Axillary node dissection determines whether the patient requires adjuvant systemic treatment because of nodal metastasis. Extensive intraductal carcinoma *in situ* may be a contraindication to breast conservation because of a higher risk of recurrence in the treated breast.

The most common but not necessarily the preferred approach to the primary management of a Stage I or Stage II breast cancer is total mastectomy and axillary lymph node dissection. Postoperative radiation therapy is an individualized rather than "standard" therapy. It is employed when narrow resection margins, extensive nodal disease, the presence of residual tumor, or other high-risk factors for local recurrence are present. With the advent of adjuvant systemic therapy for Stage II disease (see below), there may be even fewer indications for adjuvant radiation therapy, because drug treatment alone decreases the local failure rate.

Clinically suspicious nodes are pathologically negative for tumor 25 to 30% of the time, and, conversely, clinically negative nodes are positive histologically with an equal frequency. With a proper axillary dissection, radiation to the axilla is not usually necessary (and increases the risk for arm edema). Although positive axillary nodes increase the likelihood of subclinical supraclavicular and internal mammary node metastases, no evidence indicates that adjuvant radiation to those areas improves survival.

Standard pretreatment evaluation for any of these techniques includes a complete blood count, a profile of serum chemistries with particular reference to studies suggestive of liver or bone involvement, and a chest radiograph. The yield of positive bone or liver scans is extremely low in the absence of symptoms or signs suggesting metastatic disease. On the other hand, with locally advanced tumor (Stage III), the yield of screening bone scans is sufficiently high (about 30%) to warrant their use. Likewise, with abnormal blood chemistries suggestive of liver involvement or with symptoms such as bone pain, scans would be required to avoid inappropriate use of a definitive local procedure in a patient with advanced, incurable disease.

Stage III Disease and Inflammatory Breast Cancer

If a patient's disease is Stage III solely on the basis of tumor size (tumor >5 cm), but the tumor appears to be as resectable as that of a Stage I or II patient, mastectomy has historically been the primary treatment. Recent studies have also shown satisfactory local control with the use of primary chemotherapy and breast conservation ther-

apy. For patients with locally advanced but unresectable disease (i.e., invasion of chest wall, fixation of axillary nodes, or positive supraclavicular nodes), control of persistent or recurrent regional disease as well as latent distant metastases is the dominant problem. Inflammatory breast cancer is aggressive locally as well as metastatically. It is properly considered a systemic disease from the outset, even though it appears to be confined to the breast. The treatment plan for the latter two presentations involves an individualized approach using chemotherapy to reduce the tumor volume, followed by radiation therapy and possibly resection of the breast and draining nodes. This strategy requires close consultation from the outset between surgeons, radiation oncologists, and medical oncologists. Prolonged remissions can be obtained in a fraction of patients.

Metastatic Breast Cancer

CLINICAL FEATURES. Breast cancer most frequently metastasizes to lymph nodes, skin, lung, pleura, bone, liver, brain, and pericardium. In autopsy series, the adrenals are involved in up to half the patients, but adrenal insufficiency is rarely seen. Likewise, the ovaries contain tumor in up to one quarter of patients at autopsy. Rarely metastatic breast cancer may be found incidentally at oophorectomy in a patient whose first sign of breast cancer is an involved ovary presenting as a pelvic mass. Breast cancer is the most common source of metastases to the eye in women.

PATIENT ASSESSMENT. Once a metastatic focus is found, routine studies to map tumor extent include a complete blood count (which can reflect myelophthisis secondary to marrow metastases) and the measurement of serum levels of liver enzymes, bilirubin, and calcium. The carcinoembryonic antigen titer and the CA 15-3 antigen titer can be useful markers for following response to therapy. A chest radiograph is indicated and can reveal lung nodules, mediastinal or hilar node involvement, or a pleural effusion. A bone scan is also mandatory, and positive areas, especially those that are symptomatic or in weight-bearing bones, require follow-up radiographs to distinguish metastatic involvement from coexisting benign bony disease and to determine whether radiation is needed to prevent collapse or pathologic fracture. If physical findings or laboratory studies suggest hepatic involvement, a radionuclide liver scan, a sonogram of the liver, or a liver CT scan confirms the presence of metastatic disease, gauges its extent, and allows comparison with follow-up studies during treatment. "Routine" liver imaging is widely employed, but its yield and cost-effectiveness in the absence of signs suggesting liver metastasis are open to question. The same statement applies to "routine" studies of the brain, although they are clearly indicated in the presence of neurologic symptoms or signs.

COMPLICATIONS. Certain complications occur with some frequency and require urgent attention in patients with metastatic breast cancer: hypercalcemia, metastases to weight-bearing bones, and metastases to the nervous system (the epidural space, the leptomeninges, or the brain).

Hypercalcemia requires standard methods of therapy, such as saline and furosemide, along with treatment of the breast cancer itself (see Ch. 214). Pamidronate and gallium nitrate are new effective agents for the treatment of hypercalcemia which function as potent inhibitors of bone resorption. A positive bone scan, especially in the femur or vertebral column, or bone pain in these areas requires radiographic analysis of the extent of structural damage. Femoral lesions may necessitate orthopedic stabilization and radiation therapy to prevent pathologic fractures. Vertebral body lesions may require radiation to diminish pain and avoid further collapse.

Patients with persistent back pain are at greater risk for *epidural metastases* and possibly cord compression. Motor or sensory changes in a segmental distribution greatly increase the possibility of an epidural lesion. However, in the presence of back pain, their absence does not exclude an epidural lesion. Magnetic resonance scanning is useful in establishing or excluding the presence of epidural lesions. Pain without a neurologic deficit means that there is still time to treat an epidural lesion with radiation before the cord becomes ischemic and permanently damaged.

Leptomeningeal metastases present with headache and focal sensory or motor changes suggestive of single or multiple nerve root involvement. The diagnosis depends upon the demonstration of breast cancer cells in the cerebrospinal fluid and may require multi-

---

TABLE 208–18. REQUIREMENTS FOR LIMITED SURGERY AND RADIATION THERAPY FOR EARLY BREAST CANCER

	Comments
Patient Selection	
Adequate resection of tumor without major cosmetic deformity	This requires a single discrete tumor, moderate sized breast, tumor diameter <4–5 cm.
Surgical Criteria	
Wide resection with specimen orientation	Grossly negative surgical margins are essential—re-resection may be required if margins are microscopically involved.
Hormone receptor analysis	
Separate axillary incision	
Radiation Therapy	
4500–5000 rad to entire breast ± boost to tumor bed	
Treatment of the Axilla	
Level I *and* Level II axillary dissection* (*not* an informal "sampling")	Permits adequate node sampling, controls local tumor, and obviates the need for axillary radiation. Does not impose a major risk for arm edema.

Sources: Harris et al., 1985; Danoff et al., 1985.
* Level I = Complete removal of nodes lateral to the pectoralis minor muscle.
Level II = Removal of nodes beneath the pectoralis minor.

ple spinal taps to yield a diagnosis (with appropriate studies beforehand, if indicated, to rule out a mass lesion in the brain). Intrathecal or intraventricular chemotherapy is usually necessary.

TREATMENT. The two major types of therapy for disseminated breast cancer are hormonal and cytotoxic. Hormonal therapy is less toxic but can require as long as 8 to 12 weeks to produce maximal benefit. The impact of chemotherapy is more rapid. Responses to all these treatments last a median of 6 to 18 months, and responders have a significantly prolonged survival compared with nonresponders. Whether the response itself is responsible or response to therapy identifies a more favorable subgroup of patients is uncertain.

The menopausal status of the patient and the hormone receptor profile of the tumor are the major determinants of whether to employ an endocrine maneuver and which particular therapy to use. Other important considerations are the tempo of the disease, the performance status of the patient, and the sites of metastases. A long interval between mastectomy and recurrence suggests indolent disease and would, along with a good performance status, permit the longer observation period needed to gauge response to an endocrine therapy. Bone, soft tissue, and limited pulmonary metastases may respond to hormonal therapy, whereas extensive lung or liver metastases greatly decrease the probability of a response and therefore require chemotherapy. Because treatment for metastatic disease is palliative, it may reasonably be delayed in the absence of symptoms or visceral metastases.

Premenopausal Patients. For premenopausal patients with ER-positive tumors, hormonal therapy is first-line treatment in the absence of the contraindications mentioned above. Oophorectomy is generally recommended as the first endocrine treatment. A good, probably equivalent, alternative is the antiestrogen tamoxifen. Most premenopausal women continue to menstruate while receiving tamoxifen, but its mechanisms of action are diverse. LHRH agonists are currently being examined as an alternative to oophorectomy. Oophorectomy produces tumor regression in 50 to 75% of patients with ER-positive tumors. Other surgical endocrine ablative procedures, such as adrenalectomy and hypophysectomy, are considered obsolete forms of therapy for metastatic breast cancer due to the availability of newer medical endocrine treatments. If a patient progresses after initial response to oophorectomy, then antiestrogens, progestins, or aminoglutethimide can be used in sequence until there is no longer a response. At that point, the patient should receive chemotherapy. The major source of estrogen following oophorectomy or in postmenopausal women is the adrenal gland, which produces androstenedione that is converted by an aromatase reaction in peripheral tissues to estrone and estradiol. Aminoglutethimide produces a medical adrenalectomy that is reversible once the drug is stopped. Patients receiving aminoglutethimide experience rash and somnolence 10 to 40% of the time, although these side effects wane after several weeks of treatment. The drug blocks all adrenal steroidogenesis by inhibiting conversion of cholesterol to pregnenolone. In peripheral tissue, it also blocks the conversion of androstenedione to estrone, a precursor of estradiol. Aminoglutethimide therapy at moderate to high dose requires replacement corticosteroid treatment with hydrocortisone, which also suppresses the increase in pituitary ACTH secretion produced by aminoglutethimide inhibition of cortisol production, an increase that could otherwise override the blockade. A periodic check of plasma dehydroepiandrosterone levels confirms the adequacy of adrenal suppression.

Premenopausal patients with RP-negative tumors, or those originally RP-positive who have become refractory to endocrine treatment, require chemotherapy. Drug classes active against breast cancer include alkylating agents (typically cyclophosphamide), antimetabolites (5-fluorouracil, methotrexate), antimicrotubule agents such as vinca alkaloids (vincristine, vinblastine) and paclitaxel, anthracyclines (doxorubicin), and mitomycin-C. In various combinations, these agents effect responses in 60 to 70% of patients, with 10 to 15% achieving a complete remission. However, these responses have a median duration of only 6 to 12 months. Studies are in progress using high-dose chemotherapy and autologous bone marrow rescue to see if selected patients can achieve permanent ablation of metastatic disease. Although this approach has produced high complete response rates (35 to 50%) among highly selected patients with Stage IV disease, the duration of response has not yet

TABLE 208-19. INDICATIONS FOR ADJUVANT SYSTEMIC THERAPY

Axillary lymph node metastases not present
1. Tumors ≤1 cm—no adjuvant therapy (risk of relapse <10%)
2. Tumors >1 cm and especially with adverse prognostic features (see Table 208–17)—consider adjuvant tamoxifen if receptor positive or chemotherapy if receptor negative

Axillary lymph node metastases present
1. Premenopausal, receptor positive or negative—combination chemotherapy
2. Postmenopausal, receptor positive—tamoxifen
3. Postmenopausal, receptor negative—consider chemotherapy

---

been convincingly shown to be prolonged over that with conventional treatments.

Postmenopausal Patients. For RP-positive tumors in postmenopausal patients who are candidates for endocrine therapy, the antiestrogen tamoxifen has replaced estrogen therapy (diethylstilbestrol, DES) as initial treatment. Tamoxifen has few side effects, in contrast to DES, which much more frequently produces nausea, anorexia, and salt retention. Both drugs have been associated with a tumor "flare" consisting of increased bone pain and hypercalcemia. This occurs in patients with skeletal metastases during the initial weeks of treatment, more commonly with DES. These reactions usually herald an antitumor effect and do not necessitate cessation of therapy as long as symptoms and calcium levels are controlled by standard supportive treatments. Withdrawal of DES, once the tumor progresses, produces further regression of tumor in 20 to 30% of patients (withdrawal effect is less common with tamoxifen). Once the disease progresses after this initial therapy, serial endocrine maneuvers are used, as discussed for premenopausal patients, until the tumor becomes refractory to hormonal therapy. Oophorectomy has no role in the treatment of postmenopausal patients. Again, for RP-negative tumors or for tumors resistant to endocrine treatment, chemotherapy becomes the treatment of choice.

Adjuvant Systemic Therapy

The goal of adjuvant systemic therapy after mastectomy is to control any micrometastases present and thus improve survival. Combination chemotherapy, tamoxifen, and ovarian ablation are all effective in subsets of patients. Table 208–19 summarizes the present indications for adjuvant systemic therapy. Ongoing clinical trials are likely to modify these guidelines in the near future. Currently available adjuvant therapy produces an overall reduction in the risk of death of at least 25% in the first 10 years following treatment. Thus, the absolute improvement in survival for a given patient depends on that patient's risk of death due to breast cancer. Consideration of the need for adjuvant systemic therapy should be a routine part of every patient's initial management. The decision should be based upon the individual risk of recurrence, the characteristics of the tumor, and the anticipated extent of improvement with the therapy selected.

The following points should be kept firmly in mind: (1) *Optimal* treatment for any subset of patients has yet to be defined, (2) physicians should continue to enroll their patients in controlled trials, and (3) the studies to date in axillary lymph node–negative patients show a statistically significant improvement in relapse-free survival and overall survival with adjuvant drug therapy. Because 70% of node-negative women survive 10 years or more following primary treatment, the challenge remains to identify and treat only the subset at high risk.

The best choice of drugs, dose, schedule, and duration for adjuvant treatment continues to evolve. The major delayed toxicity of adjuvant chemotherapy is irreversible amenorrhea. Severe long-term sequelae of chemotherapy are rare but include cardiomyopathy affecting <1% of patients receiving doxorubicin and acute leukemia in approximately 5 of 10,000 patients treated with cyclophosphamide-based regimens, especially higher dose or longer duration regimens.

NEW DRUGS AND TREATMENTS

TAXOL. Taxol, a mitotic spindle poison, is the most promising new drug for the treatment of breast cancer. Single-agent taxol has produced overall response rates of 55% as initial therapy for metastatic breast cancer and 26% among heavily pretreated patients with advanced disease, with median response durations ranging from 8 to 12 months. Taxol appears to merit broad investigation at the Phase III level both as a single agent and in combination.

AUTOLOGOUS BONE MARROW TRANSPLANTATION. Multiple Phase II studies in patients with Stage IV disease achieving a partial response to low-dose chemotherapy have demonstrated complete remission rates of 35 to 50% following high-dose chemotherapy with autologous bone marrow rescue. Approximately 20% of these patients remain disease-free without further therapy for several years. Despite the favorable impact on survival and quality of life achieved in this highly selected minority of patients, there is no evidence that broader application of this form of therapy will provide results superior to conventional drug treatments. Evaluation of high-dose chemotherapy with autologous bone marrow rescue in patients with advanced primary breast cancer (Stage III or Stage II with ≥10 positive axillary lymph nodes) is the subject of three national, randomized Phase III trials currently under way. Interim analysis of these trials is not planned until 1999.

SPECIAL CONSIDERATIONS

Male Breast Cancer

Carcinoma of the male breast occurs with 1% the frequency of female breast cancer. Its clinical presentation and primary therapy are similar to those in women. Abnormalities of estrogen metabolism are cited as a possible causative factor. The vast majority of tumors that have been examined are estrogen RP-positive. Orchiectomy and tamoxifen have similar efficacy for the initial management of metastatic disease. Responses to progestins, LHRH agonists, and aminoglutethimide have been reported. The approach to chemotherapy for these patients is similar to that used for women.

Breast Cancer and Pregnancy

Breast cancer complicates approximately one of every 3000 pregnancies. It has been held for some time that pregnancy adversely affects the outcome of breast cancer, with studies citing a high frequency of axillary lymph node metastases and shortened survival when the diagnosis is made during pregnancy. To some extent, these poor results may have related to a delay in diagnosis and in the initiation of treatment rather than inherently different biologic factors. The treatment considerations are the same as for the non-pregnant patients, and a standard surgical approach poses a ≤1% risk to the developing fetus. When patients present with disseminated disease in the first or second trimester, cytotoxic drug treatment may pose a significant risk to the fetus. If clinical considerations permit, treatment can be delayed to the third trimester to permit delivery of a viable fetus.

Patients who develop cancer during pregnancy tend to present with more advanced stages of disease than nonpregnant patients. However, when compared stage for stage, pregnant women have only a slightly less favorable prognosis than nonpregnant women. In a woman who has had successfully treated breast cancer, subsequent pregnancy is not associated with an excessive risk of recurrence. Patients with early stage breast cancer who bear children appear to have a survival equal to that of women who do not become pregnant. A 3-year interval between primary treatment of early breast cancer and a subsequent pregnancy has been advocated.

Beahrs O, Henson D, Hutter R, Myers M: Staging for cancer of the breast. *In* Beahrs O, Henson D, Hutter R, Myers M (eds.): Manual for Staging of Cancer, 3rd ed. Philadelphia, JB Lippincott, 1988, p. 145.

Bonadonna G: Evolving concepts in the systemic adjuvant treatment of breast cancer. Cancer Res 52:2127, 1992.

Dupont WD, Page DL: Menopausal replacement therapy and breast cancer. Arch Intern Med 151:56, 1991. *This important, authoritative review of a large number of studies concludes that menopausal therapy consisting of ≤ 0.625 mg or less of conjugated estrogens daily does not increase the risk of breast cancer.*

Early Breast Cancer Trialists' Collaborative Group: Systemic treatment of early breast cancer by hormonal, cytotoxic or immune therapy: 133 randomised trials involving 31,000 recurrences and 24,000 deaths among 75,000 women. Lancet 339:1, 1992. *This comprehensive meta-analysis of breast cancer trials worldwide provides the basis for current recommendations regarding adjuvant therapy of breast cancer.*

Fisher B, Costantino J, Redmond C, et al.: Lumpectomy compared with lumpectomy and radiation therapy for the treatment of intraductal breast cancer. N Engl J Med 328:1581, 1993. *This article, plus the reference by Veronesi, establishes the value of radiation therapy to reduce the risk of local recurrence following breast-preserving surgery.*

Friedman LS, Ostermeyer EA, Lynch ED, et al.: Special lecture. The search for BRCA1. Cancer Res 54:6374, 1994. *An overview of breast cancer susceptibility genes and their role in hereditary breast cancer.*

Harris JR, Morrow M, Bonadonna G: Cancer of the breast. *In* DeVita VT, Hellman S, Rosenberg SA (eds.): Cancer: Principles and Practice of Oncology. Philadelphia, JB Lippincott, 1993. *A comprehensive treatise detailing areas such as surgical technique, pathology, and chemotherapy.*

Miki Y, Swensen J, Shattuck-Eidens D, et al.: A strong candidate for the breast and ovarian cancer susceptibility gene BRCA1. Science 266:66, 1994. *A detailed description of the breast cancer susceptibility gene BRCA1 and its role in hereditary breast cancer.*

Seshadri R: Clinical significance of HER-2/neu oncogene amplification in primary breast cancer. J Clin Oncol 11:1936, 1993. *This report establishes HER-2/neu oncogene amplification as a significant prognostic factor in breast cancer.*

Spielmann M: Taxol in patients with metastatic breast carcinoma who have failed prior chemotherapy: Interim results of a multinational study. Oncology 51 (suppl) 1:25, 1994.

Veronesi U, Luini A, Del Vecchio M, et al.: Radiotherapy after breast-preserving surgery in women with localized cancer of the breast. N Engl J Med 328:1587, 1993.

209 ENDOCRINOLOGIC DISEASES UNIQUE TO MEN

209.1 The Testis

Alvin M. Matsumoto

The testis has three major physiologic functions: (1) During embryogenesis, testosterone and müllerian inhibiting substance produced by the fetal testis play vital roles in normal male sexual differentiation (see Ch. 207). (2) Beginning at the time of puberty and continuing into adulthood, testosterone produced by the testis is necessary for the development and maintenance of secondary sexual characteristics (virilization) and sexual functioning (libido and potency). (3) Production of spermatozoa by the testis is required for fertility.

Disorders of the testis are common and have profound effects on patients. Infertility due to disordered sperm production affects approximately 5 to 6% of all men wishing to father children. Klinefelter's syndrome, which results in permanent androgen deficiency and infertility, affects approximately one in 400 to 500 males. Testicular dysfunction occurs commonly as a result of systemic illness, malnutrition, and medications. Impotence and gynecomastia, which often result from testicular dysfunction, are very common complaints for which men seek medical attention. Finally, cancer of the testis remains one of the most common fatal neoplasms of young men.

Many disorders of the testis can be treated effectively. Testosterone replacement therapy in androgen-deficient men results in the development or restoration of secondary sexual characteristics and normal sexual functioning. Gonadotropin treatment of hypogonadotropic men often stimulates spermatogenesis and induces fertility in addition to restoring androgen secretion. Finally, seminomas are exquisitely responsive to radiation therapy, and the treatment of nonseminomatous testicular cancers with multidrug chemotherapy has markedly improved survival and cure rates.

TESTICULAR STRUCTURE AND PHYSIOLOGY

Functional Anatomy

The normal adult testis normally measures 3.5 to 5.5 cm in length and 2.0 to 3.0 cm in width and has a volume between 15 and 30 ml. About 90% of the volume of the testis is composed of seminiferous tubules, where spermatozoa are produced. Therefore, any significant reduction in testicular size is likely to be reflected in a decrease in total sperm production.

During fetal development, the testes descend from an intra-abdominal position into the scrotum. The scrotal location of the testes allows them to function at a temperature approximately 2°C lower than that of the abdomen. The pampiniform plexus of veins surrounds the testicular artery and cools the arterial blood supply to the testes. The lower testicular temperature is necessary for normal spermatogenesis in man. Failure of the testes to descend into the scrotum (cryptorchidism) or an abnormality in the venous cooling mechanism (varicocele) impairs sperm production.

The testis is composed of two structurally distinct compartments: the *interstitial* or *Leydig cell compartment* and the *seminiferous tubule compartment* (Fig. 209–1). These compartments are responsible for the two major products of the testis, testosterone and spermatozoa.

The interstitial compartment is composed of *Leydig cells* that produce sex steroid hormones, primarily testosterone. Leydig cells are in close proximity to seminiferous tubules, a location that facilitates delivery of high concentrations of testosterone to the seminiferous tubule compartment which is important in stimulating spermatogenesis.

The seminiferous tubule compartment is composed of developing *germ cells* and *Sertoli cells.* Spermatogenesis involves the differentiation and maturation of spermatogonia, the most primitive germ cell, into spermatozoa. In humans, spermatogenesis takes approximately 74 days. Sperm transport through the epididymis and vas deferens takes another 12 days. Therefore, processes that adversely affect early spermatogenesis may not be manifest by reduced sperm counts in the ejaculate until 2 to 3 months after the insult.

Sertoli cells play an important role in the development of germ cells and regulation of spermatogenesis. They maintain the structural integrity and compartmentalization of seminiferous tubules, deliver nutrients and produce proteins that support spermatogenesis, and regulate the movement and release of maturing sperm within the tubule. Sertoli cells also produce *müllerian inhibiting substance* (see Ch. 207), and *inhibin,* a glycoprotein that inhibits follicle-stimulating hormone secretion from the pituitary gland.

Central Nervous System Regulation of Gonadotropin Secretion

Normal testicular function depends on adequate stimulation by the gonadotropins, *luteinizing hormone (LH),* and *follicle-stimulating hormone (FSH),* that are secreted by the anterior pituitary gland (Fig. 209–1). Like thyroid-stimulating hormone and human chorionic gonadotropin (hCG), both LH and FSH are glycoprotein hormones composed of an α and a β subunit. The α subunits of all four glycoprotein hormones are identical and biologically inactive, whereas the β subunits are unique for each hormone and determine their biologic activity.

Measurements of serum gonadotropin levels are usually performed by immunoassays (e.g., immunofluorometric assays). In normal young men, LH and FSH levels range from 0.5 to 10 mIU per milliliter depending on the specific assay used. Many gonadotropin assays cannot distinguish between low and low-normal gonadotropin levels. Therefore, a hormonal profile of low-normal gonadotropin levels and low testosterone levels is consistent with secondary hypogonadism (see below). Free α subunit is normally synthesized and secreted into the circulation by the pituitary. Gonadotropin-secreting pituitary adenomas and α subunit–secreting tumors, such as pancreatic islet cell tumors, secrete excessive amounts of free α subunit that can be measured using specific immunoassays.

Both LH and FSH are secreted into the peripheral circulation from the anterior pituitary in an episodic fashion (Fig. 209–2). Pulsatile gonadotropin secretion begins during sleep in early puberty, and by adulthood it is present throughout the day. The pulsatile secretion of gonadotropins is regulated primarily by the central nervous system through episodic stimulation of the pituitary by *LH-releasing hormone (LHRH)* (also known as *gonadotropin-releasing hormone [GnRH]*). LHRH, a decapeptide synthesized by hypothalamic neurons, stimulates release of both LH and FSH from the pituitary gland (see Fig. 209–1). Low-dose pulsatile LHRH administration is used to induce normal testicular function in patients with hypogonadotropic eunuchoidism, who lack endogenous LHRH. By contrast, administration of high-dose, continuous LHRH or potent LHRH agonists results in marked suppression of gonadotropin and testicular function. This paradoxic action of LHRH agonists has been used clinically to suppress endogenous testosterone production in the treatment of androgen-dependent tumors, such as prostate cancer.

The hypothalamic LHRH neuronal system plays an important integrative role in the regulation of testicular function (see Fig. 209–1). It receives input both from higher neural centers, such as the limbic system, through numerous stimulatory and inhibitory neurotransmitter and neuropeptide systems and from testicular feedback signals, primarily sex steroid hormones. The input from these sources alters LHRH output, which, in turn, regulates pituitary gonadotropin secretion and testicular function. Knowledge of how the central nervous system regulates LHRH secretion has clarified the mechanisms by which stress, malnutrition, and certain pharmacologic agents (such as opiate drugs) affect testicular function (see Ch. 201).

Gonadotropin Regulation of Testicular Function

LH REGULATION OF TESTOSTERONE PRODUCTION. LH binds to specific membrane receptors on Leydig cells of the testis and stimulates testicular steroidogenesis and secretion of *testosterone,* the major steroid product of the testis (see Fig. 209–1). Testosterone is secreted both locally within the testes and into the peripheral circulation. Healthy young men secrete approximately 5 to 7 mg of testosterone daily. Total plasma testosterone concentrations as determined by radioimmunoassay (RIA), range from 3 to 10 ng per milliliter. Like gonadotropins, testosterone is secreted in a pulsatile fashion (Fig. 209–2).

In early puberty, testosterone secretion increases from very low to near adult levels during sleep in response to sleep-associated rises in LH levels. In adults, testosterone secretion occurs throughout the entire day. In young healthy men testosterone levels exhibit a circadian variation of about 1.5 ng per milliliter, with maximal levels occurring at 8 A.M. and minimal levels occurring at 9 P.M.

Under LH stimulation, Leydig cells also convert testosterone to *estradiol.* However, secretion of estradiol by the testis accounts for only about 15% of the daily production of estradiol. The remainder of estradiol in blood is produced from testosterone and androstenedione (an adrenal androgen) by the enzyme aromatase in peripheral tissues.

TESTOSTERONE TRANSPORT. Like other steroid hormones, the majority of testosterone secreted into the circulation is bound to plasma proteins, primarily albumin and *sex hormone–binding globulin (SHBG).* Approximately 30 to 40% of total testosterone is bound to SHBG and is not biologically available. Only 1 to 2% is free (i.e., unbound to plasma proteins) and physiologically active. Albumin-bound testosterone is also available to act on many target organs. Therefore, measurement of non–SHBG-bound testosterone may provide the best estimate of biologically available testosterone. In certain clinical situations, alterations in SHBG levels result in total testosterone measurements that do not reflect bioavailable testosterone levels. SHBG (and total testosterone) levels are decreased with obesity, hypothyroidism, androgens, nephrotic syndrome, Cushing's disease, and acromegaly and increased with hepatic cir-

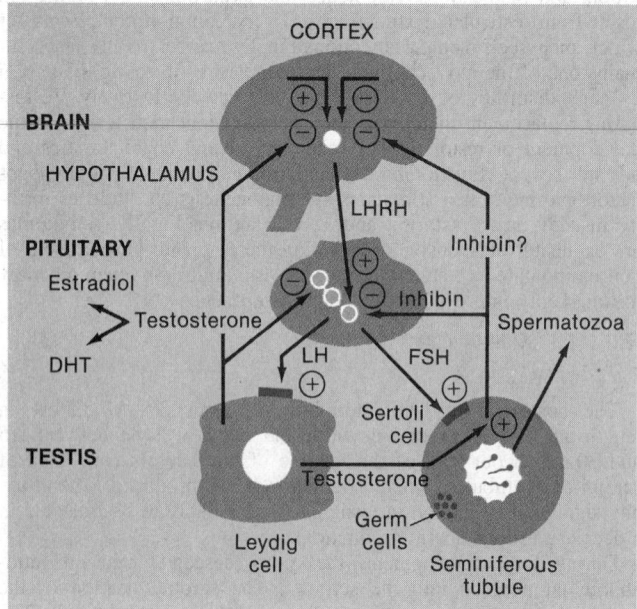

FIGURE 209–1. Diagram of the normal physiology of the hypothalamic-pituitary-testicular axis. (Adapted from Matsumoto AM, Bremner WJ: Endocrinology of the hypothalamic-pituitary-testicular axis with particular reference to the hormonal control of spermatogenesis. Bailliere's Clin Endocrinol Metab 1:71, 1987.)

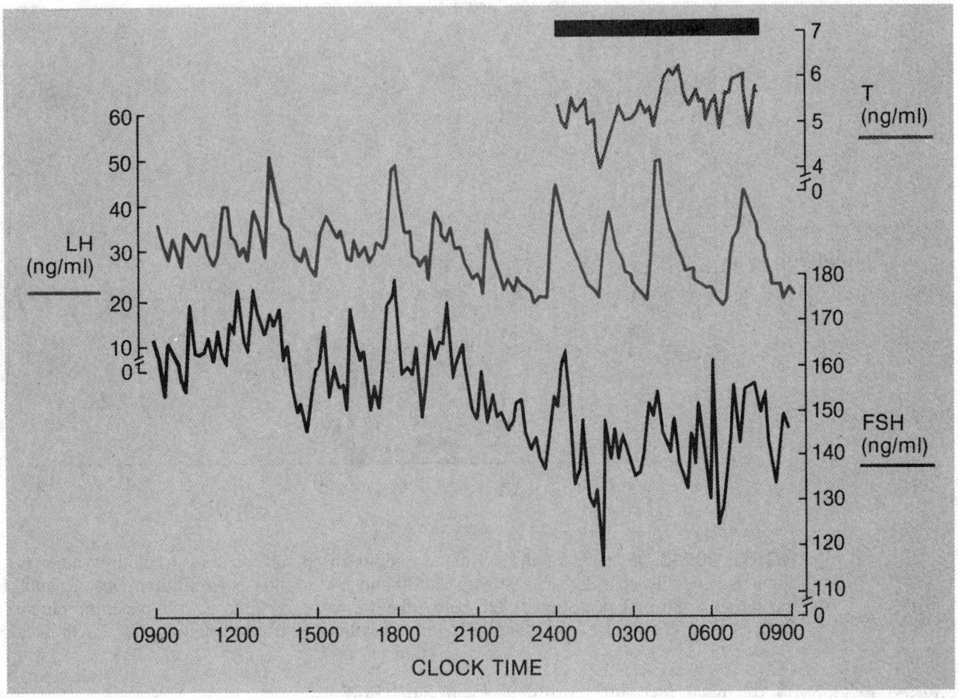

FIGURE 209-2. Example of pulsatile LH and FSH secretion throughout a 24-hour day and episodic testosterone secretion at night in a healthy young man. Blood samples were drawn at 10-minute intervals. Black bar denotes sleep, as documented by electroencephalogram.

rhosis, hyperthyroidism, and estrogens. In these situations, free or non–SHBG-bound testosterone levels should be obtained.

PERIPHERAL METABOLISM OF TESTOSTERONE. The metabolism of circulating testosterone plays a very important role in its biologic actions on target tissues. Testosterone may be converted in peripheral tissues to either *dihydrotestosterone (DHT)* or *estradiol,* which mediates many of the physiologic actions of testosterone (see Fig. 209–1).

In many androgen-dependent target tissues, testosterone is converted intracellularly to a more potent androgen, DHT, by the enzyme 5α-reductase. This conversion is required for normal male sexual differentiation (see Ch. 207). DHT mediates the androgenic effects of testosterone on skin and the prostate gland. In many peripheral tissues, especially in adipose tissue, testosterone is aromatized to estradiol, a potent estrogen. Obesity therefore results in increased peripheral estrogen formation. In men estrogens have diverse physiologic actions that may be agonistic or antagonistic to those of androgens. Therefore, the physiologic effects of testosterone result from the interactions of testosterone with its active metabolites, DHT and estradiol.

Circulating testosterone and its active metabolites are metabolized to inactive metabolites, mostly in the liver, and these metabolites are excreted primarily in the urine. In sexual tissue (including skin and prostate), DHT is efficiently metabolized to 3α-androstanediol and then to *3α-androstanediol glucuronide (3α-diol G).* Blood and urine measurements of 3α-diol G are useful markers of peripheral androgen action. In disorders in which DHT formation is reduced (such as 5α-reductase deficiency), 3α-diol G levels are reduced (see Ch. 207).

ANDROGEN ACTION AND FUNCTIONS. At the target cell, testosterone and DHT bind to intracellular androgen receptors, which interact with specific chromosomal sites to alter gene transcription and protein synthesis, resulting in expression of androgen action (see Ch. 199). Quantitative or qualitative abnormalities of the androgen receptor, resulting in impaired androgen action, cause varying degrees of male pseudohermaphroditism (see Ch. 207).

The major functions of androgens are the differentiation of male internal and external genitalia (primary sexual characteristics) during embryogenesis; the development and maintenance of secondary sexual characteristics, sexual functioning (libido and potency), certain behavioral characteristics (such as motivation), and feedback regulation of gonadotropins; and the initiation and maintenance of spermatogenesis.

FSH REGULATION OF SERTOLI CELL FUNCTION. FSH binds to specific membrane receptors on Sertoli cells of the seminiferous tubule compartment of the testis and stimulates the production of seminiferous tubule fluid and a variety of proteins thought to be important in regulating spermatogenesis (e.g., ABP, transferrin, plasminogen activator) and in feedback control of pituitary FSH secretion (inhibin and activin) (see Fig. 209–1). Testosterone produced by adjacent Leydig cells also regulates Sertoli cell functions through androgen receptors.

HORMONAL CONTROL OF SPERMATOGENESIS. Both FSH and LH stimulation are required for the initiation of spermatogenesis at the time of puberty. At this time, LH causes the differentiation of Leydig cells from interstitial connective tissue precursors and stimulates them to produce high intratesticular levels of testosterone, which are essential for sperm production. By stimulating Sertoli cell function, FSH also plays an important role in initiating spermatogenesis. In contrast to the hormonal requirements for sperm production at the time of puberty, normal levels of either FSH or LH do not appear to be absolute requirements for the maintenance of spermatogenesis in adult men.

Clinically, replacement of both FSH and LH activity is generally required to initiate sperm production in prepubertal hypogonadotropic hypogonadal patients. In contrast, initiation and maintenance of spermatogenesis in postpubertal men with acquired hypogonadotropic hypogonadism can usually be achieved with replacement of LH activity alone.

Seminal fluid analysis is used to evaluate the function of the seminiferous tubules. It is performed on seminal fluid samples obtained by masturbation after 48 hours of abstinence from ejaculation. Normal ejaculate volume ranges from 2 to 6 ml. Although the normal range of sperm concentration is generally considered to be 20 to 200 million per milliliter, sperm concentrations below 20 million per milliliter may be sufficient for fertility. In addition to determining sperm count, a careful microscopic examination of the seminal fluid is performed to assess sperm motility and morphology. Normally, >50% of sperm examined within 1 hour after ejaculation are motile, and >30% have a normal oval head morphology using stricter World Health Organization criteria.

The minimal levels of sperm concentration, motility, and oval forms compatible with fertility are not clearly defined. In any individual, sperm counts normally exhibit extreme variability (Fig. 209–3) and are often temporarily suppressed by illness. Therefore, estimates of sperm production require at least three seminal fluid analyses performed over approximately 2 months. Functional tests of sperm penetration into cervical mucus of various mammalian species or zona pellucida–free hamster ova may be helpful in assessing fertilizing capability of spermatozoa.

Testicular Feedback Regulation of Gonadotropin Secretion

Both steroid and nonsteroidal products of the testis are involved in negative feedback control of pituitary gonadotropin secretion. In-

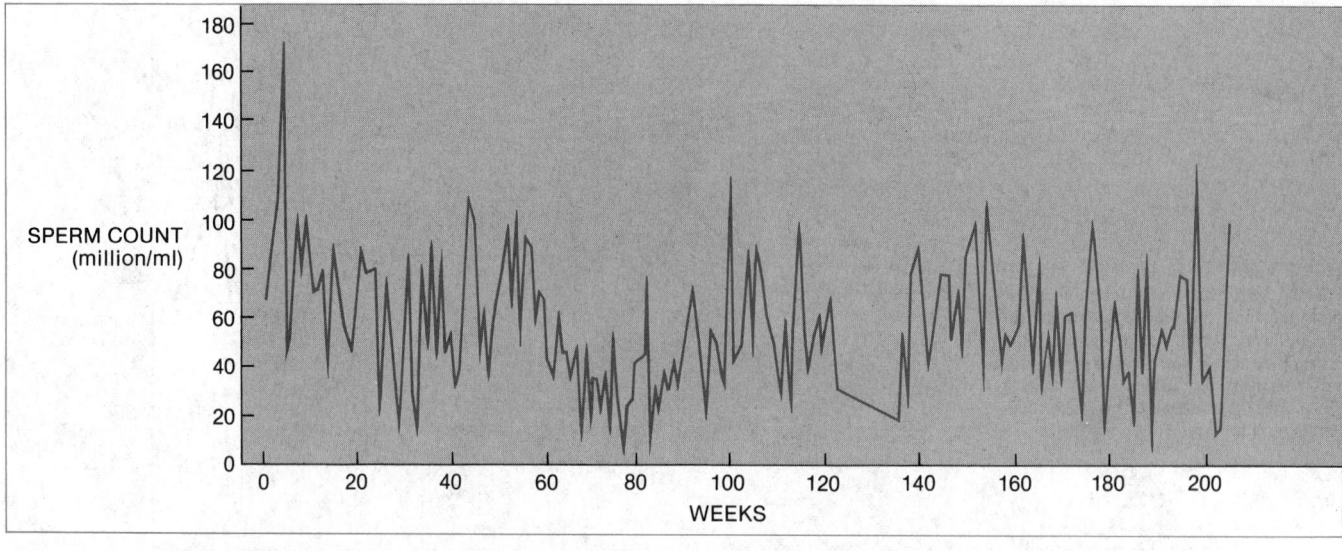

FIGURE 209–3. Example of the normal variations in sperm count in a healthy young man. Normal range of sperm count is generally considered to be between 20 and 200 million per milliliter. Despite good health and no medications, the sperm count may occasionally fall below the normal range, into the oligospermic range. (Adapted from Bardin CW, Paulsen CA: The testes. *In* Williams RH [ed.]: Textbook of Endocrinology, 6th ed. Philadelphia, WB Saunders, 1981.)

creased production of these testicular products results in suppression, whereas decreased production of these factors results in stimulation of gonadotropin secretion (see Fig. 209–1). Testosterone and its active metabolites, DHT and estradiol, exert profound inhibitory effects on both LH and FSH secretion, although the relative roles of these steroids are not clearly defined. Inhibin selectively inhibits FSH secretion. At present, the physiologic significance of inhibin is unclear. Knowledge of these negative feedback relationships is clinically useful in the diagnosis of hypogonadal states (see below).

Matsumoto AM, Bremner WJ: Endocrinology of the hypothalamic-pituitary-testicular axis with particular reference to the hormonal control of spermatogenesis. Bailliere's Clin Endocrinol Metab 1:71, 1987. *This paper reviews the normal physiologic regulation of testicular function, which forms the basis for understanding the pathophysiology and treatment of testicular disorders. An up-to-date discussion of the hormonal regulation of human spermatogenesis is also provided.*
Veldhuis J: The hypothalamic-pituitary-testicular axis. *In* Yen SCC, Jaffe RB (eds.): Reproductive Endocrinology: Physiology, Pathophysiology and Clinical Management, 3rd ed. Philadelphia, WB Saunders, 1991, p 409. *This chapter provides an excellent, detailed, and current discussion of the physiology and pathophysiology of the male reproductive axis.*

PHYSIOLOGY OF MALE SEXUAL FUNCTION

Normal male sexual function requires coordinated regulation of the following physiologic events: *libido* or sexual desire, sustained penile tumescence or *erection, ejaculation, orgasm,* and *detumescence.*

Libido

Libido is generated in the central nervous system (CNS) and stimulated by a variety of visual, tactile, imaginative, auditory, and gustatory stimuli. These stimuli are received in a number of cortical and subcortical regions of the brain, including the limbic system, and relayed via the preoptic–anterior hypothalamic area to spinal cord centers that control penile erection. Therefore, disturbances in libido are nearly always accompanied by disturbed erectile function or impotence.

Libido is regulated primarily by psychic factors and the sex steroid milieu, in particular serum testosterone concentrations. Thus, psychological disturbances of all degrees (from stress to major psychiatric illnesses), CNS lesions, drugs that alter brain function, and androgen deficiency may disturb normal libido and potency. Occasionally, castrated males maintain sexual desire and erectile function for long periods, suggesting that the requirement for androgens may be quite variable.

Erection

Erections are generated by two separate but synergistic mechanisms, one involving sensory stimulation of the genitalia, mediated through a spinal reflex arc (reflexogenic erections), and another involving psychogenic stimuli from higher brain centers (psychogenic erections). In reflexogenic erections, afferent sensory fibers from the penis travel in the pudendal nerve to the sacral spinal erection center (S2 to S4). Efferent parasympathetic fibers arising from this center travel in the nervi erigentes and innervate the blood vessels of the corpora cavernosa of the penis; efferent somatic fibers traveling in the pudendal nerve innervate the pelvic floor (ischiocavernosus and bulbocavernosus) muscles. Sympathetic fibers originating in the thoracolumbar spinal erection center (T12 to L1) innervate the muscles of the vas deferens, accessory sex glands, and internal sphincter of the bladder. In psychogenic erections, projections from higher brain centers descend in the lateral spinal columns and regulate both the thoracolumbar and sacral spinal erection centers.

Penile erectile tissue consists of paired corpora cavernosa on the dorsum of the penis and the corpus spongiosum that surrounds the urethra and forms the glans penis. The corpora are composed of spongelike, interconnected trabecular spaces lined by vascular epithelium and smooth muscle and are surrounded by a thick fibrous sheath, the tunica albuginea. Activation of the spinal erection centers results in relaxation of the penile smooth muscle and vasodilation of the cavernosal arteries (branches of the internal pudendal arteries). These actions are mediated by cholinergic and noncholinergic (e.g., vasoactive intestinal peptide) neurotransmitters, and endogenous vasodilators (e.g., nitric oxide). As a result, blood flow into the trabecular spaces of the corpora is increased, causing engorgement of the penis (tumescence). Expansion of the trabecular walls against the tunica albuginea compresses subtunical venules and impedes venous outflow, resulting in sustained tumescence, i.e., an erection.

Failure to achieve an adequate erection or impotence has many potential causes, including androgen deficiency, central and peripheral nervous system diseases, vascular disorders, and penile abnormalities. Impotence as it relates to the differential diagnosis of hypogonadism is discussed in a subsequent section of this chapter.

Ejaculation

Ejaculation is stimulated by sympathetic nervous system activation, which results in contractions of the vas deferens and accessory sex glands and emission of seminal fluid into the urethra. Emission is followed by reflex rhythmic contractions of the ischiocavernosus and bulbocavernosus muscles and expulsion of semen from the urethra, i.e., ejaculation. Like erection, the ejaculatory reflex is under considerable control by higher CNS centers. Sympathetic activation also stimulates closure of the internal urethral sphincter, thereby preventing retrograde ejaculation.

Premature ejaculation is usually due to performance anxiety or an emotional disorder and rarely has an organic cause. Retrograde ejaculation into the bladder usually occurs in patients with sympathetic neuropathy (e.g., with diabetes) or after bladder neck surgery. Reduced or absent ejaculation may occur with androgen deficiency, sympatholytic drugs, sympathectomy, or extensive retroperitoneal/pelvic surgery.

Orgasm

Orgasm, the pleasurable sensation that usually accompanies ejaculation, is primarily a CNS-mediated phenomenon that, under normal circumstances, is influenced by ascending pathways associated with ejaculation. However, orgasm can occur in the absence of erection or ejaculation (e.g., with temporal lobe lesions). Conversely, normal libido, erection, and ejaculation can occur without orgasm; this is nearly always due to a psychological disorder.

Detumescence

Detumescence results from contraction of the penile smooth muscle and α-adrenergic vasoconstriction of the cavernosal arteries, which reduce arterial blood flow into the penis. As a result, the trabecular spaces of the corpora collapse, subtunical venules are decompressed, venous outflow is increased, and the penis becomes flaccid. In many cases, premature detumescence may contribute to the pathophysiology of impotence (e.g., venous leak or incompetence). Failure of detumescence, priapism, is often painful and unrelated to sexual intercourse. It is commonly idiopathic but may be associated with spinal cord injury, sickle cell disease, chronic myelogenous leukemia, drugs (e.g., trazodone), and intracorporal injection of vasodilatory substances used in the treatment of impotence.

Korenman SG: Sexual dysfunction. *In* Wilson JD, Foster DW (eds.): Williams' Textbook of Endocrinology, 8th ed. Philadelphia, WB Saunders, 1992, p 1030. *This chapter contains a well-organized, clear, and comprehensive discussion of the physiologic and anatomic basis of male sexual function and dysfunction.*

HYPOGONADISM

Hypogonadism is the most common disorder of testicular function. The clinical manifestations of male hypogonadism differ depending on (1) whether there is *impairment of testosterone production,* which is nearly always accompanied by impairment of sperm production, or *isolated impairment of sperm production,* with normal testosterone production; (2) whether androgen deficiency occurs *during embryogenesis, before puberty,* or *after puberty;* and (3) whether testicular hypofunction is the result of a *primary* defect in the testis or is *secondary* to hypothalamic-pituitary dysfunction.

Androgen Deficiency

The clinical presentation of androgen deficiency depends on the stage of sexual development in which it occurs.

During early fetal development, testosterone and its active metabolite, DHT, mediate the differentiation of male internal and external genitalia. Androgen deficiency (e.g., due to a genetic androgen biosynthetic enzyme defect) or impaired androgen action (androgen resistance) occurring during this period of development results in varying degrees of ambiguous genital development, or *male pseudohermaphroditism* (see Ch. 207).

During puberty, testosterone is responsible for the development of male secondary sexual characteristics, such as (1) the growth of the penis and scrotum, (2) the development of accessory sexual organs (prostate and seminal vesicles) necessary to produce an ejaculate, (3) a male pattern of hair growth (face, external ear canals, chest, lower abdomen, pubis, perianal area, legs, and inner thighs) and frontal scalp regression, (4) the enlargement of the larynx and thickening of the vocal cords with consequent deepening of the voice, (5) the development of skeletal musculature and increase in strength (especially in the shoulder and pectoral muscles), (6) a redistribution of body fat, and (7) stimulation of erythropoiesis. Testosterone also stimulates the pubertal spurt of long bone growth and, eventually, the closure of long bone epiphyses, which results in cessation of bone growth. Finally androgens stimulate libido, potency, aggressive behavior, and motivation, and play an important role in initiation of spermatogenesis.

Patients who develop androgen deficiency before puberty usually present to physicians as adolescents or young adults with delayed puberty or poor male sexual development. Prepubertal testosterone deficiency results in *eunuchoidism* (Fig. 209–4), characterized by infantile genital development, failure to develop accessory sexual glands and an ejaculate (aspermia), lack of male hair pattern, high-pitched voice, poor muscular development and strength, lower abdominal–pelvic girdle fat distribution, and excessive

long bone growth (due to lack of closure of long bone epiphyses). The testes are small, usually <2 cm in length or 2 ml in volume. A eunuchoidal body habitus is characterized by excessively long arms and legs in proportion to height. Although there are racial differences in body proportions, eunuchoidal body measurements consist of an arm span that exceeds height, or a distance from the floor to symphysis pubis that exceeds that from the symphysis to the crown of the head by >5 cm. Patients with prepubertal androgen deficiency fail to develop normal sexual functioning (libido and potency), are infertile, and may occasionally have gynecomastia (benign enlargement of breast tissue).

In the adult, testosterone is responsible for the maintenance of libido, potency, secondary sexual characteristics, and spermatogenesis. The major complaints of men with adult-onset androgen deficiency are poor sexual performance, as a result of diminished libido and/or impotence; infertility, as a result of impaired sperm production; and gynecomastia. Rapid development of severe androgen deficiency (e.g., with surgical castration) may also cause vasomotor instability or hot flushes, similar to those that many women develop at the time of menopause. Androgen deficiency may also result in behavioral changes, such as passivity, lack of motivation, and irritability.

Secondary sexual characteristics do not regress to the prepubertal state in men who develop testosterone deficiency as adults. However, with longstanding androgen deficiency, there may be significant loss of hair in androgen-dependent areas of the body, fine wrinkling of skin (most noticeable around the eyes and mouth), diminished muscle strength and mass, osteoporosis, and altered fat distribution. In hypogonadal men, pubic hair may assume a female type, inverted triangular pattern (female escutcheon), in contrast to the male type, diamond-shaped distribution, with hair extending to the umbilicus (male escutcheon). The testes are usually small in hypogonadal states. However, depending on the specific cause and severity of the disorder, testis size may be normal. For example, men with recent onset of gonadotropin deficiency from a destructive pituitary tumor may have normal size testes, despite severe testosterone deficiency.

Serum testosterone levels are low in states of androgen deficiency. Routinely available assays measure total testosterone and may give falsely low values in clinical states in which sex hormone–binding globulin is reduced (e.g., obesity). In these instances serum free or non–SHBG-bound testosterone levels should be measured.

Testosterone helps to maintain quantitatively normal spermatogenesis in man; androgen deficiency, therefore, almost always results in reduced sperm production. Impaired spermatogenesis is confirmed by a low sperm count on seminal fluid analysis. Because sperm counts are highly variable and often suppressed by illness, at least three sperm counts obtained over 2 months while patients are well should be performed before a diagnosis of oligospermia (low sperm counts) is made.

Isolated Deficiency in Sperm Production

In contrast to patients with androgen deficiency, men with an isolated deficiency of sperm production present postpubertally with infertility as their major complaint, without symptoms of testosterone deficiency. Testis size may be reduced or normal and an undescended testis or *varicocele* (varicose dilatation of the pampiniform venous plexus of the scrotum) may be found. The remainder of the physical examination is usually unremarkable. Sperm counts are usually low (<20 million per milliliter) or zero (azoospermia), and there may be associated or isolated abnormalities of sperm motility and/or morphology on seminal fluid analysis. Serum testosterone levels are normal in disorders causing isolated impairment of sperm production.

Differential Diagnosis

The major manifestations of androgen deficiency in adults are impotence, infertility, and gynecomastia. Although hypogonadism resulting in testosterone deficiency is a major cause of these clinical manifestations, there are many other causes.

IMPOTENCE. Impotence is defined as a consistent inability to achieve or maintain penile erection that is adequate for completion of sexual intercourse. It is a commonly encountered complaint in

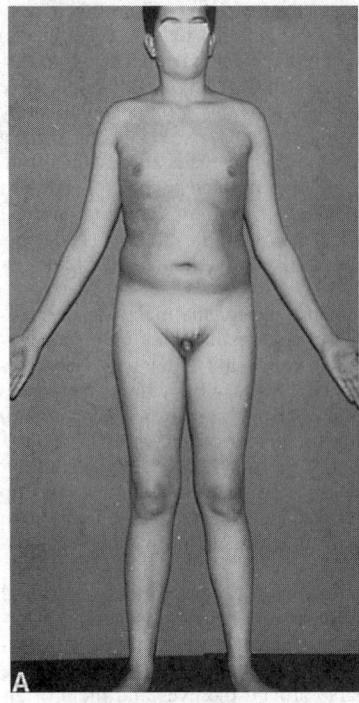
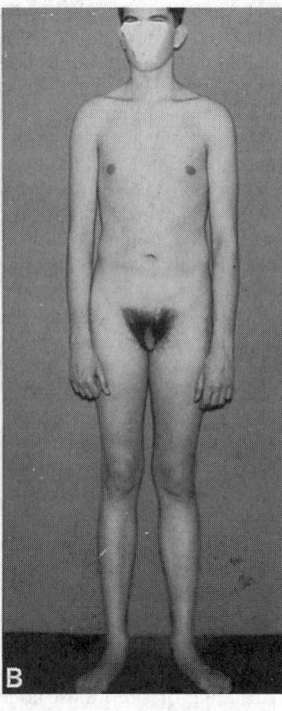
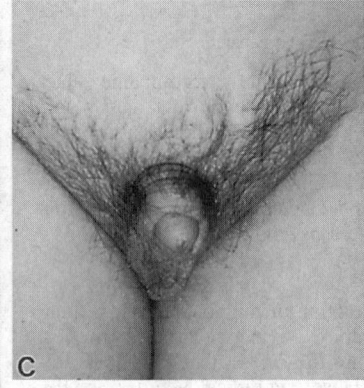
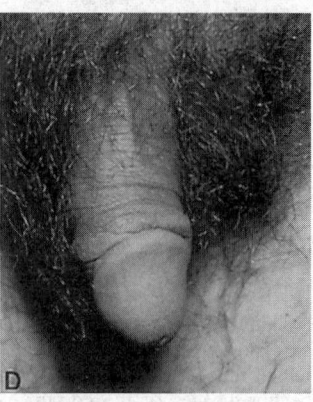

FIGURE 209–4. Example of eunuchoidism as a result of prepubertal androgen deficiency due to functional prepubertal castrate syndrome. *A* and *C*, Before androgen therapy, note the eunuchoidal features of infantile genital development, lack of male hair pattern, poor muscular development, pelvic girdle and lower abdominal fat distribution, and disproportionately long arms and legs. No testicular tissue was identified at the time of surgical exploration. *B* and *D*, After 18 months of testosterone treatment, scalp hair recession, penile development, and pubic hair growth have occurred. A masculine body habitus has developed, with an increase in pectoral and shoulder muscle development and loss of pelvic girdle and lower abdominal fat. (From Bardin CW, Paulsen CA: The testes. *In* Williams RH [ed.]: Textbook of Endocrinology, 6th ed. Philadelphia, WB Saunders, 1981.)

medical practice, occurring in 10 to 35% of adult men with medical problems and increasing in prevalence with advancing age. Impotence is often underdiagnosed because of reluctance of patients and physicians to discuss sexual dysfunction as a medical problem. Although psychogenic impotence is common, the majority of men with impotence who are followed in a general medical clinic have one or more organic causes of erectile dysfunction. Organic causes of impotence often result in performance anxiety and secondary psychogenic sexual dysfunction.

Penile erection sufficient to complete intercourse requires (1) normal *CNS* and thoracolumbar sympathetic and sacral parasympathetic *spinal cord* outputs to the penis; (2) an intact *arterial supply* and *venous drainage* of the penis; and (3) an *anatomically normal penis*. Dysfunction of any of these components interferes with normal initiation and maintenance of penile erection (Table 209–1).

Normal CNS function is necessary to produce adequate penile erections. *Libido* or sexual desire, mediated by the cerebral cortex and limbic system, has a profound influence on erectile function. In most CNS disorders that cause sexual dysfunction, reduced libido is usually associated with impotence. All degrees of *psychiatric disturbance,* from minor stress and performance anxiety to major psychiatric illness, such as depression and schizophrenia; *chronic debilitating illness,* such as cardiac, respiratory, renal, or liver disease or malignancy; and *drugs* that affect CNS function (sedatives, antipsychotics, antidepressants, centrally acting antihypertensive agents, and alcohol), are CNS causes of impotence that also generally reduce libido. *Androgen deficiency, hyperprolactinemia,* and *thyroid dysfunction* (hyperthyroidism and hypothyroidism) also impair libido and potency. Elevated prolactin levels may cause impotence by inducing secondary hypogonadism and androgen deficiency. In contrast to these disorders, *destructive or infiltrative diseases* of certain regions of the *brain* (such as tumor or infarction of the temporal lobe or limbic system) or *spinal cord diseases* (such as injury, tumor, multiple sclerosis, or syphilis) may cause impotence without associated loss of libido. Patients with high spinal cord lesions (above T11) usually retain the ability to have reflexogenic erections.

In addition to intact CNS functioning, normal penile erection requires intact peripheral nervous system function, adequate blood flow to the penis, and normal erectile structures within the penis. *Disorders of peripheral autonomic nerve function* that cause impotence include extensive pelvic surgery, such as aortoiliac bypass, pelvic lymph node dissection, abdominoperineal resection of the rectum, lumbar sympathectomy, and prostatectomy; diabetes; and other conditions causing peripheral autonomic and sensory neuropathy. Atherosclerotic *peripheral vascular disease* involving the distal

aortoiliac arteries and *trauma* to these vessels are the most common causes of vascular impotence. These patients usually have diminished or absent femoral pulses and may present with *Leriche's syndrome,* although claudication may be absent in some cases. In addition, autonomic neuropathy and atherosclerotic macro- and microvascular disease are major factors contributing to erectile dysfunction in the 30 to 50% of diabetic men who develop impotence. Penile venous incompetence (venous leak) resulting in inadequate

TABLE 209–1. CAUSES OF IMPOTENCE

I. Disorders of Central Nervous System Control	II. Disorders of Peripheral Erectile Response
Psychiatric Illness	Drugs
Stress	Anticholinergic drugs
Performance anxiety	Antidepressants
Depression	Antihistamines
Major psychiatric illness	β-Adrenergic blockers
Chronic Illness	Sympathomimetic
Cardiac disease	drugs
Respiratory disease	α-Adrenergic agonists
Renal disease	Antihypertensive
Liver disease	agents
Malignancy	Autonomic Neuropathy
Central Nervous System–	Pelvic surgery
Active Drugs	Diabetes
Sedatives	Other peripheral
Antipsychotics	neuropathies
Antidepressants	Vascular Disease
Central antihyper-	Distal aortoiliac
tensives	atherosclerosis
Alcohol	Diabetes
Endocrine Disorders	Trauma
Hypogonadism (andro-	Venous incompetence
gen deficiency)	Penile Abnormalities
Hyperprolactinemia	Peyronie's disease
Thyroid disease	Chordee
Central Nervous System	Priapism
Disease	Trauma
Temporal lobe dis-	Microphallus or
orders	micropenis
Limbic system dis-	
orders	
Spinal Cord Disease	
Trauma	
Multiple sclerosis	
Syphilis	
Other spinal cord lesions	

veno-occlusion to sustain an erection is an uncommon cause of impotence. *Penile abnormalities,* such as Peyronie's disease, chordee, priapism, and microphallus, may also cause erectile dysfunction. *Drugs* may cause erectile dysfunction by inhibiting penile smooth muscle relaxation and arterial vasodilation (anticholinergic drugs, antidepressants, antihistamines, β-adrenergic blockers) or by inducing premature detumescence (sympathomimetic drugs, α-adrenergic agonists). The mechanism of impotence associated with certain antihypertensive agents (e.g., diuretics, vasodilators, sympatholytic agents) is unclear.

Normal testosterone levels are necessary for maintenance of libido and potency. Hypogonadism resulting in androgen deficiency is a cause of impotence in approximately 15 to 20% of men complaining of sexual dysfunction in a general medical clinic. Therefore, all impotent patients should have serum testosterone and gonadotropin levels measured as part of their diagnostic workup.

A thorough history and physical examination provide invaluable clues to the cause of impotence. Erectile dysfunction that occurs abruptly and is transient, intermittent, or temporally associated with stress is usually psychogenic in origin. Men with psychogenic impotence often have spontaneous nocturnal or morning erections and are able to achieve normal erections with some partners but not with others or with masturbation but not during sexual intercourse. Patients with impotence related to central or peripheral nervous system or vascular disease or penile abnormalities usually demonstrate clinical manifestations of the underlying disorder. A careful drug history may reveal offending medications that cause impotence.

Measurement of nocturnal penile tumescence (NPT) and buckling pressure may be used to differentiate psychogenic from organic impotence. NPT is usually present in psychogenic impotence but abnormal or absent if there is an organic cause of erectile dysfunction. Formal evaluation is done in a sleep laboratory with EEG monitoring to detect sleep disturbances that may disturb NPT. Resistance of the penis to buckling is also measured; this measurement correlates better than NPT alone with ability to have sexual intercourse. A simpler assessment of NPT can be made by wrapping the shaft of the penis with a snap gauge; NPT is detected by breaking of wires of different tensile strength.

Doppler determination of the ratio of supine penile systolic blood pressure to brachial systolic blood pressure (penile/brachial index) may be useful in diagnosing patients with penile arterial vascular insufficiency. An index > 0.75 is normal; one between 0.75 and 0.60 is indeterminate; and one < 0.6 is suggestive of arteriovascular impotence, which may be confirmed by arteriography. Recently, intracavernosal injection of vasodilatory agents with and without duplex ultrasonography or direct pressure monitoring has been used in the evaluation of impotence. Development of a sustained erectile response implies normal vascular status, whereas a short-lived, partial, or absent response suggests a hemodynamic abnormality. Corporal veno-occlusion is usually evaluated by cavernosometry and cavernosography following intracavernosal injection of a vasodilating drug. In the absence of neurogenic bladder dysfunction, electromyographic determination of the bulbocavernosus reflex latency and somatosensory evoked response of the dorsal nerve may be useful in detecting peripheral and sacral spinal abnormalities contributing to impotence.

Treatment of impotence is directed at the underlying causes of erectile dysfunction. Psychosexual education, counseling, and therapy are very successful in restoring sexual function in many men with psychogenic impotence. Testosterone therapy should be reserved for hypogonadal men with androgen deficiency in whom libido and potency are restored with adequate androgen replacement. Men with impotence and hypogonadism due to hyperprolactinemia may require agents to lower prolactin levels (e.g., bromocriptine) in addition to testosterone replacement to improve potency. Self-administration of intracavernosal injections of vasodilatory drugs (e.g., prostaglandin E, papaverine and/or phentolamine) induces penile erections sufficient for sexual intercourse in many patients with impotence. In general, it is very effective and well tolerated. Patients with severe arterial insufficiency or venous leaks are least likely to respond to this therapy. Select patients with vascular impotence are candidates for corrective surgical procedures.

In patients for whom effective therapy is not available, surgical implantation of a penile prosthesis offers rigidity sufficient for sexual intercourse without interfering with ejaculation or orgasm. Recently, vacuum-constriction devices have been introduced as a non-surgical alternative to penile prostheses for the treatment of impotence. A condom-like cylinder is placed over the flaccid penis; a vacuum is applied to generate negative pressure, drawing blood into the penis and resulting in an erection. A constrictive band is then placed around the base of the penis to prevent the drainage of blood from the penis, maintaining tumescence for the duration of intercourse.

INFERTILITY. Infertility is defined as the inability of a couple to achieve a pregnancy after 1 year of unprotected intercourse. An estimated 5 to 6% of men in the reproductive age group are infertile. Most causes of male infertility result in abnormal sperm count or semen quality, as reflected by an abnormal seminal fluid analysis. About 90% of male infertility is caused by hypogonadism resulting in impaired spermatogenesis; and 80 to 90% of these men have isolated deficiency of sperm production with normal androgen production of unclear origin, i.e., *idiopathic oligospermia or azoospermia* (see below). Other causes of male infertility include *coital disorders, ductal obstruction, ejaculatory dysfunction,* and *disorders of accessory sexual organs* (Table 209–2). Even if a cause of male infertility is diagnosed, the female partner should undergo diagnostic evaluation because a concomitant female factor causing infertility is found in 30% of infertile couples.

Although uncommon, *defects* in the *coital technique,* such as timing of intercourse during menses, rather than at the time of ovulation near mid-cycle, premature withdrawal of the penis, prior ejaculation, and infrequent intercourse are causes of male infertility. They are important to remember because they are potentially reversible with proper patient education. Basal body temperature measurements or rapid immunoassay kits measuring urinary LH levels are methods often used to estimate the timing of ovulation in the partner's menstrual cycle. *Erectile dysfunction* from any cause may result in unsuccessful intercourse and infertility.

Impediment of sperm transport from the testis to the urethra results in azoospermia and infertility. Causes of *ductal obstruction* include congenital absence of the vas deferens or seminal vesicles often associated with cystic fibrosis; congenital defects of the epididymis or vas, e.g., as a consequence of diethylstilbestrol exposure *in utero;* fibrosis as a complication of genitourinary infection, especially epididymitis; Young's syndrome, in which thickened, inspissated mucous secretions lead to blockage of the epididymis and vas deferens; and vasectomy.

Obstructive azoospermia must be differentiated from a severe defect in spermatogenesis. Measurement of a serum FSH level is often helpful because elevated levels generally indicate disordered seminiferous tubular function. Normal FSH levels may occur in either obstructive azoospermia or seminiferous tubule dysfunction. In obstructive azoospermia, radiologic examination, i.e., a vasogram, demonstrates the ductal obstruction, and a testicular biopsy reveals normal spermatogenesis. Evaluation of azoospermia is one of the few indications for performing a testicular biopsy. Vasectomy has been used widely and successfully to induce infertility in men who desire fertility control, without deleterious effects on the hypothalamic-pituitary-testicular axis or general health. Using microsurgical

TABLE 209–2. CAUSES OF MALE INFERTILITY

Coital Disorders
  Defects in Technique
    Poor timing with menses
    Premature withdrawal
    Infrequent intercourse
  Impotence
Hypogonadism (Deficiency of Sperm Production)
Ductal Obstruction
  Congenital Defects of Vas Deferens, Epididymides, or Seminal Vesicles
  Postinfectious Obstruction
  Cystic Fibrosis/Young's Syndrome
  Vasectomy
Ejaculatory Dysfunction
  Premature Ejaculation
  Retrograde Ejaculation
Disorders of Accessory Glands
  Epididymitis/Seminal Vesiculitis/Prostatitis
  Immunologic

techniques, vasovasostomy has been used successfully to restore fertility in vasectomized men. Despite return of sperm in the ejaculate in 80 to 90%, fertility is restored in only 30 to 50% of men after vasovasostomy.

Ejaculatory dysfunction, such as premature or retrograde ejaculation, can cause infertility by preventing the normal deposition of sperm into the female genital tract. Premature ejaculation is often successfully treated by sex therapy techniques. Retrograde ejaculation most commonly results from diabetic autonomic neuropathy, prostatic resection, pelvic surgery, or administration of sympatholytic drugs. It is suspected if orgasm produces little or no ejaculate and is confirmed by the presence of large numbers of sperm in a postejaculation urine sample. Sympathomimetic drugs, imipramine, and harvesting and concentrating of sperm from the urine for artificial insemination have been used to treat retrograde ejaculation.

Disorders of the *accessory sexual organs* result in infertility by a number of mechanisms. Infections of the epididymis, seminal vesicles, and/or prostate have been reported to cause infertility by affecting sperm maturation or function directly or by inducing antisperm antibodies that, in turn, affect sperm function. Offending organisms include *Neisseria gonorrhoea, Chlamydia trachomatis,* coliforms, *Ureaplasma urealyticum,* and *Mycobacterium tuberculosis.* Antisperm antibodies present in the semen may cause sperm agglutination and reduce sperm motility. Induction of these antibodies after vasectomy may be responsible for the discrepancy between the success rate for return of sperm in the ejaculate and restoration of fertility after vasectomy reversal. Glucocorticoid therapy can lower antisperm antibody titers and improve fertility in some patients.

GYNECOMASTIA. Gynecomastia, a benign glandular enlargement of the male breast, is usually asymptomatic, but its rapid development may cause pain and tenderness. It is often very difficult to distinguish between true gynecomastia and an increase in adipose tissue in obese boys or men. In order to adequately detect gynecomastia, fingers should be used to grasp the tissue surrounding the areola in a pinching action.

Although usually bilateral, gynecomastia may be markedly asymmetric or rarely unilateral. In these instances, gynecomastia must be distinguished from other benign chest wall tumors and male breast cancer. In contrast to benign lesions, breast carcinoma is usually eccentric in location, hard, and associated with skin or nipple retraction and bloody discharge; lymphadenopathy due to metastatic disease may also be found.

Gynecomastia usually occurs when the breast is exposed to a hormonal milieu of increased estrogen relative to testosterone concentration or action, i.e., an increased estrogen/testosterone ratio. An increased ratio may result from pathologic conditions or drugs that either increase estrogen or reduce testosterone levels or action of these hormones. Because both of these hormonal alterations commonly result in primary or secondary hypogonadism, hypogonadal states are major causes of gynecomastia. Unless hyperprolactinemia induces androgen deficiency by inhibiting gonadotropin secretion, elevated prolactin levels do not usually cause gynecomastia. The clinical causes of gynecomastia are summarized in Table 209–3.

Gynecomastia may sometimes be *physiologic* rather than pathologic. Transient gynecomastia is usually seen in neonatal boys, as a result of exposure *in utero* to high maternal estrogen concentrations. At the time of puberty, gynecomastia is observed in 60 to 70% of boys. Pubertal gynecomastia usually lasts for months to years and does not persist into adulthood. Finally, small amounts of palpable breast tissue (2 to 3 cm in diameter) can be detected by careful examination in 40% of healthy normal adult men, increasing in prevalence with advancing age.

In addition to *androgen deficiency* and *disorders of androgen action,* gynecomastia may be caused by a number of *drugs.* Gynecomastia may result from exposure to exogenous estrogen, e.g., from diethylstilbestrol treatment of metastatic prostate cancer, or accidental ingestion, use, contact, or occupational exposure. Excessive circulating estrogens inhibit endogenous gonadotropin secretion, resulting in secondary hypogonadism and reduced testosterone production that contributes to the development of gynecomastia. Administration of high doses of aromatizable androgens, especially to prepubertal boys or severely hypogonadal men, may induce gy-

TABLE 209–3. CAUSES OF GYNECOMASTIA

I. Physiologic Gynecomastia	**V. Tumors**
Neonatal	Estrogen-Secreting
Pubertal	Tumors
Adult	Adrenal carcinoma
	Leydig cell or Sertoli
II. Hypogonadism (Deficiency of Androgen Production)	cell tumor of testis
	Gonadotropin-Secreting
III. Androgen Resistance Syndromes	Tumors
	Testicular carcinoma
	Lung carcinoma
IV. Drug-Induced Gynecomastia	Liver carcinoma
Hormones	
Estrogens	**VI. Systemic Disorders**
Aromatizable androgens	Hepatic Cirrhosis
hCG	Renal Failure
Drugs Interacting with	Thyrotoxicosis
Estrogen Receptor	
Marijuana	**VII. Miscellaneous**
Digitalis	Refeeding Gynecomastia
Drugs Altering Androgen	Familial
Production or Action	Increased Peripheral
Spironolactone	Aromatization
Cimetidine	Local Chest Trauma
Ketoconazole	
Cytotoxic agents	
Central Nervous System–	
Active Drugs	
Antihypertensive agents	
Tranquilizers	
Sedatives	
Antidepressants	
Amphetamines	

necomastia analogous to that which occurs at puberty. hCG binds to LH receptors on Leydig cells, stimulates relatively greater testicular production of estradiol than testosterone, and may cause gynecomastia. Certain drugs result in breast enlargement by interacting with the estrogen receptor (marijuana, digitalis) or by interfering with androgen production or action (spironolactone, cimetidine, ketoconazole, certain cytotoxic agents). Finally, many CNS-active drugs, such as certain antihypertensives, sedatives, tranquilizers, antidepressants, and amphetamines, are associated with gynecomastia.

Although very uncommon, gynecomastia may be the initial manifestation of an *estrogen-secreting tumor* of the adrenal gland or testis. Feminizing adrenal tumors are usually malignant and present with a palpable abdominal mass. In contrast, estrogen-secreting tumors of the testis are often small and benign. *hCG-secreting tumors,* such as testicular, lung, and hepatic carcinoma, may cause gynecomastia by stimulating excessive estrogen relative to testosterone secretion by Leydig cells. A specific β-hCG assay should be used to confirm the diagnosis of an hCG-secreting tumor.

Certain *systemic disorders* are associated with gynecomastia. In hepatic cirrhosis, gynecomastia is associated with increased estrogen production, primarily as a result of accelerated peripheral conversion of adrenal androgens (androstenedione) to estrone. In addition, serum SHBG levels are elevated, and bioavailable serum testosterone levels are low, contributing to an increased estrogen/testosterone ratio. The gynecomastia observed in patients with renal failure is associated with androgen deficiency resulting from testicular failure, and estrogen production is not usually increased. High estradiol levels and relatively reduced bioavailable testosterone levels (as a result of increased SHBG levels) are commonly found in patients with thyrotoxicosis and contribute to the development of gynecomastia in this condition.

Gynecomastia is often associated with nutritional repletion and weight gain after a period of starvation and weight loss. This *refeeding gynecomastia* was originally described in former prisoners of war who developed tender gynecomastia following their liberation and resumption of a normal diet. A similar condition may occur upon recovery from any prolonged, severe illness associated with malnutrition and weight loss. Refeeding gynecomastia may contribute to the gynecomastia associated with hemodialysis in chronic renal failure patients. Malnutrition results in severe suppression of the hypothalamic-pituitary-testicular axis. Restoration of nutrition rapidly restores gonadal function ("second puberty") and may explain the gynecomastia associated with refeeding. *Familial gynecomastia, chest wall trauma and pain,* and *idiopathic increase in peripheral aromatase activity* are very rare causes of gynecomastia.

Treatment of gynecomastia should focus on the correction of the underlying disorder or withdrawal of the offending drug. Prophylactic low-dose irradiation of the breast prior to diethylstilbestrol treatment in men with prostatic carcinoma prevents gynecomastia. Testosterone treatment of androgen deficiency may occasionally result in resolution of gynecomastia. Experience with the estrogen antagonists (such as tamoxifen), nonaromatizable androgens (such as dihydrotestosterone), and aromatase inhibitors in treating gynecomastia has been limited and variably effective. Severe, longstanding gynecomastia of any cause is usually associated with increased fibrous tissue stroma and requires surgical reduction mammoplasty.

Braunstein GD: Gynecomastia. N Engl J Med 328:490, 1993. *A well-organized, clearly written, concise review of the causes, pathogenesis, evaluation, and treatment of gynecomastia.*

Dial LK (ed.): Geriatric sexuality. Clin Geriatr Med 7:1, 1991. *The entire issue is devoted to sexuality in older adults, with very good chapters on sexuality and impotence in aging men, urologic and endocrine considerations in geriatric sexual dysfunction, and the impact of medications and chronic diseases on sexual function in the elderly.*

Lipshultz LI (eds.): Male infertility. Urol Clin North Am 21:1, 1994. *An excellent, comprehensive discussion of the evaluation and treatment of male infertility by several authors.*

Morley JE, Kaiser FE: Impotence: The internist's approach to diagnosis and treatment. Adv Intern Med 38:151, 1993. *An excellent review of the etiology, diagnosis, and treatment of erectile dysfunction from an internist's perspective.*

NIH Consensus Development Panel on Impotence: Impotence. JAMA 270:83, 1993. *A consensus statement by an interdisciplinary panel of experts that reviews current knowledge regarding the epidemiology, etiology, risk factors, pathophysiology, diagnosis, management, and consequences of impotence.*

Skakkebaek NE, Giwercman A, deKretser D: Pathogenesis and management of male infertility. Lancet 343:1473, 1994. *An updated, concise review of the causes and treatment of male infertility.*

CAUSES OF MALE HYPOGONADISM

Once the diagnosis of male hypogonadism is suspected, the diagnosis is confirmed by measurement of serum testosterone level and sperm count.

The majority of hypogonadal men with *androgen deficiency* also have impairment in sperm production. Once androgen deficiency is diagnosed (low serum testosterone and sperm count), an effort should be made to distinguish between disorders that result from primary testicular disease *(primary hypogonadism)* and those that are secondary to inadequate gonadotropin stimulation of the testis *(secondary hypogonadism),* as a result of either pituitary or hypothalamic disease.

In addition to helping to determine the specific cause of androgen deficiency, the distinction between primary and secondary hypogonadism may have practical therapeutic implications. For example, regardless of the specific cause, primary hypogonadism is usually treated with androgen replacement. In the majority of cases, the infertility in primary hypogonadism is not treatable. However, secondary hypogonadism may result from destruction of pituitary gonadotropin-secreting cells, for example by a pituitary tumor. In this instance, in addition to androgen deficiency, the space-occupying effects of the tumor mass on brain function (such as visual fields and cerebroventricular flow) and alterations (both increase and decrease) in the secretion of other anterior pituitary hormones (such as ACTH, TSH, growth hormone, and prolactin) need to be considered in formulating a therapeutic plan (see Ch. 202.1). Furthermore, because the testes usually function normally in response to adequate gonadotropin stimulation in patients with secondary hypogonadism, gonadotropins (or LHRH for hypothalamic hypogonadism) may be administered in these patients to stimulate spermatogenesis and induce fertility.

The negative feedback relationship between gonadotropin secretion and circulating testosterone levels (see Fig. 209–1) provides the physiologic basis and rationale for the use of serum gonadotropin levels to distinguish between primary and secondary testicular disorders that result in androgen deficiency. Because the negative feedback effect of testosterone on gonadotropin secretion is reduced, men with *primary hypogonadism* have reduced serum testosterone and elevated serum LH and FSH levels; i.e., they have *hypergonadotropic hypogonadism.* Not uncommonly, serum FSH levels may be disproportionately elevated compared with LH levels, especially with severe seminiferous tubule dysfunction.

In contrast to primary testicular dysfunction, men with *secondary hypogonadism* are not able to increase gonadotropin secretion ap-

propriately in the presence of reduced testosterone negative feedback and have inadequate gonadotropin stimulation of the testis. These men have a hormonal pattern of reduced serum testosterone and low to low normal serum LH and FSH levels; i.e., they have *hypogonadotropic hypogonadism.* Gonadotropin levels are often in the low normal range in men with secondary hypogonadism because most clinically available gonadotropin assays lack sufficient sensitivity to distinguish low from low normal values.

The majority of hypogonadal patients with *isolated impairment of sperm production* have primary testicular disease. These patients generally present with infertility and have no clinical manifestations of androgen deficiency. Serum testosterone and gonadotropin levels are usually normal. Infertile patients who present with no sperm in their ejaculate, i.e., azoospermia, may have either severe seminiferous tubule failure or obstruction of the genital tract. Measurement of serum FSH level may be helpful in evaluation of these patients. A selective elevation of serum FSH with normal LH levels in a patient with azoospermia implies severe germ cell dysfunction and poor prognosis for fertility. No further workup is usually necessary. A normal serum FSH level in an azoospermic patient leaves open the possibility of a surgically correctable ductal obstruction, and ultrasonography or vasography, and occasionally a testicular biopsy are performed. Selective elevation in serum FSH levels may also be observed in patients with gonadotropin-secreting pituitary adenomas. Uncommonly, isolated deficiency of sperm production results from inadequate gonadotropin stimulation of the testis. In these instances, serum gonadotropin levels are generally reduced, and very rarely selective FSH deficiency may occur.

The vast majority of adults with male hypogonadism have either primary or secondary testicular failure. Very rarely, *disorders of androgen action* may present in adults with a clinical picture of hypogonadism. Unlike the severe androgen resistance syndromes, which present at birth with male pseudohermaphroditism (see Ch. 207), these disorders are characterized by mild defects in androgen action, resulting in a nearly normal male phenotype (frequently with varying degrees of hypospadias). Both serum testosterone and gonadotropin levels are usually elevated.

In summary, clinical manifestations combined with measurements of serum testosterone, sperm count, and basal serum gonadotropin levels permit a physiologic classification of the causes of male hypogonadism into *primary* and *secondary hypogonadism* and subclassification into disorders that result in *deficiency of both sperm and androgen production,* and those with *isolated deficiency in sperm production* with normal androgen production (Table 209–4).

Primary Hypogonadism

DEFICIENCY OF SPERM AND ANDROGEN PRODUCTION. *Congenital or Developmental Disorders.* *Klinefelter's syndrome* is the most common cause of primary testicular failure resulting in impairment of both spermatogenesis and testosterone production. The syndrome is characterized by small, firm testes, azoospermia, gynecomastia, varying degrees of eunuchoidism and testosterone deficiency, and elevated gonadotropin levels. Klinefelter's syndrome is a very common disorder, affecting 1 in every 400 to 500 men. The incidence of Klinefelter's syndrome increases to 5% when maternal age is over 45 years. The fundamental defect in Klinefelter's syndrome and its variants is the presence of one or a number of extra X chromosomes.

Classically, the karyotype in Klinefelter's syndrome is 47 XXY, resulting from meiotic nondisjunction in either the maternal or paternal gamete. Variants of the syndrome demonstrate a variety of karyotypes, including XXYY, more than two X (poly X) plus Y, and mosaicism. In classic Klinefelter's syndrome (47 XXY), the presence of an extra X chromosome is responsible for the presence of a sex chromatin or Barr body in the nucleus of epithelial cells obtained on buccal smear, a normal finding in females, who carry two X chromosomes. The diagnosis of Klinefelter's syndrome is confirmed by karyotyping of lymphocytes or testicular tissue.

Clinical features of Klinefelter's syndrome are not evident prior to puberty. At the time of puberty, the testes fail to increase in size and become firmer in consistency. This is a result of fibrosis of the seminiferous tubules. The most remarkable clinical feature of Klinefelter's syndrome is the very small size of the testes, rarely exceeding 2 cm in length, in contrast to a lower limit of 3.5 cm in the nor-

TABLE 209-4. CAUSES OF MALE HYPOGONADISM

I. Primary Hypogonadism

Deficiency of Sperm and Androgen Production

Congenital or Developmental Disorders

Klinefelter's syndrome and variants

Functional prepubertal castrate syndrome

Noonan (Bonnevie-Ullrich) syndrome

Myotonic dystrophy

Polyglandular autoimmune disease

Complex genetic disorders

? Normal aging

Acquired Disorders

Orchitis (mumps, leprosy, etc.)

Surgical or traumatic castration

Drugs (spironolactone, ketoconazole, H_2-receptor blockers, alcohol, marijuana, digitalis, cytotoxic drugs)

Irradiation

Systemic Disorders

Chronic liver disease

Chronic renal failure

Malignancy (Hodgkin's, testicular)

Sickle cell disease

Paraplegia

Vasculitis (periarteritis)

Infiltrative disease (amyloidosis)

Isolated Deficiency of Sperm Production

Congenital or Developmental Disorders

Germinal cell aplasia (Sertoli cell–only syndrome)

Cryptorchidism

Varicocele

Immotile cilia syndrome (Kartagener's syndrome)

Myotonic dystrophy

Acquired Disorders

Orchitis (mumps, leprosy, etc.)

Thermal trauma

Irradiation

Cytotoxic drugs

Environmental toxins

Systemic Disorders

Acute febrile illness

Paraplegia

Idiopathic Oligospermia or Azoospermia

II. Secondary Hypogonadism

Deficiency of Sperm and Androgen Production

Congenital or Developmental Disorders

Hypogonadotropic eunuchoidism (Kallmann's syndrome)

Hemochromatosis

Complex genetic syndromes

? Normal aging

Acquired Disorders

Hypopituitarism

Hyperprolactinemia

Estrogen excess

Progestins

Androgenic anabolic steroids

Opiate-like drugs

Systemic Disorders

Glucocorticoid excess (Cushing's syndrome)

Acute stress or illness

Nutritional deficiency (protein-calorie malnutrition, anorexia nervosa)

Chronic illness

Massive obesity

Isolated Deficiency of Sperm Production

Androgen Excess

Congenital adrenal hyperplasia (21- and 11β-hydroxylase deficiency)

Androgenic anabolic steroids

Androgen-secreting tumors

Hyperprolactinemia

Isolated FSH Deficiency

III. Androgen Resistance Syndromes

Reifenstein's Syndrome

Idiopathic Oligospermia or Azoospermia

? Celiac Disease

---

mal adult. Clinical androgen deficiency is usually present but variable in degree, resulting in varying degrees of eunuchoidism (Fig. 209–5). In contrast to other conditions that result in eunuchoidism, Klinefelter's syndrome often results in a disproportionate increase in lower compared with upper extremity long bone growth. Careful palpation usually reveals bilateral gynecomastia in 80 to 90% of patients. Although the incidence of mental retardation is greater, the majority of patients with Klinefelter's syndrome have normal intelligence. Most patients exhibit character and personality disorders that may be related, in part, to the psychosocial consequences of androgen deficiency. There is a slightly increased incidence of certain systemic diseases in Klinefelter's syndrome. These include diabetes, chronic obstructive pulmonary disease, autoimmune disorders (e.g., systemic lupus erythematosus, Hashimoto's thyroiditis), malignancy (breast cancer, lymphoma, germ cell neoplasms), and varicose veins.

The clinical manifestations of Klinefelter's syndrome variants differ from those of the classic 47 XXY syndrome. In general, the presence of more than two extra X chromosomes results in a much higher incidence of mental retardation and somatic abnormalities, such as hypospadias, cryptorchidism, and bony abnormalities of the radius and ulna. The majority of patients with mosaic Klinefelter's syndrome exhibit less severe clinical manifestations, particularly if a normal XY cell line is present. Indeed, fertility in patients with mosaic Klinefelter's syndrome (XXY/XY) has been documented. Patients with an additional Y chromosome tend to be tall and have extremely aggressive, antisocial behavioral abnormalities. Very rarely, a patient exhibits the classic features of Klinefelter's syndrome with a normal (46 XY) karyotype, a so-called mutant phenocopy. Finally, phenotypic males with a 46 XX karyotype may demonstrate the typical clinical manifestations of Klinefelter's syndrome, except for having shorter stature and a higher incidence of hypospadias. In some patients with this condition, Y chromosomal material is translocated onto the X chromosome (see Ch. 207).

Azoospermia is present in >95% of patients with classic Klinefelter's syndrome. Serum testosterone levels are usually low but may be in the low normal adult range. However, free testosterone levels are reduced in most patients with Klinefelter's syndrome. Serum estradiol levels are often elevated, resulting in elevated SHBG concentrations and contributing to the development of gynecomastia. Serum gonadotropin levels, especially serum FSH levels, are uniformly elevated.

Treatment of Klinefelter's syndrome is aimed primarily at correction of the androgen deficiency with testosterone replacement therapy. The infertility is irreversible. Gynecomastia may be a source of great social embarrassment, in which case reduction mammoplasty should be performed.

The *functional prepubertal castrate* or *vanishing testes syndrome (congenital anorchia)* is characterized by bilateral absence of functioning testes, occasionally associated with absent epididymides, in a genotypic man. The presence of otherwise normal male internal and external genitalia, without müllerian duct derivatives, and descent of the vas and testicular blood vessels into the scrotum imply that a normally functioning testis was present during fetal life. It is hypothesized that testicular damage during the fetal or prepubertal period results in atrophy of the testes. Patients with this syndrome usually present with delayed puberty, eunuchoidal features, absence of palpable testes, and short stature (see Fig. 209–4). Congenital anorchia must be distinguished from bilateral abdominal cryptorchidism, which also presents with absent scrotal testes. Because of the increased risk of malignancy, intra-abdominal testes require orchiectomy or orchiopexy. The absence of a testosterone response to exogenous hCG in patients with congenital anorchia may be helpful in distinguishing it from bilateral abdominal testes. However, laparoscopy or surgical exploration is often necessary to confirm the diagnosis. Treatment of this syndrome consists of androgen replacement therapy to induce full sexual maturation. Insertion of testicular prostheses may be of psychological value.

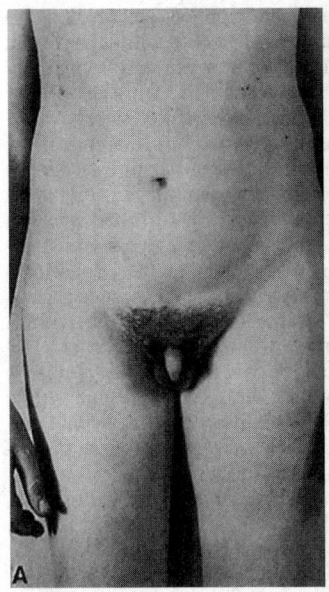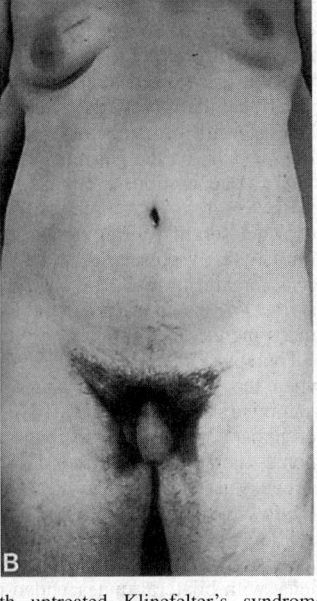

FIGURE 209–5. Two patients with untreated Klinefelter's syndrome, demonstrating the variability in degree of androgenization in this disorder. *A,* The small penis, diminished pubic hair with a female escutcheon, and sparse body hair indicate severe androgen deficiency. *B,* Normal penile development and adequate pubic and body hair indicate nearly normal androgen production by the testes. Gynecomastia is present in both patients, although only visible in the patient shown in *B.* The testes in both subjects were less than 2 cm in length. (From Bardin CW, Paulsen CA: The testes. *In* Williams RH [ed.]: Textbook of Endocrinology, 6th ed. Philadelphia, WB Saunders, 1981.)

Noonan (Bonnevie-Ullrich) syndrome, an autosomal recessive disorder, occurs in karyotypically normal males and females. It is characterized by a number of clinical features similar to those of females with Turner's syndrome. Characteristic findings include short stature, typical facies (hypertelorism, antimongoloid eye slant, ptosis, low-set ears, micrognathia, high-arched palate, and dental malocclusions), webbed neck, shield-like chest, pectus excavatum, cubitus valgus, mental retardation, cardiovascular anomalies (pulmonic stenosis and atrial septal defects), and lymphedema. Males with Noonan syndrome (also called male Turner's syndrome) exhibit primary testicular dysfunction with impairment of both sperm and androgen production and elevated serum gonadotropin levels. Cryptorchidism is frequently present. Treatment of this disorder consists of testosterone replacement to correct the androgen deficiency and orchiopexy for associated cryptorchidism, both for psychological reasons and to monitor the testes for malignancy.

Myotonic dystrophy (see also Ch. 454) is an autosomal dominant disorder characterized by progressive weakness and atrophy of muscles, especially those of the face, neck, and distal extremities. An important diagnostic feature in this disorder is the presence of myotonia, or prolonged contraction of muscles. Other characteristic findings include cataracts, cardiac arrhythmias, dysphagia, premature frontal balding, mild intellectual deterioration, and gonadal atrophy. Testicular atrophy that occurs in middle age is found in about 80% of men affected by myotonic dystrophy. The majority of these men have isolated impairment of spermatogenesis with normal androgen production. However, approximately 20% of men with myotonic dystrophy exhibit androgen deficiency. In addition to treating the androgen deficiency, testosterone replacement therapy may help to maintain or improve muscle function in these men.

Polyglandular autoimmune disease (see also Ch. 210.1) is a disorder in which there is concurrence of organ-specific autoimmune disease involving several endocrine and nonendocrine organs, associated with the presence of circulating autoantibodies to these organs. Specific conditions that occur in association with each other in this disorder are Addison's disease, Hashimoto's disease, insulin-dependent diabetes, pernicious anemia, ovarian failure, hypoparathyroidism, vitiligo, mucocutaneous candidiasis, Graves' disease, hypopituitarism, and alopecia. Although much less common than primary ovarian failure, primary testicular failure, associated

with antitesticular antibodies and resulting in androgen deficiency, may occur in males with polyglandular autoimmune disease.

Normal aging in healthy men is associated with significant reductions in testosterone and sperm production. Serum total and free testosterone levels in elderly men often fall below the normal range for younger men in association with slightly elevated or normal gonadotropin levels. Thus, a hormonal pattern suggesting either mild primary or secondary hypogonadism may be found in elderly men. The physiologic significance of reduced testosterone levels in aging men, however, is unknown. Normal aging in men is also accompanied by reductions in muscle mass and strength, bone mass, sexual interest and function, sleep, and vigor, and alterations in mood and cognition. Whether these changes in body function with aging are related to the reduction in testosterone levels remains to be determined.

Primary hypogonadism may present in a number of *complex genetic disorders,* such as *Alström ataxia-telangiectasia, POEMS, Sohval-Soffer, Weinstein,* and *Werner* syndromes. Rarely, patients with *Prader-Labhart-Willi* and *Laurence-Moon-Biedl* syndromes demonstrate primary, rather than the more commonly associated secondary, hypogonadism.

Acquired Disorders. In general, seminiferous tubule function and spermatogenesis are much more sensitive to external or environmental influences (such as irradiation, cytotoxic agents, or heat) than is Leydig cell production of testosterone. This greater sensitivity is due, in large part, to the fact that spermatogenesis involves active and coordinated cellular division and differentiation. As a result, most acquired primary testicular disorders causing hypogonadism result more commonly in isolated impairment of spermatogenesis (see below) than in androgen deficiency.

Viral orchitis, most frequently due to *mumps,* is a very common cause of acquired primary testicular failure. Approximately 15 to 25% of males with mumps develop acute orchitis. Acute mumps infection of the testes in prepubertal boys or adults usually results in permanent seminiferous tubule damage and, in severe cases, Leydig cell loss and androgen deficiency. Although clinical mumps orchitis is unilateral in the majority of cases, degenerative changes can occur in the clinically uninvolved testis. The use of mumps vaccine has significantly reduced the incidence of mumps orchitis. Orchitis may also complicate infections with viruses such as *echoviruses* and *arboviruses.* Uncommon causes of orchitis include *gonorrhea, leprosy, tuberculosis, brucellosis, glanders, syphilis,* and certain parasitic infections such as *filariasis* and *bilharziasis.* As in mumps, orchitis complicating these disorders results more commonly in isolated impairment of sperm production, although in severe cases androgen deficiency may develop.

Bilateral surgical or traumatic castration results in acute androgen deficiency. Castration after puberty often causes hot flushes and irritability, similar to women undergoing menopause.

Certain *drugs* may produce androgen deficiency by inhibiting testosterone biosynthesis and/or by blocking androgen action. *Spironolactone* inhibits testosterone synthesis and interferes with androgen action by competitively binding to the androgen receptor. *Ketoconazole* inhibits testosterone synthesis. H_2 *receptor blockers* (e.g., cimetidine) are weak androgen antagonists. *Alcohol* and *marijuana* (tetrahydrocannabinol) have direct toxic effects on both spermatogenesis and testicular steroidogenesis in addition to their CNS effects. *Digitalis* elevates serum estradiol, reduces testosterone levels, and interacts with both the estrogen and androgen receptors. A number of *cytotoxic drugs* used in cancer chemotherapy interfere with spermatogenesis and, rarely, with androgen production. In some *malignancies,* androgen deficiency occurs in the absence of exposure to chemotherapeutic agents (e.g., Hodgkin's disease or testicular cancer). Androgen deficiency may result from general debilitation and malnutrition associated with some malignancies. Exposure of the testes to very large doses of *irradiation* (over 600 to 800 rad) may compromise Leydig cell function.

Systemic Disorders. A number of systemic diseases cause deficiencies in sperm and androgen production, primarily by affecting testicular function directly, although gonadotropin secretion may also be affected in many of these conditions. In patients with *chronic liver disease* (cirrhosis), gynecomastia and testicular atrophy are commonly present (in 50 to 75%). Total serum testosterone levels are low or low normal. Because SHBG levels are elevated, free and non–SHBG-bound testosterone levels are low. Serum LH levels are usually elevated but may fall in the high normal range. Increased estrogen concentrations result from impaired hepatic clearance of adrenal androgens (androstenedione), leading to an increased substrate for peripheral aromatization to estrone and estradiol. The increased estrogen/testosterone ratio may contribute to the formation of gynecomastia. Treatment of androgen deficiency in patients with cirrhosis with an aromatizable androgen may result in worsening of gynecomastia.

Chronic renal failure usually causes reductions in both sperm and androgen production. LH and FSH levels are elevated, as a result of increased production as well as reduced renal clearance. The response of testosterone levels to hCG stimulation is impaired. Elevated serum prolactin levels and zinc deficiency may also contribute to testicular dysfunction in uremia. Hemodialysis does not significantly improve testosterone production. However, successful renal transplantation may result in some return of testicular function, which may be tempered by chronic immunosuppressive therapy to prevent graft rejection. In addition to treating androgen deficiency, testosterone replacement therapy may also improve the anemia of renal failure.

Sickle cell disease often results in primary testicular dysfunction with low serum testosterone and elevated serum gonadotropin levels. *Paraplegia* may result in a transient reduction in serum testosterone levels that return to normal in the chronic paraplegic state unless malnutrition is present. *Vasculitis* involving the testis (e.g., periarteritis nodosa) or *infiltrative diseases* (e.g., amyloidosis, leukemia) may also result in primary testicular failure.

ISOLATED DEFICIENCY OF SPERM PRODUCTION.
Congenital or Developmental Disorders. *Germinal cell aplasia, or Sertoli cell–only syndrome,* is an uncommon condition characterized on testicular biopsy by seminiferous tubules of moderately reduced size, lined with Sertoli cells but devoid of germ cells and having little or no tubular fibrosis. Patients with this syndrome are normally androgenized but infertile. They have slightly smaller than normal testes, azoospermia, and elevated serum FSH levels, indicative of severe seminiferous tubule dysfunction. Serum testosterone levels are normal, and LH levels are normal or slightly elevated. Congenital absence of germ cells is thought to be the basis for this syndrome. However, other gonadal disorders causing severe seminiferous tubule damage (such as mumps orchitis, cryptorchidism, irradiation, or cytotoxic drugs) may result in Sertoli cell–only syndrome. In these acquired causes, however, the tubules are usually extensively sclerosed and the testes are much smaller. Infertility in congenital germinal cell aplasia is irreversible.

In *cryptorchidism* the testes fail to descend normally into the scrotum and are usually located in the abdomen or inguinal canal. *Ectopic testes* are located outside the normal pathway of testicular descent and may be found in the perineal, femoral, or superficial inguinal areas. To avoid unnecessary treatment, cryptorchid testes must be distinguished from *retractile testes,* which are located in the scrotum but are withdrawn into the inguinal canal or abdomen with minimal stimulation.

The testes usually descend into the scrotum about the eighth month of fetal life. Undescended testes are found in approximately 3 to 4% of full-term newborn males, but the testes descend during the first year in all but 0.7 to 0.8%. The prevalence of cryptorchidism in adult males is about 0.3 to 0.4%. Inguinal hernia is associated with cryptorchidism in 50 to 80% of cases.

Bilateral cryptorchidism is associated with a number of disorders that cause androgen deficiency or resistance. When cryptorchidism is not associated with other hypogonadal disorders, it rarely affects Leydig cell function and usually causes isolated impairment of spermatogenesis. Even when cryptorchidism is unilateral, testicular dysfunction is very common, suggesting that both testes have altered function. In rare instances, normal testicular descent may be impeded by anatomic abnormalities along the pathway of descent, e.g., external inguinal hernias. In these instances, orchiopexy before puberty usually results in preservation of normal testicular function.

Careful physical examination of the scrotum should be performed to distinguish cryptorchidism from retractile testes, which is a more common condition. The diagnosis is particularly difficult in obese patients. Examination should be performed in the standing, squatting, and recumbent positions, and observation in warm water may

be helpful. The Valsalva maneuver and applied pressure to the lower abdomen are useful procedures to detect a mobile testis. In patients with retractile testes, elicitation of a cremasteric reflex may result in a localized puckering of the scrotal skin. Ultrasonography or CT scan may be helpful in localizing nonpalpable testes.

As a result of exposure to higher extrascrotal temperatures at the time of puberty, the germinal epithelium of cryptorchid testes shows severe degeneration, eventually resulting in seminiferous tubule fibrosis. Bilateral cryptorchidism causes infertility. Sperm counts are low, and serum FSH levels are usually elevated. Leydig cell function is usually preserved, and serum testosterone and LH concentrations remain normal. The risk of malignancy in undescended testes is five to nine times greater than in scrotal testes, and the risk remains increased even after orchiopexy.

Therapy for cryptorchidism should be instituted before puberty, when the degenerative changes of the germinal epithelium occur. Administration of hCG or LHRH to prepubertal boys with cryptorchidism may cause testicular descent in some patients. If hormonal therapy is unsuccessful in causing testicular descent, orchiopexy is performed in an attempt to preserve testicular function, to allow easier examination of the testis for malignant degeneration, and for cosmetic reasons. Despite orchiopexy, fertility rates in patients with cryptorchidism are usually reduced, particularly in patients with bilateral undescended testes.

A *varicocele* is an abnormal dilatation of the pampiniform plexus of veins surrounding the spermatic cord, caused by retrograde blood flow into the internal spermatic vein. Palpable varicocele occurs in about 10% of men and 30% of men with infertility. Although varicocele is clearly associated with infertility, approximately 50% of men with varicocele have normal seminal fluid analyses, and some men with varicocele and abnormal seminal fluid parameters are fertile. About 90% of varicoceles occur on the left side, as a result of valvular incompetence between the left internal spermatic vein and the renal vein. Occurrence of an isolated right-sided varicocele may be an early clue to venous obstruction by malignancy or to situs inversus. Varicoceles may affect testicular function by a variety of mechanisms, including increasing testicular temperature and blood flow. Seminal fluid analysis usually shows low sperm concentration with reduced motility and increased numbers of sperm with abnormal morphology. Testicular size and serum testosterone, LH, and FSH levels are usually normal. Surgical repair of varicoceles in infertile men has been reported to improve semen quality and fertility, although well-controlled clinical studies have not been performed.

Immotile cilia syndrome, or *Kartagener's syndrome,* is characterized by sinusitis, bronchiectasis, and situs inversus. Patients usually suffer from chronic respiratory infections because of impaired mucociliary clearance in the respiratory tract. In addition, these patients produce nonmotile spermatozoa. Cilia in the respiratory tract and the sperm tail are immotile in Kartagener's syndrome because of an abnormality in *dynein,* a protein that is important in microtubular filament movement. Other patients have a *deficiency of protein carboxyl methylase,* an enzyme that is important in sperm motility. Infertility in this syndrome is not treatable.

The majority of patients with *myotonic dystrophy* (see above) may have isolated impairment of spermatogenesis with normal androgen production.

Acquired Disorders. The majority of adults who develop mumps *orchitis* and orchitis due to other infectious agents sustain severe germ cell damage and isolated impairment of spermatogenesis with normal Leydig cell function (see above). Seminiferous tubule function is much more sensitive to damage from external or environmental agents than is Leydig cell function. Therefore, exposure of the testis to *thermal trauma, irradiation, cytotoxic drugs,* and *environmental toxins* often results in deficiency of sperm production without androgen deficiency. Even relatively minor thermal trauma, such as that induced by hot tubs, may result in suppression of sperm production.

The human testis is very sensitive to irradiation. Only 15 rad of x-irradiation may suppress spermatogenesis temporarily; >600 rad usually produces permanent infertility. Doses of radiation used in therapy of malignant lymphoma may result in permanent germ cell damage and infertility, despite shielding of the testis. Spermatogenesis is also very sensitive to damage by cytotoxic cancer chemotherapeutic agents, especially to alkylating agents. The likelihood of severe seminiferous tubule damage and permanent infertility is greater with combination chemotherapy regimens, such as

MOPP for Hodgkin's disease. Despite being very sensitive to radiation and cytotoxic drugs, the germinal epithelium has remarkable regenerative properties, and recovery of spermatogenesis may occur despite very severe germ cell loss. Both irradiation (> 800 rad) and cytotoxic agents occasionally produce androgen deficiency. Sperm banking offers some hope of fertility for patients who will develop permanent infertility as a result of irradiation or chemotherapy for malignant disease. Sulfasalazine has been reported to cause oligospermia, reduced sperm motility, and infertility.

Damage to the germinal epithelium has been reported in workers exposed to carbon disulfide, a solvent used in production of rayon, and to dibromochloropropane, an insecticide. A number of other chemical agents used in industry and laboratories have been implicated as direct testicular toxins (e.g., lead, deuterium oxide, cadmium, fluoroacetamide, nitrofurans, dinitropyrroles, diamines, α-chlorhydrin, other insecticides, and rodenticides).

Systemic Disorders. Minor *acute febrile illnesses* may result in temporary suppression of sperm production (e.g., minor viral infections). Over 50% of men with spinal cord lesions resulting in *paraplegia* exhibit diminished testicular function, the majority demonstrating impaired sperm production with normal androgen production. Reduced spermatogenesis may be a result of elevated testicular temperature, caused by loss of lumbar sympathetic innervation and the cremasteric reflex.

Idiopathic Oligospermia or Azoospermia. In most men who present with infertility and isolated impairment of spermatogenesis, no apparent cause can be found, leading to the diagnosis of *idiopathic oligospermia or azoospermia.* Because of the high prevalence of male infertility (5 to 6% of reproductive age men), idiopathic oligospermia or azoospermia is the most common cause of male hypogonadism. Because the pathogenesis of impaired sperm production is not known, therapy has been largely empiric and unsuccessful in improving fertility rates over those achieved by placebo or in untreated patients, who have a 20% fertility rate in 1 year. At present, infertility in these patients should be considered irreversible and couples should be offered artificial insemination using donor semen or adoption as alternatives. Recently, assisted reproductive technology using *in vitro* fertilization and intracytoplasmic sperm injection has been used successfully to achieve pregnancy in partners of men with idiopathic oligospermia and/or severely abnormal sperm function.

Secondary Hypogonadism

Secondary hypogonadism is testicular failure due to inadequate gonadotropin secretion as a result of either hypothalamic or pituitary dysfunction. In the majority of cases, both LH and FSH secretion are diminished, resulting in impairment of both sperm and androgen production. Rarely, there may be isolated deficiency of sperm production.

DEFICIENCY OF SPERM AND ANDROGEN PRODUCTION. Congenital or Developmental Disorders. *Hypogonadotropic eunuchoidism,* or *Kallmann's syndrome,* is a congenital and often familial disorder, characterized by isolated hypogonadotropic hypogonadism, eunuchoidism, and anosmia or hyposmia. Gonadotropin deficiency in this disorder is caused by a deficiency of LHRH, and chronic exogenous LHRH administration results in stimulation of normal testicular function. A developmental failure of the olfactory lobes is responsible for absent or reduced sense of smell. There is considerable genetic heterogeneity in Kallmann's syndrome, and inheritance may be autosomal dominant with male-predominant expression, autosomal recessive, or X-linked recessive.

Usually, patients with Kallmann's syndrome present with delayed puberty. They exhibit eunuchoidal features and prepubertal size testes. An early prepubertal manifestation of Kallmann's syndrome is micropenis. In addition to anosmia or hyposmia (present in approximately 80%), these patients may also exhibit other midline defects (e.g., cleft-lip or -palate, color blindness, renal agenesis, nerve deafness), cryptorchidism, and skeletal abnormalities (e.g., syndactyly, short fourth metacarpals, craniofacial asymmetry). Patients with Kallmann's syndrome are often aspermic (i.e., have no ejaculate). Serum testosterone, LH, and FSH levels are low, while other anterior pituitary functions are normal. The degree of gonadotropin deficiency, however, is highly variable.

The differentiation between Kallmann's syndrome and constitutional delayed puberty is very difficult in the absence of anosmia or hyposmia and cannot be reliably made in the prepubertal age range.

Usually, androgen therapy is initiated to induce sexual maturation in both of these conditions and is intermittently stopped to determine whether spontaneous onset of puberty occurs. Patients with Kallmann's syndrome continue to require androgen therapy to achieve and maintain sexual maturation, whereas patients with constitutional delayed puberty do not require treatment after spontaneous endogenous gonadotropin and testosterone secretion begin. When fertility is desired in men with Kallmann's syndrome, androgen treatment is stopped, and spermatogenesis may be induced with gonadotropin or LHRH therapy.

A variant of Kallmann's syndrome is *isolated LH deficiency,* also known as the *"fertile" eunuch syndrome.* In this syndrome, selective deficiency in LH secretion results in prepubertal androgen deficiency and eunuchoidism. Because FSH secretion is preserved, testis size is nearly normal and spermatogenesis is present. However, sperm production is not normal in these patients, and they are not fertile, as the name of the syndrome would imply. Treatment with hCG, which contains predominantly LH-like hormonal activity, stimulates Leydig cell production of testosterone, ameliorates androgen deficiency, and increases spermatogenesis.

Hemochromatosis is an autosomal recessive disorder in which there is parenchymal iron deposition in a variety of tissues, most prominently in the liver, skin, pancreas, and heart (see Ch. 189). Iron deposition in the pituitary gland selectively inhibits gonadotropin production without significantly affecting other anterior pituitary hormone secretion. The resulting hypogonadotropic hypogonadism and androgen deficiency are responsible for the common complaint of impotence in this disorder. Frequent phlebotomies or treatment with desferrioxamine to decrease iron overload may restore gonadotropin secretion in some patients. Even in the presence of significant iron overload, administration of gonadotropins can stimulate testicular function, including induction of spermatogenesis. Parenchymal iron deposition resulting in hypogonadotropic hypogonadism may also occur in patients with conditions that require frequent blood transfusions, such as thalassemia.

Secondary hypogonadism may be present in a number of *complex genetic syndromes,* such as *Prader-Labhart-Willi, Laurence-Moon-Biedl, Biemond, Carpenter, familial cerebellar ataxia, dyskeratosis congenita, familial ichthyosis, Börjeson, Kraus-Rupert, Lowe, steroid sulfatase deficiency, Rud, CHARGE, LEOPARD, Moebius, POEMS, Martsolf, Rothmund-Thomson,* and *Richards-Rundle* syndromes.

Acquired Disorders. *Hypopituitarism.* Any destructive or infiltrative lesion of the hypothalamus and/or pituitary may cause impairment of gonadotropin secretion, either selectively or in conjunction with deficiency of other anterior pituitary hormones (see Ch. 202.1). Specific pathologic conditions include functioning and nonfunctioning pituitary adenomas; suprasellar tumors, such as craniopharyngioma, meningioma, optic glioma, or astrocytoma; metastatic neoplasms; lymphoma; surgical ablation or irradiation of the pituitary; infarction; vasculitis; apoplexy; hypophysitis; aneurysm; abscess; trauma; granulomatous disease, such as tuberculosis, sarcoidosis, fungal disease, and histiocytosis X; and transfusional iron overload.

Usually, destructive processes involving the pituitary gland result in progressive loss of anterior pituitary function in the following order: Gonadotropin and growth hormone secretion are the first to be affected, followed by TSH production, and finally ACTH secretion. The combination of gonadotropin and growth hormone deficiency is important to recognize in prepubertal children with growth retardation. In adults, clinical secondary hypogonadism, in the absence of other anterior pituitary dysfunction, may be the initial manifestation of a hypothalamic or pituitary process. Because loss of TSH and ACTH secretion is associated with greater degrees of pituitary destruction, secondary hypothyroidism and hypoadrenalism usually do not occur without concurrent secondary hypogonadism.

Serum testosterone levels and sperm counts are low. Serum LH and FSH levels are low or in the low normal adult range. The gonadotropin response to single-dose LHRH administration does not reliably differentiate hypothalamic and pituitary causes of gonadotropin deficiency and is not a clinically useful test. Clinical evaluation of patients with secondary hypogonadism should include anatomic studies (such as CT scan and visual field examination) to determine the presence of hypothalamic or pituitary tumor and tumor mass effects, and investigation of other anterior pituitary hormone functions.

Treatment is aimed at the process causing hypopituitarism and correction of androgen deficiency with testosterone replacement therapy. If fertility is desired, androgens are discontinued and gonadotropin therapy is instituted.

Hyperprolactinemia, resulting from a pituitary adenoma, CNS-active drugs (such as phenothiazines and other antipsychotics, opiates, sedatives, antidepressants, stimulants), or adrenergic or dopaminergic antagonist drugs (antihypertensives, metoclopramide) may cause secondary testicular failure. Prolactin-secreting pituitary adenomas in men are usually large (macroadenomas), and gonadotropin deficiency results, in part, from destruction of pituitary gonadotrophs. Even in the absence of a tumor, prolactin has an inhibitory effect on gonadotropin secretion, resulting in secondary hypogonadism. Bromocriptine and other dopamine agonist drugs (such as pergolide) decrease pituitary prolactin secretion and are used to treat hyperprolactinemia. These agents may result in restoration of normal gonadotropin secretion and testicular function, and shrinkage of prolactinomas.

Estrogen excess in men causes inhibition of gonadotropin secretion and secondary hypogonadism. Estrogen excess may result from either exogenous administration of estrogens or estrogenic substances (e.g., diethylstilbestrol administration in men with prostate cancer) or endogenous secretion from an estrogen-producing neoplasm (e.g., feminizing adrenal carcinoma). Patients with estrogen excess usually manifest varying degrees of gynecomastia. *Progestins* (e.g., medroxyprogesterone or megestrol acetate), *androgenic anabolic steroids,* and *opiate-like drugs* (e.g., morphine, methadone, and heroin) also inhibit gonadotropin production and may cause secondary hypogonadism.

Systemic Disorders. *Glucocorticoid excess,* as a result of either Cushing's syndrome or high-dosage glucocorticoid administration, suppresses gonadotropin secretion, resulting in secondary testicular failure with loss of libido, impotence, and oligospermia. Activation of the hypothalamic-adrenal axis resulting in high circulating levels of endogenous glucocorticoids may contribute to the reduction in serum testosterone, LH, and FSH levels observed with *acute stress or illness,* such as emotional stress, trauma, myocardial infarction, surgery, burns, and sepsis. *Nutritional deficiency,* such as that associated with protein-calorie malnutrition or anorexia nervosa, inhibits gonadotropin production and may cause secondary hypogonadism. Concurrent primary testicular dysfunction may also be caused by inadequate nutrition. Malnutrition may contribute to the secondary testicular failure associated with a number of *chronic illnesses,* such as malignancy, AIDS, and chronic heart, respiratory, liver, and kidney disease. Moderate obesity results in reduction in SHBG and total testosterone levels, with normal free testosterone levels. Some men with *massive obesity* demonstrate clinical androgen deficiency with low free testosterone concentrations and reduced gonadotropin levels.

ISOLATED DEFICIENCY OF SPERM PRODUCTION. *Congenital adrenal hyperplasia* caused by either 21-hydroxylase or 11β-hydroxylase deficiency results in excessive production of adrenal androgens. Androgen excess suppresses gonadotropin secretion and sperm production. Excessive adrenal androgen production causes premature virilization and precocious pseudopuberty, rather than androgen deficiency. Secondary hypogonadism is therefore manifested by isolated impairment of spermatogenesis. Glucocorticoid treatment of some patients with congenital adrenal hyperplasia may result in true precocious puberty, with premature activation of the hypothalamic-pituitary-gonadal axis. Androgen excess caused by administration of *testosterone* or large doses of *androgenic anabolic steroids* or *androgen-secreting tumors* (e.g., Leydig cell tumors) also result in secondary hypogonadism presenting with isolated deficiency in sperm production. High doses of testosterone have been administered to normal men to suppress gonadotropin and sperm production in male contraceptive development trials.

Rarely, *hyperprolactinemia* impairs sperm production despite normal gonadotropin and testosterone levels. *Isolated FSH deficiency* is an extremely rare condition that causes impaired spermatogenesis.

Androgen Resistance Syndromes

Androgen resistance syndromes are caused by defects in androgen action (see Ch. 207). The severity of androgen insensitivity determines the clinical presentation of these disorders. With severely defective androgen action, patients present at birth as either phenotypic females (testicular feminization) or with ambiguous genitalia (male pseudohermaphroditism). Men with mild, incomplete androgen insensitivity or *Reifenstein's syndrome* present as adults with mild androgen deficiency and a nearly normal male phenotype. Patients with Reifenstein's syndrome may have hypospadias, gynecomastia, varying degrees of virilization, a small prostate gland, impaired spermatogenesis, and cryptorchidism. They have elevated serum testosterone, LH, and FSH levels. Some men with very mild androgen resistance present with only oligospermia or azoospermia. Some men with celiac disease are infertile and have elevated serum testosterone and LH levels, suggesting androgen resistance.

Delayed Puberty

Puberty in boys usually begins between the ages of 9 and 14 years. With the maturation of the CNS mechanisms that regulate LHRH production, pulsatile gonadotropin and testosterone secretion begin, initially during sleep and then throughout the day. The first clinical indications of the onset of puberty are an increase in testicular size (>3 ml) and wrinkling and pigmentation of the scrotal skin. Subsequently, there are increases in penile length and appearance of pubic hair, followed by increasing long bone growth and development of other secondary sexual characteristics. The increase in testicular size precedes the appearance of pubic hair by about 2 years and the peak velocity in growth of height by 3 years. The onset and duration of puberty and the degree to which secondary sexual characteristics develop vary considerably and are largely attributable to the genetic background of an individual.

Delayed puberty is the lack of sexual maturation by 14 years of age. A number of the disorders that cause *hypogonadism* may result in delayed sexual maturation. *Severe systemic illnesses* (such as malabsorption, asthma, diabetes, malignancy) that also cause growth retardation and *thyroid hormone deficiency* may also cause delayed puberty. The majority of boys with delayed puberty, however, have physiologic or *constitutional delayed puberty.* This is a benign, frequently familial form of delayed adolescence that represents a normal variation in the onset of puberty. These boys eventually undergo a delayed but normal puberty and attain normal sexual maturation and height.

The diagnosis of constitutional delayed puberty can be strongly suspected in a healthy boy with retardation of growth and bone age, normal growth velocity in relation to bone age, a bone age between 12 and 13 years, a family history of delayed adolescence, and a testicular volume >2 ml. These clinical features are often not present and the diagnosis can be very difficult. Diagnostic evaluation should exclude organic causes of delayed puberty, i.e., hypogonadism, systemic illness, and hypothyroidism. In the absence of anosmia or other morphologic manifestations, constitutional delayed puberty cannot be distinguished from hypogonadotropic eunuchoidism.

Delayed sexual maturation often results in severe psychosocial distress to both the patient and his parents. Therefore, after systemic and endocrine disorders are excluded, boys with delayed puberty are usually treated with androgen replacement therapy to induce sexual maturation coincident with that of their contemporaries.

Handelsman DJ: Testicular dysfunction in systemic disease. Endocrinol Metab Clin North Am 23:839, 1994. *An excellent review of the effects of systemic illness on testicular function.*

Kletter GB, Kelch RP: Disorders of puberty in boys. Endocrinol Metab Clin North Am 22:455, 1993. *An excellent overview of delayed and precocious puberty in boys.*

Lee PA, St L O'dea L: Primary and secondary testicular insufficiency. Pediatr Clin North Am 37:1359, 1990. *A well-organized and well-written review of the diagnosis and treatment of primary and secondary testicular failure in the pediatric age group.*

Plymate SR: Hypogonadism. Endocrinol Metab Clin North Am 23:749, 1994. *An excellent, comprehensive discussion of disorders causing primary and secondary hypogonadism.*

Rosenfeld RL: Diagnosis and management of delayed puberty. J Clin Endocrinol Metab 70:559, 1990. *A concise review of the diagnosis and treatment of delayed sexual development.*

Wang C, Swerdloff RS: Evaluation of testicular function. Bailliere's Clin Endocrinol Metab 6:405, 1992. *A very complete review of the clinical and laboratory evaluation of testicular function.*

TREATMENT OF HYPOGONADISM

Androgen Therapy

Androgens are principally used to treat testosterone deficiency in hypogonadal men. In prepubertal androgen-deficient boys, the aim of androgen replacement is to stimulate and maintain male secondary sexual characteristics, somatic development, and sexual function without compromising adult height by premature closure of long bone epiphyses. In adult androgen deficiency, the objective of therapy is to restore and maintain libido, potency, and secondary sexual characteristics.

The long-acting 17β-hydroxyl esters of testosterone, *testosterone enanthate* and *cypionate,* are the most effective, safest, and most practical preparations currently available to treat androgen deficiency. In adults with androgen deficiency, replacement therapy is usually initiated with either testosterone enanthate or cypionate at a dose of 150 to 200 mg intramuscularly every 2 weeks. At these dosages, testosterone administration generally stimulates libido and potency, improves energy level, and social drive, restores male hair growth, and increases hemoglobin concentration.

In elderly androgen-deficient men, it is wise to begin testosterone therapy gradually at a reduced dosage. In elderly men who are not concerned about normal sexual functioning, low-dose androgen supplementation (e.g., testosterone enanthate or cypionate, 100 mg intramuscularly every 2 to 4 weeks) may suffice.

Recently, a transdermal delivery system consisting of a testosterone-containing scrotal skin patch was approved for androgen replacement therapy of hypogonadal men. Daily application of this patch maintains serum testosterone levels within the normal range; however, DHT levels are elevated (probably as a result of high 5α-reductase activity in scrotal skin). Except for minor skin irritation, the testosterone patch is tolerated well and offers an alternative to testosterone esters for replacement therapy of selected androgen-deficient men.

Androgen therapy is more complicated in boys with delayed puberty. Although testosterone is very effective in inducing secondary sexual characteristics and stimulating long bone growth, overly aggressive androgen therapy can result in premature closure of long bone epiphyses and compromise final adult height. Furthermore, it is often not possible to differentiate patients with constitutional delayed puberty, who require only temporary androgen replacement, from those with permanent hypogonadotropic hypogonadism. Therefore, in boys with delayed puberty whose height is far below the expected adult height, androgen therapy is begun with testosterone enanthate or cypionate, 50 to 100 mg intramuscularly every 2 to 4 weeks, and gradually increased to full adult replacement doses over several years. Androgen therapy is intermittently stopped for 3 to 4 months to determine whether spontaneous pubertal development will occur.

Androgen therapy is absolutely contraindicated in men with androgen-sensitive cancers, i.e., prostatic carcinoma and male breast carcinoma. Excessive stimulation of libido and erections by androgens is rare, usually occurring in prepubertal boys or in men with longstanding androgen deficiency given large doses of testosterone. These symptoms resolve with time or reduction in dosage. Acute urinary retention as a result of androgen replacement therapy is very uncommon in the absence of underlying prostatic carcinoma. Patients given testosterone to induce puberty may develop acne or gynecomastia, similar to that observed during normal puberty. Adult hypogonadal men develop acne less commonly and rarely develop gynecomastia, except when a predisposing condition such as hepatic cirrhosis exists. Androgens may cause mild weight gain as a result of sodium retention and protein anabolic effects, and patients with underlying edematous states may develop worsening edema during therapy. Erythropoiesis is stimulated by androgen administration. Occasionally, significant erythrocytosis occurs, requiring phlebotomy and reduction of testosterone dosage. Testosterone may also worsen or induce obstructive sleep apnea.

All oral androgens available in the United States are 17α-alkylated derivatives of testosterone. These oral preparations are weak androgens and have the potential for serious hepatotoxicity. They may cause hepatic cholestasis and occasionally clinical jaundice. Although rare, more serious and potentially life-threatening complications of oral androgens are the development of peliosis hepatis (blood-filled cysts in the liver), hepatic adenoma, hepatoma, or hepatic angiosarcoma. Hepatotoxicity does not result from replacement dosages of parenteral 17β-hydroxyl esters of testosterone. Because they carry greater risk, have reduced clinical efficacy, and are more expensive, oral androgen preparations should not be used for the treatment of androgen deficiency.

Androgens have also been used in the treatment of anemias related to renal and bone marrow failure, micropenis and microphallus, hereditary angioneurotic edema, female breast cancer, lichen sclerosus, endometriosis, and osteoporosis. Androgen administration may induce virilization in women, manifested by acne, hirsutism, and menstrual dysfunction, and in severe cases frontal balding, voice changes, breast atrophy, and clitoral hypertrophy. The use of androgenic steroids has not been demonstrated to be of long-term value in promoting protein anabolism in catabolic states associated with a variety of acute and chronic illnesses.

Androgenic anabolic steroids are commonly used by competitive athletes with the hope of improving endurance, strength, and performance and increasingly by boys to improve their appearance. Androgens are of dubious value in increasing strength and performance, in the absence of intensive training and high-protein diets. Athletes often take multiple androgenic anabolic agents (including 17α-alkylated agents) in very high doses and in combination with other agents (e.g., growth hormone, hCG) with little regard for potentially serious side effects. Hepatotoxicity (including hepatoma) and impaired spermatogenesis resulting in infertility have been reported in athletes abusing androgenic steroids. Furthermore, the long-term sequelae of taking massive doses of 17β-hydroxyl ester preparations are unknown. The potential risks of high-dose anabolic steroid use far outweigh the potential benefits to athletic performance, and their use should be strongly discouraged.

Gonadotropin and LHRH Therapy

The aim of gonadotropin therapy is to stimulate spermatogenesis and establish or restore fertility in gonadotropin-deficient hypogonadal patients. The gonadotropin preparations usually used for this purpose are *hCG* that contains LH-like biologic activity almost exclusively; and *human menopausal gonadotropin (hMG,* Pergonal) that contains both FSH and LH activity. A more purified preparation of *human FSH (hFSH,* Metrodin) is also available for clinical use. Both hCG and hMG are expensive and require multiple injections per week. Therefore, testosterone, rather than gonadotropin therapy, is used to induce and maintain androgenization in patients with hypogonadotropic hypogonadism when fertility is not desired.

Initiation of spermatogenesis in prepubertal hypogonadotropic hypogonadism usually requires treatment with both hCG and hMG. Treatment is initiated with hCG alone, at a dosage of 1000 to 2000 IU subcutaneously or intramuscularly two to three times weekly for 6 to 12 months. Clinical evidence of sexual maturation and the increase in serum testosterone levels are monitored to determine the need for adjustments in dose. During hCG treatment, Sertoli cells mature and spermatogenesis is initiated to varying degrees of completeness. Occasionally, hCG alone stimulates spermatogenesis sufficiently for sperm to appear in the ejaculate. However, the majority of patients with prepubertal hypogonadotropic hypogonadism require FSH activity, in the form of hMG, in addition to hCG to complete spermatogenesis and induce fertility. Therefore, hMG, at a dosage of 75 to 150 IU subcutaneously or intramuscularly three times weekly, is administered together with hCG if there is no evidence of sperm in the ejaculate with hCG alone. Gonadotropin induction of sperm production may take as long as 2 to 3 years. Even with combined hCG and hMG treatment, sperm output in the ejaculate may not be normal. Despite very low sperm counts, fertility may be induced, however.

Once initiated, spermatogenesis may be maintained with hCG treatment alone in patients with prepubertal hypogonadotropic hypogonadism. In adults with acquired hypogonadotropic hypogonadism, sperm production may also be restored with hCG treatment alone. Previous androgen treatment does not alter testicular responsiveness to subsequent gonadotropin therapy. The presence of primary testicular disease, such as cryptorchidism, worsens the prognosis for induction of sperm production and fertility by gonadotropin treatment.

In patients with Kallmann's syndrome, pulsatile administration of low doses of LHRH may be used to stimulate endogenous gonadotropin secretion and spermatogenesis to induce fertility. Pulsatile administration more closely mimics the normal physiologic situation; however, a portable infusion pump must be used to deliver small doses of LHRH every few hours (5 to 20 μg subcutaneously every 2 hours) throughout the day, making LHRH therapy a much more complex management problem than gonadotropin therapy. The cost and effectiveness of LHRH and gonadotropin therapy to stimulate spermatogenesis in men with Kallmann's syndrome are comparable.

Matsumoto AM: Clinical use and abuse of androgens and antiandrogens. *In* Becker KL (ed.): Principles and Practice of Endocrinology and Metabolism. Philadelphia, JB Lippincott, 1990, p 991. *This chapter reviews the pharmacology of androgen preparations, their clinical use in treatment of male hypogonadism and other conditions, the inappropriate use of androgens, and their potential side effects.*

Matsumoto AM: Hormonal therapy of male hypogonadism. Endocrinol Metab Clin North Am 23:857, 1994. *An up-to-date review of androgen, gonadotropin, and gonadotropin-releasing hormone treatment of male hypogonadal states.*

PRECOCIOUS PUBERTY

Isosexual precocity is defined as the development of sexual maturation before the age of 9 years. In boys, premature development of secondary sexual characteristics results in virilization. This is accompanied by accelerated skeletal maturation and linear growth and premature closure of long bone epiphyses, resulting in short stature as an adult. *True precocious puberty* is caused by premature secretion of gonadotropins. Testicular androgen and sperm production are stimulated by gonadotropins, resulting in virilization and increased testis size. *Precocious pseudopuberty* results from secretion of androgens from the adrenal gland or testis. Androgen excess results in virilization, but normal sperm production is not stimulated and the testes remain small.

True Precocious Puberty

In the majority of cases of true precocious puberty no identifiable cause for premature activation of gonadotropin secretion is found. This condition is called *idiopathic precocious puberty*. It is often inherited as a male-limited autosomal dominant or X-linked recessive trait. Patients have an increased incidence of seizure disorders and abnormal electroencephalograms. The remaining cases of true precocious puberty are primarily caused by *CNS lesions* involving the posterior hypothalamus. Lesions include hypothalamic and pineal tumors, craniopharyngioma, hamartomas, hydrocephalus, postencephalitic lesions, congenital brain defects, neurofibromatosis, and tuberous sclerosis. CNS lesions may also result in disturbances of other hypothalamic functions, causing diabetes insipidus, eating disorders, somnolence, emotional lability, and altered temperature regulation, as well as mental and psychomotor retardation and seizures. Precocious puberty may precede the onset of a clinically detectable neurologic lesion. Therefore, a prolonged period of follow-up observation with repeated neurologic evaluation is necessary to exclude CNS lesions. Rarely, an *hCG-secreting tumor* (e.g., hepatoblastoma) or *hCG administration* for cryptorchidism (iatrogenic precocious puberty) causes true precocious puberty.

Precocious Pseudopuberty (see Ch. 207)

Adrenocortical hyperfunction, either from congenital adrenal hyperplasia (21-hydroxylase or 11β-hydroxylase deficiency) or a virilizing adrenocortical tumor, is the most common condition causing precocious pseudopuberty in boys. Patients with congenital adrenal hyperplasia caused by 21-hydroxylase deficiency usually have markedly elevated serum 17-hydroxyprogesterone and urinary pregnanetriol levels. Rarely, *Leydig cell tumor* of the testis, autonomous Leydig cell function *(testotoxicosis),* and administration of *androgenic steroids* may cause precocious pseudopuberty.

Treatment of these conditions is directed at the underlying cause. For idiopathic precocious puberty, drugs to inhibit pituitary gonadotropin secretion (medroxyprogesterone acetate, LHRH analogues), or androgen synthesis (spironolactone, ketoconazole), or to block androgen action (flutamide, cyproterone acetate) have been used with varying success to prevent further sexual maturation. With the exception of LHRH analogues, these treatments do not usually prevent premature closure of long bone epiphyses.

Kaplan SL, Grumbach MM: Pathophysiology and treatment of sexual precocity. J Clin Endocrinol Metab 71:785, 1990. *A concise and up-to-date review of the pathophysiology and management of precocious pubertal development.*

Wheeler MD, Styne DM: Diagnosis and management of precocious puberty. Pediatr Clin North Am 37:1255, 1990. *This is an excellent, comprehensive review of the diagnosis and treatment of sexual precocity.*

TUMORS OF THE TESTIS

Tumors of the testis are uncommon, representing about 1% of all cancers in men. They occur more commonly in white than in black males. The annual incidence of testicular tumors is 6 per 100,000 males. About 95% of testicular tumors are malignant and derive from the germ cells. The remaining 5% are non-germ cell or stromal tumors derived mostly from Leydig and Sertoli cells and are usually benign. Gonadoblastoma is a rare testicular neoplasm containing both germ cell and stromal elements, arising in dysgenetic testes containing a Y chromosome. The peak age of incidence of testicular cancer is 20 to 35 years. It is the most common malignancy in this age group. Advances in treatment have transformed testicular cancer from the most common cause of cancer death in this age group 20 years ago into one of the most curable of all cancers today.

The most significant risk factor for developing testicular cancer is cryptorchidism. In unilateral cryptorchidism, the contralateral, normally descended testis also carries an increased risk of malignant degeneration. Orchiopexy at an early age (2 to 3 years) permits easier palpation and detection of testicular cancer and may reduce the risk of neoplasm. Carcinoma *in situ* has been found in men with oligoazoospermia presenting with infertility and in the contralateral testes of patients with presumed unilateral testicular cancer, suggesting that these conditions may also carry an increased risk for testicular neoplasm.

Germ Cell Tumors

Germ cell cancers may be classified according to their pathologic characteristics into *seminoma* and *nonseminoma. Nonseminomatous cancers* include *embryonal cell carcinomas, choriocarcinomas,* and *teratomas.* Forty per cent of germ cell cancers contain a mixture of seminomatous and nonseminomatous elements. The presence of any nonseminomatous element in a tumor that is predominantly seminoma dictates its classification as a nonseminoma. The distinction between seminoma and nonseminoma is important for staging and subsequent therapy. Seminomas usually metastasize via regional lymph nodes to retroperitoneal, mediastinal, and supraclavicular lymph nodes and are very sensitive to radiation therapy. On the other hand, nonseminomas metastasize by both lymphatic and hematogenous routes (especially to liver and lungs) and are radioresistant.

Most patients with germ cell tumors present with a painless mass in the testis. A testicular mass in a patient over 50 years is more likely to be a lymphoma than a germ cell tumor. Rapid onset of a painful testicular mass is usually caused by bleeding into the neoplasm. Ultrasonography or MRI may be helpful in defining a mass in the testis. Back or abdominal pain (from retroperitoneal lymphadenopathy), shortness of breath (from diffuse pulmonary metastases), gynecomastia (from hCG secretion), supraclavicular lymphadenopathy, or ureteral obstruction may also be present.

Germ cell tumors, especially nonseminomatous cancers, often secrete biologic markers (see Ch. 158.2). Embryonal cell cancers may secrete *α-fetoprotein.* Pure seminomas never elaborate α-fetoprotein, and its presence in serum implies the presence of nonseminomatous elements in the tumor. hCG is secreted by nearly all choriocarcinomas, a third of embryonal cell carcinomas and teratocarcinomas and, rarely, by pure seminomas. This marker may be detected using a specific β-hCG assay. Both of these tumor markers may be used to monitor response to therapy. They may precede clinically detectable disease by weeks to months.

In seminoma, orchiectomy and radiation therapy to the periaortic and iliac lymph nodes or combination chemotherapy (for advanced disease) have resulted in cure rates of 80 to 95%. In nonseminomatous testicular cancer, the addition of cisplatin to aggressive, multiple-drug chemotherapeutic regimens following orchiectomy (and retroperitoneal lymph node dissection for more advanced disease) has resulted in response rates of >90% and long-term remission in 50 to 90% of patients.

Non–Germ Cell Tumors

Non–germ cell tumors are rare tumors that develop from the two major elements of testicular stroma, the *Leydig* and *Sertoli cells.* They are usually benign, but about 10% are malignant and metastasize via regional lymphatics. Both Leydig and Sertoli cell tumors may secrete a variety of steroid hormones, primarily androgens or estrogens, that may result in virilization or feminization, respectively. These tumors are usually small and difficult to diagnose; selective venous catheterization and sampling to determine the site of increased steroid production are often helpful. Gynecomastia is present in about 30% of patients with non-germ cell tumors. Children may present with either isosexual (virilizing) or heterosexual (feminizing) precocious pseudopuberty. Treatment consists primarily of orchiectomy.

Ozols RF, Williams SD: Testicular cancer. Curr Probl Cancer 13:285, 1989. *An excellent comprehensive review of the classification, epidemiology, staging, treatment, and prognosis of testicular cancer (98 references).*

Roth BJ, Nichols CR (eds.): Testicular cancer. Semin Oncol 19:1, 1992. *An up-to-date review of the treatment of testicular cancer, including therapeutic strategies, current controversies, and the direction of future research by several authors.*

209.2 DISEASES OF THE PROSTATE

Gary D. Steinberg and Charles B. Brendler

This chapter discusses three common disorders of the prostate: prostatitis, benign prostatic hyperplasia, and adenocarcinoma of the prostate. A brief review of the normal anatomy, physiology, and biochemistry of the prostate is provided first.

THE NORMAL PROSTATE

ANATOMY. The normal adult prostate, a firm, elastic organ weighing about 20 grams, is located caudad to the base of the bladder and is traversed by the first portion of the urethra. It is bordered anteriorly by the symphysis pubis and posteriorly by the rectum. The paired seminal vesicles are attached to the prostate and are located posterior to the bladder (Fig. 209–6).

The human prostate has two concentric anatomic regions: an inner periurethral zone composed of short glands and an outer peripheral zone composed of longer, branched glands. These regions are separated by a thin layer of fibroelastic tissue, the so-called surgical capsule (Fig. 209–7). Benign prostatic hyperplasia (BPH) arises within the inner periurethral zone in a specific region near the verumontanum, called the transition zone. In contrast, prostatic carcinoma usually arises in the outer peripheral zone.

PHYSIOLOGY. The secretions of the prostate and other sex accessory organs presumably protect or enhance the functional properties of the spermatozoa. Of the total average human ejaculate volume of 3.5 ml, the prostate secretes 0.5 ml and the seminal vesicles secrete 2.0 to 2.5 ml.

The concentration of zinc is higher in the prostate than in any other organ in the body. Its function is uncertain, but it may protect the prostate against infection. Two other components of prostatic secretion, acid phosphatase and prostate-specific antigen (PSA), are important serum markers for prostate cancer. An elevated serum

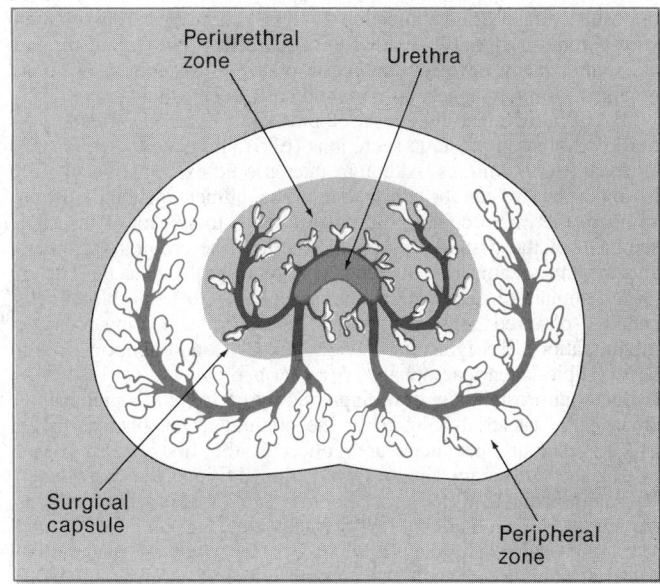

FIGURE 209–7. A coronal section through the prostate demonstrating the anatomic relationships among the urethra, periurethral tissue, surgical capsule, and peripheral tissue. (After Brendler H: *In* Glenn JF [ed.]: Urologic Surgery, 3rd ed. Philadelphia, J. B. Lippincott Company, 1983.)

prostatic acid phosphatase level, measured by enzymatic assay, is virtually diagnostic for metastatic prostate cancer. PSA is a serine protease that helps liquefy the ejaculate. The concentration of PSA is about 10-fold greater in prostate cancer than benign tissue. Since its discovery in 1979, PSA has emerged as the most important marker for prostate cancer. Serum PSA is useful in screening and staging prostate cancer, and it is the most sensitive indicator for monitoring response to treatment.

BIOCHEMISTRY. The growth and secretory function of the prostate depend on functioning testes; prostatic maturation does not occur in a male castrated before puberty. Testosterone, the major circulating androgen, is converted to dihydrotestosterone (DHT) by the enzyme 5α-reductase in prostatic epithelial cells. DHT, the major active androgenic metabolite within the prostate, binds to a cytoplasmic receptor, is transported to the nucleus, and there initiates RNA synthesis, protein synthesis, and cell replication.

Estrogens inhibit prostatic growth, largely by blocking the release of luteinizing hormone from the pituitary, thus inhibiting testicular synthesis of testosterone. If castrated animals are given both estrogens and androgens, normal prostate growth occurs, indicating that estrogens do not block androgen-induced growth in the prostate itself.

PROSTATITIS

INCIDENCE AND ETIOLOGY. About 50% of men experience symptoms of prostatic inflammation during adult life. Only about 5% of these cases are due to bacterial infection of the prostate. The etiology of these symptoms in the remaining 95% of patients is unclear.

Most bacterial infections of the prostate are caused by gram-negative organisms, most commonly *Escherichia coli.* Enterococci, staphylococci, and streptococci are rare causes of prostatic infection. *Chlamydia trachomatis* and *Ureaplasma urealyticum* probably cause prostatitis infrequently, but this topic remains controversial.

PATHOGENESIS. Most episodes of bacterial prostatic infection are due to a previous urethral infection with direct ascent of bacteria from the urethra through the prostatic ducts into the prostate. The organisms that cause bacterial prostatitis are the same as those that produce bacteriuria, and chlamydial and gonococcal infections of the urethra may involve the prostate.

Prostatic infection may also result from impairment of host defense mechanisms. The concentrations of prostatic antibacterial factor and magnesium, zinc, calcium, citric acid, spermine, cholesterol, and lysozyme are decreased in the prostatic fluid of men with chronic bacterial prostatitis. Whether these alterations contribute to

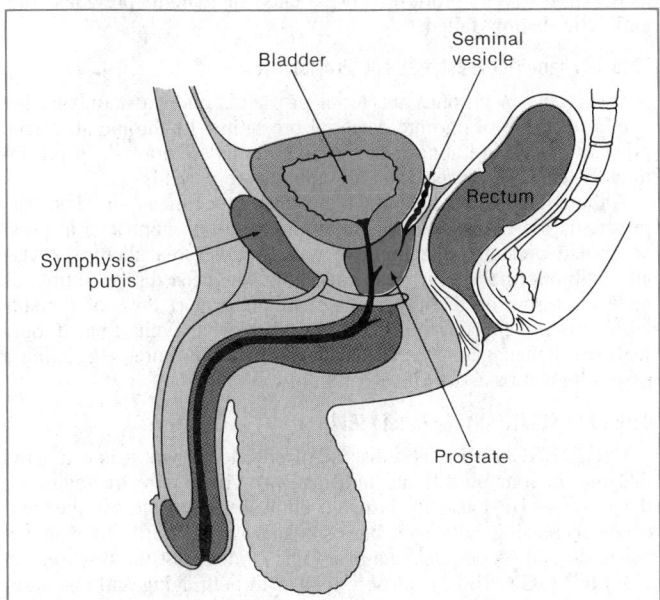

FIGURE 209–6. The anatomic relationship of the prostate to adjacent structures. (After Brendler H: *In* Glenn JF [ed.]: Urologic Surgery, 3rd ed. Philadelphia, J. B. Lippincott Company, 1983.)

or result from prostatic infection is unknown. About 10% of men with chronic bacterial prostatitis have more than one organism, and after cure, many develop reinfection of the prostate by a different organism, further suggesting impaired host defense function.

DIAGNOSIS. The diagnosis of prostatitis is based on examination of expressed prostatic secretions (EPS) and quantitative bacterial localization cultures. Although microscopic examination of EPS is important, it can be misleading. The clinician should always compare the microscopic appearance of EPS to smears of the spun sediment of the first voided 10 ml of urine (the urethral specimen) and the midstream urine (bladder specimen) to localize the site of the inflammatory response. The presence of > 20 white blood cells per high-powered field (hPF) in EPS is abnormal. During prostatic inflammation, EPS typically contain leukocytes and abnormal numbers of lipid-laden macrophages (oval fat bodies).

Bacterial prostatitis is best diagnosed by performing simultaneous quantitative bacterial cultures of the urethral urine, bladder urine, and EPS. Four specimens are collected: the first voided 10 ml (VB1), the midstream aliquot (VB2), the EPS, and the first voided 10 ml immediately after prostatic massage (VB3). All specimens are cultured quantitatively by surface streaking onto blood and MacConkey agar. The diagnosis is confirmed when the quantitative bacterial colony counts of the prostatic specimens (EPS and VB3) significantly exceed those of the urethral (VB1) and bladder (VB2) specimens by at least 1 logarithm. Based on these diagnostic maneuvers, the inflammatory diseases of the prostate have been subdivided into four categories: (1) acute bacterial prostatitis, (2) chronic bacterial prostatitis, (3) nonbacterial prostatitis, and (4) prostatodynia.

DIFFERENTIAL DIAGNOSIS. A full urologic evaluation is required in all patients with lower urinary tract complaints. The differential diagnosis in patients with lower urinary tract irritative symptoms should include upper urinary tract infection with secondary colonization of the bladder, carcinoma of the bladder, neurogenic bladder, prostatic obstruction, and urethral stricture. Because the irritative urinary symptoms in men with prostatitis are identical to those in patients with carcinoma *in situ* of the bladder, urinary cytology and cystoscopy should be carried out in these patients to exclude the presence of bladder carcinoma.

Acute Bacterial Prostatitis

Acute bacterial prostatitis is a fulminant condition that occurs mainly between the ages of 20 and 40. There is acute onset of fever, chills, and malaise associated with marked urinary irritative and obstructive symptoms. Pain may be experienced in the suprapubic region, lumbar spine, and perineum.

On physical examination, patients frequently have a temperature as high as 39 to 40° C. Patients may have marked suprapubic tenderness if prostatic infection results in urinary retention. Rectal examination to rule out a prostatic abscess should be done very carefully, as it is extremely uncomfortable for the patient and may result in septicemia or secondary epididymitis if the prostate is massaged too vigorously. The prostate is variably enlarged, markedly tender, and hot to palpation. A prostatic abscess should be suspected if an abnormally fluctuant area is palpated within the prostate.

Patients with acute bacterial prostatitis almost always have associated bacteriuria, and therefore urinalysis and urine culture are helpful in establishing the diagnosis and identifying appropriate antibiotic therapy. With recurrent bacterial prostatitis, intravenous pyelography or abdominal ultrasonography should be done to rule out upper urinary tract pathology. Pelvic ultrasonography or computed tomography may be helpful in diagnosing a prostatic abscess.

Patients with acute bacterial prostatitis are frequently quite ill and need to be hospitalized for their initial treatment. Urinary retention may necessitate placement of a temporary suprapubic cystostomy or urethral catheter. Intravenous antibiotics are usually given; a combination of gentamicin to cover gram-negative organisms and ampicillin to cover enterococci should be used. Supportive measures include hydration, analgesics, and stool softeners. Following initial intravenous therapy, antibiotic therapy should be started with broad gram-negative coverage that diffuses readily into the prostatic fluid. Trimethoprim, trimethoprim-sulfamethoxazole, and the quinolone derivatives are the usual choices. Because bacterial infections may be difficult to eradicate, oral antibiotics should be continued for 4 to 6 weeks after the acute episode. It is worthwhile to examine EPS and VB3 6 to 12 weeks after the start of therapy to be sure that the infection has resolved.

Granulomatous lesions of the prostate, observed in about 1% of tissue specimens obtained either by biopsy or by partial prostatectomy, usually result from previous bacterial infection or prior transurethral resection of the prostate. Systemic diseases commonly associated with granuloma formation, such as tuberculosis, account for only a small minority of cases. Granulomatous prostatitis may cause induration that mimics prostatic carcinoma, requiring a biopsy to distinguish the two conditions. Granulomatous prostatitis may result in irritative and obstructive urinary symptoms that usually resolve spontaneously. The value of antibiotics in this condition is controversial.

Chronic Bacterial Prostatitis

Chronic bacterial prostatitis is one of the most common causes of recurrent urinary tract infection in men. The symptoms, similar to but milder than those of acute bacterial prostatitis, include urinary frequency and dysuria along with vague lower abdominal, lumbar, and perineal pain. Fever and urethral discharge are uncommon. The diagnosis is made by examination of EPS and quantitative bacterial cultures. EPS should be considered abnormal if there are > 10 leukocytes per hPF and more than one or two lipid-laden macrophages per hPF. Men with chronic bacterial prostatitis may have normal EPS while receiving antibiotic therapy, but may continue to have recurrent infections once antibiotics have been discontinued. Furthermore, 5% to 10% of men with no symptoms of prostatic inflammation have > 10 leukocytes per hPF in their EPS.

An alternative approach to quantitative bacterial cultures, which are expensive and time consuming, is to obtain a quantitative culture of the bladder urine (VB2) and a nonquantitative culture of EPS on the first office visit. If these cultures are both negative, the prostate is probably not infected. Recovery of gram-negative bacteria from either of these specimens identifies patients who might have chronic bacterial prostatitis and provides a rationale for conventional bacterial localization cultures on the second office visit.

Chronic bacterial prostatitis is frequently difficult to treat. Antibiotic therapy alone eradicates only about 30 to 50% of the infections, but suppressive antimicrobial therapy usually results in complete symptomatic relief and reduces the risks of serious illness. The usual antibiotics used in this condition are trimethoprim-sulfamethoxazole, carbenicillin, or one of the quinolones, such as ciprofloxacin or norfloxacin, in a 4- to 12-week course of therapy. Suppressive antibiotic therapy with trimethoprim, trimethoprim-sulfamethoxazole, and nitrofurantoin is effective. Experimentally, direct injection of antibiotics, such as thiamphenicol and aminoglycosides, has given promise in patients in whom previous oral antibiotic therapy failed.

Chronic Abacterial Prostatitis and Prostatodynia

Symptoms of chronic abacterial prostatitis and prostatodynia are similar to those of chronic bacterial prostatitis. In chronic abacterial prostatitis, EPS are abnormal, but all cultures are normal. In prostatodynia, EPS are normal, and all cultures are normal.

Although cultures of prostatic biopsy specimens in abacterial prostatitis are rarely positive, some patients with nonbacterial prostatitis and prostatodynia improve with antimicrobial therapy. Overall, antibiotic therapy in these conditions has been disappointing, as have all forms of therapy to date. In one report 86% of patients with chronic abacterial prostatitis and prostatodynia treated only with stress management reported improvement or cure, suggesting a psychological basis for these conditions.

BENIGN PROSTATIC HYPERPLASIA (BPH)

INCIDENCE. BPH is a disease of advancing age; it is estimated that one in four men living until age 80 will require treatment for this disease. BPH usually is noted clinically after age 50, the incidence increasing with age, but as many as two thirds of men between 40 and 49 demonstrate histologic evidence of the disease.

ETIOLOGY. BPH is closely related to both aging and age-associated changes in circulating hormones. Circulating androgens clearly play a role; BPH does not develop in men who are castrated or who lose testicular function before puberty. Castration causes atrophy of prostatic epithelium.

With aging, serum testosterone levels decline while serum estrogen levels increase, resulting in an increase in the ratio of plasma estrogens to plasma testosterone. It is unclear, however, whether these shifts in circulating hormone levels are directly involved in the pathogenesis of BPH. Androgens and estrogens seem to act synergistically in the development of BPH in the dog, estrogens increasing prostatic androgen receptors by twofold. Levels of DHT are not actually elevated in BPH tissue, but enzymatic changes occur within the hyperplastic gland that would tend to favor the accumulation of DHT.

PATHOGENESIS. As the hyperplastic prostate enlarges, it compresses the urethra, producing symptoms of urethral obstruction that ultimately may progress to urinary retention. Urethral obstruction may cause incomplete emptying of the bladder, giving rise to urinary stasis, urinary tract infection, and bladder calculi. Furthermore, hypertrophy of the bladder muscle may cause hydronephrosis and bladder diverticula. The natural history of BPH is quite variable. In general, 1 to 2% per year of men with symptoms of BPH develop urinary retention.

SYMPTOMS. Symptoms due to BPH are either obstructive or irritative. *Obstructive symptoms* include hesitancy to initiate voiding, straining to void, decreased force and caliber of the urinary stream, prolonged dribbling after micturition, a sensation of incomplete bladder emptying, and urinary retention. These symptoms result directly from narrowing of the bladder neck and prostatic urethra by the hyperplastic prostate.

Irritative symptoms include urinary frequency, nocturia, dysuria, urgency, and urge incontinence. These symptoms may result from incomplete emptying of the bladder with voiding or may be due to urinary tract infection secondary to prostatic obstruction. More commonly, irritative symptoms result from reduced bladder compliance as a result of prostatic obstruction. It is important to recognize that irritative symptoms may be caused by other conditions such as bladder carcinoma, neurogenic bladder, and urinary tract infection unrelated to prostatic obstruction. All too frequently, patients with irritative urinary tract symptoms are presumed to have prostatic obstruction without an adequate diagnostic evaluation, resulting in delayed and sometimes inappropriate therapy.

PHYSICAL EXAMINATION. Other than a distended bladder, the usual physical findings in BPH are confined to the prostate. Examination of the prostate should be performed with the patient in either the knee-chest position or bent over the bed with his chest touching his elbows. The examining glove should be well lubricated, and the index finger should be inserted slowly into the rectum to allow the anal sphincter time to relax.

The normal prostate, the size of a walnut, has the consistency of a pencil eraser. The hyperplastic prostate is variably enlarged, usually no more than two or three times normal, but occasionally exceeding the size of a lemon. The consistency remains rubbery but is somewhat more fleshy, particularly in the larger glands. Rectal examination affords only a rough estimate of prostatic size and should never be relied upon to rule out prostatic obstruction. A much more accurate anatomic appraisal of the prostate can be obtained with transrectal ultrasonography and cystourethroscopy. The combination of a digital rectal examination (DRE) and serum PSA determination is the most effective means of screening for prostate cancer.

DIAGNOSTIC TESTS. The most valuable test for documenting urinary obstruction is measurement of the urinary flow rate. Inexpensive flowmeters allow accurate determination of the patient's voided volume and peak urinary flow rate, which can be plotted against the patient's age on a nomogram. A decreased flow rate *per se* is never an indication for prostatectomy, but, when used and interpreted correctly, uroflowmetry is an excellent physiologic test for prostatic obstruction.

An abdominal ultrasound examination is useful to rule out associated upper tract pathology, such as hydronephrosis, as well as to detect renal masses. Furthermore, ultrasound measurement of postvoid residual urine volumes and prostatic size is extremely accurate.

Cystourethroscopy, although often employed, may be misleading as a diagnostic test for prostatic obstruction. An anatomically small prostate may produce significant obstruction during voiding, while an anatomically large prostate may produce little or no obstruction. The place for cystourethroscopy is in making the decision whether the prostate is small enough to be resected transurethrally or sufficiently large to require open surgical removal. Before prostatec-

tomy, a careful inspection of the bladder is made to rule out bladder diverticula, stones, and most importantly tumors.

A retrograde urethrogram may be helpful in evaluating symptoms of BPH when a urethral stricture is suspected. Formal urodynamic pressure-flow studies may be indicated in patients with complex voiding symptomatology or suspected neurogenic bladder.

TREATMENT. Indications for treatment of BPH include (1) voiding symptoms that are troublesome to the patient; (2) urinary retention; (3) recurrent urinary tract infections caused by postvoid residual urine; (4) compromised renal function due to hydronephrosis from prostatic obstruction; (5) recurrent gross hematuria with no other explanation; and (6) urge incontinence due to prostatic obstruction.

Historically the most common treatment for BPH has been partial prostatectomy. The goal of partial prostatectomy is to re-establish a wide-open bladder neck and prostatic urethra by selectively removing all of the hyperplastic prostatic tissue down to the so-called surgical capsule, leaving the peripheral prostate intact (see Fig. 209–7). This is accomplished either by transurethral resection or by open surgical enucleation of the adenoma, depending usually on the size of the gland. Adenomas < 70 grams are usually approached transurethrally.

Transurethral prostatectomy (TURP) is generally regarded as a safe and effective procedure. Because of improvements in endoscopic instrumentation, antibiotics, anesthesia, and intraoperative management, most patients tolerate TURP well. The overall morbidity, however, is about 18% and mortality about 1%. Risk factors include age > 80 years, prostate size > 45 grams, surgical time > 90 minutes, and preoperative urinary retention. Although 80% of men report significant improvement in their symptoms following surgery, the morbidity of the procedure has stimulated interest in alternative treatments.

Alternative treatments for BPH include: (1) transurethral incision of the bladder neck, (2) α-adrenergic blockers, (3) 5α-reductase inhibitors, (4) aromatase inhibitors, and (5) laser or hyperthermic ablation of the prostate.

Transurethral incision is done by making one or two longitudinal incisions with an endoscope through the muscular fibers of the bladder neck and prostatic urethra to spring open the prostate and thus enlarge the caliber of the prostatic urethra. Transurethral incision can be performed as an outpatient procedure under local anesthesia, and operative time and blood loss are greatly reduced. Transurethral incision is probably as effective as transurethral resection in treating small prostates (< 20 grams) but appears less effective for larger, bulkier glands.

α-Adrenergic blockers relieve prostatic obstruction by decreasing α-adrenoreceptor-mediated smooth muscle tone of the prostatic capsule and bladder neck. Selective α_1-blockers, such as terazosin and doxazosin, have fewer side effects than nonselective α-blockers. Terazosin has the additional advantage of once-daily dosing. The response rate to these agents appears to be about 70%.

5α-Reductase inhibitors block the conversion of testosterone to DHT, the most active prostatic androgen, resulting in atrophy of the prostatic epithelium. Prostate size decreases an average of 30% after 3 to 6 months of therapy, but the prostate quickly regrows to its original size after cessation of therapy. Significant improvement in symptom score and urinary flow rate is achieved in about 30% of patients.

Multiple clinical trials have been performed in Europe using aromatase inhibitors to test the hypothesis that increased estrogen levels contribute to BPH in men. To date, no study has demonstrated efficacy of these agents in the treatment of BPH.

Transurethral laser ablation and transrectal hyperthermia are new treatments for BPH. The morbidity of these procedures appears to be markedly reduced from standard surgical intervention. Early results indicate, however, that laser ablation and hyperthermia may not be as effective as TURP. In addition, the instrumentation is expensive, and prostatic tissue is not obtained for pathologic examination to rule out unsuspected prostatic carcinoma.

For patients with urinary retention who are poor surgical candidates and in whom medical management is unlikely to be successful, options include either clean, intermittent urethral catheterization or long-term use of an indwelling urethral catheter. Alternatively these patients may benefit from placement of an intraurethral metal alloy prostatic stent. These stents serve to maintain an adequate channel in the prostatic urethra. They are initially associated with a high percentage of irritative voiding symptoms, but most patients ultimately tolerate them fairly well. At present, stents are available only at a limited number of investigational centers.

CARCINOMA OF THE PROSTATE

INCIDENCE. Carcinoma of the prostate is rare before age 50, but the incidence subsequently increases steadily with age. Overall, it is the most common malignant disease in United States men and the second most common cause of cancer deaths in men. Carcinoma of the prostate is more common among black American men (22 deaths per 100,000 men) than white American men (14 deaths per 100,000 men).

ETIOLOGY. The etiology of prostatic carcinoma is unknown. The disease does not occur in men castrated before puberty and partially regresses following castration or estrogen therapy, but a hormonal etiology has not been established. BPH does not appear to be causally related. Environmental factors may be involved, since men migrating from areas where prostatic cancer is uncommon to areas where it is more common develop the disease with increased frequency. The only known risk factor for prostate cancer is a positive family history. Men with a first-degree relative with prostate cancer have a twofold increased risk of developing the disease. The pattern of inheritance appears to be autosomal dominant, similar to hereditary breast cancer and nonpolyposis colon cancer.

PATHOGENESIS. Ninety-five per cent of prostatic cancers are adenocarcinomas, with the remainder being transitional cell carcinomas, squamous cell carcinomas, and sarcomas. Adenocarcinoma of the prostate usually arises in the posterior peripheral region of the prostate (Fig. 209–7), although it commonly invades the periurethral tissue where BPH originates, subsequently producing urethral obstruction. Prostate cancer may produce ureteral obstruction either by direct extension into the bladder or by spreading behind the bladder through the seminal vesicles. Distant spread occurs through lymphatic and hematogenous routes. Prostatic cancer most commonly metastasizes to the pelvic lymph nodes and skeleton, especially the pelvis and lumbar spine. Visceral metastases, which occur later and less commonly, most frequently involve the lungs, liver, and adrenals.

Prostate cancer has an extremely variable and largely unpredictable natural history. In some men the disease progresses very slowly, and they may do very well for 10 years without treatment. In others, the disease exhibits rapid metastatic spread, leading to early death.

SYMPTOMS. Early carcinoma of the prostate is asymptomatic. As the disease spreads into the urethra, it may cause symptoms of urinary obstruction indistinguishable from those produced by BPH. If the tumor has progressed to obstruct the ureters, the patient may have symptoms of uremia. Skeletal pain and pathologic fractures caused by metastatic disease may be the initial symptoms of advanced disease.

PHYSICAL EXAMINATION. The patient may have lymphadenopathy, signs of uremia, congestive heart failure, or urinary retention with a distended bladder. More commonly, the pathologic physical findings are confined to the prostate. On rectal examination the prostate feels harder than the normal or hyperplastic prostate, and the normal boundaries of the gland may be obscured. Approximately 50% of localized indurated areas within the prostate are malignant, with the remainder due to prostatic calculi, inflammation, prostatic infarction, or postsurgical change in a patient having previously undergone TURP or open prostatectomy for BPH. If induration is detected that is suggestive of carcinoma, the examiner should determine whether it is focal or diffuse in nature and whether it seems to extend beyond the border of the prostate.

DIAGNOSIS. As stated earlier, screening for prostate cancer is most effectively done by a combination of DRE and serum PSA determination. If the DRE is normal the chances of having prostate cancer are about 2%, 15%, and 35% for a serum PSA of <4, 4 to 10, or >10 ng per milliliter, respectively. If the DRE is abnormal the risks of having prostate cancer are about 10%, 35%, and 67% for a serum PSA of <4, 4 to 10, and >10, respectively. As a screening tool, transrectal ultrasound (TRUS), is relatively inaccurate, in that only 30% of the abnormal lesions detected on TRUS

are malignant. In men with an abnormal DRE and/or PSA, however, TRUS is much more accurate than digitally guided, "blind" biopsy in establishing the diagnosis of prostate cancer.

STAGING CLASSIFICATION. The treatment of prostatic carcinoma depends primarily on the stage of the disease, as illustrated in the TNM staging system (Fig. 209–8).

Stage T1 prostatic carcinoma refers to tumors that are discovered incidentally on histologic examination of prostatic tissue that has been removed for presumed BPH or by transrectal ultrasonography done because of an abnormal serum PSA. Stage T1 tumors are subdivided into stage T1a, which are well- or moderately-differentiated tumors involving <5% of the removed tissue; stage T1b lesions, which are either poorly differentiated or involve >5% of the removed tissue; and stage T1c lesions, which are detected because of an abnormal serum PSA. Stage T2 tumors are palpable on rectal examination and are confined within the boundaries of the prostate. Stage T2a and T2b include tumors involving less than one lobe of the prostate. Stage T2c includes tumors that involve one whole or both lobes. Stage T3 tumors have extended through the prostatic capsule and may involve the seminal vesicles. Stage T4 tumors have invaded other adjacent structures, such as the bladder neck or external urethral sphincter, or have extended laterally to involve the levator muscles and/or pelvic sidewall. Stage N+ and M+ tumors have metastasized—N+ to regional lymph nodes, and M+ distantly.

STAGING EVALUATION. The treatment of prostatic carcinoma is predicated largely on the stage of the tumor; accurate staging is therefore essential. The DRE is valuable in assessing the local extent of tumor, but transrectal ultrasonography and magnetic resonance imaging of the prostate may be useful when the findings on physical examination are not definitive.

Historically, enzymatic determination of serum prostatic acid phosphatase has been the basic screening test for metastatic prostate cancer, with an elevated value being about 70% sensitive and virtually 100% specific for metastatic disease. Because of its far greater specificity, however, serum PSA has replaced prostatic acid phosphatase in staging prostate cancer. Seventy per cent of prostate cancer patients who have a serum PSA < 10 ng per milliliter will have organ-confined disease, in contrast to only 35% of men with PSA levels between 10 and 20 ng per milliliter and only 20% with a

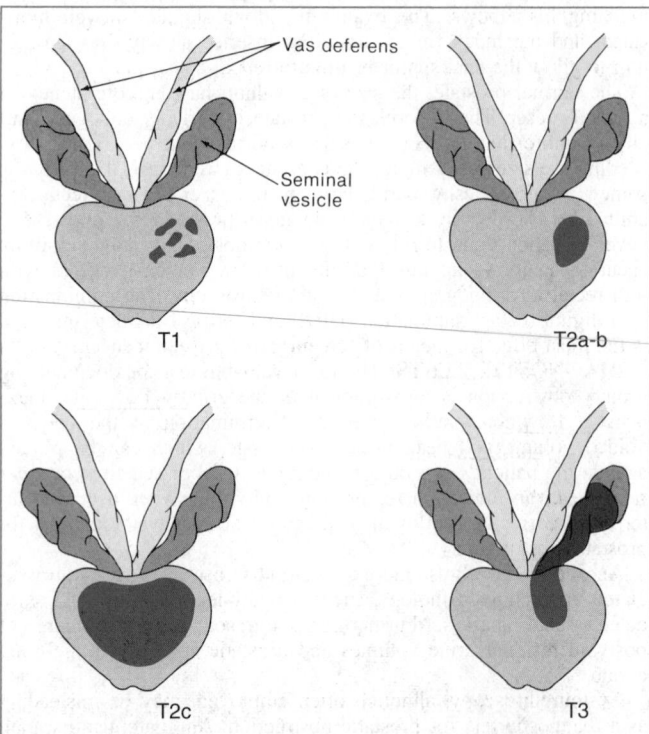

FIGURE 209–8. Whitmore staging classification of prostatic carcinoma. T1 = Microscopic disease in a clinically benign gland. T2a–b = Nodule involving less than one posterior lobe. T2c = Nodule involving one entire lobe or both posterior lobes. T3 = Extension beyond the peripheral capsule of the prostate.

PSA >20 ng per milliliter. In general, the higher the serum PSA level, the greater the likelihood of advanced disease.

Similarly, PSA is extremely useful in evaluating response to therapy, particularly radical prostatectomy. Since PSA is produced only in the prostate, serum PSA levels following successful radical prostatectomy should be undetectable. A measurable level of PSA postoperatively is thus essentially diagnostic of residual or recurrent disease and is almost always the first indicator of treatment failure.

The radionuclide bone scan is highly accurate and far more sensitive than conventional skeletal radiography in detecting osseous metastases. Pelvic lymph node metastases in prostatic carcinoma are more difficult to detect. Neither pedal lymphangiography nor pelvic computed tomography (CT) can reliably detect pelvic lymph node metastases. Neither technique is able to demonstrate microscopic nodal disease, and neither technique consistently demonstrates the obturator and hypogastric lymphatic chains, which are the primary sites of lymphatic drainage from the prostate. In patients with otherwise localized disease, a staging pelvic lymphadenectomy is usually done prior to performance of radical prostatectomy, either in conjunction with the operation, relying on a frozen-section evaluation of the lymph nodes, or several days earlier to allow a full histologic evaluation of the nodal tissue. Pelvic lymphadenectomy has a low morbidity rate and seems justified as a staging procedure to spare those patients with positive lymph nodes from a radical prostatectomy.

TREATMENT. Watchful Waiting. Since most prostate cancers are slow growing, watchful waiting with no immediate therapy may be appropriate. Watchful waiting is probably the best treatment for men with a life expectancy of less than 10 years who have well- or moderately-differentiated tumors. We believe, however, that watchful waiting is not appropriate for younger, healthier men or for those with more advanced or aggressive tumors. Patients with moderately differentiated tumors who are initially untreated have a 40 to 50% chance of developing metastatic disease within 10 years, compared with <10% of similar patients treated by radical prostatectomy.

Surgery. Radical prostatectomy is the most effective way of curing localized prostate cancer. In radical prostatectomy, the entire prostate and both seminal vesicles are removed through either a perineal or retropubic approach. The overall 10-year actuarial cure rate defined by an undetectable serum PSA is 70% following radical prostatectomy, and increases to more than 85% in men with clinical stages T1a–T2a disease. The major complications of radical prostatectomy are urinary incontinence and impotence. Recent advances in surgical technique, however, have reduced the risk of significant urinary incontinence to <5% and have allowed preservation of sexual function in the majority of men undergoing this procedure.

Radiation. Radiation therapy is administered either via external beam or via interstitial radioactive seeds that are implanted surgically into the prostate. Although the issue remains controversial, radiation therapy seems most appropriate in patients with localized disease who either are unwilling to undergo radical prostatectomy or are not surgical candidates for reasons of age and health. Radiation therapy also is the treatment of choice for patients with clinical stage T3 disease that has extended beyond the borders of the prostate and is therefore not curable surgically.

Endocrine. Hormonal therapy, the mainstay of treatment for patients with advanced disease, attempts to deprive prostatic tumors of circulating androgens and thereby produce regression of both primary and metastatic lesions. Hormonal ablation can be achieved either by medical or surgical castration. Historically, diethylstilbestrol (DES) was used to achieve medical castration, but has mostly been abandoned because of gynecomastia and cardiovascular complications. Medical castration is presently achieved with luteinizing hormone releasing hormone (LHRH) agonists that inhibit testosterone alone or in combination with antiandrogens that block androgen action in the prostate itself. These agents appear as effective as conventional hormone therapy with estrogens or orchiectomy, and the addition of an antiandrogen may provide an additional survival advantage of several months. Relapse following hormone therapy is due to continued growth of hormone-insensitive cells, and further attempts to lower serum testosterone levels provide little, if any, additional palliation.

Patient response to hormonal therapy varies considerably; 10% of patients live less than 6 months, 50% survive less than 3 years, and only 10% live longer than 10 years. The timing of endocrine therapy also appears to make little difference in the course of the disease. Initiation of treatment at the time of diagnosis may provide a longer symptom-free interval but little in the way of effective palliation once relapse has occurred. For this reason, it may be preferable to delay hormonal therapy until the patient has become symptomatic in the hope of providing increased long-term palliation.

Chemotherapy. Cytotoxic chemotherapy for carcinoma of the prostate has so far yielded discouraging results. A major goal for the future is to develop new forms of therapy that will be effective against the hormone-resistant cell population. The discovery of such agents will represent a major advance in the treatment of this disease.

Catalona WJ, Smith DS, Ratliff TL, et al.: Measurement of prostate-specific antigen in serum as a screening test for prostate cancer. N Engl J Med 324:1156, 1991. *This large study concluded that measurement of serum PSA levels is a useful addition to screening by rectal examination alone.*

Coffey DS: The molecular biology, endocrinology and physiology of the prostate and seminal vesicles. *In* Walsh PC, Retik AB, Stamey TA, et al. (eds.): Campbell's Urology, 6th ed. Philadelphia, WB Saunders, 1992, pp 221–266. *Excellent review of prostate biochemistry and physiology.*

Cooner WH, Mosley BR, Rutherford CL, Jr, et al.: Prostate cancer detection in a clinical urological practice by ultrasonography, digital rectal examination and prostate specific antigen. J Urol 143:1146, 1990. *Practical approach to detection of prostate adenocarcinoma.*

Fowler JE, Jr: Bacteriuria and associated infections of the reproductive system in men. *In* Urinary Tract Infection and Inflammation. Chicago, Year Book, 1989, pp 92–123. *Review of etiology, diagnosis, and treatment of male genital tract infections.*

Gittes RF: Medical progress: Carcinoma of the prostate. N Engl J Med 324:236, 1991. *Excellent review.*

McConnell JD, Barry MJ, Bruskewitz RC, et al.: Benign prostatic hyperplasia: Diagnosis and Treatment. Clinical Practice Guideline, Number 8, AHCPR publication No. 94-0582, Rockville, Md: Agency for Health Care Policy and Research, Public Health Service. U.S. Dept. of Health & Human Services, February, 1994. *Excellent recent review of diagnosis and treatment of benign prostatic hyperplasia.*

Osterling JE: Benign prostatic hyperplasia. Medical and minimally invasive treatment options. N. Engl J Med 332:99, 1995. *A comprehensive, highly readable review of the subject.*

Stamey TA, McNeal JE: Adenocarcinoma of the prostate. *In* Walsh PC, Retik AB, Stamey TA, et al. (eds.): Campbell's Urology, 6th ed. Philadelphia, WB Saunders, 1992, pp 1159–1221. *Provides a comprehensive review of all aspects of diagnosis and treatment of prostate carcinoma.*

210 MULTIPLE-ORGAN SYNDROMES

210.1 Polyglandular Disorders
Henry M. Kronenberg

Internists need to recognize diseases that involve independent abnormalities of more than one endocrine gland for a number of reasons: First, the known patterns of multiglandular disease can alert the clinician to look for a second disorder when one is diagnosed. Second, the treatment of many of the individual diseases in polyglandular disorders may differ from the treatment appropriate for the same diseases when they present in isolation. Third, because many of these diseases appear in characteristic familial patterns, the recognition of the syndromes can lead to useful family screening. Fourth, an understanding of the pathogenesis of these unusual disorders is likely to clarify the pathogenesis of more common single-gland disorders as well. This chapter discusses the best-characterized polyglandular disorders with these four considerations as the primary focus. Other chapters should be consulted for more detailed discussion of the diseases of individual glands.

POLYGLANDULAR NEOPLASIA

Three mechanistically distinct neoplastic syndromes involve more than one endocrine gland. Although given a variety of different names in the past, they are now most frequently called multiple endocrine neoplasia type 1, multiple endocrine neoplasia types 2a and 2b, and McCune-Albright syndrome.

MULTIPLE ENDOCRINE NEOPLASIA TYPE 1. Multiple endocrine neoplasia type 1 (MEN 1) is an autosomal dominant disorder involving characteristically the parathyroid glands, the pancreatic islets, and the anterior pituitary. Less commonly, adrenal gland neoplasia, foregut carcinoids (primarily of thymus and lung), and lipomas occur. Because thyroid neoplasms are so common in the general population, their true association with MEN 1 is debated.

Parathyroid Disease. Hyperparathyroidism is the most common abnormality in MEN 1, found in more than 90% of patients. Elevation of blood calcium generally first appears between the ages of 20 and 40, considerably earlier than in sporadic primary hyperparathyroidism; this is not a disease of children, however. At first, the disease is asymptomatic but then can lead to all the expected consequences of primary hyperparathyroidism. Unlike sporadic hyperparathyroidism, the disease is relentlessly progressive and, with prolonged follow-up, always involves all four parathyroid glands. The involvement is characteristically asymmetric and asynchronous. This pattern can lead to inappropriately limited parathyroid surgery. If fewer than three parathyroid glands are removed, hypercalcemia always recurs, although not necessarily immediately. Surgical results in MEN 1 are generally less satisfactory than in sporadic four-gland parathyroid disease. At some centers all four glands are removed, and a portion of one gland is reimplanted in the easily accessible forearm in an attempt to avoid the hazards of too much or too little surgery. The difficulty in attaining long-term normocalcemia has led many clinicians to postpone surgery when the disease is asymptomatic. This strategy may need to be modified if the patient develops Zollinger-Ellison syndrome (see below), because hypercalcemia can dramatically increase the gastrin levels in such patients.

Pancreatic Islet Disease. As many as 80% of patients have pancreatic abnormalities at autopsy; a large number correspondingly have increased blood levels of gastrin, insulin, pancreatic polypeptide, somatostatin, vasoactive intestinal polypeptide, or glucagon during stimulation or suppression tests. The pancreas is often diffusely involved with microadenomas and macroadenomas and apparently hyperplastic lesions. Characteristically, more than one islet hormone is secreted from these multiple tumors. Despite this underlying pattern of multiple cellular involvement, patients characteristically present with symptoms of only one hormonal disorder. The most common disease is Zollinger-Ellison syndrome, peptic ulcer disease associated with gastrin-producing tumors. Identification of disease-causing tumors has proven difficult. The gastrinomas in MEN 1 are often multiple, very small, and found in the duodenal wall. Macroadenomas observed in the pancreas by computed tomography (CT) or intraoperative ultrasonography may well synthesize hormones other than gastrin. Although some centers continue to experiment with aggressive attempts at surgical cure, the high recurrence rate after surgery has limited the role for surgery in this disease. Medical therapy with H_2 receptor antagonists and H^+,K^+-ATPase inhibitors can usually adequately control the secretion of stomach acid. The tumors are slow-growing but frequently metastasize locally and to the liver. Chemotherapy is only partially effective and never cures the disease.

Insulinomas are the second most common clinically important islet tumor in MEN 1. These tumors are often small and multiple and are much less frequently malignant than the gastrinomas. Despite the frequently diffuse nature of the disease, dominant insulin-producing tumors can often be identified by selective portal venous sampling. Removal of the dominant tissue, or, if necessary, subtotal (80%) pancreatectomy is the primary therapeutic strategy.

Pituitary Disease. As in sporadic disease, pituitary disease can present with a hypersecretion syndrome or with symptoms due to a sellar mass or hypopituitarism. Pituitary tumors occur in more than half of MEN 1 patients. Prolactinomas are the most common tumors. Adrenocortical hyperfunction can result from a pituitary adenoma or from production of ACTH or corticotropin-releasing hormone by a foregut carcinoid. Although nonfunctioning adrenal neoplasms are common in MEN 1, primary adrenal neoplasms causing glucocorticoid excess are rare. Acromegaly can result from a pituitary neoplasm or as a consequence of production of growth hormone–releasing hormone by pancreatic islet tumors. After con-

sideration of ectopic hormone and releasing hormone production by nonpituitary tumors, the course and treatment of pituitary disease in MEN 1 resemble those of sporadic pituitary disease.

Pathogenesis. Family studies have mapped the gene responsible for MEN 1 to the long arm of chromosome 11, band 11q13. In addition to this genetic abnormality, inherited by all cells in the body, MEN 1 tumors harbor other tumor-specific genetic changes. In the majority of parathyroid and islet tumors studied, these additional genetic abnormalities consist of loss or mutation of DNA at loci that include 11q13. Strikingly, in every case, the loss of genetic information at 11q13 in tumors always involves the chromosome inherited from the normal parent rather than the chromosome carrying the inherited MEN 1 genetic mutation. This pattern strongly suggests that loss of function of both copies of the MEN 1 gene (one from the inherited mutation and one from the mutation found in the tumor) makes tumor formation likely. The tumors are thus clonal expansions that may result from loss of function of a so-called tumor suppressor gene. The gene involved in MEN 1 may be involved in the pathogenesis of sporadic parathyroid adenomas because 25% of such neoplasms also involve somatic (not inherited) abnormalities at 11q13. Still unclear are the direct consequences of the single inherited abnormality at 11q13 in MEN 1. A second, somatic mutation may be required for tumor formation in MEN 1. Alternatively, it is possible that the inherited abnormality alone can cause hyperplasia of the involved glands, which then evolves by clonal expansion. The two-hit, tumor suppressor model can explain many of the features of MEN 1. Clinical presentation of an inherited disorder in adulthood can be explained by the requirement for second mutations before clonal expansion. The asymmetric but relentless nature of the parathyroid disease may be explained by asynchronous but inevitable somatic mutations in each of the parathyroid glands. Multiple islet tumors might result from the same process. Definitive explanations of the pathogenesis of MEN 1 await the expected isolation of the MEN 1 gene.

Without identification of the gene, the identification of affected family members relies primarily on clinical screening. The most useful single test to complement a thorough history and physical examination is measurement of blood calcium, particularly ionized calcium, at intervals after age 15. Prolactin, gastrin, and fasting blood sugar measurements can also be useful. Research laboratories can identify affected family members by characterizing closely linked genetic markers in blood cells if specimens from more than one affected family member are available.

MULTIPLE ENDOCRINE NEOPLASIA TYPES 2A AND 2B. Multiple endocrine neoplasia type 2a is an autosomal dominant disease that presents with medullary carcinoma of the thyroid (MCT), pheochromocytoma, and, less commonly, hyperparathyroidism. Multiple endocrine neoplasia type 2b is closely related to MEN 2a because it also presents with medullary carcinoma of the thyroid and pheochromocytoma and because both diseases map to the same genetic region—the pericentromeric region of chromosome 10. MEN 2b presents with a number of abnormalities not found in MEN 2a, however. These include mucosal neuromas of the tongue, lips, eyelids, and gastrointestinal tract and a marfanoid habitus. Hyperparathyroidism rarely occurs in MEN 2b. MEN 2b is less common than MEN 2a; both diseases are rarer than MEN 1.

In MEN 2a and 2b, the medullary cancers and the pheochromocytomas often present bilaterally. Careful prospective analysis of MEN 2a families has demonstrated that diffuse C cell hyperplasia precedes clinically obvious appearance of medullary cancer by decades. C cell hyperplasia can be detected by measurement of calcitonin after administration of gastrin. With current sensitive assays, the median age of presentation with C cell hyperplasia is 8 or 9. Virtually all MEN 2a patients eventually develop C cell disease. Complete thyroidectomy of patients with C cell hyperplasia has dramatically decreased the incidence of medullary cancer, which has been the major cause of death in MEN 2a.

Half the patients with MEN 2a develop pheochromocytomas. Family screening allows the detection of pheochromocytoma before the development of hypertension. The first laboratory abnormalities noted include an increase in urinary epinephrine and in the ratio of epinephrine to norepinephrine in the urine. Increases in urinary metanephrine and norepinephrine come later. The tumors are usually found in the adrenal glands and can be documented preoperatively by CT, magnetic resonance imaging, and [^{131}I]-metaiodobenzylguanidine scanning.

Most patients with MEN 2a have been found to harbor point mutations in the *RET* proto-oncogene. *RET* encodes a member of the tyrosine protein kinase family of cell surface receptors. The gene is expressed in spinal cord, in certain cultured blood cell lines, and in all tested medullary cancer and pheochromocytoma lines (both from MEN 2 patients and from sporadic tumors). The first characterized mutations have been found in four different cysteines located in the portion of the receptor predicted to form the extracellular, ligand-binding domain. In contrast to the pattern in MEN 1, no evidence for somatic mutations in the RET region of chromosome 10 have been found in MEN 2a tumors. It is likely that the mutant RET gene signals in a ligand-independent manner, thereby acting as an oncogene. The mutant RET genes can transform cultured cells, and the mutant ret protein can act as a ligand-independent protein kinase. The mutant RET genes are, therefore, likely to be inherited oncogenes.

The transition from diffuse hyperplasia of C cells or adrenal medullary cells to clonal neoplasms of the thyroid or adrenal probably requires subsequent somatic mutations. Such mutations include the loss of genetic markers on chromosomes 1p, 3p, 3q, and 22q that frequently occur in these tumors.

Patients with MEN 2b harbor a point mutation that changes methionine-918 to a threonine within the ret protein's intracellular kinase domain. Studies suggest that this mutation activates the kinase and may change its substrate specificity.

Carriers of the MEN 2 genes can best be identified by serial measurement of stimulated blood calcitonin levels, starting at an early age. Rapid progress in defining the *RET* lesions in MEN 2a (and perhaps 2b) now allows direct genetic testing, replacing calcitonin testing as a screening tool.

McCUNE-ALBRIGHT SYNDROME. The McCune-Albright syndrome is a noninherited disorder consisting of the triad of polyostotic fibrous dysplasia, light brown pigmented skin lesions (café-au-lait spots), and endocrinopathy, usually precocious puberty. Multiple endocrine abnormalities can occur. The precocious puberty, more often seen in girls than boys, is gonadotropin-independent. Hyperthyroidism is caused by autonomous thyroid nodules. Acromegaly is caused by pituitary adenomas that produce growth hormone and, usually, prolactin. Adrenocortical hyperfunction is caused by ACTH-independent adrenal adenomas. Hypophosphatemic rickets, with normal blood calcium, phosphate wasting, and low or inappropriately normal levels of $1,25(OH)_2D_3$, may result from release of a humoral factor from the dysplastic fibrous tissue.

This somewhat bewildering array of endocrine abnormalities has been rationalized by the observation that cells in the involved tissues harbor mutations in the α subunit of the G_S protein. The G_S protein links cell surface receptors to the activation of adenylate cyclase. The mutations in McCune-Albright syndrome are point mutations at arginine-201 in the G_S α subunit; these mutations lead to prolonged activity of G_S and inappropriate activation of adenylate cyclase. Increased levels of cyclic AMP lead to cellular proliferation and hormone secretion. McCune-Albright patients are genetic mosaics. Presumably, at an early stage in embryonic development, a point mutation occurs in the G_S α gene of a cell that then proliferates, differentiates, and variably populates normal bone, skin, and endocrine tissues. In cell types in which elevations in cyclic AMP lead to proliferation, abnormal cells become predominant and lead to disease. Because the disease is never inherited, the mutation is presumably lethal when present in all cells of the embryo. In contrast, the very same mutations at arginine-201 have been found in cases of isolated acromegaly and autonomous thyroid nodules. One can, therefore, speculate that McCune-Albright syndrome is the most dramatic example of a spectrum of disorders that vary in severity and presentation depending on the stage of development of the original mutant cell.

AUTOIMMUNE POLYGLANDULAR DYSFUNCTION

Organ-specific autoimmune disease, characterized by lymphocytic infiltration and organ-specific autoantibodies, commonly results in endocrine hypofunction or hyperfunction. Clinical manifestations of disease are usually limited to one gland. Not uncommonly, however, disorders of more than one endocrine gland appear in families or in individual patients. Characteristic patterns of disease presentation and genetic inheritance allow the definition of two syndromes with overlapping manifestations (Table 210–1).

TABLE 210–1. CLINICAL FEATURES OF AUTOIMMUNE POLYGLANDULAR SYNDROMES

	Type 1	Type 2
Mucocutaneous candidiasis	Very common	Not seen
Hypoparathyroidism	Common	Rare
Addison's disease	Common	Common
Primary hypogonadism	Common	Occurs
Autoimmune thyroid disease	Rare	Common
Autoimmune diabetes	Occurs	Common
Hypophysitis	Occurs	Occurs
Autoimmune hepatitis	Occurs	Not seen
Pernicious anemia	Occurs	Occurs
Vitiligo	Occurs	Occurs
Malabsorption syndrome	Occurs	Occurs in celiac disease
Alopecia	Common	Occurs
Myasthenia gravis	Not seen	Occurs
Keratopathy	Common	Not seen
Tympanic membrane calcification	Common	Not seen
Inheritance	Autosomal recessive	HLA association
Age of onset	Usually childhood	Usually adulthood

AUTOIMMUNE POLYGLANDULAR SYNDROME TYPE 1. This rare disease presents typically in early childhood. Mucocutaneous candidiasis occurs in virtually all patients and is usually the first manifestation of disease. Hypoparathyroidism and Addison's disease are the most common endocrine manifestations; each of these diseases occurs in 70 to 80% of patients. Hypoparathyroidism usually precedes Addison's disease; both diseases typically present before age 15. Premature ovarian failure (in 60% of affected women) usually presents as secondary amenorrhea; testicular failure occurs less frequently. Insulin-dependent diabetes mellitus occurs in 12% of patients, usually in adulthood; hypothyroidism is uncommon.

Nonendocrine components of this syndrome, in addition to the mucocutaneous candidiasis, include alopecia, vitiligo, corneal opacities, autoimmune hepatitis, enamel hypoplasia of teeth, tympanic membrane calcification, nail dystrophy that correlates only loosely with obvious candidiasis, parietal cell atrophy and vitamin B_{12} malabsorption, and more general intestinal malabsorption with steatorrhea. Asplenism, with Howell-Jolly bodies on peripheral blood smears, has been noted in several patients.

Each of the disease components should be sought when any patient presents with hypoparathyroidism, primary adrenal insufficiency, or mucocutaneous candidiasis. The hypoparathyroidism is treated like the sporadic disease with oral calcium and 1,25-dihydroxyvitamin D, although variable intestinal malabsorption can present a particular therapeutic challenge. The candidiasis can be satisfactorily controlled with ketoconazole.

Autoimmune polyglandular syndrome type 1 is an autosomal recessive disorder. The appearance of organ-specific autoantibodies precedes disease presentation and predicts the development of specific end-organ damage. The role of these antibodies and the precise pathogenesis of the syndrome are unknown, however.

AUTOIMMUNE POLYGLANDULAR SYNDROME TYPE 2. This syndrome is considerably more common than the type 1 syndrome and typically presents in adulthood. Insulin-dependent diabetes mellitus and thyroid dysfunction—either autoimmune hypothyroidism or Grave's disease—are the most frequent manifestations. Addison's disease is the third major endocrine component of this disorder. Although most patients who present with autoimmune diabetes or thyroid disease have clinical involvement of only one gland, a large fraction of patients with autoimmune Addison's disease develop clinically evident disease in other endocrine glands. Less common components of the type 2 polyglandular syndrome include primary hypogonadism and hypophysitis. Pernicious anemia, vitiligo, celiac disease, alopecia, and myasthenia gravis are also associated with this syndrome.

The treatment of each component of this syndrome is identical to the treatment of each disorder in isolation, although possible clustering of diseases must be kept in mind during the evaluation and follow-up of all patients with each individual component disorder. Thyroid hormone therapy can precipitate symptoms of adrenal insufficiency in patients with both disorders, for example. Consequently, careful history, including family history, physical examination, and a low threshold for specific laboratory testing for adrenal insufficiency should be part of the evaluation of every patient with autoimmune hypothyroidism. Further, combinations of hypothyroidism, adrenal insufficiency, and hypogonadism can mimic hypopituitarism, although specific hormonal testing can easily distinguish these disorders. Because multiple components of the syndrome can present asynchronously, periodic evaluation for early appearance of further disease components is indicated.

Autoimmune polyglandular syndrome type 2 is usually inherited in families with characteristic HLA associations. The HLA associations do not predict disease absolutely, even in identical twins, so environmental factors must contribute to disease presentation. Typically, several different autoimmune diseases occur in each family. Autoimmune vulnerability rather than specific organ disease is inherited. Diabetes, as part of the polyglandular syndrome, usually presents at an older age and develops more slowly than isolated autoimmune diabetes. The characteristic pattern of association with specific DQ loci does not differ between polyglandular and isolated diabetes, however. Presumably, genes not linked to the HLA complex modify the presentation of diabetes.

Organ-specific antibodies appear before clinical disease and predict subsequent disease. The role of these antibodies in organ hypofunction has not been established, however.

Ahonen P, Myllärniemi S, Sipilä I, et al.: Clinical variation of autoimmune polyendocrinopathy–candidiasis–ectodermal dystrophy (APECED) in a series of 68 patients. N Engl J Med 322:1829, 1990. *A large series with prolonged follow-up that presents a thorough summary of the clinical features of autoimmune polyglandular syndrome type 1.*

Eisenbarth GS, Jackson RA: The immunoendocrinopathy syndromes. *In* Wilson JD, Foster DW (eds.): William's Textbook of Endocrinology, 8th ed. Philadelphia, WB Saunders, 1992, p 1555. *An excellent general review stressing immune mechanisms.*

Gagel RF, Jackson CE (eds.): Proceedings of the fourth international workshop on multiple endocrine neoplasia. Henry Ford Hosp Med J 40:158, 1992. *A large collection of papers discussing both clinical and genetic aspects of MEN 1 and 2.*

Lips CJM, Landsvater RL, Höppener JWM, et al.: Clinical screening as compared with DNA analysis in families with multiple endocrine neoplasia type 2A. N Engl J Med 331:828, 1994. *The first "field" demonstration of the advantage of using DNA testing instead of calcitonin testing in MEN 2a families.*

Mignon M, Ruszniewski P, Podevin P, et al.: Current approach to the management of gastrinoma and insulinoma in adults with multiple endocrine neoplasia type I. World J Surg 17:489, 1993. *A useful survey of the varied surgical approaches to pancreatic islet disease in MEN 1.*

Santoro F, Carlomagno F, Romano A, et al.: Activation of RET as a dominant transforming gene by germline mutations of MEN 2A and MEN 2B. Science 267:381, 1995. *Elegant demonstration that mutant RET genes are the first inherited disease-causing oncogenes.*

Schwindinger WF, Levine MA. McCune-Albright syndrome. Trends Endocrinol Metab 4:238, 1993. *A succinct and thorough summary of the clinical and molecular aspects of the disease.*

210.2   Carcinoid Syndrome
John A. Oates

Carcinoid syndrome incorporates the constellation of signs and symptoms associated with malignant neoplasms of enterochromaffin cells. Cutaneous flushing, diarrhea, and cardiac valvular lesions are the most common endocrine consequences of these tumors.

THE NEOPLASMS

Tumors that cause the carcinoid syndrome have the characteristics of neuroendocrine cells of the enterochromaffin type. These tumors typically contain 5-hydroxytryptamine (serotonin) and tachykinins such as substance P. The metastatic tumors associated with carcinoid syndrome usually arise from primary tumors in the ileum. The syndrome also can be produced by neoplasms arising from the remainder of the small intestine, from organs derived from the embryonic foregut (e.g., bronchus, stomach, pancreas, and thyroid), and from ovarian or testicular teratomas. The usual carcinoid

tumor arising from the ileum has the histologic pattern of dense nests of cells with uniform size and nuclear appearance. Histochemically, they typically exhibit an argentaffin reaction in which the cells convert a silver salt to metallic silver. A positive argentaffin reaction is not required for the diagnosis, however, as carcinoid tumors arising from organs of the embryonic foregut may contain few if any argentaffin cells. Ultrastructural examination of carcinoid tumors reveals electron-dense secretion granules.

Carcinoid tumors have a proclivity to metastasize to the liver and may involve this organ extensively and predominantly. Extrahepatic metastases occur in bone, where they are often osteoblastic, and in the lung, pancreas, spleen, ovaries, adrenals, and other organs.

Primary carcinoid tumors of the appendix are common, but they rarely metastasize. Those from the large intestine may metastasize but almost never exhibit endocrine effects.

CLINICAL MANIFESTATIONS

Carcinoid tumors typically have a slow rate of growth, and many patients with carcinoid syndrome survive for a decade after the disease is recognized. For much of the duration of the illness, morbidity results largely from the endocrine functions of the tumor. Death usually is caused by cardiac or hepatic failure and by complications associated with tumor growth.

VASODILATOR PAROXYSMS. Cutaneous flushing is the most common clinical feature. The typical flush is erythematous and involves the head and neck (blush area). Some patients exhibit vivid color changes from red to violaceous to pallor. Prolonged flushing attacks may be associated with lacrimation and periorbital edema. The flush may be accompanied by tachycardia, and the blood pressure usually falls or does not change. A rise in blood pressure during flushing is rare, and carcinoid syndrome is not a cause of sustained hypertension. Flushing may be provoked by excitement, exertion, eating, and ethanol ingestion.

TELANGIECTASIA. In addition to paroxysms of cutaneous vasodilatation, some patients also develop telangiectasia, primarily on the face and neck and most marked in the malar area.

GASTROINTESTINAL SYMPTOMS. Intestinal hypermotility with borborygmi, cramping, and explosive diarrhea may accompany the episodic flushes. Chronic diarrhea is more common and may have a secretory component. When this is severe, malabsorption may occur.

CARDIAC MANIFESTATIONS. Plaquelike thickening of the endocardium of the valvular cusps and cardiac chambers occurs primarily on the right side of the heart but may involve the left side to a minimal degree. The endocardial thickening is composed of smooth muscle cells embedded in a stroma rich in mucopolysaccharides. The thickening and deformation of the valve cusps, chordae tendineae, and papillary muscles interfere with valvular function and may lead to regurgitation, stenosis, or combined functional lesions. There is a tendency for the fibrosing process to produce incompetence of the tricuspid valve and stenosis of the smaller pulmonary orifice, a deleterious hemodynamic combination. Cardiac dysfunction may be further compromised by impaired atrial and ventricular compliance and by the occasional occurrence of a high cardiac output that probably results from continuing release of a vasodilator.

PULMONARY. Bronchoconstriction, usually most pronounced during flushing attacks, is a less common feature of the syndrome, but it may be severe.

GENERAL. Intestinal obstruction may result from the primary tumor or from the desmoplastic reaction in the surrounding mesentery; infrequently, the primary tumors cause gastrointestinal bleeding. Necrosis of hepatic tumor masses may produce an acute syndrome of abdominal pain, tenderness, fever, and leukocytosis. Hepatomegaly from the metastatic disease is usually present, but extensive metastatic involvement of the liver by the slowly growing tumors may occur before liver function tests become abnormal. Generalized fatigue and debilitation are underappreciated features of carcinoid syndrome.

THE ENDOCRINE FUNCTION OF CARCINOID TUMORS

SEROTONIN. The most constant biochemical feature of carcinoid tumors is the presence of tryptophan hydroxylase, which catalyzes the formation of 5-hydroxytryptophan (5-HTP) from tryptophan (Fig. 210–1). The typical ileal carcinoid tumor also contains aromatic L-amino acid decarboxylase, which catalyzes the conver-

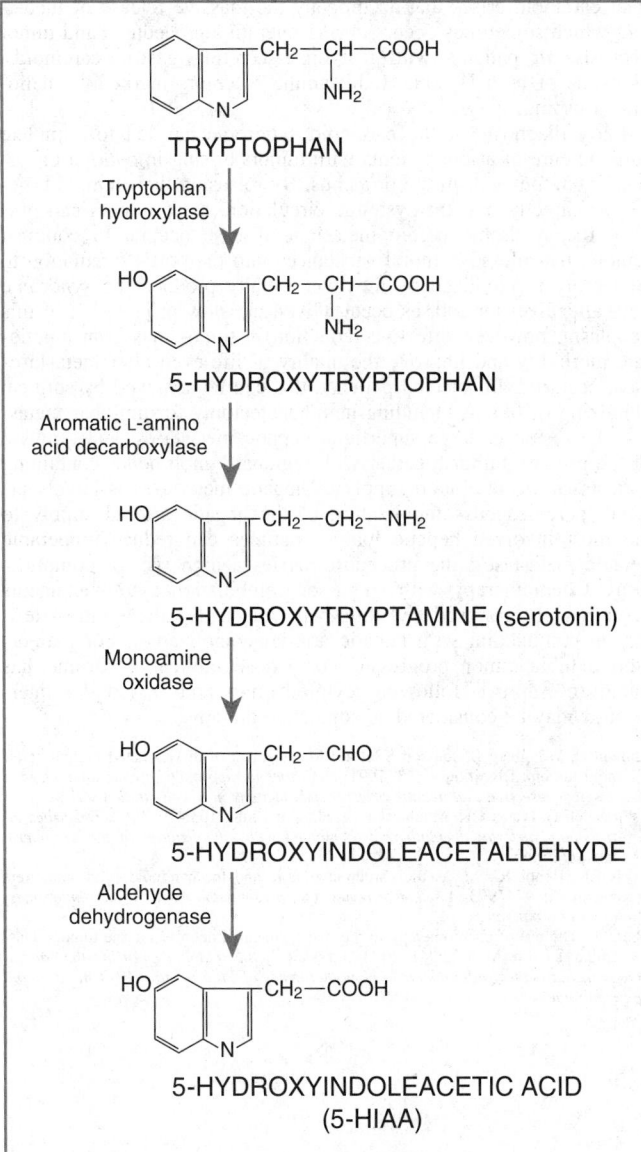

FIGURE 210–1. Synthesis and degradation of serotonin.

sion of 5-HTP to 5-hydroxytryptamine (serotonin). Gastric carcinoids, however, are frequently deficient in this decarboxylase and release 5-HTP from the tumor.

Following its release from the tumor, serotonin is inactivated primarily by monoamine oxidase; uptake in the platelets also contributes to removal of free serotonin from blood. Monoamine oxidase oxidizes serotonin to 5-hydroxyindoleacetaldehyde, which is rapidly converted to 5-hydroxyindoleacetic acid (5-HIAA) by aldehyde dehydrogenase (Fig. 210–1). This acid is rapidly excreted into the urine, and almost all circulating serotonin can be accounted for as urinary 5-HIAA.

TACHYKININS. Peptides of the tachykinin family are stored in carcinoid tumors and are released during flushing. Several tachykinins are derived from a common precursor β-preprotachykinin; of these, neuropeptide K, neurokinin A, and substance P have been identified in tumors and blood from patients with the carcinoid syndrome.

OTHER BIOLOGICALLY ACTIVE SUBSTANCES. Some carcinoid tumors, particularly those of gastric origin, release excessive amounts of histamine. This can be detected by an increased urinary excretion of histamine or its metabolite, N-methylhistamine.

Carcinoid tumors have been associated with a number of ectopic endocrine syndromes, including hyperadrenocorticism that results from ectopic production of adrenocorticotropic hormone and acromegaly due to secretion of growth hormone–releasing hormone by the tumor.

MECHANISM OF THE FLUSH. Flushing can be triggered by catecholamines, and this probably accounts for the association of flushing with exercise and emotional stimuli. For experimental induction of flushing, injection of isoproterenol in amounts of as little as 0.5 μg may be effective. Pentagastrin, in doses as small as 0.25 μg, also can trigger flushing, an action that may explain the provocation of flushes by eating in some patients. As the hemodynamic changes associated with such pharmacologically induced attacks can be severe, epinephrine and other β-adrenergic amines as well as pentagastrin should be administered with great caution. Flushing episodes can be blocked by somatostatin.

Most of the evidence points to the tachykinins as mediators of the carcinoid flush. Tachykinins, particularly neuropeptide K, can be identified in plasma during flushing. Tachykinin levels have been shown to be increased during pentagastrin-induced flushing, and when pentagastrin-induced flushing is inhibited by somatostatin, the rise in tachykinin levels also is blocked. Tachykinins are known vasodilators.

Serotonin does not cause flushing. In patients with gastric carcinoids that secrete histamine, the flushing attacks can be attributed to histamine.

PATHOPHYSIOLOGY OF SEROTONIN OVERPRODUCTION. Serotonin contributes to the intestinal hypermotility and diarrhea. A secondary effect of serotonin overproduction occurs when a large fraction of dietary tryptophan is shunted into the hydroxylation pathway, leaving less tryptophan available for the formation of nicotinic acid and protein. When urinary excretion of 5-HIAA exceeds 100 mg daily, low levels of plasma tryptophan and evidence of nicotinic acid deficiency are seen.

DIAGNOSIS

When all of its clinical features are present, carcinoid syndrome is easily recognized. The diagnosis also must be considered when any one of its clinical manifestations is present.

The diagnostic hallmark consists of overproduction of 5-hydroxyindoles accompanied by increased excretion of urinary 5-HIAA. Normally, excretion of 5-HIAA does not exceed 9 mg daily. Ingestion of foods containing serotonin may complicate the biochemical diagnosis of carcinoid syndrome; both bananas and walnuts contain enough serotonin to produce abnormally elevated urinary excretion of 5-HIAA after their ingestion. When dietary 5-hydroxyindoles are excluded, urinary excretion of 25 mg of 5-HIAA daily is diagnostic of carcinoid. Elevation in the range of 9 to 25 mg may be seen with carcinoid syndrome, nontropical sprue, or acute intestinal obstruction. Measurement of serotonin in blood or platelets is of interest but has less diagnostic value than assay of the major metabolite of serotonin in the urine.

DIFFERENTIAL DIAGNOSIS. Attacks of flushing in a patient with normal urinary excretion of 5-HIAA raises other diagnostic possibilities. Systemic mastocyte activation disorders, including systemic mastocytosis, produce flushing and diarrhea and should be considered when 5-HIAA excretion is not elevated. Flushing also occurs in genetically predisposed individuals following ethanol ingestion, in the postmenopausal state, and in conjunction with other neuroendocrine tumors such as VIPomas and medullary carcinoma of the thyroid.

VARIANTS OF THE CARCINOID SYNDROME. The origin of the tumor influences the biologically active substances produced and their storage and release. The typical carcinoid syndrome usually results from tumors of midgut origin, which almost invariably secrete serotonin. Tumor serotonin content is likely to be high, and the tumor usually contains dense nests of argentaffin-positive cells. In contrast, tumors arising from the embryonic foregut contain fewer argentaffin cells, have lower serotonin content, and may secrete 5-HTP. Ectopic hormone production (e.g., Cushing's syndrome and acromegaly) and multiple endocrine adenomas are more likely to be associated with tumors of embryonic foregut.

Patients with gastric carcinoids frequently exhibit unique flushing, which begins as a bright, patchy erythema with sharply delineated serpentine borders; these patches tend to coalesce as the blush heightens. Food ingestion is especially likely to produce flushes. The tumors are usually deficient in decarboxylase enzyme and secrete 5-HTP; histamine secretion is also common, as is a high incidence of peptic ulceration. In these patients, histamine is the principal factor causing flushing.

With carcinoid tumors arising from the bronchus, attacks of flushing tend to be prolonged and severe and may be associated with periorbital edema, excessive lacrimation and salivation, hypotension, tachycardia and tachyarrhythmias, anxiety, and tremulousness. Nausea, vomiting, explosive diarrhea, and bronchoconstriction may progress to a severe degree. This group is therapeutically unique in that severe flushes often can be prevented by corticosteroids.

TREATMENT

Treatment of the carcinoid syndrome is directed toward (1) pharmacologic therapy for humorally mediated symptoms and (2) the reduction of tumor mass.

The discovery that somatostatin can prevent the flushing and other endocrine manifestations of the carcinoid syndrome provided the basis for a major advance in the treatment of these patients. The development of analogues of somatostatin, with longer biologic half-lives than the native hormone, made subcutaneous administration a feasible route of therapy. One of the somatostatin analogues, octreotide, has been found to markedly improve the flushing and other endocrine manifestations of most patients with carcinoid syndrome. This is frequently associated with a reduction in urinary 5-HIAA excretion and in tachykinin levels in blood. With the improvement of these endocrine symptoms, including fatigue, a considerable improvement in quality of life may be achieved. Octreotide is administered subcutaneously at intervals of approximately 8 hours, usually beginning with 75 to 150 μg and titrating upward until maximum inhibition of flushing and other symptoms is achieved, which usually occurs at single doses of 750 μg or less. An uncommon but severe adverse effect of octreotide is hypoglycemia, probably as a result of the inhibition of glucagon and growth hormone secretion; the suppression of pancreatic exocrine function by octreotide can cause steatorrhea. In patients receiving octreotide, about 5% achieve tumor regression, and in the group as a whole there is less tumor progression and a longer median survival compared with historical controls. Octreotide can prevent or treat carcinoid crises that accompany the massive release of mediators which sometimes occurs during operative procedures and tumor necrosis. In patients with histamine-secreting gastric carcinoids, blockade of both H_1 and H_2 histamine receptors markedly ameliorates flushing.

Early diagnosis of the carcinoid syndrome has led to complete surgical cure of a few patients with tumors arising in ovarian or testicular teratomas or in the bronchus. By releasing their humoral mediators directly into the systemic circulation, these tumors can produce the syndrome before metastatic disease occurs. In contrast, tumors that release humoral substances into the portal circulation to be largely metabolized by the liver usually produce the syndrome only after liver metastases occur. Given the slow progression of this neoplasm, however, effective reduction in tumor mass can ameliorate morbidity and improve the quality of life even after metastases have occurred. In selected patients, this can be achieved by surgical debulking of tumor, including hemihepatectomy for unilobar metastases, excision of large superficial hepatic metastases, and removal of the primary tumor together with regional lymph nodes containing metastases. As the blood supply of hepatic metastases is largely arterial, percutaneous embolization of the hepatic arterial supply to the most involved hepatic lobe sometimes can reduce inoperable hepatic metastases; the procedure carries a high risk of complications. Chemotherapy with single or combination cytotoxic agents given acutely has produced little benefit except perhaps intra-arterially in conjunction with hepatic arterial embolization. For patients who exhibit tumor progression or whose clinical syndrome has failed to improve following cytoreduction and octreotide, interferon-α may be considered as adjunctive therapy.

Ahlman H, Wängberg B, Jansson S, et al.: Management of disseminated midgut carcinoid tumors. Digestion 49:78, 1991. *Describes an approach to cytoreduction with surgical resection and hepatic arterial embolectomy in a well-studied series.*

Hajarizadeh H, Ivancev K, Mueller CR, et al.: Am J Surg 163:479, 1992. *Describes intrahepatic arterial chemotherapy combined with embolization of the peripheral hepatic artery.*

Kvols LK, Reubi JC: Metastatic carcinoid tumors and the carcinoid syndrome. Acta Oncol 32:197, 1993. *A selective review that presents the results of octreotide therapy in 66 patients.*

Öberg K: The use of chemotherapy in the management of neuroendocrine tumors. Gastrointest Horm Med 22:941, 1993. *A review of the studies supporting the conclusion that acutely administered chemotherapy is of little or no benefit in carcinoid syndrome.*

PART XVIII

DISEASES OF BONE AND BONE MINERAL METABOLISM

211 MINERAL AND BONE HOMEOSTASIS

Stephen J. Marx

Calcium, phosphorus, and magnesium, three of the principal body elements, have diverse roles. The calcium ion is particularly versatile. In the crystalline phase, it contributes to the varied structural roles of bone. In a supersaturated solution in blood, it contributes to plasma membrane excitability, plasma enzyme activities, and accretion of all minerals in extracellular matrix of bone. In the cytoplasmic fluid, its extraordinarily low concentrations allow rapid rises of its local concentrations to transmit information among cell compartments via its interactions with high-affinity calcium-binding proteins, such as calmodulin or protein kinase C. Phosphate is the principal intracellular anion, with central roles in cytoplasm as a buffer, energy carrier (mainly via the high-energy phosphate bonds of adenosine triphosphate [ATP]), and molecular switch (through phosphorylation and dephosphorylation). Magnesium is the principal cation in cytoplasm, functioning as a cofactor in many chemical reactions (for example, as an Mg-ATP complex or as a cofactor in many steps of DNA or RNA metabolism).

MINERALS IN BLOOD

THE STATE OF CALCIUM, PHOSPHATE, AND MAGNESIUM IN BLOOD. Total calcium concentration is tightly regulated, so that typical diurnal fluctuations are not more than 5% from the mean value. Calcium in blood is divided among protein-bound, complexed, and ionized or free fractions (Table 211–1). Protein binding of calcium in blood is principally to albumin, and this binding is decreased by acid pH. The ionized calcium fraction is the focus for metabolic control by the parathyroid gland, and measurements of ionized calcium in blood give the most valid index of pathologic disruptions of calcium homeostasis.

Phosphate and magnesium in blood are principally unbound (Table 211–1), and the concentration of each is regulated over a broader relative variation from its mean than that for calcium. Neither phosphate nor magnesium has a unique endocrine system dedicated to its control. Rather, their blood concentrations are sustained indirectly by the hormones directed at calcium control and directly by poorly understood local processes in bone, kidney, and other organs.

STEADY-STATE FLOW OF MINERALS TO AND FROM BLOOD. Only 0.1% of the total body calcium is in blood and extracellular fluid (Table 211–2). This calcium pool is in a rapidly exchanging equilibrium with large calcium pools controlled by three organs (bone, intestine, and kidney), each of which is an important site for the regulation of mineral metabolism. The rate of these daily fluxes (Fig. 211–1) is sufficiently large that disturbance of mineral flux to or from any of these organs can result in abnormally high or low concentrations of one of these minerals in blood.

ORGANS EXCHANGING MUCH MINERAL WITH BLOOD

Bone

BONE FUNCTION AND ARCHITECTURE. Major functions of bone include support, locomotion, encasement of hematopoietic tissue, and reservoir for calcium, phosphate, and magnesium. The architecture of bone responds dynamically to changes in mechanical load. The mechanisms whereby the signals from altered load are transduced are poorly understood. Mature bone adopts one of two macroscopic organizations (Fig. 211–2). The cortices of all bones and the interior of certain bones have a continuous structure termed cortical or lamellar bone. Lamellar bone, which is predominant in the long bones, is characterized by little metabolic activity and few cells. It has a highly organized extracellular matrix of mineral and parallel bundles of type I collagen. During embryonic development or in states with pathologic increase of bone turnover, bone assumes a less organized "woven" architecture. Within the vertebral bodies and in portions of the interior of other bones, bone is organized as a series of thin, interdigitating plates; this is termed trabecular, cancellous, or spongy bone. Its ratio of surface to volume is higher than that found in cortical bone and is thus better suited to rapid turnover.

TABLE 211–1. CONCENTRATIONS AND STATES OF CALCIUM, MAGNESIUM, AND PHOSPHATE IN NORMAL HUMAN PLASMA OR SERUM*

State	Calcium (mM)	Magnesium (mM)	Phosphate (mM)
Protein bound	1.15 (47)	0.26 (31)	0.15 (13)
Filterable or free†			
Complexed	0.25 (10)	0.06 (7)	0.40 (35)
Ionized	1.06 (43)	0.52 (62)	0.60 (52)

* Number in parentheses indicates percentage of total for that mineral.
† Filterable or free = complexed + ionized.

TABLE 211–2. DISTRIBUTION OF CALCIUM, MAGNESIUM, AND PHOSPHATE IN THE BODY OF A 70-KG ADULT*

Compartment	Calcium (g)	Magnesium (g)	Phosphate (g)
Bones and teeth	1300 (99)	14.0 (54)	600.0 (86)
Extracellular fluid	1 (0.1)	0.3 (1)	0.2 (0.03)
Cells	7 (1.0)	12.0 (46)	100.0 (14)

* Most of calcium is in bone; almost half of magnesium is in cells. Phosphate, as the principal counterion to calcium and magnesium in their dominant pools, has an intermediate proportional distribution. Number in parentheses is the percentage of total for that mineral.

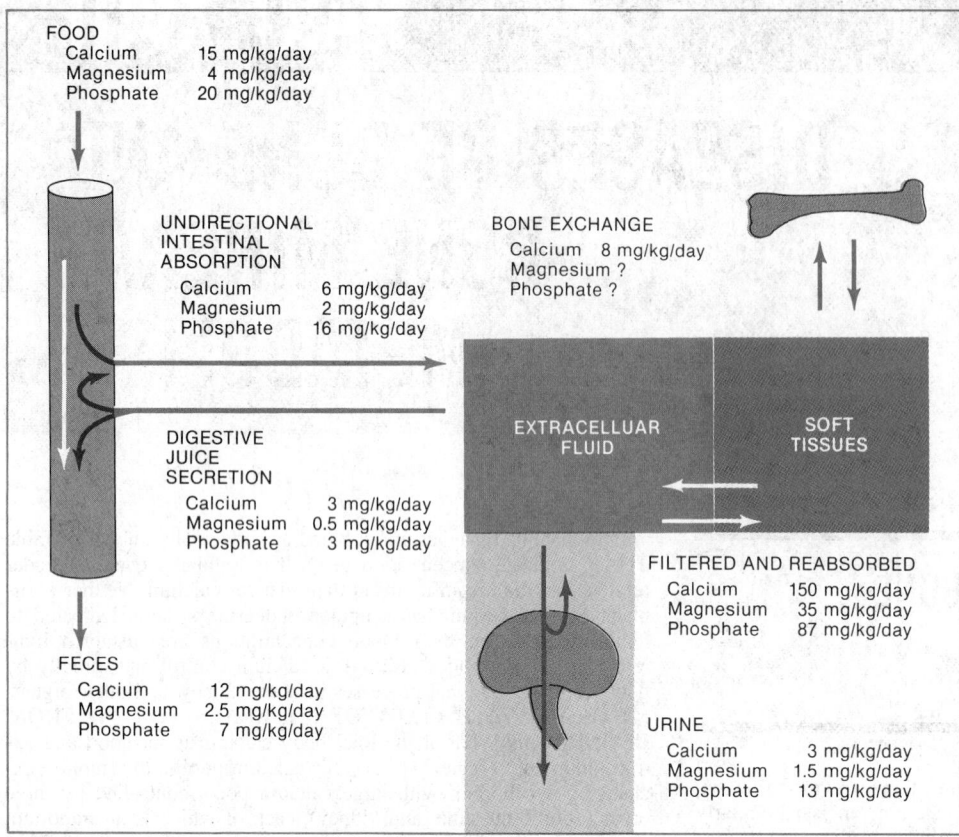

FOOD
Calcium   15 mg/kg/day
Magnesium   4 mg/kg/day
Phosphate   20 mg/kg/day

UNDIRECTIONAL
INTESTINAL
ABSORPTION

Calcium   6 mg/kg/day
Magnesium   2 mg/kg/day
Phosphate   16 mg/kg/day

BONE EXCHANGE
Calcium   8 mg/kg/day
Magnesium ?
Phosphate ?

DIGESTIVE
JUICE
SECRETION

Calcium   3 mg/kg/day
Magnesium   0.5 mg/kg/day
Phosphate   3 mg/kg/day

EXTRACELLUAR
FLUID

SOFT
TISSUES

FECES
Calcium   12 mg/kg/day
Magnesium   2.5 mg/kg/day
Phosphate   7 mg/kg/day

FILTERED AND REABSORBED
Calcium   150 mg/kg/day
Magnesium   35 mg/kg/day
Phosphate   87 mg/kg/day

URINE
Calcium   3 mg/kg/day
Magnesium   1.5 mg/kg/day
Phosphate   13 mg/kg/day

FIGURE 211–1. Typical mineral fluxes in adults. (Modified from Aurbach GD, Marx SJ, Spiegel AM: Parathyroid hormone, calcitonin, and the calciferols. *In* Wilson JD, Foster DW [eds.]: Williams Textbook of Endocrinology. 7th ed. Philadelphia, WB Saunders, 1985, p 1144.)

EXTRACELLULAR MATRIX. Newly deposited osteoid must undergo a poorly understood maturation process for 1 to 3 weeks until it is able to accumulate minerals. The mineral phase of bone extracellular matrix is a mixture of multiple amorphous and crystalline states, the latter principally as hydroxyapatite crystals $(Ca_5(OH)(PO_4)_3)$. Ninety to 95% of osteoid, the organic component of the extracellular matrix, is composed of bundles of type I collagen, a long triple helix of two alpha$_1$ (type I) chains and one alpha$_2$ (type I) chain. The principal collagen of cartilage matrix is type II as a homotrimer of three alpha$_1$ (type II) chains. Fibrils of collagen play a major role in the strength of bone (type I collagen), cartilage (type II collagen), and elastic tissues (type III collagen). Their disruption results in characteristic disturbances (osteogenesis imperfecta [type I collagen], chondrodysplasia [type II collagen], Ehlers-Danlos syndrome or arterial aneurysms [type III collagen], and even certain variants of familial osteoarthritis [type II collagen]). The second most prominent protein in bone matrix is osteocalcin (or bone gla-protein); it has a molar content of three residues of gamma-carboxyglutamic acid, an unusual amino acid that confers to the molecule high affinity for calcium on bone crystals. The roles of osteocalcin are unknown, but its concentration in blood is a potential index of osteoblast activity. Several other proteins, phosphoproteins, glycoproteins, and so on, in bone matrix have been identified in the search for molecules regulating bone mineral accumulation and bone growth.

BONE CELLS. Several cells are highly characteristic of bone. A flat bone-lining cell (perhaps derived from marrow stroma) with few organelles covers many bone surfaces thought not to be undergoing modification. This cell is perhaps one precursor of the osteoblast. The osteoblast is a cuboidal bone matrix-synthesizing cell. It lines any periosteal, endosteal, or trabecular surface at which bone formation takes place. Its plasma membrane is highly enriched with a bone-specific isoform of the alkaline phosphatase enzyme. This enzyme is believed to promote bone mineralization by catalyzing in supersaturated extracellular fluid of bone the hydrolysis of pyrophosphate and other inhibitors of calcium-phosphate crystallization. The osteocyte is the principal stable cell inside mature bone. It is probably derived from an osteoblast that has encased itself in bone. Osteocytes are interconnected with one another via long processes that traverse bone canaliculi. The role of the osteocyte is

unknown, but it is appropriately located to modulate local mineral fluxes. The chondrocyte is the dominant cell of cartilage; it releases to the extracellular matrix type II collagen and vesicles that are rich in alkaline phosphatase and that may be a central organelle for accumulating calcium in preparation for mineralizing cartilage. The osteoclast is the main bone-resorbing cell. It is derived from precursors of the premonocyte lineage. It is a highly motile, multinucleated giant cell, with several specialized features for bone. These include organelles that mediate cell attachment to bone surface (podosomes), a strikingly redundant ruffled border at the bone face for ion transport, many enzymes that can function in bone resorption, and a high concentration of carbonic anhydrase II, which helps acidify the extracellular pocket between the osteoclast ruffled border and the skeletal resorption surface.

LOCAL REGULATORS OF BONE CELLS. Bone cells are under systemic and local regulation. Known systemic regulators include parathyroid hormone (PTH), calcitonin, and calcitriol, which are considered later in this chapter. There is also a highly complex network of local controls. The term "osteoclast-activating factors" was applied in the 1980's to components in incompletely characterized fluids that could activate bone resorption *in vitro*. Some of their active components have been identified. For example, interleukin-1 and lymphotoxin/tumor necrosis factor-beta are potential stimulators of bone resorption that seem to be released locally by some tumors in bone. They cannot act directly on mature osteoclasts but can act, rather, through nearby cells, such as osteoblasts or marrow stromal cells, that communicate with osteoclasts. Like the activators of bone resorption, the activators of bone formation are poorly understood, particularly because this process involves a complex interplay of osteoblast proliferation and differentiation. Some contributors to this process include type 1 insulin-like growth factor (IGF-1) and transforming growth factor-beta (TGF-β); the latter is present selectively and at high concentrations in osteoblasts and osteocytes. In addition, several newly identified proteins (osteogenesis-inducing factor, bone morphogenetic proteins [some of which are homologues of TGF-β], and so forth) can induce bone formation in soft tissue sites. Prostaglandins can stimulate bone formation or bone resorption, and they may be important mediators in inflammatory processes of the skeletal system.

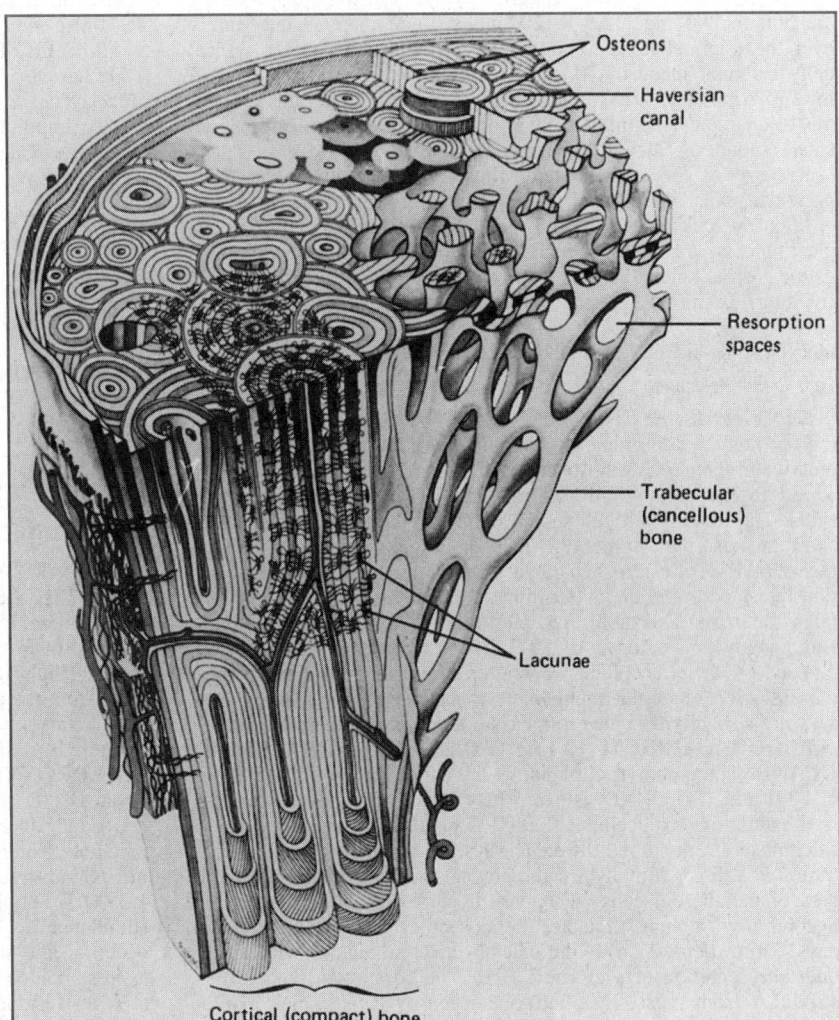

FIGURE 211-2. Bone organization. Microstructure of mature bone; areas of cortical (lamellar) and trabecular (cancellous) bone are shown. The central area in the transverse section shows differences in mineral density as degrees of shading. Note the organization of osteons, the distribution of osteocyte lacunae, and the organization of bone lamellae. (Adapted from Warwick R, Williams PL [eds.]: Gray's Anatomy. 35th ed. Edinburgh, Churchill Livingstone, 1973, p 217.)

BONE REMODELING. Bone growth or modeling occurs initially within a membrane or along the edge of cartilage (e.g., periosteum or epiphyseal growth plate). Although it contains few cells, cortical bone is constantly going through slow and orderly cycles of localized resorption and then rebuilding. This process is mediated by the local remodeling unit (alternately termed osteon or basic multicellular unit). Remodeling begins with osteoclasts excavating a cavity; as the resorption front advances, osteoclasts are replaced by other cells. Over an interval of several months, new bone is deposited in cylindrical lamellae around the rim of the cavity until it is refilled to complete this cycle. This cycle is an important example of the normal, coordinated relation between the bone resorption and bone formation processes. Most perturbations that modify one component of these two processes also modify the other in the same direction. The determinants of this coupling between bone resorption and formation are not known, but they probably include a host of growth factors present at high local concentrations in bone extracellular matrix and exposed or released by the skeletal resorption process.

Intestines

MINERAL ABSORPTION. The intestinal absorption of magnesium and phosphate is not subject to fine regulation and has not been studied intensively. By contrast, intestinal absorption of calcium is tightly regulated, and its quantitation has been analyzed in detail. Most calcium absorption is accomplished in the small bowel. Over a wide range of intakes, approximately 10% of dietary calcium is absorbed passively; the remainder of net intestinal absorption of calcium is regulated by active vitamin D metabolites, especially $1\alpha,25(OH)_2D$, in blood. With a normal diet, approximately 30% of calcium is absorbed. With low dietary calcium, the secon-

darily high blood $1\alpha,25(OH)_2D$ level can drive fractional calcium absorption to approach 90%.

Kidney

ION FILTRATION AND REABSORPTION. The non-protein-bound fractions of calcium, magnesium, and phosphate from plasma cross the glomerulus. The distal portions of the nephron have efficient and selective systems that can complete the reabsorption from tubular fluid of more than 99% of any one of these minerals. Tubular calcium reabsorption is stimulated principally by (PTH); thiazides or lithium can also increase tubular calcium reabsorption. Saline loading with or without loop diuretics can inhibit this. Tubular phosphate reabsorption is mainly under negative influence by PTH. The determinants of tubular reabsorption of magnesium are incompletely understood.

Integrated Fluxes: Mineral Balance and Nutrition

Skeletal growth is maximal throughout childhood, nearing completion during adolescence. Until this time, the rate of skeletal calcium accretion is typically 200 to 400 mg (5 to 10 mmole) per day. Fetal mineralization during the last trimester or milk secretion during lactation imposes similar daily increments on calcium efflux from maternal blood. The skeleton remains in a state of approximate zero mineral balance between ages 20 and 35, after which it slowly loses mass. This loss is greatest in the trabecular bone of the vertebrae, attaining peak rates about the menopause (3 to 10% per year during the first 1 to 4 years after surgically induced menopause).

Normal adults can sustain zero calcium balance with daily calcium intakes between 400 and 1500 mg (10 to 37.5 mmole), mainly as dairy products. Typical daily calcium intakes in the United States are 500 to 800 mg (12.5 to 20 mmole), and there is uncertainty over the minimal level for optimal skeletal health. With a typical daily calcium intake of 700 mg (17.5 mmole), one fourth, or 175 mg (43.7 mmole), is absorbed; during skeletal balance, this amount must equal the amount lost in urinary excretion (disregarding the small amount of calcium lost from skin).

Because of the large mineral fluxes between blood and three principal pools (bone, renal tubular lumen, and intestinal lumen), it is often difficult to assign mild disruptions to one pool. For example, there is uncertainty whether the slow bone losses with idiopathic age-associated osteoporosis reflect primary disturbances of calcium flux in bone, the intestine, or combinations of these.

HORMONAL REGULATORS OF MINERAL HOMEOSTASIS

Parathyroid Hormone

SYNTHESIS, SECRETION, AND METABOLISM. PTH is a rapidly regulated hormone that sustains calcium and $1,25(OH)_2D$ in blood and depresses phosphate in blood (Table 211–3). PTH is stored in the parathyroid cell mainly as a peptide of 84 amino acids. The parathyroid cell secretes PTH as the native molecule or as fragments, only some of which are biologically active. Fragments of PTH are also generated from its metabolism after secretion into blood. The amino terminus of PTH (residues 1 to 34) contains the requirements for receptor binding and biologic activity. Biologically active forms of PTH are cleared rapidly from blood, perhaps by their receptors, whereas inactive fragments are cleared more slowly, rendering them likely to be measured in immunoassays not specially designed to measure the intact molecule.

BLOOD CALCIUM EFFECT ON THE PARATHYROID GLAND. The parathyroid gland, as the coordinator of blood levels of PTH and $1,25(OH)_2D$, is exquisitely sensitive to changes of ionized calcium in extracellular fluid. The parathyroid cell responds to calcium in at least three different ways. First, low calcium concentration is a direct stimulus for the gradual increase in size and numbers of parathyroid cells (secondary hypertrophy and hyperplasia). Second, low calcium stimulates the biosynthesis of PTH over 1 to 2 days. Third, depression of the calcium level stimulates within seconds the secretion of preformed PTH. The parathyroid cell differs strikingly from most other hormone secretory cells, which exhibit accelerated secretion in response to increases of extracellular calcium.

PARATHYROID HORMONE MECHANISMS OF ACTION. PTH binds to a plasma membrane receptor; the PTH receptor then causes a rise of cyclic $3',5'$-adenosine monophosphate (cAMP) and other second messengers in the cytoplasm of its target cells. The consequence is rapid effects of PTH on the target cells in bone and kidney. A different peptide, termed "parathyroid hormone-related peptide," with homology to PTH at the amino terminus, is secreted by many cancers, causing hypercalcemia through its interactions with PTH receptors.

PARATHYROID HORMONE ACTION IN BONE. PTH in bone stimulates osteoblasts and osteoclasts. The effects on osteoclasts are indirect because these cells lack receptors for PTH. Very high PTH levels result in clear excess of bone resorption over bone formation. Controversy exists over whether mild PTH excess might have a net anabolic effect selectively in trabecular bone.

PARATHYROID HORMONE ACTION IN KIDNEY. PTH acts in the kidney to stimulate the synthesis of $1,25(OH)_2D$ by increasing the activity of $25OHD_3$ 1α-hydroxylase in the proximal tubules. PTH acts in the distal portions of the nephron to increase tubular reabsorption of calcium. In addition, PTH inhibits phosphate reabsorption in the distal, and perhaps also the proximal, tubules. PTH also inhibits bicarbonate reabsorption.

PARATHYROID HORMONE ACTION ON INTESTINE. PTH has no important direct action on the intestine. However, the direct renal effect of PTH to increase serum $1,25(OH)_2D$ causes highly important secondary effects in the intestine (see Intestinal Actions of Calcitriol, further on).

Calcitonin

CALCITONIN SYNTHESIS AND SECRETION. Calcitonin is a peptide of 32 amino acids that is normally synthesized and secreted by the parafollicular or C cells, which are neuroectodermal cells within the thyroid gland. Its secretion is stimulated by calcium and also by certain intestinal peptides (gastrin and glucagon) (see Ch. 215).

CALCITONIN ACTIONS. Calcitonin, at high concentrations, can directly inhibit osteoclast function. Calcitonin also can act in the kidney to cause mild natriuresis. These calcitonin actions have not been shown to be important in normal physiology. For the present, the principal interests in calcitonin are as a tumor marker, particularly for familial C cell neoplasia, or as a pharmacologic agent to treat bone disorders, such as Paget's disease.

Vitamin D and Its Metabolites

SYNTHESIS OF VITAMIN D. Vitamin D_3 is a seco-steroid (i.e., a steroid with one ring opened) synthesized from 7-dehydrocholesterol in the skin (Fig. 211–3), in a reaction catalyzed by ultraviolet light derived from the sun. Vitamin D_2, produced synthetically from the plant sterol ergosterol, is a vitamin D_3 analogue used as a dietary supplement or drug. The metabolism of vitamin D_3 and vitamin D_2 is similar in humans (see Ch. 212).

HYDROXYLATIONS OF VITAMIN D METABOLITES. Vitamin D ("D" refers to combinations of the D_3 and D_2 isoforms) is converted to 25OHD in hepatocytes. This reaction is not under metabolic control and is determined principally by the serum levels of its substrate, vitamin D. 25OHD is normally converted to $1,25(OH)_2D$ only in the renal proximal tubule by an enzyme system stimulated by PTH. A similar PTH-independent 1α-hydroxylation occurs in the normal placenta and abnormally in granuloma tissues, as in sarcoidosis. 25OHD and $1,25(OH)_2D$ can also be hydroxylated at other residues (C-23, C-24, C-26), but these and other conversions probably serve mainly to inactivate vitamin D metabolites.

ABSORPTION AND TRANSPORT OF VITAMIN D METABOLITES. Vitamin D metabolites enter the bloodstream like other sterols, and a small fraction of all vitamin D metabolites undergoes an enterohepatic recirculation. When cutaneous synthesis of vitamin D is marginal, any cause of intestinal malabsorption can result in vitamin D deficiency. Vitamin D metabolites are lipid soluble; they circulate in plasma bound to a specific 25OHD binding protein and, to a lesser degree, to other carriers.

MECHANISM OF ACTIONS OF VITAMIN D METABOLITES. Vitamin D is an inactive precursor; 25OHD and $1,25(OH)_2D$ are both active. Although the concentration of 25OHD is about 1000-fold higher than that of $1,25(OH)_2D$ in blood, the latter has far higher affinity for the vitamin D receptor and normally determines the degree of vitamin D receptor activation. Calcitriol binds to intracellular receptors in target cells and causes gradual changes in the nuclei of those cells. The vitamin D receptor is highly homologous to the receptors for other steroids and to those for thyroid hormone and retinoic acid. Although vitamin D receptors are present in many organs, only those in duodenal mucosa have been established as important in normal physiology.

TABLE 211–3. EFFECTS OF PRINCIPAL CALCIOTROPIC HORMONES

Hormone	Principal Target Tissues	Action
Parathyroid hormone	Renal proximal convoluted tubule	Increase serum $1,25(OH)_2D$
	Renal distal convoluted tubule	Increase calcium reabsorption
	Renal proximal and distal convoluted tubules	Decrease phosphate reabsorption
	Bone	Increase calcium and phosphate resorption
Calcitonin	Bone	Decrease calcium and phosphate resorption
$1,25(OH)_2D$	Small bowel	Increase calcium absorption
	Bone	Increase calcium and phosphate resorption
	Parathyroid gland	Decrease release of PTH

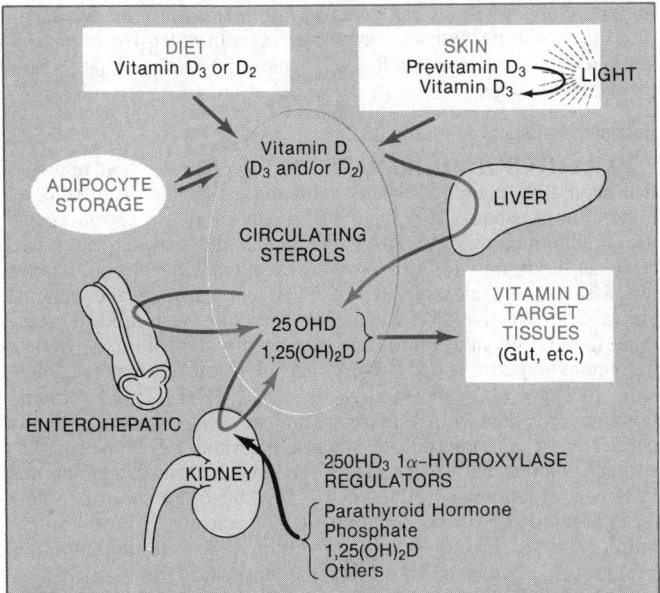

FIGURE 211-3. The vitamin D activation pathway. This involves steps in many different organs. Dysfunction at any step can have clinically important consequences.

INTESTINAL ACTIONS OF CALCITRIOL. Calcitriol $(1,25(OH)_2D)$ increases the flux of calcium from the intestinal lumen to blood. Calcitriol, to a much lesser extent, increases the flux of phosphate and magnesium from intestinal lumen to blood. Calcium, magnesium, and phosphate ions have specific processes for their intestinal transport. Calcitriol induces in duodenal mucosa high concentrations of an intracellular calcium-binding protein, termed calbindin. Calbindin belongs to the calmodulin protein family, but its role, if any, in intestinal calcium transport is unknown.

SKELETAL EFFECTS OF CALCITRIOL. The principal effects of calcitriol on bone (antirachitic effects) are indirect results of its action to promote calcium influx from intestinal lumen to blood. The deficient mineralization in vitamin D deficiency states is the consequence of the combination of low calcium in blood and low phosphate in blood, the latter resulting from the renal phosphate-wasting effects from secondary hyperparathyroidism.

The supraphysiologic concentrations of vitamin D metabolites sometimes reached during pharmacotherapy can raise blood calcium in part by increasing osteoclast numbers and activity.

OTHER EFFECTS OF CALCITRIOL. Calcitriol can inhibit PTH biosynthesis and secretion; the direct negative effects of calcitriol might contribute a form of short-loop negative feedback to parathyroid function. Calcitriol exerts direct effects on the renal enzymes that hydroxylate 25OHD; calcitriol inhibits the 25OHD$_3$ 1α-hydroxylase and stimulates the other hydroxylases that catabolize 25OHD in the renal tubule and in other tissues. Possibly important effects of calcitriol in skin and hair are suggested by its protective effect on psoriatic skin at pharmacologic doses and by the striking association of total alopecia with the rare syndrome of severely defective vitamin D receptors. Vitamin D receptors are present in many additional organs, but no role for them has been identified in normal physiology.

Other Hormones

SEX STEROIDS. Sex steroids, particularly estrogens, have slow but extremely important anabolic effects on bone. The effects are exerted directly on the bone organ, perhaps through receptors in the osteoblast. Estrogen deficiency results in accelerated bone remodeling with disproportionate bone resorption, particularly in trabecular bone.

GLUCOCORTICOIDS. Glucocorticoids affect many of the cells that contribute to mineral metabolism. The most striking effect is bone thinning that results from high glucocorticoid concentrations. This thinning is probably a consequence mainly of inhibited osteoblasts. In addition, glucocorticoids antagonize the actions of vitamin D metabolites by unknown mechanisms.

THYROID HORMONE. Thyroid hormones also have direct effects on bone cells. Excess of thyroid hormones causes increased release of calcium from bone. The skeletal consequences of deficient thyroid hormone are most evident in the disordered growth of cartilaginous epiphyses associated with congenital hypothyroidism.

GROWTH HORMONE. Growth hormone stimulates the growth of bone and cartilage, in part by stimulating local production of IGF-1 by osteoblasts and chondrocytes.

ADAPTATIONS TO DISRUPTIONS OF MINERAL METABOLISM

Two principal calciotropic hormones, PTH and $1,25(OH)_2D$, interact with each other and with multiple target tissues to control the metabolism of calcium, phosphate, and, to a lesser degree, magnesium (Fig. 211–4 and Table 211–3). These hormones allow for adaptations over time intervals that are short (minutes) or long (months).

Blood levels of ionized calcium are sustained at nearly invariant levels, with minimal diurnal changes reflecting mainly the sudden rises of calcium influx with meals. Serum levels of PTH and $1,25(OH)_2D$ also show only modest diurnal changes under normal conditions. Serum phosphate typically has broad diurnal fluctuations, with a nadir around 9:00 A.M. and peaks at around 6:00 P.M. and 4:00 A.M.

CALCIUM EXCESS STATES. States with long-term excess or deficiency of calcium are associated with deviations at multiple steps of the integrated mineral homeostasis system. The most common calcium excess state in adults is primary overfunction of the parathyroid gland. Of course, this has the potential to distort most of the normal calcium regulatory processes. Primary hyperparathyroidism results in high blood levels of PTH and often of $1,25(OH)_2D$ as well. The results are combinations of increased calcium influx to blood dependent upon the evoked dysfunctions in intestinal, skeletal, and renal pools of calcium. A very different integrated metabolic pattern results when calcium excess is caused by dysfunction outside the parathyroid—for example, with osteolytic metastases, skeletal immobilization, or dietary calcium overload (milk-alkali syndrome). In the latter disturbances, the parathyroid gland reacts appropriately and becomes suppressed by the increase of ionized calcium in blood; blood concentrations of PTH and $1,25(OH)_2D$ become low. The abnormally high filtered load of calcium without the anticalciuric effects of PTH results in severe hy-

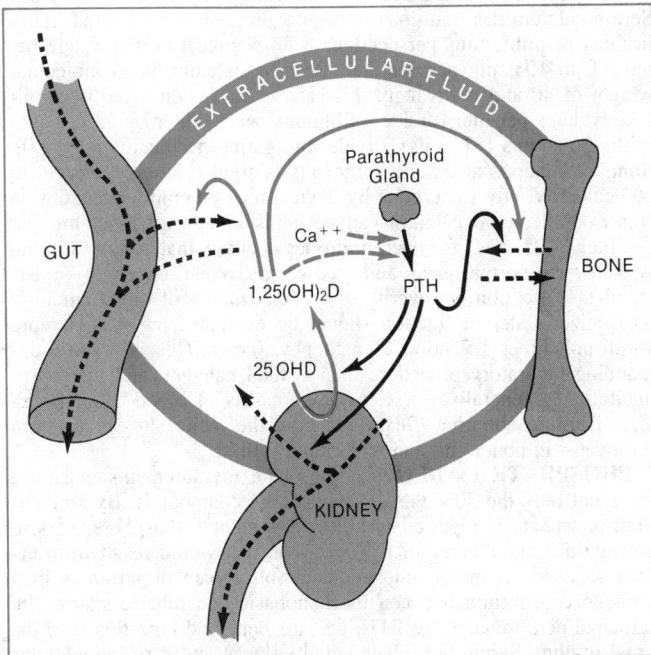

FIGURE 211-4. Integrated control of secretion and actions of parathyroid hormone (PTH) and calcitriol ($1,25(OH)_2$ vitamin D = $1,25(OH)_2D$) with emphasis on calcium fluxes. Solid black lines show secretion of PTH and calcitriol. Interrupted black lines are calcium fluxes. Solid red lines show stimulatory effects; interrupted red lines show inhibitory effects.

percalciuria; irreversible renal damage can occur over a period of only a few weeks.

CALCIUM DEFICIENCY STATES. Calcium deficiency states generally result in the parathyroid gland's recognizing the signal of a low ionized calcium level in blood. Increased PTH secretion (within seconds), increased PTH biosynthesis (within days), and parathyroid cell hyperplasia (within weeks) activate the response pathways. The consequences of this secondary hyperparathyroidism are increased renal tubular secretion of 1,25(OH)$_2$D (if there is not underlying deficiency of 25OHD or 1α-hydroxylase) and increased net calcium flux into blood from the intestinal lumen, from bone, and from the renal tubular lumen. The relative contribution of each calcium pool to this integrated response depends in part on the chronic state of that pool and on the relative levels of PTH and calcitriol. Serum calcium typically begins to fall below normal only when the osteolytic response to PTH or 1,25(OH)$_2$D becomes weakened (from depletion of readily exchangeable calcium pools or other types of tachyphylaxis). Secondary hyperparathyroidism has important effects on phosphate homeostasis by directly affecting bone and kidney, increasing phosphate influx from bone and causing a similar increase in phosphate efflux into urine. With forms of hypoparathyroidism, some residual components of mineral homeostasis can be sustained despite a deficiency of PTH and secondarily of 1,25(OH)$_2$D.

METABOLIC BONE DISEASES. Certain forms of metabolic bone disease are associated with dramatic imbalances in mineral flux to or from blood; these include increased calcium influx with aggressive osteolytic processes and decreased calcium influx with many forms of osteomalacia. Others, because they do not dramatically compromise the readily exchangeable pools of bone mineral, may have little or no long-term impact on the blood homeostatic system. For example, idiopathic osteoporosis has been categorized into two major forms (perimenopausal and aging associated), but no clear-cut changes in blood PTH or 1,25(OH)$_2$D as adaptations to altered serum calcium levels have been identified in either form.

USES OF LABORATORY TESTING

Electrolytes in Blood

CALCIUM IN BLOOD. To stabilize blood albumin concentration, total calcium should be measured in the fasting patient who is seated or recumbent. Most laboratories measure it inexpensively and with high precision. A high or low calcium value during multichannel screening is often the first indication of a treatable disorder. Serum calcium has traditionally been expressed in the United States in units of milligrams per deciliter, with a typical normal range being 8.8 to 10.2 mg per deciliter. Because calcium has a molecular weight of 40 and is divalent, this can be easily converted into milliequivalents per liter (divide milligrams per deciliter by 2.0) or into millimolar units (SI units); divide milligrams per deciliter by 4.0). Simple equations allow measurements of total calcium in serum to be "corrected" for distortions by deviation of albumin concentration (for example, total calcium can be adjusted upward by 1 mg per deciliter [0.25 mM] for each gram per deciliter that serum albumin is below the normal mean and vice versa). When uncertainty exists about the direction or severity of an abnormality of blood calcium, the ionized calcium fraction should be evaluated, as it is a more valid and direct reflection of pathophysiology. This is a more demanding laboratory procedure than is total calcium, and the reproducibility is generally worse. An abnormality of blood calcium can arise from an abnormal flux to or from the major sites of calcium turnover—in bone, gut, and renal tubular fluid.

PHOSPHATE IN BLOOD. Phosphate measurements in serum represent only the 30% that is in inorganic compounds. By convention, phosphate is reported in units of elemental phosphorus. These conventions avoid some of the confusion that would result from efforts to consider molar anion content (phosphate in serum is in a variable equilibrium between its monobasic and dibasic states). Its principal determinants are PTH, age, gender, food ingestion, and diurnal rhythm. Serum phosphate is only a weak index of intracellular phosphate stores. Its normal range is far wider than that for calcium.

MAGNESIUM IN BLOOD. Serum magnesium, like phosphate, is determined by its threshold for renal excretion and by total body pools. Primary disturbance of magnesium in blood is unusual, but

important abnormalities can occur during major illnesses; for example, in association with chemotherapy or with extensive burns, tissue necrosis may increase blood magnesium levels, or large fluid losses could depress it.

Hormones in Blood

PARATHYROID HORMONE. PTH is often the first regulator that should be examined when evaluating a possible disturbance of mineral homeostasis. Two types of immunoassay are in widespread use. Radioimmunoassay (RIA) directed at the mid-region or carboxy terminus of PTH can provide excellent clinical correlations; this assay is an index equally of PTH secretion rate and of renal clearance of inactive PTH fragments. Therefore, with mild to severe renal failure, the values must be interpreted with caution. A two-site immunoradiometric assay (IRMA) can give a result that is a more valid indicator of intact, biologically active PTH. Clinical correlations are excellent with this assay, and no adjustment is generally needed for renal compromise. Because the intact PTH molecule has a much shorter half-time than do its inactive fragments, normal PTH concentrations with the "intact" IRMA are far lower than with the mid-region or carboxy terminus RIA (typically, 10 to 60 pg per milliliter versus 100 to 400 pg per milliliter, the latter normal range being especially dependent on the laboratory standard).

CALCITONIN. Calcitonin is measured by RIA. Clinical uses are limited. When the RIA is used in family screening for early stages of C cell neoplasia, it is particularly important that the laboratory provide normal ranges adjusted for the selected C cell challenge protocol and the patient's age.

25-HYDROXYVITAMIN D. Vitamin D itself is rarely measured in clinical settings. Two different vitamin D metabolites can be measured by most laboratories. It is essential to understand that these two metabolites, 25OHD and 1,25(OH)$_2$D, are usually indicators of two entirely different types of process. Serum 25OHD is a useful index of vitamin D nutritional status. It is also a good index of sterol absorption. Low levels can arise from deficiency of sunlight, from deficiency of vitamin D nutritional supplementation, from fat malabsorption, and from accelerated hepatic catabolism of vitamin D metabolites. Because the body easily compensates for concentrations above normal, dangerously high levels occur only when consuming pharmacologic doses of vitamin D or of 25OHD.

1,25-DIHYDROXYVITAMIN D. 1,25(OH)$_2$D measurement in serum gives an index of the steroid hormone whose renal production is usually finely regulated by blood PTH. Even with vitamin D intoxication, the serum levels of 1,25(OH)$_2$D may be appropriately low because of this regulatory system. Serum 1,25(OH)$_2$D has only limited diagnostic use. However, certain states can be associated with otherwise unexplainable mineral disturbances that reflect high levels of 1,25(OH)$_2$D (sarcoidosis and other granulomas) or low levels (certain renal tubular disorders, such as X-linked hypophosphatemia).

Blood Indices of Bone Disturbance

Alkaline phosphatase enzyme in serum is an index of its sources in bone, liver, and placenta and of its excretion by the biliary tree. With increased osteoblastic activity, the amount of skeletal alkaline phosphatase enzyme in serum can rise dramatically. Skeletal alkaline phosphatase can be measured selectively through its physicochemical properties (it is the heat-labile component of total alkaline phosphatase) or otherwise (e.g., by RIA, a topic for research in several centers). High skeletal alkaline phosphatase levels can point to high bone turnover (hyperparathyroidism, Paget's disease). Specific portions of procollagen type I and other bone-specific proteins are also under investigation as possible specific indicators of skeletal processes. Osteocalcin (sometimes called bone gla-protein) is another osteoblast-specific protein that has been useful in some long-term studies of bone turnover, but its insensitivity to diffuse bone pathology has compromised its broad clinical use.

Measurements on the Skeleton

BONE RADIOGRAPHS AND SCANS. Standard radiography is often the starting point in evaluating bone disorders. Images can be specific for numerous conditions or can direct further diagnostic procedures (i.e., bone biopsy) to sites of focal disturbance. A bone scan with technetium-99m diphosphonate may identify a local disturbance that is not accompanied by radiographic change; the label adsorbs to bone mineral, and increased local blood flow without fracture is sufficient to give a positive signal.

BONE MASS INDICES. Bone mass can be measured noninvasively with a variety of techniques. These include dual-channel radiographs, single- and dual-channel photon absorptiometry, radiographs with computed tomography (CT), and other methods under development. The choice of one over another should depend largely on local expertise. For sequential studies in a patient, these methods are compromised, to varying degrees, by high cost and lack of precision.

BONE BIOPSY. Bone biopsy can be the final diagnostic tool in identifying local or generalized bone disturbances. It can be particularly useful in distinguishing osteomalacia from osteoporosis. Maximal information about the bone formation process can be obtained by prior administration of two pulses of tetracyclines 14 days apart (tetracyclines selectively adsorb to the mineralization front of osteoid and provide a fluorescent signal in the biopsy). When considering this test, the clinician should consult persons knowledgeable about its indications and the details of its processing.

Analyses of the Intestines in Mineral Metabolism

Specific tests of intestinal function are rarely used in current clinical practice. Metabolic balance studies are time consuming and expensive. Calcium absorption studies with radioactive or stable isotopes are not applied outside research settings. General indices of intestinal function are considered in other chapters.

Analyses of the Kidney and Urine

Renal biopsy should be done only for the standard indications related to intrinsic or systemic diseases in the kidney. Urinary excretion of hydroxyproline and other collagen metabolites is a useful index of bone resorption rates because 60% of urinary hydroxyproline is normally derived from collagen in bone. Pyridinum crosslinks, another collagen by-product in urine, may prove to be a more useful index of bone resorption.

Urinary excretion of calcium, magnesium, or phosphate is useful in screening for total body excess or deficiency of any of these minerals. Urinary excretion of calcium is central in the evaluation of urolithiasis. More detailed discussion of the workup of urolithiasis is presented elsewhere (see Ch. 88).

Aurbach GD, Marx SJ, Spiegel AM: Parathyroid hormone, calcitonin, and the calciferols. *In* Wilson JD, Foster DW (eds.): Williams Textbook of Endocrinology. 8th ed. Philadelphia, WB Saunders, 1991. *Detailed review of mineral metabolism with emphasis on calciotropic hormones. Other major textbooks of endocrinology have similar chapters.*

Avioli LV, Krane SM (eds.): Metabolic Bone Diseases and Clinically Related Disorders. 2nd ed. Philadelphia, WB Saunders, 1990. *A detailed review of the entire field from multiple authors.*

Favus MJ (ed.): Primer on Metabolic Bone Diseases and Disorders of Mineral Metabolism. Kelseyville, Calif., American Society for Bone and Mineral Research, 1990. *Concise chapters that quickly advance the reader to research on a topic.*

212 VITAMIN D
Bess Dawson-Hughes

Vitamin D, originally described as a fat-soluble vitamin that would prevent rickets, is a steroid hormone. Natural forms of the vitamin include cholecalciferol or vitamin D_3, produced in skin of humans and other vertebrates, and ergocalciferol or vitamin D_2, derived from plants and fungi. These forms are metabolized similarly in humans, and the term *vitamin D* in this chapter applies to both forms. To become biologically active, vitamin D is hydroxylated first in the liver to 25-hydroxyvitamin D (25(OH)D) and then in the kidney to form 1,25-dihydroxyvitamin D (1,25(OH)$_2$D).

SOURCES. Rich dietary sources of vitamin D include fish oil, cod liver oil, egg yokes, and fortified milk. Vitamin D from food and supplements is absorbed in the distal ileum by a process that requires bile salts. Gastrointestinal disorders of mixing and fat emulsification, decreased transit time, and fat malabsorption reduce vitamin D absorption. Aging also reduces vitamin D absorption effi-

ciency by about 40%, and about half of this loss may occur after age 65. Adults in the United States, Europe, and Japan typically consume 100 to 150 IU of vitamin daily. Although the US recommended dietary allowance is 200 IU per day, 400 to 800 IU is increasingly recommended.

Vitamin D_3 is produced in the epidermal layer of the skin upon exposure to ultraviolet sunlight of wavelength 294 to 310 nm by photoconversion of the prohormone 7-dehydrocholesterol to previtamin D. The latter spontaneously isomerizes to vitamin D_3 over the 3 or 4 days following sun exposure and enters the circulation bound to vitamin D binding protein. Sun screens and the skin pigment melanin reduce cutaneous production of vitamin D_3 because they absorb solar ultraviolet light, leaving fewer photons available to initiate photosynthesis. Photoproduction declines with aging because of a twofold age-related reduction in epidermal 7-dehydrocholesterol concentration. Thinning of the skin and reduced sun exposure may also contribute to decreased vitamin D_3 production in the elderly.

In the heavily populated temperate zone, season and latitude regulate cutaneous vitamin D_3 production because they determine the intensity of ultraviolet rays reaching earth's surface. At 42 degrees North, the latitude of Boston, very little photosynthesis occurs between October and March and, in the winter, 25(OH)D levels typically decline by about 30% in ambulatory adults. This decline is accompanied by an increase in circulating levels of the bone-resorbing agent, parathyroid hormone (PTH).

METABOLISM. *Liver.* Vitamin D is hydroxylated by an hepatic microsomal cytochrome P-450 mixed-function oxidase to form 25(OH)D. This process is not tightly regulated and depends on the combined skin and dietary supplies of vitamin D. Several medications and diseases alter 25(OH)D metabolism. Anticonvulsants, rifampin, primidone, and other drugs that induce microsomal enzymes accelerate metabolism of 25(OH)D to inactive metabolites, thereby increasing the requirement for vitamin D. Cholestyramine increases the vitamin D requirement by binding 25(OH)D in the gut. Production of 25(OH)D is compromised by liver disease only when the disease is advanced.

Renal. In the final step of activation, 25(OH)D is 1α-hydroxylated in the proximal renal convoluted tubule to form 1,25(OH)$_2$D. Extrarenal production occurs in the normal placenta and sometimes in sarcoid and other granulomas. PTH and low blood levels of calcium and phosphorus promote renal 1,25(OH)$_2$D production. High blood levels of calcium and phosphorus and also 1,25(OH)$_2$D itself limit 1,25(OH)$_2$D production (Fig. 212–1). When 1α-hydroxylase is inhibited, 25(OH)D is metabolized by an alternate renal pathway to 24,25-dihydroxyvitamin D, a compound with no established function in humans. Advanced renal disease compromises 1α-hydroxylase, but the stage in renal failure at which 1,25(OH)$_2$D production starts to decline varies with calcium and phosphorus intake levels.

ACTIONS OF 1,25(OH)$_2$D. This hormone is part of the vitamin D/endocrine system that regulates blood calcium and bone mineralization by its actions on the intestine, bone, kidney, and other tissues (Fig. 212–2). 1,25(OH)$_2$D promotes absorption of intestinal calcium and phosphorus by acting on mucosal cell nuclear receptors to initiate the production of separate calcium- and phosphorus-binding proteins. These proteins ferry calcium and phosphorus across the intestinal mucosa. 1,25(OH)$_2$D is essential for both the formation and resorption components of bone remodeling. In concert with

TABLE 212–1. PHARMACOLOGIC PROPERTIES OF VITAMIN D METABOLITES

Metabolite	Time to Peak Serum Concentration	Onset of Hypercalcemic Action	Duration of Action
Ergocalciferol or cholecalciferol	—	12–14 hr*	6 mo or more
Calcifediol [25(OH)D]	4 hr	12–24 hr	15–20 days†
Calcitriol [1,25(OH)$_2$D]	2 hr	2–6 hr	1–2 days

* Therapeutic effect may take 10 to 14 days.
† Increased two to three times in renal failure.
From Dawson-Hughes B: Metabolic bone disease. *In* Bayliss TM (ed.): Current Therapy in Gastroenterology and Liver Disease. 3rd ed. Ontario, BC Decker, 1990.

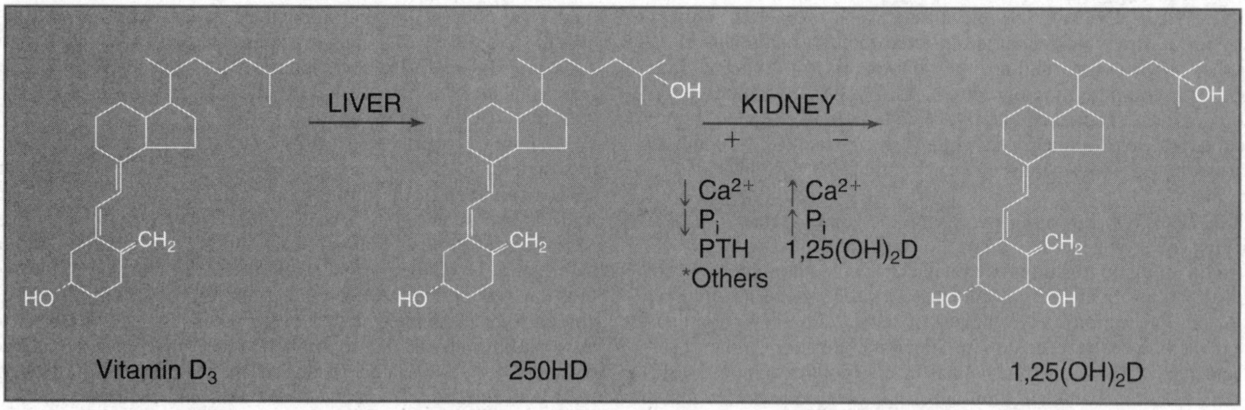

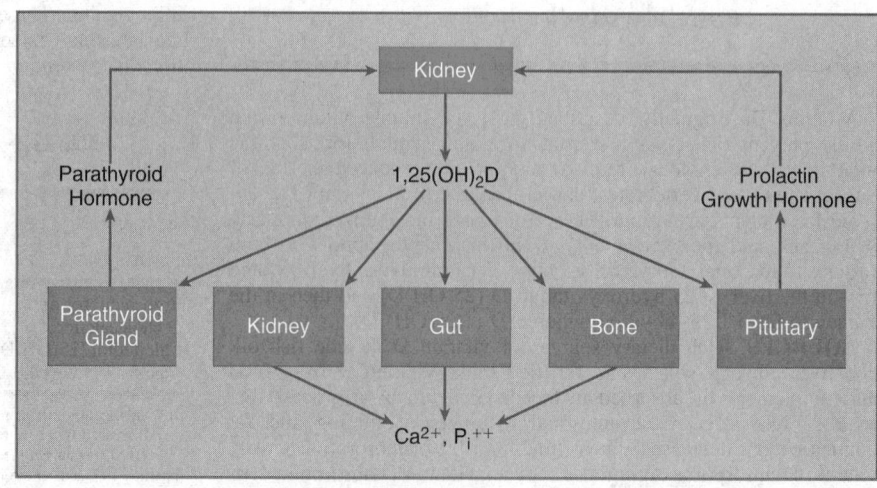

FIGURE 212–1. Activation of vitamin D. Estrogen, growth hormone, prolactin, placental lactogen, calcitonin, and insulin stimulate 1α-hydroxylase, but their role in the day-to-day regulation of 1,25(OH)₂D production is uncertain.

PTH, 1,25(OH)₂D stimulates bone resorption, perhaps by increasing the number of osteoclasts that are formed from macrophage stem cells. In addition to providing calcium for bone mineralization through increased intestinal absorption, 1,25(OH)₂D may also play a role in regulating osteoblast function. *In vitro*, 1,25(OH)₂D acts on osteoblast receptors to enhance production of alkaline phosphatase, osteocalcin, and several bone growth factors. In other actions, an elevated 1,25(OH)₂D level decreases PTH synthesis and release, and in concert with PTH, 1,25(OH)₂D reduces renal excretion of calcium.

PHARMACOLOGY. Selected properties of the major vitamin D metabolites are given in Table 212–1. Up to 99% of these three compounds circulates bound to vitamin D–binding protein, an α-globulin that protects them from rapid renal clearance. In nephrotic syndrome, the bound portion of each metabolite is reduced. Serum 25(OH)D reflects the solar and dietary contributions of vitamin D and is the best clinical measure of vitamin D status. Serum levels vary with sun exposure and intake, but typical values are vitamin D—1.5 ng per milliliter, 25(OH)D—35 ng per milliliter, and 1,25(OH)₂D—30 pg per milliliter.

HYPOVITAMINOSIS D. Vitamin D insufficiency contributes to osteoporosis (see Ch. 217), and more severe deficiency results in osteomalacia (see Ch. 213).

HYPERVITAMINOSIS D. Vitamin D toxicity causes hypercalcemia and/or hypercalciuria because of increased calcium absorption. In animals vitamin D also enhances bone resorption, but this has not yet been confirmed in people. The clinical manifestations of vitamin D intoxication are associated with hypercalcemia (see Ch. 214). Hypervitaminosis D can result from excess intake or from altered metabolism of the vitamin.

Excess Intake. Long-term ingestion of 60,000 IU of vitamin D or more per day is required to produce hypercalcemia or hypercalciuria in healthy individuals. Toxicity may result from dietary excess but more often occurs when vitamin D is given therapeutically, as for hypoparathyroidism. A study of six patients with vitamin D intoxication from drinking overfortified milk revealed that the homeostatic regulation of 1α-hydroxylase is sometimes overridden by very high levels of the substrate 25(OH)D. Two of the six patients had elevated and four maintained normal serum levels of 1,25(OH)₂D. The basis for hypercalcemia/hypercalciuria in the latter four is uncertain, although these findings demonstrate that at least one other vitamin D metabolite, perhaps 25(OH)D in very large amounts, influences calcium metabolism.

Altered Vitamin D Metabolism. Disordered calcium homeostasis sometimes occurs in granulomatous diseases, especially sarcoidosis, as a result of 1,25(OH)₂D production by macrophages in the granulomas. This hormone production is not regulated by factors that modulate renal synthesis of 1,25(OH)₂D. Hypercalcemia occurs in about 10% of patients with sarcoidosis and can be the presenting feature. Sun exposure produces more substrate for 1,25(OH)₂D synthesis and can exacerbate the hypercalcemia.

Treatment. Hypervitaminosis D of any origin is treated by restricting calcium intake, rehydration, and administration of glucocorticoids. Up to 60 mg of prednisone per day may be needed to normalize serum calcium in vitamin D intoxication. If fat stores of vitamin D are large, toxicity can persist for well beyond 1 year. Intoxication from treatment with excess 25(OH)D or 1,25(OH)₂D resolves more rapidly. Glucocorticoids in low to moderate doses inhibit 1,25(OH)₂D production in granulomas and promptly reverse hypercalcemia in sarcoidosis and related diseases.

Jacobus CH, Holick MF, Shao Q, et al.: Hypervitaminosis D associated with drinking milk. N Engl J Med 326:1173, 1992. *A careful documentation of clinical and biochemical aspects of vitamin D intoxication.*

Reichel H, Koeffler HP, Norman AW: The role of the vitamin D endocrine system in health and disease. N Engl J Med 320:980, 1989. *An extensive review of the vitamin D endocrine system.*

FIGURE 212–2. The vitamin D/endocrine system. The hormone 1,25(OH)₂D acts principally on the gut, bone, and kidney but also on other tissues to help regulate calcium (Ca²⁺) and phosphorus (Pᵢ) homeostasis. Parathyroid hormone regulates Ca⁺⁺ and Pᵢ homeostasis by direct actions on bone and kidney.

213 OSTEOMALACIA AND RICKETS

Marc K. Drezner

DEFINITION. Rickets and osteomalacia are diseases characterized by defective bone and cartilage mineralization in children and bone mineralization in adults. The abnormal calcification of cartilage occurs at epiphyseal growth plates, which also exhibit delayed maturation of the cartilage cellular sequence and disorganization of cell arrangement. The resultant profusion of disorganized, nonmineralized, degenerating cartilage causes widening of the epiphyseal plates with flaring or cupping and irregularity of the epiphyseal-metaphyseal junctions. The abnormal calcification of bone is restricted to the organic matrix at the bone-osteoid interfaces of remodeling tissue. The insufficient mineralization of newly formed matrix paradoxically results in enhanced bone volume and increased susceptibility to fractures or bone deformities. The various disorders associated with rickets and osteomalacia that have been identified and characterized to date are numerous (Table 213–1). Although the phenotypic expression of the defective bone and cartilage mineralization is similar in each of these, the associated biochemical abnormalities and the therapeutic approaches differ according to the pathogenetic defect. Therefore, when diagnosing rickets and/or osteomalacia, further systematic analysis is needed in order to determine cause and appropriate therapy for the disorder.

ETIOLOGY AND PATHOGENESIS. Mineralization of cartilage and bone is a complex process in which the calcium-phosphorus inorganic mineral phase is deposited in an organic matrix in a highly ordered fashion. Such mineralization depends on (1) the availability of sufficient calcium and phosphorus from the extracellular fluid; (2) adequate metabolic and transport function of chondrocytes and osteoblasts to regulate the concentration of calcium, phosphorus, and other ions at the mineralization sites; (3) the presence of collagen with unique type, number, and distribution of

TABLE 213–1. THE RICKETS AND OSTEOMALACIA SYNDROMES

I. Disorders of the vitamin D endocrine system
  A. Decreased bioavailability of vitamin D
    1. Deficient endogenous production
      a. Inadequate sunlight exposure
      b. Aging
    2. Nutritional deficiency
    3. Loss of vitamin D metabolites
      a. Nephrotic syndrome
      b. Peritoneal dialysis
  B. Vitamin D malabsorption
    1. Gastrointestinal disorders
      a. Partial/total gastrectomy
      b. Small bowel disease (e.g., celiac disease)
      c. Intestinal bypass
    2. Pancreatic insufficiency
    3. Hepatobiliary disease
      a. Biliary atresia
      b. Biliary obstruction
      c. Biliary fistula
      d. Cirrhosis
  C. Abnormal vitamin D metabolism
    1. Impaired hepatic 25-hydroxylation of vitamin D
      a. Liver disease
      b. Anticonvulsant therapy
    2. Impaired renal 1α-hydroxylation of 25-hydroxyvitamin D
      a. Hereditary vitamin D–dependent rickets type 1 (pseudo–vitamin D deficiency)
      b. Chronic renal failure
      c. Pseudohypoparathyroidism
  D. Target organ resistance to vitamin D and metabolites
    1. Hereditary vitamin D–dependent rickets type 2
      a. Hormone binding negative
      b. Defect in hormone-binding capacity
      c. Defect in hormone-binding affinity
      d. Deficient hormone-receptor nuclear localization
      e. Decreased affinity of the hormone-receptor complex
II. Disorders of phosphate homeostasis
  A. Dietary
    1. Low phosphate intake
    2. Ingestion of phosphate-binding antacids
  B. Impaired renal tubular phosphate reabsorption
    1. Hereditary
      a. X-linked hypophosphatemic rickets/osteomalacia
      b. Hereditary hypophosphatemic rickets/osteomalacia with hypercalciuria
      c. Autosomal dominant hypophosphatemic rickets
      d. Hypophosphatemic bone disease (nonrachitic hypophosphatemic osteomalacia)
      e. Adult-onset hypophosphatemic rickets
    2. Acquired
      a. Tumor-induced osteomalacia (oncogenous osteomalacia)
        (1) Mesenchymal, epidermal, and endodermal tumors
        (2) Fibrous dysplasia of bone
        (3) Neurofibromatosis
        (4) Linear nevus sebaceous syndrome
        (5) Light chain nephropathy
      b. Sporadic hypophosphatemic osteomalacia

C. General renal tubular disorders
  1. Fanconi's syndrome type 1
    a. Hereditary
      (1) Familial idiopathic
      (2) Cystinosis (Lignac-Fanconi disease)
      (3) Hereditary fructose intolerance
      (4) Tyrosinemia
      (5) Galactosemia
      (6) Glycogen storage disease
      (7) Wilson's disease
      (8) Oculocerebral renal syndrome (Lowe's syndrome)
    b. Acquired
      (1) Renal transplantation
      (2) Multiple myeloma
    c. Intoxication
      (1) Cadmium
      (2) Lead
      (3) Tetracycline (outdated)
  2. Fanconi's syndrome type 2
III. Metabolic acidosis
  A. Distal renal tubular acidosis
    1. Primary
      a. Sporadic
      b. Familial
    2. Secondary
      a. Galactosemia (after galactose ingestion)
      b. Hereditary fructose intolerance with nephrocalcinosis (after chronic fructose ingestion)
      c. Hypergammaglobulinemic states
      d. Medullary sponge kidney
    3. Acquired
      a. Ureterosigmoidostomy
      b. Drug-induced
        (1) Acetozolamide
        (2) Ammonium chloride
IV. Disorders of calcium homeostasis
  A. Dietary calcium deficiency
V. Abnormal bone matrix
  A. Fibrogenesis imperfecta ossium
  B. Axial osteomalacia
VI. Primary mineralization defects
  A. Hereditary
    1. Hypophosphatasia
      a. Perinatal disease
      b. Infantile disease
      c. Childhood disease
      d. Adult-onset disease
      e. Pseudohypophosphatasia
VII. Mineralization inhibitors
  1. Etidronate
  2. Fluoride
  3. Aluminum

cross-links; remarkable patterns of hydroxylation and glycosylation; and abundant phosphate content which collectively permit and facilitate deposition of mineral at gaps, "hole zones," between the distal ends of two collagen molecules; (4) maintenance of an optimal pH (approximately 7.6) for deposition of calcium-phosphorus complexes; and (5) low concentration of calcification inhibitors (e.g., pyrophosphates, proteoglycans) in bone matrix.

Many of the disorders of mineralization occur secondary to known defects in these control steps. In this regard, most disorders resulting in rickets and/or osteomalacia result from disorders in the vitamin D endocrine system (see Ch. 212). Traditionally, a direct role has been assumed for vitamin D or more properly its active metabolite, 1,25-dihydroxyvitamin D, on production of normal collagen matrix and regulation of bone mineralization. However, more likely the abnormal mineralization in these disorders results from an associated calcium and phosphorus deficiency that diminishes the driving force for calcification. Primary disorders of phosphate homeostasis also underlie a large number of the rachitic/osteomalacic disorders. Diminished gastrointestinal absorption or renal wasting of phosphorus limits this essential mineral in such disorders. The isolated deficiency of phosphorus alone or in conjunction with a frequently occurring aberration in vitamin D metabolism underlies defective mineralization. In accord with the complex regulation of bone mineralization, however, decreases in calcium or phosphorus do not account for the rickets and osteomalacia in all forms of the disease. Indeed, certain forms of rickets and osteomalacia occur in spite of a normal or even elevated calcium-phosphate product. In such diseases, altered pH, abnormal collagen matrix, or excessive concentration of calcification inhibitors underlies the abnormal mineralization. In other forms of the disease, the precise mechanism causing the defective mineralization remains unknown.

Inadequate mineralization in rickets occurs in the matrix of cartilage in the growing epiphyseal plate. These characteristic changes are confined to the maturation zone of the cartilage, whereas the resting and proliferative zones of the epiphyses exhibit normal histologic features. In the maturation zone, the height of the cell columns is increased and the cells are closely packed and irregularly aligned. Moreover, calcification in the interstitial regions of this hypertrophic zone is defective.

In bone, the abnormal mineralization results in accumulation of excess osteoid, a *sine qua non* for the diagnosis of osteomalacia in most instances (Fig. 213–1). A supranormal amount of osteoid, however, may also occur in disease states associated with accelerated bone turnover, such as hyperparathyroidism. In addition, reduced mineralization activity may be observed without hyperosteoidosis in osteoporosis. Establishing the diagnosis of osteomalacia histopathologically, therefore, requires documenting abnormal mineralization with excess osteoid. These defects are manifest in bone by an increase in the forming surface covered by incompletely mineralized osteoid, an increase in osteoid volume and thickness, and a decrease in the mineralization front (the percentage of osteoid-covered bone-forming surface undergoing calcification) or the mineral apposition rate. The amount of osteoid in bone and the mineralization dynamics are determined in 3- to 5-μm-thick sections of undecalcified bone by special stains and the fluorescence of previously ingested tetracycline that is deposited at calcification fronts (Fig. 213–1).

CLINICAL MANIFESTATIONS. The clinical features of rickets, although variable to some degree according to the underlying disorder, are primarily related to skeletal pain and deformity, bone fractures, slipped epiphyses, and abnormalities of growth. In addition, hypocalcemia, when present, may be severe enough to produce tetany, laryngeal spasm, and seizures.

In infants and young children, symptoms include listlessness, irritability, and, in some forms of metabolic rickets, profound hypotonia and proximal muscle weakness. Indeed, as the disease progresses and muscle weakness is present, children often are unable to walk without support. Throughout early life, classic skeletal deformities appear. By age 6 months, frontal bossing with flattening at the back is evident. Later, a lateral collapse of both chest walls (Harrison's sulcus) and rachitic rosary may appear. If untreated, progressive bony deformities result in bowing—particularly in the tibia, femur, radius, and ulna—and fractures. In addition, dental eruption may be delayed and, in those forms of the disease with

hypocalcemia or hereditary hypophosphatemia, enamel defects and inadequate dentin calcification occur, respectively.

In contrast, clinical signs of osteomalacia are nondescript. Indeed, the disease-specific abnormalities may be overlooked and features of an underlying disorder (e.g., malabsorption) may predominate. Symptoms, when present, may include diffuse skeletal pain and muscular weakness. The pain, often described as dull and aching, is generally worsened by activity and prominent around the hips, resulting in an antalgic gait. The muscle weakness is primarily proximal and frequently associated with wasting, hypotonia, and a waddling gait. This myopathy is seen in almost all forms of rickets and osteomalacia, X-linked hypophosphatemic rickets/osteomalacia notably excepted. Clinical improvement in the myopathy usually results from specific therapy such as vitamin D repletion in nutritional osteomalacia, phosphate supplementation in disorders marked by renal phosphate wasting, or correction of acidosis. Fractures of the ribs, vertebral bodies, and long bones may occur and lead to progressive deformities, as well as point tenderness on palpation.

The radiographic abnormalities in both rickets and osteomalacia reflect the histopathologic changes. In rickets, alterations are most evident at the growth plate, which is wide and flared and displays an irregular hazy appearance at the diaphyseal line secondary to uneven invasion of the recently calcified cartilage by adjacent bone tissue. The trabecular pattern of the metaphyses is also abnormal, the cortices of the diaphyses are thinned, and the shafts frequently are bowed.

In osteomalacia, there is usually a moderate decrease in bone density associated with coarsening of trabeculae and blurring of their margins. When secondary hyperparathyroidism is present, subperiosteal resorption in the phalanges and metacarpals, erosion of the distal ends of the clavicles, and bone cysts may be observed. A more specific radiographic abnormality is the presence of Looser's zones, also called pseudofractures or milkman's fractures, in the shafts of long bones. These are ribbon-like zones of rarefaction, ranging from a few millimeters to several centimeters in length and usually oriented perpendicular to the bone surface. Often, they occur symmetrically and most commonly are present at the medial aspect of the femurs near the femoral heads, in the metatarsals, or in the pelvis. Long-standing osteomalacia may also result in additional characteristic radiographic abnormalities, including biconcave collapsed vertebrae and a trefoil (or triangular) pelvis.

In patients with renal tubular disorders (see Ch. 82), increased rather than decreased bone density may be present. In spite of the increased bone mass, histopathologic evaluation of biopsies reveals an abundance of unmineralized osteoid, and bones remain subject to fracture. Thus, the increased density likely reflects replacement of marrow air space with osteoid.

Biochemical abnormalities in patients with rickets and osteomalacia vary with the cause of the disorder. However, the rachitic and osteomalacic syndromes may be divided into calciopenic and phosphopenic forms, as well as those in which mineral availability is apparently normal. In general, patients with the calciopenic diseases exhibit a low or marginally normal serum calcium level, a decreased serum phosphorus concentration, and (secondary) hyperparathyroidism. If vitamin D deficiency prevails, the serum 25(OH)D levels are characteristically low, generally < 3 ng per milliliter. In contrast, the serum 1,25(OH)$_2$D concentration may not be overtly decreased secondary to the prevailing hyperparathyroidism. Alternatively, a defect in vitamin D metabolism often results in an isolated deficiency of 1,25(OH)$_2$D while end-organ resistance to this active vitamin D metabolite increases the circulating level of calcitriol.

A primary abnormality of transepithelial phosphate transport in the nephron, resulting in renal phosphate wasting, underlies the majority of the phosphopenic disorders. As a rule, patients with these disorders maintain a normal serum calcium concentration, whereas the serum phosphorus is characteristically low. In contrast to the calciopenic forms of disease, the serum 25(OH)D and parathyroid hormone levels are normal in patients with hypophosphatemic disease. Moreover, affected subjects commonly maintain a normal (or mildly decreased) serum 1,25(OH)$_2$D level in spite of the prevailing hypophosphatemia, which should increase production of this active vitamin D metabolite. However, an elevated serum 1,25(OH)$_2$D concentration was recently reported in two rare genetic phosphopenic disorders, hereditary hypophosphatemic rickets with hypercalciuria and Fanconi's syndrome, type 2. Whereas the elevated cal-

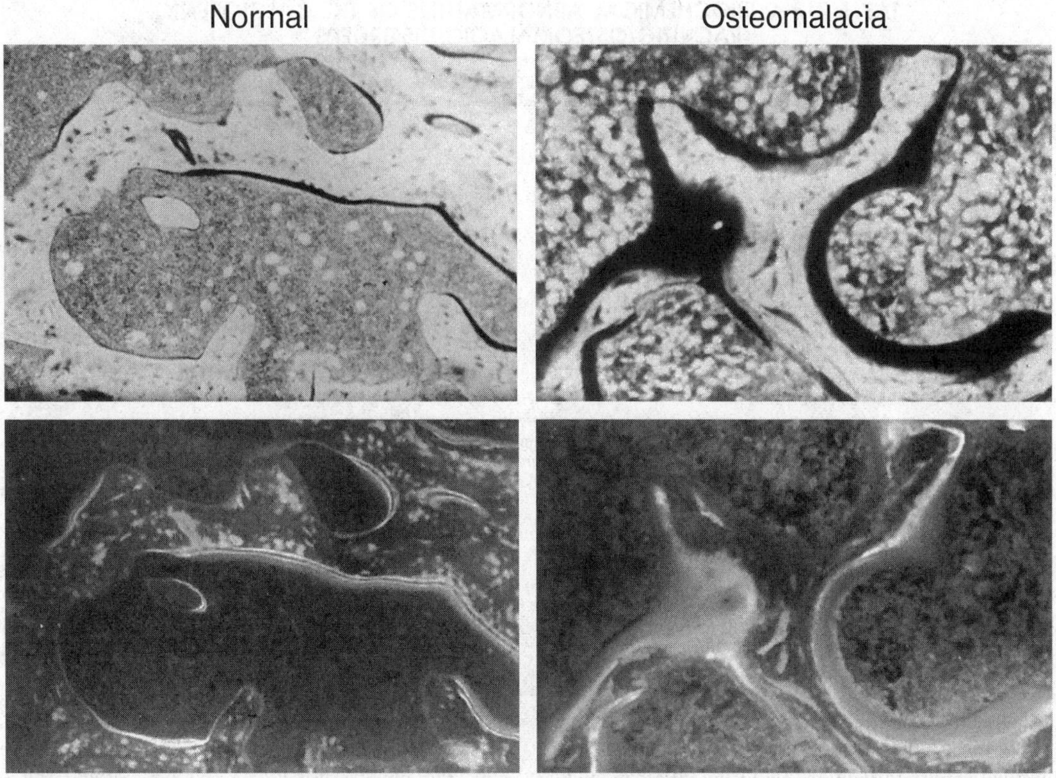

Normal

Osteomalacia

FIGURE 213–1. Microscopic appearance of bone biopsy sections from a normal and osteomalacic patient. In the upper panels the Villanueva-stained sections exhibit mineralized bone (white tones) covered by unmineralized osteoid seams (black tones). Normal bone has thin osteoid seams distributed over a limited portion of the bone surface. In contrast, osteomalacic bone is covered almost completely with thick osteoid seams. In the lower panels, the same bone sections are viewed under ultraviolet light in order to estimate mineralization activity by visualizing tetracycline labels. The normal bone reveals that the majority of the osteoid has crisp double tetracycline labels, indicative of normal mineralization activity. The osteomalacic bone, however, has evidence only of smeared tetracycline labels without the double label. Moreover, the tetracycline labels do not occupy the majority of the osteoid-bone interface. Such observations are representative of the abnormal mineralization that characterizes the osteomalacic bone disorder.

citriol level underlies increased gastrointestinal absorption of calcium and hypercalciuria in these diseases, the impact of abnormal vitamin D metabolism on the phenotypic expression of the phosphopenic disorders is less certain.

In those diseases with normal serum calcium and phosphorus concentrations, laboratory abnormalities are unique to each form of the disease. Nevertheless, alkaline phosphatase activity in plasma is generally elevated in all forms of rickets and osteomalacia. Even severe forms of disease, however, particularly those due to renal tubular disorders, may be associated with normal or only marginally elevated enzyme activity.

DIFFERENTIAL DIAGNOSIS AND THERAPY OF RACHITIC AND OSTEOMALACIC DISORDERS

Disorders of the Vitamin D Endocrine System

Rickets and osteomalacia due to disorders of the vitamin D endocrine system comprise a wide variety of calciopenic diseases. The variable biochemical abnormalities associated with these disparate disorders are summarized in Table 213–2. Although many of these diseases are no longer common causes of rickets and osteomalacia, others are often hidden causes of bone disease in a varying population of patients.

DECREASED BIOAVAILABILITY OF VITAMIN D. *Inadequate Sunlight and Nutritional Vitamin D Deficiency.* Adequate exposure to sunlight and fortification of dairy products with vitamin D have eliminated vitamin D deficiency secondary to inadequate endogenous production or nutrition in the majority of countries. However, in several populations, such as Asian immigrants in Britain, rickets and osteomalacia secondary to vitamin D deficiency occurs in neonates and infants, adolescents during pubertal growth, and less frequently among adults. Insufficient vitamin D intake secondary to using unfortified foods, racial pigmentation (which interferes with ultraviolet transmission through the skin), genetic factors, and social customs (such as avoiding sun exposure) contribute to

the development of disease in these subjects. Moreover, in the United States and other developed countries, a surprisingly frequent occurrence of vitamin D–deficiency osteomalacia has been recently recognized in alcoholics, institutionalized patients, and the elderly. Poor diet, in some cases including avoiding milk and milk products due to lactose intolerance, lack of sunlight exposure, and an age-related decline in the dermal synthesis of 7-dehydrocholesterol are among the factors predisposing to the vitamin D deficiency and consequent bone disease.

The clinical sequelae of decreased vitamin D bioavailability are generally preceded by a fall in circulating 25(OH)D levels. Measurement of this metabolite therefore serves to identify populations at risk for and facilitates early detection of vitamin D deficiency rickets and osteomalacia. Introducing vitamin D supplements (400 units per day) may, under these circumstances, prevent development of clinically significant disease.

Regardless, treating clinically evident vitamin D–deficient rickets and osteomalacia invariably results in healing of the bone disease. The disorder is best treated with vitamin D and restoration of normal dietary calcium and phosphorus intake. Ergocalciferol (vitamin D_2) is preferred because it provides the missing substrate that submits to physiologic regulation of vitamin D metabolite production.

Vitamin D Malabsorption. Gastrointestinal malabsorption associated with diseases of the small intestine, hepatobiliary tree, and pancreas may result in decreased absorption of vitamin D and/or depletion of endogenous 25(OH)D stores due to abnormal enterohepatic circulation. In general, malabsorption of vitamin D occurs as a consequence of steatorrhea, which disturbs fat emulsification and chylomicron facilitated absorption (see Ch. 103). Such abnormalities often are associated with rickets and/or osteomalacia. However, most affected patients are asymptomatic, and many exhibit only reduced bone volume rather than evidence of defective bone mineralization. Intestinal bypass surgery and adult celiac disease are common examples of disorders in which vitamin D malabsorption

TABLE 213–2. BIOCHEMICAL ABNORMALITIES OF THE CALCIOPENIC RACHITIC/OSTEOMALACIC DISORDERS

	VDDR	CRF	HVDDR 1	HVDDR 2	HP	PSH
Biochemistries						
Calcium	⇓	⇓	⇓	⇓	⇓	⇓
Phosphorus	N/⇓	⇑	N/⇓	N/⇓	⇑	⇑
Alkaline phosphatase	⇑	⇑	⇑	⇑	N/⇑	N/⇑
Parathyroid hormone	⇑	⇑	⇑	⇑	⇓	⇓
25(OH)D	⇓	N/⇓	N	N	N	N
1,25(OH)$_2$D	⇑	⇓	⇓	⇑	⇓	⇓
Renal function						
Urinary phosphorus	⇑	⇓	⇑	⇑	⇓	⇓
Urinary calcium	⇓	⇓	⇓	⇓	⇓	⇓
Gastrointestinal function						
Calcium absorption	⇓	⇓	⇓	⇓	⇓	⇓
Phosphorus absorption	⇓	⇓	⇓	⇓	⇓	⇓

VDDR = vitamin D–deficiency rickets (including sunlight or nutritional deficiency, vitamin D malabsorption, inhibition of 25-hydroxylation); CRF = chronic renal failure; HVDDR 1 = hereditary vitamin D–dependent rickets type 1; HVDDR-2 = hereditary vitamin D–dependent rickets type 2; HP = hypoparathyroidism; PSH = pseudohypoparathyroidism.
N = normal; ⇓ = decreased; ⇑ = increased; N/⇓ = normal or decreased; N/⇑ = normal or increased.

occurs and in which the suspicion for osteomalacia should remain high. In contrast, patients with cholestatic liver disease, extrahepatic biliary obstruction, and diseases of the distal portions of the small intestine, such as regional enteritis, may develop bone disease secondary not only to poor vitamin D absorption but to disruption of enterohepatic circulation as well.

Osteomalacia may also develop in patients who have had partial or total gastrectomy for peptic ulcer disease or other indications. Loss of gastrointestinal acidity or malfunction of the proximal small bowel underlies the vitamin D malabsorption in such circumstances. Absence of sufficient absorbing surface or failure of intestinal mucosal cells to respond to vitamin D or its metabolites may also cause vitamin D malabsorption and consequent bone disease.

The prevalence of osteomalacia in patients with gastrointestinal malabsorption varies widely from country to country. However, as many as 25 to 50% of British and European patients with partial gastrectomy, inflammatory bowel disease, and cholestatic liver disease have bone biopsy–proven osteomalacia.

Treatment of established disease generally requires pharmacologic amounts of vitamin D or its metabolites to overcome the defective absorption and the aberrant enterohepatic circulation or to offset end-organ resistance at the intestinal mucosa. Most patients respond well to calcium supplements, 1 to 1.5 grams per day, and ergocalciferol, 1250 to 5000 μg per day. If the severity of malabsorption makes oral vitamin D ineffective, parenteral ergocalciferol, 12,500 to 25,000 μg intramuscularly once a month is a practical alternative. Because magnesium deficiency often co-exists in malabsorptive diseases and may slow healing of the osteomalacia, adjunctive therapy with magnesium oxide may facilitate bone mineralization.

ABNORMAL VITAMIN D METABOLISM. *Liver Disease.* Because vitamin D is hydroxylated in the liver to form 25(OH)D, patients with severe parenchymal or obstructive hepatic disease (see Ch. 114) may have reduced production of this metabolite. These patients, however, rarely manifest biochemical or histologic evidence of osteomalacia. Indeed, an overt decrease of 25(OH)D generally requires concomitant nutritional deficiency or interruption of the enterohepatic circulation. Consequently, therapy for biopsy-proven osteomalacia, when present, is similar to that secondary to malabsorption of vitamin D.

Drug-Induced Disease. Decreased circulating levels of 25(OH)D may also occur in patients treated with drugs such as phenytoin or phenobarbital. This defect in vitamin D metabolism is due to induction of hepatic microsomal enzymes that metabolize 25(OH)D to inactive metabolites. Secondary to this abnormality and/or to the direct inhibitory effects of these drugs on intestinal calcium absorption and parathyroid hormone (PTH)–mediated calcium mobilization from bone, treated subjects often exhibit a decreased level of ionized calcium. These multiple influences commonly result in a bone disorder that may be mild osteomalacia or hyperparathyroid bone disease. Treatment of the bone disease and hypocalcemia generally requires modest vitamin D supplementation (150 to 400 μg per week).

Vitamin D–Dependent Rickets Type 1 (Pseudovitamin D Deficiency). Limited production of 1,25(OH)$_2$D due to hereditary or acquired diseases represents another abnormality of vitamin D metabolism that invariably results in rickets or osteomalacia. Vitamin D–dependent rickets type 1 is such a genetic disorder, transmitted as an autosomal recessive trait and characterized by hypocalcemia, hypophosphatemia, and elevated alkaline phosphatase activity. As a result of the hypocalcemia, PTH levels are elevated and consequently urinary excretion of amino acids and phosphate enhanced. In addition to these biochemical abnormalities, within the first year of life patients exhibit muscle weakness and hypotonia, motor retardation, and stunted growth. With progression patients develop the classic radiographic signs of vitamin D deficiency rickets and bone biopsy evidence of osteomalacia. Further, affected subjects have a decreased serum 1,25(OH)$_2$D concentration, likely due to an inherited deficiency of 25(OH)D-1α-hydroxylase activity, which limits production of this active vitamin D metabolite. This presumed abnormality has been substantiated by (1) experiments in humans that demonstrate serum calcitriol levels do not increase in response to classic stimuli of enzyme activity and (2) the absence of enzyme activity in renal cortical homogenates from the porcine homologue of this disease. Consistent with these observations, a physiologic dose of calcitriol (1 μg per day) generally promotes complete healing of the bone disease and resolution of the biochemical abnormalities, whereas a pharmacologic dose of vitamin D (20,000 to 100,000 U per day) or 25(OH)D (0.1 to 1.0 mg per day) is required to achieve similar effects. Regardless of the therapy used, in the majority of affected patients, therapy with vitamin D or its metabolites must be continued for life in order to prevent relapse. However, in a minority of subjects with a syndrome clinically identical to vitamin D–dependent rickets type 1, stopping treatment does not result in reappearance of biochemical or radiographic signs of the disease.

Chronic Renal Failure. Osteomalacia is common in patients with chronic renal failure and often tends to be the predominant type of renal osteodystrophy in younger patients (see Ch. 77). The defect in mineralization almost certainly results in part from a decreased conversion of 25(OH)D to 1,25(OH)$_2$D. Such abnormal vitamin D metabolism occurs secondary to either insufficient viable renal cortical tissue or the inhibitory effects of hyperphosphatemia on renal 25(OH)D-1α-hydroxylase activity. In addition, in some patients aluminum accumulated in bone underlies the abnormal mineralization. Indeed, the presence of aluminum may render the bone abnormality vitamin D resistant. Under such circumstances treatment with deferoxamine may be necessary to mobilize the aluminum from bone and other tissues and improve mineralization.

Hypoparathyroidism. Osteomalacia only rarely occurs in patients with hypoparathyroidism (see Ch. 214). Hypocalcemia and low or low-normal serum 1,25(OH)$_2$D are usually present and appear important in the pathogenesis of the bone disease. However, the underlying reason for the variable occurrence of bone pathology remains uncertain. The low serum 1,25(OH)$_2$D concentration results from the PTH deficiency. Bone pain suggests the diagnosis and generally the diagnosis depends on histomorphometric analysis of a bone biopsy. The majority of patients respond well to treatment with vitamin D and calcium supplements, but for unclear reasons some require therapy with $1,25(OH)_2D$.

Pseudohypoparathyroidism. In pseudohypoparathyroidism apparent bone and kidney resistance to PTH results in hypocalcemia, retention of phosphate, and low serum $1,25(OH)_2D$ (see Ch. 214). Surprisingly, however, affected patients often manifest bone disease marked by increased resorptive activity and osteomalacia. Indeed, severe demineralization, including frank osteitis fibrosa cystica and occasionally rickets or osteomalacia has been observed in 24 patients with pseudohypoparathyroidism. More commonly, the bone disease is silent and diagnosis often depends on histomorphometric analysis of a bone biopsy. Undoubtedly, hypocalcemia, secondary hyperparathyroidism, and low serum $1,25(OH)_2D$ are important cofactors in the pathogenesis of the disease. Patients respond well to pharmacologic amounts of vitamin D or replacement doses of $1,25(OH)_2D$.

TARGET ORGAN RESISTANCE TO CALCITRIOL. Vitamin D–Dependent Rickets, Type 2. Patients with clinical and biochemical abnormalities similar to those of subjects with vitamin D–dependent rickets type 1, but elevated $1,25(OH)_2D$ levels have recently been described. They have not only calciopenic rickets and/or osteomalacia but variably associated abnormalities, including alopecia, in 60% of patients, and in a minority of subjects additional ectodermal anomalies such as multiple milia, epidermal cysts, and oligodontia. The disease results from a group of genetic disorders that through heterogeneous mechanisms cause a decreased target organ responsiveness to $1,25(OH)_2D$. The defects identified to date are (1) failure of $1,25(OH)_2D$ binding to available receptors; (2) a reduction in $1,25(OH)_2D$ receptor–binding sites; (3) abnormal binding affinity of $1,25(OH)_2D$ to receptor; (4) inadequate translocation of $1,25(OH)_2D$-receptor complex to the nucleus; and (5) diminished affinity of the $1,25(OH)_2D$-receptor complex for the DNA-binding domain secondary to changes in the structure of receptor zinc-binding fingers. Effective treatment of this disease likely depends on the nature of the underlying abnormality. Thus, patients with deficient affinity of $1,25(OH)_2D$ to receptor and inadequate nuclear translocation respond to high-dose vitamin D or $1,25(OH)_2D$ with complete clinical and biochemical remission. In contrast, patients with other forms of the disease generally remain refractory to treatment with vitamin D or its analogues. However, every patient should receive a 6-month trial of therapy with supplemental calcium (1 to 3 grams per day) and vitamin D (400,000 to 1,200,000 U per day), 25(OH)D (0.05 to 1.5 mg per day), or, in more severe cases, $1,25(OH)_2D$ (5 to 60 μg per day). If the abnormalities of the syndrome do not normalize in response to this treatment, clinical remission may be achieved by administering high-dose oral calcium or long-term intracaval infusion of calcium.

Disorders of Phosphate Homeostasis (see Ch. 190)

Rickets and osteomalacia occur in association with a variety of disorders in which phosphate depletion predominates. Most typically, these diseases have in common abnormal proximal renal tubular function, which results in an increased renal clearance of inorganic phosphorus and hypophosphatemia. However, the biochemical abnormalities characteristic of these disorders are quite variable (Table 213–3).

IMPAIRED RENAL TUBULAR PHOSPHATE REABSORPTION. X-Linked Hypophosphatemic Rickets/Osteomalacia. X-linked hypophosphatemic (XLH) rickets/ostemalacia represents the prototypic phosphate-wasting disorder, characterized in general by progressively severe skeletal abnormalities, growth retardation, and X-linked dominant inheritance. However, the clinical expression of the disease varies widely. The mildest abnormality is hypophosphatemia without clinically evident bone disease, and the most common clinically evident manifestation is short stature. Nevertheless, the majority of children with the disease exhibit enlargement of the wrists and/or knees secondary to rickets, as well as bowing of the lower extremities. Additional early signs of the disease may include late dentition, tooth abscesses secondary to poor mineralization of the interglobular dentine, and premature cranial synostosis. In spite of marked variability in the clinical presentation, bone biopsies in affected children and adults invariably reveal osteomalacia, the severity of which has no relationship to gender, the extent of the biochemical abnormalities, or the severity of the clinical disability. In untreated youths and adults, the serum 25(OH)D levels are normal and the concentration of $1,25(OH)_2D$ is in the low-normal range. The paradoxical occurrence of hypophosphatemia and normal serum calcitriol levels is due to aberrant regulation of renal 25(OH)D-1α-hydroxylase activity, most likely caused by the abnormal phosphate transport. Indeed, studies in Hyp-mice, the murine homologue of the human disease, have established that defective regulation is confined to enzyme localized in the proximal convoluted tubule, the site of the abnormal phosphate transport.

A primary inborn error that results in an expressed abnormality in the renal proximal tubule (and perhaps the intestine), which impairs phosphate reabsorption (and absorption), underlies the pathogenesis of XLH. Although controversy exists regarding the character of the inborn error, studies in Hyp-mice suggest that elaboration of a humoral factor underlies the observed inhibition of phosphate transport in affected patients.

Choice of therapy for this disease has been remarkably influenced by an increased understanding of the pathophysiologic factors that affect its phenotypic expression. Thus, current treatment strate-

---

TABLE 213–3. BIOCHEMICAL ABNORMALITIES OF THE PHOSPHOPENIC RACHITIC/OSTEOMALACIC DISORDERS

	XLH	HHRH	ADHR	AHR	FS I	FS II	TIO
Biochemistries							
Calcium	N	N	N	N	N	N	N
Phosphorus	⇓	⇓	⇓	⇓	⇓	⇓	⇓
Alkaline phosphatase	⇑	⇑	⇑	⇑	⇑	⇑	⇑
Parathyroid hormone	N	⇓	N	N	N	⇓	N
25(OH)D	N	N	?	N	N	N	N
$1,25(OH)_2D$	(⇓)	⇑	?	(⇓)	(⇓)	⇑	⇓
Renal function							
Urinary phosphorus	⇑	⇑	⇑	⇑	⇑	⇑	⇑
Urinary calcium	⇓	⇑	?	⇓	⇓	⇑	⇓
Gastrointestinal function							
Calcium absorption	⇓	⇑	?	⇓	⇓	⇑	⇓
Phosphorus absorption	⇓	⇑	?	⇓	⇓	⇑	⇓

XLH = X-linked hypophosphatemic rickets; HHRH = hereditary hypophosphatemic rickets with hypercalciuria; ADHR = autosomal dominant hypophosphatemic rickets; AHR = adult onset hypophosphatemic rickets/osteomalacia; FS I = Fanconi's syndrome type I; FS II = Fanconi's syndrome type II; TIO = tumor-induced osteomalacia (Oncogenous osteomalacia).

N = normal; ⇓ = decreased; ⇑ = increased; (⇓) = decreased relative to the serum phosphorus concentration.

Modified from Econs MJ, Drezner MK: Bone disease resulting from inherited disorders of renal tubule transport and vitamin D metabolism. In Coe FL, Favus MJ: Disorders of Bone and Mineral Metabolism. New York, Raven Press, 1992, p 937.

gies for children directly address the combined calcitriol and phosphorus deficiency characteristic of the disease. Generally, the regimen includes a period of titration to achieve a maximum dose of calcitriol, 40 to 60 ng per kilogram per day in two divided doses and phosphorus, 1 to 2 grams per day in four or five divided doses. Although youths occasionally prove refractory to such therapeutic intervention, combined therapy often improves growth velocity, normalizes lower extremity deformities, and induces healing of the attendant bone disease. Of course treatment involves a significant risk of toxicity that is generally expressed as abnormalities of calcium homeostasis and/or detrimental effects on renal function. Therapy in adults is reserved for episodes of intractable bone pain and refractory nonunion of bone fractures.

Hereditary Hypophosphatemic Rickets with Hypercalciuria (HHRH).

This rare genetic disease is marked by hypophosphatemic rickets with hypercalciuria. In contrast to other diseases in which renal phosphate transport is limited, patients with HHRH exhibit increased $1,25(OH)_2D$ production. The resultant elevated serum calcitriol levels enhance the gastrointestinal calcium absorption, which in turn increases the filtered renal calcium load and inhibits parathyroid secretion. The clinical expression of the disease is heterogeneous, although initial symptoms generally consist of bone pain and/or deformities of the lower extremities. Additional features of the disease include short stature, muscle weakness, and radiographic signs of rickets or osteopenia. These various symptoms and signs may exist separately or in combination and may be pres-ent in a mild or severe form. Relatives of patients with evident HHRH may exhibit an additional mode of disease expression. These subjects manifest hypercalciuria and hypophosphatemia, but the abnormalities are less marked and occur in the absence of discernible bone disease. The majority of evidence indicates that HHRH is inherited by autosomal recessive transmission.

Patients with HHRH have been treated successfully with high-dose phosphorus (1 to 2.5 grams per day in five divided doses) alone. In response to therapy, bone pain disappears and muscular strength improves substantially. Moreover, the majority of treated subjects exhibit accelerated linear growth, and radiologic signs of rickets are completely absent within 4 to 9 months. Despite this favorable response, limited studies indicate that such treatment does not heal the associated osteomalacia. Therefore, further studies are necessary to determine if phosphorus alone is truly sufficient for this disorder.

Autosomal Dominant Hypophosphatemic Rickets (ADHR).

Although many investigators assume that all familial renal phosphate wasting disorders are X-linked, several studies have documented an autosomal dominant inheritance of a hypophosphatemic disorder similar to XLH. The phenotypic manifestations of this disorder include the expected hypophosphatemia due to renal phosphate wasting, lower extremity deformities, and rickets/osteomalacia. However, long-term studies indicate that a few of the affected female patients demonstrate delayed penetrance of clinically apparent disease and an increased tendency for bone fracture, uncommon occurrences in XLH. Limited information is available regarding other aspects of the disease, and no data exist regarding localization of the genetic defect.

An apparent *forme fruste* of ADHR—(autosomal dominant) hypophosphatemic bone disease—has many of the characteristics of XLH and ADHR, but recent reports indicate that affected children display no evidence of rachitic disease. Because this syndrome is described in only a few small kindreds and radiographically evident rickets is not universal in children with familial hypophosphatemia, these families may have ADHR. Further observations are necessary to discriminate this possibility.

Adult-onset Hypophosphatemic Rickets.

In some patients older than 15, an acquired form of hypophosphatemic rickets and osteomalacia occurs. Presenting symptoms in affected patients include debilitating bone pain, a significant myopathy, and Looser's zones on bone radiographs. The pathogenesis of the disorder involves renal phosphate loss due to abnormal proximal tubule function. Usually the inheritance is sporadic, but a propositus occasionally passes the disease in an X-linked dominant mode, suggesting that spontaneous mutation may cause expression of the disease. Al-

ternatively, the disorder may represent tumor-induced osteomalacia in a patient with an undetected benign tumor or malignancy.

Tumor-induced Osteomalacia (Oncogenous Osteomalacia).

Since initial recognition of this disease, there have been reports of approximately 70 patients in whom rickets and/or osteomalacia have been associated with a coexisting tumor. The coexistent tumors have been of mesenchymal origin in the majority of patients. The cardinal feature of this disease is remission of the unexplained bone disease after tumor resection. In general, affected patients present with bone and muscle pain, muscle weakness, and occasionally recurrent fractures of long bones. Biochemical abnormalities include renal phosphate wasting marked by an abnormally low renal tubular maximum for the reabsorption of phosphate per liter of glomerular filtrate, decreased gastrointestinal absorption of phosphate, and consequent hypophosphatemia. In general, serum 25(OH)D levels are normal and serum calcitriol is profoundly decreased or inappropriately normal relative to the hypophosphatemia. Generalized osteopenia, pseudofractures, and coarsened trabeculae, as well as widened epiphyseal plates in children, comprise the common radiographic abnormalities of the syndrome.

Most investigators agree that tumor production of a humoral factor(s) that may affect multiple functions of the proximal renal tubule underlies the pathogenesis of this syndrome. This possibility is supported by (1) the presence of phosphaturic activity in tumor extracts from two of three patients with tumor-associated osteomalacia; (2) the coincidence of amino aciduria and glycosuria with renal phosphate wasting in some affected subjects, indicative of complex alterations in proximal renal tubular function; and (3) diminished renal 25(OH)D-1α-hydroxylase activity in heterotransplanted tumor-bearing athymic nude mice and in renal tubule cell cultures exposed to tumor extracts.

In contrast to these observations, patients with tumor-associated osteomalacia secondary to hematogenous malignancy exhibit abnormalities of the syndrome secondary to a distinctly different mechanism. In these subjects the nephropathy associated with light-chain proteinuria results in decreased renal phosphate reabsorption and consequent hypophosphatemia. At least 15 patients with this form of the disorder have been reported.

The primary treatment of this disorder is complete resection of the associated tumor. However, recurrence or metastases of tumors often preclude such definitive therapy. In such cases, calcitriol (1.5 to 3.0 μg per day) alone or combined with phosphorus supplementation (2 to 4 grams per day) completely heals the attendant bone disease or significantly improves the biochemical and histologic abnormalities. Careful serial assessment of parathyroid function, serum and urinary calcium, and renal function are essential to ensure safe therapy in affected subjects.

Fanconi's Syndrome (see Ch. 82).

Rickets and osteomalacia are frequently associated with Fanconi's syndrome, a disorder characterized by phosphaturia and consequent hypophosphatemia, amino aciduria, renal glycosuria, albuminuria, and proximal renal tubular acidosis. Although a wide diversity of congenital and acquired diseases are associated with this syndrome (see Table 213–1), damage to the proximal renal tubule represents the common underlying mechanism of disease (see Ch. 175). Resultant dysfunction results in renal wasting of those substances primarily reabsorbed at the proximal tubule. The associated bone disease in this disorder is likely secondary to hypophosphatemia and/or acidosis, abnormalities that occur in association with aberrantly (Fanconi's syndrome type 1) or normally regulated (Fanconi's syndrome type 2) vitamin D metabolism.

Metabolic Acidosis

Osteomalacia occurs secondary to renal tubular acidosis and the acidosis that follows ureterosigmoidoscopy. The bone disease results from the multifactorial influence of acidosis, which decreases the conversion of amorphous calcium phosphate to hydroxyapatite at the mineralization front, induces renal phosphate wasting, and possibly interferes with calcitriol production. Systemic acidosis also enhances dissolution of bone and results in hypercalciuria. Affected patients have a normal serum calcium, a low normal or decreased serum phosphorus, and an elevated alkaline phosphatase. Secondary to hypercalciuria, nephrocalcinosis and renal lithiasis often occur. Bicarbonate therapy alone effectively treats the osteomalacia associated with metabolic acidosis, although administering vitamin D and calcium when starting therapy facilitates healing of the bone disease.

Primary Disorders of Bone Matrix

Intrinsic disorders of bone in which apparently abnormal matrix is produced but not normally mineralized are extremely rare and poorly understood. These diseases may result from presumed abnormalities of collagen or other proteins in the matrix or aberrant enzyme activity essential for normal mineralization.

ABNORMAL BONE MATRIX. *Fibrogenesis Imperfecta Ossium.* Fibrogenesis imperfecta ossium is a rare, sporadically occurring disorder characterized by the gradual onset of intractable skeletal pain in middle-aged men and women. Pathologic fractures are a prominent clinical feature, and patients typically become bedridden. Although the serum calcium and phosphorus are normal, alkaline phosphatase is invariably elevated. The bones have a dense, amorphous, mottled appearance radiologically and a disorganized arrangement of collagen with decreased birefringence histologically. Most likely, the disorganized collagen matrix limits normal bone mineralization.

Axial Osteomalacia. Axial osteomalacia is another unusual sporadically occurring disorder that generally affects only middle-aged men. The majority of patients present with only vague, dull, chronic axial discomfort that typically affects the cervical region most severely. Abnormal radiographic findings are limited to the pelvis and spine, where the coarsened trabecular pattern is characteristic of osteomalacia. Although the alkaline phosphatase may be increased, histopathologic studies reveal a normal lamellar pattern of collagen. However, the osteoblasts appear flat and inactive, suggesting that an osteoblastic defect and perhaps attendant abnormal matrix inhibit normal mineralization.

ABNORMAL ENZYME ACTIVITY. *Hypophosphatasia.* Hypophosphatasia is an heritable disorder characterized by a deficiency of the tissue nonspecific (liver/bone/kidney) isoenzyme of alkaline phosphatase, increased urinary excretion of phosphorylethanolamine, and skeletal disease that includes osteomalacia and rickets. The severity of clinical expression is remarkably variable and spans intrauterine death from profound skeletal hypomineralization at one extreme to lifelong absence of symptoms at the other. As a consequence, six clinical disease types are distinguished (see Table 213–1). The age at which skeletal disease is initially noted delineates, in large part, the perinatal (lethal), infantile, childhood, and adult variants of the disorder. However, affected children and adults may manifest only the unique dental abnormalities of the syndrome and accordingly are classified as having odontohypophosphatasia. Finally, patients with the rare variant, pseudohypophosphatasia, have the clinical/radiologic/biochemical features of the classic disease without a decrease in the circulating levels of alkaline phosphatase. These individuals have defects in cellular localization and substrate specificity of the enzyme.

Affected infants exhibit hypercalcemia, hypercalciuria, enlarged sutures of the skull, craniostenosis, delayed dentition, enlarged epiphyses, and prominent costochondral junctions. Genu valgum or varum may develop subsequently. In older children disease may be limited to rickets. Surprisingly, the disorder in adults is mild despite the presence of osteopenia. Indeed, the disease may be limited to slowly healing metatarsal fractures or loss or fracture of teeth. Nevertheless, 50% of patients have an history of early exfoliation of deciduous teeth and/or rickets, and disease may reflect re-expression of the childhood disorder.

The perinatal and infantile forms of disease are inherited as autosomal recessive traits. The mode(s) of inheritance for odonto-, adult, and childhood hypophosphatasia remains unclear, although an autosomal dominant disease transmission has been described in some kindreds with mild disease. The physiologic basis for the bone disease likely relates to the role of alkaline phosphatase in cleaving pyrophosphate, an inhibitor of bone mineralization. Failure to hydrolyze this physiologic substrate results in inorganic pyrophosphate elevated to levels sufficiently high to inhibit the mineralization process.

Therapy of this disease has been generally unrewarding. Thus, supportive treatment is important and may include craniotomy in children (to manage craniosynostosis) and, in adults, insertion of load-sharing intramedullary rods to treat fractures. Expert dental care is also crucial to minimize tooth loss and prevent consequent malnutrition in youths.

Mineralization Inhibitors

DRUGS. *Etidronate.* Disturbances in mineralization may be seen in patients consuming etidronate daily at doses >5 mg per kilogram body weight. The etidronate is deposited at the bone surface and inhibits osteoblast function, as well as directly inhibits calcium-phosphate crystallization.

Fluoride. Although multiple studies document that fluoride stimulates new bone formation, administering the drug in high doses without adequate calcium supplementation results in poorly mineralized bone, consistent with osteomalacia. The mechanism(s) by which fluoride alters osteoblast function and/or directly inhibits mineralization remains unknown.

Aluminum. Excess aluminum accumulation in bone inhibits mineralization and is a potential mechanism for the osteomalacia observed in patients with chronic renal failure, as discussed above. In addition, accumulation of aluminum in bone likely underlies the osteomalacia observed in patients treated with total parenteral nutrition. In such cases aluminum contamination of casein hydrolysate, as well as albumin, phosphate, and calcium solutions, provides the major source of the mineral. Changing total parenteral nutrition solutions from those with casein hydrolysate to those with purified amino acids has markedly reduced the incidence of clinically evident bone disease.

Brenner RJ, Spring DB, Sebastian A, et al.: Incidence of radiographically evident bone disease, nephrocalcinosis, and nephrolithiasis in various types of renal tubular acidosis. N Engl J Med 307:217, 1982. *Discussion of the relationship between rickets and metabolic acidosis in youths.*

Cai Q, Hodgson SF, Kao PC, et al.: Inhibition of renal phosphate transport by a tumor product in a patient with oncogenic osteomalacia. N Engl J Med 330:1645, 1994. *Presentation of evidence that tumor-induced osteomalacia is caused by ectopic secretion of a heat-labile factor with a mass between 8000 and 25,000 which inhibits renal tubular reabsorption of phosphate.*

Econs MJ, Drezner MK: Bone disease resulting from inherited disorders of renal tubule transport and vitamin D metabolism. *In* Coe FL, Favus MJ: Disorders of bone and mineral metabolism. New York, Raven Press, 1992, p 935. *Extensive review of the classic vitamin D–resistant rachitic and osteomalacic disorders. The subjects discussed include clinical features, differential diagnosis, genetics, and therapy.*

Friedman NJ, Drezner MK: Osteomalacia, genetic. *In* Bardin CW: Current therapy in endocrinology and metabolism. 4th ed. Philadelphia, B.C. Decker, Inc. 1991, p 421. *Review of the concepts underlying and the specific details of treatment for hypophosphatemic rickets in all its varieties of clinical presentation.*

Tieder M, Arie R, Modai D, et al.: Elevated serum 1,25-dihydroxyvitamin D concentrations in siblings with primary Fanconi's syndrome. N Engl J Med 319:845, 1988. *First report and discussion of Fanconi's syndrome type 2.*

214 THE PARATHYROID GLANDS, HYPERCALCEMIA, AND HYPOCALCEMIA
Allen M. Spiegel

THE PARATHYROID GLANDS

EMBRYOLOGY AND ANATOMY. Normally, there are four parathyroids, averaging 120 mg in total weight, but as many as 5% of normal individuals may have more than four glands. The superior parathyroids are derived from the fourth (more caudal) branchial pouches and remain almost stationary during embryologic development. Their typical final location is near the upper poles of the thyroid. Aberrant locations include the tracheoesophageal groove and the retroesophageal space. The inferior parathyroids develop (in association with the thymus) from the third branchial pouches. During normal development, they migrate caudally, assuming a final position near the lower poles of the thyroid. The inferior parathyroids may fail to descend, remaining near the angle of the jaw or, at the other extreme, may descend into the anterior mediastinum in association with the thymus.

SYNTHESIS AND SECRETION OF PARATHYROID HORMONE. Parathyroid hormone (PTH), together with vitamin D (see Ch. 212), is the principal regulator of ionized calcium in extracellular fluid. PTH is synthesized in the parathyroid glands as "preproparathyroid hormone," a precursor composed of 115 amino acids. A hydrophobic "leader" peptide of 25 amino acids is first cleaved from the amino-terminus to yield the prohormone, followed by cleavage of a basic, amino-terminal hexapeptide to yield the mature 84-amino-acid hormone. The latter is the principal secreted form of the hormone. There is no evidence for secretion of either the preprohormone or the prohormone. The prohormone possesses <0.2% of the biologic activity of the native 84-amino-acid hormone. The full biologic activity of the intact hormone resides within the amino-terminal 1–34 fragment, whereas fragments from the midregion and carboxy-terminal regions lack biologic activity (Fig. 214–1).

Secretion of PTH is regulated primarily by the concentration of ionized calcium in the extracellular fluid. Normally, PTH secretion is regulated at a "setpoint" that maintains serum ionized calcium within a relatively narrow range. Deviations below the setpoint stimulate, and deviations above the setpoint inhibit, hormone secretion. Effects of calcium on hormone secretion occur acutely (within minutes); low calcium levels have a slower stimulatory action on hormone synthesis. At high calcium concentrations, there is evidence for intracellular degradation of synthesized hormone and possible release of biologically inactive fragments. High magnesium ion concentrations in extracellular fluid, like high calcium concentrations, inhibit PTH secretion, but hypomagnesemia, unlike hypocalcemia, may inhibit hormone secretion and action. The active metabolite of vitamin D, $1,25(OH)_2D$ (dihydroxycholecalciferol), suppresses both secretion and synthesis of PTH. Reduction in $1,25(OH)_2D$ is a major factor contributing to increased PTH secretion in renal failure.

FORMS OF PARATHYROID HORMONE IN PLASMA. PTH circulates in plasma as the intact hormone secreted from the gland and as fragments derived either from glandular secretion (particularly in hypercalcemic states) or from peripheral metabolism of the intact hormone. Most, if not all, of these fragments lack biologic activity but may, depending on antibody specificity, contribute to immunoreactivity in plasma (Fig. 214–1).

PARATHYROID HORMONE ACTION. PTH acts directly on kidney and bone, and indirectly on the gut, to maintain the normal concentration of serum ionized calcium (see Ch. 211 for a complete discussion of mineral homeostasis). In the kidney, PTH (1) enhances reabsorption of calcium, and also magnesium, from the glomerular filtrate; (2) increases excretion of phosphate and of bicarbonate; (3) activates the enzyme (1α-hydroxylase) that forms the active metabolite, $1,25(OH)_2D$, of vitamin D. In bone, PTH causes the release of calcium and phosphate into the extracellular fluid. The hormone acts directly on osteoblasts, which secondarily affect osteoclast activity. The hypercalcemic action on bone and the anticalciuric action on kidney combine to raise the serum calcium level. The phosphatemic action on bone tends to blunt the hypercalcemic effect of the hormone owing to formation of calcium phosphate complexes, but the phosphaturic action counteracts the tendency to hyperphosphatemia. Stimulation of $1,25(OH)_2D$ formation promotes enhanced intestinal absorption of calcium, which also serves to maintain a normal serum calcium level (see Ch. 212). The clinical consequences of PTH excess (or in the opposite direction, hormone deficiency) follow directly from the actions of the hormone: (1) hypercalcemia, (2) a tendency to hypophosphatemia, (3) a tendency to reduced serum bicarbonate levels and hyperchloremia, (4) increased serum levels of $1,25(OH)_2D$, and (5) relative reduction in urinary calcium excretion and increase in urinary phosphate excretion for a given filtered load.

MECHANISM OF PARATHYROID HORMONE ACTION. The first step in PTH action is binding to specific plasma membrane–bound receptors on target cells in bone and kidney. Such receptors are coupled to guanosine triphosphate (GTP)–binding proteins—in particular, the Gs protein that links receptors to stimulation of adenylyl cyclase (for a more general description of the mechanism of polypeptide hormone action, see Ch. 199). Adenylyl cyclase catalyzes the formation of the "second messenger," cyclic adenosine monophosphate (cAMP), which mediates hormone action by stimulating the phosphorylation of critical intracellular proteins. A diagnostically useful peculiarity of PTH action on proximal renal tubular cells is that not only are cAMP levels increased intracellularly but, because of overflow into the extracellular fluid, urinary cAMP excretion is also increased. "Second messengers" other than cAMP may also mediate certain actions of PTH.

ASSAY OF PARATHYROID HORMONE IN PLASMA. Normally, the concentration of biologically active PTH circulating in

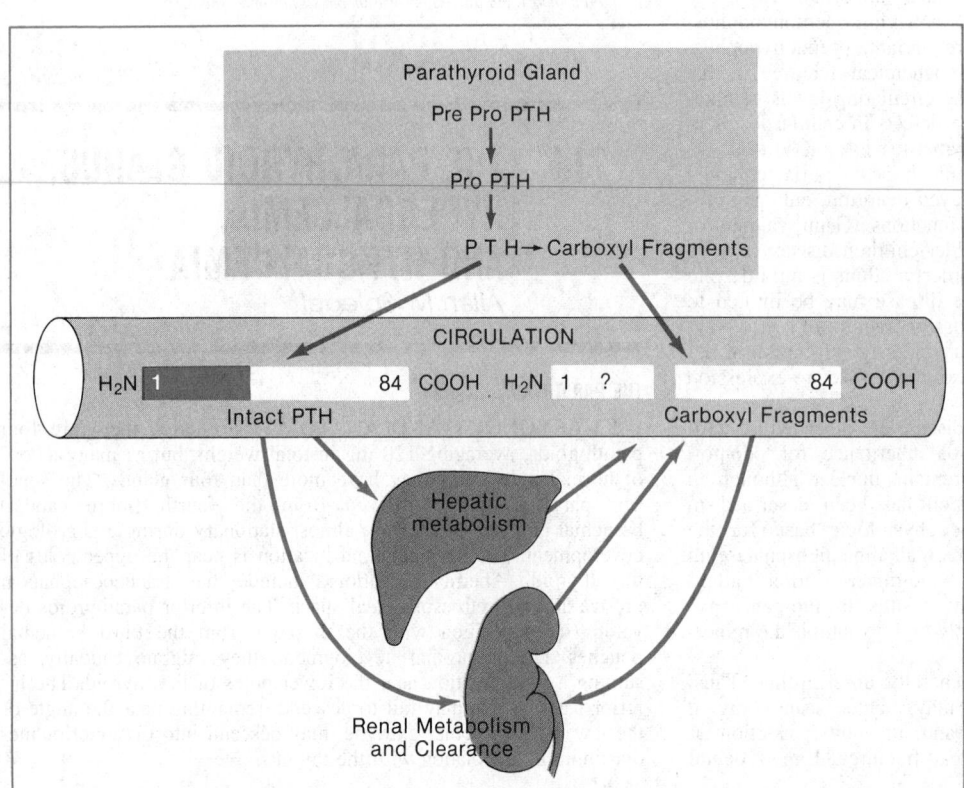

FIGURE 214–1. Secretion, metabolism, and clearance of PTH. *Top,* PTH is synthesized as a preprohormone and undergoes successive cleavages within the parathyroid to the mature (1–84), major secreted form of the hormone. Under certain conditions (e.g., hypercalcemia), some of the hormone is cleaved intracellularly into biologically inactive, carboxy-terminal fragments, which are also secreted. *Middle,* The major circulating forms of the hormone are the intact 1–84 species (the shaded region corresponds to the amino-terminal 1–34 portion possessing full biologic activity) and biologically inactive carboxy-terminal fragments. The presence of amino-terminal fragments in the circulation is unclear (indicated by "?"). *Bottom,* Peripheral metabolism of the hormone occurs in liver and kidney. The kidney also clears intact hormone and carboxy-terminal fragments from the circulation. (From Endres DE, Villanueva R, Sharp CF Jr, et al.: Measurement of parathyroid hormone. Endocrinol Metab Clin North Am 18:611, 1989.)

Figure labels: Parathyroid Gland / Pre Pro PTH / Pro PTH / P T H → Carboxyl Fragments / CIRCULATION / H_2N 1 — 84 COOH H_2N 1 ? — 84 COOH / Intact PTH / Carboxyl Fragments / Hepatic metabolism / Renal Metabolism and Clearance

plasma is quite low (<50 pg per milliliter). Bioassays sensitive enough to detect such low levels include a renal cytochemical assay and several assays based on stimulating cAMP formation in bone or kidney cells. Unfortunately, such assays are too cumbersome for routine clinical use. Total urinary cAMP excretion (normalized to creatinine clearance by simultaneously measuring serum and urinary creatinine) is an easily measured and sensitive index of circulating PTH bioactivity. It is elevated in primary hyperparathyroidism, is low in hypoparathyroidism, and falls within 1 hour of successful parathyroidectomy in patients with hyperparathyroidism. Increased urinary cAMP excretion, however, is not absolutely specific for PTH hypersecretion; parathyroid hormone-related peptide, secreted by many malignancies, similarly increases urinary cAMP excretion, and this must be taken into account when interpreting urinary cAMP measurements in subjects with hypercalcemia (see Hypercalcemia Associated with Malignancy, below).

Radioimmunoassays are sufficiently sensitive and practical for routinely measuring circulating PTH. Interpretation of assay results requires an understanding of what a particular antiserum is measuring. Immunoreactivity need not correlate with biologic activity. Indeed, the bulk of circulating PTH consists of biologically inactive mid-region and carboxy-terminal fragments. Because such fragments are cleared by the kidney, renal impairment causes them to accumulate at even higher concentrations (Fig. 214–1). Antisera with predominant specificity for mid-region and carboxy-terminal regions, therefore, measure predominantly biologically inactive hormone fragments. Such assays are reasonably useful for discriminating normal from hyperparathyroid subjects, but their utility is much more limited in subjects with renal failure. Even with normal renal function, such assays may show considerable overlap between patients with parathyroid-mediated hypercalcemia and those with non-parathyroid-mediated hypercalcemia. In part, this may reflect the parathyroid gland's release of inactive hormone fragments in non-PTH-mediated hypercalcemic states.

Most of these problems have been circumvented by the development of highly sensitive "two-site" immunoradiometric assays. Such assays employ two distinct antibodies, one against the amino-terminal region and one against the carboxy-terminal region. Effectively, only intact, biologically active hormone is measured. Such assays allow measurement of circulating hormone in most normal individuals, are scarcely affected by renal impairment, and allow excellent discrimination between PTH-mediated and non–PTH-mediated causes of hypercalcemia (Fig. 214–2).

Aurbach GD, Marx SJ, Spiegel AM: Parathyroid hormone, calcitonin, and the calciferols. In Wilson JD, Foster DW (eds.): Williams Textbook of Endocrinology. 8th ed. Philadelphia, WB Saunders, 1992, p 1406. Detailed description of basic aspects of PTH synthesis, secretion, action, and assay.
Endres DB, Villanueva R, Sharp CF Jr, et al.: Measurement of parathyroid hormone. Endocrinol Metab Clin North Am 18:611, 1989. Complete discussion of methods for PTH assay, including comparison of two-site versus mid-region immunoassays.
Juppner H, Abou-Samra A, Freeman M, et al.: A G protein–linked receptor for parathyroid hormone and parathyroid hormone–related peptide. Science 254:1024, 1991. Describes cloning of receptor that helps define mechanism of action of parathyroid hormone.

HYPERCALCEMIA

DEFINITION. Hypercalcemia is defined as an abnormal elevation in serum ionized calcium concentration.* Because total, rather than ionized, calcium is generally measured, one must be aware of factors that influence the fraction of total serum calcium that is ionized. Of these, serum albumin concentration is of greatest clinical relevance because albumin is the chief circulating calcium-binding protein. "Normal" total serum calcium concentration associated with a significant reduction in serum albumin (e.g., in patients with malignancy) may actually represent abnormally elevated levels of serum ionized calcium. Acid-base status also influences the proportion of total serum calcium that is protein bound (alkalosis decreases the ionized calcium concentration, and acidosis increases it).

ETIOLOGY. Many different diseases are potential causes of hypercalcemia. Of these, the most common are primary hyperparathyroidism (particularly in asymptomatic individuals whose hypercalcemia is detected by routine serum chemistry measurement) and malignancy (particularly in hospitalized individuals). These disorders, as well as some of the rarer causes of hypercalcemia, are considered in separate sections below.

PATHOGENESIS. Hypercalcemia results from excessive calcium influx into the extracellular fluid from bone and decreased efflux from the kidneys into the urine. Calcium mobilization from bone is mediated by activators of bone resorption. These activators include systemic factors (e.g., PTH, $1,25(OH)_2D$) and locally acting factors, such as various lymphokines. Reduced renal calcium excretion may lead to hypercalcemia, particularly in states of increased

---

* See Ch. 211 and Part XXVIII for calcium and phosphorus reference range values in serum and urine.

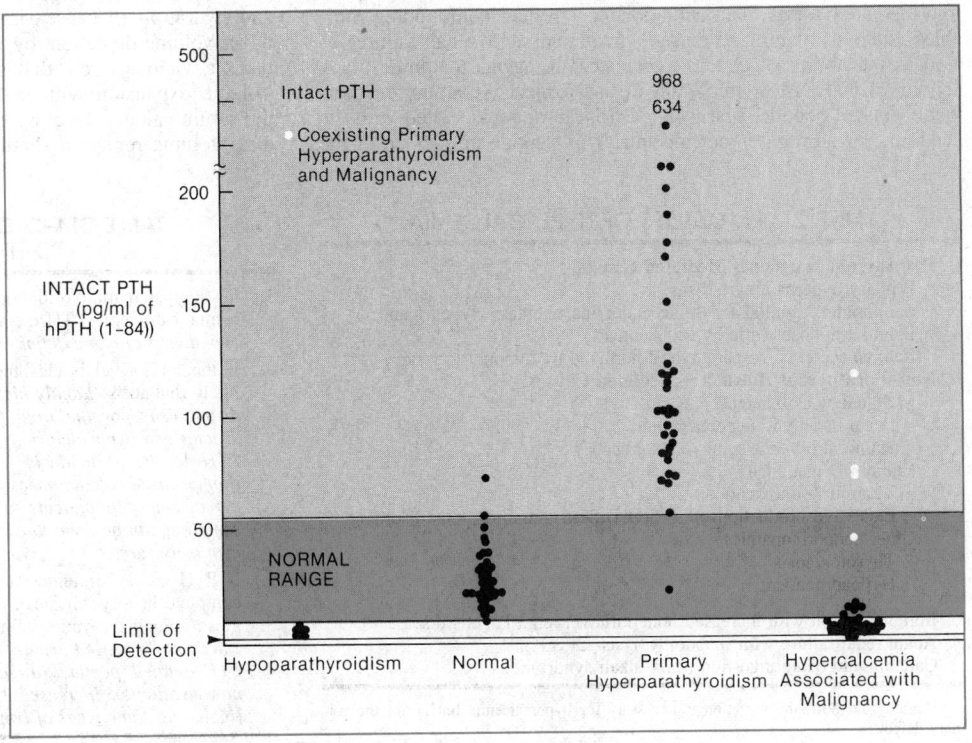

FIGURE 214–2. Two-site immunoassay for PTH in serum. The two-site method measures exclusively intact PTH. The hormone is detectable in the majority of normal subjects and undetectable in patients with various forms of hypoparathyroidism. Almost all patients with primary hyperparathyroidism show values outside the normal range. In contrast, values are low to undetectable in patients with malignancy-associated hypercalcemia, except for four individuals with coexistent primary hyperparathyroidism. (From Endres DB, Villanueva R, Sharp CF Jr, et al.: Measurement of parathyroid hormone. Endocrinol Metab Clin North Am 18:611, 1989.)

bone turnover. Renal impairment, volume depletion, and anticalciuretic agents, such as thiazide diuretics and PTH, are clinically relevant factors that can reduce renal calcium excretion and provoke hypercalcemia.

CLINICAL MANIFESTATIONS. Many manifestations are not specific to the underlying cause (specific disease manifestations are discussed under individual disease headings). Extreme hypercalcemia leads to coma and death. Neurologic manifestations in less severe cases may include confusion, lethargy, weakness, and hyporeflexia. Hypercalcemia may be detected by shortening of the QT interval on the electrocardiogram. Arrhythmias are rare, but bradycardia and first-degree heart block have been reported. Acute hypercalcemia may be associated with significant hypertension. Gastrointestinal manifestations include constipation and anorexia; in severe cases, there may be nausea and vomiting. Acute pancreatitis has been reported in association with hypercalcemia of various causes. Hypercalcemia interferes with antidiuretic hormone action, thereby leading to polyuria and polydipsia. Reversible reduction in renal function associated with significant hypercalcemia is followed by more permanent damage if hypercalcemia persists. Particularly if serum phosphorus is also increased, hypercalcemia can lead to nephrocalcinosis and interstitial nephritis. Hypercalciuria and nephrolithiasis may also occur. Deposition of calcium in other soft tissues, including skin and cornea, is most likely to occur in patients with associated hyperphosphatemia.

DIFFERENTIAL DIAGNOSIS. Potential causes of hypercalcemia are listed in Table 214–1. These may be divided into PTH-mediated (primary hyperparathyroidism) and non–PTH-mediated diseases (all others). Although ectopic secretion of PTH by tumors was long considered a potential cause of PTH-mediated hypercalcemia, there is now general agreement that ectopic secretion of authentic PTH (as opposed to PTH–related peptides; see below) by tumors is extremely rare. The first step in the differential diagnosis of hypercalcemia is to establish whether or not PTH hypersecretion is present because subsequent diagnostic maneuvers and definitive therapy critically depend on this distinction.

Readily measured blood and urine chemistries may offer some clues to diagnosis. In theory, PTH hypersecretion should be reflected by hypophosphatemia, hyperchloremia, hypobicarbonatemia, increased urinary phosphate excretion, and urinary calcium excretion that is relatively low for the filtered load. PTH secretion suppressed by hypercalcemia of non-parathyroid etiology should, in theory, reverse these parameters. In practice, there is considerable overlap in each of these parameters between patients with parathyroid-mediated forms of hypercalcemia and those with non–parathyroid-mediated forms. This situation may reflect confounding variables, such as vomiting, diuretic treatment, and renal failure, as well as the ability of certain hypercalcemic agents to mimic many actions of PTH. Most important in this respect is parathyroid hormone–related peptide, first isolated from tumors associated with the syndrome of humoral hypercalcemia. This peptide mimics all of the known actions of PTH on kidney and bone, including increasing urinary cAMP excretion and stimulating renal formation of $1,25(OH)_2D$. Decreased urinary cAMP excretion (with normal renal function) strongly suggests non–PTH-mediated hypercalcemia, but increased urinary cAMP excretion is compatible with both primary hyperparathyroidism and tumor secretion of parathyroid hormone–related peptide. Serum $1,25(OH)_2D$ concentration also does not allow definitive diagnosis. It may be elevated in primary hyperparathyroidism and vitamin D–related causes of hypercalcemia and may be reduced in other non–parathyroid-mediated causes of hypercalcemia. For reasons that are not entirely clear, the serum $1,25(OH)_2D$ level is often low in patients with malignancies secreting parathyroid hormone–related peptide, despite the ability of the peptide to stimulate $1,25(OH)_2D$ formation.

Definitive distinction between parathyroid- and non–parathyroid-mediated causes of hypercalcemia relies primarily on PTH immunoassay. As discussed earlier, this distinction is best made with the two-site type of assays that measure intact PTH and are un-affected by renal function (Fig. 214–2). An elevated PTH level secures the diagnosis of primary hyperparathyroidism. In selected cases with coexistent malignancy, the unlikely possibility of ectopic PTH secretion may be excluded by selective venous sam-pling and assay of PTH, but generally this testing is unnecessary. Hormone levels in the normal range suggest the possibility of familial hypocalciuric hypercalcemia. This entity is discussed further in the section on hyperparathyroidism. Low to undetectable values for PTH place the patient in the non–parathyroid-mediated category. Additional testing is necessary to establish a specific diagnosis within this group. Immunoassays for parathyroid hormone–related peptide have been developed, and these may allow the diagnosis of hypercalcemia caused by a tumor secreting this agent. Complete clinical evaluation, including history (e.g., vitamin ingestion, chronicity of symptoms), physical examination (masses, lymphadenopathy), radiologic studies, and other blood tests (e.g., thyroid and adrenal function), may point to a diagnosis. The diagnostic approach to hypercalcemia is summarized in Table 214–2.

TREATMENT. The definitive treatment of hypercalcemia depends on the specific diagnosis and treatment of the underlying disease, e.g., parathyroidectomy for primary hyperparathyroidism, chemotherapy for a malignancy. The initial treatment of hypercalcemia can be instituted (and in acute hypercalcemic crisis, often *must* be instituted) without a specific diagnosis, but cumulative toxicity and loss of efficacy preclude long-term nonspecific treatment. Measures aimed at reducing the serum calcium level act by increasing urinary calcium excretion and by decreasing bone resorption. General measures applicable to every patient include mobilization as soon as feasible (because immobility increases bone resorption) and hydration (because significant hypercalcemia causes dehydration). Volume depletion, by limiting renal calcium excretion, perpetuates a vicious circle that can lead to acute hypercalcemic crisis. Volume expansion with isotonic saline often significantly reduces the serum calcium level by enhancing renal calcium excretion. Only after volume repletion should diuretics be used to enhance sodium

---

TABLE 214–1. CAUSES OF HYPERCALCEMIA

Parathyroid Hormone–Mediated Causes
  Primary hyperparathyroidism
    Sporadic, familial (multiple endocrine neoplasia types I and II)
  Familial hypocalciuric hypercalcemia*
  Ectopic secretion of parathyroid hormone by tumors (very rare)
Non–Parathyroid Hormone–Mediated Causes
  Malignancy associated
    Local osteolytic hypercalcemia
    Humoral hypercalcemia of malignancy
  Vitamin D mediated
    Vitamin D intoxication
    Excessive production of $1,25(OH)_2D$ in granulomatous disorders
  Other endocrinopathies
    Thyrotoxicosis
    Hypoadrenalism

  Immobilization with increased bone turnover, e.g., Paget's disease
  Acute renal failure with rhabdomyolysis
  Calcium carbonate ingestion (milk-alkali syndrome)

* Parathyroid hormone secretion is necessary for hypercalcemia but is not the primary defect.

TABLE 214–2. DIAGNOSTIC APPROACH TO HYPERCALCEMIA

1. Distinguish parathyroid hormone (PTH)–mediated forms of hypercalcemia from non–PTH-mediated forms: *PTH immunoassay (preferably two-site type) is the definitive test.*

2. If the PTH level is elevated, primary hyperparathyroidism is the most likely diagnosis: *Family history for hypercalcemia should be checked to distinguish sporadic from familial (multiple endocrine neoplasia syndromes and hypocalciuric hypercalcemia) disease. Marginal elevation in PTH levels, particularly in young, asymptomatic individuals, should prompt urine calcium measurement to exclude familial hypocalciuric hypercalcemia. In patients with coexisting malignancy, selective venous sampling can be done to exclude ectopic PTH secretion, but the latter is extremely rare.*

3. If PTH is low or undetectable, further laboratory tests (in addition to complete history, physical, and radiologic studies) are needed to distinguish among the various forms of non–PTH-mediated forms of hypercalcemia: *Increased urinary cAMP excretion suggests tumor secretion of PTH–related peptide (direct radioimmunoassays for this peptide are now available). Increased $1,25(OH)_2D$ suggests granulomatous disease (including some types of lymphoma).*

and thereby calcium excretion. With a vigorous saline diuresis, calcium excretion in the range of 1 to 2 grams per day can be achieved as a temporary measure to reduce the serum calcium level. In patients with renal failure, dialysis can be employed almost as effectively to remove calcium from extracellular fluid. Careful monitoring of cardiac function and serum electrolytes is necessary with both saline diuresis and dialysis treatment.

Measures aimed at reducing bone resorption by inhibiting osteoclast function are most effective in treating hypercalcemia, irrespective of the specific factor causing increased bone resorption. Available agents include calcitonin, bisphosphonates (diphosphonates), plicamycin (mithramycin), and gallium nitrate. Calcitonin has low toxicity and acts most rapidly, but even in doses up to 32 MRC units per kilogram per day by intravenous infusion, lowering of serum calcium is generally limited and transient. Bisphosphonates must be given parenterally, and their effect is both significant and often prolonged (days). Initially, only etidronate (7.5 mg per kilogram per day intravenously) was available, but this is being replaced by pamidronate (dose 30 to 90 mg intravenously over 24 hours), which is more potent and effective. Plicamycin (25 μg per kilogram intravenously) quite effectively lowers serum calcium, but it has cumulative toxicity in liver, kidney, and platelets and can no longer be justified as initial therapy. Gallium nitrate is an effective calcium-lowering agent and has recently been approved by the FDA, but it has potential nephrotoxicity and its place in treating hypercalcemia is not yet clear. Intravenous phosphate poses a serious danger of metastatic calcification in the hypercalcemic patient and should probably no longer be used, given availability of other safer and effective agents. Oral phosphate is safer and useful in patients with significant hypercalcemia who are awaiting definitive treatment and in whom hypercalcemic crisis should be prevented. Dosages in the range of 2 grams of elemental phosphorus (10 grams of phosphate salts) per day in divided doses can be given. Serum phosphate and renal function should be carefully monitored.

Glucocorticoids are highly effective in treating hypercalcemia caused by vitamin D–related mechanisms (vitamin D intoxication, overproduction of 1,25(OH)$_2$D in granulomatous disorders) and by certain malignancies (cytokine release associated with myeloma) but are ineffective in most other forms of hypercalcemia, including hyperparathyroidism and most malignancies. Forty to 100 mg per day of prednisone or the equivalent is the usual dose range.

PRIMARY HYPERPARATHYROIDISM

DEFINITION. Primary hyperparathyroidism is a disorder in which hypercalcemia is due to hypersecretion of PTH.

ETIOLOGY. In most cases (about 85%), hyperparathyroidism is caused by sporadic, solitary adenomas. Hyperplasia of all four glands occurs in about 10% of cases, and these are most often familial, in the context of three distinct autosomal dominant inherited diseases: multiple endocrine neoplasia (MEN) types I and II and familial hypocalciuric hypercalcemia. Carcinoma occurs rarely (<5% of cases). The gene for MEN type I has been linked to chromosome 11q13. Enlarged glands in this disease are monoclonal tumors, with a high percentage showing loss of alleles at 11q13. This suggests that the MEN type I gene may be a "tumor suppressor" whose loss leads to tumorigenesis. A significant percentage of sporadic parathyroid tumors also show allele loss at this locus, suggesting a similar pathogenesis. The gene for MEN type II has been identified as the *RET* proto-oncogene on chromosome 10q11. This facilitates genetic diagnosis and studies of pathogenesis. Very rarely, a rearrangement involving the PTH gene on the short arm of chromosome 11 and a cell cycle control gene termed cyclin D or PRAD 1 on the long arm of chromosome 11 appears to cause parathyroid adenoma formation. Epidemiologic evidence suggests that a history of neck irradiation predisposes to parathyroid tumor formation. Specific molecular defects have not been identified. Finally, longstanding secondary hyperparathyroidism (e.g., in response to renal failure) may evolve into autonomous hypersecretion, so-called tertiary hyperparathyroidism. Loss of tumor suppressor gene(s) on 11q13 may be involved in some of these cases.

INCIDENCE. The incidence of hyperparathyroidism has increased substantially, largely as a result of routine blood calcium measurement. Age-adjusted incidence rates are between 25 and 50 per 100,000, based on recent surveys. A prevalence between 0.1 and 0.5% has been estimated, with females affected about twice as commonly as males. The incidence rises sharply after age 40.

PATHOLOGY. Microscopic distinction between adenoma and hyperplasia is difficult, if not impossible. The distinction between single-gland and multigland disease relies on gross surgical identification of more than one enlarged gland. In MEN types I and II, there is always multigland involvement, although asymmetric gland enlargement is often present. The chief cell generally predominates in parathyroid tumors; oxyphil cell tumors are much rarer.

PATHOPHYSIOLOGY. The primary disturbance is inappropriate secretion of PTH for the level of serum calcium. Studies *in vitro* with isolated parathyroid cells show that most adenomas either fail to suppress secretion at high calcium levels or show an altered setpoint, i.e., a higher calcium level is required to suppress secretion than for normal cells. Cells from hyperplastic glands may show a normal calcium setpoint for secretion. Hypersecretion of PTH in such cases may be due to a primary defect causing cellular proliferation and to an inability to suppress hormone secretion completely because of increased cell mass.

Slight increases in PTH secretion act on bone to increase turnover and may reduce cortical rather than trabecular bone density. At very high levels, PTH causes radiographically detectable subperiosteal bone resorption and, eventually, marrow fibrosis and cystic, reparative bone lesions termed "brown tumors." This is the classic form of the disease called "osteitis fibrosa cystica." PTH increases renal calcium reabsorption, but nonetheless, at high filtered loads of calcium, hypercalciuria develops. Enhanced 1,25(OH)$_2$D formation by the kidneys is prominent in some patients and is associated with increased intestinal calcium absorption. Such patients may be at particular risk for renal stones.

CLINICAL MANIFESTATIONS. Most patients either are asymptomatic at presentation (discovered through incidental blood calcium measurement) or have vague, nonspecific symptoms, such as fatigue, weakness, and mental disturbance. Patients with significant hypercalcemia show many of the signs and symptoms of hypercalcemia discussed above. Nephrolithiasis, with or without renal colic, is not specifically associated with hyperparathyroidism but is most commonly seen in this setting. Subperiosteal bone resorption is rarely seen, and osteitis fibrosa cystica even less commonly. Neuromuscular abnormalities, particularly proximal muscle weakness affecting the lower limbs, may be prominent. Joint manifestations include chondrocalcinosis that may lead to pseudogout. It has been claimed that hypertension, peptic ulcer disease, and osteoporosis are manifestations of hyperparathyroidism, but these are all common, and there is no firm evidence for a causal relationship. No specific physical findings are present in hyperparathyroidism. A neck mass, if present, most commonly represents a coincidental thyroid nodule, less commonly a benign or malignant parathyroid tumor. "Band keratopathy," calcification at "3 and 9 o'clock" of the cornea, is best seen by slit-lamp examination and occurs most often when hypercalcemia is accompanied by hyperphosphatemia—thus less commonly in hyperparathyroidism than in other hypercalcemic disorders. Radiologic findings include subperiosteal resorption, which, when present, is best seen at the radial sides of the phalanges, distal phalangeal tufts, and distal clavicles. Lucent bone lesions, representing brown tumors, are seen in rare, severely affected patients. Soft tissue calcification may be evident in the joints, kidneys, and lungs. The calcification is best appreciated on bone scans.

DIAGNOSIS. The differential diagnosis of hypercalcemia is discussed above. PTH immunoassay, preferably one of the newer two-site assays, is the key to diagnosis. In distinguishing between hyperparathyroid and normal states (e.g., in patients presenting with nephrolithiasis), repeated careful serum calcium and PTH (including the mid-region type of assay) measurements are most useful. Hypercalcemic subjects taking lithium or thiazides should be retested for hyperparathyroidism after discontinuing the drug (this may not be feasible in some patients on lithium), because both drugs may alter serum calcium and PTH secretion. In relatively young, asymptomatic individuals, or if the serum PTH level is marginally elevated, hypercalcemia may be due to familial hypocalciuric hypercalcemia rather than hyperparathyroidism (see discussion below under Familial Hypocalciuric Hypercalcemia).

PROGNOSIS AND TREATMENT. Surgical parathyroidectomy is the only definitive treatment for hyperparathyroidism. Oral phosphate treatment can lower the serum calcium level, but the long-term safety and efficacy of this approach are unclear. In mildly affected, older women, estrogen treatment has been advocated, particularly to blunt bone resorption, but, again, long-term efficacy is unknown. Thus, the only alternative to surgery at present is conservative medical follow-up. Most experts recommend surgery for all patients with symptomatic disease and even for asymptomatic patients meeting other, somewhat arbitrary, criteria, such as age below 40 or a serum calcium level >11.5 mg per deciliter. The appropriate management of patients not fitting any of these criteria is controversial; some advocate surgery for all, and others conservative follow-up. The long-term course of untreated hyperparathyroidism is unknown. Controlled studies comparing surgery versus medical follow-up have not been performed. Small series of patients followed conservatively for several years suggest that mild biochemical disease rarely progresses to severe symptomatic disease, but it is difficult to exclude subtle abnormalities, such as reduced bone density. Because definitive treatment recommendations are not possible, therapy must be individualized. The author personally follows a policy of recommending surgery for all but older patients with only mild biochemical disease.

If the decision is to perform surgery, a highly experienced parathyroid surgeon must be found. A success rate as high as 95% can be expected for initial neck exploration by a skilled surgeon. The success rate is substantially lower with inexperienced surgeons. Preoperative localization is not needed by the skilled surgeon performing initial exploration. Neither localization studies nor neck exploration itself should serve as *diagnostic* maneuvers. Only after the diagnosis has been established biochemically (by PTH assay) should one recommend surgery. In patients undergoing repeat neck exploration for recurrent or persistent disease, localization studies are extremely helpful. Noninvasive studies include ultrasonography, technetium-99m-sestamibi scanning, computed tomography (CT), and magnetic resonance imaging. Invasive techniques include fine-needle aspiration of imaged lesions for PTH assay, selective arteriography, and selective venous catheterization for hormone assay. The latter techniques are best performed by radiologists with specialized experience.

After successful surgery, hypocalcemia is generally mild and transient and rarely requires treatment. In the rare case of subjects with extensive bone disease, severe, prolonged hypocalcemia secondary to "bone hunger" occurs. Persistent relative hypophosphatemia suggests that bone hunger, rather than hypoparathyroidism, is the cause of hypocalcemia in this setting. Acute treatment with calcium infusions and long-term treatment with vitamin D and oral calcium may be needed. Eventually, treatment can be discontinued if normal parathyroid tissue remains. In patients without residual normal parathyroid tissue, lifelong vitamin D therapy is necessary. Autotransplantation of parathyroid tissue in the forearm is an experimental alternative in such cases. Successful surgery generally halts formation of renal stones in patients with nephrolithiasis and allows skeletal remineralization in patients with bone disease. There is no definitive evidence that surgery corrects hypertension or other nonspecific manifestations of hyperparathyroidism.

FAMILIAL HYPOCALCIURIC HYPERCALCEMIA

DEFINITION. This is an autosomal dominant genetic disease with essentially complete penetrance that causes hypercalcemia and relatively low urinary calcium excretion for the filtered load.

ETIOLOGY. The disease is caused by mutations in a gene on the long arm of chromosome 3 encoding a calcium-sensing receptor. In some families, the disease may be caused by a gene localized to a different chromosome.

INCIDENCE. The disorder is relatively rare, but it is over-represented among patients presenting with unsuccessful neck exploration because of the difficulty in achieving normocalcemia by surgery.

PATHOPHYSIOLOGY. The primary disturbance appears to be in divalent cation transport and/or "sensing" in at least the kidneys and parathyroids. The kidneys show an exaggerated reabsorption of filtered calcium (and magnesium) that leads to hypercalcemia. The parathyroids, however, fail to suppress fully hormone secretion despite hypercalcemia. The process is PTH-dependent because totally parathyroidectomized subjects become hypocalcemic, but even small amounts of parathyroid tissue are sufficient to maintain hy-

percalcemia. Parathyroid gland mass is generally only mildly increased.

CLINICAL MANIFESTATIONS. The disease leads to few, if any, clinical manifestations—hence its other name, "familial benign hypercalcemia." Nephrolithiasis and bone disease are, in general, not seen. Pancreatitis has been reported, but the specificity of this association is unclear. Hypercalcemia is present at birth. In some neonates, a clinically severe form of the disease is present. This severe form may be due to inheritance of a double dose of the abnormal gene. Otherwise, the main morbidity is that resulting from unsuccessful neck exploration that has failed to distinguish this disorder from conventional hyperparathyroidism. There is no evidence of associated endocrinopathies, as in the MEN syndromes.

DIAGNOSIS. A high index of suspicion is needed to recognize this disease. Hypercalcemia associated with relatively young age, with only slight elevation in the serum PTH level, or with a family history of unsuccessful neck exploration should trigger further evaluation. Hypermagnesemia is suggestive; urinary calcium-creatinine ratios <0.01:1 strongly support the diagnosis. Screening first-degree relatives for hypercalcemia may also be helpful. For those families in which the disease gene is localized to chromosome 3q, specific genetic diagnosis is possible by screening for mutations in the calcium-sensing receptor gene. Distinct mutations in this gene have already been identified in several kindreds.

PROGNOSIS AND TREATMENT. Because the disease is compatible with normal life expectancy and is associated with little, if any, morbidity, neck exploration appears to be contraindicated. Successful surgical treatment, moreover, is quite difficult, with permanent hypoparathyroidism or, more commonly, recurrent hypercalcemia, the usual result.

HYPERCALCEMIA ASSOCIATED WITH MALIGNANCY

ETIOLOGY AND PATHOGENESIS. Malignancies can cause hypercalcemia through two non–mutually exclusive mechanisms. First, local osteolytic hypercalcemia is caused by tumor metastatic to bone. Tumor cells may release bone-resorbing factors or so-called osteoclast-activating factors, which indirectly lead to bone resorption. Cytokines such as lymphotoxin and interleukin-1 are potent osteoclast-activating factors. Second, humoral hypercalcemia of malignancy is caused by tumor-secreting factors into the circulation that act systemically to increase bone resorption. Such factors may show other PTH-like actions, including increasing urinary cAMP and phosphate excretion and decreasing renal calcium excretion. This condition leads to a syndrome with biochemical features closely resembling those of primary hyperparathyroidism. One such factor commonly associated with many tumors has recently been identified as a polypeptide roughly twice as large as PTH and homologous in amino acid sequence to the biologically active amino-terminus of PTH. This so-called parathyroid hormone–related peptide may also be secreted by tumors metastatic to bone, so that humoral and local osteolytic mechanisms may combine to cause hypercalcemia. Some tumors cause hypercalcemia through excessive synthesis of $1,25(OH)_2D$, in a manner analogous to that seen in sarcoidosis (see below). A role for additional, as yet unidentified, bone-resorbing agents secreted by tumors has not been excluded.

INCIDENCE. Malignancy-associated hypercalcemia occurs most commonly in patients with bone metastases. Breast carcinoma is one of the most frequent causes. Most subjects with bone metastases are not hypercalcemic because of adequate renal compensatory mechanisms. Slight renal impairment may then provoke hypercalcemia. Treatment of women with breast cancer metastatic to bone with tamoxifen has been associated with acute sharp increases in the serum calcium level. Certain hematogenous neoplasms, such as myeloma and human lymphotropic virus type I–associated leukemia/lymphoma, are frequently associated with hypercalcemia. Humoral hypercalcemia of malignancy is much rarer. It is seen most frequently with squamous carcinomas, but biochemical evidence indicates that almost any tumor type, including breast carcinoma, can produce PTH-related peptide.

CLINICAL MANIFESTATIONS. Malignancy-associated hypercalcemia often develops acutely, may be quite severe (hypercalcemic crisis), and is frequently a grave prognostic sign. In most cases, particularly of the local osteolytic hypercalcemia variety, the underlying neoplasm is clinically evident. An otherwise occult neoplasm may occasionally manifest with humoral hypercalcemia of malignancy. Accurate and rapid diagnosis is critical in such cases because successful tumor removal may be feasible.

DIAGNOSIS. As discussed earlier, PTH radioimmunoassay is the crucial test for excluding coexistent primary hyperparathyroidism. PTH-related peptide fails to cross-react in such assays. Recently, specific immunoassays for this peptide were developed, and these facilitate diagnosis of tumor secretion of the peptide. Increased urinary cAMP excretion (coupled with low or undetectable PTH measurement) also favors tumor secretion of PTH-related peptide. If both PTH and urinary cAMP levels are low, one is dealing with a vitamin D–mediated or local osteolytic hypercalcemia.

TREATMENT AND PROGNOSIS. Acute, nonspecific treatment of hypercalcemia is instituted if the diagnosis is unclear (see Ch. 163). Definitive treatment must be directed at the underlying neoplasm, if feasible. When tumor treatment is not possible, vigorous treatment of hypercalcemia may be irrelevant. In those cases mediated by vitamin D or lymphokine release, glucocorticoids are often uniquely effective in lowering the serum calcium level.

HYPERCALCEMIA DUE TO GRANULOMATOUS DISEASES

ETIOLOGY AND PATHOGENESIS. Hypercalcemia is caused by unregulated formation of $1,25(OH)_2D$ in granuloma-associated macrophages. Normally, 1-hydroxylation takes place in the kidney and is sensitive to feedback suppression by high serum calcium levels. Unregulated synthesis of $1,25(OH)_2D$ in patients with granulomatous diseases renders them hypersensitive to vitamin D (from the diet or through sun exposure).

INCIDENCE AND PREVALENCE. This form of hypercalcemia has been observed in almost any disease capable of causing granulomas. These diseases include sarcoidosis, tuberculosis and fungal infections, berylliosis, and some lymphomas, such as Hodgkin's disease. Overt hypercalcemia may be seen in only about 10% of patients with sarcoidosis, but hypercalciuria and intestinal hyperabsorption of calcium may occur in almost half of such individuals.

CLINICAL FEATURES. Manifestations are those of the underlying disease, as well as the superimposed effects of hypercalcemia. Because this form of hypercalcemia often coexists with relatively higher serum phosphorus levels than those seen in hyperparathyroidism, soft tissue calcification, nephrocalcinosis, and renal impairment are more common. Patients may present with hypercalcemia and relatively few other findings (e.g., subtle hilar adenopathy in sarcoidosis).

DIAGNOSIS. PTH and urinary cAMP are suppressed. The serum level of $1,25(OH)_2D$ is elevated (in cases of vitamin D intoxication, the serum $1,25(OH)_2D$ level may be normal and only serum $25(OH)D$ is increased).

TREATMENT AND PROGNOSIS. The prognosis depends on that of the underlying disease. Glucocorticoids are extremely effective in lowering the serum calcium level in such cases. Chloroquine has been used effectively in subjects who cannot tolerate glucocorticoid treatment.

Aurbach GD, Marx SJ, Spiegel AM: Parathyroid hormone, calcitonin, and the calciferols. *In* Wilson JD, Foster DW (eds.): Williams Textbook of Endocrinology. 8th ed. Philadelphia, WB Saunders, 1992, p 1429. *Detailed description of primary hyperparathyroidism and malignancy-associated and other forms of hypercalcemia, including differential diagnosis and treatment.*

Bilezikian JP: Management of hypercalcemia. J Clin Endocrinol Metab 77:1445, 1993. *Concise review focusing on treatment of mild, moderate, and severe hypercalcemia.*

Broadus AE, Mangin M, Ikeda K, et al.: Humoral hypercalcemia of cancer. N Engl J Med 319:556, 1988. *Review of pathogenesis of this syndrome and discovery of parathyroid hormone-related peptide.*

Deftos LJ, Parthemore JG, Stabile BE: Management of primary hyperparathyroidism. Annu Rev Med 44:19, 1993. *Brief review focusing on managing "asymptomatic" patients. Encompasses recommendations from 1991 Consensus Conference on hyperparathyroidism.*

Heath H III: Primary hyperparathyroidism: Recent advances in pathogenesis, diagnosis, and management. Adv Intern Med 37:275, 1991. *More detailed review on all aspects of the disease.*

Pollak MR, Brown EM, Chou YW, et al.: Mutations in the human Ca^{2+}-sensing receptor gene cause familial hypocalciuric hypercalcemia and neonatal severe hyperparathyroidism. Cell 75:1297, 1993. *Evidence that distinct mutations in this receptor gene cause familial hypocalciuric hypercalcemia in heterozygotes and that neonatal severe hyperparathyroidism can be caused by mutations in both alleles of the same gene.*

Singer FR, Adams JS: Abnormal calcium homeostasis in sarcoidosis. N Engl J Med 315:755, 1986. *Review of derangements in vitamin D metabolism causing hypercalcemia and hypercalciuria in granulomatous disorders.*

HYPOCALCEMIA

DEFINITION. Hypocalcemia is an abnormal reduction in serum ionized calcium concentration.* Reduction in total serum calcium, as may occur in patients with hypoalbuminemia, does not necessarily reflect a reduction in ionized calcium. Ionized, not total, serum calcium affects neuromuscular function and is therefore the clinically relevant parameter.

ETIOLOGY AND PATHOGENESIS. Normal serum ionized calcium concentration is maintained by the direct actions of PTH on kidney and bone and by the indirect actions (through $1,25(OH)_2D$) on the intestine (see Ch. 211). Hypocalcemic disorders can be divided according to pathogenesis into two broad categories: (1) primary hypoparathyroidism, in which hypocalcemia is due to deficient secretion and/or action of PTH (specific subtypes are discussed under individual headings below); and (2) hypocalcemia due to target organ malfunction (e.g., renal failure, intestinal malabsorption, vitamin D deficiency). Hypocalcemia occurs in this category despite normal or even increased PTH secretion (secondary hyperparathyroidism). In hypoparathyroidism, there is reduced mobilization of calcium from bone, reduced renal reabsorption of calcium, lowered phosphaturia, and reduced $1,25(OH)_2D$ formation with a resultant decrease in intestinal calcium absorption. The end results are hypocalcemia and hyperphosphatemia. Renal failure (see Ch. 216) and acute phosphate loads (as may occur with chemotherapy of certain tumors such as Burkitt's lymphoma) are other causes of hypocalcemia with hyperphosphatemia. With vitamin D deficiency or malabsorption, hypocalcemia occurs with normal or low serum phosphorus levels (the latter reflecting secondary hyperparathyroidism). Hypocalcemia with low or normal serum phosphorus levels is also seen in acute pancreatitis (attributed to calcium soap formation, but this is unproved) and in some patients with osteoblastic tumor metastases. Table 214–3 summarizes the causes of hypocalcemia.

CLINICAL MANIFESTATIONS. Hypocalcemia of any cause is associated with certain typical signs and symptoms. Most prominent among these is increased neuromuscular excitability. Paresthesias of the fingers, toes, and circumoral region are mild manifestations; in more extreme cases there may be muscle cramping, carpopedal spasm, laryngeal stridor, and convulsions. Symptoms reflect not only the degree of hypocalcemia but also the acuteness of the fall in serum calcium concentration. Patients with longstanding severe hypocalcemia may show surprisingly few symptoms. Factors that acutely alter the balance between ionized and protein-bound calcium may precipitate symptoms. For example, alkalosis lowers ionized calcium; thus hyperventilation may provoke symptoms of tetany. Signs of latent tetany include Chvostek's sign (twitching of the upper lip after tapping on the facial nerve below the zygomatic arch) and Trousseau's sign (carpal spasm after inflating a cuff on the upper arm above systolic blood pressure for 2 to 3 minutes).

Various mental disturbances, such as irritability, depression, and even psychosis, have been attributed to hypocalcemia. Papilledema and other signs of increased intracranial pressure have been reported. Intracranial calcifications, particularly of the basal ganglia, may be seen on plain radiographs and even more frequently on CT. Increased sensitivity to the dystonic effects of phenothiazines has been attributed to basal ganglia calcification. Longstanding hypocalcemia may lead to cataract formation. Cardiac effects of hypocalcemia include a prolonged QT interval and, rarely, congestive heart failure. Dental anomalies depend on age of onset; in children hypocalcemia can cause enamel hypoplasia and failure of the adult teeth to erupt.

DIFFERENTIAL DIAGNOSIS. Measuring serum calcium, phosphorus, and creatinine levels allows one to categorize the form of hypocalcemia. Hypocalcemia and hyperphosphatemia with normal renal function are pathognomonic of hypoparathyroidism. Low or undetectable PTH by immunoassay despite hypocalcemia confirms the diagnosis. (Rare forms of PTH-resistant hypoparathyroidism show elevated levels of PTH and are discussed further below.) Hypocalcemia and hyperphosphatemia caused by renal failure pose no diagnostic problem. Hypocalcemia with normal or low

---

* See Ch. 211 and Part XXVII for calcium and phosphorus reference range values.

TABLE 214-3. CAUSES OF HYPOCALCEMIA

Hypoparathyroidism
    Deficient parathyroid hormone secretion
        Idiopathic (autoimmune)
        Parathyroid hormone gene mutation
        Surgical
        Infiltrative (iron overload, Wilson's disease)
    Functional
        Hypomagnesemia
        Transient postoperative
    Deficient parathyroid hormone action (hormone resistance)
        Pseudohypoparathyroidism types Ia and Ib
Normal or Increased Parathyroid Hormone Function
    Renal failure
    Intestinal malabsorption
    Acute pancreatitis
    Osteoblastic metastases
    Vitamin D deficiency or resistance

serum phosphorus levels should prompt measurement of vitamin D metabolites and assessment of gastrointestinal function to check for vitamin D deficiency and malabsorption, respectively. Measurements of PTH should show increased values in such patients, as the normal parathyroids attempt to compensate for hypocalcemia.

TREATMENT. Acute, symptomatic hypocalcemia requires emergency treatment in the form of intravenous calcium infusion. Ten to 20 ml of 10% calcium gluconate solution (contains 10 mg of elemental calcium per milliliter) may be given over 10 to 20 minutes (this may be hazardous in patients taking cardiac glycosides). In less urgent settings, a slow intravenous infusion (over 4 to 8 hours) of 20 mg of elemental calcium per kilogram of body weight may be given. As with hypercalcemic disorders, definitive resolution of hypocalcemia requires treating the underlying disease. In patients with hypoparathyroidism, lifelong therapy with vitamin D (with or without oral calcium) is required. This is discussed further under treatment of hypoparathyroidism, below.

HYPOPARATHYROIDISM

DEFINITION. Hypoparathyroidism is defined as deficient PTH secretion and/or action. This condition may lead to overt hypocalcemia and hyperphosphatemia, as discussed above, or may only predispose to hypocalcemia (decreased parathyroid reserve) in times of increased calcium demand, such as pregnancy.

ETIOLOGY AND PATHOGENESIS. *Permanent Deficiency in Parathyroid Hormone Secretion.* This deficiency may result from surgical removal of the parathyroids, from glandular destruction by iron overload (e.g., transfusions in thalassemia) or copper overload (Wilson's disease), and from glandular destruction through a presumed autoimmune mechanism. The latter often has a genetic basis. The parathyroids may fail to develop as part of the DiGeorge syndrome. Some cases termed "idiopathic hypoparathyroidism" may be due to inherited mutations in the PTH gene that prevent synthesis and secretion of PTH.

Transient Deficiency in Parathyroid Hormone Secretion. Reversible hypoparathyroidism can be caused by hypomagnesemia. The latter may compromise both PTH secretion and action. Magnesium replacement corrects the defect. Transient hypoparathyroidism may also result from suppression of normal parathyroids by parathyroid adenomas or other causes of hypercalcemia. This condition rarely lasts more than 1 week. Surgical injury to the parathyroids is another postulated cause of transiently reduced hormone secretion.

Deficiency in Parathyroid Hormone Action. Secretion of a biologically inactive form of PTH is a theoretical, but unproven, cause of deficient PTH action. Target organ resistance to PTH appears to be the major cause of this form of hypoparathyroidism, which was termed "pseudohypoparathyroidism" by Albright, who described it as the first example of a hormone-resistance disorder. Subsequent studies indicated that the defect in this disease occurs before formation of cAMP (a second messenger of PTH action) because affected subjects lack the normal brisk increase in urinary cAMP excretion observed after infusing PTH in normal individuals. There are at least two forms of pseudohypoparathyroidism. In type Ia disease, a 50% deficiency has been found in the Gs protein that couples PTH (and many other) receptors to the enzyme that forms

cAMP, adenylyl cyclase. This deficiency may limit normal cAMP production in response to PTH as well as to other hormones, such as thyroid-stimulating hormone. As a result, patients with this form of the disease show many abnormalities (e.g., hypothyroidism, hypogonadism) in addition to hypoparathyroidism. In affected subjects from several families with type Ia disease, distinct mutations that prevent synthesis of normal Gs protein have been found in the gene encoding the Gs protein. Inheritance of the mutation is autosomal dominant. In subjects with type Ib disease, the Gs protein is normal, and resistance is limited to PTH. A defective PTH receptor is a likely, but unproven, basis for this disease. In some subjects, hypocalcemia and hyperphosphatemia are associated with radiographically evident osteitis fibrosa cystica. This finding suggests selective renal, as opposed to skeletal, resistance to PTH action. The pathogenesis is unclear.

INCIDENCE. All forms of hypoparathyroidism are relatively rare. The incidence of surgical hypoparathyroidism varies widely as a function of the skill of the surgeon.

CLINICAL MANIFESTATIONS. The manifestations generally associated with hypocalcemia have been discussed above. The clinical features unique to each form of hypoparathyroidism reflect the underlying disease. In autoimmune forms, there may be associated endocrine deficiency, most frequently Addison's disease, as well as a T cell defect predisposing to mucocutaneous candidiasis. Alopecia and vitiligo may also be seen. In pseudohypoparathyroidism type Ib, the appearance is normal, but in type Ia disease, affected individuals show a constellation of abnormal physical findings termed Albright's hereditary osteodystrophy (Fig. 214–3). These findings include obesity, short stature, round face and short neck, metacarpal and metatarsal shortening (most often fourth and fifth) as well as shortening and broadening of the distal phalanges, and subcutaneous calcifications. Such individuals often show slight mental retardation and associated endocrine abnormalities, most commonly

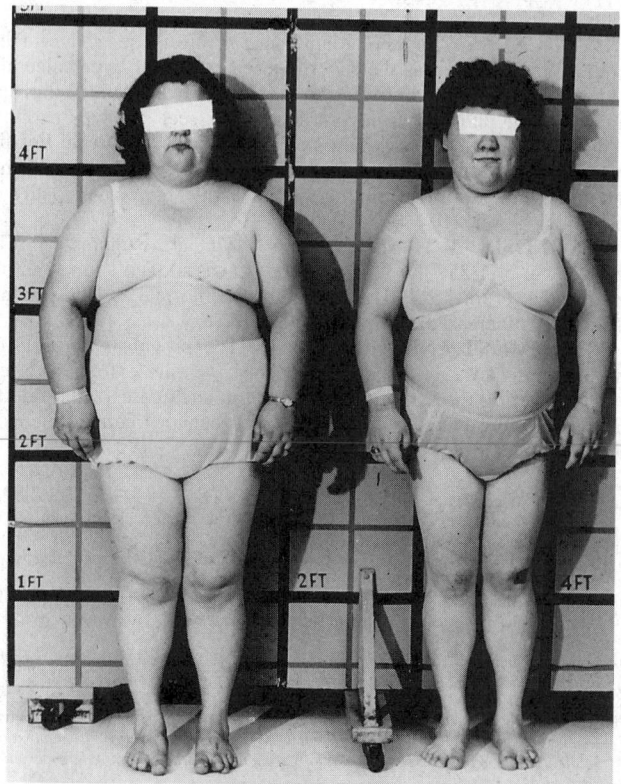

FIGURE 214–3. Phenotypic features of Albright's hereditary osteodystrophy. A mother *(left)* and daughter display many of the features of Albright's osteodystrophy, including obesity, short stature, round face, and short neck. Metacarpal and metatarsal shortening manifest as shortened fourth and fifth fingers (right hands of both subjects) and shortened fourth toes (left feet of both subjects), respectively. Both subjects show resistance to PTH and thyroid-stimulating hormone, as well as deficient Gs protein activity, characteristic of pseudohypoparathyroidism type Ia. (From Spiegel AM: Pseudohypoparathyroidism. *In* Scriver CR, Beaudet AL, Sly WS, Valle D [eds.]: The Metabolic Basis of Inherited Disease. 6th ed. New York, McGraw-Hill, 1989, p 2013; with permission.)

hypothyroidism (without goiter) and hypogonadism. First-degree relatives of patients with pseudohypoparathyroidism type Ia may show the physical features of Albright's osteodystrophy without evidence of hormone resistance. This condition has been termed pseudopseudohypoparathyroidism. Rarely, individuals with pseudohypoparathyroidism (more often of the Ib type) have radiographic evidence of osteitis fibrosa cystica and elevated serum levels of bone-derived alkaline phosphatase.

DIFFERENTIAL DIAGNOSIS. Low or undetectable serum PTH in the face of hypocalcemia, hyperphosphatemia, and normal renal function establishes the diagnosis of hormone-deficient hypoparathyroidism. Diagnosis of the underlying disease depends on history (e.g., neck surgery), physical findings (e.g., candidiasis, alopecia), and additional laboratory tests (e.g., evidence for hypoadrenalism). Antibodies to parathyroid antigens have been detected in the autoimmune form of the disease, but this test is not available for routine clinical use. An elevated level of serum PTH measured by immunoassay in a subject with hypocalcemia, hyperphosphatemia, and normal renal function suggests hormone-resistant hypoparathyroidism. PTH infusion (at present with commercially available synthetic 1–34 peptide) and measurement of urinary cAMP excretion can be performed to confirm PTH resistance. Physical appearance can help distinguish type Ia from type Ib pseudohypoparathyroidism, as can testing for other endocrinopathies, such as hypothyroidism. Measurement of Gs protein and detection of mutations in the corresponding gene are not routinely available tests.

TREATMENT. Transient forms of hypoparathyroidism may not require treatment. Reversible forms should be treated appropriately, i.e., magnesium replacement for hypomagnesemia. In permanent hormone-deficient hypoparathyroidism, hormone replacement therapy is not practical. Parathyroid autografting is effective in some patients with surgical hypoparathyroidism. When this is not feasible, and also in subjects with pseudohypoparathyroidism, lifelong treatment with oral vitamin D is required. Vitamin D_2, ergocalciferol (generally 50,000 units per day), is inexpensive by comparison with the active metabolite, $1,25(OH)_2D$ (generally 0.25 μg per day). The latter has the theoretical advantage of more rapid onset (and in case of toxicity, offset) of action, but with appropriate monitoring, vitamin D_2 can be used very effectively. Oral calcium salts (1 to 2 grams of elemental calcium per day in divided doses) may be added for individuals whose dietary calcium intake is highly variable or inadequate. The goal of treatment is the lowest serum calcium concentration compatible with avoidance of symptoms, because without PTH, urinary calcium excretion (and the possibility of nephrolithiasis) is increased at any filtered load of calcium. Both serum and urine calcium levels, as well as renal function, must be monitored. In forms of hypoparathyroidism that have associated endocrinopa-thies, appropriate hormone replacement therapy should be instituted.

Aurbach GD, Marx SJ, Spiegel AM: Parathyroid hormone, calcitonin, and the calciferols. *In* Wilson JD, Foster DW (eds.): Williams Textbook of Endocrinology, 8th ed. Philadelphia, WB Saunders, 1992, p 1456. *Detailed description of clinical and pathophysiologic features of hypocalcemic disorders and the multiple forms of hypoparathyroidism.*

Mallette L: Synthetic human parathyroid hormone 1–34 fragment for diagnostic testing. Ann Intern Med 109:800, 1988. *Description of use of this commercially available peptide in the differential diagnosis of hypoparathyroidism.*

Spiegel AM: Pseudohypoparathyroidism. *In* Scriver CR, Beaudet AL, Sly WS, et al. (eds.): The Metabolic Basis of Inherited Disease. 6th ed. New York, McGraw-Hill, 1989, p 2013. *Extensive discussion of clinical features and pathogenesis of hormone-resistant forms of hypoparathyroidism.*

215 CALCITONIN AND MEDULLARY THYROID CARCINOMA

Leonard J. Deftos

Calcitonin (CT) is a 32-residue peptide secreted primarily by the thyroidal C-cells in mammals and by the embryologically related ultimobranchial gland in submammals. The main biologic effect of CT is to decrease bone resorption by inhibiting the osteoclast. This effect decreases the concentration of blood calcium, with a nadir di-

rectly related to bone turnover; thus, the hypocalcemia may be slight in normal adults but considerable when bone resorption is increased pathologically in disease states or physiologically during bone growth. This property of CT makes it an effective drug for hyperresorptive diseases, such as Paget's disease, osteoporosis, and hypercalcemia. The physiologic significance of other reported effects of CT is not well established. The calciuric effect of CT is seen primarily with pharmacologic doses of the hormone. A stimulatory effect on bone formation may be attributed to a CT-related molecule rather than to CT itself. However, an analgesic effect of CT continues to receive considerable attention and may be related to neuroendocrine features of the hormone. In addition to its role in skeletal physiology and treatment, CT is a serum and tumor marker for medullary thyroid carcinoma (MTC), which is the signal tumor of multiple endocrine neoplasia (MEN) type II.

CALCITONIN

BIOCHEMISTRY. The 32-residue structure of CT, determined for nine species, reveals a common 1,7 amino-terminal disulfide bridge and carboxy-terminal proline. Seven of the nine amino-terminal residues are identical in all CT molecules. The interspecies structural differences in the rest of the molecule cause the submammalian (ultimobranchial) CT molecules to be more potent in mammals than the mammalian CT molecules. Thus, the potent salmon form of the hormone is widely used for treatment in humans. The greater chemical basicity of these submammalian CT species probably accounts for their increased potency. In contrast to the other major skeletal peptide hormone, parathyroid hormone (PTH), a biologically active fragment of CT has not been identified, and the entire molecule seems to be necessary for biologic activity.

SECRETION AND PRODUCTION. The most important secretory regulation of CT is mediated by ambient calcium. An acute increase in blood calcium concentration increases the secretion of CT, and an acute decrease in blood calcium level decreases the secretion of CT. The effects of chronic changes in blood calcium concentration on secretion have not been as well defined. Chronic hypercalcemia may stimulate CT production, but this compensatory response may be limited. Chronic hypocalcemia seems to increase CT storage in C-cells. Although a variety of other factors have been reported to stimulate CT secretion, only pentagastrin and its related peptides are consistent additional secretagogues. The high concentration of pentagastrin necessary to stimulate secretion does not support the presence of a normal entero–C-cell secretory pathway. Nevertheless, pentagastrin and calcium are clinically important agents for evaluating CT secretion by both normal and malignant C-cells.

The effect of gonadal steroids and age on CT production remains controversial. It is well established that blood concentrations of CT are higher in males than females and in children than adults. Some studies report a decline in CT secretion during adulthood and a stimulation of CT secretion by estrogens and testosterone. These observations have led to the hypothesis that age- and menopause-related declines in CT production contribute to the corresponding declines in bone mass seen in the elderly, especially postmenopausal women. These observations support the use of CT in treating osteoporosis, but more complex hormonal abnormalities underlie this skeletal disorder.

MEDULLARY THYROID CARCINOMA

Medullary thyroid carcinoma is a tumor of the CT-producing C-cells of the thyroid gland. These cells migrate from the neural crest to the thyroid gland and to other sites of the diffuse neuroendocrine system during embryogenesis in mammals. In submammals, these cells form their own distinct organ, the ultimobranchial gland. The neural crest origin of C-cells accounts for their production of a variety of biologically active substances. This embryologic origin may also explain the common association of MTC with other neuroendocrine tumors. Thus, MTC can occur as part of MEN type II or sporadically.

PATHOLOGY. A palpable tumor is the most common physical finding in the patient with MTC. The tumor is usually firm and located in the middle or upper lobes of the gland. Bilateral tumors are common in MEN. Calcification can be present in the tumor, and this may result in a radiographic pattern that is characteristic enough to help diagnose it clinically. Similarly, amyloid present in the tumor can assist in histologic diagnosis. However, cytologic diagnosis is made difficult by the fact that the cells of MTC can be arranged in a variety of patterns. Therefore, the diagnosis of MTC is conclusively made by demonstrating CT in the tumor by immunohistology. Hyperplasia of the C-cells antedates the frank malignancy of MTC, especially in the familial forms of the tumor. C-cell hyperplasia is often too subtle to be appreciated by light microscopy, and immunohistology for CT is necessary to make this diagnosis. The advent of genetic testing for MEN provides additional impetus for distinguishing MTC from other thyroid tumors.

TUMOR BEHAVIOR. The clinical behavior of MTC is usually intermediate between that of aggressive anaplastic thyroid cancer and that of indolent papillary and follicular thyroid cancer. Local lymph node spread is common, and metastases to lung and bone can occur. MTC in which all or most of the cells produce CT may have a better prognosis than a more heterogeneous tumor in which CT production is not uniform. Even in the most aggressive tumors, CT production is usually sufficient to serve as a specific marker for this thyroid cancer. However, there may be rare instances in which CT production has ceased. The 5-year survival of those with MTC approximates 50%. Survival can vary from several months to three decades after diagnosis. Patients under age 2 with metastatic disease and over age 50 with only localized disease have been reported. C-cell hyperplasia can occur in those as young as age 2 and as old as 45. Therefore, the tumor can be rapidly aggressive, leading to death within months after diagnosis, or it can be indolent and compatible with survival for decades.

PATHOGENESIS. MTC is preceded by C-cell hyperplasia, especially in the familial form of the disease. This progression from hyperplasia to cancer is best documented for MTC in the clinical setting of MEN type II. C-cell adenomas have also been observed. The progression of unregulated growth from hyperplasia to malignancy is similar to that seen in the progression of mucosal cells to a frankly malignant state in other tumors in which an oncogene cascade contributes to pathogenesis. It is thus interesting to speculate that an oncogene cascade is responsible for the progression of normal C-cells through hyperplasia to cancer in MTC. In the familial form of the tumor, an oncogene abnormality may be related to the chromosome 10 site, to which MEN type IIA and IIB have both been mapped. Abnormalities in expression of the *RET* oncogene have been observed in MTC, but the role in pathogenesis of this tyrosine kinase has not yet been elucidated. Abnormalities in this oncogene have recently been reported in familial MTC and Hirschsprung's disease. It is notable that this same progression of normal cells to hyperplastic and then neoplastic cells is also observed for the other two endocrine components of heritable MTC, pheochromocytoma and parathyroid neoplasia. Thus, the genetic abnormality on chromosome 10 may result in the overexpression (or undersuppression) of an endocrine cell growth factor.

DIAGNOSIS. Overexpression of the CT gene is the molecular hallmark of MTC. This overexpression results in the increased production of CT by the tumor and increased secretion of the hormone into blood. As a result, most patients with MTC have an increased circulating concentration of CT that can be detected by radioimmunoassay and increased tumor concentrations that can be demonstrated directly by immunohistology or through increased messenger RNA (mRNA) expression by *in situ* hybridization. Usually, the basal blood concentration of CT is sufficiently elevated to be diagnostic of the presence of the tumor. In the early stages of the diseases, however, the basal concentrations of CT cannot be readily distinguished from normal. In these circumstances, provocative testing of CT secretion can reveal the presence of the abnormal C-cells. Such testing is also clinically indicated for the relative of a patient with familial MTC when early diagnosis is sought. Screening is also recommended for apparently sporadic tumors because family history can be unreliable. The two most commonly used provocative agents for CT secretion are calcium and the synthetic gastrin analogue pentagastrin, alone or in combination. Most tumors respond to either agent with a diagnostic increase in CT secretion. CT blood measurements can also be used to evaluate therapy and monitor tumor recurrence. Interpretation must be made according to the specific parameters of the procedure used.

The primary genetic abnormality in MEN type IIA and IIB have been localized to chromosome 10. For MEN IIA, the genetic defect

has been localized to the *RET* oncogene, which encodes a tyrosine kinase. Molecular genetic techniques allow gene carrier status to be assigned in a patient at risk and with a well-documented pedigree. However, confounding factors such as mistaken diagnoses and nonpaternity can complicate genetic analysis. The ethical considerations that surround all genetic screening should be considered in the light of the effective and curative treatment that is available for the components of MEN type IIA and IIB. Nevertheless, genetic diagnosis represents a substantial advance in management of the inherited forms of MTC.

CT GENE EXPRESSION. A variety of bioactive substances are overproduced by MTC. Some can be attributed to the neural crest origin of the C-cells and some to deregulated CT gene expression. This gene encodes peptides in addition to CT. The CT gene consists of six exons that generate—through differential mRNA splicing—two distinct mRNA's, one of them the CT precursor and the other a precursor for calcitonin gene–related peptide (CGRP). The CT precursor is processed into three peptides: CT; its amino-terminal flanking peptide, N-pro CT; and its carboxy-terminal flanking peptide, C-pro CT. The CGRP precursor is similarly processed. Thus, the CT gene encodes at least six peptides. The peptides derived from the CT precursor, including CT, act on the skeletal system, and the peptide derived from the CGRP precursor acts as a neurotransmitter. This remarkable genetic economy produces two CT precursor–derived peptides that have opposite skeletal effects, with CT inhibiting bone resorption and N-pro CT, its amino-terminal relative, promoting bone cell mitogenesis. Human CT gene expression and processing are summarized in Figure 215–1.

MULTIPLE ENDOCRINE NEOPLASIA (MEN)

MTC can occur in association with other endocrine tumors as part of a multiple endocrine neoplasia, designated MEN type II, to distinguish it from MEN type I, which consists of parathyroid, pancreatic, and pituitary tumors. MEN type II is an autosomal dominant syndrome that can be clinically classified into two subtypes, type IIA and IIB (Table 215–1).

PHEOCHROMOCYTOMA. Pheochromocytoma is a component of MEN type IIA and IIB. Bilateral and multifocal pheochromocytomas are very common in this clinical setting, with an incidence of >70%. This figure contrasts with a bilateral incidence of usually <10% for sporadic pheochromocytomas and only 20 to 50% for familial pheochromocytomas. Adrenal medullary hyperplasia is a predecessor of the pheochromocytomas seen with MTC. The increase in adrenal medullary mass results from diffuse or multifocal proliferation of adrenal medullary cells, primarily those found within the head and body of the glands. The biochemical as well as clinical manifestations of this tumor may be subtle, so diagnostic tests for pheochromocytoma should be pursued vigorously in MEN type II.

HYPERPARATHYROIDISM. Hyperparathyroidism is much more common in MEN type IIA than in MEN type IIB (and it also occurs in MEN type I). The presence of hyperparathyroidism thus should always make one consider the possibility of MEN. Parathyroid hyperplasia is more common than adenoma, an important consideration for surgical treatment. Although a calcium-mediated functional relationship between hyperparathyroidism and MTC has been suggested, the two neoplasias are probably linked to the same gene.

MULTIPLE MUCOSAL NEUROMAS. The presence of neuromas with a centrofacial distribution is the most consistent component of MEN type IIB. The most common location of neuromas is the oral cavity. The oral lesions are almost invariably present by the first decade and in some cases even at birth. Mucosal neuromas can also be present in the eyelid, conjunctiva, and cornea. The most prominent microscopic feature of neuromas is an increase in the size and number of nerves. These hypertrophied nerve fibers are readily seen with a slit lamp and occasionally by direct ophthalmologic examination.

Gastrointestinal tract abnormalities are part of the multiple mucosal neuroma syndrome. The most common of these is gastrointestinal ganglioneuromatosis, which usually occurs in the small and large intestines but has also been noted in the esophagus and stomach. The lesions are sometimes associated with swallowing abnormalities, megacolon, diarrhea, and constipation. The diarrhea may also be due to excess production of bioactive substances by the MTC. In any case, diarrhea is the most common symptom of MTC.

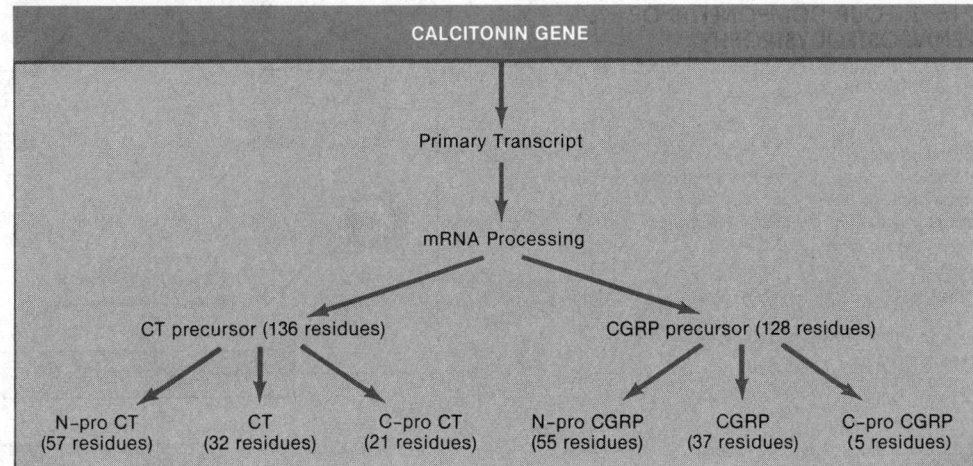

FIGURE 215–1. Summary of human calcitonin (CT) gene expression. The CT pathway occurs primarily in endocrine tissue (e.g., C-cells) and the calcitonin gene–related peptide (CGRP) pathway primarily in neural tissue. The gene has six exons whose primary RNA transcript is differentially spliced into an mRNA for the CT precursor and one for the CGRP precursor. A common 25-residue leader sequence is removed, and these two polypeptide precursors are each processed into their three respective peptide products. (Alternative designations for some of these peptides are as follows: for N-pro CT, PAS-57; for C-pro CT, PDN-21 and katacalcin; for N-pro CGRP, PAS-55). The functions of these other peptides are not firmly established.

MARFANOID HABITUS. Patients with this component have a tall, slender body with long arms and legs, an abnormal ratio of upper to lower body segments, and poor muscle development. Other features associated with the marfanoid habitus may include dorsal kyphosis, pectus excavatum or pectus carinatum, pes cavus, and high-arched palate. In contrast to patients with true Marfan's syndrome, these patients do not have aortic arch abnormalities, ectopia lentis, homocystinuria, or mucopolysaccharide abnormalities.

TREATMENT AND CLINICAL MANAGEMENT. Surgery is the treatment of choice for the three neoplasias in MEN type II. All are potentially lethal—especially MTC and pheochromocytoma—but all can be cured in their early stages by surgery. Aggressive therapy is thus warranted. Managing the individual components of MEN syndromes generally follows the accepted procedures for each of the neoplasias. However, the sequence of treatment is guided by the presence of multiple endocrine tumors. Pheochromocytomas, which are commonly bilateral, should be treated first because they can be life-threatening and pose risks for surgery of the other tumors. Thyroid and parathyroid surgery must be aggressive because all glandular tissue may be involved.

Evaluating family members is an essential feature of appropriate clinical management in MEN type II, because these tumors are transmitted in an autosomal dominant pattern. Family members must be re-evaluated periodically because of the varying penetrance of the component tumors. CT measurement remains the diagnostic procedure of choice. Genetic diagnostic techniques are being continually refined and are increasingly used to identify individuals at risk for the syndrome, especially now that the genetic abnormality has been identified for MEN IIA. Although such procedures may supplant CT measurement for diagnosis, measurement of the hormone will be useful for documenting the presence of neoplasia and monitoring therapy.

CALCITONIN AS A DRUG

CT's primary biologic effect of inhibiting osteoclastic bone resorption makes it useful for treating disorders characterized by increased bone resorption and certain forms of hypercalcemia. Thus, CT can be prescribed for treating Paget's disease, osteoporosis, and the hypercalcemia associated with malignancy. Both salmon CT and human CT are available, the former being more potent and the latter being less antigenic. Calcitonin is safer than most treatment alternatives, but its effects can be transient. The inconvenience of repeated parenteral administration may be avoided by transmucosally administering the peptide. In fact, a nasally administered preparation of CT has been recently approved by the FDA for treatment of osteoporosis.

Burns DM, Birnbaum RS, Roos BA: A neuroendocrine peptide derived from the amino terminal half of rat procalcitonin. Mol Endocrinol 3:140, 1989. *An exposition of the complexities of CT gene expression.*

Cance WG, Wells SA Jr: Multiple endocrine neoplasia. Curr Prob Surg 22:1, 1985. *A discussion of the surgical problems encountered in the treatment of multiple endocrine tumors.*

Deftos LJ: Radioimmunoassay for calcitonin in medullary thyroid carcinoma. JAMA 227:403, 1974. *Early study of the application of CT radioimmunoassay to the diagnosis of MTC.*

Deftos LJ, Roos BA: Medullary thyroid carcinoma and calcitonin gene expression. Bone Miner Res 6:267, 1989. *A detailed exposition of multiple endocrine neoplasia and the regulation of calcitonin-gene products.*

Gagel RF, Robinson MF, Donovan DT, et al.: Medullary thyroid carcinoma: Recent progress. J Clin Endocrinol Metab 76:809, 1993. *A recent review of the clinical features and molecular genetics of MTC.*

Mulligan LM, Kwok JBJ, Healey CS, et al.: Germ-line mutations of the *RET* proto-oncogene in multiple endocrine neoplasia type 2A. Nature 363:458, 1993. *Identification of the genetic abnormality in MEN IIA.*

Sobol H, Narod SA, Nakamura Y, et al.: Screening for MEN Type IIA with DNA-polymorphism analyses. N Engl J Med 321:996, 1989. *The application of RFLP to genetic analyses in MEN.*

van Heyningen V: One gene—four syndromes. Nature 367:319, 1994.

---

216 RENAL OSTEODYSTROPHY

Eduardo Slatopolsky

The main components of renal osteodystrophy are osteitis fibrosa and osteomalacia (Table 216–1). A lesser role is played by osteosclerosis and osteoporosis. Osteitis fibrosa, a consequence of an increased parathyroid hormone, is characterized by an increase in the number of osteoclasts and an increase in bone resorption and marrow fibrosis. Osteomalacia results from a decreased mineralization of osteoid tissue (shown histologically by an abnormal calcification front in bone). Osteosclerosis is due to localized areas of mineralized woven bone which appear as increased bone density on radiographic studies. Osteoporosis, defined as a decrease in the mass of normally mineralized bone, is an infrequent and minor component of renal osteodystrophy.

TABLE 215–1. COMPONENTS OF MULTIPLE ENDOCRINE NEOPLASIA TYPE II AND THEIR FREQUENCY BASED ON AVERAGE FIGURES FROM THE LITERATURE

Component	MEN Type IIA (%)	MEN Type IIB (%)
Medullary thyroid carcinoma	97	90
Pheochromocytoma	30	45
Hyperparathyroidism	50	Rare
Mucosal neuroma syndrome	—	100

TABLE 216-1. FOUR COMPONENTS OF RENAL OSTEODYSTROPHY

1. Osteitis fibrosa (high bone turnover)
   a. Phosphate retention
   b. Altered metabolism of vitamin D
   c. Skeletal resistance to PTH
   d. Decreased number of calcitriol receptors in parathyroid glands
   e. Unpaired degradation of PTH
   f. Altered feedback regulation of PTH by Ca^{2+}
2. Osteomalacia (low bone turnover)
   a. Altered metabolism of vitamin D
   b. Altered synthesis and maturation of collagen
   c. Acidosis
   d. Increased bone magnesium
   e. Increased pyrophosphate
   f. Retention of aluminum
   g. Retention of iron
3. Osteosclerosis ⎫
              ⎬ of lesser quantitative importance
4. Osteoporosis ⎭

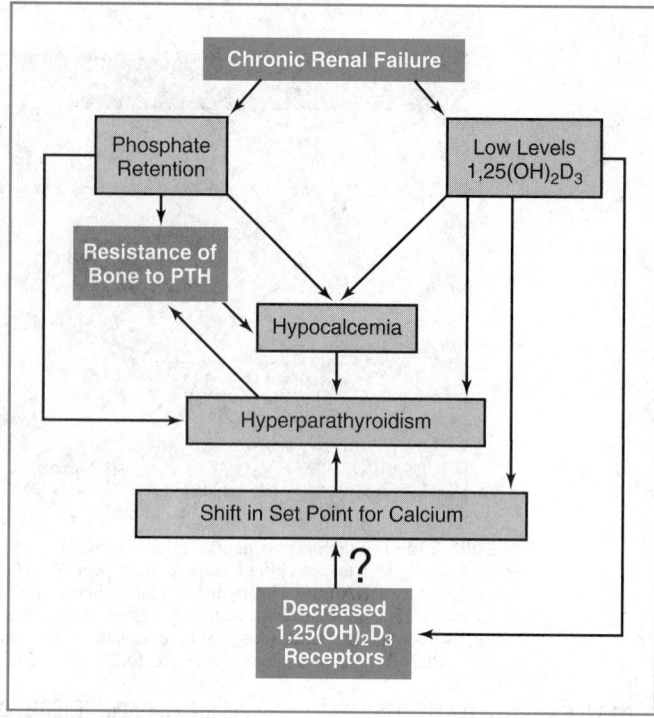

FIGURE 216-1. Diagrammatic representation of the factors involved in the pathogenesis of secondary hyperparathyroidism. (Modified from Slatopolsky E, Coburn J: Renal osteodystrophy. In Avioli L, Krane SM [eds.]: Metabolic Bone Disease, 2nd ed. Orlando, FL, Grune & Stratton, 1990.)

OSTEITIS FIBROSA (High-Turnover Bone Disease)

Chief cell hyperplasia of the parathyroid glands and high levels of immunoreactive parathyroid hormone (i-PTH) are among the earliest findings affecting mineral metabolism in most patients with chronic renal failure. Several factors contribute to the development of secondary hyperparathyroidism in renal insufficiency (Table 216-1 and Fig. 216-1).

THE ROLE OF PHOSPHATE RETENTION. Phosphorus retention plays an important role in the genesis of hyperparathyroidism. The mechanisms considered include (1) phosphorus-induced hypocalcemia, (2) phosphorus-induced decrease in the levels of calcitriol, and (3) other unknown factors. These mechanisms are closely interrelated and are not mutually exclusive.

PHOSPHORUS RETENTION AND HYPOCALCEMIA. A rise in serum phosphorus can evoke an increase in PTH secretion. An oral phosphorus load leads to an increase in serum phosphorus, a fall in ionized calcium, and increased levels of PTH in normal human subjects. Whether this sequence of events occurs in early renal failure has been questioned in that fasting or even postprandial levels of serum phosphorus are not consistently elevated. In fact, low levels of serum phosphorus are not uncommon. By contrast, in advanced renal failure, hyperphosphatemia plays a key role in the development of hypocalcemia, metastatic calcifications, peripheral vascular insufficiency, pruritus, and worsening of secondary hyperparathyroidism.

PHOSPHORUS RETENTION AND CALCITRIOL. Because phosphorus regulates the production rate of calcitriol by altering the activity of the enzyme 1α-hydroxylase, it is possible that the effects of phosphorus retention are mediated by a decrease in the synthesis of calcitriol. Conversely, the beneficial effects of phosphorus restriction in ameliorating hyperparathyroidism could be explained by increased levels of calcitriol. In patients with moderate renal insufficiency, dietary phosphorus restriction significantly increases plasma calcitriol levels with a concomitant normalization of plasma PTH. This occurs despite a lack of change in serum phosphorus levels.

OTHER MECHANISMS OF THE EFFECT OF PHOSPHORUS RETENTION. Although many investigators have focused their attention on the effects of phosphorus being mediated by changes in serum levels of calcium and/or calcitriol, there is evidence that phosphorus *per se* directly or indirectly may be involved. Several investigators have demonstrated that phosphorus restriction corrects secondary hyperparathyroidism in patients and dogs with advanced renal insufficiency. These studies suggest that a reduction in dietary phosphorus in advanced renal failure improves secondary hyperparathyroidism by a mechanism that is independent of the levels of calcitriol or serum ionized calcium.

In addition to the well-known effects of phosphorus in the regulation of calcitriol, a low-phosphorus diet may have an effect on the secretion of PTH. Although the mechanism of this effect is not yet known, phosphorus may potentially affect phospholipid composition of the parathyroid cell membrane, calcium fluxes in the parathyroid

cells, and/or regulation of calcitriol receptors in the parathyroid cell (see Ch. 214).

ALTERATIONS IN VITAMIN D METABOLISM (see Ch. 212). Because the kidney is the major site of calcitriol production, it follows that a loss of renal mass, as renal disease progresses, may decrease the ability of the diseased kidneys to produce the active metabolite of vitamin D. PTH and low-phosphate or low-calcium diets stimulate the activity of the 1α-hydroxylase; lack of PTH, hyperphosphatemia, or hypercalcemia decreases the activity of the 1α-hydroxylase. Intestinal absorption of calcium is reduced in patients with far-advanced renal insufficiency, and low levels of calcitriol are found in serum as the probable cause.

SKELETAL RESISTANCE TO THE ACTION OF PARATHYROID HORMONE. Skeletal resistance to the calcemic action of PTH may also play a role in the development of hypocalcemia seen in patients with renal insufficiency. This supports the concept of desensitization/down-regulation of the PTH receptor-effective mechanisms and minimizes the direct role of calcitriol. Thus, higher circulating levels of PTH may be needed to maintain a normal serum calcium in patients with renal failure.

IMPAIRED DEGRADATION OF PTH SECONDARY TO REDUCED RENAL FUNCTION. PTH is metabolized by the liver and the kidney. The liver takes up the intact hormone exclusively; it does not remove either amino-terminal or carboxy-terminal PTH fragments from the circulation. In chronic renal insufficiency, therefore, the high levels of carboxy-terminal circulating i-PTH result both from increased PTH secretion due to chief cell hyperplasia and from a decreased catabolism of the hormone.

ALTERED FEEDBACK REGULATION BETWEEN IONIZED CALCIUM AND THE SECRETION OF PARATHYROID HORMONE (see Ch. 214). The control of PTH secretion by ionized calcium in extracellular fluid may be blunted in patients with chronic renal insufficiency (Fig. 216-1).

OSTEOMALACIA (Low-Turnover Bone Disease) (see Ch. 211 and 212)

Although the plasma levels of calcitriol are reduced in patients with far-advanced renal insufficiency, overt osteomalacia is found in only a small fraction of such patients and may be absent even in anephric patients. Thus, other factors could also participate in the pathogenesis of osteomalacia in uremic patients—the plasma level of phosphate, for example. Hypophosphatemia *per se* can produce severe osteomalacia even in patients with normal renal function. Additional factors include altered collagen synthesis and maturation, defective bone crystal maturation, increased bone magnesium, elevated levels of pyrophosphate, and diminished calcium carbonate. The combination of these factors may influence the maturation of bone and potentially contribute to osteomalacia. Acidosis also contributes to the skeletal disease. In chronic renal insufficiency the skeleton assists in buffering the retained acids. Administering bicarbonate and correcting the acidosis in azotemic patients can reduce fecal calcium excretion.

Another type of osteomalacia in renal insufficiency, and likely the most common one, that is resistant to vitamin D therapy results from excess aluminum. Patients with osteomalacia secondary to aluminum have pathologic fractures, severe bone pain, and characteristically have low levels of PTH. High aluminum content in the water and/or the ingestion of phosphate binders containing aluminum may be the causes. The aluminum is deposited in the interface between the osteoid tissue and the calcification front and is toxic to the osteoblast. Severe iron retention can induce a similar form of osteomalacia.

More recently, a form of low bone turnover called "adynamic" or aplastic bone disease has been described. Patients maintained on continuous ambulatory peritoneal dialysis (CAPD) suffer from this more commonly than those maintained on chronic dialysis. Aluminum accumulation has been implicated in approximately 50% of these patients. In the remainder, diabetes, aging, high calcium in the dialysate, and low levels of PTH have been implicated in the pathogenesis of this condition. Histologically, this lesion is characterized by a significant decrease in the amount of osteoid tissue and lack of osteoblasts. The clinical consequences of this lesion are as yet unclear.

CLINICAL MANIFESTATIONS

The symptoms related to renal osteodystrophy usually appear only when renal failure is advanced. On the other hand, certain biochemical alterations may appear much earlier. Detecting these alterations may direct the physician to early treatment and prevent severe complications in bone and mineral metabolism.

Bone pain can progress inexorably to a point where the patient becomes bedridden, without regard to whether the bone disease is predominantly osteitis fibrosa or osteomalacia. The bone pain is characteristically vague and commonly located in the lower back, hips, knees, and legs. Low back pain may result from the collapse of a vertebral body. Sharp chest pain may indicate spontaneous rib fracture. Physical findings are frequently lacking.

Muscular weakness, when present, is usually proximal, appears slowly, and progresses with time. Plasma levels of creatine phosphokinase and transaminases are usually normal, and the electron micrographic changes are nonspecific. The pathogenesis of this muscular weakness is uncertain. In patients with myopathy, the myofibrils are disorganized in a patchy fashion and the Z-band material may be dispersed. These changes revert to normal following treatment with $25(OH)D_3$. *Pruritus* due to calcium deposition in skin is a common symptom in uremic patients, particularly with severe secondary hyperparathyroidism.

Vascular calcification and peripheral ischemic necrosis may occur, producing lesions of the tips of the digits and violaceous discoloration of the skin. Ulcerations and scarring may occur, with clear demarcation of the lesions from the surrounding skin. Acute pain and swelling around one or more joints may also develop in uremic patients. The syndrome of *calcific periarthritis,* which may be caused by deposition of hydroxyapatite crystals, is accompanied by marked hyperphosphatemia.

Skeletal deformities are common in azotemic children who are growing. Bowing of the tibia and femur and deformities from slipped epiphyses are not uncommon. Children with renal rickets sometimes exhibit typical radiographic findings of vitamin D deficiency. In adults with renal failure, particularly those with osteomalacia, marked skeletal deformities with lumbar scoliosis, thoracic kyphosis, and deformity of the thoracic cage may be observed. Growth retardation is usually seen in young children before and during maintenance hemodialysis. See Ch. 213 for a further discussion of osteomalacia and rickets.

Many patients maintained on dialysis for ≥ 10 years may develop severe bone and joint pain secondary to amyloidosis. β_2-Microglobulins have been implicated in the pathogenesis of this condi-

tion. The presence of bone cysts in the hands, the head of the humerus, and other large joints is characteristic of this condition.

Another clinical manifestation of renal osteodystrophy may occur in some after renal transplant is aseptic necrosis of the femoral head. This condition is more frequently seen in patients with severe bone disease (osteitis fibrosa) before renal transplant and in those who receive large doses of glucocorticoids.

BIOCHEMICAL FEATURES

Circulating i-PTH is elevated early in the course of renal insufficiency (glomerular filtration rate [GFR] 60 to 80 ml per minute). As the disease progresses (GFR < 40 ml per minute), hypocalcemia and low levels of calcitriol appear. With advanced renal insufficiency, however, the serum calcium may remain close to normal and values < 7.5 mg per deciliter are infrequent. Usually hypocalcemia is more marked in severe osteomalacia or with profound metabolic acidosis. Occasionally, hypercalcemia may be observed in uremic patients, particularly in those undergoing long-term dialysis. This complication can arise from (1) severe hyperparathyroidism, (2) ingesting large amounts of calcium and vitamin D, (3) the presence of unrelated diseases such as sarcoidosis or malignancies, or (4) a "pure" mineralizing defect, as may occur in osteomalacia secondary to aluminum retention, and (5) adynamic bone lesion. Hyperphosphatemia is usually present in patients with GFR < 25 ml per minute. The degree of hyperphosphatemia depends on the amount of phosphate ingested, the fraction absorbed in the intestine, and the amount excreted in the urine. If the patient ingests phosphate binders, the serum phosphate may remain normal despite advanced renal insufficiency. Patients with severe hyperparathyroidism and advanced renal insufficiency usually have higher concentrations of serum phosphate in plasma.

Advanced renal insufficiency (GFR < 15 ml per minute) may be associated with hypermagnesemia and increased bone content of magnesium. This may adversely affect crystal formation.

Total serum alkaline phosphatase levels and osteocalcin (both markers of bone formation) are commonly higher in uremic patients with osteitis fibrosa than in those with osteomalacia. Coexistent liver disease should be excluded as a cause of an elevated alkaline phosphatase.

RADIOGRAPHIC FEATURES

Secondary hyperparathyroidism increases bone resorption, most commonly evident on the subperiosteal surfaces of bone. Erosions in conjunction with formation of new bone may appear as cysts or osteoclastomas (brown tumors). The presence of subperiosteal erosion correlates with serum i-PTH and with the histomorphometric features of osteitis fibrosa on bone biopsy. Subperiosteal resorption of the phalanges may be the most sensitive radiographic sign of secondary hyperparathyroidism (Fig. 216–2). The tuft of the terminal phalanx of the second or third digit commonly shows resorption. With severe tuft erosion the soft tissue may collapse and change of the contour of the tuft so that the finger appears to show clubbing. Bone erosions may also occur at the upper end of the tibia, the neck of the femur or the humerus, and the lower surface of the medial end of the clavicle. In the skull, resorption leads to the mottled and granular appearance commonly associated with altering areas of osteosclerosis.

Osteosclerosis is thought to be another feature of osteitis fibrosa arising from an increase in the thickness and number of trabecula in spongy bone. Osteosclerosis can lead to a typical "rugger jersey" appearance of the spine.

Osteomalacia is far less distinctive radiographically than is secondary hyperparathyroidism. The Looser zone or pseudofracture is the only pathognomonic radiographic finding of osteomalacia in the adult. Rickets, i.e., widening of the epiphyseal growth plate, cannot develop after epiphyseal closure and hence is limited to children. With mechanical stress following severe prolonged deficiency of vitamin D, a Looser zone may extend across the full width of the bone and produce a true fracture with displacement of fragments. In uremia, osteomalacia is commonly associated with secondary hyperparathyroidism with radiographic features of both. The diagnosis of osteomalacia rests on histologic examinations and can be established with certainty only by bone biopsy.

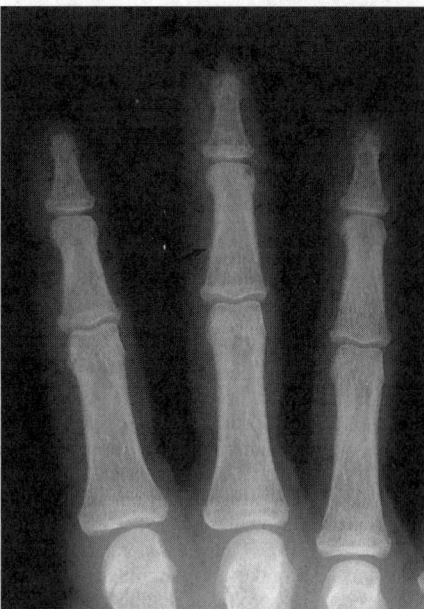

FIGURE 216–2. Radiographic manifestations of osteitis fibrosa. There are subperiosteal erosions of the phalanges and tuft of the terminal phalanx.

Soft-tissue calcification is presumed to be influenced by an increase in the calcium phosphate product in plasma, the degree of secondary hyperparathyroidism, the magnitude of alkalosis, and local tissue injury. Three major varieties include (1) calcification of the medium-size arteries, (2) articular or tumoral calcifications, and (3) visceral calcifications affecting the heart, lung, and kidney.

TREATMENT

The objectives of treating patients with renal osteodystrophy are (1) to return the blood levels of calcium and phosphate to normal, (2) to suppress secondary hyperparathyroidism, (3) to reverse the histologic abnormalities in the skeleton, and (4) to prevent and reverse extraskeletal deposits of calcium and phosphate. Guidelines for the management of renal osteodystrophy are summarized in Table 216–2.

CONTROL OF PHOSPHATE AND CALCIUM. To control phosphate, dietary phosphate intake should be reduced to 700 to 800 mg per day (determined as phosphorus) by restricting dairy products and by decreasing the amount of protein in the diet. In advanced renal failure, in addition to dietary control, phosphate binders are usually required to reduce its intestinal absorption. Phosphate binders should be ingested along with the meal in order to increase their efficiency. Aluminum-containing gels carry the potential of excessive aluminum absorption and accumulation. If the patient develops symptoms and signs suggesting aluminum-induced osteomalacia, this drug should be discontinued. Calcium carbonate (1 to 4 grams with each meal) helps bind phosphate and thereby reduces the amount of aluminum binders needed to treat hyperphosphatemia. During treatment with oral calcium carbonate, it is important to determine the amount of phosphate ingested in 24 hours and during each meal. In this way, the relative amount of calcium carbonate given can be adjusted to the phosphate-binding requirements of specific meals. Calcium carbonate also provides a calcium supplement that helps correct the negative calcium balance secondary to the calcium malabsorption of advanced renal insufficiency. The serum phosphorus should be maintained at normal or nearly normal levels, between 3.5 and 4.5 mg per deciliter, if the patient is not yet on dialysis. The serum calcium should be maintained in the upper limits of normal. Severe hyperphosphatemia should be corrected before administering calcium to reduce the risk of metastatic calcification. Supplemental calcium should be discontinued if the serum calcium increases above 11.0 mg per deciliter.

USE OF VITAMIN D AND ITS METABOLITES. Despite dietary control of phosphate using phosphate binders, adequate dietary calcium, and appropriate levels of calcium in the dialysate,

uremic patients may still develop skeletal disease. Thus, vitamin D and its metabolites are important agents for treating renal osteodystrophy. Calcitriol, the most active metabolite of vitamin D, is the drug of choice for treating hypocalcemia and secondary hyperparathyroidism (see Ch. 214). The usual dose is 0.5 to 1 μg per day. Recent evidence suggests that "oral pulse" (2 to 4 μg twice weekly) is more effective than the usual small dose (0.5 to 1.0 μg) given daily. Calcitriol, given intravenously during dialysis, at the dose of 1 to 3 μg three times per week, is the best approach to suppress secondary hyperparathyroidism. With the intravenous preparation of calcitriol, high concentrations of 1,25-$(OH)_2D_3$ can be obtained in serum. This is important because the low number of receptors in the parathyroid gland make the hyperplastic tissue more resistant to the action of calcitriol. Moreover, calcitriol can upregulate its own number of receptors.

PARATHYROIDECTOMY. The regimen outlined above can lead to improved homeostasis of calcium and phosphorus and reverse the symptoms of bone disease and suppression of PTH secretion. Such measures may not be entirely successful, however, and parathyroidectomy may be required. Indications for parathyroid surgery include severe secondary hyperparathyroidism (bone erosions and high levels of i-PTH) in the presence of any of the following: (1) persistent hypercalcemia, particularly when symptomatic; (2) intractable pruritus that does not respond to dialysis or other medical treatment; (3) progressive extraskeletal calcification in conjunction with a high calcium-phosphorus product that is consistently about 75 to 80 despite appropriate phosphate restriction; and (4) the appearance of ischemic lesions of soft tissues. Because of a lack of compliance, many patients are unable to control their serum phosphorus levels. In these cases, neither calcium supplements nor vitamin D or its metabolites can be recommended safely. Such patients are more likely to develop severe secondary hyperparathyroidism and require parathyroidectomy. Postoperative hypocalcemia may pose a problem if the remaining parathyroid tissue is inadequate and if severe osteitis fibrosa is present preoperatively. Preoperative treatment of such patients with calcitriol (1 to 2 μg per day) may obviate such problems. Serum levels of phosphorus and magnesium sometimes decrease after parathyroidectomy. Phosphate binders should be withheld if the serum phosphorus falls below 3.0 mg per deciliter. Rapid remineralization of the skeleton occurs during this period, but once the "hungry bones" have been

TABLE 216–2. GUIDELINES FOR MANAGING RENAL OSTEODYSTROPHY

Early treatment
It is important to begin treatment early, i.e., when the GFR is 30–40 ml/min, especially for the control of serum phosphate.

Control of serum phosphate (P) (3.5–4.5 mg/dl)
Restrict phosphorus intake in diet to 600–800 mg/day
Phosphate-binding antacids: aluminum carbonate or hydroxide; individualize dosage: Basaljel, Dialume, Alucap, Amphogel, 1–4 capsules with each meal. *Minimize the use of aluminum binders. Preferentially use:*
Calcium carbonate; 1–4 grams with each meal
Calcium acetate 0.5–3 grams with each meal
Hypophosphatemia should be avoided
Predialysis phosphorus: 4.5–5.5 mg/dl

Adequate calcium intake
Oral calcium supplements providing 1–2 grams/day when serum P is controlled: Os-Cal, Titralac, Tums
Dialysate Ca, 5.0–5.5 mg/dl (2.5–2.75 mEq/liter)

Use of vitamin D sterols
Vitamin D_2 or D_3, 50,000 to 250,000 IU (1.25–6.25 mg)/day
25-Hydroxyvitamin D_3 (calcifediol), 20–100 μg/day (Calderol)
1,25-Dihydroxyvitamin D_3 (calcitriol), 0.5–1.0 μg/day (Rocaltrol)
1,25-Dihydroxyvitamin D_3 (calcitriol) ("oral pulse") 2.0–4.0 μg twice a week (Rocaltrol)
1,25-Dihydroxyvitamin D_3 (calcitriol) IV, 1.0–3.0 μg three times a week (Calcijex)

Parathyroidectomy
Severe secondary hyperparathyroidism (bone erosions and increased i-PTH) plus any of the following:
Persistent hypercalcemia (serum Ca >11.5–12.0 mg/dl)
Progressive or symptomatic extraskeletal calcification
Persistently elevated serum calcium-phosphorus product
Pruritus not responsive to medical treatment
Calciphylaxis (ischemic ulcers and necrosis)
Symptomatic hypercalcemia after renal transplantation

mineralized, serum calcium levels rise. A fall in a previously elevated serum alkaline phosphatase toward normal may indicate that rapid skeletal remineralization is nearly complete and that calcium supplements and vitamin D therapy may be reduced or discontinued. In the past, removing three and a half parathyroid glands was the procedure of choice. More recently, total parathyroidectomy followed by autotransplantation of some of the parathyroid tissue into the patient's forearm has been used. The transplanted tissue is more accessible if subsequent surgical removal is necessary. Total parathyroidectomy without autotransplantation has no place in managing renal osteodystrophy because it may predispose to the development of an isolated mineralization defect or osteomalacia in uremic patients. Cryopreservation of removed parathyroid tissue is a useful precaution so that hypoparathyroidism may be treated by reimplantation of parathyroid tissue.

Occasionally after a successful renal transplant, the patient may develop hypercalcemia. Usually this is due to persistent hyperparathyroidism and increased renal production of calcitriol. In the majority of cases, the hypercalcemia subsides several months after renal transplantation. In a few patients, however, severe hypercalcemia (calcium 12 to 13 mg per deciliter) may persist for several months and may affect renal function. In these patients, a subtotal parathyroidectomy is recommended.

TREATMENT OF ALUMINUM TOXICITY. If the patient has aluminum-induced osteomalacia, phosphate binders containing aluminum should be discontinued at once. Phosphate should be controlled by using a more restrictive phosphate diet, and serum phosphorus may be allowed to increase to 6 mg per deciliter. If the patient is not extremely symptomatic, discontinuing aluminum binders will greatly improve the skeletal abnormalities after a period of 6 to 18 months. Symptomatic patients bedridden with severe bone pain and pathologic fractures should receive desferoxamine, 0.5 to 1.0 grams once per week.

SECONDARY AMYLOIDOSIS. No specific treatment is available for this condition. Renal transplantation greatly improves symptoms.

Coburn JW, Slatopolsky E: Vitamin D, parathyroid hormone and renal osteodystrophy. *In* Brenner BM, Rector FC (eds.): The Kidney. 4th ed. Philadelphia, WB Saunders, 1990. *Comprehensive review of renal osteodystrophy.*

Delmez JA, Tindira C, Grooms P, et al.: Parathyroid hormone suppression by intravenous 1,25-dihydroxyvitamin D: A role for increased sensitivity to calcium. J Clin Invest 83:1349, 1989. *Demonstrates that administering IV calcitriol partially corrects the resistance of the parathyroid glands to calcium in uremic patients.*

Korkor AB: Reduced binding of [3H] 1,25-dihydroxyvitamin D_3 in patients with renal failure. N Engl J Med 316:1573, 1987. *Describes for the first time the decreased number of calcitriol receptors in the parathyroid glands of uremic patients.*

Slatopolsky E: Vitamin D. Semin Nephrol 14:99, 1994. *Comprehensive review (several papers) of vitamin D, vitamin D receptor, and analogues. Molecular interactions between vitamin D and PTH.*

Slatopolsky E, Weerts C, Lopez-Hilker S, et al.: Long-term effects of calcium carbonate and 2.5 mEq/liter calcium dialysate on mineral metabolism. Kidney Int 36:897, 1989. *Describes the effectiveness of calcium carbonate as a phosphate binder.*

Szabo A, Merke J, Beier E, et al.: 1,25(OH)$_2$ vitamin D_3 inhibits parathyroid cell proliferation in experimental uremia. Kidney Int 35:1049, 1989. *Demonstrates the antiproliferative effect of calcitriol on the parathyroid glands of uremic rats.*

217 OSTEOPOROSIS
Joel S. Finkelstein

Osteoporosis, the most common type of metabolic bone disease, is characterized by a parallel reduction in bone mineral and bone matrix so that bone is decreased in amount but is of normal composition. Osteoporosis affects 20 million Americans and leads to approximately 1.3 million fractures in the United States each year. During the course of their lifetime, women lose about 50% of trabecular bone and 30% of cortical bone, and 30% of all postmenopausal Caucasian women eventually sustain osteoporotic fractures. By extreme old age, one third of all women and one sixth of all men have a hip fracture. The annual cost of health care and lost productivity due to osteoporosis exceeds $10 billion in the United States.

ETIOLOGY AND PATHOGENESIS

At any point in time, bone density depends on both the peak bone density achieved during development and the subsequent adult bone loss (Fig. 217–1). Thus, osteopenia can result either from deficient pubertal bone accretion, accelerated adult bone loss, or both.

DETERMINANTS OF PEAK BONE DENSITY. Bone density increases dramatically during puberty in response to gonadal steroids and eventually reaches values in young adults that are nearly double those of children. Other factors that influence peak bone density are listed in Table 217–1. Of these, genetic factors account for up to 80% of the variance in peak bone mass. The impact of genetic factors on bone density has been demonstrated in several ways. For example, bone density is lower in the daughters of women with osteoporosis than in those without osteoporosis. Moreover, the concordance of bone density is much higher among monozygotic than dizygotic twins. Recent data suggest that most of the genetic differences in bone density can be accounted for by a gene closely linked to the vitamin D receptor gene, perhaps the receptor gene itself. A large cross-sectional analysis of Caucasian men and women revealed that allelic variations of the vitamin D receptor gene are associated with absolute differences in bone density of 10 to 12%, an effect as large as that caused by 10 years of estrogen deficiency. It is not known whether the differences in bone density associated with variations in vitamin D receptor genotypes reflect differences in bone accretion during development or in the rate of subsequent bone loss.

Men have higher bone density than women and blacks have higher bone density than Caucasians. These differences may account for a lower incidence of osteoporotic fractures in men and in blacks. Men with histories of constitutionally delayed puberty have decreased peak bone density, a finding that may be important in the pathogenesis of osteoporosis in some men. Similar findings have been reported in women with delayed menarche. Studies in identical twins suggest that moderate calcium supplementation can enhance prepubertal bone accretion. Associations between peak bone density and physical activity have also been reported.

PHYSIOLOGIC CAUSES OF ADULT BONE LOSS. After peak bone density is reached, bone density remains stable for years and then declines. Considerable evidence suggests that bone loss begins before menses cease in women and in the third to fifth decades in men. Once the menopause is established, the rate of bone loss is accelerated several-fold in women. During the first 5 to 10 years of the menopause, trabecular bone is lost faster than cortical bone with rates of approximately 2 to 4 and 1 to 2% per year, respectively. A woman can lose 10 to 15% of her cortical bone and 25 to 30% of her trabecular bone during this time, a loss that can be prevented by estrogen replacement therapy. Furthermore, rates of

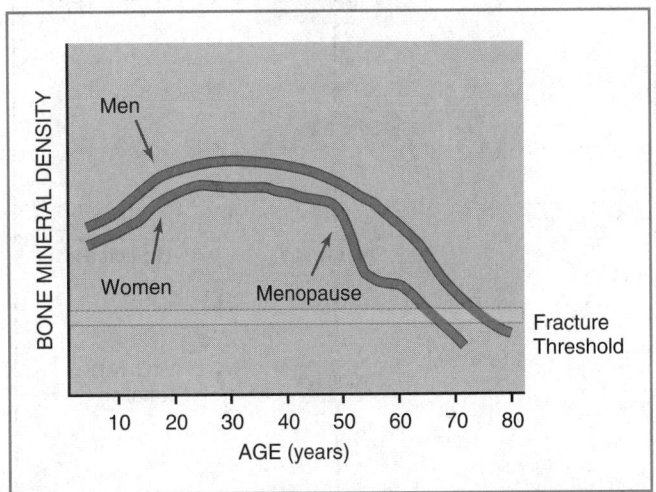

FIGURE 217–1. Cortical bone mineral density versus age in men and women. Women have lower peak cortical bone density than men and experience a period of rapid bone loss at menopause, thus reaching the fracture threshold (the level of bone density at which the risk of developing osteoporotic fractures begins to increase) earlier than men.

TABLE 217-1. FACTORS THAT MAY AFFECT PEAK BONE MASS

Gender
Race
Genetic factors
Gonadal steroids
Growth hormone
Timing of puberty
Calcium intake
Exercise

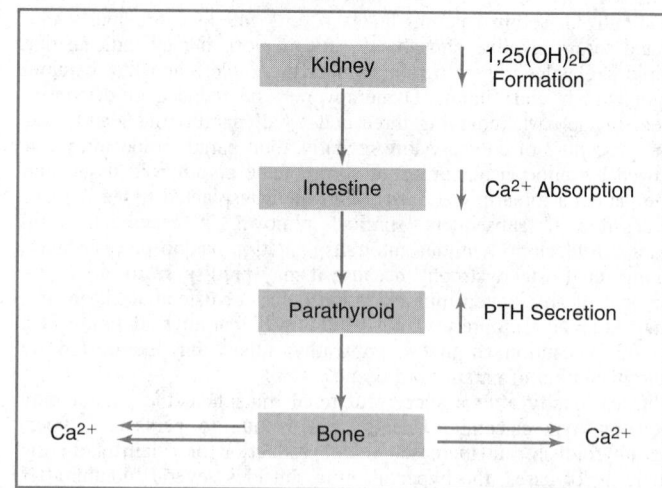

FIGURE 217-3. Physiologic alterations in women with type II ("senile") osteoporosis.

bone loss vary considerably among women. It is not clear why some postmenopausal women are "fast losers" of bone. A subset of women in whom osteopenia is more severe than expected for their age are said to have type I or "postmenopausal" osteoporosis (Fig. 217–2). Clinically, type I osteoporosis often presents with vertebral "crush" fractures or Colles' fractures. The mechanism whereby estrogen deficiency leads to bone loss is still not established. Recent evidence suggests that estrogen deficiency may increase local production of bone-resorbing cytokines such as interleukin-1 (IL-1), IL-6, and tumor necrosis factor. Bone resorption associated with estrogen deficiency can be attenuated by administering an IL-1 receptor antagonist or by knocking out the IL-6 gene, findings consistent with this hypothesis. Because estrogen also increases local production of growth factors that stimulate bone formation such as insulin-like growth factor-1 (IGF-1) and transforming growth factor-β (TGF-β), estrogen deficiency might diminish bone formation. Estrogen deficiency increases the skeleton's sensitivity to the resorptive effects of parathyroid hormone (PTH). Estrogen deficiency therefore leads to a small increase in serum calcium levels. According to one hypothesis, increased calcium levels suppress PTH secretion, thereby decreasing renal 1,25-(OH)$_2$ vitamin D formation, which then limits intestinal calcium absorption (Fig. 217–2). Finally, the discovery of estrogen receptors on osteoblasts suggests that estrogen deficiency may also alter bone formation directly.

Once the period of rapid postmenopausal bone loss ends, bone loss continues at a more gradual rate throughout life. The osteope-

nia that results from normal aging, which occurs in both women and men, has been termed type II or "senile" osteoporosis (Fig. 217–3). Some data suggest that trabecular bone loss ceases after many years of estrogen deficiency but that slow cortical bone loss continues. Because type II osteoporosis is associated with a more balanced decrease in cortical and trabecular bone mass, fractures of the hip, pelvis, wrist, proximal humerus, proximal tibia, and vertebral bodies all occur commonly. Factors that may be important in the pathogenesis of type II osteoporosis include (1) a primary defect in the ability of the kidney to make 1,25-(OH)$_2$D and/or decreased intestinal sensitivity to 1,25-(OH)$_2$D, leading to diminished calcium absorption and mild secondary hyperparathyroidism; and (2) a decrease in osteoblastic bone formation with aging. Finally, the distinctions between type I and type II osteoporosis are often quite arbitrary, and there may be considerable overlap between these syndromes.

SECONDARY CAUSES OF ADULT BONE LOSS. Many disorders can lead to osteoporosis independent of the normal effects of the menopause in women and aging in both women and men (Table 217–2). For example, young women who develop estrogen deficiency due to hyperprolactinemia, anorexia nervosa, or hypothalamic amenorrhea frequently lose bone. Hypogonadism is also an important secondary cause of osteoporosis in men. Other endocrine disorders such as hyperthyroidism, hyperparathyroidism, hypercortisolism, and growth hormone deficiency can cause osteoporosis primarily due to increased bone resorption in the former two disorders and decreased bone formation and intestinal calcium absorption in the latter. Patients with gastrointestinal and hepatobiliary disorders most often have low-turnover osteoporosis, although some have osteomalacia or secondary hyperparathyroidism owing to calcium and/or vitamin D malabsorption. The osteoporosis in patients with marrow-related disorders may be due to local effects of cytokines on bone remodeling or to the release of systemic factors that activate bone resorption. Peak adult bone mass is compromised in certain connective tissue disorders such as osteogenesis imperfecta. Many drugs such as ethanol, heparin, glucocorticoids, suppressive doses of thyroxine, and anticonvulsants can cause osteoporosis. Ethanol is toxic to osteoblasts, whereas heparin increases osteoclastic bone resorption. In patients receiving anticonvulsant therapy, the combined effects of reduced 25(OH)D levels, secondary hyperparathyroidism, direct inhibition of intestinal calcium transport, and suppression of osteoblast function can lead to osteoporosis and/or osteomalacia. Bone resorption is accelerated in patients who are immobilized and in patients with rheumatoid arthritis. Finally, bone formation may be diminished in individuals with insulin-dependent diabetes mellitus.

CLINICAL MANIFESTATIONS

Osteoporosis is asymptomatic unless it results in a fracture—usually a vertebral compression fracture or a fracture of the wrist, hip, ribs, pelvis, or humerus. Vertebral compression fractures often occur with minimal stress, such as with sneezing, bending, or lift-

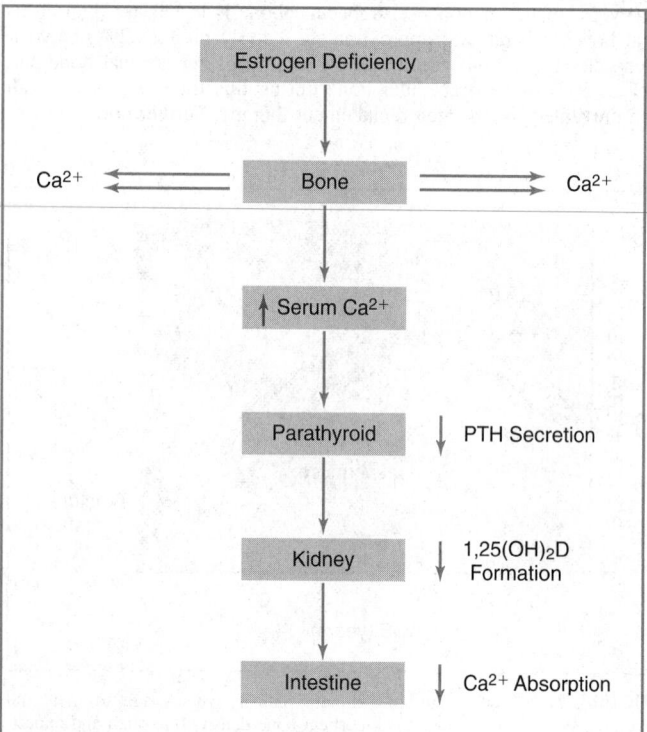

FIGURE 217-2. Physiologic alterations in women with type I ("postmenopausal") osteoporosis.

TABLE 217–2. SECONDARY CAUSES OF OSTEOPOROSIS

217 OSTEOPOROSIS / 1381

Endocrine diseases
  Female hypogonadism
    Hyperprolactinemia
    Hypothalamic amenorrhea
    Anorexia nervosa
    Premature and primary ovarian failure
  Male hypogonadism
    Primary gonadal failure (e.g., Klinefelter's syndrome)
    Secondary gonadal failure (e.g., idiopathic hypogonadotropic hypogonadism)
    Delayed puberty
  Hyperthyroidism
  Hyperparathyroidism
  Hypercortisolism
  Growth hormone deficiency
Gastrointestinal diseases
  Subtotal gastrectomy
  Malabsorption syndromes
  Chronic obstructive jaundice
  Primary biliary cirrhosis and other cirrhoses
  Alactasia
Bone marrow disorders
  Multiple myeloma
  Lymphoma
  Leukemia
  Hemolytic anemias
  Systemic mastocytosis
  Disseminated carcinoma
Connective tissue diseases
  Osteogenesis imperfecta
  Ehlers-Danlos syndrome
  Marfan's syndrome
  Homocystinuria
Drugs
  Alcohol
  Heparin
  Glucocorticoids
  Thyroxine
  Anticonvulsants
  GnRH agonists
  Cyclosporine
  Chemotherapy
Miscellaneous causes
  Immobilization
  Rheumatoid arthritis

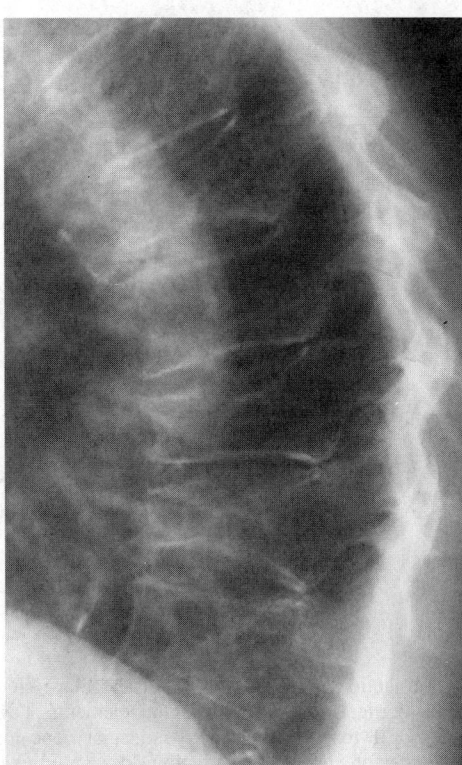

FIGURE 217–4. Radiograph showing radiolucency, compression fractures, and kyphosis in the spine of an osteoporosis patient.

ing a light object. The middle and lower thoracic and upper lumbar regions are most frequently involved. Back pain usually begins acutely and often radiates laterally to the flanks and anteriorly. The pain subsides gradually over a period of several weeks and recurs with the occurrence of new fractures. Patients with multiple fractures that result in spinal deformity may have a chronic backache that is made worse by standing. Such patients lose height and may develop the characteristic dorsal kyphosis and cervical lordosis known as the "dowager's hump." In some patients, vertebral collapse can occur slowly and without symptoms. Hip fractures are the most devastating complication of osteoporosis. They are of the femoral neck and intertrochanteric types, and the type is best predicted by the bone density of the trochanter. Hip fractures are associated with falls, occurring either as a result of modest trauma, or, in some instances, prior to the fall. The likelihood of suffering a hip fracture during a fall is also related to the direction of the fall so that fractures are more likely to occur in falls to the side, probably because less soft tissue is available to dissipate the impact. Secondary complications of hip fractures, such as pulmonary thromboembolism or nosocomial infections, carry a mortality rate of 15 to 20% in elderly patients and an additional 30% of hip fracture victims require long-term nursing home care.

RADIOGRAPHIC FINDINGS

A characteristic radiograph of osteoporosis of the spine is shown in Figure 217–4. With the loss of trabecular bone in the vertebral bodies, the vertebral end-plates appear to be accentuated. Loss of horizontal trabeculae causes the vertical trabeculae to be more prominent. The normal contrast between the radiodensity of the spinal column and the adjacent soft tissues also may be lost. Vertebral deformity may take the form of collapse (reduction in both anterior and posterior height), anterior wedging (reduction in anterior height), or the so-called codfish deformity (due to weakening of the subchondral plates and expansion of the intervertebral discs). Protrusion of the intervertebral discs in the vertebral bodies produces "Schmorl's nodules." In the absence of fractures, radiographs are insensitive indicators of bone loss because a substantial reduction in bone mass is required before it is visible on radiographs.

DIAGNOSIS

The diagnosis of osteopenia can be made by either documenting a typical fragility fracture or measuring bone mineral density, in which case a bone density value below the lower limit of normal for sex-matched young adults establishes the diagnosis. Most individuals with osteopenia have osteoporosis, although only a histomorphometric analysis of bone can distinguish osteoporosis from osteomalacia with certainty. Several techniques are available for measuring bone mineral density in the axial and appendicular skeleton (Table 217–3). Large prospective studies have demonstrated that bone density measurements of the distal and proximal radius, os calcis, proximal femur, or spine can predict the development of the major types of osteoporotic fractures, including hip fractures. However, the techniques differ greatly in their sensitivity for detecting osteopenia, reproducibility, radiation exposure, examination time, and cost. Because it measures trabecular bone in the vertebral bodies, quantitative computed tomography (QCT) of the spine is the most sensitive method for diagnosing osteopenia. However, because the expense and radiation dose of QCT are high and its reproducibility is relatively poor, it is not an ideal technique when repeat measurements aimed at detecting small changes in bone density are needed. Single-photon absorptiometry of the proximal forearm has good precision and low radiation exposure but is relatively insensitive for detecting osteopenia because it measures cortical bone, which is lost more slowly than trabecular bone in the early menopause. Dual-photon absorptiometry (DPA), which measures bone density in the axial skeleton and proximal femur, is limited by poor reproducibility, long examination times, and artifacts caused by vascular calcifications and changes in the radioactive source. For most patients, dual energy x-ray absorptiometry (DXA) of the lumbar spine is currently the method of choice for measuring bone mineral density. Because DXA scans of the spine in the an-

TABLE 217–3. TECHNIQUES FOR MEASURING BONE MINERAL DENSITY

Sites Measured	Precision (%)	Accuracy (%)	Scan Time (minutes)	Radiation Dose (mrem)
Quantitative computed tomography (QCT)	2–10	5–20	10–15	100–1000
Lumbar spine				
Proximal radius				
Distal radius				
Single-photon absorptiometry (SPA)	1–3	4–6	3–5	10–20
Proximal radius				
Distal radius				
Calcaneus				
Dual-photon absorptiometry (DPA)	2–6	4–10	20–40	10–15
Lumbar spine anteroposterior				
Lumbar spine lateral				
Proximal femur				
Total body				
Dual-energy x-ray absorptiometry (DXA)	1–2	3–5	2–8	1–3
Lumbar spine anteroposterior				
Lumbar spine lateral				
Proximal radius				
Distal radius				
Proximal femur				
Total body				

* For SPA, numbers refer to measurements of the proximal radius. For QCT, numbers refer to measurements of the lumbar spine. For DPA and DXA, numbers refer to AP measurements of the lumbar spine.

teroposterior projection include both the trabecular-rich vertebral bodies and the cortical-rich posterior spinal elements, DXA is not as sensitive as QCT for detecting early trabecular bone loss. However, its far greater precision, low radiation dose, rapid examination time, and lower cost make DXA preferable to QCT in most situations. Newer DXA scanners can measure spinal bone mineral density in both the anteroposterior and lateral projections. Lateral spine DXA is more sensitive than anterior-posterior spine DXA for detecting osteoporosis and has similar reproducibility.

Secondary causes of osteoporosis should be sought in patients with an established diagnosis of osteoporosis, particularly when the bone density is significantly lower than that of age- and sex-matched individuals. A history and physical examination that focus on the factors that may affect peak bone mass (see Table 217–1) and secondary causes of osteoporosis (see Table 217–2) and selected laboratory tests are sufficient in most patients. Levels of serum calcium, inorganic phosphate, and alkaline phosphatase are usually normal in patients with osteoporosis, although the latter may be transiently elevated after a fracture. A sustained elevation of the alkaline phosphatase level, in the absence of liver disease, may suggest osteomalacia, Paget's disease, or skeletal metastases. Other routine chemistries can help exclude renal or hepatic diseases, and a complete blood count may help uncover a hematologic or myeloproliferative disorder. Because multiple myeloma can mimic involutional osteoporosis, it should be considered when evaluating patients with osteoporosis, particularly those with severe disease. Measuring serum PTH and 25(OH)D levels is recommended to exclude hyperparathyroidism and vitamin D deficiency. A serum thyroid–stimulating hormone level should be checked when thyroid disease is suspected. In men with unexplained osteoporosis, a serum testosterone level should be measured. The clinical utility of measuring biochemical markers of bone formation (serum osteocalcin, bone-specific alkaline phosphatase, or type 1 procollagen carboxy-terminal propeptide) and bone resorption (urine hydroxyproline, urine pyridinium cross links, or urine cross linked N-telopeptides of type 1 collagen) has not been established. However, it is possible that these markers may help classify patients into high and low bone turnover states in the future and thereby provide a more rational basis for selecting therapies. Finally, in selected patients, iliac crest bone biopsy after double tetracycline labeling may be useful, particularly for distinguishing osteoporosis from osteomalacia.

TREATMENT

At present, it is not possible to reverse established osteoporosis. However, early intervention can prevent osteoporosis in most people, and later intervention can halt its progression once it has developed. The choice of treatment for osteoporosis depends on its cause

and the stage of the illness. If a secondary cause of osteoporosis is present, specific treatment should be aimed at correcting it. During the acute phase of vertebral compression, attention is directed toward relieving pain with analgesics, muscle relaxants, heat, massage, and/or rest. Many patients with discomfort related to osteoporotic fractures or deformity benefit from a well-designed program of physical therapy. Some patients appear to benefit from a corset or an orthopedic back brace. Both weight-bearing and non–weight-bearing exercises appear to have beneficial effects on bone mass. For most patients, exercises to strengthen the abdominal and back muscles are appropriate and referral to a physical therapist with expertise in treating osteoporotic patients is often helpful. Precautions to prevent falls should be taken. Pharmacologic therapy is aimed at preventing further bone loss and decreasing the likelihood of future fracture.

CALCIUM. Both dietary calcium intake and fractional intestinal calcium absorption decrease with age. Most postmenopausal women consume <500 mg of calcium each day, far below the U.S. recommended dietary allowance (RDA) of 800 to 1000 mg. The effects of calcium supplementation on bone mass in early menopausal women have been examined in several prospective, randomized trials. The results are inconsistent. In general, it appears that calcium can retard, but not arrest, cortical bone loss from the forearm in women who are within the first several years of the menopause. However, calcium supplementation is clearly less effective than estrogen. Most studies have failed to demonstrate a protective effect of calcium on spinal bone loss in early menopausal women. Calcium therapy appears to be more effective in arresting bone loss in late menopausal women, although some studies indicate that administering calcium does not halt their bone loss completely. Overall, it appears that calcium therapy is somewhat beneficial in both early and late menopausal women. However, additional therapy clearly is needed if the goal of therapy is to prevent bone loss completely. Most experts recommend that postmenopausal women consume between 1000 and 1200 mg of calcium per day, either in their diet or from supplements. Because calcium may enhance peak bone mass, the RDA for adolescents and young adults in the United States is 1500 mg of calcium per day.

ESTROGEN. Estrogen replacement therapy inhibits osteoclastic bone resorption. It prevents both cortical and trabecular bone loss in estrogen-deficient women and is effective if administered orally or topically. Estrogen replacement therapy prevents bone loss in both early and late menopausal women, although its efficacy has not been tested adequately in women over age 75. Because bone loss is most rapid in the first years of the menopause, the benefits of estrogen therapy probably are greater if started before a substantial amount of bone loss has occurred. Case-control studies suggest that estrogen therapy significantly reduces the risk of forearm, vertebral, pelvic, and hip fractures in postmenopausal women. The minimally effective doses of estrogen to prevent bone loss are 0.625 mg per day of conjugated estrogens, 2 mg per day of estradiol, 25 μg per day of ethinyl estradiol, or 50 μg per day of transdermal estrogen, although some studies have shown that lower doses of conjugated estrogens (0.3 mg per day) prevent bone loss when combined with sufficient calcium intake. How long a women should remain on estrogen replacement therapy has not been established.

Although the beneficial effects of estrogen replacement therapy on bone mass are well established, <15% of postmenopausal women in the United States take estrogen replacement. The decision to treat with estrogen is influenced by several other factors and should be individualized. In some women, estrogen is prescribed to alleviate menopausal symptoms. In others, the prospect of adhering to a treatment program that will produce cyclic menstruation is unacceptable. The relationships between estrogen replacement therapy and endometrial cancer, breast cancer, and ischemic heart disease have been the subjects of numerous investigations. When given without concomitant progestin, estrogen replacement therapy increases the risk of endometrial carcinoma. Thus, in the woman whose uterus is intact, estrogen replacement therapy should be combined with a progestin, administered either cyclically (e.g., 5 to 10 mg medroxyprogesterone acetate for 10 to 14 days each month) or continuously (e.g., 2.5 mg medroxyprogesterone acetate per day). The latter regimen often eliminates menstrual bleeding after an initial period of 3 to 6 months during which irregular bleeding may occur. Progestins may also enhance the osteoprotective effect of estrogens. In the woman who has had a hysterectomy, unopposed estrogen should be given daily. Estrogen therapy is contraindicated in women with a history of endometrial cancer.

The relationships between estrogen replacement therapy and breast cancer or cardiovascular disease have been the subject of many case-control and cohort studies yet they remain unclear. Although authors of one meta-analysis concluded that long-term (> 15 years) estrogen use is associated with an increase in the risk of breast cancer, other large cohort studies have failed to detect such a relationship. It has also been suggested that the risk of developing breast cancer is increased in women who take higher doses of estrogen (at least 1.25 mg of conjugated estrogen) and among women with a family history of breast cancer. Because the relationship between estrogen replacement therapy and breast cancer remains uncertain, estrogen replacement therapy is contraindicated in women with a history of breast cancer, and all postmenopausal women receiving estrogen therapy should have regular breast examinations and annual mammograms. Numerous case-control and cohort studies have reported that estrogen replacement therapy decreases the risk of major coronary disease by approximately 50%. However, the potential for bias due to patient selection or uneven diagnostic surveillance in these nonrandomized studies cannot be excluded completely. The potential beneficial effect of estrogen on coronary heart disease is often attributed to its ability to lower LDL cholesterol and raise HDL cholesterol. Still, because the reduction in cardiac events appears to be limited to current estrogen users and is independent of the duration of estrogen use, other mechanisms, including direct effects of estrogens on vascular wall function and coagulation factors, may be important.

CALCITONIN. Calcitonin inhibits osteoclastic bone resorption and is approved by the Food and Drug Administration (FDA) for treating postmenopausal osteoporosis. The effects of calcitonin therapy on bone loss in women who are within 5 years of the menopause have been inconsistent. Some groups have demonstrated that nasal calcitonin prevents spinal bone loss for up to 3 years while others have been unable to demonstrate such an effect. The reasons for these disparities are unclear. Calcitonin appears to prevent spinal bone loss in late menopausal women, although appendicular (i.e., cortical) bone loss continues. The effect of calcitonin therapy on the rate of osteoporotic fractures has not been well studied. At the present time, calcitonin is available only for parenteral use in the United States, although it is available as a nasal spray in some other countries. The recommended dose is 100 IU subcutaneously daily, given with adequate calcium and vitamin D, but it is possible that lower doses are equally effective. Side effects of parenteral calcitonin administration, including nausea, flushing, and local inflammatory reactions, occur in 10 to 15% of patients and can often be minimized by administering the medication at bedtime, starting at low doses (i.e., 25 IU) and increasing the dosage gradu-

ally over a period of several weeks. Calcitonin also appears to produce significant analgesic effects. Thus, it may be particularly useful in patients with osteoporosis who have chronic pain related to fractures or skeletal deformity.

BISPHOSPHONATES. Like calcitonin, bisphosphonates inhibit osteoclastic bone resorption. The only bisphosphonate that is currently available for oral administration in the United States is etidronate, although it has not yet been approved by the FDA for treating osteoporosis. Several other bisphosphonates are currently under investigation. Prospective studies have demonstrated that cyclic etidronate increases spinal bone mineral density slightly and decreases the incidence of vertebral fractures in late menopausal women when given for 2 to 3 years. However, further follow-up of these patients indicates that the previously reported beneficial effect of etidronate on fracture rate may be restricted to a subgroup of women at particularly high risk for fracture. Because the total number of fractures in these studies was small, it is difficult to draw firm conclusions regarding the effect of cyclic etidronate on osteoporotic fractures. The most commonly employed dose of etidronate is 400 mg per day for the first 2 weeks of every 3-month period. To ensure adequate absorption, it must be taken on an empty stomach.

The effects of bisphosphonates on bone loss in early menopausal women are less well studied. Short-term studies suggest that oral alendronate, tiludronate, and etidronate administration can prevent spinal bone loss in recently menopausal women.

VITAMIN D AND ITS METABOLITES. Calcium absorption decreases with age, especially after age 70. Because of low vitamin D intake, insufficient exposure to sunlight, and reduced ability to synthesize vitamin D in the skin, many elderly people are at risk for vitamin D deficiency. Furthermore, the ability to convert 25(OH)D to 1,25-(OH)$_2$D is impaired in many elderly people. Decreased vitamin D formation and calcium absorption in the elderly may lead to secondary hyperparathyroidism and accelerated bone loss.

Small doses of vitamin D (800 IU per day) plus calcium dramatically reduce the incidence of hip fractures and other nonspine fractures in elderly women. Because toxicity from such doses of vitamin D has not been reported, this therapy can be recommended to virtually all postmenopausal women. The role of 1,25-(OH)$_2$D therapy in postmenopausal osteoporosis is more controversial. At high doses (0.8 μg per day), 1,25-(OH)$_2$D plus calcium increases bone mass, but most patients develop hypercalciuria and/or hypercalcemia. At doses of 0.5 to 0.6 μg per day, 1,25-(OH)$_2$D plus calcium preserves spinal bone mass and decreases the rate of both vertebral and nonvertebral fractures with little toxicity. However, it is unclear whether 1,25-(OH)$_2$D therapy is superior to treatment with small doses of vitamin D. Because the therapeutic index of 1,25-(OH)$_2$D therapy is small, its use should probably be reserved for patients who are not candidates for other forms of pharmacologic therapy.

FUTURE THERAPIES. Several new types of therapeutic agents are currently in clinical trials. Antiestrogens such as tamoxifen can prevent spinal bone loss in postmenopausal women. Newer antiestrogens, which may have bone-sparing effects without causing endometrial hyperplasia, are being investigated. It is well known that sodium fluoride increases spinal bone density. However, the newly formed bone is qualitatively abnormal and cortical bone density sometimes decreases. A randomized controlled trial demonstrated that sodium fluoride therapy failed to reduce the risk of vertebral fractures and actually increased the incidence of fractures of the appendicular skeleton. However, lower doses of fluoride therapy and sustained-release preparations hold more promise and are under investigation. PTH, when given intermittently in low doses, is a potent stimulator of osteoblastic bone formation. In contrast to sodium fluoride, the bone formed in response to administered PTH is histologically normal and its strength is increased. Many animal studies have demonstrated that PTH can prevent or reverse estrogen-deficiency osteoporosis. Similar data have now been obtained in early human studies. Further investigation of the therapeutic potential of PTH is needed.

OSTEOPOROSIS IN MEN

Although osteoporosis is less common in men, men lose about 30% of trabecular bone and 20% of cortical bone during the course of their lifetime. By extreme old age, one in every six men has a hip fracture. Between 15 and 25% of men with hip or vertebral fractures are androgen deficient. Androgens have important effects on skeletal development. Peak bone mass is reduced in men who were androgen deficient during adolescence due to idiopathic hypogonadotropic hypogonadism or Klinefelter's syndrome and in men with histories of constitutionally delayed puberty (see Ch. 209). In adult men, castration or induction of androgen deficiency with long-acting GnRH analogues increases bone resorption and leads to rapid bone loss. Osteoporosis is also frequently observed in men with primary gonadal failure, hemochromatosis, hyperprolactinemic hypogonadism, or other disorders of the pituitary-hypothalamic axis.

Androgens may stimulate bone formation directly because osteoblastic cells possess androgen receptors. Androgens stimulate osteoblastic cell proliferation and differentiation, an effect that may be mediated by TGF-β or fibroblast growth factor. Like estrogens, androgens may inhibit bone resorption through mechanisms that involve alterations in the local production of bone-resorbing cytokines such as IL-1 and IL-6. In the majority of eugonadal osteoporotic men, bone formation and osteoblastic cell proliferation are decreased.

Other than androgen deficiency, secondary causes of osteoporosis in men are similar to those in women. Epidemiologic studies suggest that prior glucocorticoid use, gastric resection, and ethanol abuse are among the most common identifiable causes of osteoporosis in men.

In men with androgen-deficiency osteoporosis, androgen replacement is usually indicated, although beneficial effects on bone mass have been demonstrated only in men with hyperprolactinemic hypogonadism and idiopathic hypogonadotropic hypogonadism. A notable exception, however, is men with prostatic carcinoma in whom androgen replacement is contraindicated. In men with primary gonadal failure, testosterone replacement can be administered either parenterally or transdermally. In men with secondary hypogonadism, treatment with human chorionic gonadotropin or pulsatile GnRH may also be considered. The efficacy of antiresorptive agents such as calcitonin or bisphosphonates has not been investigated.

GLUCOCORTICOID-INDUCED BONE LOSS

Bone loss is a common complication of glucocorticoid excess, whether due to endogenous Cushing's syndrome or exogenous glucocorticoids. The most important adverse effects of glucocorticoids on bone metabolism appear to be suppressed osteoblast activity and a vitamin D–independent inhibition of intestinal calcium absorption. Enhanced osteoclastic activity may also be important. The ability of glucocorticoids to suppress bone formation appears to be mediated, at least in part, by suppression of local secretion of IGF-1 in bone.

The predominant effect of glucocorticoids on the skeleton is a loss of trabecular bone, although cortical bone mass also decreases. Bone loss is most rapid in the first 6 to 12 months of therapy, but accelerated bone loss appears to continue as long as therapy is continued.

Because the bone loss associated with glucocorticoids is largely irreversible, the decision to administer them should be made carefully. The dosage should be maintained as low as possible. If glucocorticoid therapy is expected to continue for several months or longer, treatment to prevent bone loss should be considered, particularly in estrogen-deficient women and when a high dosage of glucocorticoids is needed. Small studies have suggested that either calcitonin or bisphosphonates may prevent spinal bone loss in patients receiving long-term glucocorticoid therapy. Studies of the effects of vitamin D and its metabolites on glucocorticoid-induced bone loss have produced inconsistent results. Nonetheless, a recent controlled study demonstrated that 0.5 to 1.0 μg of calcitriol plus 1000 mg of calcium per day can prevent spinal bone loss for at least 1 year in patients who are starting treatment with glucocorticoids. However, because of the potential for hypercalciuria and/or hypercalcemia, patients receiving calcitriol therapy require careful monitoring. Calcitriol therapy seems most logical in patients with low urinary calcium excretion, suggesting poor intestinal absorption of calcium, and should be avoided in patients with hypercalciuria. Physiologic vitamin D replacement (400 IU per day) can be safely recom-

mended in all patients receiving glucocorticoids. Calcium supplementation (1000 mg per day) should be added unless the urinary calcium excretion is excessive.

Christiansen CC (ed.): Consensus Development Conference on Osteoporosis. Am J Med 95(5A):1S, 1993. *Short, current reviews on such important issues in osteoporosis as the value of bone densitometry and use of biochemical markers of bone turnover in assessing osteoporosis, and reviews of major current therapies as well as potential future treatment strategies.*
Jackson JA, Kleerekoper M: Osteoporosis in men: Diagnosis, pathophysiology and prevention. Medicine 69:137, 1990. *The only comprehensive review of this topic.*
Lukert BP, Raisz LG: Glucocorticoid-induced osteoporosis: Pathogenesis and management. Ann Intern Med 112:352, 1990. *A thorough, well-balanced review of the pathogenesis and management of glucocorticoid-induced osteoporosis. Most important references are cited.*
Neer RM: Osteoporosis. *In* DeGroot LJ (ed.): Endocrinology. Philadelphia, WB Saunders, 1994, pp 1228–1258. *A thorough, scholarly review that carefully discusses the limitations of many prior studies. Virtually every significant reference is cited.*
Riggs BL, Melton LJ III: The prevention and treatment of osteoporosis. N Engl J Med 327:620, 1992. *A concise, up-to-date review of practical therapeutic options for women with postmenopausal osteoporosis.*

218 PAGET'S DISEASE OF BONE (Osteitis Deformans)
John A. Kanis

DEFINITION. Paget's disease of bone is a focal disorder of skeletal metabolism in which all the elements of skeletal remodeling (resorption, formation, and mineralization) are increased. Increased bone formation results in the disorganized assembly of collagen, giving rise to bony enlargement and deformity.

ETIOLOGY. The cause is unknown. A viral infection of osteoclasts is postulated on the basis of finding viral nucleocapsids of the paramyxoviridae in affected osteoclasts. Such findings are, however, not specific and are seen in some other rare disorders of bone turnover (pycnodysostosis and some cases of osteopetrosis [see Ch. 219]). Canine distemper is one of the paramyxoviridae, and an association between owning dogs and Paget's disease has been reported. A positive family history in approximately 10% of patients suggests a dominant pattern of susceptibility, with weak associations with the HLA Dqw1 antigens in the United States and with A9 and B15 in the United Kingdom (see Ch. 229).

PREVALENCE AND EPIDEMIOLOGY. Paget's disease is the second most common disorder of bone, outstripped only by osteoporosis. It is most commonly found in the United Kingdom, where the prevalence is 5% of the population over age 55 and is roughly equal between genders. The frequency of symptomatic disease rises with age. There is, however, little evidence for the occurrence of new lesions in symptomatic disease. This suggests a high modal incidence in early middle-age, which declines rapidly thereafter, but with a variable latency between the onset of the disorder and its radiographic or clinical expression.

Although most common in the United Kingdom, it is also common in countries such as Australia, New Zealand, South Africa, and the United States, where significant British immigration occurred in the past, but occurs with a lower frequency in native-born individuals than in immigrants. The disorder is extremely rare in the Nordic countries, the Arab Middle-East, China, and Japan and among Australian Aboriginals. Intermediate rates are found in France, Germany, Italy, and Spain. There is some evidence that the incidence of Paget's disease is falling in the United Kingdom and in the United States.

PATHOPHYSIOLOGY AND HISTOPATHOLOGY. The disease is characterized by increased metabolic activity of bone surfaces. Bone remodeling normally occupies 10 to 15% of bone surfaces, and at affected sites this may be increased 5- to 10-fold. Osteoclast numbers are increased, as is their size, and they may contain up to 100 nuclei. Osteoclast competence is decreased, but their plethora result in an increase in bone resorption with crenated resorption cavities subsequently in-filled by the activity of osteoblasts. The irregular cement lines give rise to a mosaic patchwork appearance at bone histology. New bone that is formed is often woven rather than lamellar and is structurally less competent and occupies more space. Mineralization rates are normal, but because abnormally large volumes of bone are undergoing mineralization, the surface covered with unmineralized osteoid is increased. Marrow fibrosis and hypervascularity are also features.

Remodeling throughout the cortex increases its porosity and blurs the distinction between cortical and cancellous bone. An imbalance between formation and resorption characteristically results in increased bone size and deformity.

CLINICAL AND LABORATORY MANIFESTATIONS. The extent of disease involvement is markedly heterogeneous. It may involve only one bone. More frequently, multiple sites are involved, typically in an asymmetric distribution. The most common sites are the pelvis, lumbar spine, and femur; one or more of these sites are affected in more than 75% of cases.

More than 95% of patients with Paget's disease are asymptomatic. The most common problems encountered are bone pain, skeletal deformity, and fracture (Table 218-1). Apart from fracture, the onset is insidious and 30% of patients have had symptoms at presentation for more than 10 years. It may be difficult to distinguish bone pain arising from Paget's disease from that due to arthritis, particularly of the hip and the spine. Deformity is a presenting complaint in one fifth of patients. Obvious bone enlargement is seen, particularly in the limbs and also in the skull and facial bones. Bone enlargement contributes significantly to the neurologic complications and more uncertainly to joint disease. The most frequent deformity of long bones is bowing, which is characteristically lateral in the case of the femur and anterior in the case of the tibia.

The incidence of fissure fractures is significantly greater in patients with bowing. Fissure fractures may be symptomatic and may herald complete fractures, but many patients have indolent pain, particularly on weight bearing associated with local tenderness. Complete fractures of the long bones occur most commonly in the femur, followed by the tibia and the forearm, which together account for up to 90% of pathologic fractures of long bones. They commonly follow trivial injury, and, unlike in osteoporosis, femoral fractures are less frequently cervical and more usually subtrochanteric or involve the shaft.

Neurologic complications are common and are among the more serious clinical problems. A variety of neurologic problems arise from platybasia. Cranial disease also results in deafness, vertigo, and tinitus. Spinal syndromes most frequently occur when Paget's disease affects the thoracic spine. They are usually associated with enlarged vertebrae and decreased diameter of the spinal canal with cord or root compression. Also, the highly vascular pagetic bone may divert the blood supply from neural tissue.

Cardiac output may be increased and give rise to high-output failure in patients with extensive disease when ≥30% of the skeleton is involved. Sarcoma arising in pagetic bone is rare but is a serious complication of the disorder, accounting for most cases of sarcoma in the population aged 50 or older. The pelvis and femora are common sites followed by the humerus, face, and skull. Benign and malignant giant cell tumors may also occur. New pain developing in a patient with long-standing Paget's disease not attributable to microfractures should arouse a high degree of suspicion. Other presentations include the development of a large mass or pathologic fracture.

Radiographic Features. The early phase of osteolytic activity is sometimes seen clearly in the skull as osteoporosis circumscripta or as a V-shaped advancing front in a long bone. A second mixed phase shows evidence of patchy osteolysis and sclerosis which is the most common radiographic finding. The third phase is that of predominant bone sclerosis (Fig. 218-1). Thickening of the cortices is characteristic with enlargement of the long bones (Fig. 218-2). Intracortical resorption results in a loss of the corticomedullary junction and accentuation of trabecular markings. The combination of all these features is virtually diagnostic, so that bone biopsy is rarely required. The average patient has six lesions affecting 14% of the skeleton. In approximately 10 to 20% of symptomatic patients, the disorder is mono-ostotic. As a general rule, scintigraphy is more sensitive than radiography, but 2 to 3% of radiographically overt lesions may not be associated with increased scintigraphic uptake (so-called burnt-out Paget's disease).

The pelvis is the most common site affected; evidence is found in approximately two thirds of patients. Narrowing of the joint space of the hip is common. Most patients show medial or concentric narrowing of the joint space; degenerative osteoarthrosis more frequently causes narrowing of the superior aspect. Computed tomography is also useful to assess the cause of pain at the spine and in the investigation for osteosarcoma.

Biochemical Manifestations. Extracellular calcium homeostasis is almost invariably normal, despite the massive increase in bone turnover. Hypercalciuria and more rarely hypercalcemia may occur with prolonged immobilization or fracture. Serum activity of alkaline phosphatase, in part derived from osteoblasts, is most often used to measure the extent of skeletal involvement. Increased bone resorption can be assessed by the urinary excretion of hydroxyproline, which in Paget's disease is derived largely from the collagen destruction of bone. The urinary excretion of pyridinoline cross-links is a more specific and sensitive marker. In untreated patients there is a close correlation between serum activity of alkaline phosphatase and urinary excretion of hydroxyproline, and both correlate

TABLE 218-1. CLINICAL FEATURES AND COMPLICATIONS OF PAGET'S DISEASE

Common
  Bone pain—pagetic, articular
  Fracture—long bones, vertebral bodies
  Neurologic—deafness
  Deformity and enlargement of bones
Uncommon
  Pain—fissure fracture
  Spinal neurologic syndromes
  Hypercalciuria of immobilization or fracture
  Vascular bleeding from bone during surgery
  Extraskeletal (aortic) calcification
  Osteosarcoma and other bone tumors
Rare
  Cardiovascular disease
  Cranial nerve lesions (except VIII)
  Brain stem and cerebellar lesions
  Hypercalcemia of immobilization
  Extramedullary hematopoiesis
  Epidural hematoma
Significance uncertain
  Gout
  Pseudogout
  Angioid streaks
  Hyperparathyroidism
  Urolithiasis

From Kanis JA: Pathophysiology and Treatment of Paget's Disease of Bone. London, Martin Dunitz, 1991.

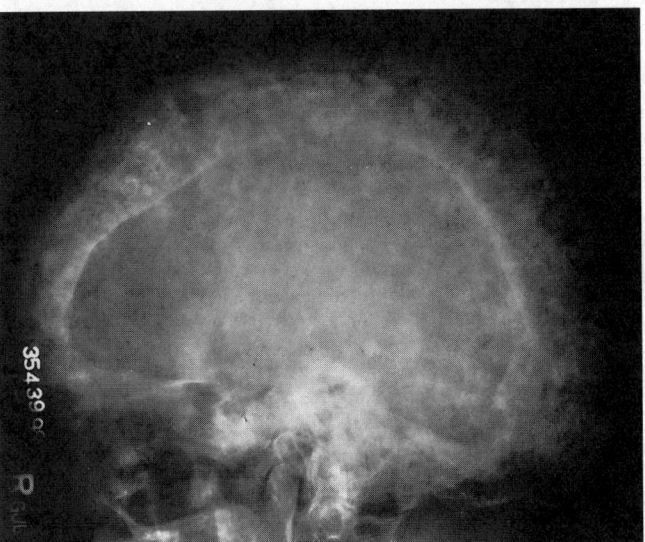

FIGURE 218-1. Advanced involvement of the skull with marked thickening of the entire vault, areas of osteolysis, and patchy new bone formation resulting in a "cotton-wool" appearance.

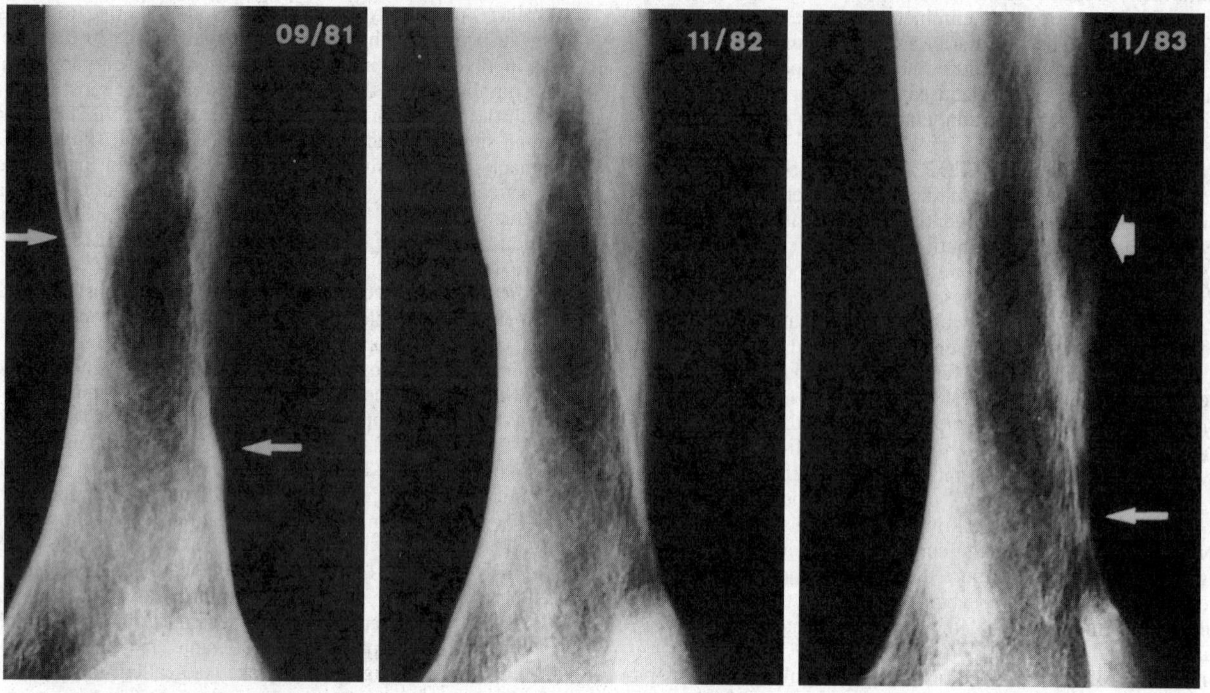

FIGURE 218–2. Sequential radiographs of the distal femur at the dates shown. *Left,* The distinction between Paget's and normal bone *(arrows),* the osteolytic front, and the expansion of bone diameter at the affected site. Treatment with a bisphosphonate–induced *(center)* infilling of the resorption front. Relapse after treatment *(right)* was associated with a new area of osteolysis *(thick arrow)* and progression of the resorption front. (From Kanis JA: Pathophysiology and Treatment of Paget's Disease of Bone. London, Martin Dunitz, 1991.)

with the extent of disease. Up to 10% of patients with symptomatic Paget's disease have values of alkaline phosphatase within the laboratory reference range, and this figure is even higher in the case of hydroxyproline.

TREATMENT. Data are insufficient to recommend medical treatment to asymptomatic patients, except in the presence of rapidly advancing osteolytic disease in the long bones of the lower limb where the risk of pathologic fracture is high. Medical treatment has centered on specific inhibitors of osteoclast-mediated bone resorption, including the bisphosphonates, calcitonins, mithramycin, and gallium nitrate.

Calcitonins. A variety of calcitonins have been used. The most common is synthetic salmon calcitonin (salcatonin), which may be given by subcutaneous injection, 50 to 100 units daily or on alternate days. In several European countries salcatonin is available as a nasal spray. Treatment results in an early decrease in bone resorption, which can be monitored by the fall in urinary excretion of hydroxyproline, and after several weeks a decrease in the serum activity of alkaline phosphatase. On average, these indices fall to 40 to 50% of pretreatment values. Treatment is associated with relief of bone pain, healing of osteolytic lesions, decreased cardiac output, and improvement of neurologic disease. Deafness is rarely reversed, but progression may be prevented.

Disease activity recurs once treatment is stopped, so if long-term control is required, calcitonin must be given indefinitely. In the case of bone pain, relief may occur for many months or years after treatment is stopped, so intermittent treatment is worthwhile. The escape phenomenon describes failure to maintain a biochemical response despite continued treatment or even increasing the dose. In some cases this acquired resistance appears to be associated with the development of salcatonin antibodies, in which case a biochemical response is elicited with an alternative calcitonin. No serious side effects of calcitonin are reported, but up to one third of patients develop transient nausea or flushing, and in 5 to 10% of patients long-term treatment cannot be tolerated.

Bisphosphonates. These pyrophosphate analogues are adsorped onto hydroxyapatite, particularly at sites of resorption. As with calcitonin, an early effect of treatment is to decrease bone resorption, followed by a later decrease in bone formation, as marked by alkaline phosphatase. Etidronate is widely available and used at a dose of 5 mg per kilogram of body weight daily for up to 6 months. Disease activity is suppressed by approximately 50% from

initial values. Pain relief occurs, but radiographic improvement is unusual. Higher than recommended doses induce more complete responses but increase the risk of impairing mineralization of bone and should be avoided. Occasionally, bone pain may be associated with recommended doses, in which case treatment should be stopped. Intravenous treatment regimens with etidronate and other bisphosphonates are widely available in Europe. These include clodronate, alendronate, and pamidronate, but these drugs have not been approved by the FDA as of publication. They have, however, no adverse effect on the mineralization of bone, and their effects on disease activity, symptoms, and radiographic abnormalities (see Fig. 218–2) are more complete than in the case of the calcitonins or etidronate. Other nonapproved treatments include mithramycin, gallium nitrate, and the combination of calcium with thiazide diuretics.

Surgical Management. Elective surgery is often undertaken with effective medical treatment because this decreases bone vascularity and provides a more normal environment for prosthetic implants. Apart from fractures, the most common indication for surgery is joint disease at the hip. In the case of hip pain and some of the spinal neurologic syndromes, surgery can be avoided by medical treatment. Osteotomy has a role in managing deformities or the pain associated with fissure fractures in the presence of deformity.

PROGNOSIS. Pagetic bone pain almost invariably responds to medical treatment. In practice it may be difficult to distinguish pain due to Paget's disease from pain due to coexisting osteoarthropathy or joint pain arising from deformity. In patients in whom pain at the hip is not controlled by analgesics or specific treatment, replacement arthroplasty is the treatment of choice.

Long-term treatment results in the resumption of lamellar bone formation, and in the case of the calcitonins and newer bisphosphonates, more normal radiographic appearances. Overall, there appears to be a good correlation between the degree of biochemical control and attaining clinical improvement, so that biochemical monitoring of disease activity is of value. Decreased bone enlargement and deformity have been reported following long-term treatment with the bisphosphonates. Effective medical management improves spinal neurologic syndromes when these are slowly progressive. The long-term results are as good as those from surgery without the mortality of the latter. The rate of neurologic improvement seen with drug treatment is often more rapid than can be accounted for by remodeling of bone but is due to a decrease in soft tissue swelling and a redistribution of blood flow.

No good evidence indicates that medical treatment significantly alters the natural history of fissure fractures. These may be indolent, occasionally giving rise to pain and complete fracture. Limited experience suggests that in these patients pain decreases following osteotomy. Pathologic fractures of long bones generally heal well, but there is a higher than normal incidence of delayed union and nonunion. The occurrence of fracture provides an opportunity to correct deformity when managed either conservatively or with surgery. Long-term treatment may decrease the frequency of pathologic fracture, but this has not been assessed by long-term prospective studies.

The prognosis of patients with osteosarcoma is extremely poor, and no evidence indicates that medical treatment alters its natural history. Indeed, the role of radiation therapy, chemotherapy, or surgical intervention is not established except for symptomatic treatment.

Anderson DC: Paget's disease. *In* Mundy GR, Martin TJ (eds.): Physiology and Pharmacology of Bone. New York, Springer-Verlag, 1993, p 419. *A general account of Paget's disease.*

Kanis JA: Pathophysiology and Treatment of Paget's Disease of Bone. London, Martin Dunitz, 1991. *A comprehensive monograph of Paget's disease of bone.*

Singer FR, Wallach S (eds.): Paget's Disease of Bone: Clinical Assessment, Present and Future Therapy. New York, Elsevier, 1991. *A collection of review articles and recent abstracts of scientific contributions.*

219 OSTEONECROSIS, OSTEOSCLEROSIS, AND OTHER DISORDERS OF BONE

Michael P. Whyte

OSTEONECROSIS

Osteonecrosis (ischemic, aseptic, or avascular necrosis of bone) refers to skeletal *infarction*. Bone infarcts may be asymptomatic, cause self-limited discomfort, or engender painful collapse of subarticular bone and lead to joint destruction.

ETIOLOGY. Many conditions are associated with osteonecrosis (Table 219–1). In adults, the most common causes are long-term glucocorticoid therapy and ethanol abuse, which manifest dose-dependent effects.

PATHOGENESIS. Certain skeletal sites (often subarticular) are susceptible to osteonecrosis but differ for traumatic and nontraumatic processes and in children and adults. *Osteochondrosis* refers to necrosis of ossification centers; more than 50 eponymic types are recorded. The susceptibility of children to osteochondrosis and its pathogenesis are poorly understood. At all ages, the femoral head is especially prone to infarction. Nontraumatic osteonecrosis also commonly affects the femoral condyles, distal tibia, humeral head, and talus. Skeletal infarction may result from blood vessel destruction (e.g., joint dislocation, fracture), obstruction (e.g., thromboemboli, sickle cell disease, fat emboli, caisson disease), or, hypothetically, compression from local expansion of fatty tissue (e.g., ethanol abuse, glucocorticoid treatment, diabetes mellitus). However, symptoms may not occur unless, weeks later, resorption of dead bone during skeletal repair leads to pathologic fracture.

CLINICAL MANIFESTATIONS. Pain occurs acutely when there is skeletal collapse. Chronic arthralgia results from desquamated necrotic tissue and articular destruction.

DIAGNOSIS. Magnetic resonance imaging (MRI), demonstrating marrow edema, is especially sensitive for detecting early osteonecrosis. Bone scintigraphy discloses skeletal reconstitution with or without fracture. Relatively late in the process, radiographs first show patchy areas of osteopenia and osteosclerosis that reflect skeletal repair. A linear subchondral radiolucency (crescent sign) indicates bony collapse.

TREATMENT. Non–weight-bearing is advisable for an affected limb. Decompression by trephine insertion is used for some sites.

TABLE 219–1. CAUSES OF ISCHEMIC NECROSIS OF CARTILAGE AND BONE

Endocrine/Metabolic
  Ethanol abuse
  Glucocorticoid therapy
  Cushing's disease
  Diabetes mellitus
  Hyperuricemia
  Osteomalacia
  Hyperlipidemia
Storage diseases (e.g., Gaucher's disease)
Hemoglobinopathies (e.g., sickle cell disease)
Trauma (e.g., dislocation, fracture)
Dysbaric conditions (e.g., caisson disease)
Collagen vascular disorders
Irradiation
Pancreatitis
Organ transplantation
Hemodialysis
Idiopathic, familial
Burns
Intravascular coagulation

Arthrotomy to remove debris, transpositional osteotomy, arthroplasty, or joint replacement may be necessary.

OSTEOSCLEROSIS

Many conditions are associated with radiographic evidence of increased bone density, i.e., osteosclerosis. Skeletal dysplasias, metabolic disturbances, and a variety of other conditions can cause generalized or focal increases in bone mass (Table 219–2). Osteosclerosis is classified as affecting predominantly trabecular versus cortical bone or both Osteosclerosis can occur with disturbances in bone growth, modeling (shaping), and/or remodeling (turnover).

Trabecular Osteosclerosis

Neoplastic, hematologic, and metabolic disorders may preferentially sclerose trabecular bone because it houses marrow and remodels more rapidly than cortical bone.

Cortical Osteosclerosis

PROGRESSIVE DIAPHYSEAL DYSPLASIA (CAMURATI-ENGELMANN DISEASE). This developmental disorder affects all races and is transmitted as an autosomal dominant trait with variable penetrance. New bone formation gradually involves both the periosteal and endosteal surface of long bone diaphyses. With severe disease, osteosclerosis also affects the axial skeleton.

Etiology and Pathogenesis. The gene defect has not been mapped. Osteoblast differentiation may be abnormal.

Clinical Presentation. During childhood there is limping or a broad-based and waddling gait. Muscular dystrophy can be diagnosed erroneously. Severely affected persons have a characteristic body habitus featuring an enlarged head with prominent forehead, proptosis, and thin limbs with little subcutaneous fat or muscle mass and tender thickened bones. Cranial nerve palsies and raised intracranial pressure can occur. Some patients have hepatosplenomegaly, Raynaud's phenomenon, and additional findings suggestive of vasculitis. Symptoms sometimes remit during or after puberty.

Diagnosis. Somewhat symmetric and irregular cortical hyperostosis of major long bone diaphyses slowly develops from periosteal and endosteal new bone formation. Femora and tibiae are most commonly affected. Metaphyses may become involved. Age of onset, rate of progression, and severity are variable. Clinical, radiologic, and bone scan findings are generally concordant. Routine biochemical parameters of bone and mineral metabolism are typically normal. Serum alkaline phosphatase activity, urinary hydroxyproline levels, and the erythrocyte sedimentation rate can be elevated. Histopathologic study reveals newly formed woven bone that matures and is incorporated into cortical bone. Electron microscopy of muscle may show myopathic changes and vascular abnormalities.

TABLE 219-2. DISORDERS THAT CAUSE OSTEOSCLEROSIS

Dysplasias
Craniodiaphyseal dysplasia
Craniometaphyseal dysplasia
Dysosteosclerosis
Endosteal hyperostosis
   van Buchem disease
   Sclerosteosis
Frontometaphyseal dysplasia
Infantile cortical hyperostosis (Caffey disease)
Melorheostosis
Metaphyseal dysplasia (Pyle disease)
Mixed sclerosing-bone dystrophy
Oculodento-osseous dysplasia
Osteodysplasia of Melnick and Needles
Osteoectasia with hyperphosphatasia (hyperostosis corticalis)
Osteopathia striata
Osteopetrosis
Osteopoikilosis
Progressive diaphyseal dysplasia (Engelmann disease)
Pyknodysostosis

Metabolic
Carbonic anhydrase II deficiency
Fluorosis
Heavy metal poisoning
Hypervitaminosis A, D
Hyperparathyroidism, hypoparathyroidism, and pseudohypoparathyroidism
Hypophosphatemic rickets or osteomalacia
Milk-alkali syndrome
Renal osteodystrophy

Other
Axial osteomalacia
Fibrogenesis imperfecta osseum
Intravenous drug abuse
Ionizing radiation
Lymphomas
Mastocytosis
Multiple myeloma
Myelofibrosis
Osteomyelitis
Osteonecrosis
Paget's disease
Sarcoidosis
Skeletal metastases
Tuberous sclerosis

From Whyte MP, Murphy WA: Osteopetrosis and other sclerosing bone disorders. *In* Avioli LV, Krane SM (eds.): Metabolic Bone Disease, 2nd ed. Philadelphia, WB Saunders, 1990.

Treatment. Glucocorticoid therapy (typically a low dose of prednisone on alternate days) can relieve bone pain and may normalize skeletal histology.

ENDOSTEAL HYPEROSTOSIS. Sclerosteosis and van Buchem disease, autosomal recessive disorders, are the principal types of endosteal hyperostosis.

Etiology and Pathogenesis. Sclerosteosis and van Buchem disease appear to reflect the same genetic defect in which differences are explained by the epistatic effects of modifying genes. The molecular basis is unknown. Enhanced osteoblast activity with failure of osteoclasts to compensate for the increased bone formation appears to explain the osteosclerosis.

Clinical Features. Sclerosteosis (cortical hyperostosis with syndactyly) occurs primarily in the Afrikaners of South Africa. Elsewhere, Dutch ancestry is also common. Gender distribution appears equal. Patients are tall and heavy beginning in childhood, and experience deafness and facial nerve palsy as a result of cranial nerve entrapment and have a prominent mandible of square configuration. Raised intracranial pressure and headache may reflect a small cranial cavity that shortens life expectancy. In van Buchem disease, progressive asymmetric enlargement of the jaw occurs during puberty, but there is no prognathism. Patients may be symptom free or suffer recurrent facial nerve palsy, deafness, and optic atrophy from narrowing of cranial foramina beginning as early as infancy. Long bones may hurt with applied pressure, but are not fragile.

Diagnosis. Radiologically in sclerosteosis, the skeleton is normal in early childhood except when syndactyly is present. Progressive bony thickening widens the skull and causes prognathism. Long bones have thickened cortices. Syndactyly, most often involving the index and third fingers, is common. Vertebral pedicles, ribs, pelvis, and other tubular bones may become dense. Computed tomography has shown fusion of ossicles and narrowing of the internal auditory canals and cochlear aqueducts. In van Buchem disease, endosteal thickening homogeneously widens diaphyseal cortices and narrows medullary canals. Bones are properly modeled. Osteosclerosis also affects the skull base, facial bones, vertebrae, pelvis, and ribs.

Serum alkaline phosphatase activity may be increased from enhanced skeletal production.

Treatment. Surgical decompression of narrowed foramina may alleviate cranial nerve palsies.

PACHYDERMOPERIOSTOSIS. Pachydermoperiostosis (hypertrophic osteoarthropathy, primary or idiopathic) is an autosomal dominant disorder that features clubbing of the digits, hyperhidrosis, and thickening of the skin (especially of the face), and periosteal new bone formation prominently in the distal limbs. Autosomal recessive transmission also seems to occur.

Etiology and Pathogenesis. No gene defect has been identified. A controversial hypothesis suggests that some circulating factor acts on the vasculature initially to cause hyperemia and thereby alters soft tissues, but later blood flow is reduced.

Clinical Presentation. Men appear to be more severely affected than women, and blacks more commonly than whites. Symptoms typically begin during adolescence, intensify during a decade, but then become quiescent. Arthralgias and fatigue are common. Stiffness and limited mobility affect both the appendicular and the axial skeleton. Progressive gradual enlargement of the hands and feet cause a pawlike appearance. Cutaneous changes include thickening, furrowing, pitting, and oiliness, especially of the scalp and face. Not all patients manifest all three principal features.

Radiologic Features. Periostitis thickens the distal portions of the tibia, fibula, radius, and ulna. Clubbing is obvious, and acro-osteolysis can occur. Ankylosis of joints, especially in the hands and feet, may affect older patients. Periosteal proliferation is exuberant and irregular and often involves epiphyses. Secondary hypertrophic osteoarthropathy (pulmonary or otherwise) typically causes a smooth, undulating periosteal reaction. Bone scanning in either condition reveals symmetric, diffuse, regular uptake along the cortical margins of long bones, especially in the legs. This feature results in a "double stripe" sign.

Treatment. Painful synovial effusions may respond to nonsteroidal anti-inflammatory drugs. Colchicine reportedly improved arthralgias, clubbing, folliculitis, and pachyderma in one patient. Contractures or neurovascular compression by osteosclerotic lesions may require surgical intervention.

Cortical and Trabecular Osteosclerosis

OSTEOPETROSIS. Osteopetrosis (marble bone disease) occurs in two major clinical forms—the autosomal recessive or "malignant" type that kills during infancy or early childhood if untreated, and the autosomal dominant or "benign" type that causes few or no symptoms. Other autosomal recessive types feature intermediate severity, neuronal storage disease, stillbirth, or renal tubular acidosis with cerebral calcification due to carbonic anhydrase II (CA II) isoenzyme deficiency.

Etiology and Pathogenesis. The defective gene loci are unknown except for CA II deficiency in which CA II gene mutations have been identified.

Histopathologic studies show that all true forms of osteopetrosis feature profound deficiency of osteoclast action. Primary spongiosa (calcified cartilage deposited during endochondral bone formation) occurs away from growth plates and constitutes the pathognomonic finding. Defective endosteal bone resorption precludes formation of marrow space. Quiescent skeletal remodeling leads to bone fragility from impaired interconnection of osteons and defective conversion of immature (woven) bone to mature (compact) bone. Hypothetically the various types of osteopetrosis could reflect abnormalities as distal as the microenvironment of osteoclast precursor cells in the marrow, or as proximal as bone tissue itself that is refractory to resorption. Viral-like inclusions in osteoclasts are of uncertain significance. Neuronal storage disease (ceroid lipofuscin) may reflect a lysosomal defect. Deficient superoxide production (necessary for bone resorption) can be a pathogenetic factor.

Clinical Manifestations. Malignant osteopetrosis presents during infancy with nasal "stuffiness" from malformed mastoid and paranasal sinuses. Small cranial foramina compress optic, oculomotor, and facial nerves. Failure to thrive, delayed dentition, and fracture are characteristic. Hypersplenism and recurrent infection, bruising, and bleeding reflect myelophthisis. There are short stature, frontal bossing, large head, nystagmus, hepatosplenomegaly, and genu valgum. Untreated children usually die during the first decade of life from hemorrhage, pneumonia, severe anemia, or sepsis. Benign osteopetrosis occasionally causes fracture, and there may be facial palsy, deafness, mandibular osteomyelitis, impaired vision or hearing, psychomotor delay, carpal tunnel syndrome, and osteoarthritis. CA II deficiency has considerable clinical variability, including failure to thrive, fracture, developmental delay, mental subnormality, and short stature. Cerebral calcification develops during childhood, but defective skeletal modeling and osteosclerosis may correct spontaneously. Both proximal and distal renal tubular acidosis have been described.

Diagnosis. Generalized symmetric osteosclerosis is the radiologic hallmark. In severe disease, modeling defects in long bones produce an "Erlenmeyer flask" deformity (Fig. 219–1). Alternating dense and lucent bands commonly occur in the pelvis and metaphyses. The cranium is usually thickened and dense, especially at the base, and the paranasal and mastoid sinuses are underpneumatized. Vertebrae may show, on lateral view, a "bone-in-bone" (endobone) configuration or end plate sclerosis causing a "rugger-jersey" appearance. Skeletal scintigraphy can disclose fractures and osteomyelitis. MRI helps to assess bone marrow transplantation, since successful engraftment normalizes marrow signals.

Serum levels of acid phosphatase and creatine kinase (brain isoenzyme), apparently from osteoclasts, are increased. In malignant osteopetrosis, hypocalcemia with secondary hyperparathyroidism and increased serum levels of calcitriol can accompany rachitic radiologic changes. In benign osteopetrosis, biochemical indices of mineral homeostasis are typically unremarkable, though serum parathyroid hormone levels may be increased.

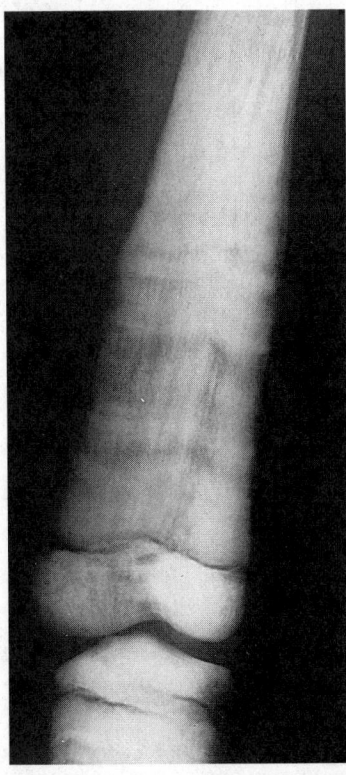

FIGURE 219–1. Osteopetrosis. Anteroposterior radiograph of the distal femur shows widened metadiaphyseal region with characteristic alternating dense and lucent bands. (From Whyte MP, Murphy WA: Osteopetrosis and other sclerosing bone disorders. In Avioli LV, Krane SM [eds.]: Metabolic Bone Disease, 2nd ed. Philadelphia, WB Saunders, 1990.)

Treatment. Since the etiology, pathogenesis, and prognosis for osteopetroses differ, correct subclassification is crucial before treatment is attempted. It may be necessary to evaluate the family and disease progression. For the malignant form, HLA-identical bone marrow transplantation has remarkably benefited some children. Calcium-deficient diets have been helpful, but may be limited by hypocalcemia and rickets. Massive oral doses of calcitriol together with dietary calcium restriction (to prevent hypercalciuria/hypercalcemia), as well as human interferon-γ, that enhances superoxide production, stimulate osteoclast activity. Prednisone with a low-calcium/high-phosphate diet may be effective. High-dose glucocorticoid therapy stabilizes pancytopenia and hepatomegaly. Hyperbaric oxygenation helps treat osteomyelitis. Surgical decompression of optic and facial nerves can be beneficial. Early prenatal diagnosis by radiographs or ultrasound has not been successful.

PYKNODYSOSTOSIS. Pyknodysostosis is believed to have affected the French impressionist painter Henri de Toulouse-Lautrec (1864–1901). Most descriptions have come from Europe and the United States, but the disorder appears to be especially common in Japan.

Etiology and Pathogenesis. The molecular basis for this autosomal recessive condition is unknown. Diminished rates of bone resorption and skeletal turnover are reported. Degradation of collagen may be defective. In chondrocytes and osteoblasts, abnormal inclusions have been described.

Clinical Presentation. During infancy or early childhood there are disproportionate short stature, fronto-occipital prominence, dental malocclusion with retention of primary teeth, proptosis, bluish sclerae, a beaked and pointed nose, as well as a relatively large cranium, obtuse mandibular angle, small facies and chin, and high-arched palate. Cranial sutures remain open. Fingers are short and clubbed from acro-osteolysis or aplasia of terminal phalanges, and the hands are small and square. Recurrent fractures cause genu valgum deformity. Mental retardation affects about 10% of patients. Adult height ranges from 4 feet 3 inches to 4 feet 11 inches. Recurrent respiratory infections and right-sided heart failure from chronic upper airway obstruction due to micrognathia may shorten life expectancy.

Laboratory Findings. Osteosclerosis is uniform, first becoming apparent in childhood and increasing with age. Skeletal modeling defects do not occur, although long bones have thick cortices from narrow medullary canals. Clavicles are gracile and hypoplastic at their lateral segments. The calvarium and base of the skull are sclerotic, orbital ridges are dense, and wormian bones are present. Serum calcium and inorganic phosphate levels and alkaline phosphatase activity are typically normal. Anemia is not a problem.

Treatment. There is no effective medical therapy. Fractures of the long bones usually mend satisfactorily. Internal fixation of long bones is formidable because of their hardness. Tooth extraction is difficult. Osteomyelitis of the mandible may require antibiotic, surgical, and/or hyperbaric therapy.

FIBROGENESIS IMPERFECTA OSSIUM. This rare, sporadic disorder manifests generalized osteopenia, but features coarsening of remaining trabeculae. Thus it is included among osteosclerotic disorders.

Etiology and Pathogenesis. The etiology is unknown. Subperiosteal bone formation and collagen synthesis in nonosseous tissue appear to be normal.

Clinical Presentation. Typically, intractable skeletal pain begins gradually during middle age or later and rapidly progresses with a debilitating course and immobility. Spontaneous fractures are a prominent complication. Physical examination reveals marked bony tenderness.

Diagnosis. Only the skull is spared. Initially, osteopenia and a slightly abnormal appearance of trabecular bone are noted. Subsequently the changes suggest osteomalacia. Corticomedullary junctions become indistinct as cortices are replaced by an abnormal trabecular bone pattern. The generalized osteopenia causes the remaining trabeculae to appear coarse and dense in a fish-net pattern. There is a mixed lytic and sclerotic appearance.

Alkaline phosphatase activity in serum is increased.

Histopathologic Findings. The skeletal lesion is a form of osteomalacia that varies considerably in severity from area to area. In diseased regions, polarized light microscopy shows collagen fibrils that lack birefringence, and electron microscopy reveals thin and randomly organized collagen fibrils.

Focal Osteosclerosis

OSTEOPOIKILOSIS. Osteopoikilosis ("spotted bones") is a radiologic curiosity transmitted as a highly penetrant autosomal dominant trait. The bony lesions are asymptomatic. Incorrect diagnosis may lead to studies for other serious conditions, including metastatic disease. Some patients have connective tissue nevi called dermatofibrosis lenticularis disseminata, i.e., Buschke-Ollendorff syndrome.

Radiologic Features. Numerous small round or oval foci of bony sclerosis appear in cancellous bone in the tarsal, carpal, pelvic, and metaepiphyseal regions of tubular bones.

OSTEOPATHIA STRIATA. This autosomal dominant curiosity features linear striations in metaphyseal regions of long bones and in the ilium. Clinically important syndromes include osteopathia striata with cranial sclerosis or with focal dermal hypoplasia (Goltz's syndrome)—a serious X-linked recessive condition in which affected boys have widespread linear areas of dermal hypoplasia and various bony defects in the limbs.

MELORHEOSTOSIS. Melorheostosis causes changes likened to melted wax dripping down a candle. No mendelian basis for this disorder has been found. The anatomic distribution suggests a segmentary embryogenetic defect.

Clinical Presentation. Usually there is monomelic involvement; bilateral disease is generally asymmetric. Cutaneous changes over affected bones are not uncommon (e.g., linear scleroderma-like areas and hypertrichosis). Soft tissue abnormalities are often noted before the hyperostosis. Symptoms typically begin during childhood. Pain and stiffness are the major complaints. Joints may become contracted and deformed. Inequality of leg length results from soft tissue contractures and premature fusion of epiphyses. Skeletal changes appear to progress most rapidly during childhood. During adulthood, melorheostosis may or may not gradually extend. Pain is, however, more frequent.

Radiologic Features. Irregular, very dense, eccentric hyperostosis affects the cortex and medullary canal of a single bone or several adjacent bones. The lower limbs are most commonly involved. Endosteal thickening predominates during infancy and childhood and periosteal new bone formation during adulthood. Ectopic bone formation may occur, particularly near joints.

Treatment. It is difficult to surgically correct contractures; recurrent deformity is common.

MIXED SCLEROSING-BONE DYSTROPHY. This typically sporadic disorder features combinations of osteopoikilosis, osteopathia striata, melorheostosis, cranial sclerosis, or additional skeletal defects in one individual. Patients may experience the problems associated with the individual patterns of osteosclerosis, e.g., nerve palsy with cranial sclerosis, bone pain with melorheostosis.

OTHER DISORDERS OF BONE

FIBROUS DYSPLASIA. This sporadic, developmental, skeletal disorder features an expansile fibrous lesion(s) that can fracture, deform, or occasionally entrap nerves. Polyostotic disease typically presents before the age of 10 years; monostotic disease begins in adolescence or early adulthood. McCune-Albright syndrome refers to polyostotic fibrous dysplasia, café au lait spots (see Color Plate 10*D*), and endocrine hyperfunction (typically pseudoprecocious puberty in girls).

Etiology and Pathogenesis. Somatic mosaicism for activating mutations in the gene that codes for the alpha subunit of the receptor/adenylate cyclase–coupling G protein causes the McCune-Albright syndrome. Endocrinopathy generally results from end-organ hyperactivity. Imperfect bone forms because mesenchymal cells do not fully differentiate to osteoblasts.

Clinical Presentation. Monostotic fibrous dysplasia is more common than polyostotic disease. The skull and long bones are affected most often. Sarcomatous degeneration, affecting usually the facial bones or femur, occurs more frequently when there is polyostotic disease but is rare (incidence < 1%). Pregnancy may "reactivate" previously quiescent lesions. McCune-Albright syndrome usually is associated with pseudoprecocious puberty in girls. Less commonly there is thyrotoxicosis, Cushing's disease, acromegaly,

hyperprolactinemia, hyperparathyroidism, or pseudoprecocious puberty in boys. In some patients, renal phosphate wasting causes superimposed hypophosphatemic rickets or osteomalacia.

Radiologic Features. In the long bones, lesions are found in either the metaphysis or diaphysis. They are typically well defined with thin cortices and have a ground-glass appearance (Fig. 219–2). Occasionally they are lobulated with trabeculated areas of radiolucency.

Treatment. With mild disease, bone defects may not change. In severe cases, individual lesions can progress and new ones appear. Spontaneous healing does not occur. Pathologic fractures generally mend well. Stress fractures, however, can be difficult to detect and treat. When the skull is involved, nerve compression may require surgical intervention. In the McCune-Albright syndrome the aromatase inhibitor testolactone appears to help control the precocious puberty of affected girls.

HEREDITARY MULTIPLE EXOSTOSES. This relatively common, highly penetrant, autosomal dominant disorder features irregular bony excrescences that protrude from expanded metaphyses of long bones. There is evidence for a gene defect on chromosome 8 in some affected families. Osteocartilaginous exostoses arise from growth plates and expand until growth ceases. They may or may not become isolated from the parent bone. Their structure is relatively unremarkable with an outer cortex and an inner spongiosa. Disability results primarily from limb-length discrepancies; linear bone growth suffers at the expense of transverse growth. Compression of the nerve, spinal cord, and vascular system occasionally develops. Sarcomatous degeneration (0.5 to 2% of patients) must be suspected when a lesion enlarges rapidly, especially during adulthood.

ENCHONDROMATOSIS (DYSCHONDROPLASIA, OLLIER'S DISEASE). This sporadic condition features cartilaginous masses within the trabecular bone that arise from growth plates. The disorder occurs in childhood with swelling and interference with linear bone growth. At puberty, growth of cartilage masses ceases, and they can be replaced by mature bone. Enchondromas appear radiologically as radiolucent defects in metaphyses of tubular or flat bones, often with central calcific stippling. When enchondromatosis occurs with multiple hemangiomas (Maffucci's syndrome), the enchondromas or hemangiomas undergo malignant transformation in about 15% of cases.

ACHONDROPLASIA. Chondrodystrophies are disorders of cartilage growth that result in disproportionate short stature. Achon-

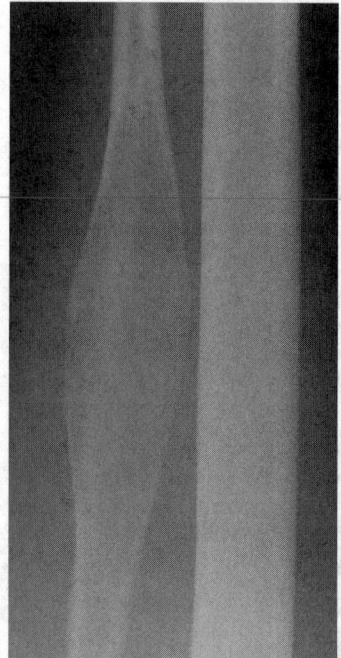

FIGURE 219–2. Fibrous dysplasia. A characteristic expansile lesion with ground-glass appearance has caused thinning of the cortex in the mid diaphysis of the fibula. (From Whyte MP: Fibrous dysplasia. *In* Favus MJ [ed.]: Primer on the Metabolic Bone Diseases and Disorders of Mineral Metabolism, 2nd ed. New York, Raven Press, 1993.)

droplasia is the most common. Mutations in the gene that encodes fibroblast growth factor receptor-3 cause achondroplasia. About 80% of cases are new mutations for this autosomal dominant trait. The mutation rate increases with paternal age. Short, tubular bones result from abnormal endochondral ossification in the limbs. A similar disturbance of the chondrocranium leaves membranous ossification undisturbed—thus the skull vault is normal. However, the cranial base and foramen magnum are small. Also, lumbar lordosis is greatly exaggerated, and the spinal canal narrows from the upper to lower lumbar spine, as revealed radiologically by decreasing interpeduncular distance. There is a notchlike sacroiliac groove. The head is large with frontal bossing and midface hypoplasia. The trunk is of relatively normal length, but the limbs have rhizomelic shortening and the hands have a trident configuration. The long bones appear massive, owing to their disproportionately normal width. Surprisingly, growth plates are not grossly disorganized, and chondrocytes appear normal. Complications can include brain stem compression, hydrocephalus, and spinal cord and root compression. Minimal impingement by a disc or osteophyte upon the small spinal canal can engender neurologic disturbances. Despite its problems, achondroplasia is compatible with good health and a normal lifespan.

Chang CC, Greenspan A, Gershwin ME: Osteonecrosis: Current perspectives on pathogenesis and treatment. Semin Arthritis Rheum 23:47, 1993. *Detailed overview of osteonecrosis.*

Horton WA, Hecht JT: The Chondrodysplasias. *In* Royce RM, Steinmann, B (eds.): Connective Tissue and Its Heritable Disorders, Somerset, NJ, Wiley-Liss, 1993. *Current, comprehensive description of connective tissue disorders including chondrodysplasias.*

McKusick VA: Mendelian Inheritance in Man: Catalogs of Autosomal Dominant, Autosomal Recessive and X-Linked Phenotypes, 11th ed. Baltimore, Johns Hopkins University Press, 1994. *Clinical features, patterns of inheritance, and molecular basis of heritable diseases in humans.*

Whyte MP: Genetic, Developmental, and Dysplastic Skeletal Disorders (Section VI) and Acquired Disorders of Cartilage and Bone (Section VII). *In* Favus NJ (ed.): Primer on the Metabolic Bone Diseases and Disorders of Mineral Metabolism, 2nd ed. New York, Raven Press, 1993. *General summary of metabolic bone diseases and disorders of mineral metabolism.*

Whyte MP, Murphy WA: Osteopetrosis and other sclerosing bone disorders. *In* Avioli LV, Krane SM (eds.): Metabolic Bone Disease, 2nd ed. Philadelphia, WB Saunders, 1990. *Detailed description of heritable disorders that increase bone mass.*

220 BONE TUMORS
Daniel I. Rosenthal

Tumors may involve bone as the result of (1) neoplastic transformation of bone or bone marrow cells, (2) metastatic dissemination of neoplasms arising in other organs, or (3) local invasion from contiguous tissues. Of these three mechanisms, metastatic involvement is by far the most frequent.

METASTATIC TUMOR

Several common cancers frequently involve the skeleton. In women, breast cancer is the most common primary tumor to result in skeletal metastases. Lung cancer is a distant second, although increasing in frequency. In men, prostate cancer is the most common primary tumor, followed by tumors arising in lung, kidney, gastrointestinal tract, and thyroid.

Whenever a destructive lesion of the skeleton is encountered, an effort should be made to determine whether it is primary or secondary. Metastatic bone lesions usually (but not always) produce an infiltrative pattern of bone destruction on radiography or other imaging studies. Compared with primary tumors, metastatic disease is usually accompanied by little or no soft tissue mass. Cancers arising in breast or prostate usually produce mixed lytic and blastic change within bone, whereas lung and renal cancers are purely lytic. A radioisotope bone scan is recommended to determine whether the lesion is solitary, as metastatic lesions are often multiple at presentation. Isotope bone scans are generally more sensitive than plain films for detecting metastasis; magnetic resonance imaging (MRI) is probably even more sensitive. Unfortunately, imaging of the entire skeleton by this modality is currently not practical. When more than one focus is present, the primary tumor is proba-

bly extraskeletal. Although bone sarcomas may metastasize to other parts of the skeleton, this phenomenon generally occurs late in the course of the disease, after lung metastases are present.

If multiple lesions are present and the primary tumor is not apparent, it may be desirable to consider biopsy for diagnosis rather than engage in an extended search for the primary. Needle biopsy can be done safely for most skeletal sites and is the most direct approach to diagnosis. Unfortunately, in a certain percentage of cases presenting as metastatic carcinoma, the primary tumor remains unknown despite all efforts.

Whether chemotherapy or hormonal therapy is useful in treating metastatic disease depends upon the primary tumor. Most metastatic lesions can be palliated with radiation. If there is important structural compromise of the skeleton and the patient's life expectancy justifies it, surgical stabilization should be considered to preserve function.

DIRECT INVASION

Direct invasion of bone by contiguous visceral or soft tissue tumors is uncommon. The most frequent cause of this complication is lung cancer invading ribs or vertebrae (see Ch. 62). Paravertebral lymphadenopathy may sometimes invade the vertebrae. Deeply situated soft tissue sarcomas may also invade bone, but this is relatively rare considering the frequent proximity of these lesions to the skeleton. The radioisotope bone scan is useful to exclude bone involvement. However, a positive bone scan must be viewed with caution, as reactive changes at the margins of the tumor may cause the bone scan to be "hot." Confirmation of involvement by computed tomography (CT) scan or MRI is desirable.

PRIMARY BONE TUMORS

Primary bone tumors may arise from any of the cellular elements that are present. Tumors may be either malignant or benign. However, tumors of the mesenchymal tissues usually fall into a more or less continuous spectrum from benign to malignant. Not all lesions are clearly characterizable as either one or the other. For this reason, adequate diagnosis of most lesions requires not only the name of the tumor but its histologic grade. Further, individual tumors commonly exhibit a variety of cell types and grades. Features on imaging studies reflect the most abundant histologic elements, whereas clinical behavior is shaped by the most aggressive or malignant components. Generally speaking, the better differentiated the lesion (lower grade), the more it resembles the tissue from which it arose. Highly malignant lesions exhibit considerable similarity to each other on imaging studies.

Tumors may arise sporadically, as part of a generalized (and sometimes inherited) tendency to neoplasia, or as degenerations of precursor lesions. Almost any condition that causes a prolonged period of accelerated bone remodeling may lead to tumor formation, including Paget's disease, infections, radiation, bone infarctions, and benign bone lesions.

Adequate staging requires four pieces of information: tumor type, histologic grade, local extent, and presence of metastases. Tissue type and grade are learned from biopsy. Biopsy of these lesions requires considerable sophistication to avoid complicating future therapy. Biopsy should be performed in such a way as to obtain representative tissue, preserve structural integrity, and permit curative resection should that prove to be desirable. The latter usually requires that the biopsy track be excised along with the tumor.

Local extent can be determined by imaging studies. Plain radiographs are important in all cases. Either CT scan or MRI may be used to evaluate soft tissue and marrow extent. If the lesion is suspected of being malignant, a radioisotope bone scan is used to determine whether the lesion is solitary, and either chest radiography or CT is desirable to exclude pulmonary metastases.

Benign bone tumors are usually relatively small and often painless. Of these the most common (and least significant) is the *bone island*. These asymptomatic lesions arise during adult life, may slowly enlarge, and eventually regress. They are usually incidental findings on radiographs. Bone islands are not usually detected on isotope scans, although large lesions may show some uptake. Benign cartilage tumors, including osteochondroma and enchondroma, are next in order of frequency. These lesions are not generally painful unless complicated by pathologic fracture, adjacent soft tissue inflammation (bursitis), or malignant degeneration. Some painful benign tumors include osteoid osteoma, chondroblastoma, giant cell tumor, and chondromyxoid fibroma. Treatment by limited resection is adequate for these tumors. If the diagnosis is certain from imaging studies and resection is not required to relieve symptoms, observation may be adequate.

The most common malignant bone tumor is multiple myeloma, which is considered separately elsewhere (see Ch. 149). Osteosarcoma (or osteogenic sarcoma) is next in order of frequency and much more common than any of the others. Osteosarcoma exhibits two age incidence peaks—one in the second decade of life and another in the fifth and sixth decades, when it frequently represents a complication of a precursor lesion such as Paget's disease. It is most common in the distal femur and proximal tibia. Although low-grade osteosarcoma exists, most lesions are highly malignant. Ten per cent of patients have metastases at the time of presentation, and, if untreated, death ensues in less than 1 year. The alkaline phosphatase is usually elevated, and levels correlate with prognosis. In contemporary treatment a combination of chemotherapy, amputation, or if possible, limb-sparing surgery is used. With this approach survival rates of 85 to 90% are possible. Even for those patients presenting with pulmonary metastases, a combination of resection of the pulmonary lesion and chemotherapy may produce a 20% salvage rate.

Ewing's sarcoma is classified in a group of round cell lesions because of similar histologic and radiographic features. Lymphoma is another member of this group. Ewing's sarcoma tends to occur in children and young adults, whereas primary lymphoma of bone (usually non-Hodgkin's type) is seen in older individuals. The two entities may be difficult to differentiate. Ewing's sarcoma is of unknown pathogenesis and is highly malignant. It is remarkable for a tendency to produce both local and systemic symptoms that may simulate infection, including fever, malaise, and chills. Chemotherapy and surgery produce 60% cure rates.

Chondrosarcoma is usually a disease of people in the fourth, fifth, and sixth decades of life. Unlike osteosarcoma and Ewing's sarcoma, chondrosarcoma is of more variable grade, with most lesions of low or intermediate malignancy. Radiation and chemotherapy are relatively ineffective, but surgery may produce cure rates of 85%.

Goorin AM, Anderson JW: Experience with multi-agent chemotherapy for osteosarcoma. Clin Orthop Rel Res 270:22, 1991. *Current status of chemotherapy.*

O'Connor MI, Pritchard DJ: Ewing's sarcoma: Prognostic factors, disease control and the re-emerging role of surgical treatment. Clin Orthop Rel Res 262:78, 1991. *Improvements in survival related to local and systemic treatment.*

Schajowicz F: Tumors and Tumorlike Lesions of Bone and Joints. New York, Springer-Verlag, 1981. *A good general textbook providing incidence and age distribution for most lesions.*

Springfield DS (ed.): Limb salvage in the treatment of musculoskeletal tumors. Orthoped Clin North Am 22:1, 1991. *A comprehensive multiauthor review of the status of limb-sparing surgery.*

PART XIX

DISEASES OF THE IMMUNE SYSTEM

221 APPROACH TO THE PATIENT WITH IMMUNE DISEASE

J. Claude Bennett

The immune system consists of an integrated constellation of various cell types, each with a specifically designated functional role (Fig. 221–1). In addition, secreted molecules (cytokines) are responsible for interactions, modulations, and regulation of the system. These molecules and cells participate in specific interactions with immunogenic epitopes present on foreign materials, i.e., antigens introduced from the exterior world and foreign to the host. Recognition events are the beginning of the physiologic steps that make up the immune response; they initiate a series of processes causing a wide range of effects within the host. These include the pathways through which inflammation takes place, the killing of in-

vading microbial agents, and the disposal of foreign toxic compounds.

Events leading to specific molecular interactions depend upon the differentiation and expansion of the cell clones that are involved. These include production of specific cell-bound receptor molecules (TCR, T-cell receptors) and secreted or cell-bound immunoglobulins (antibodies). The cellular network (Fig. 221–1) results in an enormous array of specific molecular events. Abnormal regulation of the immune system may prevent the host from handling antigenic stimuli, resulting in a state of immune deficiency (see Ch. 223). At the other extreme it may allow the host to react to its own tissues, resulting in an autoimmune process (see Ch. 240).

In an immunocompetent individual, the immune response is initiated when introduced to an external agent that possesses an immunogenic structural epitope. The appropriate response depends upon the recognition by surface receptors of B and T lymphocytes of the foreignness of the introduced agent. These interactions lead to events that allow proliferation and differentiation of the antigen-stimulated cells. In order to appreciate the exquisite degree of specificity expressed by this remarkable system, one must understand the molecular interactions that result in antigen processing,

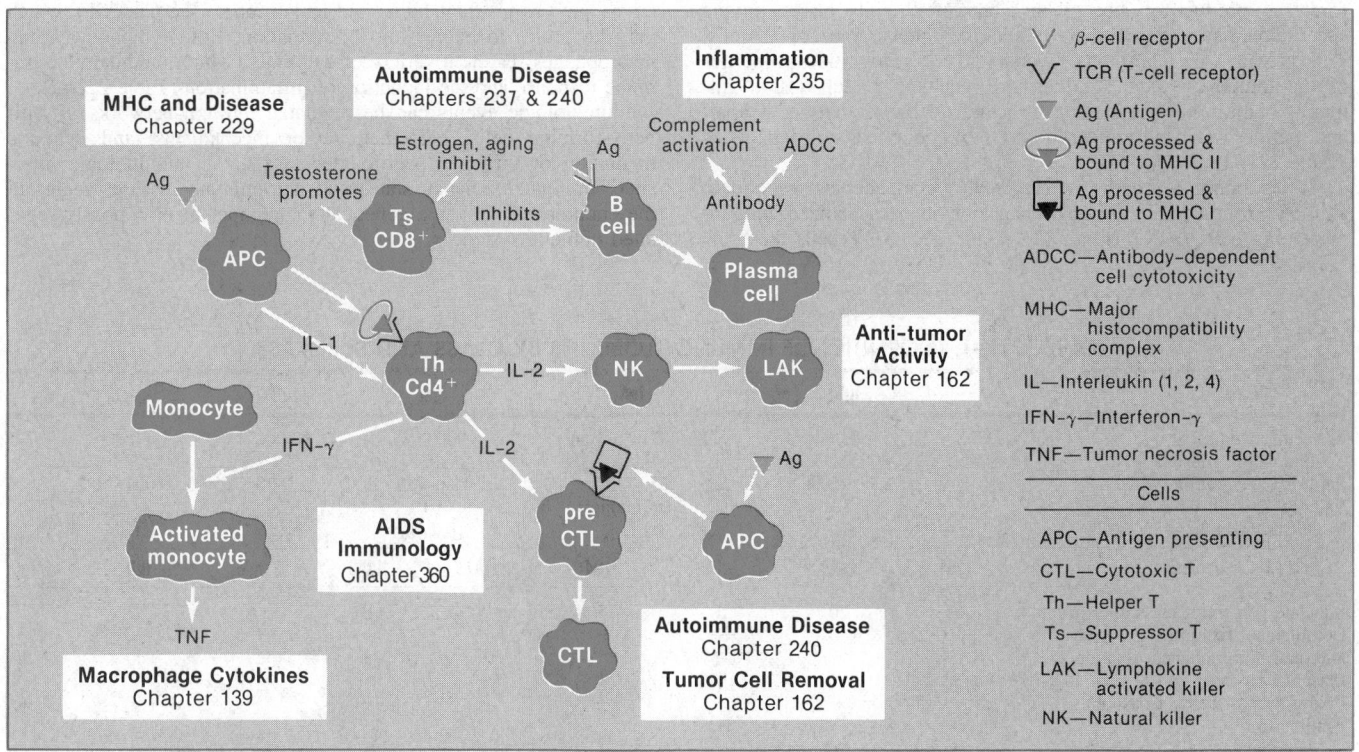

FIGURE 221–1. Schematic diagram of some of the major interactions among various cell types and secreted molecules of the immune system. Definitions of symbols are given on the right of the figure. The blocks at various stages in the pathways and their outcomes indicate their potential significance and refer to chapters elsewhere in this textbook for further reading and in-depth study.

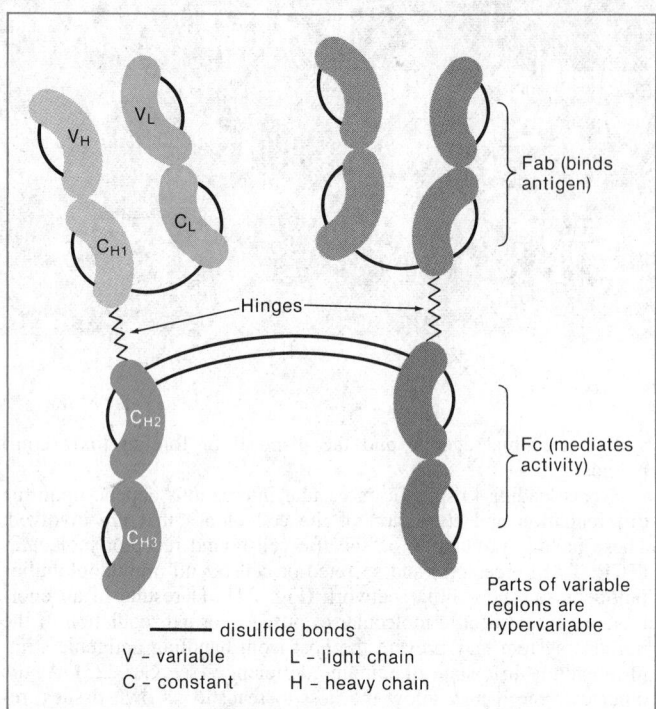

FIGURE 221–2. Diagram of the overall structure of immunoglobulin G, which is the basic structural pattern for all immunoglobulins (see text), drawn to highlight the various reactive areas and to emphasize the globular domain features of the immunoglobulin molecule.

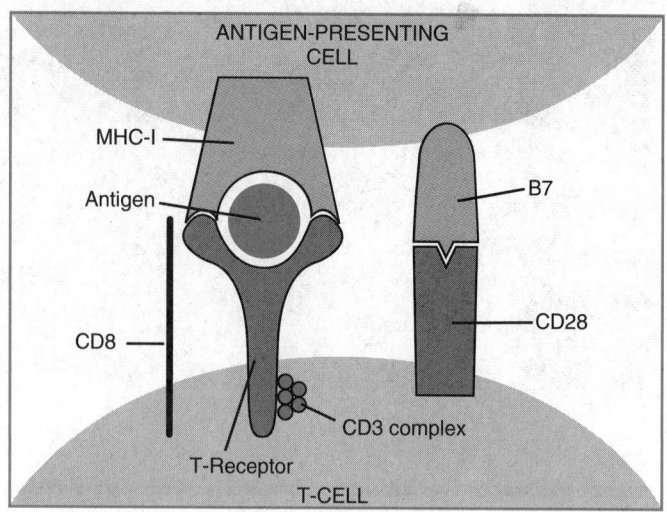

FIGURE 221–3. The molecular events involved in antigen presentation to the T cell. Shown are the interactions among the various molecules, including the major histocompatibility complex (MHC-I), the T-cell receptor, the CD8 or CD4 molecules, and the CD3 complex. Second signal events in the case of cytotoxin (CD8) T cells is shown by the interactions of B7 and CD28. See text for description of the polypeptide chain composition of the various molecules.

presentation, and cellular proliferation. B lymphocytes differentiate to produce specifically directed immunoglobulins (antibodies). All such immunoglobulins share an overall structure, but each contains its own antigen-binding area (Fab region) and within any class (e.g., IgG, IgM) a similar constant region (Fc) (Fig. 221–2). Therefore, the product of any given clone of B cells has a unique specificity distinct from that of all other clonal lines of B cells. This provides the enormous diversity in the recognition properties of the immune system. Furthermore, each of the classes of immunoglobulins is imbued with structural elements that set it apart and define its distinct function in biologic effector mechanisms (Table 221–1).

As the immune process is triggered, T lymphocytes respond to antigen on the surface of macrophages or other specialized antigen-presenting cells (APC) (Figs. 221–1 and 221–3). T cells then dif-

ferentiate as they express various functions, such as cytotoxic potential, enhanced expression of immunity (helper T cells), or down-modulation of the immune response. Therefore, the T lymphocyte becomes pivotal in the development of both *humoral immunity* by way of its stimulation of B lymphocytes and the development of *cellular immunity* and regulation by virtue of its own intrinsic properties and its role in elaborating cytokines for cellular communication processes.

Reactions of the immune system may activate the complement cascade (see Ch. 222) and the production of arachidonic acid derivatives such as prostaglandins and leukotrienes (see Ch. 235), which play key roles in expressing inflammation. Both lymphocytes and macrophages secrete a variety of cytokines, which modulate the immune response and the induction of inflammation (Table 221–2).

Immunologic events can be regulated through networks of antibody-forming cells, helper/suppressor mechanisms, and cytokine mediation or through specific mechanisms of immunologic tolerance. Immunodeficiency states and autoimmune diseases represent the endpoints of either a genetically incompetent or a poorly regulated immune system.

TABLE 221–1. PROPERTIES OF IMMUNOGLOBULINS BY CLASS AND SUBCLASS

Class	IgG	IgA	IgM	IgD	IgE
Molecular weight	160,000	17,000 or polymer	900,000	80,000	90,000
Sedimentation constant	7S	7S (9, 11, 13)	19S	7S	8S
Serum concentration	1000–5000	250–300	100–150	0.3–30	0.0015–0.2
Valence	2	2 (monomer)	10	2	2
Molecular formula	$\gamma_2 L_2$	$(\alpha_2 L_2)_n$	$(\mu_2 L_2)_5$	$\delta_2 L_2$	$\epsilon_2 L_2$

Subclass	IgG1	IgG2	IgG3	IgG4	IgA1	IgA2	IgM	IgD	IgE
Subclass percent of class, in serum	65	20	10	5	90	10			
Complement fixation	++	+	++	−	−	−	++	−	−
Alternative complement fixation					+	+		±	±
Placental passage	+	+	+	+	−	−	−	−	−
Fixing to mast cells or basophils	−	−	−	−	−	−	−	−	+
Binding to									
Macrophages	+	±	+	±	−	−	−	−	−
Neutrophils	+	+	+	+	+	+	−	−	−
Platelets	+	+	+	+	−	−	−	−	−
Lymphocytes	+	+	+	+	−	−	+	−	−
Half-life (days)	23	23	8–9	23	6	6	5	3	2.5
Synthesis rate (mg/kg/day)	25	?	3.5	?	44	22	7	0.4	0.02

TABLE 221-2. CYTOKINES AND THEIR BIOLOGIC ACTIVITIES

Cytokines Interleukin	Cell Source			Major Activities
	T	Macrophages	Other	
Interleukin-1α and β (IL-1α and β)		+	+	Fever; bone resorption; prostaglandin release; stimulate cytokine production by macrophages and T cells.
IL-1α		+		
IL-1β			+	Some
IL-2	+			Activates cytotoxic T cells and NK cells. Stimulates proliferation of T cells and NK cells. Stimulates differentiation of T cells and LAK cells. Costimulates proliferation of B cells and antibody secretion.
IL-3	+	+	+	Supports proliferation of mast cells and pre-B cells. Supports differentiation of stem cells.
IL-4	+		+	Activates resting B cells and macrophages. Induces IgG and IgE secretion in LPS-activated B cells. Stimulates proliferation of T cells and mast cells. Suppresses TNF-α, IL-1, IL-6 in monocytes.
IL-5	+			Induces IgA production and IgM secretion from LPS-activated B cells. Proliferation of eosinophils; supports differentiation of cytotoxic T cells.
IL-6	+	+	+	Induces antibody secretion; differentiation of cytotoxic T cells; proliferation of megakaryocytes. Promotes myeloma cell growth.
IL-7			Thymic strand cells	Proliferation and differentiation of pre-B cells. Proliferation of thymocytes.
IL-8		+		Neutrophil and T-cell chemotaxis.
IL-9	+			Growth of T-helper cell clones.
IL-10	+	+	+	Inhibits production of (IFN-γ and TNF-α) and B-cell growth and differentiation.
IL-11			+	Proliferation and development of B cells, macrophages, and megakaryocytes.
IL-12			B cells	Proliferation of activated T cell induction of IFN-γ.
Tumor necrosis factor-α (TNF-α) (cachectin)	+	+		Fever; shock; activates macrophages; stimulates PMN chemotoxin; angiogenesis, bone resorption; cytotoxic to many cells. Activates endothelial cells, granulocytes, and B cells.
Tumor necrosis factor-β (TNF-β) (lymphotoxin)	+			Inhibits angiogenesis; cytotoxic to many cells.
Inteferon-γ (IFN-γ)	+		NK cells	Activated NK cells, cytotoxic T cells, endothelial cells, and macrophages. Has antitumor activity. Stimulates LAK activity; costimulates B-cell proliferation; inhibits T-cell proliferation.

B LYMPHOCYTE LINEAGE AND ANTIBODY PRODUCTION

Secreted antibodies are produced by plasma cells, which represent the terminal phase of differentiation of B lymphocytes. The latter are found in all peripheral lymphoid tissues and also in the circulating pool of lymphocytes. Within their surface membranes, B cells have receptors that allow them to recognize foreign antigenic determinants. These receptors are immunoglobulin molecules, and in the initial stages of differentiation are generally of the IgM and IgD classes. When stimulated by a specific antigen, in conjunction with appropriate cytokines, these B cells proliferate and secrete antibody (see Fig. 221–1).

In the earliest stages of differentiation (Fig. 221–4), B lymphocytes lack membrane immunoglobulin (mIg). However, these cells begin to express in their cytoplasm the μ chain, which is the heavy (H) chain of IgM. Later they produce the light (L) chain (either kappa [κ] or lambda [λ]) which allows IgM molecules to be expressed on the surface. The binding region on the mIg of each cell line is unique in its specificity and is identical to that of the antibody molecule that is to be secreted. This means that at a very early developmental stage, a given cell is locked into its own specificity. This process involves several gene rearrangements (see below).

B-cell activation, proliferation, and differentiation require a variety of cytokines. Perhaps the most important in humans is interleukin-2 (IL-2), which seems to play a central role in these events and thus facilitates the production of immunoglobulins of all isotopes. Although other cytokines (e.g., IL-4 and TGF-β) are identified as being able to amplify and modify antibody production, generally they cannot do this unless IL-2 is present (Table 221–2).

IMMUNOGLOBULIN FUNCTION AND STRUCTURE

The basic structure of all immunoglobulin molecules (see Fig. 221–2) is similar among the various classes. Essentially they consist of two types of polypeptide chains—the larger called the heavy (H) chain, the smaller known as the light (L) chain. Each immunoglobulin subunit consists of two identical H and two identical L chains and would therefore have the molecular formula H_2L_2. The H and L chains are connected to each other by disulfide bonds, and similarly there are disulfide bridges between the two H chains (which vary in number for the different classes and subclasses). They are generally located in the center of the H chain region, known as the "hinge" region, which is unusually rich in cysteine and proline. The L chain has a molecular weight of about 25,000 daltons; the H chain varies between 50,000 and 65,000 daltons. H chain size is related to differences in the structure of the hinge region or to the presence of an extra globular domain, as in the case of the μ and ε H chains (in IgM and IgE, respectively). Globular domains, formed by intrachain disulfide bonds, each consist of about 110 amino acid residues; and there are four or five such domains in each H chain and two in each L chain. The domains are separated by extended regions known as interdomain stretches. These domain structures may have evolved to execute specialized biologic functions.

The amino terminal 110 to 120 residues of each immunoglobulin chain are known as the *variable* (V) region because the amino acid sequences of those molecules produced from a single clonal line differ from those of other lines. The remaining part of the immunoglobulin chain is identical for any given class and is referred to as the *constant* (C) region. Many direct lines of evidence indicate that the variable region contains the antibody-binding site into which antigen fits and that "hypervariable regions" are in the most intimate contact with the structural elements of the antigen. X-ray crystallography has confirmed these three-dimensional structures. The hypervariable regions are also largely responsible for the *idiotypic* determinants on an antibody molecule and tend to be similar on all antibodies that share specificities. The structures throughout the remainder of the V segments, which show less sequence variability, are referred to as the "framework" areas.

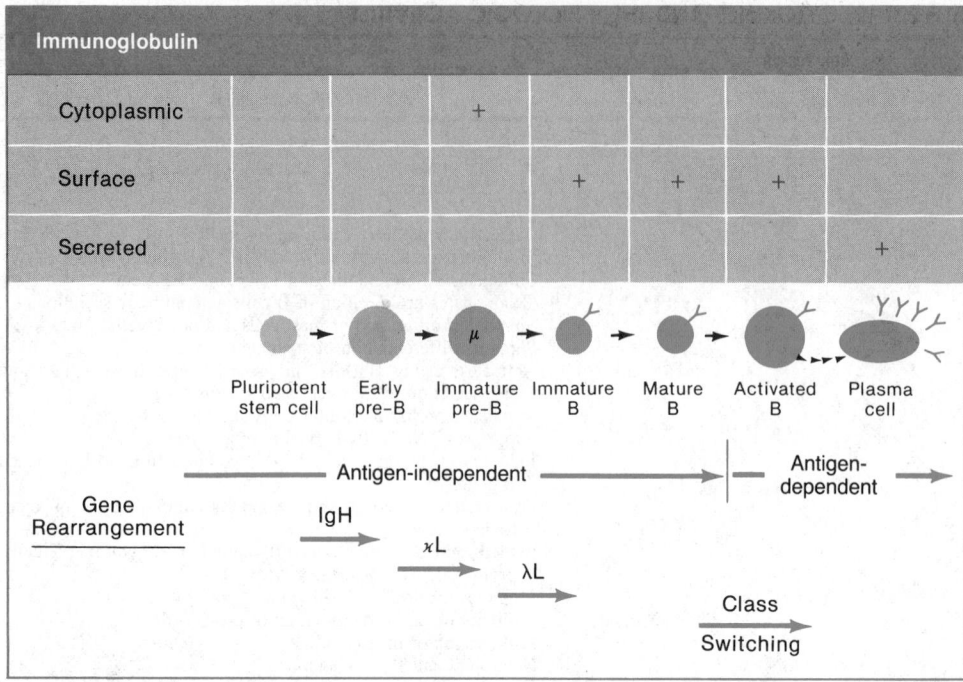

FIGURE 221–4. Presentation of B-cell pathway development in a sequential form showing when immunoglobulin appears in the cytoplasm or on the surface or is secreted. The gene rearrangements that take place at various stages of the differentiation pathway are indicated.

Although the amino acid sequences of the constant regions of the H chains show homologies among the Ig classes and subclasses, there are also very significant differences. The structural features appear to be important in giving the molecule its particular biologic function that distinguishes one class from another. Complement fixation, for example, seems to depend upon a structural determinant in the IgG CH2 domain, whereas features of the CH3 domain seem to be important for interacting with a variety of cells by way of the Fc receptors. More than one domain in the Fc region of the IgG H chain is required to react with the binding sites on rheumatoid factors (see Ch. 237).

Since Porter's original work on the structure of antibodies, much has been learned about their molecular structure by using proteolytic enzymes. For example, papain cleaves IgG into an Fc fragment and two Fab fragments, whereas pepsin degrades the Fc fragment and yields the two Fab fragments still joined by a disulfide bridge (Fab)$_2$ (see Fig. 221–2). Different enzymes cleave the various classes in different ways, and this approach has been important in defining structural corollaries to biologic properties.

Comparisons among the various classes of immunoglobulin are shown in Table 221–1. Certain immunoglobulins appear very different from IgG. For example, IgM is a large molecule but consists of five subunits of the same basic immunoglobulin pattern. It has 10 H and 10 L chains and, therefore, 10 antibody-binding sites per molecule. However, because of steric factors, when IgM reacts with large protein antigens, it tends to bind with a valence of five. This can best be seen in the case of IgM rheumatoid factor binding to IgG, which yields a 22 S complex with a formula $(\mu_2 L_2)5$-$(IgG)5$.

TABLE 221–3. CHROMOSOMAL LOCATIONS OF THE HUMAN IMMUNOGLOBULIN AND T-CELL RECEPTOR GENES

Chain	Symbol	Locus
Immunoglobulin		
Heavy chain	H	14q32
Kappa light chain	κ	2p12
Lambda light chain	λ	22q11
T-cell receptor		
Alpha and delta chains	α, δ	14q11–12
Beta chain	β	7q32–35
Gamma chain	γ	7p15

IMMUNOGLOBULIN GENETICS AND GENE ORGANIZATION

Human immunoglobulin genes are contained on chromosomes 2, 14, and 22 (Table 221–3). Several sequences of events must take place for immunoglobulin genes to be expressed. This requires a random process of gene reorganization. As shown in Figure 221–5, each C region is coded by a single gene, but many gene segments are necessary to form the repertoire of V genes. The latter are formed by rearrangement of DNA to bring one V gene into proximity with a J (junction) gene in the case of the L chains; and in the case of the H chains, the V must be brought into proximity with a D (diversity) region and a J region. For any given H-chain gene, the total V region is formed from a single V region, a single D, and a single J (Fig. 221–5). Combination with a given constant region would determine the Ig class. Recombination activating genes (RAG) facilitate the V-D-J recombination, and this suggests that they may encode enzymes that have the properties of being V-D-J recombinases. The C region genes are located in tandem, so a switching process must occur in order to allow a given assembled V-D-J region to attach to any constant region. This process deletes

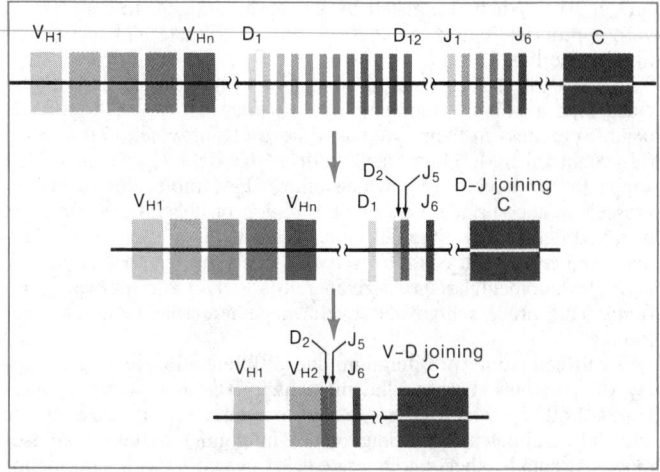

FIGURE 221–5. The mechanisms for DJ and VD joining to form the entire variable region of the heavy chain. Note that intervening gene sequences at each step of joining are deleted, giving rise to the final finished product of an entire V region with the constant region at some distance. This event would be followed by a messenger RNA developing and splicing to form the entire translatable message sequence (see text for details).

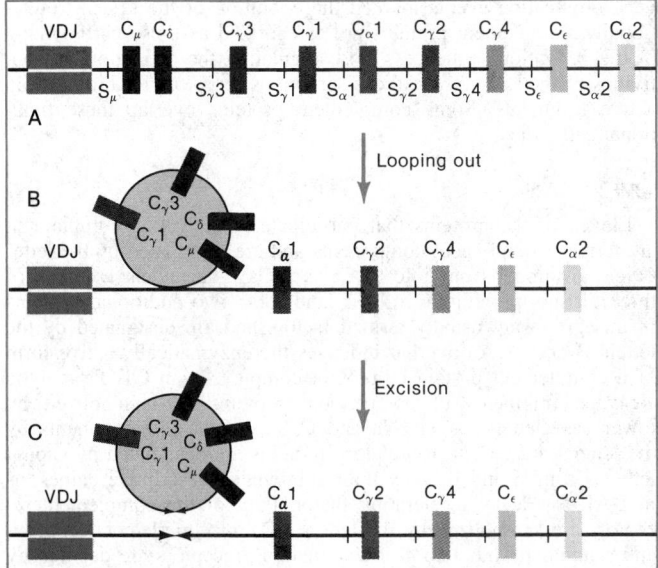

FIGURE 221–6. A diagrammatic representation of class switching to produce IgA_1. The switch sequence regions (S) identify places where looping can occur. This results ultimately in excision of the loop containing $C\mu$, $C\delta$, $C\gamma_1$, and $C\gamma_3$ and brings $C\alpha_1$ into close juxtaposition to the rearranged VDJ regions. (Adapted with permission from von Schwedler et al.: Nature 345:452–454, 1990. Copyright © 1990 Macmillan Magazines Limited.)

all intervening genes from that particular clone (Fig. 221–6). In some B lymphocytes both IgD and IgM are present on the cell membrane at the same time, and this occurs through alternative RNA splicing.

There are several mechanisms that generate antibody diversity which are inherent in the somatic process of forming Ig genes.

1. *Combinatorial diversity,* which results from the combination of various gene segments as described above
2. *Junctional diversity,* which results at the joining site because of some imprecision in codon formation
3. *Junctional insertion,* by which diversity may arise because of insertion of extra nucleotides
4. *Somatic mutational events*
5. *Exchange rearrangement* of the H segments
6. The *combination of associated H and L chains*

This process allows an essentially random extrapolation of combinations into the millions of possibilities; i.e., it *generates* antibody diversity.

T LYMPHOCYTES

T-Cell Receptors

The most common form of T-cell receptor consists of a disulfide-linked heterodimer of α and β chains. Both of these chains contain amino-terminal *variable* regions and carboxy-terminal *constant* regions, just as occur in immunoglobulins. These chains contain carbohydrate and are bound within the surface of the T cell with membrane-spanning regions. A subset of T cells possesses similar receptors made up of γ and δ chains that seem to be highly specialized and located in certain regions of the body, such as the gastrointestinal tract. A molecule called the T3 complex bears the CD3 determinant and is noncovalently linked to the T-cell receptor heterodimer (see Fig. 221–3). It is of special note that variable regions of the T-cell receptor genes are assembled from V-D-J segment joining just as the immunoglobulin V region genes are assembled. Much less if any somatic hypermutation occurs in the T-cell receptor V region genes. Thus, rearrangement occurs during the process of differentiation, and once it has occurred it produces a stable clone with a fixed specificity.

ANTIGEN PRESENTATION AND THE MAJOR HISTOCOMPATIBILITY COMPLEX

Certain cell types such as macrophages, dendritic cells, and epidermal Langerhans cells are able to take up antigens nonspecifically and, when they express major histocompatibility class I or II (MHC

I or II) molecules, present antigen to T cells (see Fig. 221–3). In some cases other cells, including activated B cells that may express class II MHC molecules, may also act as antigen-presenting cells. The antigen presented has often been processed so that only a relatively small peptide determinant is bound to the MHC for presentation. This event appears to involve the MHC molecule in conjunction with the processed antigen peptide on the surface of the antigen-presenting cell so that it can react with the T-cell receptor, and the CD4 molecule in the case of MHC-II, or with CD8 in the case of MHC-I, on the membrane of the T cell (see Ch. 229).

Similar membrane recognition events take place when cytotoxic T cells recognize and interact with cells bearing specific foreign antigens. In this case, the cytotoxic T cell may recognize the foreign antigen in conjunction with a class I MHC molecule, and it does so by virtue of its T-cell receptor in the presence of the CD8 molecule. Activation requires a second signal via B7 on the antigen-presenting cell and CD 28 on the T-cell surface. Such activated cytotoxic T cells can then destroy their target cells by a lytic process.

REGULATION AND MODULATION OF THE IMMUNE PROCESS

Complement

The complement cascade is important to modify the effector arm of the immune system. Activating complement allows important events such as removing infectious agents and expressing the inflammatory response to take place. These involve active fragments of the pathway that enhance chemotaxis of macrophages, alter blood vessel permeability, change blood vessel diameters, cause lysis to cells, alter blood clotting, and cause numerous other subtle points of modification. Complement is discussed in greater detail in Ch. 222.

IDIOTYPIC NETWORKS

As indicated previously, antibody molecules express unique antigenic determinants on their variable regions, thereby allowing secondary antibodies to be produced against them. Such determinants are designated *idiotopes.* Therefore, an idiotope of immunoglobulin is functionally equivalent to the *clonotypic* antigenic determinant of a clonal line of T cells. The idiotypic network concept (Fig. 221–7) holds that the immune system is in a dynamic regulatory equilibrium so that members of each clone within the system are recognized by members of other clones through these anti-idiotope interactions. Conceptually, this interrelated system provides mechanisms for regulation based on recognition of receptors without need for exogenous antigen. This method of regulation may allow certain idiotopes to become dominantly expressed and may be operative with unique *clonal markers,* such as those that are observed due to clonal expansion in malignant lymphoid diseases.

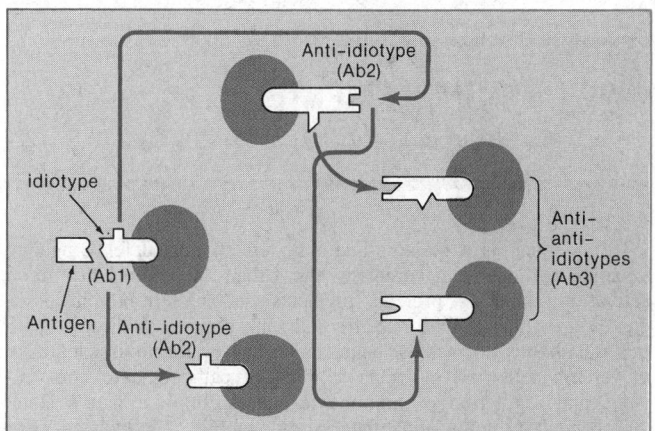

FIGURE 221–7. Diagrammatic representation of the idiotypic network showing the development of anti-idiotypes and anti-anti-idiotypes in sequential processes. This complementary fit mechanism provides the structural basis for the feedback network.

HELPER T-CELL SYSTEM

Helper T-cells may be divided into Th1 and Th2 populations. There is a feedback control mechanism for regulation of these subsets. Generally, Th1 cytokines promote Th1 activity and inhibit Th2 activity. The reverse is also true. Th1 cytokines are IL-1, IL-12, and IFN-γ and enhance the cellular immune response. Th2 cytokines are IL-4, IL-5, and IL-6 and enhance the humoral immune response.

SUPPRESSION

Regulating responses to antigenic stimulation and also controlling potential immune responses against self components are essential ingredients of a smoothly operating immune system. Suppressor T cells and the suppressor system represent a series of cell types that act in a highly complex fashion. Several distinct types of suppressor systems have been described, and their sequential action appears to have an amplification effect so that direct and graded regulation can take place. Suppressor effector cells can act on antibody-secreting cells and on T cells to downregulate their expression.

CYTOKINES

A growing array of molecules have been identified as products of cells that serve to regulate the immune system and to evoke responses in other cells, such as blood vessel endothelial cells and precursor cells in the bone marrow. Cytokines can regulate levels of response or induce differentiation and proliferation of cells. Table 221–2 summarizes the properties of some of these molecules which may be encountered in immune regulation (see also Ch. 235 and 264).

SUMMARY

The immune system is a highly orchestrated and coordinated system that allows a rapid response to foreign substances in a highly specific manner. The organization occurs at the level of the gene, the cell, and the mediator. Therefore, any qualitative or quantitative change in this system can produce profound effects. This is evident as one examines diseases of the immune system, such as those that occur as the result of altered immune regulation (see Ch. 237 and 240).

Inflammation, often immunologically mediated and often resulting in tissue damage, is a key feature of diseases of virtually any organ system. Therefore, a knowledge of basic immunology is critical to a clear understanding of the nature of these abnormalities. A student of medicine must be prepared to apply immunology to every branch of internal medicine and to recognize its importance in understanding disease and, hence, the care of the patient.

Engelhard VH: How cells process antigens. Sci Am 271:54, 1994. *Newest information on antigen breakdown and cell processing for presentation.*
Immunology Today 15:393–453, 1994 [entire issue]. *Ten papers bring together all the latest information on B-cell activation and regulation.*
Roitt IM: Essential Immunology. 8th ed. London, Blackwell Scientific, 1994. *An excellent introductory textbook of immunology; easy-to-read with good visual aids.*

222 COMPLEMENT
John E. Volanakis

Complement is a major effector system of host defense against invading pathogens. It comprises more than 30 proteins that upon activation elaborate protein fragments and protein-protein complexes that interact with specific cellular receptors or directly with cell membranes to mediate acute inflammatory reactions, clearance of foreign cells and molecules, killing of pathogenic microorganisms, and regulation of immune responses. In their native state, complement proteins are either serum soluble or associated with cell membranes (Table 222–1). Most of the serum-soluble proteins are synthesized in the liver. Complement proteins exhibit extensive structural homologies among themselves, remarkably conserving a small number of repeated structural motifs, indicating that multiple gene duplication events marked the evolution of the system. Functionally, complement proteins are categorized as those participating in the activation sequences, those regulating the activation and activities of the system, and those serving as receptors for biologically active fragments. Some complement proteins overlap these functional categories.

NOMENCLATURE

Eleven of the proteins that participate in activating complement are termed complement components and are designated by the letter C and a number from 1 to 9. C1 is a Ca^{2+}-dependent complex of three distinct proteins, C1q, C1r, and C1s. Two additional proteins in this group are usually termed factors and are designated by the letters B and D. An overbar indicates the enzymatically active form of a complement protein or protein complex, as in $\overline{C1}$. Proteolytic cleavage fragments of complement proteins are symbolized by lower case letters, as in C2a and C2b, and inactive fragments by the letter i, e.g., C2ai. Regulatory proteins are designated by capital letters, as in H and I, or by their abbreviated descriptive names, as in DAF for decay-accelerating factor. Four of the complement receptors are symbolized by the letters CR, for complement receptor, and a number from 1 to 4. The remaining receptors are denoted by the symbol of the protein or protein fragment they bind followed by the letter R, as in C5aR.

COMPLEMENT ACTIVATION

The complement system must be activated to express biologic activity and is characterized by operational simplicity and economy of design. The most important host defense activities are derived from two proteins, C3 and C5, that are structurally homologous and probably represent gene duplication products. Expression of activity requires that C3 and C5 be cleaved by highly specific proteases, termed *convertases* (Fig. 222–1). There are two C3 and two C5 convertases. One of each is assembled during activation of the two pathways of complement, which are termed *classic* and *alternative*. The two activation pathways use different proteins to form these enzymes. In addition, the assembly of the convertases is initiated by different activators in the two pathways. However, the resulting enzymes have identical substrate and peptide bond specificity, giving rise to identical biologically active fragments. Characteristic of the simplicity and economy of design of complement activation is the fact that C5 convertases are derivatives of C3 convertases (Fig. 222–1). Furthermore, C3 and C5 are activated by their respective convertases in similar fashion: A single peptide bond near the NH_2 terminus of the α polypeptide chain of either C3 or C5 is cleaved to generate a small peptide, C3a or C5a, and a large two-polypeptide fragment, C3b or C5b. Each of these four fragments, as well as

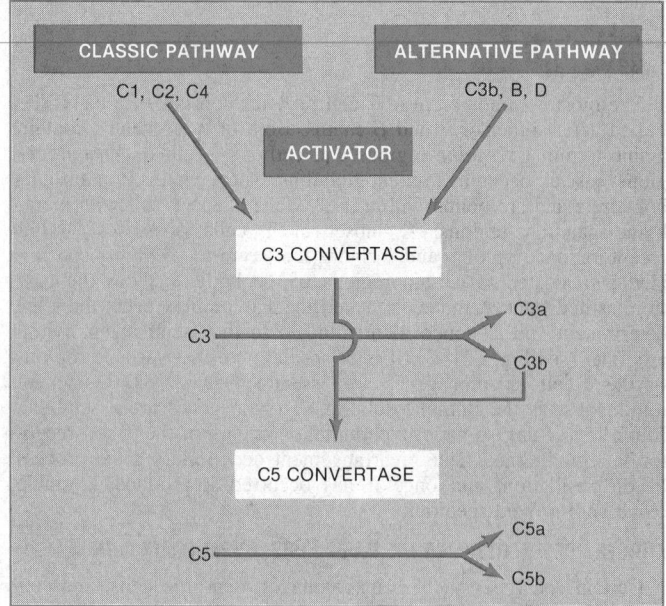

FIGURE 222–1. Activation of the complement system.

TABLE 222–1. PROTEINS OF THE COMPLEMENT SYSTEM*

	Functional Group		
Prevalent Form in Native State	*Participating in Activation Sequences*	*Regulatory*	*Receptors*
Serum soluble	Clq, Clr, Cls, D MBP, MASP C4, C3, C2, B C5, C6, C7, C8, C9	Cl INH C4bp, H, I, P C3a/C5a INA S protein	
Membrane associated		CR1 DAF, MCP HRF, CD59	ClqR, C3aR, C5aR CR1, CR2 CR3, CR4

* Established symbols have been used for most complement proteins. In addition, the following generally accepted abbreviations have been used: INH, inhibitor; C4bp, C4b-binding protein; INA, inactivator; R, receptor, e.g., CRI, complement receptor type 1; MBP = mannose-binding protein; MASP = MBP-associated serine protease; DAF = decay-accelerating factor; MCP = membrane cofactor protein; HRF = homologous restriction factor.

further cleavage fragments of C3b, expresses at least one activity important to host defense.

ASSEMBLY OF COMPLEMENT CONVERTASES

CLASSIC PATHWAY. In the classic pathway, assembly of the convertases is usually initiated by antibodies of the IgG or IgM class complexed with antigen. Several other substances, including CRP complexes, certain viruses, and gram-negative bacteria, can also activate this pathway. Activators are recognized by C1q, one of the three proteins in the C1 complex. Binding to an activator induces a change in the conformation of C1q that causes the autoactivation of C1r, which in turn activates proenzyme C1s to enzymatically active $\overline{C1s}$ (Fig. 222–2). In the next step, $\overline{C1s}$ cleaves C4, resulting in the covalent attachment of its major fragment, C4b, to the surface of the activator. C4b is attached through a transacylation reaction similar to that leading to covalent binding of C3b to activating surfaces (see below). C2 binds to C4b and is also cleaved by $\overline{C1}$ into two fragments, the larger of which, C2a, remains bound to C4b, completing the assembly of the $\overline{C4b2a}$ complex, which is the C3 convertase of the classic pathway. Cleavage of C3 by the C3 convertase results in the covalent binding of many C3b fragments to the surface of the activator and the eventual binding of one C3b to the C4b subunit of the C3 convertase. This leads to the formation of the $\overline{C3b4b2a}$ complex, which is the C5 convertase of the classic pathway. A novel C1-independent mechanism for activating the classic pathway was described recently. It uses mannose-binding protein (MBP), an acute-phase serum lectin with binding specificity for terminal mannose and *N*-acetylglycosamine. MBP binding to bacterial pathogens displaying these sugar residues results in activation of an associated protease, which in turn cleaves C4 and C2, leading to the assembly of a C3 convertase.

ALTERNATIVE PATHWAY. Alternative pathway activation is initiated by a variety of cellular surfaces, including those of certain bacteria, parasites, viruses, and fungi. Antibodies can also activate

this pathway, but they are not usually required. Assembly of the convertases is intimately related to certain structural features of the multifunctional protein C3. C3 is the most abundant complement protein in blood and is characterized by the presence on its α-chain of an unusual, for blood proteins, thioester bond. Under physiologic conditions, this bond is relatively stable, being hydrolyzed at very slow rates to give rise to C_{H_2O}, which can initiate the formation of the short-lived *initiation* C3 convertase. This is accomplished by the formation of a complex between $C3_{H_2O}$ and B and the subsequent cleavage of B by D to generate the $\overline{C3_{H_2O}Bb}$ complex, the initiation C3 convertase (Fig. 222–3). This series of reactions, starting with the hydrolysis of the thioester bond in native C3 and concluding with the cleavage of C3 into C3a and C3b by the initiation C3 convertase, is considered to occur in the blood continuously at slow rates. Thus, a constant supply of small amounts of freshly generated C3b is available at all times. The initiation C3 convertase is quickly inactivated by the control proteins H and I.

C3 cleaved by a C3 convertase induces a pronounced change in the conformation of C3b associated with an extremely labile (metastable) thioester bond that reacts either with water or with hydroxyl or amino groups on the surface of cells or proteins. Thus, C3b becomes covalently attached via an ester or amide bond to surfaces in the immediate vicinity of its generation. The fate of surface-bound C3b depends entirely on the chemical nature of the surface. C3b bound to a nonactivator of the alternative pathway, e.g., host's red cells, is quickly inactivated by the action of control proteins. In contrast, C3b bound to an activator, e.g., *Escherichia coli* cells, preferentially binds B, which is then cleaved by D, generating the $\overline{C3bBb}$ complex, which is the C3 convertase of the alternative pathway. This enzyme is stabilized by the binding of P and is termed the *amplification* C3 convertase because it generates many C3b fragments and thus additional molecules of C3 convertase. Binding of a single C3b molecule to the C3 convertase gives rise to

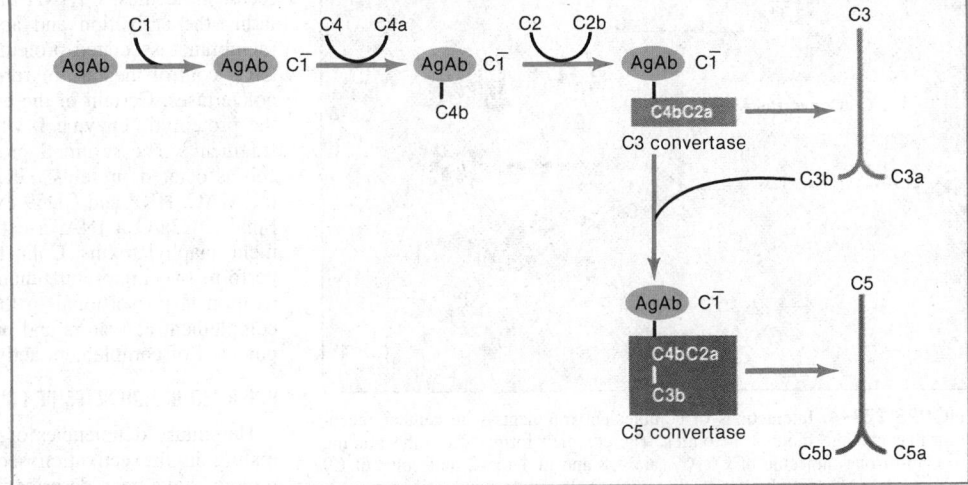

FIGURE 222–2. Formation of complement convertases in the classic pathway of activation.

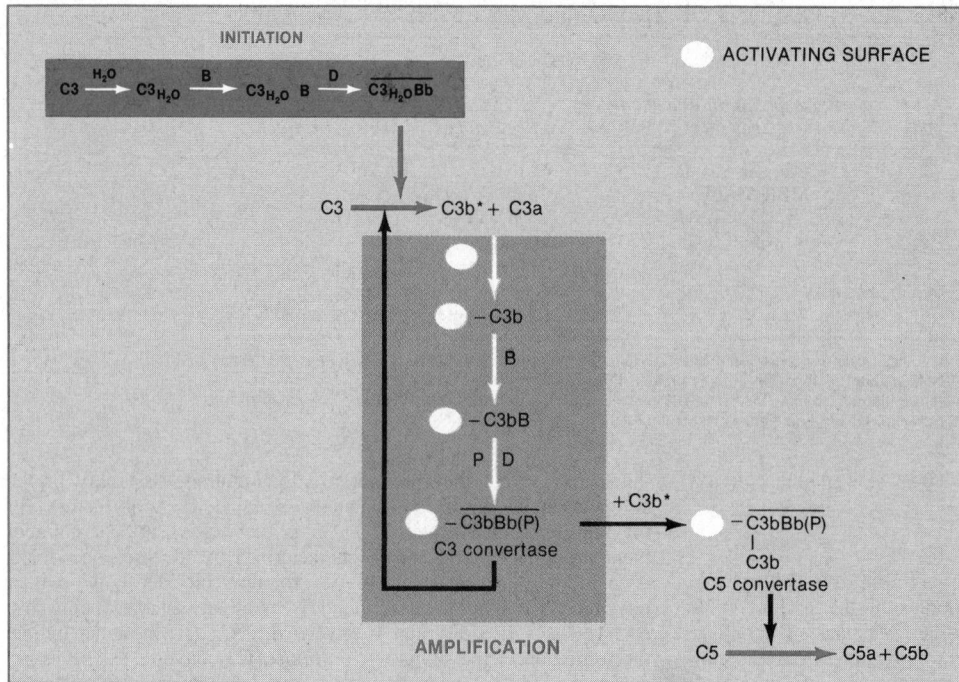

FIGURE 222–3. Formation of complement convertases in the alternative pathway of activation. Assembly of the *initiation* C3 convertase occurs at low levels continuously. When an activator is present, metastable C3b (C3b*) binds covalently to the activating surface and, because it is protected from the action of the regulatory proteins, initiates the assembly of the stable, *amplification* C3 convertase, which forms additional C3 convertase complexes and also the C5 convertase.

the $\overline{(C3b)_2Bb}$ complex, which is the C5 convertase of the alternative pathway (Fig. 222–3).

BIOLOGIC ACTIVITIES OF COMPLEMENT

With the exception of C5b, the fragments produced by the action of the convertases carry out their biologic functions by interacting with specific cellular receptors (Fig. 222–4). The complement *anaphylatoxins*, C3a and C5a, react with specific receptors to stimulate the release of histamine from mast cells and basophils mediating smooth muscle contraction and increased vascular permeability. In the presence of interleukin-3 (IL-3) or IL-5, C5a also causes release of leukotrienes from basophils. In addition, C5a evokes neutrophil and monocyte responses, including up-regulation of cellular receptors, adherence to vascular endothelia, chemotaxis, release of lysosomal enzymes, and generation of oxygen free radicals. Collectively, the anaphylatoxins allow for the recruitment of host defense molecules and cells to tissue sites invaded by pathogens. C3b and its further cleavage fragments, C3bi and C3dg, react with multiple receptors distributed in a variety of cells (Table 222–2). C3b covalently attached to immune complexes binds to CR1 receptors on erythrocytes which transport the complexes to the liver where they are taken up by Kuppfer cells and cleared from the circulation. C3b and C3bi interact with CR1 and CR3, respectively, on phagocytic cells to promote ingestion of foreign cells and particles. Reaction of C3bi and C3dg with CR2 on B lymphocytes helps regulate immune responses. C5b initiates the assembly of a large protein-protein complex, termed membrane attack complex (MAC), by interacting sequentially with a single molecule of C6, C7, and C8 and with 1 to 12 molecules of C9. The MAC interacts directly with the lipid bilayer of biologic membranes through hydrophobic domains of the participating proteins and eventually forms a transmembrane channel that leads to killing of susceptible cells.

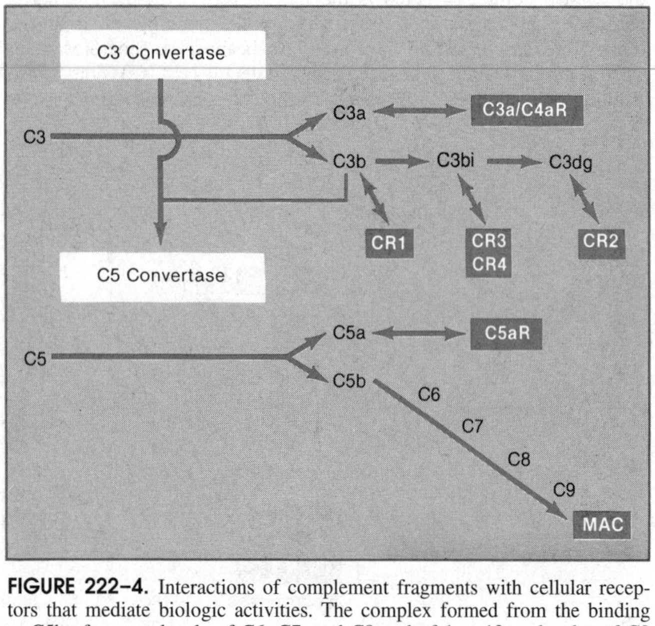

CONTROL OF COMPLEMENT ACTIVATION

The multiplicity and potency of the biologic activities generated when complement is activated and particularly the ability of complement to mediate acute inflammatory reactions and to produce lethal lesions in cell membranes present a threat not only to invading pathogens but also to the cells and tissues of the host. This self-damaging potential of complement activation is normally kept under effective control by a number of inhibitors and inactivators that act at points of enzymatic amplification and also at the level of effector molecules. C1 INH binds to and inhibits $\overline{C1r}$ and $\overline{C1s}$, regulating the activation and action of C1. A number of plasma and membrane-associated proteins, including C4bp, H, DAF, MCP, and CR1, control the rate of formation and the activity of complement convertases. Certain of these proteins act as obligatory cofactors for the proteolytic enzyme I, which cleaves C4b and C3b into smaller fragments. The serum S protein, also termed vitronectin, and two cell-associated proteins, HRF and CD59, inhibit the formation of the MAC. HRF and CD59 exhibit species specificity in their action. Finally, C3a/C5a INA, a carboxypeptidase, inactivates the complement anaphylatoxins. Collectively, the complement control proteins perform two important functions: They ensure that complement activation is proportional to the amount and duration of presence of complement activators and protect the host's cells from the harmful potential of complement activation products.

INHERITED DEFICIENCIES OF COMPLEMENT PROTEINS (Table 222–3)

Hereditary deficiencies of almost all complement proteins participating in the activation sequences and of several of the control proteins have been described. With two exceptions, complement deficiencies are inherited as autosomal recessive traits. C1 INH

FIGURE 222–4. Interactions of complement fragments with cellular receptors that mediate biologic activities. The complex formed from the binding to C5b of one molecule of C6, C7, and C8 and of 1 to 12 molecules of C9 is termed MAC (membrane attack complex). It forms transmembrane pores by interacting directly with the lipid bilayer of biologic membranes.

TABLE 222-2. RECEPTORS FOR C3b AND ITS FRAGMENTS

Receptor	Ligands	Cellular Distribution	Functions
CR1	C3b, C4b, C3bi	Erythrocytes, neutrophils, eosinophils, monocytes, macrophages, B cells, T cell subsets, follicular dendritic cells, glomerular podocytes	Immune complex clearance, endocytosis, phagocytosis
CR2	C3dg, C3bi, Epstein-Barr virus	B cells, thymocytes, follicular dendritic cells, pharyngeal epithelial cells	Immunoregulation
CR3	C3bi	Neutrophils, monocytes, macrophages, large granular lymphocytes	Phagocytosis, leukocyte adhesion, enhanced cytotoxicity
CR4	C3bi	Neutrophils, monocytes, macrophages	Unknown

deficiency is inherited as an autosomal dominant and P deficiency as an X-linked trait. A rather limited number of clinical syndromes are associated with complement deficiencies. Deficiencies of C1q, C1r, C1s, C4, and C2 are associated with diseases of immune origin, including systemic lupus erythematosus (SLE), discoid lupus, glomerulonephritis, and nonspecific vasculitis. The underlying mechanisms are unclear, but impaired processing and clearance from the circulation of immune complexes and aberrant immunoregulation have been implicated in the pathogenesis of these syndromes. Clinically, SLE in complement-deficient individuals is characterized by early onset, extensive skin lesions, absent or mild renal involvement, and low levels of antinuclear and anti-DNA antibodies. Deficiencies of C3, H, I, or P predispose to severe recurrent infections with encapsulated pyogenic bacteria. Lack of or inefficient opsonization of the bacteria by C3b/C3bi apparently causes the susceptibility to infection. Individuals deficient in C5, C6, C7, or C8 are susceptible to disseminated neisserial infections. Direct lysis by complement is probably required for effective defense against gonococci and meningococci. Curiously, individuals with C9 deficiency are usually asymptomatic. Heterozygous deficiency of C1 INH results in hereditary angioedema (see Ch. 224), characterized by episodic attacks of circumscribed, nonpruritic edema of the skin or the mucosa of the respiratory or gastrointestinal tract.

Pathophysiology

In certain human diseases, uncontrolled or aberrant activation of complement plays an important pathogenetic role. The classic pathway activated at tissue sites by autoantibodies against tissue antigens or by immune complexes deposited at basement membranes results in accumulation of inflammatory cells and tissue damage. The former mechanism is exemplified by the renal lesions of Goodpasture's syndrome and the second by the vascular and renal lesions in SLE and other immune complex diseases. Hypocomplementemia is often present in patients with immune complex diseases, particularly SLE, but also in various other clinical syndromes. Measurement of serum complement levels thus provides a simple and widely used tool to diagnose and manage human diseases. The most commonly used assays in clinical practice are total hemolytic complement, C4, and C3. Total hemolytic complement, expressed in CH_{50} units, reflects the activity of all complement components. C4 and C3 are usually measured by immunochemical assays. Low complement levels by all three assays are often but not always seen in SLE, particularly in patients with renal involvement and during acute exacerbations of the disease. In patients with partial lipodystrophy with or without glomerulonephritis and in some patients with membranoproliferative glomerulonephritis, levels of total complement and C3 are very low, whereas C4 is usually normal. This is due to the presence of an IgG autoantibody, termed C3 nephritic factor, with specificity for the amplification C3 convertase. This au-

toantibody binds to C3bBb and creates a stable complex that is not regulated by control proteins and thus continuously cleaves C3. The alternative pathway is also activated during circulation of the blood through pump oxygenators or hemodialysis machines. The C5a generated during these procedures causes aggregation of neutrophils, leading to their sequestration in the pulmonary vasculature. In some patients this is manifested by symptoms of pulmonary dysfunction and hypoxemia. Complement activation may also play a role in the pathogenesis of myocardial reperfusion injury.

Ahearn JM, Fearon DT: Structure and function of the complement receptors CR1 (CD35) and CR2 (CD21). Adv Immunol 46:183, 1989. *Molecular biology, structure, and function of two important cellular receptors for C3 fragments.*
Campbell RD, Law SKA, Reid KBM, Sim RB: Structure, organization, and regulation of the complement genes. Annu Rev Immunol 6:161, 1988. *A review of the genetics and structure of complement proteins.*
Colten HR, Rosen FS: Complement deficiencies. Annu Rev Immunol 10:809, 1992. *An excellent review of genetic abnormalities of the complement system.*
Hebert LA, Cosio FG: The erythrocyte–immune complex–glomerulonephritis connection in man. Kidney Int 31:327, 1987. *Discusses immune complex processing, disposal, and tissue deposition.*
Volanakis JE, Fearon DT: The molecular biology of the complement system. *In* McCarty DJ, Koopman WJ (eds.): Arthritis and Allied Conditions. 12th ed. Philadelphia, Lea & Febiger, 1993 p 455. *A comprehensive description of the biochemistry and biology of the complement system.*

223 PRIMARY IMMUNODEFICIENCY DISEASES
Rebecca H. Buckley

Since the first genetic defect in immunity was described in 1952, more than four dozen different primary immunodeficiency syndromes have been reported. Such diseases may involve any component of the immune system, including lymphocytes, phagocytic cells, and the complement proteins. This chapter focuses on abnormalities of lymphocytes. Deficiencies of the complement system (see Ch. 222) are mentioned briefly. A review of neutrophil dysfunction syndromes is presented in Ch. 139.1, and an overall review of the compromised host is given in Ch. 266. The acquired immunodeficiency syndrome (AIDS) is described in Part XXII.

Several of the primary immunodeficiency diseases have been mapped to specific chromosomal locations, and the fundamental biologic errors have been identified in a growing number of diseases (Table 223–1). Most are recessive traits, some of which are caused by mutations in genes on the X chromosome, others on autosomal chromosomes. Examples of the latter include an adhesion protein deficiency, now known to be due to mutations in the gene on chromosome 21q22.3 encoding the 95-Kd beta chain (CD18) common to three different leukocyte surface glycoprotein heterodimers, and combined immunodeficiencies due to abnormalities of purine salvage pathway enzymes, either adenosine deaminase (ADA, encoded by a gene on chromosome 20q13-ter) or purine nucleoside phosphorylase (PNP, encoded by a gene on chromosome 14q13.1) (see Ch. 181).

The faulty genes in many other immunodeficiencies are known to be on the X chromosome (Table 223–1). They have been localized

TABLE 222-3. DISEASES ASSOCIATED WITH INHERITED COMPLEMENT DEFICIENCIES

Deficient Protein	Diseases
C1q, C1r, C1s, C4, C2	SLE, SLE-like syndrome, discoid lupus, glomerulonephritis, vasculitis
C3, H, I, P	Recurrent pyogenic infections
C5, C6, C7, C8	Recurrent disseminated neisserial infections
C1 INH	Hereditary angioedema

TABLE 223-1. CHROMOSOMAL MAP LOCATIONS FOR FAULTY GENES IN PRIMARY IMMUNODEFICIENCY DISEASES

Chromosome	Disease
1q25	Chronic granulomatous disease (gp67^{phox})*
2p11	Kappa chain deficiency*
2g12	CD8 lymphocytopenia (ZAP70)*
6p21.3	(?)Common variable immunodeficiency and selective IgA deficiency
7q11.23	Chronic granulomatous disease (gp47^{phox})*
11	CD3 gamma chain deficiency*
11q22.3	Ataxia-telangiectasia
14q13.1	Purine nucleoside phosphorylase deficiency*
14q32.3	Immunoglobulin heavy chain deletion*
16q24	Chronic granulomatous disease (gp22^{phox})*
20q13-ter	Adenosine deaminase deficiency*
21q22.3	Leukocyte adhesion deficiency (CD18)*
22q11.2	DiGeorge syndrome
Xp21.1	Chronic granulomatous disease (gp91^{phox})*
Xp11.22–p11.23	Wiskott-Aldrich syndrome (proline-rich protein-WASP)*
Xq13	Severe combined immunodeficiency (gamma chain of IL-2R)*
Xq22	X-linked agammaglobulinemia (Bruton tyrosine kinase, BTK)*
Xq24–26	X-linked lymphoproliferative syndrome
Xq26	Immunodeficiency with hyper-IgM (CD40 ligand—gp39)*

* Gene cloned and sequenced, gene product known

to specific sites in the case of X-linked agammaglobulinemia, X-linked severe combined immunodeficiency, the Wiskott-Aldrich syndrome, X-linked lymphoproliferative disease, X-linked hyper-IgM, properdin deficiency, and X-linked chronic granulomatous disease (CGD). Until recently, there was little insight into the fundamental problems underlying most of these conditions. Recently, however, the molecular bases of four X-linked immunodeficiency disorders have been reported. These include X-linked immunodeficiency with hyper-IgM, X-linked agammaglobulinemia, X-linked severe combined immunodeficiency, and the Wiskott-Aldrich syndrome. Immune deficiency can also be associated with broad deficiencies of HLA class I and II antigens, and these have been shown to be due to different mutations in transactin factors governing the surface expression of these molecules. Table 223–2 lists the most prominent functional abnormalities and the presumed cellular level of the defect in 19 primary immunodeficiency syndromes.

In contrast to AIDS, which has a new case acquisition rate of more than 2500 per week, primary immunodeficiency diseases are rare. The incidence of agammaglobulinemia is estimated at 1 in 50,000. Selective absence of serum and secretory IgA, the most common, has a reported prevalence of 1 in 333 to 1 in 700.

APPROACHES TO THE PATIENT WITH SUSPECTED IMMUNODEFICIENCY

The number of patients suspected of having primary immunodeficiency will far exceed the incidences of these diseases. So it is important that the tests selected for immunologic assessment be broadly informative, reliable, and cost effective. Familiarity with certain clinical guidelines aids in the initial selection. Patients with antibody-, phagocytic-cell–, or complement deficiencies have recurrent infections with high-grade encapsulated bacteria. Therefore, those with only repeated viral respiratory infections are not likely to have any of these disorders. By contrast, patients with deficiencies in T-cell function usually manifest opportunistic infections. Most defects can be ruled out at little cost to the patient if the proper choice of screening tests is made. Among the most informative are the complete and differential blood counts and the sedimentation rate. Examining red cells for Howell-Jolly bodies helps exclude asplenia. A normal platelet count rules out Wiskott-Aldrich syndrome. If the sedimentation rate is normal, chronic bacterial infection is unlikely. If the absolute neutrophil count is normal, congenital and acquired neutropenia and severe chemotactic defects are eliminated. If the absolute lymphocyte count is normal, a severe T-cell defect is unlikely. Beyond this, it is good to keep in mind that tests of immune function are far more informative and cost effec-

tive than those measuring immunoglobulin concentrations or enumerating lymphocyte subpopulations.

In assessing B cell function, determinations of antibody titers to proteins (such as tetanus and diphtheria toxoids) and polysaccharides (such as pneumococcal antigens) following immunization are the most useful tests. As a rule, patients with B-cell defects for which there is an effective or indicated treatment do not produce antibodies normally. However, the presence of such antibodies does not exclude IgA deficiency, which would also be missed on a serum electrophoretic analysis. Immunoelectrophoresis is not quantitative and, for that reason, is not useful in evaluating immune competence. The quantification of serum IgA is particularly cost effective. If the IgA concentration is normal, this rules out not only IgA deficiency but all of the permanent types of agammaglobulinemia, because IgA is usually very low or absent in those conditions as well. A particularly uneconomical study is IgG-subclass measurement. It is far more helpful to know the results of antibody titer measurement because there are well-documented cases of antibody deficiency despite normal concentrations of all immunoglobulin classes and subclasses.

The most cost-effective test for assessing T-cell function is an intradermal skin test with 0.1 ml of a 1:1000 dilution of a known potent *Candida albicans* extract. If the test is positive, as defined by

TABLE 223-2. CHARACTERISTICS OF SOME PRIMARY IMMUNODEFICIENCY DISORDERS

Disorder	Functional Deficiencies	Molecular Defect
X-linked agammaglobulinemia	Antibody	Mutations in Bruton tyrosine kinase, BTK
Common variable immunodeficiency (CVID "acquired" hypogammaglobulinemia)	Antibody	Unknown, ? in MHC Class III region
Selective IgA deficiency	IgA antibody	Unknown, ? in MHC Class III region
Immunodeficiency with elevated IgM	IgG and IgA antibodies	Mutations in CD40 ligand on activated T cells
Transient hypogammaglobulinemia of infancy	None; immunoglobulins low, but antibodies present	Unknown
Antibody deficiency with near-normal immunoglobulins	Antibody	Unknown; ? related to CVID
X-linked lymphoproliferative disease	Anti-EBV nuclear antigen antibody	B cell; ? also T cell
DiGeorge syndrome	T cellular; some antibody	Microdeletions in chromosome 22q11
Nezelof syndrome (including PNP deficiency)	T cellular; some antibody	Unknown; PNP deficiency
Severe combined immunodeficiency syndromes (autosomal recessive; ADA deficiency; X-linked recessive; defective expression of HLA antigens; reticular dysgenesis)	Antibody and T cellular; phagocytic in reticular dysgenesis	ADA deficiency; mutations in gamma chain of the IL-2 receptor; other unknown defects
Wiskott-Aldrich syndrome	Antibody; T cellular	Mutations in a proline-rich protein, WASP
Ataxia-telangiectasia	Antibody; T cellular	Unknown
Cartilage-hair hypoplasia	T cellular	Unknown
Immunodeficiency with thymoma	Antibody; some T cellular	Unknown
Hyperimmunoglobulinemia E syndrome	Specific immune responses; excessive IgE	Unknown
Chronic mucocutaneous candidiasis	Variable cellular	Unknown
Leukocyte adhesion deficiency 1	Cytotoxic lymphocytes; phagocytic cell adhesion	Mutations in CD18
Leukocyte adhesion deficiency 2	Phagocytic cell adhesion	Unknown

erythema and induration of ≥10 mm at 48 hours, virtually all primary T-cell defects are excluded and the need for more expensive *in vitro* tests, such as lymphocyte phenotyping or assessments of responses to mitogens, is obviated. Killing defects of phagocytic cells, which should be suspected if the patient has problems with staphylococcal or gram-negative infections, can be screened for by tests measuring the neutrophil respiratory burst after phagocytosis or phorbol ester stimulation. Complement defects can be most effectively screened for in a CH50 assay, which measures the intactness of the entire complement pathway. If these tests are abnormal, or even if they are normal and clinical features of the patient still strongly suggest a host defect, the patient should be evaluated at a center where more definitive immunologic studies can be done before any type of immunologic treatment is begun.

ANTIBODY DEFICIENCY DISORDERS

Antibody deficiency may occur either as a congenital or an "acquired" abnormality, although in both situations it appears to be genetically determined. Most patients are recognized because they have recurrent infections, but some individuals with selective IgA deficiency or infants with transient hypogammaglobulinemia may have few or no infections.

X-LINKED AGAMMAGLOBULINEMIA (XLA). A majority of boys afflicted with this malady remain well during the first 6 to 9 months of life by virtue of maternally transmitted immunoglobulin. Thereafter, they repeatedly acquire infections with high-grade extracellular pyogenic organisms such as pneumococci, streptococci, and *Haemophilus* unless given prophylactic antibiotics or gammaglobulin therapy. The most common types of infections include sinusitis, pneumonia, otitis, septic arthritis, meningitis, and septicemia. Chronic fungal infections are usually not present, and *Pneumocystis carinii* pneumonia rarely occurs unless there is an associated neutropenia. Viral infections and live virus vaccines are also usually handled normally, with the notable exceptions of hepatitis and enterovirus infections. Several cases of paralysis after receiving polio vaccine have occurred, presumably because of muta-

tion of persistent vaccine virus to a more neurotropic form. In addition, a dermatomyositis-like syndrome accompanied by chronic, eventually fatal central nervous system disease caused by various echoviruses has occurred in more than 40 patients.

The diagnosis of XLA is suspected if serum concentrations of IgG, IgA, and IgM are below the 95% confidence limits for appropriate age- and race-matched controls (usually there is <100 mg per deciliter total immunoglobulin). Demonstrated antibody deficiency in serum and in external secretions is of great importance in distinguishing this disorder from transient hypogammaglobulinemia of infancy. Tests for natural antibodies to blood group substances, for antibodies to antigens given during standard courses of immunization, and for antibodies to and ability to clear bacteriophage $\phi \times 174$ are markedly abnormal. Polymorphonuclear functions are usually normal, but some patients with this condition have had transient, persistent, or cyclic neutropenia.

Lymphopenia is uncommon, and the percentages of T cells and T cell subsets have been found to be normal or elevated in most instances. In contrast, blood lymphocytes bearing surface immunoglobulin, "Ia-like" antigens, or the EBV receptor, or reacting with a specific anti-B cell serum are absent or present in very low numbers. Hypoplasia of adenoids, tonsils, and peripheral lymph nodes is the rule; germinal centers are not present, and plasma cells are rarely found. Conversely, normal numbers of pre-B cells are found in the bone marrow. The abnormal gene in XLA was recently discovered by two groups, one using the technique of positional cloning and the other by seeking and finding a tyrosine kinase important in B-cell signaling that proved to be encoded by a gene on the X chromosome in the region where Bruton's disease had been mapped (see Tables 223–1 and 223–2 and Fig. 223–1). The tyrosine kinase has been named Bruton tyrosine kinase (or BTK) in honor of Dr. Bruton. BTK is a member of the Src-related nonreceptor cytoplasmic tyrosine kinase family, which includes Lck, Fyn, and Lyn, thought to be involved in signal transduction in many

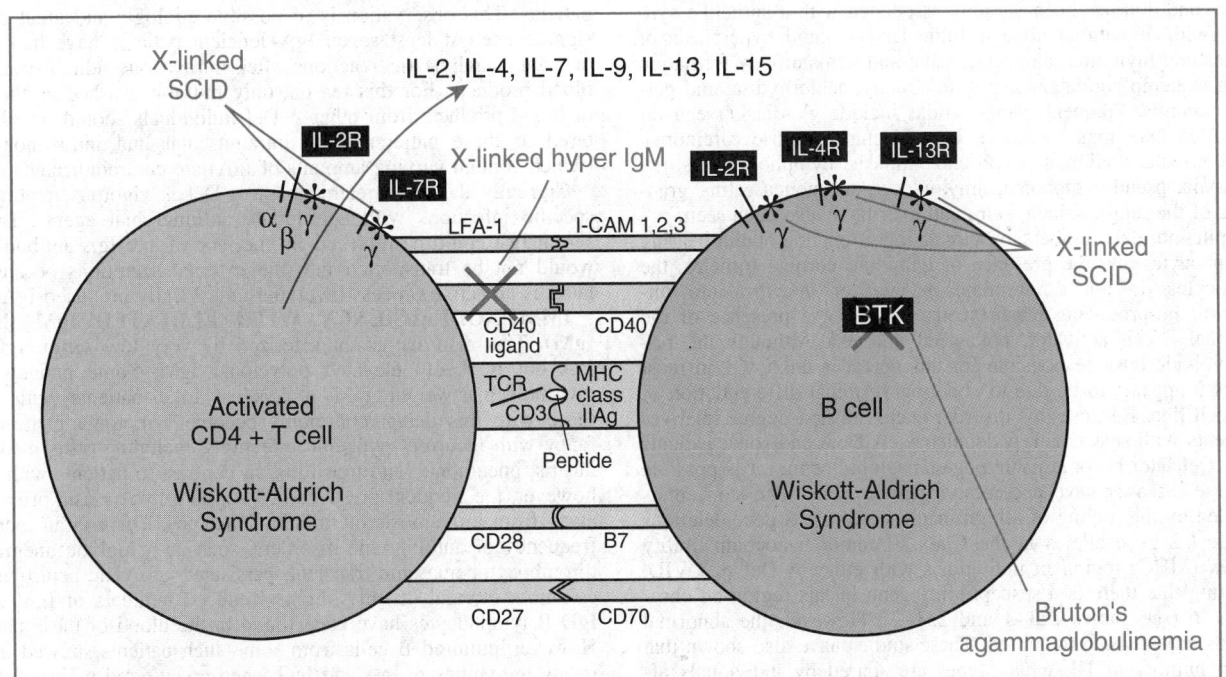

FIGURE 223–1. Schematic of molecules involved in T- and B-cell interaction and signal transduction, showing the location of newly defined molecular defects in four X-linked primary immunodeficiency diseases. Mutations in the gene encoding the cytoplasmic nonreceptor tyrosine kinase lead to Bruton's or X-linked agammaglobulinemia by preventing B-cell maturation beyond the pre–B cell stage. Mutations in the gene for the CD40 ligand, or gp39, prevent expression of this crucial molecule necessary for T cells to activate B cells by interacting with CD40 on their surface. These mutations are responsible for the defect in X-linked immunodeficiency with hyper-IgM that prevents the B cells from isotype-switching. Mutations in the interleukin-2 (IL-2) receptor gamma chain (IL-2Rγ) prevent the binding of not only IL-2 but of several other cytokines necessary for T- and B-cell development and function (IL-4, IL-7, IL-9, IL-13, and IL-15) because the IL-2Rγ chain is also a component of those cytokine receptors. IL-2Rγ mutations are thus responsible for the profound deficiencies in T, B, and natural killer (NK) cell function present in infants with X-linked severe combined immunodeficiency disease (XSCID). Finally, mutations in a novel gene encoding a 501–amino acid proline-rich protein (WASP) limited expression to lymphocytic and megakaryocytic cell lineages, resulted in the Wiskott-Aldrich syndrome.

hematopoietic cells. BTK is expressed at high levels in all B-lineage cells, including pre-B cells; it has not been detected in any cells of T lineage, but it has in cells of the myeloid series. Thus far, most males with known XLA (by family history) have had low to undetectable BTK mRNA and kinase activity due to point mutations in the catalytic (kinase) domain in BTK. Mixed lymphocyte responsiveness and lymphocyte responses to antigens and mitogens are normal. Cell-mediated immune responses can be detected *in vivo,* and the thymus has appeared normal in all autopsied cases.

Except in those unfortunate patients who develop polio, persistent echovirus infection, or lymphoreticular malignancy, the overall prognosis is reasonably good if humoral replacement therapy is instituted early. Systemic infection can be prevented by administering intravenous immune serum globulin (ISG, primarily IgG) at a dose of 400 mg per kilogram every 3 to 4 weeks. Such preparations are known to be free of the AIDS virus. Many patients go on to develop crippling sinopulmonary disease despite this therapy because no effective means exist for replacing secretory IgA at the mucosal surface. Chronic antibiotic therapy is also usually necessary for managing such patients.

COMMON VARIABLE IMMUNODEFICIENCY (CVID). Patients with this condition (formerly known as acquired hypogammaglobulinemia) may appear similar clinically in many respects to those with XLA. Although this disorder may occur in infants and young children, most patients present with a history of recurrent infection beginning several years after birth. CVID is distinguished from XLA by later age of onset, somewhat less severe susceptibility to infections, and almost equal gender distribution. In contrast to patients with the X-linked form, patients with CVID may have normal sized or enlarged tonsils and lymph nodes, and the latter may have cortical follicles. Additionally, such patients often have normal or nearly normal numbers of circulating immunoglobulin-bearing B lymphocytes. Nevertheless, the serum immunoglobulin and antibody deficiencies are usually just as profound, and the bacterial etiologic agents are the same as in the X-linked disorder. Echovirus meningoencephalitis is rare in patients with CVID.

This condition has been variably associated with a spruelike syndrome, with or without nodular follicular lymphoid hyperplasia of the intestine; thymoma; alopecia areata; and autoantibody formation leading to hemolytic anemia, gastric atrophy, achlorhydria, and pernicious anemia. Frequent complications include giardiasis (seen far more often here than in XLA), bronchiectasis, gastric carcinoma, lymphoreticular malignancy, and cholelithiasis. Lymphoid interstitial pneumonia, pseudolymphoma, amyloidosis, and noncaseating granulomas of the lungs, spleen, skin, and liver have also been seen.

Despite normal numbers of circulating immunoglobulin-bearing B lymphocytes and the presence of lymphoid cortical follicles, the lymphocytes do not differentiate *in vivo* or *in vitro* into immunoglobulin-producing plasma cells, even in the presence of the polyclonal B-cell activator, pokeweed mitogen. Although the primary biologic error responsible for this defect is unknown, in most patients it appears to be due to abnormal terminal differentiation of the B-cell line. Because this disorder occurs in first degree relatives of patients with selective IgA deficiency (A Def) and some patients with A Def later become panhypogammaglobulinemic, it is possible that these diseases have a common genetic basis. This concept is supported by the finding of a high incidence of C4-A gene deletions and rare C2 gene alleles in the Class III major histocompatibility complex (MHC) region in individuals with either A Def or CVID, suggesting that there is a susceptibility gene in this region on chromosome 6 (see Tables 223–1 and 223–2). However, the abnormal gene has not yet been identified. These studies have also shown that a small number of HLA haplotypes are shared by individuals affected with CVID and A Def, with at least one of two particular haplotypes being present in 77% of those affected. In one large family with 13 members, 2 had A Def and 3 had CVID. All of the immunodeficient patients in the family had at least one copy of an MHC haplotype shown to be abnormally frequent in A Def and CVID: HLA-DQB1 *0201, HLA-DR3, C4B-Sf, C4A-deleted, G11-15, Bf-0.4, C2a, HSP70-7.5, TNFα-5, HLA-B8, and HLA-A1. However, four immunologically normal members of the pedigree also possessed this haplotype, indicating that its presence alone is not sufficient for expression of the defects. Environmental factors, particularly drugs such as phenytoin, have been suspected to provide the triggers for disease expression in individuals with the permissive genetic background. The treatment of CVID is the same as that for the X-linked disorder.

SELECTIVE IGA DEFICIENCY (A Def). An isolated near-absence (i.e., < 10 mg per deciliter) of serum and secretory IgA is the most common primary immunodeficiency disorder, with a frequency of 1:333 being reported among some blood donors. Although A Def has been observed in apparently healthy individuals, it is commonly associated with ill health. The kinds of health problems experienced often reflect the type of clinic from which the patients are drawn. Among 75 from an allergy-immunology clinic, there were high frequencies of chronic or recurrent respiratory tract infection and atopic diseases. In contrast, 30 A Def patients drawn from a rheumatology clinic had a high frequency of autoimmune and/or collagen vascular disease.

IgA is the major immunoglobulin of external secretions. As would be expected, its deficiency is associated with infections occurring predominantly in the respiratory, gastrointestinal, and urogenital tracts. Bacterial agents responsible are essentially the same as in other types of antibody deficiency syndromes. There is no clear evidence that patients with this disorder have an undue susceptibility to viral agents. Serum concentrations of other immunoglobulins are usually normal in patients with A Def, although an IgG_2 subclass deficiency has been reported in some, and IgM (usually increased) may be of the low-molecular-weight variety. The defect may not always be permanent. Studies of T-cell function have been normal in most patients.

In addition to limiting the attachment of infectious agents to mucosal surfaces, secretory IgA antibodies probably act to prevent absorption of other foreign antigens, such as those in the diet. There is a high incidence of allergy and of IgG antibodies against cow's milk and ruminant serum proteins in patients with IgA deficiency. The antiruminant antibodies often falsely detect "IgA" in immunoassays that use goat (but not rabbit) antisera. Intestinal nodular hyperplasia has been seen in a few such patients. A spruelike syndrome may occur in adults with selective IgA deficiency and sometimes responds to a gluten-free diet.

Serum antibodies to IgA are found in as many as 44% of such patients. This observation is of possible etiologic and great clinical significance. At least seven IgA-deficient patients have had severe or fatal anaphylactic reactions after intravenous administration of blood products. For this reason, only multiply washed erythrocytes or blood products from other A Def individuals should be administered to these patients; both intramuscular and intravenous ISG (which contain varying amounts of IgA) are contraindicated.

Currently the only treatment for A Def is vigorous treatment of specific infections with appropriate antimicrobial agents. Even if serum IgA could be replaced (in the face of anti-IgA antibodies), it would not be transported into the external secretions because the latter is an active process involving only locally produced IgA.

IMMUNODEFICIENCY WITH ELEVATED IgM (hyper-IgM). This disorder is characterized by very low serum IgG and IgA but markedly elevated polyclonal IgM. Some patients have low-molecular-weight IgM molecules. Like patients with XLA, those with this defect commonly become symptomatic during infancy with recurrent pyogenic infections, including otitis media, sinusitis, pneumonia, and tonsillitis. In contrast to patients with XLA, however, the frequent presence of lymphoid hyperplasia often leads away from a diagnosis of immunodeficiency. There is an increased frequency of autoimmune disorders, such as hemolytic anemia and thrombocytopenia, and transient, persistent, or cyclic neutropenia is common. Normal or only slightly reduced numbers of IgM and/or IgD B lymphocytes have been found in the blood of these patients. However, cultured B cells from some such patients showed the capacity to synthesize IgA and IgG when co-cultured with a "switch" T cell line, suggesting that, in those patients, the defect lay in T lineage cells. A sex-linked mode of inheritance has been noted in many pedigrees. The abnormal gene in the X-linked type has been localized to Xq26 (see Table 223–1), and was recently isolated. The gene product is the gp39 ligand (CD40L, on activated T cells) (see Fig. 223–1) for CD40 on B cells (see Tables 223–1 and 223–2 and Fig. 223–1). Cross-linking of CD40 on either normal or hyper-IgM B cells by reacting them with a monoclonal antibody to CD40 or allowing CD40 to interact with normal T cell CD40L in the presence of certain cytokines (IL-2, IL-4, or IL-10) causes the B cells to undergo proliferation and isotype switching and to secrete various types of immunoglobulins. CD40L is a type II integral membrane glycoprotein with significant sequence homology to TNF; it is found only on activated T cells, primarily of the CD4 phenotype. Mutations in the CD40L on activated T cells from hyper-IgM patients result in failure of signaling of B cells to undergo isotype switching; thus, they produce only IgM. However, the facts that not all males with hyper-IgM have had a mutation in the CD40L, that B cells from such patients fail to isotype switch with monoclonal antibodies to CD40, and that there are several examples in females suggest that this condition has more than one genetic cause.

Because these patients are unable to make IgG antibodies, the treatment is the same as for agammaglobulinemia.

TRANSIENT HYPOGAMMAGLOBULINEMIA OF INFANCY. Unlike patients with XLA or CVID, those with this condition can synthesize antibodies to human type A and B erythrocytes and to diphtheria and tetanus toxoids normally, usually by age 6 to 11 months, well before immunoglobulin concentrations become normal. The finding of only 11 cases of transient hypogammaglobulinemia of infancy among > 10,000 sera tested by the author over a 12-year period suggests that this is not a common entity.

Gammaglobulin replacement therapy is not indicated in this condition. In addition to the known risks of inducing anti-IgG allotype antibodies, passively administered antibodies could block endogenous primary antibody formation in the same manner that RhoGAM suppresses anti-D antibodies in Rh-negative mothers delivering Rh-positive infants.

ANTIBODY DEFICIENCY WITH NEAR-NORMAL IMMUNOGLOBULINS. The author and her associates have studied the antibody-forming capacities of 12 patients with deficient antibody responses despite apparently normal T-cell function and normal or nearly normal immunoglobulin concentrations. This problem would not be detected unless functional tests of antibody-forming capacity are conducted. It may represent an early stage of "acquired" agammaglobulinemia (or CVID). Patients with this disorder are candidates for immunoglobulin replacement therapy.

X-LINKED LYMPHOPROLIFERATIVE DISEASE. This disorder, also referred to as *Duncan's disease* (after the original kindred in which it was described), is characterized by an impaired immune response to Epstein-Barr virus (EBV) (see Ch. 341). Affected persons are apparently healthy until they experience infectious mononucleosis. Two thirds of the more than 100 patients studied thus far died of overwhelming EBV-induced B-cell proliferation during mononucleosis. A majority of the survivors developed hypogammaglobulinemia or B-cell lymphomas or both. Such individuals have marked impairment in production of antibodies to the EBV nuclear antigen, whereas titers of antibodies to the viral capsid antigen have ranged from zero to markedly elevated. Antibody-dependent cell-mediated cytotoxicity against EBV-infected cells and natural killer function are depressed, and there is a deficiency in long-lived T-cell immunity to EBV. Despite normal numbers of B and T cells, there is an elevated percentage of lymphocytes of the suppressor (CD8$^+$) phenotype. In addition, lymphocyte immunoglobulin synthesis in response to polyclonal B-cell mitogen stimulation *in vitro* is markedly depressed. Thus, both EBV-specific and nonspecific immunologic abnormalities occur in these patients.

CELLULAR IMMUNODEFICIENCY DISORDERS

In general, patients with partial or absolute defects in T-cell function have infections or other clinical problems for which there is no effective treatment or which are often of a more severe nature than in those with antibody deficiency disorders. It is therefore rare that such individuals survive beyond infancy or childhood.

THYMIC HYPOPLASIA (DIGEORGE'S SYNDROME). This condition results from dysmorphogenesis of the third and fourth pharyngeal pouches, leading to hypoplasia or aplasia of the thymus and parathyroid glands. Other structures forming at the same age are also frequently affected, resulting in anomalies of the great vessels (right-sided aortic arch), esophageal atresia, bifid uvula, congenital heart disease (atrial and ventricular septal defects), a short philtrum of the upper lip, hypertelorism, an antimongoloid slant to the eyes, mandibular hypoplasia, and low-set (often notched) ears. The diagnosis is usually first suggested by the presence of hypocalcemic seizures during the neonatal period. DiGeorge's syndrome has occurred in both males and females, and consistent deletions and microdeletions of 22q11 have been found in a majority of cases

(see Tables 223–1 and 223–2). Familial occurrence is rare but has been reported.

A variable degree of hypoplasia is more frequent than total aplasia of the thymus and parathyroid glands. Some children with the features of this syndrome have little trouble with infections and show evidence of some cell-mediated immunity. They are often referred to as having partial DiGeorge's syndrome. Those with marked thymic hypoplasia may resemble infants with severe combined immunodeficiency in their susceptibility to infection with low-grade or opportunistic pathogens (i.e., fungi, viruses, and *Pneumocystis carinii*) and to graft-versus-host (GVH) disease from nonirradiated blood transfusions.

Serum immunoglobulins are usually normal for age, but some fractions, particularly IgA, may be diminished and IgE may be elevated. T-cell numbers are decreased, and there is an increased number of B cells. Responses of peripheral blood lymphocytes following mitogen stimulation, like the intradermal delayed hypersensitivity response, have been absent, reduced, or normal. Careful postmortem studies have sometimes revealed tiny nests of thymic tissue containing Hassall's corpuscles and a normal density of thymocytes. Lymphoid follicles usually appear normal, but lymph node paracortical areas and thymus-dependent regions of the spleen show variable degrees of depletion, depending upon the degree of thymic hypoplasia. Because of variability in the severity of the immunodeficiency, it is difficult to evaluate claimed benefits of fetal thymus transplantation.

CELLULAR IMMUNODEFICIENCY WITH IMMUNOGLOBULINS (NEZELOF'S SYNDROME). This syndrome is characterized by lymphopenia, diminished lymphoid tissue, abnormal thymus architecture, and the presence of normal or increased immunoglobulins. Children with this condition may have recurrent or chronic pulmonary infections, failure to thrive, oral or cutaneous candidiasis, chronic diarrhea, recurrent skin infections, gram-negative sepsis, urinary tract infections, severe varicella, or combinations of these. An autosomal-recessive pattern of inheritance has been suggested in some cases, but an X-linked mode seemed more likely in others. Other findings include neutropenia and eosinophilia.

Studies of cellular immune function have shown delayed cutaneous anergy to ubiquitous antigens and low to absent *in vitro* lymphocyte responses to mitogens and allogeneic cells. Such patients have profound deficiencies of total T cells and T-cell subsets. Peripheral lymphoid tissues demonstrate paracortical lymphocyte depletion. The thymuses are very small and have a paucity of thymocytes and usually no Hassall's corpuscles; however, in contrast to AIDS, thymic epithelium is present. This is the primary immunodeficiency disorder most likely to be confused with AIDS. Fatal or serious infections have included varicella, vaccinia, *Pneumocystis carinii*, cytomegalovirus, rubeola, *Pseudomonas,* and *Mycobacterium kansasii.* Some patients have been reconstituted by bone marrow transplantation, but most other forms of therapy have been unsuccessful.

With Purine Nucleoside Phosphorylase Deficiency. More than 35 patients with Nezelof's syndrome have been found to have purine nucleoside phosphorylase (PNP) deficiency. In contrast to patients with adenosine deaminase (ADA) deficiency, serum and urinary uric acid are markedly deficient, and no characteristic physical or skeletal abnormalities have been noted. Some patients have suffered from a progressive neurologic disorder with spastic tetraplegia, some developed autoimmune hemolytic anemia, and others idiopathic thrombocytopenic purpura. Deaths have occurred from generalized vaccinia, varicella, lymphosarcoma, and GVH disease following blood transfusions. There is profound lymphopenia due to a marked deficiency of T cells and T-cell subsets, but there is usually an increased percentage of cells with natural killer (NK) phenotype and function. Attempts to correct the immunologic and enzymatic deficiencies of PNP-deficient patients by enzyme replacement or deoxycytidine therapy have not been successful. Some patients have been treated successfully with HLA-identical bone marrow transplants.

SEVERE COMBINED IMMUNODEFICIENCY (SCID) DISORDERS

The syndromes of SCID are characterized by their apparent congenital absence of all adaptive immune function and a great diversity of genetic, enzymatic, hematologic, and immunologic features. Unless immunologic reconstitution can be achieved through immunocompetent tissue transplants or enzyme replacement therapy or unless gnotobiotic isolation can be carried out, death usually occurs before the patient's first birthday. The major subcategories of this disorder are discussed below.

AUTOSOMAL RECESSIVE SEVERE COMBINED IMMUNODEFICIENCY DISEASE. Within the first few months of life, infants affected with this first-described SCID syndrome have frequent episodes of otitis, pneumonia, sepsis, diarrhea, and cutaneous infections. Growth may appear normal initially, but extreme wasting soon develops. Persistent infections with opportunistic organisms such as *Candida albicans, Pneumocystis carinii,* varicella, measles, parainfluenza 3, cytomegalovirus, and BCG frequently lead to death. These infants also lack the ability to reject foreign tissue and are therefore at risk for GVH disease. GVH reactions can result from maternal immunocompetent cells crossing the placenta or from the administration of blood products containing viable histoincompatible lymphocytes.

Immunologic evaluation reveals serum immunoglobulin concentrations to be diminished, and no antibody formation occurs following immunization. There is a lack of cellular immune function, with lymphopenia and absence of lymphocyte responses to mitogens or allogeneic cells, delayed cutaneous anergy, and inability to reject foreign tissues. Marked heterogeneity of lymphocyte subpopulations exists among SCID patients. Despite the uniformly profound lack of T- or B-cell function, some patients have had low numbers of both B and T lymphocytes, whereas others have had elevated numbers of B cells, and most of the lymphocytes of other infants with SCID are large granular lymphocytes with NK cell phenotype and function. Typically, these patients have very small thymuses (<1 gram), which usually fail to descend from the neck, contain few thymic lymphocytes, lack corticomedullary distinction, and lack Hassall's corpuscles. Despite the profound thymocyte depletion in SCID patients, thymic epithelium is present. Tonsils, adenoids, lymph nodes, and Peyer's patches are absent or extremely underdeveloped.

ISG fails to halt the progressively downhill course of SCID. Transplantation of bone marrow cells from HLA genotypically identical or D locus-compatible donors has resulted in apparent complete correction of the immunologic defect in >90 of these patients. For the past 12 years techniques to deplete all post-thymic T cells from donor marrow have also allowed the use of haploidentical (half-matched) bone marrow cells for correction of SCID. These employ either a combination of soy lectin agglutination and sheep erythrocyte rosetting (the most successful method) or incubation with monoclonal antibodies to human T cells and complement. Both methods leave the stem cells intact. To date, >200 infants with SCID who would have otherwise died because of lack of an HLA-identical donor have been treated successfully with T cell-depleted haploidentical bone marrow with few signs of GVH reaction.

With Adenosine Deaminase (ADA) Deficiency (See also Ch. 181). Absence of the enzyme ADA has been observed in approximately 40% of patients with the autosomal recessive form of SCID. Marked accumulations of adenosine, 2'-deoxyadenosine, and 2'-O-methyladenosine directly or indirectly lead to lymphocyte toxicity, which causes the immunodeficiency. Adenosine and deoxyadenosine are apparent suicide inactivators of the enzyme S-adenosylhomocysteine (SAH) hydrolase, resulting in the accumulation of SAH. SAH is a potent inhibitor of virtually all cellular methylation reactions. Although most such patients have had profound lymphopenia from the earliest age studied, a few have had early normal or fluctuating lymphocyte counts that declined by ages 6 weeks to 2 years. In contrast to "classic" SCID, ADA-deficient patients have been found to have rib cage abnormalities similar to a rachitic rosary and multiple skeletal abnormalities of chondroosseous dysplasia on radiographic examination.

Both matched sibling and haploidentical post-thymic T cell-depleted bone marrow transplants have resulted in lymphocyte chimerism and partial or complete correction of the immunologic defect in ADA-deficient SCID. Enzyme replacement therapy with irradiated packed normal erythrocytes or polyethylene-glycol–modified bovine ADA on a continuing basis has resulted in improvement in some patients. This condition was the first in which somatic cell gene therapy was attempted, but to date there has been only limited success.

X-LINKED RECESSIVE SEVERE COMBINED IMMUNODEFICIENCY DISEASE (XSCID). This is thought to be the most common form of SCID in the United States. Clinically, immunologically, and histopathologically, these patients appear similar to those with the autosomal recessive form except for uniformly low percentages of T and NK cells and an elevated percentage of B cells. The abnormal gene in XSCID was mapped by RFLP and linkage analysis to Xq13 (see Table 223–1). Recently, it was identified as the gene encoding the gamma chain of the IL-2 receptor (IL-2R). IL-2, formerly known as T-cell growth factor, plays a key role in intracellular signaling in T cells and, consequently, in the function and regulation of the immune system. Because genetically engineered IL-2–deficient mice and humans have T cells and a much less severe immunodeficiency, it was initially difficult to see how abnormalities in the IL-2R could lead to the devastating immunodeficiency of XSCID. However, the γ chain of the IL-2R has recently been shown to be a component of the receptors for several other cytokines that regulate the function and development of the immune system, IL-4, IL-7, and probably IL-9, IL-13, and IL-15 (see Fig. 223–1). One chain of each of the IL-2, IL-4, and IL-7 receptors is unique for each receptor, whereas the shared γ chain functions both to increase the affinity of the receptor for the respective cytokine and to enable the receptors to mediate intracellular signaling. IL-2, IL-4, and IL-7 are all facilitators of different stages of the growth and development of both T and B cells. Therefore, incapacitation of the receptors for all of these developmentally crucial cytokines by genetic mutations in their common γ chain provides an explanation for the severity of the immunodeficiency in XSCID. All XSCID infants reported thus far have been found to have point mutations in the IL-2R gamma chain. Carriers can be detected by demonstrating nonrandom X-chromosome inactivation in their T lymphocytes. Results of X-chromosome inactivation studies in obligate carrier mothers also suggest that the genetic defect affects their B and NK lineage cells, as well as their T cells. This is in keeping with the author's personal observations of very poor B- and NK-cell function in infants with X-linked SCID following nonablated bone marrow cell transplantation, despite excellent reconstitution of T-cell function by donor-derived T cells.

DEFECTIVE EXPRESSION OF MAJOR HISTOCOMPATIBILITY COMPLEX (MHC) ANTIGENS. There are two main forms: MHC class I antigen deficiency ("bare lymphocyte syndrome") and MHC class I antigen deficiency plus absence of MHC class II antigens. These autosomal recessive conditions are due to mutations in X-box binding proteins that result in failure of surface membrane expression of the HLA antigens. Sera from affected individuals contain normal quantities of MHC class I antigens and β_2 microglobulin. Patients (usually of North African descent) present with persistent diarrhea in early infancy and have oral candidiasis, bacterial pneumonia, pneumocystosis, septicemia, and undue susceptibility to enteroviruses, herpes, and other viral agents. Those with both class I and II antigen deficiencies also have malabsorption. There is variable hypogammaglobulinemia with decreased serum IgM and IgA and poor to absent antibody production. B-cell percentages are usually normal, but plasma cells are absent in tissues. Lymphopenia is only moderate; T-cell functions *in vivo* and *in vitro* are decreased but not absent. The thymus and other lymphoid organs are severely hypoplastic. A majority of affected infants die in the first 3 years of life. The associated defects of both B- and T-cell immunity and HLA expression reinforce the important biologic role for HLA determinants in effective immune cell cooperation.

SEVERE COMBINED IMMUNODEFICIENCY WITH LEUKOPENIA (RETICULAR DYSGENESIS). In 1959, identical twin male infants were described who exhibited a total lack of both lymphocytes and granulocytes in their peripheral blood and bone marrow. Seven of eight infants reported died between ages 3 and 119 days from overwhelming infections; the eighth underwent complete immunologic reconstitution from a bone marrow transplant. Autosomal inheritance seems likely from reports of familial occurrences.

IMMUNODEFICIENCY WITH THROMBOCYTOPENIA AND ECZEMA (WISKOTT-ALDRICH SYNDROME). This X-linked recessive syndrome is characterized clinically by the triad of eczema, thrombocytopenic purpura, and undue susceptibility to infection. Often there is prolonged oozing from the circumcision site or bloody diarrhea during infancy. Atopic dermatitis and recurrent infections usually develop during the first year of life. Infections are caused by pneumococci and other bacteria with polysaccharide capsules, resulting in episodes of otitis media, pneumonia, meningitis, and sepsis. Later, infections with *Pneumocystis carinii* and the herpesviruses become more frequent. Survival beyond the teens is rare; major causes of death are infections or bleeding, but a 12% incidence of fatal malignancy also occurs in this condition. A papovavirus has been recovered from a reticulum cell sarcoma of the brain and from the urine of patients with this syndrome.

The earliest evidence of immunodeficiency is an impaired humoral immune response to polysaccharide antigens. Absent or markedly diminished isohemagglutinin titers are uniformly found, and poor or no responses are seen following immunization with polysaccharide antigens. Antibody titers to protein antigens also fall with time, and anamnestic responses are often poor or absent. Studies of immunoglobulin metabolism have shown an accelerated rate of synthesis—as well as hypercatabolism—of albumin, IgG, IgA, and IgM, resulting in highly variable immunoglobulin concentrations. The predominant dysgammaglobulinemias are a low IgM, elevated IgA and IgE, and a normal or slightly low IgG concentration. Lymphocyte responses are moderately depressed, and cutaneous anergy is a frequent finding. Analyses of blood lymphocytes with monoclonal reagents have revealed moderately reduced percentages of cells reacting with antibodies to all T cells and to the helper (CD4+) and suppressor (CD8+) subsets. The molecular basis of this defect, which had been mapped to Xp11.22-p11.23, has been recently found to be mutations in a gene encoding a proline-rich protein restricted to cells of lymphocytic megakaryocyte lineages. This protein, named WASP, is likely to be a key regulator of lymphocyte and platelet function (see Fig. 223–1).

The thrombocytopenia is due to an intrinsic platelet abnormality because antiplatelet antibodies are not usually demonstrated, and survival times of allogeneic but not autologous ^{51}Cr-labeled platelets have been normal. Megakaryocytes are present in normal number in the bone marrow, but platelet size is small.

Treatment has been directed primarily toward controlling bleeding with platelet transfusions, splenectomy, or both and controlling infections by intravenously administering ISG. Several patients have had complete corrections of both the platelet and immunologic abnormalities by HLA-matched sibling bone marrow transplants after being conditioned with irradiation or busulfan and cyclophosphamide.

ATAXIA-TELANGIECTASIA. This is a complex syndrome with neurologic, immunologic, endocrinologic, hepatic, and cutaneous abnormalities. The most prominent clinical features are progressive cerebellar ataxia, oculocutaneous telangiectasias, chronic sinopulmonary disease, a high incidence of malignancy, and variable humoral and cellular immunodeficiency. Ataxia typically becomes evident soon after the child begins to walk. Telangiectasias usually develop by age 3 to 6. Recurrent, usually bacterial, sinopulmonary infections occur in roughly 80% of these patients; common viral exanthems have not usually resulted in untoward sequelae, but varicella was fatal in one of the author's patients.

The malignant tumors reported have usually been of the lymphoreticular type, but others have been seen. Cells from patients and heterozygous carriers have increased sensitivity to ionizing radiation, defective DNA repair, and frequent chromosomal abnormalities. The abnormal gene has been mapped to the long arm of chromosome 11 (11q22.3). An autosomal recessive mode of inheritance seems operative.

The most frequent immunologic abnormality is selective absence of IgA, found in 50 to 80% of these patients. IgG$_2$ or total IgG may also be decreased. IgE concentrations are usually low, and IgM may be of the low-molecular-weight variety. Specific antibody levels may be decreased or normal. *In vivo,* there is impaired but not absent cell-mediated immunity, as evidenced by delayed cutaneous anergy and prolonged allograft survival. Death from GVH disease has

not been reported. Enumeration of blood T cells and subsets reveals reduced percentages of total T cells and T cells of the helper (CD4) phenotype, with normal or increased percentages of cells of the suppressor (CD8) phenotype. An increase in T cells bearing the γ/δ T-cell receptor has been reported. *In vitro* studies of lymphocyte function have shown moderately depressed proliferative responses to mitogens, decreased T-helper cell function, and an intrinsic defect in B-cell IgA synthesis. The thymus is very hypoplastic and lacks Hassall's corpuscles. No satisfactory treatment has been found.

CARTILAGE HAIR HYPOPLASIA. An unusual form of short-limbed dwarfism with frequent and severe infections has been reported among the Amish. Features include short and pudgy hands; redundant skin; hyperextensible joints of hands and feet but an inability to completely extend the elbows; and fine, sparse light hair and eyebrows. Severe and often fatal varicella infections appear to be a particular hazard. Progressive vaccinia and vaccine-associated poliomyelitis have also been observed.

The severity of the immunodeficiency varies; in one series, 11 of 77 patients died before age 20, but two were still alive at age 76. Three patterns of immune dysfunction have emerged: defective antibody-mediated immunity, defective cellular immunity, and severe combined immunodeficiency. The most striking abnormality appears to be one of defective cell proliferation due to an intrinsic defect related to the G1 phase, resulting in a longer cell cycle for individual cells. The trait appears to be autosomal recessive with variable penetrance.

IMMUNODEFICIENCY WITH THYMOMA. These patients are adults who almost simultaneously develop hypogammaglobulinemia, deficits in cell-mediated immunity, and benign thymoma (see Ch. 232). The thymomas are predominantly of the spindle cell variety. Eosinophilia or eosinopenia, aregenerative or hemolytic anemia, thrombocytopenia, or pancytopenia may also occur. Antibody formation is poor, although percentages of immunoglobulin-bearing B lymphocytes are normal, and progressive lymphopenia develops.

HYPERIMMUNOGLOBULINEMIA E SYNDROME. The hyper-IgE syndrome is a primary immunodeficiency characterized by recurrent staphylococcal abscesses and markedly elevated serum IgE concentrations. The disorder was first reported by the author and her co-workers in two young boys in 1972. These patients all have lifelong histories of severe recurrent staphylococcal abscesses involving the skin, lungs, joints, and other sites. Persistent pneumatoceles develop as a result of their recurrent pneumonias. The pruritic dermatitis that occurs is not typical atopic eczema and does not always persist; respiratory allergic symptoms are usually absent. An autosomal-dominant form of inheritance with incomplete penetrance seems possible. Laboratory features include exceptionally high serum IgE concentrations but usually normal IgG, IgA, and IgM concentrations; pronounced blood and sputum eosinophilia; abnormally low anamnestic antibody responses; and poor antibody and cell-mediated responses to neoantigens. *In vitro* studies have shown normal percentages of CD2-, CD3-, CD4-, and CD8-positive lymphocytes, and there is no increase in the percentage of IgE-bearing B lymphocytes. Lymphocyte responses to mitogens are normal, but responses to antigens or to related allogeneic cells have been absent or very low. Histologic sections of lymph nodes, spleen, and lung cysts show striking eosinophilia.

Phagocytic cell ingestion, metabolism, and killing mechanisms and total hemolytic complement have been normal in all patients. Defects of mononuclear and/or polymorphonuclear chemotaxis are present in some but not most patients and thus are not the basic problem in this syndrome. Indeed, the fundamental biologic error remains to be identified in this condition.

The most effective therapy is chronic administration of therapeutic doses of a penicillinase-resistant penicillin, with adding other antibiotic or antifungal agents as required for specific infections.

CHRONIC MUCOCUTANEOUS CANDIDIASIS. This clinical syndrome, probably of multiple causes, is associated with chronic candidal infection of the skin and mucous membranes but only rarely life-threatening systemic infections of the types seen in patients with severe T-cell dysfunction. Some patients have endocrinopathies involving the parathyroid, thyroid, adrenal, and/or pancreatic glands (see Ch. 210.1); however, many have neither associated endocrinopathy nor any demonstrable immunologic abnormality. Ketoconazole (Nizoral) or fluconazole (Diflucan) have been found to be effective in controlling the fungal infection.

LEUKOCYTE ADHESION DEFICIENCY 1 (LAD 1 OR CD11/CD18 DEFICIENCY). This condition is due to an autosomal or recessively inherited mutation in the gene encoding the 95-Kd MW β subunit (CD18) shared by three adhesive heterodimers: LFA-1 on B, T, and NK lymphocytes; complement receptor type 3 (CR3) on neutrophils, monocytes, macrophages, eosinophils, and NK cells; and p150,95 (function unknown). Because these cells cannot adhere to vascular endothelium, there is a significant leukocytosis, even in the absence of infection. Patients have histories of delayed separation of the umbilical cord, omphalitis, gingivitis, recurrent skin infections, repeated otitis media, pneumonia, peritonitis, perianal abscesses, and impaired wound healing. Severe widespread and life-threatening bacterial and fungal infections account for the high mortality. All cytotoxic lymphocyte functions are markedly impaired due to a lack of the adhesion protein LFA-1; deficiency of LFA-1 also interferes with immune cell interaction and immune recognition. CR3 binds fixed iC3b fragments of C3 and β glucans; its absence causes abnormal phagocytic cell adherence and chemotaxis and a reduced respiratory burst with phagocytosis. Blood neutrophil counts are usually elevated. Deficiencies of these glycoproteins can be screened for by cytofluorography of blood leukocytes with appropriate monoclonal antibodies to CR3 (OKM1, MO1, MAC-1). The disease can be corrected by bone marrow transplantation.

LEUKOCYTE ADHESION DEFICIENCY 2 (LAD 2). Very recently, another adhesion molecule deficiency state has been described, designated LAD type 2, which is due to the absence of the neutrophil Sialyl-Lewis X ligand of E-selectin on vascular endothelium (see Table 223–2). This disorder was discovered in two unrelated Israeli boys, aged 3 and 5, each the offspring of consanguineous parents. Both have severe mental retardation, short stature, a distinctive facial appearance, and the Bombay (hh) blood phenotype, and both are secretor- and Lewis-negative. They both have had recurrent severe bacterial infections similar to those seen in patients with LAD type 1, including pneumonia, peridontitis, otitis media, and localized cellulitis. Similar to patients with LAD 1, their infections have been accompanied by marked leukocytosis (30,000 to 150,000 per cubic millimeter) but an absence of pus formation at sites of recurrent cellulitis. *In vitro* studies revealed a marked defect in neutrophil motility. Because the genes for the red cell H antigen and for the secretor status encode for distinct α1,2-fucosyl transferases and the synthesis of Sialyl-Lewis X requires an α1,3-fucosyl transferase, the authors have postulated a general defect in fucose metabolism as the basis for this disorder.

T-CELL ACTIVATION DEFECTS. These conditions are characterized by the presence of T cells that appear phenotypically normal by many criteria but fail to proliferate or produce cytokines in response to stimulation with mitogens, antigens, or other signals delivered to the T-cell antigen receptor (TCR). Recently a number of these have been characterized at the molecular level, including patients who had either (1) defective surface expression of the CD3/TCR complex, due to a selective deficiency of the CD3-γ subunit or to a mutation in the CD3 gene, leading to the synthesis of an abnormal and unstable CD3 subunit; (2) defective signal transduction from the TCR to intracellular metabolic pathways; (3) pretranslational defects in the synthesis of interleukin-2 (T-cell growth factor) and/or of multiple other cytokines due to a defective NFAT-1 transcriptional complex; and (4) CD8 lymphocytopenia due to mutations in a non–SRC-related protein tyrosine kinase, ZAP 70. These patients have clinical problems similar to those of other severely T cell-deficient individuals.

PRIMARY DEFICIENCIES OF THE COMPLEMENT SYSTEM

In addition to congenital or hereditary disorders of lymphoid cells, there are several well-defined primary immune defects involving the complement system. Genetically determined deficiencies have been described for all of the components of complement, and undue susceptibility to infection is a characteristic of deficiencies of C2, C3, C5, C6, and C7. The types of infections experienced in C2, C3, and in some with C5 deficiency are with gram-positive encapsulated organisms, whereas those in patients with deficiencies of the terminal components are usually meningococcal or gonococcal. A normal CH50 would exclude all heritable complement deficiencies. The complement system is discussed in detail in Chapter 222.

Anonymous: Primary immunodeficiency diseases—report of a WHO Scientific Group meeting. Immunodef Rev 3:195, 1992. *The most recent published report of the World Health Organization's classification and discussion of the diagnosis and treatment of primary immunodeficiency diseases.*

Arnaiz-Villena A, Timon M, Corell A, et al.: Brief report: Primary immunodeficiency caused by mutations in the gene encoding the CD3 subunit of the T lymphocyte receptor. N Engl J Med 327:529, 1992. *An excellent introduction to the concept of T-cell activation defects.*

Buckley RH: Breakthroughs in the understanding and therapy of primary immunodeficiency. Pediatr Clin North Am, 41:665, 1994. *A review of recent discoveries of the fundamental causes of four X-linked and seven autosomal recessively inherited immunodeficiency diseases and of advances in therapy.*

Buckley RH, Schiff RI: The use of intravenous immunoglobulin in immunodeficiency diseases. N Engl J Med 325:110, 1991. *A discussion of intravenous immunoglobulin preparations available in the United States, indications for their use, recommended doses, and adverse effects.*

Buckley RH, Schiff SE, Schiff RI, et al.: Haploidentical bone marrow stem cell transplantation in human severe combined immunodeficiency. Semin Hematol 30:92, 1993. *An update on the use of T-cell depletion techniques that allow non–HLA-identical bone marrow to immunologically reconstitute infants with severe combined immunodeficiency disease without lethal graft-versus-host disease.*

Derry MJ, Ochs HD, Francke U: Isolation of a novel gene mutated in Wiskott-Aldrich syndrome. Cell 78:635, 1994. *The latest discovery of the molecular basis for an x-linked immunodeficiency disorder.*

Elder ME, Lin D, Clever J, et al.: Human severe combined immunodeficiency due to a defect in ZAP-70, a T cell tyrosine kinase. Science 264:1596, 1994. *The latest discovery of the molecular basis for a T cell signaling defect.*

Puck JM: Molecular and genetic basis of X-linked immunodeficiency disorders. J Clin Immunol 14:81, 1994. *An excellent review of X-linked recessive immunodeficiency diseases and the molecular bases for their defects.*

224 URTICARIA AND ANGIOEDEMA
Michael M. Frank

DEFINITION

Urticaria (Table 224–1) is defined as the transient appearance of elevated, erythematous pruritic wheals (hives) or serpiginous exanthem, usually surrounded by an area of erythema. It commonly involves the trunk and extremities, sparing palms and soles, but may involve any epidermal or mucosal surface. The wheals are thought to result from local subcutaneous and intradermal leakage of plasma filtrate from postcapillary venules. In most cases there is associated increased blood flow to the localized area of swelling, resulting in a surrounding erythema. The lesions blanch on pressure, reflecting this pathogenetic process. The appearance of urticaria is thought to reflect an ongoing immediate hypersensitivity reaction.

Angioedema is formed by a similar extravasation of fluid, but in this case the leakage of fluid involves deeper structures, including dermal and subdermal sites. Because of its location in deeper cutaneous structures, it appears as brawny nonpitting edema, usually without well-defined margins. Although urticaria is almost always pruritic, indicating stimulation of nociceptive nerves supplying deeper cutaneous structures, angioedema may be unassociated with itching. Unlike other forms of edema, angioedema is not commonly distributed in dependent areas of the body. Angioedema often involves the lips, tongue, eyelids, genitalia, or dorsum of the hands or feet but also may involve any epidermal or mucosal surface. The transient nature of involvement is important in defining both urticaria and angioedema; these manifestations appear and peak in minutes to hours and disappear over hours to days.

INCIDENCE AND PREVALENCE

Acute episodes of urticaria/angioedema are arbitrarily defined as those lasting less than 6 weeks. More prolonged episodes are defined as chronic. Acute urticaria and angioedema are very common clinical problems occurring in as many as 10 to 20% of the population at one time or another. They may occur at any age and are the most common form seen in childhood. They occur in persons of all sexes, races, and occupations and at all seasons of the year. Chronic

TABLE 224-1. CLASSIFICATION OF URTICARIA/ANGIOEDEMA

I. Manifestation of hypersensitivity to a defined agent
   A. Drug reactions
   B. Foods and food additives
   C. Inhaled and contact allergens
II. Presumed immune complex–induced
   A. Collagen disease
   B. Endocrine disease (thyroid disorders)
   C. Serum sickness
   D. Transfusion-induced
   E. Malignancy (tumor antigen–induced)
   F. Infectious agents
   G. Urticarial vasculitis
III. Physical urticarias
   A. Dermatographism
   B. Familial and acquired cold urticaria
   C. Localized heat urticaria
   D. Cholinergic urticaria
   E. Exercise-induced anaphylaxis/urticaria
   F. Delayed pressure urticaria/angioedema
   G. Familial and acquired vibratory angioedema
   H. Solar urticaria
   I. Aquagenic urticaria
IV. Urticaria pigmentosa and systemic mastocytosis
V. Chronic urticaria and angioedema
VI. Defined complement-related disorders
   A. Hereditary angioedema
   B. Acquired Cl inhibitor deficiency
   C. Complement Factor I deficiency
VII. Angioedema induced by angiotensin-converting enzyme (ACE) inhibitors and IL-2

urticaria/angioedema also can occur in individuals of any age, but the peak incidence is noted in young adults. In general, symptoms of urticaria are more striking and are more easily recognized than those of angioedema, and these symptoms are often the presenting complaint. At presentation about 50% of patients are found to have both urticaria and angioedema, approximately 40% have urticaria alone, and about 10% only angioedema. Although the majority of patients clear their lesions spontaneously or respond rapidly to treatment with H_1 antihistamines, a minority of patients continue to have lesions over a period that may last years. It has been reported that of patients with chronic urticaria and angioedema, 75% have symptoms for longer than 1 year, 50% symptoms for longer than 5 years, and 20% symptoms for decades. At times these can be quite debilitating. This clinical syndrome represents a final common pathway of multiple initiating stimuli, and the natural course of disease undoubtedly reflects these multiple initiating factors.

PATHOGENESIS AND PATHOLOGY

Urticaria/angioedema appears to result from dilatation of small vessels with associated leakage of plasma from local postcapillary venules. Experimentally such leakage can be induced by multiple stimuli. Degranulation of cutaneous mast cells is thought to be the most frequent cause of disease. Mast cells are found in high frequency within the subcutaneous tissues and dermis. Their distribution is particularly rich around blood vessels. These cells stain poorly with the commonly used histopathologic stains and often must be visualized by specific staining techniques. Upon being activated by any of a number of stimuli, these cells degranulate, releasing preformed mediators present in the granules like histamine that induce capillary permeability and also synthesize various mediators in response to the activation signal that induce capillary permeability, including prostaglandins, HETES, leukotrienes C, D, and E, and platelet-activating factor (PAF). With appropriate stimuli, cellular regulatory factors like cytokines can be released without degranulating and releasing preformed mediators; these may control the function of other cells within the lesion. Under controlled conditions, triggering of cutaneous mast cells in normal volunteers induces a typical pruritic hive, lending support to the suggestion that these cells are crucial in urticarial reactions in humans.

Many stimuli induce mast cells to degranulate. Probably most important is the interaction of mast cell membrane–bound IgE antibody with specific antigen. Mast cells have on their surface a high-affinity receptor for IgE and in tissues are found coated with IgE antibody derived from plasma. Interaction of IgE antibody with its antigen cross-links IgE receptors, a required step in initiating the degranulation process by antigen-mediated cell activation. However, not only IgE meeting its antigen but also a series of peptides derived from various plasma mediator molecules can trigger degranulation. For example, peptides derived from activated complement proteins including C3a, C4a, and C5a and small fragments of C2 can induce mast cell degranulation. Similarly, peptides like bradykinin, derived from activation and cleavage of proteins of the kinin-generating system and neuropeptides like substance P can induce mast cell degranulation. Incompletely defined cellular products derived from circulating mononuclear cells and neutrophils can cause mast cell degranulation as well. Moreover, toxic products from neutrophils and monocytes, whose release is induced by many factors including mast cell products, can on injection induce a typical hive.

Inducing an immediate hypersensitivity response in an allergic individual by intradermally injecting a sensitizing antigen leads to rapid mast cell degranulation and the immediate appearance of a wheal and flare response that gradually fades. In many individuals 4 to 6 hours later a "late-phase" response is noted with an increase in local inflammation and swelling. Biopsy of such a late-phase reaction reveals that neutrophils and eosinophils are accumulated in the inflamed area and later they are gradually replaced by mononuclear cells. The factors that induce the late-phase reaction are not completely defined, but the recent demonstration that chemotactic cytokines are produced some hours after mast cell triggering suggests that these factors may contribute to late-phase inflammation.

An understanding of these experimental findings helps explain biopsy findings in patients with acute and chronic urticaria/angioedema. It should be emphasized that although the disease may be chronic, individual lesions may be quite evanescent, lasting hours to days. On biopsy, subcutaneous edema is prominent with flattened rete pegs, widened dermal papillae, and swollen collagen fibers. There is an increased number of cutaneous mast cells noted when compared with normal individuals. Even uninvolved skin from a patient with urticaria shows more mast cells than does the skin of normals. Some mast cell degranulation is seen on biopsy of lesions, and in chronic urticaria a modest mononuclear cell infiltrate around vessels containing lymphocytes (predominantly CD4+ helper T cells) and relatively few monocyte/macrophages are noted. An increase in eosinophils may be seen. Patients with the physical urticaria tend to have more neutrophils and eosinophils on biopsy than are observed in chronic urticaria/angioedema. In a minority of cases with typical urticarial lesions a typical leukocytoclastic vasculitis is observed. This latter finding, reported to be associated with the formation of IgG–anti-Clq autoantibody, indicates that the underlying diagnosis is vasculitis and places the patient in a different diagnostic and therapeutic group.

It must be emphasized that in most cases the cause of urticaria/angioedema is never found. In several large series ~70% of all cases remained in the idiopathic group after all other urticarial syndrome complexes were eliminated. These cutaneous manifestations appear, often are treated, and disappear with no cause ever defined. It is believed that most urticaria/angioedema cases represent hypersensitivity reactions to drugs, foods, or less commonly inhalants, because when a cause is defined it commonly involves one of these sensitizing agents. Penicillin is the drug still most commonly associated with acute urticaria, but aspirin and other nonsteroidal anti-inflammatory agents (NSAID's) may exacerbate urticaria, possibly by inhibiting prostaglandin synthesis, and diuretics, radiocontrast dyes, food additives, sulfonamides, and muscle relaxants all are associated with acute urticaria. Opioids can trigger direct mast cell release of histamine and cause urticarial lesions. Among foods, nuts, milk, eggs, chocolate, citrus fruits, tomatoes, fish, shellfish, and food dyes have all been associated with onset of urticaria in some individuals. Nevertheless, so many different antigens, including food additives, drugs, foods, and food contaminants, have been defined as causative in individual cases, and so little antigen may be required to precipitate attacks that it may be difficult or impossible to define the causative agent. In many patients in whom the disease becomes chronic, the patient is asked to keep a diary to determine whether a particular food or commercial product is involved with an attack. If it proves impossible to define the precipitating agent by this means, a severely restricted elimination diet, limiting foods to boiled rice and lamb, may be tried for several weeks to see if eliminating an offending ingested agent will terminate attacks. Too often these attempts are unsuccessful.

There are defined clinical situations in which urticaria and/or angioedema is a common presenting problem: Patients undergoing immune complex–mediated reactions, as occur in active systemic lupus erythematosus and serum sickness, may experience waves of urticarial lesions, in this case thought to be due to activation of mediator pathways by circulating immune complexes with generation of kinins and complement-derived anaphylatoxins.

Autoantibodies of various sorts interacting with antigen may induce urticarial reactions. IgG anti-IgE autoantibodies have been suggested as a major cause of chronic urticaria, and a recent study suggests that IgG-anti IgE receptor antibody is found in a subset of these patients. Thyroid autoantibodies have been singled out as a cause of urticaria; in one study 90 of 624 patients with chronic urticaria were found to have thyroid autoimmunity, being either hyperthyroid or hypothyroid. Similarly, blood transfusions and infusions of fresh frozen plasma are often associated with hives caused by antibodies in the infused materials encountering host antigen or circulating host antibodies binding antigens in the blood products. Similarly, some cancers, for example lymphomas, may be associated with urticarial lesions, thought to be due to an immunologic response to tumor antigens. A similar mechanism is clearly responsible for the hives that may be associated with many infectious agents, particularly viral agents. Here antigens on or released from the infectious agent are bound to antibodies induced in the patient and hives result. Hives are a frequent response to the antibodies formed in the early response to hepatitis A and B and Epstein-Barr virus infection. Rarely fungal antigens like those derived from *Candida albicans* may precipitate hives or angioedema. Given the rarity of this latter observation, it is inappropriate to treat patients with chronic urticaria/angioedema with nystatin unless a clear association with a hypersensitivity response to candidal antigens can be demonstrated. Although rare in the United States, many parasitic diseases can at times be associated with urticaria/angioedema with or without hypereosinophilia. Presumably the presence of the urticaria/angioedema reflects an ongoing immediate hypersensitivity reaction to parasite antigens.

The complex of urticaria, bone pain, and lymphadenopathy is termed Schnitzler's syndrome. Affected patients often have greatly increased IgM levels suggesting an ongoing immunologic reaction, but the cause of the syndrome is unknown.

PHYSICAL URTICARIAS AND ANGIOEDEMAS. It is important to consider the physical urticaria/angioedema complex when evaluating patients with chronic recurrent urticaria or angioedema because in one large series these represent 16% of all chronic urticaria/angioedema patients seen. In some patients a highly specific diagnosis can be made, a clear precipitating factor can be defined, and the patient can learn to avoid attacks. Moreover, specific therapy may be available. When one lists these causes of urticaria/angioedema, they appear to be so easily defined that it appears unlikely that they could be missed. However, in practice this is not the case; a detailed history is required to identify these factors. Indeed it is common for these patients to go years before a correct diagnosis is made. The physical urticarias have in common urticaria/angioedema precipitated by a known physical cause. This response may follow exposure to cold, heat, elevated body temperature, pressure, vibration, specific wave length ultraviolet rays, or rarely even water to the skin. In some cases these reactions are thought to be IgE mediated, as they can be passively transferred with serum of an affected donor to the skin of an unaffected recipient. In other cases the cause is unknown.

SYMPTOMATIC DERMATOGRAPHISM. As many as 2 to 5% of the general population may be dermatographic, with the appearance of blanching followed by a linear streak of edema and erythema within 2 to 5 minutes of stroking the skin. A small proportion of such individuals have sufficiently severe dermatographism that they become symptomatic. In some cases the symptoms can be transferred to a normal recipient by passive transfer of plasma, suggesting that in some way IgE antibody plays a

role. In general these individuals can be treated successfully with H_1 and H_2 antihistamines.

COLD URTICARIA. These patients experience urticaria/angioedema on exposure to cold and may become hypotensive on diving into a cold swimming pool. Careful studies have shown that mast cell degranulation with histamine release occurs in these patients on cold exposure. Degranulation may be even more extensive when the patient's tissues are warmed following cold exposure. Placing an ice cube on the skin for 5 minutes and then removing it reveals an area of blanching in the shape of the cube followed by edema formation in the same area surrounded by an erythematous flare caused by local hyperemia. Under appropriate conditions blood histamine is elevated. In some of these patients passive transfer to the skin of normals has been demonstrated. It has been suggested that upon cold exposure, certain dermal antigens undergo a conformational change that allows specific IgE autoantibody to bind and initiate mast cell degranulation. These patients are typically treated with cyproheptadine, sometimes with the addition of hydroxyzine. Cold urticaria has been described in a number of diseases associated with pathologic globulins, such as cryoglobulins, or cryofibrinogens. The symptom complex, however, is not associated with the presence of cold agglutinins. When cold urticaria is associated with underlying disease, treatment of those diseases is an essential part of therapy.

In some patients the disease is atypical in that the patient gives a history of typical urticarial symptoms but the ice cube test is negative. In occasional patients dermatographism is brought out by cold exposure; in others exercise-induced urticaria is noted only in the cold. There is a rare familial type of cold urticaria inherited as an autosomal dominant trait in which patients develop urticarial lesions 9 to 18 hours after cold exposure. This cannot be passively transferred with plasma and the cause is unknown.

Similarly, localized heat urticaria has been described with a wheal and flare response noted 2 to 5 minutes after applying localized heat to the skin.

CHOLINERGIC OR GENERALIZED HEAT URTICARIA. Typically these patients, representing about 4% of all patients with chronic urticaria, develop small (several millimeters), intensely pruritic wheals on an erythematous base on their upper trunk and arms following exercise with sweating or following hot showers. A rise in core body temperature is essential to develop lesions. It is generally believed that the parasympathetic nervous system supply to cutaneous vessels releases acetylcholine as well as a neuropeptide such as vasoactive intestinal peptide, causing mediator release. There is no evidence of an IgE-mediated reaction. In support of this hypothesis is the fact that some of these patients (30 to 50%) develop typical lesions as well as a series of local satellite lesions when intracutaneously injected with Mecholyl. Atropine may inhibit the skin test but does not successfully treat the disease. These patients are typically highly responsive to hydroxyzine therapy. There is a subset of patients who respond to heat exposure, developing large urticarial lesions rather than the typical lesions of cholinergic urticaria. These patients tend not to develop their hives with exercise and are less responsive to hydroxyzine therapy.

EXERCISE-INDUCED URTICARIA/ANAPHYLAXIS. These patients note urticarial lesions appearing 5 to 30 minutes after the onset of exercise. They last for 1 to 3 hours. In severe cases anaphylactic reactions may be noted. This is an illness generally of young adults. At times symptoms are difficult to distinguish from those of cholinergic urticaria; however, these patients do not develop urticaria on raising core body temperature as in a hot bath and tend to respond poorly to antihistamines.

PRESSURE-INDUCED URTICARIA. For unknown reasons, urticarial lesions are common at pressure points on the body, e.g., where clothing is tight. Some patients note that marked urticarial lesions develop 4 to 6 hours after pressure is applied to the body. For example, these individuals may note urticarial lesions on buttocks after sitting for a long time on a hard chair or angioedema or urticaria on their feet after prolonged standing in one place. The lesions may be provoked by placing over the shoulders for 20 minutes a 1-inch strap weighted at the ends with 15-pound weights. A systemic response with malaise and even fever is often noted. The response to antihistamines is often poor. The urticaria but not the systemic toxicity may respond to antihistamine therapy. The most severely affected of these patients may require every-other-day glucocorticoid administration for partial relief. They are reported to be unresponsive to NSAID's.

Similarly, some patients respond to local vibration by developing urticarial lesions. Typically symptoms are induced by placing a vibrator or vortex mixer on the arm for 5 minutes. Urticaria appears in 1 to 5 minutes.

SOLAR URTICARIA. In general these patients develop urticarial responses shortly after exposure to sunlight; the patients are divided into groups by the wavelength of light that provokes attacks. Patients whose attacks are provoked by light at 280 to 320 nm (type 1) and 400 to 500 nm (type 4) typically have disease that can be passively transferred with serum to nonaffected recipients. This observation suggests the presence of an IgE-dependent mechanism in these cases. Type 6, provoked by light at 400 nm, is present in some patients with erythropoietic protoporphyria. Glass absorbs light with wavelength below 320 nm, and patients with urticaria in response to light wavelengths below 320 nm can be protected easily. The erythema-causing band of the solar spectrum, UVB, is at wavelength 290 to 320 nm, and these patients can sometimes be helped considerably by PABA-containing sunscreens, which absorb light in this range. However, many are not protected by the PABA sunscreens. A sunscreen preparation, butyl methoxydibenzoyl methane, absorbs light in the UVA range and may be more useful for this patient group. There are many types of light sensitivity, and sorting these out may be confusing. They range from metabolic abnormalities (erythrogenic porphyria), in which products of metabolism absorb light energy and undergo chemical alteration, developing toxic products, to photoallergic reactions in which skin- sensitizing drugs induce allergic reactions when acted upon by sunlight, to phototoxic reactions in which drugs localized in cutaneous tissues directly cause tissue-damaging reactions when exposed to light of the proper wavelength. In many of these cases the light energy is absorbed by a complex ring structure in the drug, which subsequently releases photons and electrons that lead to local generation of toxic products such as singlet oxygen, hydrogen peroxide, and chloramines. Obviously in each case one attempts to identify the cause of the urticaria and eliminate the offending agent if it can be defined.

AQUAGENIC URTICARIA. These patients respond within 2 to 30 minutes with urticaria when water is applied to the skin. Typically this is noted in the course of baths or showers, even with water at tepid temperature. In many cases these individuals are probably exquisitely sensitive to additives in the water, e.g., chlorine, but it is reported that rare individuals develop urticaria in response to distilled water.

CHRONIC URTICARIA/ANGIOEDEMA. It should be clear from the material presented that chronic urticaria/angioedema can be caused by many agents, and identifying the agent may be difficult or impossible. Often after attempts at identifying the cause of the urticaria have failed, we are left with a patient who requires treatment. H_1 antihistamines are usually the agents of first choice. Some examples of therapeutic agents are listed earlier in the chapter; in patients with chronic disease, high-dose hydroxyzine and cyproheptadine are often effective. These agents make patients drowsy and may not be well tolerated initially, but drowsiness may pass if the drug is continued. Optimally the dose is increased until drowsiness persists and then the dosage is reduced slightly. It is common to find patients who, because the drugs have not been used properly, claim to have been unresponsive to these agents. Many more conveniently used and less sedating antihistamines have become available in the last few years and have been shown in controlled studies to be effective in chronic angioedema/urticaria. These include terfenadine, astemizol, loratidine, and cetirizine. H_2 inhibitory drugs are often added to H_1 inhibitors if the clinical response is not adequate. Other agents have also proven to be beneficial, including doxepin, a tricyclic antidepressant with anti-H_1 and anti-H_2 properties; nifedipine, a calcium channel blocker; and ketotifen, a drug shown to be efficacious in the physical urticarias. If these agents fail, a course of glucocorticoids may be required. In general one begins with 40 to 60 mg of prednisone per day in divided doses for 1 week. The dosage is then consolidated to a single dose a day, and then the drug is rapidly tapered on an every-other-day schedule until the patient is receiving glucocorticoids once every other day. The dose of glucocorticoids should be tapered to

the lowest dose that will maintain the patient with minimal symptoms. Following a course of glucocorticoid therapy, patients often remain in remission for a prolonged time. The illness may recur at a later time or when glucocorticoids are tapered.

DIFFERENTIAL DIAGNOSIS

This set of diseases is multifactorial. Usually the diagnosis of urticaria/angioedema does not present a problem in the patient with clear episodes of pruritic wheals or localized brawny edema. Because many agents can cause these lesions, considerable detective work is required to define these diseases and to develop a suitable specific therapy. During the initial evaluation a number of points must be explored. A history of a fixed rather than evanescent eruption, burning, bruising, or vesiculating lesions must lead one to early biopsy. Similarly, fever or systemic signs and symptoms, including arthralgias, pulmonary symptoms, and abdominal pain, suggest that further exploration is needed. Patients with idiopathic chronic urticaria typically have a normal sedimentation rate, white cell count, and differential, and these should be examined. In appropriate cases, ANA, heterophile, STS, rheumatoid factor level, cryoglobulins and cryofibrinogen, cold hemolysin, C4, and C1 inhibitor levels should be studied for further clues to the underlying diagnosis. In the patient who responds poorly to therapy or who has atypical disease, a biopsy is clearly indicated. Patients with urticarial vasculitis are treated for the underlying vasculitis.

THERAPY

The use of antihistamines and glucocorticoids is discussed under the various entities and in the section on chronic urticaria/angioedema. Epinephrine is clinically useful in acute management of urticaria/angioedema. In this case the drug is administered as a series of injections (0.2 to 0.3 ml) of 1:1000 dilution subcutaneously, repeated at half-hour intervals two or three times until symptoms are controlled. Obviously the use of epinephrine is contraindicated in certain patient groups such as patients with severe cardiovascular disease. Longer-acting epinephrine preparations such as epinephrine in oil (Sus-Phrine) may be useful.

URTICARIA PIGMENTOSA AND SYSTEMIC MASTOCYTOSIS

Urticaria pigmentosa is characterized by the local accumulation of intradermal masses of infiltrating mast cells (see Ch. 231). The lesions may resemble freckles superficially but are raised, as might be expected of infiltrative lesions, and may be somewhat erythematous. They may urticate when stroked (Darier's sign). Systemic mastocytosis is associated with massive accumulation of mast cells in other organs, particularly the bone marrow and gastrointestinal tract. Although some affected patients may present with acute or chronic urticaria, that presentation is quite rare; systemic signs of histamine toxicity, gastrointestinal disorders, or disorders consequent to destruction of bone marrow or bone are more common.

HEREDITARY ANGIOEDEMA

Hereditary angioedema (HAE) presents clinically as episodic attacks of brawny nonpitting edema that usually involve the extremities but may affect any external body surface including the genitalia. Mucosal surfaces are affected as well and patients frequently have attacks of severe abdominal pain due to swelling of the submucosa of the gastrointestinal tract. On rare occasions attacks may affect the airway, where they can cause respiratory obstruction and asphyxiation. Although attacks are sporadic, about half of the patients note that trauma, particularly associated with local pressure, precipitates an attack, and half the patients note a marked increase in attack frequency at times of emotional stress. About one third of patients note an erythema marginatum–like rash at the onset of attacks which they often describe as nonraised, nonpruritic circles on the skin. In general, attacks become progressively more severe over about 1.5 days and then regress over a similar time period. Swelling of the gastrointestinal mucosa may be associated with exquisite abdominal pain.

Although relatively rare (incidence about 1:10,000), this disease has received a great deal of attention because of the high incidence of lethal complications, because its pathophysiologic basis is best understood of all of the angioedemas, and because adequate therapy is available for most patients. Presence of this disease is associated with either low levels or abnormal function of a plasma regulatory protein, the C1 inhibitor (see Ch. 222). This protein controls activation of the complement, kinin-generating, fibrinolytic, and intrinsic clotting pathways. Although the precise cause of the capillary leakage is unknown, it is believed that a peptide formed during activation of either the complement or the kinin-generating mediator pathway is the responsible factor. HAE has an autosomal dominant inheritance pattern, affecting 50% of the offspring of a patient and occurring with equal frequency in males and females. This autosomal dominant inheritance reflects the presence of one abnormal gene for C1 inhibitor on chromosome 11. This gene may yield no gene product (85% of patients; type 1) or may code for a nonfunctional protein (15% of patients; type 2).

HAE tends to be mild in childhood, becoming more severe at puberty. The factors that initiate attacks are unknown. There is no relationship between the level or activity of C1 inhibitor and the severity of disease. Patients are described who presumably had the defect from birth but whose attacks began at age 70. Diagnosis is established by finding low levels of C1 inhibitor antigen or function and low levels of the complement protein C4 and/or C2. C1 inhibitor inhibits the function of activated C1 of the classic complement pathway. C1 INH acts by binding to the substrate to be inhibited, and the product of one normal gene is insufficient to control mediator activation. When activated, C1 cleaves the next two proteins in the cascade, C4 and C2. Because the function of activated C1 is unregulated in the presence of a relative C1 inhibitor deficiency, C1 continues to cleave C4 and C2. Patients have low levels of circulating C4 and C2 during attacks and usually have low levels between attacks. Interestingly, because of the presence of other control proteins, the levels of C3, the most commonly measured complement protein, are almost always normal. Presumably because of the constant complement activation present in these patients, they have an immune dysregulation shown by the higher-than-normal incidence of autoimmune diseases. These include endocrinopathies, granulomatous bowel disorders, arthritides, and SLE.

Patients' angioedema attacks respond poorly to epinephrine, antihistamines, and glucocorticoids, the mainstays of treatment of urticaria and angioedema caused by immediate hypersensitivity reactions. Nevertheless, acute attacks are treated with epinephrine, both nebulized racemic epinephrine in the airway (1:1000 given by nebulization) and subcutaneous injections (0.2 to 0.3 ml 1:1000 SQ repeated q 20–30 min × 3). Epinephrine administered very early in an attack often produces some improvement. Patients also receive antihistamines for sedation. Patients often relate that intravenously administered FFP to supply the missing inhibitor proteins terminates attacks. Nevertheless, a rare patient becomes more edematous following FFP, presumably reflecting increased availability of mediator substrates, and FFP therefore is not recommended for treating life-threatening laryngeal edema. In this circumstance nasotracheal intubation in the operating room under conditions where tracheostomy can be performed is indicated. FFP can be given in nonemergency situations such as in preoperative patients to prevent attacks. The usual dose of FFP is 2 units, an arbitrary amount that has been used extensively and has proven to be effective. Evidence suggests that infusions of purified C1 inhibitor reliably terminate attacks; it is likely that this protein will be available for treatment of acute attacks within the next several years. Although short-term therapy and therapy of acute attacks of HAE have not been generally satisfactory, long-term therapy has been quite successful. Patients respond to all of the acetylated artificial androgens with increased C1 INH levels that in some cases approach normal values, a correction of serum C4 and C2, and a marked amelioration of symptoms. In the rare patient in whom the drug is ineffective or in whom drug toxicity is a problem, plasmin inhibitors such as ϵ-aminocaproic acid, have also been found to be effective. Their mechanism of action is unknown, and there is no change in the amount of C activation reflected in the persistent reduction in the serum level of C4 and C2. With all of these agents there is a high degree of patient-to-patient variation in dosage, and the lowest dose that controls symptoms is chosen. Women are often treated with danazol (200 to 400 mg per day), an impeded androgen that has

few masculinizing side effects. Men are often treated with the less expensive but more androgenic agent methyltestosterone (10 to 30 mg per day orally).

ACQUIRED C1 INHIBITOR DEFICIENCY

A number of syndromes have been recognized that are associated with a typical HAE symptom complex but are a reflection of acquired disease. A decade ago it was recognized that certain patients with malignancies, including lymphosarcoma, leukemia, lymphoma, and paraproteinemia, developed circulating or cellular factors that could activate C1 and deplete all the C1 inhibitor activity in serum. Later it was noted that rare patients with autoimmune disease also induced massive activation of the complement cascade with C1 inhibitor utilization and an HAE-like clinical picture. More recently, patients have been described with multiple myeloma and anti-idiotypic antibody causing the same symptom complex. Perhaps the most common of these rare individuals are recently described patients who form monoclonal or polyclonal autoantibodies to the C1 inhibitor, which destroy its activity. Clinically these patients cannot be distinguished from patients with HAE. However, their laboratory tests are unique. All of these patients have profound depressions in functional C1, C4, and C2. Patients with HAE commonly have normal C1 levels. Although their plasma C1 inhibitor antigen level may be normal, they have marked depression of C1 INH function. Their treatment focuses on the underlying disease where possible. Some of these patients respond to danazol or other anabolic steroids. Several of the patients with the anti–C1 INH autoantibody have responded to glucocorticoid therapy, and at least one of these patients has responded to cytotoxic therapy.

FACTOR I DEFICIENCY WITH CHRONIC URTICARIA

Factor I is one of the control proteins of the complement activation pathway. The rare individuals with an inherited deficiency of this protein continuously activate and cleave C3, generating the anaphylatoxins C3a and perhaps C5a. *In vitro* these cleavage peptides induce mast cell degranulation and cause chronic urticaria that disappears when the patient is infused with Factor I. In general, this form of urticaria is relatively mild and is treated symptomatically with antihistamines.

ANGIOEDEMA INDUCED BY ANGIOTENSIN-CONVERTING ENZYME (ACE) INHIBITORS AND INTERLEUKIN-2. Within hours to 1 week of therapy with ACE inhibitors, patients may note angioedema that becomes life-threatening. ACE plays an important role in the degradation of bradykinin and the neuropeptide substance P, and these mediators may be important in forming angioedema. Patients are treated with antihistamines and/or epinephrine as appropriate and the ACE inhibitor is discontinued. It has also been noted that systemic capillary leak or angioedema may follow the systemic infusion of IL-2 used to treat malignancy. It is reported that this cytokine activates both the complement- and kinin-generating pathways. It activates T cells, and it has been suggested that these activated cells directly damage the endothelium.

Casale TB, Sampson HA, Harrifin J, et al.: Guide to physical urticarias. J Allergy Clin Immunol 82:758, 1988. *Tables of information on the physical urticarias.*

Champion RH: Urticaria: Then and now. Br J Dermatol 119:427, 1988. *A report of the evaluation of 2300 cases and comments on the literature.*

Champion RH, Greaves MW, Kobza A, et al.: The Urticarias. Edinburgh, Churchill Livingstone, 1985. *The proceedings of a symposium on urticaria-angioedema.*

Frank MM: Hereditary angioedema. *In* Bayless TM, Brain MC, Cherniack RM (eds.): Current Therapy in Internal Medicine 2. Philadelphia, BC Decker, 1987, p 42. *Complete discussion of treatment.*

Frank MM, Gelfand JA, Atkinson JP: Hereditary angioedema: The clinical syndrome and its management. Ann Intern Med 84:580, 1976. *Although old, this represents the classic clinical review of this syndrome.*

Hide M, Francis DM, Grattan CE, et al.: Autoantibodies against the high-affinity IgE receptor as a cause of histamine release in chronic urticaria. N Engl J Med 328:1599, 1993. *First presentation of hypothesis that chronic urticaria is due to anti-IgE receptor autoimmunity.*

Leznoff A, Sussman GL: Syndrome of idiopathic chronic urticaria and angioedema with thyroid autoimmunity. A study of 90 patients. J Allergy Clin Immunol 84:66, 1989. *The best review of this patient group.*

Mehregan DR, Hall MJ, Gibson LE: Urticarial vasculitis, a histopathologic and clinical review of 72 cases. J Am Acad Dermatol 26:441, 1992. *Excellent clinical review.*

Monroe EN: Chronic urticaria. Review of nonsedating H₁ antihistamines in treatment. J Am Acad Dermatol 19:842, 1988. *Comparison of various H₁ agents and review of published studies.*

Wanderer AA: Cold urticaria syndromes. Historical background, diagnostic classification, clinical and laboratory characteristics, pathogenesis and management. J Allergy Clin Immunol 88:965, 1990. *A thorough review of this syndrome.*

225 ALLERGIC RHINITIS

Richard D. deShazo

DEFINITION

Allergic rhinitis is a symptom complex characterized by paroxysms of sneezing; itching of the eyes, nose, and palate; rhinorrhea; and nasal obstruction. It is often associated with postnasal drip, cough, irritability, and fatigue. Symptoms develop when persons inhale airborne antigens (allergens) to which they have been previously exposed and have made IgE antibodies. These IgE antibodies bind to IgE receptors on mast cells in the respiratory mucosa and to basophils in the peripheral blood. When IgE molecules on their surface are bridged by allergen, mast cells release pre-formed and granule-associated chemical mediators. They also generate other mediators and cytokines that lead to nasal inflammation and, with continued allergen exposure, chronic symptoms.

EPIDEMIOLOGY

Allergic rhinitis is common, accounting for at least 2.5% of all physician visits, 2 million lost school days per year, 6 million lost work days, and 28 million restricted work days per year. At least $1 billion is spent annually on prescription and over-the-counter medications for allergy. Between 10% and 20% of the United States population is affected, and the prevalence in urban areas is increasing. The prevalence is lowest in children under age 5, rises to a peak in early adulthood (as high as 24% in the U.S.), and declines thereafter. The 4-year remission rate is reported to be 10% in males and 5% in females.

PHYSICAL FINDINGS AND ASSOCIATIONS

The swollen nasal mucosa of patients with acute allergic rhinitis is pale and blue but becomes erythematous and indurated with chronic allergen exposure. Clear rhinorrhea may be visible anteriorly or, with nasal obstruction, dripping down a cobblestone-appearing posterior pharynx. Giemsa or Hansel's stains of these nasal secretions show cell populations to be predominantly eosinophils. A transverse nasal crease, a highly arched palate, mouth breathing, and dental malocclusion are common, especially in children. Venous dilation of the subcutaneous skin beneath the eyes may produce "allergic shiners."

Chronic allergic rhinitis may be associated with sleep disorders, sinusitis, secretory otitis media, and anosmia. Allergic rhinitis is also associated with other common allergic conditions, including allergic conjunctivitis, allergic asthma, and atopic dermatitis (eczema). Twenty-eight to 50% of patients with asthma and up to 30% with eczema have allergic rhinitis. These conditions have been termed "atopic diseases" and patients who have them are often called "atopic."

DIFFERENTIAL DIAGNOSIS

Syndromes of rhinitis may be divided into allergic, infectious, perennial nonallergic, and miscellaneous categories (Table 225–1). Allergic rhinitis should be differentiated from other forms of rhinitis, as the approach to management is different. Episodic exposure to inhaled allergens such as cat salivary proteins, horse dander, murine urinary proteins, pollen, or house dust mite feces may provoke acute allergic symptoms that are easily diagnosed as *acute allergic rhinitis*. If allergen exposure is seasonal—for instance, tree and grass pollen in the spring (rose fever) or ragweed pollen exposure in the fall (hay fever)—symptoms are predictable and reproducible and, thus, *seasonal allergic rhinitis* may be diagnosed by history (Fig. 225–1). When allergen exposure is chronic, *perennial allergic rhinitis* may result. This is common in subtropical regions with long pollinating seasons and ever-present mold and dust mite allergens and with occupational allergen exposure. This form of rhinitis may be difficult to distinguish from nonallergic forms of *perennial nonallergic rhinitis* and may require certain testing (discussed later) to diagnose accurately. Of all patients with rhinitis, 11% have seasonal symptoms, with 78% of these having an apparent allergic cause. Thirty-three percent of patients with rhinitis have perennial symptoms with a seasonal exacerbation, and 68% of these

TABLE 225–1. CLASSIFICATION OF RHINITIS

Allergic
  Seasonal
  Perennial
  Occupational
Infectious
  Acute: Viral, bacterial
  Chronic: Specific: Bacterial, fungal
      Nonspecific: Associated with immune deficiency (antibody deficiency, ciliary abnormalities)
Perennial nonallergic
  Idiopathic (vasomotor rhinitis)
  Nonallergic rhinitis with eosinophilia (NARES)
Miscellaneous forms
  Hormonal: pregnancy, hypothyroidism, etc.
  Drug-induced: Associated with aspirin and antihypertensives, rhinitis medicamentosa
  Food: gustatory, IgE-mediated, preservative-induced
  Atrophic rhinitis: *(Klebsiella ozenae)*
  Mechanical: hypertrophied turbinates, deviated nasal septum, foreign body, nasal polyps

patients have a probable allergic cause. Fifty-six percent of patients with rhinitis have perennial symptoms alone, and only about 50% of these have symptoms that can be attributed to allergens. Most patients with allergic rhinitis have allergic symptom triggers, eosinophil-rich nasal secretions, allergen-specific IgE to inhalant allergens, and a family history of allergic disease.

Nasal eosinophilia is not diagnostic for allergic rhinitis because nasal eosinophilia occurs in the *nonallergic rhinitis with nasal eosinophilia syndrome (NARES)*. This occurs in as many as 15% of patients with rhinitis and is characterized by perennial symptoms, an older average age than in patients with allergic rhinitis (39 versus 25 years), and milder symptoms of nasal itching and sneezing. The clear nasal secretions contain >25% eosinophils, but the role of eosinophils in the disorder is unclear. Fifty percent of patients with NARES have sinusitis, 33% have nasal polyps, and 14% have asthma. IgE to inhalant allergens is usually absent. Another common form of perennial nonallergic rhinitis is commonly called *vasomotor rhinitis*. Patients with this disorder complain predominantly of chronic nasal congestion intensified by rapid changes in temperature and relative humidity, odors, or alcohol. Several lines of evidence suggest that they have nasal autonomic nervous system dysfunction. For instance, they have abnormal nasal responses to temperature stimuli applied to the skin and excess nasal sensitivity to topically applied acetylcholine congeners. They have little nasal itching or sneezing, but headaches, anosmia, and sinusitis are common. A family history of allergy or allergic symptom triggers is uncommon. Positive immediate hypersensitivity skin tests to inhalant allergens and nasal eosinophilia are unusual. *Atrophic rhinitis* is a syndrome of progressive atrophy of the nasal mucosa in elderly patients who report chronic nasal congestion and constantly perceive a bad odor. *Rhinitis medicamentosa* is a complication of chronically using vasoconstrictor nasal sprays. Patients develop chronic nasal obstruction and nasal inflammation manifest as beefy red nasal membranes on physical examination. *Rhinitis of pregnancy* and rhinitis associated with birth control pills or hypothyroidism reflect nasal obstruction that occurs on a hormonal basis. Nasal obstruction may also be a side effect of antihypertensive drugs. Unilateral rhinitis or nasal polyps are uncommon in uncomplicated allergic rhinitis. Unilateral rhinitis suggests the possibility of nasal obstruction by foreign body, tumor, or polyp, and the presence of nasal polyps suggests chronic sinusitis, aspirin hypersensitivity, or cystic fibrosis.

MECHANISMS OF ALLERGIC REACTIONS

The expression of allergic diseases reflects an autosomal dominant pattern of inheritance with incomplete penetrance. This is manifested as a propensity to respond to inhalant allergen exposure by producing high levels of allergen-specific IgE. The IgE response appears to be controlled by immune response genes located within the major histocompatibility complex (MHC) on chromosome 6 (see Ch. 229). The immunologic mechanisms for atopy have been studied in murine models and in humans and appear to center on the

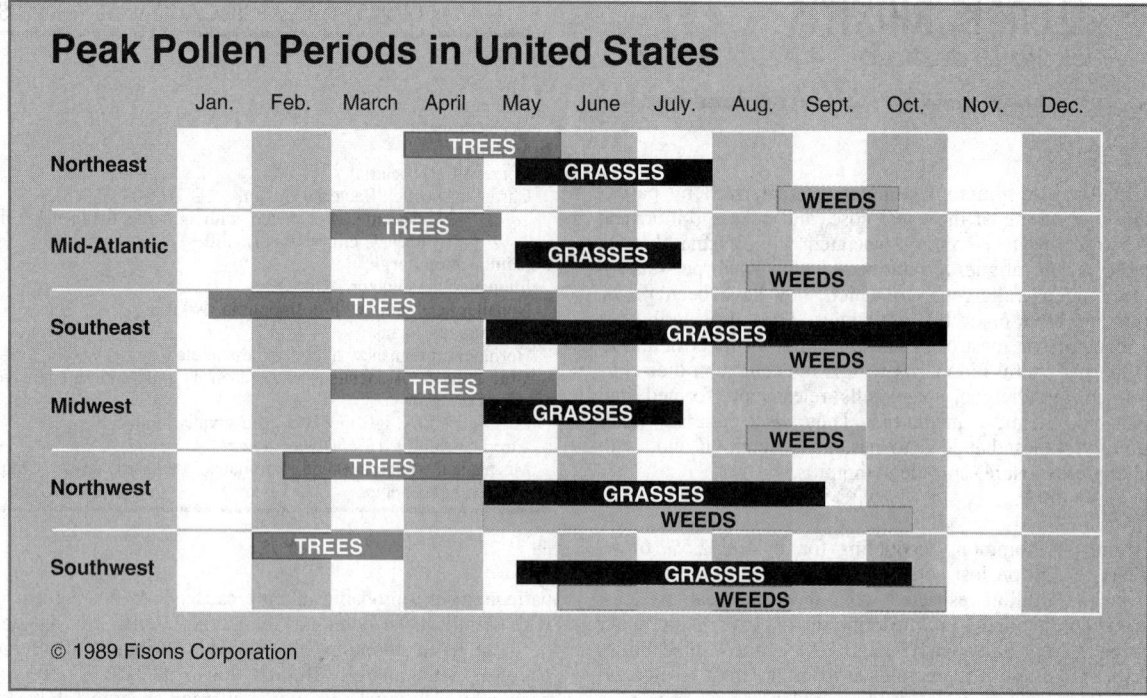

FIGURE 225–1. Peak pollen periods in the United States. (Reproduced with permission from Fisons Pharmaceuticals. © 1989, Fisons Corporation.)

expression of a repertoire of responses associated with the T_H2 type T-helper lymphocyte summarized below.

PRODUCTION OF IgE

Sensitization to allergen is necessary to elicit an IgE response (Fig. 225–2). After inhalation, the allergen must first be internalized by antigen-presenting cells, which include macrophages, dendritic cells, activated T lymphocytes, and B lymphocytes. After allergen processing, peptide fragments of the allergen are presented with class II (MHC) molecules of the host antigen-presenting cells to CD4+ T lymphocytes. These lymphocytes have receptors specific for the particular MHC-peptide complex. This interaction results in the release of cytokines by the CD4+ cell.

T-helper lymphocytes (CD4+) appear to be of two classes: T_H1 and T_H2. If the CD4+ cells that recognize the allergen are of the T_H2 class, a certain repertoire of mediators including granulocytemacrophage colony-stimulating factor (GM-CSF), interleukin (IL)-3, IL-4, IL-5, and IL-6, are released. IL-4, IL-5, and IL-6 are cytokines involved in B-cell proliferation and differentiation. Activated B lymphocytes, having bound allergen via their allergen-specific IgM-variable region binding sites, are stimulated by these cytokines to proliferate and secrete IgM. IL-4 from T_H2 cells promotes B-cell isotype switching to IgE antibody synthesis. Thus, atopy appears to be the result of a predisposition toward T_H2-type responses, which result in the formation of large quantities of allergen-specific IgE.

MAST CELLS AND EOSINOPHILS. After IgE antibodies specific for a certain allergen are synthesized and secreted, they bind to mast cells and basophils. When allergen is inhaled into the nose, the allergen or a hapten-allergen complex cross-links these allergen-specific cell-bound IgE antibodies on the mast cell surface, whereupon rapid degranulation and mediator release occur.

Mast cell mediators are either pre-formed, granule-associated, formed during degranulation, or generated after transcription (Fig. 225–3). The most important pre-formed mediator is histamine, which reproduces all of the symptoms of acute allergic rhinitis when sprayed nasally into normal volunteers. Histamine causes vasodilation that leads to nasal congestion, mucus secretion, and increased vascular permeability, which in turn leads to tissue edema and sneezing through stimulation of sensory nerve fibers. The cross-linking of IgE antibody on mast cells also initiates the release of arachidonic acid from cell membrane substrates. Mast cells then metabolize arachidonic acid—either via the cyclo-oxygenase pathway to form prostaglandin and thromboxane mediators or via the

lipoxygenase pathway to form leukotrienes. Prostaglandin D_2 (PGD_2), the sulfidopeptide leukotrienes LTC_4, LTD_4, and LTE_4 (SRS-A), platelet-activating factor (PAF), and bradykinin are formed during degranulation. PGD_2 is synthesized by mast cells but not basophils and appears more potent than histamine in causing nasal congestion. PAF is a potent chemotactic factor, and the sulfidopeptide leukotrienes and bradykinins are vasoactive. One leukotriene, LTB_4, is the most potent chemotactic factor in humans.

Mast cells are present in concentrations of 7000 per cubic millimeter in the normal nasal submucosa but only 50 per cubic millimeter in the nasal epithelium. The total number of nasal epithelial mast cells remains constant during the allergy season. However, the superficial nasal epithelium in allergic rhinitis patients has 50-fold more basophilic cells (mast cells and basophils) per specimen than the epithelium from nonallergic subjects. Increased concentrations of mast cells are found near postcapillary venules, where they increase vascular permeability; near sensory nerves, where they initiate the sneeze reflex; and near glands, where they facilitate secretion.

Once allergic reactions begin, mast cells amplify them by releasing not only vasoactive agents but also cytokines including GM-CSF, tumor necrosis factor-α (TNF-α), and IL-1 to -6. These cytokines further promote IgE production, mast cell growth, and eosinophil growth, chemotaxis, and survival. For instance, IL-5, TNF-α, and IL-1 promote eosinophil movement by increasing the expression of adhesion receptors on endothelium. In turn, eosinophils secrete IL-1, which favors T_H2 cell proliferation, and the mast cell growth factor, IL-3. Eosinophils release oxygen radicals and proteins, including eosinophil major basic protein, which are toxic to the nasal epithelium.

MECHANISMS OF NASAL ALLERGIC REACTIONS

ANATOMY AND PHYSIOLOGY OF THE NOSE. Under normal conditions, the nose accounts for nearly 50% of the resistance to airflow in the airway. It is lined by pseudostratified epithelium resting on a basement membrane, separating it from deeper submucosal layers. The submucosa contains mucous, seromucous, and serous glands. The small arteries, arterioles, and arteriovenous anastomoses determine regional blood flow. Capacitance vessels, consisting of veins and cavernous sinusoids, determine nasal patency. The cavernous sinusoids lie beneath the capillaries and venules, are most dense in the inferior and middle turbinates, and contain smooth muscle cells controlled by the sympathetic nervous system. Withdrawal of sympathetic tone or, to a lesser degree, cholinergic

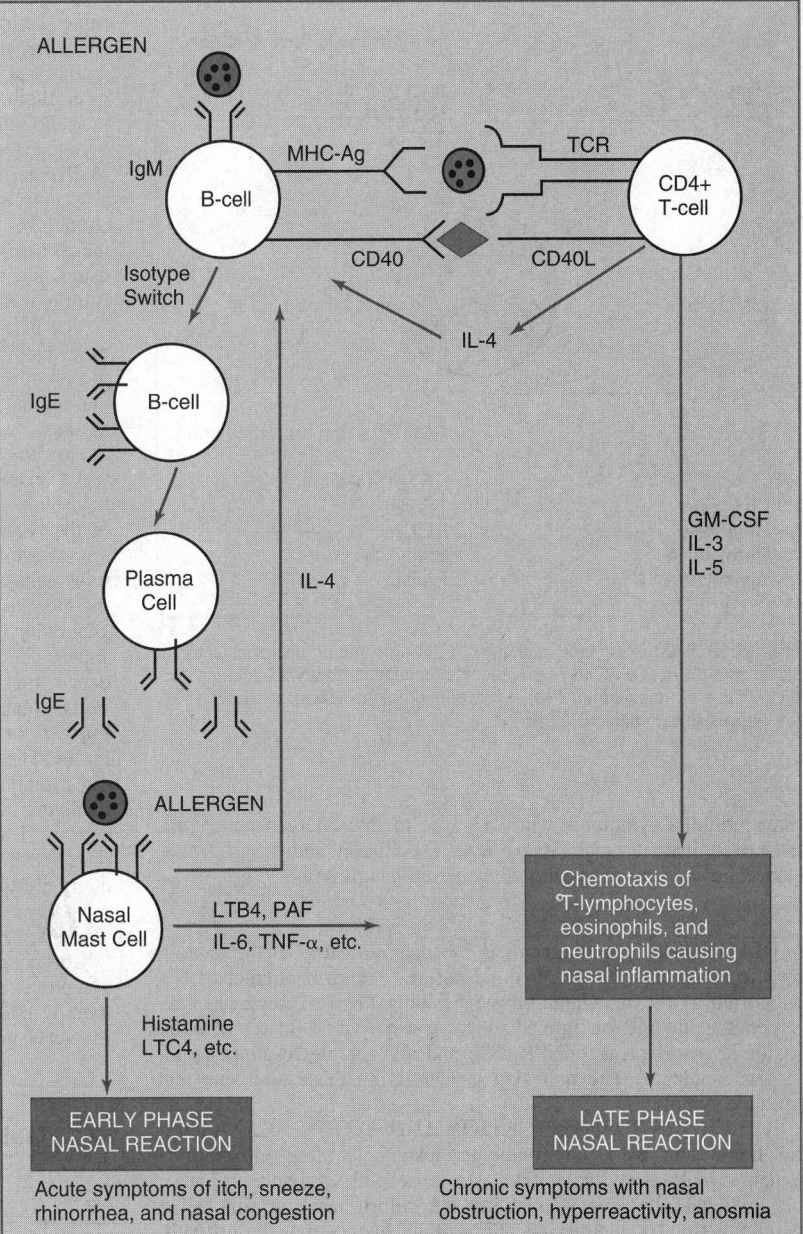

FIGURE 225–2. Pathophysiology of allergic rhinitis. Allergen is presented to T$_H$2 helper T lymphocytes by antigen-presenting cells (such as macrophages or B lymphocytes) in the context of major histocompatibility proteins. In atopic individuals, this leads to the production of cytokines including IL-4, GM-CSF, IL-3, and IL-5. The IL-4 from these T$_H$2 lymphocytes induces B-cell isotype switching to IgE. This isotype switch requires contact-dependent help from T cells via the interaction of the CD40 molecule on B cells and the CD40 ligand (CD40L) on T cells. B cells that produce allergen-specific IgE mature into plasma cells that produce IgE, which binds to mast cells in the nasal mucosa. When inhaled allergens bridge IgE molecules on mast cells, mast cell degranulation occurs, releasing pre-formed mediators. These mediators induce the *early phase nasal reaction,* characterized by rhinorrhea, sneezing, itching, and nasal obstruction. A second release of mast cell mediator may occur 2 to 6 hours later, leading to a recurrence of symptoms. This late-phase reaction is associated with an inflammatory response in the nose and the ongoing symptoms. Inflammation is promoted by the release of mast cell chemotactic factors such as LTB4 and cytokines from mast cells and T$_H$2 lymphocytes. These cytokines promote eosinophil differentiation, activation, and survival. (GM-CSF = granulocyte-monocyte colony-stimulating factor; IL = interleukin; MHC = major histocompatibility complex; TNF = tumor necrosis factor; TCR = T-cell receptor.)

stimulation causes this sinusoidal erectile tissue to become engorged. Cholinergic stimulation causes arterial dilation and promotes the passive diffusion of plasma protein into glands and the active secretion by mucous glands in cells.

Novel neurotransmitters, including substance P, calcitonin gene-related peptide, and vasointestinal peptide, have been detected in nasal secretions after nasal allergen challenge of patients with allergic rhinitis. Because they can produce changes in regional blood flow and glandular secretion, their role in rhinitis may be important.

IMMEDIATE AND LATE NASAL REACTIONS. Exposing the nasal mucosa to ragweed in ragweed-sensitive subjects (nasal challenge) provokes the immediate onset of sneezing and nasal itching associated with significantly increased concentrations of inflammatory mediators. Histamine, PGD$_2$, the kininogen product tosylarginine-methylester (TAME-esterase), tryptase, kinins, and sulfidopeptide leukotrienes are present in nasal washes. After about half an hour, PGD$_2$ and histamine levels return to baseline, whereas TAME-esterase concentrations remain elevated. Sneezing correlates with the appearance of measurable histamine, TAME-esterase, and PGD$_2$ in nasal washes. Biopsy specimens of the nasal mucosa at this time show an increased number of degranulated mast cells.

Two to 6 hours after the initial allergen challenge, symptoms recur with a second release of mast cell mediators at the time of max-

imum mast cell cytokine production. This *late-phase nasal allergic reaction* occurs in approximately 50% of patients with seasonal rhinitis undergoing nasal challenge with allergen. This is associated with elevated levels of the same mediators noted in the immediate reaction except that PGD$_2$ is not detected. Thus, basophils appear partly responsible for such late-phase reactions because histamine is generated by both mast cells and basophils, whereas only mast cells can produce PGD$_2$. In support of this, a marked basophil influx into the nasal mucosa has been noted 3 to 11 hours after allergen challenge. Large numbers of neutrophils, mononuclear cells, and eosinophils also migrate into the nasal mucosa at this time. This inflammatory response is thought to cause the recurrence of symptoms and to induce chronic ones.

After allergen challenge, lymphocytes remain the predominant cells in the nasal mucosa. These cells actively transcribe messages for IL-3, IL-4, IL-5, and GM-CSF and have increased expression of the IL-2 receptor. Interleukins 1 through 5 and GM-CSF have been recovered from nasal washes after allergen challenge.

PRIMING AND NASAL HYPERREACTIVITY

When a patient is continually exposed to pollen, persistent nasal mucosal inflammation develops. In such patients, symptoms of rhinitis occur on exposure to lower doses of allergen (priming) and to nonspecific irritants (hyperreactivity). The clinical result is con-

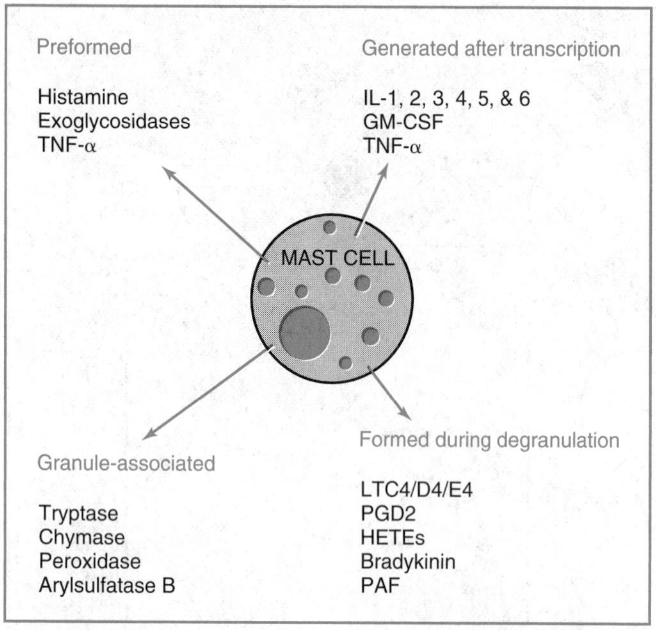

FIGURE 225–3. Mast cell mediators. (TNF-α = tumor necrosis factor-α; IL = interleukin; GM-CSF = granulocyte-monocyte colony-stimulating factor; PG = prostaglandin; PAF = platelet-activating factor; HETE = hydroxyeicosatetraenoic acid.)

tinued rhinitis symptoms with exposure to low allergen concentrations and irritants such as particulate pollution and volatile substances, even after the peak pollen season has passed.

MANAGING ALLERGIC RHINITIS

DIAGNOSIS. The diagnosis is based on a history of the characteristic symptoms that occur on exposure to known allergens. It is supported by the associated physical findings, by the presence of allergen-specific IgE on immediate hypersensitivity skin tests, or by radioallergosorbent testing (RAST) and a favorable response to allergen avoidance. The first step is identifying those allergens that produce symptoms.

ALLERGEN IDENTIFICATION AND AVOIDANCE. A careful home and work environmental history is often informative. When symptoms occur acutely, like those with exposure to cat or occupational allergens, identifying the culprit may be simple. In perennial rhinitis, identifying allergens by history may be difficult. In these circumstances, carefully performed immediate hypersensitivity skin testing (prick skin tests) is a quick, inexpensive, and safe way to identify the presence of allergen-specific IgE. In sensitive patients, testing with selected extracts of tree, grass, or weed pollen, mold, house dust mites and/or animal allergens results in a wheal and flare reaction at the skin test site within 20 minutes. A surrogate test, the RAST, although less sensitive and more expensive, gives similar information from a serum sample. Neither total serum IgE levels, elevated in only 30 to 40% of patients, nor peripheral blood eosinophil counts are sensitive enough to routinely diagnose allergic rhinitis. Stained nasal smears detect eosinophilia, helpful in narrowing the diagnosis to allergic rhinitis or NARES syndrome, and neutrophilia (>50%) associated with sinusitis.

Simple measures to avoid allergens include maintaining the relative humidity at 50% or less to limit house dust mite and mold growth and avoiding exposure to irritants such as cigarette smoke. Air conditioners decrease concentrations of pollens, molds, and dust mite allergens in indoor air. Avoiding exposure to the feces of the house dust mite—the most common cause of perennial allergic rhinitis—is facilitated by covering mattresses, box springs, and pillows with plastic and washing bedding in water hotter than 70°F once weekly. Synthetic pillows should also be used. Furry pets should be removed from the home unless testing shows they are not the source of symptoms.

PHARMACOLOGIC TREATMENT

If avoiding allergens does not result in improvement, antihistamine therapy is a reasonable next step. Antihistamines help control sneezing, rhinorrhea, and itching but may provide inadequate relief from nasal obstruction (Table 225–2). In this case, an oral antihistamine that contains a decongestant such as pseudoephedrine, phenylpropanolamine, or phenylephrine has been shown to be of added benefit. Because the latter agents may cause palpitations, insomnia or irritability, exacerbation of glaucoma, and urinary retention and are contraindicated in patients on monoamine oxidase therapy, they should be used cautiously. With use for more than 5 to 7 days, tachyphylaxis develops to nasal (decongestant) sprays of these drugs and rebound nasal congestion results. Continued use leads to rhinitis medicamentosa.

The first-generation H_1-receptor antagonists produce sedation and other CNS symptoms in 20% of patients and may cause drying of the mouth and urinary hesitancy. Newer second-generation antihistamines have sedative effects comparable to those of placebo. Two of these, terfenadine and astemizole, have been associated with inducing the complex ventricular tachyrhythmia, torsades de pointes, when used concomitantly with ketoconazole, itraconazole, or macrolide antibiotics that share hepatic metabolic pathways. Some of the second-generation H_1 antihistamines inhibit mast cell mediator release and inflammatory cell movement and function. This feature makes them effective in inhibiting not only the immediate but the late nasal reaction to allergen challenge. However, these second-generation agents have not yet been demonstrated to be clinically superior to other second-generation antihistamines. There is no evidence that pharmacologic tolerance develops to antihistamines. Thus, rotating from one antihistamine to another is not beneficial. Furthermore, clinical studies do not support using combinations of H_1 and H_2 antagonists to treat allergic rhinitis.

Cromolyn and nedocromil inhibit mast cell degranulation and mediator release from mast cells and have other anti-inflammatory actions. They thus inhibit both the immediate and late-phase nasal reaction. Both appear to be as effective as antihistamines in treating allergic rhinitis, with nedocromil the more effective. Both agents must be used frequently (three or more times a day), take 2 to 6 weeks to reach full efficacy, and have few side effects.

Corticosteroids given orally or parenterally usually abolish all symptoms of allergic rhinitis. The potential complications of such therapy make them unacceptable for treating allergic rhinitis except in very unusual circumstances. By contrast, topical intranasal

TABLE 225–2. REPRESENTATIVE ANTIHISTAMINES*

	Sedative Effects	Antihistamine Effects	Dosing Intervals (hr)
Ethanolamines			
Clemastine (Tavist)	2 +	1–2 +	12
Diphenhydramine (Benadryl)	3 +	1–2 +	6–8
Ethylenediamines			
Pyrilamine (Histadyl)	1 +	1–2 +	6–8
Alkylamines			
Chlorpheniramine (Chlor-Trimeton)	1 +	2 +	4–6
Phenothiazines			
Promethazine (Phenergan)	3 +	3 +	6–24
Piperidines			
Astemizole (Hismanal)	±	2–3 +	24
Loratadine (Claritin)	±	2–3 +	24
Terfenadine (Seldane)	±	2–3 +	12–24
Azatadine (Optimine)	2 +	2 +	12
Cyproheptadine (Periactin)	3 +	2 +	8
Piperazines			
Hydroxyzine (Atarax)	3 +	3 +	12
Cetirizine (Reactine)	1 +	2–3 +	24
Miscellaneous			
Azelastine† (inves. drug)	±	2–3 +	12
Levocabastine† (orphan drug)	±	2–3 +	12

©1993 by Facts and Comparisons. Used with permission from Drug Facts and Comparisons. 1993 ed. St. Louis, Facts and Comparisons, a division of the JB Lippincott Company. Effects were graded 1–4+.

*Antihistamines in this listing have specific contraindications that require review prior to prescribing.

†Nasal spray.

TABLE 225–3. INTRANASAL STEROIDS AVAILABLE IN THE UNITED STATES

Name/Trade Name	Dose/Max. Dose	Approved for Children
Dexamethasone sodium phosphate (Decadron Turbinaire*)	2 sprays (168 μg) into each nostril 2–3/day; max = 1008 μg/day	>6
Flunisolide (Nasalide)	2 sprays (50 μg) into each nostril 2–3/day; max = 400 μg/day	>6
Beclomethasone dipropionate (Beconase, Vancenase, Beconase AQ, Vancenase AQ)	1 spray (42 μg) in each nostril 2–4/day; max = 336 μg/day	>6
Triamcinolone acetonide (Nasacort)	2 sprays (110 μg) in each nostril once a day; max = 440 μg/day	>6
Budesonide (Rhinocort)	2 sprays (64 μg) in each nostril twice a day; max = 256 μg/day	

©1993 by Facts and Comparisons. Used with permission from Drug Facts and Comparisons. 1993 ed. St. Louis, Facts and Comparisons, a division of the JB Lippincott Company.

*For short-term use only.

steroid therapy causes few side effects when used at recommended doses (Table 225–3). In experimental nasal allergen challenges, they decrease the amount of histamine release in the early nasal response to allergen by 75% and increase the threshold dose for a positive response to allergen. With regular use, they inhibit both the immediate and late-phase nasal reactions. Their maximal therapeutic effects are seen as quickly as 3 to 5 days. Corticosteroids have both vasoconstrictor and anti-inflammatory effects, including inhibiting mediator release and inflammatory cell chemotaxis. Topical nasal steroids are more effective than cromolyn and improve the symptoms of seasonal asthma in patients with both seasonal allergic rhinitis and seasonal allergic asthma. These preparations are available in both aqueous and Freon-propelled preparations. The aqueous preparations may be particularly useful in patients in whom Freon preparations cause mucosal drying, crusting, or epistaxis. Rarely, nasal steroids are associated with nasal septal perforation, probably secondary to nasal septal wall damage from inappropriately using the pressurized aerosol. Mucosal atrophy has not been noted even after years of usage. Treatment failures occur if mucus or other debris is not cleaned from the nose prior to their application. This cleaning can be facilitated by saline nasal sprays or washes.

Ipratropium bromide, a congener of atropine, has been found to reduce rhinorrhea when used intranasally. It does not block sneezing or nasal obstruction and thus is of greater use in nonallergic rhinitis with predominant rhinorrhea.

ALLERGEN IMMUNOTHERAPY

Allergen immunotherapy is the subcutaneous administration of increasing concentrations of allergen to which the patient has demonstrated sensitization and symptoms by skin test (or RAST) and history, respectively. Immunotherapy should be considered when pharmacotherapy and avoiding allergens fail to resolve symptoms or when pharmacotherapy produces unacceptable side effects or is not cost-effective. High-dose immunotherapy for allergic rhinitis has been shown to effectively relieve symptoms of allergic rhinitis in controlled studies. It should be strongly considered in patients with perennial symptoms, perennial rhinitis with seasonal exacerbations, constitutional symptoms (such as severe fatigue) or associated sinusitis, allergic conjunctivitis, or asthma. It is time-consuming and associated with a risk of anaphylaxis, especially when administered by health care professionals not properly trained in its use.

Allergen immunotherapy blocks both the immediate and the late-phase nasal reaction. The specific mechanism by which it relieves symptoms is unclear, although it increases allergen-specific IgG, reduces allergen-specific IgE, decreases allergen-induced mediator release, decreases eosinophil chemotaxis, and appears to favor a shift to cytokine profiles associated with T_H1 responses to allergen.

Badhwar AK, Druce HM: Allergic rhinitis. Med Clin North Am 76:789, 1992. *A practical and well-written review of the diagnostic approach and treatment of allergic rhinitis.*

Creticos P: Immunotherapy with allergens. JAMA 268:2834, 1992. *A well-written review of the rationale for allergen immunotherapy in allergic respiratory disease.*
Kaliner M, Lemanske R: Rhinitis and asthma. JAMA 268:2807, 1992. *An excellent review article with an extensive discussion of the pathophysiology of allergic disease.*
Mosimann BL, White MV, Hohman RJ: Substance P, calcitonin gene-related peptide, and vasoactive intestinal peptide increase in nasal secretions after allergen challenge in atopic patients. J Allergy Clin Immunol 92:95, 1993. *Provides evidence that neural reflexes and neurotransmitters play a role in allergic rhinitis.*
Naclerio RM: Allergic rhinitis. N Engl J Med 325:860, 1991. *An excellent review article covering all aspects of the topic.*
Naclerio RM, Proud D, Togias AG, et al.: Inflammatory mediators in late antigen-induced rhinitis. N Engl J Med 313:65, 1985. *A report on nasal allergen challenge studies that provided strong support that allergic rhinitis results from inflammatory processes.*
Pipkorn U, Proud D, Lichtenstein LM, et al.: Inhibition of mediator release in allergic rhinitis by pretreatment with topical glucocorticosteroids. N Engl J Med 316:1506, 1987. *Reports the results of corticosteroid administration on the production of the chemical mediators of allergic rhinitis.*
Sibbald B: Epidemiology of allergic rhinitis. *In* Burr ML (ed.): Monographs in Allergy. Basel, Karger, 1993, p 61. *A concise review of the epidemiology of allergic rhinitis.*

226 ANAPHYLAXIS

Allen P. Kaplan

The term *anaphylaxis* arose from the experiments of Richet and Portier in the early 1900's and meant the opposite of prophylaxis, i.e., a lack of protection rather than the expected immunity. Nevertheless, the reaction is indeed immune in nature and depends upon formation of IgE antibody, the immunoglobulin responsible for typical allergic reactions. The initial sensitization step induces formation of IgE specifically directed to the initiating substance. In anaphylaxis, the reaction is systemic in nature, occurs rapidly upon administration of minute concentrations of the offending material, and is potentially fatal. How the allergen is given can dictate the manifestations and magnitude of the ensuing allergic reaction; although all routes can lead to anaphylaxis, parenteral administration is more likely than inhaled or ingested allergens to cause elevated circulating levels of unaltered allergen and a systemic reaction. Thus, parenteral administration of medication and insect sting reactions (injected into cutaneous vessels) are among the most common causes of anaphylaxis. Anaphylactoid reactions are defined as systemic reactions that have the same symptoms as anaphylaxis but are not due to an IgE-dependent mechanism and are usually not immune. Examples include reactions to radiographic contrast agents and nonsteroidal anti-inflammatory drugs (e.g., acetylsalicylic acid, indomethacin, ibuprofen).

EPIDEMIOLOGY AND ETIOLOGY. The occurrence of anaphylaxis in the early 1900's was largely due to the use of serum from animals immunized with various toxins or bacteria to treat human illness. Most were due to diphtheria antitoxin injection. In the antibiotic era penicillin and sulfa drugs have become the leading causes of fatal anaphylaxis. In recent years, there have been between 100 and 500 deaths per year in the United States due to penicillin. The insect order Hymenoptera is responsible for about 40 deaths each year and is estimated to cause one significant reaction per 10,000 individuals per year, with a mortality of 0.2 per million in the United States. Estimates of penicillin-induced anaphylaxis are 10 to 40 per 100,000 injections. Most recently allergy to latex in surgical gloves is seen in health care workers or patients undergoing frequent procedures, e.g., children with meningomyelocele or spina bifida or congenital urogenital anomalies.

Although a history of atopy (allergic rhinitis, extrinsic asthma, atopic dermatitis) might be expected to be associated with an increased likelihood of anaphylactic reactions, atopic individuals appear to have, at worst, only a slightly greater risk than nonatopics. Thus, anyone can manifest an IgE response and clinical symptoms to the agents responsible for anaphylaxis. There is also no evidence that race, gender, age, occupation, or season intrinsically predisposes an individual to anaphylaxis.

TABLE 226–1: AGENTS CAUSING ANAPHYLAXIS

Type	Common	Rare
Proteins	Venoms (Hymenoptera)	Hormones (insulin, ACTH, vasopressin, parathormone)
	Pollens (ragweed, grass, etc.)	Enzymes (trypsin, penicillinase)
	Foods (eggs, seafood, nuts, grains, beans, cottonseed oil, chocolate)	Human proteins serum proteins, seminal fluid)
	Horse and rabbit serum (antilymphocyte globulin)	
	Latex	
Haptens and other low molecular weight substances	Antibiotics (penicillins, sulfonamides, cephalosporins, tetracyclines, amphotericin B, nitrofurantoin, aminoglycosides)	Vitamins (thiamine, folic acid)
	Local anesthetics (lidocaine, procaine, etc.)	
Polysaccharides		Dextrans, iron-dextran

Proteins, polysaccharides, and haptens are capable of eliciting systemic reactions in humans (Table 226–1). Proteins are the largest and most diverse group and include antiserum, hormones, seminal plasma, enzymes, Hymenoptera venom (e.g., phospholipase A_2), pollen allergens administered for immunotherapy ("allergy shots"), and foods. Polysaccharides such as dextrans are rarer causes. The most common etiologic agents are drugs, low molecular weight substances that are not antigenic themselves but act as haptens and become antigenic upon reaction with host proteins. These include antibiotics, local anesthetics, vitamins, and diagnostic reagents. Although the most common anaphylactic reactions are due to parenteral administration, food-induced anaphylaxis and anaphylactic reactions to an orally administered drug can occur in very sensitive individuals.

CLINICAL MANIFESTATIONS. IgE-mediated reactions can cause symptoms that include the cutaneous, respiratory, cardiovascular, gastrointestinal, and hematologic systems (Fig. 226–1). The onset and manifestations vary depending on route of administration, dose, release of and sensitivity to vasoactive substances, and differ-

ing sensitivities of the organs to these substances. These parameters can vary from person to person, and individuals tend to react in a characteristic pattern. The initial manifestations can begin in seconds or take as long as an hour to develop; in severe reactions the onset is usually within 5 to 10 minutes. Initial manifestations often include skin erythema, pruritus, a generalized feeling of warmth and/or impending doom, light-headedness, shortness of breath, nausea, vomiting, or a lump in the throat. Urticaria is the most common manifestation of anaphylaxis. The rash is generalized, intensely pruritic, and consists of well-circumscribed, erythematous, raised wheals with serpiginous borders and blanched centers. Angioedema may accompany urticaria and typically manifests as swelling of face, eyes, lips, tongue, pharynx, or extremities. The respiratory tract is commonly involved in fatal anaphylaxis. The early stages of upper airway edema consist of hoarseness, stridor, and/or dysphoria. Angioedema of the epiglottis and larynx can cause mechanical obstruction and death by suffocation. The swelling can extend to the hypopharynx and trachea. Between 25 and 50% of patients dying of anaphylaxis have pathologic changes consistent with severe asthma. There is pulmonary hyperinflation, peribronchial congestion, submucosal edema, edema-filled alveoli, and eosinophilic infiltration. The patient experiences shortness of breath, chest tightness, and wheezing. Severe hypoxemia and hypercarbia can manifest themselves rapidly.

Cardiovascular collapse is among the most severe clinical manifestations of anaphylaxis. The exact extent of fatal anaphylaxis is unknown, as anaphylaxis can be associated with myocardial ischemia and ventricular arrhythmias, each of which can cause or be caused by hypotension. Decreased blood pressure may be caused by diffuse peripheral vasodilatation due to release of vasodilatory mediators, decreased effective blood volume due to leakage of fluid into tissues, hypoxemia, or primary cardiac dysfunction.

Gastrointestinal manifestations can include nausea, vomiting, cramps, and diarrhea. Central nervous system abnormalities can include delirium and seizures, each of which may be due to hypoxemia and/or hypotension.

DIFFERENTIAL DIAGNOSIS. The diagnosis of systemic anaphylaxis may be obvious when there is a typical history of antecedent exposure to foreign antigenic material and a sequence of events consistent with the syndrome. Confirmation usually requires demonstration of IgE antibody to the substance by skin testing or by RAST (radioallergosorbent test). When the history is absent or when only a portion of the full syndrome is present, it may be difficult to exclude a vascular, cardiac, or neurologic disorder. Possibilities to be considered include acute myocardial infarction, pulmonary embolism, acute asthma, hereditary angioedema, cold urticaria, seizure disorder, anaphylactoid or idiosyncratic reaction, transfusion reaction, or vasovagal reaction. Vasovagal reactions may occur after an injection (e.g., penicillin, xylocaine) and include

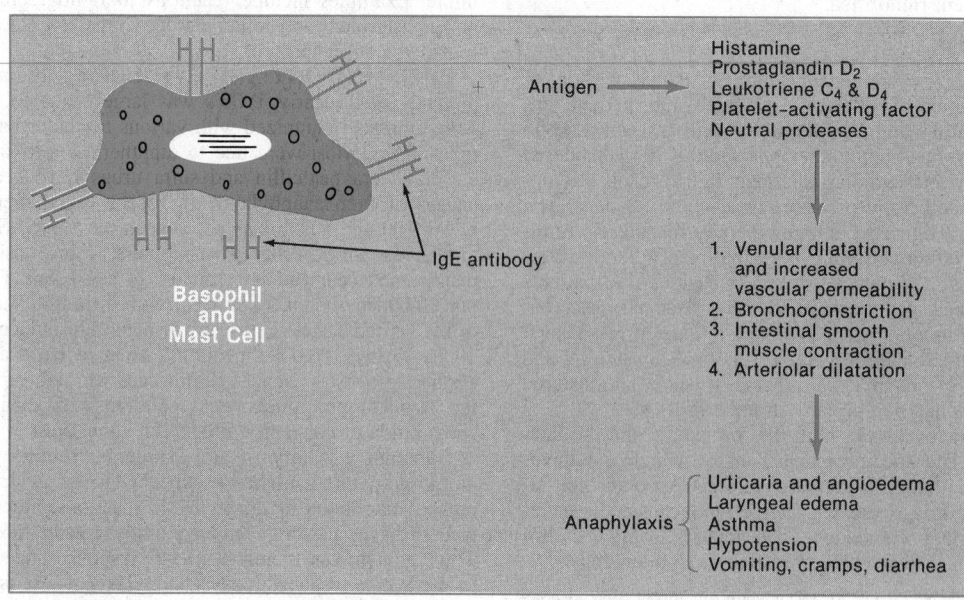

FIGURE 226–1. Acute anaphylaxis.

symptoms such as pallor, sweating, bradycardia, nausea, and hypotension, which can be confused with anaphylaxis. There is absence of any cutaneous manifestations or evidence of respiratory difficulty, and the diagnosis hinges on the cause of the hypotension. In such instances, skin testing is negative. Hereditary angioedema is due to absence or dysfunction of C1 inhibitor and is associated with laryngeal edema, peripheral angioedema, and acute abdominal pain. It is typically an autosomal dominant disorder with a family history or prior history of typical episodes. Trauma and infections may precipitate attacks of swelling. Patients with cold urticaria may have systemic symptoms due to water immersion such as while swimming; diffuse urticaria, angioedema, and hypotension may ensue. Anaphylactoid reactions can occur by substances causing direct nonimmune release of mast cell products (opiates, tubocurare, dextrans, sulfobromophthalein), which can cause urticaria, angioedema, chest tightness, wheezing, and hypotension. Aspirin and other nonsteroidal agents can cause upper and lower airway obstruction, urticaria, and/or angioedema with no IgE involvement. These agents all inhibit prostaglandin synthetase (cyclooxygenase). IgG–anti-IgA immune complexes may cause anaphylaxis-like symptoms when IgA-deficient patients receive blood. Complement activation appears to have a major role in such instances. Finally, radiocontrast media reactions occur in about 1% of studies that use them. The mechanism is unknown but may relate to their osmolarity. Newer agents seem to markedly diminish the incidence.

PATHOGENESIS. Antigenic induction of IgE formation requires antigenic processing (see Ch. 221) by dendrite cells or macrophages, T-cell help, and switching of B lymphocytes from IgG synthesis to IgE synthesis. Interleukin-4 may be critical for the latter switch and functions as a T-cell helper factor for IgE formation. Subsequent combination of antigen with IgE bound to high-affinity receptors on mast cells and basophils (see Fig. 225–2) causes secretion of a variety of vasoactive substances that may be responsible for the symptoms of anaphylaxis (Fig. 226–1). These include histamine, prostaglandin D_2, leukotrienes C_4 and D_4, and platelet-activating factor (PAF) (1-0-alkyl-2-sn-3 phosphorylcholine). Histamine is the major secretory product of basophils and mast cells. It causes venular and arterial vasodilation, increases vascular permeability, and causes a decrease in diastolic blood pressure when systemic levels of approximately 2.5 ng per milliliter are reached. Histamine has direct inotropic and chronotropic action when injected directly into cardiac muscle, effects that are prevented by H_1 plus H_2 receptor antagonists. Prostaglandin D_2 is synthesized by mast cells but not by basophils. It is a peripheral vasodilator. Leukotrienes C_4 and D_4 are produced by basophils and mast cells and profoundly constrict peripheral arterial and coronary circulations and cause bronchoconstriction and decreased dynamic compliance. They also cause venular dilation and increase vascular permeability. PAF is synthesized by mast cells but not basophils and causes venular dilatation and an increase in cutaneous vascular permeability. When infused into rabbits, it causes profound hypotension, increased pulmonary resistance, pulmonary hypertension, cardiac arrhythmias, and decreased lung compliance, all manifestations of anaphylaxis.

Bradykinin is a nine–amino acid peptide that may also contribute to the symptoms of anaphylaxis and is generated by kininogen cleaved by enzymes known as *kallikreins*. Kinins are peripheral vasodilators, cause systemic hypotension, and constrict coronary vessels. Basophils and mast cells have a kallikrein-like enzyme; organs containing glands (lung, nasal mucosa) secrete a tissue kallikrein that digests low molecular weight kininogen to release bradykinin. Plasma kinin formation is associated with contact activation of Hageman factor, conversion of plasma prekallikrein to kallikrein, and digestion of high molecular weight (HMW)-kininogen.

Anaphylaxis is associated with depletion of clotting Factors V, VII, and fibrinogen, activation of complement, and depletion of HMW-kininogen consistent with acute intravascular coagulation. Clotting defects such as a prolonged partial thromboplastin time are commonly seen. Activation or depletion of these proteins is likely caused by enzymes released from cells that include not only mast cells and basophils but also monocyte/macrophages, eosinophils, and platelets. The latter group of cells possess low-affinity receptors for IgE (CD23) which may mediate cell secretion upon contact with antigen. The participation of these cells in allergic reactions is an area of current investigation.

PREVENTION AND TREATMENT. Patients who have previously experienced anaphylactic episodes should wear a Medic-Alert bracelet and be instructed regarding the importance of relating details of their specific drug reactions before taking medications. The medical history and medical record must include not only the allergic history but a description of the associated symptoms. The physician must be aware of drugs containing cross-reacting antigens. For example, patients with allergy to sulfa-containing antibiotics should avoid other sulfa-containing substances such as chlorthiazide diuretics, furosemide, sulfonylureas, and dapsone.

There is a 15% incidence of a reaction if a cephalosporin is substituted for penicillin because they share the presence of a β-lactone ring. Reactions with second- and third-generation cephalosporins may also occur, but aztreonam is an exception.

When the patient has a history of drug allergy or of taking a drug suspected of causing a reaction, it is appropriate to substitute another non–cross-reacting therapeutic agent whenever possible. Penicillin causes more anaphylactic reactions than any other drug, yet the history of "allergy" is unreliable because close to 80% of patients with such a history have negative skin tests to the major determinant (penicillin polylysine) or a minor determinant mixture (penicillin, penicilloic acid, penicillioylamine) and can tolerate the drug with impunity. Anaphylaxis is highly associated with IgE antibody directed to these minor determinants. Thus, a negative skin test to the commercially available major determinant is insufficient testing to administer the drug given a positive history. The addition of testing for minor determinants with negative results renders anaphylaxis or even any allergic reaction rare indeed. The number of alternative antibiotics that can be used in place of penicillin is ever increasing, and avoidance, in the sensitive patient, is the best approach. Nevertheless, there are circumstances in which use of penicillin or other agents by a known or suspected sensitive patient is necessary. In this circumstance, the patient can be desensitized by gradually administering increasing concentration of the drug—first intradermally, then subcutaneously, and finally parenterally. Such a procedure should be carried out by experienced personnel in an intensive care unit setting in which anaphylactic reactions can be effectively treated.

When an anaphylactic reaction is encountered, epinephrine given early quickly reverses most manifestations. Administered at a 1:1,000 dilution (0.01 ml per kilogram with a maximum dose of 0.5 ml subcutaneously repeated every 20 minutes as necessary), it is initial treatment once an adequate airway is in place. Further exposure to the inducing substance should be limited. When an anaphylactic reaction is initiated by an injection into the arm or leg, a tourniquet may be applied to limit antigen absorption. In the case of a honeybee sting, care should be taken to remove the stinger without compressing the venom sac. Upper airway obstruction must be differentiated from asthma because laryngeal and epiglottic edema may require endotracheal intubation or emergency tracheostomy to provide an airway. Asthma can be treated with epinephrine, administering an inhaled β_2 sympathomimetic, and/or intravenous aminophylline at a 6 mg per kilogram loading dose over 20 to 30 minutes, followed by 0.5 to 1 mg per kilogram per hour.

If any respiratory, vascular, or cardiac complications occur, an intravenous line should be placed promptly and a sample of arterial blood obtained for pH, P_{O_2}, and P_{CO_2}. Supplemental oxygen should be given to reduce hypoxemia. Pulse, blood pressure, and respiratory rate are monitored, and an electrocardiogram is obtained. Hypovolemic shock requires rapid intravenous fluid administration. Additionally, 5 ml of a 1:10,000 solution of epinephrine repeated every 5 to 10 minutes can be given intravenously in severe shock. A vasopressor such as dopamine (2 to 20 μg per kilogram per minute) is indicated to manage hypotension unresponsive to volume expansion. This may increase cardiac output and improve blood flow to coronary, cerebral, renal, and mesenteric vascular beds. Higher doses of dopamine or norepinephrine yield significant α receptor stimulation, which may increase blood pressure but constrict distal vascular beds. In case of significant cardiac dysfunction, an arterial line and a Swan-Ganz catheter should be placed.

Giving antihistamines at the onset of the acute episode may relieve pruritus, urticaria, and angioedema. Once an intravenous line is placed, 50 to 100 mg of diphenhydramine can be given slowly as a bolus. An H_2-receptor blocker may aid in the therapy of hypotension. Corticosteroids have no value during the acute episode, yet steroids are often also administered intravenously. It takes many hours before their first effect is seen. Thus, administration of steroids helps treat protracted asthma and late reactions that can ensue 1 to 2 days beyond the initial insult.

Bochner BS, Lichtenstein LM: Anaphylaxis—current concepts. N Engl J Med 324:1785, 1991. *An additional review including approaches to therapy.*

Dattwyler R, Kaplan AP, Austen KF: Human anaphylaxis. *In* Kaplan AP (ed.): Allergy. New York, Churchill Livingstone, 1985, p 559. *A textbook review of etiology, pathogenesis, and therapy.*

Gold M, Swartz JS, Braude BM, et al.: Intraoperative anaphylaxis: An association with latex sensitivity. J Allergy Clin Immunol 87:662, 1991. *A description of an increasingly recognized cause of anaphylactic reactions—namely, exposure to latex products.*

Sampson HA, Mendelson L, Rosen JP: Fatal and near fatal anaphylactic reactions to foods in children and adolescents. N Engl J Med 327:380, 1992. *Description of dangerous anaphylactic reactions to foods in children describing course and confirmation with assay of tryptase.*

227 INSECT STING ALLERGY
Lawrence M. Lichtenstein

The stings of insects of the order Hymenoptera have long been recognized as a potential cause of severe, often life-threatening reactions in susceptible individuals. These reactions are unrelated to the toxic chemicals in the venoms, being due to allergic sensitization. Insect sting allergy has recently become the most intensely studied model of anaphylaxis in humans, resulting in important advances that have had rapid clinical applications.

EPIDEMIOLOGY. The incidence of immediate hypersensitivity to insect stings based on history is 3%; more than 20% of the population, however, has positive skin test reactions to insect venoms. Other allergies do not seem to predispose to insect sting sensitivity. The frequency varies with exposure and is therefore greater in children and males as well as those inclined to outdoor activities. Systemic reactions to insect stings cause few fatalities, but the morbidity, fear, and change in life style caused by these reactions is significant. A large number of people suffer prolonged and unusually severe local inflammatory reactions to insect stings, which are allergic in nature. As with other allergies, there appears to be an inherited predisposition, since multiple family members are often affected.

ETIOLOGY. The only insects possessing true stingers are those of the order Hymenoptera. There are two families of importance, the bees (honeybees, bumblebees) and the vespids (yellow jackets, hornets, wasps). The bees have barbed stingers that remain in the skin after a sting. Yellow jackets are the most common culprits, but honeybees are more commonly implicated in the western United States. Wasps are more common in the south central United States (especially Texas). Sensitivity develops to antigens in the insect venom, most of which have enzymatic activity. A major allergen in both insect families is phospholipase A, but they do not cross-react with one another.

PATHOGENESIS. The injection of foreign proteins commonly causes the production of specific antibodies of the IgE and IgG classes. Individuals may develop venom-specific IgE antibodies after any sting, this response sometimes persisting for less than 3 months and in other instances persisting for more than 25 years. Tissue mast cells and circulating basophils bind IgE antibody, thereby becoming sensitized so that a repeat encounter with the offending allergen triggers release of the mediators of anaphylaxis (see Ch. 51). The initiation and persistence of this sensitization are related to inheritable and other unknown determinants. Sensitization may occur at any time in life, even after many uneventful stings. The sensitizing sting itself causes no unusual reaction and is often so remote as to evade recollection.

Generalized mediator release from sensitized basophils and mast cells (see Table 231–2) causes the many manifestations of anaphylaxis. Localization of symptoms to specific target tissues is not well understood. The pathology observed in fatal cases includes upper airway edema and obstruction, the visceral consequences of hypotension, or occasionally no discernible abnormality (see Ch. 226 for a discussion of anaphylaxis).

Large local reactions are IgE dependent; their prolonged time-course is characteristic of the so-called late phase response to antigen. These reactions involve a cascade of events beginning with mediator release from mast cells and culminating with local inflammation involving many cell types and numerous mechanisms. The potential roles of eosinophils, basophils, lymphocytes, and cytokines and chemokines are being elucidated.

The venom-specific IgG antibody response to a sting is usually short lived, lasting only a few months. Repeated stings (as in beekeepers) are associated with high titers of IgG antibodies, which protect against allergic reactions. Beekeepers who do not have anaphylactic reactions have high IgG titers, as do affected individuals immunized with venoms. Passive transfer of these IgG antibodies protects sensitive patients from a sting. These protective antibodies are thought to block the allergic reaction by competing with IgE for the allergenic venom proteins and have therefore been termed "blocking" antibodies.

CLINICAL MANIFESTATIONS. Allergic reactions to insect stings are either generalized (systemic) or large local reactions. *Systemic sting reactions* present the classic manifestations of anaphylaxis described in Ch. 226. The observed frequency of the most common symptoms in adult patients is presented in Table 227–1. The risk of a fatal outcome increases, as might be expected, with age and the use of certain drugs, especially antagonists of β-adrenergic receptors. Fatal anaphylaxis may occur without a history of sting allergy.

The onset of systemic symptoms is rapid, within 2 to 3 minutes, and rarely occurs more than 30 minutes after a sting. Symptoms presenting hours later (except large local reactions) are not usually associated with immediate hypersensitivity or IgE antibodies. Unusual reactions such as vasculitis, nephropathies, encephalitis, and other neurologic manifestations have been reported, but no causal relationship has been established. Allergic respiratory symptoms may occur in beekeepers and their families owing to sensitization to the dust in the hives that contain bee body proteins. This sensitivity is unrelated to sting reactions.

Large local reactions are slow in onset and occur with or without concomitant early systemic reaction. The area of induration increases in size progressively for the first 24 to 48 hours and then resolves gradually over several days. These reactions may be so large as to immobilize an entire limb and are a significant cause of morbidity in sensitive individuals. Red streaks resembling lymphangitis may be observed and are often treated with antibiotics despite a lack of evidence for true cellulitis.

NATURAL HISTORY. The natural history of insect sting allergy has been incompletely documented. The prevalence of venom sensitization in the general population was noted above. It is estimated that about 20% of those at risk by virtue of positive skin tests (but with no history of a systemic reaction) will react on sting. There is considerable variability in the reaction to a sting among those who are clearly allergic as demonstrated by positive skin tests and a history of a previous reaction. Recent studies indicate that 25 to 60% of adults had a systemic reaction when stung by the appropriate insect. In children, on the other hand, a repeat sting causes a reaction in only 8%. The incidence in adolescents and young adults must lie between these extremes. This variability confounds the prediction of risk associated with sensitization.

Although many patients and physicians believe that allergic sting reactions become progressively more severe with every sting, this is not true. Most of those affected maintain a similar pattern of symptoms with every sting. Factors favoring a systemic reaction include

TABLE 227–1. SYMPTOMS REPORTED BY 245 PATIENTS

Symptom	Percentage
Cutaneous only	14
Urticaria-angioedema	78
Dizziness-hypotension	61
Dyspnea-wheezing	53
Throat tightness-hoarseness	40
Loss of consciousness	33

multiple stings, or stings in close temporal proximity (only weeks apart).

Sensitization generally decreases or disappears in time. This is far more common in children than in adults. However, resensitization has been observed upon re-sting.

DIAGNOSIS. The acute presentation of anaphylaxis is easily diagnosed by the presence of classic symptoms and signs. The insect sting may be inapparent. Differential diagnosis is more difficult in localized reactions such as acute chest pain and dyspnea or syncope without urticaria.

The diagnosis of insect sting allergy currently rests on a convincing history and positive skin tests. Demonstration *in vitro* of venom-specific IgE by the radioallergosorbent test (RAST) is less sensitive than skin tests but is equally accurate when positive.

Skin tests are performed intradermally with venoms diluted to concentrations in the range of 1 to 1000 ng per milliliter. Five venoms are used: honeybee (HB), yellow jacket (YJ), yellow hornet (YH), white-faced hornet (WH), and *Polistes* wasp (POL). Positive intradermal skin tests, a wheal >5 mm in diameter with at least 20 mm of erythema, develops within 20 minutes. The degree of skin test sensitivity does not correlate with clinical sensitivity. Within a few months after a systemic sting reaction, skin tests are almost uniformly positive. Stings more remote in time are more commonly associated with an apparent loss of sensitivity (similar to the situation in penicillin-related anaphylaxis).

Honeybee venom sensitivity occurs independent of other venom allergies, but about 10% of patients are sensitive to both bee and vespid venoms. The vespid venoms are highly cross-reactive, so that almost all vespid-sensitive patients have positive YJ, YH, and WH skin tests even though most have been stung only by YJs. Half of these patients are also sensitive to POL venom. Very few individuals are allergic to only one or two of the vespid venoms. *In vitro* RAST inhibition techniques are useful to distinguish cross-reactivity from specific sensitivity. This is clinically relevant in patients with a positive skin test to *Polistes,* which is often due to cross-reactivity, and the patient may be spared considerable expense and unnecessary immunization by RAST inhibition analysis.

TREATMENT. The treatment of choice for anaphylactic reactions is subcutaneous epinephrine 1:1000, 0.5 ml initially and repeated twice at 10-minute intervals, if necessary, to reverse the progression of symptoms. Antihistamines and glucocorticoids do not contribute to the management of life-threatening symptoms but may reduce the duration and severity of cutaneous manifestations. Their use should not be considered until the acute episode has ended. Intravenous volume expansion or airway maintenance may be necessary. In a few individuals, the process is resistant to epinephrine; in such instances an α-adrenergic agent (i.e., norepinephrine) may be tried. Affected persons not yet protected by immunotherapy are advised to carry, and are instructed in the use of, a kit containing a syringe device preloaded with one or two recommended doses of epinephrine.

Venom immunotherapy is successful in virtually all patients. Less than 2% of those immunized have any systemic symptoms after a challenge sting, and these are uniformly less severe than their previous reactions. The indications for venom immunotherapy are now based on an improved understanding of the natural history of the disease. Those with a history of life-threatening reactions should be treated. The risk of progression from strictly cutaneous to life-threatening respiratory or vascular reactions is rare (<1%) in adults and children. Cutaneous reactors who are more likely to be stung in their daily activities or who for a variety of reasons (location, age, cardiovascular disease) can ill afford a reaction should be treated. The cost and inconvenience of treatment may deter other cutaneous reactors from undergoing immunotherapy. Children, much more commonly than adults, have cutaneous symptoms only. These children may be left untreated. Venom immunotherapy is usually contraindicated in the absence of positive venom skin tests or RAST. Although there are rare individuals who are sensitive without positive tests, treatment is currently recommended using all venoms that cause a positive skin test (for *Polistes,* see above). While other mechanisms may contribute, the induction of increased serum levels of venom-specific IgG antibodies is the most apparent mechanism of protection for venom immunotherapy; <3 μg per milliliter is associated with increased risk of sting anaphylaxis. In many European centers, the patient is re-stung in the hospital before therapy is begun.

Rapid immunization in six to eight weekly visits is recommended, since it is associated with a significantly greater and more rapid immune response and with fewer adverse reactions than a slower (>20 weeks) regimen. The maintenance dose of 100 μg of each venom is repeated monthly for at least 6 months, and is then continued at 6- to 8-week intervals for 5 years. If treatment is interrupted for more than 3 months, it is likely that protection will diminish to inadequate levels. Loss of venom sensitivity during maintenance immunotherapy occurs in some patients during the first 3 to 5 years of treatment. Skin tests should, therefore, be repeated every 2 years. After 5 years it appears that patients can stop therapy and suffer a sting without serious sequelae. Possible exceptions include patients with extremely severe reactions or those with complicating medical conditions. After stopping venom immunotherapy, venom sensitivity continues to decline and is not increased even after stings.

Adverse reactions to venom immunotherapy may be early or late. Immediate reactions include all the manifestations of anaphylaxis. During the initial course of treatment, 10 to 15% of patients report systemic complaints, only half of which require epinephrine. At maintenance doses, systemic reactions occur rarely. After a systemic reaction, the dose should be reduced by up to 50% on the subsequent visit and then increased gradually toward 100 μg again.

Large local reactions occur frequently—50% of treated patients experience at least one such reaction. These occur after 10 of every 100 injections in the induction phase, most commonly in the midrange of doses (10 to 50 μg) and much less often at maintenance doses. Large local reactions do not presage systemic reactions and require a reduction of dose only for the most severe reactions. Long-term side effects have not been observed with venom immunotherapy or in beekeepers stung frequently for over 30 years.

Golden DBK, Addison BI, Gadde J, et al.: Prospective observations on patients who discontinue Hymenoptera venom immunotherapy. J Allerg Clin Immunol 88:162, 1989. *Studies of when and how to discontinue venom immunotherapy.*

Golden DBK, Lawrence ID, Hamilton RH, et al.: Clinical correlation of the venom-specific IgG antibody level during maintenance venom immunotherapy. J Aller Clin Immunol 90:386, 1992. *The relevance of IgG "blocking" antibodies in venom immunotherapy.*

Golden DBK, Marsh DG, Kagey-Sobotka A, et al.: Epidemiology of insect sting allergy. JAMA 262:240, 1989. *A review of diagnostic and therapeutic problems in insect allergy.*

Hunt KJ, Valentine MD, Sobotka AK, et al.: A controlled trial of immunotherapy in insect hypersensitivity. N Engl J Med 299:157, 1978. *A comparison of venom immunotherapy with whole body extract and placebo. Demonstrates efficacy of venom therapy and the clinical consequences of challenge stings.*

Valentine MD, Schuberth KC, Kagey-Sobotka A, et al.: The value of immunotherapy with venom in children with allergy to insect stings. N Engl J Med 323:1601, 1990. *A prospective study of the epidemiology and immunology of insect sting allergy in children, indicating that repeat reactions are rare and virtually never of increased severity.*

228 IMMUNE COMPLEX DISEASES

Richard D. deShazo

DEFINITION. Immune complex diseases are a group of conditions resulting from inflammation induced in tissues where immune complexes are formed or deposited. Clinical consequences may be local when immune complexes form in the tissues of a specific organ or systemic when complexes circulate and deposit widely. A variety of antigens have been associated with the induction of immune complex disease in humans (Table 228–1) (see Ch. 221).

PATHOPHYSIOLOGY. In their studies, von Pirquet and Schick observed that some children developed a "serumkranheit" (serum sickness) 1 to 2 weeks after being injected subcutaneously with horse-derived diphtheria antiserum. The syndrome is characterized by fever, lymphadenopathy, arthralgias or arthritis, leukopenia, proteinuria, and cutaneous findings including urticaria. They postulated that the illness was caused by newly formed host antibody reacting to horse serum and resulting in the deposition of antigen-antibody

TABLE 228-1. REPRESENTATIVE ANTIGENS KNOWN TO CAUSE IMMUNE COMPLEX DISEASE IN HUMANS

Antigens	Syndrome
Therapeutic Agents	
Horse serum products: antilymphocyte globulin, snake venom antiserum, streptokinase, monoclonal antibody products	Serum sickness
Drugs: cephalosporins, penicillin, amoxicillin, trimethoprim-sulfamethoxazole, fluoxetine, iron-dextran, carbamazepine, and others	
Drugs: quinidine, chlorpromazine, sulfonamides	Hemolytic anemia (innocent bystander reaction)
Autologous (self) Antigens	
DNA	Vasculitis and glomerulonephritis of systemic lupus erythematosus
IgG, IgM	Vasculitis of rheumatoid arthritis and mixed cryoglobulinemia
Tumor antigens: Colon carcinoma (carcinoembryonic antigen)	Glomerulonephritis
Microbial Antigens	
Hepatitis B	Systemic vasculitis
Plasmodium malariae	
Schistosoma mansoni	Glomerulonephritis
β-Hemolytic streptococci	
Staphylococcus epidermidis	

complexes in tissue. Much later, Germuth and Dixon developed rabbit models of serum sickness that confirmed this hypothesis.

In the model of acute serum sickness, rabbits receive a single injection of radiolabeled foreign serum, e.g., bovine serum albumin. Initially, levels of antigen measured in the serum decrease rapidly as the antigen equilibrates in the animal's intravascular and extravascular fluid compartments over several days. Thereafter, serum antigen concentration falls at a steady rate associated with degradation. About 10 to 12 days after injection, there is a second rapid decrease in the concentration of free antigen in the serum. This coincides with the development of host antibody to the antigen and the formation and clearance of antigen-containing immune complexes by the reticuloendothelial system. At this time, serum complement levels drop, proteinuria develops, and histopathologic studies show inflammation in the rabbit's glomeruli, synovium, and arteries. Host immunoglobulin, complement, and antigen are deposited in a granular pattern along the glomerular basement membrane and near the internal elastic lamina of the coronary arteries. These findings occur when immune complexes of relatively high weight ($>19S$) are present in serum and resolve rapidly after these complexes are no longer detectable. If additional doses of antigen are given, chronic symptoms develop.

The relative amounts of antigen and antibody detectable in this model of serum sickness form a "precipitin curve" (Fig. 228–1). The curve may be divided into zones of "free antigen" on the left, "equivalence" in the center, and "antibody excess" on the right. In antigen excess, the very small antigen complexes produced ($Ag_1 : Ab_{1-3}$) do not activate complement or induce inflammation. In antibody excess, the very large complexes present have difficulty diffusing across the endothelial barrier and are rapidly cleared by the reticuloendothelial system. Near the point of equivalence and in the area of slight antigen excess, little if any noncomplexed antigen or antibody is detectable and intermediate-size ($Ag_{2-3} : Ab_{2-6}$) ($>19S$) soluble immune complexes circulate. At this point, a lattice of antigen and antibody molecules forms. This results from noncovalent bonding between antigen and antibody and between Fc portions of adjacent antibody molecules. The structure of this lattice depends on the valence of the antibody and the number of antigenic determinants on the antigen. In general, low-affinity antibodies form smaller immune complexes than do higher affinity antibodies.

BIOLOGIC PROPERTIES OF IMMUNE COMPLEXES. The biologic properties of antigen-antibody complexes depend on the nature of the antibodies and the degree of lattice formed and include (1) their ability to activate the complement system, (2) their ability to interact with cell receptors, and (3) their propensity to deposit in tissues.

Immune complexes may fix complement by either the classic or alternate complement pathway (see Ch. 222). Immune complexes that contain antibodies of the IgG (usually IgG_1 or IgG_3) or IgM class in an appropriate lattice structure activate the classic complement pathway by binding C1q, the first subunit of the first component of complement. Antibodies of the IgG_4 subclass are less efficient at activating complement than those of the other three subclasses. Immune complexes containing IgA may activate the alternate complement pathway but not the classic one.

Phagocytic cells and certain lymphocytes possess receptors for antibody molecules. Of these, the Fcγ receptors on these cells react with IgG molecules. The Kupffer cells of the liver possess a specific type of Fcγ receptor (Fcγ RIII), which helps remove IgG-containing immune complexes from the serum. Very large latticed immune complexes containing IgG may bind to this Fcγ receptor without activating complement. Once bound, they condense or rearrange to form even larger lattices that are phagocytosed.

Human erythrocytes have receptors for C3b, called *complement receptor type I* (CR1). The CR1 binds to immune complexes that contain molecules of C3b, iC3b, or C4b. When these erythrocytes circulate through the liver, the Kupffer cells effectively remove the

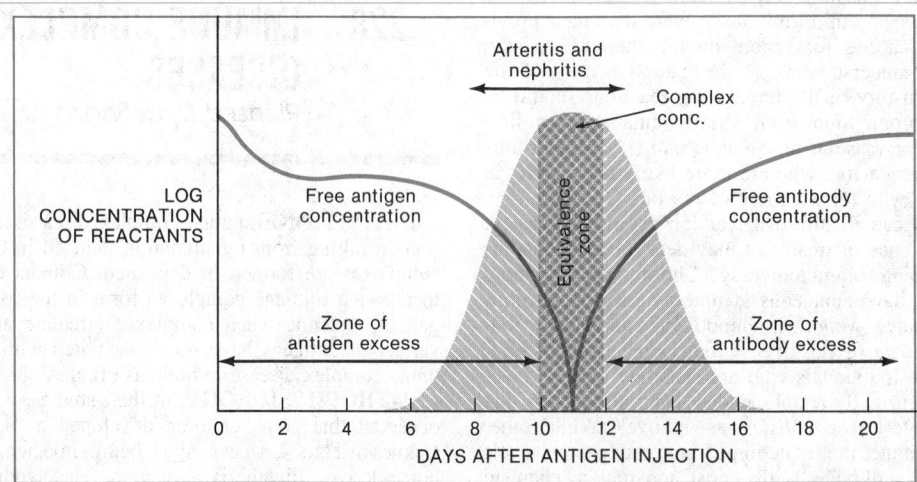

FIGURE 228-1. Natural history of acute serum sickness in rabbits following a single injection of radiolabeled bovine serum albumin (BSA) as antigen. The disease occurs when large quantities of soluble immune complexes are present in the circulation. (From Rich RR: Immune Complex Diseases. *In* Wyngaarden JB, Smith LH Jr, Bennett JC [eds.]: Cecil Textbook of Medicine. 19th ed. Philadelphia, WB Saunders, 1992, p 1468.)

large, complement-containing immune complexes without damaging the erythrocytes. This is accomplished by using their Fc receptors, which have a greater affinity for the complexes than does CR1 (Fig. 228–2).

The fate of immunocomplexes that contain IgA is less clear in humans. In experimental animals, immune complexes containing eight or more IgA antibodies are rapidly taken up by the liver.

FACTORS AFFECTING HOW IMMUNE COMPLEXES DEPOSIT. Experimental studies suggest that a number of factors determine the fate of immune complexes. These include the lattice structure, the presence of complement in the complex, the characteristics of antibodies and antigen in the complex, the numbers and functions of receptors on reticuloendothelial and other cells, and the charge of the immune complex. So far as *antibodies* are concerned, positive charges seem to facilitate deposition of immune complexes in the glomeruli. Moreover, certain nonglomerular cationic antigens like DNA appear to bind to glomeruli. They then serve as a nidus for immune complexes to form locally and deposit in the subepithelial area of the glomerular capillary membrane. IgA nephropathy (see Ch. 87) is a condition in which IgA-containing immune complexes deposit in the glomeruli, resulting in a focal glomerulonephritis. This form of glomerulonephritis, often subsequent to an infectious illness, may reflect the less efficient clearance of IgA-containing immune complexes that are unable to activate the classic complement pathway.

In respect to *complement,* patients with systemic lupus erythematosus (SLE) (see Ch. 240) have fewer CR1 receptors for C3b on their erythrocytes, a factor that may predispose them to immune complex disease. The presence of complement deficiency syndromes (C1q, C1r, C1s, C4, C2, and C3) is associated with lupuslike syndromes. This reflects, in part, the fact that complement components are not only proinflammatory in immune complex disease but also can inhibit immune complex deposition and resolubilize complexes from their sites of deposition. For instance, C1q fixation by immune complexes inhibits Fc-Fc interactions between IgG molecules and inhibits complex precipitation. Complex formation is inhibited, and deposited complexes are solubilized by the co-valent attachment of C3b to antigen-antibody complexes. That Fc receptors can bind immune complexes to reticuloendothelial cells appears to influence their rate of clearance. In immune complex disease, Fc receptor function is often diminished. Finally, certain cells have receptors that facilitate interaction with immune complexes. Glomerular epithelium has receptors for C3; endothelial cells have receptors for C1q; renal interstitial cells, damaged endothelial cells, and platelets have Fc receptors.

INDUCTION OF INFLAMMATION BY IMMUNE COMPLEXES. Inflammation associated with immune complexes results when circulating phagocytic cells move into tissue sites where the complexes deposit. This movement is influenced by several processes. Tissue mast cells release vasoactive amines after antigen reacts with IgE or on contact with the anaphylatoxins C3a and C3b. These amines increase vascular permeability, which facilitates the movement of phagocytes responding to the chemotactic and adhesion-promoting factors, including C5a, that are released when immune complexes activate complement. This may explain why antihistamines may attenuate some of the cutaneous findings in experimental and human serum sickness. Subsequently, immune complexes binding to neutrophils and/or monocytes by their C3b and Fcγ receptors result in cell activation and the phagocytosis of the immune complexes. The activated phagocytes degranulate and release proteolytic enzymes and oxygen-derived free radicals. Cellular damage and loss of blood to local tissues result, and ischemic injury follows.

IMMUNE COMPLEX DISEASES IN HUMANS. Serum sickness occurs in humans, and the clinical and laboratory findings are much like those seen in the rabbit model. This most commonly occurs after using horse serum products, including Antivenin, used to treat rattlesnake bites, and antithymocyte globulin, used to treat aplastic anemia. The first sign of the syndrome in patients with serum sickness from antithymocyte globulin is a curious band of erythema located laterally on the hands, feet, fingers, and toes. Circulating immune complexes and decreases in serum C3, C4, and CH50 concentrations occur at the time of symptoms of serum sickness. Serum sickness also occurs with certain drugs, including β-lactam antibiotics, sulfonamides, thiouracil, hydantoin, thiazide diuretics, and para-aminosalicylic acid. Patients develop fever, malaise, arthralgia and arthritis, abdominal pain sometimes associated with melena, and urticaria and/or urticarial vasculitis. Similar symptoms may be noted in patients with mixed cryoglobulinemia, rheumatoid arthritis with high titers of rheumatoid factor, and SLE with high titers of antibody to double-stranded DNA.

Another immune complex disease in humans is the syndrome of leukocytoclastic (hypersensitivity) vasculitis. It is associated with the characteristic physical finding of recurrent episodes of palpable purpura. Findings are usually, but not always, limited to the skin and may occur as a reaction to drugs or in association with specific infections like hepatitis B, in certain connective tissue diseases like SLE, in cryoglobulinemia, or for no distinguishable cause. The histopathologic feature of a predominant polymorphonuclear cell infiltrate in postcapillary venules is associated with "nuclear dust" from leukocytoclasis, endothelial cell damage and proliferation, and distal infarction of tissues. Subendothelial electron-dense deposits in postcapillary venules appear in association with circulating immune complexes, which are detectable in a high percentage of patients.

TESTS TO DETECT CIRCULATING IMMUNE COMPLEXES. No available laboratory test detects all circulating immune complexes. *Complement assays,* including CH50, C3, and C4, are depressed only when large quantities of immune complexes that activate the complement system are present. *Physical methods,* such as precipitation, are laborious because they require separating immune complexes from other serum components. Each physical method has problems specific to it; e.g., cryoprecipitation is not a property of all immune complexes. *Biologic methods* depend on the interaction of immune complexes with complement components or receptors on cells. The binding and subsequent precipitation of radiolabeled C1q with immune complexes by polyethylene glycol is a widely used method that detects as little as 10 μg of aggregated IgG. Conglutinin assays detect only those immune complexes that contain C3bi. The most commonly used assay for immune complexes employs lymphoblastoid B cells, called *Raji cells.* These cells were derived from a patient with Burkitt's lymphoma. They

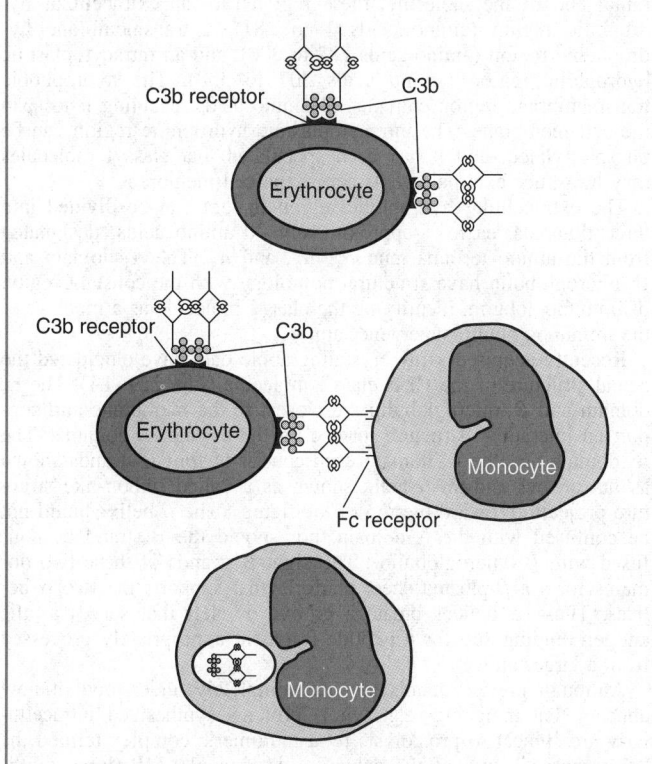

FIGURE 228–2. The role of hepatic mononuclear phagocytes (Kupffer cells) in removal of immune complexes from the circulation. Circulating complexes are bound to erythrocytes by the CR1 receptors for C3b. The complexes are removed from the erythrocytes by the Fc receptors of Kupffer cells, which have a greater affinity for the complexes. (From Virella G: Immunol Ser 58:379, 1993.)

lack surface immunoglobulins and have low-affinity receptors for IgG and high-affinity receptors for complement components.

Because immune complex assays are not antigen specific, they provide little insight into the cause of various immune complex diseases and do not provide a specific diagnosis. Some reports suggest that the presence of concentrations of immune complexes may correlate with the activity or prognosis of some diseases. Others suggest that they may be useful in the diagnosis of clinical diseases when immune complex deposition is a prominent component.

TREATMENT OF IMMUNE COMPLEX DISEASE. As with all diseases, the seriousness of the clinical syndrome determines the therapy. If the particular antigen that causes immune complex disease can be identified and avoided, for instance a drug, immune complex disease can be expected to resolve. When immune complex disease is a feature of an autoimmune disease such as SLE, controlling the disease with anti-inflammatory and/or immunosuppressive therapy usually resolves the related symptoms.

Serum sickness following drug therapy or therapeutic use of autologous serum proteins, such as rattlesnake horse antiserum, usually resolves spontaneously over 7 to 14 days. Symptoms usually respond to antihistamine therapy with or without corticosteroid treatment. Although controlled treatment studies are not available, moderate doses of prednisone (20 to 40 mg) given twice a day for 3 to 5 days followed by a tapering dose of corticosteroids over 10 to 14 days usually resolve symptoms in severe cases. The utility of plasmapheresis in immune complex disease is unproven.

Gauthier VJ, Abrass CK: Circulating immune complexes in renal injury. Semin Nephrol 12:379, 1992. *An extensive review of the mechanisms of immune complex–mediated renal disease.*

Hebert LA: The clearance of immune complexes from the circulation of man and other primates. Am J Kidney Dis 17:352, 1991. *A review of studies pertaining to the fate of immune complexes.*

Mannik M: Characteristics of immune complexes and principles of immune complex disease. *In* Arthritis and Allied Conditions: A Textbook of Rheumatology. 12th ed. Philadelphia, Lea & Febiger, 1993, p 495.

Virella G: Immune complex disease. Immunol Ser 58:379, 1993. *Two detailed reviews of the pathophysiology and clinical aspects of immune complex disease.*

229 THE MAJOR HISTOCOMPATIBILITY COMPLEX AND DISEASE SUSCEPTIBILITY

Benjamin D. Schwartz

The proper functioning of the immune system depends on its ability to distinguish "self" from "nonself." This crucial distinction is achieved via the molecules determined by the major histocompatibility complex (MHC), or HLA complex as it is known in humans. It is now clear that both foreign and self antigens are recognized by the T lymphocytes of the immune system only in conjunction with HLA molecules. During embryogenesis, a process of T-cell "education" takes place in the thymus whereby T cells recognizing self antigens (in the context of HLA molecules) are normally eliminated and T cells potentially capable of recognizing foreign antigens in the context of self HLA molecules are selected.

For a protein antigen to be recognized by the T lymphocytes of the immune system, it must undergo "processing." During processing, the protein is partially degraded into peptides, some of which are bound by HLA molecules. The peptide and HLA molecule form a complex that is the ligand recognized by the receptor on the T lymphocyte. There are two processing pathways used by the immune system. Intracellular antigens, such as viruses, are processed through the endogenous pathway and are presented by HLA class I molecules to CD8+ (generally cytotoxic) T lymphocytes. In contrast, extracellular antigens are processed through the exogenous pathway and are presented by HLA class II molecules to CD4+ (generally helper) T lymphocytes. Thus, HLA molecules are crucial in the recognition of antigen by the immune system.

HISTORY

The existence of a human MHC was first suggested in the mid 1950's when leukoagglutinating antibodies were discovered in the sera of multiparous women and multiply transfused leukopenic patients. Analysis of these sera indicated that these antisera were detecting alloantigens (i.e., antigens that were present on the cells of some individuals of a given species) which were the products of a polymorphic genetic locus. It was discovered shortly thereafter that these human leukocyte antigens (HLA) had a major role in determining the success of organ transplants, and this finding spurred the initial study of these antigens. In 1973, certain HLA antigens were found to be associated with specific diseases. In addition, at around the same time it was appreciated that the HLA complex regulates several aspects of the human immune response. These findings provided a second impetus for the study of the HLA complex. The application of molecular biology technology to the study of the HLA complex over the past 15 years has allowed additional HLA loci and alleles to be delineated and the sequence of many HLA genes to be determined. Most recently, x-ray crystallographic analysis of HLA molecules has allowed insight into their physiology. Together these findings have suggested how changes in the sequence of an HLA molecule may lead to predisposition to disease.

TISSUE DISTRIBUTION, FUNCTION, AND STRUCTURE

The HLA complex determines two distinct classes of cell surface glycoprotein molecules, designated class I and class II, with distinct structures, functions, and tissue distributions.

CLASS I MOLECULES. The HLA class I molecule consists of an HLA-encoded polymorphic glycoprotein of 44,000 molecular weight (MW) known as the heavy chain, in noncovalent association with a 12,000 MW nonpolymorphic protein known as β_2-microglobulin (Fig. 229–1A). The β_2-microglobulin is encoded by a gene on chromosome 15 and not by the HLA complex. The entire class I molecule is anchored in the cell membrane only by the heavy chain. This chain contains approximately 338 amino acids and can be divided into three regions. Starting from the amino terminal end of the molecule, these regions are an extracellular hydrophilic region (amino acids 1 to 281), a transmembrane hydrophobic region (amino acids 282 to 306), and an intracytoplasmic hydrophilic region (amino acids 307 to 338). The hydrophobic transmembrane region contains 24 amino acids, enabling it to span the cell membrane. The intracytoplasmic hydrophilic region can be phosphorylated, and it has been speculated that class I molecules may transduce external events across the cell membrane.

The extracellular hydrophilic region in turn can be divided into three domains, each of approximately 90 amino acids, designated from the amino terminal end α_1, α_2, and α_3. The α_3 domain and β_2-microglobulin have structural homology with the constant region of immunoglobulin, identifying the class I molecule as a member of the immunoglobulin supergene family.

Recently acquired x-ray crystallographic data have elucidated the actual structure of the HLA class I molecule (Fig. 229–1A). The α_3 domain and β_2-microglobulin are closest to the membrane and support an interactive structure formed by the α_1 and α_2 domains. The α_1 domain and the α_2 domain each consist of four β strands shown as flat arrows and an α helix shown as a coiled ribbon-like structure projecting toward the top of the figure. (The α helix should not be confused with the α domain, nor should the β strand be confused with β_2-microglobulin.) The eight β strands of these two domains form a β-pleated sheet platform that supports the two α helices. These α helices create a groove or cleft that serves as the antigen-binding site for a peptide fragment appropriately processed from a larger antigen.

Although precise details are not completely understood, it now appears that antigenic (e.g., viral) proteins synthesized intracellularly are subject to proteolysis by a multimeric complex termed the "proteasome." Two of the subunits, designated LMP (large multifunctional protease)-2 and LMP-7 proteins, are determined by genes within the HLA complex (see below). The resulting antigenic peptide fragments are then transported into the endoplasmic reticulum by a heterodimeric ATP-binding protein known as the transporter associated with antigen processing (TAP), whose subunits are determined by the TAP-1 and TAP-2 genes, also both within the HLA

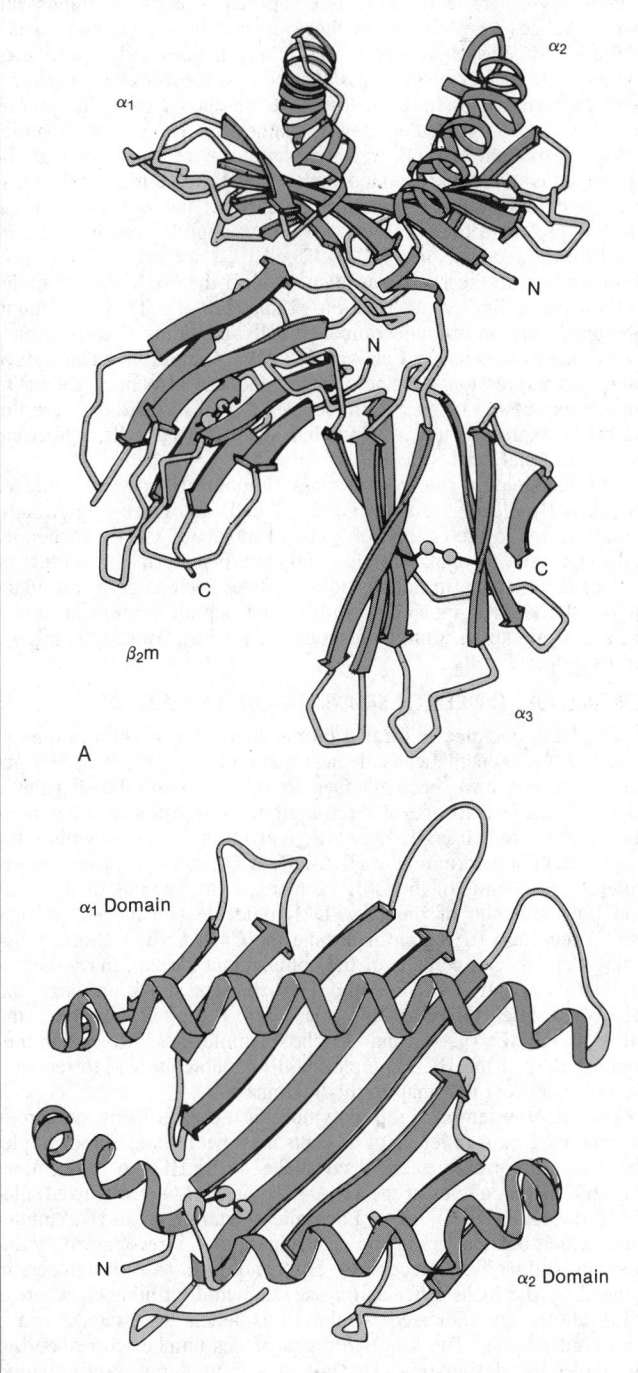

FIGURE 229–1. The HLA class I molecule crystal structure shown in both side view *(A)* and top view *(B)*. The molecule consists of an α chain which anchors the molecule in the membrane, noncovalently associated with β_2-microglobulin (β_2m). The α_1, α_2, and α_3 domains and β_2m are labeled. β strands are depicted as thick arrows in the amino to carboxy direction, and α helices are represented as helical ribbons. Connecting loops are shown as thin lines. Disulfide bonds are two connected spheres. *A,* Side view. The molecule is shown with the α_3 domain and β_2-microglobulin at the bottom, and the α_1 and α_2 domains at the top. The β-pleated sheet is seen edge on. The α helices form the cleft into which peptide can fit. *B,* Top view. The α_1 and α_2 domains are seen from above. The β-pleated sheet platform and the cleft formed by the α helices are again visible. (*A* and *B* adapted by permission from Nature, Vol 329, p 506. Copyright © 1987 Macmillan Magazines Limited.)

complex (see below). In general, antigenic peptide fragments of 8 to 9 amino acids bind to the HLA class I molecule while all components are still in the endoplasmic reticulum, and the binding of peptide is necessary for the class I molecule to be transported to the cell surface. Once at the cell surface, the two α helices of the class

TABLE 229–1. COMPARISON OF HLA CLASS I AND CLASS II MOLECULES

	Class I	Class II
Molecules included	HLA-A, B, C	HLA-DR, DQ, DP
Structure	44,000 MW heavy chain	~34,000 MW α chain
	12,000 MW β_2-microglobulin	~29,000 MW β chain
Tissue distribution	On virtually every cell	Normal limited to immunocompetent cells, particularly B cells, macrophages, activated T cells
Function	Bind and present antigenic peptides to CD8+ T cells	Bind and present antigenic peptides to CD4+ T cells

I molecule together with the bound antigenic fragment comprise the ligand recognized by the T-cell receptor on a CD8+ T cell.

A top view of the class I molecule as it would appear to the T-cell receptor of a CD8+ T lymphocyte is shown in Figure 229–1*B*. The β strands of the α_1 and α_2 domains form the floor of the cleft, and the α helices of the same domains form the sides of the cleft. The majority of alloantigenic determinants recognized both by antibodies and by T cells have been shown to be located in the α_1 and α_2 domains.

The HLA class I molecules have been divided into the classic (class I-a) molecules and the nonclassic (class I-b) molecules. The majority of our knowledge pertains to the class I-a molecules, which are designated HLA-A, -B, and -C. The class I-a molecules are found on virtually every human cell (Table 229–1). This tissue distribution is well suited to the physiologic role of the class I molecules to present foreign antigenic peptides such as viral antigenic peptides to cytotoxic T lymphocytes (CTL's). Precursors of CTL's are specific for a particular viral antigenic peptide in the context of a particular class I molecule. When the precursors encounter this particular combination of the viral antigenic peptide and the class I molecule, they proliferate and differentiate to mature CTL's. The mature CTL's are restricted in their killing to those target cells that bear both the same viral peptide and the same class I molecule as were present on the sensitizing cells. That particular CTL does not kill a target cell with the same class I molecule infected with a different virus; neither does it kill a target cell with a different class I molecule infected with the same virus. Thus, CTL killing is both antigen-specific and class I restricted. In the nonphysiologic situation of a tissue or organ graft, the class I molecules, with bound peptide, on the graft are the principal antigens recognized by the host's CTL's during graft rejection.

The HLA class I-b molecules include HLA-E, -F, and -G. These molecules are associated with β_2-microglobulin and have a similar structure to class I-a molecules, but their tissue distribution and function appear to be different. HLA-G is found on trophoblast cells and may play a role in maternal-fetal interactions during pregnancy. The function of other class I-b molecules is not entirely defined, but recent data indicate that they play a role in host defenses against prokaryotes.

CLASS II MOLECULES

Each class II molecule consists of two glycoprotein chains, an α chain of approximately 34,000 MW, and a β chain of approximately 29,000 MW. Both of the chains span the membrane and therefore serve to anchor the molecule. Each chain can be divided into three regions. Beginning at the amino terminal end, there is an extracellular hydrophilic region, a transmembrane hydrophobic region, and an intracytoplasmic hydrophilic tail. Each extracellular region has been further divided into two domains of approximately 90 amino acids each. For the α chain these are designated α_1 and α_2, and for the β chain, β_1 and β_2. The α_2 and β_2 domains, like the α_3 domain of the class I molecule and β_2-microglobulin, show homology with the constant region domain of immunoglobulin, thus indicating that class II molecules are also members of the immunoglobulin supergene family. The crystallographic structure of an

HLA class II molecule has recently been delineated (Figure 229–2) and confirms that the class II α_2 and β_2 domains comprise the portion of the molecule proximal to the cell membrane which supports the distal interactive portion formed by the α_1 and β_1 domains. Somewhat surprisingly, the crystal structure demonstrated dimers of class II molecules, suggesting that a tetramer may be the natural state of class II molecules in the cell membrane. However, the existence of such a tetramer *in vivo* has not yet been proven or refuted.

A top view of the class II α_1 and β_1 domains, as they would appear to the T-cell receptor on a CD4+ T lymphocyte, is shown in

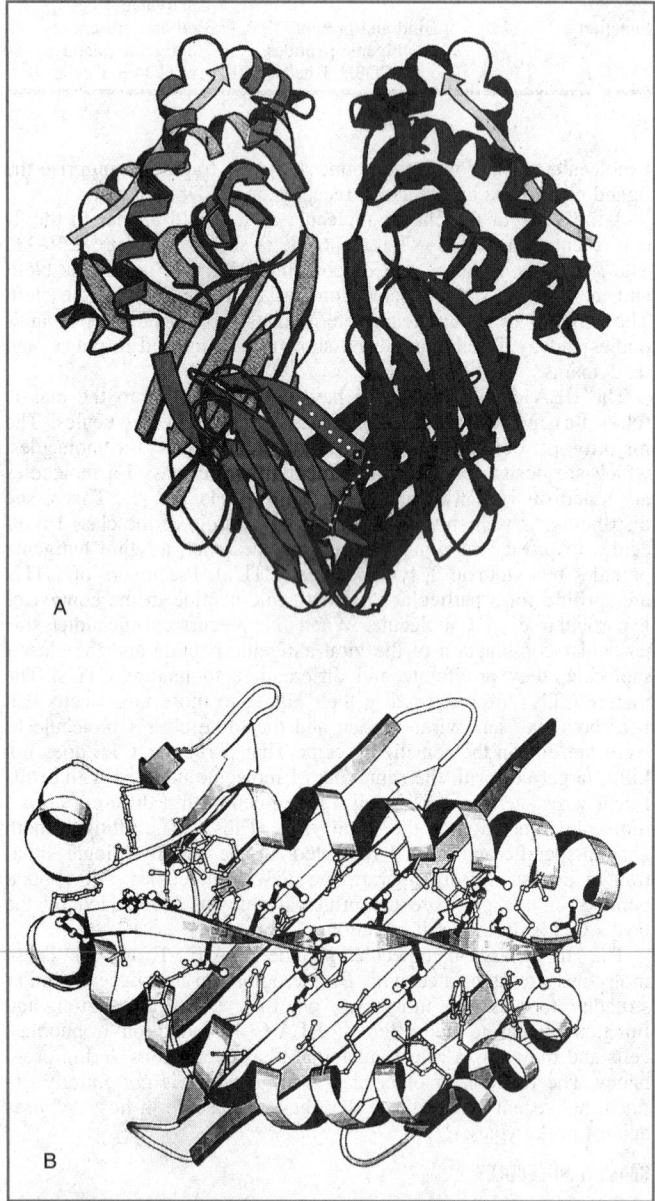

FIGURE 229–2. The HLA class II crystal structure shown in side *(A)* and top *(B)* views. The molecule consists of an α chain noncovalently associated with a β chain. Both chains anchor the molecule in the membrane. The α_1, α_2, β_1, and β_2 domains are indicated. The β strands are depicted as thick arrows in the amino to carboxy direction, and the α helices are represented as helical ribbons. *A,* The molecule is shown as a class II dimer (i.e., two class II molecules noncovalently associated), the form found in the crystal structure, although there is no evidence that this dimeric form does or does not exist *in vivo.* (In this view, the class II molecule is rotated approximately 90 degrees around the vertical axis from the side view shown of the class I molecule in Figure 229–1.) *B,* The cleft is very similar to that seen for the class I molecule. The α helices and a portion of the β-pleated sheet from the groove in which the peptide, shown as a twisted ribbon binds. (From Nature, Vol 364, p 33 Copyright © 1993, and Vol 368, p 215, Copyright © 1994, Macmillan Magazines Limited.)

Figure 229–2*B*. The structure is composed of eight β strands and two α helices very similar to those created by the α_1 and α_2 domains of the class I molecule. The two α helices and a portion of the β-pleated sheet of the class II molecule form a cleft or groove with characteristics similar to those of the class I cleft. In contrast to HLA class I molecules, newly synthesized HLA class II molecules are thought to bind processed antigenic peptides of 10 to 14 amino acids in an acidic endosomal compartment during their transport to the cell surface. On the cell surface, the α helices of the class II molecule together with the bound peptide constitute the ligand for the receptor on a CD4+ T cell.

In contrast to the HLA class I molecules, the HLA class II molecules have a limited distribution (Table 229–1). They are found predominantly on immunocompetent cells, including B cells, monocytes, dendritic cells, and activated T cells. Interferon-γ can induce increased expression on macrophages and has also been shown to induce expression of class II molecules on cells where they are not normally expressed, e.g., endothelial cells, thyroid cells, epidermal cells, and renal cells.

The physiologic role of the class II molecules parallels that of the class I molecules. Just as CD8+ T cells recognize foreign antigenic peptide in the context of a class I molecule, CD4+ (generally helper) T cells recognize foreign antigenic peptide in the context of a class II molecule. In nonphysiologic states such as graft transplantation, the class II molecules with bound peptide present on donor cells can initiate an immune response in the host by stimulating the host's helper T cells.

NOMENCLATURE AND GENETIC ORGANIZATION OF THE HLA COMPLEX

The HLA complex is located on the short arm of chromosome 6. Figure 229–3 schematically depicts many of the more than 100 genetic loci that have been mapped to this complex. These genetic loci are localized to one of three regions, designated in order from the centromere: class II, class III, and class I. Genes within the class II region determine the HLA-DR, -DQ, and -DP class II molecules, two subunits of the LMP complex, both subunits of the TAP, and both subunits of the HLA-DM molecule (see below). Genes within the class III region determine the C4A, C4B, C2, and properdin factor B components of the complement system, tumor necrosis factors α and β (TNF-α and TNF-β), heat shock proteins, and 21-hydroxylase. Genes within the class I region determine the HLA-A, -B, -C, -E, -F, and -G class I molecules. Molecular biologic studies of the HLA complex will undoubtedly lead to recognition of other loci that map to this region.

The HLA system is highly polymorphic. At each locus, numerous alternative forms (alleles) of a gene may be found. For example, there are 25 currently recognized alleles at the HLA-A locus, more than 60 distinct alleles at the HLA-B locus, and 60 recognized alleles at the HLA-DRB1 locus. Each allele determines an HLA molecule, which bears an antigenic determinant that is recognized by antibodies and/or T-cell receptors. HLA molecules are designated in general by the locus letter and a one- or two-digit number, whereas HLA alleles are indicated by the locus letter, an asterisk, and a four-digit number. The first two digits of this number correspond to the molecular designation. The last two digits allow discrimination among several distinct alleles that determine distinct molecules, all of which display a common antigenic determinant. Thus, for example, HLA-B27 refers to any of seven distinct HLA molecules, differing in 1 to 8 amino acids, all of which display the common antigenic determinant HLA-B27, but each of which is determined by a distinct allele, designated HLA-B*2701 through HLA-B*2707. A complete listing of the currently recognized HLA antigenic determinants is found in Table 229–2.

FIGURE 229–3. The current concept of the HLA complex, depicting the major HLA loci. The complex is divided into the class II, class III, and class I regions, in order, from the centromere, spanning approximately 4000 Kb. The designations of each region derive from the class of HLA genes that were first mapped to it. The types of loci are shown by different shadings. The insets indicate the different possible configurations of DRB genes and complement genes, respectively. (Adapted from Campbell RD, Trowsdale J: Map of the human major histocompatibility complex. Immunol Today 14:349, 1993.)

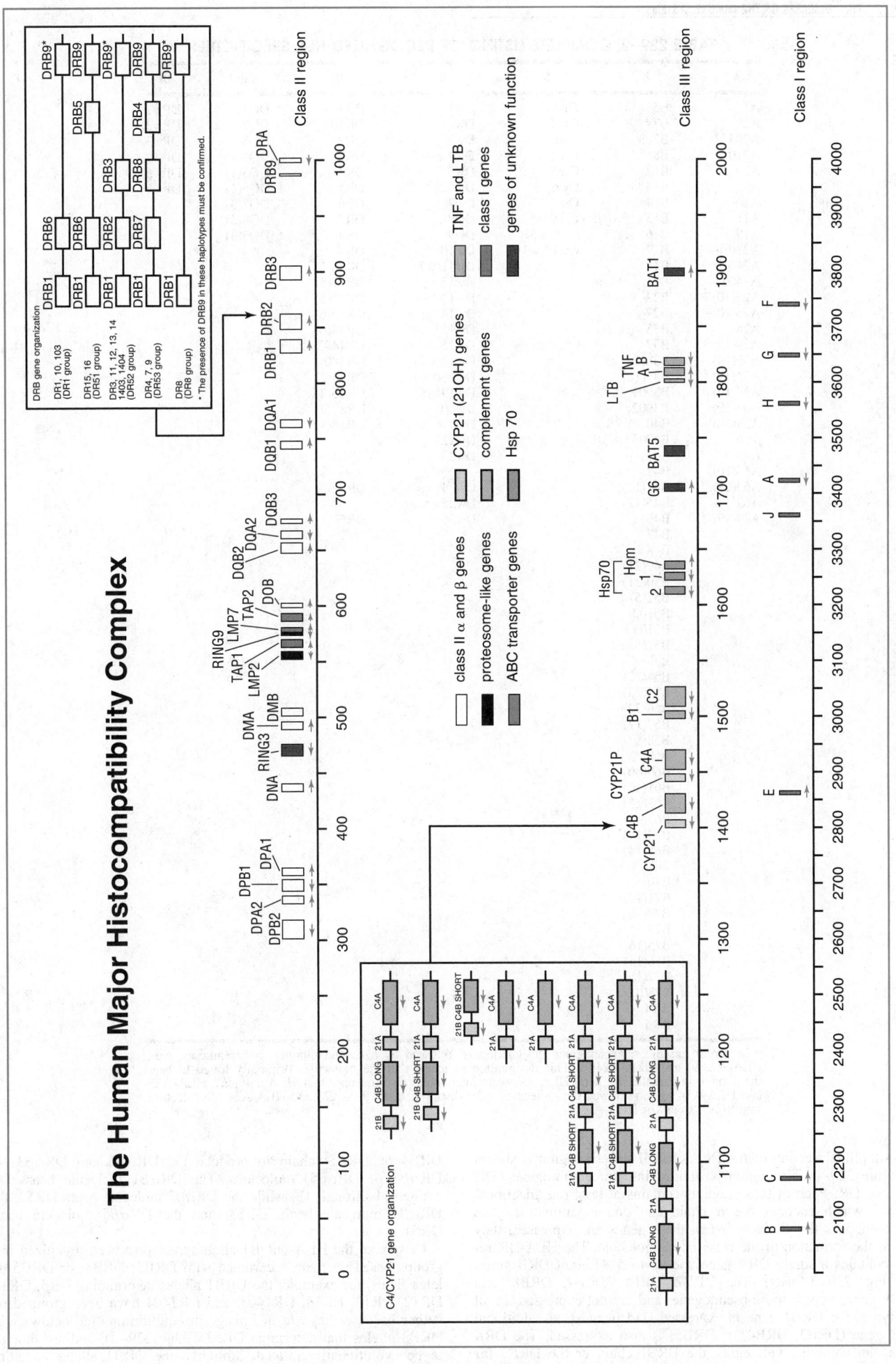

FIGURE 229–3 *See legend on opposite page*

TABLE 229–2. COMPLETE LISTING OF RECOGNIZED HLA SPECIFICITIES

A	B	C	D	DR	DQ	DP
A1	B5	Cw1	Dw1	DR1	DQ1	DPw1
A2	B7	Cw2	Dw2	DR103	DQ2	DPw2
A203	B703	Cw3	Dw3	DR2	DQ3	DPw3
A210	B8	Cw4	Dw4	DR3	DQ4	DPw4
A3	B12	Cw5	Dw5	DR4	DQ5(1)	DPw5
A9	B13	Cw6	Dw6	DR5	DQ6(1)	DPw6
A10	B14	Cw7	Dw7	DR6	DQ7(3)	
A11	B15	Cw8	Dw8	DR7	DQ8(3)	
A19	B16	Cw9(w3)	Dw9	DR8	DQ9(3)	
A23(9)	B17	Cw10(w3)	Dw10	DR9		
A24(9)	B18		Dw11(w7)	DR10		
A2403	B21		Dw12	DR11(5)		
A25(10)	B22		Dw13	DR12(5)		
A26(10)	B27		Dw14	DR13(6)		
A28	B35		Dw15	DR14(6)		
A29(19)	B37		Dw16	DR1403		
A30(19)	B38(16)		Dw17(w7)	DR1404		
A31(19)	B39(16)		Dw18(w6)	DR15(2)		
A32(19)	B3901		Dw19(w6)	DR16(2)		
A33(19)	B3902		Dw20	DR17(3)		
A34(10)	B40		Dw21	DR18(3)		
A36	B4005		Dw22			
A43	B41		Dw23	DR51		
A66(10)	B42					
A68(28)	B44(12)		Dw24	DR52		
A69	B45(12)		Dw25			
A74(19)	B46		Dw26	DR53		
	B47					
	B48					
	B49(21)					
	B50(21)					
	B51(5)					
	B5102					
	B5103					
	B52(5)					
	B53					
	B54(22)					
	B55(22)					
	B56(22)					
	B57(17)					
	B58(17)					
	B59					
	B60(40)					
	B61(40)					
	B62(15)					
	B63(15)					
	B64(14)					
	B65(14)					
	B67					
	B70					
	B71(70)					
	B72(70)					
	B73					
	B75(16)					
	B76(15)					
	B77(15)					
	B7801					
	Bw4					
	Bw6					

In certain instances, an antigenic designation is followed by a second number in parentheses, e.g., HLA-A23(9) and HLA-A24(9). This designation indicates that the molecules originally found to bear the antigen in parentheses, here, HLA-A9, were later found also to bear other HLA antigens, HLA-A23 and HLA-A24, which allowed the molecules to be distinguished. HLA-A23 and HLA-A24 are therefore said to be "splits" of HLA-A9.

A simplified version of the HLA class II genetic region is shown in Figure 229–4. The region is divided into three subregions: DP, DQ, and DR. Each of these regions contains at least one functional A gene which encodes the α chain and one functional B gene which encodes the β chain. When these genes are expressed, they lead to the formation of the class II $\alpha\beta$ molecule. The HLA-DR region contains a single DRA gene and up to 5 different DRB genes (see Fig. 229–3 inset). The DRB2, DRB6, DRB7, DRB8, and DRB9 genes appear to be pseudogenes and are not expressed. In all DR types, the DRB1 gene is expressed, and in most, an additional DRB gene (DRB3, DRB4, or DRB5) is also expressed. The DRα chain can combine with either the DRβ1 chain or the DRβ3 (or

DRβ4 or DRβ5) chain to produce the DR$\alpha\beta$1 and DR$\alpha\beta$3 (or DR$\alpha\beta$4 or DR$\alpha\beta$5) molecules. The DR$\alpha\beta$1 molecule bears DR antigens 1 through 18, while the DR$\alpha\beta$3 molecule bears DR52, the DR$\alpha\beta$4 molecule bears DR53, and the DR$\alpha\beta$5 molecule bears DR51.

Certain of the HLA-DR B1 allele types have been organized into groups based on their occurrence with DRB3, DRB4, or DRB5 alleles. Thus, for example, the DRB1 alleles determining DR3, DR11, DR12, DR13, DR14, DR1403, and DR1404 have been grouped together because they are in linkage disequilibrium (see below) with DRB3 alleles that determine DR52 (Table 229–3), and are thought to be evolutionarily related. Similarly, the DRB1 alleles encoding

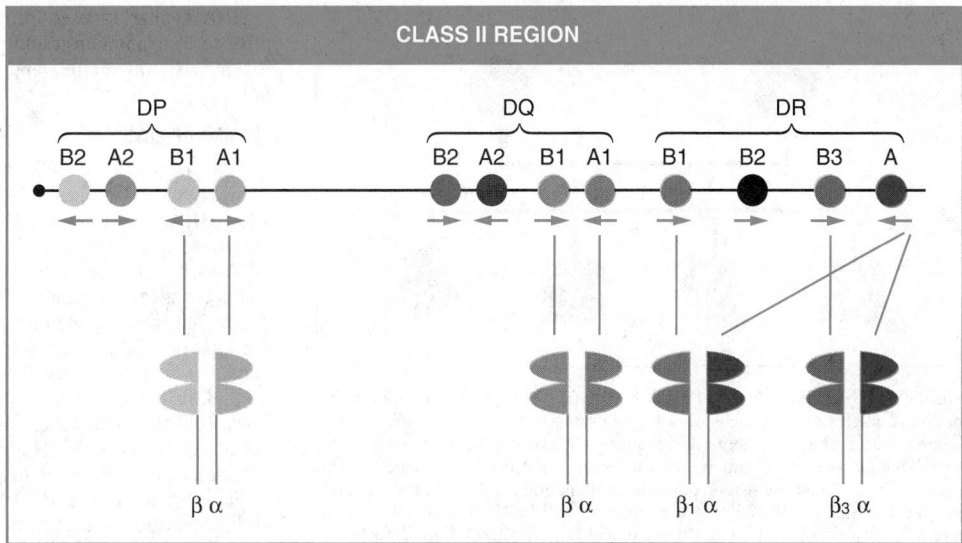

FIGURE 229–4. A simplified concept of the HLA-D region, showing the organization of the three subregions, DP, DQ, and DR. DPA2, DPB2, DQA2, DQB2, and DRB2 are pseudogenes and are not expressed. Pairs of expressed genes (DPA1 and DPB1; DQA1 and DQB1; DRA and DRB1; and DRA and DRB3) which encode class II molecules are indicated. (In other haplotypes, DRA and DRB4 or DRA and DRB5 would be the pair expressed in place of DRA and DRB3.) Arrows under genes give the direction of transcription (5′ to 3′).

DR4, DR7, and DR9 are grouped together because they are in linkage disequilibrium with DRB4 which encodes HLA-DR53, and are also evolutionarily related. Finally, the DRB1 alleles determining DR2 all are in linkage disequilibrium with DRB5. Linkage disequilibrium is also responsible for the association of particular DR antigens with particular DQ antigens (Table 229–4).

The DQ subregion contains two pairs of A and B genes. One pair, designated DQA2 and DQB2, are pseudogenes and are not expressed. The other pair, designated DQA1 and DQB1, are expressed and result in the formation of the DQ αβ molecule. Likewise, the DP subregion contains two pairs of A and B genes. One pair, designated DPA2 and DPB2, contain pseudogenes. The other pair, designated DPA1 and DPB1, encode the DPα and β chains that form the DPαβ molecule.

The polymorphism of the class II molecules (DR, DQ, and DP) varies somewhat for each set. For the DR molecules, the DRα chain is essentially nonpolymorphic between different DR types, whereas the DRβ chains are highly polymorphic. For the DQ molecules, both the DQα and DQβ chains demonstrate a high degree of polymorphism. For the DP molecules, the DPα chain shows relatively limited polymorphism, whereas the DPβ chains are again highly polymorphic.

Several additional genes have been mapped to the HLA class II region. These genes include the LMP (formerly low molecular weight polypeptide) genes, LMP-2 and LMP-7, which determine two subunits of the proteasome that digests protein antigens to peptides with the potential to bind to class I molecules; the TAP genes, TAP-1 and TAP-2, which encode proteins that transport proteasome-generated peptides from the cytoplasm to the endoplasmic reticulum; and the DMA and DMB genes, which are class II–like genes whose products have been implicated in processing antigen to peptides with the potential to bind to DR, DQ, and DP class II molecules.

It should be noted that there is no HLA-D locus or HLA-D molecule *per se*. The HLA-D antigens are defined and detected solely by a cellular reaction known as the mixed leukocyte reaction (MLR). Responder cells in the MLR appear to be detecting an array of antigenic determinants present on the HLA-DR, DQ, and/or DP molecules. In most cases, it is thought that antigenic determinants on HLA-DR molecules contribute most significantly to the MLR. As a result, HLA-D types tend to be most highly correlated with HLA-DR types.

HAPLOTYPE

Because of their close linkage, the alleles at each locus on a single chromosome are usually inherited in combination as a unit. This combination is referred to as the *haplotype*. Because each individual inherits one set of chromosomes from each parent, each individual has two HLA haplotypes. HLA genes are codominant; therefore, both alleles at a given HLA locus are expressed, and two complete sets of HLA antigens can be detected on cells. By simple mendelian genetics, there is a 25% chance that two siblings will share both haplotypes and be fully HLA compatible, a 50% chance that they will share one haplotype, and a 25% chance that they will share no haplotype and thus will be completely HLA incompatible (Fig. 229–5).

LINKAGE DISEQUILIBRIUM

Because of random matings, the frequency of finding a given allele at one HLA locus associated with a given allele at a second HLA locus should simply be the product of the frequencies of each allele in the population. However, certain combinations of alleles are found with a frequency greater than expected. This phenomenon is termed "linkage disequilibrium" and is quantitated as the difference (Δ) between the observed and expected frequencies. For example, the HLA-A*0101 allele, which determines HLA-A1, and the HLA-B*0801 allele, which determines HLA-B8, are found in the Caucasian population with frequencies of 0.161 and 0.104, respectively. Thus, the expected frequency with which the HLA-A*0101, B*0801 haplotype should be found is 0.161×0.104, or 0.0167. However, this haplotype is found with a frequency of approximately 0.0592, almost four times the expected frequency, for a $\Delta = 0.0592 - 0.0167 = 0.0425$. Table 229–5 lists some common exam-

TABLE 229–3. ASSOCIATIONS OF DRB1-ENCODED ANTIGENS WITH MOLECULES ENCODED BY DRB3, DRB4, OR DRB5 ALLELES

DRB3	DRB4	DRB5
DR3	DR4	DR15
DR5	DR7	DR16
DR6	DR9	
DR8		
DR11(5)		
DR12(5)		
DR13(6)		
DR14(6)		
DR17(3)		
DR18(3)		

TABLE 229–4. DQ ASSOCIATED HLA-DR ANTIGENS

HLA-DQ Antigens	Associated HLA-DR Antigens
DQ1	DR1, DR10, DR13(6), DR14(6), DR15(2), DR16(2)
DQ2	DR3, DR7
DQ3	DR4, DR7, DR9, DR11(5), DR12(5)
DQ4	DR8, DR15
DQ5	DR1, DR10, DR14(6), DR16(2)
DQ6	DR15(2), DR13(6)
DQ7	DR11(5), DR12(5), DR4
DQ8	DR4
DQ9	DR7, DR9

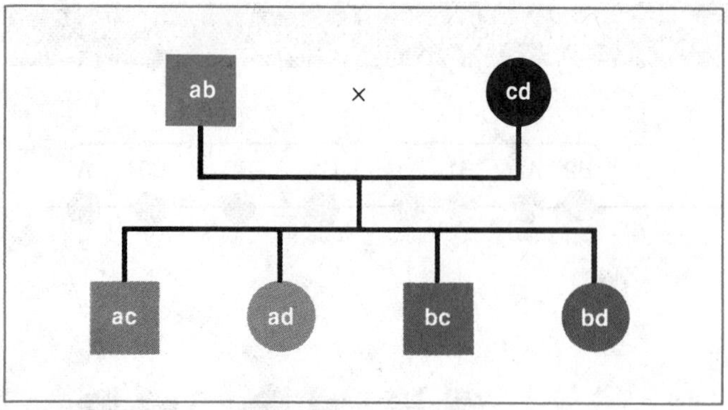

FIGURE 229–5. Inheritance of HLA haplotypes. A haplotype is the combination of alleles at each locus on a single chromosome and is almost always inherited as a unit. Haplotype designations are given by a, b, c, and d. Paternal haplotypes are a and b, and maternal haplotypes are c and d. The mating ab × cd can yield four possible combinations of haplotypes—ac, ad, bc, and bd. Statistically, 25% of the offspring will be HLA identical (e.g., ac and ac), 25% will be total HLA nonidentical (e.g., ac and bd), and 50% will be HLA-haploidentical (e.g., ac and ad).

ples of linkage disequilibrium. Several hypotheses have been put forth to explain linkage disequilibrium: (1) a selective advantage of a given haplotype, and (2) recent admixture of two inbred populations.

HLA TYPING

All HLA class I and class II antigens are present on the class I and class II molecules but are defined and detected by different methods. The HLA-A, -B, -C, -DR, and -DQ antigens are defined, detected, and typed serologically by the microlymphocytotoxicity assay. Although some monoclonal antibodies are available for particular HLA antigens, the majority of serologic typing is still done with sera obtained from multiparous women. Typing for the HLA class I antigens is done on purified populations of lymphocytes. Typing of the HLA-DR and -DQ class II antigens is performed on purified populations of B lymphocytes. Alternatively, a two-color dye procedure is used which allows B cells to be distinguished from T cells. HLA-DP antigens are defined and typed by a cellular reaction known as the primed lymphocyte test (PLT), but DP molecules can be detected by monoclonal antibodies. As noted above, HLA-D antigens are defined and typed by the mixed leukocyte reaction (MLR).

Molecular biologic techniques applied to HLA typing have made possible new and more precise methods. The most promising technique is the polymerase chain reaction (PCR) combined with oligonucleotide typing. The PCR is used to amplify the HLA gene(s) to be typed. Because each HLA allele has a unique nucleotide sequence that differentiates it from every other allele, it is possible to synthesize an oligonucleotide (or in some cases, a pair of oligonucleotides) which hybridize only to this unique sequence. A set of tagged oligonucleotides corresponding to various alleles can therefore be used for HLA typing at the DNA level. Oligonu-

TABLE 229–5. EXAMPLES OF LINKAGE DISEQUILIBRIUM IN CAUCASIANS

Haplotypes (listed as antigen phenotypes)	Δ (× 10⁻³)
HLA-A1, B8	53.2
HLA-A2, B44 (12)	14.8
HLA-A3, B7	32.4
HLA-B8, DR3	61.3
HLA-B7, DR2	36.8
HLA-DR2, DQ1	93.6
HLA-DR3, DQ2	37.4
HLA-DR7, DQ2	96.7
HLA-DR4, DQ3	87.5
HLA-A1, B8, DR3	28.0
HLA-A3, B7, DR2	11.5

cleotide typing is still in its infancy, and the vast majority of clinical HLA typing is currently done by conventional methodologies.

HLA typing is used primarily to determine HLA compatibility prior to transplantation and platelet transfusion, for paternity testing, for forensic medicine, and for establishing HLA disease associations.

HLA AND DISEASE

The discovery in 1973 that ankylosing spondylitis (see Ch. 238) is highly associated with HLA-B27 stimulated an intense search for other HLA-disease associations. Well over 100 diverse types of disease have now been associated with HLA. Despite this broad range, HLA-associated diseases for the most part share certain common characteristics. In general, these diseases have an hereditary tendency but weak penetrance and do not follow simple mendelian segregation. They lack a known causative agent and have an unknown pathophysiology. They are associated with immunologic abnormalities, and many of them are characterized as autoimmune. They follow subacute or chronic courses. Finally, they usually do not affect an individual's ability to bear offspring, thus allowing the HLA-associated diseases to persist.

The association of HLA and disease has been demonstrated by both population and family studies. These two types of studies provide different information. Population studies allow a statistically significant correlation between a particular HLA marker gene and a particular disease state. They do not constitute proof of genetic linkage between a disease susceptibility gene and the HLA marker gene because correlation does not necessarily imply genetic linkage. For example, if a disease susceptibility gene were not linked to HLA but required the presence of a particular HLA molecule for its expression, then an HLA-disease association would be demonstrated in population studies. In contrast, family studies provide an opportunity to determine linkage between a disease susceptibility gene and the HLA marker gene. Because population studies are easier to conduct, the majority of data on HLA and disease derives from this type of study.

It should be noted that no HLA-disease association is absolute. The majority of individuals with a given disease-associated HLA molecule do not contract the disease, and a given HLA-associated disease can occur in individuals who lack the usual disease-associated HLA molecule. It is now widely accepted that a combination of a particular HLA molecule, other genetic influences, and environmental agents is necessary for the disease to be manifest.

The strength of the association of a particular disease with a particular HLA molecule is quantitated by calculating the relative risk (Table 229–6). The relative risk (RR) is defined by the formula $RR = (P^+ \times C^-)/(P^- \times C^+)$, where P^+ is the number of patients possessing the disease-associated HLA molecule, C^- is the number of controls lacking that particular HLA molecule, P^- is the number of patients lacking that HLA molecule, and C^+ is the number of controls possessing that HLA molecule. The higher the relative risk above 1, the stronger the association between the HLA molecule and the disease. The relative risk can be stated as the chance of developing the HLA-associated disease for an individual with the disease-associated HLA molecule compared with an individual without that HLA molecule. Because there is usually a significant difference in the frequency of a given molecule among different racial groups, it is mandatory to compare a patient group with a control population of the same race. Thus, for example, HLA-B27 is found in 88% of American white patients with ankylosing spondylitis and approximately 8% of American white controls, yielding a relative risk of approximately 90. In contrast, HLA-B27 is found in 48% of American black patients with ankylosing spondylitis but in only 2% of American black controls, giving a relative risk of 37. Table 229–6 gives the relative risks for selected significant HLA-disease associations.

Because of the phenomenon of linkage disequilibrium and the order in which the HLA class I and class II molecules were defined, a particular disease may have appeared to be associated with a particular molecule determined by an allele at a given HLA locus when in actuality it is more highly associated with a particular molecule determined by an allele at a different HLA locus. Thus, for example, the alleles encoding HLA-DQ2, -DR3, and -B8 are known to be in linkage disequilibrium. Before any of the HLA class II molecules were well defined, celiac disease was associated with HLA-B8. The definition of the DR antigens allowed a stronger associa-

TABLE 230–4. β-LACTAM DESENSITIZATION

Penicillin Oral Desensitization Protocol*

Dose*	Penicillin V Elixir (U/ML)	Amount ML	Amount UNITS	Cumulative Dose (UNITS)
1	1000	0.1	100	100
2	1000	0.2	200	300
3	1000	0.4	400	700
4	1000	0.8	800	1500
5	1000	1.6	1600	3100
6	1000	3.2	3200	6300
7	1000	6.4	6400	12,700
8	10,000	1.2	12,000	24,700
9	10,000	2.4	24,000	48,700
10	10,000	4.8	48,000	96,700
11	80,000	1.0	80,000	176,700
12	80,000	2.0	160,000	336,700
13	80,000	4.0	320,000	656,700
14	80,000	8.0	640,000	1,296,700

Patients should be observed for 15 minutes between doses and for 30 minutes after the last dose prior to parenteral drug administration.

β-Lactam Intravenous Desensitization Protocol†

Dose No.	Concentration of Stock Solution (mg/ml)	Concentration of Infused Solution (mg/ml)	Amount of Antibiotic Administered (mg)
1	0.0005	0.00001	0.0005
2	0.005	0.0001	0.005
3	0.05	0.001	0.05
4	0.5	0.01	0.5
5	5	0.1	5
6	50	1	50
7	500	10	500

Stock solution is prepared by solubilizing the antibiotic with nonbacteriostatic saline to a final concentration of 500 mg/ml. Dilutions are prepared by adding 1 ml of each preceding dilution to 9 ml of diluent. One milliliter of stock solution is further diluted into 50 ml of saline and infused over 20 minutes.

* From Wendel GD Jr, Stark BJ, Jamison RB, et al.: Penicillin allergy and desensitization in serious infections during pregnancy. N Engl J Med 312:1229, 1985.

† From Borish L, Tamir R, Rosenwasser LJ: Intravenous desensitization to beta-lactam antibiotics. J Allergy Clin Immunol 80:314, 1987.

reported, and therapy with alternative ACE inhibitor drugs should not be attempted. The angioedema associated with these drugs is unrelated to ACE inhibitor–induced cough.

ASPIRIN AND OTHER NONSTEROIDAL ANTI-INFLAM-MATORY DRUGS (NSAID's) (see Ch. 19). Two to 6% of asthma patients have a history of aspirin-induced symptoms, and challenge studies have demonstrated airflow obstruction in up to 20% of unselected asthmatics. Asthma patients with chronic rhinosinusitis and nasal polyps are at particularly high risk for aspirin sensitivity. Aspirin can also cause symptom exacerbation in patients with chronic urticaria. Aspirin-sensitive patients with asthma or chronic urticaria also react to most other NSAID's. This cross-reactivity between drugs with chemically different structures and similar pharmacologic action suggests that these reactions are not immunologically mediated. The reactions in asthmatics may be related to inhibition of cyclo-oxygenase with concomitant enhancement of leukotriene synthesis or to hyperresponsiveness to leukotrienes, which are potent bronchoconstrictors (see Ch. 19 for a description of the pharmacologic actions of NSAID's). Desensitization regimens have been effective for patients with aspirin-induced bronchospasm and produce cross-desensitization to other NSAID's. For most sensitive asthma patients, aspirin and NSAID's are easily avoided. Patients with both asthma and chronic rhinosinusitis/polyposis should probably avoid these drugs regardless of past history of aspirin sensitivity. NSAID's have been associated with other idiosyncratic inflammatory reactions including acute aseptic meningitis and hypersensitivity pneumonitis.

DeSwarte RD: Drug allergy. In Patterson R, Grammer LC, Greenberger PA, Zeiss CR (eds.): Allergic Diseases Diagnosis and Management. 4th ed. Philadelphia, JB Lippincott, 1993, p 395. A comprehensive review with 621 references.

Shepherd GM: Allergy to β-lactam antibiotics. Immunol Allergy Clin North Am 11:611, 1991. A good review and one of several useful articles on this monograph on drug allergy.

231 MASTOCYTOSIS
Dean D. Metcalfe

Mastocytosis is a rare disease characterized by an abnormal increase in mast cells in the bone marrow, liver, spleen, lymph nodes, gastrointestinal tract, and skin. Mastocytosis may present in any age group and demonstrates a slight male predominance (1.5 : 1.0). The prevalence of the disease is unknown. Familial occurrence is unusual.

The disease is divided into four categories on the basis of clinical presentation, pathologic findings, and prognosis (Table 231–1). Patients in the first category have a good prognosis, whereas patients in the other three groups do poorly. *Indolent mastocytosis* is divided into two subgroups: those with isolated skin involvement and those with systemic disease. In most cases such patients gradually accrue more mast cells with progression of symptoms but can be managed successfully for decades using medications that provide symptomatic relief. The second most common form of mastocytosis is that associated with a *hematologic disorder,* in which examination of the bone marrow and peripheral blood reveals the hematologic abnormality. The prognosis in these patients is determined by the associated hematologic disorder. The third category of mast cell disease is *mast cell leukemia;* it is the rarest form and has the most fulminant behavior. Mast cell leukemia is distinguished by its unique pathologic and clinical picture. The peripheral blood smear shows immature mast cells. The fourth category of patients has an *aggressive form* of mastocytosis; these individuals experience a rapid increase in mast cell numbers and have poor prognostic features but do not have a distinctive hematologic disorder or mast cell leukemia.

ETIOLOGY AND PATHOGENESIS. Mast cells originate from pluripotent bone marrow stem cells and migrate through the bloodstream and lymphatics to specific sites, where they mature into fully granulated cells. The targeting of mast cells to defined locations is determined by the sequential expression of cell surface adhesion molecules. Mast cells are often found along endothelial and epithelial basement membrane, along nerves, and around glandular structures. Tissues at interfaces between the external and internal environment, i.e., the skin and gastrointestinal tract, are particularly rich in mast cells.

Mast cell number and differentiation are regulated by factors produced both in the hematopoietic marrow and by cells in the tissues in which mast cells finally reside. Early mast cell differentiation depends on the colony-stimulating factor interleukin-3 (IL-3) and is inhibited by granulocyte-macrophage colony-stimulating factor (GM-CSF). Final maturation depends on the production of specific growth factors by fibroblasts and stromal cells such as c-kit ligand, or stem cell factor.

Regardless of the cause of the increased burden of mast cells, the pathogenesis of the disease is largely the result of the increased pro-

TABLE 231–1. CLASSIFICATION OF MASTOCYTOSIS

Indolent mastocytosis
  Skin only
    Urticaria pigmentosa
    Diffuse cutaneous mastocytosis
  Systemic
    Marrow
    Gastrointestinal
    ± Urticaria pigmentosa
Mastocytosis with an associated hematologic disorder (± urticaria pigmentosa)
  Dysmyelopoietic syndrome
  Myeloproliferative disorders
  Acute nonlymphocytic leukemia
  Malignant lymphoma
  Chronic neutropenia
Mast cell leukemia
Aggressive mastocytosis

duction of mast cell mediators, which have effects both at the site of their production and at remote sites. Mast cell mediators are of three categories, all of which produce biologic effects typical of those observed in patients with mastocytosis (Table 231–2).

CLINICAL FEATURES. The categories of mastocytosis in general share similar clinical features, although some patterns of disease may predominate in a specific category. The skin, gastrointestinal tract, liver, spleen, lymph nodes, bone marrow, and skeletal system yield the most significant management problems. The respiratory tract and endocrine system are generally spared. Patients with mastocytosis do not suffer from recurrent infections.

The most common skin manifestation of mastocytosis is urticaria pigmentosa (Fig. 231–1). It is seen in >90% of patients with indolent mastocytosis and in <50% of patients with mastocytosis with an associated hematologic disorder or those with aggressive mastocytosis. The lesions of urticaria pigmentosa appear as scattered small reddish-brown macules or slightly raised papules. Scratching or rubbing the lesions usually causes urtication and erythema around the macules; this is known as Darier's sign. Urticaria pigmentosa is associated with pruritus, which may be exacerbated by changes in climatic temperature, skin friction, ingesting hot beverages or spicy foods, ethanol, and certain drugs. The diagnosis is confirmed by characteristic skin histopathology. Diffuse cutaneous mastocytosis consists of a diffuse mast cell infiltration of the skin. Solitary lesions called *mastocytomas* do occur but are quite rare. Young children with urticaria pigmentosa or diffuse cutaneous mastocytosis may have bullous eruptions.

Gastrointestinal disease often develops in patients with mastocytosis. The most common problem is gastric hypersecretion due to elevated plasma histamine with resultant gastritis and peptic ulcer disease. Diarrhea and abdominal pain are common and are followed by the onset of malabsorption in approximately one in three patients. Roentgenographic abnormalities fall into three major categories: peptic ulcers; abnormal mucosal patterns such as mucosal edema, multiple nodular lesions, coarsened mucosal folds, or multiple polyps; and motility disturbances. Histopathology of jejunal biopsies has shown moderate blunting of the villi; however, significant mast cell hyperplasia is uncommon.

Hepatic and splenic involvement in indolent systemic mastocytosis is relatively common, although liver function tests are usually normal. The most common chemical abnormality is an elevated alkaline phosphatase; this must be distinguished from bone-derived alkaline phosphatase, which may also be elevated. The most serious manifestation of hepatic and splenic involvement is portal hypertension and ascites associated with fibrosis of the liver and spleen. These conditions appear most commonly in patients who have mastocytosis with an associated hematologic disorder or in those with aggressive mastocytosis.

Bone marrow lesions consist of focal aggregates of spindle-shaped mast cells, often mixed with eosinophils, lymphocytes, and

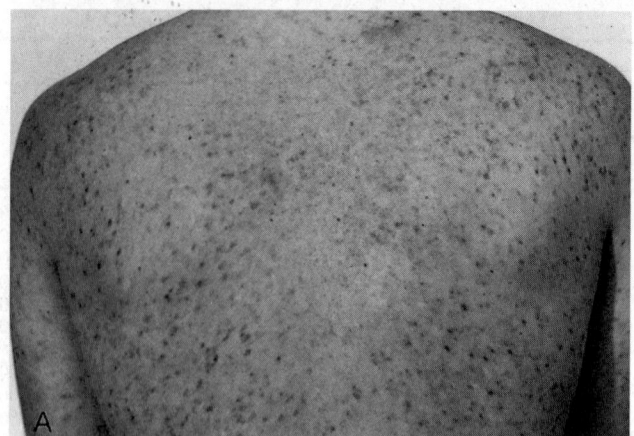
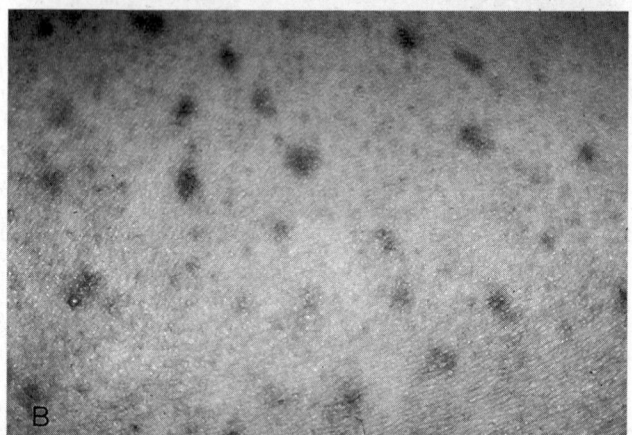

FIGURE 231–1. *A*, Urticaria pigmentosa in a patient with indolent systemic mastocytosis. *B*, Close-up view of urticaria pigmentosa.

occasional plasma cells, histiocytes, and fibroblasts (Fig. 231–2). Anemia, leukopenia, thrombocytopenia, and eosinophilia may occur in association with systemic disease. Bone marrow infiltration with mast cells may induce bone changes that cause radiographically detectable lesions in up to 70% of patients. The proximal long bones are most often affected, followed by the pelvis, ribs, and skull. Bone pain is the most common symptom and is present in 19 to 28% of patients. Skeletal scintigraphy (bone scans) is more sensitive than radiographic surveys in detecting and locating active lesions. In severe or advanced disease, pathologic fractures do occur.

Patients in every category of mastocytosis sometimes experience flushing or frank anaphylaxis. In occasional patients, anaphylaxis may be provoked by alcohol, aspirin, exercise, or infections.

Neuropsychiatric abnormalities have been reported. Problems include a decreased attention span, memory impairment, and irritability. Depression as a consequence of chronic disease or possibly mediated by mast cell products is a possibility.

DIAGNOSIS. The diagnosis of mastocytosis rests on histology, supported by clinical, biochemical, and radiographic data. Mast cells may be overlooked on histologic sections depending on the fixation and/or stain used. The most useful stains for mast cells include metachromatic stains, such as toluidine blue and Giemsa, and enzymatic stains, such as chloroacetate esterase and aminocaproate esterase. These procedures highlight the granules in the cytoplasm of the mast cell. In trephine core bone marrow biopsies, decalcification interferes with subsequent attempts to visualize mast cell granules.

The majority of patients with mastocytosis have urticaria pigmentosa. This diagnosis should be confirmed by skin biopsy. Blind skin biopsies are not recommended, as other skin conditions including eczema are associated with an increase in dermal mast cells.

In the absence of skin lesions, mastocytosis may be suspected in patients with one or several of the following: unexplained ulcer disease or malabsorption, radiographic or ^{99m}Tc bone scan abnormalities, hepatomegaly, splenomegaly, lymphadenopathy, peripheral blood abnormalities, and unexplained flushing or anaphylaxis. Ele-

TABLE 231–2. REPRESENTATIVE MAST CELL PRODUCTS AND THEIR BIOLOGIC EFFECTS

Granule-associated

Histamine	Pruritus, increased vasopermeability, gastric hypersecretion, bronchoconstriction
Heparin	Local anticoagulation
Tryptase, chymotryptic proteases	Degradation of local connective tissues

Lipid-derived

Sulfidopeptide leukotrienes	Increased vasopermeability, bronchoconstriction, vasoconstriction (LTC_4); increased vasopermeability, bronchoconstriction, vasodilation (LTD_4 and LTE_4)
Prostaglandin D_2	Vasodilation, bronchoconstriction
Platelet-activating factor	Increased vasopermeability, vasodilation, bronchoconstriction

Cytokines

Proinflammatory factors	Fibrosis (TGF-β); activation of vascular endothelial cells, cachexia (TNF-α); IgE synthesis (IL-4)
Growth enhancing	Colony-stimulating factor (IL-3); eosinophilia (IL-5)

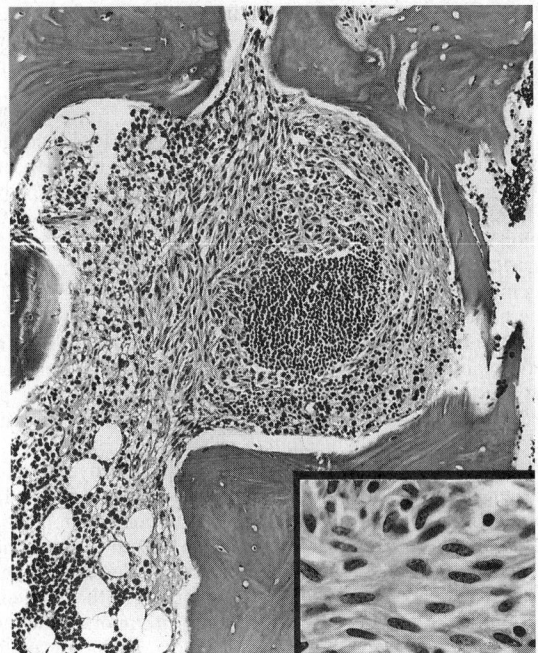

FIGURE 231–2. Bone marrow biopsy shows a characteristic lesion of systemic mastocytosis with nodular, paratrabecular infiltrate of mast cells surrounding a lymphoid aggregate. *Inset:* The mast cells are spindle-shaped, resembling fibroblasts or histiocytes. (Courtesy of W. D. Travis, Bethesda, MD.)

vated levels of plasma or urinary histamine or histamine metabolites, prostaglandin D_2 metabolites in the urine, or plasma mast cell tryptase are not diagnostic but do raise the index of suspicion of mastocytosis. Reliable tests for these substances, however, are not generally available except in research laboratories.

Patients suspected of having mastocytosis in the absence of skin lesions should have a bone marrow biopsy and aspirate for diagnosis. Patients with urticaria pigmentosa or diffuse cutaneous mastocytosis should also have this procedure if they have peripheral blood abnormalities, hepatomegaly, splenomegaly, or lymphadenopathy, to determine if they have an associated hematologic disorder. Other tissue specimens, such as lymph nodes, liver, and gastrointestinal mucosa, define the extent of mast cell involvement but are obtained only as necessary.

Patients suspected of having mastocytosis should have 24-hour urine 5-hydroxyindoleacetic acid (5-HIAA) measured to help eliminate the possibility of a carcinoid tumor. Patients with mastocytosis do not excrete increased amounts of 5-HIAA. Idiopathic anaphylaxis and flushing must also be considered. Patients with these disorders do not have histologic evidence of significant mast cell proliferation.

TREATMENT. In all categories of mastocytosis, a primary objective of treatment is to control mast cell mediator–induced signs and symptoms such as anaphylaxis, gastrointestinal cramping, and pruritus. H_1-receptor antagonists such as hydroxyzine and doxepin are helpful in reducing pruritus, flushing, and tachycardia. If insufficient relief occurs, adding an H_2 antagonist such as ranitidine or cimetidine may be beneficial. However, many patients continue to complain of bone pain, headaches, and flushing, resulting in part from the inability to block other mast cell mediators. Disodium cromoglycate (cromolyn sodium) inhibits degranulation of mast cells and may have some efficacy in the treatment of mastocytosis. Epinephrine is used to treat episodes of anaphylaxis. Patients should be prepared to self-administer this drug. If subcutaneous epinephrine is insufficient, intensive therapy for anaphylaxis should be instituted. Patients with recurrent episodes of anaphylaxis may be placed on H_1 and H_2 antihistamines to lessen the severity of attacks. Episodes of profound anaphylaxis may be spontaneous but have also been observed following stings from insects or administration of radiocontrast media.

Treatment of gastrointestinal disease is directed at controlling peptic symptoms, diarrhea, and malabsorption. Gastric acid hypersecretion leading to peptic symptoms and ulcerations is controlled with H_2 antagonists. Diarrhea is difficult to manage, and H_2 antagonists are generally not effective. Anticholinergics may give partial relief. In patients with severe malabsorption, systemic steroids have been shown to be effective. Ascites is also difficult to manage. One patient with portal hypertension was successfully managed with a portacaval shunt. Another patient with exudative ascites was treated successfully with systemic steroid therapy.

Patients with mastocytosis and an associated hematologic disorder are treated as dictated by the specific hematologic abnormality. In mast cell leukemia, chemotherapy has not yet been shown to produce remissions. Chemotherapy has no place in the treatment of indolent mastocytosis. A recent study suggested that splenectomy may improve survival in patients with poor prognostic forms of mastocytosis.

PROGNOSIS. Prognosis must be addressed separately for each category of mastocytosis. One study found seven variables that were strongly associated with poor survival. These included constitutional symptoms, anemia, thrombocytopenia, abnormal liver function tests, lobated mast cell nucleus, a low percentage of fat cells in the bone marrow biopsy, and an associated hematologic disorder. Other poor prognostic variables include absence of urticaria pimentosa, male gender, absence of skin and bone symptoms, hepatomegaly, splenomegaly, and normal bone radiographic findings.

As a group, patients with indolent mastocytosis and skin involvement alone have the best prognosis. Among children with isolated urticaria pigmentosa, at least 50% improve by adulthood. Adults with urticaria pigmentosa usually progress gradually to systemic disease and rarely may convert to type II disease. Diffuse cutaneous mastocytosis is usually associated with indolent systemic disease. Patients with mastocytosis with an associated hematologic disorder have a variable course, depending on the prognosis of their hematologic disorder. With mast cell leukemia, mean survival is less than 6 months. Survival with lymphadenopathic mastocytosis with eosinophilia is 2 to 3 years without therapy. The prognosis appears to improve with aggressive symptomatic management.

Cherner JA, Jensen RT, Dubois A, et al.: Gastrointestinal dysfunction in systemic mastocytosis: A prospective study. Gastroenterology 95:657, 1988. *Describes patterns of gastrointestinal disease in mastocytosis and the implications for clinical management.*

Garriga MM, Friedman MM, Metcalfe DD: A survey of the number and distribution of mast cells in the skin of patients with mast cell disorders. J Allergy Clin Immunol 82:425, 1988. *A study of the value of determining mast cell numbers in skin biopsies.*

Horny H-P, Kaiserling E, Campbell M, et al.: Liver findings in generalized mastocytosis: A clinicopathologic study. Cancer 63:532, 1989. *A survey of liver histopathology in mastocytosis.*

Lawrence JB, Friedman BS, Travis WD, et al.: Hematologic manifestations of systemic mast cell disease. A prospective study of laboratory and morphologic features and their relation to prognosis. Am J Med 91:612, 1991. *An excellent review of the histopathologic and clinical features of mastocytosis.*

Mekori YA, Oh CK, Metcalfe DD: IL-3–dependent murine mast cells undergo apoptosis on removal of IL-3. J. Immunol 151:3775, 1993.

Schwartz LB, Metcalfe DD, Miller JS, et al.: Tryptase levels as an indicator of mast cell activation in systemic anaphylaxis and mastocytosis. N Engl J Med 316:1622, 1987. *Demonstration of mast cell tryptase in the serum of mastocytosis patients.*

232 DISEASES OF THE THYMUS
Max D. Cooper

NORMAL DEVELOPMENT AND FUNCTION. The essential role of the thymus is to generate clonally diverse T lymphocytes that can recognize a vast array of foreign proteins presented as peptides on host cells. An essential parallel thymic function is eliminating self-reactive T-cell clones that could damage normal tissues.

The embryonic thymus is formed initially from epithelial cells lining the third and fourth pharyngeal pouches. These specialized epithelial cells migrate through the neck region to form bilateral thymic lobes in the upper anterior mediastinum. The epithelial thymus begins to attract hemopoietic stem cells from the circulation around the eighth week of fetal life. Within the thymus these precursor cells are influenced to proliferate and differentiate along T-lymphocyte lines. This lifelong process begins in the outer cortex of the thymus, and the immature thymocytes migrate toward the medullary region as they proliferate and mature. Cortical regions of the lobules that collectively form the bilateral thymic lobes thus become filled with immature T lymphocytes, the extraordinary clonal diversity of which is manifested by differences in their T-cell receptor (TCR) specificities. Each developing T cell is selected for survival or death depending on the affinity of its receptor for self-peptides, which are presented initially on the surface of cortical epithelial cells. As maturing thymocytes approach the corticomedullary junction, they encounter macrophages or dendritic cell immigrants that can also present peptide fragments of antigenic proteins. Thymocytes that fail to receive any TCR-mediated signal are programmed to die. Immature thymocytes also receive a death signal if their TCR has relatively high affinity for a self-peptide, whereas moderate affinity for a self-peptide selects for survival. Only 1% or so of the thymic T cells survive this selection process to seed the peripheral lymphoid tissues.

Thymocytes also possess an array of non-TCR cell surface glycoproteins that they use to interact with their environment. Progression of thymocyte maturation can be conveniently monitored by the expression of the CD4 and CD8 molecules. The most immature thymocytes lack detectable CD4 and CD8. Intermediate-stage thymocytes express both CD4 and CD8; these double-positives predominate in the thymic cortex. Clonal selection occurs during this stage of differentiation, and the CD4 and CD8 molecules play key roles in the selection process. The peptide fragments of antigenic proteins are presented within the α-helical grooves of the major histocompatibility complex (MHC) class II and class I molecules. CD4 has an affinity for MHC class II molecules on specialized antigen-presenting cells, whereas the CD8 molecules can bind class I molecules present on all nucleated cells. The CD4 or CD8 molecules thus serve as co-receptors in the positive clonal selection, which leads to the development of either mature CD4+ cells with helper potential or CD8+ T cells with cytotoxic potential. Most of the positively selected helper or cytotoxic T cells exit the thymus via the small blood vessels in the corticomedullary region, and only a few settle within the thymic medulla. The cellular debris of dying thymocytes is apparently swept up by macrophages, perhaps aided by the epithelial cell whirls called *Hassall's bodies* that are located in the thymic medulla.

The lymphoid thymus reaches its maximal size of approximately 30 grams by around age 1, and it gradually decreases in size thereafter to ≤3 grams in most older individuals. Because the thymus-derived T-cell clones may have lifespans of several decades, normally there is little need for constant thymic replenishment. Nevertheless, thymocyte differentiation persists throughout life, albeit usually at low levels, which may vary according to an individual's hormonal balance and need for T-cell replenishment.

DEVELOPMENTAL DEFECTS OF THE THYMUS. *DiGeorge syndrome,* also called the third and fourth pharyngeal pouch syndrome, features hypoplastic thymus and parathyroid development in addition to facial and cardiac abnormalities, which may include a ventricular septal defect and aortic abnormalities. DiGeorge syndrome occurs in both males and females, a majority of whom may have submicroscopic deletions of chromosome 22q11. The initial clinical manifestations are neonatal seizures due to hypocalcemia, or cyanosis and other signs of cardiac insufficiency. Immunodeficiency is a later manifestation, the severity of which depends on the degree of thymic hypoplasia. Most affected individuals have a small ectopic but functionally normal thymus that can seed T cells to the periphery in numbers that may or may not be sufficient for immune defense. In rare instances, affected infants have no detectable thymus or peripheral T cells, and thymic transplantation must be considered in these cases. Thymic grafts and all blood products given to these patients need to be rigorously depleted of donor T cells by high-dose irradiation or other means because of the threat of lethal graft-versus-host disease.

Ataxia-telangiectasia is a hereditary disorder in which thymic hypoplasia and variable T-cell deficiency are seen in association with oculocutaneous telangiectasia and truncal ataxia (see Ch. 223).

ACQUIRED ABNORMALITIES OF THYMIC FUNCTION. *Infection.* Human immunodeficiency virus (HIV) can drastically affect thymic development and function. First, massive thymocyte destruction occurs because most thymocytes express the CD4 molecules that serve as HIV receptors. In addition, thymic epithelial components are damaged by the HIV-induced inflammation, which results in scarring and loss of thymopoietic activity. The capacity for thymic production of CD4+ T cells is thus severely compromised and may be lost entirely in AIDS patients. Consequently, severe immunodeficiency may occur relatively early in congenital HIV infections. In contrast, individuals infected with HIV later in life usually experience a latency period of 8 to 10 years before AIDS develops because of the gradual attrition of established CD4+ T-cell clones in the periphery.

Thymectomy. Removal of the thymus after the peripheral lymphoid compartments have been seeded with T-cell clones may have no discernible effects for many years, presumably because T-cell clones normally have very long lifespans. Thymectomy is rarely complete, moreover, in part because approximately 30% of individuals have extramediastinal thymic arrests. Nevertheless, the potential need for thymic function later in life dictates careful consideration before undertaking thymectomy.

Thymic Hyperplasia. Striking variability of thymic size can occur in apparently normal adults. The physiologic basis for thymic enlargement may include hormonal influences on thymopoietic activity. Pituitary hormones that can enhance thymic growth include growth hormone, luteinizing hormone, and follicle-stimulating hormone, whereas thyrotropin may inhibit thymic growth. Interleukin-7 (IL-7), a product of thymic stromal cells, is an important thymocyte growth factor. Other locally produced factors, including epithelial growth factor and transforming growth factor-α, may regulate thymic epithelial cell production of cytokines, such as IL-1 and -6, that can affect T-cell proliferation. Thymic enlargement can occur in adults without demonstrable pathology and rarely in patients with thyrotoxicosis, Addison's disease, or following orchidectomy.

Thymic Involution. This is a well-known consequence of stressful illnesses, including severe infections, burns, and other conditions that result in elevated levels of adrenal corticosteroids. The involution is due to the relative susceptibility of immature thymocytes to lysis by corticosteroids of endogenous or exogenous origin. Temporary thymic involution also occurs as a consequence of irradiation or treatment with cytotoxic drugs. Thymic involution is a physiologic consequence of pregnancy and elevated levels of estrogen.

Myasthenia Gravis and the Thymus. Myasthenia gravis is characterized by muscle weakness attributable to an autoimmune response against the acetylcholine receptors (see Ch. 459). Improvement in this disease is frequently observed after thymectomy, thus implying a causal link between the thymus and the autoreactive T- and B-cell clones. Germinal center formation is seen in the thymic cortex of most myasthenia gravis patients, and one hypothesis is that the autoimmune response is initiated by the acetylcholine receptors present on a minor population of thymic myeloid cells. Thymic tumors are diagnosed in approximately 10% of individuals with myasthenia gravis.

Thymoma. The term *thymoma* is usually reserved for thymic epithelial cell tumors which, although rare, are the most commonly diagnosed tumors of the anterior superior mediastinum. Thymomas are frequently associated with myasthenia gravis. They also occur in rare individuals with acquired hypogammaglobulinemia who stop producing B-lineage cells; bone marrow insufficiency in these individuals may also extend to the erythroid and myeloid lineages.

The diagnosis of thymoma is suggested when these associated conditions occur or when an anterior mediastinal mass is detected, which may be an incidental finding because approximately one third of affected individuals are asymptomatic. Others with thymoma may have chest pain, dysphagia, signs of tracheal impingement, or superior vena caval obstruction. The extent of the tumor mass can be estimated by imaging procedures, but accurate diagnosis depends on obtaining thymic tissues for histologic assessment. Even when an adequate sample is available, the diagnosis may be difficult, however. There are no reliable markers for neoplastic epithelial clones, and thymomas are rarely composed of obviously neoplastic epithelial cells. Instead they are usually formed by a mixture of apparently normal lymphoid thymocytes and epithelial cells that are either spindle-shaped or ovoid. Consequently, the most reliable prognostic indication is evidence for or against invasiveness by the epithelial tumor. For this reason, direct tumor visualization by thoracotomy is favored for both diagnosis and treatment. In the case of well-encapsulated thymomas, tumors rarely occur after surgical removal. When the thymoma has invaded the capsule or surrounding tissues, surgical removal and irradiation or intensive chemotherapy may prevent 5-year recurrences in more than half of the affected patients.

Other Tumors of the Thymus. **Lymphomas.** Thymic involvement may be a prominent feature in lymphoblastic neoplasms of T-cell origin. Hodgkin's disease, usually of the nodular sclerosing type, may primarily affect the thymus. Histiocytic lymphomas may also present as an anterior mediastinal mass in adults.

Carcinoid Tumors (see Ch. 210.2). These rarely arise in the thymus; those associated with elevated levels of ACTH-like hormones and Cushing's syndrome (approximately one third) are particularly invasive. Complete excision may be curative.

Germ Cell Tumors. These occur rarely in the thymus. These include seminoma, teratoma, embryonal cell carcinoma, and choriocarcinoma.

Day DL, Gedgudas E: The thymus. Radiol Clin North Am 22:519, 1984. *A review of thymic anatomy and function emphasizing evaluation with imaging techniques such as CT scans, sonography, and magnetic resonance imaging.*

Haynes BF: Human thymic epithelium and T cell development: Current issues and future directions. Thymus 16:143, 1990. *An analytic review of the different cellular elements that form the human thymus.*

Levine GD, Rosai J: Thymic hyperplasia and neoplasia: A review of current concepts. Hum Pathol 9:495, 1978. *A thoughtful consideration of normal thymic variation and neoplasias.*

Schnittman SM, Denning SM, Greenhouse JJ, et al.: Evidence for susceptibility of intrathymic T-cell precursors and their progeny carrying T-cell antigen receptor phenotypes $TCR\alpha\beta^+$ and $TCR\gamma\delta^+$ to human immunodeficiency virus infection: A mechanism for CD4+ (T4) lymphocyte depletion. Proc Natl Acad Sci 87:7727, 1990. *Infection of early stages of the T-cell lineage via the CD4 molecule may explain the inability of the T-cell pool to regenerate in HIV-infected individuals.*

PART XX

MUSCULOSKELETAL AND CONNECTIVE TISSUE DISEASES

233 APPROACH TO THE PATIENT WITH MUSCULOSKELETAL DISEASE

Duncan A. Gordon

Diseases of the musculoskeletal (MSK) system are common, disabling, and costly to the economy. This chapter provides a guide for approaching the patient with MSK symptoms by outlining the components necessary for identifying the patient's problems, formulating the diagnosis, and initiating treatment.

The pain, stiffness, and joint swelling of MSK disorders may be inflammatory, metabolic, degenerative, or combinations thereof. For the patient, however, it is the functional interference with daily activities that determines the impact of the condition. The value of a general medical approach to the patient with MSK complaints is paramount, keeping specialized assessment in perspective. At times, a limited workup may suffice, while in other instances, assessment by a number of laboratory, imaging, and other disciplines may be necessary. Before clinical approaches are considered, it is helpful to review the anatomy and pathophysiology of the structures affected.

ANATOMY. Knowledge of the anatomic structures will answer the question, "Where is the lesion?" In the case of MSK diseases, the joints are primarily affected. The structures that may be involved are shown in Figure 233–1 *(left),* the articular structures of the MSK system. Foremost is the joint cavity and lining membrane known as the synovium. Hyaline cartilage overlying the bony end-plates provides the lubricating surface for the joint. An intact bony end-plate is required to support the cartilage. The joint capsule and ligaments provide further support and blend with the periosteum.

The nonarticular anatomy of the MSK system is equally important (Fig. 233–1, *left).* This includes local structures such as tendons, bursae, or muscles associated with various joint regions or, more generally, the collagen, elastin, and ground substance known as the connective tissue system. These latter tissues are so widespread that any organ system of the body may be involved.

PATHOPHYSIOLOGIC PROCESS. After determining which anatomic structures of the MSK system are involved, one must answer the question, "What is the lesion?" The usual pathology is either inflammatory, metabolic, degenerative, or some combination thereof (Fig. 233–1, *right).* Joint neoplasms are exceptional. With inflammatory disorders such as rheumatoid arthritis (RA) or septic arthritis, the joint cavity and synovial membrane are primarily affected, whereas with degenerative conditions such as osteoarthritis (OA) the cartilage is primarily affected. Cartilage loss also may be secondary to synovial inflammation or trauma. Metabolic crystal deposition disorders such as gout or pseudogout also cause articular inflammation, whereas avascular necrosis of bone is associated with

cartilage damage after bony end-plate collapse. Moreover, the same pathologic processes noted above may affect extra-articular systems such as skin, muscle, and vasculature.

ROLE OF THE CLINICIAN. *History.* The interview should provide a detailed chronology of the illness: anatomic location of the pain, whether local or referred; its occurrence with activity, rest, or sleep; type of onset, whether sudden or insidious; the pattern of joint involvement, symmetric or not, and whether predominantly upper or lower limbs; influence of previous and current treatments; systemic symptoms such as fatigue, weight loss, or fever and duration of morning stiffness; an up-to-date account and systematic review of all the joints of the body; and a psychosocial history. A nonrestorative sleep pattern may be associated with morning stiffness and other diffuse aching. Symptoms should be interpreted in terms of the patient's functional ability to perform self-care and other daily activities. General weakness and fatigue may reflect that many MSK conditions affect the patient's body as whole and not just the joints.

Functional Disability Indices. A number of self-report questionnaires such as the Stanford Health Assessment Questionnaire (HAQ), Functional Disability Index (FDI), Arthritis Impact Measurement Scales (AIMS), or modifications of these have been developed for ongoing evaluation of patients with arthritis (Table 233–1). These instruments document the patient's functional status with results comparable with traditional measures of joint disease activity such as tender joint count, radiographic joint erosion score, and erythrocyte sedimentation rate.

Demography. An appreciation of the age, gender, marital status, and occupation of the patient is helpful. The age of the patient is relevant to developmental and heritable disorders of connective tissue. For example, arthritis is a major manifestation of hemophilia with onset during childhood. Juvenile RA refers to polyarthritis coming on before age 16. In young adults, seropositive, seronegative, and septic arthritic conditions may arise, whereas OA is exceptional. The onset for RA is the middle years, whereas the elderly are more prone to OA. RA and the collagen diseases are more common in women, whereas ankylosing spondylitis and the other B27 spondyloarthropathies are more common in men. Gouty arthritis is more common in men and rarely attacks women before the menopause. Arthritis in the elderly is often assumed to be degenerative, when in fact the patient may suffer from an inflammatory process such as polymyalgia rheumatica, RA, or systemic lupus erythematosus. Occupation is also important because of associated physical and psychological stresses. The clinician should find out exactly what the patient does to determine how demanding the job is. Occupational factors are important with repetitive joint trauma in individuals susceptible to OA. Symptoms may be associated with jogging or trauma from sports activities.

Physical Examination. Because many MSK/rheumatic disorders are systemic, physical examination may document the presence of extra-articular features. In RA these include subcutaneous nodules, digital vasculitis, and other systemic features described in Ch. 237. Any one of these may be mistaken for a nonrheumatic condi-

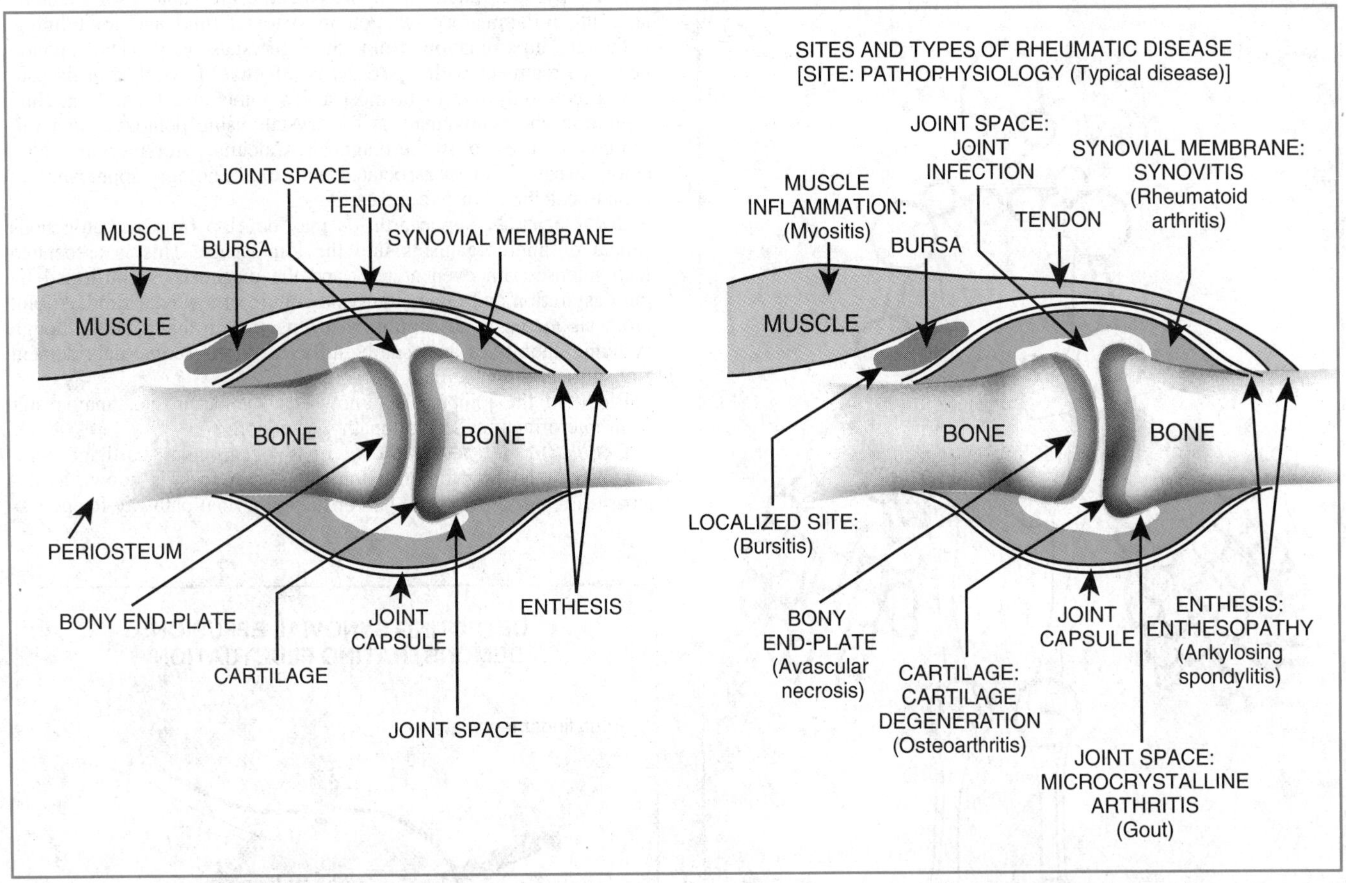

FIGURE 233–1. *Left,* Anatomic structures of the MSK system. *Right,* Location of MSK disease processes.

tion, and their presence may indicate more ominous disease. Any number of systemic features may be the result of an adverse drug reaction. The joints shown in Figure 233–2 should be examined systematically to determine if any are inflamed or damaged. The pattern of joint involvement, whether symmetrical, axial, or peripheral, should be recorded using the diagram.

Joint Inflammation. Key signs are tenderness and swelling. These may be associated with local heat, but erythema is not a feature of rheumatoid inflammation, whereas tenderness, heat, and erythema may be seen with septic or gouty arthritis. A joint is considered *active* if it is tender on pressure or passive movement with stress. Joint swelling may be periarticular or intra-articular. The latter is associated with a joint effusion detected by showing fluctua-

tion (see Fig. 233–3). It is important to note the difference between *tender joints* and deep referred *tender points* characteristic of a non-articular syndrome known as "fibromyalgia" (see Ch. 258).

Joint Damage and Destruction. This may be assessed clinically or radiologically. Common observations include loss of range of movement, collateral instability, malalignment, subluxation, or cartilage loss causing bone-on-bone crepitus. Record a separate count of damaged joints, as with actively inflamed joints.

DIAGNOSTIC CONSIDERATIONS. Clinical evaluation enables us to establish which MSK structures are inflamed, which are damaged, and how function is impaired. Nine specific types of MSK involvement can be identified as a framework for various diagnostic possibilities or hypotheses to be considered (Fig. 233–1,

TABLE 233–1. SELF-REPORT QUESTIONNAIRE FOR ARTHRITIS

Please check (✓) the ONE best answer for your abilities.

At this moment, are you able to:	Without Any Difficulty	With Some Difficulty	With Much Difficulty	Unable to Do
a. Dress yourself, including tying shoe-laces and doing buttons?				
b. Get in and out of bed?				
c. Lift a full cup or glass to your mouth?				
d. Walk outdoors on flat ground?				
e. Wash and dry your entire body?				
f. Bend down to pick up clothing from the floor?				
g. Turn regular faucets (taps) on and off?				
h. Get in and out of a car?				

From Pincus T, Callahan LF, Brooks RH, et al.: Self-report questionnaire scores in rheumatoid arthritis compared with traditional physical, radiographic, and laboratory measures. Ann Intern Med 100:259, 1989.

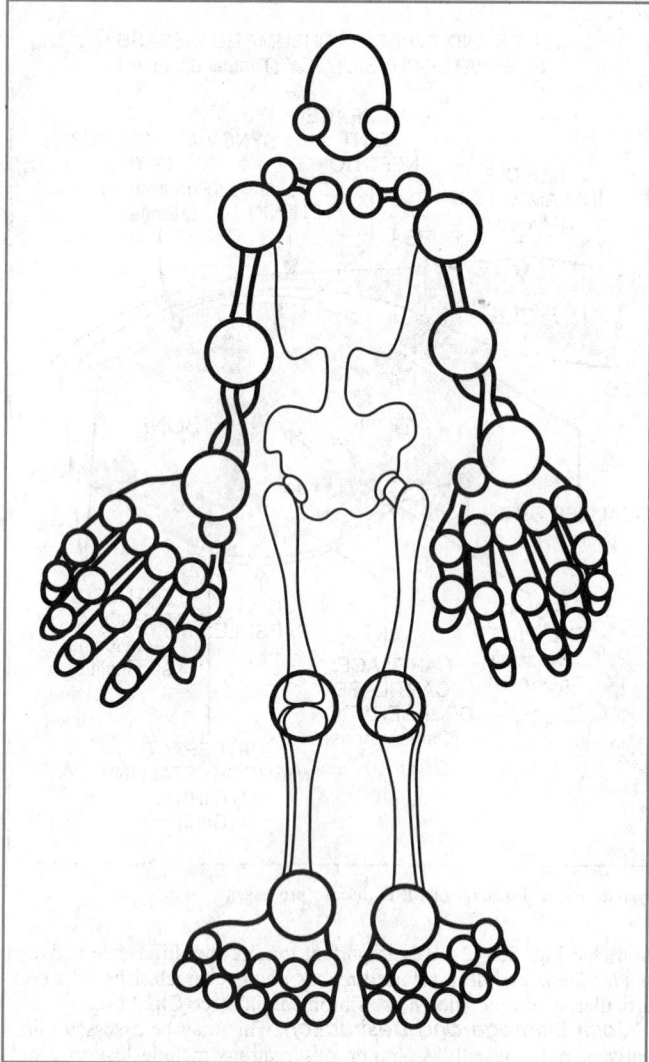

FIGURE 233–2. A pictorial method for indicating joint disease activity or destruction. The sketch may be used on a printed form or rubber stamp to chart which joints are active or deformed at the time of each assessment. (Courtesy Dr. Hugh A. Smythe, Toronto.)

right). The nine categories presented in the following paragraphs are listed in Table 233–2 along with typical diseases, examples of laboratory tests, and treatments. Table 233–2 and the descriptions below provide the basis for more detailed information contained in the following chapters of this section.

Synovitis. Inflammation of the synovial membrane lining of the joint is typical of inflammatory polyarthritis such as RA. If synovitis is persistent, irreversible joint damage results. The polyarthritis of RA is like that found in the diffuse connective tissue diseases associated with autoantibodies. These autoimmune collagen disorders include lupus, scleroderma, polymyositis, vasculitis, and Sjögren's syndrome. When these conditions are progressive or life-threatening, disease-modifying immunosuppressive drugs and/or corticosteroids are appropriate.

Enthesopathy. The enthesis is the anatomic transition zone where ligament attaches to bone. Inflammation in this region is the hallmark of a family of seronegative rheumatic diseases, of which ankylosing spondylitis is the prototype. Other members of this group include Reiter's syndrome, reactive arthritis, psoriatic arthritis, and the arthropathy associated with inflammatory bowel disease. All these conditions share in common the presence of the human leukocyte antigen HLA-B27. In ankylosing spondylitis, the sacroiliac joints and apophyseal joints of the spine show characteristic inflammation with a tendency to bony ankylosis. Nonsteroidal antiinflammatory drugs (NSAID's) are usually effective, whereas prednisone is rarely needed.

Crystal-Induced Synovitis. Crystals of monosodium urate, calcium pyrophosphate, or hydroxyapatite are capable of inducing an acute inflammatory reaction in synovial fluid and joint lining. Although inflammation from these crystals may clear spontaneously, treatment with NSAID's is effective. Crystal arthritis usually affects only one or at most a few joints at a time. Joint fluid aspiration and synovianalysis for crystals using polarized light microscopy will establish the diagnosis. Calcium pyrophosphate deposition disease is often associated with the radiologic appearance of chondrocalcinosis of hyaline cartilage.

Joint Space. Septic arthritis may develop from hematogenous spread of microorganisms into the joint space. This is associated with intense pain even at rest, and the diagnosis is confirmed by joint aspiration and Gram stain and culture of synovial fluid. A joint prothesis increases susceptibility to infection in that joint. Although systemic antibiotics are usually sufficient, arthroscopic debridement and surgical drainage may be required.

Blood in the joint space, known as "hemarthrosis," may result from microfractures, coagulopathy, or tumor.

Cartilage Degeneration. Loss of articular cartilage with bony repair leading to formation of osteophytosis is known as osteoarthritis (OA). It should be considered a final pathway for persis-

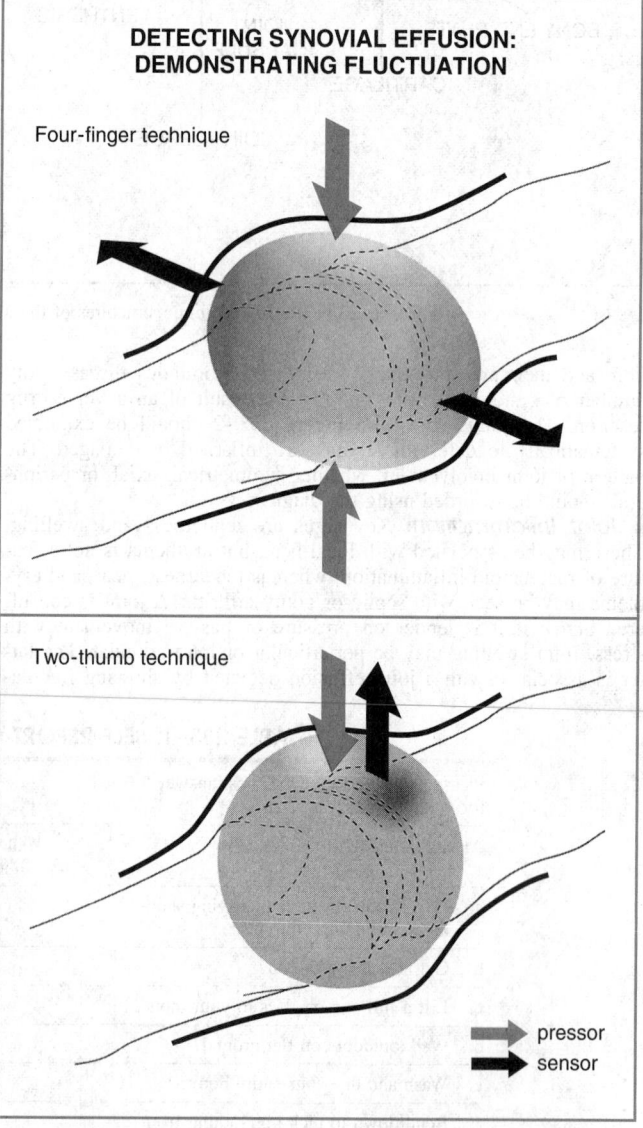

FIGURE 233–3. A demonstration of fluctuation for detecting a synovial effusion. An increase in fluid tension induced by finger pressure in one area is transmitted so that the sensor fingers can detect it elsewhere. In the two-thumb or four-finger technique, the pressure should be in a slightly different direction to the sensor finger to avoid false-positive results. (Reprinted courtesy Klippel JH, Dieppe PA: Rheumatology. London, Mosby–Year Book Europe, 1994, section 3, p 4.4.)

TABLE 233-2. CLASSIFICATION OF RHEUMATIC DISEASE

Category	Prototypes	Useful Tests	Treatments
Synovitis	Rheumatoid arthritis	Latex, erythrocyte sedimentation rate	Methotrexate
	Autoimmune collagen diseases	ANA test	Prednisone
Enthesopathy	Ankylosing spondylitis B27 spondyloarthropathies	Sacroiliac radiographs	Indomethacin
Crystal-induced synovitis	Gout	Joint fluid crystal examination	Indomethacin
	Pseudogout	Radiographic chondrocalcinosis Joint fluid crystal examination	Indomethacin
Joint space	Septic arthritis	Joint fluid culture	Antibiotics
Cartilage degeneration	Osteoarthritis	Radiographs of affected area	Physical therapy
			Analgesics
Osteoarticular	Avascular necrosis bone	Radiographs, magnetic resonance imaging	Prosthetic joint replacement
Polymyositis	Dermatomyositis Inclusion body myositis	Muscle enzymes, EMG, muscle biopsy	Corticosteroids
Local conditions	Tendinitis	None, radiographs of affected area	Local
General conditions	Fibromyalgia	Erythrocyte sedimentation rate	Fitness exercises

tent inflammatory conditions such as RA, ankylosing spondylitis, septic arthritis, and metabolic disorders with chondrocalcinosis. Joint hypermobility and previous trauma are other mechanical factors that may predispose to OA. Although hereditary OA may affect the distal interphalangeal (DIP) joints of the fingers, it usually only involves one or two larger joints such as a hip or knee. For this reason, OA disability can be more readily controlled by physical or orthopedic measures than RA. While NSAID's and analgesics may provide pain relief, they are largely palliative.

Osteoarticular Conditions. Avascular necrosis results after collapse of the bony end-plate from vascular insufficiency. The consequence is collapse and fragmentation of cartilage. Avascular necrosis may be associated with systemic conditions such as sickle cell disease or fatty liver after high-dose corticosteroids.

Inflammation of the periosteum, known as "periostitis," may be associated with hypertrophic pulmonary osteoarthropathy and clubbing. This syndrome may be a clue to underlying lung cancer.

Polymyositis. Inflammation and weakness of the proximal skeletal muscles are characteristic of polymyositis; with rash, it is called dermatomyositis. Elevated creatine kinase, electromyographic abnormalities, and histologic abnormalities of muscle biopsy are characteristic. Corticosteroids and immunosuppressives may control polymyositis, but older patients with dermatomyositis may have hidden malignancy and steroid resistance.

Local Conditions. Nonarticular disorders such as tendinitis, bursitis, and low-back strain are common medical problems. Local signs of inflammation are characteristic of these conditions that usually respond to physical therapy, protective splints, or injection of corticosteroids.

General Conditions. These nonarticular or extra-articular disorders are not usually associated with arthritis. This group includes polymyalgia rheumatica, sympathetic reflex dystrophy, and fibromyalgia. Polymyalgia rheumatica affects the elderly with persistent neck, shoulder, and hip pain; chronic fatigue; and high erythrocyte sedimentation rate. Sometimes it is associated with underlying giant cell and temporal arteritis. In the latter case, corticosteroids are mandatory because of the risk of blindness from ophthalmic arteritis.

"Fibromyalgia" refers to a common syndrome of widespread polyarthralgias associated with chronic fatigue and a nonrestorative sleep pattern. It is characterized by the presence of deep referred tender points described in Ch. 258.

TREATMENT CONSIDERATIONS. Treatment should be based on a correct diagnosis, which may not be initially obvious (see Table 233-2). Also important is whether the patient's problem is urgent, or whether treatment can be postponed until the diagnosis is established. For example, acute monarthritis due to sepsis or gout

requires immediate attention, whereas widespread smouldering polyarthritis does not. However, a patient with polyarthritis who is systemically ill requires prompt investigation to exclude a diffuse connective tissue disease, underlying infection, or hidden malignancy.

Regardless of the diagnosis, educating the patient and family is crucial to successful management of any chronic MSK illness. The informed patient is more likely to comply with treatment and hold realistic expectations of outcome. For the patient with MSK disease, the goal of management is to maintain independence. For this reason, treatment should be individualized, based on early identification of problems, a firm diagnosis, and continued monitoring of response to treatment.

Gordon DA, Inman RD: Musculoskeletal disability and rheumatology. J Rheumatol 21:387, 1994. *This editorial draws attention to the frequency, types, risk factors, and economic impact of MSK disorders in the general population.*

Pincus T, Callahan LF, Brooks RH, et al.: Self-report questionnaire scores in rheumatoid arthritis compared with traditional physical, radiographic, and laboratory measures. Ann Intern Med 100:259, 1989. *Illustrates the value of self-report questionnaires in providing quantitative data that reflect traditional disease activity measures in arthritis patients.*

Schumacher HR (ed.): Primer on the Rheumatic Diseases. 10th ed. Atlanta, Arthritis Foundation, 1993. *Classic, authoritative, current descriptions of all rheumatic diseases and of all rheumatology, available as a public service at nominal cost.*

234 CONNECTIVE TISSUE STRUCTURE AND FUNCTION
Steffen Gay and Renate E. Gay

One of the fundamental characteristics of all connective tissues is the relatively large proportion of extracellular matrix in relation to cells. Until recently, the extracellular matrix was viewed as a passive framework serving mainly as an inert scaffolding for stabilization of the physical structure of tissues. In addition to maintaining this three-dimensional form during morphogenesis and tissue repair, it is now recognized as a dynamic milieu in which cells become organized, exchange signals, and differentiate. Study of these processes has led to discovery of a plethora of new matrix components, matrix receptors, and cell-matrix interactions. The extracellular matrix is composed of multidomain macromolecules that are linked together by covalent and noncovalent bonds to form a highly intricate composite. Two major types of matrices exist: the *interstitium,* which is synthesized by mesenchymal cells and forms the stroma of organs, and the *basement membranes,* which are produced by epithelial and endothelial cells. These matrices comprise four major classes of extracellular macromolecules: (1) the collagens, (2) elastin, (3) noncollagenous glycoproteins, and (4) glycosaminoglycans, which are usually covalently linked to proteins to form proteoglycans.

COLLAGENS. The collagens are the most abundant class of proteins in the human organism, constituting almost 30% of its total protein. The central feature of all collagen molecules is the stiff structure resulting from lengthy domains of triple-helical conformation. Three polypeptide chains, called α chains, are wound around one another to generate a ropelike fold. An absolute requirement for the formation of this triple helix, as well as the most distinctive feature of the α chains, is the presence of lengthy sequences of repeating Gly-X-Y triplets in which the X and Y positions are frequently occupied by prolyl and hydroxyprolyl residues.

Studies based on protein chemistry and complementary DNA (cDNA) sequencing have revealed a genetically determined heterogeneity with as many as 19 homopolymeric or heteropolymeric collagen types. As of this writing, 30 unique polypeptide chains have been identified. It is of interest that genes coding for the different chains are distributed among at least 12 chromosomes in the human genome (Table 234–1). Even simultaneously expressed genes, such as those coding for the two $\alpha_1(I)$ and one $\alpha_2(I)$ chains of the heteropolymeric type I molecule, are located on different chromosomes.

Functional diversity of the various collagen types is accomplished by formation of distinct extracellular aggregates. The most obvious are the interstitial linear polymers of fibrils, derived from collagen types I, II, and III. These fibrils with characteristic banding patterns can be visualized readily by electron microscopy. Type I collagen fibers are found in supporting elements of high tensile strength (e.g., tendon and cornea), whereas fibers formed from type II collagen molecules are restricted to cartilaginous structures. The fibrils derived from type III collagen are prevalent in more distensible tissues, such as blood vessels and parenchymal organs. In addition, collagen types V, VI, IX, and XII are also involved in fiber formation, but largely as adducts. This finding is illustrated by the association of collagen types IX, X, and XI with type II collagen in hyaline cartilage. Knockout experiments of the $\alpha_1(IX)$ gene in transgenic mice indicate that a lack of functional type IX collagen results in the development of a mild chondrodysplasia and osteoarthritis in these animals. Adaptation for a special function is shown by type VII collagen molecules, which aggregate as antiparallel overlapping dimers to form the anchoring fibrils required to stabilize the dermoepithelial junction of the skin. In contrast to the interstitial types of collagen, type IV molecules form large polygonal aggregates fulfilling the structural and support requirements of basement membranes.

ELASTIN. Elastic fibers are composed of two morphologically and structurally distinct components: elastin and the microfibrils. Elastin, whose gene has now been characterized, is an insoluble protein polymer. The biosynthetic precursor of elastin, tropoelastin, is a linear polypeptide composed of about 700 amino acids and is rich in nonpolar amino acids: glycine (> 30%), valine, leucine, isoleucine, and alanine. Tropoelastin is synthesized by vascular smooth muscle cells and skin fibroblasts and subsequently incorporated into elastic fibers. Elastic fiber formation involves lysyloxidase-mediated formation of intermolecular crosslinks, called *desmosine* and *isodesmosine*. Since these crosslinks do not exist in other proteins and therefore are elastin-specific, determination of these two amino acid derivatives in tissue sample reflects the amount of elastin present. The microfibrillar components of interstitial elastic fibers are not fully characterized. However, disulfide-rich glycoproteins, such as *fibrillin* and *microfibril-associated glycoprotein* (MAGP) have been identified and may serve as a scaffold onto which tropoelastin is deposited.

STRUCTURAL GLYCOPROTEINS. The major noncollagenous glycoprotein present in the extracellular matrix is *fibronectin*. Fibronectins are dimeric cell adhesion glycoproteins composed of two disulfide-bonded subunits and found in rather large quantities in blood plasma (~0.3 mg per milliliter). The functions of fibronectin in cell adhesion are illustrated in Figure 234–1. Some of these functions can be mimicked by synthetic peptides that contain the sequence Arg-Gly-Asp (RGD sequence). Similar sequences are found in other cell adhesion proteins, such as vitronectin, laminin, and collagen type VI. Since fibronectin plays a major role in morphogenesis and tissue remodeling, the regulation of fibronectin biosynthesis by growth factors and cytokines has been

TABLE 234–1. POLYMORPHISM OF THE COLLAGEN TYPES

Type	Chain(s)	Major Molecular Species	Major Distribution
I	$\alpha_1(I)$ $\alpha_2(I)$	$[\alpha_1(I)]_2\alpha_2(I)$	Skin, tendon, bone, organ capsules
II	$\alpha_1(II)$	$[\alpha_1(II)]_3$	Hyaline cartilage
III	$\alpha_1(III)$	$[\alpha_1(III)]_3$	Blood vessels, parenchymal organs
IV	$\alpha_1(IV)$ $\alpha_2(IV)$ $\alpha_3(IV)$ $\alpha_4(IV)$ $\alpha_5(IV)$	$[\alpha_1(IV)]_2\alpha_2(IV)$	Basement membranes
V	$\alpha_1(V)$ $\alpha_2(V)$ $\alpha_3(V)$	$[\alpha_1(V)]_2\alpha_2(V)$	Smooth muscle
VI	$\alpha_1(VI)$ $\alpha_2(VI)$ $\alpha_3(VI)$	$[\alpha_1(VI),\alpha_2(VI),\alpha_3(VI)]$	Minor collagen of stroma matrices
VII	$\alpha_1(VII)$	$[\alpha_1(VII)]_3$	Anchoring fibrils of the dermoepidermal junction
VIII	$\alpha_1(VIII)$	$[\alpha_1(VIII)]_3$	Descemet's membrane, sclera, dura mater
IX	$\alpha_1(IX)$ $\alpha_2(IX)$ $\alpha_3(IX)$	$[\alpha_1(IX),\alpha_2(IX),\alpha_3(IX)]$	Hyaline cartilage
X	$\alpha_1(X)$	$[\alpha_1(X)]_3$	Hypertrophic cartilage
XI	$\alpha_1(XI)$ $\alpha_2(XI)$ $\alpha_1(II)$	$[\alpha_1(XI),\alpha_2(XI),\alpha_3(XI)]$	Hyaline cartilage
XII	$\alpha_1(XII)$		Tendons, ligaments, periosteum, skin, cartilage
XIII	$\alpha_1(XIII)$		Skin, gut
XIV	$\alpha_1(XIV)$		Skin, tendon, placenta, fetal cartilage
XV	$\alpha_1(XV)$		Fibroblasts
XVI	$\alpha_1(XVI)$		Placenta, fibroblasts
XVII	$\alpha_1(XVII)$		BP180 autoantigen in bullous pemphigoid
XVIII	$\alpha_1(XVIII)$		Liver, kidney, placenta

FIGURE 234-1. Multiple cell recognition sites in fibronectin. The fibronectin molecule contains a series of functional domains that bind the indicated ligands. The thick vertical bars indicate cell adhesive recognition sequences. SS = putative synergistic second site; RGD = Gly-Arg-Gly-Asp-Ser site; H = putative sites in the heparin-binding domain; CS1 = the CS1 site in the alternatively spliced IIICS region; REDV = the Arg-Glu-Asp-Val site. (Reprinted with permission from Yamada KM: Fibronectins: Structure, functions and receptors. Curr Opin Cell Biol 1:956–963, 1989. Copyright 1989 by Current Science.)

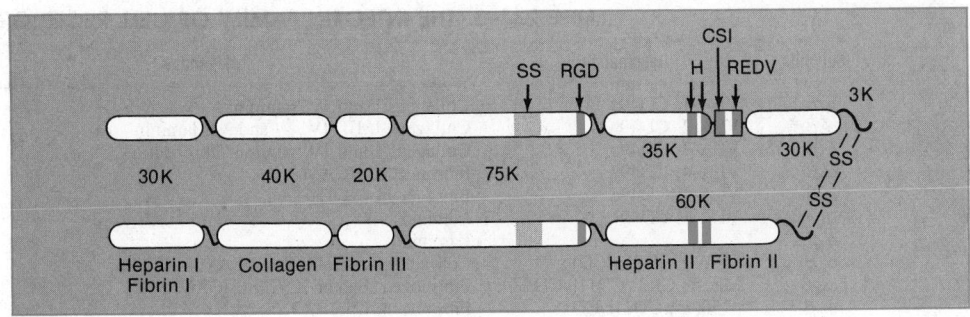

studied. For example, it is established that γ-interferon and transforming growth factor β (TGF-β) stimulate fibronectin synthesis, whereas tumor necrosis factor (TNF) and interleukin-1 (IL-1) inhibit synthesis.

Vitronectin is a 75-kD protein, which is considerably smaller than the 250-kD fibronectin polypeptide present in plasma and tissue. Vitronectin, also termed "serum spreading factor" and "complement S-protein," promotes cell attachment and spreading, inhibits cytolysis by the complement C5b–9 complex, and modulates antithrombin III–thrombin action in blood coagulation.

Tenascin is another large glycoprotein of the extracellular matrix. The previous other name *hexabrachion* refers to the disulfide-linked six-armed structure. Tenascin mediates cell attachment through an RGD-dependent receptor and is expressed in association with mesenchymal-epithelial interactions during morphogenesis and development of undifferentiated tumors. The same protein also has been referred to as myotendinous antigen, GP 250 protein, glial mesenchymal extracellular matrix protein, cytotactin, J1-protein, and brachionectin. As the names suggest, tenascin has been identified in tendons, development of smooth muscle, cartilage, and gut and in neuromuscular and neuronal-glial interactions. On the other hand, gene knockout experiments suggest that tenascin might be a superfluous nonfunctional protein and that other tenascin-like proteins, such as MHC-tenascin encoded in the human MHC class III regions, may compensate for the absence of tenascin.

Cartilage Glycoproteins. Several structural glycoproteins have been isolated from various cartilages. They include a 550-kD disulfide-bonded cartilage matrix glycoprotein (CMGP) composed of cartilage oligomeric protein (COMP) as well as two distinct 58-kD and 36-kD proteins. Fibromodulin, a 59-kD protein, and a 21-kD cell surface cartilage protein called "anchorin" are also localized in articular cartilage. In contrast, a 148-kD cartilage matrix protein (CMP) is prominent in adult tracheal cartilage but not present in articular cartilage.

PROTEOGLYCANS. Proteoglycans are proteins that carry one or more glycosaminoglycan side chains. Glycosaminoglycans are long, unbranched polysaccharide chains composed of repeating disaccharide units. One of the two sugar residues in the repeating disaccharide is always an amino sugar (N-acetylglucosamine or N-acetylgalactosamine). Glycosaminoglycans are highly negatively charged owing to the presence of sulfate and carboxyl groups on multiple sugar residues. In contrast, hyaluronic acid, also called *hyaluronan,* is a polymer of glucuronic acid and glucosamine that is not sulfated and not attached covalently to a protein core connected via a link protein. Proteoglycans of almost all sizes and shapes have been biochemically identified. Nevertheless, since cloning and sequence analysis have often identified the same core proteins, the number of distinct proteoglycans is limited (Table 234–2). With respect to their function, they have been referred to as a "multipurpose glue." Proteoglycans not only bind extracellular matrix components together and mediate cell binding to the matrix but also restrain soluble molecules such as growth factors in the matrix and at cell surfaces. Heparan sulfate proteoglycan, for example, binds basic fibroblast growth factor released from injured endothelial cells. The role of proteoglycans in cell

adhesion is best exhibited by a membrane-intercalated proteoglycan termed *syndecan.* This molecule binds to collagen and fibronectin through its heparan sulfate chains and mediates cell adhesion. Certain proteoglycans contain functional domains that are common for all the members of the aggrecan/versican family. These domains share further functional domains with other important proteins and include an immunoglobulin-like, epidermal growth factor–like, and complement regulatory protein–like sequence.

BASEMENT MEMBRANES. Basement membranes are thin, sheetlike structures deposited by endothelial and epithelial cells but also found surrounding nerve and muscle cells. They provide mechanical support for resident cells, function as a semipermeable filtration barrier for macromolecules in organs such as the kidney and the placenta, and act as regulators of cell attachment, migra-tion, and differentiation. The major constituents are collagen type IV, laminin, entactin (nidogen), and heparan sulfate proteoglycans. Collagen type IV molecules are $[\alpha_1(IV)]_2$ $\alpha_2(IV)$ heterotrimers comprising an N-terminal rod 30 μm long (7S), a linear triple helix containing over 20 noncollagenous sequences, and a C-terminal globular domain (NC1). These molecules can spontaneously aggregate into a network consisting of N-terminal tetramers (7S), lateral associations between the triple-helical rods, and C-terminal dimers (NC1). The network is eventually stabilized by disulfide- and lysyl oxidase–derived intramolecular and intermolecular crosslinks, which may provide the scaffold for basement membrane formation. Self-assembly also has been observed with *laminin,* a major basement membrane–associated glycoprotein. The typical features of the laminin molecule are a threadlike long arm terminating in a globular domain and three short arms, each con-sisting of two globular domains separated by short linear segments. Collagen type IV and laminin appear highly integrated in the basement membrane matrix and are closely associated with a 150-kD, sulfated glycoprotein called *entactin*

TABLE 234–2. STRUCTURAL FEATURES OF PROTEOGLYCANS

Location	Proteoglycan	GAG* (Number)
Extracellular matrix	Aggrecan	CS/KS (> 100)
	Versican	CS/DS (20)
	Decorin	CS or DS (1)
	Biglycan	CS or DS (2)
	Fibromodulin	KS (4)
Cell surface	Syndecan	HS/CS (4)
	Betaglycan	HS/CS (2)
	CD44	HS or CS
	Glypican	HS
	Fibroglycan	HS
Intracellular	Serglycin	CS or Hep (8)
Basement membrane	Perlecan	HS (3)
Brain	Brevican	CS/DS (3)
	Neurocan	CS (7)
	Cerebroglycan	HS (5)

* Glycosaminoglycan (GAG) chains: HS = heparan sulfate; CS = chondroitin sulfate; Hep = heparin; KS = keratan sulfate; DS = dermatan sulfate.

TABLE 234–3. THE INTEGRIN FAMILY OF CELL RECEPTORS*

Subunits	Designation	Ligands	Distribution
$\alpha_1\beta_1$	VLA-1; CD49a	Collagens I and IV, laminin	F, BM, aT
$\alpha_2\beta_1$	VLA-2; CD49b	Collagens I, III, IV, V, and VI, laminin	F, En, Ep, aT, Pl
$\alpha_3\beta_1$	VLA-3; CD49c	Collagens I and IV, laminin, fibronectin	F, Ep
$\alpha_4\beta_1$	VLA-4; CD49d	Fibronectin, VCAM-1	F, Nc, T, B, M
$\alpha_5\beta_1$	VLA-5; CD49e	Fibronectin (RGD)	F, En, Ep, aT, Th
$\alpha_6\beta_1$	VLA-6; CD49f	Laminin	En
$\alpha_7\beta_1$		Laminin	En
$\alpha_L\beta_2$	LFA-1; CD11a/CD18	Cell adhesion molecules (ICAM-1, 2)	T, B, M, G
$\alpha_M\beta_2$	Mac-1; CR3; CD11b/CD18	Fibrinogen, Factor X, C3bi, ICAM-1	M, G
$\alpha_X\beta_2$	p150,95; CD11c/CD18	Fibrinogen, C3bi	M, G
$\alpha_{IIb}\beta_3$	gpIIb, IIIa; CD41/CD61	Fibronectin, fibrinogen, von Willebrand factor, thrombospondin	Pl
$\alpha_V\beta_3$	VNR; CD51/CD61	Fibrinogen, von Willebrand factor, vitronectin, thrombospondin	En
$\alpha_6\beta_4$	CD104	—	Ec
$\alpha_V\beta_5$	CD51/CD-	Vitronectin (RGD)	Ca

* Cloning of the α and β subunits has revealed cell surface proteins on other cells. These include the very late activation (VLA) antigens and the lymphocyte function–associated antigen 1 (LFA-1)/Mac-1/p 150.95 on leukocytes and the platelet IIb/IIIa glycoprotein.

F = fibroblasts; BM = basement membrane associated; aT = activated T lymphocytes only; En = endothelial cells; Ep = epithelial cells; Pl = platelets; Nc = neural crest melanocytes; T = T lymphocytes; B = B lymphocytes; M = monocytes; Th = thymocytes; G = granulocytes; Ca = UCLA-P3 lung adenocarcinoma cells.

Data from Springer TA: Adhesion receptors regulate antigen-specific interactions, localization, and differentiation in the immune system. Prog Immunol Springer 7:121–130, 1989; Hynes RO: Integrins: Versatility, modulation, and signaling in cell adhesion. Cell 69:11–25, 1992; and Schlossman SF, et al.: CD antigens 1993. J Immunol 52:1, 1994.

(nidogen) in a stable noncovalent complex. Amino acid sequence data of entactin have revealed epidermal growth factor (EGF)–like cysteine-rich motifs, segments showing homology to the EGF precursor, the low-density lipoprotein (LDL) receptor, and thyroglobulin. *Heparan sulfate proteoglycans* occur as an integral component in all basement membranes but play different roles in specific tissues. They control permeability of the glomeru-lar basement membranes and also have been implicated in the anchorage of acetylcholinesterase to the neuromuscular junction.

CONNECTIVE TISSUE MATRIX IN CELL REGULATION

It is well established that matrix components influence the maintenance of cellular phenotypes mediated through matrix receptors.

RECEPTORS FOR EXTRACELLULAR MATRIX COMPONENTS. Adhesive interactions between cells and their surrounding extracellular matrix are not only important in most developmental events but also essential for maintaining the fundamental life processes. Cell proliferation, polarization, migration, differentiation, and protein synthesis depend on interactions between cells and supporting matrix. Diverse families of structurally similar receptors for matrix components have been identified. They include the transmembrane integrin superfamily, peripheral membrane glycoproteins, glycosyltransferases, and proteoglycans. *Integrins* are a group of α/β heterodimers involved in cell binding, some of which involve recognition of an RGD sequence present in their ligands. The integrins consist of an α subunit with a molecular mass of 130 to 210 kD and noncovalently associated β subunits (95 to 130 kD). The cytoplasmic domain of the β subunit reveals homologies to the EGF, the insulin receptor, and the *neu* oncogene protein. Both subunits define the integrin subfamilies described in Table 234–3.

Since integrins localize in known junctional regions where actin bundles and myofibrils terminate at the cell surface, the major function of integrin receptors appears to be the linkage of extracellular matrix molecules with the intracellular cytoskeletal network. The connection is thereby mediated through the cytoplasmic domain of the subunits. That extracellular matrix components may influence gene expression by signal transduction is shown by the finding that fibronectin degradation products induce, via the fibronectin receptor, collagenase and stromelysin gene expression. The latter pathway may play a major role in inflammatory tissue destruction. The pivotal role of these receptors related to infectious diseases is further illustrated by the observation that bacteria use specific receptors to adhere to host connective tissue. For example, it has been shown that certain strains of *Es-*

cherichia coli express a fibronectin receptor that is involved in colonization.

The most provoking question remains: How do matrix receptors transmit information from the extracellular structure to affect gene expression? Figure 234–2 illustrates a model of "dynamic reciprocity," in which the extracellular matrix is postulated to influence gene expression at all levels, including transcription, messenger RNA (mRNA) processing, and translation, via transmembrane and cytoskeletal components. Elucidating the molecular mechanisms of this message system remains one of the key challenges in cell biology.

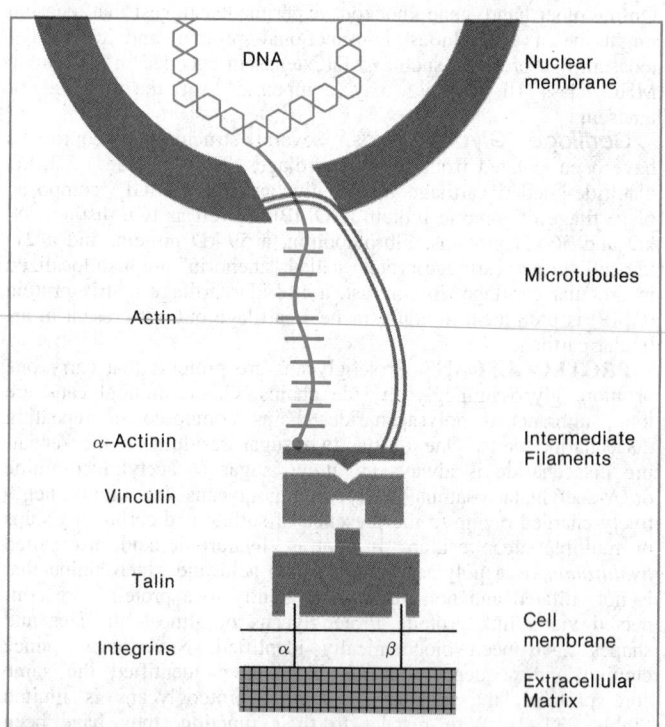

FIGURE 234–2. This refined model for the ultrastructural interaction of cells with extracellular matrix is based on a model of "dynamic reciprocity" whereby the extracellular matrix is postulated to exert an influence on gene expression via transmembrane proteins and cytoskeletal components, proposed originally by Bissell and Carcellos-Hoff (J Cell Sci Suppl 8:?27, 1987).

Some confusion remains about the role of collagen in a variety of diseases involving the connective tissues. Historically, the term "collagen disease"—describing a heterogeneous group of acute and chronic diseases, including rheumatoid arthritis, systemic lupus erythematosus, progressive systemic sclerosis, polymyositis, dermatomyositis, Sjögren's syndrome, arteritis, rheumatic fever, ankylosing spondylitis, and amyloidosis—was based on the erroneous notion that "collagen" was equivalent to "connective tissue." However, as outlined above, the different types of collagen and the macromolecular aggregates derived from them are now recognized as distinct structural and histologic entities that exist within a meticulously intercalated connective tissue matrix along with structural glycoproteins and proteoglycans. Consequently, no justification exists for using the anachronistic term "collagen disease" to encompass a group of such diseases initiated by vastly different pathomechanisms and affecting distinct connective tissue entities. The term "collagen diseases" now exclusively pertains to those inherited conditions in which the primary defect has been demonstrated to be at the gene level and to affect collagen biosynthesis, posttranslational modification, or extracellular processing directly. Recent technologies of gene cloning and gene analysis have led to the delineation of mutations in the fibrillar collagen genes. Collagen type I is the target of certain genetic mutations associated with classic clinical variants of dwarfing syndromes, osteogenesis imperfecta, and Ehlers-Danlos syndrome (types IV and VII) (see Ch. 182, 184, and 185). Moreover, polymerase chain reaction amplification of a series of overlapping segments encoding for the entire helical and telepeptide regions of the human $\alpha_1(I)$ collagen cDNA is expected to identify potentially all mutations and polymorphisms.

The acquired disorders of connective tissue involving collagen include conditions that result in repair from overt trauma; in diseases characterized by an excessive deposition of collagenous matrix, i.e., fibroproliferative disorders, or in pathologic loss of tissue matrix, including the breakdown of basement membranes in tumor invasion and rheumatoid joint destruction.

Although connective tissue repair after trauma largely depends on the type of injury and is, therefore, quite variable, the repair of various connective tissue lesions in wound healing follows a characteristic sequence of events. The initial events involve the synthesis of pericellular and basement membrane collagens in the proliferating epithelial and/or endothelial cells. Subsequently, a loose fibrillar network largely comprising fibronectin and collagen types III and V and single interspersed fibers derived from type I collagen are deposited. Finally, with the formation of scar tissue, the lesions become more fibrous and dense owing to a deposition of collagen fiber bundles derived largely from type I molecules. It is striking that the patterns of collagen deposition in fibroproliferative diseases show certain similarities. For example, liver damage is characterized by an initial accumulation of basement membrane collagens in the sinusoidal space of Disse, followed by a fine fibrillar material composed largely of type III collagen and, subsequently, in the case of the development of hepatic fibrosis (cirrhosis, Ch. 122), by an augmented deposition of type I collagen. A similar pattern appears in the development of fibrotic plaques in atherosclerosis (Ch. 40) or of cyclosporine-induced myocardial fibrosis in the transplanted human heart.

The major disease affecting almost exclusively the matrix of basement membranes is diabetes mellitus (Ch. 205). The histopathologic hallmark of diabetic microvascular disease is generalized basement membrane thickening. In the kidney, these changes include an increase in glomerular basement membrane permeability followed by decreased glomerular filtration. Evidence exists that accelerated nonenzymatic glycosylation (glycation) plays an important role in the development of diabetic microangiopathy.

The loss of a specialized connective tissue matrix plays a pivotal role in tumor progression and metastasis. With proliferation, malignant tumor cells acquire the capability to invade basement membranes actively and to migrate through the interstitial stroma. Despite the fact that tumor invasion requires a complex sequence of steps, such as the expression of receptors for basement membrane components by the malignant cells, invasion ultimately results in a loss of basement membrane integrity (Fig. 234–3). Severe recessive dystrophic epidermolysis bullosa features a loss of collagen type

VII anchoring filaments, which normally connect the epidermal basement membrane to the interstitial matrix of the dermis. In Goodpasture's syndrome, basement membranes are damaged by circulating autoantibodies against basement membrane collagen (Ch. 79). The Goodpasture antigen has been mapped to the C-terminal globular domain of type IV collagen, which explains the high cross-reactivity of the anti–glomerular basement membrane antibodies with alveolar basement membranes.

CONNECTIVE TISSUE MARKERS. The enormous progress in our knowledge of the structure and biology of the connective tissue matrix has caused considerable interest in the development of assays for diagnosis and monitoring therapy in diseases involving connective tissue. Historically, the determination of hydroxyproline as a measure of total collagen content or turnover has been a useful technique in connective tissue research. However, with the discovery of collagen polymorphism and a variety of molecules containing collagenous sequences, the measurement of hydroxyproline now appears to be of only limited value. This observation is based on the fact that there are varying levels of hydroxylation of the different collagens. For example, the type III collagen molecule contains about 30% more hydroxyproline than does type I, and other proteins such as C1q, acetylcholinesterase, and elastin also contain hydroxyproline. Specific immunohistologic and immunoserologic assays have been used to evaluate the complexity of collagenous proteins in normal and pathologic samples. As illustrated in Figure 234–3, using a monoclonal antibody specific for collagen type IV has been advantageous in studies assessing the integrity of basement membranes in neoplastic lesions. Several markers of collagen assembly and turnover have been employed to detect injury to a specific parenchymal organ or to diagnose organ fibrosis by noninvasive immunoserologic assays. The most widely applied test so far has been a radioimmunoassay to detect the N-terminal propeptide of type III procollagen in body fluids. The utility of this test was based on the notion that the propeptide is removed from type III procollagen molecules after synthesis to form new collagen fibrils. However, procollagen molecules may retain their propeptide as a part of the normal extracellular matrix. Thus the presence of the propeptide in serum may be related not only to neosynthesis but also to degradation from a preexisting matrix. Since both processes affect the results of this assay, increased levels of type III procollagen peptide have been reported in fibrotic diseases, i.e., liver cirrhosis, myelofibrosis, and lung fibrosis, and also have been correlated with destructive inflammation, such as that in acute viral hepatitis.

The development of molecular markers for joint diseases has focused on the immunochemical quantification of cartilage compo-

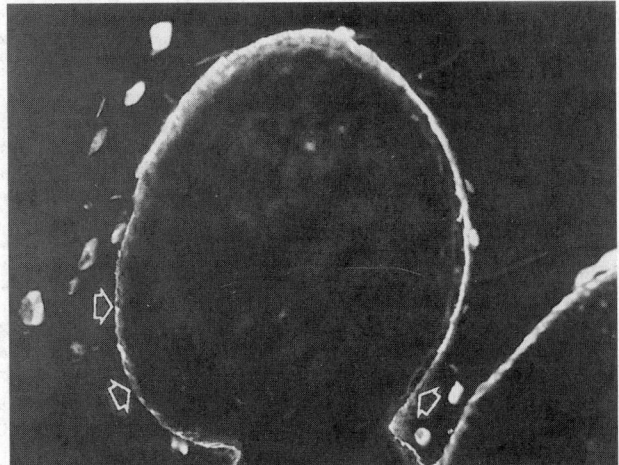

FIGURE 234–3. Frozen section of carcinoma *in situ* of the breast stained with monoclonal antibodies against human collagen type IV and fluorescence-labeled immunoglobulin antimouse G (IgG). In contrast to other atypical hyperplastic lesions, a thinning and focal loss of basement membrane integrity *(arrows)* is frequently observed in carcinoma *in situ* and suggests foci of preceding microinvasion.

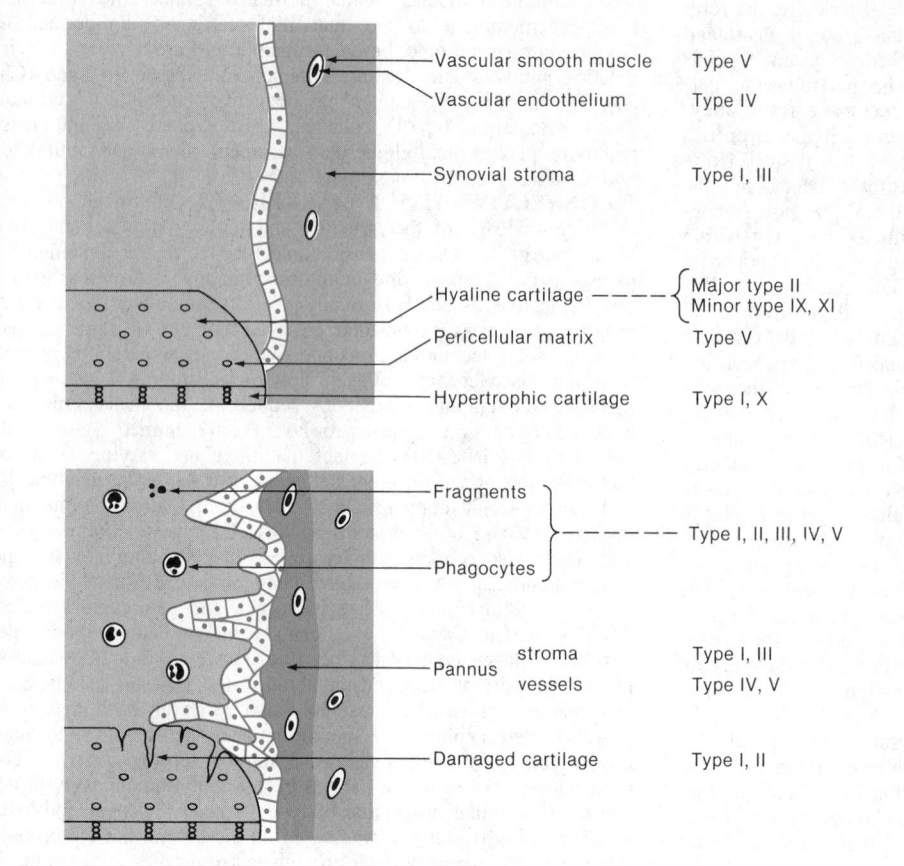

Vascular smooth muscle — Type V
Vascular endothelium — Type IV

Synovial stroma — Type I, III

Hyaline cartilage — { Major type II / Minor type IX, XI }
Pericellular matrix — Type V
Hypertrophic cartilage — Type I, X

Fragments —
— Type I, II, III, IV, V
Phagocytes —

Pannus   stroma — Type I, III
         vessels — Type IV, V

Damaged cartilage — Type I, II

FIGURE 234–4. Distribution of collagen types in a normal and rheumatoid joint. The normal synovial lining cell layer is supported by a loose fibrillar network composed of interstitial collagen types I and III, but lacking a continuous basement membrane. Basement membrane collagen type IV is restricted to the vascular endothelium. Vascular smooth muscle cells and pericytes are surrounded with fine, filamentous collagen type V, which is further associated with the interstitial fibers. The vast majority of the interstitial cartilaginous matrix is derived from type II collagen. Collagen types V, IX, and XI are distinctly associated with the hyaline articular interstitium. Synovial fluid normally does not contain collagen. Therefore, detection of collagen in synovial fluid and phagocytes indicates erosive and/or inflammatory joint disease. Detection of type IV collagen suggests endothelial damage and, if found concomitantly with type V collagen, implicates actual necrosis of the vessel walls, i.e., vasculitis. The detection of type I collagen indicates a high level of proteolytic breakdown of synovial stroma and/or bone matrix. Since type II collagen is restricted to the cartilage, the appearance of type II collagen epitopes in synovial fluid and serum represents a sensitive indicator of cartilage destruction and may serve as a tool for monitoring the effects and side effects of antirheumatoid drug therapy. (Reprinted with permission from Gay S, Gay RE: Cellular basis and oncogene expression of rheumatoid joint destruction. Rheumatol Int 9:105–113, 1989.)

nents using specific antibodies. In this regard, cartilage proteoglycan core protein and glycoproteins have been studied in serum and synovial fluid from patients with various arthritides. Keratan sulfate has been assayed as a marker of cartilage metabolism, and collagen type II as a marker of cartilage destruction (Fig. 234–4).

Bernfield M, Kokenyesi R, Kato M, et al.: Biology of the syndecans: A family of transmembrane heparan sulfate proteoglycans. Annu Rev Cell Biol 8:365, 1992. *This review article on a specialized novel structural proteoglycan supplements the review by Hardingham and Fosang.*

Christiano AM, Uitto J: Molecular pathology of the elastic fibers. J Invest Dermatol 103:55 (Suppl), 1994. *Provides the most updated information on structure and pathology of elastin.*

Hardingham TE, Fosang AJ: Proteoglycans: Many forms and many functions. FASEB J 6:861, 1992. *A concise survey of proteoglycans as modifiers of the organization of the extracellular matrices and modulators of the processes that occur there.*

Kivirikko KL: Collagens and their abnormalities in a wide spectrum of diseases. Ann Med 25:113, 1993. *Reviews mutations of the distinct collagen types and their putative role in connective tissue diseases.*

Lin CQ, Bissell MJ: Multifaceted regulation of cell differentiation by extracellular matrix. FASEB J 1993;7:737. *Summarizes the current data in which the extracellular matrix has been shown to be a crucial regulator of tissue-specific gene expression.*

Mayne R, Brewton RG: New members of the collagen superfamily. Curr Opin Cell Biol 5:883, 1993. *A concise review of previously described new collagen types XII–XIX.*

Miller EJ, Gay S: Collagen structure and function. *In* Wound Healing—Biochemical and Clinical Aspects. Philadelphia, WB Saunders, 1992, pp. 130–151. *An in-depth review on the biochemistry of collagens.*

Williams MJ, Hughes PE, O'Toole TE, Ginsberg MH: The inner world of cell adhesion: Integrin cytoplasmic domains. Trends Cell Biol 4:109, 1994. *A novel presentation of the integrin family of transmembrane receptors for transfer of signals across the cell membrane.*

Yamada H, Watanabe K, Shimonaka M, Yamaguchi Y: Molecular cloning of brevican, a novel brain proteoglycan of the aggrecan/versican family. J Biol Chem 269: 10119, 1994. *An example of the kind of experimental approaches currently applied to discover novel matrix components such as brevican and neurocan of the brain.*

235 TISSUE INJURY IN RHEUMATIC DISEASES

Gerald Weissmann

Acute inflammation and tissue injury in the rheumatic diseases are caused by host defense mechanisms that are designed to attack bacteria or viruses but become diverted instead into attacking the tissues of the host. The two major inflammatory diseases of rheumatology are rheumatoid arthritis (RA) and systemic lupus erythematosus (SLE), and we understand their pathophysiology thanks to three well-studied models of experimental pathology. Whereas some of their *acute* lesions resemble the Arthus and the Shwartzman reactions, in which neutrophils play the key role, the *chronic* features of RA mimic another model of experimental pathology, the tuberculin reaction and its late granuloma formation, in which cytokines, growth factors, and activated macrophages predominate. Joint injury and cartilage degradation result when synovial cells with activated proto-oncogenes form an invasive lesion called *pannus.*

THE ARTHUS LESION AS A MODEL FOR RHEUMATOID ARTHRITIS. Following the prescient observation of Magendie in 1839 that the second and third intravenous (IV) injections of foreign proteins into rabbits were followed by increasing distress, Richet coined the word "anaphylaxis" in 1902 to describe acute catastrophes mediated by repeated IV injections of antigens. Arthus, in 1903, then provoked "local anaphylaxis" in rabbits by repeated injections of antigen intradermally; inflammation and necrosis resulted. Opie, in 1924, confirmed that the lesions of Arthus were local antigen-antibody reactions in which inflammation was mediated by white cells and that proteolysis was crucial. Indeed, it was found that the Arthus lesions also could be provoked by planting antigen in the skin followed by specific antibody intravenously (the "passive Arthus reaction") or by injecting antibody in the skin followed by antigen intravenously (the "reversed passive Arthus reaction") (Fig. 235–1). In each case, one was dealing with the interactions at a surface of neutrophils that had been attracted by immune complexes localized beneath the endothelium of blood vessels. Comple-

ment, activated by immune complexes, releases anaphylatoxins (C5a and C3a), which liberate histamine. Histamine, in turn, causes reversible gaps to appear between endothelial cells, and once breached, the junctions permit egress of neutrophils. Stimulated by discrete receptors for C5a, C3a, and IgG's (FcγRII, FcγRIII), neutrophils release mediators of inflammation: reactive oxygen-derived products (O_2^-, H_2O_2), eicosanoids (see Ch. 19), and lysosomal enzymes. These products—especially superoxide (O_2^-), peroxide (H_2O_2), and proteases—cause irreversible tissue injury. Predictably, Arthus reactions can be abolished by rendering animals deficient in complement or in neutrophils. Antiproteases or antihistamines are somewhat less effective inhibitors of the Arthus lesion; antiplatelet agents or anticoagulants are useless. It is generally agreed that the local Arthus lesion is one model for immune complex vasculitis in humans, which is also due to interactions of neutrophils with immune complexes and complement. In generalized vasculitis of the Arthus type, the *homotypic* clumping of neutrophils to each other and their *heterotypic* sticking to endothelial cells are mediated by receptors for iC3b (CD11b/CD18), whereas the secretory responses of neutrophils are triggered by receptors for C5a and FcγRII.

The central role of neutrophils in this lesion is mirrored by their abundance in the synovial fluid of patients with RA. Their role in *periarteritis nodosa, leukocytoclastic vasculitis,* some of the *vasculitides of SLE,* and *allergic angiitis* is equally important. Although the *raison d'être* for the preponderance of neutrophils in rheumatoid synovial fluid is not yet clear, their sheer number is impressive. Neutrophils comprise over 90% of cells found in the synovial fluid of patients with RA, and it has been estimated that the daily turnover of neutrophils in 30 ml of a rheumatoid joint effusion is greater than a billion cells per joint. The cells take up self-associating complexes of IgG–IgG rheumatoid factor as well as the more common IgM/IgG complexes; complement is, predictably, activated. *Rheumatoid vasculitis* is another extra-articular problem mediated by neutrophils in seropositive *RA* patients.

THE SHWARTZMAN PHENOMENON AS ANOTHER MODEL OF VASCULITIS. Culture filtrates of gram-negative bacteria injected into the skin of rabbits prepare the site for hemorrhagic necrosis when similar filtrates are injected intravenously, a finding first made by Gregory Shwartzman in 1937. The two lesions require a latent, or "preparatory," period of 6 to 24 hours, and the second injection need not be of the same filtrate (Fig. 235–1). The systemic or generalized Shwartzman phenomenon provokes variable degrees of pulmonary or systemic vasculitis and bilateral renal cortical necrosis as its signature. Like the local lesion, it can be faithfully reproduced by purified endotoxins. Locally or systemically, the "preparatory" injection of endotoxin promotes modest adhesion of neutrophils to postcapillary venules with escape of some of the white cells from the vessels. The second, or "provocative," injection leads to microclumps of platelets and leukocytes within the circulation, and these tend to be sequestered in peripheral capillary beds or to attach to the sticky endothelium of venules of the prepared skin site.

The Shwartzman phenomenon can be elicited by second injections not only of endotoxin but also of various polyanions, glycogen, or antigen/antibody complexes, all of which share with endotoxin the capacity to activate complement via the alternative pathway. Moreover, local and systemic Shwartzman reactions can be prevented by rendering animals deficient in complement or neutrophils. In contrast to their inefficacy in the Arthus lesion, anticoagulants and antiplatelet drugs block the local and systemic Shwartzman phenomena. The final Shwartzman lesion is an intravascular insult with secondary damage to endothelial cells. It should be emphasized that the Shwartzman lesion is therefore an exception to the usual circumstances in which neutrophils fail to injure the endothelial cell layer from which they escape in response to chemoattractants.

Our modern interpretation of the Shwartzman phenomenon is based on recent studies with endotoxin tumor necrosis factor alpha (TNF-α) and cellular adhesive molecules displayed by activated endothelial cells and neutrophils. Both in the local and the systemic lesion, endotoxin elicits the formation of interleukin-1 (IL-1) by Langerhans cells, endothelial cells, or tissue histiocytes and of IL-1 and TNF-α from macrophages. These cytokines render venous en-

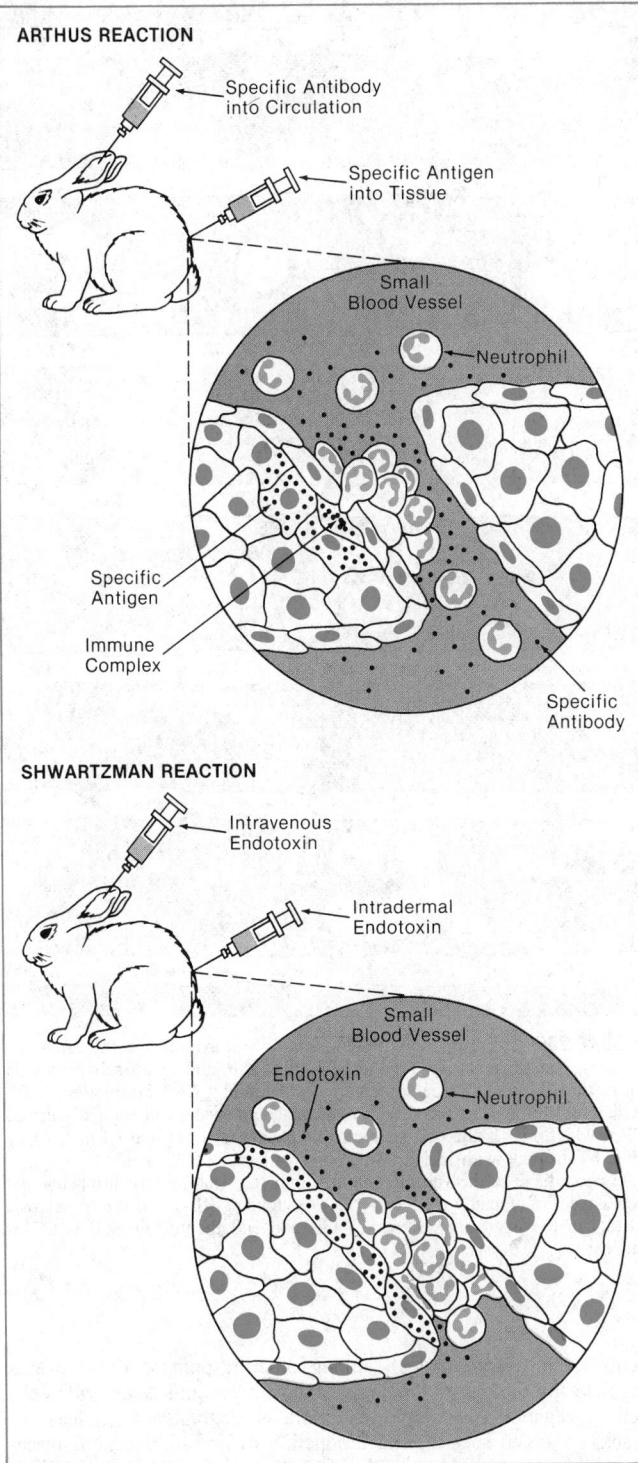

ARTHUS REACTION

Specific Antibody into Circulation

Specific Antigen into Tissue

Small Blood Vessel

Neutrophil

Specific Antigen

Immune Complex

Specific Antibody

SHWARTZMAN REACTION

Intravenous Endotoxin

Intradermal Endotoxin

Small Blood Vessel

Endotoxin

Neutrophil

FIGURE 235–1. In the Arthus model of vascular injury in SLE *(top),* intradermal injection of an antigen following intravenous injection of specific antibody leads to immune complex (IC) deposition in vessel walls at the intradermal injection site, which triggers local complement activation, inflammation, neutrophil infiltration, and tissue destruction. In the Shwartzman model *(bottom),* an intradermal injection of the antigen leads to intravascular alternate pathway complement activation. Antibody is not required, and no IC's are formed. Instead, neutrophils, primed by endotoxin and activated by complement, aggregate within small blood vessels at the intradermal injection site, plugging them and causing distal ischemia.

dothelium sticky—"prepared" in Shwartzman's terms—by inducing the display of adhesive, ligand-like molecules such as endothelial leukocyte adhesion molecule (ELAM-1) and by enhancing the procoagulant activity of endothelial surfaces (see below). The enhanced stickiness of endothelial cells induced by endotoxin, TNF, or IL-1 leads to *heterotypic* cell-cell adhesion of neutrophils by activating and upregulating the adhesive integrin CR3 (CD11b/CD18) on the neutrophil surface.

The second, provocative injection of endotoxin, glycogen, or immune complexes now causes massive *homotypic* neutrophil clumping. With C5a as the major culprit, neutrophils release inflammatory mediators such as hydroxl radical (OH⁻), H_2O_2, eicosanoids, platelet activating factor (PAF), and lysosomal enzymes. As when complement is activated in experimental and clinical examples of the adult respiratory distress syndrome (ARDS) (Ch. 65 and 68), leukoaggregates become enmeshed in small capillaries, where the procoagulant effects of endotoxin (via platelets and Factor X) contribute to plugging of the vessels (Fig. 235–2). Tissue injury has been chiefly attributed to H_2O_2 and elastase. Neutrophils adhering to endothelial cells—as provoked by TNF, for example—are antagonized by another cytokine: transforming growth factor beta (TGF-β), which in turn is the most potent chemoattractant yet described.

It has now been appreciated that complement-mediated neutrophil aggregation may contribute not only to tissue injury in such diverse conditions as *ARDS, acute pancreatitis, Purtscher's retinopathy, acute thermal injury,* and the *extension of myocardial infarction* but also—especially in SLE—to florid vascular crises. Sera from patients with active SLE contain several factors (among them C5a) that cause normal neutrophils to aggregate. Neutrophil aggregating activity correlates with the activity of the disease and is most pronounced in patients with central nervous system (CNS) involvement. The availability of radioimmunoassays specific for complement split products permitted documentation of elevated levels of circulating C3a, C5a, and the C5b-9 membrane attack complex in patients with active SLE. Indeed, elevated C3a levels may predict flares of SLE, rising 2 months before disease becomes clinically apparent. Moreover, complement split products Ba and Bb (generated exclusively by the alternative pathway) are also elevated in active SLE; elevated levels of Ba and Bb are better predictors of clinical disease than conventional assays of total C3 and C4 or CH_{50}. In the course of SLE, microthrombosis without inflammation of the vessel wall (i.e., "vasculitis") has been described in lung, kidney, and brain, and histologic evidence has been found of intravascular leukoaggregation associated with elevated levels of circulating complement split products.

With C5a and C3a active in plasma, it is not surprising that cell receptors for complement become activated and upregulated: CR3 (CD11/CD18; see below) has been best studied. As expected, increases in CD11b/CD18 correlate with increased levels of circulating C5a and C3a. Increased expression of CD11b/CD18 on neutrophils has, again, been demonstrated in patients with active, but not inactive, SLE. The highest levels of neutrophil CD11b/CD18 are found in patients with the most severe disease, especially *cerebritis,* a group that had the highest levels of circulating C3a. CD11b/CD18 expression returns to control levels with improvement of clinical disease after these episodes of the "acute cerebral distress syndrome." In sum, whereas the normal emigration of neutrophils from endothelium does little injury to the vessel wall, the unique circumstances of the Shwartzman lesion—in which C3a and C5a are activated in the circulation—permit cytokine-activated endothelial cells to become susceptible to damage by complement-activated neutrophils.

RELEASE OF MEDIATORS OF INFLAMMATION FROM THE NEUTROPHIL. After engagement of its surface receptors by immune complexes (via FcγRII and FcγRIII receptors, CD32, and CD16, respectively) or chemottractants (receptors for C5a, and others), this motile, postmitotic cell becomes equipped to seek and destroy microbes by chemotaxis and phagocytosis. After neutrophils are engaged by membrane receptors, they (1) activate phospholipases and turnover of membrane phospholipids, (2) alter ion fluxes and membrane potential, (3) increase cytosolic calcium, (4) phosphorylate cellular proteins, and (5) assemble cytoskeletal compo-

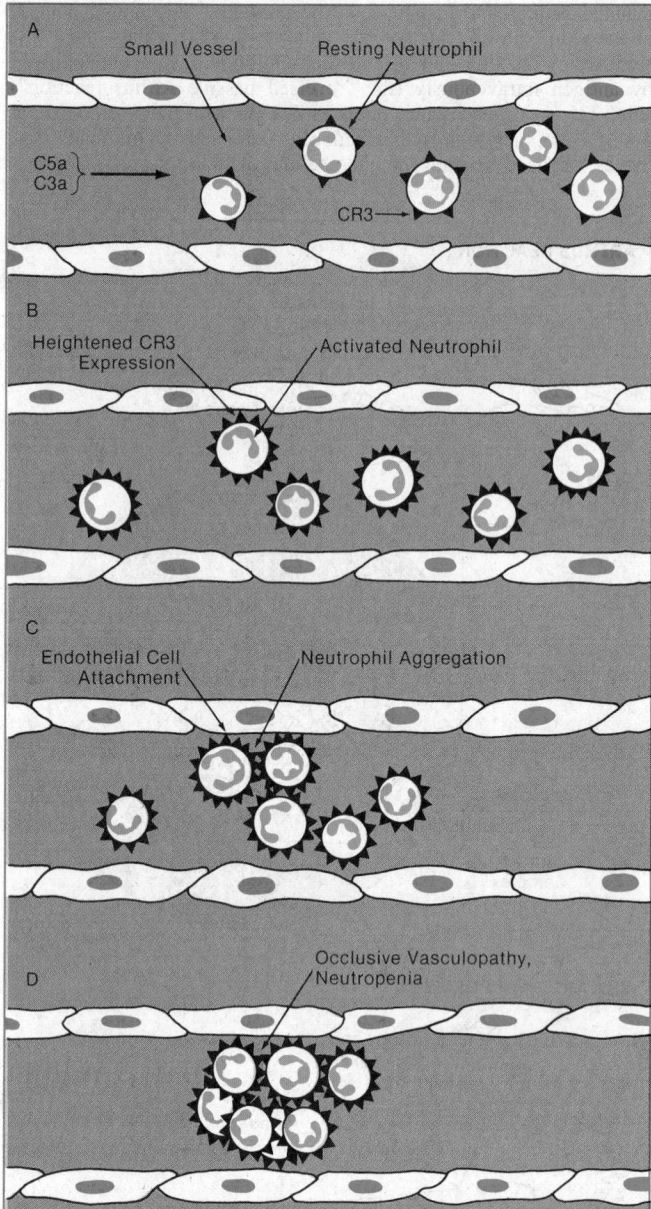

FIGURE 235–2. In active SLE, the process of intravascular complement activation, complement split product (CSP) release, and neutrophil activation may critically involve C5a stimulation of neutrophil CR3 expression (A, B). A hallmark of the activated neutrophil is heightened expression of surface CR3, which makes the cell stickier; this change can be induced *in vitro* by C5a. Neutrophils with increased numbers of surface CR3 would then aggregate and adhere to the vascular endothelium (C), leading to neutropenia and occlusive vasculopathy (D). The role of cytokines (IL-1 and tumor necrosis factor) in the interaction of neutrophils and endothelium in SLE is as yet unclear.

nents (actin, microtubules), among other responses. These events regulate the biological functions of *homotypic* and *heterotypic* cell-cell aggregation (see above), chemotaxis, degranulation, release of reactive oxygen species, and production of lipid-derived inflammatory substances such as platelet-activating factor (PAF), leukotriene B_4 (LTB_4), and lipoxin A.

Degranulation. During their maturation in the bone marrow, neutrophils acquire their characteristic populations of intracellular granules. These reservoirs, essentially lysosomes, serve as the main sources of enzymes responsible for destroying foreign substances and—by error, as it were—the tissue injury of inflammation. As they mature, neutrophils also acquire the enzymatic equipment with which to produce superoxide anion (O_2^-) and other mediators of tissue injury such as PAF or LTB$_4$. Primary (azurophil) granules, so named because of their early appearance in neutrophil maturation (or staining properties), contain myeloperoxidase, lysozyme, acid hydrolases, and several serine proteases, including elastase. Elastase is particularly important in connective tissue degradation because it is capable of breaking down not only elastin but also proteoglycans and collagen types III and IV. Secondary or specific granules are acquired later in maturation. These granules, like primary granules, also contain lysozyme, vitamin B$_{12}$–binding protein, lactoferrin, and the neutral proteinase collagenase. They also contain a reservoir of surface integrins (CD11b/CD18) and low-molecular-weight quanosine triphosphate (GTP)–binding proteins that bear homologies to the *ras* proteins of oncogenesis (see below). Collagenase has been detected in rheumatoid synovial fluid and degrades collagen types I, II, and III. Gelatinase, a third collagenolytic enzyme released by the neutrophil, has been localized to the C-particle compartment, an additional granule subclass. Gelatinase can degrade types IV, V, $1\alpha2\alpha3\alpha$, and denatured collagen. Thus neutrophil granules contain three enzymes—elastase, collagenase, and gelatinase—each with different substrate specificity and intracellular origin, which are capable of destroying collagen.

Neutrophils can discharge the contents of their intracellular granules either *overtly* or *covertly*. During uptake of particles, the neutrophil plasma membrane first invaginates to engulf particles such as immune complexes into a phagocytic vacuole. The vacuole then fuses with lysosomal granules to form a chamber called the "phagolysosome," and the granule contents are released into this chamber in the process called "covert degranulation." Sometimes, however, if the particle is too large, or if the opening of the chamber has not yet closed, lysosomal enzymes are freely discharged into the extracellular milieu, where they may attack host tissues. This "overt degranulation," a mechanism for extracellular secretion, has been termed "regurgitation during feeding," or when the material is too large to be ingested (e.g., immune complexes trapped in the matrix of cartilage), it has been given the picturesque name of "frustrated phagocytosis" (Fig. 235–3).

Antiproteases, such as α_2-macroglobulin and α_1-antitrypsin may prevent tissue damage caused by degradative proteases released inappropriately during overt degranulation. However, the effects of these antiproteases is readily overcome when they are exposed to hypochlorous acid, which inactivates them. Since hypochlorous acid (HClO$_3$) is formed in the neutrophil after interaction of myeloperoxidase, chloride anion, and H$_2$O$_2$ derived from O$_2^-$ via the NADPH oxidase of the cell, HClO$_3$ is an important mediator not only of bacterial killing (see Ch. 139) but also of tissue injury. The unfortu-nate interaction of granule enzymes and oxygen metabolites released by neutrophils permits proteases to act unopposed and to elicit the inadvertent tissue injury that accompanies brisk phagocytosis.

Release of Toxic Oxygen Products and Lipid Mediators. The H$_2$O$_2$ used in the reaction just described is one of several oxygen metabolites, including O$_2^-$ and OH$^-$, released during neutrophil activation. The generation of these toxic compounds is governed by the membrane-associated NADPH oxidase system. In addition to contributing to the formation of hypochlorous acid, oxygen metabolites also can damage connective tissue directly. For example, OH$_2^-$ is capable of degrading bovine synovial fluid and depolymerizing purified hyaluronic acid.

Neutrophils respond to engagement of receptors for chemoattractants or immune complexes by mobilizing arachidonate from the sn-2 position of phospholipids. Arachidonate—a fatty acid abbreviated as 20:4 because of its 20 carbons and 4 unsaturated double bonds—is mobilized from membrane stores directly via a phospholipase A$_2$ (PLA$_2$) or indirectly via a phospholipase C (PLC) and followed by the action of a diacylglycerol lipase on diacylglycerol (DAG). PLA$_2$'s, which are associated both with neutrophil granules and the plasma membrane, have two pH optima (5.5 and 7.5). Purified preparations of PLA$_2$'s require high concentrations of calcium for activity. Neutrophils appear to contain at least two PLC's, one which acts specifically on phosphatidylinositol (PI) and a second which acts on phosphatidylcholine (PC) to yield DAG. Data on the remodeling of lipids show that not only PLA$_2$ activity but also the activity of PLC and PLD can explain these changes (see below). After treatment with calcium ionophore or zymosan particles opsonized by C3b, neutrophils release 20:4 from PI and PC to an almost equivalent extent.

Once released from neutrophil phospholipids, 20:4 is transformed to *eicosanoid* metabolites (*eicosa* = "twenty") such as 5-HPETE by 5-lipoxygenase; the peroxide of 5-HPETE spontaneously forms 5-hydroxyeicosatetraenoic acid (or 5-HETE) or reacts further with the 5-lipoxygenase to form LTA$_4$, which has an epoxide at the 5,6 position. The 5-lipoxygenase has been purified, sequenced, and cloned. It is a complex enzyme assembly that requires an activation step. LTA$_4$ is then acted on by LTA$_4$ hydrolase (LTB$_4$ synthetase) to form 5S, 12R, 6,14-*cis,* 8,10-*trans*-dihydroxyeicosatetraenoic acid, or LTB$_4$. Alternatively, LTA$_4$ made by the neutrophil can be processed by other cells as well; transcellular metabolism is a rule with eicosanoids (see Ch. 19). LTA$_4$ can break down nonenzymatically to 5S, 6S, or 5S, 6R-6,8,10-*trans* 14-*cis*-dihydroxyeicosatetraenoic acid. These nonenzymatic metabolites have, at best, one tenth the activity of LTB$_4$ in activating neutrophils. In the presence of exogenous arachidonic acid, neutrophils also show 15-lipoxygenase activity, which, in a parallel manner, produces 15-HPETE and 15-HETE. These products, in turn, are acted on by an LTA$_4$ synthetase–like enzyme to make a 14,15-dihydroxy product and finally, in concert with 5-lipoxygenase, to yield the trihydroxy compounds lipoxins A and B. Mononuclear cells, in contrast, produce stable prostaglandins (PGE$_2$) and the sulfidopeptide leukotrienes LTC$_4$, LTD$_4$, and LTE$_4$.

Two major candidates as inflammatory mediators made from neutrophils are LTB$_4$ and lipoxin A. LTB$_4$ is a potent chemoattractant that promotes adhesion of neutrophils to endothelial cells from a variety of arterial and venous sites of several species—an effect not shared with other eicosanoids. Prostacyclin from endothelial cells (PGI$_2$) does not inhibit LTB$_4$-stimulated adhesion. Finally, lipoxin A has potent vasodilating effects *in vivo* (but not *in vitro*) and does not mimic the action of EDRF (nitric oxide). Lipoxin A only has modest effects on neutrophil chemokinesis; since its major biological action appears to be inhibiting natural killer (NK) cell activity, lipoxin A may chiefly regulate IgG receptor (FcγRIII)–mediated signal transduction.

STIMULUS-RESPONSE COUPLING: THE BASIS OF CELL ACTIVATION IN INFLAMMATION. *Phospholipids and Intracellular Calcium.* When chemoattractants such as formyl-methionyl phenyl alanine (fMLP), C5a, C3a, or LTB$_4$ engage their receptors, neutrophils respond by generating inositol trisphosphate (IP$_3$) and DAG. Although signaling via Fc receptors and receptors for chemoattractants (Fig. 235–4) differs with respect

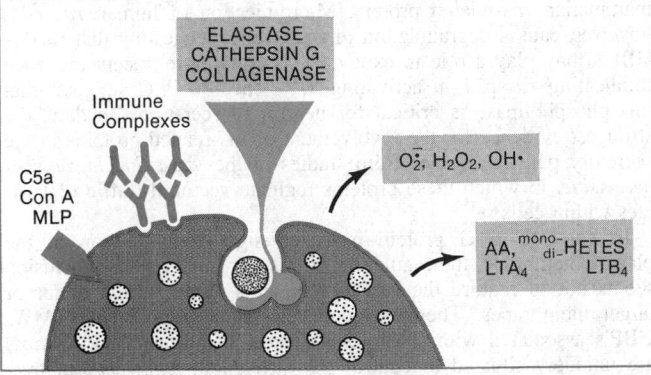

FIGURE 235–3. Release of mediators of inflammation by the human neutrophil. When neutrophils are engaged by chemoattractants of bacterial origin (fMLP, a bacterial peptide analogue), from the complement sequence (C5a), or by lectins (concanavalin A)—or by immune complexes—they release lysosomal enzymes from intracellular granules to the outside (overt degranulation), assemble and *activate* the NADPH oxidase that forms toxic oxygen species (O$_2^-$, H$_2$O$_2$, etc.), and turn over membrane phospholipids. These are the precursors for arachidonic acid (AA), which is transformed by an *activated* 5-lipoxygenase to the intermediate LTA$_4$, which can be used by neutrophils or other cells to form potent mediators: the leukotrienes (e.g., LTB$_4$).

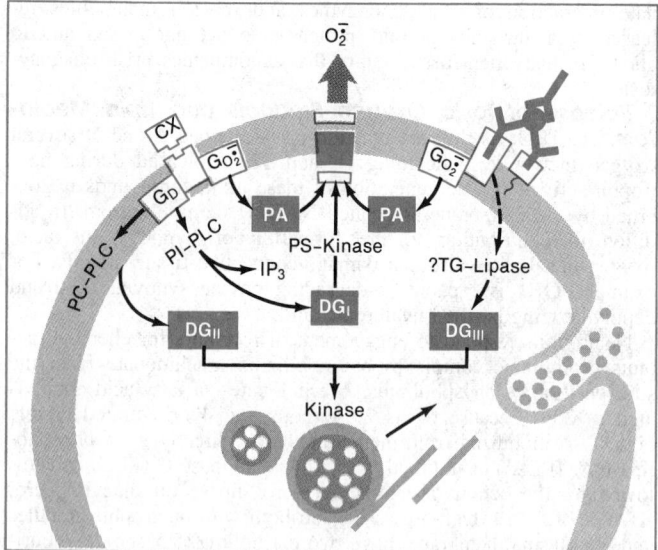

FIGURE 235–4. Stimulus-response coupling in the human neutrophil. Pathways for release of mediators of inflammation by chemoattractants (CX) on the left-hand side of the diagram differ from those launched by immune complexes (YY) on the right-hand side of the diagram. Three pools of diacylglycerol (DAG) are mobilized, only *one* of which (DAG III) is critical for secretion of lysosomal enzymes. Whereas CX-mediated generation of O_2^- is completely inhibited by pertussis toxin–sensitive G proteins, only some of the O_2^- assembly in response to immune complexes requires this intermediate. Phosphatidic acid (PA) seems to be the main intracellular messenger for assembly of the NADPH oxidase.

to some details, the *general* outline of stimulus-response coupling is similar, and neutrophils do not differ in these *general* pathways from other cells of inflammation.

Cellular IP_3 and DAG concentrations substantially increase within seconds after the fMLP receptor is engaged. By 5 seconds, IP_3 levels begin to decline. In contrast, both DAG and phosphatidic acid (PA) continue to increase over the course of the next 120 to 300 seconds. Although the exact sequence of enzyme reactions whereby the neutrophil generates these elevated levels of DAG and PA is not yet understood, it is likely that both PA and diglycerides play a crucial role in maintaining activation of the neutrophil. In order for neutrophils or macrophages to respond, over time and in space, two signals must be generated: a short "triggering" signal with an immediate increase in intracellular messengers (e.g., IP_3) and sustained "activation" signals (e.g., DAG or PA) required for the longer processes of chemotaxis and phagocytosis.

But lipid remodeling provides only *some* of the messengers needed for signal transduction. Calcium plays another key role. When treated with chemoattractants such as C5a or fMLP, neutrophils increase their levels of cytosolic calcium $[Ca]_i$, reaching a peak by 2 to 5 seconds. Over the next 2 minutes, $[Ca]_i$ slowly decreases and then returns *toward*—but not *to*—baseline. The peak levels (from 300 to 500 nM) are achieved primarily by IP_3-induced mobilization from intracellular stores, since similar levels are achieved in the absence of extracellular Ca. Influx of extracellular Ca begins approximately 5 seconds after Ca has been released from intracellular sites and while IP_3 levels are still dropping. Although IP_4 may in part regulate Ca channels, it is also possible that phosphatidic acid helps maintain Ca-dependent Ca influx.

Neutrophils break down PI to form DAG and PA within the first 5 seconds after chemoattractants or immune complexes engage receptors. Suggestions that one or another molecule in the PI-PA cycle mediate these changes in Ca permeability include the influx via PA-activated "Ca gates" or formation of IP_4 from inositol IP_3 by specific kinases. However, the turnover of IP_3/IP_4 as a consequence of specific phosphatases is extremely rapid (5 to 15 seconds), while DAG and PA continue to accumulate (30 to 120 seconds) after treating neutrophils with chemoattractants. In contrast, formation of DAG proceeds in a biphasic fashion. The first peak is at 2 to 5 sec-

onds, consistent with release of the "triggering" messengers IP_3 and DAG by the hydrolysis of polyphosphoinositides. Before this first wave is completed—by 15 to 30 seconds after treatment with fMLP—a second, more sustained wave of DAG formation commences. In contrast, PA rises throughout the time course of activation. Both PLC's and PLD's are involved in PA function. The concentration of DAG and PA remain elevated, compared with those of resting neutrophils, for more than 300 seconds in what has been called the "activation phase" of neutrophil responses. Although the evidence is by no means complete, it appears likely that the second wave of DAG is important in degranulation, whereas the increased levels of PA are important for assembly of the NAPH oxidase that is responsible for generating O_2^-.

GTP-Binding Proteins and Signal Transduction. The superfamily of GTP-binding proteins includes (1) the heterotrimeric proteins which transduce hormonal and sensory signals across the plasma membrane, (2) tubulin (each dimer binds 1 mole of GTP strongly and 1 mole loosely), (3) the elongation and initiation factors of protein synthesis, (4) products of the *ras* oncogene, and (5) putative GTP-binding proteins of cellular secretion. Whereas neutrophils clearly have GTP-binding proteins at their plasmalemma, the protein is neither a classic G_s or G_i protein and appears instead to be at least one novel G protein: G_n. In turn, at least one function of G_n is to couple receptors for chemoattractants to PLC. Composed of typical β/γ membrane components and an α subunit of the cytosol, 33 to 50% of the G_n protein is complexed to the β/γ dimer in the membrane, while the remainder is free in the cytosol. Pertussis toxin (PT) binds to the α subunit at sites distinct from the GTP site. Ribosylation by PT of the soluble α subunit is enhanced 12-fold by addition of β/γ subunits, whereas PT-ribosylation of membrane G_n is only modestly enhanced. G_n comprises between 1 and 3% of membrane proteins; no great excess of these molecules (10^6 per cell) is present over possible receptors (e.g., receptors for IgG and C5a). The neutrophil G protein (α subunit) is a substrate for ADP ribosylation both by pertussis and by cholera toxins (CT); both toxins inhibit high-affinity fMLP binding, and the protein is antigenically distinct not only from G_s and G_i proteins of other sources but also from the common G_o protein of brain. Predictably, for G protein–mediated functions, treatment of intact neutrophils with pertussis toxin inhibits ligand-mediated O_2^- generation, degranulation, chemotaxis, phospholipid turnover, high-affinity fMLP binding, release of eicosanoids, and Ca fluxes.

However, the G proteins of signal transduction are not the only G proteins of inflammatory cells; a rapidly growing family of "low-molecular-weight GTP-binding proteins" (LMW-GBP's) with molecular weights in the range of 20,000 to 30,000 are also present. These proteins are characterized by marked sequence homology to the *ras* oncogene product (*ras* p21). Unlike their high-molecular-weight counterparts, no clear function has been attributed to any mammalian *ras*-related protein. Microinjection of human *ras* p21, however, causes degranulation of mast cells, suggesting that LMW-GBP's may play a role in exocytosis. Furthermore, recent evidence implicating *ras* p21 in activating a PC-specific PLC suggests that this phospholipase is critical for neutrophil secretion. To date, the strongest evidence for the involvement of *ras*-related proteins in the secretory pathway comes from studies of the yeast *Saccharomyces cerevisiae*, in which these proteins regulate vectorial traffic of vesicles within cells.

In contrast to G protein–mediated signal transduction at the plasma membrane, the regulation of vesicular movement and fusion seems not to require the transduction of a signal across donor or target membranes. There is good reason to suspect that LMW-GBP's associated with neutrophil granule membrane GBP's *(rabs)* are uniquely situated to control the differential and vectorial trafficking of secretory granules in inflammatory cells. Indeed, these proteins can be considered as regulators of intracellular "docking" of secretory granules in the course of the inflammation.

SIGNALING VIA FC RECEPTORS: THE RESPONSE TO IMMUNE COMPLEXES. Three major classes of receptors have been described for the constant Fc region of human IgG's. FcγRI is *a high-affinity receptor* for monomeric IgG (K_a = approx. 10^{-8} M, 72 kDa) found mainly on mononuclear cells; recognized by monoclonal antibody 32, it is upregulated in response to interferon (IFN). Neutrophils also have *two low-affinity receptors* ($K_a = \sim 10^{-6}$ M) that bind aggregated IgG's or immune complexes much more avidly than monomeric IgG. FcγRII (or CD32) of approximately 40 kDa is present at 15,000 sites per cell (as recognized by monoclonal antibody IV-3) and is also present on B cells, macrophages, and platelets. FcγRII (1) is resistant to elastase, (2) is not linked to the plasmalemma via PI, (3) is present on neutrophils from patients with paroxysmal nocturnal hemoglobinuria (PNH), (4) appears to mediate O_2^- generation and degranulation, and (5) transduces all the signal for O_2^- generation and some of the signal for degranulation by means of a pertussis-sensitive G protein.

FcγRIII (or CD16) also prefers multimeric IgG and is expressed in heterogeneous fashion on neutrophils, macrophages, and NK cells. FcγRIII has a broad molecular weight range of 50,000 to 70,000, is present at approximately 120,000 sites per neutrophil, and is recognized by monoclonal antibody 3G8. The FcγRIII's on neutrophils and NK cells differ with respect to mass and are products of different but very homologous genes. FcγRIII's of the neutrophil are (1) elastase-sensitive, (2) linked to the external plasmalemma via PI, (3) reduced to 90% of controls at the plasmalemma—but not the Golgi region—of cells from patients with PNH, (4) an ineffective trigger of cells for O_2^- or enzyme release, and (5) polymorphic with respect to structure and antigenicity because there are two alleles (CNA1 and NA2). FcγRIII's are shed into the supernatant of neutrophils exposed to fMLP, whereas macrophages and NK cells—in which FcγRIII is a transmembrane structure—do not shed this receptor.

Since cells from patients with paroxysmal nocturnal hemoglobinuria respond as well as normal cells to IgG-opsonized particles by O_2^- generation and all O_2^- generating activity in response to IgG is PT-sensitive, we must conclude that the FcγRII is linked to GTP-binding proteins, whereas FcγRIII is not (see Fig. 235–4). Recent evidence shows that whereas stimulus-response coupling induced by immune complexes in the bulk phase is largely sensitive to PT, degranulation and O_2^- generation induced by immune complexes on a surface are relatively insensitive to PT. From these observations, it appears that FcγRIII may accumulate at the interface between neutrophils and the immune complexes trapped in the subendothelium. Moreover, signaling via Fc receptors *differs* from signaling via chemoattractant receptors in that the former is dependent on the integrity of cytoplasmic microtubules, whereas chemoattractant-induced signaling is independent of microtubules. *Colchicine therefore inhibits FcγR signaling.* FcγRIII receptors may serve to cluster Fc receptors in the service of "frustrated phagocytosis" when discharge of neutrophil contents is launched by an IgG-opsonized particle too large to digest. Therefore, of the two neutrophil Fc receptors for IgG, it appears that FcγRII triggers cells via classic G protein–mediated signal transduction as in synovial fluid. In contrast, FcγRIII receptors unlinked to G proteins mediate neutrophil discharge in vascular lesions where IgG's are trapped at subendothelial sites, as in vasculitis when release of mediators of inflammation is by "frustrated phagocytosis."

THE INTEGRINS AND INFLAMMATION. The adhesion of formed elements of the blood to endothelium and to each other is mediated by a superfamily of membrane proteins called "integrins." Three major families of mammalian integrins have been described: (1) receptors for extracellular matrix molecules such as fibronectin and T lymphocyte receptors known as "very late appearing antigens" (VLA's), (2) platelet surface glycoprotein IIb/IIIa and the vitronectin receptor, and (3) the LFA-1 family of leukocyte adhesion molecules. The most striking characteristic shared by these molecules is their noncovalently linked α/β heterodimer configuration in which the same β subunit is shared by all members of a family. In addition, many, but not all, integrins contain a domain that recognizes an Arg-Gly-Asp (RGD) sequence present in their respective ligands.

The LFA-1 family of leukocyte adhesion molecules includes three heterodimeric glycoproteins that share a common 95-kDa β chain (CD18): LFA-1, Mac-1 (also called Mo1, gp165/95, and CR3), and gp150/90, whose α chains have been designated CD11a, 11b, and 11c, respectively. The expression of these three molecules varies according to lineage and stage of maturation of various hematopoietic cells. In addition to mediating cell-cell adhesion, CD11b/CD18 functions as a receptor for iC3b (CR3) and thereby mediates phagocytosis of opsonized particles.

CD11b/CD18 is probably the major neutrophil adhesion molecule involved in *heterotypic* (neutrophil-endothelium) and *homotypic* (neutrophil-neutrophil) adhesion. A group of children genetically deficient in all three LFA-1 family adhesion molecules suffers from recurrent bacterial infections, impaired pus formation, delayed wound healing, and poor separation of the umbilical cord. Neutrophils from these patients are defective in functions related to adhesion such as aggregation, spreading on surfaces, directed migration, and attachment to endothelial monolayers. Normal human neutrophils treated *in vitro* with a subset of available anti-CD11b/CD18 monoclonal antibodies exhibit defects indistinguishable from those of neutrophils from patients with deficiency.

Although CD11b/CD18 is clearly implicated in the events of neutrophil adhesion, the molecular mechanisms are unclear. Under normal circumstances, neutrophil sticking must be suppressed to permit cells to circulate. Once they encounter ligands, cell activation is required to render neutrophils sticky. In heterotypic adhesion, the other agonist is the endothelial cell. The endothelial cell plays an active role in adhesion and displays to inflammatory cells an inducible endothelial surface glycoprotein designated ELAM-1 that partially mediates adhesion of leukocytes including neutrophils. Interleukin-1 (IL-1), tumor necrosis factor (TNF), lymphotoxin (LT), and endotoxin induce the expression of ELAM-1 on endothelial cells. Intercellular adhesion molecule 1 (ICAM-1), a similar but distinct antigen found on a variety of cells including endothelial cells, is the ligand for LFA-1 and is therefore one of several molecules that direct lymphocyte binding to high endothelial cells, especially those of the chronically inflamed rheumatoid joint. On the other hand, the endothelial side of the equation can be modified by transforming growth factor β (TGF-β). TGF-β inhibits the adherence of human neutrophils not only to normal endothelium but also to endothelial cells rendered sticky by ELAM-1, as induced by TNF-α.

In *homotypic* adhesion (neutrophil-neutrophil), the Cd11b/CD18 heterodimer receptor engages an as yet unknown ligand on an adherent neutrophil. The putative ligand is unlikely to be adsorbed iC3b, nor is the adhesive ligand likely to be CD11b/CD18 itself because normal neutrophils are capable of aggregating with neutrophils from CD11b/CD18-deficient patients.

CD11b/CD18 is constitutively expressed on the surface of resting neutrophils at a density of 10,000 to 20,000 molecules per cell. Upon activation by a number of stimuli, including especially chemoattractants, neutrophils upregulate their surface expression 5- to 10-fold. Since mature neutrophils synthesize few new proteins, it is not surprising that upregulation of CD11b/CD18 is due to translocation of preformed receptor to the plasma membrane from an intracellular source that co-sediments with specific granules.

Because each stimulus that enhances neutrophil adhesion also induces Mac-1 upregulation, it was widely believed that these two phenomena were causally related, but recent studies have dissociated neutrophil-neutrophil aggregation from upregulation of CD11b/CD18. Indeed, whereas the constitutive presence on the cell surface of CD11b/CD18 is *required* for neutrophil adhesion, regulation of cell-cell adhesion appears to involve a structural change in each receptor molecule rather than a quantitative change in the number of receptors.

RHEUMATOID ARTHRITIS AS A FORM OF THE TUBERCULIN REACTION. The histopathology of RA can be divided into two phases: (1) the acute inflammatory lesion—the Arthus-type lesion discussed earlier—and (2) the more chronic, mononuclear, cell-mediated, granulomatous disease proceeding in the deeper layers. This lesion—pannus—is marked by (1) focal collections of B lymphocytes and plasma cells that synthesize rheumatoid factors locally, (2) various subsets of T lymphocytes, (3) activated macrophages (Fig. 235–5), and (4) the proliferation of other mesenchymal cells of the synovium where genes for proto-oncogenes have been activated. The two types of activated cells, macrophages and synoviocytes, generate cytokines that cause chondrocytes to participate in their own destruction by releasing proteases and specific collagenase.

The lesions resemble those found in the tuberculin reaction, save for the clusters of B lymphocytes and plasma cells with rheumatoid factor. Indeed, for many years RA was thought to be a form of tu-

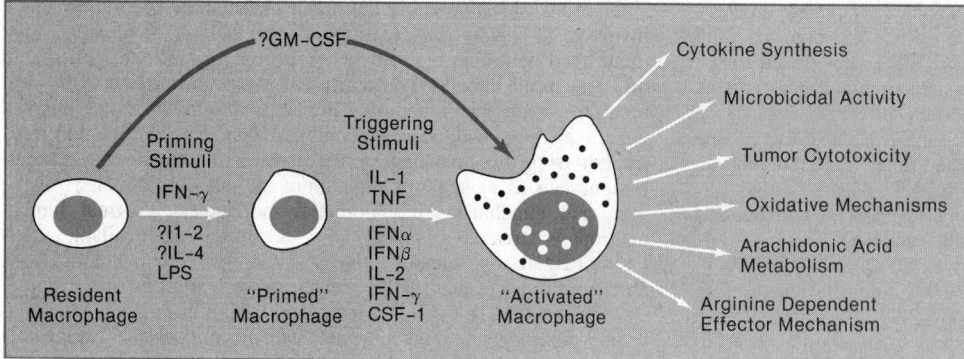

FIGURE 235–5. Schematic depiction of the role of cytokines in the two-stage hypothesis of macrophage activation. Unstimulated cells are primed by treatment with low-dose LPS, IFN-γ, and possibly IL-2. Primed macrophages can be triggered to an activated state by many other cytokines. Activation of the macrophages has classically been defined by demonstrating augmented effector functions as shown.

berculosis, and the gold salts that were used for treatment in the 1920's were first used for RA on this basis of this fuzzy correspondence. We may note that the earliest editions of this text classified RA as a form of "infectious arthritis."

Whereas the offending agent of RA is unknown, most modern speculation centers on the likelihood that one or another self-antigen looks very much like the product of a bacterium or virus. The major candidates have been (1) the Epstein-Barr virus (EBV), (2) type II collagen, (3) cartilage proteogylcan, and (4) heat shock (stress) proteins—especially a 65-kDa species against which many patients with RA mount a humoral and cellular immune response. Indeed, there is good evidence that stress proteins are present at the surface of antigen-presenting cells, and recently, it was found that a helper T-cell clone derived from a patient with tuberculous leprosy reacted with a synthetic peptide found in the third type variable region of the major histocompatability complex—DR2 β chain. The observation that cartilage proteoglycans share epitopes with acetone-extracted fractions of the tubercle bacillus suggests that when humans get RA, they respond to their own tissues as if these were products of the tubercle bacillus or EBV.

Whatever the offending antigen proves to be, the mediators released by T and B lymphocytes, by activated macrophages, and by activated synovial cells are the usual battery of cytokines found in chronic inflammation (Table 235–1). These cytokines in turn influence neutrophil function. Indeed, IL-1 (a pro-inflammatory cytokine produced chiefly by mononuclear cells but also by neutrophils) is capable of promoting thymocyte proliferation and synovial fibroblast activation and proliferation. Neutrophils display enhanced adherence to endothelial cells treated with IL-1. Among its many

other properties, IL-1 also induces production of PGE$_2$ and type II collagenase by chondrocytes. These actions are regulated by an IL-1 inhibitor, which appears to be constitutively present in cartilage cells and in the neutrophil.

Treatment of neutrophils with the lymphokines, IFN-γ, or TNF-β augments neutrophil phagocytic capacity, especially when PMN's are at the surface of cartilage. TNF-β, the most potent chemoattractant, also promotes neutrophil adherence to endothelial cells and stimulates hydrogen peroxide release and degranulation. Granulocyte macrophage colony-stimulating factor (GM-CSF), produced largely by fibroblasts, facilitates phagocytosis by neutrophils, possibly by increasing Fc receptor expression. Although many cytokines have no effect on neutrophil chemotaxis, etc., IL-8, a macrophage-derived neutrophil chemotactic factor, is one of the most potent neutrophil activators yet found.

TABLE 235–1. CELLULAR SOURCES AND TARGETS OF MAJOR CYTOKINES

Cytokine	Source	Target
IL-1α	Mφ, EC, fibroblasts	Lymphocytes, EC, HC, Mφ, fibroblasts, others
IL-1β	Mφ	Lymphocytes, EC, HC, Mφ, fibroblasts, others
IL-2	T cells	Lymphocytes, Mφ, others
IL-4	T cells	B cells, T cells, others
IL-8	Macrophages	PMN's
IFN-α	Lymphocytes	Multiple nucleated cells
IFN-β$_1$	Mφ	Multiple nucleated cells
IFN-β$_2$(IL-6)	Fibroblasts, Mφ	HC, lymphocytes, others
IFN-γ	T lymphocytes	Mφ, lymphocytes, others
M-CSF, CSF-1	Mφ	Bone marrow, Mφ, fibroblasts
GM-CSF	Fibroblasts	Mφ, PMN's
TNF-α	Mφ, fibroblasts	PMN's, Mφ others
TNF-β	Lymphocytes, Mφ	Multiple cells
TGF-β	T lymphocytes	PMN's, fibroblasts, Mφ
MDNCF	Mφ	PMN's

IFN = interferon; TNF = tumor necrosis factor; IL = interleukin; CSF = colony-stimulating factor; GM-CSF = granulocyte macrophage colony-stimulating factor; TGF-β = transforming growth factor β; Mφ = macrophage; PMN = polymorphonuclear neutrophil; EC = endothelial cell; HC = hepatocyte.

Abramson SB, Weissmann G: Complement split products and the pathogenesis of SLE. Hosp Pract 23:45, 1988. *How the Arthus phenomenon and the Shwartzman reaction apply to vasculitis in SLE.*

Bokoch GM: Signal transduction by GTP-binding proteins during leukocyte activation: Phagocytic cells. *In* Grinstein S, Rotstein OD (eds.): Mechanisms of Leukocyte Activation. New York, Academic Press, 1990, pp. 65–101. *A modern discussion of how the molecular biology of G proteins has permitted understanding of signal transduction control.*

Crofford LJ, Wilder RL, Ristimake AP, et al.: Cyclooxygenase-1 and -2 expression in rheumatoid synovial tissues: Effects of interleukin-1β, phorbol ester, and corticosteroids. J Clin Invest 93:1095, 1994. *How the two cyclo-oxygenases are influenced by interleukins and anti-inflammatory drugs in inflammation.*

Cronstein BN, Kimmel SC, Levin RI, et al.: A mechanism for the anti-inflammatory effects of corticosteroids: The glucocorticoid receptor regulates leukocyte adhesion to endothelial cells and expression of ELAM-1 and ICAM-1. Proc Nat'l Acad Sci USA 89:9991, 1992. *A modern view of how corticosteroids influence the display of adhesive molecules.*

Haines KA, Reibman J, Weissmann G: Triggering and activation of human neutrophils: two aspects of the response to transmembrane signals. *In* Poste G, Crooke ST (eds.): Cellular and Molecular Aspects of Inflammation. New York, Plenum Press, 1988, pp. 31–40. *A detailed analysis of the differences between immediate and prolonged responses to signals at the surface of inflammatory cells.*

Harris ED Jr: Pathogenesis of rheumatoid arthritis: A disorder associated with dysfunctional immunoregulation. *In* Gallin JI, Goldstein IM, Snyderman R (eds.): Inflammation. New York, Raven Press, 1985, pp. 751–774. *A review of rheumatoid inflammation with an emphasis on cell-cell interaction in chronic inflammation and cartilage destruction.*

Krane SM, Amento EP, Goldring SR, et al.: ML modulation of matrix synthesis and degradation in joint inflammation. *In* AM Glauert (ed.): The Control of Tissue Damage. Amsterdam, Elsevier, 1990, pp. 179–195. *How IL 1 appears to be crucial for the self-induced destruction in RA as mediated by prostaglandin E$_2$ and collagenase.*

Spaethe SM, Needleman P: Biosynthesis and release of lipid mediate of inflammation. *In* Poste G, Crooke ST (eds.): Cellular and Molecular Aspects of Inflammation. New York, Plenum Press, 1988, pp. 153–170. *A review of the cyclo-oxygenase and lipoxygenase pathways in inflammation, with a discussion of the role of essential fatty acid.*

Weissmann G: The role of neutrophils in vascular injury: Signal transduction mechanisms in cell/cell interactions. Springer Semin Immunopathol 11:235, 1989. *A review of the Arthus and Shwartzman models and how they relate to the vascular lesions of rheumatic diseases.*

West MA: Role of cytokines in leukocyte activation: Phagocytic cells. *In* Grinstein S, Rotstein OD (eds.): Mechanisms of Leukocyte Activation. New York, Academic Press, 1990, pp. 537–570. *A summary of the effects of cytokines—which are released in rheumatoid inflammation—on the activation of neutrophils and macrophages.*

Winfield JB: Stress proteins and autoimmunity. Arthritis Rheum 32:1497, 1989. *How heat shock proteins may be the link between autoantigens and microbial products in the perpetuating RA.*

236 SPECIALIZED PROCEDURES IN THE MANAGEMENT OF PATIENTS WITH RHEUMATIC DISEASES

Robert W. Ike and William J. Arnold

Rheumatic diseases can account for an array of clinical presentations that range from signs and symptoms reflecting multiorgan involvement to pain and compromised function in a single anatomic area. Correct diagnosis of a suspected rheumatic process and optimal management of the patient with an established rheumatic disease rest on the physician's ability to identify the site(s) from which the patient's symptoms arise, ascertain the pathologic process affecting the identified site(s), determine why the process is occurring, and find measures to gauge the activity of the disease so that response to treatment can be followed. A directed history and physical examination provide the bedrock for this exercise, with suspicions regarding anatomy, process, and diagnosis supported or refuted by appropriate laboratory tests, imaging modalities, and invasive procedures. The number of specialized procedures applicable to rheumatic diseases continues to grow. Testing for relevant immunologic phenomena becomes ever more complex as newer tests, such as those for the antineutrophil cytoplasmic antibody (ANCA) system, join established tests that have become subdivided as the molecular bases for the measured phenomena become appreciated, as for the many specific target antigens in the antinuclear antibody (ANA) reaction. Certain anatomic abnormalities that had escaped detection previously can now be identified by newer imaging procedures—both direct (arthroscopy) and indirect (ultrasound, magnetic resonance imaging)—although these procedures present hurdles of cost, availability, and operator expertise. These new tests and the other procedures discussed below must always be interpreted in the context of a thorough, comprehensive, multifaceted evaluation.

ASPIRATION OF SYNOVIAL JOINTS AND BURSAE. In any patient with undiagnosed arthritis and an associated joint effusion, examination of the synovial fluid is mandatory. Gross appearance of the synovial fluid can provide an initial clue to the underlying process, and certain disorders such as crystalline arthropathies and bacterial infection are quickly confirmed by specialized microscopic examination. Successful joint or bursal aspiration depends on a thorough familiarity with certain principles.

Both the physician and the patient must be comfortable. The physician should have some experience and confidence concerning the particular joint to be tapped. Although most general internists can aspirate the knee or the olecranon bursa, other commonly inflamed structures, such as the shoulder, ankle, elbow, first metatarsophalangeal joint, and subdeltoid bursa, require special expertise for successful aspiration. The patient should be positioned to allow relaxation of muscles on both sides of the joint to be aspirated. For the knee, the patient should be supine with the knee in slight flexion, accomplished by resting it on a pillow. Palpation identifies landmarks for entry, discerns the region of the largest "bulge" in the joint capsule (crucial for small joints), and confirms relaxation of periarticular muscles. If the patella cannot be moved side to side, entry to the knee will be painful and difficult if not impossible.

After preparing the skin with iodine solution, the gloved aspirating hand determines point of entry. Most physicians find the knee easiest to enter from the medial aspect, just inferior to midpoint of the patella edge. Except for very large effusions that can be entered quickly with the aspirating needle, the skin and subcutaneous path to the joint capsule should be anesthetized with lidocaine, delivered while advancing slowly with the smallest-gauge needle available. This promotes patient comfort and marks the path to be taken into the joint. The joint space is entered with an 18-gauge needle to which a syringe of up to 20 ml is attached, depending on the size of the effusion. Failure to obtain fluid from a clinically swollen joint space can result from several processes, including presence of synovial fluid too thick to be withdrawn through the needle used, presence of intra-articular debris clogging the needle, a swollen space comprised mainly of tissue, or sequestration of fluid away from the needle point. When aspiration of fluid is critical, such as in suspected septic arthritis, ultrasound or arthrography can help guide the needle to the fluid-containing section of the joint. A 5-ml sample of synovial fluid is more than adequate for all routine studies, including cultures.

Synovial fluid analysis begins with a look at the fluid in the heparinized tube. Fluid that transmits light and can be read through (determined by holding the tube in front of a sample of printed text) will generally prove to have <2000 white blood cells (WBC's) per milliliter and is associated with "noninflammatory" disorders, most commonly osteoarthritis (OA) (Table 236–1). Translucent fluid that blurs print will have >2000 WBC's per milliliter but $<100,000$ WBC's per milliliter and is associated with a wide array of "inflammatory" conditions, such as rheumatoid arthritis (RA). Opaque fluid, usually quite thick, carries the usual concerns of pus obtained from any other body cavity and should place acute infection as the leading diagnosis until proven otherwise. Usually, such fluid will show 50,000 to 100,000 WBC's per milliliter, but other compounds in high concentrations (cholesterol, monosodium urate) can produce opaque synovial fluid that is relatively acellular. Bloody-appearing fluid carries a specific differential diagnosis but does not always connote true hemarthrosis, since it takes but a small amount of blood within the joint space to make

TABLE 236–1. SYNOVIAL FLUID ANALYSIS

	Noninflammatory (Group I)	Inflammatory (Group II)	Purulent (Group III)	Hemorrhagic (Group IV)
Color	Yellow	Yellow	Yellow-green	Red
Clarity	Transparent	Translucent	Opaque	Opaque
Leukocyte count (WBC/ml)	<2000	2000–50,000†	$>50,000$	†
% Polymorphonuclear leukocytes	$<25\%$	$>50\%$	$>75\%$	†
Disease examples	Osteoarthritis	Rheumatoid arthritis	Bacterial infections	Trauma
	Trauma	Reiter's syndrome	Tuberculosis	Neuropathic joint
	Osteochondritis dessicans	Crystal synovitis, acute (gout, pseudogout)	RA (rare)	Coagulation disorders
	Osteonecrosis		Reiter's (rare)	Hemophilia
	Amyloidosis	Psoriatic arthritis	Pseudogout (rare)	von Willebrand's
	Scleroderma	Viral arthritis		Heparin or warfarin
	Systemic lupus*	Rheumatic fever		Sickle cell disease
	Polymyalgia rheumatica*	Behçet's syndrome		Chondrocalcinosis
	Hypertrophic pulmonary osteoarthropathy	Lyme disease		Scurvy
		Some bacterial infections		Tumor, especially pigmented villonodular synovitis, hemangioma

* Sometimes inflammatory.
† Wide range; WBC count should be interpreted in light of peripheral blood WBC and RBC counts.

synovial fluid appear bloody. Viscosity of the joint fluid is determined largely by molecular weight and concentration of hyaluronate, a proteoglycan polymer. Elaboration of enzymes that depolymerize hyaluronate can accompany synovial tissue inflammation in the absence of fluid phase inflammation. Hence "noninflammatory fluid" that appears "thin" and leaves a very short "string" when dripped from syringe into test tube can be due to synovitis that has not produced fluid phase inflammation and cloudy fluid. Bursal fluid cannot be classified by the same parameters as joint fluid. As a rule of thumb, the WBC count from bursal fluid is about one-tenth the WBC count that would be expected from a joint given the same phlogistic agent. For example, in gouty bursitis, an average bursal fluid leukocyte count is 2800 per milliliter compared with an average of 21,000 WBC's per milliliter in synovial fluid from an acute gouty joint. Thus bursal fluid with a leukocyte count of only a few hundred per milliliter should raise the same concerns—including the possibility of infection—as a joint fluid with several thousand WBC's per milliliter.

Examining synovial fluid under a polarized light microscope is essential for the diagnosis of crystal-associated arthropathies (see Color Plate 3C) and should be performed initially in all patients. Needle-shaped, negatively birefringent intracellular crystals of monosodium urate (MSU) confirm the diagnosis of gouty arthritis. Rhomboidal, positively birefringent intracellular crystals of calcium pyrophosphate dihydrate (CPPD) define the pseudogout syndrome. Intracellular CPPD and MSU crystals may be sparsely distributed on the microscope slide, and they are often identified only after a careful, thorough search guided by someone well versed in using the polarized microscope. Because other processes such as infection can "liberate" crystals into the joint fluid, identifying crystals in an acutely inflamed joint should not be taken as a complete explanation, particularly when CPPD is present. Other crystals and compounds identified by the polarized microscope include calcium oxalate (a positively birefringent tetrahedron found in some dialysis patients), corticosteroids from previous intra-articular injections (small and bright with variable birefringence characteristics), talc (positively birefringent clumps transferred from gloved hand to slide), lipid (round "maltese crosses" derived from bone marrow fat and indicative of fracture), and cholesterol (plate-like and brilliantly birefringent without a definite axis, associated with long-standing inflammatory effusions, especially when accompanied by bleeding as in hemophilia).

Bacterial infection should be considered in all patients with acute arthritis and in patients with established rheumatic disorders with exacerbation in one or several joints. Purulent, opaque synovial fluid is not present in all cases, and early-stage bacterial arthritis may not even produce "inflammatory" fluid. The most common pathogen is *Staphylococcus aureus*. Findings on Gram stain of synovial fluid can help guide initial therapy, but a negative study does not rule out infection. When clinical suspicion of septic arthritis is strong but not confirmed by initial studies of synovial fluid, empirical antibiotics should be given until culture results are available.

Arthritis due to other infectious agents may be more difficult to confirm. *Neisseria gonorrheae* is the most common gram-negative organism associated with infectious arthritis but is identified by Gram stain of synovial fluid in only a minority of cases. Chances for isolation of the gonococcus are improved if synovial fluid is plated directly onto chocolate agar and similar cultures are made from swabs of any skin lesions and of all potential portals of entry for the organism (urethra, cervix, anus, throat). *Mycobacteria* (*tuberculosis* and others) can cause an indolent monarthritis from which an inflammatory, mainly monocytic synovial fluid is obtained. Synovial fluid cultures are usually sterile, and signs of active extra-articular disease are minimal. A prompt, accurate diagnosis of tuberculous arthritis requires a high degree of suspicion and culture of synovial biopsy specimens. Extensive joint destruction is often present before a diagnosis of tuberculous arthritis is made.

Reduction in synovial fluid glucose to less than 50% of simultaneous serum measurement should raise suspicion for the diagnosis of infectious arthritis. In a patient with infectious arthritis, serial measurements of synovial fluid glucose levels can be one of the several parameters used to gauge the effectiveness of therapy.

ERYTHROCYTE SEDIMENTATION RATE AND ACUTE PHASE RESPONSE PROTEINS. The systemic response to tissue injury, regardless of cause, is characterized by a cytokine-mediated alteration in the hepatic synthesis of a number of different plasma proteins, known collectively as "acute phase reactants." These proteins, which include fibrinogen, haptoglobin, ceruloplasmin, α_1-antitrypsin, complement components C3 and C4, serum amyloid A protein, and C-reactive protein (CRP), rise in proportion to the severity of tissue injury, although the magnitude of rise in each component varies. Because some systemic rheumatic disorders cause chronic tissue inflammation and injury, assessment of the acute phase response is an important facet of rheumatic disease diagnosis and management (because the effectiveness of treatment is gauged by the extent to which the acute phase response is suppressed).

Measuring the *erythrocyte sedimentation rate (ESR)* has been a time-honored and simple method to approximate the acute phase response. "Extreme" elevation of the ESR (> 100 mm per hour) has come to have diagnostic significance, associated with polymyalgia rheumatica, giant cell arteritis, multiple myeloma, lymphoma, metastatic cancer, severe chronic infections such as subacute bacterial endocarditis and tuberculosis, and chronic renal failure. Reduction or normalization of the ESR is a goal of treatment for those treatable disorders associated with a rapid ESR. Sedimentation of erythrocytes is facilitated by certain plasma proteins that neutralize the negative charge on the erythrocyte surface, thus permitting the erythrocytes to aggregate and "fall" as a clump rather than as individual cells. Fibrinogen is among the plasma proteins capable of this action; thus the level of fibrinogen—which varies according to the intensity of the acute phase response—substantially affects the ESR. However, other proteins not associated with the acute phase response—notably immunoglobulin (particularly when present as a single paraprotein) and certain "middle molecules" in patients with chronic renal failure—also accelerate the ESR. Normal values for ESR span a wide range, slightly higher in women than in men and increasing with age in both sexes. Many individuals aged 70 and over may have ESR's in the range of 40 to 50 mm per hour without apparent inflammation or tissue injury. This confounds the utility of the ESR in supporting a suspected rheumatic disease diagnosis such as polymyalgia rheumatica in an elderly person. Finally, not all patients with clinically active rheumatic diseases have raised ESR's because of individual differences in hepatic function, alterations in erythrocytes, or abnormalities of other plasma proteins that counteract effects of acute phase reactants that speed the ESR.

Of the several acute phase reactants that can be measured directly, *C-reactive protein (CRP)*, named for its binding of pneumococcal C-polysaccharide, is the most extensively studied and clinically useful. Most rheumatic diseases, including RA, juvenile chronic arthritis, ankylosing spondylitis, polymyalgia rheumatica, systemic vasculitis, Behçet's syndrome, Reiter's disease, and psoriatic arthritis, are associated with high levels of CRP (1 to 10 mg per deciliter) when they are active, with falling or undetectable levels when improving or inactive. For diseases in the spondyloarthropathy family (ankylosing spondylitis, Reiter's, psoriatic arthritis), the CRP is far more sensitive to fluctuations in disease activity than is the ESR. Systemic lupus erythematosus (SLE) disease activity, in the majority of patients, raises the CRP only slightly if at all (1 to 3 mg per deciliter); concurrent infection in SLE will raise the CRP, and extreme CRP elevation (> 10 mg per deciliter) in a lupus patient should provoke a hunt for infection.

AUTOANTIBODIES. *Rheumatoid factors* are immunoglobulins directed against the Fc portion of immunoglobulin G (IgG) (see Ch. 237). Measuring rheumatoid factor by tests that determine the highest dilution of serum capable of agglutinating IgG-coated latex particles is being replaced in many laboratories by automated methods such as nephelometry and enzyme-linked immunosorbent assay (ELISA). Thus the reporting of rheumatoid factor "titer" is often replaced by reporting an absolute concentration. Rheumatoid factor positivity with titers up to 1:320 may be found in otherwise normal people over age 70. While rheumatoid factor can be found in 70 to 80% of patients with RA, it is also present in other rheumatic diseases (Sjögren's syndrome, cryoglobulinemia, SLE) and nonrheumatic diseases, such as chronic infections (hepatitis, subacute bacterial endocarditis). In patients with RA, the presence of rheumatoid factor is associated with more severe disease, manifested by rheumatoid nodules, rheumatoid vasculitis, and bone erosions.

Testing serum for presence of *antinuclear antibodies (ANA's)* is useful primarily in the evaluation of suspected SLE (see Ch. 240). Many different antigen-antibody reactions underlie the various patterns detected by the ANA test, and identification of antibody to a specific antigen is diagnostically useful in several instances (Table 236–2). Antibodies to double-stranded DNA (particularly if raised one or more standard deviations above normal test range) and to the Smith (Sm) antigen are highly specific for lupus but not present in all cases. Antibodies to U1-nRNP, particularly if high titer, identify "mixed connective tissue disease" (MCTD), an overlap syndrome in which features of lupus, scleroderma, and myositis are likely to persist. An ANA pattern displaying fluorescence over centromeres in dividing cells associates with a range of scleroderma syndromes, usually with the milder CREST variant (Table 236–2) (but also with diffuse scleroderma), and sometimes identifies patients with isolated Raynaud's who will progress to a scleroderma syndrome. Tests for specific antibodies that associate with subsets of polymyositis (such as Jo-1) or scleroderma (ScL-70) should prove useful if diagnostic specificity holds as the tests become more widely available.

Most positive ANA's occur for reasons other than a rheumatic disease, since 1 to 2% of the normal population shows a positive, if low-titer, test. The frequency increases with age, with 20 to 25% of persons age 60 or older showing a positive test, and is higher in family members of patients with a rheumatic disease. Many drugs can produce a positive ANA test without inducing a lupus-like syndrome, although the list of responsible agents is similar for both. Chronic liver diseases, pulmonary disorders (pulmonary fibrosis, primary pulmonary hypertension), and endocrine syndromes (type I diabetes mellitus, autoimmune thyroid disease) show positive ANA's in a high proportion in patients, which in some instances can be taken as an overlap with a *forme fruste* rheumatic disorder (such as the patient with primary biliary cirrhosis and a positive ANA test). Certain leukemias, lymphomas, and solid tumors can be associated with ANA's. Because paraneoplastic phenomena can mimic rheumatic disease, the diagnosis of malignancy should be kept in mind when serologic tests suggest a rheumatic disorder in a perplexing multisystem illness that does not fit well with any

TABLE 236–2. ASSOCIATIONS BETWEEN SELECTED NUCLEAR AND CYTOPLASMIC AUTOANTIBODIES AND CERTAIN RHEUMATIC DISEASES

Substrate Immunofluorescence Pattern	Antibody	Antigen	Disease Association(s)	Comments
Human epithelial cells (Hep-2)				
Homogeneous ANA	Antihistone	Histones H1, H2A, H2B, H3, H4	Drug-induced lupus (>95%), infectious mononucleosis (5–10%), normals (1–2%)	Low titer (<1:320) in "normals"
Rim ANA	Anti-native DNA	Double-stranded DNA	SLE (50%)	Antibodies to *double-stranded DNA* highly specific for SLE; "Rim ANA" is rare pattern on Hep-2 cells
Speckled ANA	Anti-Sm	Nonhistone proteins DEFG complexed with small nuclear RNA's	SLE (30%)	Highly specific for SLE
	Anti-U1-nRNP	U1 small nuclear ribonucleoprotein	SLE (35%); MCTD (>95%)	High titer in MCTD
	Anti-Ro (SS-A)	Two proteins complexed with small RNA's Y1-Y5	SLE (35%); Sjögren's (70–80%)	Often missed on Hep-2 ANA; common in "ANA-negative" lupus
	Anti-La (SS-B)	Single protein + RNA polymerase III transcript	SLE (15%); Sjögren's (50–70%)	
	Anti-Ku	DNA binding protein	SLE (10%)	May identify SLE/PSS/myositis overlap
	Anti-Scl-70	DNA topoisomerase I	PSS (40–70%); CREST (10–20%)	
Nucleolar ANA	Anti-PM-Scl	Nucleolar protein complex	PSS (3%); PM (8%)	May identify "sclerodermatomyositis" overlap
	Anti-Mi-2	Nuclear protein complex	DM (15–20%)	Rare in PM
	Anti-RNA polymerase I	Subunits of RNA pol I	PSS (4%)	
Dividing cell-specific patterns	Anticentromere	Centromere/kinetochore protein	CREST (80%); PSS (30%)	In patients with isolated Raynaud's, may predict progression to CREST
	Anti-proliferating cell nuclear antigen	Auxiliary protein of DNA polymerase δ	SLE (3%)	
Cytoplasmic staining	Antisynthetases:			
	Anti-Jo-1	Histidyl tRNA synthetase	PM/DM (18–25%)	Often with ISLD
	Anti-PL-7	Threonyl tRNA synthetase	PM/DM (3%)	Often with ISLD
	Anti-PL-12	Alanyl tRNA synthetase	PM/DM (3%)	Often with ISLD
	Anti-SRP	Signal recognition particle	PM (4%)	No Raynaud's, rare ISLD, poor prognosis
	Antiribosomal P	Large ribosomal subunit	SLE (10%)	May associate with CNS manifestations
	Antimitochondrial	E2 component of pyruvate dehydrogenase complex at inner mitochondrial membrane	Primary biliary cirrhosis (PBC: 90–95%); normals (<1%)	PBC may show CREST, Sjögren's features
Alcohol-fixed human neutrophils				
Cytosol staining	C-ANCA	Neutrophil serine protease	Wegener's granulomatosis (90%)	
Perinuclear staining	P-ANCA	Myeloperoxidase	Microscopic polyarteritis (glomerulonephritis with or without extrarenal small vessel vasculitis); Churg-Strauss syndrome; miscellaneous vasculitides	

ANA = antinuclear antibody; SLE = systemic lupus erythematosus; MCTD = mixed connective tissue disease; PSS = progressive systemic sclerosis (diffuse scleroderma); CREST = calcinosis, Raynaud's phenomenon, esophageal dysmotility, sclerodactyly, and telangectasias; PM = polymyositis; DM = dermatomyositis; ISLD = interstitial lung disease.

rheumatic disease diagnosis. Finally, a number of infections raise ANA's, including malaria, schistosomiasis, trypanosomiasis, and liver flukes, along with tuberculosis, leprosy, and certain bacterial infections due to *Salmonella* and *Klebsiella*. In many patients, classic Epstein-Barr virus infection (infectious mononucleosis) shows ANA's that disappear with resolution of the illness. Some human immunodeficiency virus (HIV)–infected patients have ANA's, but the prevalence and significance of this phenomenon remain to be determined.

Use of human granulocytes as substrates for immunofluorescence testing has identified a group of antibodies directed against particles in the neutrophil cytoplasm (*anti-neutrophil cytoplasmic antibodies,* or *ANCA's*) that are of growing diagnostic significance. Antibodies against a serine protease contained in cytoplasmic granules (c-ANCA) can be found in 90% of patients with Wegener's granulomatosis (WG) (see Ch. 245) and in patients with chronic inflammation isolated to one or a few sites (e.g., sinuses, lung, or kidney) who do not have full-blown WG. While ANCA disappears in some WG patients with successful treatment and may reappear prior to a clinically evident flare, these fluctuations have not proved sufficiently reliable to guide treatment. Other ANCA patterns, mostly due to reaction with myeloperoxidase, are associated with a range of nephritic and vasculitic syndromes. However, these associations are not strong enough for ANCA's to be considered a "vasculitis test," and a positive ANCA test should not be substituted for biopsy confirmation of WG or vasculitis when cytotoxic therapy is being considered.

Antiphospholipid antibodies are encountered in many SLE patients and can be detected in patients without SLE but with sequelae of thrombosis in vessels of different sizes (e.g., livedo reticularis, gangrene, venous thrombosis, pulmonary emboli, strokes, transverse myelitis, recurrent spontaneous abortions). Results of several other tests in which phospholipids play an important role can be altered by antiphospholipid antibodies. The partial thromboplastin time (PTT) is prolonged by interference with the prothrombin activator complex (coagulation Factors V and Xa, platelet factor 3, and calcium), and this *in vitro* anticoagulation is not completely corrected by normal plasma (defining the "lupus anticoagulant"). Recognizing the phospholipid-rich cardiolipin–cholesterol–phosphatidyl choline target antigen in the venereal disease research laboratory (VDRL) turns this (and other tests for syphilis) falsely positive. Thrombocytopenia and a positive Coombs' test may be seen. A solid phase immunoassay for IgG and IgM antibodies to cardiolipin is the most widely used test for antiphospholipid antibodies.

IMAGING TECHNIQUES. *Plain radiographs* of the joints are relatively inexpensive and widely available. For many rheumatic diseases, information on plain radiographs—such as the presence, character, and distribution of bone erosions, soft tissue calcification, or swelling, alignment of bones, reaction of bone adjacent to joint surfaces, and space between joint surfaces indicating cartilage space—can define the problem and help in judging response to treatment of a chronic process. Plain radiographs may be normal or nonspecific at baseline yet become diagnostic as characteristic features evolve. However, the pathologic processes of many rheumatic disorders often occur in structures for which other means of imaging must be employed. *Arthrography* has mostly been replaced by less invasive techniques for investigating suspected loose bodies, meniscal derangements, or abnormalities of the rotator cuff; however, the technique still provides the standard for determining intra-articular volume and can help in entering a difficult-to-aspirate joint.

Computed tomography (CT) provides excellent spatial resolution of bone and soft tissue structures in an axial plane and is most useful in defining abnormalities of the spine, including herniated discs, sacroiliac joint abnormalities, narrowing of the spinal canal or neural foramina by bony outgrowths (spinal stenosis), and trauma. *Magnetic resonance imaging (MRI)* also provides superb spatial resolution of anatomic structures and characterizes tissue according to its morphologic appearance and physical properties. MRI has become the procedure of choice to delineate abnormalities of intra-articular and periarticular soft tissue structures in large joints, especially the shoulder (rotator cuff tears, glenoid labrum abnormalities) and knee (derangements of menisci and ligaments). For disorders of the spine, MRI can show structural abnormalities and their effect on

the adjacent spinal cord. Although most bony abnormalities are better shown by plain radiographs or CT, MRI can show features of *osteonecrosis* (dead marrow secondary to ischemia) and *osteomyelitis* (increased focal marrow signal indicating edema) before they can be seen on any other imaging study. Because of the high cost and limited availability of MRI, it should be used only when management will be significantly altered by possible findings.

Scintigraphy differs from other imaging techniques by providing information that pertains more to function than to structure. The distribution of tracer is a function of local blood flow, vascular permeability, and tissue uptake. ^{99}Tc-pyrophosphate is taken up by metabolically active bone and thus localizes where this is increased (fractures, blastic skeletal metastases, Paget's disease, periostitis, and "actively" degenerating joints). Because initial distribution of this radionucleide depends on blood flow, scintigraphy that measures activity at several time points ("triple-phase scan") will show uptake initially at sites of increased vascularity—such as synovitis, infection, or neoplasia—and then localize to bone later. While ^{99m}Tc-scanning is nonspecific, it can image the entire skeleton at modest cost and be used to screen for bone and joint abnormalities and metastatic disease. Gallium 67 binds to serum and cellular transferrin and lactoferrin and is preferentially taken up by neutrophils and some neoplastic tissues (e.g., lymphoma). Indium 111–labeled leukocyte scans permit more specific assessment of focal bone or joint infection. Site of tracer localization can be determined with some precision by subjecting the scanned image to single photon emission computed tomography (SPECT), which generates a virtual three-dimensional reconstruction of the image.

Ultrasonography (US) can discern boundaries between the various soft tissue structures comprising the musculoskeletal system and can evaluate pathology within these structures. Its ability to localize a fluid-containing structure can be useful in identifying a joint or bursa for aspiration that would have been difficult to enter using standard landmarks. Lesions of tendons, ligaments, and muscle can be identified and characterized. US is more operator-dependent than other imaging modalities but in experienced hands is the procedure of choice for defining the pathologic anatomy of a painful periarticular region when physical examination and plain radiography are not explanatory.

ARTHROSCOPY. Direct inspection of the joint interior for diagnostic and therapeutic purposes has grown in 25 years from a rarely utilized novelty to the major procedure most commonly performed on the musculoskeletal system (other than casting for fractures). Identifying and repairing traumatic injuries to specific intra-articular structures remain the major focus of arthroscopy. However, the use of arthroscopy in investigating and treating rheumatic disorders could increase as more rheumatologists take up the procedure by using smaller "needle" arthroscopes that can be employed in an office setting.

Arthroscopy has three generic capabilities: direct inspection of intra-articular anatomy, visually guided sampling (biopsy) of tissues, and modification/resection of pathologic tissue under direct visualization using specially designed instruments. During the procedure, the joint is distended and irrigated with a physiologic saline solution to clear away blood and debris. Conventional arthroscopy is usually done in a sterile operating room using a rigid glass lens magnifying scope coupled to a small camera that projects the intra-articular view to a videoscreen. Other instruments placed into the joint through additional punctures can be used to manipulate, cut, shave, and remove various tissues. Virtually all major joints can be arthroscoped, with the knee by far the most commonly entered, followed by the shoulder, ankle, elbow, wrist, and hip. "Needle" arthroscopy employs instruments about one-third the size of conventional arthroscopes (as small as a 16-gauge needle) and can be performed under only local and intra-articular anesthesia.

Some differential diagnostic possibilities that can be confirmed or ruled out by arthroscopy include processes that are treatable but lead to joint destruction if undetected, such as tuberculosis. Arthroscopy should be considered when these processes are even remotely possible. Closed synovial biopsy can be used if arthroscopy is not available but may miss areas of pathology sparsely distributed in the joint.

Arthroscopy can be used for patients with a diagnosed inflammatory arthropathy (such as RA) who have persistent knee symptoms not responding to conventional medical management. Patients with persistent synovitis can be treated by removing visibly inflamed or proliferative synovial tissue from all compartments of the knee under arthroscopic guidance (arthroscopic synovectomy). In other patients features do not suggest ongoing synovitis (pain with minimal swelling, "locking" or "giving way"), yet arthroscopy shows pathology—focal collections of proliferative synovium, areas of synovial scarring, or other consequences of prior inflammation such as softened and torn menisci or attenuated and eroded cruciate ligaments—for which arthroscopically guided resection often can be therapeutic.

In contrast to the "inflamed" knee, the painful knee with noninflammatory synovial fluid usually is diagnosed by defining a particular derangement of the intra-articular anatomy. The most common "derangement" is that of the articular cartilage surface, often suggested by grating, or *crepitus,* of the joint surfaces moving past one another and confirmed with some certainty by other features of OA found on plain radiographs (osteophytes, joint space narrowing, subchondral sclerosis). Other intra-articular abnormalities—torn or degenerated meniscal cartilage, loose bodies, focal synovial collections—can be identified and treated by arthroscopy. Some processes that disrupt joint surfaces through changes in underlying bone cannot be seen or modified at arthroscopy; these processes—osteonecrosis, stress fracture, malignancy—are often not apparent on plain radiographs and thus require more extensive imaging, such as MRI.

Adler RS, Martel W: Imaging techniques in the assessment of rheumatic diseases. *In* Schumacher HR (ed.): Primer on the Rheumatic Diseases, 10th ed. Atlanta, Arthritis Foundation, 1993, pp 74–81. *Concise, well-illustrated synopsis of capabilities and limitations of available imaging procedures.*
Kushner I: C-reactive protein in rheumatology. Arthritis Rheum 34:1065, 1991. *A succinct review of the CRP biology and clinical utility of its measurement, particularly in managing rheumatic diseases.*
O'Rourke KS, Ike RW: Diagnostic arthroscopy in the arthritis patient. Rheum Dis Clin North Am 20:321, 1994. *A review of the various situations in rheumatology when diagnostic arthroscopy—particularly with the "needle" arthroscope—can be useful, and why.*
Shmerling RH, Delbanco TL, Tosteson AN, et al.: Synovial fluid tests: What should be ordered? JAMA 264:1009, 1990. *Prospective analysis of 100 consecutive arthrocenteses judging contribution to diagnosis from several tests. Only WBC count and percent polys discriminated between "inflammatory" and "noninflammatory" diagnoses as determined independently.*
Tan EM: Molecular biology of nuclear autoantigens. Adv Nephrol 22:213, 1993. *Recent comprehensive review of identified autoantigens and corresponding autoantibodies, discussing clinical associations as well as known function of autoantigen.*

237 RHEUMATOID ARTHRITIS
Frank C. Arnett

Rheumatoid arthritis (RA) is a chronic systemic inflammatory disease predominantly affecting diarthrodial joints and frequently a variety of other organs. The American College of Rheumatology (ACR) revised classification criteria for RA to guarantee uniformity in investigative and epidemiologic studies (Table 237–1). Although these seven items include the most characteristic clinical features of RA, a variety of other disorders may mimic the disease (see Differential Diagnosis and Table 237–3).

RA occurs worldwide in all ethnic groups. Prevalence rates range from 0.3 to 1.5% in most populations, but frequencies of 3.5 to 5.3% have been found in several Native American tribes (Yakima, Chippewa, Inuit). The peak incidence of onset is between the fourth and sixth decades, but RA may begin at any time from childhood (see Juvenile Chronic Arthritis) to later life. Females are two to three times more likely to be affected than males.

ETIOLOGY. Despite intensive research over many decades, the cause of RA remains unknown. Three areas of interrelated research are currently most promising: (1) host genetic factors, (2) immunoregulatory abnormalities and autoimmunity, and (3) a triggering or persisting microbial infection.

Genetic susceptibility to RA has been clearly demonstrated. The disease clusters in families and is more concordant in monozygotic (30%) than in dizygotic (5%) twins. Certain major histocompatibility complex (MHC) class II alleles (and their encoded HLA, or human leukocyte antigens) occur with increased frequencies in affected individuals. Among Caucasians of western European origin,

TABLE 237–1. CLASSIFICATION CRITERIA FOR RHEUMATOID ARTHRITIS (RA)*

1. Morning stiffness (≥ 1 hr)
2. Swelling (soft tissue) of three or more joints
3. Swelling (soft tissue) of hand joints (PIP, MCP, or wrist)
4. Symmetric swelling (soft tissue)
5. Subcutaneous nodules
6. Serum rheumatoid factor
7. Erosions and/or periarticular osteopenia, in hand or wrist joints, seen on radiograph

* Criteria 1 to 4 must have been continuous for 6 weeks or longer and must be observed by a physician. A diagnosis of rheumatoid arthritis requires that four of the seven criteria be fulfilled.
PIP = proximal interphalangeal; MCP = metacarpophalangeal.

HLA-DR4 occurs in 60 to 70% of seropositive patients with RA compared with 25 to 30% of normal individuals. HLA-DR1 is found in the majority of HLA-DR4–negative patients and is most strongly associated with the disease in several other ethnic groups (Israelis, Asian Indians). Several subtypes of HLA-DR4 were defined initially by mixed lymphocyte culture (MLC) and more recently by DNA sequencing (Table 237–2). Only certain HLA-DR4 subtypes predispose to RA (Dw4 or DRB1*0401, Dw14 or DRB1* 0404, and Dw15 or DRB1*0405), while others do not (Dw10 or DRB1*0402 and Dw13 or DRB1*0403). HLA-DR4 subtypes result from only a few amino acid differences in the third hypervariable region of the HLA-DR beta chain. HLA-DR1 shares this same amino acid sequence as do several other HLA alleles that have more recently been associated with RA in some populations (see Table 237–2). Thus a "shared epitope" among several MHC class II molecules appears to predispose to RA. Moreover, homozygosity for the amino acid sequence, especially if carried on HLA-DR4 molecules, has been shown to correlate with disease severity, including more destructive joint disease, subcutaneous nodules, and the extra-articular manifestations, especially rheumatoid lung disease and Felty's syndrome. The crucial region for the shared epitope on HLA-DR molecules appears to be a combining site for the T-cell antigen receptor (TCR). Since MHC class II molecules present processed antigen to the TCR on helper (CD4+) T lymphocytes (see Ch. 221), it appears likely that an abnormal antigen-specific cellular and/or humoral immune response is inherent to the etiology of RA. The nature of the antigen, whether self or foreign, remains unknown, although candidates include type II collagen, proteoglycans, heat shock proteins, and immunoglobulins. Other genes also are probably necessary for RA, perhaps TCR and/or immunoglobulin loci.

RA appears to be an "autoimmune" disease, similar to other MHC class II–associated disorders (see Ch. 229). Autoantibodies to the Fc portion of immunoglobulin G (IgG) molecules, or RF's, are produced by B lymphocytes in the blood and synovial tissues of 80% of RA patients. Such cases are termed "seropositive." High titers of serum RF, typically of the IgM isotype when detected by the usual clinical methods, are associated with more severe joint disease and with extra-articular manifestations, especially subcutaneous nodules.

Despite the extremely strong association of RF's with RA, they clearly do not cause the disease. Production of RF occurs commonly in other disorders in which there is chronic antigenic stimulation, such as bacterial endocarditis, tuberculosis, syphilis, kala-azar, viral infections, intravenous drug abuse, and cirrhosis. Normal individuals occasionally produce RF, especially with increasing age.

An infectious origin for RA has been a continuing hypothesis. Streptococci, diphtheroids, mycoplasmas, and *Clostridium perfringens* have all been proposed and later discarded because of lack of definitive evidence. Viral infections such as rubella, Ross River virus, and more recently, parvovirus B19 have been shown to produce an acute polyarthritis, but no evidence exists that they initiate chronic RA. The Epstein-Barr virus (EBV) remains a viable but unproven candidate for a pathogenetic role. The EBV is a polyclonal B cell activator capable of stimulating autoantibody production, including RF. Increased numbers of EBV-infected B cells have been found in the blood but not the synovial tissue of RA patients. Anti-

TABLE 237-2. HLA ASSOCIATIONS WITH RA

	HLA Types (Alleles) and Methods of Detection			Third Hypervariable Region Amino Acid Sequences					Most Common Ethnic Groups
	Alloantisera (DR)	*MLC (Dw)*	*DNA (DRB1)*	70	71	72	73	74	
Associated with RA	DR4	Dw4	*0401	Q	K	R	A	A	Caucasians (West Europe)
	DR4	Dw14	*0404	•	R	•	•	•	Caucasians (West Europe)
	DR4	Dw15	*0405	•	R	•	•	•	Japanese, Chinese
	DR1	Dw1	*0101	•	R	•	•	•	Asian Indians, Israelis
	DR6 (14)	Dw16	*1402	•	R	•	•	•	Yakima Native Americans
	DR10	—	*1001	R	R	•	•	•	Spanish, Greeks, Israelis
Not associated with RA	DR4	Dw10	*0402	D	E	•	•	•	Caucasians (East Europe)
	DR4	Dw13	*0403	•	R	•	•	E	Polynesians
	DR2	Dw2	*1501	D	A	•	•	•	Caucasians
	DR3	Dw3	*0301	•	•	•	G	R	Caucasians

Abbreviations for amino acids: Q = glutamine, K = lysine, R = arginine, A = alanine, D = aspartic acid, E = glutamic acid.
• = the same amino acid in that position as DRB1*0401.

bodies against a nuclear antigen (EBNA) expressed in EBV-infected cells occur in the majority of RA patients, and a variety of other unusual immune responses to EBV are found in RA patients. More recently, an EBV protein has been shown to share the same five amino acids as the HLA-DR4 (Dw14) and HLA-DR1 molecules, which are implicated in susceptibility to RA, thus raising the possibility of "molecular mimicry" as a mechanism. A similar homology with an *E. coli* heat shock protein also has been found.

PATHOLOGY AND PATHOGENESIS. The pathologic hallmark of RA is synovial membrane proliferation and outgrowth associated with erosion of articular cartilage and subchondral bone. Often likened to a malignant tumor, proliferating inflammatory tissue (pannus) may lead subsequently to destruction of intra-articular and periarticular structures and may result in the joint deformities and dysfunction seen clinically.

The events initiating the process are unknown (Fig. 237-1). The earliest findings include microvascular injury and proliferation of synovial cells accompanied by interstitial edema and perivascular infiltration by mononuclear cells, predominantly T lymphocytes. Polymorphonuclear leukocytes and plasma cells are infrequent. As the process continues, there is further hyperplasia of lining cells, both DR-positive type A (macrophage-like) and DR-negative type B (fibroblast-like), and the normally acellular subsynovial stroma becomes engorged with mononuclear inflammatory cells, which may collect into aggregates or follicles, especially around postcapillary venules. The composition of cellular infiltrates varies, with some being predominantly T cells, usually CD4+ (helper/inducer), and others having a mixed population of lymphocytes (often CD8+ cytotoxic T cells), plasma cells, macrophages, and interdigitating (dendritic) cells. Mast cells are also commonly present. Occasionally, germinal centers rich in B lymphocytes can be seen. The proliferating synovium (pannus) becomes villous and is vascularized by arterioles, capillaries, and venules.

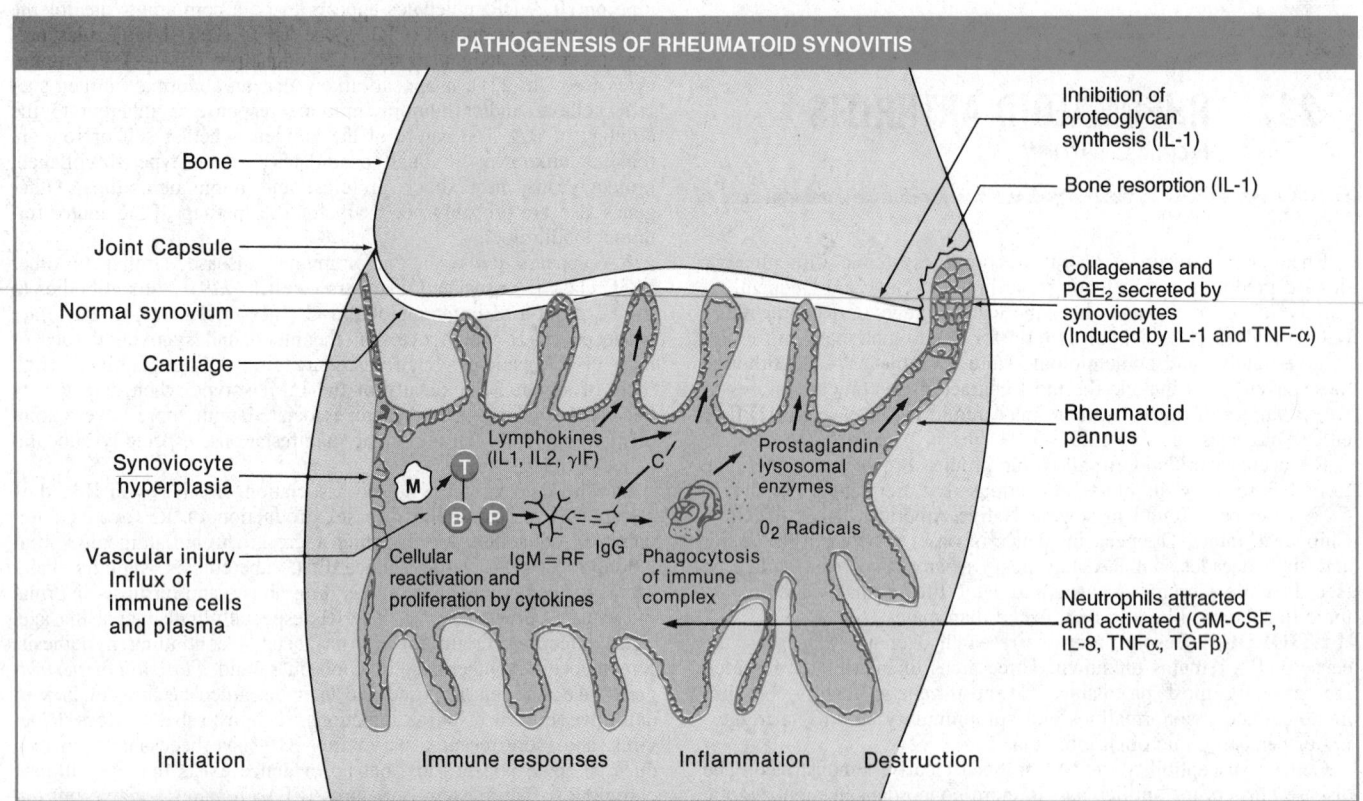

FIGURE 237-1. Events involved in the pathogenesis of rheumatoid synovitis progress from left to right. M = macrophage; T = T lymphocyte; B = B lymphocyte; P = plasma cell; Il = interleukin; TNFα = tumor necrosis factor alpha; TGFβ = transforming growth factor beta; GM-CSF = granulocyte-macrophage colony stimulating factor; γ If = gamma-interferon; RF = rheumatoid factor; PGE₂ = prostaglandin E₂; IgM = immunoglobulin M; IgG = immunoglobulin G; C = complement.

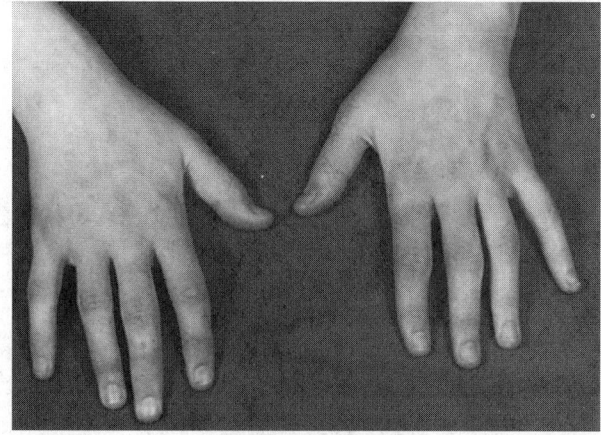

FIGURE 237–2. Early rheumatoid arthritis manifests as symmetric swelling and slight flexion deformities of proximal interphalangeal joints of the hands. Roentgenograms were normal except for evidence of soft tissue swelling.

Roles for both *cellular* and *humoral* immune mechanisms in the rheumatoid synovium are supported by molecular and immunopathologic findings. T lymphocytes appear to be activated, presumably by some unknown antigen(s) presented by DR-positive cells (type A synoviocytes, macrophages, dendritic cells, B lymphocytes). Studies of TCR gene expression suggest restricted Vβ usage and oligoclonality, but this area is controversial. Collectively, these interacting immune cells produce a variety of cytokines that promote further synovial proliferation and inflammation, as well as bone and cartilage destruction. Some of the cytokines that appear to play important and multiple roles include interleukins- (IL) 1, 2, 6, and 8, tumor necrosis factor α (TNFα), granulocyte-macrophage stimulating factor (GM-CSF), and transforming growth factor β (TGFβ). For example, IL-1 induces production of metalloproteinases (collagenase and stromelysin) and prostaglandin E_2 by synoviocytes. This cytokine also promotes degradation and inhibits synthesis of proteoglycan by chondrocytes, as well as enhances resorption of calcium from bone.

Humoral mechanisms are supported by the demonstration of local RF production within the synovium, the formation of IgM-activated B cells and IgG immune complexes, and activation and consumption of complement via the classic pathway. The sequelae of complement activation include increased vascular permeability and phagocytosis of the immune complexes by phagocytic cells. Aggregates of immune complexes within polymorphonuclear leukocytes are often seen in rheumatoid synovial fluid and have been termed "RA cells" or "ragocytes." Antigen-antibody complexes formed within the joint cavity can become trapped in hyaline cartilage and fibrocartilage, where they cause changes in matrix macromolecules. Within the synovial fluid, immune complexes activate the complement system, kinins, phagocytic cells, and the release of lysosomal enzymes and oxygen free radicals. Mediators produced in this process stimulate synovial cells to proliferate and to produce proteinases and prostaglandins. These products cause dissolution of the connective tissue macromolecules, as well as articular cartilage. They also may activate fibroblasts to produce a denser connective tissue matrix (fibrosis).

The ultimate destruction of cartilage, bone, tendons, and ligaments probably results from a variety of proteolytic enzymes, metalloproteinases, and soluble mediators. Collagenase, produced at the interface of pannus and cartilage, is probably largely responsible for the typical erosions.

CLINICAL FEATURES. The mode of onset of RA is highly variable. In the majority of cases, joint pain and/or stiffness develops insidiously over several weeks to months. One or more small joints of the hands, wrists, shoulders, or knees and/or the metatarsophalangeal (MTP) joints are frequently the first symptomatic areas. Malaise and fatigue, occasionally with low-grade fever, may accompany musculoskeletal discomfort. As the disease progresses, joint swelling, tenderness, and a red or bluish discoloration become apparent (Fig. 237–2). The pattern of joint involvement is typically polyarticular and symmetric, involving the proximal interphalangeal (PIP), metacarpophalangeal (MCP), wrist, elbow, shoulder, knee, ankle, and MTP joints. Distal interphalangeal (DIP) joints of the fingers are usually spared. Joint stiffness, especially if lasting more than 1 hour in the morning and after inactivity, is prominent. So characteristic is this symptom that the duration of morning stiffness is often used as a quantitative guide to the activity of the inflammatory process in both clinical practice and research studies. Over time the patient may experience increasing difficulty with pain and stiffness, as well as impaired joint function. The simple activities of daily living may be severely compromised, and the ability to continue a productive occupation is threatened. Sleep habits become disturbed, and the patient may experience depression and weight loss.

An "acute" onset occurring over 1 or several days is seen in about 20% of patients. Occasionally, an individual retires in the evening with no symptoms and awakens with acute, generalized RA. Such a rapid onset of pain involving joints, surrounding soft tissues, and muscle can mimic and must be differentiated from acute myositis, viral syndromes, or, if focal, even septic or crystal-induced arthritides. Rare patients experience recurrent (palindromic) episodes of acute monoarthritis, often so severe as to mimic gout, yet lasting only 24 to 48 hours. Such patients, especially if seropositive, eventually develop the typical chronic, symmetric polyarthritis of RA.

The course of RA, like its onset, varies widely. Fluctuating disease activity early in the disease process is usual. Ultimately, joint deformities and variable degrees of disability occur in most patients (Fig. 237–3). Some patients have a relentlessly progressive course leading to early disability or even death, but repeated periods of some degree of remission are the rule. The ACR has proposed criteria for clinical remission in RA. At least five of the following requirements must be fulfilled for at least 2 consecutive months: (1) duration of morning stiffness not exceeding 15 minutes, (2) no fatigue, (3) no joint pain (by history), (4) no joint tenderness or pain

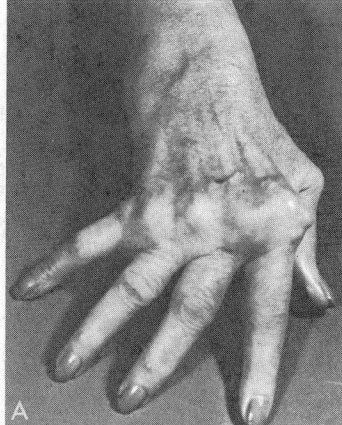
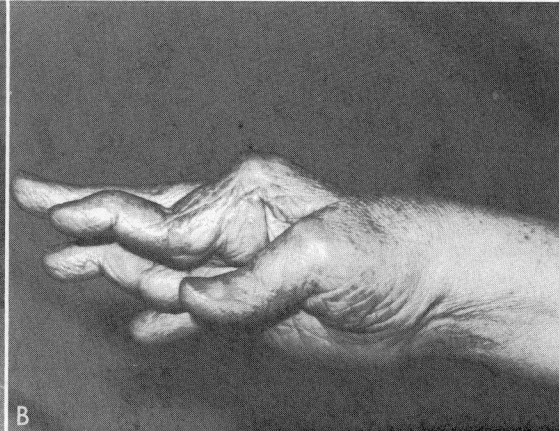

FIGURE 237–3. Hand deformities characteristic of chronic rheumatoid arthritis. *A,* Subluxation of metacarpophalangeal joints with ulnar deviation of digits. *B,* Hyperextension ("swan neck") deformities of proximal interphalangeal joints.

on motion, (5) no soft tissue swelling in joints or tendon sheaths, (6) an erythrocyte sedimentation rate (Westergren) <30 mm per hour for females or 20 mm per hour for males.

The assessment of functional capacity is frequently necessary in the RA patient. Although various schemes have been proposed, the simple classification that follows serves well in most situations:

Class I: No restriction of ability to perform normal activities.
Class II: Moderate restriction, but with an ability to perform most activities of daily living.
Class III: Marked restriction, with an inability to perform most activities of daily living and occupation.
Class IV: Incapacitation with confinement to bed or wheelchair.

DIFFERENTIAL DIAGNOSIS. Considerations in the differential diagnosis of RA are numerous (Table 237–3). Early RA, especially that of acute onset, is more difficult to diagnose than is the typical established case. The finding of subcutaneous nodules and the presence of RF are useful but are not absolutely specific differential features. Therefore, a complete medical evaluation, often including synovial fluid analysis, is indicated in all patients with significant joint manifestations.

ARTICULAR MANIFESTATIONS. RA can affect any diarthrodial joint. Those most commonly involved are the small joints of the hands, wrists, knees, and feet. With time, the disease also may affect the elbows, shoulders, sternoclavicular joints, hips, and ankles. The temporomandibular and cricoarytenoid joints are less frequently involved. Spinal involvement in RA is generally limited to the upper cervical articulations. In contrast to the spondyloarthropathies, RA does not cause sacroiliitis or clinically significant disease in the lumbar or thoracic spinal areas.

Hands. Swelling of the PIP joints, giving a fusiform or spindle-shaped appearance to the fingers, is one of the most common early signs. Bilateral and symmetric swelling of the MCP joints is also frequent (see Fig. 237–2). The DIP joints are usually spared, which is a useful sign in discriminating RA from osteoarthritis and psoriatic arthritis. Soft tissue laxity gives rise to ulnar deviation of the fingers at the MCP joints (Fig. 237–3A). Swan-neck deformities develop from hyperextension of the PIP joints in conjunction with flexion of the DIP joints (Fig. 237–3B). Boutonnière (buttonhole) deformities result from flexion contractures of the PIP joints associated with hyperextension of the DIP joints. These changes result in a loss of strength and dexterity in the hands, as well as the ability to maintain a good pinch. Synovial erosions of extensor tendons, usually at the dorsum of the wrist, may lead to sudden rupture and loss of the ability to extend one or more fingers.

TABLE 237–3. DIFFERENTIAL DIAGNOSIS OF RA

	Subcutaneous Nodules	Rheumatoid Factor (RF)
Acute viral arthritis (rubella, hepatitis B, parvovirus)	–	–
Bacterial endocarditis	+/–	+
Acute rheumatic fever	+	–
Serum sickness	–	–
Sarcoidosis	+	+
Reactive arthritis (Reiter's disease)	–	–
Psoriatic arthritis	–	–
Inflammatory bowel disease	–	–
Whipple's disease	–	–
Systemic lupus erythematosus	+	+
Sjögren's syndrome	–	+
Systemic sclerosis (scleroderma)	–	+/–
Polymyositis	–	+/–
Vasculitis syndromes	–	+
Polymyalgia rheumatica	–	–
Polyarticular gout	+ (tophi)	–
Calcium pyrophosphate disease	–	–
Amyloidosis	+/–	–
Paraneoplastic syndromes	–	–
Multicentric reticulohistiocytosis	+	–
Osteoarthritis (erosive)	–	–

– = not present; + = frequently present; +/– = occasionally present.

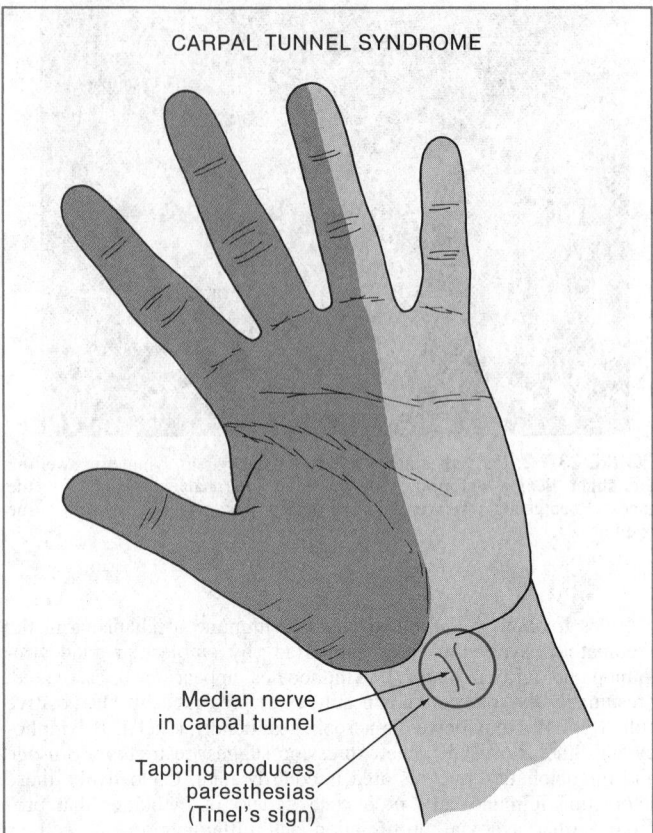

CARPAL TUNNEL SYNDROME

Median nerve in carpal tunnel

Tapping produces paresthesias (Tinel's sign)

FIGURE 237–4. Distribution of pain and/or paresthesias *(shaded area)* when the median nerve is compressed by swelling in the wrist (carpal tunnel).

Wrists. The wrists are almost invariably involved in RA and frequently demonstrate easily palpable, boggy synovium, especially over the ulnar styloid. Loss of wrist motion, both flexion and extension, usually occurs to some degree. The median nerve on the volar side often becomes compressed by proliferating synovium, resulting in a carpal tunnel syndrome (Fig. 237–4). The patient notes paresthesias or pain in the thumb, second and third digits, and radial side of the fourth digit. Symptoms are typically worse at night or with other activities associated with sustained flexion of the wrist. *Tinel's* (Fig. 237–4) and *Phalen's* (Fig. 237–5) signs can usually be elicited, and thenar muscle wasting may be evident.

Knees. Synovial proliferation and effusion are common in these weight-bearing joints. Effusions may be detected by performing ballottement on the patella or by observing a "bulge sign" along the medial aspect of the patella when fluid is pushed into the suprapatellar pouch and then expressed back into the joint. Quadriceps atrophy may occur, and a flexion contracture of the knee may compromise walking. Eventually, destruction of soft tissue around the knee can produce marked joint instability. Popliteal (Baker's) cysts may form owing to effusion or synovial proliferation into the semimembranous bursa (Fig. 237–6). Such synovial cysts may dissect or rupture into the calf, producing symptoms and signs mimicking those of thrombophlebitis. Sonograms are useful to confirm the diagnosis. Venograms also may be necessary because venous occlusion by the cyst can occur.

Feet and Ankles. The MTP joints are the most commonly involved sites. Subluxation of the metatarsal heads into the soles, often with cock-up and valgus deformities of the toes, results in painful walking and difficulty with footwear.

Neck. Neck pain and stiffness are common. As in other joints, the rheumatoid process can lead to erosion of bone and ligaments in the cervical spine. Atlantoaxial subluxation (C1 on C2) can be seen radiographically in up to 30% of cases (Fig. 237–7). Spinal cord compression with neurologic manifestations occurs infrequently but is a neurosurgical emergency. Occipital and/or frontal headache is a common premonitory sign of weakness in the extremities, bladder or bowel incontinence, or frank quadriplegia. Vertebral arteries also may be compressed, resulting in vertebrobasilar insuffi-

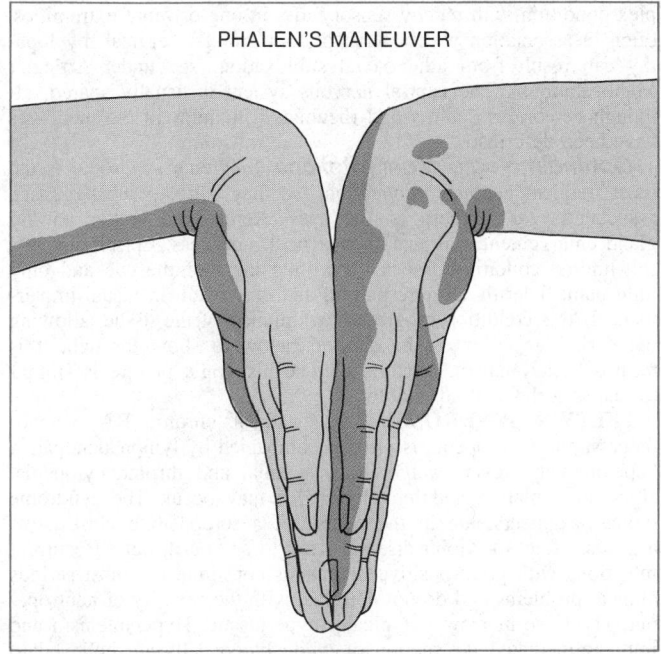

PHALEN'S MANEUVER

FIGURE 237–5. Pain and/or paresthesias are produced in the distribution of the median nerve (Fig. 237–4) when hands are held in forced flexion for 30 to 60 seconds (Phalen's maneuver).

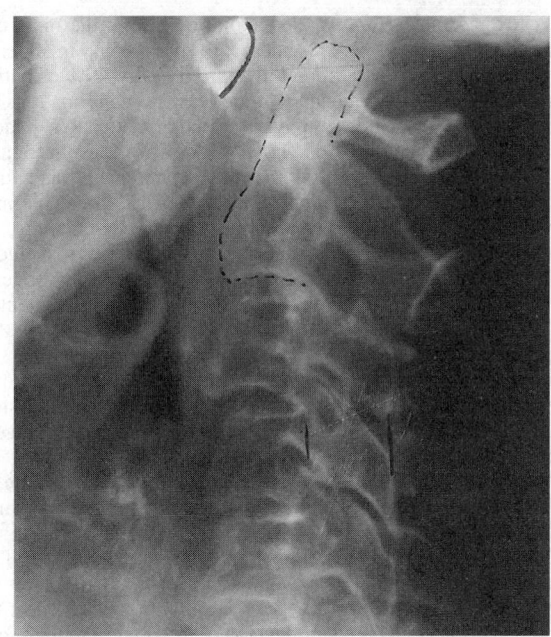

FIGURE 237–7. Lateral roentgenogram of the cervical spine in flexion. The body of C2 and its odontoid process are outlined by broken lines, and the posterior aspect of the anterior segment of C1 is indicated by a solid line. Normally, a space of only 2 to 3 mm separates C1 from C2. The space between C1 and the odontoid of C2 is markedly increased, indicating subluxation of C1 on C2. At a lower level, C3 is also displaced anteriorly owing to rheumatoid erosion of articular and ligamentous structures.

ciency with vertigo or syncope, especially on downward gaze. Head tilt may occur from lateral mass collapse of the C1 and C2 vertebrae.

Elbows. Proliferative synovitis in the elbow often causes flexion contractures, even early in the disease. Supination of the hand may be impaired, especially if shoulder motion is concomitantly decreased. Rarely, ulnar or radial nerves may become entrapped.

Shoulders. Involvement of the glenohumeral, acromioclavicular,

and thoracoscapular joints is common in advanced but not early RA. Limited motion and tenderness just below and lateral to the coracoid process are typical symptoms. Noticeable swelling is rare; however, large synovial cysts may occur (see Color Plate 3D). Joint destruction usually involves rupture of the joint capsule and subluxation of the humerus.

Hips. Pain in the groin, lateral buttock, or lower back may indicate hip involvement. Because the hip joint capsule has poor distensibility, severe pain can result if a large effusion occurs. Arthrocentesis should be done to relieve pain and to exclude infection in such cases. Rarely, extreme hip destruction results in protrusion of the femur into the pelvis.

Cricoarytenoid Joints. Synovitis of the cricoarytenoid joints may result in dysphagia, hoarseness, or anterior neck pain. The sudden onset of stridor and dyspnea in a patient with RA is an emergency. Prompt administration of intra-articular or parenteral corticosteroids and/or tracheostomy may be necessary.

EXTRA-ARTICULAR MANIFESTATIONS. Constitutional symptoms, including malaise, fatigue, weakness, low-grade fever, and mild lymphadenopathy, are common in RA. All the extra-articular complications occur almost exclusively in seropositive patients.

Skin. Subcutaneous nodules occur in 20 to 25% of RA patients and are almost always associated with serum RF and more severe articular disease. They occur most commonly in periarticular structures and areas subject to pressure, such as the elbows, extensor and flexor tendons of the hands and feet, Achilles tendons, and less commonly, occipital and sacral areas. They may occasionally become infected but are usually asymptomatic.

Palmar erythema and fragility of the skin, resulting in easy bruising, are common manifestations. Rheumatoid vasculitis occurs in two major forms. The first is manifested by small, splinter-shaped brown infarcts in the nail folds and digital pulp, often also present over subcutaneous nodules (see Color Plate 3E). Histologic examination may reveal leukocytoclastic vasculitis or a mild venulitis. This is a benign process in most patients and does not indicate serious systemic vasculitis. The second form is a severe necrotizing vasculitis of small and medium arteries indistinguishable from periarteritis nodosa. Digital infarcts, mononeuritis multiplex, fever, and other manifestations of systemic disease should prompt aggressive therapy.

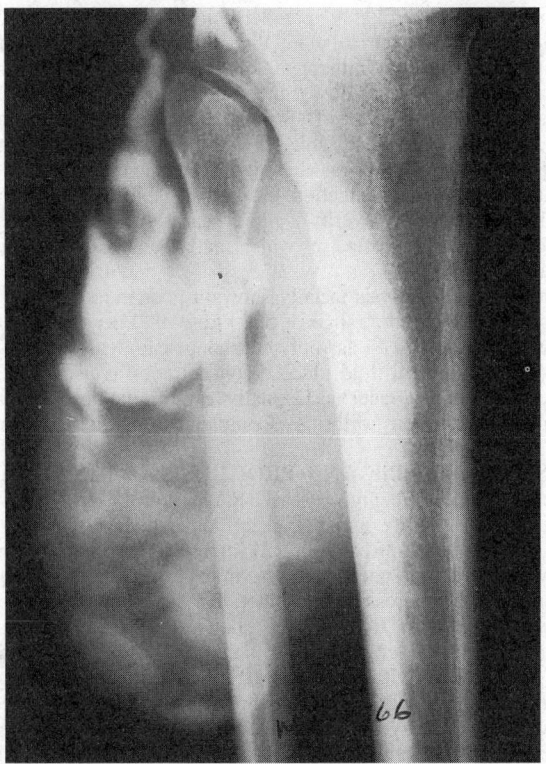

FIGURE 237–6. Arthrogram using a radiocontrast agent injected into the knee. The dye flows into the popliteal space and through a narrow channel into a large synovial cyst (Baker's cyst), which has dissected into the soft tissues of the calf.

Cardiac Manifestations. Pericardial disease is the most common cardiac feature of RA. Evidence of pericardial involvement with old fibrinous lesions is found in approximately 40% of patients at autopsy. A similar frequency of pericardial abnormalities can be detected by echocardiography in asymptomatic RA patients. Clinically evident pericarditis in RA, however, is infrequent. Large pericardial effusions with cardiac tamponade and death are rare. Constrictive pericarditis is somewhat more common and typically presents as dyspnea, right-sided heart failure, and peripheral edema. The pericardial fluid characteristics include a low glucose concentration, increased level of lactate dehydrogenase (LDH), elevated immunoglobulin levels, and low complement activity.

Rheumatoid nodules may develop occasionally in the myocardium or heart valves, and vasculitis may involve the coronary arteries. Conduction abnormalities, valvular incompetence or stenosis, and myocardial infarction are all rare clinical sequelae of rheumatoid heart disease.

Pulmonary Manifestations. Rheumatoid pleural disease, although frequently found at autopsy, is most commonly asymptomatic. Occasionally, a pleural effusion may cause respiratory limitation. Neoplasm and infection should be ruled out by a pleural tap. Typically, the pleural fluid is exudative, and white cell counts vary greatly but generally are <5000 per microliter. Glucose levels tend to be low, and the LDH enzyme level is high. Total hemolytic complement, C3, and C4 levels are low. Immune complexes and RF are frequently found in the pleural fluid.

Intrapulmonary nodules may also be seen (Fig. 237–8). Although they are usually asymptomatic, they may become infected and cavitate or rupture into the pleural space, producing a pneumothorax. Malignancy must be excluded in the RA patient, as in any other patient, with a solitary lung nodule. Similar but distinct nodular infiltrates also may be seen in rheumatoid lungs in association with pneumoconiosis (Caplan's syndrome).

Finally, a diffuse interstitial fibrosis with pneumonitis may progress to a honeycomb appearance on the roentgenogram, bronchiectasis, chronic cough, and progressive dyspnea. Pulmonary function tests show a diminished compliance and a restrictive ventilatory pattern. Large airways are not involved. An irreversible combination of respiratory insufficiency and resultant right-sided cardiac failure is possible. Rarely, small airway obstruction may develop into a necrotizing bronchiolitis. This complication also may result from therapies with gold and D-penicillamine.

Neurologic Manifestations. Peripheral neuropathies can be produced by proliferating synovium causing compression of nerves. Carpal tunnel syndrome (median neuropathy) (see under Articular Manifestations) is common, and a similar entrapment of the anterior tibial nerve (tarsal tunnel syndrome) can result in paresthesias with a foot drop. Rheumatoid vasculitis may cause a mononeuritis multi-

plex condition with patchy sensory loss in one or more extremities, often in association with a wrist or foot drop. A cervical myelopathy can result from atlantoaxial subluxation (see under Articular Manifestations). The central nervous system is usually spared, although cerebral vasculitis and rheumatoid nodules in the meninges have been described.

Ophthalmologic Manifestations. Sjögren's syndrome is the most frequent ocular complication and may cause corneal damage associated with dryness of the eyes. Xerostomia and/or parotid gland enlargement may accompany ocular dryness. Episcleritis is a self-limited condition associated with redness of the eye and only mild pain. Scleritis is more painful and may result in visual impairment. If this condition progresses to thinning of the tissue, allowing the dark blue color of the choroid below to show through, it is termed "scleromalacia perforans." The histologic picture is similar to that of a rheumatoid nodule.

FELTY'S SYNDROME. This triad of chronic RA, splenomegaly, and neutropenia is often accompanied by lymphadenopathy, hepatomegaly, fever, weight loss, anemia, and thrombocytopenia. Hyperpigmentation and leg ulcers also may occur. The syndrome typically appears late in the course of a seropositive, destructive arthritis, often after joint disease is felt to be "burnt out." Recurrent infections with gram-positive organisms constitute the most serious clinical problems and do not correlate with the severity of neutropenia. The bone marrow is typically hyperplastic. Hypersplenism and immune-mediated destruction of white blood cells are believed to cause the neutropenia. Splenectomy may correct the neutropenia and prevent further infections in some patients, but many do not improve. The "large granular lymphocyte syndrome," which is probably a premalignant disorder of T lymphocytes, may mimic Felty's syndrome in RA patients. Splenectomy should not be performed for this disorder because it may hasten the onset of malignancy.

LABORATORY FEATURES. A chronic normocytic, normochromic anemia with hematocrit values from 30 to 35% is usual. Typically, both serum iron levels and iron-binding capacity are low. The anemia does not respond to administration of iron, but erythropoietin may be effective when anemia is severe. The white blood cell count and differential are typically normal, but eosinophilia may occur in severe systemic disease. The platelet count may be moderately elevated owing to chronic inflammation. The erythrocyte sedimentation rate is elevated in most patients but only roughly parallels disease activity. The presence of RF is detected in more than 80% of cases and is useful in clinical diagnosis. Antinuclear antibodies detected by immunofluorescence, usually in low titer, can be found in 30 to 40% of cases. DNA typing of RA-associated HLA-DRB1 alleles (DR4, DR1, others; see Table 237–2) has no diagnostic utility because these genes occur in high frequencies in the normal population. However, detection of patients homozygous for these DRB1 "susceptibility/severity" alleles early in disease may predict the worst prognosis, in which early, aggressive therapy is indicated.

Synovial fluid analysis usually shows a poor mucin clot test and white cell counts in the range of 5000 to 20,000 per cubic millimeter, with 50 to 70% as polymorphonuclear leukocytes (Table 237–4). The synovial fluid glucose concentration is usually normal, but very low values occur occasionally, even in the absence of a superimposed infectious arthritis. Complement levels are typically low.

DISEASE COURSE AND PROGNOSIS. Although once considered a relatively benign disease, RA is now known to result in considerable disability and a higher than expected mortality rate. Approximately 20% of patients will improve spontaneously or even achieve remission, especially in the first year of disease; however, chronic disease progression and functional deterioration occur in the majority. Long-term studies have shown RA patients to have 6 times the probability of severe limitations of activities, 4 times as many restricted activity days, and 10 times the work disability rate as the general population, and approximately 50% are forced to stop working within 10 years of diagnosis. A higher mortality rate also correlates with the degree of disability and results from infections, systemic manifestations, and gastrointestinal bleeding or perforation. The economic impact on the health care system is also substantial.

THERAPEUTIC MANAGEMENT. Objectives of management include (1) relief of pain and stiffness, (2) reduction of inflamma-

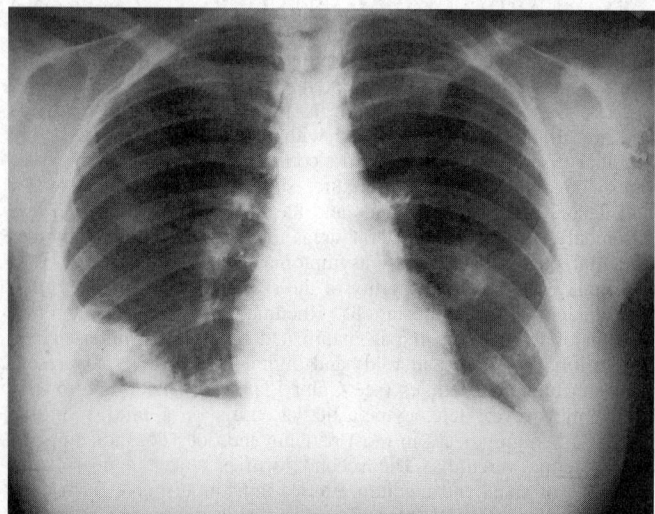

FIGURE 237–8. Chest roentgenogram demonstrating discrete rheumatoid nodules in both right and left lower lobes of the lungs. (Courtesy of Dr. Martin Lidsky, Houston, Texas.)

TABLE 237–4. SYNOVIAL FLUID FINDINGS IN RHEUMATOID ARTHRITIS AND OTHER FORMS OF ARTHRITIS

Synovial Characteristics	Rheumatoid Arthritis	Gout/Pseudogout	Reiter's/Psoriatic Arthritis	Septic Arthritis	Osteoarthritis, Traumatic Arthritis
Color	Yellow	Yellow-white	Yellow	White	Clear, pale yellow, or bloody
Clarity	Cloudy	Cloudy-opaque	Cloudy	Opaque	Transparent
Viscosity	Poor	Poor	Poor	Poor	Good
Mucin clot	Poor	Poor	Poor	Poor	Good
White blood cell count/mm^3	3000–50,000	3000–50,000 or higher	3000–50,000 or higher	50,000–300,000	< 3000
% polymorphonuclear leukocytes	> 70	> 70	> 70	> 90	< 25
Glucose levels	10–25% less than serum*	10–25% less than serum	10–25% less than serum	70–90% less than serum	5–10 less than serum
Total protein	> 3.0 grams/dl	> 3.0 grams/dl	> 3.0 grams/dl	> 3.0 grams/dl	1.8–3.0 grams/dl
Complement	Low	Normal	High	High	Normal
Microscopic features	"RA cells"†	MSU and CPPD crystals	"Reiter's cells"†	Microbes (Gram stain)	Cartilage fibrils†
Culture	Negative	Negative	Negative	Positive	Negative

* Rarely, glucose levels are very low, as in rheumatoid pleural effusions.
† These are not disease specific or diagnostic.
MSU = monosodium urate; CPPD = calcium pyrophosphate dihydrate.

tion, (3) minimizing undesirable drug side effects, (4) preservation of muscle strength and joint function, and (5) maintenance of as normal a lifestyle as possible. The basic initial program that achieves these objectives for the great majority of patients consists of (1) adequate rest, (2) adequate anti-inflammatory therapy, and (3) physical measures to maintain joint function. An additional objective, (6) to attempt to modify disease course with early, aggressive drug therapies, recently has been advocated because of the prognosis studies and the findings that rheumatoid pannus invades and irreversibly damages articular cartilage within 1 to 2 years of disease onset. Identification of patients at highest risk for a poor outcome may be possible using high serum levels of RF and DNA typing of HLA-DRB1 alleles; however, this approach is currently unproven. Moreover, it is unclear that the current armamentarium of disease-modifying drugs can achieve this goal.

Any confusion arising from the complementary requirements of rest and exercise should be promptly dispelled. Bed rest tends to decrease the general systemic inflammatory response, and most patients soon learn that their midafternoon fatigue is significantly reduced by a period of rest. During acute attacks, longer rests and perhaps even remaining in bed for the duration of the attack may be required to treat the inflammation.

At the same time, the full range of joint motion should be maintained. This usually can be accomplished by the patient through graded exercise programs. However, during acute attacks, passive range-of-motion exercises by a physical therapist or instructed layperson may be indicated. Physical overexertion increases synovitis and inflammation in the joint affected by RA, but this does not contradict the usefulness of appropriate exercise. Exercise, as well as heat treatments such as showers, baths, warm pools, paraffin baths, or hot packs, should be used to loosen the joints and relieve stiffness. Exercise following the heat treatment maintains the motion of affected joints and prevents muscle atrophy.

NONSTEROIDAL ANTI-INFLAMMATORY DRUGS (NSAID's). Anti-inflammatory therapy is crucial to the basic program. Salicylates are inexpensive, generally well tolerated, and demonstrably effective in controlling RA inflammation. The patient needs to understand that this requires a larger dose than would be used for analgesia alone. A constant blood level of 20 to 30 mg per deciliter is required. For most patients, this requires between 3 and 6 grams of aspirin per day. All patients should be monitored for toxic levels by blood tests and should be alerted to report deafness, ringing in the ears, or gastrointestinal intolerance. With the availability of buffered and coated aspirin, a suitable salicylate preparation can be found for almost any patient.

Many other NSAID's that are effective against pain, fever, and inflammation in RA are available. These include derivatives of propionic acid (ibuprofen, ketoprofen, flurbiprofen, oraprozin), naphthalene acetic acids (naproxen, nabumetone), pyrrolealkanoic acid (tolmetin), indoleacetic acid (indomethacin, sulindac), a halogenated anthranilic acid (meclofenamate sodium), piroxicam, diclofenac, di-

flunisal, and etodolac. Most of these drugs are beneficial in RA. They are generally no more effective than aspirin but may be tolerated in cases in which aspirin is not. Clinical experience suggests an occasional need to change from one to another of these drugs to minimize side effects and to give maximal benefit to the individual patient. Nonacetylated salicylates (sodium or choline) may be useful at times in patients intolerant of other NSAID's or those with aspirin hypersensitivity.

The NSAID's often cause silent gastrointestinal bleeding. Fortunately, this is usually minimal and tolerable. Overt gastrointestinal tract hemorrhage or ulceration is rare, but if this occurs or gastrointestinal bleeding is contributing to a constant anemia, the therapeutic regimen should be modified. NSAID's should be used cautiously or avoided in patients with impaired renal function.

DISEASE-MODIFYING THERAPIES. The more slowly acting drugs include antimalarials, gold, penicillamine, sulfasalazine, and methotrexate. Antimalarials are usually given as hydroxychloroquine (Plaquenil), 200 mg once or twice daily. This, or chloroquine, may cause retinal lesions and loss of vision; therefore, the patient should be examined by an ophthalmologist at least twice a year.

Gold salts, especially weekly intramuscular injections, produce remission in many cases. An oral gold salt, auranofin, appears to be therapeutically effective and to have less toxicity than do intramuscular injections. A dose of 3 mg two to three times per day is recommended. A therapeutic effect should not be expected before 4 to 6 months. Many patients have been on oral or intramuscular gold therapy for a number of years. Common side effects include pruritic skin rashes and painful mouth ulcers. Severe manifestations include bone marrow suppression, usually leukopenia or thrombocytopenia, renal damage with proteinuria, and rarely a nephrotic syndrome. Therefore, frequent urinalysis and blood counts must be done, especially during early phases of treatment.

Penicillamine is also effective in inducing improvements and sometimes even remissions. Like gold, however, its effects are slow in coming, and it may affect both the bone marrow and the kidneys, so careful monitoring for toxicity is required. In addition, it may induce other autoimmune diseases, such as myasthenia gravis, Goodpasture's syndrome, or lupus erythematosus.

Sulfasalazine, given in a dose of 2 to 3 grams daily, may be effective in some patients. Headache and gastrointestinal upset are the most common side effects.

Immunosuppressive agents such as azathioprine, cyclophosphamide, chlorambucil, and methotrexate have been used to treat especially severe, unremitting RA. Currently, the most widely used and effective form of immunosuppressive therapy for RA appears to be methotrexate. An oral dosage of 7.5 to 15 mg one time per week is usually efficacious, and a therapeutic response can be anticipated in several weeks. Side effects include hepatotoxicity and possibly cirrhosis, bone marrow suppression, oral ulcers, and a potential life-threatening pneumonitis. Methotrexate also may cause a leukocytoclastic vasculitis and may promote the formation of rheumatoid nodules, including systemic nodulosis. Concomitant treatment with folic acid, 1 mg per day, reduces toxicity from metholrexate without impairing efficacy. Sulfonamides must be avoided because of potentiation of hematologic side effects.

Because of its side effects, long-term corticosteroid therapy should be reserved for patients with unresponsive and aggressive joint disease whose ability to function is threatened. When necessary, the smallest possible dose should be used, i.e., prednisone, 5 mg to 10 mg every other day or daily. Higher doses are necessary for patients with neuropathy, vasculitis, pleuritis, pericarditis, scleritis, and related conditions. Local steroid injections can sometimes be helpful for relieving persistent effusions and are the treatment of choice for a Baker's cyst of the knee.

Finally, reconstructive orthopedic surgery is of very great importance. Prosthetic devices for hip and knee joints have given excellent results, and devices for ankle, elbow, and shoulder replacement are improving.

JUVENILE CHRONIC ARTHRITIS. A chronic arthritis beginning in childhood and for which no underlying cause is apparent has been termed *juvenile rheumatoid arthritis*. Because the majority of these cases do not resemble adult RA, the term *juvenile chronic arthritis* (JCA) is a more appropriate designation. Several subgroups of JCA are recognized on the basis of modes of onset, other clinical features, and immunogenetic differences.

Arthritis of systemic onset, or Still's disease, accounts for about 20% of patients. It can begin at any age. Rheumatoid factor and antinuclear antibodies are generally not found. Clinical characteristics include high, spiking daily fevers; an evanescent, salmon-colored rash usually appearing with fever; lymphadenopathy; hepatosplenomegaly; polyserositis; leukocytosis; thrombocytosis; and anemia. Serum ferritin levels may be extremely high. Although the disease is rarely life threatening, it can be confused with leukemia or infection. It tends to run a self-limited course in the majority of patients but may recur. Chronic polyarthritis and joint deformities occur in only about 10% of patients.

Disease with a polyarticular onset occurs in approximately 40% of patients. There is a female predominance. The majority of patients are seronegative. Seropositive patients have the worst prognosis, and the disease usually follows a chronic course similar to that in adult RA. HLA-DR4 is strongly associated with seropositive disease, but HLA-DR8 and DP3 are significantly increased in the seronegative group.

Disease with a pauciarticular onset accounts for the remaining 40% of JCA patients. There are at least two subgroups within this group. One is characterized by early age of onset and female predominance. The serum is usually positive for antinuclear antibodies but not RF. Patients in this subgroup are at risk for chronic iridocyclitis, which may progress to blindness. Therefore, frequent ophthalmologic evaluations should be performed. The arthritis usually resolves without deformity. HLA-DR5, HLA-DR8, and HLA-DP2 are significantly increased in this subgroup. A second subgroup with pauciarticular onset has a strong male predominance and later age of onset. HLA-B27 occurs in the majority of these patients. The disease in these children follows a course consistent with spondyloarthropathy.

Treatment must be determined on the basis of disease severity. Aspirin is a basic standby, but tolmetin and naproxen can be used safely in children. Physical therapy and psychosocial support are also indicated.

ADULT-ONSET STILL'S DISEASE. Still's disease is one form of juvenile-onset chronic arthritis that may begin in adulthood. Cases have been recognized that span the entire adult age spectrum, including the elderly. The clinical features are the same as described above. Acute symptoms often respond to salicylates or other NSAID's, but prednisone may be necessary for short periods. The prognosis for complete recovery is good in the majority of patients.

Arnett FC, Edworthy SM, Block DA, et al.: The American Rheumatism Association 1987 revised criteria for the classification of rheumatoid arthritis. Arthritis Rheum 31:315, 1988. *An in-depth discussion of the development, recommended uses, and potential pitfalls of criteria for RA.*

Felson DT, Anderson JJ, Meenan RF: The comparative efficacy and toxicity of second-line drugs in rheumatoid arthritis. Arthritis Rheum 33:1449, 1990. *Large meta-analyses of clinical trials of most of the disease-modifying agents.*

Firestein GS: Mechanisms of tissue destruction and cellular activation in rheumatoid

arthritis. Curr Opin Rheumatol 4:348, 1992. *An excellent review of molecular events in the rheumatoid synovium.*

Gregersen PK, Silver J, Winchester RJ: The shared epitope hypothesis: An approach to understanding the molecular genetics of susceptibility to rheumatoid arthritis. Arthritis Rheum 30:1205, 1987. *A well-written discussion of the molecular basis for different HLA associations with RA.*

Harris ED Jr: Rheumatoid arthritis: Pathophysiology and implications for therapy. N Engl J Med 322:1277, 1990. *An excellent review and extensive bibliography of current knowledge.*

Larsen EB: Adult Still's disease: Evolution of a clinical syndrome and diagnosis, treatment, and follow-up of 17 patients. Medicine 63:82, 1984. *An excellent clinical discussion.*

Pincus T: The paradox of effective therapies but poor long-term outcomes in rheumatoid arthritis. Semin Arthritis Rheum 21(Suppl 3):2, 1992. *An analysis of morbidity and mortality in RA patients.*

Weyand CM, Hicok KC, Conn DL, Goronzy JJ: The influence of HLA-DRB1 genes on disease severity in rheumatoid arthritis. Ann Intern Med 117:801, 1992. *A clinical-molecular study showing homozygosity for disease-associated HLA alleles correlates with RA severity.*

Wilske KR, Healey LA: Challenging the therapeutic pyramid: A new look at treatment strategies for rheumatoid arthritis. J Rheumatol 17(Suppl 25):4, 1990. *Advocacy for more aggressive treatment early in the course of RA.*

238 THE SPONDYLARTHROPATHIES

John J. Cush and Peter E. Lipsky

The spondylarthropathies are a heterogeneous group of disorders that share a number of clinical, radiographic, and genetic features. These disorders include ankylosing spondylitis, Reiter's syndrome, reactive arthritis, psoriatic arthritis, and the enteropathic arthropathies.

The spondylarthropathies share a constellation of characteristic clinical, radiographic, and immunogenetic manifestations that suggest a common or related etiopathogenesis (Table 238–1). Distinctive features include a propensity for axial arthritis (sacroiliitis and spondylitis), peripheral arthritis (often asymmetrical and oligoarticular), inflammation at tendinous, ligamentous, or fascial insertions (enthesitis), and a familial pattern of inheritance based on the presence of the class I major histocompatibility complex (MHC) antigen HLA-B27. These disorders can manifest extra-articular features that suggest a particular spondylarthropathy. Extra-articular manifestations may involve periarticular structures (enthesitis), eyes (uveitis), gastrointestinal tract (oral ulcerations, asymptomatic gut inflammation), genitourinary tract (urethritis), heart (aortitis, heart block), skin (keratoderma blennorrhagicum), or nails (onycholysis). Occasionally, patients with overlapping features of more than one condition or with HLA-B27(+) unclassifiable disease may be encountered. Thus approaching these conditions as a group of related disorders is important in understanding their pathologic consequences and in diagnosing them accurately.

New diagnostic criteria for the spondylarthropathies have been proposed (Table 238–2), because previous diagnostic criteria have been shown to exclude many spondylarthropathy patients. Broader definitions used in these criteria allow for earlier diagnosis and more liberal inclusion of many spondylarthropathy patients.

HLA-B27. The human leukocyte class I MHC antigen HLA-B27 was first linked with ankylosing spondylitis in 1973. This genetic marker is found in nearly 8% of North American Caucasians. The actual risk of developing ankylosing spondylitis by an HLA-B27(+) person is estimated to be 1 to 2%. Only 20% of HLA-B27(+) individuals infected with arthritogenic bacteria (Table 238–3) will develop a reactive arthropathy. Moreover, only 20% of HLA-B27(+) first-degree relatives of HLA-B27(+) spondylitis patients will develop ankylosing spondylitis, suggesting that factors other than HLA-B27 must play a crucial role in determining disease susceptibility. The prevalence of HLA-B27 varies greatly among different ethnic groups. A higher prevalence is seen in the Haida and Pima Indians, and the lowest prevalence is seen among Africans and Asians. When North American Caucasians are compared with African-Americans, HLA-B27 is found in 90 versus 60% of ankylosing spondylitis and 75 versus 50% of Reiter's syndrome patients, respectively.

TABLE 238-1. COMPARISON OF THE SPONDYLARTHROPATHIES

	Ankylosing Spondylitis	Posturethral Reactive Arthritis	Postdysenteric Reactive Arthritis	Enteropathic Arthritis	Psoriatic Arthritis
Sacroiliitis	+++++	+++	++	+	++
Spondylitis	++++	+++	++	++	++
Peripheral arthritis	+	++++	++++	+++	++++
Articular course	Chronic	Acute or chronic	Acute > chronic	Acute or chronic	Chronic
HLA-B27	95%	60%	30%	20%	20%
Enthesopathy	++	++++	+++	++	++
Common extra-articular manifestations	Eye Heart	Eye GU Oral/GI Heart	GU Eye	GI Eye	Skin Eye
Other names	von Bechterev's, Marie-Strümpell	Reiter's syndrome, SARA, NGU, chlamydial arthritis	Reiter's syndrome	Crohn's disease, ulcerative colitis	

Seven serologically defined subtypes of HLA-B27 have been defined, and five of these (B*2701, B*2702, B*2704, B*2705, and B*2707) are associated with ankylosing spondylitis. Other class I MHC antigens are termed the HLA-B27 cross-reactive antigens and include HLA-B7, -Bw22, -B40, -B42, and -B60, which are often present in HLA-B27(−) spondylarthropathy patients.

HLA-B27 has been shown to influence disease expression for most of the spondylarthropathies. HLA-B27(+) individuals are more likely to manifest an earlier disease onset, sacroiliitis, spondylitis, a severe clinical course, or acute anterior uveitis. By contrast, HLA-B27(−) patients are more likely to develop peripheral arthropathy, skin and nail disease, and inflammatory bowel disease or undifferentiated spondylarthropathy.

Strong evidence for the role of HLA-B27 in disease pathogenesis has been derived from experiments in which human HLA-B27 has been transfected into rats. These transgenic rats spontaneously develop typical features of spondylarthropathy, including gut inflammation, spondylitis, peripheral arthritis, psoriasiform skin and nail changes, uveitis, and orchitis. The role of environmental factors in disease pathogenesis is emphasized by the observation that many of these features do not develop when these animals are bred in a germ-free environment.

ANKYLOSING SPONDYLITIS. Ankylosing spondylitis is the most common inflammatory disorder of the axial skeleton. Epidemiologic studies have suggested that the prevalence of ankylosing spondylitis in a Caucasian population is 0.02 to 0.23%. Ankylosing spondylitis commonly affects young men more frequently than women, with an estimated male/female ratio ranging from 2.5 to 5:1. Ankylosing spondylitis in women is often underdiagnosed primarily because of milder axial disease and occult extra-articular manifestations. Women with ankylosing spondylitis tend to have a delayed disease onset, less hip involvement, less aggressive axial disease, more peripheral arthritis, severe osteitis pubis, and a higher incidence of isolated cervical spine disease.

Ankylosing spondylitis often begins in young adulthood. Up to 15% of children with juvenile chronic arthritis are classified with juvenile spondylitis. These children between ages 9 and 16 are often HLA-B27(+) and manifest low back pain or an asymmetrical oligoarthritis years before developing a fully expressed spondylarthropathy. In contrast, late-onset spondylarthropathy has been described in several HLA-B27(+) individuals over age 50 who developed sacroiliitis (without spondylitis), oligoarticular arthritis, an elevated erythrocyte sedimentation rate (ESR), and evidence of skeletal hyperostosis. This constellation of manifestations has been designated as the "RS3PE syndrome" ("remitting seronegative symmetrical synovitis with pitting edema").

The insidious onset of low back pain and/or stiffness is often the initial symptom of ankylosing spondylitis. The hallmark of ankylos-

TABLE 238-2. DIAGNOSTIC CRITERIA FOR THE SPONDYLARTHROPATHIES

Rome Criteria for Ankylosing Spondylitis (1961)	1981 ARA Criteria for Reiter's Syndrome
1. Low back pain and stiffness > 3 months, not relieved by rest	Peripheral arthritis > 1 month, in association with:
2. Pain and stiffness in the thoracic region	Urethritis and/or cervicitis
3. Limited motion of the lumbar spine	
4. Limited chest expansion	
5. History of iritis	
6. Radiographic evidence of bilateral sacroiliitis	

Diagnosis requires four of the first five criteria or sacroiliitis plus one of clinical criteria

ESSG Criteria for Spondylarthropathy (1992)	Criteria for Diagnosing Spondylarthropathies by Amor et al. (1993)	Score
Inflammatory spinal pain *or* peripheral synovitis (asymmetrical or lower limbs)	Lumbar pain at night or morning stiffness	1
	Asymmetrical oligoarthritis	2
Plus one or more of the following:	Buttock pain (or bilateral or alternating buttock pain)	1
Alternate buttock pain		
Sacroiliitis	Sausage-like toe or digit(s)	2
Enthesopathy	Heel pain or enthesitis	2
Positive family history	Iritis	2
Psoriasis	Nongonococcal urethritis/ cervicitis within 1 month of onset	1
Inflammatory bowel disease		
Urethritis, cervicitis, or acute diarrhea occurring within 1 month of the onset of arthritis	Psoriasis, balanitis, or inflammatory bowel disease	1
	Sacroiliitis (bilateral grade 2 or unilateral grade 3)	2
	HLA-B27(+) or (+) family history of a spondyloarthropathy	2
	Rapid (< 48 hours) response to NSAID's	2
	Diagnosis requires score ≥ 6	

TABLE 238-3. INFECTIOUS ORGANISMS ASSOCIATED WITH THE ONSET OF REITER'S SYNDROME

Enteric Pathogens	Urogenital Pathogens
Shigella flexneri (serotypes 2a, 1b)	*Chlamydia trachomatis*
Salmonella typhimurium	*Chlamydia psittaci*
Salmonella enteritidis	*Ureaplasma urealyticum*
Salmonella paratyphi	
Salmonella heidelberg	
Yersinia enterocolitica (serotypes 0:3, 0:8, 0:9)	
Yersinia pseudotuberculosis	
Campylobacter jejuni	
Campylobacter fetus	

Note: Older criteria *(top)* are being replaced by newer, more liberal criteria *(bottom)* for the spondylarthropathies.

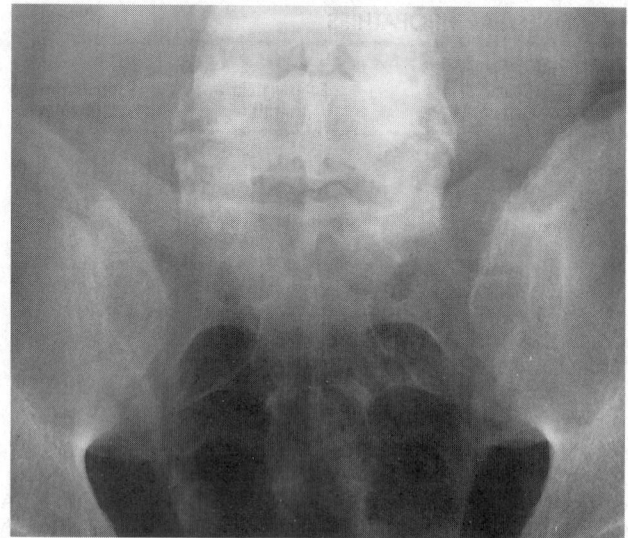

FIGURE 238–1. Bilaterally symmetrical sacroiliitis in ankylosing spondylitis.

ing spondylitis is symmetrical sacroiliitis that is often bilateral (Fig. 238–1). Sacroiliitis develops early but may take 7 to 10 years to become evident by conventional radiography. Pain is anatomically localized over the sacroiliac joints and less commonly radiates down the posterior thigh. Patients usually complain of prolonged morning stiffness that is relieved only by increased activity or anti-inflammatory therapy. Other constitutional features (e.g., fever, anorexia, weight loss) are not uncommon at the onset. With progressive axial involvement, pain and stiffness result in difficulty with ambulation and activities of daily living. The cervical spine is involved late in the disease.

A peripheral asymmetrical oligoarthropathy is seen in 30% of ankylosing spondylitis patients. Synovitis of the hip can be destructive and may lead to concentric loss of joint space, especially in men. Other involved joints include the ankles, wrists, shoulders, elbows, and small joints of the hands or feet.

Extra-articular disease in ankylosing spondylitis primarily affects the eye. Ocular involvement is seen in up to 40% of patients and is more frequently observed in HLA-B27(+) individuals. Uveitis presents as acute, unilateral orbital pain accompanied by photophobia and progressive loss of vision if untreated. Aortitis, aortic insufficiency, and conduction defects are uncommon. Other uncommon manifestations include mitral valve disease, myocardial dysfunction, pericarditis, pulmonary fibrosis, and amyloidosis.

Restricted spinal movement results from axial stiffness and paraspinal muscular spasm that accompanies inflammatory spondylitis, with or without intervertebral or zygapophyseal ankylosis. A loss of normal lumbar lordosis is a frequent observation in early disease. Fixed forward flexion, especially at the hip and neck, is seen after years of progressive disease. Chest expansion, as measured by the inspiratory minus expiratory chest circumference, is normally > 5 cm. Ankylosing spondylitis patients demonstrate diminished expansion (< 4 cm). Schober's test is performed to examine lumbar spine mobility. While the patient stands upright with heels together, a 10-cm span is marked from the fifth lumbar vertebrae cephalad. Upon maximal forward flexion, the distance between marks is remeasured. Normal spinal flexion expands the skin surface area over the flexed spine to > 15 cm. Flexion in patients with spondylitis and limitation of spinal motion measures ≤ 14 cm.

Laboratory tests support the inflammatory nature of the disease with an elevated ESR or C-reactive protein, anemia of chronic disease, or mild elevations of the alkaline phosphatase. Elevated IgA may be present, but other autoantibodies are noticeably absent. HLA-B27 determination is seldom necessary to establish the diagnosis. However, in questionable cases without distinctive radiographic changes, the presence of HLA-B27 may be of diagnostic value.

Radiographs demonstrate normal mineralization before the onset of ankylosis. Once present, ankylosis results in marked immobility and subsequent generalized osteoporosis. Sacroiliitis is indicated by erosions (leading to "pseudowidening"), ileal sclerosis, or fusion of the inferior synovial-lined portion of the sacroiliac joint (see Fig. 238–1). These findings are easily observed on plain radiographs of the pelvis and seldom require computed tomography (CT) or magnetic resonance imaging (MRI) for diagnosis. In selected instances, MRI may accurately diagnose periarticular disease, such as plantar fasciitis. Axial radiographic findings also include marginal bridging syndesmophytes, interapophyseal joint fusion, and "squaring" of lumbar and thoracic vertebrae. Collectively, these findings may produce the classic appearance of a "bamboo spine" (Fig. 238–2).

The clinical course and disease severity are highly variable. Inflammatory back pain and stiffness are prominent early in the disease, whereas chronic, aggressive disease may produce pain and marked axial immobility or deformity. An earlier age of onset and

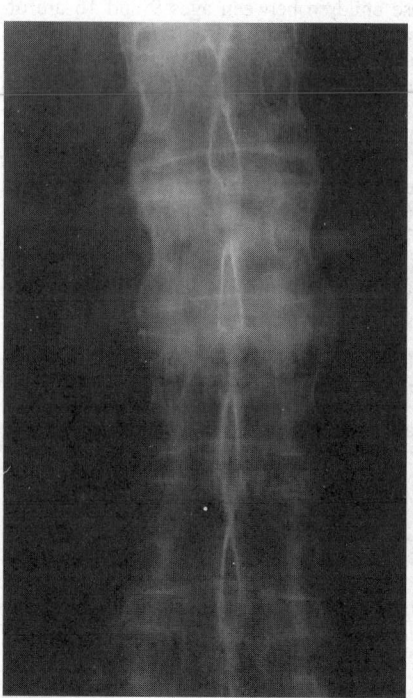
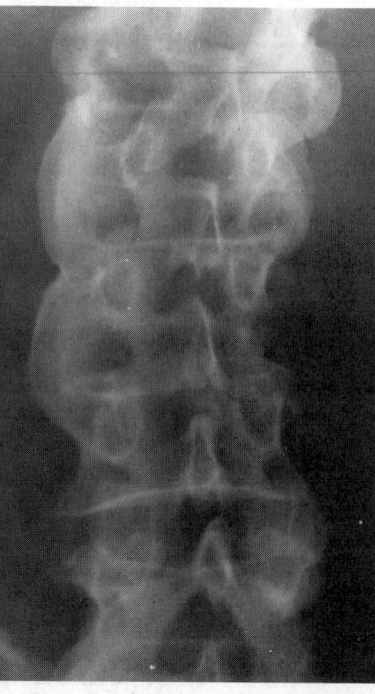

FIGURE 238–2. *(Left)* Lumbar spondylitis in ankylosing spondylitis with symmetrical, marginal bridging syndesmophytes and calcification of the spinal ligament. *(Right)* The bulky, nonmarginal, asymmetrical syndesmophytes of Reiter's syndrome with lumbar spondylitis.

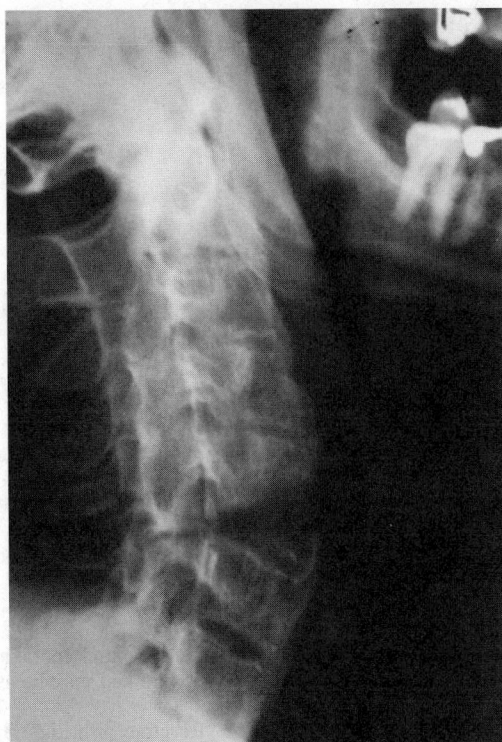

FIGURE 238–3. Posttraumatic fracture through the fifth cervical vertebrae in an ankylosing spondylitis patient with severe cervical ankylosis, interapophyseal ankylosis, and bridging syndesmophytes.

diagnosis portends a more severe outcome. Moreover, ankylosing spondylitis patients are at risk for complications, some of which may be life-threatening. These include restrictive lung disease, cauda equina syndrome, posttraumatic intervertebral fractures (Fig. 238–3), osteoporotic compression fractures, or spondylodiscitis.

Ankylosing spondylitis must be distinguished from other causes of mechanical or degenerative low back pain. The diagnosis of ankylosing spondylitis is suggested by (1) young age of onset, (2) strong family history of low back pain, (3) low back pain lasting more than 3 months, (4) prolonged morning stiffness, and (5) symptomatic improvement with activity or exercise. The differential diagnosis also includes other spondylarthropathies, osteitis condensans ilii, diffuse idiopathic skeletal hyperostosis (DISH), and other causes of hyperostosis (Table 238–4).

REITER'S SYNDROME. Reiter's syndrome is defined by the classic triad of arthritis, urethritis, and conjunctivitis. It most often affects young people, with a peak onset during the third decade of life. Like ankylosing spondylitis, however, it also has been reported in children and the elderly. Although men are most commonly affected, this predominance is often overestimated, because Reiter's syndrome in women may be associated with asymptomatic genitourinary disease and milder disease expression. Whereas postvenereal Reiter's syndrome is more common in males, postdysenteric Reiter's syndrome affects the sexes equally. Reiter's syndrome is

TABLE 238–4. CAUSES OF SKELETAL HYPEROSTOSIS

Spondyloarthropathies (ankylosing spondylitis, Reiter's syndrome, psoriatic arthritis, reactive arthritis)
Diffuse idiopathic skeletal hyperostosis (Forestier disease)
Vitamin A intoxication, retinoid therapy (i.e., etretinate)
Hypoparathyroidism
Familial hyperphosphatemia
SAPHO (synovitis, acne, pustulosis, hyperostosis, osteitis) syndrome
Pachydermoperiostitis
Hypertrophic osteoarthropathy
Plasma cell dyscrasia (POEMS syndrome)
Neurofibromatosis
Melorheostosis
Infantile cortical hyperostosis (Caffey's disease)
Fluorosis

one of the most common causes of acute inflammatory arthritis in young men. Case studies of epidemic dysentery suggest an estimated incidence of Reiter's syndrome of approximately 4 cases per 1000 dysenteric subjects per year. Analysis of epidemic dysentery secondary to arthritogenic bacteria suggests that Reiter's syndrome develops in 2 to 3% of infected individuals, whereas as many of 20% of the HLA-B27(+) infected individuals may develop arthritis. Similarly, 1 to 3% of patients with nongonococcal urethritis (NGU) secondary to *Chlamydia trachomatis* infection will develop a chronic arthritis. In Houston, the point prevalence of Reiter's syndrome was reported to be 33 per 100,000 men, and in Rochester, Minnesota, the age-adjusted incidence rate for males under age 50 was noted to be 3.5 cases per 100,000 per year.

The clinical triad of urethritis, conjunctivitis, and arthritis is observed in only 33% of patients with Reiter's syndrome. Thus many will not have evidence of prodromal enteric or urethral inflammation. Such patients are often designated as "incomplete Reiter's" or "sexually acquired reactive arthritis" (SARA). The remaining individuals can be diagnosed on the basis of an acute, additive lower extremity oligoarthritis that is accompanied by extra-articular features. The earliest features of Reiter's syndrome most frequently appear within 1 to 4 weeks of a putative microbial exposure. Disease onset is usually heralded by the development of one or more of the extra-articular features. Early genitourinary tract involvement may manifest as dysuria, urethral discharge, prostatitis in men, or cervicitis or vaginitis in women. Fever, malaise, fatigue, anorexia, weight loss, and ocular symptoms (e.g., conjunctivitis) are also common at the onset.

The arthritis is often the last feature to appear and manifests as an acute asymmetrical or ascending inflammatory oligoarthritis. Involvement of the lower extremity (first metatarsophalangeal joints, ankles, knees, and toes) is most common. Upper extremity involvement is rarely present at the onset. However, with chronicity, upper extremity involvement may occur. Involvement of the toes and fingers may result in dactylitis or the so-called sausage digit. Dactylitis is the net result of inflammatory changes affecting the joint capsule, entheses, periarticular structures, and/or periosteal bone.

Low back pain and other axial findings are present in up to 50% of individuals with Reiter's syndrome. However, radiographic evidence of sacroiliac or axial involvement is observed only with chronic and severe disease. About 20% of the most severely affected individuals demonstrate radiographic sacroiliitis.

Extra-articular Manifestations. Extra-articular manifestations are frequently seen in Reiter's syndrome. *Enthesitis* most commonly affects the insertion of the Achilles tendon and/or plantar fascia on the calcaneus with resultant heel pain. *Mucocutaneous features* may affect the genitourinary or gastrointestinal tract. Genitourinary involvement includes transient mucopurulent urethral discharge, urethritis, circinate balanitis, cervicitis, and/or vaginitis. Circinate balanitis appears as painless vesicles or large, shallow, serpiginous ulcerations or plaques on the glans or shaft of the penis. Painless lingual or palatal oral ulcerations may be seen in up to 50% of patients. Keratoderma blennorrhagicum is the most common of the cutaneous manifestations and presents as a painless papulosquamous eruption frequently found on the soles or palms and uncommonly on the penis, trunk, extremities, or scalp (Fig. 238–4). Patients with chronic disease may demonstrate nail changes of onycholysis or subungual hyperkeratosis. *Ocular manifestations* occur early in the disease and include conjunctivitis, uveitis, and rarely, keratitis. Conjunctivitis tends to be bilateral, painful, and recurrent and lasts days rather than weeks. Acute uveitis most often presents with unilateral ocular pain. *Other uncommon features* may include an asymptomatic conduction disturbance, prolonged PR interval, complete heart block, aortitis, aortic regurgitation, amyloidosis, central nervous system (CNS) involvement, serositis, or pulmonary infiltrates.

Radiographic abnormalities in Reiter's syndrome are commonly seen in the peripheral joints, primarily in an asymmetrical distribution affecting the feet, ankles, and knees. The sacroiliac and hip joints are less frequently involved. Soft tissue swelling, juxta-articular osteopenia, joint space narrowing, and/or ill-defined erosions are seen. Areas of periostitis or reactive new bone formation are common. Although bilaterally asymmetrical sacroiliitis is common (Fig. 238–5), unilaterally symmetrical inflammatory changes or ankylosis

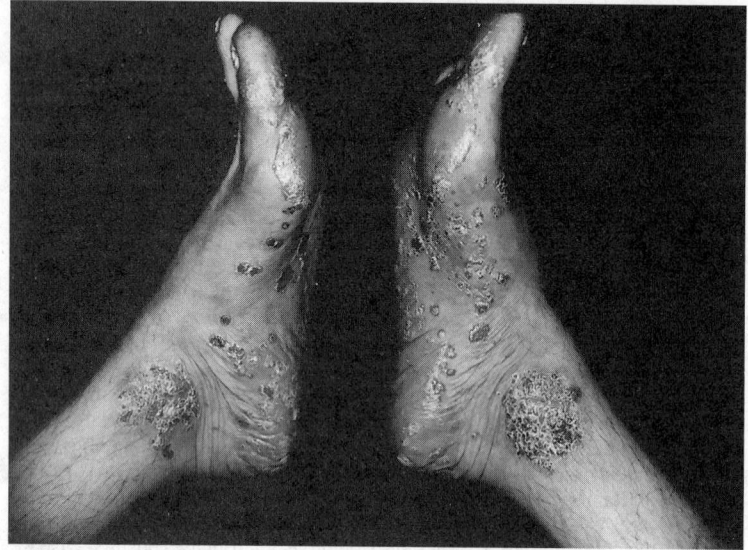

FIGURE 238–4. Keratoderma blennorrhagicum of the feet in Reiter's syndrome.

also has been observed. Involvement of the lumbar spine differs from ankylosing spondylitis with the presence of nonmarginal syndesmophytes or "bulky" osteophytes that are often unilateral or asymmetrical and tend to spare the anterior surface of the spine (see Fig. 238–2). Involvement of the cervical spine is uncommon in Reiter's syndrome.

Reiter's syndrome usually can be distinguished from rheumatoid arthritis (see Ch. 237) by the evolution, pattern of involvement, associated extra-articular features, clinical course, and absence of serum rheumatoid factor. Reiter's syndrome also should be distinguished from septic arthritis (especially gonococcal arthritis), crystal-induced arthritis, sarcoidosis, and erythema nodosum on clinical grounds and after appropriate laboratory and synovial fluid analyses. It is more difficult to distinguish Reiter's syndrome from the other spondylarthropathies and other reactive arthritides, such as that seen with *Yersinia, Chlamydia,* or AIDS-associated reactive arthritis. In such instances, a diagnosis of Reiter's syndrome is made after a careful history, identification of extra-articular features, and appropriate use of serologic testing and, most important, observation over time.

The prognosis and course of Reiter's syndrome are varied and unpredictable. The majority of patients demonstrate an initial episode usually lasting 2 to 3 months, but it may last up to a year. Recurrent attacks and prolonged disease-free intervals are common. A chronic peripheral arthropathy is observed in 20 to 50% of patients. These individuals have the greatest potential for axial progression and spondylitic changes. Death is rare and may be ascribed to cardiac complications or amyloidosis.

REACTIVE ARTHROPATHIES. "Reactive arthritis" refers to the occurrence of an acute, nonsuppurative, sterile inflammatory arthropathy arising after an infectious process but at a site remote from the primary infection. Reiter's syndrome is one of the most common examples of reactive arthritis. The microbial pathogens commonly associated with reactive arthritis are *Shigella, Salmonella, Yersinia, Campylobacter,* and *Chlamydia.* The reactive nature of these arthritides has been debated, since *Chlamydia, Yersinia,* and *Salmonella* microbial antigens have been identified at sites of tissue inflammation, suggesting that an ongoing immune response to disseminated material, rather than a reactive condition, may be the pathogenic mechanism. Many reactive arthritides occur after a known infection and therefore have been termed "postinfectious." Although the pathologic processes appear to be similar, this distinction may be important with regard to potential responsiveness to antibiotic therapy.

Reactive arthritis begins as an asymmetrical oligoarthritis, often preceded by an identifiable infectious event by one to four weeks. The temporal sequence suggests that these reactive disorders are triggered by an antecedent infectious process. Many patients without an identifiable infectious trigger have a similar constellation of signs and symptoms. The findings of sterile inflammatory synovial effusions, lymphocytes at sites of tissue inflammation, responsiveness to anti-inflammatory and immunosuppressive regimens, and the association with HLA-B27 suggest a common immunopathogenesis. A prominent feature of the reactive arthropathies is the inflammatory extra-articular process. Although frequently self-limiting, these disorders have the potential for chronicity and serious articular damage to the peripheral or axial joints.

Shigella. The occurrence of reactive arthritis following epidemics of *Shigella* dysentery has documented the arthritogenicity of this organism. Several reports suggest that 0.2 to 2% of infected individuals develop Reiter's syndrome following epidemic shigellosis. Infections with *S. flexneri* trigger Reiter's syndrome, whereas the more frequent *S. sonnei* does not. In most cases, the diarrheal illness resolves before the articular symptoms appear.

Salmonella. *S. typhimurium* is the most common *Salmonella* species inducing reactive arthritis. As many as 6 to 10% of infected individuals will develop a sterile arthropathy within 3 weeks of a *Salmonella* outbreak. Nearly 60% of patients will possess HLA-B27 or one of the cross-reactive antigens (HLA-B7 or HLA-B60). No clinical differences between *Shigella-* and *Salmonella-*induced reactive arthritis have been observed.

Yersinia. *Y. enterocolitica* is a common cause of reactive arthritis in endemic areas such as Scandinavia but is rarely encountered in England or the United States. *Yersinia* arthritis most commonly affects young adults as an acute, self-limiting gastrointestinal illness that may have associated joint complaints in 50% of cases.

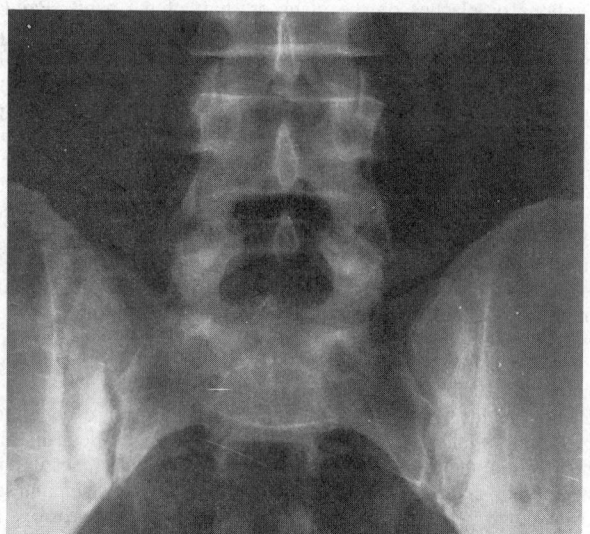

FIGURE 238–5. Bilaterally asymmetrical sacroiliitis in Reiter's syndrome. Erosions, pseudowidening, and ileal sclerosis are present.

Chronicity, severity, sacroiliitis, and ocular inflammation are more likely in HLA-B27(+) individuals. The arthritis is predominantly oligoarticular, affecting the lower extremities and hands, and may run a chronic or relapsing course. Chronic low back pain and sacroiliitis are seen in one third of patients, but severe spinal ankylosis is rare. Extra-articular features occur in 20 to 30% of individuals. Erythema nodosum and glomerulonephritis have been described in HLA-B27(−) individuals. Sustained elevations of IgA antibody titers correlate with persistent infection, chronic arthritis, and occult enteritis. Treatment is similar to that for other reactive arthropathies. However, appropriate antibiotic therapy should be used in patients with persistently positive stool cultures for *Yersinia.*

Chlamydia. *C. trachomatis* is thought to be responsible for as many as 10% of all cases of early inflammatory arthritis (see Ch. 323). As many as 1 to 3% of patients with chlamydial urethritis will develop arthritis. The incidence of *Chlamydia*-induced arthritis has been estimated to be 5 cases per 100,000 per year. Diagnosis is suggested by the presence of persistent arthritis in at least one joint, symptoms of genitourinary infection, detection of IgG or IgA anti-*Chlamydia* antibodies, or *Chlamydia* found in genitourinary swabs or urine culture. More than half of patients with Reiter's syndrome, NGU, or SARA will have antibodies to *C. trachomatis,* although positive cultures are seldom observed in patients with active disease.

The manifestations of *Chlamydia*-related reactive arthritis are similar to those described for classic Reiter's syndrome. However, only 20% of patients meet criteria for the diagnosis of Reiter's syndrome. Up to 15% of patients, especially women, have no urogenital manifestations at all. More than half develop a chronic arthropathy, with nearly one third having inflammatory low back pain, enthesitis, or radiographic sacroiliitis. Less than 50% of patients are HLA-B27(+). *Chlamydia*-induced arthritis apparently responds to antibiotic therapy, which is indicated in culture-positive or antibody (IgM or IgA)–positive patients. A prolonged course (i.e., 12 weeks) of doxycycline, minocycline, or lymecycline may improve symptoms.

ACQUIRED IMMUNODEFICIENCY SYNDROME (AIDS) AND REACTIVE ARTHRITIS (see Ch. 370). AIDS patients may develop an aggressive form of Reiter's syndrome. Early reports suggested that many of HIV(+) individuals developed Reiter's syndrome upon becoming profoundly immunosuppressed. Although it has been suggested that AIDS patients are at increased risk to develop reactive arthritis, a number of prospective analyses of HIV(+) populations failed to reveal an increased incidence or prevalence of Reiter's syndrome compared with that observed in an HIV(−) population matched for other risk factors. Each group, however, appeared to have a much higher prevalence of reactive arthritis than previously reported for young heterosexual males. Nevertheless, it seems clear that HIV infection alters the clinical expression of Reiter's syndrome. The vast majority of AIDS patients with Reiter's syndrome are HLA-B27(+) and present with incomplete symptoms and signs of Reiter's syndrome. The arthritis evolves in two main patterns: (1) an additive, asymmetrical polyarthritis or (2) an intermittent oligoarthritis that most commonly affects the lower extremities. Enthesitis, fasciitis, conjunctivitis, and urethritis are early and prominent symptoms. Although sacroiliitis does occur, HIV-associated reactive arthritis is rarely associated with axial disease or uveitis. HIV-associated disease also differs from classic Reiter's syndrome in the severity and chronicity of disease, prominent enthesitis, and a poor response to nonsteroidal anti-inflammatory drugs (NSAID's). Therapeutic options are somewhat limited in HIV(+) Reiter's patients, although some patients have responded to isotretinoin.

PSORIATIC ARTHRITIS. Psoriatic arthritis develops in roughly 5% of patients with cutaneous psoriasis. Although most cases arise in patients with established, active cutaneous disease, other patients (especially children) manifest articular disease that antedates the development of psoriasis. While the extent of psoriatic skin disease correlates poorly with the onset of arthritis, the risk of psoriatic arthritis increases with a family history of spondylarthropathy or extensive nail pitting. The age of onset is usually between 30 and 55 years, and psoriatic arthritis has been shown to affect men and women equally. Psoriatic spondylitis, however, has a male/female ratio of 2.3:1.

The genetic associations with psoriatic arthritis are heterogeneous. Cutaneous psoriasis is associated with HLA-B13, HLA-Bw17, and HLA-Cw6. By contrast, HLA-B39 and -B27 have been associated with sacroiliitis and axial involvement, and HLA-Cw6, HLA-Bw38, HLA-DR4, and HLA-DR7 have been associated with peripheral arthropathy. No etiologic agent or reactive process has been proven, although stress, trauma, the expression of heat shock proteins, and antecedent infection with *Streptococcus* or *Staphylococcus* have been suggested to play a role. Histopathology of psoriatic synovitis is similar to that seen in other inflammatory arthritides, with a notable lack of intrasynovial immunoglobulin and rheumatoid factor production and a greater propensity for fibrous ankylosis, osseous resorption, and heterotopic bone formation. Like HIV-associated Reiter's syndrome, disease severity in psoriatic arthritis is enhanced by coexistent HIV infection.

Psoriatic arthritis has an insidious onset and a progressive course. Five major variants of psoriatic arthritis have been described. These variants are not mutually exclusive, and patients may progress from one form to another. The first form is an asymmetrical oligoarthritis that is observed in 30 to 50% of patients and may involve both large and small joints. Dactylitis, or "sausage digits," may be seen in the fingers or toes. In this group, cutaneous features may be minimal and are often missed. The second variant involves the distal interphalangeal (DIP) joint and is seen in 10 to 15% of patients. It is strongly associated with nail changes of pitting, onycholysis, subungual hyperkeratosis, transverse ridging, and/or leukonychia (Fig. 238–6). Periungual erythema may reflect the extent of nail and joint disease. The third variant is a rheumatoid arthritis–like symmetrical polyarthritis that usually lacks serum rheumatoid factor or rheumatoid nodules. The fourth variant is psoriatic spondylitis, which is seen in approximately 20% of psoriatic arthritis patients, 50% of whom are HLA-B27(+). Finally, arthritis mutilans is seen in 5% of patients and presents as a destructive, erosive, polyarticular arthritis affecting the hands, feet, and spine. It often leads to progressive deformity and substantial disability.

Extra-articular features and laboratory findings are similar to those seen in Reiter's syndrome, although keratoconjunctivitis sicca, myopathy, and mitral valve prolapse are less common. Hyperuricemia may be found and often correlates with the severity of cutaneous psoriasis.

Radiographic changes in psoriatic arthritis are similar to those seen in Reiter's syndrome and include soft tissue swelling ("sausage digits"), erosions, periostitis, asymmetrical sacroiliitis, and spondylitis with asymmetrical nonmarginal bulky syndesmophytes (see Fig. 238–2). Patients with distal interphalangeal joint disease or arthritis mutilans may develop the typical "pencil and cup" deformity. Acro-osteolysis, paravertebral ossification, and pericapsular calcification also have been described.

The diagnosis of psoriatic arthritis depends on finding typical cutaneous or nail changes in association with one of the recognized articular variants. Cutaneous psoriasis should be distinguished from

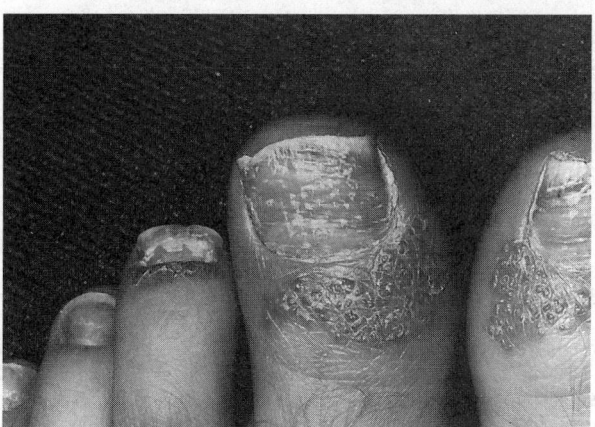

FIGURE 238–6. Nail pitting, onycholysis, and transverse ridging in psoriatic arthritis. Dactylitis of the second toe is present.

seborrheic dermatitis, fungal infection, exfoliative dermatitis, eczema, keratoderma blennorrhagicum, and palmoplantar pustulosis. The arthritis of psoriasis is often misinterpreted as erosive osteoarthritis, gout, rheumatoid arthritis, pauciarticular juvenile arthritis, ankylosing spondylitis, or Reiter's syndrome. A minority of psoriatic arthritis may exhibit clinical and radiographic features of Reiter's syndrome.

ENTEROPATHIC ARTHROPATHIES. "Enteropathic arthritis" refers to the arthropathies associated with Crohn's disease or ulcerative colitis (see Ch. 104). These disorders are unified by clinical and histologic gut inflammation, altered intestinal permeability, and the development of an inflammatory peripheral or axial arthritis. Peripheral arthritis is observed in nearly 20% and axial arthritis in 10 to 15% of patients, respectively. Peripheral arthropathy more frequently occurs in those with extraintestinal manifestations (i.e., erythema nodosum). Peripheral arthritis affects men and women equally. All age groups are affected, and while the onset of arthritis follows established intestinal inflammation in adults, the converse is true in children. Disease onset is sometimes heralded by low-grade fever, painful oral ulceration, ocular manifestations, cutaneous manifestations (i.e., erythema nodosum, pyoderma gangrenosum), or enthesitis. Rarely, a patient may have occult high fever, anemia, or weight loss. Peripheral arthritis manifests as an inflammatory, nonerosive, asymmetrical oligoarthritis or monarthritis affecting large joints (i.e., knees, ankles, elbows). Initially, the arthropathy may be migratory and may resolve in weeks or months. Peripheral articular activity often parallels gut inflammation. Thus measures to control colitis may prove beneficial for managing peripheral arthritis. With chronicity, peripheral arthritis may be misdiagnosed as seronegative rheumatoid arthritis, particularly when symmetrical joint disease or quiescent gut inflammation is present.

In contrast, with peripheral arthritis, axial disease may precede or coincide with the onset of colitis and is more common in men. Axial arthropathy is clinically and radiographically indistinguishable from ankylosing spondylitis. The course of sacroiliitis and spondylitis is independent of active bowel inflammation. Whereas no association between HLA-B27 and colitic peripheral arthritis has been noted, HLA-B27 is found in 50% of patients with spondylitic colitis. Therefore, inflammatory bowel disease should be considered in the setting of HLA-B27(−) ankylosing spondylitis.

The association between enteritis and arthritis is supported by the findings of ileocolonoscopic evidence of subclinical gut inflammation in a variety of spondylarthropathies. Histologic evidence of "acute" colitis (similar to bacterial enteritis) or "chronic" colitis (resembling chronic idiopathic inflammatory bowel disease) is commonly observed. Acute intestinal changes are commonly found in patients with postdysenteric reactive arthritis, whereas chronic lesions are more typical of ankylosing spondylitis and patients who will ultimately be diagnosed with enteropathic arthritis.

THERAPY OF THE SPONDYLARTHROPATHIES. Current therapies cannot cure the spondylarthropathies; therefore, treatment should be aimed at reducing pain and stiffness. An aggressive approach to patient education and joint protection will contribute to the maintenance of optimal function and the patient's sense of well-being and may slow progression to immobility, joint deformity, or axial malalignment. All patients should be counseled regarding a rational program of exercise, rest, physical therapy, diet, and vocational counseling. Patients with axial disease should engage in lifelong physical therapy to maintain posture and prevent slow deformity. Once the diagnosis has been established, specific treatment can be initiated. Therapeutic options are largely the same for most of the spondylarthropathies and, as such, are considered together.

NSAID's. NSAID's have replaced the use of salicylates, since they have more convenient dosing and are more efficacious. NSAID's effectively control the pain, stiffness, and/or joint swelling. While these agents modify symptoms, they are not thought to retard the underlying inflammatory disease or suppress disease progression. NSAID's are the mainstay of therapy in ankylosing spondylitis, Reiter's syndrome, reactive arthritis, and psoriatic arthritis. Their use in the enteropathic arthropathies is infrequently hampered by their potential to alter bowel permeability and/or induce exacerbations of colitis.

Although all NSAID's are potentially useful in the spondylarthropathies, only a few are of proven benefit and are FDA-approved for use in ankylosing spondylitis and/or Reiter's syndrome. These include indomethacin, diclofenac, naproxen, sulindac, and phenylbutazone. Of these, indomethacin, especially the sustained-release formula (1 to 2 mg per kilogram per day) is recommended because of its prolonged duration of effect and anti-inflammatory potency. Other NSAID's are used according to individual tolerability and efficacy. Phenylbutazone is a very effective agent but is reserved for intractable cases, primarily because of the risk of aplastic anemia.

Corticosteroids. Systemic corticosteroids are seldom used in the spondylarthropathies. They are most effective for controlling localized disease. They are used primarily as local therapy by intra-articular injection (i.e., mono- or oligoarthritis), topical management of ocular complications (conjunctivitis or uveitis), and on occasion intralesionally to control enthesitis. Systemic low-dose or high-dose "pulse" corticosteroids should be reserved for severe disease flares.

Slow-Acting Antirheumatic Drugs (SAARD's). When chronic, NSAID-unresponsive disease exists, adding certain SAARD's (e.g., sulfasalazine, methotrexate) should be considered. These agents have a delayed onset of action (2 to 6 months), and their efficacy in the spondylarthropathies is based on limited numbers of controlled trials and numerous anecdotal reports.

Placebo-controlled trials of sulfasalazine indicate that efficacy is greatest in patients with peripheral arthropathy and enthesopathy. Equivocal results have been observed in patients with longstanding disease and evidence of severe radiographic destruction or ankylosis. At a dose of 2 to 4 grams per day, it is most effective in patients with Reiter's syndrome, reactive arthritis, and enteropathic arthritis. The value of sulfasalazine in treating inflammatory axial disease has not been established but warrants consideration in poorly controlled spondylitis patients.

Methotrexate (7 to 15 mg per week) also may be effective in many spondylarthopathy patients. It is particularly effective for treating both cutaneous and articular disease in psoriasis, but higher doses and prolonged use may be associated with unacceptable hepatotoxicity. Azathioprine (1 to 2 mg per kilogram per day) should be reserved for those unresponsive to or intolerant of other SAARD's.

Additional therapeutic options exist for patients with psoriatic arthritis. Both methotrexate and sulfasalazine may be effective for managing articular and skin disease associated with psoriasis. Other patients may benefit from therapy with gold salts, antimalarials, etretinate, or cyclosporine. Although immunosuppressive regimens should be avoided in HIV-associated arthritis, agents such as sulfasalazine or etretinate may be considered.

Surgery. Surgery should be considered when pain and immobility markedly interfere with patient lifestyle. Total joint replacement is commonly performed in the hip or knee. The success of arthroplasty may be limited by postoperative heterotopic bone formation. Surgically correcting spinal deformities and/or fractures should be undertaken with extreme caution.

Arnett FC: Seronegative spondylarthropathies. Bull Rheum Dis 37:1, 1987. *An insightful overview of the clinical features of the spondylarthropathies and potential etiologic considerations.*

Bardin T, Enel C, Cornelis F, et al.: Antibiotic treatment of venereal disease and Reiter's syndrome in a Greenland population. Arthritis Rheum 35:190, 1992. *Suggested guidelines and treatment outcomes of Reiter's patients treated with antibiotics.*

Cush JJ, Lipsky PE: Reiter's syndrome and reactive arthritis. *In* McCarty DJ, Koopman WJ (eds.): Arthritis and Allied Conditions: A Textbook of Rheumatology. 12th ed. Philadelphia, Lea & Febiger, 1992, pp. 1061–1078. *A comprehensive overview of Reiter's and reactive arthropathies.*

Hammer RE, Malka SD, Richardson JA, et al.: Spontaneous inflammatory disease in transgenic rats expressing HLA-B27 and human β2m: An animal model of HLA-B27–associated human disorders. Cell 63:1099, 1990. *Describes the spectrum of clinicopathologic manifestations induced by introducing HLA-B27 into transgenic rats.*

Khan MA, van der Linden SM: A wider spectrum of spondylarthropathies. Semin Arthritis Rheum 20:107, 1990. *Clinical and pathologic similarities among the spondylarthropathies are described.*

Khan MA: Pathogenesis of ankylosing spondylitis: recent advances. J Rheumatol 20:1273, 1993. *Editorial review of the current understanding of the pathogenesis of HLA-B27–related disorders.*

Thomson GTD, DeRubeis DA, Hodge MA, et al.: Post-*Salmonella* reactive arthritis: Late clinical sequelae in a point source cohort. Am J Med 98:13, 1995. *Describes the incidence and long-term clinical consequences of reactive arthritis following epidemic dysentery caused by* Salmonella typhimurium.

239 INFECTIOUS ARTHRITIS
Luis R. Espinoza

Infectious or septic arthritis is a topic of increasing relevance in view of the continuous spread of the human immunodeficiency virus (HIV), Lyme disease, and gonorrhea and syphilis and the resurgence in recent years of more virulent strains of *Streptococcus* species and acute rheumatic fever.

In order of frequency, bacterial-nongonococcal and bacterial-gonococcal, viral, and fungal infections are the most common causes of inflammatory articular disease.

NONGONOCOCCAL BACTERIAL ARTHRITIS (Table 239–1). *Staphylococcus aureus* is the most common infectious agent in both adults and children over age 2. This is of extreme importance, since almost all strains of *Staphylococcus* are now resistant to penicillin and methicillin. Non-group A beta-hemolytic streptococci and *Streptococcus pneumoniae* are also common causative gram-positive microorganisms. Infections due to gram-negative microorganisms and anaerobes occur for the most part in patients with some degree of immunosuppression, prior joint damage (as in rheumatoid arthritis (RA), osteoarthritis, or a prosthetic joint), and underlying malignancy. *Hemophilus influenzae* is the most common infectious agent in bacterial arthritis occurring in children younger than age 2.

Most cases of bacterial arthritis result from hematogenous spread. Other routes of joint involvement include direct inoculation during diagnostic or therapeutic arthrocentesis or arthroscopies and by contiguous osteomyelitis, cellulitis, abscesses, tenosynovitis, and/or septic bursitis. Regardless of the route of infection, however, the histopathologic and biochemical changes are the same and include infiltration by polymorphonuclear (PMN) cells of the subsynovial space, neovascularization, synovial proliferation, granulation tissue, and if untreated, cartilage and bone destruction. Phagocytosis of microorganisms by PMN and/or synovial lining cells also may be found. As the inflammatory reaction progresses, increased amounts of synovial fluid, with inflammatory cells, predominantly polymorphonuclear, will be observed. The degree of synovial, cartilage, and bone destruction depends on multiple factors, including the direct toxic effect of the microorganisms or their products, the host response to the infection, and more important, the rapidity with which an accurate diagnosis and appropriate therapy are instituted.

Clinical Manifestations. The great majority of cases (80 to 90%) are monarticular, with the knee joint being affected most commonly. Polyarthritis may occur in patients with underlying connective tissue diseases or an immunosuppressed state and carries a worse prognosis, with a mortality rate of approximately 30%.

Most patients have constitutional complaints, including chills, fever, and general malaise. On physical examination, the affected joint(s) can be extremely painful, warm, and with fluid. These inflammatory signs, however, may be masked in debilitated, severely

TABLE 239–1. MICROORGANISMS IN ACUTE NONGONOCOCCAL BACTERIAL ARTHRITIS

Microorganism	%
>Age 2	
Gram-positive	50–90
Staphylococcus aureus	40–60
Non-group A beta-hemolytic streptococci	15–30
Gram-negative	5–25
Escherichia coli	
Salmonella	
Pseudomonas spp.	
Anaerobes	1–2
Fusobacterium necrophorum	
Anaerobic cocci	
Bacteroides fragilis	
<Age 2	
Haemophilus influenzae	>90

ill patients or in those receiving corticosteroids or immunosuppressive agents.

Diagnosis. The most important diagnostic test—to be performed as soon as possible—is arthrocentesis. This procedure is mandatory. Particular attention should be paid to performing the arthrocentesis through an area of uninvolved skin in patients with cellulitis or other skin involvement. In the presence of polyarticular involvement, all affected joints should be tapped. Joint aspiration should be followed immediately by Gram stain and culture of synovial fluid, leukocyte count with differential, and examination of a wet preparation for crystals. The findings of very high white blood cell count, usually over 100,000 per cubic millimeter, with a predominance of PMN's (> 90 to 95%), low glucose levels, and high protein content are characteristic of bacterial arthritis. However, similar findings can be observed in other nonseptic inflammatory articular disorders, including "pseudoseptic" arthritis seen in patients with RA, Reiter's disease, and other arthritides.

Bacteriologic studies—cultures and Gram stains—of blood, skin lesions, cervical, urethral, and/or rectal swabs, urine, and any other sources of microorganisms should be part of the diagnostic workup of patients suspected of having bacterial arthritis. Imaging studies are helpful only in certain situations. Plain radiographs are seldom useful early on, although they may reveal joint abnormalities, i.e., loss of articular cartilage and bone erosions in untreated patients or in patients with aggressive disease. In patients suspected of deep-seated joint infections such as sacroiliac or facet joint involvement, scintigraphy with leukocytes labeled with technetium-99m diphosphonate or technetium-99m diphosphonate, computed tomography or magnetic resonance may be helpful.

Management. Treatment for nongonococcal arthritis includes appropriate antibiotics and joint drainage. Antibiotic therapy should be given to all patients suspected of septic arthritis until bacteriologic studies are completed. Otherwise normal individuals should be treated initially for infections due to gram-positive organisms, while treatment for both gram-positive and gram-negative microorganisms is indicated in debilitated, severely ill, immunocompromised individuals. Parenteral, not intra-articular antibiotics, often in high doses, should be given for two or four weeks or more. Methicillin or another penicillinase-resistant synthetic penicillin is the drug of choice. Vancomycin should be used to treat methicillin-resistant *S. aureus* infections. Gram-negative organisms should be treated with either a first- or third-generation cephalosporin or an aminoglycoside. Long-term administration of oral antibiotics is recommended in patients with chronic bone and joint infections (i.e., prosthetic joints). Closed-needle aspiration on a daily basis or as often as necessary is an important part of the medical management of bacterial arthritis. Most patients can be treated in this manner, although in certain situations—hip or shoulder involvement, joints anatomically altered by underlying pathology, joints not responding to appropriate antibiotic therapy, loculated synovial fluid, or contiguous osteomyelitis—surgical drainage is indicated. Arthroscopic surgery rather than open surgery is becoming the procedure of choice. Joint immobilization is not indicated, except in cases of incapacitating pain or following surgical drainage. Joint mobilization and functional splinting of the affected joint are recommended to prevent muscle atrophy and contracture and preserve joint function.

GONOCOCCAL ARTHRITIS. Disseminated gonococcal infection (DGI) (Table 239–2) is the most frequent type of septic arthritis among young adults of low socioeconomic status and accounts for up to two thirds of septic arthritis and tenosynovitis seen in the country. Women are affected two to three times as often as men.

DGI is always preceded by mucosal infection with *Neisseria gonorrhoeae*. This commonly involves the endocervix or urethra but may involve the pharynx and rectum and may or may not be symptomatic.

Clinical Manifestations. Mono-, oligo-, or polyarthralgia is the most common symptom of DGI, occurring in a diffuse, migratory, or additive pattern within a few days of the onset. Two thirds of patients develop tenosynovitis with or without arthritis, commonly affecting the wrists, fingers, ankles, or toes. Any joint may be involved, but the knees, wrists, hands, and ankles are usually affected. Fever and chills are common. Skin involvement occurs in approximately two thirds of patients with DGI. Rash is nonpainful, infrequent, and commonly found on the extremities. Rash presents

TABLE 239–2. RISK FACTORS FOR DISSEMINATED GONOCOCCAL INFECTION (DGI)

Women during menses
Pregnancy
Immediate postpartum period
Homosexual men with asymptomatic pharyngeal or rectal infection
Inherited deficiency of complement (C5 to C8)
Human immunodeficiency virus infection(?)

as macules, papules, or pustules. They may progress to central necrosis and may develop up to 48 hours after starting antibiotics. Unusual clinical manifestations include pericarditis, meningitis, aortitis, endocarditis, myocarditis, and osteomyelitis.

Most patients with DGI have asymptomatic primary gonococcal infection of the genitourinary tract. The major differential diagnoses include Reiter's syndrome, bacterial arthritis, rheumatic fever, juvenile arthritis, bacterial endocarditis, hepatitis B infection, and meningococcemia.

Diagnosis. A definite diagnosis of DGI is established by identifying the rarely found *N. gonorrhoeae* in the synovial fluid, blood, or skin lesions. In most patients, the diagnosis is made indirectly by finding positive cultures from the genitourinary tract or, much less frequently, from the rectum or pharynx. If Gram stains and cultures are negative, a presumptive diagnosis is made by the typical clinical presentation associated with a rapid response to antibiotics.

Other laboratory findings may include leukocytosis, elevated sedimentation rate, and inflammatory synovial fluid, but they are nonspecific.

Management. Response to antibiotic therapy is excellent in most patients. Hospitalization may be indicated if endomyopericarditis and meningitis are present. Ceftriaxone, 1 gram intramuscularly or intravenously (IV) every 24 hours, or another β-lactamase–resistant cephalosporin is initially recommended because of the increasing number of penicillin (β-lactamase)–resistant strains. Penicillin G, 10 million units IV daily, or ampicillin 1 gram IV every six hours, can be administered when penicillin sensitivity is demonstrated. Parenteral therapy should be given until there is evidence of clinical improvement, 2 to 4 days, and then oral antibiotics may then be substituted; a penicillin derivative and cephalosporin should be given for another 7 to 10 days.

Joint effusions should be tapped on a daily basis with a large-bore needle. Open drainage is rarely indicated. Following completion of therapy, patients should be evaluated, repeat cultures obtained, and tests for syphilis and HIV infection considered.

***MYCOPLASMA* ARTHRITIS.** *Mycoplasma*-induced mono- or oligoarthritis is not an uncommon occurrence, especially in agammaglobulinemic individuals. *Mycoplasma*-related superantigens also may induce arthritis in animal models.

VIRAL ARTHRITIS. The most important viral infections associated with a rheumatic syndrome are hepatitis viruses, rubella virus, parvovirus, and HIV. Hepatitis B virus (HBV) infection and to a lesser extent HCV and HAV may cause immune complex–mediated rheumatic syndromes. Acute and less commonly chronic arthritis and vasculitis, including that with essential mixed cryoglobulinemia, have all been described during the course of hepatitis infection. In HBV infection, acute arthritis is seen in the prodromal phase and is usually accompanied by fever and urticarial rash. As many as 40% of patients with HBV infection develop arthritis, and the joints most commonly affected are the small hand joints in a symmetrical fashion. Arthritis follows a migratory pattern and can be either additive or nonadditive, usually lasting an average of three weeks. In general, the inflammatory articular disease subsides as jaundice appears. Polyarteritis nodosa and mixed essential cryoglobulinemia are well-defined syndromes that may occur in patients with HBV and HCV infection and much less commonly HAV infection. Arthralgia and arthritis respond for the most part to conventional analgesic and/or anti-inflammatory therapy. Prednisone, cytotoxic therapy, and interferon-α with or without plasma exchanges have been shown to be beneficial for the most serious rheumatic syndromes.

Infection with HIV causes a wide clinical spectrum ranging from no symptoms to the acquired immunodeficiency syndrome (AIDS).

Rheumatic manifestations are an important part of the clinical findings of HIV infection (see Ch. 370). Arthralgia, usually of moderate intensity, intermittent and oligoarticular, is the most frequent rheumatic manifestation of HIV. It occurs in 35% of cases and predominantly affects knees, shoulders, and elbows. Other distinct rheumatic syndromes may be seen including Reiter's syndrome, psoriatic arthritis, vasculitis, myositis, Sjögren's syndrome, and fibrositis.

Any of these rheumatic disorders may occur in an otherwise completely asymptomatic HIV(+) individual but most often occur in late stages of the disease. HIV-induced "painful articular syndrome" and arthropathy also may occur. Septic complications in joint, bursa, bone, and muscle may occur rarely, usually in IV drug users. The pathogenic mechanisms underlying the rheumatic manifestations of HIV infection are not well understood. Their treatment includes conventional anti-inflammatory therapy. Antiretroviral therapy, particularly zidovudine (AZT), can effectively ameliorate some of the rheumatic manifestations, particularly psoriatic rash and myositis. It may induce a toxic mitochondrial myopathy, however, with the appearance of "ragged red fibers." Rapid improvement of the proximal muscle weakness seen in these patients follows AZT withdrawal. Methotrexate and other immunosuppressive drugs may be indicated in patients with refractory arthritis, myositis, and/or vasculitis. These agents always should be used in combination with antiretroviral therapy and antimicrobial prophylaxis to minimize the likelihood of serious complications, including the precipitation of AIDS and Kaposi's sarcoma. Rheumatic manifestations also have been recognized in association with human T-cell leukemia virus type I (HTLV-I) and HTLV-II infection.

Rubella-associated arthritis has a predilection for adolescent and adult women, but it can occur at all ages. Joint manifestations occur within days of the appearance of skin rash in natural rubella infection or 2 to 4 weeks after vaccination. The pattern of joint involvement is frequently that of a migratory polyarthralgia and less often polyarthritis. It may mimic RA, and wrists, small joints of the hands, and knees are affected most commonly. Synovial fluid, when obtained, is inflammatory in nature, and mononuclear cells are predominant. The acute episode usually lasts 3 to 21 days, but it may persist for several months. Rubella virus has been isolated from peripheral blood and synovial fluid in both the natural and the vaccine-induce syndrome. Its role as an etiologic agent in RA is questionable, however.

Human parvovirus B19 is a DNA virus that frequently causes widespread infection in the community. In adults, especially women, B19 infection causes adult erythema infectiosum, which may be associated with a rheumatoid-like syndrome of symmetrical polyarthralgia and polyarthritis. In most patients, joint symptoms subside in a few weeks without sequelae, but in a few, they may last for several months. In the latter situation, differential diagnosis with RA can be difficult, but B19 infection is seldom accompanied by a positive rheumatoid factor, subcutaneous nodules, or joint erosions. Elevated titer of specific IgM antibodies confirms the diagnosis, and treatment is symptomatic.

Other viruses less commonly causing arthralgia and polyarthritis include herpes zoster, cytomegalovirus, Epstein-Barr virus, echovirus, adenovirus, and coxsackieviruses. Chikungunya, O'nyong-nyong, and Ross viruses and Mayaro, Sindbis, and Barmah Forest viruses are all alphaviruses responsible for major epidemics of febrile polyarthritis in other parts of the world, especially Africa, Australia, Europe, and Latin America (see Ch. 346).

MISCELLANEOUS FORMS OF INFECTIOUS ARTHRITIS. *Lyme Disease* (see Ch. 321). Lyme disease is a systemic inflammatory tick-borne disorder caused by the spirochete *Borrelia burgdorferi*. Arthritis, usually monarticular or oligoarticular, with a tendency to involve large joints in a remitting fashion lasting for months or years, is the most common manifestation of late (persistent) infection, or stage 3. It may be seen in earlier stages but much less frequently. The knee joint is involved in almost all cases. Lyme arthritis seldom presents in a symmetrical or RA-like fashion, fails to respond to antibiotic therapy, and is associated with HLA-DR4. The diagnosis of Lyme disease is facilitated when patients in endemic areas exhibit the characteristic clinical picture. Laboratory diagnosis is based on serologic techniques, but interpretation of test results is often difficult. Treatment with appropriate antibiotics is effective in most patients with the correct diagnosis. However, some patients are refractory to conventional therapy, and in these, newer modalities (i.e., vaccination) may need to be tried.

Syphilis (see Ch. 318). Joint involvement may occur at any stage of congenital, secondary, and tertiary syphilis. It is extremely important to recognize the musculoskeletal manifestations of syphilis with its reported resurgence in recent years and because of its association with HIV infection. A variety of musculoskeletal manifestations may occur, including osteochondritis, periostitis, bilateral hydrarthrosis, usually involving knees and painless joints (Clutton's joints) in children with congenital syphilis, polyarthralgias, polyarthritis, tenosynovitis (not as common or as painful as in DGI), unilateral sacroiliitis, spondylitis, osteitis and periostitis in patients with secondary syphilis, and Charcot's joints, gummatous arthritis and osteitis, and chronic arthritis in patients with tertiary syphilis. Diagnosis can be difficult, especially in the setting of HIV infection, in which repeated serology testing is often necessary. Penicillin remains the agent of choice, and when appropriately given, results are excellent.

Tuberculous Arthritis (see Ch. 311). Tuberculosis is a rare cause of arthritis in industrialized countries. The recent increase in the incidence of pulmonary tuberculosis and its association (including the atypical forms) with HIV infection compel one to consider this etiology, especially in patients with chronic indolent mono- or oligoarthritis. Active pulmonary involvement is often not detected. The skin test is usually positive in most cases, but direct histologic evidence and cultures of synovial tissue are required for diagnosis. Joint involvement with atypical *Mycobacterium* infection should be considered in immunocompromised patients, after repeated intra-articular steroid injection, and in certain occupations, e.g., fishermen. Long-term therapy with isoniazid, ethambutol, and/or rifampin is indicated.

Fungal Arthritis (see Ch. 347 through 358). Musculoskeletal involvement secondary to fungal infection is rarely seen, although there is evidence of an increasing incidence of pathogenic and opportunistic fungal infections and emergence of new species of disease-causing fungi, particularly in immunosuppressed patients. Distribution is worldwide, clinical signs of infections can be mild, and chronic evolution as well as delayed diagnosis are common.

The most frequent species affecting the musculoskeletal system are *Coccidioides immitis, Histoplasma capsulatum, Blastomyces dermatitides,* and *Sporothrix schenckii* and in immunocompromised patients *Candida, Aspergillus, Cryptococcus,* and *Histoplasma.* For diagnosis, the organism must be identified in the synovial tissue or cultured from synovial fluid or tissue. Long-term therapy with amphotericin B and the newer antimycotic agents, with or without surgical debridement, is often effective.

Cuéllar ML, Silveira LH, Espinoza LR: Fungal arthritis. Ann Rheum Dis 51:690, 1992. *Comprehensively covers the rheumatic disorders caused by fungi.*

Espinoza LR, Cuéllar ML: AIDS and other immunodeficiency diseases. *In* Schumacher HR, Klippel JH, Koopman WJ (eds.): Primer on the Rheumatic Diseases. Atlanta, GA. Arthritis Foundation, 1993, pp. 258–261. *An overview of retrovirus-associated rheumatologic complications.*

Mikhail IS, Alarcón GS: Nongonococcal bacterial arthritis. Rheum Dis Clin North Am 19:311, 1993. *An excellent review of the clinical, diagnostic, and therapeutic aspects of nongonococcal bacterial arthritis.*

Scopelitis E, Martínez-Osuna P: Gonococcal arthritis. Rheum Dis Clin North Am 19:363, 1993. *Another good review of gonococcal arthritis, emphasizing pathogenesis and newer therapeutic modalities.*

240 SYSTEMIC LUPUS ERYTHEMATOSUS

Peter H. Schur

Systemic lupus erythematosus (SLE) is a disease of unknown cause that may produce variable combinations of fever, rashes, hair loss, arthritis, pleuritis, pericarditis, nephritis, anemia, leukopenia, thrombocytopenia, and central nervous system (CNS) disease. The clinical course is characterized by periods of remissions and acute or chronic relapses. Patients with SLE develop characteristic immune abnormalities, especially antibodies to a number of nuclear and other cellular antigens. The diagnosis is facilitated by determining whether the patient has 4 of the 11 clinical and/or laboratory criteria developed for the classification of SLE (Table 240–1).

EPIDEMIOLOGY. SLE can occur at any age but has its onset primarily between ages 16 and 55. It occurs more frequently in women. In children, the female:male ratio is 1.4 to 5.8:1; in adults, it ranges from 8:1 to 13:1; in older individuals, the ratio is 2:1. The prevalence of SLE is estimated to be between 4 and 250 cases

TABLE 240–1. CRITERIA FOR CLASSIFICATION OF SYSTEMIC LUPUS ERYTHEMATOSUS*

Criterion	Definition
1. Malar rash	Fixed erythema, flat or raised, over the malar eminences, tending to spare the nasolabial folds
2. Discoid rash	Erythematous raised patches with adherent keratotic scaling and follicular plugging; atrophic scarring may occur in older lesions
3. Photosensitivity	Skin rash as a result of unusual reaction to sunlight, by patient history or physician observation
4. Oral ulcers	Oral or nasopharyngeal ulceration, usually painless, observed by a physician
5. Arthritis	Nonerosive arthritis involving two or more peripheral joints, characterized by tenderness, swelling, or effusion
6. Serositis	a. Pleuritis—convincing history of pleuritic pain or rub heard by a physician or evidence of pleural effusion *OR* b. Pericarditis—documented by electrocardiogram or rub or evidence of pericardial effusion
7. Renal disorder	a. Persistent proteinuria >0.5 gram per day or >3+ if quantitation not performed *OR* b. Cellular casts—may be red cell, hemoglobin, granular, tubular, or mixed
8. Neurologic disorder	a. Seizures—in the absence of offending drugs or known metabolic derangements, e.g., uremia, ketoacidosis, or electrolyte imbalance *OR* b. Psychosis—in the absence of offending drugs or known metabolic derangements, e.g., uremia, ketoacidosis, or electrolyte imbalance
9. Hematologic disorder	a. Hemolytic anemia—with reticulocytosis *OR* b. Leukopenia—<4000/mm³ total on two or more occasions *OR* c. Lymphopenia—<1500/mm³ on two or more occasions *OR* d. Thrombocytopenia—<100,000/mm³ in the absence of offending drugs
10. Immunologic disorder	a. Positive LE cell preparation *OR* b. Anti-DNA: antibody to native DNA in abnormal titer *OR* c. Anti-Sm: presence of antibody to Sm nuclear antigen *OR* d. False-positive serologic test for syphilis known to be positive for at least 6 months and confirmed by *Treponema pallidum* immobilization or fluorescent treponemal antibody absorption test
11. Antinuclear antibody	An abnormal titer of antinuclear antibody by immunofluorescence or an equivalent assay at any point in time and in the absence of drugs known to be associated with "drug-induced lupus" syndrome

* The classification is based on 11 criteria. For the purpose of identifying patients in clinical studies, a person shall be said to have systemic lupus erythematosus if any 4 or more of the 11 criteria are present, serially or simultaneously, during any interval of observation.

per 100,000 population. In the United States, the highest incidence is among Asians in Hawaii, black Americans, and certain Native Americans (Sioux, Crow, Arapahoe). The risk to a black American female for developing SLE has been estimated to be 1:250. The prevalence is about the same worldwide; the disease appears to be common in China, Southeast Asia, and among blacks in the Caribbean but is seen infrequently in blacks in Africa. Limited observations suggest that the incidence of discoid lupus erythematosus is the same as that for SLE.

ETIOLOGY. The cause of SLE remains unknown, although many observations suggest a role for genetic, hormonal, immune, and environmental factors. The evidence for a genetic role is summarized in Table 240–2. Some of these genetic marker associations are found more frequently in SLE patients of different races and ethnicities. It has been calculated that at least four genes are involved in predisposing individuals to SLE. Each gene presumably affects some aspect of immune regulation, protein degradation, peptide transport across cell membranes, immune responses, complement, the reticuloendothelial system (including phagocytosis), immunoglobulins, apoptosis, and sex hormones. Thus combinations of dissimilar gene defects may result in distinct abnormal responses, producing separate pathologic processes and different clinical expression.

The evidence for hormonal abnormalities is based primarily on the observation that SLE is much more common among women in their childbearing years. In addition, SLE has been observed in some males with Klinefelter's syndrome, and some abnormalities of estrogen metabolism have been noted in both men and women with SLE. However, the clinical expression of SLE is the same in men and women. Furthermore, a lupus-like disease of New Zealand mice is more common, more severe, and has an earlier onset in females—and is ameliorated by oophorectomy or treatment with male hormones. However, in other strains of mice with a lupus-like disease, this gender difference is not noted.

Numerous immune abnormalities occur in patients with SLE, the etiology of which remains unclear; neither do we know which are primary and which are secondary. Some of these immune defects are episodic, and some correlate with disease activity. SLE is primarily a disease with abnormalities of immune regulation. These are thought to be secondary to a loss of "self" tolerance; that is, SLE patients (either before or during disease evolution) are no longer totally tolerant of all their "self" antigens and consequently develop an immune response to them. The number of suppressor T cells also decreases; these would normally be down-regulating (maintaining homeostasis) immune responses. Furthermore, mice with lupus and possibly humans with SLE have a (genetic) defect in apoptosis, resulting in abnormal programmed cell death. As a result of these defects, cells break down abnormally; certain (especially nuclear) antigens are processed by antigen-presenting cells (i.e., macrophages, B lymphocytes, dendritic cells) into peptides. The peptide–major histocompatibility complex (MHC) stimulates the expansion of helper (i.e., CD4) autoreactive T cells which, through release of cytokines (i.e., interleukin-6 [IL-6], IL-4), cause autoreactive B cells to become activated, proliferate, and differentiate into antibody-producing cells and make an excess of antibodies to many nuclear antigens (Fig. 240–1). Thus a characteristic immune profile develops in the SLE patient—the development of elevated levels of antinuclear antibodies (ANA's), especially to DNA,

TABLE 240-2. GENETIC RISK FACTORS FOR SLE

High concordance rate (14–57%) in monozygotic twins
Increased frequency (5–12%) of LE, autoantibodies, suppressor cell defects in first-degree relatives
Increased frequency: HLA-B8, DR2, DR3, DQA1, DQB1
　　　　　　　　　C2, C4 (especially C4A), CR1 deficiency
　　　　　　　　　Certain Gm markers
　　　　　　　　　T-cell receptor (TCR) genes
Anti-DNA associated with DR2, DR3, DR7, DQB1
Anti-Sm associated with DR4, DR7, DQw6
Anti-RNP associated with DQw5, DQw8
Anti-Ro (SS-A) associated with DR2, DR3, DQA1/DQB1, C2D
Anti-La (SS-B) associated with DR3, DQw2.3
Antiphospholipid associated with DR4, DR7, DR53, DQw7

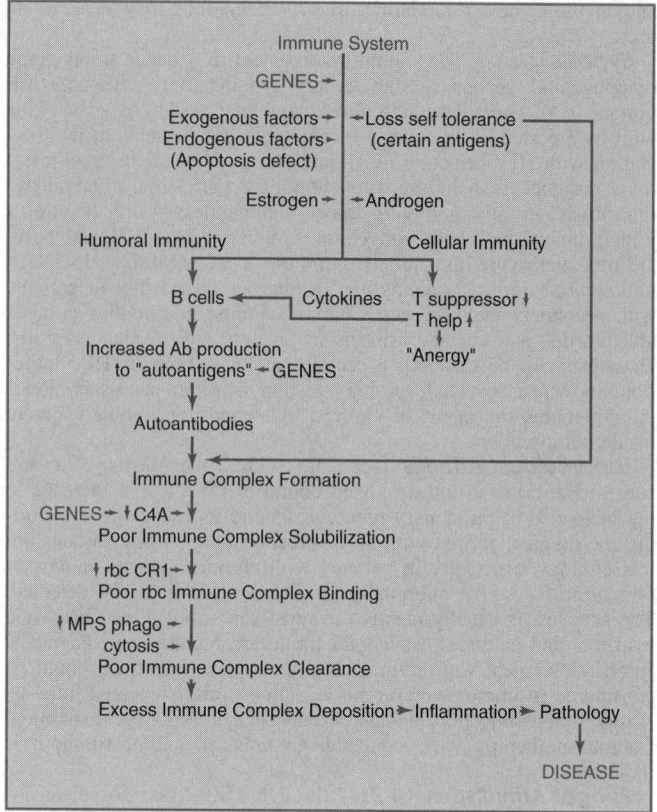

FIGURE 240–1. Pathogenetic events in SLE.

Sm, RNP, Ro, La, and others (see Ch. 236) (Table 240–3). ANA's are made to molecules involved in essential cellular functions (i.e., RNA splicing); antigens are active sites on these molecules. With continued pressure over time from "self" antigens, the immune response switches from low-affinity, highly cross-reactive IgM antibodies—via somatic (hyper)mutation—to high-affinity IgG antibodies and to more limited epitopes on "self" antigens. Unique idiotypes of antibodies may stimulate autoreactive T cells to expand, thereby helping unique clones of B cells to expand and thus making more specific ANA's with unique idiotypes. Female hormones promote B-cell hyperactivity, while androgens may have the opposite effect. Environmental factors such as microorganisms (i.e., viruses) may stimulate specific cells in this immune network. Furthermore, ultraviolet (UV) light—known to exacerbate lupus skin lesions—may stimulate keratinocytes to secrete more IL-1, which in turn stimulates B cells to make more antibody. Not all autoantibodies cause disease. In fact, all normal individuals make autoantibodies, albeit in low levels. The variability in clinical disease (different organs in specific patients) may thus reflect variability in the

TABLE 240-3. AUTOANTIBODIES IN PATIENTS WITH SLE

Test	Sensitivity (%)	Specificity (%)	Predictive Value (%)
ANA	99	80	15–35
dsDNA	70	95	95
ssDNA	80	50	50
Histone	30–80	Moderate	Moderate
Nucleoprotein	58	Moderate	Moderate
Sm	25	99	97
RNP (U1-RNP)	50	87–94	46–85
Ro (SS-A)	25–35		
La (SS-B)	15		
PCNA	5	95	95

Cytoplasm: mitochondria, lysosomes, microsomes, ribosomes. RNA: dsRNA, ssRNA, rRNA. Cell membranes: red cells, white blood (T&B) cells, platelets, brain. Other: clotting factors (APL), thyroid, rheumatoid factors, BFP-STS. In SLE, anti-DNA and anti-Sm are associated with renal disease, anti-RNP with Raynaud's, and anti-Ro with photosensitivity. Anti-RNP is seen in SLE, RA, scleroderma, Sjögren's syndrome, and MCTD. Anti-Ro (SS-A) is seen in SLE, Sjögren's syndrome, primary photosensitivity, and primary biliary cirrhosis. Anti-La (SS-B) is seen in SLE and Sjögren's syndrome.

quality and quantity of the immune response. While these observations suggest possible triggering factors for disease, it remains unclear what causes exacerbations—although clinically they often follow infections and other stressful events—and what causes perpetuation of the immune abnormalities and waxing and waning of the disease.

PATHOGENESIS. Many manifestations are mediated by antibodies. The classic example is that of diffuse proliferative glomerulonephritis. Immune complexes (IC's), consisting of nuclear antigens (especially DNA) and high-affinity complement-fixing IgG (especially IgG1 and IgG3), ANA's (especially antibodies to DNA), form in the circulation and deposit in the glomerular basement membrane (GBM) or form *in situ;* histone may facilitate IC deposition. The complement system is then activated; chemotactic factors are generated, resulting in the attraction and infiltration of leukocytes, which then phagocytose IC's and release mediators (such as activators of the clotting system), which further perpetuate the glomerular inflammation. With continuing IC deposition, chronic inflammation may ensue, ultimately leading to fibrinoid necrosis and scarring (crescents) and loss of renal function. In lupus membranous glomerulonephritis, similar mechanisms occur, although IC-containing, poorly complement-fixing IgG2 and IgG4 form primarily *in situ* on the GBM; there is no cellular infiltrate. The mechanism for the GBM protein leakage, resulting in the nephrotic syndrome, is not clear. In lupus mesangial glomerulonephritis, mesangial cells (macrophage-like cells) have phagocytosed IC's, preventing them from depositing on the GBM. IC's also have been detected (by immunofluorescence and/or electron microscopy) at the dermal-epidermal junction in both skin lesions and normal skin, in the choroid plexus, in the pericardium, and in the pleural cavity. The pathogenic potential of IC's depends on the antibody (its specificity, affinity, charge, ability to activate complement or other mediators of inflammation), the nature of the antigen (size, charge), the ability of the IC to be solubilized by complement or bound to red blood cells (both systems may be defective in SLE), the clearance ability of the mononuclear phagocytosis system, as well as other factors.

SLE patients also make antibodies to cell surface antigens. Red blood cells (RBC's), white blood cells (WBC's), and platelets coated with such antibodies are cleared from the circulation either through (Fc) receptors on macrophages of the reticuloendothelial system, by complement-mediated cytotoxicity, or by antibody-dependent cellular cytotoxicity (ADCC)—resulting in (hemolytic) anemia, leukopenia, and thrombocytopenia. Antibodies to endothelial cells have been implicated in vasculitis, to neuronal cells in organic brain disease, and to renal glomerular and tubular antigens in lupus nephritis. Of recent particular interest are the antibodies to the phospholipid–β_2-glycoprotein I complex. These antibodies appear to interfere with the normal anticoagulant effect of β_2-glycoprotein I and are thus implicated in the arterial and venous thromboses (causing strokes and thrombophlebitis) and placental infarcts (causing miscarriages) complicating SLE.

Skin lesions are thought to be multifactorial in origin. UV light (1) damages DNA (the patient makes antibodies to DNA, IC's form, complement is activated, and a local inflammatory response ensues), (2) increases binding of anti-Ro, anti-La, and anti-RNP to UV-activated keratinocytes, (3) alters cellular membrane phospholipid metabolism, (4) increases IL-1 release from cutaneous keratinocytes and Langerhans cells, and (5) affects suppressor T cells.

PATHOLOGY. There are few unique pathologic features of SLE. In those patients with arthritis, the synovial histopathology tends to be nonspecific with superficial fibrin-like material and local or diffuse cell lining proliferation. Vascular changes include perivascular mononuclear cells, lumen obliteration, enlarged endothelial cells, and thrombi, but fibrinoid necrosis is uncommon. Biopsies of the malar erythema may reveal some minor basal layer abnormalities as well as IC deposits at the dermal-epidermal junction. Discoid skin lesions are characterized by hyperkeratosis, follicular plugging, and more basal cell layer changes, including IC's at the dermal-epidermal junction. Pleura and pericardium are infiltrated by mononuclear cells. Lupus pneumonitis is characterized by alveolar wall injury, hemorrhage, and edema, hyaline membrane formation, and IC deposits. Coronary arteries often demonstrate premature-onset atherosclerosis. Libman-Sacks endocarditis is characterized by the accumulation of IC's, mononuclear cells, hematoxylin bodies, and fibrin and platelet thrombi. Pathologic examina-

tion of the spleen often reveals an "onion skin" appearance of the splenic arteries, thought to represent healed arteritis.

Renal Disease. Minimal disease (type IIA mesangial disease) of glomeruli has IC deposits only in mesangial cells. Type IIB mesangial nephritis also has mesangial hypercellularity. Focal proliferative nephritis has segmental proliferation in glomerular tufts and in the mesangium and IC deposits in the mesangium and scattered granular deposits in the subendothelial, subepithelial, and intrabasement GBM. Active diffuse proliferative glomerulonephritis affects >50% of glomeruli with cellular proliferation, necrosis, "wire loops," subendothelial deposits, and hematoxylin bodies. When chronic, the process involves sclerosis, adhesions, crescents, and (tubular) atrophy. There are extensive "lumpy and bumpy" deposits of IC's. In membranous nephritis, diffuse, uniform thickening of the GBM is seen, with a fine granular deposition of IC's in the subendothelial region beneath fused foot processes. Tubular degenerative changes with interstitial mononuclear cells are not uncommon. Extensive crescent formation, representing scarring, indicates a poor prognosis.

The brain is notable for the paucity of pathologic changes. Some minor blood vessel abnormalities, an occasional microinfarct, and some perivascular infiltration have been noted.

CLINICAL MANIFESTATIONS. SLE is highly variable in onset as well as course. The initial symptoms may be nonspecific (Table 240–4) and include myalgia, nausea, vomiting, headaches, depression, easy bruising, or more specific symptoms or any combination thereof. These symptoms may be mild or severe, fleeting or persistent.

General Symptoms. Fatigue occurs in virtually all SLE patients. Fatigue may parallel the onset of SLE or its relapse but should be distinguished from the fatigue associated with other factors such as increased workload, sleep disturbance, depression, unhealthful habits, stress, deconditioning, anemia, the use of certain medications (including prednisone), and any intercurrent disease.

TABLE 240–4. CLINICAL FEATURES IN SLE

Manifestation	Approximate Frequency (%)	
	At Onset	At Any Time
Nonspecific:		
Fatigue	—	90
Fever	36	80
Weight loss	—	60
Arthralgia/myalgia	69	95
Specific:		
Arthritis	—	
Skin		
Butterfly rash	40	50
Discoid LE	6	20
Photosensitivity	29	58
Mucous ulcers	11	30
Alopecia	—	71
Raynaud's	18	30
Purpura	—	15
Urticaria	—	9
Renal	16	50
Nephrosis	—	18
Gastrointestinal	—	38
Pulmonary	3	50
Pleurisy	—	45
Effusions	—	24
Pneumonia	—	29
Cardiac	—	46
Pericarditis	—	48
Murmurs	—	23
ECG changes	—	34
Lymphadenopathy	7	50
Splenomegaly	—	20
Hepatomegaly	—	25
Central nervous system	12	75
Functional	—	Most
Psychosis	—	20
Seizures	—	20
Hematologic	—	90

Fever is seen in 80% of patients; it is usually episodic. Infections, which occur commonly in SLE patients, always must be considered.

Musculoskeletal Manifestations. Arthralgia and arthritis have been noted in 95% of SLE patients. Symptoms tend to be asymmetric and migratory, with complaints in a particular joint often gone in 1 to 3 days. Fingers, hands, wrists, knees, and less frequently, ankles, elbows, shoulders, and hips are affected. Morning stiffness is generally measured in minutes, in contrast to hours in rheumatoid arthritis (RA). Although joint deformities are considered to be more a feature of RA, damage to periarticular tissue can cause flexion deformities, ulnar deviation, soft tissue laxity, and swan neck deformities, particularly in those with longstanding disease receiving corticosteroids. Joint erosions are rare. Tenosynovitis is noted in 10 to 13% of patients. Synovial effusions are infrequent and usually small.

Avascular necrosis may occur, especially in the femoral head and less frequently in the humeral head, tibial plateau, and scaphoid naviculare. Involvement is often bilateral. High prednisone dosage, prolonged use, and pulse steroids are risk factors. The first symptom of hip involvement may be groin pain. Radiography may be negative or equivocal, but magnetic resonance imaging (MRI) is usually diagnostic. Osteoporosis is common, especially of the trabecular bones, which may not be worsened by corticosteroids. Muscle weakness may represent myositis (uncommon) or be due to medications (corticosteroids, antimalarials). Myalgia is very common.

Mucocutaneous Lesions. Photosensitivity, implying a rash after exposure to UVB light (e.g., sunlight, fluorescent light), occurs in >50% of patients. Some patients are also sensitive to UVA light—the clue, rash after exposure to sun filtered through glass. Fair-skinned individuals tend to be more susceptible. Photosensitivity may develop at any time or vary in intensity during the course of SLE. The classic butterfly rash, i.e., erythema over the cheeks and nose, develops after UV exposure in >50% of patients. The skin may feel warm and slightly edematous. Application of alcohol, found in many sunscreens, may cause vasodilation and thereby more erythema. The rash may last for hours or days and often recurs. A maculopapular eruption with fine scaling may ensue and last longer, although generally healing without residue.

Discoid lesions develop in 25% of patients with SLE but also may occur in the absence of any other feature of SLE. Discoid lesions are characterized by discrete round, annular, erythematous, slightly infiltrated plaques covered by a well-formed adherent scale that extends into dilated hair follicles. Follicular plugging is prominent. Lesions slowly expand with active inflammation at the periphery, leaving depressed scars, telangiectasia, and depigmentation; central scarring with atrophy is characteristic. Lesions tend to occur on the face, scalp, neck, ears, and around the shoulders. Some lesions may be hyperkeratotic and thus be confused with psoriasis. Patients with isolated discoid lupus have about a 10% chance of eventually developing SLE.

Subacute cutaneous lupus erythematosus (SCLE) occurs in about 10% of SLE patients. The lesions are small, erythematous, slightly scaly papules that evolve into annular or psoriasiform forms. Lesions appear typically on the forearms and upper torso; atrophy or scarring rarely develops, although telangiectasia does. There is a strong association with HLA-DR3 and anti-Ro antibodies.

Lupus profundus/panniculitis is a rare manifestation of SLE. Typically, painful nodules develop under a skin lesion on the scalp, face, arms, chest, back, thighs, and buttocks, resolving as a depression. Ulcerations are uncommon. The presence of IC deposits at the dermal-epidermal junction helps to distinguish lesions from those of the Weber-Christian syndrome. Bullous lesions are rare and can be distinguished from other bullous diseases by the difference in serum antibodies and dermal immune deposits.

Hair loss, on the scalp or elsewhere, occurs in 71% of SLE patients. The most common is premature hair loss (telogen effluvium), characterized by a diffuse thinning of the scalp. This may follow a flare of SLE, stress, pregnancy, or the use of steroids; hair generally grows back. Some patients have "lupus hair," hair that easily fractures and is thin and unruly. Discoid lesions of the scalp usually result in permanent hair loss.

Mucous membranes are frequently affected. Discoid lesions may appear on the lip. The soft or hard palate may be involved by discoid plaques, areas of erythema, and especially by painful ulcers. These lesions should be distinguished from lichen planus, candidiasis, aphthous stomatitis, bites, leukoplakia, and malignancy—by biopsy. Nasal ulcers have been noted in 20% of patients.

Vascular Lesions. Livedo reticularis, secondary to spasm of the dermal ascending arterioles, is often seen in the forearms, legs, and even the torso. Occlusion may result in ulcers. A strong association is seen with Raynaud's phenomenon and with antiphospholipid antibodies. Telangiectasias are found commonly on the face and elsewhere. They represent dilated blood vessels and *not* an active inflammatory lesion. Telangiectasias appear more prominent when the patient blushes, is in a hot environment (shower), or takes a vasodilator (e.g., alcohol, calcium channel blocker). Telangiectasias also may be associated with solar damage, aging, hypertension, diabetes, and other rheumatic diseases.

Raynaud's phenomenon occurs in 17 to 30% of patients. It is characterized by blanching of nail beds, fingers, toes, and occasionally ears, nose, and tongue. The vasospasm of small to medium-sized arteries may be induced by cold, cigarette smoke, caffeine, decongestants, stress, and other factors. Following ischemia, there may be bluing and graying followed by vasodilation with warming and reddening. Gangrene is rare.

Vasculitis of postcapillary venules with neutrophil or lymphocyte accumulation develops in 20% of patients, presenting as urticaria or purpura. When small arteries are affected, microinfarcts of fingertips, toes, nail cuticles, forearms, or about the ankle may develop; the lesions about the ankle may ulcerate. The blood vessels typically have fibrinoid necrosis, thrombosis, and a variable cellular infiltrate. Patients with vasculitis have low serum complement and high serum IC levels and may have antiphospholipid antibodies.

Other less common vascular lesions include Janeway's spots on the palms, Osler's nodes on fingertips, atrophie blanche lesions, and chilblain lupus (pernio) on fingers and toes.

Pulmonary Manifestations. Pulmonary involvement occurs in most patients, manifesting as pleurisy, coughing, dyspnea, abnormal pulmonary function tests, or chest radiography abnormalities. Pleurisy occurs in >50% of patients; the most common cause is chest wall pain on local pressure and/or movement. Pleuritis (inflammation of the pleura) also causes pleurisy. It is diagnosed by the presence of a pleural friction rub and/or the radiographic presence of a pleural effusion. Effusions typically have low complement and protein levels, few WBC's (the pleura has mononuclear cells), glucose levels approximating plasma levels (by contrast, they are low in RA), and LE cells. Cough usually represents an infection, but pulmonary edema secondary to cardiac or renal failure or fluid overload in a patient receiving corticosteroids should be considered.

Acute lupus pneumonitis occurs in 5 to 12%; it is characterized by fever, cough (even hemoptysis), pleurisy, and dyspnea. Radiography shows diffuse acinar infiltrates, especially in lower lobes. Subsequently, interstitial infiltrates and fibrosis may develop, with pulmonary function abnormalities. The prognosis is poor.

Pulmonary hypertension may complicate SLE but is more frequent with scleroderma or mixed connective tissue disease (MCTD). Raynaud's phenomenon is common. Late findings include dyspnea, hypoxemia, restricting lung disease, and reduced CO_2-diffusing capacity.

The shrinking or vanishing lung syndrome has been described in some patients. It is believed to result from weakening and elevation of the diaphragm (lung fields are radiographically clear).

Cardiovascular Manifestations. Pericardial effusion is observed by echocardiography in most patients, and clinical pericarditis, manifested as substernal chest pain, a pericardial rub, and electrocardiographic (ECG) changes, has been noted in up to 48% of patients. Tamponade and restrictive pericarditis are rare. The fluid has characteristics similar to SLE pleural fluids.

Myocarditis, characterized by resting tachycardia, arrhythmias, ECG nonspecific ST/T-wave abnormalities, and unexplained cardiomegaly with congestive heart failure (CHF), has been noted in 8 to 78% of large series.

Coronary artery disease is being recognized increasingly, particularly in patients with longstanding disease, especially those receiving chronic corticosteroids. As a result, more younger patients with angina, myocardial infarctions, and CHF are being seen. The cause of the premature atherosclerosis remains unclear, but steroid-induced lipid abnormalities, IC deposition along blood vessels, and hypertension may all play a role. Hypertension is common, especially with flares of nephritis, chronic renal disease, and steroid use.

Valvular disease has been noted in up to 25% of patients; most common is mitral valve prolapse. Murmurs are even more common and may represent valvular disease or be due to anemia, fever, and/or cardiomegaly. Echocardiography is very useful to detect Libman-Sacks verrucous endocarditis. Verrucae are typically near the edge of the valve. Bacterial endocarditis may develop on damaged valves.

Thrombophlebitis occurs in > 10% of SLE patients. It most commonly affects the lower leg and is often associated with antiphospholipid antibodies and oral contraceptives. The renal veins and inferior vena cava are rarely involved; their involvement may cause nephrotic syndrome—pulmonary embolisms are uncommon.

Hematologic Considerations.
Abnormalities of the formed elements of blood and the clotting and fibrinolytic systems are common. Anemia occurs in at least 50% of patients. The most common cause is chronic disease; red cells are normochromic and normocytic, the reticulocyte count is low, and iron stores are adequate. Anemia may reflect chronic gastrointestinal blood loss secondary to the use of nonsteroidal anti-inflammatory drugs (NSAID's) and/or steroids—or secondary to excessive menstrual bleeding. Hemolytic anemia frequently occurs, and the reticulocyte count is elevated, haptoglobin levels are low, and the Coombs' test is positive. A positive Coombs' test with both immunoglobulin and complement on RBC's is associated with hemolysis, while only a positive complement Coombs' test rarely features hemolysis. Antibodies are usually anti-Rh and are "warm." Medications, especially immunosuppressives, may induce anemia—here, reticulocyte counts will be low and haptoglobin levels normal.

Leukopenia, with a WBC count under 4500, has been noted in over 50% of patients, while counts under 4000 occur in only 17%. Granulocytes are affected more than lymphocytes. Leukopenia usually results from immune mechanisms (i.e., antineutrophil antibodies, IC's) or medications. Lymphocytopenia (which may be due to complement-fixing IgM or cold-reactive antibodies) may occur during active disease. Leukocytosis or an excess of neutrophils generally reflects infection or steroid use. There is an increase in activated T cells and a decrease in natural killer cells, especially during active disease.

Thrombocytopenia, with platelet counts under 150,000 per cubic millimeters, has been noted in >50% of patients, while counts under 50,000 have been noted in only 10%. Thrombocytopenia may reflect myeloproliferative diseases, ineffective thrombopoiesis (e.g., megaloblastic anemia), abnormal platelet distribution (e.g., splenomegaly), and abnormal immune mechanisms (antiplatelet antibodies, disseminated intravascular coagulation, and idiopathic thrombocytopenic purpuria, or ITP). ITP may be the first manifestation of SLE. Most patients with both hemolytic anemia and ITP (Evans' syndrome) have SLE. In SLE ITP, platelets are sensitized by IgG antibodies, which then bind to (splenic) macrophage Fc receptors with resulting phagocytosis—thrombocytopenia ensues when production fails to keep up with accelerated destruction. Platelet counts under 50,000 may rarely cause symptomatic bleeding, while counts under 20,000 per cubic millimeter may cause petechiae, purpura, nose bleeds, and gum bleeding.

Lymphadenopathy occurs in 50% of patients, especially during active disease. Nodes are typically small, soft, nontender, and discrete in the neck, axillary, and inguinal areas. Biopsies may reveal follicular hyperplasia. Infection and malignancy should always be considered. When in doubt, a biopsy should be done.

Splenomegaly occurs in 10 to 20% of patients, especially during active disease, and in association with lymphadenopathy. Splenomegaly does not necessarily cause hemolytic anemia but is usually associated with leukopenia. There is no apparent increase in lymphoproliferative malignancies in patients with SLE.

Antibodies to many clotting factors have been described in patients with SLE, including Factors VIII, IX, XI, XII, and XIII. These antibodies may induce bleeding. Antiphospholipid antibodies (APL's) are found in about 25% of SLE patients (see Ch. 236). They should be suspected when the patient has a prolonged partial thromboplastin time with arterial and venous thromboses, thrombocytopenia, false-positive tests for syphilis, and recurrent midtrimester miscarriages. Weaker associations have been noted with livedo reticularis, renal disease, pulmonary hypertension, and cardiac valvular disease. Some individuals with APL's do not have SLE. APL's can be detected as a lupus anticoagulant and as anticardiolipin antibodies. Clinical risks increase with higher titers.

False-positive tests for syphilis have been noted in 25% of SLE patients and in fact may precede SLE by years. The "false" nature is confirmed when a *Treponema pallidum* immobilization test (TPI) or fluorescent *Treponema* antibody absorption test (FTA-ABS) is negative. There is no rationale for performing tests for syphilis in patients with SLE unless syphilis is suspected.

The erythrocyte sedimentation rate is elevated in most patients with SLE and is thought by some observers to correlate with clinical activity (see Ch. 236).

Renal Manifestations.
Clinical lupus nephritis is observed in about 50% of SLE patients and is characterized by either urinary or functional (e.g., clearance) abnormalities. Also, many more patients have electron microscopic and/or immunofluorescence evidence of IC deposits in the glomeruli, even in the absence of light microscopic abnormalities. The presence of clinical lupus nephritis is of concern because of its potential for morbidity and mortality.

About 24% of patients develop minimal or mesangial nephritis (type II). Patients may have some urinary abnormalities, GFR is usually normal, complement levels may be somewhat depressed, and anti-DNA antibodies may be somewhat elevated. The prognosis is very good. Fifteen per cent of patients develop focal proliferative nephritis; the clinical picture is similar to that of mesangial (type IIB) disease but is somewhat more severe. Prognosis is good.

Diffuse proliferative glomerulonephritis occurs in about 43% of patients. There is an active urinary sediment, proteinuria may be marked, glomerular clearance is diminished, complement levels are significantly diminished, anti-DNA antibody and IC levels are elevated (especially during active nephritis), and patients are usually hypertensive. Initial creatinine levels > 1.2 mg per deciliter have a poor prognosis with regard to long-term renal function.

Membranous glomerulonephritis occurs in about 15% of patients. There is marked proteinuria; little urinary sediment; complement, anti-DNA antibody, and IC levels are normal; the glomerular filtration is normal; lipid levels are elevated; and hypertension is a late event. Mild proteinuria has a good prognosis, but nephrotic syndrome with persistent edema and high lipid levels has a poor prognosis.

Biopsies are useful in patients with clinical nephritis to determine the pathologic type of nephritis, whether there is active inflammation (which has the potential for reversal) versus fibrosis and sclerosis, and to distinguish lupus nephritis from other forms of renal disease.

Urinary tract infections are common. Azotemia (slight) may result from NSAID's.

Gastrointestinal Manifestations.
The gastrointestinal tract may be involved in 50% of patients. Up to 25% of patients have esophageal complaints, including difficulty swallowing. The lack of radiographic abnormalities suggests stress, while, if positive, scleroderma-overlap syndrome should be considered. Dysphagia also may result from hiatal hernia and gastric reflux. Dyspepsia is common, especially with stress and with NSAID and steroid use. Abdominal pain, nausea, and vomiting are also common. In the absence of peptic ulcers and adverse medication effect, a cause is rarely determined. On the other hand, one should always consider mesenteric vasculitis, characterized by intermittent lower abdominal pain eventually progressing to an acute abdomen. Diagnosis is usually confirmed by angiography. Pancreatitis (8% of patients) also should be considered in the presence of upper abdominal pain, nausea, and vomiting. Pancreatitis may reflect vasculitis and/or the use of steroids. Hepatomegaly is uncommon, but liver chemistry abnormalities (lactic dehydrogenase [LDH], serum glutamate pyruvate transferase [SGPT]) are common, especially in patients with active disease or those taking NSAID's. Persistent liver chemistry abnormalities may suggest cirrhosis; chronic, active, or persistent hepatitis; granulomatous hepatitis; cholestasis; infection (e.g., hepatitis); or drug toxicity—and may warrant a liver biopsy.

Neuropsychiatric Manifestations.
These symptoms occur in virtually all patients (Table 240–5). Many patients manifest anxiety and/or depression, often in response to their illness and the threat of loss of health, family, and job, disfigurement, disability, dependency, and death. Symptoms may include psychosomatic complaints, such as insomnia, anorexia, constipation, myalgia, arthral-

TABLE 240–5. NEUROPSYCHIATRIC MANIFESTATIONS— DIAGNOSTIC MANEUVERS

Functional Etiology	Functional or Organic	Organic Etiology
Depression	Psychosis	Seizures
Hypomania/mania	Cognitive defects	Neuropathy
Anxiety	Dysesthesia	Stroke
Conversion reaction	Headache	Movement disorder
Affective disorder		Organic brain syndrome
Mood swings		Coma
Adjustment disorder		Transverse myelitis
		Meningitis
Psych testing	EEG—evoked potentials	MRI
	CT	Angiography
	Brain scan	Antineuronal Ab
		Antiphospholipid Ab
		Lumbar puncture

gia, fatigue, palpitations, diarrhea, dizzy spells, hyperventilation, memory loss, emotional lability, confusion, decreased concentration, headaches, and cognitive defects. Frank psychosis may develop with compulsive-obsessive behavior, phobias, and even suicide. These symptoms also may precede a diagnosis of SLE for years, leading to frustration by the patient and physician regarding correct diagnoses. These psychological responses to illness should be differentiated from organic brain disease—which may cause the same symptoms. Most useful in discriminating functional from organic disease are tests of cognitive function and psychological tests (e.g., the Minnesota Multiphasic Personality Inventory [MMPI]); other tests such as MRI, electroencephalograph with evoked potentials, positron emission tomographic scans, SPECT scans, and antibrain and antiribosomal P-protein antibody determinations also may be useful. Cerebrospinal fluid (CSF) analysis is most useful to exclude infection, although some physicians note correlation of complement, anti-DNA, IC's, IL-6, elevated protein levels, and antineuronal antibodies with CNS activity.

Psychosis is said to occur in about 24% of patients. Psychosis also can be caused by renal failure (uremic encephalopathy), hypertension (with multiple cerebral infarcts), metabolic abnormalities, infection, or drugs (tranquilizers, antidepressants, narcotics, β blockers, NSAID's, cimetidine, antimalarials, alcohol, caffeine, benzodiazepine, and others). Steroids may cause or help clear a psychosis, suggesting that the psychosis had an organic etiology. Medications may cause other problems: aseptic meningitis from azathioprine, ibuprofen, and other NSAID's and, rarely, headaches, hallucinations, mental confusion, psychosis, seizures, and neuromyopathy from antimalarials.

Headaches are a frequent complaint and are usually due to stress and tension; migraine has been noted in 10 to 37% of patients. Other causes of headache include cold food, hangover, nitrites, monosodium glutamate, hunger, sinusitis, dental or eye disease, and malignancies.

Seizures are said to occur in 15 to 20% of patients, including grand mal, petit mal, temporal lobe, focal, and jacksonian. Seizures may reflect an old scar or an acute inflammatory episode or may be due to metabolic imbalances, uremia, hypertension, infections, tumors, head trauma, or vasculopathy. When associated with other aspects of a lupus exacerbation, a CNS etiology should be suspected. CNS vasculitis is rare.

Cranial or peripheral neuropathies develop in 10 to 15% of patients. They usually occur coincident with a lupus exacerbation. Cranial neuropathies include those affecting eye muscles, trigeminal neuralgia, facial weakness, and vertigo. Peripheral neuropathy is usually asymmetric and mild and affects more than one nerve (mononeuritis multiplex).

Stroke has been noted in up to 15% of patients secondary to hemorrhage or thrombosis, APL's, hypertension, ITP, and thrombocytopenia. Less common are movement disorders (e.g., ataxia, choreoathetosis, hemiballismus) and transverse myelitis. Meningitis is not uncommon and may be due to either microorganisms or medication.

The eye is frequently involved by rash involving the eyelid, conjunctivitis, or keratoconjunctivitis. A characteristic finding is retinal "cotton wool" exudates (cytoid bodies), usually near the disc. They reflect a microangiopathy of retinal capillaries and localized microinfarction of the superficial nerve fiber layers of the retina. While old textbooks cited a frequency of 10 to 25%, they are now only seen rarely.

Menses and Pregnancy. Some patients think that their SLE flares with menses. Some patients have heavy menses, which may reflect lupus anticoagulants, the use of NSAID's or steroids, or hormonal abnormalities. Lupus often becomes less active after menopause.

Approximately 25 to 30% of SLE pregnancies result in miscarriage; overall fetal loss approaches 50%, and patients are more likely to have a premature delivery. An increased fetal mortality is more likely (3×) to occur in the presence of major organ involvement, especially renal disease. APL's predispose to recurrent midtrimester fetal loss. Pre-eclampsia is a frequent complication and is difficult to distinguish from a lupus flare.

Neonatal lupus is a rare condition characterized by typical skin lesions shortly after exposure to UV light in a nursery. The rash generally clears within months; SLE rarely develops later in life. Sera from the infants (and their mothers) have antibodies to Ro and La. The risk of developing neonatal lupus is about 1 to 5% in those mothers with anti-Ro antibodies. If the mothers have other specific antibodies, hemolytic anemia or thrombocytopenia may ensue. Congenital heart block is very rare but is associated with anti-Ro, anti-La, and HLA-DR3 antibodies in the mother.

Drug-Induced Lupus. Some medications, such as sulfonamides, penicillin, and oral contraceptives, may exacerbate lupus. Hydralazine and procainamide can induce a lupus-like disease, especially in those who are slow acetylators and/or HLA-DR4 +. Other medications may possibly induce lupus, or just ANA's, but the evidence is less convincing (Table 240–6). The symptoms and serology of drug-induced lupus are quite similar to those of SLE, with notable differences (Table 240–7). Furthermore, the disease tends to be mild, is not life-threatening, and is reversible. Between 50 and 100% of patients taking procainamide develop ANA's, while only 25% of those develop lupus. Therefore, the presence of a positive ANA test does not preclude continuing these medications. The mechanism for drug-induced lupus is unknown.

DIFFERENTIAL DIAGNOSIS. SLE usually begins with the nonspecific or specific symptoms and signs listed in Table 240–4, as well as easy bruising, splenomegaly, peripheral neuritis, myo- and endocarditis, interstitial pneumonitis, aseptic meningitis, or a positive Coombs' test. The presence of anemia (71%), leukopenia (56%), thrombocytopenia (11%), proteinuria, hematuria/pyuria,

TABLE 240–6. LUPUS-INDUCING DRUGS

Definite	Possible	Unlikely
Hydralazine	Phenytoin	Griseofulvin
Procainamide	Penicillamine	Phenylbutazone
	Isoniazid	Oral contraceptives
	Chlorpromazine	Gold salts
	Alpha-methyldopa	Penicillins
	Quinidine	Hydrazine
	Sulfonamides	L-Canavanine
	Propylthiouracil	Aminosalicylic acid
	Practolol	Streptomycin
	Acebutolol	Tetracyclines
	Lithium carbonate	Methylthiouracil
	P-Aminosalicylate	Oxyphenisatine
	Nitrofurantoin	Tolazamide
	Tartrazine	Methysergide
	Atenolol	Reserpine
	Metoprolol	Isoquinazepan
	Oxprenolol	
	Mephenytoin	
	Primidone	
	Trimethadione	
	Ethosuximide	
	Methimazole	
	Captopril	
	Chlorthalidone	
	Carbamazepine	
	Phenylethylacetylurea	

TABLE 240–7. CLINICAL AND LABORATORY FEATURES OF DRUG-INDUCED LUPUS

Clinical Features	Spontaneous SLE (%)	Drug-Induced Lupus (%)
Age	20–40	50
Sex (F:M)	9	1
Race	All	"No blacks"
Acetylation type	Slow-fast	Slow
Onset of symptoms	Gradual	Abrupt
Constitutional symptoms (fever, malaise, myalgia)	90	50
Arthritis/arthralgia	95	95
Pleuropericarditis	50	50
Skin rash	74	10–20
Renal disease	50	5
CNS disease	75	0
Hematologic disease	Common	Unusual
Immune abnormalities		
ANA	95	95
LE cells	90	90
Anti-dsDNA	80	Rare
Anti-ssDNA	80	Common
Anti-histone	25	90
Anti-Sm	20–30	Rare
Anti-RNP	40–50	Rare
Complement	Reduced	Normal
Immune complexes	Elevated	Normal

TABLE 240–9. CONDITIONS ASSOCIATED WITH ANA'S

Lupus erythematosus
Sjögren's syndrome
Rheumatoid arthritis
Juvenile arthritis
Leprosy
Infectious mononucleosis
Scleroderma
Liver disease
Primary pulmonary fibrosis
Vasculitis
Dermatomyositis/polymyositis
Mixed connective tissue disease
Mixed cryoglobulinemia
Aging
Medications

azotemia, hypergammaglobulinemia, IC's, cryoglobulins, APL's, and the Biologic False-Positive Serologic Test for Syphilis (BFP-STS) also should make one suspect SLE. On first examination, patients are often thought to have other connective tissue, rheumatic, or immune disorders (Table 240–8). Children tend to have more renal disease; older-onset patients have less rash, arthritis, and renal disease but more sicca; males tend to have more serositis and less arthritis.

Most physicians use the American Rheumatism Association (ARA) criteria for the classification of SLE (see Table 240–1) to help make a diagnosis—it should be noted that these criteria were developed for the *classification* of SLE, not for individual diagnoses. The sensitivity and specificity of these criteria are approximately 96% when compared with other rheumatic syndromes when patients have four of these criteria; however, their predictive value is less. Diagnosis in patients with three criteria should be "probable" SLE, and in those with two criteria, "possible" SLE.

The ANA test is a useful screening test. If the test is negative, the patient has a 0.14% probability of having SLE. A positive test has a 15 to 35% predictive value for SLE (see Table 240–3)—see Table 240–9 for a list of other diseases associated with a positive ANA test. Low titers (i.e., 1/40 to 1/80) have less predictive value. If the ANA test is positive, it is useful to test for antibodies to double-stranded DNA (dsDNA) and the Sm, RNP, Ro (SS-A), and La (SS-B) nuclear RNA proteins. Their sensitivity, specificity, and predictive value for SLE (as well as for some other specific ANA's) are detailed in Table 240–3.

Determining serum complement levels is also often helpful, both diagnostically and to assess lupus activity. Complement levels are rarely depressed in other rheumatic diseases. Levels of CH50 (total hemolytic complement), C4, and C3 tend to parallel or even precede activity, especially renal disease.

THERAPY. Treatment must be individualized for each patient. Not all patients require steroids; steroids have the potential of doing more harm than good. The goals for each therapy and the potential of each for benefit and risk should be considered carefully. The goal is to maintain organ function and prevent permanent organ injury. The threat of a chronic disease can be very stressful, as can visiting a physician frequently and having many laboratory tests—and waiting for the results. Thus emotional support is essential, as well as counseling and the provision of written (and other) material. Patients should be assured that SLE is mild in most patients, that it is rarely life-threatening, and that serious organ involvement usually can be prevented. Support by family, friends, and organizations such as the Lupus Foundation of America and the Arthritis Foundation is often helpful.

It is important to determine whether symptoms and signs are due to SLE or something else (Table 240–10). For instance, fever is more likely to be due to an infection and fatigue due to lack of sleep. Low complement levels, high anti-DNA levels, and/or high IC levels suggest active SLE.

Preventive measures are useful. Patients should avoid using sulfonamides, penicillin, and (high-dosage) birth control pills, which may exacerbate lupus. Exercise has been demonstrated to ameliorate the fatigue of SLE. Patients should be questioned regarding their degree of photosensitivity; not all have this, and the degree may vary, including over time. Photosensitive patients should use sunscreens with an SPF of at least 15 daily—and for those who are very photosensitive, twice daily. Photosensitizing medications (e.g., tetracyclines, psoralens) should be avoided. In postmenopausal women, estrogen is recommended for its benefit regarding osteoporosis and coronary artery disease—SLE women are at excess risk for these—unless there are contraindications or the patient's SLE relapses. Immunization with flu and pneumococcal vaccines is advisable.

TABLE 240–8. DISORDERS RESEMBLING SLE

Common	Less Common
Drug-induced lupus	Polymyositis/dermatomyositis
Scleroderma	Rheumatic fever
Wegener's granulomatosis	Sarcoidosis
Cutaneous (discoid) lupus	Relapsing polychondritis
Rheumatoid arthritis	Weber-Christian disease
Chronic active hepatitis (lupoid hepatitis)	Mixed cryoglobulinemia
Vasculitis	Whipple's disease
Felty's syndrome	Familial Mediterranean fever
Juvenile (rheumatoid) arthritis	
Sjögren's syndrome	
Mixed connective tissue disease	
Fibromyalgia chronic fatigue syndrome	

TABLE 240–10. SIGNS AND SYMPTOMS SUGGESTING ACTIVE SLE

Malaise	Anemia
Poor appetite	Leukopenia
Weight loss	Thrombocytopenia
Fatigue	Hematuria
Pallor	Pyuria
Abnormal menses	Proteinuria
Fever	Azotemia
Arthritis	ESR elevation
Seizures	
Chest pain	
Edema	Decreased complement (C3, C4, CH50)
Hair loss	Immune complexes
Oliguria	Anti-dsDNA
Rashes	
Mouth sores	

TABLE 240–11. TREATMENT OF SPECIFIC PROBLEMS IN LUPUS

Fever: NSAID's → antimalarials → steroids
Arthralgia/myalgia: NSAID's → acetaminophen → amitriptyline
Arthritis: NSAID's → antimalarials → steroids (alternate day) or methotrexate
Rashes: Sunscreens → topical steroids → antimalarials → injection
Oral ulcers: Antimalarials
Raynaud's: No smoking, caffeine, decongestants → warm clothing → biofeedback → (long-acting) nifedipine → prazosin
Serositis: Indomethacin → steroids
Pulmonary: Steroids
Hypertension: Diuretics → ACE inhibitors → calcium channel blockers → β blockers → vasodilators
Thrombocytopenia/hemolytic anemia: Steroids → IV gamma globulin → immunosuppressives → splenectomy
Renal disease: Steroids → pulse steroids → immunosuppressives
CNS disease
   Organic: Steroids → antiseizure → immunosuppressives
   Functional: Antianxiety/depression

In treating SLE, one should consider which organ is involved and to what degree ("severity"). Table 240–11 provides an outline of therapy based on organ involvement; treatment starts conservatively and, if there is an inadequate response, becomes more aggressive.

Treatment of lupus nephritis (Table 240–12) should be based on whether the disease is considered active, the type of nephritis (see above), and the severity. The goal of treatment should be to improve, maintain, and prevent deterioration of renal function. For mesangial or focal glomerulonephritis, bed rest or a short course of prednisone (30 mg per day) will usually suffice to clear the urinary and serologic abnormalities. For diffuse proliferative glomerulonephritis, more vigorous treatment is usually given. Patients are generally treated with 1 mg per kilogram of prednisone. If there is azotemia (especially if the creatinine level is >1.2 mg per deciliter), an immunosuppressive should be added, either azathioprine in doses of 50 to 200 mg per day (a dose to achieve slight leukopenia) or cyclophosphamide. Pulse steroids may be useful acutely until the immunosuppressives start working (which may be 7 to 10 days). Cyclophosphamide given intravenously (in the morning) once monthly (×6) and then every 3 months (×8) appears to be as effective as and less toxic than the same drug given by mouth. The risks of this therapy (malignancy, infections, hair loss, infertility) should be discussed with patients. The initial dose is 0.85 gram per 1.7 square meters of body surface. The WBC count is determined 7 to 10 days later, and the next dose is adjusted (to a maximum of 2 grams per 1.7 square meter) so as to achieve a WBC count of about 4000. Acute membranous glomerulonephritis usually responds to high doses of prednisone or pulse steroids. If not, a trial of immunosuppressives should be instituted. Hypertension should be treated vigorously; angiotensin-converting enzyme (ACE) inhibitors appear to help proteinuria. Diuretics are useful to control edema and hypertension. There is no evidence that plasmapheresis benefits the management of lupus nephritis. For active renal disease, patients should be monitored once a week with urinalysis, serum creatinine determination, and immune function tests (complement, anti-DNA). When the disease becomes inactive, monitoring will be less frequent, depending on the degree of residual damage—patients with nephrotic-range proteinuria or those with azotemia need to be followed more closely.

Acute organic brain disease should be treated aggressively and quickly, in hopes of reversing the process. This usually means high doses of prednisone (1 to 2 mg per kilogram) as well as antipsychotics. Once the psychosis has cleared, the dosage of steroids should be tapered rapidly, because patients are at high risk for infection; adding immunosuppressives, particularly cyclophosphamide, may be beneficial. Steroids themselves may induce psychosis; therefore, it is important to serially monitor the patient with objective measures, including EEG, MRI, SPECT scans, and some antibrain antibodies, as well as CSF protein. However, often one must rely on clinical judgment. Seizure disorders are treated with anticonvulsants (e.g., phenytoin, phenobarbital, carbamazepine); no evidence exists that these medications exacerbate SLE. Multiple small strokes may be due to APL's.

Treatment of the APL syndrome remains controversial. Low levels of this antibody rarely cause symptoms. Patients with high levels without symptoms should be treated with low-dose aspirin; with symptoms, chronic Coumadin therapy is used.

Patients started on prednisone should be kept on high doses only until inflammation has subsided—thus the patient should be assessed frequently regarding specific organ function as well as the immune status (complement, anti-DNA antibodies). For acute, severe lupus, split doses are recommended, then a switch to a daily morning dose. For long-term management, the benefit:risk needs to be discussed. Prednisone dosage should then be tapered—the rate depending on the severity of organ inflammation and damage, the maximum dose, and side effects from prednisone (i.e., psychological changes, insomnia, weight gain, hypertension, diabetes, peptic ulcer, infections such as acne, cushingoid features, adrenal suppression, osteonecrosis, myopathy, impaired wound and fracture healing, skin atrophy, cataracts, atherosclerosis, growth retardation). Once a dose of about 10 to 20 mg per day is achieved and the disease is "quiet," the patient can be put onto every other day prednisone by decreasing the dosage progressively on alternate days. Patients on antimalarials should have an ophthalmologic examination every 6 months; those on NSAID's should be watched for gastrointestinal and renal toxicity.

PROGNOSIS. The prognosis for SLE patients in the United States has improved dramatically since the 1950's, when the life expectancy was approximately 50% at 5 years; in 1994, it was approximately 90% at 10 years. Prognosis is worse for those with CNS involvement, hypertension, azotemia, and early age of onset. The major cause of death is infection. While there is an impression of a greater awareness of the disease, the clinical expression has not changed in 20 years; neither is there evidence that it is being diagnosed earlier.

TABLE 240–12. TREATMENT OF RENAL LUPUS

Pathology	Symptoms	Urine	GFR	Complement	Treatment	Goal
Mesangial	0	RBC, WBC, protein	nl	± ↓	Monitor	Watch for progression
Membranous	Edema	Protein	nl	nl	Trial prednisone Immunosuppressive Diuretic	Decrease proteinuria and edema
Focal ⌐Active	0	RBC, WBC, protein	↓	↓	Prednisone	Improve renal function
└Chronic	BP ↑	Protein	↓	nl	Antihypertensive	
Proliferative						
Diffuse ⌐Active	Edema BP	RBC, WBC, protein	↓↓	↓↓	Prednisone (pulse) Azathioprine, 200 mg Cyclophosphamide, 1 mg/m²	Improve renal function
└Chronic	Uremia	Protein	↓↓	nl	Antihypertensive	Prevent deterioration of renal function
Failure	Uremia	None	0	nl	Dialysis transplant	Decrease uremia

nl = normal.

Cervera R, Khamashta MA, Font J, et al.: Systemic lupus erythematosus: Clinical and immunologic patterns of disease expression in a cohort of 1000 patients. Medicine 72:113, 1993. *The largest cohort described in a cooperative European anthology—percentages of clinical and immunologic features.*

Hahn B, Wallace D (eds.): Dubois' Lupus Erythematosus. Malvern, PA, Lea & Febiger, 1993. *An excellent source.*

Lahita RG (ed.): Systemic Lupus Erythematosus. New York, Churchill Livingstone, 1992. *A comprehensive series of chapters on both mechanism and treatment divided up by organ systems.*

Schur PH (ed.): The Clinical Management of Systemic Lupus Erythematosus. New York, Grune & Stratton, 1983. *A book for internists and generalists on practical management of SLE patients.*

241 SYSTEMIC SCLEROSIS (SCLERODERMA)

E. Carwile LeRoy

Scleroderma (hard skin) is an uncommon disease marked by increases in connective tissue of skin and several visceral organs. It varies widely in extent and severity from isolated hardened skin patches of largely cosmetic importance to a life-threatening generalized condition that can restrict movement "by an ever-tightening case of steel" (Osler) and lead to insufficiency of the peripheral circulation, the lungs, the gut, the heart, and/or the kidneys. Fortunately, most persons with scleroderma are not at risk for the most severe of its consequences. Since the cause is unknown and no cure is available, the physician must distinguish as early as possible the attendant risks for each patient and manage these prospectively.

Distinctions between localized (skin only) and generalized scleroderma and the conditions that mimic each are shown in Table 241–1. Subsets of generalized scleroderma (systemic sclerosis, or SSc) are outlined in Table 241–2. SSc is a multisystem, multistage disorder in which each target organ progresses through stages of inflammation, induration (fibrosis), and atrophy, not always at the same pace.

DEFINITION. SSc is a generalized autoimmune disorder of small arteries, microvessels, and the diffuse connective tissue characterized by scarring (fibrosis) and vascular obliteration of the skin, gastrointestinal tract, lungs, heart, and kidneys, with hidebound skin as the clinical hallmark and organ compromise as the prognostic keystone.

PATHOGENESIS AND PATHOLOGY. *Fibrotic Events.* The mechanism(s) of fibrosis in SSc is (are) not understood. Mesenchymal cells (fibroblasts, smooth muscle cells, and endothelial cells) become activated by unknown stimuli, resulting in increased amounts of the usual components of connective tissue (types I, III, V, VI, and VII collagen, proteoglycans, fibronectin) being deposited in the interstitium and in the intima of small arteries. Endothelial cell changes, vasomotor and permeability changes, platelet activation, and perivascular mononuclear cell infiltrates are present in target tissues before fibrosis is prominent.

In SSc scar tissue, lesional fibroblasts can be shown to produce increased quantities of these connective tissue components (see above) on a per-cell basis even after being removed from the patient and propagated *in vitro*. One recognized profibrotic cytokine cascade playing at least a partial role in SSc is transforming growth factor beta (TGFβ) activation of fibroblasts with coordinate upregulation of the platelet-derived growth factor AA (PDGF-AA) and its alpha receptor. The features of activation of the SSc lesional fibro-blast are outlined in Table 241–3. Understanding the regulatory defect of fibroblast growth may be the key to understanding the fibrosis in SSc and perhaps also in liver cirrhosis, atherosclerosis, and other examples of unregulated fibrosis.

Vascular Events. Prominent vascular and microvascular lesions dominate the early stages of both limited and diffuse cutaneous forms of SSc (see Table 241–2). The unusual cyclic vasoconstrictive-vasodilatory features of Raynaud's phenomenon are present in >90% of SSc patients. Edema is prominent, often occurring episodically, especially in the patient with diffuse involvement. Circulating evidence of endothelial cell perturbation (elevated levels of plasma Factor VIII–von Willebrand factor) and of platelet activation is present in many, but not all, patients. Histologically, vascular lesions are widespread.

TABLE 241–1. DIFFERENTIAL DIAGNOSIS OF SYSTEMIC SCLEROSIS

Vascular Changes

Peripheral vasospasm
Primary Raynaud's phenomenon
Occupational Raynaud's phenomenon
  Vibration and physical trauma (e.g., jackhammer operator)
  Chemical exposure
    Vinyl chloride (plastics industry)
    Mining exposure (coal, silicates, gold, heavy metals)
    Organic solvents (trichloroethylene, others)
Environmental and drug-associated Raynaud's phenomenon
  Toxic oil syndrome (ingestion of adulterated rapeseed oil, Madrid, 1982)
  Arsenic
  Bleomycin
  Cisplatin
  Ergotamine
  β blockers (high dose)
  5-Hydroxytryptophan and carbidopa → L-tryptophan and contaminants
Reflex sympathetic dystrophy (shoulder-hand, thoracic outlet)
Other diffuse connective tissue diseases (SLE, polyarteritis nodosa, DM/PM)
Intravascular causes (cryoglobulinemia, cold agglutinins, nondistensible RBC's, intravascular coagulation)
Telangiectasia
  Hereditary telangiectasia (Osler-Weber-Rendu syndrome)
  Hepatic and hormonal spiders (cirrhosis, contraceptives)

Skin Changes

Localized scleroderma
  Morphea (circumscribed, guttate)
  Generalized morphea
  Linear (with hemiatrophy)
  Other localized hamartomas (collagenoma, tuberous sclerosis, keloids, hypertrophic scars)
  En coup de sabre (with or without facial hemiatrophy)
Scleroderma-like skin changes
  Inflammatory-immunologic
    Undifferentiated connective tissue syndrome (mixed)
    Eosinophilic fasciitis (including diffuse fasciitis with eosinophilia and eosinophilia myalgia syndrome)
    Overlap syndromes (SSc with SLE, RA, DM/PM, Sjögren's syndrome [sicca complex and its overlaps])
    Chronic graft-vs-host disease (CGVHD)
  Occupational, enviromental, and drug-associated (see Vascular Changes above)
  Metabolic-genetic (pseudosclerodermas)
    Porphyrias
    Phenylketonuria
    Carcinoid syndrome
    Scleredema with or without paraproteinemia
    Scleromyxedema with or without paraproteinemia
    Lichen sclerosis et atrophicus
    Insulin-dependent diabetes mellitus (digital sclerosis)
    Acromegaly
    Amyloidosis
    Heritable premature aging syndromes (Werner's, progeria, Rothmund's)

Visceral Disease

Esophageal hypomotility (diabetes mellitus, aging)
Idiopathic pulmonary fibrosis
Sarcoidosis
Amyloidosis
Infiltrative cardiomyopathies
Intestinal hypomotility syndromes (pseudo-obstruction)
Malignant hypertension (hyper-reninemic, accelerated)
Occupational, environmental, and drug-associated interstitial pulmonary disease (see Vascular Changes above) (see also Ch. 54)

RBC's = red blood cells; SLE = systemic lupus erythematosus; RA = rheumatoid arthritis; DM = dermatomyositis; PM = polymyositis.

Immune Events. As in the other rheumatic or diffuse connective tissue disorders that show manifestations of autoimmunity, antinuclear antibodies (ANA's) are prominent in SSc (see Ch. 236) (Table 241–4).

Immunogenetic associations with SSc include loci of class II and III major histocompatibility regions (human leukocyte antigens [HLA's] in humans). DR associations include 1, 3, 5, 8, and 52; since these DR loci are in linkage disequilibrium with DQ loci,

TABLE 241-2. SUBSETS OF SYSTEMIC SCLEROSIS (SSc)

Diffuse Cutaneous SSc (dcSSc)

Onset of Raynaud's phenomenon within 1 year of onset of skin changes (puffy or hidebound)
Truncal and acral skin involvement
Presence of tendon friction rubs
Early and significant incidence of interstitial lung disease, oliguric renal failure, diffuse gastrointestinal disease, and myocardial involvement
Absence of anticentromere antibodies (ACA)

Limited Cutaneous SSc (lcSSc)*

Isolated Raynaud's phenomenon for years (occasionally decades)
Skin involvement limited to hands, face, feet (acral)
A significant late incidence of pulmonary hypertension, trigeminal neuralgia, skin calcifications, telangiectasia
A high incidence of anticentromere antibodies (ACA, 60%)
Dilated nailfold capillary loops without capillary dropout

Systemic Sclerosis *sine* Scleroderma (ssSSc)

Visceral disease without cutaneous involvement
Examples: (1) esophageal hypomotility, duodenal dilatation with malabsorption, wide-mouthed colonic sacculations; (2) Raynaud's phenomenon, dilated nailfold capillary loops, esophageal hypomotility, oliguric renal failure; (3) Raynaud's phenomenon, dilated nailfold capillary loops, esophageal hypomotility, pulmonary hypertension and/or interstitial lung disease

* Also termed CREST syndrome, i.e. *c*alcinosis, *R*aynaud's phenomenon, *e*sophageal hypomotility, *s*clerodactyly, and *t*elangiectasia.

TABLE 241-4. SSc AUTOANTIBODIES IN CAUCASIAN, AFRICAN-AMERICAN, AND JAPANESE PATIENTS

Present in 1 in 3 SSc patients (>33%)
   Anti-U1-RNP; Japanese, African-American
   Anti-U3-RNP (fibrillarin), African-American
Present in 1 in 5 SSc patients (<33, >20%)
   Anti-RNAP (RNA polymerase I, II, III), Caucasian*
   Antitopoisomerase I; Caucasian, Japanese*
Present in 1 in 10 SSc patients (<20, >10%)
   Anticentromere; Caucasian, Japanese†
   Antitopoisomerase, African-American*
   Anti-RNAP, African-American
   Anti-Ku, African-American
Present in <1 in 20 SSc patients (<5%)
   Anticentromere, African-American
   Anti-RNAP, Japanese
   Antifibrillarin; Japanese, Caucasian
   Anti-Ku; Japanese, Caucasian
   Anti-Th RNP in all
   Anti-PM-Scl in all
   Anti-Ro (SS-A)
   Anti-La (SS-B)
   Anti-Jo-1 (and other synthetases)

* Prevalence enriched in diffuse cutaneous SSc.
† Prevalence enriched in limited cutaneous SSc.
Adapted from Kuwana M, Okano Y, Kaburaki J, et al.: Racial differences in the distribution of systemic sclerosis–related serum antinuclear antibodies, Arthritis Rheum 37:902, 1994.

stronger associations with SSc and DQB1 alleles were suspected and have been observed. Strong associations between anticentromere serology and the presence of polar tyrosine or glycine at position 26 of a hypervariable region of the DQB1 chain, as well as a specific sequence at positions 67–71 of the same chain in association with antitopoisomerase serology, strengthen the case that an immunogenetic propensity to develop SSc exists and can be measured. The possibility of a gene dose effect (homozygosity) and preliminary evidence for a class III association with alleles of the fourth component of complement remain to be fully documented.

THE PATIENT. *Diffuse Cutaneous SSc.* The usual age of onset is the fourth decade but may range from the first to the eighth. There is no ethnic or geographic predilection; females outnumber males only slightly. The onset may be abrupt, with swollen hands, face, and feet associated with Raynaud's phenomenon (episodic pallor of the digits, nose, or ears following cold exposure or stress associated with cyanosis and followed by erythema, suffusion, tingling, and pain). Fatigue is common; overt weakness may be present. Skin examination reveals a nonpitting fullness, an inability to pinch skin folds, and the loss of skin lines and creases in involved areas. These changes may evolve over 12 to 18 months to include the fingers, hands, forearms, arms, face, thorax, and abdomen, as well as the toes, feet, legs, and thighs (Fig. 241–1). The fingers and toes may be dusky or overtly cyanotic and are usually cool to the touch. Blood pressure and pulse may be elevated, and evaluation of swallowing, breathing, urinary excretory, and cardiac function may reveal abnormalities. Patients with diffuse SSc should be followed closely for visceral involvement (see Table 241–2). The cumulative survival rate is reduced in diffuse SSc compared with limited SSc (Fig. 241–2).

Limited Cutaneous SSc. The typical patient with limited cutaneous SSc is a woman (or a man who has worked with vibrating machines, plastics, or in mining), aged 30 to 50, who presents with a 10- to 15-year history of numbness and a "dead" or "wooden"

TABLE 241-3. CHARACTERISTICS OF ACTIVATION OF SSc FIBROBLASTS

1. Increased expression of extracellular matrix genes
   [collagens α1 (1), α2 (I), α1 (III), α3 (VI), α1 (VII); proteoglycans; fibronectin]
2. Increased expression of cytokine receptors
   (interleukin-1α, PDGFRα and β, TGFβR)
3. Increased expression of cell adhesion proteins
   (ICAM-1, B_1 and B_2 integrins)

sensation associated with color changes (often pallor only) of at first the second and third fingers of the dominant hand. Full-fledged Raynaud's phenomenon usually develops symmetrically in both hands, fingers 2 to 5, with increasing frequency, especially in winter; there may be a history of hard crusting lesions on the fingertips, initially healing in warm weather. General stamina may be decreased, and there may be breathlessness with minimal exertion (see Table 241–2). Taut skin, often limited to the digits (sclerodactyly), may not be detectable until years after the onset of Raynaud's phenomenon.

DIAGNOSIS. The annual incidence of Raynaud's phenomenon is substantially greater than the incidence of all diffuse connective tissue syndromes combined (Table 241–5). When a careful history and physical examination reveal no features of connective tissue disease, including no signs of peripheral ischemia, the single best test to select those Raynaud's patients destined to develop scleroderma and related disorders is wide-field nailfold capillaroscopy, a noninvasive, reproducible, cost-effective, permanent identification of the connective tissue–prone patient that should be coupled with ANA testing.

The diagnosis of diffuse SSc is straightforward. A previously well person is now sick with the triad of Raynaud's phenomenon, nonpitting edema, and hidebound skin that may eventually cover virtually the entire body, sparing only the back and buttocks. There are very few alternative diagnoses that must be seriously entertained. Other causes of Raynaud's phenomenon are not usually accompanied by edema, and other causes of edema are not usually associated with Raynaud's phenomenon. The key questions in such patients are (1) Are features of other connective tissue diseases present? (2) Which internal organs are affected?

If symmetric, erosive polyarthritis is present, an overlap between SSc and rheumatoid arthritis (RA) should be considered; if fever and a characteristic malar rash are present, overlap with systemic lupus erythematosus (SLE) is likely. Most often these features are not present, and the second question becomes the primary focus. Each visceral target organ (esophagus, lungs, kidneys, heart) of SSc deserves screening.

Abnormal skin texture provides the definitive diagnostic criterion of SSc in >90% of patients. When distal to the metacarpophalangeal (MCP) joints only, it is called "sclerodactyly" and is *not* diagnostic of SSc. Firm, taut, hidebound skin proximal to the MCP joints represents the major diagnostic criterion. Skin biopsy is usually *not* more sensitive diagnostically than the experienced touch. Skin changes also distinguish the three prognostically different subsets. If truncal skin changes are present, the patient has diffuse cutaneous SSc, and systematic surveillance of visceral function is indicated. If skin changes are limited to the hands, fingers, and face,

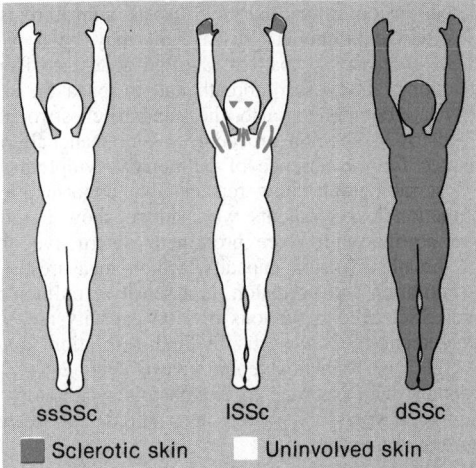

ssSSc   lSSc   dSSc

■ Sclerotic skin   □ Uninvolved skin

FIGURE 241-1. A pictorial representation of skin involvement in SSc. Note that the limited cutaneous SSc patient (see Table 241-2) may have subtle skin thickening of eyelid, neck fold, and armpit skin. ssSSc = systemic sclerosis *sine* scleroderma; lSSc = limited cutaneous systemic sclerosis; dSSc = diffuse cutaneous systemic sclerosis. (Adapted from Giordano M, Valentini G, Migliaresi S, et al.: Different antibody patterns and different prognoses in patients with scleroderma with various extent of skin sclerosis. J Rheumatol 13:911, 1986.)

limited cutaneous SSc is present, infrequent evaluation is adequate, and management should focus on the Raynaud's phenomenon. If the skin is of normal texture, two possibilities are suggested: The patient formerly had abnormal skin changes, either diffuse or limited in distribution, which have subsided (regressive systemic sclerosis), or the patient has visceral disease in the absence of skin changes, which occurs in approximately 5% of SSc patients (see Table 241-2, SSc *sine* scleroderma).

DIFFERENTIAL DIAGNOSIS. Connective tissue disorders are constellations of organ system involvement (skin, lungs, intestinal tract, serosal surfaces, joints, heart, central nervous system); each system involved can present immune-inflammatory, proliferative-erosive, or fibrotic-atrophic-insufficiency changes at different stages of the syndrome or disorder. Virtually none of the systems involved or the stages of involvement of those systems are entirely specific for the particular syndrome or disorder. It is not surprising, therefore, that the nomenclature is confusing. Terms such as "early," "mixed," or "undifferentiated connective tissue disease," as well as overlap syndromes, have emerged to describe the same patients.

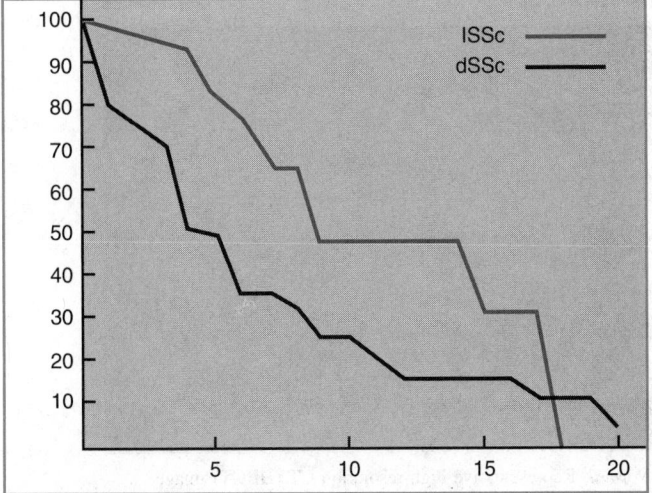

FIGURE 241-2. The cumulative survival rate (CSR, age-adjusted survival) in percent plotted against time in years for diffuse cutaneous SSc and limited cutaneous SSc patients showing the substantially reduced survival of diffuse cutaneous SSc patients (see Table 241-2). lSSc = limited cutaneous systemic sclerosis; dSSc = diffuse cutaneous systemic sclerosis. (Adapted from Giordano M, Valentini G, Migliaresi S, et al.: Different antibody patterns and different prognoses in patients with scleroderma with various extent of skin sclerosis. J Rheumatol 13:911, 1986.)

The time-honored term "overlap syndrome" remains the preferred term for established, stable connective tissue disorders with features of more than one traditional disorder (such as RA-lupus overlap). In the early-stage patient with inflammatory or edematous features that are insufficient for an established diagnosis, the term undifferentiated connective tissue disease (UCTD) is preferred.

Diffuse fasciitis with eosinophilia (also called eosinophilic fasciitis) is a syndrome which, when acute, is distinct from scleroderma and, when chronic, blends into the scleroderma spectrum of disorders. Occasionally after strenuous exertion, young, vigorous persons note the onset of swelling and tautness of the skin of the trunk and proximal extremities with a brawny texture that may be tender. Raynaud's phenomenon is consistently absent, the hands and feet are usually spared, and nailfold capillaroscopy is normal. Initially, visceral disease is absent. Deep skin and subcutaneous biopsies show inflammatory changes including the deep fascia, the subcutis, and the lower dermis. Eosinophilia is present, and eosinophils may or may not be present in the skin lesions. Symptoms subside with glucocorticoid therapy and also with no therapy over time. Eosinophilic fasciitis has been associated with aplastic anemia. In a substantial proportion of chronic patients, the visceral involvement of systemic sclerosis has been documented. In the tryptophan-associated epidemic variety of diffuse fasciitis, as well as the toxic oil syndrome, a fibrotic peripheral neuropathy may be present. Neuropathy is distinctly uncommon in SSc.

CLINICAL MANIFESTATIONS. *Peripheral Vascular System.* Pallor is the most definitive of the episodic triphasic responses of Raynaud's phenomenon (pallor, cyanosis, rubor). The circumstances that provoke pallor and the "dead" sensation of the fingers are usually reproducible in the individual patient (handling cold or frozen items, emotional disturbances). Persistent Raynaud's attacks may lead to a webbing phenomenon (as in the frenulum of the tongue), binding the fingernail to the fingertip skin of involved fingers. This is evidence of structural vascular and persistent ischemic disease, as are the more obvious fingertip calluses, digital ulcerations (of fingertips or over dorsal proximal interphalangeal joints), overt ischemic tissue, or calcification; the toes, the nose, and the ears may participate in Raynaud's attacks as well. The more widespread the areas involved, the more likely is systemic disease.

The Skin. The skin is the most distinctive diagnostic feature of SSc; the diagnosis can be made unequivocally by the texture and location of hidebound skin. In patients with diffuse SSc, skin tautness can limit movement at the wrists, elbows, shoulders, mouth, and thorax (less frequently the hips, knees, and ankles). When fully hidebound, the skin appears to become paper thin over points of bony protrusion, such as the proximal interphalangeal joints, the ulnar styloid process, the olecranon process, the bridge of the nose, and the cheek bones. Gentle pressure over these areas removes all blood from the capillaries; the refilling time can be used as a rough approximation of the degree of ischemia and the propensity to ulcerate.

Gastrointestinal System. If sensitive diagnostic techniques are used, esophageal hypomotility, by far the most common manifestation of gastrointestinal SSc, can be documented in over 90% of patients with both diffuse and limited cutaneous SSc. Many patients do not notice the subtle symptoms of esophageal SSc, which include a vertical substernal burning pain particularly at night, the occasional sense that a pill or large bit of meat "has not gone down," or "heartburn" on lying down soon after a full meal. The single best screening test for esophageal hypomotility is the radionuclide esophageal transit time; it is noninvasive, safe, and can be relied on when negative. Patients with slow transit times should be further studied with both barium swallow (using light barium and the re-

TABLE 241-5. POPULATION INCIDENCE OF MUSCULOSKELETAL DISEASE

Raynaud's phenomenon	1000*
Rheumatoid arthritis	750
Systemic lupus erythematosus	75
Systemic sclerosis	10
Dermatomyositis, polymyositis	10

* New cases per million adults per year.

From Kammer GM: Raynaud's phenomenon. *In* Andreoli TE (ed): Cecil Essentials of Medicine. Philadelphia, WB Saunders, 1990, p 657, with permission.

cumbent position) to detect structural abnormalities (hiatus hernia) and with esophageal motility studies, the definitive procedure for esophageal SSc. The earliest detectable abnormality is a reduction in resting lower esophageal sphincter (LES) pressure, which may be an isolated early finding or may be associated with reduced smooth muscle contraction (secondary and tertiary waves) of the distal two thirds of the esophagus. Upper third striated muscle dysfunction suggests an overlap syndrome with dermatomyositis. If peptic esophagitis with mucosal ulceration is well established, LES pressure may be increased, and the diagnosis of achalasia could be incorrectly entertained. The presence of other features of SSc and reduced LES pressure after treatment are helpful. Barrett's metaplasia and esophageal carcinoma are risks for all long-lived SSc patients.

Gastric hypomotility may be present but is not often of clinical significance. Small intestinal hypomotility, determined by upper gastrointestinal series with small bowel follow-through, occurs in 10 to 20% of patients, all of whom have esophageal hypomotility; this may occur in the absence of cutaneous scleroderma. It need not be searched for in the asymptomatic patient because it consistently declares its presence by postprandial bloating, abdominal distention with diffuse pain, intermittent diarrhea with or without steatorrhea, and weight loss from malabsorption (pseudo-obstruction). Abdominal attacks that mimic mechanical obstruction may lead to surgical intervention, from which some patients recover poorly and slowly, if at all.

Pulmonary System. Although renal failure was formerly the major threat to life in SSc, the combined impact of several pulmonary abnormalities now seems to be the number one cause of fatal involvement in this disease. Pleurisy and pleural effusions, pul-

monary hypertension, interstitial lung disease with fibrosis, and ultimately obstructive pulmonary disease all may be a part of pulmonary SSc. Because the patient is often sedentary from skin or joint restrictions, shortness of breath and dyspnea on exertion are surprisingly late complaints; also, the standard chest roentgenogram is not a sensitive screening procedure. More than half of SSc patients selected for the absence of pulmonary symptoms and for a normal chest radiograph show reproducible abnormalities on pulmonary function tests. Patients who smoke show a much higher positive proportion with more prominent obstructive phenomena. The single-breath diffusion capacity, which measures the balance between ventilation and perfusion, is a sensitive pulmonary screening tool for SSc. Mild reductions in vital capacity are common as well. The detection of alveolitis by high-resolution computed tomography (CT) or bronchoalveolar lavage (Fig. 241–3) identifies the SSc patient who is prone to demonstrate ventilatory deterioration over 4 to 6 years and who is a candidate for aggressive immunosuppressive therapy.

Pleural effusions are usually silent and noninflammatory. They take on clinical significance primarily in the patient with established restrictive lung disease (decreased vital capacity), in whom the aspiration of an effusion may improve ventilation. They are present in two thirds of patients at autopsy. In the immunosuppressed patient, infection may present with "silent" empyema.

Pulmonary hypertension, usually sudden in onset, constitutes a medical emergency. All patients with SSc should be followed closely for changes in the second heart sound over the pulmonic area and for the pulmonic valve closure component of that second sound, detected by the splitting of S_2 on deep inspiration. The appearance of tricuspid regurgitation or right ventricular enlargement is evidence of established pulmonary hypertension. The chest radi-

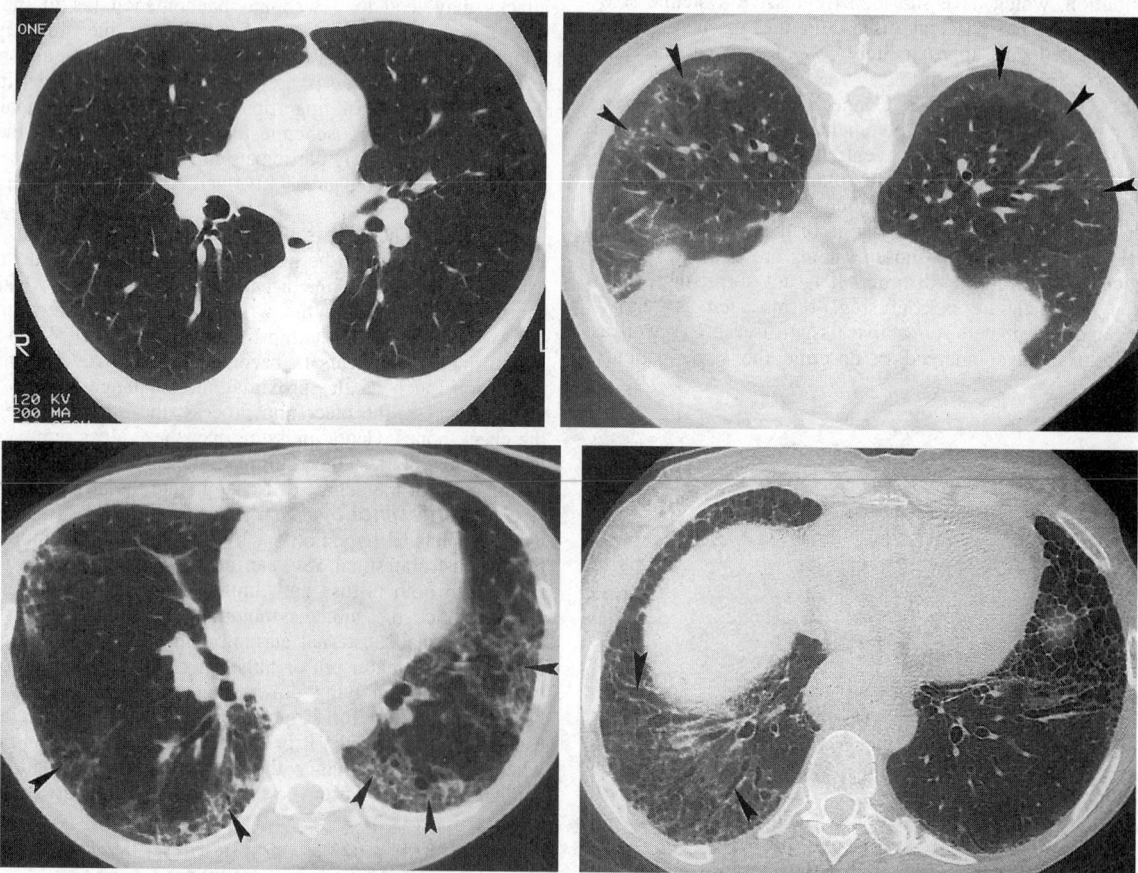

FIGURE 241–3. Computerized tomography of lung in SSc. *A, Normal.* Representative high-resolution CT (HRCT) image of normal lungs demonstrates branching pulmonary vessels tapering in diameter as they extend peripherally. With the available resolution, small vessels can only be visualized 3 to 4 mm deep to, but not extending out to, the pleural surface of the lung. *B, Alveolitis.* HRCT of a patient with early SSc shows subpleural "ground glass" opacities *(arrowheads)* in both lungs associated with and diagnostic of alveolitis. Unlike airspace opacities, these do not obscure the visibility of the small vessels. *C,* HRCT in SSc showing reticular opacities in the subpleural lung *(arrowheads)* caused by thickened intralobular and interlobular septa. Note that these are nontapering and extend all the way out to the pleural surface. Reticulonodular changes are associated with fibrosis. *D,* HRCT in advanced SSc showing honeycombing due to cystic distention of small airspaces of the lung, as well as traction bronchiectasis *(arrowheads)* caused by interstitial fibrosis. (Courtesy of M. Bhalla, M.D., Department of Radiology, Harvard University, Massachusetts General Hospital, Boston.)

ograph may provide evidence of enlarged pulmonary arteries but often does not; the echocardiogram has been useful in detecting pulmonary hypertension. Doppler techniques measuring tricuspid insufficiency (present in most patients with increased right ventricular pressures) in combination with echocardiography are promising for detecting pulmonary hypertension early. Aggressive attempts to lower pulmonary artery pressure should be instituted (see Ch. 38).

Renal System. At one time, the abrupt onset of accelerated hypertension and oliguria ("scleroderma renal crisis") accounted for the majority of deaths in SSc. Fortunately, with early identification and treatment with inhibitors of angiotensin-converting enzymes (ACE) (captopril, enalapril), the incidence of renal involvement and its consequences have been greatly reduced. All patients fulfilling the criteria for diffuse SSc should be suspected of having renal involvement and should be followed with 24-hour urine collections for protein excretion and creatinine clearance at least yearly. Excretions of >750 mg of protein per 24 hours or clearances of <60 ml per minute, or distinct changes in either proteinuria or glomerular filtration rate (GFR), should initiate measurements of resting renin level and, if elevated, treatment. The single most sensitive and cost-effective screening strategy is frequent blood pressure determinations at home, with patients asked to report a 20% increase in either systolic or diastolic level. Such increases in blood pressure and pulse rate, accelerated increases in edematous skin tightening (rapidly increasing skin score), or the appearance of microangiopathic hemolytic anemia or disseminated intravascular coagulation (see Ch. 153) also may herald the onset of renal involvement. The keys to managing renal SSc successfully are to identify the population at risk (those with diffuse SSc), to detect declining GFR early, and to treat expectantly. One remarkable feature of renal SSc is the ability of some patients to regain renal function after months to years (up to 4 years) of end-stage renal disease (ESRD) and hemodialysis. Very little is known about the mechanisms of this slow reparative process. Whatever the reason, it stays the hand that would undertake nephrectomy.

Cardiac System. More than 90% of patients with diffuse SSc (truncal skin involvement) have some form of cardiac involvement. Rarely, acute pericarditis with a friction rub is present; more frequently, a silent pericardial effusion appears slowly, with ankle edema and shortness of breath as presenting features. Echocardiography is the diagnostic procedure of choice. Pericardial effusions may predispose to renal failure by unknown mechanisms. By electrocardiographic monitoring and electrophysiologic studies, 80% of diffuse SSc patients *without* cardiovascular symptoms were found to have cardiac involvement; in more recent studies, 95% show reperfusion abnormalities of the intramyocardial circulation by thallium scanning. Most, but not all, of these patients have normal coronary arteries by coronary angiography.

Articular and Musculoskeletal Systems. Approximately 10% of SSc patients present with a symmetric small joint polyarticular synovitis initially indistinguishable from RA. Within a year, the pattern changes abruptly with subsidence of joint complaints and the appearance of Raynaud's phenomenon, edema, and diffuse cutaneous SSc. The presence of scleroderma-pattern nailfold capillary changes and a positive ANA pattern can identify these patients during their polyarticular phase, before cutaneous changes appear, as destined to develop SSc.

About one half of SSc patients develop stiffness and swelling of the fingers, wrists, knees, and ankles concomitant with cutaneous changes. Morning stiffness may be present. Signs of inflammation are usually mild. Polymorphonuclear leukocytes are usually present in synovial fluid. On biopsy, the synovium is mildly inflamed with a distinctive deposition of fibrin throughout the synovium. Obliterative microvascular disease and diffuse fibrotic changes occur at a later stage.

Indolent myopathy is common in SSc. It is difficult to distinguish from atrophy caused by taut skin. Most patients show diffuse atrophy of the extremities with slight elevations of muscle enzyme levels (creatine kinase and aldolase); these features are refractory to glucocorticoids or to immunosuppressive therapy. Mild SSc myositis is best left untreated. Less frequently, abrupt proximal muscle weakness develops and is associated with 10- to 50-fold increases in muscle enzymes, electromyographic features of acute myositis, and lymphoid cell infiltration with muscle fiber necrosis on biopsy. These patients generated the initial confusion regarding mixed, overlap, or undifferentiated connective tissue syndromes; they usually respond to glucocorticoid therapy. Rarely, their myositis is refractory, and methotrexate is warranted.

Other. In the second and third decades following the onset of Raynaud's phenomenon, a small but significant proportion of patients with limited cutaneous SSc develop unilateral or bilateral trigeminal neuralgia that can be disabling. Other entrapment peripheral neuropathies are less frequent and more subtle.

An increasing number of male SSc patients, especially those with diffuse disease, experience impotence, which is thought to be on an organic neurovascular basis because of diminished or absent nocturnal tumescence. It is refractory to treatment.

Dry eyes (keratoconjunctivitis sicca), dry mouth (xerostomia), or both occur in approximately one fourth of SSc patients. Salivary gland biopsies may show mononuclear cell infiltrates or replacement fibrosis. Supportive care with secretion substitution (artificial tears) and stimulation (lemon candy) provides some relief.

TREATMENT. No therapy has been shown to halt the progression of cutaneous or visceral SSc in a controlled, prospective study. A major source of confusion in assessing therapy is the dependence on softening skin as a key outcome measurement and the natural tendency for hidebound skin to soften after several years. Skin changes cannot be used as indications of the lessening of the critical vascular and microvascular disease.

The most distinctive change in the natural history of diffuse cutaneous SSc in the last decade is that fewer patients with SSc develop renal failure. This change has occurred with the advent of more powerful agents to control the accelerated hypertensive phase of renal failure, especially ACE inhibitors. Indications for immediate treatment are hypertension (an increase of 30 mm Hg systolic or 15 mm Hg diastolic blood pressure, no matter what the absolute level), a reduction in creatinine clearance of 30 ml per minute or to a clearance below 60 ml per minute, and microangiopathic anemia. If the serum creatinine value is < 4.0 mg per deciliter, ESRD can often, but not always, be averted. Continued intensive treatment is indicated even if hemodialysis is instituted, since some patients can regain function sufficient to discontinue dialysis after as long as 4 to 5 years.

D-Penicillamine has been advocated on the basis of retrospective studies that showed skin softening after 2 years. It probably functions as a mild immunosuppressant. The proportion of patients that develops significant side effects is 30 to 40%. Colchicine also has been proposed as capable of influencing cutaneous changes in SSc. Brief crossover studies were inconclusive, and longer open studies were promising but uncontrolled. It is better tolerated than D-penicillamine.

The management of Raynaud's phenomenon has improved in recent years (see Ch. 46); nonetheless, even the most successful management of vasoactive features does not affect the continuing appearance of new fibrotic or visceral manifestations. Sometimes a change in lifestyle is sufficient. Clothing should protect the trunk to encourage heat dissipation via peripheral vasodilatation. Extremes of cold, exhaustion, or stress should be avoided. Nitroglycerin ointment applied locally along the course of the digital arteries to only those fingers showing severe ischemia is helpful. Also, postganglionic alpha blockade with prazosin usually reduces symptoms but may be difficult to tolerate due to palpitation and orthostatic hypotension. Inhibitors of the slow calcium channels of cell membranes have been a significant advance for managing Raynaud's phenomenon. At present, nifidepine in gradually increasing doses is popular, and verapamil, diltiazem, and nicardipine have their proponents as well. When tissue necrosis is present (gangrene), prompt hospital admission for epidural sympathetic blockade is indicated.

Bronchoalveolar lavage and, more recently, high-resolution chest CT are useful to quantify the prefibrotic alveolitis in the interstitial lung disease of SSc; alveolitis is a consistent finding in SSc patients who gradually lose lung volume but not in pulmonary function–stable SSc patients. Furthermore, prednisone and cyclophosphamide, in open trials, seem to stabilize lung function in alveolitis-positive SSc patients. Defining alveolitis is key in selecting patients for aggressive immunosuppressive therapy (see Fig. 241–3).

Black C: The aetiopathogenesis of systemic sclerosis. J Intern Med 234:3, 1993. *A discussion of pathogenetic mechanisms in SSc with emphasis on immunogenetic association.*

Gay S, Trabandt A, Moreland LW, et al.: Growth factors, extracellular matrix, and oncogenesis in scleroderma. Arthritis Rheum 35:304, 1992. *A new hypothesis for the pathogenesis of SSc.*

LeRoy EC: A brief overview of the pathogenesis of scleroderma (systemic sclerosis). Ann Rheum Dis 51:286, 1992. *A concise discussion of our limited understanding of the pathogenesis of SSc with references for further study.*

LeRoy EC (ed.): Scleroderma. Rheum Dis Clin North Am 16:1, 1990. *A multiauthor and multifaceted group of reviews of many aspects of SSc.*

Rothfield NF: Autoantibodies in scleroderma in antinuclear antibodies. Rheum Dis Clin North Am 18:483, 1992. *An excellent summary of the immunology and clinical relevance of autoantibodies in SSc.*

242 SJÖGREN'S SYNDROME

Marc C. Hochberg

DEFINITION. Sjögren's syndrome (SS) is a chronic immune-mediated inflammatory disorder characterized by lymphocytic infiltration of the lacrimal and salivary glands associated with the clinical features of keratoconjunctivitis sicca and xerostomia. SS exists in both a primary and secondary form; the former comprises keratoconjunctivitis sicca and xerostomia with tissue confirmation of lymphocytic infiltration of the minor salivary glands, while the latter is either keratoconjunctivitis sicca or xerostomia occurring with a well-defined connective tissue disease, usually rheumatoid arthritis, systemic lupus erythematosus (SLE), systemic sclerosis, or polymyositis.

HISTORY. In 1933, Henrik Sjögren, a Swedish ophthalmologist, reported keratoconjunctivitis sicca with detailed histopathologic studies of the involved glands, the common occurrence of the disorder in postmenopausal women, the relationship with rheumatoid arthritis, and the ability to measure tear secretion with Schirmer's test.

EPIDEMIOLOGY. *Classification.* Numerous criteria were proposed for the classification of SS at the First International Conference on Sjögren's syndrome in 1986; however, none of these was universally accepted. In 1993, the European Community Study Group proposed preliminary criteria to classify SS (Table 242–1); the presence of four or more of six clinical and laboratory features classifies primary SS with a sensitivity of 93.5% and a specificity of 94%, while use of an algorithm has a sensitivity of 93.3% and specificity of 92.2% (Fig. 242–1). These preliminary criteria are currently undergoing validation.

Prevalence. The results of four small surveys suggest that between 2 and 5% of people aged 60 and above have primary SS. A large population-based study is currently in progress to estimate the prevalence of and investigate risk factors for the syndrome.

PATHOGENESIS AND PATHOLOGY. SS is an autoimmune disorder with a multifactorial etiology. Immunogenetic studies of patients with primary SS suggest a role for the HLA class II alleles DR3 and DQw2/DQw6 and a disease-associated haplotype DRB1*0301, DRB3*0101, DQA1*0501, DQB1*0201 in Caucasians, especially in those with antibodies to Ro(SS-A) and La(SS-B). Although different genes may be involved in patients of other racial/ethnic groups, they share a sequence homology in the first hypervariable region of the DQB1 gene from positions 58 to 69.

The role of viral infection as a trigger for the development of primary SS remains controversial; candidate viruses include Epstein-Barr virus and retroviruses, including a human intracisternal A-type particle and human T-cell lymphotropic virus type 1. Increased attention has been directed to this area because an SS-like illness, diffuse infiltrative lymphocytosis syndrome (DILS), was recognized in patients infected with human immunodeficiency virus (HIV). Patients with DILS differ from those with primary SS in that they are more likely to be male, have an absence of characteristic autoantibodies, have CD8+ rather than CD4+ T cells in biopsy specimens of lacrimal and minor salivary glands, and have an increased frequency of the HLA class II alleles DR5 and DRw6 and DRB1*1102 and *1301.

Studies of biopsies from lacrimal and minor salivary glands of patients with SS demonstrate infiltration by lymphocytes, predominantly the CD4+ subset of T cells bearing the CD45RO phenotype and expressing the $\alpha\beta$ T-cell antigen receptor, which is associated with destruction of acinar tissue and the resulting decrease in tear and saliva production, respectively. Based on the frequent discordance between the amount of acinar damage on biopsy and the physiologic decrease in fluid production, there appears to be a role for antisecre-

TABLE 242–1. PRELIMINARY CRITERIA FOR THE CLASSIFICATION OF SJÖGREN'S SYNDROME, EUROPEAN COMMUNITY STUDY GROUP

1. Ocular symptoms: A positive response to at least one of these questions:
   a. Have you had daily, persistent, troublesome dry eyes for more than 3 months?
   b. Do you have a recurrent sensation of sand or gravel in the eyes?
   c. Do you use tear substitutes more than three times a day?
2. Oral symptoms: A positive response to at least one of these questions:
   a. Have you had a daily feeling of dry mouth for more than three months?
   b. Have you had recurrent or persistently swollen salivary glands as an adult?
   c. Do you frequently drink liquids to aid in swallowing dry foods?
3. Ocular signs: Objective evidence of ocular involvement, determined on the basis of a positive result on at least one of the following tests:
   a. Schirmer 1 test (≤ 5 mm in 5 minutes).
   b. Rose Bengal score (≥ 4, according to the van Bijsterveld scoring system).
4. Histopathologic features: Focus score of 1 or more on minor salivary gland biopsy (focus defined as an agglomeration of at least 50 mononuclear cells; focus score defined as the number of foci per 4 sq mm of glandular tissue).
5. Salivary gland involvement: Objective evidence of salivary gland involvement, determined on the basis of a positive result on at least one of the following tests:
   a. Salivary scintigraphy
   b. Parotid sialography
   c. Unstimulated salivary flow (≤ 1.5 ml in 15 minutes)
6. Autoantibodies: Presence of at least one of the following serum autoantibodies:
   a. Antibodies to Ro(SS-A) or La(SS-B) antigens
   b. Antinuclear antibodies
   c. Rheumatoid factor

Exclusion criteria: Pre-existing lymphoma, acquired immunodeficiency syndrome, sarcoidosis, or graft-versus-host disease.

Modified from Vitali C, Bombardieri S, Moutsopoulos HM, et al.: Preliminary criteria for the classification of Sjögren's syndrome: Results of a prospective concerted action supported by the European Community. Arthritis Rheum 36:340, 1992.

tory cytokines produced by these T cells. In addition, a neurogenic component is suggested by the presence of nerve fibers containing vasoactive intestinal peptide that innervate the acini and the therapeutic efficacy of pilocarpine, which augments neural stimulation.

CLINICAL MANIFESTATIONS. The typical patient with primary SS is a peri- or postmenopausal Caucasian woman; however, the disease affects both sexes and all ages and races.

Ophthalmologic. Patients usually complain of dry eye symptoms, including burning, itching, or a foreign body (gritty, sandy) sensation; this is worse at the end of the day rather than on awakening. Patients also may notice blurred vision, redness of the eye, ocular discomfort, photophobia, and a mucinous discharge.

Salivary. Oral dryness may range in severity; many patients describe difficulty in chewing and swallowing, oral soreness, changes in tasting or smelling, fissures of the tongue and lips (angular cheilitis), and an increase in dental caries. Often patients carry a bottle of water with them during the day and keep a glass of water or other liquid at their bedside at night. A helpful finding on history is a positive "cracker test," i.e., the patient reports difficulty chewing and swallowing a packet of Saltine crackers without fluids. Bilateral parotid and submandibular gland enlargement may be present.

Other. Dryness also may affect other mucous membranes, including the nose, pharynx, tracheobronchial tree, and larynx; skin; and vulva and vagina. Involvement of pancreatic exocrine glands may lead to a decrease in pancreatic secretions and intestinal malabsorption; acute pancreatitis is rare. Dysphagia and noncardiac chest pain from gastroesophageal reflux are presumably due to decreased salivary production and, possibly, altered esophageal motility.

Joint involvement, particularly arthralgias and nondeforming arthritis, is common. Symmetric inflammatory polyarthritis with deformity and radiographic erosions implies the existence of rheumatoid arthritis with concomitant secondary SS rather than primary SS.

Extraglandular manifestations of SS are more common in patients with primary than secondary SS, especially those with antibodies to Ro(SS-A) and La(SS-B); the spectrum of extraglandular manifestations is summarized in Table 242–2. Skin features include nonthrombocytopenic palpable purpura of the lower extremities, some-

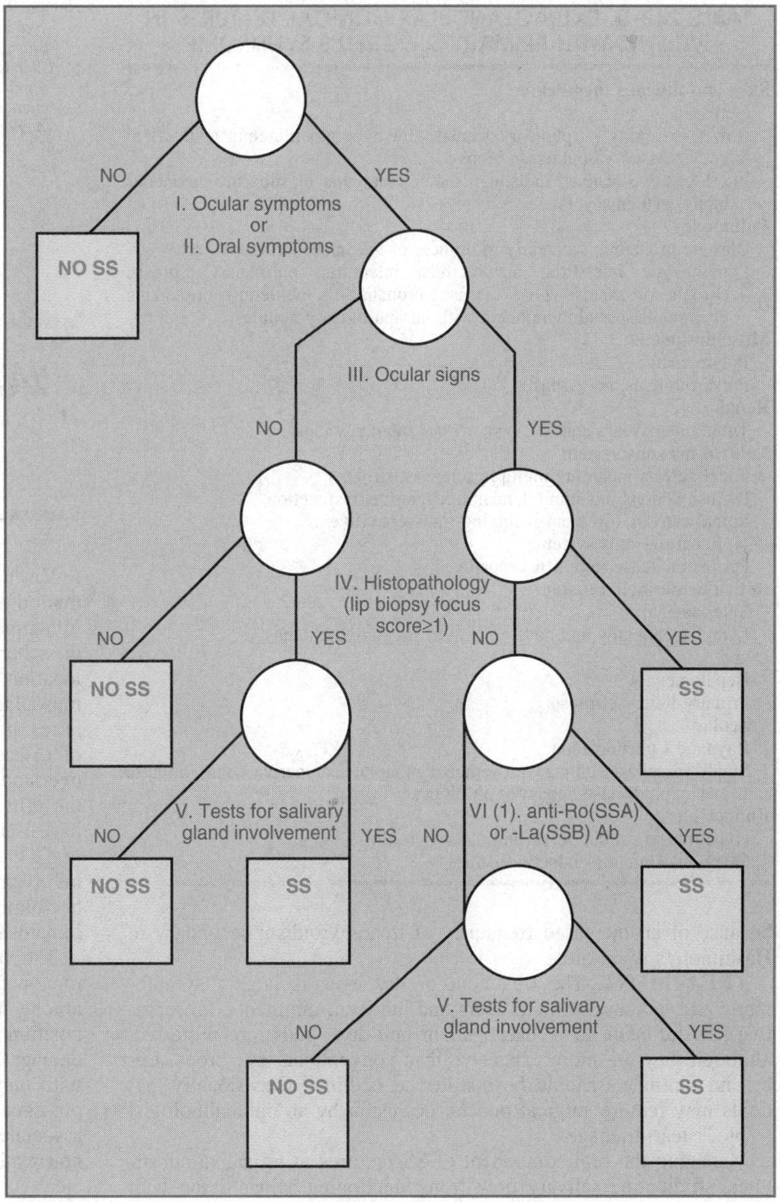

FIGURE 242-1. Algorithm for the classification of primary Sjögren's syndrome. The overall sensitivity was 93.3% in 149 patients with primary SS and the specificity was 92.2% compared with 90 control patients without connective tissue disease. See Table 242-1 for definitions of variables. (Modified with permission from Vitali C, Bombardieri S, Moutsopoulos HM, et al.: Preliminary criteria for the classification of Sjögren's syndrome: Results of a prospective concerted action supported by the European Community. Arthritis Rheum 36:340, 1993.)

times with leukocytoclastic vasculitis on biopsy, and photosensitive lesions indistinguishable from those of subacute cutaneous lupus erythematosus. Raynaud's phenomenon affects about one fifth of patients. Pulmonary features include lymphocytic pneumonitis, interstitial pulmonary fibrosis, and pseudolymphoma; pleurisy and pulmonary vasculitis are rare. Renal involvement, due to lymphocytes infiltrating the cortex, is manifest as type 1 distal renal tubular acidosis; the finding of glomerulonephritis should raise the question of coexistent SLE or cryoglobulinemia. Central nervous system involvement has been recognized only over the past decade, and its true frequency varies according to definition and referral patterns. Reported features include focal and diffuse defects, including multiple sclerosis, progressive dementia, and cognitive dysfunction, and spinal cord involvement similar to transverse myelitis. SS also has been associated with the liver secondary to primary biliary cirrhosis and, recently, hepatitis C infection.

DIAGNOSIS. *Ophthalmologic.* Keratoconjunctivitis sicca is demonstrated by decreased tear production with 5 mm or less wetting on Schirmer's test and the finding of devitalized cells and conjunctival and corneal defects with Rose Bengal staining observed during slit-lamp examination by an ophthalmologist. Other ocular tests, including measuring tear lysozyme and lactoferrin and impression cytology, have only a limited role in routine clinical diagnosis. The main differential diagnosis for the ocular findings is blepharitis; other conditions include reduced tear production after using antihistamines, diuretics, and antidepressant medications.

Oral. Salivary production can be evaluated by measuring unstimulated or stimulated flow rates; however, these tests lack specificity for SS because many conditions cause decreased production. Salivary gland scintigraphy, secretory sialography, ultrasound, and magnetic resonance imaging of the parotid glands, although useful for demonstrating glandular function and anatomy, have only a limited role in routine clinical practice. The major diagnostic tool is the labial salivary gland biopsy; the characteristic finding is focal lymphocytic infiltration. This is measured semiquantitatively by the number of foci, defined as 50 or more round cells, and a score of greater than one focus per 4 sq mm of tissue is diagnostic of SS. The biopsy is also useful in excluding other conditions that can cause xerostomia and bilateral glandular enlargement, including sarcoidosis, amyloidosis, hemochromatosis, and DILS.

Laboratory. Abnormalities in the complete blood count are common and include normochromic, normocytic anemia, leukopenia, and an elevated erythrocyte sedimentation rate; these are all nonspecific. Rheumatoid factor is present in one half to three quarters of patients, especially with secondary SS. Antinuclear antibodies are present in over three quarters of patients, and antibodies to Ro(SS-A) and La(SS-B) are found in about one-half to two thirds and one quarter to one third of patients with primary SS, respectively. Other immunologic abnormalities include a polyclonal hyperglobulinemia and positive tests for cryoglobulins; these cryoglobulins may contain monoclonal IgM_K proteins. Patients with myalgias and fatigue should have thyroid function tests performed

TABLE 242–2. EXTRAGLANDULAR CLINICAL FEATURES IN PATIENTS WITH PRIMARY SJÖGREN'S SYNDROME

Skin and mucous membranes
Xerosis
Lower extremity purpura, associated with hyperglobulinemia and/or leukocytoclastic vasculitis on biopsy
Photosensitive lesions, indistinguishable from that of subacute cutaneous lupus erythematosus
Pulmonary
Chronic bronchitis secondary to dryness of the tracheobronchial tree
Lymphocytic interstitial pneumonitis, interstitial pulmonary fibrosis, chronic obstructive lung disease, bronchiolitis obliterans organizing pneumonia, pseudolymphoma with intrapulmonary nodules
Musculoskeletal
Polymyositis
Polyarthralgias, polyarthritis
Renal
Tubulointerstitial nephritis, type 1 renal tubular acidosis
Central nervous system
Focal defects including multiple sclerosis, stroke
Diffuse deficits including dementia, cognitive dysfunction
Spinal cord involvement including transverse myelitis
Peripheral nervous system
Peripheral sensorimotor neuropathy
Reticuloendothelial system
Splenomegaly
Lymphadenopathy and development of pseudolymphoma
Liver
Hepatomegaly
Primary biliary cirrhosis
Vascular
Raynaud's phenomenon
Small vessel vasculitis, with either a mononuclear perivascular infiltrate or leukocytoclastic changes on biopsy
Endocrine
Hypothyroidism due to Hashimoto's thyroiditis
Other autoimmune endocrinopathies

---

because of an increased frequency of hypothyroidism secondary to Hashimoto's thyroiditis.

TREATMENT. The treatment of dry eyes is largely symptomatic and includes artificial tears and lubricant ointments. Preservative-free artificial tears, packaged in unit-dose vials, are preferred, although they are more expensive than conventional eye drops. Lubricant ointments should be instilled at bedtime. Occasionally, patients may require surgical punctal occlusion by an ophthalmologist to block tear drainage.

Managing the oral component of SS requires using saliva substitutes, stimulating salivary flow from functioning acinar tissue with pilocarpine hydrochloride at doses of 5 mg three times daily, treating oral candidiasis (a frequent complication of dry mouth) with nystatin or clotrimazole vaginal troches three times daily, and aggressively managing dental caries through both prevention and treatment.

Patients with extraglandular manifestations are usually treated with systemic corticosteroids, although no placebo-controlled studies have been conducted; hydroxychloroquine has been shown to be superior to placebo in these patients. Patients with secondary SS should receive appropriate therapy for their associated connective tissue disease. Patients with lymphoma should be treated in consultation with an oncologist.

PROGNOSIS. The ophthalmologic and oral manifestations of SS are generally nonprogressive. Patients with primary SS are at increased risk of developing lymphoproliferative disorders, including non-Hodgkin's lymphoma; in one study, the relative risk was estimated to be greater than 40. Patients with splenomegaly, bilateral parotid enlargement, and a history of radiation treatment to shrink these enlarged glands were at especially high risk. The lymphomas are B cell–derived, and the majority are IgM_K; recent studies have demonstrated a translocation of the *bcl*-2 t(14;18) proto-oncogene.

Young women with primary SS, especially those with antibodies to Ro(SS-A), should be counseled about the increased risk of delivering a child with neonatal SLE and congenital complete heart block; such women when pregnant should be followed closely by an obstetrician expert in high-risk pregnancies.

Fox RI (ed.): Sjögren's syndrome. Rheum Dis Clin North Am 18:507, 1992. *Covers the history, pathology, immunopathogenesis, clinical features, and management of SS.*

Homma M, Talal N (eds.): Proceedings IVth International Symposium on Sjögren's Syndrome. Amsterdam, Kluger Publications, 1994. *Includes manuscripts of symposium papers of August 1993 in Tokyo.*

St. Clair EW: Sjögren's syndrome and autoimmunity. *In* Cruse JM, Lewis RE (eds.): Clinical and Molecular Aspects of Autoimmune Disease. Concepts in Immunopathology. Basel, Karger, 1992, p 161. *This chapter reviews SS immunopathogenesis.*

Vitali C, Bombardieri S, Moutsopoulos HM, et al.: Preliminary criteria for the classification of Sjögren's syndrome: Results of a prospective concerted action supported by the European Community. Arthritis Rheum 36:340, 1993. *Presents the results of the European Community Study Group's evaluation of criteria for the classification of both primary and secondary SS.*

---

243 THE VASCULITIC SYNDROMES

Lanny J. Rosenwasser

Vasculitis is a clinicopathologic process characterized by inflammation and necrosis of the blood vessel wall. Associated with this inflammation may be compromise of the vessel lumen that results in ischemic changes in the tissues supplied by the vessel. Any size, location, and type of blood vessel may be involved, including large muscular arteries, medium-sized and small arteries, arterioles, capillaries, postcapillary venules, and veins. This heterogeneous category of diseases comprises unique syndromes as well as diseases with overlapping clinical and pathologic features. The vasculitis may be the primary process, or it may be a component of another underlying disease. Rarely, certain vasculitic disorders are life threatening (e.g., the hypersensitivity vasculitic syndromes in which cutaneous involvement usually predominates). Other vasculitic syndromes may be fulminant and, if untreated, rapidly fatal (e.g., Wegener's granulomatosis and polyarteritis nodosa).

The vasculitic syndromes are generally thought to result from immunopathogenic mechanisms; however, the evidence for this varies among the different syndromes. Among these mechanisms, the deposition of circulating immune complexes with subsequent vessel damage has emerged as a major immunopathologic event associated with most of the vasculitic syndromes (see Ch. 221 and 228). The presence of circulating immune complexes does not prove that the associated vasculitis is caused by them, and complexes *per se* need not result in vasculitis, even in diseases in which vasculitis is present.

The mechanism of tissue damage from immune complexes is thought to be similar to serum sickness. In this model, soluble immune complexes are formed in antigen excess and deposited in blood vessel walls in areas of increased vascular permeability. The increased permeability is attributed to release of vasoactive amines from platelets or mast cells under the influence of specific immunoglobulin E (IgE). Following deposition of complexes, various components of complement are activated, particularly C5a, which is strongly chemotactic for neutrophils. The neutrophils infiltrate the vessel wall at the site of immune complex deposition and release intracytoplasmic enzymes such as collagenase and elastase that directly damage the vessel wall. Compromise of the lumen occurs with resulting ischemic changes.

Certain of the vasculitides are characterized by granulomatous inflammation in and around the blood vessels. Although granulomatous responses are generally of the delayed hypersensitivity type, immune complexes themselves can trigger granuloma formation and thereby produce granulomatous vasculitis. Recently it has been found that the vessel wall itself, in addition to being a target for immune complex deposition, may actively participate in inflammation in the blood vessel by producing, locally, cytokines that are proinflammatory and that will attract other inflammatory cells, including cells that are involved in cell-mediated immunity. Hence, the mechanisms by which granulomatous inflammation may occur on the basis of immune complex initiation clearly will still involve the potential role of T cells, macrophages, and cytokines usually associated with delayed-type hypersensitivity.

The heterogeneity and the obvious overlap among the vasculitic syndromes have led to difficulties in classification of this group of diseases. The first report of a vasculitic syndrome was in 1866 by Kussmaul and Maier, who described the clinicopathologic features in a patient with what is now recognized as classic polyarteritis nodosa. It became evident that there were numerous vasculitic syndromes with diverse clinical and pathologic manifestations, but diagnostic criteria were controversial. More precise and accurate classification schemes now have emerged, based upon re-examination of clinical, pathologic, and immunologic features, as well as responses to certain therapeutic regimens. Table 243–1 is one such classification scheme.

The first group of vasculitides is the polyarteritis nodosa group. This syndrome is described in detail in Ch. 244. It is the prototype of the serious systemic necrotizing vasculitides and manifests features such as small and medium-sized muscular artery involvement, hypertension, visceral vessel involvement, and a noticeable lack of lung involvement. Eventually physicians recognized a systemic vasculitis that resembled classic polyarteritis nodosa except that lung involvement was a prominent feature and the patients generally manifested eosinophilia, granulomatous reactions, and a strong allergic diathesis, usually severe asthma. Most of these patients had what is now referred to as allergic angiitis and granulomatosis of the Churg-Strauss type. This disease is quite similar to classic polyarteritis nodosa except for the divergent features just mentioned. Many systemic necrotizing vasculitides manifest clinicopathologic characteristics that overlap these two syndromes as well as the hypersensitivity group of vasculitides (discussed below). This subgroup has been referred to as the overlap syndrome of systemic necrotizing vasculitis.

In addition to the polyarteritis nodosa group of systemic necrotizing vaculitides, certain other vasculitides are systemic and involve multiple organ systems. However, they are referred to by different names, since they possess characteristic clinical and/or pathologic features. This is true of diseases such as Wegener's granulomatosis (see Ch. 245), lymphomatoid granulomatosis, and the giant cell arteritides. In the last group, the two major subcategories—cranial or temporal arteritis (see Ch. 246) and Takayasu's arteritis—are systemic diseases involving large muscular arteries with mononuclear cell and often giant cell infiltration within the walls of the involved arteries. Despite the predisposition for certain vessels in these diseases (temporal artery in cranial arteritis and subclavian artery in Takayasu's arteritis), these are systemic diseases that involve multiple arteries. Lymphomatoid granulomatosis is generally considered in the differential diagnosis of systemic necrotizing vasculitis with lung involvement such as Wegener's granulomatosis. However, it is not, strictly speaking, an inflammatory response in vessels, but an infiltration of blood vessel walls with atypical and often neoplastic-looking lymphoid cells. Lymphomatoid granulomatosis will often evolve into a lymphoma, and it has been suggested that these cases should be classified as angiocentric proliferative lesions.

Other vasculitic syndromes can be considered under the category of miscellaneous, for want of a better term. These include Kawasaki's disease and Behçet's disease, the major pathologic feature of which is a true vasculitis (see Ch. 249), and thromboangiitis obliterans, which is an inflammatory and occlusive disease of arteries and veins, although its true vasculitic character has been questioned. In addition to the granulomatous vasculitis of the central nervous system (CNS), which is seen in association with certain lymphoproliferative malignant neoplasms, there is also a rare syndrome of isolated vasculitis of the CNS that occurs in the apparent absence of systemic vasculitis or other systemic disease. Finally, erythema nodosum, erythema multiforme, and erythema elevatum diutinum are dermal vasculitides in this category.

HYPERSENSITIVITY VASCULITIS

Hypersensitivity vasculitis is a term applied to a heterogeneous group of disorders that are thought to represent a hypersensitivity reaction to an antigenic stimulus such as a drug or an infectious agent; hence the word hypersensitivity. Although the antigenic stimuli associated with this group are heterogeneous, these disorders generally involve the small vessels. They can be subdivided into two basic groups. The vast majority of patients manifest involvement of the postcapillary venules, and hence have a venulitis. A smaller group of patients falls into the second category, in which arterioles are predominantly involved (arteriolitis). Most important, there is predominant and often exclusive involvement of the vessels of the skin. Confusion in the literature generally resulted from grouping this category of vasculitis with the more serious systemic varieties, such as classic polyarteritis nodosa and related diseases. It is true that the hypersensitivity vasculitides may have variable degrees of organ system involvement other than of the skin. However, this is usually less severe than that of typical systemic vasculitis of polyarteritis nodosa and Wegener's granulomatosis. Most frequently the skin is exclusively involved, or if other organ systems are involved, the cutaneous disease still dominates the clinical picture.

ETIOLOGY. As indicated by the terminology, the cause is usually a recognizable antigenic stimulus, such as a drug, microbe, toxin, or foreign or endogenous protein. Etiologically the hypersensitivity vasculitides segregate into two distinct groups, depending on the source of the sensitizing antigen. In the classic original group, the antigen is foreign to the host. In the second group the antigen is endogenous.

INCIDENCE AND PREVALENCE. It is difficult to determine an accurate incidence for the hypersensitivity group of vasculitides owing to the marked heterogeneity among these diverse syndromes. However, the hypersensitivity group of vasculitides is much more common than the polyarteritis group and other syndromes such as Wegener's granulomatosis and Takayasu's arteritis. The disease can be seen at any age and in both genders; however, this varies considerably with the particular subgroup in question.

PATHOLOGY AND PATHOGENESIS. The histopathologic hallmark of the hypersensitivity vasculitides is leukocytoclastic venulitis. The term leukocytoclasis refers to nuclear debris derived from the neutrophils that have infiltrated in and around the involved vessels. In skin biopsies, this type of involvement is most common in the postcapillary venules just beneath the epidermis. When biopsies are obtained in the acute phase of active disease, the typical pattern of neutrophil infiltration is readily observed. In the subacute or chronic stages, biopsies often reveal mononuclear cell infiltration. In the second and smaller category of hypersensitivity vasculitis, arterioles and capillaries are predominantly involved. In the typical case of hypersensitivity vasculitis with a predominance of cutaneous involvement, the lesions are usually found in the lower extremities or in the dependent areas such as the sacrum in supine patients. This is most likely due to the increase in hydrostatic pressure within the postcapillary venules in these areas.

TABLE 243–1. THE CLINICAL SPECTRUM OF VASCULITIS

Polyarteritis Nodosa Group

Classic polyarteritis nodosa
Allergic angiitis and granulomatosis (Churg-Strauss disease)
Overlap syndrome

Hypersensitivity Vasculitis

Henoch-Schönlein purpura
Serum sickness and serum sickness–like reactions
Vasculitis associated with infectious diseases
Vasculitis associated with neoplasms
Vasculitis associated with connective tissue diseases
Vasculitis associated with other underlying diseases
Congenital deficiencies of the complement system

Granulomatous Vasculitides

Wegener's granulomatosis
Angiocentric immunoproliferative lesions (lymphomatoid granulomatosis)
Giant cell arteritides
　　Cranial or temporal arteritis
　　Takayasu's arteritis

Other Vasculitic Syndromes

Mucocutaneous lymph node syndrome (Kawasaki's disease)
Behçet's disease
Vasculitis isolated to the central nervous system
Thromboangiitis obliterans (Buerger's disease)
Erythema nodosum
Erythema multiforme
Erythema elevatum diutinum
Miscellaneous vasculitides

Although immune complex deposition is widely considered to be the pathogenic mechanism of this group of vasculitides, not every case of hypersensitivity vasculitis has had immune complexes demonstrated, even when carefully sought, as mentioned above.

CLINICAL MANIFESTATIONS. Just as the broad group is etiologically heterogeneous, so too are the clinical manifestations. However, the hallmark of the group is the predominance of cutaneous involvement. The skin lesions may appear as the classic palpable purpura, which results from the extravasation of erythrocytes into the tissue surrounding the involved venules. In addition, one may see macules, papules, vesicles, bullae, subcutaneous nodules, ulcers, and even recurrent or chronic urticaria.

Even though skin lesions generally dominate, various organ system involvement can be seen. Certain constellations of clinicopathologic findings define relatively distinct syndromes. For example, in Henoch-Schönlein purpura the typical syndrome consists of palpable purpura (usually over the buttocks), arthralgias, gastrointestinal symptoms, and glomerulonephritis. Henoch-Schönlein purpura is usually seen in children; however, adults of any age may be affected. The disease usually remits spontaneously after 1 week. However, the disease is remarkable for its tendency to recur a number of times over weeks to months before remission is complete. The characteristic skin lesions are present in virtually all patients, with most having arthralgias involving multiple joints, but frank arthritis is rare. The gastrointestinal involvement is usually manifested as colicky abdominal pain that may mimic an "acute surgical abdomen." Patients may experience nausea, vomiting, diarrhea, constipation, and occasionally the passage of blood and mucus per rectum. In the more severe and rare case, bowel intussusception may occur. Renal disease is a glomerulitis (see Ch. 79) that is usually expressed as microscopic hematuria without significant renal functional impairment. However, in rare cases, renal failure can occur. Most frequently, patients recover spontaneously and completely.

Other groups within the hypersensitivity category include serum sickness and serum sickness–like reactions. The classic manifestations are fever, urticaria, arthralgias, and lymphadenopathy occurring 7 to 10 days after primary exposure to the antigen in question, which for serum sickness is usually a heterologous serum protein and for serum sickness–like reactions is usually a drug such as penicillin. Very careful studies of serum complement levels demonstrate consumption of serum complement components C3 and C4 during the height of heterologous protein-related serum sickness. This depression of serum C3 and C4 is associated with increases in plasma level of C3a and other products that are indicative of complement activation. These alterations in serum complement correlate with the presence of immune complexes in the serum in these models of serum sickness. In addition, cases may occasionally progress to a typical systemic necrotizing vasculitis involving multiple organ systems.

A number of disorders have vasculitis as a manifestation of an underlying primary disease. Included in these diseases are systemic lupus erythematosus (SLE), rheumatoid arthritis, mixed cryoglobulinemia, and other connective tissue diseases. In these disorders the manifestations of the underlying disease usually predominate. When vasculitis is observed it is generally of the small vessel cutaneous type, which is virtually indistinguishable from the vasculitis seen in the hypersensitivity group with recognized exogenous antigens. However, patients with these disorders, particularly SLE and rheumatoid arthritis, may also develop a systemic necrotizing vasculitis that closely resembles the polyarteritis nodosa group in manifestations and severity. Nevertheless, in the typical case, the cutaneous vasculitis usually dominates the clinical picture with respect to the vasculitic process.

Other diseases that may fall into this category are the vasculitis associated with congenital deficiencies of various complement components, such as C1r, C1s, and C2, erythema elevatum diutinum; hypocomplementemic vasculitis; the vasculitis associated with certain neoplasms, particularly of the lymphoid type; and the vasculitis associated with other primary disorders such as ulcerative colitis, Crohn's disease, biliary cirrhosis, and retroperitoneal fibrosis.

DIAGNOSIS. The diagnosis of hypersensitivity vasculitis rests on demonstration of vasculitis on biopsy. Since the predominant organ involved is the skin, histopathologic material is usually readily available. Because cutaneous involvement is often present in severe systemic vasculitides, one should undertake a systematic workup of other organ systems in patients with apparently isolated cutaneous

vasculitis. Recently it has been suggested that the presence of antibodies against the cytoplasm of neutrophils (c-ANCA) is supportive evidence for a diagnosis of Wegener's granulomatosis (see Ch. 236 and 245).

TREATMENT AND PROGNOSIS. Therapy of the hypersensitivity group of vasculitides has in general been unsatisfactory. Since most cases resolve spontaneously, the lack of response to therapeutic regimens is of less importance. However, in those patients who develop persistent cutaneous disease or serious organ system involvement, several regimens have been tried with variable results. In cases in which a recognized antigenic stimulus is present, the sensitizing drugs or responsible organisms should be removed by appropriate antibiotic therapy when possible. In situations in which disease appears to be self-limited, no specific therapy is indicated. However, when disease persists or results in organ system dysfunction, a glucocorticoid is the drug of choice. Prednisone is usually administered in doses of 1 mg per kilogram per day with rapid tapering when possible, in some instances directly to discontinuation or initially to an alternate-day regimen followed by ultimate discontinuation. In cases that prove refractory to corticosteroid therapy, cytotoxic agents such as cyclophosphamide have been used. The efficacy of these regimens has not yet been fully evaluated in hypersensitivity vasculitis.

The prognosis of most of these diseases is generally excellent, with spontaneous and complete remissions in most patients. However, certain patients may develop persistent and debilitating cutaneous disease, and some cases may evolve into typical systemic vasculitis with a serious prognosis.

Calabrese LH, Michel BA, Bloch DA, et al.: The American College of Rheumatology 1990 criteria for the classification of hypersensitivity vasculitis. Arthritis Rheum 33:1108, 1990. *This paper is from an issue of Arthritis and Rheumatism that identified the American College of Rheumatology criteria for diagnosis of vasculitis using algorithms for patient symptoms and pathologic findings.*

Cupps TR, Fauci AS: The Vasculitides. Philadelphia, WB Saunders, 1981, pp. 1–21. *Comprehensive treatise on the entire spectrum of the vasculitis syndromes, discussing pathogenesis, clinicopathologic manifestations, and updated therapeutic approaches.*

Fries JF, Hunder GG, Bloch DA, et al.: The American College of Rheumatology 1990 criteria for the classification of vasculitis: Summary. Arthritis Rheum 33:1135, 1990.

Hiltz RE, Cupps TR: Cutaneous vasculitis. Curr Opinion Rheumatol 6:20, 1994. *Reviews in detail the various mechanisms and forms of cutaneous vasculitis and provides an interesting summary of cutaneous manifestations of hypersensitivity vasculitis.*

Lawley TJ, Bielory L, Gascon P, et al.: A prospective clinical and immunologic analysis of patients with serum sickness. N Engl J Med 311:1407, 1984. *Elegant description of changes in immune complexes and serum complement levels associated with horse antithymocyte globulin–induced serum sickness.*

Lipford EH Jr, Margolick JB, Longo DL, et al.: Angiocentric immunoproliferative lesions: A clinicopathologic spectrum of post-thymic T-cell proliferations. Blood 72:1674, 1988. *Detailed description of various stages of lymphomatoid granulomatosis.*

Michel BA: Classification of vasculitis. Current Opinion Rheumatol 4:3, 1992. *Provides algorithms and overviews necessary for differential diagnosis of a number of vasculitic syndromes and gives a very concise overview of all the vasculitic syndromes.*

244 POLYARTERITIS NODOSA GROUP

Lanny J. Rosenwasser

DEFINITION. In 1866 Kussmaul and Maier described a patient with polyarteritis nodosa and introduced the term *periarteritis nodosa* to describe segmental nodules of medium-sized muscular arteries. Because swelling of the arterial walls often leads to occlusion, many of the clinical manifestations are secondary to necrosis. Hence, polyarteritis nodosa is often classified as one of the systemic necrotizing vasculitides. Classic polyarteritis does not involve the lung, as do allergic angiitis and granulomatosis of Churg-Strauss (see Ch. 54). Polyarteritis associated with hepatitis B antigenemia was described in 1970 by Gocke and colleagues. The association of hepatitis B antigen-antibody complexes and polyarteritis provides strong support for the hypothesis that the vasculitides in general are secondary to the deposition of soluble immune complexes.

Some patients have manifestations of both classic polyarteritis nodosa and allergic angiitis and granulomatosis of Churg-Strauss. Such patients are classified in the group with the so-called overlap syndrome. Diagnosis, workup, and management are no different from those in other patients in the polyarteritis nodosa group. Polyarteritis nodosa occurs from infancy to old age, with a peak incidence in the fifth and sixth decades of life; the male-female ratio has been estimated to be 2 to 3 : 1.

PATHOLOGY. The lesions of polyarteritis affect arteries of medium and small caliber, especially at bifurcations and branchings. The segmental process involves the media, with edema, fibrinous exudation, fibrinoid necrosis, and infiltration of polymorphonuclear neutrophils, and extends to the adventitia and intima. Thrombosis and infarction or hemorrhage occur at this stage. Subsequently the regions of fibrinoid necrosis are replaced by granulation tissue, and the intima proliferates. Finally the involved segment is replaced by scar tissue with associated intimal thickening and periarterial fibrosis. These changes produce partial occlusion, thrombosis and infarction, and palpable or visible aneurysms with occasional rupture.

In allergic angiitis and granulomatosis the acute fibrinoid necrosis with cellular infiltration involves arterioles and venules as well as medium-sized muscular arteries. It is characteristic of the polyarteritis nodosa group for the vascular lesions to be in different stages of evolution, i.e., acute, subacute, and healed. In allergic angiitis and granulomatosis, the pulmonary granulomatous lesions in vascular and extravascular sites are accompanied by intense eosinophilic infiltration.

In patients with polyarteritis associated with hepatitis B antigenemia, the specific antigen has been recognized in immune complexes present in the circulation and deposited in affected vessels along with complement proteins. It is presumed that this pathogenetic mechanism prevails in the entire polyarteritis nodosa group, but the basis for arterial deposition is unknown. The deposition of immune complexes in venules and glomeruli is attributed to changes in permeability and to physical trapping.

CLINICAL MANIFESTATIONS AND DIAGNOSIS. The widespread distribution of the arterial lesions produces diverse clinical manifestations, which reflect the particular organ systems in which the arterial supply has been impaired. Among the early symptoms and signs of polyarteritis nodosa are fever, weight loss, and pain in viscera and/or the musculoskeletal system. Striking and specific presenting signs may relate to abdominal pain, acute glomerulitis, polyneuritis on occasion, or myocardial infarction. Pulmonary manifestations, especially intractable bronchial asthma, would indicate allergic angiitis and granulomatosis rather than classic polyarteritis nodosa.

Renal. Renal involvement in two forms, renal polyarteritis and glomerulitis, may occur separately or together. Approximately 70% of patients with polyarteritis nodosa and renal disease have renal vasculitis, whereas the other 30% have glomerulitis. Renal polyarteritis is the most common lesion seen at postmortem examination. Manifestations of the renal involvement include intermittent proteinuria and microscopic hematuria with occasional hyaline and granular casts. The glomerulitis is manifested by microscopic and even macroscopic hematuria, proteinuria, cellular casts, and progressive renal failure. Hypertension is common. Renal involvement is the cause of death in about two thirds of patients with classic polyarteritis nodosa and about one third with allergic angiitis and granulomatosis.

Gastrointestinal. Arterial lesions are commonly found in one or more abdominal viscera. The principal manifestation is pain; anorexia, nausea, and vomiting are less prominent. Impaired arterial blood supply to the bowel can produce mucosal ulcerations, perforation, or infarction with melena or bloody diarrhea. Involvement of appendix, gallbladder, or pancreas can simulate appendicitis, cholecystitis, or hemorrhagic pancreatitis. Liver involvement can range from hepatomegaly with or without jaundice to the signs of extensive hepatic necrosis. Splenomegaly is uncommon. No consistent relationship has been seen between the development of necrotizing vasculitis and the appearance of liver disease in patients with hepatitis B antigenemia. Some of the observed combinations include necrotizing vasculitis as the initial clinical finding, superimposed on chronic active hepatitis or appearing simultaneously with acute hepatitis.

Central and Peripheral Nervous System. Central nervous system (CNS) manifestations are generally late occurrences in the course of polyarteritis nodosa, and their particular presentation reflects the specific area of the brain that is compromised. Headache, seizures, and retinal hemorrhages and exudates occur with or without localizing signs referable to the cerebrum, cerebellum, or brain stem; meningeal irritation may occur as a result of subarachnoid hemorrhage. Multiple mononeuropathy, i.e., involvement of several or even many individual nerves at the same or different times, is common and is attributed to arteritis of the vasa nervorum. The peripheral neuropathy is usually asymmetric, with both sensory and motor distribution. The former can be extremely painful, but the latter has attendant muscular degeneration, which can be so severe as to dominate the clinical presentation.

Articular and Muscular. Arthralgias and myalgias are frequent in polyarteritis nodosa. Arthralgias are migratory, generally without swelling, and thought to be due to small, localized arterial lesions. Muscle pain or weakness reflects either direct involvement of the arterial supply or a peripheral neuropathy.

Cardiac. Polyarteritis of the coronary arteries and their branches has a frequency approaching that of renal polyarteritis, and heart failure is responsible for or contributes to death in one sixth to one half of the cases. Clinical manifestations are partial or complete arterial occlusion, as modified by the superimposition of renal hypertension and an appreciable incidence of acute pericarditis without effusion. Whereas the combination of infarction and hypertension commonly leads to left-sided failure, an occasional patient with allergic angiitis and granulomatosis has predominantly right-sided decompensation.

Genitourinary. Involvement of the ovaries, testes, and epididymis is frequent, though usually asymptomatic. Mucosal ulceration in the bladder can occasionally precipitate gross hematuria with dysuria.

Cutaneous. Cutaneous involvement of some form is believed to occur in >25% of those affected. The acute cutaneous manifestations include polymorphic exanthemas—purpuric, urticarial, and multiform in character—and severe subcutaneous hemorrhage, resulting from necrotizing arteritis, with secondary gangrene. Ulcerations and a persistent livedo reticularis are associated with the more chronic stage. A most characteristic but uncommon finding is cutaneous and subcutaneous nodules; these occur at any time in the disease course. The nodules tend to group, appear in crops, are usually movable, may regress in days or persist for months, range in size from a pea to a walnut, and may cause the overlying skin to become reddened or to ulcerate.

Pulmonary. Although the bronchial arteries can be involved in classic polyarteritis, only allergic angiitis and granulomatosis that involves the pulmonary arteries and parenchyma with granulomatous lesions give rise to clinical manifestations. Asthma, when present, is intractable and associated with marked peripheral eosinophilia. Pneumonic episodes are transient or progressive and may be accompanied by hemoptysis and/or pleuritic pain. Respiratory involvement accounts for about 50% of deaths, with the remainder being attributable to the arteritis in other organs.

COURSE UNTREATED. The course of polyarteritis nodosa is progressive with destruction of vital organs. Intermittent acute episodes resulting from thrombosis of vital or nonvital structures are prominent. Death is most frequently attributed to renal involvement in cases of classic polyarteritis nodosa and to pulmonary lesions in those cases classified as allergic angiitis with granulomatosis. Cardiac failure caused by a combination of infarction and renal hypertension is an additional frequent cause of death in both groups, and acute vascular accidents of the gastrointestinal tract or CNS account for much of the remaining mortality. In the retrospective postmortem study of Rose and Spencer, the 5-year survival rate was about 10% in classic polyarteritis nodosa and about 25% in allergic angiitis and granulomatosis if onset was dated from the start of respiratory symptoms. The report of the British Medical Research Council in 1960 placed the 54-month survival rate in polyarteritis nodosa at nearly 50%. Rare patients with polyarteritis limited to nonvital sites have been reported to experience an unusually long course or even a lasting remission.

LABORATORY FINDINGS. Leukocytosis, predominantly polymorphonuclear, is apparent in >75% of the cases of polyarteritis nodosa or allergic angiitis and granulomatosis, eosinophilia often being marked in the latter group. Hypocomplementemia, which has not been observed in classic polyarteritis nodosa, has been present in patients with hepatitis B antigenemia. The erythrocyte sedimentation rate is customarily elevated. Abnormalities in the urine sediment, especially hematuria and proteinuria, reflect renal involvement. Abnormalities of the electrocardiogram and electroencephalogram are those common to arterial occlusive disease or secondary to the metabolic disturbances of uremia. Lesions apparent on chest roentgenograms are the rule in patients with allergic angiitis and granulomatosis. The findings range from transient or progressive infiltration to consolidation, cavitation, or scarring; upper and lower lobes are involved with equal frequency. As none of these findings is specific, antemortem diagnosis of polyarteritis depends on biopsy. Since the arterial involvement is segmental and spotty in distribution, it is advisable to obtain tissue from a symptomatic site, and it is essential to section the entire specimen completely. A deep, open surgical biopsy, including subcutaneous tissue and underlying muscle, should be obtained whenever possible from a skeletal muscle exhibiting pain and tenderness. Involvement of the epididymis and testes is sufficiently common to make this a useful biopsy site if palpation reveals the typical nodularity of segmental vascular lesions. Needle and surgical biopsies of internal organs with clinical involvement, such as liver or kidney, are gaining in favor. As an alternative or additional procedure, angiography to detect aneurysms of medium-sized muscular arteries in renal, hepatic, or intestinal sites may be helpful.

DIFFERENTIAL DIAGNOSIS. This includes not only the constituent syndromes but also all those conditions associated with systemic necrotizing vasculitis. The key differences between classic polyarteritis nodosa and other causes of necrotizing vasculitis include the absence of extravascular granulomas, sparing of the pulmonary arteries, failure of venous involvement except by contiguous spread, and predilection for medium-sized arteries. For allergic angiitis and granulomatosis the striking granulomatous response excludes all but Wegener's granulomatosis. The prominence of bronchial asthma, peripheral eosinophilia, and the usual absence of necrotizing lesions in the upper respiratory tract permit tentative clinical distinction between allergic angiitis and granulomatosis and Wegener's granulomatosis. Underlying connective tissue diseases are still recognized by their clinical characteristics even when necrotizing arteritis becomes prominent. For example, patients with

rheumatoid arthritis with ulcerating cutaneous lesions and peripheral neuropathy often exhibit prominent rheumatoid nodules and a high titer of rheumatoid factor. The specificities of the immunoglobulins that accompany active systemic lupus erythematosus or mixed cryoglobulinemia are distinctive; in addition, in the presence of active renal disease both entities manifest a reduced serum complement level not generally observed in classic polyarteritis nodosa. The giant cell arteritides (i.e., temporal arteritis, Takayasu's arteritis) lack the glomerulitis, peripheral neuropathy, and cutaneous manifestations notable in polyarteritis nodosa. The combination of progressive nephritis and pulmonary hemorrhage seen in Goodpasture's syndrome is unlike polyarteritis nodosa. The drug-induced hypersensitivity vasculitis group may be difficult to separate on purely clinical grounds, although a history of antecedent drug administration, infrequency of gastrointestinal manifestations, and absence of nodules along arteries are useful points. The clinical presentation in Henoch-Schönlein purpura is distinctive.

TREATMENT. The commonly used nonsteroidal anti-inflammatory agents have no specific therapeutic role in polyarteritis nodosa; thus, corticosteroids have been employed most widely. Large doses, in the range of 40 to 60 mg of prednisone per day, afford symptomatic relief but probably have little effect on the 1-year survival statistics. In a series of 17 patients within the polyarteritis group, including 2 with allergic angiitis and granulomatosis and 6 with hepatitis B–associated polyarteritis, 14 experienced dramatic remission with 2 mg per kilogram per day of cyclophosphamide. It was subsequently possible to reduce the cyclophosphamide and to taper the steroid dose to every other day and yet maintain remission, and in some instances resolution of microaneurysms was noted on repeat celiac axis angiography (Fig. 244–1).

In patients who have polyarteritis nodosa associated with hepatitis B virus infection, recent reports from a European collaborative group have identified significant responses to treatment regimens that include the cytokine, interferon α2b, and plasma exchange. When these approaches are taken in conjunction with short-term steroid therapy and potential antiviral treatment with Vira-a, a sig-

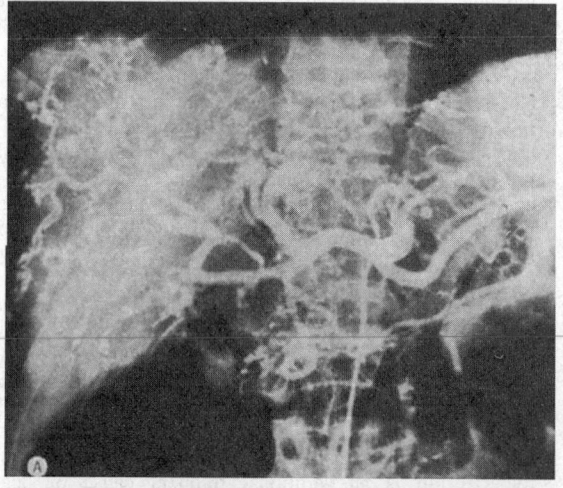

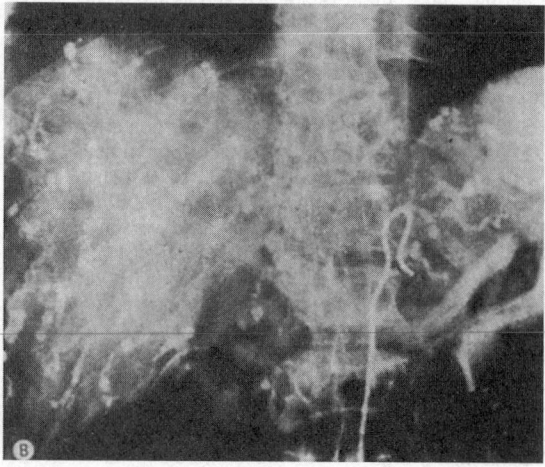

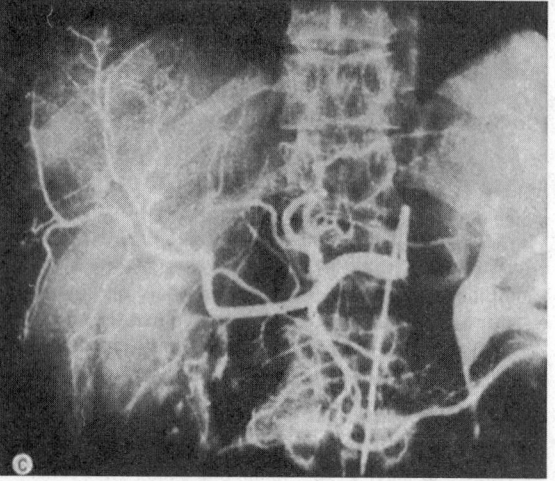

FIGURE 244–1. Selective celiac arteriogram demonstrates large hepatic arteries *(A)* and multiple aneurysms *(A and B)* throughout the liver. Resolution of aneurysms is seen after therapy *(C)*. (From Fauci AS, Doppman JL, Wolff SM: Cyclophosphamide-induced remissions in advanced polyarteritis nodosa. Am J Med 64:891, 1978.)

nificant number of patients had long-term remission and seroconversion in terms of hepatitis. Obviously, initial interest in treating this subgroup of PAN patients, those who have documented hepatitis B virus infection, with alternative treatments to cytotoxic drugs and steroids, is promising.

Fauci AS, Katz P, Haynes BF, et al.: Cyclophosphamide therapy of severe systemic necrotizing vasculitis. N Engl J Med 301:235, 1979. *Most important contribution dealing with cyclophosphamide therapy effectiveness in management of a series of patients within the polyarteritis group and including such subgroups as allergic angiitis and granulomatosis and hepatitis B–associated polyangiitis.*

Guillevin L, Lhote F, Leon A, et al.: Treatment of polyarteritis nodosa related to hepatitis B virus with short term steroid therapy associated with antiviral agents and plasma exchanges. A prospective trial in 33 patients. J Rheumatol 20:289, 1993.

Guillevin L, Lhote F, Sauvaget F, et al.: Treatment of polyarteritis nodosa related to hepatitis B virus with interferon-alpha and plasma exchanges. Ann Rheum Dis 53:334, 1994. *This and the preceding report identify prospectively the response of patients with interferon-α2b and plasma exchange. The data suggest in these two trials that cytokine and antiviral therapy as well as plasmapheresis may have a role as a potential first-line treatment in proven virus-induced vasculitis and polyarteritis nodosa.*

245 WEGENER'S GRANULOMATOSIS
Nancy B. Allen

Wegener's granulomatosis (WG) falls within the spectrum of systemic vasculitides as a clinicopathologic syndrome involving upper and lower respiratory tract and kidneys and less commonly the eyes, joints, skin, and neurologic and cardiac tissues. Described in 1931 and 1936 by H. Klinger and F. Wegener, respectively, necrotizing granulomatous vasculitis is the hallmark disorder in the lower respiratory tract, and focal, segmental glomerulonephritis and small vessel or granulomatous vasculitis are found elsewhere. The disease is now known to be associated with the cytoplasmic pattern of antineutrophil cytoplasmic antibody (c-ANCA) and more specifically with antibodies against proteinase 3 (PR-3), a serine protease found in neutrophils.

ETIOLOGY. The cause of WG is not yet known, but much research is being done. Because of the almost universal upper and/or lower airway involvement, inhaled antigen(s) stimulating granuloma formation and altered immune reactivity with features of immune complex deposition and altered cellular immune responses are believed to play significant roles, along with host factors and/or genetic predisposition. As of this writing no single genetic marker, environmental agent, microorganism, or other factor can be identified as initiating this syndrome. Rare familial reports of WG in first-degree relatives exist.

INCIDENCE AND PREVALENCE. The demographics of WG may be changing with the presence of new laboratory markers (c-ANCA), enhanced education of physicians regarding this diagnosis, and expansion of the spectrum of clinical features and presentations. In the United States, the disease frequency is approximately 1 in 30,000. In recent studies, mean age of onset is approximately 40, equal in men and women, predominant in Caucasians, and occurring from childhood into older adulthood.

PATHOLOGY AND PATHOGENESIS. Classical histopathology in WG is necrotizing granulomatous vasculitis involving small arteries and veins, most reliably found on biopsies of the lung (Table 245–1). This typical pathology has been seen in many other tissues, including unusual clinical locations, such as muscle, prostate, and breast. Upper respiratory tract biopsies including nasal septum, sinus, and trachea most often show nonspecific acute and chronic inflammation with or without giant cells and generally without true vasculitis.

Renal biopsies typically show focal segmental glomerulonephritis, with crescent formation and necrosis in more severe forms. Generally, immunofluorescent staining yields pauci-immune deposits, but these findings are not specific to WG, as they can be seen in polyarteritis nodosa, other vasculitides, and some nonvasculitic conditions. Biopsy does help to exclude other conditions such as systemic lupus erythematosus (SLE), post-streptococcal disease, Goodpasture's syndrome, and cryoglobulinemia.

TABLE 245–1. PATHOLOGIC FINDINGS IN WEGENER'S GRANULOMATOSIS

Location	Pathology
Upper airways (sinus, nasal septum)	Acute and chronic inflammation, giant cells, necrotizing granulomas, rarely vasculitis
Lung	
Transbronchial	Acute and chronic inflammation, giant cells, granuloma, rarely vasculitis
Thorascopic or open	Necrotizing, granulomatous vasculitis[*] (negative special stains and cultures), eosinophils, hemosiderin-laden macrophages, capillaritis
Kidney	Focal segmental glomerulonephritis with or without crescent formation, pauci-immune deposits, rarely vasculitis ($<1\%$)
Orbital/ocular	Acute and chronic inflammation with or without granuloma and/or vasculitis
Skin	Leukocytoclastic vasculitis, occasionally granulomatous vasculitis with or without necrosis
Sural nerve/muscle	Acute axonopathy, denervation and/or renervation, occasionally vasculitis of vasa nervorum; myopathy, with or without inflammation
Liver/spleen	Granulomatous hepatitis, triaditis; granulomatous vasculitis in spleen
Cardiac	Pericardial inflammation; rarely true coronary arteritis or granulomatous inflammation in myocardium or conduction system

[*] "Diagnostic" pathologic triad in WG.

In the initial phase of WG, bronchoalveolar lavage shows neutrophilic alveolitis, phagocytosis of neutrophils by monocytes, and higher levels of c-ANCA in lavage fluid than in serum. A current theory about the pathogenesis of WG involves a stimulus (inhalant) of some type, activation of neutrophils, transfer of PR-3 to cell membrane, and increased levels of c-ANCA, rheumatoid factor, gammaglobulins, and circulating immune complexes. Both cellular and humoral immune factors then lead to vasculitis, tissue destruction, and granuloma formation, contributing to the clinical features of the disease.

CLINICAL MANIFESTATIONS. The spectrum of clinical presentations and organ system involvement in WG is broad (Table 245–2). As a multisystem disorder involving predominantly the upper and lower respiratory tracts and the kidneys, presentations vary from "classic," with sinusitis, serous otitis media, rhinitis with nasal ulcerations, cough, hemoptysis, and constitutional symptoms, to "fulminant," with rapidly progressive renal failure and respiratory failure requiring intensive care unit management, to "mild," with arthralgias, polymyalgia rheumatica–type symptoms, or inflammatory eye disease as examples. Astute clinicians must carry WG as a potential diagnosis in their differential diagnosis list for multisystem disease or unexplained illness, much as one keeps SLE or subacute bacterial endocarditis in mind. With greater understanding of systemic vasculitic syndromes and education of primary care providers, this diagnosis may be considered in more individuals than previously, leading to earlier diagnosis and selection of appropriate management.

Nearly three fourths of patients eventually diagnosed with WG initially seek help due to upper and/or lower respiratory complaints. These include seasonal allergic rhinitis symptoms, recurrent epistaxis, oral or nasal ulcerations, ear pain, cough, fever, or hearing abnormalities. Some patients experience months or years of these symptoms before diagnosis. Constitutional symptoms with fevers, weight loss, anorexia, fatigue, arthralgias, and myalgias, although nonspecific, are common in this condition.

Lung involvement may be symptomatic with cough, dyspnea, pleuritic chest pain, and hemoptysis or may be totally asymptomatic with abnormalities found only on chest radiographs. Fleeting or persistent pulmonary infiltrates are more commonly found in the upper lobes and may be due to pulmonary hemorrhage or granulomatous inflammation along with vasculitis (see Ch. 54). Solitary or multiple pulmonary nodules and, less commonly, bibasilar interstitial changes, may be seen. Some patients with lower respiratory symptoms but normal chest radiographs may have endobronchial lesions found only at bronchoscopy.

TABLE 245–2. CLINICAL MANIFESTATIONS OF WEGENER'S GRANULOMATOSIS

Region/Organ	Sign or Symptom
Upper airway (90–95%)	Sinusitis, serous otitis media, rhinitis, nasal ulcerations/septal perforation, epistaxis, oral ulcerations, saddle-nose deformity (later), headaches
Lower airway (90–95%)	Cough, dyspnea, hemoptysis; pulmonary infiltrates (may be fleeting or persistent), nodules, cavities, pleural effusions/pleuritis, subglottic stenosis, endobronchial lesions, interstitial lung disease
Kidneys (75%)	Urinary sediment abnormalities (microscopic hematuria, casts, proteinuria), with or without renal insufficiency, nephrotic syndrome, hypertension
Musculoskeletal (70–90%)	Polyarthalgias, myalgias, mono-, oligo-, or polyarthritis (may be in rheumatoid pattern), myositis, muscle weakness
Eye (50–65%)	Conjunctivitis, scleritis/episcleritis, uveitis, proptosis, nasolacrimal duct obstruction, orbital mass lesions, retinal vasculitis, corneoscleral ulceration
Skin (50%)	Palpable purpura, subcutaneous nodules, petechiae, vesicles, ulcers, Raynaud's phenomenon, digital ischemia, livedo reticularis, necrotic papules, pyoderma gangrenosum–type lesions (rare)
Neurologic (20–25%)	Mononeuritis multiplex, peripheral neuropathy, cranial neuropathy, central nervous system vasculitis (cerebral hemorrhage, cerebritis, syncope, diabetes insipidis)
Cardiac (20%)	Pericarditis, pancarditis, cardiomyopathy, arrhythmias, coronary arteritis
Gastrointestinal (15–30%)	Alkaline phosphatase and/or aminotransferase elevations, granulomatous hepatitis/triaditis, small bowel vasculitis, ascites, splenic granulomatous vasculitis
Miscellaneous (<1–5%)	Breast, prostate, testicle, pinnae, urethra, ureter, lymph nodes, parotid, pulmonary or temporal artery, vagina, other
Constitutional	Fatigue, weight loss, fever, malaise, anorexia

Renal involvement is certainly one of the most serious clinical aspects of WG. This may be asymptomatic, such that urinalysis and serum creatinine measurements are important and must be followed closely in patients suspected to have WG. Rapidly progressive renal insufficiency with or without hypertension, edema, and nephrotic syndrome requires prompt evaluation and management. Irreversible renal failure requiring dialysis may be part of the initial clinical presentation or may slowly develop during therapy or with recurrent disease.

Musculoskeletal manifestations occur in the majority of patients. Observations have included diffuse polyarthralgias, an arthritis ranging from monoarticular to oligoarticular, and a rheumatoid arthritis–like picture with polyarthritis involving wrists, metacarpophalangeal and proximal interphalangeal joints, knees, ankles, and other large or small joints. When rheumatoid factor occurs along with symmetric polyarthritis, the initial diagnosis may be rheumatoid arthritis; however, attention to extra-articular symptoms and/or signs and laboratory data may lead to a diagnosis of WG instead. Diffuse myalgias are often present, and in patients over age 50 a polymyalgia rheumatica–type onset of WG and/or overlap of WG and temporal arteritis has been described. True myositis, with creatine phosphokinase, aldolase, or aminotransferase elevations, proximal muscle weakness, and finding of granulomatous vasculitis or less specific myositis, has been observed in WG.

Ocular involvement occurs in one half to two thirds of patients with WG on the basis of either vasculitis or tracking granulomatous tissue through the lamina papyracea into the medial aspect of the orbit. Vasculitis is responsible for conjunctivitis, scleritis-episcleritis, uveitis, retinal vasculitis, and corneoscleral ulcerations. Granulomatous mass lesions contribute to proptosis, orbital masses, optic nerve compression, diplopia, and nasal lacrimal duct obstruction.

Cutaneous involvement is most typically seen as palpable purpura, predominantly in the lower extremities, but may occur in upper extremities and over bony prominences. Vesicles, verrucous/necrotic papular lesions, subcutaneous nodules, petechiae, and more severe pyoderma gangrenosum–type lesions have been described. Raynaud's phenomenon, digital ischemia/necrosis, and livedo reticularis are present in some patients with acute and fulminant disease, with small vessel vasculitis with or without vasospasm being the predominant cause. Biopsy of the skin most commonly shows leukocytoclastic vasculitis.

Neurologic involvement is most typical with mononeuritis multiplex, foot drop and/or wrist drop or both, with patchy sensory and/or motor abnormalities. A diffuse peripheral neuropathy and cranial neuropathy, particularly of cranial nerves I, VII, and VIII, have been described. Headaches, hypothalamic or pituitary disease with clinical diabetes insipidus, and cerebral or subarachnoid hemorrhage have been reported infrequently.

Cardiovascular manifestations include pericarditis, pericardial effusions, rarely coronary vasculitis, myocarditis, congestive heart failure (other than observed secondary to acute renal failure), valvular abnormalities, and arrhythmias. Miscellaneous clinical features are listed in Table 245–2.

DIAGNOSIS. The diagnosis is based on supportive clinical, pathologic, and laboratory confirmation. The diagnosis should be strongly suspected when a patient presents with multisystem illness

TABLE 245–3. LABORATORY ABNORMALITIES IN WEGENER'S GRANULOMATOSIS

	Typical	Occasional	Rare
Hematologic	Normochromic, normocytic anemia Leukocytosis Eosinophilia Elevated erythrocyte sedimentation rate	Thrombocytosis	Microangiopathic hemolytic anemia
Urine sediment	Microhematuria Proteinuria Cellular casts	Sterile pyuria	
Chemistries	Hypoalbuminemia Renal insufficiency (mild to severe)	Elevated alkaline phosphatase +/or aminotransferases; elevated creatine phosphokinase, aldolase	
Serologic	Positive c-ANCA Positive rheumatoid factor Hypergammaglobulinemia Elevated c-reactive protein	Positive ANA (any pattern) Positive p-ANCA Elevated circulating immune complexes	

involving upper and/or lower respiratory tract disease, glomerulonephritis, and vasculitis in any organ system. (See Table 245–3 for a listing of typical, occasional, and rare laboratory abnormalities in WG.) The gold standard for a diagnosis of WG has been pathologic finding of necrotizing granulomatous vasculitis, particularly at open lung biopsy. However, active lung involve-ment is not always present initially. Localized disease may lead the clinician to entertain biopsy of other tissues, and thus knowledge of the array of pathologic findings in other organ systems is necessary.

Until relatively recently, laboratory features of WG were relatively nonspecific. A typical laboratory profile included normocytic normochromic anemia, elevated erythrocyte sedimentation rate, leukocytosis, and positive rheumatoid factor in 30 to 40% of patients, with or without urine sediment abnormalities or elevated serum creatinine. In the past 10 years, c-ANCA and its relationship to WG has been studied. Clearly, this is a helpful test in WG, particularly during active generalized disease, and may be confirmatory. Because reports of false positives are increasing and because sensitivity varies from 30 to 90% in a clinician's diagnosis of WG, depending on extent of disease and disease activity level, the test cannot be used as a sole diagnostic criterion for WG. c-ANCA and more specific antibodies against PR-3 are somewhat analogous to a combination of antinuclear antibodies in SLE as a disease marker and anti-DNA in lupus as a disease activity marker. This topic continues to attract much attention.

Radiologic imaging studies are helpful in diagnosing WG, including chest, sinus radiographs, and computed tomography. The differential diagnosis is quite broad and depends on the patient's presentation. When the classic triad of involvement occurs, with confirmatory tissue biopsy and a positive c-ANCA, the diagnosis is easy. When the process is early and/or limited to upper airway or kidney, clinical challenge occurs. Destructive upper airway disease needs to be differentiated from infection such as fungal, mycobacterial, staphylococcal, syphilitic, substance abuse (particularly cocaine), malignancy (particularly T-cell lymphoma and squamous cell carcinoma), or rarely self-mutilating trauma. In the past, *idiopathic midline granuloma* or idiopathic midline destructive disease was included in the differential diagnosis. Current investigators place this in the spectrum of *angiocentric immunoproliferative lesions (AIL),* believed to be a prelude to lymphoma (see Part XIII).

Differential diagnosis of pulmonary involvement is broad but, particularly in combination with renal disease, should include Goodpasture's syndrome, SLE, lymphomatoid granulomatosis (also in the spectrum of AIL), infection (fungal, mycobacterial, bacterial), and malignancy.

TREATMENT AND PROGNOSIS. Optimal treatment for active WG, particularly with multisystem involvement including renal disease, includes cyclophosphamide and corticosteroids. Cyclophos-

TABLE 245–4. TREATMENT OF WEGENER'S GRANULOMATOSIS

	Indications	Initial dose	Monitoring	Duration
Cyclophosphamide	Moderate to severe	1–2 mg/kg/day (po)	CBC weekly; keep WBC >3000, PMN >1000 and monitor liver tests; urine cytology and/or cystoscopy if prolonged therapy	Approximately 1 year beyond clinical remission
	Fulminant	3–4 mg/kg/day IV for 2–3 day, then reduce to 2 mg/kg/day po or IV		
Corticosteroids	Moderate to severe	1 mg/kg/day prednisone equivalent (IV initially or po)	Glucose, lipids, bone density	Taper to low dose (5–10 mg/day) or alternate-day therapy over 2 months
Methotrexate	Mild to moderate; upper airway; or diffuse disease without significant renal involvement	Up to 15–25 mg once weekly	Monitor CBC and liver tests q 4–8 weeks	Taper to lowest dose controlling features; ? trial off 1 year past clinical remission; close follow-up
Antibiotics	Adjunctive, not primary, to treat secondary bacterial infections; consider chronic suppression in chronic upper airway disease (sulfa may be contraindicated with methotrexate)			Intermittent or chronic low-dose "prophylaxis"
Cyclosporine	Refractory disease; dialysis dependent; patients awaiting renal transplant	3–5 mg/kg/day	BP, chemistries (Cr, Mg)	1 year beyond clinical remission or until transplant

phamide is initiated in a dose of 1 to 2 mg per kilogram per day, with initially weekly monitoring of complete blood counts to keep total white count above 3.0 and neutrophil count above 1.0 to limit complications of infection due to neutropenia. The dose is adjusted based on blood counts, particularly as corticosteroids are tapered. The drug is generally continued for approximately 1 year beyond clinical remission, followed by discontinuation and close observation of the patient's clinical status, laboratory features, including blood counts, erythrocyte sedimentation rate, renal parameters, chest radiographs, and c-ANCA. This drug or alternative therapy is reinstituted in the case of recurrence or relapse. Complications include hemorrhagic cystitis (and thus patients should be instructed to drink at least 1.5 liters of liquids per day), bone marrow toxicity, infections, hair loss, nausea, infertility, and increased risk of malignancy (bladder carcinoma, leukemia, lymphoma).

Corticosteroids are used at the time of diagnosis for severe disease, initially at 1 mg per kilogram per day (may be used in divided dose, intravenous methylprednisolone for fulminant disease, followed by consolidation to daily or alternate-day therapy). Prednisone equivalent doses of 60 mg per day are then tapered to alternate-day therapy over 1 month and then to the lowest possible level to control upper airway and/or musculoskeletal symptoms, preferably discontinuing this drug by 3 to 6 months. The complications and side effects of corticosteroids are well known and provided elsewhere (see Ch. 18).

Whereas WG was once an invariably fatal disease, the combination of cyclophosphamide and prednisone has provided remission in 75% of all patients and improvement in 90%, as evidenced in the NIH series long-term follow-up studies. However, relapses occur in at least 50% of those achieving remission, at any time from several months to 15 to 20 years after stopping cytotoxic therapy. Thus, WG is a chronic disease and patients deserve close follow-up, patient and provider education, and sometimes creative therapeutic strategies.

Even though mortality due to WG and/or its therapy has improved significantly, disease-related morbidity occurs in the majority of patients, with chronic renal insufficiency, hearing loss, nasal deformity, tracheal stenosis, and ocular abnormalities leading the list. These also are reviewed thoroughly in the NIH series. More recently, alternative treatment strategies have been reported. Weekly low-dose (15 to 25 mg) oral or intramuscular methotrexate has provided hope and, owing to experience in the management of rheumatoid arthritis, may provide a less toxic alternative to cyclophosphamide in patients who relapse, particularly with significant upper airway disease. Azathioprine, pulse monthly cyclophosphamide, intravenous immunoglobulin, cyclosporine, and immune modulators have all been used in individual cases. Because of the relative infrequency of the disease, controlled, double-blind studies have not yet been performed.

An overview of treatment strategies is listed in Table 245–4. Antibiotic therapy has a role, but at present this is considered adjunctive, not primary therapy. Because of necrotic upper airway tissue, staphylococcal and other infections are quite common and could be part of the "chicken and egg" perpetuation of this condition. In WG patients taking immunosuppressives, fever, new pulmonary infiltrate, new headache, hematuria, and pyuria deserve careful evaluation for infection before symptoms are ascribed to disease flare.

Thus, WG is a multisystem, inflammatory, autoimmune disorder with a spectrum of clinical, laboratory, radiographic, and pathologic features, in which c-ANCA has been helpful diagnostically. Careful diagnosis, thoughtful management, and close follow-up are necessary for optimal outcome.

Gross WL (ed.): ANCA-Associated Vasculitides: Immunologic and Clinical Aspects. New York, Plenum Press, 1993. *Compilation of papers presented at the 2nd International Colloquium on Wegener's Granulomatosis and Vasculitic Disorders in Lubeck, Germany, in May 1992.*

Hoffman GS, Kerr GS, Leavitt RY, et al.: Wegener's granulomatosis: An analysis of 158 patients. Ann Intern Med 116:488, 1992. *Updated review of NIH series on WG, focusing on clinical manifestations, disease spectrum, chronicity, and morbidity/mortality issues.*

Hoffman GS, Leavitt RY, Kerr GS, et al.: The treatment of Wegener's granulomatosis with glucocorticoids and methotrexate. Arthritis Rheum 35:1322, 1992. *First article reviewing significant number of WG patients treated with MTX.*

Jennette JC, Falk RJ, Andrassy K, et al.: Nomenclature of systemic vasculitides. Arthritis Rheum 37:187, 1994. Lie JT: Nomenclature and classification of vasculitis:

Plus ca change, plus c'est la meme chose. Arthritis Rheum 37:181, 1994. *This pair of references provides point and counterpoint discussion of the classification of vasculitides. They are thought-provoking and interesting, providing perspective on Wegener's and other vasculitides in relation to diagnostic testing, particularly ANCA.*

Lieberman K, Churg A: Wegener's granulomatosis. *In* Churg A, Churg J (eds.): Systemic Vasculitides. New York, Igaku-Shoin, 1991, p 77. *A concise review of the topic with emphasis on pathologic findings. Beautiful color photomicrographs.*

246 POLYMYALGIA RHEUMATICA AND GIANT CELL ARTERITIS
Gene G. Hunder

Polymyalgia rheumatica and giant cell arteritis are common rheumatic diseases of middle-aged and older persons. Although the etiology of these conditions is unknown and their pathogenesis is poorly understood, it is clear that they are closely related. Some believe that a single agent causes both conditions and that host and other unknown factors determine whether a patient will develop one or both processes. A strong association with HLA-DR4 has been observed, indicating a hereditary link.

POLYMYALGIA RHEUMATICA

Polymyalgia rheumatica is characterized by aching and morning stiffness in the shoulder and hip girdles, the proximal extremities, the neck, and the torso. Usually, it is accompanied by evidence of an inflammatory reaction. The mean age at onset is about age 70, and it nearly always occurs after age 50, with women affected twice as commonly as men.

CLINICAL FINDINGS. Polymyalgia rheumatica may begin abruptly but usually develops gradually over a number of weeks. In mild or early cases, the symptoms may subside 1 to 2 hours after the patient arises in the morning, only to return later after a period of inactivity. Generally, the discomfort becomes severe enough to interfere with usual activities and may confine the patient to bed. Fatigue, loss of weight, and a low-grade fever may be present. Joint inflammation has been demonstrated in some cases, which supports the contention that polymyalgia rheumatica is a form of synovitis of the proximal joints and periarticular structures. Upon careful testing, muscle strength is found to be normal or nearly normal.

LABORATORY TESTS. A normochromic anemia is typical. Usually, the erythrocyte sedimentation rate is markedly elevated, averaging 70 to 80 mm in 1 hour (Westergren). Other acute-phase protein levels also are elevated. Some patients have mild hepatic dysfunction that reverts to normal with treatment. Other tests are normal.

INCIDENCE. Caucasians appear to be affected more frequently than other groups. The highest recorded incidence rates are from northern Europe and the northern United States. In one population study, the prevalence found was approximately 1 in 200 persons in the population aged 50 or older. Recent reports on incidence rates in Europe show similar findings.

DIAGNOSIS. Several criteria sets for diagnosing polymyalgia rheumatica have been suggested. Most are similar to those in Table 246–1. Morning stiffness should last at least one-half hour. The erythrocyte sedimentation rate is an indicator of systemic inflammation. An additional criterion of rapid response to 10 to 20 mg of prednisone per day is suggested by some. These criteria are only

TABLE 246–1. POLYMYALGIA RHEUMATICA: DIAGNOSTIC CRITERIA

>Age 50
Aching and morning stiffness in at least two of the following areas:
  Neck
  Shoulder girdle
  Pelvic girdle
Erythrocyte sedimentation rate (ESR) >40 mm in 1 hr
Duration of symptoms for 1 mo
No other disease present

TABLE 246–2. DIFFERENTIAL FEATURES IN POLYMYALGIA RHEUMATICA AND SIMILAR DISORDERS

	Polymyalgia Rheumatica	Giant Cell Arteritis	Rheumatoid Arthritis	Dermatomyositis	Fibromyalgia
Morning stiffness > 30 minutes	+	±	+*	±	Variable
Headache and/or scalp tenderness	0	+	0	0	Variable
Pain with active joint movement	+	0	+*	0	Inconstant
Tender joints	±	0	+*	0	Tender spots
Swollen joints	±	±	+	0	0
Muscle weakness	±†	0	+*	+	0
Normochromic anemia	+	+	+	0	0
Elevated ESR	+	+	+	±	0
Elevated serum creatine kinase	0	0	0	+	0
Serum rheumatoid factor	0	0	70%	0	0
Distinct electromyographic abnormality	0	0	0	+	0
Response to nonsteroidal anti-inflammatory drug (NSAID)	±	0	+	0	0

0 = absent, + = present, ± = present in minority of cases.
* = Associated with affected joints.
† = Pain inhibits movement. Disuse atrophy may occur.

guidelines, since patients occasionally have normal sedimentation rates at onset and may develop symptoms slightly before age 50.

DIFFERENTIAL DIAGNOSIS (Table 246–2). Some patients with early rheumatoid arthritis lack the more characteristic distal joint involvement and serum rheumatoid factor and have prominent proximal symptoms. In polymyositis, limitation is due to a lack of muscle strength; in polymyalgia rheumatica, limitation is due to pain. In polymyositis, muscle biopsy shows an inflammatory myopathy; in polymyalgia rheumatica, biopsy is normal or shows only atrophy.

Fibromyalgia usually affects younger individuals and tends to be associated with tender spots; laboratory tests are normal. When encouraged to do so, patients with fibromyalgia can move the joints through a full range of motion without great difficulty. Wakefulness in polymyalgia rheumatica is due to discomfort caused by movement in bed. In fibromyalgia, however, there is a more generalized, persistent discomfort that is less tangible.

Other conditions that occasionally need to be distinguished from polymyalgia rheumatica include chronic infections, such as subacute bacterial endocarditis or viral infections, malignancies, hypothyroidism, and other connective tissue diseases.

GIANT CELL ARTERITIS

Giant cell (temporal) arteritis affects large and medium-sized arteries, especially those branching from the proximal aorta that supply the neck and the extracranial structures of the head and arms. The lesions tend to be scattered irregularly along the involved vessels. A focal or diffuse granulomatous inflammatory infiltration is present with multinucleated histiocytic and foreign body giant cells, histiocytes, lymphocytes, and fibroblasts. Lymphocytes tend to be predominantly helper T cells.

CLINICAL FINDINGS. This disease affects the same population as polymyalgia rheumatica. The manifestations of giant cell arteritis are diverse, and many presentations have been described.

In most patients, symptoms or signs related to the vascular system develop at some time during the course of the disease (Table 246–3). Headache may be mild or severe. Scalp tenderness may be over the arteries of the head or at other sites.

Visual symptoms are present in about one third of patients; half are transient, and half are permanent. The former includes amaurosis fugax or diplopia. Permanent visual loss may be partial or complete and may occur without warning; about half are unilateral, and half are bilateral. The vision loss is due to narrowing or occlusion of the ophthalmic or posterior ciliary arteries.

Intermittent claudication occurs in about one half of patients, with the jaw muscles most frequently involved. During chewing of firm foods such as meat, fatigue or discomfort is noted. In a small percentage of patients, claudication of the tongue or throat develops with eating and repeated swallowing. Nervous system alterations are found in up to 30%; 14% have either mononeuritis or polyneuropathy, and 7% have transient ischemic attacks or strokes.

Polymyalgia rheumatica occurs in about 40% of patients with giant cell arteritis. It may precede other symptoms or become manifest only during the withdrawal of corticosteroid therapy given for the arteritis. Diffuse or asymmetric myalgias, arthralgias, or joint swelling may be present in other patients with giant cell arteritis.

PHYSICAL EXAMINATION. The temporal, occipital, or other scalp or cervical arteries may be enlarged, tender, and erythematous. Bruits or pulse deficits may be present over the carotid, subclavian, or brachial arteries. Large artery involvement may be present initially or later, as part of an exacerbation. Findings in the eyes of patients with recent visual loss include papilledema, hemorrhages, and exudates; later, optic atrophy develops.

LABORATORY TESTS. Blood tests are similar to those seen in polymyalgia rheumatica. The platelet count is generally increased. The erythrocyte sedimentation rate averages 80 to 100 mm in 1 hour (Westergren) but is occasionally normal.

INCIDENCE. Reported annual incidence rates have varied considerably and are highest (20 per 100,000) in persons age 50 and older in northern Europe and the United States. Although the reasons for the variable rates are unknown, ethnic and geographic factors have been suggested. Familial cases of giant cell arteritis and polymyalgia rheumatica have been reported. Giant cell arteritis appears to be one third as common as polymyalgia rheumatica.

DIAGNOSIS. Giant cell arteritis should be considered in any older person who has developed transient or sudden visual changes, unexplained fever, polymyalgia rheumatica or new headaches, and an elevated erythrocyte sedimentation rate. The arteries of the head, neck, and extremities should be examined carefully. Distinct tenderness, redness, and a palpable but nonpulsatile temporal artery are important clues to the presence of arteritis. In the absence of similar changes in the lower extremities, pulse changes or bruits over the

TABLE 246–3. GIANT CELL ARTERITIS: CLINICAL FINDINGS IN 94 PATIENTS*

Clinical Manifestation	Frequency (%)
Headache	77
Abnormal temporal artery	53
Jaw claudication	51
Scalp tenderness	47
Constitutional symptoms	48
Polymyalgia rheumatica	34
Fever	27
Respiratory symptoms	23
Facial pain	14
Diplopia/blurred vision	12
Transient vision loss	5
Blindness (partial or complete)	13
Hemoglobin < 11.0 gram/dl	24
Erythrocyte sedimentation rate > 40 mm/hr	97

* After Machado EBV, Michet CJ, Ballard DJ, et al.: Trends in incidence and clinical presentation of temporal arteritis in Olmsted County, Minnesota, 1950–1985. Arthritis Rheum 31:745–749, 1988.

axillary and brachial arteries are more likely to be caused by vasculitis than by arteriosclerosis.

A temporal artery biopsy is recommended for all patients suspected of having giant cell arteritis. A biopsy should be performed on the most clinically abnormal artery segment. When the arteries appear normal on examination, a segment several centimeters long should be removed from one temporal artery, and histologic sections should be examined at multiple levels in an effort to find an involved area. In the author's experience, if the first temporal artery biopsy is normal, the second side will yield approximately 10 to 15% additional positive cases.

Some patients with polymyalgia rheumatica may be followed carefully without a temporal artery biopsy. If polymyalgia rheumatica is of recent onset or has been present for a year or more in the absence of signs or symptoms of vasculitis, biopsy may be deferred and the patient should be followed closely.

DIFFERENTIAL DIAGNOSIS. Conditions that have been confused with giant cell arteritis include systemic infections, amyloidosis with prominent vascular involvement, neoplasms, arteriosclerotic vascular disease in patients with an elevated erythrocyte sedimentation rate that is due to some other cause, arteriovenous fistulas, and other forms of vasculitis.

Follow-up studies of patients who have had a negative temporal artery biopsy have shown that only approximately 10% develop findings of giant cell arteritis and require long-term corticosteroid therapy.

MANAGEMENT

Therapy for polymyalgia rheumatica is aimed at alleviating systemic symptoms and musculoskeletal discomfort. Corticosteroids are recommend for most patients with an initial daily dose of 10 to 20 mg of prednisone (or the equivalent dose of another corticosteroid). Prednisone acts rapidly, and the patient should notice significant improvement within 24 hours. The corticosteroid dose can be reduced as tolerated after one month or earlier. Nonsteroidal anti-inflammatory drugs may be added to control mild discomfort that may occur while corticosteroids are being withdrawn and discontinued.

In giant cell arteritis, the recommended dosage of prednisone is 40 to 60 mg per day. Vascular complications seldom occur after corticosteroids have been started. If the response to the initial dose of prednisone is incomplete, the dosage should be increased by 20 to 30 mg per day. Usually, if symptoms subside and laboratory values return to normal with a given dose, the disease process is adequately suppressed. Prednisone for both conditions may be administered as a single morning dose or in two to three divided doses per day.

The overall goal of therapy is to administer the lowest dose of corticosteroid that adequately controls the arteritis and prescribe it for the shortest necessary time. The dose needed to achieve control varies among patients and must be determined empirically. There is no evidence that corticosteroid therapy alters the natural course of the disease.

In a small proportion of cases, the corticosteroid dose cannot be reduced without an exacerbation of the disease. Cyclophosphamide, azathioprine, dapsone, and methotrexate have been reported as steroid-sparing drugs in some instances. However, no controlled studies of these drugs have been done. The average duration of both polymyalgia rheumatica and giant cell arteritis is about 2 years, during which time the intensity of the process may flare up at times but appears to resolve slowly. The course in individual patients, however, varies considerably, and some may continue with active symptoms for several years. Aortic aneurysm is a late complication of giant cell arteritis.

Aiello PD, Trautmann JC, McPhee TJ, et al.: Visual prognosis in giant cell arteritis. Ophthalmology 100:550, 1993. *A study of the ocular effects and outcome of vision in giant cell arteritis.*

Hunder GG, Lie JT, Goronzy JJ, Weyand CM: Pathogenesis of giant cell arteritis. Arthritis Rheum 36:757, 1993. *A critical review of factors involved in giant cell arteritis development.*

Weyand CM, Hicok KC, Hunder GG, Goronzy JJ: The HLA-DRB1 locus as a genetic component in giant cell arteritis. J Clin Invest 90:2355, 1992. *A disease-linked gene sequence is mapped to the binding site of the HLA-DR molecule.*

247 IDIOPATHIC INFLAMMATORY MYOPATHIES

Robert L. Wortmann

DEFINITION. The term "idiopathic inflammatory myopathy" represents a group of rare diseases of unknown cause that are characterized by symmetrical proximal muscle weakness and nonsuppurative inflammation of skeletal muscle. Specific diagnoses characterized by this term include polymyositis, dermatomyositis, cancer-associated myositis, myositis associated with another connective tissue disease (overlap syndromes), and inclusion-body myositis. Patients with any idiopathic inflammatory myopathy generally fulfill the criteria used to define polymyositis originally proposed in 1975 by Bohan and Peter (Table 247–1).

INCIDENCE. The idiopathic inflammatory myopathies are rare conditions, with an annual incidence ranging between 0.5 and 8.4 cases per 1 million population. The incidence is highest in blacks and lowest in Japanese. Women are generally more affected than men, with female predominance most pronounced between the ages of 15 and 44 and in persons having myositis associated with other connective tissue diseases. The gender ratio is equal in older age groups and in myositis associated with malignancy but is reversed in inclusion body myositis. Overall, the age of onset has a bimodal distribution with peaks in children between 10 and 14 and in adults between 45 and 54. The mean age of onset for the subset of myositides with other connective tissue diseases is similar to that for the associated condition. Individuals with myositis associated with malignancy or inclusion body myositis have a mean age over 60.

PATHOLOGY AND PATHOGENESIS. Abnormalities in skeletal muscle indicative of an idiopathic inflammatory myopathy include muscle fiber degeneration, regeneration, necrosis, phagocytosis, and mononuclear cell infiltration. In polymyositis, necrosis of single muscle fibers is common, and some non-necrotic fibers are invaded by T cells and macrophages. Collections of lymphocytes, plasma cells, and histiocytes are found primarily in the endomysium. Inflammatory aggregates contain high percentages of T cells but few B cells. Over time, fiber diameter variation increases, and interstitial fibrosis develops. Although abnormalities in muscle from patients with dermatomyositis may be similar to those in polymyositis, more commonly the inflammatory cells are grouped in the perimysium with a perivascular distribution and contain a higher percentage of B cells. In the childhood variety of dermatomyositis, vasculopathy, including endothelial hyperplasia, infarction, and perifascicular atrophy, is common, and deposition of IgG, IgM, and C3 occurs, particularly within the walls of intramuscular arteries and veins. In inclusion body myositis, light microscopy reveals inflammatory changes similar to those in polymyositis with the additional feature of characteristic intracellular vacuoles. The vacuoles are lined with basophilic granules on cryostat sections and eosinophilic material on paraffin sections. Intracytoplasmic or intranuclear

TABLE 247–1. CRITERIA USED TO DEFINE IDIOPATHIC INFLAMMATORY MYOPATHY*

1. Symmetrical weakness of limb girdle muscles and anterior neck flexors with or without dysphagia.
2. Elevation in serum of skeletal muscle enzymes, especially creatine phosphokinase (CPK).
3. Electromyographic changes consistent with inflammatory myopathy: short, small polyphasic motor units; fibrillations; positive waves; and bizarre high-frequency repetitive discharges.
4. Muscle biopsy evidence of fiber necrosis, phagocytosis, and regeneration; variation in fiber size; and inflammatory exudate.

Note: Patients are classified as having definite disease with four, probable disease with three, and possible disease with two.

* These criteria were originally proposed in 1975 by Bohan and Peter to define polymyositis. At that time, the term "polymyositis" was used to represent a specific disease as well as a general term representing all the recognized forms of inflammatory myopathy.

tubulofilamentous inclusions are also seen with electron microscopy. These inclusions are straight, rigid, and have periodic striations resembling paramyxovirus. Using immunolocalization techniques, ubiquitin and β-amyloid protein (two proteins that have been identified in the plaques in brains from patients with Alzheimer's disease) have been observed in the vacuoles and tubulofilamentous inclusions.

The idiopathic inflammatory myopathies are believed to be immune-mediated processes that are triggered by environmental factors in genetically susceptible individuals. This is in part based on the prevalence of autoantibodies, inflammatory pathology, association with other autoimmune diseases, and response to corticosteroid therapy.

Many patients with idiopathic inflammatory myopathies have circulating autoantibodies (Table 247–2). Some are termed "myositis-specific autoantibodies" (MSA's) and are seen only in patients with polymyositis or dermatomyositis; others are those associated with other connective tissue diseases. Most MSA's are directed against cytoplasmic antigens and bind to evolutionary conserved epitopes. The percentage of patients with polymyositis and dermatomyositis who have circulating MSA's is uncertain, but estimates range between 10 and 50%. Eight different MSA's have been described. No more than one MSA has been found in an individual patient. The more common MSA's are directed against aminoacyl-tRNA (transfer RNA) synthetases and inhibit the activity of the respective antigenic enzyme protein *in vitro*. The most prevalent antisynthetase antibody is directed against histidyl-tRNA synthetase and is called "anti-Jo-1." Certain picornaviruses can substitute for tRNA and interact with aminoacyl-tRNA synthetase enzymes. Interestingly, there is some homology between amino acid sequences near the active site of histidyl-tRNA synthetase (Jo-1) and some capsid proteins in encephalomyocarditis virus, a picornavirus that induces a mouse model of polymyositis. Thus antibodies initially directed against virus or a virus-enzyme complex could cross-react with homologous areas of host proteins or the enzyme itself. This process is termed "molecular mimicry" and could explain the autoantibody production.

Several observations emphasize the importance of genetic factors in general and class II antigens in particular in the pathogenesis of inflammatory myopathy (see Ch. 229). Almost 50% of patients with polymyositis and dermatomyositis have the HLA-DR3 (HLA, human leukocyte antigen) phenotype. This is almost always linked with HLA-B8 and is most common in patients with anti-Jo-1 antibodies. HLA-DR52 is found in over 90% of patients who have myositis and anti-Jo-1 antibodies. The prevalence of the DR1 phenotype is increased compared with controls in inclusion body myositis.

Viruses, particularly picornaviruses, have been implicated as causes of myositis. Several viruses, especially coxsackie A9, have been associated with myositis in individual cases; elevated titers to coxsackievirus have been found in childhood dermatomyositis; mumps virus antigen has been demonstrated in inclusions in inclusion body myositis; and certain viral infections can induce inflammatory myopathy in mice, with inflammation persisting long after virus can be detected.

The pathologic changes in polymyositis and inclusion body myositis appear to result from cell-mediated, antigen-specific cytotoxicity. In these disorders, non-necrotic muscle fibers are found surrounded by and invaded by CD8+ mononuclear cells, with cytotoxic cells outnumbering suppresser cells by a ratio of 4:1. Studies of circulating mononuclear cells reveal decreased percentages of cells expressing CD8 and increases in those expressing the class II HLA antigen DR, as well as other T-cell activation antigens (interleukin-2 receptors; Ta-1, an activation marker also associated with anamnestic responses; and TLiSA-1, a late marker associated with cytotoxic T-cell differentiation). Different immune mechanisms are evident in dermatomyositis. Mononuclear cell invasion of non-necrotic fibers is rare, cellular infiltration is predominantly perivascular, B cells outnumber T cells, and the CD4/CD8 ratio is higher. In the circulation, DR+ cells and B cells (CD20+ cells) are increased, whereas T cells (CD3+ cells) are decreased. These findings indicate that humoral mechanisms play a significant role in the pathogenesis of dermatomyositis.

Loss of muscle fibers as a result of the immune response may contribute to muscle weakness in some patients with an idiopathic inflammatory myopathy. However, other factors also must be involved because weakness occurs in the presence of histology that has no inflammatory infiltrate or fiber necrosis. These observations suggest that abnormalities of the contractile process may underlie the muscle weakness. Energy (ATP) is required for normal muscle contraction and relaxation as well as the maintenance of membrane integrity. Altered muscle energy metabolism has been demonstrated *in vitro* using a coxsackievirus B1–induced mouse model of inflammatory myopathy. Muscles from these mice have increased glycolytic activity compared with controls as well as decreased activities of myophosphorylase and myoadenylate deaminase. A secondary deficiency of myoadenylate deaminase activity has been observed in muscle from some patients with polymyositis. *In vivo* ^{31}P magnetic resonance spectrographic studies of patients with polymyositis and dermatomyositis have shown lower levels of high-energy phosphate–containing compounds at rest, faster depletion of ATP with exercise, and slower recovery rates compared with normal individuals. These abnormalities reverse as patients improve with therapy, particularly in dermatomyositis. These studies support the hypothesis that metabolic changes contribute to the muscle weakness in the inflammatory myopathies.

CLINICAL MANIFESTATIONS. The onset of an idiopathic inflammatory myopathy is usually insidious, with no identified precipitating event. The cardinal feature of any inflammatory myopathy is symmetrical muscle weakness of shoulder and pelvic girdles, at times accompanied by mild pain and tenderness. Weakness of proximal leg and arm muscles, neck flexors, and pharyngeal muscles may follow. Early symptoms include difficulty getting up from a chair, climbing stairs, and using one's hands above shoulder level. Dysphagia, dysphonia, and dysarthria may develop when the disease affects the pharynx. Morning stiffness, fatigue, and other systemic symptoms are common. Arthralgias are noted with active disease, but frank synovitis is quite rare. With progression, weakness can become so severe that patients cannot lift their extremities against gravity, involved muscles become atrophic, and contractures develop. An explosive onset with rhabdomyolysis, myoglobinuria, and renal failure is rare. Typically, the neurologic examination is normal except for the motor component. Deep tendon reflexes are normal or appear slightly decreased because of muscle weakness. Cranial nerve function is normal. Dysphagia is primarily due to weakness of striated musculature in the posterior pharynx and is often associated with a poor prognosis. Patients may have difficulty swallowing liquids, are prone to aspiration, and may have nasal

TABLE 247–2. AUTOANTIBODIES FOUND IN PATIENTS WITH IDIOPATHIC INFLAMMATORY MYOPATHY

Autoantibody	Clinical Association
Myositis-specific autoantibodies	
Anti-tRNA synthetases	PM with interstitial
Anti-Jo-1	lung disease, arthritis,
Anti-PL-7	and fever; less
Anti-PL-12	common in DM
Anti-OJ	
Anti-EJ	
Anti-SRP	PM with poor prognosis
Anti-MAS	PM after alcoholic rhabdomyolysis
Anti-Mi-2	DM
Antinuclear antibodies associated with other connective tissue diseases	
Anti-SM	SLE
Anti-RNP	SLE, MCTD
Anti-SSA (anti-Ro)	SLE, Sjögren's syndrome
Anti-SSB (anti-La)	SLE, Sjögren's syndrome
Anti-centromere	CREST syndrome
Anti-SCL70	Scleroderma
Anti-PM-1	Scleroderma
Anti-Ku	Scleroderma

Anti-SRP = anti-signal recognition particle; PM = polymyositis; DM = dermatomyositis; SLE = systemic lupus erythematosus; MCTD = mixed (undifferentiated) connective tissue disease; CREST = *c*alcinosis, *R*aynaud's *e*sophageal dysmotility, *s*clerodactyly, *t*elangiectasia.

speech. These symptoms may be accentuated by spasm or fibrosis of cricopharyngeal muscles and may require surgical treatment. Esophageal dysfunction may occur but is not often clinically insignificant.

Pulmonary manifestations develop in some patients due to hypoventilation secondary to muscle weakness, swallowing abnormalities with aspiration, and infection. Approximately 5 to 10% develop interstitial lung disease (see Ch. 54). Some patients with interstitial pneumonitis have no respiratory symptoms, but others experience nonproductive cough and dyspnea, which may precede the onset of muscle weakness. The restrictive lung disease is associated with bibasilar fine crackles on chest auscultation and reduced diffusion capacity. Symptomatic cardiac problems are unusual, although conduction abnormalities and tachyarrhythmias may be seen on electrocardiograms. Congestive heart failure can result from hypoxemia, pulmonary hypertension, or cardiomyopathy. Raynaud's phenomenon is reported in a small percentage of patients (see Ch. 46).

Patients with polymyositis may develop periorbital edema. When other cutaneous manifestations are seen, the disease is termed "dermatomyositis." Typically, the rash is erythematous and appears on the face, neck, chest, and extensor surfaces of the extremities. The name "Gottron's patches" is given to raised, red to violet, scaly patches seen over the knuckles, elbows, and knees. A heliotrope rash on the upper eyelids is very characteristic. The term "mechanic's hands" is applied to the darkened or dirty-appearing horizontal lines that develop across the lateral and palmer aspects of the fingers (because of the similarity to changes seen in hands of people who do manual labor). Capillary nailfold changes are present in some individuals, especially those with Raynaud's phenomenon. These include dilated or distorted capillary loops sometimes alternating with avascular areas. Dermatomyositis in children is sometimes referred to by the specific term "childhood dermatomyositis." Childhood dermatomyositis is similar to dermatomyositis in adults, except that vascular involvement is more prominent. Fever, weight loss, and subcutaneous calcifications are more common, and gastrointestinal tract hemorrhage or perforation may occur.

When myositis occurs in association with another connective tissue or autoimmune disease, the associated conditions may dominate the clinical picture. The most frequently associated disease is systemic lupus erythematosus (SLE), but others include scleroderma, rheumatoid arthritis, polyarteritis nodosa, giant cell arteritis, autoimmune thyroid disease, insulin-dependent diabetes mellitus, dermatitis herpetiformis, myasthenia gravis, and primary biliary cirrhosis.

Approximately 20% of adults with polymyositis or dermatomyositis also have cancer. Although this may seem higher than expected for the general population, there appears to be no significant difference in the frequency of malignancy when compared with appropriate age-matched control populations. Most often the myositis and malignancy are diagnosed within a year of each other. In general, the type of the neoplasm is that expected for the patient's age. Overall, the most commonly associated tumors are of breast and lung. Ovarian and stomach cancers occur more frequently than in the general population; rectal and colon cancers are less frequent. Neoplastic disease is less common in patients with interstitial lung disease or in those with an associated connective tissue disease.

Inclusion body myositis occurs most commonly in older men and can differ from polymyositis by the additional features of distal muscle weakness, asymmetrical muscle involvement, and neuropathic findings or physical examination and electromyography.

CLINICAL COURSE AND PROGNOSIS. The overall 5-year survival rate is approximately 80%, with children having the best prognosis. About half of surviving patients with polymyositis or dermatomyositis essentially recover completely. Older patients, those with associated neoplasms, or those with significant pulmonary, cardiac, and gastrointestinal involvement have a poorer prognosis. Patients with antibodies to aminoacyl-tRNA synthetases (i.e., anti-Jo-1) have a very high prevalence of interstitial lung disease, arthritis, and fever and do not respond well to therapy. Those with circulating anti-SRP (SRP, signal recognition particle) antibodies have a high prevalence of Raynaud's and the worst prognosis of any subset. Although most patients with inclusion body myositis do not improve with therapy, their survival appears to be good. Typically, the weakness progresses very slowly and may become fixed in some cases.

LABORATORY DATA. Serum levels of muscle-derived enzymes are elevated at some time during the course of the disease in 99% of patients. Creatine phosphokinase (CPK) levels are the most sensitive, but levels of aldolase, aminotransferase (AST and ALT), and lactate dehydrogenase (LDH) are also useful. CPK levels can be used as an index of disease activity or therapeutic response in some but not all patients. When normal CPK values are encountered in the presence of active disease, possible explanations include circulating enzyme inhibitors, a possible associated malignancy, or longstanding disease with severe muscle atrophy. The MB isoenzyme of CPK may be increased in the absence of cardiac involvement due to the expression of that isoform in regenerating skeletal muscle fibers.

The erythrocyte sedimentation rate remains normal in over half the patients and when elevated does not correlate with the degree of weakness. Complete blood count, urinalysis, and other chemistries are usually normal unless there is an associated connective tissue disease or neoplasm.

Circulating autoantibodies are common in patients with idiopathic inflammatory myopathies (see Table 247–2). The most common MSA, anti-Jo-1, is found in polymyositis and less commonly in dermatomyositis. Certain antinuclear antibodies may herald an associated connective tissue disease: anti-SM and anti–double-stranded DNA for SLE; anti-SSA and anti-SSB for Sjögren's syndrome; anticentromere for CREST syndrome; and anti-PM-1, anti-Ku, and anti-SCL70 for scleroderma.

The electromyogram (EMG) is abnormal in 90% of patients. Classic changes include the triad of (1) small-amplitude, short-duration, polyphasic motor unit potentials; (2) fibrillation, positive waves, and increased insertional irritability; and (3) spontaneous bizarre high-frequency discharges. The complete triad may be found in only 40% of patients and in some patients changes are restricted to paraspinal muscles.

DIAGNOSIS AND DIFFERENTIAL DIAGNOSIS. Criteria are useful in establishing the diagnosis of an idiopathic inflammatory myopathy (see Table 247–1). These criteria can be used only after other causes are excluded, because no change or test is specific for the diagnosis. CPK elevation can occur in a wide number of conditions, as well as with blunt or sharp trauma, aerobic exercise, EMG studies, muscle biopsies, or drugs such as barbiturates or narcotics that retard the elimination of CPK from the serum. Normal blacks have higher levels of CPK than whites, frequently with values above the normals established for large populations. The EMG changes seen in polymyositis are not specific. Even in the classic case, the change can only be considered myopathic and consistent with inflammation. The EMG is useful in identifying areas of abnormality to be biopsied, but biopsy should not include the actual site of EMG needle insertion. Because of the symmetrical nature of this disease, it is best to limit the EMG to one side of the body and biopsy the other side. Magnetic resonance imaging (MRI) may provide an effective, noninvasive means for identifying the site for biopsy and for following the course of the disease, especially in dermatomyositis. Although the possibility of malignancy should be considered in each patient with myositis, extensive undirected testing is not advised. Clues to the coexistence of neoplastic disease are almost always apparent on history, physical examination, or routine laboratory tests. Routine screening should be that which is appropriate for the patient's age and sex.

A variety of other diseases may cause muscle weakness (Table 247–3), and patients with these may fulfill some or all four criteria for polymyositis (see Table 247–1); thus these diagnoses must be excluded before the diagnosis of an idiopathic inflammatory myopathy can be made. A careful history and physical examination coupled with the judicious use of laboratory tests allow one to sort through the extensive differential list efficiently. For example, a careful review of medication use may reveal an agent that induces muscle injury such as alcohol, chloroquine, corticosteroids, cimetidine, colchicine, lovastatin, penicillamine, or zidovudine (AZT). On physical examination, asymmetrical weakness and distal extremity involvement, as well as abnormal reflexes, altered sensation, or cranial nerve abnormalities, should suggest a neurologic disease. Patients with inclusion body myositis may prove the exception, because a subset may have distal or asymmetrical muscle involvement. Inclusion body myositis also may be difficult to separate from some cases of muscular dystrophy, but in the latter, family history is usually present, symptoms begin earlier in life, and the muscles involved differ.

TABLE 247–3. DIFFERENTIAL DIAGNOSIS OF MUSCLE WEAKNESS

Collagen-Vascular	Neurologic
Polymyositis	Denervating disorders
Dermatomyositis	Amyotrophic lateral
Inclusion body myositis	sclerosis
Polymyalgia rheumatica	Neuromuscular
Temporal arteritis	junction disorders
Rheumatoid arthritis	Myasthenia gravis
Systemic lupus erythematosus	Eaton-Lambert syndrome
Polyarteritis nodosa	Muscular dystrophies
Scleroderma	Limb-girdle
Adult Still's disease	Becker's syndrome
Eosinophilic fasciitis	Duchenne's syndrome
	Neuropathies
Endocrine	Guillain-Barré syndrome
	Diabetes mellitus
Hypothyroidism	Porphyria
Hyperthyroidism	
Hyperparathyroidism	**Metabolic-Nutritional**
Hypocalcemia	
Cushing's disease	Uremia
Addison's disease	Hepatic failure
Aldosteronism	Hypercalcemia
Malabsorption	Hypocalcemia
Diabetic amyotrophy	Hyperkalemia
	Hypokalemia
Infectious	Hypernatremia
	Hyponatremia
Influenza, coxsackie, HIV,	Hypomagnesemia
and other viruses	Hypophosphatemia
Infectious mononucleosis	Periodic paralysis
Rickettsia	Vitamin D deficiency
Toxoplasmosis	Vitamin E deficiency
Trichinella	
Schistosomiasis	**Carcinomatous**
Bacterial toxins	
Staphylococcal	Neuropathy
Streptococcal	Neuromyopathy
Clostridial	Myositis
	Microembolization
Toxic (Drug-Related)	Eaton-Lambert syndrome
Alcohol	**Inherited Deficiency States**
Chloroquine/hydroxychloroquine	
Clofibrate	Glycogen storage diseases
Cocaine	McArdle's syndrome
Colchicine	(myophosphorylase)
Cromolyn	Phosphofructokinase
Cyclosporine	Debrancher enzyme
Emetine	Brancher enzyme
Gemfibrozil	Phosphoglycerate kinase
L-Tryptophan	Phosphoglycerate mutase
Lovastatin	Lactate dehydrogenase
Penicillamine	Acid maltase
Zidovudine (AZT)	Lipid disorders
	Carnitine (primary and
Psychosomatic	secondary)
	Carnitine palmitoyl-
Hysterical (?)	transferase
	Purine disorders
Miscellaneous	Myoadenylate deaminase
	Mitochondrial myopathies
Hypereosinophilic syndromes	
Rhabdomyolysis	
Sarcoidosis	
Fibromyalgia	

Serum electrolytes (sodium, potassium, calcium, phosphorous, and magnesium) should be measured. An abnormality of any electrolyte may interfere with the normal function of muscle fibers and result in weakness or myalgias. Uncovering an electrolyte abnormality usually reveals a reversible myopathy, especially if the cause of the electrolyte disturbance is identified. Some inherited metabolic myopathies can mimic inflammatory myopathy. Individuals with glycogen storage diseases such as myophosphorylase deficiency (McArdle's disease) or phosphofructokinase deficiency, as well as some with carnitine deficiency or myoadenylate deaminase deficiency, have proximal muscle weakness, elevated CPK levels, and myopathic EMG abnormalities. A forearm ischemic exercise test can be used to screen for the glycogen storage diseases and myoadenylate deaminase deficiency (Table 247–4).

TABLE 247–4. PROTOCOL FOR FOREARM ISCHEMIC EXERCISE TESTING

Procedure

Venous blood samples are drawn for ammonia and lactate levels from nondominant arm, preferably without a tourniquet.
A sphygmomanometer is inflated around the upper dominant arm to at least 20 mm HG above systolic pressure.
The subject then squeezes the dominant hand as vigorously as possible at a rate of one squeeze every 2 seconds for 2 minutes.
After 2 minutes of exercise, the cuff is deflated.
Two minutes after the cuff is deflated, venous samples are taken from the dominant arm for lactate and ammonia levels.

Interpretation

Normal individuals exercising with maximal effort increase lactate and ammonia levels at least threefold over baseline values. Individuals with a glycogen storage disease elevate ammonia levels normally but cannot raise lactate levels. Myoadenylate deaminase-deficient individuals raise lactate levels, but ammonia levels remain at baseline values. Falsely abnormal results may be obtained if the subject does not exercise with sufficient intensity. Abnormal results must be confirmed by a muscle biopsy to confirm the putative diagnosis.

TREATMENT. During the active stage of the disease, bed rest is essential, and physical therapy with passive range-of-motion exercises should be performed to maintain function and avoid contractures. Smoking is prohibited, and the head of the bed should be elevated in patients at risk for aspiration. Antacids or H_2 antagonists also may be useful to raise the pH of gastric fluids.

Treatment with corticosteroids is empiric but the standard. Initially, prednisone is used in single daily doses of 1 to 2 mg per kilogram. In responsive patients, muscle strength usually improves in 1 to 2 months, and the CPK normalizes in 3 months. Daily high-dose prednisone should be continued until strength has remained normal for 3 to 6 weeks. Once remission is attained, steroids are tapered very gradually, a process that may require up to 2 years. Alternate-day steroid use is recommended only when the disease is under excellent control.

Steroid failures may be attributed to inadequate initial dosage, tapering too quickly, inaccurate diagnosis, or an associated malignancy, refractory disease, or coincident steroid myopathy. An improvement in muscle strength when the steroid dose is raised indicates active disease; improved strength with a lower dose of steroid implicates steroid myopathy. Immunosuppressive agents are used in patients who do not respond adequately to corticosteroids. Daily oral azathioprine and weekly oral or parenteral methotrexate are the usual next choices. Cyclophosphamide, chlorambucil, cyclosporine, and intravenous immunoglobulin have been used in refractory cases. Only a small percentage of patients with inclusion body myositis achieve remission with steroid or other immunosuppressive therapy. Despite this poor prognosis, a therapeutic trial is indicated because remission occurs in some cases and progression may be delayed in others. However, if some benefit is not observed, drug therapy should be discontinued in order to avoid side effects and toxicity.

Love LA, Leff RL, Fraser DD, et al.: A new approach to the classification of idiopathic inflammatory myopathy: Myositis-specific autoantibodies define useful homogeneous patient groups. Medicine 70:360, 1991. *Review of 212 patients with idiopathic inflammatory myopathies, comparing them when classified by the traditional scheme versus when classified on the basis of myositis-specific antibodies.*
Plotz PH: Not myositis: A series of chance encounters. JAMA 268:2074, 1992. *Describes six cases that were confused with myositis, emphasizing the large number of conditions to be considered in the differential diagnosis of the idiopathic inflammatory myopathies.*
Sayers ME, Chou SM, Calabrese LH: Inclusion body myositis: Analysis of 32 cases. J Rheumatol 19:1385, 1992. *Review of clinical finding in larger series of this rare disease and discussion of expectations for therapy.*
Targoff IN: Autoantibodies in polymyositis. Rheum Dis Clin North Am 18:455, 1992. *Detailed review of the myositis-specific antibodies as well as autoantibodies associated with other connective tissue diseases.*
Wortmann RL: Inflammatory diseases of muscle. *In* Kelley WN, Harris ED Jr, Ruddy S, et al. (eds.), Textbook of Rheumatology. 4th ed. Philadelphia, WB Saunders, 1993, p 1159. *In-depth review of the inflammatory myopathies.*
Wortmann RL: Inflammatory muscle disease. *In* Weisman M, Weinblatt M (eds.), Drug Therapy for the Rheumatic Diseases. Philadelphia, WB Saunders, 1994. *Current status of treatments used.*

248 THE AMYLOID DISEASES

Louis W. Heck

DEFINITION. Amyloidosis is not one clinical entity but a group of diverse structurally driven protein deposition diseases. They are similar in that protein deposition occurs extracellularly and these deposits stain eosinophilic using standard tissue histologic stains, bind Congo red dye, and emit an apple-green birefringence using polarized light microscopy; exhibit metachromasia with crystal violet; and have an array of 75- to 100-Å nonbranching fibrils by electron microscopy and a twisted β-pleated sheet antiparallel configuration by x-ray crystallography. They differ, however, in the biochemical nature of the proteinaceous deposits, the "etiology" of the associated diseases (neoplastic, inflammatory, degenerative, hereditary), the tropism of protein deposition, and the spectrum of disease manifestations. Thus amyloidosis is not a single disease but a variety of diseases ranging from the asymptomatic patient who has a focal deposit discovered as an incidental finding to generalized involvement with severe multiorgan failure.

Prior to the early 1970's, all amyloid deposits were thought to be chemically identical despite the clinical observations that systemic amyloidosis occurred in certain patients with either plasma cell myeloma or diverse chronic inflammatory states such as tuberculosis, osteomyelitis, rheumatoid arthritis (RA), ankylosing spondylitis, and Crohn's disease. The major breakthrough in the physicochemical characterization of amyloid proteins resulted from the discovery that many of the nonamyloid proteins in amyloid-laden tissue could be extracted using physiologic saline and the insoluble amyloid fibrils solubilized using dilute aqueous solutions and/or chemotropic agents such as urea and guanidine, isolated using column chromatography, and biochemically defined using amino acid sequence analysis. By studying amyloid-laden tissues and using the aforementioned techniques, many different amyloid proteins and precursor proteins associated with clinical syndromes or specific diseases have been identified (Table 248–1).

All the monomeric amyloidogenic proteins have a β-pleated sheet conformation in solution, and many have been demonstrated to form insoluble β-pleated sheet fibrils *in vitro*. The known properties of tissue amyloid deposits such as binding to Congo red, resistance to proteolysis, and insolubility in physiologic solutions are directly attributed to the periodic β-pleated sheet motif. The formation of β-pleated sheets *in vivo* is an extremely complex process involving crucial ion concentrations and hydrogen bonding between many similar monomeric polypeptide chains at high focal concentrations as well as molecular interactions with the myriad extracellular matrix components. Furthermore, most amyloid deposits contain P-component, an acute-phase circulating serum protein.

There is no satisfactory clinical classification of the amyloidoses. One method is to consider three major systemic forms—AA, AL, and ATTR; two major localized forms—$A\beta_2$ and $A\beta$; and several miscellaneous forms (Table 248–1). There are many clinical features of each form.

PATHOGENESIS AND CLINICAL MANIFESTATIONS. *Primary (AL) Amyloidosis.* This was the first amyloid protein defined biochemically and shown to be identical to the variable region of immunoglobulin light chain (Bence Jones protein). It is the most common of the systemic amyloidoses in the United States and is associated with plasma cell myeloma (20%) or plasma cell dyscrasias (80%) with involvement of skin and subcutaneous tissue, nerve, liver, spleen, heart, kidney, and lung. In a large retrospective series of AL patients, approximately 50% had presenting symptoms of fatigue and weight loss; less frequent symptoms included peripheral edema, dyspnea, paresthesias, lightheadedness, and hoarseness. Initial physical findings revealed a palpable liver and peripheral edema in one third to one half of the patients. Orthostatic hypotension, purpura, macroglossia, palpable spleen, skin papules, ecchymoses, and lymphadenopathy were found less commonly. The signs and symptoms result from amyloid infiltration of organs and tissues with subsequent dysfunction. Examples of syndromes include those related to nerve tissue such as carpal tunnel syndrome, peripheral neuropathy with paresthesias of the fingers and toes, and sympathetic dysfunction manifested by orthostatic hypotension, impotence, sweating abnormalities, and gastrointestinal disturbances due to autonomic nerve involvement and those related to congestive heart failure with either predominant right-sided failure with restrictive cardiomyopathy (see Ch. 43) with stiff, noncompliant ventricles and thick intraventricular septum (multiple discrete 3- to 5-mm highly refractile echoes with a "speckled" pattern on two-dimensional echocardiogram) or, rarely, a dilated cardiomyopathy with biventricular failure. Both forms may be associated with conduction disturbances. Renal involvement with albuminuria and the full expression of nephrotic syndrome (see Ch. 79), and slow progressive renal failure may be seen. Finally, ecchymoses and "pinch purpura" may result from minor skin trauma due to increased fragility from amyloid infiltration of the small blood vessels.

Secondary (AA) Amyloidosis. This was the second systemic type of amyloidosis shown to be due to protein deposition—in this case the precursor protein is a serum component (SAA) synthesized in the liver that may increase 100- to 200-fold following an inflam-

TABLE 248–1. NOMENCLATURE AND CLASSIFICATION OF THE AMYLOIDOSES, 1990

		Amyloid Protein	Clinical State(s)	Major Organ/Tissue Involvement*
Major systemic amyloidoses	1.	AA	1. Chronic inflammatory conditions	K, L, S, GI, Sc
			a. Infectious: tuberculosis, osteomyelitis, etc.	H, unusual
			b. Noninfectious: juvenile rheumatoid arthritis, ankylosing spondylitis, Crohn's disease, etc.	N, rare
			2. Familial Mediterranean fever	
	2.	AL	Plasma cell dyscrasia	H, L, S, T
			10% multiple myeloma/macroglobulemia	N, GI, Sc
			90% idiopathic, "primary"	
	3.	ATTR	Various familial polyneuropathies and cardiomyopathies	N, H, K, E, GI, Sc
Major localized amyloidoses	4.	$A\beta_2M$	Chronic dialysis usually greater than 8 years	B, Sy, Ts
	5.	$A\beta$	1. Alzheimer's disease	
			2. Down syndrome	
			3. Hereditary cerebral hemorrhage, Dutch	C, CV
			4. Nontraumatic cerebral hemorrhage of elderly	
Miscellaneous amyloidoses	6.	A Apo AI	Familial polyneuropathy, Iowa	N, K
	7.	A Gel	Familial amyloidosis, Finnish	CN, E, Skin
	8.	A Cys	Hereditary cerebral hemorrhage, Icelandic	C, CV
	9.	A Scr	Creutzfeldt-Jakob disease	C
	10.	A Cal	Medullary carcinoma of thyroid	Th
	11.	AANF	Atrial amyloid	H
	12.	AIAPP	Diabetes mellitus, insulinomas	P

* B = bone; C = cerebrum; CN = cranial nerves; CV = cerebral vessels; E = eye; GI = gastrointestinal; H = heart; K = kidney; L = liver; N = nerve; P = pancreas; S = spleen; Sc = subcutaneous tissue; T = tongue; Th = thyroid; Ts = tenosynovium; Sy = synovium.

matory stimulus. Certain monocyte/macrophage cytokines such as interleukin-1 (IL-1), tumor necrosis factor, and IL-6 may up-regulate hepatic gene expression of this protein. Secondary amyloidosis usually involves the liver, spleen, and kidneys; heart involvement is less frequent than seen in primary amyloidosis; and nerve involvement is very infrequent. Some of the associated infectious diseases include osteomyelitis, tuberculosis, and bronchiectasis, and some of the noninfectious inflammatory states include RA, juvenile rheumatoid arthritis, ankylosing spondylitis, Crohn's disease, and familial Mediterranean fever. Curiously, the renal disease may be slow and indolent, with progressive proteinuria evolving into nephrotic syndrome and persisting for 5 to 10 years before end-stage renal disease. In Europe, renal amyloidosis has been reported as the major cause of death in juvenile rheumatoid arthritis patients, but this associated complication has not been seen in the United States. Another interesting observation is that AA may be resorbed *in vivo*, as manifested by reduction of an enlarged liver or spleen or reduction in proteinuria without defined treatment of the underlying disorder. Finally, the successful use of colchicine to reduce the attacks and development of amyloidosis in familial Mediterranean fever patients and decrease proteinuria and improve renal function in some cases mandates that AA be considered carefully and ruled out in all amyloid patients.

Familial (ATTR) Amyloidosis.
This was the third systemic amyloidosis to be defined and shown to be associated with the presence of an abnormal plasma prealbumin protein, which normally functions to transport thyroxine and retinol-binding protein and subsequently was termed *transthyretin*. It was defined originally as an autosomal dominant inherited peripheral neuropathy (see Ch. 451) occurring in middle to late life that was progressive over the next several decades with additional autonomic neuropathy and variable organ involvement, primarily in Portuguese patients. Subsequently, many clinical manifestations defining different kindred in Europe and the United States have resulted from mutations in the gene for transthyretin with amino acid substitutions in this transport molecule, which have been associated with variable amyloid infiltration in heart, bowel, and kidney.

Dialysis-Related (β_2-Microglobulin) Amyloidosis (AB$_2$M).
This localized amyloidosis occurs in most patients on maintenance hemodialysis or peritoneal dialysis for longer than 8 years and is due to the deposition of β_2-microglobulin amyloid in the periarticular, joint, bone, and carpal tunnel tissue. Some of the rheumatic complaints/findings include chronic shoulder pain with tenderness over the subacromial bursae, pain and swelling of the wrist and finger joints, proliferative tenosynovium over the wrist extensor tendons, and radiographic evidence of subchondral erosions of the carpal bones, femur, and humerus. Pathologic fractures of the humerus and femur have been described.

β_2-microglobulin is the noncovalently associated β chain of class I MHC molecules, which is present on virtually all human nucleated cells. The catabolism of this small protein depends on normal kidney filtration and excretion. In dialysis patients and those with end-stage renal disease, plasma levels of β_2-microglobulin are elevated. Efforts to effectively remove this protein using conventional dialysis membranes of cellulose acetate or cuprophane have not been successful owing to poor protein clearance. Furthermore, these membranes induce complement activation and generation of IL-1, which may result in β_2-microglobulin accumulation.

Beta Protein (Alzheimer's Disease) Amyloidosis (AD).
Alzheimer's disease (AD) is the most common cause of dementia in elderly patients, afflicting 5 to 10% of the population over 65 (see Ch. 400). In neuropathologic studies of the brains of AD patients, neurofibrillary tangles and neuritic plaques are frequently found in the amygdala, hippocampus, and frontal, temporal, and parietal lobes. In addition, acellular thickening of the small and medium-sized arteries of the leptomeninges and cerebral cortex have been seen in AD and aged patients. By standard histologic techniques, the amorphous material in the walls of meningeal vessels and the central region of the neuritic plaques has the characteristic staining property for amyloid. The chemical nature of both amyloid deposits has been identified as a novel 40-amino-acid protein (β protein) that is generated by proteolysis of a much larger transmembrane glycoprotein termed "β amyloid precursor protein." In some forms of familial AD, point mutations have resulted in single amino acid substitutions in this precursor protein. Recent studies have reported that most patients with late-onset

sporadic AD have a strong association of ApoE$_4$ alleles and A$_\beta$ deposits within the cerebrum and cerebral vessels, which suggest the possibility that bimolecular complexes between ApoE$_4$ and A$_\beta$ may be important in the extracellular deposition and formation of cerebral amyloid.

There is evidence that the cerebrovascular deposition of β protein amyloid is an important etiology of nontraumatic/nonhypertensive brain hemorrhage in the elderly, usually presenting as cerebral lobe hemorrhage involving the cortex and subcortical white matter. In addition, a familial syndrome defined in a Dutch kindred in which certain family members died in their 40's or 50's from cerebral hemorrhages (hereditary cerebral hemorrhage with amyloidosis, Dutch type) has been shown to be due to an amino acid substitution in the β protein.

The suggestive signs and symptoms of the amyloidoses result directly from tissue/organ infiltration with subsequent dysfunction. As can be seen in Table 248–1, multiple organ involvement is common but variable in degree. This necessitates formulating a list of differential diagnoses to exclude other localized or systemic diseases. For example, carpal tunnel syndrome is a common clinical entity and is seen very frequently in patients on hemodialysis for longer than 8 to 10 years; it is due to Aβ_2M deposition in the tenosynovium of the carpal tunnel. This is also commonly found in the AL and ATTR forms and in nonamyloid diseases such as hypothyroidism, RA, and diabetes mellitus. Thus many disorders must be considered and subsequently excluded. The AA, AL, and ATTR forms may be associated with significant proteinuria or nephrotic syndrome, and many primary glomerular diseases must be excluded. AL and ATTR forms also may be the cause of vexing unexplained congestive heart failure with cardiomyopathy in patients who have had repeated heart catherization and coronary angiography without a clear answer. Clues to cardiac amyloidosis may be present on the standard 12-lead electrocardiogram, such as decreased QRS voltage, first-degree AV block with intraventricular conduction defects, and Q waves in precordial leads V_1 to V_3 (pseudoinfarction) or two-dimensional echocardiographic findings of a "speckled" pattern of intraventricular septum/myocardium. Peripheral neuropathies may be the initial and dominant expression primarily in the ATTR and other familial forms (see Table 248–1). Generally, the onset of symptoms occurs in early middle age (30 to 40 years old) in the lower extremity with progressive sensorimotor involvement including the proximal and truncal sensory nerves. Foot ulcers with secondary infections may occur. An autonomic neuropathy with orthostatic hypotension, impotence, and diminished peristalsis with pseudo-obstruction, diarrhea, or malabsorption may be present. Gastrointestinal bleeding and/or perforation may be associated with amyloid infiltration of the lamina propria and submucosal blood vessels. Often there are many interacting variables; for example, orthostatic hypotension in the amyloid patient may result from the combination of restrictive cardiomyopathy with diastolic dysfunction, diminished intravascular volume, and sympathetic dysfunction.

Two uncommon syndromes may be easily confused with amyloidosis. The POEMS syndrome (see Ch. 149) (*p*olyneuropathy, *o*rganomegaly, *e*ndocrinopathy, *m*onoclonal gammopathy, *s*kin findings) is a plasma cell dyscrasia with a constellation of diverse features similar to the systemic/localized amyloid syndrome, but no amyloid deposits have been described in these patients. Immunotactoid glomerulopathy (fibrillary renal deposits) is characterized by progressive proteinuria, microscopic hematuria, and hypertension. The renal biopsy tissue has variable glomerular deposits containing IgG, IgM, C_3, C_4, and λ and κ light chains (immunotactoid). On electron microscopy, fibrillary material is deposited within the mesangium and capillary walls and can be differentiated from the typical amyloid fibrils in that the fibrils are thicker and do not stain with Congo red.

DIAGNOSIS. *The diagnosis is made by detecting amyloid deposits in tissue preparations stained with Congo red and emitting an apple-green birefringence using polarized light microscopy.* If a patient is suspected of having one of the systemic amyloidoses (AL, AA, ATTR), aspiration and staining of abdominal subcutaneous fat tissue should be done, since this can be done rapidly and safely at the bedside. Fat tissue is obtained using a 16-gauge needle fixed to a 20- to 30-ml syringe—repeated movements of the needle with gentle pulling of the syringe barrel to produce a negative pressure is done to obtain fragments of the fatty tissue. The fatty fluid and fragments are placed on alcohol-cleaned glass slides, air-dried, and submitted for Congo red staining. Because variable false-negative results have been reported, a repeat biopsy of the subcutaneous tissue or of an alternative site such as the rectal mucosa is warranted. The redundant mucosal folds (valves of Houston) may be visualized directly and tissue (including the vascular submucosa) obtained by pincer forceps with bleeding controlled by cautery. Other biopsy sites include carpal tunnel tissue, kidney, sural nerve, heart (endomyocardial biopsy of right ventricle), bone, and synovium. Staining of amyloid deposits in synovial fluid of AL and $A\beta_2M$ patients has been described. In general, biopsy of the liver should be avoided due to the risk of bleeding. *Attempts to define the chemical amyloid type should be made.* For example, specific antisera to λ and κ light chains, SAA, β_2 microglobulin, and transthyretin are commercially available to stain the tissue using immunofluorescent or immunoperoxidase methods.

In patients with suspected AL with or without myeloma, agarose gel electrophoresis of serum and concentrated urine may be done easily. The monoclonal paraprotein is separated from other serum components by electrophoresis, interacted with separate antisera to λ and κ light chains, IgM, IgA, and IgG (immunofixation), and identified by protein staining. Bone marrow aspiration and biopsy are usually done to quantify the number of plasma wells and can be stained for amyloid. Scintigraphy using radiolabeled P-component, which binds to all amyloid types, remains experimental and cannot be justified as a screening or routine test.

TREATMENT. AL is treated with chemotherapy as a plasma cell neoplasm, even though only 10 to 20% of patients have plasma cell myeloma. The Mayo Clinic has used a treatment protocol of mephalan 0.15 mg per kilogram per day in two divided doses and prednisone 0.8 mg per kilogram per day in four divided doses. The duration of each treatment was 7 days with repeated cycles every 6 weeks. Diuretics may be necessary to treat fluid retention. Every patient with AL should be given a trial with this regimen, even though the response rate is disappointingly low at approximately 20%. However, dramatic resolution of multiorgan dysfunction/amyloid infiltration using cyclic prednisone and mephalan treatment has been reported.

The successful prevention and treatment of amyloidosis of familial Mediterranean fever with low-dose colchicine 0.6 mg once or twice daily has been a dramatic treatment development for AA. If the amyloidosis is related to an infectious process such as tuberculosis, it must be defined and treated aggressively. Likewise, any noninfectious inflammatory condition should be treated and patients given colchicine concomitantly.

Unfortunately, no standard treatment regimen for ATTR has been defined. The liver synthesizes the abnormal transthyretin protein in afflicted patients, and a small number of liver transplants have been performed but no results have been published. Furthermore, no guidelines for hepatic transplantation have been defined.

$A\beta_2M$ is a very common localized amyloidosis that is thought to result from poor clearance of β_2M by conventional dialysis membranes leading to high levels of this protein in serum and tissues enhancing fibril formation. A new group of synthetic high-flux, highly permeable dialysis membranes (polycarbonate, polymethyl methacrylate, polyacrylonitrile) is currently available but very expensive. Long-term studies are necessary to determine if these new synthetic membranes prevent dialysis-related $A\beta_2M$.

Finally, the loss of physical independence in older, frail patients with AD is devastating both emotionally and economically for these patients and their families. No preventative treatment is currently available. Much research is currently being performed to understand the mechanism(s) of $A\beta$ formation and the role of $ApoE_4$-$A\beta$ complexes in the formation of neuritic plaques.

Benson, MD: Amyloidosis: *In* Beaudet AL, Scriver CR, Sly WS: The Metabolic Basis of Inherited Disease. New York, McGraw-Hill, 1994. *A superb review of amyloidosis focusing primarily on the ATTR forms.*

Kyle RA, Griepp PR: Amyloidosis (AL): Clinical and laboratory features in 229 cases. Mayo Clin Proc 58:665, 1983. *Excellent reference for those interested in the various manifestations of AL.*

Natvig JB, Førre Ø, Husby G (eds.): Amyloid and Amyloidosis, 1990. New York, Kluwer Academic Publishers, 1991. Published proceedings of the VIth International Symposium on Amyloidosis, in Oslo, Norway. *Current status on nomenclature and scientific study of amyloidosis. Many references.*

Zemer D, Pras M, Sohar E, et al.: Colchicine in the prevention and treatment of the amyloidosis of familial Mediterranean fever. N Engl J Med 314:1001, 1986. *A review of 1070 patients on colchicine for 4 to 11 years with convincing evidence that long-term colchicine therapy prevents amyloidosis development and in some cases ameliorates already existing amyloid kidney involvement.*

249 BEHÇET'S DISEASE

Eugene V. Ball

Although there is no invariable feature of Behçet's disease (BD), certain features occur often enough to constitute a definable syndrome and serve as the basis for diagnostic criteria. One set in common use requires the presence of recurrent oral ulcers and any two of the following: genital ulcers, uveitis, cutaneous or large vessel vasculitis, arthritis, and meningoencephalitis. An "incomplete" form has been defined as recurrent aphthous ulcers and any one of the other features. Although oral ulcers are the linchpin of diagnostic criteria, a diagnosis of probable BD is tenable when several of these features occur together in the absence of aphthous ulcers, and other known causes can be excluded. Diagnosis has been possible in some patients only after as many as 20 years of minor symptoms.

CLINICAL MANIFESTATIONS. Table 249–1 lists manifestations of the disease in one group of 60 patients. Constitutional signs such as fever and weight loss were noted in 63%. Other significant manifestations include meningoencephalitis and abdominal pain. At least 24 patients from Mediterranean areas have had both BD and secondary (AA) amyloidosis.

Oral ulcers are painful, are round or oval, are usually multiple, and may be the only sign of BD; on the other hand, isolated genital ulcers are seldom indicative of BD. Ulcers occur elsewhere, as in the gut and on the skin, as do an assortment of nonulcerative skin lesions, such as erythema, erythema nodosum, photosensitivity, and spontaneous pustules. The pustular reaction of the skin to intradermal needle prick (sometimes referred to as "pathergy") denotes increased neutrophil chemotaxis and was once thought to be pathognomonic of BD, but this reaction occurs in no more than 70% of patients, usually in those with extensive disease. Furthermore, it is nonspecific, occurring in 7% of one group of healthy control subjects.

Ten to 15% of acquired blindness among Japanese is thought to be due to the uveoretinitis of BD. Decreased visual acuity results from inflammation, secondary glaucoma, cataracts, or vitreous hemorrhage; retinal vein thrombosis leading to sudden blindness is not rare.

Phlebitis or arteritis occurs in as many as a quarter of all patients and predisposes to thrombosis or aneurysms. For example, 10% of a group of 450 Tunisians had aneurysms, large artery occlusions, or both. Aneurysms are particularly common in pulmonary arteries and are most often single, but as many as 14 have occurred in one pa-

TABLE 249–1. MAJOR MANIFESTATIONS OF BEHÇET'S DISEASE

Manifestation	Prevalence (%)
Mouth ulcers	97
Genital ulcers	83
Cutaneous lesions	75
Uveitis	48
Joint pain	48
Phlebitis	17

tient in less than 1 year. Pulmonary vasculitis produces dyspnea, chest pain, cough, or hemoptysis and is a significant cause of death. Its radiographic signs include scattered infiltrates and pleural effusions.

The arthritis of BD is usually intermittent, self-limited, and localized to the knees and ankles; however, erosive changes have been observed in hip, heel, wrist, knee, ankle, and foot radiographs.

Aseptic meningitis occurs in almost all cases of neurologic BD; other manifestations include encephalopathy, seizures, corticospinal abnormalities, bulbar palsy, ataxia, transient ischemic attacks, strokes, and pseudotumor cerebri. These may be acute or gradual in onset, and they may resolve completely or cause death. Focal intracranial abnormalities are detected by imaging studies.

Small and large ulcers in the gut produce symptoms of inflammatory bowel disease and perforation and are more common in Japanese than in Turkish patients.

PREVALENCE. BD is rare in the Americas and Europe. It is more prevalent, as well as more virulent, in Turkey and the Middle and Far East. Evidence of BD was found in 19 of 1531 persons aged 10 or older in a field survey conducted in rural Turkey; on Hokkaido, Japan, its estimated prevalence was 1 in 1000 persons, but BD is less common in ethnic Japanese living in Hawaii. Its prevalence was estimated at 1 in 25,000 in Olmsted County, Minnesota.

GENETICS AND PATHOLOGY. Although not considered hereditary, BD was present in members of four HLA (human leukocyte antigen) B51–positive families. HLA-B51 has been detected in 51% of BD patients versus 16% of control subjects in Japan and in 62% with BD versus 29% of control subjects in Iraq. The HLA-B5101 allele of B51 was found in all 46 HLA-B51–positive Japanese BD patients. Histopathologic characteristics of BD are nonspecific. Despite its classification as vasculitis, fibrinoid necrosis of vessels is not usually found. Mononuclear cells, found in the epidermis and around small vessels in early lesions, are later replaced by neutrophils and plasma cells. Arteritis, which may be catastrophic, is due to inflammation of the vasa vasorum. Abnormalities of the immune system are inconstant, providing no clues to the cause and pathogenesis of BD, which remain unknown. The possible "cure" of retinitis by oral doses of retinal protein S supports the concept of autoimmunity to retinal-specific antigens in the pathogenesis of eye inflammation in BD.

TREATMENT. Numerous medications have been tried for symptomatic treatment as well as for prevention. Patients with thromboses of major vessels should receive anticoagulants. Corticosteroids are given in doses up to 1000 mg of prednisone or prednisolone per day for serious problems, such as central nervous system disease. Cyclosporine appears to be superior to colchicine in reducing the frequency and severity of ocular attacks. Other immunosuppressive drugs have been used with variable effectiveness and toxicity. Chlorambucil (0.1 mg per kilogram per day) moderates disease expression; however, long-term use is worrisome with respect to oncogenesis. Azathioprine (2.5 mg per kilogram per day) is superior to placebo in preserving visual acuity in patients with eye disease and in reducing the frequency of oral and genital ulcers and arthritis, and methotrexate may have a role in treatment of BD. Retinitis has been treated successfully with oral retinal protein S (personal communication).

Dilsen N, Konice M, Aral O, et al.: Behçet's disease associated with amyloidosis in Turkey and in the world. Ann Rheum Dis 47:157, 1988. *The features of 8 Turkish and 16 other patients with BD and amyloidosis are described.*

Hamza M: Large artery involvement in Behçet's disease. J Rheumatol 14:554, 1987. *Clinical descriptions of 10 of 450 patients evaluated over 20 years who had arterial aneurysms (7) and occlusion (3).*

Masuda K, Urayama A, Kogure M, et al.: Double-masked trial of cyclosporin versus colchicine and long-term open study of cyclosporin in Behçet's disease. Lancet 1:1093, 1989. *A randomized, 16-week, double-blind study comparing colchicine and cyclosporine in 49 and 47 patients, respectively. Thirty-six patients were enrolled in a long-term study of mean duration of 44 weeks.*

Mizuki N, Inoko H, Ando H, et al.: Behçet's disease associated with one of the HLA-B51 subantigens, HLA-B*5101. Am J Ophthalmol 116:406, 1993. *Of three HLA-B51 alleles, only B5101 was found in 46 HLA-B51–positive BD patients.*

Raz I, Okon E, Chajek-Shaul T: Pulmonary manifestations in Behçet's syndrome. Chest 95:585, 1989. *Seven of 72 patients had pulmonary vascular disease manifested as dyspnea, cough, chest pain, and hemoptysis. The clinical and radiographic data of these and 42 other patients were reviewed.*

250 PANNICULITIS AND DISORDERS OF THE SUBCUTANEOUS FAT

Gerald S. Lazarus

The subcutaneous tissue is a fibrofatty layer spread between skin and muscles. It functions not only as a thermal and mechanical insulator but also as an active metabolic organ. The characteristic "signet ring" lipocytes are organized into lobules by fibrous septa, which are continuous with the dermis and contain the blood and lymph vessels and reticuloendothelial cells.

The diagnosis of panniculitis frequently requires deep skin biopsy. The most important histologic characteristic is the location of the inflammatory process. Inflammation primarily in the septa is designated *septal panniculitis,* whereas inflammation primarily of the fat lobules is called *lobular panniculitis.* The presence or absence of vasculitis further differentiates panniculitis into four major groups.

LOBULAR PANNICULITIS WITHOUT VASCULITIS. *Nodular Panniculitis—Weber-Christian Disease.* Nodular panniculitis describes a group of syndromes or diseases characterized by subcutaneous nodules and inflammatory cells in the fat lobules. The term Weber-Christian disease is applied when cutaneous lesions are associated with systemic complaints; this eponym should be abandoned because lobular panniculitis includes a variety of distinctive disease entities.

The etiology of this group of diseases is unknown. In the early stages, the fat lobules are infiltrated with polymorphonuclear leukocytes. Later, macrophages appear and ingest fat, producing the characteristic lipophagic granuloma. The lesions heal with lobular fibrosis. Modest septal vasculitis may be observed.

Lobular panniculitis most commonly occurs in women between the ages of 30 and 60, although cases have been reported in all age groups. The lesions begin as red, slightly tender nodules deep in the skin. They appear more or less in symmetric crops on thighs and lower legs, but lesions also may occur on arms, trunk, and face. The number of lesions may vary enormously. The lesions become firmer, less red, and less tender over a period of weeks. They heal, leaving a depressed, hyperpigmented scar. *Liquefying panniculitis* is a variant in which the lesions become necrotic and drain an oily, yellow-brown fluid. Biopsy reveals polymorphonuclear leukocytes in the deep reticular dermis as well as in the fat. As many as 15% of patients with this clinical picture may have α_1 proteinase deficiency.

Systemic nodular panniculitis is a widespread process affecting cutaneous and visceral fat. Patients usually present with unequivocal cutaneous nodules and arthralgias, malaise, fatigue, weight loss, and abdominal pain. Involvement of the bone marrow may produce anemia, leukocytosis or leukopenia, and bone pain. Hepatomegaly, steatorrhea, and intestinal perforation also have been reported. Inflammation may occur in other internal organs, such as lungs, pleura, pericardium, spleen, kidney, and adrenal glands. Visceral involvement may be confined to the retroperitoneal space, producing abdominal pain, nausea, and vomiting. Mesenteric panniculitis resulting in abdominal pain, diarrhea, constipation, and occasional mass lesions may occur without cutaneous findings. Histiocytic cytophagic panniculitis is a disease characterized by panniculitis, fever, serositis, reticuloendotheliomegaly, hemorrhagic complications, and a poor prognosis; it is diagnosed by the presence of nonneoplastic T lymphocytes and histiocytosis with phagocytosis of erythrocytes, leukocytes, and platelets.

The prognosis of nodular panniculitis is good in patients with only cutaneous involvement. Remissions and exacerbations of the lesions are frequent. Some patients recover after a few months, and permanent remission is usual after several years. On rare occasions, visceral involvement may be fatal.

No specific therapy exists for this disease. Saturated potassium iodide, increasing by 1 drop per day from 5 drops three times per day to 30 drops three times per day, has been suggested. Hydroxychloroquine,* 200 mg two times per day, and cimetidine also have been advocated as treatment. High-dose prednisone, 40 to 60 mg for 1 to 2 weeks, with gradual tapering over 6 to 8 weeks, also has been reported to be of value in patients with severe disease; steroids should be used *only for acute* attacks and for limited periods. There are anecdotal reports that cyclosporine may be of value in patients with severe panniculitis.

Lobular Panniculitis Associated with Pancreatic Disease. The diagnosis is made by skin biopsy, which discloses acute fat necrosis with characteristic ghost cells. These patients often have associated arthritis, ascites, and eosinophilia. Acute pancreatitis, trauma to the pancreas, chronic pancreatitis, pancreatic cysts, and pancreatic carcinoma have been reported to be associated with this syndrome. Diagnosis depends on the histologic findings at skin biopsy and documentation of a specific pancreatic abnormality. Therapy is directed at the underlying pancreatic disease.

Poststeroid Lobular Panniculitis. Children who receive large doses of steroid for a short period, followed by abrupt discontinuance, may develop lobular panniculitis. Lesions may occur in the viscera, and a fatal case has been reported.

Physical Lobular Panniculitis. Physical trauma of any kind and cold injury, especially in children, can produce lobular panniculitis. A unique traumatic panniculitis occurs in the breasts of obese women in their 50's. Injection of silicone or other foreign materials into female breasts or buttocks and into the male genitalia may induce a granulomatous foreign body nodular panniculitis. Similar inflammatory lesions may be seen following injection of pentazocine (Talwin).

Lobular Panniculitis Associated with Systemic Disease. Lupus erythematosus, sarcoidosis, granuloma annulare, Sweet's disease, acute sudden weight loss from gastrointestinal surgery, and infections, including those caused by deep fungi, mycobacteria, and pyogens, may present as lobular panniculitis. Any patient with acquired immunodeficiency syndrome (AIDS) who has panniculitis must have a biopsy performed and the tissue sent for histologic study and culture to rule out infectious agents. Lymphoma or leukemia also may present as panniculitis; histologically, these lesions demonstrate malignant cells in the fat lobules. Lupus erythematosus confined primarily to the fat is known as "lupus profundus." The skin may be exclusively involved, or the panniculitis may be associated with systemic disease. Diagnosis is suggested by characteristic histology and the deposition of immunoglobulin at the dermal-epidermal interface.

Lobular Panniculitis with Vasculitis. This category of disease includes *nodular vasculitis* and *erythema induratum.* The eruption consists of recurring, tender, painful nodules on the calves, which often ulcerate and heal with scarring. It is much more common in females than in males. Increased erythrocyte sedimentation rate and hypertension have been associated with this syndrome. Bazin gave the name "erythema induratum" to this disease when histologic examination revealed caseation necrosis. These lesions may be associated with tuberculosis and especially a positive skin test.

Most patients experience remission of lesions with bed rest. Severe cases have been successfully treated with nonsteroidal anti-inflammatory drugs (NSAID's), dapsone, and prednisone. In cases of nodular vasculitis associated with a positive tuberculin skin test, appropriate antituberculous therapy is indicated.

SEPTAL PANNICULITIS WITHOUT VASCULITIS. This histologic picture in a patient with nodular, painful, tender lesions, especially on the anterior leg, is diagnostic of *erythema nodosum,* which is discussed in Ch. 475. A chronic disease similar to erythema nodosum clinically and histologically except that the lesions spread peripherally over months, forming rings, is called *subacute migratory panniculitis.* This disease responds to therapy with increasing doses of saturated potassium iodide as described for nodular panniculitis. Septal panniculitis without vasculitis also can be seen in scleroderma, dermatomyositis, and necrobiosis lipoidica diabeticorum. Eosinophilic fasciitis can mimic septal panniculitis. In-

gestion of pharmacologic doses of tryptophan for pain or depression has produced a syndrome mimicking acute scleroderma or eosinophilic fasciitis. These diagnostic possibilities should be investigated in all patients.

SEPTAL PANNICULITIS WITH VASCULITIS. *Thrombophlebitis* may present with subcutaneous nodules. Histology reveals inflammation of veins with adjacent panniculitis (see Ch. 46).

Cutaneous polyarteritis is a chronic recurring painful nodular eruption, primarily of the legs. An associated mottled livedo vascular pattern is often present. Cutaneous polyarteritis is associated with myalgias, arthralgias, and increased erythrocyte sedimentation rate. Histologic examination demonstrates leukocytoclastic vasculitis of medium-sized arterioles. This disease is not usually associated with systemic involvement. It has a benign course, but lesions may recur for years.

Therapy includes NSAID's and short courses of corticosteroids. Cutaneous polyarteritis associated with granulomatous bowel disease has responded to short courses of cyclophosphamide (Cytoxan).

LIPOATROPHY. Subcutaneous tissue can be lost as a consequence of healing in almost any of the panniculitides described previously. The most common diagnosable cause of lipoatrophy is recurrent insulin injection. Insulin lipoatrophy is usually associated with repetitive injections of high doses of insulin in exactly the same location in females. Injections of pentazocine (Talwin) also may produce panniculitis and severe lipoatrophy.

Total lipoatrophy associated with diabetes may occur in children and adults. The clinical picture is dramatic, and there is almost complete loss of subcutaneous fat. Partial lipoatrophy usually begins in children or young adults. It is five times more common in females than in males. Patients often lose the fat in the face and the upper half of the body. In some cases, there is hypertrophy of the fat on the lower half of the body. Patients with partial lipodystrophy often develop progressive mesangiocapillary glomerulonephritis and hypocomplementemia. Diabetes develops in one third of these patients. Retinitis pigmentosum has also been reported with this disease. The prognosis depends upon the severity of the renal disease.

Ackerman AB: Panniculitis. *In* Ackerman AB (ed.): Histologic Diagnosis of Inflammatory Skin Diseases. Philadelphia, Lea & Febiger, 1978, pp 779–826. *An outstanding review of the classification and histology of panniculitis.*
Alegre VA, Winkelmann RK: Clinical and laboratory studies: Histiocytic cytophagic panniculitis. J Am Acad Dermatol 20:177, 1989.
Bondi EE, Lazarus GS: Panniculitis. *In* Fitzpatrick TB, Eisen AZ, Wolff K, et al. (eds.): Dermatology in General Medicine, 4th ed. New York, McGraw-Hill, 1993, pp 1329–1344. *A complete overview of panniculitis emphasizing clinical descriptions, mechanisms, and treatment.*
Peters MS, Su WP: Lupus erythematosus panniculitis. Med Clin North Am 73:1113, 1989. *An excellent review of this disease.*
Rademaker M, Lowe DG, Munro DD: Erythema induratum (Bazin's disease). J Am Acad Dermatol 21:740, 1989. *Correlation of erythema induratum with hypersensitivity to tuberculin.*
Smith KC, Su WP, Pittelkow MR, Winkelmann RK: Clinical and pathologic correlations in 96 patients with panniculitis, including 15 patients with deficient levels of alpha,-antitrypsin. J Am Acad Dermatol 21:1192, 1989. *Clinical and pathologic correlations in 96 patients with panniculitis, including 15 with α₁-antitrypsin deficiency.*

251 GOUT AND URIC ACID METABOLISM
Michael S. Hershfield

Gout refers to the *inflammatory arthritis* induced by microscopic *crystals* of monosodium urate monohydrate (MSU) and to the pathognomonic deposition of aggregated MSU crystals (*tophi*) in various tissues and some organs. Chronic *hyperuricemia* is necessary for the development of gout, though not sufficient. *Urolithiasis* (renal stones composed of undissociated uric acid) may accompany gout or occur independently when renal urate excretion is excessive. Gout is chiefly a disease of adult men. It is mostly *idiopathic* and multifactorial in etiology. A few rare, inherited metabolic disorders markedly enhance urate production, causing urolithiasis and gout as primary manifestations. Other genetic and acquired disor-

---

* This use is not listed in the manufacturer's directive.

ders and some drugs cause secondary hyperuricemia and gout by impairing renal urate excretion or by indirectly increasing urate production (Table 251–1).

If untreated, gout can lead to painful, destructive arthropathy, and urolithiasis to renal failure. Correcting hyperuricemia and hyperuricosuria prevents these consequences and is achievable in most cases. However, because most hyperuricemic individuals will develop neither gout nor renal insufficiency and because therapy is not without risk and expense, *asymptomatic hyperuricemia per se* generally does not require therapy; observation and in some cases a search for a contributing, treatable disease are warranted.

PREVALENCE AND INCIDENCE. Surveys made in the 1960's estimated the prevalence of gout at about 0.5 to 0.7% for men and about 0.1% for women. Prevalence has been increasing over the past two decades. Gout is the most common inflammatory arthritis in men over 40 in the United States. A 1986 U.S. Health Interview Survey estimated 2.2 million cases of self-reported gout, about twice the physician-reported prevalence.

As Hippocrates observed, gout rarely occurs before puberty in males and seldom before menopause in females. Trends in serum urate values are consistent with this pattern. In normal children, serum urate averages 3.6 mg per deciliter in both genders. Levels rise at puberty, more so in males than in females. In the United States, the central 95% segment of the serum urate distribution ranges from 2.2 to 7.5 mg per deciliter in adult men and from 2.1 to 6.6 mg per deciliter in adult premenopausal women. Serum urate values increase with age; after menopause, mean values in women approach levels in men. Epidemiologic surveys have noted a trend toward increasing serum urate values in the United States in recent decades and significant variations among population groups, which reflect genetic and environmental factors. Obesity, alcohol consumption, and diuretic use are associated with hyperuricemia.

The incidence of gout increases with the degree and duration of hyperuricemia; age, obesity, hypertension, and alcohol intake show much weaker relationships when serum urate is factored out. Although lower levels are occasionally found during an attack, serum urate exceeds 7 mg per deciliter at some time in virtually all patients with gout. Nevertheless, the risk of gout is modest, even at higher serum urate levels. Among about 2000 initially healthy white males followed over a 15-year period, annual incidence rates for gout were 0.1% at <7 mg per deciliter, 0.5% at 7.0 to 8.9 mg per deciliter, and 4.9% at ≥9 mg per deciliter. At levels over 9 mg per deciliter (the highest 1.8% of values observed), the cumulative incidence of gout after 5 years was 22%. Incidence rates were about threefold higher for hypertensive than for normotensive men in all age groups, reflecting the hyperuricemic effect of diuretics. Convincing studies have shown that hyperuricemia is not a risk factor for either renal failure or coronary artery disease.

PATHOGENESIS AND PATHOLOGY. Serum urate levels are very low, and gout is nonexistent, in nonhuman primates and other species that possess urate oxidase *(uricase),* a hepatic peroxisomal enzyme that converts urate to allantoin. The latter is 80- to 100-fold more soluble than urate and much more efficiently excreted by the kidneys. Mutational inactivation of the uricase gene occurred during evolution of *Homo sapiens* and a few other hominoid species. From this perspective, *uricemia per se* in humans is the abnormal result of an inborn error of urate catabolism. In terms of the pathogenesis of gout, which is caused by urate crystals rather than urate in solution, "hyperuricemia" is defined by the solubility of urate in body fluids, not by statistical distributions of urate levels. More urate produced than can be disposed of or maintained in solution leads over time to extracellular deposition of MSU crystals; urate solubility is much lower at the temperature of peripheral joints (about 32°C in the knee and 29°C in the ankle). Gout ensues when an inflammatory response is triggered.

Urate Production and Elimination. The total-body urate pool, with which sodium urate in plasma is miscible, is determined by rates of uric acid production and disposal and is expanded in patients with gout (Table 251–2A). Urate arises from the action of *xanthine oxidase* on its substrates, the purine bases hypoxanthine and xanthine (Fig. 251–1). Dietary purines are largely degraded to urate by catabolic enzymes, including xanthine oxidase, located in the intestinal epithelium. Purine restriction can modestly reduce serum urate by 0.6 to 1.8 mg per deciliter, but variation in absorption has not been implicated as a cause of hyperuricemia. The majority of urate is produced by hepatic xanthine oxidase acting on hypoxanthine and xanthine derived from the degradation of nucleic acids of senescent cells and from the metabolic turnover of cellular purine nucleotides. The latter arise from two biosynthetic pathways, termed *"de novo"* and *"salvage"* (or *"reutilization"*) (see Fig. 251–1).

TABLE 251–1. CLASSIFICATION OF HYPERURICEMIA AND GOUT

Type	Disturbance in Uric Acid, Purine Metabolism	Inheritance
Primary		
I. Idiopathic (>99% of primary gout)		
A. Normal urinary excretion (80–90% of primary gout)	Decreased renal clearance ± overproduction of urate	Polygenic
B. Increased urinary excretion (10–20% of primary gout)	Overproduction ± decreased renal clearance of urate	Polygenic
II. Due to specific inherited metabolic defects (<1% of primary gout)		
A. PP-ribose-P synthetase over-activity	Increased *de novo* purine synthesis	X-linked
B. Hypoxanthine-guanine phosphoribosyltransferase deficiency	Impaired purine salvage + increased *de novo* purine synthesis	X-linked
Secondary		
I. Glucose-6-phosphatase deficiency (Gierke's glycogen storage disease)	Increased catabolism of adenine nucleotides + secondary increase in purine synthesis *de novo*	Autosomal recessive
II. Chronic hemolysis; erythroid, myeloid, and lymphoid proliferative disorders	Increased cell and nucleic acid turnover	
III. Renal mechanisms		
A. Familial progressive renal insufficiency	Reduced renal functional mass and various defects in renal tubular function	Variable
B. Acquired chronic renal insufficiency	Reduced renal functional mass	
C. Drugs (diuretics, cyclosporine, toxins, including lead)	Inhibit urate secretion or enhance reabsorption	
D. Endogenous metabolic products (lactate, ketoacids, β-hydroxybutyrate)	Inhibit urate secretion	

TABLE 251–2. URIC ACID PRODUCTION AND ELIMINATION

A. Urate Kinetics	Milligrams (mmol)
Total miscible pool	1200 (7.2)
Daily turnover	600–900 (3.6–5.4)
Daily production	750 (4.5)
Daily intestinal uricolysis	100–365 (0.6–2.2)
Daily urinary excretion	500–1000 (3–6) on normal diet
	420 ± 75 (2.5 ± 0.5)
	on purine restricted diet

B. Renal Clearance (Four-Component, Bidirectional Transport Model)	Relative Amount
1. *Glomerular filtration* • Complete • ↓ By diuretics, renal failure	100
2. *Tubular reabsorption* • Active, linked to Na⁺ reabsorption • Inhibited by *uricosuric drugs:* probenecid, sulfinpyrazone, benzbromarone, high-dose aspirin (> 2 grams/d)	98–100
3. *Tubular secretion* • Active process • Inhibited by agents that cause *hyperuricemia:* pyrazinamide, low-dose aspirin, lactate, β-hydroxybutyrate, branched-chain ketoacids	50
4. *Postsecretory reabsorption*	40–44
Net clearance	**6–10**

Note: Gouty individuals have shown enlarged urate pools and in some cases increased urate turnover. Daily urinary excretion of uric acid is an index of urate production, provided renal function is normal. About 10% of patients with idiopathic gout are "urate overexcretors," defined as a daily urinary excretion exceeding the normal mean + 2 SD (i.e., >600 mg on a purine-restricted diet or >800 mg on an ordinary diet).

Most urate is eliminated by renal excretion (Table 251–2B). About one third is degraded by bacteria in the gut; this increases substantially in renal insufficiency. Uricosuric agents act by blocking urate reabsorption, while other drugs and weak organic acids raise serum urate by blocking renal urate secretion (see Table 251–2B). The latter mechanism contributes to the hyperuricemia associated with fasting, alcohol metabolism, and ketoacidosis.

Mechanisms of Hyperuricemia. About 10% of patients with gout show evidence of urate overproduction, as indicated by urinary excretion of uric acid exceeding the normal mean plus two standard deviations (>600 mg per 24 hours on a purine-restricted diet, >800 mg on an ordinary diet). The highest overproduction occurs in patients with either of two rare inherited defects in the regulation of purine nucleotide synthesis, deficiency of the salvage enzyme hypoxanthine-guanine phosphoribosyltransferase (HPRT) and overactivity of phosphoribosylpyrophosphate (PP-ribose-P) synthetase (see Fig. 251–1).

In the majority of patients with idiopathic gout, renal function is normal, but clearance of filtered urate is reduced, resulting in hyperuricemia. No specific renal abnormality has been identified to account for this.

Urate excretion diminishes with the onset of renal insufficiency, but in general, gout is uncommon in patients with chronic renal failure. However, several kindreds have been reported in which early-onset hyperuricemia, gout, and progressive renal failure (with or without hypertension), are associated (see Table 251–1). Other factors that have been implicated in causing hyperuricemia and gout through a renal mechanism include chronic lead nephropathy, alcohol abuse, and certain drugs (see Tables 251–1 and 251–2B). Hyperuricemia and idiopathic gout are associated with both obesity

and hypertriglyceridemia. In some gouty patients, weight reduction and abstinence from alcohol reverse hypertriglyceridemia, hyperuricemia, and evidence of both overproduction and impaired renal clearance of urate.

Mechanism of the Acute Gouty Attack. A. B. Garrod noted correctly in 1859 that ". . . true gouty inflammation is always accompanied with a deposition of urate of soda in the inflamed part. . . . The deposited urate of soda may be looked upon as the cause, and not the effect, of gouty inflammation." The neutrophil is an essential mediator of acute inflammation in gout (Fig. 251–2). Ingestion of MSU crystals causes neutrophils to release leukotrienes, interleukin-1, and a glycoprotein "crystal chemotactic factor," which further amplify neutrophil infiltration into the involved joint. Activated neutrophils also produce superoxide and release lysosomal enzymes, owing to crystal-induced rupture of lysosomal membranes and to cell lysis. The resulting cleavage of complement peptides and kinins from precursors induces pain, vasodilation, and vascular permeability. Released lysosomal and cytoplasmic enzymes, as well as collagenase and prostaglandins produced by joint mesenchymal cells, contribute to chronic articular destruction and tissue necrosis.

Extracellular urate crystals are often found in asymptomatic joints of gouty individuals. Attacks may be initiated and terminated by plasma proteins that selectively adsorb to crystals and modify their interaction with neutrophils. Early in an attack, IgG antibody, possibly induced by MSU crystals acting as antigens, may serve as a nucleating agent that promotes MSU crystallization and increases their phagocytosis by neutrophils, enhancing release of lysosomal enzymes. Late in an attack, lipoproteins containing apoprotein B (Apo B) enter the inflamed joint from plasma and coat MSU crystals, inhibiting phagocytosis, neutrophil oxidative metabolism, superoxide production, and cytolysis. Qualitative and quantitative differences in protein modulators may account for the variable inflammatory response to urate crystals in gouty and nongouty individuals.

Tophi. A tophus is a deposit of fine, needle-shaped MSU crystals, surrounded by a chronic mononuclear cell reaction and a foreign body granuloma of epithelial and giant cells, which may be multinucleate (see Fig. 251–2). Tophi are commonly found in articular and other cartilage, synovia, tendon sheaths, bursae and other periarticular structures, epiphyseal bone, subcutaneous tissues, and the kidney interstitium.

Compared with the acute gouty attack, tophi evoke little inflammatory response and generally develop silently. In bone and articular cartilages they may be detected radiographically in gouty individuals who lack tophi in subcutaneous tissues and who rarely experience acute attacks of arthritis. In the joint, tophi gradually enlarge, causing degeneration of cartilage and subchondral bone, proliferation of synovium and marginal bone, and sometimes fibrous or bony ankylosis. The punched-out lesions of bone commonly seen on radiograph represent marrow tophi, which may communicate with the urate crust on the articular surface through defects in the cartilage. In vertebral bodies, urate deposits involve the marrow spaces adjacent to the intervertebral disks.

The Gouty Kidney. Interstitial deposits of MSU crystals in the medulla or pyramids, with surrounding mononuclear and giant cell reaction, are found commonly in gouty patients at autopsy and have been referred to as "urate nephropathy." Crystalline deposits of uric acid (not urate) within distal tubules and collecting ducts may occur and lead to dilatation and atrophy of the more proximal tubules. Renal disease is common in gout but generally mild and slowly progressive. Interstitial nephropathy may be due to urate deposits but also can be present in their absence. Other possible causes include nephrosclerosis due to hypertension, uric acid stone disease, infection, aging, and lead toxicity.

Uric Acid Nephrolithiasis. About 10 to 25% of gouty patients experience renal stones, over 200-fold higher than in the general population. The incidence of stones exceeds 20% when daily uric acid excretion >700 mg (see Table 251–2A) and is about 50% at 1100 mg. Prevalence of stones is also related to hyperuricemia and reaches 50% at serum urate levels > 12 mg per deciliter. Over 80% of the stones are uric acid (not sodium urate); the remainder are mixtures of uric acid and calcium oxalate or calcium oxalate or phosphate alone.

For reasons that are unclear, both gouty and nongouty uric acid stone formers exhibit persistently low urinary pH, which favors uric

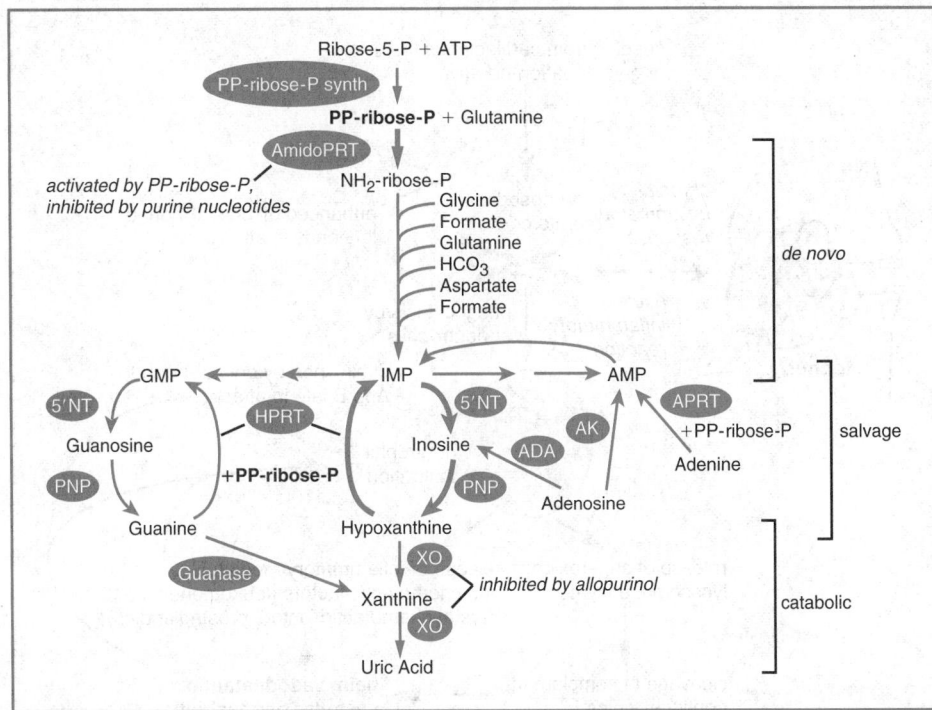

FIGURE 251–1. Intracellular purine metabolism and the basis for "metabolic" hyperuricemia. In the *"de novo"* pathway, the purine ring (hypoxanthine) of inosinic acid (IMP) is constructed from precursors on a ribose-5′-phosphate backbone derived from PP-ribose-P. At IMP the pathway branches, giving rise to AMP and GMP and their derivatives. In the "salvage" pathway, the preformed purine bases hypoxanthine, guanine, and adenine, derived from turnover of IMP, GMP, and AMP, are directly condensed with PP-ribose-P by HPRT and APRT to regenerate these ribonucleotides. Some of the hypoxanthine formed by nucleotide turnover is diverted to the liver and catabolized by XO to uric acid; the remainder is salvaged by HPRT.

Operation of the salvage pathway (the more economical in terms of energy required) reduces *de novo* activity because (1) HPRT and APRT have greater affinity for PP-ribose-P than amidoPRT (the first committed enzyme of the *de novo* pathway), (2) base salvage lowers the concentration of PP-ribose-P, which converts amidoPRT to an inactive form, and (3) the nucleotide endproducts of the HPRT and APRT reactions directly inhibit amidoPRT. Allopurinol, by blocking XO, enhances salvage of hypoxanthine, further inhibiting *de novo* activity; this reduces purine excretion more than is expected from inhibition of uric acid formation alone.

Deficiency of HPRT causes an obligatory loss of all hypoxanthine and guanine as urate. This also allows a compensatory increase in *de novo* pathway activity owing to reduced formation of inhibitory nucleotides and increased concentration and availability of PP-ribose-P for the amidoPRT reaction. In individuals with inherited "overactive" variants of PP-ribose-P synthetase, increased formation of PP-ribose-P stimulates amidoPRT, markedly enhancing *de novo* purine synthesis. The excess IMP formed is degraded to urate.

Increased nucleotide breakdown can cause hyperuricemia by increasing the production of XO substrates and by releasing inhibition of amidoPRT. This biphasic mechanism has been implicated in the hyperuricemia and gout associated with glucose-6-phosphatase deficiency (glycogen storage disease type I); glucose-6-phosphate accumulates at the expense of hepatic ATP, with degradation of AMP to urate. Hyperuricemia may occur acutely in various conditions that result in nucleotide catabolism: hypoxia, metabolism of some sugars, vigorous exercise in normal individuals, and moderate exercise in patients with metabolic myopathies. (PP-ribose-P synth = phosphoribosylpyrophosphate synthetase; AmidoPRT = amidophosphoribosyl transferase; 5′NT = 5′-nucleotidase; HPRT = hypoxanthine-guanine phosphoribosyltransferase; APRT = adenine phosphoribosyltransferase; PNP = purine nucleoside phosphorylase; ADA = adenosine deaminase; AK = adenosine kinase; XO = xanthine oxidase.)

acid stone formation. At pH 5 and 37°C, free uric acid has a solubility of only 15 mg per deciliter. Thus supersaturation is required to excrete an average uric acid load in a normal urine volume. The solubility increases more than 10-fold at pH 7 and more than 100-fold at pH 8.

CLINICAL MANIFESTATIONS. The peak age of onset of gout is about 45 in men, by which time the average gouty male has been exposed to 20 or 30 years of asymptomatic hyperuricemia and to varying degrees of tissue urate deposition. In predisposed women, gout usually occurs some years after menopause, when they become hyperuricemic.

Acute Gouty Arthritis. Gout usually presents as a fulminating arthritic attack affecting the lower extremity. Over 75% of first attacks are monarticular; at least half involve the metatarsophalangeal joint of the great toe (podagra). Next in order are the instep, ankle, heel, knee, wrist, finger, and elbow. Tenosynovitis, bursitis, or cellulitis also may occur. Minor episodes of "ankle sprain" or twinges of pain in the great toe may precede the first attack, sometimes by several years. More often the attack occurs explosively during apparent good health, often at night. Within minutes to hours the affected joint becomes hot, dusky red, and exquisitely tender and

painful. With very severe attacks, there may be fever, leukocytosis, and increased erythrocyte sedimentation rate, suggesting infection. The course of an untreated attack is variable, resolving in hours or a few days when mild and lasting many days to several weeks when severe. As the attack subsides, desquamation of inflamed skin over the affected joint may occur. Once the attack has broken, recovery is generally rapid and complete. The patient then re-enters an asymptomatic phase, often termed "intercritical" or "interval" gout.

The subsequent course is variable, but commonly a pattern of recurrences develops. Attacks often follow a precipitating event such as a long walk, trauma, surgery, alcohol or dietary overindulgence, starvation, infection, or the start of hypouricemic drug therapy. In the untreated patient, attacks often increase in frequency, and they may become more severe, last longer, and are more often polyarticular. Later attacks may involve the shoulder or hip or rarely the sacroiliac, sternoclavicular, or mandibular joints or even the spine. The more distal the site, the more typical is the attack. Eventually, attacks may be refractory to usually effective measures; they resolve incompletely, and disability may become permanent.

Chronic Tophaceous Gout. Progressive inability to dispose of urate results insidiously in tophaceous crystal depositing in and

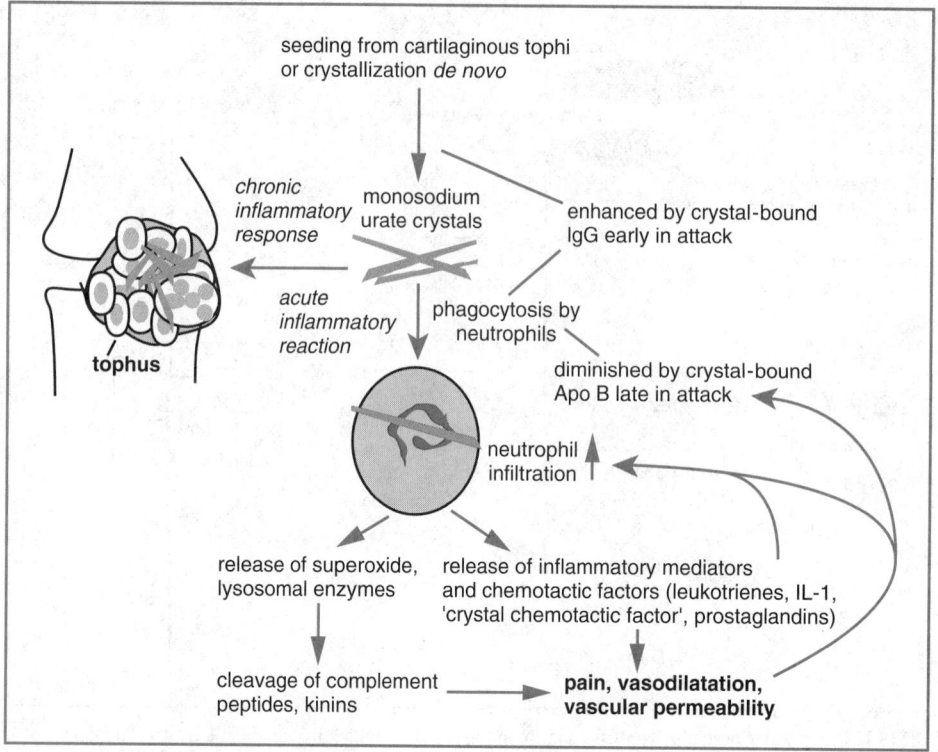

FIGURE 251-2. Inflammatory responses to monosodium urate crystals.

around joints. Tophi may first appear as superficial yellowish-white infiltrates on the fingertips, palms, and soles and later as irregular, asymmetric enlargement of joints, fusiform or nodular enlargements of the Achilles tendon, or saccular distensions of the olecranon bursa (Fig. 251–3). A classic, though relatively infrequent, site of tophi is the helix or anthelix of the external ear. Visible tophi develop in 10 to 25% of gouty patients and in >50% of those who are noncompliant; time of appearance after the initial attack is correlated with the degree and duration of hyperuricemia and with renal insufficiency. In rare patients, often those with gout secondary to a myeloproliferative disease, tophi are present at the time of the initial attack.

Although tophi themselves are relatively painless, they often result in stiffness and persistent aching that limit use of affected joints. Destruction of cartilage and bone by tophi leads to radiolucent "punched-out" lesions and to cortical erosions with characteristic "overhanging margins" (see Fig. 251–3). Eventually, extensive destruction of joints may be disabling, and large subcutaneous tophi may cause grotesque deformities. The stretched, thin skin over tophi may ulcerate and extrude white chalky or pasty "milk of urate" composed of myriads of fine, needle-like crystals. The olecranon bursa may be massively distended with this material, which may be mistaken for pus if not examined by polarized light microscopy. Rarely, tophi may involve the tongue, larynx, corpus cavernosum and prepuce of the penis, aortic or mitral valves, and cardiac conducting system, causing rhythm disturbances. They do not involve the liver, spleen, lungs, or central nervous system.

Gouty Nephropathy. Progressive renal failure due to urate nephropathy may occur in patients with inherited metabolic disorders that cause extreme urate overproduction and possibly in rare forms of inherited renal disease and chronic lead poisoning. Isosthenuria and mild intermittent proteinuria occur in about one third of patients with idiopathic gout. Decline in renal function is correlated with aging, hypertension, renal calculi, pyelonephritis, or independently occurring nephropathy. Hyperuricemia *per se* is not a risk factor for renal insufficiency.

Acute oliguric renal failure can result from bilateral tubular obstruction by uric acid crystals. This occurs in several clinical settings, including untreated leukemia and lymphoma, during chemotherapy for these disorders (tumor lysis syndrome), and in the presence of severe dehydration and acidosis. This condition is preventable by maintaining a high urine volume, with alkalinization, and by pretreating with allopurinol.

DIAGNOSIS. The sudden onset of severe inflammatory arthritis in a peripheral joint, especially of the lower extremity, suggests gout. A history of discrete attacks separated by completely asymptomatic periods is helpful for diagnosis. The diagnosis is established by demonstrating brilliant, negatively birefringent, needle-shaped MSU crystals by polarized light microscopy in the leukocytes of synovial fluid (see Ch. 236) (Fig. 251–4). The synovial fluid leukocyte count ranges from 5000 to over 50,000 per cubic millimeter, depending on the acuteness of inflammation. A Gram stain and culture of synovial fluid should always be obtained to evaluate infection, which may coexist.

Determining the 24-hour urinary excretion of uric acid can be informative, particularly in the young, markedly hyperuricemic patient in whom a metabolic etiology may be suspected. The sample should be collected after 3 days of moderate purine restriction, during an intercritical period. Values >600 mg per 1.72 square meters per day under these conditions suggest overproduction, and those >800 mg per day warrant additional studies for a specific subtype of primary gout, such as HPRT deficiency or PP-ribose-P synthetase overactivity, or of secondary gout, such as a myeloproliferative disorder. Elevated urinary uric acid excretion also predicts a higher risk for renal stones and is an indication for allopurinol rather than uricosuric drug therapy for gout.

DIFFERENTIAL DIAGNOSIS. Acute gout must be differentiated from pseudogout, acute rheumatic fever, rheumatoid arthritis, traumatic arthritis, osteoarthritis, pyogenic arthritis, sarcoid arthritis, cellulitis, bursitis, tendinitis, and thrombophlebitis. Gout can coexist with most of these conditions. Podagra, the most common initial presentation of gout, can be mimicked by trauma, degenerative arthritis, acute sarcoidosis, psoriatic arthritis, pseudogout, Reiter's syndrome, infection, and in the immediate postoperative period following parathyroidectomy can be caused by hydroxyapatite crystals. Pseudogout (see Ch. 252), which is manifested by acute attacks of arthritis of knees and other joints, is often accompanied by calcification of joint cartilage; the synovial fluid contains nonurate crystals of calcium pyrophosphate. When gout and pseudogout coexist, both types of crystals will be found in synovial leukocytes.

TREATMENT. Understanding the rationale for treatment by both the physician and patient is essential for long-term success. One aspect is aimed at terminating the acute inflammatory gouty attack, and the other is aimed at correcting the underlying metabolic problem (Table 251–3).

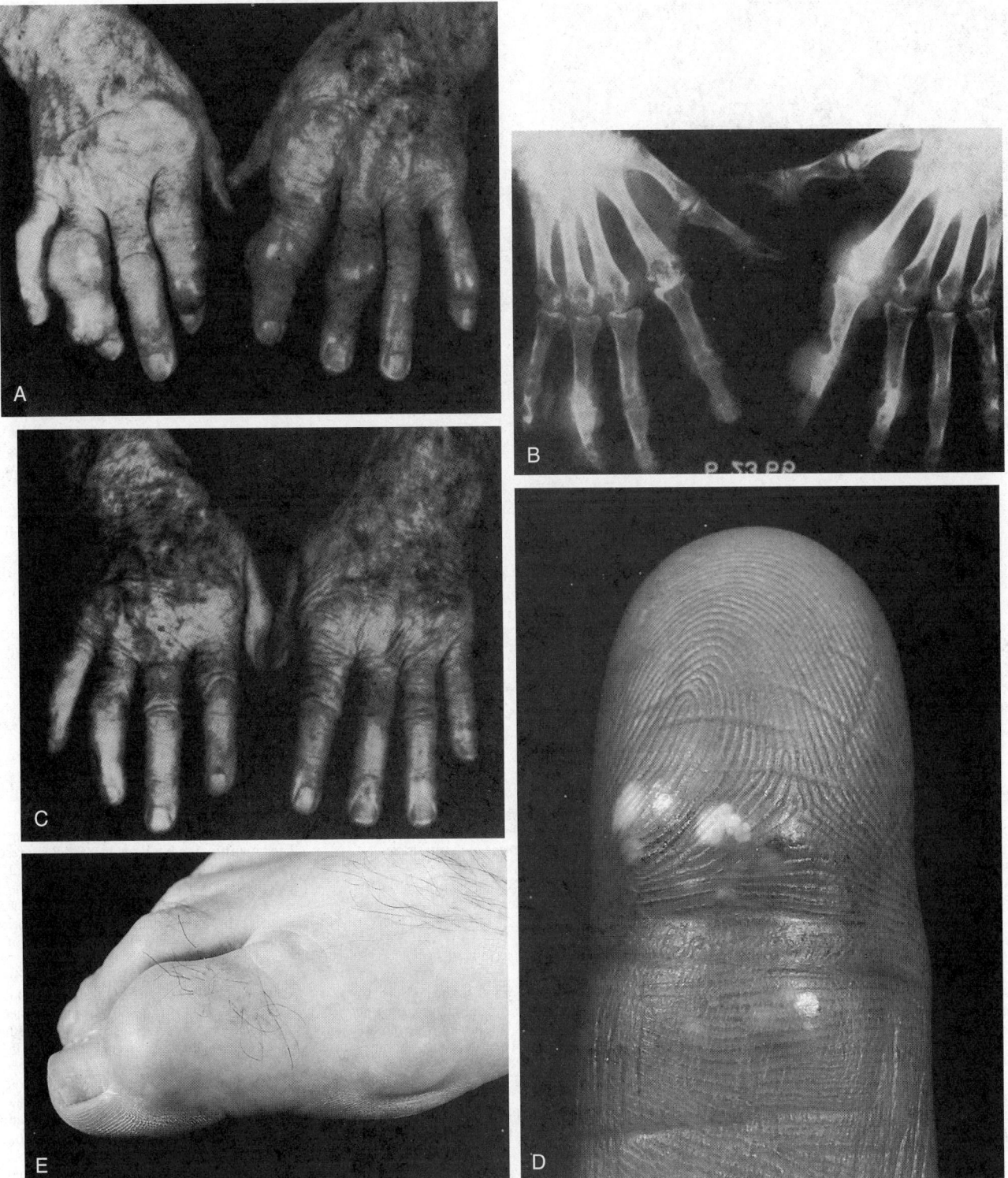

FIGURE 251–3. Tophaceous gout. *A–C,* Chronic gouty arthritis with tophaceous destruction of bone and joints *(A, B)* and improvement after 3 years of treatment with allopurinol, prophylactic colchicine, and a moderately low purine diet *(C). D,* Tophaceous deposits in digital pad of a 28-year-old man with systemic lupus erythematosus under treatment with diuretics. A single attack of gout had occurred 2 years earlier. *E,* Tophaceous enlargement of the great toe in a 44-year-old man with a 4-year history of recurrent gouty arthritis.

Acute Attack. The affected joint(s) should be kept at rest and therapy begun promptly with full doses of an oral nonsteroidal anti-inflammatory drug (NSAID). Salicylates should not be used because of their effects on urate excretion (see Table 251–2). The typical monarticular acute attack responds within 24 hours and resolves in 48 to 72 hours; established or polyarticular attacks may require longer treatment. Once the attack subsides, the NSAID is tapered over several days and discontinued. Hypouricemic therapy should not be initiated during an acute attack because it is ineffec-

tive in relieving inflammatory symptoms and may induce a recurrent attack by mobilizing urate from tissues.

Oral colchicine is effective therapy for acute gout but has a low therapeutic index; relief of pain often coincides with gastrointestinal toxicity. If an attack does not respond in 48 hours, alternative therapy should be used. If oral medication is precluded, intravenous colchicine may be used *with caution.* Colchicine is a microtubule poison; it is retained in cells (half-life about 30 hours) and is not dialyzable. Dose-related toxicity includes alopecia, bone marrow

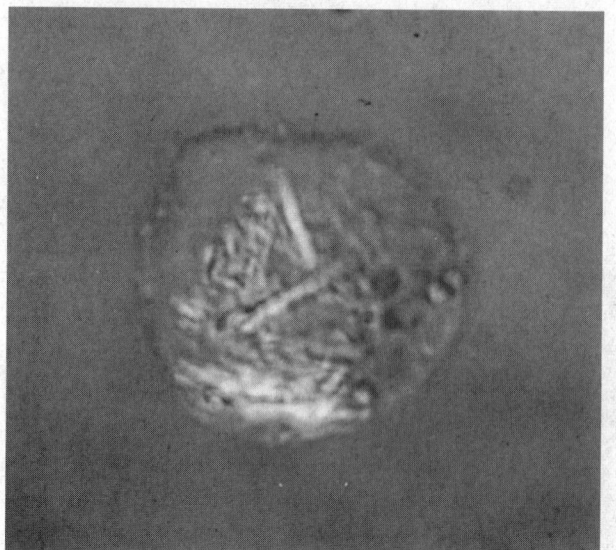

FIGURE 251–4. Sodium urate monohydrate crystals phagocytosed by leukocyte in synovial fluid from acute gouty arthritis, examined by polarized light.

suppression, and hepatocellular damage. Deaths from overdosage have been reported. Blood counts should be monitored during intravenous use of colchicine and periodically during long-term oral therapy. Dosage should be reduced in the presence of renal or hepatic disease, and it should not be used in patients with advanced disease. Reversible myopathy has occurred in elderly patients on daily colchicine prophylaxis who have been treated with larger doses for an acute attack.

Interval Phase. Patients should be warned that acute attacks

may still occur, particularly in the first 6 months or so after beginning hypouricemic therapy. Oral colchicine is effective prophylaxis to prevent recurrent attacks, but an NSAID should be taken at the first sign of prodromal symptom, if recognizable. Although hypouricemic therapy should not be initiated during an acute attack, once begun, it should *not* be interrupted during subsequent attacks. Hypertension should be treated vigorously; if hyperuricemia worsens, antihyperuricemic drug therapy can be initiated or appropriately increased.

Long-Term Management. Use of a drug to lower the serum uric acid level to ≤6 mg per deciliter is indicated in all patients with visible tophi or radiographic evidence of urate deposits or with a history of two or more major attacks of gouty arthritis. Allopurinol is preferred unless the patient is already well managed with a uricosuric agent. With either type of agent, the number of acute attacks may increase during the first few months unless prophylactic colchicine is given; after 12 to 18 months, the frequency of attacks should decline.

Allopurinol reduces urate production by inhibiting xanthine oxidase, with secondary reduction of *de novo* purine synthesis (see Fig. 251–1). Its major active metabolite, oxypurinol, has a long half-life (28 hours) and is primarily responsible for these effects during maintenance. In contrast with uricosuric agents, allopurinol reduces urinary uric acid excretion, is effective in renal failure and very useful in controlling urolithiasis, and its action is not blocked by salicylate. In the presence of renal insufficiency, the maintenance dose of allopurinol should be reduced, since the half-life of oxypurinol is prolonged. Allopurinol-induced xanthinuria has resulted in xanthine renal stones on rare occasions in patients with HPRT deficiency and during chemotherapy for leukemias.

Allopurinol is well tolerated but may cause gastric irritation, diarrhea, or skin rash in about 3% of patients. In about 0.4%, allopurinol causes a serious hypersensitivity syndrome, with worsening renal function, hepatitis, and severe dermatologic injury (epidermal necrolysis, exfoliative dermatitis, erythema multiforme, Stevens-Johnson syndrome), often with fever, leukocytosis, and eosinophilia. Patients with renal insufficiency are at higher risk, particularly if dosage has not been appropriately reduced. Allopuri-

TABLE 251–3. TREATMENT OF GOUT

Acute Gout	Interval Gout	Long Term
Therapeutic goal: Terminate acute inflammatory attack	**Therapeutic goal:** Prevent recurrent attacks	**Therapeutic goals:** Prevent attacks; resolve tophi; maintain serum urate at ≤6 mg/dl
NSAID's *(preferred):* Indomethacin 50 mg qid *or* ibuprofen 800 mg tid (or other NSAID's in full doses) *(lower dose in renal insufficiency; contraindicated with peptic ulcer disease).* *OR*	**Colchicine, oral:** 0.6–1.2 mg daily as prophylaxis against recurrent attacks.	**Colchicine, oral:** 0.6–1.2 mg daily for 1–2 weeks before initiating hypouricemic therapy and for several months afterwards to prevent recurrent attacks during initial period of hypouricemic therapy.
Colchicine, oral *(used infrequently:* 0.6–1.2 mg (1–2 tablets), then 0.6 mg (1 tablet) q1–2h until attack subsides, *or* until nausea, diarrhea, or GI cramping develops. Maximum total dose 4–6 mg. If ineffective in 48 hr, do not repeat *(see text for discussion of colchicine toxicity).*	Start hypouricemic agent if indicated by frequent attacks, severe hyperuricemia, presence of tophi, urolithiasis, or urate overexcretion.	**Allopurinol:** Dose variable; usually 300 mg once daily, but up to 900 mg may be needed in occasional patient; dose should be reduced to 100 mg daily or every other day in patients with renal insufficiency *(see text for discussion of allopurinol hypersensitivity).* *OR*
Colchicine, IV *(only if oral medication is precluded):* 1–2 mg in 20 ml 0.9% saline infused slowly *(extravasation causes tissue necrosis);* dose may be repeated once in 6 hr. Few GI symptoms with IV use. Maximum total dose 4 mg per attack. Monitor blood counts.	High fluid intake to promote uric acid excretion in a dilute urine. Diet—moderate protein, low fat; avoid excessive alcohol. Treat hypertension if present.	**Uricosuric agent** (reduced efficacy if creatinine clearance <80 ml; ineffective if <30 ml): Probenecid 0.5–1 gram bid or sulfinpyrazone 100 mg tid or qid; usually well tolerated but may cause headache, GI upset, rash.
Steroids *(only if oral medication is precluded and NSAID's or colchicine are contraindicated, e.g., postoperatively):* Prednisone, 20–40 mg daily, or ACTH 25 U by slow IV infusion. Intra-articular steroids may be used to treat a single inflamed joint: triamcinolone hexacetonide 5–20 mg or dexamethasone phosphate 1–6 mg.		High fluid intake, particularly at night, to promote uric acid excretion in a dilute urine. Acetazolamide 250 mg at bedtime may be used to keep urine pH >6. Diet—moderate protein, low fat; avoid excessive alcohol. Treat hypertension if present.
Hypouricemic agents of no benefit for inflammatory attack and may initiate recurrent attack. Should not be started until attack has resolved, but *ongoing use should not be interrupted during an attack.*		

nol interferes with the metabolism and increases the half-life of azathioprine and 6-mercaptopurine used to treat leukemia and to prevent allograft rejection, conditions in which significant hyperuricemia and gout may be associated with renal insufficiency.

If the serum urate level can be maintained below saturating levels, some tophi resolve, and bone erosions may be reduced. In selected patients, surgical treatment of chronically draining tophi or removal of large extra-articular urate deposits may be advisable. Effective treatment of severe gout is difficult in certain situations, particularly in patients with renal failure and allopurinol hypersensitivity and if allopurinol may interfere with drug therapy necessary for allograft rejection or malignancy. Desensitization to allopurinol has been used in some patients with mild allergic reactions but is considered dangerous in those who have had severe hypersensitivity reactions.

Asymptomatic Hyperuricemia. Asymptomatic hyperuricemia is frequent in family members of patients with gout and in the general population. Less than a fifth of hyperuricemic individuals ever develop gout, and effective therapy can be begun when attacks do occur. In patients with a strong family history of tophaceous diseases or gout and renal problems, treatment with allopurinol should be begun before articular or renal complications develop.

Arellano F, Sacristan JA: Allopurinol hypersensitivity syndrome: A review. Ann Pharmacother 27:337, 1993. *Reviews over 100 reports of a serious potential complication of allopurinol therapy.*

Delaney V, Sumrani N, Daskalakis P, et al.: Hyperuricemia and gout in renal allograft recipients. Transplant Proc 24:1773, 1992. *Analyzes the risk of hyperuricemia and gout in over 200 renal transplant patients.*

Gaudry M, Roberge CJ, de Medicis R, et al.: Crystal-induced neutrophil activation: III. Inflammatory microcrystals induce a distinct pattern of tyrosine phosphorylation in human neutrophils. J Clin Invest 91:1649, 1993. *Signal transduction pathways involved in triggering the inflammatory response to urate crystals.*

Wallace SL, Singer JZ: Review: Systemic toxicity associated with the intravenous administration of colchicine—guidelines for use. J Rheumatol 15:495, 1988. *Provides guidelines for the cautious use of colchicine for treating gout.*

252 OTHER CRYSTAL DEPOSITION ARTHROPATHIES

H. Ralph Schumacher, Jr.

At least three different calcium-containing crystals are now known to deposit in joints and to be associated with a variety of patterns of arthritis in much the same way as urate crystals cause the various features of gouty arthritis. Calcium pyrophosphate and occasionally calcium oxalate produce linear or punctate calcifications in menisci and articular cartilage that can be readily seen on roentgenograms (Fig. 252–1). These calcifications are termed "chondrocalcinosis." Both these crystals and calcium apatite also can deposit diffusely in synovium and periarticular tissues, giving a soft tissue pattern on roentgenograms. Radiographs may not show obvious calcifications when crystals are relatively few. Definitive diagnosis is made only by aspiration of synovial fluid for identification of the crystal type. In addition to the crystals discussed below, others of various implications may be seen in joint fluids (Table 252–1).

Schumacher HR, Reginato AJ: Atlas of Synovial Fluid Analysis and Crystal Identification. Philadelphia, Lea & Febiger, 1991. *An extensively illustrated compendium of all joint fluid findings, including less common crystals and artifacts.*

CALCIUM PYROPHOSPHATE DIHYDRATE (CPPD) CRYSTAL DEPOSITION DISEASE (Pseudogout Syndrome)

CPPD crystals are rod- or rhomboid-shaped 2- to 20-μm-long, weakly birefringent crystals with positive elongation. CPPD crystals can be present without symptoms or can cause several patterns of arthritis. They are most frequent in the elderly. Up to 27% of nursing home patients in their 80's have radiographic evidence of chondrocalcinosis. Familial cases have been described in populations of various ethnic origins. Both genders are affected.

The cause of CPPD crystal deposition is not established, but local overproduction of pyrophosphate related to excessive activity of

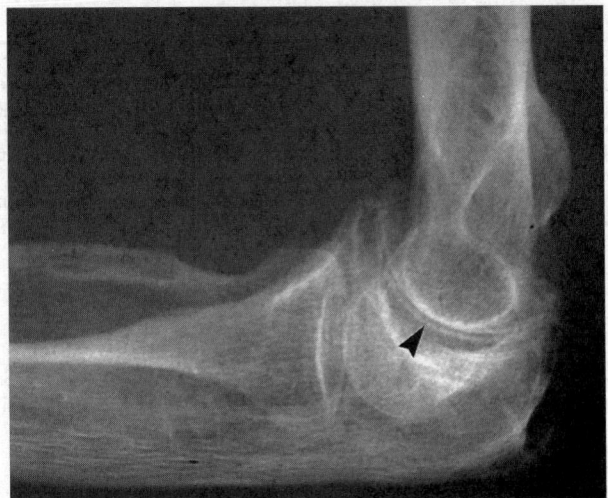

FIGURE 252–1. Chondrocalcinosis *(arrow)* at the elbow joint of a patient with CPPD deposition disease.

nucleoside triphosphate pyrophosphohydrolase, deficiency of phosphatases, and local changes in matrix proteoglycans and collagen are probably important. CPPD crystals deposit only in joints and adjacent tendons or bursae, where they produce hematoxyphilic clumps replacing the normal tissue. Virtually any joint can be involved, but knees, wrists, and second and third metacarpophalangeal joints are most common, so chronic cases can be confused with rheumatoid arthritis. Acute bouts of crystal-induced arthritis at one or more joints can mimic gout and lead to "pseudogout." Fever with bouts can mimic infection. CPPD crystal deposition often complicates osteoarthritis; this association is more prominent at knees than at hips. Whether crystals contribute to cartilage degeneration in osteoarthritis or are purely an epiphenomenon is not yet clear. Occasional severe arthritis mimics the destruction seen in neuropathic joints. Radiographic evidence of calcification can be present in some cases for years without inducing any symptoms. Others may have crystals in joint fluid with osteoarthritis-like radiographic changes but no visible chondrocalcinosis.

Synovial effusions may have leukocyte counts up to 100,000 per cubic millimeter and with 80 to 90% neutrophils during acute attacks. Between attacks or in osteoarthritis, crystals can be seen in clear, noninflammatory joint effusions.

CPPD crystal deposition can be an important clue to a number of associated diseases, many of which have specific treatments that can control systemic features if not the arthropathy. Some clearly associated diseases are shown in Table 252–2. CPPD crystal deposition is increased in knees after meniscectomy and may complicate advanced arthritides.

Treatment of inflammatory episodes with thorough aspiration and use of nonsteroidal anti-inflammatory drugs (NSAID's) is generally successful. Intra-articular steroid injections may provide relief in refractory involvement of individual joints. Intravenous colchicine may also be helpful. Chronic therapy with 0.6 to 1.2 mg of colchicine per day can decrease the frequency of attacks. Otherwise the prognosis is for slow progression. Joint replacement has been successful when needed.

Alvarellos A, Spilberg I: Colchicine prophylaxis in pseudogout. J Rheum 13:804, 1986. *Colchicine seems well worth trying to prevent acute exacerbations.*

Rachow JW, Ryan LM: Partial characterization of synovial fluid nucleotide pyrophosphohydrolase. Arthritis Rheum 28:1377, 1985. *Overproduction of pyrophosphate by this soluble extracellular enzyme is one possible factor in CPPD crystal deposition.*

Rahman MU, Shenberger KN, Schumacher HR: Initially unrecognized calcium pyrophosphate dihydrate deposition disease as a cause of fever. Am J Med 89:115, 1990. *Even mild crystal-induced joint findings can cause potentially confusing fever.*

APATITE CRYSTAL DEPOSITION DISEASE

Individual apatite crystals can be seen only by electron microscopy, but clumps of these crystals appear as 2- to 25-μm shiny (but not generally birefringent) globules that can suggest the diag-

TABLE 252–1. DIFFERENTIAL DIAGNOSTIC FEATURES FOR SOME OF THE CRYSTAL-ASSOCIATED ARTHROPATHIES

	Crystal Size (μm)	Crystal Shape	Crystal Birefringence and Elongation	Other Points	X-ray Findings
Calcium pyrophosphate	2–20	Rods, rhomboids	Weak positive	Elderly and consider associated metabolic diseases	Chondrocalcinosis, bony sclerosis
Apatite	2–25	Chunks or globules*	Nonbirefringent	Clumps stained with alizarin red S	Soft tissue calcification
Oxalate	2–15	Rods, bipyramids	Positive	Renal failure	Chondrocalcinosis or soft tissue calcification
Monosodium urate	2–20	Rods, needles	Bright negative	Middle-aged men and elderly women	Cysts and erosions; tophi may calcify
Liquid lipid crystals	2–12	Maltese crosses	Positive	Unexplained acute arthritis	
Cholesterol	10–80	Notched rectangles	Positive or negative	May complicate RA and OA	
Depot corticosteroids	4–15	Irregular or rods	Bright positive or negative	Can cause iatrogenic inflammation	
Immunoglobulins, other proteins	3–60	Rods or irregular	Positive or negative	Cryoglobulinemia	
Charcot-Leyden	10–25	Spindles	Positive or negative	Eosinophilic synovitis	

* Aggregates are seen by light microscopy. Individual needle-shaped crystals are seen only by electron microscopy.

nosis. Apatite crystal deposition and crystal-induced inflammation are common factors in bursitis and periarthritis. Apatites also occur in some otherwise unexplained acute arthritis, and in osteoarthritic joint effusions. Most joints or bursae can be involved, with more common sites including shoulders, hips, knees, and digits (including the first metatarsophalangeal joint). Joint or periarticular inflammation can be acute or chronic. An extremely destructive arthritis has been noted especially at shoulders ("Milwaukee shoulder"), hips, and knees in elderly patients. Radiographs can show soft tissue calcifications with or without bone erosions. Definitive diagnosis of the crystal type is only by electron microscopy with electron probe elemental analysis, x-ray diffraction, or infrared spectroscopy. Other calcium phosphates, such as octacalcium phosphate, can be seen along with the apatite; the significance of amounts of other associated calcium phosphates is not known. Synovial or bursal effusions can have many or few leukocytes. Serum studies are generally normal except that phosphate levels are often elevated in renal dialysis patients, who are at high risk of apatite deposition, and in tumoral calcinosis due to renal retention of phosphate.

Apatite deposition also can be associated with scleroderma and the other connective tissue diseases, repeated depot corticosteroid injections, central nervous system injury, and high-dose vitamin D therapy. In most instances, the cause of soft tissue apatite deposition is not known. Treatment for acute arthritis or periarthritis is with NSAID's or colchicine. Aspiration of crystals and local injection with depot corticosteroids also can be effective.

Doherty M, Holt M, MacMillan P, et al.: A reappraisal of "analgesic" hip. Ann Rheum Dis 45:272, 1986. *Destructive hip arthritis like the "Milwaukee shoulder" is felt to be related to apatite crystal deposition.*
Paul H, Reginato AJ, Schumacher HR: Alizarin red S staining as a screening test to detect calcium compounds in synovial fluid. Arthritis Rheum 26:191, 1983. *This describes a simple office screening test for apatite and other calcium-containing crystals.*
Pinals RS, Short CL: Calcific periarthritis involving multiple sites. Arthritis Rheum 9:566, 1966. *This recurrent calcific periarthritis is related to apatite crystals.*

OXALATE CRYSTAL DEPOSITION DISEASE

Calcium oxalate deposition can occur in joints along with other tissues of patients with renal failure who are on chronic hemodialysis or peritoneal dialysis, producing radiographic evidence of soft tissue calcification or chondrocalcinosis. Acute or chronic joint effusions with intracellular crystals can be seen. Masses of vertebral ox-

TABLE 252–2. SYSTEMIC CONDITIONS ASSOCIATED WITH CPPD DEPOSITION DISEASE

Hyperparathyroidism
Hemochromatosis
Hypophosphatasia
Hypomagnesemia
Myxedematous hypothyroidism
Ochronosis

alates can cause spinal cord compression. Diagnosis is made by identification of typical bipyramidal crystals in joint fluid or biopsy specimens. When less characteristic crystals are seen, other techniques as described under apatite deposition can be used. Vitamin C may potentiate oxalate deposition, so this might be avoided.

Hoffman EC, Schumacher HR, Paul H, et al.: Calcium oxalate microcrystalline-associated arthritis in end stage renal disease. Ann Intern Med 97:36, 1982. *Three cases with oxalosis and arthritis are described. Methods to identify oxalate crystals are included.*
Reginato AJ, Kurnik BRC: Calcium oxalate and other crystals associated with kidney disease and arthritis. Semin Arthritis Rheum 18:198, 1989. *Extensive oxalosis can involve skin, bursae, tendon sheaths, vessel walls, and joints, as well as kidneys and various viscera.*

GOUT

Monosodium urate (MSU) crystal deposition (see Color Plate 3*C*) in joints and other connective tissues accounts for the most frequent clinical manifestations of gout. The complex genetic, metabolic, and renal factors that interact to produce hyperuricemia and eventually gout are described in detail in Ch. 251. Gouty arthropathy and the gross tophaceous deposits in chronic gout are also described in Ch. 251 but are summarized here, as gout is the most common and prototypical of the crystal deposition diseases.

MSU crystals are rods or needles up to 15 to 20 μm in length and are brightly birefringent with negative elongation when viewed with compensated polarized light. Those from visible tophi or synovial microtophi tend to be more often needle-like, while some in acute arthritis can be very short. At least some crystals are intracellular during gouty arthritis. Leukocyte counts during attacks usually range from 10,000 to 50,000 per cubic millimeter, with 80 to 90% neutrophils. Gout is most common in middle-aged men but is increasingly seen in women after the menopause. It is very rare in premenopausal women but may occur with chronic renal failure. A variety of lower extremity joints are commonly involved, in addition to the classic first metatarsophalangeal joint, but any joint or bursa, including those in the upper extremities, can be affected by either acute or chronic arthritis. Chronic or recurrent acute gout can be polyarticular, can mimic rheumatoid arthritis, and may be misdiagnosed, especially if the typical dramatic early short-lived attacks are not appreciated and synovial fluid is not examined. Tophaceous gout can slowly destroy joints. Crystals are often present in joint fluids even between attacks and may contribute to low-grade inflammation and joint damage.

Radiographs show only soft tissue swelling early in gout but later can reveal cystic erosions with thin, overhanging edges of bone suggestive of gout. Soft tissue tophi are common around joints, in bursae, in Achilles tendons, and at the extensor surface of the forearm; ear tophi appear to be less common than in the past. Gout should be recognized as a syndrome resulting from the many possible causes noted in Ch. 251.

Treatment of acute gouty arthritis can be with NSAID's (although relatively high doses are needed), oral or intravenous colchicine, adrenocorticotropic hormone (ACTH), or prednisone. The latter two agents may be needed in complicated patients with renal failure, liver disease, or gastrointestinal disease. Colchicine is most effective early in attacks (see also Ch. 251). Joint aspiration with instillation of depot corticosteroids also may be used if a single joint is involved and infection is excluded. If recurrent attacks develop, chronic low doses of NSAID's or colchicine can suppress inflammation, but crystal accumulation will likely continue. Thus, with more frequent attacks or visible tophi, patients should be considered for long-term lowering of urate levels with a uricosuric agent such as probenecid (if renal function is good and the patient is not overexcreting uric acid) or, in other cases, allopurinol, a xanthine oxidase inhibitor.

Lawry GV, Fan PT, Bluestone R: Polyarticular versus monoarticular gout. A prospective, comparative analysis of clinical features. Medicine 67:335, 1988. *Polyarticular gout and other crystal-associated diseases continue to be misdiagnosed without synovial fluid analysis. Fever and other constitutional symptoms are common.*

Moreland LM, Ball GV: Colchicine and gout. Arthritis Rheum 34:782, 1991. *Some of the complex situations involved in colchicine use for acute and chronic gout are reviewed. There are risks both from disease progression and from drug toxicities. Colchicine, NSAID's, and allopurinol all require care in appropriate use.*

253 RELAPSING POLYCHONDRITIS

H. Ralph Schumacher, Jr.

This uncommon disease is characterized by recurrent inflammation and destruction of cartilaginous and other connective tissue structures. Frequently involved cartilages are the pinnae of the ears, nasal cartilages, and tracheal rings. Polychondritis occurs nearly equally in both genders and at any age, but with a peak of onset between the ages of 40 and 60.

The pathologic lesion seen by light microscopy consists of loss of matrix staining, predominantly superficial infiltration with polymorphonuclear neutrophils or lymphocytes, and eventual destruction of normal structures followed by fibrosis. Electron microscopy in addition shows alterations of superficial chondrocytes, matrix, and elastic fibers. The cause of polychondritis is unknown, but the location of lesions and frequency of associated systemic diseases suggest the importance of systemic factors. Antibodies to types II, IX, and X collagen and the presence of cell-mediated immunity to proteoglycan and type II collagen are evidence of immunologic aberrations. An association with HLA-DR4 has been noted.

Inflammation of the cartilaginous structures of the ears is the most common initial finding (see Color Plate 10*C*). There may be acute onset of pain and tenderness with erythema and swelling of one or both helices. The lobe is spared. Inner and middle ear involvement can occur, causing hearing loss or vertigo. Nasal cartilage involvement can produce a saddle nose. Laryngeal and tracheal disease can cause hoarseness or life-threatening upper respiratory obstruction. Ocular manifestations are common and include conjunctivitis, episcleritis, iridocyclitis, proptosis, and rarely other problems, such as optic neuritis. Antigens in the eye that are crossreactive with cartilage proteoglycans and their link protein have been identified.

Cardiac involvement, especially of the aortic root with aortic insufficiency, is seen in up to one fourth of cases. There also may be aortic aneurysms. Arthritis is reported in about three fourths of cases. This is generally nondestructive. Fever, rashes, oral or genital ulcers, and neurologic and renal disease can occur. Renal involvement can include glomerulonephritis and immunoglobulin A (IgA) nephropathy.

There are no diagnostic laboratory tests, although the erythrocyte sedimentation rate is often elevated. Antineutrophil cytoplasmic antibodies (ANCA's) have been reported. There may be anemia and leukocytosis. Roentgenograms can detect advanced tracheal narrowing. Computed tomographic (CT) scans and pulmonary function tests can detect more subtle airway obstruction.

Relapsing polychondritis is associated with other diseases in one third or more of cases. These include rheumatoid arthritis, systemic lupus erythematosus, Sjögren's syndrome, thyroid disease, ulcerative colitis, psoriasis, spondylarthropathies, Behçet's disease, vasculitis of various types, cryoglobulinemia, diabetes mellitus, biliary cirrhosis, panniculitis, malignancies, myelodysplastic syndromes, sinusitis, and mastoiditis. Wegener's granulomatosis and infections can cause potentially confusing chondritis.

In mild cases, nonsteroidal anti-inflammatory agents can be used for symptomatic treatment, although adrenocorticosteroids in the range of 30 to 60 mg of prednisone per day are generally needed for acute inflammatory episodes and severe respiratory involvement. Immunosuppressives and cyclosporine have been used with apparent benefit. Dapsone has been used with variable results in several series. Tracheostomy or stents may be life-saving if tracheal collapse occurs.

The course is unpredictable, with about 55% of subjects surviving for 10 years. Infection and systemic vasculitis caused more deaths than did airway obstruction in a recent series. Remissions do occur. Aortic valve disease has required surgery.

Chang-Miller A, Okamura M, Torres VE, et al.: Renal involvement in relapsing polychondritis. Medicine 66:202, 1987. *Glomerulonephritis often responds to corticosteroids or cytotoxic agents.*

Lang B, Rothenfusser A, Lanchbury JS: Susceptibility to relapsing polychondritis is associated with HLA-DR4. Arthritis Rheum 36:660, 1993. *HLA-DR4 was seen in 56% of 41 cases, suggesting similarities to rheumatoid arthritis, which is also DR4-associated.*

Michet CJ, McKenna CH, Luthra HS, et al.: Relapsing polychondritis. Survival and predictive role of early disease manifestations. Ann Intern Med 104:74, 1986. *Anemia, saddle nose deformity, and vasculitis appear to be poor prognostic signs.*

Pazirandeh M, Ziran BH, Khandelwal BK: Relapsing polychondritis and spondylarthropathies. J Rheum 15:630, 1988. *In addition to the many associated autoimmune diseases, one must also consider a possible relationship to psoriasis and spondylarthropathy.*

Yang CL, Brinkmann J, Rui HF, et al.: Autoantibodies to cartilage collagens in relapsing polychondritis. Arch Dermatol Res 285:245, 1993. *Immune mechanisms appear to be important.*

254 OSTEOARTHRITIS (Degenerative Bone Disease)

Thomas J. Schnitzer

Osteoarthritis (OA) is a disorder of diarthrodial joints characterized clinically by pain and functional limitations, radiographically by osteophytes and joint space narrowing, and histopathologically by alterations in cartilage integrity. The most common of all joint diseases, its importance derives from its economic impact, in terms of both productivity (single greatest cause of days lost from work) and cost of treatment (chronic use of analgesics and anti-inflammatory drugs). Although the etiology of the disorder is still not clearly understood, OA has been shown to be a family of disorders with cartilage as a target organ in which biomechanical factors play a central role and with risk factors such as age, weight, and occupation also of major importance. Since there is currently no treatment to prevent or ameliorate the basic disease process, medical treatment is aimed primarily at relieving pain, with orthopedic intervention largely reserved for those situations which cannot be controlled with more conservative therapy.

EPIDEMIOLOGY. OA is by far the most common joint disorder, one of the most common chronic diseases in the elderly, and a leading cause of disability. Because OA can be defined both radiographically and clinically and because there is little correlation between the two, the prevalence of this condition has been variously estimated in epidemiologic studies. Using radiographic criteria, prevalence of the joint findings steadily increases from <2% in women under age 45 to 30% in those aged 45 to 64 and to 68% in those older than 65. Prevalence in men is slightly higher in the younger age groups (younger than 45), while women are affected more commonly at ages over 55, except for disease of the hip.

The pattern of joint involvement in OA is strikingly affected by age, gender, and previous occupational history. Prior to age 55, there is little difference in joint pattern between men and women. In older men, hip OA is more common, while older women tend to have more involvement of the proximal interphalangeal (PIP) joints and the base of the thumb. Joints subjected to repeated trauma or overuse demonstrate a higher prevalence of OA. Cotton and mill workers have increased OA of the hand and involved fingers, miners demonstrate increased knee and spine involvement, and pneumatic drill workers experience increased elbow and wrist disease.

Racial and genetic factors are also important in OA prevalence and pattern. Chinese, Jamaican blacks, South African blacks, and Asian Indians have been shown to have a lower incidence of OA of the hip than Caucasians, while Japanese have an increased incidence, apparently related to the more frequent occurrence of congenital hip dysplasia. African-American women have a higher prevalence of knee OA than Caucasian women but a lower prevalence of involvement of the distal interphalangeal (DIP) joints of the hand (Heberden's nodes). Involvement of the DIP joints of the hands is particularly common in women and is often found to have a familial pattern of inheritance, with the female relatives of the proband having similar joint findings with a two- to fivefold increased prevalence.

Additional modifiable risk factors for OA also have been identified in recent studies. Weight demonstrates by far the strongest association with OA; and importantly, weight reduction has been shown to correlate with a reduction in the risk of later OA. Certain types of repetitive activities have been correlated with increased OA in the stressed joint (see above), while, interestingly, others have not. In particular, there appears to be no increased prevalence of knee OA in marathon runners, but this may be due to a self-selection process, with those experiencing knee pain unable to continue the activity. Smoking and osteoporosis have both been shown to be negatively associated with OA, but the explanation for this association is unknown.

PATHOLOGY. The hallmarks of OA on gross or arthroscopic examination are focal ulcerated areas of cartilage exposing underlying eburnated (ivory-appearing) bone that occur at the load-bearing areas of the joint surface as well as the juxta-articular osteophytes that grow at the joint margins. It is important to understand that these states represent the end stage of a continuum and that OA is a pathologic *process*. At its earliest stage, it presents as softening of the cartilage surface, progressing to fibrillation of the surface layers, loss of cartilage thickness, the development of clefts into the depth of cartilage, and eventual loss of cartilage integrity with release of shards of cartilage. Bone participates in this process as well, with reactive changes (bony sclerosis) underlying the areas of cartilage loss, the development of subchondral bone cysts that may communicate with the joint space and expand into geodes, and marginal osteophytes (new cartilage and bone growth) at non–weight-bearing areas.

The earliest histologic changes reveal loss of extracellular cartilage matrix, loss of chondrocytes in the surface layers of articular cartilage, and reactive changes in the deeper chondrocytes manifested by cellular division and "cloning" in an apparent attempt at repair. Later, there is progressive loss of chondrocytes at all levels, with marked thinning of the cartilage matrix and, in some instances, the development of fibrocartilage in place of lost hyaline cartilage. The surrounding synovium is largely unaffected, although in later disease cartilage fragments may incite focal inflammatory lesions without the progressive and destructive pannus seen in typical inflammatory arthropathies.

PATHOGENESIS. Articular cartilage serves two major functions: (1) to permit nearly frictionless joint motion and (2) to act as a "shock absorber" and transmit loads across joint surfaces to the surrounding tissues. The requisite properties of elasticity and high tensile strength are imparted by proteoglycans and collagen of the extracellular matrix that comprise over 90% of the cartilage substance. The proteoglycan elements of the matrix are actively being metabolized and turned over with a half-life of weeks. The highly negatively charged sulfated glycosaminoglycan components of the proteoglycans impart the elastic properties to cartilage. The collagen component is characterized by a unique structure (type II collagen), provides the tensile strength, and tightly constrains the proteoglycan molecules in a three-dimensional framework. The collagen fibers are covalently linked by other matrix molecules believed to provide the "glue" to hold the matrix intact. Collagen itself is extremely slowly metabolized (half-life of many years) in the normal state.

In OA, there is chondrocyte "exhaustion" with loss of matrix and cells, loss of cartilage integrity, and eventual ulceration. The reasons for failure of collagen repair are unknown but may relate to the role of mechanical factors preventing appropriate apposition of cartilage matrix or the inability to re-form the complex three-dimensional architecture in mature individuals.

The processes responsible for degrading collagen and proteoglycans in OA are driven by proteolytic enzymes being synthesized and released from the chondrocytes themselves. Although chondrocytes can respond to cytokines released from inflammatory cells in synovial fluid, in OA it appears that chondrocytic chondrolysis is initiated primarily by changes in mechanical properties of the surrounding matrix. The release of potent proteolytic enzymes and their subsequent activation in the matrix overwhelm the natural matrix defenses and ultimately result in collagen breakdown and proteoglycan cleavage. Fragments from these molecules are then released into the synovial fluid and enter the circulation, where they provide "markers" and can be used as a means to detect and measure the degradative process.

The factors responsible for activating chondrocytes to degrade matrix in OA are not known but in most instances may relate to changes in mechanical forces on the cartilage itself. Those conditions causing biomechanical alteration of cartilage are known to lead to OA: joint injury, abnormal joint loading due to neuropathic changes (Charcot joint) or ligamentous damage (ACL or meniscus injuries), altered joint surface congruity as in dysplasias, and muscle atrophy in the elderly. A number of metabolic conditions are known to predispose to the early onset of OA: ochronosis with the deposition of homogentisic acid and hemochromatosis with the deposition of iron. Gene defects affecting matrix structures would be expected to possibly lead to OA, but thus far genetic factors have played a role only in the development of dysplasias with secondary OA changes. The pathogenetic mechanisms and feedback loops associated with altered cartilage structure and biomechanics are demonstrated in Figure 254–1.

CLINICAL FEATURES. The initial stages of the OA process are clinically silent, which explains the high prevalence of radiographic and pathologic signs of OA in patients who exhibit no clinical symptoms of the disease. Even in later stages of OA, there is a poor correlation between clinical symptoms and alterations in cartilage and bone integrity, defined arthroscopically or by indirect imaging techniques (radiography, magnetic resonance imaging [MRI]). The factors or events that make the OA process clinically apparent are unknown but are likely to be heterogeneous in nature and invoke processes within the synovium, bone, and surrounding supporting structures (muscle, ligaments) that produce pain rather than involve cartilage itself, a completely aneural tissue.

Pain is the predominant symptom that prompts the diagnosis of OA, initially often involving only one joint, with others becoming painful subsequently. The pain is most often described as a deep ache, accompanied frequently by joint stiffness that follows periods of inactivity (upon arising in the morning, after sitting). Pain is aggravated by using the involved joints, may radiate or be referred to surrounding structures, and in the early stages of the disease is commonly relieved by rest. With more severe disease, pain may be persistent, interfering with normal function and preventing sleep, even with medical management. Such patients are candidates for surgery. Even in severe disease, systemic manifestations such as fever, weight loss, anemia, and elevated erythrocyte sedimentation rate (ESR) are not present.

The joints most commonly involved in OA are the metatarsophalangeal (MTP) joint of the great toe (hallux valgus or "bunion"), the proximal (PIP) and distal (DIP) interphalangeal joints, the carpometacarpal (CMC) joint of the thumb, hips, knees, and both lumbar and cervical spine. Interestingly, other joints, even major weight-bearing joints such as the ankle, are regularly spared unless involved in secondary forms of OA (Table 254–1). On physical examination, the joints may demonstrate tenderness, crepitus, and a limited range of motion. Joint swelling may be due to an accompanying synovial effusion or bony enlargement and osteophytes. Joint instability is seen only in severe disease or after internal derangement of the knee with disruption of one or more of the major supporting structures (e.g., anterior cruciate ligament, medial collateral ligament). Patients with far-advanced disease exhibit gross defor-

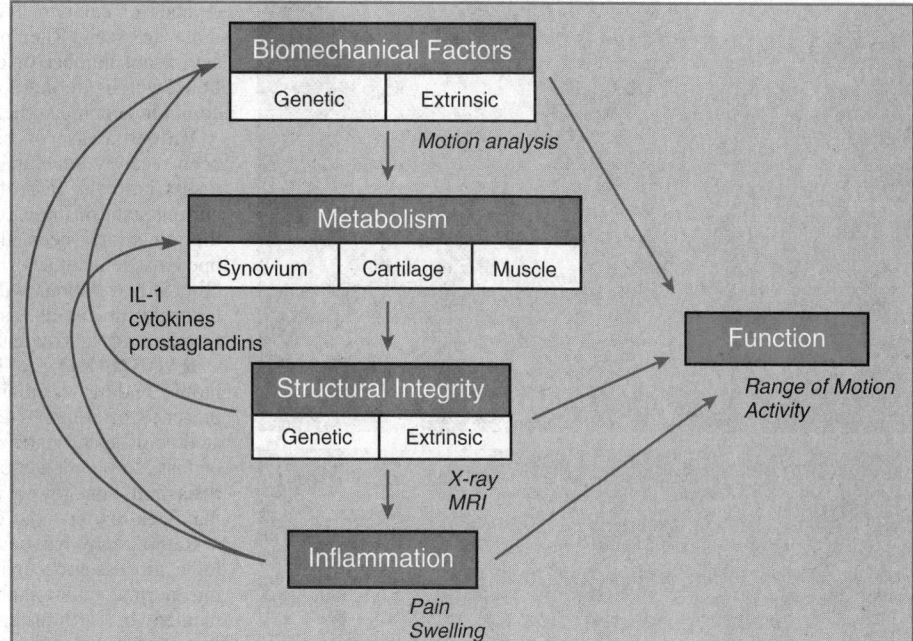

FIGURE 254–1. Pathogenetic pathways in osteoarthritis.

mity with subluxation of involved joints. Although OA is thought to be a uniformly progressive disease that invariably leads to joint replacement, this is not the case. The disease appears to stabilize in many patients with no worsening of signs or symptoms and actual improvement in some.

SPECIFIC JOINT INVOLVEMENT. Hand. Firm, slowly progressive bony enlargements of the DIP joints are called Heberden's nodes and represent marginal osteophytic spurs. Occasionally, the onset of symptoms is acute with sudden redness and tenderness in the involved joint. These changes can lead to deformity at these

TABLE 254–1. ETIOLOGIC CLASSIFICATION OF OSTEOARTHRITIS*

Idiopathic (primary)

Localized
 Hands: Heberden's nodes, erosive interphalangeal arthropathy
 Feet: hallux valgus, hammer toes; talonavicular osteoarthritis
 Knees: medial, lateral, patellofemoral compartments
 Hips: sites of cartilage loss—eccentric (superior), concentric (axial, medial), diffuse
 Spine: zygoapophyseal joints, osteophytes, intervertebral discs (spondylosis); ligaments, e.g., disseminated idiopathic skeletal hyperostosis
 Other single sites: shoulder, temporomandibular, carpometacarpal joints
Generalized—Includes three or more areas listed above
Mineral deposition diseases
 Calcium pyrophosphate deposition disease
 Hydroxyapatite arthropathy
 Destructive disease (e.g., Milwaukee shoulder)

Secondary

Post-traumatic
Congenital or developmental
 Legg-Calvé-Perthes hip dislocation
 Epiphyseal dysplasias
 Articular cartilage disorders associated with a gene deficiency (e.g., association with type II procollagen gene mutation)
Disturbed local tissue structure by primary disease, e.g., ischemic necrosis, tophaceous gout, hyperparathyroid cysts, Paget's disease, rheumatoid arthritis, osteopetrosis, osteochondritis
Miscellaneous additional diseases
 Endocrine: diabetes mellitus, acromegaly, hypothyroidism
 Metabolic: hemochromatosis, ochronosis, Gaucher's disease
 Neuropathic arthropathies
 Miscellaneous: frostbite, Kashin-Beck disease, caisson disease
 Mechanical: obesity, unequal lower extremity length; valgus/varus deformities, ligamentous laxity (including associations with type I procollagen gene mutations of Ehlers-Danlos syndrome).

*Compiled in part by Osteoarthritis Diagnostic Criteria Committee, American Rheumatism Association, 1983.

joints with lateral and flexor deviation. A related disorder, erosive OA, similarly produces repetitive episodes of acute symptoms and is differentiated by the additional finding of erosive changes on radiographs of the involved joints and a tendency to bony ankylosis. A genetic basis for Heberden's nodes appears to exist, the condition demonstrating a distinct female-dominant familial tendency (women are affected 10 times more commonly than men) (Fig. 254–2). Changes similar to those in the DIP joints occur in the PIP joints and are termed Bouchard's nodes. The only other joint to be commonly involved is the CMC joint of the thumb, often eliciting complaints of pain on use (wringing out clothes [washerwoman's hands] and grasping objects such as screwdrivers and doorknobs) and leading to a squared appearance of the base of the hand.

Knee. Idiopathic knee OA is a leading cause of painful ambulation and is directly related to weight; it is more common in women than in men. The medial compartment of the femorotibial joint space is most commonly affected, resulting in varus deformity (bow legs). Lateral compartment disease may lead to valgus (knock-knee) deformity. Patellofemoral disease has been shown recently to be common and may represent a substantial portion of knee pathology in patients presenting with knee pain. It is important to exclude other causes of knee pain such as internal derangements of the knee (which may lead to secondary knee OA), soft tissue sprains, bursal inflammation, and Baker's cysts (which may coexist with knee OA). In young women, the possibility of chondromalacia patellae should always be considered. Its cause is not known; it is almost always self-limited and is not thought to lead to OA. In idiopathic knee OA, physical examination of the involved joint often elicits crepitus, pain, and decreased range of motion. Effusions are not infrequently present but are often small and may be difficult to appreciate.

Hip. Although congenital (Legg-Calvé-Perthes disease) and developmental (slipped femoral capital epiphysis) abnormalities have long been implicated in secondary hip OA, the majority of primary hip OA is now believed to be the consequence of mild dysplasia of the femoral head and/or acetabulum resulting in incongruity of the articulating surfaces. With use of the joint, there is progressive cartilage degeneration and secondary bony productive changes typical of OA. Pain is typically referred to the groin, with anterior thigh and knee symptoms occasionally predominant. The majority of patients presenting with pain in their "hip" are suffering from OA of the lumbar spine. The earliest physical finding in hip OA is loss of internal rotation; with progressive disease, range of motion is limited further in all directions, and significant functional limitation occurs, often necessitating surgery.

Foot. The first MTP joint is the primary joint involved with associated bony swelling and deformity (bunion). Significantly more common in women than men, these changes have been attributed to

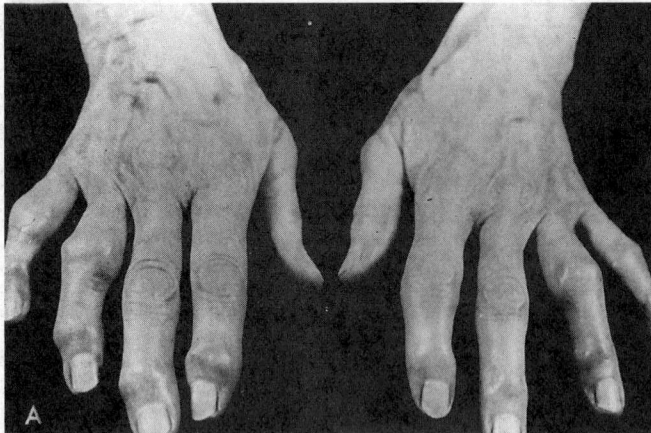

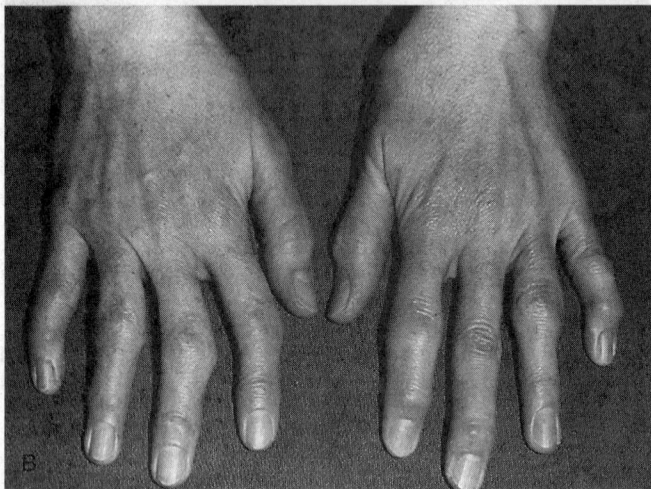

FIGURE 254–2. Typical hand deformities in osteoarthritis. *A,* Typical Heberden's and Bouchard's nodes comprise hypertrophic joint capsular and bony enlargement of the distal and proximal interphalangeal joints, respectively. *B,* Prominent Bouchard's nodes and minor subluxations may cause misdiagnosis of rheumatoid arthritis.

abnormal stresses imposed on the joint by footwear. In extreme cases, the joint space may be destroyed, leading to a condition known as "hallux rigidus," which may interfere with normal ambulation and necessitate surgical correction.

Spine. Technically, OA of the spine relates strictly to changes in synovial-lined joints (apophyseal and uncovertebral joints) that can lead to localized pain as well as irritation of adjacent nerve roots with referred pain in the form of radiculopathy. Nerve root compression resulting from apophyseal joint subluxation, prolapse of an intervertebral disc, or osteophytic spurring may occur and present with muscle weakness, hyporeflexia, and paresthesia or hypesthesia. In the cervical region, spinal involvement can lead to cord impingement with long tract signs or may affect the vertebral artery, producing posterior circulation insufficiency with associated symptoms. OA of the spine should be differentiated from diffuse skeletal hyperostosis (DISH), in which there is marked calcification of the paraspinous ligaments and sparing of the arthrodial spinal joints.

Primary Generalized OA. The pattern of involvement of three or more joints or joint groups with OA has been given this name and is seen most commonly in older women. Typically, the DIP and PIP joints of the hand, the knees, and the spine are involved. Whether this represents a distinct subset of OA is not known but has been suggested.

LABORATORY FINDINGS. OA involves a pathologic process that appears largely limited to cartilage and surrounding tissues with no evidence of systemic involvement. Typically, the ESR is normal, and there is no elevation of acute-phase reactants. The hemoglobin and leukocyte counts remain within normal limits. The synovial fluid itself demonstrates no evidence of an inflammatory

reaction with few leukocytes (typically < 3000 per cubic millimeter) and good viscosity. Occasionally, fragments of cartilage and crystals of calcium hydroxyapatite or calcium pyrophosphate dihydrate are seen. Rheumatoid factor is absent in the majority, but a significant number of older individuals will exhibit low titer elevations which are not diagnostic of rheumatoid arthritis but are a common accompaniment of aging.

Various assays of biochemical markers of disease activity have been recently developed and hold great promise to more accurately assess both the rate of progression of the disease process and the current state of the cartilage. Cartilage matrix components unique to the joints have been identified, and sensitive tests have been developed to detect them in synovial fluid, serum, and urine. Further clinical correlations will need to be performed to determine their relationship to the disease process, activity, and state and their utility for earlier diagnosis and management of OA.

RADIOLOGY AND IMAGING TECHNIQUES. Pathognomonic findings on plain radiography of involved joints include the presence of osteophytes at the margins of involved joints, associated joint space narrowing representing areas of cartilage thinning or loss, and evidence of bony reaction marked by subchondral sclerosis and bone cysts in more progressive disease. Some patients may lack one or more of these findings.

Radiography has been shown to be very insensitive to the pathologic processes occurring in the cartilage, with many patients having normal radiographs but destructive cartilage changes documented by arthroscopy. Other techniques have therefore been developed with greater potential sensitivity to detect cartilage change. In particular, MRI has the advantage of demonstrating cartilage as a positive image and has been used widely to document major cartilage injury such as meniscal tears. Further refinement of this technology will enhance the resolution possible as well as increasing sensitivity to detect changes in hydration, which mark the earliest changes in OA. It is anticipated that such technology will be important in assessing disease progression in the future.

Other technologies being developed to evaluate the OA joint include scintigraphy and ultrasound.

TREATMENT. People with OA seek pain relief and improvement in their physical function. Because there is no known therapy in humans that affects the basic disease process (inhibits cartilage degradation or enhances synthesis), medical therapy has focused on providing symptomatic relief. Largely because of ease of administration and acceptance by patients, an unwarranted reliance has been placed on pharmacologic intervention, particularly nonsteroidal anti-inflammatory agents (NSAID's), as initial therapy at the expense of physical measures that have less morbidity and may provide longer-term benefit.

Pharmacologic Therapy. Symptomatic relief of pain in patients with OA is best achieved with simple analgesic agents such as acetaminophen. The effectiveness of NSAID's is due primarily to their analgesic rather than anti-inflammatory properties. Recent controlled studies have demonstrated that acetaminophen is as effective as NSAID's with considerably fewer serious side effects. Particularly in the elderly with decreased renal reserve and an increased incidence of upper gastrointestinal bleeding, acetaminophen and other simple analgesics should be the drugs of initial choice. If inflammation is present (erosive OA) or symptoms are not well controlled with simple analgesics, lower doses of NSAID's may prove to be effective. Intra-articular injection of various steroid preparations also can control joint symptoms. Controlled studies have demonstrated only short-term relief of symptoms, although some patients with OA may derive longer-term (months) benefit. Intra-articular injections should not be repeated more than three to four times per year in any given joint because of the possibility of the steroids potentiating cartilage breakdown. Systemic use of steroids has no place in the treatment of OA.

Other approaches to therapy are under investigation. Topical treatment with capsaicin, a substance-P inhibitor, has been shown to relieve pain in some patients with OA. The intra-articular injection of hyaluronan is undergoing clinical trials. The development of agents that can stimulate cartilage synthesis or prevent degradation is being actively pursued and should provide the next generation of agents used to treat this condition.

Physical Measures. Although often overlooked, physical therapy and exercise programs can provide important benefit to patients with OA. Muscle atrophy commonly accompanies OA. Because muscles serve to reduce load on cartilage, maintaining muscle function is crucial for cartilage integrity and can reduce pain. Both muscle strength and range of motion can be improved with appropriate physical therapy. Isometric exercises are preferred to isotonic because they place less stress on the involved joint.

Heat and cold are both used with varying effectiveness to provide symptomatic relief to patients and as an important adjunct to physical therapy regimens. Using transcutaneous nerve stimulation (TENS), particularly to relieve back pain, is effective in some patients and provides an attractive alternative to pharmacologic intervention.

Periods of rest throughout the day may be an important adjunct in the routine of patients with OA. Reduction in joint loading, either by resting or appropriately using a cane, often will permit increased periods of activity with reduced pain. Using cushioned shoes (commercial running or walking shoes) also may help lower extremity joint symptoms. Back pain may be reduced by muscle-strengthening exercises as well as a well-fitted brace.

Orthopedic Surgery. Joint replacement surgery has been the single biggest advance in the treatment of OA in the past half century. Patients in whom optimal medical management has failed and who continue to have pain that interferes with sleep or activity or have significant limitations of joint function are candidates for an operation. Some individuals, those with altered limb alignment and early OA of a hip or knee, may benefit from osteotomy. Most patients have more advanced disease and require total joint replacement. Ideal candidates for total joint arthroplasty have well-maintained muscle strength and should be older than age 60. Younger patients are discouraged from undergoing joint replacement because of the small but real incidence of long-term failure of joint implants, mainly due to loosening. Revision arthroplasty is possible but has a higher failure rate and can be avoided by delaying initial arthroplasty as long as possible and putting less load on the replaced joint.

Arthroscopic surgery is useful for removing loose bodies and repairing intrinsic defects of the knee as well as shoulder (rotator cuff) and ankle pathology. Arthroscopic lavage (flushing of saline to remove cartilage debris) in patients with knee OA may provide pain relief. Abrasion arthroplasty (chondroplasty) has been widely used in patients with knee OA, but no data exist to demonstrate its efficacy, and it cannot be recommended currently.

Kuettner KE, Schleyerbach R, Peyron JG, et al.: Articular Cartilage and Osteoarthritis: Workshop Conference Hoechst Werk Kalle-Albert, Wiesbaden. New York, Raven Press, 1991. *Current understanding of cartilage biology and the pathogenesis of OA.*

McCarthy DJ: Arthritis and Allied Conditions. Philadelphia, Lea & Febiger, 1989. *Comprehensive overview of all aspects with illustrations.*

Moskowitz W, Howell DS, Goldberg VM, et al.: Osteoarthritis: Diagnosis and Medical/Surgical Management. Philadelphia, WB Saunders, 1992. *In-depth coverage of all aspects of OA.*

Silman AJ, Hochberg MC (eds.): Epidemiology of the Rheumatic Diseases. New York, Oxford Press, 1993. *A comprehensive review of definition, incidence, and prevalence of disease.*

255 THE PAINFUL SHOULDER

Dennis W. Boulware

Shoulder pain is a frequent complaint among adults and is likely to increase in prevalence as the population ages and active lifestyles remain popular. Pain can originate from many anatomic sites, including the glenohumeral joint, the periarticular soft tissue structures, or referred from the cervical spine, the thorax, the diaphragm, and the upper abdominal cavity. Although nonmusculoskeletal causes of shoulder pain are important, this chapter will focus on the musculoskeletal causes of isolated shoulder pain.

Most causes of shoulder pain are due to pathology involving the surrounding periarticular soft tissue structures: the *tendons* of the biceps and rotator cuff, the subacromial and subdeltoid *bursae,* and the *articular capsule* (Fig. 255–1). Infrequently, diseases of the *bone* and the *glenohumeral joint* can be responsible for shoulder pain. A basic knowledge of the anatomy of the shoulder joint and

the physical examination of these specific structures are essential for proper diagnosis and management.

TENDONS. In general, tendon lesions are painful only during active use. A bicipital tendinitis will hurt during active flexion of the elbow or forward flexion of the shoulder, and a rotator cuff lesion will cause pain on abduction of the shoulder. On examination, active testing of the myotendinous unit results in more tenderness than passive range of motion.

The Rotator Cuff. All *lesions of the rotator cuff* will precipitate pain on active abduction of the shoulder, particularly the initial 90 degrees of motion. This pain is usually focused over the lateral aspect of the shoulder and frequently a problem at night. On examination of the shoulder, active abduction will elicit more tenderness than passive abduction done by the examiner. A "drop sign" is helpful in identifying the rotator cuff as the source of pain. With the patient's arm passively placed at full abduction, the patient will experience severe pain when the arm is slowly adducted from 120 to 60 degrees and the arm will reflexively "drop."

Rotator cuff tendinitis is the most common cause of shoulder pain and is usually due to overusing the arm in overhead activities. This abducted position impinges the cuff between the acromian and the humeral head. Chronic impingements also can occur from inferior osteophytes of the acromioclavicular joint encroaching into the acromiohumeral space. With time, chronic impingements can result in attenuation of the rotator cuff and an eventual tear.

Injury, overuse, or degenerative processes can lead to *rotator cuff tears* in the shoulder. The tear can exist as a complete rupture of the rotator cuff or as incomplete tears. The pain is worse with active abduction of the shoulder, particularly the initial 90 degrees. A complete tear of the cuff will make abduction of the initial 90 degrees impossible.

The diagnosis of *calcific tendinitis* is made in the clinical setting of a rotator cuff tendinitis coupled with the radiographic appearance of calcification of the rotator cuff, usually the supraspinatus tendon near its insertion on the humerus (Fig. 255–2).

Diagnostic plain radiography is helpful in chronic rotator cuff lesions. Chronic impingements with tendinitis will reveal sclerotic and cystic changes of the humeral greater tuberosity. Significant attrition or complete tears of the cuff will be demonstrated as narrowing or obliteration of the acromiohumeral space. *Magnetic resonance imaging* and *ultrasonography* are useful but expensive and difficult to interpret except by experienced musculoskeletal radiologists. *Arthrography* is the best study to document complete ruptures and often can detect incomplete tears (Fig. 255–3).

The *diagnosis of a rotator cuff lesion* often can be made by instilling an intralesional local anesthetic agent. When 2 to 4 ml of a local anesthetic is properly placed inferolaterally to the acromial process in the subacromial bursa, the patient should experience significant relief of pain and be capable of active, painless abduction. The exception will be the complete rupture of the rotator cuff, which will have pain relief but still be incapable of unassisted abduction.

The *treatment of lesions of the rotator cuff* is similar for all types of problems except a complete tear, which will require a surgical referral. Initial management with heat, physical therapy, and nonsteroidal anti-inflammatory drugs (NSAID's) is more effective when prescribed early. If ineffective, intralesional corticosteroid agents placed in the subacromial bursa may be required. Recalcitrant cases of impingement may eventually require surgery in the form of acromioplasty. Job modification for individuals with chronic impingement from occupational overuse will be essential.

Bicipital Tendon. In *bicipital tendinitis,* the tendon of the long head of the biceps becomes inflamed as it traverses the bicipital groove of the humerus. Clinically, the patient experiences pain in the anterior aspect of the shoulder, especially upon actively using the biceps. Clinical examination can confirm the presence of bicipital tendinitis by one of several techniques. Directly palpating the tendon within the bicipital groove will result in tenderness, which can be accentuated by passively rotating the shoulder while maintaining pressure over the tendon. Alternatively, the patient can be placed in the initial position of maximal elbow flexion and wrist supination and asked to resist an attempt to suddenly extend the elbow and pronate the wrist. Tenderness in the anterior shoulder would be indicative of bicipital tendinitis (Yergason's sign).

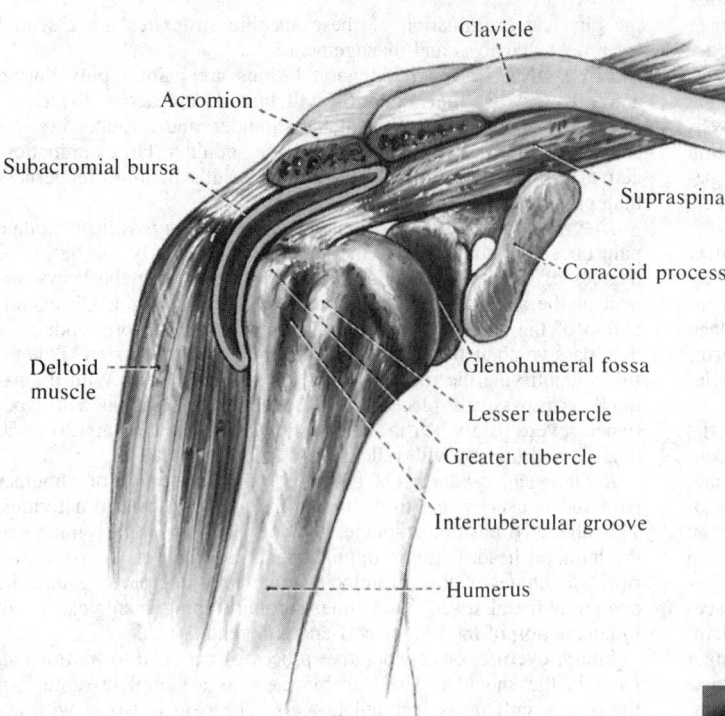

FIGURE 255–1. Anterior aspect of the shoulder joint showing palpable landmarks and their relationship to the subacromial bursa. (From Polley HF, Hunder GG [eds.]: Rheumatologic Interviewing and Physical Examination of the Joints, 2nd ed. Philadelphia, WB Saunders, 1978, p 63.)

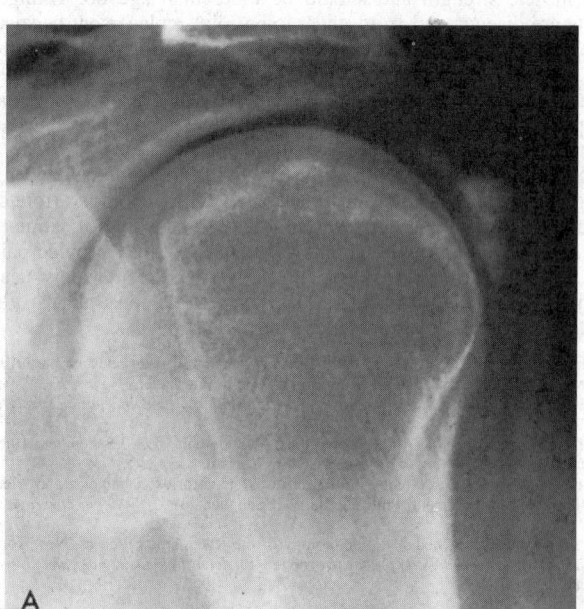

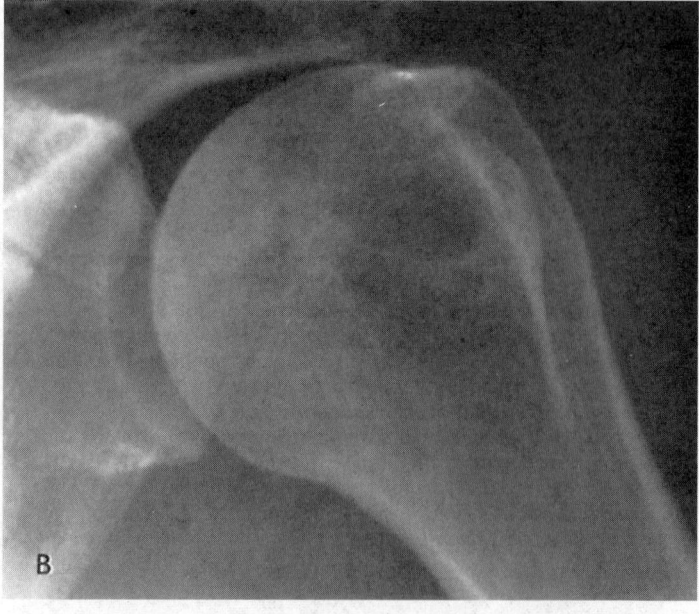

FIGURE 255–2. Calcific tendinitis. A, Two distinct deposits of calcium are present on the internal rotation view. B, External rotation projects the supraspinatus calcification above the greater tuberosity and superimposes the larger collection (within the infraspinatus tendon) over the humeral head. (From Forrester DM, Brown JC: The Radiology of Joint Disease, Vol 2. Philadelphia, WB Saunders, 1987, p 364.)

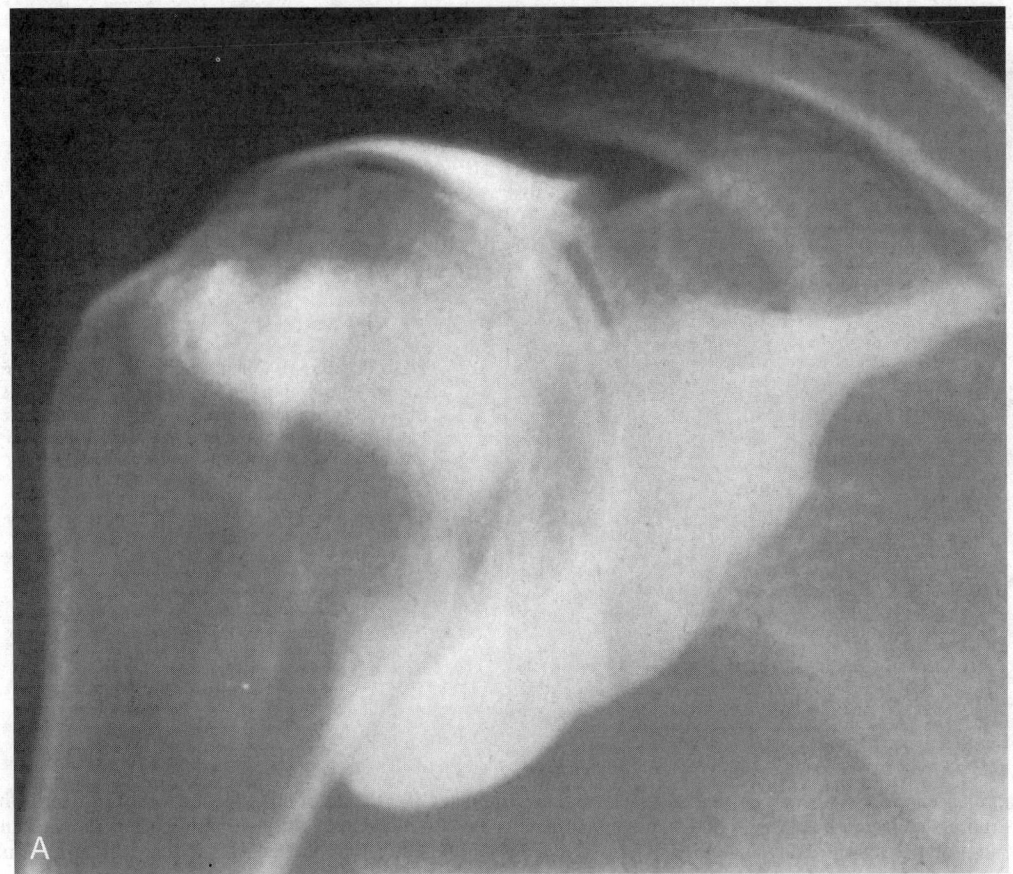

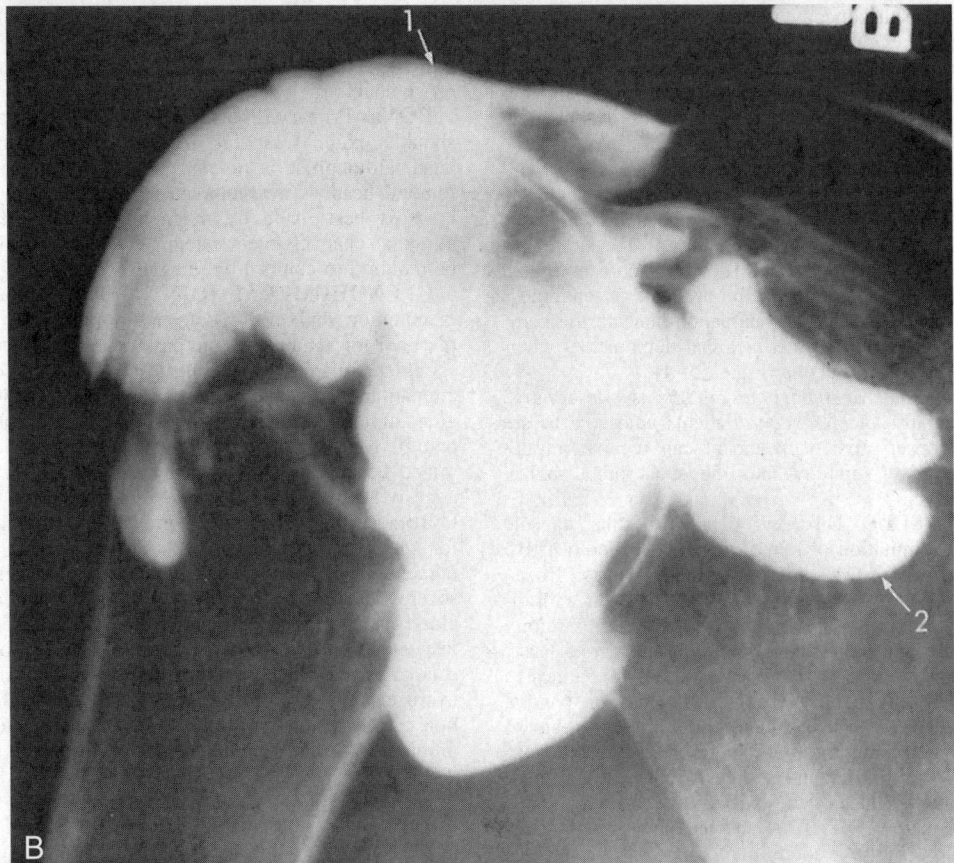

FIGURE 255–3. *A*, Arthrogram of normal shoulder. The extent of the joint capsule is delineated by contrast material. A prominent subscapular extension of the capsule is seen projecting toward the axilla. Filling of the subacromial bursa may occasionally occur normally. Extension of the capsule as a pouch around the long head of the biceps demarcates the intertubercular groove. *B*, Rotator cuff tear. Filling of (1) the subacromial bursa superiorly and (2) the subcoracoid bursa inferiorly indicates tear of the rotator cuff. The normal hyaline articular cartilage is seen as a radiolucent crescent over the head of the humerus. (From Forrester DM, Brown JC: The Radiology of Joint Disease, Vol 2. Philadelphia, WB Saunders, 1987, pp 362, 363.)

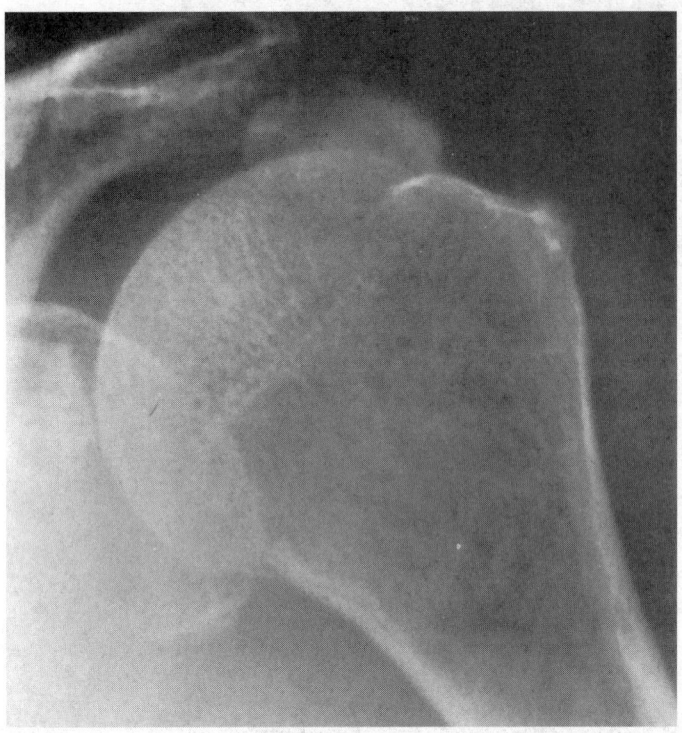

FIGURE 255–4. Calcific bursitis. A large amorphous collection of calcium lies within the subacromial bursa. In addition, a small fleck of calcium just above the greater tuberosity represents supraspinatus tendinitis. (From Forrester DM, Brown JC: The Radiology of Joint Disease, Vol 2. Philadelphia, WB Saunders, 1987, p 369.)

Chronic problems can cause attrition of the tendon and eventual rupture. Complete rupture will cause mild weakness of the biceps and a prominent bulge of the muscle belly. Integrity of the rotator cuff should be assessed in chronic bicipital tendinitis, because the two entities frequently occur concomitantly.

Treatment of bicipital tendinitis is initially conservative with rest and NSAID's. Physical therapy and intralesional corticosteroids are reserved for refractory cases. Successful treatment is more likely when initiated early. Surgery is essential for complete rupture and may be required for intractable cases of tendinitis.

BURSAE. The subacromial or subdeltoid bursa is the largest and most frequently inflamed bursa of the shoulder. Located beneath the acromian process between the rotator cuff and the deltoid muscle, *subacromial* or *subdeltoid bursitis* will cause pain in the lateral aspect of the shoulder similar to that caused by rotator cuff tendinitis. It differs from a rotator cuff tendinitis by the presence of tenderness upon passive abduction and upon direct palpation beneath the acromian process. *Plain radiography* sometimes can demonstrate calcification in chronic subacromial bursitis (Fig. 255–4).

Treatment of subacromial or subdeltoid bursitis is conservative with rest, physical therapy, and NSAID's. Patients whose cases are refractory to initial conservative management can receive intralesional corticosteroids given directly into the subacromial bursa, which are quite effective.

ARTICULAR CAPSULE. Disorders of the articular capsule will be evident by the limitation of range of motion by both active and passive abduction. *Adhesive capsulitis,* also known as "frozen shoulder," is a common entity that can occur in association with diabetes mellitus, tuberculosis, cervical spine disease, upper extremity injuries, coronary artery disease, and chronic pulmonary disease. Initially a painful condition, it will proceed through an adhesive phase characterized by the painless progressive loss of passive range of motion in all directions. Eventually, the shoulder "thaws" with the return of range of motion after several years. The diagnosis is best confirmed by arthrography, which reveals a contracture of the articular volume and loss of the axillary pouch. Pain is best managed by physical therapy, NSAID's, and judicious use of intra-articular corticosteroids. Early restoration of range of motion has been uniformly unsuccessful even when attempted by physical therapy, closed manipulation under general anesthesia, and hydraulic distention using large-volume intra-articular injections.

Reflex sympathetic dystrophy syndrome is similar to adhesive capsulitis except for more diffuse involvement with pain and vasomotor instability of the hand, wrist, and arm. More commonly seen after trauma of the upper extremity, it is seen in association with clinical situations similar to adhesive capsulitis. This condition can occur bilaterally and responds more favorably to early therapy. Treatment should include aggressive physical therapy to maintain range of motion, non-narcotic analgesia for pain management, and a short, rapidly tapering course of corticosteroids. Best results have occurred when steroids are started at 40 to 60 mg of prednisone per day and tapered over a 3-week period. Stellate ganglion blocks and intra-articular corticosteroids are used but with less uniform improvement.

BONE. Primary diseases of the bone can manifest themselves as shoulder pain. *Avascular necrosis of bone* can affect the humeral head, although it is not as common as avascular necrosis of the femoral head. If avascular necrosis of bone is suspected, the *diagnosis* is best made by magnetic resonance imaging. Plain radiographic changes occur late in the disease process and should not be required to confirm the diagnosis.

GLENOHUMERAL JOINT. Arthritis of the glenohumeral joint is common and easily detected on physical examination by the presence of tenderness on passive rotation of the fully adducted shoulder. Soft tissue swelling is not to be perceived on routine examination, and tenderness on active rotation will not discriminate glenohumeral arthritis from lesions of the rotator cuff. Although painful for the patient, passive range of motion should be determined because it will be near normal in acute arthritis but not in adhesive capsulitis.

Because the glenohumeral joint is a common site of involvement for many forms of the polyarthritides, most episodes of glenohumeral arthritis are part of a polyarthritis. Alternatively, an isolated severe destructive degenerative glenohumeral arthritis seen in the elderly should make the clinician suspect *Milwaukee shoulder.* Predisposing factors for this condition include chronic renal failure, local calcium pyrophosphate dihydrate deposition, chronic joint overuse, and large tears of the rotator cuff. The long-term disruption of the rotator cuff seems to be the key factor in allowing this problem to occur.

Biundo JJ, Torres-Ramos FM: Common shoulder problems. Primary Care Rheumatol 4:1, 1991. *A practical approach to examination of the shoulder and diagnosing common problems.*

Boublik M, Hawkins RJ: Clinical examination of the shoulder complex. J Orthop Sports Phys Ther 18:379, 1993. *A comprehensive approach to the examination of the shoulder.*

Kozin F: Painful shoulder and the reflex sympathetic dystrophy syndrome. *In* McCarty DJ, Koopman WJ (eds.): Arthritis and Allied Conditions, 12th ed. Philadelphia, Lea & Febiger, 1993, pp 1643–1676. *A detailed and comprehensive resource of etiology, diagnosis, and treatment; 301 references.*

Thornhill TS: Shoulder pain. *In* Kelley WN, Harris ED, Ruddy S, et al. (eds.): Textbook of Rheumatology, 4th ed. Philadelphia, WB Saunders, 1993, pp 417–440. *A detailed and comprehensive resource of etiology, diagnosis, and treatment; 160 references.*

256 SYSTEMIC DISEASES IN WHICH ARTHRITIS IS A FEATURE

Eugene V. Ball

Eleven per cent of adult Americans interviewed in the National Health Survey claimed to have had one or more episodes of painful joints over a period of six weeks. Much of this pain was probably due to soft tissue rheumatism and common rheumatic diseases, such as osteoarthritis and rheumatoid arthritis (RA), that are defined by their own attributes and not by associated signs. The arthralgias of a fraction of these persons might have represented early symptoms of systemic diseases diagnosable only by the later appearance of other clinical signs or by laboratory testing. Table 256–1 illustrates the applicability of general medical laboratory tests to the evaluation of nonspecific joint symptoms. The tests afford significant diagnostic clues for certain systemic diseases in which arthralgias can be the earliest and only symptoms. Brief descriptions of musculoskeletal manifestations of a few systemic disorders follow.

PRIMARY BILIARY CIRRHOSIS (see Ch. 122). More than half of women with primary biliary cirrhosis (PBC) may have serologic abnormalities, such as rheumatoid factors and antinuclear antibodies, in addition to antimitochondrial antibodies. A large number, primarily in this group, have joint pains or outright rheumatic disease, mainly RA, Sjögren's syndrome, or limited scleroderma (CREST syndrome: *c*alcinosis, *R*aynaud's phenomenon, *e*sophageal dysfunction, *s*clerodactyly, and *t*elangiectasia). An asymmetric, non-deforming arthritis has been described in as many as 30% of patients. Other defined causes for bone or joint pains in PBC include osteomalacia and hypertrophic osteoarthropathy.

HEMOCHROMATOSIS (see Ch. 189). Arthritis is frequently the first sign of hemochromatosis and eventually develops in as many as half of all persons with the disease. Typically occurring between the ages of 40 and 50, the arthritis of hemochromatosis has been reported in persons younger than age 30 and is easily overlooked or confused with primary osteoarthritis, even though their distributions often differ. It also may be dismissed as idiopathic tendinitis or bursitis. Pain and stiffness frequently appear first in the metacarpophalangeal joints; other joints involved commonly include the wrists, hips, and knees. Signs of inflammation are negligible except during episodes of pseudogout. Chondrocalcinosis is common on radiographs, as are subchondral cysts, sclerosis, and joint space narrowing. The arthritis is not altered by phlebotomy; treatment is symptomatic and may necessitate arthroplasties, particularly in the hips.

SICKLE CELL DISEASE AND OTHER HEMOGLOBINOPATHIES (see Ch. 136). Almost all persons with sickle cell disease experience musculoskeletal symptoms. Large joint arthritis lasting a few days to a few weeks results from small vessel occlusion caused by local sickling. The aseptic bone infarcts of SC (or less often SS) disease resemble osteomyelitis, which is far more common in persons with sickle cell disease than in normal persons and is often caused by *Salmonella*. Osteonecrosis occurs in both SS and SC disease, often in the head of the femur; however, multiple areas may be infarcted. Hyperuricemia attributable to SS disease has culminated in gout in older patients. Pain due to microfractures in the lower leg, ankle, or foot, lasting up to 1 to 2 years, has been described in almost one half of a group of 50 patients with beta-thalassemia.

HYPOGAMMAGLOBULINEMIA (see Ch. 223 and 266). Arthritis as a complication of hypogammaglobulinemia is most typical of the X-linked variety (Bruton's disease) in children; however, it also occurs in other types of primary hypogammaglobulinemia. Septic arthritis is caused by common pathogens or by mycoplasmal organisms such as *Ureaplasma urealyticum*. Nonerosive arthritis, without evidence of infection or other demonstrable cause, often resolves following institution of immunoglobulin therapy. Its resolution with treatment does not necessarily constitute *a priori* evidence of an infectious etiology. Intravenous gamma globulin treatment might suppress arthritis through its complex modulating effect on the immune system (e.g., it has been shown to increase suppressor T-cell functional activity).

WHIPPLE'S DISEASE (see Ch. 103). The arthritis of Whipple's disease mimics that of rheumatic fever in some respects. It is painful; there is often warmth, redness, and swelling; it favors large joints; subcutaneous nodules have been noted in a few patients; recurrences are common; and it can be migratory. Less often, small joints of the hands and feet are inflamed, and the arthritis becomes chronic and resembles RA. The synovial fluid white cell count is sometimes elevated to 50,000 per cubic millimeter, and rod-shaped bacilli may be identified, usually by electron microscopy, in synovial biopsies. These organisms are also seen attached to circulating erythrocytes. Rheumatoid factors and antinuclear antibody are not features of Whipple's disease. The arthritis may antedate gastrointestinal symptoms by years, making diagnosis difficult.

HYPERLIPOPROTEINEMIA (see Ch. 173). An association exists between type II familial hypercholesterolemia (both homozygous and heterozygous forms) and musculoskeletal symptoms such as Achilles tendinitis, oligoarthritis, and polyarthritis. Transient pain in the Achilles tendon appears to be more common than frank inflammatory tendinitis, which can last a few days and recur two or three times yearly. A few patients have acute painful monoarthritis or pauciarthritis of the knees, ankles, or small joints that lasts a week or more and recurs frequently. Less common is an incapacitating polyarthritis resembling rheumatic fever, persisting a month or more. In one study, 40% of 73 heterozygous patients were symptomatic; articular manifestations appeared at times before the xanthomas that are the major diagnostic sign of familial hypercholesterolemia.

ENDOCRINE DISORDERS (see Ch. 202, 203, and 214). Aches and stiffness simulating fibromyalgia may appear early in hypothyroidism; untreated, this may progress to proximal myopathy with elevated creatine kinase levels, simulating polymyositis, or to a syndrome of synovial thickening and joint effusions, simulating RA. There also appears to be an association of hypothyroidism with calcium pyrophosphate deposition disease. Carpal tunnel syndrome is a more common manifestation of hypothyroidism. Hyperthyroidism may cause myopathy without elevations of the creatine kinase level but with muscle wasting, which may be severe. Thyroid acropachy, seen rarely in association with pretibial myxedema and Graves' disease, is characterized by diffuse swelling of the fingers and clubbing.

Hyperparathyroidism is another cause of diffuse, vague musculoskeletal pains resembling those of fibrositis. The other musculoskeletal complications of hyperparathyroidism include back pain due to vertebral body fractures, an erosive arthritis predominantly in the hands and wrists, and chondrocalcinosis (with pseudogout occurring most often after parathyroidectomy).

Carpal tunnel syndrome has been reported in almost one-half of persons with acromegaly. Raynaud's phenomenon is rare. The

TABLE 256–1. LABORATORY TESTS IN THE EVALUATION OF NONSPECIFIC JOINT SYMPTOMS

Test	Disease
Liver function tests	Primary biliary cirrhosis; chronic active hepatitis
Calcium and phosphorus	Hyperparathyroidism
Serum protein electrophoresis	Hypogammaglobulinemic arthritis; primary amyloidosis
Serum iron and total iron-binding capacity; ferritin	Hemochromatosis
Lipase or amylase	Pancreatic-arthritis syndrome
Thyroid-stimulating hormone (TSH); thyroxine	Thyroid myopathy or arthritis
Complete blood count	Leukemia; sickle cell disease
Lipid analysis	Hyperlipidemia-associated arthritis
Partial thromboplastin time; rapid plasma reagin (RPR) or VDRL	Vasculopathy; hemophilia Vasculopathy; syphilis
Anti-HIV (human immunodeficiency virus)	HIV arthritis
Antiparvovirus antibody	Parvovirus arthritis

arthritis of acromegaly is clinically indistinguishable from osteoarthritis.

SARCOIDOSIS (see Ch. 61). Joint or juxta-articular pains are experienced by as many as one third of patients with acute sarcoidosis and may be the only symptom of the disease; however, erythema nodosum often accompanies the arthritis and, together with hilar adenopathy, suggests the diagnosis (one should be aware that arthritis may accompany erythema nodosum of any cause). Arthritis often begins in the ankles and spreads symmetrically. The distal interphalangeal joints are typically spared, but any of the other peripheral joints, as well as the heels, may be painful out of proportion to signs of inflammation, which are meager. Episodes last a few days to a few months, and the arthritis usually resolves completely. The erythrocyte sedimentation rate is often elevated; antinuclear antibodies and rheumatoid factors may be present. Treatment with salicylates, nonsteroidal anti-inflammatory drugs (NSAID's), or prednisone is based on the severity of the arthritis. Progressive, deforming arthritis is a feature of chronic sarcoidosis, as are bone lesions, both lytic and sclerotic. Clinically significant sarcoid myopathy is rare.

FAMILIAL MEDITERRANEAN FEVER (see Ch. 139.2). Serositis, fever, and arthritis are the major signs of familial Mediterranean fever (FMF). Arthritis occurs in as many as one half of patients; it is usually monoarticular and confined to large joints in the lower extremities. Although it usually lasts < 1 week, arthritis has been reported to persist for several months. Synovial fluid contains large numbers of granulocytes, and there is intense infiltration of granulocytes and hyperemia in synovial tissue. Diagnosis is suggested by demographic and other clinical features of the disease. In the absence of these, FMF can be easily confused with juvenile RA. Colchicine most often prevents recurrent arthritis as well as amyloidosis.

257 MISCELLANEOUS FORMS OF ARTHRITIS

Eugene V. Ball

NEUROPATHIC JOINT DISEASE (CHARCOT'S JOINTS). Recognition of neuropathic joint disease and its association with syphilis preceded reports of its association with diabetes mellitus by 64 years, but syphilis has been superseded by the latter as the leading cause of this disorder. In syphilis, subacute combined degeneration of the spinal cord, paraplegia, and Charcot-Marie-Tooth disease, weakness, decreased pain sensation, and impaired position sense contribute to the massive destruction of the knee (or less often the hip or ankle) that typifies the disorder. In syringomyelia, upper limb involvement is typical. Neuropathic disease of the knee or ankle is suggested by effusions, crepitus, enlargement, and relatively little pain, although pain may become worrisome late in the disease. Neuropathic joint disease in diabetes mellitus (Fig. 257–1) is more likely to cause painless swelling of one or both feet in a patient with longstanding disease and sensory neuropathy. For mechanical reasons, the joints most frequently involved are the tarsometatarsals and the metatarsophalangeals. Destruction also occurs in the talus, the calcaneus, the ankle joints, and the distal tibia. Radiographs characteristically show loss of joint space, sclerosis, multiple irregular bodies representing chip fractures, and new bone formation; analogous changes are seen in osteomyelitis and malignancy. (Less severe, but similar, changes have been reported in calcium pyrophosphate deposition disease.) Attempts at stabilizing the involved joint with various orthotic devices are often unsatisfactory, and surgical fusion is difficult.

HEMARTHROSIS. Hemophilia (see Ch. 153) is the major medical cause of hemarthrosis, which (with muscle bleeding) accounts for > 90% of all bleeding episodes in patients with hemophilia. The severity of hemarthrosis is related directly to the levels of clotting factors. For example, infants with severe factor deficiencies often experience hemarthrosis before the age of 1. By age 15, virtually all persons with severe, inadequately treated factor deficiencies have some form of chronic joint impairment.

Acute bleeding into a joint (most often the knees, elbows, or ankles) is frequently signified by stiffness or discomfort, followed by pain, swelling, and redness. The joint should be immobilized, and adequate factor replacement should be started as early as possible, preferably during the prodromal phase. The joint changes stimulated by repeated intra-articular bleeding resemble those of rheumatoid arthritis (RA). Hyperplastic synovium appears to be the source of proteases and other enzymes that destroy cartilage and bone, culminating in the absence of articular cartilage, joint disorganization, and fibrous contractures. Education of the patient and family, as well as home treatment, prevents or attenuates chronic, destructive arthritis. Joint replacements have been done successfully to relieve pain and restore function.

Bleeding into a muscle, which also should be treated with replacement factor, can lead to necrosis and fibrotic scarring. Pseudotumors are cystic bone swellings resulting from intraosseous bleeding and necrosis.

Von Willebrand's disease can produce hemarthrosis and joint destruction comparable to that of hemophilia.

Painful but nondestructive intra-articular bleeding is a common feature of scurvy, and intra-articular tumors such as pigmented villonodular synovitis frequently cause monoarticular bleeding.

MULTICENTRIC RETICULOHISTIOCYTOSIS. The chief manifestations of multicentric reticulohistiocytosis are arthritis and red to purple skin nodules varying in size from 1 to 10 mm. The nodules are found in any part of the skin but tend to concentrate on the face and hands and uncommonly coalesce. The arthritis is most often symmetric and polyarticular. Unlike adult RA, it does not spare the distal interphalangeal joints. It can be severely destructive and, in one third of cases, progresses to arthritis multilans. Systemic signs include fever and weight loss; less often, pericarditis and myositis are present, and it is frequently associated with a malignancy.

The disorder also has been termed "lipoid dermatoarthritis" because of the lipids contained within the histiocytes and granulomas that constitute the basic lesion. In the absence of a serum or lesional lipid abnormality, lipid deposition is now thought to be nonspecific. Improvement has been reported more consistently with alkylating agents than with prednisone. Methotrexate also has been used.

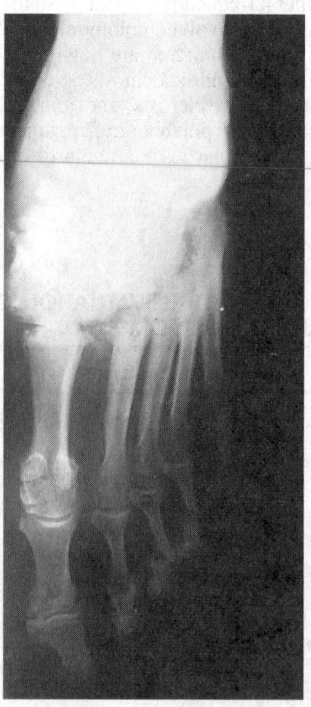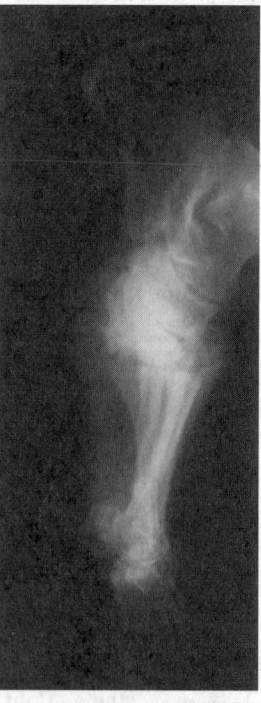

FIGURE 257–1. Diabetes mellitus and neuropathic arthritis. Note lateral displacement of metatarsals *(left)* and fragmentation and osseous debris *(right)*.

HYPERTROPHIC OSTEOARTHROPATHY AND CARCINOMATOUS POLYARTHRITIS.

Hypertrophic osteoarthropathy (HO) is a systemic disorder distinguished by periostitis of the distal ends of tubular bones. The lesions presumably begin with increased blood flow and periosteal edema, followed by new bone formation. Isotopic bone scans are positive at an early stage, often preceding radiographic evidence of periosteal new bone. Hypertrophic osteoarthropathy is often manifested as digital clubbing and frequently involves the tibiae, ulnae, radii, femora, metatarsals, and metacarpals. Painful articular swelling appears in approximately 30% of patients and may be debilitating; other variable features of the syndrome include gynecomastia and thickening and furrowing of the facial skin. Intrathoracic malignancies, especially squamous cell carcinoma, have supplanted pulmonary infections as the most common cause of HO. Pleural and diaphragmatic neoplasms and nasopharyngeal carcinomas are strongly associated with HO. Less common causes include chronic liver disease, inflammatory bowel disease, and cyanotic heart disease. There is also a hereditary form termed "pachydermoperiostosis," with strong male predominance and a curious bimodal distribution of disease onset during the first year of life or the midteens. No satisfactory unifying theory of pathogenesis exists. Successful treatment of the underlying disorder results in regression of HO. In fact, thoracotomy for cancer-causing pulmonary hypertrophic osteoarthropathy may result in a marked decrease in pain and swelling within 24 hours.

The "sudden" onset of polyarthritis resembling RA in an older adult should prompt suspicion of an associated malignancy. Carcinomatous polyarthritis may appear months before, or after, detection of malignancy of many types. Its incidence is unknown; in one small series it was almost as common as carcinomatous hypertrophic osteoarthropathy and more common than cancer-related dermatomyositis. Palmar fasciitis has been noted in association with ovarian cancer.

Ginsburg WW, O'Duffy JD, Morris JL, et al.: Multicentric reticulohistiocytosis: Response to alkylating in six patients. Ann Intern Med 111:384, 1989. *Five of six patients with multicentric reticulohistiocytosis manifesting as skin nodules and polyarthritis were treated with cyclophosphamide. The sixth was given chlorambucil. All had complete or near-complete remissions lasting as long as 32 months after cessation of treatment.*

Hoyer LW: Hemophilia A. N Engl J Med 330:38, 1994. *A review of the structure and function of Factor VIII, the molecular genetics of hemophilia A, its clinical manifestations, and treatment.*

Slowman-Kovacs SD, Braunstein EM, Brandt KD: Rapidly progressive Charcot arthropathy following minor joint trauma in patients with diabetic neuropathy. Arthritis Rheum 33:412, 1990. *This report of neuropathic arthropathy progressing rapidly after minor trauma in three patients is based on the authors' research in experimental arthritis.*

258 NONARTICULAR RHEUMATISM

Eugene V. Ball

FIBROMYALGIA (FIBROSITIS). Primary fibromyalgia (FM) has been defined as chronic, widespread musculoskeletal pain and tenderness at multiple sites, e.g., at 11 of 18 specific sites in the criteria of the American College of Rheumatology. Implicit in this definition is the absence of signs of connective tissue or other musculoskeletal disease. Because of its subjective nature and its frequent association with disturbed sleep, chronic fatigue, headaches, and irritable bowel syndrome, the validity of classifying FM as a disease rather than a "syndrome of being out of sorts" has been challenged. Patients often appear anxious and depressed, and studies have shown that they may feel dissatisfied with all aspects of their lives. Nevertheless, the specific characteristics of anxiety and depression have not been identified consistently on psychological testing, and it has been suggested that chronic pain and fatigue of any cause can engender anxiety and depression. Despite their subjectivity, symptoms of FM tend to be constant over many years; exceptionally, FM has been found to be premonitory of psychosis or hypothyroidism. There are no consistent biochemical, immunologic, or anatomic abnormalities in FM. Decreased threshold to pain on pressure over certain sites and increased skin fold tenderness have led to numerous unsuccessful attempts to demonstrate localized peripheral abnormalities and to speculation that FM is a disorder of pain modulation.

Functional disability in FM may exceed that of rheumatoid arthritis, and in 1989, FM was the most frequent single reason for disability pensions among women in Norway, accounting for 7.2% of new pensions. Patients whose FM begins acutely after a specific traumatic event are more likely to be disabled than those in whom the disorder evolves insidiously. FM is significantly less common in men than in women and is either underreported or uncommon in developing countries. Treatment should emphasize its nondestructive nature, and the physician should be wary of overusing drugs to allay anxiety or induce sleep. Low-dose amitryptyline has been found to be valuable for decreasing pain and improving sleep in some patients.

BURSITIS. Bursae are small, synovial-lined, fluid-filled sacs located between tendons and bones which serve to reduce friction between opposing muscles or tendons. Most bursae are present from birth; however, others form in response to repeated pressure.

Of the approximately 80 bursae located on each side of the body, only a few are common sources of pain. The subdeltoid is the largest of the bursae around the shoulder; it is located between the deltoid muscle and the shoulder capsule and extends under the acromion. Acute inflammation of this or nearby bursae and tendons is apt to be exceedingly painful, resulting in restricted shoulder movement and tenderness over the rotator cuff. Intrabursal injection of lidocaine is diagnostic and often curative; however, recurrences are common. Bursal calcification predisposes to more frequent attacks. Infection is most common in the olecranon bursa.

Trochanteric bursitis is thought to occur as a result of chronic strain on weak quadricep muscles or overuse of hip and thigh muscles. Pain is often perceived to be in the lateral aspect of the thigh and the low back and is aggravated by abducting the affected leg and by lying on the affected side. Tenderness is present at the edge of the greater trochanter. Injections of lidocaine often abolish the pain.

TENDINOUS LESIONS. Tendinous lesions include tenosynovitis, a lesion of the gliding surfaces of a tendon and its sheath; tendinitis, painful scarring within a tendon; and trigger lesions, which are localized enlargements of the tendon that engage a constricted part of the sheath (as in "trigger finger"). Tendinous lesions are common, occurring in many areas of the musculoskeletal system. An example is de Quervain's disease, which is stenosing tenosynovitis of the abductor pollicis longus and extensor pollicis brevis at the medial styloid. Pain can localize or radiate into the hand or back to the shoulder. This and carpal tunnel syndrome occur frequently during pregnancy.

CARPAL TUNNEL SYNDROME. The symptoms of carpal tunnel syndrome are paresthesias and pain in the palmar side of the first three fingers and at times the radial half of the fourth finger; the pain may radiate proximally to the shoulder, creating confusion with a cervical disc syndrome. Physical findings include sensory loss, weakness on abduction and opposition of the thumb, and atrophy of the thenar eminence. Carpal tunnel syndrome is caused by an array of conditions that result in pressure on the median nerve as it passes through the bony flexor compartment of the wrist. Some of these are listed in Table 258–1.

Diagnosis is confirmed by electrophysiologic nerve tests. (The clinical tests commonly used are of questionable value.) Magnetic resonance imaging may be useful in defining the cause and thus directing treatment, which might include splinting of the wrist, corticosteroid injections, and surgical release of the transverse carpal ligament. Oral pyridoxine is of questionable value.

TENNIS ELBOW. "Tennis elbow" refers to a lesion of the wrist extensor muscles causing pain at the outer elbow, along the back of the forearm, or less commonly, into the shoulder. The burning or aching pain is produced by resisted extension of the wrist, as in grasping and lifting, and rarely is felt as sudden, searing twinges of intensity sufficient to cause momentary grip paralysis. Tennis elbow usually results from repeated forceful extension of the wrist. A tear or area of degeneration most often occurs at the origin of the common extensor tendon from the lateral humoral epicondyle; much less frequently, the tear is in the muscle belly. Treatment includes

TABLE 258–1. CONDITIONS CAUSING CARPAL TUNNEL SYNDROME

1. Trauma
2. Occupation
3. Infections: for example, Lyme disease and rubella
4. Rheumatoid arthritis and gout
5. Pregnancy
6. Hypothyroidism and acromegaly
7. Amyloidosis
8. Median artery aneurysm
9. Ganglion cyst, increased fat, hypertrophy of abductor pollicis muscle

injection of triamcinolone into the painful scar, manipulation, or partial tenotomy.

Like tennis elbow, "golfer's elbow" is a misnomer in that both conditions occur frequently in people who play neither sport. Golfer's elbow is less painful than tennis elbow; it represents a lesion of the common flexor tendon at the medial epicondyle. Pain is usually localized to the inner side of the elbow and is produced by resisted flexion of the wrist. Treatment includes triamcinolone injection or massage.

TIETZE'S SYNDROME. Tietze's syndrome is an uncommon cause of chest pain that can be mistaken for visceral pain. There is tender, most often unilateral, swelling at one or more costosternal junctions. Biopsy samples of involved areas have revealed chronic inflammatory fibrosis. The syndrome may result from prolonged coughing or hyperventilation, but it is often idiopathic. Injections into the painful area with triamcinolone are sometimes curative. Tietze's syndrome may be differentiated from the more common costochondritis, in which there are no signs of inflammation.

Bennett RM: Fibromyalgia and the facts: Sense or nonsense. Rheum Dis Clin North Am 19:45, 1993.
Block SR: Fibromyalgia and the rheumatisms: Common sense and sensibility. Rheum Dis Clin North Am 19:61, 1993. *These papers present opposing points of view concerning fibromyalgia as a distinctive syndrome with distinctive diagnostic criteria.*

259 ARTICULAR TUMORS
Eugene V. Ball

Articular tumors can be classified as those which arise within the synovium; those which arise from cartilage, bone, or contiguous structures; and neoplasms that are nonarticular in origin but which metastasize to joints or develop in multiple areas, including joints.

The most common of these are probably synovial chondromatosis and osteochondromatosis, which develop as cartilaginous synovial plaques that sometimes ossify. These cause episodic pain or swelling in a knee, hip, elbow, or shoulder. The joint may lock if the plaques become detached, forming loose bodies. Radiographs reveal multiple opacities if ossification has occurred; arthroscopy may be useful for both diagnosis and treatment.

Pigmented villonodular synovitis (PVNS) is a nonmalignant proliferative disorder of unknown cause that usually affects the entire synovium of a single joint. This condition occurs most often in early middle age and in the knee in 80% of cases. Uncommonly, two or more joints are involved; similar lesions occur in tendons and bursae. Pain and swelling are characteristic, as is serosanguineous synovial fluid. Radiographic signs include soft tissue swelling, subchondral cysts (particularly in the hip), and pressure erosions. Treatment is synovectomy. Hemangiomas, lipomas, and xanthomas may simulate PVNS.

Synoviomas (synovial sarcomas) are rare, aggressive tumors of young adults. They usually originate in the extremities adjacent to, but not within, a joint. Primary tumors histologically identical to synoviomas have been found in the head and neck, abdominal wall, retroperitoneum, heart, and mediastinum, supporting the view that the tumor originates from mesenchyme rather than synovium. Detection within tumor cells of both cytokeratin (an epithelial intermediate filament) and vimentin (a mesenchymal intermediate filament) has led to the suggestion that the synovioma is a carcinosarcoma. Synoviomas are usually discovered as deep swellings within a tendon sheath, a bursa, or a joint capsule. Pain and tenderness are variable, as are effusions. They metastasize early to lungs, bone, and lymph nodes. Tumor size > 4 cm, a high mitotic rate, and local recurrence after excision convey a poor prognosis.

Chondrosarcomas and fibrosarcomas are other malignancies arising within or near joints, and intrasynovial myeloma and lymphoma are rare causes of a swollen or painful joint.

Thorough investigation is required for unexplained pain or swelling within or adjacent to a single joint.

260 ERYTHROMELALGIA
Eugene V. Ball

Erythromelalgia (see Ch. 46) is a syndrome of episodic burning pain and redness in the extremities. Attacks may be confined to feet and, if severe and prolonged, may spread to the hands, or they may begin simultaneously in hands and feet. They are most often provoked by increasing environmental temperatures, although a few persons experience attacks only with febrile illnesses. The combination of increasing ambient temperatures and exercise often induces symptoms. Some persons maintain environmental temperatures at levels that are uncomfortably low for themselves, as well as others, to avoid attacks of erythromelalgia. Some sleep bundled up against the cold of an unheated room but with feet protruding uncovered from the blankets. Relief may require immersing the feet in ice water. The feet appear normal between attacks, except in those persons who habitually walk barefoot because attacks are provoked by wearing shoes.

Erythromelalgia is sometimes familial. In one remarkable kindred, the disorder is autosomal dominant, afflicting 29 members. Most often beginning between ages 2 and 8, it has been responsible for severe adjustment problems in youth, engendered in part by an inability to sit comfortably in a heated classroom or to participate in physical activities. In this kindred, the disorder has been frequently misdiagnosed as arthritis, reflex sympathetic dystrophy, or Raynaud's phenomenon; its pathogenesis is unknown, but it is not related to thrombocythemia.

By far the most common recognized cause of nonfamilial erythromelalgia is thrombocythemia, usually a feature of a myeloproliferative disorder. Erythromelalgia was the presenting symptom in 26 of 40 patients with platelet counts in excess of 500×10^9 per liter. Arteriolar inflammation and thrombotic occlusions were found on skin punch biopsy samples. Erythromelalgia disappeared for three or four days after a single dose of aspirin, which is the duration of its inhibition of platelet aggregation. In the absence of thrombocythemia, aspirins are likely to be ineffective for treating or preventing erythromelalgia.

Other reported associations with erythromelalgia include diabetes mellitus. In addition, nifedipine and bromocriptine can cause an erythromelalgia-like disorder.

Finley WH, Lindsey JR, Fine J-D, et al.: Autosomal dominant erythromelalgia. Am J Med Genet 42:310, 1992. *Clinical description of erythromelalgia in a large kindred.*
Michiels JJ, van Joost T, Vuzevski VD: Idiopathic erythromelalgia: A congenital disorder. J Am Acad Dermatol 21(S pt. 2):1128, 1989. *A brief report of idiopathic erythromelalgia in a female whose symptoms began at 2 years of age and increased in severity until age 14, by which time she was sleeping with her feet immersed in ice water.*
Millard FE, Hunter CS, Anderson M, et al.: Clinical manifestations of essential thrombocythemia in young adults. Am J Hematol 33:27, 1990. *Essential thrombocythemia was identified in 13 patients whose median age was 26. Erythromelalgia was the most common complication, occurring in 7 of the 13, of whom 7 were males.*

261 MULTIFOCAL FIBROSCLEROSIS

H. Ralph Schumacher, Jr.

In rare instances the delicate fibrous areolar tissue in a certain anatomic region becomes the site of a chronic low-grade inflammatory process, leading to deposition of dense sclerotic plaques, which may obstruct or limit the movement of adjacent viscera. When the process is in the active phase, there are characteristic findings of chronic or granulomatous inflammation, featured by mononuclear cell infiltration, plasma cells, some eosinophils, and occasional giant cells. Macrophage infiltration has recently been emphasized in retroperitoneal fibrosis. In the end stages, the pathologic lesion is simply that of scar tissue so that by the time this process causes clinical manifestations there may be little evidence of the initial inflammatory reaction. In at least some cases there is an accompanying vasculitis. As a general rule the process tends to originate in the midline, around the great vessels, and then to spread laterally. In most cases a clue to the inciting mechanism is lacking.

Syndromes that have been considered as manifestations of multifocal fibrosclerosis include retroperitoneal fibrosis, mediastinal fibrosis, sclerosing cholangitis (see Ch. 126), Riedel's thyroiditis (see Ch. 203), pseudotumor of the orbit, Peyronie's disease (a sclerotic induration of the corpora cavernosa of the penis), and sclerosing peritonitis. Other sites of a similar fibrosis, such as the testes, vagina, and suprasellar area, also have been reported. Pulmonary and myocardial fibrosis syndromes generally have not been seen as related to multifocal fibrosclerosis, although pleural fibrosis along with retroperitoneal fibrosis can be seen with ergotamine use.

Although most of these syndromes have been described as separate entities, several anatomic areas may become affected in one person. For example, retroperitoneal fibrosis and sclerosing mediastinitis may be present at the same time along with varying combinations of sclerosing cholangitis, Riedel's thyroiditis, and pseudotumor of the orbit. A possible genetic predisposition is suggested by familial cases and by an association between fibrosing syndromes and α_1-antitrypsin deficiency. Familial mediastinal or retroperitoneal fibrosis also may be associated with HLA (human leukocyte antigen)-B27 and seronegative spondylarthropathies.

Comings DE, Skubi KB, Van Eyes J, et al.: Familial multifocal sclerosis. Ann Intern Med 66:884, 1967. *Description of multiple sites of fibrosis in two brothers.*

Goldbach P, Mohsenifar Z, Salick AI: Familial mediastinal fibrosis associated with seronegative spondyloarthropathy. Arthritis Rheum 26:221, 1983. *Two siblings with both diseases.*

RETROPERITONEAL FIBROSIS. In retroperitoneal fibrosis, the process usually begins over the promontory of the sacrum and extends laterally across the ureters and as high as the second or third lumbar vertebra. Less commonly, the lesion develops in other extraperitoneal areas, e.g., contiguous with the kidneys, duodenum, descending colon, or urinary bladder. In some cases there has been an associated vasculitis in the skin and subcutaneous tissue, manifested by the formation of nodules, erythematous discolorations, and ulcerations. Similarly, inflammatory changes in small vessels at the sites of the sclerosis have been noted. Glomerulonephritis has been seen in a few patients.

The occurrence of retroperitoneal fibrosis in patients taking methysergide for migraine has been reported with greater frequency than could be due to chance. Occasional cases have been reported after use of other drugs such as ergotamine, various β-adrenergic blocking agents, hydralazine, and methyldopa. Associated diseases in patients with retroperitoneal fibrosis have included systemic lupus erythematosus; vasculitis; scleroderma; eosinophilic fasciitis; biliary cirrhosis; rubella-associated arthritis; renal, uterine, and other cancers; and carcinoid. Trauma, surgery, and occasionally ruptured echinococcal cysts have been reported as apparent causes. One patient with associated periarticular fibrosis had elevated plasma levels of a platelet-derived growth factor.

The disorder is about twice as common in males as in females, and the peak incidence is in the fifth and sixth decades. Cases have been reported in children. The manifestations are variable, depending on the anatomic location of the process. Pain is the most common symptom; it tends to be located in the low back and may be accompanied by symptoms referable to the gastrointestinal tract. The patient is likely to lose weight and have low-grade fever. There may be some anemia and an elevated erythrocyte sedimentation rate. Although the ureter is the structure most often affected, symptoms referable to the urinary tract are uncommon until obstructive uropathy has led to azotemia and other clinical manifestations of renal insufficiency. The fibrosing process may surround the inferior vena cava, but obstruction of that vessel is uncommon. Thromboembolism and hypertension can be complications. Arterial invasion has been described. Portal hypertension may occur. Retroperitoneal fibrosis occasionally develops in association with definable abdominal aortic aneurysm or aortitis and is considered in some cases to begin as a periaortitis. A possible element of reaction to atheromatous components has been described.

Diagnosis of retroperitoneal fibrosis has been most often suggested by the findings at intravenous pyelography: displacement of the ureters toward the midline and evidence of obstruction, usually at the level of the pelvic brim. One or both ureters may be affected. In rare instances a mass can be palpated in the pelvis or on the posterior abdominal wall. Ultrasonography, computed tomographic (CT) scanning, and magnetic resonance imaging (MRI) also can identify the fibrosing masses. Once a mass has been disclosed, the main problem in differential diagnosis lies in distinguishing retroperitoneal fibrosis from retroperitoneal tumor. Multiple deep biopsies should be made at the time of laparotomy.

Surgical treatment, if used before severe renal damage, is often highly successful. Inasmuch as the fibrosing process is seldom invasive, the constricted organ usually can be freed by blunt dissection so that normal movement or flow is restored. Relief of ureteral obstruction is usually achieved by bringing the ureter out on the anterior surface of the sclerotic mass. Occasionally, however, the obstruction recurs months or years after such treatment. Some surgeons wrap the ureters in omentum to decrease recurrent obstruction. Steroid therapy may be helpful in the rare case detected early or may be employed as an adjunct to surgical measures. Azathioprine has been used successfully in a few cases. Other drugs such as penicillamine, colchicine, and gamma-interferon, with theoretical ability to limit clinical fibrosis, have not been studied in this disease. Progesterone and tamoxifen have been reported to produce regression of fibrosis. When the inferior vena cava is obstructed, surgical relief is technically difficult and risky; here it may be preferable to temporize in the hope that development of collateral pathways may alleviate the circulatory block.

The long-term outlook is fairly good if the disease is recognized and if its obstructive consequences can be treated by surgical means. The disease often tends to run its course and subside. Most deaths have been caused by renal failure.

Benson JR, Baum M: Tamoxifen for retroperitoneal fibrosis. Lancet 341:836, 1993. *Regression of fibrosis also has been described with desmoid tumors.*

Cohle SD, Leil JT: Inflammatory aneurism of the aorta, aortic and coronary arteritis. Arch Pathol Lab Med 112:1121, 1988. *Inflammatory aneurisms of the aorta and other vasculitis may be associated with retroperitoneal fibrosis.*

Ewald EA, Gikas PW, Castor CW: Periarticular fibrosis associated with idiopathic retroperitoneal fibrosis. J Rheum 15:1443, 1988. *Elevated plasma platelet-derived growth factor is proposed as a possible pathogenetic mechanism.*

MEDIASTINAL FIBROSIS. Taut bundles of collagenous tissue form in the superior and anterior mediastinum, with impingement on the aorta, trachea, bronchi, esophagus, and pericardium. Patients may have thoracic pain, but the predominant manifestations are those caused by obstruction of the superior vena cava: puffy, suffused appearance of the face and conjunctivae; nonpitting edema of the face, neck, and upper extremities; and distended veins in the neck and upper extremities. Rarely, the principal vessels affected are the pulmonary arteries, causing pulmonary hypertension. More frequently, the pulmonary veins are involved, and here severe hemoptysis may be the most prominent manifestation. Pericardial fibrosis can lead to constrictive pericarditis. The main task in differential diagnosis is to distinguish this relatively benign condition from obstruction caused by tumor. Roentgenographic examination of the chest may reveal little or no abnormality or some pleural thickening. Angiographic studies show obstruction of the affected vessels. Thoracotomy may be required for histologic diagnosis.

Histoplasmosis and possibly tuberculosis may cause some mediastinal fibrosis. Mediastinal hemorrhage can lead to fibrosis, and cases have been associated with methysergide use. An interesting recent association has been with the SAPHO syndrome (*s*ynovitis, *a*cne, *p*ustulosis, *h*yperostosis, and *o*steomyelitis). Some patients with this syndrome have shown gradual improvement over months or years, presumably because of development of collateral circulation. Successful superior vena cava bypass surgery has been described. Corticosteroid therapy was ineffective in some reported cases.

Cunningham T, Farrell J, Veale D, et al.: Anterior mediastinal fibrosis with superior vena caval obstruction complicating the synovitis-acne-pustulosis-hyperostosis-osteomyelitis syndrome. Br J Rheumatol 32:408, 1993. *This idiopathic sterile inflammatory reaction most often involves the anterior chest wall.*

Mathiesen DJ, Grillo HC: Clinical manifestation of mediastinal fibrosis and histoplasmosis. Ann Thorac Surg 54:1053, 1992. *Histoplasma were still stainable in some resected specimens.*

Papandreou L, Panagou P, Bouros D: Mediastinal fibrosis and radiofrequency radiation exposure: Is there an association? Respiration 59:181, 1992. *Hemoptysis can be a presenting symptom. This and other reports raise the question of radiation as a cause.*

SCLEROSING PERITONITIS.

A fibrotic syndrome has been observed in patients treated for prolonged periods with the now withdrawn β-adrenergic blocking drug practolol. Only a few cases have been reported with propranolol or other β blockers. Some cases have developed years after cessation of therapy. The peritonitis consists of a thick fibrous encasement of the small intestine, and the symptoms include abdominal fullness, back pain, ascites, weight loss, and signs of subacute obstruction. Surgery may be needed to peel away the fibrous tissue. Sclerosing peritonitis with many similarities also has been seen in idiopathic forms in association with systemic conditions, including drug abuse, sarcoidosis, and sicca syndrome, and now most importantly in patients treated with continuous ambulatory peritoneal dialysis (CAPD). A variety of factors used in dialysis have been suggested to contribute. Hemoperitoneum and peritoneal calcification have been reported in recent cases along with intestinal obstruction and ultrafiltration failure. Ultrasound findings can suggest the diagnosis.

Lo WK, Chan KT, Leung AC, et al.: Sclerosing peritonitis complicating prolonged use of chlorhexidine in alcohol in the connection procedure for continuous ambulatory peritoneal dialysis. Peritoneal Dialysis Int 11:166, 1991. *A mechanism is suggested and improvement noted with continued CAPD without the chlorhexidine.*

Pusateri R, Ross R, Marshall R, et al.: Sclerosing encapsulating peritonitis; report of a case with small bowel obstruction managed by long term hyperalimentation, and a review of the literature. Am J Kidney Dis 8:56, 1986. *This is a serious complication of peritoneal dialysis. Improvement in this patient occurred during parenteral nutrition.*

262 INTRODUCTION TO MICROBIAL DISEASE

Gerald L. Mandell

Infectious diseases have profoundly influenced the course of human history. The black plague (caused by *Yersinia pestis*) changed the social structure of medieval Europe. The outcomes of military campaigns have been altered by outbreaks of diseases such as dysentery and typhus. Malaria influenced the geographic and racial pattern of distribution of hemogloblins and erythrocyte antigens. The development of *Plasmodium falciparum* is inhibited by the presence of hemoglobin S, and Duffy blood group–negative erythrocytes are resistant to infection with *Plasmodium vivax*. Thus populations with these erythrocyte factors are found in areas where malaria is common. Infections are the major cause of morbidity and mortality in the developing world. AIDS threatens to disrupt the social fabric in some countries of Africa and is severely stressing the health care system in the United States and other parts of the world.

Infection may be defined as multiplication of microbes (viruses, bacteria, fungi, protozoa, or multicellular parasites) in the tissues of the host. The host may or may not be symptomatic. For example, infection with the human immunodeficiency virus (HIV) may cause no overt signs or symptoms of illness or tissue damage for years. The definition of infection probably also should include instances of multiplication of microbes on the surface or in a lumen of the host, causing signs and symptoms of illness or disease. Certain strains of *Escherichia coli* may multiply in the gut and cause a diarrheal illness without invading tissues. This is also considered an infection. Microbes can cause diseases without actually infecting the host by virtue of toxin production. *Clostridium botulinum* may grow in certain improperly processed foods and produce a toxin that can be lethal upon ingestion. At no time does the microbe grow in or on the host. A relatively trivial infection such as that caused by *Clostridium tetani* in a small puncture wound can cause devastating illness because of a toxin released from the organism growing in the tissues.

We live in a virtual sea of microorganisms, and all our body surfaces have an indigenous bacterial flora. This normal flora actually protects us from infection. Reduction of gut colonization increases susceptibility to infection by pathogens such as *Salmonella typhimurium*. The normal florae are thought to exert their protective effect by several mechanisms: (1) utilizing nutrients and occupying an ecologic niche, thus competing with pathogens; (2) producing antibacterial substances that inhibit the growth of pathogens; and (3) inducing host immunity that is cross-reactive and effective against pathogens. In addition to the normal flora, transient colonization may be seen with known or potential pathogens. This may be a special problem in hospitalized patients (see Ch. 267).

Only a very small proportion of microbial species may be considered to be principal or professional pathogens, and even among these species only a relatively small number of clones have been shown to cause disease. This supports the concept that pathogenic organisms are highly adapted to the pathogenic state and have developed a set of characteristics which enables them to be transmitted, to attach to surfaces, to invade tissue, and to cause disease. In contrast, opportunistic pathogens cause disease principally in impaired hosts. Organisms that may be harmless members of the normal flora in healthy people may act as virulent invaders in patients with severe defects in host defense mechanisms. Pathogenic organisms may be acquired by several routes. Direct contact has been implicated in the acquisition of staphylococcal disease. Airborne spread, usually by droplet nuclei, is seen in respiratory diseases such as influenza. Contaminated water is the usual vehicle in *Giardia* infection and typhoid fever. Food-borne toxin illnesses may be caused by extracellular toxins produced by *Clostridium perfringens* and *Staphylococcus aureus*. Blood and blood products may be vectors for transmitting hepatitis B virus and HIV. Sexual transmission is also important for these latter two agents and for a variety of pathogens including *Treponema pallidum* (syphilis), *Neisseria gonorrhoeae* (gonorrhea), and *Chlamydia trachomatis* (nonspecific urethritis). The fetus may be infected *in utero*, and this may be devastating with rubella virus and cytomegalovirus. Insect vectors may be important, as illustrated by mosquitoes for malaria, ticks for Lyme disease, and lice for typhus.

Pathogens are able to cause disease because of a finely tuned array of adaptations. These include the ability to attach to appropriate cells, often mediated by specialized structures such as the pili on gram-negative rods. Microbes such as *Shigella* species have the ability to invade cells and cause damage in that way. Toxins may act at a distance or may intoxicate only infected cells. Pathogens have the ability to thwart host defenses by a variety of ingenious maneuvers. The antiphagocytic capsular coat of the pneumococcus is an example. Organisms may change their surface antigen display so as to outmaneuver the host immune system. This can be seen with influenza virus and trypanosomes. Certain pathogens have the ability to inhibit the respiratory burst of phagocytes (*Toxoplasma gondii*), and others can destroy phagocytic cells that have engulfed them (*Streptococcus pyogenes*). The environment plays an important role in infection, both in transmission and in the ability of the host to combat the invader. The humidity and temperature of air may affect the infectivity of airborne pathogens. The sanitary state of food and water is an important factor for the acquisition of enteric pathogens. The "bad air" of swamps associated with malaria turned out to be due to the mosquitoes, but the environmental association was appropriate. The nutritional status of the host clearly is a significant factor in certain infectious diseases. The establishment of infection is a complicated interplay of factors involving the microbe, the host, and the environment.

With rare exceptions, infections are treatable and often curable diseases. Thus it is important to make an accurate etiologic diagnosis and promptly institute appropriate therapy. In acute infections such as pneumonia, meningitis, or gram-negative sepsis, rapid institution of therapy may be life-saving, and thus a *presumptive* etiologic diagnosis should be established prior to a *definitive* diagnosis. This presumptive diagnosis can be based on the history, physical examination, epidemiology of illness in the community, and rapid techniques such as microscopic examination of appropriate gram-stained specimens. Antimicrobial therapy can then be instituted for the presumptive etiologic agents but must be re-evaluated as more definitive diagnostic information becomes available (see Ch. 270 and 327).

263 THE FEBRILE PATIENT
David C. Dale

Fever, or "pyrexia," is an elevation of body temperature to a level above normal, i.e., to $> 37.5°C$ (99.5° F), due to resettings of the thermoregulatory center in the medulla. To detect fever, oral, rectal, tympanic membrane, and pulmonary artery measurements are more reliable than axillary temperatures. Fever is a useful marker of inflammation; usually the height of the fever reflects the severity of the inflammatory process. Anorexia, malaise, myalgias, headache, and other constitutional symptoms often occur concomitantly. When the body temperature changes rapidly, chills and sweats are also observed. Fever with night sweats is a feature of many chronic inflammatory conditions. *Hyperthermia* is a term for fever due to a disturbance of thermal regulatory control: excessive heat production (e.g., with vigorous exercise or as a reaction to some anesthetics), decreased dissipation (e.g., with dehydration), or loss of regulation (e.g., due to injury to the hypothalmic regulatory center).

Most febrile patients have pain, tenderness, redness, and swelling at the site of inflammation, and the cause of the fever is readily identified. In a general medical practice, the most common causes of fever are upper respiratory illnesses, urinary tract infections, cellulitis, superficial abscesses, and pneumonia. In otherwise healthy individuals, fever alone is not a cause for hospitalization unless it is quite high ($> 39°$ C, or 102° F) or accompanied by shaking, chills, hypotension, a change in the sensorium, or other symptoms suggesting bacteremia. However, in immunosuppressed individuals, the elderly, and patients with recent surgery, greater caution is indicated.

FEVER OF UNKNOWN ORIGIN (FUO). An FUO is usually defined in adults as an illness lasting more than 3 weeks with temperatures $> 101°$ F (38.3° C) in which a diagnosis has not been made despite a good hospital or office evaluation. Ordinarily by this time the workup has included a history, physical examination, routine blood and urine tests and cultures, radiographs, and some specialized serologic tests. With careful further evaluation a diagnosis can be made in 70 to 90% of these cases.

Diagnoses for FUO's fall into six general categories: infections, noninfectious inflammatory conditions, neoplastic diseases, drug fevers, factitious illnesses, and a group of less common causes (Table 263–1). The pattern of fever is only occasionally helpful in pointing to a specific diagnosis, e.g., the alternate-day fever in established *Plasmodium vivax* infections, the sustained fever in untreated *Salmonella typhi* infections and other continuous bacteremias, and the relapsing (Pel-Ebstein) fever in Hodgkin's disease and other lymphomas.

Evaluation of the FUO Patient. In patients with persisting fevers, it is important first to carefully review the medical history and repeat the physical examination. New clues may be found in the social, occupational, travel, and medication history. On physical examination, special attention should be given to the skin, lymph nodes (including epitrochlear, postauricular, axillary), mucous membranes (including the conjunctivae), and abdominal region (masses, tenderness, and size of the liver and spleen). Usually the basic laboratory tests—CBC, differential, sedimentation rate, urinalysis, liver function tests, skin tests for delayed hypersensitivity (e.g., PPD, mumps), and stool for occult blood—should be repeated. Most patients with active inflammation are anemic, and the leukocyte dif-

ferential can provide valuable clues. Neutrophilia suggests an occult bacterial infection. Monocytosis suggests tuberculosis, brucellosis, inflammatory bowel disease, or other chronic inflammatory conditions. Severe lymphopenia suggests immunodeficiency or a malignancy. A very elevated sedimentation rate suggests giant cell/temporal arteritis, polymyalgia rheumatica, Still's disease, bacterial endocarditis, or other occult infections, and a normal test rarely occurs with any of these illnesses. If the alkaline phosphatase is elevated, obstructive or infiltrative disease of the liver is the most likely cause, although nonspecific elevation is not uncommon. Other tests, e.g., antinuclear antibodies, febrile agglutinins, complement assays, may be positive but are rarely helpful in the FUO evaluation.

A definitive diagnosis is usually made through a combination of imaging studies, microbiologic tests, and/or biopsies. Previous radiographs should be reviewed carefully for evidence of sinusitis, apical inflammation or small nodules in the lungs, hilar adenopathy, or an intra-abdominal mass. Abdominal ultrasonography, gallium and radioisotopically labeled leukocyte scans, computed tomography (CT), and magnetic resonance imaging (MRI) are very helpful to examine the liver, gallbladder, spleen, and pelvic areas for tumors and abscesses. These tests have reduced, but not completely eliminated, the need for exploratory laparotomies.

Cultures of blood (including for *Myobacterium avium* in HIV patients), urine (including mycobacterial cultures if tuberculosis is suspected), and other bodily fluids (e.g., cerebrospinal, peritoneal, pleural) should be obtained if at all suggested by the clinical examination. It is useful to do anaerobic cultures of materials from suspected abscess cavities and to examine blood cultures for fastidious bacteria, yeast, and fungi in difficult cases. A tissue diagnosis often can be made from a biopsy of abnormal skin or lymph nodes or the bone marrow. Biopsies or needle aspirations of liver, lung, bone, or other deep tissue sites are also valuable when abscesses or tumors are suspected.

THERAPY. Therapeutic trials with antibiotics, corticosteroids, or antipyretics before the diagnosis is clear can confuse the evaluation. In some instances, a trial may be justified but should be time limited, i.e., about 2 weeks. In patients with deep tissue abscesses,

TABLE 263–1. CAUSES OF FEVER OF UNKNOWN ORIGIN

Infections

Abscesses—hepatic, subhepatic, gallbladder, subphrenic, splenic, periappendiceal, perinephric, pelvic, and other sites
Granulomatous—extrapulmonary and miliary tuberculosis, atypical *Mycobacteria,* fungal infection
Intravascular—catheter-related endocarditis, meningococcemia, gonococcemia, *Listeria, Brucella,* rat-bite fever, relapsing fever
Viral, rickettsial, and chlamydial—infectious mononucleosis, cytomegalovirus (CMV), human immunodeficiency virus (HIV), hepatitis, Q fever, psittacosis
Parasitic—extraintestinal amebiasis, malaria, toxoplasmosis

Noninfectious Inflammatory Disorders

Collagen vascular diseases—rheumatic fever, systemic lupus erythematosus, rheumatoid arthritis (particularly Still's disease), vasculitis (all types)
Granulomatous—sarcoidosis, granulomatous hepatitis, Crohn's disease
Tissue injury—pulmonary emboli, sickle cell disease, hemolytic anemia

Neoplastic Diseases

Lymphoma/leukemia—Hodgkin's and non-Hodgkin's lymphoma, acute leukemia
Carcinoma—kidney, pancreas, liver, gastrointestinal tract, lung, especially when metastatic
Atrial myxomas

Drug Fevers

Sulfonamides, penicillins, thiouracils, barbiturates, quinidine, laxatives (especially with phenolphthalein)

Factitious Illnesses

Injections of toxic materials, manipulation or exchange of thermometers

Other Causes

Familial mediterranean fever, Fabry's disease, cyclic neutropenia

fever usually persists despite antibiotics. In patients with noninfectious inflammatory diseases, e.g., sarcoidosis, Still's disease, or vasculitis, a good clinical diagnosis usually can be made before such therapies are begun. In patients with malignancies, rational therapy depends on a tissue diagnosis. Patients with factitious illness often have serious underlying psychiatric disorders. Care in confrontation is essential to prevent desperate acts including suicide.

Extensive workups of FUO's can be very expensive. In every patient the need for hospital care and testing should be continuously reassessed. When the patient is not severely ill, it is frequently worthwhile to use observation alone as a diagnostic tool. Sometimes even a short period of observation allows an obscure diagnosis to become obvious. In other cases, the fever disappears without the necessity for further diagnostic tests.

Bor DH, Makadon HJ, Friedland G, et al.: Fever in hospitalized medical patients: Characteristics and significance. J Gen Intern Med 3:119, 1988. *A careful review of the frequency and outcome of illnesses with fever in an acute care hospital.*

Kazanjian PH: Fever of unknown origin: Review of 86 patients treated in community hospitals. Clin Infect Dis 15:968, 1992. *FUO series from community hospitals, emphasizing the value of careful physical examination of the patient.*

Knockaert DC, Vanneste LJ, Bobbaers HJ: Recurrent or episodic fever of unknown origin: Review of 45 cases and survey of the literature. Medicine 72:184, 1993. *Episodic fever series, most cases with a long course before a diagnosis was made.*

Knockaert DC, Vanneste LJ, Vanneste SB, Bobbaers HJ: Fever of unknown origin in the 1980s: An update of the diagnostic spectrum. Arch Intern Med 152:51, 1992. *A series of 199 cases from the 1980's diagnosed using CT, ultrasound, and other newer modalities. Reference list includes many classic reports.*

Mackowiak PA, LeMaistre CF: Drug fever: A critical appraisal of conventional concepts: An analysis of 51 episodes in two Dallas hospitals and 97 episodes reported in the English literature. Ann Intern Med 106:728, 1987. *Illustrates the causes and courses of drug fevers in 51 cases, with a review of the literature.*

Rowland MD, Del Bene VE: Use of body computed tomography to evaluate fever of unknown origin. J Infect Dis 156:408, 1987. *Outlines the usefulness of CT for FUO patients.*

264 THE PATHOGENESIS OF FEVER

Bruce Beutler and Steven M. Beutler

DEFINITION. *Fever* (pyrexia) is defined as an elevation of core body temperature above the level normally maintained by the individual. Under normal circumstances, core body temperature (the temperature of blood in the right atrium) is tightly regulated, exhibiting circadian variations over a range that usually does not exceed $1°F$ ($0.6°$ C), with a mean value of $98.6°$ F ($37°$ C) (the normal "setpoint"). An array of thermoregulatory mechanisms, described in detail below, ensures that this temperature is maintained. During episodes of fever, the thermoregulatory setpoint is shifted such that the same thermoregulatory mechanisms are employed to maintain an abnormally elevated temperature.

It is important to realize that fever is not equivalent to an elevated core temperature but to an elevated setpoint. Under many circumstances, ranging from intense physical exertion to immersion in hot liquids, core temperature may be elevated yet fever does not exist, because the body is attempting to cope with the departure from homeostasis. Failure of thermoregulation also may be associated with elevated core temperature; this problem too (which occurs in malignant hyperthermia) is distinct from fever.

THERMOREGULATORY MECHANISMS. Core body temperature is determined by two opposing processes, each of which is regulated by the central nervous system (CNS). On the one hand, energy in the form of heat is generated by living tissues ("thermogenesis"). Energy may be passively absorbed from the environment as well. On the other hand, energy is inevitably lost to the environment, chiefly through the emission of infrared radiation and through transfer of energy to a surrounding medium. The temperature at which tissues are maintained is related to heat capacity (e.g., to the amount of energy required to elevate temperature by a defined increment) and to the quantity of energy lost or gained by the system.

Metabolic reactions proceed more rapidly at an elevated temperature. Therefore, the passive warming effect of a febrile state leads to accelerated energy production in the form of heat: for each temperature increment of $1°$ F ($0.6°$ C), basal metabolic rate increases by approximately 10%. This may, at times, be quite significant from a nutritional point of view.

Muscle is a particularly flexible transducer of chemical energy. "Shivering thermogenesis" refers to the unconscious process whereby muscles are recruited to produce energy through the exercise of activity, leading to an enhanced metabolic demand. This is one mechanism responsible for the rise in body temperature in fever. Hence a sharp "chill" often heralds the onset of fever.

Conservation of energy is effected through piloerection in mammals other than humans. In humans, "gooseflesh" is the equivalent response. "Flushing" represents a redistribution of circulation to dermal vessels and facilitates heat loss; a blanched appearance of the skin indicates an attempt to conserve heat.

INITIATION OF FEVER. The neural pathways responsible for thermoregulation originate in the hypothalamus. A local sensing mechanism exists wherein the temperature of blood is coupled to the development of autonomic discharge. Elevation of body temperature depends primarily on sympathetic outflow, leading to shivering thermogenesis and dermal vasoconstriction, whereas cooling mechanisms (sweating and dermal vasodilation) involve a mixture of sympathetic and parasympathetic pathways.

Certain neurotropic drugs can disrupt the hypothalamic thermosensory mechanism, or blunt the hypothalamic response, and so may interfere with the development of fever. Among these, phenothiazines are the best known for their "poikilothermic" effect. These agents are not specifically active in febrile states; rather, they act to disable thermoregulatory mechanisms.

CLINICAL MANIFESTATIONS. Although fever patterns tend to be nonspecific, they may sometimes provide diagnostic clues (Table 264–1). Intermittent fevers are seen in many conditions and are therefore of little help in discriminating between various disorders. Intermittent fever also may be caused when a continuous fever is interrupted with antipyretics or cooling measures; such interventions must be taken into account in analysis of a temperature curve.

In addition to considering patterns of pyrexia, it is worthwhile to note the relationship between core temperature and other vital signs. For example, a dissociation between the temperature and pulse is sometimes seen in cases of typhoid fever, Legionnaire's disease, psittacosis, and brucellosis. Factitious fever is also accompanied by an inappropriately low pulse. In addition, the respiratory rate may remain unchanged and normal superimposed diurnal variations in temperature may be absent in factitious fever.

Drug fever may occur in association with nearly any medication (see Ch. 10). There is no characteristic fever pattern. Fevers due to drug allergy tend to be well tolerated and may be accompanied by other allergic phenomena such as rash, nephritis, or neutropenia in 20 to 60% of patients.

Extreme pyrexia (characterized by a core temperature $> 106°$ F) often indicates failure of a distal mechanism of thermoregulation, occurring alone or in combination with infection. Examples of noninfectious causes of such extreme pyrexia include heat stroke (see Ch. 71), neuroleptic malignant syndrome (see Ch. 457), and malignant hyperthermia associated with succinylcholine.

CYTOKINES AND FEVER. Hypothalamic dysregulation and fever are triggered by proteins released from cells of the immune system (Fig. 264–1). This communication between the immune system and the nervous system is perhaps the most thoroughly studied "neuroimmunoendocrine" link. In response to invasive stimuli, including components of various microorganisms (e.g., lipoteichoic

TABLE 264–1. FEVER PATTERNS AS DIAGNOSTIC CLUES

Fever Pattern	Cause
Alternate-day fever	*Plasmodium vivax, P. ovale*
Fever every third day	*P. malariae*
Relapsing fever: daily for 3–6 days; fever-free interval for about 1 week supervenes	*Borrelia sp*, rat bite fever (*Streptobacillus moniliformis; Spirillum minus*)
Continuous "undulating fever"	Brucellosis; typhoid
Periodic pyrexia (Pel-Ebstein phenomenon) with variable cycles	Hodgkin's disease

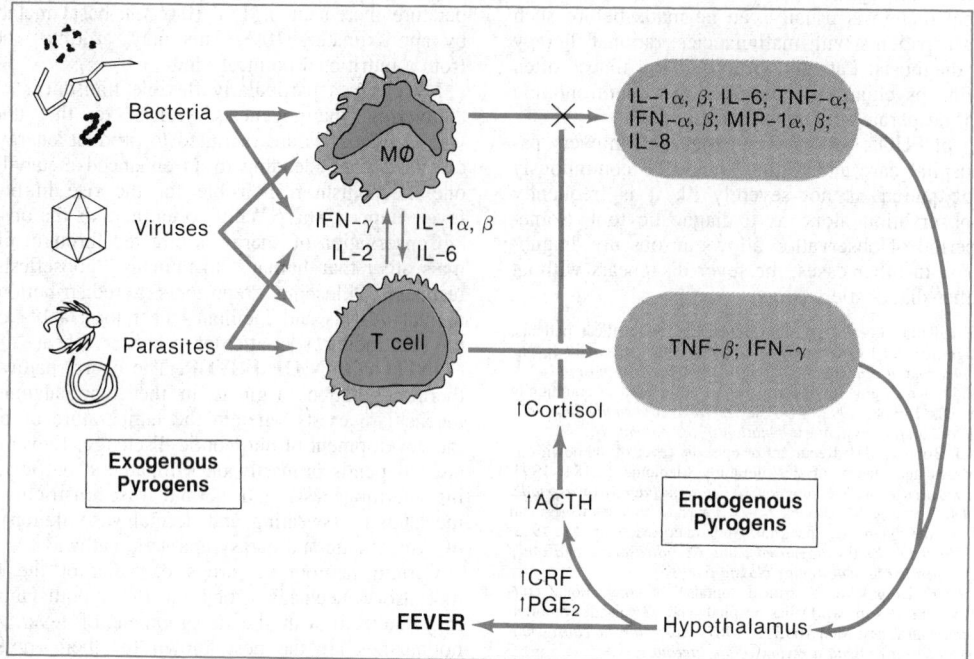

FIGURE 264–1. Production of endogenous pyrogens by macrophages and T lymphocytes. A variety of microbial pathogens produce molecules that function as exogenous pyrogens, triggering the release of endogenous pyrogens from mononuclear cells. ACTH = Adrenocorticotropic hormone; CRF = corticotropin-releasing factor; PGE$_2$ = prostaglandin E$_2$; other abbreviations are defined in the text and Table 264–2.

acid, lipopolysaccharides, and other collectively termed constituents ["exogenous pyrogen"]) or certain chemical agents (e.g., amphotericin and perhaps other drugs), cells of the immune system (principally macrophages and, to a lesser extent, lymphocytes) produce proteins that behave as "endogenous pyrogens." These proteins are designated as "monokines" and "lymphokines," respectively, and are often denoted under the more general heading of "cytokines." During the past decade, several of the cytokines active in the pathogenesis of fever have been isolated, and their structures have been determined by molecular cloning. As of this writing, 11 proteins with pyrogenic activity have been identified (Table 264–2); it is likely that many others exist. While mononuclear phagocytes comprise the principal source of pyrogenic cytokines, the same proteins may sometimes originate from nonimmune cells of neoplastic tissue, in which autonomous production and secretion may occur.

The pyrogenic cytokines are structurally diverse proteins with well-established effects in hematopoiesis, inflammation, and the regulation of cell metabolism. Individual agents are often markedly pleiotropic in their actions. In addition to their involvement in mediating fever, cytokines mediate the "acute phase response" (see Ch. 265), which is characterized by increased production of "acute phase reactants" in the liver (fibrinogen, C-reactive protein, complement proteins B, C3, C4, α_2 acid glycoprotein, serum amyloid A, and a variety of proteinase inhibitors among them), decreased production of albumin and transferrin, hypoferremia, hypertriglyceridemia, and other metabolic changes.

Pyrogenic cytokines are presumed to bind to receptors present on vascular endothelial cells that lie within the hypothalamus. They act to reset the hypothalamic thermoregulatory center, prompting an elevation of core body temperature. The resetting is believed to depend largely on endothelial cells producing prostaglandins (PGE$_2$ and perhaps PGF$_{2\alpha}$). Thromboxanes and lipoxygenase products also may affect the setpoint. Cytokines also may interact directly with neural tissues; there is evidence to suggest that the release of corticotropin-releasing factor (CRF) may trigger thermogenesis in response to at least one cytokine (interleukin-1β, or IL-1β).

Although no single cytokine is capable of provoking fever of a magnitude equivalent to that elicited by endotoxin, it is probable that combined production of several cytokines is sufficient to explain most fevers.

One monokine known as tumor necrosis factor-α (TNF-α) seems capable of reproducing many of the physiologic derangements ob-

served in septic shock and thus appears to mediate most of the deleterious effects of bacterial endotoxin, including fever. A lymphokine known as lymphotoxin (also referred to as tumor necrosis factor-β) is homologous to TNF-α, binds to the same receptor as TNF-α, and elicits many of the same effects. Two other cytokines (IL-1α and IL-1β), while incapable of causing shock by themselves, produce many effects similar to those of TNF-α, and in some instances, synergistic responses have been noted.

Many of the cytokines are mutually inducing, and the concept of a "cytokine cascade" has been offered to describe the production of several factors occurring in response to the elaboration of one member of the group. The temporal sequence of induction may be reflected in the course of fever *in vivo*. For example, injecting a bolus of TNF-α into a rabbit will immediately raise body temperature and cause a delayed rise, apparently related to secondary production of IL-1.

MECHANISMS OF ANTIPYRESIS. Nonsteroidal antipyretic agents inhibit fever by blocking the synthesis of prostaglandins (see Ch. 13) within the endothelium of the hypothalamic vasculature, which is accomplished through inhibition of cyclo-oxygenase. However, they do not diminish the elaboration of endogenous pyrogens and may actually increase the production of some of these proteins (notably TNF-α). Nonsteroidal antipyretics do not produce poikilothermic effects; they can reduce fever but cannot lower body temperature beneath its normal setpoint. It may reasonably be inferred from this observation that prostaglandins do not normally act to maintain core body temperature.

Glucocorticoid hormones directly impede the production of endogenous pyrogens by mononuclear phagocytic cells. Cytokine synthesis is inhibited at more than one level and has been studied most thoroughly in the case of TNF-α biosynthesis. Both transcription of the TNF-α gene and translation of the TNF-α mRNA are down-regulated by glucocorticoid agonists.

The cyclic (often circadian) course followed in many febrile illnesses has not been fully explained. In some instances (e.g., in malaria), a clear relationship to the life cycle of the pathogen has been demonstrated. Cyclicity may, in other cases, follow from the fact that cells comprising the chief source of endogenous pyrogens are rendered refractory by continued exposure to the stimulatory agent and must recover or be replaced.

TREATMENT. In the absence of specific knowledge concerning the benefits of fever, a conservative approach to the treatment of

TABLE 264–2. PROTEINS WITH PYROGENIC ACTIVITY

Endogenous Pyrogen	Other Names/ Abbreviations	Principal Source	Induced by	Principal Effects in Addition to Pyrogenesis	Physical Characteristics
Cachectin/tumor necrosis factor-α	TNF-α	Macrophages	LPS, other microbial products	Fever, shock, anorexia, wasting, tumor necrosis, bone resorption, $\downarrow$ adipocyte lipoprotein lipase, neutrophil activation, $\uparrow$ endothelial cell adhesiveness/procoagulant effect	Homotrimer; 17 kDa subunit size (nonglycosylated) $\updownarrow$ 26% identity
Lymphotoxin/tumor necrosis factor-β	TNF-β; LT	Lymphocytes (T & B)	Antigenic/mitogenic stimulation		Homotrimer; 20–25 KDa subunit size (glycosylated)
Interleukin-1α (IL-1α)	Leukocyte activity factor (LAF), leukocyte endogenous mediator (LEM), mononuclear cell factor (MCF), endogenous pyrogen (EP)	Macrophages and many other cell types	LPS, other microbial products, TNF	Fever, IL-2 production, bone resorption, pannus formation, neutrophil activation, $\uparrow$ endothelial cell adhesiveness/procoagulant effect	Monomer; 17 KDa (glycosylated) $\updownarrow$ 26% identity
Interleukin-1β (IL-1β)					Monomer; 17 KDa (glycosylated)
Interferon-α	IFN-α; leukocyte interferon	Leukocytes (esp. monocyte-macrophages)		Induction of antiviral state	22 KDa (glycosylated) $\updownarrow$ 23% identity
Interferon-β	IFN-β; fibroblast interferon	Fibroblasts	LPS, viral infection, double-stranded RNA		22 KDa (glycosylated)
Interferon-γ	IFN-γ; immune interferon; type 2 interferon	T lymphocytes		Macrophage activation Upregulation of Class I and Class II MHC molecules	20–25 KDa (glycosylated)
Interleukin-6 (IL-6)	Interferon-β_2, hepatocyte-stimulating factor (HSF), B-cell stimulating factor-2 (BSF-2), B-cell differentiation factor (BCDF)	Many cell types	LPS, TNF	$\uparrow$ Synthesis of acute phase reactants Weak antiviral effect Terminal differentiation of B cells; T-cell activation	21–26 KDa (glycosylated)
Macrophage inflammatory protein 1α	MIP 1α	Macrophages	LPS	Neutrophil chemotaxis	7.9 KDa (nonglycosylated) $\updownarrow$ 57% identity
Macrophage inflammatory protein 1β	MIP 1β				7.8 KDa (nonglycosylated)
Interleukin-8 (IL-8)	Monocyte-derived neutrophil chemotactic factor (MDNCF)		LPS, TNF, IL-1		8.0 KDa (nonglycosylated)

fever is advisable. Core temperatures beneath 105° F are well tolerated by most individuals. Moreover, when its source has been defined, fever often serves as an important indicator of therapeutic effect.

Under certain circumstances, aggressive treatment of fever is warranted. Patients with myocardial ischemia, patients predisposed to seizures, and pregnant women may require treatment with antipyretics, since elevation of core temperature increases cardiac output and myocardial oxygen demand, increases the likelihood of seizures, and may exert a teratogenic effect. Acetaminophen or nonsteroidal anti-inflammatory agents prove adequate for this purpose in the majority of cases. Physical methods for increasing heat dissipation also may be employed.

Temperatures that exceed 106° F are life-threatening and must be lowered immediately. Antipyretics are often ineffective in such instances, since pyrexia of this degree does not result from an aberrant hypothalamic setpoint. It is advisable, in such cases, to lower temperature by any means possible; the most effective action to be taken is to immerse the patient in ice water while monitoring core temperature to be certain that a state of hypothermia is not induced.

Moltz H: Fever: causes and consequences. Neurosci Biobehav Rev 17:237, 1993. *An excellent review analyzing the neurochemistry and neuroanatomy of fever.*
Rothwell NJ: CNS regulation of thermogenesis. Crit Rev Neurobiol 8:1, 1994. *A current appraisal of the pyrogenicity of various cytokines.*

265 THE ACUTE PHASE RESPONSE
Charles A. Dinarello

ACUTE PHASE CHANGES. Infections, trauma, inflammatory processes, and some malignant diseases induce a constellation of host responses collectively referred to as the "acute phase response." The response is associated with characteristic metabolic changes in liver protein synthesis, but on closer examination, changes also occur in several other systems that include hematologic, endocrinologic, and immunologic dysfunctions. These changes are called "acute" because most are observed within hours or days following the onset of infection or injury, although some acute phase changes also indicate chronic disease. The full spectrum of the response includes dramatic increases in the synthesis of several unique hepatic proteins that are not produced in health. One of these, C-reactive protein, is a marker of the acute phase response and can be used to indicate disease. The increased plasma concentrations of acute phase hepatic proteins, glycoproteins, and globulins are responsible for elevated erythrocyte sedimentation rates. Although the liver is producing increasing amounts of a variety of proteins, hepatic albumin synthesis is decreased. Increases in gluconeogenesis, energy expenditure, and muscle proteolysis occur and contribute to weight loss. However, anorexia is often present and may account for most of the weight loss. Fever may be present, and increased sleep and lethargy are frequent clinical complaints. Leukocytosis with increased numbers of circulating immature neutrophils is common, and serum iron and zinc levels are depressed, while increased ceruloplasmin levels result in elevated serum copper. Thyroid dysfunction can be present, and there is often abnormal glucose tolerance and lipid metabolism. In addition, anemia develops despite adequate stores of iron, and hypergammaglobulinemia often occurs.

Although the most florid presentation of the acute phase response is observed in patients with bacterial infections, burns, or multiple injuries, clinicians also encounter acute phase changes in patients with occult infections or chronic illnesses such as rheumatoid arthritis, Crohn's disease, and several autoimmune diseases. The presence of acute phase changes also can serve as an indicator of silent disease and some cancers, particularly renal cell carcinoma and Hodgkin's disease. The acute phase response has the outstanding characteristic of being a generalized host reaction irrespective of the localized or systemic nature of the inciting disease. The various components of the response are remarkably consistent despite the considerable variety of pathologic processes that induce it. For example, plasma levels of several acute phase proteins are elevated following myocardial infarction, fracture of a bone, or bacterial pneumonia.

INDUCTION OF ACUTE PHASE CHANGES. How are infections, injuries, and immunologic and inflammatory reactions able to elicit acute phase changes in the host? The initiation of the acute phase response is linked to the production of hormone-like polypeptide mediators, now called cytokines. Several cytokines induce acute phase changes: interleukin 1 (IL-1), tumor necrosis factor, interferon-γ, interleukin 6 (IL-6), leukemia inhibitory factor, ciliary neurotropic factor, oncostatin M, and interleukin-11 (IL-11). This last five cytokines induce hepatic acute phase protein synthesis via the glycoprotein cell receptor 130. The ability of microbial and inflammatory substances to stimulate the production of these mediators in strategically located, specialized cells appears to be part of local pathologic changes in many diseases, as well as the systemic characteristics of the acute phase response.

Interferon-α is produced primarily during viral infections. Although it shares with IL-1 and tumor necrosis factor the ability to produce fever, sleep, and lethargy, interferon-α does not induce certain other acute phase changes, and hence elevated erythrocyte sedimentation rates and neutrophilia are not commonly observed during viral infections.

The patient with a localized bacterial infection represents an excellent example of the development of the acute phase response. At the onset of the infection, blood monocytes and tissue macrophages become activated either by phagocytosis of the invading microbe or by exposure to its products or toxins; the process results in the synthesis and release of various cytokines within 1 to 2 hours. These mediators enter the circulation and reach the brain where they initiate fever. Whereas fever is clearly one of the most obvious signs of the acute phase response, other components of the response can be present without apparent clinical manifestations. One of the most sensitive measures of the acute phase response is an increase in the number and immaturity of circulating neutrophils. In human subjects injected with small doses of IL-1 or related cytokines, neutrophilia can be measured in the absence of fever. Although not routinely measured, serum zinc and iron levels are depressed. Low serum iron associated with anemia in the face of adequate iron stores is characteristic of the acute phase response.

Within 8 to 12 hours after the onset of infection or trauma, the liver increases the synthetic rate of the so-called acute phase proteins. The response includes increases in proteins normally found in health as well as the appearance of new proteins that serve as markers of a pathologic event. Several normal plasma proteins increase several-fold during the acute phase response. These include haptoglobin, certain protease inhibitors, complement components, ceruloplasmin, and fibrinogen. However, true acute phase reactants increase several hundredfold. These include serum amyloid A protein, a precursor of the amyloid fibril in secondary amyloidosis, and C-reactive protein. C-reactive protein was named for its ability to interact with the C-polysaccharide of pneumococci and was the first acute phase protein described. Table 265–1 lists the characteristic pattern of increased plasma proteins observed during the acute phase response. Note one exception: The plasma concentration of albumin is decreased.

Of all the acute phase proteins, C-reactive protein is clinically the most important because its presence serves as an indicator of disease. C-reactive protein is particularly useful as a marker of the hepatic acute phase protein response and can be measured easily in most hospital clinical laboratories.

Despite the anabolic processes of the liver, the acute phase response is accompanied by a pronounced catabolism of muscle protein associated with loss of body weight and overall negative nitrogen balance. Fever increases oxygen and caloric demands (usually 7% per degree F), and most of the negative nitrogen balance results from oxidation of amino acids from skeletal muscle, which contributes to wasting. These amino acids are largely used for gluconeogenesis. Although the metabolic demands of elevated temperature contribute to the increased need for energy substrates, the host also requires a large supply of amino acids to synthesize new protein at a time when food intake may be impaired or appetite reduced. Amino acids are required for immunologic and reparative processes such as the clonal expansion of lymphocytes and the proliferation of fibroblasts. Also, they are needed for synthesis of hepatic acute phase proteins, immunoglobulins, and collagen. The mechanism of providing ample amino acids for these cellular functions seems to be well orchestrated during the acute phase response. The catabolism during infection and inflammation differs from that of starvation. Unlike starvation, in which large amounts of ketones are spilled into the urine, an individual with an infectious or inflammatory disease excretes protein with small amounts of ketones. IL-1, tumor necrosis factor, and IL-6 the primary mediators of acute phase changes, inhibit lipoprotein lipase and suppress appetite. In addition, these cytokines and interferons directly stimulate hepatic lipogenesis, contributing to the hypertriglyceridemia observed in patients with either acute or chronic disease.

MEASUREMENT OF ACUTE PHASE CHANGES IN CLINICAL MEDICINE. The acute phase response is nonspecific. However, the presence of certain acute phase changes in an otherwise healthy individual can alert the physician to hidden disease. Increased peripheral neutrophils and erythrocyte sedimentation rate are often used to detect an acute phase response. Measurement of C-reactive protein can help the physician determine the presence of disease in patients with vague, constitutional complaints. C-reactive protein levels are usually $< 100 \mu$g per liter but increase within hours 10- to 1000-fold. In severe bacterial infections, the serum level can rise from undetectable to over 100 mg per liter in 48 hours. The presence of elevated levels of C-reactive protein or serum amyloid A protein, even in the absence of fever or neutrophilia, may indicate occult infection or malignant change. Increases in C-reactive protein and serum amyloid A protein occur in

TABLE 265–1. PLASMA PROTEINS THAT INCREASE DURING THE ACUTE PHASE RESPONSE

C-reactive protein
Serum amyloid A protein
α_1-Glycoprotein
Ceruloplasmin
α-Macroglobulins
Complement components (C1–C4, factor B, C9, C11)
α_1-Antitrypsin
α_1-Antichymotrypsin
Fibrinogen
Prothrombin
Factor VIII
Plasminogen
Haptoglobin
Ferritin
Immunoglobulins
Lipoproteins

patients of any age and also in immunocompromised patients with opportunistic infections.

Not all inflammatory diseases are associated with elevated C-reactive protein. A refractory state can develop in certain diseases such as scleroderma, ulcerative colitis, and lupus erythematosus. Failure to develop hepatic protein changes and the neutrophilia of the acute phase response seems to be related to the presence of circulating inhibitors of cytokines, e.g., the IL-1 receptor antagonist.

TREATMENT OF ACUTE PHASE RESPONSES. Measurements of fever, acute phase plasma proteins, and peripheral leukocyte numbers are well-established procedures for monitoring many disease states. Although nonsteroidal anti-inflammatory agents are used to treat the fever and associated myalgias of acute phase responses, these drugs do not affect other acute phase changes in the liver, various endocrinologic parameters, or the bone marrow response. Antipyretic blood levels of aspirin and therapeutic concentrations of drugs such as indomethacin or ibuprofen do not reduce production of cytokines. On the other hand, corticosteroids are highly effective in reducing cytokine synthesis as well as the effect of these mediators on various tissue targets. Patients receiving therapeutic doses of corticosteroids have blunted acute phase responses with ongoing infections, inflammatory processes, or immunologic reactions.

The role of acute phase proteins in host defense and repair is not entirely clear. Studies suggest that the major role of C-reactive protein is to bind serum lipids or opsonize pneumococci, whereas serum amyloid A is thought to be immunosuppressive. Ceruloplasmin scavenges toxic free oxygen radicals that are injurious to many tissues. What is clear, however, is that the production and physical structure of these acute phase proteins have been conserved through 400 million years of evolution, and therefore they have presumably been useful to the host. The *Limulus* crab and fish make C-reactive protein that is nearly identical to human C-reactive protein. This argues that the acute phase response plays a role in survival.

Beisel WR: Magnitude of the host nutritional responses to infection. Am J Clin Nutr 30:1236, 1977. *Discussion of the metabolic imbalances seen in patients with infection and injury.*

Dinarello CA, Wolff SM: The role of interleukin-1 in disease. N Engl J Med 328:106, 1993. *Clinical role for IL-1 and IL-1 receptor antagonist in disease.*

Feingold KR, Soued M, Serio MK: Multiple cytokines stimulate hepatic lipid synthesis *in vivo*. Endocrinology 125:267, 1989. *Evidence that interleukin-1, tumor necrosis factor, and interferon may account for the hyperlipidemias observed in patients with acute or chronic inflammatory disease.*

Kushner I, Gewurz H, Benson MD: C-reactive protein and the acute-phase response. J Lab Clin Med 97:739, 1981. *A brief discussion of the usefulness of measuring C-reactive protein levels in clinical practice.*

Pepys MB, Baltz ML: Acute phase proteins with special reference to C-reactive protein and related proteins (pentaxins) and serum amyloid A protein. *In* Dixon FJ, Kunkel HG (eds.): Advances in Immunology, Vol 34. New York, Academic Press, 1983, pp 141-211. *A comprehensive discussion of the hepatic acute phase protein pattern observed during the acute phase response, with special attention to various autoimmune diseases.*

266 THE COMPROMISED HOST
Philip A. Pizzo

"Compromised host" is used to describe patients who have an increased risk for infectious complications as a consequence of a congenital or acquired qualitative or quantitative abnormality of one or more components of the host defense matrix (Table 266–1). Until the early 1980's, this term was largely restricted to patients with congenital immunodeficiencies (see Ch. 223) or to those who became immunocompromised as a consequence of cancer or its treatment, bone marrow failure, or treatment with immunosuppressive therapy. The advent of the acquired immunodeficiency syndrome (AIDS) has given the term "compromised host" a new meaning and relevance. The compromised host with AIDS is discussed in detail in Part XXII. In this chapter, the focus is on non-AIDS patients with altered immune defenses. However, many of the complications and approaches to diagnosis and management are generic.

PHYSICAL DEFENSE BARRIERS

The skin and mucosal surfaces represent the primary defense against both endogenous and exogenous sources of infection. Disruption of skin and mucosa may result from trauma, tumor invasion, the cytotoxic effects of chemotherapy or radiotherapy, the use of invasive diagnostic or therapeutic procedures (e.g., intravenous catheters), and effects of locally destructive infections such as oral herpes simplex. Such mucosal alterations provide a nidus for microbial colonization, a focus for localized infection, and a portal of entry for systemic invasion.

The skin and various mucosal surfaces are normally colonized by aerobic and anaerobic bacteria. However, in patients who have been hospitalized, who are neutropenic, or who have received prior broad-spectrum antibiotics, the normal gram-positive flora of the skin can be replaced by other gram-positive organisms such as CDC group JK *Corynebacterium* or *Bacillus* species or by gram-negative organisms (e.g., pseudomonads, enteric gram-negative rods), fungi (e.g., *Candida albicans* or *Aspergillus* species), and atypical *Mycobacterium* species such as *M. chelonei* or *M. fortuitum.*

Similarly, the gastrointestinal tract is normally colonized by an array of aerobic and anaerobic bacteria as well as some fungi, and disruption of its mucosa may lead to infections by a variety of pathogens including polymicrobial infections. A common cause for disruption of the gastrointestinal mucosal integrity is cytotoxic chemotherapy to patients with malignancy, particularly cytarabine (ara-C), the anthracyclines (daunorubicin and doxorubicin), methotrexate, 6-mercaptopurine, and 5-fluorouracil. Although stomatitis is usually the most clinically recognizable manifestation of gastrointestinal toxicity, diffuse gastrointestinal involvement is also likely. Frequently, the differentiation between chemotherapy-induced stomatotoxicity and localized infection (e.g., necrotizing gingivitis due to anaerobic bacteria or mucosal lesions due to herpes simplex virus) can be difficult, particularly in the neutropenic patient.

In addition to mucosal breakdown, mechanical obstruction of body passages also can increase the risk of serious localized infection due to stasis of local body fluids and resultant overgrowth of potentially pathogenic colonizing organisms. Common sites of secondary infection due to obstruction include the lung, urinary tract, biliary tract, and eustachian tube. One should consider an obstructive process when infection at any of these sites fails to respond to appropriate antibiotics.

Anatomic changes also can contribute to the risk of infection. For example, in patients with sickle cell disease, macrophage and splenic dysfunction predispose to the development of certain bacteremias, especially by *Streptococcus pneumoniae* and *Salmonella* species. Anatomic abnormalities of bones and joints as a result of vaso-occlusive crises caused by infarction of bone marrow, bony cortex, or synovium in patients with sickle cell disease also can predispose to development of infections such as osteomyelitis or arthritis caused by these organisms.

PHAGOCYTE DEFECTS

The polymorphonuclear leukocyte (PMN) and the monocyte are the two most important components of cellular host defense that protect against invasive bacteria and fungi. Both quantitative and qualitative defects affecting PMN's and monocytes may occur in compromised patients.

Quantitative Abnormalities of Phagocytes

Granulocytopenia is among the most important risk factors for serious infection in the compromised host. However, it is important to keep in mind that except for congenital neutropenias, there are often other alterations of the host defense matrix that occur in concert with granulocytopenia and can further alter the risk for infection as well as the types of infectious complications that occur.

Granulocytopenia is most commonly associated with malignant disease and its treatment with cytotoxic therapy. This includes patients with hematologic malignancies and lymphomas as well as the increasing number of patients with solid tumors who receive cytotoxic chemotherapy. Patients with primary or secondary bone marrow failure also have neutropenia as their predominant risk for infection. In addition to the neutropenia *per se,* the patterns of infection are also influenced by the other disease- or treatment-related immune abnormalities. For example, despite equivalent degrees of granulocytopenia, the patient with acute myelogenous

TABLE 266–1. PREDOMINANT PATHOGENS IN COMPROMISED PATIENTS; ASSOCIATION WITH SELECTED DEFECTS IN HOST DEFENSE

Host Defense Impairment	Bacteria	Fungi	Viruses	Other

Neutropenia	Gram-negative
	  Enteric organisms
	    (*E. coli, K. pneumoniae, Enterobacter* spp., *Citrobacter* spp.)
	    Pseudomonas aeruginosa
	Gram-positive
	  Staphylococci
	    (coagulase-negative, coagulase-positive)
	  Streptococci, including viridans strep
	    (enterococci)
	  Anaerobes
	    (anaerobic streptococci, *Clostridia* spp., *Bacteroides* spp.)
		Candida species
		  (*C. albicans* > *C. tropicalis* > other species)
		Aspergillus species
		  (*A. fumigatus, A. flavus*)		

Abnormal cell-mediated immunity	*Legionella* *Nocardia asteroides* *Salmonella* spp. Mycobacteria (*M. tuberculosis* and atypical mycobacteria) Disseminated infection from live bacteria vaccine (BCG)	*Cryptococcus neoformans* *Histoplasma capsulatum* *Coccidioides immitis* *Candida*	Varicella-zoster virus Herpes simplex virus Cytomegalovirus Epstein-Barr virus Herpesvirus 6 Disseminated infection from live virus vaccines (vaccinia, measles, rubella, mumps, yellow fever, live polio)	*Pneumocystis carinii* *Toxoplasma gondii* *Cryptosporidium* *Strongyloides stercoralis*

Immunoglobulin abnormalities	Gram-positive
	  Streptococcus pneumoniae, S. aureus
	Gram-negative
	  Haemophilus influenzae
	  Neisseria spp., enteric organisms
			Enteroviruses
			Disseminated infection from live virus vaccines (vaccinia, measles, rubella, mumps, yellow fever, polio)
				Giardia lamblia

Complement abnormalities
  C3, C5
	Gram-positive
	  S. pneumoniae, staphylococci
	Gram-negative
	  H. influenzae, Neisseria spp., Enteric organisms			

C5–C9	*Neisseria* species (*N. gonorrheae, N. meningitides*)			

Anatomic disruption
  Oral cavity
	α-Hemolytic streptococci, oral anaerobes
	  (*Peptococcus, Peptostreptococcus*)
		Candida	Herpes simplex virus	

Esophagus	Staphylococci, other colonizing organisms	*Candida*	Herpes simplex virus Cytomegalovirus	

Lower gastrointestinal tract	Gram-positive
	  Enterococci
	Gram-negative
	  Enteric organisms
	Anaerobes (*B. fragilis, C. perfringens*)
		Candida		*Strongyloides stercoralis*

Skin (IV catheter)	Gram-positive
	  Staphylococci, streptococci
	  Corynebacteria, Bacillus spp.
	Gram-negative
	  P. aeruginosa, enteric organisms
	Mycobacteria
	  M. fortuitum, M chelonei
		Candida
		Aspergillus		

Urinary tract	Gram-positive
	  Enterococci
	Gram-negative
	  Enteric organisms
	  P. aeruginosa
		Candida		

Splenectomy	Gram-positive
	  S. pneumoniae
	Gram-negative
	  Capnocytophaga
	  H. influenzae
	  Salmonella (sickle cell disease)
				Babella

From Rubin M, Walsh TJ, Pizzo PA: Clinical approach to the compromised host. *In* Hoffman R, Benz EJ Jr, Shattil SJ, et al. (eds.): Hematology: Basic Principles and Practices, 2nd Ed. New York, Churchill Livingstone, 1994.

leukemia (AML) may have a different pattern of infection than the patient with aplastic anemia. The disruption of a mucosal defense barrier occurring in the patient with AML who is receiving cytotoxic therapy appears to increase the risk for infection with enteric gram-negative bacteria, α-streptococci, or anaerobes. In contrast, the patient with aplastic anemia who does not have impaired mucosal integrity may be able to sustain longer periods of granulocytopenia without developing a systemic bacterial infection. On the other hand, if the patient with aplastic anemia is treated with steroids or cyclosporine, the risk for viral or fungal infection may be increased.

Regardless of these modifying factors, the relationship between granulocytopenia and serious infection has been established unequivocally by the classic study of Bodey and colleagues (Table 266–2). This study demonstrated that the risk of infection begins to increase significantly when granulocyte counts fall below 1000 per

TABLE 266–2. ASSOCIATION OF GRANULOCYTE LEVEL AND CHANCE OF DEVELOPING SIGNIFICANT INFECTION

Granulocyte Level (per cu mm)		Percentage of Serious Infections (Duration of Granulocytopenia in Weeks)							
Initial	Change	1	2	3	4	6	10	12	14
Any level	Any fall	12							
Any level	Fall to 2000	2							
Any level	Fall to 1500	5							
Any level	Fall to 1000	10	30	45	50	65	70	85	100
Any level	Fall to 500	19							
Any level	Fall to < 100	28	50	72	85	100			

Adapted from Bodey GP, Buckley M, Sathe YS, Freireich EJ: Quantitative relationships between circulatory leukocytes and infection in patients with acute leukemia. Ann Intern Med 61:328, 1966.

microliter and is most marked when the counts are ≤ 100 per microliter. In addition to the absolute granulocyte count, the duration of granulocytopenia is also directly related to the direction of granulocytopenia as well as to whether the counts are rising or falling.

For practical purposes, granulocytopenia is usually defined as a count of ≤ 500 PMN's and band forms per microliter. However, a patient with an absolute granulocyte count of 500 to 1000 per microliter that is rapidly falling is probably at greater risk for infection than a patient with a count of 200 per microliter that is rising. Thus the absolute granulocyte count, the duration of granulocytopenia, and whether the neutrophil count is falling or rising must all be considered when assessing the risk to any individual patient. Some clinicians also include the monocyte count in this equation to generate an absolute phagocyte index.

Granulocytopenia primarily predisposes patients to bacterial and fungal infection and does not of itself appear to increase the incidence or severity of viral and parasitic infections. In the 1950's and 1960's, when cytotoxic therapy was first being developed, gram-positive bacteria (especially *Staphylococcus aureus*) predominated. In the early 1970's, with the availability of antibiotics to control gram-positive bacteria (e.g., methicillin), gram-negative organisms (e.g., *Escherichia coli, Klebsiella, Pseudomonas aeruginosa*) emerged as the predominant pathogens in neutropenic patients, perhaps because of the increasing use of more aggressive chemotherapy regimens and the use of broader-spectrum antibiotics. During the 1980's, gram-positive organisms re-emerged as common bacterial isolates, and at many centers they now represent the most frequently encountered organisms.

In addition to these changes in the pattern of infection, institutional variations in the causes of infection and the antibiotic sensitivity patterns of isolates cannot be overemphasized, making it imperative for physicians to have a working knowledge of the specific isolates encountered at their own clinical setting.

The gram-negative organisms encountered most commonly in granulocytopenic patients are *E. coli, K. pneumoniae,* and *P. aeruginosa.* Together, these have generally accounted for approximately 90% of the gram-negative isolates at most centers. A precise source for gram-negative bacteremia is identified in only a minority of cases, but the gastrointestinal tract, respiratory tract soft tissue, and urinary tract are the most probable sources for infection. Of these three organisms, *P. aeruginosa* is often the most virulent in neutropenic hosts, although in most developed countries the incidence of infection due to *Pseudomonas* declined in neutropenic patients during the 1980's. But as a general rule, virtually any organism can be pathogenic if the host defenses are severely impaired. *Enterobacter* species, *Citrobacter* species, and *Serratia marcescens* are less frequently encountered but are notable because they rapidly become resistant to β-lactam antibiotics through the induction of chromosomally mediated β-lactamases. Of concern, an increase in *Enterobacter* sepsis has been observed at a number of treatment centers. Other less common gram-negative isolates include *Acinetobacter* species, *Haemophilus* species (usually nontypable *H. influenzae*), and nonaeruginosa pseudomonads (often catheter-related and antibiotic-resistant).

The gram-positive organisms most frequently encountered are the coagulase-negative staphylococci (most commonly *S. epidermidis*), coagulase-positive staphylococci *(S. aureus),* enterococci, and α-hemolytic streptococci (e.g., *S. mutans* or viridans group streptococci). Both coagulase-positive and -negative staphylococci are most commonly isolated from the blood, often from patients with indwelling intravenous catheters, or from those with foreign bodies such as prosthetic heart valves or orthopedic implants. *S. aureus* tends to be significantly more virulent and its sensitivity to β-lactam antibiotics (e.g., methicillin, oxacillin, or nafcillin) can vary from center to center, making it imperative for physicians to be aware of the frequency of methicillin-resistant *S. aureus* (MRSA) at their institutions. In contrast, the coagulase-negative staphylococci tend to be relatively indolent. During the last decade, the coagulase-negative staphylococci have become increasingly resistant to β-lactam antibiotics, and the majority (50 to 80%) are methicillin-resistant and generally require treatment with vancomycin. Notable are the recent reports of α-hemolytic viridans streptococci that have been associated with septic shock and the adult respiratory distress syndrome (ARDS) in patients who are receiving high-dose cytosine arabinoside and who develop oral mucosal disruption. Other gram-positive bacteria that may be encountered in neutropenic patients include *Bacillus* species (often catheter-related), group CDC-JK *Corynebacterium* (often catheter-related and relatively antibiotic-resistant), *Enterococcus faecium* (may be resistant to vancomycin), and *Lactobacillus* (may also be resistant to vancomycin).

Infections due solely to anaerobic bacteria are less common and are usually associated with a concomitant abnormality in gastrointestinal mucosal integrity. While *B. fragilis* and *Clostridium perfringens* are the most common organisms, other *Bacteroides* species, as well as other *Clostridium* species (e.g., *C. tertium, C. septicum*), which are often clindamycin-resistant, can be clinically important. Anaerobes are frequent components of intra-abdominal infections, including peritonitis, intra-abdominal abscesses, and perirectal cellulitis or abscesses. *C. difficile* is a common cause of colitis in neutropenic patients treated with antibiotics or cytotoxic agents.

Although infections due to *Mycobacterium tuberculosis* have not been dominant in non-AIDS immunocompromised hosts, the rising incidence of tuberculosis (especially with multidrug-resistant strains) in homeless persons and people with AIDS increases the likelihood that these infections will occur in other immunocompromised hosts. Patients with hairy cell leukemia (HCL), who have profound monocytopenia in addition to neutropenia, appear to have an increased risk for developing atypical mycobacterial infection (e.g., *M. kansasii, M. fortuitum, M. chelonei,* and *M. avium-intracellulare* complex). Rapidly growing mycobacteria (*M. fortuitum* and *M. chelonei*) also may cause exit-site infections in patients with indwelling intravenous catheters, or wound infections following surgery.

In contrast to the bacterial infections, which are often associated with the onset of fever in neutropenic patients, fungal infections only rarely cause primary infection (i.e., initial infection in patients not yet receiving antibiotics). More commonly, fungal infections occur as a secondary process in patients receiving antibacterial agents. Although a variety of fungal infections may be encountered in the neutropenic host, *Candida* and *Aspergillus* species predominate.

The vast majority of infections due to *Candida* are caused by *C. albicans,* with other potential pathogens including *C. tropicalis, C. parapsilosis, C. krusei,* and *C. glabrata* (also known as *Torulopsis glabrata*). In neutropenic patients, *Candida* infections may include candidemia, catheter-related infections, invasive mucosal infections (e.g., oral, esophageal, or lower gastrointestinal), and disseminated disease, in which the most commonly affected organs are the liver and spleen (so-called hepatosplenic candidiasis), the eye (endophthalmitis), and the skin.

Aspergillosis is usually due to *A. fumigatus* and *A. flavus,* although *A. niger* and *A. terreus* also can result in infection. The upper airways (e.g., oral cavity, nasal cavity, or sinuses) and lung are the primary sites involved with *Aspergillus,* and spread is usually by direct invasion into contiguous areas, although widespread dissemination has been described in various sites including brain, liver and spleen, gastrointestinal tract, heart, and kidneys. However, positive blood cultures virtually never occur.

Other fungal pathogens that may occur in neutropenic patients include the Mucoraceae species (*Mucor, Rhizopus, Absidia,* and *Cunninghamella*—often clinically resembling *Aspergillus* infections), *Trichosporon beigelii* (which may cause disseminated visceral and cutaneous disease), *Fusarium, Drechslera, Pseudallescheria boydii,* and *Malassezia furfur.*

Qualitative Abnormalities of Phagocytes

The microbicidal activity of granulocytes and monocytes involves complex interactions between the cell and the organism or inflammatory site. Some of the major functions important for microbicidal activity include migration of the cell to the inflammatory site (or chemotaxis), cell activation, phagocytosis, and intra- and extracellular killing via both oxygen-dependent and -independent pathways. These qualitative abnormalities can be operationally divided into the following categories: (1) those associated with malignant or myeloproliferative disease itself, (2) those associated with diseases that do not primarily affect the leukocytes, (3) iatrogenic causes (such as administration of pharmacologic agents or radiation), and (4) primary disorders of phagocytes.

PATIENTS WITH MALIGNANT DISORDERS AND MYELODYSPLASIA. Significant functional defects in mature PMN's can occur in patients with AML and acute lymphoblastic leukemia prior to therapy. Although it has been largely assumed that granulocytes from patients with chronic myelogenous leukemia have normal microbicidal activity, some studies have documented significant impairment in neutrophil function of morphologically mature PMN's from patients with chronic myelogenous leukemia, including abnormalities in phagocytosis, random migration, chemotaxis, and bactericidal activity. Nevertheless, during the stable chronic phase of the disease, infectious complications are rarely seen in these patients.

In addition to immunoglobulin deficiencies that impair opsonization, patients with chronic lymphocytic leukemia and multiple myeloma also may have such abnormalities as defective granulocyte adherence, decreased granulocyte migration, a decrease in the number of granulocyte receptors for C3b and IgG, and decreased chemotaxis of monocytes.

Significant defects in granulocyte function also have been found in PMN's from patients with myelodysplastic syndromes and preleukemic states. The clinician should probably assume that neutrophils from patients with myelodysplastic syndromes or preleukemia are functionally defective, and thus patients with "borderline" granulocyte counts should be approached as if they had an absolute neutropenia.

NONMALIGNANT HEMATOLOGIC DISEASE. Although the predominant defect in host defense in most patients with aplastic anemia is neutropenia, followed by immune suppression as a result of therapy (e.g., steroids, antithymocyte globulin, or cyclosporine), deficient production of superoxide and a deficiency of myeloperoxidase can sometimes be observed. Patients with paroxysmal nocturnal hemoglobinuria (PNH) appear to have an increased susceptibility to bacterial infection. Impaired chemotaxis despite normal phagocytosis and bacterial killing has been described in PNH, and the Fc receptor type III (the major Fc receptor in blood and on neutrophils) also has been shown to be deficient in PNH.

In addition to splenic dysfunction, abnormal complement activation, and defective serum opsonizing capacity, defective phagocytic function has been described in patients with sickle cell anemia, although the significance of this is unclear. Neutrophils from infection-prone children with sickle cell disease have been shown to have defective bactericidal activity, perhaps secondary to zinc deficiency.

Some patients with severe G6PD deficiency appear to have an increased susceptibility to infections caused by catalase-positive bacteria. The clinical picture resembles that of chronic granulomatous disease of childhood, although only rarely are infections reported in the first decade of life. The granulocytes show normal phagocytosis and chemotaxis but defective bactericidal activity.

Although most studies address disseminated intravascular coagulation (DIC) secondary to overwhelming bacterial infection, the potential role of fibrinogen degradation products (FDP's) in modifying PMN function has been suggested by the finding that two FDP's (FDP D and FDP E) can cause substantial *in vitro* inhibition of PMN chemotaxis, oxidative metabolism, and killing of *E. coli.* DIC associated with infection, then, may represent a vicious circle in which the organism triggers the coagulation abnormalities, which in turn may result in neutropenia and defective PMN function, thus worsening the infection.

PHARMACOLOGIC AGENTS AND RADIOTHERAPY. Most cytotoxic drugs used for treatment of malignant and autoimmune diseases or transplantation have antiproliferative effects, resulting in neutropenia and monocytopenia. Among the antineoplastics, the most commonly implicated agents include methotrexate, 6-mercaptopurine, vincristine, vinblastine, anthracyclines, cyclophosphamide, carmustine, and platinum compounds.

Glucocorticoids are associated with increased susceptibility to infection. As a general rule, the signs and symptoms of even severe infections may be masked or greatly reduced in patients receiving steroids. Steroids impair neutrophil chemotaxis, and at high dosages, PMN phagocytosis, microbicidal activity, and antibody-dependent cytotoxicity also may be altered. In addition, steroids may cause monocytopenia as well as defects in monocyte chemotaxis, phagocytosis, and killing of bacteria and fungi. In addition to their action on granulocytes and monocytes, steroids may enhance susceptibility to infection by impairing wound healing, increasing skin fragility, and depressing lymphocyte function, the production of cytokines, and humoral immune responses.

Biologic agents (e.g., colony-stimulating factors [CSF's], interleukins, interferons) are being employed increasingly in clinical medicine. Studies to date suggest that granulocyte-macrophage (GM)-CSF or granulocyte (G)-CSF not only may increase cell number but also may enhance a number of neutrophil functions, including oxidative metabolism, phagocytosis, microbicidal activity, and antibody-dependent cytotoxicity. At the same time, in adults undergoing autologous bone marrow transplant, there appeared to be the unanticipated finding of a marked decrease in migration of PMN's toward a sterile, artificially created inflammatory site on the skin during periods of GM-CSF administration. Although the clinical significance of any of these effects has not yet been established, these data underscore the importance of carefully evaluating biologics as they are introduced into the therapeutic armamentarium. For example, although interleukin-2 (IL-2) appears promising in mediating tumor lysis (with either lymphokine-activated killer [LAK] cells, tumor infiltrating lymphocytes [TIL's], or interferon-α), impaired granulocyte function, decreased chemotaxis, and decreased Fc receptor γ-III expression have been noted in some patients receiving high doses of IL-2 and may be associated with an increased incidence of significant infections due to *S. aureus.* In contrast, other biologic agents such as interferon-γ may increase phagocyte function and decrease the risk for infection (e.g., in patients with chronic granulomatous disease).

PRIMARY DISORDERS OF PHAGOCYTE FUNCTION. Chronic granulomatous disease (CGD) has served as a prototype for diseases characterized by defective oxidative metabolism of phagocytes. Although CGD represents a heterogeneous group of disorders from a molecular and genetic perspective, the common denominator is that phagocytes lack essential components of oxidative metabolism and fail to generate the respiratory burst in response to various stimuli, including certain pathogenic organisms. The organisms that cause serious infections in patients with CGD are most often those which contain the enzyme catalase. In the absence of cellular production of H_2O_2, the peroxide generated by non–catalase-containing organisms is enough to ameliorate the neutrophil deficiency and allow microbicidal activity. However, if the organism also contains catalase, the H_2O_2 it produces is rapidly degraded and is not available for participation in oxidative-based killing. The majority of infections in patients with CGD are caused by *S. aureus,* although serious infections also can result from enteric gram-negative bacilli (*E. coli, K. pneumoniae,* or *Serratia* species), *P. cepacia, Nocardia asteroides,* and *Aspergillus* species.

Serious recurrent infections usually begin in the first year of life in children with CGD. The lung is the most common site of infection (pneumonias and abscesses), with other common infections including skin and soft tissue abscesses, visceral abscesses (particularly hepatic), osteomyelitis (especially of the small bones in the hands and feet), and suppurative lymphadenopathy. Uncommonly, CGD can present in adolescence or adulthood, although with careful history, infectious complications often date back to childhood.

Prophylactic antibiotics, with trimethoprim-sulfamethoxazole, have been advocated by many investigators. Interferon-γ also has been shown to reduce the incidence of serious infection and the number of hospital days for patients with CGD.

Myeloperoxidase (MPO) deficiency is perhaps the most common of all granulocyte disorders, with an estimated frequency ranging from 1 in 2000 to 1 in 4000. MPO is a lysosomal enzyme that catalyzes the formation of hypochlorous acid from H_2O_2 produced in the respiratory burst. Interestingly, most individuals identified with

MPO deficiency are healthy, and infectious complications are exceedingly rare. Systemic *Candida* infections have occurred in a small number of MPO-deficient patients who also had diabetes mellitus.

Chédiak-Higashi syndrome (CHS) is a rare disorder characterized by autosomal recessive inheritance, recurrent infections, partial oculocutaneous albinism, central and peripheral neuropathy, and increased bleeding time. Neutropenia also can be present. Infections result from combined effects of neutropenia and functional defects in phagocytes, which include impaired degranulation and defective chemotaxis. Infections frequently involve the skin, respiratory tract, and mucous membranes and are most commonly caused by *S. aureus* or gram-negative bacilli. Deficiency of the iC3b receptor (also known as CR3, Mo1, and MAC-1), which is important for adherence and phagocytosis, is a rare disorder. Accordingly, neutrophils demonstrate defects in aggregation, margination, chemotaxis, and phagocytosis. The most common infections are skin and subcutaneous tissue infections, otitis, mucositis, gingivitis, and periodontitis.

A number of disorders have been described that are characterized by defects in chemotaxis of granulocytes and/or monocytes. Infections in these patients tend to be cutaneous, and the most common pathogens are *S. aureus*, streptococci, *C. albicans*, *E. coli*, and *Trichophyton rubrum*. Depending on the specific syndrome, deep-seated infections also may occur. The "lazy leukocyte" syndrome also may be associated with neutropenia and is characterized by gingivitis, recurrent otitis media, rhinitis, and stomatitis. Hyperimmunoglobulin E syndrome (Job's syndrome) is usually associated with multiple cutaneous abscesses caused by staphylococci, but deep-seated infections and infections due to other organisms such as pseudomonads and *Candida* have also been reported. Wound healing does not appear to be a problem, as it is in CGD. Chemotaxis defects have been reported in patients with congenital ichthyosis and recurrent *T. rubrum* infections.

DEFECTS IN CELL-MEDIATED IMMUNITY (CMI)

Cellular immune dysfunction either may be primary, as in a number of congenital immunodeficiency states, or may occur secondary to other disorders or therapeutic interventions. Defective CMI may lead to infections caused by bacteria, fungi, viruses, and protozoa. The predominant pathogens are intracellular organisms (those microbes which survive inside of macrophages) and include mycobacteria (both *M. tuberculosis* and atypical mycobacteria), *Legionella*, *N. asteroides*, *Salmonella* species, *Cryptococcus neoformans*, *Histoplasma capsulatum*, *Coccidioides immitis*, varicella-zoster virus (VZV), herpes simplex virus (HSV), cytomegalovirus (CMV), Epstein-Barr virus (EBV), *Pneumocystis carinii*, *T. gondii*, *Cryptosporidium*, and *Strongyloides stercoralis*.

Patients with Malignant Disorders

Hodgkin's disease and the non-Hodgkin's lymphomas are associated with altered CMI not only when the malignancy is active but in some instances even when the malignancy is in remission.

CMI defects have been postulated to help explain the incidence of atypical mycobacterial infections in patients with hairy cell leukemia and also occur in relatively rare T-cell malignancies such as mycosis fungoides and T-cell chronic lymphocytic leukemia (CLL). CMI defects exist in children with ALL, as evidenced by their increased susceptibility to infections due to *P. carinii* or disseminated VZV, but it is likely that concurrent therapy plays a major role. Clinically significant impairment of CMI has not been well established for other malignancies.

Patients with Nonmalignant Hematologic Disorders

Impaired CMI is not a prominent feature of nonmalignant hematologic disorders unless associated with therapy or acquisition of HIV-1 infection. Abnormalities in CMI have been best described in patients with hemophilia who have received Factor VIII concentrates even in the absence of apparent HIV-1 infection. Patients with sickle cell anemia have been found to be anergic in association with zinc deficiency and decreased nucleoside phosphorylase activity.

A number of infections may produce impaired CMI either directly (e.g., by infecting key cellular components such as T lymphocytes or macrophages) or by affecting other immunoregulatory mechanisms. The most notable viral infection associated with impaired CMI is HIV-1. Other viral infections that also are associated with CMI defects include CMV, EBV, RSV, hepatitis B, and influenza. Other nonviral infections that have been variably associated with impaired CMI by *in vitro* testing have included tuberculosis, leprosy, bacterial pneumonia, brucellosis, typhoid fever, coccidioidomycosis, syphilis, and a variety of parasitic diseases.

Noninfectious conditions that have been linked to abnormal CMI include chronic protein-calorie malnutrition, uremia, diabetes mellitus, surgery, anesthesia, sarcoidosis, and cystic fibrosis.

Pharmacologic Agents

Corticosteroids are the pharmacologic agents most often associated with CMI abnormalities, although they also may cause immune suppression due to effects on other host defense mechanisms. The degree of immunosuppression and the relative risk of infection depend on the dose and duration of corticosteroids as well as the underlying disease. Patients receiving pharmacologic doses of steroids (e.g., brain tumor patients, those with inflammatory bowel disease, and with autoimmune disorders) may have impaired CMI and should be considered at risk for mycobacterial, viral, and parasitic infections. Patients to be treated with corticosteroids with a known history of tuberculosis or a positive PPD skin test should be given prophylactic isoniazid (INH) to prevent reactivation and potential dissemination of disease.

A number of cytotoxic agents are also associated with impaired CMI, including methotrexate, cyclophosphamide, 6-mercaptopurine, and azathioprine. Cyclosporine is an immunosuppressant used to suppress transplant rejection and is associated with alterations in helper T cells, effector T cells, and natural killer (NK) cells. It has not been established, however, that cyclosporine *per se* is associated with an increased risk of infection.

Radiotherapy also may result in impaired CMI, especially when used in combination with other immunosuppressive agents or to treat patients with underlying diseases associated with intrinsic CMI defects (e.g., as a component of the preparatory regimen for bone marrow transplantation or for treatment of Hodgkin's disease).

Primary Disorders of Cell-mediated Immunity (see Ch. 223)

Defects in CMI are found as components of mixed primary B- and T-cell abnormalities, including severe combined immunodeficiency disease (SCID), Wiskott-Aldrich syndrome, ataxia-telangiectasia, and certain purine pathway enzyme deficiencies. Infections in patients with these disorders tend to begin early in life and may be caused not only by pathogens associated with CMI abnormalities but also by those seen with humoral defects such as the encapsulated bacteria.

SCID is associated with a marked decrease in both B- and T-cell numbers and extremely low levels of immunoglobulins. Patients fail to react to skin tests and have a negligible antibody response following immunizations. Failure to thrive and recurrent infections are seen within the first few months of life. Infections are due to *S. aureus*, *S. pneumoniae*, *H. influenzae*, *P. carinii*, *Candida*, and herpes group viruses. Affected infants usually die by 2 years of age. A variant of SCID has been described that is associated with chronic skin eruption, hepatosplenomegaly, eosinophilia, and histiocytic infiltration of the lymph nodes (Omenn's disease). *P. carinii* pneumonia may be a common presenting symptom in this disorder.

In patients with Wiskott-Aldrich syndrome, the major abnormality is an inability to respond to polysaccharide antigens. Infections are caused by polysaccharide-encapsulated bacterial pathogens such as *S. pneumoniae* and *H. influenzae*. However, patients also may lose T-cell functions and may have increased susceptibility to pathogens such as HSV and certain fungi and protozoa.

Ataxia-telangiectasia is associated with absent serum and secretory IgA. The thymus is hypoplastic, and thymus-dependent zones in lymph nodes are empty or unoccupied. Infection with encapsulated bacteria predominates, especially recurrent sinopulmonary infections. Many patients progressively lose T-cell function over time and may become susceptible to associated pathogens.

Purine pathway enzyme deficiencies (adenosine deaminase deficiency or nucleoside phosphorylase deficiency) may be associated with either combined B- and T-cell defects or isolated B- or T-cell abnormalities. The type of infection depends on the predominant immune defect. Infections may not appear until 6 to 12 months of age.

The primary cellular immunodeficiencies associated with T-cell abnormalities include thymic hypoplasia (DiGeorge's syndrome), combined immunodeficiency with predominant T-cell defect (Nezelof's syndrome), purine nucleoside phosphorylase deficiency, and chronic mucocutaneous candidiasis.

DiGeorge's syndrome develops when the third and part of the fourth pharyngeal pouches fail to develop during embryogenesis, resulting in absence of the thymus and parathyroid glands. Children with DiGeorge's syndrome lack T lymphocytes and have severe depression of CMI, making them susceptible to overwhelming infections due to a variety of organisms, including HSV, VZV, *C. albicans,* and *P. carinii.* Nezelof's syndrome can be differentiated from DiGeorge's syndrome by the absence of parathyroid and cardiac involvement.

Cartilage-hair hypoplasia is a form of short-limbed dwarfism associated with a virtual absence of T-cell function. Interestingly, susceptibility to infection is not as pronounced as in other T-cell deficiencies. Overwhelming viral infections due to vaccinia or varicella viruses may occur.

Chronic mucocutaneous candidiasis involves impairment in CMI, and infection is almost always limited to the skin and mucous membranes.

ABNORMALITIES OF HUMORAL DEFENSE MECHANISMS—IMMUNOGLOBULINS AND COMPLEMENT

Immunoglobulins and complement are among the most important components of the humoral immune system, and defects or deficiencies in either may be associated with serious infections. Other proteins that have been classified as part of the humoral defense system include lysozyme, lactoferrin, tuftsin, and fibronectin. Immunoglobulins may be opsonic (enhance phagocytosis), neutralizing (inhibit replication of viruses), or with complement mylyse microbes or cells. The humoral system functions predominantly against bacterial infections. Patients with either primary or secondary defects or deficiencies in these proteins are at highest risk for developing serious infections due to the encapsulated bacteria and to a lesser extent the enteroviruses and *Giardia lamblia.*

Patients with Malignant Disorders

The degree of humoral impairment in multiple myeloma appears to be related to the stage of the disease, primarily due to malignant plasma cell induction of a protein that is synthesized by macrophages and that selectively suppresses B-cell function. Myeloma patients are most susceptible to recurrent infections from encapsulated bacteria such as *S. pneumoniae* or *H. influenzae* early in the course of the disease. Infections due to enteric gram-negative rods and staphylococci are also encountered, especially in patients with refractory or advanced disease. Recurrent infection most often occurs in the upper respiratory tract, urinary tract, or skin.

Patients with B-cell CLL appear to have an unbalanced immunoglobulin chain synthesis and resultant hypogammaglobulinemia. The incidence of infection correlates with the duration and stage of the disease as well as the serum levels of immunoglobulins (particularly IgG). Encapsulated bacteria predominate, although infections due to staphylococci and enteric gram-negative bacilli also occur. Upper and lower respiratory tract infections are encountered most commonly, although other sites such as urinary tract and skin are frequently involved.

Nonmalignant states (e.g., nephrotic syndrome, burns, protein-losing enteropathy) can be associated with increased immunoglobulin catabolism or loss and may lead to decreased antibody levels and enhanced susceptibility to infection. Clinically significant acquired complement defects are unusual.

Primary Deficiencies

Isolated B-cell immunodeficiency states and their associated risks for infection in children include transient hypogammaglobulinemia of infancy, which is not usually associated with serious infections; sex-linked hypogammaglobulinemia, which is associated with recurrent pyogenic infections and septicemia due to *S. pneumoniae, H. influenzae, S. aureus, N. meningitidis,* and *P. aeruginosa;* hypogammaglobulinemia associated with hyperimmunoglobulin M, in which patients have recurrent respiratory, soft tissue, and gastrointestinal infections; selective IgM deficiency, in which patients have severe recurrent infections due to pyogenic bacteria; and selective IgA deficiency, in which certain patients may have increased numbers of upper respiratory tract infections, whereas others appear not to be at increased risk. Chronic diarrhea due to *G. lamblia* is also associated with IgA deficiency. Common variable hypogammaglobulinemia is associated with respiratory tract infections due to *S. pneumoniae, H. influenzae,* and *S. aureus.* Diarrhea due to *G. lamblia* also occurs.

Many patients with B-cell deficiencies, particularly those with congenital hypogammaglobulinemia, appear to be at risk for developing chronic central nervous system infections due to enteroviruses.

A number of primary defects in complement components also have been described. Although deficiencies of the early classic pathway components (C1, C2, C4) have been reported, associated infection is rare, probably because the alternative pathway remains functional and is able to compensate. Deficiencies of C3 or C5, on the other hand, often lead to severe infections due to encapsulated organisms, enteric gram-negative bacteria, and staphylococci. Absence of the later components (C5b, C6, C7, C8, C9) leads to an increase in infections, primarily due to *Neisseria* species, both *N. gonorrhoeae* and *N. meningitidis.* Although the defects in these later components may be present from birth, infectious episodes do not typically begin until the teenage years. Indeed, any patient with recurrent infections due to *Neisseria* species should be investigated for complement deficiency.

SPLENECTOMY AND SPLENIC DYSFUNCTION

Splenectomy may be performed either as a part of staging or as a therapeutic intervention in a number of disorders, including Hodgkin's disease, agnogenic myeloid metaplasia, paroxysmal nocturnal hemoglobinuria, hereditary spherocytosis, thalassemia, and a variety of autoimmune disorders.

The spleen probably plays an adjunctive role in host defense by removing organisms from the blood that have been ineffectively opsonized by complement. In addition, it participates in the primary immunoglobulin response and is involved in regulation of the alternative complement pathway, with low levels of immunoglobulins and properdin reported in patients following splenectomy. A decrease in the opsonic peptide tuftsin also has been reported following splenectomy, and alternative pathway defects may be important in patients with sickle cell disease and splenic dysfunction.

The risk of developing serious infection, as well as the types of infections, may vary depending on the reason for abnormal splenic function and the presence or absence of other immune abnormalities. Patients who undergo post-traumatic splenectomy appear to be at a lower risk for infection. An increased risk of *Salmonella* infections appears to be unique for the sickle cell population. Most asplenic patients or patients who have undergone splenectomy are at increased risk for serious bacterial infections, primarily due to *S. pneumoniae* and *H. influenzae,* as well as *Neisseria* species and *Capnocytophaga.* The initial presentation of even overwhelming infection may be deceptively subtle, with fever often being the only sign of infection. Asplenic patients with an underlying hematologic disease who present with fever should be managed initially as potentially septic.

EVALUATING AND MANAGING THE FEBRILE GRANULOCYTOPENIC PATIENT: A PARADIGM FOR THE COMPROMISED HOST

A classic tenet of infectious disease is that antibiotic therapy is based on isolating and identifying a specific organism or on reliably predicting a specific organism from a clinically involved site of infection. The overall management of neutropenic patients is based on use of empirical antibiotics directed against a wider array of potential pathogens. Indeed, it is well accepted that when a neutropenic patient develops a new fever (usually defined as one oral temperature $\geq 38.5°C$ or more than two successive readings of $\geq 38°$ C in a 12-hour period), an empirical broad-spectrum antibacterial regimen should be started expeditiously. The rationale for this approach evolved from the observation that bacteremias in neutropenic patients were rapidly lethal, especially those due to gram-negative organisms, if antibiotic therapy was delayed until an organism was isolated or a site of infection identified. Although the goal of the preantibiotic evaluation of a newly febrile neutropenic patient is to identify potential sources, the majority of patients will not have a source of infection identified to explain the fever.

The standard initial evaluation should include a careful physical examination with particular attention to areas that may "hide" an infection, notably the oral cavity and the perianal area. Examination of the perirectal area, including deep palpation, should be performed, and only if there are findings suggestive of a localized inflammatory site (e.g., pain or fluctuance) should a judicious digital examination be performed. At a minimum, two sets of blood samples for culture should be obtained. If the patient has an indwelling intravenous catheter, then at least one set should be drawn through the catheter and another from a peripheral vein. For patients with multilumen intravenous catheters, a culture should be obtained through *each* lumen and the specific lumen clearly identified on the culture bottle. This is important, because catheter infection may be limited to a single lumen. Because of the absence of granulocytes, microscopic examination of the urine may be normal even in the presence of a urinary tract infection. A chest radiograph can serve as a valuable baseline, although some investigators have questioned the use of this procedure in patients without pulmonary symptoms. In addition, accessible sites of potential infection should be aspirated or biopsied, with appropriate material sent for Gram stain, culture, and histologic examination.

Even with a comprehensive evaluation, an infectious cause for the fever is found in only 30 to 50% of patients. Nonetheless, even subtle indications of inflammation must be considered as sites of potential infection in the presence of granulocytopenia. For example, minimal perirectal erythema and tenderness may be harbingers of a perirectal cellulitis. Minimal erythema or serous discharge at the exit site of an indwelling intravenous catheter may herald a tunnel or exit-site infection.

Colonization with microorganisms often precedes development of significant infection. However, routine "surveillance" cultures are not of practical benefit in a neutropenic patient, since colonization of a single body site is not consistently predictive and multiple potential pathogens are usually isolated from any single site, making it difficult to predict the organism responsible for infection. Moreover, since empirical broad-spectrum antibiotics are administered under any circumstance, the expense of routine surveillance cannot be justified.

Tests such as nuclear scanning also have been used to define occult sites of infection. Although gallium citrate accumulates in inflammatory lesions because of its avid binding to lactoferrin, this test has not been shown to be useful in granulocytopenic patients. Autologous or allogeneic leukocytes labeled *in vitro* with indium-111 or indium-111 linked to IgG have been used with some success in the evaluation of febrile granulocytopenic patients.

Because of these diagnostic difficulties, even fevers that are temporally associated with the administration of blood products or with fever-producing antineoplastic agents should be considered potentially infectious and treated as such. In sum, virtually all new fevers in the neutropenic population warrant careful clinical and microbiologic evaluation, followed by prompt initiation of empirical antibiotic therapy. Conversely, any clinically evident site of potential infection mandates expeditious broad-spectrum therapy, even in the absence of fever.

Since the goal of empirical antibiotic therapy is to protect against the early morbidity and mortality that result from untreated bacterial infections, regimens have been formulated to maximize activity against commonly encountered organisms that are particularly virulent. However, empirical regimens cannot realistically be designed to cover every potential bacterial pathogen. Moreover, no regimen is capable of completely eliminating the risk of subsequent infections in persistently neutropenic patients.

Management of Indwelling Intravenous Catheters

Although gram-positive bacterial infections (especially staphylococcal) are the most frequent causes of catheter-related infections, other bacterial and nonbacterial species can be encountered, particularly in the neutropenic patient. These include resistant *Corynebacterium*, *Bacillus* species, gram-negative organisms, and fungi. In approaching the patient with a catheter-related infection, it is important to consider the specific type of infection, its location (i.e., bacteremia versus exit site versus tunnel), the type of access device (e.g., Hickman versus implantable subcutaneous reservoir), and the duration of symptoms.

In general, the vast majority of simple catheter-related bacteremias and exit-site infections can be cleared using appropriate antibiotics and do not require catheter removal. This applies to both neutropenic and non-neutropenic patients. If multilumen devices are used, the antibiotic infusion should be rotated among the ports, since infection may be limited to one lumen (failure to do so can be a cause of persistent infection despite antibiotics). If there is persistent bacteremia after 48 hours of appropriate therapy, the catheter should be removed. Failures of therapy are more common when the infections are due to certain organisms, such as *Bacillus* species or *C. albicans,* and when these are isolated, the catheter usually should be removed.

Infections extending to involve the tunnel of a Hickman catheter also mandate prompt removal of the device, because antibiotics alone rarely cure this "closed-space" infection, particularly in the granulocytopenic host. Likewise, infections around the reservoir of an implantable subcutaneous device may be difficult to eradicate without catheter removal. Patients with recurrent catheter infections (despite a history of appropriate therapy) are also candidates for prompt catheter removal.

It is unresolved whether a non-neutropenic patient with an indwelling catheter who becomes newly febrile should receive antibiotics empirically. The safest policy is to begin antibiotics (using a third-generation cephalosporin such as ceftriaxone or an aminoglycoside plus vancomycin) and continue them pending culture results and clinical response. This approach protects against rapid progression of undetected yet virulent infections (such as *S. aureus*) and may minimize the need for ultimate catheter removal. If by 72 hours the cultures are negative and the patient is stable, antibiotics can be discontinued.

Initial Management of the Neutropenic Patient Who Becomes Febrile

Although gram-negative bacteria still predominate at some institutions, there has been a trend in recent years toward more gram-positive infections, and these now comprise the majority of isolates at many centers. In general, the gram-negative infections tend to be more virulent, and early empirical regimens have been formulated to provide protection primarily against these organisms while maintaining a broad spectrum of activity against other potential pathogens. Indeed, adequate coverage of these gram-negative organisms is still an essential property of any empirical regimen.

Although there is no single best regimen or recipe, there are a number of appropriate options. The selection of a specific antibiotic regimen depends on many factors, including institutional sensitivity patterns, individual and institutional experience, and clinical parameters.

The standard approach to the empirical management of the febrile neutropenic patient has been to use combination antibiotic regimens. Until recently, this has been the only way to provide coverage broad enough to encompass the predominant gram-positive and gram-negative organisms. Moreover, some combinations have been considered to provide synergy and to have the potential for decreasing the emergence of resistant isolates. Aminoglycoside–β-lactam combinations were the first empirical regimens with acceptable efficacy in the setting of fever and neutropenia. Such combination regimens are still widely used and represent a standard against which newer regimens are tested. Many variations have been studied and include aminoglycosides combined with either an extended-spectrum penicillin or a cephalosporin, or as a component of a triple-drug regimen. If an aminoglycoside-containing combination regimen is to be employed, the choice of specific antibiotics should be based primarily on the institutional antibiotic sensitivity patterns and secondarily on toxicity and cost differences.

Non–aminoglycoside-containing combination regimens also have been studied. These have consisted of combinations of two β-lactam antibiotics, or so-called double β-lactam regimens, usually consisting of an expanded-spectrum carboxy- or ureidopenicillin plus a third-generation cephalosporin (e.g., piperacillin and ceftazidime).

New or Novel Antibiotics for Neutropenic Patients

The advent of β-lactam antibiotics with broad-spectrum activity which achieve high serum bactericidal levels has made monotherapy another option for the initial empirical therapy of the febrile neutropenic patient (Table 266–3). The third-generation cephalosporins and the carbapenems are the two classes that include potential candidates for empirical single-agent therapy. Ceftazidime

TABLE 266–3. MEDICATIONS IN PATIENTS WITH NEUTROPENIA AND FEVER

Agent	Comments
Antibiotic	
Third-generation cephalosporins	Only ceftazidime and cefoperazone are appropriate for coverage of *P. aeruginosa.*
Carbapenems	If *P. aeruginosa* is suspected or cultured, an aminoglycoside should be added.
Extended-spectrum penicillins	Because of the potential for resistance, piperacillin, azlocillin, or mezlocillin should be administered with either an aminoglycoside or a third-generation cephalosporin.
Monobactams	Aztreonam is an important alternative for patients allergic to β-lactam antibiotics, but it should be combined with vancomycin for empirical therapy.
Quinolones	Important for gram-negative infection and possibly for use in low-risk patients with neutropenia; to avoid resistance, do not use for prophylaxis.
Vancomycin	Pathogen-directed therapy generally suffices. Empirical use can be restricted to centers with a high incidence of methicillin-resistant *S. aureus.* Of concern, strains of vancomycin-resistant enterococci have been described.
Antifungal	
Amphotericin B	Still the best treatment. A dose of 0.6 mg per kilogram of body weight per day suffices for *C. albicans* and cryptococcus; 1 mg/kg/day is preferred for *C. tropicalis;* and 1.5 mg/kg/day is preferred for aspergillus.
Ketoconazole	Not an alternative to amphotericin B for empirical therapy. Useful for thrush or esophagitis.
Fluconazole	Very effective for thrush or esophagitis. Value for systemic mycoses, including hepatosplenic candidiasis, requires additional study.
Antiviral	
Acyclovir	Oral therapy is not advised for severely immunocompromised patients with varicella-zoster infections. For such patients parenteral therapy (1500 mg per square meter of body-surface area per day in 3 divided doses) is indicated. For patients with herpes simplex, oral or parenteral therapy (750 mg/m²/day in 3 divided doses) is satisfactory.
Ganciclovir	Of value for cytomegalovirus retinitis, prevention of pneumonitis, and combined with an intravenous immunoglobulin for pneumonitis.
Antiparasitic	
Trimethoprim-sulfamethoxazole	Best drug for *Pneumocystis carinii* prophylaxis. Not required in all cancer patients. Thrice-weekly schedule is satisfactory (150 mg of trimethoprim/m²/day in 2 divided doses).
Aerosolized pentamidine	Expensive and not as effective as trimethoprim-sulfamethoxazole in adults with HIV infection.

From Pizzo PA: Management of fever in patients with cancer and treatment-induced neutropenia. N Engl J Med 328:1323, 1993. Copyright by the Massachusetts Medical Society.

has been the most extensively studied of the third-generation cephalosporins as monotherapy because of its superior activity against *P. aeruginosa.*

A large, randomized study evaluating 550 consecutive episodes of fever and neutropenia was conducted at the National Cancer Institute (NCI). In this study, patients with fever and granulocytopenia underwent a standard initial evaluation and then were randomized to receive either a combination of antibiotics (cephalothin, gentamicin, and carbenicillin) or ceftazidime as a single agent. The overall results show that monotherapy compared favorably with a standard combination regimen. Approximately two thirds of the episodes in both groups were treated successfully for the entire duration of their granulocytopenia, without requiring *any* changes in their initial regimen. Another one third of the episodes required some change or modification (such as addition of an antibacterial,

antifungal, or antiviral drug) to ensure a successful outcome (see indications for modifications below), and an equally low number in both groups (about 5%) died of infection. None of the deaths was attributable to a specific deficiency in one regimen that was not present in the other.

Two subgroups of patients were identified who required more frequent modifications of the initial regimen in order to achieve a successful outcome: (1) those presenting with a documented source of infection to account for the initial fever and (2) those having relatively protracted periods of granulocytopenia (>1 week). The need for modification in these subgroups was identical for those episodes treated with monotherapy and those treated with combination therapy. In this study, these modifications did not represent a failure of either regimen *per se* but instead were reflective of the limitations of any regimen in treating patients who are at high risk for development of subsequent infections.

Results of an international cooperative study, which enrolled 876 episodes of fever and neutropenia (in 676 patients, 83% with acute leukemia) in a recently reported randomized trial comparing ceftazidime monotherapy with the combination of piperacillin and tobramycin, demonstrated comparable efficacy with both regimens but less toxicity with ceftazidime monotherapy.

Concerns regarding the use of ceftazidime as a single agent for fever and neutropenia include the lack of synergy against documented gram-negative infections, lack of activity against certain gram-positive isolates, poor antianaerobic activity, and the potential for developing resistance.

In addition to the third-generation cephalosporins, other antibiotics are also being evaluated in neutropenic patients. Imipenem, for example, is a member of the carbapenem class of antibiotics. It is formulated in fixed combination with cilastatin, which inhibits a renal enzyme that can degrade imipenem. Overall, it has the broadest spectrum of activity of any available antibiotic. Of note is its excellent *in vitro* activity against enterococci as well as many anaerobes.

Results of two randomized studies appear to corroborate its efficacy in this setting—one comparing it with an aminoglycoside-containing combination and another performed at the NCI comparing it with monotherapy with ceftazidime. Interestingly, neither of these studies appears to demonstrate superior efficacy for imipenem. Two potential drawbacks to its use include a relatively high incidence of the development of resistant *P. aeruginosa,* as well as its potential to decrease the seizure threshold in patients with central nervous system pathology. In addition, in the ongoing NCI trial, a higher than expected frequency of nausea has been found with imipenem.

Because of the increasing incidence of gram-positive infections in cancer patients during the 1980's and their increased resistance to β-lactam antibiotics, some authorities have recommended that vancomycin be added to empirical regimens. Conversely, it has been argued that since many of these organisms are of relatively low virulence, vancomycin may be safely withheld until the gram-positive isolate has been identified microbiologically.

At the present time, it seems reasonable not to routinely include vancomycin in all empirical antibiotic regimens. Its use, however, should be guided by institutional experience and sensitivity patterns. For example, in a center with a high incidence of methicillin-resistant *S. aureus,* routine use of vancomycin is clearly warranted, since this may be a particularly virulent organism if not treated. In addition, fluctuations in patterns of infecting microorganisms may occur over time. For example, penicillin-resistant α-hemolytic streptococci have recently been identified as particularly virulent pathogens in some centers (perhaps related to the use of high-dose cytosine arabinoside). Clearly, the emergence of new pathogens or pathogens with altered sensitivity profiles may force dramatic changes in how we use antibiotics in the future.

The appropriate role for the quinolones in the neutropenic patient has yet to be defined. Because of their relatively poor activity against certain gram-positive organisms, they should not be used for empirical therapy alone. They may, however, be useful to complete therapy in patients who initially respond to intravenous antibiotics and who have had either a fever of undetermined origin or a susceptible bacterial isolate.

A particularly useful feature of aztreonam is its apparent lack of cross-reactivity with the other β-lactams in patients who have penicillin or β-lactam allergies. In this group of patients, empirical therapy might begin with a combination of vancomycin, aztreonam, and an aminoglycoside.

Also recently introduced are combinations of β-lactams with β-lactamase inhibitors (i.e., clavulanic acid and sulbactam). Three preparations are now available, including amoxicillin + clavulanic acid (oral formulation only), ticarcillin + clavulanic acid, and ampicillin + sulbactam. A number of studies have documented the efficacy of ticarcillin + clavulanic acid combined with aminoglycoside for initial empirical therapy of fever in neutropenic patients. The expanded gram-positive coverage may obviate additional anti–gram-positive agents.

APPROACH TO THE PATIENT WITH PROLONGED GRANULOCYTOPENIA

How Long Should Antibiotics Be Continued?

A question of practical importance is how long empirical antibiotics should be continued in persistently neutropenic patients. Should they always be continued until the granulocyte count recovers, or can they be safely discontinued before that?

The question of duration of therapy can be approached by placing patients in two categories: those whose initial workup (at the time of presentation with fever and neutropenia) did not reveal a source of infection (i.e., a fever of undetermined origin, or FUO; see Ch. 263), and those whose initial workup revealed an infection to account for the fever (i.e., a positive culture, or clinically infected site, or both). Approximately 60% fall into the FUO category, although this varies with the institution, the therapy, and the patient population (Fig. 266–1).

FUO PATIENTS. There are only limited data that specifically address the issue of duration of empirical therapy in neutropenic patients presenting with an FUO. For patients with an expected short duration of granulocytopenia (e.g., < 1 week) and those with evidence of hematologic recovery, abbreviated courses of empirical therapy are safe and appropriate. However, the real dilemma arises in the population with more prolonged granulocytopenia.

In a study from the NCI, patients with FUO and persistent granulocytopenia were randomized either to discontinue antibiotics on day 7 of therapy or to continue them until the resolution of the neutropenia. Nearly 40% of afebrile patients in whom antibiotics were stopped developed recurrent fever, and 38% of febrile patients whose antibiotics were discontinued developed hypotensive episodes. It was concluded that day 7 was too early to discontinue antibiotics in this group.

A subsequent study randomized persistently neutropenic, afebrile patients to continue or discontinue antibiotics on day 14. Preliminary analysis showed no difference between the two groups: Approximately one third of patients became febrile again regardless of whether they stopped or continued antibiotics. However, those whose fevers recurred following discontinuation of antibiotics responded to a reinstitution of their initial regimens, whereas those remaining on antibiotics required addition of amphotericin B. On this basis, it seems reasonable to discontinue antibiotics and carefully observe FUO patients who are predicted to have a long duration of neutropenia and who have remained afebrile after 14 days of therapy.

PATIENTS PRESENTING WITH DOCUMENTED INFECTIONS. There are even fewer data that address the issue of duration of antibiotics in patients with defined sites of infection. For persistently neutropenic patients who have had clinical and microbiologic resolution of their infection and who are afebrile at day 14 (for a minimum of 7 days), antibiotics should be discontinued. The ultimate decision of whether to continue or discontinue rests on a number of clinical parameters, such as the degree of or potential for antibiotic toxicity, the predicted duration of neutropenia, the seriousness of the initial infection, and the presence or absence of a continued site of infection or other factors predisposing to subsequent infection. It should be emphasized that any neutropenic patient whose antibiotics are discontinued requires careful, meticulous follow-up in order to quickly detect new fevers or infection.

Modifications of Antibiotic Therapy During the Course of Granulocytopenia

Empirical antibiotics have their greatest impact early in the course of neutropenia. However, it is during a prolonged granulocytopenic episode when the patent is at highest risk for developing multiple types of secondary infections or superinfections. Many of these dictate specific modifications of the initial regimen (Table 266–4).

Bacterial isolates that are resistant to the initial empirical regimen are invariably encountered when managing neutropenic patients. For example, at most centers, the majority of coagulase-negative staphylococci are resistant to β-lactams, and breakthrough infec-

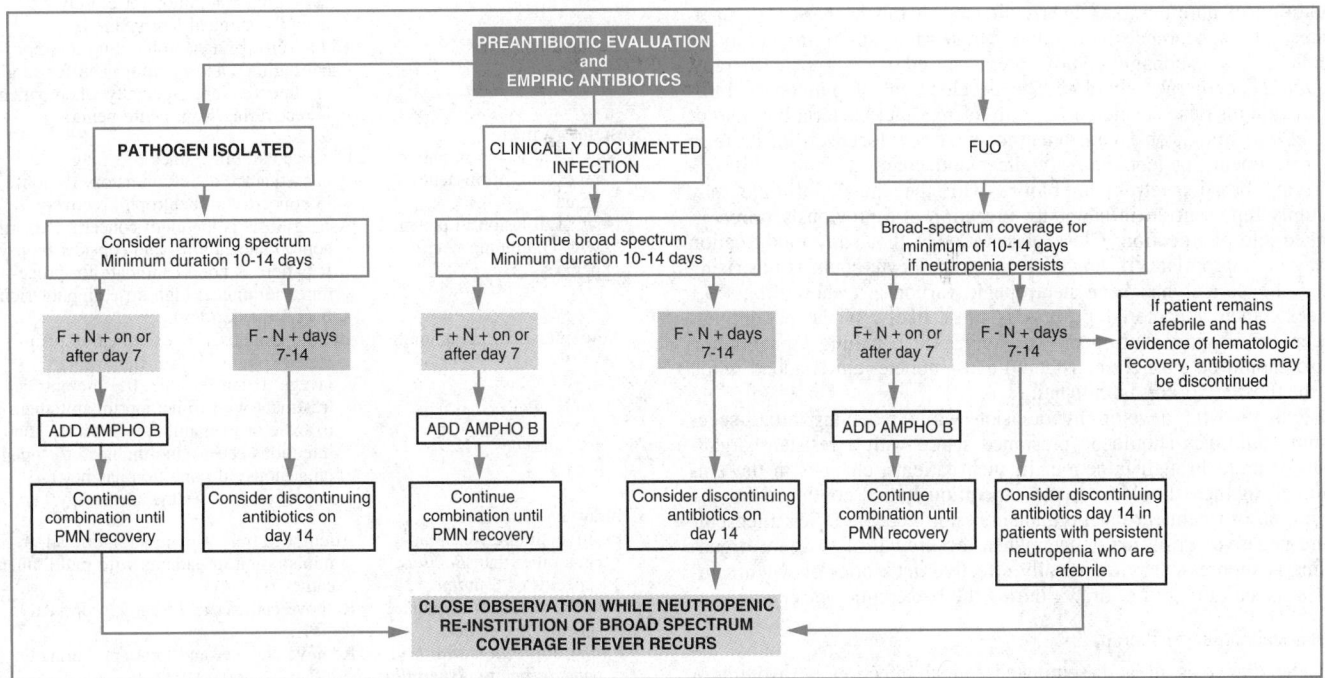

FIGURE 266–1. Management of fever and neutropenia. F + N + = Febrile, neutropenic. F − N + = Afebrile, neutropenic. FUO = No source for fever on preantibiotic evaluation. AMPHO B = Amphotericin B. (From Rubin M, Walsh TJ, Pizzo PA: Clinical approach to the compromised host. *In* Hoffman R, Benz EJ Jr, Shattil SS, et al. [eds.]: Hematology: Basic Principles and Practices, 2nd ed. New York, Churchill Livingstone, 1994.)

tions might be anticipated. Fortunately, coagulase-negative staphylococci are relatively indolent, and the risk for secondary infection can be balanced accordingly. Thus, for the patient who develops evidence of gram-positive infection while receiving β-lactam or who has evidence of a catheter site infection, vancomycin is an appropriate addition to the initial antibiotic regimen. Similarly, if the coverage of the initial regimen has limited antianaerobic activity, secondary infection with anaerobics might be anticipated.

The appearance of "secondary" resistance is seen more frequently with certain organisms. For example, Enterobacter species, Citrobacter species, and Serratia have inducible β-lactamases, and the appearance of a clinically significant clustering of resistant Enterobacter in a neutropenic population has been observed recently. Accordingly, when these organisms are isolated from a patient, careful observation for emergence of resistance is warranted, and for patients receiving monotherapy with a broad-spectrum β-lactam, an aminoglycoside should be added. P. aeruginosa may develop resistance to imipenem through a relatively novel mechanism involving a change in the porins. Hence patients receiving single-agent therapy for P. aeruginosa infection also should have an aminoglycoside added to their regimens. Secondary development of resistance by gram-positive organisms is somewhat rarer, although it has been increasingly described. Of note, recent studies have documented the emergence of vancomycin-resistant coagulase-negative staphylococci and enterococci in patients receiving vancomycin.

The appearance of a new site of infection (e.g., cellulitis or pneumonia) or the progression of a previously documented site of infection is an additional reason for changes or modifications of the antimicrobial regimen. For example, the development of marginal or necrotizing gingivitis is relatively common in patients who have received intensive cytotoxic therapy. Anaerobic organisms contribute to this process, and an antianaerobic agent such as clindamycin or metronidazole should be added to the empirical regimen if gingivitis is diagnosed.

The most common pathogens contributing to perianal cellulitis are the aerobic gram-negative bacilli, enterococci, and bowel anaerobes. Therefore, when it occurs in a patient already receiving broad-spectrum antibiotics, the addition of an antianaerobic agent as well as a change in the broad-spectrum coverage may be necessary. Similarly, any suspected intra-abdominal site of infection should prompt addition or inclusion of antibiotics active against aerobic gram-negative bacilli, enterococci, and bowel anaerobes.

The development of a new site of infection also may warrant the addition of antimicrobial agents directed at fungi, viruses, or parasites. The appearance of burning retrosternal pain is frequently an indicator of esophagitis, most often caused by cytotoxic therapy, Candida, or herpes simplex. The development of pulmonary infiltrates might raise suspicion not only of resistant bacteria but also of P. carinii, fungi, or a viral pneumonia. A new localized infiltrate in a neutropenic patient whose white blood count is rising while receiving broad-spectrum antibiotics with the "new" infiltrate may simply represent an inflammatory reaction at a previously unrecognized site of infection. Close observation without any modification may be appropriate. If, however, the granulocyte count is not rising and the patient has been neutropenic for only a short time (≤ 1 week), then a bacterial process is most likely. If the patient has been persistently neutropenic for longer, then a fungal pneumonia also should be strongly considered and amphotericin B added while a diagnostic workup is initiated.

Patients who develop hypotension while receiving broad-spectrum antibiotics should be presumed septic with a resistant organism or breakthrough infection. In such patients, changes in the empirical regimen should be made expeditiously and continued for the duration of treatment if an organism is not recovered. So-called culture-negative sepsis may occur when the growth of resistant organisms is suppressed by marginally effective antibiotics or when samples for culture are not drawn during the bacteremic episode.

Empirical Antifungal Therapy

The diagnosis of a disseminated fungal infection is difficult in an immunocompromised patient. Neutropenic patients who remain persistently febrile despite a 4- to 7-day trial of broad-spectrum antibacterial therapy are particularly likely to have a fungal infection. Empirical antifungal therapy might be expected to have a dual ef-

TABLE 266–4. COMMON MODIFICATIONS OR ADDITIONS TO INITIAL EMPIRICAL ANTIBIOTIC THERAPY IN PATIENTS WITH NEUTROPENIA AND FEVER

Status or Symptoms	Modifications of Primary Regimen
Fever	
Persistent for > 1 week	Add empirical antifungal therapy with amphotericin B.
Recurrence after 1 week or later in patient with persistent neutropenia	Add empirical antifungal therapy.
Persistent or recurrent fever at time of recovery from neutropenia	Evaluate liver and spleen by CT, ultrasonography, or MRI for hepatosplenic candidiasis, and evaluate need for antifungal therapy.
Bloodstream	
Cultures before antibiotic therapy	
Gram-positive organism	Add vancomycin pending further identification.
Gram-negative organism	Maintain regimen if patient is stable and isolate is sensitive. If *P. aeruginosa*, *Enterobacter*, or *Citrobacter* is isolated, add an aminoglycoside or an additional β-lactam antibiotic.
Organism isolated during antibiotic therapy	
Gram-positive organism	Add vancomycin
Gram-negative organism	Change to new combination regimen (e.g., imipenem plus gentamicin or vancomycin, or gentamicin plus piperacillin).
Head, eyes, ears, nose, throat	
Necrotizing or marginal gingivitis	Add specific antianaerobic agent (clindamycin or metronidazole) to empirical therapy.
Vesicular or ulcerative lesions	Suspect herpes simplex infection. Culture and begin acyclovir therapy.
Sinus tenderness or nasal ulcerative lesions	Suspect fungal infection with *Aspergillus* or *Mucor*.
Gastrointestinal tract	
Retrosternal burning pain	Suspect *Candida*, herpes simplex, or both. Add antifungal therapy and, if no response, acyclovir. Bacterial esophagitis also a possibility. For patients who do not respond within 48 hours, endoscopy should be considered.
Acute abdominal pain	Suspect typhlitis, as well as appendicitis, if pain in right lower quadrant. Add specific antianaerobic coverage to empirical regimen and monitor closely for need for surgical intervention.
Perianal tenderness	Add specific antianaerobic drug to empirical regimen and monitor need for surgical intervention, especially when patient is recovering from neutropenia.
Respiratory tract	
New focal lesion in patient recovering from neutropenia	Observe carefully, since this may be a consequence of inflammatory response in concert with neutrophil recovery.
New focal lesion in patient with continuing neutropenia	Aspergillosis is the chief concern. Perform appropriate cultures and consider biopsy. If patient is not a candidate for procedure, administer high-dose amphotericin B (1.5 mg/kg/day).
New interstitial pneumonitis	Attempt diagnosis by examination of induced sputum or bronchoalveolar lavage. If not feasible, begin empirical treatment with trimethoprim-sulfamethoxazole or pentamidine. Consider noninfectious causes and the need for open-lung biopsy if condition has not improved after 4 days of therapy.
Central venous catheters	
Positive culture for organisms other than *Bacillus* species or *Candida*	Attempt to treat. Rotate antibiotic administration in patients with multilumen catheters.
Positive culture for *Bacillus* species or *Candida*	Remove catheter and treat appropriately.
Exit-site infection with *Mycobacterium* or *Aspergillus*	Remove catheter and treat appropriately.
Tunnel infection	Remove catheter and treat appropriately.

From Pizzo PA: Management of fever in patients with cancer and treatment-induced neutropenia. N Engl J Med 328:1323, 1993. Copyright by the Massachusetts Medical Society.

fect: preventing a fungal overgrowth in patients with prolonged neutropenia and treating "subclinical" fungal disease early.

To date, the only proven agent for empirical therapy has been amphotericin B. Amphotericin B should be begun at 0.5 mg per kilogram per day and administered along with antibiotics until the resolution of neutropenia. If *Aspergillus* or *Mucor* is suspected, the dosage of amphotericin should be increased to 1 to 1.5 mg per kilogram per day. A number of new azole and triazole antifungal agents (fluconazole, itraconazole) offer less toxic alternatives to amphotericin B for certain patients.

Patients who remain febrile after the resolution of neutropenia should be evaluated for hepatosplenic candidiasis. The diagnosis is suggested by "bull's-eye" lesions on CT scan or ultrasonography of the liver and spleen. MRI scanning of the liver may be even more sensitive. Biopsy and histologic examination are essential. Patients with hepatosplenic candidiasis may require extended courses of antifungal therapy. The average amount of amphotericin B required to resolve these lesions is approximately 5 grams, often in conjunction with 5-flucytosine (100 mg per kilogram per day).

PREVENTION OF INFECTIONS

Because bacteria account for the majority of infections in compromised patients, prophylactic strategies have focused on these pathogens. The strategies that have been explored include mechanical techniques to prevent acquisition of new pathogens, absorbable or nonabsorbable oral antibiotic regimens to either prevent acquisition or decrease the number of potentially pathogenic colonizing organisms, and methods to improve the host defense matrix, including immunization and, more recently, biologic agents (e.g., the colony-stimulating factors) (Table 266–5).

Perhaps the most important infection prevention strategy of all, however, is handwashing. Although taken for granted, this simple procedure is frequently overlooked to the detriment of the patient.

Neutropenic Patients

MECHANICAL TECHNIQUES. Reverse isolation (i.e., single room with gowns, masks, and gloves) following the onset of neutropenia does not prevent infection. This is so because most of the infections arise from the patient's endogenous microbial flora. In addition, having patients wear a surgical mask outside of their room does little to protect against subsequent infection. Although some authorities have recommended that all foods be thoroughly cooked and that fresh fruits and vegetables be avoided to decrease the acquisition of gram-negative bacteria, the value of these measures in preventing infection remains unproven.

TABLE 266–5. METHODS STUDIED FOR PREVENTING INFECTION IN HIGH-RISK PATIENTS

Prevent Acquisition and/or Suppress or Eliminate Microbial Flora	Improve or Modify Host Defenses
Isolation	Immunization
Simple or reverse isolation	Active
Isolation with HEPA air filtration	*Pneumococcus*
Prophylactic antibiotics	VZV
Nonabsorbable antibiotics	Passive
Trimethoprim-sulfamethoxazole,	J-5 core glycolipid
erythromycin	Pooled immunoglobulins
Selective decontamination	Hyperimmune globulins
Quinolones	Monoclonal antibodies
Prophylactic antivirals	Cell-component replacement
Acyclovir	Leukocyte transfusions
Amantadine	Accelerate granulocyte recovery
Prophylactic antifungals	G-CSF
Nystatin	GM-CSF
Imidazoles	Immunomodulations
Triazoles	Interferons
Amphotericin B	Interleukins
Prophylactic antiparasitics	
Thiabendazole	
Trimethoprim-sulfamethoxazole	
Combination-comprehensive	
Total protective isolation	

Modified from Pizzo PA: Considerations for the prevention of infectious complications in patients with cancer. Rev Infect Dis 11:S1551, 1989.

The total protective environment (TPE) is a comprehensive regimen designed to reduce the patient's endogenous microbial burden as well as the acquisition of new organisms. The TPE includes a HEPA-filtered laminar airflow room together with an aggressive program of surface decontamination, including the sterilization of all objects that enter the room, and an intensive regimen to disinfect the microbial diet. A number of studies have documented that TPE can reduce infections in profoundly granulocytopenic individuals. However, TPE is expensive, and because of the improvement in treating established infections, it does not offer a current survival advantage to most patients. Thus TPE is not necessary for the routine care of the majority of granulocytopenic patients.

ORAL ANTIBIOTIC REGIMENS. Numerous studies have evaluated both nonabsorbable antibiotics (such as gentamicin, vancomycin, polymyxin, or colistin) and antibiotics that are absorbed from the gastrointestinal tract (e.g., trimethoprim-sulfamethoxazole, erythromycin, or quinolones). The goal of antibiotics has ranged from "total decontamination" of the alimentary tract with oral nonabsorbable antibiotics to "selective decontamination," in which the goal is to eliminate the potentially pathogenic aerobic flora (mostly the enteric gram-negative bacteria) while preserving the majority of anaerobic organisms and thus preserving "colonization resistance." Although the introduction of each new prophylactic regimen has been met with enthusiasm, over time these strategies have failed because of the emergence of resistant organisms.

The fluoroquinolones (mostly norfloxacin and ciprofloxacin) have been used in recent years for prophylaxis in neutropenic patients. These agents are well absorbed, and their use may really represent "early treatment" rather than prophylaxis. Although studies evaluating quinolones have demonstrated a reduction in gram-negative infections in the patients who receive them, caution about the widespread use of quinolones for prophylaxis should be underscored. Organisms resistant to the quinolones have been increasingly described, and the indiscriminate use of these agents only accelerates this process. Since the quinolones are useful for the treatment of both immunocompromised and immunocompetent individuals, the use of these antibiotics for prophylaxis should be discouraged.

PATIENTS WITH SICKLE CELL ANEMIA. Since patients with sickle cell anemia are prone to infections with encapsulated organisms (e.g., *S. pneumoniae, H. influenzae*), especially in young children, the pneumococcal vaccine and prophylactic penicillin have been used to prevent these infections. Unfortunately, the vaccination has not resulted in an effective antibody response. Prophylactic penicillin can, however, significantly reduce the incidence of infection, and it is recommended that penicillin prophylaxis be begun by 4 months of age in children with sickle cell anemia and that it be continued beyond the third birthday.

Prevention of Fungal Infections

Although the increasing incidence of fungal infection makes a preventive strategy desirable, to date no clear evidence of benefit has been demonstrated. It is hoped that newer azole and triazole antifungal agents may improve the ability to control these opportunistic pathogens.

Prevention of Viral Infections

HERPES SIMPLEX. Herpes simplex is a frequent cause of morbidity in compromised patients, particularly in association with bone marrow or renal transplantation or intensive chemotherapy regimens. Several studies have demonstrated that acyclovir administered either orally or intravenously at dosages of 250 mg per square meter every 8 hours can reduce the incidence of herpetic gingivostomatitis. Accordingly, it seems reasonable to administer prophylactic oral or intravenous acyclovir in patients who are HSV seropositive (titers ≥ 1:16) or who have a prior history of infection and are undergoing bone marrow transplantation or intensive therapy for acute leukemia.

VARICELLA-ZOSTER VIRUS. One of the most important ways to prevent VZV transmission is to prevent contact of immunosuppressed individuals with infected individuals. This includes patients with either primary VZV (chicken pox) or secondary VZV (zoster). If a seronegative individual has had contact with an infected individual, passive immunization with ZIG (zoster-immune globulin) has been shown to reduce the incidence of pneumonitis and encephalitis. Administration of ZIG (1 vial per 15 kg) must occur within 72 hours after exposure.

A varicella vaccine has been shown to reduce infection in children with leukemia. The live vaccine may be released soon for administration in normal healthy children and if effective should reduce the overall population of infected individuals.

CYTOMEGALOVIRUS. Successful strategies aimed at preventing CMV infection have included use of seronegative blood products in seronegative patients, passive immunization, and chemoprophylaxis with acyclovir or ganciclovir.

Prevention of Parasitic Infections

Pneumocystis carinii pneumonia can be largely prevented with trimethoprim-sulfamethoxazole. The decision to administer prophylaxis for *P. carinii* should be influenced by the patient's underlying disease, the intensity or immunosuppression of the therapy being delivered, and the center where treatment is being administered. Recent studies have demonstrated that trimethoprim-sulfamethoxazole can be effective and safe at a dosage of 75 mg per square meter twice a day given on 3 consecutive days each week. Alternatives include aerosolized pentamidine or atovaquone.

Improving Host Defense

Immunization against bacterial and viral pathogens has played an extremely important role in decreasing the incidence and/or severity of many infectious diseases. Unfortunately, active immunization is generally unsuccessful in immunocompromised hosts, since they are unable to mount or to sustain an antibody response to most vaccines.

Passive immunization, on the other hand, involves administration of preformed antibodies to high-risk patients. ZIG, for example, is effective in preventing infection and decreasing the incidence of morbidity and mortality associated with primary chicken pox in susceptible hosts. Another "hyperimmune" preparation that has been investigated in high-risk patients is the so-called J-5 antisera, collected from patients with high titers of antibody directed against the core glycolipid of Enterobacteriaceae. The results of early clinical trials with the J-5 antisera appeared encouraging, although confirmatory studies have not been consistent. Pooled immunoglobulin preparations do not appear to offer benefit for neutropenic hosts but are of benefit to patients who have either congenital or acquired (e.g., CLL, multiple myeloma) hypogammaglobulinemia. Monoclonal antibodies have been recently evaluated but were accompanied by unanticipated toxicity, impeding the use of current formulations.

Perhaps the most exciting new developments will be the therapeutic use of cytokines and lymphokines to enforce the host defense repertoire. Several studies have demonstrated that both GM- and G-CSF can shorten the duration of chemotherapy-induced neutropenia, abbreviate the durations of hospitalization, and decrease the need for antimicrobial therapy. The American Society of Clinical Oncology has recommended, on the basis of published data, that hematopoietic cytokines be used when the likelihood of a chemotherapy regimen resulting in fever and neutropenia > 40%; when the interest is not in reducing the dose intensity of chemotherapy after a prior episode of fever and neutropenia; and when they are needed following autologous bone marrow transplantation. Conversely, these colony-stimulating factors are not indicated for patients with low-risk (i.e., short-duration) neutropenia. Clearly, as new factors become defined, the prospect for restoring function in the compromised host stands as the opportunity for the 1990's.

Ambrosino DM, Molrine DC: Critical appraisal of immunization strategies for prevention of infection in the compromised host. Hematol Oncol Clin North Am 7:1027, 1993.

Chanock SC: Evolving risk factors for infectious complications of cancer therapy. Hematol Oncol Clin North Am 7:771, 1993.

Freifeld AG, Hathorn JW, Pizzo PA: Infectious complications in the pediatric cancer patient. *In* Pizzo PA, Poplack DG (eds.): Principles and Practice of Pediatric Oncology, 2nd ed. Philadelphia, JB Lippincott, 1993, pp 987–1020.

Hathorn JW: Critical appraisal of antimicrobials for prevention of infections in immunocompromised hosts. Hematol Oncol Clin North Am 7:1051, 1993.

Heimenz JW, Greene JN: Special considerations for the patient undergoing allogeneic or autologous bone marrow transplantation. Hematol Oncol Clin North Am 7:961, 1993.

Pizzo PA: Management of fever in patients with cancer and treatment induced neutropenia. N Engl J Med 328:1323, 1993.

Roilides E, Pizzo PA: Biologicals and hematopoietic cytokines in prevention or treatment of infections in immunocompromised hosts. Hematol Oncol Clin North Am 7:841, 1993.

Rubin RH, Ferraro MJ: Understanding and diagnosing infectious complications in the immunocompromised host: Current issues and trends. Hematol Oncol Clin North Am 7:795, 1993.

Sloas M, Rubin M, Walsh TJ, et al.: Clinical approach to infections in the compromised host. *In* Hoffman R, Benz EJ Jr, Shattil SJ, et al. (eds.): Hematology. Basic Principles and Practices, 2nd ed. New York, Churchill-Livingston, 1994.

Walsh TJ: Management of immunocompromised patients with evidence of an invasive mycosis. Hematol Oncol Clin North Am 7:1003, 1993.

Weinberger M: Approach to the management of fever and infection in patients with primary bone marrow failure and hemoglobinopathies. Hematol Oncol Clin North Am 7:865, 1993.

267 PREVENTION AND CONTROL OF HOSPITAL-ACQUIRED INFECTIONS

William Schaffner

HISTORY. Hospitals are viewed today as institutions where scientific advances are used to provide the most up-to-date diagnostic and therapeutic services for patients. This optimistic view is tempered, however, by the realization that the hospital also can be a dangerous place for patients. The application of technology is not without hazards, and among these hospital-acquired infection has the longest history. When hospitals first were established in Europe during the Middle Ages, they were primarily places where the gravely ill were taken to die. Because facilities were primitive, infections that prompted the admission of some patients were readily spread to others. Hospital typhus and typhoid were commonplace, for example, and hospitals acquired the reputation of pest houses.

These circumstances remained basically unchanged until the mid-nineteenth century, when a Hungarian physician, Ignaz P. Semmelweis, was appointed to direct the obstetric service of the prestigious Allgemeines Krankenhaus (General Hospital) in Vienna. Semmelweis encountered a puzzling situation concerning the hospital's two obstetric wards. They were ostensibly similar and admitted patients on alternate days. Yet the mortality rates on the two wards were strikingly different. Semmelweis performed a seemingly elementary exercise but one that was unique in his time. He tabulated the monthly mortality rates on the two wards and documented that on Ward I the rates regularly were 8 to 10% or even higher, whereas on Ward II they rarely rose above 2%. The cause of this extraordinary mortality was puerperal sepsis (childbed fever), a rapidly fatal septic illness. Semmelweis worked before the formulation of the germ theory of disease, but we now know puerperal sepsis to be caused by the group A β-hemolytic streptococcus. He systematically examined a series of hypotheses attempting to explain the disparate mortality rates, but none proved valid. Among the more far-fetched notions was that the disease was psychosomatic and that intense anxiety was provoked when monks made their rounds, tolling hand-bells in mourning for those recently dead. Semmelweis persuaded the monks not to ring the bells and, of course, the occurrence of puerperal sepsis continued unaffected.

At that point a pathologist cut his finger while performing an autopsy of a woman who had died of puerperal sepsis. He soon developed a fatal illness with a clinical course that was entirely similar to puerperal sepsis. Because the pathologist had been inoculated with trace amounts of material during the autopsy, Semmelweis drew an insightful analogy: Perhaps the obstetric patients also were being inoculated with infectious material. It was then that a seemingly trivial difference between the two obstetric wards became important. The deliveries on the low-mortality ward were performed by midwives; on the high-risk ward they were performed by medical students and physicians. Furthermore, the autopsy room was directly adjacent to the ward, and Semmelweis deduced that the unwashed contaminated hands of students and physicians going from autopsies to the delivery room were the vehicles for transmitting infection to patients. Despite protestations from the medical staff, Semmelweis then insisted upon hand-washing after autopsies and before the examination of each patient. The mortality rate on Ward I promptly fell to levels even lower than those on the other ward.

Semmelweis is honored as the originator of hospital infection control efforts. His process of systematically gathering data, performing an analysis, and instituting control measures still is followed today. Furthermore, his emphasis on the hands of caregivers as the means for carrying pathogens from patient to patient remains valid. Unfortunately, as in the last century, contemporary physicians still require constant reminders to wash their hands during their patient care duties.

After the acceptance of the germ theory of disease, rapid advances in microbiology, disinfection, and aseptic technique around the turn of the century substantially enhanced the safety of patient care in hospitals. Starting in the 1930's, the introduction of antimicrobials made possible the development of progressively more elaborate surgery. However, predictions that hospital infections soon would become inconsequential have not come true. Rather, the types of hospital infection have changed in response to advancing medical science.

The 1950's and 1960's witnessed a global pandemic of hospital infections caused by *Staphylococcus aureus*. Previously very susceptible to penicillin, the new penicillin-resistant epidemic strain (phage type 80/81) became the scourge of hospitals worldwide. It stimulated research into all aspects of hospital-acquired infection and persuaded authorities that every hospital should have a formal infection-control program. For reasons still not clear, the staphylococcal pandemic waned in the 1970's and gram-negative bacilli, often antibiotic resistant, became the dominant nosocomial pathogens. In the 1980's there again was a shift; staphylococci returned (now methicillin resistant), enterococci rose in importance, and *Candida* and other yeast infections caused a larger proportion of nosocomial infections in seriously ill patients. During the 1990's, antibiotic-resistant organisms of all kinds assumed even greater importance in hospitals. Thus it seems that there will be no infection-free utopia; each era presents infection control challenges anew as yesterday's saprophyte becomes tomorrow's pathogen.

THE PROBLEM OF NOSOCOMIAL INFECTIONS. Infections that are acquired during hospitalization and are neither present nor incubating at the time of hospitalization are defined as *nosocomial* * infections. The occurrence of a nosocomial infection does not *per se* indicate that the hospital or its personnel were at fault or committed an error in patient care. Current preventive measures still cannot prevent many nosocomial infections. Medicolegal liability regarding a nosocomial infection occurs when it can be demonstrated that physicians or hospital personnel have been negligent in not adhering to appropriate standards of care and that an infection resulted from the failure to perform consistent with the standard.

It is estimated that 5 to 8 nosocomial infections occur for every 100 admissions to acute-care hospitals in the United States, resulting in 2 to 4 million such infections annually. Some nosocomial infections are more serious than others, but taken together they are estimated to require over 6 million days of excess hospital stay a year and contribute to the deaths of many patients (Table 267–1).

Most studies of nosocomial infections have been performed in the high-technology hospitals of the developed countries. Although less attention has been given to delineating nosocomial infections in developing countries, it is clear that they are an important problem there as well. Hospital outbreaks of measles and shigellosis, as well as infections related to a lack of disinfectants and other supplies, occur regularly. Because developing countries have only modest re-

sources, it is especially unfortunate that their efforts to provide medical care are so often thwarted by nosocomial infections. The World Health Organization has acknowledged that nosocomial infections are a substantial international public health issue.

PREDISPOSING FACTORS. All patients do not have an equal risk of developing a nosocomial infection. The inherent resistance of the patient to infection is probably the most important determinant of risk. The extremes of age, poor nutritional status, severity of underlying diseases, and breaks in the integrity of the skin and mucous membranes all increase a patient's risk of nosocomial infection.

The second strong influence on risk of nosocomial infection is the array of diagnostic and therapeutic manipulations undertaken for the patient's benefit. Every invasive procedure carries some risk of infection because it violates either a cutaneous or mucosal barrier to microbial invasion. The risk varies with the degree of invasiveness. For example, an intramuscular injection usually has virtually no risk of infection, whereas 15 to 20% of colorectal operations are complicated by wound infections despite meticulous surgical technique, preoperative bowel preparation, and appropriate antibiotic prophylaxis. Thus, physicians should weigh every invasive procedure's potential benefits against potential risks. Medical therapy also can make patients extremely susceptible to nosocomial infections. Cancer chemotherapy eliminates virtually all of a patient's circulating neutrophils, and the immunosuppressive regimens used in organ transplantation ablate the normal immune response to invading microorganisms (see Ch. 266). Infection control measures are designed to protect the patient until periods of such exquisite vulnerability have passed and the patient again has normal or nearly normal phagocytic and immune functions. In addition, the antibiotics used to combat infection can be considered a two-edged sword. Although their use does not generally confer an increased risk of complicating infection, when new infections occur in the face of antibiotic therapy, the pathogens often are resistant to the antibiotics being used (so-called suprainfections). Lastly, it follows that the longer a patient remains in the hospital, the more likely it is that a nosocomial infection will occur.

MODES OF TRANSMISSION. Nosocomial pathogens can be found in both the animate and inanimate environment of the hospital. It is not generally appreciated how clean the hospital's inanimate environment has become. The furniture, bedclothes, curtains, and other inanimate surfaces in the hospital only very rarely harbor microorganisms that cause infections in patients. Nevertheless, reservoirs of nosocomial pathogens still can be established in inanimate areas of the hospital occasionally, especially in specialty care areas. For example, if the countertop in the intensive care unit where urine specific gravity determinations are performed remains wet, it may harbor multiresistant gram-negative bacilli. Nurses' hands then become contaminated, and the organisms can be carried back to patients in the unit. Although similar infection hazards in the inanimate environment are detected periodically and need to be remedied, we cannot look to enhanced housekeeping of the general hospital environment to reduce nosocomial infection rates further.

Whereas the hospital's general inanimate environment has receded as a source of nosocomial infections, the role of contaminated medical devices has increased substantially; more than 100,000 device-related infections are estimated to occur each year. Medical devices are examples of imaginative medical technology that offer new benefits to patients. However, manufacturers often do not consider the potential infection risks of new devices fully, and physicians often employ devices in ways that were not initially anticipated. For example, when intravascular pressure transducers first

---

* *Nosocomial* is a new word constructed from Greek roots to define an event, such as an infection, originating in the hospital or other health care facility.

TABLE 267–1. IMPACT OF HOSPITAL-ACQUIRED INFECTIONS IN ACUTE-CARE HOSPITALS

Anatomic Site	Number of Infections per 100 Admissions	Proportion of All Hospital-Acquired Infections (%)	Estimated Direct Mortality (%)	Estimated Number of Excess Hospital Days per Infection	Proportion of All Excess Hospital Days (%)
Urinary tract	2.5	30–40	<1	2	19
Postoperative wound	1.5	20–25	1–2	7	33
Pulmonary	1	10–20	5–10	8	21
Bloodstream	0.5–1	5–15	25	14	16
Others	1	20–25	Varies with site	2	12

were introduced, their use was associated with outbreaks of bacteremia. Investigations revealed that instruments were being inadequately disinfected because the instruments were very fragile. When appropriate disinfection protocols were developed, this new infection risk associated with technologic innovation was virtually eliminated.

The animate hospital environment consists of the patients and their caregivers. These humans are the sources of most nosocomial pathogens, and the intimacies of patient care often result in their sharing their microbial flora.

A familiar scenario involves *Staphylococcus aureus,* a classic hospital pathogen. Hospital personnel have a higher rate of asymptomatic carriage of *S. aureus* (often >30%) than does the general population. Staphylococci may be transmitted from hospital workers to patients, in whom they later can produce, for example, postoperative wound infections. Such "hospital staph" pathogens often are more antibiotic resistant than community-acquired *S. aureus,* providing a distinctive marker that enables their movement to be readily traced. However, hospital personnel are not the only source of resistant microbial flora. Studies have demonstrated that when admitted to the hospital, some patients already may be colonized with small numbers of resistant bacterial strains. After antibiotic treatment, these resistant strains have a survival advantage and multiply to potentially cause nosocomial infection. Indeed, the endogenous flora is the major source of both the bacterial and viral pathogens that cause nosocomial infections in patients who receive organ transplants and are immunosuppressed for long periods.

More than 100 years have passed since Semmelweis implicated the hands of the students and physicians as the means of spreading pathogens to patients. Nevertheless, such direct contact continues to be the most common way patients are colonized with microorganisms of exogenous origin. At times the microorganisms may be from the caregiver's own flora. Usually, however, the hands of nurses or doctors are contaminated transiently while caring for one patient, and the pathogens then are carried over to the next patient (this process is aptly called cross-infection in Britain). Gram-positive skin flora (*S. aureus* and *S. epidermidis*), many gram-negative bacilli (*Enterobacter* and *Serratia*) and even viruses (respiratory syncytial virus, rotavirus) are spread by this means. Over a century ago Semmelweis introduced the most effective way to interrupt transmission by contaminated hands: hand-washing. To promote hand-washing after every patient contact, modern hospitals have located sinks conveniently and have provided disinfectant soap wherever patient examinations and manipulations take place, with special attention to intensive care areas, treatment rooms, and the like. However, persuading medical staff, especially physicians, to routinely wash their hands remains a challenge, especially in the hectic environment of the intensive care unit (ICU).

Airborne transmission once was thought to have an important role in the spread of pathogens in the hospital. Today this seems not to be the case, although occasional explosive outbreaks of tuberculosis and chickenpox strongly suggest airborne transmission from a source patient. *Aspergillus* infections have occurred in immunosuppressed patients whose rooms drew air from the vicinity of major construction sites in or adjacent to the hospital. Likewise *Legionella* infections have been produced by the contaminated water spray from an air conditioning cooling tower. Concern about the role of airborne infection in the operating room continues to influence the design and construction of these areas. Most studies indicate that the bacteria causing wound infections originate from the resident flora of either the patients themselves or the operating team. This suggests that transmission likely occurs by direct contact or droplet spread. Nevertheless, because only a few bacteria can incite infection in certain elaborate procedures that implant foreign bodies (such as total joint replacements), such procedures are performed in laminar airflow facilities where the airstream is designed to flow away from the operative field.

ANTIMICROBIAL RESISTANCE. Since the pandemic of the 1950's and 1960's caused by staphylococcal strains newly resistant to penicillin, it has become axiomatic that antibiotic resistance has been a major feature of nosocomial infections. Although antibiotic-resistant bacteria are not inherently more virulent than their susceptible counterparts, they reduce the physician's therapeutic options and often require the use of more expensive antibiotics.

Currently, both gram-positive and gram-negative hospital pathogens have developed patterns of antimicrobial resistance. *S. aureus* infections are resurgent, and many strains now have developed resistance to methicillin and other similar β-lactam antibiotics that have been mainstays of therapy until recently. Many physicians turned to the quinoline antibiotics as alternate therapy, but quinoline-resistant strains were recovered with extraordinary rapidity in hospitals where these drugs were used widely. *S. epidermidis* has become a notable nosocomial pathogen in some ICU's; these organisms have a very diverse pattern of antibiotic resistance. Likewise, gram-negative bacilli have developed distinctive resistance profiles in some hospitals; *Enterobacter cloacae, Pseudomonas aeruginosa,* and *Acinetobacter calcoaceticus* particularly have been involved. It has become clear that genes determining antibiotic resistance are often carried on extrachromosomal plasmids that can be transferred among bacterial species. Thus, some medical centers have had years-long outbreaks of resistant gram-negative bacillary infections. The distinctive antibiotic resistance pattern first was detected in one bacterial species (among *Serratia,* for example) and then over time also was found among other gram-negative nosocomial pathogens (among *Enterobacter* and *Klebsiella* sequentially). Investigations that combine studies of infections in hospital populations with molecular biologic studies of the pathogens have been called "molecular epidemiology."

During the early 1950's bacterial pathogens isolated from infections virtually anywhere in the United States had essentially identical antibiotic susceptibility patterns. Shortly after antimicrobial resistance was recognized, however, it became apparent that different hospitals began to develop antibiotic resistance patterns among their hospital pathogens that were distinctive and different from each other. Thus, one hospital might have a problem with multiresistant *Serratia,* whereas another directly across the street might encounter almost no such isolates. Although never precisely explained, these differences have been attributed to factors of patient populations, severity of illness, length of stay, and, most importantly, patterns and intensity of antibiotic use. Physicians needed to be aware of these differences, so clinical microbiology laboratories maintained surveillance of resistance patterns and reported them periodically to the medical staff. The more sophisticated surveillance systems were able to distinguish resistance patterns between community-acquired and hospital-acquired infections. More recently it has become clear that such hospital-wide surveillance is insufficient in large, complex medical centers. Rather than a uniform hospital-wide nosocomial flora, there are a number of independent subpatterns that are specific to each special care area. Thus, the burn unit, neonatal ICU, and surgical ICU each may have a distinctive nosocomial flora, each with its own localized resistance problem. Laboratories have started to adapt their computerized data management systems so that specialty unit–specific surveillance data can be provided to the physicians who practice in each unit.

COMMON NOSOCOMIAL INFECTIONS, BY ANATOMIC SITE (See Table 267–1)

URINARY TRACT INFECTIONS. Urinary tract infections (UTI's) continue to be the most common nosocomial infection, accounting for 30 to 40% of all hospital-acquired infections. They occur so frequently because almost all are linked to prior urinary tract instrumentation, most often with the seemingly innocuous bladder catheter. Even single in-and-out catheterization is associated with 2 to 3% bacteriuria in otherwise healthy persons. The urethral meatus is colonized with bacteria, and even after appropriate cleansing, some are inoculated into the bladder during the catheterization process. The healthy bladder almost always rids itself of small numbers of introduced bacteria. If the bladder and urethra are traumatized, however, an infection is more likely to be established. After complicated labor with its associated urethral and bladder trauma, 23% of postpartum women develop UTI after only a single catheterization.

Given these risks, the use of indwelling Foley catheters is preferred, and 10 to 20% of hospitalized patients are treated with these devices. Because of their frequent use, Foley catheters are the leading factor predisposing to nosocomial UTI's. The longer the catheter is in place, the more likely it is that an infection will occur; approximately 5% of patients with a catheter develop bacteriuria per day. The infecting strains colonize the urethral meatus. Through movement of the catheter as well as their own motility they gain entrance to the bladder. Contemporary urinary drainage systems are well designed so that ascending infection from the reservoir bag now is quite uncommon.

Most nosocomial UTI's are asymptomatic or mild, clear with little or no therapy after catheter removal, and do not prolong hospital stay very much (an average of 1 to 2 days only). They are important, however, for two reasons. They are occasionally severe, and 1 of every 200 nosocomial UTI's results in bacteremia. In addition, many nosocomial UTI's are caused by antibiotic-resistant bacterial strains. Thus, the infected catheter systems become reservoirs of resistant gram-negative bacilli, especially in ICU's where they can be spread easily to other very ill patients. The most common organisms producing nosocomial UTI's include *E. coli* (30%), enterococci (16%), *Pseudomonas* (12%), and *Klebsiella* (6%). Pseudomonads and other multiresistant gram-negative bacteria account for a gradually increasing proportion of these infections as the hospitalized population becomes older, is more severely ill, and receives more intensive antibiotic treatment.

The prevention of nosocomial UTI's has received sustained attention and considerable success. Of course, assuring that catheters are used only for patients who genuinely require continuous bladder drainage is the first guiding principle. It follows that catheters should be removed as soon as possible when patients no longer need them. Industry has been very responsive by producing reliable, sturdy, closed drainage systems. In the past, catheters were disconnected from drainage bags to empty the bags, obtain diagnostic urine specimens, and the like. Every such interruption was an opportunity to introduce bacteria into the catheter system. Contemporary designs maintain the system's integrity by allowing the catheter to be aspirated with a needle and syringe.

These systems work so well that catheters need not be changed routinely, nor is catheter irrigation required unless the catheter becomes obstructed. The use of triple-lumen catheters with a closed prophylactic antibiotic irrigation system has been proposed, but these systems offer no great advantage in preventing infection and are difficult to manage by ward nurses. They may be useful in some patients after urologic surgery to prevent obstruction by blood clots and proteinaceous debris. There is no need to culture the urine routinely when removing the catheter; the practice of cutting off the catheter tip and culturing it has no value.

Regular perineal hygiene and antibiotic-containing creams have not proven to reduce infection; neither have catheters impregnated with antibacterial materials. Use of prophylactic systemic antibiotics to "cover" an indwelling catheter has been decried for 30 years, yet some data suggest they may be efficacious for the first 4 days of catheterization. A serious prospective trial has not been undertaken, perhaps because of the fear of selecting antibiotic-resistant strains.

BACTEREMIA. If UTI's are the most frequent nosocomial infections, nosocomial bacteremias are the most serious. Bacteremias may be secondary to recognized infection at some site, or they may be primary and cannot be attributed to an obvious infection in another anatomic location. Identifying the source of secondary bacteremia permits one to treat it as well as the bacteremia and prevent recurrences.

The occurrence of primary bacteremia should always prompt a thorough review of all the patient's intravenous infusions as well as other intravascular devices, as they are frequent sources of bloodstream infections. More than 25% of hospitalized patients receive intravenous fluids. Other diagnostic and therapeutic procedures require access to the venous or arterial systems for either brief or prolonged periods. An intravenous pyelogram and cardiac catheterization are examples of abbreviated procedures, whereas intra-arterial pressure monitoring may continue for days. Although all these procedures create an access for bacteria to enter the bloodstream, they are remarkably safe. Nevertheless, the history of intravascular technology is punctuated with many studies of endemic and epidemic bloodstream infections. The procedures that offer assurance of reasonable safety today were hard won, and any lapse in appropriate care can result in a device-related bacteremia. As more patients have required admission to ICU's, the rate of nosocomial bacteremia gradually rose during the 1980's and 1990's.

Intrinsic contamination of intravenous fluid by the manufacturer is fortunately a rare event. Most episodes of infusion-related sepsis are caused by microorganisms that enter the system during its use (extrinsic contamination). The major locus of contamination is the cannulation site. The longer the catheter is left in place, the more

likely it is that infection will occur. The catheter site may be purulent, and phlebitis may be evident, but these overt clinical manifestations frequently are not present. Suppurative thrombophlebitis is an unusual event in which a substantial segment of vein becomes a linear abscess, the entire lumen being filled with pus. *S. aureus* and *S. epidermidis* are the most frequently isolated pathogens, but an array of gram-negative bacilli and *Candida* species also regularly are associated with catheter sepsis.

Any indwelling vascular access device can be associated with infection. Hickman-Broviac catheters that are tunneled under the skin of the anterior chest wall before they enter the subclavian vein were developed to provide long-term vascular access (as for cancer chemotherapy) and minimize the risk of infection. They have been largely successful. When infection does occur, it often is possible to treat the infection, leaving the catheter in place. Although such catheters have an enhanced risk for developing another infection, enough time is often gained to complete a course of chemotherapy.

The essentials of prevention begin with meticulous aseptic catheter insertion technique. Because the risk of infection increases with increasing duration of use, strict nursing protocols exist to ensure that use of all catheters is discontinued on a regular rotation and that new catheters are inserted at different sites. As a reminder, the dressings at the insertion site are dated; peripheral catheters should be left in place no longer than 72 hours unless there is no alternative. If a catheter must remain in place, a note providing the reasons should be written in the chart. Likewise, the infusions themselves also must be changed regularly; infusions should hang no longer than 24 hours. Because most infections originate at the insertion site, in-line filters have not reduced infection rates; they add expense without increasing safety. The catheter insertion site is protected by a single dressing for the duration of the catheter's routine use; daily dressings and antibiotic ointments are no longer considered useful.

NOSOCOMIAL PNEUMONIA. Hospital-acquired lower respiratory tract infections (including pneumonia and bronchitis) account for 10 to 15% of nosocomial infections. Almost 1% of patients admitted to the hospital develop pneumonia. Elderly patients with serious underlying illnesses are at risk, as are all patients receiving mechanical ventilation. These infections usually extend a patient's hospital stay for 7 days or more, produce substantial morbidity, and contribute to the deaths of already seriously ill patients.

In contrast to community-acquired pneumonia in younger patients, nosocomial pneumonia usually is a mixed infection involving more than one organism. Although a hospital's ICU may develop a dominant bacterial respiratory tract pathogen, the list of bacteria associated with nosocomial pneumonia is large. Aerobic gram-negative bacilli are associated with more than half the cases, including *P. aeruginosa, Enterobacter, Klebsiella, E. coli,* and *Acinetobacter,* among others. *Acinetobacter* particularly is associated with ventilated patients in busy ICU's. Among gram-positive organisms, *S. aureus* is isolated with regularity, but may not always have a major pathogenic role. Pneumococci contribute to about 3% of nosocomial pneumonias, usually in elderly patients with predisposing lung disease. Most clinical laboratory routines do not process respiratory tract specimens anaerobically, and even research methods have limitations in ascribing a role for anaerobes in lower respiratory tract infections. Although aerobic pathogens clearly are dominant, most authorities believe that anaerobes are involved in about one third of nosocomial pneumonias. *Legionella pneumophila* can be a vexing problem in some hospitals, where it can be isolated from the water supply. Viral respiratory infections are increasingly recognized as causes of nosocomial pneumonia and as infections predisposing to subsequent bacterial invasion. Respiratory syncytial virus, influenza, and cytomegalovirus are the viruses most commonly identified.

Endotracheal tubes and tracheostomies bypass the upper respiratory tract defense mechanisms and can traumatize mucous membranes. When managed improperly, these devices can provide direct access for hospital pathogens to be introduced on the hands of personnel or by contaminated suction tubing. Ventilator machines often produced contaminated aerosols in past years, but current maintenance protocols have made nosocomial pneumonia due to the machine itself an unusual event.

Aspiration of oropharyngeal secretions is the principal initiating event in nosocomial pneumonia. Patients who have an impaired gag reflex, are sedated, or have altered consciousness are more likely to aspirate. The volume and pH of the aspirate as well as its bacterial population contribute to the likelihood of lung injury. The bacterial population is determined by the organisms colonizing the oropharynx. The flora of the normal pharynx is largely gram-positive. Gram-negative bacillary colonization occurs in older persons with a variety of underlying diseases, after antibiotic therapy, and in patients who are leukopenic.

Gastric alkalinization can permit gram-negative bacteria to multiply in the stomach. These bacteria can then become the source of oropharyngeal colonization. Antacids and histamine type-2 (H_2) blockers are often given to patients in ICU's who are being ventilated to prevent stress ulcers. Because they raise gastric pH, these drugs promote the growth of bacteria in the stomach and increase the risk of nosocomial pneumonia. Because it does not neutralize gastric acidity, sucralfate is preferred for stress ulcer prophylaxis.

The prevention of nosocomial pneumonia is a daunting challenge. Positioning patients with their heads raised may reduce somewhat the occurrence of aspiration. Scrupulous hand-washing inhibits the transmission of nosocomial pathogens. Meticulous maintenance of ventilatory equipment and assiduous pulmonary toilet by nurses reduce risks. The role of selective decontamination of the gastrointestinal tract with combinations of oral and systemic antibiotics currently is being studied.

SURGICAL WOUND INFECTIONS. Postoperative wound infections account for 20% of nosocomial infections. These infections account for a substantial amount of morbidity, increase hospital stay considerably, and are costly. Some postoperative infections extend down from the skin incision to the depths of the surgical field where they can destroy vascular anastomoses or disrupt an implanted prosthetic device. Bacteremia may accompany such infections. The extent of the surgical procedure and its anatomic location, the severity of the patient's underlying illness, and the surgeon's skill are all important determinants of risk. When surgery involves tissues that normally are not subjected to a large microbial population during the procedure ("clean" operations), wound infection rates often are <2%. Such operations include inguinal herniorrhaphy and vascular surgery in the neck, for example. When procedures transect mucosal surfaces, as in a colectomy ("contaminated" operations), up to 20% of patients have a postoperative wound infection. If patients are malnourished, at the extremes of age, or have serious underlying diseases, wound infections are more likely to occur. The longer the operation, the more likely that postoperative infection will occur. A surgeon's skill is critical. If tissues are traumatized, the vascular supply is unnecessarily interrupted, devitalized tissue or blood clots are left in the wound, or wound layers are not realigned properly, the risk of wound infection increases.

S. aureus and *S. epidermidis* are the most commonly isolated pathogens from wound infections, reflecting their common residence on human skin. A wide variety of other organisms contribute to these infections, including enterococci, *E. coli, P. aeruginosa,* and *Bacteroides,* largely determined by the organ undergoing surgery. The infecting bacteria most often originate in the patient's own endogenous microbial flora, whether on the skin or on a mucosal surface. A smaller contribution comes from the bacterial flora of the surgeon and other members of the operating team. Even clean wounds are not truly sterile; small numbers of bacteria can be recovered from virtually all wounds at the time of wound closure. Thus, for the most part, the infecting bacteria are in the wound when the patient leaves the operating room, unless there is a drain or packing in the incision. Occasionally bacteria originating from another infected site implant at the operative site; there have been a few well-described instances in which a wound was infected during postoperative care.

A whole array of techniques are used to minimize the occurrence of wound infection. The architecture, air handling, and housekeeping in the operating room have made the physical environment very clean. Special laminar flow rooms are used for some procedures, such as implantation of an artificial joint. An elaborate ritual of aseptic practice involves both the patient (shaving the surgical area, baths with disinfectant soap, skin preparation just before surgery, among others) and the surgeon (precise hand scrubbing, operating room gowns and masks, use of sterile gloves, and the like). The importance of the appropriate use of antibiotic prophylaxis cannot be overemphasized. Indeed, some medical historians suggest that the most important consequence of the discovery of antibiotics was that their use permitted the development of the technologically adventurous procedures that characterize contemporary surgery. In recent years it has been amply confirmed that for antibiotics to be effective in preventing wound infection they need to be given only briefly, chosen to be effective against the most commonly expected pathogens at the surgical site, and given in amounts sufficient to provide killing concentrations in the tissues. The brevity of their use (often no longer than 24 hours) results in very little drug toxicity or development of bacterial resistance.

MISCELLANEOUS SITES. In addition to the most commonly occurring infections discussed above, nosocomial infections also occur in numerous other sites and circumstances. The extent of nosocomial infectious diarrhea is only now being recognized. Among children, the most common pathogen is rotavirus; among adults, *Clostridium difficile* colitis is a complication of antibiotic therapy. Epidemics of keratoconjunctivitis due to adenoviruses can be propagated by the contaminated hands of ophthalmologists as well as contaminated tonometers. Meningitis, usually caused by *S. epidermidis,* can follow the placement of shunts in the cerebral ventricles. Meningitis also can occur in immunocompromised organ transplant recipients. In renal transplant patients *Cryptococcus* and *Listeria* are the most frequent pathogens. Transfusions of blood and blood products have resulted in the transmission of hepatitis B virus and human immunodeficiency virus (HIV) as well as other viruses and bacteria.

INFECTION CONTROL PROGRAMS

Although many efforts were being made to prevent infections in hospitals, most institutions did not have a formal organized program until the 1960's. At that time it became apparent that the previous focus by hospitals on environmental hygiene was insufficient. Strongly influenced by the Centers for Disease Control, the American Hospital Association, and the Joint Commission on Accreditation of Health Care Organizations, every hospital now must have an active infection control program to secure accreditation. Central to the program is an Infection Control Committee whose members are broadly representative of hospital administration and the professional disciplines. A physician knowledgeable about infection control is designated the Hospital Epidemiologist. It is recommended that the hospital employ one infection control practitioner (usually a nurse with special infection control training) for every 250 beds. These practitioners organize a variety of infection control activities, but all who work in hospitals must realize that the practitioners alone cannot produce the safest milieu for patients. Rather, all who work in hospitals must assume responsibility: Infection control is everyone's business.

A critical element of the program is a system of surveillance for detecting nosocomial infections, analyzing the data, and reporting on distinctive events. Surveillance may involve reviewing microbiology laboratory reports, visiting wards, inspecting surgical wounds, and the like. It now has been well demonstrated that such surveillance provides more pertinent information than routinely culturing features of the environment, a practice that has largely ceased.

The infection control practitioners also orchestrate the institution's control measures, ranging from appropriate isolation systems to responses when an epidemic is detected. Each unit in the hospital contributes its own section of procedures to a hospital-wide infection control manual. Its procedures are reviewed on 1- to 2-year cycles and as needed when new developments occur.

Sophisticated support from the clinical microbiology laboratory is necessary for a successful infection control program. The laboratory provides its routine data for surveillance purposes, may be asked to process extra cultures when an outbreak is under investigation, and may undertake special studies with nosocomial pathogens.

Other hospital service units also provide critical support for the infection control program. Although the role of the inanimate environment has been de-emphasized, the housekeeping department must maintain a high level of cleanliness throughout the institution. They also are responsible for managing and disposing of the hospital's solid waste. Heavily contaminated wastes (as from the microbiology laboratory) must be incinerated. Solid waste disposal has become a major political issue over the last several years and has become very expensive, so this function has grown in importance.

The central supply operation cleans and either disinfects or sterilizes reusable materials that are used in the diagnosis and therapy of patients. The laundry collects and launders soiled linen. Linen need be sterilized only for use in operative procedures. The hospital kitchen or outside food service must adhere to strict hygiene standards in preparing the many and varied diets for patients. Fortunately, foodborne outbreaks in hospitals are not common.

The occupational health service has special responsibilities to protect hospital personnel from acquiring an infection from patients while performing their patient-care duties, and, in turn, also to prevent employees from transmitting their own infections to patients. In this regard, several diseases have assumed particular importance.

AIDS (see Part XXII). Although the risk of acquiring HIV infection from occupational exposure is very low, this disease has received great attention from hospital infection control programs over the past several years. AIDS has raised a number of scientific, ethical, social, and legal issues that have had an impact on the ability of the infection control team to devise solutions. Not every issue has as yet been adequately addressed, largely because certain essential data are lacking.

Because HIV is not transmitted through casual contact, routine interactions with patients are not hazardous. Exposures that are associated with a risk of acquiring HIV infection are injuries by "sharps" (needles and scalpels, primarily) contaminated with the body fluid (blood, most commonly) or tissue of an HIV-infected patient. A number of studies have indicated that approximately 1 of every 300 such exposures results in transmission of HIV infection to the health care worker. Transmission is more likely to occur when the exposures are multiple and deep and when a substantial volume of blood is inoculated during the injury. The prospective studies of exposures on skin or mucous membranes have not shown any seroconversions, but there have been anecdotal reports suggesting that such exposures rarely might result in transmission. Much remains to be learned in this regard.

Standard protocols have been developed to manage the hospital worker who sustains an occupational injury involving a patient's blood or other body fluid. These include testing the source patient for HIV infection (if the patient can be identified), counseling the hospital worker, and possibly offering zidovudine prophylaxis. Such injuries often are major anxiety-provoking events, and cooperation of the occupational health service and the infection control team in supportive counseling of the hospital worker is extremely important. See Ch. 363 for additional discussion of AIDS prevention and control.

TUBERCULOSIS (see Ch. 311). Health care workers have always been at greater risk than the general population for acquiring tuberculosis. The patient in whom tuberculosis is diagnosed is only a modest hazard. Respiratory isolation techniques and antituberculosis therapy quickly reduce the hazard of nosocomial transmission. Rather, the risk is from the cryptic case, the patient with as yet undiagnosed tuberculosis. After a steady decline for years, tuberculosis is again resurgent because of the recent wave of immigrants from Southeast Asia and Central America and the frequency with which tuberculosis complicates HIV infection.

All hospitals are obliged to have a tuberculosis control program. All personnel receive a tuberculin skin test on employment. Those who are skin test-negative are followed by periodic skin testing, usually at yearly intervals, although high-risk persons may be tested at shorter intervals. Those in whom the skin test converts to positive are evaluated for active disease and are candidates for isoniazid (INH) preventive therapy. There is no place for annual chest roentgenograms, a now discarded practice.

HEPATITIS B (see Ch. 117). Like HIV infection, hepatitis B is transmitted in the hospital by exposure to blood and other body fluids that contain the virus. Hospital personnel who are exposed to blood and use needles, scalpels, and other sharp objects are at increased risk of hepatitis B infection. Programs to prevent hepatitis B infection are two-pronged. First, strong attempts must be made to reduce injuries through education, designing safer devices, and providing for the secure disposal of sharps in impervious containers. These precautions help avert not only hepatitis B infections, but all other blood-borne pathogens, including retroviruses and other viral hepatitis agents. Secondly, hepatitis B vaccine must be offered to all workers at potential risk. Ideally, all students of the health care professions should be immunized early in their training. In addition, insistent attempts to immunize current health care workers, including physicians and nurses, must continue. After an injury, standard protocols are used by the occupational health service to evaluate the health worker and the source patient and to offer appropriate prophylaxis.

In addition to providing hepatitis B vaccine, hospitals should provide other vaccines for the protection of personnel. Measles, mumps, and rubella have produced outbreaks in hospitals resulting in a great deal of unnecessary illness, turbulence, and expense. In these outbreaks, hospital workers have both acquired these viral infections and transmitted them to patients. It now is recommended that hospital workers born since 1957 receive a second dose of measles vaccine. If this is provided as the combined measles-mumps-rubella (MMR) vaccine, protection is achieved against all three diseases.

Finally, as the United States population ages, as hospitals care for increasingly sicker patients, and as medical technology continues its aggressive advances in organ transplantation and other invasive therapy, the importance of nosocomial infections will likely continue to increase. Infection control programs must be alert to these changes and be prepared to respond to them with equally new and innovative preventive measures.

Centers for Disease Control and Prevention: Public health focus: Surveillance, prevention, and control of nosocomial infections. Morb Mortal Wkly Rep 41:783, 1992. *Examines knowledge about effectiveness of nosocomial infection surveillance, prevention, and control and their cost-benefits.*

Evans RS, Burke JP, Classen DC, et al.: Computerized identification of patients at high risk for hospital-acquired infection. Am J Infect Control 20:4, 1992. *Statistical method to predict risk—based on guidelines of the Study of Efficacy of Nosocomial Infection and the CDC—identified more nosocomial infections than did traditional methods. Computerized equations that can help identify patients at risk of having nosocomial infections can help focus prevention efforts.*

Goldrick B, Larson E: Assessment of infection control programs in Maryland skilled-nursing long-term care facilities. Am J Infect Control 22:83, 1994. *The CDC Infection Surveillance and Control Questionnaire is a reliable instrument to assess infection control programs in long-term care facilities. Nationwide study is planned to examine relationship between control activity and risk of nosocomial infection among US skilled-nursing long-term care facilities.*

Nathens AB, Chu PT, Marshall JC: Nosocomial infection in the surgical intensive care unit. Infect Dis Clin North Am 6:657, 1992. *ICU infections are commonly caused by endogenous organisms of low intrinsic pathogenicity, and contributions of these infections to the ICU outcome is controversial. Prevention is based on timely and definitive surgical therapy, judicious use of invasive devices and antibiotics, and early enteral feeding. Infection-control measures aimed at endogenous reservoirs show preliminary promise for certain subsets of patients but remain experimental; 85 references.*

Sepkowitz KA: AIDS, tuberculosis, and the health care worker. Clin Infect Dis 20:232, 1995. *HIV infection and tuberculosis, alone and together, pose increasing risks to health care workers. The hazards of occupationally acquired tuberculosis are described as well as methods used in hospitals to promote a safe working environment.*

268 ADVICE TO TRAVELERS
Richard D. Pearson

International travel has become increasingly common over the past three decades. Millions of North Americans and Europeans visit developing areas each year for business, vacation, study, or religious activities. Modern air transportation has brought even the most exotic locations within easy reach. In addition, hundreds of thousands of troops have been deployed at various times in Southeast Asia, the Middle East, Africa, and other areas.

The risks associated with international travel vary with the locations visited, the duration of the trip, and the traveler's health, age, and activities while abroad. In general, persons going to Australia, Canada, Europe, Japan, New Zealand, and the United States require no special prophylactic measures. In contrast, visitors to developing areas, especially in the tropics, may be exposed to serious and at times life-threatening infections, as well as significant noninfectious problems.

There is no typical traveler. The usual duration abroad is 1 to 3 weeks, but some stay longer and a few reside overseas for extended periods. Pretravel medical preparation should be tailored to the traveler's individual needs. The major issues to be addressed are immunizations, malaria prophylaxis, traveler's diarrhea, and other hazards that can be avoided or minimized. Travelers to developing areas should obtain advice on the ever-changing international health requirements and the epidemiology of diseases abroad. Detailed information about specific geographic areas can be obtained from the Centers for Disease Control and Prevention (CDC) through its publications (see bibliography) or by calling the CDC International Travelers Hotline [(404) 332-4559], through publications of the World Health Organization (WHO) and the American Society of Tropical Medicine and Hygiene, or through commercially available computer programs.

IMMUNIZATIONS (See Ch. 10)

GENERAL CONSIDERATIONS. Before travel, vaccines can be administered that are routinely recommended for residents of North America, that are needed to protect travelers against infectious diseases in developing or tropical areas, or that are legally required for entry into countries (Table 268–1). A number of countries require the yellow fever vaccine. Some apply these regulations to all entering travelers, even those arriving directly from the United States, while others require them only of travelers who have visited areas where yellow fever is endemic. They are listed in the CDC publications. A few local authorities require documentation of cholera immunization, although it is marginally effective. No immunizations are required for citizens returning to the United States. Required vaccines and other immunizations should be documented in the yellow booklet entitled, "International Certificate of Vaccination," as approved by the WHO.

Pregnant travelers and those immunocompromised by human immune deficiency virus (HIV), neoplasms, or chemotherapy present special challenges. Most live viral and bacterial vaccines are contraindicated in these persons, although there are exceptions. For example, the measles vaccine is safe in persons with HIV infection, while other live vaccines such as yellow fever, oral polio, and oral typhoid should be avoided. Inactivated vaccines can be used in immunocompromised travelers, but the immune responses they elicit may be impaired, leaving the traveler at increased risk.

With a few exceptions, vaccines can be given simultaneously without adversely affecting the immune responses they elicit. Exceptions include the cholera and yellow fever vaccines, which inhibit antibody responses to each other, and immune globulin, which can inactivate some live viral vaccines. Immune globulin should be

TABLE 268–1. IMMUNIZATION OF INTERNATIONAL TRAVELERS

Routine Vaccines that Should Be Up-to-Date in All Travelers

Tetanus
Diphtheria
Pertussis (children <7 years)
Poliomyelitis
Measles
Mumps
Rubella
Haemophilus influenzae (children)
Hepatitis B

Routine Vaccines Indicated in Special Populations

Influenza
Pneumococcal

Vaccines Potentially Indicated for Travelers to Developing Areas*

Immune globulin (hepatitis A)
Typhoid
Yellow fever†
Meningococcal
Rabies
Japanese B encephalitis
Cholera†

* The choice of specific vaccines depends on the itinerary, activities, and duration of travel as well as cost, efficacy, and potential side effects of the vaccines.
† Required for entry by some countries. See Centers for Disease Control and Prevention: Health Information for International Travel and "Summary of Health Information for International Travel" for a listing of countries requiring vaccination for entry.

given at least 2 weeks after or 3 months before administering measles, mumps, and rubella vaccines. It has no apparent adverse effect on the oral polio vaccine or the yellow fever vaccine, but when possible, immune globulin should be given at a separate time. If live viral vaccines are not administered simultaneously, it is recommended that they be separated by at least 3 weeks. Immune globulin is given close to the time of departure because it has a limited duration of effectiveness.

Before vaccination, a thorough history should be obtained to identify allergies. A history of hypersensitivity reactions to egg proteins is important because many viral vaccines (e.g., yellow fever, mumps, measles, and influenza) are prepared in embryonated hen's eggs or chicken embryo cell culture. On rare occasions, there is hypersensitivity to thimerosal, neomycin, or other trace vaccine contaminants.

IMMUNIZATIONS TO PROTECT INTERNATIONAL TRAVELERS. *Cholera* (see Ch. 296). The currently available, nonviable, parenteral cholera vaccine provides approximately 50% protection for 3 to 6 months. Few experts recommend the vaccine, but travelers are strongly urged to follow food and water precautions (see below) and to institute rehydration and antibiotic treatment immediately if diarrhea develops. Cholera immunization is no longer required for entrance into any country, but documentation of immunization may be required by some local officials. In those circumstances, one dose of the vaccine properly recorded and given at least 6 days before travel is adequate.

***Hepatitis A* (see Ch. 117).** Hepatitis A constitutes a major risk for travelers to areas where sanitation and hygiene are poor. The likelihood of acquiring hepatitis A has been estimated to be as high as 1 in 1000 travelers per 2- to 3-week trip in some areas. Hepatitis A infection can be prevented or rendered asymptomatic by immune globulin 2 ml given intramuscularly to adult travelers who will be in endemic areas less than 3 months and 5 ml to travelers going for 3 to 5 months. Transmission of HIV is not a concern with immune globulin preparations manufactured in North America.

It is worthwhile to determine the antibody status of travelers who may have been previously infected with hepatitis A. The presence of anti-hepatitis A IgG antibodies indicates that travelers do not need immune globulin. Several active hepatitis A vaccines are under development.

***Japanese B Encephalitis* (see Ch. 346).** The Japanese B encephalitis vaccine is indicated for travelers who have intense and/or prolonged (>4 weeks) exposure in rural endemic areas in China, Korea, Southeast Asia, India, the lowlands of Nepal, Sri Lanka, and, to a limited degree, Japan. This mosquito-borne disease is most common in rural rice and pig farming areas. It occurs from June through September in temperate regions and throughout the year in tropical areas. Travelers to urban sites are usually at low risk of infection. Unfortunately, the vaccine is not without side effects. Allergic reactions, including rash, urticaria, anaphylaxis, and on rare occasions sudden death, occur in 0.1 to 10 per 100,000 vaccines. Persons with a history of hypersensitivity responses to other allergens seem to be at greatest risk. Vaccine recipients should be observed in the office for 30 minutes after immunization; however, reactions can occur days to weeks later, most within 10 days of immunization.

***Meningococcal Disease* (see Ch. 281).** The quadrivalent meningococcal vaccine (A/C/Y/W-135) should be considered for travelers going to northern India, Nepal, Saudi Arabia during the Moslem Hajj, Kenya, Tanzania, Burundi, sub-Saharan Africa, or other sites where travel advisories have been issued.

***Rabies* (see Ch. 427).** Rabies is endemic in many areas. Travelers should be warned about the disease and advised to avoid dogs and other animals. In general, long-term travelers (30 days or more) who live in areas where rabies is a threat should receive pre-exposure immunization with the human diploid cell rabies vaccine. Any short-term traveler who plans to have close contact with dogs, wild animals, or bat-infested caves also should be immunized. Simultaneous administration of chloroquine, and possibly mefloquine, can decrease the immunogenicity of intradermally administered rabies vaccine. If the drug cannot be stopped, the vaccine should be given intramuscularly. The high cost of the rabies vaccine has limited its use for pre-exposure prophylaxis.

All persons, whether or not they have received pre-exposure immunization, who are bitten by a potentially rabid animal should be advised to wash the site thoroughly with water and detergent and to seek medical care. Those who have received pre-exposure prophy-laxis need additional doses of the human diploid cell vaccine; those who have not been previously immunized require full immunization plus human rabies immune globulin.

Typhoid (see Ch. 292). Typhoid is common in developing areas where sanitation is poor. The risk is relatively low among short-term travelers to urban areas who adhere to food and water precau-tions. The oral, live Ty21a typhoid vaccine has largely replaced the killed vaccine for adults and children older than 6. The oral vaccine has fewer side effects than the killed, parenteral vaccine, which can cause severe local pain, erythema, and constitutional symptoms. The oral typhoid vaccine should not be given to HIV-infected per-sons or those taking antibiotics or mefloquine, which can inactivate it. It is recommended that the oral series be repeated at 5-year inter-vals; the inactivated vaccine is boosted with a single dose at 3-year intervals.

Yellow Fever (see Ch. 345). Yellow fever is endemic in tropical areas of Africa and Latin America in a band ranging from approxi-mately 15° north to 15° south of the equator. The yellow fever vac-cine is a live, attenuated strain (17D). It is available only at li-censed centers, which can be identified by calling local or state health offices. The vaccine is boosted at 10-year intervals. The yel-low fever vaccine should not be given to HIV-infected travelers. They should be advised to avoid endemic areas. If they must travel, they should do all that they can to minimize mosquito bites and carry with them written evidence of medical exemption.

Other Vaccines (see Ch. 300). The plague vaccine is not available in the United States. It has been used for persons with in-tense field exposure in endemic areas, but it is seldom recom-mended for travelers. There are currently no vaccines to protect against a number of important viral diseases, including dengue, and parasitic diseases such as malaria.

TRAVELER'S DIARRHEA (See Ch. 298)

Traveler's diarrhea is the most common problem encountered by North Americans who visit developing areas. The incidence is as high as 40 to 60% in some areas of Latin America, Africa, and In-dia if appropriate food and water precautions are not followed.

The risk of traveler's diarrhea can be reduced approximately fourfold by following the commandment, "Cook it, boil it, peel it, or forget it" and by eating only foods served piping hot. Even when these recommendations are followed, diarrhea may occur. The dura-tion and severity can be reduced by early self-treatment. Travelers should be instructed in oral rehydration with solutions containing glucose and electrolytes. They also should have available and take an appropriate antibiotic; ciprofloxacin is widely used in adults. Use of an antimotility agent such as loperamide can further reduce the duration of secretory diarrhea, but it should not be taken by chil-dren or by adults with bloody diarrhea, high fever, or other evi-dence of inflammatory colitis.

PREVENTING MALARIA (See Ch. 374)

Malaria is a major health hazard for travelers to endemic tropical areas. The risk of exposure varies greatly throughout the tropics. The frequency of transmission is particularly high in sub-Saharan Africa. More than 80% of the cases of falciparum malaria diag-nosed in the United States are acquired in East Africa. The mortal-ity of falciparum malaria in returning travelers and immigrants to the United States is approximately 4%. Fortunately, malaria trans-mission is infrequent in most urban areas of Latin America and Asia.

Every effort should be made by travelers to minimize contact with *Anopheles* mosquitoes—the vector of malaria—which prefer to feed in the evening, at night, and in the early morning. Travelers outdoors at those times should wear long-sleeved clothing and ap-ply insect repellents that contain *N,N*-diethylmethyltoluamide (DEET) at a concentration of 30 to 35% to exposed skin. DEET should be used cautiously in young children because of the poten-tial for seizures and other neurologic side effects due to percuta-neous absorption. Clothing and mosquito netting can be treated with permethrin, which confers further protection against mosqui-toes for weeks.

Even with these measures, chemoprophylaxis is necessary (Table 268–2). For a full discussion of the efficacy and toxicity of these drugs, see Ch. 374.

✔ TABLE 268–2. CHEMOPROPHYLAXIS FOR MALARIA*

Travelers to areas with chloroquine-sensitive Plasmodium *species:*

Chloroquine phosphate, 300 mg base (500 mg salt) orally once a week[†]

Travelers to areas with chloroquine resistance:

Mefloquine, 250 mg orally once a week[†]
or
Doxycycline, 100 mg orally daily[†]

Alternative

Chloroquine phosphate as above[†]
plus
Presumptive treatment with pyrimethamine-sulfadoxine (Fansidar), 3 tablets self-administered for a febrile illness when medical care is not immediately available
or
Proguanil, 200 mg orally daily[†‡]
(in sub-Saharan Africa)

Prevention of late relapses with P. vivax *and* P. ovale[§]

Primaquine phosphate, 15 mg base (26.3 mg salt) orally each day for 14 days

* Based on recommendations of The Medical Letter on Drugs and Therapeutics (35:111, 1993). Insect repellents, insecticide-impregnated bed nets, and proper clothing are important adjuncts for preventing malaria. The potential toxicities and contraindica-tions of antimalarial medications are discussed in Ch. 374 and should be reviewed be-fore use. Chloroquine has been used extensively and safely in pregnancy, but other pro-phylactic medications are either contraindicated during pregnancy or their safety is uncertain. No prophylactic regimen guarantees protection, and travelers should be warned about the possibility of a relapse of malaria months to a year or more after re-turning.
† Adult dose; start 1 week prior to departure with chloroquine and mefloquine, 1–2 days with doxycycline, continue during travel, and for 4 weeks after return.
‡ Not available in the United States. Failures have been reported with chloroquine and proguanil in persons with chloroquine-resistant falciparum malaria in Kenya.
§ Some relapses have been reported with this regimen. Some experts prescribe pri-maquine during the last 2 weeks of malaria prophylaxis for travelers with presumed ex-posure to P. vivax or P. ovale. Others avoid primaquine and rely on early detection and treatment of P. vivax or P. ovale malaria if it occurs.

BEHAVIORAL MODIFICATIONS

INFECTIOUS DISEASES TO BE AVOIDED. Sexually Transmitted Diseases (STD's) (see Ch. 314–318, and Part XXII). A surprising number of U.S. and European travelers have sexual relations with local residents or casual contacts among other travelers while abroad, risking HIV infection and other STD's. These risks must be explicitly discussed with all travelers. Absti-nence is the only fully effective way to avoid STD's. Travelers who choose to have sex abroad should use latex condoms. They should purchase them prior to departure because condoms manufactured abroad may not be protective. Some countries now require HIV testing before granting entrance visas.

Arthropod-Borne Diseases (see Ch. 345, 346, 374–377). A number of infectious diseases can be avoided by taking appropriate precautions. Every effort should be made to minimize exposure to arthropod vectors with clothing, insect repellents, and mosquito nets. Travelers to Latin America should not sleep in mud or adobe dwellings where reduviid bugs can transmit *Trypanosoma cruzi,* the cause of Chagas' disease.

Helminthic Infections (see Part XXIII). Travelers should not walk barefoot where hookworms and *Strongyloides stercoralis* are endemic. Persons visiting areas where *Schistosoma* species are found should avoid swimming or bathing in fresh or brackish water. People should not lie directly on beaches where dogs may have defecated leaving *Ancylostoma braziliensis,* the cause of cutaneous larva migrans.

OTHER IMPORTANT ISSUES. Chronic Medical Prob-lems. Special attention should be directed to patients with chronic medical problems. They should wear medical alert identification. Travelers requiring medications should always keep these with them, since luggage may be unavailable, lost, or stolen. It is wise to keep a list of all medications. An extra set of glasses often comes in handy.

Jet Lag. When travelers cross multiple time zones, the follow-ing few days are frequently disrupted by jet lag. Dietary measures have not been rigorously evaluated, but it is thought that the symptoms may be minimized by avoiding excessive amounts of alcohol and food during flight. Short-acting benzodiazepines have been recommended by some to help with the adaptation to new time zones, but they can result in confusion.

Motion Sickness. Travelers with motion sickness may gain relief with short-term, over-the-counter preparations of diphenhydramine. For longer trips or cruises, sustained-release transdermal scopolamine may be preferred.

Altitude Sickness. Travelers to high elevations are at risk of acute mountain sickness, particularly if they ascend rapidly to heights greater than 9000 feet. Gradual ascent over a period of days is the best way to acclimatize. Acetazolamide, 250 mg two or three times a day, has been recommended for those who do not have time to acclimatize, but it is a diuretic, causes tingling and paresthesias that may interfere with climbing, and is contraindicated in persons with sulfonamide allergies. If mountain sickness develops, the safest course of action is to descend. Steroids and pressurizing bags are helpful. Anyone going to extreme elevations should seek advice from a mountaineering expert before the trip.

Venomous Snakes, Spiders, and Scorpions. In tropical areas it is advisable to hike on clear paths, to avoid thick grass or brush, and to check the inside of shoes, closets, and drawers before

extending feet or hands into them. Hikers should always wear shoes or boots.

Accidents. Travelers frequently have a false sense of security. They should inquire about potential risks to their safety before exploring new areas or swimming, particularly in the ocean where tides may be dangerous. Information about civil unrest and political instability can be obtained from the Department of State [(202) 647-5225].

Centers for Disease Control and Prevention: CDC Health Information for International Travel 1994 [HHS Publication No. (CDC) 94-8280]. Atlanta, U.S. Department of Health and Human Services, Public Health Service, 1994. For sale by the US Government Printing Office, Superintendent of Documents, Washington, DC 20402-9328. *This is an excellent source of information on health risks in overseas locations as well as key information on vaccines and drugs. It is updated yearly.*
Centers for Disease Control and Prevention: Summary of Health Information for International Travel (HHS Publication No. 396). Atlanta, U.S. Department of Health and Human Services. *Published biweekly, listing countries or areas reporting yellow fever, cholera, and plague.*
Gardner P (ed.): Health issues of international travelers. Infect Dis Clin North Am 6:275, 1992. *This review summarizes preparations for international travel as well as the evaluation of returning travelers who are ill.*
Health Hints for the Tropics. 11th ed. Washington, American Society of Tropical Medicine and Hygiene, 1993. *A comprehensive review of health issues related to international travel.*
International Travel and Health. Vaccination Requirements and Health Advice. Geneva, World Health Organization, 1994. *Summarizes the WHO recommendations for vaccinations and malaria prophylaxis as well as other health advice for travelers.*

Bacterial Diseases

269 INTRODUCTION TO BACTERIAL DISEASE
Gerald L. Mandell

Bacteria are classified in the kingdom Procaryotae and contain DNA in a double-stranded loop not bounded by a membrane. The success of bacteria as life forms can be illustrated by the fact that fossils of bacteria 3.5 billion years old have been found. Bacteria are ubiquitous and can grow at temperatures as low as 0° C and as high as 110° C. All bacteria have a bilayered cytoplasmic membrane, and most bacteria (*Mycoplasma* are exceptions) have an outer cell wall containing muramic acid. Morphologic features are often used to categorize bacteria. Bacilli are rods or cylinders, with

about half the species being motile, while cocci are spherical and nonmotile. It is useful to distinguish bacteria by their ability to retain a basic dye (crystal violet) after iodine fixation and alcohol decolorization (the Gram reaction). Gram-positive organisms retain the dye and contain techoic acids in their cell walls (Fig. 269–1), whereas gram-negative bacteria have an additional outer membrane containing lipopolysaccharide (endotoxin) (Fig. 269–2). Capsules may serve as major virulence factors by interfering with the ability of phagocytes to ingest the encapsulated organisms. The capsules of the pneumococcus and *Haemophilus influenzae* are important factors for the virulence of the organisms. Other virulence factors include exotoxins released from the microbe, such as tetanus toxin

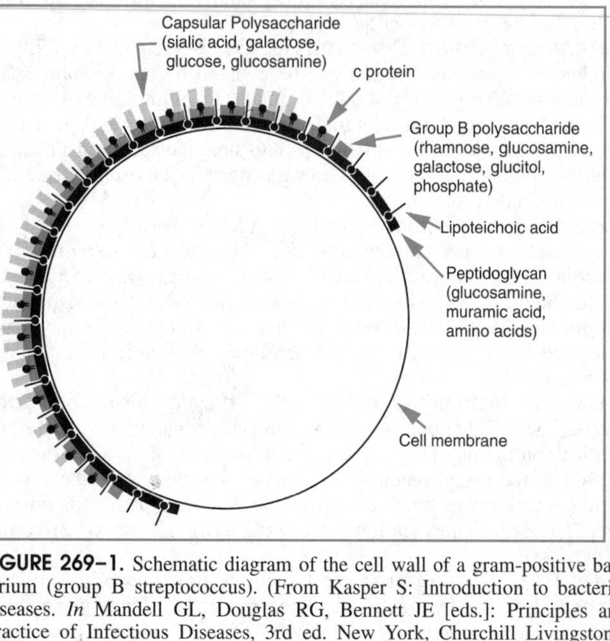

FIGURE 269–1. Schematic diagram of the cell wall of a gram-positive bacterium (group B streptococcus). (From Kasper S: Introduction to bacterial diseases. *In* Mandell GL, Douglas RG, Bennett JE [eds.]: Principles and Practice of Infectious Diseases, 3rd ed. New York, Churchill Livingstone, 1990, pp 1484–1489.)

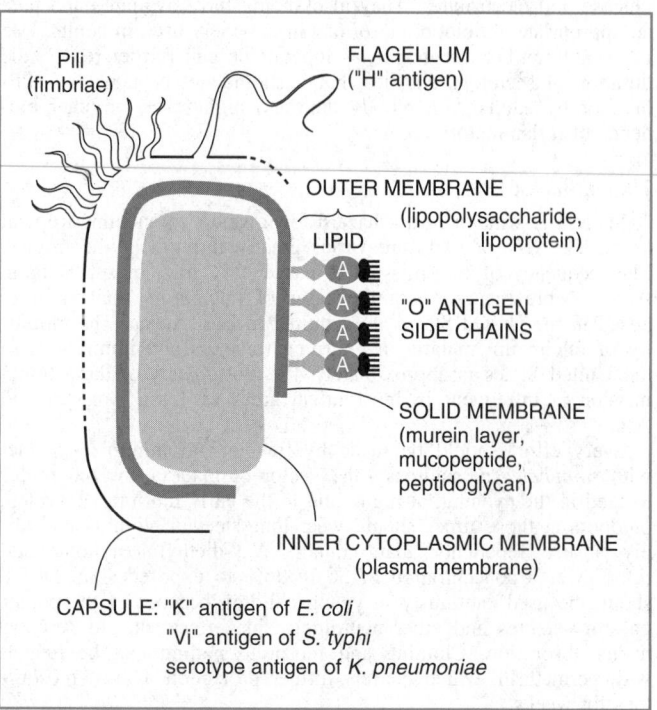

FIGURE 269–2. Schematic diagram of a gram-negative bacillus. (From Young L: Gram-negative sepsis. *In* Mandell GL, Douglas RG, Bennett JE [eds.]: Principles and Practice of Infectious Diseases, 3rd ed. New York, Churchill Livingstone, 1990, pp 611–636.)

and cholera toxin. Some bacteria, such as *Shigella flexneri,* can invade and damage host cells. Many gram-negative bacteria contain potent endotoxins that are important mediators of the sepsis syndrome. Pili or fimbriae are smaller hairlike structures that mediate bacterial attachment to various tissues and body surfaces. Only a very small proportion of species are pathogenic for humans, and new data suggest that even among those pathogenic species only certain clones are true pathogens.

Bacteria may be separated by their ability to reside and replicate intracellularly. Examples of intracellular bacteria include *Salmonella typhi, Legionella* species, mycobacteria, and chlamydiae. Extracellular pathogens include streptococci (including pneumococci), staphylococci, and most gram-negative enteric rods such as *Escherichia coli, Klebsiella* species, and *Pseudomonas* species. The main technique used for identification of bacteria in patient specimens is culture on artificial media. The ability to grow on the surface of such media in air defines aerobic organisms. Anaerobes cannot grow under such conditions, and facultative organisms can grow either aerobically or anaerobically. Microscopy can be a very useful technique, especially when combined with appropriate staining procedures such as acid-fast stains for mycobacteria or Gram stain to differentiate gram-positive from gram-negative organisms. Newer techniques use direct immunofluorescence (e.g., for *Chlamydia trachomatis*), DNA probes (e.g., for *Legionella* species), and latex agglutination tests to detect antigen (e.g., for pneumococcal capsular antigen in spinal fluid). Assays using the polymerase chain reaction are now employed. Tests for antibodies are less useful but may be helpful in some diseases (e.g., Lyme disease).

Classification of bacteria has a historic basis and is based in large part on morphology and Gram-stain reaction. Genetic studies result in frequent changes in nomenclature. Table 269–1 is a much-abbreviated summary of potentially pathogenic microbes.

TABLE 269–1. CLASSIFICATION OF SELECTED BACTERIA THAT CAUSE DISEASE IN HUMANS

Aerobes
Gram-positive cocci
  Catalase-positive
    Staphylococcus aureus
    Staphylococcus epidermidis
    Other coagulase-negative staphylococci
  Catalase-negative
    Enterococcus faecalis
    Enterococcus faecium
    Leuconostoc sp.
    Streptococcus agalactiae
      (group B streptococcus)
    Streptococcus bovis
    Streptococcus pneumoniae
    Streptococcus pyogenes
      (group A streptococcus)
    Viridans group streptococci
      S. anginosus
      S. mutans
Gram-negative cocci
  Moraxella catarrhalis
  Neisseria gonorrhoeae
  Neisseria meningitidis
Gram-positive bacilli
  Bacillus anthracis
  Corynebacterium diphtheriae
  Corynebacterium jeikeium
  Erysipelothrix rhusiopathiae
  Gardnerella vaginalis
  Acid-fast organisms
    Mycobacterium avium-complex
    Mycobacterium kansasii
    Mycobacterium leprae
    Mycobacterium tuberculosis
    Nocardia sp.
Gram-negative rods
  Enterobacteriaceae
    Citrobacter sp.
    Enterobacter aerogenes
    Escherichia coli
    Klebsiella sp.
    Morganella morganii
    Proteus sp.
    Providencia rettgeri
    Salmonella sp.
    Salmonella typhi
    Serratia marcescens
    Shigella sp.
    Yersinia enterocolitica
    Yersinia pestis
  Fermentive non-enterobacteriaceae
    Aeromonas hydrophila
    Chromobacterium violaceum
    Plesiomonas shigelloides
    Pasteurella multocida
    Vibrio cholerae
    Vibrio vulnificus

Nonfermentive non-enterobacteriaceae
    Acinetobacter calcoaceticus
    Alcaligenes xylosoxidans
    Eikenella corrodens
    Flavobacterium meningosepticum
    Pseudomonas aeruginosa
    Pseudomonas sp.
Gram-negative coccobacilli
  Actinobacillus actinomycetemcomitans
  Bartonella bacilliformis
  Brucella sp.
  Bordetella sp.
  Campylobacter sp.
  Haemophilus sp.
  Haemophilus influenzae
  Helicobacter pylori
  Legionella sp.
  Rochalimaea sp.
  Chlamydiae
    Chlamydia trachomatis
    Chlamydia pneumoniae
    Chlamydia psittaci
  Rickettsiae
    Rickettsia prowazekii
    Rickettsia rickettsii
  Myoplasmas
    Mycoplasma pneumoniae
  Treponemataceae (spiral organisms)
    Borrelia burgdorferi
    Leptospira sp.
    Treponema pallidum

Anaerobes
Gram-negative bacilli
  Bacteroides fragilis
  Bacteroides
  Fusobacterium sp.
  Prevotella sp.
Gram-negative cocci
  Veillonella sp.
Non–spore-forming gram-positive bacilli
  Actinomyces sp.
  Bifidobacterium sp.
  Eubacterium sp.
  Proprionibacterium sp.
Endospore-forming gram-positive bacilli
  Clostridium botulinum
  Clostridium perfringens
  Clostridium tetani
  Clostridium sp.
Gram-positive cocci
  Peptostreptococcus sp.
  Gemella morbillorum
  Peptococcus niger

Adapted from Bruckner DA, Colonna P: Nomenclature for aerobic and facultative bacteria. Clin Infect Dis 16:598, 1993, and Summanen P: Microbiology terminology update: Clinically significant anaerobic gram-positive and gram-negative bacteria (excluding spirochetes). Clin Infect Dis 16:606, 1993.

270 ANTIBACTERIAL THERAPY

Adolf W. Karchmer

The introduction of sulfonamides in the mid-1930's and of penicillin and streptomycin a decade later marked the beginning of the major developments in modern medicine. Subsequently there has been an expanded array of antimicrobics with increased potency and activity against the major bacterial pathogens. Not only has modern antibacterial therapy markedly reduced the morbidity and mortality of infections, but the judicious use of antimicrobics has also prevented disease and has contributed significantly to the development of modern surgery, trauma therapy, and organ transplantation. The broad application of antimicrobial agents in modern medicine has not, however, been problem free. These agents occasionally cause major adverse reactions among patients or untoward reactions when interacting with other classes of pharmacologic agents, and are a selective pressure for the increasingly widespread antimicrobial resistance among bacteria.

MECHANISMS AND TYPES OF ANTIBACTERIAL ACTIVITY

An effective antimicrobic should kill or inhibit the growth of a bacterium and not injure the human host. This selectivity results from targets that are either absent from mammalian cells or are more vulnerable to inhibition by the antimicrobic than are the analogous targets in mammalian cells. For example, the peptidoglycan rigid cell wall is unique to bacteria and thus a target for selective activity by β-lactam antibiotics. In contrast to humans who can use exogenous folic acid, bacteria cannot use exogenous tetrahydrofolic acid (folinic acid) in the synthesis of nucleic acids and must synthesize folinic acid from para-aminobenzoic acid. Inhibition of this pathway by sulfonamides or trimethoprim, independently or together, thus results in selective antibacterial activity. Antimicrobial agents that merely inhibit the growth of microorganisms are *bacteriostatic*, while those that kill bacteria at physiologically achievable concentrations are *bactericidal*. Growth inhibition and killing in general are the product of the drug's mechanism of action, but on occasion are concentration-dependent or unique to the interaction of a drug and a particular bacterial species. For example, chloramphenicol, which is generally bacteriostatic even at high concentrations, is bactericidal for *Haemophilus influenzae* at concentrations achieved in patients with standard doses. Conversely, penicillin G is generally bactericidal for susceptible organisms but is only bacteriostatic against *Enterococcus faecalis* and *E. faecium*. The site of action and antibacterial effect of major classes of antimicrobial agents are shown in Table 270–1. Combinations of antibiotics may produce an antibacterial effect greater than the sum of their independent activities; this is called *synergism*. The sequential inhibition of tetrahydrofolic acid by a sulfonamide and trimethoprim may cause synergism. Also, facilitated penetration of aminoglycosides into enterococci by penicillin, ampicillin, or vancomycin can result in bactericidal synergism.

MECHANISMS OF BACTERIAL RESISTANCE TO ANTIMICROBICS

In considering bacterial resistance to antimicrobial agents, it is useful to consider both the mechanisms of action of individual antibacterial compounds and the general properties of antibiotics that are necessary for efficacy. Antimicrobics must be able to (1) reach the molecular targets, which are primarily intracellular, in sufficient amounts; (2) interact with a target molecule in a manner that initiates an antibacterial effect; and (3) avoid inactivation by drug-modifying enzymes in the extracellular environment or within the bacterial cell. The molecular mechanism used by individual bacteria to resist specific antimicrobics can be viewed as a strategy to subvert one of these requirements for antimicrobial efficacy (Table 270–2). Frequently bacteria use more than one strategy; multiple mechanisms acting in concert may produce markedly enhanced antimicrobial resistance. Resistance to an antimicrobial agent may be an intrinsic property of a bacterial species or an acquired capability. To acquire resistance a bacterium must alter its DNA by mutating native DNA or by introducing foreign DNA. Resistance genes are often part of extrachromosomal plasmid DNA, which can transfer among organisms by conjugation, transduction, or transformation. Some resistance genes are part of DNA units called *transposons* that move between chromosomes and transmissible plasmids. Foreign DNA may be acquired through transformation, resulting in ex-

TABLE 270–1. MECHANISMS OF ACTION OF ANTIMICROBIAL AGENTS

Agent	Site of Action	Effect	Cidal	Static
Penicillins, cephalosporins, other β-lactams	Penicillin-binding proteins (peptidoglycan synthetic enzymes)	Inhibits cross-linking of peptidoglycan (transpeptidation), impairs cell wall synthesis	+	Occasionally
Vancomycin, teicoplanin	Terminal D-ala-D-ala of pentapeptide, peptidoglycan, precursor	Inhibits polymerization of disaccharide precursors to peptidoglycan (transglycosylation), impairs cell wall synthesis	+	Occasionally
Polymyxin B, colistin	Cytoplasmic membrane	Binds to phospholipid cytoplasmic membrane, disrupts membrane function	+	
Aminoglycosides	Ribosome, 30S subunit	Complex; inhibits peptide elongation, causes misreading of genetic code	+	
Tetracycline	Ribosome, 30S subunit	Inhibits binding of transfer RNA, inhibits protein synthesis		+
Chloramphenicol	Ribosome, 50S subunit	Blocks transfer of amino acids to peptide chains, inhibits protein synthesis	Occasionally	+
Erythromycin	Ribosome, 50S subunit	Inhibits translocation of ribosome on messenger RNA, inhibits protein synthesis	Occasionally	+
Clindamycin	Ribosome, 50S subunit	Blocks transfer of amino acids to peptide chain, inhibits protein synthesis	Occasionally	+
Rifampin	DNA-dependent RNA polymerase	Impairs RNA synthesis	+	
Metronidazole	Nucleic acids	Damages nucleic acid structure	+	
Quinolones	DNA topoisomerase (gyrase)	Impairs supercoiling in DNA synthesis	+	
Sulfonamides	Dihydropteroate synthetase	Competitive inhibition of synthesis of dihydrofolate from para-aminobenzoic acid		+
Trimethoprim	Dihydrofolate reductase	Inhibits reduction of dihydrofolate to tetrahydrofolic acid		+

TABLE 270–2. MECHANISMS OF ANTIBIOTIC RESISTANCE

Antimicrobic	Mechanism	Representative Organism
β-Lactam (penicillins, cephalosporins, carbapenems, carbacephems, monobactams)	Altered target (penicillin-binding protein)	*Enterococus faecium, Streptococcus pneumoniae,* methicillin-resistant *Staphylococcus aureus*
	Reduced permeability	*Enterobacter* species, *Pseudomonas aeruginosa*
	β-Lactamase	*S. aureus,* gram-negative bacilli, *Haemophilus influenzae, Neisseria gonorrhoeae, Enterococcus faecalis*
Aminoglycosides	Modifying enzymes (acetylation, adenylation, phosphorylation)	*S. aureus,* enterococci, *P. aeruginosa,* Enterobacteriaceae
	Reduced permeability or energy-dependent uptake	Enterobacteriaceae, *P. aeruginosa, S. aureus* (small cell variant), enterococci
	Decreased ribosomal binding	*S. aureus, E. faecalis* (streptomycin)
Chloramphenicol	Active efflux	*H. influenzae*
	Reduced permeability	Enterobacteriaceae
	Inactivating enzyme (acetylation)	*S. aureus,* enterococci, Enterobacteriaceae
Erythromycin, clindamycin	Decreased ribosomal binding (methylation of ribosomal RNA)	*S. aureus, S. pneumoniae,* streptococci, *Bacteroides fragilis*
	Reduced permeability	Enterobacteriaceae, *Staphylococcus epidermidis*
	Modifying enzymes	*E. coli, Klebsiella pneumoniae, S. aureus*
Quinolones	Target alteration (DNA gyrase)	Enterobacteriaceae, *S. aureus*
	Reduced permeability	Enterobacteriaceae, *P. aeruginosa*
	Active efflux	*Escherichia coli*
Tetracyclines	Altered target (ribosome)	*N. gonorrhoeae,* streptococci
	Active efflux	*E. coli*
	Permeability barriers	Enterobacteriaceae
	Drug detoxification	*B. fragilis*
Rifampin	Reduced RNA polymerase binding	*E. coli, S. aureus*
Sulfonamides, trimethoprim	Altered dihydropteroate synthetase or dihydrofolate reductase	Enterobacteriaceae, *Moraxella catarrhalis*
	Increased para-aminobenzoic acid	*S. aureus, N. gonorrhoeae*
	Reduced permeability	*P. aeruginosa,* Enterobacteriaceae
Vancomycin	Altered peptidoglycan precursor-binding site	*E. faecium*

changes of chromosomal DNA among species and subsequent interspecies recombination. Genetic mechanisms of resistance function constitutively (at a constant rate) or may be induced upon exposure to antimicrobial agents, which may confound detection of resistance by laboratory tests.

Exclusion of effective amounts of an antibiotic from intracellular compartments is a common mechanism of intrinsic resistance. Limited permeability is a property of the lipopolysaccharide outer cell membrane of gram-negative bacteria. The permeability of this membrane resides in special proteins, *porins,* which provide specific channels through which substances can pass to the periplasmic space and thereafter into the cell. Limited permeability accounts for the intrinsic resistance of gram-negative bacilli to penicillin, erythromycin, clindamycin, and vancomycin and that of *Pseudomonas aeruginosa* to trimethoprim. Similarly, the relative exclusion of aminoglycosides from the intracellular milieu of streptococci and enterococci accounts for intrinsic resistance of these organisms to this class of antimicrobics. Additionally, bacteria use this strategy in acquiring resistance. Thus, a mutational change in the specific porin of the outer cell membrane of *P. aeruginosa* through which imipenem usually diffuses can exclude the antibiotic from its target and render the *P. aeruginosa* resistant to imipenem. In general, however, mutations to decrease porin channels and reduce permeability are inefficient mechanisms for bacterial resistance and require a second mechanism, e.g., a coexisting β-lactamase, to generate higher-level resistance. The active pumping of antimicrobials from the intracellular milieu, i.e., active efflux, in effect excludes antibiotics from their targets and causes bacterial resistance. Plasmid-encoded resistance to tetracyclines among *Escherichia coli* results from active efflux.

Alteration of the target site at which an antimicrobic acts, such that an inhibitory or killing effect no longer occurs, constitutes a second major mechanism of resistance. Bacteria may acquire a gene that encodes a new antibiotic-resistant product that now substitutes for the original target. Thus, new forms of dihydropteroate synthetase and dihydrofolate reductase with lower affinity to sulfonamides and trimethoprim, respectively, mediate resistance to these drugs. Methicillin-resistant *Staphylococcus aureus* and coagulase-negative staphylococci have acquired the chromosomal gene *mecA* and produce a β-lactam–resistant penicillin-binding protein (PBP), called 2a or 2′, which is sufficient to maintain cell wall integrity during growth when other essential PBP's are inactivated by β-lactam antibiotics. Alternatively, a newly acquired gene may act to modify a target, rendering it less vulnerable to an antimicrobic. Thus, a plasmid- or transposon-borne gene encodes an enzyme that methylates the 23S rRNA of the 50s ribosome and impairs the binding of erythromycins and clindamycin to their target. The resulting resistance to these antimicrobics, which has been noted in *S. aureus,* streptococci, pneumococci, clostridia, and *Bacteroides fragilis,* may be constitutive or inducible. Mutations in existing genes or homologous DNA acquired by transformation may result in antibiotic-resistant targets. Mutations leading to amino acid changes in RNA polymerase decrease the binding of rifampin to this enzyme and result in rifampin resistance. Similarly, mutations in the *gyrA* gene that alter amino acids in the A subunit of DNA gyrase have resulted in resistance to the fluoroquinolones among methicillin-resistant *S. aureus.* Perhaps the most striking alterations of native targets resulting in antibiotic resistance are those that occur among the various essential high molecular mass PBP's of gonococci, meningococci, *E. faecium,* and pneumococci and result in the decreased binding of penicillin to these targets. Alterations of PBP's in pneumococci have also resulted in the resistance of pneumococci to third-generation cephalosporins. In these naturally transformable bacteria, the acquisition of homologous DNA has resulted in mosaic genes, which in turn give rise to the penicillin-resistant hybrid PBP's. Pneumococci with relative and high-level resistance to penicillin due to PBP alterations are now widely distributed in the world and are an increasingly common cause of disease.

The third, and perhaps the most commonly used, mechanism by which bacteria are resistant to antibiotics entails the enzymatic alteration and inactivation of an antimicrobic. β-Lactamases hydrolyze the amide bond of the β-lactam ring, thus destroying the site at which β-lactam antibiotics bind to bacterial PBP's and through which they exert their antibacterial effect. Many different β-lactamases have been described. These enzymes are encoded chromosomally or extrachromosomally through plasmids or transposons and may be either produced constitutively or induced. The almost universal resistance of *S. aureus* to penicillin, ampicillin, the carboxypenicillins, and the ureidopenicillins is mediated by a plasmid-encoded, inducible β-lactamase. Staphylococcal β-lactamase, which is secreted into the surrounding environment, does not inactivate the penicillinase-resistant penicillins (oxacillin, nafcillin), the cephalosporins, or the carbapenems (imipenem, meropenem). Although occasionally hyperproduction of β-lactamase by *S. aureus* has engendered borderline resistance to oxacillin and nafcillin, these antibiotics retain antistaphylococcal activity in the presence of this β-lactamase. β-Lactams with minimal antibacterial activity that can bind irreversibly and inhibit β-lactamases have been developed. These compounds (clavulanic acid, sulbactam, tazobactam) have been combined with the penicillins to restore their activity despite the presence of staphylococcal β-lactamase. In gram-negative bacteria the role of β-lactamases in bacterial resistance is both complex and extensive. There are an abundance of structurally unique enzymes; many inactivate a broad range of β-lactam antibiotics; and the genes encoding these β-lactamases are subject to mutations that expand enzymatic activity and are both relatively easily transferred and widely distributed. In addition, in gram-negative bacteria β-lactamases are secreted into the limited confines of the periplasmic space where they act in concert with the permeability barrier of the outer cell wall to produce clinically significant antibiotic resistance. Among the more common of the plasmid-mediated β-lactamases are the TEM-1 and TEM-2 enzymes, the SHV-1 of *Klebsiella pneumoniae,* and the PSE-1 of *P. aeruginosa.* These confer resistance to penicillin, ampicillin, carbenicillin, ticarcillin, cephalothin, and cefamandole but not to the cephamycins (cefoxitin, cefotetan), third-generation cephalosporins, monobactams, or carbapenems. Plasmid-mediated, extended-spectrum β-lactamases (ESBL's) that inactivate third-generation cephalosporins and monobactams result from mutations in the TEM and SHV genes leading to amino acid substitutions in their products. Overproduction of TEM-1 β-lactamase by genes on multicopy plasmids have been encountered in *E. coli* that are resistant β-lactam/β-lactamase inhibitor combinations. Chromosomally mediated β-lactamases are produced at low levels by *P. aeruginosa, Enterobacter cloacae, Serratia marcescens,* and other gram-negative bacilli; when these organisms are exposed to β-lactam antibiotics, high levels of β-lactamase are induced, causing resistance to the broad-spectrum cephalosporins, cephamycins, and the β-lactam/clavulanic acid or sulbactam combinations. The third-generation cephalosporins are relatively resistant to hydrolysis by these enzymes. However, the limited entry of these cephalosporins into the periplasmic space allows even these β-lactamases to effectively mediate resistance. Some strains undergo a mutation resulting in fixed derepression of the chromosomal gene and constitutively produce these β-lactamases. Fortunately, β-lactam/β-lactamase inhibitor combinations and cephamycins remain active against organisms producing ESBL's, and imipenem remains active against organisms producing either ESBL's or chromosomal-type β-lactamases.

Resistance can result from constitutively produced modifying enzymes that acetylate amino groups and phosphorylate or adenylate hydroxyl groups on aminoglycosides. Permeability barriers to aminoglycosides may enhance this type of resistance. Several genes that encode different aminoglycoside-modifying enzymes may exist simultaneously in a bacterium. They are commonly on a plasmid, the chromosome, or a transposon. Modifying enzymes commonly cause aminoglycoside resistance in gram-negative bacilli. A bifunctional acetylating and phosphorylating enzyme that results in resistance to all clinically available aminoglycosides except streptomycin has been found increasingly in *Staphylococcus aureus* and coagulase-negative staphylococci, and enterococci. In enterococci this enzyme prevents the combination of penicillin, ampicillin, or vancomycin plus any aminoglycoside, except streptomycin, from exerting a bactericidal effect. The frequent coexistence in enterococci of this enzyme and streptomycin-adenylating enzyme renders strains resistant to all bactericidal combinations.

To effectively treat infection, physicians must be aware of resistance profiles for pathogens generally as well as in their immediate environment. For example, ceftriaxone has superseded penicillin as the drug of choice for gonorrhea because the frequency of penicillin-resistant strains in national surveillance data indicates unacceptable failure rates with continued penicillin therapy. In contrast, in any given hospital a physician must know the frequency with which wound infections are caused by methicillin-resistant *S. aureus* to choose between vancomycin and oxacillin as empiric therapy for the patient with apparent staphylococcal wound infection and bacteremia. Additionally, physicians must attempt to reduce the emergence of antimicrobial resistance among bacteria. Treatment with multiple antimicrobials, an effective strategy to decrease muta-

tional resistance among *Mycobacterium tuberculosis,* is less applicable to controlling antibiotic resistance among bacteria because bacteria become resistant to the multiple antimicrobials through acquiring a single plasmid or transposon rather than by multiple mutations. Antibiotics do not cause mutations and create resistant bacteria; nevertheless, their indiscriminate use provides enormous selective pressure to sustain and enrich resistant bacteria. Expanded antibiotic use is followed by increased frequency of resistant bacteria, which are then disseminated by poor sanitation and hygiene. Improved sanitation and hygiene and enhanced infection control in hospitals can reduce the dissemination of resistant organisms. While antimicrobic use cannot be eliminated, optimal antibiotic use not only requires judicious selection of an agent and duration of therapy but also avoidance of inappropriate use.

SELECTING ANTIMICROBIAL THERAPY

IDENTIFYING THE INFECTING AGENT. Effective therapy requires that the causative agent either be recovered and its antimicrobial susceptibility identified or reliably anticipated on the basis of the clinical presentation. Recovering the pathogen(s) by culture and subsequently determining antimicrobial susceptibility is highly desirable. Culture results, however, are usually not available when initial therapy is being selected, particularly for patients with more acute or severe infections. There are a few non–culture-based tests used to identify bacterial pathogens, e.g., group A streptococci in the pharynx, gonococci from genital secretions, pneumococci and *H. influenzae* in cerebrospinal fluid (CSF), and *Legionella pneumophila* antigen in urine. Examination of a Gram stain, or acid-fast stain, of material obtained from an infected site allows rapid assessment of bacterial content (semiquantitative) and the types of bacteria, and awareness of the local inflammatory response.

Physicians commonly initiate antimicrobial therapy empirically, and even when knowing the pathogen, must select antibacterial therapy without having specific antimicrobial susceptibility information. Various scenarios prompt empiric therapy: (1) The infection is immediately life threatening; (2) a less threatening infection is likely to worsen if therapy is delayed until culture results become available; (3) considering the predictability of the pathogens causing a syndrome, the inconvenience or hazards of acquiring a culture are unjustified; (4) the causative agent is predictable, therapy relatively simple, and the hazards of failed therapy are low. Meningitis with a polymorphonuclear CSF response (presumably bacterial) or clinical findings suggestive of septic shock mandate empiric therapy immediately after cultures are obtained. In contrast, pneumonia, even when not life threatening, is likely to progress if therapy is delayed. Hence, it is prudent to obtain blood and sputum cultures, examine a sputum Gram stain, and initiate empiric therapy. In contrast, the treatment of otitis media or acute bacterial sinusitis is initiated empirically based on the high probability that the bacterial infection is likely to be caused by pneumococci, *H. influenzae, Moraxella catarrhalis,* or less commonly, group A streptococci. Tympanocentesis or aspiration of the sinus for material to culture is reserved for patients in whom empiric therapy fails. Empiric treatment of recurrent uncomplicated cystitis in a young, otherwise healthy woman is an example of the fourth scenario. Although urine is easily cultured, the infection is probably due to *E. coli* or *Staphylococcus saprophyticus,* and successful empiric therapy with trimethoprim-sulfamethoxazole or a fluoroquinolone for 3 days will have been completed before culture results are available.

Culture results must be interpreted in the clinical context. Does the *E. coli* recovered from an abscess due to a ruptured appendix reflect the true microbiology or were the anticipated anaerobic bacteria not isolated because the specimen was mishandled? Furthermore, all isolates are not necessarily causing the infection; some may be contaminants or reflect colonizing flora. Thus, interpretation of the culture results is important, particularly if the specimen has been obtained across nonsterile surfaces. Some isolates from normally sterile material must be questioned. The coagulase-negative staphylococcus or *Corynebacterium* species recovered from a blood culture is possibly a contaminant, but in the patient with indwelling vascular catheters or leukopenia and fever after cancer chemotherapy, these isolates may be pathogens. Repetitive isolation or isolation of large numbers of organisms commonly considered contaminants, e.g., *S. epidermidis,* suggests that the bacteria are causing infection and warrants careful assessment.

Whether one is treating an infection empirically or on the basis of microbiologic data, the antimicrobial regimen should be as targeted as possible. The uncertainty inherent in empiric therapy necessitates broader-spectrum antimicrobial therapy. Nevertheless, judgment must be exercised to focus initial and subsequent (after culture data are available) antimicrobial therapy as much as the clinical syndrome allows. Using multiple antimicrobics or broad-spectrum therapy where more narrow spectrum therapy will suffice inevitably exposes the patient to increased risks of adverse effects and selects for increasingly resistant organisms.

EVALUATING ANTIMICROBIAL SUSCEPTIBILITY. Appropriate antimicrobial therapy is founded upon laboratory-documented inhibition of growth or actual killing of the organism by concentrations of antibiotics that can be achieved in a patient's serum using acceptable doses. Excretion by the kidney results in striking urine concentrations for some antibiotics; for an agent used only to treat urinary tract infection, e.g., nitrofurantoin, susceptibility is based on concentrations achieved in urine.

For most bacteria, antibiotic susceptibility cannot be adequately predicted and should be determined with *in vitro* tests. The predictable susceptibility of a few organisms obviates the need for their testing. Group A streptococci are universally susceptible to penicillin and cephalosporins, and *Neisseria meningitidis* is susceptible to penicillin, ampicillin, and chloramphenicol. These species do not require testing against those specific antibiotics. The susceptibility of these organisms to other antimicrobials is less predictable, and if other agents were used for therapy, testing would be required (e.g., erythromycin or tetracycline against group A streptococci or sulfonamides against meningococci). Resistance to penicillin has been noted among *Streptococcus pneumoniae* recovered worldwide. As a consequence, the antibiotic susceptibility of pneumococci isolated from blood or CSF must be evaluated as a guide for therapy.

PHARMACOLOGIC AND PHARMACODYNAMIC CONSIDERATIONS. Successful therapy requires that an antibiotic with *in vitro* activity be delivered to the site of infection in adequate concentration without inducing adverse reactions. Knowledge of the major pharmacologic and pharmacokinetic properties of the antimicrobic is necessary. The major pharmacologic properties of commonly used antibiotics are shown in Table 270–3. Penetration of antibiotics into some tissues and fluids is limited and drug specific. Lipid-soluble agents such as chloramphenicol, rifampin, sulfonamides, trimethoprim, ciprofloxacin, ofloxacin, metronidazole, and isoniazid penetrate into the CSF well, whereas penicillins, third-generation cephalosporins, and vancomycin penetrate adequately only when there is meningeal inflammation. Treatment of infection occurring in the CNS or other sites where antibiotic penetration is limited, e.g., the prostate or vitreous humor of the eye, requires special consideration and, on occasion, direct instillation. Most antibiotics are excreted primarily through the kidneys. Biliary excretion can be an advantage in treatment of biliary tract infection; however, excretion is markedly reduced if the biliary tract is obstructed. To achieve meaningful serum concentrations, aminoglycosides, carbapenems, and glycopeptides (vancomycin and teicoplanin) must be administered parenterally. Although parenterally administered antimicrobics are preferred for treatment of severe infections, the availability of well-absorbed potent penicillins, cephalosporins, quinolones, macrolides, and metronidazole allows early transition from parenteral to less costly oral therapy in many patients (exceptions include those with endocarditis, meningitis, or CNS infection).

Antibiotic penetration into cells, particularly polymorphonuclear leukocytes and macrophages, and intracellular antibacterial activity are necessary to effectively treat some infections (e.g., *M. tuberculosis, L. pneumophila, Listeria monocytogenes, Brucella* species, and *Salmonella typhi*).

The serum and tissue concentrations over time of an antimicrobic administered by a given route and the microbiologic activity of that antimicrobic when viewed together describe the pharmacodynamic properties of the agent. Bacterial killing by β-lactam antibiotics and vancomycin does not increase after antibiotic concentrations exceed an organism's minimum inhibitory concentration (MIC) by several multiples. Also, the postantibiotic effect (inhibition of an organism's growth resulting from immediately prior exposure to an antibiotic) of these antimicrobics is negligible. These interactions suggest that administration of β-lactam antibiotics and vancomycin to achieve sustained concentrations (four to five times the MIC) over longer periods is likely to result in more profound antibacterial action than

transient higher concentrations. Sustained concentrations may be achieved by more frequent dosing, by using higher doses, by using antibiotics with a long half-life, or by continuous infusion. Aminoglycosides and quinolones exhibit concentration-dependent killing wherein higher concentrations exert an increasingly bactericidal effect and cause a prolonged postantibiotic effect. These interactions suggest that larger doses administered less frequently provide greater antibacterial activity. Increasing numbers of controlled studies report that aminoglycoside therapy given as a single daily dose is as effective and less ototoxic and nephrotoxic than the same quantity of aminoglycoside divided in the standard multiple daily-dose regimen.

PATIENT-RELATED CONSIDERATIONS. Unique aspects of the patient and site of the specific infection are important in selecting an optimal antimicrobial agent, as well as the appropriate dose, route of administration, and duration of therapy. Recent treatment with an antibiotic, for example, increases the risk that the subsequent infection is caused by residual antibiotic-resistant bacteria. Residing in an environment that has an extensive antibiotic-resistant flora, e.g., an intensive care unit, a skilled nursing care facility, or a day care center, increases the risk for colonization and subsequent infection by antibiotic-resistant bacteria.

The patient's physiologic and metabolic status must be considered when therapy is selected. Premature infants and neonates have incompletely developed renal function, requiring adjustment of antibiotic doses. The hepatic glucuronyl transferase pathway through which chloramphenicol is metabolized is immature in newborns. As a result, chloramphenicol is likely to accumulate and cause circulatory collapse—the gray baby syndrome. Because tetracyclines deposit in growing bones and teeth and quinolones may damage cartilage, they are not used in children. Genetically determined drug metabolism also affects antibiotic selection. Antimicrobics, including sulfonamides, sulfones (dapsone), nitrofurantoin, chloramphenicol, and pyrimethamine, may cause hemolysis in patients with deficient glucose-6-phosphate dehydrogenase. Pridoxine is routinely given with isoniazid treatment or prophylaxis of tuberculosis to prevent the peripheral neuropathy that occurs among those who are "slow" acetylators of isoniazid.

Hypersensitivity to one member of an antibiotic class usually extends to all other compounds in that class, and if the reaction was severe, contraindicates their use. However, if the hypersensitivity reaction to penicillin, for example, was not an immediate or accelerated anaphylactic or urticarial reaction, cautious treatment with a cephalosporin is acceptable. From 3 to 7% of patients with a history of penicillin allergy experience an allergic reaction when treated with a cephalosporin, a rate 1.5 to 2 times that noted among patients who do not report a penicillin allergy.

Most antimicrobics cross the placenta and reach therapeutic concentrations in fetal tissues; thus, antibiotics, in general, should be administered during pregnancy only if absolutely required. The fetus should not be exposed to trimethoprim or rifampin, both of which are teratogens in animals; to metronidazole, which is mutagenic; or to clarithromycin, which has been associated with fetal toxicity in primates. Tetracyclines cause fetal bone changes, and in pregnant women are associated with increased risk for hepatotoxicity. If antimicrobial therapy is required during pregnancy, penicillins, β-lactam/β-lactamase inhibitor combinations, cephalosporins, and erythromycin are preferred. Data indicating safety during pregnancy are insufficient for clindamycin, vancomycin, azithromycin, and the aminoglycosides; hence these agents should be avoided, if possible. Many antibiotics appear in breast milk; antibiotics that pose a risk to the neonate or infant (chloramphenicol, sulfonamides, tetracyclines, and quinolones) must not be administered to nursing mothers. Generally, mothers are advised to temporarily discontinue nursing during periods of antimicrobial therapy.

The pharmacokinetics of antibiotics that are primarily excreted by the kidneys are significantly altered in patients with moderate to severe renal dysfunction. If antibiotic accumulation and potential toxicity are to be avoided, dosage adjustments, after an initial standard dose, are necessary when the antibiotics are administered to patients with renal dysfunction (Table 270–3).

Antibiotics that are metabolized in the liver or excreted in the bile should be used with caution when treating patients with severe liver failure (Table 270–3). The potential for antibiotics to interact

✓ **TABLE 270–3. DOSAGE, PHARMACOLOGIC FACTORS, AND ADJUSTMENT IN RENAL AND HEPATIC FAILURE**

Class/Agent	Dose* Systemic Infection	Oral Formu-lation	Peak Serum Con-centration μg/ml	Protein Binding (%)	Normal Serum Half-Life (hr)	Dose Adjustment Hepatic Failure	Dose Adjustment Renal Failure	Serum Levels Affected by Dialysis‡
Aminoglycosides								
Amikacin	5–7 mg/kg/q8	—	35	0	2–3	No	Major	Yes (H, P)
Gentamicin	1.7 mg/kg/q8	—	7	0	2–3	No	Major	Yes (H, P)
Netilmicin	1.7 mg/kg/q8	—	7	0	2–3	No	Major	Yes (H, P)
Tobramycin	1.7 mg/kg/q8	—	7	0	2–3	No	Major	Yes (H, P)
Antituberculous Agents								
Ethambutol	15 mg/kg/d (PO)	Yes	2	10	1.5	No	Major	Yes (H, P)
Isoniazid	5 mg/kg/d (PO)	Yes	4.5	10	3	Yes	Minor	Yes (H, P)
Pyrazinamide	10 mg/kg/q8h (PO)	Yes	39	—	10	Yes	Yes	Yes (H)
Rifampin	10 mg/kg/d (PO)	Yes	7	70	3	Yes	Minor	No (H)
First-Generation Cephalosporins								
Cefadroxil	15 mg/kg/q12h (PO)	Yes	16	20	1.2	No	Yes	Yes (H)
Cefazolin	15 mg/kg/q8	—	80	80	2	No	Major	Yes (H) No (P)
Cephalexin	7 mg/kg/q6	Yes	18	15	1	No	Yes	Yes (H, P)
Cephalothin	30 mg/kg/q6	—	65	70	0.7	Minor	Yes	Yes (H, P)
Cephapirin	30 mg/kg/q6h	—	150	50	0.6	No	Yes	Yes (H, P)
Cephradine	30 mg/kg/q6h	Yes†	140	10	0.7	No	Yes	Yes (H, P)
Second-Generation Cephalosporins								
Cefaclor	7 mg/kg/q6 (PO)	Yes†	13	20	1	No	Yes	Yes (H)
Cefamandole	30 mg/kg/q6	—	150	70	1	No	Yes	Yes (H) No (P)
Cefmetazole	30 mg/kg/q12h	—	140	65	1.1	No	Yes	Yes (H)
Cefotetan	30 mg/kg/q12	—	230	85	3	No	Major	Yes (H)
Cefoxitin	30 mg/kg/q6	—	150	70	0.7	No	Yes	Yes (H) No (P)
Cefprozil	15 mg/kg/q12h (PO)	Yes	10	42	1.2	No	Yes	Yes (H)
Cefuroxime	15–20 mg/kg/q12h	—	100	50	1.5	No	Yes	Yes (H, P)
Cefuroxime axetil	7.5 mg/kg/q12h (PO)	Yes	9	50	1.2	No	Yes	Yes (H, P)
Third-Generation Cephalosporins								
Cefepime	30 mg/kg/q12h	—	193	20	2.1	No	Yes	Yes (H, P)
Cefixime	8 mg/kg/d (PO)	Yes	3.9	67	3.7	No	Yes	No (H, P)
Cefoperazone	30 mg/kg/q8–12	—	250	90	2	Some	No	Yes (H)
Cefotaxime	30 mg/kg/q6	—	130	50	1.2	Some	Minor	Yes (H) No (P)
Cefpodoxime proxetil	3–6 mg/kg/q12h (PO)	Yes	3.9	25	2.5	No	Yes	Yes (H)
Ceftazidime	30 mg/kg/q8	—	160	60	2	No	Major	Yes (H, P)
Ceftizoxime	30 mg/kg/q6–8	—	130	50	1.3	No	Minor	Yes (H) No (P)
Ceftriaxone	30 mg/kg/q12–24	—	250	90	8	No	No	No (H)
Penicillins								
Amoxicillin	7 mg/kg/q6 (PO)	Yes	6	20	1	No	Yes	Yes (H) No (P)
Ampicillin	30 mg/kg/q6	Yes†	100	20	1	No	Yes	Yes (H) No (P)
Azlocillin	50 mg/kg/q6	—	220	50	1	Minor	Major	Yes (H) No (P)
Carbenicillin	70 mg/kg/q4	—	300	50	1	Minor	Major	Yes (H, P)
Cloxacillin	7 mg/kg/q6 (PO)	Yes†	9	95	0.5	No	No	No (H, P)
Dicloxacillin	7 mg/kg/q6 (PO)	Yes†	18	97	0.5	No	No	No (H, P)
Methicillin	30 mg/kg/q4–6	—	100	30	0.5	No	Minor	No (H, P)
Mezlocillin	50 mg/kg/q6	—	260	50	1	Yes	Major	Yes (H) No (P)
Nafcillin	30 mg/kg/q4–6	—	160	90	0.5	Yes	No	No (H, P)
Oxacillin	30 mg/kg/q4–6	—	200	90	0.5	Yes	No	Yes (H, P)
Penicillin G	3–4 million U q4–6	Yes†	60	60	0.5	No	Yes	Yes (H) No (P)
Penicillin V	7 mg/kg/q6 (PO)	Yes	4	80	1	No	No	Yes (H) No (P)
Piperacillin	40 mg/kg/q6	—	240	50	1	Minor	Major	Yes (H)
Ticarcillin	40 mg/kg/q4–6	—	220	50	1	Minor	Major	Yes (H, P)
Quinolones								
Ciprofloxacin	7 mg/kg/q12 (PO)	Yes†	2–2.8	30	3		Yes	No (H, P)
Lomefloxacin	6 mg/kg/q24h	Yes	4	10	8		Yes	No (H, P)
Norfloxacin	6 mg/kg/q12 (PO)	Yes†	1.4–1.8	15	3	No	Yes	No (H, P)
Ofloxacin	6 mg/kg/q12h	Yes†	3–5	30	7		Yes	No (H, P)
Tetracyclines								
Doxycycline	1.5 mg/kg/q12–24	Yes	1.8–2.9	90	15–20	Avoid	No	No (H, P)
Minocycline	1.5 mg/kg/q12–24	Yes	2.2	90	15	No	Avoid	No (H, P)
Tetracycline	7 mg/kg/q6	Yes†	4	50	7	Avoid	Avoid	No (H, P)
Sulfonamides								
Sulfadiazine	15 mg/kg/q6	Yes	30	50	3	Avoid	Avoid	Unknown
Sulfamethoxazole	12 mg/kg/q8 (IV)	Yes	100	50	6	Avoid	Major	Yes (H) No (P)
Trimethoprim (used with sulfamethoxazole)	2.3 mg/kg/q8–12 (IV)	Yes	3–9	60	10	No	Avoid	Yes (H) No (P)
Sulfisoxazole	15 mg/kg/q6	Yes	60	50	6	Avoid	Major	Yes (H, P)
Macrolides-Lincosamides								
Azithromycin	4 mg/kg/q24h (PO)	Yes†	0.4	50	57 (tissue)	Unknown	Unknown	Unknown
Clarithromycin	7.5 mg/kg/q12h (PO)	Yes	2–3	70	7	No	Yes	Yes (H) No (P)
Clindamycin	7 mg/kg/q6	Yes	15	90	2.5	Some	No	No (H, P)
Erythromycin	7 mg/kg/q6 (PO)	Yes†	1.8	20	1.5	Some	No	No (H, P)
Other Agents								
Aztreonam	30 mg/kg/q8	—	250	60	2.0	No	Major	Yes (H, P)
Chloramphenicol	7–15 mg/kg/q6 (PO)	Yes	8–14	30	1.5	Some	No	Yes (H) No (P)
Imipenem	7.5 mg/kg/q6	—	40	15	1	No	Avoid	Yes (H)
Loracarbef	15 mg/kg/q12h (PO)	Yes†	18	25	1.2	No	Yes	Yes (H)
Meropenem	15 mg/kg/q8h	—	40		1.0	Unknown	Yes	Yes (H)
Metronidazole	7 mg/kg/q6	Yes	25	20	8	Yes	No	Yes (H) No (P)
Nitrofurantoin	1 mg/kg/q6 (PO)	Yes	nil	60	0.3	No	Avoid	Yes (H)
Spectinomycin	30 mg/kg/d	—	100	0	2	No	Avoid	Unknown
Vancomycin	15 mg/kg/q12h	Yes§	35	10	6	No	Major	No (H, P)

* mg/kg body weight at hour interval in patients with normal renal function; all doses are parenteral unless specified PO.
† Do not administer with food—absorption is decreased or delayed.
‡ H = hemodialysis; P = peritoneal dialysis.
§ Orally administered vancomycin is not absorbed; gastrointestinal tract lumen therapy only.

with other drugs that the patient is receiving is yet another important consideration that affects the selection of antimicrobial therapy (Table 270–4).

SPECIFIC ANTIMICROBIAL AGENTS

Although oversimplifying the process of selecting appropriate therapy, Table 270–5 lists the agents of choice and some of the alternative agents recommended for the treatment of infections caused by specific bacteria. Penicillin G remains the agent of choice for treatment of all stages of syphilis. Table 270–6 details the relative antibacterial activity of specific antimicrobics against organisms that commonly cause infections. Because gram-negative bacilli commonly acquire resistance genes, antimicrobial susceptibility testing is required when treating serious infection caused by these organisms.

BROAD-SPECTRUM PENICILLINS AND RELATED COMPOUNDS. Selected side chains added to the β-lactam ring of the penicillin nucleus result in broad-spectrum penicillins that, while still inactivated by staphylococcal β-lactamase, possess enhanced activity against gram-negative bacilli. The aminopenicillins—ampi-

TABLE 270–4. IMPORTANT ANTIBIOTIC-DRUG INTERACTIONS*

Antimicrobial Agent	Interacting Drug	Effect
Aminoglycosides	Amphotericin B, cyclosporin A, vancomycin	Increased nephrotoxicity
	Loop diuretics (bumetanide, furosemide, ethacrynic acid)	Increased ototoxicity (avoid)
	Carboxy/ureidopenicillins	Decreased aminoglycoside activity (renal failure only)
Cephalosporins		
MTT side chain	Warfarin, dicumarol	Increased anticoagulation, bleeding
MTT side chain	Alcohol	Disulfiram-like reaction
All	Loop diuretics	Nephrotoxicity
Chloramphenicol	Warfarin	Increased warfarin activity, increased anticoagulation
	Phenytoin	Increased serum phenytoin, phenytoin toxicity
	Sulfonylureas	Increased sulfonylurea, hypoglycemia
Clarithromycin,† erythromycin	Carbamazepine	Increased serum carbamazepine (avoid)
	Cyclosporin A	Increased serum cyclosporin A, nephrotoxicity
	Digoxin	Increased serum digoxin, toxicity
	Terfenadine, astemizole, loratadine	Increased antihistamine level, arrhythmia (avoid)
	Theophylline	Increased theophylline level, toxicity
Isoniazid	Warfarin	Increased warfarin activity, increased anticoagulation
	Alfentanil	Prolonged alfentanil activity
	Phenytoin	Increased serum phenytoin, phenytoin toxicity
	Disulfiram	Psychosis, behavioral change (avoid)
	Carbamazepine	Increased carbamazepine, toxicity (avoid)
	Rifampin	Additive hepatotoxicity
Metronidazole	Alcohol	Disulfiram-like reaction
	Disulfiram	Psychosis (avoid)
	Warfarin, dicumarol	Increased anticoagulation
	Phenobarbital	Decreased metronidazole
Penicillins		
Ampicillin/amoxicillin	Allopurinol	Increased rash
Ampicillin/carboxy-, ureidopenicillins	Oral contraceptives	Decreased contraceptive effect
	Probenecid	Increased serum penicillins
Fluoroquinolones		
All	Cimetidine	Increased antibiotic concentration
	Cyclosporin A	Increased serum cyclosporin A, nephrotoxicity
	Multivalent cations (Ca, Mg, Fe, Zn, Al orally)	Decreased absorption of quinolones
	Sucralfate	Decreased absorption of quinolones
	Warfarin	Increased anticoagulation
	Probenecid	Increased fluoroquinolone
Ciprofloxacin, enoxacin	Theophylline	Increased serum theophylline, toxicity
Norfloxacin, pefloxacin	Caffeine	Increased serum caffeine, insomnia, restlessness
Enoxacin	Fenbufen	Seizures
Rifampin‡	Corticosteroids	Decreased corticosteroid, supplement dose
	Cyclosporin A	Decreased cyclosporin A
	Methadone	Decreased serum methadone, withdrawal
	Phenytoin	Decreased serum phenytoin
	Warfarin, dicumarol	Decreased anticoagulation, need large doses
	Oral contraceptives	Decreased contraceptive effect
	Sulfonylureas	Decreased sulfonylurea, hyperglycemia
	Theophylline	Decreased serum theophylline
	Quinidine, β-blocker	Decreased quinidine, β-blocker
Rifabutin	Clarithromycin	Uveitis
Sulfonamides	Cyclosporin A	Decreased serum cyclosporin A
	Phenytoin	Increased serum phenytoin, toxicity
	Warfarin	Increased warfarin effect
	Sulfonylureas	Increased sulfonylurea, hypoglycemia
Trimethoprim	Azathioprine	Increased leukopenia
	Dapsone	Increased serum dapsone and trimethoprim, increased methemoglobinemia
Tetracycline	Multivalent cations (Ca, Al, Mg, Bi, Zn, Fe)	Decreased tetracycline absorption
	Barbiturates, carbamazepine	Decreased doxycycline
	Digoxin	Increased digoxin, toxicity
	Phenytoin	Decreased doxycycline
	Methoxyflurane (Penthrane)	Severe nephrotoxicity (avoid)

* Not all interactions have been listed.
† Interactions with azithromycin not adequately studied.
‡ Multiple other rifampin interactions mediated through cytochrome system.
MTT = methylthiotetrazole ring (cefamandole, cefotetan, cefmetazole, cefoperazone, moxalactam, cefmenoxime).

✔ **TABLE 270–5. ANTIBACTERIAL DRUGS OF CHOICE FOR INFECTIONS CAUSED BY SELECTED BACTERIA**

Infecting Organism	Agent of Choice*	Alternative Agent†
Gram-Positive Cocci		
S. aureus/coagulase-negative staphylococci		
Nonpenicillinase producing	Penicillin G or V	Cephalosporin§, vancomycin, clindamycin, erythromycin
Penicillinase producing	Nafcillin, oxacillin	Cephalosporin§, vancomycin, clindamycin, erythromycin, imipenem, β-lactam/β-lactamase inhibitor combinations
Methicillin resistant‡	Vancomycin	Trimethoprim-sulfamethoxazole, minocycline, teicoplanin (investigational)
β-hemolytic streptococci (groups A, B, C, G)	Penicillin G or V	Cephalosporin§, erythromycin, vancomycin, clindamycin
Viridans streptococci, *Streptococcus bovis*	Penicillin G	Cephalosporin§, vancomycin, erythromycin
Enterococci‡		
Uncomplicated urinary tract infection	Ampicillin, amoxicillin	Nitrofurantoin, quinolone¶
Moderately severe wound infection	Ampicillin	Penicillin G, vancomycin
Serious infection: Endocarditis or meningitis	Ampicillin plus gentamicin or streptomycin	Vancomycin plus gentamicin or streptomycin (test for high-level aminoglycoside resistance)
Streptococcus pneumoniae‡		
Pneumonia, upper respiratory tract infection	Penicillin G, amoxicillin	Cephalosporin, erythromycin, clindamycin, vancomycin
Meningitis	Ceftriaxone, cefotaxime	Ceftriaxone plus vancomycin ± rifampin, vancomycin + rifampin, penicillin G (if MIC < 0.1 μg/ml)
Gram-Negative Cocci		
N. gonorrhoeae	Ceftriaxone, cefixime	Second- or other third-generation cephalosporins**, quinolones¶, spectinomycin, trimethoprim-sulfamethoxazole, azithromycin (choices vary by sites of infection)
N. meningitidis	Penicillin G	Third-generation cephalosporin**, chloramphenicol, sulfonamide (if susceptible)
Moraxella catarrhalis	Trimethoprim-sulfamethoxazole	Amoxicillin/clavulanate, third-generation cephalosporin**, cefuroxime, clarithromycin
Gram-Positive Bacilli		
Bacillus anthracis (anthrax)	Penicillin G	Erythromycin, tetracycline
Corynebacterium diphtheriae	Erythromycin	Penicillin G
Corynebacterium species	Penicillin + gentamicin	Vancomycin
Listeria monocytogenes	Ampicillin or penicillin G ± gentamicin	Trimethoprim-sulfamethoxazole, vancomycin, tetracycline
Clostridium perfringens	Penicillin G	Metronidazole, chloramphenicol, imipenem, tetracycline
Clostridium difficile	Metronidazole	Vancomycin (oral only), bacitracin
Gram-Negative Bacilli‡		
Acinetobacter species	Imipenem ± gentamicin	Ureidopenicillin; aminoglycoside
Bordetella pertussis (pertussis)	Erythromycin	Trimethoprim-sulfamethoxazole, ampicillin
Brucella species (brucellosis)	Tetracycline + gentamicin or streptomycin	Tetracycline + rifampin, chloramphenicol ± streptomycin, trimethoprim-sulfamethoxazole
Campylobacter fetus spp. *jejuni*	Erythromycin, quinolone¶	Tetracycline
Enterobacter species	Imipenem, aminoglycoside††	Quinolone¶, third-generation cephalosporin**, cefepime, trimethoprim-sulfamethoxazole
Eikenella corrodens	Penicillin G, ampicillin	Trimethoprim-sulfamethoxazole, tetracycline, cefoxitin, third-generation cephalosporin**
E. coli		
Uncomplicated urinary tract infection	Trimethoprim-sulfamethoxazole	Ampicillin, cephalosporin§, trimethoprim, quinolone¶, tetracycline
Systemic infection	Third-generation cephalosporin**	Aminoglycoside††, β-lactam/β-lactamase inhibitor, aztreonam, trimethoprim-sulfamethoxazole

cillin and amoxicillin—have expanded the penicillin spectrum to include many of the gram-negative bacilli. However, subsequent acquisition of β-lactamase genes by many of these species, except *P. mirabilis,* has limited the use of aminopenicillins. Notably, 25% of *E. coli* and at least 15% of *H. influenzae* are resistant to these agents. Bacteria that are susceptible to penicillin G remain susceptible to ampicillin and amoxicillin. Although the *in vitro* antibacterial spectra of amoxicillin and ampicillin are equivalent, amoxicillin is more fully absorbed from the gastrointestinal tract than ampicillin. Amoxicillin is the recommended antimicrobic for prophylaxis against endocarditis at the time of dental procedures. Aminopenicillins are effective therapy for early Lyme disease (*Borrelia burgdorferi* infection) as are doxycycline, cefuroxime axetil, clarithromycin, and azithromycin.

The carboxypenicillins—carbenicillin and ticarcillin—and the ureidopenicillins—azlocillin, mezlocillin, and piperacillin—comprise the remaining broad-spectrum penicillins available in the United States. Carbenicillin and ticarcillin extended the antibacterial spectrum of penicillins to include indole-positive *Proteus* species, some *Enterobacter* species, *Acinetobacter,* and importantly *Pseudomonas aeruginosa.* The spectra of antibacterial activity of carbenicillin and ticarcillin are similar; however, the potency of ticarcillin against *P. aeruginosa* is twice that of carbenicillin. Mezlocillin and piperacillin are more active against the Enterobacteriaceae than are carbenicillin, ticarcillin, and azlocillin. While the

activity of mezlocillin against *P. aeruginosa* is similar to that of ticarcillin, piperacillin and azlocillin are more potent antipseudomonas agents than either ticarcillin or mezlocillin. The carboxypenicillins and ureidopenicillins are important agents for treating serious gram-negative infection; however, in this setting they are combined with an aminoglycoside because of their inactivation by various β-lactamases and the potential emergence of resistance.

To further expand their antimicrobial activity, agents from each group of broad-spectrum penicillins have been combined with a β-lactamase inhibitor. The β-lactamase inhibitors, which exert only weak antibacterial activity themselves, irreversibly bind and inhibit staphylococcal β-lactamase, many plasmid-mediated β-lactamases of gram-negative bacilli, the ESBL's, and the chromosomal β-lactamases of *Klebsiella* spp. and *Bacteroides* spp. Unfortunately, they do not inhibit the Bush class I chromosomal β-lactamases of *Enterobacter* spp., *Serratia,* and *P. aeruginosa.* Among the penicillin/β-lactamase inhibitor combinations, ampicillin-sulbactam, ticarcillin-clavulanate, and piperacillin-tazobactam are available for parenteral use, and amoxicillin-clavulanate is available for oral administration.

CEPHALOSPORINS. The cephalosporins contain a nucleus in which the β-lactam ring is fused to a six-membered dihydrothiazine ring (in contrast to the five-membered thiazolidine ring in the analogous position in penicillins). Substituent side chains are added to the β-lactam ring to alter antimicrobial activity and to the dihydrothiazine ring to alter metabolic and pharmacokinetic properties.

✔ **TABLE 270–5. ANTIBACTERIAL DRUGS OF CHOICE FOR INFECTIONS CAUSED BY SELECTED BACTERIA** Continued

Infecting Organism	Agent of Choice*	Alternative Agent†
Helicobacter pylori	Tetracycline + metronidazole + bismuth subsalicylate	Amoxicillin + metronidazole + bismuth subsalicylate, tetracycline + clarithromycin + bismuth subsalicylate
Francisella tularensis (tularemia)	Streptomycin, gentamicin	Tetracycline, chloramphenicol
H. influenzae		
Meningitis, bacteremia	Ceftriaxone, cefotaxime	Trimethoprim-sulfamethoxazole, ampicillin (if β-lactamase negative)
Other infection	Ampicillin/clavulanate, amoxicillin/clavulanate	Trimethoprim-sulfamethoxazole, cefuroxime, quinolone,¶ third-generation cephalosporin**
Haemophilus ducreyi (chancroid)	Ceftriaxone	Azithromycin, erythromycin, amoxicillin/clavulanate, quinolone¶
Klebsiella pneumoniae/oxytoca	Aminoglycosides††, third-generation cephalosporin**	First- or second-generation cephalosporin, quinolone¶, ureidopenicillin, imipenem, aztreonam, β-lactam/β-lactamase inhibitor
Legionella pneumophila	Erythromycin ± rifampin	Quinolone¶ ± rifampin
Nocardia asteroides	Sulfonamides (high dose)	Trimethoprim-sulfamethoxazole, minocycline, amoxicillin/clavulanate
Pasteurella multocida	Penicillin G	Tetracycline, amoxicillin/clavulanate, third-generation cephalosporin**
Proteus mirabilis	Ampicillin	Cephalosporin†, trimethoprim-sulfamethoxazole, aminoglycoside††
Proteus (indole positive)	Third-generation cephalosporin	Imipenem, aminoglycoside††, trimethoprim-sulfamethoxazole, quinolone¶
Rochalimaea (Bartonella) henselae/quintana	Erythromycin	Tetracycline, clarithromycin
Salmonella spp.	Ceftriaxone, quinolone¶	Chloramphenicol, trimethoprim-sulfamethoxazole
Serratia marcescens	Aminoglycoside††, third-generation cephalosporin**	Imipenem, quinolone,¶ aztreonam
Shigella spp.	Quinolone¶, norfloxacin	Trimethoprim-sulfamethoxazole, ceftriaxone, chloramphenicol
Pseudomonas aeruginosa		
Urinary tract infection	Quinolone¶, ureidopenicillin	Aminoglycoside††, ceftazidime, imipenem, aztreonam
Pneumonia, bacteremia	Aminoglycoside†† + ureidopenicillin or ceftazidime	Imipenem + aminoglycoside††, aztreonam + aminoglycoside††
Vibrio vulnificus	Tetracycline + ceftazidime	Chloramphenicol
Xanthomonas multiphilia	Trimethoprim-sulfamethoxazole	Ticarcillin/clavulanate, quinolone¶
Yersinia pestis (plague)	Streptomycin, gentamicin	Tetracycline, chloramphenicol
Anaerobic Gram-Negative		
Bacteroides spp.		
Oropharyngeal isolates	Penicillin G	Metronidazole, clindamycin, cefoxitin, cefotetan, cefmetazole, chloramphenicol, β-lactam/β-lactamase inhibitor
Bacteroides fragilis group	Metronidazole	Cefoxitin, cefotetan, clindamycin, imipenem, β-lactam/β-lactamase inhibitor, chloramphenicol

* Dose and route of administration must be adjusted for severity of illness and host characteristics (organ dysfunction, allergy).
† List of alternative agents is not fully inclusive; confirm susceptibility *in vitro*.
‡ Must test susceptibility; resistant strains are increasingly frequent.
§ First-generation cephalosporin preferred (cephalothin, cephapirin, cephradine, cephalexin, cefazolin).
¶ Ciprofloxacin, lomefloxacin, ofloxacin (or for urinary tract infection, norfloxacin).
** Third-generation cephalosporins for this indication include ceftriaxone, cefotaxime, ceftizoxime.
†† Aminoglycosides for this indication include gentamicin, tobramycin, netilmicin, amikacin.

A widely accepted system classifies the cephalosporins into "three generations" on the basis of their spectrum of microbiologic activity. With each successive generation, cephalosporins have increasing antibacterial activity against gram-negative bacilli, and to a degree, decreasing activity against gram-positive bacteria. For treatment of serious *S. aureus* infections in patients intolerant of antistaphylococcal penicillins, first-generation cephalosporins are preferred. The cephamycins (cefoxitin, cefotetan, and cefmetazole) are grouped with the second-generation cephalosporins and are active against many gram-negative anaerobic bacteria, including many *B. fragilis*. All cephalosporins are inactive against enterococci, methicillin-resistant staphylococci, and *L. monocytogenes*. Only ceftazidime and cefepime possess significant antipseudomonal activity, and only cefepime is active against *Enterobacter* spp. and related organisms that have been induced to produce Bush I chromosomal β-lactamases. ESBL production by *Klebsiella* spp. renders these organisms resistant to third-generation cephalosporins. Among the cephalosporins, only the third-generation agents retain clinically relevant activity against *S. pneumoniae* that are resistant to penicillin. Some strains of pneumococci have become resistant to third-generation cephalosporins. Cefazolin, the "workhorse" first-generation cephalosporin, is widely used for perioperative prophylaxis in surgical procedures involving foreign body implantation and for many clean and clean-contaminated operations, except those involving the colon. Cefotaxime, ceftriaxone, and ceftizoxime are the agents of choice for treatment of meningitis due to enteric gram-negative bacilli (except *Enterobacter* spp.) and are used widely in initial empiric therapy for meningitis in children (after the neonate period) and adults. Ceftazidime is the agent of choice for meningitis caused by *P. aeruginosa*. Ceftriaxone is the drug of choice for treatment of late stages of Lyme disease.

Adverse reactions caused by the cephalosporins are independent of their antibacterial spectra. Hypersensitivity cross-reactions between cephalosporins are not universal; nevertheless, they occur more frequently than penicillin-cephalosporin cross-reactions. There are no skin test reagents that predict cephalosporin hypersensitivity, and testing with the drug in question is not recommended. Whereas aztreonam can be administered to most patients with hypersensitivity to penicillins and cephalosporins, use of imipenem may result in cross-reactions. A methylthiotetrazole moiety on the dihydrothiazine ring (cefamandole, cefoperazone, cefotetan, moxalactam, cefmenoxime, and cefmetazole) is associated with unique reactions (Table 270–7).

COMBINATION ANTIMICROBIAL THERAPY

There are several rationales for administering antibiotics in combination: (1) A broader, more comprehensive antibacterial effect when treating a severe infection of unknown cause may be achieved; (2) the bacteria causing mixed infection may exceed the antibacterial range of a single agent; (3) combination therapy may

TABLE 270–6. ACTIVITY OF MAJOR ANTIBIOTICS AGAINST SELECTED ORGANISMS*

	Streptococci	Streptococcus pneumoniae†	Enterococci‡	Staphylococcus aureus (MS)	Staphylococcus aureus (MR)	Coagulase-negative staphylococci§	Listeria monocytogenes	Neisseria gonorrhoeae	Neisseria meningitidis	Moraxella catarrhalis	Haemophilus influenzae	Escherichia coli	Enterobacter spp.	Klebsiella spp.	Proteus mirabilis	Proteus vulgaris	Salmonella spp.	Serratia spp.	Shigella spp.	Acinetobacter spp.	Pseudomonas aeruginosa	Xanthomonas maltophilia	Pasteurella multocida	Vibrio vulnificus	Legionella spp.	Chlamydia spp.	Mycoplasma pneumoniae	Rickettsia spp.	Bacteroides fragilis group#	Clostridium spp. (not C. difficile)	Prevotella melaninogenicus	Actinomyces spp.
Penicillin G	+	+	+	0	0	0	+	±	+	0	0	0	0	0	±	0	0	0	0	0	0	0	+	±	0	0	0	0	0	+	+	+
Oxacillin[1]	+	±	0	+	0	±	0	0	0	0	0	0	0	0	0	0	0	0	0	0	0	0	0	+	0	0	0	0	0	0	0	0
Ampicillin[2]	+	+	+	0	0	0	+	±	+	0	±	±	0	0	+	0	+	0	±	0	0	0	+	+	0	0	0	0	0	+	+	+
Ampicillin-sulbactam[2]	+	+	+	+	0	±	+	±	+	+	+	+	±	+	+	+	+	0	±	0	0	0	+	+	0	0	0	0	+	+	+	+
Ticarcillin	+	+	+	0	0	±	0	+	+	0	±	±	±	0	+	+	+	+	+	+	+	±	+	+	0	0	0	0	0	+	+	+
Ticarcillin-clavulanate	+	+	+	+	0	±	0	+	+	+	+	+	±	+	+	+	+	+	+	+	+	±	+	ND	0	0	0	0	+	+	+	+
Piperacillin	+	+	+	0	0	±	+	+	+	0	±	+	±	±	+	+	+	±	+	+	+	±	+	+	0	0	0	0	±	+	+	+
Piperacillin-tazobactam	+	+	+	+	0	±	+	+	+	+	+	+	±	+	+	+	+	±	+	+	+	±	+	+	0	0	0	0	+	+	+	+
Aztreonam	0	0	0	0	0	0	0	+	+	+	+	+	+	+	+	+	+	+	+	0	+	0	0	ND	0	0	0	0	0	0	0	0
Imipenem	+	+	±	+	0	±	+	±	+	+	+	+	+	+	+	+	+	+	+	+	+	0	+	ND	ND	0	0	0	+	+	+	+
Cefazolin[3]	+	+	0	+	0	±	0	+	+	+	±	+	0	+	+	0	+	0	+	0	0	0	0	0	0	0	0	0	0	+	+	+
Cefotetan[4]	+	+	0	±	0	±	0	+	+	+	+	+	±	+	+	+	+	+	+	0	0	0	0	+	0	0	0	0	±	0	+	+
Cefoxitin	+	+	0	+	0	±	0	+	+	+	±	+	0	+	+	+	+	0	+	0	0	0	0	0	0	0	0	0	+	+	+	+
Cefuroxime	+	+	0	+	0	±	0	+	+	+	+	+	±	+	+	+	+	+	+	0	0	0	+	+	0	0	0	0	0	+	+	+
Cefotaxime	+	+	0	+	0	±	0	+	+	+	+	+	±	+	+	+	+	+	+	±	0	0	+	+	0	0	0	0	±	+	+	+
Ceftriaxone	+	+	0	+	0	±	0	+	+	+	+	+	±	+	+	+	+	+	+	±	0	0	+	+	0	0	0	0	0	+	+	+
Ceftazidime	+	+	0	±	0	±	0	+	+	+	+	+	±	+	+	+	+	+	+	±	+	±	+	+	0	0	0	0	±	+	+	+
Cefepime	+	+	0	+	0	±	0	+	+	+	+	+	+	+	+	+	+	+	+	+	+	0	ND	ND	0	0	0	0	0	ND	ND	ND
Cephalexin[3]	+	+	0	+	0	±	0	0	+	±	±	+	0	+	+	0	+	0	+	0	0	0	0	ND	0	0	0	0	0	ND	ND	+
Cefuroxime axetil	+	+	0	+	0	±	0	+	+	+	+	+	0	+	+	0	+	0	+	0	0	0	+	ND	0	0	0	0	0	+	+	+
Loracarbef	+	+	0	+	±	±	0	+	+	+	+	+	±	+	+	+	+	0	ND	0	0	0	ND	ND	0	0	0	0	0	ND	+	ND
Cefixime	+	+	0	0	0	0	0	+	+	+	+	+	0	+	+	+	+	0	+	0	0	0	+	ND	0	0	0	0	0	0	+	+
Cefpodoxime proxetil	+	+	0	+	0	±	0	+	+	+	+	+	0	+	+	±	+	0	+	0	0	0	0	ND	0	0	0	0	0	ND	ND	ND
Gentamicin[5]	C/S	0	C/S	C/S	±	C/S	C/S	0	0	+	+	+	+	+	+	+	0	+	+	+	+	0	0	0	0	0	0	0	0	0	0	0
Clindamycin	+	+	0	+	±	±	±	0	0	+	0	0	0	0	0	0	0	0	0	0	0	0	0	0	0	0	0	0	±	+	+	+
Clarithromycin[6]	+	+	0	±	0	±	ND	+	+	+	+	0	0	0	0	0	0	0	0	0	0	0	0	±	+	+	+	ND	0	±	+	+
Erythromycin	+	+	±	±	0	±	±	+	+	+	+	0	0	0	0	0	0	0	0	0	0	0	0	0	+	+	+	±	0	+	+	+
Doxycycline[7]	±	±	±	±	±	±	±	+	+	+	+	±	±	±	0	0	0	+	+	±	0	0	+	+	+	+	+	+	0	±	+	±
Vancomycin	+	+	±	+	+	+	+	0	0	ND	ND	0	0	0	0	0	0	0	0	0	0	0	0	±	0	0	0	0	0	+	0	0
Ciprofloxacin	±	±	±	±	0	±	±	+	+	+	+	+	+	+	+	+	+	+	+	±	+	0	0	0	+	+	0	+	0	0	0	ND
Ofloxacin	±	+	±	±	0	±	±	+	+	+	+	+	+	+	+	+	+	+	+	±	±	0	0	±	+	+	+	ND	0	0	0	ND

TABLE 270–6. ACTIVITY OF MAJOR ANTIBIOTICS AGAINST SELECTED ORGANISMS* *Continued*

	Streptococci	Streptococcus pneumoniae†	Enterococci‡	Staphylococcus aureus (MS)	Staphylococcus aureus (MR)	Coagulase-negative staphylococciø	Listeria monocytogenes	Neisseria gonorrhoeae	Neisseria meningitidis	Moraxella catarrhalis	Haemophilus influenzae	Escherichia coli	Enterobacter spp.	Klebsiella spp.	Proteus mirabilis	Proteus vulgaris	Salmonella spp.	Serratia spp.	Shigella spp.	Acinetobacter spp.	Pseudomonas aeruginosa	Xanthomonas maltophilia	Pasteurella multocida	Vibrio vulnificus	Legionella spp.	Chlamydia spp.	Mycoplasma pneumoniae	Rickettsia spp.	Bacteroides fragilis group#	Clostridium spp. (not C. difficile)	Prevotella melaninogenicus	Actinomyces spp.
Metronidazole	+	0	0	0	0	0	+	0	±	0	0	0	0	0	0	0	0	0	0	0	0	0	0	0	0	0	0	0	+	+	+	0
Trimethoprim-sulfamethoxazole	+	+	0	+	±	±	+	±	+	+	+	+	±	+	+	0	+	+	+	0	0	+	±	+	+	0	0	0	ND	ND	ND	ND
Chloramphenicol	+	+	0	±	0	C/S	±	+	+	+	+	ND	0	±	ND	±	+	0	0	0	0	ND	+	+	ND	+	+	+	+	+	+	+
Rifampin⁸	ND	C/S	ND	C/S	C/S	C/S	C/S	ND	+	ND	+	ND	0	ND	ND	ND	ND	0	ND	ND	0	ND	ND	ND	C/S	ND	ND	±	ND	ND	ND	ND

* Activity estimate is based on *in vitro* susceptibility and, where available, the results of treatment; activity against individual gram-negative facultative bacilli within a given species is difficult to predict. Discrepancies may exist between *in vitro* antimicrobial activity and clinical efficacy (especially for intracellular pathogens); review of disease-specific therapeutic recommendations is advised.

0 = uniformly or frequently resistant.

+ = usually susceptible.

± = variable susceptibility.

C/S = used in combination or for synergy.

ND = insufficient or no data.

¹ Similar activity for methicillin, nafcillin, cloxacillin, dicloxacillin.

² Similar activity for amoxicillin and amoxicillin/clavulanate, respectively.

³ Similar activity for other first-generation cephalosporins.

⁴ Similar activity for cefmetazole.

⁵ Similar activity against gram-negative bacilli for tobramycin, netilmicin; resistance of gram-negative rods to amikacin less frequent.

⁶ Similar activity for azithromycin.

⁷ Similar activity for other tetracyclines.

⁸ Broad spectrum of activity, but resistance emerges rapidly; limit use to combination therapy or eradication of meningococcal and *H. influenzae* pharyngeal carriage.

† Relative and full resistance to penicillin increasingly prevalent; resistant to first- and second-generation cephalosporins parallels that to penicillin.

‡ *E. faecium* intrinsically more resistant than *E. faecalis*; resistance to penicillin, ampicillin, vancomycin, and aminoglycosides (high level) increasingly frequent.

ø Many nosocomially acquired strains are methicillin resistant.

Some of the *Bacteroides fragilis* group (*B. thetaiotaomicron, B. distasonis, B. ovatus, B. vulgatus*) are more resistant than *B. fragilis*.

1567

TABLE 270–7. UNTOWARD EFFECTS OF ANTIMICROBIAL AGENTS*

Agent	Target—Manifestation						
	General	Skin	GI Tract	Blood Cells	Kidney	Nervous System	Other
Sulfonamides	Hypersensitivity, anaphylaxis, serum sickness; fever	Rash, Stevens-Johnson syndrome, photosensitivity	Hepatitis	Hemolysis (G-6-PD deficiency), agranulocytosis, marrow suppression	Crystalluria	Neuropathy	Vasculitis
Trimethoprim with/without sul-famethoxazole†	Fever	Rash, erythema multiforme, Stevens-Johnson syndrome, TEN‡	Hepatitis, pancreatitis	Marrow suppression	Hyperkalemia, acute renal failure		
Penicillin	Hypersensitivity, anaphylaxis, Jarisch-Herx-heimer reaction (syphilis), serum sickness	Rash, urticaria, erythema multiforme	Diarrhea (ampicillin, amoxicillin/ clavulanate), hepatitis (oxacillin)	Coombs' test positive, impaired platelet function (carbenicillin, ticarcillin), leukopenia, thrombocytopenia	Nephritis (methicillin), hypokalemia, alkalosis (carboxy-, ureidopenicillins)	Seizures, twitching (high doses, renal failure)	Inactivate aminoglycosides when admixed, possible with concurrent ther-apy in renal failure
Cephalosporins	Serum sickness (cefaclor), hypersensitivity, anaphylaxis (rare)	Rash, urticaria	Diarrhea (cefoperazone), hepatic dys-function, pre-cipitates in bile (ceftriaxone), mild increase in LFT‡	Neutropenia, increased pro-thrombin time–bleeding (relates to MTT‡ side chain), impaired platelet function (moxalactam), Coombs' test positive	Enhance amino-glycoside toxicity, acute renal failure (rare), nephritis		Disulfiram-like reaction with concurrent al-cohol use (MTT‡ side chain)
Carbapenems	Hypersensitivity	Rash, urticaria, erythema multiforme	Nausea, vomiting, abnormal LFT‡	Bone marrow suppression, Coombs' test positive	Renal dysfunction	Seizures, myoclonus	
Chloramphenicol	Fever			Marrow suppres-sion (dose related), aplastic anemia		Optic neuritis, neuropathy	Circulatory collapse (gray baby syndrome–neonate)
Tetracyclines	Allergy	Photosensitization (doxycycline, demeclocycline)	Hepatotoxicity in azotemia or pregnancy, GI discomfort		Catabolic aggravation of azotemia (except doxycycline)	Vertigo (minocycline)	Deposition in bone (dysplasia) and teeth (staining)
Erythromycin	Fever	Rash	GI discomfort, nausea, cholestatic jaundice (erythromycin estolate)			Decreased hearing	Phlebitis if given through periph-eral veins
Metronidazole	Headache, allergy		Nausea, metallic taste, pancreatitis	Leukopenia		Peripheral neu-ropathy, ataxia	Mutagenic, carcino-genic in rodents; disulfiram-like reaction with alcohol
Vancomycin	Allergy, fever	Rash		Leukopenia, throm-bocytopenia	Nephrotoxic with aminoglycoside	Decreased hearing (serum > 50 µg/ml), neuropathy	Histamine release with flushing and hypotension (infusion < 1 hr–antihistamines prevent)
Aminoglycosides	Fever	Rash			Renal failure	Irreversible vestibular toxic-ity (streptomy-cin, gentamicin, tobramycin), irre-versible auditory damage (kana-mycin, netilmicin, amikacin), neuro-muscular block-ade (with anes-thetics and myasthenia–calcium reverses)	
Quinolones	Headache, allergy, anaphylaxis (rare)	Rash, photosensi-tization (peflox-acin, fleroxacin), urticaria	GI distress, LFT‡ abnormalities			Dizziness, insomnia, nervousness, tremors, visual changes, seizures, pseudotumor cerebri	Cartilage deposition and arthropathy (animal studies)

* Not all reactions are listed; check other sources for unusual reactions.
† Reactions to sulfonamides are not repeated.
‡ TEN = toxic epidermal necrolysis; MTT = methylthiotetrazole ring; LFT = liver function tests.

decrease the opportunity for the emergence of resistant bacteria; and (4) antibiotics administered concurrently may interact to exert an enhanced (synergistic) or additive antibacterial effect. An im-provement in outcome of infection achieved by the enhanced an-tibacterial effect of combination therapy is seen in ampicillin-gen-tamicin therapy of enterococcal endocarditis, antipseudomonal penicillin-tobramycin therapy of *P. aeruginosa* endocarditis, and the synergistic β-lactam plus aminoglycoside therapy of bacterial infec-tion in the neutropenic patient.

In spite of laudable goals, the end result of the combination ther-apy is not always favorable. Antibiotics administered as combina-tion therapy may interact in antagonistic fashion (the net effect of the combination is less than that of the most effective of the agents acting individually). Antagonism was demonstrated clinically with penicillin and tetracycline treatment of pneumococcal meningitis. Antagonism is difficult to demonstrate clinically, but must remain a concern when antibiotics are used in combination. Additionally, administering multiple antibiotics may increase the risk for adverse events, especially unanticipated drug-drug interactions. Therapy with multiple antibiotics may increase selective pressure, leading to emergence of resistant bacteria or to colonization by fungi. For these reasons it is desirable to use targeted single-antibiotic therapy whenever possible.

DURATION OF THERAPY

There is no easy formula to determine optimal duration of therapy. One must weigh the site of infection, the patient as a host, the pathogen involved and its antimicrobial susceptibility, the response to treatment, the toxicity of the regimen, and the hazards of failure occasioned by terminating therapy prematurely. When the infecting organisms are vegetative, as in the vegetation of endocarditis, more prolonged therapy is required to eradicate the bacteria. Patients with impaired host defenses are treated with longer courses of therapy, assuming that host defenses will play less of a role in terminating infection. Superficial mucosal infection can be cured by single-dose therapy as noted with ceftriaxone, cefixime, or fluoroquinolone treatment of uncomplicated genitourinary gonorrhea. Single-dose therapy was also effective for bacterial cystitis, although 3-day short-course therapy is now preferred. Decisions regarding duration of therapy often are based on published trials and studies in which the goal was not to examine the impact of duration of therapy on outcome but rather to assess a predefined regimen. It is likely that antibiotic therapy is often excessive in length. This is not desirable in that it exacerbates cost of treatment, increases the risks of adverse events, and exerts unnecessary selective pressure on bacteria to become resistant.

ANTIBIOTIC TOXICITY AND UNTOWARD REACTIONS

Antibiotics commonly cause adverse drug reactions (Table 270–7). The majority of adverse events are mild, short lived, and resolve when the offending drug is withdrawn. Increasingly, untoward reactions are the manifestation of interactions between an antimicrobic and another medication that the patient is receiving (see Table 270–4).

FAILURE OF THERAPY

The persistence of fever and other signs of infection during antibiotic therapy calls for careful reassessment of the patient. The physician must reconsider the antimicrobials that have been administered in the light of available microbiologic data and seek new culture data that would explain the failure of therapy. Alternative explanations for fever must be considered; these range from a new superimposed infection, e.g., nosocomial intravenous catheter-related bacteremia, to a noninfectious complication, e.g., a pulmonary embolus, or a drug reaction. If the reassessment suggests that the diagnosis is correct, if the microbiology and clinical sequence of events support the antibiotic therapy given, and if no other explanations are noted, reasons for failure of appropriate therapy must be considered. These include (1) the presence of anatomic abnormalities or an obstructed drainage system; (2) an undrained abscess; (3) the presence of a foreign body or the equivalent (renal calculus, osteomyelitic sequestrum) at the site of infection; (4) infection in infarcted tissue; (5) emergence of resistance in the original pathogen or a resistant superinfecting organism; and (6) suboptimal effect of antibiotic therapy because of atypical disposition of the antibiotic, poor penetration to the site, or inactivation of the antibiotic. The physician must search diligently to explain and correct the antibiotic failure.

Bennett WM, Swan SK: Drug therapy in renal disease (chronic renal failure, appendix A). *In* Rubenstein E (ed.): Scientific American Medicine. New York, Scientific American, 1994, pp. A2–11. *Highly practical guide to dose reduction of antibiotics in renal failure. Updated annually.*

Davies J: Inactivation of antibiotics and the dissemination of resistance genes. Science 264:375, 1994. *Detailed discussion of the major mechanisms whereby bacteria inactivate antibiotics. The original sources of the genes conveying these abilities are considered.*

Mandell GL, Sande MA: Antimicrobial agents: Penicillins, cephalosporins, and other beta-lactam antibiotics. *In* Gilman AG, Rall TW, Nies AS, Taylor P (eds.): The Pharmacologic Basis of Therapeutics. Elmsford, NY, Pergamon Press, 1990, pp. 1065–1097. *Scholarly authoritative review of β-lactam antibiotics. This is best suited for reader seeking fundamental rather than clinical view of this core group of antibiotics.*

Neu HC: Pathophysiologic basis for use of third-generation cephalosporins. Am J Med 88:3S, 1990. *Detailed consideration of sophisticated clinical use of broad-spectrum cephalosporins.*

Neu HC: Quinolone antimicrobial agents. Ann Rev Med 43:465, 1992. *This well-referenced review of this important class of agents addresses chemistry, antibiotic activity, pharmacology, and appropriate clinical use.*

Neu HC: The crisis in antibiotic resistance. Science 257:1064, 1992. *Excellent review of mechanisms and epidemiology of antibiotic resistance, viewed from organism-by-organism perspective.*

Nightingale CH, Quintiliani R, Nicolau DP: Intelligent dosing of antimicrobials. *In* Remington JS, Swartz MN (eds.): Current Clinical Topics in Infectious Diseases. Boston, Blackwell Scientific Publications, 1994, vol. 14, pp. 252–265. *Clinically oriented, detailed discussion of pharmacodynamics and pharmacodynamic strategies for antibiotic dosing at one hospital. An important view of antibiotic dosing that may gain increasing support.*

Nikaido H: Prevention of drug access to bacterial targets: Permeability barriers and active efflux. Science 264:382, 1994. *Detailed consideration of permeability and active efflux mechanisms as used by bacteria in resisting antibiotics. Special attention is directed toward active efflux systems increasingly recognized as important in antibiotic resistance.*

Sande MA, Mandell GL: Antimicrobial agents: The aminoglycosides. *In* Gilman AG, Rall TW, Nies AS, et al. (eds.): The Pharmacologic Basis of Therapeutics. Elmsford, NY, Pergamon Press, 1990, pp. 1098–1116. *Provides a thorough consideration of this important class of antibiotics; other chapters on antibiotics are equally well written.*

Sanford JP, Gilbert DN, Gerberding JL, Sande MA: Guide to Antimicrobial Therapy 1994. Dallas, Antimicrobial Therapy, Inc., 1994. *Pocket guide to antibiotic use.*

Spratt BG: Resistance to antibiotics mediated by target alterations. Science 264:388, 1994. *Readable discussion of antibiotic resistance that results from changes in targets and resulting reductions in the affinity of antibiotics for their sites of action. Major focus is alterations in penicillin-binding proteins.*

271 PNEUMOCOCCAL PNEUMONIA

Richard J. Duma

DEFINITION. Pneumococcal pneumonia is an acute, suppurative infection of the lungs produced by an encapsulated bacterium, *Streptococcus pneumoniae* (pneumococcus). It is the most commonly occurring bacterial pneumonia in the world; in the United States, an estimated 150,000 to 570,000 cases occur annually.

MICROBIOLOGY. Virulent *S. pneumoniae* organisms are encapsulated, gram-positive cocci about 0.8 μm in diameter that occur in chains (streptococci) or pairs (diplococci) (see Color Plate 9E). When in pairs, cocci are characteristically lancet shaped; i.e., each coccus is pointed at the end like the tip of a lance, and the bases are in juxtaposition. The capsule, which is a complex polysaccharide and which varies in chemical composition and thickness, is not seen with Gram stain but may be recognized by negative staining (e.g., with India ink or methylene blue). In purulent clinical specimens, some pneumococci stain negatively rather than positively on the Gram stain, since aging, exposure of the cell wall to a variety of destructive host enzymes (e.g., lysozyme), and/or inhibition of cell wall synthesis by antibiotics (e.g., penicillin) result in incomplete or abnormal bacterial cell walls that no longer retain the iodine-fixed crystal violet stain.

Pneumococci are fastidious, facultative bacteria that grow best in the presence of blood or serum and in air supplemented with 10% carbon dioxide. Since they are fermentative and lactic acid is the usual end-product, concentrations of glucose in the culture media must be controlled and should not exceed 1%. In addition, since they produce hydrogen peroxide (H_2O_2) but not catalase, the addition of a catalase source (e.g., red blood cells) enhances growth. Viability is reduced by drying, a low pH (< 6.5), and prolonged incubation.

On blood agar after overnight incubation at 37°C, colonies generally appear mucoid, glistening, and dome shaped and are surrounded by an area of greening (α-hemolysis) within the blood agar. With continued incubation, as aged bacteria undergo autolysis, the colony domes of highly encapsulated strains collapse centrally and appear umbilicated. An important biologic feature that distinguishes *S. pneumoniae* from other streptococci is its bile solubility or susceptibility to surface-active agents, such as sodium deoxycholate and ethyl hydrocuprein chloride (optochin). The latter agent (optochin) is incorporated into a standardized 5-μg disc and is used worldwide to identify pneumococci rapidly. However, since optochin-resistant pneumococci occur, and since some nonpneumococcal, α-hemolytic streptococci are optochin sensitive, for purposes of species determination, the usefulness of this biologic property may be questioned.

Pneumococcal virulence is often studied in the mouse, since this animal is highly sensitive to encapsulated pneumococci (with the exception of type 14). Indeed, the sensitivity of mice to encapsulated pneumococci may be used for rapidly and selectively isolating virulent pneumococci from sputum specimens or from clinical materials containing other bacteria. If injected into the peritoneal cavity of the mouse, an exudate containing pneumococci may be harvested in 24 hours.

Unlike many other streptococci, particularly those belonging to Lancefield group A, and unlike other pyogenic bacteria that produce pneumonia, *S. pneumoniae* do not produce any major toxins, and particularly none that are tissue destructive. Some strains may elaborate hyaluronidase, and all contain pneumolysin, a hemolytic cytotoxic protein released when the organism undergoes autolysis, which disrupts the respiratory epithelium and slows ciliary movement.

The most important factor defining virulent *S. pneumoniae* is the presence of a high molecular weight complex polysaccharide capsule, which is a potent inhibitor of neutrophil phagocytosis. At least 84 different immunogenic types of capsules exist, and two different nomenclatures (Danish and American) are used to number them (which is often a source of confusion). Antigenically distinct capsules are easily identified with polyvalent antisera in an agglutination or precipitin test or by the Neufeld quellung reaction, a rapid test based on visualization of refractile swelling of the capsule after application of a polyvalent or monovalent type-specific antiserum to the bacterium in question. Nonencapsulated pneumococci, which are generally avirulent, do not react with antipolysaccharide antisera. Although the identification of pneumococcal capsular antigen in certain body fluids or secretions may suggest active pneumococcal infection (see below), immunologic tests to detect such antigens must be interpreted with caution, since antibodies against some pneumococcal capsular serotypes cross-react with polysaccharides of other streptococci (particularly group B), *Haemophilus influenzae* type B, *Escherichia coli*, *Klebsiella pneumoniae*, *Salmonella* species, and even human ABO blood group isoantigens.

Capsular polysaccharides consist of repeating di- or penta-oligosaccharides, some of which contain large proportions of acid constituents such as cellobiuronic, hexuronic, and pyruvic acid. Most are linear, although some are branched, and their antigenicities result principally from oligosaccharide epitopes of no more than six or seven sugar residues. The frequency of capsular types observed varies with time, geography, and the age of the patient; for example, types 6, 14, 18, 19, and 23 are common in infants and children, while types 1, 2, 3, 5, and 8 are common in adults.

The susceptibility of pneumococcus to most chemotherapeutic antibacterials is generally excellent; however, this may be changing. Noteworthy among antipneumococcal drugs are the β-lactams, especially penicillins, cephalosporins, cephamycins, and carbapenems (but *not* monobactams). In addition, erythromycins, lincosines (e.g., clindamycin), vancomycin, chloramphenicol, and teicoplanins are usually effective. For penicillin G, the antibiotic against which all other antipneumococcal agents are compared, *susceptibility* is defined as inhibiting the growth of pneumococci at a concentration of < 0.1 μg per milliliter (referred to as the *minimal inhibitory concentration*, or MIC). Indeed, the MIC of penicillin G worldwide for the majority of pneumococcal strains is predictably ≤ 0.1 μg per milliliter. However, since 1968, when penicillin-resistant strains were first identified in Australia, a significant but variable percent is now intermediately (i.e., the MIC is 0.1 to < 2.0 μg per milliliter) or highly resistant (i.e., the MIC is ≥ 2.0 μg per milliliter). Isolates that are highly resistant are usually resistant to other antibacterials (Table 271–1), although such bacteria are uniformly susceptible to vancomycin and occasionally to third-generation cephalosporins or carbapenems. The resistance of pneumococci to β-lactams is *not*

due to bacterial production of a β-lactamase and is *not* plasmid mediated, but rather it results from chromosomal point mutations that dictate the production of aberrant target membrane penicillin-binding proteins (PBP's); it is the lack of affinity of these PBP's for penicillin G that distinguishes the penicillin-resistant strains from the penicillin-susceptible ones.

Pneumococci are relatively resistant to aminoglycosides; in fact, gentamicin may be incorporated into primary culture media for selective isolation of pneumococci from sputum, since it suppresses the growth of concurrent bacteria. Similarly, quinolones at low or clinically achievable concentrations are generally ineffective in inhibiting the growth of most pneumococci; further, in some studies, > 50% of pneumococcal isolates are resistant to tetracyclines.

EPIDEMIOLOGY. Pneumococcal pneumonia is a sporadic disease that occurs most often during the coldest months of the year. The vast majority of cases occur after aspiration of "normal" oropharyngeal secretions that may contain encapsulated pneumococci, followed by an inability to clear such secretions; thus oropharyngeal carrier rates of pneumococci are important in the dynamics of acquiring pneumococcal pneumonia, its spread, and its frequency of occurrence within a population.

Since most data referable to oropharyngeal carrier rates were obtained prior to the use of pneumococcal vaccine, colonization rates with (or carriage of) certain serotypes and the relative importance of factors that impact on carriage must be interpreted with caution. Nevertheless, in longitudinal, prevaccine studies of pneumococcal oropharyngeal carriage by people living in temperate zones, serotypes with USA numbers of 23 or less are most frequently encountered, further suggesting that humans are infected by their own endogenous flora, since more than half the cases of pneumococcal pneumonia and bacteremia are caused by these strains. Clustering of one serotype within a family commonly occurs, and carriage rates do not appear to be affected by gender. Rates of carriage are higher in children, particularly those of a preschool age, than in adults; and among adults, rates are highest in those intimately exposed to preschool children. Oropharyngeal carriage appears to be highest during the coolest months of the year (fall, winter, and early spring), when respiratory infections are common, and spread may be enhanced during respiratory tract infections due to the pneumococcus or to certain respiratory viruses, such as the rhinovirus. Although the prevalence of oropharyngeal carriage in the surrounding community or within households affects the risk of individual acquisition, crowding does not appear to be important. The duration of oropharyngeal carriage of a particular serotype ranges from

TABLE 271–1. MIC$_{90}$ OF SOME COMMONLY USED BETA-LACTAM ANTIBIOTICS AGAINST PENICILLIN-RESISTANT PNEUMOCOCCI

Antibiotic	MIC$_{90}$ (μg/ml)*	
	Intermediate Penicillin Resistance	*High-Level Penicillin Resistance*
Ampicillin	0.5	8
Oxacillin	4.0	31
Methicillin	—	64
Carbenicillin	32.0	64
Ticarcillin	64.0	128
Piperacillin	1.0	8–16
Mezlocillin	1.0–2.0	8–15
Azlocillin	1.0	16
Cephalothin	1.0	8–31
Cefaclor	4.0–16.0	16
Cefonicid	16.0	16
Cefoxitin	4.0–8.0	32–125
Cefamandole	0.5–2.0	8–31
Cefuroxime	0.25–0.44	—
Cefotaxime	0.125–1.0	1–4
Ceftriaxone	0.12–0.5	1
Ceftazidime	3.2–32.0	64
Cefoperazone	1.0–2.0	2–16
Moxalactam	2.0–4.0	128
Imipenem	0.06–1.0	1–2

* MIC$_{90}$ = Minimal inhibitory concentration at which 90% of strains are susceptible.
Adapted with permission from Klugman KP: Pneumococcal resistance to antibiotics. Clin Microbiol Rev 3:171, 1990.

TABLE 271–2. RISK FACTORS OR UNDERLYING CONDITIONS PREDISPOSING TO THE DEVELOPMENT OF PNEUMOCOCCAL PNEUMONIA OR SERIOUS PNEUMOCOCCAL INFECTIONS

Age (extremes)
Alcoholism
Bone marrow transplantation
Bronchiectasis
Cerebrovascular occlusions or severe neurologic impairment
Chronic bronchitis
Chronic lymphocytic leukemia
Chronic obstructive pulmonary disease (COPD)
Cirrhosis or chronic liver disease
Complement deficiency (particularly C′3)
Conditions associated with aspiration (e.g., seizures)
Congestive heart failure
Dementia
Diabetes mellitus
Immunologic deficiencies (acquired, hereditary, or iatrogenic)—humoral (IgG or IgA) or cellular (e.g., AIDS)
Institutionalization, homelessness, day care centers
Malignancy (particularly solid tumors of the lung)
Multiple myeloma
Nephrotic syndrome
Neutropenia
Smoking
Splenic dysfunction (e.g., in sickle cell disease) or asplenia
Viral diseases, especially influenza

2 weeks to years, the mean being 6 to 8 weeks. Reacquisition of the same serotype commonly occurs. In children, but usually not adults, initial acquisition within a family setting is frequently associated with rises in homotypic serum antibody and occasionally with illness.

Although epidemics of pneumococcal pneumonia may occur, they are *rare* and generally appear in special populations at high risk for pneumococcal disease, such as domiciliary populations of alcoholics, institutionalized elderly, Navajo Indians, New Guinea highlanders, Alaskan natives, and South African gold miners. In studies of ambulatory adult populations, a variety of risk factors appear to predispose to the development of pneumococcal infections (Table 271–2).

IMMUNOLOGY. In nonimmunized, untreated patients, specific anticapsular humoral antibody (immunoglobulin M [IgM] and immunoglobulin G [IgG]) can be detected in the blood 5 to 10 days after infection and correlates with the clearance of pneumococci and eventual recovery. Both classic and alternate pathway complement (C′3) and type-specific, opsonizing antibody, principally IgG (IgG1 in children and IgG2 and IgG4 subclasses in adults), enhance phagocytosis and intracellular killing of pneumococci by polymorphonuclear leukocytes and alveolar macrophages, the major host defense mechanism for eradicating pneumococci. Patients with deficiencies of biologically active IgM, IgG, and, to a lesser degree, IgA (particularly secretory) are more susceptible to developing pneumococcal pneumonia and other pneumococcal infections than are normal persons without such deficiencies. In normal persons, once specific anticapsular antibodies form, they generally persist for life.

If pneumococci escape this host defense mechanism, they may enter the bloodstream via lymph channels and the thoracic duct and produce bacteremia. Clearance from the blood also depends on opsonization via type-specific antibodies and activated complement; however, liver and spleen macrophages are principally responsible for removing pneumococci from the blood rather than polymorphonuclear leukocytes. Thus splenectomy or cirrhosis of the liver rather than neutropenia increases the risk for pneumococcal bacteremia, dissemination, and death.

PATHOGENESIS AND PATHOLOGY. Most cases of pneumococcal pneumonia result from the aspiration of oropharyngeal material containing indigenous, virulent pneumococci into terminal bronchioles and alveoli, followed by atelectasis and the inability to clear bacteria from these sites. Although microaspiration is a natural event that occurs commonly, pneumonia in normal individuals seldom results, because pulmonary bacterial clearance and/or local host defense mechanisms are adequate and intact and are not defec-

tive or suppressed. These important defense mechanisms, which serve as either a barrier against or a clearance for bacteria, are the epiglottic reflex, ciliary escalator and mucous blanket, secretory and humoral immunoglobulins, surfactant, alveolar macrophage and polymorphonuclear leukocyte activity, and lymphatic drainage. When these mechanisms are blunted or overwhelmed by aspirated noxious material, by large inocula of pneumococci, by a highly virulent strain, and/or by material containing additional pathogens, pneumonia may result. In addition, once infection occurs, further atelectasis from inspissated material may result.

After pneumococci establish themselves in the lung, the first visible evidence of an inflammatory response is localized capillary dilatation and hyperemia, the appearance of serous edema within alveoli, followed by margination, diapedesis, and chemotaxis of polymorphonuclear cells induced by immunoglobulins and/or activated complement. Fluid-filled alveoli enhance the passage of bacteria through the pores of Kohn and into terminal bronchioles, with spread to contiguous, uninfected alveoli, forming the advancing margins of the disease. If clearance and host immune mechanisms are adequate at this stage, the infection may resolve. However, if not, the disease may spread until the pleura and interlobar fissures are reached and consolidation with dense infiltrates of polymorphonuclear leukocytes and extravasated red blood cells occurs (see Color Plates 9A to 9C).

Pneumococcal pneumonia may involve an entire lobe (lobar pneumonia), multiple lobes (multilobar pneumonia), or just segments of a lobe, producing a patchy area (or areas) of pneumonia (pneumonitis). At times, infection spreads concentrically from bronchi (bronchopneumonia), a pattern occasionally seen in infants and in the elderly. In the central and oldest portions of infection, consolidation with massive numbers of polymorphonuclear leukocytes predominates, while peripheral to this are new areas of hemorrhage, infiltrating polymorphonuclear cells, and edema. Early pathologists referred to these areas in the lung as "gray hepatization" and "red hepatization," respectively, because of the gross resemblance of involved lung to liver tissue (see Color Plate 9A). In fully developed, untreated pneumococcal pneumonia, all stages of the cellular inflammatory process may be present.

In 5 to 10% of patients, infection may extend into the pleural space, resulting in an *empyema,* or in 15 to 25% of patients, bacteria may enter the bloodstream *(bacteremia)* via the lymphatics and thoracic duct. Invasion of the bloodstream by pneumococci may lead to serious metastatic disease at a number of extrapulmonary sites (Table 271–3), the most important and most frequent of which is the subarachnoid space *(meningitis).* Other infections that may occur from bacteremic spread are *septic arthritis, pericarditis, endocarditis* (infection of the heart valves), and, in patients with ascites, *peritonitis (spontaneous bacterial peritonitis,* or SBP). In addition, pneumococci may infect concurrently other tissues or organs, such as the sinopulmonary system, air sinuses *(sinusitis),* mastoids *(mastoiditis),* ears *(otitis media),* conjunctivae (pyogenic *conjunctivitis),* epiglottis *(epiglottitis,* particularly in infants), or rarely the soft tissues of the neck or retropharyngeal area *(Ludwig's angina).*

CLINICAL FINDINGS. The presentation of acute bacterial pneumonia due to *S. pneumoniae* may be highly variable, depend-

TABLE 271–3. CONCURRENT OR COMPLICATING PNEUMOCOCCAL INFECTIONS OCCURRING IN PNEUMOCOCCAL PNEUMONIA

Otitis media
Sinusitis/mastoiditis
Conjunctivitis (suppurative)
Epiglottitis
Tracheobronchitis
Pleuritis (empyema)
Soft tissue cellulitis (Ludwig's angina)
Pericarditis*
Endocarditis*
Meningitis*
Arthritis (septic)*
Peritonitis (in presence of ascites)*

* Usually blood borne.

ing on when the patient presents to the physician in the course of the disease, the patient's age, whether or not effective antibiotics were previously administered, the presence or absence of satisfactory host defenses, and the existence of risk factors for dissemination of pneumococci (e.g., asplenia, neutropenia, and agammaglobulinemia). The presentation may be mild or explosive and rapidly lethal. Classically, the onset of acute pneumococcal pneumonia is sudden and is characterized by an abrupt occurrence of cough, chills, high fever (up to 40°C), myalgias, tachypnea, shallow respirations, tachycardia, weakness, and often frank rigors. Initially, the cough may be productive of scant mucopurulent or blood-streaked sputum; later (after 24 to 48 hours), it may be thick, purulent, frankly bloody or rust-colored, and consistent with an alveolar, hemorrhagic, exudative process. If the infecting pneumococcus is highly encapsulated, a gelatinous, blood-tinged sputum may be seen. The presence of pleuritic pain is specific clinical evidence that the pneumonia is probably bacterial and, in the presence of most of the above findings, probably pneumococcal.

The patient with pneumococcal pneumonia is generally diaphoretic and, in addition, may be dehydrated and hypotensive. Anorexia, nausea, and vomiting are common. If allowed to continue untreated, single-lobe disease may progress to multilobe involvement, and the patient may become dusky, cyanotic, and confused. If bacteremia occurs, chills and rigors may persist, and rarely shock, a disseminated intravascular coagulopathy (DIC), and/or an adult respiratory distress syndrome (ARDS) may supervene and ultimately lead to the patient's death.

A history is frequently elicited of a recent upper respiratory or viral-like illness that has occurred prior to the appearance of clinical pneumonia, especially during the winter months, when influenza is common. Risk factors for aspiration, such as alcoholism, seizures, or vomiting, or for acquiring pneumococcal pneumonia may be present (see above).

On physical examination, the acutely ill patient is tachypneic and may be observed to use accessory muscles for respiration (intercostal, abdominal, and sternocleidomastoid) and even to exhibit nasal flaring. If pleuritic pain is severe, reflex splinting of the ipsilateral thorax is observed. Fever and tachycardia are present, and although hypotension may occur, frank shock is unusual, except in the later stages of infection or DIC.

Auscultation of the chest reveals bronchovesicular or tubular breath sounds and wet rales over the involved lung. As consolidation occurs, vocal and tactile fremitus is increased; however, if a concurrent pleural effusion is present, breath sounds and fremitus may be diminished or absent. A localized, grating pleural friction rub may occasionally be heard.

Examination of the upper respiratory passages may be helpful in suggesting a diagnosis of pneumococcal pneumonia. For example, in children, the absence of an exudative pharyngitis and the presence of otitis media might suggest pneumococcal involvement. In older children and adults, the air sinuses and/or mastoids may be acutely infected. (But these infections also can occur with streptococcal, staphylococcal, and H. influenzae pneumonia.)

Evidence of extrapulmonary infections may be present, particularly in untreated disease lasting more than 48 hours; for example, signs of meningeal irritation (stiff neck, Kernig's or Brudzinski's sign) with abnormalities in mentation may suggest meningitis; the appearance of pathologic heart murmurs, splenomegaly, and heart failure may be evidence of endocarditis; or the presence of pain, swelling, tenderness, heat, and possibly redness in one or more joints may point toward a septic arthritis of hematogenous origin.

Additional findings unrelated to pneumonia per se but related to sepsis and/or toxicity may be noted: a paralytic ileus with abdominal pain, distention, and loss of bowel sounds; mild jaundice due to a reactive hepatitis or to intrapulmonary hemorrhage; frank shock; purpuric lesions resulting from DIC; or symmetric gangrene and purpura of the fingers and/or toes (purpura fulminans) associated with bacteremia.

LABORATORY FINDINGS. The peripheral white blood cell (WBC) count is often two to three times the normal value; however, in alcoholics or immunosuppressed patients, it may be normal or low. Of more value is the WBC differential, which consists predominantly of bands and polymorphonuclear leukocytes (left shift). If DIC is suspected, thrombocytopenia, pleomorphism of red blood cells (schistocytes and helmet cells), prolonged prothrombin and partial thromboplastin times, and hypofibrinogenemia and circulating fibrin-split products may be present.

In some patients, the total bilirubin and hepatic cellular enzyme levels may be slightly elevated. Since dehydration and hypovolemia commonly occur (owing to fever, diaphoresis, nausea, and vomiting), the hemoglobin, hematocrit, and serum sodium level may be elevated. When pneumonia is the dominant clinical event, arterial blood gas studies, which reflect pulmonary function and compensatory events, usually reveal hypoxemia (low Po_2), hypocarbia (low Pco_2), and alkalosis (blood pH > 7.4) resulting from hyperventilation and shunting. However, if frank shock intervenes, a metabolic acidosis may result (blood pH < 7.4); if it is not corrected, death may follow.

Good posteroanterior and lateral chest roentgenograms are important to obtain, first to confirm the presence and to ascertain the extent and radiographic character of the pneumonia and second to determine if underlying predisposing pulmonary diseases are present, such as bronchiectasis, bronchial obstruction, emphysema, tumor, or tuberculosis. In severely dehydrated or profoundly neutropenic or immunodeficient patients, early inflammatory infiltrates may not be seen radiographically or may be patchy and irregular in appearance, but after hydration or restoration of circulating levels of inflammatory cells, patterns of lobar consolidation may become apparent.

Characteristically, in immunocompetent patients with untreated, frank pneumococcal pneumonia, chest roentgenograms reveal a lobar distribution and an air space (or alveolar exudative) pattern of disease with an air bronchogram effect. However, if prior, partially effective antibiotic usage has occurred, the pattern may be atypical, and a lobar distribution may be the exception rather than the rule. Interlobar fissures may bulge, owing to considerable fluid content within the involved lung associated with large amounts of capsular material. In severe cases, more than one lobe may be involved (multilobar pneumonia). In 30% of cases, a pleural effusion may be present and may be readily detected by a lateral decubitus film. Such effusions may be sterile and represent parapneumonic collections of fluid, or occasionally they may be infected with pneumococci, in which case they are called empyemas.

If blunting of the costophrenic angle is noted radiographically, and the finding is believed to represent an effusion, then at least 300 to 500 ml of fluid is probably present, and a thoracentesis is indicated. Unless contraindicated, every pleural effusion associated with an acute bacterial pneumonia in which the etiology of the pneumonia is unclear should be tapped and the fluid studied for microorganisms (see Color Plate 9D). Ordinarily, fluid removed from the pleural space is sterile, so any bacteria seen on a Gram stain or cultured from the fluid represent pathogens until proved otherwise.

Other important laboratory studies that must be obtained early in the patient's workup are routine cultures of the blood, a microscopic examination of a Gram stain and a culture of purulent material from the site of infection (alveoli, bronchi, or lung), and an examination of any infected material that can be removed from a secondarily infected extrapulmonary focus. Results of blood cultures may not be available for 18 to 24 hours and thus cannot assist the physician in making a presumptive diagnosis or in selecting appropriate initial chemotherapy. Often, in asplenic patients, a high-grade bacteremia occurs, so examination of the peripheral WBC smear or of the buffy coat for pneumococci may be useful.

Microscopic examination and cultures of expectorated purulent sputum from a patient with acute bacterial pneumonia are essential if a correct presumptive etiologic diagnosis is to be made and an appropriate antibiotic is to be given. Ideally, these tests should be done before therapy is initiated; however, a significant delay in instituting therapy should not be permitted. Attention must be given to obtaining a diagnostically useful sputum sample; that is, material must be purulent to be presumed to be from the site of infection. Saliva or oropharyngeal contamination of the sample should be avoided.

In a patient with the clinical picture of acute bacterial pneumonia, the finding of gram-positive diplococci in expectorated sputum that contains many (≥ 50 bacterial cells per $100 \times$ field) polymorphonuclear cells (purulent sputum) and few (< 10 squamous cells per $100 \times$ field) or no squamous epithelial cells (which indicates little or no oropharyngeal contamination of the specimen) is strong presumptive evidence of pneumococcal pneumonia.

Cultures of expectorated sputum are also important but are not without problems; for example, since *S. pneumoniae* is fastidious, it may fail to grow in culture, but this does not exclude its presence. In addition, pneumococci may be overlooked, since they may be overgrown by other organisms or mixed with similar-appearing, nonpneumococcal, α-hemolytic streptococci, which are normally present in oropharyngeal secretions. On the other hand, since *S. pneumoniae* is often present normally in the oropharynx, its growth from sputum, especially from that which is expectorated, may not be indicative of pneumococcal disease. Perhaps the main value of securing a sputum culture is to confirm or question observations made from the Gram stain and, if pneumococci (and/or other bacteria) are ultimately isolated, to perform antibiotic susceptibility testing.

If the patient is unable to expectorate purulent sputum for microscopic examination and culture, and if other infected materials (e.g., pleural or joint fluid) are not available or are negative for pneumococci, various procedures for obtaining pus from the infected lung must be considered. Cough can be induced by having the patient inhale an aerosol of warm 3% NaCl; a plastic catheter can be inserted into the trachea via the nose or throat and suction applied; a direct transtracheal needle and catheter aspiration may be performed (a procedure not without complications); the patient may undergo endoscopy (provided the arterial Po_2 is ≥ 50 mm Hg), and alveolar washings or bronchial brushings may be obtained; or rarely, direct aspiration of the pneumonic infiltrate through the chest wall with a long, "skinny" needle (22 gauge) may be employed (a procedure also not without risks). Open-lung biopsies for pneumococcal pneumonia are not indicated, although they may be for certain complications, ill-defined superinfections, or underlying diseases. In any acute bacterial pneumonia, the guiding principles for deciding what procedure, if any, to use for obtaining purulent sputum from the involved lung are as follows: (1) If expectorated sputum is satisfactory (i.e., purulent and relatively free of contaminating oropharyngeal material), further efforts to obtain pus from the deeper recesses of the lung are probably not necessary; (2) if additional procedures are necessary, one should select first the procedure that is least traumatic and invasive and is risk free and then proceed, if necessary, in a stepwise fashion to the next least invasive, risk-free procedure until satisfactory material is obtained; (3) one should not delay more than several hours before beginning chemotherapy, and if the patient is extremely ill, one must rely on clinical judgment and not delay treatment at all; and (4) one must make every effort to identify the etiologic agent (or agents) responsible for the pneumonia early in the course of the illness, since once this goal is realized, the chances of managing the patient successfully are markedly enhanced.

A variety of other tests may be applied to sputum specimens to identify pneumococci in acute bacterial pneumonia; but in skilled hands, few, if any, are better, less costly, easier to do, and more informative than the Gram stain. All tests done on sputum possess a similar problem in interpretation, namely, determining whether or not bacteria present in the sample are responsible for the pneumonia observed. If blood or pleural fluid cultures are subsequently positive for *S. pneumoniae*, the etiologic agent is confirmed, although the presence of additional pathogenic bacteria within the lung may not be entirely excluded, as, rarely, blood or pleural fluid cultures may yield other bacteria (polymicrobial infection) in addition to pneumococci.

Detection of pneumococcal capsular antigen generally requires the presence of approximately 10^5 bacteria per milliliter, about the same concentration as required to observe an average of one bacterium per $1000 \times$ field (or an oil-immersion field on a standard light microscope) on a Gram stain. Cross-reactions with other antigens of other bacteria are frequent, and with certain serotypes, false-negative results are common. Perhaps the greatest value of capsular antigen detection is to confirm the presence of pneumococci in those patients who have been partially treated and in whom sputum cultures may be negative and a Gram stain may reveal few, if any, intact bacteria.

Colony counts of bacteria from bronchoalveolar lavage (BAL) washings obtained during endoscopy are seldom available early in the course of illness. Specimens must be obtained with a special cuffed endoscope so that oropharyngeal contamination does not occur with insertion of the scope. Generally, counts of colony-forming units (CFU's) of bacteria higher than 10^3 to 10^5 per milliliter

of fluid removed are considered significant, but this is not invariably so.

DNA hybridization studies may be performed, but as with capsular antigen detection, adequate numbers of bacteria must be present for the test to be positive. Use of the polymerase chain reaction (PCR) may amplify pneumococcal DNA and improve the potential for detection; however, such enhanced sensitivity may lead to false-positive results caused by very small numbers of contaminating pneumococci.

Elastase or elastin fibers in sputum may suggest the presence of a gram-negative bacillary necrotizing pneumonia, particularly that due to *Pseudomonas,* but this test is of little value in the diagnosis of pneumococcal pneumonia (other than the test should be negative), since necrosis of tissue is not produced by pneumococci.

DIFFERENTIAL DIAGNOSIS (see also Ch. 55 and chapters dealing with specific organisms). The clinical picture and many of the routine laboratory and roentgenographic features associated with pneumococcal pneumonia are often indistinguishable from those of other acute bacterial pneumonias. Thus collecting appropriate microbiologic data is essential if the correct etiologic diagnosis is to be made.

In adults, the second most common community-acquired, acute bacterial pneumonia is that caused by *H. influenzae.* The Gram stain of purulent sputum from such patients often reveals myriads of tiny gram-negative coccobacilli, with the observation of an occasional filamentous form. Such an infection often occurs in a patient with chronic bronchitis or chronic obstructive pulmonary disease and usually is due to nonencapsulated *H. influenzae* (as opposed to highly encapsulated, serotype B strains commonly infecting young children).

Staphylococcus aureus is another bacterium occasionally producing acute pneumonia, but when this kind of pneumonia is community acquired, it usually occurs during or just after an epidemic of viral influenza. In the hospital setting, *S. aureus* may be seen year round, because it is a commonly occurring nosocomial infection. If a highly virulent, toxin-producing strain is responsible, the "toxic shock syndrome" may be observed. On a Gram stain of purulent sputum, clusters and characteristic tetrads of gram-positive cocci are seen. Late in the clinical course, abscess formation or destruction of the lung occurs.

Group A streptococci *(S. pyogenes)* also produce acute pneumonia, and in such instances, the patient may be more toxic-appearing than the extent of involvement of the lung might suggest. Classically, a small, peripherally located, wedge-shaped infiltrate is seen, and a thin, watery, serosanguineous, pleural effusion is present. A roentgenogram of the chest may suggest a pulmonary infarction. An upper respiratory tract infection, particularly an exudative or erythematous pharyngitis or tonsillitis (especially in children), may be present, and an erythematous rash produced by streptococcal erythrogenic toxin (scarlet fever) may be seen. A Gram stain of purulent sputum usually reveals numerous short chains of gram-positive cocci or diplococci. Thus the Gram stain may not differentiate group A streptococcal from pneumococcal pneumonia.

Branhamella catarrhalis may produce acute pneumonia, but usually this occurs in the elderly and particularly in those with chronic bronchitis or obstructive lung disease. It is a relatively benign infection, compared with those produced by other pyogenic bacteria, and is rarely, if ever, associated with bacteremia. A Gram stain of purulent sputum is again important, and the diagnosis should probably be made only when numerous gram-negative diplococci, in the absence of other potentially pathogenic bacteria, are seen. *N. meningitidis* (meningococci) are morphologically similar to *B. catarrhalis* and must be included in the differential diagnosis. However, in such instances, patients are generally young adults, and the infection is associated with significant toxicity.

Gram-negative bacilli, particularly those belonging to the family Enterobacteriaceae (e.g., *E. coli, Klebsiella, Enterobacter, Serratia,* and *Proteus*), also must be considered as causative agents in the differential diagnosis of pneumococcal pneumonia, particularly if the patient is debilitated and is residing in a nursing home or similar institution, and certainly if the patient is hospitalized. Aerobic gram-negative bacilli are often responsible for nosocomial but infrequently for community-acquired pneumonias. This is so because gram-negative bacilli rarely colonize the oropharynx of otherwise healthy people in the community, but they are common oropharyngeal residents in debilitated, hospitalized, or institutionalized patients. In addition, the patient in question may exhibit certain risk factors associated with invasion by gram-negative bacilli, such as the receipt of prior antibiotics, corticosteroids, inhalation therapy, or tracheostomy and the existence of profound neutropenia or severe debilitation. The pneumonic process is usually necrotizing, and gas formation may be detected on roentenograms. A Gram stain of purulent sputum usually reveals many large, bipolar-staining gram-negative rods. Elastin fibrils also may be seen on a KOH preparation of sputum from the site of infection.

Anaerobic bacteria also may produce acute suppurative pneumonia. Those most frequently involved are *Bacteroides* species (usually *B. melaninogenicus*), *Peptostreptococcus,* and *Fusobacterium.* Frequently, anaerobic infections are polymicrobial and may include bacteria other than strict anaerobes (e.g., *S. aureus*). The occurrence of anaerobic infection is usually preceded by gross aspiration and is enhanced if the individual has anaerobic oral infections or solid tumors of the oropharyngeal structures or tracheobronchial tree. The clinical presentation of anaerobic pleuropneumonic disease may be indolent rather than abrupt, and it may be accompanied by pus that has a fetid and nauseating odor. Necrosis of the lung with gas formation is often noted.

Mycoplasma pneumoniae, Chlamydia, and *Legionella* also may produce acute pneumonias, which are usually best described as atypical. With mycoplasmal pneumonia, patients are ordinarily young, and prolonged communicability, especially within households, may often be documented. The clinical, radiographic, and pathologic features are usually those of an interstitial pneumonia, rather than lobar consolidation and an alveolar exudative process. Serum cold agglutinin levels may be elevated, and the disease is rarely, if ever, fatal. Chlamydial pneumonia, especially that due to *C. psittaci,* is contracted from infected psittacine birds, while *C. pneumoniae* or the TWAR agent is acquired from other infected humans. *C. pneumoniae* is the most common species producing chlamydial pneumonia in humans, and the clinical picture is usually that of pharyngitis, often with laryngitis, and segmental pneumonia of a single lobe without pleural effusion. Seroepidemiologic studies reveal a higher prevalence of antibodies in males than females and in older adults than children. Legionnaires' disease, which may be produced by a variety of *Legionella* species but principally by *L. pneumophila,* is associated with considerable systemic toxicity (nausea, vomiting, and diarrhea) and may be very difficult to differentiate from pneumococcal pneumonia. However, in the temperate zones, community-acquired Legionnaires' disease usually occurs in the warmer months or summer; patients are typically male construction workers and smokers in their 50's whose clinical manifestations include fever, chills, myalgias, headache, dry cough, and nonspecific pulmonary infiltrates. Anti-*Legionella* fluorescein-labeled antibodies, which may be employed to examine sputum for *Legionella,* as well as antigen detection techniques applied to the urine, may be helpful in the early diagnosis of this disease.

Patients with the acquired immunodeficiency syndrome (AIDS) and acute pneumonia present considerable diagnostic problems. Although pneumococcal pneumonia and infections from encapsulated bacteria occur with greater frequency in patients with AIDS than in normal individuals, pneumocystosis and cytomegalovirus pneumonia occur frequently and thus must be excluded.

Finally, not only does pneumonia due to microbes other than the pneumococcus have to be considered in a differential diagnosis, but also a variety of noninfectious conditions may mimic the clinical picture of pneumococcal pneumonia. Pulmonary infarction, with emboli (e.g., in right-sided endocarditis) or without emboli (e.g., in sickle cell anemia), may present a considerable diagnostic challenge, even after differential lung scanning and pulmonary angiography. Chemical pneumonitis, localized or diffuse (Mendelson's syndrome), often caused by aspiration of gastric juice of low pH, also may be difficult to differentiate from pneumococcal or other bacterial pneumonias; however, in the absence of antibiotic therapy, a Gram stain of purulent sputum consistently reveals few or no bacteria.

TREATMENT. All patients with suspected pneumococcal pneumonia should be treated as promptly as possible with an effective antimicrobial agent. One should not wait for cultural confirmation of the diagnosis to initiate therapy. Although many patients may recover without antibacterial therapy, effective antimicrobial agents reduce morbidity, mortality, and complications.

At present, *penicillin G* is the therapy of choice, and it is the standard against which all other antipneumococcal agents are compared. Susceptible strains exhibit an MIC of < 0.1 μg per milliliter, levels that are easily achieved in a variety of tissues with therapeutic dosing of 1.2 to 2.4 million units per day. If complicating pneumococcal bacteremia occurs, only 10 to 15% of untreated patients may be expected to survive, while this figure increases to 85 to 90% with penicillin G treatment. A variety of other β-lactam antibiotics are also effective and may be used in special circumstances, such as when bacteria other than or in addition to pneumococci are considered in the differential diagnosis or when penicillin-resistant pneumococci are present. Ideally, initial therapy should be parenteral to ensure delivery and adequate serum and tissue levels. If the patient is in shock or has heart failure, the route of delivery should be intravenous. Later in the course of therapy, if the patient's progress is good, the route of administration may be changed to oral. Treatment with any effective agent should be for at least 5 to 7 days.

For patients who are believed to be allergic to penicillin, a variety of other antibacterial agents may be used. Usually, a first-generation cephalosporin is selected, since its molecular configuration is slightly different from that of penicillin G (a six-membered thiazole ring rather than a five-membered one) and since the frequency of serious reactions due to cross-allergenicity appears to be low. However, careful observation of the penicillin-allergic patient during the initial use of a cephalosporin must still be made. If the patient has a clear history of a type I (immediate) hypersensitivity reaction, all β-lactams should be avoided. For such patients, erythromycin is an excellent choice, even though an increasing frequency of resistance (MIC ≥ 1.0 μg per milliliter) to erythromycin is being observed worldwide. Tetracyclines should be avoided because the frequency of resistant strains is often widespread and high (up to 80% of isolates in some parts of the world). Similarly, quinolones also should not be used routinely because levels of susceptibility of most strains are often too high to predict a satisfactory outcome.

With the advent of penicillin-resistant pneumococci (see above), different strategies of therapy may have to be devised on the basis of susceptibility or resistance to other agents (Table 271–4). In the United States, such strains, although sporadic, localized to certain geographic areas, and generally of intermediate resistance (MIC between 0.1 and 2.0 μg per milliliter), appear to be increasing in frequency (up to $> 30\%$ in some locales). Nevertheless, each locale or hospital needs to monitor its own isolates, and therapeutic strategies should be based on these results. If strains are intermediate in resistance, simply increasing the dose of penicillin G to 6 million units per day will suffice (unless the complication of meningitis or endocarditis exists). However, if strains highly resistant to penicillin G (MIC ≥ 2.0 μg per milliliter) are repeatedly or frequently isolated, then penicillin G should not be routinely employed as initial therapy. In fact, such highly resistant isolates are generally resistant to most other β-lactam antibiotics (see Table 271–1), as well as to many other antimicrobials, so agents such as vancomycin, teicoplanin, clindamycin, fluoroquinolones, or rifampin may have to be used (with or without empirical penicillin) until the results

TABLE 271–4. CRITERIA FOR RESISTANCE OF *STREPTOCOCCUS PNEUMONIAE* TO SOME COMMONLY USED ANTIBIOTICS*

Antibacterial Agent	MIC (μg/ml)†
Penicillin G	
Intermediate	≥ 0.1 to < 2.0
High level	≥ 2.0
Erythromycin	≥ 1.0
Trimethoprim-sulfamethoxazole	≥ 1.19
Rifampin	≥ 2.0
Chloramphenicol	≥ 8.0

* Based on criteria established by the National Committee for Clinical Laboratory Standards (NCCLS).

† MIC = minimal inhibitory concentration.

of susceptibility studies are available. Among currently available β-lactams, cefotaxime, ceftriaxone, cefepime, and the carbapenems are active against many highly resistant pneumococci (see Table 271–1).

If effective antibacterial therapy is employed, the patient's temperature usually falls to or below normal by crisis within 24 hours. However, in some instances, perhaps because of the nature of the pathology or complications that occur (e.g., pleural effusion), the patient's temperature may fall by lysis over 2 to 3 days. Resolution and recovery from pneumococcal pneumonia generally result in restoration of normal pulmonary architecture. Occasionally, healing may be via fibrosis, in which instance persistence of pulmonary infiltrates on roentgenograms may be evident for months after clinical recovery.

In addition to effective antibacterial therapy, a variety of supportive measures are generally used in the initial management of acute pneumococcal pneumonia; these include bed rest, monitoring vital signs and urine output, inserting a Swan-Ganz catheter to monitor cardiac output, administering an occasional analgesic to relieve pleuritic pain to permit effective breathing and coughing, replacing fluids if the patient is dehydrated, correcting electrolytes, oxygen therapy, and relieving an ileus with nasal gastric suctioning. In relieving pleuritic pain or in providing sedation in situations requiring it (e.g., in delirium tremens), care should be taken not to use excessively high doses of analgesics or sedatives that might depress the respiratory center. Intercostal nerve blocks, which do not interfere with respiratory drive, may be used. If possible, antipyretics also should be avoided, since these agents interfere with the evaluation of fever as a measurement of the patient's progress (or lack of).

COMPLICATIONS. Approximately 5% of patients with pneumococcal pneumonia develop an empyema, although a larger percentage (up to 30%) commonly develop sterile pleural effusions. Most effusions resolve with successful antibacterial therapy, although empyemas often require drainage. Empyemas usually consist of thick pus composed of fibrin, serous proteins, large numbers of leukocytes and/or their products, and pneumococci. Initially, such collections may be drained by needle aspiration; however, later, as loculations occur, drainage via chest tubes is usually necessary. Chest roentgenograms with lateral decubitus films are often useful in the early recognition of pleural effusions; however, at a later time and in the course of removal and follow-up, ultrasonography and/or computed tomography (CT) may be necessary. In any acute bacterial pneumonia, pleural fluid that is removed should be subject to a Gram stain, aerobic and anaerobic cultures, pH determination, cell count and differential, protein and sugar analysis, and a lactate dehydrogenase test to determine whether or not an empyema is present.

If pneumococcal bacteremia occurs, extrapulmonary complications, such as *meningitis, septic arthritis,* and *endocarditis,* must be excluded, since their therapy generally requires higher dosages of penicillin G and, in the case of septic arthritis, may require drainage. A spinal tap with examination of cerebrospinal fluid (CSF) should be done if meningitis is suspected, and multiple pretreatment blood cultures and echocardiography of the heart valves should be obtained if endocarditis is suspected. Other complications that might occur are *pyogenic pericarditis,* which may produce tamponade and require drainage, and *peritonitis* in those with ascites (e.g., cirrhosis or nephrotic syndrome).

PROGNOSIS. The case fatality rate for untreated pneumococcal pneumonia is about 25%, whereas in those treated promptly with penicillin G, it may be <5%. Fatality rates differ considerably among patient groups, depending on such factors as presence or absence of bacteremia, multilobe or single-lobe involvement, presence or absence of neutropenia or asplenism, underlying diseases (particularly of the heart or lung), age of the patient (the prognosis being poor at the extremes), complicating extrapulmonary pneumococcal infections (e.g., meningitis), the occurrence of shock, the serotype of pneumococcus responsible (type 3 being highly virulent), delayed therapy, penicillin susceptibility or resistance, and prior immunization with polyvalent pneumococcal vaccine. However, since the advent of penicillin G in the 1940's, the case fatality rate of pneumococcal pneumonia and bacteremia remains essentially unchanged.

PREVENTION. The most important preventive tool available is polyvalent pneumococcal vaccine. This type-specific vaccine contains 23 antigenic capsular polysaccharides, which in the United States account for up to 90% of bacteremic infections. In immunocompetent populations, it is estimated to be 79% protective, inducing antibodies of the IgG2 and IgG4 subclasses in adults, which enhance opsonization, phagocytosis, and killing of pneumococci by polymorphonuclear leukocytes and fixed macrophages. It is virtually free of life-threatening side effects and obviously cannot produce a pneumococcal infection, since it contains no viable, intact pneumococci. About 15 to 30% of patients who receive the vaccine may develop fever, localized swelling, and/or pain at the injection site. As with all polysaccharide vaccines, it is not immunogenic below ages 18 to 24 months and is poorly immunogenic in the very elderly and in those with a variety of conditions generally associated with decreased vaccine responsiveness. In normal individuals, if antibodies result from vaccination, colonization, or natural infection, they usually persist for several years, and then progressively decline. The vaccine is not associated with a booster effect, probably because it functions as a thymus-independent type 2 antigen. At present, highly immunogenic vaccines in which the capsular antigens are conjugated to proteins are under development. Revaccination of the elderly and other high-risk groups needs to be considered at 3- to 5-year intervals.

The U.S. Public Health Service specifically recommends the currently available pneumococcal vaccine for patients with underlying conditions that are associated with increased susceptibility to pneumococcal infections or increased risk of mortality from such infections, namely, healthy adults 65 years or older and those with chronic cardiac or pulmonary diseases, anatomic or functional asplenia, chronic liver disease, alcoholism, diabetes mellitus, and CSF leaks. Perhaps the greatest value of vaccination against pneumococci is to reduce bacteremia, dissemination, and mortality, especially in those with hepatic or splenic dysfunction. Type-specific antibody can be elicited with pneumococcal polysaccharides by subcutaneous vaccination even in splenectomized patients. In addition, recommendations for receiving the vaccine also are made for those with chronic renal failure or those on hemodialysis; for those with Hodgkin's disease, chronic lymphocytic leukemia, multiple myeloma, and AIDS; or for those receiving or about to receive chemotherapy for cancer, organ transplantation, or splenectomy.

Antibiotic prophylaxis with penicillin G or similar agents in otherwise healthy patients with viral upper respiratory infections is not routinely indicated, is not cost-effective, and may only lead to superinfections with antibiotic-resistant bacteria or to adverse side effects from the antibiotic itself. However, in individuals with seriously compromised pulmonary, cardiac, or immune function, a narrow-spectrum agent, such as penicillin G, may be given in low dosages during a viral syndrome for a limited time to reduce the risk of morbidity and mortality from potentially invasive pneumococci. Such prophylaxis may especially apply to those in households where pneumococcal infections recently occurred.

Finally, it should be appreciated that pneumococcal infections, including pneumonia, are generally not acquired by otherwise normal people from exposure to other patients with pneumococcal pneumonia; thus patients with pneumococcal pneumonia do not require isolation, and prophylaxis for medical staff exposed to such infections is not indicated.

Austrian R: Life with the Pneumococcus. Notes from the Bedside, Laboratory, and Library. Philadelphia, University of Pennsylvania Press, 1985. *An array of interesting observations, both clinical and laboratory, on pneumococcal infections by an outstanding authority and the father of the modern capsular polysaccharide pneumococcal vaccine.*

Austrian R, Gold J: Pneumococcal bacteremia with especial reference to bacteremic pneumococcal pneumonia. Ann Intern Med 60:759, 1964. *A landmark clinical study that clearly points out the major risk factors involved in pneumococcal pneumonia and bacteremia.*

Bruyn GAW, Zegers BJM, van Furth R: Mechanisms of host defense against infection with Streptococcus pneumoniae. Clin Infect Dis 14:251, 1992. *A thorough, up-to-date review of virulence factors of, and humoral and cellular mechanisms against, pneumococci.*

Friedland IR, McCracken GH Jr: Management of infections caused by antibiotic-resistant Streptococcus pneumoniae. N Engl J Med 331:337, 1994. *An excellent review of clinical responsiveness of infections due to penicillin-resistant pneumococci to various antibiotics with suggested therapeutic strategies.*

Hook EW III, Horton CA, Schaberg DR: Failure of intensive care unit support to influence mortality from pneumococcal bacteremia. JAMA 249:1055, 1983. *A clinical study that reveals that even intensive care and special units have not influenced the survival rate in pneumococcal pneumonia and bacteremia since the advent of penicillin, thus further emphasizing the need for prevention.*

Klugman KP: Pneumococcal resistance to antibiotics. Clin Microbiol Rev 3:171, 1990.

A complete, in-depth microbiologic, epidemiologic, and clinical review, evaluation, and update of the problem of penicillin resistance by an authority with considerable experience with such isolates.

Musher DM, Groover JE, Rowland JM, et al.: Antibody to capsular polysaccharides of Streptococcus pneumoniae: Prevalence, persistence and response to revaccination. Clin Infect Dis 17:66, 1993. Presents new and reviews previously published data on the appearance, persistence, and fall of anticapsular antibodies against pneumococci after colonization, natural infections, and immunization.

272 MYCOPLASMAL INFECTION
David Schlossberg

BACKGROUND. The mycoplasmas associated with humans include species from the genera *Mycoplasma, Ureaplasma,* and *Acholeplasma.* Since these genera all belong to the order Mycoplasmatales in the class Mollicutes, they are called collectively "mollicutes" or, more commonly, "mycoplasmas." There are over 150 species, and they are found in humans, animals, plants, and insects. Most of these organisms are commensals, but some of the human strains are pathogenic; rarely, some of the animal strains infect humans as well.

The mycoplasmas are the smallest free-living organisms. At 200 nm, they approximate the size of the larger viruses. Bound by a triple-layered cell membrane, they have no cell wall (thus the name "mollicute," Greek for "soft skin") and therefore are not seen on Gram stain and cannot be treated with cell wall–active antibiotics such as the β-lactams or vancomycin. Their small genome limits their genetic information, so mycoplasmas usually require media enriched with nucleic acid precursors and cholesterol.

Most mycoplasmas are facultative anaerobes. They grow down into agar and produce a dark center with a light periphery on the surface, the so-called fried-egg colonies. Mycoplasmas are distinguished from bacteria because they lack a cell wall and cannot produce cell wall precursors and from viruses, chlamydiae, and rickettsiae because the mycoplasmas can grow on cell-free media.

The mycoplasmas of humans are listed in Table 272–1. Some are established pathogens, some are commensals, and some infect immunocompromised patients.

IMMUNOLOGY. The mycoplasmas have a wide range of immunomodulatory effects. These include stimulating proliferation of T and B lymphocytes, inducing cytolytic activity of macrophages and cytotoxic T cells, stimulating cytokine production, inducing expression of major histocompatibility complex in macrophages and B cells, and producing chemotactic factors, Fc factors, Fc receptors, superantigens, and immunoglobulin proteases. This explosive and varied immunologic activity may contribute to disease expression. It is well known that rheumatoid factor, biologic false-positive tests for syphilis, antinuclear antibodies (ANA's), and other antibodies sometimes appear in the course of mycoplasmal infection.

MYCOPLASMA PNEUMONIAE. Mycoplasma pneumoniae accounts for 10 to 20% of all pneumonias and for at least half of all pneumonias in children and young adults. Although most cases occur in the first two decades of life, mycoplasmal infection is seen at all ages.

Infection with *M. pneumoniae* can occur in any season, with a 4-year periodicity for outbreaks. Since epidemics of pneumonia due to other agents usually peak in the winter, it is diagnostically help-

TABLE 272–1. HUMAN MYCOPLASMAS

Established Pathogens	Opportunists	Commensals
M. pneumoniae	M. salivarium	M. buccale
M. hominis	M. ovale	M. faucium
M. fermentans	M. genitalium	M. lipophilum
M. urealyticum	M. pirum	M. primatum
	M. penetrans	M. spermatophilum
	M. arginini	A. laidlawii
		A. oculi

ful when *Mycoplasma* pneumonia occurs in other seasons. College epidemics of *Mycoplasma,* for example, tend to peak in the fall.

The incubation period for *M. pneumoniae* averages $2\frac{1}{2}$ weeks but ranges from 4 days to over 3 weeks. This longer incubation period furnishes an important diagnostic clue, since incubation periods for most of the respiratory viruses are measured in days, not weeks. Because of the long incubation period and the lower efficiency of spread of *M. pneumoniae,* this infection spreads slowly through a population group or family. For example, several passages are needed to infect a large family, as opposed to the explosive swath through a household made by the influenza virus. Spread is person-to-person via droplet nuclei after close and prolonged contact. Patients shed the organism 2 to 8 days prior to the onset of clinical illness. They then transmit the disease during the acute phase of illness; patients with asymptomatic infection are not efficient transmitters of disease.

The attack rate of *M. pneumoniae* diminishes with age. Second infections can occur (especially if a patient is immunocompromised), but the second case is usually milder than the first. Extremely severe disease is seen in patients who have SS or SC hemoglobinopathy, Down syndrome, and hypogammaglobulinemia. Further, patients with humoral deficiency are more likely to become chronic carriers; normal patients shed the organism by 6 weeks, but immunodeficient patients may carry it for 4 months.

CLINICAL FINDINGS (Fig. 272–1). Most patients with *M. pneumoniae* infection are older children, adolescents, and young adults who develop a minor respiratory illness. In general, 75% of patients have a tracheobronchitis, 5% have an atypical pneumonia, and 20% are asymptomatic. Children under age 5 tend to have coryza and wheezing. Asthmatics may develop bronchospasm. In many patients, a sequence of symptoms occurs: The illness begins insidiously over days or a week with constitutional symptomatology (e.g., fever, myalgias, headache, and malaise); then upper respiratory signs and symptoms appear, with combinations of sore throat, cervical adenopathy, hoarseness, earache, coryza, and nonproductive cough; less commonly, croup or bronchiolitis may supervene, and in a small percentage, pneumonia ensues. At this point, the cough becomes productive.

Many patients report chilliness but not rigors. Protracted coughing results in tracheal tenderness and a sore chest, but actual pleuritic pain is rare. Signs include fever, an erythematous pharynx without exudate, and rarely, bullae on the tympanic membrane. The illness is usually self-limited and mild.

The insidious onset is usually followed by a gradual recovery. The upper respiratory symptoms may last for 2 to 3 weeks, and signs of pneumonia may persist for 4 to 6 weeks. Laboratory abnormalities are not specific; a slight leukocytosis (< 15,000 per cubic millimeter) is seen in 25% of patients, with a normal differential count. Sputum Gram stain is very helpful in demonstrating inflammatory cells (polys or lymphs) but a paucity of bacteria.

Radiographic findings are manifold. Most patients have unilateral lower lobe segmental abnormalities on the right. The earliest signs are an interstitial accentuation of markings with subsequent patchy airspace consolidation and thickened bronchial shadows. Additional findings are platelike atelectasis, Kerley B lines, perihilar accentuations of markings, and nodular infiltrates. Hilar adenopathy is seen only occasionally in the adult but in 30% of children and may be unilateral or bilateral. A small effusion is seen in one-fourth of patients, but even in these patients pleuritic pain is rare. Complications seen on chest radiograph include pneumothorax, pneumatoceles, abscess, and in the rare case of fulminant disease, changes compatible with respiratory distress syndrome (see Ch. 65). In convalescence, an area of hyperlucent lung may persist on chest radiograph, but most of the changes resolve. Rarely, bronchiectasis, bronchiolitis obliterans, and progressive fibrosis are permanent sequelae.

Pathology of pulmonary involvement includes peribronchial and peribronchiolar mononuclear inflammatory infiltrates with intraluminal polymorphonuclear leukocytes. Occasionally seen are hyaline membrane formation and organizing pneumonia, with alveolar hemorrhage or proteinaceous material and, rarely, interstitial fibrosis.

Extrapulmonary complications are common and are usually superimposed on pulmonary disease so that a mycoplasmal etiology can be suspected. The most frequent extrapulmonary complication is neurologic.

Neurologic symptoms are seen as early as several days after the onset of respiratory symptoms or 2 weeks or more after the respira-

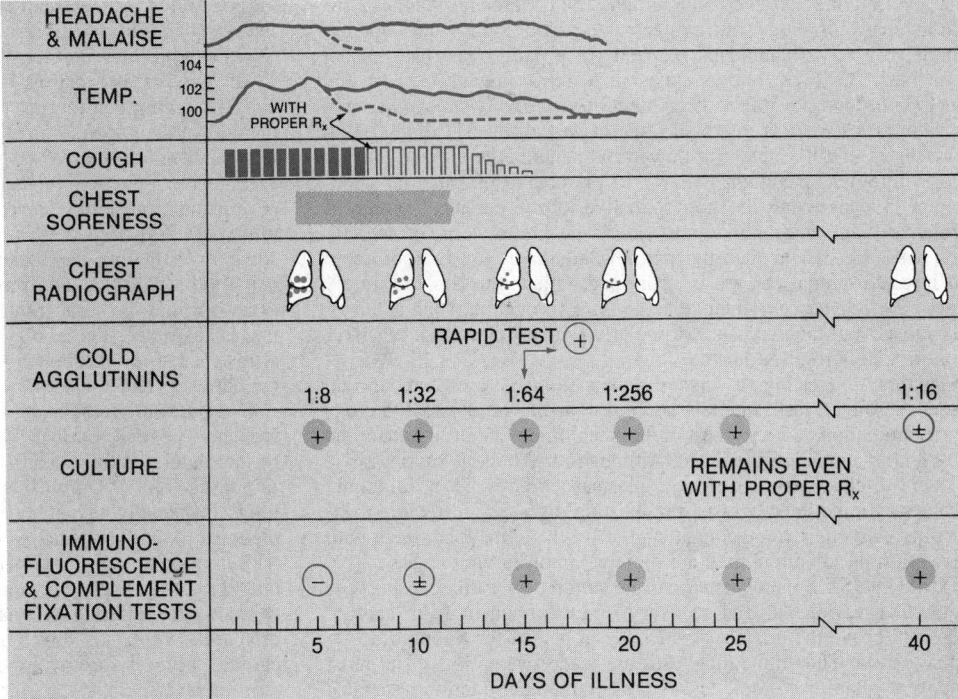

FIGURE 272-1. Major clinical and laboratory manifestations of mycoplasmal pneumonia.

tory symptoms subside. Thus both infectious and postinfectious mechanisms seem to be involved. Respiratory disease may be absent in as many as 50% of patients at presentation. Most neurologic complications occur in children, and mycoplasmal infection accounts for 10 to 15% of childhood encephalitis. Cerebrospinal fluid typically displays a small number of lymphocytes (50 to 100) with normal or slightly elevated protein and occasionally lowered glucose.

Encephalitis may result in coma or psychosis or more focal phenomena such as stroke, ataxia, and choreoathetosis. A postinfectious leukoencephalitis has been described. Patients also may present with clinically characteristic meningitis. A number of types of myelitis are seen, including transverse myelitis and a polio-like syndrome. Finally, peripheral neuropathy may involve peripheral or cranial nerves; it is felt that M. pneumoniae accounts for 5% of cases of Guillain-Barré syndrome. Sequelae of neurologic involvement range from mental retardation to movement disorders and epilepsy. Corticosteroids and plasma exchange have been used as therapy, in addition to antibiotics, but there is no consensus on these additional modalities.

Rashes are seen in 10 to 20% of patients. Most are maculopapular, but they also may be vesicular, petechial, or urticarial, most commonly on the trunk and extremities. Less frequently, the face, buttocks, genitalia, hands, and feet are included. Rash usually begins during the acute illness but may precede or follow it. Most patients have obvious respiratory disease, and some have an associated conjunctivitis or an exanthem in the oropharynx. Other exanthemata associated with M. pneumoniae infection include pityriasis rosea, toxic epidermal necrolysis, erythema nodosum, and erythema multiforme or Stevens-Johnson syndrome. In fact, 15 to 20% of patients with erythema multiforme have been shown to have M. pneumoniae infection.

M. pneumoniae is the most common cause of rash and pneumonia, a combination also produced by viruses (herpes simplex, varicella-zoster, Epstein-Barr virus, enterovirus, adenovirus, and measles), Chlamydia psittaci, Mycobacterium tuberculosis, fungi (histoplasma, cryptococci, coccidioides), and meningococci.

Hematologic complications are well-known features of mycoplasmal infection. Anemia, hemolytic anemia, thrombocytopenia, disseminated intravascular coagulation, thromboembolism, thrombotic thrombocytopenic purpura, Pelger-Huët abnormality (polymorphonuclear leukocytes with monolobed or bilobed appearance), and hemophagocytic histiocytic syndrome are all described, but the most common hematologic complication is formation of cold agglutinins. These antibodies agglutinate red blood cells and are seen in

a variety of infections (influenza, mononucleosis, psittacosis, rubella, adenovirus, measles, and others) but usually occur at higher titer in mycoplasmal infection. If the titer is high enough, they may bind complement and cause hemolysis. These cold agglutinins are IgM antibodies directed against the I antigen of the red blood cell. They are seen in up to 70% of patients, especially those with severe disease. Appearing in the second week of illness, they peak at 4 weeks and disappear by 2 months. Thus, at the time the cold agglutinin titer is highest and hemolysis most likely to occur, the clinical disease is abating. A simple bedside test may be performed by adding 1 to 2 ml of the patient's blood to an anticoagulated tube. This tube is placed in a cup of ice water and tilted after 2 to 3 minutes to detect clumping, which represents agglutination of red blood cells. The tube is then warmed by holding it in the hands, and if the clumps redissolve, the test is positive and correlates with a titer of cold agglutinins of 1:64 or greater. Hemolysis is treated with corticosteroids as well as antibiotics; the role of plasmapheresis is uncertain, but patients (and any blood that is transfused) should be kept warm.

Cardiac complications include pericarditis with occasional hemopericardium and myocarditis, which can result in complete heart block or congestive heart failure. A migratory arthritis may be seen, involving medium-sized joints and occasionally resembling rheumatoid arthritis. Ophthalmologic complications include iritis and conjunctivitis, as well as optic neuritis with optic nerve atrophy. On occasion, retinal hemorrhages and exudates are seen. A number of other organ systems may be involved, with resultant bullous myringitis, glomerulonephritis, hepatitis, pancreatitis, splenomegaly, polymyositis, and Raynaud's phenomenon.

The differential diagnosis of M. pneumoniae infection includes most causes of the atypical pneumonia syndrome (Table 272-2). This syndrome refers to a generally benign febrile illness with prominent systemic complaints, nonproductive cough, and intersti-

TABLE 272-2. DIFFERENTIAL DIAGNOSIS OF *M. PNEUMONIAE* INFECTION

Common	Rare
Chlamydia pneumoniae pneumonia	Q fever
Legionnaires' disease	Psittacosis
Viral pneumonia	Acute fungal infection
Early bacterial pneumonia	Tularemia
	Tuberculosis

tial abnormalities on chest radiograph. The differential diagnosis includes many diseases with clinical or epidemiologic clues. For example, psittacosis should be suspected if a patient has had contact with birds, Q fever follows exposure to farm animals or cats, and *Legionella* tends to infect older men who smoke. *Chlamydia pneumoniae* (see Ch. 323) infection often causes a biphasic illness, with sore throat and hoarseness followed by cough. True viruses cause a more fulminant pneumonia. Early in the course of bacterial pneumonia, a cough may be nonproductive, but eventually sputum is produced with neutrophils and bacteria on Gram stain, in association with rigors and pleuritic pain. Tularemia follows exposure to an infected animal carcass or arthropod. Other illnesses that rarely mimic *M. pneumoniae* include acute fungal infection, such as histoplasmosis, and tuberculosis, particularly primary disease or reactivation in a compromised host.

Factors suggesting a mycoplasmal etiology are sore throat, headache, fever, rash, indolent course, a paucity of physical findings on examination, and a chest radiograph more abnormal than the physical examination predicted. Although rare, bullous myringitis is a helpful clue. *Against* a mycoplasmal etiology is a fulminant course, extreme leukocytosis, pre-existing disease, and recurrent infection. Although both coryza and hoarseness may be seen with mycoplasmal infection, they are more common in viral disease.

DIAGNOSIS. *Mycoplasma* can be cultured, but this capability is not widely available, and recovery of the organism from sputum does not prove the diagnosis, since it can persist for a long time after infection. Thus most diagnoses are made by serology. The most widely available serologic test is the complement fixation test (CF). Ninety percent of patients have either a fourfold rise in the CF titers (2 to 3 weeks apart) or a single titer of 1:32 or greater. There are problems with this test, however: First, the CF titer can remain elevated for a year after the infection. Second, the glycolipid antigen used in the test is not specific for *Mycoplasma* and is found in a variety of tissues, including human heart muscle, brain, and pancreas, as well as in some streptococci and leafy vegetables. Thus false-positive results may be seen, for example, in certain neurologic syndromes and pancreatitis. Third, there are false-negative reactions.

Other serologic tests include the ELISA, which can readily detect IgM as well as IgG antibody; this test is promising but is not as widely available as the CF. Other diagnostic tests that identify antibody in blood or nucleic acid in clinical samples (e.g., polymerase chain reaction [PCR]) are presently either under investigation or not widely available. Thus diagnosis is generally *proven* by a fourfold rise in CF titer or by a single IgM determination, and diagnosis is strongly *supported* by a single CF titer ≥ 1:32 or a titer of cold agglutinins ≥ 1:64.

THERAPY. From a practical standpoint, therapy for *M. pneumoniae* infection is empirical because culture takes time and may be misleading and serologic investigation is not diagnostic early in the course. Thus a compatible illness in a susceptible patient should be treated on the basis of clinical suspicion. There is a definite clinical response to tetracyclines and erythromycin, although treatment does not influence the carrier state, and the organism may persist in respiratory secretions despite appropriate antibiotic therapy.

Currently, erythromycin or tetracycline (either as 2 grams daily in divided doses) is standard therapy (Table 272–3). Doxycycline and the newer macrolides (azithromycin and clarithromycin) can probably substitute for tetracycline and erythromycin, respectively, and offer the advantage of greater patient convenience but at increased cost. Although most recommendations are for 10 to 14 days of therapy, longer courses of treatment (e.g., 2 to 3 weeks) may avoid the relapse that occurs in 5 to 10% of patients. Prophylaxis of contacts does not prevent infection but can prevent clinical disease. Tetracyclines should be avoided in children under the age of 8 and pregnant patients but are preferable if the differential diagnosis includes psittacosis, Q fever, or *M. fermentans* (see below). Correspondingly, erythromycin is preferred if the differential diagnosis includes legionellosis.

M. hominis is a commensal of the genitourinary tract, especially in women. It is seen in up to 50% of sexually active women and 30% of sexually active men. Occasionally, it is found in the pharynx. *M. hominis* may produce several different syndromes. It is a known pathogen of the female urogenital tract, causing Bartholin's

gland abscess, pelvic inflammatory disease (PID), and pyelonephritis. It also causes postabortal and postpartum fever and wound infection following cesarean section. *M. hominis* can infect the fetus *in utero* or during birth, resulting in neonatal infection and stillbirth. Scalp wound infection may complicate fetal monitoring devices.

M. hominis also causes extragenital infection in the adult, typically following genitourinary manipulation in an immunosuppressed patient. Infection of surgical wounds should be suspected if a purulent exudate is negative on Gram stain and culture. Other sites of extragenital infection include brain, lung, prosthetic devices, skin, peritoneum, and joints (especially in patients with hypogammaglobulinemia). Although these organisms are not visible on Gram stain, some investigators have identified them in infected joint fluid by using the acridine orange stain and immunofluorescent staining. The organism may grow on routine media but is easily overlooked, and if it is suspected, the laboratory should be alerted. Since *M. hominis* is resistant to erythromycin, tetracycline is the drug of choice, with clindamycin and the quinolones as alternatives (see Table 272–3).

Ureaplasma urealyticum colonizes the genital tract of 75% of women and 45% of men who are sexually active (see Ch. 314). In the adult, it may cause nongonococcal urethritis as well as salpingitis and PID; outside the genitourinary tract, it can infect joints (especially in patients with hypogammaglobulinemia), transplant sites, and surgical wounds. In the neonate, it is associated with chorioamnionitis and with chronic lung disease of prematurity, but is not strongly associated with prematurity, and treatment to eradicate it during pregnancy does not reduce the incidence of premature birth or low birth rate. Tetracyclines are agents of choice, with erythromycin or possibly quinolones as alternatives (see Table 272–3).

Another definite pathogen has been recognized in *M. fermentans*. This organism has been recovered from the lower genital tract of men and women, the oropharynx, and the lower respiratory tract. Although associated with immunosuppression (leukemia, AIDS, and chemotherapy), it also has been described in normal patients who develop a febrile illness with fever, vomiting, and diarrhea and progress to fulminant disease with respiratory distress syndrome, multiple organ failure, and death. This organism is resistant to erythromycin and should be treated with doxycycline or a quinolone (see Table 272–3).

. A variety of other mycoplasmas possibly cause disease, especially in immunosuppressed patients; *M. orale* has been isolated from the blood and marrow of children with leukemia; *M. pirum* has been recovered from lymphocytic cells from patients with AIDS; *M. genitalium* may cause urethritis or arthritis in hypogammaglobulinemic patients; *M. penetrans* is strongly associated with homosexual activity and has been isolated from the urine of patients with AIDS; *M. salivarium* causes periodontitis and septic arthritis in hypogammaglobulinemic patients; and *M. arginini*, an animal strain of *Mycoplasma*, has caused septicemia and pneumonia in an immunocompromised patient with lymphoma. Like *M. fermentans*, this strain of *Mycoplasma* is resistant to erythromycin and should be treated with tetracycline if suspected (see Table 272–3). Other human mycoplasmas, as noted in Table 272–1, are presently considered commensals.

Recent interest has focused on the relationship between mycoplasmas and human immunodeficiency virus (HIV) infection. It is possible that in patients with infection due to HIV-1, coincident infection with mycoplasmas may lead to accelerated disease via enhanced viral replication or cytopathic effects. This role of cofactor with HIV has been suggested for several strains of mycoplasmas, including *M. fermentans, M. pirum,* and *M. penetrans,* all of which

TABLE 272–3. ANTIBIOTIC SUSCEPTIBILITY*

	ERY	TCN	CLN	QUN
M. pneumoniae	sens	sens		
M. fermentans	res	sens	sens	sens
M. hominis	res	sens†	sens	
U. urealyticum	sens†	sens†	res	sens
M. arginini	res	sens		

* ERY = erythromycin; TCN = tetracycline; CLN = clindamycin; QUN = quinolones; sens = sensitive; res = resistant.
† Some resistance seen.

have been isolated from HIV-infected patients and are potent immunomodulators.

Couch RB: *Mycoplasma pneumoniae* (primary atypical pneumonia). *In* Mandell GL, Douglas RG Jr, Bennett JE (eds.): Principles and Practice of Infectious Diseases, 3rd ed. New York, Churchill-Livingstone, 1990. *A good general reference for all aspects of* Mycoplasma *infection.*

Koskiniemi M: CNS manifestations associated with *Mycoplasma pneumoniae* infections: Summary of cases at the University of Helsinki and review. Clin Infect Dis 17(suppl 1):S52, 1993. *An excellent and thorough review of neurologic complications.*

Lo S-C, Wear DJ, Green SL, et al.: Adult respiratory distress syndrome with or without systemic disease associated with infections due to *Mycoplasma fermentans.* Clin Infect Dis 17(suppl 1):S259, 1993. *Excellent clinical and laboratory description of this infection.*

McMahon DK, Dummer JS, Pasculle AW, et al.: Extragenital *Mycoplasma hominis* infections in adults. Am J Med 89:275, 1990. *Good concise review with helpful references.*

273 PNEUMONIA CAUSED BY AEROBIC GRAM-NEGATIVE BACILLI

Waldemar G. Johanson, Jr.

Over the past 30 years, the group of organisms known collectively as "aerobic gram-negative bacilli" (GNB) has assumed an increasing importance in clinical respiratory infections. There is no evidence that this phenomenon is due to increasing virulence of these organisms. Rather, it is due to changes in the human hosts they infect and, to some degree, to changes in the environment induced by antibiotics and other factors, especially in hospitals. Each of the GNB has its place (or places) in nature. Many are regular inhabitants of the human gastrointestinal tract, while others are found in water or other sites in the environment. None is especially virulent for the respiratory tract of healthy mammalian hosts; all are distinctly inferior to the pneumococcus, for example, in that regard. A careful review of the preantibiotic literature reveals that the presence of these organisms in the respiratory tracts of seriously ill patients is not a recent occurrence; rather, their presence was disregarded for many years, an approach that was not unjustified, considering the preeminence of the pneumococcus as a cause of fatal pneumonia before highly efficacious antibiotics were available. The emergence of GNB as respiratory pathogens in recent years is the result of more aggressive organisms being suppressed by effective therapy and the long-term survival of people who would have succumbed to other infections or other processes in an earlier era.

PATHOGENESIS. Pneumonias due to GNB are caused by one of three mechanisms: inhalation of contaminated aerosols, hematogenous infection of the lungs from another primary source of infection, or aspiration of oropharyngeal secretions that are colonized by these organisms.

Contamination of respiratory therapy equipment by GNB, usually *Pseudomonas aeruginosa,* was recognized as a major cause of nosocomial pneumonias in the 1960's. With the advent of disposable nebulizers and other control strategies, this problem has been largely eliminated.

Most instances of bacteremia from a nonpulmonary source, such as the gastrointestinal or urinary tract, associated with pulmonary infiltrates, fever, and hypoxemia, represent noncardiogenic pulmonary edema, or the "adult respiratory distress syndrome" (see Ch. 65 and 68), and not actual pneumonia. In fact, pneumonia due to this cause is sufficiently uncommon that the presence of gram-negative bacteremia in association with new pulmonary infiltrates should initiate a vigorous search for a primary site of infection outside the lungs before it is concluded that pneumonia is responsible.

Aspiration of oropharyngeal secretions that contain GNB is the usual event leading to pneumonia caused by these organisms. Colonization of the upper respiratory tract with GNB occurs in 10% or fewer of normal people but is markedly increased among patients with acute or chronic diseases. Colonization rates among populations with chronic disease, such as alcoholics and residents of

skilled nursing facilities, and previously healthy individuals with acute but severe illnesses or trauma approach 50%. Colonization of the oropharynx by GNB among healthy persons undergoing elective surgical procedures rises from essentially zero to 35 to 50% within 24 hours following surgery. The organisms responsible for colonization vary from one study to another, but only rarely can this sudden acquisition of GNB be attributed to demonstrable environmental sources. Instead, colonization appears to be caused by a translocation of the patient's fecal flora or the transfer of organisms from one patient to another on the hands of personnel. However, the root cause of this colonization is the great susceptibility of ill patients to acquire GNB from the immediate environment.

Once established in the oropharynx, GNB multiply, achieve high concentrations in secretions, and are aspirated in small liquid boluses into the lungs (see Ch. 55). Since lung defenses are often impaired by the same underlying conditions that promote changes in cell resistance to adherence and colonization, the ability of the lungs to handle this bacterial inoculum is insufficient, and pneumonia results. The specific lung defense mechanism that might be impaired in a given patient varies with the nature of underlying illness. For example, patients with chronic airway obstruction have impaired mucociliary transport and alveolar hypoxia that hinders the effectiveness of phagocytic cells. Some data suggest that the bronchial abnormalities in these patients allow persistent colonization of the distal airways by potentially pathogenic bacteria, a factor that affords the bacteria the advantage of access to the distal lung. Patients who are neutropenic are remarkably predisposed to develop pneumonias with GNB, a clinical observation that correlates nicely with the experimental finding that swift recruitment of circulating neutrophils into the lungs is a crucial aspect of host defense against *Pseudomonas* infection. Alcoholism seems to predispose to GNB pneumonias in several ways. Malnutrition promotes colonization of the upper tract by GNB, aspiration is facilitated by episodes of impaired consciousness, and acute alcohol intoxication hinders the ability of phagocytes to migrate to the site of inflammation.

Of the many species of gram-negative aerobic bacilli that colonize human hosts, only *Haemophilus influenzae* can be classified as a true respiratory pathogen, if the ability of the organism to produce infections in previously normal individuals is accepted as a reasonable criterion of pathogenicity. All the others together, including Enterobacteriaceae (*Escherichia coli, Klebsiella, Enterobacter, Serratia,* and *Proteus*), *Pseudomonas,* and *Acinetobacter,* account for 10 to 20% of community-acquired pneumonias, and these occur almost exclusively in patients with serious underlying disease. The genus *Klebsiella* contains four species, of which only *K. pneumoniae* and *K. oxytoca* cause pneumonia; infections due to *K. pneumoniae* are by far the most common.

Pneumonia caused by *Klebsiella* has been held separate from that caused by other gram-negative bacilli largely for historical reasons. It was the first such organism to be recognized as a pulmonary pathogen, and the pneumonia it caused was distinct from that caused by the pneumococcus, especially in its lack of response to early forms of treatment and its predilection to cause upper lobe pneumonias in alcoholic men. However, the classic features of *Klebsiella* pneumonia as described in the earlier literature, such as "currant jelly" sputum (a mixture of blood and mucus), the bulging fissure associated with upper lobe consolidation, and the syndrome of "chronic cavitary pneumonia," are rarely observed today. While *Klebsiella* remains an important pulmonary pathogen, the illness it causes cannot be clinically differentiated from that caused by other aerobic gram-negative bacilli, and its treatment is similar.

CLINICAL MANIFESTATIONS. Pneumonias caused by GNB may be community acquired or hospital acquired (nosocomial). Virtually all patients with community-acquired pneumonias caused by GNB have serious underlying chronic illnesses, especially chronic obstructive pulmonary disease (COPD), alcoholism, or malignancy. Nosocomial pneumonias resulting from GNB occur principally in patients with severe, acute illnesses whether or not they have underlying chronic disease as well. Thus these infections are most likely to be found in postoperative patients or patients who require intensive care for other reasons. The clinical manifestations of infection are influenced by the nature of the associated processes.

Community-acquired gram-negative bacillary pneumonias share the common features of all bacterial pneumonias—fever, cough productive of purulent sputum, chest pain, and shortness of breath. The illness tends to be abrupt and associated with prominent systemic signs and symptoms, such as mental confusion, vomiting, and hypotension. Physical examination reveals rales in most patients, but the classic findings of dense consolidation are uncommon. Pleural effusion is present in 15 to 20% of patients. Radiographic infiltrates may involve any lobe and are bilateral in about one third of patients. Although cavitation is most likely to occur in pneumonia caused by *Klebsiella,* it also occurs commonly with *Pseudomonas* infections and occasionally with other organisms. Laboratory features include leukocytosis or leukopenia, either of which is characteristically associated with a marked left shift. Leukopenia is a poor prognostic sign.

Nosocomial pneumonia produced by GNB can be an explosive illness similar to the community-acquired form but frequently proceeds with a more indolent but seemingly inexorable course. Often the patient is in respiratory failure, intubated, and receiving mechanical ventilation. GNB are initially found colonizing the oropharynx, and over the subsequent few days appear in tracheal secretions, followed by increasing numbers of neutrophils. Finally, the patient becomes febrile and develops new radiographic infiltrates and worsening hypoxemia. Another common presentation is fever on the second or third postoperative day. Postoperative pneumonias are most common after lateral thoracotomies (especially combined thoracoabdominal procedures) and upper abdominal incisions. When nosocomial GNB pneumonia complicates the course of an already seriously ill patient, it is frequently associated with evidence of multiple organ failures.

DIAGNOSIS. Confirmation that GNB are responsible for pneumonia is a difficult clinical problem created largely by colonization of proximal airways by these organisms. Thus GNB are often present in the secretions of ill patients whether they have pneumonia or not and whether or not the GNB are the cause of pneumonia. Blood cultures are positive in 20 to 30% of patients with community-acquired infections but in as few as 8% of those with nosocomial pneumonias. Nevertheless, because the information gained from a positive blood culture regarding the causative organism and its antimicrobial susceptibility is so important in patient management, blood cultures should always be obtained when GNB pneumonia is suspected. Similarly, while pleural effusion is usually not present, the yield of positive cultures from such fluid when it is present is about 30%, and a diagnostic thoracentesis should be performed if a sufficient volume of fluid is identified radiographically.

The usefulness of invasive sampling remains somewhat controversial. Transthoracic needle aspiration is rarely used in critically ill patients because of concern about complications, especially pneumothorax. Sampling via the fiberoptic bronchoscope using either bronchoalveolar lavage (BAL) or the protected specimen brush (PSB) technique offers a safe alternative. Both techniques have been studied extensively and accurately portray the lung's bacterial flora in the absence of antibiotic therapy. Using a cutoff of at least 10^3 bacteria by PSB to diagnose infection, over 50% of patients suspected of having nosocomial pneumonia on the basis of new-onset fever, leukocytosis, and radiographic infiltrates have been shown not to be infected. However, in patients who have received prior antimicrobial therapy, both techniques lose sensitivity and, in some studies, specificity. BAL has the added advantage of providing specimens for special staining and cytology and is especially useful in the diagnosis of infections in immunocompromised hosts. Despite the ready availability of bronchoscopy, the etiology of nosocomial pneumonias is often frustratingly difficult to establish with certainty.

TREATMENT. Recommendations for the antimicrobial treatment of pneumonia due to GNB are changing rapidly as new drugs aimed at this group of organisms are entering clinical practice. It must be remembered that GNB are relatively poor respiratory pathogens and that patients susceptible to infection by them are at even greater risk of pulmonary infection by more virulent organisms, such as the pneumococcus, *Haemophilus,* and *Staphylococcus aureus.* Thus, despite the presence of GNB in sputum, initial treatment of these pneumonias—particularly those acquired outside the hospital or in the absence of concomitant antibiotic therapy—should include coverage of the usual respiratory pathogens.

TABLE 273–1. EMPIRICAL ANTIBIOTIC THERAPY OF AEROBIC GRAM-NEGATIVE BACILLARY PNEUMONIA

Combination Therapy

Cefuroxime 1.5 grams every 8 hours + gentamicin 1.5 mg/kg every 8 hours*

Cefotaxime 2 grams every 8 hours + gentamicin 1.5 mg/kg every 8 hours*

Piperacillin 4 grams every 6 hours + gentamicin 1.5 mg/kg every 8 hours*

Monotherapy

Cefotaxime 2 grams every 8 hours

Ticarcillin/clavulanate 3.1 grams every 6 hours

Piperacillin/tazobactam 4.5 grams every 6 hours

Imipenem/cilastatin 500 mg every 6 hours

High Likelihood of *Pseudomonas aeruginosa*

Ceftazadime 2 grams every 8 hours + amikacin 7.5 mg/kg every 12 hours*

Ticarcillin 3 grams every 4 hours + amikacin 7.5 mg/kg every 12 hours*

Imipenem/cilastatin 500 mg every 6 hours + amikacin 7.5 mg/kg every 12 hours*

* Recommendations for adults with normal renal function; serum levels should be monitored.

Table 273–1 provides therapeutic options for the patient with a pneumonia suspected to be of GNB etiology. Agents must be given parenterally and in adequate dosage. Traditionally, therapy has consisted of broad-spectrum combination antibiotic therapy with an aminoglycoside in conjunction with a β-lactam agent. The rationale behind this approach has been (1) the identification and susceptibility of the infecting organism are unknown, and two agents allow better coverage, (2) emergence of resistance may be prevented by combining antibiotics, and (3) additive or synergistic effects may result from a two-drug combination. There is increasing evidence that monotherapy with a third-generation cephalosporin, imipenem/cilastatin, or a drug combining a β-lactam antibiotic with a β-lactamase inhibitor, such as ticarcillin/clavulanate or piperacillin/tazobactam, may be as efficacious as combination therapy.

Treatment of nosocomial infection is often made more difficult by previous antimicrobial therapy, and drug susceptibility studies are critically important. However, empirical therapy usually must be initiated before the results of such studies are available. Factors to consider when selecting appropriate therapy include knowledge of local resistance patterns, previous culture results, and prior treatment. For example, resistance of *P. aeruginosa* to gentamicin may approach 50% in some hospitals. If *P. aeruginosa* is strongly suspected on the basis of previous cultures or the clinical setting (respiratory failure, neutropenia), a β-lactam agent with antipseudomonal activity should be combined with an aminoglycoside (see Table 273–1). Amikacin is often used in this setting because of less frequent resistance to this agent. Because the pharmacokinetics of aminoglycosides vary widely, adjustments in dosing must be determined from peak and trough serum levels in the individual patient. Improved clinical outcomes in the treatment of pneumonia caused by GNB have been associated with peak plasma levels of 6 μg per milliliter for gentamicin or tobramycin and 24 μg per milliliter for amikacin.

When the pathogenic organisms have been identified and the susceptibility patterns are known, modifications can be made to optimize antibiotic therapy. Ideally, antibiotics with the narrowest spectrum of activity, the least toxicity, and the best lung penetration should be chosen. In neutropenic patients and in seriously ill patients with pneumonia caused by resistant organisms such as *P. aeruginosa, Serratia marcescens,* and *Acinetobacter,* continued combination therapy with an appropriate β-lactam agent and an aminoglycoside is recommended. Duration of therapy should be based on clinical response, but a minimum of 2 to 3 weeks is usually required.

PROGNOSIS. The mortality of GNB pneumonias remains high—in the range of 30 to 50%. It has been argued that this is the result of the underlying disease usually present in patients who develop these pneumonias. This notion could lead to therapeutic nihilism. Other data clearly indicate that GNB pneumonias increase hospital mortality among patients who have nonlethal disease processes, a finding that would support an aggressive diagnostic and treatment approach. It is probable that both conclusions could be correct, depending on the population of patients studied. There is little doubt that GNB pneumonias represent the terminal event for a number of patients with irreversible and lethal diseases and that such patients form a large fraction of all hospital patients. On the other hand, there is reason to expect recovery rates of 80% or more among patients who develop GNB pneumonias in the context of acute, severe, but nonlethal disease processes, and in these patients, aggressive diagnostic maneuvers and intensive therapy are clearly indicated.

COMPLICATIONS. Pneumonias caused by GNB are more likely than other pneumonias to be complicated by one or another adverse event. Important complications include empyema, lung necrosis, superinfections, and multiple organ failure; metastatic seeding of infection to other sites is an uncommon complication.

Empyema occurs in perhaps as many as 30% of patients with GNB pneumonias. Criteria for the diagnosis of empyema, besides the presence of gross pus, include the presence of bacteria on Gram stain, a pleural fluid pH ≤ 7.2, or a pleural fluid white cell count $> 30,000$ per deciliter. Each of these criteria indicates a condition that is unlikely to respond to antimicrobials alone, but that usually requires drainage of the pleural space as well. Thus the term "complicated effusion" has gained favor over "empyema" to identify pleural fluid collections for which drainage needs to be considered. The occurrence of a complicated effusion generally prevents the recovery of the patient until it is recognized and effectively treated. Signs and symptoms of continuing illness, such as fever, persistent leukocytosis, and the onset of multiple organ failure, in a patient undergoing treatment for a GNB pneumonia should raise suspicion of a complicated effusion. If pleural fluid is identified on upright posteroanterior and lateral chest radiographs, thoracentesis should be performed; useful studies of the fluid obtained include measurements of pH and glucose, white cell count, Gram stain, and cultures for aerobic and anaerobic organisms.

If the fluid qualifies as a complicated effusion, most authorities recommend prompt placement of a thoracostomy tube and drainage. Alternative approaches, principally repeated thoracentesis, are less successful owing to loculation of the pleural space. Surgical drainage of the pleural space, using localized resection of an overlying rib with creation of a larger drainage tract, is reserved for patients who do not respond to tube drainage. Decortication of the pleura may be necessary if the clinical signs of uncontrolled infection are not ameliorated by simple drainage plus antimicrobial therapy. In such patients, radiographic evidence of effusion persists, along with continued fever and leukocytosis. At surgery, the pleural space is found to contain numerous loculated pockets of pus. The timing of intervention with these techniques requires excellent clinical judgment, because the patients are usually seriously ill and poor candidates for surgical treatment of any kind; on the other hand, they will not recover unless the pleural space is adequately drained.

Extensive lung necrosis has been termed "lung gangrene" because of the rapid occurrence of pulmonary cavitation associated with marked systemic toxicity and the appearance of extensive devitalization of lung tissue at necropsy. Occasionally, an entire lung appears to dissolve within a few days, leaving multiple cavities with air-fluid levels. This complication occurs with all of the common GNB, although perhaps more commonly in infections produced by *K. pneumoniae* and *P. aeruginosa*. Lung necrosis may be caused by the extracellular products of these organisms. *P. aeruginosa* makes a number of "virulence factors," including exotoxin A, exoenzyme S, elastase, and a neutral protease. However, *K. pneumoniae* makes none of these, and the propensity of this organism to cause lung necrosis remains unexplained.

Extensive lung necrosis may be followed by massive hemoptysis, continued suppuration because of inadequate drainage of the massively disrupted lung parenchyma, or bronchopleural fistula caused by extension of the necrotizing process through the pleura. The last must be promptly treated by placing a chest tube because of the attendant pneumothorax. However, the definitive treatment of extensive lung necrosis is surgical resection of the involved lobe or lobes. As with management of complicated effusion, the timing of such an intervention must be carefully considered in light of the control of the underlying infection, the severity of complicating problems (hemoptysis, air leak, and so on), and the patient's general condition.

Assessment of the patient with multiple organ failure in the context of a serious illness complicated by a GNB pneumonia is always difficult. The major question is usually whether a new complication such as oliguria is due to the underlying disease, to the current treatment, or to the infection. Each of the common manifestations of multiple organ dysfunction—altered liver function, acute renal failure, hematopoietic abnormalities, upper gastrointestinal bleeding, and altered mental state—may be multifactorial in etiology, and the antimicrobial agents used to treat GNB pneumonia may cause most of them. The guiding principles are to treat the infection aggressively and to correct life-threatening complications as they occur.

Superinfections may develop during the treatment of GNB pneumonia, just as GNB pneumonia may occur as a superinfection of a previous pneumonia. Unfortunately, treatment of the patient's pneumonia does not prevent colonization of the oropharynx and tracheobronchial tree by additional GNB or fungi. Thus the clinician is often faced with evaluating a new set of microorganisms recovered from the patient's secretions. The guiding principle here is to treat patients, not culture results. If the patient is responding well and appears to be improving, the new cultures can be disregarded for the time being. On the other hand, if the new cultural data correspond to a worsening clinical course, the process of evaluation and revision of treatment must be begun again.

Dever LL, Johanson WG Jr: Nosocomial pneumonia. *In* Simmons DH, Tierney DE (eds.): Current Pulmonology, vol. 13, St. Louis, Mosby–Year Book, 1992, pp 1–28. *This review provides a current bibliography of 140 references with sections on pathogenesis, diagnosis, etiologic agents, therapy, and prevention.*

Dotson RG, Pingleton SK: The effect of antibiotic therapy on recovery of intracellular bacteria from bronchoalveolar lavage in suspected ventilator-associated nosocomial pneumonia. Chest 103:541, 1993. *This article highlights the difficulty encountered when patients have received antibiotic therapy.*

Fagon J, Chastre J, Hance AJ, et al.: Nosocomial pneumonia in ventilated patients: A cohort study evaluating attributable mortality and hospital stay. Am J Med 94:281, 1993. *Whether patients die of nosocomial pneumonia or with it has been controversial. This study found that nosocomial GNB pneumonias added significantly to patient mortality and length of hospital stay.*

Kollef MH: Ventilator-associated pneumonia. JAMA 270:1965, 1993. *Understanding risk factors for pneumonia might lead to effective forms of prevention. This study examines risk factors in a large group of patients who developed pneumonia in a university ICU setting.*

274 ASPIRATION PNEUMONIA
Waldemar G. Johanson, Jr.

Categorization of the various syndromes associated with aspiration of liquids into the tracheobronchial tree is not an area distinguished by precise terminology or even consistency in the use of terms. Most of the important syndromes are dealt with elsewhere in this volume: gastric acid aspiration (see Ch. 54.2), anaerobic pneumonias and lung abscess (see Ch. 56), lipoid pneumonia (Ch. 60), and hydrocarbon aspiration (see Ch. 54.2). In this chapter we concentrate on an infrequent but difficult problem: that of recurrent bacterial pneumonias associated with aspiration. Such pneumonias are defined as recurring clinical illnesses characterized by fever, purulent sputum, and new radiographic infiltrates in the lungs in a patient with known or suspected chronic aspiration of oropharyngeal contents.

ETIOLOGY. Most patients afflicted with this problem have serious problems with swallowing for one or another reason. Common predisposing conditions are carcinoma of the esophagus with obstruction, tracheobronchial fistula (usually following treatment for cancer), and neurologic diseases affecting deglutition. Strokes are certainly the most common cause of the latter, but amyotrophic lateral sclerosis (including bulbar palsy), multiple sclerosis, and the myopathies may be responsible. Recurrent nocturnal aspiration of gastric contents by patients with esophageal reflux represents the one situation in which the swallowing mechanism may be intact in this syndrome.

Impaired swallowing having neural or myopathic causes is most pronounced when the patient attempts to swallow liquids. By contrast, dysphagia caused by obstruction is always worst with solid foods. Thus it is not surprising that the patient with myoneural deficits of the pharyngeal musculature repeatedly aspirates oropharyngeal secretions. In patients with esophageal obstruction, secretions accumulate proximal to the obstruction, especially at night, and are aspirated. Gastric contents are normally sterile. However, as the patient with reflux aspirates gastric contents, a certain volume of oropharyngeal secretions is necessarily carried along.

Oropharyngeal secretions are massively contaminated, containing 10^6 to 10^8 aerobic bacteria per milliliter and about 10 times as many anaerobic organisms. Although the majority of organisms composing the normal flora of this region have little invasiveness for the normal host, highly pathogenic organisms, including *Streptococcus pneumoniae, Staphylococcus aureus,* and *Haemophilus influenzae,* may be present in the secretions of normal people. Since most of the patients susceptible to recurrent aspiration have serious underlying diseases, their upper respiratory tracts are likely to be colonized by enteric gram-negative bacilli and *Pseudomonas* as well.

Normal individuals aspirate small volumes of oropharyngeal secretions during sleep but do not develop recurrent pneumonias. The difference between normal people and those who do develop recurrent pneumonias is probably the volume of material aspirated and the underlying chronic illnesses of the latter patients; differences in the bacterial flora of secretions may play a role as well.

CLINICAL MANIFESTATIONS. Episodes of recurrent pneumonia associated with aspiration tend not to be acute, fulminant illnesses but rather are characterized by progressive fever, purulent sputum production, shortness of breath, and systemic symptoms (such as loss of appetite and malaise) over a period of days. The frequency of such episodes in an individual prone to recurrent aspiration varies widely. In patients with tracheobronchial fistulas, the episodes are essentially continuous until an effective preventive measure can be implemented or the patient dies. By contrast, patients with esophageal reflux may go years between episodes. The frequency of episodes is usually directly related to the frequency and volume of material aspirated and thus is increased in conditions in which aspiration is a daily event, especially if coupled with a decreased level of awareness, as occurs in some patients following strokes.

Physical findings include those related to the underlying illness and the presence of coarse rhonchi over dependent lung zones. Rales and signs of consolidation may or may not be present. Fever and leukocytosis are regularly present. Radiographs of the chest reveal infiltrates of varying intensity, with a preponderance of change in the dependent zones, i.e., posterior aspects of the lower lobes and posterior segments of the upper lobes. Pleural effusion is uncommon unless anaerobic infection is present.

DIAGNOSIS. Examination of expectorated sputum helps confirm the suspicion of aspiration pneumonia but is of little help in defining a specific bacterial etiology. Typically, the sputum of such patients is intensely purulent, with a wide spectrum of bacterial forms present on Gram stain. Culture of this material yields the same flora as in upper respiratory secretions, and the clinical problem consists of trying to discern which of several pathogenic organisms should be treated. Cultures should be obtained, however, since knowledge of the sensitivity of the organisms present may be needed to guide therapy. Blood cultures are rarely positive. The presence of food particles in tracheal secretions is clear evidence of aspiration. In patients receiving enteral feedings, the presence of glucose in secretions may be demonstrable by bedside tests. Since normal secretions contain an undetectable level of glucose, a positive result is highly specific for aspiration. Dietary lipids form large intracellular deposits when ingested by phagocytic cells, and examination of sputum with a lipid stain may confirm the clinical impression of chronic aspiration. The microscopic appearance of the large lipid deposits is important in differentiating this type of lipid inclusion from the foamy deposit that occurs in macrophages owing to the accumulation of endogenous lipid distal to an obstructing lesion in the airways.

When the diagnosis of recurrent aspiration is in doubt, cineradiographic studies of the patient swallowing a thin, water-soluble contrast material is usually definitive. Thick barium should be avoided because aspiration of this material compounds the patient's problems and a thick solution is less likely to identify the swallowing difficulty. In questionable cases, the procedure may need to be repeated with the patient in the supine position. Follow-up films of the chest reveal the presence of contrast material in the airways.

Patients with infrequent episodes of recurrent pneumonia caused by esophageal reflux and nocturnal aspiration represent a somewhat different problem. The presence of a hiatus hernia or the demonstration of reflux during an upper gastrointestinal contrast study does not necessarily prove that pneumonia was caused by this mechanism, although that would be a reasonable presumption if other aspects of the patient's presentation were compatible with the diagnosis. One diagnostic test in uncertain circumstances is to monitor the pH in the upper esophagus during sleep. Reflux into the upper esophagus is marked by a sudden fall in pH, an event that is easily captured on a long-term strip chart recorder for review the next morning. Recent refinements in technique have improved the sensitivity of radioisotopic methods, which may become the diagnostic procedure of choice.

TREATMENT. Initial antibiotic therapy should provide coverage for gram-positive and gram-negative organisms as well as anaerobes. Pending the results of culture and susceptibility studies, empirical therapy with intravenous penicillin or clindamycin and an aminoglycoside is reasonable. Alternatively, monotherapy with a second- or third-generation cephalosporin, imipenem, or a drug combining a β-lactam antibiotic with a β-lactamase inhibitor such as ampicillin-sulbactam, ticarcillin-clavulanate, or piperacillin-tazobactam can be used. Supportive care, including aggressive tracheobronchial toilet, is required. Nutrition must not be overlooked despite the difficulties encountered in many of these patients. If swallowing is impossible and a small feeding tube cannot be placed in the intestinal tract via the nose or mouth, parenteral nutrition should be provided while a long-term solution to the patient's problem is sought. Failure to address the nutritional deficits of these patients is a common cause of protracted and often lethal complications.

Surgical intervention to prevent esophageal reflux is indicated for the patient in whom recurrent pneumonia can be reasonably attributed to this mechanism. Long-term solutions for the other patients with this syndrome often involve difficult choices. Bypassing the mouth to facilitate feeding can be accomplished with a feeding gastrostomy or enterostomy. The former can be performed noninvasively via fiberoptic gastroscopy, with the feeding tube being passed percutaneously into the stomach. In some patients, cessation of swallowing food diminishes the frequency and severity of aspiration and successfully ameliorates the clinical problem. However, in many it does not because patients must still handle their own secretions. Drug therapy aimed at reducing the volume of secretions in this situation is usually not successful. The only certain preventive measure is tracheostomy with all its complications. Even tracheostomy does not negate the possibility of aspiration around the tube unless the larynx is removed or the vocal cords are sewn together. The latter can be undone at a later date if the patient's condition improves. These procedures should not be contemplated in all patients with the syndrome of recurrent aspiration, since many patients have underlying conditions that will be lethal in a short time. However, if the patient has a reasonable chance of long-term survival in the absence of recurrent episodes of pneumonia, these steps should be considered.

Johnson ER, McKenzie SW, Sievers A: Aspiration pneumonia in stroke. Arch Phys Med Rehabil 74:973, 1993. *This study found that nearly 50% of stroke victims with dysphagia developed aspiration pneumonia within the first year. Pharyngeal transit time, as assessed by videofluoroscopy, was the best predictor of the subsequent development of pneumonia.*

Ruth M, Carlsson S, Mansson I, et al.: Scintigraphic detection of gastropulmonary aspiration in patients with respiratory disorders. Clin Physiol 13:19, 1993. *This carefully done study examined and corrected for artifacts produced by instilling radiolabeled materials into the stomach and demonstrated that aspiration could be detected in 20% of patients with a variety of pulmonary complaints, including asthma, chronic laryngitis, and recurrent infections. If properly controlled, this technique may be the method of choice for demonstrating aspiration because it is easily tolerated by patients.*

Torres A, Serra-Batlles J, Ros E, et al.: Pulmonary aspiration of gastric contents in patients receiving mechanical ventilation: The effect of body position. Ann Intern Med 116:540, 1992. *Aspiration occurs regularly in intubated patients receiving mechanical ventilation and is associated with the development of nosocomial pneumonia. Not surprisingly, nursing the patient supine, as contrasted with semirecumbent, promotes aspiration.*

275 LEGIONELLOSIS

Paul H. Edelstein

DEFINITION. "Legionellosis" is the term used to describe infections caused by bacteria of the genus *Legionella*. The most important of these diseases is pneumonia, called "legionnaires' disease." Either as part of legionnaires' disease or distinct from it, the legionellae may cause infections elsewhere in the body, usually in the form of abscesses. Pontiac fever, which is a self-limited mild febrile illness, is assumed to be caused by legionellae, although this is unproven.

HISTORY. Legionnaires' disease was first recognized when it caused epidemic pneumonia among members of the American Legion attending a convention in Philadelphia in 1976; this resulted in 29 deaths and in 182 cases of pneumonia. Charles McDade and William Shepard, of the United States Centers for Disease Control and Prevention, determined that this disease was caused by an ostensibly newly discovered bacterium, which was named *Legionella pneumophila*. Neither the disease nor the bacterium is new. The first documented epidemic of legionnaires' disease occurred in a meat packing plant in Minnesota in 1957, and the first recorded isolation of the bacterium was in 1943. In fact, three different *Legionella* species had been isolated from humans prior to 1976, although they were thought to be rickettsia-like agents. Several unsolved epidemics of pneumonia, including one in Philadelphia in 1974, were recognized to have been due to legionnaires' disease.

BACTERIOLOGY. Thirty-nine *Legionella* species have been recognized to date. About half of these have been isolated from patients with legionnaires' disease, and about half have been isolated only from the environment. The species that most commonly cause disease are *L. pneumophila*, *L. micdadei*, *L. bozemanii*, *L. dumoffii*, and *L. longbeachae*. Fifteen serogroups are recognized for *L. pneumophila*, while several other species contain up to two serogroups. *L. pneumophila* serogroup 1 causes up to 90% of cases of legionnaires' disease in nonimmunocompromised individuals. *L. micdadei* is probably the second most common cause of legionnaires' disease and commonly causes legionnaires' disease in immunocompromised patients.

The legionellae are small, gram-negative, obligately aerobic bacilli. *Legionella* requires complex growth media, having an absolute nutritional requirement for L-cysteine. Optimal growth occurs on a buffered charcoal yeast extract medium supplemented with iron, L-cysteine, and α-ketoglutarate (BCYEα). These bacteria do not grow on conventional bacteriologic media, such as tryptic soy blood agar, MacConkey's agar, or unsupplemented chocolate agar. Their usual habitat is natural and treated waters, such as lakes, ponds, and tap water. Legionellae are found in highest concentration in warm water, especially in water heaters, hot water plumbing fixtures, and cooling towers. They appear to be obligate or facultative parasites of freshwater amoebae, such as *Hartmannella* and *Acanthamoeba*. Humans are very likely accidental hosts of these bacteria.

Virulence factors have been examined for relatively few strains each of *L. pneumophila* and *L. micdadei* and are not well understood. The bacteria produce endotoxins and exotoxins, which may cause tissue damage independently or in concert with the host immune system.

PATHOGENESIS. Legionnaires' disease is acquired by inhaling aerosolized water containing *Legionella* organisms or possibly by pulmonary aspiration of contaminated water. The contaminated aerosols are derived from humidifiers, shower heads, respiratory therapy equipment, industrial cooling water, and cooling towers. Aerosols formed by contaminated water in plumbing systems and in cooling towers are the most common sources of infection. Inhaled organisms are phagocytosed by pulmonary alveolar macrophages, which are unable to kill the bacteria. The bacteria multiply within the phagosome. Eventually, the multiplying bacteria, which produce cytotoxins, kill the macrophage and are released extracellularly. The intracellular infection cycle is reinitiated in another macrophage. Continuing bacterial multiplication and consequent lung damage produce symptoms 2 to 14 days after initiation of infection.

Bacterial uptake and multiplication are curtailed by the action of cytokines (e.g., γ-interferon), which are produced by macrophages and lymphocytes. Natural killer and lymphokine-activated killer cells probably lyse infected macrophages, aborting the intracellular infection cycle. The role of polymorphonuclear phagocytes is unclear, although they probably have some part in eliminating bacteria, especially after activation by interleukin-2 and tumor necrosis factor. Antibody appears to have little function in host immunity or defense, whereas T lymphocytes play a major role in the immune process. The actual mechanism of pulmonary damage is not well understood and could be due to bacterial toxins, immune reactions to infection, or both. The bacteria may spread to extrapulmonary sites via the lymphatic system and bloodstream; they are likely transported in the blood by infected blood mononuclear cells. The mechanism whereby the pneumonia exerts systemic effects is unknown but could be the result of disseminated bacterial infection, the effect of toxin, or the production of host factors such as tumor necrosis factor.

The pathogenesis of Pontiac fever is a mystery. Inhalation of water contaminated with many different types of bacteria, including *Legionella* species, produces the disease. The incubation period of the disease, 12 to 36 hours, is too short to allow for bacterial infection and multiplication. It is possible that bacterial or fungal toxins present in the water produce this illness, as has been hypothesized for a closely related disease, "humidifier fever." Another possibility is an immune response to one or more of the multiple microorganisms found in the water. Antibody to *Legionella* species found in the contaminated water is present in most disease victims, but it is unclear what this means.

EPIDEMIOLOGY. Legionnaires' disease occurs worldwide but is primarily a disease found in technically advanced countries. Case reports from underdeveloped countries are rare, perhaps because of limited diagnostic facilities and also perhaps because of the infrequent use of air conditioning and complex plumbing systems. Normal children have this disease very rarely. Cigarette smokers, especially those 50 years of age or older, are at increased risk. The presence of chronic lung or heart disease may also increase risk. Glucocorticosteroid administration or its endogenous production is the major risk factor for legionnaires' disease. OKT3 administration also may predispose to this illness, but cyclosporine administration probably does not. Administration of cytotoxic agents is not a risk factor, nor are hematologic malignancies (except hairy cell leukemia) or neutropenia in the absence of glucocorticoid administration. Patients with the acquired immunodeficiency syndrome (AIDS) are at increased risk, although legionnaires' disease is an uncommon disease in such patients. Patients in the immediate postoperative period are at increased risk of acquiring legionnaires' disease, because of inhalation of contaminated water aerosols during anesthesia, transient paralysis of local lung defenses, or both. Males get legionnaires' disease about twice as often as females, although this does not hold true for several epidemics of legionnaires' disease. No good evidence exists for person-to-person spread of legionnaires' disease.

Legionnaires' disease may occur in epidemics originating in a single building or area. Outbreaks of the disease have occurred among hotel guests, hospital inpatients and outpatients, office building workers, and factory workers. There appears to be little, if any, increased risk of disease acquisition among people with occupational water exposure. The majority of Legionnaires' disease cases are nonepidemic in nature. Of these, perhaps 10% may be acquired in the home and the remainder through other exposures.

It is estimated that from 1 to 5% of all pneumonias in adults are due to legionnaires' disease. In some geographic regions, community-acquired legionnaires' disease is more common, with average prevalence rates of 10 to 20% of all pneumonias. When the disease occurs in endemic or epidemic nosocomial form, 1% to as many as 20% of hospitalized patients with pneumonia have this disease.

Pontiac fever has been recognized primarily as an epidemic illness, with attack rates in excess of 90%. It has been noted to occur in office and factory workers and in recreational bathers using spa or Jacuzzi-type baths. The disease very likely has a sporadic form, but the lack of specific diagnostic tests makes diagnosing this form very difficult.

TABLE 275–1. EXTRAPULMONARY INFECTIONS CAUSED BY *LEGIONELLA*

Dialysis shunt infection
Sinusitis
Pericarditis
Prosthetic valve endocarditis
Peritonitis
Abscesses
    Skin
    Brain
    Bowel
    Rectum
    Kidney
    Myocardium

PATHOLOGY. Specific pathologic changes are found only in the lung in the vast majority of fatal cases of legionnaires' disease. Intense inflammation is present in the alveolus, alveolar ducts, respiratory bronchioles, and alveolar septa. The inflammatory process consists of bacteria, polymorphonuclear leukocytes, and macrophages. On occasion, pleuritis, pleural empyema, pericarditis, and cavitary lung disease are found. Very rarely, abscess formation occurs outside the chest cavity.

CLINICAL PRESENTATION. Legionnaires' disease manifests as a febrile systemic illness with pneumonia. Several prospective and retrospective studies of patients with different types of pneumonia have shown that legionnaires' disease has few, if any, characteristic clinical features and that it cannot be distinguished clinically from pneumococcal pneumonia. However, clinical observations during epidemics of legionnaires' disease have often documented characteristic clinical findings. It is probable that the spectrum of clinical presentations is wide, ranging from a "typical" form of legionnaires' disease to one indistinguishable from other causes of pneumonia. This chapter describes the "typical" form of legionnaires' disease, which in reality may be present in the minority of patients. A prodromal illness consisting of malaise, low-grade fever, and anorexia may develop several days before the onset of more severe symptoms. Myalgia, extreme fatigue, and high fever then develop. Gastrointestinal complaints are common, such as generalized or localized abdominal pain, nausea, vomiting, and diarrhea; the diarrhea is generally watery and not dehydrating. Recurrent rigors and prostration may occur. Symptoms referable to the respiratory tract may not develop until later. It is this paucity of respiratory tract symptoms, despite evidence of a systemic febrile illness, that can either be a clue to diagnosis or mislead clinicians. When the patient is pressed for details regarding symptoms, a history of a nonproductive cough, or one productive of nonpurulent, sometimes bloody, secretions, is usually obtained. Production of large amounts of grossly purulent sputum is unusual. Pleuritic chest pain, sometimes in concert with hemoptysis, is present and may mislead the clinician into considering pulmonary infarction. Mental confusion is reported commonly in some series; obtundation, seizures, and focal neurologic findings may also occur less frequently.

Fever is almost uniformly present in cases of legionnaires' disease, although there are reports of short (days) afebrile periods in some immunosuppressed patients with *L. micdadei* pneumonia. Chest examination early in the disease may reveal only scattered rales or evidence of pleural effusion. However, later in the course, most patients have classic findings of consolidating pneumonia. Abdominal examination may reveal generalized or local tenderness and, in rare cases, evidence of peritonitis. Splenomegaly is uncommon. Findings of pericarditis, myocarditis, and focal abscesses are rare. No rash is associated with this disease, except that caused by other factors, such as drug therapy.

The fatality rate of untreated legionnaires' disease is about 3 to 30% in nonimmunosuppressed patients and up to 80% in immunocompromised ones. The majority of previously healthy people recover from untreated legionnaires' disease after 7 to 10 days of severe illness; those who do not recover die of progressive respiratory and multisystem failure.

Clinically significant extrapulmonary infection in patients with legionnaires' disease is quite rare (Table 275–1).

Pontiac fever is a nonfatal influenza-like disease, with symptoms of myalgia, fever, headache, and malaise occurring in 60 to 90% of patients. Arthralgia occurs with variable frequency, as do cough, anorexia, and abdominal pain. The illness is generally not severe enough nor long enough in duration to cause most patients to seek medical attention. Not much is known about physical findings early in the disease; findings after 3 to 5 days of illness are generally normal except for fever and possibly tachypnea. Pneumonia does not occur. The illness lasts about 3 to 5 days, although some patients may have persistent fatigue or nonfocal neurologic complaints for weeks to months afterward.

CHEST ROENTGENOGRAPHIC FINDINGS. Legionnaires' disease causes alveolar filling infiltrates that usually eventuate in consolidation. Interstitial infiltrates are rare, although they may occur early in the course of disease and then progress to consolidating infiltrates. The infiltrates may be unilateral or bilateral and can spread very quickly to involve the entire lung. Pleural effusion, usually small in volume, occurs commonly and may be the sole abnormal radiographic finding in early disease.

DIAGNOSIS. The results of multiple nonspecific laboratory tests may be abnormal in patients with legionnaires' disease. These abnormal findings include proteinuria, pyuria, hematuria, leukocytosis, leukopenia, and thrombocytopenia. Disseminated intravascular coagulation may be seen in patients with respiratory failure caused by legionnaires' disease. Hyponatremia, hypophosphatemia, hyperbilirubinemia, and elevated serum alanine transaminase (ALT), serum aspartate transaminase (AST), and alkaline phosphatase concentrations may also be found. Elevation of creatine kinase (MM

TABLE 275–2. SPECIFIC DIAGNOSTIC TESTS FOR *LEGIONELLA*

Type	Suitable Specimens	Sensitivity* (%)	Specificity (%)	Notes
Culture	Sputum, lung, pleural fluid, blood, abscess contents	—	100	Use of special and selective media required; 3 to 5 days required for growth
Immunofluorescent microscopy	Sputum, lung, pleural fluid, abscess contents	25–75	95–99.9	Species-specific monoclonal antibody available; not helpful for diagnosis of all species; highest specificity for *L. pneumophila;* relatively low specificity for other species; 2 to 3 hours required for testing
DNA probe	Sputum, lung	50–60	99.1–99.9	Genus specific; may have lower sensitivity for detection of some species and for detection of organism in pleural fluid and transtracheal aspirates; 2 to 3 hours required for testing
Urine radioimmunoassay (RIA)	Urine	90–95	99.9	Useful only for detection of *L. pneumophila* serogroup 1, the most common cause of legionnaires' disease; 2 to 3 hours required for testing
Antibody	Serum	60–70	90–99	Requires testing of paired specimens; seroconversion may not occur until 2 to 3 months after infection; most specific for *L. pneumophila* serogroup 1; cross-reactions e.g., with antibodies to many other bacteria.

* Sensitivity versus culture. Culture is the most sensitive diagnostic technique, but its absolute sensitivity is unknown; reasonable estimates are 80 to 90%.

TABLE 275–3. ANTIMICROBIAL DRUG THERAPY OF LEGIONNAIRES' DISEASE*

Drug	Route	Dosage	Duration (days)
First choice			
Erythromycin ± rifampin	Oral	500 mg four times daily	14–21
	IV	500 mg to 1 gram every 6 hours	
Second choices			
Azithromycin	Oral	500 mg daily	3–5
or			
Clarithromycin	Oral	500 mg twice daily	10–14
or			
Ciprofloxacin	Oral	500 mg twice daily	10–14
	IV	400 mg every 12 hours	
or			
Ofloxacin	Oral or IV	500 mg twice daily	10–14
or			
Doxycycline ± rifampin	Oral or IV	200 mg load, then 100 mg twice daily	14–21
or			
Cotrimoxazole ± rifampin	Oral or IV	5 mg per kilogram of trimethoprim three times daily	14–21
Rifampin†	Oral or IV	600 mg twice daily	3–5

* Only erythromycin is FDA-approved for the treatment of legionnaires' disease.
† Rifampin is administered only in combination with another antimicrobial agent.

isoenzyme) is common, and some patients develop myoglobinuria and renal failure. The cerebrospinal fluid is usually normal, although rare patients may have 25 to 100 white blood cells per microliter of cerebrospinal fluid.

Legionnaires' disease can be diagnosed using specific laboratory tests (Table 275–2). The most sensitive and specific test is culture of respiratory tract secretions, such as sputum. Sputum culture for *Legionella* should be performed on every patient suspected of having this disease. Serologic testing is more useful to epidemiologists than to clinicians, because of cross-reactions with antibodies to unrelated organisms. No laboratory test currently available is 100% accurate for the diagnosis of legionnaires' disease. Thus empirical therapy must be considered in appropriate clinical settings.

The diagnosis of Pontiac fever is based on demonstration of legionellae in water to which the patient was exposed, significant increases in antibody to the isolated *Legionella* species, and a clinical course compatible with this diagnosis. To be certain about the diagnosis of Pontiac fever, it is almost always necessary to perform extensive studies of unaffected people and their environments. This is so because recovery of legionellae from water and the elevation of antibodies to *Legionella* are relatively common events. Thus it is nearly impossible to diagnose nonepidemic cases of Pontiac fever specifically.

The differential diagnosis of legionnaires' disease is broad, since the disease usually presents as a nonspecific pneumonia. Mycoplasmal pneumonia is generally much less severe and causes significant respiratory system complaints. Pneumococcal pneumonia, in contrast to legionnaires' disease, is usually penicillin-responsive. Psittacosis and Q fever can have clinical presentations quite similar to that of legionnaires' disease.

THERAPY. Erythromycin (Table 275–3) is considered the drug of choice for this disease on the basis of retrospective studies, which show that the case-fatality rate is lowered about fivefold by prompt administration of erythromycin. Alternative drugs are listed in Table 275–3; there is not substantial clinical experience with any of these drugs. Intravenous drug therapy should be given until there is clinical improvement, which usually occurs in 2 to 4 days. After this, oral drug therapy is continued. Mild cases of legionnaires' disease can be treated with oral therapy exclusively. Quinolone antimicrobials (ciprofloxacin, ofloxacin) and the newer macrolide antimicrobials (azithromycin, clarithromycin) are more effective than are erythromycin, doxycycline, or cotrimoxazole (Septra or Bactrim) in experimental laboratory studies; with further clinical experience

they will likely become the drugs of choice. The quinolone drugs are preferred for organ transplant patients because of their lack of interference with cyclosporine levels. Because of its potent activity in experimental legionnaires' disease, many clinicians add rifampin for treatment of severe cases of legionnaires' disease. There are no clinical data indicating the superiority of such combination therapy. Penicillins, cephalosporins (first, second, and third generation), and aminoglycosides are ineffective for the therapy of legionnaires' disease. In fact, the failure of pneumonia to respond to these agents should prompt consideration of legionnaires' disease and perhaps initiation of erythromycin therapy. No effective therapy for Pontiac fever is known.

Most patients with legionnaires' disease respond within 1 to 4 days to specific antimicrobial therapy. The symptoms clearing most rapidly are rigors, mental confusion, myalgia, anorexia, fatigue, and abdominal complaints. Fever may persist for a week after initiation of therapy but starts a downward trend within a few days. Despite this clinical evidence of improvement, other findings may falsely imply disease progression, such as evidence of increased pulmonary consolidation on physical examination and on roentgenography. Weeks to months are required for the resolution of pulmonary infiltrates. Patients with respiratory failure have a relatively poor prognosis and tend to have a much slower response to therapy.

Barbaree JM, Breiman RF, Dufour AP (eds.): *Legionella:* Current Status and Emerging Perspectives. American Society for Microbiology, Washington, D.C. 1993. *Comprehensive reviews and experimental reports from a recent international meeting.*
Edelstein PH: Legionnaires' disease. Clin Infect Dis 16:741, 1993. *More extensive discussion of treatment and clinical diagnosis.*
Fang GD, Fine M, Orloff J, et al.: New and emerging etiologies for community-acquired pneumonia with implications for therapy: A prospective multicenter study of 359 cases. Medicine 69:307, 1990. *Excellent survey of community-acquired pneumonia, including legionnaires' disease.*

276 STREPTOCOCCAL INFECTIONS

Dennis L. Stevens

CLASSIFICATION AND IDENTIFICATION OF STREPTOCOCCI

Streptococci are gram-positive globular or coccoid bacteria that grow in chains. Streptococci colonize the mucous membranes of animals, produce catalase, and may be aerobic, anaerobic, or facultative. Streptococci require complex media containing blood products for optimal growth. On blood agar plates, streptococci may cause complete (β), incomplete (α) or no hemolysis (γ). The exhaustive work of Rebecca Lancefield has allowed hemolytic streptococci to be classified into types A through O based on acid-extractable antigens of cell wall material. Availability of rapid latex agglutination kits provides even small clinical laboratories with the means to identify streptococci according to Lancefield group. Bacitracin susceptibility, bile esculin hydrolysis, and the CAMP test (flame-type synergistic hemolysis on a *Staphylococcus aureus* blood agar streak) are useful presumptive tests for classifying groups A, D, or B streptococci, respectively. Modern schemes of classification of hemolytic and nonhemolytic streptococci use complex biochemical and genetic techniques.

GROUP A STREPTOCOCCAL INFECTIONS

EPIDEMIOLOGY. *Host Range.* The concept of group A streptococcus as a pure human pathogen is supported by the observations that (1) natural group A streptococcus infection in animals is rare; (2) laboratory animals are not useful models of streptococcal pharyngitis, scarlet fever, erysipelas, rheumatic fever, or poststreptococcal glomerulonephritis; (3) the inoculum needed to cause infection in laboratory animals is orders of magnitude greater than that estimated to cause infection in humans; and (4) streptococci have developed highly sophisticated defensive molecules which bind, inactivate, or destroy human immune response molecules (e.g., IgG antibody and complement [C5a]).

Age-Related Attack Rates. All group A streptococcal infections have the highest incidence in children younger than age 10. The asymptomatic prevalence is also higher (15 to 20%) in children compared with adults (< 5%). Age is not the only factor, because crowded conditions in temperate climates during the winter months are associated with epidemics of pharyngitis in school children as well as military recruits. Impetigo is most common in children from ages 2 to 5 and may occur year-round in tropical areas but largely in the summer in temperate climates. Similarly, 90% of cases of scarlet fever occur in children 2 to 8 years and, like pharyngitis, is most common in temperate regions during winter. An experiment of nature in the Faeroe Islands (Denmark) suggested that susceptibility to scarlet fever is not dependent on young age *per se*. Briefly, scarlet fever had disappeared from that isolated island group for several decades until it was reintroduced by a visitor with unsuspected scarlet fever. An epidemic of scarlet fever ensued, with significant attack rates in all age groups, suggesting that other factors, such as the lack of protective antibody against scarlatina toxin or the introduction of a new strain, rather than age predisposed those individuals to clinical illness.

In contrast to pharyngitis, impetigo, and scarlet fever, bacteremia has had the highest age-specific attack rate in the elderly and in neonates. Between 1986 and 1988, the prevalence of bacteremia increased 800 to 1000% in adolescents and adults in Western countries. Although some of this increase is attributable to intravenous drug abuse and puerperal sepsis, most of the increase is due to cases of streptococcal toxic shock syndrome (strepTSS).

Transmission of Group A Streptococcus. Human mucous membranes and skin serve as the natural reservoirs of *S. pyogenes.* Pharyngeal and cutaneous acquisition is by person-to-person spread via aerosolized microdroplets or direct contact, respectively. Epidemics of pharyngitis and scarlet fever also have occurred after consumption of contaminated nonpasteurized milk or food. Epidemics of impetigo have been reported, particularly in tropical areas, in day care centers, and among underprivileged children. Group A streptococcal infections in hospitalized patients occur during childbirth (puerperal sepsis), times of war (epidemic gangrene), surgical convalescence (surgical wound infection, surgical scarlet fever), or as a result of burns (burn wound sepsis). Thus, in most clinical streptococcal infections, the mode of transmission and portal of entry are easily ascertained. In contrast, among patients with strepTSS, the portal of entry is obvious in only 50% of cases.

PATHOGENESIS. Adherence of cocci to the mucosal epithelium is necessary but not sufficient to cause disease in all cases, since prolonged asymptomatic carriage is well documented. Complex interactions between host epithelium and streptococcal factors such as M-protein, lipoteichoic acid (LTA), and fimbriae are necessary for adherence. Fibronectin-binding protein (protein F) also contributes to adherence, because protein F–deficient mutants are incapable of binding to epithelial cells.

Within the tissues, streptococci may evade opsonophagocytosis by destroying or inactivating complement-derived chemoattractants and opsonins (C5a peptidase) and by binding immunoglobulins. Expression of M-protein, in the absence of type-specific antibody, also protects the organism from phagocytosis by polymorphonuclear leukocytes (PMN's) and monocytes. In tissues, streptolysin O (SLO) secreted in high concentration destroys approaching phagocytes. Distal to the focus of infection, lower concentrations of SLO stimulate PMN adhesion to endothelial cells, effectively preventing continued granulocyte migration and promoting vascular damage. In the nonimmune host, SLO, streptococcal pyrogenic exotoxin (SPE) type A, and other streptococcal components stimulate host cells to produce tumor necrosis factor (TNF) and interleukin-1 (IL-1), cytokines that mediate hypotension and stimulate leukostasis, resulting in shock, microvascular injury, multiorgan failure, and if excessive, death. A unique feature of the pyrogenic exotoxins and some M-protein fragments is their ability to interact with certain V_β regions of the T cell receptor in the absence of classic antigen processing by antigen-presenting cells (Fig. 276–1). This results in massive clonal proliferation of T lymphocytes. SPE type B is related to the proteinase precursor and may play a role in the pathogenesis of necrotizing fasciitis and myositis and may contribute to shock in

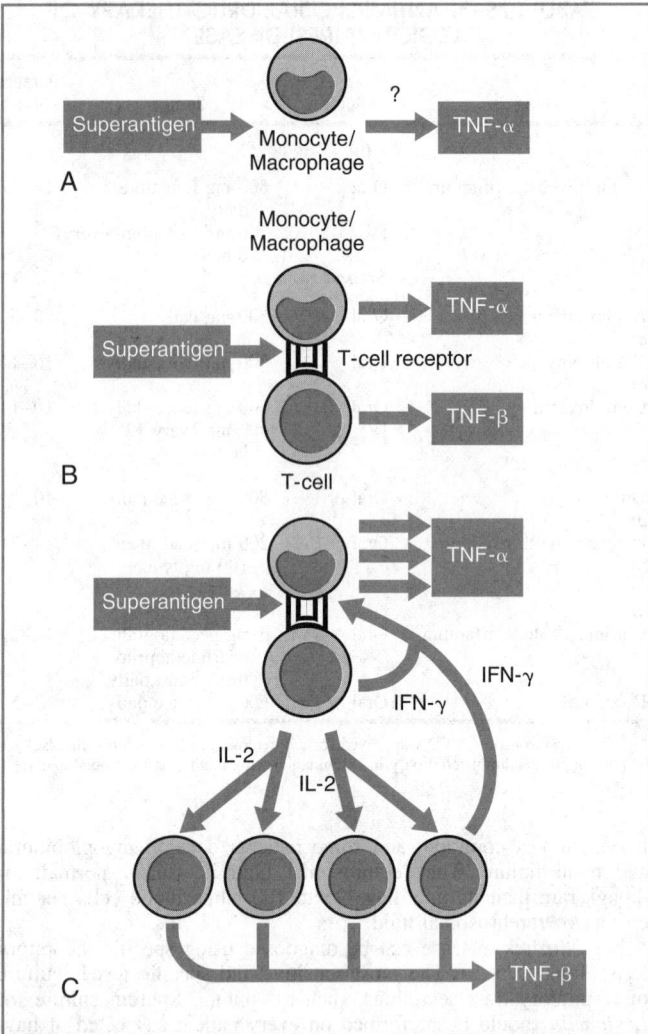

FIGURE 276–1. Superantigen-induced production of tumor necrosis factor-α (TNF-α) and lymphotoxin (TNF-β) by periperal blood mononuclear cells. *A,* Superantigens induce human monocytes to produce TNF-α; however, it is unclear whether such production results solely from direct stimulation of the monocyte by the superantigen. *B,* In mixed mononuclear cell populations, superantigens stimulate TNF-α synthesis in monocytes and, by binding to specific V_β regions of the T cell receptor, induce synthesis of lymphotoxin (TNF-β) from T cells. *C,* The T cell response to superantigen stimulation includes production of interleukin-2 (IL-2), resulting in clonal proliferation with concordant production of interferon-gamma (IFN-γ) and TNF-β. IFN-γ can then amplify monocyte synthesis of TNF-α, IL-1, and IL-6. (From Stevens DL, Bryant AE, Hackett SP: Sepsis syndromes and toxic shock syndromes: Concepts in pathogenesis and a perspective of future strategy. Current Opin Infectious Dis 6:374, 1993.)

strepTSS through its ability to cleave pre-IL-1β into active IL-1β. Thus, in strepTSS, lymphokines such as TNF-β, interferon-γ, and IL-2 may be crucial in the mediation of shock and microvascular injury.

BACTERIAL CELL STRUCTURE AND EXTRACELLULAR PRODUCTS. Capsule. Some strains of *S. pyogenes* possess luxuriant capsules of hyaluronic acid, resulting in large mucoid colonies on blood agar. Luxuriant production of M-protein also may impart a mucoid colony morphology, and this trait has been associated with M-18.

Cell Wall. The cell wall is composed of a peptidoglycan backbone with integral LTA components. The function of LTA is not well known, but both peptidoglycan and LTA have important interactions with the host.

M-Proteins. Over 80 different M-protein types of group A streptococci are currently described. The protein is a coiled coil consisting of four regions of repeating amino acids (A–D), a proline/glycine-rich region that serves to intercalate the protein into the bacterial cell wall, and a hydrophobic region that acts as a membrane anchor. Region A near the *N* terminus is highly variable, and antibodies to this region confer type-specific protection. Within the more conserved B–D regions lies an area that binds one of the complement regulatory proteins (factor H), stearically inhibiting antibody binding and complement-derived opsonin deposition and effectively camouflaging the organism against humoral immune surveillance. M-protein inhibits the phagocytosis of *S. pyogenes* by PMN's, though this property can be overcome by type-specific antisera. Observations by Lancefield suggest that the quantity of M-protein produced decreases with passage on artificial media and conversely increases rapidly with passage through mice. The quantity of M-protein produced by an infecting strain progressively decreases during convalescence and during prolonged carriage.

Streptolysin O. Streptolysin O (SLO) belongs to a family of oxygen-labile, thiol-activated cytolysins (TAC) and causes the broad zone of β hemolysis surrounding colonies of *S. pyogenes* on blood agar plates. TAC toxins bind to cholesterol on eukaryotic cell membranes, creating toxin-cholesterol aggregates that contribute to cell lysis via a colloid-osmotic mechanism. Cholesterol inhibits toxicity in isolated myocytes and hemolysis of red blood cells *in vitro*. In situations where serum cholesterol is high, i.e., nephrotic syndrome, falsely elevated ASO titers may occur because both cholesterol and anti-ASO antibody will "neutralize SLO." Striking amino acid homology exists between SLO and other TAC toxins.

Streptolysin S. Streptolysin S is a cell-associated hemolysin that does not diffuse into the agar media. Purification and characterization of this protein have been difficult, and its only role in pathogenesis may be in direct or contact cytotoxicity.

Deoxyribonucleases A, B, C, and D. Expression of deoxyribonucleases (DNases) *in vivo* elicits production of anti-DNase antibody following both pharyngeal and skin infection; this is most true for DNase B with group A streptococci.

Hyaluronidase. This extracellular enzyme hydrolyzes hyaluronic acid in deeper tissues, facilitating the spread of infection along fascial planes. Antihyaluronidase titers rise following *S. pyogenes* infections, especially those involving the skin.

Pyrogenic Exotoxins. SPE types A, B, and C, also called scarlatina toxin and erythrogenic toxins, induce lymphocyte blastogenesis, potentiate endotoxin-induced shock, induce fever, suppress antibody synthesis, and act as superantigens. The identification of these three different types of SPE's may in part explain why some individuals may have multiple attacks of scarlet fever. The gene for pyrogenic exotoxin A *(speA)* is transmitted by bacteriophages, and stable production depends on lysogenic conversion in a manner analogous to diphtheria toxin production by *Corynebacterium diphtheriae*. Control of SPE A production is not yet understood, though the quantity of SPE A produced varies dramatically from decade to decade. Historically, SPE A–producing strains have been associated with severe cases of scarlet fever and, more recently, with strepTSS.

Although all strains of group A streptococci are endowed with genes for SPE B *(speB)*, like SPE A, the quantity of toxin produced varies greatly.

Pyrogenic exotoxin type C (SPE C), like SPE A, is bacteriophage-mediated, and expression is likewise highly variable. Recently, mild cases of scarlet fever in England and the United States have been associated with SPE C–positive strains.

CLINICAL INFECTIONS. Pharyngitis and the Asymptomatic Carrier. Patients with streptococcal pharyngitis have abrupt onset of sore throat, submandibular adenopathy, fever, and chilliness but usually not frank rigors. Cough and hoarseness are rare, but pain on swallowing is characteristic. The uvula is edematous, tonsils are hypertrophied, and the pharynx is erythematous with exudates that may be punctate or confluent. Acute pharyngitis is sufficient to induce antibody against M-protein, SLO, DNase, hyaluronidase, and if present, pyrogenic exotoxins. Depending on the infecting strain, pharyngitis may progress to scarlet fever, bacteremia, suppurative head and neck infections, rheumatic fever, poststreptococcal glomerulonephritis, or strepTSS. Pharyngitis is usually self-limited, and pain, swelling, and fever resolve spontaneously in 3 to 4 days even without treatment.

Definitive diagnosis is difficult based only on clinical parameters, especially in infants, in whom rhinorrhea may be the dominant manifestation. Even in older children with all the preceding physical findings, the correct clinical diagnosis is made in only 75% of patients. Absence of any one of the classic signs greatly reduces the

specificity. Rapid antigen detection tests in the office setting have a sensitivity and specificity of 40 to 90%. A popular approach in clinical practice is to obtain two throat swab samples from the posterior pharynx or tonsillar surface. A rapid strep test is performed on the first, and if it is positive, the patient is treated with antibiotics and the second swab discarded. If the rapid strep test is negative, the second is sent for culture, and treatment is withheld pending a positive culture.

Scarlet Fever. During the last 30 to 40 years, outbreaks of scarlet fever in the Western world have been notably mild, and the illness has been referred to as "pharyngitis with a rash" or "benign scarlet fever" (see Color Plate No. XXI-0-1). In contrast, in the latter half of the nineteenth century, mortalities of 25 to 35% were common in the United States, western Europe, and Scandinavia. The fatal or malignant forms of scarlet fever have been described as either septic or toxic. "Septic scarlet fever" refers to patients who develop local invasion of the soft tissues of the neck and complications such as upper airway obstruction, otitis media with perforation, meningitis, mastoiditis, invasion of the jugular vein or carotid artery, and bronchopneumonia. "Toxic scarlet fever" is rare today, but historically patients initially developed severe sore throat, marked fever, delirium, skin rash, and painful cervical lymph nodes. In severe toxic cases, fevers of 107° F, pulses of 130 to 160 beats per minute, severe headache, delirium, convulsions, little if any skin rash, and death within 24 hours were common. These cases occurred before the advent of antibiotics, antipyretics, and anticonvulsants, and sudden deaths were the result of uncontrolled seizures and hyperpyrexia. In contrast, children with septic scarlet fever had prolonged courses and succumbed 2 to 3 weeks after the onset of pharyngitis. Complications of streptococcal pharyngitis and malignant forms of scarlet fever have been less common in the antibiotic era. Even before antibiotics became available, necrotizing fasciitis and myositis were not described in association with scarlet fever.

Erysipelas. Erysipelas is caused exclusively by *S. pyogenes* and is characterized by an abrupt onset of fiery red swelling of the face or extremities. Distinctive features are well-defined margins, particularly along the nasolabial fold, scarlet or salmon-red rash, rapid progression, and intense pain. Flaccid bullae may develop during the second to third day, yet extension to deeper soft tissues is rare. Surgical debridement is not necessary, and treatment with penicillin is effective. Swelling may progress despite treatment, although fever, pain, and the intense redness diminish. Desquamation of the involved skin occurs 5 to 10 days into the illness. Infants and elderly adults are most commonly afflicted, and historically erysipelas, like scarlet fever, was more severe before 1900.

Streptococcal Pyoderma (Impetigo Contagiosa). Impetigo is most common in patients with poor hygiene or malnutrition. Colonization of the unbroken skin occurs first, and then intradermal inoculation is usually initiated by minor abrasions or insect bites. Single or multiple thick crusted, golden-yellow lesions develop within 10 to 14 days. Penicillin orally or parenterally and bacitracin or mupuricin topically are effective treatments for impetigo and also reduce transmission of streptococci to susceptible individuals. None of these treatments, including penicillin, prevents poststreptococcal glomerulonephritis.

Cellulitis. Group A streptococcus is the most common cause of cellulitis; however, alternative diagnoses may be obvious when associated with a primary focus such as an abscess or boil (*Staphylococcus aureus*), dog bite (DF-2), cat bite (*Pasteurella multocida*), freshwater injury (*Aeromonas hydrophila*), seawater injury (*Vibrio vulnifica*), and so on (see Ch. 325 and 391). Clinical clues to diagnosis are important because aspiration of the leading edge or punch biopsy yields a causative organism in only 15 and 40% of cases, respectively. Patients with lymphedema of any cause such as lymphoma, filariasis, or after regional lymph node dissection (as in mastectomy or carcinoma of the prostate) are predisposed to developing streptococcal cellulitis, as are patients with chronic venous stasis. Recently, recurrent saphenous vein donor-site cellulitis has been attributed to group A, C, or G streptococci. Group A streptococci may invade the epidermis and subcutaneous tissues, resulting in local swelling, erythema, and pain. The skin becomes indurated and, unlike the brilliant redness of erysipelas, is pinkish. Streptococcal cellulitis responds quickly to penicillin, although when staphylococcus is of concern, nafcillin or oxacillin may be a better choice. If fever, pain, or swelling increases, if bluish or violet bullae or discoloration appears, or if signs of systemic toxicity develop, a deeper infection such as necrotizing fasciitis or myositis should be considered (see Necrotizing Fasciitis). When an elevated serum creatine phosphokinase level suggests deeper infection, prompt surgical inspection and debridement should be performed.

Lymphangitis. Cutaneous infection with bright red streaks ascending proximally is invariably due to group A streptococcus. Prompt parenteral antibiotic treatment is mandatory, because bacteremia and systemic toxicity develop rapidly once streptococci reach the bloodstream via the thoracic duct.

Necrotizing Fasciitis. Necrotizing fasciitis, originally called "streptococcal gangrene," is a deep-seated infection of the subcutaneous tissue that results in progressive destruction of fascia and fat but may spare the skin itself. Subsequently, "necrotizing fasciitis" has become the preferred term, since *Clostridium perfringens, C. septicum,* and *S. aureus* can produce a similar pathologic process. Infection may begin at the site of trivial or inapparent trauma. Within the first 24 hours, swelling, heat, erythema, and tenderness develop and rapidly spread proximally and distally from the original focus. During the next 24 to 48 hours, the erythema darkens, changing from red to purple and then to blue, and blisters and bullae form that contain clear yellow fluid. On the fourth or fifth day, the purple areas become frankly gangrenous. From the seventh to the tenth days, the line of demarcation becomes sharply defined, and the dead skin begins to reveal extensive necrosis of the subcutaneous tissue. Patients become increasingly prostrated, emaciated, and may become unresponsive, mentally cloudy, or even delirious. Aggressive fasciotomy and debridement ("bearclaw fasciotomy") and irrigations with Dakan's solution achieved mortality rates as low as 20%, even before antibiotics were available. The increased morbidity and mortality of necrotizing fasciitis could be due to increased virulence of streptococci (see section on Streptococcal Toxic Shock Syndrome).

Myositis. Historically, streptococcal myositis has been an extremely uncommon infection, only 21 cases being documented from 1900 to 1985. Recently, the prevalence of streptococcal myositis has increased in the United States, Norway, and Sweden. Translocation of streptococci from the pharynx to the deep site of trauma (muscle) must occur hematogenously. Symptomatic pharyngitis or penetrating trauma are uncommon. Severe pain may be the only presenting symptom, and swelling and erythema may be the only signs of infection. In most cases a single muscle group is involved; however, because patients are frequently bacteremic, multiple sites of myositis or abscess can occur. Distinguishing streptococcal myositis from spontaneous gas gangrene due to *C. perfringens* or *C. septicum* may be difficult, although the presence of crepitus or gas in the tissue would favor clostridial infection. Myositis is easily distinguished from necrotizing fasciitis anatomically by surgical exploration or incisional biopsy, although clinical features of both conditions overlap. In published reports, the case-fatality rate of necrotizing fasciitis is between 20 and 50%, whereas that of streptococcal myositis is between 80 and 100%. Aggressive surgical debridement is extremely important because of the poor efficacy of penicillin described in human cases, as well as in experimental models of streptococcal myositis (see section on antibiotic efficacy).

Pneumonia. Pneumonia caused by group A streptococcus is most common in women in the second and third decades of life and causes large pleural effusions and empyema. Chest tube drainage is mandatory even though management is complicated by multiple loculations and fibrinous effusions resulting in restrictive lung disease. Prolonged penicillin therapy, thoracoscopy, and decortication of the pleura may be necessary.

Streptococcal Toxic Shock Syndrome (strepTSS). Epidemiology. In the late 1980's, invasive group A streptococcal infections occurred in North America and Europe in previously healthy individuals ages 20 to 50. This illness is associated with bacteremia, deep soft tissue infection, shock, multiorgan failure, and death in 30% of cases. Although strepTSS occurs sporadically, minor epidemics have been reported. Most patients have either a viral-like prodrome, history of minor trauma, recent surgery, or varicella infection. The prodrome may be due to a viral illness predisposing to strepTSS, or these vague early symptoms may be related to the evolving infection. In cases associated with necrotizing fasciitis, the infection begins deep in the soft tissue at a site of minor trauma that frequently did not result in a break in the skin. Although surgical procedures and viral infections such as varicella and influenza may provide portals of entry, no portal can be ascertained in 45% of cases. Preceding symptomatic pharyngitis is rare.

Symptoms and Physical Findings. The abrupt onset of severe pain is a common initial symptom of strepTSS (Table 276-1). The pain most commonly involves an extremity but also may mimic peritonitis, pelvic inflammatory disease, acute myocardial infarction, or pericarditis. Treatment with nonsteroidal anti-inflammatory agents may mask the presenting symptoms or predispose to more severe complications such as shock.

Fever is the most common presenting sign, although some patients present with profound hypothermia secondary to shock (see Table 276-1). Confusion is present in over half the patients and may progress to coma or combativeness. On admission 80% of patients have tachycardia, and over half have systolic blood pressure < 110 mm Hg. Of those with normal blood pressure on admission, most become hypotensive within 4 hours. Soft tissue infection evolves to necrotizing fasciitis or myositis in 50 to 70% of patients, and these require emergent surgical debridement, fasciotomy, or amputation. An ominous sign is progression of soft tissue swelling to violaceous or bluish vesicles or bullae. Many other clinical presentations may be associated with strepTSS, including endophthalmitis, myositis, perihepatitis, peritonitis, myocarditis, meningitis, septic arthritis, and overwhelming sepsis. Patients with shock and multiorgan failure without signs or symptoms of local infections have a worse prognosis, because definitive diagnosis and surgical debridement may be delayed.

Laboratory Abnormalities. Hemoglobinuria is present and serum creatinine is elevated in most patients at the time of admission. Serum albumin concentrations are moderately low (3.3 grams per deciliter) on admission and drop progressively over 48 to 72 hours. Hypocalcemia, including ionized hypocalcemia, is detectable early in the hospital course. The serum creatinine kinase level is a

TABLE 276-1. CLINICAL AND LABORATORY FEATURES OF THE STREPTOCOCCAL TOXIC SHOCK SYNDROME

Symptoms
  Viral-like prodrome
  Severe pain
  Confusion
  Nausea
  Chills

Signs
  Fever
  Soft tissue swelling and tenderness
  Tachycardia
  Tachypnea
  Hypotension

Laboratory Findings
  Hematologic tests
    Marked left shift
    Red cell hemolysis
    Thrombocytopenia
  Chemistry tests
    Azotemia
    Hypocalcemia
    Hypoalbuminemia
    Creatine phosphokinase elevation
  Urinalysis
    Hematuria
  Blood gases
    Hypoxia
    Acidosis
  Radiographic
    ARDS
    Soft tissue swelling

Complications
  Profound hypotension
  ARDS
  Renal failure
  Liver failure
  Necrotizing soft tissue infections
  Bacteremia
  Death (30%)

TABLE 276–2. ANTIBIOTIC THERAPY OF GROUP A STREPTOCOCCAL INFECTIONS

Condition	Route	Dosages
I. Pharyngitis and impetigo		
Benzathine penicillin	IM	1.2 million units (>27 kg)
Penicillin G (or V)	PO	200,000 units q.i.d. for 10 days
Erythromycin	PO	40 mg/kg/day (up to 1 gram per day)
II. Recurrent streptococcal pharyngitis/tonsillitis Same as I above, *or*		
Ampicillin plus clavulinic acid	PO	20–40 mg/kg/day
Oral Cephalosporin		Check *PDR*
Clindamycin	PO	10 mg/kg/day
III. Cellulitis and erysipelas		
Penicillin G or V	PO	200,000 units q.i.d. for 10 days
Dicloxacillin*	PO	500 mg q.i.d. for 10 days (adults)
IV. Necrotizing fasciitis/ myositis/streptococcal toxic shock syndrome		
Clindamycin	IV	1800–2100 mg daily (adults)
Penicillin	IV	2 million units q4h (adults)
V. Prophylaxis for rheumatic fever (see Ch. 277)		

* Alternative to penicillin if *S. aureus* is of concern. Cephalosporins could be used; however, most (except ceftriaxone) have less activity than penicillin G against streptococci.

useful test to detect deeper soft tissue infections, such as necrotizing fasciitis or myositis.

The initial hematologic studies demonstrate only mild leukocytosis, but a dramatic left shift (43% of white blood cells may be band forms, metamyelocytes, and myelocytes). The mean platelet count is normal on admission but may drop rapidly by 48 hours, even in the absence of criteria for disseminated intravascular coagulopathy.

Clinical Course. Shock is apparent early in the course, and fluid management is complicated by profound capillary leak. Adult respiratory distress syndrome occurs frequently (55%), and renal dysfunction that precedes hypotension in many patients may progress in spite of treatment. In patients who survive, serum creatinine levels return to normal within 4 to 6 weeks; many require dialysis. Overall, 30% of patients die despite aggressive treatment including intravenous fluids, colloid, pressors, mechanical ventilation, and surgical interventions such as fasciotomy, debridement, exploratory laparotomy, intraocular aspiration, amputation, and hysterectomy.

Characteristics of Clinical Isolates. Group A streptococcus is isolated from blood in 60% of cases and from deep tissue specimens in 95% of cases. M types 1, 3, 12, and 28 are the most common strains isolated. Pyrogenic exotoxins A and/or B have been found in isolates from the majority of patients with severe infection. Infections in Norway, Sweden, and Great Britain have been primarily due to M type 1 strains that produce pyrogenic exotoxin B. Other novel pyrogenic exotoxins are being described that also may explain the recent enhanced virulence of group A streptococcus.

NONSUPPURATIVE COMPLICATIONS. The nonsuppurative complications of streptococcal disease are acute rheumatic fever and acute glomerulonephritis. These are discussed in Ch. 277 and 79, respectively.

TREATMENT OF GROUP A INFECTIONS. Prophylaxis. During epidemics, particularly when rheumatic fever or a poststreptococcal glomerulonephritis are prevalent, treatment of asymptomatic carriers may be necessary. Studies by the U.S. military have shown that monthly injections of benzathine penicillin greatly reduce the incidence of streptococcal pharyngitis and rheumatic fever in young soldiers living in crowded conditions.

Emergence of Resistance. Erythromycin resistance of *S. pyogenes* is currently 4% in Western countries; however, in Japan in 1974 the rate reached 72%. Sulfonamide resistance currently is reported in <1% of group A streptococcal isolates.

Therapeutic Failure of Penicillin. The recommended antibiotic therapies for group A streptococcal diseases are shown in Table 276–2. Resistance to penicillin has not been described, yet in some settings there is a lack of *in vivo* efficacy despite *in vitro* susceptibility to penicillin. Three mechanisms may explain this lack of efficacy.

1. *β-Lactamase production by co-infecting organisms.* Penicillin failure in pharyngitis, tonsillitis, or mixed infections may be due to inactivation of penicillin *in situ* by β-lactamases produced by co-colonizing organisms such as *Bacteroides fragilis, Haemophilus influenzae,* or *S. aureus.* For example, the failure rate of penicillin treatment of group A streptococcal pharyngitis may approach 25%, and if such patients are treated with a second course of penicillin, the failure rate may approach 80%, perhaps due to selection of β-lactamase–producing bacteria. In contrast, cures of 90% have been achieved when treatment consisted of amoxacillin plus clavulanate or clindamycin.

2. *Genotypic tolerance.* Genotypic tolerance to penicillin also may contribute to penicillin's lack of efficacy in tonsillitis or pharyngitis. In fact, penicillin-tolerant strains also have caused epidemics of pharyngitis. Tolerant strains demonstrate a slower rate of growth, a slower rate of bacterial killing by penicillin, and an absence of β-lactam–induced cell lysis. The role of tolerance in antibiotic treatment failure is not fully understood.

3. *Inoculum effect.* Studies in animals infected with group A streptococcus demonstrate that penicillin is effective only if given early or if small numbers of streptococci are used to initiate infection. It is likely that streptococci are not in a logarithmic phase of growth at the time the clinical diagnosis of necrotizing fasciitis or myositis is made. Penicillin is most effective against streptococci in log phase growth, a stage in their life cycle when five penicillin-binding proteins are expressed. Conversely, during stationary phase, the two penicillin-binding proteins with the greatest affinity for penicillin are absent. In contrast, clindamycin has much greater efficacy than penicillin even if treatment is delayed up to 16 hours. Clindamycin's greater efficacy could be due to its ability to suppress M-protein synthesis, its longer postantibiotic effect, an indifference to *in vivo* inoculum effect, or its effects on the host's immune system.

NON–GROUP A STREPTOCOCCAL INFECTIONS (Table 276–3)

Enterococcus faecalis. These gram-positive, facultatively anaerobic bacteria are usually nonhemolytic but may demonstrate α or β hemolysis. Enterococci were previously classified as group D streptococci because they hydrolyze bile esculin and possess the group D antigen. Based on nucleic acid hybridization studies, they

TABLE 276–3. NON-GROUP A STREPTOCOCCAL INFECTIONS

Organism	Lancefield Group	Type of Infection	Therapy
S. agalactiae	B	Neonatal sepsis Postpartum sepsis Septic arthritis Soft tissue infection Osteomyelitis	Ampicillin or penicillin
Enterococcus faecalis	D	Endocarditis Bacteremia UTI Abscesses, GI	Ampicillin + gentamicin
S. milleri	A, C, F, G, and nontypable	Abscesses Bacteremia	Penicillin
S. bovis	D	Bacteremia Abscesses	Penicillin
S. equi	C	Bacteremia Cellulitis Pharyngitis	Penicillin
S. canis	G	Bacteremia Cellulitis Pharyngitis	Penicillin
"Viridans"	Nontypable		
S. salivarius		Nonpathogen	
S. mutans		Endocarditis Caries	Penicillin
S. sanguis		Endocarditis	Penicillin
S. mitior		Endocarditis	Penicillin

are now designated *Enterococcus*. Enterococci are commonly isolated from stool, urine, and sites of intra-abdominal and lower extremity infection. Enterococci cause subacute bacterial endocarditis and have become an important cause of nosocomial infection, not because of increased virulence but because of antibiotic resistance. First, person-to-person transfer of multidrug-resistant enterococci is a major concern to hospital epidemiologists. Second, superinfections and spontaneous bacteremia from endogenous sites of enterococcal colonization are described in patients receiving quinolone or moxalactam antibiotics. Lastly, conjugational transfer of plasmids and transposons between enterococci in the face of intense antibiotic pressure within the hospital mileu have created multidrug-resistant strains, including those with vancomycin and teicoplanin resistance. Serious infections with enterococci such as endocarditis or bacteremia require a synergistic combination of antimicrobials such as ampicillin or vancomycin, together with an aminoglycoside. β-Lactamase–positive (Nitrocefin disc positive) strains can be treated with ampicillin and sulbactam.

Streptococcus bovis. *S. bovis* is also a cause of subacute bacterial endocarditis and bacteremia in patients with underlying gastrointestinal malignancy. Unlike enterococcus, it remains highly sensitive to penicillin.

Group C and G Streptococci. These organisms may be isolated from the throats of both humans and dogs, produce SLO, and resemble group A in colony morphology and spectrum of clinical disease. Before rapid identification tests were developed, many infections caused by groups C and G were mistakenly attributed to group A, such as pharyngitis, cellulitis, skin and wound infections, endocarditis, meningitis, osteomyelitis, and arthritis. Rheumatic fever following group C or G infection has not been described. These strains also cause recurrent cellulitis at the saphenous vein donor site in patients who have undergone coronary artery bypass surgery. Both organisms are susceptible to penicillin, erythromycin, vancomycin, and clindamycin.

Streptococcus milleri. *S. milleri* are usually β hemolytic and produce minute colonies on blood agar plates. They are found in the oropharynx, upper gastrointestinal tract, and appendix. Infections are most commonly related to contiguous abscess formation such as tooth abscess, periapendiceal abscess, and so on. Primary bacteremia with or without endocarditis and metastatic abscesses of the brain, lung, bone, joints, liver, and spleen are characteristic of *S. milleri*.

Streptococcus agalactiae. *S. agalactiae* (group B streptococci) colonize the vagina, gastrointestinal tract, and occasionally the upper respiratory tract of normal humans. They are recognized as gray-white colonies, slightly larger than group A streptococci, but with a narrower zone of hemolysis. They are resistant to bacitracin, do not hydrolyze bile esculin, demonstrate a positive CAMP test, and hydrolyze sodium hippurate. Definitive identification is made using group-specific antiserum or commercial kits that use agglutination endpoints. There are currently six different capsular polysaccharide types of group B designated Ia, Ib, II, III, IV, and V. Immunity results from the development of opsonic type-specific antibody.

Group B streptococci are the most common cause of neonatal pneumonia, sepsis, and meningitis in the United States and western Europe, with an incidence of 1.8 to 3.2 cases per 1000 live births. Preterm infants born to mothers colonized with group B streptococci and premature rupture of the membranes are at highest risk for early-onset pneumonia and sepsis. The mean time of onset is 20 hours, and symptoms are respiratory distress, apnea, fever, and hypothermia. Ascent of the streptococcus from the vagina to the amniotic cavity causes amnionitis. Infants may aspirate streptococci either from the birth canal during parturition or from amniotic fluid *in utero*. Radiographic evidence of pneumonia and/or hyaline membrane disease is present in 40% of neonates with infection, and meningitis occurs in 30 to 40% of cases. Type III group B streptococcus causes most cases of meningitis.

Late-onset neonatal sepsis occurs 7 to 90 days postpartum, with symptoms of fever, poor feeding, lethargy, and irritability. Bacteremia is common, and meningitis occurs in 80% of cases.

Adults with group B infections include postpartum women and patients with peripheral vascular disease, diabetes, or malignancy. Soft tissue infection, septic arthritis, and osteomyelitis are the most

common presentations. Although penicillin is the treatment of choice, in practice many neonates are empirically treated with ampicillin (300 to 400 mg per kilogram per day) plus gentamicin. Once the diagnosis is established, penicillin at 200 to 500,000 units per kilogram per day should be given. Adults should receive 10 to 12 million units of penicillin per day for bacteremia, soft tissue infection, or osteomyelitis, but the dose should be increased to 18 or 24 millions units per day for meningitis. Vancomycin and a first-generation cephalosporin are alternatives for the penicillin-allergic patients. Intrapartum administration of ampicillin to women colonized with group B streptococcus who also had premature labor or prolonged rupture of the membranes prevents group B neonatal sepsis. Infants should continue to receive ampicillin for 36 hours postpartum. It is imperative that women during the third trimester be screened for risk factors for premature labor, and those at high risk should be cultured. Women presenting in labor without such definition could be screened with a rapid antigen detecting kit, even though the false-negative rate may be 10 to 30%. Passive immunization with IVIG or active immunization with multivalent polysaccharide vaccine shows promise and will likely be the best approach to prevent neonatal sepsis as well as postpartum infection of the mother.

Anthony B: Group B streptococcal infections. *In* Feign R, Cherry J (eds.): Textbook of Pediatric Infectious Diseases. 2d ed. Philadelphia, WB Saunders, 1987, p 1322. *A thorough review of the epidemiology, microbiology, and clinical aspects of group B neonatal infections, including medical management.*

Baker CJ, Edwards MS: Group B streptococcal infections. *In* Remington JS, Klein JO (eds.): Infectious Diseases of the Fetus and Newborn Infant. 3rd ed. Philadelphia, WB Saunders, 1991, p 820. *An excellent review of the clinical infections, virulence factors, and therapeutic approaches to group B streptococcal infections.*

Bisno AL: Group A streptococcal infections and acute rheumatic fever. N Engl J Med 325:783, 1991. *An excellent review article with emphasis on rheumatic fever; there are sections on virulence factors, epidemiology, and streptococcal infections in general.*

Cone LA, Woodard DR, Schlievert PM, et al.: Clinical and bacteriologic observations of a toxic shock–like syndrome due to *Streptococcus pyogenes*. N Engl J Med 317:146, 1987. *Case report of an early case of streptococcal toxic shock syndrome.*

Gossling R: Occurrence and pathogenicity of the *Streptococcus milleri* group. Rev Infect Dis 10:257, 1988. *An excellent review of the distribution of* S. milleri *in the human host. The types of human infection, the virulence factors of the organism, and its susceptibility to antimicrobial agents are discussed in detail.*

Herman DJ, Gerding DN: Screening and treatment of infections caused by resistant enterococci. Antimicrob Agents Chemother 35:215, 1991. *An excellent review of screening parameters and treatment regimens for infections caused by antibiotic-resistant enterococci.*

Martin PR, Hoiby PR: Streptococcal serogroup A epidemic in Norway 1987–1988. Scand J Infect Dis 22:421, 1990. *An excellent population-based study demonstrating a remarkable increase in bacteremia in age groups from 18 to 50.*

Murray BE: The life and times of the enterococcus. Clin Microbiol Rev 3:46, 1990. *Reviews recent changes in clinical findings, biochemical properties, and antibiotic resistance associated with the enterococcus.*

Schwartz B, Facklam RR, Breiman RF: Changing epidemiology of group A streptococcal infection in the USA. Lancet 336:1167, 1990. *A survey of group A streptococcal isolates sent to the CDC over the last decade. A clear indication that invasive infections are currently associated with M types 1 and 3.*

Stevens DL: Invasive group A streptococcus infections. Clin Infect Dis 14:2, 1992. *A review article describing the changing epidemiology of scarlet fever, necrotizing fasciitis, myositis, bacteremia, and the streptococcal toxic shock syndrome.*

Stevens DL, Bryant AE, Hackett SP: Sepsis syndromes and toxic shock syndromes: Concepts in pathogenesis and a perspective of future treatment strategies. Curr Opin Infect Dis 6:374, 1993. *Compares the cellular basis of cytokine- and lymphokine-mediated shock caused by gram-negative and gram-positive bacteria.*

Stevens DL, Tanner MH, Winship J, et al.: Severe group A streptococcal infections associated with a toxic shock-like syndrome and scarlet fever toxin A. N Engl J Med 321:1, 1989. *Reports clinical and laboratory features and complications of 20 patients with streptococcal toxic shock syndrome. An analysis of strains reveals that most were M types 1 and 3 and most strains produced pyrogenic exotoxin type A.*

277 RHEUMATIC FEVER
Alan L. Bisno

DEFINITION. Rheumatic fever is an inflammatory disease that occurs as a delayed, nonsuppurative sequel of upper respiratory infection with group A streptococci. The clinical manifestations include polyarthritis, carditis, subcutaneous nodules, erythema marginatum, and chorea in varying combinations. In its classic form, the disorder is acute, febrile, and largely self-limited. However, damage to heart valves may be chronic and progressive, causing cardiac disability or death many years after the initial episode.

ETIOLOGY. The development of acute rheumatic fever (ARF) requires antecedent infection with a specific organism, the group A *Streptococcus,* at a specific body site, the upper respiratory tract. Cutaneous streptococcal infection, a precursor of poststreptococcal acute glomerulonephritis, has never been shown to cause rheumatic fever.

Strains representing a number of the more than 80 M-protein serotypes of group A streptococci can cause ARF. There is a substantial body of evidence to indicate, however, that group A streptococci vary in their rheumatogenic potential. Strains causing clusters or epidemics usually belong to a limited number of serotypes (e.g., 3, 5, 18, 24, and others) and are often heavily encapsulated, as evidenced by their growth as mucoid colonies on blood agar plates. Streptococci epidemiologically associated with ARF outbreaks occurring during the 1980's in the United States exhibited these characteristics.

PATHOGENESIS. The mechanism by which group A streptococci elicit the connective tissue inflammatory response that constitutes ARF remains unknown. Various theories have been advanced, including (1) toxic effects of streptococcal products, particularly streptolysins S and O, both of which can initiate tissue injury; (2) inflammation mediated by antigen-antibody complexes, perhaps localized to sites of tissue injury; and (3) "autoimmune" phenomena induced by the similarity of certain streptococcal and human tissue antigens.

Efforts to discriminate among these potential pathogenetic mechanisms have been hampered by the lack of an animal model of rheumatic fever. Most authorities currently favor the theory that ARF is an "autoimmune" disorder in which tissue damage is mediated by the host's own immunologic responses to the antecedent streptococcal infection. This theory is rendered more credible by the relatively long latent period between the onset of pharyngitis and ARF and by the demonstration of numerous examples of antigenic similarity between somatic constituents of the group A *Streptococcus* and human tissues. The most intensively studied of these cross-reactions is that between streptococci and human heart. Many patients with ARF (as well as patients with uncomplicated streptococcal infections) have in their sera antistreptococcal antibodies that cross-react with heart tissue in a variety of test systems. Components of the streptococcal cell wall (including group A carbohydrate and M-protein) and of the cell membrane contain epitopes that share antigenic determinants with certain constituents of the human heart.

Antibodies to the cytoplasm of neurons located in the caudate and subthalamic nuclei of the brain have been identified in sera of patients with Sydenham's chorea, and such antibodies cross-react with group A streptococcal membranes. Streptococcal extracellular products appear to be present in immune complexes circulating in the blood of ARF patients. Taken together, these and other reported immunologic cross-reactions and toxic phenomena could theoretically account for most of the manifestations of ARF. As yet, however, there is no direct evidence that any of them is pathogenetically significant.

Patients with ARF have, on average, higher titers of antibodies to streptococcal extracellular and somatic antigens than do patients with uncomplicated streptococcal infections. Data relating to cellular immunity are more limited. ARF patients exhibit an exaggerated cellular reactivity to streptococcal cell membrane antigens, as demonstrated by inhibition *in vitro* of migration of peripheral blood lymphocytes.

Several observations suggest that development of rheumatic fever may be modulated, at least in part, by the specific genetic constitution of the host. These include (1) the tendency of rheumatic fever to affect more than one member of a given family, (2) the fact that only a small percentage of all individuals experiencing an immunologically significant streptococcal infection develop ARF, (3) the tendency of rheumatic individuals to experience recurrent attacks, (4) the propensity of rheumatic subjects to exhibit exaggerated immunologic responses to streptococcal antigens, and (5) the fact that certain class II histocompatibility antigens are encountered significantly more frequently in ARF patients than in controls. Recently, a unique antigen has been found to be strongly expressed on the B cells of virtually all ARF patients but in <20% of controls.

EPIDEMIOLOGY. The epidemiology of ARF mirrors that of streptococcal pharyngitis. The peak age of incidence is 5 to 15 years, but both primary and recurrent cases occur in adults. ARF is rare in children younger than age 4, a fact that has led some observers to speculate that repetitive streptococcal infections are necessary to "prime" the host for the disease. There is no clear-cut gender predilection, although females are more likely to develop certain manifestations such as Sydenham's chorea and mitral stenosis.

The frequency with which ARF develops following untreated group A streptococcal upper respiratory infection differs with the prevalence of highly rheumatogenic strains in the population and the epidemiologic circumstances. In the years following World War II, careful prospective studies were conducted among personnel in military camps suffering from exudative tonsillitis or pharyngitis caused by M-typable group A streptococci. Under such circumstances, in which cases of streptococcal pharyngitis tend to be clinically severe and to appear in epidemics, approximately 3% of untreated patients developed ARF. Studies of endemically occurring streptococcal infection among open populations of children are complicated by the difficulties of differentiating cases of streptococcal pharyngitis from viral pharyngitis occurring in streptococcal carriers; nevertheless, the ARF attack rate in such circumstances is clearly lower than in the military experience, with an overall attack rate of <1%.

Certain features of the antecedent streptococcal infection are associated with an increased risk of ARF. Among these are the magnitude of the antistreptolysin O (ASO) titer rise and the persistence of the infecting organism in the pharynx. Although ARF is more likely to occur following clinically severe exudative pharyngitis than following mild nonexudative illness, one third or more of cases occur after streptococcal infections that are asymptomatic or so mild as to have been forgotten by the patient.

Patients with a history of ARF are at greatly increased risk of recurrent disease following an immunologically significant streptococcal infection. In one long-term prospective study of rheumatic subjects at a rheumatic fever sanitarium, one of every five documented streptococcal infections gave rise to a recurrence of ARF. The risk of recurrence is greater in patients with pre-existing rheumatic heart disease and in those experiencing symptomatic throat infections; the risk declines with advancing age and with increasing interval since the most recent rheumatic attack. Nevertheless, rheumatic patients remain at increased risk well into adult life, perhaps indefinitely.

Rheumatic fever occurs in all parts of the world; there is no known racial predisposition. In temperate climates, ARF peaks in the cooler months of the year, in the winter and early spring or shortly after schools open in the fall. The major environmental factor favoring occurrence appears to be crowding, as in military barracks or similar closed institutions and large households. Crowding favors interpersonal spread of group A streptococci and perhaps enhances streptococcal virulence by frequent human passage.

ARF remains rampant in developing areas such as the Middle East, the Indian subcontinent, and many nations of Africa and South America. It has been estimated that rheumatic heart disease causes 25 to 40% of all cardiovascular disease in the Third World. In striking contrast, the incidence of ARF and the prevalence of rheumatic heart disease have declined both in North America and in western Europe during the course of the twentieth century. Rates of fewer than 2 per 100,000 school children have been reported from several areas of the United States. The disease has become extremely uncommon in the affluent suburbs of many U.S. cities, while persisting among lower socioeconomic groups, particularly in the densely populated core areas of major urban centers. The higher incidence rates reported for African-Americans than Caucasians thus appears to be due to socioeconomic rather than genetic factors.

The mid-1980's, however, witnessed some startling developments in the epidemiology of ARF in the United States. Outbreaks of the disease were reported in Salt Lake City, Utah, Columbus and Akron, Ohio, Pittsburgh, Pennsylvania, Nashville and Memphis, Tennessee, and a number of other communities. The largest outbreak was in Salt Lake City and its environs, where approximately 200 cases occurred between 1985 and 1989. Equally surprising was the fact that, in many of these outbreaks, the victims were predominantly white, middle-class children dwelling in the suburbs. Moreover, ARF epidemics occurred in military training bases in Missouri and California, a phenomenon that had not been observed for two decades. Group A streptococci recovered from ARF patients, their families, and community and training camp surveys were generally highly mucoid and belonged to well-established rheumatogenic serotypes (e.g., serotypes 3 and 18). There is as yet no evidence that these events presage a major national resurgence of ARF.

PATHOLOGY. ARF is characterized by exudative and proliferative inflammatory lesions in the connective tissues, especially those of heart, joints, and subcutaneous tissues. The early lesions consist of edema of the ground substance, fragmentation of collagen fibers, cellular infiltration, and fibrinoid degeneration. In the heart, diffuse degeneration and even necrosis of muscle cells may be observed. At a slightly later stage, focal perivascular inflammatory lesions develop. These so-called Aschoff nodules (Fig. 277–1), considered virtually pathognomonic of rheumatic fever, consist of a central area of fibrinoid surrounded by lymphocytes, plasma cells, and large basophilic cells, some of them multinucleate. Many of these cells have elongated nuclei with a distinctive chromatin pattern, sometimes called "caterpillar" or "owl-eye" nuclei, depending on their orientation in microscopic cross section. Cells containing these nuclei are called "Anitschkow myocytes," despite the fact that most authorities believe them to be of mesenchymal origin.

Cardiac findings may include pericarditis, myocarditis, and endocarditis. Foci of coronary arteritis also may be observed. A thickened and roughened area ("MacCallum's patch") is frequently present in the left atrium above the posterior leaflet of the mitral valve. Valvular lesions appear early as small verrucae along the line of closure. Later, as healing occurs, the valves may become thickened and deformed, the chordae shortened, and the commissures fused. These changes result in valvular stenosis or insufficiency. The mitral valve is involved most commonly, followed by the aortic, the tricuspid, and rarely, the pulmonic valves.

Pathologically, the arthritis of ARF is characterized by a fibrinous exudate and sterile effusion without erosion of the joint surfaces or pannus formation. Subcutaneous nodules have many histologic features in common with the Aschoff nodules. These consist of central zones of fibrinoid necrosis surrounded by histiocytes, fibroblasts, occasional lymphocytes, and rare polymorphonuclear cells. Inflammation of the smaller arteries and arterioles may occur throughout the body. Despite pathologic evidence of diffuse vasculitis, aneurysms and thrombosis are not typical features of ARF.

CLINICAL MANIFESTATIONS. Rheumatic fever may involve a number of different organ systems, most notably the heart, joints, skin, subcutaneous tissues, and central nervous system. The clinical picture of the disease may thus be quite variable (Table 277–1), depending on which systems are attacked, whether they are involved

TABLE 277–1. THE MANY FACES OF ACUTE RHEUMATIC FEVER: POSSIBLE PRESENTATIONS

High fever, prostration, crippling polyarthritis
Lassitude, tachycardia, new cardiac murmurs
Acute pericarditis
Fulminant heart failure
Sydenham's chorea, without fever or toxicity
Acute abdominal pain, mimicking appendicitis
Varying combinations of the above

singly or in combination, and the severity of the involvement. Five clinical features of the disease are so characteristic that they are recognized as "major manifestations" according to the revised Jones criteria (see below) for the diagnosis of ARF: carditis, polyarthritis, chorea, subcutaneous nodules, and erythema marginatum. Certain other findings, frequently present but nonspecific, have been designated "minor manifestations." These include arthralgia, fever, and certain laboratory findings (see below).

In cases in which it can be determined, the latent period between the antecedent streptococcal infection and the onset of symptoms of ARF ranges between 1 and 5 weeks. The average latent period is 19 days for both primary and recurrent attacks. When acute polyarthritis is the presenting complaint, the onset is often rather abrupt and may be marked by high fever and toxicity. If isolated carditis is the initial manifestation, the onset may be insidious or even subclinical. Between these two extremes, diverse gradations exist in the initial presentation of ARF (see Table 277–1). In most attacks, fever and joint involvement are the earliest clinical manifestations, although occasionally they may be preceded by abdominal pain localized to the periumbilical or infraumbilical areas. At times, the location and severity of the pain, as well as fleeting signs of peritoneal inflammation, may lead to a misdiagnosis of acute appendicitis. Carditis, if it is to appear, usually does so within the first 3 weeks of the illness. In contrast, chorea tends to occur later in the course of the disease, sometimes after all other manifestations have subsided. Fortunately, chorea and polyarthritis almost never occur simultaneously. Epistaxis may be a feature of ARF, occurring both at the onset and throughout the acute phase of the illness; it may be quite severe.

The incidence of major manifestations varies in reported series. Overall, however, arthritis occurs in approximately 75% of first attacks of ARF, carditis in 40 to 50%, chorea in 15%, and subcutaneous nodules and erythema marginatum in <10%. The frequency of individual manifestations varies with age. Carditis is more frequent in the youngest age groups and is relatively uncommon in first attacks occurring in adults. Chorea occurs primarily in persons between age 5 and puberty. It is seen more frequently in females and virtually never occurs in adult males. Thus the majority of ARF attacks occurring in adults are manifested primarily by arthritis.

Arthritis. Joint involvement ranges from arthralgia alone to acute, disabling arthritis, characterized by swelling, warmth, erythema, severe limitation of motion, and exquisite tenderness to pressure. The larger joints of the extremities are usually involved— most frequently the knees and ankles but also the wrists and elbows. The hips and small joints of the hands and feet are affected occasionally. Involvement of shoulders and lumbosacral, cervical, sternoclavicular, and temporomandibular joints occurs in a relatively small percentage of cases. The synovial fluid contains thousands of white blood cells, with a marked preponderance of polymorphonuclear leukocytes; bacterial cultures are sterile. Characteristically, the articular involvement in ARF assumes a pattern of migratory polyarthritis. This does not mean that inflammation in one joint disappears before the next is attacked. Rather, a number of joints are affected in succession, and the periods of involvement overlap. Inflammation in one joint may subside while another is becoming symptomatic so that the process seems to migrate from joint to joint. In untreated cases, as many as 16 joints may be affected, and about half the patients develop arthritis in more than 6 joints. When effective anti-inflammatory therapy is administered early in the course of the disease, the involvement not infrequently remains monarticular or pauciarticular.

In most instances, inflammation in any one joint begins to subside spontaneously within a week, and the total duration of involvement is no more than 2 or 3 weeks. The entire bout of polyarthritis

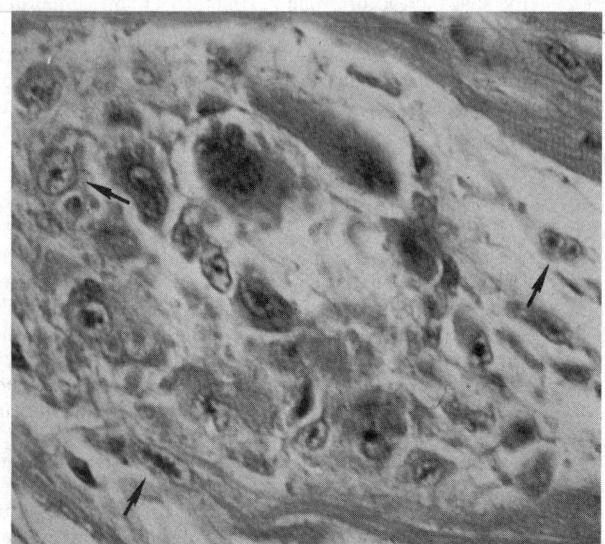

FIGURE 277–1. Myocardial Aschoff nodule demonstrates areas of fibrinoid degeneration and numerous large cells with polymorphous nuclei; several of the nuclei have "owl-eye" or "caterpillar" configurations *(arrows)*. X 630. (Courtesy of Robert Peace, M.D.)

rarely lasts more than 4 weeks and resolves completely, leaving no residual joint damage. Some authors have described the rare occurrence of Jaccoud's arthritis, so-called chronic post-rheumatic fever arthropathy of the metacarpophalangeal joints, following repetitive bouts of rheumatic polyarthritis. This entity is not a true arthritis but a form of periarticular fibrosis; its relationship to rheumatic fever remains unresolved.

Carditis. Rheumatic fever may involve the endocardium, myocardium, and pericardium (Table 277–2), and thus the disease is capable of inducing a true pancarditis. Carditis is the most important manifestation of ARF because it is the only one that can cause significant permanent organ damage or death. Although the clinical picture may at times be fulminant, it is more frequently mild or even asymptomatic and may escape notice in the absence of more obvious associated findings, such as arthritis or chorea. The diagnosis of carditis requires the presence of one of the following four manifestations: (1) organic cardiac murmurs not previously present, (2) cardiomegaly, (3) pericarditis, or (4) congestive heart failure. In practice, the characteristic murmurs of ARF are almost always present in cases of rheumatic carditis, unless the ability to hear them is obscured (e.g., loud pericardial friction rub, large pericardial effusion, low cardiac output, severe tachycardia). The diagnosis of carditis should be made with caution in the absence of one of the following three murmurs: apical systolic, apical mid-diastolic, and basal diastolic. Such murmurs, if they are destined to develop, do so usually within the first week and almost always within the first 3 weeks of illness. (An exception to this rule may occur in the patient with "pure" chorea; see later discussion.) The apical systolic murmur of relative or actual mitral regurgitation encompasses most of systole. It is blowing, relatively high pitched, and heard best at the apex; it radiates to the axilla and at times to the base of the heart or the back. It must be distinguished carefully by quality, location, and radiation from a variety of functional precordial systolic murmurs heard in normal individuals, especially in children. The apical mid-diastolic (Carey-Coombs) murmur is a low-pitched sound replacing or immediately following the third heart sound and ending distinctly before the first heart sound. It may be heard in a variety of conditions associated with increased flow across the mitral valve and is thus not pathognomonic of ARF. It may be differentiated from the diastolic rumble of mitral stenosis by the absence of an opening snap, presystolic accentuation, or accentuated first sound at the mitral area. The high-pitched, decrescendo basal diastolic murmur of aortic regurgitation is best heard along the upper left sternal border or over the aortic area. It may be brief and faint, best heard after expiration with the patient leaning forward. The prognostic significance, if any, of echocardiographically recorded valvular regurgitation in the absence of audible murmurs remains to be determined.

Other prominent auscultatory findings in patients with active rheumatic carditis include tachycardia, which persists during sleep; protodiastolic, presystolic, or summation gallops; an indistinct or "mushy" quality to the first heart sound (resulting in some cases from first-degree heart block); pericardial friction rub; or muffling of heart tones caused by pericardial effusion. In the early stages of congestive heart failure, rapid distention of the hepatic capsule may lead to right upper quadrant aching and tenderness over the liver. All the usual clinical findings of pericarditis or congestive failure may be observed.

A number of different rhythm disturbances may occur during the course of ARF. By far the most common is first-degree atrioventricular block. Second- and third-degree heart block, nodal rhythm, and premature contractions also may be observed; atrial fibrillation, on the other hand, is usually a feature of chronic rather than acute rheumatic involvement. Conduction disturbances do not in themselves indicate acute carditis, and their presence or absence is unrelated to the subsequent development of rheumatic heart disease.

In cases of ARF with severe carditis, areas of patchy pneumonitis are sometimes seen. Many observers feel that these pulmonary infiltrates represent a specific rheumatic pneumonia. The case is difficult to prove, however, because of the confusion induced by such confounding clinical entities as pulmonary edema, pulmonary embolization, superimposed bacterial pneumonia, and the acute respiratory distress syndrome in these severely ill and toxic patients.

Sydenham's Chorea (Chorea Minor, "St. Vitus' Dance"). This neurologic syndrome occurs after a latent period that is variable but on average longer than that associated with the other manifestations of ARF. It frequently occurs in "pure" form, either unaccompanied by other major manifestations or, after a latent period of several months, at a time when all other evidence of acute rheumatic activity has subsided. Chorea is characterized by rapid, purposeless, involuntary movements, most noticeable in the extremities and face. The arms and legs flail about in erratic, jerky, uncoordinated movements that may sometimes be unilateral (hemichorea). Facial tics, grimaces, grins, and contortions are evident. The speech is usually slurred or jerky. The tongue, when protruded, retracts involuntarily, while asynchronous contractions of lingual muscles produce a "bag of worms" appearance. The involuntary motions disappear during sleep and may be partially suppressed by rest, sedation, or volition.

Patients with chorea display generalized muscle weakness and an inability to maintain a tetanic muscle contraction. Thus, when the patient is asked to squeeze the examiner's fingers, a squeezing and relaxing motion occurs that has been described as "milkmaid's grip." The knee jerk may have a pendular quality. There is no cranial nerve or pyramidal involvement, and sensory modalities are unaffected. The electroencephalogram may display abnormal slow wave activity.

Emotional lability is characteristic of Sydenham's chorea and often may precede other neurologic manifestations, leaving teachers and parents puzzled over apparently inexplicable personality changes.

Subcutaneous Nodules. These are firm, painless subcutaneous lesions that vary in size from a few millimeters to approximately 2 cm. The skin overlying them is freely movable and is not inflamed. The lesions tend to occur in crops over bony surfaces or prominences and over tendons. Sites of predilection include the extensor surfaces of the elbows, knees, and wrists, the occiput, and spinous processes of the thoracic and lumbar vertebrae (Fig. 277–2). Nodules are virtually never the sole major manifestation of ARF; they almost always appear in association with carditis, and the cardiac involvement in such cases tends to be clinically severe. Nodules ordinarily do not appear until at least 3 weeks after the onset of an attack, usually lasting 1 to 2 weeks. They may appear in repeated crops in patients with protracted carditis. Similar nodules may be seen in systemic lupus erythematosus (SLE) and in rheumatoid arthritis. Subcutaneous nodules in the latter disease are larger and more persistent than those in rheumatic fever.

Erythema Marginatum. The rash begins as an erythematous macule or papule which then extends outward while the skin in the center returns to normal. Adjacent lesions coalesce, forming circinate or serpiginous patterns. The lesions may be raised or flat, are neither pruritic nor indurated, and they blanch on pressure. They vary greatly in size and appear mostly on the trunk and proximal extremities, sparing the face. The lesions are evanescent, migrating from place to place, at times changing before the observer's eyes, and leaving no residual scarring. The erythema may be brought out by applying heat. Individual lesions may come and go in minutes to hours, but the process may go on intermittently for weeks to months uninfluenced by anti-inflammatory therapy; its persistence is not necessarily an adverse prognostic sign. In the great majority of cases, erythema marginatum is accompanied by carditis; it also tends to be associated with subcutaneous nodules.

LABORATORY FINDINGS. No specific laboratory test is diagnostic of ARF. Usually there is a leukocytosis with an increase in the proportion of polymorphonuclear leukocytes. A mild to moderate normocytic, normochromic anemia is the rule. In some patients,

---

TABLE 277–2. CLINICAL MANIFESTATIONS OF CARDITIS IN ACUTE RHEUMATIC FEVER

Murmurs*
  Apical systolic
  Apical mid-diastolic (Carey-Coombs murmur)
  Basal diastolic
Pericarditis
Cardiomegaly
Congestive heart failure

* At least one of the characteristic murmurs is almost always present in acute rheumatic carditis (see text for details).

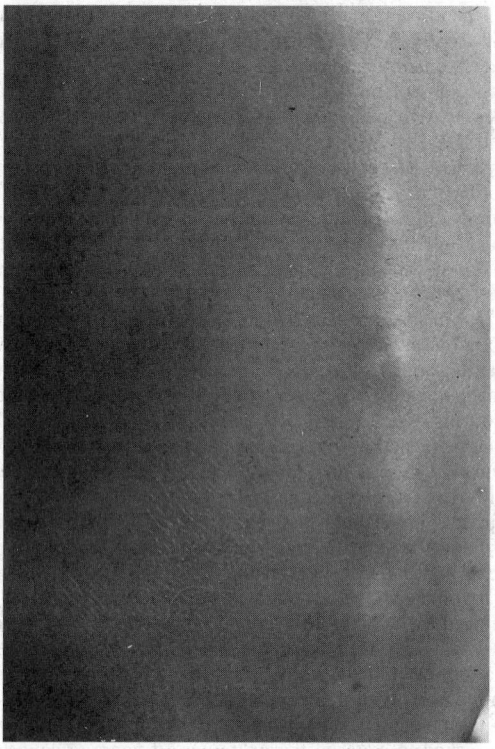

FIGURE 277–2. Subcutaneous nodules over spinous processes on the back of a patient with acute rheumatic carditis. (Courtesy of S. Levine, M.D.)

the serum aspartate aminotransferase (AST) level is elevated. Evidence of acute inflammation is prominent, including readily detectable quantities of C-reactive protein in the blood and elevation of the erythrocyte sedimentation rate. An exception is "pure" chorea, which may appear long after indices of inflammation have returned to normal.

The urine may contain protein, white cells, and red cells. Biopsy studies have revealed a variety of renal abnormalities, but the classic proliferative glomerular abnormalities that characterize post-streptococcal acute glomerulonephritis occur quite rarely in ARF. Electrocardiographic and radiographic studies may reveal evidence of rhythm disturbances, pericarditis, or congestive heart failure. Echocardiography may document myocardial and valvular dysfunction and pericardial effusion.

The major laboratory contribution to the diagnosis of ARF is the documentation of recent group A streptococcal infection. Throat culture should always be performed but is positive in only a minority of cases. The low rate of culture positivity remains unexplained, although it may be due in part to the time lapse of several weeks between the onset of the pharyngeal infection and the throat culture. The serum titer of ASO is elevated in 80% or more of ARF patients. If two streptococcal antibody tests, e.g., ASO plus either anti-DNase B or antihyaluronidase, are performed, an elevated titer of at least one will be found in 90% of ARF patients. A battery of three tests establishes the presence of recent, immunologically significant streptococcal infection in >95% of individuals experiencing an acute rheumatic attack. The definition of an "elevated" titer varies, depending on the test used, the patient's age, and geographic locale. ASO titers of at least 240 Todd units per milliliter in adults and 320 Todd units in children are generally considered elevated. At times, serial sampling may detect a rising titer of streptococcal antibodies in patients seen early in the course of a rheumatic attack.

COURSE AND PROGNOSIS. The average duration of an untreated attack of ARF is approximately 3 months. The duration tends to be longer, up to 6 months, in patients with severe carditis. Fewer than 5% of patients have continuing rheumatic activity for longer than 6 months. In a few of these the disease is limited to chorea and is otherwise benign. Other patients exhibit evidence of persistent inflammatory activity, including arthritis, carditis, and subcutaneous nodules. "Chronic rheumatic fever" occurs more frequently in patients who have had one or more previous attacks; cardiac involvement in chronic rheumatic fever tends to be frequent and severe.

Death from intractable myocarditis during the acute phase of ARF is now very rare. Once the acute attack has subsided, the only long-term sequel is that of rheumatic heart disease, manifested primarily by scarring and/or calcification (Fig. 277–3) of the mitral and aortic valves (see Ch. 42) and leading to insufficiency and/or stenosis. The prognosis from a cardiac standpoint very much depends on the clinical findings when the patient is first seen. In one large study, for example, 347 patients were examined during an acute rheumatic attack and again 10 years later. Among patients who had been free of carditis during their acute attack, only 6% had residual heart disease on follow-up. Patients with no pre-existing heart disease and with mild carditis during their acute attack (i.e., apical systolic murmur without pericarditis or heart failure) had a relatively good prognosis in that only approximately 30% had heart murmurs 10 years later. About 40% of subjects with apical or basal diastolic murmurs and 70% of subjects with failure and/or pericarditis during their acute attacks had residual rheumatic heart disease. The prognosis was worse in patients with pre-existing heart disease and in those who had experienced recurrent attacks of ARF in the 10-year interval.

These data indicate that patients who do not develop carditis during an acute attack and are protected from ARF recurrences are most unlikely to suffer from rheumatic heart disease. The patient with "pure" chorea represents an exception to this rule. A significant proportion of such patients who have no evidence of carditis when first examined may develop rheumatic valvular disease on prolonged follow-up. Although the explanation for this phenomenon is unknown, it is conceivable that in view of the long latent period associated with chorea, signs of carditis might have been present earlier but subsided by the time the neurologic abnormality became evident.

DIAGNOSIS. Although ARF is readily recognized in the individual who presents with multiple major manifestations or in epidemic circumstances, at other times the disease may be extraordinarily difficult to diagnose with confidence. This is so because of the variability of its clinical presentation, the frequency with which only a single major manifestation is detected, and the fact that there is no definitive diagnostic laboratory test. Nevertheless, precise diagnosis is especially important in this disease because of the need to advise the patient regarding prolonged antimicrobial prophylaxis (see below).

The diagnostic criteria of T. Duckett Jones, initially proposed in 1944 and subsequently modified by committees of the American Heart Association, attempt to minimize overdiagnosis and underdiagnosis (Table 277–3). The most recent (1992) revision specifies that the guidelines are designed to assist in the diagnosis of the initial ARF attack. Although most patients with recurrent ARF fulfill the criteria, in some cases the diagnosis of a recurrence may be less apparent.

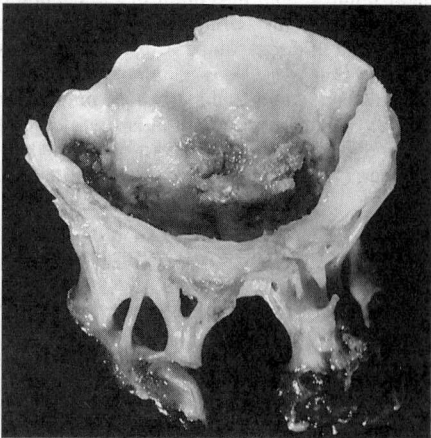

FIGURE 277–3. Calcified mitral valve from a patient with rheumatic heart disease. (Courtesy of A. Morales, M.D. From Bisno AL: Rheumatic fever. *In* Kelley WN, et al. [eds.]: Textbook of Rheumatology, 4th ed. Philadelphia, WB Saunders, 1993, p 1214.)

Two major manifestations, or one major and two minor manifestations, indicate a high probability of ARF, provided that there is supporting evidence of recent streptococcal infection. Although a positive throat culture or rapid antigen test for group A streptococci technically satisfies this requirement, streptococcal carriage rates of 15% are not uncommon among school-aged children during the fall and winter. Elevated titers of antibodies to streptococcal extracellular products, although not diagnostic of ARF, do indicate a recent, immunologically significant streptococcal infection. Conversely, if a battery of streptococcal antibody tests fails to reveal any evidence of recent infection, the diagnosis of ARF must be considered unlikely.

The modified Jones criteria are, of course, only guidelines. They are most difficult to apply confidently when polyarthritis is the single major manifestation. Under such circumstances, the diagnosis of ARF should be made only after excluding other causes of polyarthritis, such as rheumatoid arthritis, Still's disease, Lyme disease, viral arthritides (e.g., rubella, hepatitis B), the early prepurpuric phase of Henoch-Schönlein purpura, and septic arthritis, including gonococcal arthritis. The latter diagnosis cannot be excluded unequivocally by negative cultures of blood and synovial fluid. Therefore, if the clinical and epidemiologic picture is compatible with disseminated gonococcal infection, a trial of antigonococcal therapy should precede initiation of treatment with anti-inflammatory drugs.

Some patients have been described as manifesting polyarthritis that is atypical in time of onset and duration, does not respond dramatically to salicylate therapy, and is unassociated with other clinical features of ARF. Such individuals have on occasion been categorized as having "post-streptococcal reactive arthritis." The existence of this entity as a distinct syndrome, however, and its relationship to rheumatic fever remain uncertain. Pending further clarification, such individuals should be considered to have ARF if they fulfill the Jones criteria and alternative diagnoses have been excluded.

Serum sickness is frequently a serious consideration, particularly if the patient has received penicillin or other antibiotics for a preceding respiratory infection. SLE, sickle cell hemoglobinopathies, and infective endocarditis may involve the joints and the heart. Other differential diagnostic considerations include congenital heart lesions, viral and idiopathic forms of myocarditis and pericarditis, and functional heart murmurs. Nonfamilial forms of chorea have been described in SLE and rarely in association with the use of birth control pills. It remains uncertain how often episodes of chorea occurring during pregnancy ("chorea gravidarum") represent attacks of rheumatic fever. Other disorders that may at times be confused with ARF are gout, sarcoidosis, Hodgkin's disease, and acute leukemia.

There are certain circumstances in which ARF can be diagnosed even when the guidelines set forth in Table 277–3 have not been met. Patients whose only rheumatic manifestation is Sydenham's chorea may not fulfill the Jones criteria. Because of the long latent period between the antecedent streptococcal infection and the appearance of the neurologic abnormalities, evidence of inflammation encompassed in the minor manifestations may no longer be present, and previously elevated antibody titers may have declined to normal. A similar situation occasionally occurs in patients with indo-lent carditis, who may not come to medical attention until months after the onset of rheumatic fever. In patients with established rheumatic heart disease, it may be difficult to distinguish new from pre-existing cardiac involvement unless the patient has been under careful prospective follow-up, a previously undamaged valve is involved, or pericarditis is evident. Thus the diagnosis of recurrent ARF must be strongly entertained in the presence of suggestive clinical findings, provided there is evidence of recent group A streptococcal infection.

TREATMENT. Antibiotics neither modify the course of a rheumatic attack nor influence the subsequent development of carditis. Nevertheless, it is conventional to give a course of antibiotics designed to eradicate any rheumatogenic group A streptococci remaining in the tonsils and pharynx, in order to prevent spread of the organism to close contacts. The recommended regimens are those conventionally used for treatment of acute streptococcal pharyngitis (see Ch. 276). Benzathine penicillin G is preferred in non–penicillin-allergic patients. Following completion of this therapy, continuous antistreptococcal prophylaxis should commence (see below).

Treatment with anti-inflammatory agents is effective in suppressing many of the signs and symptoms of ARF. These agents do not "cure" the disease, nor do they prevent the subsequent evolution of rheumatic heart disease. They should be avoided in very mild or equivocal cases because, by suppressing the clinical manifestations, they may obscure the diagnosis. The two drugs most widely used are aspirin and corticosteroids. The former is used in patients with acute polyarthritis, provided that carditis is either absent or mild and there is no evidence of congestive heart failure. Aspirin is very effective in decreasing fever, toxicity, and joint inflammation. It should be given in a dosage of 90 to 100 mg per kilogram per day in children and 6 to 8 grams per day in adults. This is administered in equally divided doses, every 4 hours for the first 24 to 36 hours; thereafter it may be given in four doses during waking hours. A salicylate level of 25 mg per deciliter is usually satisfactory. The incidence of nausea and vomiting may be minimized by starting somewhat below the optimal dosage level and gradually increasing over a few days. The patient should be observed for evidence of significant gastrointestinal bleeding and for signs and symptoms of salicylism (see Ch. 19). After 2 weeks, the dosage is reduced to 60 to 70 mg per kilogram per day for an additional 6 weeks. These dosage schedules represent general guidelines only. The precise aspirin dose must be determined by the patient's clinical response, blood salicylate levels, and tolerance of the drug.

Corticosteroids are generally reserved for patients who have severe carditis manifested by congestive heart failure, who are unable to tolerate large doses of salicylates, or whose signs and symptoms are inadequately suppressed by aspirin. As with aspirin, the dosage must be individualized. Prednisone, 40 to 60 mg per day in divided doses, may be used initially. After 2 to 3 weeks it should be withdrawn slowly over an additional 3-week period. In cases of fulminating carditis with profound heart failure, intravenous corticosteroids may be used. As is the case for other patients receiving corticosteroids, the physician should be alert to problems such as

TABLE 277–3. GUIDELINES FOR THE DIAGNOSIS OF INITIAL ATTACK OF RHEUMATIC FEVER (JONES CRITERIA, UPDATED 1992)*

Major Manifestations	Minor Manifestations	Supporting Evidence of Antecedent Group A Streptococcal Infections
Carditis	Clinical findings	Positive throat culture or rapid streptococcal antigen test
Polyarthritis	Arthralgia	Elevated or rising streptococcal antibody titer
Chorea	Fever	
Erythema marginatum	Laboratory findings	
Subcutaneous nodules	Elevated acute-phase reactants	
	Erythrocyte sedimentation rate	
	C-reactive protein	
	Prolonged PR interval	

* If supported by evidence of preceding group A streptococcal infection, the presence of two major manifestations or of one major and two minor manifestations indicates a high probability of acute rheumatic fever.

Reprinted from Special Writing Group of the Committee on Rheumatic Fever, Endocarditis and Kawasaki Disease, American Heart Association. Guidelines for the diagnosis of rheumatic fever: Jones Criteria, 1992 update. JAMA 268 15:2069, 1992 with permission. Copyright, 1992, American Medical Association.

gastrointestinal bleeding, sodium and water retention, and impaired glucose tolerance. Suppression of the pituitary-adrenal axis or of the host immune system is a potential problem but not ordinarily a major one during this relatively short course of treatment. The role of nonsteroidal anti-inflammatory agents in managing ARF remains to be defined.

After cessation of anti-inflammatory therapy, clinical or laboratory evidence of ARF may reappear. Such therapeutic "rebounds" occur more frequently after corticosteroid therapy than after treatment with aspirin. They may be minimized by prolonging salicylate therapy for 9 to 12 weeks and, when corticosteroids have been required, by continuing aspirin for a month after corticosteroids have been discontinued. Congestive heart failure is managed by conventional measures. If digitalis is used, the potential risk of drug-induced arrhythmias in the patient with active myocarditis must be kept in mind. Patients with Sydenham's chorea require a quiet environment, and sedatives such as phenobarbital may be helpful.

Once the acute attack has subsided completely, the patient's subsequent level of physical activity depends on cardiac status. Patients without residual heart disease may resume full and unrestricted activity. It is important that patients not be subjected to unwarranted invalidism, because of either their own inaccurate perceptions of the nature of the rheumatic process or those of parents, teachers, or employers.

PREVENTION. "Primary prevention" of ARF consists of accurate diagnosis and appropriate treatment of streptococcal sore throat (see Ch. 276). Although straightforward in theory, primary prevention is often frustratingly difficult to achieve. In many of the densely populated indigent communities in which the risk of ARF is greatest, children with self-limited illnesses such as sore throats may never come to medical attention, and throat culture services are usually unavailable to aid in diagnosis. Moreover, in one third or more of cases, ARF may arise after a clinically inapparent streptococcal infection.

Perhaps the most effective strategy for avoiding the mortality and chronic cardiac disability associated with ARF is that of "secondary prevention." This strategy focuses on the group of persons who have already suffered a rheumatic attack and who are inordinately susceptible to a recurrence following an immunologically significant streptococcal upper respiratory infection. Recurrent attacks tend to be mimetic in nature, so patients who have suffered carditis with their previous attack are likely to have repetitive cardiac involvement and progressive cardiac damage. Because even patients who experienced only arthritis or chorea may develop carditis with recurrent attacks of ARF, all patients who have experienced a documented attack of ARF should receive continuous antimicrobial prophylaxis to prevent either symptomatic or asymptomatic streptococcal infections. The specific regimens to be used are indicated in Ch. 42 and 276. By far the most effective of these is intramuscular benzathine penicillin G every 4 weeks. Rheumatic recurrences are very unusual in patients faithfully adhering to this regimen. In areas of the world where the incidence of ARF and the risk of recurrence are extremely high, however, injections every 3 weeks may provide more complete protection.

The total duration of intramuscular or oral rheumatic fever prophylaxis remains unresolved. The risk of rheumatic recurrence is known to diminish with increasing age and increasing interval since the most recent rheumatic attack. Patients who escape carditis during their initial attack are less likely to experience rheumatic recurrences and less likely to develop carditis if a recurrence does ensue. These facts suggest that prophylaxis need not be perpetual for all rheumatic subjects. Continuous prophylaxis should be maintained indefinitely for those with clinically significant rheumatic heart disease. Other rheumatic subjects should be protected until reaching adulthood, for at least 5 years after their most recent attack, and if they are in an epidemiologic circumstance that places them at high risk of streptococcal acquisition (e.g., parents of small children, school teachers, military recruits, nurses, pediatricians, or residents of areas with a high incidence of ARF). The decision to remove a rheumatic subject from continuous prophylaxis should be an individualized one, based on the physician's assessment of the risk and likely consequences of recurrence, and taken with the patient's informed consent. Patients taken off prophylaxis must be instructed to

return immediately for medical follow-up whenever symptoms of pharyngitis occur.

Patients with rheumatic valvular heart disease must receive prophylaxis designed to avoid bacterial endocarditis whenever they undergo dental or surgical procedures likely to evoke bacteremia. This is not necessary in the rheumatic subject who is free of residual heart disease. The regimens to prevent endocarditis (see Ch. 278) are different from those prescribed for preventing ARF, and the fact that a patient is receiving rheumatic fever prophylaxis does not exempt him/her from endocarditis prophylaxis. This is a frequent point of confusion not only among patients but among physicians and dentists as well.

Berrios X, Del Campo E, Guzman B, Bisno AL: Discontinuance of rheumatic fever prophylasis in selected adolescents and young adults. Ann Intern Med 118:401, 1993. *Presents new data, along with a review of previous studies, on the circumstances under which rheumatic fever prophylaxis might be discontinued.*

Bisno AL: Group A streptococcal infections and acute rheumatic fever. N Engl J Med 325:783, 1991. *Review of the biology of the group A streptococcus as it relates to civilian and military outbreaks of ARF in the 1980's and the more recent resurgence of life-threatening streptococcal infections.*

Stollerman GH: Rheumatic Fever and Streptococcal Infection. New York, Grune & Stratton, 1975. *A comprehensive, extremely readable summary of rheumatic fever. Detailed descriptions of clinical manifestations will be particularly valuable to physicians unfamiliar with the disease.*

Veasy LG, Tani LY, Hill HR: Persistence of acute rheumatic fever in the intermountain area of the United States. J Pediatr 124:9, 1994. *A summary of the demographic and clinical data on 274 cases of ARF hospitalized in Salt Lake City between 1985 and 1992.*

278 INFECTIVE ENDOCARDITIS
Matthew E. Levison

Endocarditis is characterized by the vegetation, a lesion that results from deposition of platelets and fibrin on the endothelial surface of the heart. Infection is the most common cause, the usual pathogen being one of a variety of bacterial species, microscopic colonies of which are buried beneath the surface of fibrin. However, other types of microorganisms, such as rickettsia, chlamydia, and fungi, may be involved, so that the more general term *infective,* rather than *bacterial,* endocarditis is preferred. Usually the heart valve is the site of the vegetation, but in certain instances vegetations may occur on other parts of the endocardium. Involvement of extracardiac intravascular sites, which can produce an illness clinically similar to endocarditis, is properly termed *endarteritis.*

PATHOGENESIS

Endocarditis is the result of the interaction among (1) host factors that predispose the endothelium to infection, (2) circumstances that lead to transient bacteremia, and (3) the tissue tropism and virulence of the circulating bacteria.

HOST. In population-based studies, the age- and gender-adjusted incidence of endocarditis is about 5 per 100,000 person-years. Advancing age and male gender are significant risk factors; the incidence rate ratio for those age 65 or older is almost 9 times that of those under 65 and for males 2.5 times that of females. The greater frequency in the aged is due in part to the increased prevalence of predisposing cardiac lesions (e.g., degenerative cardiac lesions and prosthetic cardiac valves) and circumstances that may lead to bacteremia (e.g., invasive urologic procedures, anorectal and colonic disease, and intravascular catheterization) in this age group, and in males, the increased prevalence of certain cardiac lesions, such as bicuspid aortic valves.

Local Host Factors. **Nonbacterial Thrombotic Endocarditis (NBTE).** The normal endothelium is nonthrombogenic, but when damaged or denuded the endothelium is a potent inducer of blood coagulation. Certain types of congenital or acquired heart disease can result in a high-velocity jet stream from a high to low pressure chamber (aortic or mitral insufficiency, ventricular septal defect, or patent ductus arteriosus), or create a pressure gradient across a narrowed orifice between two chambers (aortic stenosis or coarctation of the aorta). The high-velocity jet stream can lead to turbulent blood flow distal to the pressure gradient, which is thought to damage the valvular and endocardial endothelium in a predictable pattern distal to the pressure gradient (Fig. 278–1). Damage to the endothelium can be induced in an experimental animal by passing a catheter into the heart across the aortic or tricuspid valves, and intracardiac catheters can induce similar lesions in humans. Platelets are deposited on the surface of the damaged endothelium. The adherent platelets then degranulate and stimulate local deposition of fibrin. In the process, a sterile thrombus is formed on the endothelial surface, the so-called NBTE. For unknown reasons, NBTE are also found in some patients with chronic wasting illnesses (marantic endocarditis) and systemic lupus erythematosus (SLE) (Libman-Sacks endocarditis). NBTE can dislodge fibrin, embolize to block peripheral arteries, and produce sterile infarction of distal organs. The resultant clinical manifestations of NBTE in cachetic illnesses or SLE may simulate those of infective endocarditis (see below).

NBTE is the point of attachment and subsequent proliferation for certain microorganisms once they have gained access to the circulation. Following induced bacteremia in experimental animals without pre-existing NBTE, the endothelial surface is resistant to bacterial attachment and the subsequent development of infective endocarditis. The left side of the heart is apparently more susceptible to infection than the right side. For example, the left side is infected more readily with relatively avirulent microorganisms, such as α-hemolytic streptococci, whereas the right is infected only by virulent pathogens, such as *Staphylococcus aureus;* bacteria reach higher densities on the left side (e.g., 10^{10-11} colony-forming units [CFU] per gram) than on the right (e.g., 10^8 CFU per gram). Right-sided lesions tend to respond more readily to antimicrobial therapy than do left-sided lesions; right-sided lesions may even heal spontaneously, in contrast to persistence of infection on the left. Responsible factors may include differences between the left and right side of the heart in blood P_{O_2} and intracardiac pressures. Spontaneous resolution of right-sided endocarditis is probably also a consequence of bacterial clearance on the right side by polymorphonuclear leukocytes, a factor not operative to the same extent on the left for unknown reasons. Pre-existing cardiac lesions that are believed to promote the formation of NBTE are identified in about two thirds of patients with infective endocarditis. The cardiac defects most frequently found in patients with endocarditis are mitral valve prolapse (MVP), degenerative heart disease, congenital heart disease, rheumatic heart disease (RHD), and prosthetic cardiac valves. However, the degree of risk that each type of cardiac lesion poses for subsequent endocarditis cannot be inferred from their relative frequency because the prevalence of these cardiac defects in the general population varies widely. The absolute risk is indicated by incidence rate of endocarditis for each cardiac lesion (when the frequency of the cardiac defect in the general population is known) and the relative risk by the incidence rate ratio with reference to the incidence rate of endocarditis in the general population (Table 278–1).

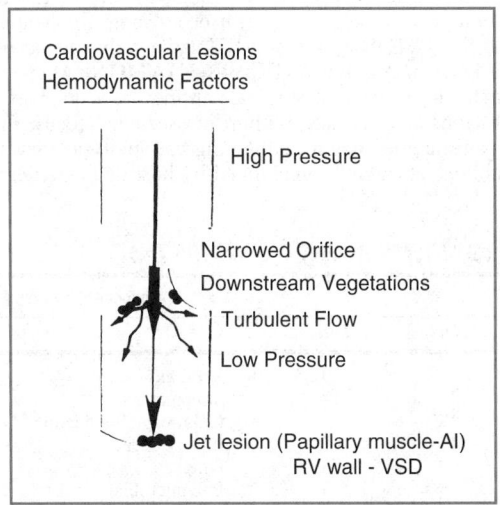

FIGURE 278–1. A schematic diagram of the hemodynamic factors favoring development of nonbacterial thrombotic endocarditis.

TABLE 278–1. ABSOLUTE AND RELATIVE RISK FOR ENDOCARDITIS AMONG VARIOUS CARDIAC LESIONS (INCIDENCE RATE, CASES PER 100,000 PATIENT-YEARS)

Prosthetic valves	308–630	(63–129)*
Prior native valve endocarditis, non-IVDU	300–740	(61–151)
Rheumatic heart disease	380–440	(78–90)
Congenital heart disease	120	(25)
Coarctation of the aorta		
Tetralogy of Fallot		
Bicuspid aortic valve		
Transposition of the aorta		
Patent ductus arteriosus		
Ventricular septal defect		
Mitral valve prolapse with regurgitant murmur	52	(11)
Hypertrophic cardiomyopathy		
Other acquired valvular dysfunction (e.g., degenerative heart diseases)		
Marfan's syndrome		

*Incidence rate relative to rate of endocarditis in normal population, 4.9/100,000 patient years.

IVDU = Intravenous drug user.

Prosthetic cardiac valves are a major risk factor for endocarditis. Endocarditis occurs in 1 to 5% of patients with prosthetic valves over the lifetime of the valve, with an incidence rate of about 300 to 600 per 100,000 patient-years. Mechanical prosthetic cardiac valves probably have about the same risk as bioprostheses (e.g., porcine heterografts), and risk probably does not vary by site of prosthetic valve replacement but is greater when valves are placed in the presence of active endocarditis. Prior native valve endocarditis poses a significant risk factor for subsequent episodes as a consequence of both the continued presence of the risk factors that contributed to the initial episode (e.g., intravenous drug use or periodontitis) and the additional risk posed by the damage to the valve sustained in the initial episode. The decreasing relative frequency of RHD among patients with endocarditis in the United States reflects the decreasing prevalence of RHD in this country. Nevertheless, RHD is a major risk factor for endocarditis, with an incidence rate only slightly lower than that for prosthetic valves. RHD remains a frequent predisposing lesion for endocarditis in the developing world because of persistence of RHD in those populations. Congenital defects at increased risk for endocarditis are shown in Table 278–1. Although surgical correction of congenital defects such as ventricular septal defect lowers risk, it does not eliminate it. Nevertheless, the American Heart Association does not recommend preventive antibiotic therapy for patients 6 or more months after corrective surgery with prosthetic devices. As a general rule, cardiac lesions not associated with turbulent blood flow, such as cardiac lesions in a relatively low pressure system (e.g., on the right side of the heart) or abnormal flow through a wide orifice (e.g., secundum type of atrial septal defect) are less likely to be complicated by endocarditis. Because of its high prevalence in the population, MVP is the most frequent lesion predisposing to endocarditis. However, the absolute risk for endocarditis among patients with MVP and an audible murmur of mitral insufficiency is considerably lower than that of other cardiac abnormalities. Cardiac lesions that rarely predispose to endocarditis are shown in Table 278–2. Endocarditis can occur on structurally normal native valves in ≥25% of patients. In these patients, endocarditis is more likely to be nosocomial or

TABLE 278–2. CARDIAC LESIONS THAT RARELY PREDISPOSE TO ENDOCARDITIS

Isolated secundum type of atrial septal defect
Syphilitic aortitis
Previous coronary artery bypass graft
Mitral valve prolapse without murmur
Previous rheumatic heart disease without valvular dysfunction
Permanent cardiac pacemakers and implanted defibrillators
Surgical repair, without residua, of secundum atrial septal defect, ventricular septal defect, patent ductus arteriosus after 6 months

Adapted from Dajani AS, Bisno AL, Chung KJ, et al.: Prevention of bacterial endocarditis. Recommendations by the American Heart Association. JAMA 264:2919, 1990. Copyright, 1990, American Medical Association.

TABLE 278–3. CIRCUMSTANCES LIKELY TO LEAD TO TRANSIENT BACTEREMIA THAT CAN PRECEDE ENDOCARDITIS

Dental and periodontal procedure known to induce mucosal bleeding
Tonsillectomy and adenoidectomy
Bronchoscopy with rigid scope
Surgical procedure on the respiratory or intestinal mucosa
Gallbladder surgery
Esophageal dilatation and sclerotherapy for esophageal varices
Prostatic surgery
Vaginal hysterectomy
Cystoscopy or urethral dilatation
In the presence of infection, urethral catheterization or urologic surgery
In presence of infection, vaginal delivery, dilatation and curettage, therapeutic abortion, insertion and removal of intrauterine devices, sterilization procedures
Incision and drainage of infected tissue

Adapted from Dajani AS, Bisno AL, Chung KJ, et al.: Prevention of bacterial endocarditis. Recommendations by the American Heart Association. JAMA 264:2919, 1990. Copyright, 1990, American Medical Association.

caused by more virulent organisms, such as *S. aureus,* or the patient is more likely to be an intravenous drug user (IVDU).

Systemic Host Factors. Systemic host defenses (e.g., granulocytes, T lymphocytes, antibody, complement) most likely play a minor role in development or maintenance of endocarditis, except perhaps for granulocytes in right-sided endocarditis. Various immunodeficiency states, including HIV infection, do not seem to place the patient at increased risk for endocarditis.

CIRCUMSTANCES THAT LEAD TO TRANSIENT BAC-TEREMIA. Transient bacteremia is a common event and occurs as a consequence of trauma to skin or mucosal surfaces that are normally laden with an endogenous flora. The bacteremia is characterized by a low number of organisms per milliliter of blood (usually < 10 CFU per milliliter) and very short duration (15 to 30 minutes). The intensity of the bacteremia is related directly to the magnitude of the trauma, the density of the microbial flora, and the presence of inflammation or infection at the site of skin or mucosal injury. Mucosal sites that have a dense endogenous flora include the gingival crevice, oropharynx, terminal ileum and colon, distal urethra, and vagina. Minor trauma to the gingival crevice as routine as brushing teeth or chewing hard candy may account in part for the 75% of patients with viridans streptococcal endocarditis who fail to recall any unusual circumstance that could have resulted in an episode of transient bacteremia preceding the onset of endocarditis. Transient bacteremia likely to lead to endocarditis can also result from illicit intravenous drug use and nosocomial procedures. Circumstances known to predispose to transient bacteremia that can precede endocarditis are shown in Table 278–3.

A history of such procedures is obtained in only about 25% of patients with viridans streptococcal endocarditis, 40% of patients with enterococcal endocarditis, and 30 to 40% of patients with community-acquired staphylococcal endocarditis, but nevertheless this history is more frequent among patients with endocarditis than among matched controls without endocarditis. The source of bacteremia can be identified in >90% of cases of nosocomial endocarditis. However, some of these procedures may be associated with subsequent endocarditis only in the presence of high-risk underlying cardiac lesions, such as prosthetic valves or previous native valve

endocarditis. The prosthetic valve is usually infected at the time of surgical insertion of the valve or at any time following transient bacteremia in the postoperative period. Rarely the source is a prosthetic valve that was contaminated before insertion.

INFECTING MICROORGANISMS. Trauma to the skin or mucosal surfaces that harbor a prolific endogenous flora releases into the bloodstream many different microbial species. The array of microorganisms entering the circulation varies with the unique endogenous microflora at the particular traumatized site. Staphylococci and diphtheroids are characteristic for skin; oral anaerobes and streptococci for the oropharyngeal mucosa; and colonic anaerobes, enteric aerobic gram-negative bacilli, and enterococci for the genitourinary and lower intestinal mucosa. However, only a few of these species, e.g., most commonly oral streptococci, staphylococci, and enterococci, are likely to cause endocarditis. The frequency with which a particular organism causes endocarditis depends on the how frequently it can gain access to the circulation and its ability to survive in the bloodstream and adhere to components of NBTE, exposed subendothelial structures, or the endothelial surface itself.

A predictable array of microorganisms cause endocarditis for each of the specific conditions that predispose the patients to develop infective endocarditis (Table 278–4). For example, in community-acquired endocarditis in non-IVDU's, a variety of α-hemolytic streptococci (*S. mitis, S. sanguis, S. mutans,* and *S. intermedius*) and enterococci are the usual pathogens. *S. bovis,* a streptococcal species that contains group D polysaccharide capsular material, as does enterococci, causes endocarditis in patients who are likely to have an underlying gastrointestinal lesion. Isolating *S. bovis* from blood cultures should prompt a complete evaluation of the gastrointestinal tract, especially the colon, in that patient. Less frequent are fastidious gram-negative bacilli, the so-called HACEK microorganisms (*Haemophilus* species, *Actinobacillus, Cardiobacterium, Eikenella,* and *Kingella*). The *Haemophilus* species are usually *H. aphrophilus, H. paraphrophilus,* or *H. parainfluenzae,* and rarely *H. influenzae. S. aureus* causes >50% of cases of endocarditis occurring in IVDU's, and in many geographic locations the strains of *S. aureus* are resistant to all β-lactam antibiotics (i.e., usually designated as methicillin-resistant strains). Streptococci and enterococci are less frequent pathogens in IVDU. Gram-negative bacilli (usually *Pseudomonas aeruginosa, P. cepacia,* and *Serratia marcescens*) and fungi (usually non-albicans *Candida* species), unusual in non-IVDU native valve endocarditis, occur in about 8 and 5% of cases of IVDU endocarditis, respectively. Although uncommon in patients without prosthetic valves, coagulase-negative staphylococci, usually of the methicillin-resistant variety, are the predominant pathogen of prosthetic valve endocarditis (PVE) within 2 months after surgery, designated as early PVE. Indeed, the frequency of methicillin-resistant coagulase-negative staphylococci remains constant over the entire first 12 months, which suggests that a similar pathogenesis may extend over the first year after surgery, not just the first 2 months. After the first year, the array of organisms in PVE tends to resemble that of native valve endocarditis (NVE), i.e., streptococci. However, fungi, usually *C. albicans,* and aerobic enteric gram-negative bacilli occur more frequently in both early and late PVE than in non-IVDU native valve endocarditis.

DEVELOPMENT OF THE VEGETATION. Microorganisms adherent to the vegetation stimulate further deposition of platelets and fibrin on their surface. Within this secluded focus, the buried microorganisms then begin multiplying as rapidly as they would in broth cultures, apparently uninhibited by host defenses, e.g., phago-

TABLE 278–4. FREQUENCY OF INFECTING MICROORGANISMS IN ENDOCARDITIS (%)

Native Valve		PVE			Endocarditis in IVDU	
			Early	Late		
Streptococci	50	Coagulase-negative staphylococcus	33	29	*S. aureus*	57
Enterococci	10	*S. aureus*	15	11	Streptococci	13
Staphylococcus aureus	20	Gram-negative bacilli	17	11	Gram-negative bacilli	8
HACEK	5	Fungi	13	5	Enterococci	7
Other	10	Streptococci	9	36	Fungi	5
Culture-negative	5	Diphtheroids	9	3	Polymicrobial	5
		Other	4	5	Culture-negative	5

IVDU = Intravenous drug user.

cytes, antibody, and complement, to reach maximally dense populations of 10^{8-11} CFU per gram of vegetation. Over 90% of the microorganisms in these established vegetations are metabolically inactive and nongrowing, i.e., in a phase least susceptible to the bactericidal effects of β-lactam and aminoglycoside antibiotics.

Sustained bacteremia that is characteristic of endocarditis results from an equilibrium between the rate of release of microorganisms as the vegetation fragments and the rate of clearance of the circulating microorganisms by the reticuloendothelial system in the liver, spleen, and bone marrow. The vegetation enlarges as circulating bacteria are redeposited on the surface of the vegetation, which in turn stimulates further deposition of fibrin on the surface (Fig. 278–2). The resultant vegetation is composed of successive layers of fibrin and clusters of bacteria, with rare red cells and leukocytes, almost always covered by a layer of fibrin on the luminal surface. Enlargement of the vegetation tends to be counterbalanced by continued fragmentation. The ultimate size of the vegetation can vary from small sessile granular protuberances to a large pedunculated mass. The size of the vegetation itself and the fragments that break off depend to some extent on the type of infecting microorganism; e.g., *H. parainfluenzae* and *C. albicans,* tend to produce large friable vegetations and large emboli.

With effective antimicrobial therapy the vegetation becomes progressively organized as the edematous, vascular, and fibrogenic granulation tissue grows in from the base and is replaced by mature fibrous tissue with varying degrees of calcification. Healed vegetations are re-endothelialized, but the associated valve leaflet may become progressively more distorted as the healing proceeds. Thus, despite bacteriologic response, distortion of the healing valve may lead to hemodynamic decompensation and a highly susceptible site for development of repeated episodes of infective endocarditis in the future.

CLINICAL PRESENTATIONS (see Color Plates 11*A* through 11*D*)

Clinical manifestations include fever and cardiac and extracardiac findings that are the result of either (1) the valvular infection itself, (2) embolization of fragments of the vegetation, (3) suppurative complications on the basis of hematogenous spread of infection, or (4) immunologic response to the infection in the form of immune complex vasculitis.

NATIVE VALVE ENDOCARDITIS. Symptoms usually begin within 2 weeks of the inciting bacteremia. In the preantibiotic era, when endocarditis was uniformly fatal, a short duration of illness of < 6 weeks prior to death was used to characterize acute endocarditis; in contrast, subacute and chronic endocarditis had a more indolent course until death of 6 weeks to 2 years. Chronicity is now used in reference to the duration of illness prior to presentation. Acute endocarditis is usually (50 to 70%) caused by *S. aureus,* especially when accompanied by marked signs of general infection and suppurative embolic phenomena and has a rapidly fatal course if treatment is delayed. Infection may develop on a previously normal valve. In the non-IVDU, the aortic valve is usually involved. Therefore, a diagnosis of acute endocarditis can serve as an effective guide to empiric antibiotic therapy, even before results of blood cultures are available. Subacute endocarditis, commonly caused by streptococci and enterococci, in contrast often develops on previously damaged endocardium, has less dramatic clinical manifesta-

tions of general infection, and is characterized by nonsuppurative peripheral vascular phenomena.

Systemic manifestations of endocarditis include fever most commonly and other symptoms that may accompany fever, such as drenching night sweats, arthralgias, myalgias (especially in the low back and thighs), and weight loss. Fever is usually low grade, the temperature peaks rarely exceeding 39.4° C. Fever may be absent in a few patients, e.g., those who are very elderly or severely debilitated, have significant renal or heart failure, or are taking antipyretics or antibiotics.

Cardiac manifestations include: (1) murmurs of valvular insufficiency due to a destroyed or distorted valve and its supporting structures, or valvular stenosis due to large vegetations. (2) Valve ring abscess due to local extension of the infection from the valve ring of the noncoronary cusp of the aortic valve. Valve ring abscesses can lead to persistent fever despite appropriate antimicrobial therapy, heart block as a result of destroyed conduction pathways in the area of the atrioventricular node and bundle of His in the upper interventricular septum, pericarditis or hemopericardium as a result of burrowing abscesses into the pericardium, or shunts between cardiac chambers or between the heart and aorta as a result of burrowing abscesses into other cardiac chambers or aorta. (3) Myocardial infarction from coronary artery embolization. (4) Myocardial abscess as a consequence of bacteremia. (5) Diffuse myocarditis possibly as a consequence of immune complex vasculitis. Murmurs are likely to be absent in tricuspid endocarditis or may be absent when a patient is first seen with acute endocarditis. Congestive heart failure (CHF) is the most common complication of endocarditis, developing in about 60% of patients as a consequence of valvular or myocardial involvement, or may precede the onset of endocarditis as a consequence of the underlying cardiac lesion. CHF is usually present on admission in patients with subacute or streptococcal endocarditis but may develop dramatically in patients with acute *S. aureus* endocarditis with an aortic diastolic murmur or sudden rupture of mitral valve chordae. CHF occurs more frequently with left-sided than right-sided endocarditis and with aortic more than mitral involvement.

Extracardiac manifestations include (1) embolic events that result in infarction of numerous organs, such as the lung in right-sided endocarditis or the brain, spleen, or kidneys in left-sided endocarditis; (2) suppurative complications that include abscesses, septic infarcts, and infected mycotic aneurysms; and (3) immunologic reactions to the valvular infection including glomerulonephritis, sterile meningitis, and polyarthritis, and a variety of vascular phenomena, such as mucocutaneous petechiae (Color Plates 11*A* and 11*C*), splinter hemorrhages, Roth spots (see Color Plate 11*B*), and Osler's nodes. Systemic embolization, often a devastating complication when it involves the cerebral circulation, occurs in about 20 to 40% of patients with left-sided endocarditis. Frank cerebral abscess is rare, except in *S. aureus* endocarditis, when it occurs in 1 to 5% of patients. Septic pulmonary emboli commonly occur in patients with right-sided endocarditis. On chest radiograms, these emboli appear as multiple round infiltrates that may undergo cavitation or be complicated by empyema. Emboli can occur at any time during the course of illness, even after an otherwise successful course of antibiotic therapy is completed, although the frequency of embolization decreases as the vegetation heals. Mycotic aneurysms are an unusual but important complication of endocarditis. Mycotic aneurysms (see Color Plate 11*D*) are commonly asymptomatic but can become clinically evident in 3 to 5% of patients, even months or years after completion of successful therapy. These aneurysms characteristically develop at arterial bifurcations, e.g., in the middle cerebral, splenic, superior mesenteric, pulmonary, coronary, and extremity arteries, the abdominal aorta, and the sinus of Valsalva. In a patient with endocarditis, unremitting headache, visual disturbance, or cranial nerve palsy suggests an impending rupture of a cerebral mycotic aneurysm. Signs of blood loss at any site in a patient with endocarditis should suggest rupture of a mycotic aneurysm once the aneurysm has enlarged beyond a critical size, probably about 1 cm in diameter. The development of clinically apparent splenomegaly and many of the various nonsuppurative peripheral vascular phenomena is related to the duration of illness prior to presentation. The frequency of these clinical manifestations (< 50%) is currently less than in

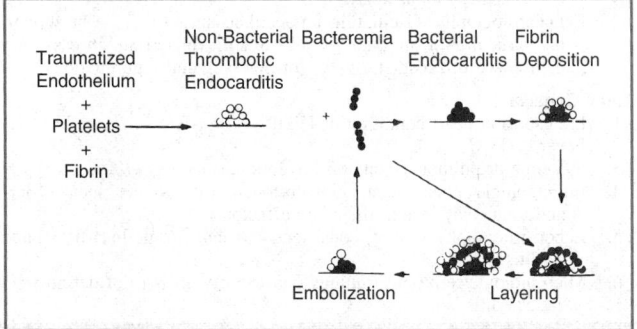

FIGURE 278–2. A schematic diagram of the pathogenetic events leading to development of infective endocarditis.

the past as a result of shorter durations of illness before antimicrobial therapy is given.

ENDOCARDITIS IN IVDU's. IVDU's with endocarditis tend to be younger than non-IVDU's with endocarditis, the disease is usually acute, and a previously normal tricuspid valve is usually involved. In tricuspid endocarditis, murmurs and heart failure are usually absent, but septic pulmonary complications occur in about 75% of these patients and *S. aureus* is the usual pathogen. Left-sided endocarditis in IVDU's resembles that in non-IVDU's, manifested by aortic or mitral murmurs, heart failure, neurologic damage, systemic embolization, peripheral mucocutaneous stigmata of endocarditis, or systemic metastatic infection such as osteomyelitis and septic arthritis. The pathogens isolated from IVDU's with left-sided endocarditis are similar those isolated from non-IVDU's, although *S. aureus* is probably disproportionately involved in IVDU's. Fever, the usual initial manifestation of endocarditis in the IVDU, also accompanies other major and minor illnesses in this population. Indeed only about 10% of febrile IVDU presenting to the emergency room have endocarditis. In most febrile IVDU's with a major infectious diseases such as cellulitis, endocarditis, pneumonia, or osteomyelitis, the cause of the patient's fever is obvious on presentation. However, in about one third of febrile IVDU's with endocarditis the cause of the patient's fever will be not apparent on presentation.

NOSOCOMIAL ENDOCARDITIS. Nosocomial endocarditis, which is defined as being due to a hospital-based procedure performed within 4 weeks preceding the onset of symptoms, accounts for 10 to 30% of cases of endocarditis, the frequency varying with the types of patients. Patients with nosocomial NVE tend to be elderly and have predisposing cardiac lesions, usually on the left-side of the heart. The major predisposing cardiac lesion for nosocomial endocarditis is a prosthetic cardiac valve (present in up to 50% of cases). The most important bacteremia-inducing event during hospitalization which results in endocarditis is use of an intravascular device, present in up to 50% of cases. Nosocomial *S. aureus* bacteremia is much more frequently complicated by endocarditis (5 to 10% of the time) than is enterococcal bacteremia (< 1%). The clinical presentation of nosocomial endocarditis is similar to that of community-acquired endocarditis. In patients with PVE, fever is usually present, although the classic clinical features of endocarditis, such as peripheral vascular phenomena, are frequently absent, especially in early infection. Although blood cultures are usually positive, the diagnosis is frequently delayed owing to failure to recognize the significance of the positive blood cultures.

ELECTROCARDIOGRAPHIC MANIFESTATIONS. A baseline electrocardiogram (ECG) should be obtained to assess the presence of conduction abnormalities that develop in about 10 to 20% of patients with endocarditis as a consequence of burrowing valve ring abscesses. A prolonged PR interval may be the initial indication of the sudden development of more severe conduction abnormalities, such as complete heart block. Other abnormalities that can be detected by ECG include myocardial infarction and pericarditis.

HEMATOLOGIC MANIFESTATIONS. Progressive anemia of chronic disease with normochromic, normocytic indices routinely develops in subacute endocarditis with relatively normal platelet, white blood cell, and differential counts. In acute endocarditis of short duration due to *S. aureus,* anemia may initially be absent, although the white blood cell count is usually elevated with a shift to the left and the platelet count is often low. PVE with an unstable prosthesis may cause acute hemolysis. The erythrocyte sedimentation rate is routinely elevated in endocarditis except when there is hypofibrinogenemia secondary to disseminated intravascular coagulation or congestive heart failure.

RENAL MANIFESTATIONS. Proteinuria and microscopic hematuria are common findings, occurring in up to 50% of patients. Renal emboli or focal glomerulonephritis can cause microscopic hematuria, but gross hematuria usually indicates renal infarction. Renal failure that develops in a patient with endocarditis is usually due to diffuse immune complex glomerulonephritis (see Color Plate 11*E*).

OTHER LABORATORY MANIFESTATIONS. Serologic evidence of circulating immune complexes (CIC) may by found in endocarditis, the frequency of which is related to the duration of illness. Occasional false-positive nontreponemal serologic tests for syphilis occur. The cerebrospinal fluid may show polymorphonuclear leukocytes and moderately elevated protein concentration in

up to 15% of patients. Frank bacterial meningitis, although unusual, occurs in *S. aureus* endocarditis.

DIAGNOSIS

Definitive diagnosis depends on microbiologic or pathologic proof of infection by histology or culture of vegetations obtained at surgery or autopsy or when an arterial embolus is surgically removed. In lieu of surgery or autopsy, definitive diagnosis can be established by demonstrating (1) a characteristic vegetation, valve ring abscess, or new prosthetic valve dehiscence with echocardiography and (2) intravascular infection with multiple blood cultures obtained over an extended period of time that are positive for a microorganism consistent with endocarditis. However, a blood culture or echocardiography is usually obtained only after the diagnosis is suspected based on history and physical findings. The diagnosis can be ranked in order of probability that endocarditis is present by distinction between major and minor criteria, which allows for weighting of clinical findings, echocardiographic findings, the type of microbial species isolated from blood, the frequency of positive blood cultures, and the absence of another source of infection (Table 278–5).

MICROBIOLOGIC INVESTIGATION. Isolating a pathogen from several blood cultures that are obtained over an extended period is important both to confirm the diagnosis of endocarditis and to enable determination of the antibiotic regimen that is optimal for therapy. Bacteremia in endocarditis is characterized by a constant number of organisms per milliliter of blood (usually 20 to 200 CFU per milliliter), unrelated to the height of the patient's temperature or the site of blood sampling (e.g., arterial versus venous blood), except for a slight fall in numbers across the hepatic or splenic circulation. Less than 5% of patients with endocarditis have sterile blood cultures if adequate blood culture methods are used. Three blood cultures should be obtained at least 1 hour apart to demonstrate that the bacteremia is continuous. If the cultures remain negative for 48 hours, two additional cultures should be obtained. However, in the absence of prior antibiotic therapy, the first three blood cultures are

---

TABLE 278–5. CRITERIA FOR THE DIAGNOSIS OF INFECTIVE ENDOCARDITIS (DUKE UNIVERSITY ENDOCARDITIS SERVICE)

1. Definitive diagnosis
   a. Pathology/microbiology of vegetations obtained at surgery or autopsy
   b. Two major criteria
   c. One major/three minor criteria
   d. Five minor criteria
2. Possible diagnosis: Findings consistent with but fall short of definitive diagnosis of endocarditis
3. No endocarditis: No pathology at surgery or autopsy or clinical resolution with 3 days of antimicrobial therapy; firm alternate diagnosis

Major Criteria
1. Blood culture
   a. 2 separate blood cultures positive for:
      i. Viridans streptococci, *S. bovis,* HACEK
      ii. Community-acquired *S. aureus* or enterococci, in absence of primary focus
   b. Positive blood cultures > 12 hours apart
   c. Positive blood cultures: 3 of 3, majority of ≥ 4 with 1st and last ≥ 1 hour apart
2. Echocardiography: Oscillating intracardiac mass on valve or supporting structure or in path of jet stream, valve ring abscess, new dehiscence of prosthetic valve, or new valvular regurgitation

Minor Criteria
1. Predisposing heart condition or IVDU
2. Fever ≥ 38°C
3. Systemic or pulmonary emboli, mycotic aneurysm
4. Immunologic phenomena: glomerulonephritis, Roth's spot, Osler's node, Janeway lesion, rheumatoid factor
5. Echocardiography finding consistent with but not definitive of endocarditis
6. Microbiologic/serologic findings consistent with but not definitive of endocarditis

Adapted from Durack DT, Lukes AS, Bright DK, et al.: New criteria for diagnosis of infective endocarditis: Utilization of specific echocardiographic findings. Am J Med 96:200, 1994.

IVDU = Intravenous drug user.

expected to be positive in >95% of patients with positive cultures. Prior antibiotic therapy, fastidious bacteria (such as the nutritionally deficient streptococci, the HACEK group of organisms, *Neisseria, Brucella,* and *Legionella*), fungi, chlamydia, and rickettsia can result in negative cultures. In acute endocarditis, when empiric antibiotic therapy should be initiated as soon as possible, two or three blood cultures should be drawn 1 hour apart before starting empiric therapy. In the face of a preceeding course of antibiotics, further antibiotic therapy should be held and blood cultures repeated until positive, if clinical conditions permit. The longer the time since the last dose of antibiotic or the shorter the preceding course of antibiotic, the more likely it is that the blood cultures will be positive. When fastidious bacteria and fungi are suspected, the clinical microbiology laboratory should be consulted for advice on the optimal methods to isolate these microorganisms, which may require more prolonged incubation (e.g., up to 3 weeks) or special media for isolation. Gram stain of the cultures may identify some pathogens not otherwise apparent in the blood cultures. Fungal endocarditis, which is likely to have negative blood cultures, tends to be complicated by large vegetations and embolization, in which case the organisms can be identified by Gram stain and culture of the surgically removed emboli. Serology techniques are needed to diagnose endocarditis due to *Chlamydia psittaci, C. trachomatis,* or *Coxiella burnetti* and may be helpful for *Brucella* endocarditis. Bacteriuria with either enterococci or *S. aureus* occurs in endocarditis due to the respective organism. Several *in vitro* tests must be done on the pathogen isolated from blood to assess susceptibility to potential bactericidal drugs (Table 278–6).

CARDIAC IMAGING PROCEDURES. Echocardiography has become second only to culture of blood for investigating patients who clinically are suspected to have endocarditis. Echocardiography can visualize valvular vegetations, satellite vegetations, flail valves, ruptured chordae, perivalvular abscesses, fistulas, valvular perforations, and mycotic aneurysms. Echocardiography can also identify predisposing cardiac lesions. Two-dimensional transthoracic echocardiography (TTE) and transesophageal echocardiography (TEE), the two currently performed types of echocardiography, are safe and portable to the bedside. TTE is rapid, noninvasive, and relatively inexpensive (see Ch. 33.3).

OTHER INVESTIGATIVE PROCEDURES. Although other studies may be suggestive, angiography is required for the definitive antemortem diagnosis of a mycotic aneurysm. Cardiac catheterization can provide important information and should not be avoided when indicated in selected patients with endocarditis for fear of dislodging emboli. Coronary angiography is used to assess the presence of significant coronary artery disease before elective placement of prosthetic cardiac valves in patients who are over age 40 and have additional atherogenic risk factors. Computed tomography is used to define the cause of focal neurologic findings and identify metastatic suppurative infection or embolic events that can impede clinical or bacteriologic therapeutic response.

DIAGNOSTIC STRATEGIES IN SPECIAL SITUATIONS. *IVDU* (see Ch. 12). Since outpatient follow-up in this population is rarely possible, admitting febrile IVDU's without a clinically apparent source for their fever is indicated for at least 1 week until results of blood culture are available. Blood cultures become positive within 1 week in most patients if fungi, fastidious gram-negative bacilli or streptococci, or anaerobes are involved or the patient has recently taken antibiotics. After obtaining blood cultures, empiric antimicrobial therapy should be initiated. Once the blood cultures are found to be positive, evidence of endocarditis should be sought initially by TTE, and if the TTE is negative, by TEE. If echocardiography reveals vegetations, valvular destruction or its hemodynamic effects, valve ring abscess or fistula, or predisposing valvular lesion and/or clinical evidence of left-sided or right-sided endocarditis (e.g., septic pleuropulmonary complications) exists, the diagnosis of endocarditis is made. Vegetations detected by TTE indicate a group of patients at greater risk of morbidity, i.e., prolonged fever or development of CHF. Evidence of CHF on echocardiogram defines a group of patients who may subsequently require valve replacement. Even if there is another potential source for the bacteremia and no echocardiographic or clinical evidence of endocarditis, but the organism isolated is likely to cause endocarditis, such as *S. aureus* or a streptococcus, the diagnosis of endocarditis should nevertheless be suspected. If there is no apparent source for the bacteremia, even if echocardiographic and clinical evidence is lacking, the patient should still be considered to possibly have endocarditis. With negative echocardiography, if the clinical course dictates and another diagnosis is still not apparent, the TEE should be repeated in about 1 week. If blood cultures remain negative after 1 week of incubation, the patient may be discharged from the hospital without echocardiography, unless there is clinical evidence of left-sided or right-sided endocarditis, in which case the diagnosis of endocarditis should nevertheless be suspected.

NOSOCOMIAL NATIVE VALVE ENDOCARDITIS. In patients with bacteremia related to intravascular devices, such as an arteriovenous fistula or graft for hemodialysis, indwelling central intravenous line, cardiac assist balloon pump, or pacemaker wire, the device should be removed, especially with *S. aureus* bacteremia or fungemia, or if an indwelling catheter is associated with a tunnel or exit site infection. In patients with clinical evidence of endocarditis, echocardiography should be done to confirm the diagnosis and to assess local complications. Catheter-associated coagulase-negative staphylococcal nosocomial bacteremia, which rarely eventuates in NVE, should not be investigated with echocardiography after antibiotics are begun unless a prosthetic cardiac valve is present. Indeed, catheter removal may not be necessary to cure coagulase-negative staphylococcal catheter-associated bacteremia. Catheter-associated nosocomial fungemia probably should be investigated with echocardiography after the catheter is removed and an-

TABLE 278–6. *IN VITRO* ASSAYS

Viridans streptococcus	Broth dilution test	Penicillin MIC
Enterococcus	Broth dilution test	Penicillin MIC
		Vancomycin MIC
	Growth in	High-level resistance to:
	500 μg/ml	gentamicin
	1000 μg/ml	streptomycin
	Nitrocephin	β-Lactamase production
Staphylococcus aureus,	Nitrocephin	β-Lactamase production
coagulase-negative	Oxacillin/methicillin	MRSA/MRSE
staphylococcus	sensitivity	
	Broth dilution test	Vancomycin MIC
		Rifampin MIC
		TMP-SMX MIC
Other pathogens	Broth dilution tests	Antibiotic MIC/MBC
All pathogens	Serum bactericidal activity*	Bactericidal activity at peak
	Serum antibiotic level	Peak and trough gentamicin and vancomycin levels

*May be useful for nonstandard antimicrobial regimens or unusual pathogens.
MIC = Minimal inhibitory concentration; MBC = minimal bactericidal concentration; MRSA = methicillin-resistant *S. aureus;* MRSE = methicillin-resistant coagulase-negative staphylococci; TMP-SMX = trimethoprim-sulfamethoxazole.
From Levison ME: *In vitro* assays. In Kaye D (ed.): Infective Endocarditis. 2nd ed. New York, Raven Press, 1992, p 151.

tifungal chemotherapy begun, whether or not clinical evidence of endocarditis is present.

PROSTHETIC VALVE ENDOCARDITIS. The diagnosis of PVE is usually suspected because of fever and confirmed by the presence of multiple blood cultures positive for the same microorganism. In a recent study, 43% of patients with a prosthetic valve who developed fever and bacteremia had or developed PVE. Any organism in blood cultures in these patients must be taken seriously as potential causes of endocarditis. In those presenting with clinical evidence suggestive of PVE, empiric antibiotic therapy can be initiated after three or four sets of blood cultures are obtained. After antimicrobial therapy is started, blood cultures should be repeated to assess for clearance of bacteremia. In bacteremic patients with no evidence of endocarditis despite these studies, antimicrobial therapy has traditionally been recommended for 2 weeks, but new data suggest that even therapy continued beyond 2 weeks may not prevent PVE from occurring as a result of the initially transient bacteremia.

ANTIBIOTIC THERAPY

PRINCIPLES. Effective antimicrobial therapy of endocarditis optimally requires identification of the specific pathogen and assessment of its susceptibility to various antimicrobial agents. Therefore, every effort must be made to isolate the pathogen before initiating antimicrobial therapy, if clinically feasible. In those patients who are in immediate danger of death, empiric antibiotic therapy should be started as soon as possible after obtaining blood cultures. Empiric therapy should be targeted at the most likely pathogens in that particular clinical setting (see Table 278–4). The minimal requirements for an effective antimicrobial regimen include the following:

1. Bactericidal Activity. Bacteriostatic agents are not able to clear the pathogen from infected tissues unaided by host defenses, such as polymorphonuclear leukocytes, antibody, and complement. Because host defenses are thought not to operate within vegetations (except in tricuspid valve vegetations, in which polymorphonuclear leukocytes may aid the effect of an antimicrobial agent) clearing bacteria from these vegetations requires bactericidal action from the antibiotics. In fact, complete eradication of pathogens from the vegetation is thought to be essential to cure endocarditis. If any bacteria remain after completion of antibiotic therapy, the residual organisms regrow and result in relapse. If the pathogen cannot be eliminated completely by antimicrobial therapy, e.g., if relapse occurs or the patient has persistent bacteremia, the infected vegetation may need to be excised surgically for cure. Table 278–7 shows the various antimicrobial agents that have bactericidal activity. For microorganisms without predictable susceptibility, bactericidal activity of an antimicrobial agent for the particular patient's pathogen must be assessed by determination of the minimal inhibitory (MIC) and minimal bactericidal concentrations (MBC) of the antimicrobial agents *in vitro* (see Table 278–6).

The enterococcus illustrates the problems in selecting appropriate bactericidal therapy for endocarditis. Enterococci are relatively resistant to penicillin. In contrast to viridans streptococci, which are inhibited by 0.1 μg per milliliter of penicillin G, most *E. faecalis* require up to 6.3 μg per milliliter to be inhibited. Unlike viridans streptococci that are killed by relatively low concentrations of penicillin, penicillin G alone, even at concentrations of up to 1000 μg

per milliliter, is only inhibitory or at best slightly bactericidal against enterococci. The aminoglycosides are also poorly effective at low concentrations (< 500 to 1000 μg per milliliter) owing to inadequate permeability. Antibiotic synergism does occur, however, as the result of enhanced intracellular uptake of the aminoglycoside in the presence of a β-lactam (such as penicillin, ampicillin, or piperacillin) or a glycopeptide (such as vancomycin or teicoplanin), the so-called cell wall–active antibiotics. The definition of synergism requires that the reduction in bacterial count at 24 hours with the drug combination be at least 100-fold greater than that with the cell wall–active antibiotic alone. Synergism is predicted on routine screening of strains by inhibition of growth with 500 μg per milliliter of gentamicin or 1000 μg per milliliter of streptomycin (see Table 278–6). No bactericidal therapy exists for strains that exhibit high-level resistance to both gentamicin and streptomycin or strains that exhibit high-level resistance to both β-lactam and glycopeptide antibiotics.

2. High Concentrations of the Antimicrobial Agent in the Vegetation. Doses of the antimicrobial agent must achieve blood concentrations of the antimicrobial agent high enough to facilitate passive diffusion of the antimicrobial agent into the depths of the vegetation where the microcolonies of the pathogen are located. Dosing sufficiently large to attain bactericidal activity in a $\geq 1:8$ dilution of the patient's serum against the patient's pathogen at the peak time after administrating the antimicrobial agent has traditionally guided therapy (although more recent data suggest that dilutions of $\geq 1:64$ have more predictive accuracy for bacteriologic cure).

3. Prolonged Duration of Antimicrobial Therapy. Over 90% of the microbial population in the vegetation is nongrowing and metabolically inactive once the infection has become well established. Nongrowing organisms are more likely to be found in the central portions of the microcolonies in the deeper regions of the vegetation. As a result, microorganisms in vegetations for the most part are not susceptible to commonly used antibiotics that are effective only against actively growing bacteria, such as the β-lactams and aminoglycosides. Optimally the antimicrobial agent should be active against nongrowing microorganisms. However, when the drug is active only against growing microorganisms, each dose of the bactericidal drug is able to effect a reduction in the microbial count only in that minor portion (< 10%) of the population that happens to be growing at the time of drug administration. The duration of drug therapy therefore must be prolonged in order to completely clear the pathogen from the vegetation.

Duration of therapy varies with the specific pathogen, the site of the infection, and the type of antibiotic. For example, bacterial clearance is more rapid for viridans streptococci than for staphylococci, in tricuspid than in aortic vegetations, with antistaphylococcal β-lactams than with vancomycin, or with combinations of cell wall–active agent plus aminoglycoside than with single drugs. More rapid clearance in these special circumstances may permit a shorter course of therapy to achieve cure.

4. Dosing Should Be Frequent Enough to Prevent Regrowth of Microorganisms Between Doses. The organisms that remain after a brief *in vitro* exposure to an aminoglycoside or a β-lactam antibiotic frequently exhibit a postexposure delay in further *in vitro* growth, the so-called postantibiotic effect. Unfortunately, no such effect occurs with some organisms, such as enterococci or *P. aeruginosa* in vegetations. Thus, even though a bactericidal effect can be achieved in the vegetation in the early portions of a dosing interval when levels of the drug are high, if antibiotic levels are not maintained in the vegetation at least above the MIC during the rest of the dosing interval, the residual organisms may regrow and efficacy may be compromised.

Standardized regimens have been recommended for the most common pathogens—viridans streptococci, enterococci, and staphylococci on native and prosthetic valves (Table 278–8). Standardized regimens are not available for more unusual pathogens, including strains of *E. faecalis* that both produce β-lactamase and are highly aminoglycoside-resistant; strains of enterococci that exhibit high-level resistance to vancomycin, ampicillin, and aminoglycosides; and gram-negative bacilli, anaerobes, and diphtheroids. *In vitro* susceptibility testing should be performed for these organisms and the patient treated with the regimen that demonstrates the best bactericidal activity. Bactericidal activity for anaerobic gram-negative bacilli can frequently be achieved with metronidazole, for HACEK organisms with ceftriaxone, for aerobic enteric gram-negative bacilli

---

TABLE 278–7. BACTERICIDAL AGENTS

β-lactams	Penams (e.g., penicillin, ampicillin, amoxicillin, nafcillin, ticarcillin)
	Penems (none as yet marketed)
	Carbapenem (imipenem)
	Cephems (cephalosporins, cefoxitin)
	Carbacephems (loracarbef)
	Monobactam (aztreonam)
Aminoglycosides	E.g., gentamicin, tobramycin, amikacin
Quinolones	E.g., ciprofloxacin, ofloxacin, norfloxacin, enoxacin
Glycopeptides	Vancomycin, teicoplanin
Other	Trimethoprim-sulfamethoxazole
	Metronidazole
	Rifampin

Adapted from Levison ME: *In vitro* assays. *In* Kaye D (ed.): Infective Endocarditis. 2nd ed. New York, Raven Press, 1992, p 151.

or *P. aeruginosa* with a cell wall–active agent–aminoglycoside combination or ciprofloxacin, for diphtheroids with a vancomycin-aminoglycoside combination, and for methicillin-resistant coagulase-negative staphylococci causing PVE with vancomycin-aminoglycoside-rifampin combination.

SURGICAL THERAPY (see Ch. 41.3)

Prosthetic valve surgery is indicated in the following situations: (1) Increasing or refractory CHF secondary to valvular dysfunction. In those patients who are hemodynamically unstable, emergency cardiac valve replacement should not be delayed to allow further antibiotic therapy. Although operative mortality and PVE are higher in this situation than when a prosthetic valve is placed in the absence of active infection, the overall outcome is better if the prosthesis is replaced promptly, the patient's clinical condition permitting, despite active infection. If the patient is hemodynamically stable, prosthetic valve replacement is best delayed until a course of antimicrobial therapy is completed or has been given for at least 7 days. (2) Multiple clinically significant emboli, despite antibiotic therapy for 2 weeks. (3) Infection due to certain pathogens such as fungi, which rarely respond to medical therapy, high level ampicillin/aminoglycoside/vancomycin-resistant enterococci, β-lactamase producing/high-level aminoglycoside–resistant *E. faecalis,* and β-lactam or quinolone resistant gram-negative bacilli. Surgical indications for valve ring abscess, which may heal with antimicrobials alone, include extension of infection, development of prosthetic valve dehiscence, heart block, or CHF, and persistence of infection despite medical therapy. Patients with valve ring abscess should be monitored for conduction abnormalities, which may require placing a transvenous pacemaker because of the risk of high-grade heart block.

 TABLE 278–8. ANTIBIOTIC THERAPY (ADULT DOSES) FOR INFECTIVE ENDOCARDITIS

Regimen	Dose and Duration

Highly penicillin-susceptible streptococci (MIC ≤ 0.1 μg/ml)
1. Aqueous penicillin G, 10–20 million U daily IV for 4 weeks
2. Aqueous penicillin G, 10–20 million U daily IV
   plus
   Streptomycin, 7.5 mg/kg (maximum 500 mg) q12h IM[a]
   or
   Gentamicin, 1 mg/kg (maximum 80 mg) q8h IV/IM[b] for 2 weeks
3. Aqueous penicillin G, 10–20 million U daily IV for 4 weeks
   plus
   Streptomycin, 7.5 mg/kg (maximum 500 mg) q12h IM[a]
   or
   Gentamicin, 1 mg/kg (maximum 80 mg) q8h IV/IM[b] for the first 2 weeks
4. Ceftriaxone, 2 grams q24h IV for 4 weeks

Highly penicillin-susceptible streptococci in penicillin-allergic patients
1. Cefazolin,[c] 1 gram q8h IV/IM
   or
   Ceftriaxone, 2 grams q24h IV for 4 weeks
   or
2. Vancomycin,[d] 30 mg/kg daily (maximum 2 grams/day unless serum levels are monitored) divided q6h or q12h IV for 4 weeks

Streptococci relatively resistant to penicillin (MIC > 0.1 and < 0.5 μg/ml)
Aqueous penicillin G, 20 million U daily IV for 4 weeks
   plus
Streptomycin, 7.5 mg/kg (maximum 500 mg) q12h IM[a]
   or
Gentamicin, 1 mg/kg (maximum 80 mg) q8h IV/IM[b] for the first 2 weeks

Enterococci or other streptococci (MIC ≥ 0.5 μg/ml)
Aqueous penicillin G, 20–30 million U daily IV, or ampicillin, 12 grams daily IV
   plus
Gentamicin, 1 mg/kg (maximum 80 mg) q8h IV/IM[be]
   or
Streptomycin, 7.5 mg/kg (maximum 500 mg) q12h IM[ae] for 4 to 6 weeks

Enterococci or other streptococci in penicillin-allergic patients (MIC ≥ 0.5 μg/ml[f])
Vancomycin,[g] 30 mg/kg daily (maximum 2 grams/day unless levels are monitored) divided q6h or q12h IV
   plus
Gentamicin, 1 mg/kg (maximum 80 mg) q8h IV/IM[be]
   or
Streptomycin, 7.5 mg/kg (maximum 500 mg) q12h IM[ae] for 4 to 6 weeks

 TABLE 278–8. ANTIBIOTIC THERAPY (ADULT DOSES) FOR INFECTIVE ENDOCARDITIS *Continued*

Regimen	Dose and Duration

Methicillin-susceptible staphylococci
Nafcillin, 2 grams q4h IV
   or
Oxacillin, 2 grams q4h IV for 4 to 6 weeks
   with or without
Gentamicin,[h] 1 mg/kg (maximum 80 mg) q8h IV/IM for first 3 to 5 days only

Methicillin-susceptible staphylococci in penicillin-allergic patients
Cefazolin, 2 grams q8h IV
   with or without
Gentamicin,[h] 1 mg/kg (maximum 80 mg) q8h IV/IM for first 3 to 5 days only
   or
Vancomycin,[d] 30 mg/kg daily (maximum 2 grams/day unless serum levels are monitored) divided q6h or q12h IV for 4 to 6 weeks

Methicillin-resistant staphylococci
Vancomycin,[g] 30 mg/kg daily (maximum 2 grams/day unless serum levels are monitored) divided q6h or q12h IV for 4 to 6 weeks

Methicillin-resistant staphylococci in the presence of a prosthetic device
Vancomycin,[g] 30 mg/kg daily (maximum 2 grams/day unless serum levels are monitored) divided q6h or q12h IV
   plus
Rifampin,[i] 300 mg q8h PO for 6 weeks or longer
   plus
Gentamicin, 1 mg/kg (maximum 80 mg) q8h IV/IM[b] for first 2 weeks

Methicillin-susceptible staphylococci in the presence of a prosthetic device
Nafcillin,[j] 2 grams q4h IV
   or
Oxacillin, 2 grams q4h IV for 6 weeks or longer
   plus
Gentamicin, 1 mg/kg (maximum 80 mg) q8h IV/IM[b] for the first 2 weeks
   with or without
Rifampin,[k] 300 mg q8h PO for 6 weeks or longer

[a]Peak serum levels should be approximately 20 μg/ml.
[b]Peak serum levels should be approximately 3 μg/ml.
[c]Streptomycin or gentamicin may be added for the first 2 weeks as in Regimen 3.
[d]Vancomycin is preferred if immediate-type hypersensitivity is suspected. The dose should be infused over 1 hour, and peak levels at 1 hour after the end of infusion should be approximately 30 to 45 μg/ml when given every 12 hours or 20 to 35 μg/ml when given every 6 hours.
[e]Choice of an aminoglycoside should be based on *in vitro* susceptibility testing. Enterococci should be tested for high-level resistance.
[f]Penicillin desensitization should be considered. Cephalosporins are not acceptable alternatives.
[g]Vancomycin should be infused over 1 hour, and peak levels at 1 hour after the end of infusion should be approximately 30 to 45 μg/ml when given every 12 hours or 20 to 35 μg/ml when given every 6 hours.
[h]The benefit of additional aminoglycoside has not been established.
[i]Rifampin should be added in cases of coagulase-negative staphylococci; its use for coagulase-positive staphylococci is controversial.
[j]Cefazolin or vancomycin should be used in penicillin-allergic patients. Vancomycin is preferred if there is immediate-type hypersensitivity.
[k]The use of rifampin for methicillin-susceptible staphylococci is controversial.
Adapted from Bisno AL, Dismukes WE, Durack DT, et al.: Antimicrobial treatment of infective endocarditis due to viridans streptococci, enterococci and staphylococci. JAMA 261:1471, 1989.

The surgical indications for PVE are the same as those outlined for NVE and include relapse after a course of appropriate antibiotic therapy. To avoid the complications of prosthetic valve replacement (e.g., PVE, bleeding, thromboembolic events, and valve deterioration), new surgical options, which have been proposed as an alternative to a prosthetic valve, include valve debridement, valvuloplasty, and repair or replacement of the paravalvular structure with pulmonary root autograft. Prosthetic valve replacement in an IVDU is problematic, because the prosthetic valve places the patient at continued risk of PVE. Alternatively for tricuspid valve endocarditis, tricuspid valve resection without prosthetic replacement can be tolerated hemodynamically for extended periods of time in many of these patients.

Intrathoracic, intra-abdominal, or peripheral mycotic aneurysms usually require surgical excision. Cerebral aneurysms may heal on medical therapy alone. If symptomatic, cerebral aneurysms should be followed closely with serial angiography and may require surgery if enlarging or bleeding.

Myocardial revascularization should be performed at the time of elective valve surgery if significant coronary artery disease is present. However, patients who require emergency placement of the

TABLE 278-9. REASONS FOR INADEQUATE CLINICAL RESPONSE

1. Inadequate therapy: wrong drug, wrong dose
2. Infarcts secondary to emboli
3. Metastatic abscesses of the spleen, kidney, brain, etc., that may require surgical drainage
4. Suppurative thrombophlebitis at site of an IV catheter, with or without superinfecting endocarditis
5. Other superinfections: e.g., *Clostridium difficile* colitis, urinary tract infection
6. Febrile reaction to the antimicrobial agent or another drug
7. Another unrelated febrile illness

TABLE 278-10. CURE RATES (ANTIMICROBIAL THERAPY + SURGERY) (%)

Native valve endocarditis	
Non-IVDU	
Viridans streptococci*	> 90
Vancomycin, ampicillin, aminoglycoside– susceptible enterococci*	75–90
*Staphylococcus aureus**	60–75
Fungi	40–50†
IVDU	
S. aureus, left-sided	50
S. aureus, right-sided	95
Prosthetic valve endocarditis	
Early onset	12–44
Late onset	47–70

*Deaths due to complications, not failure of antibiotic therapy.
†Antimicrobial therapy plus surgery.
IVDU = Intravenous drug user.

✔ TABLE 278-11. PROPHYLACTIC REGIMENS FOR BACTERIAL ENDOCARDITIS

Genitourinary/gastrointestinal procedures*

Standard regimen

Ampicillin, gentamicin, and amoxicillin	IV or IM administration of ampicillin, 2.0 g, plus gentamicin, 1.5 mg/kg (not to exceed 80 mg), 30 min before procedure; followed by amoxicillin, 1.5 g, orally 6 hr after initial dose; alternatively, the parenteral regimen may be repeated once 8 hr after initial dose.

Ampicillin/amoxicillin/penicillin–allergic patients

Vancomycin and gentamicin	IV administration of vancomycin. 1.0 g, over 1 hr, plus IV or IM administration of gentamicin, 1.5 mg/kg (not to exceed 80 mg), 1 hr before procedure; may be repeated once 8 hr after initial dose.

Alternate low-risk patients

Amoxicillin	3.0 g orally 1 hr before procedure; then 1.5 g 6 hr after initial dose.

Dental, oral, or upper respiratory tract procedures in patients who are at risk*

Standard regimen

Amoxicillin	3.0 g orally 1 hr before procedure; then 1.5 g 6 hr after initial dose

Amoxicillin/penicillin–allergic patients

Erythromycin	Erythromycin ethylsuccinate, 800 mg, or erythromycin stearate, 1.0 g, orally 2 hr before procedure, then half the dose 6 hr after initial dose
or	
Clindamycin	300 mg orally 1 hr before procedure and 150 mg 6 hr after initial dose

Patients unable to take oral medications

Ampicillin	IV or IM administration of ampicillin, 2.0 g, 30 min before procedure; then IV or IM administration of ampicillin, 1.0 g or oral administration of amoxicillin, 1.5 g, 6 hr after initial dose

Ampicillin/amoxicillin/penicillin–allergic patients unable to take oral medications

Clindamycin	IV administration of 300 mg 30 min before procedure and IV or oral administration of 150 mg 6 hr after initial dose

Patients considered high risk and not candidates for standard regimen†

Ampicillin, gentamicin, and amoxicillin	IV or IM administration of ampicillin, 2.0 g, plus gentamicin, 1.5 mg/kg (not to exceed 80 mg), 30 min before procedure; followed by amoxicillin, 1.5 g, orally 6 hr after initial dose; alternatively, the parenteral regimen may be repeated 8 hr after initial dose

Ampicillin/amoxicillin/penicillin–allergic patients considered high risk†

Vancomycin	IV administration of 1.0 g over 1 hr, starting 1 hr before procedure; no repeat dose necessary

*Initial pediatric doses are as follows: ampicillin or amoxicillin, 50 mg/kg; erythromycin ethylsuccinate or erythromycin stearate, 20 mg/kg; clindamycin, 10 mg/kg; gentamicin, 2.0 mg/kg; and vancomycin, 20 mg/kg. Follow-up doses should be one half the initial dose. *Total pediatric dose should not exceed total adult dose.* The following weight ranges may also be used for the initial pediatric dose of amoxicillin: < 15 kg, 750 mg; 15 to 30 kg, 1500 mg; and > 30 kg, 3000 mg (full adult dose). Follow-up amoxicillin dose is 25 mg/kg.
†Includes those with prosthetic heart valves and other high-risk patients.
Adapted from Dajani AS, Bisno AL, Chung KJ, et al.: Prevention of bacterial endocarditis. Recommendations by the American Heart Association. JAMA 264:2919, 1990.

prosthetic valve for hemodynamic decompensation secondary to acute endocarditis usually cannot tolerate the dye load necessary for coronary angiography and the additional bypass surgery.

Anticoagulant therapy, although it may impede further enlargement of a vegetation, is relatively contraindicated in endocarditis due to conversion of a unsuspected cerebral infarct into an intracerebral bleed.

SHORTER INPATIENT THERAPY

Shorter courses of antibiotic therapy, oral regimens, and parenteral antibiotic therapy administered at home have been investigated in selected patients to shorten the course of hospitalization. Having a focal infection that would require more than 2 weeks of antimicrobial therapy, PVE, and significant renal or eighth nerve impairment precludes use of short-course β-lactam–aminoglycoside combination therapy. Absorption of orally administered agents may be unreliable, and oral therapy is generally not recommended. Patients can be selected for parenteral therapy at home by their being at low risk for complications of endocarditis, the most frequent of which are CHF and emboli. In streptococcal endocarditis, heart failure, if not present on admission, rarely first develops during therapy. Emboli most often occur before or within the first few days of antimicrobial therapy. Before considering outpatient therapy, most patients should first be evaluated and stabilized in the hospital, although some patients may be managed entirely as outpatients. The standard regimens used to treat penicillin-sensitive streptococci require either continuous infusion of penicillin or frequent intravenous administration. A single daily dose of ceftriaxone is an attractive alternate to penicillin for antibiotic therapy at home. Because of its long half-life and good potency against these streptococci, serum levels of ceftriaxone remain well above the MIC and MBC for over 24 hours.

RESPONSE TO THERAPY

Once on appropriate antimicrobial therapy, most patients note a sense of well-being, less fatigue, and improved appetite, and their temperature usually falls to normal levels within 2 to 5 days. However, the erythrocyte sedimentation rate, anemia, and renal function may take weeks to months to improve. CIC and related serologic findings that include hypocomplementemia, mixed cryoglobulinemia, and rheumatoid factor also tend to resolve with effective antibiotic therapy. Blood cultures for streptococci and enterococci should become sterile after 1 to 2 days of appropriate therapy and for *S. aureus,* after 3 to 5 days; however, with vancomycin therapy, blood cultures for *S. aureus* may take 10 to 14 days to become sterile. Blood cultures are obtained daily until sterile. If no organism is isolated from blood, but there is a good clinical response to an empiric antimicrobial regimen, empiric therapy should be continued. If no organism is isolated and there is no clinical response to empiric therapy after 1 to 2 weeks, endocarditis due to a fastidious pathogen, e.g., fungi or anaerobes, or a diagnosis other than endocarditis should be considered. If the pathogen is initially isolated from blood and appropriate antimicrobial therapy started but fever persists or recurs, blood cultures should be repeated to assess persistent or relapsing infection, among other possibilities, which include most commonly pulmonary or systemic embolization (Table 278–9). For nonstandard regimens or unusual pathogens, peak serum bactericidal activity may be assayed against the patient's pathogen early in the course of therapy, and if inadequate the dose of the antibiotic is increased (although not at the cost of toxicity) and the serum retested. Measuring vancomycin or aminoglycoside serum levels may be helpful to ensure adequate but nontoxic antibiotic levels. Blood cultures are repeated 2 and 4 weeks after therapy has been completed, relapse being most common within 1 month. The relapse organism should be evaluated for the development of antibiotic resistance.

OUTCOMES (Table 278–10)

Factors that affect mortality include the infecting organism (the mortality of endocarditis due to fungi and aerobic enteric gram-negative bacilli > staphylococci > enterococci > streptococci), the site of infection (aortic > mitral and left-sided > tricuspid infection), NVE versus PVE (early onset PVE > late onset PVE > NVE), age (higher in the elderly and very young), gender (men > women), and the presence of certain complications, such as heart or renal failure, rupture of a mycotic aneurysm, cardiac arrhythmias and

conduction abnormalities, and cerebral emboli. Heart failure remains the leading cause of death. However, with increasing use of prosthetic valve replacement for heart failure, the leading cause of death may shift to neurologic complications due to embolic episodes or mycotic aneurysms or uncontrolled infection due to antibiotic-resistant microorganisms. Following cure of one episode of endocarditis, patients remain at increased risk for reinfection.

PREVENTION

The effect of endocarditis prophylaxis with antimicrobial agents has been estimated to be modest; i.e., < 10% of all cases are preventable by prophylaxis. For example, only about one half of cases have recognizable predisposing cardiac lesions, most cases do not follow an invasive procedure, and only about two thirds of cases are due to microorganisms (viridans streptococci and enterococci) against which prophylactic regimens are directed. However, in those patients who are known to have a risky cardiac lesion (see Table 278–1) and are to undergo a procedure that is likely to induce bacteremia (see Table 278–3), with organisms having predictable susceptibility to antibiotics with minimal inconvenience, toxicity, and cost, the American Heart Association has made the recommendations shown in Table 278–11. Additional preventive measures are minimizing invasive procedures, avoiding intravascular catheters (a major predisposing event for PVE), aggressively treating focal infections, and maintaining good dental hygiene in patients at increased risk for endocarditis.

Durack DT: Prevention of infective endocarditis, N Engl J Med 332:38, 1995. *Discusses prevention as a complex issue involving diverse aspects of medicine, microbiology, dentistry, surgery, epidemiology, and decision analysis.*
Durack DT, Lukes AS, Bright DK, et al.: New criteria for diagnosis of infective endocarditis: Utilization of specific echocardiographic findings. Am J Med 96:200, 1994.
Kaye D (ed.): Infective Endocarditis. 2nd ed. New York, Raven Press, 1992. *This multiauthored text is a thorough, up-to-date review of every aspect of infective endocarditis, written by experts.*
Wilson WR, Steckelberg JM (eds.): Infective endocarditis. Infect Dis Clin North Am 7:1, 1993. *This issue highlights important new developments in pathogenesis, diagnosis, and treatment.*

279 STAPHYLOCOCCAL INFECTIONS
Gordon L. Archer

Staphylococcus aureus has been recognized as one of the most important and lethal human bacterial pathogens since the beginning of this century. Until the antibiotic era, >80% of patients growing *S. aureus* from their blood died; most of those dying had been healthy with no underlying disease. Though infections caused by coagulase-positive *S. aureus* were generally known to be potentially lethal, coagulase-negative staphylococci had been dismissed as avirulent skin commensals incapable of causing human disease. However, over the past 20 years, coagulase-negative staphylococcal infections have emerged as one of the major complications of medical progress. They are currently the pathogens most commonly isolated from infections of indwelling foreign devices and are the leading cause of hospital-acquired bacteremias in United States hospitals. This ascendancy of staphylococci as pre-eminent nosocomial pathogens also has been associated with a major increase in the proportion of these isolates that are resistant to multiple antimicrobial agents. If the trend continues, we may be forced to revisit the serious staphylococcal infections of the preantibiotic era that textbooks had long since relegated to medical history.

BACTERIOLOGY. The name staphylococcus means "bunch of grapes" and describes the clusters and clumps of gram-positive cocci seen on Gram stain of both infected material and organisms recovered from culture bottles and agar plates. Staphylococci produce catalase, breaking down hydrogen peroxide to H_2O and O_2; streptococci do not. This is the definitive test for separating the two

TABLE 279–1. STAPHYLOCOCCAL SPECIES FOUND ON HUMAN SKIN AND MUCOUS MEMBRANES

Coagulase-positive	Coagulase-negative	
S. aureus	S. epidermidis	S. cohnii
	S. saprophyticus	S. xylosus
	S. haemolyticus	S. auricularis
	S. warneri	S. similans
	S. capitis	S. schleiferi
	S. hominis	S. lugdanensis
	S. saccharolyticus	

genera of gram-positive cocci. Staphylococci are nonmotile and are facultative anaerobes. The latter characteristic predicts that these organisms should grow equally well in both aerobic and anaerobic media. The coagulase test identifies the exoenzyme produced by *S. aureus* that interacts with a prothrombin-like plasma factor, converting fibrinogen to fibrin and causing plasma to clot. This is the test that traditionally separates the pathogenic species, *S. aureus,* from the numerous nonpathogenic staphylococci, collectively referred to as "coagulase-negative staphylococci." However, in current practice, many clinical microbiology laboratories use rapid tests for identifying *S. aureus* that rely on the clumping of latex beads coated with plasma factors that interact with *S. aureus* cell-surface components rather than coagulase.

S. aureus comprises a homogeneous species, as determined by biochemical testing and nucleic acid analysis, while coagulase-negative staphylococci are sufficiently varied to be assigned to numerous species. Coagulase-negative staphylococci are found as normal skin flora on all mammals, and currently, 30 different and distinct species are recognized. Of these, 14 species are found colonizing the cornified squamous epithelium and mucous membranes of humans. Each species has a unique niche on the body, but *S. epidermidis* is the predominant species in terms of numbers and different colonization sites. Since many laboratories report specific species of coagulase-negative staphylococci to clinicians, a list of the most prevalent human pathogenic species is shown in Table 279–1. Because only 60 to 70% of coagulase-negative species identified from specimens processed by the clinical laboratory are *S. epidermidis,* it is clearly improper to refer to coagulase-negative staphylococci as "*S. epidermidis.*" However, since no specific pathogenic potential has been recognized for one coagulase-negative staphylococcus versus another, routine species identification of these organisms is useful only for purposes of epidemiology.

EPIDEMIOLOGY. *S. aureus* is carried asymptomatically on the mucous membranes in the anterior nares, nasopharynx, vagina, and/or rectum in 20 to 40% of normal, healthy adults without underlying diseases. Carriage can be transient, lasting hours to days; intermittent, lasting weeks to months; and recurring or chronic, persisting for months to years despite attempts at eradication. Intact cornified squamous epithelium will not support intermittent or chronic carriage of *S. aureus* for reasons that are not clear but may involve bacteriostatic skin lipids, absence of *S. aureus*–specific receptors, or interference by colonizing coagulase-negative staphylococci. However, transient hand carriage clearly occurs and is an important means of exchange between patients and hospital personnel. Certain conditions have been described, however, that markedly increase skin carriage as well as nasal carriage of *S. aureus.* These include a variety of acute and chronic skin conditions, most prominently burn injuries, atopic dermatitis, eczema, psoriasis, and decubitus ulcers. In addition, needle use by insulin-dependent diabetics and intravenous drug abusers has been associated with increased *S. aureus* carriage; health care workers have been found to have a higher prevalence of nasal colonization that those individuals not involved with patients or hospitals; and patients on chronic hemodialysis have a higher-than-expected colonization rate.

S. aureus is extremely hardy and can survive drying, extremes of environmental temperature, wide ranges of pH, and high salt. It can therefore survive in the hospital on inanimate objects such as pillows, sheets, and blood pressure cuffs (called "fomites") for some time. However, the major reservoir of *S. aureus,* in both hospitals and nature, is humans (see Ch. 267).

In certain cases, *S. aureus* infections result when patients who are carriers infect themselves. This has been shown to be true for most hemodialysis shunt and peritoneal dialysis catheter infections, for infective endocarditis in intravenous drug abusers, and for both individuals and families who suffer from recurrent staphyloccal furunculosis. Eradicating nasal carriage in patients by using topical mupirocin ointment has been shown to reduce the incidence of shunt infections and recurrent furunculosis in hemodialysis patients.

Coagulase-negative staphylococci colonizing the skin and mucous membranes of hospitalized patients and some hospital personnel have been shown to be more resistant to antimicrobial agents than staphylococci found on the skin of outpatients or hospital personnel not working on inpatient units. The alteration in skin flora is associated with antimicrobial use that selects more resistant organisms on patient skin. This comprises a huge hospital reservoir for multiple-antibiotic-resistant coagulase-negative staphylococci that can be transferred among patients, can be acquired by hospital personnel, and may eventually be inoculated into wounds in association with implanted, indwelling foreign devices.

IMMUNITY AND PATHOGENESIS OF INFECTIONS. *S. aureus* causes disease syndromes by two different mechanisms. The organism can become locally or systemically invasive by producing molecules that thwart host defense mechanisms, or it can elaborate toxins that cause disease without the need for the organism itself to invade tissue (toxinoses).

Local Infection. The hallmark of the localized staphylococcal infection is an abscess—a walled-off lesion consisting of central necrosis and liquefaction and containing cellular debris and multiplying bacteria surrounded by a layer of fibrin and intact phagocytic cells. The abscess may be superficial, in skin (furuncle), or deep, in organs (renal carbuncle), as a result of bacteremic dissemination. The factors that result in initial *S. aureus* infections are not clear; normal individuals seem to be fairly resistant to local infection. Intact cornified squamous epithelium is normally a barrier both to colonization and infection by *S. aureus,* and even injecting virulent organisms into the skin will cause infection only if a foreign body (e.g., suture) is also present. Furthermore, most adult serum contains both heat-labile and heat-stable opsonins (complement and specific antibody) that are highly efficient at mediating the phagocytosis and killing *S. aureus* by neutrophils. Since humoral immunity and opsonophagocytosis are the body's major defense against pyogenic microorganisms such as *S. aureus,* most individuals are well equipped to resist infection. The role of neutrophils and opsonophagocytosis as the primary antistaphylococcal host defense is illustrated by patients with neutrophil defects (see Ch. 139.1 and 266) who have an increase in *S. aureus* infection. These include defects in intracellular killing (chronic granulomatous disease and Chédiak-Higashi syndrome) and impaired neutrophil chemotaxis and humoral immunity (Job's syndrome). Once the balance is tipped in favor of the organism, *S. aureus* possesses a number of factors that may produce an abscess and promote its survival inside the lesion. While no single factor has been shown to be the major abscess-forming virulence factor and mutants deficient in each of the factors have been recovered from full-blown infections, there is a general feeling that, since most of these factors differentiate the pathogenic *(S. aureus)* from nonpathogenic (coagulase-negative staphylococci) members of the genus, they probably play some coordinate role in initiating and maintaining of infection. Table 279–2 outlines *S. aureus* factors that may contribute to the establishment of local infections.

Disseminated Infection. A small percentage of local infections progress to dissemination, where *S. aureus* gains access to the blood. Dissemination is characterized by *bacteremia* and *metastatic infection.* The factors leading to dissemination and the type and appearance of local infections that are more likely to disseminate are not known.

S. aureus produces such enzymes as *staphylokinase* (a fibrinolysin), *hyaluronidase,* and various *proteases* that may enable it to escape the abscess, invade tissue, and eventually enter the blood. Once in the blood, the most lethal immediate consequence is *sepsis* or *septic shock* (see Ch. 70). This syndrome is mediated chiefly by *enterotoxins* and *toxic shock syndrome toxin* (TSST-1), all of which contain similar motifs (superantigens) that enable them to bind to T cells and macrophages, stimulating the production of such sepsis-associated cytokines such as interleukin-1, tumor necrosis factor, and interleukin-6. Approximately 60% of *S. aureus* isolates contain a gene for one of the five serotypes of enterotoxin (A to E) or TSST-1.

TABLE 279-2. *S. AUREUS* FACTORS THAT MAY PROMOTE LOCAL INFECTIONS BY THWARTING HOST DEFENSE

Factor	Proposed Mechanisms for Interfering with Host Defense
Coagulase	Prevents neutrophil access to infection site
Microcapsule	Inhibits phagocytosis
Protein A	Inhibits IgG-mediated opsonization (binds Fc fragment)
Clumping factor (fibrinogen receptor)	Inhibits opsonization (fibrin coating)
Catalase	Interferes with intracellular killing
Proteases, nuclease, lipase, and cytolysins (alpha, beta, and delta)	Liquefaction necrosis and phagocyte dysfunction
Leucocidin and gamma toxin	Neutrophil cytolysis
Fatty acid metabolizing enzyme	Inactivates bactericidal lipids

One of the target cells for bacteremic *S. aureus* is the endothelial cell. Organisms adhere to and are internalized by endothelial cells, where, by releasing cytolysins, the bacteria can disrupt the endothelial cell layer and invade underlying tissue. *S. aureus* also can exist inside intact endothelial cells. The ability for the organisms to survive inside phagocytes and endothelial cells may explain their propensity to cause recurrent and refractory bacteremia despite seemingly appropriate therapy.

Toxinoses. *S. aureus* produces three toxins, or classes of toxin, that produce specific syndromes without the need for the organism itself to invade and disseminate. *Staphylococcal food poisoning* occurs when a preformed, heat-stable *enterotoxin* is ingested and interacts with parasympathetic ganglia in the stomach, producing vomiting. Five closely related toxin serotypes (A to E) can all produce the characteristic symptoms. *Staphylococcal scalded skin syndrome* results from the production of *exfoliative toxin* by *S. aureus* isolates that colonize or infect the skin of newborns. The characteristic exfoliation of the superficial stratum granulosum layer of the epidermidis is due to the action of the toxin on desmosomes that hold the cells of this skin layer together. There are two exfoliating serotypes, A and B. The variety of *toxic shock syndrome* associated with tampon use in young women is due to TSST-1 entering into the blood through the vagina, produced by *S. aureus* that colonize the mucosa.

DIAGNOSIS. The diagnosis of staphylococcal infections requires that the organism be seen on Gram stain of an infected specimen and be grown on artificial media, preferably in pure culture. Since coagulase-negative staphylococci are the most common contaminants of any culture obtained by crossing skin, it is important that multiple cultures grow the same organism. This is a major reason for drawing blood cultures in pairs from two different sites. While various tests for serum antibody to *S. aureus* antigens (e.g., teichoic acid antibody) have been evaluated for their ability to differentiate serious, deep-seated infection from trivial infections or self-limited bacteremia, none has proved to have a sensitivity or specificity sufficient to warrant its use as a basis for making clinical decisions.

CLINICAL MANIFESTATIONS: *S. AUREUS* INFECTIONS.
Skin and Soft Tissue Infections. The most common *S. aureus* infections are *folliculitis* and the *furuncle*, or boil (Table 279-3). These infections involve a single hair follicle or a localized area of the epidermidis and dermis. While most *S. aureus* furuncles are without systemic symptoms, those on the face should be treated aggressively because of their potential to migrate directly to the brain via the venous circulation. Furuncles can coalesce and spread through deeper skin layers or extend down to and along a fascial plane causing a much more extensive and serious infection called a "carbuncle." Carbuncles are most common over the upper back and back of the neck, where they can form multiple draining sinuses; bacteremia results in approximately one-quarter of patients. A boil or furuncle also may be called a skin abscess if it becomes large but remains circumscribed, confined to one area, and fluctuant. A nonlocalized *S. aureus* skin infection is called "cellulitis" and may resemble the skin infections caused by *Streptococcus pyogenes*, the most common cause of cellulitis (see Ch. 276). *S. aureus* cellulitis also can lead to bacteremia, proving the staphylococcal etiology of

some of these infections. *S. aureus* cellulitis is particularly common in individuals with pre-existing chronic skin disease such as stasis dermatitis and diabetic, trophic, or decubitus ulcers. Adults also can develop a form of impetigo, called "bullous impetigo." The lesions are characterized by erythema with a crusty surface and small or large bullous lesions. The bullae are thought to be the result of the elaboration of exfoliative toxin and are the localized, adult equivalent of the scalded skin syndrome (Ritter's disease) seen in infants.

The most common nosocomial *S. aureus* skin and soft tissue infection is the *wound infection,* where surgical or catheter exit-site wounds are contaminated with *S. aureus* and become erythematous, draining purulent or serosanguineous fluid. *S. aureus* is the most common and most serious cause of hospital-acquired wound infections, leading to local, deep-wound infections and systemic, metastatic infections due to bacteremia.

Recurrent furunculosis can occur in members of families, usually due to persistent nasal or perineal carriage in family members with autoinoculation of skin due to scratching. The infections are commonly superficial and without systemic symptoms but are painful and annoying. Interruption is not possible until the carrier state is eradicated in all family members. While most individuals with recurrent furunculosis have normal immune systems, a syndrome called Job's syndrome (see Ch. 139.1) is recognized in individuals with recurrent *S. aureus* furunculosis. In addition to recurrent furunculosis, patients have high levels of serum IgE, neutrophil chemotactic defects, and a generalized disorder of immunoregulation. Adults with this syndrome usually not only describe a long history of recurrent skin infections since childhood but often also have had recurrent sinopulmonary infections as well.

Pleuropulmonary Infections. *S. aureus* is an uncommon cause of pneumonia in otherwise healthy, unhospitalized adults, accounting for <10% of community-acquired pneumonia. However, following influenza A infections, the incidence of *S. aureus* pneumonia markedly increases. Chest radiographs of patients with community-acquired *S. aureus* pneumonia may show abscesses and thin-walled cysts, resembling the pneumatocoeles seen in infants.

In contrast to community-acquired pneumonia, *S. aureus* is a prominent cause of nosocomial pneumonia, particularly in intubated patients on mechanical ventilation. Cultures obtained from intubated patients by techniques designed to minimize contamination of specimens by organisms colonizing the upper airway have found *S. aureus* in up to a third of patients. Pneumonia in ventilator-dependent patients is a particularly lethal event, with one-quarter to one-half of the patients dying as a direct result of their pulmonary infection. There seems to be nothing that distinguishes the radiographic appearance of nosocomial *S. aureus* pneumonia from that of pneumonia due to other nosocomial pathogens. *S. aureus* bacteremia due solely to nosocomial pneumonia also is uncommon.

Septic pulmonary emboli in patients with right-sided *S. aureus*

TABLE 279-3. INFECTIONS CAUSED BY *S. AUREUS*

Common or Usual Etiologic Pathogen	Less Common Etiologic Pathogen	Uncommon or Rare Etiologic Pathogen
Furuncle or skin abscess	Cellulitis	Community-acquired pneumonia
Bullous impetigo	Hospital-acquired pneumonia	Ascending urinary tract infection
Surgical wound infection	Brain abscess	Meningitis
Hospital-acquired bacteremia	Empyema	Enterocolitis
Acute or right-sided bacterial endocarditis		
Hematogenous osteomyelitis		
Septic arthritis		
Pyomyositis		
Renal carbuncle		
Scalded skin syndrome		
Toxic shock syndrome		
Food-borne gastroenteritis (short incubation)		
Botryomycosis		
Paraspinous or epidural abscess		

endocarditis (see below) also can present like a primary pneumonia. However, these patients will all have *S. aureus* bacteremia and usually have discrete lesions in multiple lobes, often accompanied by hemoptysis and chest pain.

S. aureus is cultured from the pleural space in up to 15% of adults with empyema, but it is found in pure culture in fewer than 10%. The incidence of *S. aureus* as a cause of empyema seems to have decreased overall in the past 20 years but is still a prominent etiologic pathogen in patients with nosocomial empyema.

Endocarditis (see also Ch. 278). There are two different and distinct populations who develop endocarditis caused by *S. aureus;* these are compared in Table 279–4. One group consists of older patients with underlying diseases who develop primarily left-sided endocarditis and have a high mortality rate (20 to 30%). Approximately half will develop heart failure, half will have central nervous system (CNS) manifestations, and 40 to 50% will have had either a skin infection or an intravenous catheter as the presumed portal of entry. Although it is important to realize that patients with left-sided *S. aureus* endocarditis can present acutely, with symptoms compatible with the sepsis syndrome, and that *S. aureus* can infect previously normal valves, the majority of patients will have had more subacute symptoms of fever, malaise, and fatigue for 1 to 2 weeks, and three quarters will have evidence by history or echocardiography of previously damaged or abnormal valves. An increasing proportion of patients in this category infect cardiac valves as a result of a hospital-acquired bacteremia (see below). Patients with nosocomial *S. aureus* endocarditis may be infected with methicillin-resistant staphylococci.

The second population developing *S. aureus* endocarditis consists of those who inject illicit drugs intravenously. These individuals are younger, healthier, usually have no known valvular heart disease, and infect the tricuspid valve in 80 to 90% of cases. The patient is the source of the infecting organism. The major presenting symptoms in these patients are those of septic pulmonary emboli. The chest film typically shows multiple nodular infiltrates in various lobes that often cavitate and occasionally form pneumatocoeles. Most of these patients have pure right-sided endocarditis and only rarely will have any peripheral left-sided manifestations. However, a murmur of tricuspid insufficiency is heard in less than half the cases. The mortality rate is extremely low for these patients, usually only 2 to 5%, but recurrence is relatively common, given the individuals' proclivity for continued drug abuse.

Bacteremia. *S. aureus* is second only to coagulase-negative staphylococci as a cause of hospital-acquired bacteremia. The usual source of nosocomial bacteremia is intravenous catheters. The consequences of nosocomial bacteremia are usually only fever and malaise, but they can include endocarditis, osteomyelitis, metastatic abscesses in various organs, and death from overwhelming sepsis. Treatment, therefore, is prolonged in order to eradicate the organism from tissues and organs. Bacteremia caused by *S. aureus* is usually high-grade, with the organism grown from all blood cultures drawn over a period of time even if there is no endocarditis or infected foreign body present. Furthermore, bacteremia may persist for several days even with appropriate therapy and removal of an infected catheter. This is felt to be due to the organism's ability to survive host phagocytic defense and to be sequestered inside cells.

In contrast to nosocomial *S. aureus* bacteremia, the source of community-acquired bacteremia is often obscure. It may originate from a skin infection, intravenous injection of illicit drugs, or an infected focus in the heart or at a peripheral site. In all patients with community-acquired *S. aureus* bacteremia, a diligent search should be made for an infected source. If none is found, patients should be treated as if they have endocarditis.

Osteomyelitis (see also Ch. 283). *S. aureus* is the most common cause of acute hematogenous osteomyelitis. While most cases occur in children, adults are also at risk, particularly those who have had documented *S. aureus* bacteremia. Children develop osteomyelitis almost exclusively in long bones, while in adults from a third to a half of the cases of hematogenous osteomyelitis are in the lumbar or thoracic vertebrae. Vertebral osteomyelitis results when *S. aureus* initially seeds the intervertebral disc space and then spreads from the disc space to involve contiguous veretebrae. A paraspinous or epidural abscess frequently occurs as an extension of the initial intervertebral focus. Patients present with fever and back pain and may have neurologic symptoms from cord compression. Radiographs typically show narrowing of one or more intervertebral disc spaces with collapse of adjacent vertebrae. A magnetic resonance imaging scan is particularly helpful in defining the extent of vertebral osteomyelitis. Long bones may be involved following hematogenous dissemination of *S. aureus,* but osteomyelitis in these locations is more typically the result of contiguous spread from an infected decubitus, trophic ulcer, or traumatic wound. One of the most common causes of *S. aureus* osteomyelitis of the foot bones is infection of ulcers in diabetics with vascular disease. Occasionally, hardware used to repair long bone fractures will become infected with *S. aureus*. These infections are particularly refractory to therapy without removal of the foreign body.

Septic Arthritis (see also Ch. 239). *S. aureus* is a common cause of acute septic arthritis, although spontaneous *S. aureus* septic arthritis in otherwise normal joints is usually seen in children rather than adults. In adults, *S. aureus* septic arthritis typically occurs in joints that previously have been damaged by a chronic inflammatory arthritis or osteoarthritis; that have been violated by needle aspiration, injection, or surgery; or that contain a prosthetic device. Occasionally, an otherwise normal joint will be seeded by the hematogenous route or the joint space will be invaded from a contiguous focus of osteomyelitis. These infections need to be differentiated from such other causes of acute monarticular arthritis in adults as gout and gonococcal infection. In all cases of septic arthritis, arthrocentesis should be performed before beginning therapy so that a specific cultural diagnosis can be made. *S. aureus* pyarthrosis can be present with relatively little systemic toxicity in patients with chronic inflammatory arthritis taking large doses of anti-inflammatory medication; this may be particularly difficult to diagnose. One unique form of *S. aureus* septic arthritis is infection of the sternoclavicular joint usually seen in intravenous drug users or in patients who have had subclavian intravenous catheters.

Genitourinary Tract Infections. The only important *S. aureus* infections of the genitourinary tract are those which result from hematogenous dissemination. These include microabscesses, renal carbuncles, and perinephric abscesses. The presence of *S. aureus* in the urine, therefore, is either the result of contamination in individuals asymptomatically colonized in the vagina and/or rectum or an indication that the kidney has been infected during an episode of *S. aureus* bacteremia. The absence of cells in the urine should suggest contamination. However, if *S. aureus* is repeatedly cultured from urine or present in the urine together with pyuria or hematuria, the patient should be evaluated for bacteremia, for a deep focus that might have caused disseminated infection, and for an intrarenal or perinephric abscess. The presence of *S. aureus* in the urine should *never* be assumed to be secondary to an ascending urinary tract infection.

Central Nervous System Infections. While brain abscess and meningitis can be caused by *S. aureus,* they are relatively rare. Fewer than 10% of cases of meningitis and 20 to 30% of cases of brain abscess are caused by *S. aureus*. They are usually due to metastatic seeding as a result of bacteremia from an identified focus, to direct inoculation following trauma or a neurosurgical proce-

TABLE 279–4. *S. AUREUS* ENDOCARDITIS IN DIFFERENT PATIENT POPULATIONS

Patient and Disease Characteristics	Intravenous Drug Abusers	Nonintravenous Drug Abusers
Mean age (yr)	30	50
Underlying disease	No	Yes
Portal of *S. aureus* entry	Skin (IV injection)	Skin (infection or IV catheter)
Valves involved	Tricuspid	Mitral, aortic
Pre-existing valve abnormality	No	Yes
Presentation	Chest pain, fever hemoptysis	Fever, fatigue, malaise; sepsis (less common)
Peripheral manifestations	Septic pulmonary emboli	Skin manifestations; central nervous system abnormalities; metastatic infection in bone, kidney, and spleen
Heart failure	Rare	Common
Mortality	<5%	20–30%
Treatment duration	2–3 weeks	4–6 weeks

TABLE 279-5. DIFFERENTIATION OF DESQUAMATING SYNDROMES

	Staphylococcal Scalded Skin Syndrome	Toxic Epidermal Necrolysis
Etiology	*S. aureus* exfoliative toxin	Drug hypersensitivity
Pathology	Intraepidermal cleavage plane; no inflammatory cells	Involvement of entire epidermis; infiltration with inflammatory cells
Clinical appearance	Involvement of epidermis only; positive Nikolsky's sign	Involvement of skin, mucous membranes, and multiple organs; negative Nikolsky's sign
Outcome	Low mortality; heals without scarring	High mortality; often heals with scarring

dure, or to infection of an indwelling foreign body, such as a ventricular shunt. The prognosis of patients infected as a result of metastatic seeding is particularly poor, with a mortality rate of 30 to 50%. The one infection associated with the CNS that is uniquely caused by *S. aureus* is a paraspinous or epidural abscess, usually secondary to vertebral osteomyelitis.

Pyomyositis. Infection of the large skeletal muscles is due to *S. aureus* in >80% of cases. It is prevalent in tropical countries, giving it the name "tropical pyomyositis," but it is being increasingly described in temperate climates. Patients in tropical countries usually are adults who have no underlying disease and present with fever, pain, and swelling in the involved muscle, but there is often little evidence of local inflammation. Diagnosis is made by needle aspiration of pus. Because eosinophilia is common in patients in tropical countries who have pyomyositis, parasites are felt to have a role in the pathogenesis of this disease. Pyomyositis in temperate climates presents in much the same manner but more often is seen in children or in adults with underlying diseases, is associated with muscle trauma in more than half of patients, and more frequently involves more than one noncontiguous muscle group.

Toxinoses. *Staphylococcal scalded skin syndrome,* also known as Ritter's or Lyell's syndrome, is usually a disease of neonates and is due to the action of the exfoliative toxins, A and B. This syndrome results from *S. aureus* colonization or local infection, usually of the umbilical stump, and results in generalized desquamation of the superficial granulosum cell layer of the epidermis. The adult equivalent is bullous impetigo, associated with localized skin involvement, but adult cases of more generalized desquamation have been described. However, it is important to differentiate staphylococcal scalded skin syndrome from toxic epidermal necrolysis (TEN). Table 279-5 contrasts the two syndromes.

The *toxic shock syndrome* was initially described in young, menstruating women and was associated with tampon use in women vaginally colonized with *S. aureus* that produced TSST-1. However, the number of tampon-associated cases has decreased markedly in recent years. The majority of cases are now secondary to *S. aureus* infections of skin or other sites, and the etiologic toxin is often one of the enterotoxins rather than TSST-1. The criteria for the diagnosis of staphylococcal toxic shock syndrome are shown in Table 279-6. Staphylococcal toxic shock syndrome has a relatively low mortality and is a true toxinosis; bacteremia is rare.

Gastroenteritis or *staphylococcal food poisoning* is due to ingesting preformed staphylococcal enterotoxin. Enterotoxin-producing *S. aureus* are inoculated into food by a colonized food handler. If the food sits at room temperature before being cooked, the organism

TABLE 279-6. DIAGNOSTIC CRITERIA FOR STAPHYLOCOCCAL TOXIC SHOCK SYNDROME

1. Fever (usually ≥ 38.9°C, or 102°F)
2. Rash (diffuse macular erythroderma, sunburn or scarlet fever–like)
3. Desquamation, 1 to 2 weeks after onset of illness, particularly of palms and soles
4. Hypotension (systolic blood pressure < 90 mm Hg or orthostatic syncope)
5. Involvement of three or more of the following organ systems: gastrointestinal (nausea and vomiting), muscular (myalgias), mucous membrane (hyperemia), renal, hepatic, hematologic (↓ platelets), central nervous system, or pulmonary (ARDS)
6. *S. aureus* infection or mucosal colonization

TABLE 279-7. CHARACTERISTICS OF COAGULASE-NEGATIVE STAPHYLOCOCCAL INFECTIONS

1. Hospital-acquired
2. Caused by species *S. epidermidis* (70–80%)
3. Resistant to multiple antimicrobial agents (> 80% methicillin resistant)
4. Involve indwelling foreign devices (catheters, prosthetic heart valves and joints, vascular grafts)
5. Exhibit a long latent period between device contamination and clinical presentation

will multiply and produce toxin. Subsequent cooking will not inactivate the heat-stable toxin, and ingestion will produce symptoms predominantly of vomiting after a short (2 to 8 hours) incubation period.

Miscellaneous Infections. The older literature describes "botryomycosis," a chronic *S. aureus* infection of skin, lung, or bone that produces granules resembling those seen in actinomycosis, and "enterocolitis," a necrotizing infection of bowel in surgical patients associated with sheets of organisms seen on Gram stain of stool. These infections are rarely seen today.

CLINICAL MANIFESTATIONS: COAGULASE-NEGATIVE STAPHYLOCOCCAL INFECTIONS. The major infections caused by coagulase-negative staphylococci are hospital-acquired and involve indwelling foreign devices. Table 279-7 outlines the characteristics of these infections. In general, coagulase-negative staphylococci are of low virulence, rarely causing metastatic infections, even though they are the most common cause of hospital-acquired bacteremia. Bacteremia is usually the result of intravascular catheter infection. However, coagulase-negative staphylococci can be lethal when they infect prosthetic cardiac valves. They are the most common cause of prosthetic valve endocarditis, presenting in the first year after surgery, presumably inoculated into the area of the sewing ring during valve implantation. Valve dysfunction results from dehiscence or obstruction of the valve orifice, and most patients require surgery for cure. The exception to infections described in Table 279-7 are those caused by *S. saprophyticus*. This organism is second only to *Escherichia coli* as a cause of ascending urinary tract infections in young, sexually active female outpatients, implicated in 15 to 20% of cases in this population. In addition, low colony counts of this staphylococcal species have been recovered from urine obtained by suprapubic aspiration in some women with the anterior urethral syndrome or symptomatic abacteriuria.

THERAPY. Antimicrobial agents effective for treating *S. aureus* infections are listed in Table 279-8. Treatment of hospital-acquired infections is limited by resistance to many of these agents. Methicillin-resistant isolates are *cross-resistant* to *all* β-lactams (penicillins, cephalosporins, and imipenem) and are usually also resistant to at least three additional classes of antimicrobial agents (multiresistant). However, while only 20 to 30% of nosocomial *S. aureus* isolates are methicillin-resistant, >70% of nosocomial coagulase-

TABLE 279-8. ANTIMICROBIAL AGENTS EFFECTIVE FOR TREATING *S. AUREUS* INFECTIONS

Agents	Resistance*	
	Hospital-Acquired	Community-Acquired
Penicillin G	>90	>90
Antistaphylococcal penicillins and cephalosporins	30	S
Erythromycin	40	10
Clindamycin	40	10
Sulfamethoxasole-trimethoprim	20	S
Tetracycline	20	10
Minocycline	S	S
Rifampin	S	S
Gentamicin	30	S
Quinolones	30	S
Vancomycin	S	S

* Numbers are percentage of isolates from patients with hospital-acquired or community-acquired infections resistant to each agent; S = >95% susceptible

negative staphylococci are methicillin-resistant and multiresistant. Thus, while the treatment of hospital-acquired *S. aureus* infections should be guided by susceptibility testing, infections caused by nosocomial coagulase-negative staphylococci are usually treated with vancomycin.

Treating staphylococcal infections usually consists of administering antimicrobial agents, surgical or catheter drainage of abscesses, and removal of foreign bodies. The duration of therapy is usually 1 to 2 weeks for localized, drained infections not associated with bacteremia or a foreign body. In general, infections can rarely be cured if the foreign material is left in place. Infections requiring more specialized therapeutic decisions are detailed below.

Bacteremia and Endocarditis. For *S. aureus,* all patients with community-acquired bacteremia who have evidence of a metastatic infection or who have no obvious source for bacteremia should be treated as if they have endocarditis. For intravenous drug abusers with right-sided endocarditis: 2 to 3 weeks of an antistaphylococcal penicillin (nafcillin or oxacillin) or vancomycin, plus gentamicin for the entire treatment period; for left-sided endocarditis: 4 to 6 weeks of an antistaphylococcal penicillin or vancomycin, with gentamicin for the first week. However, in patients with hospital-acquired *S. aureus* bacteremia from a removable focus (usually an intravascular catheter), the decision becomes more difficult. Those patients whose fever and bacteremia resolve within 3 days after removing the infected focus, those who have no complications or evidence of metastatic infection, and those who have no abnormality of cardiac valves can receive 2 weeks of therapy. All other patients with nosocomial bacteremia who do not meet all the exclusions should be treated as if they have endocarditis (see Ch. 278).

Osteomyelitis. Patients with *S. aureus* osteomyelitis require a minimum of 6 weeks of therapy, with the initial 2 to 4 weeks being parenteral. Therapy of osteomyelitis of long bones often will be unsuccessful if sequestra are left in place.

PREVENTION. Preventing hospital-acquired infections is accomplished by paying attention to tenets of infection control. These include handwashing and regloving between patients and strict adherence to aseptic technique when creating or caring for any kind of wound. Patients undergoing procedures that may result in wound or implanted device infections also should receive prophylactic antibiotics before and during the procedure. Patients with recurrent *S. aureus* infections of skin, catheters, or dialysis shunts should have their nares cultured, and if they are *S. aureus* carriers, they should be treated with topical mupirocin ointment. Chronic carriers resistant to topical *S. aureus* eradication may be given oral rifampin plus sulfamethoxazole-trimethoprim, a fluoroquinolone (ofloxacin or ciprofloxacin), or minocycline.

Chambers HF: Methicillin-resistant staphylococci. Clin Microbiol Rev 1:173, 1988. *A good overview of antibiotic resistance among staphylococci.*

Novick RP: Staphylococci. *In* Davis BD, Dulbecco R, Eisen HN, et al. (eds.): Microbiology. 4th ed. Philadelphia, JB Lippincott, 1990, pp 539–550. *An excellent summary of basic staphylococcal biology and pathogenic factors produced by* S. aureus.

Raad LI, Sabbagh MF: Optimal duration of therapy for catheter-related *Staphylococcus aureus* bacteremia: A study of 55 cases a review. Clin Infect Dis 14:75, 1992. *An excellent study and review of a difficult problem.*

Rupp ME, Archer GL: Coagulase-negative staphylococci: Pathogens of medical progress. Clin Infect Dis 19:231, 1994. *The most recent review of infections caused by coagulase-negative staphylococci.*

Bacterial Meningitis

280 BACTERIAL MENINGITIS
Morton N. Swartz

Meningitis is an inflammation of the arachnoid, the pia mater, and the intervening cerebrospinal fluid (CSF). The inflammatory process extends throughout the subarachnoid space about the brain and spinal cord and regularly involves the ventricles. Pyogenic meningitis, considered in this chapter, is usually an acute infection with bacteria that evoke a polymorphonuclear response in the CSF. One of its major forms, that caused by meningococci, is considered in Ch. 281; less acute forms of bacterial meningitis, characterized by a mononuclear cell response in the CSF, are discussed in Ch. 311 and 406.

ETIOLOGY AND INCIDENCE. In the 1970's and 1980's, 20,000 to 25,000 cases of bacterial meningitis occurred annually in the United States. If all cases are included regardless of the age of patients, data from the Centers for Disease Control and Prevention indicate that *Haemophilus influenzae* type b was the most frequent bacterial cause (45%), followed by *Streptococcus pneumoniae* (18%) and *Neisseria meningitidis* (14%). About 70% of all cases occurred in children under age 5. The relative frequencies with which the different bacterial species cause meningitis are age related (Table 280–1). In the newborn, group B streptococci and gram-negative bacilli (most frequently *Escherichia coli,* but also other enteric bacilli and *Pseudomonas*) are the principal causes. Beyond the first month of life and extending through childhood, *H. influenzae* and *N. meningitidis* have been the most frequent causes of bacterial meningitis. The pre-eminent position of *H. influenzae* as a cause of meningitis in infants and young children (and as the leading cause of bacterial meningitis overall) has changed dramatically since immunization with the *H. influenzae* type b conjugate vaccines was introduced in the late 1980's. Whereas the rate of *H. influenzae* meningitis in the United States had been about 40 per 100,000 children under age 5 in the mid-1980's, it had fallen to about 2 per 100,000 in this age group by 1993. Consequently, the relative frequencies of *S. pneumoniae* and *N. meningitidis* have increased among children. In adults, *S. pneumoniae, N. meningitidis,* and *Listeria monocytogenes* are responsible for most cases of community-acquired bacterial meningitis. Meningococcal meningitis is the only type that occurs in outbreaks; its relative frequency among the meningitides depends on whether statistics have been gathered in a hyperendemic area or during an epidemic period. In about 10% of patients with pyogenic meningitis, the bacterial cause cannot be defined. Simultaneous mixed meningitis is rare, occurring in the setting of neurosurgical procedures, penetrating head injury, erosion of the skull or vertebrae by adjacent neoplasm, or intraventricular rupture of a cerebral abscess; the isolation of anaerobes should strongly suggest the latter two of these.

Important changes have occurred in the frequencies of several types of bacterial meningitis over the past 25 years. Gram-negative bacillary meningitis has doubled in frequency in adults, reflecting more frequent and extensive neurosurgical procedures as well as other nosocomial factors. *L. monocytogenes* has increased eight- to tenfold as a cause of bacterial meningitis in urban general hospitals, reflecting the enlarging immunosuppressed population at particular

TABLE 280–1. BACTERIAL CAUSES OF MENINGITIS*

	Neonates (≤ 1 month) (%)	Children (1 month– 15 years) (%)	Adults† (> 15 years) (%)
S. pneumoniae	0–5	10–20	40–50
N. meningitidis	0–1	25–40	15–30
H. influenzae	5	40–60¶	2–4
Streptococci	40–50‡	2–4	5–10
Staphylococci	5	1–2	5–10
Listeria	5–10	1–2	5–10
Gram-negative bacilli	30–45§	1–2	5

* In the United States in the 1980's.
† These represent cases of community-acquired meningitis.
‡ Almost all isolates from neonatal meningitis are group B streptococci.
§ Of all cases of neonatal meningitis, *E. coli* accounts for about 40% and *Klebsiella-Enterobacter* for about 8%.
¶ Markedly lower in the 1990's.

risk. *Listeria* infections appear to be foodborne (dairy products, un-cooked vegetables) and involve particularly organ transplant recipients, patients in hemodialysis units, other patients receiving corticosteroids and cytotoxic drugs, patients with liver disease, pregnant women, and neonates. Meningitis due to coagulase-negative staphylococci, essentially unheard of 30 years ago, now represents about 3% of cases in large urban hospitals. It occurs as a complication of neurosurgical procedures and may present a particular therapeutic problem due to methicillin resistance of many of the involved strains.

In large urban tertiary-care general hospitals, the distribution of bacterial etiologies of adult meningitis differs from that in smaller community hospitals, where community-acquired disease predominates. For example, at the Massachusetts General Hospital about 40% of cases of bacterial meningitis in adults are of nosocomial origin. In this category, the leading etiologies are gram-negative bacilli (primarily *E. coli* and *Klebsiella*), accounting for about 40% of nosocomial episodes, and various streptococci, *Staphylococcus aureus,* and coagulase-negative staphylococci, each responsible for 10% of nosocomial cases.

CLINICAL SETTINGS. The clinical setting in which meningitis develops may provide a clue to the specific bacterial cause. Meningococcal disease, including meningitis, may occur sporadically and in cyclic outbreaks. In the past, military recruits were particularly susceptible, but now meningococcal vaccine (polysaccharides of groups A, C, Y, and W135) is employed for protection. Large urban outbreaks can occur.

Certain predisposing factors are frequently associated with the development of *pneumococcal meningitis. Acute otitis media* (±*mastoiditis*) occurs in about 20% of adult patients. *Pneumonia* is present in about 15% of patients with pneumococcal meningitis, a much higher frequency than in meningitis caused by *H. influenzae* or *N. meningitidis. Acute pneumococcal sinusitis* is occasionally the initial focus from which infection spreads to the meninges. A significant head injury (recent or remote) has occurred in about 10% of patients with pneumococcal meningitis. CSF rhinorrhea (usually caused by a defect or fracture in the cribriform plate) is present in about 5% of patients with pneumococcal meningitis. Meningitis occurring in young children with sickle cell anemia is most likely to be caused by *S. pneumoniae.* A variety of defects in host defenses (primary or acquired immunoglobulin deficiencies, the asplenic state) may predispose to severe pneumococcal disease, particularly bacteremia and meningitis. Alcoholism is an underlying problem in 10 to 25% of adults with pneumococcal meningitis in urban hospitals.

S. aureus meningitis is seen most commonly as a complication of a neurosurgical procedure, following penetrating skull trauma, or occasionally secondary to staphylococcal bacteremia and endocarditis. Meningitis caused by *gram-negative bacilli* takes one of three forms: neonatal meningitis, meningitis following trauma or neurosurgery, or spontaneous meningitis in adults (e.g., bacteremic *Klebsiella* meningitis in a patient with diabetes mellitus). The most common causes of gram-negative bacillary meningitis in the adult are *E. coli* (about 30%) and *Klebsiella-Enterobacter* (about 40%). The most frequent causes of bacterial meningitis in patients with neoplastic disease are gram-negative bacilli (particularly *Pseudomonas aeruginosa* and *E. coli*), *L. monocytogenes, S. pneumoniae,* and *S. aureus.* Meningitis caused by *group A streptococci* is uncommon but occasionally occurs following acute otitis media.

The age-related incidence (children under 5 years) of *H. influenzae* type b meningitis has been so striking that the occurrence of this disease in an adult should raise the question of the presence of an underlying anatomic or immunologic defect, circumventing the usual barrier interposed by serum bactericidal mechanisms.

Neonatal Meningitis. The incidence of meningitis is higher in the first month of life than in any other single month. In the newborn, the group B *Streptococcus* can produce either an "early-onset" (occurring within 8 days of delivery and characterized by a fulminant illness with septicemia, severe respiratory distress, and sometimes meningitis) or a "late-onset" (occurring 10 days to 2 months after delivery and presenting a more insidious, slowly progressive illness which usually includes meningitis) infection. The second leading cause, *E. coli* strains containing K1 capsular antigen, is usually acquired by the neonates from their mothers, who carry the organism in their stool.

The clinical signs in neonatal meningitis suggest sepsis but not necessarily central nervous system (CNS) involvement: fever (in only 60%), jaundice, diarrhea, lethargy, poor feeding or vomiting, respiratory distress (including apnea), seizures, irritability, bulging fontanel (in only 30%), and nuchal rigidity (15%). Frequently, only by examining the CSF can the presence of meningitis be ruled in or out.

PATHOLOGY. The purulent exudate is distributed widely in the subarachnoid space, most abundant in the basal cisterns and about the cerebellum initially, but also extending into the sulci over the cerebrum. There is no direct invasion of cerebral tissue by the infecting organism or the inflammatory exudate, but the subjacent brain becomes congested and edematous. The effectiveness of the pial barrier accounts for the fact that cerebral abscess does not complicate bacterial meningitis. Indeed, when these two processes coexist, the sequence usually has been that of an initial abscess subsequently leaking its contents into the ventricular system, producing meningitis. There are two possible exceptions to the aforementioned generalization: (1) neonatal meningitis due to *Citrobacter,* in which the organisms appear to invade the brain after producing a necrotizing vasculitis of small penetrating blood vessels, and (2) *Listeria* rhombencephalitis, a very rare process in which brain stem infection can occur simultaneously with *Listeria* meningitis (or alone). Structures adjacent to the meninges may show a variety of pathologic changes secondary to bacterial meningitis. *Cortical thrombophlebitis* results from venous stasis and adjacent meningeal inflammation. Infarction of cerebral tissue may follow. *Involvement of cortical and pial arteries* with peripheral aneurysm formation and vascular occlusion occurs occasionally in bacterial meningitis. Rarely, narrowing of the supraclinoid portion of the internal carotid artery at the base of the brain occurs as a result of arteritis and arterial spasm. In fulminating cases (particularly meningococcal meningitis), *cerebral edema* may be marked even though the pleocytosis is only moderate. Rarely such patients develop temporal lobe and cerebellar herniation, resulting in compression of the midbrain and medulla. *Damage to cranial nerves* occurs in areas where dense exudate accumulates; the third and sixth cranial nerves are also vulnerable to damage by increased intracranial pressure. *Ventriculitis* probably occurs in most cases of bacterial meningitis; rarely this progresses to the accumulation of pus, *ventricular empyema. Hydrocephalus* can develop during meningitis from obstruction to CSF flow within the ventricular system (obstructive hydrocephalus) or extraventricularly (communicating hydrocephalus). *Subdural effusions* are sterile transudates that develop over the cerebral cortex in about 15% of infants with bacterial meningitis. Rarely such effusions become infected, producing a subdural empyema. In the past the diagnosis was made almost exclusively in infants, in whom abnormal transillumination or increasing head size can be detected. Now, sterile or infected (showing peripheral contrast enhancement) subdural collections can be demonstrated readily by computed tomographic scan as low-density areas about the cerebrum.

PATHOGENESIS. Bacteria may reach the meninges by several routes: (1) systemic bacteremia, (2) direct ingress from the upper respiratory tract or skin through an anatomic defect (e.g., skull fracture, eroding sequestrum, meningocele), (3) passage intracranially via venules in the nasopharynx, or (4) spread from a contiguous focus of infection (infection of the paranasal sinuses, leakage of a brain abscess). Bacteremic spread to the meninges is probably the most frequent path of infection. However, not all bacteremic organisms have the same likelihood of causing meningitis. Bacteremia with *H. influenzae* and *N. meningitidis* is usually initiated by pharyngeal adhesion and colonization by an infecting strain. Adhesion of such strains, as well as of *S. pneumoniae,* to mucosal surfaces is abetted by their capacity to produce IgA proteases (cleaving this antibody in the hinge region) and thus inactivating this local antibody defense. *N. meningitidis* adhesion to nasopharyngeal cells is effected by fimbriae or pili. In an *in vitro* nasopharyngeal organ culture these organisms injure ciliated epithelial cells and induce ciliostasis, selectively adhering to nonciliated epithelial cells. Meningococci invade the nasopharyngeal mucosal cells via endocytosis and are transported to the abluminal side in membrane-bound vacuoles. *H. influenzae,* in contrast, invades intercellularly by causing separation of apical tight junctions between columnar epithelial cells. When these meningeal pathogens gain access to the bloodstream, their intravascular survival is aided by the presence of polysaccharide capsules that inhibit phagocytosis and confer resistance to complement-mediated bactericidal activity.

Following entry into the bloodstream, CNS invasion occurs, but the mechanisms by which and sites at which this occurs are unclear. A high-grade and sustained bacteremia appears necessary. An important role for specific bacterial adhesion to elements of the blood-brain barrier is likely, as indicated by the preferential binding of fimbriated strains of *E. coli* to the endothelial cell surface of cerebral capillaries and the epithelial cell surface of the choroid plexus and ventricles. Evidence from animal models suggests that CNS invasion sites following bacteremia may develop at foci of nonspecific sterile inflammation above the cribriform plate and through the choroid plexus.

Most bacterial species causing meningitis (*H. influenzae* type b, *N. meningitidis, S. pneumoniae, E. coli* K1, group B *Streptococcus*) are antiphagocytic. Whether the capsular polysaccharide confers some special meningeal tropism, possibly through surface receptors, is not known. Although the primary focus initiating the bacteremia is usually in the upper respiratory tract or lung (pneumonia), it may be in the heart (endocarditis) or the gastrointestinal or urinary tracts. Once established in any part of the meninges, infection quickly extends throughout the subarachnoid space. Bacterial replication proceeds relatively unhindered, since CSF levels of complement are low early in meningeal inflammation, resulting in minimal opsonic and bactericidal activity (or none), and since surface phagocytosis of unopsonized organisms is meager in such a fluid environment. A secondary bacteremia may follow meningeal infection and itself contribute to continuing further inoculation of the CSF.

PATHOPHYSIOLOGY. Current experimental evidence suggests that meningeal inflammation follows bacterial entry and growth in the CSF and that specific bacterial components (e.g., pneumococcal cell walls or lipoteichoic acid, *H. influenzae* lipopolysaccharide [LPS]) are major eliciters of this response by causing release into the subarachnoid space of various pro-inflammatory cytokines such as interleukin-1 (IL-1) and tumor necrosis factor (TNF) from endothelial and meningeal cells. These cytokines increase adherence and transendothelial movement of neutrophils, as has been shown in endothelial cell monolayers in culture. Cytokines appear to enhance this passage of leukocytes by inducing several families of adhesion molecules that interact with corresponding receptors on leukocytes. The three likely families mediating endothelial-leukocyte adhesion are the (1) immunoglobulin superfamily, e.g., intercellular adhesion molecules (ICAM) 1 and 2; (2) integrins, e.g., CD11/CD18 subfamily; and (3) selectins, e.g., endothelial-leukocyte adhesion molecule (ELAM-1). Cytokines also can act to increase the binding affinity of a leukocyte selectin, leukocyte-adhesion molecule (LAM-1), for its endothelial cell receptor, contributing further to neutrophil trafficking into the subarachnoid space.

Once within the subarachnoid space, neutrophils are further activated to release products such as prostaglandins and toxic oxygen metabolites that increase local vascular permeability and may cause direct neurotoxicity. Evidence of breaching of the blood-brain barrier is found in animal models of meningitis where endothelial intercellular tight junctions are disrupted, where increased pinocytotic vesicles appear in endothelial cells, and where albumin escapes across postcapillary venules into the subarachnoid space.

The foregoing inflammatory changes can contribute to development of increased intracranial pressure and alterations in cerebral blood flow. Cerebral edema is commonly due to increased permeability of the blood-brain barrier (vasogenic), may be due to cellular

swelling in the brain as a result of toxic molecules released by bacteria and neutrophils (cytotoxic), and sometimes increased CSF pressure may result primarily from obstruction to CSF outflow due to inflammation at the level of the arachnoidal villi (interstitial). Whereas cerebral blood flow appears to be increased in the early stages of meningitis, subsequently it decreases, mirroring the severity of the disease. Localized regions of marked hypoperfusion (attributable to focal vascular inflammation or thrombosis) can occur in patients with normal blood flow. Impairment of autoregulation of cerebral blood flow may be a factor in cerebral edema or ischemia in some patients due to altered cerebral perfusion pressure.

CLINICAL MANIFESTATIONS. History. An acute onset of fever, generalized headache, vomiting, and stiff neck are common to many types of meningitis. The majority of patients with pyogenic meningitis of the three common causes have had an antecedent or accompanying upper respiratory tract infection or nonspecific febrile illness, acute otitis (or mastoiditis), or pneumonia. Myalgias (particularly in meningococcal disease), backache, and generalized weakness are common symptoms. The illness usually progresses rapidly, with development of confusion, obtundation, and loss of consciousness. Occasionally the onset may be less acute, with meningeal signs present for several days to a week.

General Physical Findings. Evidences of meningeal irritation (drowsiness and decreased mentation, stiff neck, Kernig's and Brudzinski's signs) are usually present. In certain patients, the findings of meningitis may be easily overlooked; infants, obtunded patients, or elderly patients with congestive failure or pneumonia may develop meningitis without prominent meningeal signs. Their lethargy should be investigated carefully, and meningeal signs should be sought; if any doubt exists, examination of the CSF is indicated.

The presence of a petechial, purpuric, or ecchymotic rash in a patient with meningeal findings almost always indicates meningococcal infection and requires prompt treatment because of the rapidity with which this infection can progress (see Ch. 281). Rarely, extensive petechial and purpuric lesions occur in meningitis caused by *S. pneumoniae* or *H. influenzae*. Very rarely skin lesions almost indistinguishable from those of meningococcal bacteremia occur in patients with acute *S. aureus* endocarditis who also have meningeal signs and a pleocytosis (secondary either to staphylococcal meningitis or to embolic cerebral infarction). Usually one or two of the lesions in such a patient are those of purulent purpura; aspiration of material reveals staphylococci on Gram stain. In the summer months, viral aseptic meningitis may produce meningeal signs, macular and petechial skin lesions, and a pleocytosis of several hundred cells, sometimes with neutrophils predominating initially.

Neurologic Findings and Complications. *Cranial nerve abnormalities,* involving principally the third, fourth, sixth, or seventh nerves, occur in 5 to 10% of adults with community-acquired meningitis. These usually disappear shortly after recovery. Persistent sensorineural hearing loss occurs in 10% of children with bacterial meningitis. In another 16% a transient conductive hearing loss develops. The most likely sites of involvement in persistent sensorineural deafness appear to be the inner ear (infection or toxic products possibly spreading from the subarachnoid space along the cochlear aqueduct) and the acoustic nerve. In children, permanent hearing impairment is more common following meningitis due to *S. pneumoniae* than to *H. influenzae* or *N. meningitidis*.

Seizures (focal or generalized) occur in 20 to 30% of patients and may result from readily reversible causes (high fever in infants; penicillin neurotoxicity when large doses are administered intravenously in the presence of renal failure) or, more commonly, from focal cerebral injury. Seizures can occur during the first few days or

TABLE 280–2. CENTRAL NERVOUS SYSTEM FINDINGS IN COMMUNITY-ACQUIRED BACTERIAL MENINGITIS IN ADULTS*

| Time of Onset of Findings | Percentage of Episodes of Meningitis | | | | | |
	Hemiparesis	Aphasia	Visual-Field Defect	Gaze Preference	Seizures	Other
Early (≤ 24 h)	9	6	2	10	15	5
Late (> 24 h)	2	1	0.3	0	8	1
Total†	11	7	2.3	10	23	6

* Based on data of Durand et al.
† Total percent of 279 episodes in which individual finding occurred (some episodes involved more than one finding).

can appear with associated focal neurologic deficits caused by vascular inflammation some days after the onset of the meningitis (Table 280–2). In adults with seizures accompanying meningitis, *S. pneumoniae* is more commonly the cause, but alcoholism is a confounding factor.

Brain swelling and increased CSF pressure are associated with seizures, third nerve dysfunction, abnormal reflexes, coma, hypertension, and bradycardia. In approximately one-quarter of fatal cases of community-acquired meningitis in adults, cerebral edema accompanied by temporal lobe herniation is observed at autopsy.

Papilledema is rare (1%) in bacterial meningitis even with high CSF pressures, probably because the patient is seen early in the process before changes have occurred in the nerve head. Its presence should indicate the possibility of some other associated or independent suppurative intracranial process (subdural empyema, brain abscess). Marked central hyperpnea sometimes occurs in patients with severe bacterial meningitis; CSF acidosis (principally caused by increased lactic acid levels) provides much of the respiratory stimulus.

Focal cerebral signs (principally hemiparesis, dysphasia, visual field defects, and gaze preference) occur in about 25% of adults with community-acquired bacterial meningitis (Table 280–2). They may develop during early meningitis secondary to occlusive vascular processes or some days later. Also, cerebral blood flow velocity may be decreased in the presence of increased intracranial pressure and lead to temporary or lasting neurologic dysfunction. It is important to distinguish lateralizing findings resulting from postictal changes (Todd's paralysis), which usually persist for no more than several hours.

Prompt treatment of bacterial meningitis usually results in rapid recovery of neurologic function. Persistent or late-onset obtundation and coma without focal findings suggests development of brain swelling, subdural effusion (in the infant), hydrocephalus, loculated ventriculitis, cortical thrombophlebitis, or sagittal sinus thrombosis. The last three are commonly associated with fever and continuing pleocytosis.

Residual neurologic damage remains in 10 to 20% of patients who recover from bacterial meningitis. Developmental delay and speech defects are each observed in about 5% of children. In infants surviving neonatal meningitis, significant sequelae are much more frequent (15 to 50%).

LABORATORY DIAGNOSIS. *Cerebrospinal Fluid Examination.* Initial CSF pressure is usually moderately elevated (200 to 300 mm H$_2$O in the adult). Striking elevations (> 450 mm H$_2$O) occur in occasional patients with acute brain swelling complicating meningitis in the absence of an associated mass lesion.

Gram-Stained Smear. By the time of hospitalization, most patients with pyogenic meningitis have large numbers (at least 10^5 per milliliter) of bacteria in the CSF. Careful examination of the Gram-stained smear of the spun sediment of CSF reveals the etiologic agent in 60 to 80% of cases. In most instances when gram-positive diplococci (or short-chaining cocci) are observed on stained CSF smear, they are pneumococci. In certain clinical settings it is important to distinguish this organism from the relatively penicillin-resistant *Enterococcus,* which would require adding an aminoglycoside to penicillin in treatment. This can be done by identifying pneumococcal polysaccharide in the CSF by latex particle agglutination (or by employing the quellung reaction). Rarely, three species may morphologically mimic *Neisseria* in the CSF or suggest a mixed infection with short gram-negative rods and meningococci: *Acinetobacter calcoaceticus, Moraxella* spp., and *Pasteurella multocida.* Culture of the CSF reveals the etiologic agent in 80 to 90% of patients with bacterial meningitis.

Special Immunologic and Serologic Procedures. In patients in whom the etiologic agent is not identified on Gram-stained smear of the CSF, rapid diagnosis may often be made by detection of specific bacterial antigens by latex agglutination (LA). This technique has been employed most extensively in the rapid diagnosis of meningitis caused by *H. influenzae* type b but also has been used in diagnosing meningococcal (groups A, B, C, and Y) and pneumococcal meningitis and meningitis due to group B streptococci. Since *E. coli* K1 and *N. meningitidis* serogroup B share a common antigenic determinant, immunologic cross-reactivity may cause a false-positive reaction with the group B meningococcal reagent. Since the bacterial cause can be found on Gram-stained smear in most cases

of bacterial meningitis, the role of LA appears to be as an adjunct in rapid diagnosis when no organisms are observed or in providing a specific rather than a morphologic (Gram stain) diagnosis.

The limulus gelation assay for endotoxin is positive in the CSF of patients with meningitis caused by gram-negative but not by gram-positive bacteria.

Cell Count. The cell count in untreated meningitis usually ranges between 100 and 10,000 per cubic millimeter, with polymorphonuclear leukocytes predominating initially ($\geq$ 80%) and lymphocytes appearing subsequently. Extremely high cell counts (> 50,000 per cubic millimeter) may occur rarely in primary bacterial meningitis but also should raise the possibility of intraventricular rupture of a cerebral abscess. Cell counts as low as 10 to 20 may be observed early in bacterial meningitis (particularly that caused by *N. meningitidis* and *H. influenzae*). Occasionally, in granulocytopenic patients or in the elderly with overwhelming pneumococcal meningitis, the CSF may contain very few leukocytes and yet may appear grossly turbid because of the presence of myriads of organisms. Meningitis caused by several bacterial species (*Mycobacterium tuberculosis, Borrelia burgdorferi, Treponema pallidum*) characteristically produces a lymphocytic pleocytosis. *L. monocytogenes* meningitis in infants may produce a primarily lymphocytic response in the CSF; in the adult there is usually a polymorphonuclear response, but rarely lymphocytes predominate.

Glucose. The CSF glucose is reduced to values of 40 mg per deciliter or below (or < 50% of the simultaneous blood level) in 50% of patients with bacterial meningitis; this finding can be very valuable in distinguishing bacterial meningitis from most viral meningitides or parameningeal infections. A normal CSF glucose does not exclude the diagnosis of bacterial meningitis. The simultaneous blood glucose level should be determined, because patients with diabetes mellitus (or those who are receiving intravenous glucose infusions) have an elevated level of glucose in the CSF, and its significance can be appreciated only on comparison with the simultaneous blood level. However, it may take 90 to 120 minutes for equilibration to occur after major shifts in the level of glucose in the circulation. The hypoglycorrhachia characteristic of pyogenic meningitis appears to be due to interference with normal carrier-facilitated diffusion of glucose and to increased utilization of glucose by host cells.

Protein. The level of protein in the CSF is usually elevated above 100 mg per deciliter, and the higher values are more commonly observed in pneumococcal meningitis. Extreme elevations, 1000 mg per deciliter or more, indicate subarachnoid block secondary to the meningitis.

Other Abnormalities in the CSF. Elevated levels of lactic acid occur in pyogenic meningitis. Although lactic dehydrogenase levels are higher in patients with bacterial meningitis than in those with viral infections of the CNS, these alterations are not of help in determining the specific etiologic agent involved. C-reactive protein is increased in about 95% of patients with bacterial meningitis and is not increased in most patients with viral meningitis. However, it does not seem to provide more information than the CSF cell count, is not helpful in diagnosing bacterial meningitis in newborns, and does not provide clues to the bacterial species involved.

***Other Laboratory Tests.* Blood and Respiratory Tract Cultures.** Bacteremia is demonstrable in about 80% of patients with *H. influenzae* meningitis, 50% of those with pneumococcal meningitis, and 30 to 40% of those with meningococcal meningitis. Cultures of the upper respiratory tract are not helpful in establishing an etiologic diagnosis. Determining serum creatinine and electrolytes is important in view of the gravity of the illness, the occurrence of specific abnormalities secondary to the meningitis (syndrome of inappropriate secretion of antidiuretic hormone), and problems in therapy in the presence of renal dysfunction (seizures and hyperkalemia with high-dose penicillin therapy). In patients with extensive petechial and purpuric skin lesions, evaluation for coagulopathy is indicated.

Radiologic Studies. In view of the frequency with which pyogenic meningitis is associated with primary foci of infection in the chest, nasal sinuses, or mastoid, roentgenograms of these areas should be taken at the appropriate time after antimicrobial therapy begins when clinically indicated. Computed tomographic (CT) scans are not indicated in most patients with bacterial meningitis. If a mass lesion (cerebral abscess, subdural empyema) is suspected by history, clinical setting, or physical findings (papilledema, focal cerebral signs), then CT scans should be performed. *Bacterial meningitis is a medical emergency requiring immediate diagnosis and rapid institution of antimicrobial therapy.* Delay in performing a diagnostic lumbar puncture in order to obtain a CT scan should be avoided except on the basis of findings indicative of a parameningeal collection or other intracranial mass lesions, and in that case it would be reasonable to initiate antimicrobial therapy aimed at meningitis of unknown etiology or brain abscess before performing the CT scan. Changes may be observed on CT scan during meningitis itself: cerebral edema and enlargement of the subarachnoid spaces, contrast enhancement of the leptomeninges and the ependyma, or patchy areas of diminished density owing to associated cerebritis and necrosis. Patients with meningitis rarely have significant CT abnormalities in the absence of focal neurologic findings. In the patient with meningitis whose clinical status deteriorates or fails to improve, the CT scan may help demonstrate suspected complications: sterile subdural collections or empyema, ventricular enlargement secondary to communicating or obstructive hydrocephalus, prominent persisting basilar meningitis, extensive areas of cerebral infarction resulting from occlusion of major cerebral arteries, veins, or venous sinuses, or marked ventricular wall enhancement, suggesting ventriculitis or ventricular empyema. In about 10% of adults with bacterial meningitis, cranial CT scan findings (mastoid or sinus wall defect, eroding retrobulbar mass, pneumocephalus) are indicative of disruption of the dural barrier.

DIAGNOSIS. Diagnosis of bacterial meningitis is not difficult in a febrile patient with meningeal symptoms and signs developing in the setting of a predisposing illness. The diagnosis may be less obvious in the elderly, obtunded patient with pneumonia or the confused alcoholic patient in impending delirium tremens. Examination of the CSF should be carried out promptly whenever there is any question of meningitis.

Headache, fever, vomiting, stiff neck, and pleocytosis are features of meningeal inflammation and are common to many types of meningitis (e.g., bacterial, fungal, viral) and also to some parameningeal processes. The CSF findings are most helpful in distinguishing among these processes (see Ch. 421). In the patient with meningitis whose CSF does not reveal the etiologic agent on Gram-stained smear, particularly when the CSF glucose is normal and the polymorphonuclear pleocytosis is atypical, certain treatable processes which can mimic bacterial meningitis should be considered in differential diagnosis: (1) *Parameningeal infections.* The presence of infections (chronic ear or nasal accessory sinus infections, lung abscess) predisposing to brain abscess, epidural (cerebral or spinal) abscess, subdural empyema, or pyogenic venous sinus phlebitis should be sought. Neurologic findings may appear in the course of primary bacterial meningitis, but their presence should alert the physician to the need for close scrutiny for the presence of a space-occupying infectious process in the CNS. Neurologic symptoms or findings antedating the onset of meningeal symptoms should suggest the possibility of a parameningeal infection. The isolation of an anaerobic organism should suggest the possibility of intraventricular leakage of a cerebral abscess. (2) *Bacterial endocarditis.* Bacterial meningitis may occur during bacterial endocarditis caused by pyogenic organisms such as *S. aureus* and enterococci. In subacute bacterial endocarditis, sterile embolic infarctions of the brain may occur and produce meningeal signs and a pleocytosis containing several hundred cells, including polymorphonuclear leukocytes. A history of dental manipulation, fever, and anorexia antedating the meningitis should be sought; careful examination for heart murmurs and peripheral stigmata of endocarditis is indicated. (3) *"Chemical" meningitis.* The clinical and CSF findings (polymorphonuclear pleocytosis and even reduced glucose level) of bacterial meningitis may be produced by chemically induced inflammation. Acute meningitis following a diagnostic lumbar puncture or spinal anesthesia may be due to bacterial or chemical contamination of equipment or anesthetic agent. Chemical meningitis, characterized by a polymorphonuclear pleocytosis, hypoglycorrhachia, and a latent period of 3 to 24 hours, may occur following 1% of metrizamide myelograms. Endogenous chemical meningitis resulting from material from an epidermoid tumor or a craniopharyngioma leaking into the subarachnoid space can produce a

polymorphonuclear pleocytosis and hypoglycorrhachia. Birefringent material may be seen on polarizing microscopy of the CSF sediment.

Rarely, a patient develops meningitis characterized by subacute onset and persistent neutrophilic CSF pleocytosis lasting weeks or months without ready bacteriologic diagnosis. The etiologic agent in such cases of *chronic neutrophilic meningitis* has usually been either a fungus *(Aspergillus, Candida, Blastomyces)* or a bacterium such as *Nocardia* or *Actinomyces* species.

NON-NEUROLOGIC COMPLICATIONS. *Shock.* When shock occurs in pyogenic meningitis, it is usually a manifestation of an accompanying intense bacteremia, as in fulminant meningococcemia, rather than of the meningitis itself. Management is guided by the principles of septic shock therapy with appropriate modifications for myocardial failure (see Ch. 281).

Coagulation Disorders. Coagulopathies are frequently associated with the intense bacteremias (usually meningococcal, occasionally pneumococcal) and hypotension which can accompany meningitis. The changes may be mild, such as thrombocytopenia (with or without prolongation of prothrombin and partial thromboplastin times), or more marked, with clinical evidences of disseminated intravascular coagulation (see Ch. 281).

***Septic Complications.* Endocarditis.** Previously, 5 to 10% of patients with pneumococcal meningitis, particularly those with bacteremia and pneumonia as well, developed acute endocarditis, most commonly on the aortic valve. The incidence is currently much lower, as a result of earlier treatment of the initiating infection. In such patients, febrile relapse and a new murmur may appear shortly after completion of antimicrobial therapy for meningitis.

Pyogenic Arthritis. Septic arthritis may result from the bacteremia associated with meningitis caused by *S. pneumoniae, N. meningitidis,* or *H. influenzae.*

Prolonged Fever. With appropriate antimicrobial treatment of meningitis of the three most common bacterial causes, patients become afebrile within 2 to 5 days. Sometimes fever persists beyond this or recurs after an afebrile period. In the patient with persisting headache, obtundation, and cerebral findings, inadequate drug therapy or neurologic sequelae (cortical venous thrombophlebitis, ventriculitis, subdural collections) are important considerations. Re-evaluation of the CSF, particularly Gram-stained smear and culture, is essential under these circumstances. Drug fever may be responsible in the patient who continues to show clinical improvement in all other respects. Metastatic infection (septic arthritis, purulent pericarditis, thoracic empyema, endocarditis) may be the cause of continuing or recurrent fever.

A syndrome consisting of fever, arthritis, and pericarditis 3 to 6 days after initiation of effective antimicrobial therapy of meningococcal meningitis occurs in about 10% of patients (see Ch. 281).

RECURRENT MENINGITIS. Repeated episodes of bacterial meningitis generally indicate a host defect, either in local anatomy or in antibacterial and immunologic defenses (e.g., recurrent *N. meningitidis* infections in patients with congenital or acquired deficiencies of complement, particularly late-acting components). Eleven percent of adults with pneumococcal meningitis have had more than one episode, whereas 0.5% of patients with meningitis caused by other organisms have had recurrent attacks. *S. pneumoniae* is the cause of one third of episodes of community-acquired recurrent meningitis; various streptococci, *H. influenzae,* and *N. meningitidis* are the causes of another one third of episodes. In contrast, in nosocomial recurrent meningitis, gram-negative bacilli and *S. aureus* are the causes of about 60% of episodes. A history of head trauma is much more frequent in patients with recurrent meningitis. Organisms may enter the subarachnoid space directly, through a defect in the cribriform plate (the most common site), in association with the empty sella syndrome, via a basilar skull fracture, through an erosive sequestrum of the mastoid, through congenital dermal defects along the craniospinal axis (usually evident before adult life), or as a consequence of penetrating cranial trauma or neurosurgical procedures. The anatomic defect may produce a frank CSF leak (rhinorrhea or, less commonly, otorrhea) or may entrap a vascular cuff of meninges which might subsequently serve as a direct route for organisms to reach the meninges. CSF rhinorrhea may be intermittent, and meningitis may occur months or years after head injury.

Any patient with bacterial meningitis, particularly if meningitis is recurrent, should be evaluated carefully for any congenital or post-traumatic defects. The presence of CSF rhinorrhea should be sought at admission and subsequently (rhinorrhea may clear during active meningitis only to recur when inflammation has resolved). Clinical clues suggesting the presence of a CSF fistula through the cribriform plate, pericranial air sinuses, or temporal bone include (1) salty taste in the throat, (2) positionally dependent rhinorrhea (rhinorrhea only in the lateral recumbent or prone position suggests an otic or sphenoid origin), (3) anosmia (cribriform plate leak), (4) hearing loss or full feeling in the ear, often with a finding of fluid or bubbles behind the tympanic membrane (leakage into the middle ear). Demonstration of glucose in nasal secretions with glucose oxidase "sticks" (Dextrostix) suggests the presence of CSF. Quantitative determination of glucose and chloride content of nasal secretions and detection by protein electrophoresis of transferrin bands unique to CSF can definitively establish the presence of CSF rhinorrhea.

Recurrent pneumococcal meningitis may occur without apparent predisposing circumstances, and cryptic CSF leaks should be sought actively in such patients by CT scanning of the frontal and mastoid regions and by radioisotope techniques. (Radioiodine-labeled albumin is introduced intrathecally, and pledgets of cotton placed in the nares are subsequently examined for the radionuclide. Radioisotopic cisternography has been used successfully.) Intrathecal introduction of fluorescein as a visual tracer (under ultraviolet light) can be employed similarly to detect active leaks. Surgical closure of CSF fistulas should be carried out to prevent further episodes of meningitis. Newer extracranial approaches via the ethmoid sinuses to repair cribriform plate or sphenoid sinus dural defects are successful and avoid the higher morbidity associated with craniotomy.

In most patients with CSF otorrhea and rhinorrhea following an acute head injury, the leak ceases in 1 or 2 weeks. *Persistent rhinorrhea for more than 4 to 6 weeks is an indication for surgical repair.* Prolonged administration of penicillin does not prevent pneumococcal meningitis and may encourage infection with more drug-resistant species.

Rarely, recurrent meningitis of nonbacterial etiology may mimic bacterial meningitis. *Mollaret's meningitis* consists of repeated febrile episodes of mild meningeal symptomatology, usually without neurologic abnormalities. Initially, large "endothelial" cells may be seen in the CSF along with polymorphonuclear leukocytes, which subsequently are replaced by lymphocytes. *Behçet's syndrome,* characterized by relapsing oral and genital ulcers and ocular lesions (hypopyon), may exhibit a variety of neurologic abnormalities, including recurrent meningitis.

PROGNOSIS. The introduction of antimicrobial agents has converted bacterial meningitis from a disease that was almost always fatal to one that the majority of patients survive without significant neurologic residua. The mortality rate for community-acquired bacterial meningitis varies with the etiologic agent and the clinical circumstances. With current antimicrobial therapy the mortality rate for *H. influenzae* meningitis is below 5% and that for meningococcal meningitis is about 10%. The highest mortality is with pneumococcal meningitis, in which the rate is about 25%. The mortality rate for gram-negative bacillary meningitis, commonly nosocomial in origin, in adults has been 20 to 30%, but it appears to be decreasing in the past 5 to 10 years. The mortality rate for recurrent community-acquired meningitis in adults (about 5%) is strikingly lower than the 25% rate for nonrecurrent episodes. Poor prognostic factors include advanced age, presence of other foci of infection, underlying diseases (leukemia, alcoholism), obtundation, seizures within the first 24 hours, and delay in instituting appropriate therapy.

TREATMENT. Antimicrobial Agents. Antimicrobial therapy should be begun promptly in this life-threatening emergency. Treatment should be aimed at the most likely causes based on clinical clues (age of the patient, presence of a purpuric rash, a recent neurosurgical procedure, CSF rhinorrhea). If the infecting organism is observed on examination of the Gram-stained smear of the CSF sediment, specific therapy is initiated. If the etiologic agent is not seen on smear (or not detected by LA), treatment for bacterial meningitis of unknown etiology should be carried out (see below).

With the exception of chloramphenicol, the commonly used antimicrobial agents do not readily penetrate the normal blood-brain barrier, but the passage of penicillin and other antimicrobials is enhanced in the presence of meningeal inflammation. Antimicrobial drugs should be administered intravenously throughout the treatment period; reducing dosage as the patient improves should be avoided, because normalization of the blood-brain barrier during recovery reduces the CSF levels of drug that are achievable. Bactericidal drugs (penicillin, ampicillin, third-generation cephalosporins) are preferred whenever possible in the treatment of meningitis caused by susceptible bacteria. In animal models of bacterial meningitis, CSF levels of antibiotics at least 10 to 20 times the minimal bactericidal concentration appear to be needed for optimal therapy. Several antimicrobial drugs (first- or second-generation cephalosporins, clindamycin) do not provide effective levels in the CSF and should not be used.

Meningitis of Specific Bacterial Cause. The treatment of choice for pneumococcal meningitis in the adult has been penicillin (Table 280–3). For patients allergic to penicillin, chloramphenicol has been a reasonable alternative (see below). However, problems have developed because of the emergence of penicillin resistance in some pneumococcal isolates. Such resistance has arisen as a result of successive stepwise chromosomal mutations in genes for penicillin-binding proteins and is not due to β-lactamase production. Penicillin-resistant isolates are either relatively resistant (minimum inhibitory concentration [MIC] of 0.1 to 1.0 μg per milliliter) or highly resistant (MIC > 1.0 μg per milliliter). Penicillin-resistant pneumococcal strains have been found worldwide: 44% of isolates in parts of Spain, 45% in regions of South Africa, and almost 60% of isolates in Hungary. In the United States, currently almost 7% (range 0 to 32%) of pneumococcal isolates are penicillin-resistant, with higher percentages being noted in certain geographic areas such as Nashville, Tennessee, and parts of Texas and Kentucky. Cases of pneumococcal meningitis due to moderately and highly penicillin-resistant strains (some multiple antibiotic resistant) have now emerged in this country. Thus antimicrobial susceptibilities should be determined for all pneumococcal isolates from CSF, blood, or sterile body fluids (Table 280–3). Worrisome has been the recent appearance of cefotaxime resistance in pneumococcal isolates from children in South Africa and Texas. Since commercial MIC panels may not detect resistance to third-generation cephalosporins, it is necessary to determine the MIC to these drugs by means other than using such a panel. If the MIC for cefotaxime or ceftriaxone (< 1.0 μg per milliliter) indicates a highly susceptible isolate, cefotaxime or ceftriaxone would be the drug of choice. If the isolate is highly penicillin-resistant or is resistant to 1.0 μg per milliliter of ceftriaxone or cefotaxime, alternative therapy (vancomycin with or without rifampin intravenously) is indicated. If the patient has pneumococcal meningitis and comes from an area where highly resistant strains are known to occur, then initial therapy (pending susceptibility testing) with cefotaxime (or ceftriaxone) plus vancomycin intravenously is reasonable.

Although resistance to chloramphenicol is unusual among pneumococcal isolates from the United States, chloramphenicol has shown poor bactericidal activity against penicillin-resistant isolates from children with meningitis in South Africa. The relative chloramphenicol resistance of such strains may not be discerned on usual laboratory testing but is revealed when the minimum bactericidal concentration is determined. In areas where highly penicillin-resistant or chloramphenicol-resistant pneumococci are found, vancomycin replaces chloramphenicol in initial treatment of pneumococcal meningitis in the highly penicillin-allergic patient.

Penicillin G or ampicillin intravenously, in the dosage used to treat meningitis due to penicillin-susceptible pneumococci, is used to treat *N. meningitidis* meningitis. Recently, meningococci resistant to penicillin have been isolated occasionally in Spain, South Africa, Canada, and rarely the United States. Most of these isolates have been relatively resistant to penicillin (MIC 0.1 to 1.0 μg per milliliter), although a rare strain has had high-level resistance due to β-lactamase production. The latter-type strains require the use of third-generation cephalosporins, but "meningitis dosages" of penicillin or ampicillin may provide CSF levels that are sufficient for infections due to some strains of relatively penicillin-resistant *N. meningitidis.*

At present, 30 to 35% of isolates of *H. influenzae* type b in the United States are β-lactamase producers and ampicillin resistant; cefotaxime is the initial therapy of choice (see Table 280–3). Chloramphenicol combined with ampicillin is an acceptable alternative. If the isolate proves susceptible to ampicillin, the chloramphenicol

TABLE 280-3. THERAPY FOR MENINGITIS WITH KNOWN BACTERIAL CAUSE*

Therapy of Choice†	Penicillin Susceptibility	Alternative Therapy†
Pneumococcal Meningitis		
Penicillin, 24 million units qd in divided doses q2–4h	MIC <0.1 μg/ml	If penicillin allergic: chloramphenicol, 4–6 grams qd; cefotaxime or ceftriaxone; vancomycin
_or_		
Ampicillin, 12 grams qd in divided doses q2–4h		
Cefotaxime, 2 grams q4–6h	MIC 0.1–1.0 μg/ml	Vancomycin
_or_		
Ceftriaxone, 2 grams q12h		
Vancomycin, 2–3 grams‡ qd in divided doses q8–12h ± rifampin	MIC >1.0 μg/ml	
Haemophilus influenzae Meningitis		
For child: Cefotaxime, 180 mg/kg qd in divided doses q4–6h		Chloramphenicol, 100 mg/kg qd
_or_		_plus_
Ceftriaxone, loading dose of 100 mg/kg followed by 50 mg/kg q12h (not to exceed 4 grams/d)		Ampicillin, 300–400 mg/kg until β-lactamase status known
For adult: Cefotaxime, 2 grams q4h		Chloramphenicol, 4–6 grams qd
		plus
		Ampicillin, 12 grams qd until β-lactamase status known
Staphylococcus aureus Meningitis		
Methicillin-susceptible		
Nafcillin, 10–12 grams qd in divided doses q4h; in difficult cases may add rifampin, 600 mg qd IV or PO		If penicillin allergic: vancomycin, 2–3 grams qd in divided doses q8–12h
Methicillin-resistant		
Vancomycin, 2–3 grams‡ qd in divided doses q8–12h; in difficult cases may add rifampin, 600 mg qd IV or PO		
Listeria monocytogenes Meningitis		
Penicillin§, 24 million units qd in divided doses q2–4h		If penicillin allergic: trimethoprim-sulfamethoxazole (20 mg/kg of trimethoprim component qd in divided doses q6–12h)
_or_		
Ampicillin, 12 grams qd in divided doses q2–4h		
Meningitis Due to Susceptible Enterobacteriaceae		
Cefotaxime, 12 grams qd in divided doses q4h		Aztreonam; trimethoprim-sulfamethoxazole; ciprofloxacin
_or_ (if susceptibilities not known)		
Ceftazidime, 6 grams qd in divided doses q8h and an aminoglycoside (e.g., gentamicin, 5 mg/kg qd in divided doses q8h) (if no response to initial therapy, consider adding intrathecal gentamicin, 3–5 mg dose q24h for first few days)		
Pseudomonas aeruginosa Meningitis		
Ceftazidime, 6–8 grams qd in divided doses q6–8h and an aminoglycoside (tobramicin or gentamicin); (if no response to initial therapy, consider adding intrathecal gentamicin)		Antipseudomonal penicillin (piperacillin or azlocillin) plus tobramicin (or gentamicin); ciprofloxacin; aztreonam

* All doses are intravenous for adults unless otherwise indicated.
† Dosages are for patients with normal renal function.
‡ Higher of the suggested vancomycin doses considered when serum levels inadequate on lower dose.
§ Addition of gentamicin may be considered.

may be discontinued. Although in areas of Spain >50% of isolates are chloramphenicol resistant, <1% have been resistant in the United States. Cefuroxime, a second-generation cephalosporin, has been used extensively in the past 8 years, but the third-generation cephalosporins are preferable because of reports indicating slower sterilization of CSF and a higher incidence of sensorineural hearing loss with cefuroxime.

Treatment for adult meningitis caused by methicillin-sensitive _S. aureus_ is listed in Table 280–3. For the penicillin-allergic, vancomycin is the alternative of choice. Since penetration of vancomycin into the CSF is limited, adjunctive intrathecal (or intraventricular) therapy with vancomycin* (without preservative) has occasionally been resorted to when CSF cultures have remained positive after 48 hours of intravenous therapy alone and where CSF levels can be monitored. For adult meningitis due to methicillin-resistant _S. aureus_, intravenous vancomycin (with adjunctive intrathecal vancomycin as needed) is the treatment of choice. In refractory cases, adding another drug for systemic therapy (rifampin or gentamicin) may be warranted.

Cefotaxime (see Table 280–3) is used to treat meningitis known

to be due to susceptible gram-negative bacilli (_E. coli, Klebsiella, Proteus,_ and so forth). It should not be used to treat meningitis due to less susceptible species such as _Pseudomonas aeruginosa_ and _Acinetobacter._ Initial treatment (on the basis only of findings on Gram-stained smear of CSF) of adults with gram-negative bacillary meningitis is listed in Table 280–3. After identifying the specific pathogen and determining its drug susceptibilities, alterations in antimicrobial therapy may be indicated. If the organism is _P. aeruginosa,_ use a third-generation cephalosporin with antipseudomonal activity (see Table 280–3).

Bacterial Meningitis of Unknown Etiology. Initial treatment of meningitis when the etiologic agent cannot be identified on Gram-stained smear of CSF is based on available clinical clues. _In the neonate,_ a wide range of gram-positive (group B streptococci, _Listeria_) and gram-negative organisms (_E. coli, Klebsiella, H. influenzae_) may be the cause, indicating the intravenous use of combined therapy with drugs such as ampicillin with gentamicin (or amikacin), or ampicillin with cefotaxime (the combination favored by most pediatric infectious disease specialists), until results of cultures become available. _In children,_ therapy is directed at the three most frequent pathogens: _H. influenzae, S. pneumoniae,_ and _N. meningitidis._ The appearance of ampicillin resistance among strains of _H. influenzae_ two decades ago necessitated the shift from single-drug therapy (ampicillin) to a two-drug approach (ampicillin-chloramphenicol) in the treatment of meningitis of unknown cause in

---

* Intrathecal use is not mentioned in the manufacturer's package insert approved by the U.S. Food and Drug Administration. Therefore, its use in these circumstances must be considered investigational.

this age group, pending results of culture. Now, ceftriaxone (same dosage as for *H. influenzae* meningitis) or cefotaxime is most commonly used in pediatric centers. *In adults,* therapy with ampicillin in combination with a third-generation cephalosporin (cefotaxime or ceftriaxone) is employed in view of the role of *L. monocytogenes* (susceptible to ampicillin but not to third-generation cephalosporins) in meningitis of older adults and in previously noted high-risk groups, the emergence of infections due to relatively penicillin-resistant pneumococci, and the increased frequency of aerobic gram-negative bacilli in nosocomial meningitis and meningitis in immunocompromised patients. In the penicillin-allergic individual, trimethoprim-sulfamethoxazole is a suitable alternative in the treatment of *Listeria* meningitis. In special settings (nosocomial meningitis or presence of endemic highly penicillin-resistant pneumococci) where more resistant species (resistant gram-negative bacilli, *S. aureus,* coagulase-negative staphylococci, or highly penicillin-resistant *S. pneumoniae*) are likely to be involved, broader initial therapy (addition of vancomycin) may be indicated.

Duration of Therapy. The frequency of CSF examinations depends on the clinical course, but a repeat examination should be done in 24 to 48 hours if there has not been satisfactory improvement. Routine "end-of-treatment" CSF examination is unnecessary in most patients with the common types of community-acquired bacterial meningitis. Meningococci are rapidly eliminated from the circulation and CSF with appropriate antimicrobial therapy, which should be continued for 5 to 7 days after the patient becomes afebrile. If the patient has responded well, a follow-up lumbar puncture is not necessary. *H. influenzae* meningitis should be treated for 10 days (at least for 7 days after the patient becomes afebrile). Follow-up CSF examination may be omitted in those patients who have responded with rapid clinical resolution of the meningitis. In pneumococcal meningitis, antimicrobial treatment should be continued for 10 to 14 days, and follow-up examination of the CSF should be done. More prolonged therapy is indicated with concomitant parameningeal infection. Treatment of gram-negative bacillary meningitis with parenteral antimicrobials is prolonged, usually for a minimum of 3 weeks (particularly in patients with a recent neurosurgical procedure) in order to prevent relapse. Repeated examinations of the CSF are necessary both during and at the conclusion of treatment to determine whether bacteriologic cure has been achieved.

Other Aspects of Treatment. Occasional patients with acute bacterial meningitis develop marked brain swelling (CSF pressure >450 mm H_2O), which may lead to temporal lobe or cerebellar herniation following lumbar puncture. To decrease the possibility of this complication of increased pressure, only a small amount of CSF should be removed for analysis (the amount present in the manometer) and a 20% solution of mannitol (0.25 to 0.5 gram per kilogram) infused intravenously over 20 to 30 minutes, monitoring (if possible) the decline of CSF pressure to a lower level before the spinal needle is removed. Continued control of increased intracranial pressure, if needed thereafter, may be effected with mannitol, dexamethasone (10 mg intravenously, followed by 4 mg every 6 hours), or both. Brain swelling is about the only current indication for the use of corticosteroids in treating pyogenic meningitis in adults; they should be employed only when the appropriate antimicrobial drugs are administered. In the stuporous patient or one with respiratory insufficiency and markedly increased intracranial pressure, use of a ventilator to reduce the arterial PCO_2 to between 25 and 32 mm Hg is reasonable. Intravenous lidocaine can be used to block increased intracranial pressure associated with intubation, and subsequent transient increases associated with hyperactive airway reflexes can be mitigated by intratracheal instillation of lidocaine prior to vigorous suctioning. With continued elevations of intracranial pressure, a continuous intracranial monitoring device may be warranted.

Initial hypotension, if present, should be treated with fluid resuscitation in keeping with shock management principles. Over the next 24 to 48 hours, fluid limitation (1200 to 1500 ml daily in adults) to prevent brain swelling from the effects of inappropriate antidiuretic hormone secretion, sometimes associated with meningitis (particularly in children), is advisable.

Four prospective, controlled trials in children of the routine use of dexamethasone to reduce the pathophysiologic CNS conse-

quences of the inflammatory response during bacterial meningitis have been performed. Dexamethasone was administered intravenously (either 0.15 mg per kilogram every 6 hours for 4 days or 0.4 mg per kilogram every 12 hours for 2 days) either at the time of or 10 to 20 minutes before initiating antimicrobial therapy (third-generation cephalosporin). Corticosteroid use had no effect on mortality but did reduce the incidence of neurologic sequelae (primarily bilateral sensorineural hearing loss). Complicating gastrointestinal bleeding (usually occult) has been observed rarely but merits caution. On the basis of these studies, most pediatric infectious disease programs surveyed in 1992 used dexamethasone in bacterial meningitis of children over 2 months of age. Most of the children in the studies had *H. influenzae* meningitis, the most common type at the time, and the results reflect primarily the effects of dexamethasone on this form. Currently, *H. influenzae* meningitis has been sharply reduced in incidence by the use of protein-conjugate vaccines, but whether dexamethasone will have a similar effect in reducing neurologic sequelae of meningitis due to *S. pneumoniae* and *N. meningitidis* in children has not yet been established. As of this writing, use of adjunctive dexamethasone in cases of severe *H. influenzae* meningitis seems indicated, but whether adjunctive corticosteroid use will have a similar salutary effect in reducing the incidence of sensorineural hearing loss or neurologic sequelae in adults is not known and awaits results of a multicenter trial.

Patients with acute bacterial meningitis should receive constant nursing attention to ensure prompt recognition of seizures and to prevent aspiration. If seizures occur, they should be treated acutely with diazepam (Valium) administered slowly intravenously in a dose of 5 to 10 mg in the adult. Maintenance anticonvulsant therapy can be continued thereafter with intravenous phenytoin (Dilantin) until the medication can be administered orally. Sedation should be avoided because of the danger of respiratory depression and aspiration.

Surgical treatment of an accompanying pyogenic focus such as mastoiditis should be carried out when complete recovery from the meningitis has occurred, but under continuing antibiotic administration. Rarely, the mastoid infection (e.g., Bezold abscess) is so hyperacute that early drainage may be required after 48 hours or so of antibiotic therapy when the acute meningeal process has subsided somewhat.

Durand ML, Calderwood SB, Weber DJ, et al.: Acute bacterial meningitis in adults: A review of 493 episodes. N Engl J Med 328:21, 1993. *A detailed review of an extensive experience in adults between 1962 and 1988 in a large urban general hospital. Community-acquired, nosocomial, and recurrent forms of bacterial meningitis are categorized; the bacteriologic, clinical, CSF, and neurologic findings are well described.*

Feigin RD, McCracken GH Jr, Klein JO: Diagnosis and management of meningitis. Pediatr Infect Dis J 11:785, 1992. *A comprehensive review of bacterial meningitis in children (from neonate to adolescent). Epidemiology, bacteriology, pathogenesis and pathophysiology, neurologic features, CNS complications, and current treatment are emphasized.*

Odio CM, Faingezicht I, Paris M, et al.: The beneficial effects of early dexamethasone administration in infants and children with bacterial meningitis. N Engl J Med 324:1525, 1991. *This study showed that adjuvant dexamethasone treatment resulted at 12 hours in lowered CSF pressures and improved cerebral perfusion pressures and at follow-up, after 15 months, in decreased sensorineural hearing loss or neurologic sequelae.*

Pfister H-W, Feiden W, Einhaupl K-M: Spectrum of complications during bacterial meningitis in adults. Arch Neurol 50:575, 1993. *In this thorough prospective evaluation of 86 adults with bacterial meningitis, neurologic complications (cerebrovascular injury, brain swelling, cerebral herniation, hydrocephalus) are described. This study describes features helpful for identification of these complications and, particularly, their temporal relationships.*

Quagliarello V, Scheld WM: Bacterial meningitis: Pathogenesis, pathophysiology, and progress. N Engl J Med 327:864, 1992. *In this insightful and comprehensive review, particular attention is given to the role of bacterial components, cytokines and other mediators, and endothelial and leukocyte adhesins in the generation of the inflammatory response in the subarachnoid space.*

Roos KL, Tunkel AR, Scheld WM: Acute bacterial meningitis in children and adults. In Scheld WM, Whitley RJ, Durack DT (eds): Infections of the Central Nervous System. New York, Raven Press, 1991. *A thorough, particularly well illustrated consideration of all aspects of bacterial meningitis, including pathology, pathogenesis, clinical features, epidemiology, and treatment. Includes a helpful section on neuroimaging changes.*

Swartz MN, Dodge PR: Bacterial meningitis—A review of selected aspects. N Engl J Med 272:725, 1965. *Detailed account of Massachusetts General Hospital experience. Particularly good on clinical aspects, neurologic complications, and differential diagnosis.*

281 MENINGOCOCCAL INFECTIONS

Michael A. Apicella

Meningococcal infections are a major cause of mortality and morbidity in developed and developing nations. *Neisseria meningitidis* is the causative agent in meningococcal infections. It has become the most common cause of bacterial meningitis in United States children since using the *Haemophilus influenzae* type b protein-capsular polysaccharide conjugate vaccine in infants has dramatically reduced their incidence of meningitis due to this organism. Considerable progress has been made in managing and preventing infections due to *N. meningitidis* since the organism was first described in 1887 (Table 281–1). Because the meningococcal vaccine has limited effectiveness in the group at greatest risk for infection, children younger than age 2, meningococcal infection is still a major worldwide problem. The devastating nature of systemic meningococcal infection makes it imperative that preventive measures be developed to fully control this disease. In addition, an effective vaccine against meningococcal serogroup B infection has not been developed. Until this goal is realized, it is crucial that the clinician recognize and be able to successfully treat the infection as early as possible in its course to ensure an outcome with minimal mortality and morbidity.

MICROBIOLOGY AND PATHOGENESIS. *N. meningitidis* is a gram-negative diplococcus. Meningococci are considered a fastidious species, and media containing appropriate supplementation must be used to ensure reliable growth from clinical samples. Selective media such as Thayer-Martin medium have allowed the organism to be isolated from sites that contain diverse background flora, such as the nasopharynx. The organism grows best between 35 to 37° C in an atmosphere of 5% carbon dioxide. The organism will not grow below 32° C or above 41° C. Laboratory confirmation of the presence of the organism depends on the metabolism of glucose and maltose with the production of acid. Gas is not produced during this metabolic process.

The meningococcus has a very narrow environmental niche. It is a strict human pathogen that has only been isolated from human mucosal surfaces or body fluids. A number of factors contribute to the organism's ability to colonize and cause infection. The meningococcus has a typical gram-negative cell wall containing lipopolysaccharide or endotoxin, which is the primary toxin of the meningococcus. Meningococci express pili (attachment organelles) which they need to adhere to nasopharyngeal epithelial cells. Meningococci can express polysaccharide capsules; this is probably the most important virulence factor associated with this species.

TABLE 281–1. ADVANCES IN THE DIAGNOSIS, MANAGEMENT, AND PREVENTION OF MENINGOCOCCAL INFECTION

Year	Advance
1805	Epidemic cerebrospinal fluid fever (meningococcal meningitis) described in Geneva.
1885	Causative organism identified.
1904	Distinct serotypes of *N. meningitidis* described.
1909	Asymptomatic nasopharyngeal carrier state recognized.
1911	Use of serotherapy for management of meningococcal infection.
1933	Use of sulfonamides to treat meningococcal meningitis.
1942	Sulfonamide prophylaxis used in military camps to prevent epidemics.
1950	High-dose penicillin used successfully to treat meningococcal meningitis.
1963	Sulfonamide-resistant meningococci identified at Fort Ord, CA.
1971	Meningococcal capsular C polysaccharide used to successfully prevent meningococcal disease to prevent disease in U.S. Army recruits.
1989	*N. meningitidis* resistant to penicillin C first reported.

Thirteen serologically distinct encapsulated forms have been implicated in infection. Immunochemical differences in these capsules are the basis for the principal system used to serogroup encapsulated meningococci. Over 98% of cases are caused by five serogroups: A, B, C, W-135, and Y. Meningococci that lack capsular polysaccharides can be cultured. Called "nonencapsulated strains," they are frequently identified in nasopharyngeal cultures during screening in endemic periods. They have not been isolated from body fluids of patients with systemic meningococcal disease. In addition to serogrouping based on capsular antigens, meningococci also can be serotyped based on antigenic differences in their outer membrane proteins and lipopolysaccharides. These serotypes have become important in studies of the epidemiology of infection and in the development of new vaccines.

The pathogenesis of meningococcal infection is now beginning to be understood. The factors involved in colonization and invasion of the nasopharyngeal surface are shown in Figure 281–1A. The meningococcus can adhere to and enter the nonciliated cells of the nasopharyngeal mucosa. Organisms are able to transmigrate through these cells to the submucosal space, where they have access to enter capillaries and arterioles. If the organism can invade the vascular system, the capsular polysaccharide (in the absence of specific antibody) provides an antiphagocytic barrier that protects the organism against normal host clearing mechanisms. Figure 281–1B outlines the process by which endotoxin (lipo-oligosaccharide, or LOS), through the release of cytokines, leads to shock and disseminated intravascular coagulation (DIC) in meningococcal sepsis. Endotoxin and cytokine levels in meningococcal sepsis have been measured and high tumor necrosis factor alpha (TNFα) and interferon-γ levels correlate with a poor prognosis.

The propensity of the meningococcus to invade the central nervous system (CNS) and cause meningitis is poorly understood. The organism probably gains entry through the arachnoid villi. The release of endotoxin and peptidoglycan in the cerebrospinal fluid (CSF) evokes inflammatory factors that are chemoattractive for polymorphonuclear leukocytes (PMN's). Enzymes released by PMN's intensify the meningeal inflammation, leading to increased cerebral vascular permeability and brain edema.

EPIDEMIOLOGY. *N. meningitidis* can cause endemic and epidemic infection. At present, meningococcal infection is endemic in the United States, with approximately 2500 cases per year reported to the Centers for Disease Control and Prevention. This gives a case rate of approximately 1 in 10^5 total population. The fatality rate is approximately 12%. Disease rates in children younger than age 2 are approximately 10 times higher than in the overall population. Seasonal variation occurs, with the highest attack rates in February and March and the lowest in September. The male-to-female patient ratio is approximately equal. The predominate serogroups causing infection in the United States currently are serogroups B and C.

Before World War II, periodic epidemics of meningococcal infection ravaged American cities. These were caused primarily by the serogroup A meningococcus. With increasing standards of living, these epidemics have abated in this country, and infection due to the serogroup A has virtually disappeared in the United States.

Large-scale epidemics still occur with a deadly frequency in Africa, parts of Asia, South America, and the countries of the former Soviet Union. These epidemics are most commonly caused by serogroup A meningococcus and occasionally by the serogroup C meningococcus. In an area appropriately named "the meningitis belt" because it crosses the waist of sub-Saharan Africa, epidemics of meningococcal infection occur every 7 to 10 years. The case rate during these epidemics can be as high as 1 in 1000 total population. Case rates in children younger than 2 can be 1 in 100. In the developed nations of western Europe, epidemics due to serogroup B meningococcus have occurred over the past decade. Norway suffered such an epidemic with case rates of 1 in 10,000; a high attack rate was seen among teenagers.

The reason for the epidemic spread of the meningococcus is not known. The organism is considered a respiratory pathogen, and spread is most likely by the aerosol route. It is clear that the high attack rates seen in developing countries is in part due to poverty and the consequences of crowding, poor sanitation, and malnutrition. Factors such as herd immunity and specific virulence factors associated with "epidemic strains" have been implicated in the rapid spread of infection in these situations. Predisposition to meningococcal infection has been associated with preceding respiratory tract infection, particularly influenza.

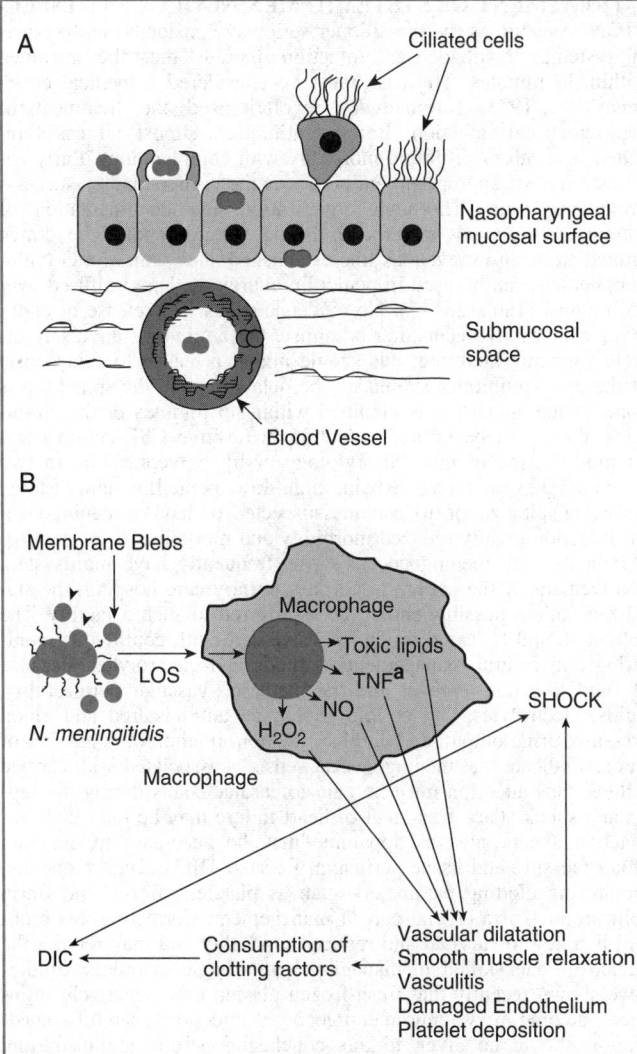

FIGURE 281–1. *A,* A schematic representation of nasopharyngeal invasion by the meningococcus. The process involves attachment to surface of nonciliated cells by meningococcal pili. Short-range attachment factors (meningococcal surface components) are probably involved in the endocytotic engulfment process as microvilli of the nasopharyngeal cell surround the organism. The nonciliated cells through which the organisms transmigrate do not appear to sustain damage. By contrast, the ciliated mucosal cells die and are extruded from the mucosal surface. Meningococcal lipooligosaccharide, peptidoglycan, and possibly other toxins are thought to be responsible for this cytolytic activity. Organisms in the submucosal space then have access to entry into capillaries and arterioles and can invade the vascular system. (Data from Stephens DS: Gonococcal and meningococcal pathogenesis as defined by human cell, cell culture, and organ culture assays. Clin Microbiol Rev 2:S104, 1989.) *B,* The rapid doubling time of the meningococcus and its ability to shed large amounts of endotoxin by a process called "blebbing" rapidly lead to a high-grade septic state with shock. Endotoxin (lipo-oligosaccharide, or LOS) interacts with macrophages to release cytokines, vasoactive lipids (prostaglandins), and free radicals such as H_2O_2, O^-, and NO. These substances damage vascular endothelium, resulting in platelet deposition and vasculitis. This leads to vascular disruption and the petechiae and ecchymoses that are frequently seen during meningococcal infection. Clotting factors are consumed, and DIC ensues, which is an ominous consequence of delayed treatment. Occasionally, the intravascular clotting can lead to occlusion of major arterial vessels in the extremities, requiring amputation. The most dire consequence of all these vascular effects is Waterhouse-Friderichsen syndrome, which is multiorgan failure due to shock and hemorrhagic diathesis. (Data from Brandtzaeg P, Ovstebo R, Kierulf P: Compartmentalization of lipopolysaccharide production correlates with clinical presentation in meningococcal disease. J Infect Dis 166:650, 1992.)

Epidemic infections in American military recruit camps were a major problem before vaccination was introduced. Throughout the nineteenth century, the unique susceptibility of military recruits can be attested to by the clinical descriptions of this infection that can be found in the records of the Crimean and American Civil Wars.

Since vaccinating recruits started in 1972 with a tetravalent vaccine containing serogroup A, C, Y, and W-135 polysaccharides, epidemics have not occurred.

Intimate contacts of cases, including family members, college roommates, and nursery school classmates are at 100- to 1000-fold increased risk of acquiring meningococcal infection. Such individuals should be told about the increased risk and monitored closely for emergence of co-primary cases (cases that arise within 48 hours of the primary case) and given chemoprophylaxis (see treatment section below) to prevent secondary cases of infection. Hospital personnel who care for patients with meningococcal disease are not at increased risk of acquiring infection. Exceptions would include individuals who suffer needle sticks contaminated with body fluids from untreated patients and health care personnel who give mouth-to-mouth resuscitation to infected individuals. It may be wise to manage such individuals with parenteral therapy rather than using chemoprophylaxis. Isolating patients in hospitals is a common practice—limited to respiratory isolation and terminated 24 hours after instituting appropriate antibiotic therapy.

CLINICAL SYNDROMES. *The Carrier State.* There are several different meningococcal infection syndromes. In the early twentieth century, the ability to isolate meningococci from the nasopharynx of otherwise healthy individuals led to the concept of asymptomatic carriage of bacterial pathogens. The observation that increased carriage rates coincided with onset of epidemics among military recruits during World War I first linked the relationship of the carrier state to disease. The nasopharyngeal carrier state is considered an active infection, because some individuals have symptomatic pharyngitis and develop rises in serologic titers to the infecting organism. It is considered that all cases of acute systemic meningococcal infection are preceded by recent nasopharyngeal colonization. Studies have shown that the carrier state can persist for long periods, with about 5% of the population carrying the meningococcus in their nasopharynx during endemic periods. The majority of these isolates are unencapsulated. During epidemics, the carrier rate can rise to over 30%, with the majority of individuals carrying the epidemic strains in their nasopharynx. Generally, most individuals who become carriers are asymptomatic. Evidence exists that the systemic immune system is primed during the period of nasopharyngeal carriage, since antibodies to the infecting strains can be shown to evolve concordant with colonization.

In a study of an epidemic among military recruits, it has been shown that nasopharyngeal colonization by the meningococcal strain responsible for the epidemic resulted in a 40% incidence of systemic infection if the person colonized also lacked bactericidal antibodies to the epidemic strain. This study confirmed the role of nasopharyngeal carriage as the source of systemic infection and the importance of the serum antibody in protecting against systemic meningococcal infection.

Meningitis and Meningococcemia. Acute systemic infection can be manifest clinically by three syndromes: meningitis, meningitis with meningococcemia, and meningococcemia without obvious signs of meningitis. Typically, an otherwise healthy patient develops sudden onset of fever, nausea, vomiting, headache, decreased ability to concentrate, and myalgia. The patient frequently tells the physician that this is the sickest he/she has ever felt. Many have an impending feeling of death. In children, the infection is rarely seen below age 6 months because they are protected by placentally transferred antibodies. Because children younger than age 2 cannot relate many symptoms, sudden onset of fever, leukocytosis, and lethargy become important findings. Initially, the physical examination may be unrevealing, with the exception of an acutely ill patient. The preceding symptoms of pharyngitis which may be associated with nasopharyngeal carriage can lead to a preliminary diagnosis of streptococcal infection. This frequently results in treatment with low-dose penicillin, which has little effect on the emerging meningococcal sepsis. Alternatively, the diagnosis of influenza is assigned to the patient because of complaints of fever, chills, and myalgia. In general, patients with meningococcal infection present considerably sicker than the majority of patients with streptococcal or viral infections. The vital signs will show a low blood pressure with an elevated pulse rate. Diaphoresis is common. In such patients, an intensive search for petechiae should be mounted (see Color Plate 10*A*). A complete examination of the skin with the patient completely undressed is essential. The physical examination should include provocative tests of meningeal irritability, the Kernig and Brudzinski signs. It must be remembered that patients with meningococcemia may not necessarily have meningeal signs but that from 50 to 80% will have petechiae upon presentation. An examination of the mucosal surfaces of the soft palate and ocular and palpabral conjunctivae for petechiae must be done.

The infection can progress rapidly. Depending on the patient's presentation, a critical situation can occur very quickly. Profound shock with DIC is the most ominous development in these patients. Coagulopathy, defined as a partial thromboplastin time of >50 seconds or a fibrinogen concentration of >150 μg per deciliter, is an excellent predictor of poor prognosis. A number of studies have demonstrated that myocardial dysfunction can occur in meningococcal sepsis. Signs of heart failure, including gallop rhythms and congestive heart failure with pulmonary edema, are not uncommon. In one large series, 15% of pediatric patients were admitted to intensive care units because of cardiovascular manifestations. Approximately 25% of patients who died of meningococcal sepsis had evidence of myocarditis. In France, a group of severely ill patients with meningococcal sepsis showed low stroke volume indices (29 ml per square meter) and tachycardia (>135 beats per minute), a profile suggesting a greater myocardial depression than usually observed in gram-negative sepsis. In infection due to meningococcal serogroup C, pericarditis with tamponade can seriously complicate the course of treatment unless recognized and managed. When DIC occurs, persistent bleeding at intravenous sites and sites of arterial punctures can complicate management of the tamponade.

Neurologic complications include signs of meningeal irritation, an encephalopathic state, and coma. Seizures can occur but are less common than in other forms of bacterial meningitis. In general, patients surviving meningococcal CNS infection have remarkably few sequelae (see Ch. 421), but cerebrovascular accidents secondary to intracranial bleeding can lead to paresis. Cases of posterior pituitary insufficiency have been reported in patients recovering from meningococcal infection.

Prognosis can vary depending on the presentation of the patient, the skill and completeness of the physician, and the nature of the facility. At tertiary care hospitals during endemic periods of infection, mortality rates as low as 8% have been reported. Patients who present with meningococcemia alone tend to have a higher mortality rate (up to 20%). During World War II, meningococcal mortality rates using sulfonamides were as low as 2%. Many of these patients were hospitalized and treated as soon as symptoms began. Recent studies in Norway and Africa have supported the concept that early onset of therapy significantly reduces mortality.

LABORATORY DIAGNOSIS. The laboratory diagnosis is based on isolating N. meningitidis from blood cultures or CSF. Blood cultures will be positive in 60 to 80% of untreated patients, while CSF cultures will be positive in 50 to 70%. Gram stain analysis of CSF requires a skilled patient observer but it can provide diagnostic results rapidly. Gram stain of the CSF can be useful as a rapid diagnostic tool, especially in patients with meningococcal meningitis. Approximately 50% of these patients will have a positive Gram stain. In cases of meningococcemia without overt meningitis, the CSF Gram stain will be positive in <25% of patients. Recent studies have suggested that Gram stain analysis of punch biopsy or needle aspiration of hemorrhagic skin lesions in meningococcal sepsis without clinical evidence of meningitis can lead to rapid diagnosis; approximately 70% of such skin lesions were positive. The tinctorial results for punch biopsy specimens were not affected by antibiotics, because Gram staining gave positive results up to 45 hours after antibiotic therapy was started. Cultures of these biopsies or aspirates also were useful diagnostically for as long as 13 hours after instituting antibiotic therapy. Detecting meningococcal capsular polysaccharide in CSF also can be used for rapid diagnosis; the test is most sensitive for the A and C polysaccharides and considerably less sensitive for serogroup B polysaccharide. In meningococcemia without clinically apparent meningitis, the antigen detection methods can be negative despite profound sepsis. Recently, polymerase chain reaction (PCR) has been demonstrated as a potentially rapid method for diagnosing CSF infection and serum. Further testing must be done to confirm the specificity and sensitivity of this technique.

TREATMENT OF SYSTEMIC MENINGOCOCCAL INFECTION. As soon as the practitioner seriously considers the diagnosis of systemic meningococcal infection, therapy must be instituted within 30 minutes. The case must be considered a medical emergency. In 1933, sulfonamides revolutionized the treatment of meningococcal infection. Before antibiotics, almost all cases resulted in death or profound morbidity with complications. Early administration of appropriate antibiotics is the cornerstone of successful management. Thorough organization and documentation of patient management are crucial. Blood cultures should be drawn immediately, an intravenous line established, and penicillin G (chloramphenicol can be used in penicillin-allergic patients) infused over 15 minutes (Table 281–2). No evidence exists that release of endotoxin which may occur after administering antibiotics adversely effects outcome; therefore, this should not be a reason to delay onset of therapy. Antibiotics should not be delayed while the spinal tap is done. If the spinal tap is obtained within 45 minutes of the antibiotics, there will be limited reduction in positive CSF cultures and no modification of the CSF cytology or hypoglycoracchia. In two recent studies in Great Britain, high-dose penicillin administered before hospitalization to patients suspected of having meningococcal infection greatly reduced morbidity and mortality.

Patients with meningococcal sepsis frequently have multisystem involvement. If the patient is not at a tertiary care hospital, the stabilized patient possibly should be transferred to such a facility. The patient should be cared for in intensive care with continuous monitoring and careful management of fluids and electrolytes. Because of fluid loss due to fever and the increased vascular permeability, fluids, electrolytes, and colloid should be administered and blood pressure, urine output, and cardiac function monitored. A number of studies indicate that meningococcal sepsis is associated with cardiac failure; thus attention must be paid to cardiac status during the sepsis and shock state. Treatment of heart failure may be indicated. Vasoactive agents such as dopamine may be necessary to maintain blood pressure and tissue perfusion. Because DIC occurs frequently, monitoring clotting parameters such as platelets, fibrin, and fibrin split products is a crucial part of management. Correcting this problem is a key to survival and reduced morbidity and may require the advice of one skilled in managing hemorrhagic disorders. Studies have shown recently that fresh-frozen plasma may negatively influence outcome in systemic meningococcal infections; careful consideration should be given to this conclusion before administration. Recent studies have suggested that exchange transfusion may improve the survival rate among patients with fulminant meningococcal sepsis. The beneficial effect is most likely not based on the elimination of endotoxin. One of the most serious causes of morbidity in fulminant meningococcal sepsis is skin necrosis and loss of distal digits and limbs. It has been suggested that epidural sympathetic blockade may preserve the lower extremities of such patients. Skin necrosis can be managed by debridement, grafting, and nutritional support after the patient has been stabilized.

Penicillin remains the cornerstone of therapy. The meningococcus is sensitive to a wide range of antibiotics, including third-generation cephalosporins and quinolones. Ampicillin is equivalent to penicillin G and can be used if there is uncertainty about the etiologic diagnosis at the time that therapy is instituted. Recent reports from southern Europe (primarily Spain and Greece) of the isolation of penicillin-resistant meningococci could have ominous consequences if epidemics occur due to these organisms. In Spain, the prevalence of N. meningitidis isolates that are moderately susceptible to penicillin and ampicillin has increased to almost 50%. These strains do not produce β-lactamase. In these strains, the basis of meningococcal resistance to penicillin is alteration in a group of inner membrane enzymes, the penicillin-binding proteins (PBP's), which are

TABLE 281–2. ANTIBIOTIC MANAGEMENT OF SYSTEMIC MENINGOCOCCAL INFECTION

Antibiotic	Dosage
Penicillin G	300,000 units/kg/d IV, up to 24 million units/day
Ampicillin	150–200 mg/kg/d IV, up to 12 grams/day
Ceftriaxone	2 grams/day IV
Chloramphenicol	For use in penicillin-allergic patients, 100 mg/kg/day IV, up to 4 grams/d

responsible for cell wall synthesis. Specifically, alterations in the PBP 2 result in decreased binding affinity of penicillin and ampicillin to these enzymes. Third-generation cephalosporins are usually effective against organisms that are resistant on this basis. However, careful antibiotic sensitivity testing should be performed to ensure that this is the case, since some third-generation cephalosporins also may not bind efficiently to these modified penicillin-binding proteins. Disk diffusion methods can still be used to analyze such strains, although plate dilution methods are preferred. Sulfonamide-resistant meningococci are still common in the United States; hence sulfonamides should not be used to treat acute infections.

Complement Deficiency and Meningococcal Sepsis.
Individuals with deficiencies in complement components appear to be uniquely susceptible to meningococcal infection. In properdin-deficient patients, fulminant meningococcal sepsis is a frequent cause of death. Families of such individuals should be investigated for a history of sudden septic death in relatives. Such families should be managed closely and undergo vaccination with the tetravalent meningococcal vaccine.

In patients with the late complement component deficiencies (LCCD), meningococcal infection occurs in older individuals (mean age 17) and tends to be milder (mortality ~ 2%) and caused by less common serogroups (serogroup Y and W-135) than occurs in the general population. LCCD patients respond normally to meningococcal capsular polysaccharide vaccine with the development of antibodies that are functional in both complement-dependent bactericidal assays and opsonophagocytic assays. These patients have a more rapid decline in capsular antibody than that seen in normal individuals, suggesting that LCCD patients are critically dependent on capsular antibody for protection against meningococcal disease. Vaccination, probably on a recurrent basis, is an important component in preventing meningococcal disease in LCCD patients.

OTHER CLINICAL SYNDROMES. Chronic Meningococcemia.
Chronic meningococcal sepsis, which is indistinguishable from the gonococcal dermatitis-arthritis syndrome, can occur. These patients have typical painful skin lesions usually on the extremities with migratory polyarthritis and tenosynovitis (see Ch. 239). This form of meningococcal sepsis can persist for weeks if untreated. This syndrome responds promptly to antibiotic therapy.

Respiratory Tract Infection.
Pneumonia due to *N. meningitidis* has been reported since the 1930's. In a recent study of community-acquired infections in Finland, *N. meningitidis* was implicated as the etiologic agent in 6%. Epidemic pneumonia due to serogroup Y strains has occurred at a military training center. Patients presented with chills, chest pain, and cough; rales and fever occurred in almost all patients, and infections were frequently multilobar (40%). The incidence of sepsis associated with these infections is quite low, and the diagnosis is usually made with transtracheal aspirations. There was no mortality, and all patients responded well to treatment with penicillin.

Meningococcal Pericarditis.
Pericarditis is usually associated with infections due to *N. meningitidis* serogroup C. It has been reported associated with meningococcemia and as an isolated syndrome. Patients can present with chest pain and signs of tampanode, but relatively asymptomatic disease can occur with detection made by sonography. Treatment with antibiotics and removal of the pericardial fluid usually results in a successful outcome. Pericarditis can occur in patients convalescing from meningococcal sepsis. It should be considered if fever and shortness of breath on minimal exertion occur when the patient is recovering from meningococcal sepsis. Echocardiogram will result in rapid diagnosis of this complication of infection. In convalescent patients, antibiotic therapy should be continued, and pericardiocentesis may be indicated. There is no evidence that steroids or anti-inflammatory agents have a role in management.

Meningococcal Urethritis.
Meningococci have been isolated from the urethra and can cause clinical urethritis. In a recent study of over 5000 urethral cultures from homosexual men, the isolation rate was 0.2%, compared with 4.7% for *N. gonorrhoeae* among the same population. Eight of these patients had symptomatic urethritis. In the same study, there were no isolates among almost 9000 urethral cultures from heterosexual males or almost 16,000 cervical cultures. This study strongly suggests that there is an association between orogenital sex and urethral acquisition of the meningococcus. Meningococcal urethritis has been managed successfully with penicillin and/or tetracycline.

CHEMOPROPHYLAXIS. The observation that sulfonamides could clear the nasopharynx carriage of meningococci for weeks after a single day of therapy led to the concept of chemoprophylaxis for preventing secondary infection in hyperepidemic situations. However, because of the profligate use of sulfonamides for chemoprophylaxis in the 1950's, the meningococcus developed resistance to these agents, and in 1963 epidemics were occurring on Vietnamese military bases. Military studies to find alternatives to sulfonamides resulted in an effective anticapsular vaccine in 1971 and use of minocycline and rifampin for chemoprophylaxis. Eradication of the carrier state in intimate contacts of index cases with chemoprophylaxis is an effective way to prevent secondary cases. The concept behind successful prophylaxis is the use of short-term antibiotic therapy (one to two doses) to achieve long-term (3- to 4-week) eradication of the meningococcus from the nasopharynx. Although physicians realize that prophylaxis is necessary, they fail to appreciate that specific antibiotics must be used for effective management. Penicillin, penicillin derivatives, and first- and second-generation cephalosporins are not effective for prophylaxis because they do not eradicate the meningococcus during the short courses of therapy. Rifampin and ceftriaxone have been shown to be effective agents for prophylaxis (Table 281–3). Recently, quinoline derivatives also have been shown to be effective for chemoprophylaxis.

PREVENTION. The immunologically different meningococcal serogroups were identified in the early 20th century, which led to the use of capsular-specific serotherapy to manage meningococcal infection before effective chemotherapy was developed. The ability of these polysaccharides to evoke a protective immune response is the basis for the meningococcal vaccines. An effective tetravalent capsular polysaccharide vaccine (containing A, C, Y, and W-135 polysaccharides) is available to prevent meningococcal infections in people older than age 2. Over 100 million doses of this vaccine have been given worldwide, with no serious side effects reported. Tetravalent vaccine should be administered to all intimate contacts of index cases at the start of chemoprophylaxis. This vaccine also has been used effectively in the U.S. military and in aborting epidemics caused by serogroup strains represented in the vaccine. A principal drawback of the vaccine is the lack of immunogenicity in children younger than age 2, limiting widespread application of the current vaccine in countries with recurrent epidemic infections. These children respond poorly to polysaccharides for reasons that are not clearly understood. Recent successes in vaccinating young children with *H. influenzae* polysaccharide conjugated to proteins suggest that a similar strategy might be useful for meningococcal polysaccharides. Such a vaccine is not currently available.

In addition, the lack of an antigen that can elicit protection against meningococcal serogroup B infection has limited the vaccine's use. The serogroup B polysaccharide is a poor immunogen, even in adults, perhaps because it resembles "self" antigens. Vaccine development in serogroup B strains has focused on other meningococcal subcapsular surface antigens (proteins and possibly lipopolysaccharide). These vaccines are based on serotypic protein antigens, and the vaccine must be tailored to the serotype of the specific meningococcal strain causing the epidemic. A recent noncapsular serogroup B vaccine has been tested in an epidemic in Brazil, and the results indicate that there was vaccine efficacy in children older than age 2.

TABLE 281–3. CHEMOPROPHYLAXIS FOR PREVENTING MENINGOCOCCAL INFECTION

Antibiotic	Dosage
Rifampin	Adults, 600 mg q12h for 2 days. Children, 10 mg/kg q12h for 2 days.
Ceftriaxone	Single 250-mg dose for adults, single 125-mg dose for children. Limited experience and at present should only be used if rifampin is contraindicated.
Ofloxacin	400 mg as a single dose. Limited experience and should be used only if rifampin is contraindicated. No experience in children.

Apicella MA: *Neisseria meningitidis. In* Mandell GL, Douglas RG, Bennett JE (eds.): Principles and Practices of Infectious Diseases, New York, Churchill Livingstone, 1990, pp 1600–1612. *Complete description of the biology and pathogenesis of* N. meningitidis *infection.*

Cartwright K, Reilly S, White D, et al.: Early treatment with parenteral penicillin in meningococcal disease. Br Med J 305:143, 1992. *Description of the improved outcome in meningococcal infection if therapy is instituted early.*

Densen P: Complement deficiencies and meningococcal disease. Clin Exp Immunol 86(suppl 1):57, 1991. *Review of the role of complement deficiencies and susceptibility to meningococcal infection.*

Durand ML, Calderwood SB, Weber DJ, et al.: Acute bacterial meningitis in adults. N Engl J Med 328:21, 1993. *Recent review of bacterial meningitis in an American hospital.*

Gilja HO, Halstensen A, Digranes A, et al.: Single-dose Ofloxacin to eradicate tonsillopharyngeal carriage of *Neisseria meningitidis.* Antimicrob Agents Chemother 37:2024, 1993. *This article demonstrates the usefulness of quinolones for meningococcal prophylaxis.*

McGee ZA, Baringer JR: Acute meningitis. *In* Mandell GL, Douglas RG, Bennett JE (eds.): Principles and Practices of Infectious Diseases. New York, Churchill Livingstone, 1990, pp 741–761. *Detailed discussion of the differential diagnosis and management of bacterial meningitis.*

Ni H, Knight AL, Cartwright K, et al.: Polymerase chain reaction for diagnosis of meningococcal meningitis. Lancet 340:1432, 1992. *Description of PCR to diagnosis meningococcal infection from clinical materials.*

Schwartz B: Chemoprophylaxis for bacterial infections: Principles of and application to meningococcal infection. Rev Infect Dis 13(suppl 2):S170, 1991. *Review of the concepts and strategies in chemoprophylaxis of meningococcal infection; studies validating using ceftriaxone.*

282 INFECTIONS CAUSED BY *HAEMOPHILUS* SPECIES

Michael S. Simberkoff

DEFINITION. The name *Haemophilus* is derived from the Greek nouns *haima,* meaning "blood," and *philos,* meaning "lover." *Haemophilus* species primarily infect the respiratory tract, skin, or mucous membranes of humans. From these sites, organisms can invade to cause bacteremia, meningitis, epiglottitis, endocarditis, septic arthritis, or cellulitis.

MICROBIOLOGY. The *Haemophilus* species are small, nonmotile, aerobic or facultative anaerobic, pleomorphic, gram-negative bacilli. The prototype of this genus, *H. influenzae,* was originally recovered from patients with influenza by Richard Pfeiffer in 1893, and it was considered the etiology of that disease for many years. The growth requirements of important *Haemophilus* species are summarized in Table 282–1. Primary isolation of *Haemophilus* species is best accomplished on chocolate agar medium in a CO_2-enriched atmosphere.

INFECTIONS CAUSED BY *H. INFLUENZAE*. General Considerations and Laboratory Characterization. *H. influenzae* is the most important pathogen in this genus. It can be recovered from sites where it colonizes, such as the nasopharynx and upper respiratory tract, and from sites where it causes disease, such as the blood, cerebrospinal fluid (CSF), sputum, pleura, middle ear, and joints (Table 282–2).

H. influenzae consists of encapsulated (typable) and nonencapsulated (nontypable) strains. The former are responsible for most of

TABLE 282–1. GROWTH REQUIREMENTS AND HEMOLYTIC PROPERTIES OF *HAEMOPHILUS* SPECIES

Species	X	V	CO_2	Hemolysis
H. influenzae	+	+	–	–
H. influenzae, b. *aegyptius*	+	+	–	–
H. parainfluenzae	–	+	–	–
H. aphrophilus	+*	–	+	–
H. paraphropilus	–	+	+	–
H. haemolyticus	+	+	–	+
H. parahaemolyticus	–	+	–	+
H. ducreyi	+	–	–	+†

* Hematin needed for primary isolation.
† Delayed hemolysis occurs in 11 to 89% of strains.

TABLE 282–2. SITES OF COLONIZATION AND INFECTIONS BY *H. INFLUENZAE*

Species	Normal Flora	Associated Disease(s)
H. influenzae	Nasopharynx Upper respiratory tract	Meningitis Epiglottitis Sinusitis Otitis Pneumonia Cellulitis Arthritis Osteomyelitis Obstetric infections Endocarditis
H. influenzae b. *aegyptius*	No	Purulent conjunctivitis Brazilian purpuric fever

the invasive infections in children, while the latter cause respiratory mucosal infections, including sinusitis and pneumonia, as well as invasive disease in adults. The capsules of *H. influenzae* consist of polysaccharide antigens. Six capsular serotypes (a through f) exist in the species.

Factors Affecting Virulence. The capsules of *H. influenzae* are important virulence factors that inhibit opsonization, clearance, and intracellular killing of the organisms. *H. influenzae* type b, the most common cause of meningitis in infancy and childhood worldwide, contains a pentose capsular polysaccharide consisting of polyribosyl-ribitol phosphate (PRP). Other serotypes contain hexose polysaccharides. It is believed that *H. influenzae* type b is more virulent than other serotypes because it is highly resistant to clearance once bacteremia has been initiated.

Fimbriae are important virulence factors that enhance the adherence of *H. influenzae* to mucosal surfaces. Both typable and nontypable *H. influenzae* isolates contain fimbriae. The lipo-oligosaccharides (LOS's) of *H. influenzae* also contribute to their virulence. LOS's appear to play a crucial role in facilitating the survival of *H. influenzae* on mucosal surfaces within the nasopharynx and in initiating invasive disease (bloodstream invasion) from these sites.

Outer membrane proteins (OMP's) also serve as virulence factors in *H. influenzae* disease. At least 15 different *H. influenzae* OMP's have been identified. One of these OMP's (P2, 39 to 40 kDa) functions as a porin, and others are associated with iron binding. Successful scavenging of iron within the human host is crucial for *H. influenzae* to multiply.

Host Defenses. Antibodies have been recognized for decades as an important part of the host defenses against *H. influenzae* diseases. The classic studies of Fothergill and Wright (1933) demonstrated that most cases of *H. influenzae* meningitis occurred in children during the ages between their losing passively acquired maternal antibodies and developing active humoral immunity to the organism. It is now recognized that these protective antibodies function primarily to opsonize and facilitate *H. influenzae* clearance rather than to directly kill virulent organisms.

Complement is also an essential component of the host defenses against some *H. influenzae* diseases. Children with congenital deficiencies of C2, C3, and Factor I have an increased incidence of *H. influenzae* infections. Patients who lack a functional spleen or who have undergone splenectomy also are at risk for developing overwhelming infection with *H. influenzae* type b.

Prevalence, Incidence, and Epidemiology. The precise prevalence and incidence of *H. influenzae* infections are unknown. This organism can be detected frequently in the nasopharynx of both children and adults. Between 3 and 5% of infants harbor *H. influenzae* type b in their nasopharynx. Nontypable *H. influenzae* can be detected in the nasopharyngeal culture of >70% of young children. Infections, however, occur in only a small fraction of colonized patients. The risk of infection in nonimmune household contacts of a patient with invasive *H. influenzae* disease is approximately 600-fold greater than the risk in the age-adjusted general population.

H. influenzae type b was the most common cause of meningitis in young children before effective vaccines were introduced in the 1980's. Vaccination dramatically reduced the incidence of this infection in young children. In a recent population-based study in Atlanta, Ga., over a 1-year period, invasive *H. influenzae* disease occurred in only 5.6 per 100,000 children and 1.7 per 100,000 adults. Forty of the 47 strains associated with invasive disease from adult patients in this study were serotyped. Twenty of these isolates (50%) were *H. influenzae* type b, 19 (47.5%) were nontypable, and 1 (2.5%) was a type f.

Patients with human immunodeficiency virus (HIV) infection are at increased risk for *H. influenzae* infection. Rates of invasive *H. influenzae* infection among men aged 20 to 49 with HIV infection and the acquired immunodeficiency syndrome (AIDS) were 14.6 and 79.2 per 100,000, respectively. The majority of these infections were caused by nontypable *H. influenzae* strains, although in a second study, 10 of 15 bacteremic *H. influenzae* type b infections observed in adults occurred in patients at risk for HIV infection, and AIDS was documented in 7 of these patients.

Other factors also increase the risk of *H. influenzae* infections. These include globulin deficiencies, sickle cell disease, splenectomy, malignancy, pregnancy, CSF leaks, head trauma, alcoholism, and race. Eskimo, Navajo, and Apache children have *H. influenzae* type b infection rates which are significantly greater than those in comparable non-native populations. In addition, day care attendance, crowding, presence of siblings, previous hospitalizations, and previous otitis media have been shown to increase the risk *H. influenzae* type b disease in young children, while breast-feeding decreases this risk.

Pathogenesis. *H. influenzae* is spread from person to person. Colonization of an individual depends on the virulence factors described above. When *H. influenzae* translocates across damaged epithelial cells, it invades the blood stream. Encapsulated organisms, particularly *H. influenzae* type b, are especially resistant to clearance.

The central nervous system (CNS) is primarily invaded via the choroid plexus. *H. influenzae* and its LOS's initiate an inflammatory process within the subarachnoid which is typical of pyogenic meningitis. This process can be transiently accelerated by using antibiotics that liberate LOS's from organisms if corticosteroids are not administered simultaneously.

Clinical Syndromes. Meningitis. *H. influenzae* meningitis commonly occurs in children under age 5 and in adults with histories of skull trauma or CSF leaks. *H. influenzae* type b strains cause the overwhelming majority of cases. A review of 493 episodes of acute bacterial meningitis in adults over a 27-year period showed that 19 cases (4%) were due to *H. influenzae*.

H. influenzae meningitis is clinically indistinguishable from other forms of acute bacterial meningitis. Most patients with *H. influenzae* meningitis have CSF white blood counts > 1000 per cubic millimeter and hypoglycorrhachia. The CSF Gram stain shows pleomorphic gram-negative bacilli in 60 to 70% of untreated cases. In some patients, however, the bipolar staining may result in a mistaken diagnosis of pneumococcal meningitis. Thus Gram stain is neither sensitive nor specific for diagnosing *H. influenzae* meningitis.

A diagnosis of *H. influenzae* type b meningitis can be rapidly and reliably established by detecting PRP capsular antigens in CSF. The diagnosis can be established in most cases even when antibiotics have been given before CSF is obtained.

Epiglottitis. *H. influenzae* type b is the most common cause of acute epiglottitis in both children and adults. Epiglottitis is a life-threatening infection in children which usually occurs in patients younger than age 5. The symptoms are fever, drooling, dysphagia, and respiratory distress or stridor, which appear over the course of hours. In adults, fever, sore throat, dysphagia, and odynaphagia occur. Cervical tenderness and lymphadenopathy can be found at all ages. Laryngoscopy demonstrates a swollen, cherry-red epiglottis. However, this procedure should be avoided or undertaken only by experts, since it may precipitate an acute airway obstruction and thus make an emergency tracheotomy necessary. The diagnosis of acute epiglottitis is more safely confirmed by a lateral x-ray of the neck. The patient must be maintained in an upright position during this procedure, however, in order to avoid additional compromise of the airway. The etiology is usually established by blood culture. Cultures of the pharynx and other mucosal surfaces are less useful because *H. influenzae* may be part of the normal flora. A recent review suggests that while vaccination has effectively reduced the incidence of this disease in children, it is increasingly observed in adults.

Pneumonia. *H. influenzae* is a common cause of pneumonia in both children and adults. Nosocomial infections, including ventilator-associated pneumonia, also can be caused by these organisms. The clinical features of *H. influenzae* pneumonia include fever, cough, and signs and radiographic findings of lobar consolidation. Parapneumonic effusions or empyema occur commonly in patients with *H. influenzae* pneumonia. Gram-negative bacilli in sputum suggest the diagnosis, but isolation of *H. influenzae* from sputum culture alone is inadequate to prove an etiology because of the high frequency with which this organism colonizes the respiratory tract. A diagnosis can be established by isolating *H. influenzae* from either the blood or pleural fluid.

Tracheobronchitis. Tracheobronchitis is a condition characterized by fever, cough, and purulent sputum that occurs in the absence of radiographic infiltrates suggestive of pneumonia. It frequently occurs in patients with known chronic lung disease. Blood cultures are rarely positive. A combination of pleomorphic gram-negative bacilli predominating in purulent sputum, antibody titers to *H. influenzae* that rise following infection, and the response, at least transiently, to treatment for *H. influenzae* infection strongly suggest this diagnosis.

Sinusitis. *H. influenzae* and *Staplylococcus pneumoniae* are the most frequent bacterial isolates from antral punctures or surgical specimens of patients with acute purulent sinusitis. Most *H. influenzae* isolates are nontypable. While patients may respond initially to treatment directed against *H. influenzae,* the response is transient if sinus obstruction is not relieved. *H. influenzae* is not an important pathogen in patients with chronic sinusitis.

Otitis Media. *H. influenzae* is the most frequent cause of otitis media in young children. Approximately 90% of the *H. influenzae* isolates obtained by tympanocentesis are nontypable; *H. influenzae* type b causes most of the remaining 10% of infections. Patients with otitis media may present with ear pain or irritability. Drainage can be present. An inflamed, opaque, bulging or perforated tympanic membrane is usually demonstrated. The etiology can be proven by Gram stain and culture of purulent fluid obtained by tympanocentesis. Otitis caused by *H. influenzae* type b may occur in association with bacteremia and meningitis.

Cellulitis. *H. influenzae* type b is the cause of 5 to 15% of the cases of cellulitis in young children. Most of the infections occur on the face or neck. *H. influenzae* cellulitis is often described as causing a distinctive blue or violaceous discoloration of the skin. However, the fever, erythema, and tenderness observed may not be distinguishable from other causes. Diagnosis is established by culture of blood and/or tissue aspirates from the involved area.

Bacteremia Without a Primary Focus of Infection. *H. influenzae* causes primary bacteremia in both children and adults. In infants or children, occult meningitis or epiglottitis can be present. A rigorous clinical and laboratory evaluation is essential to avoid missing diagnoses of life-threatening focal infections in these patients. In adults, primary *H. influenzae* type b bacteremia often occurs in patients with underlying diseases such as lymphoma, leukemia, or alcoholism.

Obstetrical Infection. Pregnancy is associated with a significant risk for *H. influenzae* infection. In the Atlanta study, 7 of 47 adult *H. influenzae* invasive infections occurred in pregnant women.

Pericarditis. *H. influenzae* type b is an important cause of primary bacterial pericarditis in children. It rarely causes this infection in adults; however, pericarditis can occur in association with pneumonia, probably as a result of contiguous spread of the infection.

Endocarditis. *H. influenzae* is a very unusual cause of endocarditis, considering the frequency with which invasive disease occurs. Most infections occur in patients with pre-existing valvular heart disease. Because of its slow initial growth in blood culture media, the diagnosis of this infection may be delayed or missed. Patients with *H. influenzae* endocarditis are at high risk for arterial embolic phenomena.

Septic Arthritis. *H. influenzae* type b is a common cause of septic arthritis in young children; it is rare in adults. *H. influenzae* type b arthritis is clinically indistinguishable from other cause of pyogenic arthritis.

Treatment. Third-generation cephalosporins are currently considered to be the treatment of choice for serious *H. influenzae* infections, such as meningitis or epiglottitis. Treatment with ceftriaxone (adult dose: 1 gram IV every 12 hours) or cefotaxime (adult dose: 2 grams IV every 8 hours) should be started for patients with proven or suspected *H. influenzae* infection, and this should be continued at least until the full susceptibility data are available.

Ampicillin was considered to be the treatment of choice for all *H. influenzae* infections until the mid-1970's. Since the first reports of ampicillin-resistant *H. influenzae* isolates in 1972, however, this problem has been increasing. At present, 30% of *H. influenzae* type b isolates and 15% of nontypable *H. influenzae* isolates are resistant to ampicillin. The majority contain a plasmid-mediated, R-factor enzyme (TEM-1) β-lactamase, which can be detected rapidly in the laboratory. A small number of isolates, however, have altered penicillin-binding proteins. These proteins bind penicillin and other β-lactam antibiotics poorly. As a consequence, the isolates may be resistant to some cephalosporins such as cefaclor, cefamandole, and cefuroxime in addition to ampicillin. Therefore, patients with proven or suspected *H. influenzae* infections should not be treated with ampicillin or with second-generation cephalosporins until susceptibilities to these antibiotics are proven. Chloramphenicol resistance also occurs in *H. influenzae;* resistance is caused by an inactivating enzyme, chloramphenical acetyl transferase. A small number of *H. influenzae* isolates are resistant to both ampicillin and chloramphenicol.

Amoxicillin can be used for otitis media in children because of the lower prevalence of β-lactamases in nontypable *H. influenzae* isolates. Bactrim is also effective for most isolates. A combination of erythromycin and sulfisoxazole can be used in patients with documented penicillin allergy.

Prevention. The first *H. influenzae* type b vaccines were licensed for use in the United States in 1985. These contained purified PRP antigens. However, postlicensing studies of PRP vaccines in the United States showed variable efficacy. The PRP vaccines elicit a type 2, thymus-independent B-cell response, generate few (if any) memory B cells, and fail to stimulate a response in neonates and infants.

Protein-conjugated PRP vaccines were developed to overcome the problem of the lack of immune response in the most susceptible infants and some young children. Several are now licensed for use in infants. At present, protein-conjugated PRP vaccines are recommended for use in all infants over age 2 months, but not earlier than age 6 weeks. However, all patient populations are not equally protected. Additional studies are necessary to determine the optimal vaccine preparations and dosage schedules for the infants at greatest risk for *H. influenzae* type b disease.

Antibiotic prophylaxis should be used for unimmunized household or day care contacts of a patient with invasive *H. influenzae* type b disease. Rifampin is the treatment of choice. It should be given in a dose of 10 mg per kilogram once daily for 4 days to neonates younger than 1 month, 20 mg per kilogram (up to a maximum of 600 mg) once daily for 4 days to older children, and 600 mg daily for 4 days to adults.

INFECTIONS CAUSED BY *H. INFLUENZAE*, BIOGROUP *AEGYPTIUS* (PURULENT CONJUNCTIVITIS AND BRAZILIAN PURPURIC FEVER). *H. influenzae,* biogroup *aegyptius* (Koch-Weeks bacillus) causes epidemic purulent conjunctivitis in children. This disease commonly occurs in hot climates or in the summer season. The infection causes conjunctival erythema, edema, mucopurulent exudate, and varying discomfort in the eyes. An unusually virulent clone of *H. influenzae,* biogroup *aegyptius,* causes an invasive infection called Brazilian purpuric fever (BPF). BPF is characterized by petechial or purpuric skin lesions and vascular collapse, which occur days to weeks after an initial episode of conjunctivitis in infants and children younger than 10 years. BPF is usually fatal.

INFECTIONS CAUSED BY OTHER *HAEMOPHILUS* SPECIES. *H. parainfluenzae.* *H. parainfluenzae* can be found as part of the normal flora of the mouth and pharynx (Table 282-3). It is a rare cause of meningitis in children and an even rarer cause of meningitis in adults. It may cause dental infections or dental abscesses. Cases of brain abscess, epidural abscess, liver abscess, osteomyelitis, pneumonia, empyema, epiglottitis, peritonitis, septic arthritis, and septicemia caused by this organism have been reported. *H. parainfluenzae* also causes subacute endocarditis, often in young adults. *Haemophilus* species cause approximately 1% of cases of infective endocarditis in non–drug-abusing patients. *H. parainfluenzae* and *H. aphrophilus* (see below) are the species most frequently recovered from these patients. *H. parainfluenzae* forms

TABLE 282-3. SITES OF COLONIZATION AND INFECTIONS BY OTHER *HAEMOPHILUS* SPECIES

Species	Normal Flora	Associated Disease(s)
H. parainfluenzae	Mouth and pharynx	Endocarditis, brain abscess, liver abscess, pneumonia, epiglottitis, arthritis, osteomyelitis
H. aphrophilus	Mouth	Endocarditis, brain abscess, periodontal abscess, osteomyelitis
H. paraphrophilus	Mouth and pharynx	Endocarditis, brain abscess, liver abscess
H. haemolyticus	Nasopharynx	?
H. parahaemolyticus	Mouth and pharynx	Endocarditis, empyema of gallbladder, ? pharyngitis
H. ducreyi	No	Chancroid

bulky vegetations on heart valves. Arterial embolization is common in patients with *H. parainfluenzae* endocarditis. Most isolates are sensitive to ampicillin, but some produce β-lactamases. Pending sensitivity reports, patients should be treated with a drug that combines a β-lactam antibiotic and a β-lactamase inhibitor (such as ampicillin/sulbactam; adult dose: 3 grams IV q6h) with ampicillin plus an aminoglycoside or with a third-generation cephalosporin.

H. aphrophilus. *H. aphrophilus* can be found as part of the normal oral flora (see Table 282-3). Like *H. parainfluenzae, H. aphrophilus* grows very slowly on primary isolation from blood cultures. It frequently causes bulky vegetations, and arterial emboli are common. *H. aphrophilus* is also a rare cause of brain abscess, periodontal abscess, meningitis, osteomyelitis, and suppurative pulmonary infections. Ampicillin or ampicillin plus an aminoglycoside should be used to treat infections.

H. paraphrophilus. *H. paraphrophilus* can be found as part of the normal flora of the mouth and pharynx (see Table 282-3). *H. paraphrophilus* is a rare cause of endocarditis, and arterial emboli have been observed in 50% of the cases *H. paraphrophilus* endocarditis. It is also a rare cause of brain abscess and liver abscess. Ampicillin is the treatment of choice for this infection.

H. parahaemolyticus. *H. parahaemolyticus* is an important pathogen in domestic animals, causing porcine pleuropneumonia. The organism can be found in the human mouth and pharynx. It is a rare cause of human subacute endocarditis and of empyema of the gallbladder (see Table 282-3). *H. parahaemolyticus* has been isolated from throat cultures of patients with pharyngitis. Animal isolates of *H. parahaemolyticus* are sensitive to tetracycline and sulfa drugs. There is insufficient information about human isolates to permit recommendations for therapy.

H. ducreyi. See Ch. 314.

Adams WG, Keaver KA, Cochi SL, et al.: Decline of childhood *Haemophilus Influenzae* type b (Hib) disease in the Hib vaccine era. JAMA 269:221, 1993. *Shows that, in children < age 5, there was a 71 to 82% reduction in* H. influenzae *type b meningitis in the year following licensing of the Hib conjugate vaccines in the U.S.*

Centers for Disease Control and Prevention. Recommendations for use of the *Haemophilus* b conjugate vaccines and a combined diphtheria, tetanus, pertussis, and *Haemophilus* b vaccine. Recommendations of the Advisory Committee on Immunization Practices (ACIP). MMWR 42 (No.RR-13):1, 1993. *Contains recommendations for use of* Haemophilus b *conjugate vaccines for infants beginning at age 2 months (but not earlier than age 6 weeks); also describes the safety, immunogenicity, efficacy, adverse reactions, contraindications, and precautions for vaccine use.*

Durand ML, Calderwood SB, Weber DJ, et al.: Acute bacterial meningitis in adults: A review of 493 episodes. N Engl J Med 328:21, 1993. *Summarizes data from a large series of adults with acute bacterial meningitis seen over 27 years.* H. influenzae *caused acute bacterial meningitis in 19 (4%) of the adults. Thirteen of these patients had community-acquired infections and six developed nosocomial* H. influenzae *meningitis after neurosurgery.*

Farley MM, Stephens DS, Brachman PS, et al.: Invasive *Haemophilus influenzae* disease in adults. Ann Intern Med 116:806, 1992. *A population-based study showing that 47 cases of invasive* H. influenzae *disease occurred in adults in metropolitan Atlanta from December 1988 through May 1990 (incidence 1.7 per 100,000 adults per year).*

Fothergill LD, Wright J: Influenzal meningitis: The relation of age incidence to the bactericidal power of blood against the causal organism. J Immunol 24:273, 1993. *The classic study showing that* H. influenzae *meningitis occurs in children during the ages between the loss of passively acquired maternal antibodies and the development of active immunity to this organism.*

Liu VC, Smith A: Molecular mechanisms of *Haemophilus influenzae* pathogenicity. Antibiot Chemother 45:30, 1992. *Reviews the virulence factors that have been associated with invasive* H. influenzae *infections, including the capsule, outer membrane proteins, fimbria, and lipo-oligosaccharides of the organism.*

Moxon ER: Pathogenesis of invasive *Haemophilus influenzae* disease. Molecular basis of invasive *Haemophilus influenzae* type b disease. J Infect Dis 165(Suppl 1): S77, 1992. *Studies of mutant strains of* H. influenzae *have clarified the mechanisms of colonization, mucosal damage, translocation, and multiplication of the*

organism within the vascular system to reach concentrations necessary for CNS invasion.

Steinhart R, Reingold AL, Taylor F, et al.: Invasive *Haemophilus influenzae* infection in men with HIV infection. JAMA 268:3350, 1992. *A population-based study shows that the rates of invasive* H. influenzae *among men aged 20 to 49 with HIV infection without AIDS and with AIDS were 14.6 and 79.2 in 100,000 respectively.*

Osteomyelitis

283   OSTEOMYELITIS
Barry D. Brause

DEFINITION. Osteomyelitis is an infection by microorganisms that invade bone. Three pathogenetic routes of infection define the major forms of osteomyelitis, with pathogens reaching osseous tissue by (1) hematogenous seeding, (2) contamination accompanying surgical and nonsurgical trauma (termed "introduced" infection), or (3) spread from infected contiguous tissue.

ETIOLOGY. Although virtually all microorganisms can infect bone, bacteria are the usual pathogens, and staphylococci are the most prominent etiologic agents. *Staphylococcus aureus* causes ap-

proximately 60% of hematogenous and introduced infections and is a principal agent when osseous sepsis spreads by contiguity. *S. epidermidis* has become a major pathogen in bone infections associated with indwelling prosthetic materials, such as joint implants and fracture fixation devices, responsible for 30% of these cases. Streptococci, gram-negative bacilli, anaerobes, mycobacteria, and fungi are etiologic agents in a variety of clinical settings (Table 283–1).

INCIDENCE, PREVALENCE, AND EPIDEMIOLOGY. The anatomic location of hematogenous osteomyelitis is age-dependent (Table 283–1). From birth to puberty the long bones of the extremities are the most frequently involved. In adults blood-borne osteomyelitis generally affects the spine, because vertebrae become more vascular than other skeletal tissue with maturation. Seventy percent of compound fractures are contaminated, but because of effective debridement and perioperative antibiotic therapy only 2 to 9% develop infection. Osteomyelitis develops by contiguous spread in 30 to 68% of diabetic patients with foot ulcers, and it is notable

TABLE 283–1. PREDISPOSITIONS, ANATOMIC SITES, AND PROMINENT PATHOGENS IN FORMS OF OSTEOMYELITIS

Form of Osteomyelitis	Predisposing Condition	Site	Prominent Pathogens
Hematogenous			
Childhood	None	Long bones	*S. aureus*
			Streptococci
			Hemophilus
	Sickle cell hemoglobinopathy	Multiple	*Salmonella*
Adult	Urinary tract infection or instrumentation	Vertebral	GNB
			Streptococci
	Skin infection	Vertebral	*S. aureus*
			Streptococci
	Respiratory infection	Vertebral	Streptococci
	IV drug abuse, or vascular catheters	Vertebral	GNB
			Staphylococci
			Candida
	AIDS	Multiple	Fungi
			Mycobacteria
Introduced type	Fractures	Fracture site	*S. aureus*
			S. epidermidis
			GNB
	Prosthetic joint	Prosthesis	*S. epidermidis*
			S. aureus
Contiguous spread	Skin ulcer	Foot, leg	Polymicrobial
			Staphylococci
			Streptococci
			GNB
			Anaerobes
	Sinusitis	Skull	Streptococci
			Anaerobes
	Dental abscess	Mandible Maxilla	Streptococci
			Anaerobes
	Human or animal bites	Hand	Streptococci
			Anaerobes
			Pasturella
	Felon	Finger	*S. aureus*
	Gardening	Hand	*Sporothrix*

GNB = gram-negative bacilli.

that more in-hospital days are spent treating foot infections than any other complication of diabetes.

PATHOGENESIS. In childhood hematogenous osteomyelitis the initial infective site is the long bone metaphysis due to its large blood flow. In adults bacteremias seed vertebral bodies preferentially at the more vascular anterior end-plates. Osteomyelitis commonly involves two adjacent vertebral bodies and the intervertebral disc space. Infection compromises the nutrient supply to the intervertebral disc, resulting in disc necrosis and disc space narrowing, which is often the earliest sign of vertebral osteomyelitis (Fig. 283–1). Table 283–1 lists examples of clinical conditions that predispose to the development of blood-borne bone infection.

With the introduced form of osteomyelitis, direct septic trauma breaches all protective tissue around the bone, allowing microorganisms into the osseous matrix. The risk of infection is increased further when metallic fixation devices or prosthetic joints are implanted. Indwelling foreign bodies decrease the quantity of bacteria necessary to establish infection in bone and permit pathogens to persist on the surface of the avascular material, sequestered from circulating immune factors and systemic antibiotics. Osteomyelitis is caused by contiguous extension from infected, adjacent soft tissue when the soft tissue process is sufficiently chronic or uncontrolled (see Table 283–1).

Once infection becomes established in bone, the microorganisms induce local metabolic changes and inflammatory reactions that increase necrosis. As the septic process spreads, local thrombophlebitis develops, further increasing ischemia, which results in necrosis of large areas of bone called "sequestra" (Fig. 283–2). When the osseous cortex is breached, subperiosteal abscesses can develop with periosteal inflammation that induces new bone formation in adjacent soft tissue.

CLINICAL MANIFESTATIONS. In the classic presentation of childhood hematogenous osteomyelitis, fever, chills, and malaise are present but are frequently absent in the other forms of bone infection. Localized pain is a characteristic feature of osteomyelitis, with overlying erythema, warmth, and swelling variably observed. Limb motion may be limited if infection is near an articulation, and joint effusions can occur but are usually sterile when the epiphyseal cartilage is intact.

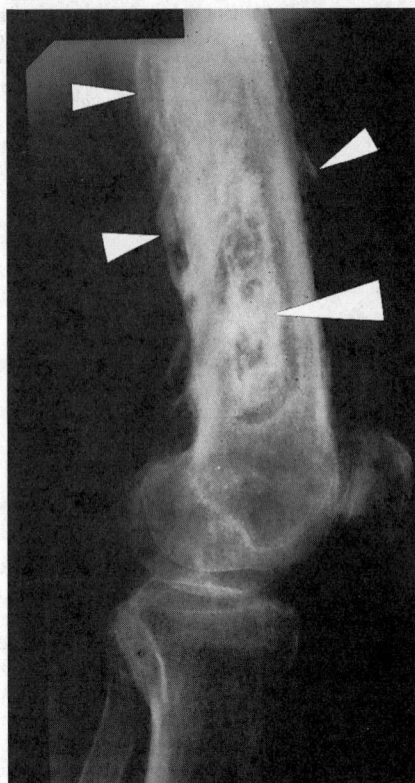

FIGURE 283–2. Femoral osteomyelitis. Hyperdense central zone is a sequestrum *(large arrowhead)*, and peripheral linear densities are areas of periosteal elevation with periosteal new bone formation *(small arrowheads)*.

Hematogenous vertebral osteomyelitis often presents with back pain, spine tenderness, and low-grade fever following urinary tract instrumentation or infection (30%), skin infection (13%), or respiratory infection (11%). The septic process extending beyond the vertebral column produces suppuration at the particular spinal level of infection such as retropharyngeal abscess, mediastinitis, empyema, subdiaphragmatic and iliopsoas abscesses, as well as meningitis. If paresis, sensory deficits, or bowel or bladder dysfunction develop, spinal epidural abscess—the most feared complication—should be suspected and evaluated immediately. *Mycobacterium tuberculosis* should be considered in relatively indolent infections of vertebrae (as well as at the hip and knee) (Table 283–1).

Osteomyelitis after trauma or bone surgery is usually associated with persistent or recurrent fevers, increasing pain at the operative site, and poor incisional healing, which is often accompanied by protracted wound drainage or dehiscence. Prosthetic joint infection presents with joint pain (95%), fever (43%), or cutaneous sinus drainage (32%).

Bone involvement by contiguous spread from an overlying chronic ischemic or neuropathic foot ulcer typically occurs in patients with longstanding insulin-dependent diabetes or other vascular disease and involves the metatarsals or the proximal phalanges. It is characterized by local cellulitis with inflammation and necrosis, but pain is only variably found due to the frequent presence of sensory neuropathy. Additional examples of osteomyelitis from contiguous spread of infection are listed in Table 283–1.

DIAGNOSIS. Diagnosis requires both confirming the osseous site of involvement and identifying the etiologic microbes. Bone infection must be differentiated from septic arthritis and bursitis, cellulitis and soft tissue abscesses, bone fractures, and neoplasms, as well as bone infarcts seen with sickle cell hemoglobinopathy and Gaucher's disease. Anatomic delineation of bone infection depends largely on radiologic techniques. In hematogenous infection, the earliest osseous changes by radiography are osteopenic or lytic lesions. They require 30 to 50% decalcification to be seen and take 2 to 4 weeks to develop. With further progression, periosteal elevation, thickening, and new bone formation are seen with sequestra and sclerotic changes occurring in chronic infection (see Fig. 283–2). Vertebral osteomyelitis appears initially as disc space nar-

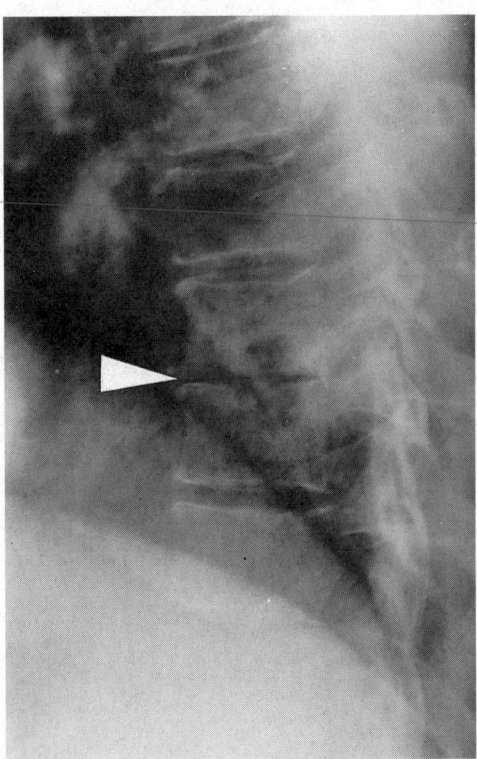

FIGURE 283–1. Vertebral osteomyelitis. Lateral view of spine illustrating disk space narrowing *(arrowhead)* and cortical destruction at the vertebral end-plates.

rowing followed by cortical destruction at the adjacent end-plates (see Fig. 283–1). Computed tomography (CT) is helpful to identify small osseous alterations and sequestra.

Technetium diphosphonate bone scans, gallium-citrate scans, and indium-labeled leukocyte scintigraphy are far more sensitive than radiography and usually reveal increased radionuclide uptake when symptoms begin. However, these techniques are plagued by inadequate specificity and spatial resolution, so they are not conclusively diagnostic. Inflammatory and degenerative processes in adjacent tissues, recent orthopedic surgery, bone fractures, and neoplasms produce abnormal scans in the absence of osteomyelitis. Magnetic resonance imaging (MRI) can detect osteomyelitis earlier than roentgenograms or CT scans with equivalent or greater sensitivity, specificity, and spatial resolution when compared with scintigraphic methods.

The exact microbial etiology of osteomyelitis should be determined, because it is never sufficiently predictable to permit routine presumptive therapy (see Table 283–1). Blood cultures are positive in 25 to 50% of acute childhood hematogenous osteomyelitis but are helpful in < 10% of the other forms of bone infection. When septic arthritis or soft tissue abscess accompanies the osseous process, arthrocentesis or abscess aspiration cultures can be diagnostic. However, superficial cultures of open wounds or skin ulcers and cultures of cutaneous sinus tracts do not delineate the true bone pathogen(s). In patients with deep chronic skin ulcers from which infection has spread to bone, curettage cultures from the base of the ulcer correlate with osseous tissue 75% of the time. Bone aspirate and biopsy cultures are positive in 70 to 93% of cases and should be sought (percutaneously or by operative debridement) when there is no overlying skin ulcer and the microbiologic diagnosis has not been otherwise established. Specimens for mycobacterial, fungal, and anaerobic cultivation should be considered when routine bacterial cultures are negative.

TREATMENT. Acute osteomyelitis is curable with adequate antimicrobial therapy and surgical debridement when necessary. Parenterally administered antibiotics are usually employed, but oral therapy is also effective when the pathogen is sufficiently susceptible and gastrointestinal absorption is ensured. The exact potency and duration of therapy required to eradicate bone infections are not known. Antibiotics that produce trough serum bactericidal activity at a 1:2 titer have been associated with high cure rates. Treatment should be given for 4 to 6 weeks. Surgery is indicated to drain abscesses, debride necrotic tissues, and remove foreign materials.

PROGNOSIS. Inadequate therapy of acute osteomyelitis results in relapsing infection and progression to chronic osteomyelitis; therefore, definitive treatment of acute infection is obligatory. Due to the presence of gross and microscopic foci of avascular bone, chronic osteomyelitis is not curable except by radical resection (occasionally amputation). Acute exacerbations of these chronic, recurrent infections can be suppressed successfully by debridement of identifiable sequestra followed by protracted courses of parenteral and oral antimicrobial agents.

Brause BD: Infected orthopedic prostheses. *In* Bisno AL, Waldvogel FA (eds.): Infections Associated with Indwelling Medical Devices. Washington, American Society for Microbiology, 1989, pp 111–127. *Detailed summary of the pathogenesis, microbiology, diagnosis, and treatment of osteomyelitis associated with prosthetic joints.*

Gold RH, Hawkins RA, Katz RD: Bacterial osteomyelitis: Findings on plain radiography, CT, MR, and scintigraphy. AJR 157:365, 1991. *Pictorial essay comparing all the different imaging techniques useful in diagnosing osteomyelitis.*

Norden CW (ed.): Osteomyelitis. Infect Dis Clin North Am 4:361, 1990. *A current and comprehensive evaluation of the epidemiology, clinical presentation, diagnosis, and therapy of osteomyelitis.*

Waldvogel FA, Medoff G, Swartz MN: Osteomyelitis: A review of clinical features, therapeutic considerations and unusual aspects, parts I, II, and III. N Engl J Med 282:198, 1970. *This detailed clinical description of the pathogenetic features of osteomyelitis remains best for in-depth understanding of the nature of these infections.*

Weinstein M, Stratton C, Hawley HB, et al.: Multicenter collaborative evaluation of a standardized serum bactericidal test as a predictor of therapeutic efficacy in acute and chronic osteomyelitis. Am J Med 83:218, 1987. *The best data collection for defining quantitatively effective antibiotic therapy for osteomyelitis.*

Whooping Cough

284 WHOOPING COUGH (Pertussis)
Richard B. Johnston, Jr.

DEFINITION. Whooping cough (synonym, pertussis) is a noninvasive, highly communicable bacterial respiratory illness. It occurs at all ages but is most common and most severe in infants and young children. The etiologic agent of the syndrome is usually *Bordetella pertussis*. The descriptive name derives from a distressing, prolonged inspiratory effort that follows paroxysmal coughing. Whooping cough is estimated to cause 500,000 deaths yearly, primarily in infants.

ETIOLOGY. When first isolated, *B. pertussis* is a small, nonmotile, weakly staining, gram-negative coccobacillus, 0.5 to 1.0 μ in length. Capsules can be demonstrated by special procedures, and bipolar metachromatic granules are present. The complex medium containing blood originally employed by Bordet and Gengou is still used (in modified form) for cultivation. *Primary isolates do not grow on conventional laboratory media.*

An estimated 5 to 10% of clinical whooping cough is caused by *B. parapertussis*. The animal pathogen *B. bronchiseptica* is responsible for a minor percentage of cases. These organisms can be differentiated from *B. pertussis* by growth requirements, enzyme production, and presence of species-specific antigens. It has been suggested that adenoviruses, alone or in concert with *B. pertussis*, and *Chlamydia trachomatis* may play an etiologic role in some cases of whooping cough.

EPIDEMIOLOGY. In nonimmune households the attack rate is 80 to 90%. Transmission is by droplet infection. Carriers of *B. per-tussis* are found infrequently, but persons previously immunized have been shown during outbreaks of disease to excrete the organism in the absence of clinical symptoms or in the presence of mild or atypical illness.

The mortality rate from whooping cough has fallen since the beginning of the twentieth century owing to improved supportive therapy. The incidence of whooping cough, however, did not change until after the 1940's, when immunization of young children became standard practice. In the 1940's, approximately 200,000 cases of pertussis were reported annually in the United States, compared with about 5000 cases annually in recent years. Most deaths occur in children under 1 year of age. The case fatality rate in infants under 6 months of age is 1%.

Neither immunization against pertussis nor natural disease provides lifelong protection. In the case of immunization, an attack rate greater than 50% has been reported when the interval after immunization exceeds 12 years. Adolescents and adults represent a large reservoir of susceptibles who can transmit the disease to unimmunized infants, and pertussis is an important cause of persistent cough in adults.

PATHOGENESIS. *B. pertussis* adheres to ciliated epithelial cells of the respiratory tract and multiplies there without invading the tissues. Yet this colonization leads to profound changes in tissues which persist long after the responsible bacteria have been cleared. Such observations suggest that a toxin or toxins from the bacteria play an important part in the pathogenesis of the syndrome. A variety of biologic activities have been demonstrated by injecting *B. pertussis* products into experimental animals. An endotoxin and a heat-labile toxin that can cause tissue necrosis have been identified among these bacterial factors, but the exotoxin *pertussis toxin* (PT) is the best candidate at the moment for a major virulence factor. Immunization with chemically detoxified PT appears to prevent severe whooping cough with an efficacy similar to that achieved with the standard cellular vaccine. PT is believed to be responsible for the characteristic lymphocytosis of whooping cough.

PT is a protein composed of five noncovalently linked subunits (S1–S5). The subunits S2–S5 form a nontoxic unit that binds to the cell membrane; toxicity is mediated by the enzymatically active subunit, S1. Activity of S1 inhibits a subclass of guanosine triphosphate (GTP)–binding proteins (G proteins) that are essential for transmembrane signaling and, thus, certain types of receptor-mediated cell functions.

Adherence of *B. pertussis* to respiratory epithelium is required for the pathogenesis of whooping cough. Adherence appears to involve a bacterial outer membrane protein with a molecular weight of 69 kilodaltons, termed pertactin. An antigenically similar protein exists on *B. parapertussis* and *B. bronchiseptica.* Injection of this protein into mice or humans elicits agglutinating antibody to *B. pertussis* and protects the mice against lethal *B. pertussis* respiratory challenge. Synthesis of pertactin is controlled by a regulatory gene at the *vir* (virulence) locus, which modulates synthesis of PT and additional factors that may contribute to pathogenesis, including filamentous hemagglutinin.

PATHOLOGY. Lesions caused by *B. pertussis* are found principally in the bronchi and bronchioles, but changes are also seen in the nasopharynx, larynx, and trachea. Masses of bacteria and mucopurulent exudate are intertwined with the cilia of the columnar epithelium. There is necrosis of the midzonal and basilar epithelium with infiltration of polymorphonuclear leukocytes and macrophages. The most frequent findings in the lung are bronchopneumonia, interstitial pneumonitis, and numerous small areas of atelectasis. The brain can show edema and scattered petechiae at autopsy.

CLINICAL MANIFESTATIONS. The incubation period lasts 7 to 14 days (rarely over 2 weeks). It is customary to divide the clinical course into three stages.

Catarrhal Stage. Whooping cough begins with symptoms indistinguishable from those of a mild viral upper respiratory infection. Sneezing is frequent, conjunctivae are injected, and a nocturnal cough appears. The temperature may be slightly elevated. Infectivity is greatest at this stage.

Paroxysmal Stage. Seven to 14 days after onset, the cough becomes more frequent, then paroxysmal. In a typical paroxysm there is a series of 5 to 20 short coughs of increasing intensity and then a deep inspiration, making the "whoop." A tenacious mucus plug is usually expelled, and vomiting frequently follows. Paroxysms may occur as often as every half hour and are accompanied by signs of increased venous pressure, including deeply engorged conjunctivae, periorbital edema, petechial hemorrhages, particularly about the forehead, and epistaxis. During the attack, the infant may be cyanotic until the crowing whoop occurs. Between paroxysms, the child usually feels well, although justifiably apprehensive. This phase lasts 2 to 4 weeks.

Physical examination of the chest is often unremarkable except for scattered rhonchi. The chest roentgenogram sometimes reveals hilar and mediastinal nodal enlargement. The presence of fever should immediately suggest the development a secondary infectious process.

Convalescent Stage. Gradually the paroxysms become less frequent and less intense; vomiting ceases, and slow recovery ensues. Convalescence requires 4 to 12 weeks. For many months even a mild, unrelated respiratory infection can induce a return of paroxysmal cough and whoop.

In infants younger than 6 months old, the paroxysms and the whoop are often absent; choking spells and apneic episodes may be the major manifestations. Second attacks of whooping cough as well as disease occurring in previously immunized individuals often present simply as an upper respiratory illness or bronchitis.

Complications. Recurrent vomiting can lead to metabolic alkalosis or malnutrition. Central nervous system changes can result from cerebral anoxia or hemorrhages consequent to the elevated venous pressure. Rarely, cortical degeneration occurs, but the exact pathogenesis of the encephalopathy is unknown. A serous meningitis with lymphocytosis of the cerebrospinal fluid has been described. Pneumothorax and interstitial emphysema are infrequently seen. Secondary bacterial otitis media occurs frequently. The major cause of death in whooping cough is pneumonia, either primary or caused by other bacteria or viruses.

DIAGNOSIS. There is little difficulty in making the clinical diagnosis of whooping cough in a patient who, after a period of coryzal symptoms, develops paroxysmal coughing with a terminal inspiratory whoop. Lymphocytosis often occurs toward the end of the catarrhal stage or early in the spasmodic phase. Characteristically the leukocyte count ranges from 15,000 to 30,000 per microliter or higher, and 80% of the cells are small lymphocytes. Polymorphonuclear leukocytosis suggests a secondary bacterial complication.

Microbiologic identification of the organisms may be required to make the diagnosis in abortive or mild cases or in young infants. During the early stages, *B. pertussis* can be isolated from approximately 90% of patients. By the third or fourth week, the organism can be recovered in only 50% of cases, and in the convalescent stage it is unusual to obtain a positive culture.

Specimens for culture are best obtained by pernasal swab rather than by the cough plate method. A sterile cotton swab wrapped about a flexible copper wire is passed through the nares, and mucus is obtained from the posterior pharynx. *B. pertussis* is readily killed by desiccation, so the specimen should be quickly plated onto fresh medium, to which antibiotic has been added to prevent overgrowth of adventitious organisms.

A fluorescent antibody staining procedure can be applied directly to clinical specimens or organisms grown in culture, but false-positive and false-negative results are relatively common. Probes for *B. pertussis* DNA are available.

Serologic procedures are of little help in diagnosing whooping cough because a rise in titer of most antibodies does not occur until at least the third week of illness. Tests have not been well standardized.

TREATMENT. *Supportive Therapy.* Young infants, particularly those younger than 6 months of age, should be hospitalized. Supportive measures combined with careful nursing care are of paramount importance. Specific attention must be devoted to the maintenance of proper water and electrolyte balance, adequate nutrition, and sufficient oxygenation. Constant alertness for the presence of secondary infectious complications such as pneumonia is required. Mild cases require only supportive treatment.

Antimicrobials. Specific therapy of severe whooping cough has been disappointing despite the *in vitro* susceptibility of *B. pertussis* to various antimicrobial agents. Antimicrobials given in the catarrhal stage may ameliorate the disease. In the established paroxysmal stage, the organisms can be readily eliminated by antimicrobials, but the course of the illness is unaltered. Antibiotics may be justified in order to render the patient noninfectious. Erythromycin is the drug of choice. The daily dose is 50 mg per kilogram of body weight given in four divided doses. The organism is eliminated after a few days of therapy, but because bacteriologic relapse may occur, treatment should be continued for 14 days. Trimethoprim-sulfamethoxazole (8 mg per kilogram and 40 mg per kilogram per day in two doses) is a possible alternative for patients who do not tolerate erythromycin.

PREVENTION. Unfortunately, the diagnosis is usually not made until the end of the catarrhal stage, and by then, spread of the disease has already occurred. Exposed susceptibles should receive erythromycin prophylaxis for 14 days, and close (household, day care, classroom) contacts younger than 7 who have been previously immunized should receive a booster dose of vaccine in addition to erythromycin. Booster doses of vaccine or erythromycin chemoprophylaxis have been used to protect adults, such as hospital staff.

Active Immunization. Women of childbearing age generally do not have significant levels of protective antibody in their sera, and most newborns have received no passive protection. Consequently, active immunization is begun as early as is practicable. At present, it is recommended that the infant receive three injections of pertussis vaccine (inactive *B. pertussis* organisms) at 8-week intervals commencing at age 2 months. The pertussis suspension is mixed with alum-precipitated diphtheria and tetanus toxoids (DTP). A fourth injection is given 6 to 12 months after the third dose (15 to 18 months of age), and a booster is given before entering kindergarten. Administration of pertussis vaccine to those over age 6 is not generally recommended.

As previously noted, immunization does not confer lifelong protection. Approximately 80% of those vaccinated within 4 years of exposure are protected, whereas 80 to 90% of a matched unimmunized group with similar exposure contract pertussis. The prophylactic efficacy of pertussis vaccine was clearly demonstrated when epidemics occurred in the United Kingdom in 1977–79 and

1982 following a 3- to 5-year period during which vaccine acceptance had declined to very low levels. More than 170,000 cases of whooping cough were reported, including 42 deaths, principally among children under age 5. Similar outbreaks have followed diminished vaccine utilization in Japan and Sweden.

Reactions at the injection site as well as fever and hyperirritability occur commonly after injection of whole-cell pertussis vaccine. The incidence of postinjection acute encephalopathy is uncertain but apparently rare, and it is not clear whether administering DTP vaccine increases the overall risk in children of chronic nervous system dysfunction. It is clear that the risk of neurologic complications from pertussis immunization is far less than the hazards of whooping cough in the young child. Nevertheless, in infants with a personal history of convulsions or other neurologic disorders, pertussis immunization should be deferred until the condition has stabilized.

Acellular vaccines containing various combinations of pertussis toxin, pertactin, filamentous hemagglutinin, or other *B. pertussis* products are being studied for use in infants and adults, and one has been approved for the fourth and fifth injections. Acellular vaccines cause far fewer reactions than does the whole bacterial cell vaccine. If tests currently under way of their immunogenicity and prophylactic efficacy are convincing in field use, acellular vaccines should replace the killed whole-cell vaccine.

Edwards KM, Decker MD, Graham BS, et al.: Adult immunization with acellular pertussis vaccine. JAMA 269:53, 1993. *A report of the immunogenicity and safety of the new vaccine in adults.*

Gale JL, Thapa PB, Wassilak SGF, et al.: Risk of serious acute neurological illness after immunization with diphtheria-tetanus-pertussis vaccine. JAMA 271:37, 1994. *A careful (and unrevealing) population-based case-control study. Accompanying editorial on page 68.*

Howson CP, Howe CJ, Fineberg HV (eds.): Adverse Effects of Pertussis and Rubella Vaccines. Washington, National Academy Press, 1991. *A scientific, fully referenced review by the Institute of Medicine of DTP immunization and possible adverse events.*

Pittman M: The concept of pertussis as a toxin-mediated disease. Pediatr Infect Dis J 3:467, 1984. *A thorough, now classic review of pathogenesis, immunity, and immunization.*

Stratton KR, Howe CJ, Johnston RB Jr (eds.): DPT Vaccine and Chronic Nervous System Dysfunction: A new Analysis. Washington, National Academy Press, 1994. *A re-evaluation of this relationship by the Institute of Medicine.*

Diphtheria

285 DIPHTHERIA
Iain R. B. Hardy

Diphtheria is an acute communicable disease caused by *Corynebacterium diphtheriae.* The organism chiefly infects the respiratory tract, where it causes tonsillopharyngitis and/or laryngitis, classically with a pseudomembrane, and the skin, causing a variety of indolent lesions. If the infecting strain produces exotoxin, myocarditis and neuritis may ensue.

ETIOLOGY. *C. diphtheriae* is an aerobic, nonmotile, unencapsulated, nonsporulating, pleomorphic gram-positive bacillus. Its name comes from the Greek *korynee* ("club"), describing the shape of the organism on stained smears, and *diphtheria* ("leather hide"), for the characteristic adherent membrane. Both nontoxigenic and toxigenic strains exist. Toxigenicity is conferred when a nontoxigenic organism is infected by a β-phage carrying the gene for the toxin *(tox)*. *C. diphtheriae* has three biotypes, *gravis, mitis,* and *intermedius,* which are distinguished by colonial morphology and varying biochemical and hemolytic reactions. Strains may be distinguished for epidemiologic purposes by molecular techniques. There are a few reports of classic diphtheria, including toxic complications, due to infection with *C. ulcerans.*

EPIDEMIOLOGY. Humans are the only natural reservoir of *C. diphtheriae.* Spread occurs in close-contact settings via respiratory droplets or by direct contact with respiratory secretions or skin lesions. The organism survives for weeks on environmental surfaces and in dust, and fomite transmission may occur. Approximately one in seven individuals with nasopharyngeal infection develops clinical disease; asymptomatic carriers are important in transmission. Diphtheria immunization protects against disease but does not prevent carriage. In the prevaccine era, respiratory disease dominated in temperate climates, with a fall/winter peak in incidence, and most individuals developed natural immunity by adulthood. Cutaneous disease was primarily a problem in tropical countries, but over the last two decades, outbreaks of this form of diphtheria have occurred in the United States and Europe, typically among homeless and alcoholic inner-city adults.

Vaccination with diphtheria toxoid (formalin-treated toxin) was introduced in the 1920's and 1930's. Immunization of children in an era when the majority of older individuals had natural immunity resulted in a dramatic drop in diphtheria incidence and an even more rapid decline in the proportion of toxigenic strains isolated. This is believed to be because the selective advantage of the *tox* gene—promotion of greater replication and spread of the organism—is lost in the immune host. Currently in most Western countries, toxigenic *C. diphtheriae* has been virtually eliminated. In the United States, reported cases fell from 147,991 in 1920, to 15,536 in 1940, to a total of 40 cases from 1980–1993. Since 1988, all culture-confirmed cases have been caused by imported strains.

Vaccine-induced immunity to diphtheria wanes with time, and there is a growing cohort of individuals with no natural diphtheria immunity. Serosurveys indicate that 20 to 60% of adults in developed countries have antitoxin levels below 0.01 IU per milliliter, which is considered the lower limit of protection. As long as a high proportion of the population remains susceptible, the danger of reintroduction or re-emergence of toxigenic strains exists. Since 1990 there has been a major resurgence of diphtheria in several countries of the former Soviet Union. In Russia, the number of reported cases rose from 603 in 1989 to approximately 40,000 in 1994, with over two-thirds of cases among adults.

PATHOGENESIS. In classic diphtheria, *C. diphtheriae* colonizes the mucosal surface of the nasopharynx and multiplies locally without bloodstream invasion. Released toxin causes local tissue necrosis, and a tough, adherent pseudomembrane forms, composed of a mixture of fibrin, dead cells, and bacteria. The membrane usually begins on the tonsils or posterior pharynx. In more severe cases it spreads, extending progressively over the pharyngeal wall, fauces, soft palate, and into the larynx, which may result in respiratory obstruction. Toxin entering the bloodstream causes tissue damage at distant sites, particularly the heart (myocarditis), nerves (demyelination), and kidney (tubular necrosis). Nontoxigenic strains may cause mild local respiratory disease, sometimes including a membrane.

Diphtheria toxin is an extremely potent inhibitor of protein synthesis, with an estimated human lethal dose of 0.1 μg per kilogram of body weight. The extent of toxin absorption varies with site of infection, being much less from skin or nose than from the pharynx.

CLINICAL MANIFESTATIONS. *Respiratory Diphtheria.* Infection limited to the anterior nares manifests as a chronic serosanguineous or seropurulent discharge without fever or significant toxicity. A whitish membrane may be observed on the septum. The faucial (pharyngeal) form is most common. After an incubation period of from 1 to 7 days, the illness begins with a sore throat, malaise, and mild to moderate fever. There is initial mild pharyngeal erythema, usually followed by progressive formation of a whitish tonsilar exudate, which over 24 to 48 hours changes into a grayish membrane that is tightly adherent and bleeds on attempted removal. In more severe cases, the patient appears toxic, and the membrane is more extensive. Cervical adenopathy and soft-tissue edema may occur, resulting in the so-called bull neck and stridor. Laryngeal involvement, which may occur on its own or as a result of membrane extension from the nasopharynx, presents with hoarseness, stridor, and dyspnea.

The likelihood of toxic complications depends on the severity of disease at presentation and the interval between disease onset and administration of antitoxin. Myocarditis typically occurs between 1 and 2 weeks after the onset of respiratory symptoms and presents either suddenly or insidiously with signs of low cardiac output and congestive failure. Conduction disturbances, which may occur without other signs of myocarditis, include ST-T wave abnormalities, arrhythmias, and heart block. Neurologic impairment manifests as cranial nerve palsies and peripheral neuritis. Palatal and/or pharyngeal paralysis occurs during the acute phase; peripheral neuritis, symmetrical and predominantly motor, occurs from 2 to 12 weeks after disease onset. Motor deficit may range from minor proximal weakness to complete paralysis. Complete recovery is the rule. In fulminant, sometimes called "hypertoxic," diphtheria, toxic circulatory collapse with hemorrhagic features occurs.

In the United States, the diphtheria case-fatality rate has remained 5 to 10% over recent decades.

Cutaneous diphtheria lesions are classically indolent, deep, punched-out ulcers, which may have a grayish white membrane. However, the lesions may be indistinguishable from impetigo, or *C. diphtheriae* may infect chronic dermatoses, such as stasis dermatitis. There is frequently coinfection with *Streptococcus pyogenes* and/or *Staphylococcus aureus*. Toxic complications are rare.

Uncommonly, *C. diphtheriae*, both toxigenic and nontoxigenic, may cause *invasive disease*, including endocarditis, osteomyelitis, septic arthritis, and meningitis. Frequently, but not always, these patients have predisposing factors such as a prosthetic cardiac valve or underlying immunosuppression.

DIAGNOSIS. The decision to initiate therapy should be made on clinical grounds, since delayed treatment is associated with worse outcomes. A high index of suspicion is required. Cultures should be taken from beneath the membrane, from the nasopharynx, and from any suspicious skin lesions. Because special media are required, the laboratory should be alerted to the concern about diphtheria. *C. diphtheriae* is best isolated on selective media that inhibit the growth of other nasopharyngeal organisms; generally one containing potassium tellurite is used. Based on colonial morphology and Gram stain appearance, a presumptive diagnosis may be possible within 18 to 24 hours. Cultures may be negative if the patient received previous antibiotics. Toxigenicity testing should be performed on all *C. diphtheriae* isolates. Because both nontoxigenic and toxigenic strains may be isolated from the same patient, more than one colony should be tested. Traditional methods include guinea pig inoculation and the Elek test, where the isolate and appropriate controls are streaked on a culture plate in which a filter strip soaked with antitoxin has been embedded; toxin production is confirmed by an immunoprecipitation line in the agar. A recently developed polymerase chain reaction (PCR) test may allow both detection of the organism and determination of toxigenicity.

The differential diagnosis includes streptococcal and viral tonsillopharyngitis, infectious mononucleosis, Vincent's angina, candidiasis, and acute epiglottitis. A history of travel to a region with endemic diphtheria or of contact with a recent immigrant from such an area increases the possibility of diphtheria, as does a pre-antitoxin treatment serum antitoxin level of < 0.01 IU per milliliter.

TREATMENT AND PREVENTION. Treatment goals are to neutralize toxin, eliminate the infecting organism, provide supportive care, and prevent further transmission. The mainstay of therapy is equine diphtheria antitoxin. Because only unbound toxin can be neutralized, treatment should commence as soon as the diagnosis is suspected. A single dose is given, ranging in quantity from 20,000 units for localized tonsillar diphtheria up to 100,000 units for extensive disease with severe toxicity. Antitoxin may be given intramuscularly or intravenously; particularly for more severe cases, the intravenous route is preferred. Tests for sensitivity to antitoxin should be performed before administering it and desensitization performed if necessary. Antibiotic therapy, by eliminating the organism, halts toxin production, limits local infection, and prevents transmission. Parenteral penicillin (4 to 6 million units per day) and erythromycin (40 mg per kilogram per day in 4 divided doses; maximum, 2 grams per day, usually orally if the patient can swallow) are the drugs of choice. General supportive care includes ensuring a secure airway, electrocardiographic monitoring for evidence of myocarditis, treating heart failure and arrhythmias, and preventing secondary complications of neurologic impairment such as aspiration pneumonia. The patient should be in strict isolation until follow-up cultures are negative. Convalescing patients should receive diphtheria toxoid.

The local health department must be notified. Close contacts should be cultured and commenced on prophylactic antibiotics. A positive culture in a contact may confirm the diagnosis if the patient is culture-negative. All contacts without full primary immunization and a booster within the preceding 5 years should receive diphtheria toxoid.

Immunization with diphtheria toxoid is the only effective means of prevention. The primary series is four doses of diphtheria toxoid (given with tetanus toxoid and pertussis vaccine) at 2, 4, 6, and 12 to 18 months; a booster is given at ages 4 to 6 years. Thereafter, Td (tetanus and diphtheria toxoid for adults) boosters should be given every 10 years, from the fifteenth birthday.

Dixon JMS, Noble WC, Smith GR: Diphtheria; other corynebacterial and coryneform infections. *In* Topley WWC, Parker MT, Collier L, et al. (eds.): Topley and Wilson's Principles of Bacteriology. 8th ed. Philadelphia, BC Becker, 1990, pp 56–75. *A useful review with especially comprehensive epidemiologic data.*

Farizo KM, Strebel PS, Chen RT, et al.: Fatal respiratory disease due to *Corynebacterium diphtheriae:* Case report and review of guidelines for management, investigation, and control. Clin Infect Dis 16:59, 1993. *Includes latest recommendations of the United States Centers for Disease Control and Prevention for case and contact management.*

Harnisch JP, Tronca E, Nolan CM, et al.: Diphtheria among alcoholic urban adults: A decade of experience in Seattle. Ann Intern Med 111:71, 1989. *Summary of last major outbreak of diphtheria in the United States.*

Pappenheimer AM: Diphtheria: Studies on the Biology of an Infectious Disease. The Harvey Lectures. New York, Academic Press, 1982, series 76, pp 45–73. *Detailed description of the cellular and molecular biology of diphtheria toxin.*

Clostridial Disease

286 CLOSTRIDIAL MYONECROSIS AND OTHER CLOSTRIDIAL DISEASES

Dennis L. Stevens

The genus *Clostridium* encompasses over 60 species of gram-positive anaerobic spore-forming rods that cause a variety of infections in humans and animals by virtue of a myriad of proteinaceous exotoxins (Table 286–1). *C. tetanii* and *C. botulinum* manifest specific clinical disease by elaborating single, but highly potent, toxins.

Though botulism is usually the result of ingestion of preformed toxin, tetanus requires the bacteria to proliferate at the site of penetrating injury (see Ch. 288 and 289). Frequently, signs of infection are not apparent even with lethal exotoxinemia. In contrast, other strains of clostridia, such as *C. perfringens* and *C. septicum,* cause aggressive necrotizing infections, attributable, in part, to bacterial proteases and cytotoxins.

CLOSTRIDIAL GAS GANGRENE

TYPES. Clostridial gas gangrene, or myonecrosis, occurs in three different settings. First, and most commonly, traumatic gas gangrene develops after deep, penetrating injury that compromises the blood supply (e.g., knife or gunshot wound, crush injury), creating an anaerobic environment ideal for clostridial proliferation. *C. perfringens* accounts for 80% of such infections. The remaining cases are caused by *C. septicum, C. novyii, C. histolyticum,*

TABLE 286–1. CLINICAL DISEASES CAUSED BY CLOSTRIDIA

Organism	Clinical Diagnosis	Clinical Features	Laboratory Features	Toxins
		Invasive Infections		
C. perfringens type a	Traumatic gas gangrene	Pain, necrotizing infection, renal impairment, shock	• Renal failure • ↑CPK • Gas in tissues	α toxin θ toxin
C. septicum	Spontaneous gas gangrene	Pain, necrotizing infection, bowel portal	• Renal failure • ↑CPK • Gas in tissues	α toxin
C. sordellii	Malignant edema	No pain, no fever, massive third spacing	• Leukomoid reaction • Hemoconcentration	?
C. tertium	Bacteremia in compromised hosts receiving antibiotics	Bacteremia, shock	• Positive blood cultures	?
		Gastrointestinal		
C. perfringens type a	Food poisoning	Nausea, vomiting, watery diarrhea	None	Enterotoxin
C. perfringens type c	Necrotizing enterocolitis	Bloody diarrhea, ruptured bowel	None	β toxin
C. septicum	Neutropenic enterocolitis, "typhlitis"	RLQ pain, abdominal distention	• Low white count	Unknown
C. difficile	Pseudomembranous colitis	Water, bloody diarrhea	• Stools positive for organism, toxin, blood and leukocytes	Toxin A Toxin B
		Neurologic		
C. tetanii	Tetanus	Spastic paralysis	None	Tetanospasmin
C. botulinum	Botulism	Flaccid paralysis	None	Botulinum toxin (A,B,E,F,G)

C. bifermentans, and *C. fallax.* Other conditions associated with traumatic gas gangrene are bowel and biliary tract surgery, criminal abortion, and retained placenta; prolonged rupture of the membranes; or intrauterine fetal demise or missed abortion in postpartum patients. Secondly, spontaneous or nontraumatic gas gangrene is most commonly caused by the more aerotolerant *C. septicum.* Lastly, recurrent gas gangrene caused by *C. perfringens* has been described in individuals with nonpenetrating injuries at sites of previous gas gangrene, where spores of *C. perfringens* remain quiescent in tissue for periods of 10 to 20 years and then germinate when minor trauma provides conditions suitable for growth.

TRAUMATIC GAS GANGRENE

CLINICAL MANIFESTATIONS. The first symptom is usually sudden and severe pain at the site of surgery or trauma. The mean incubation period is less than 24 hours but ranges from 6 to 8 hours to several days, probably depending on the degree of soil contamination or bowel spillage and degree of vascular compromise. The skin may appear pale initially but quickly changes to bronze and then purplish red and becomes tense and exquisitely tender. Bullae develop; they may be clear, red, blue, or purple. Gas present in tissue may be obvious by physical examination, soft tissue radiographs, or computed tomographic (CT) scan. Signs of systemic toxicity develop rapidly, including tachycardia, low-grade fever, and diaphoresis, followed by shock and multiorgan failure. Bacteremia occurs in 15% of patients and is usually associated with brisk hemolysis. Patients have been described with hematocrits of 0% for as long as 24 hours. Complications include jaundice, renal failure, hypotension, and liver necrosis. Renal failure is largely due to hemoglobinuria and myoglobinuria but complicated by acute tubular necrosis following hypotension. Renal tubular cells are likely directly affected by toxins, but this has not been proven.

DIAGNOSIS. Increasing pain at the site of prior injury or surgery, together with signs of systemic toxicity and gas in the tissue, supports the diagnosis. Definitive diagnosis rests on demonstrating large, gram-variable rods at the injury site. Note that although clostridia stain gram-positive when obtained from bacteriologic media, when visualized from infected tissues, they appear both gram-positive and gram-negative. Surgical exploration is essential and demonstrates muscle that does not bleed or contract when stimulated. Grossly, muscle tissue is edematous and may have a reddish blue to black coloration. Usually, necrotizing fasciitis and cutaneous necrosis are also present. Microscopic evaluation of biopsy material invariably demonstrates organisms among degenerating muscle bundles and, characteristically, an absence of acute inflammatory cells.

PATHOGENESIS. The initiating trauma introduces organisms (either vegetative forms or spores) into the deep tissues and produces an anaerobic niche with a sufficiently low redox potential and acid pH for optimal clostridial growth. Necrosis progresses within hours. At the junction of necrotic and normal tissues, no polymorphonuclear leukocytes (PMNL's) are present, yet pavementing of PMNL's is apparent within capillaries and in small arterioles and postcapillary venules, followed later in the course by leukostasis within larger vessels. Thus the histopathology of clostridial gas gangrene is completely opposite to that seen in soft tissue infections caused by organisms such as *Staphylococcus aureus,* in which an early luxuriant influx of PMNL's localizes the infection without adjacent tissue or vascular destruction.

Recent studies suggest that theta toxin, when elaborated in high concentrations at the site of infection, destroys host tissues and inflammatory cells. As the toxin diffuses into surrounding tissues or enters systemic circulation, it promotes dysregulated PMNL–endothelial cell adhesive interactions and primes leukocytes for increased respiratory burst activity. These actions lead to vascular leukostasis, endothelial cell injury, and regional tissue hypoxia. Such perfusion deficits expand the anaerobic environment and contribute to the rapidly advancing margins of tissue destruction that are characteristic of clostridial gangrene.

Shock associated with gas gangrene may be attributable, in part, to direct and indirect effects of toxins. Alpha toxin directly suppresses myocardial contractility *ex vivo* and may contribute to profound hypotension via a sudden reduction in cardiac output. Theta toxin contributes indirectly by inducing endogenous mediators that cause relaxation of blood vessel wall tension such as nitric oxide or the lipid autocoids, prostacyclin, or platelet-activating factor. Reduced vascular tone develops rapidly, and in order to maintain adequate tissue perfusion, a compensatory host response is required which either increases cardiac output or rapidly expands the intravascular blood volume. Patients with gram-negative sepsis markedly increase cardiac output; however, this may not be possible in *C. perfringens*–induced shock due to direct suppression of myocardial contractility by alpha toxin. The role of other endogenous mediators such as cytokines (e.g., tumor necrosis factor, interleukin-1, interleukin-6), as well as the potent endogenous vasodilator bradykinin, has not been elucidated.

TREATMENT. Penicillin, clindamycin, tetracycline, chloramphenicol, metronidazole, and a number of cephalosporins have excellent *in vitro* activity against *C. perfringens* and other clostridia.

No clinical trials have been conducted to compare the efficacy of these agents in humans. Experimental studies in mice suggest that clindamycin has the greatest efficacy and penicillin the least. Slightly greater survival was observed in animals receiving both clindamycin and penicillin; in contrast, antagonism was observed with penicillin plus metronidazole. Resistance of some strains to clindamycin suggests a combination of penicillin and clindamycin is warranted.

Aggressive surgical debridement is mandatory to improve survival and prevent complications. The use of hyperbaric oxygen (HBO) is controversial, though some nonrandomized studies have reported excellent results with HBO therapy when combined with antibiotics and surgical debridement. Experimental studies demonstrate slight benefit of HBO when combined with penicillin, though survivals were greater with clindamycin alone.

Therapeutic strategies directed against toxin expression *in vivo*, such as neutralization with specific antitoxin antibody or inhibiting toxin synthesis, may be valuable adjuncts to traditional antimicrobial regimens. Future strategies may target endogenous proadhesive molecules such that toxin-induced vascular leukostasis and resultant tissue injury are attenuated.

PROGNOSIS. Patients presenting with gas gangrene of an extremity have a better prognosis than those with truncal or intra-abdominal gas gangrene, largely because it is difficult to adequately debride such lesions. HBO could be useful in such patients, yet there are little data on this subject. In addition to truncal gangrene, patients with associated bacteremia and intravascular hemolysis have the greatest likelihood of progressing to shock and death.

PREVENTION. Aggressive debridement of devitalized tissue, as well as rapid repair of compromised vascular supply, greatly reduces the frequency of gas gangrene in contaminated deep wounds. Intramuscular epinephrine, prolonged application of tourniquets, and surgical closure of traumatic wounds should be avoided. Patients with contaminated wounds should receive prophylactic antibiotics.

SPONTANEOUS, NONTRAUMATIC GAS GANGRENE DUE TO *CLOSTRIDIUM SEPTICUM*

CLINICAL MANIFESTATIONS. The onset of disease is abrupt, often with excruciating pain, although the patient may sense only heaviness or numbness. The first symptom may be confusion or malaise. Extremely rapid progression of gangrene follows. Swelling advances, and blisters appear filled with clear, cloudy, hemorrhagic, or purplish fluid. The skin around such bullae also has a purple hue, perhaps reflecting vascular compromise resulting from bacterial toxins diffusing into surrounding tissues. Histopathology of muscle and connective tissues includes cell lysis and gas formation; inflammatory cells are remarkably absent.

Predisposing factors include colonic carcinoma, diverticulitis, gastrointestinal (GI) surgery, leukemia, lymphoproliferative disorders, and either chemotherapy or radiation therapy. Cyclic neutropenia is also associated with spontaneous gas gangrene due to *C. septicum,* and in such cases, necrotizing enterocolitis, cecitis, or distal ileitis are commonly found. These GI pathologies permit bacterial access to the bloodstream; consequently, the aerotolerant *C. septicum* can become established in normal tissues. Patients surviving bacteremia or spontaneous gangrene due to *C. septicum* should have appropriate diagnostic studies of the GI tract to rule out pathology in this area.

DIAGNOSIS. Unlike traumatic gas gangrene, bacteremia precedes cutaneous manifestations by several hours, causing delays in the appropriate diagnosis and, as a consequence, an increase in the mortality rate.

PATHOGENESIS. *C. septicum* produces four toxins—alpha toxin (α, lethal, hemolytic, necrotizing activity), beta toxin (β, DNase), gamma toxin (γ, hyaluronidase), and delta toxin (Δ, septicolysin, an oxygen-labile hemolysin)—as well as a protease and a neuraminidase. This alpha toxin does not possess phospholipase activity and is thus distinct from the alpha toxin of *C. perfringens.* Active immunization against alpha toxin significantly protects against challenge with viable *C. septicum.* The mechanism by which alpha toxin contributes to *C. septicum* pathogenesis is unknown; however, the recent cloning and sequencing of this toxin should facilitate studies in this area.

TREATMENT. Though no comparative human trials have evaluated the efficacy of antibiotics or HBO for treating clinical cases of spontaneous gas gangrene, *in vitro* data suggests that *C. septicum* is uniformly susceptible to penicillin, tetracycline, erythromycin, clindamycin, chloramphenicol, and metronidazole. The aerotolerance of *C. septicum* may reduce the efficacy of HBO therapy.

PROGNOSIS. The mortality of spontaneous clinical gangrene ranges from 67 to 100%, with the majority of deaths occurring within 24 hours of onset. Risk factors include underlying malignancy and compromised immune status.

OTHER CLOSTRIDIAL DISEASES

FOOD POISONING (ENTEROTOXEMIA) CAUSED BY *CLOSTRIDIUM PERFRINGENS* (see Ch. 109). *C. perfringens* accounts for nearly 20% of all reported cases of food poisoning. Ingesting large numbers of vegetative cells from inadequately prepared and stored food leads to multiplication and sporulation in the intestine. When mature spores are released, enterotoxin is liberated into the lumen of the GI tract. The alkaline environment of the proximal small intestine and the presence of trypsin (a pancreatic enzyme found in the gut lumen) cause a 2.5-fold increase in biologic activity of enterotoxin. Histologically, enterotoxin causes bleb formation and desquamation of the microvillus tips of the brush border. Physiologically, such cells are incapable of glucose and ion absorption. The net effect is loss of electrolytes and fluid across the brush border, with resultant diarrhea. Other symptoms that manifest 5 to 24 hours after ingesting contaminated food are nausea, vomiting, and abdominal cramping. The definitive diagnosis rests on demonstrating enterotoxin in stool samples. Reliable biologic tests, radioimmunoassays, and ELISA tests have been developed, though the ELISA is favored due its sensitivity, cost, and quick results.

NECROTIZING ENTERITIS. Neutropenic enterocolitis is a fulminant form of necrotizing enteritis that occurs in neutropenic patients. Neutropenia is often profound and may be related to cyclic neutropenia, leukemia, aplastic anemia, or chemotherapy. Symptoms include abdominal pain, chills, and malaise. Copious watery diarrhea, abdominal distention, and pain localizing to the right lower quadrant develop, followed rapidly by signs of toxicity, such as tachycardia, fever, and delirium. Radiographic examinations may reveal thickening of the wall of the colon or cecum and, in advanced cases, gas in the wall of the colon. Anecdotal reports suggest that CT scanning may be a superior means of diagnosing this condition. Complications include rupture of the bowel with peritonitis, bacteremia, and death in 100% of cases. Aggressive supportive measures, surgical intervention, and appropriate antibiotics (see section on Spontaneous Gas Gangrene) have reduced the mortality to 25%.

Postmortem examinations reveal that among children dying of leukemia, localized infection of the ileocecal region (typhilitis) is extremely common and may have contributed to death in nearly 40%. *C. septicum* is the most common organism isolated from the blood of such patients, and Gram stain and immunofluorescence studies demonstrate that these bacteria invade the bowel wall in most cases.

Other forms of necrotizing enteritis have occurred endemically in New Guinea (pigbel), in epidemic proportion in Germany following World War II (Darmbrand), and sporadically in Africa, Southeast Asia, and the United States. All cases are associated with ingesting meats contaminated with *C. perfringens* type c. Clinical courses vary between abdominal pain, fever, and diarrhea, which resolve spontaneously, to bloody diarrhea, ruptured bowel, and death. Beta toxin from *C. perfringens* type c has been implicated as causing these infections. Beta toxin paralyzes the intestinal villi and causes friability and necrosis of the bowel wall. Predisposing factors include malnutrition, specifically in those with diets low in protein and rich in trypsin inhibitors such as sweet potato or soy bean. In addition, *Ascaris lumbricoides* is found commonly in such patients, and it, too, secretes a trypsin inhibitor. These protease inhibitors protect beta toxin from intraluminal proteolysis.

Medical management should include aggressive fluid and electrolyte replacement, bowel decompression, and antibiotic treatment with penicillin or chloramphenicol. Surgical resection of necrotic bowel is necessary in 50% of patients, and mortality rates as high as 40% have been described. If peritonitis develops, broader antibiotic coverage may be necessary. Immunization of children in New Guinea with a beta toxoid vaccine has dramatically reduced the incidence of this disease.

C. SORDELLII INFECTION. Patients with *C. sordellii* infection present with unique clinical features including edema, absence of fever, leukemoid reaction, hemoconcentration, and later shock and multiorgan failure. Often *C. sordellii* infections develop after childbirth or after gynecologic procedures, though some cases involve sites of minor trauma such as lacerations. Unlike *C. perfringens* and *C. septicum* infections, pain may not be a prominent feature. The absence of fever and paucity of signs and symptoms of local infection make early diagnosis difficult. The mechanisms of diffuse capillary leak, massive edema, and hemoconcentration are not well established but clearly are related to elaboration of a potent toxin. Hematocrits of 75 to 80% have been described, and leukocytosis of 50 to 100,000 cells per cubic millimeter with a left shift is common.

C. TERTIUM INFECTIONS. *C. tertium* causes bacteremia in compromised hosts who have received long courses of antibiotics, thus explaining the organism's relative resistance to penicillin, cephalosporins, and clindamycin. *C. tertium* is, however, usually quite sensitive to chloramphenicol, vancomycin, and metronidazole. Because this organism can grow aerobically, it may be mistakenly disregarded as a contaminant such as a diphtheroid or bacillus species.

Farnell MB: Neutropenic enterocolitis: A surgical disease? Infect Surg 6(2):120, 1987. *Describes the clinical presentation of necrotizing lesions of the terminal ileum associated with neutropenic conditions; also describes the evidence that implicates* Clostridium septicum *as the cause of enterocolitis.*

Stevens DL, Bryant AE, Adams K, et al.: Evaluation of hyperbaric oxygen therapy for treatment of experimental *Clostridium perfringens* infection. Clin Infect Dis 17:231, 1993. *This study describes the efficacy of hyperbaric oxygen, alone and with various antibiotics, for treating experimental clostridial myonecrosis. In the same issue, editorials describe the pros and cons of hyperbaric oxygen treatment.*

Stevens DL, Laine BM, Mitten JE: Comparison of single and combination antimicrobial agents for prevention of experimental gas gangrene caused by *Clostridium perfringens.* Antimicrob Agents Chemother 31:312, 1987. *This study demonstrated superior efficacy of clindamycin alone and that neither synergy nor antagonism occurred when penicillin and clindamycin were both used to treat experimental clostridial myositis.*

Stevens DL, Musher DM, Watson DA, et al.: Spontaneous, nontraumatic gangrene due to *Clostridium septicum.* Rev Infect Dis 12(2):286, 1990. *A review article concerning clinical features of spontaneous gas gangrene (complete with color plates).*

Weinstein L, Barza M: Gas gangrene. N Engl J Med 289:1129, 1972. *A review of clinical features and management recommendations for gas gangrene.*

287 PSEUDOMEMBRANOUS COLITIS
Robert Fekety

DESCRIPTION. Pseudomembranous colitis (PMC) is a toxin-induced inflammatory process characterized by exudative plaques or pseudomembranes attached to the surface of the inflamed colonic mucosa. The disease is often referred to as "antibiotic-associated colitis" (AAC) because many patients who develop the disease after using antimicrobials have no grossly visible pseudomembranes but on biopsy have microscopically visible pseudomembranes.

ETIOLOGY. Although most patients with PMC develop it as a complication of antimicrobial therapy, the disease was recognized in the preantibiotic era. The etiologic agent in nearly all instances is *Clostridium difficile,* and the disease is caused by elaboration of two or more toxins during growth of *C. difficile.* Growth of the organism is promoted by poorly understood antibiotic-induced alterations in the normal intestinal flora. PMC is usually found in association with one or more underlying medical and surgical diseases, especially those involving the abdomen and requiring antibiotic therapy, although occasionally it occurs in healthy persons.

INCIDENCE AND EPIDEMIOLOGY. The disease occurs at all ages. The incidence of PMC depends on the frequency with which endoscopy and toxin tests on stools are performed to establish the diagnosis, on patterns of antimicrobial use, on antibiotic resistance patterns of the *C. difficile* isolates, and on epidemiologic factors favoring transmission of the organism. Nearly all antimicrobials have been implicated in PMC, but the most frequent are ampicillin, clindamycin, and the cephalosporins. Less frequent are penicillins other than ampicillin, erythromycin, aminoglycosides, and sulfamethoxazole-trimethoprim. *C. difficile*–induced colitis occurs both sporadically in hospitals and communities and in clusters within institutions. Studies indicate that *C. difficile* may be detected in the colonic flora of 3 to 5% of healthy adults and that it is widely distributed in our environment, including soil and water. It is especially common in hospitals and nursing homes, where as many as 20 to 30% of patients who have received antibiotics may be asymptomatic carriers and where spread of the organism from patients who have colitis to others treated with antibiotics is likely to occur. Spread from patients who are healthy carriers or who have colitis seems most often the result of transmission via the hands of hospital personnel, although transmission by directly contacting contaminated surfaces or objects also can occur.

MECHANISM. *C. difficile*–induced colitis is a toxin-mediated disease in which there is attachment of one or more toxins to the colonic mucosa but rarely any invasion of it by the organism. Toxin A (an enterotoxin) appears to be responsible for most of the features of the disease, while toxin B, a cytotoxin detectable in cell cultures that does not attach to the intact mucosa, may cause additional damage in severe cases. About 75% of *C. difficile* isolates produce both toxins. Isolates that do not produce toxins do not cause colitis or diarrhea.

CLINICAL MANIFESTATIONS. The disease may begin as early as 1 day after antibiotic therapy is started or as late as 6 weeks after it is discontinued. The most frequent symptoms are profuse watery diarrhea and cramping abdominal pain. Most patients also have fever (while usually low grade, it may exceed 40° C). Leukoytosis as high as 50,000 per cubic millimeter is common. In some patients, fever and leukocytosis are the *only* early clues to the disease, and diarrhea may not begin until several days later. Other findings include marked lower abdominal tenderness, hypoalbuminemia, and edema. Mild colitis is much more common than severe colitis, and many patients simply have annoying watery diarrhea resembling that seen in benign antibiotic diarrheal states. Complications in severe cases include dehydration, anasarca, electrolyte disturbances, toxic megacolon, and colonic perforation. Unusual manifestations include reactive arthritis and the development of diarrhea and enterocolitis in very young children with Hirschsprung's disease. Colitis occasionally presents with fever, leukocytosis, and marked pain and tenderness *without* diarrhea, especially after use of opiates for postoperative pain. Symptoms may begin during the course of antimicrobial treatment, but in as many as 20% of patients, they may not begin until up to 6 weeks *after* therapy is discontinued. The differential diagnosis includes acute and chronic diarrhea caused by other enteric pathogens, an adverse reaction to medications other than antibiotics, idiopathic inflammatory bowel diseases, and intra-abdominal sepsis. Diarrhea beginning 3 or more days *after* admission to the hospital is not likely to be caused by enteropathogens other than *C. difficile.*

DIAGNOSIS. The role of various studies in the diagnosis of AAC is summarized in Table 287–1. The best and most rapid way to establish the diagnosis of PMC is by endoscopy.

The "gold standard" laboratory test for establishing the diagnosis and etiology of *C. difficile* colitis is still the demonstration in filtrates of diarrheal stools, a cytopathic effect (CPE) caused by toxin B that is neutralized by antitoxin. Computed tomography (CT) may be useful in detecting evidence of PMC, especially in patients presenting with an acute abdominal syndrome without diarrhea or in early detection of complications of PMC (Figs. 287–1 and 287–2).

TREATMENT. Discontinuing all antimicrobial agents is desirable, although not essential if specific antibiotic therapy for PMC is given. Discontinuing antibiotics and replacing fluid and electrolyte losses may resolve symptoms without further specific therapy, particularly if the patient has "simple" diarrhea without colitis. Patients with severe symptoms should have stool examinations performed to implicate *C. difficile* toxins and also should promptly receive specific therapy for colitis. Antiperistaltic drugs are best avoided because they may cause worsening of the illness, even though they usually do not.

Specific therapy with metronidazole or vancomycin is usually given for about 7 to 10 days, using antibiotics orally to prevent the organism from growing and producing toxins. Metronidazole given orally, 250 or 500 mg 4 times per day, is used for colitis of mild or

TABLE 287-1. DIAGNOSING *CLOSTRIDIUM DIFFICILE* COLITIS

Test	Comments
Laboratory Tests on Feces	
Test for fecal leukocytes	A simple screening test but sensitivity only 30 to 50%. *A positive test rules out benign or simple antibiotic diarrhea.*
Stool culture for *C. difficile*	Results delayed. *Not diagnostic,* since 10 to 25% of patients in hospitals may carry the organism, and only 75% of isolates produce toxins. May be used epidemiologically.
Tests for the presence of fecal toxins	
Cytopathic effect of toxin B in tissue cultures	*"Gold standard,"* but some cell lines are not as sensitive as others, so false-negatives may occur. Time consuming, expensive, and not widely available. Requires antitoxin neutralization for specificity.
Toxin A by ELISA	*Rapid, widely available, relatively inexpensive.* Sensitivity varies and may be only fair. If cut point is chosen to minimize false-negatives, false-positives become a problem.
Latex agglutination for *C. difficile*	Rapid and inexpensive. *Detects glutamic dehydrogenase* (neither a toxin nor specific for *C. difficile*). Many false-positives and false-negatives.
Counterelectrophoresis (antigen detection)	*Nonspecific.* Many false-positives and false-negatives.
Radiologic Studies	
Plain film of the abdomen	*Nonspecific* and useful only when colitis is far-advanced or complications such as toxic megacolon or perforation are present.
Barium enema	*Nonspecific* findings. May precipitate perforation or megacolon.
Computed tomography	Safe, but expensive, and not highly specific. *Can be useful,* especially when patients present with an acute abdomen without diarrhea. May demonstrate unsuspected PMC.
Radionuclide scans (indium) (labeled WBC)	May detect inflammation, but *doesn't diagnose etiology.*
Procedures	
Flexible sigmoidoscopy	*Most rapid way to make the diagnosis.* Expensive. Misses about 10% of cases (those with only minor or proximal colonic lesions). Biopsy of minor or nonspecific lesions increases yield.
Colonoscopy	Rapid and *most sensitive way to make the diagnosis.* Expensive and may be hazardous. Biopsy of minor or nonspecific lesions increases yield.

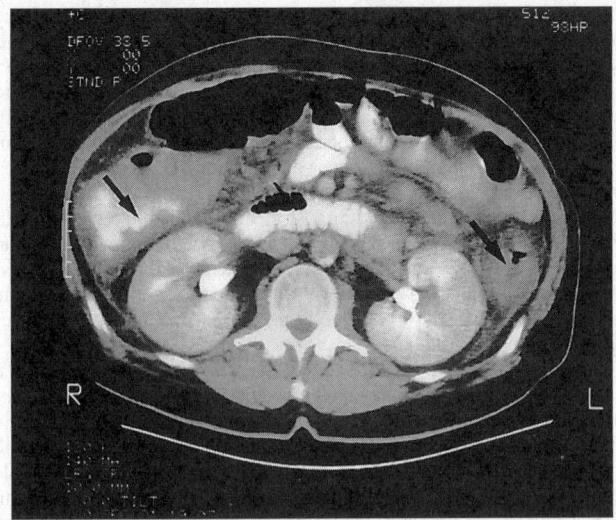

FIGURE 287-1. CT scan of abdomen of an elderly neurosurgical patient with fever and diarrhea postoperatively. Stools were positive for *C. difficile* cytotoxin. The arrow at left indicates irregularly thickened cecal mucosa; the arrow at right indicates lumenal narrowing, mucosal thickening, and edema of the descending colon. (From Fekety R: Infectious colitis. *In* Greenfield LJ et al [eds.]: Surgery: Scientific Principles and Practice. Philadelphia, JB Lippincott, 1992, p 1055.)

10 days) to bind the toxins of *C. difficile,* but they also bind vancomycin and teicoplanin. Oral bacitracin or teicoplanin has been an effective therapeutic alternate, but these drugs are not always readily available. Patients who cannot be treated orally or via a nasogastric tube should be given vancomycin in solution via a catheter passed to the cecum with a colonoscope, or via a long intestinal tube passed from above to the distal ileum, or via an ileostomy or colostomy, or if these are not possible, by colectomy. Therapy with intravenous metronidazole may be helpful in this setting, but is *not* reliable by itself.

Relapse or recurrence of colitis a few weeks or months after discontinuing antibiotic therapy occurs in 15 to 35% of successfully treated patients, whether the patient was treated with vancomycin or metronidazole. Attempts have been made recently to restore the normal fecal flora by giving live lactobacilli, mixtures of intestinal bacteria, or a live yeast (*Saccharomyces boulardii*) by mouth for a few weeks. *S. boulardii* reduced the frequency of relapses in a controlled study by about 50%, but it is not yet available in the United States.

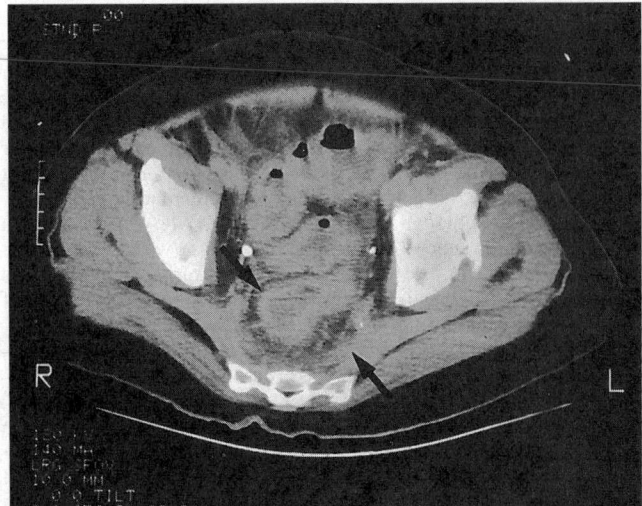

FIGURE 287-2. CT scan at another level of the patient with pseudomembranous colitis. The arrow at left points to thickening of the rectal mucosa; the arrow at right indicates edema and inflammation in the perirectal soft tissues. (From Fekety R: Infectious colitis. *In* Greenfield LJ et al [eds.]: Surgery: Scientific Principles and Practice. Philadelphia, JB Lippincott, 1992, p 1055.)

moderate severity but may produce side effects, and it should be noted that occasional isolates of *C. difficile* are resistant to metronidazole. The preferred treatment for seriously ill patients is vancomycin, 125 to 500 mg given orally 4 times per day for 7 to 14 days. Vancomycin is active against virtually all isolates of *C. difficile.* Major problems with vancomycin are its relatively high cost, bad taste, and unreliability when given intravenously to treat colitis. An alternative treatment uses anion exchange resins such as cholestyramine (4-gram packet given orally 3 times daily for 5 to

TABLE 287–2. PREVENTING *CLOSTRIDIUM DIFFICILE* COLITIS

General	Outbreak Setting
Prudent use of antibiotics (narrow spectrum, short courses)	Education about the disease
Washing hands between patients	Emphasize handwashing before and after each patient
Enteric isolation of cases: stool precautions, use of gloves	Use of gloves for handling positive patients
Oral prophylaxis with *S. boulardii* (future)	Patient cohorting
Immunization with *C. difficile* toxoids (future)	Treatment of fecal carriers with oral metronidazole, bacitracin, or vancomycin to reduce fecal shedding of *C. difficile.*
Toxin adsorbents: Cholestryramine, sucralfate (still experimental)	Disinfection of unit and fomites to kill spores and vegetative forms with 2% alkaline glutaraldehyde or hypochorite solutions (1600 ppm)
	Closure of unit (as a last resort)

PREVENTION. The most important preventive measures are careful handwashing or use of gloves after contact with patients who have the disease or who may be carriers of the organism and judicious use of antimicrobial agents (Table 287–2).

Barbut F, Kajzer C, Planas N, et al.: Comparison of three enzyme immunoassays, a cytotoxicity assay, and toxigenic culture for diagnosis of *Clostridium difficile*–associated diarrhea. J Clin Microbiol 31:963, 1993. *A good review of diagnostic laboratory tests.*

deLalla F, Nicolin R, Rinaldi E, et al.: Prospective study of oral teicoplanin versus oral vancomycin for therapy of pseudomembranous colitis and *Clostridium difficile*–associated diarrhea. Antimicrob Agents Chemother 36:2192, 1992. *Comparison of this alternate to treatment with vancomycin or metronidazole, which is available in Europe but not yet in the United States.*

Fekety R, Shah AB: Diagnosis and treatment of *Clostridium difficile* colitis. JAMA 269:71, 1993. *Reviews the disease and presents an algorithim for diagnosing and managing the disease and its complications.*

Gumerlock PH, Tang YJ, Weiss JB, Silva J Jr.: Specific detection of toxigenic strains of *Clostridium difficile* in stool specimens. J Clin Microbiol 31:507, 1993. *Describes the use of PCR in diagnosis, which may eventually be the best diagnostic laboratory test.*

Kelly CP, Pothoulakis C, Lamont JT: *Clostridium difficile* colitis. N Engl J Med 330:257, 1994. *A good recent review.*

McFarland LV, Surawicz CM, Greenberg RN, et al.: A randomized, placebo-controlled trial of *Saccharomyces boulardii* in combination with standard antibiotics for *Clostridium difficile* disease. JAMA 271:1913, 1994. *Shows relapse rate was reduced by half with the use of this yeast as an adjunct to specific therapy.*

Waler KJ, Gilliland SS, Vance-Bryan K, et al.: *Clostridium difficile* colonization in residents of long-term facilities: Prevalence and risk factors. J Am Geriatr Soc 41:940, 1993. *Reviews important epidemiologic aspects of the disease in nursing homes.*

288 BOTULISM
John G. Bartlett

DEFINITION. Botulism is a severe neuroparalytic disease caused by botulinal toxin produced by clostridial species, usually *Clostridium botulinum.* There are four recognized disease categories: (1) foodborne botulism, (2) infant botulism, (3) wound botulism, and (4) unclassified cases.

ETIOLOGY. *C. botulinum* is a gram-positive, spore-forming obligate anaerobe that is widely distributed in nature and frequently found in soil, marine environments, and agricultural products. Adults regularly ingest *C. botulinum* spores from fresh agricultural products without deleterious consequences, and this organism is not recognized as a component of the normal fecal flora. Each strain produces one of eight antigenically distinct toxins of approximately 150,000 daltons, designated A through H. Human disease is caused by types A, B, E, and rarely by F and G. *C. barati* and *C. butyricum* have been implicated in infant botulism with production of type F and E toxins, respectively. Botulinal toxins are hematogenously disseminated to peripheral cholinergic synapses, where they bind irreversibly and block acetylcholine release. The result is hypotonia with a descending symmetric flaccid paralysis. Botulinal toxin is the most potent poison in humans; it has an estimated lethal dose in the bloodstream of 10^{-9} mg per kilogram. Type A

botulinum toxin is now available for injection as treatment for ocular muscle disorders, such as strabismus and blepharospasm, and dystonias, such as torticollis and hemifacial spasm.

FOOD POISONING. Foodborne botulism results from the ingestion of preformed toxin in inadequately prepared food, although *C. botulinum* in the intestine may be responsible or may serve as a continuing source of toxin. There are an average of 15 "outbreaks" annually in the United States, most of which involve a single case. The most frequently implicated vehicle in the United States is home-canned foods, which usually have a putrefactive odor. Meat and meat products are more commonly responsible in Europe, and preserved fish is most frequent in Japan, Scandinavia, and Russia. Type A and B organisms predominate in the United States, type A west of the Mississippi River and type B in eastern states. Type E organisms are usually, but not exclusively, associated with an aquatic source in northern latitudes, where they are found in coastal waters, lakes, and intestines of fish that inhabit these areas.

CLINICAL MANIFESTATIONS. The incubation period is usually 18 to 36 hours but may be as short as 2 hours or as long as 8 days. Persons with the shortest incubation period usually have the most severe disease. The bulbar musculature is affected first, with resultant diplopia, difficulty in focusing to a near point, dysphonia, dysarthria, and dysphagia. Involvement of the cholinergic autonomic nervous system may cause decreased salivation with a dry mouth and sore throat, ileus, or urinary retention. Common gastrointestinal symptoms include nausea, vomiting, and abdominal pain. Neurologic examination shows lateral rectus muscle weakness (cranial nerve VI), ptosis, dilated pupils with sluggish reaction, decreased gag reflex, or medial rectus paresis. This is followed by descending involvement of the motor neurons to peripheral muscles, including the muscles of respiration. Some patients have only mild illness, whereas others have severe paralysis that may require intensive supportive care for weeks. Mentation remains clear, there is no fever, and neurologic dysfunction is bilateral but not necessarily symmetric. The principal causes of death are respiratory or bulbar paralysis and infectious complications during the period of supportive care.

DIAGNOSIS. The usual laboratory test in suspected cases is analysis of serum, stool, gastric contents, and/or food for botulinum toxin and analysis of stool and/or food for *C. botulinum.* The classic toxin test is a mouse assay in which specimens are injected intraperitoneally to demonstrate a lethal toxin that is neutralized by type-specific antitoxin. Alternative antigen assays, such as the enzyme-linked immunoassay, have been developed but are not widely available. Among patients with clinical evidence of botulism, the toxin is detected in sera from one third, the toxin is found in the stool from one third, and the organism is recovered in stool from 60%.

Botulism should be suspected in patients with acute flaccid paralysis, especially when there is bilateral sixth cranial nerve dysfunction, associated gastrointestinal symptoms, prior ingestion of possibly contaminated food, and typical symptoms in other persons who shared this food. The differential diagnosis includes myasthenia gravis, Guillain-Barré syndrome, tick paralysis, cerebrovascular accident involving branches of the basilar artery, trichinosis, the Eaton-Lambert syndrome, hypocalcemia, hypermagnesemia, organophosphate poisoning, atropine poisoning, paralytic poisoning caused by shellfish or puffer fish, and psychiatric syndromes. Electromyography using repetitive stimulation at 40 Hz or greater is useful in differentiating botulism from other neurologic syndromes. This shows a diminished amplitude of muscle action potentials with a single supramaximal stimulus and facilitation of action potentials using paired or repetitive stimuli. These findings do not appear until the patient develops peripheral muscle weakness and are most likely to be positive in an affected limb.

TREATMENT. Sudden respiratory arrest is the most important serious complication, so patients must be carefully observed with monitoring of vital capacity and liberal use of ventilatory support. Elimination of the toxin from the gastrointestinal tract may be facilitated using gastric lavage, cathartics, and enemas early in the course. Antitoxin is usually given irrespective of the duration of illness, since the toxin may persist in the blood for extended periods. Treatment is initiated using two vials of the trivalent antitoxin, each containing 7500 IU type A, 5500 IU type B, and 8500 IU type E antitoxin; one vial is given intravenously, one is given intramuscularly. The antitoxin is horse serum and is associated with a 9% incidence of acute (5%) or delayed (4%) hypersensitivity reactions; 2% had anaphylaxis. Efficacy of the antitoxin is most clearly established with type B and type E botulism. Other therapeutic considerations include guanidine hydrochloride (15 to 50 mg per kilogram daily) to enhance acetylcholine release, but efficacy has not been established. Some advocate penicillin to help eradicate *C. botulinum* from the intestine, since this represents a potential source of additional toxin.

PROGNOSIS. The case fatality rate for foodborne botulism has decreased from >60% to <10% due largely to improved management methods, especially for ventilatory support. Patients who survive generally have complete recovery.

PREVENTION. Foodborne botulism is caused by germination of spores in food with toxin produced by vegetative forms, although the toxin also may be produced *in vivo* by simultaneously ingesting spores. The disease may be prevented by destroying spores in the original food source, inhibiting germination, or destroying preformed toxin. Specific measures are as follows:

1. Destroying spores with heat or irradiation. Spores of types A and B may survive boiling for several hours, especially at high altitudes (such as in Colorado), where the boiling point may be substantially lower. These spores may be destroyed if kept at 120°C for 30 minutes using pressure cookers. Spores of type E are most heat-labile and are killed with heating at 80°C for 30 minutes.

2. Germination may be inhibited by reducing pH, refrigerating, freezing, drying, or adding salt, sugar, or other inhibitory substances such as sodium nitrite.

3. Inactivation of preformed toxin is accomplished by terminal heating for 20 minutes at 80°C or 10 minutes at 90°C.

INFANT BOTULISM. Infant botulism results from botulinal neurotoxin produced *in vivo* following colonization of the gastrointestinal tract in children ages 1 to 9 months. This is the most common form of botulism in the United States, with 30 to 80 reported cases annually. Spores of *C. botulinum* (but not the toxin) have been found in about 10% of honey supplies, which previously accounted for one third of cases. The disease spectrum varies considerably, including "failure to thrive," "the floppy baby syndrome" (the most commonly recognized form), and sudden infant death syndrome or "crib death." Common symptoms in the floppy baby syndrome include lethargy, diminished suck, constipation, weakness, feeble cry, and diminished spontaneous activity with loss of head control, followed by extensive flaccid paralysis. The diagnosis is established by recovering *C. botulinum* or its toxin in stool. The toxin has rarely been detected in the serum. Fecal carriage of the organism and the toxin may persist for weeks to months following clinical improvement and hospital discharge. The major therapeutic need is supportive care with special attention to nutrition and maintenance of respiratory function. The role of antitoxin, guanidine, and antibiotics in this form of botulism has not been established, and generally their use is not advised. The mortality rate for hospitalized patients given supportive care is only 2%.

WOUND BOTULISM. This is a rare form of botulism in which a traumatic wound is infected by *C. botulinum* with toxin production *in vivo*. Types A and B have been implicated, reflecting their presence in soil. Clinical features are identical to those of foodborne botulism except that the incubation period from the time of injury is 4 to 14 days and there is a paucity of gastrointestinal symptoms. The diagnosis is established by recovering *C. botulinum* from the wound or by detection of the toxin in serum. Management includes wound debridement and other treatments described for foodborne botulism except for bowel cleansing.

UNCLASSIFIED BOTULISM. This category includes persons over the age of 12 months who have typical symptoms and signs of botulism with no identifiable vehicle. It is possible that some cases result from production of toxin *in vivo* by organisms colonizing the intestine in a fashion comparable with the mechanism described for infant botulism.

SPECIAL NOTE. Physicians may contact the Centers for Disease Control and Prevention (CDC) for advice on management of patients with botulism at (404) 639-2206; to obtain botulinal antitoxin, the 24-hour CDC contact number is (404) 639-2888.

Arnon SS: Infant botulism: Anticipating the second decade. J Infect Dis 154:201, 1986. *An authoritative review of infant botulism based on the 10-year experience following its original report in 1976.*

Black RE, Gunn RA: Hypersensitivity reactions associated with botulinal antitoxin. Am J Med 69:567, 1980. *The authors review the CDC experience with 268 patients who received botulinal antitoxin.*

Chia JK, Clark JB, Ryan CA, et al.: Botulism in an adult associated with food-borne intestinal infection with *Clostridium botulinum*. N Engl J Med 315:239, 1986. *This is a case report of an adult with the infant form of botulism and an accompanying editorial that places this observation in perspective.*

Dowell VR Jr, McCroskey LM, Hathaway CL, et al.: Coproexamination for botulinal toxin and *Clostridium botulinum*. JAMA 238:1829, 1977. *Reviews methods to establish the diagnosis in foodborne botulism.*

Woodruff BA, Griffin PM, McCroskey LM, et al.: Clinical and laboratory comparison of botulism from toxin types A, B and E in the U.S., 1975–1988. J Infect Dis 166:1281, 1992. *This is a review of clinical and laboratory observations in 309 cases of botulism. Patients with type A appeared to have a more serious illness.*

289 TETANUS
John G. Bartlett

DEFINITION. Tetanus is a neurologic syndrome caused by a neurotoxin elaborated at the site of injury by *Clostridium tetani*.

ETIOLOGY. *C. tetani* is an anaerobic, gram-positive, slender, motile bacillus. The sporulated form has a characteristic drumstick or tennis racket shape with a terminal spore. The vegetative form produces tetanospasmin, a protein neurotoxin with a molecular weight of approximately 150,000. Tetanospasmin ranks with botulism toxin as the most potent known microbial toxin; 1 mg is capable of killing 50 to 70 million mice. The vegetative forms of *C. tetani* are highly susceptible to heat, disinfectants, and other adverse environmental conditions, but the spores are highly resistant and can survive in soil for months to years. Killing of spores requires boiling for at least 4 hours or autoclaving for 12 minutes at 121°C.

EPIDEMIOLOGY. *C. tetani* can be found in 20 to 65% of soil samples and in stool from a variety of animals, house dust, operating rooms, and contaminated heroin. Approximately 10% of humans harbor *C. tetani* in the colon.

Tetanus is most common in warm climates and in highly cultivated rural areas. The greatest problem is in economically deprived countries, owing to poor immunization standards and unhygienic practices. An example is the practice of dressing the umbilical stump with animal dung or "dusting powder," a local dried clay sold for cosmetic purposes, after childbirth by unimmunized mothers. It is estimated that the annual toll from neonatal tetanus in developing countries is 1 million. In the United States, the incidence of tetanus declined dramatically when tetanus toxoid became available. The national tetanus surveillance system showed a decrease from 560 reported cases in 1947 to 36 in 1993. Nearly all cases currently reported occur in inadequately immunized persons due to failure to comply with guidelines for primary childhood vaccination, for a reinforcing dose at 10-year intervals, or for postexposure prophylaxis (most did not seek medical attention for the injury). Of 117 patients with tetanus reported in 1989–90, 86 (74%) had an acute injury (44 had a puncture injury), 14 (12%) had chronic wounds (skin ulcers, abscesses, or gangrene), 5 (4%) were injection drug users, and 10 (9%) had no defined pre-existing condition. Most patients (58%) were over age 60, and 6% were younger than 20. This predilection for the disease in the elderly appears to reflect waning immunity associated with aging.

PATHOGENESIS. Clinical tetanus requires a source of the organism, local tissue conditions that promote toxin production, and immunologic naiveté. The spores are ubiquitous in the environment, and most cases reflect contamination from exogenous sources. Important factors at the site of injury are necrotic tissue, suppuration, and the presence of a foreign body. These are responsible for a reduction in the local oxidation-reduction potential (Eh), thus promoting reversion of spores to the vegetative forms that produce tetanospasmin. Tetanospasmin is taken up by the peripheral nerve terminals and carried intra-axonally within membrane-bound vesicles to spinal neurons at a transport rate of approximately 250 mm per day. Upon reaching the perikarya of the motor neurons, the toxin passes to the presynaptic terminals, where it blocks release of neurotransmitters, including glycine, which is the neurotransmitter used by group 1A inhibitory afferent motor neurons. Loss of the inhibitory influence results in unrestrained firing with sustained muscular contraction. The result with spinal cord neurons is rigidity. In severe cases there is also involvement of the sympathetic chain causing autonomic dysfunction.

CLINICAL FEATURES. Forms of tetanus include generalized, localized, cephalic, and neonatal. In the United States, these account for 87, 9, 3, and 1% of reported cases, respectively.

"Generalized tetanus" is the most common. The extent of the associated trauma varies and may be trivial and forgotten or a severe crush injury. The usual incubation period is 4 to 14 days, depending largely on the distance of the site of injury from the central nervous system. Trismus is the presenting complaint in 75% of cases. Other early features include irritability, restlessness, diaphoresis, and dysphagia with hydrophobia and drooling. Sustained trismus may result in a characteristic sardonic smile, or "risus sardonicus," and persistent spasm of the back musculature may cause opisthotonos. These early manifestations reflect involvement of the bulbar muscles and paraspinous muscles, possibly because they are innervated by the shortest axons. Waves of opisthotonos are highly characteristic of the disease. With progression, the extremities become involved in episodes characterized by painful flexion and adduction of the arms, clenched fists, and extension of the legs. Noise or tactile stimuli may precipitate spasms and generalized convulsions, although they occur spontaneously as well. Involvement of the autonomic nervous system may result in severe arrhythmias, oscillation in the blood pressure, profound diaphoresis, hyperthermia, rhabdomyolysis, laryngeal spasm, and urinary retention. In most cases the patient remains lucid. Complications include fractures from sustained contractions and convulsions, pulmonary emboli, bacterial infections, and dehydration.

"Localized tetanus" refers to involvement of the extremity with a contaminated wound and shows considerable variation and severity. In the more severe cases, there are intense, painful spasms that usually progress to generalized tetanus. Cases that remain localized have a good prognosis.

"Cephalic tetanus" generally follows a head injury or occurs with *C. tetani* infection of the middle ear. The clinical symptoms consist of isolated or combined dysfunction of the cranial motor nerves, most frequently the seventh cranial nerve. This may remain localized or progress to generalized tetanus. The incubation period is only 1 or 2 days, and the prognosis for survival is extremely poor.

"Tetanus neonatorum" refers to generalized tetanus resulting from *C. tetani* infection in neonates. This occurs primarily in underdeveloped countries where various contaminated materials are used to sever or dress the umbilical cord in newborn infants of unimmunized mothers. The usual incubation period following birth is 3 to 10 days, and it is sometimes referred to as "the disease of the seventh day," reflecting the average incubation period. The child typically shows irritability, facial grimacing, and severe spasms with touch. The mortality rate > 70%.

DIAGNOSIS. The diagnosis of tetanus is usually made clinically. The following is the case definition used by the Centers for Disease Control and Prevention (CDC): "Acute onset of hypotonia and/or painful muscular contractions (usually the muscles of the jaw and neck) and generalized muscle spasms without other apparent medical cause." *C. tetani* is infrequently recovered with cultures of the wound. A confirmed history of immunization or a serum antitoxin level of ≥ 0.01 units per milliliter makes tetanus unlikely. Spinal fluid analysis is entirely normal, and the electroencephalogram generally shows a sleep pattern. The differential diagnosis depends on the dominant clinical features and includes oculogyric crisis secondary to phenothiazine toxicity, meningitis, dental abscess, seizure disorder, subarachnoid hemorrhage, hypocalcemic or alkalotic tetany, alcohol withdrawal, and strychnine poisoning. Strychnine poisoning produces very similar symptoms but differs from tetanus in that patients usually recover rapidly following supportive care.

TREATMENT. *Surgery.* Debridement of any associated wound. (This may pose a problem in "skin poppers," who often have multiple possibly infected sites.)

Antibiotics. Penicillin G should be given parenterally in doses of 1 to 10 million units daily for 10 days; tetracycline, erythromycin, and chloramphenicol are alternative agents for penicillin-allergic patients.

Antitoxin. Human tetanus immunoglobulin (TIG) should be given as soon as possible to neutralize toxin that has not entered neurons. The dose is arbitrary but averages 3000 IU. It may be administered intramuscularly as split doses and by infiltration into the wound. Some authorities advocate intrathecal administration of 250 IU of TIG. Equine tetanus immune globulin (10,000 to 100,000 IU intravenously or intramuscularly) is equally effective, but the rate of reactions is high owing to the equine source. Epinephrine 1:1000 should be readily available for severe reactions. This preparation is far less expensive and is consequently used most extensively in underdeveloped countries.

Active Immunization. Natural infection does not result in detectable levels of circulating antibody, so a full course of immunization with tetanus toxoid in three doses should be given.

Muscle Spasms. Chlorpromazine (50 to 150 mg every 4 to 8 hours in adults), meprobamate (400 mg every 3 to 4 hours in adults*), or diazepam (2 to 20 mg intravenously every 2 to 8 hours) is given to control spasms and convulsions, and short-acting barbiturates are useful for sedation. Overuse of these agents may lead to hypoventilation. When muscle spasms are severe or interfere with ventilation, therapeutic paralysis should be introduced using pancuronium bromide or metocurine combined with mechanical ventilation.

Supportive Care. Trismus, dysphagia, laryngeal spasm, respiratory muscle spasm, and sedatives all contribute to the high frequency of pulmonary complications. Maintaining a patent airway is imperative, often with intubation followed by a tracheostomy. The patient may then be maintained with mechanical ventilation in conjunction with diazepam in intravenous doses titrated to relieve rigidity without excessive sedation.

Patients with dysphagia should be fed via a nasogastric tube. Fluid balance needs to be followed assiduously, since large losses may occur and may be difficult to measure owing to profuse sweating. Autonomic nervous system involvement may result in tachycardia and hypertension with high cardiac output and cardiac arrhythmias. α- and β-adrenergic blocking agents were used formerly, but β blockade was sometimes complicated by cardiac arrest. Other considerations with autonomic instability include morphine, epidural blockade, or magnesium sulfate infusions. Additional concerns are pulmonary emboli requiring anticoagulation, gastrointestinal bleeding that may be prevented with sucralfate, rhabdomyolysis with myoglobinuria and renal failure that may require dialysis, superimposed infections requiring judicious use of antibiotics, hyperthermia requiring a cooling blanket, and hypotension requiring pressor agents.

Prognosis. The overall mortality rate for generalized tetanus has decreased in the U.S. from 91% in 1947 to 24% for 1989–90. Important prognostic features are the form of tetanus, as described above, the incubation period, the "onset period" (the period from first clinical symptoms of tetanus to the first generalized spasm), patient's age, and severity of symptoms. Patients with mild disease have only trismus with or without minor and brief muscle spasms. Moderate disease is characterized by trismus, dysphagia, rigidity, and intermittent muscle spasms. With severe tetanus there are generalized convulsions. Patients with moderate or severe generalized tetanus generally require 3 to 6 weeks for recovery. They may require intensive care during most of this time, but if they survive their recovery is usually complete. The highest mortality rates are at the extremes of age. The most frequent cause of death is pneumonia, but many patients have no obvious findings at autopsy, suggesting that death was directly due to the neurotoxin.

PREVENTION. Nearly all cases of tetanus occur in unimmunized or inadequately immunized individuals (see Ch. 10). The Immunization Practices Advisory Committee recommends active immunization of infants and children with DPT (diphtheria and tetanus toxoids and pertussis adsorbed) at 2 months, 4 months, 6 months, 15 months, and 4 to 6 years. Tetanus vaccination of school-age children is required in 47 states. Tetanus toxoid is a highly effective antigen, and protective levels of serum antitoxin in persons who complete the primary series persist for at least 10 years. Td (tetanus and diphtheria toxoids adsorbed for adult use) is

---

* May exceed manufacturer's recommended dosage.

TABLE 289–1. GUIDELINES FOR TETANUS PROPHYLAXIS IN WOUND MANAGEMENT

History of Adsorbed Tetanus Toxoid	Clean and Minor Wounds		Other Wounds*	
Number of Doses	Td†	TIG‡	Td†	TIG‡
Unknown or less than three	Yes§	No	Yes§	Yes
Three or more	Yes if over 10 years since last dose	No	Yes if over 5 years since last dose	No

* Included but not limited to wounds contaminated with dirt, feces, soil, saliva, puncture wounds; avulsions; and wounds resulting from missiles, crushing, burns, and frostbite.

† Td: Tetanus and diphtheria toxoids adsorbed. Children under 7 should receive DPT (diphtheria and tenanus toxoids are pertussis vaccine adsorbed). Too frequents booster doses of tenanus toxoid have been associated with hypersentivity reactions.

‡ TIG: Tetanus immune globulin in a dose of 250 to 500 IU intramuscularly. The usual dose is 250 IU. The usual prophylactic dose of equine tetanus immune globulin is 1500 t0 5000 IU intramuscularly. When tetanus toxoid is given concurrently there should be separate syringes and injection sites.

§ Unimmunized or incompletely immunized persons (1 or 2 doses of toxoid) should receive complete immunization with Td at times 0, 4–8 weeks later, amd 6–12 months later

recommended every 10 years at mid-decade ages (15 years, 25 years, 35 years). This is commonly neglected, as disclosed by surveys showing only 13% of persons older than 65 had received a dose of tetanus toxoid in the past 5 years and serosurveys showing 30 to 70% of older adults lack protective antibody levels. The recommended primary immunization series for unimmunized persons older than age 7 is Td at time 0, 4 to 8 weeks, 6 to 12 months after the second dose, and then every 10 years. About 90% of cases of tetanus in the U.S. involving patients with known vaccination status are in patients who failed to receive the primary immunization series. Immunized childbearing women confer protection on their infants through transplacental maternal antibody.

Preventing tetanus after injury requires managing wounds appropriately, assuring adequate immunity, and considering antibiotic prophylaxis. The aim of surgery is to eliminate necrotic tissue, purulent collections, and foreign bodies that promote the environmental conditions necessary for spore germination. Guidelines for immunoprophylaxis based on immunization status and wound characteristics are summarized in Table 289–1. Passive immunization is recommended only for "tetanus prone" wounds, preferably with TIG prepared from plasma of adults hyperimmunized with tetanus toxoid. The alternative is tetanus antitoxin equine prepared from hyperimmunized horses. The horse serum is associated with a high reaction rate, including pain at the injection site, serum sickness, and anaphylactic shock. Equine antitoxin also generates immune complexes that are rapidly excreted so that larger doses are required to produce sustained blood levels. The definition of "tetanus-prone" depends on the interval between injury and treatment, the degree of contamination, the extent of devitalized tissue or foreign bodies within the site of injury, and the depth of the injury. Antimicrobial agents such as penicillin, erythromycin, or metronidazole may be given to inhibit replication of the vegetative forms of *C. tetani*, but immunization and wound cleansing are considered more important so the use of antibiotics is generally dictated by other considerations.

Armitage P, Clifford R: Prognosis in tetanus: Use of data from therapeutic trials. J Infect Dis 138:1, 1978. *Data for 1385 patients with tetanus in India are reviewed to propose a prognostic classification.*

Bizzini B: Tetanus toxin. Microbiol Rev 43:224, 1979. *An extensive discussion of tetanus toxin.*

Centers for Disease Control and Prevention: Tetanus surveillance—United States, 1989–90. MMWR 41(55-8):1, 1991. *A review of the clinical experience with tetanus in the United States and the guidelines for tetanus prophylaxis.*

Dowell VR Jr: Botulism and tetanus: Selected epidemiologic and microbiologic aspects. Rev Infect Dis 6(suppl 1):202, 1984. *A review of the reported experience in the United States for these neurologic syndromes.*

Faust RA, Vickers OR, Cohn L Jr: Tetanus: 2,449 cases in 68 years at Charity Hospital. J Trauma 16:704, 1976. *The authors review a large clinical experience with tetanus in a United States hospital.*

Griffin JW: Local tetanus. Johns Hopkins Med J 149:84, 1981. *A good review of local tetanus and the pathophysiology of tetanospasmin.*

Olsen KM, Hiller FC: Management of tetanus. Clin Pharm 6:570, 1987. *A review of management guidelines with emphasis on the important role of benzodiazepines.*

Schofield F: Selective primary health care: Strategies for control of disease in the developing world XXII. Tetanus: A preventable problem. Rev Infect Dis 8:144, 1986. *The author reviews the tetanus problem in the developing world.*

Anaerobic Bacteria

290 DISEASES CAUSED BY NON–SPORE-FORMING ANAEROBIC BACTERIA

Ellie J. C. Goldstein

Anaerobic bacteria are the predominant indigenous, normal flora of the human body, including the skin and oral, gastrointestinal, and vaginal mucosa (Fig. 290–1; Table 290–1). Although these organisms perform beneficial functions, they are also consummate opportunistic pathogens and can cause serious and lethal infection, often in combination with aerobic bacteria. Their role in disease was first described 100 years ago and has been increasingly appreciated during recent decades. In almost all such infections, anaerobes are mixed with aerobes. Because the flora of these infections is often complex and culture results may be delayed, knowledge of the usual flora at the location of infection is an indispensable guide in selecting and instituting empirical antimicrobial therapy.

TAXONOMY

Anaerobic bacteria range from those that die with very brief exposure to oxygen and are usually isolated only in normal flora studies to those that can survive on the surface of a fresh agar plate even in the presence of atmospheric oxygen (e.g., *Bacteroides fragilis*). Most anaerobes require an environment with a low oxidation-reduction potential (eH gradient), which can be accomplished in association with low pH, tissue destruction, by-products from aerobic bacterial metabolism, or low oxygen content. Although not true anaerobes, some organisms such as microaerophilic streptococci and other capnophilic or hard-to-grow organisms are sometimes lumped together with anaerobes owing to their fastidious nature. Some genera such as *Lactobacillus* and *Actinomyces* contain both aerobic and anaerobic species.

Recent taxonomic advances have led to reclassification of many anaerobic species (Table 290–2). The term *"Bacteroides"* will ultimately be reserved for the 10 species of the *Bacteroides fragilis* group. What were previously considered "oral" *Bacteroides* and "pigmented" *Bacteroides* species have been reclassified as *Prevotella, Porphyromonas,* and other genera. Those that are capnophilic and not true anaerobes are often more related to *Campylobacter, Capnocytophaga,* and other genera. In addition, many new genera and several new species have been created to accommodate pathogens such as *Bilophila wadsworthia* and *Wolinella* species.

VIRULENCE FACTORS

Anaerobic bacteria possess a variety of virulence factors that differ among the species (Table 290–3).

DISEASES

BACTEREMIA. Transient anaerobic bacteremia occurs in approximately 85% of patients immediately after dental cleaning or

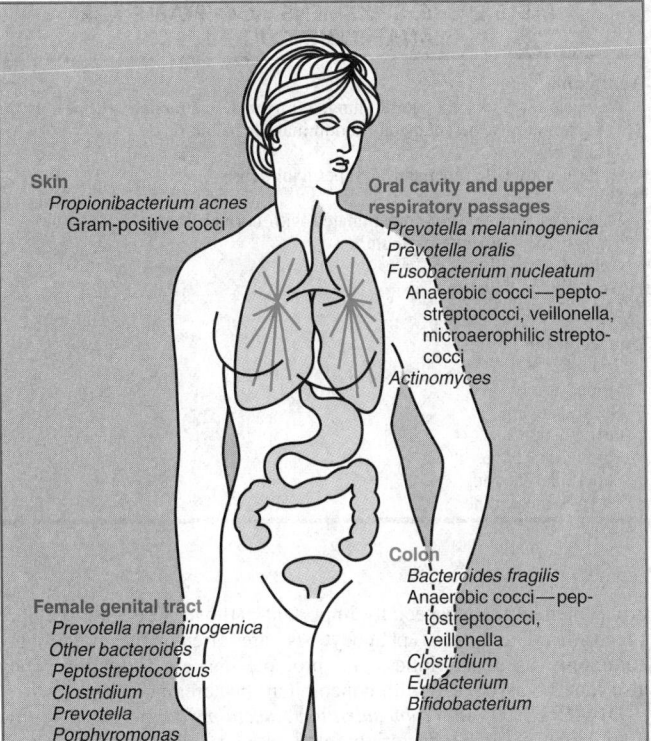

FIGURE 290–1. Anaerobes as predominant normal microflora of the human body by general anatomic location. (Adapted from Finegold SM, Sutter VL: Diagnosis and Management of Anaerobic Infections. Kalamazoo, MI, Upjohn, 1976. Copyright by Dr. Finegold.)

manipulation. More than 220 cases of endocarditis due to anaerobes have been reported and are usually associated with anatomic abnormalities or damaged valves. The majority of anaerobic bacteremias are intermittent and associated with serious intra-abdominal and female genital tract infections. Overall, it has been estimated that 10 to 20% of bacteremias are due to anaerobes, and in 80% of those anaerobes are the sole isolates.

HEAD AND NECK. Dental infections including periodontal disease, gingivitis, acute necrotizing ulcerative gingivitis, localized juvenile periodontitis, adult periodontitis, pericoronitis, endodontitis, dental abscess, and postextraction infection are associated with a variety of oral anaerobic bacteria.

Peritonsillar abscess is a deep-seated and potentially life-threatening complication of acute tonsillitis. It may extend into the various potential spaces of the neck or even the mediastinum and cause jugular vein thrombosis. Anaerobes may be isolated in >50% of such cases, usually in mixed culture with aerobes. Other regional infections include cervicofacial actinomycosis, Ludwig's angina, *Fusobacterium necrophorum* sepsis with metastatic infection (Lemiere's syndrome), and neck space infections. Whereas their

TABLE 290-1. LOCATION OF VARIOUS GROUPS OF NONSPORULATING ANAEROBES AS NORMAL MICROFLORA OF HUMANS

Organism	Skin	Oral/Respiratory	Gastrointestinal Tract	Genitourinary Tract
Actinomyces		+		
Bacteroides		+	+	
Eubacterium		+	+	
Fusobacterium		+	+	
Lactobacillus			+	+
Peptostreptococcus	+	+	+	+
Porphyromonas		+	+	
Prevotella		+	+	
Propionibacterium	+			
Veillonella		+	+	

TABLE 290-2. TAXONOMY OF ANAEROBIC BACTERIA

Current Name	Synonym/Comment
Bacteroides fragilis	⎫
Bacteroides caccae	⎪
Bacteroides distasonis	⎪
Bacteroides merdae	⎪
Bacteroides eggerthii	⎬ *B. fragilis* group
Bacteroides stercoris	⎪
Bacteroides ovatus	⎪
Bacteroides thetaiotaomicron	⎪
Bacteroides vulgatus	⎪
Bacteroides uniformis	⎭
Bacteroides gracilis	Probably new species
Bacteroides ureolyticus	Probably new species
Prevotella bivia	*Bacteroides bivius*
Prevotella buccae	*Bacteroides buccae (ruminicola)*
Prevotella denticola	*Bacteroides denticola*
Prevotella disiens	*Bacteroides disiens*
Prevotella intermedia	*Bacteroides intermedius*
Prevotella melaninogenica	*Bacteroides melaninogenicus*
Prevotella oralis	*Bacteroides oralis*
Prevotella oris	*Bacteroides oris*
Porphyromonas asacharolytica	*Bacteroides asaccharolyticus*
Porphyromonas gingivalis	*Bacteroides gingivalis*
Porphyromonas salivosa	*Bacteroides salivosus*
Fusobacterium nucleatum subspecies: nucleatum, polymorphum, fusiforme	New subspecies
Fusobacterium necrophorum	
Fusobacterium ulcerans	New species
Anaerobiospirillum succiniproducens	New species
Bilophila wadsworthia	New species
Peptostreptococcus	Now includes almost all prior *Peptococcus* species of medical importance
Actinomyces	
Eubacterium nodatum	New species

acute counterparts are usually infections due to aerobes, chronic sinusitis and chronic otitis media often involve anaerobic bacteria of the normal oral flora.

PULMONARY. Because anaerobic bacteria are the predominant normal flora of the oral cavity and upper respiratory tract and most pneumonias are due to aspiration of indigenous oral flora, it is not

TABLE 290-3. POTENTIAL VIRULENCE FACTORS IN VARIOUS ANAEROBES

Factor	Species
Adhesion	
Capsule	*B. fragilis* group
Pili/fimbriae	*B. fragilis* group, *P. gingivalis*
Hemagglutinin	*P. gingivalis*
Lectin	*F. nucleatum*
Invasion/tissue damage	
Proteases	*F. necrophorum*
	Bacteroides species
	Porphyromonas species
Hemolysins	Many species
Fibrinolysin	*B. fragilis* group
	Porphyromonas species
Heparinase	*B. fragilis* group
	Porphyromonas species
Neuraminidase	*B. fragilis* group
	Porphyromonas species
Antiphagocytic	
Capsule	*B. fragilis* group
	P. gingivalis
Lipopolysaccharide	*B. fragilis* group
	F. necrophorum, P. gingivalis
Metabolic products	Most anaerobes

Adapted from Duerden BI: Virulence factors in anaerobes. Clin Infect Dis 18 (suppl 4): 253, 1994.

TABLE 290-4. OBSTETRIC-GYNECOLOGIC INFECTIONS THAT COMMONLY INVOLVE ANAEROBES

Abscesses
Pelvic
Vulvovaginal
Vaginal cuff
Tubo-ovarian
Bartholin gland
Skenes gland
Endometritis
Myometritis
Parametritis
Pelvic cellulitis
Pelvic thrombophlebitis
Bacterial vaginosis
Salpingitis
Chorioamnionitis
IUD-associated infection
Pelvic actinomycosis
Postabortal sepsis

TABLE 290-6. SPECIMENS ACCEPTABLE FOR ANAEROBIC CULTURE

Acceptable
Any aspirate: abscess, joint, lung, empyema, suprapubic (urine), brain, myringotomy, percutaneous abdominal, or pelvic
Tissue biopsy
Cellulitis after debridement of superficial debris
Bile
Surgical specimen (not contaminated with normal flora)
Transtracheal aspirate of sputum
Culdocentesis fluid
Antral sinus puncture
Deep gingival pocket

Unacceptable
Sputum
Voided urine
Nasal discharge
Feces/diarrhea
Vaginal discharge
Superficial wounds
Mucous membrane

surprising that anaerobes are important pulmonary pathogens. They are involved in aspiration pneumonia (both community-acquired and nosocomial), necrotizing pneumonia, empyema, and lung abscess. Aspiration of oral flora may be a result of altered consciousness, dysphagia, or mechanical devices such as intubation. Poor oral hygiene is associated with an increased anaerobic bacterial burden, and the presence of aerobes or tissue necrosis leads to a lowered eH, which in turn facilitates the growth of anaerobes. In community-acquired aspiration pneumonias, anaerobes are involved in 90% of cases, and in many cases may be the sole pathogens. Anaerobes can be isolated in 35% of nosocomial aspiration pneumonias. If one forgets to treat a routine aspiration pneumonia for its anaerobic component, then one must remember the propensity for anaerobes to cause abscess.

Management involves good pulmonary toilet and antimicrobial therapy. Because of the increasing resistance of the "oral *Bacteroides* species" (*Prevotella/Porphyromonas* species), penicillin alone is no longer recommended. Alternatives include penicillin plus metronidazole, β-lactamase inhibitor combinations, second-generation cephalosporins such as cefoxitin and cefotetan, carbapenems, and clindamycin plus penicillin. In choosing coverage, one must also consider the microaerophilic streptococci and the aerobic gram-positive and locally prevalent gram-negative components of the oral flora. Nosocomial aspiration frequently is a mixture of all these components.

INTRA-ABDOMINAL. Because anaerobes outnumber aerobes by 1000:1 in the large intestine, they play an important role in almost all intra-abdominal infections. Most visceral abscesses (e.g., hepatic), chronic cholecystitis, perforated and gangrenous appendicitis, postoperative wound infections and abscesses, diverticulitis, and any infection associated with fecal contamination of the abdominal cavity involve both aerobes and anaerobes. *B. fragilis*

group members are especially important pathogens because they are encapsulated and resist phagocytosis, are often resistant to many commonly used antibiotics, and promote abscess formation. They also may be associated with concomitant bacteremia and sepsis.

DIARRHEA. *Anaerobiospirillum succiniproducens* is a motile gram-negative spiral bacterium with bipolar flagellae. It has been isolated from the feces of asymptomatic dogs and cats and has been transmitted from them to humans. It may also be associated with bacteremia.

Although *B. fragilis* is part of the normal intestinal flora, evidence incriminating enterotoxin-producing strains as a cause of diarrhea in animals and humans has mounted.

OBSTETRIC-GYNECOLOGIC. Table 290-4 lists the various obstetric-gynecologic diseases that involve anaerobes. Bacterial vaginosis has been linked to a perturbation of the normal anaerobic vaginal flora and accounts for 45% of all cases of vaginitis. It is present in approximately 20% of college women, and up to 45% of women attending STD clinics. It can be diagnosed by the presence of a foul, gelatinous vaginal discharge, a vaginal pH >4.5, the presence of "clue cells," and a fishy amine odor after 10% KOH is added to vaginal secretions. Bacterial vaginosis has also been associated with premature rupture of membranes, chorioamnionitis, postpartum endometritis, vaginal cuff cellulitis, and postabortal pelvic inflammatory disease (PID). Culture of tubo-ovarian abscess, a complication of chronic PID, grows anaerobes in up to 85% of cases.

SKIN AND SOFT TISSUE. *Diabetes.* The infected fetid foot is the most frequent infectious cause for diabetics to be hospitalized. The role of anaerobes in >50% of these infections is well established. When present, anaerobes are often associated with the more severe cases, especially with vascular insufficiency and tissue necrosis and those that ultimately require amputation. In addition, the presence of fever, longstanding wounds, crepitus, foul odor, abscess, or prior antimicrobial therapy more often involves anaerobes.

TABLE 290-5. CLUES TO THE PRESENCE OF ANAEROBIC INFECTION

Infection in proximity to a mucous membrane
Foul odor to a discharge or wound
Gas or crepitus in a tissue
Infection associated with necrotic tissue or malignancy
Bacteremia with associated jaundice
Gram stain morphology consistent with anaerobes
"Sulfur" granules (actinomycosis)
Infection following human or animal bite
Dental infection
Infection following abdominal or pelvic surgery
No growth on routine bacterial culture (especially if Gram stain shows organisms)
Fistulous tracts
Any abscess
Typical clinical picture of gas gangrene or necrotizing fasciitis

Adapted from Finegold SM: Anaerobic Bacteria in Human Disease. New York, Academic Press, 1977, p 42.

TABLE 290-7. GENERAL PRINCIPLES OF THERAPY FOR ANAEROBIC INFECTIONS

Elimination of dead space
Debridement
Drainage
Irrigation
Provide adequate circulation when possible
Remove foreign body
Antimicrobials
Activity against most likely pathogen(s): location-dependent, normal flora considered
Absorption, appropriate route of administration
Penetration into site of infection
Dosage appropriate for local tissue levels, body mass of patient, renal and liver function
Duration appropriate for condition
Susceptibility testing of isolate to guide specific therapy

TABLE 290–8. ANTIMICROBIAL SUSCEPTIBILITY PATTERNS FOR ANAEROBIC BACTERIA*

Bacteria	Drug						
	Penicillin	*β-Lactamase†*	*Cefoxitin*	*Cefotetan*	*Imipenem*	*Clindamycin*	*Metronidazole*
B. fragilis	−	+	+	+	+	v	+
B. thetaiotaomicron	−	+	v	v	+	v	+
B. fragilis group, other	−	+	v	v	+	v	+
Prevotella species	v	+	+	+	+	+	+
Fusobacterium nucleatum	v	+	+	+	+	+	+
Fusobacterium necrophorum	+	+	+	+	+	+	+
Porphyromonas species	+	+	+	+	+	+	+
Peptostreptococci	+	+	+	+	+	+	v
Propionibacterium acnes	+	+	+	+	+	+	−
Veillonella	+	+	+	+	+	+	+
Actinomyces	+	+	+	+	+	+	−

* Based on a variety of *in vitro* susceptibility studies from different laboratories and utilizing different techniques.
† β-lactamase inhibitor—β-lactam combinations, e.g., ticarcillin clavulanate, ampicillin/sulbactam, pipericillin/tazobactam.
+ = Susceptible.
− = Resistant.
v = Variable.

Bites. Anaerobes are present in approximately 35% of animal bite wound infections (see Ch. 325), especially those that are more severe or are associated with tissue necrosis or abscess formation. These anaerobes are part of the oral flora of the biting animal. Consequently, the routine bacteriology laboratory may have difficulty in identifying them. Most are penicillin/ampicillin susceptible. Besides anaerobes, *Pasteurella multocida*, *Staphylococcus intermedius*, *Staphylococcus aureus*, and streptococci should be considered potential pathogens.

Human bites, both occlusional injuries and clenched fist injuries, tend to be more serious than animal bites. Anaerobes can be isolated from 55% of human bite wounds and are more frequently β-lactamase–producing and penicillin-resistant. There is also a higher frequency of septic arthritis and osteomyelitis associated with human bite wounds. One must consider anaerobes plus *Eikenella corrodens*, streptococci, *S. aureus*, and *Haemophilus* species as potential pathogens when choosing empirical antimicrobial therapy.

Gangrenes. Gangrene indicates necrosis, most often of skin and subcutaneous tissue, and is often rapidly progressive. Several types of "infectious gangrene" have been described and may sometimes be indistinguishable on a clinical basis. These include the following:

1. *Gas gangrene*, which can incidentally involve other anaerobes besides *C. perfringens* and other clostridia.
2. *Progressive bacterial synergistic gangrene* often involves mi-croaerophilic streptococci and peptostreptococci as well as aerobic bacteria such as *S. aureus* and Enterobacteriaceae.
3. *Synergistic necrotizing cellulitis* involves a mixed aerobic and anaerobic bacteria including B. *fragilis* and peptostreptococci. Diabetic patients may be predisposed. The cellulitis is markedly painful, crepitus may be present, and the discharge has a foul odor.
4. *Fournier's gangrene* is a serious infection of the scrotum or perineum which starts with scrotal pain and erythema and rapidly progresses to necrosis and gangrene, which can lead to sloughing of tissue. It is more often seen in diabetics and can be associated with trauma.

PRINCIPLES OF DIAGNOSIS AND THERAPY

Clues as to when one should suspect anaerobic infection are listed in Table 290–5. Obtaining an appropriately collected and acceptable specimen (Table 290–6) must be an active process and specified in the orders.

General principles of therapy are listed in Table 290–7. In general, appropriate antimicrobial therapy coupled with prompt drainage and surgical debridement are essential for therapeutic success. Table 290–8 notes the susceptibility patterns of the various clinically important anaerobes.

Finegold SM, Goldstein EJC (eds.): Proceedings of the First North American Congress on Anaerobic Bacteria and Anaerobic Infections. Clin Infect Dis 16(suppl 4):159, 1993.
Finegold SM, Mulligan ME: Centennial Symposium on Anaerobes: A memorial to André Veillon, The Secret Pathogens. Clin Infect Dis 18(suppl 4):245, 1994.

Enteric Infections

291 INTRODUCTION TO ENTERIC INFECTIONS
Herbert L. DuPont

Enteric infections are second only to respiratory tract infections as common medical problems. In certain populations, enteric infections are hyperendemic: in poorly nourished children living in developing tropical countries where they are significant causes of pediatric mortality, in infants in day care centers, in residents of custodial institutions for the mentally retarded, in homosexual males, and in those who venture from industrialized to developing regions ("travelers' diarrhea").

In approaching a patient with an enteric infection, epidemiologic (Table 291–1) and clinical features (Table 291–2) are used to deter-mine the proper approach to evaluation and management. One must work through the various considerations to be certain that the proper differential diagnosis and workup are developed. Recent travel to a mountainous region of North America should raise the possibility of infection by *Giardia lamblia*. Travel to Russia, particularly St. Petersburg, is associated with an increased risk of infection by *Cryptosporidium parvum* and *G. lamblia*. When diarrhea occurs during or after travel to a developing tropical region, a bacterial enteropathogen should be suspected.

A specific food or water vehicle cannot be suspected unless multiple cases of illness with a common exposure occur. In this situation, the incubation period will often help determine the etiologic diagnosis: < 4 hours in the case of a *Staphylococcus aureus* or *Bacillus cereus* enterotoxin food poisoning or > 8 hours in the case of intestinal infection. On evaluation of the clinical expression of the illness (see Table 291–2), a tentative diagnosis may be made. In the patient who is receiving an antimicrobial drug, or who has recently completed a course of therapy, and presents with an enteric infection manifested by diarrhea with or without fever and dysenteric disease, *Clostridium difficile* should be suspected. When a per-

TABLE 291–1. EPIDEMIOLOGIC FEATURES IMPORTANT IN DETERMINING POTENTIAL CAUSES OF ENTERIC INFECTION

Epidemiologic Feature	Etiologic Agent to Suspect
Travel to mountainous areas of North America	*Giardia lamblia*
Travel to Russia (especially St. Petersburg)	*Cryptosporidium, G. lamblia*
Travel to the developing tropical/semitropical world from an industrialized region	Enterotoxigenic *Escherichia coli, Shigella, Salmonella* (including *S. typhi*), other bacterial causes, *G. lamblia,* and *Cryptosporidium*
Presence of associated cases (an outbreak)	Use incubation period and clinical features (Table 291–2) to determine probable cause
Antibiotic use in the last 2 weeks	*Clostridium difficile*
Contact with day care centers	Any enteropathogen, often *G. lamblia, Cryptosporidium, Shigella,* or rotavirus
Homosexual male with diarrhea	Any organism spread by fecal-oral route, with proctitis suspect *Neisseria gonorrhoea, Chlamydia trachomatis,* herpes simplex, or *Treponema pallidium,* with AIDS any agent, especially *Cryptosporidium, Microsporidium, Cyclospora, Salmonella, C. jejuni, C. difficile, Mycobacterium avium-intracellulare,* cytomegalovirus

son has close contact with an infant or infants attending a day care center, a number of pathogens found in this setting should be suspected. Finally, the homosexual male with an enteric infection may have acquired it through fecal-oral contamination so common in this setting (and in this case multiple pathogens may be found in stool), through receptive anal intercourse, or when intestinal immu-

TABLE 291–2. CLINICAL FEATURES OF ENTERIC INFECTION

Clinical Syndrome	Etiologic Agents Suspected	Special Considerations
Enteric or typhoid fever	*Salmonella typhi, S. enteritidis, Campylobacter, Shigella, Yersinia enterocolitica*	Blood cultures; antibiotics generally needed
Acute watery diarrhea	Any agent may be responsible. Consider: *Vibrio cholerae,* enterotoxigenic *Escherichia coli, Shigella, Salmonella, C. jejuni*	Fluid and electrolyte therapy crucial for recovery in dehydration
Gastroenteritis	Viral agents (rotavirus or small round viruses) or enterotoxin mediated disease *(Staphylococcus aureus* or *Bacillus cereus)*	In case of an outbreak, incubation period suggests the etiology
Dysentery	*Shigella, C. jejuni, Salmonella,* enterohemorrhagic (0157:H7) or enteroinvasive *E. coli, Aeromonas hydrophilia, Vibrio parahemolyticus, Yersinia enterocolitica, Entamoeba histolytica,* or inflammatory bowel disease	Stool culture and occasionally parasite exam important to determining cause; hemolytic uremic syndrome may complicate diarrheal disease caused by *E. coli* 0157:H7 or *S. dysenteriae* 1
Persistent diarrhea	*Giardia lamblia,* small bowel bacterial overgrowth, bacterial diarrhea, lactase deficiency, Brainerd diarrhea	Stool culture and parasite exam indicated; empiric anti-*Giardia* therapy may be useful; milk should not be consumed; a history of raw milk or untreated (well or surface) water consumption suggests Brainerd diarrhea

nity has become depressed as a result of the acquired immune deficiency syndrome (AIDS).

Enteric infection syndromes may be divided into five groups based on the clinical presentation, including febrile systemic disease (enteric fever), acute watery diarrhea (small bowel secretory process), profuse vomiting (gastroenteritis), the passage of many small-volume stools containing blood and mucus (dysenteric disease), and diarrhea lasting longer than 2 weeks (persistent diarrheal disease). Table 291–2 lists the major syndromes along with the expected etiology. In the majority of cases of enteric infection, it is not possible to determine the cause of illness on clinical grounds. Laboratory tests are often useful, particularly in the more severe or intensely ill patients, to help establish cause and to develop the proper plan of treatment.

Treatment of diarrhea should be tailored to clinical syndrome. Oral rehydration with fluids and electrolytes is used in acute watery diarrhea and gastroenteritis and in all forms of enteric infection when any degree of dehydration occurs. For enteric fever and dysenteric disease, antimicrobial therapy is indicated. For patients with persistent diarrhea, workup for cause is indicated before a management plan is developed.

292 TYPHOID FEVER
Thomas Butler

DEFINITION. Typhoid fever is a bacterial disease caused by *Salmonella typhi.* It is characterized by prolonged fever, abdominal pain, diarrhea, delirium, rose spots, and splenomegaly and complicated sometimes by intestinal bleeding and perforation. Enteric fever is synonymous with typhoid fever, which is occasionally caused also by *S. enteritidis* bioserotype paratyphi A or B.

ETIOLOGY. The typhoid bacillus is a motile gram-negative rod in the family Enterobacteriaceae. It possesses a flagellar (H) antigen, a cell wall (O) lipopolysaccharide antigen, and a polysaccharide virulence (Vi) antigen located in the cell capsule. The polysaccharide side chain of the O antigen confers serologic specificity to the organism and is essential in virulence because salmonellae other than *S. typhi* and *S. enteritidis* bioserotype paratyphi A or B do not produce enteric fever in humans.

INCIDENCE AND PREVALENCE. Typhoid fever has been almost eliminated from developed countries because of sewage and water treatment facilities but remains a common disease in developing countries. In 1980, the number of cases occurring yearly was estimated as about 7 million in Asia, over 4 million in Africa, and 0.5 million in Latin America. About 500 cases are diagnosed each year in the United States, and over half of these are in recently arrived travelers who contracted their infections abroad.

EPIDEMIOLOGY. Adults and children of all ages and both genders appear equally susceptible to infection. In developing countries, most cases occur in school-age children and young adults. Although acquired immunity provides some protection, reinfections have been documented. Typhoid fever occurs during all seasons.

Transmission is by the fecal-oral route through contaminated water or food. The main human sources of infection in the community are asymptomatic fecal carriers and cases during either disease or convalescence. Females and older males are prone to become chronic fecal carriers because underlying cholecystitis enables them to harbor chronic infection in the gallbladder. *S. typhi* is resistant to drying and cooling, thus allowing bacteria to survive prolonged periods in dried sewage, water, food, and ice.

Vi-phage typing of *S. typhi* is a useful epidemiologic tool to trace cases of typhoid fever to a carrier or food source. Single-source outbreaks of typhoid fever are rare. In endemic situations, multiple phage types are present, and several phage types may be responsible for an epidemic.

PATHOGENESIS AND PATHOLOGY. After *S. typhi* is ingested, the part of the inoculum that survives stomach acid enters the small intestine, where bacteria penetrate the mucosa and enter mononuclear phagocytes of ileal Peyer's patches and mesenteric lymph nodes. Inocula of at least 10^5 bacteria are necessary to initiate disease, and inocula of 10^7 and more cause disease regularly. The incubation period ranges from 8 to 28 days, depending on inoculum size and immune status of the host. Bacteria proliferate in mononuclear phagocytes and spread by way of the blood to the spleen, liver, and bone marrow, where further proliferation in macrophages occurs. The earliest symptoms of fever and chills (Table 292–1) are associated with bacteremia. Inflammatory reactions occur in the spleen, liver, bone marrow, Peyer's patches mainly in the terminal ileum, and skin, consisting of mononuclear cell infiltration, hyperplasia, and focal necrosis. Focal collections of mononuclear leukocytes are called "typhoid nodules." Fever and other constitutional symptoms are probably caused by the release of cytokines, including tumor necrosis factor and interleukin-1, from infected mononuclear phagocytes. Endotoxemia does not occur in typhoid fever. Intestinal manifestations are caused by hyperplasia of Peyer's patches with ulcerations of overlying mucosa, resulting in pain, diarrhea, bleeding, or perforation.

CLINICAL MANIFESTATIONS. In the first days of illness, the nonspecific symptoms of fever, chills, and headache are mild and in the typical case build up in intensity during the first week, resulting in prostration. The evolution of disease syndromes occurs stepwise over 1 to 3 weeks (Table 292–1) but may be variable in the time of appearance. The early symptoms of fever, abdominal pain, and prostration tend to persist throughout the illness, which in untreated cases lasts a month or longer. Abdominal pain occurs in more than half of patients and is frequently diffuse or located in the right lower quadrant over the terminal ileum. Diarrhea occurs in about a third of patients and consists of either watery stools or semisolid stools. Melena occurs less commonly. Rose spots occur in more than half of light-skinned individuals but are often not visible in dark-skinned patients. The rash is seen most commonly on the shoulders, thorax, and abdomen and rarely affects the extremities. The lesions are erythematous macules or papules about 1 to 5 mm in diameter which typically blanch with pressure but may become hemorrhagic. Many patients display abnormal behavior or altered mental status that may be out of proportion to the severity of the systemic illness. Among the common presentations are "toxic" staring, delirium, aphonia, and coma. Seizures are common in children. Patients are rarely jaundiced.

In about 5% of patients, intestinal bleeding or intestinal perforation occurs, usually after the second week of illness. Bleeding occurs from ileal ulcers and may present as melena or bright red blood in stools. Brisk bleeding develops rarely but is an occasional cause of death. Intestinal perforation presents as the sudden onset of more severe abdominal pain, distention, and tenderness. Bowel sounds are diminished, and the abdominal radiograph usually reveals free air. Perforation most often occurs unexpectedly after a few days of treatment when a patient has started to improve. Other complications of typhoid fever include pneumonia, which develops as a superinfection due to other bacteria, myocarditis, acute cholecystitis, and acute meningitis.

Relapses occur in about 10 to 20% of patients treated with chloramphenicol. Patients with relapses experience the reappearance of typical symptoms about 7 to 14 days after the end of treatment. Relapses tend to be less severe than the initial episode.

DIAGNOSIS. The preferred method of diagnosis is isolation of *S. typhi* from a blood culture, which is positive in most patients during the first 2 weeks of illness. Urine and stool cultures are positive less frequently but should be taken to increase the diagnostic

yield. The bone marrow culture is the most sensitive test, positive in nearly 90% of cases, and can be used when a bacteriologic diagnosis is crucially needed or in patients who have been pretreated with antibiotics. The duodenal string test to culture bile has also been used with success in typhoid fever.

The Widal test for agglutinating antibodies against the somatic (O) and flagellar (H) antigens of *S. typhi* is widely used for serodiagnosis. An O agglutinin titer of $\geq 1:80$ or a fourfold rise supports a diagnosis of typhoid fever, whereas the H agglutinins are more often nonspecifically elevated by immunization or previous infections with other bacteria. Serodiagnosis is of limited value because false-positive results are often obtained in endemic areas and false-negative results occur in some cases of bacteriologically proven typhoid fever.

Other laboratory findings are anemia of variable severity and a white blood cell count that is normal or decreased with an increased percentage of band forms. Platelets are often diminished, and signs of disseminated intravascular coagulation are present. Liver function tests frequently show elevated aminotransferases and bilirubin concentrations. Renal failure is an infrequent complication. In patients with diarrhea, the stool shows fecal leukocytes.

The differential diagnosis depends on infections that are endemic in the area where an individual contracted the infection. For returned travelers from developing countries, the common possibilities are malaria, hepatitis, typhus, amebic liver abscess, shigellosis, nontyphoid salmonellosis, and leptospirosis. In the United States one must consider septicemias originating from the urinary tract, gastrointestinal tract, or gallbladder as well as influenza, infectious mononucleosis, meningococcemia, miliary tuberculosis, and bacterial endocarditis.

TREATMENT. Chloramphenicol has remained the drug of choice since its introduction in 1948 because no other drug has been demonstrated to cause more rapid or consistent improvement of disease. Chloramphenicol is given orally in a dose of 50 to 60 mg per kilogram of body weight per day in four equal portions every 6 hours. After defervescence and clinical improvement the dosage can be reduced to 30 mg per kilogram per day to complete a 14-day course. In patients unable to take oral medication, the same dosage should be given intravenously until the patient can take capsules.

Alternative drugs should be considered when *S. typhi* resistant to chloramphenicol is isolated or strongly suspected. Several are nearly equal to chloramphenicol in efficacy. Trimethoprim-sulfamethoxazole is effective in a standard adult dose of 160 mg trimethoprim and 800 mg sulfamethoxazole given orally or intravenously twice a day for 14 days. Other drugs that are effective include ampicillin (intravenously), amoxicillin, cefoperazone, and ceftriaxone. In recent years, most isolates of *S. typhi* from cases in India and Pakistan have shown plasmid-mediated, multidrug resistance to chloramphenicol, ampicillin, and trimethoprim-sulfamethoxazole. These adults can be treated with ciprofloxacin, 750 mg twice daily for 7 to 14 days, or with other fluoroquinolones. Children with multidrug-resistant infections should receive ceftriaxone.

Patients who are dehydrated, anorectic, or suffering from diarrhea should receive intravenous saline with attention to electrolyte and acid-base disturbances. Patients with brisk intestinal bleeding require blood transfusion. Patients with suspected perforation should have an abdominal radiograph to look for free air and peritoneal

TABLE 292–1. EVOLUTION OF TYPICAL SYMPTOMS AND SIGNS OF TYPHOID FEVER

Disease Period	Symptoms	Signs	Pathology
First week	Fever, chills gradually increasing and persisting; headache	Abdominal tenderness	Bacteremia
Second week	Rash, abdominal pain, diarrhea or constipation, delirium, prostration	Rose spots, splenomegaly, hepatomegaly	Mononuclear cell vasculitis of skin, hyperplasia of ileal Peyer's patches, typhoid nodules in spleen and liver
Third week	Complications of intestinal bleeding and perforation, shock	Melena, ileus, rigid abdomen, coma	Ulcerations over Peyer's patches, perforation with peritonitis
Fourth week and later	Resolution of symptoms, relapse, weight loss	Reappearance of acute disease, cachexia	Cholecystitis, chronic fecal carriage of bacteria

fluid. Laparotomy should be undertaken as early as possible to suture the perforation.

In some high-risk patients with delirium, coma, or shock, high-dose dexamethasone in addition to antibiotics reduces mortality. The dose should be 3 mg per kilogram initially, followed by 1 mg per kilogram every 6 hours for 48 hours. One must be cautious with this therapy because signs and symptoms of perforation are masked by steroids. Antipyretic drugs such as aspirin should be administered with caution because they occasionally markedly reduce blood pressure.

Patients with relapses of typhoid fever should be treated the same as patients with a first attack. Chronic fecal carriers (asymptomatic excretion for a year or longer) should be given high doses of ampicillin or amoxicillin, 100 mg per kilogram per day, plus probenecid, 30 mg per kilogram per day for 4 to 6 weeks. Trimethoprim-sulfamethoxazole is also effective. Patients with multidrug-resistant infections can be treated with ciprofloxacin or other quinolones. Patients with gallstones or cholecystitis may require cholecystectomy to eradicate the carrier state. Chloramphenicol neither prevents nor effectively treats the chronic carrier state.

PROGNOSIS. Typhoid fever carried a case fatality rate of about 12% in the preantibiotic era which was reduced to about 4% after chloramphenicol became available. Case fatality rates > 10% continue to be reported in developing countries despite availability of antibiotics, whereas developed countries show case fatality rates < 1%. After treatment with chloramphenicol or other effective drug, most patients become afebrile in 4 to 7 days. In the preantibiotic era, about 10% of recovered patients had relapses, and chloramphenicol treatment has not reduced this rate. Intestinal bleeding or perforation occurs in about 5% of patients and may not be prevented by antibiotic treatment. Thus bleeding or perforation is occasionally detected after patients have defervesced during treatment. About 1 to 3% of patients become chronic fecal carriers after recovery.

PREVENTION. Travelers to developing countries should avoid consuming untreated water, drinks served with ice, peeled fruits, and other food that is not served hot. American international travelers face an overall risk of developing typhoid fever of < 1 case in 10,000 trips, but travelers to high-risk countries like India and Pakistan have a probability of about 4 in 10,000 trips of getting typhoid fever. Travelers wishing immune protection should receive either live oral vaccine Ty21a (Berna Products [305-443-2900]) given as one capsule every other day for a total of four capsules or typhoid vaccine, U.S.P., administered as two subcutaneous injections of 0.5 ml each at intervals of 4 weeks, with booster doses given every 3 years if needed. These vaccines give only partial protection, and thus vaccinated persons should still exercise dietary precautions. The traditional method of controlling typhoid is to follow stool cultures of convalescent cases and report positive cultures to the health department. The health department investigates nonimported typhoid cases to identify possible food sources or contact with a chronic carrier.

Butler T, Ho M, Acharya G, et al.: Interleukin-6, gamma interferon, and tumor necrosis factor receptors in typhoid fever related to outcome of antimicrobial therapy. Antimicrob Agents Chemother 37:2418, 1993. *Plasma concentrations of cytokines were elevated but not to the same extent as in other causes of bacteremia.*

Butler T, Islam A, Kabir I, et al.: Patterns of morbidity and mortality in typhoid fever dependent on age and gender: Review of 552 hospitalized patients with diarrhea. Rev Infect Dis 13:85, 1991. *Severe and fatal disease in Bangladesh was more common in young children and adults and was correlated with high incidences of seizures, delirium or coma, intestinal perforation, and pneumonia.*

Islam A, Butler T, Nath SK, et al.: Randomized treatment of patients with typhoid fever by using ceftriaxone or chloramphenicol. J Infect Dis 158:742, 1988. *Study of treatment in Bangladesh showed that chloramphenicol remains the treatment of choice because of low cost and rapid defervescence, but newer cephalosporins are good alternatives.*

Levine MM, Ferreccio C, Black RE, et al.: Large-scale field trial of Ty21a live oral typhoid vaccine in enteric-coated capsule formulation. Lancet 1:1049, 1987. *In Chilean school children, three capsules given every other day conferred 67% protection during 3 years; oral vaccination is preferred to parenteral vaccine because of absence of toxic reactions.*

Trujillo IZ, Quiroz C, Gutierrez MA, et al.: Fluoroquinolones in the treatment of typhoid fever and the carrier state. Eur J Clin Microbiol Infect Dis 10:334, 1991. *Ciprofloxacin, norfloxacin, ofloxacin, and pefloxacin have been effective in limited trials against typhoid fever and chronic typhoid carriers.*

293 *SALMONELLA* INFECTIONS OTHER THAN TYPHOID FEVER
Donald Kaye

DEFINITION. *Salmonella*, a genus of the family Enterobacteriaceae, can cause an asymptomatic intestinal carrier state or clinical disease in both humans and animals. In humans, the most common clinical manifestation is enterocolitis, with diarrhea as the major symptom. Some patients develop bacteremia without gastrointestinal manifestations. Localization from bacteremia may result in osteomyelitis, a mycotic aneurysm, or other localized infection. *S. typhi*, a pathogen of humans only, causes enteric fever. Enteric fever produced by *S. typhi* is called "typhoid fever," whereas enteric fever caused by other salmonellae is named "paratyphoid fever."

An asymptomatic intestinal carrier state of variable duration may follow inapparent or symptomatic infection. Most carriers are transient carriers. A chronic carrier state, defined as lasting more than 1 year, is usually permanent and is most often related to persistent infection in the gallbladder. With the exception of *S. typhi*, in which a human carrier is always implicated, most *Salmonella* infections are acquired from food products derived from infected animals (e.g., eggs, poultry, meat, milk).

ETIOLOGY. Salmonellae are motile, gram-negative, non–spore-forming bacilli. They are differentiated from other Enterobacteriaceae by biochemical tests. They ferment glucose, maltose, and mannitol but not lactose or sucrose. Almost all salmonellae produce acid and gas with fermentation. Exceptions to the rules which are helpful in identification are the following: *S. typhi* does not produce gas, and *S. gallinarum-pullorum* is nonmotile. As another confounding exception, lactose-fermenting strains of salmonellae have been isolated.

Salmonellae can be differentiated into over 2000 serotypes by their somatic (O) antigens, which are composed of lipopolysaccharides and are part of the cell wall, and flagellar (H) antigens. Proper nomenclature has divided the salmonellae into three species: *S. typhi*, *S. choleraesuis*, and *S. enteritidis*. The first two consist of only one serotype each, whereas the third contains all the rest of the serotypes. These latter serotypes are recognized as *S. enteritidis* serotype _____ (e.g., *S. enteritidis* serotype typhimurium). However, in a less confusing and cumbersome system, each serotype is commonly referred to as a separate species and is so indicated in this chapter. In this system, using common O antigens, salmonellae have been divided into five major groups, A through E. Some of the important serotypes and their groups are *S. typhi* (group D), *S. choleraesuis* (Group C₁), *S. typhimurium* (group B), and *S. enteritidis* (group D).

S. typhimurium and *S. enteritidis* are the most common causes of human disease and represented 22 and 19% of *Salmonella* isolates from human sources reported in the United States in 1991. Other common isolates are *S. heidelberg*, *S. hadar*, *S. newport*, *S. agona*, *S. montevideo*, *S. poona*, *S. javiana*, and *S. thompson*. In 1991, these 10 serotypes accounted for 68% of the human isolates. In recent years, *S. enteritidis* outbreaks related to eggs have been increasing.

EPIDEMIOLOGY. *S. typhi*, *S. paratyphi A*, *S. schottmuelleri (S. paratyphi B)*, *S. hirschfeldii (S. paratyphi C)*, and *S. sendai* are either solely or almost always pathogens in humans only, and human-to-human transmission is important.

The remaining serotypes of salmonellae are widely spread in the animal kingdom, and salmonellae have been isolated from virtually all species, including birds, poultry, mammals, reptiles, amphibians, and insects. *Salmonella* infection in humans usually occurs from ingesting contaminated animal food products, most often eggs, poultry, and meat. Eggs usually become contaminated from feces on the surface of the egg, with small cracks allowing entry into the egg. However, infection of the ovary allows primary incorporation of salmonellae into the egg. Meat and poultry become widely contaminated at the slaughterhouse with salmonellae spread from carcass to carcass, usually on the surface. *S. choleraesuis* is associated with pig products and *S. dublin* with cattle and consumption of unpasteurized milk from cattle. Salmonellae may survive cooking at relatively low temperatures in the center of eggs or turkeys, or food may be contaminated after cooking from kitchen utensils or from the hands of food preparers who handle raw food.

Salmonella infections have been acquired following contamination of food or water with feces of pet turtles, chicks, birds, dogs, cats, and many other species. These pets become infected from their food.

Salmonella infection also can be acquired by eating food or less commonly drinking water contaminated by a human carrier who has not washed his/her hands adequately. Infection has been spread by the fecal-oral route in children, by contaminated enema and fiberoptic instruments, and by diagnostic and therapeutic preparations made from animal or insect products (e.g., pancreatic extract, carmine dye). Homosexual men are prone to fecal-oral infection.

Outbreaks of salmonellosis occur in institutionalized patients, who are probably more prone to develop *Salmonella* infections for three reasons. First, there are more underlying diseases which decrease host defense mechanisms against salmonellae such as disorders of gastric acidity and intestinal motility; second, use of antimicrobial agents reduces the normal, protective intestinal flora; and third, institutional food prepared in bulk is more likely to be contaminated than individually prepared meals. Outbreaks in nurseries and in the elderly in nursing homes have the highest mortality rates (i.e., >5%). Diabetes may be an additional risk factor for *Salmonella* infection.

Most cases of *Salmonella* infection occurring in the United States are sporadic rather than related to outbreaks. However, when an infection occurs in a family, other members of the household also tend to have positive stool cultures. About 40,000 cases of *Salmonella* infection have been reported to the CDC in recent years, a marked increase over the past 30 years. However, this undoubtedly represents only a fraction of actual cases. It has been estimated that over 1 million cases actually occur each year. A disproportionate number of infections occur in July through October, probably related to the warm weather. *Salmonella* infections are most common in infants and children under 5 years of age.

Salmonellae have become increasingly resistant to antibiotics, usually by acquiring resistance transfer factors. It is believed that much of the resistance has been related to widespread use of antimicrobial agents in farm animals.

PATHOGENESIS. Following ingestion of organisms, the determinants of whether or not infection results, as well as the severity of infection, are the dose and virulence of the *Salmonella* strain and the status of host defense mechanisms. Large inocula such as 10^7 bacteria are usually required to produce clinical infection in the normal host. Smaller inocula are more likely to result in no infection or to produce a transient intestinal carrier state. Gastric acid serves as a host defense mechanism by killing many of the ingested organisms, and intestinal motility is also probably a host defense mechanism. In the absence or decrease of gastric acidity (as in the elderly, following gastrectomy, vagotomy, or gastroenterostomy, with H_2-receptor antagonists, and with antacids) and with decreased intestinal motility (as with antimotility drugs), much smaller inocula can produce infection and the infection tends to be more severe.

Administration of antimicrobial agents prior to ingestion of salmonellae can markedly reduce the size of inoculum needed to produce infection, presumably by reducing the protective bowel flora.

While any *Salmonella* serotype can produce any of the *Salmonella* syndromes (transient asymptomatic carrier state, enterocolitis, bacteremia, enteric fever, and chronic carrier state), each serotype tends to produce certain syndromes much more often than others. For example, *S. anatum* usually causes asymptomatic intestinal infection, whereas *S. typhimurium* usually causes enterocolitis. *S. choleraesuis* is more likely to produce bacteremia (often with metastatic infection) than asymptomatic infection or enterocolitis, and some serotypes such as *S. typhi* are most likely to cause enteric fever as well as the chronic carrier state. Fortunately, most *Salmonella* serotypes are of relatively low pathogenicity for humans, and therefore, although food products are commonly contaminated, large outbreaks occur only when more virulent serotypes are involved.

In order to produce infection (even asymptomatic intestinal infection), enteric pathogens (including salmonellae) must first adhere to intestinal mucosal epithelial cells. Pili on the surface of salmonellae adhere to specific receptor sites on the epithelial cells. Following adherence, invasion of the mucosal cell may result, or multiplication may occur without invasion, resulting in asymptomatic infection. When the organisms reach the lamina propria, polymorphonuclear leukocytes serve as a defense mechanism to prevent invasion of lymphatics. Certain serotypes seem more able than others to invade lymphatics and subsequently produce bacteremia. For example, *S. dublin,* which has been isolated from unpasteurized milk, commonly produces bacteremia following intestinal infection. Both the small intestine and colon are involved in the inflammatory process. The diarrhea in *Salmonella* enterocolitis results from the inflammation. In addition, watery stools may occur, apparently the result of secretion of water and electrolytes by small intestinal epithelial cells in response to an enterotoxin secreted by some of the *Salmonella* strains or in response to tissue mediators of inflammation.

Patients with diseases that impair host defense mechanisms seem to have an increased frequency of severe *Salmonella* infection. For many years, a striking association has been recognized between diseases producing hemolysis and *Salmonella* bacteremia. Specifically, *Salmonella* bacteremia is common in patients with sickle cell disorders, malaria, and bartonellosis. In fact, because of the frequency of *Salmonella* bacteremia in sickle cell diseases and the underlying bone disease in these patients to which salmonellae localize, these organisms are the most common cause of osteomyelitis in patients with sickle cell disorders. Prolonged *Salmonella* bacteremia occurs in patients with hepatosplenic schistosomiasis, probably related to localization on and in the intravascular schistosomes. Patients with lymphoma and leukemia also are more prone to develop *Salmonella* bacteremia. Recently, prolonged and recurrent refractory *Salmonella* bacteremia has been observed in patients with AIDS.

CLINICAL SYNDROMES. *Asymptomatic Intestinal Carrier State.* The asymptomatic intestinal carrier state may result from inapparent infection, which is the most common form of *Salmonella* infection, or may follow clinical disease (convalescent carrier). The carrier state is usually self-limited to several weeks to months, with the incidence of positive stool cultures rapidly decreasing. By 1 year, far less than 1% still have positive stools. The major exception is with *S. typhi:* About 3% of those infected excrete the organism for life. A patient who has had *Salmonella* in the stool for 1 year (chronic carrier) is likely to become a lifelong carrier. Patients with *Schistosoma haematobium* infections are predisposed to become chronic urinary carriers of *Salmonella.*

Enterocolitis. After an incubation period, which is usually 12 to 48 hours, the illness starts suddenly with crampy abdominal pain and diarrhea. A chill is common. Although occasional patients have nausea and vomit once or twice, vomiting is not persistent. The diarrhea may be watery and of large volume or small volume. The stools may contain mucus and occasionally blood. Polymorphonuclear leukocytes are present in the stool. Diarrhea may be mild or may be severe with up to 20 to 30 stools a day. Fever is present in most patients and may reach 40°C (104°F) or higher. The abdomen is tender to palpation. Transient bacteremia may occur and is most likely in infants, the elderly, and patients with impaired host defense mechanisms.

Symptoms usually improve over a period of days, with fever lasting no more than 2 to 3 days and diarrhea no more than 5 to 7 days. However, these symptoms may occasionally persist for up to 14 days. More severe disease is seen with malnutrition, inflammatory bowel disease, and AIDS. Reactive arthritis may follow enterocolitis in up to 7% of cases. It is especially frequent in those with the HLA-B27 phenotype.

Enteric Fever. Paratyphoid fever is an enteric fever syndrome identical to typhoid fever but produced by a serotype other than *S. typhi* (most often *S. paratyphi A, S. schottmuelleri,* or *S. hirschfeldii.* On occasion, it may immediately follow classic enterocolitis caused by the same organism. The syndrome, characterized by prolonged sustained fever, relative bradycardia, splenomegaly, rose spots, and leukopenia, is described in Ch. 292. Enteric fever produced by serotypes of *Salmonella* other than *S. typhi* is usually milder than typhoid fever, and the chronic carrier state follows less commonly than after typhoid fever.

Bacteremia. Patients with the syndrome of *Salmonella* bacteremia usually complain of fever and chills for a period of days to weeks. Gastrointestinal symptoms are unusual, but in some patients the syndrome of *Salmonella* bacteremia follows classic enterocolitis. Other symptoms are nonspecific such as malaise, anorexia, and weight loss. Metastatic infection of bones, joints, mycotic aneurysm (particularly of the abdominal aorta), meninges (mainly in infants), pericardium, pleural space, lungs, heart valves, cysts, uterine myomas, malignancies, and other sites is common, and symptoms may be related to the site of metastatic infection. Stool cultures are usually negative for *Salmonella,* but blood cultures are positive.

Although any *Salmonella* serotype can produce the syndrome of bacteremia, *S. choleraesuis* is most likely to cause this syndrome; over 50% of *S. choleraesuis* infections are bacteremic.

Salmonella bacteremia occurs with increased frequency in infants and the elderly and in patients with diseases associated with hemolysis (such as sickle cell diseases, malaria, and bartonellosis), with lymphoma, with leukemia, and perhaps with systemic lupus erythematosus. Localization to bone is common in patients with sickle cell diseases.

Prolonged *Salmonella* bacteremia lasting for months occurs in patients with hepatosplenic schistosomiasis. Patients with AIDS develop recurrent, relapsing *Salmonella* bacteremia that is difficult to cure with antibiotics.

DIAGNOSIS. The diagnosis of *Salmonella* infection is made by isolating the organism from the stool in enterocolitis, from the blood in bacteremia, from blood and stool in enteric fever, and from the local site in localized infection. Serologic studies are of little clinical value in salmonella infections other than typhoid fever, but they may be of use in epidemiologic studies. A stained smear of the stool usually demonstrates polymorphonuclear leukocytes in patients with *Salmonella* enterocolitis.

The differential diagnosis of *Salmonella* enterocolitis includes all causes of acute diarrhea, including invasive bacteria such as *Campylobacter jejuni, Shigella* species, invasive *E. coli, Yersinia enterocolitica,* and *Vibrio parahaemolyticus;* toxigenic bacteria such as *Vibrio cholerae,* enterotoxigenic *E. coli, S. aureus, B. cereus, C. perfringens,* and *C. difficile;* viruses; and protozoa such as *E. histolytica, G. lamblia,* and *Cryptosporidium* species. Invasive bacterial causes of diarrhea and *C. difficile* infection are also associated with polymorphonuclear leukocytes in the stool, whereas bacterial toxigenic causes (other than *C. difficile*), viruses, and protozoa generally are not. The bacterial toxigenic causes of diarrhea other than *C. difficile* do not produce fever.

Stool culture is definitive for the diagnosis of *Salmonella* enterocolitis, but by the time the results of the stool culture are available, most patients are recovering.

The differential diagnosis of *Salmonella* bacteremia includes all acute infectious and noninfectious causes of fever, including bacteremia caused by other organisms.

The differential diagnosis of enteric fever is the same as discussed in Ch. 292.

TREATMENT. *Enterocolitis.* The primary approach to treatment of *Salmonella* enterocolitis is fluid and electrolyte replacement. Drugs with antiperistaltic effects such as loperamide or diphenoxylate with atropine can relieve cramps but should be used sparingly because they can prolong the diarrhea.

Salmonella enterocolitis is self-limited, and the large majority of cases do not require antimicrobial therapy. However, infants, the elderly, and those with sickle cell disease, lymphoma, leukemia, or other serious underlying diseases who are severely ill and may have bacteremia may benefit from antimicrobial therapy. Amoxicillin, 1 gram every 6 hours orally, or trimethoprim-sulfamethoxazole, one double-strength tablet every 12 hours orally in adults, can be used in those who are able to take oral drugs. Ampicillin, 1 to 2 grams IV every 6 hours, and trimethoprim-sulfamethoxazole, 10 mg per kilogram per day IV of the trimethoprim component, have been used in those who are more severely ill. Antibiotic susceptibility studies should be performed on the isolates, as many strains are now resistant to ampicillin and trimethoprim-sulfamethoxazole. Therapy is continued for 5 days.

There has been a reluctance to treat *Salmonella* enterocolitis, since antibiotic therapy has been reported to have no effect on the clinical course and furthermore to prolong the period of time that salmonellae are excreted in the stool. In addition, most patients are improving by the time that salmonellae or other bacterial pathogens

are isolated from the stool. Perhaps most important, effective, single-drug therapy active against *Salmonella, Shigella, Campylobacter,* and other bacterial causes of diarrhea was lacking until the availability of the fluoroquinolones (e.g., norfloxacin, ciprofloxacin, ofloxacin). These agents are active against virtually all bacterial pathogens that cause diarrhea except for *C. difficile,* and it is reasonable to use them empirically in the early therapy of severe diarrhea of presumed bacterial etiology. Furthermore, several studies indicate that these agents may decrease the duration of the clinical course of *Salmonella* enterocolitis, although prolonging the duration of fecal excretion while others have shown no differences from placebo. At present, routine use of these agents cannot be advocated for suspected *Salmonella* enterocolitis. Further caution is warranted concerning routine use of fluoroquinolones for acute diarrheal disease of unknown etiology because *Campylobacter* has been seen to develop resistance to these agents following treatment.

Bacteremia and Enteric Fever. The major therapeutic agents have been chloramphenicol, 50 mg per kilogram per day in four equally divided doses orally or IV, or ampicillin, 2 grams IV every 6 hours. With resistant organisms or when these agents cannot be used for other reasons, trimethoprim-sulfamethoxazole IV may be substituted at a dose of 10 mg per kilogram per day of the trimethoprim component. Ampicillin is preferred when localized infection (especially intravascular) is present. After response, oral amoxacillin or oral trimethoprim-sulfamethoxazole can be given in the doses described under enterocolitis. Although experience has not been extensive, third-generation cephalosporins such as cefotaxime, ceftizoxime, ceftriaxone, and ceftazidime and the fluoroquinolones appear to be as effective as the older agents, and resistance to these newer agents is less likely. Thus, with further experience, they may become the drugs of choice. Therapy is continued for 2 weeks for enteric fever and bacteremia without localization of organisms and for much longer periods of time with localization to bone, aneurysms, heart valves, and various other sites. Surgical drainage or removal of foreign bodies is often necessary to cure localized infection.

Curing schistosomiasis in patients with *Salmonella* bacteremia may cure the bacteremia. Patients with AIDS tend to relapse repeatedly after treatment courses for *Salmonella* bacteremia. Long-term suppressive therapy has been recommended by some.

Carriers. Chronic carriers (i.e., over 1 year) of salmonellae other than *S. typhi* are rare. Stools of convalescent carriers spontaneously become negative over a period of weeks to months, and no therapy should be given. The rare chronic carrier of non–*S. typhi* serotypes (usually infected with *S. paratyphi A, S. schottmuelleri,* or *S. hirschfeldii*) may be treated with 4 to 6 grams of ampicillin plus 2 grams of probenecid orally each day in four divided doses for 6 weeks. The fluoroquinolones are probably equally effective. Patients who relapse usually have gallbladder disease (most often calculi) and will not be cured with antimicrobial therapy. Cholecystectomy plus antimicrobial therapy may cure these patients, but it is doubtful that the carrier state *per se* is a sufficient indication for cholecystectomy.

PROGNOSIS. Mortality in *Salmonella* enterocolitis is rare; infants and the elderly are at greatest risk, with death occurring from dehydration and electrolyte imbalance. Mortality from *Salmonella* bacteremia or enteric fever is not uncommon and is most likely to occur in the very young and the very old. *S. choleraesuis* bacteremia has the highest mortality rate of any *Salmonella* serotype, as high as 20 to 30%.

PREVENTION. *Salmonella* infection is best prevented by properly managing the water supply and sewage disposal, cooking and refrigerating foods made from animal products, pasteurizing milk and milk products, and handwashing before preparing foods and after handling animals and uncooked animal products. Despite these precautions, because of the widespread presence of salmonellae in the animal kingdom, it is unlikely that the frequency of *Salmonella* infections will be significantly diminished.

There is no vaccine for any salmonellae other than *S. typhi.*

Centers for Disease Control and Prevention: *Salmonella* Surveillance: Annual Summary, 1991. Washington, U.S. Public Health Service, 1991. *A compilation of the serotypes of* Salmonella *isolated from human and nonhuman sources in the United States.*

Katz SG, Andros G, Kohl RD: *Salmonella* infections in the abdominal aorta. Surg Gynecol Obstet 175:102, 1992. *A review of* Salmonella *infections of the abdominal aorta demonstrating the importance of surgical therapy.*

Mäki-Ikola O, Granfors K: *Salmonella*-triggered reactive arthritis. Scand J Rheumatol 21:265, 1992. *A review of the clinical significance of reactive arthritis triggered by* Salmonella *infection.*

Sanchez C, Garcia-Restoy E, Garau J, et al.: Ciprofloxacin and trimethoprim-sulfamethoxazole versus placebo in acute uncomplicated *Salmonella* enteritis: A double-blind trial. J Infect Dis 168:1304, 1993. *A report of use of ciprofloxacin and trimethoprim-sulfamethoxazole in* Salmonella *enterocolitis with no differences from placebo in resolution of symptoms or clearance of salmonellae from the stool.*

Telzak EE, Zweig Greenberg MS, Budnick LD, et al.: Diabetes mellitus: A newly described risk factor for infection from *Salmonella* enteritidis. J Infect Dis 164:538, 1991. *A report of an outbreak of* S. enteritidis *infection in hospitalized patients demonstrating increased susceptibility of medication-dependent diabetes.*

Winstrom J, Jertborn M, Ekwall E, et al.: Empiric treatment of acute diarrheal disease with norfloxacin. Ann Intern Med 117:202, 1992. *A report of use of norfloxacin in acute diarrheal disease demonstrating clinical response in* Salmonella *enterocolitis. However, the duration of fecal excretion of* Salmonella *was prolonged by therapy, and emergence of resistance to norfloxacin occurred among* Camplyobacter *strains.*

294 SHIGELLOSIS
Thomas Butler

DEFINITION. Shigellosis is an acute bacterial infection caused by the genus *Shigella* resulting in colitis affecting predominantly the rectosigmoid colon. "Bacillary dysentery" is synonymous with shigellosis. The disease is characterized by diarrhea, dysentery, fever, abdominal pain, and tenesmus. Shigellosis is usually limited to a few days. Early treatment with antimicrobial drugs results in more rapid recovery.

ETIOLOGY. Shigellae are nonmotile gram-negative bacilli belonging to the family Enterobacteriaceae. Four species of shigellae are recognized on the basis of antigenic and biochemical properties: *S. dysenteriae* (group A), *S. flexneri* (group B), *S. boydii* (group C), and *S. sonnei* (group D). Among these species there are over 40 serotypes, each of which is designated by the species name followed by a specific Arabic number. *S. dysenteriae* 1 is called the "Shiga bacillus" and causes epidemics with higher mortality than other serotypes. With the exception of *S. flexneri* 6, they do not ferment lactose.

Serotypes are determined by the O polysaccharide side chain of the lipopolysaccharide (endotoxin) in the cell wall. Endotoxin is detectable in the blood of severely ill patients and may be responsible for the complication of the hemolytic-uremic syndrome. To be virulent, shigellae must be able to invade epithelial cells, as tested in the laboratory by keratoconjunctivitis in the guinea pig (Sereney test) or HeLa cell invasion. Bacterial invasion of cells is genetically governed by three chromosomal regions and a 140-megadalton plasmid. Shiga toxin is produced by *S. dysenteriae* 1 and in lesser amounts by other serotypes. It inhibits protein synthesis and has enterotoxic activity in animal models, but its role in human disease is uncertain.

INCIDENCE AND PREVALENCE. In the United States there were more than 23,000 reported cases of shigellosis annually in 1990–92. The predominant species in the 1980's was *S. sonnei* (64%), followed by *S. flexneri* (31%), *S. boydii* (3%), and *S. dysenteriae* (2%). Most cases were in young children, women of child-bearing age, and low-income minority residents, and a large proportion occurred in population groups living in homes for the mentally ill or in nursing homes. A large outbreak in 1987 in Tennessee affected more than 1000 persons camping under unsanitary conditions at a mass gathering.

Worldwide, most cases of shigellosis occur in children of developing countries, where *S. flexneri* is the predominant species. During the past 20 years, major epidemics due to *S. dysenteriae* 1 have occurred in Central America, Central Africa, India, and Bangladesh.

EPIDEMIOLOGY. Shigellosis is transmitted by the fecal-oral route. Crowded living conditions, low standards of personal hygiene, poor water supply, and inadequate sewage facilities all contribute to an increased risk of infection. Transmission most often occurs by close person-to-person contact through contaminated hands. During clinical illness and for up to 6 weeks after recovery, organisms are excreted in the feces. Although the organisms are sensitive to desiccation, they may survive several months in food or water, which are occasional vehicles of transmission.

Children between 1 and 4 years old have the greatest risk of developing shigellosis. Inhabitants of custodial institutions, such as homes for retarded children, are at highest risk. Intrafamilial spread follows often when the initial case has occurred in a preschool child. In young adults, the incidence is higher in women than men, which probably reflects closer contact of women with children. The male homosexual population in the United States is at increased risk for shigellosis, which is one of the causes of the "gay bowel syndrome."

Humans and higher primates are the only known natural reservoirs of shigellosis. Transmission shows variable seasonal patterns in different regions. In the United States, the peak incidence is in late summer and early autumn.

PATHOGENESIS AND PATHOLOGY. Since the microorganisms are relatively resistant to acid, shigellae pass the gastric barrier more readily than other enteric pathogens. In volunteer studies, as few as 200 ingested bacilli regularly initiate disease in 25% of healthy adults. This contrasts strikingly with the much larger numbers of typhoid or cholera bacilli required to produce disease in normal individuals. During the incubation period, usually 12 to 72 hours, the organisms traverse the small bowel, penetrate colonic epithelial cells, and multiply intracellularly. An acute inflammatory response ensues in the colonic mucosa attended by prodromal symptoms (Table 294–1). Epithelial cells containing bacteria are lysed, resulting in superficial ulcerations and shedding of shigella organisms into stools. The mucosa is friable and covered with a layer of polymorphonuclear leukocytes. Advancing inflammation causes the formation of crypt abscesses. Initially, the inflammation is confined to the rectosigmoid colon but after about 4 days of illness may advance to involve the proximal colon also. In severe cases, there may be pancolitis with extension of inflammation into the terminal ileum; a pseudomembranous type of colitis may develop. Diarrhea results because of impaired absorption of water and electrolytes by the inflamed colon.

Although the colonic inflammation is superficial, bacteremia occurs occasionally, especially in *S. dysenteriae* 1 infections. Susceptibility of organisms to serum complement–mediated bacteriolysis may explain the infrequency of bacteremia and disseminated infec-

TABLE 294–1. EVOLUTION OF CLINICAL SYNDROMES IN SHIGELLOSIS

Stage	Time of Appearance After Onset of Illness	Symptoms and Signs	Pathology
Prodrome	Earliest	Fever, chills, myalgias, anorexia, nausea, vomiting	None or early colitis
Nonspecific diarrhea	0–3 days	Abdominal cramps, loose stools, watery diarrhea	Rectosigmoid colitis with superficial ulceration, fecal leukocytes
Dysentery	1–8 days	Frequent passage of blood and mucus, tenesmus, rectal prolapse, abdominal tenderness	Colitis extending sometimes to proximal colon, crypt abscesses, inflammation in lamina propria
Complications	3–10 days	Dehydration, seizures, septicemia, leukemoid reaction, hemolytic-uremic syndrome, ileus, peritonitis	Severe colitis, terminal ileitis, endotoxemia, intravascular coagulation, toxic megacolon, colonic perforation
Postdysenteric syndromes	1–3 weeks	Arthritis, Reiter's syndrome	Reactive inflammation in HLA-B27 haplotype

tion. Colonic perforation is a rare complication during toxic megacolon. Children with severe colitis due to *S. dysenteriae* 1 are prone to develop the hemolytic-uremic syndrome. In this complication fibrin thrombi are deposited in the renal glomeruli, causing cortical necrosis and fragmentation of red cells.

CLINICAL MANIFESTATIONS. Most patients with shigellosis begin their illness with a nonspecific prodrome (Table 294–1). The height of the temperature varies, and children may have febrile convulsions. The initial intestinal symptoms soon follow as cramps, loose stools, and watery diarrhea, which usually precede the onset of dysentery by 1 or more days. The average fecal output is about 600 grams a day for adults. The dysentery consists typically of flecks and small clots of bright red blood and mucus in stools that are small in volume. Frequency of passage is often as high as 20 to 40 times a day, with excruciating rectal pain and tenesmus during defecation. Some patients develop rectal prolapse during severe straining. The amount of blood in stools varies widely but usually is small because of the superficial colonic ulcerations. Abdominal tenderness is often most marked in the left lower quadrant over the sigmoid colon but also may be generalized. The fever is likely to abate after a few days of dysentery, making afebrile bloody diarrhea an occasional clinical presentation. After 1 to 2 weeks of untreated disease, spontaneous improvement occurs in most patients. Some patients with mild disease develop only watery diarrhea without dysentery.

Complications include dehydration, which can cause death, especially in children and the elderly. *Shigella* septicemia occurs mainly in malnourished children with *S. dysenteriae* 1 infections. The leukemoid reaction and hemolytic-uremic syndrome may develop in children late in the course after antimicrobial treatment when the dysentery has started to improve. Neurologic manifestations can be striking and include delirium, seizures, and nuchal rigidity.

The important postdysenteric syndromes are arthritis and Reiter's triad of arthritis, urethritis, and conjunctivitis (see Ch. 238). These are nonsuppurative phenomena that occur in the absence of viable *Shigella* organisms about 1 to 3 weeks after resolution of dysentery.

DIAGNOSIS. Shigellosis should be considered in any patient with acute onset of fever and diarrhea. Examination of the stool is essential. Blood and pus are grossly apparent in severe bacillary dysentery; even in milder forms of the disease, microscopic examination of the stool often reveals numerous leukocytes and erythrocytes. The fecal leukocyte examination should be performed with a portion of liquid stool, preferably containing mucus. A drop of stool is placed on a microscopic slide, mixed thoroughly with two drops of methylene blue, and overlaid with a coverslip. The presence of abundant polymorphonuclear leukocytes helps distinguish shigellosis from diarrheal syndromes caused by viruses and enterotoxigenic bacteria. The fecal leukocyte examination is not helpful in distinguishing shigellosis from diarrheal illnesses caused by other invasive enteric pathogens (nontyphoidal *Salmonella, Campylobacter,* and *Yersina*). Amebic dysentery is excluded by the absence of trophozoites on a microscopic examination of fresh stool under a coverslip. The peripheral white cell count is of little diagnostic value, since it may range from less than 3000 to more than 30,000. Sigmoidoscopic examination reveals diffuse erythema with a mucopurulent layer and friable areas of mucosa with shallow ulcers 3 to 7 mm in diameter.

Definitive diagnosis depends on isolating shigellae by selective media. A rectal swab, a swab of a colonic ulcer obtained by sigmoidoscopic examination, or a freshly passed stool specimen should be inoculated immediately on culture plates or into carrying media. Since isolation rates of shigellae from freshly passed stools of patients with shigellosis may be as low as 67%, culturing for 3 successive days is recommended. Stool cultures are generally positive within 24 hours after onset of symptoms and may remain positive for several weeks in the absence of antimicrobial therapy. Appropriate culture media include blood, desoxycholate, and *Salmonella-Shigella* (S-S) agars. Selected colonies should be diagnosed by agglutination with polyvalent *Shigella* antisera. S-S agar is inhibitory for *S. dysenteriae* 1.

Definitive bacteriologic diagnosis becomes critically important for distinguishing the more severe and prolonged cases of shigel-

losis from ulcerative colitis, with which it may be confused both clinically and on sigmoidoscopic examination. Patients with shigellosis have been subjected to colectomy because of a mistaken diagnosis of ulcerative colitis; a positive culture should prevent such a misadventure.

TREATMENT. Appropriate antimicrobial therapy instituted early may decrease the duration of symptoms by 50% and decrease the duration of excretion of shigellae (an important epidemiologic factor) by a far greater percentage. Because of the increasing frequency of plasmid-mediated antimicrobial resistance to *Shigella* infections, surveillance of drug susceptibility in an endemic area is important. In adults, ciprofloxacin given orally in a dose of 500 mg twice daily for 5 days or 1 gram as a single dose is the treatment of choice when the susceptibility of a strain is unknown. In children, treatment should be trimethoprim-sulfamethoxazole, ampicillin, or pivmecillinam, depending on susceptibilities of *Shigella* in a given location.

Fluid losses in shigellosis are qualitatively similar to those in other infectious diarrheal diseases, and the patient should be treated with appropriate intravenous or oral electrolyte repletion fluids in quantities adequate to correct clinical signs of saline depletion. The requirement for fluids is generally small, but fluid repletion is lifesaving in exceptional cases.

Agents that decrease intestinal motility should not be used. Such preparations as diphenoxylate and paregoric may exacerbate symptoms, presumably by retarding intestinal clearance of the microorganisms. There is no convincing evidence that pectin- or bismuthcontaining preparations are helpful.

PROGNOSIS. The mortality rate in untreated shigellosis depends on the infectious strain and ranges from 10 to 30% in certain outbreaks caused by *S. dysenteriae* 1 to <1% in most *S. sonnei* infections. Even with infection caused by *S. dysenteriae* 1, mortality rates should approach zero if appropriate fluid replacement and antimicrobial therapy are initiated early.

About 2% of patients may develop arthritis or Reiter's syndrome weeks or months after recovery from shigellosis.

PREVENTION. Individuals excreting shigellae should be excluded from all phases of food handling until negative cultures have been obtained from three successive stool specimens collected after completion of antimicrobial therapy. In institutional outbreaks, strict and early isolation of infected individuals is mandatory. Targeted antimicrobial chemoprophylaxis has been disappointing. The most important control measure is rigorous handwashing with soap and water by all individuals involved in handling of food or changing diapers. Reporting of shigellosis cases to health authorities should be mandatory.

For the traveler to countries with major *Shigella* problems, no chemoprophylactic agent is an adequate substitute for good personal hygiene and avoiding contaminated food and water. A variety of vaccines has been developed and tested, but no vaccine is now commercially available.

Bennish ML, Harris JR, Wojtyniak BJ, et al.: Death in shigellosis: Incidence and risk factors in hospitalized patients. J Infect Dis 161:500, 1990. *Among more than 9000 infected inpatients, 9% died, with death more likely in infants, the malnourished, and patients with low serum protein concentrations and thrombocytopenia.*

Bennish ML, Salam MA, Khan WA, et al.: Treatment of shigellosis: III. Comparison of one- or two-dose ciprofloxacin with standard 5-day therapy. Ann Intern Med 117:727, 1992. *Ciprofloxacin given as a single dose of 1 gram cured patients with infections other than* S. dysenteriae *1 as well as 500 mg given twice daily for 5 days. For* S. dysenteriae *1 infections, the 5-day treatment gave better results.*

Butler T, Islam MR, Azad MAK, et al.: Risk factors for development of hemolytic uremic syndrome during shigellosis. J Pediatr 110:894, 1987. *In children with* S. dysenteriae *1 infection, hemolytic-uremic syndrome developed after antibiotic therapy, which was usually inappropriate for the susceptibilities of the isolated bacterial strains.*

Butler T, Speelman P, Kabir I, et al.: Colonic dysfunction during shigellosis. J Infect Dis 154:817, 1986. *Studies perfusing the human colon showed diminished colonic water absorption, increased potassium secretion, and normal ileocecal flow rates.*

Tauxe RV, Puhr ND, Wells JG, et al.: Antimicrobial resistance of *Shigella* isolates in the USA: The importance of international travelers. J Infect Dis 162:1107, 1990. *In the United States, resistance of* Shigella *isolates to trimethoprim-sulfamethoxazole occurred in 4% of domestically acquired cases and 20% of travel-related cases.*

Wharton M, Spiegel RA, Horan JM, et al.: A large outbreak of antibiotic-resistant shigellosis at a mass gathering. J Infect Dis 162:1324, 1990. *Poor sanitation at a camp site in Tennessee led to an attack rate of more than 50% in several thousand attendees; disease was caused by multiresistant* S. sonnei.

295 *CAMPYLOBACTER* ENTERITIS

Richard L. Guerrant

Enteric infection with a member of the genus *Campylobacter* usually results in an inflammatory, occasionally bloody diarrhea or dysentery syndrome, in industrialized, temperate areas. *Campylobacter jejuni* is often the most commonly recognized cause of community-acquired inflammatory enteritis. The diarrhea also may be watery, especially in developing, tropical areas. An enterocolitis or protocolitis syndrome similar to that seen with *C. jejuni* is also seen in homosexual males with several "*Campylobacter*-like organisms." The other major *Campylobacter* species that infects humans is *C. fetus,* a relatively uncommon cause of bacteremia and occasional intravascular infection in immunocompromised hosts. *Helicobacter pylori* (the cause of gastritis and peptic ulcers that was previously called *Campylobacter pylori*) is now classified separately.

ETIOLOGY. *Campylobacter* (meaning "curved rod") is a curved or spiral, motile, non–spore-forming, gram-negative rod measuring 1.5 by 3.5 μm which is distinguished from Enterobacteriaceae by its inability to ferment or oxidize carbohydrates. It was formerly called a "vibrio" but is now recognized as a separate genus on the basis of its distinctive DNA content. It is both oxidase- and catalase-positive and is a microaerophilic organism that requires reduced oxygen (5 to 10%) and increased carbon dioxide (3 to 10%). The organism does not grow at either aerobic or strictly anaerobic conditions. Perhaps reflecting its avian reservoir, *C. jejuni* also requires an increased temperature to 42°C for optimal growth. *C. jejuni* is distinguished from *C. fetus* by its higher growth temperatures, cephalothin resistance, and nalidixic acid sensitivity. As shown in Table 295–1, the additional *Campylobacter* species that infect humans include *C. laridis,* a thermophilic organism commonly found in healthy sea gulls that has been reported in children with mild recurrent diarrhea and in an elderly patient with sepsis and terminal multiple myeloma. The weak or non–catalase-producing *C. upsaliensis* may cause diarrhea or bacteremia, and *C. hyointestinalis,* like *C. fetus,* causes occasional bacteremia in compromised hosts. These organisms are also inhibited by cephalothin that is in some selective culture media. Up to three distinct species of "*Campylobacter*-like organisms" (including proposed species names *C. fennelliae* and *C. cinaedi*) are associated with protocolitis in homosexual males and occasionally with bacteremia or diarrhea in women and children. Like *C. fetus,* these *Campylobacter*-like organisms do not grow at 42°C or in the presence of cephalosporin antibiotics (present in some selective media for *C. jejuni*) and may

require several days to a week or more to grow in culture. *C. jejuni* is further subdivided into over 90 serotypes on the basis of heat-stable O antigens or over 50 serotypes on the basis of heat-labile capsular and flagellar antigens, markers that are helpful in tracing the epidemiology of this common enteric pathogen.

EPIDEMIOLOGY. Although the frequency of other *Campylobacter* infections is either low or unclear, *C. jejuni* infections are extremely common throughout the world. In many studies, the frequency of *Campylobacter* enteritis exceeds that of *Salmonella* or *Shigella* infections, and it has been estimated that as many as 2 million *Campylobacter* enteritis cases occur annually in the United States. The reservoirs of *C. jejuni/coli* include a wide range of mammalian species. Between 30 and 100% of chickens, turkeys, and water fowl may be infected asymptomatically in their intestinal tracts, and commercially prepared poultry in supermarkets can often be shown to be culture-positive. In addition, swine, cattle, sheep, horses, and even household pets and rodents may carry *C. jejuni, C. coli,* or *C. fetus.* Enteric symptoms may be found, particularly in puppies, kittens, calves, or lambs, which may have diarrhea when infected. Furthermore, the organisms survive days to weeks in fresh or salt water and in milk and are killed most effectively by pasteurization, chlorination, drying, or freezing.

The transmission of *Campylobacter* infections is likely via the fecal-oral route. Fecal-oral spread may occur by contact among animals, homosexual males, and those in day care centers. Secondary transmission is relatively infrequent, and the infectious dose appears to vary from 500 to over 1 million organisms. The majority of infections are probably acquired by ingesting contaminated food, water, or milk vehicles. Many cases and outbreaks are associated with ingesting inadequately cooked poultry, unpasteurized milk, inadequately treated water, and even cake icing, salads, beef, and clams.

The majority of those infected in well-described outbreaks are symptomatic. Asymptomatic infection appears to be relatively infrequent in temperate climates and in adults. An exception is among young children in certain tropical developing areas such as Bangladesh, where as many as 39% of children under age 2 years may be infected asymptomatically (Table 295–2). These frequent asymptomatic infections in tropical areas raise important questions about possible strain differences in virulence, host susceptibility, and protective immunity against disease that might be acquired very early in developing areas.

Throughout the world, *Campylobacter* infections appear to predominate during the warmer or wet season. As with diarrheal illnesses in general, the highest age-specific attack rate is in young children. However, the greatest proportion of positive fecal cultures occurs in older children and young adults. The latter contributes a small peak in the age-specific attack rates during the "second weaning," when young adults leave home and lack experience with cooking poultry and other products. There is little, if any, sexual predominance of recognized *C. jejuni* infections.

PATHOGENESIS AND PATHOLOGY. *C. jejuni* and *C. coli* are reasonably susceptible to gastric acidity. However, the reported variation in infectious dose suggests considerable host or strain variability. After an incubation period of 1 to 7 (median 4) days, symptoms of the enteric infection begin. *C. jejuni* organisms are attracted toward mucus and fucose in bile, and the flagellae may be important in both chemotaxis and adherence to epithelial cells or mucus. Adherence also may involve lipopolysaccharide or other outer membrane components. Several laboratories around the world have documented the production by *C. jejuni* of a cholera-like, heat-labile enterotoxin that binds to ganglioside and is neutralized by anticholera toxin antiserum. However, the genetic code and role of this toxin in disease remain elusive to date. Studies from Mexico have shown that antitoxic immunity develops after infection, often with watery diarrhea, suggesting that this toxin is significant in those infections.

However, more characteristic in temperate areas is a diffuse, often bloody exudative enteritis involving the ileum and colon. These pathologic changes may include nonspecific crypt abscesses that on colonoscopy and histopathology may mimic the changes seen with inflammatory bowel disease. Such invasive pathology is also seen in rabbit, chick, mouse, dog, and monkey models of infection. Although *C. jejuni* is negative in the Sereny test for guinea pig con-

TABLE 295–1. HUMAN *CAMPYLOBACTER* INFECTIONS

Species	Growth Temperature	Reservoir	Clinical Manifestations
C. jejuni/coli	37–42°C	Poultry, mammals	Common cause of dysentery/diarrhea
C. fetus (sub sp. *fetus,* old sub sp. *intestinalis*)	25–37°C	Cattle, sheep	Uncommon, bacteremia; intravascular infections in debilitated hosts
C. laridis	30–42°C	Sea gulls	Uncommon, childhood diarrhea, one case of sepsis
C. upsaliensis	37–42°C	Dogs	Occasional diarrhea
C. hyointestinalis	37°C	Swine	Occasional bacteremia in compromised hosts
"*Campylobacter*-like organisms": (including *Helicobacter cinaedi,* *H. fennelliae*)	37°C / 37°C	?	Proctocolitis, rarely sepsis, in homosexual males
H. pylori (formerly *C. pylori*)			Histologic gastritis ulcer or gastritis symptoms

TABLE 295–2. CLINICAL PRESENTATIONS OF *CAMPYLOBACTER JEJUNI* INFECTION

	Industrialized Countries	Developing Countries
Percent of all diarrhea with *C. jejuni*	5–13	2–35
Percent of *C. jejuni* diarrhea with:		
Fecal PMN	78–93	22–46
Blood in stool	60–65	5–17
Asymptomatic infection rates (%)	<2	0–39*

* Depending on age—39% if less than 2 years old.

junctivitis, some have reported the production of cytotoxins by certain strains of *C. jejuni* that may be involved in the pathogenesis of the invasive colitis. The relative infrequency of bloodstream invasion by *C. jejuni*, compared with *C. fetus*, likely relates to the relative serum sensitivity of most *C. jejuni* strains and to the rapid development of bactericidal antibody with infection in normal individuals. Volunteer studies suggest that effective immunity develops to rechallenge with the homologous strain, and animal studies suggest that protective immunity may be transferred in immune milk to suckling offspring. Additional evidence of effective immunity comes with the decreasing illness/infection ratio among children in endemic areas as well as among regular consumers of raw milk.

Once patients are infected, they shed 10^7 to 10^9 organisms per gram of stool for a median duration of 2 to 3 weeks, if not treated with effective antibiotics. Although some may continue to excrete the organism for 2 to 3 months, chronic asymptomatic intestinal carriage is rare.

CLINICAL MANIFESTATIONS. As noted in Table 295–1, the major recognized disease with human *Campylobacter* infections is the characteristic diarrheal illness seen with *C. jejuni* or *C. coli* infections. Although asymptomatic infections and watery, noninflammatory diarrhea are seen with *C. jejuni* infections in tropical, developing areas as shown in Table 295–2, *C. jejuni* is characteristically associated with an inflammatory, febrile enteritis in industrialized countries throughout the world. After an incubation period of 1 to 7 days, a brief prodrome of fever, headache, and myalgias lasting for 12 to 24 hours is promptly followed in a case of *C. jejuni* enteritis in a child or young adult with the symptoms of acute enteritis. These characteristically include crampy abdominal pain, fever to 39 or 40°C, and diarrhea with up to 10 or more loose, often bloody bowel movements per day. Occasionally, the crampy abdominal pain may predominate as an appendicitis-like syndrome, with mesenteric adenitis or terminal ileitis being the predominant pathology. On physical examination, the abdomen is diffusely tender and may mimic appendicitis. Although the acute febrile enteritis is usually self-limited to 5 to 7 days, 10 to 20% of cases may last longer than 1 week and 5 to 20% of untreated cases may relapse with a similar illness.

Complications, particularly if antimotility agents are used, include toxic megacolon, pseudomembranous colitis, and colonic hemorrhage. In addition, hemolytic-uremic syndrome, postinfectious polyneuritis, or Guillain-Barré syndrome (GBS) may follow *C. jejuni* enteritis. Some suggest that *C. jejuni* (especially O type 19) may be a major recognized predisposing cause of GBS. As with many inflammatory colitis syndromes, reactive arthritis and full-blown Reiter's syndrome may follow weeks after *Campylobacter* enteritis. Bacteremia may occur relatively rarely (<1% of cases), particularly in the very young or the elderly, in whom meningitis, endocarditis, cholecystitis, urinary tract infections, and pancreatitis have been described. In patients with hypogammaglobulinemia or HIV infection, *C. jejuni* infections may be prolonged or severe despite appropriate antimicrobial therapy.

In striking contrast to *C. jejuni*, the slow-growing *C. fetus* is primarily an uncommon cause of bacteremia, often in immunocompromised hosts. Although *C. fetus* would be missed on most routine stool cultures for *C. jejuni*, studies with filtration methods suggest that it is a relatively infrequent cause of diarrhea. Instead, *C. fetus* tends to cause intravascular, meningeal, or localized infections such as arthritis, cellulitis, abscesses, cholecystitis, and urinary, placental,

or pleural infections, often in elderly or debilitated hosts. As it does in animals, *C. fetus* may cause stillbirth or septic abortions more often than generally recognized in humans. *C. fetus* infections are often recognized only by astute clinical microbiology technicians who methodically examine or subculture cultured specimens of blood or other body fluids after 1 week in the laboratory. The clinical course of *C. fetus* bacteremia is often related to its recognition and appropriate treatment as well as to the underlying disease.

DIAGNOSIS. The diagnosis of *Campylobacter* infections is related to a careful history for exposure or characteristic clinical syndromes, direct stool examination, and selective culture methods. *C. jejuni* enteritis should be suspected in anyone presenting with a febrile enteritis, especially if there is a history of recent ingestion of inadequately cooked poultry, unpasteurized milk, or untreated water. As suggested in Figure 295–1, such a history should prompt obtaining a fecal specimen in a cup if at all possible and direct microscopic examination using methylene blue or Gram stain for leukocytes as well as gross and/or occult blood. In many industrialized areas, the presence of blood or fecal leukocytes with fever strongly suggests the presence of a cultivable enteric pathogen such as *C. jejuni*, *Salmonella*, or *Shigella*, with *C. jejuni* being most common. Additional immediate clues to *C. jejuni* infection may be seen on dark-field or phase microscopy for characteristic darting motility or on a carbolfuchsin Gram stain of stool for characteristic curved rods or sea gull morphology. However, dark-field and Gram stains, while reasonably specific with trained observers, are each only 50 to 66% sensitive. Patients with febrile enteritis, particularly with blood and leukocytes in the stool, should be cultured for *C. jejuni*.

Additional differential diagnostic possibilities for febrile inflammatory enteritis include *Salmonella* and *Shigella* infections, for which one should seek a history of an outbreak or contact exposure (such as in day care centers or among homosexual males, respectively). If the patient has recently taken antibiotics, *C. difficile* colitis or *Salmonella* enteritis should be considered. Recent ingestion of raw seafood should prompt investigation for *Vibrio* infection that may present with either inflammatory or noninflammatory diarrhea. A history of sick pet exposure, persisting abdominal pain, or unexplained inflammatory diarrhea also should prompt consideration of *Yersinia enterocolitica* infections, and travel exposure to tropical areas or residence in an institution where careful hygiene is difficult should prompt an examination of stool and possibly rectal biopsy specimens for *E. histolytica* (which often destroys fecal leukocytes). Another frequent diagnosis that is considered, especially if *Campylobacter* enteritis has relapsed once or twice, is inflammatory bowel disease. However, it is imperative that anyone who is being considered for that diagnosis have treatable causes such as *Campylobacter* enteritis or amebiasis excluded by appropriate cultures or stains, as treatment with steroids may worsen *Campylobacter* or amebic enteritis with potentially devastating consequences. Additional noninfectious causes of bloody diarrhea with abdominal pain include intussusception and vascular insufficiency.

The diagnosis of *H. pylori* infections is best made by documenting the organism by culture and histology of gastric biopsies. Additional clues may be provided by ureases tests of biopsies, breath tests for urease degradation of ingested urea, or serologic tests for anti-*H. pylori* antibody (see Ch. 99.2).

THERAPY. The most important treatment for *Campylobacter* enteritis, as with all diarrheal illnesses, is adequate rehydration and maintenance fluid therapy, which can often be accomplished with oral glucose-electrolyte solutions. The effectiveness of specific antimicrobial therapy remains debated. Although most *C. jejuni* strains are sensitive to erythromycin as well as to tetracyclines, chloramphenicol, clindamycin, the quinolones, and aminoglycosides, they are characteristically resistant to penicillin, ampicillin, cephalosporins, and sulfamethoxazole-trimethroprim. Indications for antibiotic treatment remain controversial. Several studies have failed to show a significant reduction in the duration of illness with erythromycin treatment despite its prompt eradication of the organism from the stool. Some reserve antimicrobial treatment for those with particularly severe symptoms of high fever, bloody or severe diarrhea, young children in day care centers, or prolonged or relapsing illnesses. Antimotility agents should be avoided in *Campylobacter* enteritis, as with any inflammatory diarrhea.

It should be remembered that erythromycin orally may not be adequate for systemic *C. jejuni* or *C. fetus* endovascular infections,

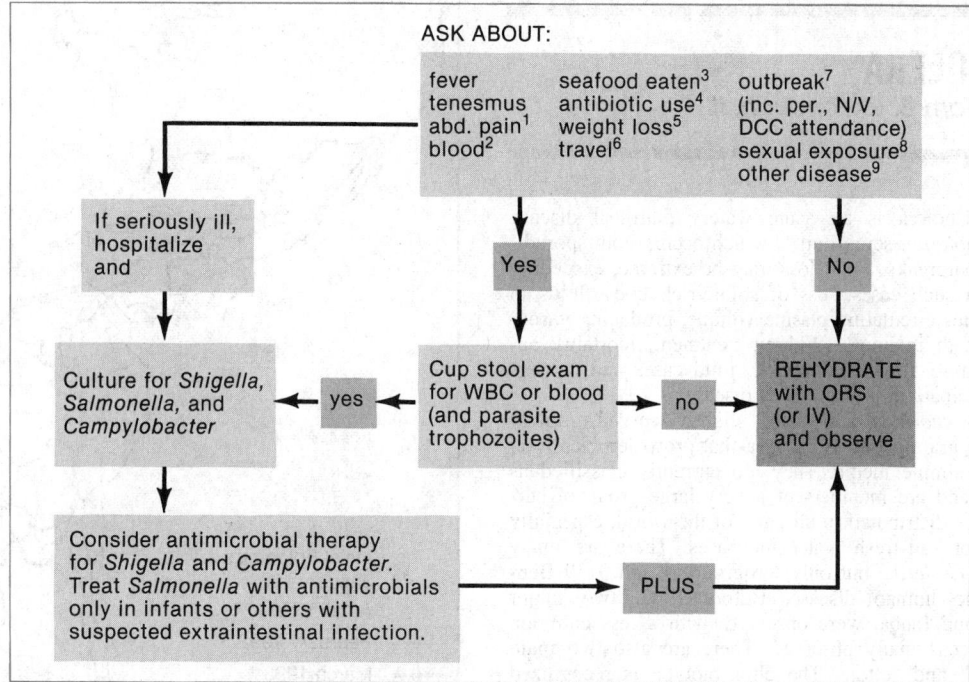

ASK ABOUT:

fever
tenesmus
abd. pain[1]
blood[2]

seafood eaten[3]
antibiotic use[4]
weight loss[5]
travel[6]

outbreak[7]
(inc. per., N/V,
DCC attendance)
sexual exposure[8]
other disease[9]

Yes   **No**

If seriously ill, hospitalize and

Culture for *Shigella*, *Salmonella*, and *Campylobacter* ← **yes** ← Cup stool exam for WBC or blood (and parasite trophozoites) → **no** → REHYDRATE with ORS (or IV) and observe

Consider antimicrobial therapy for *Shigella* and *Campylobacter*. Treat *Salmonella* with antimicrobials only in infants or others with suspected extraintestinal infection. → **PLUS**

FIGURE 295–1. Approach to the diagnosis and management of acute infectious diarrhea.
1. If unexplained abdominal pain and fever persist or suggest an appendicitis-like syndrome, culture for *Yersinia enterocolitica*.
2. Bloody diarrhea, especially if without fecal leukocytes, suggests enterohemorrhagic (*Shiga* toxin–producing) *E. coli* O157 or amebiasis (where leukocytes are destroyed by the parasite).
3. Ingestion of inadequately cooked seafood should prompt consideration of *Vibrio* infections or Norwalk-like viruses.
4. Associated antibiotics should be stopped if possible and cytotoxigenic *C. difficile* considered.
5. Persistence (> 10 days) with weight loss should prompt consideration of giardiasis or cryptosporidiosis.
6. Travel to tropical areas increases the chance of enterotoxigenic *E. coli* as well as viral (ex. Norwalk-like or rotaviral), parasitic (ex. *Giardia, Entamoeba, Strongyloides, Cryptosporidium*), and, if fecal leukocytes are present, invasive bacterial pathogens as noted in the algorithm.
7. Outbreaks should prompt consideration of *S. aureus, B. cereus, Anisakis* (incubation period <6 hours), *C. perfringens, ETEC, Vibrio, Salmonella, Campylobacter, Shigella* or EIEC infection. If unexplained, consider saving *E. coli* for LT, ST, invasiveness, adherence testing, and serotyping, and save stool for rotavirus and stool + paired sera for Norwalk-like virus testing.
8. Sigmoidoscopy in symptomatic homosexual males should distinguish proctitis in the distal 15 cm only (caused by herpesvirus, gonococcal, chlamydial, or syphilitic infection) from colitis (*Campylobacter, Shigella, C. difficile,* or chlamydial [LGV serotypes] infections) or noninflammatory diarrhea (due to giardiasis).
9. Immunocompromised hosts should have a wide range of viral (ex. CMV, HSV, coxsackie, rotavirus), bacterial (ex. *Salmonella, Mycobacterium avium-intracellulare, Listeria*), fungal (ex. *Candida*), and parasitic (ex. *Cryptosporidium, Strongyloides, Entamoeba,* and *Giardia*) agents considered.
(Adapted from Guerrant RL, Shields DS, Thorson SM, et al.: Evaluation and diagnosis of acute infectious diarrhea. Am J Med 78:91, 1985; and Guerrant RL, Bobak DA: Bacterial and protozoal gastroenteritis. N Engl J Med 325:327, 1991.)

which probably warrant 2 to 4 weeks of parenteral bactericidal antimicrobial therapy.

H. pylori infections, although difficult to eradicate with a single agent, may be eradicated by combinations of agents such as bismuth compounds plus metronidazole, provided that the organism is susceptible (see Ch. 99.1).

PROGNOSIS. The prognosis of *C. jejuni* enteritis is generally quite good, and the disease is usually self-limited with or without specific therapy.

PREVENTION. Since most *Campylobacter* infections arise from fecal contamination, often from animal reservoirs, many if not most *Campylobacter* infections are potentially preventable by education. The most common recognized vehicles of spread are inadequately cooked food, unpasteurized milk, and inadequately treated water. Consequently, thoroughly cooking meat and poultry, careful hand-washing after preparing food, pasteurizing milk, and adequately chlorinating drinking water should greatly reduce the frequency of *Campylobacter* infections. Parents should be warned that sick pet kittens or puppies may harbor potential human pathogens such as *C. jejuni* and keep them away from small children and practice careful hygienic measures in their care.

Blaser MJ, Wells JG, Feldman RA, et al.: *Campylobacter* enteritis in the United States. Ann Intern Med 98:360, 1983. *Critical analysis of the presentation of* C. jejuni *and other enteritides in the United States.*
Butzler JP, Skirrow MB: *Campylobacter* enteritis. Clin Gastroenterol 8:737, 1979.

Good review of cultivation methods, epidemiology, clinical presentation, and models of C. jejuni *infections.*
Guerrant RL, Lahita RG, Winn WC, et al.: Campylobacteriosis in man: Pathogenic mechanisms and review of 91 bloodstream infections. Am J Med 65:584, 1978. *Review of both* C. fetus *and* C. jejuni *infections and their presentations as bacteremic illnesses.*
Guerrant RL, Bobak DA: Bacterial and protozoal gastroenteritis. N Engl J Med 325:327, 1991. *Update on epidemiology and pathogenesis as well as a practical clinical approach to diagnosis and management of bacterial and other causes of diarrhea.*
Mishu B, Blaser MJ: Role of infection due to *Campylobacter jejuni* in the initiation of Guillain-Barré syndrome. Clin Infect Dis 17:104, 1993. *Excellent update of data confirming a review of over 20 reports from 1984 showing that 20 to 40% of Guillain-Barré syndrome (GBS) cases may follow* C. jejuni *infections, especially those with LPS O type 19, which has been implicated in the pathogenesis of GBS.*
Nachamkin I, Blazer MJ, Tompkins LS: *Campylobacter jejuni:* Current Status and Future Trends. Washington, DC, ASM, 1992. *An excellent compendium of multiauthored chapters on epidemiology, microbiology, clinical manifestations, pathogenesis, immunity and therapy of* Campylobacter *infections.*
Perlman DM, Ampel NM, Schiffman RB, et al.: Persistent *Campylobacter-jejuni* infections in patients infected with the human immunodeficiency virus: Association with abnormal serological response to *C. jejuni* and emergence of erythromycin resistance during therapy. Ann Intern Med 108:540, 1988. *Report of persistent, severe* C. jejuni *enteritis and occasional bacteremia in patients with HIV infection who fail to mount a serum antibody response.*
Quinn TC, Corey L, Chaffee RG, et al.: The etiology of anorectal infections in homosexual men. Am J Med 71:395, 1981. *Review of the clinical manifestations and diagnostic approach to the wide range of enteric infections commonly seen in promiscuous homosexual males.*
Walker RI, Caldwell MB, Lee EC, et al.: Pathophysiology of *Campylobacter* enteritis. Microbiol Rev 50:81, 1986. *Excellent recent review of the virulence traits, pathogenic mechanisms, and animal models of* C. jejuni *infections.*

296 CHOLERA
William B. Greenough, III

DEFINITION. Cholera is an acute watery diarrheal disease caused by *Vibrio cholerae,* serogroup 1, which occurs both sporadically and as large outbreaks. Fluid loss may be extreme, exceeding 1 liter per hour. In such cases, loss of solute-rich body fluids in stools rapidly depletes circulating plasma volume, producing vascular collapse and death in hours. Without treatment, mortality approaches 60% of those affected; however, mild cases and carriers also occur and participate in the spread of disease.

ETIOLOGY. *V. cholerae* are short, slightly curved, rapidly motile, uniflagellate gram-negative bacteria that grow aerobically at 37°C on relatively simple media. They are currently classified as Enterobacteriaceae and are members of a very large group of surface water organisms distributed in all parts of the world, especially favoring brackish or salt-fresh water interfaces. There are many O serogroups of *V. cholerae,* but only serogroups 1 and 0139 Bengal cause epidemic human disease. Before 1992, two major serotypes, Ogawa and Inaba, were observed, with a less common Hikojima variant occasionally observed. There are also two main biotypes, "classical" and "eltor." The eltor biotype is recognized by its resistance to polymyxin B and by characteristic vibriophage susceptibility. These markers are of use epidemiologically. *V. cholerae* produces a potent exotoxin (choleragen) that binds to intestinal epithelium, producing a chloride ion–driven secretion and malabsorption of sodium ion and water. Other vibrios can produce exotoxins but do not have other biologic characteristics that lead to spreading epidemic disease. However, an entirely new serogroup (0139 Bengal) is currently responsible for major epidemics.

EPIDEMIOLOGY. Cholera is thought to be a disease of antiquity, with clear written descriptions dating before 500 B.C. The present global spread (seventh pandemic) has been due to an eltor biotype first recognized in 1911 at the El Tor quarantine station in the Persian Gulf. Epidemics due to this organism first appeared in the Celebes in the 1930's, spreading westward through Southeast Asia and reaching the Mediterranean and Africa in the 1970's. However, in the Ganges delta, epidemics of classic *V. cholerae* were replaced by eltor late in the 1960's. There have been small but regular outbreaks of cholera in the United States in the Mississippi delta regions since 1973. The eltor strains isolated have not been the same as the global epidemic strain. In 1991, *V. cholerae* 01 eltor caused explosive outbreaks of cholera in Peru and have subsequently spread throughout Latin America (Fig. 296–1). The newly arisen *V. cholerae* 0139 Bengal clearly has the potential for rapid global spread. *V. cholerae* serogroup 1 can be identified by gene amplification or immunofluorescent methods in many waters often associated with phytoplankton.

Mode of Spread. During epidemics, cholera is mainly waterborne. Large numbers of vibrios enter many water sources from the voluminous liquid stools that soak clothing and linens and contaminate the environment. The setting for epidemics is often extreme poverty with lack of safe water. However, an outbreak in Portugal affected the most careful travelers who used only bottled water, which unfortunately had been supplied from a spring contaminated with *V. cholerae.* Occasionally, contaminated foods spread disease. Most often raw or undercooked shellfish or fresh vegetables washed with contaminated water are responsible. These played an important role in the recent Latin American epidemics. There is a high risk of secondary spread in families or institutions in which water and food are shared. Contamination of household food and water sources is the rule. It is easy to understand how this occurs when an adult patient may produce 30 to 50 liters of stool in 2 to 3 days and is usually too weak to use a commode or toilet. Mild cases and convalescent carriers probably spread the disease between communities. True long-term carriers are rare enough to be reportable.

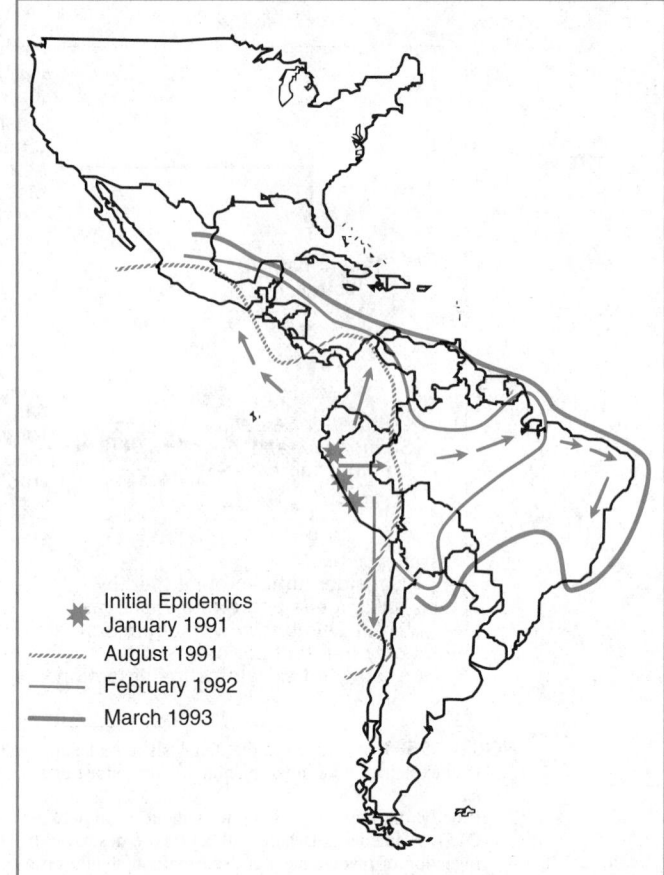

FIGURE 296–1. Geographic extent of the Latin American epidemic over time. Lines represent the advancing front of the epidemic at different times. By March 1993, all Latin American countries except Uruguay had reported cholera, and no cases had been reported from the Caribbean.

Susceptibility to Cholera. In areas where cholera occurs each year, children younger than 5 are the main victims. Older children and adults in such endemic areas have acquired a lasting and strongly protective local intestinal immunity. Breast-fed infants in such circumstances do not get cholera and are solidly protected by antibodies from their mother's milk. When cholera attacks a population that has not experienced it for many years, as was true in recent spread to the Philippines and Africa, all ages are attacked equally, but morbidity and mortality are greatest among the very young and very old. Individuals with low gastric acid production, or those who are on acid-suppressing medications, or who have had gastrectomies are especially vulnerable, since *V. cholerae* is quite sensitive to acid. Cholera tends to attack persons of blood group O more frequently and with greater severity, whereas individuals with AB blood group have less severe disease. People with a safe, piped water supply and effective disinfected waste disposal are at least risk regardless of host susceptibility.

PATHOGENESIS. After *V. cholerae* is ingested, vomiting and diarrhea may begin as early as 12 hours or not appear for more than a week. Illness occurs when viable organisms reach the duodenum and jejunum where alkaline pH, nutrients, and bile salts favor rapid multiplication. Actively motile vibrios penetrate mucous layers and attach to the brush border of the intestinal epithelium, where they secrete a potent exotoxin. This toxin is a protein of 84,000 daltons consisting of five B subunits that bind irreversibly to a specific chemical receptor on the cell surfaces (GM1-ganglioside). The toxic moiety or A subunit is linked to the B aggregate and gains entry once binding has occurred. ADP ribosylates the α subunit of G protein, producing increased adenylate cyclase activity and consequent raised cyclic AMP levels in the enterocytes or any other affected cells. The most visible result in the small intestine is the profuse watery diarrhea resulting from abolition at the villous tips of the normal absorption of sodium ion and with it anions and water, and stimulation of crypt cells to secrete chloride, drawing with them cations and water from the blood stream into the gut lumen. The resulting solute-rich stream originating in the duodenum and jejunum is profuse, eliciting vomiting as it progresses cephalad and diarrhea as it flushes through the colon. The fluid lost in cholera is a slightly fishy-smelling nonfecal whitish mucous-flecked liquid ("rice water stool"). There is no cellular damage and no inflammation or loss of plasma proteins or formed elements of the blood. There is also increased secretion of hepatic and pancreatic fluids, prostaglandins, and other intestinal hormones. All signs and symptoms of cholera derive from the fluid losses, which approach in composition an ultrafiltrate of plasma enriched in potassium and bicarbonate (Table 296–1). There is no evidence for systemic effects by cholera toxin itself, since V. cholerae does not invade the body, nor is the toxin absorbed. It exerts all its effects topically by adhering to the intestinal lining and producing toxin that is bound at cell surfaces.

CLINICAL MANIFESTATIONS. Cholera can reduce a perfectly healthy, robust adult to shock and death in 4 to 6 hours. More usually, death ensues in 18 or more hours. In rare instances, "cholera sicca" shock and death occur before diarrhea appears, the voluminous secretions pooling in distended loops of bowel and not escaping as either diarrhea or vomiting. Despite the capacity of cholera to cause severe illness, many of the infected patients have only a mild diarrhea indistinguishable from that of ordinary gastroenteritis. In epidemics, about half those infected have either no symptoms or very mild illness.

Without fluid replacement, cholera patients demonstrate signs of severe volume depletion—sunken eyes, poor skin turgor, hoarse voice, extreme thirst, faint heart sounds, weak or absent peripheral pulses, and severe muscle cramps. Patients are oriented but appear apathetic except for thirst. If patients survive and have not received adequate hydration, fever secondary to sepsis and pneumonia are common, and pulmonary edema can ensue with even modest fluid replacement.

In children, unconsciousness and/or convulsions may signal hypoglycemia. In both children and adults, adequate early volume replacement with a correctly formulated oral hydration solution can prevent all signs and symptoms except diarrhea. Initial laboratory values from depleted cholera patients (Table 296–1) reflect the loss of isotonic fluid without larger molecules such as albumen. This results in increased concentrations of plasma proteins and blood cells. Loss of bicarbonate leads to acidosis with a low arterial pH and bicarbonate. Potassium depletion, which may be severe, is not reflected by low plasma values until acidosis has been corrected.

DIAGNOSIS. Cholera should be ruled out in any patient with acute watery diarrhea. Travel to or residence in a cholera-endemic area should raise the index of suspicion. In clusters of acute watery diarrhea, particularly where sanitation is poor, it is especially important to recognize cholera early to permit advance actions to prevent deaths of large numbers of people.

Treatment does not depend on an etiologic diagnosis. Fluid replacement should be started without delay as soon as diarrhea begins. After initiating treatment, stool should be examined directly for red and white blood cells. Except in mixed infections with invasive organisms, which do occur in cholera outbreaks, fecal red and white cells are not a feature of cholera. If phase or dark-field microscopy is available, the characteristic darting motility of vibrios can be recognized in fresh wet preparations. To be certain that these motile bacteria are V. cholerae, serogroup 1 antisera can be applied to wet preparations, immobilizing the organisms in a rapid and specific diagnostic test. For greater sensitivity of this test, a stool sample or rectal swab can be incubated in an enrichment medium for vibrios, such as alkaline peptone water, for 12 to 18 hours. Stool culture is best done on a selective medium, since colonies of V. cholerae may be overgrown or are easily missed on standard enteric media. A simple method uses thiosulfate citrate–bile salt–sucrose (TCBS) agar, which is very stable and selective for vibrios. Opaque flat yellow colonies form on TCBS agar in 18 hours at 37°C. Confirmation of serogroup and serotype can be done by direct slide agglutination with specific antisera that are available commercially, including against the new 0139 Bengal strain. Biotyping requires more elaborate procedures, but resistance to polymyxin B is a quick way to recognize the eltor biotype.

Although the first line of immune defense is local at the intestinal epithelium, circulating antibodies occur to the specific O antigens. Testing for these is of use only as an epidemiologic tool to judge prevalence of disease in a specific population.

TREATMENT. Early and complete replacement of fluid losses averts death and all complications. Advanced oral hydration solutions based on rice or other starchy foods hydrate efficiently and reduce diarrhea and vomiting substantially (30 to 50%) as compared with intravenous treatment or glucose-based oral rehydration solutions. In all except the most severe cases, oral rehydration therapy is sufficient to treat cholera, especially if started as soon as diarrhea begins. All varieties of watery diarrhea lose fluid of similar composition, which varies with the rate of loss. Oral hydration therapy is the treatment of choice in all situations except when a patient is in shock or is comatose. Oral rehydration therapy should be used in hospitals, at home, or in the field, since it entails fewer risks, is much less costly, does not require trained medical personnel for administration, and is effective. The discovery that absorption of sodium by cotransport pathways in intestinal mucosa is spared during cholera and other diarrheal diseases opened the way for safe, inexpensive, and effective oral replacement solutions. Glucose, amino acids, and small peptides, when absorbed by separate cotransport pathways of the intestine, carry with them sodium ions. Water and anions follow down the osmotic and electochemical gradients from the gut lumen to the bloodstream. Originally, oral rehydration solutions were based only on glucose. These remain very effective but do not diminish diarrheal fluid losses. The composition of available oral rehydration solutions is listed in Table 296–2, together with some standard intravenous solutions.

Intravenous fluid replacement should be reserved for neglected patients who have not received oral replacement and are in shock. In a cholera epidemic it is essential that all individuals at risk be thoroughly familiar with oral rehydration therapy and use it early to minimize deaths and the need for intravenous fluids. Thirst and urination are adequate guides to oral replacement therapy even in small children. This eliminates the need for accurate intake and output measurements and weighings, which even in excellent hospitals are difficult and are out of the question under epidemic conditions. Intravenous replacement for patients who are depleted and in shock should be given rapidly through a large-bore needle to ensure infusion rates of 50 to 100 ml per minute until a strong radial pulse has been achieved. Remaining fluid deficits may then be replaced less rapidly over 2 hours. The fluid deficit in a severely depleted patient is about 10% of body weight (for a 50-kg patient—5 liters). As soon as patients are strong enough to drink, oral rehydration therapy should begin, preferably with a rice- or other cereal-based solution of the proper solute composition. If this is done adequately, no further intravenous fluids are needed. In semicomatose patients who are unable to cooperate, nasogastric intubation permits adequate enteral replacement. For both intravenous and oral solutions the composition is crucial and should be within a range to properly replace losses of solutes and water (Table 296–2). It should be noted that many drinks ordinarily given to diarrhea patients are not adequate, although they may complement oral rehydration therapy. Vomiting is not a contraindication for oral rehydration therapy. However, fluids of high osmolarity should be avoided.

TABLE 296–1. TYPICAL CHEMICAL VALUES IN STOOL AND PLASMA FROM PATIENTS WITH SEVERE CHOLERA

| | | Plasma | |
	Stool	Untreated	Treated†
Sodium*	138 (105)	141	142
Chloride*	102 (90)	107	106
Potassium*	18 (25)	4.5	3.6
Bicarbonate*	45 (30)	9	21
Arterial pH	–	7.21	7.43
Plasma specific gravity	–	1.040	1.026

*Milliequivalents per liter. Stool values in parentheses are for children less than 10 hours old.

†Four hours after water and electrolyte replacement.

TABLE 296-2. CHOLERA AND ACUTE DIARRHEA TREATMENT SOLUTIONS (ORAL AND INTRAVENOUS)

	Substrate (g/L)	Na+	K+	Base* (millimoles/L)	Cl-	Osmolality
Oral						
WHO/UNICEF	20 (glucose)	90	20	30	80	330
Pedialyte	25 (glucose)	45	20	30	65	300
Rice solution	80 (rice)	90	20	30	80	240
Infalyte‡	30 (rice digest)	50	25	34	45	200
Ceralyte‡	40 (rice digest)	90	20	30	65	235
Intravenous						
Dhaka solution	0	134	13	48 (bicarbonate)	99	294
Ringer's†	0	130	4	28 (lactate)	109	271

*Citrate is generally used but bicarbonate is equally effective, and lactate or acetate are used in intravenous solutions.
†Also contains calcium, 3.0 mEq per liter.
‡Available as dried powder in packets.

If a commercial preparation of oral rehydration salts is not available, a home solution can be prepared. The safest and most effective of these is a thick but drinkable suspension prepared from rice or other suitable ground starchy foods. If precooked products are available, these are very convenient but not essential. To a quart of water with cereal thickly suspended, a half level teaspoon (one three-finger pinch of salt) is added and the mixture cooked only long enough to soften the ground cereal powder. The mixture should be used within 6 hours and may be taken warm or cold. In cholera it may be necessary to drink a great deal of fluid every hour for the first day. The patient must be offered a small cup every few minutes to minimize overloading the stomach and consequent vomiting. This is labor intensive but does not require medical skills. Especially in epidemics, family members and friends are the backbone of a successful treatment program.

In treating either children or adults, fluid therapy should be guided by thirst, observations on the circulation, urine output, and presence of edema or rales at the lung bases. Feeding is important and should be initiated immediately. Breast feeding is especially useful in affected infants, although few breast-fed babies contract cholera except in nonendemic areas where maternal milk lacks protective antibodies. Feeding should be with appetizing complex carbohydrates and proteins culturally adapted to the taste of the patient.

Adjunctive antibiotic therapy may be indicated. This varies with the epidemic strain, but tetracycline and doxycycline have been effective when resistance is not present. As with other Enterobacteriaceae, resistance arises quickly and must be monitored to avoid wasting high-cost antimicrobics that are neither crucial nor lifesaving in cholera. Antibiotic prophylaxis has not been useful and encourages the emergence of resistant strains.

PREVENTION. Safe water supplies and appropriate disposal of human waste prevent spread of cholera but may not be achievable. Rapid loss of large volumes require the use of special beds (cholera cots) or fecal conduits that avoid widespread dissemination into surrounding areas. *V. cholerae* is a fragile organism and cannot withstand drying, mild oxidation, or acid conditions. Thus a variety of disinfectants are effective for soiled articles. Bleaching powder is frequently used. Handwashing with soap before food handling is important. Patients suspected to have cholera should be reported to state health authorities by telephone or fax because of epidemic risks.

The available injected cholera vaccine is not useful, but there are effective killed bacterial and toxoid oral vaccines as well as very promising genetically altered live vaccines. At present, none of these is available commercially.

Addressing emerging infectious disease threats: Preventive strategy for the U.S. MMWR 43:1, 1994. *Emphasizes risks of emerging infectious diseases, including V. cholerae 0139 Bengal.*

Barua D, Greenough WB III: Cholera. New York, Plenum Scientific Publishing Co., 1992. *A broad review of all aspects of cholera.*

Wachsmuth IK, Blake PA, Olsvik O: *Vibrio choleroae* and Cholera Molecular and Global Perspectives. Washington, ASM Press, 1994. *Comprehensive, current review on new epidemic strains, epidemiology, and microbiology of cholera.*

Weber JT, Levine WC, Hopkins DP, Tauxe RV: Cholera in the United States 1965–1991: Risks at home and abroad. Arch Intern Med 184:55, 1994. *Summary of risks of cholera in the United States.*

297 ENTERIC *ESCHERICHIA COLI* INFECTIONS
Richard L. Guerrant

Escherichia coli is the predominant aerobic, coliform species in the normal colon. However, *E. coli* also can be an enteric pathogen and cause intestinal disease, usually diarrhea. Diarrhea caused by *E. coli* may be watery, inflammatory, or bloody, depending on which genetic codes for virulence traits the organism happens to possess. Consequently, diarrheogenic *E. coli* must be defined more specifically according to its virulence traits. Specific virulence traits determine the type of disease the organism causes, such as enterotoxigenic, enteroinvasive, enterohemorrhagic, enteropathogenic, or enteroadherent *E. coli* diarrhea. Each of these categories is being further resolved by the type of enterotoxin (such as the cholera-like, heat-labile toxin, LT, or the heat-stable toxin, ST) or adherence (such as close, localized, epithelial cell effacing, or diffuse) it causes. Taken separately, organisms such as enterotoxigenic *E. coli* constitute major bacterial causes of diarrhea morbidity and mortality on a global scale, particularly among children in tropical, developing areas and in travelers. Taken together, the varied types of *E. coli* diarrhea not only constitute the major category of bacterial enteric pathogens but also illustrate the wide array of ways that enteric pathogens can cause disease.

As noted in Table 297–1, at least three different types of *E. coli* enterotoxins may cause intestinal secretion (ETEC), others are enteroinvasive (EIEC), still others cause foodborne hemorrhagic colitis (EHEC) and produce large amounts of Shiga-like toxin (EHEC), while the classically recognized enteropathogenic *E. coli* (EPEC) serotypes are neither enterotoxigenic nor invasive but attach and efface the epithelium. Further information is emerging on additional types of enteroadherent *E. coli* that exhibit aggregating (EAggEC) or diffuse adherence (DAEC) traits and may be associated with prolonged diarrhea among children in tropical, developing areas.

ETIOLOGY. *E. coli* is a small, catalase-positive, oxidase-negative, gram-negative bacillus in the family Enterobacteriaceae. It characteristically reduces nitrates, ferments glucose and usually lactose, and is either motile (with peritrichate flagella) or nonmotile. It gives a positive methyl red reaction and negative reactions with Voges-Proskauer, urease, phenylalanine deaminase, and citrate agents. *E. coli* constitutes the predominant facultative gram-negative bacillus in the intestinal tract of humans and other mammals. As with other gram-negative organisms, the lipopolysaccharide cell wall contains lipid A and 2-keto-3-deoxyoctanate (KDO), a core glycolipid that has been used to develop vaccines that provide cross-protection against systemic infections with other gram-negative organisms. Smooth (S) forms of *E. coli* have O-specific carbohydrate chains attached to this core glycolipid to provide 169 O serogroups as well as at least 60 heat-labile protein flagellar (H) antigens by which strains are currently serotyped. Historically, some 80 variably heat-labile capsular (K) antigens also have been described (L, B, and A), not to mention the more recently appreciated numerous adherence, enterotoxin, cytotoxin, and invasiveness factors that may be gained or lost by a particular serotype, since they are characteristically encoded on transmissible genetic elements such as plasmids or bacteriophages. Consequently, this common inhabitant of the normal human intestinal tract becomes a pathogen when it houses one or more specific traits contributing to its colonization and virulence in the intestinal tract. Other traits such as O and H serogroup also may be important for certain enteropathogenic and enteroinvasive organisms. For reasons that remain obscure, only a few O serogroups tend to predominate in the normal human colon (O groups 1, 2, 4, 6, 7, 8, 18, 25, 45, 75, and 81), while others noted in Table 297–1 tend (albeit not absolutely) to be associated with specific virulence traits and thus different types of pathogenesis in the intestine. The O antigens of invasive *E. coli* often cross-react with various *Shigella* species, suggesting further that, in addition to the 140-MDa plasmid, serotype also has a role in pathogenesis.

EPIDEMIOLOGY. Enteric *E. coli* infections are essentially acquired by the fecal-oral route, reflecting primarily a human reservoir for most recognized types of *E. coli* enteropathogens. Enterotoxigenic *E. coli* is also an important veterinary pathogen, especially in calves and piglets. However, the attachment traits of animal strains are different from those that infect humans and likely substantially influence their epidemiology.

The infectious doses of enterotoxigenic *E. coli* and enteroinvasive *E. coli* have been determined in volunteers to be 10^6 to 10^8, numbers that usually require multiplication in contaminated food or water vehicles for their transmission. Heavy contamination with enterotoxigenic *E. coli* has been documented in foods prepared in homes, restaurants, and at street vendors as well as in drinking water in many tropical areas, and contaminated water and foods likely represent the major sources of its acquisition, primarily in the warm or wet season. In the United States, major outbreaks of water- or food-borne *E. coli* diarrhea of different types have been documented in the last 10 to 15 years. A large waterborne outbreak of diarrhea at a popular national park was found to be caused by enterotoxigenic *E. coli* (ETEC), and a widespread outbreak of enteroinvasive *E. coli* (EIEC) enteritis was traced to consumption of French Camembert cheese. More recently, bloody, noninflammatory diarrhea has been increasingly associated with enterohemorrhagic *E.*

coli (EHEC) (O157) in rare hamburgers in several fast-food chains. EHEC infections are especially alarming because they are increasing in frequency and may cause hemolytic-uremic syndrome, which can be fatal despite antimicrobial therapy. Occasional nosocomial outbreaks of enterotoxigenic *E. coli* and enteropathogenic *E. coli* serotypes (EPEC) also have occurred in hospitalized infants in the United States and other industrialized countries.

As with most diarrheal illnesses, the highest age-specific attack rates of enterotoxigenic *E. coli* infections are in young children, especially at the time of weaning, when enterotoxigenic *E. coli* account for 15 to 50% of illnesses. Like immunologically inexperienced young children, the traveler visiting tropical areas has a 30 to 50% chance of acquiring travelers' diarrhea over a 2- to 3-week stay unless untreated water or ice and uncooked foods such as salads are strictly avoided. The most commonly recognized pathogen associated with travelers' diarrhea around the world is enterotoxigenic *E. coli* that produces either the STa, LT, or both enterotoxins (see Ch. 298).

Of potential immunologic significance is the continued occurrence of symptomatic infections with *E. coli* which produce the less immunogenic STa in adult residents of tropical or other areas endemic for enterotoxigenic *E. coli* infections. In contrast, adult residents in endemic areas often carry LT-producing *E. coli* asymptomatically, suggesting that they may be protected from symptoms, if not from colonization.

Limited data on invasive *E. coli* suggest that the infectious doses are relatively high. As with enterotoxigenic *E. coli* infections, such large numbers have been readily spread in food with high attack rates. Enteropathogenic *E. coli* have been recognized primarily in urban areas, especially among hospitalized infants in their first year of life, with apparent cross-infection in hospital nurseries. While sporadic cases still occur, nosocomial outbreaks of EPEC diarrhea during the summer appear to have become less common and less severe in industrialized countries in the last decade or two.

PATHOGENESIS AND PATHOLOGY. The pathogenesis of enteric *E. coli* infections begins with the ingestion of the organism in contaminated food or water, which then faces the normal gastric acid barrier. Both enterotoxigenic *E. coli* and enteroinvasive *E. coli* appear to be sensitive to gastric acid; neutralization by gastric acid

TABLE 297–1. DIFFERENT TYPES OF ENTERIC *E. COLI* INFECTIONS

Type	Mechanism	Predominant O Serogroups	Genetic Code	Detection	Clinical Syndromes
Enterotoxigenic E. coli (ETEC)					
1. Cholera-like, heat-labile toxin (LT)	Activates intestinal adenylate cyclase and adhesin fimbriae	6, 8, 11, 15, 20, 25, 27, 63, 80, 85, 139	Plasmid	ELISA, RIA, PIH, CHO, Y1 cells, 18 h loops, gene probe	Watery diarrhea, travelers' diarrhea
2. Heat-stable toxin (STa: STh or STp)	Activates intestinal guanylate cyclase and adhesin fimbriae	12, 78, 115, 148, 149, 153, 155, 166, 167	Plasmid (transposon)	ELISA, RIA, suckling mice, 6 h loops, gene probes	Watery diarrhea, travelers' diarrhea
3. Heat-stable toxin (STb)	?; Not cAMP or cGMP		Plasmid	Piglet loops, gene probe	?
Enteroinvasive E. coli (EIEC)					
4. Enteroinvasive E. coli (EIEC)	Cell invasion and spread	11, 28ac, 29, 124, 136, 144, 147, 152, 164, 167	Plasmid (140 MDa, pWR110)	Sereny test, gene probe, (lys⁻, NM, oft. lactose⁻)	Inflammatory dysentery
Enterohemorrhagic E. coli (EHEC)					
5. Enterohemorrhagic (EHEC)	Shiga-like toxin(s) and adhesin fimbriae	26, 39, 113, 121, 128, 139, 145, 157, occ 55, 111	Phage(s) & adhesin plasmid(s)	Serotype, HeLa, Vero cells, sorbitol, agar, SLT or eae gene probes	Bloody noninflammatory diarrhea; hemolytic-uremic syndrome
Enteropathogenic E. coli (EPEC)					
6. Focal attaching and effacing EPEC	Attach, then efface the mucosa	55, 111, 119, 125, 126, 127, 128, 142, 158,	Plasmid (60 MDa, pMAR2) + Chromosomal (eae and cfm)	Serotype, focal HEp2 adhesion, gene probes for EAF or eae	Infantile diarrhea
Enteroadherent E. coli					
7. Enteroaggregating E. coli (EAggEC)	Colonize (bundle-forming pili) ? toxins (EAST, EALT)	3, 15, 44, 51, 77, 78, 91	Plasmid	HEp2 cell adherence; AA probe	Persistent diarrhea
8. Diffusely adherent E. coli (DAEC)	Colonize (F 1845 fimbriate adhesin)	75 (F 1845), 15 (57-1), ? (189)	Chromosomal/ plasmid	HEp2 cell adherence; DA gene probe	Persistent diarrhea in children > 18 mos. old

reduces the infectious dose by 100- to 1000-fold. This is followed by an incubation period of 2 to 7 days, during which colonization of the involved part of the intestinal tract and enterotoxin production or invasion take place. Best characterized is the colonization by enterotoxigenic *E. coli* in the upper small bowel, which involves one of at least five major colonization factor antigen groups (which are fimbriate or fibrillar protein structures on the surface of the organism). The colonization fimbriae bind the organism to cell surface receptors in the upper small bowel where the enterotoxin is delivered to reduce normal absorption and cause net electrolyte and water secretion. The heat-labile toxin (LT) with a molecular weight of about 86,000 has a binding and active subunit that, like choleratoxin, binds to a monosialoganglioside (Gm1) receptor. Also like choleratoxin, the active subunit ADP-ribosylates the regulatory subunit of adenylate cyclase to activate adenylate cyclase. The consequently increased chloride secretion and reduced sodium absorption combine to cause net isotonic electrolyte loss that must be replaced to prevent severe dehydration and hypotension and its potential consequences. Other strains produce the heat-stable toxin (STa), a much smaller molecule of 18 to 19 amino acids (molecular weight less than 2000), which activates intestinal particulate guanylate cyclase. Like cyclic AMP, the cyclic GMP thus formed also causes net secretion. A third type of *E. coli* enterotoxin (STb) causes secretion in porcine intestine without activating adenylate or guanylate cyclase; STb has no known role in human disease. Similarly, the roles of enterotoxins such as LTII, EAST, EIET, and others seen in ETEC, EAggEC, and EIEC, respectively, are unclear at present. Both the colonization traits and enterotoxin production are encoded on transmissible plasmids. Besides the complications of dehydration, the only significant pathologic change is depletion of mucus from intestinal goblet cells.

Other *E. coli*, often of certain serogroups noted in Table 297–1, have the capacity, analogous to *Shigella*, to invade and multiply in epithelial cells, cause conjunctivitis in guinea pigs (Sereny test), and cause inflammatory colitis and dysenteric or bloody diarrhea. As seen with shigellosis, a striking inflammatory response is seen, with sheets of polymorphonuclear leukocytes in the stool. The colon shows patchy, acute inflammation in the mucosa and submucosa with focal denuding of the surface epithelium but usually without deeper invasion or systemic spread. While epithelial cell invasiveness in both enteroinvasive *E. coli* and *Shigella* appears to be encoded on a large 120- to 140-MDa plasmid, several chromosomal determinants, including the O antigen, are crucial for full invasive virulence.

Classically recognized enteropathogenic *E. coli* serotypes often fail to produce known enterotoxins or to be invasive. Nevertheless, they are well-established causes of infantile diarrhea. The majority of classically recognized EPEC serotypes such as O55 and O111 exhibit both plasmid-encoded localized adherence to epithelial cells and chromosomally mediated attachment and effacement of the microvilli. There is also villus atrophy, mucosal thinning, inflammation in the lamina propria, and variable crypt cell hyperplasia. These morphologic changes are associated with a reduction in the mucosal brush border enzymes and may contribute to the impaired absorptive function and diarrhea.

Other *E. coli*, most notably serotype O157:H7 but also serogroups O26 and 39, are associated with foodborne outbreaks of bloody, noninflammatory diarrhea and with the hemolytic-uremic syndrome. These organisms produce Shiga-like toxins that may be responsible for the characteristic colonic mucosal inflammation, edema, and hemorrhage, as well as the complication of hemolytic-uremic syndrome. Sigmoidoscopy usually reveals only moderately hyperemic mucosa, and barium enema may reveal a thumbprint pattern of submucosal edema in the ascending and transverse colon. Some patients have superficial ulceration with mild neutrophil infiltration in the edematous submucosa. The mechanisms by which EAggEC (which adhere in an aggregative pattern to the mucosa and produce heat-stable and heat-labile "toxins"), DAEC, or colonization alone may cause diarrhea remain unclear at present.

CLINICAL MANIFESTATIONS. The most common clinical manifestation of enteric *E. coli* infections is the watery diarrhea that characterizes enterotoxigenic *E. coli* infections, particularly in young children and travelers to tropical or developing areas. This may range from mild to severe, cholera-like diarrhea that may be life-threatening, especially in small children and elderly patients, who are particularly prone to suffer the most severe consequences of dehydration, undernutrition, and electrolyte imbalance (especially hypokalemia and acidosis).

The incubation period (2 to 7 days) varies with the size of the inoculum. Characteristic symptoms include malaise, abdominal cramping, anorexia, and watery diarrhea, occasionally associated with nausea, vomiting, or low-grade fever. The illness is usually self-limited to 1 to 5 days and rarely extends beyond 10 days or 2 weeks. Infections with *E. coli* which produce both ST and LT or ST alone may be more severe than those with only LT-producing *E. coli*. The persistence of impaired mucosal absorptive capacity for 1 to 3 weeks may further compound the cycle of malnutrition that complicates diarrheal illnesses in children in developing, tropical areas.

Infection with EIEC is characterized by inflammatory colitis, often with abdominal pain, high fever, tenesmus, and bloody or dysenteric diarrhea essentially like that seen with *Shigella*, to which this organism is closely related. The incubation period is usually 1 to 3 days with the duration usually self-limited to 7 to 10 days.

Outbreaks of EPEC infections in newborn nurseries have ranged from mild transient diarrhea to severe and rapidly fatal diarrheal illnesses, especially in premature or otherwise compromised infants. The more severe illnesses appear to have been more common in industrialized countries prior to 1950. However, more recent outbreaks and sporadic cases are well documented.

Hemorrhagic colitis associated with the Shiga-like toxin producing *E. coli* (EHEC) O157:H7 or O26:H11 is characterized by grossly bloody diarrhea with remarkably little fever or inflammatory exudate in the stool. Although the diarrheal illnesses have been self-limited, a significant number of children and adults have subsequently developed a potentially fatal hemolytic-uremic syndrome. Outbreaks of hemorrhagic colitis due to EHEC in nursing homes or other institutions may be quite severe and more common than previously appreciated. The incubation period in two outbreaks has been 3 to 4 days (range 1 to 7 days), and the illness is characteristically self-limited to 5 to 12 days (mean 7.8).

Enteroaggregative and diffusely adherent *E. coli* have been associated with persistent diarrhea in children in developing areas.

DIAGNOSIS. A definitive etiologic diagnosis of *E. coli* diarrhea requires the documentation of a specific virulence trait such as enterotoxin, invasiveness, enteroadherence, or serotype, which usually requires specialized immunologic, tissue culture, animal bioassay, or gene probes that are available only in research and reference laboratories. Such tests are rarely cost-effective or clinically indicated, except in outbreak or research situations. Fortunately, a likely diagnosis often can be suspected by the clinical and epidemiologic setting. For example, self-limited, noninflammatory diarrhea in tropical, developing areas is most likely due to enterotoxigenic *E. coli*, rotaviruses (young children), or Norwalk-like viruses (older children and adults). Noninflammatory diarrhea in winter months in temperate areas in older children or younger adults is more likely to be due to Norwalk-like viruses. Specific tests for the respective virulence traits of different types of *E. coli* are noted in Table 297–1. One should also consider *Vibrio* infections in areas endemic for cholera or in any coastal area where inadequately cooked seafood may be eaten. If noninflammatory diarrhea persists, especially with weight loss, one also should consider *Giardia lamblia* or *Cryptosporidium* infection. In outbreaks of food poisoning, *S. aureus*, *Clostridium perfringens*, and *Bacillus cereus* should be considered.

Inflammatory colitis with high fever, tenesmus, and leukocytes, mucus, and blood in the stool may well be due to enteroinvasive *E. coli* but should prompt a stool culture for more common invasive pathogens such as *Campylobacter jejuni*, *Shigella*, and *Salmonella* or even *Clostridium difficile*, *Yersina enterocolitica*, or noncholera *Vibrio* (see Ch. 295). On the other hand, bloody diarrhea without high fever and few, if any, fecal leukocytes should prompt consideration of the Shiga-like toxin producing enterohemorrhagic *E. coli* (EHEC) such as strain O157:H7. This organism is often suspected as a sorbitol-negative *E. coli*, which may require further study for serotype or Shiga-like toxin production.

THERAPY. As with all diarrheal illnesses, the primary treatment is replacement and maintenance of water and electrolytes. Losses of water and electrolytes may be particularly severe and even life-threatening with enterotoxigenic *E. coli* and can usually be replaced with a simple oral rehydration solution that uses the intact, sodium-coupled glucose, and/or amino acid absorption to replace fluid losses, as described in Ch. 296. This oral rehydration solution should be given *ad libitum* with free water and, in breast-fed infants, continued breast feeding and early refeeding to compensate for the nutritional losses.

Because most *E. coli* diarrhea is self-limited, the role of antimicrobial agents is debated and remains of secondary importance to rehydration. In areas where the enterotoxigenic *E. coli* remains sensitive, early initiation of sulfamethoxazole-trimethoprim, tetracycline, or new quinolone derivatives may reduce a 3- to 5-day illness to a 1- to 2-day illness if started with the first loose stool in travelers to endemic, tropical areas (see Ch. 298). The use of antimotility agents should be tempered by the potential added risk of worsening or prolonging inflammatory diarrheas and by their lack of effectiveness in reducing fluid loss even though abdominal cramping and overt diarrhea may be temporarily reduced. Because of the potential severity of the disease in infants, some pediatricians use neomycin, 100 mg per kilogram per day PO, divided into three daily doses for 5 days, for documented enteropathogenic *E. coli* infections in neonates. Bismuth subsalicylate may reduce symptoms in travelers' diarrhea but should be used with caution to avoid toxic doses of salicylate. A number of pharmacologic agents enhance absorption or reduce secretion with experimental diarrhea but remain inadequately studied or too toxic for recommended use to date.

The role of antimicrobial agents in treating EHEC infections or in preventing serious complications is controversial. The treatment of hemolytic-uremic syndrome may require plasma exchange as well.

PROGNOSIS. The overall prognosis in *E. coli* diarrheas of the various types noted, if fully and adequately treated, is generally excellent. However, the impact of *E. coli* and other common diarrheas on mortality and morbidity (particularly with repeated infections compounding malnutrition in young children) remains one of the major health problems on a global scale; this problem may actually be worsening in some transitional areas. The potentially serious complication of hemolytic-uremic syndrome may follow EHEC infection.

PREVENTION. The prevention of many *E. coli* enteric infections is ultimately related to basic economic development and adequate sanitary facilities and wide availability of sufficient quality and quantity of water. In the interim, especially in areas where adequate water supplies and sanitary facilities are not available, such measures as breast feeding for at least 6 to 12 months and hygienic measures like handwashing should reduce the likelihood of acquiring *E. coli* enteric infections. Travelers to developing or tropical areas should avoid drinking untreated or unboiled water or ice and eating uncooked fruits or vegetables that may have been "freshened" with highly contaminated water. Although a number of antimicrobial agents have been documented to be effective over short periods of time when taken prophylactically, their effectiveness is sharply limited by the rapidly emerging resistance to antimicrobial drugs as well as by the potential side effects of their indiscriminate, widespread use. For example, tetracycline resistance among enterotoxigenic *E. coli* is common, and combined sulfamethoxazole-trimethroprim resistance is rapidly emerging around the world. Finally, currently developing toxoid or colonization factor vaccines hold considerable promise for the prevention of enterotoxigenic *E. coli* diarrhea. EHEC infections can be largely prevented by adequately cooking beef, especially hamburgers, and by careful handwashing and other hygienic measures in day care centers and nursing homes.

Bhan MK, Raj P, Levine MM, et al.: Enteroaggregative *Escherichia coli* associated with persistent diarrhea in a cohort of rural children in India. J Infect Dis 159:1060, 1989. *A first report of a clinical role for new types of enteroadherent* E. coli.

Carter AO, Borczyk AA, Carlson AK, et al.: A severe outbreak of *E. coli* O157:H7 associated hemorrhagic colitis in a nursing home. N Engl J Med 317:1496, 1987. *A common source outbreak with secondary, probable person-to-person spread, of this cause of bloody diarrhea and hemolytic-uremic syndrome in the institutionalized elderly.*

Donnenberg MS, Kaper JB: Enteropathogenic *Escherichia coli.* Infect Immun 60:3953, 1992. *Excellent overview of recent advances regarding the pathogenesis of enteropathogenic* E. coli *infections.*

Griffin PM, Tauxe RV: The epidemiology of infections caused by *Escherichia coli* O157:H7 and other enterohemorrhagic *E. coli* and the associated hemolytic uremic syndrome. Epidemiol Rev 13:60, 1991. *Excellent review of the increasing problem of enterohemorrhagic* E. coli *infections and complications, often associated with rare hamburger and other foods and also seen in day care centers and institutions.*

Guerrant RL, Kirchhoff LV, Shields DS, et al.: Prospective study of diarrheal illnesses in northeastern Brazil: Patterns of disease, nutritional impact, etiologies and risk factors. J Infect Dis 148:986, 1983. *A detailed study of endemic diarrhea in a tropical area, including seasonality, risk after weaning, and nutritional impact, as well as relationship of enterotoxigenic* E. coli *to other pathogens.*

Guerrant RL, Hughes JM, Lima NL, Crane JK: Diarrhea in developed and developing countries: Magnitude, special settings and etiologies. Rev Infect Dis 12:S41, 1990. *Overview of community-based and hospital-based studies of diarrhea that reviews the relative importance of* E. coli *among other pathogens in developing and developed countries.*

Levine MM: *Escherichia coli* that cause diarrhea: Enterotoxigenic, Enteropathogenic, Enterohemorrhagic, and Enteroadherent. J Infect Dis 155:377, 1989. *A good overview of major pathogenic mechanisms of* E. coli *diarrhea.*

Microbial Toxins and Diarrheal Diseases. CIBA Foundation Symposium No. 112, 1985. *Thorough review of the mechanisms of enterotoxin action, relating the pharmacology of* E. coli *toxins (LT, STa, STb, Shiga) to those of such enteric pathogens as* V. cholerae, Shigella, *and* C. difficile.

NIH Consensus Development Conference on Traveler's Diarrhea. JAMA 253:2700, 1985. *A balanced critical appraisal of the epidemiology, etiologies, presentation, and treatment of travelers' diarrhea.*

Sansonetti PJ, Hale TL, Oaks EV: Genetics of virulence in enteroinvasive *Escherichia coli.* Microbiology, 1985, pp 67–82. *One of a series of three brief reviews that offer considerable new information on pathogenesis of the major types of* E. coli *enteric infection including ETEC, EIEC, EPEC, and EHEC.*

Thielman NM, Guerrant RL: *Escherichia coli. In* Emmerson AM, Hawkey PM, Gillespie SH (eds.); Principles and Practices of Clinical Bacteriology, New York, John Wiley & Sons, 1994. *Concise overview of 6 to 10 types of* E. coli *pathogenesis with update on new clinical and pathogenic studies of different types of* E. coli *pathogens.*

298 THE DIARRHEA OF TRAVELERS

R. Bradley Sack

Travelers from the developed world who visit the developing world are highly susceptible to an acute infectious diarrheal illness known as "travelers' diarrhea" or by more colorful names that fit the locale in which the travelers find themselves incapacitated. The etiologic agents of this syndrome are the same as those which cause endemic diarrheal illness, primarily in children, throughout the areas of the world in which sanitation is less than optimal. Travelers (see Ch. 268) from sanitized, developed countries are in a sense immunologically naive "children" who are suddenly transported to an endemic area of infection, where they are highly susceptible to the local pathogens. Other than during a common-source outbreak of diarrheal disease (such as a gross fecal contamination of a water supply), the attack rates among travelers are the highest known in any identifiable population. Approximately 25 to 50% of travelers will experience a diarrheal illness during their first 3 weeks of stay in a developing country; this will decrease markedly thereafter as immunity develops.

By way of contrast, travelers from developing countries who visit other developing countries usually have a considerably lower attack rate owing to their prior exposure and subsequent immunity to these organisms. As expected, these same visitors who visit the developed world do not develop the illness.

ETIOLOGY. Multiple studies have described the causes of this syndrome throughout the world, and it is clear that enterotoxigenic *Escherichia coli* is the most common pathogen. Other bacteria, viruses, and protozoa are also involved but with lesser frequency (Table 298–1). In certain localities and in certain seasons, the prevalence of *Campylobacter* or *Salmonella* may be particularly high. Even now, a considerable proportion of episodes (20 to 30%) cannot be diagnosed microbiologically, and new etiologic organisms continue to be discovered. Contrary to "popular" notions, relatively few cases of travelers' diarrhea are caused by *Entamoeba histolytica* or other protozoa.

PATHOGENESIS AND CLINICAL PICTURE. The clinical syndrome of travelers' diarrhea is typically that of a nonfebrile, secretory, watery diarrhea that is produced by the enterotoxins of bacteria, particularly *E. coli* (see Ch. 297). The watery diarrhea usually lasts 3 to 4 days and, when most severe, may result in 15 to 20 evacuations per day, with significant water and electrolyte loss, leading to clinical signs of dehydration. The vast majority of ill-

TABLE 298-1. ETIOLOGIC AGENTS OF TRAVELERS' DIARRHEA

Agent	Percentage
Enterotoxigenic *E. coli*	30–70
Shigella	5–10
*Salmonella**	< 5
*Campylobacter**	< 5
Enteroadherent *E. coli*	5–10
Rotavirus	< 5
Giardia lamblia	< 5
Entamoeba histolytica	< 3
Cryptosporidium	< 5
Cyclospora	< 1
Unknown agents	20–30

* May be higher in certain geographic areas.

nesses are much milder, however, consisting of only 3 to 5 diarrheal stools per day, and are important primarily because they limit the activities of the traveler. Episodes due to invasive bacteria, such as *Shigella* or *Campylobacter,* may be dysentery-like in nature, with abdominal pain, fever, and blood in the stool (see Ch. 294).

Nearly all episodes are self-limited, but a few (<1%) may become persistent and require evaluation after the return home. Some of these prolonged episodes may be due to infection with *Cyclospora,* a newly recognized cyanobacterium-like organism.

TRANSMISSION. Transmission of the enteric pathogens occurs almost exclusively through fecally contaminated food and water. Of highest risk to the traveler are foods that are not cooked or peeled, foods obtained from roadside vendors, or foods kept unrefrigerated for long periods of time.

PREVENTION. Since the modes of transmission are known, prudent attention to the ingestion of uncontaminated food and water should entirely prevent the disease. This has been shown in the military or on board cruise ships, where all food is hygienically prepared and packaged. For the usual traveler, however, food must be obtained from local sources, and contamination cannot be entirely prevented. Even the "best" hotels in the developing world may have unsanitary kitchens, and "first class" travelers are therefore not exempt.

Many studies have now shown that a number of drugs can prevent 75 to 90% of diarrheal episodes when taken regularly during short-term travel (<3 weeks). Medication is begun on the day before reaching the locale and discontinued on the day after leaving. The antimicrobials that have been well studied are shown in Table 298–2. Doxycycline, which was the earliest antimicrobial shown to be effective, is no longer recommended because of marked increase in antibiotic resistance of enterotoxigenic *E. coli.* Because the antibacterial spectrum of the fluoroquinolones includes *Campylobacter,* these drugs provide the broadest spectrum of antibacterial coverage against the disease. A nonantimicrobial drug, bismuth sub-salicylate (BSS), taken four times a day also has given a significant but lesser degree (approximately 60%) of protection. Other antimicrobial drugs also have been used successfully (erythromycin, mecillinam, trimethoprim alone) but have not been tested as extensively.

Drugs that have been tested and found to be of little or no benefit include neomycin, streptotriad, hydroxyquinolines, and *Lactobacillus* preparations.

TABLE 298-2. PREVENTION AND TREATMENT OF TRAVELERS' DIARRHEA WITH ANTIMICROBIALS

Antimicrobial	Prevention* Daily Dose (mg)	Treatment† Dose (mg)	Treatment† Duration‡ (days)
Trimethoprim-sulfamethoxazole	160/800	160–800 bid	3
Norfloxacin	400	400 bid	3
Ciprofloxacin	500	500 bid	3

* For periods up to 3 weeks.
† Loperamide given along with antimicrobials has given further improvement.
‡ Some studies have shown larger doses given as only a single dose to be effective.

THERAPY. Therapy is usually carried out by the patient, who must be able to recognize when to take the medication. Instructions for therapy should be given by the traveler's physician, who must be familiar with the disease. One aim of self-treatment is to avoid consultation by the traveler of local physicians (or diagnostic laboratories) for advice and medications. Therapy includes specific fluid replacement when indicated, specific antimicrobial therapy directed against the most likely causative agents, and, if necessary, symptomatic therapy directed at relieving the frequency of stooling and abdominal cramps.

Fluids may be replaced by increasing the amount of liquids ingested, such as soup and fruit juices, if the diarrhea is mild. For more severe diarrhea, an oral glucose electrolyte solution (ORS), which has been developed to treat all dehydrating diarrheas regardless of etiologic agent or age of the patient, should be taken. ORS is now available commercially in packets; the traveler can carry and use them as required by mixing the contents with appropriate volumes of potable water.

In many controlled studies, a short course (1 to 3 days) of appropriate antimicrobials has been shown to significantly shorten the disease to approximately 24 to 36 hours. The most widely used drugs (shown in Table 298–2) are also the ones that have been shown to be effective in prevention. In addition, some of the newer fluoroquinolones (oflaxacin, fleroxacin) and aztreonam have been shown to be equally effective.

Symptomatic therapy with antimotility agents, such as loperamide, may be useful for travelers who need to participate in certain vital events during which the need to evacuate frequently would be embarrassing and particularly inconvenient, such as during long bus rides or while giving lectures. The combination of loperamide with an effective antimicrobial has been shown to resolve the illness more quickly than would the antimicrobial alone.

BSS also has been shown to give significant but less striking symptomatic improvement, although the exact mechanism of action is unknown. Kaolin/pectin preparations are of no significant effect in treatment.

THE STRATEGY OF MANAGING TRAVELERS' DIARRHEA. Whether to give antimicrobials prophylactically or to rely on early patient-initiated treatment is the major question in management. The decisions should be based on the following considerations. It is known that all persons who travel to developing countries, regardless of whether they are taking antimicrobials, have an alteration in their microbial gut flora, which includes acquiring antibiotic-resistant bacteria. Antimicrobials are widely available without prescription in most developing countries and are used widely; therefore, the contribution of tourists taking antibiotics to the local microbial ecology is probably negligible. The real concern of giving antimicrobials prophylactically is side effects. Although adverse effects are known to be infrequent, some travelers will experience these when large numbers of persons are taking drugs. Contraindications include known allergies, pregnancy, and age. Therefore, the following suggestions are made when considering prophylaxis: Travelers should be on short-term visits (<3 weeks), they should request the use of antimicrobials, and they should be able to understand and accept the risk of side effects. Certain travelers with medical illnesses, for whom an episode of diarrhea would be particularly deleterious, also may be given special consideration for prophylaxis. The more widely recommended strategy is to have the traveler carry the medicines and self-administer them on recognition of the onset of illness.

The problem of travelers' diarrhea will continue until the general sanitation of the developing world approaches that of industrialized countries or until effective vaccines against the major diarrheal pathogens become available. Neither of these is expected soon; therefore, this common syndrome will need to be addressed for some time. Fortunately, this can now be done rationally and effectively based on our knowledge of causes and modes of transmission.

Black RE: Epidemiology of travelers' diarrhea and relative importance of various pathogens. Rev Infect Dis 12(suppl. 1):S73, 1990. *A summary of many studies worldwide on causes identified in persons with travelers' diarrhea.*

Consensus Conference: Travelers' diarrhea. JAMA 253:2700, 1985. *A summary of the NIH conference in which all aspects of the problem were reviewed; a complete publication of the conference is given in Rev Infect Dis 8(suppl. 2), 1986.*

DuPont HL, Ericsson CD: Prevention and treatment of travelers' diarrhea. N Engl J Med 328:1821, 1993. *A recent review of the problem with an extensive discussion of management options.*

299 EXTRAINTESTINAL INFECTIONS CAUSED BY ENTERIC BACTERIA

Elizabeth J. Ziegler

Bacteria constitute over half the dry weight of stool. *Bacteroides* species far outnumber other genera, at 10^{12} organisms per gram. Other anaerobes such as fusobacteria, clostridia, and peptostreptococci also are abundant. Among the facultative bacteria, members of the family Enterobacteriaceae predominate, at about 10^9 organisms per gram. Pseudomonads, enterococci, other nonhemolytic streptococci, and yeasts are present as well.

These bacteria that normally inhabit the human gastrointestinal tract perform important functions beneficial to the host. *Bacteroides fragilis,* clostridia, and enterococci deconjugate bile acids for participation in fat metabolism. Some intestinal bacteria synthesize menaquinone, or vitamin K, a cofactor for blood coagulation. Normal gut flora discourage colonization of the bowel with primary pathogens and overgrowth of bacteria usually present in small numbers. Colonization resistance is not understood completely, but it must involve bacteriocins, regulation of local oxidation-reduction potential, competition for receptors, and balance of nutrients as well as unknown factors. Breakdown of colonization resistance is illustrated by the increase in susceptibility of antibiotic-treated animals to *Salmonella* and by the emergence of fecal *Pseudomonas aeruginosa* and *Candida* in patients receiving antimicrobial agents.

PATHOGENESIS OF INFECTIONS

Enteric bacteria are not primary pathogens but cause disease when they escape from their usual gastrointestinal habitat. Direct penetration of the bowel wall by surgical, traumatic, or spontaneous rupture spills fecal contents into the peritoneal cavity and into open wounds. Gut bacteria on the perineal skin gain access to the urinary tract and proliferate there, especially when the flushing action of urine flow is disrupted by mechanical obstruction or neurologic dysfunction. When the biliary tract is obstructed by gallstones or tumor, the upper small bowel, which normally is sterile, becomes colonized with facultative bacteria (*Escherichia coli, Klebsiella,* enterococci) or, less often, with *Bacteroides* and *Clostridium,* which then infect the gallbladder and bile ducts. Intestinal flora can be introduced into the respiratory tract from contaminated skin or the environment; they proliferate there under the influence of antibiotics and loss of fibronectin and in the presence of underlying pulmonary disease and tracheal instrumentation. Penetrating foreign bodies, such as intravenous catheters and intraventricular cerebral pressure monitors, become colonized by gut flora on the skin and in respiratory secretions and then induce infection in adjacent tissues. In burns, destruction of the skin barrier, the rich culture medium of oozing tissue fluid, and a shift of surface flora by application of local and systemic antibacterial agents result in local necrotizing infection of the burn wound with gut flora and frequent secondary gram-negative bacteremia.

In the absence of mechanical and surface abnormalities such as those outlined above, systemic resistance to enteric bacteria is very strong. The mainstay of this resistance is the polymorphonuclear neutrophil, destruction or malfunction of which leads almost inevitably to bloodstream invasion by bowel bacteria. Serum complement must be protective against invasion of some organisms, since very few of the gram-negative bacilli isolated from blood are sensitive to complement-mediated bacteriolysis, whereas many enteric rods in feces are susceptible. Newborn infants, whose neutrophils and complement activity have not fully matured, are at high risk for disseminated infections with facultative enteric rods. Microbial factors are important, too. Although anaerobes predominate over facultative bacteria and aerobes in the gut, these anaerobes rarely cause bacteremia or metastatic infection even in neutropenia. The presence of certain bacterial polysaccharide capsules (e.g., *E. coli* K1) or production of large amounts of capsule (e.g., by *Klebsiella pneu-*

moniae in hyperglycemic or glycosuric diabetics) predisposes to systemic invasion by these organisms.

Infections with enteric bacteria have increased dramatically during the past four decades. The reasons should be apparent from the foregoing discussion. Advances in surgical and intensive care, trauma and burn management, blood transfusion, antimicrobial and cancer chemotherapy, transplantation, and immunosuppression all create opportunities for these infections. The average lifespan has lengthened, so that those receiving medical attention carry the added risks of advanced age. Many extraintestinal infections with enteric bacteria now arise in the hospital, and they exact a high toll in mortality and increased hospital costs. Furthermore, they jeopardize the success of the advanced treatments we have worked so hard to develop. Therefore, physicians should understand the pathogenesis of each infection so that they can effect a cure and prevent recurrence if possible.

SPECIFIC INFECTIONS WITH ENTERIC BACTERIA

The diagnosis and management of each of the following gram-negative infections are discussed in depth in the appropriate section elsewhere in the textbook. A few points are emphasized here.

PERITONITIS (see Ch. 111). It can be difficult to recover bacteria from patients with spontaneous bacterial peritonitis; large volumes of fluid should be submitted for culture. Patients undergoing chronic peritoneal dialysis frequently develop peritonitis. If the same organism is isolated from repeated episodes and especially if it is an enteric rod or *Pseudomonas,* infection of the subcutaneous catheter tunnel should be suspected. A radiolabeled white blood cell scan can be helpful in detecting such infections so that the infected catheter can be removed.

PYELONEPHRITIS (see Ch. 84). Urinary tract infections localized to the bladder or kidneys can have important implications for therapy. Symptoms may be misleading, selective ureteral catheterization carries considerable risk, and examination of urine for antibody-coated bacteria is not practical in most laboratories. A simple culture technique can differentiate between upper and lower urinary tract infections in difficult cases in which parenteral antibiotics would be required for kidney infection. In brief, the test employs a newly placed three-way bladder catheter through which a combination antibiotic and enzyme mixture (fibrinolysin and DNaase) is instilled to sterilize the bladder. Neomycin is used for most organisms; polymyxin can be used for *Pseudomonas* and amphotericin for yeast. Bladder instillation is followed by a large-volume sterile water wash. Then the catheter is clamped, and three 10-minute specimens are collected. Increasing bacterial counts after the wash point to pyelonephritis. If infection is limited to the bladder, this procedure can cure it. The test is unreliable in patients with low urinary output, and it should not be performed in those with neutropenia.

PROSTATITIS (see Ch. 209.2). Most antibiotics available for treating infections with enteric bacilli do not penetrate the prostate well. For this reason, chronic prostatitis rarely is cured. However, the role of chronic prostatitis as a nidus of recurrent acute urinary tract infection in males can be curbed by low levels of suppressive antibiotics in bladder urine, achieved by a single tablet of an oral antibiotic given daily.

MENINGITIS (see Ch. 280). Enteric rods, especially *E. coli* and *Klebsiella,* are a frequent cause of neonatal meningitis. In adults, meningitis with enteric bacilli is exceedingly rare except in cases of head trauma or neurosurgery. Bacteria may be infrequent and difficult to see on stained smears of spinal or ventricular fluid. Treatment with a third-generation cephalosporin that penetrates the blood-brain barrier at high dose may be sufficient, but infections with organisms resistant to such drugs may require chloramphenicol or a combination of intravenous and intrathecal aminoglycosides. Infected foreign bodies must be removed.

PNEUMONIA (see Ch. 19, 55, 274). Seeing gram-negative rods in respiratory secretions or growing them from the secretions does not necessarily imply infection. Susceptible patients often have severe chronic lung disease with abnormal chest radiographs. Many are on respirators with inflammation around endotracheal tubes and have abnormal gram-negative nasopharyngeal flora. Evidence of increasing infiltrates, fever, increasing leukocytosis, and/or worsening respiratory function should be sought before the diagnosis of gram-negative pneumonia is made in such cases.

INFECTIONS OF INTRAVENOUS CATHETERS. Critically ill patients may have limited numbers of sites for placing intravenous catheters. If catheter infection is suspected, it may be impractical or impossible to remove all the lines. Comparing simultaneous quantitative blood cultures drawn through each catheter and from one peripheral vein can identify the infected site and preserve the uninfected catheters in place.

INFECTIONS IN NEUTROPENIA (see Ch. 266). The most common bowel infection in neutropenia is perirectal abscess. Inflammation may be modest, but patients complain of severe pain. Examination can cause bacteremia. Surgical drainage may not be required unless neutropenia resolves and fluctuance develops. A less common but much more serious condition is typhlitis, an infection of the cecum associated with gas in the bowel wall, peritonitis, perforation, and bacteremia. This condition can be fatal within hours. Surgical resection has been helpful in a few cases, but surgical mortality is very high. Aggressive antibiotic therapy should be directed against *E. coli* and *P. aeruginosa,* the most common etiologic agents.

Necrotic skin lesions can accompany gram-negative bacteremia in neutropenic patients. These lesions are called ecthyma gangrenosum, and they are seen most frequently in *Pseudomonas* bacteremia. Cases have been reported with other gram-negative rods and with *Candida* and *Aspergillus* septicemia as well. The lesions can be scraped to search for the organism on smear. If nothing is seen, a punch biopsy for culture and histologic section can be done safely even in severe thrombocytopenia. In fungemia, the histologic section may be the only premortem specimen from which a diagnosis is obtained.

GRAM-NEGATIVE BACTEREMIA (see Ch. 70). Gram-negative bacteria gain access to the bloodstream from foci of tissue infection or, when host resistance is depressed, from sites of heavy colonization and minor trauma. Although bacteremia creates the opportunity for metastatic infections, a more immediate and serious consequence of gram-negative bacteremia is septic shock. The incidence of gram-negative bacteremia has risen steadily during the past three decades. It is estimated that at least 200,000 episodes occur in the United States each year, of which 20 to 60% are fatal. Mortality varies with the severity and nature of underlying disease, the source of bacteremia, and the incidence of serious sequelae. Rates of shock vary in different series from <20% to >50%. In comparable groups, shock is somewhat more frequent in gram-negative bacteremia than in gram-positive bacteremia or fungemia. However, gram-negative bacteremia is distinguished from the other septicemias by the fact that very small numbers of circulating bacteria are associated with hypotension. Figure 299–1 is a schematic representation of the complex relationship between sepsis, bacteremia, hypotension, and endotoxemia in gram-negative infection.

For therapeutic purposes, the diagnosis of gram-negative bacteremia cannot await the results of blood cultures but must be made on clinical grounds alone. The clinical setting is very helpful. A diagnosis of gram-negative bacteremia should be considered when sudden deterioration occurs in patients with focal infections usually caused by gram-negative bacteria (e.g., pyelonephritis, cholecystitis), in patients with significant focal infections from which gram-negative bacteria already have been isolated, and in patients with compromise in host defenses (e.g., neutropenia, burn injury), rendering them susceptible to their own bacterial flora. Neutropenic patients rarely have physical signs to localize the source of their bacteremia, but careful conversation often reveals a history of minor trauma, slight pain, or diarrhea. Gram-negative bacteremia and endotoxin infusion both cause transient neutropenia followed by neutrophilic leukocytosis. Large "toxic" vacuoles are seen. The first leukocyte count often is obtained after the leukopenic phase, but patients recovering from chemotherapy may have limited leukocyte reserves and thus exhibit only an apparent reversal of marrow recovery. Isolated thrombocytopenia or full-blown disseminated intravascular coagulopathy is not diagnostic of gram-negative bacteremia but, if present, is good supporting evidence. Arterial blood gas determinations may reveal unexplained hypoxemia without overt pulmonary disease, followed by metabolic acidosis.

TREATMENT. The correct choice of antibiotics is crucial to successful treatment of gram-negative bacteremia. When inappropriate drugs are used or the doses are too low, outcome is poor. It is never wise to give a single antibiotic to a patient at the onset of a bacteremic episode, even if the diagnosis and etiology seem certain. Many other infections can mimic gram-negative bacteremia, as discussed. Sometimes more than one bacterial species is involved. In neutropenia, the outcome of *Pseudomonas* bacteremia is much better if more than one effective antibiotic is used. The choice of empiric antibiotics should be made on the basis of the site of the focal infection (or infections) present, the known antimicrobial sensitivities of previous isolates from the patient and of agents of recent nosocomial infections in the hospital, and the patient's underlying diseases. In most patients the best regimen seems to be a combination of an aminoglycoside with a third-generation cephalosporin. An antistaphylococcal drug should be added if *S. aureus* infection is likely. If bowel perforation or infarction has occurred, *Bacteroides fragilis* must be covered. If *Clostridium perfringens* is suspected to be part of a mixed infection, concomitant high-dose penicillin should be used. (*C. perfringens* decolorizes easily in the Gram stain and may be distinguishable from gram-negative rods only by its boxlike rectangular shape.) A common mistake in use of aminoglycosides is to tailor the initial regimen to the first renal function tests. If azotemia is acute and attributable to poor perfusion, initial low doses will give inadequate levels as soon as hypotension is reversed. Renal toxicity from these drugs rarely occurs early; it is far more important to treat infection effectively in the first 24 hours than to avoid aminoglycoside toxicity.

Gram-negative bacteremia cannot be cured without eradicating the source of bacteremia. In cases of infection associated with ureteral or biliary obstruction, bacteremia and shock may persist in the face of adequate antibiotics until the obstruction is relieved. All likely sites of infection should be cultured, if possible, before antibiotics are given. However, antibiotic treatment should not be delayed for this reason. Wound cultures often remain positive after blood and urine have been sterilized. Physicians should not be content until they have found a satisfactory explanation for bacteremia. New fever or clinical deterioration can signal a new infection in a susceptible patient, the emergence of resistant bacteria, spread of the original focal infection, inadequate antibiotic levels, or a drug reaction. Such an episode requires complete re-evaluation with physical examination and repeat cultures.

Calandra T, Cometta A: Antibiotic therapy for gram-negative bacteremia. Infect Dis Clin North Am 5:817, 1991. *A good summary of recent studies.*

Kreger BE, Craven DE, Carling PC, et al.: Gram-negative bacteremia. III. Reassessment of etiology, epidemiology and ecology in 612 patients. Am J Med 68:332, 1980. *A recent classic clinical description of gram-negative bacteremia in an academic hospital setting with emphasis on the pathogenesis and the influence of the underlying condition on outcome.*

Uzun O, Akalin HE, Hayran M, Unal S: Factors influencing prognosis in bacteremia due to gram-negative organisms: Evaluation of 448 episodes in a Turkish university hospital. Clin Infect Dis 15:866, 1992. *A large recent series with good comments on prognostic factors.*

Van Deventer SJH, Buller HR, ten Cate JW, et al.: Endotoxemia: An early predictor of septicemia in febrile patients. Lancet 1:606, 1988.

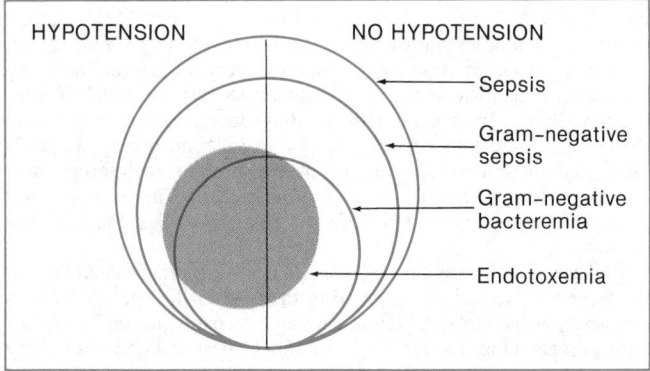

FIGURE 299–1. Schematic representation of etiologies of the sepsis syndrome. (Courtesy of Craig R. Smith.)

Other Bacterial Infections

300 *YERSINIA* INFECTIONS
J. Glenn Morris, Jr.

The genus *Yersinia* contains at least nine species which have been isolated from humans. *Y. enterocolitica, Y. pseudotuberculosis,* and *Y. pestis* (the causative agent of plague) are well-recognized human pathogens; diseases associated with each of these three species are described in detail below. Within the past 15 years, DNA hybridization and other studies have resulted in the delineation of six additional *"Y. enterocolitica*–like" species: *Y. frederiksenii, Y. kristensenii, Y. intermedia, Y. aldovae, Y. mollaretii* (formerly biogroup 3A of *Y. enterocolitica*), and *Y. bercovieri* (formerly biogroup 3B of *Y. enterocolitica*). These latter species carry antigens that in some instances are identical to those of *Y. enterocolitica* strains (allowing strains to be serotyped with *Y. enterocolitica* typing sera), and may be identified as *Y. enterocolitica* in some laboratory identification systems. Although all have been isolated from humans, these species appear to have minimal pathogenic potential.

YERSINIA ENTEROCOLITICA

DEFINITION. *Y. enterocolitica* is an enteric pathogen that can cause gastroenteritis, mesenteric adenitis and ileitis ("pseudoappendicitis"), and sepsis. Infection may also trigger a variety of autoimmune phenomena, including erythema nodosum, reactive arthritis, and possibly thyroiditis.

Y. enterocolitica is a gram-negative bacillus within the family Enterobacteriaceae; when first identified, it was designated *Pasteurella* "X."

DISTRIBUTION AND EPIDEMIOLOGY. *Y. enterocolitica* is widely distributed in the environment (especially in cooler, temperate regions of the world) and frequently colonizes wild and domestic animals. The organism is a common pharyngeal commensal in swine, with potentially pathogenic strains isolated from 25 to 90% of pork tongues after slaughter. Fifty-eight per cent of *Y. enterocolitica* infections in Belgium (which has one of the highest rates of *Y. enterocolitica* disease in the world) have been attributed to eating raw pork. *Y. enterocolitica* outbreaks have also been linked with milk, in which the organism grows at refrigerator temperatures. *Y. enterocolitica* may also be introduced into a household by pets or by symptomatic or asymptomatic human carriers. Once the organism is present within a household, infants and young children appear to be at greatest risk for infection.

In parts of Canada and western Europe, *Y. enterocolitica* rivals *Salmonella* and surpasses *Shigella* as a cause of acute diarrheal disease. In the United States, isolation rates from diarrheal stool samples are somewhat lower, generally about one third of those for *Salmonella*. However, recent studies suggest that US rates are increasing. Isolation rates tend to be much lower in tropical areas. In one study in Bangladesh, *Y. enterocolitica* was isolated from only 0.06% of diarrheal stool samples from children under age 7; this very low rate may reflect both the decreased frequency of environmental isolation outside of cold areas and the dietary restrictions limiting pork consumption in Moslem countries.

PATHOGENESIS. *Y. enterocolitica* is an intracellular pathogen. It invades and survives within macrophages and may persist and grow within lymph nodes and other lymphoid tissue for extended periods. It can also produce one or more protein enterotoxins, which may be responsible for or contribute to the diarrheal disease caused by the organism. Autoimmune phenomena occurring after *Y. enterocolitica* infections appear to be due to cross-reactivity between host and bacterial antigens; several putative target antigens are under active investigation, including bacterial antigens that may cross-react with the HLA-B27 antigen (in reactive arthritis) (see Ch. 238), or with the human thyrotropin receptor (in Graves' disease) (see Ch. 203).

Human illness is most commonly associated with a group of *Y. enterocolitica* strains which share certain virulence characteristics, especially the ability to invade epithelial cells.

CLINICAL AND LABORATORY FEATURES. The most common clinical manifestation of *Y. enterocolitica* infection is diarrhea, frequently accompanied by abdominal pain and fever; vomiting occurs in 20 to 40% of cases. Diarrhea is mild to moderate in severity and may last 1 to 2 weeks. As many as 10 to 20% of patients are reported to have bloody diarrhea. The limited available data suggest that leukocytosis is common.

Abdominal pain may be quite severe, mimicking appendicitis, and may occur in the absence of diarrhea. This has resulted in several outbreaks of "pseudoappendicitis" associated with transmission of *Y. enterocolitica* in a common food item.

Y. enterocolitica can cause pharyngitis (8% of *Y. enterocolitica* cases identified in one large, multistate outbreak), hepatic and splenic abscesses, peritonitis, and septicemia. Sepsis has been closely linked with iron overload states (and the administration of deferoxamine, used in treating iron overload), and with the presence of underlying conditions such as cirrhosis, chronic renal failure, diabetes, and immunosuppression. Recent reports suggest that very young infants (<3 months) with intestinal *Y. enterocolitica* infections have an increased susceptibility to septicemia; these infants may or may not be febrile and may have protein-losing enteropathy and failure to thrive.

Infection with *Y. enterocolitica* can trigger myriad autoimmune processes, most notably erythema nodosum and a reactive polyarthritis. Arthritis generally occurs within 1 to 2 weeks of onset of gastrointestinal symptoms, usually in HLA-B27–positive patients. Viable organisms cannot be cultured from involved joints; however, *Yersinia* antigens have been identified in synovial fluid cells. *Y. enterocolitica* infections have also been implicated in the development of Reiter's syndrome, carditis, glomerulonephritis, Graves' disease, and Hashimoto's thyroiditis.

DIAGNOSIS. Diagnosis is based on isolation of the organism from stool, blood, or other clinical specimen.

Although not generally available in the United States, serologic diagnosis of *Y. enterocolitica* infections is widely used in Europe.

TREATMENT. Currently available data do not indicate that antimicrobial therapy is efficacious in cases of uncomplicated *Y. enterocolitica* enteritis, but it is indicated in systemic disease or focal extraintestinal infection. *Y. enterocolitica* strains are susceptible *in vitro* to aminoglycosides, chloramphenicol, tetracycline, trimethoprim-sulfamethoxazole, third-generation cephalosporins, and quinolones; isolates are resistant to penicillins and first-generation cephalosporins. Recent evidence suggests that fluoroquinolones may be the drug of choice for extraintestinal *Y. enterocolitica* infections, in combination with a third-generation cephalosporin or an aminoglycoside in severe cases.

PROGNOSIS. Most cases of *Y. enterocolitica* enteritis are self-limited, and recovery is complete. Mortality rates among persons with *Y. enterocolitica* sepsis were originally reported to exceed 50%. In more recent studies, with aggressive antimicrobial therapy and supportive care, mortality has been approximately 7.5%. Arthritis may persist for a period of months (mean of 3.2 months in one study), with mild residual symptoms occurring in 50% of patients; 1 to 2% develop chronic arthritis.

YERSINIA PSEUDOTUBERCULOSIS

Y. pseudotuberculosis is most commonly recognized as a cause of mesenteric adenitis. Cases of enteritis in children have been reported from Japan (Izumi fever), and septicemia is seen in patients who have underlying liver disease or immunosuppression. The organism is widely distributed in the environment and is carried by wild and domestic animals. Secondary immunologic complications, such as erythema nodosum, arthritis, and renal insufficiency, have also been observed.

YERSINIA PESTIS (PLAGUE)

DEFINITION. *Y. pestis* is the etiologic agent for plague. The most common clinical form is bubonic plague, or acute regional lymphadenitis; septicemic and pneumonic forms also occur. Although epidemics of plague have had a major impact on human history, cases today are confined largely to isolated endemic foci. Three biovars have been described: biovar orientatis is distributed worldwide; biovar antiqua is found in Central Asia and Central Africa, and biovar medievalis is found in Iran and in the former Soviet Union.

DISTRIBUTION AND EPIDEMIOLOGY. Among rodent populations, plague is spread by transmission from rodents to fleas and back to rodents (sylvatic plague). Soil can also be contaminated by infected dead fleas and rodents; rodents coming from noninfected areas can become infected when they dig burrows in previously infected areas. This cycle may be relatively stable (enzootic) or may result in periodic epidemics (epizootics) in susceptible rodent populations. Humans are an accidental host in this natural cycle, with cases occurring when infected fleas bite people, or, occasionally, after direct inoculation of the skin by body fluids of an infected animal (often rabbits or carnivores). Direct, person-to-person transmission is seen only in the setting of pneumonic plague.

In the United States, plague is found west of the 100th meridian, which runs from North Dakota to Texas. Animals most commonly involved have included ground squirrels, rock squirrels, and prairie dogs. Between 1983 and 1992, there were an average of 16 cases of plague per year in the United States, based on reports to the Centers for Disease Control and Prevention. Approximately one third of recent cases have occurred in Native Americans; this is presumably a function of lifestyle, which may involve herding animals, assisted by dogs, in enzootic areas. Two thirds of cases occur in persons under age 25.

CLINICAL AND LABORATORY FEATURES. Plague presents most commonly as an acute regional lymphadenitis, or bubonic plague. Symptoms generally occur after an incubation period of 2 to 6 days. Illness is marked by the sudden onset of fever, chills, weakness, and headache. Then or shortly thereafter, patients note an intensely painful swelling in one region of lymph nodes, usually the groin, axilla, or neck. This swelling, or bubo, is typically oval, varying from 1 to 10 cm in length; the overlying skin is elevated and warm and may appear stretched or erythematous. The bubo itself is firm, extremely tender to palpation, and nonfluctuant. Patients with bubonic plague usually do not have skin lesions. However, in studies in Vietnam, about one fourth of patients had pustules, vesicles, eschars, or papules near the bubo or in areas drained by the affected nodes; these were presumed to represent sites of flea bite inoculations.

In the absence of therapy, disease progresses rapidly to a septicemic phase, with marked toxicity, prostration, and shock. The white blood cell count is elevated, and evidence of disseminated intravascular coagulation may appear. Purpura may be seen, associated with vasculitis and thrombosis. Some patients do not develop a bubo and progress directly to septicemia (septicemic plague). Diagnosis in these cases may be particularly difficult, as initial symptoms are relatively nonspecific (fever, headache, sore throat, malaise, myalgia, nausea, diarrhea, vomiting).

One of the feared complications of plague is plague pneumonia. Secondary pneumonia results from hematogenous spread of *Y. pestis* to the lung. Patients develop cough, chest pain, and may have hemoptysis. Radiographically, there is patchy bronchopneumonia or confluent consolidation. Sputum is purulent and contains the etiologic organism. Plague pneumonia is highly contagious by airborne transmission; persons inhaling the organism, from either an infected person or an animal, are susceptible to infection (primary plague pneumonia). Plague meningitis is a rarer complication; it typically occurs more than a week after inadequately treated bubonic plague but may be seen as a primary manifestation, without associated lymphadenopathy.

DIAGNOSIS. Plague can be diagnosed by isolating *Y. pestis* from blood, from an aspirate of a bubo, or from sputum. A presumptive diagnosis can be made in the appropriate clinical setting by demonstrating (by Gram stain or fluorescent antibody) characteristic organisms in sputum or in an aspirate of the bubo. In the absence of culture results, infection can be diagnosed by serology.

TREATMENT AND PROGNOSIS. In the absence of therapy, plague has an estimated mortality of >50%; untreated primary septicemic or pneumonic plague is invariably fatal. Fatality rates of up to 22% continue to be reported in the United States, owing primar-

ily to delays in initiation of appropriate therapy. Because of this, therapy should be started immediately if the diagnosis of plague is suspected.

Streptomycin was the first drug to be shown to have activity against plague, and, in the absence of controlled trials with other agents, it remains the drug of choice. Chloramphenicol and tetracycline are thought to be acceptable alternative therapies. Other aminoglycosides, trimethoprim/sulfamethoxazole, and the fluoroquinolones may be effective, but data on which to base a recommendation for their use are limited. Penicillin and first-generation cephalosporins are not effective, are associated with a high mortality, and should not be used. Aggressive supportive care is essential for patients in shock or with disseminated intravascular coagulation.

PREVENTION. All suspected plague cases should be reported immediately to local health authorities. Patients with bubonic plague (with no cough and a normal chest radiograph) should be placed on drainage/secretion precautions; if any evidence of pneumonic involvement is present, patients should be placed in strict isolation with precautions against airborne spread of the organism. Isolation should be maintained for a minimum of 3 days after starting appropriate antimicrobial therapy. Clinical samples must be carefully handled to minimize the risk of skin contact or aerosolization of the organism. Close contacts of suspected or confirmed plague pneumonia cases (including medical personnel) should be provided with chemoprophylaxis with tetracycline or sulfonamides.

Persons living in endemic areas should be advised to protect themselves against rodents and fleas; this includes measures designed to reduce rodent populations near homes, and applying insecticides, as necessary, to control flea populations. A formalin-killed vaccine, plague vaccine, is commercially available. Its use is recommended for persons traveling to epidemic areas, for individuals who must live and work in close contact with wild rodents, and for laboratory workers who must handle *Y. pestis* cultures.

Crook LD, Tempest B: Plague: A clinical review of 27 cases. Arch Intern Med 152:1253, 1992. *A description of 27 plague cases seen at the Gallup, New Mexico, Indian Medical Center between 1965 and 1989; 19 patients had bubonic plague and 8 septicemic plague.*

Gayraud M, Scavizzi MR, Mollaret HH, et al.: Antibiotic treatment of *Yersinia enterocolitica* septicemia. Clin Infect Dis 17:405, 1993. *A comprehensive, albeit retrospective, review of the management of* Y. enterocolitica *sepsis.*

Tacket CO, Narain JP, Sattin R, et al.: A multistate outbreak of infections caused by *Yersinia enterocolitica* transmitted by pasteurized milk. JAMA 251:483, 1984. *A description of clinical and epidemiologic features of* Y. enterocolitica *infection in one of the largest outbreaks reported to date.*

301 TULAREMIA
Richard B. Hornick

DEFINITION. Tularemia is a rare infectious disease caused by a small gram-negative pleomorphic rod, *Francisella tularensis*. This organism is acquired from an animal reservoir, frequently cottontail rabbits, by direct contact with diseased animal tissues, the bite of an infected tick or deer fly, ingestion of contaminated food or water, and inhalation of aerosolized bacteria. Clinical manifestations usually include a cutaneous ulcer with enlargement of regional lymph nodes. Rarely, a pneumonitis results from inhalation of *F. tularensis* or secondary spread from the skin ulcer and lymph nodes. Confirmation of the diagnosis by cultural technique is not advocated because of the high contagion risk to personnel handling this organism. The therapeutic response to effective antibiotic therapy is rapid.

The typhoidal form of tularemia was first described in Japan in 1818. A clear description of the organism occurred in 1906 when McCoy uncovered a "plaguelike" disease among ground squirrels in Tulare County, California. In Japan, tularemia may be referred to as Ohara's disease or Yato-byo (wild hare disease).

ETIOLOGY, SPECIFIC LABORATORY DIAGNOSIS, AND EPIDEMIOLOGY. *F. tularensis* is a small gram-negative pleomorphic rod-shaped bacterium. Organisms are not seen in smears of infected tissue unless special staining techniques are used. Fluorescent antibody conjugate staining and modified Dieterle staining are the best methods. All tularemia strains are serologically identical, but there are biochemical and virulence differences for mammals that have allowed differentiation of two strains. These are called Jellison A and B; the former, found only in North America, is lethal for domestic rabbits (*Oryctolagus*) and causes severe disease in humans. The unique biochemical capabilities of this strain—e.g., it ferments glycerol and contains citrulline ureidase—do not explain its increased virulence. Strain B lacks these biochemical features, is not lethal for cottontails, causes milder disease in humans, usually is isolated from rodents or from water, and is distributed over Europe, Asia, and North America. Reasons for the differences in virulence are unknown.

Culture Methods. The direct isolation of *F. tularensis* from blood (rarely), pus from ulcers or buboes, sputum, or pharyngeal or gastric aspirations in a patient with pneumonitis can be achieved by two methods. This is a class 4 organism requiring an effective hood or an adequate isolation laboratory to prevent human disease or epizootics. The two methods for isolation are intraperitoneal inoculation of guinea pigs and direct plating of a specimen onto glucose cysteine blood agar, cystine heart agar, or eugon agar. As few as one to five viable organisms will cause the death of guinea pigs in 5 to 10 days. Appropriate facilities are needed to prevent spread of the disease to other animals. The media used to isolate the organism usually contain drugs to suppress other flora and allow the tularemia colonies to be visible. Useful additions are 0.1 mg of cycloheximide and 20 units of penicillin per milliliter of media. The colonies are small on these media; they appear in 48 to 72 hours of incubation at 37° C.

Serologic Diagnosis. The measurement of serum agglutinating antibodies is a useful and safer method of diagnosing tularemia. Titers begin to rise in about 7 to 10 days and peak in 3 to 4 weeks. Paired serum specimens obtained 2 weeks apart and demonstrating a fourfold or greater rise are diagnostic of tularemia. However, a single specimen with a titer of 1:160 or greater in a patient thought to have tularemia on clinical grounds is diagnostic. Antibiotic therapy does not appear to dampen the antibody response. Titers remain elevated for 6 to 8 months and then decline in the subsequent 1 to 1.5 years to low or undetectable levels. There is a cross-reaction with brucella antigen during the early phase of the antibody response. The brucella titer falls off faster than and is never so high as the tularemia titer (see Ch. 308).

Skin Testing. A skin test antigen has proved to be reliable for diagnostic and epidemiologic purposes. A positive test result, similar in appearance to a tuberculin test response, is present during the first week of illness, frequently before the agglutinins are detectable, and remains positive for years. There is no known cross-reacting skin test antigen. The antigen is derived from *F. tularensis* by ether extraction; however, it is not commonly available. It can be obtained from the Centers for Disease Control and Prevention, Atlanta. In 10% of patients, the skin test antigen may boost pre-existing agglutinating antibody titers. Skin test reactivity can be shown to be associated with sensitized lymphocytes.

Epidemiology. Tularemia is a sporadic disease; humans acquire it when bitten by an infected tick or deer fly or when handling an infected animal. In the process of dressing a rabbit or skinning a muskrat, the hands may become contaminated with infected blood, subcutaneous abscesses, or liver and spleen that contain millions of organisms. The act of eviscerating the animal can create an aerosol that can be inhaled. Contaminated water or food is the least likely method of acquiring tularemia. Many carnivores such as dogs, cats, bull snakes, and others may feed on diseased rabbits, resulting in contamination of the teeth and saliva. These animals are relatively resistant to tularemia. Contact with the teeth of a pet dog or cat has resulted in ulceroglandular tularemia. Studies in volunteers have quantified the susceptibility of humans to infection and disease and the virulence of *F. tularensis* for humans. As few as 50 type A organisms injected subcutaneously cause ulceroglandular disease. Pneumonic tularemia can be induced by a similar inoculum size if the aerosolized and inhaled particles are small (<5 μm). Type B organisms require an inoculum about 1000 times larger to induce ulceroglandular or respiratory disease in humans.

The incidence of tularemia is low, 150 to 300 cases a year having been reported in each of the past 20 years. The peak incidence was in 1939, when almost 2300 cases were reported. Laws passed at that time prohibited the sale of wild rabbits, especially cottontails, and this legislation plus increased public awareness of the danger of handling sick or dying wild animals has contributed to the decline. Most cases occur in the Midwest, but the disease is not restricted to any one geographic location in the United States. Cottontail rabbits in urban and suburban areas provide the reservoir from which tularemia can occur. Epizootics among these or other animals can cause epidemics in humans. Tularemia has been reported only north of the 30th parallel. The cottontail is not found in Europe; various rodents such as voles, muskrats, and hares carry *F. tularensis* (Jellison B type) in that part of the world. Diseased jackrabbits, found west of the Mississippi River, may be an important source of contamination of ticks and deer flies.

In the summer months, most cases of tularemia are caused by tick or deer fly bites. Ulceroglandular disease begins with an ulcer at the site of the bite, e.g., groin, axilla, or scalp. In the fall during hunting season, sporadic cases, usually ulceroglandular, occur among hunters and trappers. In Scandinavia, epidemics have occurred in winter when farmers handling stored hay contaminated by diseased voles inhaled *F. tularensis* and developed pneumonic tularemia.

MECHANISMS OF INFECTION AND PATHOLOGY. The most common form of tularemia results from *F. tularensis* penetrating the skin. This penetration may be through hair follicles or minute areas of trauma. Subsequent disease develops in 2 to 6 days, depending on the number of bacteria and their virulence. The organisms multiply in the dermis and induce a marked inflammatory process consisting primarily of mononuclear cells with a perivascular distribution. This process produces an erythematous tender papule. The inflamed area continues to swell until the induced ischemia causes the skin to ulcerate. The base of the ulcer becomes black and depressed and the edges sharply demarcated. At the time of penetration, some organisms may be phagocytized and transported in the lymph to regional nodes. There is no clinically apparent lymphangitis. The nodes enlarge and become painful when caseation occurs. Histologic sections reveal geographic necrosis and disruption of the capsule. Fluctuation of the node is a late and rare event. It may then rupture. The necrotic, purulent, painful lymph node is termed a bubo. Healing of a bubo takes months even with appropriate antibiotic treatment. Aspiration of an unruptured node may lead to an indolent draining sinus tract. *F. tularensis* may remain in the necrotic tissue and purulent drainage for many weeks. The ulcer heals slowly and usually leaves a depigmented, rounded area in the skin.

Oculoglandular tularemia may occur when the conjunctival sac is infected from an ulcer or contaminated finger. Small yellowish granulomatous lesions develop on the palpebral conjunctivae, accompanied by enlargement of the preauricular lymph nodes. In untreated patients the cornea may perforate.

Inhaled small particle aerosols (<5 μm in diameter) containing *F. tularensis* (usually type A) are ultimately deposited in the terminal bronchioles and alveoli, although infection of the trachea and large bronchi also occurs. A peribronchial inflammation develops, with infiltration by neutrophils and mononuclear cells. This produces necrosis of alveolar walls and results in localized pneumonitis. In humans, small areas of pneumonitis represent the most common findings on chest roentgenograms. Often these are ill defined and difficult to interpret. Lobar consolidation or lung abscesses, infrequent in humans, represent extensive spread and necrosis. Mediastinal and peritracheal lymph nodes enlarge and may be apparent on chest films. They may be partially responsible, along with the bronchitis, for the substernal burning common with tularemic pneumonia. The incubation period for this form of tularemia varies inversely with the size and virulence of the inhaled inoculum. Following an inoculum of 10 to 50 organisms, disease appears in about 4 to 7 days in volunteers.

Typhoidal tularemia follows systemic spread of *F. tularensis* from the oropharynx and probably the gastrointestinal tract when a huge inoculum is swallowed. Enlargement of cervical lymph nodes, and presumably nodes in the mesentery, occurs. This latter process causes abdominal pain and is associated with an ileus. This is the most unusual form of tularemia in this country.

CLINICAL MANIFESTATIONS. Disease initiated by a tick bite is manifested by an ulcer at the site or adjacent to it. The tick defecates after feeding, and the infected feces may be scratched into the epidermis. Usually the lesion is in the inguinal, axillary, or scalp skin. If contact with tularemia organisms results from handling an infected animal, an ulcerative lesion evolves in the skin of the hands, frequently around a fingernail. This lesion may be so trivial that it is ignored by the patient. The ulcer is depressed into the dermis, has sharply demarcated edges, and gradually develops a black base. Initially, the lesion produces a thick, yellowish exudate. Regional lymph nodes enlarge and are tender to palpation. Fever and chills are common. The temperature curve is usually remittent or continuous in character. Without antibiotic therapy, most patients remain febrile for several weeks, the ulcer heals slowly over weeks to months, and the enlarged lymph nodes persist for months. Untreated patients may occasionally develop a secondary necrotizing pneumonia as a consequence of bacteremia, causing acute illness.

Primary tularemia pneumonia involves the sudden development of substernal burning and a nonproductive paroxysmal cough associated with fever and chills. Headache, myalgia, photophobia, malaise, and prostration are common. The temperature elevates quickly to 39.4 to 40°C and remains at that level (continuous fever curve) until antibiotic treatment is given. Sixty to 70% of patients survive without specific therapy, and in these a slow defervescence occurs over several months. Radiographs of the lungs may reveal ill-defined, scattered oval areas of infiltration, with enlarged peritracheal lymph nodes. Pleural effusions, lobar consolidation, and lung abscess are other manifestations of this form of tularemia. Cervical lymph nodes are palpable and tender.

DIAGNOSIS AND DIFFERENTIAL DIAGNOSIS. The diagnosis of ulceroglandular tularemia is made on the basis of the clinical manifestations and serologic studies. Paired serum specimens collected over a 2- to 3-week period are required to demonstrate a fourfold rise in titer. A baseline agglutinin titer of 1:160 in a patient with a history of an indolent ulcer for 2 or more weeks is diagnostic of tularemia. Culture of an ulcer and blood should be performed only if the hospital laboratory has appropriate protective isolation hoods. Patients with sporotrichosis or *Mycobacterium marinum* infections may have ulcers suggestive of tularemia but are usually afebrile. Enlarged lymph nodes extending centripetally as a beaded chain are a characteristic finding in sporotrichosis. Lesions of the fingers infected with staphylococci or β streptococci usually produce more pus and may be associated with lymphangitis. *Bacillus anthracis* can produce an ulcer (anthrax) with black-based, sharply demarcated edges similar to that initiated by *F. tularensis*. A careful history and serologic data help in the differential diagnosis. In patients in whom any form of tularemia is suspected, the skin test antigen is helpful. The test result is usually positive before agglutinating antibodies develop.

Tularemia pneumonia must be differentiated from the more common bacterial, viral, and mycoplasmal pneumonias. The history and the presence of ulceroglandular disease are helpful. Skin testing and serologic studies are diagnostic. The chest radiographs may yield suggestive findings consisting of ill-defined, small, oval, multiple infiltrates but is not diagnostic.

Patients infected with *F. tularensis* usually have a normal leukocyte count with an elevated sedimentation rate. The white count is elevated when a bubo or a lung abscess is present.

COMPLICATIONS. Pericarditis and meningitis are rare events that usually occur in patients who have been misdiagnosed and have received inappropriate treatment. Pericarditis results from direct extension of the infection from the purulent, necroic mediastinal lymph nodes or the involved lung. Constrictive pericarditis has been reported. Meningitis develops rarely, represents a seeding of the meninges during bacteremia, and is characterized by a lymphocytic pleocytosis in the cerebrospinal fluid.

TREATMENT. Patients with all forms of tularemia respond to the antibiotics streptomycin, gentamicin, tetracycline, and chloramphenicol. The aminoglycoside antibiotics are recommended; they produce a prompt cure of patients with the most severe form of tularemia. Patients with pneumonitis are afebrile within 24 to 48 hours and do not relapse. Ulcers and tender lymph nodes heal in 7

to 10 days. Gentamicin, 5 mg per kilogram per day in divided doses, is given for 10 days. Streptomycin was the principal drug for treating tularemia before gentamicin; 1 gram is given every 12 hours for 10 days. Treatment with tetracycline or chloramphenicol may produce an equally rapid response, but relapses occur in 15 to 20% of the patients. These drugs are not recommended unless gentamicin and streptomycin are contraindicated. Doses of 3 to 4 grams of tetracycline or 3 grams of chloramphenicol daily for 10 days can be used. Naturally acquired resistance to any of these antibiotics has not been found. Ceftriaxone has excellent *in vitro* inhibitory activity but in one study failed to cure eight pediatric patients. *In vitro* studies also indicate the potential antibacterial effect of the quinolones. However, no systematic *in vivo* testing has been reported.

Patients with ulceroglandular tularemia respond well to these antibiotics. Fluctuant lymph nodes should not be aspirated until the patient has finished the course of the antibiotic treatment. Isolation of patients with any form of tularemia is not required; there is no evidence of person-to-person spread.

PROGNOSIS. The mortality for untreated ulceroglandular disease is about 5%. Patients infected with type B strains and untreated probably have a mortality <1%. Many cases probably go undiagnosed, as the disease is mild and self-limiting. Treatment with antibiotics prevents death and promotes healing in a week to 10 days.

The mortality for pneumonic tularemia in the preantibiotic period was 30 to 40%. Treatment with streptomycin or tetracycline has lowered this figure to <1%. Healing occurs without residual lung damage or deficits in pulmonary function.

PREVENTION. Patients who recover from tularemia have a high degree of resistance to reinfection. If *F. tularensis* is reintroduced into the skin, a positive skin test reaction ensues without ulceration. Resistance to pulmonary disease may be associated with sensitized lymphocytes and alveolar macrophages.

A live attenuated strain of *F. tularensis* has been prepared as a vaccine. This can be administered by the acupuncture route, and it produces excellent immunity. The vaccine can be obtained from the Commander, U.S. Army Medical Research Institute of Infectious Diseases, Frederick, Maryland 21701. Its use is limited to persons considered at high risk, such as selected laboratory workers, forest rangers, game wardens, and perhaps others known to be exposed during an outbreak. The vaccine works by stimulating cellular immune mechanisms. Circulating agglutinins are not associated with resistance to disease.

Capellan J, Fong IW: Tularemia from a cat bite: Case report and review of feline-associated tularemia. Clin Infect Dis 16:472, 1993. *Summarizes literature reports of patients acquiring tularemia from cats. Offers advice on management of cat bite wounds not healing with penicillin therapy.*

Enderlin G, Morales L, Jacobs RF, Cross JT: Streptomycin and alternative agents for the treatment of tularemia: Review of the literature. Clin Infect Dis 19:42, 1994. *Compares in vitro with in vivo results. A good guide to current therapy.*

Evans ME, Gregory DW, Schaffner W, et al.: Tularemia: A 30-year experience with 88 cases. Medicine 64:251, 1985. *An excellent summary of the clinical presentations of* F. tularensis *disease.*

Penn RL, Kinasewitz GT: Factors associated with a poor outcome in tularemia. Arch Intern Med 147:265, 1987. *A retrospective study of the factors leading to poor outcomes. One significant factor was delay in diagnosis and treatment.*

Scofield RH, Lopez EJ, McNabb SJ: Tularemia pneumonia in Oklahoma, 1982–1987. J Okla St Med Assoc 85:165, 1992. *Discusses factors influencing failure to diagnose pneumonic tularemia. This form is difficult to diagnose because of few distinguishing features.*

302 ANTHRAX
Jonas A. Shulman

DEFINITION. Anthrax is a zoonotic disease caused by *Bacillus anthracis,* a large gram-positive, spore-forming bacillus transmitted to humans by contact with infected animals or contaminated animal products. Other names for anthrax include woolsorter's disease, Siberian ulcer, malignant pustule, charbon, malignant edema, and ragsorter's disease. In 1877, Koch described *B. anthracis* as one of the first microbes identified as a cause of a specific disease, thereby making anthrax the prototype for Koch's postulates and the first disease to satisfy them. Anthrax has all but disappeared from North America, Western Europe, and Australia since being nearly eradicated in livestock following extensive veterinary programs, including vaccination. The disease is still prevalent in many developing countries, however, especially Asia, Africa, and Central America, where livestock are only marginally subjected to veterinary control and where environmental conditions are favorable for an animal-to-soil-to-animal cycle.

Anthrax occurs primarily in herbivorous animals, especially cattle, goats, and sheep, but many other animals, including pigs, buffalo, and elephants, have also been infected with the disease. Cattle are particularly susceptible to the systemic form of anthrax, which clinically progresses to death in 24 to 48 hours. The large numbers of organisms found in infected cattle may contaminate not only the animal but also its products and environs, thereby allowing infection to occur in animals more resistant to anthrax, such as humans.

The primary forms of anthrax in humans are cutaneous, inhalation, gastrointestinal, and oropharyngeal. Septicemia and meningitis may occur from any of these primary foci. By far the most common form of the disease in the United States is the cutaneous lesion, which accounts for >95% of clinical cases. Inhalation anthrax has occurred only rarely in the United States in the past 25 years, and gastrointestinal anthrax has never been reported in this country.

ETIOLOGY. *B. anthracis* is a large gram-positive, nonmotile, spore-forming bacillus (1 to 1.3×3 to 8 μm). Although spores of *B. anthracis* do not form in living tissue, they are induced by aerobic conditions in the external environment and may persist for years in the soil, in animal products, or in an appropriate industrial setting. The organism grows well aerobically on ordinary laboratory media at 35° to 37° C. The colonies produced are especially sticky (positive tenacity test, positive string of pearls test) and have a tendency to stand up in stalagmite fashion when lifted with a bacteriologic loop. The colonies are nonhemolytic, rough, and flat, with many comma-shaped outgrowths on blood agar. Microscopic examination of organisms growing on artificial media shows long, parallel chains of organisms frequently described as having a rather characteristic "boxcar" appearance. Spores are oval and occur either centrally or paracentrally but cause no swelling of the bacillus. Material from fresh lesions contains single or short chains of two or three bacilli, which may appear encapsulated, the ends of which are slightly rounded.

Anthrax organisms can be differentiated from the saprophytic *Bacillus* species by fluorescent antibody staining, lysis with a specific γ bacteriophage, and virulence for mice, guinea pigs, and rabbits. Parenteral inoculation into these species results in death in 1 to 3 days.

INCIDENCE AND PREVALENCE. *B. anthracis* is a soil organism that has worldwide distribution. Animal anthrax is endemic in some areas of Asia, Africa, and Latin America, especially in rural regions that have inadequate animal vaccination programs and poor animal husbandry. These areas are more likely to have a number of human cases as well. Certain areas within the United States and other parts of the world may provide a particularly favorable environment for large numbers of resistant spores to survive in the soil for many years. In fact, a number of epizootics related to focal regions of heavily contaminated soil have occurred.

Since no reliable reporting of anthrax exists, and in many instances the diagnosis may never be made, the actual worldwide incidence of anthrax is not known. Estimates in the past have ranged between 20,000 and 100,000 human cases per year, but these figures have more recently been estimated at 2000 to 20,000 cases per annum. In the United States, approximately one case of human anthrax per year was reported between 1970 and 1985, but only three cases have been documented since 1984. Reports of human anthrax have been especially frequent in Turkey, Pakistan, Iran, Haiti, and several Asian and African countries. There are probably many parts of the world with significant endemic problems but from which data are not available.

The potential for large outbreaks in animals and humans continues to exist, especially when economic or political upheaval is present. One of the largest epidemics of anthrax was reported in Zimbabwe between 1978 and 1980, when nearly 10,000 human cases of cutaneous anthrax and a few cases of gastrointestinal anthrax occurred, resulting in approximately 100 deaths. This outbreak was related to an extensive epizootic infection in cattle. Another major outbreak of anthrax occurred in Siberia in 1979. It was initially

thought by some to be related to inhalation, but more recently the route of infection has been identified as the ingestion and handling of infected "black market" meat. The source of anthrax in the cattle in this epidemic appeared to be a single 29-ton lot of bone meal used as animal feed that likely was made from the bones of animals that had died of anthrax the previous year.

Very rare cases of inhalation anthrax have developed in workers exposed to aerosolized anthrax spores generated during the processing of contaminated materials such as woolens, hides, or bone meal, and even more rarely in people who have simply been in the vicinity of a wool-processing mill or tannery but who were not directly involved in the processing of the product. Cases have even been reported in home weavers, such as those using contaminated goat yarn, or in individuals working with contaminated bone meal fertilizer.

In the United States, the average annual occurrence has diminished. From 1977 to 1988, the number of cases was only 0.8, as opposed to 127 cases reported to occur annually between 1916 and 1925. The case fatality rate of the 221 U.S. cases of cutaneous anthrax from 1955 to 1986 was approximately 5.0% (11 of 221), whereas the case fatality rate was 82% in the patients with inhalation anthrax (9 of 11). The overall mortality rate in these 232 American cases of anthrax was 8.6%.

EPIDEMIOLOGY. Cases of anthrax are classified generally as either agricultural or industrial. Most of the agricultural cases of human anthrax result from direct contact with contaminated discharges from infected animals. Occasional human cases have been transmitted by bites of flies that have fed on the carcasses of animals dead of anthrax. Others have been caused by ingestion of poorly cooked or raw infected meat. Industrial cases usually result from contact with anthrax spores contaminating animal products, such as goat hair, wool, hides, and skin, and animal bones, especially those imported from areas of high endemicity. Transmission usually occurs during the processing of these animal products, either by direct contact with the contaminated raw material or by indirect contact with a contaminated environment; rarely, transmission may occur via airborne particles produced during the manufacturing process. Because the *B. anthracis* spores can survive for long periods, a wide variety of unusual products have been associated with human infection, such as imported bongo drums made with goat skins, shaving brushes, various leather or woolen blankets, and ivory piano keys. Laboratory-acquired infections have been reported; however, human-to-human transmission of anthrax is not thought to occur.

Most cases of anthrax in the United States are sporadic, but occasional epidemics have been reported. In 1957, the largest and most serious of these occurred in New Hampshire, where nine employees of a textile mill acquired anthrax while processing a batch of contaminated goat hair imported from Asia. This outbreak included four cutaneous cases and five inhalation cases, with four fatalities reported in the latter group.

PATHOGENESIS. The virulence of *B. anthracis* is determined by both a plasmid-mediated group of exotoxins (plasmid pX01), and another plasmid-mediated antiphagocytic polydiglutamic acid capsule (plasmid pX02). Three toxic proteins (exotoxins) have been identified and cloned, including a protective antigen (PA), an edema factor (EF), and a lethal factor (LF). A combination of two of these proteins (PA and EF) has been demonstrated to decrease polymorphonuclear neutrophil function, suggesting that this is one of the ways that host susceptibility to infection with *B. anthracis* may be increased.

Furthermore, a combination of PA and EF causes local edema, whereas the combination of PA and LF may cause death in as little as 60 minutes. None of these three toxins, when administered alone, has any biologic effect in experimental animals. Protective antigen is able to bind to cell-surface receptors, in turn enabling them to be used by both EF and LF to reach the cytoplasm. Recently, EF has been found to be related to its ability to increase cyclic AMP. EF, in fact, is a calmodulin-dependent adenylate cyclase, and it is likely that the edema is produced through this mechanism.

As noted, virulent strains of *B. anthracis* contain two large plasmids, pX01 and pX02, both of which are necessary for virulence. Strains that contain only one of these plasmids are totally avirulent.

In cutaneous anthrax, the organism is introduced either through a wound or by means of infected animal fibers that disrupt the skin.

The organism is not known to penetrate intact skin. Once in the subcutaneous tissue, the anthrax spore is thought to germinate, multiply, and produce both its exotoxin and the antiphagocytic capsular material. The toxins are capable of provoking a marked edematous response and tissue necrosis with a paucity of neutrophil invasion. Phagocytosis of the organisms by local macrophages occurs, and these bacilli are then spread to regional lymph nodes, where further production of toxins produces a hemorrhagic, necrotic, and edematous lymphadenitis. Bacilli may enter the circulation, at times producing meningitis, pneumonia, and systemic toxicity.

Inhalation anthrax is fortunately a very uncommon clinical presentation of anthrax, as it is associated with close to 100% mortality. In the United States, inhalation anthrax is now essentially obsolete, with only two cases reported during the past 25 years; however, this is still a cause of significant disease in many parts of the world. Inhalation anthrax, commonly known as woolsorter's disease, occurs not as a result of direct contact with infected animals but rather by inhalation of an aerosol of spores in particle sizes < 5 μm. These aerosols usually occur during processing of contaminated material. In humans, spores are inhaled, reach the alveoli, and may then eventually be phagocytized by macrophages and carried by these cells to the mediastinal lymph nodes. Germination, growth, and toxin formation at this site can produce severe, massive hemorrhagic lymphadenitis and mediastinitis. *B. anthracis* may also directly affect the pulmonary capillary endothelium, causing thrombosis and respiratory failure. Pleural effusion is common. Anthrax is not thought to cause primary pneumonia, but secondary bacterial pneumonia may complicate inhalation anthrax. *B. anthracis* may also enter the bloodstream from this site, with the evolution of intense bacteremia. The number of organisms per milliliter of blood may be so great that in some instances the organism may be seen on smears of the peripheral blood. Hemorrhagic meningitis may ensue. Respiratory failure, shock, and pulmonary edema are frequent causes of death.

Ingestion of markedly contaminated, poorly cooked meat may result in either the oropharyngeal or the gastrointestinal form of infection. When oropharyngeal anthrax occurs, there is localized swelling of the pharynx, sometimes causing tracheal obstruction, and marked cervical adenopathy with overlying brawny edema. Similarly, the organism may reach the small and large intestines and cause a gastrointestinal syndrome. In this case, the spores that are deposited in the submucosa of the intestinal tract may germinate, multiply, and produce toxin, again resulting in marked edema, hemorrhage, and necrosis. Regional mesenteric lymphadenopathy is common, and findings associated with the syndrome include fever, vomiting, abdominal pain and distention, massive bloody diarrhea, mesenteric adenitis, hemorrhagic ascites, and septicemia. Gastrointestinal anthrax is a very severe form of the disease, has a high mortality rate (25 to 75%), and is rarely diagnosed during life except in the setting of an epidemic.

It is important to note that although antimicrobial agents may rapidly eradicate the organism, the persistence of the toxin that has been produced may result in continued development of the disease process until the toxin is metabolized. Thus, although the mortality rate may be diminished by appropriate antibiotic therapy, especially in the cutaneous form of the disease, the clinical process may continue to progress even after the institution of antimicrobial therapy. Antitoxins have been tried by some in the past, but such antitoxins are not currently available.

CLINICAL MANIFESTATIONS. Cutaneous anthrax is the most common form of the disease in humans, accounting for >95% of cases. After an incubation period of 1 to 5 days, the infection generally begins with a small, somewhat pruritic papule at the site of an abrasion, which over the next several days develops into a vesicle containing serosanguineous fluid teeming with organisms. The lesion generally occurs on the upper extremities, especially the arms and hands, or on the face, neck, or other areas that are likely to be exposed to the contaminated animal product or infected soil. As the lesion progresses, ulceration occurs, with formation of a necrotic ulcer base frequently surrounded by smaller vesicles. The characteristic black eschar evolves over several weeks to a size of several centimeters, gradually separating and leaving a scar. This black eschar accounts for the name *anthrax*, which comes

from the Greek word for coal. The edema is frequently nonpitting, gelatinous, and brawny and is very striking. It may be quite extensive, spreading over a wide area in severe cases. With involvement near the eye, periorbital swelling may be especially intense. The edema may be so dramatic that hypotension occurs in part because of the loss of intravascular volume as fluid enters the subcutaneous tissues. This edema, in combination with the vesicle progressing to the necrotic black eschar, forms the lesion that is highly characteristic of anthrax. Despite the dramatic appearance of the lesion, it is frequently painless.

In association with the localized cutaneous lesion, most patients have minimal constitutional findings, such as fever, malaise, myalgias, and headaches. In those with extensive edema, the systemic symptoms may be more severe. Localized lymphadenopathy may occur at times and may be complicated by bacteremia and even meningitis. Death is rare if appropriate antimicrobial therapy is instituted; in untreated cases of cutaneous anthrax, however, the mortality rate remains about 25%.

Bacterial adenitis due to staphylococci and streptococci, tularemia, plague, orf, cat scratch disease, localized herpes, and ecthyma gangrenosum are diagnostic considerations, and lesions seen in these diseases may be confused with those of anthrax. The diagnosis of cutaneous anthrax will rarely be missed if the disease is considered in any patient who has had exposure to an appropriate animal or animal product and who develops a painless ulcer surrounded by small vesicles, along with marked edema and eschar formation. Gram stains of the vesicular fluid and lesion usually readily demonstrate the characteristic gram-positive bacilli, as the organisms are present in large numbers in these lesions and are readily isolated by culture. Informing the bacteriology laboratory of the possibility of the diagnosis of anthrax is important to prevent the organism from being discarded as merely a probable contaminant of *Bacillus* species, which is frequently not fully characterized. At times, secondary bacterial infection may occur in these ulcers. Rarely, more than one lesion may be present, resulting from coprimary infections.

Inhalation anthrax is very rare, usually fatal, and extremely difficult to diagnose. The incubation period in this syndrome is generally 1 to 6 days, and the illness is generally biphasic. Initially, a brief, nonspecific "influenza-like" illness occurs, manifested by high fever, fatigue, myalgias, malaise, a nonproductive cough, and at times some chest discomfort. Few physical findings are noted at this time; however, within several days after a short period of clinical improvement, the patient becomes much more ill. This second phase is manifested by severe dyspnea, cyanosis, hypoxia, hemoptysis, stridor, chest pain, and diaphoresis. Physical examination may reveal some crepitant rales and evidence of pleural effusions. Some subcutaneous brawny edema of the chest wall and neck may be noted. The chest radiograph in these patients shows a rather distinctive clinical finding, namely, a widened mediastinum. Bacteremia, shock, and meningitis are frequently present, and death generally follows within 1 to 2 days of the onset of the respiratory distress. The mortality rate is 80 to 100%, even with appropriate therapy.

Inhalation anthrax should be considered in patients with appropriate exposure to an animal product, as in a weaver using imported goat hair or a textile mill worker. The most important clue is the presence of an appropriate epidemiologic history in a patient developing severe respiratory distress and a rapidly enlarging mediastinum.

Gastrointestinal anthrax is an extremely rare disease. It has an incubation period of 2 to 5 days, although there are some cases in which a more prolonged incubation period has been postulated. The diagnosis is rarely suspected before death except in areas where anthrax is highly endemic and in which multiple human cases are occurring. The symptoms include severe abdominal pain, hematemesis, melena, rapid onset of ascites, and at times, marked diarrhea. Paracentesis may reveal hemorrhagic ascites, and sometimes these cases may simulate "acute" or "surgical abdomen." The disease usually progresses to bacteremia, toxemia, shock, and eventually death in many patients. No cases of intestinal anthrax have been reported in the United States.

Oropharyngeal anthrax presents as severe sore throat with neck swelling, adenopathy, dysphagia, and at times tracheal compression and dyspnea. Cervical and submandibular lymphadenopathy is common. Again, bacteremia and its complications may ensue.

Meningitis may be a complication of any of the forms of anthrax and almost never is found without a primary focus of infection. It is frequently hemorrhagic and most often fatal.

DIAGNOSIS. The clinician who elicits a careful epidemiologic history and who has a high index of suspicion of anthrax will not have problems establishing the diagnosis in cutaneous anthrax and will even be alert to the rarer and more difficult to recognize cases of inhalation, gastrointestinal, or oropharyngeal anthrax.

Inhalation anthrax is rarely suspected before death and only if an epidemiologic history of aerosol exposure is obtained or if an epidemic is recognized. The major finding in the clinical evaluation, other than epidemiologic history, is the presence of a widened mediastinum or at times hemorrhagic pleural effusions or associated hemorrhagic meningitis. Ordinarily, Gram stains of sputum and cultures do not demonstrate *B. anthracis*. These patients frequently do develop bacteremia, however, and in these cases the organism can be readily isolated and sometimes seen on stains of the peripheral blood.

A number of serologic tests are available to diagnose anthrax retrospectively, but many of these very ill patients die so quickly that the initial serologic studies may not be especially helpful to the clinician. In some cases, however, serology has been a helpful diagnostic tool, especially when prior antibiotics have eradicated the bacteria before cultures or smears were obtained. Current serologic tests considered valuable include an enzyme-linked immunosorbent assay (ELISA), which detects antibodies to the capsular antigen, and an electrophoretic immunotransblot test, which detects antibodies to the PA exotoxin. Both of these serologic tests are quite sensitive and specific enough to be useful, but the test for antibody to the PA exotoxin may be more specific.

TREATMENT. Penicillin G is the drug of choice for treatment of anthrax. Only a few isolates of *B. anthracis* have been identified as resistant to penicillin G. In cutaneous anthrax, cultures of the infected blisters have become negative for the organism within 5 hours of the patient's receiving 2 million units of penicillin G. As previously mentioned, however, the presence of the toxin may persist, and the cutaneous lesion frequently goes through its various phases of evolution, even though the organism has been eradicated and the mortality rate reduced.

For cutaneous anthrax, intravenous penicillin G is given, 2 million units every 6 hours for several days, followed by a 7- to 10-day course of oral penicillin G. In patients with severe, overwhelming edema, corticosteroids have been thought by some to be helpful, although no controlled studies of their use have been performed. Severe neck swelling may require intubation or tracheostomy. In patients who are allergic to penicillin, effective alternatives include streptomycin, erythromycin, tetracycline, and chloramphenicol. No local surgery should be performed on these patients, because no pus requiring drainage is usually present and excision of the lesion has been reported to increase symptoms severity and organism spread. The lesion should be covered with a sterile dressing. No definite cases have been reported of spread of anthrax from human to human.

In inhalation, gastrointestinal, or oropharyngeal anthrax or in anthrax meningitis, high dosages of intravenous penicillin G, in the range of 24 million units per day, are recommended, along with excellent supportive care for the problems of hypotension and respiratory distress. Some physicians encourage parenteral streptomycin in a dosage of 1 to 2 grams per day to the penicillin G therapy in these cases. When the patient is hospitalized, good infection control practices are required. Soiled dressings must be incinerated or autoclaved.

PROGNOSIS. Inhalation anthrax is considered to be fatal in 80 to 100% of cases, and gastrointestinal anthrax has a case fatality rate of 25 to 75%. The case fatality rate for cutaneous anthrax is about 20 to 25% without treatment but generally is < 1% with appropriate treatment.

PREVENTION. Control of anthrax in animals is essential to control of the disease in humans. All cases of anthrax—animal as well as human—should be reported to the state health department or the appropriate veterinary agency. Live avirulent animal vaccines are effective and may help control anthrax in endemic areas. Animals dead of anthrax should be cremated or buried, and care must be taken at autopsy to avoid additional environmental contamination by infected blood and tissues. Human anthrax can be partially prevented by proper disposal of the infected animals. In addition,

formaldehyde has been used successfully to decontaminate raw wool and hair. A cell-free filtrate vaccine has been shown to protect humans from anthrax and is available from the Michigan State Department of Health. This vaccine should be offered to workers likely to be exposed to contaminated animal products in high-risk industries. Newer vaccines are being evaluated, such as a PA toxoid vaccine and a PA-producing live vaccine. In the former Soviet Union, in addition to the chemical vaccine, a live anthrax spore vaccine has been widely used for prophylaxis against anthrax in both humans and animals.

Because none of the currently available vaccines is ideal, efforts at developing better agents are a major area of research. Among the newer approaches for anthrax vaccine development for human use are (1) combination of the PA with adjuvants derived from the BCG strain or killed cells of *Bordetella pertussis* and (2) PA cloned into a *Bacillus subtilis* as a recombinant vaccine that does not contain the *B. anthracis* genome.

Good personal hygiene, as well as the use of protective clothing and respirators when contaminated aerosols are likely to be encountered, may also prove to be helpful preventive measures. Gastrointestinal anthrax can be prevented by proper cooking of meat and by avoiding ingestion of potentially contaminated meat. Care must be taken by the laboratory personnel working with *B. anthracis,* since cases of anthrax have been acquired in this setting.

Farrar E: Anthrax: Virulence and vaccines. Ann Intern Med 121:379, 1994. *Excellent editorial outlining newer molecular biologic features of* B. anthracis *and the role of virulence factors in pathogenesis of the disease produced; also highlights new approaches to vaccine development.*

Harrison LH, Ezzell JW, Abshire TG, et al.: Evaluation of serologic tests for diagnosis of anthrax after an outbreak of cutaneous anthrax in Paraguay. J Infect Dis 160:706, 1989. *Serologic methods for diagnosis and detection of immunity.*

Ivins BE, Welkos SL: Recent advances in the development of an improved human anthrax vaccine. Eur J Epidemiol 4:12, 1988. *A approach to vaccines for anthrax.*

Ivins BE, Welkos SL, Little SF, et al.: Immunization against anthrax with *Bacillus anthracis* protective antigen combined with adjuvants. Infection Immunity 60:662, 1992. *Discusses the protective efficacy of immunization against anthrax with* B. anthracis *protective antigen combined with different adjuvants.*

Knudson GB: Treatment of anthrax in man: History and current concepts. Milit Med 151:71, 1986. *Reviews history of anthrax with emphasis on treatment.*

Shlyakov EN, Rubenstein E: Human live anthrax vaccine in the former USSR. Vaccine 12:727, 1994. *Describes the history of the development and use of the Soviet live spore human anthrax vaccine.*

303 DISEASES CAUSED BY PSEUDOMONADS

Stephen C. Schimpff

PSEUDOMONADS. Pseudomonads are gram-negative aerobic bacilli that prefer moist environments and are relatively noninvasive yet can cause serious and often fatal infection when the host defense mechanism is damaged or deficient. Each species is different in its pathogenic properties, each causes somewhat different types of infection, and each invades as a result of different host defense defects, but with each pseudomonad, the environmental source is usually water, moist soil, or a contaminated medical device, infusion, or injection.

Pseudomonads are divided into five major groups based on RNA homology (Table 303–1). Most human infections are caused by members of groups I, II, and V. For purposes of discussion, this chapter considers *Pseudomonas pseudomallei* (the cause of melioidosis), *Pseudomonas mallei* (the cause of glanders), *Pseudomonas aeruginosa* (which principally causes bacteremia, endocarditis, pneumonia, keratitis, and urinary tract infections), and *Pseudomonas cepacia, Pseudomonas pickettii,* and *Xanthomonas (Pseudomonas) maltophilia* (which cause bacteremia, pseudobacteremia, endocarditis, and urinary tract infections).

Pseudomonas pseudomallei. This organism causes melioidosis, often characterized as a glanders-like infectious disease. It was first described in Rangoon among debilitated morphine addicts. The term "melioidosis" means "a similarity to distemper of asses."

TABLE 303-1. CLASSIFICATION OF PSEUDOMONADS THAT HAVE BEEN ISOLATED FROM CLINICAL SPECIMENS

Group/Subgroup	Genus and Species
RNA group I	
Fluorescent group	*P. aeruginosa*
	P. fluorescens
	P. putida
Nonfluorescent group	*P. stutzeri*
	P. alcaligenes
	P. pseudoalcaligenes
RNA group II	*P. mallei*
	P. pseudomallei
	P. cepacia
	P. pickettii
RNA group III	*P. acidovorans*
	P. testosteroni
RNA group IV	*P. diminuta*
	P. vesicularis
RNA group V	*Xanthomonas maltophilia*

From Sanford JP: *Pseudomonas* species (including melioidosis and glanders). *In* Mandell GL, Douglas RG Jr, Bennett JE (eds.): Principles and Practice of Infectious Diseases, 3rd ed. New York, Churchill Livingstone, 1990, pp 1692–1696.

Despite the clinical resemblance to glanders, it has a totally different epidemiology. Melioidosis occurs in animals and humans in endemic areas of southeast Asia and northern Australia and has now been recognized to occur in epidemic-like form in specific areas, given the combination of the environment (an appropriate rainy season with water-covered rice paddies) and a susceptible host (abraded skin in barefoot farmers who have a high prevalence of diabetes mellitus, renal disease, or both).

P. pseudomallei is a gram-negative, motile, aerobic bacillus that is small and may grow in filamentous chains. Staining with methylene blue or Wright's stain shows a bipolar "safety pin" pattern. *P. pseudomallei* has a characteristic wrinkling appearance of the colonies on agar if held long enough. The organism, like most pseudomonads, can be isolated from soil and water and particularly streams, rice paddies, and ponds of the endemic areas and on plants, including commonly consumed vegetables. Most human infection probably occurs through skin abrasions. However, laboratory animals have been found to become infected by the respiratory route, so inhalation may be a possible human route of acquisition, which would explain the occurrence of primary pneumonia.

At the conclusion of United States involvement in the Vietnam war, 343 cases were reported, with 36 deaths; however, serologic surveys suggest that either mild or inapparent infection may be fairly common, with positive serologies found in 1 to 2% of healthy, nonwounded Army troops returning to the United States. This would suggest that as many as 225,000 military personnel may have had subclinical infection with *P. pseudomallei*. The importance of this observation is that recrudescence of disease has been observed many years after primary infection.

In addition to inapparent infection or asymptomatic pulmonary infection, the frequently observed forms of melioidosis are an acute, localized, suppurative soft tissue infection, an acute pulmonary infection, and an acute septicemic presentation. The localized infections are probably related to skin abrasion, with development of a nodule with secondary lymphangitis and regional lymphadenitis. An apparent primary pulmonary infection ranges from bronchitis to necrotizing pneumonia. The patient with pneumonia usually has high fever and signs and symptoms of consolidation, ordinarily in an upper lobe. It is an acute pyogenic process, frequently leading to early cavitation and giving a pulmonary appearance consistent with tuberculosis. Progression to bacteremia is rare.

Patients with the acute septic form characteristically present with a short history of fever and no clinical evidence of focal infection, although skin abrasion is the presumed site of origin. Most are profoundly ill, with signs of sepsis, such as tachypnea or Kussmaul's breathing, and occasional evidence of septic shock. Clinical and radiologic evidence frequently demonstrates progression to diffuse bilateral and patchy pulmonary infiltrate, which progresses to abscess

and cavity formation if the patient survives. Subcutaneous abscesses are relatively uncommon but can occur at multiple sites. Liver abscess, usually multiple, is not uncommon and is accompanied in more than 50% by multiple splenic abscesses, a combination unlikely for most other causes of liver abscess.

The diagnosis should be considered in any patient living in an endemic area who has a febrile illness and especially one occupationally at risk and, perhaps, at further risk of sepsis because of diabetes or renal disease. The diagnosis should be highly suspected in such an individual with a rapidly progressive, extensive pulmonary process if subcutaneous lesions are present or in one whose condition progresses to a cavitary form indistinguishable from tuberculosis. A Gram stain of pulmonary or abscess exudate shows small gram-negative bacilli, and methylene blue staining shows the characteristic bipolar "safety pin." The organism grows on standard media and is usually detected in blood cultures within 48 hours.

In northeast Thailand, a report from a hospital serving a population of nearly 2 million rural rice farming families determined that about 20% of all community-acquired bacteremias were caused by *P. pseudomallei* and that during the rainy season, when the paddy fields are under water (from June to September), *P. pseudomallei* was the single most common organism isolated from blood culture, representing nearly one half of all documented cases of community-acquired bacteremia in the month of August (Fig. 303–1). An interesting observation was the higher than expected frequency of both diabetes mellitus and renal calculi in patients with sepsis who are from this region, where both diabetes and calculi are common.

Treatment of pulmonary or suspected septic forms should probably begin with a combination of agents. The standard recommended treatment had been a combination of chloramphenicol, doxycycline, and trimethoprim-sulfamethoxazole. These agents, however, are bacteriostatic rather than bactericidal, do not represent a regimen one would wish to use for suspected community-acquired bacteremia, and are associated with a high mortality rate. The third-generation cephalosporin ceftazidime is now likely the drug of choice, with imipenem, piperacillin, or amoxicillin–clavulanic acid as reasonable alternatives. Adding an aminoglycoside during empirical therapy might be appropriate until culture results are known. Treatment apparently needs to be prolonged, including intravenous therapy (ceftazidime, imipenem, or piperacillin) for 2 to 4 weeks, followed by oral therapy (perhaps amoxicillin–clavulanic acid) for 6 months or longer to prevent recrudescence.

The prognosis for patients with localized disease should be excellent with appropriate therapy. However, those with the septicemic form are often gravely ill at the time of admission, and the mortal-

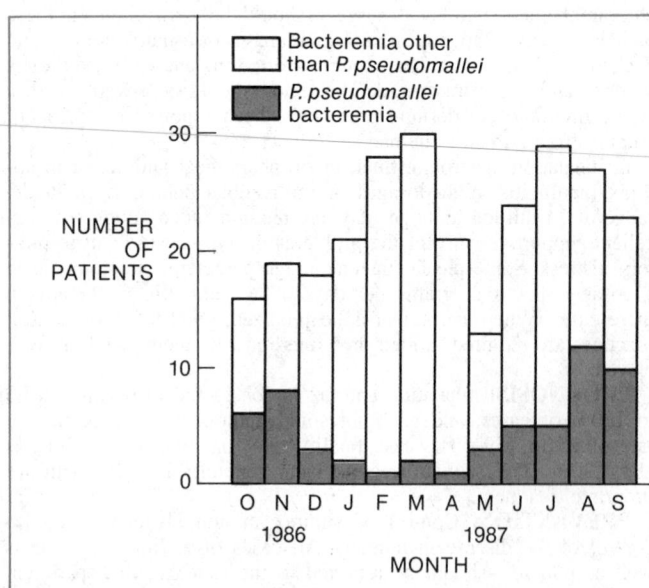

FIGURE 303-1. Number of persons with community-acquired bacteremia caused by *P. pseudomallei* and other organisms, in northeast Thailand from October 1986 to September 1987. (From Chaowagul W, White NJ, Dance DAB, et al.: Melioidosis: A major cause of community-acquired septicemia in northeastern Thailand. J Infect Dis 159:890, 1989; by permission of the University of Chicago Press, 1989.)

ity rate, even with current therapy, is about 40%. Patients with the highest mortality include those who are hypothermic, azotemic, or unable to produce a leukocytosis. Prompt early therapy with ceftazidime has now been found to reduce the mortality by 50% when historically compared with combination therapy with chloramphenicol, doxycycline, and cotrimoxazole as used before 1987. Relapses are common, perhaps 25% overall, with clinical severity and initial therapy the crucial risk factors (Fig. 303–2). Long-term oral treatment with amoxicillin–clavulanic acid appears logical to reduce relapses, since recurrence carries a high mortality rate.

Pseudomonas mallei. *P. mallei* can cause an infection in horses, mules, and donkeys that occasionally has been transmitted to humans. The name "glanders" comes from the prominent pulmonary involvement, although the infection can, instead, be characterized by subcutaneous ulcerative lesions or lymphatic thickening with nodules (known as farcy).

Glanders was never a common human infection, and with the decline in the use of horses for day-to-day activities and with improved sanitation, glanders has become a very rare disease. Apparently, there have been no naturally acquired infections in the United States since 1938, although the occasional case occurs in other countries.

Like melioidosis, glanders tends to occur as an acute localized suppurative infection, an acute pulmonary infection, an acute septicemic infection, or a chronic suppurative infection. An abraded area of skin may lead to a local nodule with acute lymphangitis. Inoculation into an abraded mucous membrane can lead to extensive ulcerating granulomatous lesions. These forms of infection seem to have an incubation period of 1 to 5 days; in contrast, after inhalation, a primary pneumonia tends to develop 10 to 14 days later. Symptoms are relatively nonspecific and include fever, occasional rigors, malaise, fatigue, and headache. Examination findings depend on the form of infection. Leukocytosis is common. Chest radiographs of the acute pulmonary form usually show densities consistent with early lung abscess; however, lobar or bronchopneumonia-type infiltrates are common. Chronic suppurative disease involves multiple subcutaneous and intramuscular abscesses, especially on the extremities, with lymphatic involvement and, in many, a nasal discharge with or without ulceration.

The organism is usually difficult to find in exudates but, when seen with a Gram stain or methylene blue, appears similar to *P. pseudomallei*. The organism is reasonably easy to cultivate.

The treatment of glanders is uncertain because of its rarity—hence the inability to carry out clinical trials. A reasonable recommendation is to initiate therapy with regimens found effective for melioidosis, recognizing that the acute septicemic form has been uniformly fatal and suggesting that full dosage of intravenous combinations of agents be given initially.

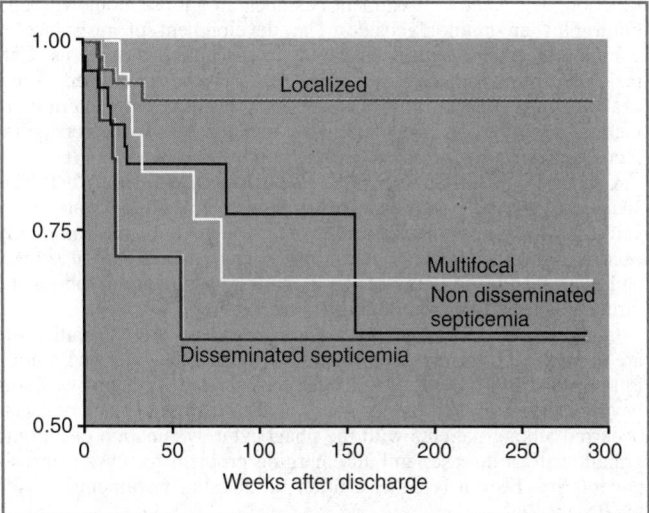

FIGURE 303–2. Relapse-free probability in survivors of acute melioidosis stratified by clinical severity on first admission. (From Chaowagul W, Suputtamongkol Y, Dance DAB, et al.: Relapse in melioidosis: Incidence and risk factors. J Infect Dis 168:1181, 1993.)

Pseudomonas aeruginosa. The name "aeruginosa" comes from the fluorescent blue-green pigment pyocyanin, produced by many, but not all, strains. Other pigments produced by *P. aeruginosa* include pyoverdin (green) and, occasionally, pyorubin (deep red) and pyomelanin (black). Like other pseudomonads, *P. aeruginosa* grows well in multiple moist settings with limited nutrients. Found in soil, in water, and on plants, it also can be a normal commensal in animals and humans. Colonization in humans usually takes place in moist areas, such as perineum, auditory canal, axillae, and the lower alimentary canal. It is commonly found in faucet aerators, sink traps, ice machines, and kitchen settings in the hospital; it can become a particular problem when it contaminates medications or medical devices with a moist environment, such as ventilators, endoscopes, pressure monitors, and the like. It can withstand many disinfectants and is resistant to a broad variety of antimicrobial agents. In the nonhospital setting, infections have been related to growth in swimming pools, contact lens solutions, and hot tubs.

Infection with *P. aeruginosa* has become, to a large degree, a byproduct of medical advances in technology. In the 20 years prior to 1960 at the Johns Hopkins Hospital, only 91 cases of *P. aeruginosa* bacteremia occurred. In recent years, *P. aeruginosa* has been the fourth most common cause of primary nosocomial gram-negative bacteremia and the fourth most frequently isolated nosocomial pathogen, having caused about 10% of all hospital-acquired infections, 13% of all nosocomial pneumonias, 12% of urinary tract infections, and 7% of surgical wound infections.

The most common infections caused by *P. aeruginosa* include nosocomial bacteremia, nosocomial pneumonia, nosocomial urinary tract infection, surgical wound infection, endocarditis related to intravenous drug abuse or placement of artificial heart valves, respiratory infection associated with cystic fibrosis, external otitis, including "malignant" external otitis (see Ch. 421), corneal keratitis, and uncommon occurrences of spinal osteomyelitis in heroin addicts (see Ch. 283) and rare cases of meningitis or brain abscess. A common origin of bacteremia in the granulocytopenic patient is infection along the alimentary canal, especially perianal cellulitis, colonic lesions, and, occasionally, pharyngitis or esophagitis. Finally, extensive burns are commonly colonized by *P. aeruginosa*, with progression to sepsis and death.

P. aeruginosa almost never causes infection in the absence of (1) damage to a normal host defense mechanism (e.g., cancer chemotherapy–induced mucosal damage to the alimentary canal, granulocytopenia, or extensive third-degree burns), (2) deficiency or alteration in a defense mechanism (e.g., the progressive respiratory tract changes of cystic fibrosis), or (3) bypass of a normal defense mechanism (e.g., respiratory assist device directly inoculating organisms into the bronchial tree while concurrently limiting or damaging the mucociliary mechanism, or insertion of an indwelling urinary catheter, circumventing the normal bladder clearance mechanism). Thus infections with *P. aeruginosa* are seen most commonly in patients with a urinary catheter; those neutropenic from disease, chemotherapy, or both; those with cystic fibrosis; those with extensive thermal injuries; those in the intensive care unit who are subjected to any number of invasive procedures; those with head trauma, allowing entry either directly or via a pressure monitoring device; those with artificial heart valves or damaged endocardium from contaminants in illicit drugs; and those who have had extensive surgery, particularly when there is consequent need for open drainage. Pulmonary infection late in the course of AIDS may present as an acute infection or as an indolent, frequently recurrent infection mimicking that seen with cystic fibrosis.

Pollack has pointed out three distinct stages of *Pseudomonas* infection: stage I—bacterial attachment and colonization; stage II—local invasion; and stage III—bloodstream dissemination and systemic disease. Stage I is a prerequisite to stage II, which, in turn, is a prerequisite to stage III, although obviously not all colonized individuals have local invasion and not all those with local invasion progress to dissemination or systemic disease. The three stages relate to the fact that this organism is both invasive and toxigenic. Colonization in a normal person is relatively uncommon at most sites, although, over time, a fair proportion of the population will have transient colonization of the colon. However, hospitalized patients have a much higher frequency of colonization, related in part to changes in host defenses, as discussed above, and partly to the frequency of hospital reservoirs of this organism. In addition, broad-spectrum antimicrobial therapy suppresses other normal microbial flora, especially along the alimentary canal. This suppression reduces the body's normal mechanism of colonization resistance so that an organism such as *P. aeruginosa* or other species resistant to the antibiotics used can more readily colonize multiple locations in high concentration. Additional specific factors further predispose to colonization by *P. aeruginosa.* These include the presence of pili for attachment, flagella for motility, and exoproducts, especially proteinases. Also involved is the secretory protease-induced loss of fibronectin from epithelial cells during serious illness (among patients hospitalized or not), which in turn allows the pili or fimbriae to adhere to the oral, pharyngeal, and respiratory epithelium. Thus the illness determinants of protease production are major modulators of the oral flora. This colonization in turn can be accentuated by local damage caused by an endotracheal tube, by viral infection (such as influenza), by thermal injury, or by cancer chemotherapy and is exacerbated by antibiotics. *P. aeruginosa,* in some settings, can help protect itself from defense mechanisms by producing a glycocalyx, a carbohydrate produced by many bacteria, which, by surrounding the cell and anchoring it to epithelial cells or invasive devices such as an intravascular or urinary catheter, protects the bacterium from antibody, complement, and polymorphonuclear leukocytes or macrophages.

After colonization, *P. aeruginosa* can invade in the appropriate setting through the effect of extracellular enzymes (toxins). These include elastase, alkaline protease, and perhaps also cytotoxin and hemolysins. Elastase and protease have been demonstrated to cause necrotizing lesions in the skin, lung, and cornea, along with small vessel necrotizing lesions, which cause the characteristic skin finding known as "ecthyma gangrenosum." It is this combination of local necrosis and blood vessel destruction that is the essence of the initial invasive characteristic of *P. aeruginosa.*

The third stage of *Pseudomonas* infection, dissemination and systemic disease, is due, in the first case, to these same extracellular enzymes and, in the second case, to *Pseudomonas* liposaccharide (endotoxin) and exotoxin A. As with other septicemias caused by gram-negative bacilli, endotoxin is thought to be a critical factor in the activation of the clotting, fibrinolytic, kinin, and complement systems, along with the production of prostaglandins and leukotrienes, the release of β-endorphins, and the release of cytokines, including tumor necrosis factor. By some interaction of many or all of these factors come fever, shock, disseminated intravascular coagulation (which is relatively uncommon with *Pseudomonas* bacteremia), and the adult respiratory distress syndrome. The other factor, exotoxin A, is similar to diphtheria toxin in that it inhibits protein synthesis. It causes local necrosis and encourages bacterial dissemination to the systemic circulation and, in itself, has been shown to produce shock in animal models.

Pseudomonas bacteremia occurs most commonly in cancer patients who are receiving intensive chemotherapy that produces granulocytopenia in patients with extensive third-degree burns and, occasionally, in patients with immunoglobulin or hypocomplementemia states. It is also a common cause of bacteremia in the patient with urinary catheterization. It is the fourth most frequent cause of primary hospital-acquired gram-negative bacteremia. Sepsis in burn patients arises from the thermally damaged skin. Bacteremia in neutropenic patients arises principally from the lower intestinal tract and occasionally from primary pneumonia. Surveillance cultures have documented that granulocytopenic patients frequently become colonized, and nearly all colonized patients will develop bacteremia if profound (< 100 per microliter) granulocytopenia persists for more than a few days. Ecthyma gangrenosum, usually a sign of fairly advanced systemic infection, is not pathognomonic but is most frequently associated with *P. aeruginosa* bacteremia. These skin lesions at first are small and indurated, and then rapidly enlarge, become necrotic, and may ulcerate. Bacteria, on histologic section, are seen to be invading small arteries and veins, with remarkably minimal evidence of inflammation. A histologically similar lesion can be found in the lungs as a secondary consequence of bacteremia. The mortality of *Pseudomonas* sepsis is high, with the underlying status of the patient's host defenses and the promptness of instituting empirical antibiotic therapy being the two

critical factors affecting survival. The presence of septic shock, the evidence of septic metastases, or both when antibiotics are started are usually considered adverse prognostic signs but, in reality, represent another measure of late institution of therapy.

The standard approach to suspected gram-negative sepsis, including that caused by *P. aeruginosa,* is a combination using an antipseudomonal β-lactam (penicillin or cephalosporin) with an aminoglycoside. Two newer drugs, imipenem and the antipseudomonal quinolones—again, in combination with an aminoglycoside—are also effective. Although in some cases, such as in the febrile neutropenic patient, monotherapy has been recommended with agents such as ceftazidime or imipenem, a two-drug regimen is advised for initial empirical therapy. Studies suggest that survival is improved when two antibiotics to which the organism is susceptible are given immediately and that survival is further improved if the two agents prove to be synergistic in activity. For example, in a study of 200 episodes of *P. aeruginosa* bacteremia, combination therapy yielded a mortality of 27%, whereas monotherapy mortality was 47%. A later study suggested that adding rifampin to the β-lactam–aminoglycoside would further improve response rates and reduce breakthrough or relapsing bacteremia, although survival was not affected. For the future, we must also look to immunologic approaches to bacteremia prevention and treatment, such as monoclonal antibodies to lipopolysaccharide.

Respiratory tract infections (see Ch. 273) can take the form of a primary pneumonia, a secondary pneumonia due to bacteremia, or a chronic infection with intermittent exacerbations. Primary pneumonia occurs almost exclusively in hospitalized patients whose oropharynx or tracheobronchial tree is colonized by *P. aeruginosa,* the latter as a result of intubation. Frequently, *Pseudomonas* pneumonia occurs in the setting of additional pulmonary damage, such as blunt trauma, substantial atelectasis, or hemothorax. Atelectasis appears to be a key contributing pathogenic factor. Early, aggressive physiotherapy for the chest sometimes clears what appears to be a pneumonia but in fact is atelectasis that has resulted in fever, purulent sputum production, and a positive chest radiograph. However, once actual pneumonia has begun, the prognosis is poor, and early empirical therapy is crucial.

The pneumonia that follows bacteremia is usually fulminant, with multiple areas of hemorrhage around small and medium-sized pulmonary arteries and lesions caused by necrosis of the small muscular arteries and veins in a fashion similar to ecthyma gangrenosum. Survival is limited even with prompt, aggressive therapy.

Chronic *Pseudomonas* respiratory infections are largely limited to patients with cystic fibrosis (see also Ch. 58), with the frequency of this infection increasing with age so that, ultimately, almost all patients will have significant *Pseudomonas* pulmonary infection. The age differential is probably related to the progressive development of airway obstruction, a crucial factor in development of *Pseudomonas* infection. This chronic infection is associated with chronic cough, nutritional losses, and progressive loss of pulmonary function. The standard treatment has been an antipseudomonal penicillin plus an aminoglycoside. The development of resistance is common, so therapy must be based on susceptibility patterns. Ceftazidime, imipenem, or a quinolone also may be considered. Acute exacerbations may be reduced or even prevented with intermittent therapy a number of times each year, irrespective of whether the infection is currently quiescent.

OTHER PSEUDOMONADS. *Pseudomonas cepacia.* This species of *Pseudomonas* can grow as well in distilled water as it can in trypticase soy broth; it is resistant to many of the commonly used hospital disinfectants; it can use penicillin as a carbon source; and it is resistant to many of the commonly used antimicrobials. Its virulence properties are not understood.

Community-acquired infections are rare. However, certain hosts are at substantially increased risk. Endocarditis has occurred among intravenous drug abusers; skin infections related to extensive burns have occurred; a necrotizing, occasionally recurrent pneumonia has occurred among patients with the phagocytic dysfunction of chronic granulomatous disease; and an emerging problem for cystic fibrosis patients has been a relentless, often fulminating pneumonia caused by *P. cepacia.*

Nosocomial infections and pseudoinfections are considered together because of a common origin and because it can be difficult to distinguish between the two. The source of hospital *P. cepacia* is usually a moist or water-based reservoir, which, given the technologic advances of medicine, suggests that *P. cepacia* has the potential to become a not infrequent cause of infection and pseudoinfection in the high-technology or intensive care setting. *P. cepacia* has been found to cause pneumonitis, endocarditis, wound infections, and urinary tract infections, along with primary bacteremia. The origins of iatrogenic bacteremia can be conveniently divided into those related to contaminated solutions, injectables, and medical devices. Among the contaminated solutions implicated in bacteremia or pseudobacteremia have been disinfectant solutions, heparinized flushing solutions, distilled water, topical anesthetics, and intravenous infusates, including human serum albumin and cryoprecipitate. Contaminated injectables have included saline, methylprednisolone, and fentanyl. The implicated devices all include a moist environment where the organism can multiply; pressure monitoring devices, respiratory assist devices, peritoneal dialysis machines, reusable hemodialysis coils, and blood gas analyzers have been documented as point sources.

Figure 303–3 shows an epidemic of *P. cepacia* bacteremia among patients at the Clinical Center of the National Institutes of Health. The figure indicates that *P. cepacia*–positive blood cultures were uncommon in the years preceding this outbreak and that the majority during the epidemic occurred within the medical intensive care unit. A blood gas analyzer in an adjoining laboratory was found to be contaminated, and this served as the point source for this series of bacteremias. Although some were apparently pseudobacteremias (i.e., the blood culture became positive owing to contamination by skin or other sources), others were true bacteremias with significant morbidity. Indeed, among those highly compromised patients, many with cancer and significant immune suppression, the mortality resulting from the *P. cepacia* infection itself was 38%. Respiratory colonization in an appropriately predisposed host can progress to pneumonia, as evidenced by 14 of 37 patients with colonization and hematologic malignancies who developed pneumonia during an 18-month outbreak. In another outbreak of 14 bacteremias among cancer patients, all had central venous lines flushed with a contaminated heparin solution.

P. cepacia is resistant to many of the commonly used broad-spectrum antibiotics but is usually susceptible to trimethoprim-sulfamethoxazole and ceftazidime.

Pseudomonas pickettii. This is an uncommon cause of infection. In the past 30 years, 49 cases of bacteremia were reported. Thirty-eight of the 49 were caused by contaminated injected solutions; 7 more were related to contaminated ventilators or dialysis equipment. Four patients had bacteremia related to indwelling intravenous catheters; all were treated at one institution over a 2-year period. *P. pickettii* is usually resistant to aminoglycosides but susceptible to cephalosporins and antipseudomonal penicillins.

Xanthomonas maltophilia (Pseudomonas maltophilia). *X. maltophilia* is atypical of the other pseudomonads in that the oxidase test is negative or equivocal. It is probably a fairly common commensal and a part of the transient flora, especially of hospitalized patients. In hospitals it is not infrequently found in moist or wet settings. The organism is resistant to most of the first- and second-generation cephalosporins, semisynthetic penicillins, and aminoglycosides, although it has variable susceptibility to the antipseudomonal penicillins. It is generally susceptible to many of the third-generation cephalosporins, trimethoprim-sulfamethoxazole, and rifampin. Synergy has been noted with trimethoprim-sulfamethoxazole plus carbenicillin and with the triple regimen of trimethoprim-sulfamethoxazole plus carbenicillin and rifampin.

X. maltophilia is an uncommon cause of a wide spectrum of diseases that, in general, are less severe than infections caused by other gram-negative bacilli in similar locations. *X. maltophilia* is susceptible to many, but not all, of the common broad-spectrum antibiotics. It is frequently resistant to cephalosporins, antipseudomonal penicillins, imipenem, and quinolones, and is usually susceptible to trimethoprim-sulfamethoxazole. The most common types of infection are pneumonia, endocarditis, urinary tract infection, and iatrogenic bacteremia or pseudobacteremia. Cholangitis and meningitis have been reported but are quite unusual, and wounds, although a common site for *X. maltophilia* isolation, are rarely infected by this organism. Pneumonias tend to occur in debilitated patients with prior antibiotic therapy in a nosocomial setting, but they are very uncommon, and the organism should be questioned as causative in the absence of a pure culture via bronchoscopy, thoracentesis, or blood. Endocarditis in the community occurs among intravenous drug abusers and in the hospital as a complication of open heart surgery, usually among those with abnormal valves. Traumatized victims, especially with contaminated wounds, develop serious infections in association with ventilatory assist and broad-spectrum antimicrobials. *X. maltophilia* is being increasingly recognized as a cause of serious infection (pneumonia, bacteremia, urinary tract and wound infection) among cancer patients who are granulocytopenic and have received broad-spectrum antibiotics, especially imipenem.

X. maltophilia bacteriuria is found occasionally in patients with indwelling long-term catheters; however, only rarely has the organism been shown to cause clinical infection. When infection has occurred, it has usually been in association with significant instrumentation, genitourinary surgery, or both. The morbidity has tended to be low, and therapy, especially with trimethoprim-sulfamethoxazole, has frequently been effective.

Iatrogenic bacteremia and pseudobacteremia caused by this organism have been reported often. In one epidemic of 25 patients with positive blood cultures, it was determined that these cases were pseudobacteremias due to contaminated blood collection tubes. In another setting, eight children were found to have bacteremia after open heart surgery, apparently as a result of contamination of the monitoring transducers in the intensive care unit. *X. maltophilia* has been found to contaminate the deionized water used for diluting disinfectants, and the organism can even survive in the diluted disinfectant. It is important to emphasize that not all of

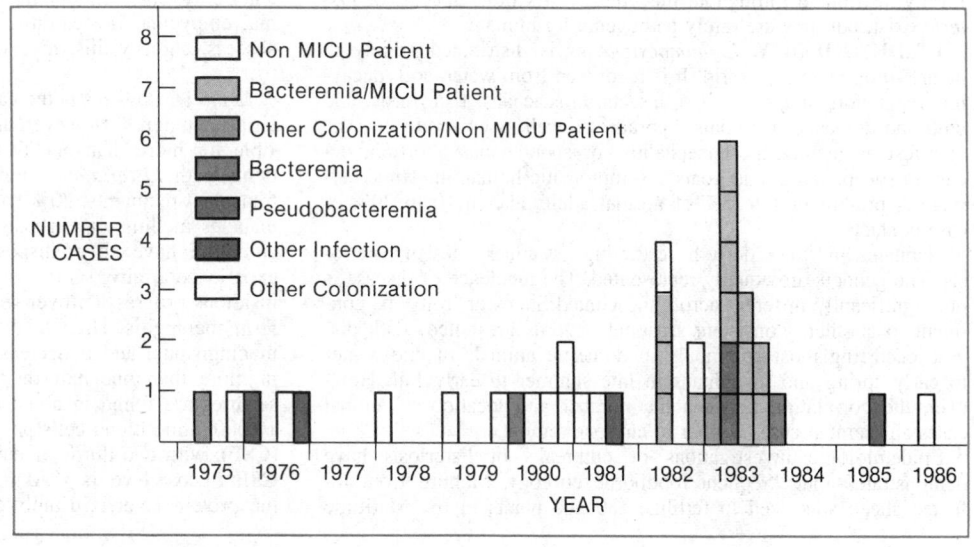

FIGURE 303–3. An epidemic of *Pseudomonas cepacia* bacteremia among patients at the Clinical Center of the National Institutes of Health. Note that the epidemic in 1982–1983 within the MICU was caused by a contaminated nearby blood gas analyzer. MICU = medical intensive care unit. (Reprinted with permission from Henderson DK, Baptiste R, Parillo J, et al.: Indolent epidemic of *Pseudomonas cepacia* bacteremia and pseudobacteremia in an intensive care unit traced to a contaminated blood gas analyzer. Am J Med 84:75, 1988.)

these bacteremias have been "pseudobacteremias"; for example, two fatal cases of endocarditis have been noted as a result of bacteremia caused by a contaminated device or solution. Permanent indwelling vascular catheters are a major source of bacteremias; imipenem therapy is an important predisposing factor.

Bodey GP, Jadeja L, Elting L: *Pseudomonas* bacteremia: Retrospective analysis of 410 episodes. Arch Intern Med 145:1621, 1985. *A review of* P. aeruginosa *bacteremia.*

Chaowagul W, Suputtamongkol Y, Dance DAB, et al.: Relapse in melioidosis: Incidence and risk factors. J Infect Dis 168:1181, 1993. *A 23% relapse rate was related to initial infection severity and therapy.*

Henderson DK, Baptiste R, Parillo J, et al.: Indolent epidemic of *Pseudomonas cepacia* bacteremia and pseudobacteremia in an intensive care unit traced to a contaminated blood gas analyzer. Am J Med 84:75, 1988. *A nice review of bacteremia and pseudobacteremia due to* P. cepacia.

Hilf M, Yu VL, Sharp J, et al.: Antibiotic therapy for *Pseudomonas aeruginosa* bacteremia: Outcome correlations in a prospective study of 200 patients. Am J Med 87:540, 1989. *A critical evaluation of antimicrobial therapy for* P. aeruginosa *bacteremia suggesting an advantage for combination therapy.*

Marshall WF, Keating MR, Anhalt JP, Steckelberg JM: *Xanthomonas maltophilia:* An emerging nosocomial pathogen. Mayo Clin Proc 64:1097, 1989. *A thorough review.*

Pollack M: *Pseudomonas aeruginosa. In* Mandell GL, Douglas RG Jr, Bennett JE (eds.): Principles and Practice of Infectious Diseases. 3rd ed. New York, Churchill Livingstone, 1990, pp 1673–1691. *A very thorough discussion of the microbiology, epidemiology, pathogenic factors, and clinical syndromes of* P. aeruginosa.

Raveh D, Simhon A, Gimmon Z, et al.: Infections caused by *Pseudomonas pickettii* in association with permanent indwelling intravenous devices: Four cases and a review. Clin Infect Dis 17:877, 1993. *A review of the few reported cases of bacteremia by this organism.*

Sanford JP: *Pseudomonas* species (including melioidosis and glanders). *In* Mandell GL, Douglas RG Jr, Bennett JE (eds.): Principles and Practice of Infectious Diseases. 3rd ed. New York, Churchill Livingstone, 1990, pp 1692–1696. *Broad discussion of melioidosis and glanders by an expert in infections of importance to the U.S. military.*

White NJ, Dance DAB, Chaowagul W, et al.: Halving of mortality of severe melioidosis by ceftazidime. Lancet 2:697, 1988. *New antibiotics have had a major impact on mortality.*

304 LISTERIOSIS
Alan M. Stamm

DEFINITION. Listeriosis is an infectious disease caused by the bacterium *Listeria monocytogenes*. The majority of afflicted patients are immunocompromised and present with meningoencephalitis.

ETIOLOGY. *L. monocytogenes* is a gram-positive bacillus but may stain unevenly and/or appear coccoid. It is facultatively anaerobic, non–spore-forming, and β-hemolytic on blood agar. It grows optimally at 35 to 37°C, grows less well at temperatures as low as 4°C, and exhibits tumbling motility at 20 to 25°C.

Although at least 16 serotypes of *L. monocytogenes* are identified, each of the types 1/2a, 1/2b, and 4b accounts for about 30% of human disease in the United States. These serotypes are uniformly distributed throughout this country. Six other species of *Listeria* exist, but they are rarely pathogenic for humans.

EPIDEMIOLOGY. *L. monocytogenes* is distributed widely in nature throughout the world. It is recovered from water, soil, decaying vegetation, silage, sewage, insects, crustaceans, fish, birds, and wild and domestic mammals. Sporadic as well as epizootic disease, manifest as meningitis, encephalitis, or spontaneous abortion, occurs in sheep, cattle, and goats. Asymptomatic human intestinal carriage is present in 1 to 5% of normal adults and in 10 to 20% of case contacts.

Neonates and the elderly have the highest attack rates of listeriosis. The genders are equally represented. The incidence of disease is not significantly different across the United States or from one continent to another. Consistent seasonal patterns are noted, with disease occurring most commonly in domestic animals in late winter to early spring and in humans in late summer to early fall. However, the correlation between the number and location of animal cases and human cases is poor in any one region.

Epidemiologic investigations of outbreaks of listeriosis have demonstrated their frequent foodborne etiology. Manure from infected sheep was used to fertilize cabbage plants in the Maritime Provinces of Canada; 41 cases of human disease in 1980–1981 were linked to the ingestion of cole slaw prepared from these cabbages. Milk from cows was pasteurized but nonetheless implicated in 49 cases of listeriosis in Massachusetts in 1983; whether the microorganism survived pasteurization or contaminated the product afterward remains controversial. The largest epidemic occurred in southern California in 1985; 142 cases were associated with the consumption of soft, Mexican-style cheese made with unpasteurized milk. Similarly, an outbreak of 122 cases in Switzerland during 1983–1987 was attributed to a soft cheese. During periods of increased disease activity, the organism causing an epidemic strain is differentiated from that causing sporadic disease by serotyping, electrophoretic enzyme typing, ribotyping, or DNA fingerprinting. All four of these outbreaks were due to *L. monocytogenes* serotype 4b.

Further evidence for foodborne acquisition of *L. monocytogenes* is provided by recent microbiologic investigations. The microorganism has been identified as a fairly common contaminant of raw and pasteurized milk; ice cream; soft cheese; raw beef, pork, and lamb; ready-to-eat meat products, including salami, sausages, paté, and hot dogs; retail poultry; cooked shrimp and crab; raw vegetables such as cabbage, cucumbers, potatoes, and radishes; and packaged salads. Although commercial food production methods may effectively kill the microorganism, products may become contaminated during subsequent processing and packaging before leaving the production facility.

PATHOGENESIS. Most adults with listeriosis have impaired cell-mediated immunity caused by cytotoxic chemotherapy for malignancy, immunosuppressive therapy for organ transplantation, or pregnancy. Both helper and suppressor T cells are centrally involved, whereas immunoglobulin and complement play lesser roles as opsonins. The gastrointestinal tract is the usual portal of entry. Bacteria are taken up from the lumen by endocytosis of epithelial cells covering intestinal villi. The inoculum required to cause disease may depend on the immunologic health and gastric acidity of the host as well as the virulence characteristics of the microorganism.

Dissemination occurs via simple bacteremia and/or circulation of infected monocytes. *L. monocytogenes* is a facultative intracellular parasite capable of multiplying within the nonimmune monocyte-macrophage. Listeriolysin O, a hemolysin structurally similar to streptolysin O, may be an important virulence factor in this process. Phagocytosis of the bacterium stimulates its production; it binds to cholesterol in cell membranes, leading to their disruption. This feature may allow the microorganism to escape from phagolysosomes but to persist and multiply within macrophages, ultimately leading to their destruction.

CLINICAL MANIFESTATIONS. The incubation period between acquiring the infection and disease onset varies from days to weeks. The clinical presentation of listeriosis is as meningitis in 50 to 60% of cases; bacteremia without evident localized disease in 25 to 30%; parenchymal disease of the central nervous system (CNS) with or without meningitis, in 10%; and endocarditis in 5%. Infrequent manifestations due to hematogenous dissemination include anterior uveitis, endophthalmitis, cervical lymphadenitis, pneumonia, empyema, myocarditis, pericarditis, peritonitis, hepatitis, liver abscess, cholecystitis, mycotic aneurysm, osteomyelitis, and arthritis.

L. monocytogenes is the cause in about 1% of cases of acute bacterial meningitis. However, among patients with cancer, it is responsible for more than one fifth of episodes. Conversely, among patients with *Listeria* meningitis, 25% have a malignancy; 25% are transplant recipients; 20% have another underlying disorder, such as diabetes mellitus or cirrhosis, or are receiving glucocorticosteroids; and 30% have no predisposing condition. Two thirds of patients experience a fairly sudden onset of symptoms, but one third note an insidious progression over several days. No features distinguish *Listeria* meningitis. High fever is almost always reported. Headache, meningismus, and a decreased level of consciousness are present in more than one half of patients. Focal neurologic deficits and seizures are found in about one fourth. Most patients have 100 to 10,000 white blood cells per cubic millimeter of cerebrospinal fluid (CSF), with two thirds of them being polymorphonuclear cells. The CSF glucose level is < 50 mg per deciliter in one half of cases, and the protein level is usually 50 to 300 mg per deciliter. The Gram stain of CSF is interpreted as revealing gram-positive bacilli in only 25% of cases. Cultures of blood are positive in 60%. The differential diagnosis includes disease due to *Streptococcus pneumoniae*, a gram-negative bacillus, or *Cryptococcus neoformans*.

Parenchymal disease of the CNS is associated with clinical and CSF findings of meningitis in only 50% of cases. Anatomically, the spectrum of disease includes diffuse and localized cerebritis, brain stem meningoencephalitis (rhombencephalitis), and macroscopic abscess formation in the brain or spine. All patients are febrile; other common symptoms and signs are decreased consciousness in two thirds of patients, headache and hemiparesis in one half, and seizures and cranial nerve palsies in one third. *Listeria* rhombencephalitis merits special mention. Eighty per cent of reported victims have been previously healthy. The illness has a biphasic course: A 3- to 10-day prodrome of fever, headache, and vomiting is terminated by the abrupt onset of asymmetric palsies of cranial nerves V, VI, VII, IX, and/or X, cerebellar signs, paresis, and hypesthesia. In patients without concurrent meningitis, the analysis of CSF is usually normal or reveals only a mild pleocytosis and increased protein; Gram stain and culture are positive in a minority. Blood cultures are positive in most patients with parenchymal CNS disease. The differential diagnosis includes tuberculosis, toxoplasmosis, nocardiosis, mycoses, and stroke.

Bacteremia without evident localized disease (primary bacteremia) occurs in patients with hematologic malignancies (33% of cases), organ transplant recipients (25%), pregnant women (13%), and individuals suffering from alcoholism or cirrhosis (11%). *Listeria* bacteremia has no distinguishing features. Up to one fourth have premonitory gastrointestinal symptoms: nausea, vomiting, abdominal pain, and/or diarrhea.

Endocarditis occurs not in immunocompromised hosts but usually in those with underlying valvular heart disease. The aortic valve is involved in two thirds of cases and the mitral valve in one third, and prosthetic valve disease is well described. The onset of illness is subacute, with a median duration of symptoms prior to hospitalization of 5 weeks. Fever is cited in 75% of reported cases, a new or changing murmur in 40%, splenomegaly in 35%, and hepatomegaly, CNS emboli, and pulmonary emboli each in 25%.

One third of all cases of listeriosis are associated with pregnancy. Most commonly, in the third trimester, the mother develops a "flu-like" illness with fever, sore throat, myalgias, crampy abdominal pain, and diarrhea. After 3 to 7 days, premature labor or abortion ensues. Transplacental transmission of disease becomes clinically evident in the newborn within hours of delivery; this severe septicemic illness is known as "granulomatosis infantisepticum." Babies also may acquire infection in the birth canal or nosocomially in the nursery; at a mean of 14 days of life, disease presents as anorexia, fever, or meningismus. *L. monocytogenes* is the third most common cause of neonatal sepsis and meningitis after *Escherichia coli* and group B streptococci.

The complete spectrum of listeriosis is seen among patients with acquired immunodeficiency syndrome (AIDS). Chemoprophylaxis of pneumocystosis with trimethoprim-sulfamethoxazole may prevent listeriosis.

DIAGNOSIS. The microbiologic diagnosis of listeriosis is established by culture of blood, CSF, or tissue. In cases of granulomatosis infantisepticum, meconium, amniotic fluid, and lochia are cultured. Initial growth in the laboratory may be slow and may require several days. Unwary technicians may misinterpret these gram-positive bacilli as diphtheroids and label them contaminants.

TREATMENT. Ampicillin is the antimicrobial agent of choice for listeriosis. Although no comparative trials have been conducted, it has an established record of efficacy and can be administered safely even during pregnancy and infancy. The standard dosage in patients with meningitis is 200 mg per kilogram per day in six divided doses given intravenously. The duration of therapy necessary for consistent cure is 3 weeks. Seriously ill and immunocompromised patients are treated with ampicillin plus gentamicin; the latter drug is administered intravenously in doses sufficient to yield peak serum concentrations of 5 to 8 μg per milliliter and predictable CSF concentrations of 1 to 2 μg per milliliter. Most *in vitro* studies and animal model trials suggest that these two drugs act synergistically against *L. monocytogenes*.

Trimethoprim-sulfamethoxazole has emerged as the preferred therapy for patients allergic to penicillins. The combination is bactericidal at achievable serum and CSF concentrations. Many case reports have appeared in the literature, including those of immunocompromised patients with CNS disease, and all were cured. Experience to date suggests an initial dosage of 160 mg of trimethoprim plus 800 mg of sulfamethoxazole given intravenously every 6 to 12 hours in adults with normal renal function.

The inordinate number of treatment failures and relapses among patients treated with cephalosporins or chloramphenicol indicates that these agents are not to be used. Newer β-lactams, including imipenem, are not as active as ampicillin against *L. monocytogenes*. The quinolones do not appear to be sufficiently active at achievable concentrations to be useful clinically. There has been no significant change in the antimicrobial susceptibility profile of *L. monocytogenes* over the past two decades.

PROGNOSIS. The overall mortality rate of *Listeria* meningitis is 30%, being higher in patients with cancer, hypoglycorrhachia, or bacteremia and lower in previously healthy individuals. Parenchymal CNS disease and endocarditis are fatal in 50% of cases.

PREVENTION. Individuals at increased risk should avoid raw milk, wash raw vegetables carefully, and cook meats thoroughly. In the hospital, patients with listeriosis should be isolated from immunocompromised hosts.

Armstrong RW, Fung PC: Brainstem encephalitis (rhombencephalitis) due to *Listeria monocytogenes*: Case report and review. Clin Infect Dis 16:689, 1993. *A detailed analysis of the clinical aspects of this syndrome of immunocompetent adults.*

Farber JM, Peterkin PI: *Listeria monocytogenes*, a food-borne pathogen. Microbiol Rev 55:476, 1991. *An extensive review of the microbiology, epidemiology, and pathogenesis of foodborne disease.*

Jurado RL, Farley MM, Pereira E, et al.: Increased risk of meningitis and bacteremia due to *Listeria monocytogenes* in patients with human immunodeficiency virus infection. Clin Infect Dis 17:224, 1993. *Incidence, demographics, and clinical outcome were assessed in a prospective, population-based survey. The estimated incidence among patients with AIDS was 150 times higher than in the general population.*

Schuchat AM, Deaver KA, Wenger JD, et al.: Role of foods in sporadic listeriosis: I. Case-control study of dietary risk factors. JAMA 267:2041, 1992. *An interesting and enlightening description of the methods used to identify contaminated foods responsible for one third of sporadic disease. Provides detailed dietary recommendations for listeriosis prevention.*

305 ERYSIPELOID
Annette C. Reboli

DEFINITION. *Erysipelothrix rhusiopathiae,* the causative agent of swine erysipelas, causes three well-defined patterns of human infection: (1) a mild, localized cutaneous form (erysipeloid of Rosenbach); (2) a severe, diffuse cutaneous form without bacteremia; and (3) a bacteremic form, with or without cutaneous involvement, usually complicated by endocarditis. Sheep and swine erysipelas and diamond skin disease are animal diseases, whereas erysipeloid, whale finger, and seal finger involve localized cellulitis of the fingers and hands, which is the most common manifestation of infection with *E. rhusiopathiae* seen in humans. The term "erysipeloid" refers to cutaneous infection caused by *E. rhusiopathiae* and should not be confused with erysipelas, which is a superficial cellulitis due to streptococci or staphylococci.

ETIOLOGY. *E. rhusiopathiae* is a thin, pleomorphic, nonsporulating, microaerophilic, gram-positive rod. It may be confused with other gram-positive bacillary organisms, in particular *Listeria monocytogenes* and *Corynebacterium* species. It can be differentiated from *L. monocytogenes* by its lack of motility, lack of catalase and coagulase production, and resistance to neomycin. Most strains of *E. rhusiopathiae* produce hydrogen sulfide on triple sugar iron agar slants. This feature distinguishes *E. rhusiopathiae* from *L. monocytogenes* and from corynebacteria. Because α-hemolysis may be seen after 48 hours of incubation of *E. rhusiopathiae,* confusion with streptococci also may occur.

EPIDEMIOLOGY. *E. rhusiopathiae* is found worldwide as a commensal or a pathogen in a variety of animals, including swine, sheep, cattle, horses, dogs, and rodents; fowl, including chickens, ducks, turkeys, and parrots; and flies, ticks, mites, and lice. The greatest commercial impact of *E. rhusiopathiae* infection is due to disease in swine, but infection of sheep and poultry is also important economically. Although the organism colonizes the mucoid surface slime of fish, it does not appear to cause disease in these animals. Environmental surfaces in contact with infected animals or their products are potential sources of *E. rhusiopathiae*. It can persist for prolonged periods in contaminated soil. Although *E. rhusiopathiae* is resistant to smoking, salting, and pickling, it is killed within 15 minutes by heating to 55°C.

Infection in humans is usually the result of contact with infected animals or their products. Persons at greatest risk for infection include fishermen, fishmongers, butchers, slaughterhouse workers, and veterinarians. The organism gains entry via cuts and abrasions on the skin. The seasonal incidence of erysipeloid parallels that of swine erysipelas and is highest in the summer and early fall.

CLINICAL MANIFESTATIONS. Because of its mode of acquisition (contact with infected animals or their products, with organisms inoculating abrasions on the skin), lesions are usually confined to the fingers and hands. A well-defined, slightly elevated, violaceous lesion, accompanied by a very painful, throbbing, burning, or itching sensation, develops within 2 to 7 days of traumatic dermal inoculation. The infected area is swollen. Vesicles may be present, but suppuration is absent. The lesion spreads slowly to other fingers but rarely involves the fingertips or the skin above the wrist. As the lesion spreads peripherally, the central area clears. Systemic signs and symptoms are rare. There may be sterile arthritis of an adjacent joint. Regional lymphadenopathy or lymphadenitis occurs in about 20% of cases, and low-grade fevers occur in approximately 10%. Because *E. rhusiopathiae* is located only in deeper parts of the skin in cases of erysipeloid, biopsy of the entire thickness of the dermis from the edge of the lesion yields maximum recovery of the organism. *E. rhusiopathiae* grows on routine laboratory media. Lesions usually resolve within 3 weeks without treatment. Relapse occurs in 1% of cases.

The diffuse cutaneous form is rare. The cutaneous lesion progresses proximally from the site of inoculation or appears at remote areas. The patients often have fever and arthralgias, but blood cultures are negative.

Systemic *E. rhusiopathiae* infection is uncommon. Approximately 60 cases of bacteremia have been reported; 90% of the patients had endocarditis. All but two cases involved native valves. In 60% of cases, infection developed on apparently normal heart valves. One third of patients had an antecedent or concurrent skin lesion of erysipeloid. Clinical manifestations of endocarditis due to *E. rhusiopathiae* and other microorganisms are similar. *E. rhusiopathiae* endocarditis correlates highly with occupation, exhibits a tropism for the aortic valve, affects more males than females, and is associated with a high mortality.

TREATMENT. Most isolates of *E. rhusiopathiae* are susceptible to penicillins, cephalosporins, imipenem, clindamycin, and ciprofloxacin. Some resistance has been observed with erythromycin, tetracycline, and chloramphenicol. *E. rhusiopathiae* is resistant to vancomycin, aminoglycosides, trimethoprim-sulfamethoxazole, and sulfonamides. Penicillin G is the treatment of choice for infections caused by *E. rhusiopathiae*. Uncomplicated cutaneous lesions usually respond well to a 5- to 7-day course of oral penicillin. Treatment hastens healing, although relapse may still occur. Bacteremia should be treated with intravenous penicillin; cases of endocarditis should be treated with 12 to 20 million units of penicillin G daily for 4 to 6 weeks. Ciprofloxacin is an alternative therapy in the penicillin-allergic patient. Valve replacement may be necessary in patients with endocarditis.

Barnett JH, Estes SA, Wirman JA, et al.: Erysipeloid. J Am Acad Dermatol 9:116, 1983. *A complete review of the clinical and pathologic features of* Erysipelothrix *infections and their treatment.*

Reboli AC, Farrar WE: *Erysipelothrix rhusiopathiae:* An occupational pathogen. Clin Microbiol Rev 4:354, 1989. *Reviews epidemiology, clinical features, and bacteriology.*

Venditti M, Gelfusa V, Tarasi A, et al.: Antimicrobial susceptibilities of *Erysipelothrix rhusiopathiae.* Antimicrob Agents Chemother 34:2038, 1990. In vitro *susceptibility data on 10 isolates of* E. rhusiopathiae *to 16 antimicrobial agents.*

306 ACTINOMYCOSIS
Ward E. Bullock

DEFINITION. Actinomycosis is a chronic bacterial infection that induces both a suppurative and a granulomatous inflammatory response. It spreads contiguously through anatomic barriers and frequently forms external sinuses, from which may extrude "sulfur granules" that are characteristic but not pathognomonic. The most common clinical forms are cervicofacial, thoracic, abdominal, and, in females, genital.

ETIOLOGY. Members of the genus *Actinomyces* are prokaryotes with cell walls that contain both muramic acid and diaminopimelic acid. Unlike the cell walls of fungi, the cell walls of these organisms do not contain sterols and are insensitive to polyene antibiotics. *Actinomyces israelii* is the species most often recovered from human cases of actinomycosis. However, *A. naeslundii, A. odontolyticus, A. viscosus, A. meyeri,* and a related genus, *Arachnia propionica,* cause identical clinical infections and bear close resemblance in primary culture. *Actinomyces bovis* produces "lumpy jaw" in cattle but is not a human pathogen. These gram-positive bacteria are filamentous (0.5 to 1.0 μm in diameter) with branching and are non–acid fast, with a tendency to break up into coccobacilli. They require anaerobic to microaerophilic conditions for growth, which is quite slow; usually, 3 to 10 or more days are required before these organisms can be macroscopically detected in culture.

EPIDEMIOLOGY. Actinomycosis is observed throughout the world, and its prevalence is unrelated to climate, occupation, race, or age. The disease has been reported more commonly in men than in women (3:1). However, since the recognition of pelvic actinomycosis in association with the use of intrauterine contraceptive devices (IUCD's), the male prevalence ratio may be decreasing. The number of cases of actinomycosis reported annually to the Centers for Disease Control and Prevention is fewer than 100. These infections are not easily recognized by clinicians, and the organisms are fastidious; therefore, it is likely that the true incidence is substantially greater. Although many animal species are susceptible to actinomycosis, infection is neither transmissible from animal to human nor transmissible from person to person. *Actinomyces* species are part of the indigenous microbiota colonizing the teeth and oral cavity. They also may be found in the tonsillar crypts of asymptomatic individuals, in the fecal flora, and within the female reproductive tract.

PATHOGENESIS AND PATHOLOGY. The *Actinomyces* species maintain their niche within the microbial community of the mouth by adherence to oral surfaces, especially to dental plaque, a thin film of salivary proteins and glycoproteins that coats the enamel surface. Adherence is achieved by complex protein-protein stereochemical interactions and by lectin-carbohydrate interactions, the latter of which also mediate cellular coaggregation of oral *Actinomyces* with *Streptococcus milleri, Streptococcus sanguis,* and other mouth flora. This propensity for coaggregation may explain, in part, why actinomycotic infections often are polymicrobic, with "associate" mouth flora frequently isolated from cervicofacial, thoracic, and central nervous system (CNS) abscesses. The associate flora may play a synergistic role in infection by maintaining the low oxygen tension necessary for *Actinomyces* growth. To cause disease, these organisms must be introduced into tissue through a break in the mucous membrane resulting from dental infections and manipulations or from aspiration of infected dental debris. They may enter the abdominal cavity by perforation of the lower gastrointestinal tract or by ascending infection of the genital tract in women.

Actinomycotic infection evokes a combination of suppurative and granulomatous inflammatory responses accompanied by intense fibrosis. Plasma cells and multinucleated giant cells often are observed within lesions, as may be large macrophages with foamy cytoplasm around purulent centers. The infection spreads through fascial planes and ultimately may produce draining sinus tracts, especially in infections of the pelvis and abdomen. Sulfur granules within lesions and sinus drainage are a typical feature, not always present. These granules are gritty aggregates of organisms measuring 1 to 2 mm in diameter; the centers have a basophilic staining property, with eosinophilic rays terminating in pear-shaped "clubs" on the surface. They contain calcium phosphate, probably as a result of phosphatase activity of both the host and the organisms.

CLINICAL MANIFESTATIONS. Cervicofacial actinomycosis comprises 50 to 60% of reported cases. Infection is usually observed in a setting of poor oral hygiene with tooth decay, periodontal disease, or gingivitis, in which mucosal integrity is disrupted by dental manipulations or other injury. The infection generally evolves as a chronic or subacute soft tissue swelling or mass involving the submandibular or paramandibular region. The swelling may have a ligneous consistency caused by tissue fibrosis. More rapidly developing lesions often simulate pyogenic infections. Trismus may be present, and advanced lesions may discharge odorless pus containing "sulfur granules" through one or more sinuses. Fever, pain, and leukocytosis may be present. The infection can extend to the tongue, salivary glands, pharynx, and larynx. Bone (most commonly the mandible) may be invaded from the adjacent soft tissue. Cervical spine or cranial bone infection may lead to subdural empyema and invasion of the CNS. The differential diagnosis includes tuberculosis (scrofula), fungal infections, nocardiosis, suppurative infections by other organisms, and neoplasms.

Thoracic actinomycosis comprises 15 to 30% of the disease spectrum and usually results from aspiration of infective material from the oropharynx. Less commonly, thoracic infection may be introduced by esophageal perforation, by extension into the mediastinum from the neck, or by spread from an abdominal site; hematogenous spread to the lung is rare. Pulmonary actinomycosis commonly spreads from an early pneumonic focus across lung fissures to involve the pleura and the chest wall, with eventual fistula formation and drainage containing sulfur granules (Fig. 306–1). Granules rarely are present in the sputum. The incidence of this complication, as well as the destruction of thoracic vertebrae and adjacent ribs, has declined in the antibiotic era.

The complaints of patients with thoracic actinomycosis are nonspecific. The most common are a productive cough, dyspnea, weight loss, fever, and chest pain. Anemia, mild leukocytosis, and an elevated sedimentation rate are relatively common. There often is a history of underlying lung disease, and patients rarely present in an early stage of infection. The pulmonary lesions may resemble tuberculosis, especially when cavity formation occurs, and blastomycosis, which may destroy ribs posteriorly but rarely form sinuses. Nocardiosis, bronchogenic carcinoma, and lymphoma can also mimic thoracic actinomycosis.

ABDOMINAL-PELVIC ACTINOMYCOSIS. Actinomycosis of the abdomen and pelvis is a chronic, localized inflammatory process that often is preceded weeks or months by surgery for acute appendicitis with perforation or for perforated colonic diverticulitis or by emergency surgery on the lower intestinal tract after trauma. Occasionally, abdominal actinomycosis may manifest without identifiable predisposing factors. The ileocecal region is involved most frequently, with the formation of a mass lesion. The infection extends slowly to contiguous organs, especially the liver, and may involve retroperitoneal tissues, the spine, or the abdominal wall. Persistent draining sinuses may form, and those involving the perianal region can simulate Crohn's disease or tuberculosis. The extensive fibrosis of actinomycotic lesions, presenting to the examiner as a mass, often suggests tumor. Constitutional symptoms and signs are nonspecific; the most common are fever, weight loss, nausea, vomiting, and pain.

An association has been recognized between long-term use of IUCD's and actinomycosis of the genital tract. Manifestations of infection may range from a chronic vaginal discharge to pelvic inflammatory disease with tubo-ovarian abscesses or pseudomalignant masses. No association exists between actinomycotic infection and the type of IUCD used. Accurate data on the prevalence and incidence of infection among IUCD users are sparse, since cytologic criteria and fluorescent antibody staining techniques are the principal means of detecting *Actinomyces* in vaginal smears and other genital tract specimens. Anaerobic cultures of the female genital tract generally are unsuccessful.

Currently, it is generally agreed that *Actinomyces* species may be part of the indigenous genital tract flora of females and that demonstrating their presence by morphologic criteria and fluorescent anti-

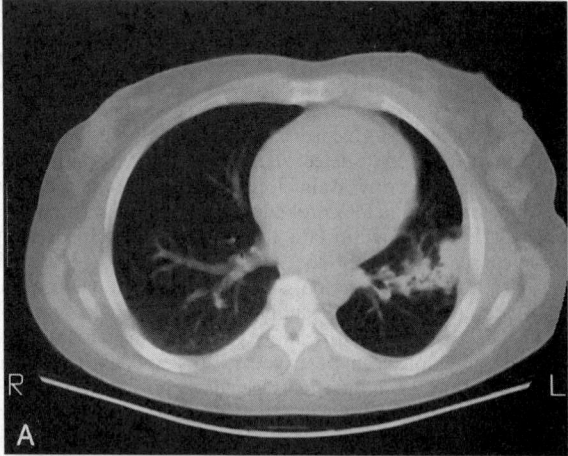
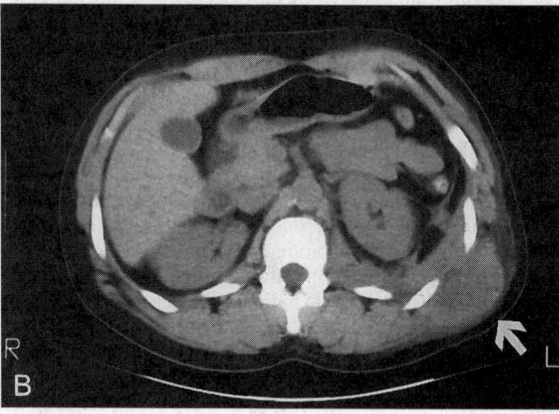

FIGURE 306–1. Thoracic computed tomographic scan of a 43-year-old woman with pulmonary actinomycosis. There is consolidation of the lung with pleural thickening adjacent to the parenchymal disease *(A)*. Abscess extended into the left breast and inferiorly to the costophrenic sulcus, to the retroperitoneum, and into the lateral abdominal wall *(B) (arrow)*.

body stains does not predict disease. However, colonization of the endometrium appears to require the presence of an IUCD. Although many cases of genital-pelvic actinomycosis associated with IUCD use have been reported, the actual incidence of disease appears to be low relative to the millions of those who use IUCD's.

CNS and disseminated actinomycosis are very uncommon. Most infections of the CNS manifest as encapsulated brain abscesses that are indistinguishable from those caused by other organisms. Most actinomycotic infections of the CNS are thought to be seeded hematogenously from a distant primary site; however, direct extension of cervicofacial disease is well recognized. Sinus formation is not a characteristic of CNS disease. The rare meningitis caused by *Actinomyces* is chronic and basilar in location, and the pleocytosis usually is lymphocytic. Thus, it may be misdiagnosed as tuberculous meningitis.

Unlike *Nocardia* species (see Ch. 307), *Actinomyces* species usually are not opportunistic in the immunocompromised host. To date, few systemic actinomycotic infections have been reported among patients with AIDS.

DIAGNOSIS. Crucial to the diagnosis is a high index of suspicion communicated to the microbiology diagnostic laboratory, along with material from draining sinuses, from deep needle aspiration, or from biopsy specimens. Anaerobic culture is required, and no selective media are available to restrict overgrowth of the slow-growing *Actinomyces* by associated microflora. The presence, in pus or tissue specimens, of non–acid-fast, gram-positive organisms with filamentous branching is very suggestive of the diagnosis. The characteristic morphology of "sulfur granules" and the presence of gram-positive organisms within are helpful. However, the granules must be distinguished from similar structures that are sometimes produced in infections and that are caused by *Nocardia, Monospo-*

rium, *Cephalosporium*, *Staphylococcus* (botryomycosis), and others. *Actinomyces* and *Arachnia* generally can be differentiated from other gram-positive anaerobes by means of growth rate (slow), by catalase production (negative, except *A. viscosus*), and by gas-liquid chromatographic detection of acetic, lactic, and succinic acids produced in peptone-yeast-glucose broth. Direct fluorescent antibody conjugates can be used to detect *Actinomyces* in clinical material or culture but are not readily available to clinical microbiology laboratories. There are no reliable serologic tests or skin tests.

TREATMENT. Penicillin G is the drug of choice for treating an infection caused by any of the *Actinomyces*. It is given in high dosage over a prolonged period, since the infection has a tendency to recur, presumably because antibiotic penetration to areas of fibrosis and necrosis and into "sulfur granules" may be poor. Most deep-seated infections can be expected to respond to intravenous penicillin G, 10 to 20 million units per day given for 2 to 6 weeks, followed by an oral phenoxypenicillin in a dosage of 2 to 4 grams per day. A few additional weeks of oral penicillin therapy may suffice for uncomplicated cervicofacial disease; complicated cases and extensive pulmonary or abdominal disease may require treatment for 12 to 18 months. To date, little evidence exists of acquired resistance to penicillin G by *Actinomyces* during prolonged therapy. Radical excision of large sinus tracts should be considered in some cases. Alternative first-line antibiotics for treating *Actinomyces* infections include tetracycline, erythromycin, and clindamycin. First-generation cephalosporins and imipenem also are highly effective. Antifungal drugs are not active against these organisms. *In vitro* antibiotic sensitivity testing of *Actinomyces* is difficult, and the results may not be predictive of antibiotic activity *in vivo*.

The need to use combination antibiotic therapy to attack microorganisms that are isolated in association with *Actinomyces* has not been established. The generally good results obtained with penicillin G alone over nearly three decades indicate that monotherapy is effective in most cases. In complicated infections of the lower abdomen, where anaerobic gram-negative organisms, among others, may be the "associates," combination antibiotic therapy is appropriate.

The presence of organisms presumed to be *Actinomyces* on a Papanicolaou smear, obtained from an asymptomatic female with or without an IUCD in place, is not an indication for therapy. When patients experience well-defined IUCD-related symptoms and Papanicolaou smears demonstrate *Actinomyces* by specific fluorescent-labeled antibody, the device should be removed. Antibiotic administration for a 2-week period may be indicated. More serious infections require prolonged therapy as recommended above.

PROGNOSIS. The advent of antibiotics has greatly improved the prognosis for all forms of actinomycosis. At present, cure rates are high, and neither deformity nor death is common.

Bennhoff DF: Actinomycosis: Diagnostic and therapeutic considerations and a review of 32 cases. Laryngoscope 94:1198, 1984. *A general review.*

Bernardi RS: Abdominal actinomycosis. Surg Gynecol Obstet 149:257, 1979. *A thorough review of all aspects of actinomycosis, with emphasis on the abdominal form.*

Cisar JO, Sandberg AL, Clark WB: Molecular aspects of adherence of *Actinomyces viscosus* and *Actinomyces naeslundii* to oral surfaces. J Dent Res 68 (special issue):1558, 1989. *A brief summary for those wishing to know more about adherence mechanisms.*

Evans DTP: *Actinomyces israelii* in the female genital tract: A review. Genitourin Med 69:54, 1993. *An up-to-date summary.*

Flynn MW, Felson B: The roentgen manifestations of thoracic actinomycosis. AJR 110:707, 1970. *An outstanding guide to roentgenographic diagnosis of pulmonary actinomycosis.*

Richtsmeier WJ, Johns ME: Actinomycosis of the head and neck. CRC Crit Rev Clin Lab Sci 11:175, 1979. *An excellent review, with an emphasis on infection of the head and neck.*

Smego RA Jr: Actinomycosis of the central nervous system. Rev Infect Dis 9:855, 1987. *A good review of 70 cases of CNS actinomycosis.*

307 NOCARDIOSIS
Ward E. Bullock

DEFINITION. Nocardiosis is a subacute or chronic bacterial infection that evokes a suppurative response. The most common sites of primary infection are, first, the lung and then the skin, from which bacteria may disseminate hematogenously to the central nervous system (CNS) and other tissues. The infection often pursues a more acute and aggressive course in immunosuppressed patients.

ETIOLOGY. The nocardiae are gram-positive, aerobic actinomycetes, many of which are weakly acid fast in tissue or on initial isolation. They reproduce by filamentous branching, with fragmentation into bacillary and coccoid forms. *Nocardia* species are distributed widely in nature and commonly are found in soil, grasses, and rotting vegetation. Of the species that cause most infections in humans, *N. asteroides* is by far the predominant pathogen. *N. caviae*, *N. farcinica*, *N. transvalensis,* and *N. brasiliensis* also produce pulmonary and disseminated infections, but much less frequently. *N. brasiliensis* is the most common cause of actinomycetoma in Latin and South America.

INCIDENCE AND PREVALENCE. A 1976 survey estimated the incidence of nocardiosis in the United States to be 500 to 1000 new cases per year. At present, the incidence undoubtedly is higher as a consequence of an expanding population of people who are immunosuppressed iatrogenically or by underlying diseases. Nocardiosis has been reported worldwide in all ages and races and is two to three times more common in men than in women. No occupational related risks have been found. Thus possible hormonal effects on bacterial growth or virulence have been postulated.

EPIDEMIOLOGY. The majority of infections caused by *N. asteroides* occur in patients with impaired cell-mediated immunity (CMI). However, the organism clearly is capable of infecting apparently normal persons. Nocardiosis presumably is acquired by inhaling airborne bacteria, since the primary site of infection is the lung in the majority of cases. Other mammals can be infected. However, no well-established evidence exists for animal-to-person transmission or for person-to-person transmission. Occasional clusters of nocardial infection have been reported among immunosuppressed hospital patients, suggesting possible nosocomial acquisition. *N. asteroides* has been recovered from the sputum, skin, and other body regions of patients who do not have apparent disease. Nevertheless, repeated isolation of *Nocardia* species from any immunocompromised person should be considered evidence of infection rather than colonization, and treatment should be initiated. Nocardiosis can manifest as a primary cutaneous infection (especially *N. brasiliensis*) after inoculation through local injury and may disseminate to other organs.

PATHOGENESIS AND PATHOLOGY. The typical nocardial lesion within the lung and other tissues is one of liquefactive necrosis with abscess formation. Polymorphonuclear leukocytes predominate in association with varying proportions of macrophages and lymphocytes. Granuloma formation is infrequent, and in contrast with actinomycotic lesions, fibrosis is rare. Confluent daughter abscesses are common. Sulfur granules are not present in visceral lesions, as they are in actinomycosis. However, they may be seen in nocardial lesions of the skin.

That CMI plays a major role in host defense against nocardiosis is suggested by the fact that immunocompromised patients are prone to this infection. The importance of antigen-specific T lymphocyte immune function is illustrated by the increased susceptibility of athymic nude mice to *Nocardia* infection and by the capacity of T lymphocytes from rabbits immunized with *N. asteroides* to augment phagocytosis and growth inhibition of these organisms by macrophages. Neutrophils exhibit poor nocardicidal activity *in vitro* but may inhibit growth of organisms during an early phase of infection prior to maturation of cellular immune responses.

N. asteroides may counter host defenses by inhibiting the phagolysosome fusion that enables phagocytic cells to kill ingested bacteria, by producing superoxide dismutase and catalase, and by blocking the acidification of parasitized phagolysosomes.

Nocardia species are not visible in tissue specimens stained by hematoxylin and eosin or by the periodic acid–Schiff procedure. They can be visualized by a tissue Gram stain or after slight overstaining by the Gomori methenamine silver method, which demonstrates the filamentous structure of the organisms. Many *Nocardia* are weakly acid fast and can be seen on a modified Ziehl-Neelsen stain.

CLINICAL MANIFESTATIONS. Pulmonary infection is the most frequent manifestation of nocardiosis (about 75% of the reported cases). The clinical manifestations are nonspecific and include fever, cough, weight loss, and dyspnea. The range of pulmonary involvement extends from transient or inapparent infection to confluent bronchopneumonia with complete consolidation. Radiographic examination of the chest may reveal one or more of the following: fluffy infiltrates, multiple abscess formation with cavitation in 10 to 20% of cases, bulging fissures, masses, nodules, and empyema. Hilar involvement and calcification are infrequent. *Nocardia* can disseminate to other organs from pulmonary lesions, especially in patients who are immunosuppressed following organ transplantation and in individuals with the acquired immunodeficiency syndrome (AIDS). Patients who have received extensive x-irradiation and chemotherapy for malignancies and those treated with high-dosage steroids also are prone to metastatic infection, and evidence thereof should be sought aggressively.

In 20 to 40% of patients with pulmonary nocardiosis, dissemination to the CNS occurs, and therefore, computed tomographic (CT) scanning of the head should be considered. Loculated brain abscesses, either singular or multiple, are common and are often accompanied by headache and focal neurologic findings; meningitis is infrequent. Other common sites of dissemination include the skin and subcutaneous tissues, kidneys, eyes, liver, and lymph nodes. In cases of apparently localized nocardial lesions of skin, it is important to distinguish between the possibilities of primary inoculation and hematogenous dissemination to the skin from another site.

DIAGNOSIS. The clinical and radiographic findings in pulmonary nocardiosis are nonspecific. Consequently, it may be confused with a variety of other bacterial infections of the lung, including actinomycosis and tuberculosis, as well as fungal infections and malignancies. Alertness to the possibility of nocardiosis can expedite the diagnostic workup, especially in immunosuppressed patients, in whom the disease may coexist with other opportunistic infections. Cultures and stains should be done on specimens of sputum, pleural fluid, bronchial lavage fluid, as well as on percutaneous lung aspirates or open lung biopsy specimens. Needle biopsy of cerebral mass lesions should be considered strongly in patients with AIDS who have pulmonary nocardiosis because of the multiplicity of infections and tumors that can manifest in a similar manner.

Skin lesions should be aspirated if fluctuant or biopsied, and specimens should be submitted for culture and the smear preparations or histologic sections examined for organisms. Nocardiosis often can be diagnosed with a high degree of confidence by direct examination of sputum or purulent material. The presence of gram-positive, filamentous branching rods that stain unevenly with crystal violet to give a beaded appearance is highly suggestive of either *Actinomyces* or *Nocardia*. If the organisms are acid fast on a modified Ziehl-Neelsen stain, the probability of *Nocardia* is high. However, lack of acid-fast staining does not exclude *Nocardia*.

Nocardia species are not fastidious and grow aerobically, though slowly, on routinely used media. Characteristic heaped, waxy colonies, often colored tan, orange, or even purple, may be seen after 2 to 7 days of culture. Longer times may be required. Thus the microbiology laboratory should be advised of possible nocardiosis to ensure that plates are held for 10 to 14 days and that steps are taken to limit overgrowth by microbial contaminants, particularly in sputum samples. The use of defined carbon-free medium to which paraffin is added may enhance the chances of isolating *N. asteroides* from sputum because it can use paraffin as a sole source of carbon, in contrast to most other organisms. Several simple tests can assist in the presumptive differentiation of *Nocardia* from other aerobic actinomycetes and from rapidly growing *Mycobacteria*, as, for example, the decomposition of casein, xanthine, and tyrosine. However, most clinical laboratories should rely on reference facilities for definitive taxonomic designations.

TREATMENT. The sulfonamides are equally efficacious and are first-line agents for treatment, as is the combination of trimethoprim-sulfamethoxazole (TMP-SMX). The dosage of sulfadiazine is 6 to 10 grams per day given in three to six divided doses, with adjustment as needed to achieve peak serum levels of 12 to 15 mg per deciliter. Dosing schedules of TMP-SMX range from 160 mg/800 mg to 320 mg/1600 mg every 6 or 8 hours. These antimicrobials penetrate the CNS and other body compartments well. A high percentage of *Nocardia* isolates are sensitive to sulfonamides and to TMP-SMX by *in vitro* testing. However, the techniques of *in vitro* sensitivity testing with *Nocardia* have not been standardized, in part because of technical difficulties created by slow growth in culture and problems in obtaining a homogeneous suspension of cells for standardization of the inoculum. Thus the results of *in vitro* tests frequently are poor predictors of *in vivo* efficacy and should be interpreted with caution.

Not all patients respond to sulfonamide or TMP-SMX therapy. Resistance developed to the sulfonamides during therapy has been documented, and metastatic lesions can appear during the course of apparently successful treatment. Hypersensitivity reactions, nephrotoxicity, or hemopoietic toxicity induced by these drugs may force discontinuation of treatment, especially in renal transplant recipients receiving cyclosporine and in patients with AIDS. The alternative antibiotics that have proved to be most efficacious, both *in vitro* and clinically, are minocycline, amikacin, and imipenem. Ceftriaxone, cefuroxime, and cefotaxime display *in vitro* activity against many, but by no means all, clinical isolates of the *Nocardia* species. However, it remains to be determined if the last-named three antibiotics will prove valuable for treating nocardiosis. Although some *in vitro* studies indicate that certain combinations of antibiotics may exert synergistic activity against *Nocardia,* no good clinical evidence exists that combination antibiotic regimens are superior to single-agent therapy.

Treatment should be prolonged, since relapse of nocardiosis is common. In patients with intact host defenses, treatment should be continued for at least 6 weeks after clinical recovery. In those who have AIDS or who are otherwise immunocompromised, treatment should be continued for a year or more. As a rule, it is necessary to perform surgical drainage of brain abscesses, empyema, and subcutaneous abscesses. Patients with cerebral nocardiosis or other deep abscesses should be monitored by serial CT scans. If patients are receiving immunosuppressive drugs, the dosage should be reduced if at all possible.

PROGNOSIS. The prognosis for clinical cure of nocardiosis is influenced by the location of the infection, by pre-existing impairment of cellular immunity from underlying disease or drug therapy, and by the aggressiveness of the patient's management. Mortality rates range from near 0% in patients with isolated skin lesions to more than 40% in cases of CNS involvement. The overall mortality rate in patients with pulmonary disease is in the range of 15 to 30%, including those who are immunocompromised.

Barnicoat MJ, Wierzbicki AS, Norman PM: Cerebral nocardiosis in immunosuppressed patients: Five cases. Q J Med 268:689, 1989. *Presentation of five cases with a good bibliography on the topic.*

Javaly K, Horowitz HW, Wormser GP: Nocardiosis in patients with human immunodeficiency virus infection: Report of 2 cases and review of the literature. Medicine 71:128, 1992. *A current discussion of nocardial infection in AIDS patients.*

Palmer DL, Harvey RL, Wheeler JK: Diagnostic and therapeutic considerations in *Nocardia asteroides* infection. Medicine 53:391, 1974. *A comprehensive literature review of 243 cases of nocardiosis (including 13 patients in the authors' own experience).*

Smego RA Jr, Moeller MB, Gallis HA: Trimethoprim-sulfamethoxazole therapy for *Nocardia* infections. Arch Intern Med 143:711, 1983. *This article provides an extensive literature review and discusses TMP-SMX in depth.*

Wallace RJ Jr, Steele LC, Sumter G, et al.: Antimicrobial susceptibility patterns of *Nocardia asteroides*. Antimicrob Agents Chemother 32:1776, 1988. *An examination of antibiotic sensitivity patterns among 78 clinical isolates of N. asteroides by a group experienced in the complexities of* in vitro *sensitivity testing with these organisms.*

Wilson JP, Turner HR, Kirchner KA, et al.: Nocardial infections in renal transplant recipients. Medicine 68:38, 1989. *A well-written review of nocardiosis, with emphasis on disease manifestations in renal transplant patients.*

308 BRUCELLOSIS
Robert A. Salata

DEFINITION. Bacteria of the genus *Brucella* cause disease with protean manifestations. Infection is transmitted to humans from animals as a consequence of occupational exposure or ingestion of contaminated milk products. Despite the attempt to institute effective control measures, brucellosis remains a significant health and economic burden in many countries.

ETIOLOGY. Brucellae are slow-growing, small, aerobic, nonmotile, nonencapsulated, non–spore-forming, gram-negative coccobacilli. *B. abortus, B. suis, B. melitensis,* and *B. canis* are known to infect humans and are typed on the basis of biochemical, metabolic, and immunologic criteria. There are differences in virulence among these four species. *B. abortus,* with a reservoir in cattle, usually is associated with mild sporadic disease; suppurative or disabling complications are rare. *B. suis* infection, resulting from swine contact, is often associated with destructive, suppurative lesions and may have a prolonged course. *B. melitensis,* with a reservoir in sheep and goats, may cause severe, acute disease and disabling complications. *B. canis,* spread to humans from infected dogs, causes disease with an insidious onset, frequent relapse, and a chronic course that is indistinguishable from infection related to *B. abortus.*

EPIDEMIOLOGY. Over 500,000 cases of brucellosis are reported yearly to the World Health Organization from 100 countries. *B. melitensis* infection, distributed primarily in the Mediterranean region (particularly Spain and Greece), Latin America, and Asia (with increased occurrences in Iraq and Kuwait), accounts for the majority of cases. *B. abortus* infection occurs worldwide but has been effectively eradicated in several European countries, Japan, and Israel. *B. suis* occurs mainly in the midwestern United States, South America, and Southeast Asia, whereas *B. canis* infection is most common in North and South America, Japan, and Central Europe.

In association with effective control programs in animals, human brucellosis has decreased dramatically in the United States, from over 6000 cases in 1947 to fewer than 200 cases since 1980. States reporting the greatest number of cases include Texas, California, Virginia, and Florida. In North America, brucellosis occurs mainly in spring and summer and is most common in adult males, usually related to occupational exposure.

Brucella infection in the United States most frequently occurs in high-risk groups, including slaughterhouse workers, farmers and dairymen, veterinarians, travelers to endemic areas, and laboratory workers handling the organisms. More than one half of reported cases occur in the meat-processing industry, particularly in the kill areas, where infection is spread through abraded or lacerated skin and the conjunctiva, possibly by aerosolization, and rarely by ingestion of infected tissue. Many cases of *B. abortus* infection in veterinarians have accidentally occurred from the strain 19 vaccine used to immunize cattle. *B. melitensis* infection, transmitted through the ingestion of goat's milk cheese, has been seen in United States travelers to and immigrants from Mexico.

Brucellosis in children accounts for only 3 to 10% of all reported cases worldwide, is common in endemic areas (may account for 20 to 25% of cases), and is often a mild, self-limited process. Infection occurs most frequently in school-age children and in familial outbreaks; no convincing evidence exists to associate *Brucella* infection with abortion in humans.

PATHOGENESIS AND IMMUNITY. After penetrating the epithelial cells of human skin, conjunctiva, pharynx, or lung, *Brucella* organisms initially induce an exuberant polymorphonuclear neutrophil response in the submucosa. Following ingestion of organisms by neutrophils and tissue macrophages, spread to regional lymph nodes occurs. If host defenses within the lymph nodes are overwhelmed, bacteremia follows. The usual incubation period between infection and bacteremia is 1½ to 3 weeks. Bacteremia is accompanied by phagocytosis of free *Brucella* organisms by neu-

trophils and localization of bacteria primarily to the spleen, liver, and bone marrow, with the formation of granulomas.

If the inoculum is large and the patient is untreated, large granulomas may form, suppurate, and serve as a source of persistent bacteremia with the potential for multiorgan spread.

Both virulent and attenuated strains of *Brucella* are readily phagocytized by neutrophils after opsonization with normal human serum. Whole bacteria and extracts of *Brucella* species may inhibit neutrophil oxidative burst activity and degranulation. Intracellular killing of ingested bacteria has been demonstrated with *B. abortus* but not *B. melitensis;* this may explain differences in pathogenicity between these species.

Humoral factors may be important in the host defense against *Brucella.* Even in the absence of specific agglutinating antibody, normal human serum is bactericidal for *Brucella* organisms; *B. abortus* is more susceptible to serum lysis than is *B. melitensis.* The intracellular location of the organism may provide a means for the bacteria to escape the lethal effects of serum. Specific serum agglutinating antibody has opsonic activity but does not correlate with the development of protective immunity.

A role for mononuclear phagocytes and cell-mediated immunity in brucellosis has been demonstrated. Protection against *Brucella* infection in animals is associated with preceding infection with *Listeria monocytogenes* or *Mycobacterium tuberculosis,* both of which stimulate cell-mediated immune mechanisms. Skin testing with *Brucella* proteins elicits a typical delayed hypersensitivity response in infected individuals. Macrophages, activated with lymphokines, kill *Brucella in vitro.* In some cases of chronic brucellosis, depressed proliferative responses to classic T-cell mitogens or to *Brucella* antigen occur.

CLINICAL MANIFESTATIONS. Clinically, human brucellosis may be conveniently divided into subclinical illness, acute/subacute disease, localized disease and complications, relapsing infection, and chronic disease (Table 308–1).

Subclinical Illness. Detected only by serologic testing, asymptomatic or clinically unrecognized human brucellosis often occurs in high-risk groups, including slaughterhouse workers, farmers, and veterinarians. More than 50% of abattoir workers and up to 33% of veterinarians have high anti-*Brucella* antibody titers but no history of recognized clinical infection. Children in endemic areas frequently have subclinical illness.

Acute and Subacute Disease. After an incubation period of several weeks or months, acute brucellosis may occur as a mild, transient illness (with *B. abortus* or *B. canis*) or as an explosive, toxic illness with the potential for multiple complications (with *B. melitensis*). Approximately 50% of patients have an abrupt onset over days, while the remainder have an insidious onset over weeks. Symptoms in brucellosis are protean and nonspecific. More than 90% of patients experience malaise, chills, sweats, fatigue, and weakness. More than 50% of patients have myalgias, anorexia, and weight loss. Fewer patients complain of arthralgias, cough, testicular pain, dysuria, ocular pain, or visual blurring. Likewise, few localizing physical signs are apparent. Fever, often >39.4°C (103°F), occurs in 95%. An undulating or intermittent fever pattern is unusual. A relative pulse-temperature deficit may occur. Splenomegaly is present in 10 to 15%, lymphadenopathy occurs in up to 14% (axillary, cervical, and supraclavicular locations are most frequent, related to hand-wound or oropharyngeal routes of infection); hepatomegaly is less frequent. Other laboratory findings in acute or subacute disease may include mild anemia, lymphopenia or neutropenia (especially with bacteremia), lymphocytosis, thrombocytopenia, or (rarely) pancytopenia. The majority of infected individuals recover completely without sequelae if the diagnosis is appropriately made and prompt therapy is initiated.

Localized Disease and Complications. *Brucella* organisms may localize in almost any organ, most commonly in bone, joints, central nervous system (CNS), heart, lung, spleen, testes, liver, gallbladder, kidney, prostate, and skin. Localized disease may occur simultaneously at multiple sites. Localized complications most often appear in association with a more chronic course of illness, although complications may occur with acute disease due to *B. melitensis* or *B. suis.* In the United States, localized disease is most frequently related to *B. suis.*

Relapsing Infection. Up to 10% of patients with brucellosis relapse after antimicrobial therapy. This probably results from the intracellular location of the organisms, which protects the bacteria

TABLE 308-1. CLINICAL CLASSIFICATION OF HUMAN BRUCELLOSIS

	Duration of Symptoms Before Diagnosis	Major Symptoms and Signs	Diagnosis	Comments
Subclinical	—	Asymptomatic	Positive (low titer) serology, negative cultures	Occurs in abattoir workers, farmers, and veterinarians
Acute and subacute	Up to 2–3 mo and 3 mo to 1 yr	Malaise, chills, sweats, fatigue, headache, anorexia, arthralgias, fever, splenomegaly, lymphadenopathy, hepatomegaly	Positive serology, positive blood or bone marrow cultures	Presentation can be mild, self-limited (*B. abortus*), or fulminant with severe complications (*B. melitensis*)
Localized	Occurs with acute or chronic untreated disease	Related to involved organs	Positive serology, positive cultures in specific tissues	Bone/joint, genitourinary, hepatosplenic involvement most common
Relapsing	2–3 mo after initial episode	Same as acute illness but may have higher fever, more fatigue, weakness, chills, and sweats	Positive serology, positive cultures	May be extremely difficult to distinguish relapse from reinfection
Chronic	Longer than 1 yr	Nonspecific presentation but neuropsychiatric symptoms and low-grade fever most common	Low titer or negative serology, cultures negative	Most controversial classification; localized disease may be associated

from certain antibiotics and host defense mechanisms. Relapses occur most frequently within months after initial infection but may occur as long as 2 years after apparently successful treatment. Relapsing infection is difficult to distinguish from reinfection in high-risk groups with continued exposure.

Chronic Disease. Disease with a duration >1 year has been called chronic brucellosis. A majority of patients classified as having chronic brucellosis really have persistent disease caused by inadequate treatment of the initial episode, or they have focal disease in bone, liver, or spleen. About 20% of patients diagnosed as having chronic brucellosis complain of persistent fatigue, malaise, and depression; in many aspects this condition resembles the chronic fatigue syndrome. These symptoms frequently are not associated with clinical, microbiologic, or serologic evidence of active infection.

DIAGNOSIS. Many more common illnesses mimic the clinical presentation of brucellosis. The most conclusive means of establishing the diagnosis of brucellosis is by positive cultures from normally sterile body fluids or tissues. Isolation of the organism can be enhanced by use of special media. The culture of *Brucella* organisms is potentially hazardous to laboratory personnel. Therefore, most cases of brucellosis are diagnosed by serologic testing.

In acute brucellosis, positive blood cultures are obtained in 10 to 30% of cases (as high as 85% with *B. melitensis*). Blood culture positivity decreases with increasing duration of illness. With *B. melitensis* infection, bone marrow cultures are of higher yield than are blood cultures. Blood cultures processed in radiometric detection or isolator systems may yield positive cultures in <10 days. With localized brucellosis (e.g., lymph nodes, spleen, liver, or skeletal system), cultures of purulent material or tissues usually yield *Brucella* organisms. Culture of cerebrospinal fluid is positive in 45% of patients with meningitis. Antibody against *Brucella* may be demonstrated in cerebrospinal fluid by enzyme-linked immunosorbent assay (ELISA).

Most patients mount significant serologic responses to *Brucella* infections. The most frequently used test is the standard tube agglutination (STA) test, measuring antibody to *B. abortus* antigen. A fourfold or greater rise in titer to 1:160 or higher is considered significant. A presumptive case is one in which the agglutination titer is positive ($\geq$1:160) in single or serial specimens, with symptoms consistent with brucellosis. By 3 weeks of illness, >97% of patients demonstrate serologic evidence of infection. This test equally detects antibodies to *B. abortus*, *B. suis,* and *B. melitensis,* but not to *B. canis.* Serologic confirmation of *B. canis* infection requires *B. canis* or *B. ovis* antigen. Despite adequate antibiotic treatment, significant STA titers can persist for up to 2 years in 5 to 7% of cases. Because the STA titer may remain elevated, it is not useful in differentiating relapsing infection from other febrile illnesses in patients with past *Brucella* infection. Individuals with subclinical infection may demonstrate significant STA titers. In chronic localized brucellosis, STA titers may appear absent or low owing to a prozone phenomenon. This prozone effect appears to be related to the presence of immunoglobulin G (IgG) or immunoglobulin A (IgA) blocking antibodies; it can be eliminated if dilutions are carried out to at least 1:1280. False-positive STA titers due to immunologic cross-reactivity have been associated with *Brucella* skin testing, cholera vaccination, or infections due to *Vibrio cholerae, Francisella tularensis,* or *Yersinia enterocolitica.*

Immunoglobulin M (IgM) is the major agglutinating antibody formed in the first few weeks following infection with *Brucella* organisms. Thereafter, IgG levels also rise. The STA test measures both IgM and IgG. With prompt and adequate therapy, IgG antibody levels usually become undetectable after 6 to 12 months. If therapy is given, those patients who develop persistent *Brucella* infection usually maintain elevated IgG agglutinins. In the absence of rising STA titers, a single elevated 2-ME *Brucella* agglutination titer ($\geq$1:160) suggests either current or recent infection. Certain

TABLE 308-2. TREATMENT FOR BRUCELLOSIS

	Treatment	Comments
Acute With no endocarditis or CNS involvement	Doxycycline (200 mg/day) plus rifampin (600 to 900 mg/day) for 6 weeks	Treatment of choice by World Health Organization
	Tetracycline, streptomycin, chloramphenicol, rifampin, trimethoprim-sulfamethoxazole	Combination therapy indicated
	Fluoroquinolones, imipenem, and a variety of antimicrobial combinations	Being evaluated in trials
	Tetracycline (2 grams/day) for 6 weeks plus streptomycin (1 gram/day) for 3 weeks	Widely used; low rate of relapse; intramuscular administration of streptomycin may be difficult
In children	Trimethoprim-sulfamethoxazole	
CNS	Third-generation cephalosporin with rifampin	
Localized	Surgically drain abscesses plus antimicrobial therapy for 6 or more weeks	
Brucella endocarditis	Bactericidal drugs; early valve replacement may be necessary	Possible aortic valve destruction and/or major arterial emboli

newer antibody tests, including an ELISA and radioimmunoassay, are more sensitive than the STA; these methods have not been widely employed, and agglutination tests remain the standard for serologic diagnosis.

TREATMENT. Antibiotic treatment of *Brucella* infections is complicated by a number of complex issues, including the requirement for antibiotics that penetrate intracellularly, for prolonged therapy to prevent relapse, and for bactericidal antibiotics in treating CNS infection and endocarditis, as well as the lack of controlled, randomized, double-blind studies comparing different antimicrobial regimens. Debate is still considerable regarding which antibiotic regimens are clearly superior. Current recommendations are given in Table 308–2.

PROGNOSIS. Brucellosis appropriately treated within the first month of symptom onset is curable. Acute brucellosis often produces severe weakness and fatigue, and patients are frequently unable to work for up to 2 months. Immunity to reinfection follows initial *Brucella* infection in the majority of individuals. With early antimicrobial therapy, cases of chronic brucellosis or localized disease and complications are rare. Of patients who die of brucellosis, 84% have endocarditis involving a previously abnormal aortic valve, often associated with severe congestive heart failure.

PREVENTION. The control of human brucellosis relates directly to prevention programs in domestic animals and avoiding unpasteurized milk and milk products. In slaughterhouses, important means of prevention include careful wound dressing, protective glasses and clothing, prohibition of raw meat ingestion, and the use of previously infected (immune) individuals in high-risk areas.

Akova M, Uzun O, Akalin E, et al.: Quinolones in the treatment of human brucellosis: Comparative trial of ofloxacin-rifampin versus doxycycline-rifampin. Antimicrob Agents Chemother 37:1831, 1993. *The quinolone-rifampin combination was as effective as doxycycline plus rifampin regardless of the complications of the disease.*

Ariza J, Pujol M, Valverde J, et al.: Brucella sacroiliitis: Findings in 63 episodes and current relevance. Clin Infect Dis 16:761, 1993. *Epidemiologic, clinical, diagnostic, and treatment aspects of sacroiliitis reviewed over a 15-year period in Spain suggest that a mild disease exists with a good outcome similar to uncomplicated brucellosis.*

Buchanan TM, Faber LC, Feldman RA: Brucellosis in the United States, 1960–1972: An abattoir-associated disease. I. Clinical features and therapy. Buchanan TM, Sulzer CR, Frix MK, et al.: II. Diagnostic aspects. Buchanan TM, Hendricks SL, Patton CM, et al.: III. Epidemiology and evidence for acquired immunity. Medicine 53:403, 415, 427, 1974. *A very complete description of all aspects of brucellosis derived from a study of 160 patients in a large Iowa slaughterhouse.*

Gazapo E, Gonzalez Lahoz J, Subiza JL, et al.: Changes in IgM and IgG antibody concentrations in brucellosis over time: Importance for diagnosis and follow-up. J Infect Dis 159:219, 1989. *Patterns of antibody responses correlating with successful treatment, chronic disease, or drug relapses and failures were followed prospectively and proved clinically useful.*

Hall WH: Modern chemotherapy for brucellosis in humans. Rev Infect Dis 12:1060, 1990. *A comprehensive analysis of the world's literature related to therapy of brucellosis that stresses that prolonged combined chemotherapy in conjunction with surgery, where indicated, is the key to successful treatment.*

309 CAT SCRATCH DISEASE AND BACILLARY ANGIOMATOSIS

David A. Relman

Cat scratch disease and bacillary angiomatosis are manifestations of infection by members of the *Bartonella* genus (formerly the *Rochalimaea* genus). Cat scratch disease has been traditionally defined on the basis of a history of intimate cat exposure, the presence of an inoculation site lesion, local or regional (granulomatous) lymphadenitis, and a positive cat scratch antigen skin test. Bacillary angiomatosis involves skin and visceral sites with angioproliferative lesions whose gross appearance may be confused with that of Kaposi's sarcoma. Despite the two different histopathologic pictures, *Bartonella (Rochalimaea) henselae* causes both cat scratch disease and bacillary angiomatosis; *B. quintana* also can cause bacillary angiomatosis.

ETIOLOGY

In 1983, small pleomorphic weakly gram-negative but strongly argyrophilic bacilli were first described in cat scratch disease and bacillary angiomatosis tissues. An organism was subsequently cultivated from a small number of cat scratch disease lymph nodes on artificial media and on tissue culture cells, and was named *Afipia felis*. However, this organism and its DNA have not been detected often or consistently in patients with this disease; hence, the clinical significance of *A. felis* is in question. In 1990, a different bacillus was identified within tissues from patients with bacillary angiomatosis. Phylogenetic analysis revealed a novel *Rochalimaea* species: *R. henselae*. The close evolutionary relationships among the *Rochalimaea* and *Bartonella bacilliformis* (the cause of another human angioproliferative disease, verruga peruana; see Ch. 310), have led to a proposal to transfer all of the former *Rochalimaea* species to the *Bartonella* genus (Fig. 309–1). *B. henselae* and *B. quintana* (the etiologic agent of trench fever; see Ch. 324) have each been cultivated directly from and detected in tissues affected by bacillary angiomatosis. The relative importance of *B. henselae* and *B. quintana* in the causation of this disease is unclear.

A variety of data strongly incriminate *B. henselae* as an etiologic agent of cat scratch disease, as well as bacillary angiomatosis. Approximately 84 to 88% of patients who meet traditional diagnostic criteria for cat scratch disease demonstrate a significant elevation of serum IgG antibodies directed against *B. henselae;* approximately 20% of asymptomatic cat owners and 3 to 4% of the general population have elevated titers. In addition, *B. henselae* antigens and DNA can be detected in tissues from these patients with the polymerase chain reaction (PCR) and *in situ* immunohistochemistry. *B. henselae* DNA has been amplified from cat scratch antigen preparations. Finally, *B. henselae* has been cultivated from blood and tissues of patients with cat scratch disease. However, Koch's postulates have not been fulfilled for this organism, and a role for organisms other than *B. henselae* and *B. quintana* in either cat scratch disease or bacillary angiomatosis has not been ruled out.

B. henselae is a slightly curved, small (0.5 × 1 to 2 mm), self-aggregating, gram-negative bacillus that is capable of twitching motility. Optimal growth occurs on enriched media supplemented with 5% sheep or rabbit blood, at 35°C in a 5 to 10% CO_2 humified atmosphere. Colonies become visible after 9 to 15 days of primary culture (two different morphologies), and after 3 to 5 days on subsequent laboratory passage. *B. quintana* grows under similar conditions, especially after co-cultivation with endothelial cell monolayers. Species identification requires using specific antisera,

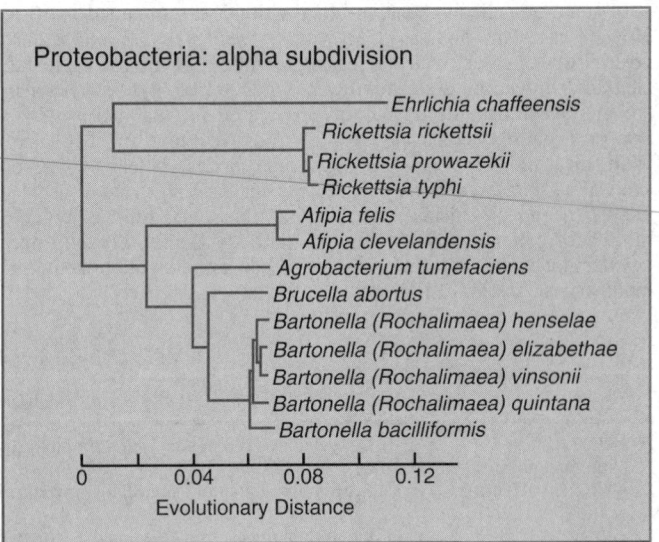

FIGURE 309–1. Phylogenetic relationships among the alpha-proteobacteria, based upon small subunit ribosomal RNA sequence analysis. Many of these organisms are endosymbiotic, and may have evolved in close association with insects or plants. Evolutionary distance is proportional to the length of horizontal line segments, and is expressed as the number of nucleotide substitutions per sequence position. (Modified from Mandell GL, Bennett JE, Dolin R [eds.]: Principles and Practice of Infectious Diseases. New York, Churchill Livingstone, 1995.)

cellular fatty acid profiles, or DNA polymorphism or sequence analysis.

EPIDEMIOLOGY

Cat scratch disease affects approximately 22,000 persons in the United States per year. The highest incidence of the disease occurs in the 5- through 14-year-old age group, and in the South. The incidence and prevalence of bacillary angiomatosis are unknown. Approximately 90% of individuals with this disease are co-infected with HIV or are otherwise immunocompromised.

Intimate or traumatic cat contacts are among the strongest risk factors for acquiring cat scratch disease and bacillary angiomatosis. In one study, 41% of cats had *B. henselae* bacteremia. Bacteremia is detected more often in younger cats, is asymptomatic, and may persist for the animal's lifetime. *B. quintana* has not been detected in cats, and cat exposure is uncommon among bacillary angiomatosis patients that are infected with this species. Unlike *B. quintana*-infected human body lice and the transmission of trench fever, it is uncertain whether arthropods play a role in either cat scratch disease or bacillary angiomatosis. Fewer than 5% of cases of cat scratch disease belong to a family cluster.

PATHOLOGY AND PATHOGENESIS

Histologic changes in lymph nodes evolve over a period of months in patients with cat scratch disease. Follicular hyperplasia and hypertrophy, and sinus histiocytosis and B cell proliferation are followed by granuloma formation and later by neutrophilic infiltration with central or stellate necrosis, and surrounding palisades of histiocytes. Microabscesses are common. Bacilli are best visualized with the Warthin-Starry silver impregnation stain early in the course of the disease.

The lesions of bacillary angiomatosis assume diverse macroscopic appearances, including an erythematous, polypoid or papular, cutaneous or mucosal pattern; deeply erythematous and indurated dermal plaques; and subcutaneous or visceral nodules. In all of these lesions, a distinctive lobular proliferation of capillaries is seen within a fibrous stroma. Hematoxylin and eosin reveal granular amphophilic material in the interstitium between vessels. This material corresponds to clumps of extracellular bacteria, as viewed with the Warthin-Starry silver stain or with electron microscopy. Bacillary peliosis is a histologic variant form of bacillary angiomatosis that is characterized by blood-filled cystic spaces, fibromyxoid stroma, and inflammatory cells; it is also associated with *B. henselae* and occurs most often within the liver and spleen.

CLINICAL MANIFESTATIONS

After an incubation period of 3 to 10 days, an erythematous papule develops at the inoculation site in more than half of those later diagnosed with cat scratch disease. These lesions may form a crust or become pustular; they resolve spontaneously in 1 to 3 weeks. Within a few weeks of inoculation, regional lymphadenopathy becomes apparent; usually a lymph node in the axillary or neck regions is found to be enlarged and tender (Table 309–1). Low-grade fever, malaise, anorexia, and nausea each occur in a minority of patients. Infrequently, inoculation of the eye results in a granulomatous lesion of the conjunctiva and in preauricular adenopathy, a condition known as the oculoglandular syndrome of Parinaud (4 to

6% of cat scratch disease patients). In a typical case of cat scratch disease, lymph nodes remain enlarged for at least 2 to 4 months.

Severe or systemic manifestations are reported in 2% of cat scratch disease patients, excluding those involving the central nervous system. These include persistent fever, weight loss, splenomegaly, diffuse papular rash, erythema nodosum, pleuritis, splenic abscess, central lymphadenopathy, osteolytic lesions, hepatitis, and thrombocytopenic purpura. An additional 2% of cat scratch disease patients experience neurologic complications. Encephalopathy or encephalitis are most common; other presentations include radiculitis, meningitis, cranial neuritis, neuroretinitis, and cerebral arteritis. Neurologic complications occur 2 to 3 weeks after onset of the initial illness.

Bacillary angiomatosis is most often manifested clinically by tender cutaneous or subcutaneous lesions. Mucosal lesions are also common. These lesions may be solitary or multiple, red, purple, or flesh-colored dome-shaped papules, nodules, polypoid tumors, or plaques. With age the lesions may ulcerate, form a crust, or develop a collarette of scale. Subcutaneous lesions sometimes erode underlying bone. In an undetermined percentage of cases, visceral bacillary angiomatosis occurs, sometimes in the absence of cutaneous disease. Visceral involvement may be asymptomatic or, as in disseminated cutaneous disease, may be associated with fever, chills, malaise, and anorexia. Liver, spleen, and internal lymph nodes appear to be the most frequent sites of extracutaneous disease. Biliary obstruction has resulted from external compression of periportal lymph nodes. Other sites affected by bacillary angiomatosis include bone marrow, lung, and brain.

A syndrome of *B. henselae* or *B. quintana* bacteremia has been reported sporadically in widespread regions of the United States. Signs of sepsis or localized (granulomatous or angioproliferative) disease are uncommon. Fever, headache, myalgias, and arthralgias may persist or recur over a period of weeks to months, despite therapy. Alcoholism and malnutrition characterize some urban clusters of *B. quintana* bacteremic disease. In addition, *B. henselae*, *B. quintana*, and *B. elizabethae* are reported agents of infective endocarditis. *B. henselae* is associated with lymphocytic meningitis.

DIAGNOSIS

The diagnosis of cat scratch disease and bacillary angiomatosis rests upon tissue examination and serologic tests in a compatible clinical setting. Typical histology in a hematoxylin and eosin-stained tissue is suggestive. Warthin-Starry stains will usually confirm a diagnosis of bacillary angiomatosis, and may confirm a diagnosis of cat scratch disease (i.e., reveal clumps of small, pleomorphic bacilli). Commercial laboratories, as well as the Centers for Disease Control and Prevention, offer an immunofluorescent or enzyme-linked immunosorbent assay for serum IgG antibodies directed against *B. henselae* and *B. quintana*. Most current assays do not distinguish between these species. Cultivation of *Bartonella (Rochalimaea)* and detection of specific genetic sequences by PCR or antigens by immunohistochemical methods are technically demanding and may currently exceed the capabilities of most clinical microbiology laboratories.

The differential diagnosis for localized cat scratch disease may include pyogenic lymphadenitis, mycobacterial infection, tularemia, brucellosis, lymphogranuloma venereum, syphilis, fungal disease, toxoplasmosis, and Epstein-Barr or Cytomegalovirus infection. Kaposi's sarcoma is the most important entity confused with bacillary angiomatosis. Visual detection of bacilli distinguishes the latter from the former. Lytic bone lesions in an HIV-infected individual should raise the possibility of bacillary angiomatosis because they are otherwise uncommon.

TREATMENT

Most patients with cat scratch disease do not require more than symptomatic support. A fluctuant or suppurative lymph node may benefit from needle aspiration. Antibiotic therapy should be reserved for immunocompromised individuals or those with evidence of severe or systemic disease. Because nearly all persons with bacillary angiomatosis fit into one of these latter categories, antibiotics should be routinely offered. *Bartonella (Rochalimaea)* bacteremia in the absence of localization also deserves antibiotic therapy.

TABLE 309–1. SELECTED CLINICAL FEATURES OF CLASSICAL CAT SCRATCH DISEASE

Feature	% of Cases
Site of lymphadenopathy	
Axilla	25–52
Neck	26–39
Groin	7–18
Elbow	2–13
Preauricular	5–7
Single node involvement	43–85
Lymphadenopathy only	48–51
Fever	31–48
Splenomegaly	11–12
Hospitalization	9–17

TABLE 309–2. TREATMENT SUGGESTIONS

Severe Cat Scratch Disease*

Trimethoprim-sulfamethoxasole	160–320 mg (TMP component) bid
Rifampin	300 mg bid
Ciprofloxacin	500 mg bid
Gentamicin sulfate	5 mg/kg qd

Bacillary Angiomatosis
B. henselae or *B. quintana* Bacteremia†

Erythromycin	250–500 mg qid
Doxycycline	100 mg bid
Azithromycin (anecdotal)	1 gram qd

* Treat for 7–14 days.

† Treat for at least 4 weeks; some patients may require more prolonged or lifelong treatment.

There are no data from prospective randomized studies to help a physician choose an antimicrobial regimen for cat scratch disease or bacillary angiomatosis. Nevertheless, *in vitro* susceptibility testing and retrospective or empiric clinical observations offer the basis for the suggested approaches in Table 309–2. Corticosteroids are not recommended for either disease.

Adal KA, Cockerell CJ, Petri WA: Cat scratch disease, bacillary angiomatosis, and other infections due to *Rochalimaea*. N Engl J Med 330:1509, 1994. *Useful review of a rapidly evolving field. Emphasizes clinical features and microbiology. Contains helpful color photographs.*

Koehler JE, Quinn FD, Berger TG, et al.: Isolation of rochalimaea species from cutaneous and osseous lesions of bacillary angiomatosis. N Engl J Med 327:1625, 1992. *First isolation of* R. henselae *directly from lesions of bacillary angiomatosis, and first definitive association of* R. quintana *with this clinical syndrome. Excellent photographs.*

Koehler JE, Glaser CA, Tappero JW: *Rochalimaea henselae* infection: A new zoonosis with the domestic cat as reservoir. JAMA 271:531, 1994. *The first definitive demonstration that* R. henselae *bacteremia is common in asymptomatic domestic cats! Even though cat fleas were implicated, the mechanism(s) of* R. henselae *transmission from the cat reservoir to humans is presumed to be direct inoculation.*

Margileth AM: Antibiotic therapy for cat scratch disease: Clinical study of therapeutic outcome in 268 patients and a review of the literature. Pediatr Infect Dis J 11:474, 1992. *A large retrospective study of antibiotic efficacy in patients with classical (lymphadenopathic) cat scratch disease.*

Relman DA, Loutit JS, Schmidt TM, et al.: The agent of bacillary angiomatosis: An approach to the identification of uncultured pathogens. N Engl J Med 323:1573, 1990. *Describes the first clinical application of a molecular approach for identifying fastidious or uncultivated microbial pathogens directly from infected host tissue. The results of this study suggested a close relationship between the agent(s) of bacillary angiomatosis and* R. quintana.

310 BARTONELLOSIS
C. Glenn Cobbs

DEFINITION. Bartonellosis (Carrión's disease) is an insect-borne bacterial disorder characterized by two well-defined clinical stages. It has a striking geographic restriction, occurring only on the western coast of South America at altitude. The first stage, Oroya fever, and the latter cutaneous stage, verruga peruana, were recognized in the nineteenth century. The common bacterial etiology of the two stages was established in 1885 when Daniel Carrión, a Peruvian medical student, died of acute hemolytic anemia 39 days after self-inoculation with material from a verruga lesion.

ETIOLOGY. In 1909, Barton described the causative microorganism, *Bartonella bacilliformis*, a small motile pleomorphic bacillus that requires enriched media for growth. It appears from recent genetic sequence analyses that *B. bacilliformis* is closely related to *Rochalimaea quintana* and *Rochalimaea henselae,* bacteria implicated in trench fever, bacillary angiomatosis, and cat scratch disease.

EPIDEMIOLOGY. Bartonellosis is generally restricted to the habitat of its main vector, the sandfly, *Phlebotomus verrucarum,*

which breeds and transmits the infection in river valleys of the Andes Mountains at an altitude between 2500 and 9000 feet. Humans provide the only known reservoir of the microorganism. Convalescent individuals may have low-grade bacteremia for months to years after infection, and *B. bacilliformis* may be recovered from 5 to 10% of apparently healthy persons in an endemic area. These carriers present the greatest transmission threat.

PATHOLOGY AND PATHOGENESIS. After inoculation by the vector, bacteria replicate, adhere to, and invade erythrocytes and endothelial cells. Red cell parasitization results in increased fragility and increased phagocytosis by the reticuloendothelial system. In severe cases, as many as 90% of the circulating erythrocytes may be parasitized. The ensuing hemolytic anemia causes fever, anemia, and weakness. Peripheral blood smears reveal a normochromic macrocytosis, striking polychromasia, Howell-Jolly bodies, Cabot rings, and nucleated erythrocytes, as well as the intracellular bacteria. The Coombs test and other assays for red cell agglutinins and hemolysins are usually negative. Reactive hyperplasia of lymphatic tissue is common.

Most untreated patients who survive the acute hemolytic episode go on to develop the chronic cutaneous lesions of verruga peruana. These hemangiomatous nodules consist of proliferating small vessels infiltrated by lymphocytes and macrophages and bear a distinct resemblance, clinically and histologically, to the lesions of bacillary angiomatosis (see Ch. 309). Verrugas also may occur in viscera, bone, and central nervous system.

CLINICAL MANIFESTATIONS. Within 2 to 6 weeks after the bite of an infected sandfly, the nonimmune host develops *Oroya fever,* characterized by the insidious onset of myalgias and low-grade fever, followed by high fever, headache, and painful muscles and joints. Tender lymphadenopathy is common, but splenomegaly is rare unless secondary infection is present. Anemia occurs rapidly, and the combination of anemia and jaundice results in a lemon color in light-skinned patients. In some, the disease is characterized by a febrile crisis, followed by rapid resolution of symptoms and signs, increased erythropoiesis, and gradual reduction in fever. Recurrence of fever after initial improvement suggests secondary infection. *Salmonella* disease is an especially important complication of bartonellosis, as it is of other hemolytic disorders.

After the febrile hemolytic anemia has resolved, immunity develops, and relapses of that syndrome are unusual. Following a latent period, which ranges in untreated patients from weeks to months, many patients manifest the second stage of bartonellosis, *verruga peruana.* This disorder is characterized by 1- to 2-cm reddish purple hemangiomatous nodules that typically evolve over 1 to 2 months in crops on exposed skin but also on mucous membranes and internal organs. The lesions are usually nontender and morphologically may vary, appearing as ulcers or secondarily infected pustules. The verrugas may persist for months to years in untreated patients.

DIAGNOSIS. The diagnosis is made by examining the peripheral blood film. There bacilli may be seen within red cells, either singly or in pairs or clusters. With a Giemsa stain, the bacilli appear as 0.3- to 1.5-μm red or reddish purple rods with some pleomorphism. The microorganism may be cultured from blood if appropriate media are used. It is difficult to identify the microorganisms in the verrucal lesion.

PROGNOSIS AND TREATMENT. Mortality in untreated Oroya fever approaches 50% and is a result of acute hemolytic anemia or secondary infectious disorders, e.g., *Salmonella* disease. Malaria, amebiasis, and tuberculosis also appear to be more common in these patients. Penicillin, chloramphenicol, and possibly tetracycline or streptomycin all appear to be effective. Because of the likelihood of associated *Salmonella* disease, chloramphenicol, at a dose of 2 to 4 grams daily for at least 7 days, is the therapy of choice. In patients so treated, fever generally disappears within 2 to 3 days, although blood smears may remain positive for some time longer. Verruga peruana may require more prolonged therapy.

PREVENTION. Insecticides are of use in eradicating the vector.

O'Connor SP, Dorsch M, Steigerwalt AG, et al.: 16S rRNA sequences of *Bartonella bacilliformis* and cat scratch disease bacillus reveal phylogenetic relationships with the alpha-2 subgroup of the class Proteobacteria. J Clin Microbiol 29:2144, 1991.

Schultz MG: A history of bartonellosis (Carrión's disease). Am J Trop Med Hyg 17:503, 1980. *A fascinating summary of the initial historical accounts, medical descriptions, and investigations into the etiology and epidemiology of the disease.*

311 TUBERCULOSIS
Michael D. Iseman

DEFINITION. Tuberculosis is an infectious disease caused by *Mycobacterium tuberculosis.* Characteristic features include a generally prolonged latency period between initial infection and overt disease, prominent pulmonary disease (although other organs can be involved), and a granulomatous response associated with intense tissue inflammation and damage.

ETIOLOGIC AGENT. Mycobacteria are small, rod-shaped, aerobic, non–spore-forming bacilli. In the genus *Mycobacterium,* there is a group of organisms so closely related that they are referred to as "the tuberculosis complex": *M. tuberculosis, M. bovis, M. africanum,* and *M. microti.* However, given the singular epidemiologic, clinical, public health, and therapeutic considerations associated with *M. tuberculosis,* the term "tuberculosis" should be reserved exclusively for infection or disease caused by this organism. Disease caused by other organisms of this genus should be referred to as "mycobacteriosis due to *M. x*" and not "atypical tuberculosis" or "tuberculosis due to . . ." (see also Ch. 312).

The mycobacteria are primarily soil or environmental organisms. However, *M. tuberculosis* has become so adapted to the human body that it has no natural reservoirs in nature other than infected/diseased persons; it is passed almost exclusively by aerosol transmission from the respiratory secretions of diseased patients to their contacts.

Mycobacterial cell walls contain high concentrations of lipids or waxes, making them resistant to standard staining techniques. They can be induced to take up a dye such as carbol fuchsin by alkalinity or by heating, and once so colored, they are resistant to the potent decolorizing agent acid-alcohol—hence the reference to "acid-fast" bacilli.

M. tuberculosis and most of the other mycobacteria grow quite slowly; their doubling time in most media is approximately 18 hours. Readily discernible colonies typically do not appear on solid media for 3 to 5 weeks; because of this, culture confirmation, speciation, and drug susceptibility testing have proven clinically problematic.

M. tuberculosis is an obligate aerobe and a facultative intracellular parasite. Tissues attacked are characterized by high regional oxygen tension. The ability to invade and spread throughout the human body has largely to do with the capacity of tubercle bacilli to survive and proliferate within mononuclear phagocytes.

TRANSMISSION. Infection is spread almost exclusively by aerosolization of contaminated respiratory secretions. Patients with *cavitary* lung disease are particularly infectious because their sputum usually contains 1 million to 100 million bacilli per milliliter, and they cough frequently.

However, the intact skin and respiratory mucous membranes of normal exposed individuals are quite resistant to invasion. For infection to occur, bacilli must be delivered to the distal air spaces of the lung, the alveoli, where they are not subject to bronchial mucociliary clearance. Once deposited in alveoli, bacilli are adapted to promote uptake by alveolar macrophages, which—depending on innate, genetically determined properties as well as immunologic experience—may be more or less permissive to bacillary proliferation (see below).

To reach the alveoli, which lie at the end of a ramifying system of progressively smaller airways, the bacilli must be suspended in very fine units that behave as the air itself and not as particles with significant mass. These units are the dehydrated residuals of the tinier particles generated by high-velocity exhalational maneuvers. These droplet nuclei are calculated to be approximately 1 to 5 μ in diameter, may remain suspended in room air for many hours, and when inhaled can traverse the airways to reach the alveoli.

Although patients with cavitary tuberculosis expectorate massive numbers of bacilli, the probability of generating *infectious* particles is relatively low. Household contacts of patients with extensive pulmonary disease who have had productive coughs for weeks or months before diagnosis have, on average, less than a 50% chance of being infected. Hence the usual case of pulmonary tuberculosis is of a low order of infectiousness compared with an airborne disease such as measles. However, infrequent cases demonstrate extremely high rates of transmission; specific factors in these instances have not been clearly elucidated.

The preponderance of transmission occurs as described above, but other mechanisms of transmission have been identified. Aerosols generated by debridement or by dressing changes of skin or soft tissue abscesses due to *M. tuberculosis* have been shown to be highly infectious. Also, tissue agitation associated with autopsies and direct inoculation into soft tissues via contaminated instruments or bone fragments also have been reported. Fomites do not play a significant role in transmission.

PATHOGENESIS AND IMMUNITY. The natural history and various clinical syndromes of tuberculosis are intimately related to the hosts' defenses. Tubercle bacilli do not elaborate classic endo- or exotoxins; rather, the inflammatory illness and tissue destruction are mediated by products elaborated by the host during the "immune" response to the infection (see Part XIX).

When an immunologically naive alveolar macrophage engulfs a tubercle bacillus, it initially provides a nurturing environment within its phagosome in which the bacilli survive and replicate. However, the infected macrophage releases a substance that attracts T lymphocytes; the macrophages then present antigens from the phagocytized bacilli to these lymphocytes, initiating a series of committed immune effector cells. The lymphocytes, in turn, elaborate cytokines which "activate" the macrophages, enhancing their antimicrobial capacity. Thus is set in motion an elaborate, delicately balanced struggle between the host and the parasite.

Among "normal" adult persons, the host initially prevails in over 95% of cases. However, this initial encounter typically extends over a few weeks to several months during which the bacillary population has proliferated massively and undergone variable degrees of dissemination. Tissues that are seeded during this bacillemia, such as the apices of the lungs, the kidneys, bones, meninges, or other extrapulmonary sites, are potential foci for subsequent "reactivation" tuberculosis. Through complex interactions involving mononuclear phagocytes and various T-cell subsets, host defenses are enhanced. This results in more competent macrophages capable of inhibiting the intracellular replication of mycobacteria. Also, disruption of permissive macrophages that support bacillary multiplication occurs in order that more competent macrophages may engulf and limit the growth of the mycobacteria. These phenomena are broadly referred to as "cell-mediated immunity" (CMI) and "delayed-type hypersensitivity" (DTH), respectively. DTH is associated clinically with the development of the tuberculin reaction, an indurated response 48 to 72 hours after the intradermal injection of tuberculosis protein antigens (such as purified protein derivative, or PPD). Skin test reactivity typically develops 4 to 6 weeks after infection, although intervals up to 20 weeks have been noted.

As these defenses gain momentum, involution of the numerous disseminated granulomatous foci in the lungs, lymph nodes, and scattered sites occurs. Typically, all that remains to overtly mark this encounter is the tuberculin skin test reactivity. In a minority of cases, a small single residual of the primary infection appears in the lung parenchyma (the Ghon focus); occasionally, this is accompanied by calcifications of the ipsilateral hilar nodes. Some patients also develop fibronodular shadowing in one or both lung apices ("Simon foci"); these presumably are the residua of subclinical disease at these sites.

The vast majority of cases occur due to late reactivation of the vestigial lesions of this primary infection, either in the lungs or in extrapulmonary sites. Rapid progression to overt disease occurs in a minority of newly infected persons who cannot mount sufficient immune responses. Groups at high risk include infants through age 4, the infirm elderly, and immunocompromised subjects, including those with human immunodeficiency virus (HIV) infection or acquired immunodeficiency syndrome (AIDS), organ transplant recipients, and those with other immunosuppressive illnesses or chemotherapy.

EPIDEMIOLOGY. Globally, tuberculosis is now the leading infectious cause of morbidity and mortality. However, in the more industrialized nations, the disease has retreated from the general populations, afflicting selected groups. Recognition of these high-risk groups is vital in terms of diagnosis, prevention, and control programs.

Global. The World Health Organization (WHO) estimated in 1990 that one third of the world's population, or 1.7 billion people, were latently infected with *M. tuberculosis.* From this pool, 8 to 10 million new active cases emerge per year, the majority of whom have communicable forms of pulmonary disease. Regions in the world where the infection and disease are most prevalent include the Pacific Rim nations (excluding Japan), Southeast Asia, Indo-Asia, sub-Saharan Africa, and Latin America. Due to delayed, inadequate, or unavailable therapy, 2 to 3 million persons die annually; indeed, WHO estimates that 26% of preventable deaths in the developing nations are attributable to tuberculosis.

United States. The United States has a considerably lower prevalence of infection, with only 4 to 6% of the population—10 to 15 million persons—harboring latent infections. From this pool, approximately 24,000 new active cases arose in 1992. These patients infected approximately 60,000 of their contacts, 3000 of whom went on to develop active disease in that same year—thus the cumulative morbidity of 27,000 cases in 1992.

Case numbers had declined steadily at 5 to 6% annually from 1953 to 1984; however, from 1985 to 1992 there has been a consistent increase in annual numbers of cases (Fig. 311–1). Indeed, from 1985 to 1992, there have been approximately 52,000 excess cases above those projected by the trend from 1953 to 1984; in 1992 alone, this "excess" constituted about 40% of the reported cases.

U.S. morbidity entails remarkable disparities according to race, age, and national origins. Among nonwhite Americans, it is largely a disease of young adults, with the peak incidence between ages 25 and 44 years; by contrast, the peak age among whites is 70 years and older, due presumably to latent early infections (Fig. 311–2). In 1992, 71% of U.S. tuberculosis cases occurred among minorities.

Immigration has contributed significantly to the upturn in morbidity. In 1992, roughly 27% of cases occurred among foreign-born persons (up 20% from 1985). Major sources of these cases include Mexico, the Philippines, Southeast Asia, the Caribbean, and Latin America, the bulk occurring within 5 years of arrival in the United States.

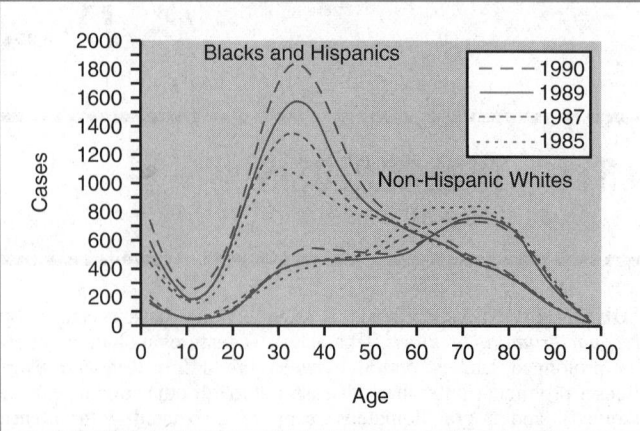

FIGURE 311–2. The majority of cases among non-Hispanic whites occurred between the ages of 60 to 90 years; the incidence declined over this interval. By contrast, the great bulk of cases among blacks and Hispanics occurred among 20- to 50-year-olds; the case numbers rose dramatically in this period. The incidence in 1992 per 100,000 population for non-Hispanic whites was 4 ($RR = 1$); for Hispanics it was 22.4 ($RR = 5.6$); for blacks it was 31.7 ($RR = 7.9$). (From Centers for Disease Control and Prevention, Division of Tuberculosis Elimination: Tuberculosis Statistics for the United States, Atlanta, 1990.)

HIV Infection/AIDS. HIV infection and AIDS have contributed to the rising case rates of tuberculosis through three broad pathways: (1) Individuals with latent tuberculosis infection who acquired HIV infection are at much greater risk of reactivation as their immune capacity diminishes; (2) persons with HIV infection or AIDS may well be at higher risk of acquiring new infections with tuberculosis, due probably to both biologic factors (they may be more prone to become infected on exposure due to impaired defenses) and situational factors (they are more likely to be exposed due to time spent in high-risk, congregate environments); and (3) young adults with HIV infection and active tuberculosis transmit it to people with whom they reside.

In the United States, the upsurge in tuberculosis from 1985 to the present has been clearly linked to the HIV epidemic, although full quantification of the association is not possible due to incomplete serologic testing. Conservatively, at least half the recent excess morbidity can be attributed to the effects of HIV. Direct evidence adduced in support of the relationship includes seroprevalence surveys in tuberculosis clinics located around the country; overall, 11% of U.S.-born tuberculosis patients were HIV-positive; these rates were higher in East Coast clinics and among persons ages 30 to 39. Inferential evidence includes temporal, geographic, and demographic associations between the two infections.

CLINICAL PRESENTATIONS. Since the primary pulmonary infection usually results in bacillemic dissemination, tuberculosis commonly entails disease in extrathoracic as well as pulmonary or pleural sites. As a generalization, hosts with more competent immunity tend to have disease limited to their lungs or other single sites, while those with less robust defenses experience multifocal or disseminated disease.

Normal Adults. Overall, excluding the influence of HIV infection, about 85% of adults present with pulmonary parenchymal disease, 15% with disease at extrapulmonary sites, and approximately 4% with simultaneously active disease at intra- and extrathoracic locations.

Two important comments should be made about clinical tuberculosis in normal adults: (1) The tuberculin skin test (TST) will be falsely negative in 20 to 25% at the time of diagnosis, and (2) although most complain of feeling "feverish," a substantial proportion do not have fever when measured. Thus a clinician should not be diverted from considering the diagnosis by nonreactive TST's or lack of fever in patients with other typical features of tuberculosis.

Pulmonary Disease. Classic symptoms include the following: Cough is nearly universal; typically, it is initially dry but then progresses with increasing volumes of purulent secretions and

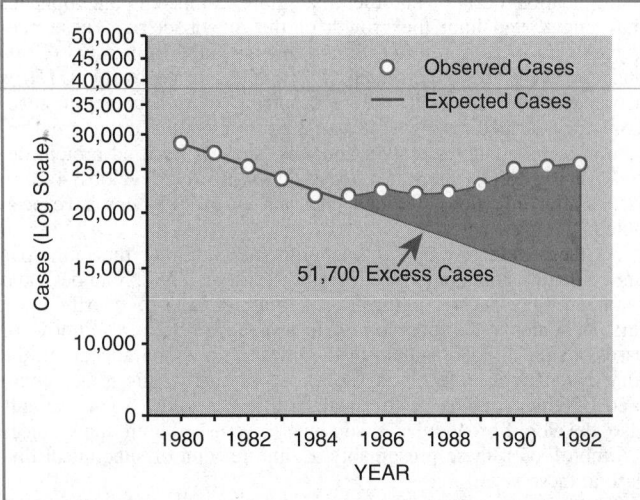

FIGURE 311–1. Excess cases, 1985–1992. CDC data indicate nearly 52,000 cases above the number anticipated based on constant decline of cases between 1953 and 1984. Major influences on this resurgence include HIV infection and immigration. (From Centers for Disease Control and Prevention: Tuberculosis morbidity, United States, 1992. MMWR 42:696, 1993.)

the variable appearance of blood streaking or gross hemoptysis. Feverishness is common as the disease advances; actual temperatures range from subnormal to extreme elevations. Sweating, including drenching night sweats, is quite typical. Other common complaints include malaise, fatigue, weight loss, nonpleuritic chest pain, and dyspnea.

Signs may be quite limited until the disease is in advanced stages. Fever with peaks as high as 40 to 41°C, typically occurring in the evening, is seen among patients with disease of various forms and extent. Localized rales are early findings; coarse rhonchi evolve as secretions become more voluminous and tenacious; signs of lung consolidation are rarely heard. Wheezing and/or regionally diminished breath sounds may be heard in cases with peri- or endobronchial airway compromise.

The chest radiograph is central to the diagnosis. Upper lung zone fibronodular shadowing involving one or both apices is seen in the majority of cases. As these lesions advance, they enlarge and become fluffy or softly margined; coalescence occurs, and cavitation devolves as intense local inflammation produces necrosis and sloughing of lung tissue. The most common sites involved in reactivation adult tuberculosis are, in descending order, the posterior and apical segments of the right upper lobe, the apical-posterior segment of the left upper lobe, and the superior segments of the lower lobes. Lower zone disease is the presenting appearance in < 15% of HIV-negative adults; it is seen somewhat more commonly in diabetics and patients with prominent peribronchial and endobronchial involvement. Pleural effusions are uncommon in adults with reactivation-type pulmonary disease.

Sputum smears and cultures are the most specific components of diagnosis. Some contemporary laboratories still use the classic acid-fast stains (Ziehl-Neelsen or Kinyoun); however, most use a modified acid-fast method, the fluorochrome technique, which relies on the uptake and acid-fast retention of auramine-O, a dye that fluoresces when excited by ultraviolet light. With the fluorochrome technique, the tubercle bacillus is more easily discernible (bright yellow contrasted to an inky black background) than the older methods (red on a blue and white background); hence the fluorochrome system is visually more sensitive. Microscopic acid-fast bacilli (AFB) found in respiratory secretions associated with suitable clinical, epidemiologic, and radiographic findings highly suggests tuberculosis. However, microscopy is not specific, because other pathogenic or saprophytic mycobacteria may be found in sputum. The test is not very sensitive; the likelihood of positive smears depends heavily on the extent of pulmonary involvement. With readily visible cavities and no prior treatment, it would be rare to have negative sputum microscopy. However, with noncavitary fibronodular or miliary patterns on chest films, negative microscopy is common. Cultures are the gold standard for diagnosis; however, current methods typically entail 3 to 6 weeks to cultivate and identify species. More rapid cultivation and identification techniques that use liquid media with radiometric, molecular biologic, or chromatographic methods have reduced the required time substantially. The diagnosis is occasionally made on the basis of symptoms, radiographic findings, and response to empirical therapy *without* culture confirmation. Because of the rising prevalence of resistance to standard drugs, susceptibility testing on all initial *M. tuberculosis* isolates is recommended.

As noted earlier, the TST will be falsely negative in 20 to 25% of HIV-negative adults with pulmonary tuberculosis. Testing with other delayed-type hypersensitivity antigens may help identify persons who are broadly anergic; however, selective anergy to tuberculin occurs.

Extrapulmonary Tuberculosis (XPTB). XPTB occurs in roughly one sixth of HIV-negative adults in the United States with active disease. The most common sites and relevant features are displayed in Table 311–1 (see also Part XXII).

Clinically, it should be noted that the severe wasting seen with advanced pulmonary diseases—consumption—is rarely seen with

TABLE 311–1. COMMON FORMS OF EXTRAPULMONARY TUBERCULOSIS IN PATIENTS WITHOUT HIV INFECTION

Organ System	Relatively High Risk Groups	Common Clinical Manifestations	Diagnosis	Management
Lymphatic	Youngsters and young adults; F > M, Asian and Indian females high-risk	Unilateral, cervical; painless; sinus tracts late	Excisional biopsy with culture; PPD usually positive	May respond slowly to medication; rarely may require excision
Pleural	Young adults with primary infection; older adults with reactivation disease	May be acute *or* indolent; severe pleurisy or asymptomatic	Lymphatic exudate; AFB smear usually negative; biopsy with culture gives best yield	Usually responds well to medication; do not drain with tube thoracostomy
Genitourinary	Rare in young; more frequent among females, foreign born, and Native Americans	May involve kidneys, ureters, bladder, testes, epididymis, uterus, fallopian tubes	Culture urine; biopsy and culture masses and uterine scrapings	Usually responds well to medication; beware of early or late obstructive uropathy
Bone-joint	More common in elderly, although seen in all ages	Lumbar and low dorsal spine common in older; high dorsal in young; weight-bearing bones/joints	Needle biopsy and aspirate for spinal lesions; synovial biopsy and culture for joints	Debride and stabilize spine; try to avoid fusing joints
Disseminated	Most frequent in very young or old; blacks and Native Americans	Chest film abnormalities may lag; progressive fever and inanition; PPD negative in 50%	Smears and cultures of involved fluids, organs, and mesothelia; smear and culture urine	Early therapy vital; steroids of uncertain value
Meninges—CNS	Most common among infants/children with XPTB; higher risk for Hispanics, blacks, and Native Americans	Three stages; early fever, headache, and malaise; later confusion, obtundation, seizures, and coma	LP: ↑ protein and cells; ↓ glucose, ↑ pressure; smears rarely positive; special tests (see text)	Prognosis related to stage; steroids indicated in most cases; drugs must penetrate CNS
Peritoneal-GI	Increases with age; higher risk among minorities	Mainly mesothelial but ileal involvement may resemble Crohn's; abdominal swelling and vague pain common	Laparoscopic biopsy ideal; smear and culture ascites; stool cultures may be useful	Beware of adhesions and obstruction; steroids may be useful
Pericardial	Rare in children; more common in blacks	Acute pain rare; cough, dyspnea, and vague discomfort	Widened cardiac silhouette; left pleural effusion; ECG low voltage and chronic ST/TW changes; ↓ heart sounds, rubs rare	Steroids ↓ effusion, improve performance; may reduce late adhesive complications; pericardiectomy for tamponade

Note: Among persons without HIV infection, roughly 16% of tuberculosis presents as extrapulmonary involvement. Lymphatic and pleural disease are the most common forms.

XPTB. Feverishness occurs with more extensive disease, prominently including miliary, pleural, and genitourinary disease.

Diagnosis is problematic in most forms of XPTB due to the relative paucity of bacilli. Histopathology of involved tissues typically shows giant cell granulomas with caseating necrosis and few, if any, demonstrable AFB. Analysis of mesothelial effusions (pleural, peritoneal, or pericardial) characteristically reveals a lymphocyte-rich exudate with low concentrations of glucose; however, the *initial* inflammatory responses in these spaces may be polymorphonuclear (PMN) leukocyte predominant. Cerebrospinal fluid (CSF) in meningitis begins with a modest leukocytosis, shifting from PMN to lymphocyte dominance; leukocyte counts typically range from 50 to 300 cells per milliliter. The CSF protein concentration is typically moderately elevated. Glucose levels are progressively depressed in relation to the degree of leukocytosis. Because of the scarcity of AFB in the CSF, sophisticated markers, including the polymerase chain reaction, tuberculostearic acid levels, or antibody assays, appear to be useful in establishing the diagnosis, although they are not widely available.

Tuberculosis in Persons with HIV Infection/AIDS.
Early in the course of HIV infection, the clinical manifestations of tuberculosis are quite similar to those in normal hosts. However, with the progressive reduction in the T lymphocyte population, the following major changes ensue: (1) a steady reduction in the proportion who react significantly to tuberculin skin testing, reaching a nadir of 10 to 20% reactors among those with advanced AIDS; (2) substantially greater extrapulmonary involvement, reaching 60 to 80% prevalence of XPTB among those with CD4 counts < 50; and (3) changing patterns of disease on chest radiography, evolving from classic upper zone fibronodular, cavitary disease to lower zone, nondescript pneumonic patterns, infrequent cavity formation, interstitial or miliary shadowing, very prominent hilar or paratracheal adenopathy, and substantial pleural effusions.

TREATMENT. One unique aspect to the care of tuberculosis patients merits emphasis before discussing specific therapy: Because of the hazard of casual, airborne transmission of infection and of the potentially morbid or lethal consequences for the recipients, there is a singular public health mandate that *persons with communicable tuberculosis must either be treated or quarantined.* U.S. public health policy throughout the 20th century has empowered governmental representatives to quarantine patients with potentially lethal infectious diseases. In the case of tuberculosis, modern chemotherapy has, in effect, become "chemical quarantine"; thus nonadherence to treatment may be seen as breaching this quarantine. Because of the consequences of inadequate or incomplete treatment, directly observed therapy (DOT) to prevent noncompliance is being employed increasingly (see the section on nonadherence below).

Indications for Commencing Treatment.
Because it usually takes 3 to 8 weeks to culture and identify species, treatment for most patients is initiated before a "definitive" diagnosis is established, based rather on an amalgam of historical, epidemiologic, radiographic, tissue or fluid analysis, and microscopic findings. Beginning empirical therapy for patients with potentially rapid, life-threatening conditions such as central nervous system (CNS) or miliary disease usually entails a low threshold of suspicion; however, care should be taken to obtain optimal diagnostic specimens before commencing medication, lest the chemotherapy suppress growth from paucibacillary material.

The Principles of Multidrug Treatment.
Patients with active tuberculosis should receive multiple agents both to prevent the emergence of drug-resistant mutants as dominant strains and to accelerate the bacterial clearance. Of these, the former is more crucial, for the emergence of a substantial population of drug-resistant bacilli may significantly and permanently compromise the treatment outcome.

Biologically, tubercle bacilli have the well-documented capacity to undergo spontaneous mutations that confer resistance to the various antituberculosis medications. These mutations occur at predictable frequencies, usually in the range of 1 in 10^8 replications, and are unlinked, resulting in resistance to only one drug or drug category. In patients with cavitary tuberculosis, the population of bacilli is so numerous that small numbers of mycobacteria exist that are resistant to each of the standard medications. However, because the mutations are unlinked, there is an extremely low probability of spontaneous resistance to two or more drugs by a single microbe; e.g., the isoniazid-resistant mutants would be killed by rifampin (RIF) and the rifampin-resistant mutants killed by isoniazid (INH). Thus, early in treatment when the mycobacterial burden is greatest, it is vital that *at least* two effective agents be employed.

If patients are nonadherent, i.e., stop one of their medications unbeknownst to their clinician, the unopposed mutants are allowed to proliferate, resulting in treatment failures or relapses associated with acquired drug resistance. When this happens serially, multidrug resistance is created. Such organisms can be transmitted then to other persons, giving rise to initial drug-resistant tuberculosis.

In addition to combating drug resistance, multidrug regimens can shorten the required duration of treatment through unique contributions by the various agents. A regimen of INH and ethambutol (EMB) requires 18 months to cure the typical case of pulmonary tuberculosis; adding RIF to INH reduces the duration to 9 months; and when an initial 2-month phase of pyrazinamide (PZA) is added to INH and RIF, cure occurs in 6 months.

Choice of Regimen.
Due to concern over the rising prevalence of drug resistance, recent Centers for Disease Control and Prevention (CDC) recommendations advocate a four-drug regimen for most cases of known or suspected tuberculosis (Table 311–2). INH and RIF are the central agents of any regimen based on their

TABLE 311–2. RECOMMENDED REGIMEN OPTIONS FOR TUBERCULOSIS, UNITED STATES

Regimen	Medications	Total Duration	Comments
ATS/CDC (as modified by ACET)	INH and RIF daily for 6 mos. PZA and SM or EMB daily for 2 mos.	6 mos.	Add SM or EMB in areas/patients at risk for initial drug resistance. Stop PZA, EMB, or SM after 2 mos. if strain susceptible; continue or modify regimen if resistance present.
Denver	INH, RIF, PZA, and SM daily for 2 weeks; then twice weekly for 6 weeks. Follow with INH and RIF twice weekly for 18 weeks.	6 mos.	Stop PZA and SM at 8 weeks if strain is susceptible; continue through 6 mos. if there is initial INH resistance. May substitute EMB for SM. 24 weeks of twice-weekly therapy facilitates DOT.
Hong-Kong	INH, RIF, PZA, and SM or EMB thrice weekly for 6 mos. (may stop PZA, SM, or EMB after 2 mos.)	6 mos.	All-intermittent. If strain is susceptible, may stop PZA and SM or EMB after 2 mos. If there is INH resistance, stop INH and add the fourth drug (EMB or SM).
Arkansas	INH and RIF daily for 1 mo.; then INH and RIF twice weekly for 8 mos.	9 mos.	This regimen should only be employed in populations with a very low prevalence of drug resistance. Initial therapy probably should include a third drug until drug susceptibility is reported.

Note: Currently, the Advisory Council for the Elimination of Tuberculosis of the CDC advocates initial four-drug therapy for cases in communities with a background prevalence of initial drug resistance of 4% or greater. If susceptibility has been demonstrated or if resistance is deemed very unlikely, initial three-drug regimens may be used. INH = isoniazid; RIF = rifampin; PZA = pyrazinamide; SM = streptomycin; EMB = ethambutol.

TABLE 311-3. DOSAGE, TOXICITY, AND SPECIAL CONSIDERATIONS FOR STANDARD ANTITUBERCULOSIS MEDICATIONS

Drug	Daily	Usual Adult Dose Thrice ‖ Twice Weekly	Toxicity	Special Considerations	Comments
Isoniazid (INH)	300 mg PO	600 ‖ 900 mg	Hepatitis, neuritis, mood/cognition, lupus reaction	Pregnancy: safe Liver disease: caution Renal impairment: ↓ dose if severe	Monitor liver function tests monthly in most patients; clinically significant interactions with phenytoin and antifungals (azols)
Rifampin (RIF)	600 mg PO 450 mg in persons < 50 kg body weight	600 ‖ (same)	Hepatitis, thrombopenia, nephritis, flu syndrome	Pregnancy: acceptable Liver disease: caution Renal impairment: safe	Key: multiple, profound drug interactions possible (see below); turns urine and fluids red
Pyrazinamide (PZA)	25–30 mg/kg PO	30–35 mg/kg ‖ (same)	Hepatitis, arthralgias and arthritis secondary to hyperuricemia, GI distress, rash	Pregnancy: unknown (avoid) Liver disease: caution Renal impairment: caution	Urate levels always rise; do not treat or stop PZA unless unmanageable gout develops
Ethambutol (EMB)	15–25 mg/kg PO	35 mg/kg ‖ 50 mg/kg	Optic neuritis	Pregnancy: safe Liver disease: safe Renal impairment: ↓ dose/frequency	Monitor visual acuity and color vision regularly
Streptomycin (SM)	12–15 mg/kg IM	15 mg/kg ‖ (same)	Vestibular and auditory, cation depletion	Pregnancy: high-risk (avoid) Liver disease: safe Renal impairment: ↓ dose/frequency	Reduce dose and/or frequency in case of renal impairment

Note: Rifampin drug interactions have been reported with oral contraceptives, anticoagulants, methadone, corticosteroids, estrogen replacement, calcium channel blockers, beta blockers, cyclosporine, antifungal azols, phenytoin, theophylline, sulfonylureas, haloperidol, and others (see *PDR*).

superior bactericidal activity and low toxicity. PZA has special utility in promoting rapid, early reduction in bacillary burden; in drug-susceptible cases, PZA need be given only for the initial 2 months to produce this effect. EMB is useful primarily to protect against the emergence of drug resistance in cases with unknown initial susceptibility patterns and large mycobacterial burdens; EMB may be terminated if susceptibility is reported or be continued throughout the duration of treatment if resistance is noted (see below). Streptomycin (SM), a parenteral agent, has found a diminishing role in modern therapy due to problems with regularly administering intramuscular injections; however, for patients with very extensive tuberculosis, SM may accelerate initial bactericidal activity. Dosage and toxicity for these agents are displayed in Table 311-3.

Does every patient need to receive such a four-drug regimen? In actual practice, clinicians should review every proven or suspected case and consider individual modifications or exemptions of this standard program. For example, (1) an elderly patient with known remote exposure to tuberculosis in the prechemotherapy era, with no recent contacts and no history of tuberculosis medical treatment, might reasonably be started on a three-drug (INH, RIF, EMB) or even two-drug (INH, RIF) regimen because of the very low likelihood of drug resistance; and (2) an injection drug–using 35-year-old HIV-positive man from the Bronx who has been hospitalized on multiple occasions over the prior 12 months might receive initial seven-drug treatment because of the substantial risk of disease due to one of the multidrug-resistant tuberculosis strains prevalent in the New York City area.

Common factors that might influence the initial choice of drugs are included in Table 311-4. Additional considerations in selecting therapy are noted below.

AIDS (see Part XXII). The most salient particular issue in patients with AIDS and tuberculosis is to ensure adequate absorption of the antituberculosis medications. Due to a variety of AIDS-associated enteropathies, there is a risk of grossly reduced serum drug concentrations, which can result in treatment failure and potentially promote acquired drug resistance. Direct determination of drug levels at some time early in treatment is the ideal means for addressing this issue. If this is not feasible, very close monitoring of responses to treatment and use of high-range drug dosing may be appropriate. Also, because of the polypharmacy typically used with AIDS, special attention should be given to the potential impact of RIF-induced hepatic catabolism of other medications (Table 311-4).

CNS Disease. Smaller un-ionized molecules such as INH and PZA cross the blood-brain barrier well, even in the absence of gross

inflammation. RIF crosses less well, although therapeutic effects are seen. EMB CSF levels are significantly lower than those in serum, and its use in meningitis is less well established. SM and the other aminoglycoside antibiotics are large, complex, and ionically charged molecules; they cross the barrier very poorly, even in the presence of inflammation.

Combating Nonadherence with Directly Observed Intermittent Chemotherapy. Treatment given intermittently, thrice or twice weekly, is generally comparable in efficacy with daily treatment. These intermittent schedules make it practical that patients either come to treatment centers or have visits by outreach workers at home or in shelters, schools, or work sites to observe ingestion or actually administer medications. Most reported regimens have begun with a daily phase of therapy and switched to an intermittent schedule after 1 or 2 months. However, effective treatment can either entail a brief (2-week) initial daily phase *or* be intermittent (thrice weekly) throughout. Not all patients need to receive directly observed therapy; many can be trusted to self-administer their drugs. However, it is extremely difficult to predict those who are likely to be compliant, and careful attention should be given to patient education and ongoing monitoring of medication-taking behavior for all patients. If nonadherence is demonstrated or reasonably anticipated (on the basis of risk factors such as homelessness, substance abuse, personality or thought disorders, language or cultural barriers), supervised treatment will benefit patients, their future contacts, and ultimately the community at large. Directly observed therapy may be the only feasible means of stemming the rising prevalence of tuberculosis in general and multidrug-resistant tuberculosis in particular in certain communities and populations.

Common Clinician Errors in Relation to Acquired Drug Resistance. Among the more common errors that contribute to the evolution of multidrug resistance are failure to recognize and cope with nonadherence in a timely manner, failure to identify an individual at high risk for pre-existing drug resistance resulting in use of an inadequate initial regimen, and adding a single drug to a failing regimen.

Monitoring for and Coping with Drug Toxicity. In the general population about a 5% incidence of significant reactions requiring transient or permanent discontinuation of one or more drugs is seen in a typical three- or four-drug regimen. Common drug toxicities are listed in Table 311-4. Vague gastrointestinal complaints are relatively common in association with all the first-line oral drugs. However, with coaching and encouragement, most patients can be induced to tolerate these drugs. Caution should be taken that pa-

TABLE 311-4. HIGH-RISK CANDIDATES FOR IPT

Candidates for preventive chemotherapy—persons at high risk for tuberculosis. Various persons with latent tuberculosis infection are at relatively great risk of developing active disease. The degree of tuberculin skin test reactivity to identify such persons varies based on epidemiologic and biologic factors. The recommended duration of therapy is 6 months for most candidates but 12 months for HIV-infected persons or patients with upper-zone fibronodular shadows on chest film.

High-Risk Groups

Certain groups within the infected population are at greater risk than others and should receive high priority for preventive therapy. *In the United States, persons with any of the following six risk factors should be considered candidates for preventive therapy, regardless of age, if they have not previously been treated:*

- Persons with human immunodeficiency virus (HIV) infection (≥ 5 mm) and persons with risk factors for HIV infection whose HIV infection status is unknown but who are suspected of having HIV infection.
- Close contacts of persons with newly diagnosed infectious tuberculosis (≥ 5 mm). In addition, tuberculin-negative (< 5 mm) children and adolescents who have been close contacts of infectious persons within the past 3 months are candidates for preventive therapy until a repeat tuberculin skin test is done 12 weeks after contact with the infectious source.
- Recent converters, as indicated by a tuberculin skin test (≥ 10 mm increase within a 2-year period for those < 35 years old; ≥ 15 mm increase for those ≥ 35 years of age).
- Persons with abnormal chest radiographs that show fibrotic lesions likely to represent old healed tuberculosis (≥ 5 mm).
- Intravenous drug users known to be HIV seronegative (≥ 10 mm).
- Persons with medical conditions that have been reported to increase the risk of tuberculosis (≥ 10 mm).

In addition, in the absence of any of the above risk factors, persons < 35 years of age in the following high-incidence groups are appropriate candidates for preventive therapy if their reaction to a tuberculin skin test is ≥ 10 mm:

- Foreign-born persons from high-prevalence countries.
- Medically underserved low-income populations, including high-risk racial or ethnic minority populations, especially blacks, Hispanics, and Native Americans.
- Residents of facilities for long-term care (e.g., correctional institutions, nursing homes, and mental institutions).

In addition to the groups listed above, public health officials should be alert for other high-risk populations in their communities. For example, through a review of cases reported in the community over several years, health officials may use geographic or sociodemographic factors to identify groups that should be targeted for intervention. Screening and preventive therapy programs should be initiated and promoted within these populations based on an analysis of cases and infection in the community. To the extent possible, members of high-risk groups and their health-care providers should be involved in the design, implementation, and evaluation of these programs. Staff of facilities in which an individual with disease would pose a risk to large numbers of susceptible persons (e.g., correctional institutions, nursing homes, mental institutions, other health-care facilities, schools, and child-care facilities) may also be considered for preventive therapy if their tuberculin reaction is ≥ 10 mm induration.

From Screening for Tuberculosis and Tuberculous Infection in High-Risk Populations and the Use of Preventive Therapy for Tuberculous Infection in the United States. Recommendation of the Advisory Committee for the Elimination of Tuberculosis. MMWR 39(No. RR-8):7, 1990.

tients, in an effort to diminish gastrointestinal intolerance, do not take their oral medications directly with meals, antacids, or H_2 blockers, any of which may substantially reduce absorption of certain of these agents. Regular monitoring of liver chemistries is indicated for all patients receiving multidrug therapy; monthly surveillance is common. In addition, patient education regarding the typical symptoms of hepatitis and regular reminders may be of major importance in preventing serious liver injury. When patients experience serious hepatitis, all potentially hepatotoxic drugs should be held until liver chemistries and symptoms normalize; then the drugs can be reintroduced one at a time at 3- to 4-day intervals, monitoring liver function tests and symptoms to identify the offending agent. Elderly patients receiving SM or other aminoglycosides should have baseline and periodic audiometry; in addition, surveillance of vestibular function is required. For younger patients who

are receiving only 2 months of SM, objective testing is generally not indicated.

Duration of Treatment and Posttreatment Surveillance. Currently, a 6-month regimen consisting of INH and RIF supplemented by an initial 2-month phase of PZA is regarded as sufficient and curative for the vast majority of cases caused by drug-susceptible strains. If these three agents cannot be used, the duration of treatment may be prolonged (see Table 311–3). Other situations in which therapy may be extended beyond 6 months include the following: *HIV infection/AIDS:* Although no well-controlled studies have demonstrated the superiority of longer therapy, some clinicians fear that impaired immunity will place these patients at higher risk of relapse. *Far-advanced, cavitary lung disease with delayed clinical response or sputum conversion:* About 95% of patients will become culture negative by 3 months of treatment; for those who remain positive longer than this, treatment for 3 months *after* conversion is recommended. *Irregular, interrupted therapy:* If patients fail to attend 10% or more of DOT encounters or are otherwise deemed to have been significantly nonadherent to their treatment, extended treatment is prudent. *Miliary or meningeal cases:* Due both to the concern that such patients may be less competent hosts and the implications of disease recurrence, therapy may be extended to 9 to 12 months.

A low and unavoidable risk of relapse exists following treatment; for the regimens described above in usual populations, the probability is < 5%. The majority of such recurrences occur within 2 years and are usually associated with the same drug susceptibility profile as pretreatment. Current guidelines do not compel posttreatment surveillance. Rather, patients should be instructed to return after treatment when there are changes in their clinical status; suitable tests including sputa, chest radiographs, or other studies should be obtained if symptoms or signs appear.

Indications for Corticosteroid Therapy. Steroids may be used to reduce acute inflammation and limit delayed fibrotic complications. Acute reductions in inflammation with significant benefits in outcome have been demonstrated in meningitis and pericarditis cases treated with corticosteroids. Prednisone, at 1 mg per kilogram of body weight, is usual. Less well proven are the benefits of such therapy in pleural, peritoneal, miliary, or extensive pulmonary disease, although salutary effects may occur in individual cases. While high-dose corticosteroids may impair immune responses, there is no evidence that they adversely affect the outcome of treatment when given for 4 to 8 weeks to patients who are receiving adequate chemotherapy.

Adrenal insufficiency due to tuberculous destruction is uncommon in this era. However, among patients with marginal cortisol production, RIF may precipitate hypocortisolism by accelerating catabolism of endogenous steroids.

Drug-Resistant Tuberculosis. In a recent CDC survey, the national prevalence of resistance to one or more drugs was 14.2%. Resistance to INH was noted most commonly: 8.2% of new cases and 21.5% of recurrent cases. Resistance to INH and RIF was noted in 3.5% of strains studied; cases with resistance to INH and RIF, with or without resistance to other drugs, are referred to as "multidrug-resistant tuberculosis" (MDR-TB). This report indicated that the regional patterns of resistance varied widely, and it is incumbent on clinicians to consider this when choosing empirical therapy. For example, in New York City, resistance to INH and RIF was found in 12.9% of isolates. The particular importance of MDR-TB is that, in the absence of INH and RIF, the period required for treatment is doubled, the probability of cure drops substantially, and the ability to provide effective preventive therapy for infected contacts is sorely compromised.

Risk markers for the likelihood of drug resistance include prior treatment for tuberculosis, close contact to such persons, and time spent in communities/countries with known high prevalence. Cases proven or suspected to involve MDR-TB should be referred with alacrity to specialty facilities for expedited laboratory studies and individualized management.

CONTACT INVESTIGATION. It is vital that clinicians realize that their responsibilities are not complete when they have established the diagnosis and initiated chemotherapy for their patient. Tuberculosis is a reportable disease in all U.S. communities and states; clinicians are obligated to promptly notify public health authorities of all cases of proven or suspected tuberculosis. Contact investigation of the home, workplace, school, or other congregate facilities may well reveal other active cases or newly infected persons who are at substantial risk for tuberculosis. Priority must be given to investigations where infants or AIDS patients have been exposed due to their compressed incubation periods for potentially lethal forms of tuberculosis. Preventive chemotherapy of infected contacts is a highly efficient means of curtailing tuberculosis morbidity (see below).

PREVENTION OF TUBERCULOSIS. Multiple modalities are involved with the efforts to control tuberculosis. In the U.S. over the past 25 years, isoniazid preventive chemotherapy (IPT) has been relied upon. For the remainder of the world, vaccination with bacille Calmette-Guérin (BCG) has been the central element. The relative merits and limitations of these methods are discussed below.

Isoniazid Preventive Therapy: Principles and Efficacy.
Because most U.S. tuberculosis cases arise from endogenous reactivation of latent infection acquired remotely in time, authorities reasoned that chemotherapy given to persons harboring such infections might be protective. In a series of randomized, placebo-controlled studies, IPT demonstrated 75% reduction of morbidity in the year of treatment and 54% protection in the posttreatment years; even higher rates of protection were shown in a large trial in Eastern Europe, ranging from approximately 70 to 90% with 6- and 12-month IPT, respectively.

Indications for IPT. The focus of IPT recommendations is on persons who are deemed to be at relatively higher risk for experiencing reactivation. Specific groups or conditions that are regarded at high risk and to be candidates for IPT are noted in Table 311–4.

In most instances, the TST is the central modality to identify latent infection. Interpretation of the TST, however, is influenced by circumstances. Thus, in some instances, IPT would be recommended despite nonreactivity, while in other cases ≥ 15 mm induration is required for significance.

Special Considerations in Preventive Therapy. HIV infection is probably the most potent risk factor for endogenous reactivation. Hence persons with positive HIV serology or strong epidemiologic or clinical markers for HIV risk should be assigned very high priority for IPT. In addition to protecting the individual patient from tuberculosis, IPT may extend survival by ameliorating the accelerated progression of HIV infection seen with active tuberculosis *and* could prevent transmission to other very vulnerable HIV-infected persons (e.g., in shared health care, social, or residential facilities).

Persons exposed to and presumed infected by resistant strains of *M. tuberculosis* pose problems for preventive therapy. If the strain from the source case is resistant only to INH, RIF likely would be a highly effective substitute. However, if the source-case strain is resistant to both INH and RIF, there are no really promising alternatives. For very high-risk persons (such as AIDS patients) exposed to an MDR-TB case, preventive therapy with ofloxacin and EMB or PZA may be indicated but should be undertaken only after expert consultation.

Monitoring for Compliance and Toxicity. Patients receiving preventive chemotherapy should be seen periodically to both provide adherence to the treatment and survey for signs or symptoms of drug toxicity. Intermittent, directly observed preventive therapy is not widely feasible; however, it may be applicable in selected circumstances such as prisoners, especially with HIV infection, or recently infected infants or children in chaotic households where reliable treatment is unlikely.

The major toxicity of INH is hepatitis, which may prove fatal if therapy is continued into the period of symptoms and gross chemical derangements. Therefore, it is important that initial education alert the patient and/or responsible family members to the early manifestations of liver injury (anorexia, nausea, malaise, loss of taste for cigarettes, dark urine) with instructions to stop the INH and report promptly for evaluation. Also, patients should have monthly communication with a health care worker, directly if possible but by telephone as an alternative, to inquire regarding their health and to reiterate the education. Biochemical monitoring of liver chemistries is indicated for persons 35 years of age or older, due to the age-related risk of hepatitis, and should be obtained at baseline and monthly intervals. Innocent increases in the transaminase levels three- to fourfold over baseline without symptoms are

noted among up to 20% of persons on IPT; this is not an indication to discontinue the drug but to maintain close surveillance. However, liver chemistries elevated to higher levels or those associated with symptoms should result in discontinuation of the INH. The decision to rechallenge with this drug or to use an alternative agent should be made after expert consultation.

Vaccination with BCG. BCG is a live vaccine prepared from an attenuated strain of *M. bovis.* It has been used widely around the world, but its efficacy and utility are debated. The performance of various strains of BCG, given to different populations over time, has ranged from 80% protection to detrimental effects (more tuberculosis in those receiving the vaccine). A recent meta-analysis of published BCG studies indicated that vaccinations offered an overall 50% protective effect, with higher levels of protection against meningeal or disseminated tuberculosis. This study revealed that the efficacy of BCG diminished at sites near the equator. Although the calculated protection in this meta-analysis reached statistical significance, no explanation was offered for the failure to show efficacy in two large, recently conducted trials.

In addition, since BCG is presumed to work by conferring tuberculoimmunity to those *not* previously infected, it is not appropriate for widespread use in the United States, where most cases arise among those already infected with *M. tuberculosis.* Some have called for BCG vaccinations for health care workers at high risk for tuberculosis infection. However, given the disputable protection afforded by the vaccines and the loss of utility of the TST (due to reactivity induced by BCG) as a tool to mark recent infection and to qualify for preventive chemotherapy—which *has* proven efficacy—this seems to be a dubious proposition.

LIMITING NOSOCOMIAL TRANSMISSION. Substantial microepidemics of tuberculosis have been documented recently in various institutions, including hospitals, clinics, residential facilities, and prisons. To prevent institutional transmission, the CDC has advocated a three-tiered system: administrative measures, environmental programs, and personal respiratory protection. These measures are currently being employed by Occupational Safety and Health Administration (OSHA) as criteria to assess institutional tuberculosis control programs. *Administrative measures* include educational programs to alert staff on how to recognize and isolate possible active cases early. Also, staff tuberculin skin testing is required to assess the risks of intrainstitutional transmission. *Engineering or environmental programs* are intended to effectively isolate proven or suspected cases by placing them in negative-pressure rooms and diluting the air in the patients' environment through six or more air changes per hour, with the options of decontamination via the adjunctive use of HEPA filtration or ultraviolet germicidal irradiation. *Personal respiratory protection* entails respirators or masks that theoretically can filter out the infectious "droplet nuclei"; presently, HEPA filtration respirators most clearly meet federal guidelines. The optimal role for personal respirators is controversial. Perhaps the most suitable role would be to protect health care workers who have unavoidable exposure to smear-positive cases during cough-inducing procedures such as bronchoscopy or intubation. Use in other circumstances depends on source case and environmental factors. For considerations of both public health concerns and regulatory oversight, all institutions that might be involved with caring for tuberculosis patients should have an active program to limit the hazard of nosocomial transmission to health care workers and other patients or clients.

American Thoracic Society: Treatment of tuberculosis and tuberculosis infection in adults and children. Am J Respir Crit Care Med 149:1359, 1994. *Most recent guidelines for treatment and prevention in adults, children, and infants. Excellent overview of contemporary issues.*
Bloch AB, Cauthen GM, Onorato IM, et al.: Nationwide survey of drug-resistant tuberculosis in the United States. JAMA 271:665, 1994. *A careful delineation of the patterns, frequencies, and special risk-factors for drug resistance in the U.S. in the '90's. Helpful in selecting empirical drug regimens and preventive chemotherapy.*
Cantwell MF, Snider DE Jr, Cauthen GM, et al.: Epidemiology of tuberculosis in the United States, 1985–1992. JAMA 272:535, 1994. *Recent trends in demographics and special risk factors. Helps quantify the impacts of HIV infection and immigration upon case rates; also targets high-risk groups for screening, case detection, and prevention.*
Iseman MD: Treatment of multidrug-resistant tuberculosis. N Engl J Med 329:784, 1993. *Reviews recent epidemiology, management, and prevention of multidrug-resistant tuberculosis; discusses use of second-line medications and resectional surgery.*

312 OTHER MYCOBACTERIOSES
Laurel C. Preheim

MICROBIOLOGY. Among the mycobacteria, *M. tuberculosis, M. bovis,* and *M. leprae* have caused most human infections. In the 1950's, however, Timpe and Runyon established that other mycobacteria could cause disease in humans and classified these organisms based on pigment production, growth rate, and colonial characteristics. Photochromogens (group I) grow slowly on culture media (>7 days). Their colonies change from a buff shade to bright yellow or orange after exposure to light. Scotochromogens (group II) also grow slowly but demonstrate pigmented colonies when incubated in the dark or the light. Group III mycobacteria grow slowly and lack pigment in the dark or light. Rapid growers (group IV) also lack pigment, but they grow in culture within 3 to 5 days. Collectively, these four groups have been called the "atypical mycobacteria," "nontuberculous mycobacteria" (NTM), "mycobacteria other than tubercle bacilli" (MOTT), or "potentially pathogenic environmental mycobacteria" (PPEM).

EPIDEMIOLOGY. The rate of isolation of NTM is increasing and has surpassed that for *M. tuberculosis* in some areas. Ubiquitous in nature, many have been isolated from ground or tap water, soil, house dust, domestic and wild animals, and birds. Despite their wide distribution, some species are more common in certain geographic locations. Most infections, including those which are hospital-acquired, result from inhalation or direct inoculation from environmental sources. Ingestion may be the source of infection for children with NTM cervical adenopathy and for patients with AIDS whose disseminated infection may begin in the gastrointestinal tract. These infections are not considered contagious, since person-to-person transmission is extremely rare.

PATHOPHYSIOLOGY. The pathogenic potential for human disease varies among NTM. As a group, these organisms are less virulent for humans than *M. tuberculosis* and may colonize body surfaces or secretions without causing disease. Tissue invasion is most likely to occur in individuals with predisposing conditions associated with impaired local or systemic host defenses. In general, disease is slowly progressive, and histopathologic findings resemble those seen in tuberculosis.

DIAGNOSIS. The steps taken to diagnose tuberculosis generally apply to NTM infections. Standardized, specific skin test antigens for NTM, however, are unavailable. In addition, colonization of asymptomatic individuals and environmental contamination of specimens can yield positive cultures in the absence of clinical disease. NTM disease can be considered present in patients with a cavitary infiltrate on chest radiograph when (1) two or more sputums (or sputum and a bronchial washing) are smear-positive for acid-fast bacilli and/or yield moderate to heavy growth on culture, and (2) other reasonable causes for the disease process have been excluded, e.g., fungal disease, tuberculosis, malignancy. An additional criterion, (3) failure of the sputum cultures to convert to negative with either bronchial hygiene or 2 weeks of specific mycobacterial drug therapy, is applied in the presence of a noncavitary infiltrate not known to be due to another disease.

The diagnosis is also established if transbronchial, percutaneous, or open lung biopsy tissue reveals mycobacterial histopathologic changes and yields the organism. Extrapulmonary or disseminated disease is confirmed by isolating the organism from normally sterile body fluids, closed sites, or lesions, and environmental contamination of specimens is excluded. Radiometric culture systems, DNA probes, and polymerase chain reaction assays have increased the speed and accuracy of laboratory diagnosis of pulmonary and extrapulmonary infections.

CLINICAL DISEASE. NTM cause a broad spectrum of diseases (Table 312–1). The following discussion includes infections caused by selected species most likely to be encountered in clinical settings. It should be noted that therapeutic approaches continue to evolve and therefore remain controversial. Most conventional antituberculous agents have little or no activity against the majority of

TABLE 312–1. NONTUBERCULOUS MYCOBACTERIAL DISEASES AND ETIOLOGIC SPECIES

Clinical Disease	Etiologic Species (Runyan Group)*	
	Common	*Less Common*
Pulmonary	*M. avium* complex (III)	*M. simiae* (I)
	M. kansasii (I)	*M. szulgai* (II)
	M. abscessus (IV)	*M. malmoense* (III)
	M. xenopi (II)	*M. fortuitum* (IV)
		M. chelonae (IV)
Lymphadenitis	*M. avium* complex (III)	*M. fortuitum* (IV)
	M. scrofulaceum (II)	*M. chelonae* (IV)
		M. abscessus (IV)
		M. kansasii (I)
Cutaneous	*M. marinum* (I)	*M. avium* complex (III)
	M. fortuitum (IV)	*M. kansasii* (I)
	M. chelonae (IV)	*M. terrae* (III)
	M. abscessus (IV)	*M. smegmatis* (IV)
	M. ulcerans (III)	*M. haemophilum* (III)
Disseminated	*M. avium* complex (III)	*M. fortuitum* (IV)
	M. kansasii (I)	*M. xenopi* (II)
	M. chelonae (IV)	
	M. abscessus (IV)	
	M. haemophilum (III)	

* I = photochromogen; II = scotochromogen; III = nonpigmented; IV = rapid grower.

these organisms. Many treatment regimens contain new agents or older antimicrobials newly found to have activity against mycobacteria. In therapeutic decisions all potential drug toxicities and interactions must be weighed.

Mycobacterium avium-intracellulare. *M. avium* and *M. intracellulare* are closely related and commonly grouped as *M. avium-intracellulare* or *M. avium* complex (MAC). Distributed worldwide, they rank first among NTM isolates in the United States. MAC causes about 80% of NTM lymphadenitis cases. *M. scrofulaceum* is responsible for most of the rest. Excisional therapy without chemotherapy is curative in about 95% of cervical adenopathy cases. Pulmonary infection usually occurs in individuals with underlying lung disease and generally follows an indolent or slowly progressive course. Differentiation between colonization and true infection may be difficult initially. Extrapulmonary or disseminated disease, infrequently seen in immunocompetent patients, occurs in up to 40% of individuals with AIDS. It usually affects patients with advanced human immunodeficiency virus (HIV) disease. Therefore, prophylaxis with rifabutin (300 mg daily) is recommended for patients with CD4+ T lymphocyte counts < 100 cells per microliter. Symptoms suggesting disseminated MAC include fever, weight loss, anorexia, abdominal pain, and diarrhea. Findings may include hepatosplenomegaly and generalized lymphadenopathy, including mediastinal adenopathy. Diagnosis of disseminated disease is commonly made by culturing the organism from blood, bone marrow, stool, or tissue biopsy.

Newer regimens for MAC infections are based on recent trials with patients with AIDS who received treatment for disseminated disease. These guidelines can be applied to patients with or without AIDS who have either pulmonary or disseminated infections. Treatment regimens should include at least two agents. Every regimen should contain either azithromycin (500 mg once daily) or clarithromycin (500 mg twice daily). Many experts prefer ethambutol (15 mg per kilogram once daily) as the second drug. One or more of the following may be added as second, third, or fourth agents: clofazimine (100 mg daily), rifabutin (300 to 600 mg daily), rifampin (600 mg daily), ciprofloxacin (750 mg twice daily), and in some situations amikacin (7.5 to 10 mg per kilogram daily). Isoniazid and pyrazinamide are not effective. No specific regimen has emerged as being superior for pulmonary or disseminated disease, and the optimal duration of therapy remains unknown. Immunocompetent patients probably should receive a minimum of 18 to 24 months of therapy. Therapy should continue for the lifetime of patients with AIDS if clinical and microbiologic improvement is observed.

Mycobacterium kansasii. *M. kansasii*, the most important photochromogen, often appears beaded or cross-barred on acid-fast stain. It ranks second among NTM in causing human infections. Most disease occurs in midwestern and southern United States. Pulmonary infection resembling tuberculosis is the usual clinical presentation. Although adult white men are most commonly affected, infection can occur in individuals of any age, gender, or race. Extrapulmonary disease can involve any organ system, and risks of dissemination are increased in immunocompromised patients.

Standard treatment of pulmonary disease is isoniazid (300 mg daily), rifampin (600 mg daily), and ethambutol (15 mg per kilogram daily) for 18 months. In patients who are unable to tolerate isoniazid, rifampin and ethambutol, with or without streptomycin for the first 3 months, is an alternative regimen. *M. kansasii* isolates are resistant to pyrazinamide. Patients with isolates resistant to rifampin can be treated with isoniazid (900 mg daily), pyridoxine (50 mg daily), ethambutol (25 mg per kilogram daily), and sulfamethoxazole (3.0 grams daily) for 18 to 24 months. This regimen can be combined with streptomycin or amikacin given daily or 5 times per week for 2 to 3 months, followed by intermittent streptomycin or amikacin for a total of at least 6 months. These treatment regimens apply to patients with pulmonary or extrapulmonary infection and have been used with some success in individuals with AIDS. The optimal agents and duration of therapy for disseminated disease in patients with AIDS are unknown.

Rapidly Growing Mycobacteria. Rapidly growing mycobacteria are acid-fast rods that resemble diphtheroids on Gram stain. Growth is rapid on subculture (1 to 3 days), but primary isolation from clinical specimens may require 2 to 30 days. Unlike other mycobacteria, they grow well on most routine laboratory media. Sporadic, community-acquired infections have been reported from most areas of the United States. The spectrum of diseases ranges from localized to disseminated, with cutaneous involvement being most common. Most infections are acquired by inoculation after accidental trauma, surgery, or injection. Nosocomial epidemics or clusters have been reported in numerous settings including augmentation mammaplasty, hemodialysis, plastic surgery, long-term venous catheter use, cardiac surgery, and jet injector use.

These NTM are highly resistant to conventional antituberculous drugs but may be sensitive to traditional antibiotics. Susceptibility testing of individual isolates is important, since resistance patterns vary by and within species subgroups. *M. fortuitum* is usually susceptible to amikacin, ciprofloxacin, sulfonamides, cefoxitin, and imipenem, and occasionally to doxycycline. *M. abscessus* is generally susceptible to amikacin and cefoxitin and occasionally erythromycin. In contrast, *M. chelonae* is most likely to be susceptible to tobramycin, amikacin, or erythromycin and occasionally to doxycycline.

Amikacin plus cefoxitin (12 grams daily) can be used for initial therapy of severe infections caused by all species except *M. chelonae*. The decision to change to oral therapy depends on clinical improvement and susceptibility testing results. Oral agents may include ciprofloxacin (500 mg twice daily), sulfamethoxazole (1 gram thrice daily), doxycycline (100 mg twice daily), and clarithromycin (500 mg twice daily). Because development of resistance has been reported during single-drug therapy with ciprofloxacin, the use of two agents should be considered. Treatment duration should be a minimum of 3 months for serious disease and 6 months for bone infections. Any regimen should include surgical débridement of infected wounds or excision of foreign bodies.

Other Nontuberculous Mycobacteria. *M. marinum* cutaneous infections commonly follow aquatic-related inoculation. Papules on an extremity, especially on the elbows, knees, and dorsum of feet and hands, may progress to shallow ulceration and scar formation. Therapeutic approaches have included simple observation for minor lesions, surgical excision, and antimicrobials. Acceptable regimens include doxycycline (100 mg twice daily), trimethoprim-sulfamethoxazole (160/800 mg twice daily), or rifampin (600 mg daily) plus ethambutol (15 mg per kilogram daily) for a minimum of 3 months. Recent studies indicate clarithromycin (500 mg twice daily) may be effective as a single agent. *M. xenopi, M. malmoense, M. szulgai, M. simiae, M. haemophilum,* and *M. terrae* are being reported with increasing frequency as causes of pulmonary or disseminated infections in Europe, England, Canada, and the United States. Patients with AIDS appear particularly prone to disseminated disease. Initial therapy for these infections should consist of isoniazid, rifampin, and ethambutol with or without streptomycin or amikacin. Optimal duration of therapy is unknown, but at least 18

to 24 months is recommended. *M. gordonae,* a scotochromogen also known as the "tap water bacillus," has been associated with nosocomial pseudo-outbreaks. It rarely, if ever, causes infection, and its isolation should suggest likely environmental contamination of a clinical specimen.

American Thoracic Society: Diagnosis and treatment of disease caused by nontuberculous mycobacteria. Am Rev Respir Dis 142:940, 1990. *Outstanding guidelines for the diagnosis and therapy of NTM.*

Centers for Disease Control and Prevention: Recommendations on prophylaxis and therapy for disseminated *Mycobacterium avium* complex for adults and adolescents infected with human immunodeficiency virus. MMWR 42(RR-9):13, 1993. *Authoritative, up-to-date therapeutic recommendations that can be applied to all types of MAC infections.*

Inderlied CB, Kemper CA, Bermudez LEM: The *Mycobacterium avium* complex. Clin Microbiol Rev 6:266, 1993. *An excellent review on the most common NTM.*

Straus WL, Ostroff SM, Jernigan DB, et al.: Clinical and epidemiologic characteristics of *Mycobacterium haemophilum,* an emerging pathogen in immunocompromised patients. Ann Intern Med 120:118, 1994. *A good description of a newly recognized NTM pathogen.*

Wayne LG, Sramek HA: Agents of newly recognized or infrequently encountered mycobacterial diseases. Clin Microbiol Rev 5:1, 1992. *An excellent, very comprehensive review; includes 244 references.*

313 LEPROSY (Hansen's Disease)

Gilla Kaplan and Zanvil A. Cohn*

DEFINITION. Leprosy is a bacterial disease of great chronicity and low infectivity that occurs worldwide. The primary host is the human, in whom the causative agent *Mycobacterium leprae* accumulates largely in the skin and peripheral nerves, leading to a variety of cutaneous lesions and loss of nerve conduction. Serious disfigurement and loss of digits may result and represent the stigmata of this biblical disease. The clinical manifestations are largely governed by the ability of the host to mount a cell-mediated immune (CMI) response to the organism and its antigens. Patients unable to generate an immune response develop widely distributed skin lesions of the "lepromatous" state and allow unrestricted growth of bacilli. In contrast, a moderate to vigorous immune response leads to the localized cutaneous lesions of the "tuberculoid" form. In addition to these polar states, there are intermediate forms that demonstrate gradations in reactivity. Spontaneous modulation of the disease toward more polar forms can occur and may lead to tissue damage via humoral (immune complex) and cellular (CMI) mechanisms. Multiple-drug therapy promptly reduces viable organisms and transmissibility but must be maintained for long periods for the disappearance of skin lesions and a reduction in bacterial load.

TRANSMISSION. Little detailed information is available about how the bacillus is transmitted from one individual to another. This deficit in our understanding is related to the long incubation period (>3 years) and the absence of adequate techniques to identify the organism in the environment. Other than in humans, the disease has been discovered in feral armadillos studied in Louisiana and Texas. These animals contain large numbers of acid-fast bacilli in parenchymatous organs, which by DNA hybridization and restriction fragment length polymorphism analysis techniques are identical to bacilli obtained from humans. The sooty mangabey, a new world monkey, can become infected naturally in the wild or when injected with human bacilli. In both armadillos and monkeys it takes 18 to 24 months for the injected bacilli to reach high numbers. These infections are quite unlike the spectrum of human disease.

How the localized lesions of tuberculoid leprosy and the generalized cutaneous distribution of lepromatous disease evolved is unclear. Direct inoculation via trauma and puncture wounds might lead to an initial focus with environmental bacilli. Some suggest that the initial route may be through the respiratory or gastrointestinal tract. Biting insects have been considered, but no clear evidence

---

* Dr. Cohn is deceased.

exists on them as an intermediate vector. It seems reasonable, however, that at some point during the infection in lepromatous leprosy patients, hematogenous spread occurs with wide seeding of the body.

The extent of contact with environmental bacilli is correlated with transmission. The incidence of the disease within a household containing an infected tuberculoid or lepromatous index patient may be four to eight times that of the general population. In particular, lepromatous patients with lesions in the nasal mucosa discharge large numbers of organisms. Bacilli recovered from dry nasal discharges retain some viability for up to 7 to 10 days, with somewhat greater viability under conditions of higher humidity. Transmission of the disease from an untreated, infected mother to an infant is not uncommon and should always be considered. In general, clinical wisdom indicates that disease transmission takes place only after years of exposure. Little likelihood of transmission is present in a ward or hospital setting, and patients are now cared for on an ambulatory basis with a minimum of precautions.

SUSCEPTIBILITY. Leprosy occurs worldwide and in individuals of all ages. It appears more frequently in young adults, but this may be related to a parental index case and the long period of incubation. A large number of studies suggest, but do not prove, that the overall susceptibility to leprosy is not controlled by immune response genes and their expressed major histocompatibility class II antigens. Early analysis of the disease incidence and susceptibility in identical twins has not been conclusive. More recent studies suggest that the type of leprosy rather than overall disease susceptibility may be controlled by HLA determinants. No clear-cut conclusions on the genetic basis of susceptibility can therefore be accepted at this time. In this context, environmental factors such as nutrition and coincident microbial and parasitic infections must be considered as unproven alternatives.

The physiologic immunodeficiency of the newborn may lead to an early colonization with the bacillus. The AIDS pandemic has been associated with a rise in the incidence of other mycobacterial diseases, and this association, although not yet observed, may become more apparent in leprosy in the future.

EPIDEMIOLOGY. The worldwide number of leprosy cases has been estimated to be about 10 million in 1991. In many countries, valid statistics are not available, and the incidence in outlying, rural areas is poorly documented. The highest prevalence rates are in Asia and Africa, followed by Central and South America and Oceania. The highest rates do not usually exceed 55 per 1000 but may be as high as 200 per 1000 in selected villages. Many accept the fact that with effective chemotherapy the worldwide prevalence is dropping and will continue to do so with advanced diagnostic and public health methods. However, incidence does not appear to be changing.

The majority of leprosy cases are found in tropical areas. Socioeconomic condition, availability of health care, and body exposure to the environment may all contribute. The disease also occurs in the colder climates of Tibet, Nepal, Korea, and Siberia. In previous centuries, the disease occurred more commonly in Scandinavia and those countries bordering the North Sea. Small numbers (300 to 500 per year) of cases currently occur in the United States. The majority of these are in immigrant groups from Asia and South America, although occasional cases are seen in the southern states and those bordering Mexico.

The nature of the disease varies considerably with geographic distribution. African and Asian countries have a predominance of tuberculoid leprosy, and 20% or fewer of the cases are of the lepromatous type. In contrast, larger numbers of lepromatous cases are

reported in Brazil and Venezuela. Early infection and/or sensitization with cross-reacting antigens of other mycobacteria have been considered as an explanation for the variation in type of leprosy with which an individual presents.

ETIOLOGIC AGENT. *M. leprae* is the causative agent of human leprosy, and no evidence of strain variation has been noted by DNA-DNA hybridization or restriction fragment length polymorphism. The organism is acid-alcohol fast when stained by the Ziehl-Neelsen method. *M. leprae* is an obligate intracellular parasite and has never been cultivated extracellularly in laboratory media. It is a resident of the phagolysosomes of macrophages, Schwann cells, and endothelial cells. *M. leprae* is classified as a mycobacterium and contains mycolic acid, arabinogalactan, and phenolic glycolipid. The latter molecule is the only *M. leprae*–specific component. Most other carbohydrates, peptidoglycans, and proteins share antigenic determinants with other mycobacterial species, making serologic diagnosis especially difficult.

The absence of a culture system for *M. leprae* has complicated any investigations of the physiology and pathogenicity of the organism. Many advances in this field have resulted from the ability of the armadillo to support the growth of the mycobacteria. Eighteen to 24 months after inoculation, large numbers of bacilli (10^9 per gram) can be purified from liver and spleen and serve as a source for antigenic and chemical analysis. Many of the metabolic activities of *M. leprae* appear to be low compared with other mycobacteria. *M. leprae* lacks catalase activity, and *de novo* purine biosynthesis appears to be missing. *M. leprae* replicates very slowly within host cells and has a doubling time of approximately 13 days. It prefers ambient temperatures below 37°C and grows selectively in cooler portions of the body such as skin, testes, and nasal mucosa.

Determining bacillary viability and resistance to chemotherapeutic agents depends on its slow growth in the foot pads of mice—a bioassay taking about 12 months. Accelerated growth occurs in the athymic nude mouse but still requires 6 or more months. These properties impose severe restrictions on rapid diagnosis. Applying the polymerase chain reaction, in which selected DNA sequences are amplified a millionfold, may lead to the specific identification of as few as 10 bacilli within a few days.

IMMUNOLOGIC CONSIDERATION. A major immunologic defect occurs in patients with lepromatous leprosy. This is expressed as a selective unresponsiveness of T cells to *M. leprae* and is evident in skin test (Mitsuda) anergy and the *in vitro* lymphocyte transformation test for *M. leprae* antigens (Table 313–1). Patients with the tuberculoid form of the disease respond normally, and in neither form of the disease are there abnormalities in humoral immunity. The association between cell-mediated cutaneous responses, T-cell accumulation in lesions, T-cell–directed immunity, and the number of *M. leprae* in the tissues is shown in Table 313–1. These parameters are inversely related. In the absence of *M. leprae*–specific T-cell reactivity, lymphokine formation is depressed or absent and tissue macrophages fail to be activated into an antimicrobial state. Normally, macrophage activation occurs largely through the local release of interferon-gamma (IFN-γ), a lymphokine that enhances the production of toxic oxygen intermediates in these cells. Bacilli taken up by "resting" and "aged" macrophages of the skin are able to multiply intracellularly, leading in the case of lepromatous disease to multibacillary vacuoles. In tuberculoid forms, the bacilli are largely destroyed, and only small numbers survive to perpetuate the cell-mediated immune reactions.

Lepromatous patients, although unresponsive to *M. leprae* antigen, develop adequate reactions to other antigens to which they have been sensitized. These include skin test antigens such as PPD, mumps, *Candida,* trichophytin, and tetanus toxoid. The highly se-

TABLE 313–1. IMMUNOLOGIC FEATURES OF LEPROSY PATIENTS

	Tuberculoid	Borderline Tuberculoid	Mid Borderline	Borderline Lepromatous	Lepromatous
Acid-fast bacilli in skin lesion	−	−/+	+	+++	+++
Lepromin (Mitsuda) reaction	+++	++	−	−	−
Lymphocyte transformation test	95%	40%	10%	1–2%	1–2%
Anti–*M. leprae* antibodies	−/+	−/++	++	+++	+++
CD4+/CD8+ T-cell ratio in lesions	1.35	1.11	NT	0.48	0.20

lective anergy of leprosy may be related to the loss of *M. leprae*-specific T cells rather than suppressor cell phenomena.

CLINICAL DIAGNOSIS. Patients with leprosy are first seen and followed by dermatologists because the anesthetic cutaneous lesions are often the presenting complaint. The range in immunity to *M. leprae* is reflected clinically by a wide variation of skin lesions and peripheral nerve involvement. In this section we review the characteristics of the major polar and borderline forms.

Polar Tuberculoid Leprosy (TT). This form presents as one to a few asymmetric plaques or macules defined by a sharp, raised border. In dark-skinned patients, they are often centrally hypopigmented with a more erythematous border. The central area is scaly, lacks hair, and is anesthetic. Nerves leading to the area of the ear, elbow, and knee may be palpably enlarged. Almost any area of the skin may be affected except for the warmer regions of the scalp, axilla, and perineum. The disease is stable.

Borderline Tuberculoid and Borderline Lepromatous Leprosy (BT and BL). As the body burden of antigen increases, in association with a partial reduction in immunity, the number, distribution, and nature of the cutaneous lesions increase in complexity and the sequelae of peripheral nerve damage increase in severity. The skin exhibits a polymorphic array of macular, erythematous, hypopigmented lesions involving the trunk, extremities, and face. These vary randomly in number and distribution. Larger nerve trunks are infiltrated with a granulomatous reaction, leading to nerve damage resulting in foot drop, flexion contractions of the digits, and corneal abrasions. The anesthesia of hands and feet and the resulting damage from burns, trauma, and secondary infection leads to loss of digits, plantar ulcerations, and blindness. These widely dispersed lesions suggest hematogenous spread and a cell-mediated reaction that is not capable of fully controlling bacillary growth. Disease is unstable and may evolve toward the polar forms. Reactional states are common.

Lepromatous Leprosy (LL). Here there is little or no CMI, and tremendous numbers of organisms are dispersed throughout the skin. Again, the lesions are pleomorphic but often are less "angry" or erythematous than in borderline disease. Macules, papules, and nodules may cover wide areas of the trunk and extremities, and lesion distribution is often symmetric. Almost any area of affected or "normal" looking skin contains bacilli. Often there are no obvious lesions, but the skin looks shiny and "full," as the dermis is expanded with macrophages containing bacilli. This is particularly prominent on the ears, eyebrows, and face, giving rise to an appearance called "leonine facies." Eyebrow loss is frequent; a saddle nose deformity may result from cartilage destruction; gynecomastia from reduced testosterone levels secondary to testicular damage may be present; and blindness and iridocyclitis, laryngeal stenosis, loss of incisor teeth, and loss of digits may occur. Nerve damage in lepromatous leprosy is more slowly progressive but is eventually severe and diffuse and leads to a sensory polyneuropathy. Rigid, swollen nerves are palpable in many locations. Disease is stable. These results of long-term untreated lepromatous leprosy are the stigmata that ostracized the leper from his/her community and necessitated custodial care. This is almost never the case today, and patients undergoing chemotherapy remain members of their households.

REACTIONAL STATES. *Erythema Nodosum Leprosum (ENL).* Patients with BL and LL disease maintain high levels of circulating anti–*M. leprae* antibodies as well as high antigen levels in tissue depots. Following effective chemotherapy, a prompt and extensive kill of bacilli takes place, and large amounts of soluble antigens are liberated extracellularly. More than 30% of such patients develop ENL and present with painful subcutaneous erythematous nodules that arise diffusely and may eventually lead to necrosis and suppuration. These symptoms, accompanied by fever and malaise, can continue for months, are extremely debilitating, and are often accompanied by acute inflammation of the eyes, testes, nerves, lymph nodes, and joints. Some patients develop glomerulonephritis with the deposition of complement and immune complexes in the glomeruli. Enhanced production of tumor necrosis factor alpha (TNFα) has been associated with ENL. This serious complication requires prompt diagnosis and therapy.

Reversal Reactions. This reactional state also may occur after chemotherapy but differs from ENL in that acceleration or decrease of the local cell-mediated reaction is observed, accompanied by widespread erythema and induration of pre-existing lesions as well

as systemic symptoms, e.g., pyrexia. The onset of this state is slower, takes weeks to months, and may persist for many months if not properly treated. Rapid progression of pre-existing peripheral nerve damage may take place. These irreversible changes in nerve conduction should be considered a medical emergency and treated accordingly.

LABORATORY DIAGNOSIS. In addition to clinical manifestations, the primary method for diagnosing leprosy is identifying acid-fast bacilli in the skin. The slit smear technique is used throughout the world. Skin is incised with a scalpel, squeezing the area to maintain a bloodless field. The edges of the slit are scraped with the edge of the scalpel, smeared on a slide, fixed, and stained by the Ziehl-Neelsen method. A microscopic logarithmic score (1 + to 6 +; 5 + equals 100 to 1000 acid-fast bacilli per high-power field) is used to quantitate the bacterial load. Usually six sites on the earlobes, elbow, knee, and a lesion are prepared. This simple method, when skillfully applied, is as sensitive as any diagnostic procedure.

A more definitive estimate of bacillary numbers in the skin comes from biopsy material. A logarithmic score is made by counting the number of bacilli in high-power fields. This ranges from 1 + to 6 + and is a useful index in following the response of patients to therapy in terms of bacillary numbers and histopathologic classification. (Bacterial index: 0—no bacilli in 100 microscopic fields ($\times$100); 1 + = 1 to 10 bacilli in 100 fields; 2 + = 1 to 10 bacilli in 10 fields; 3 + = 1 to 10 bacilli per field; 4 + = 10 to 100 bacilli per field; 5 + = 100 to 1000 bacilli per field; and 6 + = many 1000s per field.)

A skin test may be used which distinguishes the immunologically reactive (tuberculoid) and nonreactive (lepromatous) poles of the disease. A crude antigen consisting of heat-killed bacilli from lepromatous skin nodules is injected and induces local induration and the formation of granulomas in 3 to 4 weeks in most tuberculoid patients. Patients with lepromatous leprosy fail to react to the antigen and may remain unresponsive long after effective chemotherapy.

Serologic tests are useful in assaying the level of anti–*M. leprae* antibodies in multibacillary lepromatous but not in the paucibacillary tuberculoid forms. However, the many cross-reactive antigenic epitopes shared with other mycobacteria complicate interpretation and differential diagnosis. ELISA tests, which recognize antibodies against the carbohydrate moieties of the phenolic glycolipids, the only molecule that is *M. leprae*–specific, are positive in patients with lepromatous but not tuberculoid disease and decline after chemotherapy is initiated. Patients with lepromatous leprosy have a polyclonal hypergammaglobulinemia, acute phase reactants such as C-reactive protein, and immune complexes in the circulation. Ten percent give false-positive tests for syphilis and 30% have cryoglobulinemia.

HISTOPATHOLOGY AND IMMUNOPATHOLOGY. Microscopic analysis of tissue plays a primary role in diagnosing and classifying the various clinical forms of leprosy and uses the standardized classification described by Ridley and Jopling. Five groups have been defined spanning the spectrum from polar tuberculoid (TT) to polar lepromatous (LL) and include borderline (BB) as well as borderline tuberculoid (BT) and borderline lepromatous (BL). Our discussion focuses on the polar forms, and the details pertaining to the intermediate manifestations can be found in more specialized texts.

Lesions of the Skin. **Tuberculoid Leprosy.** Microscopic examination of H & E–stained sections of biopsies obtained from a TT macular plaque reveals heavy infiltration of the dermis by mononuclear leukocytes organized in well-developed granulomas. These contain large numbers of lymphocytes scattered between and surrounding other components of the granulomatous response, including macrophage-derived epithelioid cells and Langhans-type multinucleated giant cells (Fig. 313–1). Occasional plasma cells but no granulocytes are found. Langerhans cells are found within the dermal infiltrate in significant numbers. Staining with monoclonal antibodies shows that the majority of lymphocytes are T cells and that the CD4+ "helper type" phenotype predominates over CD8+ "suppressor/cytotoxic" cells.

The epidermis overlying the dermal infiltrate is thickened (two- to threefold), and individual keratinocytes are enlarged. The keratinocytes display large amounts of MHC class II determinants on

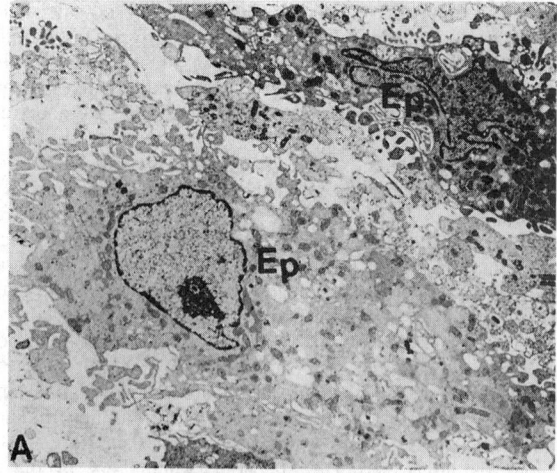

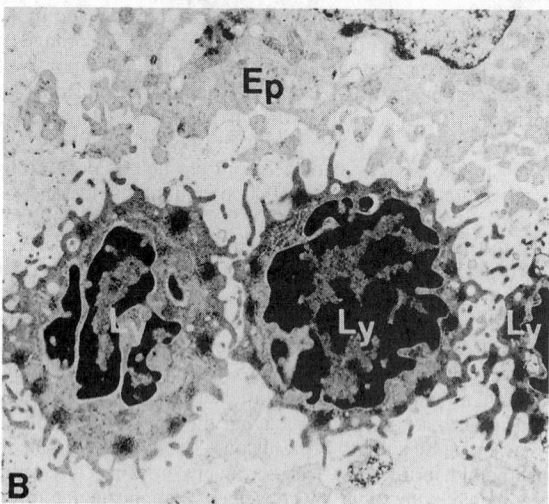

FIGURE 313–1. Transmission electron photomicrographs of cutaneous granulomas from a patient with tuberculoid leprosy. *A*, The granuloma contains large epithelioid cells (Ep) with multiple cytoplasmic organelles (×4500). *B*, Three T lymphocytes (Ly) and an epithelioid cell are observed (×9000).

their surface. This is a response to the local production of IFN-γ in the dermis and is accompanied by the expression of other IFN-γ–induced molecules by keratinocytes and other cell types.

Acid-fast staining of sections reveals an occasional bacillus or bacillary remnants within macrophages. BT lesions are similar except that acid-fast bacilli are more readily seen.

Lepromatous Leprosy. In contrast to TT lesions, the lepromatous lesion contains only small numbers of lymphocytes, predominantly of the CD8+ phenotype, scattered through a background of loosely organized dermal macrophages and collagen (Fig. 313–2). The macrophages often have a pale, foamy cytoplasm and may contain large clumps of *M. leprae* called "globi" (Fig. 313–3). By electron microscopy, these organisms are seen to reside within large cytoplasmic vacuoles, embedded in a lucent matrix that contains a phenolic glycolipid. Remnants of the osmiophilic bacilli are always present along with structurally intact organisms (Fig. 313–3*B*). A gram of skin may contain 10^9 bacilli. Langerhans cells are rarely seen in the dermis; the overlying epidermis is thin and atrophic and fails to show surface MHC class II antigens.

The loose bacilli-rich infiltrates of LL are present in almost every area of the skin, and individual infected macrophages may be observed surrounded by collagen bundles.

Lesions of Peripheral Nerve. Tuberculoid Leprosy. The paucibacillary granulomatous response is associated with significant destruction of peripheral nerve fascicles and late in the disease may lead to caseous necrosis of nerve trunks. Large numbers of T cells and mononuclear phagocytes breach the perineurium and lead to destruction of Schwann cells and axons alike. By the time the skin

lesion is apparent, nerve damage and sensory loss have occurred. The mechanism of the nerve damage in TT is unclear but is related to CMI and the granulomatous response.

Lepromatous Leprosy. Many bacilli are observed within Schwann cells and macrophages surrounding and within the perineural sheath in the majority of subcutaneously placed nerve trunks (Fig. 313–4). Nerve damage is relatively slow as compared with a TT but more extensive and insidious. Few, if any, lymphocytes are part of the lesion. Eventually, more enlargement and displacement by connective tissue result. Schwann cells are capable of taking up *M. leprae* and serve as permissive hosts for their replication (Fig. 313–4).

Other Organs. Granulomatous lesions can be seen in the lymph nodes, liver, spleen, bone marrow, endocrine organs, and eye. These contain bacilli but are not considered to be an important source of infection. Patients with untreated multibacillary disease can have a constant bacteremia of 10^5 AFB per milliliter, all of which are present within monocytes. The total body burden of *M. leprae* can reach 10^{12}.

Lesions of Reactional States. **Erythema Nodosum Leprosum (ENL).** Examination of the skin nodules of ENL shows extensive mixed leukocyte infiltration of neutrophils and mononuclear cells and tissue necrosis. Immune complexes are evident, and there is a panvasculitis of dermal arteries and veins. These are all hallmarks of an extensive acute inflammatory response resulting in tissue damage. TNFα and other monocyte cytokine–induced cell surface antigens can be demonstrated.

Reversal Reactions. Patients with BT, BB, or BL leprosy, who are partially responsive to *M. leprae* antigens, occasionally undergo an upgrading reaction after several months of therapy. This differs from ENL in the migration of a predominantly T-cell infiltrate into pre-existing inflammatory sites. Many of the T cells are of the helper phenotype and are secreting lymphokines into their environment. T-cell migration into skin lesions is associated with mononuclear phagocyte differentiation into organized granuloma and is often associated with the rapid progression of peripheral nerve damage. This enhancement of CMI leads to limited bacillary destruction. A downgrading or reduction in CMI also may occur. Such reactions may continue for weeks or months and are associated with severe morbidity leading to serious sequelae.

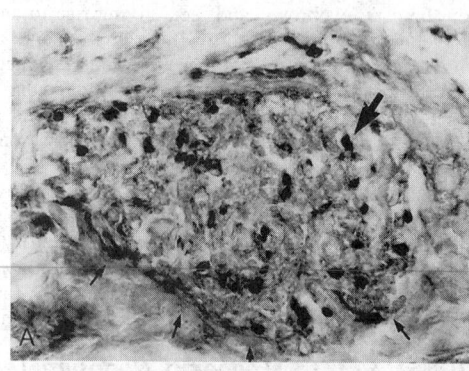

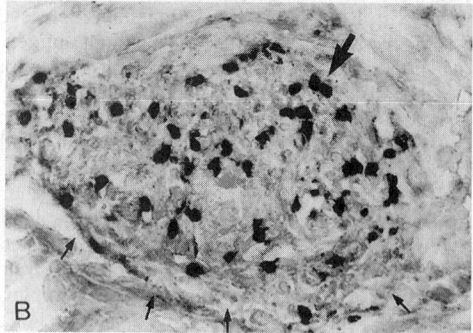

FIGURE 313–2. Lepromatous leprosy—cutaneous lesion. Frozen serial sections stained with Leu 3 (anti-CD4–helper T-cell subset) (*A*) and with Leu 2 (anti-CD8–suppressor/cytotoxic T-cell subset) (*B*). The inflammatory infiltrates (*small arrows*) contain few T cells. Cells of the CD4+ subset (*large arrow* in *A*) are less numerous than those of the CD8+ subset (*large arrows* in *B*). Immunoperoxidase, counterstained with hematoxylin (×200).

PATHOGENESIS. Recovery from infections with obligate intracellular parasites such as *M. leprae* requires the host to mount an effective CMI response. For this purpose, antigen-presenting cells must recognize and cluster with appropriate T cells, leading to T-cell stimulation, differentiation, and replication. T cells then follow two distinct pathways. In the first, helper cells synthesize and secrete a variety of hormone-like lymphokines which seem to enhance the microbicidal activity of monocytes and macrophages as well as stimulate other cells in the environment, e.g., keratinocytes, endothelial cells, and fibroblasts. A second pathway leads to the development of T cells which are of the CD4+ phenotype and are antigen specific and MHC class II restricted. Along with NK (natural killer) and LAK (lymphokine-activated killer) cells, they serve as potent specific and nonspecific cytotoxic effector cells.

In lepromatous leprosy, in the absence of local lymphokine production, bacilli multiply in macrophages that have the capacity neither to kill the organism nor to be activated by lymphokines. To modify this fertile intracellular culture environment, the host must destroy the heavily parasitized macrophage, liberating its contents into the extracellular milieu. Here, newly emigrated monocytes ingest, kill, and degrade *M. leprae* with the help of a lymphokine stimulus. This is the situation which applies in the tuberculoid form of the disease and is lacking in the lepromatous state.

RECOMMENDED TREATMENT SCHEDULES. The most commonly used drug in the therapy of leprosy is 4,4'-diaminodiphenylsulfone (dapsone, DDS). Because of the widespread emergence of dapsone-resistant strains of *M. leprae*, all patients now receive multidrug therapy. The components and schedules vary depending on the presence of dapsone-sensitive strains and the part

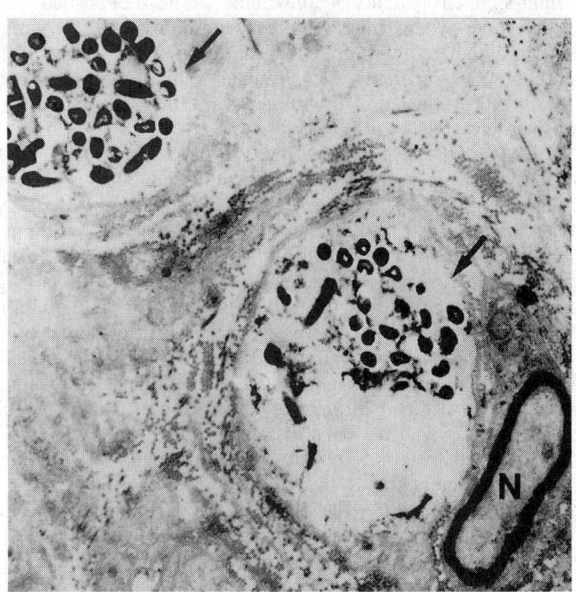

FIGURE 313-4. Transmission electron micrograph of an infiltrated peripheral nerve of a cutaneous lesion from a lepromatous leprosy patient. The myelinated neuron (N) and two *M. leprae*–infected Schwann cells *(arrows)* are observed (×9000).

of the world in which the patient resides. In the United States, the following recently modified regimens are employed:

1. *Paucibacillary disease of the TT and BT categories.*
   a. Dapsone-sensitive *M. leprae*—Dapsone is given in a daily dose of 100 mg and rifampin at a daily dose of 600 mg for 1 year.
   b. Dapsone-resistant *M. leprae*—Clofazimine at a daily dose of 50 to 100 mg is substituted for dapsone.

2. *Multibacillary disease of the BB, BL, and LL categories.*
   a. Dapsone-sensitive or dapsone-resistant *M. leprae*—Dapsone is given in a daily dose of 100 mg, rifampin is given in a dose of 600 mg per day, and clofazimine is given in a daily dose of 50 mg for 2 years.

To evaluate the dapsone sensitivity, the mouse foot pad assay must be used; this procedure is available only in specialized facilities.

A modified schedule for third world country control programs was issued in 1982 and is based on practical consideration by the World Health Organization (WHO), including the availability of slit smear facilities and financial constraints:

1. *Paucibacillary disease—a bacillary index of 0 at all six skin sites.* Dapsone is given daily at a dose of 100 mg, unsupervised. Rifampin is given at a dose of 600 mg once a month, supervised. Treatment is given for 6 months and is then discontinued.

2. *Multibacillary disease—a bacillary index of 1+ or more at any one of six skin sites.* Dapsone is given daily at 100 mg with clofazimine 50 mg daily, unsupervised. Rifampin 600 mg and clofazimine 300 mg are given once monthly, supervised. This therapy is continued for 2 years.

The WHO schedule for intermittent rifampin therapy is based in part on its expense and on clinical and laboratory trials. It should be noted, however, that many leprologists use rifampin at 450 to 600 mg daily for 2 to 3 years. Relapses under the WHO schedule are infrequent.

Rifampin is the most rapidly effective bactericidal agent and kills the majority of *M. leprae* within 2 to 3 weeks. This is evident by mouse foot pad assays. Resistance to rifampin is well known in the therapy of *M. tuberculosis* and is now becoming evident with *M. leprae*.

Therapy with clofazimine, a phenazine derivative, has certain unpleasant side effects based on its lipophilicity. The compound is a red-purple dye taken up and concentrated by macrophages of the

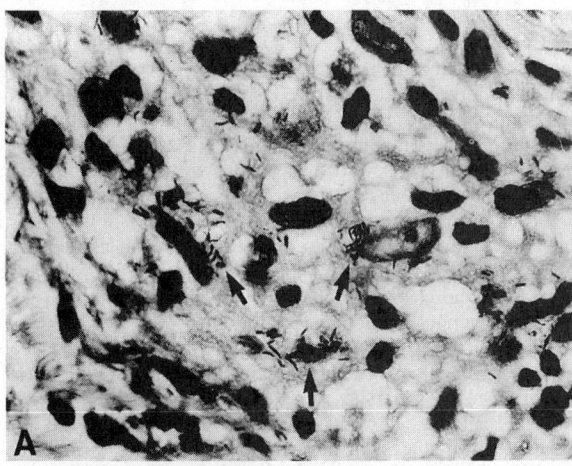

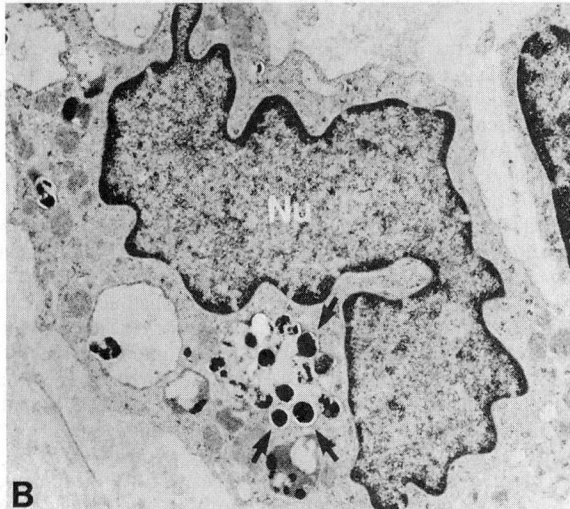

FIGURE 313-3. Lepromatous leprosy—cutaneous lesions. Acid-fast staining of histologic section *(A)* and transmission electron photomicrograph *(B)* of *M. leprae*–parasitized foamy macrophages *(arrows)*. The phagocytes have large nuclei and many light and electron lucent vacuoles containing darkly staining bacteria *(A, ×500; B, ×9000).*

skin, causing increased skin pigmentation. This is distressing to certain light-skinned patients. Clofazimine is also deposited in the small intestine, where it at high concentrations causes segmental thickening associated with crampy pain and diarrhea. If clofazimine is unacceptable to patients, the physician should consider substitution with 100 mg daily of minocycline or 400 mg daily of ofloxacin.

THERAPY OF REACTIONS. *Erythema Nodosum Leprosum.* The acute onset of ENL may be mild enough to require only salicylates or other cyclo-oxygenase inhibitors. With severe episodes, high doses of corticosteroids (prednisone 60 to 80 mg per day) are necessitated and should be tapered off as soon as feasible. However, exacerbations occur frequently, and repeated dosing is necessary. A particularly useful drug in severe ENL is thalidomide, a selective inhibitor of TNFα. It is given initially at 200 mg twice a day and then tapered to levels of 50 to 100 mg per day. Thalidomide is a potent teratogen and should be assiduously avoided if pregnancy is possible. Clofazimine also has been found useful in ENL but requires 4 to 6 weeks to achieve therapeutic effects. ENL in some patients responds poorly to thalidomide, and prednisone and/or clofazimine is employed.

Reversal Reactions. The chronicity and potential nerve damage of this cell-mediated reaction require high-dose steroids and careful evaluation of peripheral nerve condition. Thalidomide is not used in this condition, but clofazimine along with steroids allows the more rapid withdrawal of prednisone.

Other Complications. A number of surgical procedures are available at specialized leprosy hospitals to help correct foot drop, hand deformities, madarosis, and lagophthalmos. Plastic surgical procedures can replace nasal septa and help close large plantar ulcerations. On occasion, patients request the removal of glandular tissue for gynecomastia.

The presence of a cold abscess of a peripheral nerve with sudden increase in pain and functional loss requires immediate decompression by surgical drainage.

IMMUNOMODULATION. Recombinant lymphokines that can enhance the microbicidal properties of macrophages and stimulate the expression of CMI may find a place in the care of leprosy patients. Preliminary studies with the T-cell mitogen interleukin-2 (IL-2) have already been carried out in patients with lepromatous leprosy. The intradermal injection of IL-2 leads to a local cell-mediated reaction associated with induration, the destruction of parasitized macrophages, and a marked reduction in the bacillary load. Trials with more prolonged administration have demonstrated that a systemic response can be achieved.

PROGNOSIS. Tuberculoid leprosy is usually self-limited and responds well to chemotherapy. Nerve damage is, however, irreversible. In lepromatous disease, prolonged courses of multiple drugs arrest the progression of the illness when compliance is good. It is the ability of the public health infrastructure to monitor compliance that is central to effective therapy. Recurrences due to poor maintenance therapy are not infrequent.

PREVENTION AND PROPHYLAXIS. Education of the general public plays an important role in sensitizing individuals to the nature of leprosy lesions and the ability to cure the illness with medication. Once a case has been identified in a household, careful physical examination of all contacts with the biopsy of suspicious lesions should be carried out. The threat of contagion is much higher in children younger than age 16. In this adolescent category, the prophylactic use of dapsone should be considered.

A number of vaccine trials are currently underway, many sponsored by WHO. These are employing BCG vaccine with and without heat-killed *M. leprae* or other mycobacteria in highly endemic areas of Africa, Asia, and India. There is suggestive evidence that BCG alone may reduce the incidence of disease.

Cohn ZA, Kaplan G: Leprosy, cell-mediated immunity and recombinant lymphokines. J Infect Dis 163:1195, 1991. *Discussion of the regulation of CMI with cytokines.*
Guinto RS, Abalos RM, Cellona RV, Fajardo TT: An Atlas of Leprosy. Sasakawa Memorial Health Foundation, 1983. *Excellent pictorial of diagnostic signs.*
Hansen GA: Causes of leprosy. Norsk Laegevidensk 4:76, 1874. *The classic work on leprosy.*
Hastings RC, Franzblau SG: Chemotherapy of leprosy. Annu Rev Pharmacol Toxicol 28:231, 1988. *Current update of therapy and complications thereof.*
Job CK: Nerve damage in leprosy. XIII Leprosy Congress State of the Art Lectures. Int J Leprosy 57:532, 1989. *Good discussion of mechanisms of nerve damage.*
Kaplan G, Britton WJ, Hancock GE, et al.: The systemic influence of recombinant interleukin-2 on the manifestations of lepromatous leprosy. J Exp Med 173:993, 1991. *Systemic modulation of CMI with IL-2.*

Sexually Transmitted Diseases

314 INTRODUCTION TO SEXUALLY TRANSMITTED DISEASES AND COMMON SYNDROMES

P. Frederick Sparling

Sexually transmitted diseases (STD's) are a diverse group of infections, caused by biologically dissimilar microbial agents, that are grouped together because of certain common clinical and epidemiologic features. Advent of the acquired immunodeficiency syndrome (AIDS) has heightened public awareness of the importance of STD's and the dangers of unsafe sexual practices. New knowledge has accumulated rapidly about old diseases; for instance, it is now clear that cervical carcinoma is a complication of certain human papillomavirus (genital wart virus) infections. Some relatively less severe infections, such as chlamydial ones, are known to be alarmingly prevalent in young persons. This chapter discusses certain common features of some of these infections, as well as the differential diagnosis and management of several of the common syndromes of genital infections.

DEFINITIONS. Those infectious agents that are frequently transmitted by sexual contact, and for which sexual transmission is epidemiologically important, are considered STD's. In some cases, such as gonorrhea and genital herpes simplex virus infection, sexual transmission is the only important mode of transmission, at least between adults. In others, such as the hepatitis viruses, giardiasis, shigellosis, and amebiasis, there are also important nonsexual means of acquiring infection. Table 314–1 lists the important infectious agents commonly transmitted sexually, as well as their known or probable disease syndromes. "Sexual" includes the full range of heterosexual or homosexual behavior, including genital, oral-genital, oral-anal, and genital-anal contact.

EPIDEMIOLOGIC CONSIDERATIONS. Sexually transmitted infections are prevalent in many segments of society, but, for obvious reasons, are most prevalent in the groups with the most promiscuous sexual activity. It is not sexual activity *per se* but the number and type of different sexual partners that determine the risk of acquiring STD. The highest rates of gonorrhea are found in the young (15 to 30) and unmarried and in groups of low educational and socioeconomic status. Rates of gonococcal infection may be 50-fold higher in young, single inner-city persons than in married middle- to upper-middle-class persons. Decisions regarding the cost-effectiveness of screening for STD should be governed by these considerations; screening is most effective in high-risk groups.

Multiple infections are frequent in patients with sexually transmitted infection. In venereal disease clinics, about 20% of men with gonorrhea also have urethral chlamydial infection, and 30 to 50% of women with gonorrhea also have cervical chlamydial infection. In women with vaginitis, one study showed that 16% of cases were caused by mixed infection with various combinations of *Candida*, *Trichomonas*, and *Gardnerella vaginalis*. However, no convincing evidence exists that one sexually transmitted infection directly increases the risk of acquiring others. Rather, the frequent coexistence of multiple sexually acquired infections probably reflects the multiplicity of sexual partners among the subject patients.

Control of sexually transmitted infections is complicated by the frequent lack of significant symptoms. The majority of gonococcal and chlamydial infections in women probably are associated with few symptoms. From 10 to 50% of urethral gonococcal infections in men are oligo- or asymptomatic. Chlamydial infections are more common than gonococcal infections and frequently are asymptomatic. One of the crucial issues in management is proper diagnosis and treatment of the asymptomatically infected partner.

TABLE 314–1. SEXUALLY TRANSMITTED AGENTS AND THEIR SYNDROMES*

Microorganism	Syndromes
Bacteria	
Neisseria gonorrhoeae	Urethritis, cervicitis, bartholinitis, proctitis, pharyngitis, salpingitis, epididymitis, conjunctivitis, perihepatitis, arthritis, dermatitis, endocarditis, meningitis, amniotic infection syndrome
Mobiluncus species and *Gardnerella vaginalis*	"Nonspecific" vaginosis
Treponema pallidum	Syphilis (multiple clinical syndromes)
Haemophilus ducreyi	Chancroid
Calymmatobacterium granulomatis	Granuloma inguinale
Shigella species	Enteritis in homosexual men
Campylobacter species	Enteritis in homosexual men
Group B *Streptococcus*	Neonatal sepsis and meningitis
Chlamydiae	
Chlamydia trachomatis	Nongonococcal urethritis, purulent hypertrophic cervicitis, epididymitis, salpingitis, conjunctivitis, trachoma, pneumonia, perihepatitis, lymphogranuloma venereum, Reiter's syndrome
Mycoplasmas	
Ureaplasma urealyticum	Nongonococcal urethritis, ? premature rupture of membranes and abortion
Mycoplasma hominis	Postpartum fever, pelvic inflammatory disease
Viruses	
Herpes simplex virus (HSV)	Genital herpes, proctitis, meningitis, disseminated infection in neonates
Hepatitis A virus	Hepatitis in homosexual men
Hepatitis B virus	Hepatitis, ? periarteritis nodosa, hepatoma; especially prevalent in homosexual men
Cytomegalovirus	Congenital infection (birth defects, infant mortality, mental deficiency, hearing loss), mononucleosis syndrome
Human papillomavirus (HPV)	Condyloma acuminatum, cervical and perianal
Molluscum contagiosum virus	Molluscum contagiosum
Human immunodeficiency virus (HIV)	Acquired immunodeficiency syndrome (AIDS) and related illnesses
Protozoa	
Trichomonas vaginalis	Trichomonal vaginitis, occasional urethritis
Entamoeba histolytica	Enteritis in homosexual men
Giardia lamblia	Enteritis in homosexual men
Fungi	
Candida albicans	Vaginitis, balanitis
Ectoparasites	
Phthirus pubis	Pubic lice infestation
Sarcoptes scabiei	Scabies

* The relative importance of sexual transmission in the epidemiology of several of these agents remains to be defined; these include Group B streptococci, hepatitis A virus, cytomegalovirus, *Candida albicans,* and others.

INCIDENCE OF STD'S. The true incidence of STD's is not known in the United States because of serious problems of underreporting. Gonorrhea is the most common of the reported infectious diseases, with >500,000 infections reported annually. Although genital chlamydial infections generally are not reported, their prevalence certainly exceeds that of gonorrhea. Herpes simplex virus (HSV) and human papillomavirus (HPV) infections also are more prevalent than gonorrhea. The relative incidence of STD is quite variable in different areas of the world. For instance, chancroid is currently uncommon in the United States but is about as common as gonorrhea in certain areas of the Far East and Africa.

COMMON SYNDROMES *Urethritis in Males.* Urethritis in males is a very common syndrome. It is ordinarily classified as either gonococcal or nongonococcal urethritis (NGU), depending whether the presence of gonococci can be demonstrated by Gram stain or culture. In STD clinics, the prevalence of gonococcal and nongonococcal urethritis is similar, but NGU is considerably more common in private practice and in college infirmaries. Several studies of asymptomatic sexually active young persons found an incidence of up to 15% of genital chlamydial infection.

A large number of studies have established *Chlamydia trachomatis* as a cause of approximately 40% of cases of NGU. Case-control studies have provided evidence that suggests *Ureaplasma urealyticum* (formerly T-strain mycoplasma) is a significant factor in chlamydia-negative NGU. In addition, urethral inoculation of volunteers with pure cultures of *U. urealyticum* produced rather typical NGU. In practice, however, it is difficult to define the importance of *Ureaplasma* infection in patients with urethritis, because colonization of these organisms occurs in up to 70% of asymptomatic sexually active persons. A very small proportion of cases of NGU in men is due to *Trichomonas vaginalis* or HSV infection.

Diagnosis of urethritis requires demonstration of an inflammatory urethral exudate. A discharge may not be evident if the patient has recently voided, and patients preferably should be examined several hours after their last urination. The discharge may be present only in the morning, prior to urination. Demonstration of discharge often requires urethral "milking" and may require insertion of a small calcium alginate or similar swab into the anterior urethra, with examination of a direct gram-stained smear of the swab for leukocytes. Presence of an average of at least five polymorphonuclear leukocytes per high-power ($100\times$) field suggests the diagnosis of urethritis.

The patient should be questioned for past history of urethritis and for symptoms suggestive of systemic diseases such as Reiter's syndrome or disseminated gonococcal infection. Examination should be made for signs of conjunctivitis, arthritis, dermatitis, and epididymitis. Prostatitis is rarely present unless there are symptoms of perineal, suprapubic, or rectal discomfort, and rectal examination is not routinely indicated. Rectal examination and urine culture are indicated in men with dysuria but without signs of anterior urethral discharge.

Laboratory studies are ordinarily limited to a Gram stain of urethral exudate. Demonstration of typical gram-negative diplococci, many of which are inside neutrophils, establishes the diagnosis of gonococcal urethritis. A Gram stain is positive in at least 90% of men with symptomatic culture-proven urethral gonorrhea. In occasional patients, especially those with an equivocal Gram stain, it may be necessary to culture the anterior urethra or freshly voided urine sediment for gonococci. This is particularly important in asymptomatic male contacts of patients with disseminated gonococcal infection or gonococcal salpingitis, since a Gram stain of urethral contents is positive in only about 60% of men with asymptomatic urethral gonorrhea.

Diagnosis of NGU usually is made by exclusion of gonorrhea. Immunoassays and a DNA hybridization test for chlamydia are widely available and have sensitivities of 70 to 80% and specificities of >90% for polymerase chain reaction (PCR) and culture. PCR is just now becoming widely available. Although culture is the "gold standard" for diagnosis of chlamydia, it is probably not as sensitive as PCR. There is no serologic test that is clinically useful. Tests for *Ureaplasma* are not readily available and rarely are indicated. Examination of a saline suspension of urethral exudate occasionally may reveal motile trichomonads in patients with recurrent urethritis who fail to respond to appropriate therapy. A serologic test for syphilis should be obtained, but the diagnostic yield is low.

Management is outlined in Figure 314–1 and is discussed further in Ch. 315. Sexual partners of men with gonococcal or nongonococcal urethritis should be treated to prevent both reinfection of the patient and development of complications in the partners.

The syndrome of *postgonococcal urethritis* (persistence or recrudescence of urethritis after administration of therapy that has eradicated gonococcal infection) is usually due to concomitant ure-

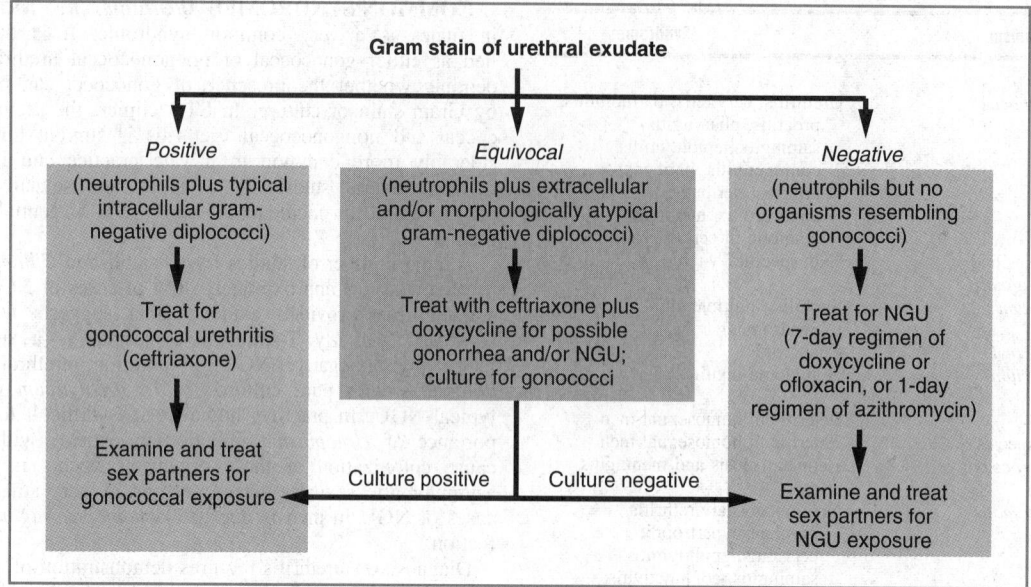

FIGURE 314–1. Management of male patients with urethritis.

thral chlamydial infection that was not eradicated by the original treatment. This syndrome is more common after therapy with a β-lactam antibiotic than after a regimen of tetracycline, undoubtedly because of the greater efficacy of tetracycline for treating chlamydial infections. Accordingly, there is considerable merit to use of oral tetracycline to follow up ceftriaxone therapy for genital gonorrhea.

Genital Ulcer Syndrome. Genital skin lesions may be either ulcerative or nonulcerative. In patients seen in a venereal disease clinic, the most common sexually transmitted nonulcerative genital lesions are due to scabies, genital warts, molluscum contagiosum, or *Candida* species, but differential diagnosis includes a long list of dermatologic conditions.

The most common cause of ulcerative genital lesions in patients in the United States is HSV, but differential diagnosis includes syphilis, chancroid, lymphogranuloma venereum (LGV), granuloma inguinale (GI), and trauma. Chancroid is becoming more common in certain cities in the United States; LGV and GI are rare. The most important distinction is among syphilis, genital herpes, and chancroid. Sometimes the appearance is virtually diagnostic: Grouped, painful, superficial vesicles are nearly diagnostic of herpes, whereas a single, clean-based, nonpainful ulcer with indurated margins suggests primary syphilis. In relatively recent studies, only about 60% of penile syphilitic chancres had this classic appearance. Painful ulcers suggest herpes or chancroid. Genital herpes may occur as a single ulcer, particularly in patients with recurrent herpes, and syphilis may occur with multiple ulcers. Secondarily infected lesions of primary syphilis may be painful.

It is a useful rule to obtain a serologic test for syphilis on all patients with genital ulcers, and, if the initial serologic findings are negative and if the diagnosis remains uncertain, to obtain a second serologic examination about 2 weeks later. A darkfield examination for syphilis should also be done, and it should be repeated twice on successive days if syphilis is seriously suspected and the initial examination is negative.

Infection by HSV may be efficiently diagnosed by viral culture or by immunofluorescent methods, but these are frequently unavailable in practice. Papanicolaou smear is suggestive of herpes in about two thirds of culture-positive cases. Giemsa's or Wright's stain of cells scraped from the base of a vesicle may reveal multinucleate giant cells (Tzanck's test), but this test is particularly insensitive in herpetic lesions that have become ulcerated. Serologic tests for herpesvirus are not helpful in management but may indicate persons with latent infection. Referral of patients to centers with capability of viral culture may be indicated in diagnostically difficult patients.

In addition to herpesvirus infection, chancroid should be suspected in patients with painful genital ulcers. Chancroid is occurring in epidemics in certain United States cities, particularly among crack house clients. Attempts should be made to isolate the causative agent, *Haemophilus ducreyi;* selective culture media are an improvement over previously available methods. No serologic tests are available.

Therapy clearly depends on the correct diagnosis. Topical antibiotics are never indicated. Initial genital herpes (first infection) is best treated with topical or oral administration of acyclovir or intravenous administration for severe infections. Therapy of chancroid is with ciprofloxacin, azithromycin, erythromycin, or ceftriaxone. Occasional empiric trials of oral ciprofloxacin, azithromycin, or erythromycin are warranted in patients with persistent genital ulcers not readily attributable to herpesvirus or syphilis, but repeated attempts to isolate *H. ducreyi* should be made in such instances. It is not possible to arrive at an unequivocal diagnosis of the cause of genital ulcers in all patients.

Lower Genital Tract Infections in Women. Infections of the female genitourinary tract produce a variety of syndromes, often with overlapping symptoms (dysuria, vaginal discharge, vulvar irritation). These infections are very common, relatively poorly understood by most physicians, sometimes difficult to treat, and often frustrating for both doctor and patient. However, the various syndromes usually can be distinguished on relatively simple clinical and laboratory grounds, and a precise microbial cause often can be established.

It is most helpful first to determine the primary anatomic site of infection: urethra or bladder, endocervix, or vagina. This can sometimes be accomplished by history; women with urinary tract infection (UTI) usually experience "internal" dysuria, whereas women with dysuria associated with vaginitis usually experience "external" dysuria owing to passage of urine over inflamed labia. Cervicitis is diagnosed by physical examination; mucopurulent secretions emanate from the endocervical canal, and there is often a hypertrophic, mucoid, reddened "cobblestone" appearance to the cervical mucosa. The cervix may appear normal in women with culture-positive gonococcal or chlamydial infection of the cervix. Patients with cervicitis may also have urethritis or vaginitis. Vaginitis is associated with increased vaginal discharge of several types, as discussed below, and frequently there are associated signs and symptoms of vaginal, vulvar, and perineal irritation (dyspareunia, external dysuria, itching, pain). In patients with lower genitourinary infection, it is important to determine whether the upper genitourinary tract is involved (pyelonephritis, salpingitis).

The Urethral Syndrome. Bacterial cystitis with or without pyelonephritis is usually diagnosed in women with dysuria, urinary frequency, and pyuria if colony counts are at least 10^5 bacteria per milliliter of urine. If similar symptoms are present but routine cultures grow $< 10^4$ bacteria per milliliter of voided urine, the "urethral syndrome" is likely.

In a study of young women with dysuria and urinary frequency, and who did not have vaginitis or active herpes simplex infection, 43% had the urethral syndrome (urethritis). Among women with urethritis, 25% had positive urethral cultures for *C. trachomatis*. Gonococci also were shown to cause this syndrome. Thus, women as well as men may have urethritis caused by gonococci and chlamydiae.

Patients with symptoms of UTI who do not have bacteriuria should have urethral and cervical cultures for *Neisseria gonorrhoeae*. If these cultures are also negative, a therapeutic trial may be made with a tetracycline, azithromycin, or ofloxacin.

Vaginitis. In a large study of women in a primary care clinic who had lower genitourinary complaints, vaginitis was more than five times as common as UTI's. In this and similar studies, there were three predominant types of vaginitis: yeast infection (*Candida albicans*), *Trichomonas* (*T. vaginalis*) infection, and bacterial vaginosis (BV) caused by organisms other than *Candida* and *T. vaginalis*. The incidence of these types of vaginitis varies in different patient populations, but in general *Candida* and BV are more common than *T. vaginalis* vaginitis.

Symptoms of vaginitis include increased volume of vaginal discharge, which is often abnormally yellow or green in appearance and may be malodorous. Vaginal and vulvar itching may be troublesome, especially in *Candida* infection. There may be vaginal tenderness and pain, dyspareunia, or dysuria.

The most common sign of vaginitis is an increased vaginal discharge. In *T. vaginalis* infections, there is often a profuse and frothy discharge. A curdlike, white discharge is common in *Candida* infections, and many patients with BV have an adherent, often gray, and frequently malodorous discharge. Microscopic examination shows many polymorphonuclear leukocytes in the discharge in all but BV. Speculum examination may show signs of endocervicitis as well, with purulent discharge issuing from the cervical os. In occasional patients, no objective signs of vaginal inflammation are found despite the presence of troublesome symptoms (Table 314–2).

Candida **Vaginitis.** Most vaginal yeast infections are due to *C. albicans*. Diagnosis is usually made by visualizing yeasts or pseudohyphae by microscopic examination of vaginal secretions suspended in normal saline or 10% potassium hydroxide (KOH). Microscopic examination is less sensitive than culture. However, many asymptomatic women have positive vaginal cultures for *C. albicans*, and therefore some authorities advocate using microscopy in preference to culture. The discharge in *Candida* vaginitis is not malodorous and has a pH of < 4.5 when a drop is applied to pH paper with a range of 4.0 to 5.5.

Therapy of *Candida* vaginitis is with one of the imidazole compounds (e.g., clotrimazole, miconazole, butoconazole, or terconazole) once each night for 3 to 7 days intravaginally, or an oral azole agent (ketoconazole, fluconazole, or itraconazole) for 1 to 5 days. The oral regimens are less well evaluated. No convincing evidence exists that attempts to eradicate yeast from the gastrointestinal tract significantly affect rates of cure or relapse of *Candida* vaginitis. There is no evidence to warrant therapy of sexual partners. Attempts should be made to correct ancillary conditions that increase susceptibility to vaginal candidiasis: antibiotic therapy, diabetes, or oral anovulatory steroids. Relapse is a significant problem in some patients. No therapy is indicated for asymptomatic vaginal carriers of *C. albicans*.

T. vaginalis **Vaginitis.** Diagnosis is made ordinarily by visualizing motile trichomonads in a normal saline suspension of vaginal secretions. The organisms are easily seen at high-dry ($100 \times$) magnification and may usually be seen under low-power magnification. The saline suspension should be examined promptly. Culture is more sensitive, but about 80 to 90% of culture-positive cases are detected by microscopy. Addition of a drop of 10% KOH to vaginal secretions usually results in liberation of a detectable fishlike odor, attributed to release of volatile amines. The pH of vaginal secretions is usually > 5.0. In these latter two respects, *T. vaginalis* vaginitis is similar to BV.

Therapy of trichomoniasis is with one of the nitroimidazoles, either metronidazole or newer compounds such as tinidazole. The latter is extensively used in Europe but is not approved in the United States. A single 2-gram oral dose of metronidazole is as effective as multiple-day regimens. Metronidazole is mutagenic, and there is evidence that it is a weak carcinogen in certain animal systems (but, so far, not in humans). Accordingly, it should be used with caution; it has been advocated for women with asymptomatic trichomoniasis, but others would reserve its use for women with symptomatic infections because of possible adverse effects. Metronidazole should not be used in the first trimester of pregnancy. Since more than one third of male sexual partners of women with trichomoniasis are asymptomatic urethral carriers of *T. vaginalis*, the male partners should also be treated with a single 2-gram dose of metronidazole.

Although *T. vaginalis* can be transmitted sexually, it probably is transmitted by other means as well. This conclusion is based on prevalence studies that show one peak in young, sexually active women and a second peak in older women who have no other evidence for sexually transmitted infection.

Bacterial Vaginosis (BV). This syndrome is probably due to infection by an organism formerly called either *Corynebacterium vaginale* or *Haemophilus vaginalis* but now termed *Gardnerella vaginalis*, in association with anaerobic bacteria, including the curved or comma-shaped rods now known as Mobiluncus species. *G. vaginalis* is a small, gram-variable coccobacillus that can be grown quite successfully on partially selective enriched media. Among women with abnormal vaginal discharge who do not have yeast infection or trichomoniasis, $> 90\%$ grow *G. vaginalis*, whereas $< 10\%$ of matched controls grow the same organism. There usually are increased numbers of anaerobic vaginal bacteria as well and decreased numbers of the normal vaginal lactobacilli. Development of full symptoms may require both *G. vaginalis* and vaginal anaerobes, although the precise pathophysiology of this syndrome is still under investigation.

Diagnosis of BV is by exclusion of trichomoniasis, candidiasis, and purulent cervicitis. Abnormal cells termed clue cells are often seen in a wet mount of vaginal secretions in normal saline; these are stippled, granular-appearing vaginal epithelial cells that contain large numbers of adherent *G. vaginalis*. Few polymorphonuclear leukocytes are present. Addition of a drop of 10% KOH usually results in production of an unpleasant fishy odor. The pH of the vaginal secretions is nearly always > 5.0.

Optimal therapy is being investigated. Metronidazole has only borderline activity *in vitro* against *G. vaginalis*, but in a dose of 500 mg by mouth twice daily for 7 days it was effective in eradicating both *G. vaginalis* and the symptoms of vaginitis from 80 of 81 patients in one trial; similar results have been obtained in other trials. This suggests that the principal cause of this syndrome is an anaerobe, since metronidazole is principally effective against anaerobes. Clindamycin (300 mg orally twice daily for 7 days) also is effective. More than 90% of male partners are urethral carriers of *G. vaginalis* and therefore probably should be treated with the same regimen as the patient, although data to support this are lacking at present.

Mixed Vaginitis. In 2 to 16% of patients, vaginitis may be due to polymicrobial infection with two or three organisms. Such mixed infection may account for some instances of treatment failure. Particular care should be given to identification of all causative organisms in patients who have recurrent or relapsing vaginitis.

Cervicitis. Two organisms are recognized as probable causes of mucopurulent endocervicitis: *N. gonorrhoeae* and *C. trachomatis*. Women who are sexual partners of men with chlamydia-positive NGU have a much higher rate of isolation of chlamydiae from the

TABLE 314–2. DIFFERENTIAL DIAGNOSIS OF VAGINITIS

Characteristics of Vaginal Discharge	Organism Causing Vaginitis		
	C. albicans	*T. vaginalis*	*BV*
pH	4.5	> 5.0	> 5.0
White curd	Usually	No	No
Odor with KOH	No	Yes	Yes
Clue cells	No	No	Usually
Motile trichomonads	No	Usually	No
Yeast cells	Yes	No	No

cervix than do women who are partners of men with chlamydia-negative NGU, and they also have significantly higher rates of mucopurulent cervicitis. HSV can also cause cervicitis, especially in primary infection. However, the clinical appearance in herpetic cervicitis is different, with cervical vesicles and ulcers rather than mucopurulent cervicitis.

True cervicitis should not be confused with cervical ectopy, which is merely the appearance of endocervical columnar epithelium on the exposed, visible exocervix. This results in a red-appearing cervix and may result in increased production of a mucoid vaginal discharge but does not require therapy.

Diagnosis of mucopurulent endocervicitis requires visualization of purulent discharge from the cervical os. There often is a roughened cobblestone appearance to the cervix. Gram stain is about 60% sensitive and >90% specific for gonorrhea if typical intracellular gonococci are seen, but cultures for N. gonorrhoeae should be taken. Tissue culture for isolation of C. trachomatis may be employed if available. Cytologic methods are not sufficiently sensitive to warrant widespread use. Several nonculture diagnostic tests for C. trachomatis allow rapid, sensitive, specific diagnosis from patient secretions and undoubtedly should be more widely used to document cause and to initiate proper treatment for cervicitis due to chlamydiae.

Antibiotic therapy appears to result in clinical improvement in mucopurulent cervicitis. Patients with negative cultures for the gonococcus should be treated with doxycycline (100 mg twice daily for 7 days); alternatives are oral azithromycin in a single dose of 1 gram or oral ofloxacin in a dose of 300 mg twice daily for 7 days. No other form of cervicitis has been shown to respond to antimicrobial therapy.

Upper Genital Tract Disease in Women: Salpingitis.

Full coverage of this important topic is precluded by space considerations. This is a very important clinical problem, resulting in considerable morbidity in the estimated 250,000 to 500,000 women who are affected yearly in the United States.

Etiology. The gonococcus accounts for 20 to 50% of cases in the United States, particularly among women with relatively severe and first-episode salpingitis. About 15 to 20% of women with gonococcal cervicitis probably subsequently develop salpingitis. Strong evidence now implicates genital chlamydial infections as another significant cause of salpingitis. Salpingitis due to genital chlamydial infections may be mild, and patients may not seek medical care. Nevertheless, complications may follow, particularly tubal scarring and infertility. There is less convincing evidence that *Mycoplasma hominis* may occasionally cause a similar syndrome. Many cases of salpingitis are caused by mixed infection with microaerophilic streptococci and enteric bacilli, often including *Bacteroides* species. These polymicrobial infections appear to be more common in recurrent attacks of salpingitis.

Diagnosis. Clinical diagnosis of salpingitis is inexact. Perhaps only 20% of patients have the classic syndrome of lower abdominal pain and tenderness, cervical tenderness, fever, leukocytosis, and elevated sedimentation rate. The most common findings are lower abdominal tenderness, which is usually bilateral, and adnexal and cervical tenderness. Patients with gonococcal salpingitis are more likely to have fever and more commonly have onset near the menses, whereas patients with nongonococcal salpingitis more commonly have adnexal masses. Laparoscopy is commonly used to diagnose salpingitis in certain countries but is invasive and requires general anesthesia. In the United States, laparoscopy is usually used only in selected patients whose differential diagnosis includes ectopic pregnancy, appendicitis, ruptured abscess, or other potential emergencies.

Complications. Complications are primarily infertility and ectopic pregnancy. Rates of involuntary infertility are about 15% after one attack of salpingitis and about 75% after three or more attacks. Total hysterectomy may eventually be necessitated by symptoms of chronic salpingitis.

Therapy. Recommendations from the Centers for Disease Control and Prevention suggest initial therapy of outpatients with cefoxitin, 2 grams intramuscularly, along with probenecid, 1 gram orally, followed by doxycycline, 100 mg orally twice daily for 10 to 14 days. There are no controlled data on efficacy of various regimens used for hospitalized patients. Current recommendations call for doxycycline, 100 mg twice daily, plus cefoxitin, 2 grams intravenously four times daily; or clindamycin, 900 mg intravenously three times daily, plus gentamicin, 1.5 mg per kilogram three times daily. After discharge, doxycycline should be given in a dose of 100 mg twice daily to complete 10 to 14 days of therapy. Patients should usually be hospitalized if they are very ill, are pregnant, or have significant adnexal masses; if previous therapy failed; or if the differential diagnosis includes a surgical emergency such as appendicitis or ectopic pregnancy.

Prevention. Sexual partners of women with gonococcal salpingitis must be identified, examined, and treated to prevent subsequent reinfection of the patient. About one half of the infected male partners of women with gonococcal salpingitis are asymptomatic. Treatment of women with tetracycline (as compared with penicillin) to eradicate chlamydiae from the cervix reduces the incidence of posttherapy salpingitis, which suggests that increased emphasis on treatment of chlamydiae in the male and female genital tract will reduce the incidence of salpingitis.

Addiss DG, Vaughn ML, Ludka D, et al.: Decreased prevalence of *Chlamydia trachomatis* infection associated with a selective screening program in family planning clinics in Wisconsin. Sex Transm Dis 20:28, 1993. *Chlamydia can be controlled by screening and treatment.*

Brunham RC, Paavonen J, Stevens CE, et al.: Mucopurulent cervicitis—the ignored counterpart in women of urethritis in men. N Engl J Med 311:1, 1984. *Genital chlamydial infection causes mucopurulent cervicitis; proper diagnosis leads to effective treatment.*

Holmes KK, Mardh P-A, Sparling PF, et al. (eds.): Sexually Transmitted Diseases, 2nd ed. New York, McGraw-Hill, 1990. *The definitive textbook on STD's; heavily referenced.*

Nettleman MD, Jones RB, Roberts SD, et al.: Cost-effectiveness of culturing for *Chlamydia trachomatis*: A study in a clinic for sexually transmitted diseases. Ann Intern Med 105:189, 1986. *Cultures most cost-effective in low-risk women. Empiric therapy suggested in high-risk groups.*

Rees E: The treatment of pelvic inflammatory disease. Am J Obstet Gynecol 138:1042, 1980. *Treatment of chlamydial infection of cervix with tetracycline compared with penicillin reduced incidence of subsequent salpingitis.*

Stamm WE, Koutsky LA, Benedetti JK, et al.: *Chlamydia trachomatis* urethral infections in men: Prevalence, risk factors, and clinical manifestations. Ann Intern Med 100:47, 1984. *Asymptomatic male urethral carriers of chlamydiae are very common.*

Stamm WE, Wagner KF, Amsel R, et al.: Causes of the acute urethral syndrome in women. N Engl J Med 303:409, 1980. *Females may also develop a form of nongonococcal urethritis resulting from infection with* Chlamydia trachomatis.

Toye B, Laferriere C, Claman P, et al.: Association between antibody to the chlamydial heat-shock protein and tubal infertility. J Infect Dis 168:1236, 1993. *Evidence that* Chlamydia *causes tubal infertility.*

Wu C-H, Lee M-F, Yin S-C, et al.: Comparison of polymerase chain reaction, monoclonal antibody based enzyme immunoassay, and cell culture for detection of *Chlamydia trachomatis* in genital specimens. Sex Transm Dis 19:193, 1992. *One of many papers suggesting that PCR is the test of choice for* Chlamydia.

315 GONOCOCCAL INFECTIONS
P. Frederick Sparling

Neisseria gonorrhoeae is a common sexually transmitted organism that causes anterior urethritis in males and endocervicitis and urethritis in females. Other types of primary infection include pharyngitis, proctitis, conjunctivitis, and vulvovaginitis; the last-named occurs principally in prepubescent females. Complications may occur by direct extension of infection, including epididymitis, prostatitis, Bartholin gland abscess, salpingitis, and perihepatitis. Bacteremia may occur, with production of characteristic cutaneous lesions, arthritis, and tenosynovitis; rare complications include endocarditis and meningitis. Conjunctival infection formerly was a common cause of blindness in neonates.

Gonorrhea is the most common reportable infectious disease in the United States, with about 500,000 cases annually. The true incidence is probably at least 1 million cases annually. Incidence has declined dramatically in much of the industrialized West in recent years.

EPIDEMIOLOGY. The only natural hosts for N. gonorrhoeae are humans. The organism normally resides on the columnar epithelium of mucosal surfaces and is usually transmitted by intimate sexual contact. The incidence of gonorrhea varies greatly in different groups. As many as 5% of persons in high-risk populations may be infected at any time. Highest incidence is found in young (15 to 30) single persons of low socioeconomic and educational status, probably because these factors correlate positively with sexual promiscuity.

The risk of acquiring infection depends on the type of contact with an infected person. About 60 to 80% of females in contact with a male with urethral gonorrhea develop gonococcal cervicitis. By contrast, it is estimated that only 20 to 30% of males having sex with an infected female develop gonorrhea. This difference may be due to exposure of females to a larger inoculum of gonococci. A person having oral sex with a male with gonococcal urethritis has considerable risk of acquiring pharyngeal gonorrhea. Transmission of infection by oral contact with the genitals of an infected female is rare. Infection is apparently efficiently spread by penile-rectal contact.

Gonococci die rapidly upon drying, and transmission by fomites is rare. Epidemics were reported in prepubertal females living in proximity in orphanages, but such episodes are now very uncommon.

Control of gonorrhea is difficult because of the frequency of asymptomatic infection. Perhaps 50% of infections in females are asymptomatic or only minimally symptomatic, and at least 10% of infected males are asymptomatic.

In past years there was considerable emphasis on case finding by endocervical culture in young, sexually active females. The merit of this strategy depends on the prevalence of infection in the community and the lifestyle of the patient. A more cost-effective method for finding infected patients is to obtain a culture in patients about 6 weeks after treatment for gonorrhea; as many as 15 to 20% of such cases are culture positive, usually because of reinfection.

THE ORGANISM. N. gonorrhoeae is a gram-negative, aerobic diplococcus. Many strains require 3 to 10% CO_2 for optimal growth. They are highly autolytic and die rapidly when outside their normal human environment. They are sensitive to fatty acids and grow best on media with added starch to inhibit fatty acids present in agar. Several partially selective media are available; most employ antibiotics to inhibit growth of other microorganisms.

Presumptive identification in vitro is made by colonial morphology, Gram stain, and a positive oxidase test. Differentiation from the closely related meningococcus and the various nonpathogenic Neisseria is ordinarily by patterns of utilization of various simple carbohydrates; gonococci use glucose but not maltose or sucrose.

Gonococci are highly variable and occur in a number of different colonial forms. Small colonial types are piliated and more virulent in humans than the larger, nonpiliated variants. Variation is also found in certain outer membrane proteins. Gonococci undergo rapid variation in the antigenic type of pilus expressed, which probably contributes to prolonged infections without treatment and to the ability of persons to acquire repeat infections after treatment. The importance of surface components of the gonococcus in the pathogenesis of infection is under intense investigation.

Gonococci can be serotyped on the basis of antigenic differences in outer membrane proteins. These tests are not routinely available.

PATHOGENESIS. Surface pili undoubtedly help to attach the bacteria to the mucosal surface, and they also help prevent ingestion and killing by polymorphonuclear leukocytes. Typical urethral infections result in moderately severe inflammation, probably due to release of toxic lipopolysaccharide from gonococci and to production of chemotactic factors that attract neutrophilic leukocytes. Certain strains can cause asymptomatic urethral infection for reasons not completely understood. These strains are usually penicillin sensitive, resistant to the bactericidal effects of normal human serum, and particularly likely to cause bacteremia and septic arthritis.

In the preantibiotic era, symptoms usually persisted for 2 to 3 months before host defenses finally eradicated the infection. Host defenses include serum opsonic and bactericidal antibodies, as well as local (mucosal) antibodies of the IgG and IgA classes. All gonococci produce an enzyme, IgA protease, that cleaves the major class of secretory IgA, perhaps contributing to persistence of local gonococcal infections.

Serum bactericidal antibodies are undoubtedly important in preventing bacteremic infection. The best evidence for this has been provided by patients who suffer from homozygous deficiency of one of the complement components C6, C7, C8, or C9. This results in deficiency of serum bactericidal activity but no alteration of serum opsonic activity. Such individuals are particularly prone to

recurrent bacteremic gonococcal infection or to recurrent meningococcal meningitis or meningococcemia.

CLINICAL PATTERNS OF DISEASE. *Gonorrhea in Males.* Gonococcal urethritis in males ("the clap" or "the strain") is characterized by a yellowish, purulent urethral discharge and dysuria. The usual incubation period is 2 to 6 days. The discharge in gonorrhea is slightly more copious and purulent than in nongonococcal urethritis (NGU). Symptoms are probably produced by 90% of infections, although asymptomatic infections do occur and may persist for many months. Males with asymptomatic infection do not seek treatment, whereas those with symptomatic infection are usually promptly treated and cured. This is the probable explanation for prevalence studies that show that up to 50% of infected males are asymptomatic. Asymptomatic infection in males and females is of great epidemiologic importance, since such carriers may continue to spread infection to new sexual partners for months if the infection is not properly diagnosed and treated.

Complications of gonococcal urethritis in males are now rare. Urethral stricture was formerly a common complication but was probably due in part to the use of caustic treatment regimens. Epididymitis and prostatitis, relatively common complications in the past, are seen only occasionally today. The principal complication is disseminated gonococcal infection, which is estimated to affect about 1% of persons with gonorrhea. This entity is discussed below. The differential diagnosis of gonococcal urethritis is discussed in Ch. 314.

Gonococcal infections of the pharynx and rectum are common problems in homosexual males. Most patients with pharyngeal infection are asymptomatic, but occasional patients have exudative pharyngitis with cervical adenopathy. Gonococcal infection of the rectum causes a wide spectrum of symptoms, ranging from no symptoms to severe proctitis with tenesmus and bloody, mucopurulent discharge. Although rectal cultures are also positive in approximately 40% of females with cervical gonorrhea, symptoms of proctitis in females are unusual. This has suggested that the trauma of rectal intercourse may contribute to the proctitis observed in males. Sigmoidoscopy may be indicated to exclude ulcerative colitis, Crohn's colitis, rectal lacerations, or other infections such as shigellosis, amebiasis, or syphilis, all of which are common in male homosexuals.

Gonococcal epididymitis is usually unilateral. Both *Chlamydia trachomatis* and the gonococcus are significant causes of epididymitis in men under 35, whereas coliform bacteria are the usual cause in older males. The differential diagnosis includes trauma, tumor, and torsion of the testicle, suggested by sudden onset and elevation of the testicle. If there is question of testicular torsion, consultation with a urologist is necessary. In epididymitis there is often a urethral exudate, which should be cultured for gonococci and other bacteria. Treatment of gonococcal epididymitis includes scrotal elevation and 7 to 10 days of appropriate antibiotics (Table 315–1).

Gonorrhea in Females. In incidence studies, approximately one half of women infected with the gonococcus are asymptomatic or have so few symptoms that they do not seek medical care. The most commonly involved site is the endocervix (80 to 90%), followed by the urethra (80%), rectum (40%), and pharynx (10 to 20%). Most pharyngeal, urethral, and rectal infections cause few or no symptoms. Cervical infection may result in vaginal discharge or abnormal menstrual bleeding. Neither of these symptoms is specific for gonococcal infection. Gonococcal urethritis may mimic cystitis caused by enteric bacilli, although standard urine cultures are negative because gonococci do not grow on culture media ordinarily used to diagnose urinary tract infection. Culture methods are discussed below under Laboratory Diagnosis. The differential diagnosis of cervicitis, vaginitis, and the urethral syndrome is discussed in Ch. 314.

The most important complication of gonorrhea is salpingitis. The less precise term "pelvic inflammatory disease" (PID) is often used synonymously. Although many other organisms can cause a similar syndrome, the gonococcus accounts for about half of the cases of PID in the United States. About 15% of women with gonococcal cervicitis develop PID, often in proximity to a menstrual period. Symptoms usually include abdominal pain, and often there is fever. Physical examination usually discloses cervical motion tenderness and bilateral adnexal tenderness; in a small proportion of cases the

TABLE 315–1. ANTIBIOTIC REGIMENS RECOMMENDED FOR GONOCOCCAL INFECTION

Diagnosis	Treatment
Uncomplicated genital, rectal, or pharyngeal infection of men and women	Ceftriaxone, 125 mg IM once, plus doxycycline, 100 mg PO twice daily for 7 days *or* Cefixime, 400 mg PO once, plus doxycycline, 100 mg PO twice daily for 7 days *or* Ciprofloxacin, 500 mg PO once, plus doxycycline, 100 mg PO twice daily for 7 days *or* Ofloxacin, 400 mg PO once, plus doxycycline, 100 mg PO twice daily for 7 days
Gonorrhea in pregnancy	Ceftriaxone, 125 mg IM once, plus erythromycin base, 500 mg PO 4 times daily for 7 days *or* Spectinomycin, 2 grams IM, plus erythromycin (as in ceftriaxone regimen)
Salpingitis—outpatient	Cefoxitin, 2 grams IM, plus doxycycline, 100 mg PO twice daily for 10–14 days *or* Ofloxacin, 400 mg PO twice daily for 14 days, plus either clindamycin, 450 mg PO 4 times daily or metronidazole, 500 mg PO twice daily for 14 days
Salpingitis—inpatient	Doxycycline, 100 mg IV twice daily, plus cefoxitin, 2 grams IV 4 times daily until improved, followed by doxycycline, 100 mg PO twice daily to complete 14 days of therapy; alternative regimens include clindamycin plus an aminoglycoside
Disseminated gonococcal infection	Ceftriaxone, 1 gram IM every 24 hours *or* Spectinomycin, 2 grams IM every 12 hours (see text)

disease may be unilateral, causing confusion with appendicitis or ectopic pregnancy. There may be signs of generalized peritonitis. Laboratory studies often show elevation of the white blood cell count and sedimentation rate. The diagnosis of PID is inexact, as shown by laparoscopic examination; many cases of PID are missed if undue reliance is placed on presence of fever or elevation of white blood cell count or sedimentation rate.

Although PID is uncommon in pregnancy, it may be particularly severe, and pregnant patients with PID should probably be hospitalized. The incidence of gonococcal PID is increased about threefold in women using an intrauterine device (IUD) for contraception.

A single attack of gonococcal PID seems to increase twofold the risk of developing another with subsequent gonococcal cervicitis. About half of the male sexual partners of women with gonococcal PID are infected, and half of these infections are asymptomatic. Failure to diagnose cases and treat properly the male partners exposes the patient to the risk of further attacks of PID. After the patient has been effectively treated, it often is wise to refer her and her sexual partners to a public health clinic for follow-up.

The major complication of gonococcal PID is tubal scarring and infertility. The incidence of involuntary infertility is estimated as 15% after one attack of PID and about 50% after three attacks. The incidence of ectopic pregnancy is increased from seven- to tenfold in women with previous salpingitis, with resultant increased fetal and maternal mortality. Treatment is indicated in Table 315–1.

Gonococci may spread upward to the liver, causing perihepatitis (Fitz-Hugh–Curtis syndrome). Gonococcal perihepatitis causes tenderness and pain in the region of the liver, mimicking acute cholecystitis. However, it resolves promptly with appropriate antibiotic therapy. Peritoneoscopy may be indicated rarely for diagnostic purposes; "violin-string" adhesions between the liver capsule and the peritoneum are seen.

Gonorrhea in Children.
Infants born to a mother with cervicovaginal gonorrhea may develop gonococcal conjunctivitis, although routine use of prophylactic 1% silver nitrate eye drops (or, in some hospitals, topical erythromycin or tetracycline) has markedly reduced the incidence of this problem. Neonates may also acquire pharyngeal, respiratory, or rectal infection and may develop gonococcal sepsis. Older children up to 1 year of age usually acquire conjunctival or vaginal infection by accidental contamination from an adult, whereas from 1 year to puberty most childhood gonorrhea is the result of purposeful sexual abuse by an adult.

Gonococcal Bacteremia.
Approximately 1% of adults with gonorrhea develop the syndrome of gonococcal bacteremia, dermatitis, and arthritis, or disseminated gonococcal infection (DGI). In most series, the majority of patients with DGI are women. The regional incidence of DGI probably varies because of geographic differences in prevalence of the usually antibiotic-sensitive, serum-bactericidal-resistant strains of *N. gonorrhoeae* that cause this syndrome. The severity of the syndrome is variable, from a slowly evolving mild illness with little or no fever, mild arthralgias, and few skin lesions to a fulminant illness with high temperature and prostration. Most episodes of DGI are relatively mild in comparison with meningococcemia.

Many patients with DGI have no local symptoms of gonococcal infection. Initial manifestations are usually migratory asymmetric polyarthralgias and skin lesions that are often accompanied by fever. Many patients have tenosynovitis, typically involving the flexor tendon sheaths of the wrist or the Achilles tendon (colloquially known as "lover's heels"). Skin lesions are few in number (< 30 usually), are acral in distribution (fingers, toes, extremities), and may be painful before they are visible. The individual lesions may be papules, pustules, or bullae on an erythematous base; less commonly seen are petechiae or necrotic lesions. The rash is not pathognomonic but is sufficiently typical that it should strongly suggest DGI when seen in young patients with polyarthralgia. Blood cultures are often positive at this stage, and circulating immune complexes may be present. Gram stain of the skin lesions is positive in only about 5% of patients, but gonococcal antigens can be detected in these lesions in about two thirds of patients by use of immunofluorescent-labeled antigonococcal antibody.

The early stage of gonococcemia may subside spontaneously or may merge indistinctly after about 1 week into a second stage of septic arthritis. Skin lesions have usually disappeared by this time, and blood cultures are nearly always negative. Septic arthritis may occur without preceding skin lesions or polyarthralgia. One large joint (elbow, wrist, hip, knee, ankle) is usually involved, although some series report involvement of two joints in a significant minority of patients. On infrequent occasions symmetric involvement of the fingers may mimic acute rheumatoid arthritis. Physical examination typically discloses a swollen, warm joint with evident intra-articular fluid. Aspiration of the joint often reveals marked neutrophilic leukocytosis (50,000 to 100,000 leukocytes per cubic millimeter), although early in the development of the septic joint the synovial leukocyte count may be much lower. Cultures of joint fluid are often positive if the leukocyte count is $\geq 80,000$, but are often negative when leukocyte counts are $\leq 20,000$.

Other complications of gonococcal bacteremia include mild hepatitis, myocarditis, the Fitz-Hugh–Curtis syndrome, meningitis, and endocarditis. In the preantibiotic era, gonococcal infection accounted for up to 10% of all endocarditis, but it is now rare. Gonococcal endocarditis is often a rapidly progressive infection with severe valvular damage; it should be suspected in patients with a new murmur, severe prostrating illness, severe myocarditis, or evidence of renal failure, or in the presence of stigmas of peripheral embolization.

The differential diagnosis of the gonococcal bacteremia arthritis syndrome includes Reiter's syndrome, rheumatic fever, rheumatoid arthritis, systemic lupus erythematosus, other infectious or postinfectious arthritis, subacute bacterial endocarditis, meningococcemia, and viral hepatitis. In young males, Reiter's syndrome is the principal consideration. Conjunctivitis is rarely seen in gonococcemia but is common in Reiter's syndrome. In the absence of typical skin lesions, DGI may not be suspected until culture results are known.

Diagnosis of DGI is secure when gonococci are recovered from the blood, skin lesions, or synovial fluid. The diagnosis of DGI is probably correct in patients in whom the only positive cultures are from local mucosal surfaces but in whom there are both typical skin lesions and a prompt response to antigonococcal therapy.

LABORATORY DIAGNOSIS. Gram stain of urethral exudate in symptomatic males has a sensitivity of 90 to 98% and a specificity of 95 to 98%. Accordingly, urethral cultures are not ordinarily indicated in untreated symptomatic males. Since the sensitivity of the Gram stain is only about 60% in asymptomatic male urethral infection, cultures of the anterior urethra or fresh urine sediment are recommended when epidemiologic evidence suggests possible asymptomatic urethral infection. Gram stain of the endocervix is about 50 to 60% sensitive and about 82 to 97% specific in women with positive cervical cultures for *N. gonorrhoeae*. Care must be taken to avoid mistaking normal endocervical flora and neutrophils for gonorrhea; only smears showing several neutrophils with multiple, typical intracellular gram-negative diplococci should be read as presumptively positive for gonorrhea. Cultures for *N. gonorrhoeae* should be obtained in all women, even if the Gram stain appears positive.

Cultures should be plated immediately if possible onto chocolate agar or chocolate agar containing selective antibiotics (e.g., modified Thayer-Martin medium [MTM]). Holding media such as Amies' or Stuart's transport media may be used if necessary, but viability of gonococci drops after 12 to 24 hours in such media. In infected women, a single endocervical culture on MTM is about 80 to 90% sensitive, as judged by yields obtained with multiple cultures from multiple sites. In about 3 to 5% of women the only positive culture is at the pharyngeal, urethral, or rectal site. The yield from these sites is too low to warrant routine pharyngeal, urethral, or rectal cultures. Urethral cultures are indicated in women with the urethral syndrome. Both cervical and rectal cultures should be obtained as part of the test of cure in women after treatment, since inclusion of the rectal culture increases the diagnostic yield of treatment failures by as much as 50%. Pharyngeal cultures should be obtained from patients with symptomatic pharyngitis or from persons exposed by fellatio to infected males. Patients with possible DGI should have culture samples taken from all possible mucosal sites (pharynx, urethra, cervix, rectum), as well as blood and synovial fluid.

Cultures of the cervix should be taken under direct visualization during speculum examination, using a cotton-tipped swab. Lubricant jellies may be deleterious to gonococci and should be avoided. Cultures of the anterior urethra of males should be obtained with calcium alginate swabs or a sterile wire loop. Immediate culture of first-voided urine is also useful.

Positive cultures from the pharynx or rectum should be carefully evaluated by the microbiology laboratory to avoid confusion between gonococci and meningococci. Meningococci are more common than gonococci in throat cultures. No serologic test available is sufficiently sensitive and specific to merit use for screening or diagnostic purposes.

TREATMENT. Gonococci frequently have chromosomal mutations that result in relative resistance to penicillin, tetracycline, and other antibiotics. Strains with chromosomally mediated resistance (CMRNG strains) have become prevalent in certain areas of the United States and are more common in parts of Asia. These strains do not respond to penicillin but do respond to spectinomycin or ceftriaxone. As many as 5 to 10% of all gonococci in the United States now are CMRNG.

Gonococci that carry a β-lactamase (penicillinase) plasmid emerged in the Far East and elsewhere in 1975 and have spread to much of the world. Penicillinase-producing gonococci (PPNG) account for 30 to 50% of all gonorrhea in certain cities in Africa and the Far East but are less common in the United States. The incidence of PPNG is about 5% in the United States but varies in different locales. The gonococcal plasmids are similar to penicillinase plasmids found in *Haemophilus* species. PPNG are resistant to clinically attainable doses of penicillins but are sensitive to spectinomycin and to certain cephalosporins (cefuroxime, cefoxitin, ceftriaxone). PPNG are known to cause DGI and salpingitis.

Plasmid-encoded tetracycline resistance, Tc^r, is a newer problem. These strains do not respond to tetracycline but do respond to spectinomycin or ceftriaxone and may respond to penicillin. Incidence of Tc^r gonococci is increasing and approximates 5 to 15% in various U.S. cities.

The antibiotic regimens recommended for gonorrhea in the United States are summarized in Table 315–1. Ceftriaxone has replaced penicillin and ampicillin, because of the prevalence of CMRNG and Pc^r strains. Tetracyclines no longer are acceptable therapy for gonorrhea because of the prevalence of Tc^r strains. Because gonococcal infections commonly are associated with genital chlamydial infection, most authorities now recommend a 7-day

course of a tetracycline (usually doxycycline) for all patients with gonorrhea as follow-up to initial ceftriaxone therapy.

Each of the recommended regimens is highly effective for genital gonorrhea. In patients who do not respond, isolates can be tested for production of penicillinase, and spectinomycin should be used for retreatment. However, most apparent failures are really reinfections. Some studies show that 15% of patients are reinfected within 6 weeks of successful therapy. On this basis, many authorities recommend that recultures should be obtained 6 weeks after treatment.

In the absence of an effective vaccine, control of this disease depends on proper diagnosis and treatment of patients' sexual contacts. If patients are given simple instructions, many bring their contacts to the physician for examination. There are sound epidemiologic reasons for treating contacts immediately. Local health departments are not utilized sufficiently for help in examination and treatment of contacts.

Treatment of salpingitis (PID) has not been studied adequately (see Table 315–1). Most authorities recommend removal of IUD's in women with PID. It is crucial to examine and treat all sexual partners of women with gonococcal PID.

Therapy of gonococcal arthritis is ordinarily highly successful with each of the recommended regimens (see Table 315–1). Failure to improve in 3 days suggests that the patient does not have DGI. Septic joints should be aspirated, both to make the initial diagnosis and to remove inflammatory exudate. Open drainage is rarely indicated, except in infection of the hip in childhood. Repeat closed aspiration may be necessary if joint fluid rapidly reaccumulates, but most patients require only one or a few joint aspirations. Antibiotics should not be injected into the joint space. Most patients with DGI should be hospitalized initially, but outpatient therapy may be used to conclude a 7-day course of treatment. Oral therapy may be used initially in carefully selected, compliant patients with a definite diagnosis and only mild infection. Antibiotics for oral use in this situation include cefixime, 400 mg twice daily, or ciprofloxacin, 500 mg twice daily. Therapy should be continued for 7 days.

Gonococcal conjunctivitis should be treated by immediate saline irrigation and intravenous ceftriaxone.

PREVENTION. Although vaccines are currently under intense study, an effective gonococcal vaccine is still only a hope. Condoms prevent most infection. Certain contraceptive foams have antigonococcal activity but are of unproven efficacy clinically.

Centers for Disease Control and Prevention: Sexually transmitted diseases treatment guidelines. MMWR 42 (RR-14):1, 1993. *Current recommendations for treatment of gonorrhea and other STD's.*

Cohen MS, Sparling PF: Mucosal infection with *Neisseria gonorrhoeae*: Bacterial adaptation and mucosal defenses. J Clin Invest 89:1699, 1992. *A review of pathogenesis with emphasis on interactions with the host.*

Handsfield HH, Sparling PF: *Neisseria gonorrhoeae. In* Mandell GL, Bennett JE, Dolin R (eds.): Principles and Practice of Infectious Diseases, 4th ed. New York, Churchill Livingstone, 1995, pp 1909–1926. *Highly referenced overview of pathogenesis, epidemiology, clinical presentation, diagnosis, and treatment.*

Hook EW, Holmes KK: Gonococcal infections. Ann Intern Med 102:229, 1985. *Excellent, clinically relevant review.*

Luciano AA, Grubin L: Gonorrhea screening: Comparison of three techniques. JAMA 243:680, 1980. *Culture of the first-voided urine in asymptomatic males shown to be highly reliable method for diagnosis.*

Sparling PF, Cohen MS, Wyrick PB, Elkins C: Vaccines for bacterial sexually transmitted infections: A realistic goal? Proc Natl Acad Sci USA 91:2456, 1994. *Discussion of immunobiology of gonorrhea and prospects for a vaccine.*

316 GRANULOMA INGUINALE (Donovanosis)
*Edward W. Hook III**

Granuloma inguinale, also known as donovanosis, is a slowly progressive ulcerative disease involving principally the skin and subcutaneous tissues of the genital, inguinal, and anal regions. It is

---

* The author acknowledges the contribution of Dr. P. Frederick Sparling on this subject in the 19th edition of the *Cecil Textbook of Medicine.*

primarily transmitted sexually but probably can be transmitted by nonsexual contact as well. Multiple sexual contacts with an infected partner seem necessary for transmission of infection. The disease is uncommon in the United States, with < 100 recorded cases annually. It is quite common, however, in certain other areas of the world, especially Papua New Guinea.

ETIOLOGY. The causative organism is *Calymmatobacterium granulomatis,* a gram-negative bacterium immunologically related to certain *Klebsiella* strains. Current evidence suggests that *C. granulomatis* is not a member of the *Klebsiella-Enterobacter-Serratia* family; its exact taxonomic status is uncertain. The organism can be grown in yolk sacs, but only with great difficulty on artificial medium. It is apparently a facultative intracellular parasite because in infected lesions it is found primarily in histiocytes or other mononuclear cells.

CLINICAL MANIFESTATIONS. The initial lesion usually appears as a subcutaneous nodule that erodes through the surface and develops into a beefy, elevated granulomatous lesion. This usually is painless and unassociated with systemic symptoms. Secondary bacterial infection may cause a necrotic painful ulcerative lesion that may be rapidly destructive. A cicatricial form may also occur with a depigmented elevated area of keloid-like scar containing scattered islands of granulomatous tissue. Lesions in the genital area are commonly associated with pseudobuboes in the inguinal region; these swellings are usually not due to involvement of the inguinal lymph nodes but rather to granulomatous involvement of the subcutaneous tissues. Metastatic infection of bones or other viscera is occasionally seen. Clinical experience suggests that secondary carcinomas may be a complication of granuloma inguinale.

DIFFERENTIAL DIAGNOSIS. The differential diagnosis includes tumor, lymphogranuloma venereum, chancroid, syphilis, and other ulcerative granulomatous diseases. Chancroid is usually differentiated by its irregular undermined borders, which are not seen in the usual cases of granuloma inguinale. Darkfield examination and serologic tests should help to distinguish syphilis. Biopsies may be necessary to distinguish granuloma inguinale from certain tumors.

DIAGNOSIS. Diagnosis is made by demonstrating intracellular "Donovan bodies" in histiocytes or other mononuclear cells from lesion scrapings or biopsies. Wright's stain and Giemsa's stain of fresh impression smears or unfixed biopsies usually demonstrate the bacilli relatively easily, although multiple biopsies may be necessary in chronic cases. Culture is not practical at present. A serologic test has been devised but is not clinically available. Histologic examination of biopsies shows mononuclear cells with some infiltration by polymorphonuclear leukocytes but no giant cells.

TREATMENT. Treatment consists of tetracycline or sulfisoxazole in a dosage of 0.5 gram four times daily for at least 3 weeks. Other regimens that have proved effective include ampicillin, chloramphenicol, gentamicin, and co-trimoxazole. Limited experience suggests that lincomycin may be used successfully. Patients should be followed for at least several weeks after treatment is discontinued because of the possibility of relapse. Although the risk of communicability appears to be low, sexual contacts should also be examined; at present, treatment of contacts is not indicated in the absence of clinically evident disease.

PREVENTION. No effective prevention is known.

Breschi LC, Goldman G, Shapiro SR: Granuloma inguinale in Vietnam: Successful therapy with ampicillin and lincomycin. J Am Vener Dis Assoc 1:118, 1975. *Ampicillin was frequently effective in patients previously unresponsive to tetracycline.*

Garg BR, Lal S, Sivamani S: Efficacy of co-trimoxazole in donovanosis. A preliminary report. Br J Vener Dis 54:348, 1978. *Trimethoprim and sulfamethoxazole were effective.*

Kuberski T: Granuloma inguinale (donovanosis). Sex Trans Dis 7:29, 1980. *An excellent short review.*

Maddocks I, Anders EM, Dennis E: Donovanosis in Papua New Guinea. Br J Vener Dis 52:190, 1976. *A description of the epidemiology and clinical manifestations in an endemic area of granuloma inguinale.*

Rosen T, Tschen JA, Ramsdell W, et al.: Granuloma inguinale. J Am Acad Dermatol 11:433, 1984. *An American epidemic of this relatively rare disease is described.*

317 CHANCROID
*Edward W. Hook III**

Chancroid is a sexually transmitted infection caused by the gram-negative bacillus *Haemophilus ducreyi.*

EPIDEMIOLOGY. Worldwide, chancroid is considerably more common than syphilis, and in parts of Africa and in Southeast Asia is nearly as great a problem as gonorrhea. In the United States it is an uncommon disease. In the mid-1980's, chancroid rates increased more than fivefold, peaking at 4986 cases in 1987. Since then rates have steadily declined. In North America there are strong epidemiologic links between chancroid and both prostitution and illegal drug use. Although all genital ulcer diseases are associated with increased risk for human immunodeficiency virus (HIV) acquisition, the association is particularly strong for chancroid. The majority of reported cases occur in males. An outbreak in Greenland was exceptional in that about 40% of cases were noted in women. It is quite likely that there has been significant underdiagnosis in women in the past.

CLINICAL MANIFESTATIONS. The usual incubation period is 2 to 5 days but may be up to 14 days. In the Greenland outbreak the incubation period averaged nearly 2 weeks in women. The clinical manifestations of chancroid are quite variable. Classically, the initial manifestation is an inflammatory macule that then becomes a vesicle-pustule and finally a sharply circumscribed, somewhat ragged, and undermined painful ulcer. The base is moist and may be covered with a grayish necrotic exudate. Removal of the exudate reveals purulent granulation tissue. There is usually surrounding cutaneous erythema. Lesions typically are single but may be multiple, possibly owing to autoinoculation of nearby tissues. There are rarely systemic symptoms. Inguinal adenopathy is noted in one half of patients, approximately two thirds of whom have unilateral adenopathy. Lesions are usually noted on the penile shaft or glans. In women lesions may occur on the cervix, vagina, vulva, or perianal area. Lesions may occasionally occur primarily on or spread to the abdomen, thigh, breast, fingers, or lips. Intraoral lesions are uncommon.

There are reports of a transient genital ulcer, followed by significant inguinal adenopathy. This may be difficult to distinguish from lymphogranuloma venereum. Other uncommon clinical variants include the *phagedenic type* of ulcer with secondary suprainfection and rapid tissue destruction; *giant chancroid,* which is characterized by a very large single ulcer; *serpiginous ulcer,* which is characterized by rapidly spreading, indolent, shallow ulcers on the groin or the thigh; and a *follicular* type with multiple small ulcers in a perifollicular distribution.

DIFFERENTIAL DIAGNOSIS. The differential diagnosis includes syphilis, herpes genitalis, lymphogranuloma venereum, traumatic ulcers, and granuloma inguinale. Of these the most commonly confused are syphilis and herpes genitalis. Multiple infections are relatively common. Outpatients with suspected chancroid should have a serologic test for syphilis and preferably a darkfield examination as well.

DIAGNOSIS. The diagnosis of chancroid is made on the basis of the clinical appearance of the lesions plus either morphologic demonstration of typical organisms in the lesions or recovery of *H. ducreyi* by culture. Culture is the preferred method, but selective culture media are often not available. Under optimal conditions, positive cultures can be obtained in > 80% of cases. Best culture results seem to be obtained with supplemented chocolate agar media containing 3 μg per milliliter of vancomycin and incubated at 33°C. Necrotic debris should be removed from the ulcer with physiologic saline. The base and edges of the ulcer should be swabbed with a cotton-tipped swab and inoculated directly onto the culture plate if possible; swabs may be put into Amies transport medium if culture plates are not immediately available. Smears obtained from the undermined edges should be gently rolled onto a slide. *H. ducreyi* is a small gram-negative bacillus with rounded ends, which

---

* The author acknowledges the contribution of Dr. P. Frederick Sparling on this subject in the 19th edition of the *Cecil Textbook of Medicine.*

typically forms chains or parallel aggregates in lesions. Typical organisms are seen in 50 to 80% of cases. Organisms may also be obtained by aspirating inguinal nodes. Nodes should be aspirated by placing the needle through normal skin to avoid formation of fistulous tracts. Nodes should not be incised. There is no commercially available serologic test for chancroid.

TREATMENT. The drug of choice is a single intramuscular dose of ceftriaxone, 250 mg. A single 1-gram dose of azithromycin, given orally, is highly effective. Erythromycin, 500 mg orally four times daily for 7 days, is also usually curative. Another effective agent is ciprofloxacin, 500 mg orally twice daily for 3 days. Ampicillin should not be used because some strains of *H. ducreyi* produce a typical TEM-type β-lactamase and are quite ampicillin resistant. Interestingly, the plasmids containing the gene for production of β-lactamase are very closely related to the penicillinase plasmids present in *H. influenzae* and *Neisseria gonorrhoeae.* Tetracycline resistance is common. Serologic testing for HIV is recommended for all patients treated for possible chancroid. All regular sexual partners should be examined and epidemiologically treated with a similar regimen.

PREVENTION. No vaccine is available. Use of a condom is presumably helpful. There are no data regarding efficacy of antibiotic prophylaxis.

Blackmore CA, Limpakarnjanarat K, Rigau-Perez JG, et al.: An outbreak of chancroid in Orange County, California: Descriptive epidemiology and disease-control measures. J Infect Dis 151:840, 1985. *A very large continental U.S. outbreak is described. Sulfa and tetracycline resistance was common, but erythromycin and cotrimoxazole were effective.*

Centers for Disease Control and Prevention: 1993 Sexually transmitted diseases treatment guidelines. MMWR 42(RR-14):20, 1993. *Current treatment and management recommendations for chancroid.*

Lykke-Olesen L, Larsen L, Pedersen TG, et al.: Epidemic of chancroid in Greenland 1977–78. Lancet 1:654, 1979. *A remarkable epidemic, affecting 3% of the adult population. Tropical climates are not necessary for disease transmission or expression.*

Schmid GP, Sanders LL, Blount JH, et al.: Chancroid in the United States: Reestablishment of an old disease. JAMA 258:3265, 1987. *A useful description of factors contributing to the chancroid resurgence in the mid-1980's.*

Taylor DN, Pitarangsi C, Echeverria P, et al.: Comparative study of ceftriaxone and trimethoprim-sulfamethoxazole for the treatment of chancroid in Thailand. J Infect Dis 152:1002, 1985. *Ceftriaxone appears to be effective for this infection as well, in a single intramuscularly administered dose of 250 mg.*

Telzak EE, Chaisson MA, Bevier PJ, et al.: HIV-1 seroconversion in patients with and without genital ulcer disease. Ann Intern Med 119:1181, 1993. *In this study of heterosexual men attending New York City STD clinics, a diagnosis of chancroid was associated with a more than threefold increased likelihood of HIV acquisition.*

318 SYPHILIS

*Edward W. Hook III**

DEFINITION. Syphilis is a chronic infectious disease caused by the bacterium *Treponema pallidum.* It is usually acquired by sexual contact with another infected individual. Syphilis is remarkable among infectious diseases in its large variety of clinical presentations. It progresses, if untreated, through primary, secondary, and tertiary stages. The early stages (primary and secondary) are infectious. Spontaneous healing of early lesions occurs, followed by a long latent period. In about 30% of untreated patients, late disease of the heart, central nervous system (CNS), or other organs ultimately develops. At one time this disease was termed "the great imitator." Although the disease is less common now than previously, it remains a great challenge to the clinician because of its protean manifestations and is of great interest to biologists as well because of the long and tenuous balance between the host and the invading spirochete.

ETIOLOGY. The cause of syphilis was discovered in 1905 by Schaudinn and Hoffman when they visualized spirochetal organisms in early infectious lesions. The causative agent of syphilis, *T. pallidum,* is closely related to other pathogenic spirochetes, including those causing yaws *(T. pertenue)* and pinta *(T. carateum).*

T. pallidum is a thin, helical cell approximately 0.15 μ wide and

6 to 50 μ long. Ordinarily there are approximately 6 to 14 spirals. The organism is tapered on either end. It is too thin to be seen by ordinary Gram stain but can be visualized in wet mounts by darkfield microscopy (see below) or by silver stains or fluorescent antibody methods.

Recent studies have described several unusual characteristics of the *T. pallidum* outer membrane that may provide clues to syphilis pathogenesis. Unlike most bacteria having protein-rich outer membranes, the outer membrane of *T. pallidum* appears to be predominantly made up of phospholipids with few surface-exposed proteins. It has been hypothesized that because of this structure syphilis can progress despite a brisk antibody response (to non–surface-exposed, internal antigens). Between the outer membrane and the peptidoglycan cell wall are six axial fibrils. The axial fibrils are attached three at each end and overlap in the center of the organism. They are structurally and biochemically similar to flagella and may be in part responsible for the motility of the organism.

It is possible to culture *T. pallidum in vitro,* but sustained *in vitro* cultivation is not yet possible and yields are very low. Culture is of limited use in research but of no use in clinical practice. *T. pallidum* can be maintained by serial passage in rabbits without loss of virulence. Only a few strains have been isolated in rabbits and carefully studied, and little evidence is available regarding the genetic diversity of the organism. All studied isolates have been susceptible to penicillin and are similar antigenically. Immunity to the homologous strain develops after prolonged infection in rabbits. The only known natural hosts for *T. pallidum* are humans and certain monkeys and higher apes.

PATHOGENESIS AND HOST RESPONSE. *T. pallidum* may penetrate through normal mucosal membranes and also through minor abrasions of epithelial surfaces. In experimental rabbit syphilis, spirochetes can be found in the lymphatic system within 30 minutes of inoculation and are found in blood shortly thereafter. There have been occasional instances in humans of transfusion syphilis resulting from use of blood from a donor who was in the incubation stage of the disease. Therefore it seems clear that syphilis is a systemic disease from the onset in humans as well. However, the first lesions appear at the site of primary inoculation, presumably because of the large numbers of treponemes implanted at this site. In laboratory animals, there is an inverse relationship between numbers of treponemes inoculated and time required for development of the primary cutaneous lesion. The minimal number of treponemes required to establish infection is not known but may be as low as one treponeme. Multiplication of organisms is very slow, with a division time in rabbits of approximately 33 hours. Similarly slow growth of treponemes in humans probably accounts in part for the protracted nature of the illness and for the relatively long incubation period.

T. pallidum is not known to produce any toxins. Treponemes are capable of specific attachment to host cells, but it is not known whether attachment results in damage to host cells. Most treponemes are found in intercellular spaces, but occasional treponemes can be seen within phagocytic cells. However, there is no evidence for prolonged intracellular survival of treponemes.

The primary pathologic lesion of syphilis is a focal endarteritis. There is an increase in adventitial cells, endothelial proliferation, and presence of an inflammatory cuff around affected vessels. Lymphocytes, plasma cells, and monocytes predominate in the inflammatory lesion, and in some cases polymorphonuclear cells are seen as well. The vessel lumen is frequently obliterated. With healing there is considerable fibrosis. Treponemes may be seen in most early lesions of syphilis and in some of the late lesions such as the meningoencephalitis of general paresis.

Granulomatous reaction is also frequent in secondary syphilis and in late syphilis. The granuloma is histologically nonspecific, and cases of syphilis have been incorrectly diagnosed as sarcoidosis or other granulomatous diseases. Human inoculation studies suggest that the pathogenesis of the gumma, which is a granulomatous lesion, involves hypersensitivity to small numbers of virulent treponemes introduced into a previously sensitized host.

Intracutaneous inoculation of patients with syphilis in various stages with partially purified antigens of *T. pallidum* showed that delayed cellular hypersensitivity developed only in late secondary syphilis but was uniformly present in latent syphilis. There may be

* The author acknowledges the contribution of Dr. P. Frederick Sparling on this subject in the 19th edition of the *Cecil Textbook of Medicine.*

temporary hyporesponsiveness of lymphocytes from patients with primary and secondary syphilis to treponemal antigens. It is possible but not proved that the unusual waxing and waning of lesions in early syphilis depend on the balance between development of effective cellular immunity and suppression of thymus-derived lymphocyte function.

The host also responds to infection with production of numerous antibodies, and in some instances circulating immune complexes may be formed. The nephrotic syndrome has been recognized occasionally in secondary syphilis, and renal biopsies from such cases have shown membranous glomerulonephritis characterized by focal subepithelial basement membrane deposits. The deposits contain both IgG and C3, and treponemal antibody.

Antibodies useful in diagnosis are discussed under Serologic Tests, below.

EPIDEMIOLOGY. Syphilis, with the exception of congenital syphilis, is acquired almost exclusively by intimate contact with the infectious lesions of primary or secondary syphilis (chancre, mucous patches, condylomata lata). This is usually through sexual intercourse, including anogenital and orogenital intercourse. Health workers have sometimes been infected during unsuspecting examination of patients with infectious lesions. Infection by contact with fomites is extremely uncommon.

Syphilis is most common in large cities and in young, sexually active individuals. The highest rate in both men and women occurs at ages 20 to 24, followed by ages 25 to 29 and 15 to 19 years. Among predominantly rural areas in the United States the disease is most prevalent in the southeast.

Syphilis spares no class, race, or group but is more prevalent in the United States among the poorly educated and economically deprived than among more prosperous groups. In 1992, U.S. syphilis rates were more than 60-fold greater among African-Americans than among non-Hispanic whites (92.4 versus 1.5 per 100,000 population). Increased numbers of different sexual partners and perhaps indiscriminate choice of partner increase the risk of acquiring sexually transmitted disease. Patients with primary and secondary syphilis name on the average nearly three different sexual contacts within the previous 90 days. A traditional cornerstone of syphilis control has been epidemiologic investigation of sexual contacts of patients with primary or secondary lesions, and of patients with early latent disease. More recently, as syphilis has been associated with drug use and anonymous sex, epidemiologic investigations have become less efficacious.

In the 1970's and 1980's male homosexuals accounted for an increasing proportion of the total cases of infectious syphilis. The ratio of male:female cases of primary and secondary syphilis in the United States rose from 1.6:1.0 in 1965 to 2.5:1.0 in 1975 and about 3:1 in the mid 1980's. Similar trends were noted in other countries. From 1986 to 1990, U.S. syphilis rates nearly doubled to reach 50,578 cases in 1990. This epidemic disproportionately affected nonwhite heterosexual men and women and occurred contemporaneously with an epidemic of crack cocaine use. Many cases were related to the exchange of sex for drugs or money to buy drugs. After 1990, syphilis rates again declined and in 1993 there were 26,498 cases of primary and secondary syphilis reported, the lowest number since 1979. This epidemic is likely to have also contributed to the spread of HIV (see Syphilis/HIV Interactions, below) and to dramatic increases in congenital syphilis.

The annual incidence of syphilis has generally declined worldwide for approximately 100 years with the exception of periods of extensive war. With the introduction of penicillin there was a rapid decline in primary and secondary syphilis after World War II, to annual rates of approximately 4 cases per 100,000 in 1957. This resulted in declining federal expenditure for syphilis control, however, and there was a subsequent resurgence in infectious primary and secondary syphilis in the United States, reaching peaks of >12 cases per 100,000 several times in the period 1965–1983. Because many cases of syphilis are not reported, the true incidence is much higher, perhaps 75,000 to 100,000 annually.

Reported deaths from syphilis declined from 2434 in 1965 to 200 in 1976. Infant deaths from syphilis fell by 98 to 99% by 1980, but rose sharply in 1988–1990. Patients with clinically manifest late syphilis, particularly those with gummas, are becoming less common, perhaps as a result of the effectiveness of penicillin therapy for early syphilis. However, surveys indicate that there still are sig-

nificant numbers of patients with untreated cardiovascular and neurologic syphilis, especially among older age groups. There is suggestive evidence that neurosyphilis may be presenting with atypical clinical manifestations and therefore may not be easily recognized.

NATURAL COURSE OF UNTREATED SYPHILIS. The incubation period from time of exposure to development of the primary lesion at the place of initial inoculation of treponemes averages approximately 21 days but ranges from 10 to 90 days. A painless papule develops and gradually breaks down to form a clean-based ulcer with raised, indurated margins. This persists for 2 to 6 weeks and then heals spontaneously. Several weeks later the patient characteristically develops a secondary stage characterized by low-grade fever, headache, malaise, generalized lymphadenopathy, and a mucocutaneous rash. There may be involvement of visceral organs. The secondary eruption may occur while the primary chancre is still healing or several months after the disappearance of the chancre. The secondary lesions heal spontaneously within 2 to 6 weeks, and the infection then enters latency. Some patients may later develop relapsing lesions similar to those of the secondary stage; rarely the relapse takes the form of recurrence of the primary chancre. About one third of untreated patients eventually develop late destructive tertiary lesions involving one or more of the eyes, CNS, heart, or other organs, including skin. These may occur at any time from a few years to as late as 25 years following infection.

The incidence of late complications of untreated syphilis is currently unknown but seems less than noted previously. Cases of gumma are at present so rare as to be reportable.

CLINICAL MANIFESTATIONS. *Primary Syphilis.* The typical lesion of primary syphilis is the chancre, a painless, clean-based, indurated ulcer. The chancre starts as a papule, but then superficial erosion occurs, resulting in the typical ulcer. The borders of the ulcer are raised, firm, and indurated. Occasionally, secondary infections change the appearance, resulting in a painful lesion. Most chancres are single, but multiple ulcers are sometimes seen, particularly when skin folds are opposed ("kissing chancres"). The untreated chancre heals in several weeks, leaving a faint scar. The chancre is usually associated with regional adenopathy, which may be either unilateral or bilateral. The regional nodes are movable, discrete, and rubbery. If the chancre occurs in the cervix or in the rectum, the affected regional iliac nodes are not palpable. See Figure 318–1.

Chancres may occur at any site of potential inoculation by direct contact. The majority of chancres occur at anogenital locations. Chancres may also be seen in the pharynx, on the tongue, around the lips, on the fingers, on the nipples, or in diverse other areas. The morphology depends in part on the area of the body in which they occur and also on the host immune response. Chancres in previously infected individuals may be small and may remain papular. Chancres of the finger may appear more erosive and may be quite painful.

The *differential diagnosis* of a genital ulcer should include genital herpes. Classically, herpetic ulcers are multiple, superficial, and, if seen early, vesicular. They are often painful. However, atypical presentations may be indistinguishable from a syphilitic chancre. Genital herpes is orders of magnitude more common than syphilis. Thus, genital herpes is now the most common cause of a "typical chancre" in North America. Herpetic ulcers, unlike syphilitic ulcers, may yield positive findings on Tzanck's test—multinucleated giant cells in the base of the ulcer. The ulcers of chancroid are usually painful, often multiple, and frequently exudative and nonindurated. Lymphogranuloma venereum may produce a small papular lesion associated with a regional adenopathy. Other conditions that must be distinguished include granuloma inguinale, drug eruptions, carcinoma, superficial fungal infections, traumatic lesions, and lichen planus. Final distinction in most cases is made on the basis of darkfield examination, which is positive only in syphilis.

Secondary Syphilis. Approximately 4 to 8 weeks after the appearance of the primary chancre, patients typically develop lesions of secondary syphilis. They may complain of *malaise, fever, headache, sore throat,* and other systemic symptoms. Most patients have generalized lymphadenopathy, including the epitrochlear nodes. Approximately 30% of patients have evidence of the healing chancre, although many patients, including male homosexuals and women, give no history of a primary lesion.

At least 80% of patients with secondary syphilis have cutaneous lesions or lesions of the mucocutaneous junctions at some point in

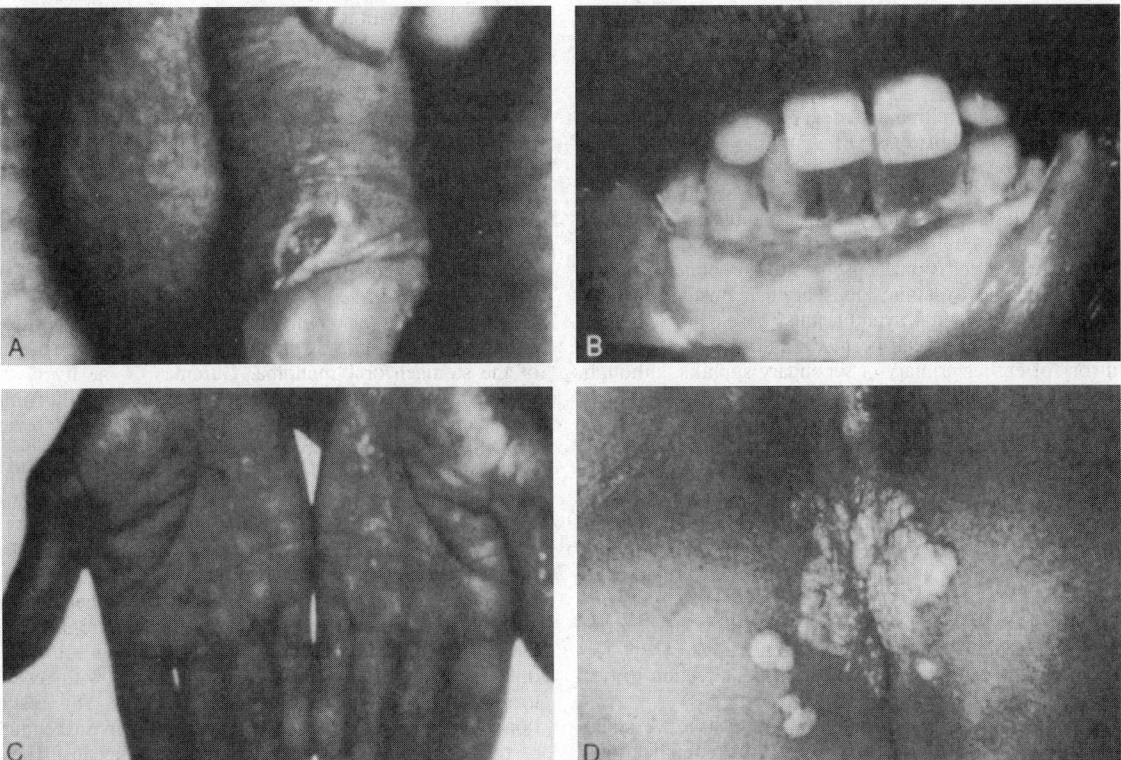

FIGURE 318–1. *A,* Primary syphilis, chancre. *B,* Secondary syphilis, mucous patch. *C,* Secondary syphilis, papulosquamous rash. *D,* Secondary syphilis, condylomata lata.

their illness. The diagnosis is usually first suspected on the basis of the cutaneous eruption. The rash is often minimally symptomatic, however, and many patients with late syphilis do not recall either primary or secondary lesions. The rashes are quite varied in their appearance but have certain characteristic features. The lesions are usually widespread and are symmetric in distribution. They often are pink, coppery, or dusky red, particularly the earliest macular lesions. They usually are nonpruritic, although occasional exceptions have been noted, and are almost never vesicular or bullous in adults. They are indurated except for the very earliest macular lesions and frequently have a superficial scale (papulosquamous lesions). They tend to be polymorphic and rounded, and on healing they may leave residual pigmentation or depigmentation. The lesions may be quite faint and difficult to visualize, particularly on dark-skinned individuals.

The earliest pink macular lesions are frequently seen on the margins of the ribs or the sides of the trunk with later spread to the rest of the body. The face is often spared except around the mouth. Subsequently a papular rash appears, which is usually generalized but is *quite marked on the palms and soles.* These rashes frequently are associated with a superficial scale and may be hyperpigmented. When the rash occurs on the face, it may be pustular, resembling acne vulgaris. On occasion the scale may be so great as to resemble psoriasis. Deep nodular lesions may cause confusion. Ulceration may occur, producing lesions resembling ecthyma. In malnourished or debilitated patients extensive destructive ulcerative lesions with a heaped-up crust may occur, the so-called rupial lesion. Lesions around the hair follicles may result in patchy alopecia of the beard or of the scalp.

Ringed or annular lesions may occur, especially around the face, particularly on black individuals. Lesions at the angle of the mouth or the corner of the nose may have a central linear erosion (the so-called split papule).

In warm, moist areas such as the perineum, large, pale, flat-topped papules may coalesce to form condylomata lata. These may also be seen in the axilla and rarely in a generalized form. They are extremely infectious. They are not to be confused with the common venereal warts (condylomata acuminata), which are small, often multiple, and more sharply raised than condylomata lata.

Other lesions of the mucous membranes are common. The palate and pharynx may be inflamed. Approximately 30% of patients develop the so-called mucous patch. This is a slightly raised oval area covered by a grayish-white membrane, which when raised reveals a pink base that does not bleed. These may be seen on the genitalia, in the mouth, or on the tongue and, like condylomata lata, are highly infectious.

Other manifestations of secondary syphilis include hepatitis, which has been reported in up to 10% of patients in some series. Jaundice is rare, but an elevated alkaline phosphatase is common. Liver biopsy reveals small areas of focal necrosis and mononuclear infiltrate or periportal vasculitis. Spirochetes can often be visualized with silver stains. Periostitis with widespread lytic lesions of bone has been reported occasionally; bone scanning appears to be a sensitive test for early syphilitic osteitis. An immune complex type of nephropathy with transient nephrotic syndrome has been rarely documented. There may be iritis or an anterior uveitis. From 10 to 30% of patients have pleocytosis in the cerebrospinal fluid (CSF), but symptomatic meningitis is seen in < 1% of patients. Symptomatic gastritis may be present.

Differential diagnosis of secondary syphilis includes a large number of diseases. The cutaneous eruptions may be mimicked by pityriasis rosea, which can be differentiated by the occurrence of lesions along lines of skin cleavage and frequently by the presence of a herald patch. Drug eruptions, acute febrile exanthems, psoriasis, lichen planus, scabies, and other diseases must also be considered in some cases. The mucous patch may superficially resemble oral candidiasis (thrush). Infectious mononucleosis may appear very similar to secondary syphilis, with sore throat, generalized adenopathy, hepatitis, and a generalized rash. Infectious hepatitis may also cause confusion. A high index of suspicion is required to make the diagnosis of syphilis in some cases. Unfortunately even classic cases with widespread, hyperpigmented, papulosquamous lesions involving the palms and the soles are not infrequently misdiagnosed today. Fortunately, if the serologic tests for syphilis are obtained, they are positive in 99% of patients. The condylomata lata and mucous patches contain large numbers of treponemes on darkfield examination. Aspiration of lymph nodes may occasionally reveal motile *T. pallidum.*

Relapsing Syphilis. Following resolution of primary or secondary syphilis skin lesions, approximately 30% of patients experience cutaneous recurrences. Recurrent lesions may be fewer or more firmly indurated than initial lesions and, like typical lesions of primary or secondary syphilis, are infectious for exposed sexual partners.

Latent Syphilis. By definition latent syphilis is that stage in which there are no clinical signs of syphilis and the CSF is normal. Latency begins with the passing of the first attack of secondary syphilis and may last for a lifetime thereafter. It is usually detected by reactive serologic tests for syphilis. The test must be shown to be reactive on more than one occasion to rule out technical errors. Diseases known to cause occasional false-positive treponemal reactions for syphilis, such as systemic lupus erythematosus, must be excluded. In addition, congenital syphilis must be excluded before the diagnosis of latent syphilis can be made. Patients may or may not have a history of earlier primary or secondary syphilis, although such history is obviously helpful in making a firm diagnosis of latent syphilis.

Latency has been divided into two stages: *early* and *late latency*. Evidence suggests that most infectious relapses occur in the first year, and epidemiologic evidence shows that the most infectious spread of syphilis occurs during the first year of infection. *Therefore early latency in the United States is defined as the first year after the resolution of primary or secondary lesions or as a newly reactive serologic test for syphilis in an otherwise asymptomatic individual who has had a negative serologic test within the preceding year.* Late latent syphilis is ordinarily not infectious except for the case of the pregnant woman, who may transmit infection to her fetus after many years.

Late Syphilis. Late, or tertiary, syphilis is the destructive stage of the disease and can be crippling. Late syphilitic complications are still important medical problems, but newly recognized cases of late syphilis have been declining steadily in the United States since World War II. Although the incidence of late syphilis is unknown, the prevalence of various types of late syphilis has been approximated (Table 318–1).

Late syphilis is usually very slowly progressive, although certain neurologic syndromes may have sudden onset owing to endarteritis and thrombosis in the CNS. Late syphilis is noninfectious. Any organ of the body may be involved, but three main types of disease may be distinguished: late benign (gummatous), cardiovascular, and neurosyphilis.

Late Benign Syphilis. Late benign syphilis, or gumma, was the most common complication of late syphilis in the Oslo Study of untreated patients (1891–1951). In the penicillin era gummas are rare. They typically develop from 1 to 10 years after the initial infection and may involve any part of the body. Although they may be very destructive, they respond rapidly to treatment and therefore are relatively benign. Histologically the gumma is a granuloma. The histologic findings are nonspecific and may be associated with central necrosis surrounded by epithelioid and fibroblastic cells and occasionally giant cells. There is sometimes vasculitis. *T. pallidum* is ordinarily not demonstrable by silver stains but can sometimes be recovered by inoculation of rabbits.

Gummas may be solitary or multiple. They are usually asymmetric and are often grouped. They may start as a superficial nodule or

TABLE 318–1. NEWLY DIAGNOSED TERTIARY SYPHILIS IN 105 PATIENTS IN DENMARK, 1961–1970

Type of Tertiary Syphilis	Number Observed*
Neurosyphilis	72
Asymptomatic	45
Tabes dorsalis	11
General paresis	13
Meningovascular	1
Optic atrophy	2
Cardiovascular syphilis	44
Aortic insufficiency	16
Aortic aneurysm	13
Uncomplicated aortitis†	15
Late benign syphilis (gumma)	4

*Some patients had more than one form of late syphilis.
†Autopsy diagnoses only.

as a deeper lesion that breaks down to form punched-out ulcers. They are ordinarily indolent and slowly progressive. They are indurated on palpation. There often is central healing with an atrophic scar surrounded by hyperpigmented borders. Cutaneous gummas may resemble other chronic granulomatous ulcerative lesions caused by tuberculosis, sarcoidosis, leprosy, and other deep fungal infections. Precise histologic diagnosis may not be possible. However, the syphilitic gumma is the only such lesion to heal dramatically with penicillin therapy. Another form of gumma is papulosquamous and may mimic psoriasis.

Gummas may also involve deep visceral organs, of which the most common are the respiratory tract, the gastrointestinal tract, and bones. In earlier centuries gummas of the nose and palate commonly resulted in septal perforations and disfiguring facial lesions. Gummas may also involve the larynx or the pulmonary parenchyma. Gumma of the stomach may masquerade as carcinoma of the stomach or lymphoma. Gummas of the liver were once the most common form of visceral syphilis, presenting often with hepatosplenomegaly and anemia, occasionally with fever and jaundice. Skeletal gummas typically produce lesions in the long bones, skull, and clavicle. A characteristic symptom is nocturnal pain. Radiologic abnormalities, when present, include periostitis and either lytic or sclerotic destructive osteitis.

Cardiovascular Syphilis. The primary cardiovascular complications of syphilis are aortic insufficiency and aortic aneurysm, usually of the ascending aorta. Less commonly other large arteries may be involved, and rarely involvement of the coronary ostia results in coronary insufficiency. These complications in all cases are due to obliterative endarteritis of the vasa vasorum with resultant damage to the intima and media of the great vessels. This results in dilatation of the ascending aorta and eventually in stretching of the ring of the aortic valve, producing aortic insufficiency. The valve cusps remain normal. Death may eventually result from congestive heart failure. There has been some success with placing prosthetic heart valves in patients with syphilitic aortic insufficiency. Aneurysms occasionally present as a pulsating mass bulging through the anterior chest wall. Syphilitic aortitis may involve the descending aorta, but this is almost always proximal to the renal arteries, unlike atherosclerotic aneurysms, which typically involve the descending aorta below the renal arteries.

The disease usually begins within 5 to 10 years after initial infection but may not become clinically manifest until 20 to 30 years after infection. Cardiovascular syphilis is thought to be more common in men than in women and possibly in blacks than in whites. Cardiovascular syphilis does not occur after congenital infection—a phenomenon that remains unexplained.

Asymptomatic aortitis is best diagnosed by visualizing linear calcifications in the wall of the ascending aorta by radiography. The signs of syphilitic aortic insufficiency are the same as for aortic insufficiency of other causes. In aortic insufficiency resulting from dilatation of the aortic ring, the decrescendo murmur is often loudest along the *right* sternal margin. Syphilitic aneurysms may be fusiform but are more typically saccular and do not lead to aortic dissection. Approximately 10 to 25% of patients with cardiovascular syphilis have coexistent neurosyphilis, and it is therefore mandatory to do a lumbar puncture in all patients with cardiovascular syphilis.

At present, syphilis is a relatively more common cause of aortic insufficiency among the elderly than among younger patients; this is due to the progressively decreasing incidence of new cases of late cardiovascular syphilis.

Neurosyphilis. Neurosyphilis may be divided into four groups: asymptomatic, meningovascular, tabes dorsalis, and general paresis. These are more fully described in Ch. 422. Division is not absolute, and overlap between syndromes is typical. Current cases of neurosyphilis are more likely than heretofore to be variants of the classic syndromes, possibly as a result of use of antimicrobials for other diseases.

Asymptomatic Neurosyphilis. Asymptomatic neurosyphilis is diagnosed when there are CSF abnormalities (pleocytosis, protein elevation, or a reactive VDRL*) in a syphilis patient in the absence of signs and symptoms of neurologic disease. Although numerous other processes may cause CSF pleocytosis or protein elevations, false-positive VDRL test results are very rare in CSF in the absence

* See Serologic Tests, p. 1710. Also refer to Table 318–2.

of a traumatic tap. The CSF usually shows an increased total protein and a lymphocytic pleocytosis. If the CSF is normal 2 or more years after the initial infection, the patient is not likely to develop a positive CSF later. Although up to 50% of patients with untreated secondary syphilis have an abnormal CSF, penicillin therapy apparently prevents progression to late symptomatic neurosyphilis. Because of this, routine lumbar punctures for examining CSF are not indicated in early syphilis unless the patient is known to have HIV infection. Unfortunately, it has become common practice to avoid lumbar punctures in later stages of syphilis as well. Instead, patients are treated with doses of penicillin thought to be effective for neurosyphilis, if present. As a result, there are few data on the present frequency and course of asymptomatic neurosyphilis.

Some laboratories perform an FTA-ABS* test on spinal fluid. Interest in tests such as this has been prompted by good evidence that patients with untreated neurosyphilis may have a nonreactive CSF-VDRL. Reports were published of positive FTA-ABS test results in the CSF of patients with otherwise normal spinal fluid, in whom there were clinical signs and symptoms compatible with neurosyphilis. However, the CSF FTA-ABS test has not been standardized, and some evidence exists that reactive CSF test results are caused by passive transfer of serum antibody into spinal fluid. At present, although a nonreactive CSF FTA-ABS may be useful to rule out the diagnosis, no diagnosis of asymptomatic (or symptomatic) neurosyphilis should be based solely on the CSF FTA-ABS* test.

Meningovascular Syphilis. An acute to subacute aseptic meningitis may occur at any time after the primary stage but usually within the first year of infection. It frequently involves the base of the brain and may result in unilateral or bilateral cranial nerve palsies. In about 10% of cases, the onset of meningitis coincides with the rash of secondary syphilis. The spinal fluid shows a lymphocytic pleocytosis with increased protein and usually normal glucose concentration. The CSF-VDRL is nearly always reactive. Rarely CSF glucose concentration is decreased. This syndrome can mimic tuberculous or fungal meningitis or nonpurulent meningitis of various causes.

In other patients, the meningeal involvement may be less prominent, but there is sufficient endarteritis and perivascular inflammation to result in cerebrovascular thrombosis and infarction. This usually occurs 5 to 10 years after the initial infection and is more common in males. There often is associated aseptic meningitis as well. Most cerebrovascular accidents are not due to syphilitic arteritis even in patients with a reactive serologic test for syphilis. However, syphilis should be considered as the cause in young patients with a history of syphilis and without other causes for cerebrovascular accidents.

Tabes Dorsalis. Tabes dorsalis is a slowly progressive degenerative disease involving the posterior columns and posterior roots of the spinal cord, resulting in progressive loss of peripheral reflexes, impairment of vibration and position sense, and progressive ataxia. There may be chronic destructive changes in the large joints of the affected limbs in far-advanced cases (Charcot's joints). Incontinence of the bladder and impotence are common. Sudden and severe painful crises of uncertain cause are a characteristic part of the syndrome. These most typically involve the lower extremities but may occur at any site. Not infrequently severe, sharp abdominal pains lead to exploratory surgery. These attacks may be triggered by exposure to cold or other stresses or may arise with no obvious precipitating cause.

Optic atrophy is seen in 20% of cases. The pupils are abnormal in 90% of cases, with bilaterally small pupils that fail to constrict further in response to light but that do constrict normally to accommodation (Argyll Robertson pupils).

The cause of tabes dorsalis is unclear. Spirochetes cannot be demonstrated in the posterior column or dorsal root.

Onset of the disease is usually delayed, often 20 to 30 years after initial infection. It is thought to be more common in whites and in men. Typical cases of patients presenting with lightning pains, ataxia, Argyll Robertson pupils, absent deep tendon reflexes, and loss of posterior column function are easy to diagnose. Atypical cases may be more troublesome, particularly because the VDRL test result in the serum is normal in as many as 30 to 40% of patients, and 10 to 20% of patients (even before the advent of penicillin)

have normal CSF-VDRL results as well. The FTA-ABS test in serum is nearly always reactive.

Treatment is unsatisfactory. Penicillin usually arrests progression but does not reverse the symptoms. Carbamazepine in doses of 400 to 800 mg per day has been reported to effectively treat the lightning pains.

Tabes dorsalis is now thought to be uncommon, although a survey of newly diagnosed late syphilis in Denmark in the decade 1961 to 1970 showed that in approximately 10% of all persons with late syphilis and 40% of all with clinical neurosyphilis there was evidence of tabes dorsalis.

General Paresis. This form of neurosyphilis is a chronic meningoencephalitis resulting in gradually progressive loss of cortical function. It typically occurs 10 to 20 years after the initial infection. Pathologically there is a perivascular and meningeal chronic inflammatory reaction with thickening of the meninges, a granular ependymitis, degeneration of the cortical parenchyma, and abundant spirochetes in the tissues.

The most devastating effect of general paresis is on the mind. With effective penicillin therapy this disease has become much less common; in the United States, first admissions to mental hospitals because of syphilitic psychosis declined from 7694 in 1940 to 154 in 1968, the last year for which definite figures are available.

In its early stages general paresis results in nonspecific symptoms such as irritability, fatigability, headaches, forgetfulness, and personality changes. Later there is impaired memory, defective judgment, lack of insight, confusion, and often depression or marked elation. The patients may be delusional, and seizures are sometimes seen. There may also be loss of other cortical functions, including paralysis or aphasia.

Physical signs are primarily those of the altered mental status. Cranial nerve palsies are uncommon. Optic atrophy is rare. The complete Argyll Robertson pupil is also uncommon, but irregular or otherwise abnormal pupils are not infrequent. Peripheral reflexes are often somewhat increased.

The CSF is nearly always abnormal, with lymphocytic pleocytosis and increased total protein. The VDRL is usually reactive in both spinal fluid and serum. The disease responds well to penicillin therapy if administered early, although as many as a third of treated patients may develop progressive neurologic decline in later years. Fever therapy induced with malaria was formerly an effective adjunct to treatment with arsenicals but has now been abandoned.

Even though classic general paresis is now infrequent, it remains reasonable to suspect syphilis as the cause of undiagnosed neurologic illness.

Syphilis/HIV Interactions. Syphilis and HIV infection interact on multiple levels. Thus, clinicians evaluating patients with newly diagnosed syphilis should consider whether coexistent HIV infection is present and how the two diseases might be interacting. Conversely, clinicians seeing patients with newly diagnosed HIV should be attuned to the possible existence of previously undiagnosed syphilis.

Syphilis, like other genital ulcer diseases, is associated with three- to fivefold increased risk for HIV acquisition. Presumably genital ulcers act as portals of entry through which HIV may more readily infect exposed individuals. In individuals with HIV infection who acquire syphilis, the natural history of the infection may be modified. HIV-infected syphilis patients are more likely to present with secondary syphilis than are non–HIV-infected patients. In addition, HIV-infected secondary syphilis patients are more likely to have coexistent chancres than are HIV-negative secondary syphilis patients, suggesting that either the healing of chancres is delayed or the appearance of secondary manifestations is accelerated in the presence of HIV coinfection.

Several reports have suggested that neurosyphilis may be more common in patients with HIV infection; however, no large or carefully controlled studies document this association. In HIV-infected syphilis patients in whom therapy fails, neurosyphilis may be a more common presenting feature than in patients without HIV infection.

Most experts agree that failure of treatment using currently recommended regimens for syphilis therapy is more common in patients with coexistent HIV infection. The magnitude of this increase, however, is probably small and as a result alternate

---

* See Serologic Tests, p. 1710. Also refer to Table 318-2.

treatment regimens are not currently recommended. Rather, closer follow-up is suggested to permit early detection of treatment failure and to help prevent disease progression or transmission of infection to others.

Congenital Syphilis. Congenital syphilis results from transplacental hematogenous spread of syphilis from the mother to the fetus. The incidence of congenital syphilis diagnoses in the United States fell below 1000 per year for the first time in 1975, and <500 cases occurred per year until 1988, when the epidemic of syphilis in adults led to similar epidemic increases in congenital infections. From 1990 through 1993 >3000 new cases of congenital syphilis have been reported each year. Each case of congenital syphilis represents a tragedy that could have been prevented by better case reporting and by proper prenatal care. A VDRL should be obtained in all expectant mothers at the beginning and near the end of pregnancy.

Spirochetes can be found in abortuses of as little as 9 to 10 weeks' gestation. The risk of fetal infection is greatest in the early stages of untreated maternal syphilis and declines slowly thereafter, but the mother may infect her fetus during at least the first 5 years of her infection. Adequate treatment of the mother prior to the sixteenth week usually prevents manifest clinical illness in the neonate. Later treatment may not prevent late sequelae of the disease in the child. Untreated maternal infection may result in stillbirth, neonatal death, prematurity, or syndromes of early or late congenital syphilis among surviving infants.

Manifestations of early congenital syphilis are often seen in the perinatal period but may not develop until the infant has been discharged from the hospital. The disease resembles secondary syphilis of the adult except that the rash may be vesicular or bullous, which is extremely rare in adults. There often is rhinitis, hepatosplenomegaly, hemolytic anemia, jaundice, and pseudoparalysis (immobility of one or more extremities) resulting from painful osteochondritis. There may be thrombocytopenia and leukocytosis. The early stages of congenital syphilis must be differentiated from rubella, cytomegalovirus infection, toxoplasmosis, bacterial sepsis, and other diseases.

Late congenital syphilis is defined as congenital syphilis of more than 2 years' duration. The disease may remain latent with no manifest late damage. Cardiovascular alterations have not been observed in congenital syphilis. Neurologic manifestations are common, and there may be eighth cranial nerve deafness and interstitial keratitis. The latter occurs in >10% of patients but may not be apparent until the tenth year of life or later. Periostitis may result in prominent frontal bones, depression of the bridge of the nose ("saddle nose"), poor development of the maxilla, and anterior bowing of the tibias ("saber shins"). There may be late-onset arthritis of the knees (Clutton's joints). The permanent dentition may show characteristic abnormalities known as Hutchinson's teeth; the upper central incisors are widely spaced, centrally notched, and tapered in the manner of a screwdriver. The molars may show multiple poorly developed cusps (mulberry molars). Some of the late manifestations such as interstitial keratitis and Clutton's joints may be due to hypersensitivity responses and are benefited by corticosteroids in some cases.

DIAGNOSIS. ***Darkfield Examination.*** The most definitive means of making a diagnosis is finding spirochetes of typical morphology and motility in lesions of early acquired or congenital syphilis. The darkfield examination is often positive in primary syphilis and in the moist mucosal lesions of secondary and congenital syphilis. It may occasionally be positive in aspirates of lymph nodes in secondary syphilis. Problems arise, however, because of false-negative results in primary syphilis owing to application by the patient of soaps or other toxic compounds to the lesions. A single negative result is therefore insufficient to exclude syphilis. Optimally, patients with suspicious lesions but with an initially negative darkfield examination should be instructed to avoid washing the lesion and to return daily for two successive examinations. In practice, however, for high-risk individuals (drug users, homosexually active men), it may be more appropriate to treat patients with suspicious lesions presumptively after obtaining serologic tests. Confusion may also arise because of the presence of spirochetes that are morphologically indistinguishable from *T. pallidum* in the mouth, particularly around the gingival margins. For lesions in these areas

diagnosis often depends on clinical appearance, history, and serologic testing.

To perform the darkfield examination, the surface of the suspected ulcerative lesion should be cleaned with saline solution and gauze without producing bleeding. The presence of red cells in the specimen makes it difficult to visualize small numbers of *T. pallidum*. Squeezing of the lesion (with gloves on) may help produce serous fluid, which is picked up on a glass slide, covered with a coverslip, and examined with the darkfield microscope. Living *T. pallidum* organisms demonstrate gradual motion to and fro, rotational movement around the long axis, and rather sudden 90-degree bending near the center of the organism. Because most physicians do not have the proper equipment and are not familiar with the techniques of darkfield microscopy, the state public health authorities can be called for assistance.

T. pallidum may also be demonstrated in biopsies or pathologic specimens by fluorescent antibody stains or by silver stains.

Serologic Tests. Two basic types of serologic tests for humoral antibody are widely used to diagnose infection with *T. pallidum*: nontreponemal tests that detect antibodies reactive with diphosphatidylglycerol (cardiolipin), which is a normal component of many tissues; and specific treponemal antibodies. Nonspecific antibodies against cardiolipin were formerly designated "reagin," a term that should be discarded to avoid confusion with another "reagin," IgE. The kinds of tests used in syphilis are summarized in Table 318–2.

Nontreponemal Tests. Anticardiolipin antibodies were first discovered by Wassermann in 1907, using extracts of congenitally syphilitic livers as the antigen for a complement fixation test. Subsequently it was shown that normal livers contained the same antigen as do many other tissues; the antigen for this class of test is now extracted from beef heart. As yet there is no convincing explanation for why patients infected with *T. pallidum* develop increasing titers of antibody against a normal tissue component.

The Wassermann test has now been replaced by related tests. The standard test in use today to detect anticardiolipin antibody is the Venereal Disease Research Laboratories (VDRL) test, which is an easily quantified slide flocculation test. Many similar tests, including the rapid plasma reagin (RPR) test and the unheated serum reagin (USR) test, are frequently used for screening for syphilis.

The VDRL and related tests are simple, well standardized, cheap, and the screening tests of choice. The VDRL is readily quantified and, for that reason, is the test of choice for following the response of patients to treatment. Because the VDRL detects antibody against a normal tissue component, it may be falsely positive in a significant number of conditions. The relative proportion of patients with a false-positive VDRL depends on the prevalence of syphilis in the community; the lower the prevalence of syphilis, the higher the proportion of reactive VDRL tests that are due to nonsyphilitic causes.

The VDRL test begins to turn positive 1 to 2 weeks after the onset of the chancre. In large series of patients with primary syphilis, approximately two thirds have had a positive VDRL test result. Obviously, then, a nonreactive VDRL test does not exclude primary syphilis, particularly if the lesion is <2 weeks old. The VDRL is positive in 99% of patients with secondary syphilis, the only exceptions being patients with such high titers of antibody that they are in antibody excess; dilution of the serum then paradoxically results

TABLE 318–2. SEROLOGIC TESTS FOR SYPHILIS

Type	Use
Nontreponemal (anticardiolipin) antibodies:	
VDRL (slide flocculation)	Screening, quantitation, following response to treatment
RPR (circle-card) (agglutination)	Screening
Specific treponemal antibodies:	
FTA-ABS (immunofluorescence with absorbed serum)	Confirmatory, diagnostic, not for routine screening
MHA-TP (microhemagglutination)	Similar to FTA-ABS but can be quantified and automated

VDRL = Venereal Disease Research Laboratories test.
RPR = Rapid plasma reagin test.
FTA-ABS = Fluorescent treponemal antibody absorption test.
MHA-TP = Microhemagglutination assay for *T. pallidum*.

in conversion of a negative test to positive. In patients with coexistent HIV infection, the serologic responses to syphilis may be modified. In large groups of syphilis patients nontreponemal test titers tend to be higher than for comparison groups of patients without HIV infection. In contrast, however, there are also case reports of patients with advanced HIV infection in whom development of a serologic response was delayed or absent and infection could be diagnosed only by biopsy. For most patients with HIV infection, however, serologic tests for syphilis remain useful for diagnosis and management. VDRL reactivity tends to diminish in later stages of the disease, and only about 70% of patients with cardiovascular or neurosyphilis have a positive VDRL test result.

The *quantitative titer* of the VDRL test is somewhat useful in diagnosis and quite useful in following therapeutic response. The titer is reported as the highest dilution that gives a positive response. Most patients with secondary syphilis have titers of at least 1:16. Most patients with false-positive VDRL tests have titers of < 1:8. No single titer is in itself diagnostic. Significant rises (fourfold or greater) in paired sera, however, are strongly indicative of acute syphilis.

Treponemal Tests. There are many varieties of specific treponemal antibody tests. The most widely used is the fluorescent treponemal antibody absorption (FTA-ABS) test. Patient serum is absorbed with extracts of nonpathogenic cultivable treponemes to remove cross-reacting group treponemal antibody. Agglutination of red cells to which *T. pallidum* antigens have been fixed is the basis of the microhemagglutination assay for *T. pallidum* (MHA-TP).

The precise nature of the antigens involved in these tests is not known. Characterization of the antigens of *T. pallidum* has been greatly hindered by inability to grow the organism in cell-free culture. Recent success in cloning *T. pallidum* antigens into *Escherichia coli* may circumvent this problem. Antibodies reactive in the various tests are found in all major immunoglobulin classes (IgG, IgM, IgA). A modification of the FTA-ABS test has been developed using fluorescein-labeled anti–human IgM (IgM FTA-ABS). The IgM FTA-ABS test is of some use in the diagnosis of early congenital syphilis but is of no use in distinguishing acute disease from old infections in adults.

The FTA-ABS test is best used as a confirmatory test. It is somewhat more difficult to perform than the VDRL test and cannot be easily quantified. It is sensitive and has a high degree of specificity, being reactive in only approximately 1% of normal individuals. It is reactive in 85% of patients with primary syphilis, 99% with secondary syphilis, and at least 95% with late syphilis. It may therefore be the only test positive in patients with cardiovascular or neurologic syphilis. In late syphilis the FTA-ABS test often remains reactive for life despite adequate therapy. It (as well as the MHA-TP) is positive in other treponemal diseases, such as pinta, yaws, and endemic syphilis (formerly bejel) (see Ch. 319).

The FTA-ABS test is reported in terms of relative brilliance of fluorescence, from borderline to 4+. Borderline reactivity has the same meaning as nonreactive for clinical purposes. Most laboratories report 1+ positive tests as reactive, but some studies have shown that such tests may be difficult to reproduce. Occasional laboratories therefore report as positive only tests with 2+ or greater reactivity. In patients lacking historical or clinical evidence of syphilis but with a reactive FTA-ABS test, one should repeat the FTA-ABS test. Use of another treponemal test such as the MHA-TP may be helpful in problem cases.

The MHA-TP test is less sensitive than either the VDRL or the FTA-ABS test in primary syphilis. Its sensitivity and specificity otherwise are nearly identical to those of the FTA-ABS test, being reactive in nearly all patients with secondary syphilis and in ≥ 95% of patients with late syphilis. The reactivity of serologic tests for syphilis in various stages of disease is shown in Table 318–3.

TABLE 318–3. FREQUENCY OF POSITIVE SEROLOGIC TESTS IN UNTREATED SYPHILIS

Stage	VDRL (%)	FTA-ABS (%)	MHA-TP (%)
Primary	70	85	50–60
Secondary	99	100	100
Latent or late	70	98	98

False-Positive Serologic Test Results for Syphilis. The VDRL or RPR test may be reactive in a variety of diseases other than syphilis. A false-positive result is defined as a reproducible positive test in a patient with no clinical or historical evidence of syphilis and whose serum FTA-ABS or MHA-TP test is negative.

"Acute" (<6 months) false-positive VDRL test results occur with low frequency in atypical pneumonia, malaria, and other bacterial or viral infections and may occur after smallpox or other vaccinations as well. *Chronic false-positive VDRL tests* (lasting >6 months) are relatively common in autoimmune disorders such as systemic lupus erythematosus (SLE), in narcotic addicts, in HIV infection, in leprosy, and in aged persons. From 8 to 20% of patients with SLE have been reported as having a false-positive VDRL test, and the false-positive result may develop many years prior to the onset of other manifestations of the disease. A chronic false-positive VDRL test in females aged 20 or younger carries a significant risk of future development of SLE, thyroiditis, or other autoimmune disorders, and such patients should be followed carefully for a considerable period of time. As many as one third of patients with narcotic addiction have a false-positive VDRL test. More than 1% of patients aged 70 and 10% of patients over age 80 have a low-titer false-positive VDRL test. Most false-positive VDRL tests have a titer of ≤ 1:8, although occasional patients with lymphoma and other diseases have been described with very high-titer false-positive VDRL tests.

A reactive FTA-ABS result is usually indicative of recent or past syphilis. However, there is an increased incidence of false-positive FTA-ABS results in SLE and in other chronic inflammatory diseases associated with hyperglobulinemia, including rheumatoid arthritis, biliary cirrhosis, and others.

Occasionally one encounters reproducible positive FTA-ABS results in patients with no clinical or historical evidence of syphilis and in whom there is no evidence of diseases associated with false-positive FTA-ABS results. It may be wise to obtain CSF for examination of total protein, cells, and VDRL reactivity in order to rule out neurosyphilis. If in doubt and if the patient is not allergic to penicillin, it is often wisest to treat such patients for possible syphilis.

IgM FTA-ABS Test for Congenital Syphilis. Mothers with a reactive VDRL or FTA-ABS deliver infants with a reactive VDRL and FTA-ABS because of passive transfer of the IgG antibodies reactive in these tests. Because many infants with congenital syphilis are clinically normal at birth but develop serious symptomatic disease some weeks later, it is important to determine whether a newborn with a reactive VDRL or FTA-ABS test has passively transferred maternal antibody or is actively infected. Because maternal IgM antibodies are not passively transferred to the fetus, an IgM FTA-ABS test has been developed to detect syphilis in the newborn. Unfortunately there is approximately a 35% incidence of false-negative IgM FTA-ABS test results in delayed-onset congenital syphilis. There also is a false-positive rate of approximately 10%. For these reasons the IgM FTA-ABS test is of limited use for diagnosing neonatal syphilis.

If the mother has been adequately treated for syphilis during pregnancy and the infant is clinically normal at birth, one may elect to follow the infant carefully by serial examination and VDRL titers. If the reactive VDRL in the infant is due to passively transferred maternal antibody, the titer of reactivity falls markedly in the first 2 months of life. A rising titer indicates active disease and the need for treatment. Many physicians are unwilling to risk failure of proper follow-up of VDRL-positive but clinically normal neonates and instead administer effective therapy immediately. The risk of penicillin allergy in neonates is very low.

TREATMENT. *T. pallidum* is highly susceptible to penicillin, being inhibited by < 0.01 μg of penicillin G. Because treponemes divide slowly and because penicillin acts only on dividing cells, it is necessary to maintain serum levels of penicillin for many days. Studies in animals and in humans show that more therapy is required as the length of infection increases. Current recommendations for treatment of syphilis are summarized in Table 318–4.

Early (< 1 Year) Infectious Syphilis. Early syphilis may be treated with a single injection of 2.4 million units of *benzathine penicillin G,* which provides low but effective serum levels for >2 weeks. Extensive studies in the 1940's and 1950's with regimens

TABLE 318–4. PENICILLIN TREATMENT PRACTICE IN SYPHILIS AS RECOMMENDED BY UNITED STATES PUBLIC HEALTH SERVICE

Indications for Syphilis Therapy†	Dosage and Administration*	
	Benzathine Penicillin G	Aqueous Benzyl Penicillin G or Procaine Penicillin G
Primary, secondary, and early latent syphilis (< 1 year); epidemiologic treatment	Total of 2.4 million units; single IM dose of two injections of 1.2 million units in one session	Total of 4.8 million units IM in doses of 600,000 units daily for 8 consecutive days
Late latent (> 1 year) or when CSF was not examined in "latency"; cardiovascular syphilis, late benign (cutaneous, osseous, visceral gumma)	Total of 7.2 million units IM in doses of 2.4 million units at 7-day intervals, over 21 days	Total of 9 million units IM in doses of 600,000 units daily over 15 days
Symptomatic or asymptomatic neurosyphilis	2 to 4 million units of aqueous (crystalline) penicillin G IV every 4 hours for at least 10 days	2 to 4 million units procaine penicillin IM daily and probenecid, 500 mg orally 4 times daily for 10–14 days
Congenital Infants	CSF normal: Total of 50,000 units per kilogram IM in a single or divided dose at one session	CSF abnormal: Total of 50,000 units per kilogram IM per day for 10 consecutive days‡
Older children	CSF normal: Same as for early congenital syphilis, up to 2.4 million units	CSF abnormal: 200,000–300,000 units per kilogram per day IV aqueous crystalline penicillin for 10–14 days

*Individual doses can be divided for injection in each buttock to minimize discomfort.

†In *pregnancy,* treatment is dependent on the stage of syphilis.

‡For aqueous penicillin, give in two divided IV doses per day; for procaine penicillin, give as one daily dose IM.

that provided similar serum levels and duration of therapy showed that approximately 95% of patients were cured by such treatment. Many of the remaining 5% who had clinical or serologic evidence of relapse may actually have been reinfected. It is not necessary to examine the CSF at this stage because penicillin prevents development of later neurosyphilis. Motile treponemes disappear from primary lesions in 24 hours.

A single injection of 2.4 million units of *aqueous procaine penicillin,* which provides relatively high serum levels for a brief period, is ineffective in established early syphilis but is curative if the disease is still in the incubating stage. The ceftriaxone regimen currently useful for gonorrhea probably is curative for incubating syphilis, but data are few, and careful follow-up is indicated if there is reason to suspect exposure to syphilis in a patient treated for gonorrhea with ceftriaxone. The incidence of incubating syphilis in gonorrhea patients is ≥ 2% in several series.

For patients allergic to penicillin, doxycyline, 100 mg twice daily for 14 days, is recommended. Particularly careful follow-up is necessary in patients treated with drugs other than penicillin, because patients may not be fully compliant with these prolonged courses of oral therapy and these regimens have been less fully evaluated clinically. Ceftriaxone, 2 grams intramuscularly daily for 10 days, may be effective but has not been well studied. Chloramphenicol is of equivocal efficacy and for this reason, as well as because of the risk of toxicity, should not be used. Spectinomycin and quinolone antibiotics have essentially no effect on syphilis. Erythromycin is of questionable efficacy.

Syphilis of > 1 Year's Duration. Larger doses of penicillin are needed for *neurosyphilis* (see Ch. 422) than for syphilis of < 1

year's duration. In general, patients with general paresis respond better to treatment than do patients with tabes dorsalis, although patients with paresis should be expected to show residual effects of the infection. This is particularly true in advanced cases. Meningovascular syphilis usually responds well, except for residual damage resulting from ischemic infarcts. Published studies show that a total of 6.0 to 9.0 million units of penicillin G results in a satisfactory clinical response in approximately 90% of patients with neurosyphilis, in the absence of HIV infection.

Benzathine penicillin regimens have received relatively little study in neurosyphilis but were previously recommended. However, there are reports of patients who have failed standard benzathine penicillin therapy for neurosyphilis but who responded to intensive intravenous therapy that provided high serum levels of penicillin. Benzathine penicillin does not provide measurable levels of penicillin in the spinal fluid or aqueous humor of the eye. There are anecdotal reports of increased treatment failures in patients with concomitant HIV infection. *Therefore there is considerable rationale to treatment with intravenous penicillin G (20 million units per day for at least 10 days in hospital).* Therapy of neurosyphilis not infrequently results in increased CSF pleocytosis for 7 to 10 days after starting treatment and may transiently convert a normal CSF to abnormal.

Limited evidence suggests that treating *latent syphilis* with 7.2 million units total dose of benzathine penicillin is curative even if the patient has asymptomatic neurosyphilis. However, because of the possible lack of the efficacy of benzathine penicillin in some patients with CNS syphilis, it is preferable to examine CSF in all patients with latent syphilis to exclude asymptomatic neurosyphilis. This is particularly important in HIV-positive patients. Alternatively, a lumbar puncture may be performed at the conclusion of the follow-up period (2 years); if the CSF is normal, the patient can be reassured that neurosyphilis will not develop.

There is no evidence that therapy with antimicrobial drugs is clinically beneficial to patients with *cardiovascular syphilis.* Nevertheless, treatment of cardiovascular syphilis is recommended in order to prevent further progression of disease and because approximately 15% of patients with cardiovascular syphilis have associated neurosyphilis.

There is no evidence regarding the efficacy of other antimicrobials in the treatment of later syphilis. Therefore if patients are allergic to penicillin, it is mandatory that the CSF be examined before therapy is undertaken. Either tetracycline or doxycycline taken for 4 weeks is probably effective.

Syphilis in Pregnancy. All pregnant women should be examined with a VDRL or RPR test during pregnancy; if they are at high risk for syphilis, a second test should be obtained before delivery. Because of the risk to the fetus, evaluation and treatment of the VDRL-positive patient should be done as rapidly as possible, particularly for patients first seen in the later stages of pregnancy. If a confirmatory FTA-ABS is positive and the patient has not been treated, penicillin should be administered in doses appropriate for early or late syphilis as outlined above. Penicillin-allergic patients should not be treated with tetracycline or erythromycin because of toxicity (tetracycline) or lack of efficacy (erythromycin). Penicillin desensitization may be considered but also carries risks. For patients who are VDRL positive but FTA-ABS negative and who have no clinical signs of syphilis, treatment may be withheld. In such patients a quantitative VDRL test and another FTA-ABS test should be repeated in 4 weeks. If the VDRL titer has risen by fourfold or more, or if clinical signs of syphilis have developed, the patient should be treated. If after repeat examination the diagnosis remains equivocal, the patient should be treated to prevent possible disease in the neonate. After treatment a quantitative VDRL titer should be followed monthly; if it rises fourfold, the patient should be treated a second time.

Congenital Syphilis. Proper treatment of the mother usually prevents active congenital syphilis in the neonate. However, infected infants may be clinically normal at birth, and the infant may be seronegative if the mother's infection was acquired late in pregnancy. The infant should be treated at birth if the mother has received no or inadequate treatment, or has been treated with drugs other than penicillin, if the mother has not yet responded to possibly effective therapy, or if the infant cannot be carefully followed up for several months after birth. The CSF should be examined before the infant is treated. If the CSF is normal, treatment may be with a single injection of 50,000 units per kilogram of benzathine penicillin G. If the CSF is abnormal, treatment should be with aqueous penicillin G, 50,000 units per kilogram intramuscularly or intravenously daily, given in two divided doses, for a minimum of 10 days. Alternatively, a single daily intramuscular injection of procaine penicillin G, 50,000 units per kilogram, may be given for 10 days. These recommendations are based upon the failure of benzathine penicillin to provide adequate treponemicidal levels in spinal fluid and on evidence that aqueous or procaine penicillin does provide adequate CSF levels of penicillin. Many experts believe that all syphilis in infected infants should be treated with either procaine or aqueous penicillin to ensure adequate CSF levels. Tetracycline should not be used to treat children younger than age 8. Antimicrobial agents other than penicillin are not recommended for treating congenital syphilis.

Follow-up Examinations. All HIV-seronegative patients with early syphilis or congenital syphilis should return for quantitative VDRL titers and clinical examination 3, 6, and 12 months after treatment. Treatment failure is somewhat more common in patients with HIV infection and although more aggressive therapy is usually not required, more aggressive follow-up is suggested. Serologic tests should be repeated at 1, 2, 3, 6, 9, and 12 months. Patients with late latent syphilis should be examined also at 24 months after therapy; if CSF was not examined prior to therapy, a lumbar puncture should be done prior to discharge to rule out inadequately treated asymptomatic neurosyphilis.

In most patients with early (primary, secondary, or early latent) syphilis, quantitative VDRL titers become nonreactive in 12 to 24 months after therapy. Prolonged reactive VDRL test results are associated with higher initial VDRL titers, prolonged infection, more advanced stage (primary < secondary < early latent), or repeated infection. In a small percentage of patients with early syphilis, the VDRL remains reactive in low titer for long periods. Chronic lowtiter VDRL reactivity after therapy is much more common in late syphilis and should not be viewed with alarm. The FTA-ABS test may remain positive for years, despite adequate therapy. A fourfold or greater rise of VDRL titer after therapy is sufficient evidence for retreatment. Patients with treated early syphilis are fully susceptible to reinfection, and many clinical and serologic relapses after therapy are probably reinfections. As such they represent failures of proper epidemiologic case finding and of preventive therapy of the patient's sexual contacts.

Patients with neurosyphilis should be followed with serologic tests for at least 3 years and with repeat examination of CSF at 6-month intervals. The CSF pleocytosis is the first abnormality to disappear, but cell counts may not be normal for 1 to 2 years. The elevated CSF protein level falls more slowly, followed by the positive CSF-VDRL test, which may take years to become negative. It is not known whether high-dose intravenous penicillin therapy accelerates the return of CSF to normal. Rising CSF cell counts, protein, and VDRL titer obtained at follow-up are an indication for retreatment.

Epidemiologic Investigation and Treatment. All patients with syphilis should be reported to public health authorities. In the absence of an effective vaccine, control of syphilis depends on finding and treating persons with infectious lesions of primary and secondary syphilis before they can further transmit the disease and on finding and treating persons with incubating syphilis before they develop infectious lesions. All patients with early syphilis (< 1 year) should be carefully interviewed by qualified persons to determine the nature of their recent sex contacts. Approximately 16% of the named recent contacts of patients with early syphilis are found to have active untreated syphilis on examination, and a similar proportion of individuals named as suspects or associates also have active syphilis.

Most authorities, particularly in the United States, recommend treating sexual contacts of patients with early syphilis even if the contacts are clinically and serologically normal on examination. This is justifiable, because 30% of clinically normal individuals named as contacts of persons with infectious lesions of syphilis within the previous 30 days go on to develop syphilis if untreated. In general, preventive treatment is given to all sexual contacts of the past 90 days, although nearly all cases of syphilis in contacts develop within 60 days of exposure.

Jarisch-Herxheimer Reactions. Up to 60% of patients with early syphilis, and a significant proportion of patients with later

stages of syphilis, experience a transient febrile reaction after therapy for syphilis. This usually occurs in the first few hours after therapy, peaks at 6 to 8 hours, and disappears within 12 to 24 hours of therapy. Temperature elevation is usually low grade, and there is often associated myalgia, headache, and malaise. The skin lesions of secondary syphilis are often exacerbated during the Herxheimer reaction, and cutaneous lesions that were not visible may become visible. It is usually of no clinical significance and may be treated with salicylates in most cases. In patients with syphilis of the coronary ostia or of the optic nerve, there is a theoretical risk that local inflammation coincident with the Herxheimer reaction could precipitate serious damage. This is the subject of much discussion in the old literature, but there is little current evidence that "local Herxheimer reactions" constitute a significant risk to the patient. Corticosteroids have been used to prevent adverse effects of the Herxheimer reaction, but there is no evidence that they are clinically beneficial (other than reducing fever) or necessary. Institution of treatment with small doses of penicillin does not prevent the Herxheimer reaction.

The pathogenesis of the Herxheimer reaction is unclear. It may be due to liberation of antigens from the spirochetes. There is evidence that the complement cascade (see Ch. 222) is activated, including transient consumption of C3, C4, C6, and C7, and of transient decrease in treponemal antibodies coincident with the Herxheimer reaction. There is also evidence for endotoxemia, obtained by positive limulus amebocyte gelatin tests, at the time of the Herxheimer reaction, although *T. pallidum* does not contain biologically active endotoxin. These seemingly contradictory observations could be explained if the reaction resulted in release of endogenous endotoxin from the gut.

Persistence of Treponemes After Treatment. Studies in humans and in rabbits have shown that spiral forms may be visualized by silver stains in lymph nodes after effective treatment. Living virulent treponemes have occasionally been recovered by rabbit inoculation from lymph nodes, CSF, or ocular fluids after effective treatment has been given. These documented cases of treponemal persistence are very rare, however. At present there is little reason to worry about persistence of virulent treponemes after therapy with penicillin, with the possible exception of CNS syphilis, which needs further evaluation. No evidence exists for selection of penicillin-resistant mutants of *T. pallidum* to date.

PROSPECTS FOR PREVENTION. Solid immunity develops in rabbits following prolonged infection with virulent *T. pallidum*. It has not yet been possible to transfer immunity passively in laboratory animals by either immune serum or immune lymphocytes alone, suggesting that both cellular and humoral systems are necessary for immunity. Rabbits have been effectively immunized with multiple injections of treponemes that have been rendered avirulent by irradiation or by exposure to cold. However, a very large number of injections and a large mass of treponemes are necessary to effect immunity in the laboratory animal. For this reason and because *T. pallidum* cannot yet be grown in a virulent state in cell-free medium, there is no immediate prospect for a vaccine. However, significant immunity does develop in humans after prolonged infection. For the present, control depends entirely on clinical awareness on the part of physicians, adequate reporting to public health authorities, and vigorous application of epidemiologic investigation and preventive treatment of sexual contacts.

Cox DL, Chang P, McDowell A, Radolf JD: The outer membrane, not a coat of host proteins, limits the antigenicity of virulent *Treponema pallidum*. Infect Immun 60:1076, 1992. *New data regarding the causative agent of syphilis and the reasons humoral antibody does not control or prevent infection.*

Drusin LM, Singer C, Valenti AJ, et al.: Infectious syphilis mimicking neoplastic disease. Arch Intern Med 137:156, 1977. *A fascinating and frightening account of diagnostic problems caused by oral, rectal, or lymphatic syphilis, nearly leading to cancer surgery.*

Feher J, Somogyi T, Timmer M, et al.: Early syphilitic hepatitis. Lancet 2:896, 1975. *A description of the frequency and histology of early syphilitic hepatitis.*

Fischer A, Kristensen JK, Husfelt V: Tertiary syphilis in Denmark 1961–1970. A description of 105 cases not previously diagnosed or specifically treated. Acta Dermatovener 56:485, 1975. *One of few studies of the prevalence of newly diagnosed late syphilis in the antibiotic era.*

Gamble CN, Reardan JB: Immunopathogenesis of syphilitic glomerulonephritis: Elution of antitreponemal antibody from glomerular immune-complex deposits. N Engl J Med 292:449, 1975. *Clear evidence for an immune-complex cause of syphilitic nephrosis.*

Gjestland T: The Oslo study of untreated syphilis: An epidemiologic investigation of the natural course of the syphilitic infection based upon a re-study of the Boeck-

Bruusgaard material. Acta Derm Venereol 35:Suppl 34, 1955. *A medical classic, in which the long-term course of untreated syphilis is evaluated.*

Holmes KK, Märdh P-A, Sparling PF, et al.: Sexually Transmitted Diseases, 2nd ed. New York, McGraw-Hill, 1990. *The definitive text on sexually transmitted diseases.*

Hook EW III, Marra CM: Acquired syphilis in adults. N Engl J Med 326:1060, 1992. *A review of syphilis in the 1990's, including syphilis-HIV interactions.*

Lee TJ, Sparling PF: Syphilis. An algorithm. JAMA 242:1187, 1979. *An algorithm for management of patients who present with a positive VDRL or similar test.*

Lugar A, Schmidt B, Spendlingwimmer I, et al.: Recent observations on the serology of syphilis. Br J Vener Dis 56:12, 1980. *An evaluation of the merits of serologic tests for syphilis.*

Magnuson HJ, Thomas EW, Olansky S, et al.: Inoculation syphilis in human volunteers. Medicine 35:33, 1956. *A classic paper, in which prison volunteers were inoculated with virulent T. pallidum. Immunity to inoculation syphilis was observed only in individuals who had congenital or late syphilis.*

Raskind MA, Eisdorfer C: Screening for syphilis in an aged psychiatrically impaired population. West J Med 125:361, 1976. *Syphilitic disease of the CNS may be more prevalent than hospital surveys suggest.*

Tramont EC: Persistence of *Treponema pallidum* following penicillin G therapy: Report of two cases. JAMA 236:2206, 1976. *At least one of the cases of neurosyphilis probably was a true penicillin treatment failure.*

Wilner E, Brody JA: Prognosis of general paresis after treatment. Lancet 2:1370, 1968. *Neurosyphilis frequently shows clinical progression despite what is probably adequate therapy.*

Spirochetal Diseases Other Than Syphilis

319 NONSYPHILITIC TREPONEMATOSES

Edward W. Hook III*

DEFINITION. The nonsyphilitic treponematoses are the skin diseases called *yaws, endemic syphilis* (previously known as *bejel*), and *pinta.* They occur predominantly in tropical regions and are transmitted by skin contact with infected persons. Disfiguring ulcerations of the skin may be produced, and invasion of bone and other tissues has been described. Treatment with benzathine penicillin G is effective, and the World Health Organization (WHO) has carried out extensive treatment campaigns in endemic areas.

ETIOLOGY. Yaws is caused by *Treponema pallidum* subspecies *pertenue;* pinta is caused by *T. carateum;* and endemic syphilis is caused by *T. pallidum* subspecies *endemicum.* The *T. pallidum* subspecies causing nonsyphilitic treponematoses are closely related to *T. pallidum* subspecies *pallidum,* which causes venereal syphilis; there is a high degree of DNA homology, and they share unique, pathogen-restricted antigens. Like *T. pallidum,* these treponemes are spirochetal bacteria with helical structures and measure about 0.2 μ in diameter and 10 μ in length. They are visible by darkfield microscopy but cannot be cultivated for prolonged periods *in vitro.*

DISTRIBUTION AND EPIDEMIOLOGY. Yaws is prevalent in rural areas of tropical Africa, the Americas, Southeast Asia, and Oceania. The highest incidence is in children between ages 2 and 5 years. Endemic syphilis occurs in Africa, in Eastern Mediterranean countries, on the Arabian peninsula, in Central Asia, and in Australia. It is most prevalent in arid regions. Pinta occurs in rural areas of tropical Central and South America. Pinta affects mostly older children and adolescents. Humans are the only known carriers of the nonsyphilitic treponematoses. The spirochete enters the skin only after it is broken, as by a scratch or insect bite. Transmission is believed to occur by contacting the skin directly or indirectly by contaminated hands or fomites and is facilitated by conditions of poor personal hygiene and crowding.

CLINICAL FEATURES. *Yaws* produces a skin papule at the inoculation site after an incubation period of 3 to 4 weeks. The most common sites are the legs and buttocks. The papule enlarges, ulcerates, and develops a serous crust from which treponemes can be recovered. Regional lymphadenitis may accompany the papule, which will heal spontaneously within 6 months. A generalized secondary rash will occur before or after the initial lesion heals, and these rashes are also papular and often covered with brown crusts. Relapsing crops of lesions can occur. Papillomas may result, and the plantar surfaces of the feet are involved with hyperkeratotic lesions. Periostitis of long bones leads to tender bones, and fever may be present. Relapsing lesions may occur over several years, resulting in chronic ulcerations and destructive gummatous lesions affecting the skin and bones.

Endemic syphilis produces patches on the mucous membranes of the oral cavity and pharynx and can cause split papules at the mucocutaneous junction of the oral angles. Anal, genital, and other intertriginous skin areas can be affected by lesions that resemble secondary syphilis. Regional lymphadenitis is common, and generalized rashes are rare. Healing of these early lesions is followed by latency manifested by seropositivity or by late lesions that resemble tertiary syphilis. These include nodular ulcers of skin, deformities of bones, and gummatous lesions that can perforate the palate.

Pinta starts similarly as a cutaneous papule with regional lymphadenitis that is followed by a generalized maculopapular eruption. One to three years after healing of the initial lesion, large hyperpigmented macules that are brown or blue develop and subsequently lose their pigment and become white. The time required for lesions to pass through these stages varies, so that the same patient may have coexisting areas of increased pigment and loss of pigment.

DIAGNOSIS. By darkfield microscopy, the causative spirochetes from early skin lesions can be observed directly. Spirochetes have been demonstrated also in lymph node aspirates. There is no specific test for any of the nonsyphilitic treponematoses. Serologic tests for syphilis detect cross-reacting antibodies in these diseases. The VDRL test, the serologic test for syphilis, and the fluorescent treponemal antibody absorption test all give positive results if serum is obtained at least 2 weeks after the lesions initially appear.

TREATMENT AND PROGNOSIS. Long-acting benzathine penicillin G given as 1.2 million units intramuscularly is the preferred treatment for patients with early lesions. For patients with late manifestations, this therapy should be repeated twice at approximately 7-day intervals. The early lesions heal rapidly, and most seropositive cases convert to seronegative status. Late destructive lesions take longer to show improvement.

PREVENTION. The prevalence of these diseases has been reduced in several areas of the world by mass treatment campaigns using penicillin. The WHO has treated about 53 million cases of yaws and 350,000 cases of pinta in the field with good results. These campaigns, however, are not adequate to eradicate the disease, and in recent years the prevalence of yaws may have increased. It has been suggested that reduction in transmission requires improvements in the sanitation and economic standards of people living in endemic areas.

Engeikens HJ, Niemel PL, van der Sluis JJ, et al.: Endemic treponematoses. Part II. Pinta and endemic syphilis. Int J Dermatol 30:231, 1991.

Guthe T: Clinical serological and epidemiological features of framboesia tropica (yaws) and its control in rural communities. Acta Dermatovener 49:343, 1969.

Hackett CJ, Lowenthal LJA: Differential Diagnosis of Yaws. WHO Monograph Series No. 45. Geneva, WHO, 1960.

Kantor I, Wilentz JM, Berger BB: Yaws. Arch Dermatol 103:546, 1971.

Koff AB, Rosen T: Nonvenereal treponematoses: yaws, endemic syphilis, and pinta. J Am Acad Dermatol 29:519, 1993. *With worldwide travel there is a need to consider diagnosis of nonvenereal treponematoses in appropriate clinical and historical situations.*

Vorst FA: Clinical diagnosis and changing manifestations of treponemal infection. Rev Infect Dis 7(suppl 2):S327, 1985. *This paper shows that yaws in populations after mass treatment with penicillin assumes attenuated forms characterized by shorter duration of papillomas and lower antibody titers.*

* The author acknowledges the contribution of Dr. Thomas Butler on this subject in the 19th edition of the *Cecil Textbook of Medicine.*

320 RELAPSING FEVER
William A. Petri, Jr.

DEFINITION. Relapsing fever is a spirochetal infection with bacteria of the genus *Borrelia*. There are two modes of transmission: epidemic louse-borne and endemic tick-borne relapsing fever.

ETIOLOGY. *Borrelia* are spirochetes that measure 0.5 μ in diameter and 5 to 40 μ in length. They are aerophilic and require long-chain fatty acids for growth. Louse-borne relapsing fever is caused by *B. recurrentis*. Tick-borne relapsing fever organisms are named after their tick vector and include the closely related species *B. duttonii* (Old World) and *B. hermsii*, *B. turicatae*, and *B. parkeri* (North America).

EPIDEMIOLOGY. Louse-borne epidemic relapsing fever is carried from person to person by the human body louse. There is no animal reservoir. The spirochete lives in the hemolymph, and infection is transmitted to humans when the louse is crushed. Epidemics have occurred at wartime when breakdown in sanitation favors transmission of body lice. Louse-borne disease remains endemic in Ethiopia, Somalia, and the Sudan.

Tick-borne endemic relapsing fever is carried by *Ornithodoros* ticks, which become infected by feeding on wild rodents. In the United States, relapsing fever is limited to mountainous areas of the West at altitudes of 1500 to 8000 feet where the tick vector *O. hermsii* resides in forests of ponderosa pine and Douglas fir. A key diagnostic clue has been a history of sleeping in rodent-infested rustic cabins in western national parks.

PATHOLOGY AND PATHOGENESIS. *Borrelia* infection begins in the skin at the site of the louse or tick bite and is followed by rapid dissemination of the spirochetes via the bloodstream. Spirochetes are visible on Wright's stained peripheral blood smears during the initial febrile episode and during each relapse in most patients. Clearance of spirochetes from the blood is associated with the production of serotype-specific immune sera; anti-*Borrelia* antibodies have been shown in animal models to be the major mechanism of immune clearance of infection.

Relapses are associated with antigenic variation in the variable major proteins (VMP's), which are the abundant outer-membrane proteins of the spirochete that carry the serotype-specific epitopes. Antigenic variation is the consequence of recombination events occurring between VMP genes at silent and expression sites on linear plasmids.

CLINICAL FEATURES. An abrupt onset of fever to 38.5 to 40°C (>39°C in most patients), headache, myalgias, and shaking chills characterize the onset of illness. Cough, nausea and vomiting, and fatigue are less frequent complaints. Signs include fever, tachycardia, lethargy or confusion, conjunctival injection, and epistaxis. Hepatosplenomegaly, jaundice, and often a truncal petechial skin rash are common signs in louse-borne relapsing fever. Untreated louse-borne disease lasts 6 days, and relapses occur once after an afebrile period of 9 days. Tick-borne relapsing fever lasts about 4 days without antibiotic treatment and an average of two relapses occur after a 10-day afebrile period.

Relapsing fever in pregnancy results in miscarriage in one third of patients. Neonatal infection presents in both the tick- and louse-borne forms with jaundice, hepatosplenomegaly, and often sepsis and hemorrhage. Fever and hepatosplenomegaly are also common signs in children.

LABORATORY FEATURES. Spirochetes can be demonstrated in the Wright's stained peripheral blood smear of most patients. The white blood count is usually normal, but platelet counts <50,000 per cu mm occur in up to 90% of cases of louse-borne disease. Prothrombin and partial thromboplastin times are often prolonged. In louse-borne disease, elevations in hepatic enzymes and blood urea nitrogen are common. The degree of spirochetemia is often 10^5 organisms per cu mm.

DIAGNOSIS. Spirochetes can be demonstrated on peripheral blood smears taken during the febrile episodes in 70% of patients. With an average incubation period of one week, relapsing fever is often diagnosed in a nonendemic area after the individual has returned from a stay in the Rocky Mountains. Only a few patients will remember tick exposure, since *O. hermsii* is a night feeder and only remains attached for 15 minutes. Culture of the organism requires a special medium and is not practical in a clinical laboratory setting. Because the number of organisms in blood is extremely high, the diagnosis is most often made by direct visualization of the organism on a blood smear.

PROGNOSIS. Epidemics of louse-borne relapsing fever have been reported, with mortalities approaching 40%. With antibiotic treatment, mortality is <5% in all recent series, with complete recovery expected. Autopsies of patients with louse-borne disease have documented intracranial hemorrhage, brain edema, bronchopneumonia, hepatic necrosis, and splenic infarcts.

THERAPY AND PREVENTION. A single 500-mg dose of tetracycline may be as effective as longer treatments in clearing spirochetemia of louse-borne disease, although many physicians still treat with 500 mg tetracycline every 6 hours for 5 to 10 days. Erythromycin is also effective and should be used in children under age 7 (in whom tetracyclines can stain the permanent teeth). Penicillin treatment has been reported to clear the spirochetemia more slowly than tetracycline.

The Jarisch-Herxheimer reaction (typically characterized by a rise in body temperature of 1°C, rigors, a slight fall followed by a rise in blood pressure, and transient leukopenia) occurs 2 to 3 hours after treatment in many patients with louse-borne disease, less commonly in tick-borne disease, and should be anticipated and managed supportively. Deaths due to shock from the Jarisch-Herxheimer reaction occur rarely. The Jarisch-Herxheimer reaction has been associated with accelerated phagocytosis of spirochetes by neutrophils and transient elevations of tumor necrosis factor, interleukin-6, and interleukin-8.

Barbour AG: Antigenic variation of a relapsing fever *Borrelia* species. Annu Rev Microbiol 44:155, 1990. *Immunology and molecular biology of antigenic variation are reviewed.*

Common source outbreak of relapsing fever—California. MMWR 39:579, 1990. *Six individuals who had at different times spent the night in the same cabin at Big Bear Lake in California all developed relapsing fever with sudden onset of high fever, severe headache, prostration, nausea, and vomiting. Inhabited ground squirrel burrows were found under the cabin.*

Perine PL, Teklu B: Antibiotic treatment of louse-borne relapsing fever in Ethiopia: A report of 377 cases. Am J Trop Med Hyg 32:1096, 1983. *Tetracycline, doxycycline, erythromycin, and chloramphenicol were all effective as single-dose therapy but are associated with a Jarisch-Herxheimer reaction within 2 hours of drug administration.*

321 LYME DISEASE
Stephen E. Malawista

Lyme disease is a tick-borne inflammatory disorder caused by a newly recognized spirochete, *Borrelia burgdorferi*. Its clinical hallmark is an early expanding skin lesion, *erythema chronicum migrans* (ECM), which may be followed weeks to months later by neurologic, cardiac, or joint abnormalities. Symptoms may refer to any one of these four systems alone or in combination. All stages of Lyme disease may respond to antibiotics, but treatment of early disease is the most successful. Although cases of the illness are concentrated in certain endemic areas, foci of Lyme disease are widely distributed within the United States, Europe, and Asia.

"Lyme arthritis" was recognized in November 1975 because of unusual geographic clustering of children with inflammatory arthropathy in the region of Lyme, Connecticut. It soon became clear that this was a multisystem disorder (Lyme disease) occurring at any age, in both sexes, and often preceded by a characteristic expanding skin lesion, ECM. In Europe ECM had been associated with the bite of the sheep tick, *Ixodes ricinus*, and with tick-borne meningopolyneuritis. In the Lyme region, a closely related deer tick, *I. scapularis* (thought until recently to represent a new species, called *I. dammini*), was implicated as the principal disease vector on epidemiologic grounds. In 1982, Burgdorfer and associates iso-

...ated a spirochete, now called *B. burgdorferi,* from *I. scapularis* and linked it serologically to patients with Lyme disease. It was soon recovered from patient specimens.

DISTRIBUTION AND EPIDEMIOLOGY. Lyme disease is widespread. In the United States there are three distinct foci: the Northeast from Massachusetts to Maryland, the Midwest in Wisconsin and Minnesota, and the West in California, southern Oregon, and western Nevada. However, the illness has been reported in 46 states, as well as throughout Europe and Asia. The earliest known cases in the United States occurred on Cape Cod in 1962 and in Lyme, Connecticut, in 1965; annual cases now number in the thousands. Disease can occur at any age and in either gender. Onset of illness is generally between May 1 and November 30, with the peak in June and July.

The primary vectors of Lyme disease are tiny ixodid ticks. Major foci of disease correspond to the distribution of *I. scapularis* (Northeast, Midwest), *I. pacificus* (West), *I. ricinus* (Europe), and *I. persulcatus* (Eurasia, Asia), but other vectors, including the Lone Star tick, *Amblyomma americanum,* are likely in some areas. In one United States study, 31% of 314 patients recalled a tick bite at the skin site where ECM developed days to weeks later. The six ticks that were saved were invariably nymphal *I. scapularis,* whose peak questing period is May through July; the nymphal stage is primarily responsible for transmission of disease. Preferred hosts for *I. scapularis* nymphs are white-footed mice and, for adults, white-tailed deer, in whose fur they mate. A less successful transmission cycle involving the dusky footed woodrat has been described in California.

The rising incidence of Lyme disease in recent years in the United States may be explained by multiple factors, including an increase in the numbers of ixodid ticks, the outward migration of residential areas into previously rural woodlands (habitats favored by ixodid ticks and their hosts), an exploding deer population, and increased recognition.

In areas endemic for Lyme disease, the prevalence of *B. burgdorferi* in nymphal *I. scapularis* ranges from about 20 to >60% (cf. *I. pacificus,* 1 to 3%). The organism has been isolated, or specific antibody found, in blood and tissues of a wide variety of large and small animals, including domestic dogs and birds. Indiscriminate feeding on a variety of animals by immature *I. scapularis* may favor the spread of infection.

In high-risk areas, vaccines based on one of the outer surface proteins (OspA) of *B. burgdorferi,* which have been shown to protect animals against infection, are currently being tested in human volunteers.

PATHOGENESIS. Recovery of *B. burgdorferi* is straightforward from the tick but difficult from patients—except from ECM lesions, where the clinical diagnosis is usually obvious—in part because of a relative paucity of organisms in specimens of tissue and fluids from the latter. Nevertheless, rare positive cultures are reported at all stages of the illness—from blood (early), secondary annular lesions, meningitic cerebrospinal fluid (CSF), heart, joint fluid, ligament, and even a late skin lesion, *acrodermatitis chronica atrophicans,* that had been present for 10 years. Spirochetes have been identified by silver stain or by immunofluorescence in some histologic sections of ECM and rarely of secondary annular lesions, synovium, brain, eye, heart, striated muscle, ligament, liver, spleen, kidney, and bone marrow.

From these data, combined with clinical (see below) and epidemiologic features of Lyme disease, the following pathogenetic sequence is likely. *B. burgdorferi* is transmitted to the skin of the host via the tick vector. After an incubation period of 3 to 32 days, the organism migrates outward in the skin (ECM), spreads in lymph (regional adenopathy), or disseminates in blood to organs (e.g., central nervous system [CNS], joints, heart, and presumably liver and spleen) or other skin sites (secondary annular lesions; see below). Maternal-fetal transmission is distinctly uncommon. Although organisms are hard to find in later stages of Lyme disease, it is entirely possible that persistent live spirochetes are driving the illness throughout its course. Evidence for this interpretation includes the responsiveness of many patients to antibiotics, the rare sightings of spirochetes in affected tissues, the variable recovery from affected tissues and fluids of spirochetal DNA amplified by the polymerase chain reaction (PCR), and an expansion of the antibody response to additional spirochetal antigens over time. If live spirochetes are invariably present, it is not yet clear how they occasionally remain out of harm's way in the face of both antibiotic therapy and the body's usual phagocytic and other immune clearance mechanisms.

In the clinical laboratory, characteristic immune abnormalities are found. At disease onset (ECM), almost all patients have evidence of circulating immune complexes. At that time, the findings of elevated serum immunoglobulin M (IgM) levels and cryoglobulins containing IgM predict subsequent nervous system, heart, or joint involvement—i.e., early humoral findings have prognostic significance. Serial determinations of serum IgM are often the single most helpful laboratory indicator of disease activity. These abnormalities tend to persist during neurologic or cardiac involvement. Later in the illness, when arthritis is present, serum IgM levels are more often normal. By then, immune complexes are usually lacking in serum but are present uniformly in joint fluid, where their titers correlate positively with the local concentration of polymorphonuclear leukocytes. Mononuclear cells from peripheral blood increase their antigen-specific proliferative response as the disease progresses, but the greatest reactivity to antigen is seen in cells from inflamed joints. Adjacent to that joint fluid, on biopsy a proliferative synovium is seen, often replete with lymphocytes and plasma cells that are presumably capable of producing immunoglobulin locally. Thus an initially disseminated, immune-mediated inflammatory disorder becomes in some patients localized and propagated in joints.

Although *B. burgdorferi* seem not to destroy tissue directly, they nonspecifically activate monocytes, macrophages, synovial lining cells, B cells, and complement, resulting in the elaboration of a host of proinflammatory materials. These spirochetes adhere to extracellular matrix proteins, to endothelial cells (and penetrate endothelial monolayers), and to neural glycolipid. They can induce the production of cross-reactive antibodies and of specific immune B and T lymphocytes that may be associated histologically with endarteritic microvascular occlusive changes (e.g., in nervous tissue, hearts, joints), but it is not clear that these phenomena persist in the absence of live spirochetes.

In addition to factors related to the pathogenicity of specific isolates of *B. burgdorferi,* immunogenetic makeup may play a role in whether infected individuals can rid themselves of spirochetes, their antigens, or their effects. Patients with treatment-resistant chronic arthritis have been reported to have an increased frequency of the B-cell alloantigen HLA DR4.

CLINICAL CHARACTERISTICS. Lyme disease is conveniently divided into three clinical stages, but the stages may overlap, most patients do not exhibit all of them, and in fact seroconversion can occur in asymptomatic individuals. The illness usually begins with ECM and associated symptoms (stage 1), sometimes followed weeks to months later by neurologic or cardiac abnormalities (stage 2) and weeks to years later by arthritis (stage 3). Chronic neurologic and skin involvement also may occur years after onset.

Early Manifestations. ECM, the unique clinical marker for Lyme disease, begins as a red macule or papule at the site where the tick vector, usually long gone, had engorged. As the area of redness expands to 15 cm or so (range 3 to 68 cm), there is usually partial central clearing (see Color Plate 10*B*). The outer borders are red, generally flat, and without scaling. The centers are occasionally red and indurated, even vesicular or necrotic. Variations may occur—multiple rings, for example. The thigh, groin, and axilla are particularly common sites. The lesion is warm to touch, but not often sore, and is easily missed if out of sight. Routine histologic findings are nonspecific: a heavy dermal infiltrate of mononuclear cells, without epidermal change except at the site of the tick bite.

Within days of onset of ECM, one half of U.S. patients develop multiple annular secondary lesions (see Color Plate 10*B*; Table 321–1). They resemble ECM itself but are generally smaller, migrate less, and lack indurated centers; they are not associated with the sites of previous tick bites. Individual lesions may come and go, and their borders sometimes merge. Other occasional skin lesions are noted in Table 321–1. In addition, benign lymphocytoma cutis has been reported in Europe. ECM and secondary lesions fade in 3 to 4 weeks (range 1 day to 14 months). They may recur.

Skin involvement is often accompanied by musculoskeletal flu-like symptoms—malaise and fatigue, headache, fever and chills, myalgia, and arthralgia (Table 321–2). Even without ECM, this syndrome in summer, in an endemic area for Lyme disease, is grounds for treatment. Some patients have evidence of meningeal

TABLE 321-1. EARLY SIGNS OF LYME DISEASE

Signs	No. of Patients N = 314	(%)
Erythema chronicum migrans	314	(100)*
Multiple annular lesions	150	(48)
Lymphadenopathy		
Regional	128	(41)
Generalized	63	(20)
Pain on neck flexion	52	(17)
Malar rash	41	(13)
Erythematous throat	38	(12)
Conjunctivitis	35	(11)
Right upper quadrant tenderness	24	(8)
Splenomegaly	18	(6)
Hepatomegaly	16	(5)
Muscle tenderness	12	(4)
Periorbital edema	10	(3)
Evanescent skin lesions	8	(3)
Abdominal tenderness	6	(2)
Testicular swelling	2	(1)

Erythema chronicum migrans was required for inclusion in this study.
From Steere AC, Bartenhagen NH, Craft JE, et al.: The early clinical manifestations of Lyme disease. Ann Intern Med 99:76, 1983.

irritation or mild encephalopathy—for example, episodic attacks of excruciating headache and neck pain, stiffness, or pressure—but typically lasting only for hours at this stage of the illness and without CSF pleocytosis or objective neurologic deficit. Except for fatigue and lethargy, which are often constant, the early signs and symptoms are typically intermittent and changing. For example, a patient may have meningitic attacks for several days, a few days of improvement, and then the onset of migratory musculoskeletal pain. This last may involve joints (generally without swelling), tendons, bursa, muscle, and bone. The pain tends to affect only one or two sites at a time and to last a few hours to several days in a given location. The various associated symptoms may occur several days before ECM (or without it) and last for months (especially fatigue and lethargy) after the skin lesions have disappeared.

Later Manifestations. **Neurologic Involvement.** Within several weeks to months of the onset of illness, about 15% of patients develop frank neurologic abnormalities, including meningitis, encephalitis, chorea, cranial neuritis (including bilateral facial palsy), motor and sensory radiculoneuritis, or mononeuritis multiplex, in various combinations. The usual pattern is fluctuating meningoencephalitis with superimposed cranial nerve (particularly facial) palsy and peripheral radiculoneuropathy, but Bell's palsy may occur

TABLE 321-2. EARLY SYMPTOMS OF LYME DISEASE

Symptoms	No. of Patients N = 314	(%)
Malaise, fatigue, and lethargy	251	(80)
Headache	200	(64)
Fever and chills	185	(59)
Stiff neck	151	(48)
Arthralgias	150	(48)
Myalgias	135	(43)
Backache	81	(26)
Anorexia	73	(23)
Sore throat	53	(17)
Nausea	53	(17)
Dysesthesia	35	(11)
Vomiting	32	(10)
Abdominal pain	24	(8)
Photophobia	19	(6)
Hand stiffness	16	(5)
Dizziness	15	(5)
Cough	15	(5)
Chest pain	12	(4)
Ear pain	12	(4)
Diarrhea	6	(2)

From Steere AC, Bartenhagen NH, Craft JE, et al.: The early clinical manifestations of Lyme disease. Ann Intern Med 99:76, 1983.

alone. By now, patients with meningitic symptoms have a lymphocytic pleocytosis (about 100 cells per cubic millimeter) in CSF and sometimes diffuse slowing on electroencephalogram. However, the neck is rarely stiff except on extreme flexion; Kernig's and Brudzinski's signs are absent. Neurologic abnormalities typically last for months but usually resolve completely (late neurologic complications are noted below).

Cardiac Involvement. Also within weeks to months of onset, about 8% of patients develop cardiac involvement. The most common abnormality is fluctuating degrees of atrioventricular block (first-degree, Wenckebach, or complete heart block). Some patients have evidence of more diffuse cardiac involvement, including electrocardiographic changes compatible with acute myopericarditis, radionuclide evidence of mild left ventricular dysfunction, or, rarely, cardiomegaly. None has had heart murmurs. Cardiac involvement is usually brief (3 days to 6 weeks), but it may recur.

Arthritis. From weeks to as long as 2 years after the onset of illness, about 60% of patients develop frank arthritis, usually characterized by intermittent attacks of asymmetric joint swelling and pain primarily in large joints, especially the knee, one or two joints at a time. Affected knees are commonly more swollen than painful, often hot, and rarely red; Baker's cysts may form and rupture early. However, both large and small joints may be affected, and a few patients have had symmetric polyarthritis. Attacks of arthritis, which generally last from weeks to months, typically recur for several years, decreasing in frequency with time. Fatigue is common with active joint involvement, but fever or other systemic symptoms at this stage are unusual. Joint fluid white cell counts vary from 500 to 110,000 cells per cubic millimeter, with an average of about 25,000 cells per cubic millimeter, mostly polymorphonuclear leukocytes. Total protein ranges from 3 to 8 grams per deciliter. The C3 and C4 levels are generally greater than one-third, and glucose levels usually greater than two-thirds, that of serum. Rheumatoid factor and antinuclear antibody are absent.

In about 10% of patients with arthritis, involvement in large joints may become chronic, with pannus formation and erosion of cartilage and bone. Synovial biopsy findings may mimic those of rheumatoid arthritis: surface deposits of fibrin, villous hypertrophy, vascular proliferation, and a heavy infiltration of mononuclear cells. In addition, there may be an obliterative endarteritis and (rarely) demonstrable spirochetes. As noted above, *B. burgdorferi* stimulates mononuclear cells to produce cytokines (e.g., interleukin-1, TNFα, interleukin-6), and elevated concentrations of inflammatory cytokines have been found in synovial fluid. In one patient with chronic Lyme arthritis, synovium grown in tissue culture produced large amounts of collagenase and prostaglandin E$_2$. Thus in Lyme disease the joint fluid cell counts, the immune reactants (except for rheumatoid factor), the synovial histology, the amounts of synovial enzymes released, and the resulting destruction of cartilage and bone may be similar to those in rheumatoid arthritis.

Other late findings (years) associated with this infection include a chronic skin lesion—*acrodermatitis chronica atrophicans*—well known in Europe but still rare in the United States. One sees violaceous infiltrated plaques or nodules, especially on extensor surfaces, that eventually become atrophic. Uncommon late chronic neurologic disease includes transverse myelitis, diffuse sensory axonal neuropathy, and demyelinating lesions of the CNS. Mild memory impairment, subtle mood changes, and chronic fatigue states may also occur.

LABORATORY TEST RESULTS. The diagnosis of Lyme disease is based on recognizing clinical features of the illness in a patient with a history of possible exposure to the causative organism. Culture of *B. burgdorferi* from patients is definitive but has rarely been successful except from skin biopsy specimens. The organism can be isolated from blood in a significant minority of patients with systemic manifestations of early disease (it grows very slowly). Special tissue staining techniques generally have a low yield and are not readily available. Determination of specific antibody titers, usually performed by enzyme-linked immunosorbent assay (ELISA), is currently the most helpful additional diagnostic test for Lyme disease. In serum, specific IgM antibody titers against *B. burgdorferi* usually reach a peak between the third and sixth weeks after the onset of disease; specific immunoglobulin G (IgG) antibody titers rise more slowly and are generally highest months later when arthritis is present (Fig. 321–1). Individuals with Lyme disease of more than 6 weeks' duration can be expected to have elevated levels of specific antibodies. However, the tests employed are not yet standardized, and results from different commercial laboratories may vary, especially for borderline elevations. The vast majority of individuals with established Lyme arthritis have elevated specific IgG titers. This finding makes antibody titers against *B. burgdorferi* particularly useful in differentiating Lyme disease from other rheumatic syndromes, especially when ECM is missed, forgotten, or absent. This antibody cross-reacts with other spirochetes, including *Treponema pallidum*, but patients with Lyme disease do not have positive VDRL test results. Western blots can be helpful when false-positive ELISA's are suspected.

Another test of diagnostic interest uses the polymerase chain reaction (PCR) to detect spirochetal DNA in host material. Although this powerful tool is notorious for false-positive results when not performed under the most stringent conditions, it shows great promise, particularly in Lyme arthritis, in which synovial fluid from the large majority of untreated patients appears to be positive.

The most common nonspecific laboratory abnormalities, particularly early in the illness, are a high erythrocyte sedimentation rate, an elevated serum IgM level, or increased serum levels of aspartate transaminase (AST). The enzyme levels generally return to normal within several weeks. Patients may be mildly anemic early in the illness and occasionally have elevated white cell counts with shifts to the left in the differential count. A few patients have had microscopic hematuria, sometimes with mild proteinuria (dipstick); values for creatinine and blood urea nitrogen have been normal. Throughout the illness, serum C3 and C4 levels are generally normal or elevated. Rheumatoid factor and antinuclear antibodies are usually absent.

DIFFERENTIAL DIAGNOSIS. ECM is the unique herald lesion of Lyme disease (see Color Plate 10B). When present in its classic form, there is little else that might be confused with it. However, some patients are not aware of having had ECM, and in others, its appearance is not always characteristic. Secondary lesions might suggest *erythema multiforme,* but blistering, mucosal lesions, and involvement of the palms and soles are not features of Lyme disease. Malar rash may suggest systemic lupus erythematosus; an urticarial rash, hepatitis B infection or serum sickness. Evanescent blotches and circles may resemble *erythema marginatum,* but those of Lyme disease do not expand.

Early musculoskeletal flulike symptoms may be misleading, especially when ECM is absent or missed or is not the first manifestation. Severe headache and stiff neck may resemble aseptic meningitis, abdominal symptoms, hepatitis, and generalized tender lymphadenopathy and splenomegaly, infectious mononucleosis. As in the last infection, fatigue in Lyme disease may be a major and persistent complaint. However, initial presentations of an isolated chronic fatigue syndrome or of fibromyalgia-like complaints (diffuse aching, trigger points, sleep disturbance) are not characteristic of Lyme disease.

In later stages, Lyme disease may mimic other immune-mediated disorders. Like rheumatic fever, Lyme disease may be associated with sore throat followed by migratory polyarthritis and carditis, but without evidence of valvular involvement or of a preceding streptococcal infection. Migratory pain in tendons and joints may also suggest disseminated gonococcal disease. An isolated facial weakness may mimic Bell's palsy of other causes. Late neurologic involvement may suggest multiple sclerosis (transverse myelitis), Guillain-Barré syndrome (symmetric peripheral neuropathy), primary psychosis, or brain tumor. In adults with Lyme arthritis, the large knee effusions can resemble those in Reiter's syndrome, and the occasional symmetric polyarthritis, that of rheumatoid arthritis. In children, the attacks of arthritis, although generally shorter, may be identical to those seen in the oligoarticular form of juvenile rheumatoid arthritis, but without iridocyclitis.

TREATMENT. The major goal of therapy in Lyme disease is to eradicate the causative organism. Like other spirochetal diseases, Lyme disease is most responsive to antibiotics early in its course. Treatment regimens have evolved over time based on both controlled clinical data and on clinical experience. Because of the difficulty in proving that bacteria have been eradicated and the common persistence of some symptoms long after treatment, the endpoint of

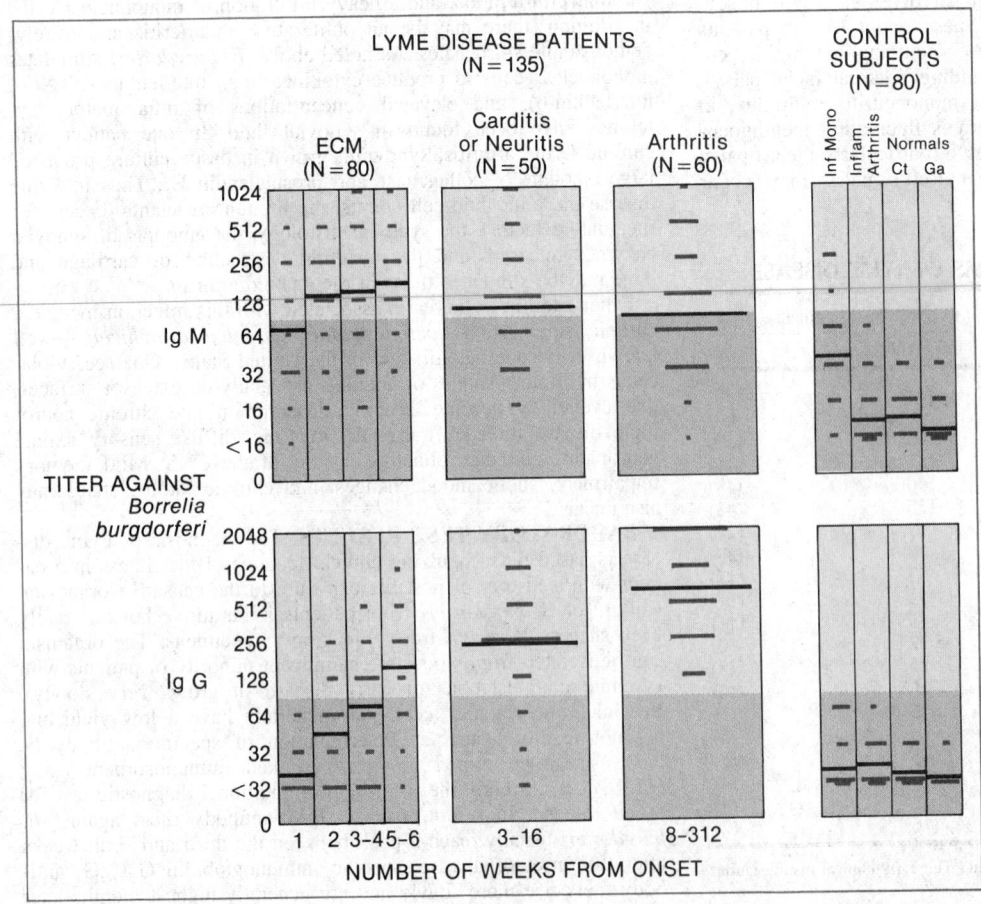

FIGURE 321–1. Antibody titers against *Borrelia burgdorferi* are shown in serum samples from 135 patients with different clinical manifestations of Lyme disease, and from 80 control subjects with infectious mononucleosis, inflammatory arthritis, or no disease (titers determined by indirect immunofluorescence). The black bar shows the geometric mean titer for each group; the pink shaded areas indicate the range of values generally observed in control subjects. Note that all patients with Lyme arthritis have elevated IgG antibody titers. (Adapted from Steere AC, Grodzicki RL, Kornblatt AN, et al: The spirochetal etiology of Lyme disease. N Engl J Med 308:733–740, 1983. Copyright 1983 Massachusetts Medical Society.)

antibiotic therapy is not always clear. The treatment regimens presented here represent guidelines that will no doubt be refined in time (Table 321–3).

Early Lyme Disease. If patients are treated early with oral antibiotics, ECM typically resolves promptly, and major later sequelae (myocarditis, meningoencephalitis, or recurrent arthritis) usually do not occur. Prompt treatment is therefore important, even though such patients may be susceptible to reinfection. For adults, antibiotic choices and doses are listed in Table 321–3; amoxicillin or doxycycline is favored. In children younger than 9, give divided doses of amoxicillin (30 mg per kilogram per day; not < 1 gram or > 2 grams per day) or, for the penicillin-allergic, erythromycin (30 mg per kilogram per day) for 10 to 20 days.

About 10% of patients with early Lyme disease experience a Jarisch–Herxheimer–like reaction (higher fever, redder rash, or greater pain) during the first 24 hours of antibiotic therapy. Whichever drug is given, 30 to 50% of patients have brief (hours to days) recurrent episodes of headache, musculoskeletal pain, and fatigue which may continue for extended periods. The etiology of these symptoms is unclear at present; they may result from undegraded spirochetal antigen(s) rather than persistence of live spirochetes. It is clear, however, that the risk of delayed resolution is greatest in individuals with disseminated manifestations of disease (multiple skin lesions, headache, fever, lymphadenopathy, or Bell's palsy) prior to the institution of antibiotics.

Later Lyme Disease. For Lyme meningitis, with or without other neurologic manifestations (cranial neuropathy or radiculoneu-

TABLE 321–3. RECOMMENDATIONS FOR ANTIBIOTIC TREATMENT OF LYME DISEASE[a]

Early Lyme Disease[b]
Amoxicillin, 500 mg three times daily for 21 days[c]
Doxycycline, 100 mg twice daily for 21 days
Cefuroxime axetil, 500 mg twice daily for 21 days
Azithromycin, 500 mg daily for 7 days[d]
    (less effective than other regimens)

Neurologic Manifestations
Bell's palsy (no other neurologic abnormalities)
    Oral regimens for early disease suffice
Meningitis (with or without radiculoneuropathy or encephalitis)[e]
    Ceftriaxone, 2 grams daily for 14–28 days
    Penicillin G, 20 million units daily for 14–28 days
    Doxycycline, 100 mg twice daily (oral or intravenous) for 14–28 days[f]
    Chloramphenicol, 1 gram four times daily for 14–28 days

Arthritis[g]
Amoxicillin and probenecid, 500 mg each, four times daily for 30 days[h]
Doxycycline, 100 mg twice daily for 30 days
Ceftriaxone, 2 grams daily for 14–28 days
Penicillin G, 20 million units daily for 14–28 days

Carditis
Ceftriaxone, 2 grams daily for 14 days
Penicillin G, 20 million units daily for 14 days
Doxycycline, 100 mg orally twice daily for 21 days[i]
Amoxicillin, 500 mg three times daily for 21 days[i]

Pregnancy
Localized early disease
    Amoxicillin, 500 mg three times daily for 21 days
Any manifestation of disseminated disease
    Penicillin G, 20 million units daily for 14–28 days
Asymptomatic seropositivity
    No treatment necessary

[a]These are guidelines, to be modified by new findings and to be applied always with close attention to the clinical context of individual patients.
[b]Without neurologic, cardiac, or joint involvement. For early Lyme disease limited to single ECM lesion, 10 days is sufficient.
[c]Some experts advise addition of probenecid 500 mg three times daily.
[d]Experience with this agent is limited; optimal duration of therapy is unclear.
[e]Optimal duration of therapy has not been established. There are no controlled trials of therapy longer than 4 weeks for any manifestation of Lyme disease.
[f]No published experience in the United States.
[g]An oral regimen should be selected only if there is no neurologic involvement.
[h]Amoxicillin is generally administered three times daily, but the only trial of this agent for Lyme arthritis employed a four times daily regimen.
[i]Oral regimens have been reserved for mild carditis limited to first degree heart block with PR ≤ .30 sec and normal ventricular function.
From Rahn DW, Malawista SE: Treatment of Lyme disease (special article). In Mandell GL, Bone RC, Cline MJ, et al. (eds.): 1994 Year Book of Medicine. St. Louis, Mosby–Year Book, 1994.

ropathy), intravenous penicillin G, 20 million units a day in six divided doses for 10 days, is effective therapy; in practice, courses are often extended to 3 weeks. Headache and stiff neck usually begin to subside by the second day of therapy and disappear by 7 to 10 days; motor deficits and radicular pain frequently require 7 to 8 weeks for complete recovery but do not require longer antibiotic courses. For Bell's palsy alone, oral regimens may suffice, but these patients may be at higher risk of later sequelae than are individuals with early disease without neurologic dissemination.

Although not studied systematically, carditis also responds rapidly (in days) to this regimen. Recovery from carditis was the rule even in the preantibiotic era, but untreated patients are at high risk for later manifestations of Lyme disease. Prednisone, 40 to 60 mg a day in divided doses, has, in the past, seemed to hasten resolution of high-grade heart block, but one should hesitate to institute glucocorticoids during antibiotic administration because they may impede eradication of infecting organisms. For patients with allergy to penicillin, doxycycline, 100 mg twice a day, is reasonable but unevaluated. If second- or third-degree heart block is present, patients should be admitted to hospital for cardiac monitoring; temporary pacing is occasionally required for complete heart block.

In clinical practice, ceftriaxone (2 grams daily for 14 to 21 days) has largely replaced penicillin for the therapy of disseminated Lyme disease. Arguments in favor of this practice are a once-daily administration schedule which is amenable to outpatient intravenous antibiotic programs and improved penetration of the CSF in comparison with penicillin. Penicillin and cefotaxime have been found equally effective for the treatment of acute neurologic Lyme disease (meningitis or radiculitis) in a group of patients studied in Germany. Ceftriaxone also appeared responsible for the complete recovery of 6 of 9 unusual Austrian patients with dilated cardiomyopathy attributed to Lyme disease.

Late Lyme Disease. Lyme arthritis has been successfully treated with both oral and parenteral antibiotics, but failures occur with any regimen chosen. Unless CNS involvement coexists, first-line treatment with a month-long course of doxycycline, 100 mg twice a day, or amoxicillin plus probenecid, 500 mg each four times a day, is recommended. The large majority of patients respond, although complete response can be delayed as long as 3 months or more after therapy is completed, and some patients may develop neurologic disease later. During treatment, the affected joint should be kept at rest and effusions drained by needle aspiration as for any infected joint. In patients who fail one or more courses of antibiotics, arthroscopic synovectomy can result in a long-term response and perhaps cure. Even without antibiotic or surgical treatment, persistent Lyme arthritis tends to resolve within several years.

Optimal therapy for the later neurologic complications of Lyme disease is also not yet clear, but 14 to 21 days of intravenous ceftriaxone or penicillin (see Table 321–3) are recommended. The frequency of subtle chronic encephalopathy and peripheral neuropathy is debated at present. These entities, when suspected, should be carefully documented through neurologic, neuropsychological, and electrophysiologic testing before aggressive or prolonged antibiotic therapy is instituted. Although some current thinking favors longer periods of the highest tolerated oral doses of amoxicillin (with probenecid), doxycycline, or even intravenous antibiotics in difficult cases, there is no controlled experience with courses of antibiotics longer than 1 month for any manifestation of Lyme disease. The infiltrative lesions of *acrodermatitis chronica atrophicans* are usually cured by 3 weeks of oral phenoxymethyl penicillin, 2 to 3 grams daily in divided doses.

Pregnancy. Because the spirochetes that cause relapsing fever and syphilis can cross the placenta, there has been concern regarding this possibility in Lyme disease. Maternal-fetal transmission of *B. burgdorferi* resulting in either neonatal death or stillbirth has been reported in rare instances in which symptomatic early Lyme disease occurred early in pregnancy and was either untreated or inadequately treated. In follow-up studies conducted by the Centers for Disease Control and Prevention, maternal Lyme disease was not directly implicated as a cause of fetal malformations. There have been no cases of fetal infection occurring when currently recommended antibiotic regimens for Lyme disease have been used during pregnancy. A lower threshold for initiating therapy for suspected Lyme disease in pregnancy is understandable, but women acquiring the illness during pregnancy should be reassured that the vast majority of infants born to women in these circumstances have been entirely well.

Tick Bites. A final treatment issue regards the advisability of administering antibiotics prophylactically to individuals sustaining ixodid tick bites in endemic areas. Studies completed to date have not supported this common practice. Because nymphal ixodid ticks must, in general, feed for a day or more before transmitting spirochetes (at least in mice), ticks removed prior to this time are unlikely to have transmitted *B. burgdorferi* even if infected. Tick bite sites should be observed for development of ECM and patients cautioned regarding the common associated symptoms of early Lyme disease. A watched tick bite allows for very early treatment of ECM in the small minority of patients in whom it will develop, and this is the stage of disease most amenable to therapy.

Barbour AG, Fish D: The biological and social phenomenon of Lyme disease. Science 260:1610, 1993. *The emergence of Lyme disease in the United States, unknown 2 decades ago, now its most common arthropod-borne illness.*

Bockenstedt LK, Malawista SE: Lyme Disease. *In* Rich RR (ed.): Clinical Immunology. St. Louis, Mosby–Year Book, 1995. *An expanded version of this chapter, with extensive recent references.*

Malawista SE, Steere AC, Hardin JA: Lyme disease: A unique human model for an infectious etiology of rheumatic disease. Yale J Biol Med 57:473, 1984. *The larger significance of Lyme disease, a disorder that is infectious in origin but inflammatory or "rheumatic" in expression.*

Rahn DW, Malawista SE: Treatment of Lyme disease (special article). *In* Mandell GL, Bone RC, Cline MJ, et al. (eds.): 1994 Year Book of Medicine. St. Louis, Mosby–Year Book, 1994. *Evolution of current recommendations for therapy, based on published studies, practical considerations, and clinical experience.*

Steere AC, Levin RE, Molloy PJ, et al.: Treatment of Lyme arthritis. Arthritis Rheum 37:878, 1994. *Oral antibiotics cured the large majority of patients with Lyme arthritis within 1 to 3 months, but a few developed neurologic disease later.*

Steere AC, Malawista SE, Snydman DR, et al.: Lyme arthritis: An epidemic of oligoarticular arthritis in children and adults in three Connecticut communities. Arthritis Rheum 20:7, 1977. *The first description of a new nosologic entity, recognized because it clusters geographically; rheumatoid arthritis does not.*

322 LEPTOSPIROSIS
William A. Petri, Jr.

DEFINITION. Leptospirosis is a spirochetal infection with bacteria of the genus *Leptospira*. The severe icteric form of infection is called Weil's disease, after the investigator who in 1886 described four men with an acute but self-limited infectious illness characterized by fever, jaundice, nephritis, and hepatomegaly and a biphasic course, with fever recurring 1 to 7 days into convalescence.

ETIOLOGY. There are two species of *Leptospira*, *L. interrogans*, which is pathogenic in humans and animals, and *L. biflexa*, which is free-living. *L. interrogans* is divided into >200 serovars grouped into 19 serogroups based on shared major agglutinins. Virulence does not in general correlate with serovars, although serovar classifications can be useful epidemiologically to identify common-source outbreaks. *Leptospira* are motile spirochetes 6 to 20 μ in length and 0.1 to 0.2 μ in diameter which are obligate aerobes with unique nutritional requirements for long-chain fatty acids.

EPIDEMIOLOGY. Leptospirosis is one of the most common, widespread, and underdiagnosed infections transmitted from animals to humans. *L. interrogans* can survive for months in the proximal convoluted tubules of the kidney in asymptomatically infected animals and upon excretion in urine survives in the environment for as long as 6 months. The optimal temperature for growth is 28 to 32°C, with slightly alkaline water ideal for growth and survival. Herbivores with alkaline urines, such as pigs, shed higher numbers of organisms than animals with acidic urine, such as dogs. The most common source of exposure in the United States is dogs, followed by livestock, rodents, and other wild animals. Humans become infected via recreational (e.g., windsurfing, kayaking, swimming) or occupational exposure to animal urine or urine-contaminated water and soil. Occupations with the greatest documented risks include New Zealand dairy farmers (incidence of 1.1 infections per 10 person-years), Glasgow sewer workers (3.7 infections per 10 person-years), and U.S. Army soldiers undergoing jungle warfare training in Panama (4.1 infections per 10 person-years). Approximately 15% of veterinarians and abbatoir workers have serologic evidence of infection. Leptospirosis is up to 10 times more frequent in rural than in urban dwellers and three times more frequent in men, with a peak incidence in men at ages 30 to 39.

PATHOLOGY AND PATHOGENESIS. *Leptospira* penetrate intact mucous membranes and abraded skin and disseminate widely via the bloodstream. In the first week to 10 days of illness, spirochetes can be cultured with special media from blood and cerebrospinal fluid (CSF). Leptospirosis is an infectious vasculitis, with damage to capillary endothelial cells responsible for the major clinical manifestations of disease, including renal tubular and hepatic dysfunction, myocarditis, and pulmonary hemorrhage. Intra- to extravascular fluid shifts secondary to endothelial damage lead to hypovolemia, which complicates renal dysfunction and can lead to shock. Fatal cases are associated with widespread hemorrhage of mucosal, skin, and serosal surfaces. Examination of the kidneys from autopsies has revealed ischemic damage, including epithelial cell necrosis in the distal convoluted tubules and the ascending loop of Henle, and interstitial nephritis but only rarely glomerular damage. Liver pathology includes disorganization of liver cell plates, marked variation in the size and shape of parenchymal cells, mitotic figures, and evidence of cholestasis but not necrosis. Muscle biopsies have demonstrated focal necrotic changes with a mild mononuclear infiltrate. Only rarely is the spirochete visualized in the infected tissue. Hemorrhagic myocarditis has been observed frequently in autopsies. The secondary "immune" phase of leptospirosis is associated with the clearance of the organism from blood and CSF and the appearance of agglutinating anti-*Leptospira* antibodies.

CLINICAL FEATURES. Symptoms develop 7 to 12 days after exposure. Most patients have an abrupt onset of a self-limited 4- to 7-day anicteric illness characterized by the sudden onset of fever, mild to severe headache, myalgias, chills, cough, chest pain, neck stiffness, and/or prostration. An estimated 10% of patients will present with jaundice, hemorrhage, renal failure, and/or neurologic dysfunction (Weil's disease). Signs of leptospirosis include fever of 38 to 40°C (97 to 100% of patients), conjunctival suffusion (40 to 100%), hepatomegaly (80% of icteric cases), splenomegaly (15 to 25%), diffuse abdominal tenderness (5 to 30%), muscle tenderness (40 to 80%), meningeal signs (12 to 40%), disturbances in sensorium (50% of icteric cases), jaundice (10%), and a truncal rash that can be macular, urticarial, or purpuric (7 to 9%). Pretibial, raised, 1- to 5-cm erythematous lesions are seen characteristically in a form of leptospirosis called "Fort Bragg fever."

Classically, leptospirosis has been considered a biphasic illness, although many patients with mild disease will not have symptoms of the secondary "immune" phase of illness, and patients with very severe disease will have a relentless progression from onset of illness to jaundice, renal failure, hemorrhage, hypotension, and coma. Overall, about half the patients with leptospirosis will have a relapse. Typically 1 week after the initial fever resolves, fever, headache, and meningeal signs return. This immune phase of the illness can last several days to a month. A late complication is anterior uveitis, which may be seen in 10% of patients during and months to years after convalescence. Leptospirosis in pregnancy is associated with spontaneous abortion; children born with congenitally acquired leptospirosis have not been described to have congenital anomalies and have been treated successfully with antibiotics.

LABORATORY FEATURES. *Leptospira* can be cultured with special media from blood and CSF early in the illness, but incubation of the cultures for 5 to 6 weeks at 28 to 30°C is often required. Mild proteinuria is seen in most patients and may be accompanied by pyuria, casts, and microscopic hematuria. In patients with renal failure, the blood urea nitrogen level rarely exceeds 100 mg per deciliter, and the creatinine concentration is usually <8 mg per deciliter. Liver function tests are usually abnormal only in icteric patients, where two- to threefold elevations in aminotransferases and alkaline phosphatase are observed (lower than the elevations commonly seen in acute viral hepatitis), and a predominantly conjugated bilirubinemia is seen. Myositis with elevated serum creatine phosphokinase (MM band) occurs in about half of patients. Thrombocytopenia (usually ≥50,000 per microliter), anemia, and leukocytosis are commonly seen. Thrombocytopenia is seen most commonly in patients with renal failure. CSF examination shows a pleocytosis (<500 cells per cu mm) with an early neutrophilic and late mononuclear cell predominance, a normal glucose level, and mildly elevated protein level (50 to 110 mg per deciliter). Chest radiographs were abnormal in the majority of patients in one study, with small nodular densities showing a tendency to consolidate. First-degree atrioventricular block and changes consistent with acute pericarditis have been documented in one third of patients.

DIAGNOSIS. The presentation of the illness in anicteric cases is nonspecific. It is important to search for an exposure history to animal urine in a patient with a flu-like illness, respiratory illness, aseptic meningitis, acute hepatitis, acute renal failure, pericarditis, atrioventricular block, or anterior uveitis. In some developing countries, leptospirosis is more common than hepatitis A as a cause of acute hepatitis. Useful means to distinguish icteric leptospirosis from acute viral hepatitis include the prominent myalgias, conjunctival suffusion, elevated serum creatine phosphokinase, and the only two- to threefold elevations in aminotransferases seen in leptospirosis. The diagnosis is usually made retrospectively by a fourfold rise in agglutinating antibody titer. Agglutinins characteristically appear within the first 1 to 2 weeks of illness and peak at three to four weeks. It is possible to grow the organism from blood and CSF collected during the first week of illness, but it may take 4 to 6 weeks for the cultures to be positive because the organism is so slow growing.

PROGNOSIS. Case fatality rates for leptospirosis are <1% in studies where aggressive surveillance has been conducted (increasing the proportion of mild cases). The illness is usually self-limited. Liver and renal dysfunction are for the most part reversible, with return to normal function over 1 to 2 months. The mortality rate for icteric disease has been reported in different studies to be 2.4 to 11.3%, with deaths occurring secondary to renal failure, gastrointestinal and pulmonary hemorrhage, and the adult respiratory distress syndrome.

THERAPY AND PREVENTION. Antibiotic treatment is most beneficial when started within 4 days of illness; unfortunately, the diagnosis of leptospirosis is rarely made this rapidly. Doxycycline, 100 mg orally twice a day for 7 days, started within 48 hours of illness, decreased the duration of illness by 2 days in one study; penicillin at a dose of 2.4 to 3.6 million units per day also has been successful early treatment. A beneficial effect of antibiotic therapy later in disease course has not been uniformly seen. While a randomized, double-blinded trial of penicillin treatment (1.5 million units intravenously every 6 hours for 7 days) started on average nine days into illness showed a decrease in fever duration from 11.6 to 4.7 days and in elevated serum creatinine level from 8.3 to 2.7 days, a second randomized trial of penicillin in patients with icteric leptospirosis and a median duration of illness of 1 week demonstrated no beneficial effect. Jarish-Herxheimer reactions (fever, rigors, hypotension, and tachycardia) rarely occur upon initiation of antibiotic therapy. Supportive care and treatment of the hypotension, renal failure (including dialysis), and hemorrhage, which can complicate leptospirosis, are crucial for a good outcome.

Immunization of animals is not necessarily effective at preventing human disease, since leptospiruria can still occur in immunized animals. Because asymptomatically infected wild animals can chronically excrete large numbers of spirochetes in their urine, controlling environmental sources of leptospirosis is difficult if not impossible. Occupationally exposed individuals (abbatoir workers, veterinarians) should wear protective clothing to prevent exposure of skin and mucous membranes to potentially infected urine. Bodies of water associated with recreational exposures to leptospirosis may need to be placed off limits. Doxycycline, 200 mg orally once a week, has been 95% effective at preventing leptospirosis in U.S. troops undergoing training in the jungle warfare school in Panama and has a place in the short-term prevention of the disease in high-risk settings. No licensed vaccine is available in the United States for humans.

Lecour H, Miranda M, Magro C, et al.: Human leptospirosis—A review of 50 cases. Infection 17:8, 1989. *Epidemiologic and clinical aspects of 50 consecutive hospitalized patients with leptospirosis.*

Shaked Y, Shpilberg O, Samra D, Samra Y: Leptospirosis in pregnancy and its effect on the fetus: Case report and review. Clin Infect Dis 17:241, 1993. *Review of 16 cases of leptospirosis in pregnancy indicates that spontaneous abortion is a common consequence.*

Watt G, Padre LP, Tuazon ML, et al.: Placebo-controlled trial of intravenous penicillin for severe and late leptospirosis. Lancet 1:433, 1988. *Demonstration of the effectiveness of intravenous penicillin in severe leptospirosis.*

323 DISEASES CAUSED BY CHLAMYDIAE

Robert C. Brunham

Chlamydiae are obligate intracellular pathogens whose extreme biosynthetic defects in intermediate metabolism and energy generation cause them to be absolutely dependent on a host cell to grow and replicate. They are among the most common of all human infectious agents and produce much disability although little mortality.

CHLAMYDIAE AS ORGANISMS

Chlamydiae are a unique monophyletic bacterial family as defined by 16S rRNA sequences with an extremely ancient origin within the bacterial domain and are composed of four species (Table 323–1).

The chlamydial bacterial cell has a gram-negative cell wall structure consisting of an outer membrane and an inner cytoplasmic membrane. However, no peptidoglycan layer is found within the periplasmic space separating these two layers. The outer membrane is extremely protein-rich, composed of a single major outer membrane protein (MOMP 40 kDa) and two minor outer membrane proteins (60 and 12.5 kDa). All three proteins are extraordinarily rich in the amino acid cysteine, and inter- and intramolecular disulfide bonding produces a supramolecular protein complex that confers structural rigidity on the bacterial cell analogous to the role played by peptidoglycan in other bacteria. Within *Chlamydia trachomatis*, MOMP variation determines the serologic types that characterize the individual serovars. As with other gram-negative bacteria, the chlamydial outer membrane also contains lipopolysaccharide (LPS). Chlamydial LPS is a rough type without O-saccharides and is composed of a trisaccharide of 3-deoxy-D-manno-octulosonic acid (KDO). Although the core KDO sequences are shared by LPS from many other gram-negative bacteria, the chlamydial LPS is unique because two of the three KDO's are bonded through a unique 2.8 instead of a 2.4 linkage. Thus antibodies to chlamydial LPS are specific. Since all four species of chlamydiae share the same LPS structure, antibodies to chlamydial LPS are genus-specific.

Chlamydiae share a common and distinctive growth cycle. Figure 323–1 shows the distinctive developmental cycle typical for all chlamydiae. The size of the chlamydial genome is small at 1045 kilobases, containing enough information to code for approximately 600 different proteins. Most strains of chlamydiae also contain a 7-kilobase cryptic plasmid. Chlamydiae absolutely depend on host cells to obtain nutrients from the extracellular environment and convert them into forms they can use. Chlamydiae are obligate energy parasites of their host cells, and no net ATP-generating reactions have been observed in the organism. In comparison with other bacteria, chlamydiae are virtually unique in being able to transport phosphorylated compounds found in the host cell cytoplasm, and this undoubtedly represents their premiere adaptation to the intracellular environment. Despite sharing many characteristics in cell architecture and in the developmental cycle, chlamydiae are remarkably diverse at the DNA level. By DNA-DNA homology, the

TABLE 323–1. CLASSIFICATION OF BIOLOGIC VARIANTS (BIOVARS) AND SEROLOGIC VARIANTS (SEROVARS) OF THE GENUS *CHLAMYDIA*

	Biovar	Serovar
C. trachomatis	Trachoma	12
	Lymphogranuloma venereum	3
	Mouse pneumonitis	1
C. pneumoniae	TWAR	1
C. psittaci	Birds, mammals	Unknown, multiple
C. pecorum	Ruminants	Unknown, multiple

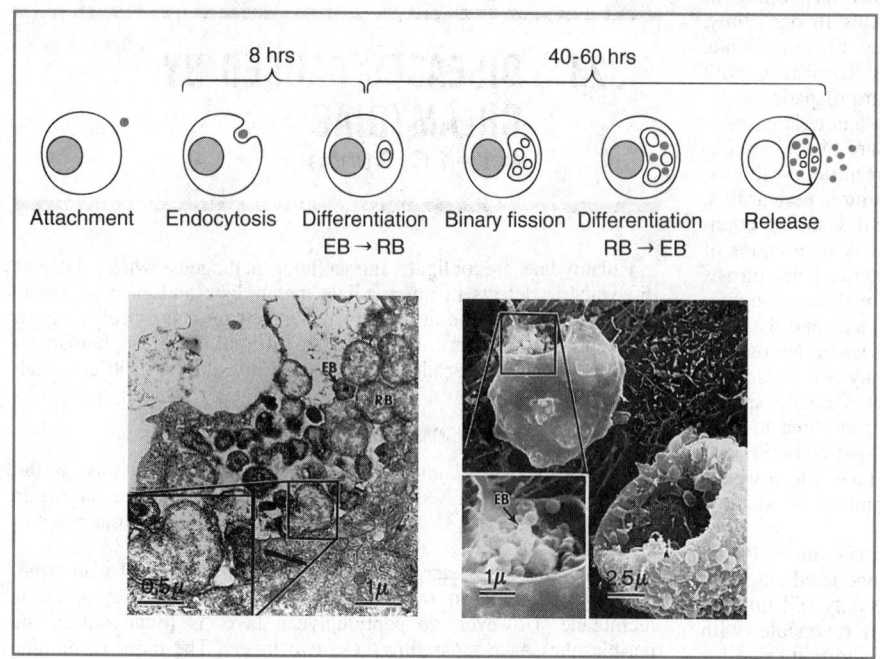

FIGURE 323–1. The top panel schematically shows the developmental cycle common to all chlamydiae. The red circles represent elementary bodies (EB's) and the open circles represent reticulate bodies (RB's). Chlamydiae infect eukaryotic cells through multiple attachment mechanisms, best understood for *C. trachomatis*. A trimolecular complex with a secreted heparan sulfate–like glycosaminogin synthesized by *C. trachomatis* acts as a bridge between ligands on the chlamydial EB and the eukaryotic cell surface. Different mechanisms exist among different chlamydial species and may explain their distinct trophism. After attachment, EB's enter the cell within a membrane-bound vacuole that remains unfused with lysosomes. EB's reorganize into RB's and asynchronously replicate 8 to 12 times with a doubling time of 2 to 3 hours. At the conclusion of the growth cycle, RB's differentiate back to EB's, and each inclusion yields 100 to 1000 new infectious EB's. The bottom left-hand panel is a transmission electron micrograph at 40 hours after infection showing the large RB's and the smaller EB's, which have a condensed nucleoid structure within their cytoplasm. The bottom right-hand panel is a scanning electron micrograph at 60 hours after infection showing a membrane-bound vacuole containing many EB's and apparently exiting from an infected HeLa cell.

chlamydial species share < 33% homology. Within each species, DNA-DNA homology varies between 14 and 95%.

CHLAMYDIAE AS PATHOGENS

Immune Responses

Chlamydiae produce intracellular infection, and, depending on the species of chlamydiae, macrophage or nonmacrophage host cells can support the organisms' replication. Macrophages appear to be the principal target cell for *C. psittaci* and *C. trachomatis* lymphogranuloma venereum (LGV) biovars. Columnar epithelial cells found in mucous membranes are the usual host cells for trachoma biovar and for *C. pneumoniae* replication. Host cell trophisms are correlated with the type of inflammation elicited by chlamydiae. LGV biovar and *C. psittaci,* which infect macrophages, produce granulomatous inflammation characteristic of delayed hypersensitivity reactions. Trachoma biovar, which infects epithelial cells, produces neutrophilic exudate during acute infection and submucosal mononuclear infiltration with lymphoid follicle formation during later stages of infection.

Chlamydiae elicit marked humoral and cellular immune responses. *C. trachomatis* elicits secretory IgA and circulatory IgM and IgG antibodies. Serum antibodies commonly recognize the chlamydial LPS as detected in the complement-fixation assay. *C. trachomatis* infection often elicits antibodies to serovar-specific epitopes on the MOMP. Women with reproductive sequelae such as tubal infertility or ectopic pregnancy due to prior *C. trachomatis* infection often have prominent antibody responses to a heat shock protein 60 antigen of chlamydiae.

Because chlamydiae produce intracellular infection, T cell–mediated immune responses are likely to be important. For chlamydiae that infect macrophages (LGV biovar and *C. psittaci*), granulomatous inflammation suggests the *in vivo* occurrence of T_h-1 activation. Interferon-gamma (IFN-γ), the principal cytokine of T_h-1 cells, has been detected in secretions from individuals infected with *C. trachomatis*. Cytotoxic T cells have not been detected during human chlamydial infection.

PATHOGENESIS AND MECHANISM OF HOST INJURY

Most animal model studies of chlamydial infection demonstrate an acute self-limited course. However, case reports of human LGV biovar and *C. psittaci* infections that last 10 to 20 years and observations from a longitudinal follow-up study of untreated cervical *C. trachomatis* infection showing that infection can last 15 months or more suggest that chlamydiae also can produce chronic persistent infection. Chronic persistent infection or repeated episodes of acute infection appear to elicit the immune mechanisms that cause host injury. Infection of a previously exposed host results in an accelerated and intensified inflammatory response, and tissue destruction appears to be directly correlated with the intensity of inflammation. This is best elucidated for *C. trachomatis* ocular infection. Inflammatory and scarring (cicatricial) trachoma are diseases of reinfection, and the more intense the initial inflammatory response, the more prominent is the late fibrotic response. Thus the mechanism for host injury with *C. trachomatis* infection is thought to be mediated by cellular immune responses.

CHLAMYDIAL DISEASES

Table 323–2 lists the most frequent chlamydial diseases.

Chlamydia trachomatis

The major diseases caused by *C. trachomatis* are trachoma produced by serovars A, B, Ba and C, sexually and perinatally transmitted diseases caused by serovars D through K, and sexually transmitted lymphogranuloma venereum caused by serovars L_1, L_2, and L_3. Trachoma and lymphogranuloma venereum are essentially restricted to developing areas of the world, whereas sexually and perinatally transmitted chlamydial infections are distributed globally. Trachoma and sexually/perinatally transmitted chlamydial infections are restricted to the mucosal surfaces of the body, and lymphogranuloma venereum causes systemic infection, principally of the lymphoid system.

TRACHOMA. *Epidemiology.* Trachoma is a distinctive ocular disease from infection by specific serovars of *C. trachomatis*. An estimated 500 million people worldwide are afflicted with trachoma, most of whom are young children. Trachoma is especially common in poor areas of sub-Saharan Africa. Trachoma is a major public health problem because 1 to 5% of infected individuals later develop scarring, which deforms the eyelid, causes inward turning of the eyelashes (entropion), and results in corneal abrasion (trichiasis). Corneal damage results in blindness. Trachoma is the most common preventable cause of blindness; an estimated 7 million people are blind as a result of trachoma. Most of these individuals are middle-aged and elderly adults. Active trachoma often occurs within the first 1 to 2 years of life but after the first month. Recurrences of active disease are common during childhood and spontaneously cease by age 10 to 15. Among children, the frequency of face washing, access to water, sharing a sleeping room with an affected individual, and intensity of eye-seeking fly exposure are important risk factors for trachoma. Active trachoma also can occur in adults, especially in mothers caring for young children with active disease. Trichiasis is related to repeated intense trachoma episodes in childhood, is more common in women than in men, and preferentially occurs in families.

The *C. trachomatis* serovars that produce trachoma are spread by direct contact with contaminated fomites such as washcloths or eye-seeking flies. Perinatal exposure to *C. trachomatis* from maternal genital tract infection is not important in transmitting trachoma.

Clinical Features. Trachoma is a chronic follicular conjunctivitis that causes macroscopically visible lymphoid follicles to form in the submucosa. These are especially apparent along the upper tarsal plate. The bulbar conjunctiva is minimally involved. Limited mucoid ocular discharge occurs; preauricular lymphadenopathy is rare and, if present, suggests other diagnoses such as adenovirus infection. The cornea may be involved with superficial vascularization and lymphocytic infiltration (pannus). Epidemic bacterial conjunctivitis due to *Haemophilus influenzae* can supervene on trachoma and cause a marked purulent conjunctivitis involving the bulbar conjunctiva. Bacterial conjunctivitis worsens the trachoma inflammatory damage. Tarsal conjunctival scarring deforms the eyelid structure and produces entropion and trichiasis in adulthood. Eventually, the corneal epithelium is eroded, and bacterial keratitis occurs. The cornea subsequently heals with opacification, resulting in blindness.

Diagnosis. Trachoma is most often a clinical diagnosis and is made if two of the following findings are observed:

1. Lymphoid follicles along the upper tarsal plate
2. Lymphoid follicles (or Herbert's pits) along the corneal limbus
3. Linear conjunctival scarring
4. Corneal pannus

Because most cases of trachoma occur in remote areas of the developing world without access to laboratory testing, most cases are diagnosed clinically. When laboratories are available, isolating *C. trachomatis* in cell culture provides definitive proof of the diagnosis. Culture is most often positive in young children with active disease and is rarely positive in adults with late scarring disease. Even in young children with active disease, culture is positive in only one-third to one-half of cases. Nonculture tests such as the direct immunofluorescent detection of elementary bodies (EB's) with monoclonal antibody or detecting chlamydial antigen by enzyme-linked immunosorbent assay (ELISA) are more frequently positive than are cultures. Detecting chlamydial DNA by the polymerase chain reaction (PCR) is the most sensitive diagnostic test, with about 70 to 80% of children with active trachoma testing positive. Few adults with late cicatricial disease are found to have positive tests for chlamydial EB's, antigen, or DNA.

Treatment and Prevention. Active trachoma in children can be treated with the topical ocular application of tetracycline or erythromycin ointment for 21 to 60 days. Because extraocular *C. tra-*

chomatis infection of the nasopharynx and gastrointestinal tract is relatively common during childhood trachoma, oral antibiotics such as erythromycin may be preferred. Single-dose oral azithromycin (20 mg/kg) seems as effective as 6 weeks of topical tetracycline. Trichiasis can be alleviated by depilation.

The prevalence of trachoma in a community responds dramatically to socioeconomic development. Mass chemotherapy for young school-aged children has a temporary impact on trachoma prevalence. No vaccine is available.

SEXUALLY AND PERINATALLY TRANSMITTED CHLAMYDIAL INFECTIONS. Epidemiology. Currently, *C. trachomatis* is the most prevalent sexually transmitted bacterial infection in the United States. More than 4 million chlamydial infections occur annually, and prevalence rates are highest (>10%) among sexually active adolescent females. Prevalence is higher in inner-city areas among lower socioeconomic status individuals and among minority ethnic groups such as African-Americans in the United States and Native Americans in Canada. Importantly, although prevalence rates are higher in these subgroups, with few exceptions, prevalences are ≥5% irrespective of geographic region, urban location, or ethnicity. In the United States, the direct and indirect costs of chlamydial disease exceed $2.4 billion annually. From a global perspective, sexually transmitted chlamydial infections are a major cause of total disease burden and healthy life years lost because of effects on the reproductive health of women.

Clinical Features. Urethritis. *C. trachomatis* causes 30 to 40% of cases of nongonococcal urethritis (NGU) in men, and an estimated 40 to 60% of urethral chlamydial infections are symptomatic with NGU. NGU is characterized by complaints of mild urethral discharge, urethral discomfort, and mild dysuria. On examination, a mild to moderate clear or cloudy urethral exudate can be detected. Often this is best observed in the morning prior to voiding. Sometimes, urethral discharge is apparent only on "milking" the urethra from the base of the penis to the glans. Gram stain of urethral exudate demonstrates ≥5 polymorphonuclear leukocytes per 1000× field and no gram-negative intracellular diplococci. Asymptomatic urethral infection is common with *C. trachomatis* infection and can be recognized by the urinary leukocyte esterase test on unspun first-void urine.

C. trachomatis urethral infection also occurs in women, in whom it produces the acute urethral syndrome. In such cases, the individual complains of dysuria, and pyuria (≥5 white blood cells per 1000× field) is found on urinalysis, but culture for uropathogens is negative. Urinary frequency and urgency are usually absent. Mild urethral exudate may be observed during pelvic examination when the urethra is compressed at the pubic ramus.

Epididymitis. In some men with urethral chlamydial infection (an estimated 1 to 3%), infection spreads from the urethra to the epididymis. This results in unilateral testicular pain, scrotal ery-

TABLE 323–2. MAJOR DISEASES CAUSED BY *CHLAMYDIA* AND CARDINAL EPIDEMIOLOGIC FEATURES

	Disease	Host Reservoir	Transmission Route	Epidemiologic Periodicity
C. trachomatis	Trachoma	Children	Fomites/flies	Endemic
	Urethritis/ cervicitis	Sexually active teenagers and adults	Direct sexual contact	
	Epididymitis/ salpingitis	Sexually active teenagers and adults	Direct sexual contact	
	Lymphogranuloma venereum	Sexually active teenagers and adults	Direct sexual contact	
	Inclusion conjunctivitis Infant pneumonia	Infected pregnant mothers	Direct perinatal contact	
C. psittaci	Atypical pneumonia Culture-negative endocarditis	Birds	Aerosol	Epidemic
C. pneumoniae	Bronchitis Atypical pneumonia	Humans	Respiratory droplet	Epidemic and endemic

thema and tenderness, or swelling over the epididymis. Epididymitis associated with urethritis is most commonly due to *C. trachomatis* or *Neisseria gonorrhoea* (see Ch. 315). Among men < 35 years of age, *C. trachomatis* is the principal cause of epididymitis. Among men > 35 years of age, complicated urinary tract infection with uropathogens is more commonly the cause of epididymitis.

Reiter's Syndrome. Reactive arthritis can complicate chlamydial infection (see Ch. 238). About 50% of men with nondiarrheal Reiter's syndrome have urethral *C. trachomatis* infection. It is estimated that approximately 1% of men with chlamydial urethritis develop Reiter's syndrome.

Mucopurulent Cervicitis. Mucopurulent cervicitis in women is the epidemiologic counterpart of NGU in men. As with NGU, *C. trachomatis* causes 40 to 50% of cases of mucopurulent cervicitis. Twenty to 50% of women with cervical chlamydial infection have mucopurulent cervicitis. Women with mucopurulent cervicitis may complain of mucoidy vaginal discharge. Unless concurrent infection with other pathogens is present, the vaginal discharge lacks odor, and vulvar pruritus does not occur. Mucopurulent cervicitis is best recognized during vaginal speculum examination with the cervix fully exposed and well illuminated. There is a yellow or cloudy mucoid discharge from the cervix, though the color may be better appreciated on the tip of a cotton swab than *in situ*. Gram stain of endocervical mucus shows > 10 polymorphonuclear leukocytes per 1000× field. Often, a red area of columnar epithelium is visible on the face of the cervix (ectopy). The area is erythematous, edematous, and bleeds easily when touched with a cotton-tipped swab.

Endometritis and Salpingitis. *C. trachomatis* infection can spread from the cervix to the endometrium to produce endometritis and to the fallopian tubes to produce salpingitis. Spread occurs in 10 to 40% of women with cervical chlamydial infection. If *C. trachomatis* spreads to the endometrium after therapeutic or postvaginal delivery, it can produce late onset postpartum or postabortal endometritis. More commonly, chlamydial infection spreads spontaneously to the upper reproductive tract. Although endometritis and salpingitis can occur subclinically, clinically patent disease includes the following features: subacute onset of low abdominal pain during menses or during the first 2 weeks of the menstrual cycle, pain on sexual intercourse (dyspareunia), and prolonged menses or intermenstrual vaginal bleeding. Fever is not a common feature of *C. trachomatis* endometritis or salpingitis.

Infant Inclusion Conjunctivitis and Pneumonia. Perinatally transmitted *C. trachomatis* infection is an important health problem for infants. Approximately, two of three infants perinatally exposed to *C. trachomatis* acquire infection. Clinically patent disease occurs in about 75% of infected infants, and 25% are subclinically infected. Inclusion conjunctivitis of the newborn develops in one in three exposed infants and a distinctive pneumonia syndrome in about one in six. Since 5 to 20% of pregnant women in the United States have *C. trachomatis* cervical infection, the morbidity due to perinatally transmitted chlamydial infection is substantial.

The distinctive pneumonia syndrome has a subacute onset in infants between ages 1 and 4 months. The natural history of illness is protracted, and importantly, fever is absent. The cardinal clinical characteristic is a distinctive staccato cough reminiscent of pertussis but without the whoop or posttussive vomiting. Hematologic examination consistently shows eosinophilia (≥ 400 eosinophils per cubic millimeter) and hypergammaglobulinemia (serum IgG ≥ 600 and IgM ≥ 110 mg per deciliter).

Lymphogranuloma Venereum. LGV is the result of sexually transmitted infection with *C. trachomatis* serovars L_1, L_2, or L_3. This is a systemic infection that involves lymphoid tissue. In the United States in 1992, 302 cases of LGV were reported to the Center for Disease Control and Prevention (CDC). In the developing world, especially sub-Saharan Africa, LGV is much more common, although accurate statistics are lacking.

The *C. trachomatis* serovars that produce LGV are much more invasive than are other *C. trachomatis* serovars. Similar to diseases due to other *C. trachomatis* serovars, LGV produces acute disease and late fibrotic complications. Among heterosexuals, primary LGV infection produces an evanescent and rarely observed genital ulcer

2 to 3 weeks after exposure. The ulcer spontaneously heals, and 2 to 4 weeks later painful bilateral inguinal lymphadenopathy develops, often associated with signs of systemic infection such as fever, headache, arthralgias, leukocytosis, and hypergammaglobulinemia. In the absence of treatment, LGV spontaneously heals, sometimes leaving lymphatic scarring. Late fibrotic complications of LGV include genital elephantiasis, strictures, and fistulas of the penis, urethra, and rectum.

In women and homosexual men, rectal infection with *C. trachomatis* L_1, L_2, or L_3 strains produces a severe febrile protocolitis illness. Patients complain of frequent painful defecation (tenesmus) with urgency and less commonly mucopurulent bloody discharge in stool. Biopsy of rectal mucosa shows submucosal granulomas, crypt abscesses, and diffuse mononuclear cell inflammation. The clinical, endoscopic, and histopathologic findings can mimic Crohn's disease of the rectum.

Laboratory Diagnosis. Empirical treatment for *C. trachomatis* infection should be initiated when a specific chlamydial syndrome is recognized. However, definitive diagnosis of *C. trachomatis* infection depends on laboratory identification of the organism. Laboratory diagnosis confirms the clinical diagnosis, assists in managing contacts of infected cases, and detects asymptomatic but infectious individuals.

The gold standard for diagnosing *C. trachomatis* infection is isolating the organism in cell culture. The development of culture-independent technologies to identify *C. trachomatis* infection was an important advancement. Culture-independent tests detect (1) *C. trachomatis* EB's in mucosal exudate by fluorescent labeled monoclonal antibody, (2) antigen (mainly lipopolysaccharide) in extracted mucosal exudate by ELISA, (3) plasmid DNA by direct probing, and (4) DNA by PCR amplification. The relative sensitivity of these tests is as follows: cell culture or PCR (capable of detecting a single EB) > LPS antigen detection by ELISA (lower limit of detection approximately 10^3 EB's) > chromosomal or plasmid DNA probe detection (lower limit of detection about 10^3 to 10^4 EB's). Because many chlamydial infections such as NGU, salpingitis, and trachoma are characterized by low numbers of organisms, amplification-based tests are preferred. At present, the higher costs of these tests will limit their widespread use, and antigen-based tests remain the most commonly used tests. Interpreting a positive ELISA test for chlamydia antigen can be difficult in situations where the prevalence of *C. trachomatis* is low (< 5%) because such tests typically have false-positive rates of 1 to 3%. For example, when an antigen-ELISA has a specificity of 98%, a sensitivity of 80%, and is used to screen 1000 individuals from a high-risk population with a *C. trachomatis* prevalence of 15%, the predictive value of a positive test is 88%. When the same test is used to screen 1000 individuals from a low-risk population with a *C. trachomatis* prevalence of 2%, the predictive value of positive tests falls to 44%. Clinicians should verify positive antigen-ELISA tests with a second *C. trachomatis* diagnostic test based on a different method if the risk of false-positive tests results in adverse medical, social, or psychological consequences.

Serology is infrequently used to diagnose *C. trachomatis* infection except in two circumstances: Specific *C. trachomatis* IgM antibody at a titer of 1:32 or more is useful to diagnose the infant pneumonia syndrome, and a complement-fixation antibody titer of 1:64 or more suggests LGV.

Treatment. *C. trachomatis* is uniformly susceptible to tetracyclines, macrolides, and sulfonamides. Recent data also suggest that selected quinolones (ofloxacin) are useful to treat *C. trachomatis* infection.

The recommended treatment for uncomplicated *C. trachomatis* urethritis and mucopurulent cervicitis is doxycycline (100 mg orally twice daily for 7 days) or azithromycin (1 gram orally in a single dose), although azithromycin is substantially more expensive than doxycycline. Alternate treatment regimens include erythromycin base (500 mg orally four times a day for 7 days), sulphisoxazole (500 mg orally four times a day for 10 days), or ofloxacin (300 mg orally twice daily for 7 days). *C. trachomatis* epididymitis and endometritis/salpingitis should be treated for 10 to 14 days. LGV should be treated for 3 weeks.

Sexual partners and parents of infants infected with *C. trachomatis* should be evaluated, tested, and empirically treated. Sexual contacts within the preceding 30 to 60 days should be seen.

In 1986, a new chlamydial pathogen was recognized—*C. pneumoniae*—which causes respiratory illness. Although initially confused with *C. psittaci*, *C. pneumoniae* is a separate species with < 10% DNA homology with the other three chlamydial species. Pneumonia and bronchitis are the most frequently identified illnesses caused by *C. pneumoniae*.

EPIDEMIOLOGY. Much of what has been learned about *C. pneumoniae* epidemiology has resulted from serologic studies. More than 50% of adults in the United States and populations from other developed countries are seropositive. Most seroconversion occurs during childhood with rates of 6 to 9% per year for the age group 5 to 14. Many seroconversions occur subclinically. *C. pneumoniae* causes both endemic and epidemic atypical pneumonia syndromes. In Seattle, the average annual endemic incidence of *C. pneumoniae* pneumonia was 1.2 per 1000 population. Approximately 10% of pneumonia illnesses were attributed to *C. pneumoniae*. Periods of increased incidence were observed at 3- to 4-year cycles. The bacteria also has been documented to produce epidemics of atypical pneumonia in closed populations such as military recruits and university students. Case-to-case transmission appears to involve respiratory droplet spread with an average case-to-case interval of 1 month. Both diseased and asymptomatically infected individuals transmit infection.

CLINICAL FEATURES. Even though most acute infections occur in children, most *C. pneumoniae* disease occurs in adults, especially the elderly. It causes an afebrile, usually relative mild pneumonia. Extrapulmonary findings are not prominent. Nonproductive cough with sore throat and hoarseness are characteristic. The time from onset of illness to clinic presentation is long. On auscultation, localized crackles are often heard. Chest radiography shows a pneumonitis, most often evident as a single subsegmental lesion. Hematologic studies show a normal leukocyte count but a high erythrocyte sedimentation rate.

C. pneumoniae also causes bronchitis and sinusitis. Bronchitis is often subacute in onset, lasting several days or weeks. Some patients with the bronchitis illness unexpectedly have pneumonia on radiography. Sinusitis is often demonstrated by sinus percussion tenderness. Isolated pharyngitis is rarely attributable to *C. pneumoniae* infection, but when pharyngitis, sinusitis, and bronchitis are observed in association with pneumonia, *C. pneumoniae* is a likely cause.

LABORATORY DIAGNOSIS. Serology, isolation, and nonculture detection are the primary methods for laboratory disease of *C. pneumoniae* infection. A complement fixation titer of 1:8 or more has been considered a test for *C. psittaci* infection, but only 25% of hospitalized patients with *C. pneumoniae* pneumonia have a positive test result. The indirect microimmunofluorescent test for *C. pneumoniae* antibodies remains the best method for laboratory diagnosis but is restricted to the research laboratory. Isolating *C. pneumoniae* in cell culture (HL cell line) is successful in 50 to 75% cases of serologically confirmed infections but is technically demanding. PCR of *C. pneumoniae*–specific DNA is about 25% more sensitive than culture and likely will become the diagnostic test of choice. At present, no effective diagnostic method for *C. pneumoniae* is commercially available.

TREATMENT. *C. pneumoniae* is susceptible to tetracycline and macrolides but not sulfonamides. Antimicrobial therapy of *C. pneumoniae* infection can be difficult, and clinical response is not dramatic. Recommended treatment includes tetracycline or erythromycin base 500 mg orally four times a day for 10 to 14 days.

Chlamydia psittaci

EPIDEMIOLOGY. Strangely, *C. psittaci* is the least common but the only reportable chlamydial infection. This is so because it can produce common-source outbreaks of serious disease often related to infected imported birds. *C. psittaci* is a heterogeneous chlamydial species that naturally infects a variety of nonhuman mammals and birds. *C. psittaci* strains appear to be host-specific, and most human psittacosis infections are linked to bird and not mammal exposure. Approximately 100 to 200 cases of psittacosis are reported annually in the United States with no apparent periodicity. The annual incidence has been stable for the past 15 years. Psittacine birds (parrots, parakeets, budgerigars) are most com-

monly implicated as source contacts, although human cases have been traced to contact with pigeons, ducks, turkeys, chickens, and other birds. Among infected birds, *C. psittaci* is present in nasal secretions, guano, and feathers. Psittacosis in birds is a mild illness manifested by ruffled feathers and anorexia. Recovered and asymptomatically infected birds can shed the organism for months.

Transmission to humans is by the aerosol route to the respiratory tract. The infectious inoculum is likely very small, and brief contact with a contaminated environment can result in transmission. Person-to-person spread of *C. psittaci* rarely occurs.

CLINICAL FEATURES. Psittacosis is a systemic infection of the reticuloendothelial system and of the interstitium and alveoli of the lung by *C. psittaci*. Seven to 14 days following aerosol exposure, an abrupt febrile illness begins with shaking chills and a fever as high as 40°C. Headache, myalgias, and arthralgias can be disabling. Cough appears early in the illness but is usually nonproductive. Auscultation may be normal or show bilateral crackles. Chest radiograph shows single or multiple localized bronchopneumonic patches. Clinically, psittacosis can resemble legionnaires' disease. In distinction to *C. pneumoniae* pneumonia, psittacosis is more severe with high fever and absent or minimal upper respiratory complaints.

Extrapulmonary findings are usual with psittacosis, and myalgias can mislead the clinician to suspect meningitis or pyelonephritis. Fulminant psittacosis can produce meningoencephalitis, hepatitis, and a faint macular rash (Horder's spots) resembling the rose spots of typhoid fever. Like typhoid fever, psittacosis may cause abdominal pain, diarrhea, constipation, and splenomegaly. Occasional patients, especially with underlying valvular heart disease, develop endocarditis, and *C. psittaci* is a recognized, if rare, cause of culture-negative endocarditis. Untreated psittacosis can be fatal, but most patients recover slowly after an illness lasting 10 to 21 days.

LABORATORY DIAGNOSIS. The diagnosis can be established by isolating the organism in cell culture or by serology. Because laboratory-acquired *C. psittaci* infections are well documented, cell culture isolation is discouraged, and serology is the preferred test method. If culture is attempted, it is essential to contain the specimen in a biosafety cabinet for processing. Blood and respiratory secretions can be used to isolate the organism during acute disease. Psittacosis is most readily diagnosed by demonstrating a rising titer of complement-fixing antibody in the serum. Acute and 3- to 6-week convalescent sera should be tested.

TREATMENT. *C. psittaci* is susceptible to tetracyclines and macrolides but resistant to sulfonamides. Tetracycline has had the greatest clinical use. Psittacosis is the most gratifying of all chlamydial diseases to treat. Defervescence and marked symptomatic relief of systemic signs occur within 24 to 48 hours after starting tetracycline 500 mg four times a day. Treatment should be continued for 10 to 14 days.

PREVENTION. Epidemic psittacosis is a preventable disease by quarantining and giving all imported psittacine birds tetracycline. Preventing psittacosis acquired from nonpsittacine birds is more problematic and will remain a continuing source for human infection. No vaccine is commercially available.

Bailey RL, Arullendran P, Whittle HC, et al.: Randomised, controlled trial of single-dose azithromycin in treatment of trachoma. Lancet 342:453, 1993. *Single-dose treatment with azithromycin is remarkably effective in curing childhood trachoma.*

Centers for Disease Control and Prevention: Recommendations for the prevention and management of *Chlamydia trachomatis* infections, 1993. MMWR 42(RR-12):1, 1993. *Review of the major clinical syndromes due to sexually and perinatally transmitted* C. trachomatis *infection and a review of available diagnostic tests and how to screen for asymptomatic chlamydial infection.*

Grayston JT: Infections caused by *Chlamydia pneumoniae* strain TWAR. Clin Infect Dis 15:757, 1992. *A succinct review of the current status of* C. pneumoniae *as a human pathogen.*

Hedberg K, White KE, Forfang JC, et al.: An outbreak of psittacosis in Minnesota turkey industry workers: Implications for modes of transmission and control. Am J Epidemiol 130:569, 1989. *An interesting epidemiologic investigation of a large outbreak of psittacosis typifying many of the clinical and epidemiologic markers of this disease.*

Moulder JW: Interaction of chlamydiae and host cells in vitro. Microbiol Rev 55:143, 1991. *A masterful review of the cellular and molecular mechanisms of chlamydiae's interaction with host cells.*

Schachter J, Dawson CR: The epidemiology of trachoma predicts more blindness in the future. Scand J Infect Dis Suppl 69:55, 1990. *A good overview of the epidemiology of childhood trachoma and its relationship to blindness in adulthood.*

324 RICKETTSIAL DISEASES

Richard B. Hornick

Introduction

The rickettsiae are small obligate intracellular, gram-negative pathogens. They do not have a symbiotic relationship with human host cells and therefore cause metabolic derangements that result in cell death. Infections with the typhus and spotted fever groups of rickettsiae involve endothelial cells. This host-pathogen interaction results in a perivasculitis. Q fever induces granulomas in the liver plus interstitial pneumonia. Ehrlichiosis is a relatively new human disease, the cause of which continues to be investigated. It is caused by rickettsial organisms that are related to ones causing infections in dogs, horses, and so on. At least two species have been identified, *Ehrlichia chaffeensis* and an organism yet to be cultured which is related to the *E. phagocytophilia/E. equi* group. They are transmitted by ticks and cause illness in areas where Rocky Mountain spotted fever (RMSF) is endemic. Trench fever and cat scratch fever and three unusual infections occurring in immunocompromised hosts—bacillary angiomatosis, bacillary peliosis of the liver, and endocarditis—are caused by small gram-negative rods formerly classified as *Rochalimaea quintana, R. henselae,* and *R. elizabethae.* They are now included in the family Bartonellaceae and no longer part of the order Rickettsiales (see Ch. 310).

Each of the rickettsiae is transmitted to humans by ticks, mites, lice, fleas, or aerosols originating from animal products (placentas, Q fever) or from feces of the aforementioned insects. In the United States, there are relatively few cases of rickettsial infections. RMSF is the most prevalent, 600 to 700 cases having been reported annually since 1985. Fewer cases of Q fever and murine typhus are identified each year. Certain other rickettsial infections are major public health problems in developing countries but are not found in the United States, e.g., scrub typhus. The potential for tourists to return to the United States with an emerging rickettsial infec-tion is increasing. Because of the rarity of rickettsial infections in this country, diagnosis may be delayed. Delays in diagnosing these illnesses can adversely affect the potential for recovery.

In this chapter three tables (Tables 324–1 to 324–3) are included that summarize, first, the epidemiologic features of rickettsial infections; second, the host cells involved in the pathogenesis of the clinical manifestations of the disease; and third, those clinical features that will assist in differentiating the various forms of rickettsial infections. Additional details on the major rickettsial infections that occur in the United States or that represent potential threats to persons traveling abroad are found under separate sections in this chapter.

324.1 The Typhus Group

This group of conditions includes three established clinical and epidemiologic entities: epidemic louse-borne typhus fever, the oldest disease known to be caused by rickettsiae; Brill-Zinsser disease, a classic example of reactivation of a latent infection; and flea-borne murine typhus. The first two conditions are induced by *Rickettsia prowazekii,* a pathogen transferred from person to person by the bite of body lice. Persons who have recovered from epidemic typhus have persistent rickettsiae in various host cells, presumably in the reticuloendothelial cells; stresses that cause a defect in the suppressive lymphocytes will, years later, permit these rickettsiae to be reactivated, resulting in a mild typhus-like illness, called Brill-Zinsser disease. In 1975, *R. prowazekii* was isolated from flying squirrels in the southeastern United States. A number of persons ac-quired typhus fever from squirrels living in their attics and probably harboring infected fleas or lice or both.

Flea-borne murine typhus, caused by *R. typhi,* is a mild form of typhus fever occurring in the U.S. and elsewhere. It is transmitted by fleas from rodents. *R. canada* is a tick-borne (mouse-rabbit reservoirs), rickettsial organism, formerly classified with the typhus group. It is distinct from the typhus, as well as the spotted fever group. Whether it is a significant human pathogen requires more study. It has been implicated by serologic means as the cause of acute febrile cerebrovasculitis in one patient.

EPIDEMIC LOUSE-BORNE TYPHUS

INTRODUCTION. Synonyms include classic, historic, and European typhus; jail, war, camp, and ship fever; *Flichfieber* (German); *typhus exanthematique* (French); and *tifus exantematico* and *tabardillo* (Spanish). Many of these names indicate the location of the outbreaks—military and concentration camps, crowded ships with poor and starved immigrants, outbreaks in persons living in occupied countries during wartime, and so forth. Each implies crowded, unsanitary living conditions where bathing and laundry facilities are inadequate. These conditions allow for body lice to breed and propagate. The impact of typhus fever on military campaigns and immigration patterns is a fascinating and provocative story. The reader is referred to Woodward (1973) for an introduction to the effects of this disease on history.

DEFINITION. Classic typhus fever is manifested by the sudden onset of headache, fever, rash, and an altered mental state. (Typhus is derived from the Greek word meaning cloudy or misty. Applied to typhus, it describes the obtunded, lethargic state of mind.) *R. prowazekii* is transmitted by human body lice *(Pediculus humanus humanus).*

ETIOLOGY. *R. prowazekii* is a small obligate intracellular, gram-negative bacillus. In cells it stains red when exposed to Gimenez's stain. Viable rickettsiae stimulate the endothelial cell to act like a phagocyte to engulf the rickettsiae in a phagosome and internalize it. If rickettsiae do not break out of the phagosome promptly they begin to disintegrate, perhaps owing to enzymatic activities. The rickettsiae have an enzyme, phospholipase A, that enables them to lyse the phagosome wall and to multiply freely in the cytoplasm. *R. prowazekii* escape from the cell by destroying it. The necrotic cell stimulates an inflammatory response that leads to the vasculitis and subsequent clotting abnormalities.

TRANSMISSION AND EPIDEMIOLOGY. The unique feature of infection with *R. prowazekii* is that no animal reservoir has been implicated, at least until its isolation from the flying squirrel *(Glaucomys volans).* It is still uncertain how significant the flying squirrel will be in amplifying the incidence of this disease. Very few, if any, cases of classic typhus occur each year in the U.S. (Centers for Disease Control and Prevention [CDC] does not have an active surveillance for it). Fifteen cases were reported in 1980 and 1981, all in persons having contact with flying squirrels.

Classic typhus is a disease of humans. An individual with rickettsemia can infect body lice. The lice acquire the organisms in their blood meal. These ectoparasites may then find another person to whom they transmit the rickettsiae via infected feces. Body lice do not survive the ingestion of rickettsiae. The organisms multiply in the gut of the louse, destroy the epithelial cells, and the louse dies (usually in 1 to 3 weeks). However, during the period of infection, the louse passes feces heavily laden with rickettsiae. Either the human host scratches the site of the bite and thereby self-inoculates the rickettsiae, or the feces and rickettsiae contaminate minute apertures in the epidermis, allowing the organisms to find cells in which to multiply. Dried, contaminated feces can also become airborne, e.g., by shaking out clothing loaded with lice and feces and thereby creating an infectious aerosol. When inhaled, the rickettsiae can penetrate the mucosal cells and enter endothelial cells. Laboratory accidents frequently generate aerosols that induce infection in technicians. Nurses and other medical personnel are at risk for inhaling airborne particles when they remove the clothing from a patient.

When the body louse obtains a blood meal containing antibody-coated rickettsiae, the louse may modify the infectivity of the rickettsiae-antibody combination by partially digesting the antibody coating of the organism in its gut. This digestion destroys the Fc portion of the antibody that would have permitted attachment to macrophages. The rickettsia is then free of the inhibiting action of the antibody when it infects the next person.

TABLE 324-1. SUMMARY OF SOME EPIDEMIOLOGIC FEATURES OF SELECTED RICKETTSIAL DISEASES OF HUMANS

Disease	Organism	Natural Cycle		Usual Mode of Transmission to Humans	Common Occupational or Environmental Association	Geographic Distribution
		Arthropod Vector	*Reservoir/ Mammalian Host*			
Typhus group						
Murine typhus	*Rickettsia mooseri* (*R. typhi*)	Flea	Rodents	Infected flea feces into broken skin or aerosol to mucous membranes	Rat-infected premises (shops, warehouses, grain elevators)	Scattered foci, worldwide
Epidemic typhus	*R. prowazekii*	Body louse	Humans*	Infected crushed louse or feces into broken skin or aerosol to mucous membranes	Lousy human population with louse transfer	Worldwide
Brill-Zinsser disease	*R. prowazekii*	Recrudescence months to years after primary attack of louse-borne typhus			Unknown; ?stress	Worldwide
Spotted fever group (selected examples)						
Rocky Mountain spotted fever	*R. rickettsii*	Ixodid ticks	Ticks/small mammals	Tick bite, mechanical transfer to mucous membranes, ?airborne	Tick-infested terrain, houses, dogs	Western hemisphere
Ehrlichiosis	*Ehrlichia chaffeensis*	Ticks	?Dogs	Tick bite	Tick-infested areas	At least 12 states in U.S., primarily southern states
	E. phagocytophilia/ E. equi group	Ticks	Ticks/Mammals	Tick bite	Tick-infested areas	Wisconsin-Minnesota
Boutonneuse fever	*R. conorii*	Ixodid ticks	Ticks/rodents, dogs	Tick bite	Tick-infested terrain, houses, dogs	Mediterranean littoral, Africa, ?Indian subcontinent
Rickettsialpox	*R. akrai*	Mouse mite	Mite/mice	Mouse mite bite	Unique mouse- and mite-infested premises (incinerators)	United States, former USSR, Korea, ?Central Africa
Scrub typhus Tsutsugamushi disease	*R. tsutsugamushi* (multiple serotypes)	Chigger	Chigger/?rodents	Chigger bite	Chigger-infested terrain; secondary scrub, grass airfields, golf courses	Asia, Australia, New Guinea, Pacific Islands
Q fever	*Coxiella burnetii*	?Ticks	Ticks/mammals	Inhalation of dried airborne infective material; ?tick bite	Domestic animals or products, dairies, lambing pens, slaughterhouses	Worldwide

* Recent isolations of putative *R. prowazekii* from flying squirrels in the eastern United States have not been evaluated as reservoirs for human infection. Previous claims of involvement of domestic animals are now largely discounted.

The louse does not transmit *R. prowazekii* transovarially to offspring and is not an amplifier for further propagation. Patients who recover from classic typhus have the opportunity to develop Brill-Zinsser disease and at that time have rickettsemia and are able again to infect body lice. However, this happens rarely, for few cases of Brill-Zinsser disease have been detected among the many hundreds of thousands of soldiers who acquired typhus in World War II; one estimate suggested a rate of 10 per 100,000 cases of primary typhus. More cases may be recognized as the geriatric population continues to increase. This group will have significant ill-

ness, surgical procedures, and chemotherapy that could cause reactivation of the latent rickettsiae.

Typhus fever remains a threat to persons living under unsanitary and deprived circumstances. As long as there are persons who are latent reservoirs for *R. prowazekii,* an epidemic can erupt. One country with persistent typhus is Ethiopia. There, prolonged drought, poverty, and malnutrition contribute to the perpetuation of the disease.

PATHOLOGY. The rickettsiae invade only endothelial cells, as described in the section on RMSF. This leads to vasculitis, with dif-

TABLE 324-2. RICKETTSIA TARGET CELL RELATIONSHIPS, PATHOLOGIC, LESIONS, AND CLINICAL MANIFESTATIONS OF HUMAN RICKETTSIOSES*

Disease	Target Cell	Host-Cell Association	Basic Lesion	Clinical Manifestations
Typhus-like fevers				
Typhus group	Endothelial	Free intracytoplasmic	Vasculitis	Acute self-limited fever
Scrub typhus	Endothelial	Free intracytoplasmic	Vasculitis	Acute self-limited fever
Spotted fever group	Endothelial, smooth muscle	Free intracytoplasmic and intranuclear	Vasculitis	Acute self-limited fever
Ehrlichiosis	Neutrophils/monocytes	Intracytoplasmic inclusion body (morulae)	Leukopenia, thrombocytopenia, liver cell damage	
Q fever	Reticuloendothelial	Intracytoplasmic vacuole	Granulomas	Acute self-limited fever, "atypical pneumonia," subacute hepatitis, subacute endocarditis

* Adapted from Stickland (ed.): Hunter's Tropical Medicine, Philadelphia, WB Saunders, 1984.

TABLE 324-3. SOME CLINICAL FEATURES OF SELECTED RICKETTSIAL DISEASES

| Disease | Usual Incubation Period (Days) | Eschar | Rash | | | Usual Duration of Disease* (Days) | Usual Severity† | Fever After Chemotherapy (Hours) |
			Onset, Day of Disease	Distribution	Type			
Typhus group								
Murine typhus	12 (8–16)	None	5–7	Trunk → extremities	Macular, maculopapular	12 (8–16)	Moderate	48–72
Epidemic typhus	12 (10–14)	None	5–7	Trunk → extremities	Macular, maculopapular, petechial	14 (10–18)	Severe	48–72
Brill-Zinsser disease	—	None		Trunk → extremities	Macular	7–11	Relatively mild	48–72
Spotted fever group								
Rocky Mountain spotted fever	7 (3–12)	None	3–5	Extremities → trunk, face	Macular, maculopapular, petechial	16 (10–20)	Severe	72
Ehrlichiosis	7–21	None	?Rare	Unknown	Petechial	7 (3–19)	Mild	72
Boutonneuse fever	5–7	Other present	3–4	Trunk, extremities, face, palms, soles	Macular, maculopapular, petechial	10 (7–14) 7	Moderate	—
Rickettsialpox	?9–17	Often present	1–3	Trunk → face, extremities	Papulovesicular	7 (3–11)	Relatively mild	—
Scrub typhus (tsutsugamushi disease)	1–12 (9–18)	Often present	4–6	Trunk → extremities	Macular, maculopapular	14 (10–20)	Mild to severe	24–36
Q fever	10–19	None		None		(2–21)	Relatively mild‡	48 (occasionally slow)

* Untreated disease.
† Severity can vary greatly.
‡ Occasionally subacute infections occur (e.g., hepatitis, endocarditis).

fering pathologic changes in various organs. There is no eschar in this disease. The rash appears to have its origin in the leakage of blood and fluid from the damaged capillaries. The damage to the endothelial cells results in cell death, and at these sites platelet-fibrin thrombi form, platelet-active substances are released, and vasoconstriction and occlusion of small vessels occur. These changes can lead to infarcts in various organs, edema of tissue, leakage of inflammatory cells around small blood vessels ("typhus nodules" of the brain, for instance), stimulation of clotting mechanisms, and the development of shock. Almost all organs are involved in patients with untreated disease. The inflammatory exudate consists of mononuclear cells, plasma cells, histiocytes, and polymorphonuclear leukocytes. Gangrene of skin and limbs occurs in the presence of extensive thrombotic activity.

CLINICAL MANIFESTATIONS AND COURSE. The incubation period averages about 7 days but can range from 6 to 15 days. The onset is abrupt with intense headache, chills, fever, and myalgia. There is back or leg pain—presumably due to the muscle damage secondary to the vasculitis. Bites of lice may cause pruritus, and persons infested with lice may have numerous scratches in the skin. Sometimes the skin has a yellow-gold hue because of frequent lice bites. The headache is described as the "worst ever," and the pain is unremitting unless treated with narcotic analgesics. The temperature rises quickly during the first 2 days and persists for about 2 weeks, maintaining a continuous fever pattern if not altered by antibiotics or antipyretic medications. During the first week, there is a bradycardia relative to the temperature elevations of 39° to 41°C. Conjunctivae are injected, and photophobia is present. Deafness, tinnitus, and sometimes vertigo are prominent features. The patient appears to be in a toxic state, with a flushed face, obtundation, and profound weakness. There may be a cough, but no rales are apparent on auscultation of the lungs. The pharyngeal mucous lining is dry and inflamed.

The rash, characteristic of the typhus group, appears on the fourth to seventh day of disease. The lesions appear first on the trunk and axillary folds (areas of skin stress) and spread to the extremities but spare the palms and soles of the feet. The lesions are reddish-pink macules that fade on pressure. With treatment or in mild cases, the rash disappears within several days. In untreated patients, it can spread and coalesce, leading to gangrene of portions of

the skin, especially over regions of bony prominences. In 5 to 10% of patients, the rash may not be present.

These and other manifestations occur because of the initial unchecked multiplication and spread of the rickettsiae, involving ever-enlarging segments of the endothelial surface. The resulting damage to the organs evolves because of the compromised circulation and the associated acute inflammatory responses. Whether rickettsial toxin or endotoxin contributes to the pathologic changes is still debated. Whatever processes are involved, certain organs are regularly involved: the skin, heart, kidneys, and skeletal muscle. In patients with severe disease, hypotension and renal failure portend a fatal outcome.

The altered mental status that occurs as the disease progresses (in untreated patients) is striking. The patient may progress from stupor to coma. The stupor may be interrupted by brief periods of delirium. Patients may have to be restrained in order to protect them from trauma. At this stage, lymphocytic pleocytosis of the cerebrospinal fluid (CSF) may be present. Despite the seriousness of the patient's condition, complete recovery can ensue. Cranial nerve lesions are common. There are also temporary mental aberrations.

Patients who have acquired typhus fever in the U.S. from flying squirrels have had signs and symptoms of the classic disease. The rash was noted in 8 of 15, and it was evanescent. Significant central nervous system involvement was reported in five patients; two had coma and three had confusion or delirium.

Death in untreated patients occurs between the ninth and eighteenth days. Recovery from the disease begins with a rapid lysis of fever after about 2 weeks of disease. When the fever disappears, mental function returns quickly. Recovery of a sense of well-being is protracted owing to the need to counter the stresses of prolonged negative nitrogen balance, inanition, and loss of muscle mass.

Brill-Zinsser disease is manifested in a manner similar to classic typhus. All signs and symptoms are milder, presumably because the host has well-developed immune mechanisms that can regain control in a short time. Serologic studies in these patients demonstrate immunoglobulin G (IgG) rather than immunoglobulin M (IgM) antibodies. Occasionally, patients with unrecognized Brill-Zinsser disease die. An underlying disease or procedure may permit activation of the latent rickettsiae, and this combination can culminate in death. Reactivation has been noted following surgical procedures and the use of immunosuppressive drugs. In experimental animals that have recovered from the primary disease, isolation of rickettsiae at a future date is facilitated by steroid administration.

PROGNOSIS. The fatality rate in untreated groups of patients with classic typhus is 10 to 60%. Children usually have a mild illness with minimal risk of death. Patients over age 60 have the highest mortality rate. Recovery is the rule with appropriate antibiotic treatment.

TREATMENT. *R. prowazekii* responds well to tetracycline and chloramphenicol antibiotics. Doxycycline, 200 mg as a single oral dose, is the treatment of choice. Tetracycline, 25 mg per kilogram daily in four doses, or chloramphenicol, 50 mg per kilogram daily in four doses, is an effective alternative. Therapy should be continued for 2 to 3 days after the fever has defervesced. Most patients are afebrile within 48 to 72 hours and improve quickly from the debilitating headache or mental aberrations or both. Relapses occur in persons who are treated early, on day 1 or 2 of illness. Such patients do not develop the required immune mechanisms to contain the proliferation of the residual rickettsiae. Furthermore, both antibiotics are rickettsiostatic and do not eradicate all of these intracellular parasites even when specific immune mechanisms are introduced. Recovery from disease without antibiotics also allows rickettsiae to remain in cells, later to be activated and cause Brill-Zinsser disease. In the severely ill patient, fluid therapy and proper nutrition are mandatory. Fortunately, antibiotic therapy has simplified the need for supportive care.

PREVENTION AND CONTROL. To prevent and control the spread of classic typhus, the body lice (and feces) associated with patients and their clothes must be destroyed. The clothing should be carefully placed in plastic bags and sealed and carefully removed only in the area where they are to be treated. Clothes that can sustain boiling are boiled, and the rest should be subjected to steam and dry heat. It is also possible to kill the lice (also the eggs present in seams and elsewhere—these eggs will hatch in a week) with insecticides. Lice now are generally resistant to 10% DDT (chlorophenothane) and 1% lindane dust. Malathion (1%) and 2% temefos (Abate) are effective in most areas. These dusts are applied to the fully clothed individual. This approach controls the acute outbreaks of disease when applied to all persons in the community. Long-time use of insecticides is not effective because resistance develops, because long-term compliance is difficult, and because the insecticides may adversely affect the ecology of the region. Control requires improvement of sanitary conditions and standards of living as well as health education.

Health personnel treating patients with classic typhus are at risk for acquiring the disease from lice picked up from the patients or their clothing. There is no risk of direct human-to-human transfer of the rickettsiae other than by aerosolized, dried, contaminated feces. Once the patient has been deloused, no isolation barriers are required.

No vaccine is currently available for preventing classic typhus.

Travelers to endemic areas are rarely at risk unless, for example, they work in camps for displaced persons or carry out relief work that brings them in contact with persons with lice. Decontaminating the clothing overnight with insecticides or wearing insect repellent-treated clothes provides some protection. Prophylactic doxycycline has been effective when given weekly to prevent scrub typhus and would be expected to be effective in preventing *R. prowazekii* infections. This drug should be used only for short periods, 2 to 4 weeks. It is important under these circumstances to monitor the temperature for 2 weeks at least, as the drug may have masked the initial infection and delayed the onset of symptoms. Retreatment with doxycycline at the onset of the fever is curative.

MURINE TYPHUS

DEFINITION. Murine typhus, a milder form of classic typhus, is caused by *Rickettsia typhi* and is transmitted from rodents to humans by means of the rat flea *(Xenopsylla cheopis)*. It is the only disease of the typhus group that occurs regularly in the United States, albeit in small numbers.

ETIOLOGY. *R. typhi* is a small gram-negative obligate intracellular pathogen. Like *R. prowazekii*, it can penetrate into endothelial cells by induced phagocytosis. Its disease potential resides in its ability to multiply in these cells, destroy them, and initiate a vasculitis. *R. typhi* is catalogued with the typhus group because it shares common antigens with *R. prowazekii* and *R. canada*. In addi-

tion, there is cross-immunity between *R. prowazekii* and *R. typhi* induced by infections. Despite these similarities, it is clear from DNA homology studies that the two are not closely related.

TRANSMISSION AND EPIDEMIOLOGY. *R. typhi* causes disease worldwide. Wherever there are large rodent populations, there is the potential for outbreaks. The rat and other small animals serve as reservoirs of this disease. *Rattus rattus* and *Rattus norvegicus* are two species of rats that can sustain the *R. typhi*, serve as a source of rickettsiae for the rat flea, and have no obvious illness from carrying this human pathogen. The rat flea disseminates the infection not through its bite but by placing contaminated feces on the skin. These may be rubbed or scratched into the skin; they can be carried to the conjunctival sac or mucous membranes on the fingers, where the rickettsiae can invade; or they can be aerosolized after drying and cause infection if inhaled. In the flea, the rickettsiae multiply in the enterocytes in the gut, do not kill the flea, and continue to be shed in the feces for the life of the flea. Transovarial transmission of *R. typhi* occurs in the oriental rat flea.

Murine typhus is a reportable disease. The CDC received 28 reports in 1992, 18 of which came from Texas. In the previous 10 years, the number ranged from 37 to 67 annually, with Texas and California having the highest numbers. Cases are probably underreported. A dramatic drop occurred in the number of reported cases after the mid 1940's. In 1944 there were over 5400 cases. By 1954 there were 163. This decline was due to intensive efforts at rodent control. Most of the cases occur in the warmer months, when rat fleas are plentiful.

PATHOLOGY. Descriptions of the pathologic lesions in this disease are few because of the rarity of fatal cases. Since the rickettsiae are known to invade endothelial cells, the pathologic consequences should mimic those seen in other rickettsial infections. The reasons for the differences in virulence of these rickettsiae and the varying severity of illnesses produced are unknown.

CLINICAL MANIFESTATIONS AND COURSE. Headache, fever, and myalgia are the principal symptoms and signs. These appear after an incubation period of about 1 to 2 weeks. A faint macular-papular pink-colored rash appears in about 80% of patients after 4 to 5 days of illness. It may be difficult to see in poor light. When present, it may be visible for 4 to 8 days before it gradually fades.

Rarely are there any significant complications of this infection, but as it is an infection of the endothelial cells, a vasculitis can cause widespread organ derangement. The patients, especially if older, are debilitated when not treated. They may remain febrile, with a temperature of 39° to 40°C for 2 weeks. This metabolic stress necessitates prolonged convalescence. Antibiotic therapy brings about a prompt recovery.

DIAGNOSIS. This disease has no distinguishing characteristics during the early days of symptoms. The rash appearing on the fourth or fifth day should alert the physician to the possibility of a rickettsial infection. The history of a possible exposure to areas where rats are known to exist, e.g., grain elevators, port facilities, and farm buildings, provides useful information. Flea bites, if seen early, are discrete and may have a central hemorrhagic punctum. The location and grouping of flea bites are important diagnostic features. They occur in covered parts of the body, in irregular groups of several to a dozen or more, in the region of the belt, shoulders, and hips, or on the legs.

Differentiating this disease from RMSF may be difficult. The rash of RMSF usually begins on the wrists and palms and on the soles of the feet and then extends to the skin of the thorax and abdomen. In murine typhus the lesions are on the skin of the chest and abdomen and rarely on the extremities. The history of a tick bite or exposure provides evidence for a clinical diagnosis of RMSF.

Serologic studies confirm the rickettsial infection. Weil-Felix OX-19 reaction is positive in most patients who have not received antibiotic treatment. This test, however, does not distinguish murine typhus from the spotted fever group of infections. The indirect immunofluorescent test can be used to identify *R. typhi* infections. However, because of the common antigens shared with *R. prowazekii,* the serum requires cross-absorption with special antigens from these two rickettsia strains. Isolating the organism is possible but should be done only in special laboratories where containment facilities are available.

PROGNOSIS AND TREATMENT. The mortality rate is < 5% in untreated patients. Appropriate antibiotic treatment results in prompt cure, and the mortality rate is reduced almost to zero. Two deaths were reported between 1982 and 1991.

Tetracycline and chloramphenicol are effective for treating this rickettsial infection. A 5- to 7-day course of either is effective. The usual dosage of 25 mg per kilogram of tetracycline per day in four doses or chloramphenicol, 50 mg per kilogram per day in four doses, effects a prompt cure. The organisms are sensitive to these antibiotics. No resistant strains have been identified. Relapses do occur when antibiotics are administered early in the course of the illness. Retreatment with the antibiotic of choice provides prompt response.

PREVENTION AND CONTROL. There is no vaccine to prevent this disease. Control of rats has been shown to be very effective. When rat control programs are instituted, appropriate insecticides should be simultaneously used to prevent the fleas from seeking humans for feeding as the rat population is decreased.

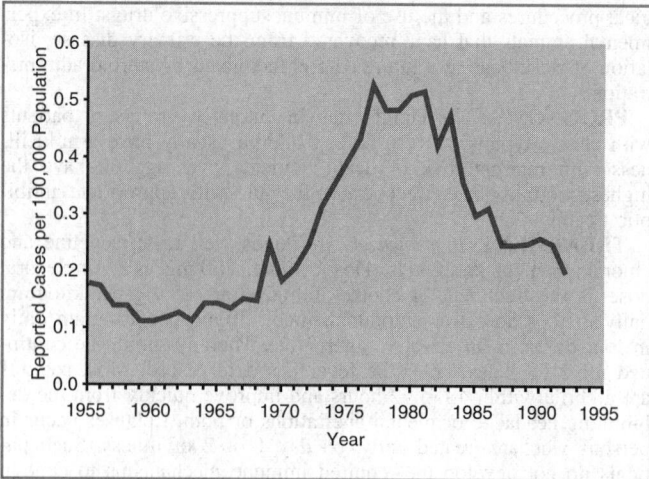

FIGURE 324–1. Rocky Mountain spotted fever in the United States, 1955 to 1992.

324.2 Rocky Mountain Spotted Fever

SYNONYMS AND DEFINITION. Rocky Mountain spotted fever (RMSF) is also known as typhus fever, tick-borne, by the CDC, *fiebre manchada* (Mexico), *fiebre petequial* (Colombia), and *febre maculosa* or Sao Paulo typhus (Brazil).

RMSF is a sometimes fatal systemic infection manifested by fever, severe headache, rash, and other organ disease caused by the vasculitis induced by *Rickettsia rickettsii*. The organism is usually transmitted to humans from animal reservoirs by a tick bite.

ETIOLOGY. *R. rickettsii* organisms are small gram-negative coccobacillary bacteria that can grow only inside eukaryotic host cells. They cannot be isolated on cell-free culture media. In human infections the rickettsiae invade and multiply within endothelial cells of arteries and veins. Different strains of *R. rickettsii* vary in virulence in human as well as animal hosts. Mortality rates appear to be higher in Montana than on the Eastern seaboard. Attempts to correlate virulence with structural components in the polysaccharide portion of the cell wall have been unsuccessful. However, two surface proteins, with molecular weights of 120,000 and 155,000, have been identified as possible virulence factors (protective antigens), and the latter has been produced from cloned genes in *Escherichia coli*. The antigenic material protects mice from lethal infection and will be studied as a potential vaccine.

DISTRIBUTION AND INCIDENCE. This disease was named for the geographic site of its original discovery; the causative agent was named for the discoverer, Howard T. Ricketts. By the 1940's the disease had become more common on the East Coast than in the West. The incidence rose sharply beginning in 1971 and peaked in 1981 at 5.2 per million population in the United States. In 1992, 502 cases were reported, for a low of 2.0 per million (Fig. 324–1). The decline occurred primarily in the southeast. Reasons for these fluctuations are unknown.

Serologic surveys in children and adults in North Carolina, the state with the highest number of reported cases, demonstrate that subclinical infections occur. Almost 20% of the children had OX-19 agglutination titers in the diagnostic range, and a smaller number had positive indirect fluorescent antibody titers, a more specific test. None of these children was previously diagnosed as having had RMSF.

TRANSMISSION AND EPIDEMIOLOGY. Ninety percent of reported cases occur between April 1 and September 30, with two thirds in May, June, and July. Children and young adults account for about 40% of cases. Ninety percent of patients give a history of a tick bite or attachment or of having been in a tick-infested area 14 days prior to onset of illness. Infected ticks are found in urban as well as rural areas. A park in New York City was the source of ticks that transmitted *R. rickettsii* to four children, one of whom died.

RMSF occurs in humans when an infected tick bites and injects *R. rickettsii* into the skin. Probably fewer than 10 organisms injected intradermally are sufficient to induce disease.

Several species of ticks are commonly involved in transmission of disease: *Dermacentor andersoni,* the wood tick, in the Rocky Mountain states; *D. variabilis,* the dog tick, in the East and Oklahoma; *Amblyomma americanum* in Texas and Oklahoma; and *Rhipicephalus sanguineus* in Texas and Mexico. These ticks feed on small mammals such as ground squirrels and rabbits as well as on larger animals such as bear and deer. Dogs serve as a reservoir to infect ticks and then other animals or humans. Figure 324–2 shows the distribution of cases of RMSF by state in the United States in 1992.

Laboratory-acquired infections have occurred in persons exposed to droplets from accidental generation of aerosols from solutions of the organism. However, even in circumstances conducive to airborne transmission, person-to-person transmission does not occur. RMSF can also be acquired by the transfusion of contaminated blood.

PATHOLOGY. The basis of the pathologic changes in this disease, as in other rickettsial infections, is the inflammatory response stimulated by the irreparable damage of the endothelial cells. In patients dying within 3 to 5 days of onset of disease, significant coagulation abnormalities are present. Causes may include damage to the endothelial cells with release of Factor VIII and stimulation of the release of platelet factors by damage to the endothelium or by activation of the kallikrein-kinin system by the Hageman factor. Microinfarcts result from occlusions of small vessels, and edema and hemorrhages occur secondary to increased permeability of the vasculature. Such lesions can be found in the heart, kidneys, adrenals, lungs, brain, skin, spleen, and subcutaneous tissues.

The rash is thought to result from the vasculitis and the associated permeability changes. Petechial lesions are caused by microhemorrhages secondary to the vasculitis and thrombocytopenia.

Patients with glucose-6-phosphate dehydrogenase (G6PD) deficiency appear to be prone to severe infections caused by *R. rickettsii* and other rickettsial agents. These patients have severe hemolytic reactions and significant thrombotic lesions in the glomeruli, resulting in oliguria.

CLINICAL MANIFESTATIONS. The incubation period of naturally acquired disease has a range of 2 to 14 days with an average of 7 days. The onset of disease in the typical case is sudden, with a severe headache, often retrobulbar in location, chills, fever, myalgia, malaise, nausea and vomiting, conjunctival injection, and photophobia. Tenderness may be present in large muscle groups. The duration of fever in untreated cases is about 2 weeks, but recovery from the debilitating effects of the disease requires several additional weeks.

Rash appears in 80 to 90% of patients—usually on the third or fourth day of fever, rarely after 5 or more days. It consists of pink macules, 2 to 5 mm, often noted first around the wrists and ankles. Lesions then spread to arms, chest, face, feet, and abdomen. Rarely does the rash involve the mucous membranes. Initially, these lesions blanch with pressure, but after 2 to 3 days they become fixed and turn dark red or purple and then slowly disappear during convalescence. The latter lesions represent microhemorrhages. Lesions

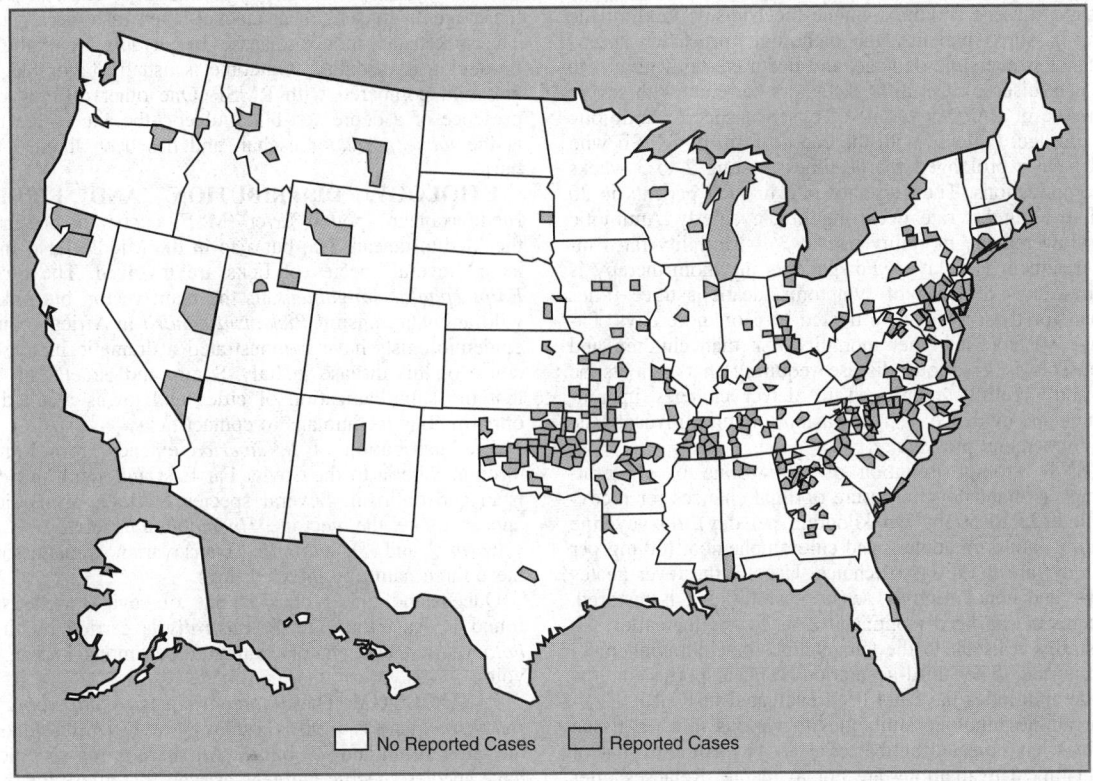

FIGURE 324–2. United States counties reporting cases of Rocky Mountain spotted fever, 1992.

No Reported Cases   Reported Cases

on the palms and soles of the feet, in conjunction with the rash elsewhere, and petechial lesions in the skin folds of the axillae and around the ankles, constitute the classic distribution of the rash. Biopsy of the rash reveals perivascular round cell infiltration. Staining of the specimens of skin with fluorescent tagged antibodies to *R. rickettsii* shows the intracellular organisms.

In patients with unrecognized and inappropriately treated disease, the rash coalesces as the spread of the infectious process involves additional and larger vessels. This can result in large ischemic and gangrenous lesions. Especially susceptible is the skin of the tip of the nose, earlobes, digits, and scrotum. Involvement of the cooler portions of the body may reflect the optimal temperature for growth of *R. rickettsii* (32°C). Thrombosis of larger arteries can cause gangrene of a limb or hemiplegia. Patients with untreated disease may die of myocarditis and pulmonary edema.

The reported incidence of pulmonary abnormalities varies from 10 to 40% in large series of patients. Respiratory symptoms and signs as part of this illness have not been emphasized sufficiently. In fact, after the spleen, the heaviest concentrations of rickettsiae can be demonstrated by fluorescent antibody staining in the endothelial cells of the pulmonary vasculature.

Edema of the brain and ring hemorrhages may cause delirium and stupor and ultimately lead to death.

DIAGNOSIS. The diagnosis of RMSF is difficult in the patient presenting with nonspecific complaints such as sudden onset of fever, headache, myalgia, and malaise. A history of travel, camping, or outdoor recreational activities where tick exposure could occur and of recent tick bites is an especially important part of any workup of a febrile patient during the warmer months. The patient complains of a severe headache, photophobia, and pain when moving the eyes. There is no meningismus. Lumbar puncture usually reveals normal CSF. Patients with stupor or coma may demonstrate elevated CSF protein and a few mononuclear cells. The presence of a faint, pink-colored rash on wrists and ankles should raise a suspicion of RMSF. The information that the rash appeared after the fever helps make the diagnosis.

A search for an attached tick should concentrate on the scalp and groin. Hard body ticks such as *D. andersoni* tend to remain attached for long periods. The finding of an engorged tick should settle the clinical diagnosis. There usually is no ulceration or scar from the tick bite.

Most patients have thrombocytopenia but not significant clotting abnormalities. In severe cases, disseminated intravascular coagulopathy (DIC) occurs with hypofibrinogenemia and prolonged prothrombin and partial thromboplastin times. Other laboratory studies are not helpful in making a diagnosis. The white blood cell count is usually normal.

RMSF is confirmed by immunofluorescence staining of tissue specimens and by serologic analyses. The detection by immunofluorescence of rickettsiae in tissues, such as skin or rash biopsies, is the one test that can provide the most rapid (4 to 6 hours) and early (day 3 to 4) diagnosis. The state health department should be contacted about the availability of this test.

Serologic tests do not provide rapid diagnostic confirmation. The Weil-Felix reaction uses the polysaccharide antigens of three *Proteus* strains (OX-19, OX-2, and OX-K) to agglutinate antibodies produced by a rickettsial infection. Serum specimens from patients with RMSF agglutinate OX-19 and OX-2, but not OX-K. The peak titer occurs at about 2 to 3 weeks and then falls rapidly. Antibiotic treatment blunts the antibody response. The test is inexpensive, and with a fourfold or greater increase in titer of OX-19 or OX-2, or both, in paired specimens (drawn 2 weeks apart) confirmation is obtained. Indirect immunofluorescent antibody (IFA) testing is the most specific and sensitive serologic test available. It has replaced the complement fixation test and, in many laboratories, the Weil-Felix reaction. The IFA is now used in epidemiologic surveys because of the persistence of these antibodies compared with the short-lived antibodies demonstrated in the Weil-Felix reaction. A diagnostic rise (fourfold or greater) in titer also takes 2 to 3 weeks.

Differentiation of this disease from other infections is difficult without the history of a tick bite or the information about the fever preceding the rash. In children measles and atypical measles (in those who received killed vaccine) can mimic the early phase of RMSF illness. The location and type of lesions making up the rash, the presence of Koplik's spots, and a history of measles-like illness in close associates should permit a differentiation. Meningococcemia with meningitis usually produces petechiae or purpura, or both, in the patient earlier in the course of the disease than expected in all but rare patients with RMSF. Furthermore, the CSF indicates the septic nature of the meningitis caused by the meningococci.

PROGNOSIS. RMSF is a serious infectious disease that involves endothelial cells throughout the host. Prompt antibiotic therapy is necessary to assist cellular immune mechanisms to eliminate the pathogen. In some patients, the pathologic processes spread rapidly and cause irreversible damage, and death ensues within 3 to 5 days (fulminant disease). Certain risk factors correlate with severe diseases: presence of G6PD/A–, time of onset of specific antibiotic therapy, and old age. Patients with the classic form of RMSF who are untreated have a prolonged febrile illness lasting 2 to 3 weeks with many complications. The mortality rate in such patients is 20 to 30%, with the highest rate occurring in the elderly. Antibiotic treatment has lowered the mortality rate to 3%. Mortality rates increase when treatment is delayed. For patients in whom therapy is started within 4 days of onset of symptoms, death is three times less likely than for those who were treated at 5 or more days. Patients over age 40 have a higher mortality risk than children and young adults. This is a serious disease requiring that patients be hospitalized and carefully monitored to detect changes in pulmonary findings and evidence of hypotension, oliguria, myocarditis, or increasing intracranial pressure.

TREATMENT. Prompt initiation of tetracycline or chloramphenicol therapy is mandatory to ensure optimal chances for recovery. Tetracycline (25 to 50 mg per kilogram per day), doxycycline (100 mg every 12 hours in adults), and chloramphenicol (50 mg per kilogram per day) are the drugs of choice. Usually the fever abates in 2 to 3 days, and concurrently a sense of well-being is restored. Antibiotic treatment can be discontinued 2 to 3 days thereafter. No instances of strains resistant to the tetracyclines or chloramphenicol have been reported. The third-generation cephalosporins or the aminoglycoside antibiotics have not been evaluated in RMSF. Evaluation of four aminoquinolone antibiotics in various infected tissue culture cell lines has revealed antibacterial activity equal to that of tetracyclines. Clinical evaluations are not available. Relapses after tetracycline or chloramphenicol treatment are uncommon.

PREVENTION AND CONTROL. Immunity to reinfection after recovery from RMSF appears to be complete. No naturally acquired second cases have been reported. There is no effective vaccine.

The best method for preventing disease is to avoid contact with ticks. Ticks are brushed off grass onto clothes or skin. Ticks usually remain stationary until the host is quiet. They then seek warm, dark areas and migrate to the groin or the scalp, where they can grasp hair shafts while inserting their mouth parts into the skin. Small barbs on each side of the mouth make it difficult to withdraw the whole tick from the skin while it is feeding; the mouth parts may remain embedded. Ticks should be searched for at the end of each day spent in tick-infested country and removed with forceps or tweezers. A drop of acetone or a lighted match brought close to the tick may ensure that the tick withdraws its mouth parts. The tick should not be removed with exposed fingers because a tick crushed between the fingers may induce disease. Prophylactic antibiotics are not indicated for persons with known tick bites. They should be advised concerning the usual incubation period and urged to watch for development of fever or headache. Oral temperature should be recorded twice a day for 2 weeks. On elevation, medical attention should be obtained promptly. Therapy begun before the onset of fever could result in a prolongation of the incubation period.

Dalton MJ, Clarke MJ, Holman RC, et al.: National surveillance for Rocky Mountain spotted fever, 1981–1982; Epidemiologic summary and evaluation of risk factors for fatal outcome. Am J Trop Med & Hyg 52:405, 1995.
Donohue JF: Lower respiratory tract involvement in Rocky Mountain spotted fever. Arch Intern Med 140:223, 1980. *This retrospective review of pulmonary findings in patients with RMSF points out the delays that occurred in making the correct diagnosis because the respiratory symptoms were not considered to be a part of the clinical picture of RMSF.*

324.3 Other Tick-borne Rickettsioses

DEFINITIONS. *Mediterranean spotted fever,* also known as North African tick typhus, Kenya tick-bite fever, Indian tick typhus, and boutonneuse fever, is caused by *Rickettsia conorii.* A second disease, called North Asian tick-borne rickettsiosis, is induced by

R. siberica. A third tick-borne rickettsial infection, called Queensland tick typhus, is caused by *R. australis.* The disease produced by these agents consists of headache, fever, rash, myalgia, and malaise. The rickettsiae induce disease by invading endothelial cells and producing a vasculitis. Outcome is usually favorable. The illnesses are mild compared with RMSF. One other difference is the usual presence of a depressed black ulcer—the site of the tick bite. This is the *tache noire,* or eschar, and has been likened to a cigarette burn.

ETIOLOGY, DISTRIBUTION, AND EPIDEMIOLOGY. Mediterranean spotted fever (MSF) occurs in countries bordering the Mediterranean Sea, but also in the Middle East, India, and Pakistan. Several species of ticks are involved. The brown dog tick, *Rhipicephalus sanguineus,* is the main vector, but ticks common to wild animals transmit *Rickettsia conorii* in African countries. Italian epidemiologists have demonstrated a dramatic increase in the incidence of this disease in Italy, Spain, and Israel. The assumption is that the suburbanization of cities and towns resulted in increased opportunities for humans to contact ticks.

The distribution of *R. siberica* extends from European Russia through Siberia to the Soviet Far East and south into the Indo-Pakistan subcontinent. Several species of hard, or ixodid, body ticks appear to be the vectors: *Haemaphysalis concinna, Dermacentor sylvarum,* and *D. nuttallii.* Transovarian transmission occurs in these three naturally infected ticks.

Queensland tick typhus is one of several rickettsial infections found in Australia. The *R. australis* is carried by the tick *Ixodes holocyclus,* and marsupial animals are among known animal reservoirs.

PATHOLOGY. These three rickettsiae are very similar to *R. rickettsii.* There is >90% homology by DNA hybridization between the latter strain and *R. conorii.* All share group-specific antigens but have species-specific antigens as well that allow for their identification. These strains invade endothelial cells and cause cell death, resulting in a vasculitis (see above). Each of these three strains produces an eschar *(tache noire)* at the site of the tick bite.

SYMPTOMS, LABORATORY FINDINGS, AND DIAGNOSIS. The onset of disease caused by each of these three rickettsiae is sudden and characterized by fever, headache, malaise, myalgia, and conjunctival injection. These symptoms and signs appear about 5 to 7 days after the tick bite. The eschar is the distinguishing sign that confirms the diagnosis. It should be looked for in the scalp, axillae, and groin area, regions of the body favored by ticks. Because of the necrotic nature of the eschar, lymph nodes draining the region of the eschar are enlarged. The lesion has been appropriately likened to a cigarette burn, about 2 to 5 mm in diameter with a black center and a raised, erythematous rim. The lesion is only mildly tender.

As with RMSF, a generalized rash appears on the fourth to fifth day, including the palms and soles of the feet. The faint pink macular-papular lesions represent small hemorrhages into the skin. The duration of the disease is about 2 weeks. Death is unusual.

The Weil-Felix reaction demonstrates agglutinating antibodies to OX-19 antigen in most patients; these appear in the second to third week of disease. The microimmunofluorescence test for antibodies to *R. conorii* is the serologic test of choice, if available.

A skin biopsy stained with immunofluorescent antibody stain is the most rapid and earliest diagnostic procedure. This is indicated only when the diagnosis of spotted fever is suspected and a *tache noire* eschar is not present.

TREATMENT AND PROPHYLAXIS. Excellent outcomes are reported in patients receiving 200 mg of doxycycline every 12 hours for two doses. Tetracycline, chloramphenicol, and rifamycin can be used. Defervescence occurs over 2 days.

Tick bites should be avoided. Travelers into wild game country of Africa should check their clothes and skin carefully for ticks. Tourists traveling to southern European countries should search for ticks if they go hiking through suburban and rural areas during the spring and summer months.

Recovery from these rickettsial infections imparts solid immunity. In experimental animals *R. conorii* is relatively avirulent compared with most strains of *R. rickettsii.* However, animals recovered from infections with the former strain are protected against challenge with virulent *R. rickettsii.* This protection is mediated by T lymphocytes that recognize antigens on other species of rickettsial agents of the spotted fever group.

HUMAN EHRLICHIOSIS (SPOTLESS ROCKY MOUNTAIN SPOTTED FEVER). The first reported case of infection with a species of *Ehrlichia* in the United States occurred in 1986. A patient was found to have intracytoplasmic inclusions (morula) in monocytes and subsequently had an antibody rise to *E. canis.* This organism is known to cause severe pancytopenia in dogs. It is one of four species known to infect animals—*E. canis, E. equi, E. risticii,* and *E. phagocytophilia.* An additional species, *E. sennetsu,* was isolated from a patient in Japan in 1954, who had an infectious mononucleosis-like syndrome. This strain has not been identified outside of the Far East. In the United States since 1986, many investigators tried to isolate *E. canis* or a similar strain from patients with clinical and serologic evidence of ehrlichiosis. In 1990, the first isolation was made on a continuous cell line of canine macrophage cells using blood drawn from a patient with a 3-day history of fever, headache, pharyngitis, nausea, and vomiting. This isolate was named *E. chaffeensis* because the patient was an Army reservist stationed at Ft. Chaffee, Arkansas. This strain is different from but closely related to *E. canis* and is now used as the antigen for serologic studies. Patients suspected of having ehrlichiosis, but with no antibodies when tested with *E. canis,* do have antibodies to this human isolate. The organism can be stained in circulating monocytes. They are found in the cytoplasm as a clump of many organisms (0.2 to 1.5 μm) enclosed in a membrane; this mass is the morula (mulberry-like). These organisms have been found in *D. variabilis* ticks, one of the same tick species that transmits *R. rickettsii.* Most cases have been identified in Oklahoma, Missouri, and Arkansas—states in which RMSF is common.

In 1994 another *Ehrlichia* species was associated with human disease. Infection with this agent was confirmed in 12 patients in Wisconsin and Minnesota by serologic studies (IFA and/or polymerase chain reaction [PCR]). Two of these 12 died of infection. This strain has not been isolated as yet; it is different from *E. chaffeensis* as demonstrated by various serologic studies and is closely related to the *E. equi/E. phagocytophilia* group. None of the 12 patients was exposed to horses, sheep, deer, bison, and cattle, animals known to be infected with these strains. Eleven of the 12 had known tick exposure. *D. variabilis* and *I. scapularis* were identified in eight instances. The unique feature of infection with this strain was the location of the morulae. They were found in granulocytes in the circulation and in the bone marrow. Because of this, the current name for the disease is human granulocytic ehrlichiosis (HGE).

The clinical symptoms of both forms of ehrlichiosis are similar and can be difficult to distinguish from those found in patients with RMSF. Fever, chills, myalgias, headaches are common. Nausea, vomiting, and asthenia add to the patient's discomfort. The physical examination usually is nonrevealing. Rash has been reported in about 20% of patients infected with *E. chaffeensis,* but not in those infected with HGE. The rash has been described with a variety of lesions—macular or papular or both, petechial or erythematous. It is seen most frequently on the thorax, legs, and arms. The rash appears after the onset of symptoms; the median day of onset was 5 days in a series of 212 patients. Striking laboratory values are leukopenia, thrombocytopenia, and abnormal liver function tests. Liver abnormalities may be due to enlargement of cells of the reticuloendothelial system compressing adjacent parenchyma. The alanine aminotransferase (ALT) and aspartate aminotransferase (AST) values peak at the end of the first week of illness. The platelet count drops to its lowest level at about the same time. The leukocyte count falls quicker, within the first 3 to 5 days of disease. The presence of the morula in lymphocytes and monocytes *(E. chaffeensis)* and in granulocytes (HGE agent) is a significant laboratory diagnostic clue. This finding needs to be identified by skilled observers.

The severity of the clinical illnesses range from mild to fatal. Serologic evidence exists to indicate that more infections with *E. chaffeensis* are asymptomatic than those requiring medical attention. The PCR assay is now available at the CDC for precise diagnosis; when widely available it will provide a rapid diagnostic test.

Elderly patients are most prone to acquire the disease and to have the most severe illnesses. In the few patients who have died, the diagnosis was usually made late in the course of the disease. Therefore, there was a delay in onset of specific therapy, and frequently life-threatening complications were seen with severe infectious diseases, e.g., renal failure, meningitis, coma, DIC. The rapid appearance of pancytopenia in the sick patients has been postulated to be due to bone marrow hypoplasia, but more recent investigations point to sequestration or destruction of various blood elements (the hemophagocytic syndrome) as the most likely explanation.

The diagnosis of ehrlichiosis is based on epidemiologic information regarding possible tick exposure in areas where the tick-borne diseases are present, plus the aforementioned clinical and laboratory features. This febrile illness needs to be differentiated from Colorado tick fever and Lyme disease (see Ch. 321). The geographic location of the patient helps determine the possibility of Colorado tick fever. Differential features of Lyme disease include the classic erythema migrans lesion and the usual lack of leukopenia and thrombocytopenia. In the small percentage of patients with a rash more typical of RMSF, a mistaken diagnosis of RMSF is possible. Confusion with *R. rickettsii* disease is not a serious clinical management problem if the patient is treated with a tetracycline antibiotic or chloramphenicol. Failure to consider either disease and administer appropriate therapy can lead to serious consequences for the patient. Prompt antibiotic treatment needs repeated emphasis since delay is associated with the poorest prognosis.

Treatment of patients infected with either of the known strains of *Ehrlichia* requires doxycycline (100 mg every 12 hours for the first day and 100 mg once daily for at least 3 days after the fever abates). Tetracycline (500 mg once daily or chloramphenicol 500 mg once daily) can also be used. With early therapy the febrile course is short. Heparin therapy is not recommended because the pancytopenia disappears promptly as the disease is brought under control with antibiotics.

Bakken JS, Dumler JS, Chen S, et al.: Human granulocytic ehrlichiosis in the upper midwest United States. JAMA 272:212, 1994. *The first report on a new disease entity, caused by another species of* Ehrlichia.

Everett ED, Evans KA, Henry B, et al.: Human ehrlichiosis in adults after tick exposure. Ann Intern Med 120:730, 1994. *Presents data on 30 patients diagnosed and followed by this group.*

Fishbein DB, Dawson JE, Robinson LE: Human ehrlichiosis in the United States, 1985 to 1990. Ann Intern Med 120:736, 1994. *This report follows Everett et al. and is the usual excellent CDC review of 237 cases garnered by a laboratory surveillance.*

324.4 Rickettsialpox

DEFINITION. Rickettsialpox is a rare mite-borne infectious disease caused by *Rickettsia akari.* This mild, self-limited illness consists of headache, fever, an eschar at the site of the mite bite, and a papulovesicular rash.

ETIOLOGY. *R. akari* is classified with the spotted fever group of rickettsiae. It is a small, gram-negative, coccobacillus-shaped, obligate intracellular organism.

DISTRIBUTION AND INCIDENCE. Rickettsialpox was first described in 1946. In the subsequent few years, more than 500 cases were diagnosed, primarily in New York City. Since the early 1950's, only one outbreak has occurred, again in New York City. The disease is virtually unknown throughout the rest of the United States.

TRANSMISSION AND EPIDEMIOLOGY. The original description included *R. akari* isolated from persons with the disease, from mites *(Allodermanyssus sanguineus)* that feed on rodents, and from house mice *(Mus musculus).* Engorged mites were occasionally found on the mice; attachment was usually around the rump. The mites remain in the nest, where access to mice is readily available. Human intrusion into this animal-ectoparasite cycle can result in an infected mite's biting and inducing disease. The ecologic range of *A. sanguineus* covers most of the United States, and mice are ubiquitous animals. Thus the elements for potential epidemics exist. Isolated cases may develop from unusual exposure to mice, as in persons working in landfills or in homeless persons sleeping in abandoned buildings.

Rickettsialpox is fairly common in some urban areas of Ukraine, where rats appear to be the animal reservoir. In Korea small field mice are infected.

PATHOLOGY. The known pathologic changes are limited to the skin, since this is a nonfatal infection. Histologic examination of the eschar (site of mite bite) reveals intense inflammation with necrosis. Other findings are similar to those in RMSF: thrombosis and necrosis of capillaries, edema, and a monocytic perivascular infiltrate. The characteristic rash in this disease is papulovesicular. The lesions contain fluid that may yield *R. akari* on culture.

CLINICAL MANIFESTATIONS AND COURSE. The bite of the mite is not painful and goes unnoticed. This site undergoes a localized inflammatory reaction over the next week to 10 days. During this time the edema and cellular components of the reaction create a slowly enlarging, firm, erythematous papule, which may reach 1 to 1.5 cm in diameter. The involved skin separates gradually, creating a vesicle that finally breaks down to form an ulcer. The base of the ulcer is usually black and is surrounded by a rim of erythematous skin. This progression occurs over 3 to 7 days, at the end of which there is the sudden onset of fever, chills, sweats, headache, backache, and malaise. The lymph nodes draining the area of the eschar enlarge but are nontender. These symptoms and signs may be present for a week if no specific antibiotic treatment is administered.

As with other members of the spotted fever group, a rash appears after 2 to 3 days of illness. Initially the lesions are maculopapular, few in number, and distributed mostly on the trunk and abdomen, rarely involving the palms or soles. The lesions evolve quickly and uniformly into vesicular lesions; the vesicle appears to sit on top of an erythematous papule. These lesions persist for about a week; the fluid in the vesicle is slowly absorbed, and a scab forms, which leaves a brownish discoloration in the skin after it falls off. This gradually clears without leaving a scar. There is no significant internal organ involvement.

DIAGNOSIS. The diagnosis is made by clinical observation; the unique lesions of the rash, the presence of the eschar, and a history that suggests contact with rodents in the past 2 weeks provide sufficient evidence to make the diagnosis. Serologic studies confirm the diagnosis; complement-fixing antibody titers have been the standard, but indirect immunofluorescent antibodies are more specific, when available. Confusion exists regarding whether the Weil-Felix reaction can be used to diagnose rickettsialpox. In about 10% of patients in small series, significant titer rises to OX-19 and OX-2 have been observed. The test lacks sensitivity for confirming the diagnosis. The organism can be isolated from the vesicular fluid or from clotted blood specimens. These materials must be injected into animals or embryonated eggs. Laboratory tests are of no diagnostic help, although leukopenia is common.

The rash may be confused with the lesions of chickenpox, but no eschar is present in chickenpox (see Ch. 336). In addition, the lesions of chickenpox are usually in various stages of maturity, whereas the character of those in rickettsialpox is more uniform. Finally, the vesicle of rickettsialpox appears to sit on a papule, whereas those of chickenpox lack such a base.

PROGNOSIS AND TREATMENT. Rickettsialpox is a benign illness, and recovery occurs without therapy.

Treatment with tetracycline or doxycycline shortens the febrile period and hastens recovery. Antibiotic treatment need only be administered for 3 to 4 days to ensure a cure. No relapse will occur.

PREVENTION AND CONTROL. Rickettsialpox is a zoonosis involving a common house pest, the mouse. Control of this reservoir through elimination of mouse harborages and use of residual acaricides to walls adjacent to mice-infested areas should control mite populations. There is no available vaccine.

324.5 Scrub Typhus

DEFINITION. Scrub typhus is an acute febrile illness caused by *Rickettsia tsutsugamushi* (from the Japanese: *tsutsuga*, "dangerous"; *mushi*, "bug"). This rickettsia is inoculated into humans during the bite by a chigger. The site of the bite develops into an eschar.

ETIOLOGY. *Rickettsia tsutsugamushi (R. orientalis)* is a small gram-negative, obligate intracellular organism. Unlike other rickettsial infections, infection with *R. tsutsugamushi* does not induce solid protection against additional bouts of scrub typhus. This results from the variable antigenic compositions of the strains.

This is the only rickettsia whose polysaccharides bear an anti-genic relationship to *Proteus* OX-K. This *Proteus* strain is used in serologic tests to confirm scrub typhus.

DISTRIBUTION. This disease occurs almost exclusively in the large triangular region extending from the northern islands of Japan southwest to Australia and southeast to the South Pacific Islands. This region contains the larval form of mites that are both vector and reservoir of rickettsiae.

TRANSMISSION AND EPIDEMIOLOGY. *R. tsutsugamushi* is transmitted to humans by the bite of the larva of trombiculid mites (chiggers). Chiggers are the only stage in the life cycle of these mites (*Leptotrombidium deliensis* and others) that can feed on humans. Chiggers are almost microscopic, often brilliantly colored (red bugs). The chiggers feed on rats and other small rodents. The word "scrub" was applied because of the type of vegetation—transitional between forests and clearings—that maintains the chigger-mammal relationship. But other regions (semiarid, sandy beaches, and so on) also support rodents and mites. Humans encounter scrub typhus when they enter such areas to build roads, to clear fields or forests, or on military expeditions. Circumscribed regions are highly endemic, a reflection of the lack of mobility of the chiggers and their rodent hosts. Mites transmit the rickettsiae to their offspring via the ova. Therefore they can serve as vector and reservoir of the etiologic agent.

This disease has been called river or flood fever because of the increased incidence during the rainy seasons. Chiggers and mites proliferate in warm, wet environments.

PATHOLOGY. *R. tsutsugamushi* invades endothelial cells to produce a vasculitis. The serious pathologic manifestations in untreated patients are predominantly myocarditis, meningoencephalitis, and pneumonitis. Coagulopathy develops but is less severe than in RMSF or typhus.

The site of the chigger bite develops into a papular lesion that ulcerates to form an eschar. This is associated with regional and later generalized lymphadenopathy.

CLINICAL MANIFESTATIONS AND COURSE. The incubation period for development of the primary papular lesion ranges from 6 to 18 days. This lesion can occur anywhere on the body. It enlarges, undergoes central necrosis, and crusts to form the eschar. As the eschar matures, the patient has the sudden onset of headache, fever, chills, and malaise. Over the next several days, these symptoms increase in severity with further elevation of the temperature. The patient, if untreated, may become stuporous as meningoencephalitis develops. Signs of cardiac dysfunction, including minor electrocardiographic abnormalities such as first-degree heart block and inverted T waves, can appear. The rash of scrub typhus appears at the end of the first week of disease. This is a faint, pink maculopapular rash appearing first on the trunk and spreading to the extremities.

Physical findings late in the first week of illness include generalized lymphadenopathy and palpable spleen and occasionally liver. Pulmonary findings are often absent despite radiographic evidence of interstitial pneumonia. In those patients with myocarditis, there may be a gallop rhythm, poor-quality heart sounds, and systolic murmurs.

Various cranial nerve deficits have been noted in untreated patients. Deafness, dysarthria, and dysphagia may occur but are usually transient, although deafness can last for several months.

All of 87 (nonimmune) soldiers in Vietnam who developed scrub typhus had fever and headache, 46% had an eschar, and 35% had a rash. Eighty-five percent had generalized lymph node enlargement. It is not surprising that many were misdiagnosed as having infectious mononucleosis.

Laboratory studies reveal leukopenia early in the disease with subsequent increase of white blood cell counts to normal levels. Coagulopathies can be demonstrated, but only rare patients develop the disseminated intravascular clotting syndrome. Liver enzyme values may be elevated, indicating hepatocellular damage. Proteinuria is common.

Patients with untreated disease remain febrile for about 2 weeks and have a long convalescence of 4 to 6 weeks thereafter.

DIAGNOSIS. The variable presentations in this disease make the clinical diagnosis difficult. The eschar and rash should suggest a rickettsial infection, but these may be found in fewer than one half of patients. Furthermore, the eschar and rash may suggest other rickettsial infections, such as tick-borne typhus. The endemic foci of scrub typhus and whether the patient has traveled or worked in such areas constitute important epidemiologic information. A therapeutic trial of tetracycline or chloramphenicol is indicated in patients in whom the diagnosis of scrub typhus is suspected. Defervescence should occur within 24 hours.

The specific serologic test is the detection of significant increases (greater than fourfold) of IFA's in paired serum specimens obtained 2 weeks apart. The *Proteus* OX-K antigen test is readily available and inexpensive, so that it is frequently employed in endemic areas. About 50% of patients have diagnostic titers. In Malaya, the sensitivity and specificity of both tests were found to be about the same, but their usefulness was enhanced when they were used concurrently.

R. tsutsugamushi can be isolated from a patient's blood by inoculating it, intraperitoneally, into white mice. The rickettsiae can be demonstrated in the tissues of the mice.

PROGNOSIS AND TREATMENT. Without treatment, the mortality rate ranges from 0 to 30% depending upon virulence and resistance factors; with treatment, survival is the expected outcome. Second or third attacks of scrub typhus, caused by different serotypes, usually result in a mild illness, usually with no eschar or rash.

Persistence of *R. tsutsugamushi* in lymph node tissues has been demonstrated 1 year after recovery. This finding raises the possibility of disease reactivating during immunosuppression.

Tetracycline, doxycycline, and chloramphenicol are all effective. The drug should be continued for at least 2 days after the patient has become afebrile.

PREVENTION AND CONTROL. Vaccines were developed and tested during and after World War II. Some were effective against homologous strains. However, no single antigen has been identified that induces protection against all of the antigenically diverse strains of *R. tsutsugamushi*. In military populations in endemic areas, weekly doses of doxycycline protect against scrub typhus.

Avoidance of chigger attachment can be accomplished by insect repellents applied to the skin and by use of protective clothing impregnated with benzyl benzoate. Diethyltoluamide preparations such as OFF and DEET are also effective if sprayed on clothing and exposed skin but are removed rapidly by water. Applying this chemical to socks is especially important in preventing chigger bites.

324.6 Q Fever

DEFINITION. Q fever is a systemic infection caused by inhaling small numbers of *Coxiella burnetii*. Domestic animals and pets are the usual sources of infection for humans. This highly infectious rickettsial agent induces mild febrile illness, occasionally associated with pneumonitis, but in a few patients causes chronic hepatitis and life-threatening endocarditis.

ETIOLOGY. *C. burnetii* is unique among the rickettsiae in the following ways: It is not transmitted to humans by arthropod vectors; rather, it is readily disseminated by aerosols. No rash ensues despite the similarity of the infection of endothelial cells (vasculitis) to that with *Rickettsia rickettsii*. The organism resides uniquely inside the phagolysosome in the cytoplasm of the infected cell. *C. burnetii* does not have cross-reacting antigens with *Proteus vulgaris,* and therefore antibodies developed during infection do not agglutinate in the Weil-Felix test. These rickettsiae are resistant to destruction by environmental stresses, e.g., sunlight, humidity.

Isolation of *C. burnetii* from pulmonary secretions, liver biopsies, and surgical cardiac valve specimens is possible but not recommended unless appropriate laboratory facilities are available. This is a highly infectious agent that can readily cause laboratory-acquired infections. These materials are injected into eggs and/or guinea pigs. In the latter, the production of agglutinating antibodies confirms the presence of the organism. *C. burnetii* can exist in two phases. Phase I organisms are usually associated with chronic, severe clinical illnesses, such as endocarditis. Phase II organisms evolve (through the loss of mono- and polysaccharide chains of the lipopolysaccharide surface antigens) following multiple transfers in eggs. Antibodies to Phase II organisms are predominant in most patients with Q fever. However, patients with endocarditis have higher titers of antibodies to Phase I organisms, specifically IgA and IgG; the latter two types of antibodies are diagnostic for this entity.

Virulence factors associated with *C. burnetii* include three plasmids. These appear to be specific for acute versus chronic disease; they control the production of proteins that may be involved in the infectious processes. The lipopolysaccharide antigen is another virulence factor. The antigen in strains causing chronic disease is different from that in strains involved in acute disease. The organism may resist destruction inside the phagolysosome by producing large quantities of acid phosphatase, which inhibits the superoxide production of the host cell, thereby avoiding lysis. In addition, its ability to survive in the acid milieu of the phagolysosome provides an environment that impairs the efficacy of most antibiotics. Raising the pH in tissue culture systems results in increased antibiotic efficacy. These virulence factors can enable *C. burnetii* to establish chronic infections.

EPIDEMIOLOGY. Human disease is acquired by inhaling aerosols containing *C. burnetii*. The organisms are disseminated from infected ruminants and pets (cats). The placentas from these animals contain huge concentrations of rickettsiae. During delivery of the placenta, aerosols are generated which may be wind borne to contaminate soil, clothing, and the wool or fur of other animals or may be transmitted hundreds of yards to susceptible persons. Trucks carrying sheep appear to disseminate organisms to persons passed on the streets. Sheep regularly transported to research laboratories through hallways in a medical center caused an epidemic that persisted for 6 months. Organisms are also found in amniotic fluid, feces, and the mammary glands and milk of sheep and cows. The ability of *C. burnetii* to form sporelike structures that resist environmental destruction allows these organisms to cause disease long after the initial contamination occurs and at sites distant from the original source.

The animals are infected by ticks. There are ticks that transmit the organisms among wild animals, such as the kangaroo in Australia. Spread to domestic animals occurs when the two populations of animals intermingle. Ticks have not been implicated in the transmission from animals to humans. Q fever is a mild and inapparent infection in animals. It may be responsible for placental deficiencies that lead to stillbirth of kittens and lambs. *C. burnetii* attach to the head of the sperm from infected mice. Males can infect female mice by sexual contact. Whether this occurs in humans is unknown.

Various volunteer studies, designed to evaluate vaccine effectiveness, have demonstrated that very few organisms, probably fewer than 10, are sufficient to induce disease. For this reason, as well as the ability to survive in most environments, *C. burnetii* is a hazardous organism with which to work. In one laboratory 21 of 50 cases diagnosed over a 15-year period occurred in persons working in laboratories (or offices) not directly involved in Q fever research. Presumably, these persons were infected by widely disseminated aerosols from laboratory accidents or from contaminated clothing of workers socializing outside their laboratory. Despite the infectious nature of the organism and its presence in sputum, human-to-human transmission does not occur and respiratory isolation for infected patients is not needed.

In the United States and Canada, *C. burnetii* (and antibodies) has been found in milk from numerous herds of cattle. Despite this evidence, documented cases of Q fever occurring after unpasteurized milk from such cows was ingested have not been identified. The ingestion of 10^5 organisms by mouth by volunteers failed to induce disease. If disease occurs, it could originate from aerosols created in the act of pouring the milk into a glass.

The incubation period varies indirectly with inoculum size. Large doses result in disease at about 7 days. Most persons develop symptoms at 13 to 18 days.

PATHOLOGY. Knowledge of the pathologic changes is greatest for the more severe form of this disease. For example, microscopic examinations of liver biopsies and autopsy material from patients dying of chronic hepatitis and from heart valves infected with *C. burnetii* are available. Patients with pneumonitis usually have a mild illness so tissue specimens are scarce. Animal studies have provided complementary pathohistologic data.

Hepatitis. Granulomas with fatty necrosis are typical microscopic findings. These granulomas are doughnut-shaped. While they are common in Q fever, they also are seen in patients with tuberculosis. Fatty metamorphosis is also seen. Patients with mild forms of Q fever may have elevated liver enzyme values indicative of minimal liver cell damage.

Subacute and Chronic Endocarditis.
This is a life-threatening disease because it is difficult to eradicate the infection. These patients may have large vegetations on the aortic valve and less likely on the mitral valve. They have negative blood cultures and frequently have a history of a febrile illness with or without pneumonitis months previously. The vegetations have a histologic picture similar to that in other forms of endocarditis, an avascular collection of fibrin and platelets. These patients also have enlarged livers and spleens, plus signs of vasculitis associated with endocarditis, e.g., splinter hemorrhages, Roth spots, and petechiae.

Pneumonitis.
In the few autopsies performed, consolidation similar to that of other bacterial pneumonias was the gross finding. The microscopic examination revealed an exudate loaded with histocytes and no polymorphonuclear leukocytes. This inflammatory response is compatible with a nonbacterial process. The histologic features have been described as those of a severe intra-alveolar, focally necrotizing, hemorrhagic pneumonia with associated necrotizing bronchitis and bronchiolitis.

The portal of entry of *C. burnetii* is the respiratory tract; small particles <3 to 5 μ in diameter can reach the terminal bronchioles. The pneumonia does not appear until the third or fourth day of fever. In a mouse model, the rickettsiae enter pneumatocytes, histocytes, and fibroblasts. The self-limiting nature of this infection is probably related to the destruction of the organisms in the macrophages. However, *C. burnetii* can persist for 2 months inside those cells. Some of the macrophages can be damaged by *C. burnetii*, leading to an inflammatory response. Cellular immune mechanisms attack these damaged cells. Numerous factors are involved in the pathogenesis of pneumonia—the number and virulence of the rickettsiae, particle size, and the functional status of the macrophages and parenchymal cells of the lung.

CLINICAL MANIFESTATIONS.
The onset of Q fever is very abrupt; the manifestations are not specific. The patient develops a high fever that is associated with headache, chills, myalgia, and malaise. This flulike syndrome differs from influenza disease because of the height of the temperature, frequently 39.4° to 40°C. The fever also persists for 10 to 14 days. No rash occurs. Retroorbital pain, common in other rickettsial infections, is reported by 10 to 15% of patients.

Patients may have a dry, nonproductive cough indicative of the bronchiolitis and the minimal pneumonitis produced by the invading *C. burnetii*. Physical findings of consolidated lung are lacking early in the course of the pneumonia. There may be decreased breath sounds, but rales are unlikely until the lesions start to resolve. The chest films reveal patchy infiltrates that frequently are multiple round, segmental opacities. These are discrete lesions. Larger areas of the lung may show consolidation, and linear atelectatic lesions occur in about half the patients with pneumonia. Resolution of the lesions is slow. The incidence of pneumonitis varies from 4 to 97% in series of cases reported from the United States (28%), Australia (4 to 75%), and Switzerland (97%). The reasons for these variations are unknown.

Most patients (85%) with Q fever have hepatic involvement as measured by abnormal liver cell enzymes. Hepatomegaly is noted in about 65% of patients, but few patients (10%) have liver tenderness. Jaundice is unlikely (about 5% of cases) unless chronic hepatitis ensues, a very rare manifestation. Liver biopsies have demonstrated, by direct immunofluorescent studies, rickettsia residing in hepatic cells. Q fever may account for a few cases of acute hepatitis. Patients with a strong exposure history should be evaluated for infection by *C. burnetii*.

The clinical manifestations of Q fever endocarditis are characteristic of those associated with the syndrome of endocarditis; e.g., splenomegaly, splinter hemorrhages, and heart murmurs. Few cases of *C. burnetii*–induced valvular infections are seen in the United States; small series are reported from countries in which Q fever is more common. Evidence of endocarditis in a patient occurs years after the acute infections. The lack of positive cultures contributes to a delay in diagnosis. The diagnosis is made by serologic means, demonstrating high (>1:800 for IgG and >1:50 for IgA) or rising titers of Phase I antibodies by indirect immunofluorescence. The

level of Phase I antibodies exceeding those for Phase II antibodies is indicative of chronic Q fever, whether it is endocarditis or a localized infection of bone, vascular prosthesis, aneurysm, liver, or joint. Phase II antibodies indicate a recent exposure or an acute infection.

PROGNOSIS.
The key to diagnosing Q fever in a patient with a debilitating febrile illness is obtaining a history of contact with sheep, cattle, goats, or cats or the skins or wool from these animals. This history should be compelling enough to initiate antibiotic treatment and to obtain acute and convalescent serum for serologic studies. These latter studies are the practical and definitive diagnostic aids. Phase II antibodies (complement fixing [CF] or IFA) are present in two thirds of patients at the end of 2 weeks of illness and in 90% at 1 month. Phase I antibodies, if present, are found in titers lower than Phase II antibodies. IFA is more sensitive than CF in detecting early antibody formation (IgM) and also in demonstrating persistence of antibody at 1 year or longer. The presence of Phase I antibodies in excess of Phase II, and specifically Phase I IgA, is diagnostic of Q fever endocarditis.

The nonspecific clinical manifestations of early symptoms and signs of Q fever, e.g., headache, fever, myalgia, suggest numerous infectious diseases. Influenza infections are seasonal, the temperature is less than that of Q fever, and liver function tests are normal. The white blood cell count is not helpful, as it is normal in both infections. Other diseases such as typhoid fever and brucellosis can be diagnosed by bacterial cultures. Viral hepatitis can be mistaken for Q fever. Appropriate serologic studies and liver biopsy provide diagnostic evidence. In those patients with pneumonitis, the differential diagnosis includes viral or mycoplasmal etiologies, tularemia, psittacosis, and *Legionella pneumophila*. Serologic and culture results identify these organisms.

TREATMENT AND PROGNOSIS.
C. burnetii is known to be susceptible to a number of antibiotics. Sensitivity studies have been conducted in eggs, guinea pigs, and in acute and chronically infected tissue culture cells. Tetracycline and doxycycline or chloramphenicol have been effective *in vitro* as well as in clinical studies. Early institution of tetracycline (within 3 days of onset) reduces the febrile course by half. Tetracycline, 500 mg four times a day, or doxycycline, 100 mg twice a day, should be continued for at least 1 week after the patient becomes afebrile (usually 2 to 3 days). The prognosis with such therapy is excellent, with no mortality expected. Those patients who receive no antibiotics also do well, with a recovery rate of >99%. If a febrile relapse occurs, retreatment with the same antibiotic is effective.

The recommended treatment of patients with Q fever endocarditis is not settled. Doxycycline and a quinolone have been somewhat effective, but cures have not been achieved even after 2 years of continuous therapy. The mortality rate remains high (24%). The location of the organism in an acid environment inside the phagolysosome interferes with the activity of antibiotics. Experimental studies designed to alkalize the fluid helped to eradicate the organisms in phagocytes. The combination of doxycycline and chloroquine in these studies was most effective and may be useful in patients with chronic Q fever. Surgical resection of infected valves is usually required because the large vegetations cause hemodynamic deficiencies in cardiac function.

PREVENTION.
There is no commercially available vaccine for Q fever. Experimental vaccines using either Phase I or Phase II organisms have been effective in preventing disease in volunteers and in several field trials. For those persons at high risk, such as researchers working with sheep, veterinarians, or exposed laboratory workers, vaccine can be obtained under an investigational new drug (IND) application.

Focusing on controlling disease in the workplace is more effective than attempting to control the disease in animals. Three recommended measures include knowing the serologic status of the employees, not permitting pregnant women or persons with valvar heart disease to be in the high-risk jobs, and confining the research on sheep to a building dedicated solely to that purpose. Vaccination of employees should also be attempted.

Brouqui P, Dupont HT, Drancourt M, et al.: Chronic Q fever: Ninety-two cases from France, including 27 cases without endocarditis. Arch Intern Med 153:642, 1993. *An excellent review of chronic Q fever.*

Yeaman MR, Roman MJ, Baca OG: Antibiotic susceptibilities of two *Coxiella burnetii* isolates implicated in distinct clinical syndromes. Antimicrob Agents Chemother 33:2053, 1989. *A new method to evaluate sensitivities of Q fever isolates to antibiotics.*

325 ZOONOSES
Stuart Levin

"Zoonoses" are most simply defined as human infections derived from animals. There are approximately 200 different infectious agents that cause disease in humans and fulfill the definition of a zoonosis. Man's so-called best friend, the dog, has been targeted as facilitating the transmission of more than 50 different infectious agents and is credited with more than one million bite injuries each year in the United States. The risk of developing a zoonosis is increased by outdoor activities, with exposure to and inhalation of infectious air particles, direct animal contact, insect bites, contact with previously infected human blood products, and contact with and ingestion of infectious agents transmitted by animal-contaminated water and insufficiently cooked meat, eggs, dairy products, fish, and shellfish. Raw shellfish are the garbage filters of the ocean and can transmit at least 25 different infectious or toxic illnesses to humans. In addition, the farmer, pet owner, hunter, laboratory researcher, and cave explorer, among others, is at higher risk than the general population to develop a zoonosis. Infective agents transmitted by these routes from animal sources essentially include members of all microbial classes: viruses, bacteria, fungi, and parasites. Immunocompromised hosts such as splenectomized patients, trans-

TABLE 325–1. RESPIRATORY TRACT ZOONOSES

Disease	Microorganism	Clinical Syndrome and Diagnosis	Reservoir and/or Vector
Psittacosis	*Chlamydia psittaci*	Pneumonia, often severe; serology	Aerosols from parrots, ducks, turkeys
Q-fever	*Coxiella burnetii*	Pneumonia, hepatitis, or myocarditis; serology	Airborne from soil contaminated by sheep, goats, and cats, particularly if parturient
Tularemia	*Francisella tularensis*	Cutaneous ulcer and regional node; pneumonia and hilar node; pleural effusion, sepsis; serology	Rabbit contact (winter) and tick bites (summer)*
Plague	*Yersinia pestis*	Inguinal nodes, bubonic plague (10% will develop basilar pneumonia); hilar node enlargement; serology	Fleas from prairie dogs, rock squirrels, rats
Hantavirus adult respiratory distress syndrome	*Hantavirus muerto canyon†*	URI to LRI to ARDS; death; serology	Deer mouse fomites: urine, feces, saliva
Rhodococcus pneumonia	*Rhodococcus equi*	Pneumonia, often cavitate, in AIDS and other immunosuppressed patients; sputum culture	Horse manure, soil
Mycoplasma arginini pneumonia	*Mycoplasma arginini*	Pneumonia, sepsis, neutropenic hosts; special culture	Sheep, goats
Foot and mouth disease	Aphthovirus	Nonspecific URI, oral vesicles; serology	Cloven-footed mammals

Note: See Table of Contents and Index for more detailed discussion of each disease.
* Occurs in more than 1000 animal species.
† Proposed name.

TABLE 325–2. CENTRAL NERVOUS SYSTEM INFECTION: ZOONOSES

Disease	Organism	Clinical Syndrome and Diagnosis	Reservoir
Listeriosis	*Listeria monocytogenes*	Purulent meningitis during pregnancy and in neonate; immunosuppression; culture	Unpasteurized cheese and other dairy products; cattle, goats
Leptospirosis	*Leptospira interrogans*	Aseptic meningitis, hepatorenal syndrome; serology, culture	Asymptomatic dogs, cattle, water source common
Herpes B encephalitis	*Herpes simiae*	Diffuse, progressive encephalitis; culture	Bites or scratches of Macaques monkey
Lyme disease	*Borrelia burgdorferi*	Lymphocytic meningitis, motorsensory neuropathy, facial palsy; serology	Tick bites, mouse hosts
Lymphocytic choriomeningitis	Lymphocytic choriomeningitis virus	Lymphocytic meningitis, occasionally with pneumonia; serology	Inhalation of mouse secretions, urine, feces, saliva
Mosquito-borne encephalitis, USA	Eastern, western equine encephalitis; St. Louis, California encephalitis	Diffuse encephalitis; least severe: California encephalitis; most severe: Eastern equine encephalitis; serology	Mosquito-borne from horses, birds
Rabies encephalitis	Rabies virus	Almost always fatal; encephalitis; serology	Bites from dogs, skunks, bats, raccoons, foxes
Toxoplasmosis	*Toxoplasma gondii*	CNS, multiple lesions, AIDS patient; CNS scan, serology, biopsy	Cat feces or ingestion of undercooked lamb, pork
Cerebral cysticercosis	*Taenia solium*	Epilepsy, CNS cysts, eosinophilic meningitis, hydrocephalus; scan, serology	Fecal-oral contamination of food; swine

Note: See Table of Contents and Index for more detailed discussion of each disease.

plant patients, and AIDS patients, as well as pregnant women and their fetuses, are at high risk of developing clinical disease when exposed to these various infectious agents.

Non–animal-associated environmental- or travel-related infectious diseases can be confused with zoonoses. The vast majority of clinical diseases caused by *Legionella pneumophila, Plasmodium falciparum, Entamoeba histolytica, Giardia lamblia, Pseudomonas pseudomallei, Chromobacterium violaceum, Aeromonas hydrophila, Francisella philomiragia,* and airborne fungi such as *Blastomyces dermatitidis, Coccidioides immitis,* and *Histoplasma capsulatum* are acquired through environmental exposure and are only rarely related to animal hosts.

Unfortunately, some descriptive disease titles can be misleading to clinicians and thus can interfere with the possible diagnoses that they consider. The transmission of tick-borne Rocky Mountain spotted fever actually occurs more commonly in the southeastern United States than in the Rocky Mountains and has even been acquired in the middle of the Bronx, New York. Vegetarians and other strict non–pork-eating persons have been seriously infected with the pig tapeworm, *Taenia solium,* as a result of fecal contamination of food from unsuspected infected human sources.

The influence of the animal host on human infection can be quite deceptive. Human influenza A is not typically considered a zoonosis; however, there is evidence that an initial incubation period within an animal host may facilitate the more dramatic antigenic change "shifts" that account for the devastating pandemics of the

TABLE 325–3. SKIN RASHES: ZOONOSES

Disease	Microorganism	Clinical Information and Diagnosis	Reservoir and/or Vector
Ehrlichiosis	*Ehrlichia chaffeensis*	Macular rash (one third of patients), central distribution; in south central U.S.; culture, serology	Tick bite
Leptospirosis	*Leptospira interrogans*	Central macular rash in 20%, with occasional enanthem; serology, culture	Urine-contaminated water, dogs, cattle
Lyme disease	*Borrelia burgdorferi*	Primary lesion is erythema chronicum migrans; 40% have multiple lesions; serology, culture	Mouse reservoir–tick bite
Rocky Mountain spotted fever	*Rickettsia rickettsii*	Acral or peripheral distribution of macular papular to hemorrhagic rash to gangrenous lesions; serology	Tick bite
Typhus (endemic)	*Rickettsia prowazeckii*	Central distribution, macular rash (can be hemorrhagic); serology	Flying squirrel fleas or fomites
Scabies	Mite *Sarcoptes scabiei*	Pruritic macules on trunk; skin burrow	Dogs—close contact. Up to one third of asymptomatic dogs have mite infection
Flea bite dermatitis	*Pulex irritans*	Pruritic papules, urticaria vesicles; fleas found on pets or in the environment	Fleas on dogs
Cat scratch disease	*Rochalimaea henselae, Afipia felis*	Large purplish skin nodules and papules in AIDS patients; bacillary angiomatosis, hepatic peliosis, cervical adenopathy, and local ulcer in normal hosts; culture, serology, silver stain biopsy	Cat scratch or bite

Note: See Table of Contents and Index for more detailed discussion of each disease.

TABLE 325–4. HIGHLY FATAL ZOONOSES

Disease	Fatality Rate (%)
Rabies	99
*Herpes simiae**	50–75
Ebola virus	70
Eastern equine encephalitis	50–70
Hantavirus pulmonary syndrome, U.S.†	60
Yellow fever‡	20–50
Lassa fever‡	15–25
Plague*	50–80
Rocky Mountain spotted fever*	20–60
East African sleeping sickness*	20–30
Anthrax*	20
Tularemia	10–15
Visceral leishmanias*	5–25
Louse-borne relapsing fever*	5–40

Note: See Table of Contents and Index for more detailed discussion of each disease.
* Fatality rate if untreated.
† If jaundiced.
‡ Case mortality of hospitalized patients.

TABLE 325–5. NEWLY CHARACTERIZED ZOONOSES

Disease	Clinical Information	Reservoir and/or Vector
Ehrlichia chaffeensis	Fever, myalgia, leukopenia	Tick bite
Cat scratch disease, *Rochalimaea henselae, Afipia felis*	Cervical lymphadenopathy in normal hosts and cutaneous and hepatic angiomatosis in AIDS patients	Cat scratch or bite
Enterohemorrhagic *Escherichia coli* 0157-H7	Rectal bleeding, dysentery, hemolytic uremia syndrome	Contaminated, undercooked meat
Hantavirus	Adult respiratory distress syndrome	Fomites of rodents
Cryptosporidium	Diarrhea	Contaminated water
Campylobacter jejuni	Dysentery, Reiter's syndrome, Guillian-Barré syndrome	Contaminated chicken
Capnocytophaga canimorsus	Sepsis, skin infection	Dog bites

Note: See Table of Contents and Index for more detailed discussion of each disease.

disease that appear every 10 to 30 years. Recent information suggests that avian (bird) influenza viruses common in domestic fowl (ducks) can intermix with human influenza A viruses in a third animal species, the domestic pig of China, leading to an antigen shift. Indeed, in areas of China the three species live together in very close quarters. This "new" influenza A virus is transmitted to the human host from the pig and then transferred rapidly from human to human around the world, with catastrophic health and economic consequences. Leprosy, a human-to-human–transmitted illness of biblical notoriety, is endemic in at least three animal species, including the armadillo, which occasionally has been implicated in the transmission of this disease to humans in the United States.

As clinicians evaluate an individual patient, they need consider only a limited number of historical details that generally will lead to an appropriate differential diagnosis. These include

1. Questions regarding direct contact with animals or animal products must be pursued. Details regarding animal bites, arthropod exposures, and food ingestion may offer clues to the correct etiology.
2. Consideration must be given to a patient's travel history, because a number of zoonoses are quite limited in their geographic distribution.
3. Details about occupational and recreational high-risk activities must be ascertained.
4. The patient's clinical presentation is used to focus simultaneously on the most likely cause and disease considerations. Tables 325–1 through 325–5 take advantage of this "syndrome" approach. Additional lists of zoonotic agents can be generated for the differential diagnoses of arthritis, jaundice, diarrhea, sepsis and shock, renal failure, fever of unknown origin, and endocarditis.

Cook GC: Canine-associated zoonoses: An unacceptable hazard to human health. Q J Med 70:5126, 1989.
Glaser CA, Angulo FJ, Rooney JA: Animal-associated opportunistic infections among persons infected with the human immunodeficiency virus. Clin Infect Dis 18:14, 1994.
Eastaugh J, Shepherd S: Infectious and toxic syndromes from fish and shellfish consumption. Arch Intern Med 149:1735, 1989.
Salgo MP, Telzak EE, Currie B, et al.: A focus of Rocky Mountain spotted fever within New York City. N Engl J Med 318:1345, 1988.
Schantz PM, Moore AC, Munoz JL, et al.: Neurocysticercosis in an orthodox Jewish community in New York City. N Engl J Med 327:692, 1992.

Viral Diseases

326 INTRODUCTION TO VIRAL DISEASES

R. Gordon Douglas, Jr.

Viruses are among the simplest and smallest of all forms of life. They are obligate intracellular parasites that require host cell structural and metabolic components for replication. They infect bacteria as well as plants and animals. More than 400 distinct viruses infect humans. They produce diseases ranging from subclinical infections and mild, self-limited, localized infections to common systemic infections and overwhelming, highly lethal infections such as meningoencephalitis or hemorrhagic fever with shock.

CHARACTERISTICS OF VIRUSES. Essentially, virus particles, or "virions," consist of nucleic acid enclosed in a protein coat. They lack metabolic activity and do not possess ribosomes or most enzymes necessary for replication. In addition, some possess a lipid envelope. Both the lipid and the protein coats protect the nucleic acid from enzymatic degradation. The nucleic acid may be either deoxyribonucleic acid (DNA) or ribonucleic acid (RNA). It may code for only a few or, in some cases, several hundred proteins. The protein coat, or "capsid," consists of repeating, identical subunits called "capsomeres." The capsid and nucleic acid together are called the "nucleocapsid." The smallest (parvoviruses) are only 18 nm in diameter; some poxviruses may be as large as 450 nm.

There are two major types of structures of virus particles. In the first type, capsomeres are arranged as a regular polyhedron with 20 triangular faces and 12 corners. Such a virus exhibits icosahedral symmetry. Many nonenveloped viruses are of this type. Other viruses exhibit helical symmetry in which a helix is formed of ribonucleoprotein and nucleic acid. Helical viruses are always enveloped, whereas icosahedral viruses may be enveloped or nonenveloped. The envelope is derived from host cell membranes and modified by insertion of one or more spikelike glycoproteins. These and other proteins on the surface of enveloped or nonenveloped viruses are important for two reasons: They provide specific interaction with receptors on host cells, and they serve as the major antigens of the virus.

Figure 326–1 demonstrates schematically the marked variety in size, shape, and structure of human viruses. In addition, there is great diversity in the structure of the viral genome: Either RNA or DNA may be single stranded or double stranded. The genome may be linear or circular and may exist as single or multiple segments.

Viruses are classified by the International Committee on Taxonomy of Viruses according to the scheme presented in Table 326–1. The following order of virion characteristics is used: nucleic acid type, presence or absence of envelope, genome replication strategy, positive- or negative-sense genome, and genome segmentation.

Because virus structure varies and genomes are complex, mechanisms of replication are diverse. Following a random collision between a virus particle and a cell surface, attachment occurs by binding of a surface protein of a virus to a host cell virus receptor. The nature of the viral attachment protein has been identified for a number of viruses. Penetration of the plasma membrane of the cell occurs by endocytosis, a process similar to receptor-mediated endocytosis of nonviral ligands, or by nonendocytic pathways such as direct translocation across the plasma membrane. Following acidification of the endosome, the viral membrane fuses with that of the vesicle, releasing the nucleocapsid. After uncoating of the viral nucleic acid, macromolecular synthesis of nucleic acid and protein occurs. The strategy for genome replication depends on the type of nucleic acid. Assembly of virus components then occurs, with release of mature viruses by budding, in the case of enveloped viruses, or by lysis of the cell, in the case of some nonenveloped viruses. Such released virions are infectious for other cells.

Viruses cause cell injury by a number of mechanisms: directly by lysis resulting from viral replication, by lysis induced by antiviral antibody and complement, or by cell-mediated immune mechanisms recognizing infected host cells. As virus infection spreads and sufficient numbers of cells are injured, disease results. A role for viral toxins has never been established, and such enzymes as are virus

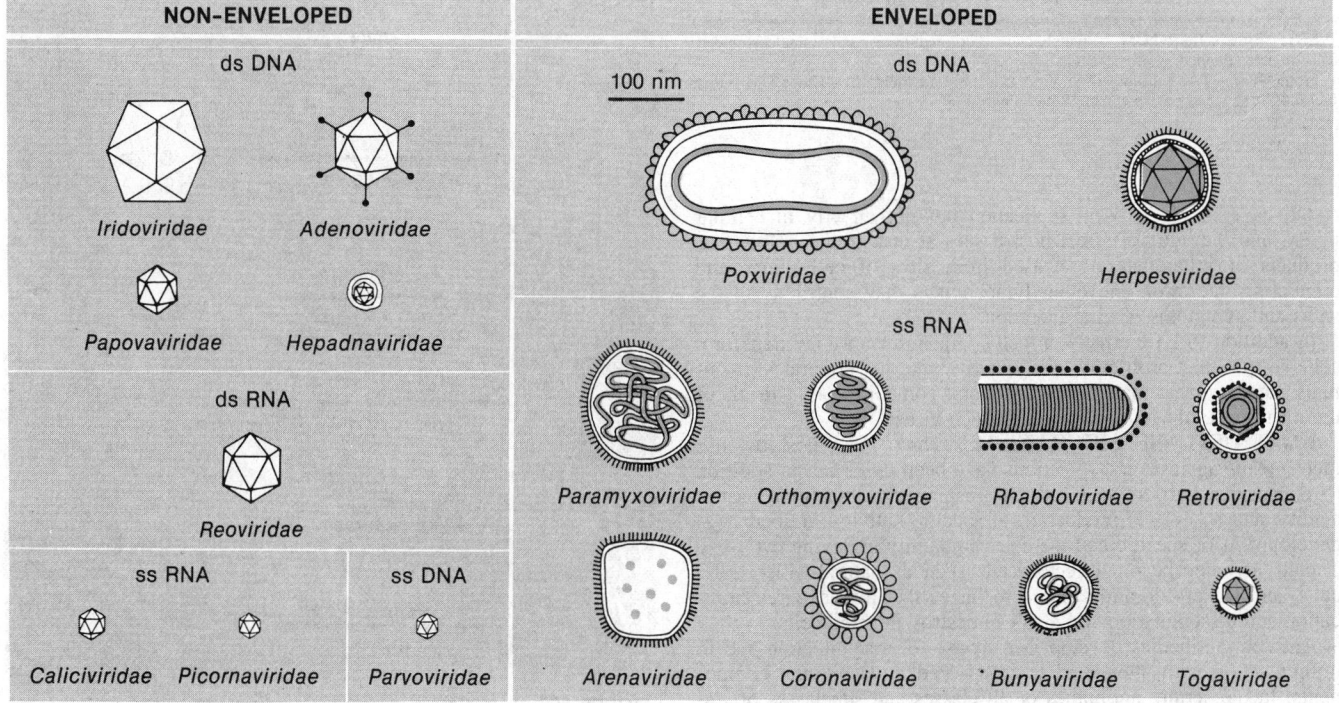

FIGURE 326–1. Structure and relative size of human virus families. (Modified from Matthews REF: Classification and nomenclature of viruses. Intervirology 12:158, 1979.)

TABLE 326-1. CLASSIFICATION OF HUMAN VIRUSES

Dividing Characteristics	Virus Families	Important Human Viruses
DNA Viruses		
dsDNA, enveloped	Poxviridae	Variola (smallpox) virus
		Vaccinia virus
	Herpesviridae	Herpes simplex virus types 1 and 2
		Varicella-zoster virus
		Human cytomegalovirus
		EB virus
		Human herpesvirus type G
dsDNA, nonenveloped	Adenoviridae	Human adenovirus
	Papovaviridae	Papillomavirus
	Hepadnaviridae	Hepatitis B virus
ssDNA, nonenveloped	Parvoviridae	Parvovirus B19
RNA Viruses		
dsRNA, nonenveloped	Reoviridae	Colorado tick fever virus
		Human rotaviruses
ssRNA, enveloped No DNA step in replication		
Positive-sense genome	Togaviridae	Alphavirus: Eastern equine encephalitis, Western equine encephalitis
		Rubivirus: Rubella virus
	Flaviviridae	Yellow fever virus
		Dengue viruses
		St. Louis encephalitis
	Coronaviridae	Human coronaviruses
Negative-sense genome		
Nonsegmented genome	Paramyxoviridae	Parainfluenza virus
		Measles virus
		Respiratory syncytial virus
	Rhabdoviridae	Rabies virus
	Filoviridae	Marburg and Ebola viruses
Segmented genome	Orthomyxoviridae	Influenza A and B virus
	Bunyaviridae	California encephalitis virus
	Arenaviridae	LCM virus
		Lassa virus
DNA step in replication	Retroviridae	HTLV I, II
		HIV I, II
ssRNA, nonenveloped	Picornaviridae	Polioviruses, coxsackieviruses, echoviruses, rhinoviruses
	Caliciviridae	Norwalk virus

EB = Epstein-Barr; LCM = lymphocytic choriomeningitis; ss = single stranded; ds = double stranded.
From Murphy FA, Kinsbury DW: Virus taxonomy. *In* Fields BN, Knipe DM (eds.): Fields Virology. 2nd ed. New York, Raven Press, 1990.

coded have a role in viral replication but not directly in cellular injury, and they do not affect host tissues at distant sites. However, products of inflammation released from sites of cell injury and circulating interferon and other lymphokines may contribute to the signs and symptoms of viral infection.

In addition to lytic effects on cells, viral infection may transform cells so that they proliferate continuously and, in vertebrates, mammals, and humans, may produce tumors, sometimes as a result of the occurrence of viral oncogenes in such viruses.

HOST DEFENSE MECHANISMS. Three main host defense mechanisms against viral infections have been described in addition to nonspecific barriers such as skin, respiratory epithelium, gastric acidity, and so on: (1) production of specific antiviral antibody, (2) development of specific cell-mediated immunity involving cytotoxic T cells and nonspecific effector cells such as natural killer (NK) cells, and (3) proliferation of macrophages that restrict virus replication and dissemination and also can destroy infected cells.

Antiviral antibodies develop in response to viral infection and to immunization with attenuated or inactivated virus or viral components. In the serum, antibodies of all classes and subclasses of immunoglobulins are found; in addition, secretory antibodies consisting predominantly of immunoglobulin A (IgA) molecules develop on mucosal surfaces in response to infection of their surfaces. They are of critical importance in diseases in which the primary site of inoculation is a mucosal surface.

The immune system may interact with extracellular (free) virus or cell-associated virus. Specific antibody inactivates (neutralizes) extracellular virus, and this activity may be enhanced by complement. Thus it can prevent initial infection or restrict cell-to-cell spread of virus through extracellular fluids. It cannot, however, penetrate into cells and neutralize intracellular virus. Thus virus may escape the effects of antibody by direct cell-to-cell transfer. Virus-infected cells possess viral antigens on their surface and may be lysed by specific antibody and complement, by specific cytotoxic T cells, or by nonspecific cells such as NK cells or macrophages. Virus released in the process may be neutralized by antiviral antibody.

Cytotoxic T cells (Tc), which are HLA class I antigen restricted, also develop in response to infection or immunization (see Ch. 221). They are important in limiting the growth of certain viruses in the infected host. This has been most clearly shown for influenza infections in mice, and Tc are undoubtedly important in a number of viral infections in humans.

NK cells are another important host defense mechanism against viral infections. During early stages of viral infection, the numbers of natural killer cells and their activity are greatly augmented by virus-induced interferon. Mice deficient in NK cells are more sensitive to cytomegalovirus infection, and NK activity has been demonstrated in a number of human infections.

Virus-induced interferons (α and β) have important roles in protection against virus infection through their ability to prevent viral replication in many cells throughout the body and by means of their regulatory function in the immune system. In experimental infections in animals in which interferon activity is neutralized by specific antibody, potentiation of viral infection occurs. In humans, in a number of infections, endogenous interferon developed in serum or secretions correlates with recovery: decreasing virus titers and amelioration of symptoms. Since administering interferon to humans produces a number of side effects, such as fever, leukopenia, and myalgias, interferon also may account, in part, for some of the systemic signs and symptoms that accompany viral infections.

Interferon-γ is induced as a result of immune stimulation. It also has antiviral effects and is a major immune regulatory protein that induces Tc, activates macrophages and NK cells, and regulates antibody production by B cells.

MECHANISMS OF PATHOGENESIS. Infection is initiated, often when one or a very few virus particles are deposited in the

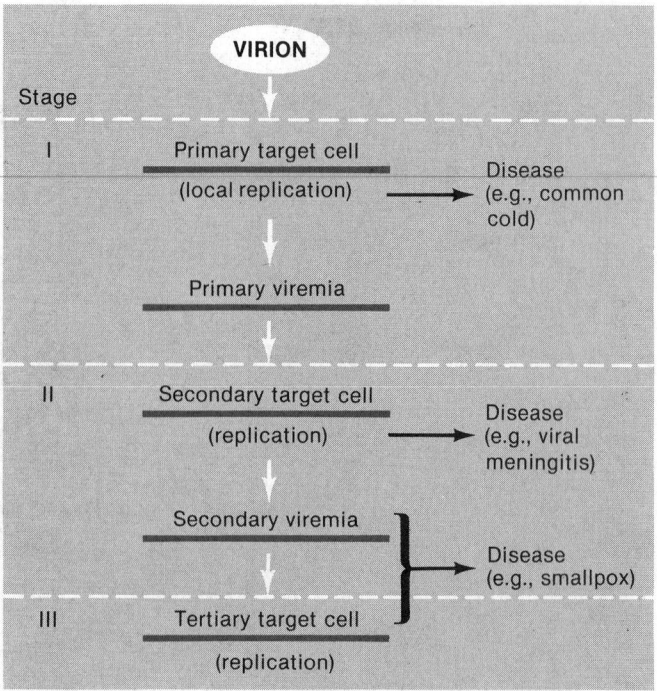

FIGURE 326-2. Stages of viral pathogenesis. Initial invasion may involve only primary target cells or may lead to secondary or tertiary target cell invasion, which results in the characteristic disease. (Courtesy of ED Kilbourne.)

TABLE 326–2. VIRUSES COMMONLY ASSOCIATED WITH DIFFERENT SYNDROMES

Disease Category	Common Associated Virus	Disease Category	Common Associated Virus
Respiratory Tract		*Gastrointestinal Tract*	
Upper respiratory infection (including common cold and pharyngitis)	Rhinoviruses Coronaviruses Parainfluenza 1–3 Influenza A, B Herpes simplex Adenoviruses Echoviruses Coxsackieviruses Epstein-Barr virus Respiratory syncytial	Gastroenteritis Hepatitis	Rotavirus Norwalk-like agents Adenovirus Hepatitis A Hepatitis B Hepatitis C Hepatitis D Hepatitis E Epstein-Barr virus Cytomegalovirus
Croup	Parainfluenza 1–3 Influenza A, B Respiratory syncytial	*Skin*	
Bronchiolitis	Respiratory syncytial Parainfluenza 1–3	Maculopapular rash	Measles Rubella Parvovirus B19 Echoviruses Coxsackievirus A16 Enterovirus 71
Pneumonia (adults)	Influenza A	Hemorrhagic rash	Herpesvirus G Alphavirus Bunyavirus Flaviviruses
Pneumonia (children)	Respiratory syncytial Parainfluenza 1–3 Influenza A	Localized lesions	Herpes simplex Human papillomavirus 1, 2, 4, 41 Molluscum contagiosum
Central Nervous System		*Neonatal*	
Aseptic meningitis	Mumps Coxsackievirus B1–5 Coxsackievirus A9 Echovirus 4, 6, 9, 11, 14, 18, 30, 31	Teratogenic effects	Rubella Cytomegalovirus
Paralysis	Polio 1–3	Disseminated disease	Coxsackievirus B1–5 Echoviruses Hepatitis B Parvovirus B19 Cytomegalovirus Herpes simplex
Encephalitis	Human immunodeficiency virus I Alphaviruses Flaviviruses Bunyaviruses Herpes simplex 1 Enterovirus 71 Mumps	Lower respiratory disease	Respiratory syncytial Influenza
Genitourinary Tract		Enteritis	Rotavirus
Vulvovaginitis, cervicitis	Herpes simplex 2	*Other*	
Penile and vulvar lesions	Herpes simplex 2 Molluscum contagiosum Human papillomavirus 6, 10, 11, 40–45, 51	Arthritis	Rubella Parvovirus B19 Hepatitis B
Acute hemorrhagic cystitis	Adenovirus 11	Myositis	Togaviruses Influenza B
Ocular		Carditis	Coxsackievirus B
Conjunctivitis	Adenovirus 3, 4, 7, 8, 19 Herpes simplex Varicella-zoster Measles	Parotitis, pancreatitis, and orchitis	Mumps
Acute hemorrhagic conjunctivitis	Enterovirus 70 Coxsackievirus A 24		
Immune System			
Acquired immunodeficiency syndrome	Human immunodeficiency virus I		

Modified from Manegus MA, Douglas RG Jr: Viruses, rickettsiae, chlamydiae, and mycoplasmas. *In* Mandell GL, Douglas RG, Jr, Bennett JE: Principles and Practice of Infectious Diseases, 3rd ed. New York, Churchill Livingstone, 1990.

respiratory, gastrointestinal, or genitourinary tract or are injected percutaneously or pass transplacentally. As shown in Figure 326–2, human viral infections may be classified according to mechanisms of pathogenesis. Many infections are limited to cells at the portal of entry, and dissemination does not occur. Conjunctivitis due to adenovirus type 8 and common colds due to rhinoviruses and to other respiratory viruses are excellent examples of this type of pathogenesis.

Other virus infections spread hematogenously to distal sites. Infection at the primary site may or may not result in symptoms, but viral replication in the distal site usually results in the characteristic illness associated with such a virus infection. Enteroviruses such as coxsackievirus and echovirus infect the gastrointestinal tract as their primary site, and this infection is usually clinically silent but produces a primary viremia, following which encephalitis, meningitis, or other central nervous system disease may occur as these tissues are infected. Other viruses reach target organs through nerves: rabies, varicella-zoster virus, and herpes simplex virus.

In other infections, viral replication in the secondary site produces a viremia that results in replication in still other sites. Such was the case with smallpox and may be the case with measles. Rash may be a manifestation of either primary or secondary viremia.

Many virus infections have clinical characteristics that permit diagnosis: measles, mumps, chickenpox, and poliomyelitis. However, many others do not, and many syndromes have multiple etiologies, as is shown in Table 326–2. In fact, as many as 200 serologically distinct viruses may cause the common cold and related disorders. In the case of some syndromes—for example, atypical pneumonia—the etiology may be shared with other infectious organisms: *Mycoplasma pneumoniae, Chlamydia pneumoniae,* and *Legionella pneumophila.* Others, however, are exclusively viral in etiology.

PREVENTION AND CONTROL. Recent advances in antiviral chemotherapy have produced a number of specific antivirals that are available and effective for prophylaxis or treatment, or both, of certain viral diseases. Drugs such as trifluridine, amantadine, ribavirin, acyclovir, vidarabine, zidovudine, ganciclovir, foscarnet, didanosine, zalcitabine, d4T, and interferon-α are available in the

United States. For many other viral infections, however, no specific therapy exists. Proper use of antivirals requires specific viral diagnosis. Fortunately, in the case of herpes zoster, the diagnosis can usually be made clinically, and in influenza, the diagnosis can often be made on clinical and epidemiologic grounds; however, for many infections, viral diagnosis is required. Viral diagnostic laboratories are more common than in the past, and rapid techniques are gaining acceptance.

Vaccines are available for a number of viral infections, and many have greatly affected morbidity and mortality due to specific infections. Antibodies induced by vaccination may block initiation of infection in a primary site, as in the case in influenza. Others, such as inactivated poliomyelitis vaccine, are designed to prevent primary viremia after initial infection has occurred. Live attenuated viruses induce cell-mediated as well as humoral immune response.

Fields BN, Knipe DM (eds.): Fields Virology, 2nd ed. New York, Raven Press, 1990. *Excellent definitive textbook of basic virology.*
Tyler UL, Fields BN: Introduction to viruses and viral diseases. *In* Mandell GL, Bennett JE, Dolin R (eds.): Principles and Practice of Infectious Diseases, 4th ed. New York, John Wiley & Sons, 1995. *Excellent detailed review of virus structure, virus-cell interactions, virus-host interactions, and virus transmission.*

327 ANTIVIRAL THERAPY (Non-AIDS)

Richard J. Whitley

Compared with the progress made in the treatment of bacterial infections over the past four decades, advances in the chemotherapy of viral diseases have come much more slowly. In the United States, only a few antiviral agents of proven clinical value are available and for a limited number of indications. The problems associated with the development of antiviral agents can be summarized as follows: (1) viruses are obligate intracellular parasites that use biochemical pathways of the infected host cell, so it is difficult to achieve clinically useful antiviral activity without also adversely affecting host cell metabolism; (2) early diagnosis of viral infection is crucial for effective antiviral therapy, yet by the time symptoms appear, several cycles of viral multiplication may have occurred and replication has begun to wane; (3) precise diagnosis is difficult for many viral infections because of the lack of specificity of symptoms; and (4) since many of the disease syndromes caused by viruses are common, relatively benign, and self-limiting, the therapeutic index (ratio of efficacy to toxicity) must be extremely high for therapy to be acceptable.

As with all infectious diseases, the effectiveness of therapy is related to host defenses. Not only is the incidence of reactivation of certain viral diseases high in the immunocompromised host, but these infections are often much more severe. These patients require high doses of antiviral agents for long periods of time and have a high morbidity and mortality with currently approved antiviral therapy.

ANTIVIRALS FOR HERPESVIRUS INFECTIONS

Acyclovir

MECHANISM OF ACTION. Acyclovir, 9-((2-hydroxyethoxy)methyl) guanine, is an acyclic analogue of guanosine. Virus-specified thymidine kinase phosphorylates acyclovir to its monophosphate derivative, an event that does not occur in uninfected cells to a significant extent. Acyclovir is then further phosphorylated by cellular enzymes to its triphosphate derivative. Acyclovir triphosphate binds viral DNA polymerase, acting as a DNA chain terminator. Because acyclovir is taken up selectively by virus-infected cells, the concentration of acyclovir triphosphate is 40 to 100 times higher in infected than in uninfected cells. Furthermore, viral DNA polymerase exhibits a 10- to 30-fold greater affinity for acyclovir triphosphate than does cellular DNA polymerases. The higher concentration in infected cells plus the affinity for viral poly-

merases results in the very low toxicity of acyclovir for normal host cells. Although Epstein-Barr virus (EBV) and cytomegalovirus (CMV) do not have virus-specific thymidine kinases, acyclovir does have minimal activity against these viruses.

LICENSED USES. Acyclovir is available in ointment, capsule, and intravenous formulations. In the topical form, acyclovir is licensed for managing primary herpes genitalis in both immunocompetent and immunocompromised hosts as well as in limited, non-life-threatening mucocutaneous herpes simplex virus (HSV) infections in immunocompromised hosts. It is less active topically than when delivered by other routes, and its use by this route should be discouraged.

Oral acyclovir is indicated in the management of most cases of primary or initial genital herpes in all patient populations and as suppressive therapy in normal hosts with frequently recurrent genital herpes (six or more recurrences a year). Oral acyclovir is also used as prophylaxis and treatment in immunocompromised patients with a history of HSV infections, e.g., herpes labialis or genital herpes. High-dose oral acyclovir (i.e., 800 mg five times per day) has recently been approved for use in immunocompetent patients with localized herpes zoster.

Intravenous acyclovir is indicated in severe initial herpes genitalis of immunocompetent patients and in the treatment of some initial and recurrent mucocutaneous infections in immunocompromised patients, as well as in the treatment of herpes simplex encephalitis (HSE). Intravenous acyclovir is approved for treatment of varicella-zoster virus (VZV) infections in immunocompromised hosts.

TOXICITY. Acyclovir has an excellent safety profile and is well tolerated. The major adverse effect of acyclovir is that it alters renal function. High-dose bolus injection of acyclovir can cause crystallization in renal tubules and subsequent acute tubular necrosis or simply a reversible elevation of serum creatinine. Dehydration, pre-existing renal insufficiency, and higher doses of acyclovir are risk factors for renal toxicity. Dosage alterations are required with renal impairment (Table 327–1). In addition, there have been a few brief reports suggesting central nervous system (CNS) toxicity after intravenous administration of acyclovir. Oral acyclovir has not been associated with renal toxicity, even when given in high doses (800 mg five times a day).

Because acyclovir is a nucleoside analogue that can be incorporated into both viral and host-cell DNA, it has been studied extensively for its potential as a carcinogen, teratogen, and mutagen. There is no significant evidence that acyclovir is a carcinogen in humans, and animal studies indicate that acyclovir is not a significant teratogen in clinically used doses. Acyclovir is not a significant mutagen *in vitro* but seems to be able to induce chromosomal events as does caffeine. Because of the many possible indications for acyclovir during pregnancy, as well as the likelihood of frequent first-trimester exposures to drug before pregnancy is established, it is extremely important to define its risk. An "Acyclovir in Pregnancy Registry" has been established to gather data on all reported prenatal exposures to oral acyclovir. Although no significant risk to the mother or fetus has been documented, the total number of monitored pregnancies remains too small to detect any risk that is not overwhelming. The safety of acyclovir in pregnancy, therefore, has not been unequivocally established. Since acyclovir crosses the placenta and can concentrate in amniotic fluid, there is valid concern about the potential for renal toxicity in the fetus.

RESISTANCE TO ACYCLOVIR. Resistance to acyclovir develops through mutations in one of two HSV genes, namely, those specifying viral thymidine kinase (TK) or DNA polymerase. Clinical isolates resistant to acyclovir are almost uniformly deficient in

TABLE 327–1. DOSAGE ADJUSTMENT FOR INTRAVENOUS ACYCLOVIR IN PATIENTS WITH IMPAIRED RENAL FUNCTION

Creatinine Clearance (ml/min/1.73 M^2)	Percentage of Standard Dose	Dosing Interval (Hours)
>50	100	8
25–50	100	12
10–25	100	24
0–10*	50	24

* Administered after hemodialysis.

TK. Until recently, such resistance has been rare; all such mutants had reduced neurovirulence and did not readily establish latency. However, acyclovir-resistant HSV mutants are being reported more frequently in the immunocompromised patient population and in one normal host. These mutants are deficient in viral TK and sensitive to vidarabine and foscarnet, drugs that do not require viral TK for activation. Some isolates are fully neurovirulent and able to establish latency in a murine model. With the growing population of immunocompromised patients (due to both HIV infection and therapeutic immunosuppression) who suffer from frequent and severe herpesvirus infections, it is expected that acyclovir resistance will become more prevalent.

Ganciclovir

MECHANISM OF ACTION. Ganciclovir, also known as DHPG, is an acyclic nucleoside analogue of acyclovir that has increased *in vitro* activity against all herpesviruses as compared with acyclovir, including an 8 to 20 times greater antiviral activity against CMV. Like acyclovir, the activity of ganciclovir in HSV-infected cells depends on phosphorylation by virus-specific TK. Also like acyclovir, ganciclovir monophosphate is further converted to its di- and triphosphate derivatives by cellular kinases. In cells infected by HSV-1 or HSV-2, the triphosphate (DHPG-TP) competitively inhibits the incorporation of guanosine-TP into viral DNA and terminates chain synthesis. The mode of action of ganciclovir against CMV and EBV (which do not produce virus-specific TK) is not entirely known, but it has been suggested that these viruses may induce a cellular TK or viral kinase that efficiently promotes the obligatory initial phosphorylation of ganciclovir to its monophosphate.

LICENSED USES. Ganciclovir has been licensed by the United States Food and Drug Administration for treating CMV retinitis and life-threatening CMV diseases in AIDS and other immunocompromised patients.

TOXICITY. The most important side effects of ganciclovir are neutropenia and thrombocytopenia. Neutropenia occurs in approximately 35% of patients and is usually (but not always) reversible with dose adjustment or discontinuation. Thrombocytopenia occurs in about 20% of patients. Numerous other side effects possibly related to ganciclovir, such as nausea, vomiting, dizziness, and headache, are usually not of clinical significance. Agents with significant myelotoxicity, such as antimetabolites or alkylating agents, cannot be used concomitantly with ganciclovir. Zidovudine (azidothymidine, or AZT) may be used cautiously in low doses in patients receiving ganciclovir, but hematologic parameters must be monitored closely.

Ganciclovir also has significant gonadal toxicity in animal screening systems, most notably as a potent inhibitor of spermatogenesis. As an agent affecting DNA synthesis, ganciclovir has carcinogenic potential.

CLINICAL USE. Ganciclovir has been the most widely tested drug for the treatment of CMV infections. There is support for clinical benefit in immunocompromised patients with CMV retinitis and gastrointestinal infection. Benefit is suggested but has been less dramatic for CMV pneumonia in AIDS patients and organ transplant recipients. Ganciclovir has effectively suppressed the reactivation of CMV infections in organ transplant recipients.

Idoxuridine and Trifluorothymidine

Idoxuridine and trifluorothymidine are analogues of thymidine. When administered systemically, these nucleosides are phosphorylated by both viral and cellular TK to active triphosphorylate derivatives that inhibit both viral and cellular DNA synthesis. The result is antiviral activity but also sufficient host cytotoxicity to prevent the systemic use of these drugs. Toxicity of these compounds is not significant, however, when applied topically to the eye in the treatment of HSV keratitis. Both idoxuridine and trifluorothymidine, as well as vidarabine, ophthalmic ointments are effective and licensed for such treatment. Acyclovir as an ophthalmic preparation also appears to be effective but is not yet licensed. Trifluorothymidine appears to be the most efficacious of these compounds. Although these agents are not of proven value in the treatment of stromal keratitis and uveitis, trifluorothymidine is more likely to penetrate the cornea. Some forms of stromal keratitis and uveitis are thought to be caused by immune mechanisms and thus would not respond to antiviral drugs. The ophthalmic preparations of idoxuridine, vidarabine, and trifluorothymidine may cause local irritation, photophobia, edema of the eyelids and cornea, punctual occlusion, and superficial punctate keratopathy.

Vidarabine

Vidarabine has been shown to be effective when administered parenterally for HSE, neonatal herpes, and VZV infections in the immunocompromised host. Because of a lower therapeutic index than acyclovir, it is only available as an ophthalmic preparation for therapy of HSV keratitis.

Foscarnet

Foscarnet, a pyrophosphate analogue of phosphonoacetic acid, has potent *in vitro* and *in vivo* activity against herpesviruses. Foscarnet inhibits the DNA polymerase of all human herpesviruses by blocking the pyrophosphate binding site and preventing chain elongation. Unlike acyclovir, which requires activation by a virus-specific TK, foscarnet acts directly on the virus DNA polymerase. TK-deficient, acyclovir-resistant herpesviruses remain sensitive to foscarnet.

Foscarnet was recently approved for the treatment of CMV retinitis in HIV-infected patients. Data collected from the Soka clinical trial indicate the equal effectiveness of foscarnet and ganciclovir therapy of retinitis in this population. However, use of foscarnet in combination with zidovidine resulted in enhanced survival. These findings remain to be confirmed in a larger study population. Foscarnet has been used for induction therapy of retinitis as well as when ganciclovir is not tolerated. However, administration of foscarnet is not without toxicity. Renal toxicity has been documented as well as hypocalcemia and altered levels of serum magnesium. Foscarnet's lack of bone marrow toxicity offers an advantage over ganciclovir. Additionally, foscarnet also has been used to treat acyclovir-resistant herpes simplex genital disease.

ANTIVIRALS FOR RESPIRATORY VIRAL INFECTIONS

It is difficult to overestimate the impact of respiratory viral illnesses on human health. Almost 90% of the population experiences one of these illnesses each year, resulting in a staggering number of days lost from work and school, as well as significant potential for serious morbidity and even death. Nonetheless, since these conditions in most patient populations are self-limited and rarely fatal, the requirements for new drugs are stringent: an extreme degree of safety, moderate to high effectiveness, ease of administration, and low cost. Accordingly, only two such antivirals are approved for use in the United States, each with fairly limited indications. Because of the number of developmental programs identifying new antivirals for treatment of respiratory viruses, it seems likely that an expanded armamentarium will be forthcoming.

Amantadine and Rimantadine

MECHANISM OF ACTION. Amantadine and rimantadine have a narrow spectrum of activity and at concentrations achievable in humans are useful only against influenza A infections. Although amantadine was the first antiviral to be approved in the United States, its mechanism of action is not yet completely understood. Influenza A viruses differ in their susceptibility to amantadine, and the drug may have different actions depending on the concentration and virus strain. Early studies indicated that amantadine acted by preventing the penetration and/or uncoating the virus. More recently, low concentrations of the drug were shown to inhibit virus assembly by interacting with hemagglutinin; high concentrations appear to inhibit an early stage of the infection involving fusion between the virus envelope and the membrane of secondary lysosomes. Rimantadine has a similar mechanism of action.

LICENSED USES. As antiviral agents, amantadine and rimantidine are licensed for both the chemoprophylaxis and the treatment of influenza A infections. Both drugs can be used for any unimmunized member of the general population who wishes to avoid influenza A, but prophylaxis is especially recommended to control presumed influenza outbreaks in institutions housing high-risk persons. High-risk individuals include adults and children with chronic disorders of the cardiovascular or pulmonary systems requiring regular follow-up or hospitalization during the preceding year, as well as nursing homes and other chronic-care facilities residents. In these instances, drugs should be administered to all residents of the institution, whether or not they received influenza vaccination the previous fall. To reduce spread of virus and to minimize disruption of patient care, it is also recommended that amantadine prophylaxis be offered to unvaccinated staff who care for high-risk patients. Amantadine prophylaxis is also recommended in the following situations:

1. As an adjunct to late immunization of high-risk individuals. Amantadine does not interfere with antibody response to the vaccine.

2. For persons who have not been immunized and who care for high-risk persons in home settings, both to reduce spread of virus and to allow persons to maintain care for high-risk persons in the home setting.

3. For immunodeficient persons, who may be expected to have a poor antibody response to vaccine.

4. For persons for whom influenza vaccine is contraindicated, e.g., for persons hypersensitive to egg protein.

Both drugs are also indicated in the treatment of uncomplicated respiratory illness caused by influenza A. Studies have shown a beneficial effect on the signs and symptoms of acute influenza, as well as a significant reduction in quantity of virus in respiratory secretions. Because of the short duration of disease, amantadine must be administered within 48 hours of symptom onset to show benefit. The effect of amantadine on the prevention of complications in high-risk groups is under evaluation.

Rimantadine is a structural analogue of amantadine, with the same spectrum of activity, mechanism of action, and clinical indications. Rimantadine is somewhat more effective than amantadine against influenza type A viruses at equal concentrations. Absorption of rimantadine is delayed when compared with amantadine, and furthermore, equivalent doses of rimantadine produce lower plasma levels than does amantadine. The lower plasma levels may explain the lower incidence of side effects at similar doses. Rimantadine has similar CNS side effects even though, unlike amantadine, this drug does not affect CNS catecholamine release and is not effective in the treatment of Parkinson's disease. The efficacy of rimantadine in both the prophylaxis and treatment of influenza A infections is similar to that of amantadine. There has been a recent report of rimantadine-resistant strains of influenza isolated from patients treated for acute influenza A.

TOXICITY. Amantadine is reported to cause side effects in 5 to 10% of healthy young adults taking the standard adult dose of 200 mg per day. These side effects are usually mild, cease soon after amantadine is discontinued, and often disappear even with continued use of the drug. CNS side effects are most common and include difficulty in thinking, confusion, lightheadedness, hallucinations, anxiety, and insomnia. Activities requiring mental alertness (e.g., driving) should be avoided until it is reasonable to assume that these symptoms will not occur. More severe adverse effects, e.g., mental depression and psychosis, are usually associated with doses exceeding 200 mg daily. About 5% of patients complain of nausea, vomiting, or anorexia. Older individuals are more likely to experience side effects. Rimantadine appears to be somewhat better tolerated.

Patients with renal disease should receive doses based on their creatinine clearance (Table 327–2). Doses for older people and children are usually lower as well. Persons with an active seizure disorder may be at increased risk for seizures when amantadine is given at standard doses.

Ribavirin

MECHANISM OF ACTION. Ribavirin is a nucleoside analogue whose mechanisms of action are poorly understood and probably not the same for all viruses; however, its ability to alter nucleotide pools and the packaging of mRNA appears to be important. This process is not totally virus-specific, but there is a certain selectivity in that infected cells produce more mRNA than noninfected cells. The capacity of viral mRNA to support protein synthesis is markedly reduced by ribavirin. High concentrations also inhibit cellular protein synthesis.

LICENSED USES. The development of a mechanism to deliver ribavirin via a small-particle aerosol greatly enhanced the potential usefulness of this drug for respiratory viral infections. At this time ribavirin is licensed for the treatment, by aerosol administration, of carefully selected hospitalized infants and young children with severe lower respiratory tract infections caused by respiratory syncytial virus (RSV). The vast majority of infants and children with RSV infection have disease that is mild and self-limited and do not require ribavirin.

TOXICITY AND CLINICAL PROBLEMS. No adverse effect has been clearly attributable to aerosol therapy with ribavirin, although reports of adverse effects during or following therapy of infants with RSV have included bronchospasm, pulmonary function test changes, pneumothorax in ventilated patients, apnea, cardiac arrest, hypotension, and concomitant digitalis toxicity. Precipitation of drug within the ventilatory apparatus of patients on mechanical ventilation can be a serious problem. When proper precautions are taken, such as frequent changes in ventilator tubing, safe delivery of ribavirin to ventilated patients can be accomplished. Reticulocytosis, rash, and conjunctivitis have been associated with the use of ribavirin aerosol. Although there are no pertinent human data, ribavirin has been found to be teratogenic and mutagenic in nearly all species in which it has been tested. This drug is therefore contraindicated in women who are or may become pregnant. Some concern has been expressed about the risk to persons in the room with infants being treated with ribavirin aerosol, particularly females of childbearing age. Although this risk seems to be minimal with limited exposure, awareness and caution are warranted.

FUTURE ANTIVIRALS

Advances in molecular virology continue to define those sites of viral replication which may be vulnerable to attack without harm to the host cell. Further characterization of the viral DNA polymerase, required for replication but not used by the host cell, is a major research focus. In addition, classes of compounds, many of them nucleoside analogues, are being systematically evaluated in order to identify more efficacious and less toxic antivirals. A description of some of the most promising drugs follows.

Several compounds have activity against the herpesviruses, including 1-β-D-arabinofuranosyl-E-5-(2-bromovinyl) arabinosyluracil (BV-araU), fluoroidoarabinosyl cytosine (FIAC), valacyclovir, famciclovir, and (S)-1-((3-hydroxy-2-phosphonylmethoxy)propyl) cytosine (HPMPC).

Bromovinyl arabinosyl uracil, BV-araU, is a potent inhibitor of HSV-1 and EBV. More important, it is exquisitely active against VZV, being over 1000 times more potent than acyclovir. Like acyclovir, the mechanism of action of BV-araU is based on the phosphorylation of the parent compound by herpesvirus TK, which restricts its action to virus-infected cells. BV-araU appears to have a favorable toxicity profile and will soon begin clinical trials in the United States.

Valacyclovir is the prodrug of acyclovir. Plasma concentrations achieved with oral valacyclovir approximate that of 5 mg per kilogram of acyclovir administered intravenously. Controlled clinical studies indicate that valacyclovir is as good as acyclovir for both the treatment of herpes zoster in the normal host and recurrent genital HSV infections.

Famciclovir is the prodrug of penciclovir. Famciclovir has been administered orally to individuals with herpes zoster as well as genital HSV infection, both primary and recurrent etiology. For patients with shingles, famciclovir therapy is as good as, if not better than,

---

TABLE 327–2. DOSAGE ADJUSTMENT FOR ORAL AMANTADINE IN PATIENTS WITH IMPAIRED RENAL FUNCTION

Creatinine Clearance (ml/min/1.73 M²)	Suggested Oral Maintenance Regimen After 200 mg (100 mg bid) on the First Day
≥ 80	100 mg bid
60–80	100 mg bid alternating with 100 mg daily
40–60	100 mg daily
30–40	200 mg (100 mg bid) twice weekly
20–30	100 mg 3 times each week
10–20	200 mg (100 mg bid) alternating with 100 mg every 7 days
< 10	100 mg every 7 days

acyclovir for managing infection. In the management of recurrent genital herpes, there appears to be accelerated healing of recurrent disease with episodic treatment. This drug was recently licensed for the treatment of shingles in the United Kingdom.

Fluoroiodoarabinosyl cytosine (FIAC) and fluoroiodoarabinosyl uracil (FIAU), its principal metabolite, are both potent selective inhibitors of herpesviruses. Like acyclovir and BV-araU, their activity depends on phosphorylation by herpesvirus TK. The parent compound is converted rapidly to the triphosphate in infected cells, selectively utilized by virus DNA polymerase, and incorporated into viral DNA, resulting in the formation of very short DNA chains. FIAU was proven to cause hepatic failure in patients with chronic hepatitis B infection.

HPMPC is a potent, broad-spectrum antiviral agent that is one of a new class of nucleotide analogues structurally characterized as phosphonylmethyl ethers of acyclic nucleoside derivatives. HPMPC has *in vitro* activity against HSV-1, HSV-2, CMV, VZV, EBV, adenovirus, and a retrovirus. The mechanism of action of HPMPC is thought to be similar to that of acyclovir, i.e., the triphosphate analogue inhibiting viral DNA polymerase. The difference, however, is that HPMPC is a monophosphate equivalent and does not require phosphorylation by a virus-specific TK, allowing HPMPC to have an expanded spectrum of activity. Of all of these compounds, HPMPC is emerging with the most clinical potential.

INTERFERONS

HISTORY AND INTRODUCTION. Interferons (IFN) are glycoprotein cytokines (intracellular messengers) with a complex array of immunomodulating, antineoplastic, and antiviral properties. The name *interferon* was derived from landmark experiments by Isaacs and Lindemann in 1957 demonstrating the existence of a biologic substance that "interfered" with viral replication in infected cells. Interferons are currently classified as α, β, or γ, with natural sources of these classes, in general, being leukocytes, fibroblasts, and lymphocytes, respectively. Each type of IFN can now be produced via recombinant DNA technology. The complexity of the response to IFN, including the variability of dose response, duration of therapy, and combination with other treatments, creates enormous challenges to determine appropriate clinical scenarios in which IFN might be a worthwhile therapeutic agent.

MECHANISM OF ACTION. Binding of IFN to the intact cell membrane is the first step in establishing an antiviral effect. Interferon binds to specific cell surface receptors; IFN-γ appears to have a different receptor from either IFN-α or β, which may explain the purported synergistic antiviral and antitumor effects sometimes observed when IFN-γ is given with either of the other two IFN species.

A prevalent view of IFN action is that following binding, there is synthesis of new cellular RNA's and proteins which mediate the antiviral effect. The antiviral state is not fully expressed until these primed cells are infected with virus. In addition to their antiviral effect, IFN's have a number of other biologic activities, including inhibition of cell proliferation and enhancement of the cytotoxic activities of lymphocytes, the expression of cell surface antigens, and the phagocytic and tumoricidal activities of macrophages. These properties may play an important role in the *in vivo* antiviral and antitumor effects of the IFN's.

LICENSED USES. Although promising for a number of viral infections and HIV-associated conditions, the only licensed use of IFN as an antiviral is its intralesional administration in the treatment of condyloma acuminatum, or genital warts, which are caused by human papillomaviruses, and therapy of chronic hepatitis B and C. Only IFN-α is licensed.

TOXICITY AND CLINICAL PROBLEMS. Side effects are frequent with IFN administration and are usually dose-limiting. Influenza-like symptoms, i.e., fever, chills, headache, and malaise, commonly occur, but these symptoms usually become less severe with repeated treatments. At doses used in the treatment of condyloma acuminatum, these side effects rarely cause termination of treatment and may be reduced in severity by pretreatment with acetaminophen. For local treatment (intralesional injection), pain at the injection site does not differ significantly from that in placebo-treated patients and is short-lived. Leukopenia is the most common hematologic abnormality, occurring in up to 26% of patients treated for condyloma. Leukopenia is usually modest, not clinically relevant, and reversible when therapy is discontinued. Increased alanine

aminotransferase levels also may occur, as well as nausea, vomiting, and diarrhea.

At higher doses of IFN, neurotoxicity is encountered, as manifested by personality changes, confusion, loss of attention, disorientation, and paranoid ideation. Early studies with IFN-γ show similar side effects as treatment with IFN-α and -β but with the additional side effects of dose-limiting hypotension and a marked increase in triglyceride levels.

CLINICAL TRIALS. IFN has potential use against virtually all viral infections. Its ultimate utility depends on a number of factors, including the acceptability of side effects, cost, and the availability of other antivirals. Of the many viral infections in which IFN has been tested, treatment of condyloma acuminatum, chronic hepatitis B, chronic hepatitis C, and recurrent respiratory papillomatosis and prophylaxis of rhinovirus and coronavirus upper respiratory infection have been promising.

Condyloma Acuminatum. Several large controlled trials have demonstrated the clinical benefit of IFN-α therapy of condyloma acuminatum. These studies have demonstrated clearance rates of treated lesions from 36 to 62%. Up to one-third of lesions treated with IFN recur. Much research remains to be done to examine the effects of different routes of administration, prolonged therapy, repeated courses of treatment, and combined treatment with other therapeutic modalities (i.e., cryotherapy podophyllin, and laser ablation).

Respiratory Papillomatosis. Recurrent respiratory papillomatosis is a disease in which squamous papillomata relentlessly recur within the larynx and trachea of both children and young adults. Standard management consists of careful microendoscopic excision, usually with a CO_2 laser. In recent years, there have been numerous case reports and uncontrolled studies supporting benefit from IFN as an adjunct to surgery. Results of placebo-controlled trials have suggested benefit.

Hepatitis. The inhibitory effect of human leukocyte IFN-α on hepatitis B virus (HBV) replication was first reported more than 10 years ago. Treatment with IFN-α in chronic hepatitis B subsequently has been investigated in several large, randomized, controlled trials. The earlier studies were encouraging, but the response rate was low at approximately 30%.

In an attempt to enhance the efficacy of antiviral therapy, combinations of IFN with other agents also have been studied. Vidarabine and acyclovir have been used in such studies with little success. It has been observed, however, that a short course of corticosteroids before treatment with IFN-α results in "immunologic rebound" after prednisone withdrawal. This phenomenon, which seems to be directed at virus-infected hepatocytes, is characterized by an acute hepatitis-like elevation of serum aminotransferases and a transient decline in levels of HBV DNA polymerase and HBV DNA. A large multicenter trial comparing patients randomly assigned to receive one of two doses of IFN-α versus prednisone followed by IFN-α or no treatment recently showed that a 4-month treatment regimen of subcutaneous IFN-α in a dose of 5 million units daily resulted in a complete response (loss of serum HBeAg and HBV DNA) in nearly 40% of patients and that reactivation of infection within 6 months after treatment was no greater than 2%. The beneficial effect of pretreatment with a tapering dose of prednisone was limited to patients with low baseline levels of alanine aminotransferase (<100 units per liter). The best predictor of response in this study was the HBV DNA level before treatment, with approximately half of the patients having levels <100 pg per milliliter experiencing a complete response. Long-term follow-up studies are required to determine the duration of antiviral effect and the impact on survival.

The efficacy IFN for treating chronic hepatitis C (non-A, non-B hepatitis) has been established. The first large, randomized, placebo-controlled study of IFN-α therapy in patients with chronic hepatitis C showed that the serum alanine aminotransferase levels declined to normal in 38% of patients treated with 3 million units of IFN-α for 6 months, compared with 4% of untreated patients. However, only 52% of the patients who initially responded to treatment remained in remission during 6 months of follow-up.

Respiratory Infections. The upper respiratory infection known as the "common cold" has a multitude of possible viral causes (see Ch. 328). It has been demonstrated that nasal spray or drops of IFN-α provide prophylaxis against the common cold caused by rhi-

TABLE 327-3. INDICATIONS FOR THE USE OF AVAILABLE ANTIVIRAL AGENTS

Indication	Antiviral Agent	Route	Dose	Comments
Respiratory syncytial virus infection (infants)	Ribavirin	Aerosol	Diluted in sterile water to a concentration of 20 mg/ml, then delivered via aerosol for 12–18 hrs/day for 3–7 days	Only for infants at high risk
Life- or sight-threatening CMV infections in immunocompromised hosts	Ganciclovir	IV	5.0 mg/kg q12h × 14 days	Maintenance therapy of 5.0 mg/kg/day recommended for AIDS patients. Leukopenia is a frequent complication; in bone marrow transplant patients with CMV pneumonia, CMV immune globulin may be a useful adjunct
	Foscarnet	IV		
Condyloma acuminatum	Interferon-α	Intralesional	1.0 million units injected into the base of each lesion, up to 3 times per week for 3 weeks	Flu-type symptoms may occur with administrations
Influenza A infection	Amantadine	Oral	Adults: 100–200 mg/day for 5–7 days Children $\leq$ 9 years: 4.4–8.8 mg/kg/day for 5–7 days not to exceed 150 mg/day	Normal person >65 years should receive 100 mg/day
Prophylaxis against influenza A virus infection	Amantadine	Oral	Adults: 100–200 mg/day Children $\leq$ 9 years: 4.4–8.8 mg/kg/day (not to exceed 150 mg/day)	Continued for the duration of the epidemic or for 2 weeks in conjunction with influenza vaccination (until vaccine-induced immunity develops); normal persons >65 years should receive 100 mg/day
	Rimantadine	Oral		
Herpes simplex virus (HSV) encephalitis	Acyclovir	IV	10 mg/kg (1 hour infusion) every 8 hours for 10–14 days	Morbidity and mortality are significantly lower in patients treated with acyclovir than with vidarabine
Neonatal herpes	Acyclovir	IV	10 mg/kg (1 hour infusion) every 8 hours for 10 days	Efficacy of vidarabine is established; vidarabine and acyclovir show equal efficacy
Mucocutaneous HSV in immunocompromised hosts	Acyclovir or	IV	250 mg/M^2 or 6.2 mg/kg (1 hour infusion) every 8 hours for 7 days	Choice of topical, oral, or intravenous preparation depends upon clinical severity and setting; topical acyclovir is appropriate only when it can be applied to all lesions; it does not affect untreated lesions or systemic symptoms
	Acyclovir or	Oral	400 mg 5 times/day for 10 days	
	Acyclovir	Topical	5% ointment; 4–6 applications/day for 7 days or until healed	Least desirable
Prophylaxis against mucocutaneous HSV during intense immunosuppression	Acyclovir or	Oral	200 mg 3–4 times/day	Oral therapy most convenient; lesions recur when therapy stops
	Acyclovir	IV	250 mg/M^2 every 8 hours or 5 mg/kg every 12 hours (1 hour infusion)	Lesions recur when therapy stops
Treatment of initial genital HSV infections	Acyclovir or	Oral	200 mg 5 times/day for 10 days	Drug of choice in most clinical settings; treatment has no effect on subsequent recurrence rates
	Acyclovir	IV	5 mg/kg (1 hour infusion) every 8 hours for 5–7 days	For patients requiring hospitalization or with neurologic or other visceral complications
Recurrent genital herpes	Acyclovir	Oral	200 mg 5 times/day for 5 days	No effect on subsequent recurrence rates; efficacy greater if used early in attack
Prophylaxis against frequently recurring genital herpes	Acyclovir	Oral	200 mg 3–5 times/day	Occasional "breaking through" attacks and/or asymptomatic virus shedding during treatment; re-evaluation every 6 months recommended
Treatment of HSV keratitis	Trifluorothymidine or	Topical	One drop of 0.1% ophthalmic solution every 2 hours while awake (up to 9 drops/day)	3% acyclovir ointment (ophthalmic) is equal or superior to idoxuridine, vidarabine, and trifluridine for treatment of HSV keratitis but is not available in the United States
	Vidarabine or	Topical	One-half-inch ribbon of 3% ophthalmic ointment 5 times/day	
	Idoxuridine	Topical	One-half-inch ribbon of 0.5% ophthalmic ointment 5 times/day	
Localized herpes zoster in immunocompetent hosts	Acyclovir	Oral	800 mg 5 times/day for 7–10 days	Shortens time to lesion healing, but not shown to decrease the incidence of postherpetic neuralgia
Chickenpox in immunocompromised hosts	Acyclovir or	IV	500 mg/M^2 (1 hour infusion) every 8 hours for 7 days	In the absence of comparative data, acyclovir is preferred because of its ease of administration and lower toxicity
	Vidarabine	IV	10 mg/kg/day (continuous infusion over 12 hours) for 5 days	
Treatment of severe localized or disseminated herpes zoster in immunocompromised hosts	Acyclovir or	IV	500 mg/M^2 or 12.4 mg/kg (1 hour infusion) every 8 hours for 5–7 days	Comparative trials in severe localized and disseminated herpes zoster are underway; pending results, acyclovir is preferred because of its ease of administration and lower toxicity
	Vidarabine	IV	10 mg/dg/day (continuous infusion over 12 hours) for 5–7 days	
Chronic hepatitis B	Interferon-α	SQ	10 × 10^6 units tiw for 16 weeks or 5 × 10^6 units daily for 16 weeks	Patients must have compensated liver disease
Chronic hepatitis C	Interferon-α	SQ	3 × 10^6 units tiw for 24 weeks	Must have compensated liver disease

novirus or coronavirus infection. Although clinical benefit was demonstrated in these studies, administration of IFN-α for 2 to 3 weeks led to hemorrhage of nasal mucosa.

IMMUNOGLOBULIN THERAPY

Efficacy has been established for prophylactic immunoglobulin administration for several viral infections, but the use of immunoglobulin alone for therapy of established disease has not been proven unequivocally beneficial for any viral infection. Benefit has been shown for the administration of intravenous immunoglobulin or CMV hyperimmune globulin when combined with ganciclovir in the treatment of CMV pneumonia in bone marrow transplant recipients. Survival was increased to 52 to 79%, which is significantly better than that of historical controls treated with either agent alone.

Currently active areas of research include the efficacy of CMV hyperimmune globulin for prevention and treatment of disease in bone marrow, kidney, and heart transplant patients, and that of CMV monoclonal antibody in the treatment of established CMV disease in AIDS patients.

Although relatively few antiviral drugs are licensed for use at this time, there is significant interest in the development of antiviral compounds. Table 327–3 summarizes the use of currently available antivirals for indications other than therapy of HIV infections. Systematic approaches have revealed a number of promising new drugs and biologic agents in various stages of evaluation. A better understanding of the molecular biology of virus replication and pathogenesis should elucidate agents with enhanced virus-specific activity.

Buhles WC, Mastre BJ, Tinker AJ, et al.: Ganciclovir treatment of life- or sight-threatening cytomegalovirus infection: Experience in 314 immunocompromised patients. Rev Infect Dis 10:495, 1988. *Describes the clinical efficacy of ganciclovir when used to treat infections of the retina, gastrointestinal tract, and lungs.*

Couch R: Respiratory diseases. *In* Galasso G, Whitley R, Merigan T (eds.): Antiviral Agents and Viral Diseases of Man, 3rd ed. New York, Raven Press, 1990, pp 327–372. *This chapter contains a summary of the published work regarding the efficacy and toxicity of amantadine, rimantadine, and ribavirin for influenza and respiratory syncytial virus infections.*

Davis GL, Balart LA, Schiff ER, et al.: Treatment of chronic hepatitis C with recombinant interferon alfa. N Engl J Med 321:1501, 1989. *The first large, randomized, placebo-controlled trial of interferon therapy of chronic hepatitis C.*

Dorsky DI, Crumpacker CS: Drugs five years later: Acyclovir. Ann Intern Med 107:859, 1987. *A detailed analysis of the chemistry, antiviral activity, and clinical efficacy of acyclovir.*

Hayden FG, Belshe RB, Clover RD, et al.: Emergence and apparent transmission of rimantadine-resistant influenza A virus in families. N Engl J Med 321:1696, 1989. *Postexposure prophylaxis with rimantadine in families was not as effective as pre-exposure prophylaxis during community outbreaks.*

Hirsch MS, Kaplan JC: Antiviral Agents. *In* Fields BN, Knipe DM (eds.): Virology, 2nd ed. New York, Raven Press, 1990, pp 441–468. *A comprehensive text which includes a detailed analysis of antiviral therapy.*

Perillo RP, Schiff ER, Davis GL, et al.: A randomized, controlled trial of interferon alfa-2b alone and after prednisone withdrawal for the treatment of chronic hepatitis B. N Engl J Med 323:295, 1990. *A multicenter study of combination therapy for chronic hepatitis B.*

Reichman RC, Oakes D, Bonnez W, et al.: Treatment of condyloma acuminatum with three different interferons administered intralesionally. Ann Intern Med 108:675, 1988. *Intralesional injections of three different interferon preparations were found to be efficacious in the treatment of condyloma acuminatum.*

Reines ED, Gross PA: Antiviral agents. Med Clin North Am 72:691, 1988. *An excellent review of the principles and applications of antiviral chemotherapy.*

Viral Infections of the Respiratory Tract

328 THE COMMON COLD
J. Owen Hendley

DEFINITION. The common cold, also known as upper respiratory infection (URI) or acute coryza, is an acute, self-limited illness caused by a virus. Nasal symptoms including rhinorrhea and nasal obstruction are invariably present; sore/scratchy throat and/or cough may be present. Many myths surround the source of the virus causing colds. There are no normal viral flora of the respiratory tract in humans (two possible exceptions are human herpesvirus type 6 in saliva and adenovirus, which can be recovered from adenoid tissue of otherwise healthy children by co-cultivation with susceptible cells). In sharp contrast, luxuriant normal bacterial flora occur in the upper respiratory tract and mouth. Because viruses are not part of normal flora, the viruses that cause colds are not present in the host ready to be activated because "resistance" has been lowered by chilling, loss of sleep, or bad diet. Instead, the virus must be *passed* from another human in order to produce the cold.

ETIOLOGY. Colds are common because the viruses with few serotypes reinfect many times, and the viruses that infect an individual only once have multiple serotypes (Table 328–1). Rhinoviruses (*rhino* = "nose") cause 30 to 50% of colds in adults, and coronaviruses (*corona* = "crown") are responsible for 10 to 15%. Each of the other virus groups listed in Table 328–1 cause <5% of colds. Adults are susceptible to respiratory syncytial virus (RSV) and parainfluenza virus, but the illness in adults is usually a cold rather than the more severe involvement seen in infants. Some of the viruses that cause colds are characteristically associated with other syndromes. Influenza viruses cause febrile respiratory disease with lower tract involvement, adenoviruses cause pharyngoconjunctival fever or acute undifferentiated febrile illness, ECHO and other enteroviruses are an important cause of aseptic meningitis, and coxsackie A viruses cause herpangina.

EPIDEMIOLOGY AND TRANSMISSION. Colds are the most frequent disease of humans and the single most common cause of absenteeism from school and work. Frequency of colds varies with age. Even before widespread day care attendance, colds were particularly common in children younger than age 6. In the Cleveland family study in the 1950's, infants under age 1 had an average of 6.7 colds per year, 1- to 5-year-olds had 7.4 to 8.3 colds per year, and teenagers averaged about 4.5 colds per year. Mothers reported 4.5 colds and fathers 3.5 colds per year. The wider exposure to other preschoolers in day care has increased the frequency of colds in children under 6 even more. The number of colds in adults may

TABLE 328–1. IMMUNITY TO COMMON COLD VIRUSES

a. *Solid immunity not produced by infection (repeated infection with same serotype usual)*

Virus	No. of serotypes
Respiratory syncytial virus	1
Parainfluenza virus	4
Coronavirus	4

b. *Immunity produced by infection (reinfection with same serotype uncommon)*

Virus	No. of serotypes
Rhinovirus	>100
Adenovirus	≥33
Influenza	3 (type A subtypes change)
Echovirus	31
Coxsackie virus	
Group A	23
Group B	6

From Hendley JO: Immunology of viral colds. *In* Veldman JE, McCabe BF, Huizing EH, Mygind N (eds.): Immunobiology, Autoimmunity, Transplantation in Otorhinolaryngology. Amsterdam, Kugler Publications, 1985, pp 257–260.

increase for several years because of exposure to young children, which highlights the fact that children commonly introduce new viruses to their families. At least with rhinovirus, the home setting is the primary site for viral transmission. Co-workers in an insurance company office with simultaneous rhinovirus colds usually were infected with different serotypes of virus, but each worker's serotype was found in his/her family contacts.

In temperate climates, colds are epidemic in the winter months (Fig. 328–1). The epidemic starts with a sharp rise in frequency in September after children have returned to school; the incidence then remains at an almost constant level until spring. This epidemic curve is produced by successive waves of different viruses moving through the community. Although rhinovirus infections occur year-round, the epidemic is initiated by a sharp rise of rhinovirus infections in early fall. Parainfluenza viruses move through in October and November, followed by RSV and coronaviruses in winter months. Influenza viruses appear later in winter, then rhinovirus has a resurgence in spring. Summer colds are usually caused by rhinovirus or one of the enteroviruses. The wave of each virus moving through is not sharp, and many times two or three viruses may be overlapping. Adenovirus and parainfluenza virus type 3 contribute to the burden of illness throughout the epidemic.

Determinants of this yearly epidemic of colds are not established but certainly include human behavior, with more virus transmitted

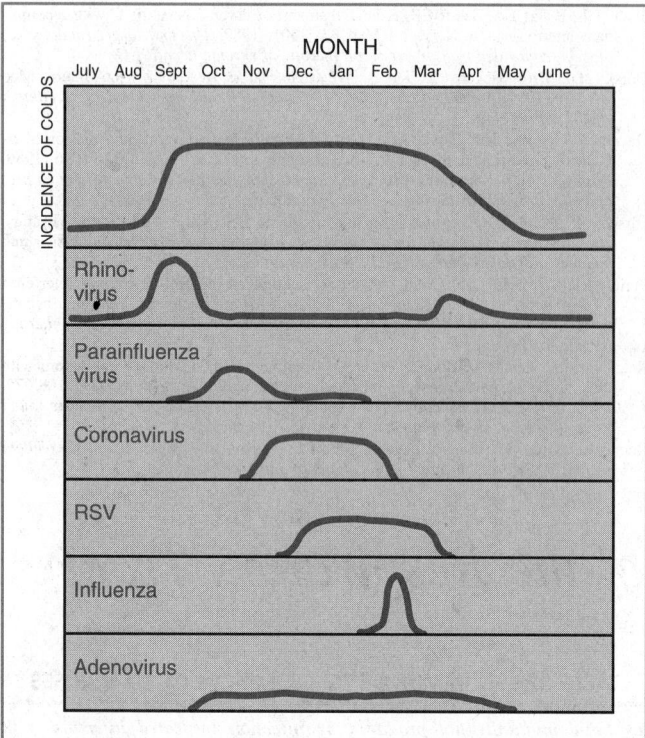

FIGURE 328–1. Schematic diagram of the incidence of colds and frequency of the causative viruses.

by higher indoor contact in colder months. Another determinant might be attributes of the viruses. Enveloped viruses, including RSV, parainfluenza virus, influenza virus, and coronavirus, may survive outside the host for longer periods in winter when the relative humidity of indoor (but not outdoor) air is very low.

Transmission of viruses causing colds could occur by one or more of three mechanisms: (1) small-particle (<5 μ in diameter) aerosol in which virus may be suspended in air for an hour and infect by inhalation, (2) large-particle (>10 μ in diameter) airborne droplets that travel <1 m and infect by landing on a mucosal surface such as conjunctiva or nasal mucosa, and (3) direct transfer of virus in secretions via hand contact from a person with a cold to a well person, who inoculates the virus onto his/her own conjunctival or nasal mucosa. Oral inoculation of rhinovirus or RSV does not result in infection, presumably because the stratified squamous epithelium of the mouth and oropharynx is not susceptible. The transmission route under natural conditions in the home has not been definitely established for any of the viruses. However, the importance of spread of colds in the home favors direct contact and/or large-droplet spread as being most likely. Influenza virus clearly can be transmitted by small-particle aerosol in some circumstances.

PATHOGENESIS. It had been assumed until recently that the symptoms of colds were produced by a viral cytopathic effect destroying the nasal mucosa. However, a recent study found that the histologic appearance of the nasal mucosa in biopsies taken during natural colds could not be distinguished from biopsies taken 2 weeks after illness except for an increased number of polymorphonuclear leukocytes (PMN's) during illness. The unexpected infiltration of PMN's in the nose in uncomplicated colds was confirmed in another study; the number of PMN's in nasal secretions increased coincidently when symptoms appeared in experimentally induced rhinovirus colds. Rhinovirus and coronavirus, in contrast to influenza virus and adenovirus, were not found to be destructive of nasal epithelium in organ cultures *in vitro.* Since mucosal damage by the virus during colds does not adequately explain the symptoms, the hypothesis that the viral infection of the nose triggers a cascade of inflammatory mediators that results in the symptoms is being explored. Support for this hypothesis was provided in volunteers with experimentally induced rhinovirus colds. Kinins (primarily bradykinin) and PMN's appeared in nasal secretions of infected volunteers at the time that they became ill, and their presence paralleled cold symptoms. Kinins sprayed into the noses of uninfected volunteers can reproduce many of the symptoms of a cold. Additional work on this hypothesis, with a focus on cytokines, is needed. How viral infection of the nose initiates the events leading to an influx of kinins, PMN's, and (possibly) cytokines into the nose and whether the sequence can be interrupted are of current research interest. However, the concept that it might be possible to ablate cold symptoms by blocking the mediators of the host response without having to kill the virus is exciting.

CLINICAL MANIFESTATIONS. The clinical manifestations of colds, which are familiar to all, are predominately subjective. In adults, rhinorrhea, nasal obstruction, and scratchy/sore throat are usually noted. The rhinorrhea is usually clear early in illness and may become white or yellow-green. Some malaise and nonproductive cough are common; sneezing is noted in some colds. Other common symptoms include sinus fullness and a "nasal" quality to the voice. Hoarseness is sometimes present. Objective findings in an adult with a cold are usually minimal. The nasal mucosa may be red but not to a degree that differs from normal. Mild erythema of the pharynx and redness around the external nares from nose blowing may be noted. Fever ($>38°C$) is uncommon in a cold in an adult; the presence of fever would suggest influenza or a bacterial complication of the cold. The symptoms of the cold usually abate in 5 to 7 days.

Colds in infants and children may be associated with more objective signs than in adults. In addition to rhinorrhea and nasal obstruction, moderate enlargement of the anterior cervical lymph nodes is frequent. Fever during the first 2 to 3 days of a cold in young children is not unusual, even when the child's parent or older sibling does not have an elevated temperature during the cold due to the same virus. In contrast to adults, the usual duration of cold symptoms in children is 10 to 14 days.

DIAGNOSIS. Self-diagnosis of a cold by the patient is usually accurate. Laboratory tests including white blood cell count and differential are not helpful. Sloughed ciliated cells may be present, and PMN's would be expected in nasal secretions during viral colds. The differential diagnosis of a cold includes an intranasal foreign body in a child and allergic or vasomotor rhinitis in adults and children. Examination of the nose should exclude a foreign body; the chronicity of symptoms with allergic or vasomotor rhinitis should differentiate these conditions from an acute cold.

Etiologic (virologic) diagnosis of a cold can be attempted by inoculation of a sample of nasal secretions into tissue cell cultures, but this is rarely needed or useful. Rhinoviruses can be grown in human embryonic lung fibroblast cultures; detection of rhinovirus using the polymerase chain reaction may soon be available. Coronaviruses cannot be detected accurately in cell cultures. Most coronavirus infections have been diagnosed by serologic titer rise in acute/convalescent paired sera. RSV in nasal secretions can be reliably detected by commercially available rapid tests. Influenza and parainfluenza viruses are usually grown in primary rhesus monkey kidney cell culture, and adenoviruses will grow in human embryonic kidney cells.

TREATMENT. Given the self-limited nature of colds, any treatment should be completely safe. Antibiotics have no place in therapy of uncomplicated colds, since they neither hasten nor delay recovery from the cold, nor do they reduce the frequency of bacterial complications.

Since the subjective symptoms of a cold disappear in 7 days without intervention, a variety of actually ineffective treatments have been reported to be effective due to inadequate blinding of placebo recipients. One example of this phenomenon was a study of large doses of vitamin C to prevent colds, in which many placebo recipients dropped out of the study because they could tell by tasting the medication that they were not receiving the vitamin C. Another example was the use of zinc gluconate lozenges as an antiviral treatment for colds. In the blinded trial, the only appropriate placebo that could be found to match the noxious taste of the zinc was denatonium benzoate, which is so bitter that it has been painted on the thumbs of children to discourage them from thumb-sucking.

No antivirals are currently available for treating colds. Individual symptoms may be treated. Malaise may be relieved by analgesics (e.g., aspirin, acetaminophen, ibuprofen). Nasal congestion may be relieved by decongestants by mouth (pseudoephedrine 60 mg, three times a day) or by topical application (oxymetazoline 0.05%, two sprays to each nostril twice daily). The benefit of oral antihistamines in colds remains controversial.

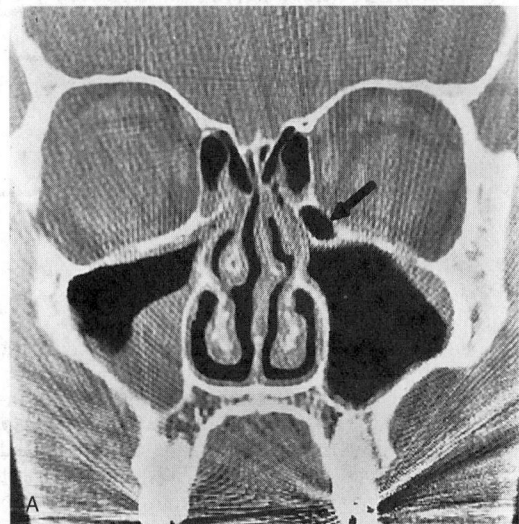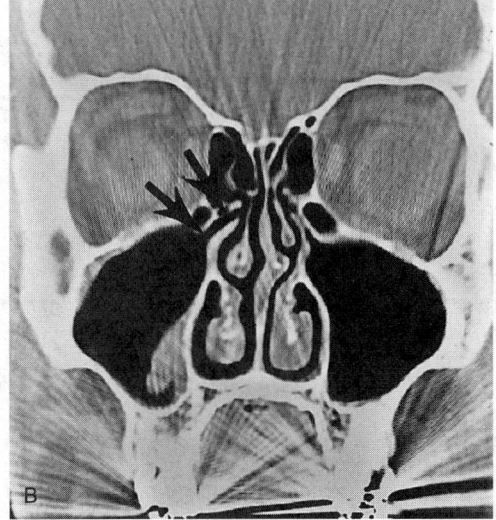

FIGURE 328–2. Sinus CT scan of adult during symptomatic cold *(left panel)* and 2 weeks later *(right panel).* Arrow in the left panel denotes an infraorbital air cell (Haller cell). Bilateral abnormalities were observed in the ethmoid and maxillary sinuses during the cold, with an air-fluid interface in the right maxillary sinus. Two weeks later, all abnormalities had cleared except for a residual density in the right maxillary sinus. The infundibulum *(two arrows)* draining the maxillary antrum was now open. (Courtesy of Dr. Jack M. Gwaltney, Jr., Department of Internal Medicine, University of Virginia School of Medicine, Charlottesville, Virginia).

COMPLICATIONS. Secondary bacterial infection may complicate viral colds. The most common is bacterial suppurative otitis media, which occurs in some 5% of colds in preschool-aged children. Otitis media may be heralded by a secondary fever with associated ear pain. Bacterial sinusitis is estimated to occur in 0.5% of colds, primarily in adults. Sinusitis would be suggested by the presence of fever and/or facial pain (see Ch. 64). Bacterial pneumonia is thought to complicate colds, but it is very uncommon.

Clinical differentiation between primary viral and secondary bacterial infection of the respiratory tract is a challenge, since respiratory viruses may involve the middle ear or paranasal sinuses in the absence of bacterial infection. Tympanocentesis or maxillary sinus puncture provides definitive information on viral versus bacterial infection, but these are too invasive for routine use. Coronal computed tomographic (CT) scan is an accurate noninvasive method for imaging the paranasal sinuses. Recent work using CT scans has demonstrated that abnormalities in the sinuses may occur in colds not complicated by secondary bacterial infection. Coronal CT scans in 27 (87%) of 31 young adults during uncomplicated colds had abnormalities in one or more sinuses (Fig. 328–2). In 11 (79%) of the 14 subjects who had repeat scans 2 weeks later, the abnormalities had cleared or were markedly improved without antibiotic therapy.

An important complication of viral colds occurs in adults and children with underlying reactive airways disease or asthma. Wheezing occurs in 30 to 50% of episodes of viral colds in prospective studies of patients with asthma. Colds in these patients produce a large burden of illness, since up to 50% of asthma exacerbations in children and up to 20% of exacerbations in adults have been associated with an identified virus.

PREVENTION. Vaccine(s) to prevent common colds are unlikely to be useful given the multiplicity of immunotypes of some of the viruses and the lack of solid immunity to reinfection with the other viruses (see Table 328–1). Prophylaxis with topical interferon applied intranasally for 5 days after one family member appears with a cold has been shown to be moderately effective in preventing other family members from acquiring a cold, particularly colds due to rhinovirus. The practicality of this preventive approach may be argued, particularly in view of the fact that prolonged use of intranasal interferon is complicated by alteration or damage of the nasal mucosa.

Probably the only practical, albeit imperfect, means of preventing colds available is to prevent virus from reaching the nasal or conjunctival mucosa by way of one's own hands. If transmission occurs by inhalation of airborne small particles or by adherence of large droplets to a mucosal surface, infection is inevitable for those

who enjoy contact with other humans. However, if transmission occurs by self-inoculation with virus on contaminated fingertips, the simple measure of ridding the fingers of viable virus before touching one's eye or nose might be helpful. The virus can be removed physically by rinsing the hands. Applying a virucide to the hands might be another approach.

Gwaltney JM Jr, Phillips CD, Miller RD, et al.: Computed tomographic study of the common cold. N Engl J Med 330:25, 1994. *Sinus CT scans during naturally acquired common colds demonstrated that one or more of the sinuses was abnormal in more than 80% of subjects. Most abnormalities had cleared on repeat scan after the cold was over.*

Hendley JO, Gwaltney JM Jr: Mechanism of transmission of rhinovirus infections. Epidemiol Rev 10:242, 1988. *Review of the various modes of transmission of rhinovirus common colds.*

Naclerio RM, Proud D, Lichtenstein LM, et al.: Kinins are generated during experimental rhinovirus colds. J Infect Dis 157:133, 1988. *Kinins, albumin, and PMN's appeared in nasal secretions of infected volunteers around the time they became ill but did not appear in secretions of subjects infected but not ill. Histamine in secretions did not correlate with illness.*

Pattemore PK, Johnston SL, Bardin PG: Viruses as precipitants of asthma symptoms: I. Epidemiology. Clin Exp Allergy 22:325, 1992. *Review of evidence incriminating viral respiratory infections as common precipitants of wheezing. Rhinovirus and RSV were most commonly associated with episodes of wheezing, but all respiratory viruses have been found.*

Winther B, Gwaltney JM, Hendley JO: Respiratory virus infection of monolayer cultures of human nasal epithelial cells. Am Rev Respir Dis 141:839, 1990. *Growth of rhinovirus and coronavirus in nasal epithelial cells produced no visible destruction of the epithelial layer, whereas influenza and adenovirus produced obvious disruption.*

329 VIRAL PHARYNGITIS, LARYNGITIS, CROUP, AND BRONCHITIS

Maurice A. Mufson

DEFINITION. Viral infections that localize to the upper and middle respiratory passages produce an acute inflammatory response and, depending on the anatomic site involved, evoke the clinical manifestations of pharyngitis, laryngitis, croup (laryngotracheobronchitis), and bronchitis. These infections do not ordinarily involve the pulmonary alveoli. Pharyngitis, laryngitis, and bronchi-

TABLE 329-1. VIRUSES THAT CAUSE PHARYNGITIS, LARYNGITIS, CROUP, AND BRONCHITIS

Virus	Serotype
Influenza	Types A, B
Parainfluenza	Types 1, 2, 3
Respiratory syncytial	Subgroups A, B1, B2
Adenovirus	Types 1, 2, 3, 4, 5, 6, 7 (also others)
Coronavirus	Types 229E, OC43 (also others)
Rhinovirus	Most or all of more than 100 serotypes
Enterovirus	At least some of more than 75 serotypes
Herpes simplex	Type 1

tis can occur in persons of any age. Croup occurs exclusively in children and mainly during the second year of life. Usually these illnesses begin abruptly with predominant upper respiratory tract signs and symptoms and limited systemic findings. The uncomplicated illness abates after 5 to 10 days.

ETIOLOGY. The major viral pathogens of the respiratory tract that can cause pharyngitis, laryngitis, croup, and bronchitis include members of the myxoviruses (influenza, parainfluenza, and respiratory syncytial viruses), adenoviruses, coronaviruses, picornaviruses (rhinoviruses and enteroviruses), and herpesviruses (Table 329–1). However, they differ in their propensity to cause these illnesses (Table 329–2). An etiologic diagnosis requires either isolation of virus or detection of viral antigen or demonstration of a rise in antibody during convalescence.

Pharyngitis also can occur as part of systemic viral illnesses associated with *Epstein-Barr virus* (see Ch. 341) or *cytomegalovirus* (see Ch. 340) infection, and laryngitis and bronchitis occur in *measles* virus infection (see Ch. 334). When coryza represents the main feature of an upper respiratory infection, the term "common cold" (see Ch. 328) prevails. When the infecting virus is an influenza virus, the designation *influenza* describes an acute respiratory tract infection with fever and prostration (see Ch. 332).

INCIDENCE AND PREVALENCE. Most children and adults experience three to five viral infections of the upper respiratory tract each year. In infants and children, croup is a serious illness that peaks in the second year of life, as high as 47 cases per 1000 children per year, and by age 4 to 5 it declines to under 15 cases per 1000 children per year.

EPIDEMIOLOGY. Viral pharyngitis, laryngitis, croup, and bronchitis occur during all months of the year, with peaks of occurrence paralleling epidemics of individual viruses. Respiratory syncytial virus, influenza A and B viruses, and parainfluenza virus type 1 occur in epidemics, mainly in the late fall, winter, and spring (see

TABLE 329-2. RELATIVE IMPORTANCE OF VIRUSES CAUSING PHARYNGITIS, LARYNGITIS, CROUP, AND BRONCHITIS

Virus	Occurrence in Indicated Illness*			
	Pharyngitis	*Laryngitis*	*Croup*	*Bronchitis*
Influenza A	+ + + +	+ + + +	+	+ + + +
B	+ +	+ +		+ +
Parainfluenza 1	+ +	+ +	+ + + +	+ +
2	+	+	+ + +	+
3	+ +	+ +	+ + + +	+ +
Respiratory syncytial	+		+	+ + +
Adenovirus	+ + + +	+ +		+ +
Coronavirus	+	+		+ + +
Rhinovirus	+ + + +	+		+
Enterovirus	+			
Herpes simplex	+ +		±	+

* Graded from minimal (+) to major (+ + + +) importance; blank means unlikely occurrence; and ± means rare occurrence.

TABLE 329-3. EPIDEMIOLOGY OF VIRUSES THAT CAUSE PHARYNGITIS, LARYNGITIS, CROUP, AND BRONCHITIS

Epidemic	Endemic	Sporadic
Parainfluenza 1*	Parainfluenza 3	Parainfluenza 2
Influenza A†	Adenovirus	Herpes simplex
Influenza B	Coronavirus	
Respiratory syncytial‡	Rhinovirus	
	Enterovirus	

* Alternate years, usually.
† Epidemic and pandemic.
‡ Annual epidemics.

Table 329–3). The other viral pathogens occur endemically or sporadically. Virus infections of the respiratory tract spread by direct person-to-person contact, by infectious aerosols, or by fomites.

CLINICAL MANIFESTATIONS. *Viral Pharyngitis.* Acute viral pharyngitis is characterized by a scratchy and sore throat, but pain upon swallowing is not a prominent or constant feature. Dysphagia occurs infrequently in viral pharyngitis. Cough is not a feature of acute viral pharyngitis. Fever and malaise accompany influenza and adenovirus infections, but these findings are infrequent with the other respiratory viral pathogens. Pharyngeal erythema and edema and enlarged and tender lymph nodes may be the only physical findings. Adenovirus pharyngitis may be associated with conjunctivitis. Exudative tonsillitis occurs in adenovirus infections, infectious mononucleosis associated with Epstein-Barr virus infection, herpetic pharyngitis (with or without vesicles or small ulcers), as well as streptococcal pharyngitis. Exudative tonsillitis alone does not distinguish these infections. Bronchospasm occurs as a feature of herpes tracheobronchitis in elderly persons.

Viral Laryngitis. In acute viral laryngitis, hoarseness predominates, associated with difficulty in talking, pain on clearing respiratory secretions, and often fever, depending on the infecting virus. Cough and pharyngitis may be present. The larynx is erythematous and edematous, and the regional lymph nodes are slightly enlarged and tender. Wheezes may be audible upon auscultation.

Viral Croup. The clinical picture of croup characteristically includes inspiratory stridor, hoarseness, and a brassy cough. This distinctive triad of symptoms reflects the acute and intense edema and mucoid exudative secretions of the larynx and associated obstruction of the subglottic portion of the upper airway. These symptoms develop acutely, accompanied by fever, cough, tachypnea, and wheezing. Retractions of the chest wall occur. Hemoptysis does not occur. Rhonchi, rales, or wheezes, alone or in combination, may be audible upon auscultation of the lungs. Radiographic examination of the neck can demonstrate subglottic narrowing, and a chest roentgenogram may show hyperinflation of the lungs. In the uncomplicated case, the findings resolve in several days, but some children develop respiratory failure and pneumonia. Children who previously experienced multiple episodes of croup manifest hyperreactive airways several years later.

Viral Bronchitis. In acute viral bronchitis, cough, with or without sputum production, and fever are the main features. The sputum is slightly mucoid or watery and white. Other common symptoms include hoarseness, nonpleuritic substernal chest pain, and malaise. Rhonchi or rales may be heard upon auscultation of the chest. The chest roentgenogram may show increased intensity of the vascular pattern, but pulmonary infiltrates do not occur. Acute bronchitis associated with influenza or coronavirus infection occurs often as an exacerbation of chronic bronchitis.

TREATMENT AND PROGNOSIS. Viral pharyngitis, laryngitis, and bronchitis are self-limited illnesses and not severe, except for herpes tracheobronchitis infections. The symptoms of these illnesses should be treated with analgesics, fluids, and rest. Persistent cough can be treated with suppressant preparations. Antibiotics are not indicated, except when secondary bacterial infection occurs; it is likely to develop mainly with influenza virus infections. In pharyngitis, pharyngeal pain or dysphagia should be treated with analgesics and fluids.

The less serious cases of croup can be managed by having the child rest in bed at home. Vaporizers that produce a mist of moist air may be beneficial. Children with severe croup require hospitalization, supportive treatment, and constant monitoring for the devel-

TABLE 329–4. ANTIVIRAL DRUG THERAPY OF VIRUSES THAT CAUSE PHARYNGITIS, LARYNGITIS, CROUP, AND BRONCHITIS

Virus	Drug	Dose (Duration)	Route
Influenza A	Amantadine*	200 mg daily (7–10 days)	Oral
	Rimantidine*	200 mg daily‡ (7–10 days)	Oral
Respiratory syncytial	Ribavirin	20 mg/ml solution (12–18 hours)	Aerosol
Herpes simplex†	Acyclovir	8 mg/kg q8hr (7–10 days)	IV

* More commonly used for prophylaxis at same daily dose over longer periods of time until the virus leaves the community.

† Herpes simplex tracheobronchitis treated with IV acyclovir.

‡ In patients with hepatic dysfunction or renal failure and elderly nursing home residents, the dose for treatment and for prophylaxis is 100 mg daily.

opment of respiratory distress. If hypoxemia develops, oxygen therapy is essential; hypoxemia requiring oxygen can develop therapy even before cyanosis becomes evident. Subglottic edema may be reduced by the administration of racemic epinephrine. Administration of corticosteroids in the treatment of croup may have limited benefit. Antiviral drug therapy is available for influenza A, respiratory syncytial, and herpes simplex viruses (Table 329–4). Ribavirin lessens the severity of serious respiratory syncytial virus infection in the infant and child. Herpes tracheobronchitis responds to treatment with acyclovir. Influenza virus vaccine must be administered to persons in the high-risk group (unless contraindicated) to diminish the chance of infection (see Ch. 10).

Avila MM, Carballal G, Rovaletti H, et al.: Viral etiology in acute lower respiratory tract infections in children from a closed community. Am Rev Respir Dis 140:634, 1989. *One fifth of 94 children with bronchitis had virus infections; respiratory syncytial virus and adenoviruses were the most common.*

Houvinen P, Lahtonen R, Ziegler T, et al.: Pharyngitis in adults: The presence of coexistence of viruses and bacterial organisms. Ann Intern Med 110:612, 1989. *About one fourth of 106 adults with pharyngitis had virus infections; respiratory syncytial and influenza A viruses were most common.*

Inglis AF Jr: Herpes simplex virus infection: A rare case of prolonged croup. Arch Otolaryngol Head Neck Surg 49:551, 1993. *Croup due to herpes simplex type 1 in two children with 3- to 4-week illness; one child treated with acyclovir had a prompt response.*

Mufson MA, Åkerlind-Stopner B, Örvell C, et al.: A single season epidemic with respiratory syncytial virus subgroup B2 during 10 epidemic years, 1978 to 1988. J Clin Microbiol 29:162, 1991. *Annual winter-spring epidemics of respiratory syncytial virus. Subgroup A predominated. One third to one half of infections were limited to the upper respiratory tract.*

330 RESPIRATORY SYNCYTIAL VIRUS

Edward E. Walsh

DEFINITION. Respiratory syncytial virus (RSV), first identified in 1957, causes yearly outbreaks of respiratory illness during the fall, winter, and early spring. It is the single most important cause of bronchiolitis and pneumonia in young infants and is a common etiology of upper respiratory symptoms in older children and young adults. In addition, RSV is increasingly recognized as a cause of serious acute respiratory infection in the elderly. The name comes from the giant syncytial cells produced when it is grown in tissue culture.

ETIOLOGY. RSV is an enveloped virus of the family Paramyxoviridae, genus *Pneumovirus*. The single-stranded negative-polarity RNA encodes 10 proteins, of which 8 are found in purified virions. Two surface glycoproteins (G, attachment protein; F, fusion protein) protrude from a lipid bilayer encompassing three nucleocapsid proteins (N, P, polymerase) complexed with the genome. At least two additional proteins (M, 22K) are associated with the viral envelope. Neutralizing antibodies are directed at F and G glycoproteins, while F, N, and 22K are targets for cytotoxic T cells. Two major strains (A and B) are distinguishable, characterized by antigenically divergent G proteins and highly conserved F proteins. The closely related animal RSV strains (bovine, ovine, caprine) cause significant illness in farm animals but no human disease.

EPIDEMIOLOGY. Uniquely among respiratory viruses, worldwide RSV outbreaks occur annually. Epidemics generally begin in late fall, lasting until early spring. In the United States, RSV causes approximately 90,000 hospitalizations and accounts for 60% of bronchiolitis and 25% of pneumonia cases in infants. In the first year of life, over half of all infants become infected, with the remainder infected the following year. Family studies suggest that school children introduce RSV into the home with subsequent spread to parents and younger siblings, with infection rates of 43% and 62%, respectively. The virus readily infects infants and staff of day care centers, with attack rates approaching 100% for children below age 1. Like rhinovirus (see Ch. 328), RSV is transmitted principally by direct contact with large-particle fomites from respiratory secretions, in sharp contrast to the mode of spread of influenza virus, aerosolization. Direct inoculation of virus into the nose or eye by the hand appears to be the principal mode of spread. Since a virus survives for hours on hard surfaces and shorter times on clothing, inanimate objects also may play a role in transmission.

Approximately 0.5% of infected infants require hospitalization, but underlying prematurity, congenital cardiac abnormalities, bronchopulmonary dysplasia, and immunosuppression significantly increase the risk of serious disease. Lower socioeconomic status and being male also adversely influence severity. Hospitalization is most frequent between the ages of 1 to 6 months, with a median age of 2 months. Maternally derived antibody appears to protect in the first month of life when serious lower respiratory symptoms are infrequent, but this benefit is rather brief. Nosocomial spread of RSV on pediatric wards is a significant problem. Up to 32% of infants admitted to pediatric floors during the RSV season become infected while in the hospital. Infection among medical staff reaches 40%, and they probably serve as vectors for transmission to other infants. Careful attention to appropriate infection-control measures can reduce nosocomial transmission. Reinfection occurs frequently throughout life, although illness is less severe and hospitalization infrequent. However, older infants with serious underlying cardiac or pulmonary conditions, such as cystic fibrosis, may require inpatient care. Although primarily considered a pediatric disease, RSV infection in adults over age 65 may be serious and require hospitalization. Nursing home outbreaks are not uncommon. Both RSV strains usually co-circulate during outbreaks, although A strains usually dominate and may be associated with worse disease. Evidence suggests that strain variation alone does not solely account for reinfections. Partial immunity to RSV develops over time, as indicated by the resistance to both infection and illness. Clinical and experimental evidence indicates that neutralizing serum antibody diminishes the severity of illness, while mucosal IgA antibody reduces infection rates. Laboratory correlates of cell-mediated immunity can be identified; however, their role in illness and infection is unclear. The virus spreads from nasal epithelium to the lower respiratory tract, infecting the epithelium of small bronchioles; allergic mediators such as IgE, histamine, and leukotrienes also may contribute to the clinical symptoms.

CLINICAL MANIFESTATIONS. Following an incubation period of 3 days, the majority of previously uninfected infants develop signs and symptoms of upper respiratory infection. Asymptomatic primary RSV infection is considered rare. Conjunctival injection, copious mucopurulent nasal discharge, cough, and low-grade fever (38°C) are typical and indistinguishable from other respiratory infections. Otitis media occurs commonly, and RSV has been isolated from middle ear effusions, generally in association with bacteria. After several days, lower respiratory tract symptoms develop in 25 to 50% of infants. Cough, wheezing, increased respiratory rate, accessory muscle use, nasal flaring, intercostal retractions, and cyanosis are seen as the disease progresses. Expiratory wheezes, rhonchi, and fine rales are the most common findings on lung examination. With lower respiratory symptoms, arterial oxygen desaturation is universal, and hypercarbia and acidosis are ominous findings, suggesting impending respiratory failure. Ventilatory support is required in approximately 8% of hospitalized infants and is disproportionately high among infants with underlying cardiopulmonary disorders. Mortality for otherwise healthy children is about 1% but can reach 37% in infants with cardiac disorders.

Hyperinflation and diffuse interstitial pneumonitis are the most frequent radiographic findings. Infiltrates are usually diffuse, but consolidation is seen in up to one quarter. Although tachypnea is a universal respiratory pattern, sudden and irregular apneic spells can occur, especially in younger infants. RSV-induced apnea has been implicated in some cases of sudden infant death syndrome.

The usual hospital stay is 3 to 5 days, but the most severely ill infants may remain confined for several weeks. Virus is shed from respiratory secretions for 7 to 10 days, although immunocompromised infants (i.e., those with HIV infection) may excrete virus for considerably longer. Interestingly, clinical symptoms may not correlate with prolonged shedding. Co-infection with other viruses, such as influenza, adenovirus, parainfluenza, and enteroviruses, is not uncommon but is usually not clinically discernible. Bacterial superinfection may develop, with *Streptococcus pneumoniae* and *Haemophilus influenzae* being the most frequent organisms isolated. Treatment with antibiotics is indicated when bacterial superinfection develops. Clinical findings in primary RSV infection above age 1 are similar to those in younger infants but, in general, are milder. Long-term sequelae of lower respiratory tract infection include development of childhood asthma, although the precise contributions of RSV infection and allergic predisposition are unknown.

Longitudinal studies indicate that reinfection occurs in up to 75% of previously infected infants between the ages of 1 and 2 years. Reinfections are less severe than primary infection, and upper respiratory symptoms typically dominate, with the exception of infants with recurrent wheezing episodes. Adults are not spared reinfections and typically manifest nasal discharge, pharyngitis, and low-grade fever. Virus is shed for an average of 3 days. The very elderly with RSV infection may develop cough, dyspnea, fever, wheezing, and, in rare cases, respiratory failure. Analogous to the young infant, elderly patients with underlying chronic pulmonary and cardiac disease are most subject to severe disease and may require hospital care.

DIAGNOSIS. In the outpatient setting, a presumptive diagnosis is often suggested by typical symptoms occurring during the epidemic season, especially if RSV is known to be circulating in the community. However, since the clinical picture of RSV is often indistinguishable from illness caused by other infectious agents of respiratory disease, laboratory confirmation of RSV infection is required, especially if antiviral therapy is contemplated. Facilities for virus culture, immunofluorescence (IF) and enzyme immunoassay (EIA), are required for optimal speed and diagnostic accuracy. RSV is readily grown from respiratory secretions on HEp-2, human diploid fibroblast, and HELA cell lines. The sensitivity of viral culture varies with the method of collection and transport and the individual laboratory but is 100% specific when RSV is isolated. RSV is relatively labile, and samples should be kept at 4°C until placed on cell lines, preferably immediately. The characteristic giant cell cytopathic effect develops on average in 4 days but may require 10 days. Rapid diagnostic tests rely on detecting viral antigen in respiratory secretions. IF is the most widely used test and has a sensitivity of about 80%, while commercial EIA is less sensitive and less specific than IF. Serologic diagnosis can be made using a variety of highly sensitive methods but is not useful in immediate diagnosis.

THERAPY AND PREVENTION. Therapy for hospitalized infants includes hydration, oxygen, bronchodilators, and specific antiviral medication. Severely ill infants are commonly dehydrated and require intravenous fluid. Supplemental oxygen, administered as a humidified mist, should be given to all infants with hypoxia. The value of brochodilators for the treatment of wheezing is controversial, since most studies have not demonstrated clear benefit, but a trial of inhaled bronchodilators is probably indicated, especially in older infants. Specific antiviral therapy is currently limited to inhaled ribavirin (1-β-D-ribafuranosyl-1,2,4-triazole-3-carboxamide), a nucleoside analogue with activity against a number of RNA viruses. Ribavirin is administered via aerosol, typically for 4 hours three times a day for 3 to 5 days, although longer therapy has been used. Placebo-controlled clinical trials demonstrate more rapid resolution of respiratory symptoms and hypoxia and are associated with diminished virus shedding. Ribavirin treatment is indicated for infants at high risk of serious disease (congenital heart disease, bronchopulmonary dysplasia, prematurity, and immunodeficiency), those who

are severely ill, and infants who require mechanical ventilation. Although short- or long-term toxicity of ribavirin has not been recognized, hospital personnel and family members of patients should minimize exposure to the drug because of possible long-term side effects. It is recommended that pregnant health care workers avoid exposure altogether. Adhering to standard infection-control principles (e.g., gloves, gowns, and frequent handwashing) can substantially reduce nosocomial spread. RSV is inactivated by common detergents, soaps, and dilute bleach solutions. Thus far, efforts to control RSV infection by immunization with killed and live virus vaccines have been unsuccessful.

Collins PL: The molecular biology of human respiratory syncytial virus (RSV) of the genus pneumovirus. *In* Kingsbury D (ed.): The Paramyxoviruses. New York, Plenum Press, 1991, pp 103–162. *Provides a detailed overview of the molecular genetics and structure of RSV.*

Committee on Infectious Diseases: Use of ribavirin in the treatment of respiratory syncytial virus infection. Pediatrics 92:501, 1993. *Recommendations by clinical virology experts on appropriate use of aerosolized ribavirin.*

Falsey AR, Treanor JJ, Betts RF, Walsh EE: Viral respiratory infection in the institutionalized elderly: Clinical and epidemiologic findings. J Am Geriatr Soc 40:115, 1992. *This prospective study of respiratory illness in a long-term care facility describes clinical features of RSV infection in the elderly with comparison with other viral pathogens.*

331 PARAINFLUENZA VIRAL DISEASE
Edward E. Walsh

DEFINITION. Parainfluenza viruses are important causes of a wide spectrum of respiratory illness in infants and young children, producing syndromes ranging from the common cold and otitis media to severe croup, bronchiolitis, and pneumonia. In older children and adults, illness is usually limited to the upper respiratory tract, although immunocompromised individuals may develop fatal respiratory failure.

ETIOLOGY. The parainfluenza viruses are enveloped single-stranded nonsegmented RNA viruses and belong to the family Paramyxoviridae, which also includes measles, mumps, and respiratory syncytial viruses. The genome encodes for six structural proteins, of which the hemagglutinin-neuraminidase (HN) and fusion proteins (F) are exposed on the bilayered lipid envelope that surrounds a helical nucleocapsid-RNA complex. The two surface proteins, which mediate attachment and penetration of the virus into susceptible mammalian cells, have retained antigenic stability for over 30 years, unlike the influenza virus hemagglutinin protein.

There are four distinct serotypes of human parainfluenza viruses, types 1 through 4, with two subgroups (A and B) of type 1 and 4 viruses. In addition, numerous animal strains of parainfluenza viruses exist, including Sendai virus, which infects mice; SV5, which causes respiratory illness in dogs; and shipping fever virus of cattle and Newcastle disease virus of chickens, important causes of lost income for the livestock industry. These viruses do not cause human illness.

EPIDEMIOLOGY. The parainfluenza viruses are ubiquitous and have worldwide geographic distribution, as determined by both virus recovery and serologic studies. Spread principally by large-particle fomites and close person-to-person contact, each of the four serotypes displays somewhat different epidemiologic features, although none is so uniquely characteristic as to allow definitive diagnosis.

Over the years, parainfluenza type 1 activity has displayed both endemic and epidemic patterns (Table 331–1). Primary infection with parainfluenza viruses begins soon after birth, with each serotype favoring different age groups and causing distinct clinical syndromes. Significant overlap exists in this regard, thus precluding specific diagnosis based on clinical and epidemiologic grounds. Among the parainfluenza viruses, type 3 infects infants first, with over 50% showing serologic evidence of infection in the first year of life. Parainfluenza virus type 3 is second only to respiratory syncytial virus (RSV) as a cause of bronchiolitis and pneumonia in this youngest age group. Parainfluenza virus type 1 and type 2 infections occur later, with specific antibody developing slowly from

TABLE 331–1. PARAINFLUENZA PATTERNS

Type	Manifestation	Season	Comments
1	Epidemic croup	Fall of odd-number years	Since 1970
2	Epidemic croup	Fall or early winter	Less predictable than type 1; less widespread
3	Endemic epidemic bronchitis and pneumonia	Late winter, early spring	Recently epidemic, often following influenza season; low levels of virus year-round
4	Unknown	?	Mild illness; frequently unrecognized

ages 2 through 6. The peak incidence of infection, manifested principally as croup, occurs between ages 1 and 2. Virtually all adults have serologic evidence of infection with each of the serotypes. The lower infection rate with parainfluenza type 1 and 2 viruses in very young infants suggests that maternally derived antibody is protective, in contrast to parainfluenza virus type 3 infection, in which maternal antibody has only limited benefit. Following primary infection, a relatively brief period of immunity against homotypic reinfection develops, mediated principally by serum IgG and mucosal IgA. The fact that reinfections are common later in childhood highlights the lack of durable immunity. Although both genders are equally susceptible to infection with the parainfluenza virus, males manifest more severe illness.

CLINICAL MANIFESTATIONS. Illness associated with primary parainfluenza virus infection varies by age and the virus serotype, although substantial overlap occurs. Underlying medical conditions, such as cardiopulmonary or immune disorders, also will influence the severity of disease. In general, parainfluenza virus types 1 and 2 are associated with croup, while parainfluenza virus type 3 causes bronchiolitis and pneumonia. However, because of the greater frequency of parainfluenza virus type 3 infections, it is a more important cause of croup than is type 2 parainfluenza. Other causes of croup include influenza A and RSV.

Infection typically starts with upper respiratory signs and symptoms, notably coryza, rhinorrhea, pharyngitis without cervical adenopathy, and fever. If croup evolves, the child then develops a raspy, barking cough with notable inspiratory stridor, dyspnea, and respiratory distress. These latter symptoms, which may be spasmodic, are due to subglottic inflammation and edema. Typically, in mild to moderate illness symptoms last 3 to 5 days but may be quite unpredictable and result in sudden respiratory failure. In hospitalized infants, hypoxia is universal, and hypercarbia is present in half. Although imperfect as a guide, respiratory rate best correlates with the degree of hypoxemia. In severe stridor, differentiation from epiglottis due to *Haemophilus influenzae* type b (see Ch. 282) may be suggested by lateral neck radiography, which can show subglottic edema and narrowing, in contrast to epiglottic swelling.

Although also a cause of croup, parainfluenza virus type 3 more commonly causes disease indistinguishable from RSV: tracheobronchitis, bronchiolitis, and pneumonia. Cough, rales, and wheezing associated with hypoxia and air trapping on radiography are common. Although virus infection of the lower airway directly contributes to symptoms, parainfluenza virus–specific IgE is found frequently in respiratory secretions in infants who wheeze.

Reinfection with the parainfluenza viruses is less severe and typically causes cold symptoms, although nursing home outbreaks with a high incidence of pneumonia have been reported. More recently, reinfection with parainfluenza virus has been implicated in severe pneumonia in immunocompromised children and adults. In a large series of bone marrow transplant recipients, 27 parainfluenza virus infections caused 6 deaths due to respiratory failure.

DIAGNOSIS. Although the clinician may suspect parainfluenza virus based on clinical and epidemiologic grounds, specific diagnosis requires isolating the virus or detecting viral antigen in respiratory secretions. Monkey kidney or human embryonic kidney cell cultures are optimal for virus recovery. Although parainfluenza virus types 1 and 3 do not produce cytopathic effect in cell culture, in contrast to syncytial giant cells caused by type 2 virus, they can generally be detected by hemadsorption with guinea pig red blood cells by day 10 of culture. Parainfluenza virus type 4 grows more slowly, often requiring up to 3 weeks in culture. Specific serologic tests are also useful to diagnose both primary and reinfections.

THERAPY AND PREVENTION. Specific antiviral treatment for parainfluenza virus is currently unavailable. Aerosolized ribavirin, approved for use in RSV infection, has *in vitro* activity against the parainfluenza viruses. Reports of ribavirin therapy of immunocompromised children and adults with severe parainfluenza virus pneumonia suggest possible benefit.

Treatment of croup, under usual circumstances, includes mist and supplemental oxygen. Aerosolized bronchodilators (racemic epinephrine) have definite but only transient benefit, while steroid use is controversial. Antibiotics are indicated only when bacterial superinfection is documented, an uncommon occurrence. Vaccination to prevent parainfluenza virus infection is under development.

Chanock RM, McIntosh K: Parainfluenza viruses. *In* Fields BN, Knipe DM (eds.): Fields Virology, 2nd ed. New York, Raven Press, 1990, pp 963–988. *Reviews the molecular biology, genetics, clinical diseases, and therapy for parainfluenza viruses.*

Denny FW, Murphy TF, Clyde WA, et al.: Croup: An 11-year study in a pediatric practice. Pediatrics 71:871, 1983. *Describes the viruses which account for 360 cases of croup in a single outpatient pediatric practice from 1964 to 1975.*

Welliver R, Wong DT, Choi T-S, Ogra PL: Natural history of parainfluenza virus infection in childhood. J Pediatr 101:180, 1982. *Describes immune response to parainfluenza virus infection in 130 infants, with correlation to protection from reinfection.*

Wendt CH, Weisdorf DJ, Jordan MC, et al.: Parainfluenza virus respiratory infection after bone marrow transplantation. N Engl J Med 326:921, 1992. *Clinical and therapeutic description of parainfluenza virus infection in bone marrow transplant recipients.*

332 INFLUENZA
Frederick G. Hayden

Influenza is an acute febrile respiratory illness that occurs in annual outbreaks of varying severity. The causative virus infects the respiratory tract, is highly contagious, and typically produces prominent systemic symptoms early in the illness. Influenza virus infection can produce various clinical syndromes in adults, including common colds, pharyngitis, tracheobronchitis, and pneumonia. Conversely, infections with other respiratory viruses, such as respiratory syncytial virus (RSV) or adenovirus, may produce influenzal illness. Influenza A viruses can cause worldwide epidemics (pandemics) and have done so four times this century (Table 332–1). The pandemic of 1918–1919 caused at least 500,000 deaths in the

TABLE 332–1. ANTIGENIC SUBTYPES OF INFLUENZA A VIRUS ASSOCIATED WITH PANDEMIC INFLUENZA

Year	Interval (Years)	Designation	Extent of Antigenic Change in Indicated Surface Protein*	Severity of Pandemic
1870	—	H2N8?	?	Moderate
1889	19	H3N8?	H + + + N ?	Severe
1918	29	H1N1†	H + + + N + + +	Very severe
1957	39	H2N2	H + + + N + + +	Severe
1968	11	H3N2	H + + + N −	Moderate‡
1977	9	H1N1	H + + + N + + +	Mild§

* Compared with antecedent or co-circulating virus: + = minor change; + + = moderate change; + + + = major change; − = no change.
† Formerly designated as H0N1 (swine virus prototype) or Hsw1N1.
‡ Population had some immunity to the N2 neuraminidase.
§ Most of population immune due to prior infection with earlier circulating identical virus.

TABLE 332–2. INFLUENZA VIRUS PROTEINS

Designation	Location (Approximate No. per Virion)	Function	Other
Hemagglutinin (HA)	Surface (500)	Cell attachment and penetration; fusion of virus and cell membranes	Subtype- and strain-specific antigens
Neuraminidase (NA)	Surface (100)	Virus release; enzymatic activity	Subtype- and strain-specific antigens
Membrane or M1 matrix	Internal (3000)	Major structural envelope protein; virus assembly	Type-specific antigen
M2 matrix	Surface (20–60)	Virus uncoating and assembly; ion channel	Site of action of amantadine/rimantadine
Nucleoprotein (NP)	Internal (1000)	Associated with RNA and polymerase proteins	Type-specific antigen
Polymerases (PB1, PB2, PA)	Internal (30–60)	RNA replication and transcription	Probable site of action of ribavirin
NS1, NS2	Nonstructural (infected cells)	Uncertain, regulation of virus replication	

Adapted from Murphy BR, Webster RG: Orthomyxoviruses. *In* Fields BN, Knipe DM (eds.): Fields Virology, 2nd ed. New York, Raven Press, 1990, p 1095.

United States and over 20 million worldwide. Influenza epidemics are associated with enormous morbidity, economic loss, and often substantial mortality. Excess deaths due to influenza average over 10,000 persons per epidemic in the United States.

ETIOLOGY. Influenza viruses belong to the family Orthomyxoviridae and are divided into three types (A, B, and C) distinguished by the antigenicity of their internal and external proteins (Table 332–2). The virion (Fig. 332–1) is a medium-sized enveloped pleomorphic particle covered with two types of surface glycoprotein spikes, the hemagglutinin (H or HA) and neuraminidase (N or NA). The envelope is composed of a lipid bilayer overlying the matrix

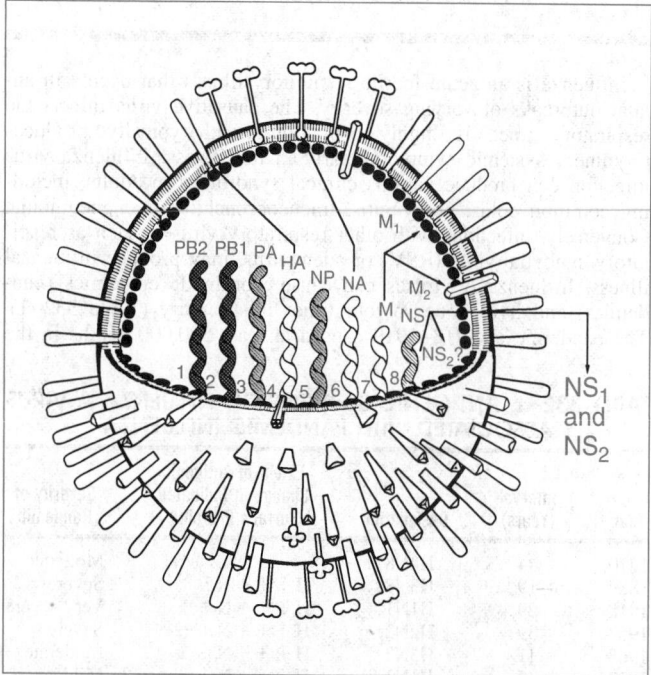

FIGURE 332–1. Diagram of influenza virus structure. Eight segments of viral RNA are contained within the envelope and matrix (M1) shell. Each codes for one or two proteins that form the virus or regtulate its intracellular replication. The presumed functions of each are listed in Table 332–2. (Courtesy of Dr. Robert G. Webster.)

(M1) protein that surrounds the segmented viral genome. The genome comprises eight segments of single-stranded RNA. Influenza C viruses have seven segments and only a single surface glycoprotein. Whereas influenza B and C viruses are principally human pathogens, influenza A viruses infect diverse animal species, including birds, horses, swine, and marine mammals. Influenza A viruses are further classified into subtypes based on their HA and NA glycoproteins. As of this writing, three hemagglutinins (H1, H2, and H3) and two neuraminidases (N1 and N2) have been recognized in human influenza A viruses. Each strain within a subtype is identified by site, number, and year of isolation.

EPIDEMIOLOGY. *Antigenic Variation.* Influenza viruses are unique among the respiratory viruses with regard to their extent of antigenic variation, epidemic behavior, and association with excess mortality during community outbreaks. The changing antigenicity of the surface glycoproteins accounts in part for the continuing epidemics of influenza in humans. Antibody to the HA neutralizes viral infectivity and thus is the major determinant of immunity. Anti-NA antibody is not neutralizing but limits viral replication and therefore the severity of infection. Variation involves either relatively minor (antigenic drift) or major (antigenic shift) changes in antigenicity. Significant antigenic variation is much less frequent with influenza B than with influenza A and may not occur with influenza C.

Antigenic drift refers to small changes that occur frequently (every year or every few years) within an influenza A or B virus. For example, the original H3N2 variant, A/Aichi/68, has undergone successive drifts resulting in epidemic strains that include the recent circulation of A/Beijing/32/92(H3N2)-like viruses. Antigenic drift results from an accumulation of point mutations in the RNA segment coding for the HA that cause amino acid substitutions in at least one of five antigenic sites on the HA. Immunologic selection favors the new variant over the old for transmission because of the less frequent presence of antibody in the population to the new virus.

Antigenic shift results from the appearance of an influenza A virus with HA or NA (or both) glycoproteins new to humans or possible reappearance of virus after decades of absence. Because of the high level of immunity to the old strain and lack of immunity to the new strain within the human population, a virulent new strain can cause pandemic disease (see Table 332–1). Infection by one subtype does not provide cross-protection against another. The origin of new pandemic strains and the basis for their apparent recirculation remain incompletely defined. Reassortment of gene segments may occur when two influenza viruses simultaneously infect a single cell. The finding of 14 H and 9 N subtypes in animal influenza A viruses has lead to the hypothesis that viruses in nature, particularly those infecting birds, serve as the reservoir of new genes for human pandemic strains.

Epidemic or Interpandemic Influenza. An "epidemic" is an outbreak of influenza confined to one geographic location. In a given community, epidemics of influenza A virus infection have a characteristic pattern. They usually begin rather abruptly, reach a sharp peak in 2 or 3 weeks, and last 6 to 10 weeks. Increased numbers of school children with febrile respiratory illness is often the first indication of influenza in a community. This is soon followed by illnesses among adults and about a week later by increased hospital admissions of patients with influenza-related complications. Hospitalization rates in high-risk persons increase two- to fivefold during major epidemics (Table 332–3). School and employment absenteeism increases, as does mortality from pneumonia and influenza, especially in older persons (see Table 332–3). The latter finding is a highly specific indicator of influenza activity.

Epidemics occur almost exclusively during the winter months. In temperate areas, it is rare to recover influenza virus during nonepidemic periods. However, in the tropics, influenza activity may continue year-round. Regional differences in the time of occurrence of influenza outbreaks are common, and major outbreaks may occur in some communities or regions while others are experiencing no activity whatsoever. During epidemics, the overall attack rates typically average 10 to 20%. Attack rates of 40 to 50% are not uncommon in closed populations, including hospital and nursing homes, and in certain highly susceptible age groups. In recent years it has been recognized that two different strains within a single subtype, two different influenza A subtypes (H1N1 and H3N2), or both influenza A and B viruses may co-circulate. In addition, simultaneous outbreaks of influenza A and RSV have been found. Strains circu-

TABLE 332–3. AGE-SPECIFIC RATES FOR ILLNESS AND MORTALITY DURING URBAN INFLUENZA EPIDEMICS

Age (years)	Physician Visits per 100	ARD Hospitalizations per 10,000	P + I Mortality per 100,000
<5	28	43	3
5–14	14	5	1
15–44	10	8	1
45–54	9	13	10
55–64	10	21	10
≥65	—	73	104

ARDS = acute respiratory disease; P + I = pneumonia and influenza; – = not stated.

Adapted from Glezen WP: Anatomy of an urban influenza epidemic. *In* Hannoun C, Kendal AP, Klenk HD, et al. (eds.): Options for the Control of Influenza II. Amsterdam, Elsevier Science, 1993, p 12.

lating at the end of one season's epidemic are likely to be responsible for the next season's outbreak (the so-called herald wave phenomenon). Furthermore, other than the association of influenza outbreaks with colder seasons, the factors are unknown that allow an epidemic to develop or those responsible for the tapering off of an epidemic, when only some susceptible persons have been infected.

Pneumonia and influenza (P + I) deaths predictably fluctuate annually, with peaks in the winter months. When such P + I deaths exceed the predicted number, this is due to influenza A or occasionally to influenza B virus or RSV activity. Although mortality is greatest during pandemics, substantial total mortality occurs with epidemics. Over 80% of P + I deaths occur among persons aged 65 and older (see Table 332–3). Other cardiopulmonary and chronic diseases also show increased mortality following influenza epidemics.

Pandemic Influenza. Pandemics of influenza A result from the emergence of a new virus to which the population contains no or limited immunity so that epidemics of influenza progress to involve all parts of the world (see Table 332–1). The pandemics of 1957, 1968, and 1977 all began in mainland China, and Southeast Asia has been postulated to be the epicenter for such strains. The interval between pandemics is variable and unpredictable. The most severe pandemics have resulted when there were major antigenic alterations in both the major surface antigens. Furthermore, it appears that intrinsic virulence is a virus-coded function that also varies among strains. The intrinsic virulence of recent H1N1 viruses appears to be milder than that of H3N2 viruses. After one or more waves of pandemic influenza, the level of immunity in the population increases. Such a chain of events provides a setting for emergence of a variant showing antigenic drift, since the level of immunity to it is less than that to the original strain. Repeated epidemics caused by strains showing antigenic drift within the subtype occur in subsequent years. After 10 to 40 years of circulation of variants within this given subtype, the population's immunity to all variants within the subtype is very high, and the conditions for the spread of a new virus are favorable.

PATHOGENESIS AND PATHOLOGY. Influenza virus infection is transmitted from person to person by virus-containing respiratory secretions. Small-particle aerosols appear most important, but transmission by other routes, including fomites, may be possible. Virtually all cells of the respiratory tract can support viral replication. Once the virus initiates infection of the respiratory tract epithelium, successive cycles of viral replication infect large numbers of cells and result in destruction of ciliated epithelium. The duration of the incubation period until onset of illness and virus shedding, which occur in close proximity, varies from 1 to 3 days. The quantity of virus in respiratory tract specimens correlates with severity of illness, which suggests that a major mechanism in producing illness is cell death resulting from viral replication. However, interferon is frequently detected in respiratory secretions and blood about a day after virus shedding and may contribute to systemic symptoms and fever. The roles of specific cytokines in producing and resolving illness are not defined. The duration of viral shedding depends on age and generally lasts for 3 to 5 days in adults and often into the second week in children. Viremia is rare.

Nasal and bronchial biopsy specimens from persons with uncomplicated influenza reveal desquamation of the ciliated columnar epithelium. Individual cells show shrinkage, pyknotic nuclei, and loss of cilia. In addition, the lungs in fatal influenza show extensive hemorrhage, hyaline membrane formation, and paucity of polymorphonuclear (PMN) cell infiltration. Secondary bacterial infections develop as a result of altered bacterial flora, damage to bronchial epithelium with depressed mucociliary clearance, decreased PMN and alveolar macrophage functions, and/or alveolar fluid.

Neutralizing, hemagglutination-inhibiting (HAI), antineuraminidase, complement-fixing, enzyme-linked immunosorbent assay (ELISA), and immunofluorescent antibodies begin to develop in the sera of persons with primary influenza virus infection during the second week after infection and reach a peak by 4 weeks. Secretory antibodies develop in the respiratory tract after influenza infection and consist predominantly of IgA antibodies that reach peak titers in 14 days. Cell-mediated immune responses also occur. Immunity to influenza appears to be subtype-specific and durable. Protection against infection is afforded by serum HAI titers of 1:40 or greater, serum-neutralizing antibody titers of 1:8 or greater, or nasal neutralizing antibody titers of 1:4 or greater.

CLINICAL FINDINGS. *Influenza Syndrome.* The abrupt onset of feverishness, chilliness, or frank rigors, headache, myalgia, and malaise is characteristic of influenza. Systemic symptoms predominate initially, and prostration occurs in more severe cases. Usually myalgia or headaches are the most troublesome early symptoms, and their severity is related to the level of fever. Arthralgia is common, and less often ocular symptoms, photophobia, tearing, burning, and pain on moving the eyes are helpful diagnostically. Respiratory symptoms, particularly dry cough and nasal discharge, are usually also present at the onset but are overshadowed by the systemic symptoms. Nasal obstruction, hoarseness, and sore throat also may be present. As systemic illness diminishes, respiratory complaints and findings become more apparent. Cough is the most frequent and troublesome and may be accompanied by substernal discomfort or burning. Nasal obstruction, discharge, pharyngeal pain, and injection are also common. Cough, lassitude, and malaise may persist for 2 more weeks before full recovery.

Fever is the most important initial physical finding. The temperature usually rises rapidly to a peak of 38 to 40° C and occasionally to 41° C within 12 hours of onset, concurrently with systemic symptoms. Fever is usually continuous but may be intermittent, especially if antipyretics are administered. As fever subsides, the systemic symptoms diminish. Typically, the duration of fever is 3 days, but it may last from 1 to 5 or more days. Uncommonly, a biphasic fever course occurs. Early in the course of illness, the patient appears toxic, the face is flushed, and the skin is hot and moist. The eyes are watery and reddened. Clear nasal discharge is common. The mucosa of the nose and throat are hyperemic, but exudate is not observed. Small, tender cervical lymph nodes are often present. Transient scattered rhonchi or localized areas of rales are found in <20% of cases.

The pattern of illness just described occurs with any strain of influenza A or B virus. Illness is more frequent and severe in smokers, and attack rates are higher in children than in adults. Maximum temperatures are higher in children, cervical adenopathy may be more frequent, and gastrointestinal symptoms of nausea, emesis, or abdominal pain more common. Older adults (≥60 years) experience muscle aches, sore throat, and headache less often but have higher rates of pulmonary complications. Influenza C virus generally causes only sporadic upper respiratory tract illness.

Respiratory Complications. Three kinds of pneumonic syndromes have been described: primary influenza viral pneumonia, secondary bacterial pneumonia, and mixed viral and bacterial pneumonia. Influenza A and B virus infections may be associated with other respiratory tract complications, including exacerbations of chronic bronchitis, asthma, or cystic fibrosis; croup and bronchiolitis in young children; and otitis media, sinusitis, and rarely parotitis or bacterial tracheitis. Apparently uncomplicated influenza is often accompanied by abnormal tracheobronchial clearance, airway hyperactivity, and small airways dysfunction lasting weeks. A syndrome mimicking pulmonary embolism with transiently altered perfusion scans also has been described.

Primary influenza viral pneumonia occurs predominantly among persons with underlying pulmonary and cardiac disorders, pregnancy, or immunodeficiency states, although up to one-half of reported cases have no recognized underlying disease. Following a typical onset of influenza, there is rapid progression of fever, cough, dyspnea, and cyanosis. Physical examination and chest roentgenograms reveal bilateral findings consistent with the adult respiratory distress syndrome. Blood gas studies show marked hypoxia. Gram stain of the sputum may show abundant PMN's but scant bacterial flora. Viral cultures of sputum or tracheal aspirates yield high titers of influenza virus. Such patients do not respond to antibiotics, and mortality is high, exceeding 50%.

Bacterial superinfection is often clinically distinguishable from primary viral pneumonia. The patients are most often elderly or have chronic pulmonary, cardiac, metabolic, or other diseases. Following a typical influenza illness, a period of improvement lasting from 1 to 4 days may occur. Recrudescence of fever is associated with symptoms and signs of bacterial pneumonia, such as cough, sputum production, and a localized area of consolidation apparent on physical and chest roentgenogram examination. Gram stain and culture of sputum reveal predominance of a bacterial pathogen, most often *Streptococcus pneumoniae, Staphylococcus aureus,* or *Haemophilus influenzae* (see relevant chapters for specific bacterial diseases). Such patients usually respond to specific antibiotic therapy, although staphylococcal infections may be particularly virulent and cause destructive pulmonary lesions. Invasive aspergillosis occurs rarely following influenza.

In addition, during an outbreak of influenza, many less distinct cases are observed that do not clearly fit into either of these categories. These patients may have viral tracheobronchitis, milder forms of localized viral pneumonia, or mixed viral and bacterial infection. Many respond to antibiotics. Such cases are more likely to be confused with a pneumonia due to *Mycoplasma pneumoniae* than to that produced by other bacterial infection.

Nonpulmonic Complications. Reye's syndrome is a well-recognized hepatic and central nervous system (CNS) complication of influenza A and B virus infections, typically in children and rarely in adults (see Ch. 430). Toxic shock syndrome due to respiratory tract infection with toxin-bearing *S. aureus* has been reported. Outbreaks of meningococcal infections have been associated with both influenza A and B virus infections. Myositis with tender leg muscles and elevated serum creatine kinase (CPK) levels may develop uncommonly, more often in children. Disseminated intravascular coagulopathy (DIC) develops rarely, as does renal failure related to DIC or myoglobinuria. Myocarditis or pericarditis has been described rarely. Aseptic meningitis, myelitis, encephalopathy associated with acute illness, and postinfluenzal encephalitis also have been described. A possible relationship to Guillain-Barré syndrome remains to be substantiated.

DIAGNOSIS. In an individual case, influenza often cannot be distinguished from infection with a number of other viruses (and occasionally streptococcal pharyngitis) that produce headache, muscle aches, fever, and/or cough. In summer, enteroviruses produce a similar clinical picture, and the acute manifestations of many other infections, such as dengue, may mimic influenza. On the other hand, when public health authorities report an epidemic of influenza A and B virus infection in a given community and a patient is seen with typical illness, it is highly likely that these symptoms are caused by an influenza virus infection.

Definitive diagnosis depends on detecting infectious virus or viral antigen in secretions from patients or detecting a serum antibody response. Influenza virus is readily isolated from throat or nasal specimens, sputum, or tracheal secretion specimens in the first 2 or 3 days of illness. Usually infectivity is detected within 48 to 72 hours in cell cultures. Commercially available EIA tests can document influenza A virus infection rapidly and have sensitivities of 70% or better. Serologic methods are less useful clinically because they require a convalescent serum obtained 10 to 14 days after the onset of infection.

TREATMENT. Oral rimantadine or amantadine therapy shortens the duration of fever and of systemic and respiratory symptoms in uncomplicated influenza A by 1 to 2 days and speeds functional recovery. The possible effectiveness of these drugs in treating pulmonary complications of influenza is unknown. The usual dosage is 200 mg per day for 5 days. A daily dose of 100 mg should be used in older adults. Rimantadine has a lower risk of the CNS side effects that occur with amantadine. Amantadine is excreted un-

changed in the urine, so dose adjustments are needed for those with modest renal impairment. These agents are ineffective for influenza B infections. Treated persons sometimes transmit virus to close contacts.

Other symptomatic measures include antipyretics and cough suppressants. Many authorities recommend that aspirin not be used, especially for persons under age 16, because of its association with Reye's syndrome.

Influenza viral pneumonia in its severe form requires intensive respiratory monitoring and support. Oral amantadine, intravenous ribavirin, and aerosolized ribavirin have been used anecdotally. Secondary bacterial pneumonia should be treated with appropriate antibiotics. When studies of the sputum do not clearly indicate an infecting bacterium, use antibiotics that are effective against the likely pathogens, including *S. aureus.*

PREVENTION. The mainstay of prevention is using inactivated influenza virus vaccines. These vaccines provide about 60 to 90% protection against influenzal illness when vaccine matches the epidemic strain. Immunogenicity and hence protection rates are often lower in the elderly, particularly in infirm nursing home residents, and immunosuppressed patients, including those with advanced HIV infection or receiving chemotherapy. Among elderly nursing home residents vaccine is approximately 50 to 60% effective in preventing hospitalization and pneumonia. The antigenic composition is reviewed annually so that the vaccine contains the most recently circulating strains, usually one or more subtypes of influenza A and an influenza B virus. Between 1 and 2% of immunized adults have fever and less than 10% systemic symptoms peaking at 8 to 12 hours after vaccination, but 25% or more may have mild local reactions at the site of injection. Persons with malignant disease should receive vaccine between chemotherapy courses.

The priority groups for vaccine include those at highest risk for influenza complications and their immediate contacts (Table 332–4), although vaccine can be safely administered to anyone trying to avoid influenza. Vaccine should be given each year in the fall before the influenza season. The vaccine is contraindicated in persons with chicken egg anaphylactic hypersensitivity. Rarely reported and unproven complications of inactivated vaccine include Guillain-Barré syndrome, systemic vasculitis syndrome, and theophylline or warfarin toxicities. Intranasal attenuated vaccines and improved adjuvants are under study.

Rimantadine and amantadine are approximately 70 to 90% effective in preventing influenza A illness and can be used to supplement vaccine programs. Persons who are not vaccinated in the fall should be placed on prophylaxis when an outbreak occurs or throughout the influenza season for the highest-risk group. If vaccine is available, persons may be vaccinated simultaneously and drug therapy stopped after 14 days. Alternatively, if vaccine is not available, administration may be continued for duration of the outbreak. When given to patients and staff alike, these drugs may be helpful in

TABLE 332–4. TARGET GROUPS FOR INFLUENZA IMMUNIZATION

Groups at Increased Risk of Complications

Persons aged 65 and older
Residents of nursing homes and other chronic care facilities
Patients with chronic pulmonary (including asthma) or cardiac disorder
Patients with chronic metabolic disease (including diabetes), renal dysfunction, hemoglobinopathies, or immunosuppression
Children and teens receiving long-term aspirin

Groups in Contact with High-Risk Persons

Physicians, nurses, and other health care providers
Employees of nursing homes and chronic care facilities
Providers of home care to high-risk persons
Household members (including children) of high-risk persons

Other Groups

Providers of essential community services (e.g., police, fire)
International travelers
Students, dormitory residents
Anyone wishing to reduce risk of influenza

Adapted from Advisory Committee on Immunization Practices, Centers for Disease Control and Prevention. MMWR 43(No RR-9):1, 1994.

managing nosocomial outbreaks. Postexposure prophylaxis in households is also effective. Hospitalized patients should be placed in respiratory isolation.

Centers for Disease Control and Prevention. Prevention and control of influenza: 1. Vaccines. MMWR 43(no. RR-9):1, 1994. *Recommendations for influenza immunization that are updated on an annual basis.*

Hannoun C, Kendal AP, Klenk HD, et al. (eds.): Options for the Control of Influenza II. Amsterdam, Elsevier Science, 1993, pp 1–468. *Compilation of review articles and papers emphasizing virologic, immunologic, epidemiologic, and public health aspects of influenza.*

Hayden FG, Couch RB: Clinical and epidemiological importance of influenza A viruses resistant to amantadine and rimantadine. Rev Med Virol 2:89, 1992. *Review article summarizing data regarding this problem and suggesting management strategies.*

Kilbourne ED (ed.): Influenza. New York, Plenum Press, 1987, pp 1–359. *Single-authored, authoritative text covering all aspects of influenza virus infections.*

Leonardi GP, Leib H, Birkhead GS, et al.: Comparison of rapid detection methods for influenza A virus and their value in health-care management of institutionalized geriatric patients. J Clin Microbiol 32:70, 1994. *Examples of commercially available rapid diagnostic assays for detecting influenza.*

333 ADENOVIRUS DISEASES

John J. Treanor

VIROLOGY

The adenoviruses are found in a variety of animal species, including humans, simians, horses, pigs, goats, and dogs. These viruses have been the subject of intense investigation for many years because of their ability to undergo latency and to induce tumors in experimental animals; consequently, the molecular biology of the adenoviruses is among the most completely known of all viruses. However, despite much effort in this regard, there is no well-documented association between adenoviruses and any human tumor.

The virus is nonenveloped, with a double-stranded DNA genome (Fig. 333–1). The human adenoviruses are grouped into six subgenera (A–F) based on differences in genome content, pattern of hemagglutination, and ability to cause tumors in experimental animals. In addition, at least 47 distinct serotypes are defined based on neutralization tests. Specific disease syndromes or hosts are often associated with specific adenovirus serotypes (Table 333–1).

CLINICAL FEATURES

DISEASE IN NORMAL HOSTS. The adenoviruses can infect and cause disease in a variety of human epithelial tissues including those of the eye, respiratory tract, gastrointestinal tract, and urinary bladder. Most infections in immunologically competent individuals are subclinical. Virus may be shed for months following infection from either the gastrointestinal or respiratory tract.

Eye Disease. **Pharyngoconjunctival Fever** (see Ch. 329). The syndrome of pharyngoconjunctival fever (PCF) is characterized by bilateral conjunctivitis accompanied by mild pharyngitis without exudate. Fever, myalgias, and malaise also may be present. The eyes are itchy but not painful, with a boggy, hyperemic conjunctiva, and

TABLE 333–1. ADENOVIRUS SEROTYPES AND ASSOCIATED SYNDROMES

Host and Disease Category	Epidemiologic Features	Associated Adenovirus Serotypes
Immunocompetent Hosts		
Pharyngoconjunctival fever	Epidemics in schools, family and the military, associated with swimming pools.	3, 7
Epidemic keratoconjunctivitis	Sporadic epidemics in schools, families, and industrial sites; may cause nosocomial outbreaks. More common in fall and winter	8, 19
Endemic upper respiratory disease	Seen predominantly in children, in families and day care setting	1, 2, 5
Acute respiratory disease of military recruits		3, 4, 7, 14 21
Acute hemorrhagic cystitis	Male predominance	7, 11, 21, 35
Gastroenteritis	Predominant in children <2	40, 41
Immunocompromised Hosts		
Transplantation		7, 11, 31, 34, 35
Acquired immunodeficiency syndrome		Multiple, 35, 42–47

watery discharge. Occasionally, the syndrome may be complicated by punctate keratitis.

PCF is highly contagious (see Table 333–1) and can be spread by contact with the eyes and mouth for 8 to 10 days after the onset of symptoms. The incubation period is 5 to 8 days. The illness is self limited, with a duration of from a few days to as long as 3 weeks. There is no specific therapy.

Epidemic Keratoconjunctivitis. In contrast to PCF, epidemic keratoconjunctivitis (EKC) presents as unilateral disease in the majority of cases and is generally not accompanied by sore throat, fever, or systemic symptoms. The patient may complain of a mild foreign body sensation with watery tearing but is not in significant discomfort. Physical findings include a swollen eyelid, conjunctival hyperemia with edema and chemosis, and tender preauricular adenopathy. Keratitis eventually develops in about 80% of patients and is usually noted on about the eighth day of illness with the onset of pain, photophobia, lacrimation, and blepharospasm. Visual acuity also may be temporarily reduced during the height of illness. Subepithelial corneal infiltrates can be detected in about one third of patients and may take weeks or months to resolve.

Many EKC outbreaks (see Table 333–1) have been attributed to contamination of ophthalmalogic equipment, such as tonometers, and stringent infection-control procedures often must be implemented to terminate nosocomial outbreaks.

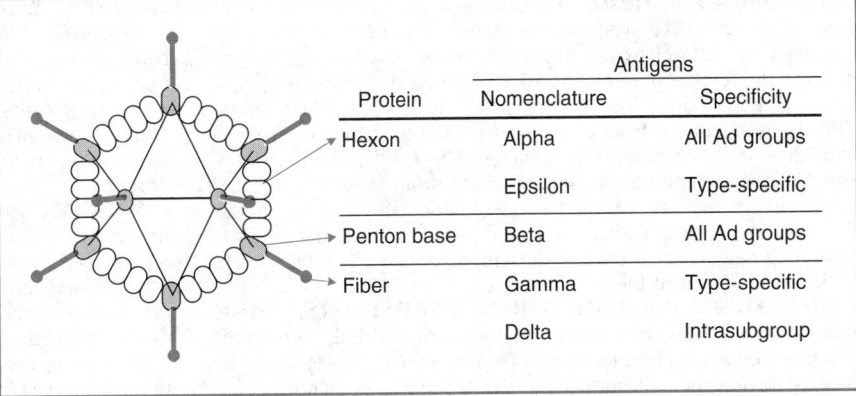

FIGURE 333–1. Structure of the capsid of adenovirus showing the major antigenic systems and capsid proteins. The viral capsid is an icosahedron composed of 252 capsomers arranged in 20 triangular faces and 12 vertices. The 12 vertex capsomers are called pentons because each is surrounded by five neighboring subunits. Each penton consists of a base and a fiber. The penton base is a toxic factor that causes cytopathology in cell culture. The nonvertex capsomers are called hexons, because each is surrounded by six neighboring subunits. (Adapted from Horwitz MS: Adenoviridae and their replication. *In* Fields BN, Knipe DM (eds.): Fields' Virology, 2d ed. New York, Raven Press, 1990, used with permission.)

Protein	Antigens	
	Nomenclature	Specificity
Hexon	Alpha	All Ad groups
	Epsilon	Type-specific
Penton base	Beta	All Ad groups
Fiber	Gamma	Type-specific
	Delta	Intrasubgroup

Respiratory Disease. **Upper Respiratory Tract Illness** (see Ch. 329). Acute pharyngitis is the most common respiratory syndrome attributed to the adenoviruses. Adenoviruses can cause an exudative tonsillitis similar to that caused by group A streptococci. In children, common associated syndromes include otitis media, coryza, and undifferentiated fever. Overall, adenoviruses are associated with about 7% of acute febrile illnesses in children, with a peak age of incidence between 6 months and 2 years. High secondary attack rates are seen in families or in the day care setting.

Lower Respiratory Tract Illness. Adenoviruses have been implicated as causing approximately 10% of childhood pneumonias. Clinical features are nondescript, and chest radiographs are similar to those in other forms of viral pneumonia, with the exception that hilar adenopathy is more common in children with adenoviral pneumonia than with other forms of viral pneumonia. Mixed bacterial/viral pneumonia is often present and may be suggested by elevations in band forms in peripheral blood.

Military recruits generally present with the atypical pneumonia syndrome (see Table 333–1), and illness clinically resembles that due to *Mycoplasma pneumoniae.* Although the illness is typically mild, more severe disseminated infections and deaths have been reported. Multiple radiographic patterns are noted; there may be large pleural effusions. Prodromal symptoms of upper respiratory infection are reported by most patients, and pharyngitis is often found on presentation. The disease is associated with the special conditions of fatigue and crowding found in military barracks and does not commonly occur in similarly crowded situations such as college dormitories. Bacterial superinfection, particularly with *Neisseria meningitidis,* may occur.

Adenoviruses rarely cause pneumonia in otherwise healthy adults, and adenovirus isolated from stool or respiratory secretions in normal adults with pulmonary infiltrates should be interpreted with caution.

Urinary Disease. **Hemorrhagic Cystitis.** Acute hemorrhagic cystitis (AHC) may be caused by adenoviruses (see Table 333–1). The patient complains of gross hematuria and dysuria. The presentation may be confused with glomerulonephritis, but laboratory tests of renal function remain normal, and fever and hypertension do not occur. AHC is generally self-limited.

Gastrointestinal Disease. **Gastroenteritis** (see Ch. 344). Although multiple adenovirus serotypes may be shed in the stool, only the so-called enteric adenoviruses, i.e., types 40 and 41, have been convincingly associated with acute gastroenteritis. These adenovirus types belong to the newly created group F and differ from other adenoviruses in being highly restricted in their ability to replicate in conventional cell culture. Development of alternative culture systems, such as use of the Ad 5–transformed HEK-293 cell line, allowed laboratory propagation of these viruses and clarification of their role in human disease.

Gastroenteritis due to enteric adenovirus is a disease predominantly of children under age 2. Clinical features include watery diarrhea and vomiting similar to those seen with infection with group A rotavirus. In contrast to gastroenteritis due to the rotaviruses and astroviruses, adenoviral gastroenteritis shows no significant seasonal variability. The frequency of illness is about 10% of that caused by rotavirus in the same age group. Adenoviruses are rarely causes of acute gastroenteritis in adults.

Other Syndromes Associated with Adenoviruses in Immunocompetent Hosts. Adenoviruses are often isolated in cases of pertussis-like syndrome, but there is no evidence that adenoviruses by themselves are important causes of whooping cough. A toxic shock–like presentation of disseminated adenovirus infection in a normal host has been reported. Adenoviruses have occasionally been isolated from cerebrospinal fluid in immunocompetent individuals with meningitis or meningoencephalitis. These viruses also have been implicated in sudden infant death syndrome (SIDS). Adenoviruses may be detected in mesenteric lymph nodes at the time of surgery for intussusception, and it is postulated that viral infection causes an acute mesenteric lymphadenitis which then leads to the development of this condition.

DISEASE IN IMMUNOCOMPROMISED HOSTS. *Transplantation.* Adenoviruses are causes of morbidity and mortality in immunocompromised patients, particularly after transplantation. In contrast to infection in normal hosts, infection in immunocompro-

mised subjects tends to be disseminated, with virus isolated from multiple body sites, including lung, liver, and gastrointestinal tract, and in urine. In addition, the spectrum of serotypes includes both those found in immunocompetent individuals and a markedly increased frequency of higher-numbered serotypes found rarely in immunologically normal subjects (see Table 333–1). The source of infection may be reactivation of latent virus; nosocomial infection has also been documented.

Adenoviruses may cause hemorrhagic cystitis in bone marrow transplant recipients, which may be confused with that due to cyclophosphamide. Differentiation between these two possibilities is generally made by virus culture and by the timing of cystitis in relationship to drug administration. Individuals with cystitis may develop pneumonia, hepatic necrosis, gastroenteritis, and encephalitis. The case-fatality rate of disseminated infection can be as high as 60%. Disseminated disease after liver transplantation can be seen and frequently leads to loss of the transplanted liver. However, this does not appear to preclude successful transplant of a new liver if one is available. Adenovirus disease in renal transplant recipients is generally not as severe as that seen in other transplants. Hemorrhagic cystitis is the most commonly seen problem, with pneumonia seen more rarely.

AIDS. Adenoviruses also have been isolated frequently from the stool and urine of individuals with the acquired immunodeficiency syndrome (AIDS), particularly those with relatively low CD4 lymphocyte counts. The most remarkable aspect of this situation is the isolation of a wide variety of serotypes in these patients (see Table 333–1), including new, higher-numbered serotypes isolated for the first time in these subjects. In addition, antigenically intermediate types have been isolated which possibly reflect recombination events made possible by prolonged virus replication in these hosts.

Because adenoviruses are almost always isolated in these patients in conjunction with multiple other opportunistic pathogens, it is difficult to ascribe specific clinical syndromes to them. Described associations include pneumonia, meningoencephalitis, hepatitis, gastroenteritis, and colitis. Adenoviruses have been detected in the large bowel of such patients in association with chronic diarrhea, but generally these have not been the enteric adenoviruses most commonly associated with gastroenteritis in immunologically normal hosts.

DIAGNOSIS

Virus can be isolated efficiently from conjunctival swabs, respiratory secretions, urine, or stool in primary cells of human epithelial origin, such as human embryonic kidney cells. However, diagnosis is complicated by the prolonged time required for isolation. Other means of directly detecting viral antigen or nucleic acid in clinical specimens are therefore widely used, including enzyme immunoassays, immunofluoresecence tests, and nucleic acid hybridization techniques. In addition, the time required to detect virus in cell culture can be shortened to as little as 2 days by applying centrifugation culture systems coupled with detection of early virus replication in culture using immunofluorescent or other means.

TREATMENT AND PREVENTION

THERAPY. *Conjunctivitis.* Therapy is generally supportive. Steroids should be avoided in mild cases of conjunctivitis, since symptoms will usually recur when steroids are discontinued. In more severe cases of keratitis, mild topical steroids may be used with cycloplegics as needed for iritis. Topical antibiotics may be administered to prevent bacterial superinfection.

Systemic Infections. There is no antiviral therapy that has been proven to be effective in any systemic adenoviral syndrome. A number of antiviral compounds are active against common adenovirus serotypes *in vitro,* and there have been uncontrolled anecdotal reports of successful treatment of AHC in immunocompromised hosts with intravenous ribavirin, a broad-spectrum antiviral drug.

VACCINATION. Live adenovirus vaccines have been developed for serotypes 4 and 7. These vaccines are administered orally in enteric-coated capsules and bypass the respiratory tract to replicate asymptomatically in the intestine. They have been shown to provide effective serotype-specific protection against adenovirus respiratory disease in high-risk military recruits, but these vaccines have not been used in civilian populations because of the plethora of additional serotypes causing severe disease in this population.

Because relatively large portions of the adenovirus genome can be replaced without affecting viral viability, adenoviruses have received considerable attention in constructing recombinant vaccines for other infectious diseases, such as hepatitis B, and as a vector for the delivery of gene therapy.

Baum SG: Adenovirus. *In* Mandell G, Dolin R, Bennett J (eds.): Principles and Practice of Infectious Diseases. 4th ed New York, Churchill-Livingstone 1995, pp 70–75. *Readily accessible, detailed review of the clinical significance of the human adenoviruses.*

Hierholzer JD: Adenoviruses in the immunocompromised host. Clin Microbiol Rev 5:262, 1992. *A complete description of reported cases of adenovirus infection in individuals with primary and secondary immunodeficiencies, including AIDS.*
Horwitz MS: Adenoviridae and their replication. *In* Fields BN, Knipe DM (eds.): Fields Virology, 2d ed. New York, Raven Press, 1990, pp 1679–1722. *Detailed description of the molecular biology of adenovirus replication.*
Liu C: Adenoviruses. *In* Belshe RB (ed.): Textbook of Human Virology, 2d ed. St. Louis, Mosby–Year Book, 1991, pp 791–803. *An excellent overall review of the biology of the adenoviruses.*

Exanthems and Mumps

334 MEASLES
Philip A. Brunell

DEFINITION. Measles is an acute, highly contagious disease characterized by fever, coryza, cough, conjunctivitis, and both an enanthem and an exanthem.

ETIOLOGY. The virus is an enveloped, negative-stranded RNA paramyxovirus (genus *Morbillivirus*) measuring 120 to 250 mm in diameter, similar to other members of the Paramyxovirus family but lacking neuraminidase. Its single antigenic serotype has been remarkably stable throughout the world for many years. The virus contains six major polypeptides, which are responsible for a number of structural and functional properties, including hemagglutination (of primate erythrocytes), hemolysis, cell fusion, and others. Isolation of virus from clinical specimens is most successful with primary kidney cell cultures of human or simian origin. Selected laboratory strains grow well in other primary and continuous cell lines of mammalian and avian origin.

EPIDEMIOLOGY. With the introduction of routine immunization against measles in the United States in 1963, the incidence of measles fell by about 99%. Smaller outbreaks have occurred at increasing intervals in 1971, 1976, and 1986. A somewhat larger outbreak appeared in 1989. Prior to the advent of measles vaccine, almost every child got measles, most before entering school. The frequency increased every other year. This pattern still is seen in developing countries, where measles in the very young is common. It is estimated that there are from 1 to 2 million deaths annually worldwide. Many developed countries have a less stringent policy toward measles immunization than does the United States.

During the 1989–1990 epidemic in the United States, the highest attack rates were in infants, followed by preschool children. The largest number of measles deaths in over a decade, 89, was reported in 1990. About 30% occurred in those over 20 years of age, many in those who were immunocompromised. Almost all the remaining deaths occurred in those under 5 years of age, most of whom were unimmunized and otherwise normal. During the past few years, however, the reported cases of measles have been at an all-time low.

Communicability. Measles is one of the most highly contagious infections. Almost all unprotected household contacts are infected. Demonstration of virus in nasopharyngeal secretions during the prodromal, pre-eruptive phase and in the first days of rash is in accord with epidemiologic evidence of contagiousness. Close physical proximity or direct person-to-person respiratory droplet contact is the usual requisite for infection, although airborne transmission has been documented.

Immunity. An unmodified attack of measles is followed by lifelong immunity. Passively transferred maternal antibody protects the young infant during the early months of life.

PATHOLOGY AND PHYSIOLOGIC RESPONSES. Pathologic changes in fatal measles usually represent the compound effect of viral and secondary bacterial infection. Pneumonia is almost invariably present; it is most frequently interstitial. More representative are changes of the uncomplicated viral diseases within the tonsillar, nasopharyngeal, and appendiceal tissue removed during the prodrome. These changes consist of round cell infiltration and the presence of multinucleated giant cells. Giant cells also are observed in tissue cultures infected with measles virus. The skin and mucous membranes contain perivascular round cell infiltrates with congestion and edema. Koplik's spots are inflammatory lesions of the submucous glands with similar microscopic features.

Simultaneous with the onset of rash, measles-specific antibodies are detectable in serum. Leukopenia is observed on the first day of rash mainly due to a decrease in lymphocytes; subsequently, granulocytopenia ensues as well. Measles virus replicates in lymphoid tissues (spleen, thymus, lymph nodes), can be isolated from monocytes and other mononuclear cells during acute infection. The virus is propagable in suspension of leukocytes *in vitro*.

Immunosuppressive Effects of Measles. It has long been known that cell-mediated immunity is impaired during measles. There is transient suppression of the tuberculin reaction (observed also with measles vaccines); improvement in eczema and allergic asthma and the induction of remissions in nephrosis have been described. In severe disease, the magnitude of depression of the total lymphocytes has been positively correlated with a lessened chance of recovery.

CLINICAL MANIFESTATIONS. After an incubation period that averages 11 days, measles becomes clinically manifest with symptoms of fever, malaise, myalgia, and headache. Within hours, *ocular symptoms* of photophobia and conjunctival injection occur. The palpebral and, to a lesser extent, the bulbar conjunctivae are involved. There is usually no exudate. Sneezing, coughing, and nasal discharge occur almost simultaneously. Less commonly, hoarseness and aphonia may reflect laryngeal involvement. In this prodromal stage of 1 to 4 days' duration, tiny white spots on the buccal mucosa may herald the appearance of skin rash. The white lesions described by Koplik characteristically occur lateral to the molar teeth and typically are mounted on a bluish red areola of injected mucosa, superimposed on a diffuse red background. They generally appear a day or so prior to rash and disappear within 2 days after its appearance. They constitute a pathognomonic diagnostic sign. The enanthem may involve other mucous membranes such as the palpebral conjunctiva and vaginal lining.

The *rash* of measles follows the prodromal symptoms by 2 to 4 days, occasionally as late as 7 days. It first appears behind the ears or on the face and neck as a blotchy erythema, spreads downward to cover the trunk, and finally is manifest on the extremities. The hands and feet may escape involvement. Initially, the eruption consists of discrete red macules that blanch with pressure. Subsequently, these lesions become papular, tend to coalesce, and may develop a red, nonblanching component. In adults, the rash generally is more extensive, with a greater tendency to become confluent and slightly raised and redder than in children. This is particularly true on the face. The rash fades in the order of its appearance; its disappearance about 5 days after onset may be attended by a fine, powdery desquamation that spares the hands and feet. In adults, malaise may continue for 1 to 2 weeks.

The *fever* of measles may persist for about 6 days and frequently reaches 40 or 41°C. Throughout the febrile period, productive cough and auscultatory evidence of bronchitis may be evident. These manifestations may persist after defervescence, and cough is often the last symptom to disappear. Bronchopulmonary symptomatology is an integral part of the primary viral infection; roentgenographic evidence of pulmonary involvement is frequently seen in the uncomplicated disease in the absence of leukocytosis and obvious bacterial infection. Generalized lymphadenopathy accompanies the acute febrile illness and may persist for several weeks thereafter. Nausea and, less commonly, emesis appear to be more common in adults and are often accompanied by elevated serum aminotransferases.

COMPLICATIONS. The persistence or recurrence of fever and development of leukocytosis are presumptive evidence of the common bacterial sequela of otitis media or pneumonia. Transtrachial aspirates in patients with pneumonia have yielded a variety of organisms.

Laryngitis of sufficient severity to embarrass respiration has been observed. Keratoconjunctivitis is part of the acute phase. Electrocardiographic abnormalities may be found. Severe measles has been described in pregnant women with hepatitis and pneumonia, the latter sometimes ending fatally. Premature labor has resulted in prematurity and stillbirths.

Encephalomyelitis. A rare (0.1%) but serious consequence of measles is a demyelinating encephalomyelitis that may appear from 1 to 14 days after the onset of infection. This complication is associated with recurrence of fever and headache, vomiting, and stiff neck. Stupor and convulsions usually follow. Localizing neurologic symptoms may be present. Death ensues in about 10% of patients; more than half of survivors suffer permanent residuals of varying severity. Abnormal electroencephalograms were recorded in about half of children with measles without clinical signs of encephalitis.

Infection of brain cells results in an incomplete viral replicative cycle with production of defective virions lacking the matrix (M) measles virus protein. Studies of patients with acute measles encephalomyelitis and those with late-onset subacute sclerosing panencephalitis show high titers in serum and cerebrospinal fluid of antibodies to all the measles virus proteins except M.

Other late sequelae of measles are thrombocytopenic purpura and exacerbation or activation of pre-existing pulmonary tuberculosis. The late complication of subacute sclerosing panencephalitis is discussed in Ch. 428.4.

Giant-Cell Pneumonia. In patients who are immunocompromised, e.g., those with AIDS, measles virus may induce an interstitial pneumonia characterized by giant cells and intracellular inclusion bodies. The disease is often fatal.

Measles Modified by Administering Antibodies. Attenuation of the natural disease by antibody prophylaxis may result in an illness of lessened severity comparable with the milder infection as seen in infants with illness modified by maternally acquired antibody. Fever alone may be observed, but some degree of exanthem is usually apparent. Koplik's spots may not appear. In general, the course is truncated and relatively uncomplicated. Lasting immunity is uncertain. Later routine immunization of these individuals is probably indicated.

Atypical Measles. From 1963 to 1967, two types of measles vaccine, one live attenuated and the other inactivated or "killed," were available in the United States. The live attenuated vaccine has been the sole product licensed and used in this country since 1967. A severe illness was reported in killed vaccine recipients after exposure to natural measles. These patients had high fever, pneumonia with pleural effusion, obtundation, and an unusual rash. The exanthem was hemorrhagic and was most marked on the extremities. In some instances, vesicular, macular, or maculopapular phases have been observed. The rash is sometimes accompanied by edema of

hands and feet. Concomitantly, these patients' sera revealed extraordinarily high titers of measles-specific antibodies.

Subsequent investigations showed that patients who had received inactivated measles vaccines failed to develop antibodies to the fusion (F) protein of the virus. Lack of antibodies to the cell fusion factor is believed to have permitted these patients to support measles infection. Thus the atypical measles syndrome is believed to be due to an anamnestic antibody response in the face of an abundance of measles antigens.

In addition to the rash and pulmonary findings, these patients may have elevated liver enzymes, disseminated intravascular coagulation, and marked myalgia. Nodular pulmonary changes have persisted in some patients. Some cases of pneumonia are reported to have occurred in the absence of rash. Initial diagnoses on presentation have included Rocky Mountain spotted fever and meningococcemia because of the similarities of rash and toxicity. Since inactivated vaccines were available only from 1963 through 1967, the past recipients are now young adults. This atypical measles syndrome is of increasing importance to the internist. Atypical measles has been reported in some patients who received live vaccine alone or after killed vaccine. Recipients of killed vaccine who later received live vaccine may have severe local and systemic reactions to reimmunization.

DIAGNOSIS. The diagnosis should be suspected during an epidemic or following history of exposure. Prior to the appearance of rash, the diagnosis may be difficult unless Koplik's spots are present. Finding an uncomfortable patient in a darkened room who has conjunctivitis, coryza, and cough should make one suspect measles. The rash in adults may be more violaceous, confluent, slightly raised, and more extensive than in children. A history of having received measles vaccine does not preclude the diagnosis, because most individuals with measles of school age or older have had the vaccine.

Differential diagnosis (Table 334-1) includes consideration of rubella, scarlet fever, infectious mononucleosis, secondary syphilis, drug eruptions, toxic shock syndrome, and Kawasaki's disease. Of value in excluding these possibilities are the milder course, postauricular nodes, and pinker rash of rubella; the sore throat, eventual desquamation, strawberry tongue, and leukocytosis of scarlet fever; and serologic tests for infectious mononucleosis. Fever, enanthem, and catarrh are uncommon with the cutaneous manifestations of drug hypersensitivity. Erythema infectiosum is usually an afebrile illness with rash on the cheeks, arms, and legs. There is no prodrome or accompanying respiratory tract involvement. Kawasaki's disease is rare in adults.

Specific Diagnosis. Virus isolation is technically difficult. Increase in specific antibody may be detected as early as the first or second day of rash. Generally acute and convalescent sera are required. Demonstration of measles IgM is available in some laboratories.

Presumptive diagnosis may be made if giant cells are detected in stained smears of nasal exudate in the pre-eruptive period.

PROGNOSIS. Uncomplicated measles is rarely fatal, and complete recovery is the rule. Fatalities are almost always the result of pneumonia, occurring in adults or children younger than age 1. Congestive cardiac failure is a common cause of death in patients over 50 years old. The prognosis is particularly poor in patients with AIDS or other immunocompromised patients (see Ch. 360).

Antimicrobial drugs effective against the usual secondary in-

TABLE 334-1. A GUIDE TO THE DIFFERENTIAL DIAGNOSIS OF MEASLES

	Conjunctivitis	Rhinitis	Sore Throat	Enanthem	Leukocytosis	Specific Laboratory Tests Available
Measles	+ +	+ +	0	+	0	+
Rubella	0	±	±	0	0	+
Exanthem subitum	0	±	0	0	0	+
Enterovirus infection	0	±	±	0	0	+
Adenovirus infection	+	+	+	0	0	+
Scarlet fever	±	±	+ +	0	+	+
Infectious mononucleosis	0	0	+ +	±	±	+
Drug rash	0	0	0	0	0	0

0 Not usually present; no test available.
± Variable in occurrence.
+ Present: test available (virus or bacterial culture, serology).
+ + Present and severe.

vaders have reduced the case fatality rate of measles sharply. They have proved effective in therapy of bacterial complications, but not in prophylaxis.

Encephalitis occurs as frequently in mild as in severe measles (i.e., about one in 1000 cases); subacute sclerosing panencephalitis occurs about 7 years after measles and has essentially disappeared with widespread vaccine use.

TREATMENT. There is no specific antiviral therapy for measles with demonstrated efficacy, although ribavirin has been used in some cases.

Symptomatic Therapy. In the absence of complications, bed rest is the essence of treatment in this self-limited disease. Codeine sulfate may be useful to ameliorate headache and myalgia and is effective for cough. Analgesics and antipyretics may be useful. Fluids should be encouraged. Bright light is not an ocular hazard, but photophobia may require darkening the patient's room.

Antimicrobial Prophylaxis. The course of uncomplicated measles is not influenced by antimicrobial drugs, and their use during the acute illness has resulted in no decrease of secondary bacterial complications (otitis, sinusitis, pneumonia). Instead, the same rates of complications (about 10 to 15%) have been observed, but with organisms resistant to the antibiotics used during the viral illness. If careful observation of the patient is possible, rational therapy is based on promptly recognizing and defining the etiology of complications, followed by starting the appropriate antimicrobial drug in proper dosage.

PREVENTION. Vaccination. A highly effective vaccine available for preventing measles is derived from the Edmonston strain of virus isolated originally in the laboratory of Dr. John Enders. This live virus vaccine produces immunity by infection. A second dose now is recommended routinely. In children over age 1, seroconversion after vaccination in recent years is about 98 to 99%. Measles vaccine usually is given as a single preparation as measles, mumps, and rubella (MMR) vaccine. Failure of measles immunization was much more common prior to 1980. The reasons for this are unclear. It may be due to poor recall or faulty documentation of immunization, age of immunization, use of immune globulin with the vaccine, receipt of killed rather than live vaccine, or the type of live vaccine.

Vaccine recommendations vary depending on the measles experience in the community (see Ch. 10). The first dose is now recommended at age 12 months as MMR. During epidemics, it may be given as monovalent measles vaccine to infants as young as 6 months of age. In the latter case, it should be repeated in combination with mumps and rubella (MMR) after the first birthday. The second routine dose of MMR is given between ages 5 and 12. All entering college students and beginning health care workers born after 1956 should show evidence of measles immunity, e.g., positive serologic test, physician-documented measles, or receipt of two doses of measles vaccine or preferably MMR. The immune status of those contemplating foreign travel should be reviewed. A large number of military personnel have been reimmunized without significant side effects.

Contraindications to live virus vaccine include pregnancy, immunodeficiency, leukemia, and other systemic malignant diseases, active tuberculosis, and administration of resistance-depressing drugs such as corticosteroids and antimetabolites.

Annunziato D, Kaplan MH, Hall WW, et al.: Atypical measles syndrome: Pathologic and serologic findings. Pediatrics 70:203, 1982. *Excellent clinical description and explanation of a syndrome now seen in young adults.*

Atmar RL, Englund JA, Hammill H: Complications of measles during pregnancy. Clin Infect Dis 14:217, 1992. *A review of the complications and the treatment of measles in pregnancy.*

Centers for Disease Control and Prevention: Measles prevention: Recommendations of the Immunization Practices Advisory Committee (ACIP). MMWR 38:1, 1989. *Everything you want to know about the use of measles vaccine.*

Gilad M: Measles in adults: A prospective study of 291 consecutive cases. Br Med J 295:1313, 1987. *A brief summary of findings in a large number of adults.*

Gremillioin DH, Crawford GE: Measles pneumonia in young adults. Am J Med 71:539, 1981. *A large series of cases of measles pneumonia in young adults and other features of measles in this group.*

Gustafson TL, Brunell PA, Lievens AW, et al.: Measles outbreak in a "fully-immunized" secondary school population. N Engl J Med 316:771, 1987. *School outbreaks are described in a presumably well-immunized population.*

Katz SL, Gellin BG: Measles Control—Resetting the Agenda: A report of the children's vaccine initiative ad hoc committee on an investment strategy for measles control. J Infect Dis 170(suppl):S1, 1994. *An all-inclusive presentation of measles and its prevention throughout the world.*

Panum PL: Observations Made During the Epidemic of Measles on the Faroe Islands. New York, Delta Omega Society, 1940. *A classic clinical epidemiologic description of measles introduced into an isolated population with disease among all susceptibles born since the previous epidemic 65 years earlier.*

335 RUBELLA (German Measles)
Philip A. Brunell

DEFINITION. Rubella is an acute, usually benign infectious disease characterized by a 3-day rash, generalized lymphadenopathy, and minimal or no prodromal symptoms. Since 1941, it has been known to cause congenital malformations when infection occurs during the early months of pregnancy.

ETIOLOGY. Rubella is a small, spherical, enveloped virus containing single-stranded RNA of positive polarity. The structural proteins consist of membrane glycoproteins and a nucleocapsid protein. The virus is classified as a togavirus, genus *rubivirus*. It multiplies in a variety of primary cell culture systems and in some continuous cell lines in most systems without detectable cytopathic effects.

EPIDEMIOLOGY. Before rubella vaccines were available, the disease was worldwide in distribution, produced major epidemics at 6- to 9-year intervals, and was recognized mainly in school-age children; it also produced outbreaks in settings such as military recruit bases and college campuses where large numbers of susceptible young adults gathered in relatively crowded conditions. Since licensure in 1969 of the vaccine in the United States, there has been strikingly altered epidemiology. There has been no major epidemic since 1964–1965. In other nations, where rubella vaccine has not been widely used, the epidemiology has remained unchanged. Because the disease may be quite nonspecific clinically, with nearly one-third of adults undergoing infection without rash, epidemiologic reporting tends to underestimate its prevalence. Since 1966, congenital rubella has been a reportable disease. It is probable that rubella is spread by the respiratory route and by close and sustained personal contact. The incubation period in experimentally infected individuals was found to be 12 to 19 days, with most cases occurring 14 to 15 days following exposure. Although virus was isolated as early as 7 days prior to and as late as 21 days following onset of rash, infectivity probably is greatest throughout the period of prodromal symptoms and for as long as 7 days after the appearance of rash. Infants with congenitally acquired infection may excrete virus in respiratory secretions and in urine for months after birth and are contagious during this time. In hospital environments, especially in nurseries, the congenital rubella baby had been a source of nosocomial infection of personnel involved in his/her care.

Immunity is lifelong after initial infection. Authenticated second attacks are exceedingly rare and require serologic documentation because of the nonspecific nature of the clinical syndrome. Subclinical reinfection demonstrated by increase in IgG serum antibody has been documented. Such reinfections are not associated with viremia and thus pose little threat to pregnant women. IgM response has been used to distinguish primary infection from reinfection. Immunity that follows artificial immunization with live virus vaccine is apparently of equal duration even though the antibody titers induced may be somewhat lower.

PATHOLOGY. Death from postnatal rubella is usually due to encephalitis. Thus most autopsies describe only the brain findings. Since 1962, it has been possible to investigate the pathogenesis and to correlate clinical findings with virologic events. After initial invasion of the upper respiratory tract, virus spreads to local lymphoid tissue, where it multiplies and initiates a viremia of approximately 7 days' duration. Respiratory tract shedding of virus and the viremia rise to peak levels until the onset of rash, at which time the latter becomes undetectable, whereas respiratory secretions contain diminishing quantities of virus over the succeeding 5 to 15 days. Specific serum antibodies can be demonstrated with the onset of rash, and circulating immune complexes are detectable soon thereafter.

Congenital Rubella. Necropsies of fetal and neonatal victims of intrauterine infection have shown a variety of embryonal defects related to developmental arrest involving all three germ layers.

The virus establishes chronic persistent infection of many tissues, with resultant intrauterine growth retardation. Delayed and disordered organogenesis produces embryopathic structural defects of the eye, brain, heart, and large arteries; continued viral infection during the fetal and postnatal period causes organ and tissue damage, e.g., hepatitis, nephritis, myocarditis, pneumonia, osteitis, meningitis, cochlear degeneration, and pancreatitis with the development of diabetes.

CLINICAL MANIFESTATIONS. *Postnatally Acquired Rubella.* Twelve to 19 days after exposure, the onset of rubella is manifested by the appearance of a rash with mild accompanying constitutional symptoms of malaise and occasionally sore throat. Enlargement of the postauricular and suboccipital nodes generally appears about a week prior to rash. Moderate fever may accompany or precede the rash. Generalized peripheral lymphadenopathy and, more rarely, splenomegaly may occur.

The exanthem of rubella is usually apparent within 24 hours of the first symptoms as a faint macular erythema that first involves the face and neck. Characterized by its brevity and evanescence, it spreads rapidly to the trunk and extremities, sometimes leaving one site even as it appears at the next. The pink macules that constitute the rash blanch with pressure and rarely stain the skin. Rubella virus has been isolated from the skin lesions as well as from uninvolved sites. The truncal rash may coalesce, but the lesions on the extremities remain discrete. The eruption usually vanishes by the third day. Rubella may occur without rash. In the absence of an epidemic and of serologic or virologic confirmation, the clinical diagnosis of rubella is not reliable.

COMPLICATIONS. Recovery is almost always prompt and uneventful. In contrast to measles, secondary bacterial infections are not encountered in rubella. Transient polyarthralgia and polyarthritis are more common among adolescents and adults with rubella, particularly females. They appear 3 or more days after onset of rash and may last 5 to 10 days. The knees and joints of the hands and wrists are most often involved. Surveys during urban epidemics have revealed rates of 5 to 15% in males and 10 to 35% in females.

Thrombocytopenia, when sought by serial platelet counts, is common but rarely of clinical consequence. A meningoencephalitis of short duration may occur 1 to 6 days after the appearance of rash. Its incidence is estimated at 1 in 5000 cases, and it is fatal in approximately 20% of those afflicted. Rubella encephalopathy is not associated with demyelinization, in contrast to other postviral encephalitides. Survivors may have electroencephalographic abnormalities, but intellectual function seems to be preserved.

Congenital Rubella. Congenital transplacental infection of the fetus occurs as a consequence of maternal infection, usually in the first 4 months of pregnancy. Virus is demonstrable in placental and fetal tissues obtained by therapeutic abortion at that time. If pregnancy is not interrupted, fetal infection persists, and on delivery of the infant, virus is recoverable from the throat, urine, conjunctivae, bone marrow, and cerebrospinal fluid of the living infant and from most organs at autopsy. From 20 to 80% of infants born to mothers infected in the first trimester of pregnancy have stigmata of infection readily recognizable in the first year of life. These include cardiac lesions and eye defects, e.g., cataracts, glaucoma, retinitis, microphthalmia. Most infants in whom virus is detectable do not have evidence of disease at birth or may simply have intrauterine growth retardation. In others, more severe disease occurs. Most prominent of these manifestations is thrombocytopenic purpura, which disappears soon after birth. Hepatosplenomegaly with active hepatitis may persist for months. Other involvement includes interstitial pneumonia, meningoencephalitis, hearing loss of varying extent, and lesions of the long bones. Recently, a progressive panencephalitis simulating subacute sclerosing panencephalitis has been observed in the second decade following congenital infection. The long-term sequelae for infants with congenital rubella include psychomotor retardation, hearing loss, retinopathy, and diabetes.

A striking finding has been the persistence of virus in the pharynx, urine, and cerebrospinal fluid for as long as 1 year after birth in 7% of infants. Infective virus was found in a congenital cataract after 3 years. This evidence of continuing viral synthesis occurs coincidentally with circulating antibody. The character of the antibody changes during the first months from maternal IgG to IgM, indicating a primary response of the infant to the persisting viral antigen. Studies of older infants and children with stigmata of congenital rubella show them to be free of demonstrable virus and to possess the IgG immunoglobulins that characteristically persist after other viral infections.

DIAGNOSIS. Rubella may be diagnosed clinically with assurance only during an epidemic. Distinction from measles may be made on the basis of fainter, nonstaining rash, the milder course, and the minimal or absent systemic complaints. Sore throat is a more prominent complaint in scarlet fever; the course of infectious mononucleosis is often more protracted, and splenomegaly is more frequent than in rubella. Specific diagnosis of rubella is made by isolating the virus in any of several cell culture systems or by demonstrating a rise in hemagglutination-inhibiting (HI), ELISA, or complement-fixing antibody during infection.

PROGNOSIS. Complete recovery from postnatally acquired rubella is almost invariable. The rare deaths attributable to rubella follow the infrequent complication of meningoencephalitis. Infection in pregnancy constitutes a grave hazard to the fetus but not to the mother.

TREATMENT. There is no specific antiviral therapy. Few patients suffer discomfort severe enough to warrant symptomatic medication. Headache and myalgia or arthritis may be controlled by analgesics.

PREVENTION. *Passive Immunization.* Administration of gamma globulin to the pregnant woman may only mask her symptoms of infection and not protect the fetus from viral invasions. Thus its use may only obscure the picture and confound decision about the need to terminate the pregnancy.

Active Immunization. Rubella may be prevented in children and adults by parenteral attenuated live virus vaccines produced in cell cultures. Seroconversion rates after immunization are at least 98% with the current RA 27/3 vaccine. Joint symptoms are less common than with the older HPV 7-DE strain, occurring in about 2.5% of adults. Arthritis occurs 13 to 19 days following immunization and lasts 2 to 11 days. The fingers are most often affected, with the wrists and knees less commonly involved. Arthralgias generally begin 10 to 25 days following vaccination and last 1 to 9 days. Joint symptoms are less common in men than in women. In children, vaccination is attended by little or no reaction.

It was initially recommended in the United States that immunization be carried out principally in childhood. There now is a more aggressive attempt to immunize those remaining susceptible women and adolescent girls. Current policy recommends vaccinating all such persons who have no history of previous rubella immunizations. Postpartum immunization of those found to be seronegative during pregnancy is encouraged. Although occasionally vaccine virus has been transmitted to the newborn by breast milk, this has proven to be of little consequence. Only nonpregnant individuals should be immunized, and contraception, when appropriate, should be carried out for at least 3 months after vaccination. Inadvertent administration of vaccine to pregnant women has occasionally resulted in attenuated vaccine viruses infection of the fetus. In more than 500 such cases studied, no infant has been observed with congenital malformations as a result. The frequency of fetal infection with the RA 27/3 vaccine currently used is less than with the previous rubella vaccine. Use of vaccine in the United States prevented a large epidemic of rubella expected in the early 1970's and has reduced the reported annual occurrence from more than 50,000 cases annually, with epidemic peaks of 200,000 to 500,000, to an all-time low in 1988 of 221 cases. A slight increase in cases of rubella accompanied by cases of congenital rubella syndrome occurred in 1990.

Burke JP, Hinman AR, Krugman S (eds.): International symposium on prevention of congenital rubella infection. Rev Infect Dis 7(Suppl):1, 1985. *Fifteen years of vaccine use summarized by investigators from the developed nations.*

Centers for Disease Control and Prevention: Rubella and congenital rubella syndrome—United States. MMWR 38:173, 1989. *A summary report of progress in rubella "eradication" in the United States.*

Gregg NM: Congenital cataract following German measles in the mother. Trans Ophthal Soc Aust 3:35, 1941. *The original "classic" report associating rubella in pregnancy with congenital malformations.*

Proceedings of the International Conference on Rubella Immunization. Am J Dis Child 118, July 1969. *A compendium on rubella and congenital rubella.*

Sherman FE, Michaels RH, Kenny FM: Acute encephalopathy (encephalitis) complicating rubella. JAMA 192:675, 1965. *A clinical, pathologic, and epidemiologic study of rubella encephalitis.*

Townsend JJ, Stroop WG, Baringer JR, et al.: Neuropathology of progressive rubella panencephalitis after childhood rubella. Neurology 32:185, 1982. *A review of the clinical and neuropathologic findings.*

Weibel RE, Vilarejos VM, Klein EB, et al.: Clinical and laboratory studies of live attenuated RA 27/3 and HPV 77-DE rubella virus vaccines (40931). Proc Soc Exper Biol Med 165:44, 1980. *A description of the clinical and serologic response to rubella vaccine.*

336 VARICELLA (Chickenpox, Shingles)

Philip A. Brunell

DEFINITION. Varicella, or chickenpox, is an acute communicable disease characterized by a generalized vesicular rash. Because it is highly contagious, most individuals contract it in childhood. Herpes zoster, due to reactivation of varicella-zoster virus (VZV), is a dermatomal cutaneous eruption.

ETIOLOGY. Varicella is caused by VZV, a member of the α-herpes virinae subfamily. This enveloped herpesvirus contains a number of glycoproteins, some of which bear some homology to those of other members of the human herpesvirus group. The double-stranded DNA has a molecular weight of approximately 80 million. There is some diversity in the restriction enzyme patterns among wild isolates; there is only a single serotype. Although the human is the only known natural host, a closely related virus has been identified in a simian species.

EPIDEMIOLOGY. Varicella is a highly contagious disease. After continuing household exposure, as would occur in a family, almost all susceptibles are infected. The subclinical attack rate is believed to be no more than 4%. The results of nonhousehold exposure are less certain. Chickenpox may be most contagious the day prior to the onset of rash. Chickenpox is contagious for no more than 5 days after the appearance of the first lesion. Children may return to school at this time or earlier if the lesions are crusted. The incubation period is usually about 14 days. Ninety-nine percent of the cases occur 10 to 20 days following exposure. The disease is known to be spread by direct contact. Airborne spread also has been demonstrated, most notably in hospitals.

Nosocomial spread of varicella has been well documented. This has occurred room to room by airborne spread as well as by patient-to-patient or staff-to-patient contact. Adults with herpes zoster who are hospitalized are less likely to cause secondary cases of chickenpox among adult contacts than among children. The reason is that hospitalized children are more likely to be susceptible to chickenpox than hospitalized adults. Strict isolation is recommended for hospitalized patients with varicella and for children or immunocompromised adults with herpes zoster. Adults with localized herpes zoster require less stringent isolation procedures.

Most cases of chickenpox occur in childhood. Most children contract chickenpox either in day care situations or shortly after they enter school. Fewer than 2% of the cases occur following the second decade. Approximately 10% of hospital workers with a negative history are seronegative. Almost all individuals with a positive history are seropositive. A single attack of chickenpox usually confers lifetime immunity.

There appears to be more efficient transmission of disease in temperate than in tropical climates. The reason for this is uncertain but may be due to temperature rather than urbanization. Varicella occurs most commonly during the late winter and spring months, the peak being about in March. Sporadic cases occur into the early summer and start in late fall.

Varicella is more common than other childhood diseases during the early months of life. In this situation the disease is generally mild. Maternal antibody transferred across the placenta may not be as effective in protecting infants against this disease as are antibodies against other viruses. However, nursery outbreaks have been rare. Children who develop varicella during the early months of life or are exposed *in utero* have a greater risk of developing herpes zoster in childhood.

PATHOGENESIS. Replication of virus is believed to occur initially in the epithelial cells of the mucosa of the upper respiratory tract. Since VZV produces a disseminated rash, one can assume that bloodstream distribution must have occurred. Virus can be isolated from white blood cells from 5 days prior to 2 days following the appearance of rash. After clinical recovery, the virus infection continues in the absence of clinical symptoms in a latent phase. During this time, messenger RNA (mRNA) can be demonstrated in non-neuronal cells in dorsal root ganglia. The segmental distribution of herpes zoster (see Ch. 426.3), which usually occurs decades after the initial VZV infection, is consistent with a dorsal root ganglion site for the latent virus. In uncomplicated chickenpox, rises in serum aminotransferases levels have been demonstrated. This suggests that there is visceral involvement in the normal course of this disease.

The vesicular lesions of varicella contain a predominance of polymorphonuclear leukocytes even during the early phase of vesicle formation. Multinuclear giant cells are occasionally found in the base of the lesions, often containing eosinophilic intranuclear inclusions. Large amounts of virus can be demonstrated in vesicular fluid by electron microscopy.

Postmortem descriptions of patients with varicella have usually involved immunocompromised subjects. In these cases, inflammatory changes are usually found in multiple organs, including the lung, liver, spleen, and skin, together with anoxic changes in the brain. Similar involvement is found in the newborn. Focal areas of necrosis and intranuclear eosinophilic inclusions in mononuclear cells are common. Changes in otherwise normal individuals usually include myocardial and pulmonary lesions. On microscopic examination, the brain has demonstrated edema with some lymphocyte cuffing around the cerebral vessels.

CLINICAL MANIFESTATIONS. Varicella is characterized by a generalized eruption that is centripetal in distribution; erythematous macules, papules, vesicles, and scabbed lesions may be present at the same time. The vesicles are superficial, with varying amounts of erythema at their bases. Adults tend to have considerably more erythema than children. During the early phase of the eruption, lesions are found on the face, scalp, and trunk. By running the fingers through the hair, one often detects lesions that were not visible. Later, new lesions appear on the extremities. By this time, the earlier lesions have dried and crusted. Excoriations are common, attesting to the pruritic nature of the lesions. Mucous membranes of the conjunctiva and oropharynx are more frequently involved in adults than in children. New lesions continue to appear over a 3- or 4-day period, after which the rate of their appearance decelerates markedly.

There is a striking variation in the extent of systemic symptoms associated with varicella. Most children have a mild illness with few systemic complaints and an average maximal temperature of about 38.3°C. It is more common for adults to have considerable malaise, muscle ache, arthralgia, and headache. These may precede the first skin lesions by 24 to 48 hours.

In the immunocompromised subject, the disease often is very severe. Approximately 30% of children with leukemia or lymphoma who get varicella and receive no prophylaxis or treatment develop "progressive varicella." Vesicles continue to erupt into the second week of illness, accompanied by high fever. Lesions tend to be deep seated rather than superficial. Toward the end of the first week and the beginning of the second week, the lesions are more common on the extremities than on the trunk. Indeed, the distribution and lesions may resemble those with smallpox. Visceral involvement occurs in about 30% of these patients. The lung, liver, pancreas, and brain may be involved. Death occurs in about 9% of immunocompromised patients who develop varicella. The death usually is due to pulmonary involvement. Patients with HIV infections may have recurrent attacks of varicella in the absence of exposure or a persistent eruption that may continue for months.

Varicella in pregnant women is believed to be more serious than in nongravid females; fatalities have been reported. The rate of fetal wastage is not increased. About 1% of infants born to mothers who have had varicella early in pregnancy, however, have been found at birth to have "varicella embryopathy." The infants are born with cerebral damage and a variety of ocular findings, and characteristically they have a scarred, atrophic limb. The children are generally small for gestational age and may have other abnormalities as well. When mothers develop chickenpox within a few days of delivery, "varicella of the newborn" may occur. If the onset of varicella is between 5 and 10 days after birth, it is associated with a higher risk of serious disease and even death.

Bacterial infections of the skin are the most common complication of chickenpox in childhood. The rate of complications is much higher in adults than in children. Although fewer than 2% of the reported cases occur after the second decade, almost 35% of the deaths occur in this group. A disproportionate rate of hospitalization also is found in adults. The major complications of varicella in adults are encephalitis and pneumonia.

Approximately 1 in 400 adults with chickenpox are hospitalized for pneumonia. In a prospective study, however, it was found that only 6% of young adults with chickenpox had respiratory symptoms, whereas 16% had roentgenographic evidence of pulmonary involvement.

Infection produces a diffuse interstitial type of pneumonia with hypoxia resulting from poor diffusion of gases. Diffuse calcification of the lung parenchyma may be found years after recovery.

Encephalitis in childhood is most commonly manifested by a cerebellitis, which usually occurs at the end of the first week or during the second week following onset of rash. This complication is almost always self-limited. In contrast, an acute form of encephalitis usually occurring soon after the onset of rash often has a fulminating course; it is characterized by severe brain swelling. It has been estimated that as many as 20% of cases of Reye's syndrome may be preceded by chickenpox. A variety of other neurologic complications, including optic neuritis, transverse myelitis, and Guillain-Barré syndrome, may be associated with chickenpox. Hemorrhagic complications of chickenpox include thrombocytopenic purpura and purpura fulminans. Nephritis, myocarditis, and arthritis also have been described.

DIAGNOSIS. There is usually little difficulty in recognizing typical forms of chickenpox, particularly if there has been a history of exposure. The diagnosis may be more difficult in immunocompromised hosts, because they may have features of progressive varicella with visceral involvement. Modified cases of chickenpox may occur following passive or active immunization. These cases may require laboratory confirmation. The most common sources of confusion are insect bites, generalized herpes in the immunocompromised host, rickettsialpox, or "hand, foot, and mouth disease" caused by an enterovirus. The differentiation of disseminated herpes zoster from chickenpox may be difficult. The former usually has dermatomal involvement initially. Generalization usually does not occur until 3 to 5 days after onset of the zosteriform rash. In severely immunocompromised patients, e.g., bone marrow recipients, generalization may occur earlier and the clinical differentiation may be difficult.

The Tzanck smear is a frequently used laboratory aid for diagnosis. Multinucleated giant cells identify the lesions as being caused by one of the herpesviruses, but this is not specific for varicella. A properly stained smear also contains eosinophilic intranuclear inclusions. Virus can usually be isolated during the first 3 or 4 days after the onset of lesions. The virus is quite labile; it must be stored at −70°C if cultures cannot be inoculated immediately. Our preference is to collect vesicular fluid in unheparinized capillary tubes and put the specimen directly into human embryonic lung fibroblasts at the bedside. Specimens from throat, urine, or stool are of little value for isolation of virus. Polymerase chain reaction (PCR) can be used to demonstrate the presence of virus in vesicular fluid and throat swabs.

Serologic confirmation of diagnosis can be made using a variety of techniques. The enzyme-linked immunosorbent assay (ELISA) and complement fixation are the most generally available. The laboratory director should be consulted regarding appropriate time of collection of specimens as well as interpretation of data. Because complement-fixing antibody generally does not persist, a single high titer often is confirmatory evidence of recent infection.

Determining the immune status of contacts can be done with the ELISA, latex agglutination test, or the fluorescent antibody test against membrane antigen (FAMA). The ELISA is a much simpler and technically less demanding test. Because complement-fixing antibody is lost rapidly after infection, it cannot be used for determining susceptibility. Fluorescence antibody test using fixed cells sometimes yields false-positive results. A number of laboratories have developed tests for VZV immunoglobulin M (IgM). It was hoped that these might differentiate varicella from herpes zoster in cases in which this was unclear. Unfortunately, these tests have not been very useful, as VZV IgM is present in the sera of many patients with acute herpes zoster.

TREATMENT. Major therapeutic objectives are the prevention of superinfection and relief of pruritus. The latter can be accomplished frequently by application of calamine lotion. Occasionally this does not suffice, and a systemic antipruritic agent such as trimeprazine may be necessary. It is advisable to trim and file nails to reduce the damage from scratching. Bacterial superinfection can best be prevented by encouraging daily bathing with an antibacterial soap. Following this with a colloidal starch bath also may be useful for relieving pruritus.

Relief of systemic symptoms may require additional medication such as acetaminophen, although this may increase pruritus. Salicylates are contraindicated, since there is an association between their use and development of Reye's syndrome in children. Special care should be taken to be certain that over-the-counter medications containing salicylates are avoided.

Some patients, particularly those who are immunocompromised, may require antiviral therapy. Intravenous acyclovir has been shown to be effective in immunocompromised children with varicella. A dose of 500 mg per square meter repeated every 8 hours has been used. VZV is generally less sensitive to acyclovir than herpes simplex. For this reason, larger doses are probably required. Studies on the use of oral antiviral drugs in the treatment of varicella have demonstrated some efficacy. Initial reports indicate that prophylaxis for 7 days starting 7 days following exposure is more effective. Patients who are sick enough to require antiviral therapy probably should be treated with parenteral rather than oral medication.

Patients on high doses of steroids or other immunosuppressive drugs who have been exposed to chickenpox are at high risk of developing progressive varicella. Steroids appear to be most deleterious when given during the incubation period. They have been used in the treatment of pneumonia after the eruption has occurred without any obvious deleterious effects.

PREVENTION. Immune serum globulin does not prevent varicella. Massive doses are required to produce measurable modification. If prevention or modification is indicated, varicella-zoster immune globulin (VZIG) should be given. Candidates are those who (1) are susceptible, (2) are at high risk of developing complicated varicella, and (3) have had an adequate exposure to the disease. Any individuals fulfilling the first two criteria who had a household exposure should receive prophylaxis. It is often difficult to judge the degree of intimacy in other types of exposure. Reference to guidelines published by the Academy of Pediatrics or Centers for Disease Control and Prevention (CDC) may be helpful.

Patients considered at high risk are (1) those who are immunocompromised by virtue of either disease or immunosuppressive therapy, (2) infants born to mothers who have had varicella less than 5 days prior to or 2 days following delivery, (3) certain premature infants, (4) bone marrow transplantation recipients regardless of susceptibility, and (5) certain adults.

A history of varicella is usually reliable in both adults and children. Children who have a negative history are usually susceptible. Serologic testing of adults who have a negative history is useful if it does not delay administration of VZIG. VZIG should be given as soon as possible following exposure and has not been shown to be effective if delayed more than 96 hours.

Nosocomial infection following herpes zoster or varicella has been well documented. These outbreaks may result in significant morbidity and cause disruption of hospital routine. These situations are best managed by serologic screening of personnel and by permitting only those who are seropositive to care for patients with varicella or herpes zoster. Patients who are hospitalized with varicella should be isolated 7 days. Susceptible persons who are exposed to active cases should be isolated from the tenth to the twenty-first day after the last exposure if they cannot be discharged. Whenever possible, patients with chickenpox should be isolated in a room with negative pressure in order to prevent dissemination of infectious virus to other patients. Airborne spread in hospitals has been documented.

An attenuated live vaccine has been licensed for use abroad and is being considered for licensure in the United States. Susceptible adults who receive the vaccine have some local reactions and occasionally develop a varicelliform rash. Protection against infection is less complete than in children. Two doses 2 months apart are recommended for adults. In normal children, the vaccine is virtually benign and appears to offer very good protection. Initial data suggest that herpes zoster would be no more frequent and perhaps less common following immunization than following natural infection.

Advisory Committee on Immunization Practice: Varicella-zoster immune globulin for the prevention of chickenpox. MMWR 33:84, 95, 1984. *Guidelines for passive immunization against chickenpox.*

Brunell PA: Varicella in pregnancy, the fetus and the newborn: Problems in management. J Infect Dis 166:542, 1992. *A comprehensive review of varicella in pregnancy.*

Brunell PA: Varicella vaccine—where are we? Pediatrics 78:721, 1986. *A symposium on the epidemiology, cost burden, and complications of varicella and on varicella vaccine.*

Brunell PA: Varicella-zoster virus. *In* Rose NR, Friedman H, Fahey JL (eds.): Manual of Clinical Laboratory Immunity, 4th ed. Washington, DC, American Society for Microbiology, 1992, pp 560–562. *A review of serologic tests for varicella-zoster antibody.*

First International Conference on Varicella. J Infect Dis 166 (Suppl 1):S1, 1992. *A comprehensive review of basic and clinical information.*

Srugo I, Israele V, Wittek, AE, et al.: Clinical manifestations of varicella-zoster virus infections in human immunodeficiency virus–infected children. Am J Dis Child 147:742, 1993. *A description of the various manifestations of VZV infection in HIV-infected children.*

Varicella-zoster infections. Report of the Committee on Infectious Diseases, 22nd ed. Evanston, IL, American Academy of Pediatrics, 1994, pp 510–517. *A useful guide to management of patients exposed to varicella, including control of nosocomial infection.*

337   VARIOLA AND VACCINIA
Donald A. Henderson

The Thirty-third World Health Assembly "declares solemnly that the world and all its peoples have won freedom from smallpox" (Resolution 33.3, May 8, 1980, Geneva, Switzerland).

This announcement was made some 30 months after the last known endemic case, in Somalia, on October 26, 1977. In 1978, two additional cases of smallpox occurred in Birmingham, England, as a result of a laboratory infection, but except for these cases, no others have been found.

To confirm that eradication had been achieved, each country where smallpox had been endemic since 1967 and those at risk of importations conducted a search for cases for at least 2 years after the last known case. At the end of this period, World Health Organization (WHO)–appointed international commissions reviewed the records of work and conducted extensive field visits to confirm the results. Between 1973 and 1979, 21 different commissions visited and certified eradication in 49 countries.

Finally, a Global Commission for the Certification of Smallpox Eradication reviewed the findings and made special field visits. After satisfying itself that eradication had been achieved, the commission reported its findings to the World Health Assembly. The assembly members concurred and recommended that "smallpox vaccination be discontinued in every country except for investigators at special risk" and advised that "an international certificate of vaccination against smallpox should no longer be required of any traveller."

Thus concluded the first successful global program to eradicate a disease—one that had proved to be one of the most devastating known to humanity.

HISTORY (Fig. 337–1). Because of the need for variola virus to spread continually from person to person to survive, historians speculate that it emerged after the first agricultural settlements, about 10,000 B.C. In ancient times, only a few populated areas, probably in India, could have sustained its transmission. In the early Christian era, descriptions suggestive of smallpox appear in historical accounts of western Asia, and by the eighth century it had established itself in Europe. Central and southern Africa were probably infected sometime later.

Case-fatality rates of 20% and greater were characteristic, and where population densities permitted the disease to become endemic, virtually all persons eventually contracted smallpox. At the end of the eighteenth century, it was killing an estimated 400,000 Europeans each year and was responsible for one third of all cases of blindness.

VACCINATION. Edward Jenner discovered in 1796 that smallpox could be prevented by "vaccination" with material from a cowpox lesion. Before his discovery, the only defense against smallpox was deliberately to inoculate (variolate) scabs or pustular material from smallpox patients into the skin of susceptible persons. The resulting infection was usually less severe than infection acquired naturally by inhalation. Although case-fatality rates among those with in-

duced infection were sometimes as low as 1%, they readily transmitted infection to others.

During the nineteenth century, vaccination was increasingly widely practiced in temperate-climate countries, but the difficulties of sustaining the virus through arm-to-arm inoculation resulted in an uncertain supply.

In the industrialized countries, smallpox incidence declined steadily, and Europe and North America succeeded in interrupting smallpox transmission after World War II. In these areas, the impetus for vaccination had diminished early in the century when a less virulent strain, variola minor, with a case-fatality rate of about 1%, replaced variola major. In most of Africa, however, 5 to 15% died of smallpox, and in Asia the virulent variola major prevailed. Neither in Africa nor in Asia was vaccination widely practiced.

ERADICATION OF SMALLPOX. Smallpox was a problem to all countries. Even those without disease feared importations and conducted vaccination programs. Although the global control of smallpox was in everyone's best interests, progress was slow. Finally, in 1959, the World Health Assembly decided that a global eradication program should be undertaken. During the succeeding 7 years, a number of countries undertook campaigns, but few succeeded in interrupting smallpox transmission (see Fig. 337–1).

In 1967, when a definitive eradication program was decided, four geographic reservoirs of smallpox were identified: (1) Africa south of the Sahara, (2) a group of Southeast Asian countries extending from Bangladesh through India, Nepal, Pakistan, and Afghanistan, (3) Indonesia, and (4) Brazil. The estimated population of these countries was more than 1 billion persons.

WHO's strategy called for each country to undertake a program of vaccination with the objective of reaching at least 80% of the population during a 2- to 3-year period. During this time, a reliable reporting system was to be developed to identify foci of smallpox that would be eliminated by isolation of patients and vaccination of contacts. Extensive vaccination was believed necessary to increase population immunity and so reduce the number of cases to permit disease surveillance and containment activities to be effective.

Experience soon showed that the surveillance-containment strategy was more effective than had been thought, and this proved to be a key to success. In part, this was due to the unique characteristics of smallpox. An infected patient was able to transmit infection only from the time of first appearance of rash until the last scabs had separated. There were no chronic carriers or individuals with latent, transmissible infection and no animal reservoir. The rash was sufficiently characteristic to be diagnosed with a high degree of accuracy. The presence or absence of smallpox in an area could thus be reliably determined without laboratory studies. Moreover, approximately two thirds of recovered patients had characteristic residual facial scars. Thus it was possible to determine both the present status of smallpox and its past history in an area.

To persist, smallpox virus had to be transmitted from patient to susceptible contact. By isolation of the patient and by vaccination of contacts, a barrier to transmission was created. In small villages and in scattered populations, chains of transmission often terminated without intervention. Because smallpox did not spread rapidly, and then only to those in close contact, secondary cases usually were found among neighbors and relatives. A patient rarely infected more than two to three others. Because of these factors, early detection of outbreaks and their containment proved effective in stopping transmission.

Smallpox vaccine that conferred excellent and durable immunity was important to success. Studies revealed vaccine efficacy ratios of >90% after 20 years. Because the lyophilized vaccine retained its potency after incubation at 37°C for at least 1 month, the logistics of vaccine storage and distribution were comparatively simple. Vaccination was greatly facilitated by the inexpensive, newly developed bifurcated needle. The technique was learned quickly and produced a high proportion of successful vaccinations.

PROGRESS IN THE PROGRAM (see Fig. 337–1). By 1969, eradication programs were in progress in all the infected and immediately adjacent countries except for Ethiopia. Four years later, smallpox had been eliminated from most of Africa and in Asia, there remained only four smallpox-endemic countries: India, Pakistan, Nepal, and Bangladesh. However, the population of these four was over 700 million, and the techniques of surveillance and con-

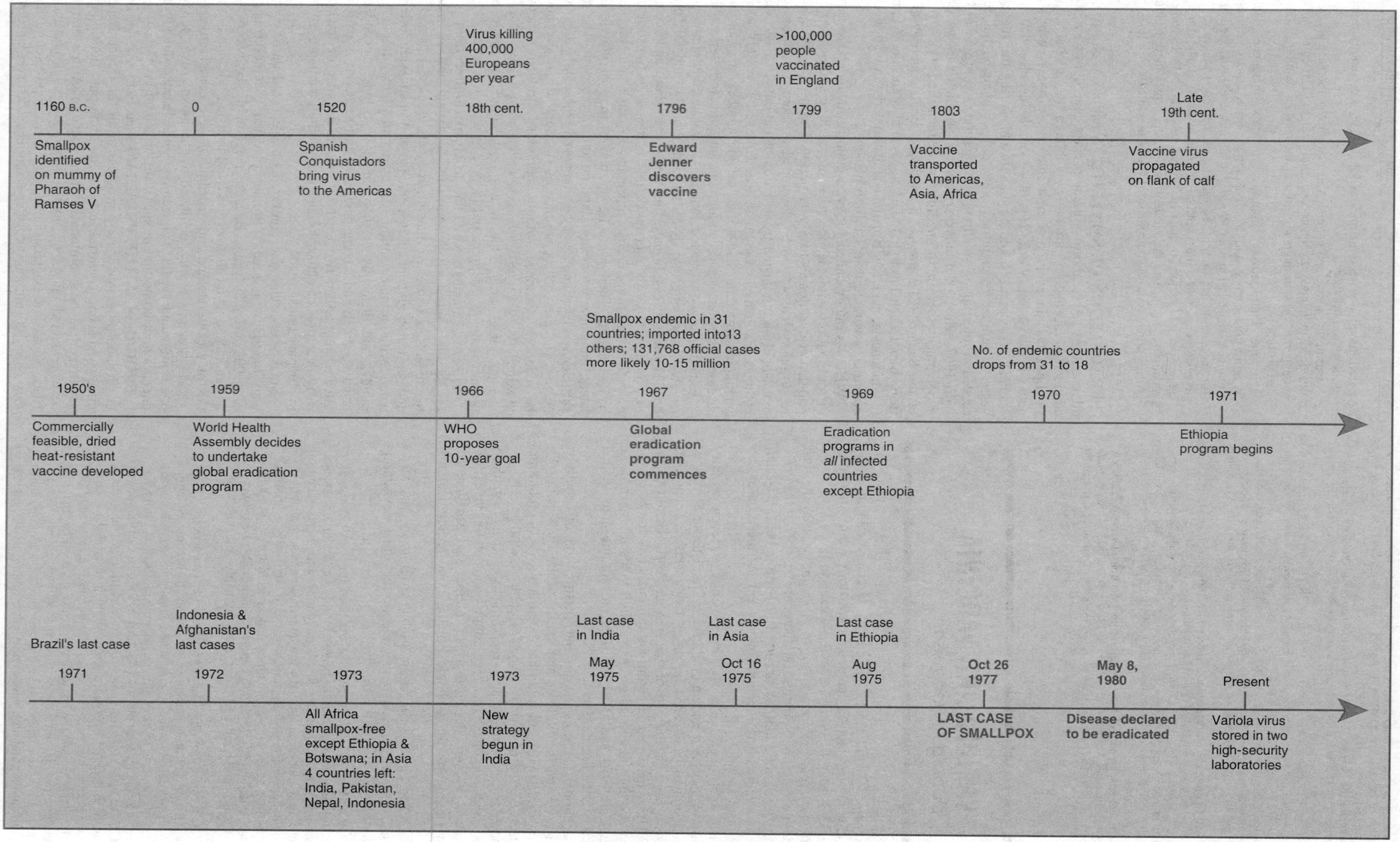

FIGURE 337–1. Smallpox timeline.

tainment that had been applied in other areas proved to be less successful.

A new strategy in India began in the autumn of 1973 (Basu and colleagues). Far more rapid case detection and more effective containment of outbreaks were required. Accordingly, for 1 week each month more than 100,000 health workers were mobilized to search house by house to detect cases. Hundreds of special teams contained the outbreaks that were found. Between searches, the teams asked questions at markets and in schools to uncover rumors of cases. By the summer of 1974, new cases began to decline, and a cash reward was offered to anyone who reported a case (see Fig. 337–1). In October 1975 the last case occurred in Asia and in October 1977 the world's last naturally occurring infection.

POSSIBLE SOURCES FOR A RETURN OF SMALLPOX. As of 1994, variola virus was known to exist in only two laboratories, where it was kept under high-security conditions.

Extensive studies had been conducted since 1967 to discover a possible animal or other natural reservoir of the virus. None was found. However, some 400 cases of a newly recognized disease that is clinically indistinguishable from smallpox but caused by the related monkeypox virus occurred in seven central and west African countries between 1970 and 1990. Genome maps of this and other animal poxviruses reveal many differences between them and variola.

The recurrence of smallpox resulting from a deliberate release of variola virus cannot be ruled out. However, the potential damage of such an act should not be exaggerated. Smallpox does not spread rapidly, and an outbreak caused in this manner should be able to be contained within 3 to 4 weeks.

Barring improbable circumstances, a human case of smallpox will never again be seen. However, the problem of mistaken diagnosis is a real one. For this reason, WHO medical officers with expertise in diagnosis remain on call to investigate rumors.

VARIOLA (Smallpox)

ETIOLOGY. Variola virus is one of a group of orthopoxviruses that includes vaccinia, monkeypox, rabbitpox, cowpox, camelpox, buffalopox, and ectromelia. The poxviruses are the largest viruses so recognized. The virions are brick-shaped structures with a diameter of about 200 μm. The genome consists of a single molecule of a double-stranded DNA.

INCIDENCE AND PREVALENCE. The disease was declared to be eradicated on May 8, 1980.

PATHOLOGY AND PATHOGENESIS. The site of entry of the smallpox virus was probably the respiratory tract. In the 12-day incubation period, the virus multiplied in the regional lymphoid tissues. Viremia occurred at the onset of fever and continued during the first 2 or 3 days of the pre-eruptive phase. During this time, the virus localized in mucous membranes, skin, and internal tissues. Virus multiplication in the epithelial cells of the skin and mucous membranes caused pustulation. Antibodies appeared as early as the fourth day of disease.

CLINICAL MANIFESTATIONS. The incubation period of smallpox was about 12 days with a range of 7 to 17 days. The illness began with severe malaise, prostration, head- and backache, and high fever lasting 2 to 5 days (Rao). Following the initial febrile period, a macular rash developed, which quickly became papular, and within 2 days the papules developed into vesicles and then pustules. On the eighth or ninth day of rash, crusting began. The scabs separated over the succeeding 2 to 3 weeks, leaving pigment-free skin. Subsequently, scarring or pitting developed. The eruption was characteristically more severe on the face and the distal parts of the arms and legs, and less severe over the trunk and abdomen. Lesions were often found on the palms of the hands and the soles of the feet.

VARIOLA MINOR AND INTERMEDIATE FORMS. In the early twentieth century, a milder clinical form of smallpox (variola minor, or alastrim) became prevalent in the Americas, Europe, and parts of southern and eastern Africa. Case-fatality rates were ≤1%. Variola major and minor were distinct, although at times coexisting. Each of the two types gave rise to illnesses with a wide spectrum of severity. There was cross-protection between each of these forms and vaccinia.

DIFFERENTIAL DIAGNOSIS. Most cases of smallpox could readily be identified by the typical deep-seated rash, the centrifugal distribution of lesions, and the fact that in any area on the body all lesions were at the same stage of development. The infrequent severe hemorrhagic cases were frequently mistakenly diagnosed as meningococcemia, acute leukemia, or drug toxicity. Mild cases with few lesions were confused with varicella. Of help in diagnosis, however, was the fact that in any outbreak ≥80% of the cases were clinically typical.

LABORATORY TESTS. Diagnosis of a poxvirus infection can be rapidly established by electron microscopic identification of virus particles in vesicular or pustular fluid or scabs. Differentiation among poxviruses requires that the virus be isolated on chick chorioallantoic membrane and its properties characterized by specific biologic tests. WHO Reference Laboratories are prepared to undertake necessary diagnostic studies.

TREATMENT. No specific treatment is available.

IDENTIFICATION OF A SUSPECT CASE OF SMALLPOX. Because smallpox has been eradicated, the occurrence of a single case has profound international implications. Should a suspect case be identified, *immediate notification of local, state, and national health officials is essential.* Most suspected cases in recent years have been cases of varicella in adults. Should a case prove to be smallpox, the source of virus must be assumed to be inadvertent or deliberate release from a laboratory. A suspect patient should be placed under strict isolation. Additional measures will be dictated by epidemiologic circumstances.

VACCINIA (Vaccination)

No countries now require international certificates of vaccination, and none conducts civilian vaccination programs. Several countries, including the United States, continue to vaccinate military personnel. Vaccination is recommended only for investigators who are working with poxviruses in the laboratory.

THE VACCINE. Vaccinia virus is grown in tissue culture or on the scarified flank of a calf. After purification and the addition of stabilizing agents, the suspension is freeze dried. Inoculated intradermally, vaccinia virus induces a mild infection and confers protection against all orthopoxviruses known to infect humans—monkeypox, variola, and cowpox.

VACCINE PROTECTION. Following successful vaccination, protection against variola is virtually complete for 5 years, but effectiveness wanes over time. In poxvirus laboratories, vaccination at least every 3 years has been customary.

RISKS OF VACCINATION. Those who are candidates for vaccination are adults, a diminishing proportion of whom have received primary vaccinations as children. Although the risk of serious complications is very low, primary vaccination of adults once had been thought to be associated with a higher incidence of serious complications. However, a special study of vaccination complications among military recruits failed to document any cases of the most important, postvaccinal encephalitis, among an estimated 2 million primary vaccinees.

FIRST VACCINATION (PRIMARY TAKE). Three days after vaccination, a papule appears at the vaccination site; the papule changes to a vesicle and by the seventh day is a fully developed pustule. It is whitish, umbilicated, and multilocular and contains clear lymph. An erythematous areola expands to reach a maximal diameter about 9 days after vaccination. A crust forms and falls off about 3 weeks after vaccination, leaving a scar.

REVACCINATION. When persons are vaccinated a second time, a gradation of cutaneous responses is observed. Individuals who have not been vaccinated for several decades may develop what appears to be a primary take. In persons with an intermediate level of immunity, development of the lesion is more rapid, and the maximal diameter of erythema is reached in 3 to 7 days. In the highly immune person, virus multiplication may not occur. In such persons, a hypersensitivity response to vaccinial protein may occur. A papule and sometimes a vesicle with erythema may develop, reaching its peak in 48 hours.

To distinguish the hypersensitivity type of reaction, which may be caused by heat-inactivated vaccine, from one in which virus multiplication has taken place, the site of inoculation is examined between the sixth and eighth days. If there is evidence of induration or congestion, virus multiplication may be assumed.

CONTRAINDICATIONS. Four groups of persons are at special risk of complications: (1) persons with eczema or other forms of chronic dermatitis; (2) pregnant women; (3) patients with leukemia, lymphoma, other reticuloendothelial malignancies, and AIDS; and (4) those receiving immunosuppressive drugs, especially glucocorticosteroids. Vaccinees in close contact with persons with eczema may infect them, sometimes with serious consequences. If vaccination is required for persons at special risk, vaccinia immune globulin (0.3 ml per kilogram intramuscularly) should be administered simultaneously.

COMPLICATIONS. *Postvaccinal Encephalitis.* Encephalitis following vaccination is a rare event and occurs between the eighth and fifteenth days. Paralysis, when it occurs, is generally spastic in type. Residual paralysis and other central nervous system symptoms may persist. There is no treatment. Studies conducted in the United States in 1963 and 1968 (Neff and colleagues, Lane and associates) revealed 28 cases, 9 fatal, among 11.3 million primary vaccinees. No cases occurred among 16.3 million revaccinees.

Progressive Vaccinia (Vaccinia Gangrenosa). Progressive vaccinia is an exceedingly rare but often fatal complication among vaccinated persons who have deficient immune responses. The initial vaccinial lesion fails to heal and progresses to involve adjacent skin with necrosis of tissue. Dissemination may result in metastatic vaccinial lesions in other parts of the skin, bones, or viscera. Treatment with vaccinia immune globulin is beneficial.

Eczema Vaccinatum. Eczema vaccinatum is sometimes a serious complication, which may occur in vaccinated persons with active or healed eczema, or in subjects in contact with recent vaccinees. The disease tends to localize at sites where eczematous lesions are or have been present. Vaccinia immune globulin is of help in therapy.

Generalized Vaccinia. Generalized vaccinia represents a secondary eruption resulting from bloodborne dissemination of vaccinia virus. Almost all cases occur after primary vaccination. The lesions become evident between 6 and 9 days after vaccination. The number of lesions may range from a few to a generalized involvement of the skin. It is a self-limited illness, and complete recovery occurs without specific therapy.

Fetal Vaccinia. Fetal vaccinia results from a bloodborne dissemination of vaccinia virus in the pregnant woman given primary vaccination. It may occur during any trimester of pregnancy and frequently results in death of the fetus.

Miscellaneous Complications. A great variety of rashes have been reported to be caused by vaccination. Most common are erythema multiforme and variously distributed urticarial, maculopapular, blotchy erythematous eruptions.

Basu RN, Jerek Z, Ward NA: The Eradication of Smallpox from India. New Delhi, India, World Health Organization, 1979. *A well-written, detailed, profusely illustrated book describing the epidemiologic and operational aspects of the program in India.*

Fenner F, Henderson DA, Jerek Z, et al.: Smallpox and its Eradication. Geneva, Switzerland, World Health Organization, 1988. *This 1400-page, extensively illustrated and referenced book is the definitive text, providing an historical account of smallpox control and eradication as well as a summary of current knowledge regarding the epidemiology, virology, and pathogenesis of the disease.*

Hopkins DR: Princes and Peasants: Smallpox in History. Chicago, University of Chicago Press, 1983. *The only comprehensive history of smallpox prepared in this century, this interesting and readable book complements that by Fenner and associates.*

Lane JM, Ruben FL, Neff JM, et al.: Complications of smallpox vaccination, 1968. N Engl J Med 281:138, 1969. *With the paper by Neff and co-workers, one of the few detailed studies of the frequency of complications following smallpox vaccination.*

Neff J, Lane JM, Pert JH, et al.: Complications of smallpox vaccination. N Engl J Med 276:1, 1967. *With the paper by Lane and associates, one of the few detailed studies of the frequency of complications following smallpox vaccination.*

Rao AR: Smallpox. Bombay, India, Kothari Book Depot, 1972. *Written by a clinician who treated more than 3000 cases, this book is an excellent reference on the clinical aspects of variola major.*

338 MUMPS

John W. Gnann, Jr.

Mumps is an acute systemic viral infection that is usually self-limited, occurs most commonly in school-aged children, and is clinically characterized by nonsuppurative parotitis.

VIROLOGY. Mumps virus is classified as a member of the Paramyxovirus family. Mumps virions are pleomorphic, roughly spherical, enveloped particles with an average diameter of 200 nm. Glycoprotein spikes project from the surface of the envelope, which encloses a helical nucleocapsid composed of nucleoproteins and linear, nonsegmented, single-stranded, negative-sense RNA. Humans are the only natural hosts for mumps virus, although infection can be induced experimentally in a variety of mammalian species. *In vitro,* mumps virus can be cultured in many mammalian cell lines and in embryonated hens' eggs.

EPIDEMIOLOGY. In unvaccinated urban populations, mumps is a disease of school-aged children, and >90% will have mumps antibodies by age 15. Before the mumps vaccine was released in the United States in 1967, mumps was an endemic disease with a seasonal peak of activity occurring between January and May. Mumps epidemics occurred at 2- to 5-year intervals. The largest number of cases reported in the United States was in 1941, when the incidence of mumps was 250 cases per 100,000 population. In 1968, when the vaccine was first entering clinical use, the incidence of mumps was 76 cases per 100,000 population. In 1985, only 2982 cases of mumps were reported, an incidence of 1.1 per 100,000 population, representing a 98% decline from the number of cases reported in 1967. Between 1985 and 1987, the incidence of mumps in the United States increased fivefold to 5.2 cases per 100,000 population. More than one third of the cases reported between 1985 and 1989 occurred in adolescents and young adults, reflecting the slow acceptance of universal mumps vaccination during the 1970's when this cohort of children grew up. Renewed emphasis on vaccination has resulted in a further decline in the annual incidence of mumps. In 1993, the Centers for Disease Control and Prevention (CDC) reported only 1640 cases of mumps in the United States, the lowest annual total ever recorded. Epidemiologic studies during the 1980's of mumps epidemics in high schools, colleges, and military units demonstrated that outbreaks were due principally to failure to vaccinate. More recent studies have attributed smaller mumps outbreaks in the 1990's to primary vaccine failure and possibly to waning vaccine immunity.

PATHOGENESIS. Mumps is highly contagious and can be transmitted experimentally by inoculation of virus onto the nasal or buccal mucosa, suggesting that most natural infections result from droplet spread of upper respiratory secretions. The average incubation period for mumps is 18 days. Primary viral replication takes place in epithelial cells of the upper respiratory tract, followed by spread of virus to regional lymph nodes and subsequent viremia and systemic dissemination. Virus can be isolated from saliva for 5 to 7 days before and up to 9 days after the onset of clinical symptoms, meaning that an infected individual is potentially able to transmit mumps for a period of about 2 weeks. An estimated 30% of mumps infections in children are subclinical or associated only with nonspecific upper respiratory infection (URI) symptoms.

CLINICAL MANIFESTATIONS. *Parotitis.* Mumps usually begins with a short prodromal phase of low-grade fever, malaise, headache, and anorexia. Young children may complain initially of ear pain. The patient then develops the characteristic parotid tenderness and enlargement, which lifts the earlobe forward and obscures the angle of the mandible. The parotid glands are involved most commonly, although other salivary glands occasionally may be enlarged. Parotitis initially may be unilateral, with swelling of the contralateral parotid gland occurring 2 to 3 days later; bilateral parotitis eventually develops in 70% of patients with symptomatic salivary gland involvement. Painful parotid gland enlargement progresses over about 3 days, followed by defervescence and resolution of parotid pain and swelling within about 7 days. Long-term sequelae of mumps parotitis are uncommon.

Aseptic Meningitis. Symptomatic meningitis occurs in 15% of cases and is the second most common manifestation of mumps. About 50% of patients with mumps parotitis have cerebrospinal fluid (CSF) pleocytosis, although many have no signs or symptoms of meningitis. Symptoms of meningeal irritation (headache, neck stiffness, vomiting, and lethargy) plus high fever usually develop 4 to 5 days after the onset of parotitis, although the meningitis may occasionally precede the parotitis. Indeed, 40 to 50% of all cases of documented mumps meningitis occur in patients who never develop clinical parotitis. Symptomatic central nervous system (CNS) involvement with mumps is two to three times more common in males than in females. Examination of the CSF usually reveals a normal opening pressure and a mononuclear cell pleocytosis with an average cell count of 450 per cubic millimeter. A polymorphonuclear leukocyte predominance may be seen in some patients early during the course of mumps meningitis. The CSF protein is usually normal or mildly elevated (< 100 mg per deciliter). Hypoglycorrhachia, which is not usually seen in viral meningitis, may be present in 10 to 30% of patients with mumps meningitis. Mumps virus can be recovered from CSF. While the symptoms of mumps meningitis usually resolve within 7 to 10 days, the CSF abnormalities may persist for up to 5 weeks. Mumps meningitis is usually benign and significant neurologic complications are rare.

Encephalitis. The spectrum of mumps-induced CNS disease ranges from mild "aseptic" meningitis (which is common) to severe encephalitis (which is rare). Some cases of encephalitis develop concurrently with the parotitis and are thought to result from direct extension of viral infection from the choroid plexus ependyma into parenchymal neurons. Other cases of mumps encephalitis occur 1 to 2 weeks after the onset of parotitis and may represent a demyelinating postinfectious encephalitis. Clinical findings in mumps encephalitis include obtundation (and less commonly delirium), generalized seizures, and high fever. Other neurologic findings can include focal seizures, aphasia, paresis, and involuntary movements. Recovery from mumps encephalitis is usually complete, although complications such as aqueductal stenosis with hydrocephalus, seizure disorders, and psychomotor retardation have been reported. The overall mortality from mumps encephalitis is 0.5 to 2.3%.

Orchitis. Epididymo-orchitis is rare in boys with mumps but occurs in 15 to 35% of postpubertal men with mumps. Orchitis is most often unilateral (bilateral involvement occurs in 17 to 38% of cases) and results from replication of mumps virus in seminiferous tubules with resulting lymphocytic infiltration and edema. Orchitis typically develops within 1 week of the onset of parotitis, although orchitis (like mumps meningitis) can develop prior to or even in the absence of parotitis. Mumps orchitis is characterized by marked testicular swelling and severe pain, accompanied by fever, nausea, and headache. The pain and swelling resolve within five to seven days, although residual testicular tenderness can persist for weeks. Testicular atrophy may follow orchitis in about 35 to 50% of cases, but sterility is an uncommon complication even among men with bilateral orchitis (see Ch. 209.1).

Other Manifestations. Mumps can cause inflammation of other glandular tissues, including pancreatitis and thyroiditis. Oophoritis and mastitis have been reported in postpubertal women with mumps. Transient renal function abnormalities are common in mumps, and virus can be isolated readily from urine; significant renal damage is rare, however. Other infrequent manifestations of mumps include sensorineural deafness (either transient or permanent), arthritis, myocarditis, and thrombocytopenia. Maternal mumps infection during the first trimester of pregnancy results in an increased frequency of spontaneous abortions, but no clear association between congenital malformations and maternal mumps has been demonstrated.

IMMUNE RESPONSE. Transient IgM antibody responses are detected early in the course of mumps infection, followed by the appearance of IgG antibody and cytotoxic T lymphocytes. Mumps-specific IgG can be detected during the first week of acute infection, peaks at 3 to 4 weeks, and persists for decades. Lifelong immunity follows natural infection. Patients who report more than one episode of mumps probably had parotitis due to another etiology.

A variety of serologic tests have been designed to determine susceptibility to mumps. The neutralizing antibody (NA) assay has been considered the "gold standard" test but is technically demanding. The hemagglutination inhibition (HAI) assay is simple to perform but less specific due to cross-reactivity with other paramyxoviruses. Detection of complement-fixing (CF) antibodies against V (hemagglutinin-neuraminidase) and S (nucleocapsid) antigens previously has been the routine method for determining immune status but has been replaced by a sensitive and specific enzyme-linked immunosorbent assay. The mumps skin test is not a reliable indicator of immune status.

DIAGNOSIS. The diagnosis of mumps is usually made on the basis of clinical findings in a child who presents with parotitis, particularly if the individual is known to be susceptible and has been exposed to mumps during the preceding 2 to 3 weeks. However, an atypical clinical presentation (e.g., meningitis or orchitis without parotitis) may require laboratory confirmation. Culturing for mumps virus is definitive but frequently not available. Testing of acute and convalescent sera should demonstrate a diagnostic fourfold rise in mumps antibody titer. Alternatively, finding mumps IgM antibody provides good evidence of recent infection. About 30% of patients will have an elevated serum amylase level that may be due to parotitis or pancreatitis.

The differential diagnosis of parotitis includes infections caused by other viruses such as influenza A, parainfluenza virus, coxsackievirus, lymphocytic choriomeningitis virus, or bacteria such as *Staphylococcus aureus*. Parotid gland enlargement also can be associated with Sjögren's syndrome, sarcoidosis, thiazide ingestion, iodine sensitivity, tumor, or salivary duct obstruction. A careful examination should distinguish parotitis from lymphadenopathy.

THERAPY. Management of the patient with mumps consists of conservative measures to provide symptomatic relief and to ensure adequate hydration and nutrition. Therapy of orchitis includes bed rest, scrotal support, analgesics, and ice packs. Patients with significant CNS involvement will require hospitalization for observation and supportive care. There is currently no established role for antiviral drugs, corticosteroids, or passive immunotherapy.

PREVENTION. The cornerstone of mumps prevention is active immunization using the live attenuated mumps vaccine. In the United States, mumps vaccine is administered in combination with the measles and rubella (MMR) vaccines to children at age 15 months and produces protective antibody levels in >95% of recipients. A second dose of MMR is recommended for children when they enter school. The mumps vaccine is also indicated for susceptible adults.

The "Jeryl-Lynn" strain of attenuated mumps virus used in the United States since 1967 is a very well-tolerated vaccine, although rare instances of fever, parotitis, and possibly aseptic meningitis have been reported following immunization. In 1988 and 1989, however, an apparent increased frequency of cases of vaccine-related mumps meningitis was recognized in Canada and Japan. These cases occurred after MMR vaccine was administered that contained the Urabe AM-9 mumps virus, and in several cases, the vaccine virus was isolated from CSF and positively identified by nucleotide sequencing. This problem has not been recognized in the United States, where the Jeryl-Lynn mumps vaccine continues to be used.

Questions regarding prevention often arise when an individual with no history of mumps (typically an adult male) is exposed to a patient with active mumps. The immune status of the exposed individual can be determined by serologic testing, although this may involve some delay. The vast majority of adults born in the United States before 1957 have been naturally infected and are therefore immune. Mumps vaccine can be safely administered to an individual of unknown immune status, although vaccine given to a susceptible individual after exposure to mumps may not provide protection.

Briss PA, Fehrs LJ, Parker RA, et al.: Sustained transmission of mumps in a highly vaccinated population: Assessment of primary vaccine induced immunity. J Infect Dis 169:77, 1994. *Investigation of a mumps outbreak attributed to vaccine failure.*

CDC: General recommendations on immunization: Recommendations of the Advisory Committee on Immunization Practices (ACIP). MMWR 43 (RR-1):1, 1994. *Current recommendations for mumps vaccination.*

The Herpes Group of Viruses

339 HERPES SIMPLEX VIRUS INFECTIONS

Richard J. Whitley

Herpes simplex virus (HSV), a member of the family Herpesviridae, has been implicated in human infections since descriptions of cutaneous spreading lesions in ancient Greek times. Scholars of Greek civilization define the word *herpes* to mean "to creep or crawl," in reference to the spreading nature of the observed skin lesions. More recently, infection has been defined by the spectrum of illnesses caused by HSV. In 1968, well-defined antigenic and biologic differences were demonstrated between herpes simplex virus type 1 (HSV-1) and herpes simplex virus type 2 (HSV-2). HSV-1 was more frequently associated with nongenital infection and HSV-2 with genital disease. Further study has revealed that, of all the herpesviruses, HSV-1 and HSV-2 are the most closely related, with approximately 60% genomic homology. These two viruses can be distinguished most reliably by DNA restriction enzyme analyses; however, differences in antigen expression and biologic properties also serve as methods for differentiation.

STRUCTURE. Membership in the family Herpesviridae is based on the structure of the virion (Fig. 339–1). HSV contains double-stranded DNA at the central core, has a molecular weight of approximately 100 million, and encodes at least 70 polypeptides. The DNA core is surrounded by a capsid that consists of 162 capsomers, arranged in icosapentahedral symmetry. The capsid is approximately 100 to 110 nm in diameter. Tightly adherent to the capsid is the tegument, consisting of amorphous material. Loosely surrounding the capsid and tegument is a lipid bilayer envelope derived from host cell membranes. The envelope consists of polyamines, lipids, and glycoproteins. These glycoproteins confer distinctive properties to the virus and provide unique antigens to which the host is capable of responding. Notably, glycoprotein G (gG) provides antigenic specificity to HSV and therefore results in an antibody response that allows for the distinction between HSV-1 (gG-1) and HSV-2 (gG-2).

A unique feature of HSV DNA is its genomic sequence arrangement. The genome consists of two components, L (long) and S (short), each of which contains unique sequences that can invert on themselves, leading to four isomers. Viral DNA extracted from virions of infected cells consists of four equimolar populations, differing only with respect to the relative orientation of the two unique components. Biologic relevance of this phenomenon is unknown.

REPLICATION. Replication of HSV is a multistep process (Fig. 339–2). Following the onset of infection, DNA is uncoated and transported to the nucleus of the host cell. This is followed by transcription of immediate-early genes, which encode for the regulatory proteins, and is followed by the expression of proteins encoded by early and then late genes. These proteins include enzymes necessary for viral replication and structural proteins.

Assembly of the viral core and capsid takes place within the nucleus. Envelopment at the nuclear membrane and transport out of the nucleus occur through the endoplasmic reticulum and the Golgi apparatus. Glycosylation of the viral membrane occurs in the Golgi. Mature virions are transported to the outer membrane of the host cell inside vesicles. Release of progeny virus is accompanied by cell death. Replication for all herpesviruses is considered inefficient, with a high ratio of noninfectious to infectious viral particles.

PATHOGENESIS AND LATENCY. A critical factor for transmission of HSV, regardless of virus type, is intimate contact between a person who is shedding virus and a susceptible host. With inoculation onto the skin or mucous membrane, HSV replicates in epithelial cells; the incubation period is 4 to 6 days (Fig. 339–3). As replication continues, cell lysis and local inflammation ensue, resulting in characteristic vesicles on an erythematous base. Regional lymphatics and lymph nodes become involved with the draining of infected secretions from the area of viral replication. Viremia and visceral dissemination may develop depending on the immunologic competence of the host. In all hosts, the virus generally ascends peripheral sensory nerves to reach the dorsal root ganglia. Replication of HSV within neural tissue is followed by spread of the virus to other mucosal and skin surfaces via the peripheral sensory nerves. Virus replicates further in epithelial cells, reproducing the lesions of the initial infection, until infection is contained through host immunity.

The histopathologic changes induced by HSV replication are similar for both primary and recurrent infection. Changes induced by

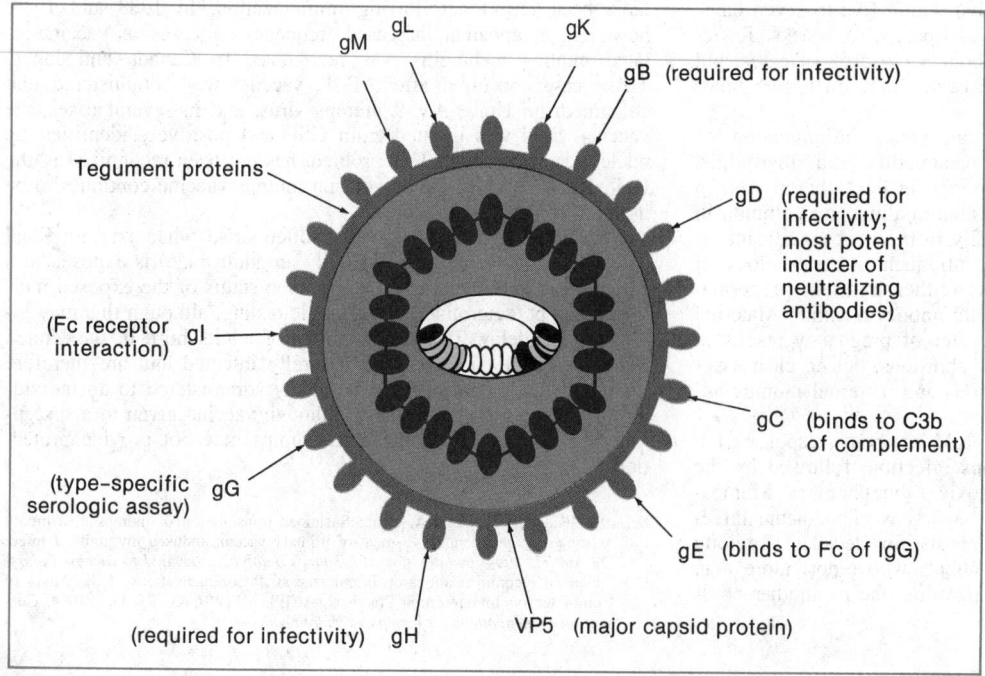

FIGURE 339–1. Schematic diagram of the HSV virion.

gM gL gK
gB (required for infectivity)
Tegument proteins
gD (required for infectivity; most potent inducer of neutralizing antibodies)
(Fc receptor interaction) gI
gC (binds to C3b of complement)
(type-specific serologic assay) gG
gE (binds to Fc of IgG)
(required for infectivity) gH VP5 (major capsid protein)

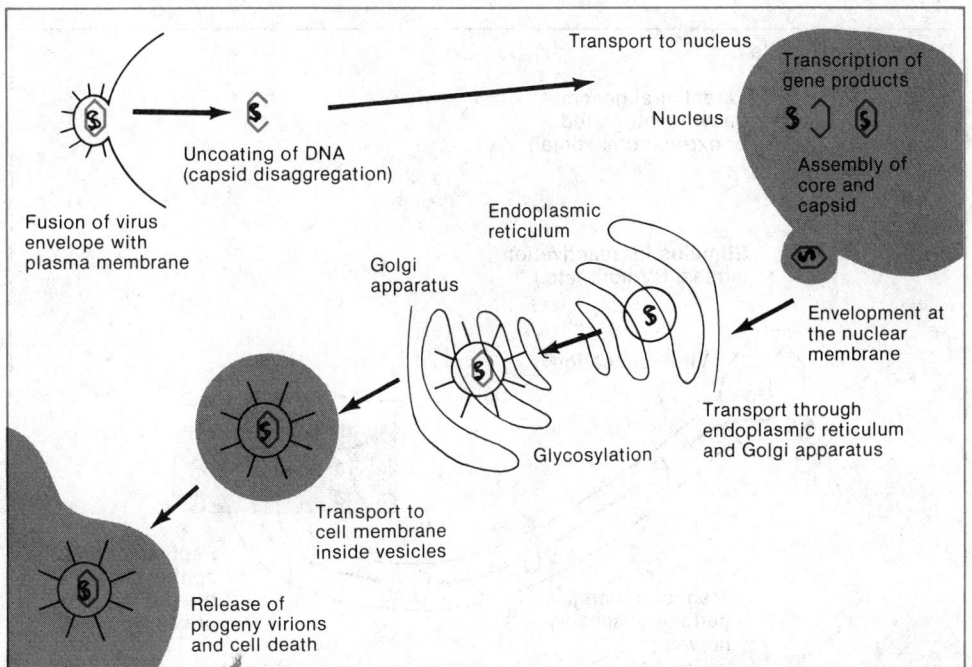

FIGURE 339-2. Schematic diagram of HSV replication.

viral infection include ballooning of infected cells and the appearance of condensed chromatin within the nuclei of cells, followed by subsequent degeneration of the cellular nuclei. Cells lose intact plasma membranes and form multinucleated giant cells. They also may demonstrate the intranuclear inclusion bodies known as Cowdry type A bodies, which are suggestive but not diagnostic of HSV infection. With cell lysis, a clear vesicular fluid containing large quantities of virus forms between the epidermis and dermal layer. The dermis reveals an intense inflammatory response, more so with primary infection than with recurrent disease. As healing progresses, the clear vesicular fluid becomes pustular with the recruitment of inflammatory cells. The pustule then forms a scab, with scarring being uncommon.

The vascular changes in the area of infection include perivascular cuffing and hemorrhagic necrosis. These changes are particularly prominent when organs other than skin are involved, as is the case with herpes simplex encephalitis or disseminated neonatal HSV in-

fection. Local lymphatics can show evidence of infection with intrusion of inflammatory cells due to the draining of infected secretions from the area of viral replication. As host defenses are mounted, an influx of mononuclear cells can be detected in infected tissue.

A unique characteristic of the herpesviruses is their ability to establish latent infection, persist in an apparently inactive state for varying amounts of time, and then be reactivated (Fig. 339–4). The latent viral genome may be either extrachromosomal or integrated into host-cell DNA.

Latency is established when HSV reaches the dorsal root ganglia after retrograde transmission via sensory nerve pathways. Latent virus may be reactivated and enter a replicative cycle at any point in time. The reactivation of latent virus is a well-recognized biologic phenomenon but not one that is understood from a molecular standpoint. Stimuli that have been observed to be associated with the reactivation of latent HSV have included stress, menstruation,

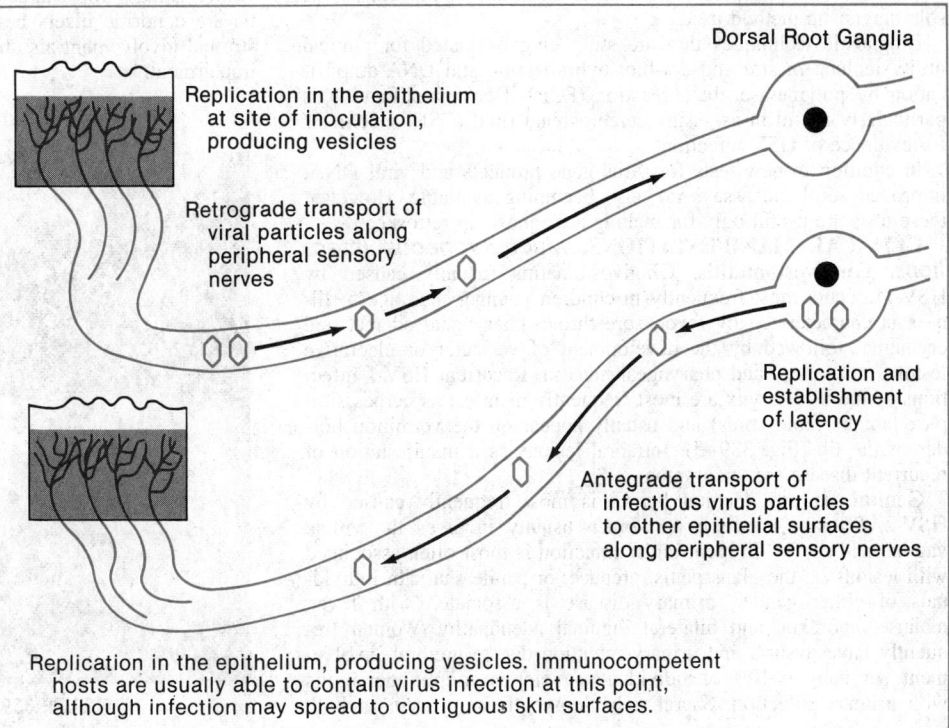

FIGURE 339-3. Schematic diagram of primary HSV infection.

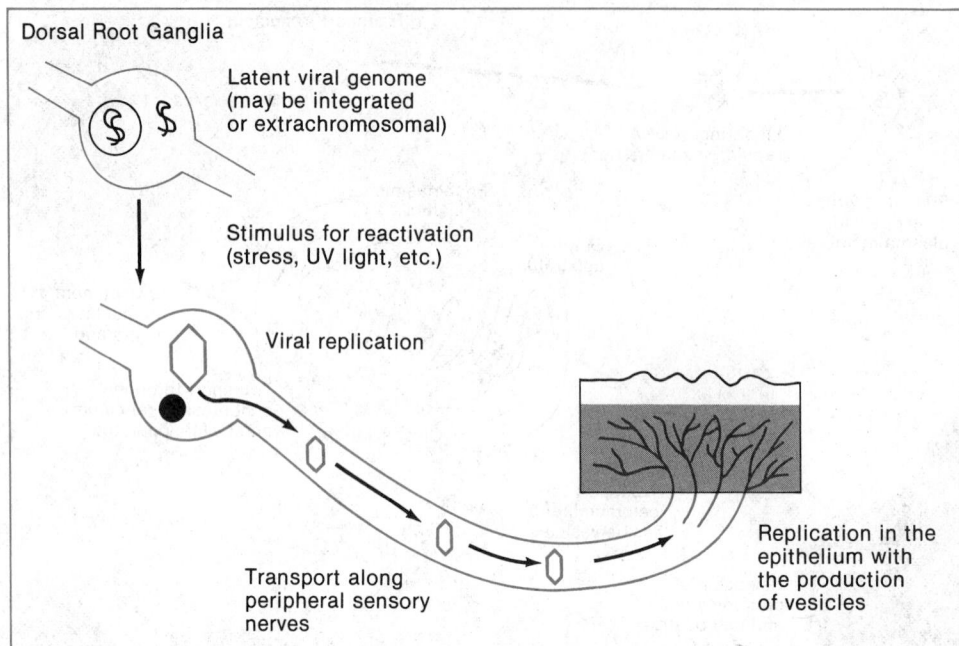

Dorsal Root Ganglia

Latent viral genome
(may be integrated
or extrachromosomal)

Stimulus for reactivation
(stress, UV light, etc.)

Viral replication

Transport along
peripheral sensory
nerves

Replication in the
epithelium with
the production
of vesicles

FIGURE 339–4. Schematic diagram of HSV latency and reactivation.

and exposure to ultraviolet light. Precisely how these factors interact at the level of the ganglia remains to be defined. Reactivation may be clinically asymptomatic, or it may produce life-threatening disease.

DIAGNOSIS. The definitive diagnosis of HSV infection requires isolation of virus. Swabs of clinical specimens or other body fluids can be inoculated into susceptible cell lines and observed for the development of characteristic cytopathic effects. This technique is very useful for the diagnosis of HSV-1 and HSV-2 infection because of the short replicative cycles.

In the absence of diagnostic virology facilities, cytologic examination of cells scraped from a clinical lesion may be useful in making a presumptive diagnosis of HSV infection. Material obtained from scraping the base of a lesion should be smeared on a glass slide and promptly fixed in cold ethanol. The slide can be stained according to the methods of Papanicolaou, Giemsa, or Wright. The presence of intranuclear inclusions and multinucleated giant cells is indicative, but not diagnostic, of HSV infection. This method has a sensitivity of only approximately 60 to 70% and should not be the sole diagnostic method used.

Diagnostic techniques that are still being evaluated for clinical utility include *in situ* and dot-blot hybridization and DNA amplification by polymerase chain reaction (PCR). DNA amplification is particularly useful in assessing cerebrospinal fluid (CSF) specimens for evidence of HSV infection.

In addition to new tests for virus gene products and viral DNA, improved serologic assays are also becoming available. However, these tests are useful only for making a diagnosis in retrospect.

CLINICAL MANIFESTATIONS. *Mucocutaneous Infections*. Gingivostomatitis. Gingivostomatitis (usually caused by HSV-1) occurs most frequently in children younger than age 5. Illness is characterized by fever, sore throat, pharyngeal edema, and erythema, followed by the development of vesicular or ulcerative lesions on the oral and pharyngeal mucosa. Recurrent HSV-1 infections of the oropharynx are most frequently manifest as herpes simplex labialis (cold sores) and usually appear on the vermilion border of the lip (Fig. 339–5). Intraoral lesions as a manifestation of recurrent disease are uncommon.

Genital Herpes. Genital herpes is most frequently caused by HSV-2. Primary infection in women usually involves the vulva, vagina, and cervix. In men, initial infection is most often associated with lesions on the glans penis, prepuce, or penile shaft. In individuals of either gender, primary disease is associated with fever, malaise, anorexia, and bilateral inguinal adenopathy. Women frequently have dysuria and urinary retention due to urethral involvement. As many as 10% of individuals develop an aseptic meningitis with primary infection. Sacral radiculomyelitis may occur in both

men and women, resulting in neuralgias, urinary retention, or obstipation. The complete healing of primary infection may take several weeks. It has been recognized that the first episode of genital infection is less severe in individuals who have had previous HSV-1 infections at other sites. Antibodies to HSV-1 appear to ameliorate the expression of HSV-2 clinical disease.

Recurrent genital infections in either men or women can be particularly distressing. The frequency of recurrence varies significantly from one individual to another. It has been estimated that one third have virtually no or few recurrences, one third have approximately three recurrences per year, and another third have more than three per year. Seroepidemiologic studies have found that between 25 and 65% of individuals in the United States in 1978 had antibodies to HSV-2 and that seroprevalence is correlated with the number of sexual partners.

Herpetic Keratitis. Herpes simplex keratitis is usually caused by HSV-1 and is accompanied by conjunctivitis in many cases. It is considered the most common infectious cause of blindness in the United States. The characteristic lesions of HSV keratoconjunctivitis are dendritic ulcers best detected by fluorescein staining. Deep stromal involvement also has been reported and may result in visual impairment.

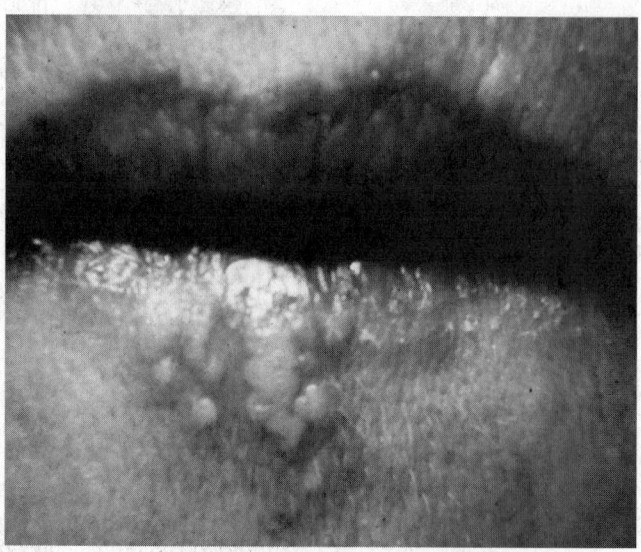

FIGURE 339–5. Herpes simplex labialis.

Other Cutaneous Manifestations. HSV infections can occur at any skin site. Common among health care workers are lesions on abraded skin of the fingers, known as herpetic whitlows. Similarly, wrestlers, because of physical contact, may develop disseminated cutaneous lesions known as herpes gladiatorum.

Neonatal Herpes Simplex Virus Infection. Neonatal HSV infection is estimated to occur in approximately 1 in 3500 deliveries in the United States each year. Approximately 70% of cases are caused by HSV-2 and usually result from contact of the fetus with infected maternal genital secretions at the time of delivery. Manifestations of neonatal HSV infection can be divided into three categories: (1) skin, eye, and mouth disease; (2) encephalitis; and (3) disseminated infection. As the name implies, skin, eye, and mouth disease consists of cutaneous lesions and does not involve other organ systems. Involvement of the central nervous system may occur with encephalitis or disseminated infection and generally results in a diffuse encephalitis. The CSF formula characteristically reveals an elevated protein and a mononuclear pleocytosis. Disseminated infection involves multiple organ systems and can produce disseminated intravascular coagulation, hemorrhagic pneumonitis, encephalitis, and cutaneous lesions. Diagnosis can be particularly difficult in the absence of skin lesions, which occurs in as many as 36% of cases. The mortality rate for each disease classification varies from zero for skin, eye, and mouth disease to 15% for encephalitis and 60% for neonates with disseminated infection, even with appropriate antiviral treatment. In addition to the high mortality associated with these infections, morbidity is significant in that children with encephalitis or disseminated disease develop normally in only 40% of cases, even with appropriate antiviral therapy.

Herpes Simplex Encephalitis. Herpes simplex encephalitis is characterized by hemorrhagic necrosis of the temporal lobe. Disease begins unilaterally, spreads to the contralateral temporal lobe, and is characterized by hemorrhagic necrosis (Fig. 339–6). It is the most common cause of focal, sporadic encephalitis in the United States today and occurs in approximately 1 in 150,000 individuals. Most cases are caused by HSV-1. The actual pathogenesis of herpes simplex encephalitis requires further clarification, although it has been speculated that primary or recurrent virus can reach the temporal lobe by ascending neural pathways, such as the trigeminal tracts or the olfactory nerves.

Clinical manifestations of herpes simplex encephalitis include headache, fever, altered consciousness, and abnormalities of speech and behavior, findings characteristic of temporal lobe involvement. Focal seizures also may occur. The CSF formula for these patients is variable but usually consists of a pleocytosis with both polymorphonuclear leukocytes and monocytes present. The protein concentration is characteristically elevated, and glucose is usually normal. Diagnosis can be achieved by PCR evaluation of CSF in experienced laboratories. The mortality and morbidity are high, even with appropriate antiviral therapy. At present, the mortality rate is ap-

proximately 30% 1 year after treatment. In addition, approximately 50% of survivors have moderate or severe neurologic impairment.

Herpes Simplex Virus Infections in the Immunocompromised Host. HSV infections in the immunocompromised host are usually due to reactivation of latent infection and are clinically more severe, may be progressive, and require a longer time to heal. Manifestations of HSV infections in this patient population include pneumonitis, esophagitis, hepatitis, colitis, and disseminated cutaneous disease. Individuals suffering from human immunodeficiency virus (HIV) infection may have extensive perineal or orofacial ulcerations. HSV infections are also noted to be of increased severity in individuals with extensive burns.

EPIDEMIOLOGY. HSV infections are distributed worldwide and have been reported in both developed and underdeveloped countries. Animal vectors for human HSV infections have not been described, and there is no seasonal variation in the incidence of HSV infections. The virus is transmitted from infected to susceptible individuals during close personal contact, and virus must come in contact with mucosal surfaces or abraded skin for infection to be initiated. Since approximately one third of the world's population has recurrent HSV infections, and because infection is rarely fatal, a large reservoir of HSV exists in the community.

Although HSV-1 and HSV-2 are usually transmitted by different routes and involve different areas of the body, there is a great deal of overlap between the epidemiology and clinical manifestations of infections caused by these viruses. The mouth and lips are clearly the most common sites of HSV-1 infection. Primary HSV-1 infection in the young child is usually asymptomatic but may be manifest as gingivostomatitis. Primary infection in young adults has been associated with pharyngitis and sometimes a mononucleosis-like syndrome. Seroprevalence studies have demonstrated that acquisition of HSV-1 infection is related to socioeconomic factors. Antibodies, which indicate past infection, are found early in life among individuals of lower socioeconomic groups. This presumably is a consequence of crowded living conditions that provide a greater opportunity for direct contact with infected individuals. As many as 75 to 90% of individuals from lower socioeconomic populations develop antibodies by the end of the first decade of life. In contrast, only 30 to 40% of persons in middle and upper socioeconomic groups are seropositive by the middle of the second decade of life.

Because infections with HSV-2 are usually acquired through sexual contact, antibodies to this virus are rarely found until the onset of sexual activity. There is a progressive increase in infection rates with HSV-2 in all populations beginning in adolescence. As with HSV-1 infections, the rate of acquisition of HSV-2 infection appears related to socioeconomic factors. The number of sexual contacts is also an important risk factor for the acquisition of HSV-2. Importantly, genital herpes infection has been found to be a risk factor for another sexually transmitted virus, HIV.

Localized, recurrent HSV-2 infection is the most common form of HSV infection during gestation. Transmission of infection to the fetus is most frequently related to the shedding of virus at the time of delivery. Since HSV infection of the fetus is usually the consequence of contact with infected maternal genital secretions at the time of delivery, the determination of viral excretion at this time is of utmost importance. The incidence of cervical shedding in pregnant women with asymptomatic HSV infection is approximately 1%. Interestingly, most infants who develop neonatal disease are born to women who are completely asymptomatic for genital HSV infections at the time of delivery and who have neither a past history of genital herpes nor a sexual partner reporting a genital vesicular rash. These women account for 60 to 80% of all women whose children develop neonatal HSV infection.

PREVENTION. At present, there are no licensed vaccines directed against HSV. However, experimental vaccines for HSV-1 and HSV-2 are being evaluated. Acyclovir is currently being given to recipients of solid organ and bone marrow transplants in the immediate post-transplant period in an effort to prevent reactivation of latent disease.

TREATMENT. Infections caused by HSV-1 and HSV-2 are amenable to therapy with antiviral drugs (see Ch. 327). Both vidarabine and acyclovir have proved useful for managing specific infections caused by these viruses. At present, acyclovir is the treat-

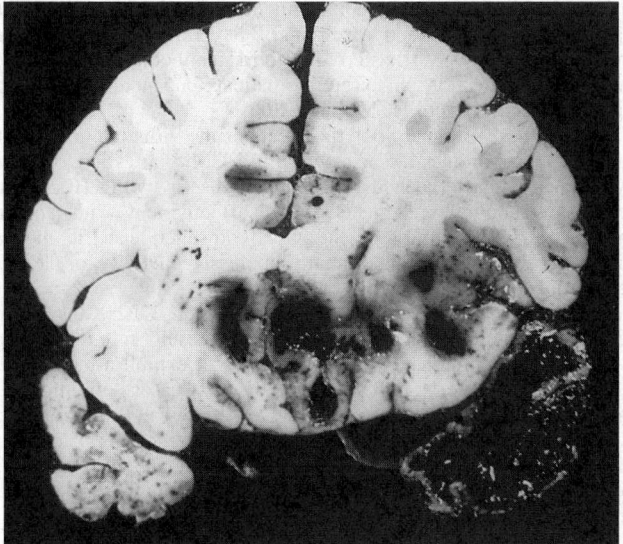

FIGURE 339–6. Hemorrhagic necrosis in herpes simplex encephalitis.

ment of choice for mucocutaneous HSV infections in the immuno-compromised host, herpes simplex encephalitis, and neonatal HSV infections. Intravenous administration is preferred for therapy of life-threatening disease. Intravenous acyclovir is also recommended for clinically severe initial genital herpes in the immunocompetent host. This includes patients with complications such as urinary retention or aseptic meningitis, and they should receive 5 mg per kilogram every 8 hours for 5 to 7 days. Caution must be exercised when acyclovir is used intravenously because it may crystallize in the renal tubules when given too rapidly or to dehydrated patients.

Immunocompromised individuals with mucocutaneous HSV infections that are not life threatening may be given oral acyclovir. Oral acyclovir is also useful in treating initial genital herpes. Recurrent episodes, however, are not as responsive to acyclovir. For individuals who experience severe or frequent recurrences of genital herpes, a "suppressive" regimen of acyclovir in doses of 600 to 800 mg per day may be useful. The efficacy of acyclovir for primary or recurrent oropharyngeal HSV in the immunocompetent host has not been well established.

Corey L, Spear P: Infections with herpes simplex viruses. N Engl J Med 314:686, 1986. *This two-article series is a concise review of herpes simplex virus infections.*
Goldsmith SM, Whitley RJ: Herpes simplex encephalitis. *In* Lambert HP (ed.): Infections of the Central Nervous System. Philadelphia, BC Decker, 1991, pp 283–299. *This chapter describes the clinical presentations, diagnostic evaluation, and treatment of herpes simplex virus encephalitis.*
Nahmias AJ, Lee FK, Bechman-Nahmias S: Sero-epidemiological and sociological patterns of herpes simplex virus infection in the world. Scand J Infect Dis 69:19, 1990. *A comprehensive analysis of herpes simplex virus seroepidemiology, utilizing new techniques for HSV-2-specific antibody.*
Roizman B: Herpesviridae: A brief introduction. *In* Fields BN, Knipe DM et al. (eds.): Fields Virology, 2nd ed. New York, Raven Press, 1990, p 1787. *This chapter provides an overview of the herpes family of viruses.*
Roizman B: New viral footprints in Kaposi's sarcoma (editorial). N Engl J Med 332:1227, 1995. *Discusses the discovery of human herpesvirus 8 by a novel technique and that the virus' footprints were found in cells affected by Kaposi's sarcoma.*
Straus SE: Clinical and biological differences between recurrent herpes simplex virus and varicella-zoster virus infections. JAMA 262:3455, 1989. *A concise article that emphasizes the distinctions between recurrent herpes simplex virus infections and recurrent varicella-zoster infections.*
Whitley RJ: Herpes simplex viruses. *In* Fields BN, Knipe DM, et al. (eds.): Fields' Virology. New York, Raven Press, 1990. *A comprehensive text that includes a detailed analysis of the molecular biology and clinical manifestations of herpes simplex virus.*

340 INFECTIONS ASSOCIATED WITH HUMAN CYTOMEGALOVIRUS

William J. Britt

Human cytomegalovirus (HCMV) is the largest and most structurally complex human herpesvirus. Its linear double-stranded DNA genome consists of 250,000 base pairs which can potentially encode over 200 different proteins. Two different types of infections have been defined, primary and recurrent. Recurrent infection may follow reactivation of previous infection or reinfection by a superinfecting viral strain. Host immunity is thought to be protective, because clinical evidence of infection rarely develops in the immunocompetent host. Abnormalities in immune responses caused by immunosuppressive drugs following allotransplantation, retroviral infections in patients with human immunodeficiency virus (HIV), or developmental immune dysfunction in the fetus predispose these unique populations to HCMV-induced disease.

EPIDEMIOLOGY. HCMV circulates within the population, and there is no evidence of epidemics or seasonal dependence. In most underdeveloped countries, HCMV is acquired early in childhood, likely as a result of either breast-feeding or secondary to crowded living conditions. Seropositivity reaches nearly 100% in these populations before childbearing age. In contrast, the seroprevalence in the United States is dependent on age and socioeconomic status. By

childbearing age, the seroprevalence often exceeds 90% in lower socioeconomic groups. In individuals of higher socioeconomic groups, approximately 50% are seropositive by early adulthood.

Several routes of virus transmission have been documented, including transmission following sexual contact. Previous studies have documented high levels of virus within semen and cervical secretions. Epidemiologic studies have demonstrated a correlation between a history of sexually transmitted disease with HCMV seropositivity. Transmission from young children represents another important source of HCMV infection. Careful epidemiologic studies within child care centers demonstrated virus transmission between young children, as well as transmission to adult caretakers and susceptible parents. The importance of children as a major source of virus can be appreciated if one considers that approximately 1% of all babies are born with HCMV infection (congenital) and that 30 to 70% of breast-fed babies of seropositive mothers will become infected. Because these infants often excrete large amounts of virus in their saliva and urine for months to years following infection, they provide an important reservoir of infectious HCMV.

Major sources of virus exposure among hospitalized patients include blood products and transplanted organs. Transfusion-acquired HCMV infection, prior to routine serologic screening of donor blood products, occurred at a consistent rate of approximately 2.5% per unit of whole blood. Numerous studies have demonstrated that leukocytes present within various blood products were responsible for the majority of transfusion-acquired HCMV infections. Measures that reduce leukocyte contamination within blood products or, alternatively, screening blood donors and matching HCMV serologic status of donor and recipient have reduced the incidence of transfusion-associated HCMV infection. Nosocomial transmission of HCMV to health workers is uncommon, even in personnel caring for patients excreting large amounts of HCMV, such as congenitally infected infants.

PATHOLOGY. Although HCMV can be consistently propagated *in vitro* only in human fibroblast cells, it can be isolated from a myriad of organs and cell types from infected humans. HCMV has been demonstrated in the endothelium of the vasculature, epithelium of almost every organ (including endocrine and exocrine organs), and neuronal cells of the central nervous system (CNS). Pathologic findings range from extensive tissue destruction to isolated cytomegalic cells. The typical cytomegalic cell consists of an enlarged cell with scant to reduced cytoplasm containing a large nucleus with prominent nucleoli and intranuclear inclusions.

PATHOGENESIS. Cellular-, antibody-, and cytokine-mediated immune responses have been proposed to limit HCMV infection, although direct evidence is lacking. A number of studies in bone marrow and solid organ allograft recipients have provided a strong correlation between the depression of HCMV-specific T lymphocyte responses and susceptibility to HCMV-associated infection and, more important, clinical disease. These responses have included both major histocompatability (MHC) class II–restricted CD4+ T lymphocytes and class I–restricted CD8+ cytotoxic T lymphocytes. Although the virus-encoded target antigens of these cellular responses are unknown, protein components of the virus itself are thought to induce protective responses. Several studies have documented that passively transferred antiviral antibodies failed to prevent HCMV infection in susceptible patients but modulated clinical disease associated with HCMV infection.

As yet poorly defined nonlytic effects of the virus may contribute to disease syndromes associated with HCMV infection. Clinical syndromes of bacterial and fungal infections following HCMV infection in allograft recipients are also consistent with an immunomodulatory activity of the virus; however, specific mechanisms accounting for this immunosuppressive activity of HCMV remain inadequately defined.

CLINICAL ASPECTS OF HCMV INFECTION. Although infection in the immunocompetent host rarely results in clinically apparent disease, infrequently, normal hosts will exhibit a mononucleosis-like syndrome. Approximately 8% of cases of infectious mononucleosis may be caused by HCMV. Clinically, this infection is indistinguishable from mononucleosis caused by Epstein-Barr virus, with the exception that it is heterophile-negative. Nonspecific constitutional symptoms predominate, including malaise, decreased appetite, and low-grade fever. Laboratory abnormalities include atypical lymphocytosis, chemical hepatitis and cholestasis, and less frequently, thrombocytopenia. Similar but often exaggerated findings have been associated with transfusion-acquired HCMV, including the previously described postperfusion syndrome that followed cardiopulmonary bypass.

Congenital HCMV infection (present at birth) is common, occurring in approximately 1% of all live births in the United States. Some 10% of these will suffer signs and symptoms of cytomegalic inclusion disease (CID), which include petechiae, hepatosplenomegaly, jaundice, and microcephaly. Thrombocytopenia, cholestasis, and evidence of hepatocellular damage are consistent laboratory findings. Although almost all end-organ disease is self-limited, CNS damage associated with congenital HCMV infection is permanent and often results in significant developmental delays, seizure activity, gross neurologic impairment, and most frequently, hearing loss. Subclinical congenital HCMV infection is less commonly associated with permanent CNS sequelae; however, up to 15% of infants with subclinical infection may exhibit evidence of CNS damage, such as sensorineural hearing loss. Both forms of congenital HCMV infection result in chronic virus excretion which may persist for years, thus providing an important source of HCMV exposure in the community.

HCMV infection following allograft transplantation is the most common infection in the post-transplant period. An estimated 60 to 100% of seropositive renal transplant recipients will excrete HCMV following transplantation. Although the vast majority of patients will not exhibit evidence of invasive HCMV infection, HCMV is a major cause of disease in heart, heart-lung, liver, and bone marrow transplant recipients. In the latter setting, HCMV pneumonia has been the leading infection-related cause of death, with mortality rates approaching 90%. Sources of HCMV infection in the allograft recipient include (1) reactivated infection of the HCMV-seropositive recipient, (2) exogenous blood products given in the post-transplant period, and (3) most commonly, from the transplanted organ obtained from an HCMV-seropositive donor. The highest risk for infection and disease is observed in the HCMV-seronegative recipient of an allograft from a HCMV-seropositive allograft donor (see Ch. 266). Other factors associated with clinically significant HCMV infections in solid organ allograft recipients include the use of cadaveric grafts, leukocyte-containing blood products, and immunosuppressive agents which deplete T lymphocytes such as antithymocyte globulin or anti-DC3 monoclonal antibodies. In bone marrow allograft recipients, the severity of HCMV infection often parallels the development of graft-versus-host disease (GVHD).

Clinical evidence of HCMV infection usually develops 4 to 6 weeks after transplantation and can present with a variety of end-organ diseases such as pneumonitis or hepatitis and more commonly as a syndrome similar to HCMV mononucleosis, which can include fever, leukopenia, thrombocytopenia, and hepatitis. Virus can be isolated from the urine in almost-infected patients and from the blood in a subset of patients. This latter finding may presage the development of invasive multiorgan disease. Potentially fatal invasive infections include pneumonitis, severe gastrointestinal ulcerative disease with perforation, and life-threatening hepatitis. HCMV pneumonitis most commonly presents insidiously as a diffuse interstitial pneumonia that progresses in the absence of specific therapy. Acute allograft loss may accompany HCMV disease either as a direct result of graft involvement, as seen in hepatic transplants, or secondary to the reduction in immunosuppression which may be necessary for treating invasive HCMV disease. Long-term allograft survival also appears to be reduced as a result of HCMV infection. In cardiac allografts this has been proposed to result from virus-associated acceleration of coronary artery atherosclerosis of the allograft, whereas in hepatic allografts it has been suggested that HCMV causes increased expression of MHC antigens resulting in enhanced immunologic recognition of the graft.

HCMV has become a major cause of morbidity and mortality in patients with acquired immunodeficiency syndrome (AIDS) (see Part XXII). Because of the importance of sexual transmission in the spread of HCMV in adult populations, it is not surprising that the rate of HCMV seropositivity approaches 100% in populations at high risk for HIV infection. Thus endogenous virus and frequent sexual exposure to reinfecting viral strains are likely sources of HCMV in these populations. The importance of HCMV coinfection to progression of AIDS has been proposed, and in vitro findings support a potential role of HCMV in HIV replication. Risk factors for the development of invasive HCMV disease in this population include a CD4+ lymphocyte count of < 50 per cubic millimeter. In

addition, it has been noted that the development of invasive HCMV disease is a grave prognostic sign, since overall survival is significantly shortened in patients with documented HCMV disease.

Invasive HCMV infections in patients with AIDS have included end-organ disease in almost all organ systems, with three systems being more frequently involved: the CNS, gastrointestinal (GI) system, and pulmonary system. HCMV infection of the CNS, although uncommon in allograft recipients, is not infrequent in HIV-infected patients. Encephalopathies, both diffuse and focal, as well as myelopathies and neuropathies, have been ascribed to HCMV. The most common and important disease associated with HCMV in this population is retinitis. It has been estimated that between 8 and 25% of long-lived patients with AIDS will develop this invasive HCMV infection. GI involvement includes both colitis and esophagitis and less frequently gastritis. Clinical and laboratory evidence of HCMV colitis is often found in association with other GI pathogens, thus raising questions about the importance of HCMV as a primary pathogen. Likewise, the significance of HCMV as a frequent cause of pneumonitis in AIDS patients has been challenged.

DIAGNOSIS. The diagnosis of HCMV has conventionally relied on isolating the virus from urine, saliva, blood, or biopsy specimens obtained from patients exhibiting symptoms compatible with HCMV infection. There is no convenient method to distinguish acute, invasive infection from peripheral shedding resulting from reactivation of a pre-existing infection. In the transplant and AIDS population, this has prompted diagnostic approaches for measuring viral burden, including HCMV blood cultures and cultures from biopsy specimens, both of which more closely correlate with invasive disease as compared with viruria. Adaptation of immunocytochemistry and centrifugation-enhanced culture techniques has shortened the time required to identify HCMV in clinical specimens to less than 24 hours.

Serologic determination of HCMV is valuable when both IgG and IgM virus-specific antibodies are measured and most frequently only in normal hosts. Measurement of IgG alone is of limited value because of the high seroprevalence of HCMV in the population and the persistence of antibody responses to the virus. Although HCMV-specific IgM antibodies persist for at least 2 to 3 months in normal individuals, their value in immunocompromised hosts is often limited.

Newer methods of diagnosis include the polymerase chain reaction (PCR) of several different body fluids as well as biopsy material. PCR has been used successfully to detect viremia and plasma HCMV DNA. Quantifying PCR results also should prove of prognostic value. A semiquantitative assay of viral burden that detects virus-encoded protein in polymorphonuclear leukocytes, the antigenemia assay, appears predictive of invasive disease in allograft recipients and patients with AIDS.

THERAPY. Until recently, effective antiviral therapy has not been available for HCMV infection. Two agents, ganciclovir and foscarnet, have been shown to be virostatic in vitro and in vivo. Clinical trials have documented efficacy of these agents in treating invasive HCMV disease in both transplant and AIDS patients. Both have significant toxicity, which often precludes their long-term administration. Ganciclovir causes dose-limiting hematopoietic toxicity, often resulting in clinically significant neutropenia. Foscarnet has significant nephrotoxicity, which limits its use in patients with azotemia. In addition, long-term therapy in immunocompromised patients has resulted in the development of viral resistance to both agents.

Perhaps the most beneficial use of these agents has been as prophylaxis in the immediate transplant period. Both foscarnet and ganciclovir have been used successfully to reduce the incidence of HCMV disease in the post-transplant period in both solid organ and bone marrow transplant recipients.

Immunoprophylaxis of HCMV infection has included passive transfer of antibody and limited clinical trials of a live-virus vaccine. The use of intravenous immunoglobulin containing anti-HCMV antibodies remains controversial, although a clinical trial in renal allograft recipients has provided evidence of its efficacy. Its use in bone marrow transplantation is contentious, but accumulating evidence suggests that any efficacy may result from poorly understood immunomodulatory properties that influence the severity of GVHD. Active immunization with a replicating HCMV virus as a means of inducing protective immunity has been attempted on a limited scale in renal transplant recipients. The results of this trial remain controversial, although there was some evidence suggesting that protective immunity was induced by the vaccine virus.

Alford CA, Britt WJ: Cytomegalovirus. *In* Roizman B, Whitley RJ, Lopez C (eds.): The Human Herpesviruses. New York, Raven Press, 1993, pp 227–255. *Discussion of biology and clinical syndromes associated with HCMV.*

Fowler KB, Stagno S, Pass RF, et al.: The outcome of congenital cytomegalovirus infection in relation to maternal antibody status. N Engl J Med 326:663, 1992. *Recent information on the importance of maternal immunity and outcome of congenital HCMV.*

Gallant JE, Moore RD, Richman DD, et al.: Incidence and natural history of cytomegalovirus disease in patients with advanced human immunodeficiency virus disease treated with zidovudine. J Infect Dis 166:1223, 1992. *Prospective study of natural history of HCMV in HIV-infected patients.*

Ho M: Cytomegalovirus Biology and Infection. New York, Plenum Press, 1991. *Monograph on the biology of HCMV.*

Mocarski ES: Cytomegalovirus biology and replication. *In* Roizman B, Whitley RJ, Lopez C (eds.): The Human Herpesviruses. New York, Raven Press, 1993, pp 173–226. *Excellent overview of molecular biology of HCMV.*

Pass RF, Britt WJ, Stagno S: Cytomegalovirus. *In* Lennette EH, Lennette DA, Lennette ET (eds.): Diagnostic Procedures for Viral, Rickettsial and Chlamydial Infections. 7th ed. Washington, APHA, 1994. *Discussion of commonly used methodologies for diagnosing HCMV.*

Schmidt GM, Horak DA, Niland JC, et al.: A randomized, controlled trial of prophylactic ganciclovir for cytomegalovirus pulmonary infection in recipients of allogeneic bone marrow transplants. N Engl J Med 324:1005, 1991. *Early randomized trial of ganciclovir treatment of HCMV pneumonia in bone marrow allograft recipients.*

Singh N, Yu VL, Mieles L, et al.: High-dose acyclovir compared with short-course preemptive ganciclovir therapy to prevent cytomegalovirus disease in liver transplant recipients. Ann Intern Med 120:375, 1994. *Prophylaxis of HCMV following liver transplantation.*

Winston DJ, Ho WG, Champlin RE: Cytomegalovirus infections after bone marrow transplantation. Rev Infect Dis 12:S776, 1990. *Review of HCMV infections in bone marrow transplant recipients.*

341 INFECTIOUS MONONUCLEOSIS: EPSTEIN-BARR VIRUS INFECTION

Elliott D. Kieff

DEFINITION. Infectious mononucleosis is a clinical syndrome characterized by malaise, headache, fever, pharyngitis, pharyngeal lymphatic hyperplasia, lymphadenopathy, atypical lymphocytosis, heterophile antibody, and mild transient hepatitis. The syndrome occurs most commonly in adolescents and young adults.

ETIOLOGY. Primary Epstein-Barr virus (EBV) infection is the cause of almost all typical infectious mononucleosis syndromes. EBV is a herpes virus. *In vitro,* it infects only human B lymphocytes. Virus infection of B lymphocytes *in vitro* results in lymphocyte proliferation and immunoglobulin secretion. EBV usually remains latent in the infected B lymphocytes and can be induced to replicate in these cells using a variety of chemicals.

EPIDEMIOLOGY. The usual mode of EBV infection is by direct contact of saliva from a previously infected person with the oropharyngeal epithelium of a nonimmune person. Infection in infancy commonly results from eating food premasticated by an infected mother, whereas infection in adolescence or as an adult is usually from salivary transfer during kissing. Virus survival in expectorated saliva is probably brief, since infection does not usually spread to susceptible roommates. Spread among young children sharing toys has not been studied.

Following oropharyngeal inoculation with infected saliva, the virus replicates in oropharyngeal epithelial cells. Although the amount of virus in saliva is highest during primary infection and for months thereafter, virus replication in the oropharynx occurs intermittently for many years, possibly for life. In the course of primary oropharyngeal infection, EBV infects tonsillar and peripheral blood B lymphocytes. Virus persists indefinitely in a small fraction of the peripheral blood B lymphocytes. Transfusion of whole blood, bone marrow, blood fractions, or tissue containing viable B lym-

phocytes to susceptible (nonimmune) persons can result in symptomatic primary infection. Following bone marrow transplantation, the donor's virus may predominate in the recipient and may emerge as the dominant virus in the oropharynx of the recipient, indicating that a bone marrow or blood cell such as B lymphocytes are a site of persistent latent infection and the source of virus for continuing infection of the epithelium. EBV has also been found in salivary gland secretions and in cervical secretions, indicating that latently infected B lymphocytes can transmit virus to other epithelial tissues.

Previously infected normal persons are immune to the development of infectious mononucleosis. In less industrialized societies or among lower socioeconomic groups in industrialized societies, most children experience primary infection in the first decade of life. Among middle and higher socioeconomic groups, primary infection usually occurs as a consequence of adolescent or postadolescent kissing. More than 90% of adults in all human populations have serologic evidence of previous primary EBV infection and are carriers of the virus. Although EBV infection is limited to humans, each Old World primate species is endemically infected with a related virus characteristic of that species. New World primates are free of EBV-related viruses and can be experimentally infected. Experimental infection of some species with a sufficient EBV inoculum results in acute fatal lymphoproliferation.

CLINICAL MANIFESTATIONS. The syndrome of infectious mononucleosis was a distinctive clinical entity for at least 40 years before the discovery of its etiologic agent. After a 2- to 5-week incubation period, most infected nonimmune adolescents and young adults develop malaise, headache, fever, pharyngitis, and lymphadenopathy lasting from 1 to several weeks. Temperatures may reach 40°C. Tonsillar or cervical lymph nodes may be quite enlarged, painful, and tender. Laboratory findings include relative or absolute lymphocytosis and a high titer of antibody to horse or ox red blood cells, referred to as a heterophile antibody. Up to 40% of the peripheral lymphocytes are atypical large cells with unusually abundant cytoplasm and a large pale pleomorphic nucleus. Other common manifestations are listed in Table 341–1. Malaise or weakness may recur over several months. Rashes are significantly more common in patients with primary EBV infection receiving penicillin or ampicillin treatment than in untreated patients or patients with other diseases who are treated with penicillin. Almost all normal people completely recover from acute infectious mononucleosis

TABLE 341–1. CLINICAL MANIFESTATIONS OF INFECTIOUS MONONUCLEOSIS

Common manifestations	(%)
Splenomegaly	50
Vomiting	20
Hepatitis	20–50
Jaundice	5
Palatal petechiae	
Skin rash	4
Albuminuria	10
Less frequent manifestations (0.5–1%)	
Cough	
Pneumonitis	
Neck stiffness	
Aseptic meningitis	
Cerebritis	
Cerebellar dysfunction	
Mononeuritis or polyneuritis	
Transverse myelitis	
Guillain-Barré syndrome	
Uveitis	
Subcapsular splenic hemorrhage or rupture	
Myocarditis	
Pericarditis	
Cardiac conduction abnormalities	
Nephrotic syndrome	
Renal dysfunction	
Diarrhea	
Hemolytic anemia with anti-i antibody	
Thrombocytopenia	
Agranulocytosis	
Pancytopenia	
Hemophagocytic syndrome	

Outside of the adolescent and young adult populations, primary EBV infection frequently does not result in the full infectious mononucleosis syndrome. In younger children, fever and pharyngitis from primary EBV infection may be clinically indistinguishable from upper respiratory tract infections caused by other viruses, mycoplasma, or streptococci. At any age cerebritis, neuritis, pneumonitis, hepatitis, carditis, autoimmune hemolytic anemia, or thrombocytopenia may be the predominant clinical manifestation. Atypical lymphocytosis or heterophile antibody may be less prominent or absent.

Severe, progressive, and sometimes fatal primary EBV infections occur in children in X-linked lymphoproliferative disease (Duncan's syndrome). Non–X-linked, sporadic cases also occur. Although these children have no obvious pre-existing immune deficiency, primary EBV infection leads to massive lymphoproliferation, fever, anemia, hepatitis, or fulminant hepatic necrosis. The proliferating B lymphocytes are EBV-infected cells that express EBV-latent-infection–associated proteins. The early proliferation is polyclonal. Fulminant hepatic failure is a frequent cause of death. Recovery may be accompanied by persistent anemia, hypogammaglobulinemia, or pancytopenia. Oligoclonal or uniclonal EBV-infected B lymphomas may occur during the primary infection or after recovery. Similar illnesses with polyclonal lymphoproliferative disease occur in other immunosuppressed patients with primary EBV infection. Administration of high-dose cyclosporine as part of immunosuppressive regimens for heart, lung, liver, or bone marrow transplantation has been associated with severe EBV infection and polyclonal lymphoproliferative disease. The lymphoproliferative process may involve cervical, abdominal, or gastrointestinal lymphatics. Moreover, children with human immunodeficiency virus (HIV) infection are also at risk for severe EBV infection and lymphoproliferative disease (see Ch. 369), and EBV-infected lymphocytes are a frequent cause of the central nervous system lymphomas that occur in AIDS or organ transplant recipients. In AIDS patients, replicating EBV has also been found in hairy leukoplakia of the tongue, a proliferative epithelial lesion.

Very rare cases of chronic progressive primary EBV infection in otherwise normal young adults have been well documented. These few patients have had severe acute mononucleosis that persists with clinical manifestations that include lymphadenopathy or visceral organ involvement and abnormally high antibody titers to EBV replicative cycle antigens. These titers are characteristically 10- to 100-fold higher than those in normal persons after primary EBV infection. Some patients have lacked antibody to EBV nuclear antigens. Most patients eventually recover without specific treatment. In one patient, acyclovir treatment produced clinical remission.

Persistent active EBV infection has been proposed to be the cause of a more common chronic mononucleosis or *chronic fatigue syndrome*. This syndrome is characterized by recurrent episodes of malaise and weakness, sometimes accompanied by myalgias, arthralgias, pharyngitis, lymphadenitis, or mild fever. The persistent lack of significant objective clinical or laboratory abnormalities distinguishes most patients with this poorly defined syndrome from those with documentable infectious, autoimmune, oncologic, metabolic, or neurologic diseases that can also occur with chronic fatigue. EBV-specific antibody titers in most patients with the chronic fatigue syndrome do not differ significantly from those of normal infected adults (see below). Thus there is little to support the initial hypothesis that EBV is a frequent cause of this syndrome.

Latent EBV infection is also associated with B lymphomas in immunosuppressed patients, with Burkitt-type lymphoma in African children, with some of the sporadic Burkitt-type lymphomas that occur in developed societies, with about 50% of cases of Hodgkin's disease, with some T cell lymphomas in adolescents or young adults, and with anaplastic nasopharyngeal carcinoma. A substantial fraction of B lymphomas occurring in immunocompromised patients have EBV DNA in the tumor cells. In B lymphomas in which the virus is latent in all of the tumor cells, the virus probably provides an initial, and in some cases an ongoing, stimulus for cell proliferation. Malignant conversion in many late postinfection lymphomas requires at least one additional factor, since these cells frequently also have a chromosome translocation that enhances *c-myc* oncogene expression. In a prospective study of African children, a correlation was noted between children with higher EBV antibody responses in the years after primary infection and tumor occurrence, suggesting that the extent of EBV replication is an important parameter in tumor induction.

In the last few years, considerable evidence has been amassed that EBV is an etiologic agent in Hodgkin's disease (see Ch. 146). EBV DNA is present in about 50% of Hodgkin's disease, with the highest incidence of EBV positivity being in younger patients, in Hispanic patients, and in patients with the mixed cellularity form of Hodgkin's disease. When present, EBV DNA is in all of the Hodgkin's disease "tumor" cells, and the cells are uniclonal with regard to EBV infection, indicating that infection did not occur after the onset of Hodgkin's disease.

EBV infection is also associated with anaplastic nasopharyngeal carcinomas. In retrospective and prospective clinical studies, high levels of IgA antibody to EBV antigens have been closely associated with anaplastic nasopharyngeal carcinoma. EBV has been uniformly found in each of the tumor cells of anaplastic nasopharyngeal carcinoma. The uniclonality of the virus genomes in these tumor cells indicates that the tumors arise in a single virus-infected cell. The virus is therefore likely to be necessary for this oncogenic conversion. Chinese and some North African and Canadian and U.S. Native American populations have a high incidence of nasopharyngeal carcinoma. Among peoples of Southern Chinese extraction, anaplastic nasopharyngeal carcinomas are the most common or second most common malignant growth. Genetic factors are therefore likely to be important determinants of tumor incidence. Other factors in the pathogenesis of nasopharyngeal carcinoma have not been defined.

PATHOLOGY AND PATHOGENESIS. EBV first infects pharyngeal epithelial cells and then spreads to subepithelial circulating B lymphocytes. The virus carries a gene similar to the human interleukin-10 gene, and the expression of this protein partially blocks the initial interferon, natural killer (NK), and T-cytotoxic responses. Infection may be confined to epithelial and B-lymphocyte tissues, since only these cells have EBV receptors. The EBV receptor is also the receptor for the C3d fragment of complement. Tonsils and regional and systemic lymph nodes enlarge because of follicular hyperplasia, due in part to virus-infected B lymphocytes and infiltration of sinuses and paracortex with reactive, atypical T lymphocytes. Loss of normal architecture and the presence of Reed-Sternberg–like cells may make EBV infection difficult to distinguish from Hodgkin's disease. Similar changes occur in the spleen. In patients with significant hepatitis, hepatic lobules or portal areas may be infiltrated with mononuclear cells. The bone marrow is usually unaffected. Early in the illness, up to 1 or 2% of the circulating leukocytes may be EBV-infected B lymphocytes. The predominant atypical lymphocytes in the peripheral blood, however, are reactive NK cells and T cells. EBV-infected B lymphocytes can be detected by their expression of EBV nuclear proteins (EBNA's) and latent infection membrane proteins or by their ability to proliferate continuously *in vitro* or in severe combined immunodeficiency (SCID) mice, a property that normal B lymphocytes lack. EBV infection of B lymphocytes stimulates both B-cell proliferation and Ig secretion, particularly IgM. The heterophile antibody may be the direct product of EBV-infected B lymphocytes, or it may be produced as a result of lymphokines produced by EBV-infected or reactive lymphocytes.

Lymphoproliferation following EBV infection of normal B lymphocytes *in vitro* is associated with the expression of six EBV nuclear proteins or EBNA's, two EBV integral membrane proteins or latent infection membrane proteins (LMP's), and two small RNA's. The same repertoire of genes is expressed in the peripheral B lymphocytes in acute infectious mononucleosis and in EBV-associated lymphoproliferative disease. The EBV-encoded nuclear proteins are transactivators of virus and cell gene expression. The virus LMP1 gene encodes the primary transforming protein of the virus. This protein is characteristically expressed in EBV-associated lymphoproliferative disease, in EBV-associated Hodgkin's disease, and in early nasopharyngeal carcinomas. The LMP2 gene encodes a protein that prevents reactivation of virus lytic infection in response to usual B-cell activators. In normal patients with primary EBV infection, the acute, non–B-lymphocyte response to EBV infection is multifunctional. Some T lymphocytes suppress both B-lymphocyte proliferation and Ig secretion. Other peripheral blood T lymphocytes and NK cells from patients with infectious mononucleosis are cytotoxic to autologous EBV-infected B cells. Most cytotoxic T lymphocytes are largely CD8+ and recognize EBNA or LMP epitopes in the context of class I histocompatibility molecules. Other T lymphocytes may augment the T- and B-lymphocyte immune responses. Two EBV types are endemic in humans. These two types differ in their EBNA proteins and in their ability to transform B lymphocytes *in vitro*. Some cytotoxic T-lymphocyte clones are specific for EBNA proteins. Some of these EBNA-specific cytotoxic T lymphocytes recognize only the EBNA protein of one virus type.

After the patient recovers from acute infectious mononucleosis, the proportion of circulating B lymphocytes infected with EBV is 1 in 10^5 to 10^6. Most of these lymphocytes express only the EBNA 1 protein, which is not usually recognized by immune cytotoxic T lymphocytes. These latently infected B lymphocytes are likely to be the site of virus persistence, since long-term suppression of virus replication in the oropharynx with antiviral chemotherapy does not decrease the number of circulating EBV-infected B lymphocytes; and after cessation of treatment, the virus rapidly returns to the oropharyngeal epithelium. Also after bone marrow transplantation, the donor's rather than the recipient's virus may persist in the oropharynx of the recipient. Long after primary EBV infection, T lymphocytes, which can suppress or kill HLA-related EBV-infected cells that express EBNA's or LMP's, continue to circulate in the peripheral blood. Cyclosporine administration for organ transplantation indirectly inhibits the EBV-specific T-lymphocyte immune response, thereby enabling EBV-infected B lymphocytes to overgrow in transplantation recipients receiving high doses of cyclosporine and other immunosuppressive drugs. In this patient group, EBV-associated lymphoproliferative diseases are a significant, albeit unusual, problem.

DIAGNOSIS. In normal adolescents the diagnosis of acute infectious mononucleosis can usually be made on clinical grounds and confirmed by the laboratory findings of atypical lymphocytosis and heterophile antibody to ox or horse erythrocytes. Bacterial throat culture should be obtained in patients with significant pharyngitis to exclude concomitant β-hemolytic streptococcal infection. The rapid heterophile tests are >95% sensitive and >95% specific in an adolescent or young adult population. Titers are substantially diminished by 3 months after primary infection and undetectable by 6 months. In patients with absence of or equivocal heterophile antibodies, EBV-specific serologic testing should be done. The differential diagnosis may include streptococcal or gonococcal pharyngitis; cytomegalovirus, hepatitis virus A or B, HIV, HHV6, adenovirus, or toxoplasma infection; leukemia, lymphoma, and Hodgkin's disease. Most heterophile-negative infectious mononucleosis with pharyngitis is also caused by EBV. In the absence of pharyngitis, however, cytomegalovirus, toxoplasma, hepatitis virus, or HIV infections are likely causes of heterophile-negative or low-titer heterophile-positive infectious mononucleosis. In some patient populations, acute HIV infection is a significant cause of typical or atypical infectious mononucleosis syndromes. HIV antigen or nucleotide sequence–specific detection may be necessary to diagnose HIV infection early in the illness. Later, seroconversion may establish the diagnosis.

Specific serologic testing for EBV infection involves determining antibody titers to latently infected (anti-EBNA), early replication cycle (anti-EA), or late replication cycle (anti-VCA) viral proteins (Fig. 341–1). This is usually done by indirect immunofluorescence microscopy or by enzyme-linked immunoassay. Infection titers are listed in Table 341–2. Those rare patients with chronically progressive EBV infection tend to have abnormally high titers of antibodies to some or many EBV antigens. On the other hand, serologic diagnosis may be misleading in immunosuppressed patients, including children with X-linked immunodeficiency. These infected children may have high or low antibody titers. EBV serologic studies are helpful in following patients with anaplastic nasopharyngeal carcinoma or in screening for early detection of this malignant disease in high-risk populations. Patients at risk for primary anaplastic nasopharyngeal carcinoma or for recurrences have high IgG or IgA EA antibody titers.

TREATMENT. No treatment is necessary for most EBV infections. Rest during the period of acute symptoms and slow return to normal activity are commonly advised, although the therapeutic efficacy of this regimen has not been firmly established. Patients with

splenomegaly should restrict their involvement in sports to avoid traumatic rupture. Acetaminophen or aspirin may be used to reduce temperature and pharyngeal pain in most patients who have normal or only slightly abnormal liver function. Very brief courses of glucocorticoid treatment (e.g., 60 mg prednisone per day for 4 days followed by rapidly decreasing doses) have been effective in shrinking obstructing tonsils, probably by ameliorating an overactive T cell response. Autoimmune hemolytic anemia, granulocytopenia, and thrombocytopenia usually respond to longer courses of glucocorticoid therapy. The use of glucocorticoids for other manifestations of EBV infection is less certain to be beneficial. Glucocorticoids have no antiviral activity and are contraindicated in most herpes virus infections. A few patients with severe hemorrhagic thrombocytopenia refractory to glucocorticoids have responded to intravenous immunoglobulin. Early plasmapheresis is indicated in patients with Guillain-Barré syndrome. Acyclovir and its derivatives have activity against EBV *in vitro* and *in vivo* but are not approved for use against EBV. These drugs should not be used in normal patients with EBV infections since they do not affect the length or severity of illness. Acyclovir can be used for AIDS patients with oral hairy leukoplakia or for patients with well-documented chronically progressive EBV infection. Acyclovir has not affected the outcome of EBV-associated lymphoproliferative syndromes in immunosuppressed patients. Partial restoration of immune function by lowering immune suppression has been beneficial. In one patient with X-linked lymphoproliferative disease, recombinant interferon-γ produced rapid clinical remission.

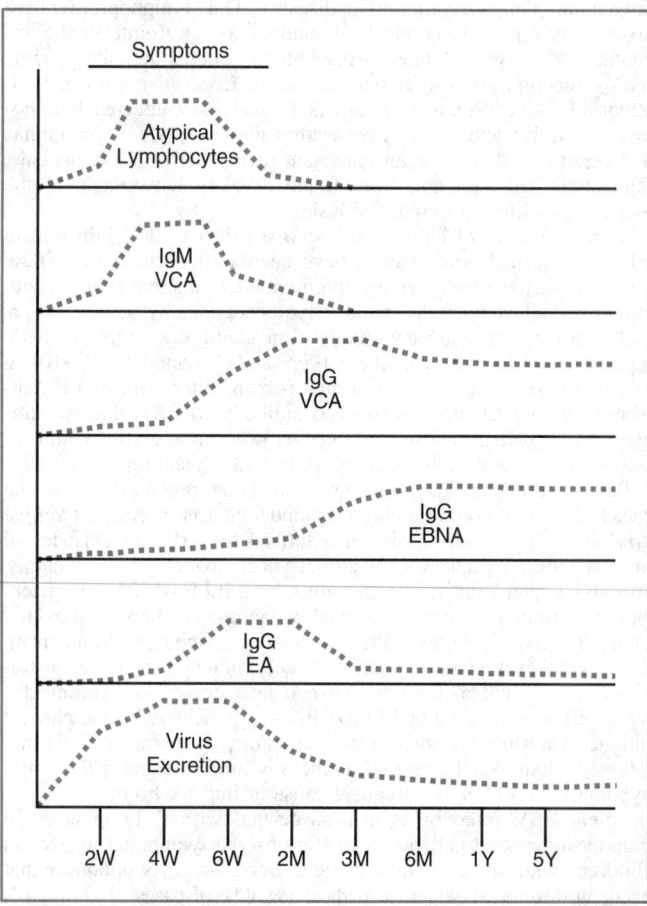

FIGURE 341–1. The usual incubation period after EBV infection is 10 days to 2 weeks. By the time headache, malaise, and fever develop there are usually a few atypical lymphocytes and the monospot or heterophile test may be slightly positive. By 4 weeks, symptoms, monospot test, atypical lymphocytosis, and IgM antibody against EBV viral capsid antigen (VCA) are usually at their maximum. They may persist for another 2 to 3 weeks. IgG anti-EBV early antigen (EA) and anti-VCA are frequently detectable at 4 weeks, but reach their maximum at 6 to 8 weeks. Anti-EBV nuclear protein (EBNA) IgG is usually not detectable until symptoms begin to resolve. Malaise may persist for 8 to 12 weeks. By 3 months, patients are usually fully recovered. IgG anti-VCA and EBNA titers persist at a high level for many years thereafter. EBV infection in normal humans is persistent but asymptomatic.

TABLE 341-2. ANTIBODY TESTS FOR EPSTEIN-BARR VIRUS

	Titers
Acute primary infection	
IgM EA and VCA	High
IgG VCA and EBNA	Low
Recovering from primary infection	
IgM EA or VCA	Lower
IgG VCA	Rising
EBNA	Low
After several months	
IgM EA and VCA	Low or normal
IgG VCA and EBNA	Persist at high for several years

Duncombe AS, Amos RJ, Metcalfe P, Pearson TC: Intravenous immunoglobulin therapy in thrombocytopenic infectious mononucleosis. Clin Lab Haematol 11:11, 1989. *Effect of Ig in two cases of refractory hemorrhagic thrombocytopenia.*

Ernberg I, Andersson J: Acyclovir efficiently inhibits oropharyngeal excretion of Epstein-Barr virus in patients with acute infectious mononucleosis. J Gen Virol 67:2267, 1986. *Effect of acycloguanosine on EBV infection.*

Kieff E: Epstein-Barr virus and its replication. *In* Fields B, Knipe D (eds.): Fields Virology, 3rd ed. New York, Raven Press, 1995. *Review of the biochemistry of Epstein-Barr virus and its effect on lymphocytes.*

Liebowitz D: Epstein-Barr virus—an old dog with new tricks (editorial). N Engl J Med 332:55, 1995.

Rickinson A, Kieff E: Epstein-Barr virus: Biology, pathogenesis and medical aspects. *In* Fields B, Knipe D (eds.): Virology, 3rd ed. New York, Raven Press, 1995. *Review of EBV-associated diseases.*

Schooley RT, Carey RW, Miller G, et al.: Chronic Epstein-Barr virus infection associated with fever and interstitial pneumonitis. Clinical and serologic features and response to antiviral chemotherapy. Ann Intern Med 104:636, 1986. *Illustrative case of chronic EBV.*

Retroviruses

342 RETROVIRUSES OTHER THAN HIV

William A. Blattner

The discovery in 1979 of human T-lymphotropic virus type I (HTLV-I) began a new age of medical virology. It resulted in discoveries that linked human retroviruses to diverse lymphoreticular and chronic degenerative conditions and to the discovery in 1983 of the human immunodeficiency virus (HIV), a lente-retrovirus, the cause of AIDS. These discoveries had scientific roots in the search for human cancer viruses in the early decades of this century; they were propelled by studies of mammalian cancer-causing retroviruses and the delineation of a replication cycle involving reverse transcriptase, which catalyzes the creation of a proviral DNA copy from a viral RNA template. This chapter focuses on the virologic, epidemiologic, and clinical correlates of the HTLV class of viruses; it reviews the distribution of HTLV-I and HTLV-II and presents the known and possible disease associations. Ch. 359 and 361 provide a comprehensive review of HIV and AIDS.

HTLV VIROLOGY

HTLV-I and -II are single-stranded RNA viruses containing a diploid genome that replicates through a DNA intermediary able to integrate into the host cell genome as a provirus. The integration process is essential to the ability of this class of virus to cause lifelong infection, evade immune clearance, and produce diseases of long latency such as leukemia and lymphoma. Morphologically, HTLV-I is approximately 100 nm in diameter with a thin electron-dense outer envelope and an electron-dense, roughly spherical core (Fig. 342–1). The genomic structure of HTLV-I is shown in Figure 342–2. The long terminal repeats (LTR) at the 5' and 3' ends of the genome contain regulatory elements that control virus expression and virion production. Retroviral genes generally code for large overlapping polyproteins that are later processed into functional peptide products by virally encoded protease and cellular proteases. The encoding genes of the virus are *gag* (group-specific antigen), *pol* (polymerase/integrase), *env* (envelope), and a series of accessory genes that regulate virus expression. The *gag* proteins function as structural proteins of the matrix, capsid, and nucleocapsid. The *pol* gene encodes for several enzymes—reverse transcriptase (involved in RNA to DNA transcription), endonuclease (ribonuclease-H), and integrase, which functions for viral integration. The *env* gene encodes the major components of the viral coat: the surface glycoprotein of 46,000 MW (gp46) and the transmembrane 21,000 MW (gp21). The regulatory region, pX, expresses *tax*, which is responsible for enhanced transcription of viral and cellular gene products; it has been postulated to play a crucial role in leukemogenesis. *Rex* (regulator of expression of virion proteins for HTLV) modulates, in a complex manner, the transport of virion components in the production of virus particles.

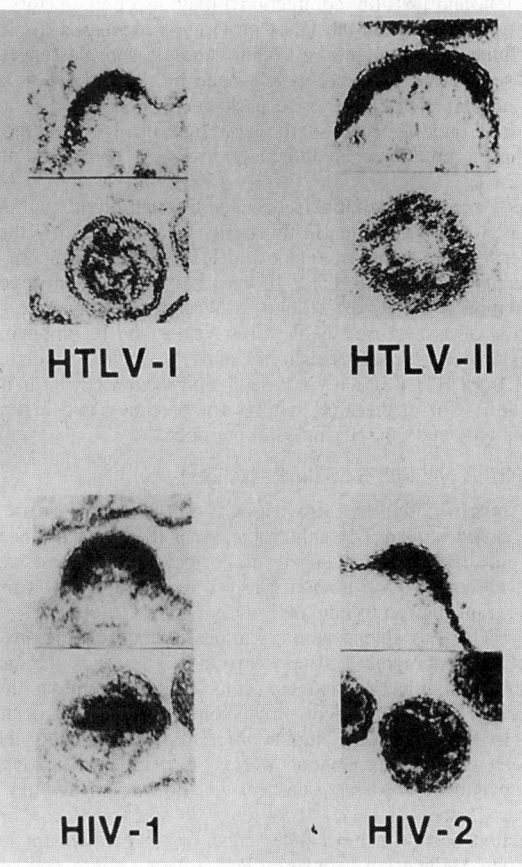

FIGURE 342–1. Morphology of human retroviruses. The budding particles are shown in the upper panel for each virus and the mature virion in the lower panel. The HTLV-I and -II viruses have a roughly spherical electron-dense core, in contrast to the more cylindrical core of human immunodeficiency virus, HIV. (From Blattner WA: Retroviruses. *In* Evans A [ed.]: Viral Infections of Humans, Epidemiology and Control, 3rd ed. New York, Plenum Publishing, 1989, p 545.)

The initial step in the life cycle of HTLV is attachment of the virus envelope glycoprotein to an unknown cell surface receptor, which results in preferential infection of CD4, T-helper cells, for HTLV-I, and CD8 cells for HTLV-II. Following uptake and uncoating, viral RNA is transcribed by *reverse transcriptase*, an RNA-dependent DNA polymerase complexed to the RNA in the core of the virus particle, into double-stranded DNA. This double-stranded viral DNA is integrated into the host cell nucleus by the virally encoded integrase, resulting in cell infection that may be lifelong.

The viral LTR elements are essential to integration: They form the sites for covalent attachment of the provirus to cellular DNA and important viral regulatory elements. The virus may remain "hidden" (unexpressed, not replicated) in cells for long periods.

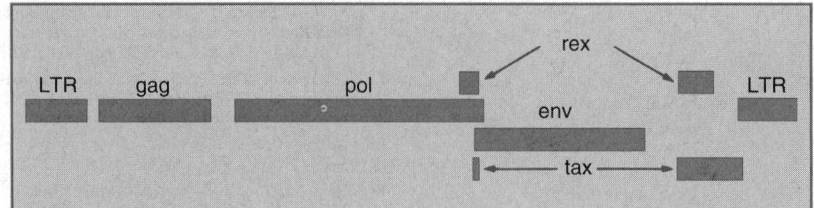

FIGURE 342–2. Genomic structure of human T-lymphotropic viruses. LTR = Long terminal repeat, which is organized into three regions: U5, R, and U3, which house the polyadenylation site; and the *rev* = response element—and the transactivating response element, which are involved in controlling virus expression. *gag* = group specific antigen, whose products form the skeleton of the virion (matrix, capsid, nucleocapsid, nucleic acid binding protein); *pol* = gene for reverse transcriptase, integrase, and protease; *env* = envelope gene; *tax* = transactivator gene; *rex* = viral regulatory gene involved in promoting genomic RNA production. (Courtesy of Dr. Robert C. Gallo.)

This may contribute to the long interval (sometimes many years to decades) between the time of infection and disease.

Factors that control viral replication (viral regulatory genes, cell stimulation, and possibly coinfections) may also be cofactors in disease progression. When the DNA provirus is expressed (transcribed by a cellular RNA polymerase), viral genomic and messenger RNA and subsequently viral proteins are made by the cell. These assemble at the cell membrane to be packaged and released (budding). During the budding process the envelope incorporates the cell's lipid bilayer, producing an infectious virion of about 100 nm (see Fig. 342–1).

HTLV-I and -II are routinely detected through blood bank screening assays that use whole HTLV-I virus lysates. Recently these assays were shown to be insensitive to HTLV-II detection, so newer test kits with enhanced HTLV-II sensitivity have been developed. Confirmation of positives is done by Western blotting. The current generation of assays uses whole virus lysates and recombinant viral antigens; these increase sensitivity and the ability to distinguish HTLV-I from HTLV-II. Polymerase chain reaction (PCR) is another technique useful in research settings for detecting and distinguishing virus type and quantifying viral presence.

EPIDEMIOLOGY AND MODES OF TRANSMISSION

The source of human retroviruses is not known. Primate retroviruses called simian T-lymphotropic virus (STLV) have been isolated from several primate species in Africa; these viruses share significant homology with human HTLV-I and raise the possibility of enzootic transmission to humans.

How HTLV has spread among various human populations is not known. The geographic distribution pattern is unusual; the inconsistent clusters of infection and molecular epidemiologic studies suggest that HTLV is an ancient virus showing patterns of occurrence similar to those of early human migrations. Clusters of HTLV-I have been detected throughout Western and Equatorial Africa and among persons of African descent in the Caribbean and South America. Clusters of HTLV-I are found in southern Japan; little or no infection occurs in most other areas of Asia except for isolated foci among Melanesian peoples in Papua New Guinea and northern Australia. The virus from Melanesia differs molecularly from the Japanese and African strains by 5 to 10%. This variability may be the result of the independent evolution of the virus in these populations of Africa and Asia, which have been separated for tens of thousands of years. A concentration of HTLV-I in northeastern Iran may have resulted from the cross-cultural migrations occurring along the trade routes from the Far East to the Middle East and Europe. HTLV-II has an equally intriguing worldwide distribution: Very limited clusters are found among Native American peoples throughout North, Central, and South America. An Asian focus was recently reported in remote areas of Mongolia, among people who share genetic links with Native American populations whose ancestors emigrated from this region during the Ice Age. HTLV-II has also been detected in Africa, originally among pygmies in Equatorial Africa but more recently in some areas of West Africa. Infections in Europe occur among injection drug users (IDU's) who may have acquired the virus via contact with US IDU's.

Table 342–1 summarizes the routes, cofactors, and viral characteristics associated with HTLV-I transmission; the basic modes of transmission for HTLV-I and HIV-1 are similar.

Sexual transmission of HTLV-I from male to female and female to male as well as from male to male has been documented. HTLV-I transmission is cell-associated and appears to be at least an order of magnitude less infectious than HIV-1. Coincidental infection with other sexually transmitted diseases, particularly those associated with ulcerative genital lesions in males and inflammatory lesions in women, amplify the risk of transmission. For HTLV-I, elevated antibody titer, which appears to correlate with elevated virus load, is linked to heightened transmission. In viral endemic regions there is a characteristic age-dependent rise in HTLV-I seroprevalence. This increase first becomes evident in the adolescent years; it is steeper in women than in men and continues in women after age 40, whereas rates in men plateau around age 40. The most plausible explanation for this pattern is more efficient male-to-female transmission. For HTLV-II the pattern differs; here, the rates for both genders are equal. This finding suggests that there may be differences between the two viruses in the kinetics of transmission.

The second major route of transmission is from mother to child. For HTLV-I, breast-feeding is more efficient than *in utero* or perinatal transmission. For example, whereas 20% of breast-fed infants on average seroconvert to HTLV-I, only 1 to 2% of bottle-fed infants of HTLV-I–positive (HTLV+) mothers become infected. In this regard HTLV-I differs significantly from HIV-1; *in utero* and perinatal transmission accounts for virtually all HIV-1 transmission in the West, where breast-feeding is discouraged. The rate of breast milk–associated HIV-1 transmission is estimated to be approximately 15%. HTLV-II has been detected in breast milk, but mother to child transmission by this route has not been documented.

The third major route of transmission is parenteral, via either transfusion or injection drug use. Surveys of blood donors in the United States document that more than half of the HTLV infections are due to HTLV-II. Among IDU's the vast majority of infections are due to HTLV-II; it is projected that HTLV-II is more efficiently transmitted by this route than is HTLV-I.

Prospective studies of transfusion transmission indicate that both HTLV-I and -II are transmitted in association with cellular components. This is in sharp contrast to HIV-1, which is transmitted by

TABLE 342–1. TRANSMISSION OF HTLV-I/II

	Modes of Transmission	
	HTLV-I	*HTLV-II*
Mother to infant		
Transplacental	Yes	Not known
Breast milk	Yes	Probable
Sexual		
Male to female	Yes	Yes
Female to male	Yes	Yes
Male to male	Yes	Not known
Parenteral		
Blood transfusion	Yes	Yes
Intravenous drug use	Yes	Yes
	Co-factors	
Elevated virus load		
Mother to infant	Yes	Not known
Heterosexual	Yes	Not known
Ulcerative genital lesions	Yes	Not known
Cellular transfusion products	Yes	Yes
Sharing of "works"	Yes	Yes

cells, plasma, or plasma products. Approximately one half of the recipients of HTLV-I and -II + blood seroconvert; the percentage for HIV-1 is > 95%.

The only documented illness linked to HTLV-I or -II transfusion transmission is the HTLV-associated demyelinating neurologic syndrome described below. Leukemia has not been associated with transfusion of HTLV+ blood. Among US blood donors who are confirmed HTLV+ (slightly less than half are HTLV-I and the others are HTLV-II), the major risk factors are intravenous drug use, birthplace in a viral endemic area, or sexual contact with a person with this profile.

Coinfection with HTLV-I and HIV-1 appears to increase the progression to AIDS through unexplained mechanisms, possibly related to the cell proliferative effects of HTLV-I on HIV-1–infected T cells. Such a relationship has not been shown for HTLV-II. Other modes of transmission involving "casual contact," mosquito transmission, and so on, do not seem to happen. Health care and laboratory workers who experience a needle stick, skin or mucous membrane exposure in the absence of protective barriers are at little or no risk for infection; a single case of such infection has been documented in a Japanese health care worker exposed to HTLV-I.

CLINICAL MANIFESTATIONS AND PATHOGENESIS

HTLV-I–associated diseases are listed in Table 342–2.

Adult T-Cell Leukemia/Lymphoma (ATL)

The most common malignancy caused by HTLV-I is ATL; this is more accurately classified as a form of peripheral T-cell lymphoma that may include peripheral blood involvement. The HTLV-associated lymphomas include several subtypes of ATL: acute, chronic, smoldering, and lymphoma-type. Their clinical features are summarized in Figure 342–3. These tumors represent high-grade lymphomas, usually of large, medium, and/or pleiotropic morphology and advanced clinical stage, and are associated with a poor prognosis.

The worldwide occurrence of these HTLV-I–associated malignancies is difficult to quantify because the incidence in any population depends on the prevalence of viral infection. In HTLV-I endemic areas such as southern Japan and the Caribbean Islands, the annual incidence of virus-associated leukemia is approximately 3 in 100,000 per year and may account for one half of adult lymphoid malignancies. The chance of an infected individual developing a malignancy over a lifetime is approximately 5%; early life exposure is associated with the greatest risk for subsequent disease.

The acute form of ATL (Fig. 342–3) is characterized by an aggressive mature T-cell lymphoma whose clinical course is often associated with high white count, hypercalcemia, and cutaneous involvement. Other cases resemble T-cell chronic lymphocytic leukemia and are termed chronic ATL. Smoldering ATL may clinically resemble mycosis fungoides/Sezary syndrome with cutaneous involvement presenting as erythema or as infiltrative plaques or tumors. Sometimes a long prodrome of symptoms is noted before transformation to an acute, rapidly fatal form of disease occurs. Sometimes ATL presents as a T-cell non-Hodgkin's lymphoma with no other clinical features of ATL except for monoclonal integration of HTLV-I in proviral DNA in the tumor cells. Most patients with acute and lymphoma-type ATL die within 6 months of diagnosis. The cause of death is usually an explosive growth of tumor cells, hypercalcemia, and various opportunistic infections including *Pneumocystis carinii* pneumonia and other infections observed in AIDS patients.

The age group ranges from adolescence to a peak in middle-aged adults. The diagnosis should be considered in an adult with mature T-cell lymphoma and hypercalcemia and/or cutaneous involvement, particularly if the individual is from a known risk group or endemic region. The diagnosis is established by testing serum for HTLV-I antibodies and finding leukemic T cells with the provirus in the blood or in biopsy specimens.

TABLE 342–2. HTLV-ASSOCIATED DISEASES

Diagnosis	Nature of Syndrome	Strength of Association
HTLV-I–associated diseases		
Adult T-cell leukemia/ lymphoma	Aggressive lymphoproliferative malignancy of mature T lymphocytes	Strong
B-cell chronic lymphocytic leukemia	Tumor-associated immunoglobulin reacts to HTLV antigen	2 cases reported
Tropical spastic paraparesis (TSP)/ HTLV-associated myelopathy (HAM)	Chronic progressive demyelinating syndrome of long motor tracks of spinal cord	Strong
Polymyositis	Degenerative inflammatory syndrome of skeletal muscles	Probable
Infective dermatitis	Chronic generalized eczema of skin in children; potential for preleukemia and immunodeficiency	Strong
Uveitis	Inflammatory infiltration of the uvea of the eye	Strong
HTLV-associated arthritis	Large joint polyarthropathy; rheumatoid factor positive with HTLV-I positive cells infiltrating the synovia	Probable
Immune deficiency	Anecdotal reports of AIDS-like illness in HTLV-I positives; subclinical (e.g., decreased PPD response) or clinical (e.g., poor response to therapy for symptomatic strongyloidiasis)	Possible
Miscellaneous clinical conditions	Case reports or case series of Sjögren's syndrome, interstitial pneumonitis, small cell lung cancer with monoclonal HTLV-I integration, and invasive cervical cancer	Uncertain
HTLV-II–associated diseases		
T-hairy cell/ large granulocytic	Case reports of T-cell malignancy with either monoclonal or polyclonal integration	Possible
Leukemia	HTLV-II integration in T cells and either T-cell, NK-cell, or B-cell proliferation	
HTLV-associated myelopathy	Case reports of TSP/ HAM in association with HTLV-II. In some cases ataxic form of neurologic involvement reported	Probable
Miscellaneous clinical conditions	Case reports or case series of HTLV-II and mycosis fungoides, asthma, glomerular nephritis, pulmonary disease	Uncertain

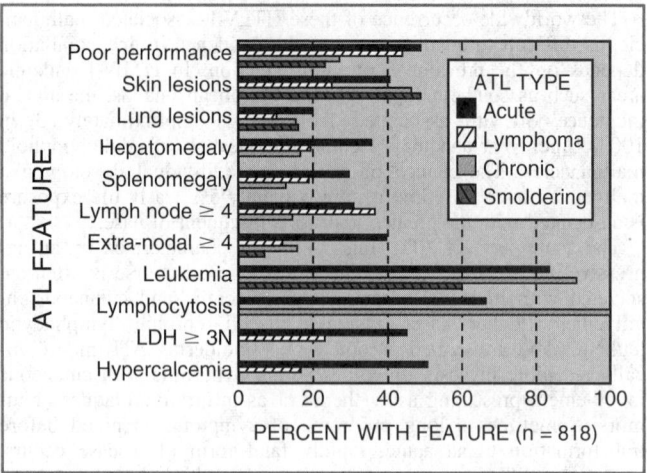

FIGURE 342–3. Features of adult T-cell lymphoma/leukemia in Japan. A combination of clinical and laboratory features is involved in defining the various subtypes of ATL (see text for details). (From Blattner W: Human T-cell lymphotropic viruses and cancer causation. *In* Devita VT, Hellman S, Rosenberg SA [eds.]: Cancer Prevention, Update. Philadelphia, JB Lippincott, 1993, p 1.)

ATL has proven refractory to most conventional and experimental chemotherapeutic regimens (Fig. 342–4). In general, smoldering ATL is the least aggressive form. The chronic type has a relatively poor prognosis with death occurring within a few years of diagnosis. Patients with chronic and smoldering ATL receive no therapy or they are treated with prednisone with or without cyclophosphamide. The more indolent forms of ATL have a high rate of complicating infections resulting from the immunosuppressive effects of aggressive therapy. Acute and lymphoma-type ATL's are aggressive high-grade lymphomas with a generally poor prognosis, although some cases do respond to multidrug regimens with prolonged remission.

Initial response rates, even for the poorest risk categories, are > 50%, and complete remissions are achieved in 20% of the cases. Relapses often occur within weeks to months after treatment, although up to 15% of the patients have extended survival beyond 2 years (Fig. 342–4). Poor prognosis is associated with poor performance status at diagnosis: age over 40, extensive disease, hypercalcemia, and high serum LDH level. Relapses in long-term survivors often occur in the central nervous system (CNS) and prove refractory to subsequent therapy. Experimental approaches under investigation include using monoclonal antibodies to the interleukin-2 (IL-2) receptor linked with cell toxins selectively targeted to the leukemic cells and a combination of zidovudine and interferon.

A possible association was reported between HTLV-I and some cases of B-cell chronic lymphotropic leukemia. In these cases, chronic stimulation of B-cell proliferation by viral antigens, coupled with virus-induced impairment of CD4 cell function, resulted in malignant transformation in B cells with HTLV-I–specific cell surface antibodies.

Tropical Spastic Paraparesis/HTLV-1–Associated Myelopathy (TSP/HAM)

HTLV-I has been linked to a neurologic syndrome known as TSP/HAM. This disease is characterized by a chronic, slowly progressive development of spastic paraparesis resulting from the demyelination of the long motor neurons of the spinal cord. Symptoms often begin with a stiff gait, progressing (usually slowly) to increasing spasticity and weakness, with incontinence and impotence developing later in the course of the illness. Sometimes ataxia develops. In some cases, isolated lesions of the CNS are detected on a nuclear magnetic resonance scan. This syndrome differs from classic multiple sclerosis because of its generally slow, progressive course and the absence of a waxing and waning symptomatology. However, some cases are acutely progressive; such cases are sometimes associated with the transfusion of HTLV-I+ blood.

The incidence of disease is approximately half of the rate for ATL. The diagnosis is suspected in unexplained CNS disease with loss of pyramidal tract functions and is confirmed by testing sera for HTLV-I antibodies. Treatment with corticosteroids benefits some patients, particularly those with rapidly progressive disease; Danazol, an androgenic steroid, improves urinary and fecal incontinence but does not affect the underlying neurologic deficit.

TSP/HAM is the prototype for a series of immune-mediated syndromes characterized by high virus load, significant immune activation, and an indirect pathogenic mechanism produced by virally induced perturbations in immune function. Examples of these conditions include polymyositis of the skeletal muscle, uveitis of the eye, a large joint arthritis, and Sjögren's syndrome. Additional oncogenic effects are suggested by a Japanese case of small cell lung cancer with monoclonal HTLV integration and association with invasive cervical cancer. HTLV-I has also been linked to immunosuppression through clinical and laboratory observations of Japanese patients with AIDS-like illnesses associated with HTLV-I (in the absence of underlying malignancy), perturbations in skin test reactivity, and the finding that parasitic infestations (e.g., strongyloidiasis) are refractory to conventional treatments. The infective dermatitis syndrome first reported in Jamaica represents the first childhood HTLV-I syndrome; immunosuppression and preleukemia are possible features.

HTLV-II AND DISEASE

At this time HTLV-II continues to be an "orphan" virus with no true disease association. The virus was originally isolated from a patient with hairy T-cell leukemia, but surveys of hairy T-cell leukemia and related entities have identified only occasional HTLV-II positives. These include one case in which the virus was polyclonally infecting T cells while causing a B-cell malignancy. Large granulocytic cell leukemia (LGL), a malignancy with a natural killer (NK) cell phenotype, has also been linked to HTLV-II in

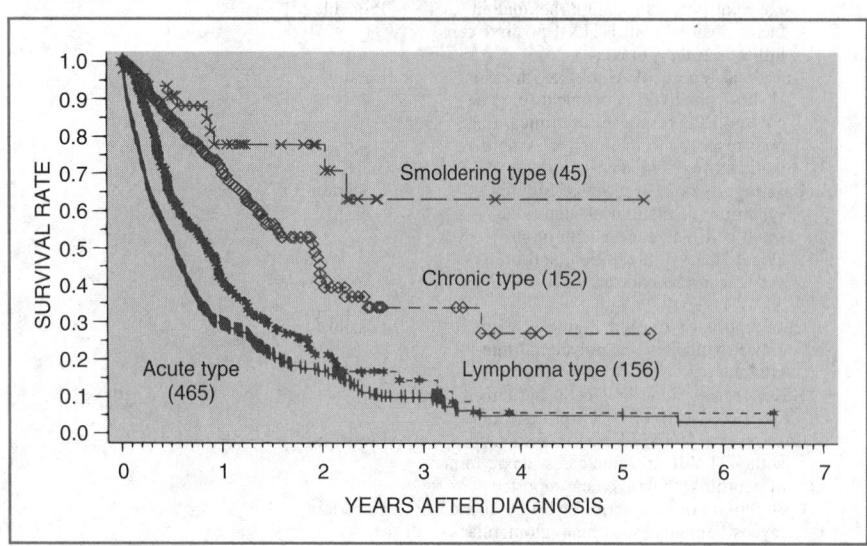

FIGURE 342–4. Survival by ATL subtype after polychemotherapy in Japan. Poorest survival is observed in patients with acute and lymphoma-type ATL. (From Tsukasaki K, Ikeda S, Murata K, et al.: Characteristics of chemotherapy-induced clinical remission in long survivors with aggressive adult T-cell leukemia/lymphoma. Leuk Res 17:157, 1993.)

some cases. In these instances, there is a pattern of polyclonal infection of T cells and malignant expansion of NK cells not infected with the virus. It has been hypothesized that in these cases HTLV-II is acting through an indirect mechanism.

Approximately a dozen TSP/HAM cases associated with HTLV-II have been reported. In some instances the clinical pattern had features of the ataxic form, but most had the more typical spastic paraparesis. Preliminary data suggest this syndrome is infrequent compared to its occurrence in HTLV-I carriers.

HTLV-I PATHOGENESIS

A great deal has been learned about the pathogenesis of HTLV-I–associated leukemia. Early in infection, HTLV-I infects only a small number of T cells and probably the monocyte/macrophage. The DNA provirus randomly integrates into the DNA of infected cells. Although HTLV-I may exist as a latent virus, the virus genes promote cell proliferation by direct and indirect mechanisms, including various lymphokine pathways. In the process they may promote the expression of additional activated target cells and thereby amplify virus spread. For example, when lymphocytes from HTLV-I–infected normal persons are placed in tissue culture, they undergo spontaneous (in the absence of exogenous antigens or mitogens) lymphocyte proliferation. Early in the infection phase, host immune responses to the virus are activated, producing viral antibodies and cytotoxic T cells targeted at viral antigens. In some cases persons with documented exposure (e.g., via blood transfusion) do not seroconvert and develop cell-mediated immune responses that presumably clear virus infection. Some healthy carriers develop T-cell polyclonal and oligoclonal proliferations that can later progress to malignancy or may disappear spontaneously. Morphologically distinct "flower cells," representing T cells with deeply lobulated nuclei resembling ATL leukemic cells, are seen on peripheral blood smears of healthy carriers but do not presage risk for subsequent disease. In ATL, the HTLV-I provirus is found integrated in the DNA of the leukemic cells in a clonal fashion with one (or occasionally two) copy of the provirus integrated in the same chromosomal location in each cell. This would indicate that ATL is tumor derived from a single transformed cell that sprouted from a virus infection before transformation and clonal expansion rather than afterwards as a passenger virus. Tumors from different patients have proviral integration in different locations. This indicates that cis-activation of a nearby cellular gene by the LTR of the virus, as occurs with some animal leukemia viruses, is not the mechanism for transformation in ATL.

The latent period for this process is years to several decades; it involves an interaction between viral expression and oncogenic mutations. For example, recent studies have identified abnormalities in the clearance of the p53 suppressor gene in HTLV-I infected cells; other studies demonstrate the binding of viral tax to a receptor on NF-kB. Immunosuppressive events may also play a role because the tumor necrosis factor-β (TNF-β) is turned on in ATL. Evidence is growing that at some stage, transformation involves the expression of the tax protein encoded by the px gene of HTLV-I. Because the tax protein induces expression of cellular genes critical for T-cell proliferation, including IL-2 and its receptor (IL-2R), an autocrine mechanism may be involved, particularly in the first steps of leukemogenesis, which involves polyclonal expansions of T cells. In order for malignancy to develop, additional genetic changes most probably take place (e.g., cytogenetic changes, oncogene alterations). Because tax gene expression is detectable in tumor samples,

even in some cases of antibody-negative ATL, this viral gene may be crucial in oncogenesis.

The pathogenesis of TSP/HAM is uncertain, but it appears to occur with a much shorter latency (sometimes acutely following transfusion-associated infection) than does ATL. Some researchers speculate a direct mechanism involving infection of nervous system cells; others conjecture an indirect mechanism involving immune- and autoimmune-mediated responses following from HTLV-I infection of regulatory T-cell populations.

PREVENTION

A major issue confronting practicing physicians is what to tell patients identified as HTLV+ based on blood bank screening. First and foremost, they must emphasize that disease complications related to HTLV-I are rare and that for HTLV-II no specific disease has been verified, and second, that the viruses are not easily transmitted. Third, the patient should be clearly counseled concerning the distinction between the HTLV and the HIV viruses because the greatest fear the patient may have is that he/she has the "AIDS virus." Recently, guidelines for prevention and counseling have been developed for HTLV-I and -II by a Centers for Disease Control and Prevention Working Group: (1) Blood for donation should be screened prior to transfusion and positive donors should be deterred from donating. (2) HTLV-I/II+ mothers should be discouraged from breast-feeding when practicable to prevent mother-to-infant transmission (except in particular settings, such as in the tropics, where diarrheal disease in non–breast-fed infants presents a high risk for morbidity and mortality). (3) Condoms should be used by discordant couples, but, given the relatively low frequency of sexual transmission per sexual encounter, couples who desire a pregnancy could time unprotected sexual intercourse to coincide with periods of maximal fertility. (Such decisions require careful discussion between physician and patient; there are no absolute guidelines in this area.)

Vaccines containing whole virus and recombinant HTLV-I envelope antigens have successfully prevented HTLV-I infection in monkeys and in a rabbit model; it is uncertain whether a vaccine for HTLV-I or -II will ever be implemented for humans. For example, in Japan epidemiologic data show that new infections are declining because of changing socioeconomic and lifestyle factors, whereas in developing countries rates as high as 1 to 1.5% per year are reported in sexually active populations. It is unclear whether the disease burden associated with these viruses warrants a vaccine.

Blattner WA (ed.): Human Retrovirology: HTLV. New York, Raven Press, 1990. *Comprehensive update of human T-cell leukemia virus including chapters on virology, immunology, epidemiology and clinical features, and management. In Devita VT, Hellman S, Rosenberg SA (eds.).*

Blattner W: Human T-cell lymphotrophic viruses and cancer causation. In Devita VT, Hellman S, Rosenberg SA (eds.): Cancer Prevention, Update. Philadelphia, JB Lippincott, 1993, p 1. *A clinically oriented review of HTLV-I and related diseases.*

Centers for Disease Control and Prevention: Guidelines for counseling persons infected with human T-lymphotropic virus type I (HTLV-I) and type II (HTLV-II). Ann Intern Med 118:448, 1993. *Presents important information to clinicians confronted with counseling persons referred with HTLV infection.*

Hall WW: Human T cell lymphotropic virus type I and cutaneous T cell leukemia/lymphoma. J Exp Med 180:1581, 1994. *A concise review of the pathogenic role of HTLV-I in the etiology of mature T-cell malignancies, including recent data exploring the role of this family of viruses in cutaneous T-cell malignancies in the United States and Europe.*

Takatsuki K (ed.): Adult T-cell Leukemia. Oxford, Oxford Press, 1994. *The most recent update of a monograph series on the subject of ATL and related diseases.*

Enteric Viral Infections

343 ENTEROVIRUSES
Michael N. Oxman

Enteroviruses, so named because they generally infect the alimentary tract and are shed in the feces, cause a variety of diseases in humans and lower animals. They comprise one of the five

major subgroups, or genera, of the Picornavirus (*pico,* small; *rna,* ribonucleic acid) family. The other Picornavirus genera are: *Rhinoviruses,* which inhabit the upper respiratory tract and include the principal recognized etiologic agents of the common cold (see Ch. 328); *Cardioviruses,* recovered chiefly from rodents and only very rarely implicated in human disease; *Aphthoviruses,* named for the vesicular lesions that they produce in cloven-footed animals; and *Hepatovirus,* a newly designated genus with human hepatitis A virus as its only currently recognized member.

Enteroviruses are differentiated from *rhinoviruses* primarily by their resistance to acid; they are fully infectious at pH 3 or even lower. Consequently, enteroviruses that have undergone limited replication in the oropharynx survive passage through the stomach and implant in the lower intestinal tract, where they undergo more extensive multiplication. In contrast, rhinoviruses are acid labile; they begin to lose infectivity at pH 6 and are completely inactivated at pH 3. They are further distinguished from enteroviruses by their lower optimal temperature of replication (33°C versus 37°C for enteroviruses) and higher buoyant density in cesium chloride. Since rhinoviruses inhabit the nasopharynx, they have no obvious need for acid stability, and preferential replication at lower than body temperature probably reflects their adaptation to the cooler nasal passages.

Hepatitis A virus was originally classified as an enterovirus and designated enterovirus 72. However, it is more resistant to inactivation by heat than enteroviruses, and its genome has relatively little nucleotide sequence homology with members of the *Enterovirus* genus. Furthermore, in contrast to enteroviruses, hepatitis A virus does not cause a rapid shut-off of host cell protein synthesis, and the infected cells are not lysed. Because of these important differences, hepatitis A virus has been accorded its own genus, *Hepatovirus*, within the Picornavirus family. Hepatitis A virus is discussed in Ch. 117.

Within the *Enterovirus* genus, species are distinguished immunologically by the ability of specific antisera to neutralize only the homotypic virus. There are now 67 recognized human enterovirus species (*serotypes* or *immunotypes*), as well as numerous enteroviruses of lower animals. Humans appear to be the only natural host for the human enteroviruses, and, in general, the enteroviruses of lower animals are not natural pathogens for humans.

Historically, human enteroviruses have been subclassified into *polioviruses,* group A and group B *coxsackieviruses,* and *echoviruses* on the basis of antigenic relationships, differences in host range, and type of disease produced (Table 343–1). By 1969, 67 species (serotypes) of human enteroviruses had been identified and classified according to these criteria, although reclassification and redundancy have reduced this number to 63. The distinguishing characteristics of these enterovirus subgroups are outlined below.

POLIOVIRUSES. The first human enteroviruses to be recognized, *polioviruses* produce characteristic lesions when inoculated into the central nervous system (CNS) of primates. Clinical isolates replicate only in primates and in primate cell cultures (see Ch. 425). There are three poliovirus serotypes.

COXSACKIEVIRUSES. In contrast to polioviruses, *coxsackieviruses* produce paralysis and death when inoculated into suckling mice. This property was responsible for their detection and differentiation from polioviruses when they were first recovered in 1948 from the feces of two children in the village of Coxsackie, New York, who were suffering from a poliomyelitis-like paralytic illness. With the isolation of additional serotypes, it was recognized that when inoculated into suckling mice, some coxsackieviruses, designated *group A coxsackieviruses,* produced generalized myositis of skeletal muscles that resulted in flaccid paralysis, whereas others,

designated *group B coxsackieviruses,* produced only focal myositis but caused an encephalitis that resulted in spastic paralysis and a generalized infection that involved the myocardium, brown fat, pancreas, and other organs. Moreover, group B coxsackieviruses could be readily propagated in primate cell cultures, whereas group A coxsackieviruses grew poorly or not at all. Twenty-three group A and six group B coxsackievirus serotypes have been identified.

ECHOVIRUSES. The use of the cell culture techniques developed by Enders and colleagues led to the recovery, from the feces of healthy children, of additional enteroviruses that produced cytopathic effects in primate cell cultures but failed to produce disease in suckling mice or in the CNS of primates. These agents, initially considered "orphan" viruses because they were unrelated to any disease, were called *echoviruses* (enteric *c*ytopathic *h*uman *o*rphan). Echoviruses have now been associated with a variety of diseases, and 31 serotypes have identified. Most echoviruses are readily propagated in primate cell cultures.

SIMPLIFIED TAXONOMIC SCHEME. The detailed comparison of enterovirus genomes supports the validity of this classification scheme. Different serotypes within the same human enterovirus subgroup, e.g., group B coxsackieviruses, generally have 30 to 50% of their nucleotide sequences in common, whereas serotypes from different subgroups generally share < 20% of their nucleotide sequences. About 5% of the nucleotide sequences are conserved among all human enteroviruses.

Over the years, however, an increasing number of enterovirus isolates were identified that could not be subclassified unambiguously by these criteria (e.g., viruses serologically related to known echoviruses but with a host range characteristic of coxsackieviruses). Consequently it was agreed in 1970 that newly recognized human enteroviruses would be classified simply as *enteroviruses* and numbered sequentially, beginning with enterovirus 68. To avoid confusion with the older literature, the original classification (*poliovirus,* group A and group B *coxsackievirus,* and *echovirus*) has been retained for the first 63 serotypes. Since adoption of this simplified taxonomic scheme, four new human enteroviruses, enteroviruses 68–71, have been recognized.

ENTEROVIRUSES 68–71. Enterovirus 68 was initially isolated from the throat of an infant with bronchiolitis and pneumonia. Few isolates have since been reported, and the agent is little studied. Enterovirus 69 was recovered from the feces of an asymptomatic child, and this serotype has not yet been associated with disease. Enterovirus 70 is the principal cause of acute hemorrhagic conjunctivitis, a disease first recognized in 1969, which has subsequently affected tens of millions of persons throughout the world. Enterovirus 70 has an unusually broad host range; it causes meningoencephalitis in humans and in experimentally infected monkeys, and it infects both primate and nonprimate cell cultures. Genome analysis and serologic surveys raise the possibility that enterovirus 70 may be a zoonotic enterovirus that has recently extended its host range to include humans. Enterovirus 71, first recognized as the cause of an outbreak of aseptic meningitis and encephalitis in California between 1969 and 1972, is neurovirulent in monkeys and produces a myositis in suckling mice that is typical of that produced by group A coxsackieviruses. Enterovirus 71 has been recovered throughout the world in association with a variety of clinical

TABLE 343–1. CLASSIFICATION OF HUMAN ENTEROVIRUSES*

Enterovirus Group	Number of Serotypes	Numerical Designation	Growth in Primate Cell Culture	Pathogenicity for Suckling Mice	Pathogenicity for Monkeys
Poliovirus	3	1–3	+	−	+
Coxsackievirus, group A	23	A1–22, A24†	+/−‡	+	−α
Coxsackievirus, group B	6	B1–6	+	+	+
Echovirus	31	1–9, 11–27, 29–34¶	+	−	−
Enterovirus	4	68–71**	+	variable††	variable‡‡

* Many enterovirus strains have been isolated that do not conform to these criteria.
† Coxsackievirus A23 has been reclassified as echovirus 9.
‡ Except for a few serotypes (e.g., A7, A9, A16), primary isolates of group A coxsackieviruses grow poorly or not at all in cell culture; virus isolation requires inoculation of suckling mice.
α Coxsackievirus A7 is neurovirulent in monkeys.
¶ Echovirus 10 has been reclassified as reovirus type 1; echovirus 28 has been reclassified as rhinovirus 1A.
** Hepatitis A virus, formally classified as human enterovirus 72, is now classified as a member of the *Hepatovirus* genus.
†† Enteroviruses 70 and 71 are pathogenic for suckling mice.
‡‡ Enteroviruses 70 and 71 are neurovirulent in monkeys.

manifestations and many fatal infections. These have included respiratory infections, aseptic meningitis, hand-foot-and-mouth disease, maculopapular exanthems, and encephalitis. In addition, enterovirus 71 has been responsible for epidemics of acute paralytic disease indistinguishable from poliomyelitis.

The discovery of the enteroviruses, as well as the origins of modern virology, were closely associated with efforts to control poliomyelitis. Poliovirus type 1 is the prototype for the *Enterovirus* genus and for the Picornavirus family. It is one of the most extensively studied and thoroughly characterized agents of disease. While a number of nonpolio enteroviruses have also been well characterized and the genomes of several have been cloned and sequenced, much of our present understanding of enterovirus structure, replication, genetics, pathogenesis, and immunology is derived from studies carried out with wild type and vaccine strains of poliovirus.

The enteroviruses have many features in common, and they will be discussed as a group before considering the special features of individual members. Since polioviruses are the subject of Ch. 425, this discussion will be limited to the nonpolio enteroviruses.

PHYSICAL AND BIOCHEMICAL CHARACTERISTICS OF ENTEROVIRUSES

The enteroviruses share with all picornaviruses certain important physical and biochemical characteristics: They are small, spherical, nonenveloped viruses approximately 30 nm in diameter. Their genome consists of a linear, single-stranded, unsegmented molecule of RNA with a molecular weight of about 2.6×10^6 daltons (approximately 7500 nucleotides) which has the same polarity as messenger RNA, i.e., it is plus (+) stranded, and is thus infectious. In fact, purified enterovirus RNA can initiate the synthesis of complete infectious virions *in vitro* in cell-free extracts from susceptible cells. The viral genome is tightly packed within an icosahedral protein shell or *capsid* composed of 60 identical subunits or *protomers,* each of which has a molecular mass of 90,000 to 100,000 daltons and is itself composed of four nonidentical virus-encoded polypeptides (VP1, VP2, VP3, and VP4). VP1, VP2, and VP3 are exposed on the virion surface, whereas VP4 lies buried in association with the RNA core. Like all picornaviruses, enteroviruses exhibit a unique pattern of replication in which the viral genome is translated into a single giant *polyprotein,* which is then cleaved by endogenous viral proteinases into the individual viral structural and nonstructural proteins.

Enteroviruses are stable over a wide range of pH (pH 3 to 10) and retain infectivity for days at room temperature, weeks at refrigerator temperature, and indefinitely when frozen at $-20°C$ or lower. They are readily inactivated at temperatures above $50°C$, but this inactivation is inhibited by molar magnesium chloride, which greatly enhances the stability of enteroviruses at all environmental temperatures. Thus, magnesium chloride is widely used as a stabilizer for oral poliovirus vaccines.

Enteroviruses are resistant to proteolytic enzymes and to inactivation by organic solvents, deoxycholate, and various detergents that destroy lipid-containing enveloped viruses such as herpesviruses, orthomyxoviruses, and paramyxoviruses. Enteroviruses are inactivated by formaldehyde, chlorination, and ultraviolet light but are protected from inactivation by dissolved organic matter, the formation of virus aggregates, and adsorption to particulate matter. Consequently, enteroviruses may survive secondary sewage treatment and chlorination as generally practiced, and are abundant in urban sewage and treated waste water. The agricultural use of treated sewage and recycled waste water may thus contaminate food and water supplies. Since sewage treatment that destroys fecal coliform bacteria does not eliminate enteroviruses, the use of fecal coliform counts to assess the sanitary quality of water is inadequate with respect to its potential for transmission of enteroviral diseases. Enteroviruses are often detectable in samples of recreational water judged acceptable on the basis of fecal coliform counts. Although person-to-person (fecal-oral) spread is the dominant mode of transmission, and water-borne outbreaks of enterovirus infection have rarely been documented, the hazard associated with the discharge of virus-laden sewage into coastal waters is demonstrated by the occurrence of shellfish-associated outbreaks of hepatitis A. Clams, mussels, and oysters are filter-feeders that concentrate virus and function as passive virus carriers. Most of the enteroviruses in sewage are associated with suspended solids, and virus adsorbed to sediment remains infectious for long periods in the marine environment. The reintroduction of specific enteroviruses into coastal populations when marine sediments are disturbed by storms, dredging, and so on, might explain the sudden occurrence of epidemics as well as the reappearance of certain enterovirus serotypes after years of absence from the human population.

EPIDEMIOLOGY

Human enteroviruses are worldwide in distributions, and humans are their only known reservoir. The prevalence of enterovirus infection varies markedly with season and climate, and with the age and socioeconomic status of the population studied. In tropical and semitropical regions, enterovirus infections are frequent throughout the year. In temperate climates, the incidence of infection is markedly increased in the summer and early fall; in Europe and North America 80 to 90% of enterovirus isolates are recovered from June through October, with peak recovery in August. Even within the United States, climatic and socioeconomic factors affect the prevalence of enterovirus infections. Enterovirus isolation rates from young children are twofold to threefold higher in southern than in northern cities, and threefold to sixfold higher in lower than in middle and upper socioeconomic districts. In developed countries, usually only one to three enterovirus serotypes are highly prevalent in a given community each year, with different serotypes prevalent in different years, and isolation rates in young children rarely exceed 10%. In developing countries with poor sanitation, a greater number of enterovirus serotypes circulate simultaneously, and isolation rates in children are regularly > 75%, with many fecal specimens yielding three or more enterovirus serotypes.

Some enteroviruses appear to be endemic, being isolated at low frequency in the same locality each year, whereas others produce local or regional epidemics and then disappear, only to return again years later. Occasionally an enterovirus will spread worldwide, infecting tens of millions of persons and producing pandemic disease. This pattern was observed with echovirus 9 in the late 1950's and with enterovirus 70, which caused a pandemic of acute hemorrhagic conjunctivitis beginning in 1969.

Enteroviruses exhibit a high rate of mutation during replication in the human gastrointestinal tract, and this can lead to the appearance of antigenic varients, as well as virus strains with altered tissue tropism and virulence. Such mutations are readily detected within days after administration of attenuated poliovirus vaccines to normal children. They have also been observed in a number of nonpolio enteroviruses. Recently isolated strains of several coxsackieviruses, echoviruses, and enterovirus 70 have been found to differ in many epitopes from the corresponding *prototype* strains isolated more than a decade earlier, a pattern of "antigenic drift" not unlike that seen with influenza viruses. In addition, recombination between the genomes of different enterovirus serotypes can be observed in multiply infected individuals, e.g., in young children in developing countries, and in recipients of trivalent oral poliovirus vaccines. Antigenic changes and alterations in cell tropism produced by mutation and recombination may help to account for the ability of individual enterovirus serotypes to persist in nature and to cause a variety of clinical syndromes.

Transmission of human enteroviruses is chiefly by the fecal-oral route directly from person to person or via fomites; spread by respiratory secretions plays a lesser role. After infection by most serotypes, virus can be recovered from the oropharynx and intestine of both symptomatic and asymptomatic individuals, but virus is shed in greater amounts and for a longer period (a month or more) in the feces.

Young children have the highest rates of infection, and enteroviruses are most efficiently disseminated by infected children younger than 2 years of age. Spread is from child to child, and then within family groups, and is facilitated by crowding and poor hygiene. Secondary attack rates of approximately 90% for polioviruses, 75% for coxsackieviruses, and 50% for echoviruses are observed in families. Middle-class parents with children in day care centers are at particular risk. Reared in circumstances that minimized their childhood exposure, they are likely to be susceptible to infection by many of the enteroviruses brought home from day care centers by their asymptomatically infected toddlers.

Although the epidemiology of most enteroviruses is similar, patterns of infection with some serotypes are distinctive. Enterovirus

70 and coxsackievirus A24, etiologic agents of acute hemorrhagic conjunctivitis, are transmitted by direct inoculation of the conjunctivae by fingers and fomites contaminated with infected tears. Replication of these viruses in the alimentary tract, if it occurs at all, is limited. Coxsackievirus A21 is shed primarily from the upper respiratory tract, where it produces a rhinovirus-like illness. It is transmitted by respiratory secretions.

The incubation period for illnesses caused by enteroviruses may vary from < 1 day to > 3 weeks, but it is generally 2 to 7 days. It is shortest when symptoms are the direct result of virus replication at the portal of entry (e.g., acute hemorrhagic conjunctivitis caused by enterovirus 70 or coxsackievirus 24) and longest when they reflect tissue injury that involves immunopathology in target organs infected following viremia (e.g., some forms of coxsackievirus myocarditis).

PATHOGENESIS OF ENTEROVIRUS INFECTIONS

The pathogenesis of enterovirus infections is understood best for polioviruses, which have been extensively studied in experimentally infected primates and in humans infected with attenuated vaccine strains. The pathogenesis of most nonpolio enterovirus infections appears to be similar, except for the principal target organs affected.

Following ingestion of fecally contaminated material, virus implants and replicates in susceptible tissues of the pharynx and distal small intestine. Within a day or two virus spreads to regional lymph nodes, and on about the third day small quantities escape into the bloodstream (the "minor viremia") and are disseminated throughout the reticuloendothelial system and to other receptor-bearing target tissues. In most cases, infection is contained at this stage by host defense mechanisms with no further progression, resulting in *asymptomatic infection*. In a minority of infected persons, replication continues in reticuloendothelial tissues producing, by about the fifth day, heavy sustained viremia (the "major viremia") that coincides with the "minor illness" of poliovirus infection (see Ch. 425) and with the "nonspecific febrile illness" caused by other human enteroviruses.

The major viremia disseminates large amounts of virus to target organs, such as the spinal cord, brain, meninges, heart, and skin, where further virus replication results in inflammatory lesions and cell necrosis. In most such patients, host defense mechanisms quickly terminate the major viremia and halt virus replication in target organs; only rarely is virus replication in target organs extensive enough to be clinically manifest. Although other host defense mechanisms (e.g., macrophages, interferon production) are doubtless involved, neutralizing antibodies play a major role in terminating viremia and limiting enterovirus multiplication in target tissues. Serotype-specific neutralizing antibodies may be detected in the serum within 4 or 5 days of the infection, and they generally persist for life. Evidence for the critical role of antibodies in terminating infection is provided by the occurrence of chronic persistent enterovirus infections in agammaglobulinemic children. Host defenses do not, however, terminate virus replication in the intestine, and fecal shedding continues for weeks after both symptomatic and asymptomatic enterovirus infections. Reinfection (i.e., virus excretion by a person with pre-existing homotypic antibodies) is relatively uncommon. When it occurs, infection is confined to the alimentary tract and is not associated with illness, and the duration of virus shedding is markedly reduced.

The clinical syndrome(s) caused by a given enterovirus reflect the particular target organs and tissues that it infects, i.e., its *cell tropism*. All of the determinants of cell tropism have not been elucidated, but a major factor is the presence on the cell surface of specific *receptor* molecules to which the virus attaches. Different groups of enteroviruses utilize different receptors, most or all of which are encoded by genes on human chromosome 19. A number of distinct receptors, each shared by multiple enterovirus serotypes, have been identified. The receptor used by all three polioviruses (PVR) and a receptor used by a subset of group A coxsackieviruses and by the majority of human rhinoviruses (ICAM-1) are both members of the immunoglobulin superfamily. A receptor used by a subset of the echoviruses (VLA-2) and another used by coxsackievirus A9 are members of the integrin family. Decay-accelerating factor (DAF), a surface glycoprotein that protects cells from complement-mediated lysis, is used as a receptor by another group of echoviruses. All six group B coxsackieviruses share the same receptor, a cell surface glycoprotein.

CLINICAL MANIFESTATIONS OF ENTEROVIRUS INFECTIONS

The majority of nonpolio enterovirus infections (50 to 80%) are asymptomatic. Most symptomatic infections consist of *undifferentiated febrile illnesses* ("summer grippe"), often accompanied by upper respiratory symptoms. These are generally mild and last only a few days. This syndrome is totally nonspecific; it can be caused by virtually any enterovirus serotype, as well as by members of a number of other virus families (e.g., adenoviruses, paramyxoviruses, orthomyxoviruses). The so-called characteristic enterovirus syndromes, such as aseptic meningitis, hand-foot-and-mouth disease, and pleurodynia, are in fact unusual manifestations of enterovirus infection. They represent the very small tip of a very large iceberg.

Some clinical syndromes are highly associated with certain enterovirus serotypes or subgroups (e.g., hand-foot-and-mouth disease with coxsackievirus A16, myopericarditis with group B coxsackieviruses), but even these associations are not specific. The same syndrome may also be caused by a number of other enterovirus serotypes. Conversely, a single enterovirus serotype may cause several different syndromes, even within the same outbreak (Table 343–2). The more important syndromes are discussed below.

CENTRAL NERVOUS SYSTEM SYNDROMES

ASEPTIC MENINGITIS. Aseptic meningitis is the most common significant illness caused by nonpolio enteroviruses, and these viruses are responsible for > 80% of the cases of aseptic meningitis in which an etiologic agent is identified. Almost every enterovirus serotype has been implicated, but those most frequently associated include coxsackieviruses A2, A4, A7, A9, A10, and B1–5, echoviruses 3, 4, 6, 9, 11, 14, 16, 17, 18, 19, 25, 30, and 33, and enteroviruses 70 and 71, all of which have been responsible for outbreaks as well as sporadic cases. Although attack rates are generally highest in children, cases also occur in adults, especially during larger outbreaks. Initial symptoms, which are typical of the *undifferentiated febrile illness* (e.g., fever, headache, malaise, myalgias, and sore throat), are followed, usually within a day, by signs and symptoms of meningitis, including a more severe headache that is often retrobulbar, photophobia, meningismus, stiffness of the neck and back, and nausea and vomiting, especially in children. The illness is sometimes biphasic like poliomyelitis. The cerebrospinal fluid (CSF) is clear and under slightly increased pressure. The total cell count, which can vary from < 10 per cubic millimeter to > 3000 per cubic millimeter, averages 50 to 500 per cubic millimeter. Initially, neutrophils may predominate (although they rarely exceed 90%), but they are quickly replaced by mononuclear cells. The glucose concentration is usually normal, although levels < 40 mg per deciliter are occasionally observed. The protein concentration is normal or slightly elevated, but rarely exceeds 100 mg per deciliter. Fever and signs of meningeal inflammation subside in 3 to 7 days, although pleocytosis may persist for an additional week or more. The great majority of children and adults recover fully without sequelae. However, enteroviral meningitis during the first year of life may, in up to 10% of affected infants, result in permanent neurologic damage as evidenced by reduced head circumference, spasticity, and impaired intellectual function.

In some cases, especially those caused by echoviruses and enterovirus 71, meningitis may be accompanied by a rash, which, if petechial, may raise the specter of meningococcemia. It is frequently necessary to distinguish enteroviral meningitis from partially treated bacterial meningitis. In bacterial meningitis, even when treated with appropriate antibiotics, the polymorphonuclear pleocytosis is usually more persistent, the protein concentration higher, and the glucose concentration lower. Aseptic meningitis may be caused by a number of other infectious and noninfectious agents, including mumps virus, arthropod-borne viruses, lymphocytic choriomeningitis virus (LCM), human immunodeficiency virus (HIV), herpes simplex virus, Lyme borreliosis, and leptospirosis. Differential diagnosis is aided by the distinct epidemiologic features and characteristic signs and symptoms of these other diseases.

PARALYTIC DISEASE. Paralytic disease may occur in the course of many nonpolio enterovirus infections. It is similar, but generally less severe, than that caused by polioviruses. Muscle weakness is far more common than frank paralysis, and recovery is nearly always complete, although occasional patients suffer cranial

TABLE 343–2. CLINICAL MANIFESTATIONS OF NONPOLIO ENTEROVIRUS INFECTIONS*

Clinical Syndrome	Group A Coxsackieviruses†	Group B Coxsackieviruses	Echoviruses	Enteroviruses
Asymptomatic infection	All serotypes	All serotypes	All serotypes	All serotypes
Undifferentiated febrile illness ("summer grippe") with or without respiratory symptoms	All serotypes	All serotypes	All serotypes	68, 70, 71
Aseptic meningitis	1, <u>2</u>, 3, <u>4</u>, 5, 6, <u>7</u>, 8, <u>9</u>, <u>10</u>, 11, 14, 16, 17, 18, 22, 24	<u>1</u>, 2, <u>3</u>, <u>4</u>, <u>5</u>, 6	1, 2, 3, <u>4</u>, 5, <u>6</u>, 7, 8, <u>9</u>, 10, <u>11</u>, 12, 14, <u>16</u>, 17, 18, 19, 20, 21, 22, 23, 25, <u>30</u>, 31, <u>33</u>	<u>70</u>, <u>71</u>
Encephalitis	2, 4, 5, 6, 7, <u>9</u>, 10, 16	1, <u>2</u>, <u>3</u>, <u>4</u>, 5	2, 3, <u>4</u>, <u>6</u>, 7, <u>9</u>, <u>11</u>, 14, 17, 18, 19, 22, 25, <u>30</u>, 33	70, <u>71</u>
Paralytic disease (poliomyelitis-like)	<u>4</u>, 5, 6, <u>7</u>, <u>9</u>, 10, 11, 14, 16, 21	1, <u>2</u>, <u>3</u>, <u>4</u>, <u>5</u>, 6	1, <u>2</u>, <u>4</u>, <u>6</u>, 7, <u>9</u>, <u>11</u>, 14, 16, 17, 18, 19, <u>30</u>	70, <u>71</u>
Myopericarditis	1, 2, <u>4</u>, 5, 7, 8, <u>9</u>, 14, <u>16</u>	<u>1</u>, <u>2</u>, <u>3</u>, <u>4</u>, <u>5</u>, 6	1, 2, 3, 4, <u>6</u>, 7, 8, <u>9</u>, <u>11</u>, 14, 16, 17, 19, <u>22</u>, 25, 30	
Pleurodynia	1, 2, 4, 6, 9, 10, 16	<u>1</u>, 2, <u>3</u>, <u>4</u>, <u>5</u>, 6	<u>1</u>, 2, 3, <u>6</u>, 7, 8, 9, 11, 12, 14, 16, 19, 23, 25, 30	
Herpangina	<u>1</u>, <u>2</u>, <u>3</u>, <u>4</u>, <u>5</u>, <u>6</u>, <u>7</u>, <u>8</u>, 9, <u>10</u>, 16, <u>22</u>	<u>1</u>, 2, 3, 4, 5	6, 9, 11, <u>16</u>, 17, 22, <u>25</u>	
Hand-foot-and-mouth disease	4, <u>5</u>, 7, <u>9</u>, <u>10</u>, <u>16</u>	2, 5		<u>71</u>
Exanthems	2, 4, 5, 6, 7, <u>9</u>, 10, <u>16</u>	1, 2, 3, 4, 5	2, 4, 5, 6, <u>9</u>, <u>11</u>, <u>16</u>, 18, 25	71
Common cold	2, 10, <u>21</u>, <u>24</u>	1, 2, 3, 4, 5	2, 4, 8, 9, 11, 20, 25	
Lower respiratory tract infections (broncheolitis, pneumonia)	7, <u>9</u>, <u>16</u>	1, 2, 3, 4, 5	4, 8, 9, 11, 12, 14, 19, 20, 21, 25, 30	68, 71
Acute hemorrhagic conjunctivitis‡	<u>24</u>			<u>70</u>
Generalized disease of the newborn	3, 9, 16	1, <u>2</u>, <u>3</u>, <u>4</u>, <u>5</u>	3, 4, 6, 7, 9, <u>11</u>, 12, 14, 17, 18, 19, 20, 21, 22, 30	

* A great many enterovirus serotypes have been implicated in most of these syndromes, at least in sporadic cases. The serotypes listed are those that have been clearly and/or frequently implicated. Serotypes with the strongest association are underlined.

† Because isolation of many of the group A coxsackieviruses requires suckling mouse inoculation, they are likely to be underreported as causes of illness.

‡ Conjunctivitis without hemorrhage is frequently seen in association with other manifestations in patients infected with many group A and group B coxsackieviruses and echoviruses, especially coxsackieviruses A9, A16, and B1–5 and echoviruses 2, 7, 9, 11, 16, and 30.

nerve palsies or severe, sometimes fatal, bulbar involvement. Frequently implicated serotypes include coxsackieviruses A7, A9, and B2–5, echoviruses 2, 4, 6, 9, 11, and 30, and enteroviruses 70 and 71. In contrast to paralytic poliomyelitis, which in the prevaccine era occurred in epidemics, cases of paralysis associated with nonpolio enteroviruses are generally sporadic. However, several nonpolio enteroviruses produce paralytic disease with sufficient frequency to cause local outbreaks and epidemics. A variant of coxsackievirus A7 has caused outbreaks, as well as numerous sporadic cases of paralytic disease. In fact, coxsackievirus A7 was once thought to be a fourth serotype of poliovirus. Paralytic disease resembling poliomyelitis, with a significant incidence of residual paralysis and muscle atrophy, has been observed in patients with acute hemorrhagic conjunctivitis caused by enterovirus 70. Enterovirus 71 has caused outbreaks and epidemics of cutaneous and CNS disease in temperate regions around the world since its initial isolation in California in 1969. These have included epidemics of poliomyelitis-like paralytic disease with residual flaccid paralysis, encephalitis, and significant mortality.

ENCEPHALITIS. Encephalitis is a well-recognized but uncommon manifestation of enterovirus infection. Thus, despite their prevalence, enteroviruses account for only 10 to 20% of the cases of encephalitis in the United States of proven viral etiology. The most frequently implicated serotypes include coxsackieviruses A9, B2, and B5, echoviruses 4, 6, 9, 11, and 30, and enterovirus 71. In most cases, encephalitis complicates the course of aseptic meningitis; parenchymal involvement is indicated by the onset of confusion, coma, abnormalities of motor function, hemiparesis, vasomotor instability, cranial nerve palsies, cerebellar ataxia, and focal or generalized seizures, singly or in various combinations. Cerebral involvement is usually generalized, but focal encephalitis does occur and may occasionally be clinically indistinguishable from herpes simplex encephalitis. Recovery is usually complete, although neurologic sequelae and deaths do occur, especially in young infants and during enterovirus 71 epidemics.

OTHER REPORTED NEUROLOGIC COMPLICATIONS. Other neurologic complications, including Guillain-Barré syndrome, transverse myelitis, Reye's syndrome, and cerebellar ataxia, have been reported in patients with enterovirus infections. However, no clear epidemiologic or etiologic linkage to enteroviruses has been established. Given the high prevalence of asymptomatic enterovirus infections, these associations may be only coincidental.

EPIDEMIC PLEURODYNIA (BORNHOLM DISEASE)

Epidemic pleurodynia is an acute febrile viral illness characterized by the sudden onset of intense paroxysmal lower thoracic or abdominal pain. Synonyms include Bornholm disease, devil's grip, epidemic myalgia, epidemic benign dry pleurisy, and Sylvest's disease. The name, pleurodynia (*pleura*, side; *odyne*, pain) reflects the characteristic intercostal location of the pain and does not connote disease of the pleura. Pleurodynia is usually an epidemic disease, but sporadic cases do occur.

ETIOLOGY. The enteroviral etiology of epidemic pleurodynia was established in 1949. Group B coxsackieviruses, especially B3 and B5, are the principal cause. Other viruses associated with epidemic disease include echoviruses 1 and 6. Sporadic cases have also been associated with these viruses, as well as with many other enteroviruses, including coxsackieviruses A1, A2, A4, A6, A9, A10, and A16 and echoviruses 2, 3, 7, 8, 9, 11, 12, 14, 16, 19, 23, 25, and 30.

EPIDEMIOLOGY. Epidemics of pleurodynia have been recognized in Scandinavian countries for more than two centuries, but the disease was little known elsewhere until 1933, when the Danish physician Ejnar Sylvest described an epidemic on Bornholm, a Danish island in the Baltic Sea. Since then, epidemics and sporadic cases have been recognized in many parts of the world. As with other enteroviral infections, the majority of illnesses occur in summer and early fall. However, in contrast to the annual outbreaks of enteroviral aseptic meningitis, epidemics of pleurodynia are much less frequent, generally occurring at intervals of 10 to 20 years.

Transmission is primarily from person to person, and multiple family members may be attacked almost simultaneously or in rapid succession at intervals of 2 to 5 days. In epidemics, disease is observed in children and adults of both genders. Although the peak age of incidence is somewhat older than with other enterovirus syndromes, the majority of cases occur in persons under 30 years of age. The incubation period is generally 2 to 5 days.

PATHOGENESIS. Pleurodynia is a disease of skeletal muscle, not of the pleura or peritoneum. As in most enteroviral diseases, infection is initiated in the alimentary tract. Skeletal muscle is probably most often infected during the primary (minor) viremia, although it may be infected later, during the major viremia in the minority of patients in whom pleurodynia is preceded by a prodromal illness. Host immune responses terminate viremia and halt virus replication in the tissues, but they also contribute to the severity of local inflammation. Histopathologic data in humans are lacking because of the benign nature of the disease, but studies in murine models of coxsackievirus infection suggest that the myositis results from a combination of direct virus-induced cytolysis and immunopathology mediated by sensitized T lymphocytes.

CLINICAL MANIFESTATIONS. Pleurodynia is characterized by the abrupt onset of fever and sharp, paroxysmal pain over the lower ribs or upper abdomen. In about 25% of patients, this is preceded by a 1- or 2-day prodrome of headache, malaise, anorexia, sore throat, and diffuse myalgia. The pain varies in intensity, but is often severe. It is accentuated, sometimes elicited, by deep breathing, coughing, and movement. The pain of pleurodynia has been described as catching (a "stitch" in the side), stabbing, knife-like, lancinating, crushing, or vise-like. In adults, the pain is primarily in muscles of the thorax, especially the intercostals. In children, abdominal muscles are more often involved. Occasionally it may involve muscles in the neck or limbs. The pain is often unilateral, and is generally experienced in only one or two locations. Muscle tenderness and, occasionally, swelling can be detected at the site of pain, and characteristic paroxysms of pain can often be elicited by pressure on the affected muscles. Pleural friction rubs are uncommon, and peritonitis has generally not been observed in patients who have come to laparotomy. The level of creatine phosphokinase in the serum may be elevated, reflecting injury to striated muscle. Other laboratory values are usually normal, although there may be mild leukopenia in some patients.

During paroxysms of severe pain, the patient lies still in bed, sweating profusely and appearing acutely ill and apprehensive. Respiration, limited by pain, is shallow, rapid, and grunting, suggesting pneumonia or pleural inflammation. A temperature of 38°C to 40°C is present at the onset of pain, reaches its peak during the episode, and resolves between paroxysms. Multiple paroxysms of pain occur, each lasting from a few minutes to several hours. The initial paroxysm is usually the most severe, and patients frequently appear relatively well between paroxysms.

The acute illness generally lasts for 2 to 6 days, with a range of 12 hours to 3 weeks. The disease is often biphasic; the initial pain and fever resolve and the patient is asymptomatic for a day or more, and then the pain and fever recur, frequently at the same site. Rarely, patients will have several recurrences over a period of several weeks or will have a late recurrence after being symptom free for a month or more.

DIFFERENTIAL DIAGNOSIS. The most useful distinguishing feature of pleurodynia is the intermittent paroxysmal character of the pain. Epidemiologic information, such as the occurrence of similar illnesses in family members or in the community, may also suggest the diagnosis. Nevertheless, depending upon the location of the pain, pleurodynia may be confused with any of a number of more serious diseases. When the pain is thoracic, these include pneumonia, pulmonary infarction, rib fracture, costochondritis, and myocardial infarction. The absence of physical and roentgenographic evidence of fracture, costochondritis, or pulmonary parenchymal disease, lack of sputum production, absence of leukocytosis, and normal electrocardiogram help to exclude these diagnoses. When the pain is abdominal, it can be difficult to differentiate pleurodynia from serious causes of acute abdominal pain, such as peritonitis, cholecystitis, appendicitis, perforated peptic ulcer, and acute intestinal obstruction. Thus, during epidemics of pleurodynia, it is com-

mon to have as many children with the disease admitted to surgical wards as to medical wards, and in one epidemic 9 of 49 of these children underwent laparotomy with normal findings before the nature of their disease was recognized. The absence of signs of peritonitis and the normal white blood cell count are helpful in excluding these diagnoses, as are normal ultrasound and roentgenographic studies. Pleurodynia may also be confused with the pain of pre-eruptive herpes zoster, herniated intervertebral disc, and renal colic. However, the pain of pre-eruptive herpes zoster is usually more constant, and the localization of pain and tenderness to the affected muscle, normal roentgenographic and neurologic examinations (except perhaps for a local area of hyperesthesia over the affected muscle), and the absence of hematuria help to exclude the other two diagnoses.

TREATMENT AND PROGNOSIS. Treatment of pleurodynia is symptomatic. Episodes of pain can usually be controlled with salicylates or other mild analgesics, but opiate analgesics are recommended for severe pain once serious intraabdominal processes have been excluded. Heat applied to affected muscles may also be useful. Despite the tendency of the disease to relapse, patients with epidemic pleurodynia eventually recover completely. Occasionally, convalescence may be prolonged, with malaise or asthenia persisting for several months. Complications, which reflect dissemination of virus to other tissues, are relatively uncommon. When they do occur, they generally become apparent within several days after the onset of the disease. Aseptic meningitis is observed in approximately 5% of cases, and orchitis in a similar proportion of postpubertal males. Pericarditis and myocarditis are rare complications of epidemic pleurodynia.

MYOCARDITIS AND PERICARDITIS CAUSED BY ENTEROVIRUSES

Myocarditis and pericarditis have long been known to occur in association with epidemic viral diseases, including measles, mumps, rubella, varicella, influenza, poliomyelitis, and pleurodynia. Because many of these diseases have been controlled with vaccines, enteroviruses have emerged as the major recognized infectious cause of myocarditis and pericarditis in North America and Western Europe. The pathogenesis, clinical manifestations, and outcome of enteroviral infections of the heart vary markedly, depending on properties of the virus and characteristics of the host, especially age. Neonatal infections frequently result in severe myocarditis, widespread involvement of other organs, and high mortality, whereas in older children and adults, pericarditis often predominates, and the disease is generally benign and self-limited. In fact, it appears that the clinical manifestations are generally so subtle that cardiac involvement during enteroviral infections is often unrecognized. However, idiopathic dilated cardiomyopathy may, in many cases, be a late sequela of both recognized and unrecognized enteroviral myocarditis.

ETIOLOGY. The evidence linking specific enteroviruses with myocarditis or pericarditis varies markedly. Proof of causation requires isolation of virus from, or demonstration of viral proteins or nucleic acids in, the myocardium, pericardium, or pericardial fluid. Except in neonatal myopericarditis, virus is rarely isolated from cardiac tissue or pericardial fluid, and detection of viral proteins has been difficult, primarily because lack of specificity has led to false positive results. However, increasing use of endomyocardial biopsy and application of new techniques such as in situ hybridization and polymerase chain reaction (PCR) for detection and amplification of enteroviral nucleic acid has substantially improved our ability to establish the etiology in cases of myocarditis and pericarditis. While these techniques are not yet widely available, their limited application has already demonstrated the presence of enteroviral RNA in 20 to 30% of tissue specimens from patients with myocarditis and up to 15% of tissue specimens from patients with idiopathic dilated cardiomyopathy. In most instances, however, the association of a particular enterovirus with myocarditis or pericarditis is based only on isolation of virus from noncardiac sources (e.g., feces) and/or serologic evidence of recent or concurrent enterovirus infection. These associations may often be coincidental rather than causal.

Coxsackieviruses B1–6, A4, and A16 and echoviruses 9, 11, and 22 have been proven to cause myopericarditis in children and adults. Coxsackieviruses A1, A2, A5, A8, A9, and A14 and echoviruses 1, 2, 3, 4, 6, 7, 8, 14, 16, 19, 25, and 30 have also been implicated. The group B coxsackieviruses are the most common etiologic agents of myocarditis and pericarditis. They appear to account for approximately 50% of sporadic cases of acute myocarditis and for virtually all cases that have occurred in epidemics. Group B coxsackieviruses also appear to account for 30% or more of sporadic cases of acute nonbacterial pericarditis.

EPIDEMIOLOGY. Enteroviral myocarditis and pericarditis occur most frequently in the summer and early fall. Idiopathic myopericarditis also peaks during this period of maximum enteroviral prevalence; this is consistent with the notion that most cases of idiopathic myopericarditis are caused by enteroviruses.

The incidence of myopericarditis during enteroviral infections depends upon the virus and characteristics of the host, especially age. Myopericarditis has been the predominant manifestation of infection in only about 3% of group B coxsackievirus infections. However, 5 to 10% of infected adults and children older than 9 who sought medical care during coxsackievirus B5 epidemics were found to have evidence of acute myopericarditis. The incidence of myocarditis and disseminated disease during group B coxsackievirus infection is very high during the neonatal period. It drops to a minimum (e.g., ≤1% of symptomatic coxsackievirus B5 infections) in children 1 to 9 years of age and then increases again in older children and adults. Thus, despite the higher frequency of enterovirus infections in younger children, enteroviral myopericarditis is primarily a disease of adolescents and young adults. At least two thirds of the cases occur in males, and the risk of cardiac involvement also appears to be increased during pregnancy and immediately post partum. Enterovirus transmission associated with myocarditis and pericarditis is the same as that of enteroviruses in general: it is primarily fecal-oral.

PATHOGENESIS. When enteroviral infections involve the heart they almost always cause an inflammatory response in both the myocardium *(myocarditis)* and the pericardium *(pericarditis)*. Although one or the other usually predominates, the term *myopericarditis* best describes the pathologic process. The hallmark of enteroviral myopericarditis is injury to myocytes with an adjacent inflammatory infiltrate. Cardiac myosites, which bear a receptor utilized by all 6 group B coxsackieviruses, are infected and lysed. The acute process may resolve completely or progress. Healing and progression are reflected by the development of interstitial fibrosis and loss of myocytes. Enteroviral pericarditis is almost always accompanied by focal subepicardial myocarditis, which has these same pathologic characteristics.

In neonatal enteroviral myopericarditis, the relatively short incubation period, the widely disseminated infection, and the presence of high titers of virus in the heart and other organs indicate that the primary pathogenic mechanism is direct cytolytic virus infection of the tissues involved. In myopericarditis in older children and adults, the longer incubation period, the presence of virus-specific antibodies and T lymphocytes at clinical presentation, the low frequency of virus isolation from the heart and pericardial fluid, and the later occurrence of relapses all suggest that immunopathologic mechanisms are involved. Patients with myocarditis have also been found to have cytotoxic T lymphocytes that react with normal cardiac myocytes, as well as high titers of antimyocyte antibodies.

Idiopathic dilated cardiomyopathy (see Ch. 43) may in many instances represent the end stage of an immunologically mediated chronic progressive enteroviral myocarditis. This notion is supported by the development of chronic cardiomyopathy in approximately 10% of patients observed long-term after group B coxsackievirus myocarditis, by demonstration of progressive fibrosis in such patients by serial endomyocardial biopsies, and by failure to isolate enterovirus from these biopsy specimens. The association of idiopathic dilated cardiomyopathy with group B coxsackievirus myocarditis has been further strengthened by the recent demonstration of group B coxsackievirus RNA in myocardial biopsies obtained from patients with the disease. These observations need to be confirmed and extended.

CLINICAL MANIFESTATIONS. Although the term *myopericarditis* best describes the pathologic process observed in enteroviral infections of the heart, *myocarditis* or *pericarditis* usually predominates, and the two syndromes are sufficiently distinct in clinical presentation and pathophysiology to warrant separate consideration. They are discussed in detail in Ch. 43 and 44.

Neonatal Myocarditis. Most severe neonatal enterovirus infections begin during the first week of life; the infant's mother has frequently been infected shortly before delivery and has transmitted the virus transplacentally or by contact during or soon after delivery. However, the disease can be present at birth or may occur at any time during the first 3 months of life following a 2- to 8-day incubation period. It is usually a manifestation of generalized enteroviral disease of the newborn.

Myocarditis and Pericarditis in Older Children and Adults. In contrast to the neonate, enteroviral infections of the heart in older children and adults often present clinically as pericarditis rather than myocarditis, although the myocardium is almost always involved to some degree. Approximately 60% of older children and adults with symptomatic group B coxsackievirus-associated heart disease have a clinical diagnosis of pericarditis; approximately 40% have a clinical diagnosis of myocarditis. More than two thirds of the patients are male. See Ch. 43 and 44 for clinical features of myocarditis and pericarditis.

TREATMENT AND PROGNOSIS. Specific antiviral chemotherapy is not yet available for enterovirus infections, and treatment of neonatal myocarditis is supportive. Infants with neonatal myocarditis are unlikely to have received transplacental antibodies to the causative virus from their mothers. Thus it seems reasonable to administer human immune serum globulin, which contains high titers of neutralizing antibodies to a number of enterovirus serotypes, in an attempt to terminate viremia and limit further virus replication in infected tissues.

Treatment of enteroviral myopericarditis in older children and adults is primarily supportive. It should include control of pain with analgesics; careful monitoring for arrhythmias, heart failure, and hemodynamic compromise; and prompt treatment of these complications if they arise. Bed rest is an important component of therapy because of clear evidence in mice with coxsackievirus B3 myocarditis that exercise markedly increases the extent of myocardial necrosis and mortality during the acute phase of the disease. Adequate oxygenation should be assured and fluid overload avoided and promptly treated if it develops. In severe cases cardiac assist devices may be lifesaving.

Corticosteroids should not be administered to patients with suspected enteroviral myocarditis or pericarditis. Their use during the acute phase of viral myocarditis has been associated with rapid clinical deterioration.

The majority of children and adults with enteroviral myopericarditis recover without obvious sequelae. Acute mortality is low (0 to 5%), and deaths occur as a result of arrhythmias or congestive heart failure in patients with myocarditis; cardiac tamponade is extremely rare in enteroviral pericarditis.

Approximately 20% of patients experience one or more episodes of recurrent myopericarditis within 1 year of their initial illness and persistent electrocardiographic (ECG) abnormalities are observed in 10 to 20% of patients. Cardiomegaly persists in 5 to 10% of patients, and long-term follow-up suggests that ≥10% may develop chronic cardiomyopathy. Constrictive pericarditis rarely occurs following enteroviral pericarditis.

MUCOCUTANEOUS SYNDROMES CAUSED BY ENTEROVIRUSES

Enteroviruses are the leading cause of exanthematous disease in the United States and most other developed countries. Almost all enteroviruses can cause maculopapular eruptions, and most serotypes are occasionally responsible for petechial or papulovesicular exanthems and enanthems, as well. Moreover, a given enterovirus may cause more than one pattern of mucocutaneous disease, even within a single infected household. Consequently, except for hand-foot-and-mouth disease, which is usually caused by coxsackievirus A16 or enterovirus 71, there are no clinical or epidemiologic characteristics of any given enteroviral rash that point to a specific enterovirus as its cause.

EPIDEMIOLOGY. The epidemiology of enteroviral exanthems and enanthems is the epidemiology of enteroviral infections in general. The vast majority occur during the summer and early fall. The incidence of enanthems and exanthems in infected persons varies among different enteroviruses and even among different strains of the same enterovirus. For example, enanthems and exanthems are often seen in >50% of infected children during outbreaks of infection caused by echovirus 9 or coxsackievirus A16, but are rare during outbreaks caused by echovirus 6 or coxsackievirus A7. Host factors, especially age, are also important; infants and young children are more likely to develop mucocutaneous lesions, whereas other manifestations of enterovirus infection, such as aseptic meningitis, are more likely to develop in older children and adults. Thus during outbreaks of echovirus 9 infection, rash is often seen in the majority of infected children younger than 5 years of age, but in <5% of infected adults, and it is not uncommon when evaluating an adult with aseptic meningitis and no rash to find that a child in the same household is convalescing from an illness characterized by a maculopapular rash. Enteroviral exanthems and enanthems occur in outbreaks and as sporadic cases. Asymptomatic infections are common and are often the source of virus for symptomatic infections. Attack rates are highest in young children, who frequently introduce the virus into households where several members may become infected simultaneously or sequentially, with an incubation period of 3 to 10 days.

PATHOGENESIS. Enteroviral lesions in the oropharyngeal mucosa and skin are manifestations of a systemic virus infection. They result from the secondary infection of endothelial cells of small vessels in the underlying lamina propria and dermis, which occurs during the viremia that regularly follows enteroviral infection and replication in the alimentary tract. Their pathogenesis thus resembles that of the mucocutaneous lesions of measles, rubella, and varicella and contrasts with the pathogenesis of the lesions of acute herpetic gingivostomatitis, human papillomavirus infections (warts), and acute hemorrhagic conjunctivitis, which are the direct result of exogenous virus infection and replication in epithelial cells at the portal of entry.

The obligatory occurrence of alimentary tract replication and viremia before mucocutaneous lesions develop explains the 3- to 10-day incubation period and the frequent occurrence of prodromal signs and symptoms. Moreover, the simultaneous dissemination of virus to a number of target organs explains the concurrent appearance of other manifestations of enterovirus infection, such as aseptic meningitis and myopericarditis.

CLINICAL MANIFESTATIONS. *Enanthems.* The oropharyngeal mucosa is involved to some degree during most symptomatic enteroviral infections. This is usually manifest by mild pharyngitis and mucosal erythema, but it may also result in a variety of enanthems. These may consist of macules, papules, vesicles, petechiae, or ulcers, and they may occur alone or in association with exanthems and other manifestations of systemic enteroviral infection. They are often transient and frequently unrecognized, but they occasionally lead to diagnostic confusion, for example, when they resemble Koplik's spots and accompany a morbilliform exanthem in a child infected by echovirus 9. Two enanthems are sufficiently unique to warrant separate description.

Herpangina (*herpes,* vesicular eruption, *angina,* inflammation of the throat) is a syndrome characterized by sudden onset of fever, sore throat, pain on swallowing, and a vesicular enanthem of the posterior pharynx. It is seen primarily in children between ages 3 and 10. The disease begins abruptly, after a 3- to 10-day incubation period, with temperature ranging from 38° C to 41° C, sore throat, and pain on swallowing. Fever tends to be greater in younger children, who may suffer febrile convulsions; older children and adults frequently complain of headache and myalgia. On examination there is pharyngeal erythema but little or no tonsillar exudate. The characteristic lesions are discrete 1- to 2-mm vesicles and ulcers surrounded by 1- to 5-mm zones of erythema. Lesions are few, averaging 4 to 5 per patient, with a range of 1 or 2 to 20. They occur most frequently on the anterior tonsillar pillars, the posterior edge of the soft palate, and the uvula, and less frequently on the tonsils, the posterior pharyngeal wall, and the posterior buccal mucosa. They begin as small papules, progress to vesicles, and ulcerate within 24 hours. The shallow ulcers, which are moderately painful, may enlarge over the next day or two to a diameter of 3 to 4 mm. Symptoms generally disappear in 3 or 4 days, but the ulcers may persist for up to a week. Most cases are mild and resolve without complications, but herpangina is occasionally associated with exanthems, aseptic meningitis, or other serious manifestations of enterovirus infection.

Outbreaks of herpangina are common during the summer, and sporadic cases are also observed. Group A coxsackieviruses (A1–6, A8, A10, and A22) account for the majority of outbreaks, but outbreaks have also been caused by other enteroviruses, including coxsackievirus B1 and echoviruses 16 and 25. In addition, these viruses, as well as coxsackieviruses A7, A9, A16, and B2–5 and echoviruses 6, 9, 11, 17, and 22, have been isolated from sporadic cases.

A variant of herpangina has been described in children infected with coxsackievirus A10. The lesions have the same distribution as typical cases of herpangina, but instead of evolving into vesicles and ulcers, they remain papular and are infiltrated with lymphocytes to form 2- to 3-mm gray-white nodules surrounded by narrow zones of erythema. The disease, which has been called *acute lymphonodular pharyngitis,* is otherwise indistinguishable from herpangina.

Hand-foot-and-mouth disease (vesicular stomatitis with exanthem) is a mild enteroviral disease characterized by a vesicular eruption in the mouth and over the extremities. It occurs most frequently in children younger than age 5. After an incubation period of 3 to 6 days, the disease begins with mild fever ranging from 38° C to 39° C, anorexia, malaise, and, often, a sore mouth. Within a day or two, vesicular lesions appear in the oral cavity, most frequently on the anterior buccal mucosa and the tongue, but also on the labial mucosa, gingivae, and hard palate. In the majority of preschool children, but in only about 10% of infected adults, the oral lesions are accompanied by vesicular skin lesions, most often on the dorsal or lateral surfaces of the hands and feet and on the fingers and toes, but not infrequently on the palms and soles. Less often, lesions occur on the buttocks or more proximally on the extremities, and rarely on the genitalia. They are generally 3 to 7 mm in diameter and surrounded by a narrow zone of erythema. They range from 2 or 3 to 30 or more and consist of subepidermal vesicles containing a mixed inflammatory infiltrate of lymphocytes, monocytes and neutrophils, and accompanied by acantholysis and cellular degeneration in the overlying epidermis. Hand-foot-and-mouth disease is caused most frequently by coxsackievirus A16, less frequently by enterovirus 71 and coxsackieviruses A5, A9, and A10, and occasionally by coxsackieviruses A4, A7, B2, and B5. Outbreaks and sporadic cases occur primarily in the summer and early fall. It may be accompanied by more serious manifestations, especially when caused by enterovirus 71.

Exanthems. Enterovirus exanthems themselves are benign, but they are clinically important for at least three reasons: (1) They constitute direct evidence of enterovirus dissemination and thus provide a clue to the presence and the etiology of coexistent disease referable to other infected target organs, such as the heart and the CNS; (2) they represent the "tip of the iceberg" of enterovirus infection in the community; and (3) they are often confused with other infectious exanthems, some of which have more serious consequences, require specific control measures, or are amenable to specific anti-infective therapy. Since enteroviral rashes are not sufficiently distinctive to permit an etiologic diagnosis to be made on clinical grounds, laboratory diagnosis is required. However, the problem of confusing enteroviral rashes with other infectious exanthems can be approached by comparing the enterovirus rashes to the nonenterovirus rashes that they resemble.

The most common cutaneous manifestation of enterovirus infection is an erythematous maculopapular rash that appears together with fever and other manifestations of systemic infection. This is also a common manifestation of infection by a variety of other organisms, but it is more often caused by enteroviruses. Only certain enteroviruses (e.g., echovirus 9) cause this syndrome with high frequency, but almost all can produce it at least occasionally. The rash begins on the face and quickly spreads to the neck, trunk, and extremities. It consists of 1- to 3-mm erythematous macules and papules that may be discrete (*rubelliform,* resembling rubella) or confluent (*morbilliform,* resembling measles). It usually lasts for 2 to 5 days and does not itch or desquamate. Enteroviral exanthems are generally not accompanied by significant posterior cervical, suboccipital, or postauricular lymphadenopathy, but there are many exceptions. For example, posterior cervical and suboccipital lymphadenopathy similar to that seen in rubella has been observed in many children with exanthems caused by coxsackievirus A9.

Enteroviral rashes are sometimes petechial and occasionally purpuric. While this pattern is seen most frequently in echovirus 9 and coxsackievirus A9 infections, it is observed occasionally with many other enterovirus serotypes.

Vesicular exanthems are most often seen as a component of

hand-foot-and-mouth disease (see above), but several enteroviruses, including echovirus 11 and coxsackievirus A9, may cause vesicular exanthems without an associated enanthem. The lesions resemble those caused by varicella-zoster and herpes simplex viruses. In contrast to varicella, however, vesicular rashes caused by enteroviruses are usually peripheral in distribution and consist of relatively few lesions that heal without crusting. When they are not associated with hand-foot-and-mouth disease, vesicular lesions caused by enteroviruses are often confused with insect bites or poison ivy. Echovirus 11 and several coxsackievirus serotypes have been associated with skin lesions resembling papular urticaria, lesions that usually result from insect bites.

Enteroviral rashes are generally accompanied by fever; they develop at or within a day or two of its onset. In some cases, however, the rash does not develop until the fever subsides, a pattern resembling that of *roseola infantum* (exanthem subitem), a benign sporadic disease of infants 6 to 24 months old now known to be caused by human herpesvirus 6. These roseola-like enterovirus infections are typified by the "Boston exanthem," caused by echovirus 16 and first described during an epidemic in Boston in 1951. It is characterized by fever (to 38° C to 39° C) lasting 2 to 4 days, followed by defervescence and then by the appearance of a salmon-pink maculopapular rash on the face and upper chest. The rash resolves in 1 to 5 days without sequelae. Frequently, multiple cases occur sequentially in households; the illness is mild in children and more severe in adults, who often develop high fever and aseptic meningitis without rash. In addition to echovirus 16, a number of other enterovirus serotypes have occasionally been associated with roseola-like illnesses.

DIFFERENTIAL DIAGNOSIS. Herpangina is most often confused with bacterial pharyngitis or tonsillitis, or with pharyngitis caused by other viruses. Other considerations include hand-foot-and-mouth disease, primary herpes simplex virus infections, particularly acute herpetic pharyngotonsillitis, and herpes zoster involving the palate.

The vesicular lesions of hand-foot-and-mouth disease resemble those caused by herpes simplex and varicella-zoster viruses. Patients with primary herpetic gingivostomatitis usually have more toxicity, cervical lymphadenopathy, and more prominent gingivitis. Their cutaneous lesions are usually perioral, but may occasionally involve a finger that has been in the mouth. Recurrent herpes simplex (herpes labialis) usually involves the vermilion border of the lip or the adjacent skin, is rarely accompanied by lesions on the hands or feet, often has a neuralgic prodome, and frequently has a history of recurrent episodes. The cutaneous lesions of varicella are generally more extensive and are centrally distributed, sparing the palms and soles. Oral lesions are far less prominent in varicella, and its prevalence in winter and spring further distinguish it from hand-foot-and-mouth disease. Aphthous stomatitis is distinguished from hand-foot-and-mouth disease by the absence of fever and other signs of systemic illness, the absence of cutaneous lesions, and often by a history of recurrence.

Maculopapular exanthems caused by enteroviruses are distinguished from measles and rubella by their summertime occurrence, the usual absence of posterior cervical, suboccipital, and postauricular lymphadenopathy, and their relatively short incubation period. The absence of significant coryza and conjunctivitis further distinguishes the typical enteroviral exanthems from measles. In addition, the probability of measles and rubella is markedly reduced in persons with a well-documented history of adequate immunization.

When enteroviral rashes are maculopapular they may be confused with drug reactions; when they are petechial they may be confused with bacterial or rickettsial rashes. When enteroviral rashes are petechial or purpuric it is impossible to rule out meningococcemia on clinical grounds alone, and when the rash is associated with aseptic meningitis (as is often the case in echovirus 9 and coxsackievirus A9 infections), it is clinically indistinguishable from meningococcal meningitis. Laboratory investigation is required, even during proven outbreaks of enteroviral disease, because concurrent enteroviral and meningococcal infections can occur.

TREATMENT AND PROGNOSIS. Enteroviral enanthems and exanthems are benign self-limited illnesses that require only symptomatic therapy for headache and sore throat. When illness mimics meningococcemia or meningococcal meningitis, antimicrobial chemotherapy should be initiated until bacterial infection is ruled out by appropriate cultures and antigen-detection assays.

RESPIRATORY TRACT DISEASE CAUSED BY ENTEROVIRUSES

A number of enteroviruses have been associated with mild upper respiratory tract illness in children and adults, especially coxsackieviruses A21, A24, and B1–5 and echoviruses 9 and 11, as well as 2, 4, 8, 20, and 25. Many of the enteroviruses, most notably coxsackievirus A21, produce illness that resembles the common cold, except for a higher incidence of fever. In contrast to most other enteroviruses, coxsackievirus A21 is shed primarily from the upper respiratory tract, rather than in feces. Enteroviruses have also been associated with lower respiratory tract illnesses in infants and children, though rarely in adults. These include tracheitis, bronchitis, croup, bronchiolitis, and pneumonia. Frequently implicated serotypes include coxsackieviruses A9, A16, and B1–5; echoviruses 4, 8, 9, 11, 12, 14, 19, 20, 21, 25, and 30; and enterovirus 68. In addition, respiratory tract symptoms frequently accompany the undifferentiated febrile illnesses (summer grippe) caused by most enteroviruses. Survillence data indicate that enteroviruses account for 2 to 10% of viral respiratory disease, and that 10 to 15% of symptomatic enterovirus infections are associated with respiratory symptoms. The respiratory illnesses caused by enteroviruses are clinically indistinguishable from similar illnesses caused by viruses more commonly considered to be respiratory tract pathogens, such as rhinoviruses, influenza viruses, parainfluenza viruses, respiratory syncytial virus, and adenoviruses. However, infections with these viruses occur most frequently during the winter, whereas enterovirus infections occur primarily in the summer and early fall. Viral respiratory tract infections are discussed in Ch. 328 through 333.

ACUTE HEMORRHAGIC CONJUNCTIVITIS

Acute hemorrhagic conjunctivitis (AHC) is an acute, highly contagious, self-limited disease of the eye characterized by sudden onset of pain, photophobia, conjunctivitis, swelling of the eyelids, and prominent subconjunctival hemorrhages. Since its first appearance in 1969, AHC has occurred in explosive epidemics throughout the world. The disease was initially nicknamed Apollo 11 disease because its appearance in Ghana coincided with the Apollo 11 moon landing.

ETIOLOGY. Enterovirus 70, a new enterovirus isolated from patients during the initial pandemic of AHC that began in Ghana in 1969, has been responsible for tens of millions of cases that have occurred in widespread epidemics during the past 25 years. A variant of coxsackievirus A24, which first appeared at about the same time as enterovirus 70, has been responsible for hundreds of thousands of cases of the disease that have occurred in a number of more circumscribed epidemics during the same period. Both viruses have been involved concurrently in some epidemics. To date, coxsackievirus A24 has been responsible for fewer cases of epidemic conjunctivitis than enterovirus 70, and it does not cause subconjunctival hemorrhages in as high a proportion of patients. Nucleic acid hybridization and serologic studies have shown that the two viruses are genetically and antigenically unrelated.

Enterovirus 70 is a most unusual enterovirus. In addition to being a naturally occurring temperature-sensitive virus that causes disease at its portal of entry and is not transmitted by the fecal-oral route, it has an exceptionally broad host range. Oligonucleotide mapping of a series of epidemic strains suggests that they all evolved from a hypothetical ancestor strain that did not exist before 1967. Serologic studies have reinforced the notion that enterovirus 70 has only recently emerged as a human pathogen; neutralizing antibodies to enterovirus 70 have generally not been found in human sera collected before 1969, even sera from elderly persons. Neutralizing antibodies to enterovirus 70 have been detected in animal sera from Japan and West Africa collected before 1969, indicating that enterovirus 70 or a very similar virus was circulating in animals before the first appearance of AHC in humans. These observations suggest that enterovirus 70 may represent a zoonotic picornavirus that extended its host range to humans, perhaps as a consequence of recombination with poliovirus type 3.

EPIDEMIOLOGY. Although mild conjunctivitis may occur as a minor manifestation of infection by many enteroviruses, especially in children, its occurrence as the major clinical manifestation of enterovirus infection was not observed until 1969, when explosive epidemics of AHC occurred in Ghana and almost simultaneously in Indonesia. Over the next 2 years the disease assumed pandemic proportions, with large epidemics occurring in many areas of Africa, Southeast Asia, the Far East, India, and Japan, and involving tens of millions of people. A number of smaller outbreaks also occurred in Europe. Scattered epidemics of AHC continued to occur in these same areas during the remainder of the decade, and the recurrence of epidemics in the same geographic areas suggests that immunity to AHC may be short-lived.

AHC is a highly contagious disease. In contrast to most enteroviral infections, it is transmitted by direct inoculation of the conjunctivae with virus-contaminated fingers or fomites (i.e., transmission is eye to finger or fomite to eye). Enterovirus 70 and the coxsackievirus A24 variant are both naturally occurring temperature-sensitive viruses that replicate optimally at 33°C to 35°C, the temperature of the conjunctivae. There appears to be little or no virus replication in the alimentary tract. Virus is abundant in the conjunctivae and in the ocular exudate, from which it can be readily isolated early in infection. During epidemics all age groups are affected; attack rates of clinical illness are highest in young adults, but infection rates are highest in children younger than 10 years, many of whom experience mild or inapparent infections. Infection rates are also substantially higher among the poor than in middle and upper socioeconomic groups. School-age children are most likely to introduce infection into households, where secondary attack rates are often > 50%.

PATHOGENESIS. In contrast to other enteroviral infections, AHC is transmitted by direct inoculation of the conjunctivae with virus on contaminated fingers or fomites (e.g., ophthalmologic instruments, shared towels). Disease results from local virus replication at the portal of entry; prior replication in the alimentary tract and viremia are not required to disseminate virus to ocular tissues. This explains the unusually short incubation period, generally lasting 24 hours or less (range, 12 to 72 hours).

The major complication of AHC is poliomyelitis-like flaccid paralysis, which occurs in a very small proportion of patients with AHC caused by enterovirus 70, but apparently not at all in patients with AHC caused by coxsackievirus A24. The pathogenesis of this AHC-associated paralytic disease is not clear, but infections and destruction of motor neurons appears to reflect axonal rather than viremic spread of enterovirus 70 to the CNS.

CLINICAL MANIFESTATIONS. AHC begins with the sudden onset of eye pain and foreign body sensation, lacrimation, photophobia, blurred vision, and bulbar conjunctivitis. Signs and symptoms rapidly increase in severity with the development of palpebral conjunctivitis, conjunctival edema, swelling of the eyelids, subconjunctival hemorrhages in the bulbar conjunctivae, and a serous or seromucoid ocular discharge containing large numbers of polymorphonuclear leukocytes. The subconjunctival hemorrhages, which are the hallmark of the disease, range from discrete petechiae to confluent hemorrhages that occupy virtually the entire bulbar conjunctiva. They are present, usually within 24 hours of onset, in 70 to 90% of patients with AHC caused by enterovirus 70, but are much less frequent in AHC caused by coxsackievirus A24. AHC often begins unilaterally, but it rapidly spreads to the other eye. Signs and symptoms peak within 24 to 36 hours of onset, by which time most patients have also developed hypertrophy of palpebral follicles and papillae, preauricular lymphadenopathy, and punctate epithelial keratitis with tiny corneal erosions that are often seen only by slit-lamp examination after fluorescein staining. Clinical improvement usually begins by the second or third day, and recovery is generally complete without sequelae within 7 to 10 days. Constitutional symptoms, including headache, low-grade fever, and malaise, occur in a minority of patients.

Poliomyelitis-like motor paralysis occurs as a rare complication of AHC caused by enterovirus 70, but not in AHC caused by coxsackievirus A24. It occurs predominantly in adult males. The neurologic disease generally does not begin until 2 to 5 weeks after AHC (range, 5 to 60 days or more), and thus its relationship to the conjunctivitis is often overlooked by physicians as well as by the patients themselves. Radicular pain and paresthesia, usually accompanied by headache, fever, and malaise, are followed in 1 to 3 days by acute asymmetric areflexic paresis or paralysis of one or more limbs. Proximal muscles are usually affected more than distal mus-

cles and lower limbs more than upper limbs. Bulbar involvement, as evidenced by paralysis of one or more cranial nerves, is observed in one third or more of affected patients. The CSF is characterized by mononuclear pleocytosis and elevated protein concentration. Permanent paralysis and muscular atrophy occur in approximately 25% of affected patients. More than 200 cases have been reported to date, and the long interval between AHC and paralysis almost certainly accentuates underreporting. Nevertheless, in view of the many tens of millions of cases of AHC that have occurred since 1969, the incidence of this neurologic complication is probably less than 1 in 10,000 cases of AHC.

DIFFERENTIAL DIAGNOSIS. During major epidemics, AHC is unlikely to be confused with other eye infections. However, small outbreaks and sporadic cases may be mistaken for adenovirus infections, either acute follicular conjunctivitis or the more severe epidemic keratoconjunctivitis.

A variety of noninfectious conditions can produce the signs and symptoms of conjunctivitis (see also Part XXV).

TREATMENT AND PROGNOSIS. AHC almost always resolves spontaneously without sequelae, and treatment is symptomatic. Topical application of antihistamine/decongestant eye drops and cold compresses may be used to reduce discomfort. Corticosteroids, a component of many topical ophthalmic preparations, are contraindicated. Transmission of AHC can be prevented by careful hand-washing, avoidance of contaminated washcloths and towels, and sterilization of all ophthalmologic instruments. These practices should be routine in eye clinics.

CHRONIC MENINGOENCEPHALITIS IN AGAMMA-GLOBULINEMIC PATIENTS. Enteroviruses, primarily echoviruses, have been responsible for a syndrome of chronic meningoencephalitis in patients with inherited or acquired defects in B lymphocyte function, most often children with X-linked agammaglobulinemia. The majority of these patients also have a dermatomyositis-like syndrome, and many have chronic hepatitis. Surprisingly, despite the presence in their CSF of abundant virus, an increased number of lymphocytes, and elevated protein concentration, these patients generally exhibit few if any clinical signs of meningitis. Enteroviruses have been recovered from many sites in addition to the CSF, including cardiac and skeletal muscle. However, the pathogenesis remains to be elucidated.

DIAGNOSIS

The enteroviral etiology of a disease may be suspected on clinical and epidemiologic grounds, but the multiplicity of agents capable of causing most clinical syndromes makes it impossible to establish a specific etiologic diagnosis on the basis of such information alone. Virus isolation and/or serologic evidence are required, with serotype-specific IgM assays and direct detection of enterovirus RNA in tissues and CSF following PCR implification.

TREATMENT AND PREVENTION

Specific antiviral chemotherapy and chemoprophylaxis are not yet available for enterovirus infections. Treatment is symptomatic and, in severe disease, supportive. Corticosteroids, which have a deleterious effect on coxsackievirus-infected mice, should not be administered during acute enterovirus infections. Strenuous exercise and intramuscular injections, both of which may precipitate paralysis of the involved muscles during poliovirus and enterovirus 70 infections, should also be avoided during the acute, presumably viremic, phase of symptomatic enterovirus infections. Intravenous immunoglobulin (IVIG), which contains high titers of neutralizing antibodies to many enteroviruses, appears to have been useful in some agammaglobulinemic patients with chronic enteroviral meningoencephalitis. IVIG may also have a role in the treatment of enteroviral infections in other patients with severely compromised B lymphocyte function. Infants with generalized neonatal enterovirus infections are unlikely to have received transplacental antibodies to the causative virus from their mothers. Consequently it would seem reasonable to administer IVIG to such infants in an attempt to terminate their viremia and limit virus replication in infected tissues. Prophylactic IVIG should also be considered for patients with severely compromised B lymphocyte function, including bone marrow transplant recipients.

Live attenuated and inactivated poliovirus vaccines have been remarkably successful in preventing paralytic poliomyelitis (see Ch. 425). However, the large number of nonpolio enterovirus serotypes, and the benign nature of most nonpolio enterovirus infections, have precluded the development of vaccines for these agents. Pre-exposure administration of immune serum globulin reduces the risk of paralytic poliomyelitis. Since immune serum globulin also contains neutralizing antibodies to many nonpolio enteroviruses, it would probably prevent many nonpolio enteroviral diseases as well. This approach has proven effective for pre-exposure and postexposure prophylaxis of hepatitis A and probably reduces the frequency of severe enteroviral infections in agammaglobulinemic patients receiving replacement therapy. However, the benign nature of most enterovirus infections, the fact that exposures are rarely recognized (most result from contact with an asymptomatically infected person), and the relatively short half-life of exogenous immune serum globulin make this approach to prevention impractical in most situations. Nursery outbreaks of severe enteroviral disease provide an exception. The administration of IVIG to all infants in the nursery offers protection to those infants without transplacentally acquired neutralizing antibody who have not yet been infected.

McKinney RE, Katz SL, Wilfert CM: Chronic enteroviral meningoencephalitis in agammaglobulinemic patients. Rev Infect Dis 9:334, 1987. *Excellent review of this interesting syndrome with thoughtful discussion of pathogenesis and management.*

Melnick JL: Enteroviruses. *In* Fields BN, et al. (eds.): Fields Virology, 3rd ed. New York, Lippincot-Raven Publishers, 1996. *Authoritative review, with emphasis on epidemiology and extensive bibliography.*

Modlin JF: Coxsackieviruses, echoviruses, and newer enteroviruses. *In* Mandell GL, et al. (eds.): Principles and Practice of Infectious Diseases, 4th ed. New York, Churchill Livingstone, 1995, p 1620–1636. *Extensive review of epidemiology and clinical manifestations of nonpolio enterovirus infections with excellent bibliography.*

Rotbard HA: Enteroviruses. In Murray PR et al: Manual of Clinical Microbiology, 6th ed. Washington, DC, ASM Press, 1995. *A comprehensive treatment of laboratory diagnosis by the leader in PCR technology applied to enteroviral infections diagnosis.*

Rueckert RR: Picornaviridae and their replication. *In* Fields BN, et al. (eds.): Fields Virology, 3rd ed. New York, Lippincott-Raven Publishers, 1996. *Detailed summary of current knowledge of picornavirus structure, replication, and virus-cell interactions.*

Ryan MD, Jenkins O, Hughes PJ, et al.: The complete nucleotide sequence of enterovirus type 70: Relationships with other members of the Picornaviridae. J Gen Virol 71:2291, 1990. *Detailed comparison of genome of enterovirus 70 to genomes of other human and animal enteroviruses, with evidence for its unique nature and origin.*

Savoia MC, Oxman MN: Myocarditis and Pericarditis. *In* Mandell GL, et al. (eds.): Principles and Practice of Infectious Diseases, 4th ed. New York, Churchill Livingstone, 1995. *Well-referenced review of etiology, pathogenesis, clinical manifestations, and diagnosis of myocarditis and pericarditis.*

344 VIRAL GASTROENTERITIS

Albert Z. Kapikian

DEFINITION

Viral gastroenteritis (acute infectious nonbacterial gastroenteritis, epidemic diarrhea, winter vomiting disease, sporadic infantile gastroenteritis) is a common acute infectious disease of all age groups, characterized by vomiting or watery diarrhea, or both, that may be accompanied by fever, nausea, anorexia, and malaise. It ranges from a mild, self-limited illness of short duration to life-threatening dehydration, especially in infants and young children.

The importance of this disease in a developed country was highlighted in the Cleveland Family Study, in which infectious gastroenteritis, presumably nonbacterial, was the second most common disease experience, accounting for 16% of approximately 25,000 illnesses in a period of almost 10 years. In developing countries the impact of diarrheal illnesses is staggering: In Asia, Africa, and Latin America, 3 to 5 billion cases of diarrhea and 5 to 10 million diarrhea-associated deaths occur annually, with the major impact in infants and young children. In addition, diarrheal illness was ranked first among infectious diseases in incidence and mortality in these developing areas.

In spite of major discoveries in bacteriology and parasitology in the past century, the etiology of most acute diarrheal illnesses remained elusive for many years. In the 1940's and 1950's, oral administration of bacteria-free stool filtrates from patients with acute diarrhea induced illness in volunteers, but the suspected viral etiologic agent could not be identified. In 1972, Kapikian and colleagues, employing immune electron microscopy (IEM), discovered the first virus-like particles that could be implicated as an important cause of acute gastroenteritis, in a stool suspension derived from a gastroenteritis outbreak in Norwalk, Ohio. In 1973, Bishop and associates, using electron microscopy (EM), discovered rotavirus particles in duodenal biopsies from infants and young children hospitalized with acute gastroenteritis. Rotaviruses have emerged as the major known cause of severe diarrhea of infants and young children worldwide.

ETIOLOGY

NORWALK VIRUS GROUP. The 27 nm Norwalk virus is the prototype strain of a group of fastidious, nonenveloped 27- to 40-nm particles usually named after the geographic location of the gastroenteritis outbreak from which they were first derived. They share these common characteristics: (1) are detected in feces of patients with gastroenteritis; (2) lack a distinctive morphologic appearance by EM; (3) have not been grown in cell culture; (4) possess an RNA genome; (5) have a buoyant density of 1:33 to 1:41 grams per cubic centimeter in cesium chloride; (6) possess a single primary virion-associated protein with a molecular weight of approximately 60,000. The Norwalk virus group includes at least four serotypes: Norwalk, Hawaii, Snow Mountain, and Taunton viruses. Related viruses include the Montgomery County (MC), Southampton, Desert Storm, Toronto (formerly minireovirus), Otofuke, and other small round-structured viruses (SRSV's). Although lacking the distinctive cup-like surface indentations of the "classical" caliciviruses (calix = cup in Latin), the Norwalk virus group is now classified definitively as a calicivirus in the family Caliciviridae. Recent molecular biologic studies established that the overall genomic organization of Norwalk and related strains was similar to that of feline calicivirus and rabbit hemorrhagic disease virus, another calicivirus. The Norwalk virus genome is composed of positive sense polyadenylated single-stranded RNA of 7642 nucleotides that encode three open reading frames. Previously, other noncultivatable human enteric viruses, which were associated with gastroenteritis in children or with outbreaks in the elderly, were considered to be "classical" caliciviruses morphologically. These viruses, which were recovered in the United Kingdom or Japan, were classified by IEM into five serotypes.

ROTAVIRUS. Rotaviruses are classified as a genus in the family Reoviridae and are etiologic agents of diarrhea in humans and in numerous animal and a few avian species. They are 70 nm in diameter, nonenveloped, and possess a distinctive double-layered capsid which surrounds the core that contains the genome consisting of 11 segments of double-stranded RNA, (Fig. 344–1). The name rotavirus (rota = wheel) was adopted because the sharply defined circular outline of the outer capsid was reminiscent of the rim of a wheel placed on short spokes radiating from a wide hub (the inner capsid). The virions have a density of 1.36 grams per cubic centimeter in cesium chloride and are antigenically distinct from the three reovirus serotypes. Rotaviruses possess three important antigenic specificities—group, subgroup, and serotype—which are mediated by different proteins: group specificity prominently by VP6 and subgroup by VP6 alone (encoded by RNA segment 6). Serotype specificity has been defined by VP7, a glycoprotein that is one of the two major neutralization antigens located on the outer capsid (encoded by RNA segment 7, 8, or 9). The other outer capsid protein VP4, which is encoded by RNA segment 4 and which protrudes from the smooth outer surface as a series of 60 short spikes of about 12 nm in length, also induces neutralizing antibodies. VP4 is the hemagglutinin in certain strains. Antibodies to both VP4 and VP7 are associated with protection against rotavirus illness. There are ten human rotavirus serotypes as defined by VP7 (also designated as "G" [for glycoprotein] serotypes), of which only four (nos. 1, 2, 3, or 4) are of epidemiologic importance. Many human and animal rotavirus strains share VP7 serotype specificity. Most animal and human rotaviruses share the common group antigen and are thus classified as group A rotaviruses, and these are further divided into subgroups. A serotyping scheme based on neutralization of VP4 (also designated "P" [for protease sensitive]) has been developed. The VP4 genotype of various strains has also been described, based on sequence analysis and/or nucleic acid hy-

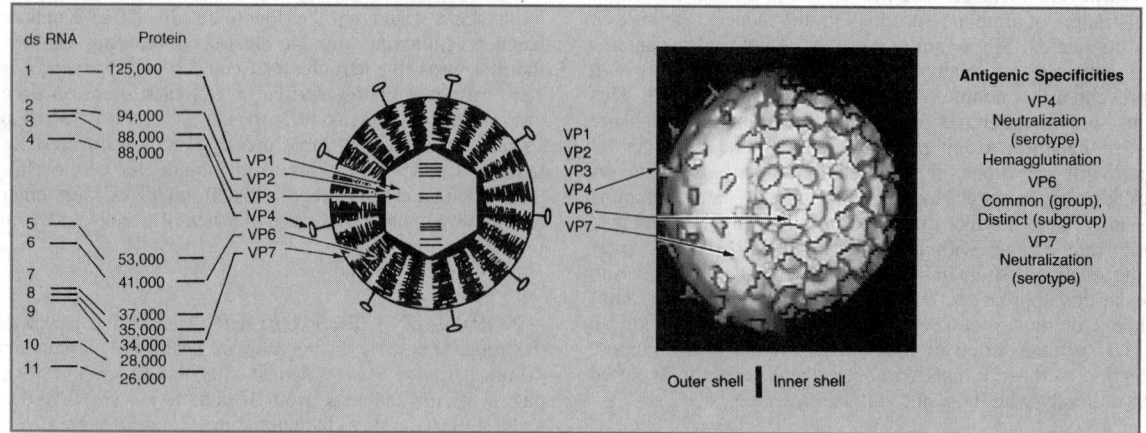

FIGURE 344–1. *Left,* Schematic representation of the rotavirus double-shelled particle. *Right,* Surface representations of the three-dimensional structures of a double-shelled particle (on the left half) and a particle (on the right half) in which most, if not all, of the outer shell and a small portion of the inner shell mass have been removed. (From Kapikian AZ, Chanock RM: Rotaviruses. *In* Fields BN, et al. (eds.): Fields Virology, 3rd ed. Philadelphia, Lippincott-Raven Publishers, 1996. Figure on right from Prasad BV, Wang GJ, Clerx JP, et al.: Three-dimensional structure of rotavirus. J Mol Biol 199:269, 1988.)

bridization of VP4. The human rotaviruses have only recently been grown efficiently in cell culture. Several human and animal rotavirus strains have been discovered that do not share the common group antigen and are classified as non-group A rotaviruses (groups B to G). In this chapter, when the term rotavirus is used, it is meant to describe only those rotaviruses belonging to group A, unless specified otherwise.

OTHER AGENTS. Other viral agents have been associated with gastroenteritis and include enteric adenoviruses belonging to types 40 and 41 (70 to 80 nm in diameter); astroviruses (28 to 30 nm); small, round viruses other than the Norwalk virus group (20 to 30 nm); putative coronavirus-like particles (100 to 150 nm); the pleomorphic, fringed, Breda or Berne virus-like particles (toroviruses) (100 to 140 nm); 35 nm "picobirnaviruses"; and a pestivirus antigen. The role of these viruses as etiologic agents of severe infantile diarrhea appears to be minor, with the exception of the enteric adenoviruses, which are associated with approximately 3 to 10% of the diarrheal illnesses of infants and young children requiring hospitalization. In addition, the role of these other agents in epidemic viral gastroenteritis appears to be minor. Additional studies are needed to assess the role of these other agents in gastroenteritis. It should be noted that about one third to one half of gastroenteritis episodes in developed countries have yet to be associated with an etiologic agent.

EPIDEMIOLOGY

NORWALK VIRUS GROUP. The Norwalk group of viruses comprises major etiologic agents of acute nonbacterial gastroenteritis, which typically occurs as a sharp outbreak affecting adults, school-age children, and family contacts. The location or source of contamination responsible for these outbreaks includes various settings such as schools, camps and recreational areas, nursing homes, swimming facilities, cruise ships, and restaurants. For example, the Norwalk virus was derived from an outbreak in an elementary school in Norwalk, Ohio, in which 50% of the students and teachers developed gastroenteritis within a 2-day period. Norwalk virus has been linked with 42% of 74 nonbacterial gastroenteritis outbreaks investigated from 1976 to 1980 and approximately 10% of all acute gastroenteritis outbreaks. In the United States, antibody to the Norwalk virus is acquired gradually in childhood and somewhat more rapidly in the adult years, so that by age 50 at least 50% of individuals have serum antibody. In developing countries, infants and young children acquire Norwalk antibody at an earlier age, and the virus is associated with mild gastroenteritis in this age group.

Norwalk virus is most likely transmitted via the fecal-oral route; however, it has also been detected in vomitus. Although sporadic cases attributed to person-to-person transmission may occur, the explosive nature of outbreaks associated with the Norwalk virus group often suggests a common source of infection, such as water or food. Common-source outbreaks have been attributed to contamination of community and noncommunity public water systems, stored water on cruise ships, or recreational swimming water and to inges-

tion of various foods, such as tainted oysters, lettuce, potato salad, cole slaw, or cake frosting. Secondary person-to-person transmission to contacts is relatively common. The incubation period ranges from 10 to 51 hours, with a mean of 24 hours, and symptoms usually last 24 to 60 hours. Norwalk virus outbreaks occur throughout the year without a peak season.

Norwalk virus infections have been detected in individuals with travelers' diarrhea. However, this agent is not considered to be an important cause of this disease.

The Norwalk virus or related agents have recently been shown to be important agents of acute gastroenteritis in military personnel deployed to different parts of the world. The "classical" caliciviruses have been associated primarily with pediatric gastroenteritis that characteristically is not severe enough to require hospitalization.

ROTAVIRUS. Rotaviruses are the major known etiologic agents of severe diarrhea in infants and young children in most areas of the world and are usually associated with sporadic infantile gastroenteritis, which differs from epidemic viral gastroenteritis associated with the Norwalk virus group in the following characteristics: (1) it usually does not occur in sharp outbreaks; (2) it can cause severe diarrheal illness in infants and young children; (3) it does not usually cause illness in adults; and (4) the attack rate among family contacts of index cases is low, although subclinical infections occur frequently in contacts. In addition, in contrast to Norwalk virus infections, about 90% of infants and young children in both developed and developing countries experience a rotavirus infection (as determined from antibody prevalence) by 3 years of age.

The most compelling evidence for the importance of rotaviruses in severe infantile gastroenteritis has emerged from numerous cross-sectional studies in developed and developing countries. In developed countries, including the United States, rotaviruses are associated with approximately 35 to 52% of acute diarrheal illness requiring hospitalization of infants and young children. The contribution of other enteric pathogens is consistently relatively minor. A similar pattern is also usually observed in developing countries, where rotaviruses are the most frequently detected pathogens in children younger than 2 who have severe gastroenteritis; however, bacterial agents also play an important role in such areas. It is estimated that in developing countries 873,000 infants and young children under age 5 die from rotavirus diarrhea each year. It should be noted that in developing countries during longitudinal studies in a community setting where all diarrheal episodes are monitored, the incidence of rotavirus diarrhea is lower than that of diarrhea caused by other pathogens, but dehydration is more often associated with rotavirus disease than with illness caused by other agents.

In temperate climates, rotavirus gastroenteritis has a characteristic seasonal occurrence during the cooler months of the year with peak prevalence in the winter months. In tropical countries it occurs throughout the year, with less pronounced peaks. Rotavirus diarrhea occurs most frequently in children between age 6 months and 24 months. Infants less than 6 months have the next highest frequency,

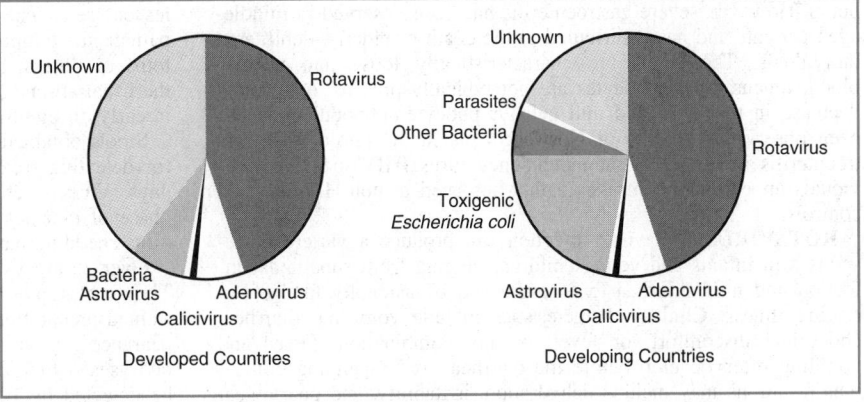

FIGURE 344-2. An estimate of the role of etiologic agents in severe diarrheal illnesses requiring hospitalization of infants and young children in developed countries *(left)* and in developing countries *(right)*. (From Kapikian AZ: Viral gastroenteritis. JAMA 269:627, 1993.)

although in certain studies the highest frequency is observed in this age group. The low frequency of clinical illness in neonates who undergo rotavirus infection is an unusual paradox that has not been explained. Rotavirus gastroenteritis occurs infrequently in adults, but subclinical infections are common.

Rotaviruses are likely transmitted by the fecal-oral route, although respiratory transmission remains a possibility, since there is such a rapid acquisition of serum antibody during the first 2 years of life regardless of hygienic conditions. Nosocomial rotavirus infections occur frequently. The incubation period of rotavirus illness is approximately 2 to 4 days. There are 10 recognized human rotavirus serotypes of which those numbered 1 to 4 appear to be clinically important. Group B rotavirus is responsible for widespread outbreaks of gastroenteritis in adults in China, and a relatively small number of group C rotaviruses have been recovered from individuals with gastroenteritis in various countries. With the exception of the group B rotaviruses in China, the role of the non–group A rotaviruses in other regions of the world appears to be relatively minor at this time.

Rotavirus infections have been observed in individuals with travelers' diarrhea. However, rotaviruses are not considered to be an important cause of this illness.

An estimate of the role of rotaviruses and other microbial agents in the etiology of severe diarrhea of infants and young children is shown in Figure 344–2. In addition, a summary of key findings regarding the epidemiology and importance of various viruses associated with acute gastroenteritis is shown in Table 344–1.

PATHOLOGY AND PATHOGENESIS

NORWALK VIRUS GROUP. Histopathologic lesions following Norwalk or Hawaii virus infection are characterized by a reversible involvement of the upper jejunum. The jejunal mucosa remains intact with marked broadening and blunting of the villi and shortening of the microvilli, along with mononuclear cell infiltration and cytoplasmic vacuolization. Functional alterations may include a transient malabsorption of fat, D-xylose, and lactose and a significant decrease in levels of small intestinal brush border enzymes (alkaline phosphatase and trehalase). Adenylate cyclase activity in the jejunum is not elevated. Delay in gastric emptying may be responsible for the nausea and vomiting associated with these agents.

The nature of immunity to Norwalk virus is perplexing, because a high percentage (~50%) of adults are susceptible to both natural and experimental illness. In addition, although immunity has been observed in approximately 50% of adults, it appears to correlate inversely with the level of serum or local jejunal antibody.

ROTAVIRUS. The major histopathologic lesions are characterized by reversible involvement of the proximal small intestine. The mucosa remains intact, with shortening of the villi, mononuclear cell infiltration in the lamina propria, distended cisternae of the endoplasmic reticulum, mitochondrial swelling, and sparse, irregular microvilli. Functional alterations may include impaired D-xylose absorption and depressed levels of disaccharidases (maltase, sucrase, and lactase).

The mechanism of immunity to human rotaviruses is not clear. Although significant levels of serum antibodies correlate with resistance to illness, the role of local intestinal immunity has not been elucidated. Animal studies indicate that antibody in the small intestine is the major determinant of resistance to illness. A high rate of subclinical infection in neonates is well documented and may be related to passively acquired maternal antibody, host factors, or naturally attenuated rotaviruses that are able to persist in newborn nurseries.

CLINICAL MANIFESTATIONS

NORWALK VIRUS GROUP. Clinical characteristics of illness induced by the Norwalk group of viruses include nausea, vomiting, diarrhea, anorexia, or abdominal discomfort, or any combination. Accompanying clinical manifestations may also include myalgias, low-grade fever, headache, and chills. In children, vomiting occurs more often than diarrhea, whereas in adults the opposite is observed. The onset of illness may be abrupt, marked by vomiting, diarrhea, or both. The illness is usually mild and lasts about 24 to 60

TABLE 344-1. VIRUSES ASSOCIATED WITH ACUTE GASTROENTERITIS IN HUMANS

Virus	Size, nm	Epidemiology	Important as a Cause of Hospitalization
Rotavirus			
Group A	70	Single most important cause (viral or bacterial) of endemic severe diarrheal illness in infants and young children worldwide (in cooler months in temperate climates)	Yes
Group B	70	Outbreaks of diarrheal illness in adults and children in China	No
Group C	70	Sporadic cases and occasional outbreaks of diarrheal illness in children	No
Enteric adenovirus	70–80	Second most important viral agent of endemic diarrheal illness of infants and young children worldwide	Yes
Norwalk virus or Norwalk-like caliciviruses	27–32	Important cause of outbreaks of vomiting and diarrheal illness in older children and adults in families, communities, and institutions; frequently associated with ingestion of food	No
Caliciviruses ("classical")	28–40	Sporadic cases and occasional outbreaks of diarrheal illness in infants, young children, and the elderly	No
Astroviruses	28	Sporadic cases and occasional outbreaks of diarrheal illness in infants, young children, and the elderly	No

Adapted from Kapikian AZ: Viral gastroenteritis. JAMA 269:627, 1993.

hours. However, severe gastroenteritis has been observed in middle-aged patients and has contributed to the death of elderly, debilitated individuals. The stools are characteristically loose and watery; blood, mucus, and leukocytes are not typically present. A transient decrease in the T, B, and null cell lymphocyte subpopulations has been observed. The role of Norwalk virus in the etiology of gastroenteritis in human immunodeficiency virus (HIV)-positive individuals appears to be similar to that observed in non-HIV infected controls.

ROTAVIRUS. Rotavirus infection can produce a variety of responses in infants and young children, ranging from subclinical infection and mild diarrhea to a severe and occasionally fatal dehydrating illness. Clinical characteristics include vomiting, diarrhea, abdominal discomfort, or fever, or any combination. Fever and vomiting often develop before the diarrhea. Accompanying clinical manifestations may include dehydration, irritability, and pharyngeal or tympanic membrane erythema. In hospitalized patients, the mean duration of confinement is 4 days, with a range of 2 to 14 days. The stools are characteristically loose and watery and only infrequently contain blood or leukocytes.

Although rotaviruses can cause severe or fatal dehydrating illnesses in developing countries, deaths have also been documented in developed countries. In a study in Canada, rotavirus gastroenteritis was implicated in the deaths of 21 children 4 to 30 months old (mean 11 months) over a period of about 5 years. Twenty children were dead or moribund upon arrival at hospital, and one child was infected nosocomially. With the exception of the latter patient and one other, each child was considered healthy prior to the rotaviral illness. Death occurred within 1 to 3 days of onset of symptoms. Dehydration and electrolyte imbalance leading to cardiac arrest were believed to be the major cause of death in 16 patients; aspiration of vomitus was the cause of death in 3 patients; and seizures were a contributing factor in the remaining 2 patients.

Rotavirus can also induce chronic symptomatic diarrhea with prolonged fecal shedding of the virus and antigenemia in patients with primary immunodeficiency diseases. Infections with rotaviruses or other viral and bacterial enteric pathogens may be especially severe in individuals who are immunosuppressed for bone marrow transplantation. In one study, 8 of 78 such patients (average age of entire group, 20.5 years) shed rotavirus in stools and 5 of the 8 died. In addition, a non–group A rotavirus was associated with severe gastroenteritis in an 8-year-old bone marrow transplant patient. Rotavirus infections have also been persistent and severe in children with severe combined immunodeficiency. Rotavirus infections have also been associated with necrotizing enterocolitis and hemorrhagic gastroenteritis in neonates.

Outbreaks of rotavirus gastroenteritis have occurred in elderly individuals in nursing homes with several fatalities.

Rotaviruses do not appear to have an important role as etiologic agents of acute diarrhea in HIV-positive adults.

DIAGNOSIS

NORWALK VIRUS GROUP. Since a specific diagnosis of infection with this group cannot be made by clinical observation, the diagnosis must be made in the laboratory and relies on detection of virus in the stool or a serologic response to a viral-specific antigen. These tests include IEM (for the entire group), radioimmunoassay (Norwalk and Snow Mountain agents), and enzyme-linked immunosorbent assay (ELISA) (Norwalk, Snow Mountain, and Hawaii viruses). These are still research procedures, because reagents are not generally available. Virus shedding is maximal at or shortly after onset of illness and minimal at 72 hours following onset. The characteristic absence of fecal leukocytes in Norwalk infection may be helpful for differentiation from *Shigella* or *Salmonella* enteritis. Recent molecular biologic advances in the study of the Norwalk group of viruses should lead to a proliferation of diagnostic assays.

Although a specific clinical diagnosis of infection with Norwalk virus cannot be made in the individual patient, a tentative diagnosis of infection can be made during an outbreak if certain criteria are met: (1) bacterial or parasitic pathogens are not detected; (2) vomiting is present in at least 50% of cases; (3) incubation period is 24 to 48 hours; and (4) mean or median duration of illness is 12 to 60 hours.

ROTAVIRUS. The clinical manifestations of rotavirus gastroenteritis are not distinctive enough to enable diagnosis. Thus, diagnosis requires either detection of the virus or demonstration of a significant serologic response to rotavirus in paired acute and convalescent sera. The epidemiologic pattern relating to the age of the patient, the temporal occurrence of illness, and the signs and symptoms of illness, however, may suggest the diagnosis. In addition, the usual absence of fecal leukocytes in rotavirus diarrhea may help in early differentiation from *Shigella* or *Salmonella* enteritis.

Stools obtained from the first to fourth day of illness are optimal for detecting rotavirus, but virus shedding may continue up to 21 days. Virus is characteristically present in stools during the early phase of diarrhea, but diarrhea may continue for 2 to 3 days after virus shedding has ceased.

Over 25 assays have been developed to detect rotavirus in stools. The most rapid method is still direct EM because in negatively stained preparations these agents have a distinctive morphologic appearance and are present in large amounts. The non–group A rotaviruses, which do not share the common group antigen, can also be detected by EM. However, an electron microscope may not be readily available, and its use may be impractical when evaluating a large number of specimens. Thus, other rapid and highly effective methods for virus detection have been developed, including ELISA, counterimmunoelectroosmophoresis (CIEOP), radioimmunoassay (RIA), reverse passive hemagglutination assay (RPHA), latex agglutination (LA), RNA electrophoresis, dot hybridization, and recently by using the polymerase chain reaction. Commercial kits are now available for the ELISA, LA, and RPHA assays. A popular method is the confirmatory ELISA because it is simple to perform, is sensitive, does not require specialized equipment, and has a negative serum antibody control for detecting nonspecific reactions. An ELISA using monoclonal anti-VP7 antibody is also available. The non–group A rotaviruses cannot be detected by these assays, because they lack the common group antigen; however, an ELISA for group B rotaviruses has been developed. Diagnosis of group A rotavirus infection by growth in cell cultures is not practical.

There are many methods for measuring a serologic response to rotavirus infection, including IEM, complement fixation (CF), immunofluorescence, immune adherence hemagglutination assay, ELISA, neutralization, hemagglutination-inhibition (HI), inhibition of RPHA, and a competition solid-phase immunoassay that measures epitope specific immune responses to individual rotavirus serotypes. Complement fixation is an efficient assay for detecting a serologic response to rotavirus in patients age 6 to 24 months but is not as effective in adults or infants younger than 6 months.

Detection of rotavirus or demonstration of a serologic response does not necessarily establish an etiologic association with the patient's illness, especially in newborns and adults, who frequently undergo subclinical infection.

TREATMENT

NORWALK VIRUS GROUP. Since the Norwalk group of viruses characteristically causes a mild, self-limited gastroenteritis, replacement of fluid and electrolyte loss with orally administered isotonic fluids is usually sufficient. However, if severe vomiting or diarrhea occurs, parenteral fluid replacement may be necessary. Oral administration of bismuth subsalicylate significantly reduces the severity of abdominal cramps, with a decrease in the median duration of gastrointestinal symptoms from 20 hours to 14 hours. However, the number, weight, and water content of stools and the level of virus excretion are not affected significantly.

ROTAVIRUS. Because rotavirus gastroenteritis may lead to severe dehydration in infants and young children, the early replacement of fluids and electrolytes is essential. Intravenous fluids have been used effectively in treating dehydration. However, in many parts of the world where such treatment is not feasible, efforts have been made to evaluate the effectiveness of an oral rehydration salts (ORS) solution. In a double-blind study comparing ORS with intravenous fluids in children with rotavirus gastroenteritis, ORS solution containing either glucose (20 grams per liter) or sucrose (40 grams per liter) plus electrolytes was found to be as effective as intravenous therapy for rehydration. Glucose electrolyte solutions are recommended for optimal results. The recommended World Health Organization (WHO) ORS solution is made by adding the following to 1 liter of water: sodium chloride, 3.5 grams; trisodium citrate, dihydrate, 2.9 grams; potassium chloride, 1.5 grams; and glucose, anhydrous, 20 grams. Sodium bicarbonate, 2.5 grams, may be substituted for the trisodium citrate, dihydrate. The efficacy of oral glucose-electrolyte solutions that contained either 90 mmol of sodium per liter (as in the WHO formula above) or 50 mmol of sodium per liter, plus additional electrolytes, was examined in well-nourished ambulatory or hospitalized children with mild or moderate dehydrating diarrheal illnesses of varied etiology (including rotavirus but excluding cholera), and each was found to be safe and effective. After the initial calculated fluid deficit is corrected by the ORS, water or fluids without added electrolytes, such as breast milk or some other form of low-solute feeding, should be given orally in addition to the ORS solution, to replace both continued diarrheal fluid and electrolyte losses and to provide normal daily fluid requirements. If oral rehydration fails to correct the fluid and electrolyte loss or if the patient is severely dehydrated or in shock, or has depressed consciousness (see below), intravenous therapy must be given.

In recent studies, rice-based ORS solutions were also found to be effective in rehydrating infants and young children hospitalized with mild to moderate dehydration caused by diarrhea associated with various pathogens, including rotavirus. Both glucose-based or rice-based ORS solutions were effective in rehydration and maintenance therapy. Oral rehydration therapy should not be given to infants and younger children with depressed consciousness because of the possibility of fluid aspiration.

In a limited study, chronic rotavirus illness in immunodeficient children has been treated effectively by oral feeding of pooled human milk that contained rotavirus antibody. Oral administration of preparations containing rotavirus antibody has produced conflicting results regarding their efficacy for treatment of normal children during episodes of rotavirus gastroenteritis.

Orally administered bismuth subsalicylate (BSS) was evaluated in a placebo-controlled study as an adjunct to rehydration therapy in children age 4 to 28 months who were hospitalized with rotavirus diarrhea. The BSS group had a shorter course of diarrhea than the placebo group. Because of the reported association between the use of salicylates and Reye's syndrome, the authors reviewed the literature regarding the possibility of such an association with BSS and other non–acetyl-salicylic acid salicylates and were unable to find any such association.

PREVENTION

NORWALK VIRUS GROUP. There are no specific methods for preventing illness by the Norwalk virus group. However, because of the extremely infectious nature of these agents, careful handwashing and proper disposal of contaminated material should minimize transmission. In addition, hygienic preparation of food and measures to decrease contamination of drinking water or swimming facilities should limit the frequency of Norwalk virus outbreaks. Active immunization against this group of viruses is not yet feasible.

ROTAVIRUS. Epidemiologic studies indicate the global need for a rotavirus vaccine to prevent rotavirus diarrhea in the first 2 years of life, when illness is most severe. Current efforts are focused on developing a live, attenuated oral vaccine that is effective against all serotypes. A promising initial strategy involved the "Jennerian" approach, in which a related rotavirus from a nonhuman host (a bovine or rhesus rotavirus strain) was used as the immunizing agent. Efficacy trials of several such candidate rotavirus vaccines gave variable results and it soon became apparent that these vaccines did not induce satisfactory heterotypic immunity in infants not primed by previous rotavirus infection. The rhesus rotavirus vaccine (a VP7 serotype 3 strain) induced protection against rotavirus diarrhea in the 1- to 4-month age group in a study in which VP7 serotype 3 was predominant, but it failed in other studies to protect unprimed infants against illnesses caused by other than serotype 3 rotaviruses. Thus, the Jennerian approach has been modified with the goal being a quadrivalent vaccine composed of rhesus rotavirus (serotype 3) and three reassortant rotaviruses each containing 10 rhesus rotavirus genes and a single human rotavirus gene that encodes VP7 serotype 1, 2, or 4 specificity. Field trials of the quadrivalent vaccine in infants and young children have been encouraging, with approximately 80% efficacy against the development of severe rotavirus diarrhea observed in two separate trials in the United States.

Breast milk is generally considered to confer some degree of protection against clinically significant rotavirus diarrhea during infancy. The prophylactic oral administration of human serum globulin containing rotavirus antibody to low birth weight neonates provides significant protection against rotavirus diarrhea. In addition, passive oral immunization of infants and young children with bovine colostrum that contained antibodies to human rotavirus was effective in preventing rotavirus illness when compared with a control group.

Bernstein DI, Glass RI, Rodgers G, et al.: Evaluation of rhesus rotavirus monovalent and tetravalent reassortant vaccines in U.S. children. JAMA 273:1191, 1995. *A placebo-controlled vaccine trial in which the tetravalent vaccine induced > 80% protection against very severe rotavirus gastroenteritis.*

Guarino A, Canini RB, Russo S, et al.: Oral immunoglobulins for treatment of acute rotaviral gastroenteritis. Pediatrics 93:12, 1994. *A study reporting the benefit of oral human serum immunoglobulin in infants and young children hospitalized with acute viral gastroenteritis.*

Hoshino Y, Kapikian AZ: Rotavirus vaccine development for the prevention of severe diarrhea in infants and young children. Trends in Microbiol 2:242, 1994. *A concise review of rotavirus vaccine strategies and an up-to-date presentation of rotavirus serotypes.*

Jiang X, Graham DY, Wang K, Estes MK: Norwalk virus genome cloning and characterization. Science 250:1580, 1990. *A study describing the cloning of the fastidious Norwalk virus.*

Kapikian AZ (ed.): Virus Infections of the Gastrointestinal Tract. New York, Marcel Dekker, Inc., 1994. *An entire volume on viral infections of the gastrointestinal tract by numerous contributors. Includes relevant data on viral agents associated with gastroenteritis with extensive references.*

Kapikian AZ, Chanock RM: Norwalk group of viruses. In Fields BN, et al. (eds.): Virology, 3rd ed. New York, Raven Press, in press. *A detailed current review of the Norwalk group of viruses from a virologic, epidemiologic, and clinical point of view. 277 references.*

Kapikian AZ, Chanock RM: Rotaviruses. In Fields BN, et al. (eds.): Virology, 3rd ed. New York, Raven Press, in press. *A detailed current review of rotaviruses from a virologic, epidemiologic, and clinical point of view. 993 references.*

Molina S, Vettorazzi C, Pearson JM, et al.: Clinical trial of glucose-oral rehydration solution (ORS), rice dextrin-ORS, and rice flour-ORS for the management of children with acute diarrhea and mild or moderate dehydration. Pediatrics 95:191, 1995. *A study evaluating the efficacy of two rice-based rehydration solutions and a conventional glucose-based solution in hospitalized infants and young children with acute diarrhea associated with various pathogens, including rotavirus.*

Soriano-Brucher H, Avendano P, O'Ryan M, et al.: Bismuth subsalicylate in the treatment of acute diarrhea in children: A clinical study. Pediatrics 87:18, 1991. *A study evaluating oral BSS as an adjunct to rehydration in infants and young children hospitalized with acute diarrhea associated with various pathogens, including rotavirus.*

Hemorrhagic Fever Viruses

345 INTRODUCTION TO HEMORRHAGIC FEVER VIRUSES
Robert E. Shope

The viral hemorrhagic fevers encompass syndromes that vary from febrile hemorrhagic disease with capillary fragility to acute severe shock leading rapidly to death. The causative agents include arthropod-borne and rodent-borne viruses. The rodent-borne viruses do not require an arthropod vector but are transmitted directly to vertebrates by aerosol spread or contact with infected excreta or body secretions of the rodent. The reservoir and natural mode of transmission for the African hemorrhagic fever viruses, Marburg and Ebola, are not known.

There are at least 18 viruses that cause human hemorrhagic fevers (see Table 345–1). They are in the families Flaviviridae, Bunyaviridae, Arenaviridae, and Filoviridae. All contain RNA, and all are zoonoses.

The hemorrhagic fevers form a special group of diseases charac-

TABLE 345-1. CLINICAL PARAMETERS OF VIRAL HEMORRHAGIC FEVERS

Disease	Viral Agent	Incubation Period (Days)	Clinical Syndromes				ARDS*	Case-Fatality Rate (%)
			Hemorrhage	Hepatitis	Encephalitis	Nephropathy		
Yellow fever	Yellow fever	3–6	major	major	absent	moderate	absent	2–20
Dengue hemmorrhagic fever	Dengue 1–4	5–8	moderate	moderate	absent	absent	absent	2–5
Rift Valley fever	Rift Valley fever	3–6	major	major	moderate	absent	absent	30–50
Crimean-Congo hemmor-rhagic fever	Crimean-Congo hemmor-rhagic fever	2–9	major	major	minor	absent	absent	30–50
Kyasanur Forest disease	Kyasanur Forest disease	3–8	minor	minor	moderate	absent	absent	5–10
Omsk hemmorrhagic fever	Omsk hemmorrhagic fever	3–8	minor	minor	moderate	absent	absent	0.4–2.5
Hemorrhagic fever with renal syndrome	Hantaan, Puumala, Dobrava, Seoul	2–42	moderate	rare	minor	major	absent	2–5
Hantavirus pulmonary syndrome	Sin Nombre Shelter Island I	12–16	minor	minor	absent	minor	major	40–50
Venezuelan hemorrhagic fever	Guanarito	7–14	moderate	rare	rare	minor	absent	60
Brazilian hemorrhagic fever	Sabiá	8–12	major	minor	minor	minor	absent	33
Argentine hemorrhagic fever	Junin	10–14	minor	rare	moderate	minor	absent	1–15
Bolivian hemorrhagic fever	Machupo	7–14	moderate	rare	moderate	minor	absent	15–30
Lassa fever	Lassa	3–16	minor	major	minor	minor	absent	10–25
African hemorrhagic fever	Marburg	3–9	major	major	minor	absent	absent	20–30
	Ebola	3–18	major	major	minor	absent	absent	60–90

* Adult respiratory distress syndrome.

terized by viral replication in lymphoid cells, followed by fever and myalgia and leading to hemorrhagic manifestations and hypovolemic shock. The basic physiologic defect in most is capillary leakage. In some, such as yellow fever, hepatocellular damage is prominent. In others, such as hemorrhagic fever with renal syndrome, renal lesions are striking. The mortality rates may be high, and the pathogenesis is poorly understood. Disseminated intravascular coagulopathy (DIC) is a feature in some cases, but probably not all. Antigen-antibody complexes may lead to release of mediators of shock in some cases, and direct effects of viral replication on capillary permeability in some have not been ruled out. It is important to understand the pathogenetic mechanism to manage the patient, but our knowledge is sparse at present.

Control can be achieved by interrupting the cycle, including peridomestic rodent control (Bolivian hemorrhagic fever), and, in those that are arboviruses, by vaccinating reservoir animals (Rift Valley fever), vector control, and education on methods to avoid the vector (dengue) or rodent reservoir (hantavirus pulmonary syndrome). Vaccines are available or under development for some of the agents such as Rift Valley fever, yellow fever, dengue, and Junin viruses. For others such as Lassa virus, we now have an antiviral drug, and for still another (Junin) pre-exposure and postexposure protection is afforded by human immune plasma.

345.1 Yellow Fever

DEFINITION. Yellow fever is an acute viral disease caused by infection with yellow fever virus. The disease is exemplary of the viral hemorrhagic fevers described in the following sections (Table 345–1). The infection is often subclinical but may lead to disease whose severity varies from mild and self-limited to a fulminant fatal outcome. Classic yellow fever is characterized by sudden onset, moderately high fever, nausea, bradycardia, prostration, vomiting of altered blood, jaundice, oliguria, and albuminuria. Natural cycles of the infection occur periodically in mosquitoes and primates of tropical South America as far north as Panama and in tropical west, central, and east Africa.

ETIOLOGY. Yellow fever virus is in the genus *Flavivirus* of the family Flaviviridae. Members of the family are single-stranded, negative-sense RNA viruses, spherical and approximately 40 nm in diameter. Particles form in the cytoplasm in close association with endoplasmic reticulum. They contain a lipid envelope and replicate in both arthropod and vertebrate cells. Other members of the Fla-

viviridae, including dengue, West Nile, and St. Louis encephalitis, cross-react with yellow fever virus in serologic tests and may confound the diagnosis. Minor antigenic differences exist between strains of yellow fever virus from Africa and South America, and among strains from different regions of Africa; however, the 17D yellow fever vaccine protects against all strains. The virus can be isolated in mosquitoes, arthropod and vertebrate tissue cultures, baby mice, and several monkey species. Rhesus monkeys regularly succumb following experimental inoculation and mimic severe human disease.

EPIDEMIOLOGY. Two epidemiologic types of yellow fever are distinguished: the urban and the sylvan (jungle) forms. Urban yellow fever is transmitted by *Aedes aegypti* mosquitoes from person to person, whereas sylvan yellow fever is maintained in a forest cycle of monkeys and forest-canopy mosquitoes; humans are infected when they enter the forest. The two types do not differ clinically.

A. aegypti is a peridomestic mosquito that breeds in abandoned tires, jars, cans, water storage containers, roof catchments, and drains in and around houses. Urban yellow fever was a major killer until the early 1900's, when mosquito control in Havana, Rio de Janeiro, Guayaquil, and the other large urban centers eliminated the disease. The last recorded urban case in the Americas was in Trinidad in 1954. *A. aegypti* continues to be prevalent in African cities, and *A. aegypti*-transmitted outbreaks still occur there. Major epidemics were recorded in Ethiopia, 1960–1962; Nigeria, 1969; Senegal, 1965 and 1979; Gambia, 1978; Ghana and Burkina Faso, 1983; and Kenya, 1993. In 1986, an epidemic involving at least 3000 persons occurred in Nigeria, in Benue and Cross River States, and extended into Oyo and Niger States in 1987. An estimated 39,000 cases, with 8400 deaths, were recorded.

Yellow fever virus in Africa is transmitted by *A. aegypti* not only in the cities but also in semirural areas. In addition, some African epidemics are maintained by other *Aedes* species, such as *bromeliae* and the tree hole-breeding *africanus, leuteocephalus,* and *furcifer-taylori,* which transmit the virus in savannah and the transition forest-savannah zones of west Africa.

Sylvan yellow fever was recognized initially in Brazil in 1932. After urban yellow fever had been controlled in the Americas, sporadic cases continued to occur in persons exposed to mosquitoes in the jungles of South America and Africa. This sylvan form is maintained in tropical America by *Haemagogus* mosquitoes and forest primates, and sometimes by other sylvan animals. Evidence favors the hypothesis that the virus moves through the forest, cycling in one place until the monkeys are immune, then dying out and moving to areas where there are susceptible monkeys. People entering the forest are at risk. Sylvan yellow fever extends periodically outside the enzootic zone into forests such as those in Panama and Central America. The virus can be maintained over dry periods by transovarial transmission in mosquitoes, although it remains to be shown whether maintenance in mosquito eggs is more than a temporary mechanism.

The sylvan cycle in Africa is more complicated than in the Americas; in tropical Africa the virus cycles between *A. africanus* and monkeys. Another African mosquito, *A. bromeliae,* which feeds on both humans and monkeys, serves in some areas as a link between primates in the deep forest and people in the African villages.

A. aegypti was once carried on sailing ships between tropical ports and into temperate-zone cities. Modern ocean-going ships no longer harbor mosquito-breeding sites, but the mosquito continues to travel by small boats, airplanes, cars, and especially in the form of dried eggs transported by used tires. Cities such as Rio de Janeiro, which were once freed of the mosquito, are now reinfested. Dengue fever reappeared there in 1986. To control the mosquito again in this area will be difficult because of insecticide resistance and the high price of labor and materials. Jungle yellow fever continues to cycle, reappearing in the same locale every 5 to 40 years. The scene is thus set again for emergence of the virus from the jungle to reinitiate the urban cycle in the Americas.

A. aegypti is easily identified. It has white thoracic scales in the shape of a lyre and black legs with white bands. Mosquitoes that have fed on a viremic vertebrate become infective after an extrinsic incubation period of 9 to 30 days, the shorter periods correlating with higher ambient temperatures. This extrinsic incubation period in the mosquito accounts for the delay from the first human infection in an urban outbreak to subsequent clusters of infection.

Yellow fever is not found in Asia, although large areas harbor *A. aegypti* that are capable of transmitting the virus, should it be introduced. India and other Asian nations require vaccination of travelers from yellow fever-endemic regions.

All age groups and races are susceptible. However, sylvan yellow fever is found almost always in young males because they are the individuals who venture into the forest. Immunity following vaccination or infection is long-lasting. During an epidemic, the population at risk, therefore, may be limited to age groups not covered by prior immunization or those born since a prior outbreak. There is also some evidence that persons may be protected by antibody to heterologous flaviviruses.

During the 24-year period from 1965 to 1988, there were 3324 cases of yellow fever reported in the Americas, and 7701 in Africa. The numbers of cases are greatly underestimated, probably by a factor of at least 10. Case-fatality rates are usually about 20%, but are higher in some epidemics. Ratios of apparent to inapparent infection, estimated at 1:10, may vary greatly.

PATHOLOGY AND PATHOGENESIS. The lesions of yellow fever involve primarily the liver, heart, kidneys, and lymphoid tissues. Grossly, the skin is icteric, and there may be multiple hemorrhages or petechiae of the skin, mucous membranes, and multiple organs. The liver is normal in size, icteric, and fatty. The heart is soft and flabby, and the kidneys are swollen and a pink-gray color. Small peritoneal and pleural effusions are sometimes observed.

Histology is often characteristic in patients who die before the ninth day of illness, but the lesions are not always pathognomonic. The most striking lesion is the eosinophilic degeneration and coagulation of hepatocytes (Councilman's bodies). Hepatocyte destruction is most marked in the midzone of the lobule, with relative sparing of the central vein and portal areas. Intranuclear eosinophilic granular inclusions or enlarged nucleoli (Torre's bodies) are also described. Both microvacuolar and multivacuolar fatty changes are prominent, especially after the first week of illness. Inflammation is uncommon, and the reticulum framework is unaffected, probably accounting for the absence of postnecrotic fibrosis in convalescence and the regeneration of hepatocytes in recovered patients. The kidneys show cloudy swelling of tubular epithelium leading to acute tubular necrosis. The glomeruli are not obviously affected, but special stains indicate Schiff-positive alterations in the basal membranes, and proteinaceous material accumulates in the capsular spaces and lumina of the proximal tubules. The myocardium is characterized by granular or fatty infiltration of muscle fibers and of the atrioventricular (AV) conduction system and cloudy swelling and degeneration of myocytes without inflammation. Large monocytes replace lymphocytic cells in the splenic follicles and lymph nodes. Encephalitis is rare, although petechial hemorrhage in the brain stem and cerebral edema are observed.

Knowledge of the pathogenesis of yellow fever is sparse. Yellow fever cases occur in remote areas, and pathophysiologic studies of yellow fever patients are usually done with only rudimentary laboratory facilities. The virus replicates in the hepatocytes and myocytes, and it is presumed that lesions in these target cells are a direct effect of the virus. Jaundice and prolonged prothrombin time can be explained by hepatocellular damage; bradycardia and arrhythmias, by myocyte and AV node perturbation. The etiology of renal tubular necrosis is not clear, but it may be secondary to hepatic changes. Some, but not all, fatal cases are associated with thrombocytopenia; increased prothrombin, partial thromboplastin, and thrombin times; diminished Factor VIII and fibrinogen; and the presence of fibrin split products. The bleeding in these cases may be secondary to disseminated intravascular coagulopathy (DIC), but this is not generally accepted by all investigators. Hypoglycemia, metabolic acidosis, and hyperkalemia characterize the terminal stage and are probably the result of multiple organ system failure.

CLINICAL MANIFESTATIONS. Severe yellow fever is a fulminant febrile illness with ≥ 50% mortality. There is a great deal of variation, however; most cases are mild with a better prognosis, and only about 10 to 20% are in the severe category. The intrinsic incubation period is 3 to 6 days, exceptionally as long as 10 days.

The clinical syndrome is classified as very mild, mild, moderately severe, or malignant. Patients with very mild cases have fever and headache, and the patient recovers in 48 hours or less. Those with mild cases have sudden fever and headache with nausea, sometimes bleeding of the gums or epistaxis, bradycardia, or albuminuria. The patient recovers in 2 or 3 days. Those with moderately severe cases have more marked manifestations of bleeding, definite bradycardia in relation to the fever, nausea and vomiting, jaundice, and striking albuminuria. The illness may be aborted after 3 to 4 days or may develop serious hemorrhagic manifestations, such as black vomit, melena, and metrorrhagia. Moderately severe yellow fever may last 1 week or even longer.

Classic yellow fever is characterized as malignant and is divided into three periods. The period of infection involves sudden onset of fever and headache, with initial rapid pulse, but by day 2, the pulse slows in spite of continued fever (Faget's sign). Headache, back, and muscle pain may be severe, blood oozes from the gums, and other signs of bleeding become prominent. The face is flushed, the tongue is reddened (strawberry tongue), and the conjunctivae are injected; the patient is irritable, unable to sleep, and frequently constipated. The temperature is often 40° C or higher. On the third day of illness, there is nausea, vomiting of coffee-ground material, and notable albuminuria. The bleeding is usually gastric, not lower intestinal. In the period of remission, often on day 4, the patient feels better, the fever drops, and headache and nausea subside. Remission lasts a few hours to 2 days. It is followed by the period of intoxication in which the classic signs of fever, epigastric tenderness with vomiting of altered blood, nosebleeds, and albuminuria leading to oliguria or anuria occur. Dehydration may predispose to suppurative parotitis; the lungs are usually normal, but bacterial pneumonia may complicate the disease. Intoxication lasts from 3 days up to 2 weeks and may be accompanied by heart failure with drop in blood pressure, hiccup, coma, and death. Sometimes the patient is lucid until the end.

The clinical syndrome may be predominantly one of hepatic, renal, or cardiac failure. Meningoencephalitis has also been recorded. Death usually occurs between the seventh and the tenth day of illness. Patients who survive generally recover completely, although the convalescence may be prolonged, and late death from cardiac failure or arrhythmias is a rare complication.

CLINICAL LABORATORY FINDINGS. Early in the course there may be leukopenia with relative neutropenia (but sometimes with normal or elevated leukocyte count), decreased prothrombin time, and elevation of the serum bilirubin level. After the third day of illness, full-blown yellow fever is associated with abnormalities referable to the liver, kidneys, and heart. The total and conjugated bilirubin concentration values are elevated and rise together. The mean bilirubin value is 9 to 10 mg per deciliter but averages 15 to 20 mg per deciliter in severe cases and may be much higher. There are increased prothrombin and partial thromboplastin times and decreased platelets, blood glucose, and clotting Factors II, V, VII, IX, and X. Alkaline phosphatase levels are normal. Aminotransferase levels are of prognostic value; serum aspartate aminotransferase and alanine aminotransferase levels are consistently elevated in jaundiced patients.

Albuminuria usually appears on the fourth day, reaching levels of 3 to 5 mg per liter (in severe cases much higher). Blood urea averages 109 mg per deciliter, and creatinine averages 5.9 mg per deciliter in fatal cases; the averages are much lower in nonfatal yellow fever. The urine may contain bile and casts. Electrocardiogram abnormalities are sometimes present, including abnormal ST-T waves and prolonged PR and QT intervals. The cerebrospinal fluid (CSF) is under increased pressure and may contain increased protein with normal cell counts.

DIAGNOSIS. Diagnosis can be made by histopathologic examination of the liver, by isolation of yellow fever virus from blood during life and from liver and other tissues post mortem, by demonstration of specific nucleic acid, or by serologic tests. Yellow fever should be suspected in any febrile patient from endemic zones of Africa and the Americas and in areas of high *A. aegypti* prevalence where yellow fever may be introduced. Diagnosis post mortem by examination of liver taken by a viscerotome was successfully used in South America routinely for many years. Liver biopsy should not be attempted because of the danger of uncontrolled bleeding.

Yellow fever virus can be isolated from serum and blood during the first 4 days of fever by inoculation intracerebrally into baby mice or onto mammalian or mosquito cell cultures. Mice are observed for death; the virus causes cytopathic effect in Vero cells and is detected by immunofluorescence tests in mosquito cells 3 to 6 days after inoculation. The most rapid method of diagnosis is detection of antigen in acute phase blood by the antigen-capture enzyme-linked immunosorbent assay (ELISA). The test can be completed in a few hours, although detection of antigen by ELISA is less sensitive than virus isolation.

Serologic diagnosis is made by demonstrating immunoglobulin M (IgM) by the antibody-capture ELISA. Since IgM is relatively specific and is detectable for only a short time after infection, this technique is reliable using a single convalescent serum specimen. Alternatively, tests of sera collected during the acute and convalescent phases are diagnostic if they show a fourfold or greater rise (or fall) of yellow fever antibody. The neutralization test is highly specific, but the complement fixation, hemagglutination-inhibition, and ELISA methods are usually used because they are quicker and lend themselves to field laboratory use. The laboratory must also rule out cross-reacting antibody by related viruses such as dengue. A radiolabeled RNA probe detected yellow fever RNA in fixed human liver stored for more than 20 years.

DIFFERENTIAL DIAGNOSIS. The mild form of yellow fever is not clinically distinguishable from other tropical fevers. Severe yellow fever simulates viral hepatitis, including hepatitis D; other hemorrhagic fevers; leptospirosis; rickettsial fevers; malignant malaria; and drug- and toxin-related conditions.

PROGNOSIS. Two to 20% of patients with clinically evident yellow fever die, although as many as 50% of severely ill patients succumb. It is not clear whether these patients would survive if they received the most modern supportive treatment, because most cases are treated in primitive clinics in Africa and South America. Patients who enter the period of intoxication have a guarded prognosis, especially if they develop anuria, high levels of albuminuria and bilirubinemia, a prothrombin time prolonged beyond 25% of normal, a rapid, weak pulse, uncontrolled bleeding, persistent hiccup, delirium, hypotension, or coma.

TREATMENT. Treatment consists of complete bed rest, fluid and blood replacement, and supportive care, including monitoring of vital signs. Analgesics and antiemetics may be useful, but aspirin is contraindicated because it may exacerbate bleeding. Patients are placed under bed nets to prevent possible mosquito transmission to other patients and to hospital personnel. Malaria and bacterial complications should be treated if diagnosed. Electrolyte imbalance should be corrected. Dialysis has not been used in cases of renal tubular damage, but on theoretical grounds may benefit patients with renal failure. If DIC is evident by laboratory tests, heparin may be used cautiously, although there is insufficient experience to date to predict its efficacy. Interferon and other antiviral substances have not been tried in patients with yellow fever.

PREVENTION AND CONTROL. Yellow fever can be prevented by inoculation of 17D attenuated vaccine. This vaccine is safe and in >90% of vaccinees induces antibody that persists at least 10 years, and usually for life. The vaccine is produced in eggs and should not be given to persons with egg allergies. Travelers should be vaccinated at least 10 days before arrival in yellow fever–endemic areas. Since the presence of yellow fever often goes undetected and unreported in tropical Africa and South America, the vaccine should be given to travelers whether or not there is known active transmission. Human immunodeficiency virus (HIV) infection is not a contraindication to vaccination. Unless the risk of exposure to yellow fever is great, vaccine is not recommended during pregnancy; however, it is not known to have caused fetal damage. In an epidemic, mosquito control measures and use of bed nets and repellents are recommended until vaccine can be obtained.

345.2 Hemorrhagic Fever Caused by Dengue Viruses

DEFINITION. Dengue hemorrhagic fever (DHF) is an acute febrile illness characterized by decreased platelet counts and hemoconcentration in patients infected with any one of the four serotypes of dengue virus. The disease affects children mainly and sometimes adults. Capillary permeability and coagulation defects lead to hemorrhagic manifestations and, in the more severe cases, to hypovolemic shock (dengue shock syndrome), with death in 40 to 50% of untreated shock syndrome patients. The disease has been endoepidemic in Southeast Asia since 1953 and is increasing in prevalence. It was restricted to Asia and the Pacific until 1981, when epidemic DHF appeared in Cuba; it reappeared in Venezuela in 1990.

ETIOLOGY. DHF is caused by infection with dengue viruses, but it is not yet established why one patient develops hemorrhagic fever and another develops classic dengue fever. Initially, it was hypothesized that strains of dengue virus that caused DHF were more virulent than others; another current theory holds that infection is enhanced and the disease is more severe when the host has been sensitized by a prior dengue infection of different serotype.

EPIDEMIOLOGY. The epidemiology of DHF is that described for dengue fever with some added features. Epidemics of DHF are limited to Southeast Asia, the Pacific Islands, and, since 1981, the Caribbean and South America. It is estimated that <5% of individuals with dengue develop DHF. The attack rate in Thailand is highest in children, with a minor peak in infants, when maternal antibody is waning, and a major peak at ages 4 to 12 years, when second dengue infections are most common; adults as well as children develop DHF in some outbreaks, such as that in Cuba in 1981. Well-nourished children in Southeast Asia appeared to be at higher risk than the undernourished, and blacks in the Cuban epidemic had milder illness than whites; well-controlled studies are needed to substantiate these observations.

PATHOLOGY. Post mortem there are focal hemorrhages, vascular congestion, and edema in multiple organs. The spleen and lymphoid tissues show marked lymphocytolysis and phagocytosis of lymphocytes, primarily in the T cell-dependent zones. There is also proliferation of lymphoblasts and young plasma cells. Monocytic and lymphocytic non-necrotizing perivascular infiltration is found in skin lesions, resembling an antibody-dependent Arthus reaction.

PATHOGENESIS. Dengue virus infects the macrophages, lymphocytes, and endothelial cells. On rare occasions, DHF occurs in primary dengue, indicating that direct infection of these cells with the virus can lead to the syndrome; however, the vast majority of cases are secondary infections. In these cases there is a rapid anamnestic antibody response, with formation of antigen-antibody complexes. Experimentally, formation of complexes enhances infectivity of the virus for monocytes through attachment of complexes at the Fc receptor site and entry of virus into the cell. Between 0.05 and 0.1% of monocytes in the peripheral blood can be visualized carrying dengue antigen. The replication of dengue virus in the monocyte is postulated to be the effector pathway leading to vascular permeability. Monocyte infection is presumably responsible for the observed complement activation and consumption via the classic and perhaps the alternate pathway. This process may result in formation of C3a and C5a, which are anaphylatoxins, or some other as yet unknown mediator of vascular permeability may be activated. Another effector pathway leads to coagulation defects, including thrombocytopenia and abnormal clotting. The entire process is rapid. It may evolve in a few hours to shock and death or, if managed effectively, to complete recovery. Although the pathogenesis is not understood, the pathophysiologic events are known and can be treated rationally.

CLINICAL MANIFESTATIONS. DHF usually starts with sudden onset of high fever and the signs and symptoms of dengue fever, which include facial flush, anorexia, headache, nausea, and pains in the muscles and joints. Hepatic tenderness, epigastric or generalized abdominal pain, and sore throat are frequent. The liver is usually palpable, and the spleen is characteristically prominent on radiographs. The temperature continues high for 2 days to a week. A positive tourniquet test result, easy bruising, and fine petechiae on the face, soft palate, and extremities indicate a hemorrhagic disorder. Sometimes gum bleeding and epistaxis are noted. The majority of cases are moderately severe or mild, and the patients recover after lysis of fever. The lysis may be associated with sweating, coolness of extremities, and transient lowering of blood pressure.

More severe cases are associated with shock. The fall in blood pressure occurs suddenly on the third to the seventh day of illness and is accompanied by cool, blotchy skin, circumoral cyanosis, and tachycardia. The patient becomes restless and may complain of acute abdominal pain. The pulse pressure drops to ≤20 mm Hg, and in severe cases the blood pressure and pulse may not be detectable. Uncorrected shock may lead to metabolic acidosis and severe bleeding from the gastrointestinal tract and other sites. Death or recovery usually occurs in 12 to 24 hours. Surviving patients do not usually have sequelae. The white blood cell count is normal or slightly elevated, with lymphocytosis and atypical lymphocytes commonly seen. There is hemoconcentration and elevated serum aspartate aminotransferase and blood urea nitrogen levels.

DIAGNOSIS. The laboratory diagnosis is that of dengue fever, which is usually made retrospectively. DHF with shock syndrome is a medical emergency, and therefore early clinical diagnosis is essential. DHF presents with (1) acute onset of fever, which is high, continuous, and lasts 2 days or more; (2) positive tourniquet test result, with spontaneous petechiae or ecchymoses; bleeding from gums or nose; hematemesis or melena; (3) hepatomegaly, observed in >90% of Asian patients; (4) hypotension with cold, clammy skin, restlessness, and pulse pressure <20 mm Hg; (5) thrombocytopenia; (6) hematocrit increased 20% over the convalescent value; and (7) radiographic evidence of pleural effusion. Fever, hemorrhagic phenomena, thrombocytopenia, and hemoconcentration are the hallmarks of DHF, and, with hypotension or narrow pulse pressure, of dengue shock syndrome (DSS). Hepatoencephalopathy sometimes develops as a late manifestation. Bacterial endotoxic shock and meningococcemia can mimic DHF/DSS.

TREATMENT. There is no specific treatment. The object of therapy is to maintain hydration, to combat acidosis, and to correct coagulation abnormalities. Salicylates may contribute to bleeding and acidosis and are contraindicated. Paracetamol may be used. Steroids should not be used. Hematocrit should be determined frequently, at least daily, to measure the degree of plasma loss and the need for intravenous fluid. Fluid should be started at 20 ml per kilogram of body weight. One third to one half of fluid should be physiologic saline and the remainder, 5% glucose in water. If acidosis is present, one quarter of fluid should be 0.167 mol per liter of sodium bicarbonate. In shock cases, one should use Ringer's lactated solution, 5% glucose in physiologic saline, 5% glucose in one-half physiological saline, 5% glucose in one-half Ringer's, or 5% glucose in one-third physiologic saline (depending on degree of dehydration and age). One should monitor for signs of cardiac failure during rapid fluid administration.

In case of shock, one should administer fluid rapidly and under pressure if necessary. One should give plasma or another volume expander if shock persists and should follow the vital signs and hematocrit. The hematocrit should decline with fluid therapy, which is continued until the hematocrit is <40%, urine output is adequate, and the appetite returns. If electrolytes and blood gases indicate acidosis, sodium bicarbonate should be administered. Heparin for intravascular coagulopathy (prolonged prothrombin and partial thromboplastin times) is usually not needed but may be used cautiously in refractory cases. Chloral hydrate for sedation, oxygen for shock, and blood should be administered as needed.

PROGNOSIS. Case fatality from DHF is 2 to 10%; deaths occur in shock cases. Most patients will survive when treated early by experienced health care workers. Recovery is rapid and without sequelae.

PREVENTION. Prevention is as described for dengue fever.

345.3 Tick-Borne Flavivirus Diseases: Kyasanur Forest Disease and Omsk Hemorrhagic Fever

DEFINITION. Kyasanur Forest disease (KFD) of India and Omsk hemorrhagic fever (OHF) of western Siberia are tick-transmitted flavivirus fevers characterized by hemorrhage or encephalitis. Some patients manifest both syndromes.

ETIOLOGY. KFD and OHF viruses belong to the tick-borne complex of flaviviruses, which also encompasses the closely related viruses of central European tick-borne encephalitis, Russian spring-summer encephalitis, and Powassan encephalitis of North America and Asia.

EPIDEMIOLOGY. KFD was originally limited to the forests of Shimoga District of Karnataka State, India, but since its discovery in 1957 it has spread in an unpredictable fashion to three other neighboring forested districts. The largest outbreak occurred during 1982–1983 in a new focus in Nidle Forest. Many tick species are involved in transmission, especially nymphal *Haemaphysalis spinigera*. Small terrestrial mammals as well as birds and bats are infected in nature. When the forest is felled for plantations, the ecology is upset. Cattle brought in to graze at the forest fringe are not infected but serve as hosts that greatly increase the numbers of ticks. Infected ticks feed on black-faced langur monkeys and South Indian bonnet macaques, which become viremic, serve as amplifiers of infection, and often die. At the same time, epidemics occur in persons with forest occupations. People are infected incidentally and do not form part of the transmission cycle.

OHF occurs in the forest-steppe areas of the lake region of western Siberia. Epidemics of as many as 600 cases were recorded in the 1940's, but in recent years the disease has virtually disappeared. Numbers of cases peak in May and again in August and September. The virus is transmitted by *Dermacentor pictus* ticks and is maintained in small-mammal populations. Muskrats, which were introduced for hunting in the 1920's, are susceptible and apparently transmit OHF virus to other muskrats and to hunters by direct contact. Lake water contaminated by dead muskrats is said to be responsible for water-borne disease. Both KFD and OHF are transmitted transovarially and trans-stadially in ticks.

CLINICAL MANIFESTATIONS AND PATHOLOGY. The incubation period is 3 to 8 days. Onset is sudden, with temperature up to 40° C, headache, papulovesicular lesions of the soft palate, myalgia, and prostration lasting 1 to 2 weeks. In more severe cases, there may be nasal, enteric, uterine, or pulmonary hemorrhage. Leukopenia, thrombocytopenia, and albuminuria are found. Some patients have a diphasic course, with a more severe illness and meningoencephalitis after a 1- or 2-week afebrile period. The second phase is characterized by fever, severe headache, meningismus, mental disturbances, and tremors. Hemorrhagic manifestations or pneumonia may also be prominent in the second phase. The case fatality rate of KFD is 5 to 10%; that of OHF is 0.4 to 2.5%. There are no sequelae. Infections in laboratory workers are common but usually mild. Histopathology is minor in comparison to the gravity of the clinical disease. Findings include extravasation of red blood cells, edema, and thrombi in the small vessels.

DIAGNOSIS AND TREATMENT. Diagnosis is by isolation of virus from the blood during the first 10 days of illness and by demonstration of antibody rise or presence of specific immunoglobulin M (IgM) during convalescence. There is no specific treatment, but fluid and electrolyte balance should be maintained and blood transfused if needed. Analgesics other than aspirin may be indicated.

PREVENTION. Tick repellents, protective clothing, and spraying of forest tracts with acaricides are the only measures available for prevention.

345.4 Crimean-Congo Hemorrhagic Fever

DEFINITION. Crimean-Congo hemorrhagic fever (CCHF) is an acute febrile hemorrhagic tick-borne disease of Asia, Europe, and Africa. Mortality is high and hospital-based outbreaks are common.

ETIOLOGY. The disease is caused by CCHF virus of the *Nairovirus* genus, family Bunyaviridae. The virus kills baby mice and replicates in CER cells and several other cell culture systems.

EPIDEMIOLOGY. CCHF virus is transmitted in nature principally by hard ticks of the genus *Hyalomma*, but also by ticks in the genera *Rhipicephalus, Boophilus,* and *Amblyomma.* Virus is maintained by transovarial and trans-stadial passage in the tick and is amplified by hares and possibly hedgehogs, sheep, and cattle. Giraffe, rhinoceros, eland, buffalo, kudu, zebra, and dogs in southern Africa have antibody to CCHF virus.

The virus or its antibody is found in the distribution of *Hyalomma* ticks. Foci occur in the former Soviet Union, the Balkan nations, Iraq, Iran, Pakistan, Afghanistan, western China, the Middle East, and most of sub-Saharan Africa, including South Africa. Outbreaks occur among military personnel, campers, and persons tending sheep and cattle. Medical workers are at high risk because of frequent spread in hospitals from infected human blood and tissues.

CLINICAL MANIFESTATIONS. The incubation period is usually between 2 and 9 days. Onset is sudden, with severe headache, fever, chills, myalgia, especially in the back and legs, sore throat, abdominal pain, nausea, vomiting, diarrhea, photophobia, and conjunctival injection. The fever is constant but may be remitting. The patient is often confused or aggressive with a marked mood change. Leukopenia and thrombocytopenia are usually observed. On days 3 to 6, hemorrhagic manifestations and a petechial rash on the trunk, limbs, and oral cavity appear. Epistaxis, hematemesis, melena, and uterine bleeding may be severe and require transfusion. The liver is sometimes enlarged and tender. In severe cases, hepatorenal failure or multiple organ system failure leads to death, usually on days 6 to 14 of illness. Death may also result from blood loss, cerebral hemorrhage, dehydration after diarrhea, or pulmonary edema. Patients recover gradually starting on day 10 when the rash fades. Asthenia may last for a month or more. Recovery is usually complete, although neuritis may persist for months. Liver function tests are abnormal, especially the aspartate aminotransferase, and serum bilirubin levels are often elevated late in the illness. Abnormal prothrombin, activated partial thromboplastin, and thrombin times, as well as increased fibrin degradation products, are indicative of disseminated intravascular coagulation (DIC).

DIAGNOSIS. Virus is easily isolated during the first 8 days of illness. Antibodies are detectable by the immunofluorescence and enzyme-linked immunosorbent assays (ELISA) in surviving patients. Specific immunoglobulin M (IgM) and immunoglobulin G (IgG) are present by days 7 to 9 of illness.

TREATMENT AND PROGNOSIS. Patients suspected of having CCHF should be housed in an isolation facility with needle and blood precautions. Health care personnel should use respirators and protective clothing. Treatment is supportive, including monitoring and correcting fluid and electrolyte imbalance and treating DIC. The vital signs and hematocrit should be tested frequently, and blood should be replaced by transfusion. Case-fatality rates range from 30 to 50%.

PREVENTION. Protection from tick bites and care in handling blood and tissues of sick sheep and cattle are the only preventive measures available in the case of exposure in natural foci.

345.5 Hemorrhagic Diseases Caused by Arenaviruses (Argentine, Bolivian, Venezuelan, and Brazilian Hemorrhagic Fevers and Lassa Fever)

DEFINITION. Argentine, Bolivian, Venezuelan, and Brazilian hemorrhagic fevers and Lassa fever are acute febrile diseases characterized by hemorrhagic diatheses, marked myalgia, and, in severe cases, shock. Case-fatality rates are between 5 and 30%.

ETIOLOGY. The diseases are caused by the viruses Junin (Argentina), Machupo (Bolivia), Guanarito (Venezuela), Sabiá (Brazil), and Lassa (West Africa) of the family Arenaviridae.

EPIDEMIOLOGY. The reservoirs are rodents that excrete virus in urine and possibly other body fluids. The rodents involved are Junin virus, *Calomys musculinus, Calomys laucha,* and *Akodon arenicola;* Machupo virus, *Calomys callosus;* Guanarito virus, *Sigmodon hispidus;* Sabiá virus, not known; and Lassa virus, *Mastomys natalensis.* People are believed to be infected by inhaling or eating contaminated excreta or by passage of virus through abraded skin or mucous membranes. In Argentina, exposure to Junin virus is primarily in workers harvesting corn in Cordoba and Buenos Aires provinces in the north. In Bolivia, domestic and peridomestic exposure to Machupo virus occurs in Beni province, and in Venezuela, similar exposure occurs to Guanarito virus in Portugesa and Barinas states. The site of exposure to Sabiá virus in São Paulo State, Brazil, is not known. Lassa virus is endemic in west and central Africa, especially in Liberia, Sierra Leone, and parts of Nigeria, where it is transmitted in and around homes that have an abundance of domestic rats.

Argentine hemorrhagic fever epidemics involving hundreds to thousands of farm workers are recorded annually. Bolivian hemorrhagic fever epidemics were common in the 1960's, but after institution of rodent control measures, the disease was not reported after 1974 until it reappeared in 1994. Lassa fever was recognized first in 1969 in a nosocomial outbreak in Nigeria. Several other nosocomial outbreaks were subsequently diagnosed, but studies in Sierra Leone established the basic endemic nature of the disease. In the eastern province, 8 to 52% of the population have antibody, and the annual seroconversion rate in susceptible subjects ranges between 5 and 22%. It is estimated that 5 to 14% of the fevers are Lassa virus infections and that Lassa fever accounts for 10 to 16% of the adult hospital admissions.

PATHOGENESIS AND PATHOLOGY. The diseases are characterized by multiple organ impairment, yet specific lesions are absent. The prominent findings are focal diapedesis and capillary hemorrhage, but inflammation is minimal. Focal areas of liver necrosis in Lassa fever are not sufficient to account for the profound shock and death. It is postulated that the virus infects cells of the reticuloendothelial system, including the B and T cells. It causes temporary inhibition of immune cell function, leading to prolonged and high-titered viremia. It is not known whether subsequent capillary damage and parenchymal edema are direct or indirect effects of the virus.

CLINICAL MANIFESTATIONS. The five diseases have many similarities. The incubation period of Lassa fever is 3 to 16 days; of Argentine hemorrhagic fever, 10 to 14 days; and of Bolivian hemorrhagic fever, 7 to 14 days. Onset is insidious, initially with fever, chills, malaise, asthenia, headache, retro-ocular pain, anorexia, nausea, vomiting, and muscle pain, (especially at the costovertebral angle in the South American forms and the legs in Lassa fever). Fever is nonremitting between 39 and 40.5° C. Sore throat is not prominent in the Argentine, Venezuelan, and Bolivian diseases, but purulent pharyngitis and aphthous ulcers are common in Lassa fever.

Signs include conjunctivitis, facial edema, exanthem with pharyngeal vesicles, exanthem of the face, neck, and upper thorax, tenderness of thighs, laterocervical and other polyadenopathy, and petechiae, especially in the axillae. There is no jaundice or hepatosplenomegaly. Leukopenia, thrombocytopenia, and albuminuria with casts are characteristic.

Late in the first week of illness, the signs and symptoms become more pronounced. Signs of dehydration, decreased blood pressure, and relative bradycardia are prominent. Hemorrhage from the gums, nose, stomach, intestines, uterus, and urinary tract indicates a severe hemorrhagic diathesis. Bleeding was observed commonly in the South American forms, but in only 17% of Lassa fever cases. Blood loss is not massive enough to account for the shock. The acute phase usually lasts 7 to 15 days. Death is the result of uremia or hypovolemic shock, usually in the second week of illness. Recovery is heralded by lysis of fever; there is usually a prolonged convalescence marked by periods of sweating, flush, and postural hypotension, but patients suffer no permanent non-neurologic sequelae.

Neurologic signs are prominent in Bolivian hemorrhagic fever; nearly 50% of patients have an intention tremor of the tongue and hands at about the fifth day of illness, and 25% of these progress to more serious encephalopathy with delirium and convulsions. The cerebrospinal fluid (CSF) is normal in these patients. A similar syndrome is occasionally seen in Lassa fever, and about 5% of patients develop unilateral or bilateral eighth cranial nerve damage, which may be permanent. Other transient complications are loss of hair and Beau's lines of the nails.

Most patients have leukopenia with depression of both lymphocytes and neutrophils; however, some Lassa fever patients have markedly elevated white counts. Thrombocytopenia is present during the first week of illness.

DIAGNOSIS. The diagnosis can be made definitively only with laboratory tests. Fever, muscle pain, and diminished white cell count in the endemic areas should alert the physician to the diagnosis. Virus can be isolated in Vero cells from blood, CSF, and throat washings during life and from most tissues at necropsy. Virus is recoverable even in the presence of antibody. Isolation of virus from Bolivian hemorrhagic fever cases is more difficult than from the Argentine or West African form. Virus isolation should be attempted only in laboratories with high biosecurity containment equipment because of the risk of infection of laboratory workers. Serologic diagnosis is made by the immunofluorescence test. Immunoglobulin G is present in 53% of Lassa fever patients on admission to hospital and immunoglobulin M (IgM), in 67%. The IgM test is useful for early and rapid diagnosis.

TREATMENT. Supportive therapy, including attention to electrolyte and fluid balance, is essential. Hematocrit and urine protein measurements aid in detection of hypovolemic shock. Plasma expanders are effective if used early, but may precipitate pulmonary edema late in the clinical course.

Specific Junin virus-immune human plasma given during the first 8 days of Argentine hemorrhagic fever reduced the case-fatality rate from 16 to 1%. A neurologic illness was observed about 3 weeks after the acute attack in some patients receiving this therapy. Most of these persons recovered completely.

Ribavirin given to Lassa fever patients early in the illness significantly reduced mortality. The drug was administered intravenously, 60 mg per kilogram per day for the first 4 days, and then orally, 30 mg per kilogram per day for 6 days more. Immune plasma was not effective in Lassa fever patients in controlled trials.

PROGNOSIS. In Lassa fever, bleeding manifestations, high levels of circulating virus in the blood, and elevated aspartate aminotransferase levels in serum are predictive of death. There are no such predictors for the South American arenavirus hemorrhagic fevers. Shock or abnormal neurologic findings indicate a poor prognosis.

PREVENTION AND CONTROL. Environmental sanitation, including rodent-proofing of homes, and proper storage of grains and other foods to diminish rodent populations are the only community control measures now available. A vaccine for Junin virus has proved efficacious in Argentina. Barrier nursing with use of gloves and gowns should be instituted in suspected cases of arenaviral

hemorrhagic fevers. Blood and other tissues are infective and should be decontaminated.

345.6 African Hemorrhagic Fever (Marburg-Ebola Disease)

DEFINITION. African hemorrhagic fever is an acute, often fatal, hemorrhagic disease. Fever, rash, hemorrhage, hepatic and pancreatic inflammation, and prostration are hallmarks of the illness.

ETIOLOGY. The disease is caused by Marburg and Ebola viruses of the family Filoviridae. The two viruses are distinct antigenically but of very similar morphology.

EPIDEMIOLOGY. Marburg disease was described in 1967 in Germany and Yugoslavia, where workers in vaccine manufacturing facilities sickened and died after they were exposed to infected tissues of African green monkeys from Uganda. Where the monkeys became infected is not known, although Marburg virus is indigenous to Africa. (Additional isolated cases in South Africa and Kenya are recorded.) Ebola virus epidemics in Sudan and Zaire in 1976 were traced to contact with infected patients and, in Zaire, to spread by needle. The disease recurred in Sudan in 1979, and there was an isolated case in Kenya in 1980. The most recent outbreak was in Zaire in 1995, and a single case in Ivory Coast followed exposure of a Swiss ethologist during necropsy of a naturally infected chimpanzee in 1994. (The ethologist recovered.) The source of the outbreaks is unknown, and the natural history remains a mystery. A third filovirus, most closely related to Ebola virus, was isolated in 1989 from sick cynomolgus monkeys recently imported to the United States from the Philippines. Animal handlers in the United States seroconverted to the virus without associated illness.

PATHOLOGY. African hemorrhagic fever is a systemic disease with multiple organ involvement, most prominently the lymphatic system, testes, ovaries, and liver. Liver cell necrosis with eosinophilic inclusions, unlike that in yellow fever, is random and focal. Fibrin deposits are found in the renal glomeruli, consistent with disseminated intravascular coagulopathy (DIC). There is edema and diffuse inflammation in the brain.

CLINICAL MANIFESTATIONS. The incubation period is 3 to 9 days for Marburg virus infection and 3 to 18 days for Ebola. Onset is abrupt, with severe headache, backache, muscle pains, and sometimes abdominal pain. At this stage, the disease is not readily differentiated from malaria, typhoid fever, and other bacterial, rickettsial, or viral illnesses. On about the third day, nausea, vomiting, and profuse watery diarrhea with mucus and blood commence. Diarrhea may continue for several days. A maculopapular rash appears on the trunk and spreads to the rest of the body. On day 4 or 5, the patient's status becomes critical, with high, unremitting fever and an altered mental state, including confusion, aggression, or lethargy. There is spontaneous bleeding from injection sites, hematemesis, melena, hemoptysis, and, in pregnant patients, abortion, often with massive blood loss. Renal failure may be a terminal event. Death occurs from day 8 to 17, often on day 8 or 9. Recovery is marked by fatigue, anorexia, weight loss, hair loss, and, sometimes, psychological problems.

The pathophysiology is characterized by leukopenia, thrombocytopenia, increased prothrombin time, and other abnormalities in the liver function tests, increased serum amylase, proteinuria, and electrocardiographic changes indicative of myocardial disease. DIC has been documented in some cases.

DIAGNOSIS. Virus is isolated from acute phase blood, liver, and other organs by inoculation into guinea pigs or cell culture. The immunofluorescence and enzyme-linked immunosorbent assays (ELISA) become positive during the second week of illness.

TREATMENT AND PROGNOSIS. There is no specific treatment. Supportive therapy consists of maintenance of fluid and electrolyte balance and administration of blood, platelets, or fresh frozen plasma to control bleeding. Peritoneal dialysis for renal failure and heparin for DIC have been recommended, but their value in

African hemorrhagic fever is not established. The presence of bleeding indicates a poor prognosis. The case-fatality rate under relatively sophisticated hospital conditions in Marburg, Germany, was 22% in 1967, and under Third World rural conditions in Zaire during 1976, it was 90%. As of this writing, at least 30% of cases in the 1995 Zaire outbreak were fatal.

PREVENTION. Control activities are not carried out because the natural reservoir is unknown. Nosocomial spread can be minimized by barrier nursing and handling of blood and tissues in isolator laboratory units with proper decontamination.

345.7 Hemorrhagic Fever with Renal Syndrome

DEFINITION. Hemorrhagic fever with renal syndrome (HFRS) is a disease of Europe and Asia characterized by fevers, capillary dilatation, leakage of blood leading to hemorrhagic manifestations, and, in severe cases, shock and renal tubular disease.

ETIOLOGY. HFRS is caused by any one of several closely related viruses of the genus *Hantavirus,* family Bunyaviridae. The prototype is Hantaan virus, originally isolated from *Apodemus agrarius* field mice in the endemic region of Korea.

EPIDEMIOLOGY. The virus is transmitted from rodents. *A. agrarius* in Korea and other parts of Asia, *Clethrionomys glareolus* in Finland and west of the Ural Mountains, and *Rattus rattus* and *R. norvegicus* in cities of Japan, Korea, and Belgium serve as reservoirs. The rodent excretes virus in urine, saliva, and feces for weeks, and sometimes for months, after infection. Transmission is presumably by respiratory spread or direct contact with fomites contaminated by rodent excretions. Persons at risk include soldiers in field operations, campers, farmers, woodsmen, and, especially in the winter, family groups in houses harboring field rodents that seek shelter from the cold. Outbreaks have also occurred in laboratories housing field rodents or housing laboratory rats that carry the virus as an inapparent infection. Nosocomial infections are not reported. Viruses of the genus *Hantavirus* have been isolated from rodents in the Americas; the American viruses are associated with *Hantavirus* pulmonary syndrome (HPS).

PATHOLOGY. Patients who die of shock in the early stages demonstrate retroperitoneal gelatinous edema. There are macroscopic hemorrhages in the pituitary and right atrium. The renal medulla is congested and hyperemic, and patients who die later in the course of the disease have marked renal tubular necrosis. Petechial hemorrhages found in the skin and in multiple organs indicate widespread capillary fragility.

CLINICAL MANIFESTATIONS AND PATHOLOGIC PHYSIOLOGY. The incubation period ranges from 2 to 42 days but is usually about 2 weeks. Eighty percent of cases are mild (demonstrating only fever, facial flush, backache, and muscle aches) or moderate (fever plus proteinuria, and petechial hemorrhages). The remaining 20% are severe. They progress through five characteristic phases: febrile, hypotensive, oliguric, diuretic, and convalescent. The febrile phase lasts about 5 days, during which fever, facial flush, conjunctival injection, and backache precede the appearance of petechial hemorrhages and albuminuria. In the hypotensive phase, the temperature returns to baseline, and the patient manifests nausea, vomiting, abdominal pain, and about 3 days of capillary leakage with a rising hematocrit, heavy proteinuria, leukocytosis, thrombocytopenia, and decreased renal clearance. This is followed for about 4 days by the oliguric phase, when extravascular fluid is resorbed, leading to relative hypervolemia, hypertension, metabolic acidosis, and sometimes pulmonary edema and/or acute renal failure. The diuretic phase is accompanied by return of renal clearance to normal, but with marked electrolyte and fluid imbalance, which may lead to death if not adequately managed. The convalescent phase may last 1 to 3 months, with slowly recovering renal function. The clinical diagnosis may be reliable during an outbreak with classic severe cases but not with mild infections; serologic confirmation is obtained by the immunofluorescence, enzyme-linked im-

munosorbent assay (ELISA), and neutralization tests, which become positive at the end of the first week of illness. Antibody titers peak at 2 weeks and last for many years.

TREATMENT AND PROGNOSIS. Management includes careful monitoring of electrolytes and fluid intake and output with correction, especially during the oliguric and diuretic phases. Plasma expanders can be used for shock, and hemodialysis in cases of renal failure with hyperkalemia. Ribavirin improves survival if given within 5 days of onset. The case fatality rate in Korea is about 5% with hospital management; the disease in northern Europe is milder with a more favorable prognosis.

PREVENTION. Rodent control should be practiced where feasible, especially in urban settings.

345.8 Hantavirus Pulmonary Syndrome

DEFINITION. Hantavirus pulmonary syndrome (HPS) is a disease of North America first recognized in the Four Corners region of New Mexico and Arizona in 1993 and characterized by fever, muscle pain, and gastrointestinal symptoms, progressing to acute respiratory failure and shock. Case fatality approaches 50%.

ETIOLOGY. HPS is caused by any one of several closely related viruses of the genus *Hantavirus,* family Bunyaviridae. The prototype is Sin Nombre virus, originally characterized from human lung by reverse transcriptase-polymerase chain reaction (RT-PCR) analysis of its RNA.

EPIDEMIOLOGY. The viruses are transmitted from Cricetid rodent excreta, presumably by inhalation and percutaneous contamination. *Peromyscus maniculatus* in New Mexico and neighboring states, *Peromyscus leucopus* in New York and *Sigmodon hispidus* in Florida serve as reservoirs of different but related viruses. Transmission, seasonality, and risk factors are very similar to those of hantaviruses in Europe and Asia. No person-to-person transmission has been documented. Patients range in age from 12 to 69 years with a median of 35. The disease has not been recognized in young children. Fifty-four percent of patients are male and 62% white. Subclinical infections are rare.

PATHOLOGY. Pleural effusions and lung edema are found at autopsy. Microscopically, alveolar edema and pulmonary interstitial infiltrates of T cells and macrophages are evident in the absence of necrosis. There may be splenomegaly, but lymph nodes and other organs appear grossly normal. Infiltrates of atypical mononuclear cells are found in the spleen, liver, and lymph nodes. The hemorrhage, retroperitoneal effusions, and kidney lesions of hemorrhagic fever with renal syndrome (HFRS) are absent.

CLINICAL MANIFESTATIONS AND PATHOLOGIC PHYSIOLOGY. A prodrome of fever and myalgia, sometimes with abdominal pain, nausea, vomiting, and dizziness, lasts 3 to 6 days. A cardiopulmonary phase follows in which the patient has fever, cough, dyspnea, hypoxia, noncardiogenic pulmonary edema, and shock. Surviving patients recover completely, usually within a week after onset of respiratory signs, although there may be some continued fever. The partial thromboplastin and prothrombin times are prolonged, and thrombocytopenia and hemoconcentration are common, as are increased aspartate aminotransferase and serum lactate dehydrogenase levels. Leukocytosis, atypical lymphocytes, and immature granulocytes are noted in the peripheral blood. Severe cases develop metabolic acidosis. The only signs of renal involvement are proteinuria and mild elevation of creatinine levels. Viral antigen has been found in capillary endothelium of several organs. Diagnosis depends on demonstration of specific antibodies by immunofluorescence, enzyme-linked immunosorbent assay (ELISA), and Western blot. IgM detected with hantavirus antigens is usually present on admission to the hospital. RT-PCR and immunohistochemistry of lung or other tissues have also been used for diagnosis.

TREATMENT AND PROGNOSIS. Management includes adequate oxygenation and monitoring of hemodynamic status. Mechanical ventilation may be needed. Invasive monitoring is required in hypotensive patients and will guide therapy with pressors and/or inotropic agents. Crystalloids are recommended instead of colloids for volume replacement because of the increased pulmonary capillary permeability. Overhydration should be avoided. Ribavirin efficacy in HPS is not established; it is effective in treatment of HFRS if given early, and is available for intravenous administration to HPS patients under an investigational protocol.

Butler JC, Peters CJ: Hantaviruses and hantavirus pulmonary syndrome. Clin Infect Dis 19:387, 1994. *State-of-the-art clinical review of hantavirus pulmonary syndrome.*

Le Guenno B, Formentry P, Wyers M, et al.: Isolation and partial characterisation of a new strain of Ebola virus. Lancet 345:1271, 1995. *Description of the 1995 outbreak in Zaire.*

Preston R: The Hot Zone. New York, Random House, 1994. *Historical novel dealing with Marburg-Ebola Disease.*

Rev Infect Dis 11(suppl 4):5669–5896, 1989. *A comprehensive compilation of reviews of the viral hemorrhagic fevers, including DHF, Crimean-Congo hemorrhagic fever, arenaviral hemorrhagic fevers, African hemorrhagic fevers, and HFRS.*

Swanepoel R, Shepherd AJ, Leman PA, et al.: Epidemiologic and clinical features of Crimean Congo hemorrhagic fever in Southern Africa. Am J Trop Med Hyg 36:120, 1987. *Clinical description and review of CCHF literature.*

WHO Expert Committee Report: Viral Haemorrhagic Fevers. WHO Tech Rep Ser No 721, 1985. *Excellent review of hemorrhagic fevers by an international group of experts with detailed guide to management of patients, investigation of outbreaks, and vector control.*

WHO Scientific Group Report: Arthropod-borne and rodent-borne viral diseases. WHO Tech Rep Ser No. 719, 1985. *Authoritative discussion of epidemiologic principles, laboratory safety, vector control, and epidemic preparedness.*

WHO Technical Advisory Group Report: Dengue haemorrhagic fever: Diagnosis, treatment and control. Geneva, World Health Organization, 1986. *A most comprehensive manual for the physician faced with management of DHF patients.*

346 OTHER ARTHROPOD-BORNE VIRUSES

R. Gordon Douglas, Jr.

Arthropod-borne viruses (arboviruses) are transmitted by an arthropod to a vertebrate host, either a human or a lower animal. During an incubation period, the viruses replicate in the arthropod, which may be a mosquito, tick, phlebotomine sandfly, or culicoid midge. The viruses are transmitted by bite to the vertebrate, which becomes viremic and then can infect another biting arthropod. Some arboviruses also are transmitted vertically through the egg of the arthropod and may be maintained this way between seasons.

There are nearly 500 arthropod-borne viruses, and at least 100 of these infect humans. Most fit into five families—Togaviridae, Flaviviridae, Bunyaviridae, Rhabdoviridae, and Reoviridae. Within each family are one or more genera, each usually corresponding to an antigenic group. These groups are important, because the clinician must rely heavily on the laboratory for a serologic diagnosis or identification of an isolate.

Most infections are inapparent. The remainder are associated with one or more of five major syndromes: (1) undifferentiated fever, (2) fever with rash and/or arthritis, (3) pulmonary disease, (4) encephalitis, and (5) hemorrhagic fever (see Ch. 345).

This chapter describes several of the more important arboviruses known to infect people. Table 346–1 lists some that cause fever, rash, or polyarthritis in humans; those which cause encephalitis in humans are listed in Table 346–2.

The diseases described here are nearly all "zoonoses" (i.e., illnesses caused by viruses transmitted from animals to humans). They are more prevalent in the tropics and subtropics and are usually focal because of ecologic restrictions on their transmission. Diagnosis depends on a careful history encompassing exposure to vertebrate animals and arthropod vectors, age, season, and travel, including geographic site of exposure. The physician must have a high index of suspicion. Fevers are often diagnosed erroneously as malaria; indeed, in malaria-endemic regions, the patient frequently has malaria concomitantly with an arboviral infection.

Laboratory confirmation of infection is essential. Classically, the virus was isolated from acute phase serum or whole blood in laboratory animals or in tissue culture. Neutralization, complement-fixation, hemagglutination-inhibition, fluorescent antibody, and enzyme-linked immunosorbent assays (ELISA) tests of acute and 3-week convalescent sera also produced the correct diagnosis. Antigen detection and IgM-capture ELISA often permit diagnosis upon initial presentation and at least within a week of illness onset in most cases.

Treatment is symptomatic and may include bed rest, antipyretics, and analgesics. Ribavirin has shown some activity against certain viruses, but controlled clinical trials have not been done.

Control can be achieved by interrupting the cycle, including vaccination of reservoir animals, vector control, and education on vector avoidance. Vaccines are available or under development for some agents such as Rift Valley fever, Venezuelan encephalitis, yellow fever, Japanese encephalitis, and dengue.

FEVER AND RASH SYNDROMES

COLORADO TICK FEVER. Colorado tick fever (CTF) is an acute, benign tick-transmitted viral infection that occurs throughout the Rocky Mountain area. It is characterized by headache, myalgia, a biphasic febrile course lasting about 1 week, and leukopenia.

Etiology. CTF virus is an RNA virus in the coltivirus genus of the Reoviridae family; it is unrelated to other major arbovirus groups. The hard-shelled wood tick, *Dermacentor andersoni,* transmits the virus to humans by bite. Human cases are limited to the combined geographic distribution of the tick vector and the major mammalian rodent reservoirs, ground squirrels and chipmunks.

Epidemiology. Exposure usually occurs during the spring and summer in mountainous terrain and high plains between 4000 and 10,000 feet. Cases occur at lower altitudes during April and May and at higher altitudes during June and July, presumably because

TABLE 346–1. ARTHROPOD-BORNE VIRUSES THAT CAUSE FEVER, RASH, OR POLYARTHRITIS

Family (*Genus*) Virus	Human Disease	Distribution	Vector
Togaviridae (*Alphavirus*)			
Mayaro	Fever, arthritis, rash	South America	Mosquito
Ross River	Arthritis, rash, sometimes fever	Australia, South Pacific	Mosquito
Chikungunya	Fever, arthritis, hemorrhagic fever	Africa, Asia, Philippines	Mosquito
O'nyong-nyong	Fever, arthritis, rash	Africa	Mosquito
Sindbis	Arthritis, rash, sometimes fever	Africa, Europe, Australia	Mosquito
Flaviviridae (*Flavivirus*)			
Dengue (4 types)	Fever, rash, hemorrhagic fever	Worldwide (tropics)	Mosquito
Yellow fever	Fever, hemorrhagic fever	Tropical Americas, Africa	Mosquito
West Nile	Fever, rash, hepatitis, encephalitis	Asia, Europe, Africa	Mosquito
Bunyaviridae (*Bunyavirus*)			
Oxopouche	Fever	Brazil, Panama	Midge
Bunyaviridae (*Phlebovirus*)			
Sandfly fever viruses	Fever	Asia, Africa, tropical Americas	Sand fly, mosquito
Rift Valley fever	Fever, hemorrhagic fever, encephalitis, retinitis	Africa	Mosquito
Bunyaviridae (*Hantavirus*)			
Muerto Canyon	Pulmonary disease	Southwest U.S.	Rodent-borne
Reoviridae (*Coltivirus*)			
Colorado tick fever	Fever	Western U.S.	Tick

Note: Shown are the most important of over 100 arboviruses that infect humans.

TABLE 346-2. ARTHROPOD-BORNE VIRUSES THAT CAUSE ACUTE CENTRAL NERVOUS SYSTEM INFECTION AND ENCEPHALITIS

Virus by Group	Mode of Transmission	Geographic Distribution	Disease in Domestic Livestock
Viruses principally associated with the encephalitis syndrome; epidemic and endemic			
Togaviridae, alphavirus			
Eastern equine encephalitis	Mosquito	Eastern North America, Caribbean, South America	Equines, penned pheasants
Western equine encephalitis	Mosquito	Western North America, South America	Equines
Venezuelan equine encephalitis	Mosquito, possibly other	Florida, Central and South America	Equines
Flaviviridae, flavivirus			
St. Louis encephalitis	Mosquito	North America, Caribbean, Central and South America	None
Japanese encephalitis	Mosquito	East and Southeast Asia, India	Equines, swine
Rocio encephalitis	Mosquito	Brazil	None
Murray Valley encephalitis	Mosquito	Australia	(Equines)*
Tick-borne encephalitides	Tick, ingestion of milk	Europe, former U.S.S.R.	None
Russian spring-summer and Central European encephalitis			
Louping ill	Tick	British Isles	Sheep, equines, cows
Powassan	Tick	North America	None
Bunyaviridae, California subgroup			
California encephalitis, LaCrosse, Jamestown Canyon, snowshoe hare	Mosquito	North America, China, former U.S.S.R.	None
Viruses principally associated with other syndromes, but occasionally causing encephalitis; epidemic and endemic			
Togaviridae, alphavirus			
Sindbis (febrile illness with rash)	Mosquito	Africa, Europe	None
Semliki Forest (febrile illness)	Mosquito	Africa, Southeast Asia	(Equines)*
Flaviviridae, flavivirus			
West Nile (febrile illness with rash)	Mosquito	Africa, Middle East	(Equines)*
Kyasanur Forest disease†	Tick	India	None
Omsk hemorrhagic fever†	Tick	Central Asia	None
Bunyaviridae, phlebovirus			
Rift Valley fever (febrile illness, hemorrhagic fever, retinitis)	Mosquito, direct contact	Africa	Sheep, cows, goats
Crimean hemorrhagic fever†–Congo	Tick	Eastern Europe, former U.S.S.R., Africa	None
Reoviridae, orbivirus			
Colorado tick fever (febrile illness)	Tick	Western North America	None
Rare and sporadic infections associated with encephalitis			
Flaviviridae, flavivirus			
Ilheus‡	Mosquito	South America	None
Negishi	Tick	Japan, China	None
Langat†	Tick	Asia	None
Orthomyxovirus			
Thogoto	Tick	Africa	None

* Disease rare or suspected but not well documented.
† Tick-borne hemorrhagic fevers.
‡ Encephalitis recorded in laboratory infections or experimental infections of cancer patients only; significance in naturally acquired infections unknown.

ticks emerge later at higher altitudes. Most patients find attached ticks, but others may have seen ticks on their body or clothing. Postexposure travel during the incubation period or accidental transportation of infected adult ticks in clothing or bedding may result in cases outside the endemic area.

CTF virus has been recovered from up to 14% of *D. andersoni* collected in endemic areas. The virus overwinters in hibernating nymphal and adult ticks and in infected hibernating rodent hosts. Infected nymphal ticks feed on ground squirrels and chipmunks in the spring, and since viremia in the rodent reservoirs lasts for weeks or months, a cycle involving larval and nymphal ticks and their rodent hosts evolves. Humans are accidental hosts, resulting from the bite of an adult tick.

Incidence and Prevalence. The disease has been reported from most states in the Rocky Mountain area and from western Canadian provinces. The several hundred cases diagnosed annually in the endemic area probably represent only a fraction of the total. Mild or wholly subclinical infections probably occur.

The virus has been isolated from other species of ticks and from numerous species of small mammals, suggesting that the disease may occur over a wider geographic area than currently appreciated.

Pathogenesis. There is no unusual local reaction to the tick bite. The virus replicates in hematopoietic stem cells, and symptoms begin 3 to 6 days after tick exposure. Viremia can be demonstrated at onset of fever and in red blood cells long after the virus

has vanished from serum and neutralizing antibody has appeared. Transfusion-transmitted CTF has been documented.

Fatal cases are rare. Occasional patients have clinical evidence of central nervous system (CNS) or meningeal involvement, and CTF virus has been recovered from cerebrospinal fluid (CSF).

Clinical Manifestations. The disease begins abruptly, with chills, fever of 38 to 40°C, myalgias (especially in the back and legs), headache, retro-orbital pain, and photophobia. Malaise and nausea may occur, but vomiting is uncommon. Physical findings during the first 2 to 3 days of illness are nonspecific. The patient may be flushed with conjunctival and pharyngeal erythema. Mild splenomegaly is sometimes present. Up to 12% of patients suffer rashes, commonly macular or macropapular and distributed over the entire body, sometimes petechial and involving primarily the extremities. Tachycardia is in proportion to the temperature elevation.

In approximately one half of cases, a distinctly biphasic illness occurs, the so-called saddleback fever. Symptoms and fever abate after 2 to 3 days, and the patient feels relatively well for 1 or 2 days, after which there is an abrupt return of fever, headache, and back pain, often more intense than in the first phase. The second phase lasts 2 to 4 days and then subsides, leaving the patient with weakness and lassitude that disappear during the succeeding week or two. A prolonged convalescence of 3 weeks or more may ensue in patients over 30 years of age. Some patients do not exhibit the typical biphasic course, experiencing only one bout of fever, three phases of fever, or a single protracted febrile illness lasting 5 to 8 days.

Children are most susceptible to CNS involvement. Findings may include aseptic meningitis with nuchal rigidity and mononuclear pleocytosis or encephalitis with a depressed sensorium or stupor. Hemorrhagic manifestations have been described in a few children with encephalitis.

Laboratory findings very early in the illness are generally not helpful, but leukopenia usually is present by the third day and becomes even more pronounced during the second phase, reaching levels as low as 1000 per cubic millimeter. The most striking decrease is in the granulocyte series, with a relative lymphocytosis, and there is frequently an accompanying thrombocytopenia. Atypical, vacuolated lymphocytes are often observed. Bone marrow examination reveals a maturation arrest in the granulocyte series.

Diagnosis. CTF should be suspected in any person with a history of tick exposure in the endemic area 3 to 7 days before the onset of a febrile illness. Findings during the first phase, however, cannot be differentiated from many other acute febrile illnesses. A brief symptom-free interval followed by a second febrile illness should strongly suggest CTF.

Isolation of the virus from serum or whole blood, via inoculation of suckling mice, confirms the diagnosis. Direct immunofluorescent staining of virus in the patient's erythrocytes may provide more rapid identification. A diagnostic rise in antibody titers can be detected by indirect immunofluorescence or by neutralization test; an ELISA is also available.

The differential diagnosis can be troublesome, inasmuch as Rocky Mountain spotted fever (see Ch. 324.2) is transmitted in the tick fever endemic area by the same vector, *D. andersoni*. Paradoxically, Rocky Mountain spotted fever is abating in the state of Colorado; CTF now outnumbers it by at least 20-fold. Nevertheless, differential diagnosis may be impossible early in the course of disease, before the characteristic rash of Rocky Mountain spotted fever appears. A relatively symptom-free interval after 2 or 3 days would be most unusual in Rocky Mountain spotted fever and strongly favors the diagnosis of CTF.

Treatment and Prognosis. Therapy is entirely supportive. The disease is almost invariably benign, and the prognosis is excellent. Severe illness, complicated by CNS involvement, is seen infrequently and only in children.

Prevention. The most effective means of preventing CTF is for people outdoors in endemic areas during the spring and summer months to wear protective clothing or use tick repellents, together with frequent body inspection and prompt tick removal. Transfusion-associated disease can be prevented by excluding convalescent donors for a minimum of 6 months.

DENGUE. Dengue is an acute arbovirus infection that presents chiefly with fever, malaise, lymphadenopathy, and rash. Epidemics occur worldwide over large areas of the tropics and subtropics, including the Pacific Basin, Southeast Asia, and Africa. Outbreaks recurred in the Caribbean, including Puerto Rico and the U.S. Virgin Islands, in 1969. For the first time in 35 years, indigenous infections were recognized in the continental United States in 1980, but they have not recurred recently.

Dengue viruses are members of the Flaviviridae family. Single-stranded nonsegmented RNA viruses, they occur in four distinct serogroups, types 1 through 4.

Epidemiology. Dengue virus is transmitted from person to person primarily by *Aedes aegypti* mosquitoes, although other species of *Aedes* are involved in Asia and the Pacific. *A. aegypti* is peridomestic, biting humans readily or even preferentially. A single mosquito can infect a number of people. Small collections of water in backyard litter, especially tires, are favored breeding sites. *A. aegypti* has reappeared along the U.S. Gulf Coast; hence the threat of dengue reemerging in the United States is real.

Dengue viruses multiply in the midgut epithelium and salivary glands of mosquitoes without producing pathologic changes. Mosquitoes remain infectious for life.

Zoonotic cycles of dengue virus transmission involving monkeys and forest *Aedes* species occur in Malaysia and West Africa. The mechanism for maintaining the virus between epidemics has not been defined, but vertical transmission in *Aedes* has been documented experimentally.

Nonimmune individuals are uniformly susceptible, and susceptibility is not influenced by age. During outbreaks, attack rates in nonimmune individuals may be high; in Puerto Rico and the U.S. Virgin Islands, the overall rate of clinical disease was 20%, with infection rates as determined by serologic surveys as high as 79%. Immunity against homotypic reinfection is complete and probably lifelong, but cross-protection between different serotypes lasts < 3 months.

Clinical Features and Treatment. Dengue virus infection is often inapparent. When disease occurs, three overlapping clinical forms are recognized: classic dengue, a mild to moderate febrile illness; dengue hemorrhagic fever (DHF), a severe form; and the dengue shock syndrome (DSS). Classic dengue (breakbone fever) occurs primarily in nonimmune individuals, often nonindigenous children and adults. Disease begins abruptly after a 2- to 7-day incubation with severe splitting headache, retro-orbital pain, backache (especially in the lumbar area), leg pain, and arthralgia. Most patients complain of pain on moving their eyes. True rigors are common during the illness but usually do not herald the onset. Other common symptoms include insomnia, nausea, anorexia with taste aberrations, cutaneous hyperesthesia, and generalized weakness. Mild rhinopharyngitis occurs in one fourth of patients. Examination reveals a relative bradycardia, scleral injection (30 to 90%), tenderness on pressure on the ocular globes, and pharyngeal injection. A transient macular rash may appear on the first or second day. Within 2 to 3 days after onset, the temperature may decrease to nearly normal and other symptoms subside. Remission in this biphasic illness typically lasts 2 days. Fever then returns, as may other symptoms, although they are generally less severe. On the third to fifth day (with the second phase), a more definite maculopapular rash usually appears on the trunk and then spreads to the arms and legs while sparing the palms and soles. The rash is often characterized by 2- to 5-mm "islands of white in a sea of red." The rash is accompanied in some cases by complaints of burning in the palms and soles. On resolution, the rash may desquamate. Concurrently, generalized nontender lymphadenopathy, typically including posterior cervical, epitrochlear, and inguinal chains, develops. The biphasic febrile course is considered characteristic but often is not encountered. The entire illness lasts 5 to 7 days and terminates abruptly. Complaints of fatigue and depression for an additional several weeks are common.

In addition to the classic syndrome, a mild illness characterized by fever, anorexia, headache, myalgia, and evanescent rashes sometimes occurs and is usually not associated with lymphadenopathy. At onset in both classic and mild dengue, leukocyte counts may be normal or low; however, by the third to fifth day leukocyte counts are decreased (< 5000 per cubic millimeter with granulocytopenia). Thrombocytopenia (< 100,000 per cubic millimeter) also may be a feature. Urinalysis may show moderate albuminuria.

A history of travel to dengue-endemic areas and occurrence of other cases in a community are important reminders to include dengue in the differential diagnosis. Specific diagnosis depends on virus isolation or serologic tests. Viremia can be detected for the initial 3 to 5 days with dengue types 1, 2, and 3 by inoculation of mosquito tissue cell cultures. Viral titers in patients with dengue 4 are considerably lower than in patients with types 1, 2, and 3, making viral isolation less common. Of serologic tests, neutralization is most specific. IgM antibodies indicate recent dengue infection but do not provide a type-specific diagnosis and cross-react with other flavivirus antibodies, including those following immunization with yellow fever vaccine.

Treatment is entirely symptomatic. In the absence of DHF or DSS, mortality is nil. Preventing epidemics relies principally on reducing or eradicating *A. aegypti* by eliminating breeding sites and using larvacides. Ultra-low-volume aerial spraying of organophosphate insecticides (malathion) to reduce the population of adult female mosquitoes has been successful in emergency control of epidemics.

WEST NILE FEVER. Like dengue, West Nile fever is a mosquito-transmitted, acute, self-limited illness that presents chiefly with fever, malaise, lymphadenopathy, and rash. A flavivirus, West Nile fever viral strains from Africa, Europe, the former U.S.S.R., and the Middle East are antigenically distinct from strains isolated in India and the Far East.

Virus transmission involves mosquitoes and wild birds, with mammals, including humans, as incidental end-stage hosts. The mosquito vector species varies: *Culex univittatus, C. pipiens,* and *C. molestus* in the Middle East and Africa, *Mansonia metallicus* in Uganda, and *C. tritaeniorhynchus* in Asia. In endemic areas, human infections are extremely common, with over 60% of young adults having antibodies; this suggests a high prevalence of inapparent or undifferentiated febrile illness in children. There is no gender predominance.

Clinical Features. Following an incubation period of 1 to 6 days, the onset is usually abrupt without prodromal symptoms. The temperature rises quickly to 38.3 to 40°C, with rigors in one third of patients. Symptoms include drowsiness, severe frontal headache, ocular pain, myalgia, and pain in the abdomen and back. A small number of patients have dryness of the throat, anorexia, and nausea. Cough is common. Examination shows facial flushing, conjunctival injection, and coating of the tongue. The predominant finding is generalized lymphadenopathy. Nodes are of moderate size and nontender and usually include the occipital, axillary, and inguinal chains. The spleen and liver are occasionally slightly enlarged. The temperature curve may be biphasic. In one-half of patients, a pale roseolar maculopapular rash, predominantly on the trunk and upper arms, appears from the second to fifth day. It may be evanescent (several hours) or persist until defervescence and does not desquamate. Vesicular lesions may occur but are rare. The illness is self-limited and lasts 3 to 5 days in 80% of patients.

Infection also may result in aseptic meningitis or meningoencephalitis, especially in the elderly. CSF examinations may reveal a lymphocytic pleocytosis with some increase in protein concentration. Other rare complications include myocarditis, pancreatitis, and hepatitis. Convalescence is often prolonged, lasting several weeks with prominent symptoms of fatigue. Lymph node enlargement requires several months to regress. Laboratory findings include leukopenia (< 4000 per cubic millimeter in one third of patients).

Clinically, West Nile fever resembles dengue. West Nile virus can be isolated from the blood of three fourths of patients on the first day, with viremia persisting but decreasing over 5 days. Serologic diagnosis is possible using a number of tests; however, cross-reactions with other flaviviruses complicate interpretation.

Treatment is symptomatic. Ribavirin has activity against West Nile fever virus, but since the disease is self-limited and almost never fatal, its use does not seem indicated.

PHLEBOTOMUS FEVER. Phlebotomus (sandfly, pappataci, or 3-day) fever is an acute, relatively mild, self-limited infection transmitted by *Phlebotomus* flies.

The sandfly fever group of viruses are enveloped, single-stranded, trisegmented RNA viruses belonging to the phlebovirus genus of the Bunyaviridae family. There are at least five immunologically distinct phleboviruses (Naples, Sicilian, Punto Toro, Chagres, and Candiru). The principal vector of Phlebotomus fever viruses in the Mediterranean, Middle East, and northwest India is *Phlebotomus paptasii,* which breeds in dry sandy areas and feeds in early evening. In Central America, *Lutzomyia,* a forest-dwelling species is the primary culprit. Although undefined, sandfly fever viruses presumably are maintained in a vector-host wildlife cycle between epidemics. During epidemics, humans may act as the major host. Transovarial transmission probably serves as an alternative mechanism for virus perpetuation. Sandflies are small (2 to 3 mm), which enables them to penetrate screens and mosquito netting. There is no pain or itching after the bite; hence only about 1% of patients remember being bitten.

Clinical Features and Treatment. After an incubation period of 2 to 6 days, symptoms develop abruptly in > 90% of patients. Temperatures rise to 37.8 to 40.1°C. Headache is nearly always present and often is accompanied by pain on ocular movement and retro-orbital pain. Myalgia is common and may be localized, for example, to the abdomen; if to the chest, it resembles pleurodynia. Other symptoms include vomiting, photophobia, alteration or loss of taste, and arthralgia. Conjunctival injection is seen in one third of patients. With severe illness, mild papilledema has been seen. Small vesicles occur on the palate. Macular or urticarial rashes may erupt. The spleen is rarely palpable, and lymphadenopathy is absent. Pulse is proportional to the temperature on the first day, followed by relative bradycardia. Fever persists for 2 to 4 days in most patients and gradually decreases. Weakness and feelings of de-

pression are common during convalescence. Second attacks occur 2 to 12 weeks after the first in 15% of cases. Aseptic meningitis may develop. In one series, 12% of patients had lumbar punctures; findings included pleocytosis (average cell counts of 90 per cubic millimeter with either mononuclear or neutrophilic leukocytes). Laboratory findings include leukopenia (< 5000 per cubic millimeter) in 90% of patients. The leukopenia may not occur until the third day. Lymphopenia with an increase in band neutrophils early in the illness is followed by a relative lymphocytosis (40 to 65%). Urinalyses are usually normal.

Diagnosis is made on clinical and epidemiologic findings. Sandfly fever viruses replicate and produce plaques in Vero cell cultures. Serologic tests are not available.

Treatment is symptomatic. No fatalities have been reported.

RIFT VALLEY FEVER. Rift Valley fever (RVF) is an acute disease principally of livestock—sheep, goats, cattle, and camels—caused by the mosquito-transmitted RVF virus. The virus is an enveloped, single-stranded, trisegmented RNA virus belonging to the phlebovirus genus and the Bunyaviridae family. The virus multiplies readily in most common cell cultures, is cytopathic, and forms plaques.

RVF virus can be transmitted by a number of mosquito species; in Egypt, *Culex pipiens,* in South Africa, *C. theileri,* and in East Africa, *Aedes* species are the major vectors. Epizootics in large domestic animals have been associated with particularly wet rainy seasons and high mosquito density. In cattle and sheep, most pregnant ewes and cows abort, and mortality in newborn lambs is > 90%. A wildlife-mosquito cycle during interepizootic periods has been postulated but not confirmed. Transovarial vertical transmission is an alternative. During an epizootic, disease occurs first in animals and then in humans. Direct transmission to humans by contact with blood or tissues of infected animals may be more frequent than mosquito transmission. Laboratory-acquired infections presumably due to aerosols are common. In addition to eastern and southern Africa, RVF virus has been isolated in western Africa. Zinga virus, a cause of sporadic human disease in central Africa, is a strain of RVF virus.

Clinical Features. After an incubation period of 3 to 6 days, illness begins with an abrupt onset, malaise, occasionally rigors, headache, myalgia, and backache. The temperature rises rapidly to 38.3 to 40°C. Later complaints include anorexia, loss of taste, photophobia, and epigastric pain. Findings may include facial flushing and conjunctival injection. Biphasic fever, with the initial elevation lasting 2 to 3 days, followed by remission and then a second febrile period, is common. Fever generally lasts a total of about 1 week. Convalescence is usually rapid. Normally a benign illness with almost no fatalities, rare cases with severe complications—meningoencephalitis, retinopathy, or hepatic or hemorrhagic manifestations—have resulted in death. Encephalitis with intense headache, confusion, and stupor may appear as the acute infection subsides. The CSF shows a lymphocytic pleocytosis with normal CSF glucose values. Ocular complications including visual loss occur 2 to 7 days after the onset. Findings on ophthalmoscopic examination include macular edema, cotton-wool exudates on the macula, hemorrhages, retinitis, and vascular occlusion. One half of such patients have some permanent loss of visual acuity. Hepatic and hemorrhagic manifestations may develop during the acute illness. Deaths from massive hepatic necrosis occur 7 to 10 days after onset. Hemorrhagic manifestations include epistaxis, hematemesis, melena, and intracranial hemorrhage. The fatality ratio in severely ill patients exceeds 50%. Laboratory findings include initial normal to increased total leukocyte counts initially, followed by leukopenia with granulocytopenia but an increase in band forms. Thrombocytopenia and clotting defects occur.

Diagnosis. Isolating virus from blood by inoculating mice confirms the diagnosis. Three fourths of patients are viremic at the onset of illness. Neutralizing antibodies appear as early as 4 days.

Treatment and Prevention. Treatment is symptomatic. In patients with hemorrhagic manifestations, transfusion of platelets and fresh frozen plasma may be beneficial. Ribavirin has been partially protective in experimentally infected animals. Thus one might consider administering ribavirin (2.0-gram loading dose IV, then 1.0 gram IV every 6 hours for 4 days, then 0.5 gram IV every 8 hours for 6 days) to patients with severe disease. Because the virus can be spread by contact with blood and tissues, and humans show high levels of viremia, blood and needle precautions are essential.

Fever, rash, and polyarthritis are caused by at least six viruses belonging to the alphavirus genus of the Togaviridae family. This group of single-stranded RNA viruses shares antigenic determinants and is transmitted by mosquitoes to vertebrate hosts.

CHIKUNGUNYA VIRUS. *Epidemiology.* Chikungunya virus (CK) is of major importance in Africa and Asia. CK virus is transmitted by *Aedes* mosquitoes in Africa; in the tropical forests of the continent, the mosquitoes belong to the subgenera *Stegomyia* and *Diceromyia*. Nonhuman primates—monkeys or baboons—serve as primary hosts, with transmission occurring mostly in the rainy season. Human involvement is largely secondary. *A. aegypti* also functions as a vector in villages and urban areas, where humans may serve as the vertebrate host. In sub-Saharan Africa, except in the dry areas and below 18 degrees latitude, antibody prevalence surveys range from 20% to > 90%. In Asia, transmission is primarily human to human via *A. aegypti*. CK virus is present in India, Southeast Asia, and the Philippines. Seroprevalence rates of 31% were observed in Bangkok. The potential exists for CK virus transmission outside the current distribution, i.e., Central and South America, as well as the southern United States.

Clinical Features. The incubation period is usually 2 to 3 days but may be as long as 12 days. The onset is usually abrupt, with temperatures rising to 38.3 to 40°C, often accompanied by rigors and incapacitating arthralgia. The arthralgias are polyarticular and migratory, involving predominantly the small joints of the hands, wrists, ankles, and toes. Pain is increased with motion and worse in the morning. Joint swelling is common, but effusions are not. The arthralgia is associated with generalized myalgia. Other symptoms include headache, photophobia, sore throat, anorexia, and vomiting. At onset there is flushing of the face and neck. Other signs include conjunctival injection and lymphadenopathy. A macropapular rash usually involving the trunk and limbs typically occurs on the second to fifth day. The rash lasts 1 to 5 days and may just fade or may desquamate. On the second or third day, the fever may remit for 1 to 2 days and then recur. However, the biphasic course is not as striking as that seen with dengue. Laboratory findings may include leukopenia with relative lymphocytosis, although leukocyte counts are usually normal. Mild thrombocytopenia may develop. The joint symptoms may persist for long periods, only one third of individuals being asymptomatic within a few weeks. About 5% of patients have persistent joint pain, stiffness, and recurrent effusions. Persistence may be more common in HLA-B27–positive patients. In African children, disease is milder, with arthralgia less prominent. In Asia, CK virus is responsible for a hemorrhagic fever syndrome closely resembling dengue hemorrhagic fever or the DSS. Other features may include encephalitis and myocarditis.

Diagnosis and Treatment. CK virus disease should be suspected clinically given the appropriate epidemiologic history and the triad of fever, acute arthralgia/arthritis, and rash. Most patients are viremic during the first 48 hours. Hemagglutination inhibition (HI) (III) antibodies appear by the fifth to seventh day. Treatment is symptomatic.

O'NYONG-NYONG VIRUS. The name *o'nyong-nyong* (in the language spoken in the Ugandan province of Acholi) means "weakening of the joints." Epidemics have occurred in Uganda and Kenya. *Anopheles funnestus* and *A. anogambiae* mosquitoes are o'nyong-nyong (ON) virus vectors.

Clinical features are similar to those of CK disease. The incubation period may be somewhat longer, at least 8 days. Fever is less prominent, exceeding 38.3°C only in one third of patients. Rash occurs in 60 to 70%. In contrast to CK virus disease, generalized lymphadenopathy is a common feature, and there appears to be less residual arthropathy. Diagnosis is based on virus isolation or seroconversion by HI assays, but cross-reactions with CK virus make interpretation difficult.

MAYARO VIRUS. Mayaro virus (MYV) has been associated with epidemics of acute polyarthritis in Brazil and Bolivia.

MYV exists in the forested areas of Central and South America with annual infection rates of 10 to 60% and a 2:1 male predominance. The vectors for MYV are *Haemagogus* mosquitoes. The virus causes high-level viremia in marmosets and other primates.

Clinical Features. After a 1-week incubation period, illness begins abruptly with fever, chills, severe frontal headache, myalgia, and dizziness. Arthralgia (which in some cases precedes the fever) is uniform, very prominent, and occasionally incapacitating, striking small joints, wrists, fingers, ankles, and toes. Temperatures usually exceed 40°C. Other initial symptoms (less than one third of patients) include nausea, vomiting, and diarrhea. Initial clinical features include occasional conjunctival suffusion, inguinal lymphadenopathy (one half of patients), and joint swelling (one quarter of patients). About the fifth day, maculopapular rash develops over the chest, back, arms, and legs. Rash appears in 90% of children and one half of adults and lasts about 3 days. MYV's clinical course is usually 3 to 5 days except for the arthralgia, which may persist for several months. Laboratory findings include leukopenia (as low as 2500 per cubic millimeter). Urinalyses revealed albuminuria (2+) in one fourth of patients. Some patients showed increases in AST levels. Occasional fatalities have been reported.

Diagnosis. Diagnosis is confirmed by virus isolation. MYV-specific IgM responses have been observed.

ROSS RIVER VIRUS. Ross River (RR) virus outbreaks occur almost entirely between December and June. RR virus infection exists in Australia, New Guinea, and the Solomon Islands, Fiji, the Samoan, Cook, and some Melanesian islands. The natural vector-reservoir relationships have not been well established. *Culex annulirostris* is probably the major vector, although other species of mosquitoes may be involved. Several mammalian species, especially the New Holland mouse and wallabies, are important hosts in Australia. In the Pacific outbreak, *Aedes vigilax* also may have been an important vector, and human-mosquito-human transmission was likely. Infection rates are equal at all ages and in both genders, but clinical disease rates are 4% in patients under age 20 and 42% in those older than 20. The clinical attack rate of males to females is 1:1.7.

Clinical Features. In Australia, incubation is 7 to 9 days, while in the Pacific the incubation period is shorter. At onset, the illness is characterized by headache, myalgia, nausea, and vomiting, and occasionally tenderness of the palms and soles. Initially, fever may be absent or minimal (highest 38°C). About one half of patients experience arthritis involving mainly the small joints, wrists, and ankles. Knee involvement also is common. The joint swelling and paresthesias may precede a rash by 1 to 15 days. In the other half of patients, the rash precedes the arthralgia. The rash, which is usually maculopapular, appears on the cheeks and forehead, occasionally spreads to the trunk, or may be restricted to extremities. The rash may be pruritic. Vesicles occur rarely. Tender lymphadenopathy occurs in one fifth of patients. Recovery is slow, only one half being able to return to work by 1 month and 10% still having joint symptoms at 3 months. Laboratory findings are not striking; leukocyte counts are normal or minimally decreased. The erythrocyte sedimentation rate is increased acutely but normalizes over several weeks even with continued joint symptoms. Antinuclear antibodies and rheumatoid factor tests are negative. Synovial fluid changes are not striking: cell counts of 1000 to 60,000, predominantly mononuclear, normal viscosity. Urinalyses are normal, although recently RR virus has been associated with segmental sclerosing glomerulonephritis.

The diagnosis is usually based on clinical features. In Australia patients seldom have viremia on presentation, while in the Pacific outbreak viremia was readily detected. HI antibodies appear early. Treatment is symptomatic.

SINDBIS VIRUS (OKELBO DISEASE, POGOSTA DISEASE, KARELIAN FEVER). Sindbis virus has caused disease in Egypt, elsewhere in Africa, in Europe, and in Australia. In the former U.S.S.R. it is known as "Karelian fever," in Sweden as "Okelbo disease," and in Finland as "Pogosta disease." *C. univittatus* is the principal vector, and birds are the major hosts. Human infection is common where birds and *Culex* mosquitoes are in close proximity. Human antibody rates are commonly 20 to 30% in the Nile Valley of Egypt. Since Sindbis and West Nile fever virus share the same transmission cycles, Sindbis transmission often parallels West Nile fever virus. In northern Europe, symptomatic disease appears in late summer between 60 and 65 degrees of north latitude, usually affecting adults with forest occupations. The virus has been isolated from *Culiseta, Aedes,* and *Culex* mosquitoes. The host has not been identified.

Clinical Features and Treatment. The incubation period for Sindbis has not been defined. The illness more closely resembles Ross River virus disease than chikungunya or o'nyong-nyong disease. Clinically, fever is low grade and accompanied by malaise, myalgia, rash, and arthralgia in wrists, ankles, knees, and elbows. Periarticular involvement and tendinitis are common. The rash begins on the trunk as scattered macules and spreads to the extremities, palms, and soles. The rash may precede or follow the joint symptoms by 1 to 2 days. Unlike that caused by other alphaviruses, the rash frequently becomes vesicular, especially on the feet and hands. The rash fades within a week. In Europe, persistence of joint complaints is a common feature. In Sweden, >20% had joint symptoms longer than 1 month after onset.

Antibodies can be detected by HI tests within 7 to 10 days of onset. Treatment is symptomatic.

PULMONARY SYNDROMES

MUERTO CANYON VIRUS. Muerto Canyon virus is a recently discovered hantavirus responsible for an outbreak in 1993 of serious pulmonary disease (hantavirus pulmonary syndrome, or HPS) in the southwestern United States. The virus belongs to the hantavirus genus of the Bunyaviridae family, a group of large enveloped, negative-sense RNA viruses with tripartite genomes. Other hantaviruses cause hemorrhagic fever (see Ch. 345.8).

Muerto Canyon virus is a parasite of the deer mouse, *Peromyscus maniculatus.* Deer mice are found over most of the United States with the exception of the southeast and eastern seaboard states. The 1993 outbreak of approximately 50 cases involved predominantly the "four corners" region (New Mexico, Arizona, Colorado, and Utah), but at least 6 cases occurred in California, Nevada, Texas, and Oregon. Abundant deer mice populations were found in the southwestern United States in the summer of 1993. Transmission is thought to occur via aerosols contaminated with infectious rodent urine or feces.

Pathology. The lungs of patients dying from HPS show interstitial infiltration of T lymphocytes and alveolar pulmonary edema without marked necrosis or polymorphonuclear leukocyte infiltration. The major abnormality is thought to be an increase in vascular permeability via an immunopathologic mechanism.

Clinical Features. The disease begins abruptly with fever and myalgias, often accompanied by gastrointestinal symptoms and headache; it is indistinguishable from other nonspecific acute febrile illnesses such as influenza. Examination is unrevealing except for fever, tachycardia, and tachypnea. The respiratory symptoms begin after 4 to 5 days. The patient first notes cough and dyspnea, but acute pulmonary edema and hypotension develop rapidly in most patients. About three fourths of patients die.

Laboratory abnormalities include elevated hematocrit, marked leukocytosis (median count 26,000 per cubic millimeter) with shift to the left, abnormal lymphocytes on smear, thrombocytopenia, prolonged prothrombin and partial thromboplastin times, and mildly elevated alananine transaminase (ALT) and lactate dehydrogenase (LDH) levels. The severe renal abnormalities seen in hemorrhagic fever with renal syndrome (HFRS), characteristic of other hantavirus infections, are not seen, although mild elevations of serum creatinine and proteinuria have been observed. Blood gases reveal marked hypoxia of adult respiratory distress syndrome (ARDS).

Diagnosis. HPS should be considered when an otherwise healthy adult develops an ARDS-like picture without any of the known causes of ARDS. The diagnosis can be confirmed serologically: Virtually all patients will have specific IgM and IgG antibodies detectable by ELISA on admission to hospital. Virus recovery

from clinical specimens is difficult. Polymerase chain reaction and immunohistochemical staining can detect virus in tissue.

Treatment and Prevention. Intravenous ribavirin has been used to treat HPS in patients, but its efficacy has not been established. Nonspecific treatment of ARDS, shock, and other complications may be helpful.

Avoiding contact with rodent urine and feces and rodent control in the home form the basis of HPS prevention.

ARTHROPOD-BORNE VIRAL ENCEPHALITIDES

Arboviral encephalitis is a significant health problem in Europe, the former U.S.S.R., parts of Asia, and Central and South America but not Africa. The disease is of particular concern in the Americas not only because of its multiple etiologic agents and widespread occurrence but also because of its concurrent affliction of domestic animals and humans and its potential for epidemic spread.

The most important arthropod-borne viruses that cause encephalitis are shown in Table 346–2. Only a small fraction of persons infected with these viruses experience severe CNS manifestations, and human infection is most often subclinical (Table 346–3). The ratio of inapparent to clinically overt infections is a distinctive, age-dependent quality of each disease. The neurologic disease usually begins after a variable period of nonspecific, systemic symptoms and may take the form of aseptic meningitis, meningoencephalitis, or encephalitis. These syndromes are not distinguishable on clinical grounds alone from similar syndromes caused by other infectious agents.

Pathology and Pathogenesis. Two pathologic processes are common to the arboviral encephalitides: (1) neuronal and glial damage mediated by intracellular viral infection and (2) migration of immunologically active cells into the perivascular space and brain parenchyma. Endothelial cell swelling and proliferation, destruction of myelin sheaths in deep white matter areas, and vasculitis are present in some arboviral encephalitides.

After a bite by an infected arthropod, viral replication occurs in local tissues and in regional lymph nodes. Viremia, which seeds extraneural tissues, occurs and persists depending on the extent of replication in extraneural sites, the rate of viral clearance by the reticuloendothelial system, and the appearance of humoral antibodies. Sites of extraneural infection vary from virus to virus. Many alpha- and flaviviruses involve striated muscle and vascular endothelium, whereas Venezuelan encephalitis virus is associated with myeloid and lymphoid tissue invasion. During this viremia, the neural parenchyma may be invaded, but the mode of penetration of virus across the blood-brain barrier is not completely understood. Possible mechanisms include passive movement of virus across vascular membranes and virus replication in cerebral capillary endothelial cells. Factors that increase vascular permeability promote neuroinvasion. In experimental animals infected with some flaviviruses, virus enters the CNS via the olfactory neuroepithelium.

The immature brain is more susceptible to damage by western equine, Venezuelan equine, and California encephalitis viruses (see Table 346–3). St. Louis encephalitis principally affects the elderly, whereas Japanese encephalitis and eastern equine encephalitis have a bimodal incidence, striking both children and elderly persons. In endemic areas, immunity accumulated with increasing age may reduce the incidence of disease in older persons for some viruses; however, the reasons for increased severity of illness with other viruses remain unknown.

Differential Diagnosis. The most important consideration in diagnosis is to differentiate arthropod-borne viral encephalitis from

TABLE 346–3. DIFFERING FEATURES OF ARTHROPOD-BORNE ENCEPHALITIDES IMPORTANT IN THE UNITED STATES

	Western Equine Encephalitis	Eastern Equine Encephalitis	Venezuelan Equine Encephalitis	St. Louis Encephalitis	California Encephalitis
Incidence	0–200/year, mostly infants and children	15/year	Rare in U.S.; mostly children	0–2000/year, mostly adults	50–100/year, mostly children
Time of year	Early or midsummer	Late summer, early fall	Summer	Mid- to late summer	July–September
Case-fatality	3–5% in children	50–70%, highest in children <15 years and adults >55 years	35% in children; <10% in older persons	9% overall; 0% <20 years, 30% >65 years	<1%
Residual damage	33% in infants	30–50%, especially in children	Frequent in children	Frequent in elderly	Probably rare
Cerebrospinal fluid	<500 cells	500–2000 cells PMN's*	<500 cells	<500 cells	<500 cells

* Polymorphonuclear leukocytes.

acute CNS infection due to treatable organisms. The early prodromata resemble influenza, dengue, or other influenza-like illnesses. Bacterial meningitis (especially early or partially treated), infective bacterial endocarditis, brain abscess, subdural empyema, and cerebral thrombophlebitis may mimic viral encephalitis, and CSF changes are sometimes similar. Other infections that occasionally cause meningoencephalitis resembling arthropod-borne viral encephalitis include tuberculosis, cryptococcosis, histoplasmosis, coccidioidomycosis, Rocky Mountain spotted fever, leptospirosis, falciparum malaria, trichinosis, *Naegleria* meningitis, typhoid fever, Lyme disease, and *Mycoplasma* pneumonia.

Acute meningoencephalitis may result from infections with other viruses, including herpesviruses, human immunodeficiency virus (HIV), mumps virus, enteroviruses, lymphocytic choriomeningitis virus, rabies, influenza, and the exanthematous viral infections of childhood. Exposure history, presence of an outbreak of similar disease in the community, and summer-fall occurrence are principal clues to an arboviral etiology. Enteroviruses also cause summer-fall outbreaks, but the predominant syndrome is aseptic meningitis, and the occurrence of rash or pleurodynia is a helpful clue. Herpes simplex encephalitis presents an important diagnostic challenge, since chemotherapy is available. The presence of localizing neurologic signs, localizing findings on computed tomography (CT) or magnetic resonance imaging (MRI) scans, or brain biopsy may help distinguish herpes simplex encephalitis from that due to arthropod-borne viral encephalitides.

Noninfectious diseases of the CNS such as *cerebrovascular accident* may be confused with viral encephalitis. For example, St. Louis encephalitis, a disease of the elderly, has been misdiagnosed as a stroke. Subarachnoid hemorrhage produces meningismus, fever, headache, and neurologic signs that mimic an infectious etiology. *Metabolic encephalopathies* may present features suggesting infectious encephalitis. *Neoplastic* or *granulomatous diseases* involving the CNS and a variety of diseases of uncertain etiology (cat scratch disease, Behçet disease, Reye syndrome, acute multiple sclerosis, and systemic lupus erythematosus) must be considered in the differential diagnosis as well.

WESTERN EQUINE ENCEPHALITIS (WEE). Etiologic Agent.
WEE virus is a member of the alphavirus genus of the Togaviridae family.

Epidemiology. Incidence and Prevalence. Since 1955, the number of cases of WEE reported annually in the United States has varied from 0 to 200. Most affected in recent years has been the area from the Mississippi River west to the Rocky Mountains. Mixed outbreaks of WEE and St. Louis encephalitis are common. Epidemics occur in early or midsummer and may follow heavy snow melt or flooding, conditions favorable for breeding of mosquitoes. Cases of encephalitis in equines often precede the appearance of human disease. The illness principally affects residents of rural communities, and the incidence is higher in males than in females. WEE is most severe in infants and young children. The case-fatality rate is between 3 and 5%. The ratio of inapparent to apparent infection is also age-dependent, ranging from about 1:1 in infants under age 1 year, to 58:1 in children aged 1 to 4 years, to over 1000:1 in persons over age 14 years.

WEE virus also occurs in South America. Equine epizootics in Argentina have been associated with human cases.

Transmission. WEE virus circulates between wild birds and *C. tarsalis* mosquitoes. *C. tarsalis* is responsible for infection of humans and equines, which develop low or undetectable viremias and do not perpetuate the chain of transmission. In temperate areas, transmission ceases during the winter months.

Clinical Features and Pathology. The disease usually begins with an influenza-like illness consisting of fever, headache, malaise, and myalgias lasting 1 to 4 days. Somnolence, lethargy, photophobia, vomiting, and neck stiffness may follow; neurologic involvement may rapidly progress to stupor, coma, and convulsions. Paresis, cranial nerve deficits, tremors, and abnormal reflexes may be present. In fatal cases, patients die 1 to 2 days after coma develops. Survivors generally experience a sudden and rapid recovery. However, about one third of surviving infants suffer retardation, cerebellar damage, choreoathetosis, and spastic paralysis. Children with protracted illnesses who develop convulsions during the acute stage are more likely to suffer long-term neurologic impairment. Adults may have a prolonged convalescent syndrome, but objective residua are rare. Congenital infections are documented and result in severe and progressive neurologic deterioration.

Leukocytosis and shift to the left are common. The CSF contains < 500 white cells (at first polymorphonuclear, then mononuclear) per cubic millimeter and elevated protein concentration (usually 90 to 110 mg per deciliter).

Pathologic examination of the brains of infants reveals massive neuroparenchymal destruction; children dying months or years after the acute insult often have large cystic lesions in many areas of the brain. In older children and adults, acute WEE is characterized by focal necrosis and perivascular cuffing, predominantly in the basal ganglia and thalamic nuclei but also in deep cerebral white matter.

Diagnosis. Viral isolation from blood or CSF is almost never successful. Diagnosis is achieved by demonstrating a rise in HI, fluorescent, complement-fixing (CF), ELISA, or neutralizing-antibody titers in appropriately timed (10 to 14 days apart) paired sera. IgM antibodies demonstrated in serum or CSF by ELISA provides a presumptive diagnosis.

Treatment. There is no specific therapy for WEE. Supportive care is essential and may reduce mortality. Control of high fever, cerebral edema, convulsions, fluid and electrolyte imbalances, and airways is critical.

Prevention and Control. An experimental formalin-inactivated vaccine grown in chick embryo cell cultures has been used to protect laboratory workers but is not indicated for others. In threatened or ongoing epidemics, residents should be advised to use protective clothing, insect repellents, and window screens and to restrict outdoor activity in the early morning, late afternoon, and evening (times of greatest mosquito activity). Public health measures include spraying insecticides aimed at the adult *C. tarsalis* vector.

EASTERN EQUINE ENCEPHALITIS (EEE). Etiologic Agent.
EEE virus is a member of the Togaviridae family, alphavirus genus.

Epidemiology. Incidence and Prevalence. The disease in humans is relatively rare, with fewer than 15 cases occurring each year in the Gulf Coast and Atlantic states, usually associated with a predominantly equine epizootic involving 100 to 300 animals. Outbreaks usually occur during the late summer and early fall. The occurrence of equine cases or outbreaks of fatal encephalitis in penned exotic birds (pheasants, chukar partridges) precedes the appearance of human cases by several weeks or more. Epizootics of EEE have been reported in the Caribbean (Hispaniola) and South America.

Despite the small size of EEE epidemics, the severity is high. The case-fatality rate is 50 to 70%. Incidence and mortality are highest in children under age 15 and in persons over 55, with no gender predilection.

Transmission. In temperate areas, EEE virus circulates between wild birds and *C. melanura* mosquitoes in freshwater swamp habitat. Equine epizootics and associated human cases result from extension of the transmission cycle to involve *Aedes* and *Coquillettidia* mosquitoes, which feed on horses and humans.

Clinical Features and Pathology. The disease is more acute and rapidly progressive than the other arboviral encephalitides. Onset is abrupt, with high fever, vomiting, and somnolence. Stupor, coma, myoclonus, and generalized convulsions appear within 24 to 48 hours. Autonomic disturbances (sialorrhea) may be prominent, and respiratory difficulty and cyanosis are frequent. In children, facial, periorbital, or generalized edema may be present. Death usually occurs during the first week; in surviving patients, recovery begins during the second week and may progress rapidly. Good functional recovery is associated with a long prodromal course and absence of coma. Residual damage, found in 30 to 50% of the patients, is often severe, especially in children, and is characterized by retardation, spastic paralyses, and atrophy of brain sustance.

A striking peripheral leukocytosis and shift to the left are frequent findings in patients with EEE. Examination of the CSF reveals 500 to 2000 white cells (predominantly polymorphonuclear) per cubic millimeter. As the total cell count falls, polymorphonuclear cells persist as a significant fraction. Red blood cells may be present, the protein is elevated, and glucose is normal.

In contrast to St. Louis encephalitis and WEE, the brain is grossly edematous and congested, and the inflammatory response is predominantly polymorphonuclear. The areas most affected are basal ganglia, thalamus, hippocampus, and frontal and occipital cortex. Focal vasculitis, endothelial cell swelling, intravenous and arteriolar thrombus formation, demyelination, necrosis, neuronolysis, and neuronophagia are prominent.

Specific Diagnosis. Isolating the virus from blood and CSF is rarely successful. Serologic diagnosis by demonstrating a rise in antibody titer using appropriately timed paired sera is the most practical and available test. Because of the rapid course of the clinical disease, sera should be obtained at 2- to 3-day intervals during the acute phase of illness.

Treatment, Prevention, and Control. Treatment is supportive (see previous discussion of WEE). An experimental formalin-inactivated chick embryo cell culture vaccine is used to protect laboratory and field workers. Reduction of mosquito populations by appropriate use of insecticides may be effective in threatened or established outbreaks.

VENEZUELAN EQUINE ENCEPHALITIS (VEE). Etiology. The causative agent of VEE is a member of the Togaviridae family and alphavirus genus. Six antigenic subtypes (I to VI) and multiple antigenic variants of subtypes I and III are recognized by serologic tests. Subtypes IAB and IC are responsible for epidemics involving humans and equines. In Florida, subtype II is enzootic and produces sporadic human disease.

Epidemiology. Incidence and Prevalence. Prior to 1973, large equine epizootics occurred at 5- to 10-year intervals in Venezuela, Colombia, Ecuador, and Peru, involving many thousands of animals and incurring mortality rates as high as 40%. Associated human morbidity also was great (up to 32,000 clinical cases). No outbreaks of equine or human disease have been recognized in over 12 years.

The predominant syndrome is a self-limited influenza-like illness; only about 4% of infected persons, principally children under age 15, develop encephalitis. Subclinical infections are rare. The case-fatality rate in children up to 5 years old with encephalitis is approximately 35%, but in older persons it is <10%. Laboratory infections are common in unvaccinated persons working with the virus or infected animals.

Transmission. A large variety of mosquito vectors, including species of the genera *Aedes, Psorophora,* and *Mansonia,* transmit subtypes IAB and IC during epizootic epidemics. Equines are the principal viremic hosts. Virus may be present in pharyngeal excretions of human patients; contact or aerosol person-to-person spread, although possible, is not epidemiologically important.

The other members of the VEE viral complex, including subtype II in Florida, have enzootic transmission cycles involving *Culex (Melanoconion)* species mosquitoes and small forest rodents and marsupials. Human disease is sporadic and relatively uncommon.

Clinical Features and Pathology. After an incubation period of 2 to 5 days, there is sudden onset of fever, chills, malaise, and headache, followed by myalgias, nausea, vomiting, and occasionally diarrhea. Physical examination reveals fever, tachycardia, conjunctival injection, and, in some cases, nonexudative pharyngitis. The acute illness generally subsides in 4 to 6 days, and convalescent symptoms may last up to 3 weeks. A biphasic course has sometimes been noted; acute symptoms reappear after a brief remission, within a week after the initial onset.

Some patients will exhibit evidence of mild CNS involvement (photophobia, somnolence, confusion) during the typical influenza-like illness. When it occurs, severe encephalitis is characterized by meningeal signs, convulsions, tremor, stupor, coma, spastic paralysis, abnormal reflexes, cranial nerve palsies, and central respiratory failure. Residual neurologic damage occurs in severe cases. Infections of pregnant women acquired during the first and second trimesters may result in fetal encephalitis and death.

The peripheral leukocyte count is often low, with decrease in both lymphocytes and neutrophils, or normal, with a relative lymphopenia. In patients with CNS signs, the CSF contains up to 500 cells, predominantly lymphocytes, per cubic millimeter. The serum LDH and glutamic-oxaloacetic transaminase levels may be elevated.

Pathologic changes in the CNS include edema, congestion, meningeal and perivascular inflammation, intracerebral hemorrhages, neuronal degeneration, and vasculitis. In addition, hepatocellular degeneration and necrosis, widespread lymphoid depletion and follicular necrosis, and interstitial pneumonitis are frequent findings. In the congenitally infected fetus, there are massive and widespread necrosis of brain tissue, hemorrhages, and resorption of brain material, resulting in hydranencephaly.

Diagnosis. In contrast to the other arthropod-borne encephalitides, VEE virus can be isolated from the blood or from throat swabs or washings during the first 3 or 4 days of illness. Serodiagnosis is usually more practical and is achieved by testing appropriately timed paired sera by HI, CF, ELISA, neutralization, or IgM immunoassay.

Treatment, Prevention, and Control. No specific therapy is available, and treatment of encephalitis cases is supportive. An experimental live, attenuated vaccine made from subtype IAB is used for adult laboratory personnel. It provides solid immunity to subtype IAB and its closest relative (IC) but incomplete protection against infection with other heterologous VEE viruses. Epidemics and epizootics can be prevented by effective vaccination of equines. Spraying insecticides to reduce adult (infective) mosquito populations is the only means of immediate control in the face of an ongoing epidemic. Individual protection against mosquitoes also is advised.

ST. LOUIS ENCEPHALITIS (SLEn). Etiology. St. Louis encephalitis virus, a member of the family Flaviviridae, shares close antigenic relationships with Japanese encephalitis, Murray Valley encephalitis, and West Nile viruses and is related to yellow fever and dengue viruses. Strains associated with *C. pipiens*–borne epidemics in the eastern United States are distinct from endemic strains transmitted by *C. tarsalis* in the western states.

Epidemiology. Incidence and Prevalence. The virus is present in all parts of the Western Hemisphere, but epidemics occur only in North America and some Caribbean islands. During epidemic years, the virus has been responsible for up to 80% of all reported cases of encephalitis of known etiology in the United States. In recent years, epidemics of up to 2000 cases have taken place, mainly in urban-suburban localities of the Ohio-Mississippi River basin, in eastern and central Texas, and in Florida. Small outbreaks also have occurred in the western United States. Epidemics usually transpire between July and September but may arise later in the year in warm areas such as Florida. Prior exposure and immunity to dengue may provide a degree of cross-protection against clinical SLEn.

The overall case-fatality rate is approximately 9%. Mortality is negligible in persons under age 20 but rises steeply after age 55 to approximately 30% in patients over age 65. The inapparent/apparent infection ratio is 800:1 in children up to age 9, 400:1 in persons aged 10 to 49, and 85:1 in persons older than 60.

Transmission. In most of the eastern United States, SLEn virus circulates between wild birds and *C. pipiens* mosquitoes, which breed in polluted water. In Florida and in parts of the Caribbean, *C. nigripalpus* is the principal vector. The cycle in the western United States also involves wild birds, but the vector is *C. tarsalis,* the vector of WEE. Because of the similar ecology of SLEn and WEE viruses in the west, mixed outbreaks occur, mostly in rural, agricultural areas.

Above-average summer temperatures and conditions such as deficient rainfall, which create stagnant pools suitable for *C. pipiens* breeding, are associated with epidemics in the eastern United States. SLEn in the western states is favored by warm spring temperatures, heavy snow melt, and flooding.

Clinical Features and Pathology. Three clinical syndromes are recognized: febrile headache, aseptic meningitis, and encephalitis. After an incubation period of 4 to 21 days, there is a variable period of nonspecific symptoms, including fever (38 to 41°C), headache, malaise, drowsiness, myalgias, and sore throat. This may be followed by the acute or subacute onset of meningeal or encephalitic signs or both. Nausea, vomiting, and photophobia are common. Neurologic abnormalities occur in up to 25% of patients. Extrapyramidal abnormalities (tremor of tongue, face, and limbs) and an altered state of consciousness are the most significant findings. Others include altered sensorium, meningismus, cranial nerve deficits (particularly N. VII), abnormal reflexes, tremors, myoclonic twitching, nystagmus, and ataxia. Motor abnormalities are infrequent and sensory changes extremely uncommon. Convulsions occur in 10% of patients and are a poor prognostic sign, as is a persistent high temperature of 40 to 41°C. Signs of markedly increased intracranial pressure are very unusual. Guillain-Barré syndrome has occasionally been associated with SLEn, both as an acute presentation and during the convalescent period. Approximately half the patients with fatal outcome succumb during the first week and 80% within 2 weeks after onset.

In uncomplicated cases of SLEn, there is a moderate peripheral neutrophilic leukocytosis and shift to the left. CSF pressure is elevated, protein mildly elevated, and sugar normal. Pleocytosis up to 500 cells per cubic millimeter is present. Polymorphonuclear cells predominate early, the change to lymphocytes occurring within several days. Serum creatinine phosphokinase, glutamic-oxaloacetic transaminase, and serum aldolase are frequently elevated. The electroencephalogram typically shows amorphous delta wave activity and diffuse generalized slowing most prominently in the frontal and temporal regions, but brain scans are normal. Inappropriate secretion of antidiuretic hormone is present in one third of patients.

Genitourinary tract symptoms (urgency, frequency, incontinence, and retention), microscopic hematuria, pyuria, and proteinuria, and elevated blood urea nitrogen are frequent. SLEn viral antigen in cells of the urinary sediment has been detected by fluorescent techniques and virus-like particles in urine by immunoelectronmicroscopy.

A convalescent syndrome characterized by weakness, fatigue, nervousness, tremulousness, sleeplessness, irritability, depression, difficulty in concentrating, and headaches occurs in 30 to 50% of older persons and clears in 80% of these within 3 years.

Pathologic changes in fatal cases are limited to microscopic findings. Leptomeningitis is characterized by lymphocytic inflammation. Parenchymal changes consist of lymphocytic perivascular cuffing, cellular nodule formation, and neuronal degeneration.

Diagnosis. SLEn virus is rarely isolated from blood or CSF obtained during the acute phase of illness. Serologic diagnosis is achieved by demonstrating changing antibody titers; the HI, fluorescent, ELISA, and neutralizing tests demonstrate antibody within the first week after onset, and titers rise during the ensuing 2 weeks. CF antibodies appear 10 to 20 days after onset. Rapid, early diagnosis is possible by detecting IgM antibodies by ELISA in serum and CSF. Serologic cross-reactions may occur in persons with prior exposures to dengue and other related flaviviruses.

Treatment, Prevention, and Control. Treatment is supportive. No vaccine is available for SLEn. Surveillance of viral activity in vectors and avian hosts is used to define the risk of human infection and initiate vector control efforts. In an established outbreak, avoiding mosquito bites and spraying to reduce infected adult mosquitoes are the only effective means of control.

CALIFORNIA ENCEPHALITIS. Etiology. At least four members of the California serogroup of the Bunyaviridae family (*Bunyavirus* genus)—LaCrosse, California encephalitis, Jamestown Canyon, and snowshoe hare virus—cause encephalitis. California encephalitis virus occurs in the western United States (California, New Mexico, Utah, Texas) and has been implicated in only three human cases. In contrast, LaCrosse virus, distributed more widely in the eastern half of the United States and southern Canada, is a major human pathogen. Recently, Jamestown Canyon and snowshoe hare viruses have been implicated in sporadic human encephalitis cases in the north central United States and Canada. California serogroup viruses have been implicated in human disease in the People's Republic of China and the former U.S.S.R.

Epidemiology. Incidence and Prevalence. California encephalitis occurs as an endemic rather than an epidemic disease, with individual or small clusters of cases scattered across the affected areas. An average of 80 cases are reported each year, generally occurring between July and September, with peak incidence in August. The virus primarily affects persons younger than 15 living in rural and suburban areas characterized by deciduous hardwood forests. It is most prevalent in the north central states, where it is responsible for as many as 20% of cases of acute CNS infection in children. Focal "hot spots" (communities, even backyards) of recurrent summertime viral activity are recognized. The case-fatality rate is less than 1%. The inapparent/apparent infection ratio has been estimated variably at between 26:1 and 157:1.

Transmission. The vector of LaCrosse virus is *A. triseriatus,* which breeds both in forest tree holes and in peridomestic artificial containers. The vector also serves as a reservoir of LaCrosse virus. Wild rodents (squirrels, chipmunks) contribute to a cycle of transmission as viremic hosts. Humans acquire the disease by being bitten by an infected mosquito.

A. communis, A. stimulans, A. triseriatus, and possibly anophe-

line mosquitoes are involved in transmitting Jamestown Canyon virus, and deer are the principal vertebrate hosts.

Clinical Features. The clinical spectrum of California virus infection includes nonspecific febrile illness, aseptic meningitis, and meningoencephalitis. The disease begins with fever, headache, sore throat, and gastrointestinal symptoms, with appearance of the neurologic disorder within 1 to 3 days. In mild cases, CNS signs appear on the third day after onset and subside within 7 to 8 days. In the more severe form, neurologic signs appear within 24 to 48 hours of onset, usually in the form of generalized seizures and altered consciousness, and are more prolonged. Papilledema or abnormal optic disc margins have been noted. Encephalitis may be quite severe in the acute stage, but the disease is almost always self-limited, and death is extremely rare. The question of permanent sequelae is unsettled. Many researchers believe LaCrosse virus infection is responsible for residual psychological problems, emotional lability, hyperkinesis, infantilism, compulsive behavior, and auditory and visual perceptual problems. There are case reports of hemiparesis and persistent seizure disorders.

The peripheral white cell count is elevated, with a predominance of polymorphonuclear cells and a shift to the left. The CSF contains up to 500 lymphocytes per cubic millimeter, normal or mildly elevated protein, and normal glucose concentrations. The electroencephalogram reveals generalized slowing in the delta and theta range, indicating diffuse cortical dysfunction. Focal delta wave activity related to cortical destruction or focal seizures is also a common finding.

Histopathologic features in the CNS are qualitatively similar to those of other viral encephalitides; however, absence of inflammatory lesions in cerebellum, medulla, and spinal cord has been postulated to be a distinguishing feature of LaCrosse infection.

Diagnosis. The virus cannot be recovered from blood or CSF obtained during the acute phase. Diagnosis is best achieved by tests for antibody in paired acute and convalescent sera using counterimmunoelectrophoresis, HI, CF, fluorescent, ELISA, and neutralization tests. The most practical, sensitive, and reliable methods are the HI test using the LaCrosse viral antigen and IgM antibody capture ELISA.

Treatment, Prevention, and Control. Treatment is supportive. There is no vaccine for California encephalitis. Vector control methods are of uncertain usefulness in this disease. In defined "hot spots" of recurrent viral activity, efforts to eliminate breeding sites for *A. triseriatus* should be made. Parents should protect children by limiting exposure and using mosquito repellents.

JAPANESE ENCEPHALITIS (JE). Etiology and Epidemiology. Incidence and Prevalence. JE virus is a member of the Flaviviridae family. It causes epizootics of clinical encephalitis in equines. The disease occurs throughout Asia, including Japan, the Korean peninsula, Taiwan, the People's Republic of China, Okinawa, Vietnam, the Philippines, Burma, Malaysia, Bangladesh, east and south India, Sri Lanka, Thailand, and Indonesia. Over 30,000 cases occur annually. JE is a summertime disease in temperate areas but occurs sporadically year-round in the tropics. Epidemics have been most frequent at the northern fringe of the tropical zone. JE is predominantly a rural disease, and the incidence in males is often higher than in females. In hyperendemic areas, over 70% of adult populations surveyed have antibodies, and children under age 15 principally are affected by the disease. In areas without a high prevalence of background immunity (e.g., northern India), however, all age groups are affected. In Japan, where school children have been protected by vaccination campaigns targeted at this age group, occurrence of encephalitis in the elderly has become prominent. The inapparent/apparent infection ratio is over 500:1 in children and decreases with age; in Korea, the ratio among American servicemen was estimated at 25:1. The case-fatality rate probably is about 25%, but rates of 50% or more have been reported, which may reflect under-recognition of nonfatal cases.

Transmission. The natural cycle involves *Culex* mosquito vectors and wild birds and swine. Humans and equines are incidental hosts.

Clinical Features and Pathology. Manifestations of JE include febrile headache, aseptic meningitis, and meningoencephalitis. Onset is abrupt, with fever, headache, and gastrointestinal symptoms. Meningeal irritation develops within 24 hours and is followed on the second or third day by the appearance of irritability, impaired consciousness, convulsions (especially in children), muscular rigidity, masklike facies, ataxia, coarse tremor, involuntary movements, cranial nerve deficits, paresis, hyperactive deep tendon reflexes, and pathologic reflexes. Weight loss and dehydration are often striking findings. In mild cases, fever subsides after the first week and neurologic signs resolve by the end of the second week after onset. In severe cases, hyperpyrexia, progressive neurologic dysfunction, and coma result in death, usually between the seventh and tenth days. About 25% of patients undergo a prolonged recovery, often leaving permanent sequelae. Cardiorespiratory complications are frequent during the acute stage in these patients. A poor prognosis is associated with protracted high fever, frequent or prolonged seizures, high protein content in the CSF, Babinski signs, and early appearance of respiratory depression. Fetal death and abortion due to transplacental JE infection have been reported.

The occurrence of sequelae correlates with severity of the acute stage of illness. Young children are most susceptible, and sequelae such as mental impairment, emotional lability, choreoathetosis, tremor, parkinsonism, autonomic disturbances, motor paralysis, and pathopsychologic syndromes (including schizophrenia) have been reported in up to 75% of patients.

A moderate peripheral leukocytosis and neutrophilia occur early in the disease. Pleocytosis, protein elevation, and normal glucose in the CSF are usual findings.

Neuropathologic changes and distribution of lesions are similar to those described for St. Louis encephalitis (see earlier discussion of SLEn).

Diagnosis. Isolating JE virus from blood is uncommon; virus may be recovered from the CSF of about one third of patients who progress to a fatal outcome but rarely from patients who live. HI and neutralizing antibodies appear during the first and CF antibodies during the second week after onset. Cross-reactions with other flaviviruses make serodiagnosis difficult. Specific IgM antibodies in serum or CSF are detectable by immunoassays in over three fourths of patients at the time of hospital admission.

Treatment, Prevention, and Control. Treatment is supportive (see WEE). Uncontrolled trials of intrathecal interferon suggest a beneficial effect but require confirmation. Inactivated, partially purified mouse brain vaccines produced in Japan are safe and effective in preschool- and school-age children. Recently licensed for use in the United States, a vaccine produced in Japan is available to U.S. citizens traveling to high-risk areas. Information should be sought from state health departments or the Centers for Disease Control and Prevention. Since three doses of the inactivated vaccine are used and approximately 1 month is required to confer protection, vaccination is not a practical measure in the face of an ongoing epidemic. Reduction of vector mosquito populations by applying insecticides may help to abort outbreaks. Immunization of swine is an ancillary control strategy.

MURRAY VALLEY ENCEPHALITIS AND ROCIO ENCEPHALITIS. Murray Valley encephalitis and Rocio encephalitis are similar to JE in pathogenesis and clinical features and are caused by closely related flaviviruses. Murray Valley encephalitis has occurred in small epidemics in the Murray and Darling River valleys of Victoria and New South Wales, Australia. The virus is endemic in northern Australia and New Guinea, where it is maintained in a bird-mosquito cycle. Rocio encephalitis has caused epidemics of 1000 cases in São Paulo State, Brazil.

TICK-BORNE ENCEPHALITIS. *Etiologic Agents.* A complex of six antigenically related tick-borne flaviviruses cause encephalitis: Powassan, tick-borne encephalitis (TBE), louping ill, Kyasanur Forest disease (KFD), Omsk hemorrhagic fever (OHF), and Langat viruses. The predominant syndrome in KFD and OHF is hemorrhagic fever (see Ch. 345.3), but meningoencephalitis may be a component of the disease spectrum. Two subtypes of TBE virus (Central European encephalitis and Russian spring-summer encephalitis) are distinguished by special serologic tests, are ecologically distinct, and differ in virulence for humans. Powassan and louping ill viruses are rare causes of encephalitis in North America and the British Isles, respectively. These viruses are serologically easily distinguished from mosquito-borne flaviviruses but induce cross-reactions within the complex.

Tick-Borne Encephalitis (TBE). TBE occurs in Europe (including Eastern Europe and Ukraine), southern Scandinavia, and far

eastern Russia during summer months, corresponding to peak tick vector populations. Several hundred to 2000 cases are reported annually, with morbidity rates of up to 20 per 100,000 inhabitants. Inapparent infections are common. Adults over age 20 are mainly affected, and persons frequenting wooded areas that are heavily tick-infested are at highest risk. In Europe, the disease is relatively mild (case-fatality rate 1 to 2%), but in the Far East, it is severe (20 to 25%).

In Europe, the vector of TBE is *Ixodes ricinus,* and in the Far East, *I. persulcatus.* The tick vector also serves as a reservoir of the virus. Larval ticks parasitize small rodents, which serve as amplifying viremic hosts during the spring and summer. Large vertebrates (goats, sheep, cattle) are hosts for nymphal and adult ticks. Outbreaks have occurred in families or groups of individuals ingesting unpasteurized milk or cheese from goats or sheep.

TBE in Europe typically (but not invariably) has a biphasic course, beginning 7 to 14 days after exposure with an influenza-like illness lasting 1 week, followed by a period of clinical remission for several days and then abrupt onset of aseptic meningitis or meningoencephalitis. The latter is usually benign, although severe paralytic illness, myelitis, myeloradiculitis, and bulbar forms may occur. Convalescence is often prolonged, and residual paralysis may follow in severe cases. In the Far East, TBE begins suddenly with fever, headache, and gastrointestinal symptoms, followed rapidly by appearance of depressed sensorium, coma, convulsions, and paralysis. Bulbar paralysis and cervical myelitis are frequent findings. In fatal cases, death occurs in the first week after onset. Survivors have a high incidence of residual paralyses, especially lower motor neuron paralysis of upper extremities or shoulder girdle. Aseptic meningitis and milder forms of encephalitis also occur. Chronic forms of TBE have been described, with active clinical and pathologic abnormalities a year or more after onset.

In TBE, virus isolation from blood is also possible during the early phase of illness. Serologic diagnosis is achieved by the HI, CF, N, or ELISA techniques.

Treatment is supportive (see WEE).

In eastern Europe and the former U.S.S.R., TBE vaccines are used in high-risk groups (forestry and agricultural workers, military personnel). In Austria, immunization of the general population has resulted in a marked decline in incidence. Avoiding tick exposure by wearing protective clothing and using repellents may be recommended in areas of high TBE activity.

Louping Ill Encephalitis. Louping ill causes encephalitis in sheep (rarely in cattle, horses, and swine) in Scotland and in northern England and Ireland. Sporadic human cases have been recognized. Louping ill virus is maintained in nature by *I. ricinus* ticks and a variety of hosts, including small mammals, ground-dwelling birds (grouse), and probably sheep. The clinical features of louping ill resemble the European form of TBE.

Powassan Virus Encephalitis. Powassan virus encephalitis has been documented in a small number of cases in the northeastern United States and eastern Canada, with a case-fatality rate of 50%. The virus is not associated with animal disease. The transmission cycle of Powassan virus involves *I. cookei, I. marxi* (and possibly other tick species), and mammals, particularly rodents and carnivores. Powassan encephalitis is characterized by fever and nonspecific symptoms, followed by encephalitic signs, which are frequently severe. Residual paralysis may occur. Peripheral blood and CSF changes are similar to those described in other forms of flaviviral encephalitis.

Duchin JS, Koster FT, Peters CJ, et al.: *Hantavirus* pulmonary syndrome: A clinical description of 17 patients with a newly recognized disease. N Engl J Med 330:949, 1994. *Detailed clinical description of the first 17 patients with hantavirus pulmonary syndrome.*

Markoff L: Alphaviruses. *In* Mandell G, Bennett J, Dolin R (eds.): Principles and Practice of Infectious Diseases, 4th ed. New York, Churchill-Livingstone, 1995. *Clear description of alphaviruses and important syndromes including fever, polyarthritis, and encephalitis in a well-referenced, easily accessible source.*

Monath TP: Colorado tick fever. *In* Mandell G, Bennett J, Dolin R (eds.): Principles and Practice of Infectious Diseases, 4th ed. New York, Churchill-Livingstone, 1995. *A current, thoroughly researched review of Colorado tick fever.*

Peters CJ, Johnson KM: Bunyaviridae: California encephalitis viruses, *Hantavirus,* and other Bunyaviridae. *In* Mandell G, Bennett J, Dolin R (eds.): Principles and Practice of Infectious Diseases, 4th ed. New York, Churchill-Livingstone, 1995. *An up-to-date, well-referenced review of important Bunyaviruses and their infections in humans.*

Spach DH, Liles WC, Campbell GL, et al.: Tick-borne diseases in the United States. N Engl J Med 329:936, 1993. *Reviews recent advances in understanding these diseases, especially their microbiology, epidemiology, diagnosis, and treatment; 145 references.*

PLATE 9   INFECTIOUS AND PROTOZOAN DISEASES

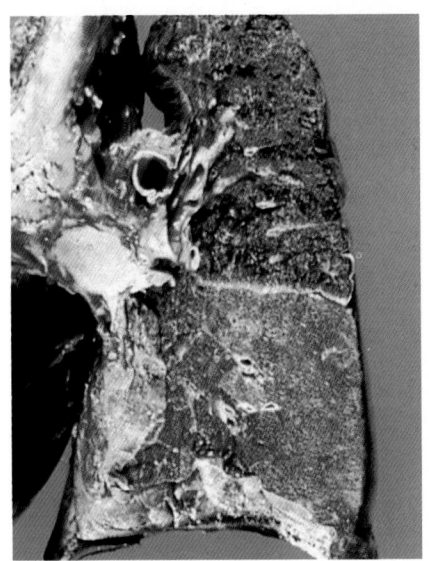

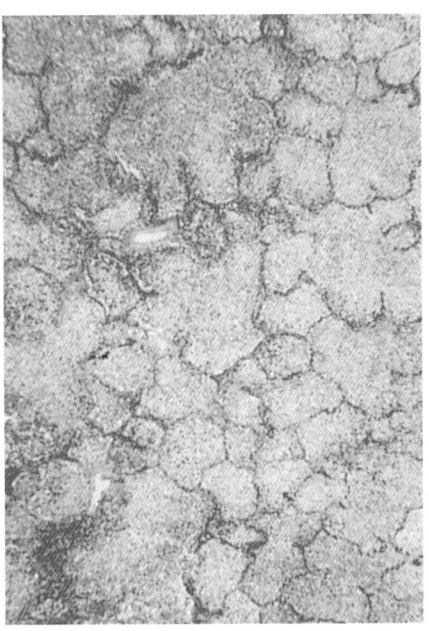

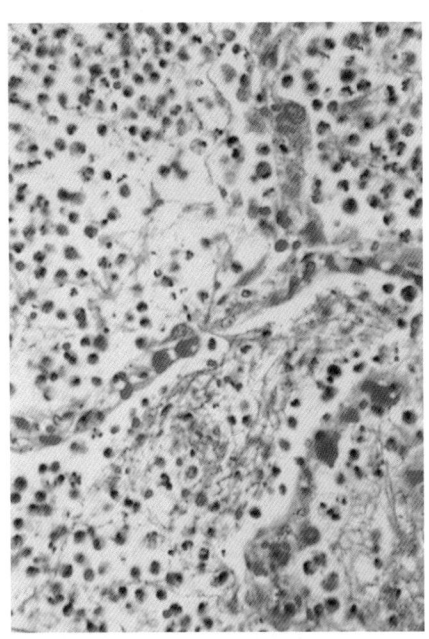

A, Autopsy specimen revealing lobar consolidation (gray and red hepatization) of the left lower lobe due to *Streptococcus pneumoniae.* Note the absence of abscess formation and the presence of dense consolidation extending from the hilum to the pleural surface.

B, Low-powered magnification (3 100) of hematoxylin and eosin (H & E) stain of tissue section from left lower lobar pneumonia pictured in *A.* Note intact alveolar walls and alveoli filled with edema and thick cellular exudate.

C, Higher magnification (3 500) H & E stain depicted in *B.* Note heavy infiltrate of polymorphonuclear cells and intact alveolar walls.

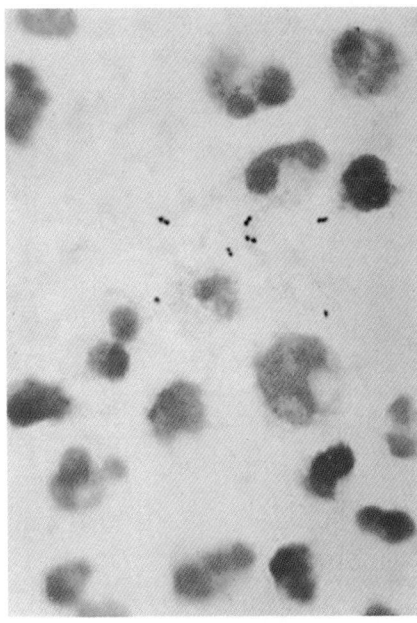

D, Fluid removed from the pleural space in a patient with early pneumococcal pneumonia and pleural effusion. The fluid may be serous, serosanguineous, green, or thick and white.

E, Gram stain of pleural fluid shown in *D,* revealing the presence of polymorphonuclear cells and typical gram-positive diplococci in pairs, consistent with pneumococci.

F, Cutaneous leishmaniasis due to *L. braziliensis.* (From Jeronimo SMB, Pearson RD: Subcell Biochem 18:1, 1992.)

G, Brazilian patient with mucosal leishmaniasis due to *L. braziliensis.* Note the destructive lesions involving the nose, nasal septum, and lips. (From Pearson RD, et al.: Rev Infect Dis 5:907, 1983.)

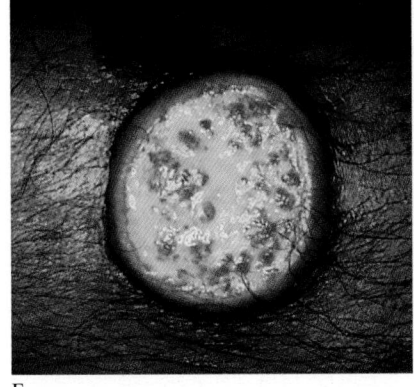

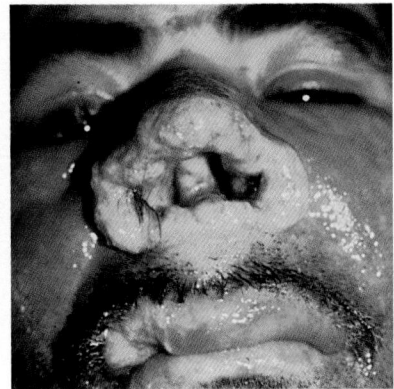

F

G

PLATE 10 INFECTIOUS, MUSCULOSKELETAL, AND PROTOZOAN DISEASES

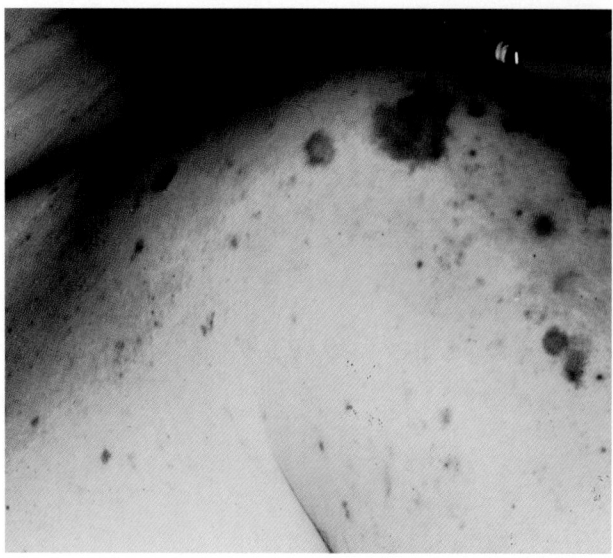

A, A patient with advanced meningococcemia who demonstrates multiple petechiae and ecchymoses on the shoulders, chest, and arm.

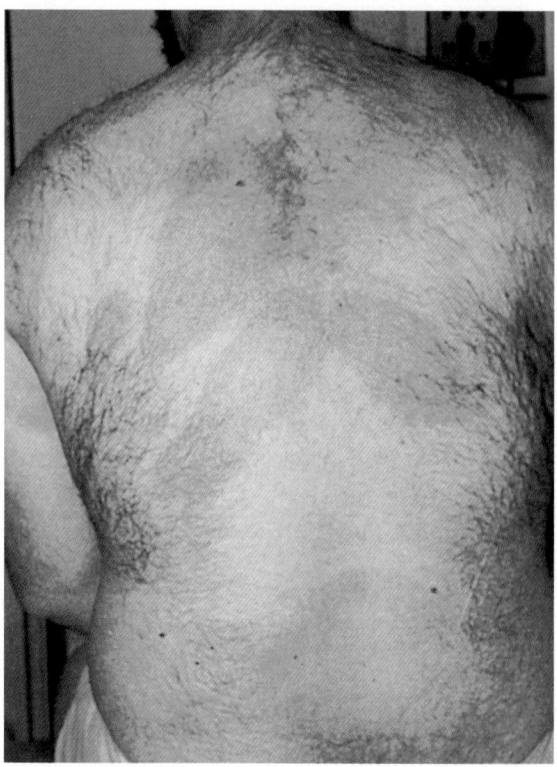

B, Erythema chronicum migrans (ECM), the major dermatologic manifestation of Lyme disease. Four days after onset of ECM, this patient has developed secondary annular lesions; some of their borders have merged. (From Steere AC, Bartenhagen NH, Craft JE, et al.: The early clinical manifestations of Lyme disease. Ann Intern Med 99:76–82, 1983; with permission.)

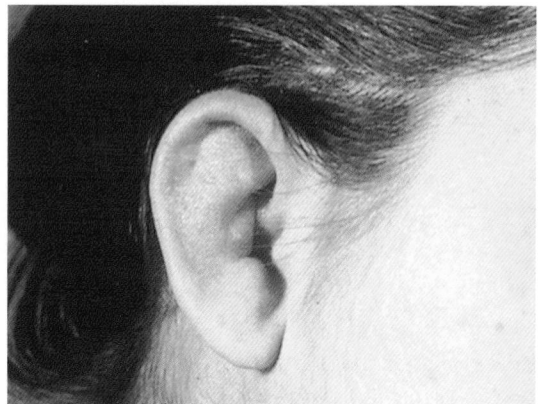

C, Polychondritis. Note nodularity of ear.

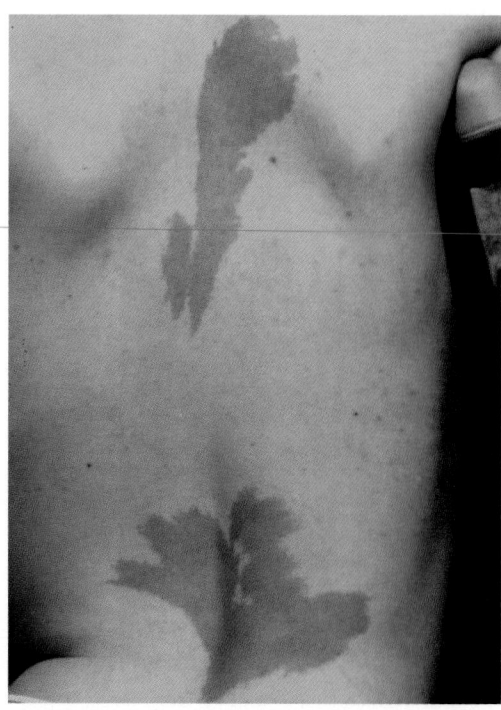

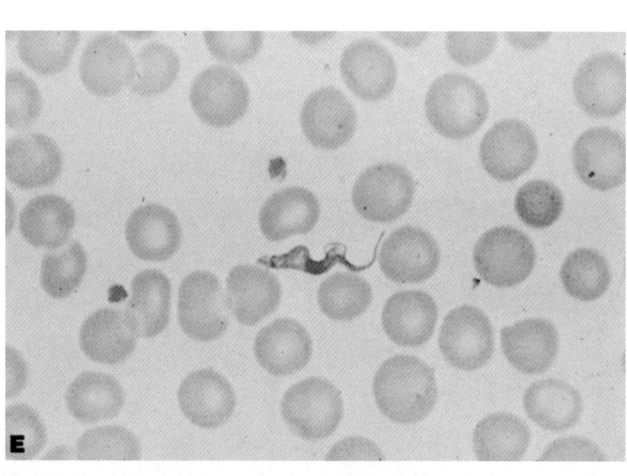

E, Trypanosoma rhodesiense in the peripheral blood. It has a nucleus, posterior kinetoplast, undulating membrane, and flagellum (× 1500).

D, McCune-Albright Syndrome. Typical rough-border ("coast-of-Maine") pigmented café au lait spot (From Whyte MP: Metabolic and dysplastic disorders. *In* Coe FL, Favus MJ [eds]: Disorders of Bone and Mineral Metabolism, New York, Raven Press, 1992.)

PLATE 11 INFECTIOUS AND PROTOZOAN DISEASES AND HIV

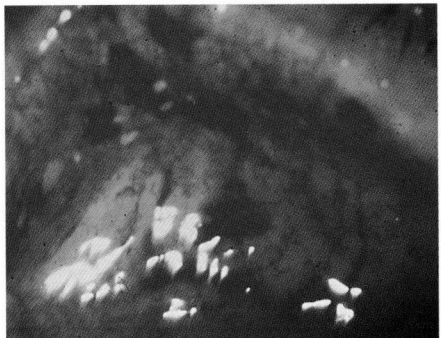

A, Conjunctival petechiae.

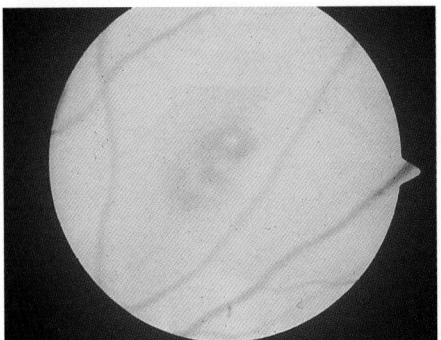

B, Roth's spots on retina.

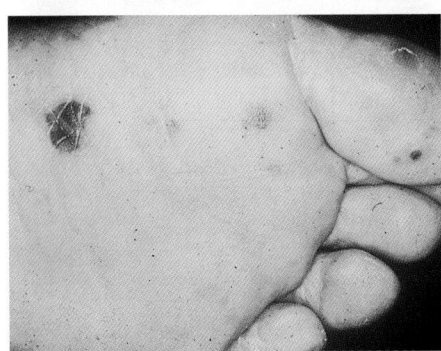

C, Janeway lesion: painless hemorrhagic macule on sole. (From Korzeniowski O, Kaye D: Infective endocarditis. *In* Braunwald E (ed.): Heart Disease, 4th ed. Philadelphia, WB Saunders, 1992.)

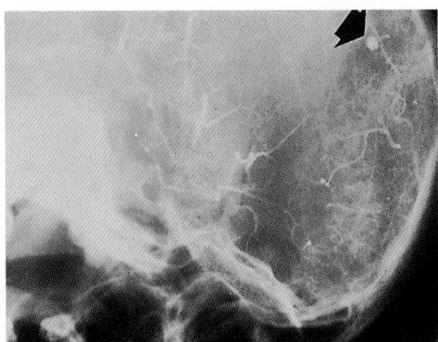

D, Cerebral angiogram illustrating a mycotic aneurysm *(arrow).* (From Kaye D [ed.]: Infective Endocarditis. Baltimore, University Park Press, 1976.)

H, Section of liver from a patient with zidovudine-induced steatosis. The hepatocytes are swollen with lipid vacuoles (mixed macrovesicular and microvesicular steatosis). A necrotic hepatocyte is seen at the center of the field (H & E, ×400). (Courtesy of Dr. D. Kleiner.)

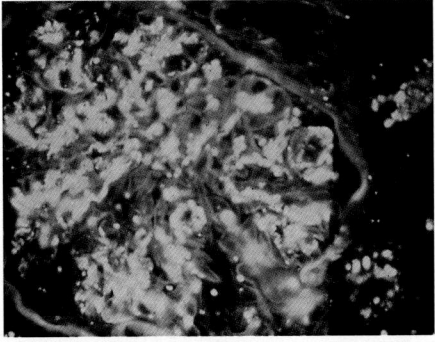

E, Fluorescent immunoglobulin staining of a glomerulus in a patient with glomerulonephritis. (From Kaye D [ed.]: Infective Endocarditis. Baltimore, University Park Press, 1976.)

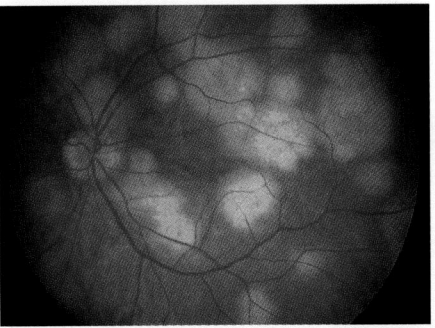

F, Photomicrograph of the indirect funduscopic examination of the left eye from a 35-year-old AIDS patient who was receiving aerosolized pentamidine for secondary prophylaxis of pneumocystis pneumonia. There is extensive choroidal exudation but, unlike CMV retinitis, there is sparing of the retina and minimal hemorrhage. (From Rao NA, Zimmermann PL, Boyer D, et al.: A clinical, histopathologic, and electron microscopic study of *Pneumocystis carinii* choroiditis. Am J Ophthalmol 107:218, 1989.)

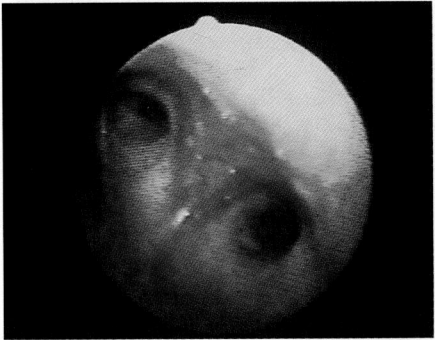

G, Bronchoscopic view of a typical endobronchial Kaposi's sarcoma lesion. The lesion is macular and bright red and straddles a carina. These lesions are sufficiently distinctive to be diagnostic of Kaposi's sarcoma.

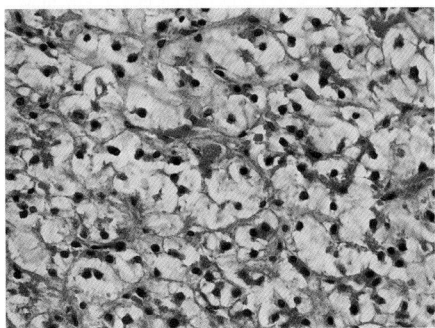

PLATE 12 HIV AND ASSOCIATED DISORDERS

A to *E* show dermatologic abnormalities in AIDS.

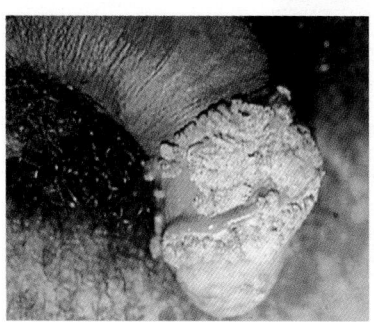

A, Prominent condyloma surrounding the corona and the shaft of the penis.

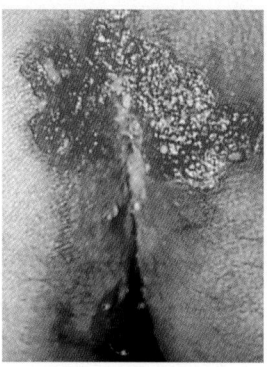

B, Chronic ulcerative herpetic infection is commonly seen in the intergluteal fold.

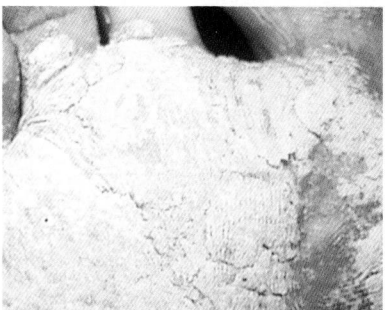

C, Marked hyperkeratosis characterizes keratoderma blennorrhagicum of Reiter's syndrome in HIV-seropositive patients.

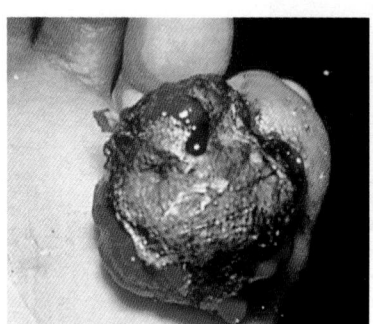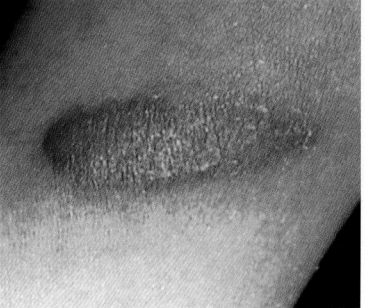

D, Left, An exophytic tumor of Kaposi's sarcoma on the sole. *Right,* Lesion demonstrating the linear configuration frequently noted in Kaposi's sarcoma of the skin in patients with AIDS.

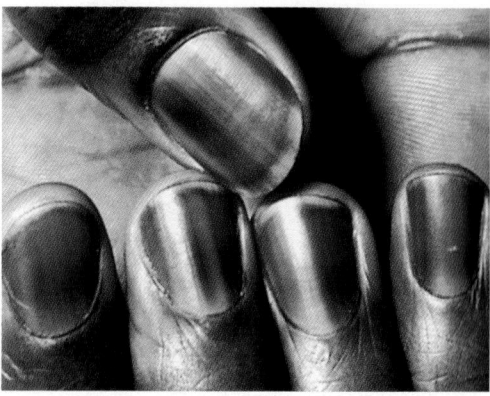

E, Bluish discoloration of the nail plates developed during treatment with AZT.

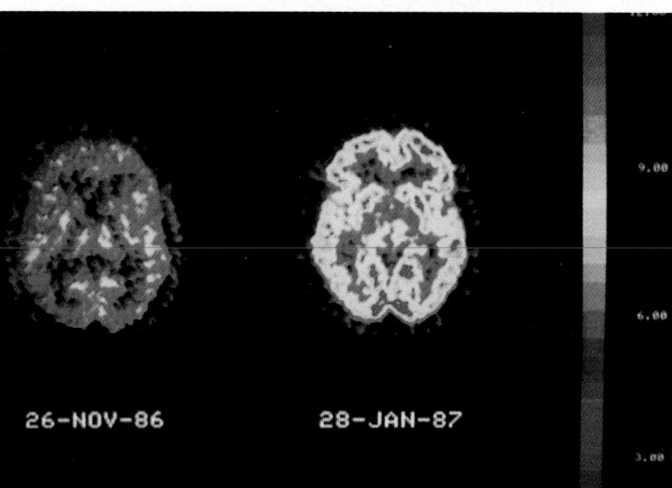

26-NOV-86   28-JAN-87

F, Positron emission tomography (PET) scan showing glucose metabolism in the brain of a patient with AIDS dementia before *(left)* and during *(right)* therapy with AZT. This patient had marked improvement in his cognitive function that was associated with a relative normalization of glucose metabolism in the brain. (Reproduced with permission from Brunetti A, Berg G, Di Chiro G, et al.: Reversal of brain metabolic abnormalities following treatment of AIDS dementia complex with 39-azido-29, 39-dideoxythymidine [AZT, zidovudine]: A PET-FDG study. J Nucl Med 30:581–590, 1989.)

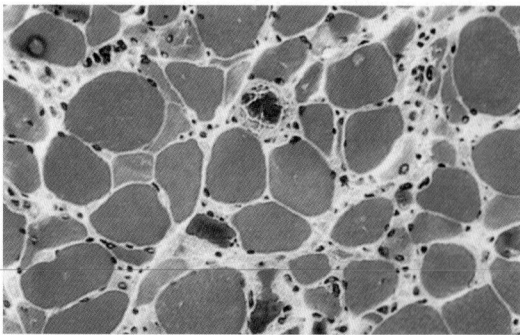

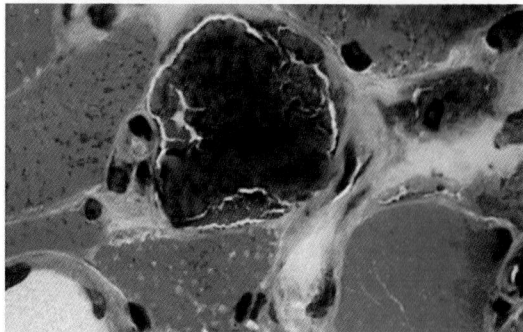

G, Pathologic findings in a patient with AZT-induced myopathy. *Top,* Destructive changes with variation in fiber size and a "ragged-red" fiber. Inflammatory changes can be seen in both AZT-induced myopathy and the myopathy of HIV infection. However, ragged-red fibers are seen only in patients receiving AZT. Transverse section, stained with the modified Gomori trichrome stain (3 320). *Bottom,* Detail showing a ragged-red fiber (3 900). (Photographs courtesy of Dr. M. C. Dalakos.)

The Mycoses

347 INTRODUCTION TO THE MYCOSES

William E. Dismukes

Fungi are classified as eukaryotic microorganisms, in contrast to bacteria, which are considered prokaryotic. Eukaryotes, such as fungi, possess a discrete nuclear membrane and a nucleus that contains several chromosomes, whereas prokaryotes have no nucleus or nuclear membrane and possess only a single chromosome. Fungi also differ from bacteria in the ability of the former to reproduce sexually or asexually. Most fungi reproduce by asexual spore formation. When sexual mating of two closely related species, e.g., *Cryptococcus neoformans,* serotypes A and D, takes place, the "perfect state" (*Filobasidiella neoformans* var. *neoformans*) is produced. Fungi for which a perfect state has not been identified are referred to as fungi imperfecti (e.g., *Candida albicans* and *Coccidioides immitis*). The cell walls of fungi are rigid, usually composed of chitin, glucan, and mannoproteins, another feature that distinguishes fungi from bacteria. In addition, the cytoplasmic membrane of fungi contains sterols, principally ergosterol, which are the target sites of action for the major classes of antifungal drugs.

The terms "fungal diseases" and "mycoses" are used interchangeably. Fungal infections that involve only the skin and its appendages are referred to as cutaneous or superficial mycoses (e.g., ringworm of the scalp or groin and tinea versicolor). By contrast, fungal infections that are acquired primarily by inhalation and spread via lymphohematogenous dissemination to involve one or more organs, such as the lungs, skin, liver, spleen, and central nervous system, are referred to as systemic mycoses (Table 347–1). Candidiasis is a mycosis that may cause superficial disease (e.g., intertrigo, oral thrush, and vaginitis) or deep organ disease (e.g., candidemia and disseminated candidiasis).

Fungi causing systemic disease may also be classified by the morphologic or structural form of the organism. For example, *Aspergillus* species and zygomycetes (*Mucor* and *Rhizopus* species) are molds that grow as a hyphal structural form both in the laboratory (and nature) and in humans. By contrast, other fungi are dimorphic; i.e., they have the ability to transform morphologically into either a mold or a yeast form, depending on the environmental conditions. *Blastomyces dermatitidis, Coccidioides immitis, Histoplasma capsulatum, Paracoccidioides brasiliensis,* and *Sporothrix schenckii* exist as hyphal or filamentous forms in nature, but as yeasts (*B. dermatitidis, H. capsulatum, P. brasiliensis, S. schenckii*) or endosporulating spherules (*C. immitis*) in humans. *Cryptococcus neoformans* is a true yeast, growing as the same spherical form in both nature and humans.

Discussions of the epidemiologic features of the major systemic mycoses are provided in the individual chapters that follow. Soil and other environmental niches are the natural reservoirs for most of the causative organisms. Infections of humans primarily result from inhaling aerosolized spores (respiratory route of transmission). Exceptions include sporotrichosis, for which most cases are acquired via cutaneous inoculation, and candidiasis, which results either from an endogenous site of colonization such as the oropharynx, skin, or vagina, or from person-to-person contact. The other systemic mycoses are not transmitted routinely from human to human. The natural habitat of several fungal pathogens is limited to specific geographic areas. Consequently, persons living in these areas are at highest risk of acquiring infection. The diseases caused by such organisms are referred to as endemic mycoses and include blastomycosis, coccidioidomycosis, histoplasmosis, and paracoccidioidomycosis. These diseases typically are associated with asymptomatic or mild pulmonary infection that heals spontaneously. Progressive pulmonary infection or spread to extrapulmonary sites occurs less frequently.

Some fungal organisms are considered opportunistic pathogens and are especially prone to cause disease in the setting of altered host defense (Table 347–2). Common predisposing conditions or factors include interruptions in anatomic barriers (burns and endotracheal tubes) or indwelling foreign bodies (arterial or central venous catheters, urinary catheters, and prosthetic heart valves or joints); granulocyte dysfunction secondary to hematologic malignancies (leukemia) or cytotoxic chemotherapy; and depressed cell-mediated immunity associated with organ transplantation, AIDS, or immunosuppressive therapy, such as corticosteroids and azathioprine. Other conditions that may predispose to systemic mycoses include diabetic ketoacidosis (rhinocerebral mucormycosis) and intravenous drug abuse (*Candida* endocarditis and basal ganglia mucormycosis).

Culture for fungus and histopathologic studies using special stains of infected body fluids (sputum, blood, urine, and cerebrospinal fluid [CSF]) and tissues (skin, lung, liver, bone marrow, and lymph nodes) are the mainstays of diagnosis of the mycoses. If fungal disease is suspected, the microbiology laboratory should be alerted to use appropriate culture media. For example, the likelihood of recovering fungi in blood cultures is enhanced by using the lysis centrifugation method. Skin testing with fungal antigens has no place in the diagnosis of individual infections, although skin tests are useful as indicators of prior infection in epidemiologic studies of prevalence. Although most serologic tests for mycoses have limited value in diagnosis because of either low sensitivity and specificity or poor standardization of assay reagents and methods, there are exceptions. A positive latex agglutination test for cryptococcal antigen in CSF or blood is a highly reliable indicator of cryptococcal disease; similarly, a positive titer for complement-fixing antibody in serum or CSF is a reliable marker of coccidioidal disease. Widely available serologic tests that are both sensitive and specific would be very useful in the diagnosis of invasive aspergillosis and candidiasis.

Table 347–3 shows the currently available classes of antifungal drugs, with examples of each class and their mechanisms of action. Although amphotericin B remains the standard of therapy for many systemic fungal diseases, especially serious life-threatening infec-

TABLE 347–1. COMMON SYSTEM MYCOSES

Disease	Causative Fungus
Aspergillosis	*Aspergillus* species
Zygomycosis (mucormycosis)	*Mucor* and *Rhizopus* species
Candidiasis	*Candida* species
Cryptococcosis	*Cryptococcus neoformans*
Blastomycosis	*Blastomyces dermatitidis*
Coccidioidomycosis	*Coccidioides immitis*
Histoplasmosis	*Histoplasma capsulatum*
Paracoccidioidomycosis	*Paracoccidioides brasiliensis*
Sporotrichosis	*Sporothrix schenckii*

TABLE 347–2. ALTERED HOST DEFENSE AND OPPORTUNISTIC FUNGAL DISEASE

Alteration in Host Defense	Opportunistic Fungal Disease
Interruption of mechanical barriers or indwelling foreign bodies	Candidiasis (invasive)
Granulocyte dysfunction (quantitative or qualitative)	Aspergillosis
	Candidiasis
	Zygomycosis
Depressed cell-mediated immunity	Aspergillosis
	Candidiasis (mucosal)
	Coccidioidomycosis
	Cryptococcosis
	Histoplasmosis

TABLE 347–3. CURRENTLY AVAILABLE DRUGS FOR THERAPY OF SYSTEMIC MYCOSES BY CLASS AND MECHANISM OF ACTION

Class of Antifungal Drug with Examples	Mechanism of Action

Polyene
  Nystatin
  Amphotericin B
	Binds irreversibly to ergosterol, resulting in increased permeability of cell membrane with leakage of intracellular contents

Azole
  Clotrimazole
  Miconazole
  Ketoconazole
  Fluconazole
  Itraconazole
	Blocks synthesis of ergosterol via inhibition of cytochrome P-450 dependent enzyme, 14α-demethylase

Substituted pyrimidine Flucytosine	Inhibits both DNA and protein synthesis

tions in immunocompromised patients, this drug has two principal disadvantages—it must be administered intravenously and it is associated with a high toxicity profile, including azotemia, hypokalemia, and bone marrow suppression. Over the past two decades, much progress in antifungal therapy has been made, especially with regard to antifungal azoles. Miconazole, the first of this class of drugs and a parenteral preparation, is highly toxic and therefore of limited usefulness. The licensing of three orally administered azoles, ketoconazole (imidazole) in 1981, fluconazole (triazole) in 1990, and itraconazole (triazole) in 1992, represented a major breakthrough. Fluconazole possesses several pharmacologic advantages over ketoconazole and itraconazole, including availability as either an oral or parenteral formulation, significant urinary excretion of active drug, and excellent penetration into CSF (60 to 80% of plasma concentrations). In addition, the two triazoles, fluconazole and itraconazole, are better tolerated and less toxic than ketoconazole and are not associated with clinically significant suppression of endogenous steroid synthesis in humans, as is ketoconazole.

The only other antifungal drug currently approved for treating systemic mycoses is flucytosine, an oral preparation, which is often used in combination with amphotericin B to provide a synergistic effect against *C. neoformans* and *Candida* species and sometimes used alone as therapy for chromomycosis. Unfortunately, flucytosine is potentially toxic to the bone marrow and liver; in addition, its use, especially as a single agent, may be associated with rapid emergence of resistant organisms.

Several lipid formulations of amphotericin B, either encapsulated in liposomes or complexed with lipids, are currently in phase II and III clinical trials; these formulations include liposomal amphotericin B (Ambisome), colloidal dispersion of amphotericin B (Amphocil), amphotericin B lipid complex (ABLC), and amphotericin B intralipid. Preliminary evidence indicates that these investigational lipid preparations may offer advantages over currently available amphotericin B (Fungizone), including less toxicity, increased tropism for reticuloendothelial organs, and increased dosing of active drug.

Como JA, Dismukes WE: Oral azole drugs as systemic antifungal therapy. N Engl J Med 330:263, 1994. *An up-to-date review of the pharmacology, spectrum of activity and resistance, adverse effects, drug interactions, and clinical indications of the available oral azole drugs (118 references).*

Gallis HA, Drew RH, Pickard WW: Amphotericin B: 30 years of clinical experience. Rev Infect Dis 12:308, 1990. *A practical review of the pharmacology, clinical uses, and adverse effects of amphotericin B, the most important intravenous antifungal agent (190 references).*

Kwon-Chung KJ, Bennett JE (eds.): Medical Mycology. Philadelphia, Lea & Febiger, 1992. *An exhaustive, well-illustrated text that considers all fungal pathogens and their diseases, including the common and uncommon.*

348 HISTOPLASMOSIS
William E. Dismukes

DEFINITION. Histoplasmosis, the most common endemic systemic mycosis in the United States, is associated with a variety of clinical syndromes, the most frequent of which is an asymptomatic or self-limited influenza-like respiratory infection. Less frequently, histoplasmosis manifests as chronic cavitary pulmonary disease, progressive disseminated disease involving multiple organs, or immune-mediated disease of the mediastinum or eye.

HISTOPLASMOSIS

Causative fungus	*Histoplasma capsulatum*
Primary geographic distribution	Worldwide; endemic in North and South Central United States
Primary route of acquisition	Respiratory (inhalation of spores)
Principal sites of disease	Lungs, lymph nodes, liver, spleen, bone marrow, adrenal glands, gastrointestinal tract
Opportunistic infection in compromised hosts	Frequent, especially in AIDS patients
Drug of choice for most patients	Itraconazole
Alternative therapy	Amphotericin B, ketoconazole, or fluconazole

ETIOLOGY. *Histoplasma capsulatum* is the imperfect state of a dimorphic fungus that grows as a mycelial form at temperatures below 35°C in the laboratory and in soil, its natural habitat, and as a yeast form at 37°C and in infected hosts. The perfect state is *Ajellomyces capsulatus.* The mycelial form bears two types of infectious spores, macroconidia and microconidia, both of which are readily airborne, but the smaller microconidia (2 to 6 μm versus 8 to 14 μm) more easily reach alveoli or small bronchioles upon inhalation. The oval yeast cells (2 to 3 × 3 to 4 μm) reproduce by single narrow-based buds, are unencapsulated, and are usually found within macrophages in viable tissue. A variant strain, *H. capsulatum* var. *duboisii*, which is found solely in Central Africa, is characterized by a larger yeast form (7 to 15 μm).

EPIDEMIOLOGY. Results of skin test surveys using histoplasmin antigen indicate that histoplasmosis is worldwide in distribution, with greatest prevalence in tropical and temperate zones. The disease is endemic in the South Central and North Central United States, especially along the Mississippi, Tennessee, Missouri, Ohio, and St. Lawrence River basins. A high prevalence has also been noted in selected areas of the eastern United States. In these endemic areas, over 80% of persons are infected by age 20. *H. capsulatum* can be readily recovered from soil, especially that enriched by bird and bat guano. Because of high body temperatures, birds are not infected, whereas bats are. Soil contaminated by chicken, pigeon, blackbird, or starling droppings and areas frequented by bats, such as caves, hollow trees, old buildings, and attics, are frequently identified sources of outbreaks. The disturbance of soil or sites by wind, bulldozing, demolition, or other construction-related activities may greatly increase the number of airborne spores and result in exposure of both nearby and distantly located persons. Although *H. capsulatum* is more prevalent in bird- or bat-related microenvironments, aerosolized microconidia are commonly present as "air pollutants" in endemic areas and may account for the majority of sporadic infections.

Pulmonary infection does not convey protective immunity; consequently, reinfection may occur. Person-to-person transmission of histoplasmosis is not known to occur. Although age, gender, and race do not significantly affect susceptibility to infection, middle-aged white men with pre-existing chronic obstructive pulmonary disease (COPD) appear to be at highest risk of developing chronic pulmonary histoplasmosis. Over recent years, *H. capsulatum* has emerged as an opportunistic fungal pathogen, especially in hosts with altered cellular immunity secondary to organ transplantation, corticosteroid or cytotoxic drugs, or infection with human immunodeficiency virus (HIV). In some endemic areas, disseminated histoplasmosis is the most common acquired immunodeficiency syndrome (AIDS)–defining opportunistic infection.

PATHOGENESIS AND PATHOLOGY. Aerosolized microconidia of *H. capsulatum,* after being inhaled into the lungs, undergo transformation into yeast forms at body temperature and are promptly phagocytized by macrophages. In nonimmune persons, macrophages are initially unable to kill the yeasts, which multiply intracellularly.

These infected macrophages migrate to the mediastinal lymph nodes and to other organs of the mononuclear phagocyte system (reticuloendothelial system) such as the spleen. Recent evidence indicates that L3T4+ cells are a critical determinant of an effective host response to *H. capsulatum.* In normal hosts, once antigen-specific cellular immunity becomes established, infection is usually contained by a sequence of events including a vasculitic response, granuloma formation with caseation necrosis, enlargement of regional lymph nodes followed by fibrosis, and ultimately, calcification. In contrast, in persons with impaired cell-mediated immunity, the mononuclear phagocyte system is unable to contain the infection and viable *H. capsulatum* organisms disseminate widely to macrophage-rich tissues, including liver, spleen, visceral lymph nodes, and bone marrow. In these individuals, because normal reaction of host tissue to parasitized macrophages is either minimal or absent, infection goes unchecked and progressive disseminated disease ensues. The pathogenesis of mediastinal fibrosis and ocular histoplasmosis, two uncommon but clinically significant complications of infection with *H. capsulatum,* is presumed to be immune mediated, at least in part. Mediastinal fibrosis appears to develop in hypersensitive persons with a large antigen load in caseous mediastinal nodes. Exuberant fibrous encapsulation of nodes and adjacent tissues may lead to bronchial or vascular occlusion or erosion.

In histopathologic specimens stained with periodic acid–Schiff (PAS), Giemsa, or Gomori methenamine silver (GMS), the characteristic ovoid yeast forms of *H. capsulatum,* surrounded by a clear space resembling a capsule but actually due to fixation artifact, are generally found in macrophages. Organisms are more difficult to visualize in tissue stained with hematoxylin-eosin. The likelihood of identifying organisms in tissue sections is directly related to the effectiveness of cellular immunity in a given host. In immune individuals with an intact host defense, fungi are rare, granuloma formation is well developed, and extent of disease is limited. By contrast, in compromised hosts with impaired cellular immunity, macrophages, including those in peripheral blood, are filled with intracellular yeasts, granulomas are poorly developed or absent, and disease is extensive.

CLINICAL MANIFESTATIONS. Pulmonary disease in histoplasmosis is conveniently classified into acute and chronic forms. Acute disease, which results from primary infection, most often resolves spontaneously but may be associated with early and late complications.

Acute Pulmonary Infection. The vast majority of primary infections with *H. capsulatum* are either asymptomatic or associated with a flulike illness, manifested by fever, chills, headache, nonproductive cough, pleuritic or substernal chest pain, malaise, and myalgias. The incubation period and severity of illness are directly related to the inoculum of inhaled spores and the prior immune status of the individual. In nonimmune persons with a heavy exposure, respiratory symptoms tend to be more severe and progressive and include severe dyspnea. A normal chest radiograph is most common, but abnormalities range from one or two patchy infiltrates, with or without mediastinal and hilar adenopathy, to diffuse miliary opacities, which frequently heal in a pattern of "buckshot" calcifications. Pleural effusion and cavitation are uncommon. Extrapulmonary symptoms and signs, including arthralgias, erythema nodosum, and erythema multiforme, may be present, especially in young women. Early and late complications of acute or primary pulmonary infection may result from vigorous host reactions causing enlarged mediastinal or hilar nodes and exuberant encapsulating fibrosis, which in turn lead to compression or erosion of adjacent mediastinal structures. These rare complications include acute peri-

carditis; tracheal, bronchial, or esophageal obstruction; esophageal diverticuli; bronchoesophageal fistula; broncholithiasis (secondary to erosion of a calcification into a bronchus); mediastinal granuloma; mediastinal fibrosis or fibrosing mediastinitis; and enlarging histoplasmoma (usually located in the peripheral lung parenchyma and recognized by concentric laminations of calcium). Mediastinal granuloma, which tends to develop more often in the right paratracheal area, is more circumscribed, smaller in size, and associated with fewer sequelae than is mediastinal fibrosis. Both entities are recognized causes of superior vena cava syndrome.

Chronic Pulmonary Infection. Chronic pulmonary histoplasmosis often resembles pulmonary tuberculosis in symptomatology and radiographic manifestations, although the course of this type of histoplasmosis tends to be milder and more indolent than that of tuberculosis. The pathogenesis and course of chronic pulmonary histoplasmosis are highly complex; pathologic studies indicate two basic lesions. An interstitial pneumonitis is characteristic of the early lesion, whereas the chronic lesion is manifested by organization of diseased tissue, with prominence of giant cells and progressive cavitation. In the thicker-walled cavities, infection is persistent, with continuing necrosis, leading to progressive cavity enlargement (marching cavity) at the expense of the surrounding lung parenchyma. In general, the symptoms and roentgenographic findings reflect the two types or stages of disease, namely, pneumonitis and progressive cavitation. Although symptoms overlap, they tend to be more abrupt in onset, with more severe constitutional symptoms, such as fever, night sweats, and malaise, in the pneumonitis stage; hemoptysis and progressive dyspnea are more typical of the cavitation stage. In 80% of cases, the pneumonitis stage tends to resolve spontaneously over 2 to 3 months, with a small fibrotic residuum, whereas the cavitation stage, especially that associated with thick-walled cavities, tends to be relentlessly progressive, leading to destruction and diminution of lung parenchyma, fibrosis, and, eventually, respiratory insufficiency.

Disseminated Histoplasmosis. This less common form of histoplasmosis develops primarily in persons with defective host immunity, including infants with immature immune systems; compromised hosts, such as corticosteroid-treated organ recipients and HIV-infected persons; and individuals with either no measurable defect or a highly selective defect, such as the failure of host lymphocytes to undergo *in vitro* blast transformation upon exposure to *H. capsulatum* antigen. The severity of the symptoms and signs of disseminated disease and the attendant histopathologic findings in a given patient mirror the level of immunocompetence of the individual. For example, in patients with the mildest and most chronic forms of disseminated disease, well-developed tuberculoid granulomas, typical of the response in normal hosts, can be found in reticuloendothelial tissues. In contrast, in patients with overwhelming multiorgan histoplasmosis superimposed on a severely immunocompromising condition, such as AIDS, the host response is suboptimal, with the pathologic findings consisting of large numbers of diffusely scattered macrophages filled with yeast forms and minimal or no granuloma formation.

Fever, chills, and other nonspecific constitutional symptoms, including malaise and weight loss, predominate. On initial presentation, many patients satisfy criteria for fever of unknown origin. Enlargement of liver and spleen is common; less frequently, peripheral lymphadenopathy is present. Mucous membrane ulceration, especially of the oropharynx, occurs in about 25 to 75% of patients with subacute disease and should alert the physician to the possibility of histoplasmosis. Laboratory clues may include anemia, leukopenia and thrombocytopenia as evidence of impaired bone marrow function or replacement of the marrow, elevated alkaline phosphatase levels, elevated erythrocyte sedimentation rate, and electrolyte abnormalities suggestive of adrenal insufficiency. In some patients, adrenal hypofunction may not be clinically manifest until years later. Chest radiographs may be normal or show findings suggestive of earlier primary infection or an interstitial pneumonitis consistent with hematogenous spread of infection. Unusual syndromes, including cardiac involvement with culture-negative endocarditis associated with large emboli, gastrointestinal involvement with bleeding secondary to mucosal ulceration, or central nervous system (CNS) involvement with chronic lymphocytic meningitis, occasionally dominate the clinical course. Cutaneous lesions, manifested by diffusely scattered papulonodules on an erythematous base, and CNS disease are more likely in HIV-positive persons. In some AIDS patients, disseminated histoplasmosis represents reactivation of dormant foci, as evidenced by the development of symptoms and signs during a period of residence in a nonendemic area, years after having lived in an endemic region.

Ocular Histoplasmosis. Vision loss associated with the triad of punched-out choroidal lesions or "spots," macular neovascular membranes, and peripapillary atrophy or scarring, in the absence of inflammatory changes in the vitreous or anterior chamber, has been labeled presumed ocular histoplasmosis syndrome (POHS). Although no direct relationship to active ongoing infection with *H. capsulatum* has been established, POHS is believed to represent a localized hypersensitivity response to *Histoplasma* antigen. In almost all instances, the syndrome occurs in young adults with no evidence of pulmonary or disseminated histoplasmosis. Antifungal therapy, either systemic or intraocular, is not indicated. Laser photocoagulation appears to be the most beneficial therapeutic modality to prevent or reduce vision impairment.

DIAGNOSIS. The diagnostic approach varies in part with the clinical syndrome under consideration. Special features or presentations that should raise suspicion of histoplasmosis include atypical pneumonia syndrome that occurs in a resident of an endemic area, right paratracheal adenopathy, superior vena cava syndrome secondary to adenopathy or a mediastinal mass, an oral ulcer resembling carcinoma, chronic progressive upper lobe cavitation associated with negative sputum smears and cultures for tuberculosis, adrenal insufficiency, "buckshot" calcifications in the lungs or spleen, and persistent unexplained fever in an HIV-infected person. In most instances, diagnosis should be based on demonstrated *H. capsulatum* by culture or by histopathologic study of involved organs. The histoplasmin skin test, although important in epidemiologic studies, is not recommended for diagnostic purposes, owing to the high positivity rate among persons residing in endemic areas. In addition, the skin test may falsely elevate titers of serum antibodies.

Among the serologic tests to detect serum antibody to *H. capsulatum,* complement fixation is the most widely used. Although a titer of 1:32 or more or a fourfold rise in titer provides presumptive evidence of active infection, a negative or lower titer does not exclude histoplasmosis. Similarly, titers do not parallel disease activity, correlate with response to therapy, or predict outcome. Testing of serum by immunodiffusion to detect precipitin bands to M and H antigens appears to be a more specific but less sensitive serologic method than complement fixation. All antibody tests are associated with frequent false-positive reactions to *Histoplasma* antigens among patients with tuberculosis and other fungal diseases, especially blastomycosis and coccidioidomycosis. On the other hand, use of radioimmunoassay to detect *H. capsulatum* polysaccharide antigen in body fluids such as serum and urine provides a relatively sensitive and specific marker of disseminated histoplasmosis. Antigen levels fall with treatment; consequently, this test is useful for both diagnosing and evaluating the response to therapy.

The diagnosis of primary pulmonary histoplasmosis should be suspected on the basis of clinical, radiographic, and epidemiologic clues, e.g., an acute febrile respiratory illness accompanied by scattered patchy infiltrates and hilar adenopathy in an individual with high risk of exposure to *Histoplasma* spores. An elevated complement fixation titer and/or precipitin bands in serum provide presumptive evidence. Whereas sputum cultures are rarely positive (only 10 to 20%) in primary pulmonary disease, the likelihood of positive sputum cultures is significantly higher in chronic pulmonary histoplasmosis. Among patients with chronic disease, about 60% with marching thick-walled cavities have positive cultures, and a significant percentage of these also have positive smears of stained sputum. Although serologic tests for antibody are only moderately helpful (positive results in only 50% of cases), an elevated complement fixation titer in a patient with characteristic radiographic findings provides strong supportive evidence. Definitive diagnosis of chronic pulmonary histoplasmosis must be based on a positive sputum culture or smear or on histopathologic studies and special stains of lung tissue obtained by bronchoscopy.

The diagnosis of disseminated histoplasmosis depends on either demonstrating intracellular yeast forms by histopathologic study or a positive culture of blood, bone marrow, lymph node, skin or mu-

cous membrane, liver, lung, or other involved site. A Wright-stained smear of peripheral blood is positive in > 50% of acute or subacute cases. If possible, serum and urine should be examined for *H. capsulatum* antigen by radioimmunoassay. The cerebrospinal fluid of patients with chronic unexplained culture-negative lymphocytic meningitis should be tested for antigen and antibodies to *H. capsulatum.*

TREATMENT. For most patients with primary pulmonary histoplasmosis, no antifungal therapy is necessary. For those with severe or progressive primary infection, short-course intravenous amphotericin B (around 1000 mg total dose), oral ketoconazole, (400 mg daily for 3 to 6 months) or oral itraconazole, (200 to 400 mg daily for 3 to 6 months) is recommended, although none of these regimens has been prospectively evaluated in this setting. The treatment of chronic pulmonary histoplasmosis is even less standardized, in large part owing to the relative difficulty in clinically and radiologically distinguishing the pneumonitic and cavitary stages of disease. Although the early pneumonitic form of chronic pulmonary disease has been reported to resolve spontaneously in 80% of cases, rest and inactivity clearly promote healing. Traditionally, antifungal therapy has been advocated only for patients with progressive or marching cavitary disease, manifested by persistent or enlarging, thick-walled, > 2 mm cavities. Amphotericin B (total dose 2.0 to 2.5 grams), ketoconazole (400 mg daily for at least 6 months), or itraconazole (200 to 400 mg daily for 6 to 9 months) is effective therapy. There may be merit in liberalizing criteria for treatment in patients with chronic pulmonary disease. Rather than reserving therapy only for patients with advanced cavitary disease, some authorities suggest that oral ketoconazole or itraconazole may be indicated for all patients with chronic pulmonary disease, regardless of the stage. Although itraconazole is better tolerated and less toxic, ketoconazole is less expensive.

In contrast to the somewhat controversial guidelines regarding therapy of pulmonary histoplasmosis, there is no question that all patients with disseminated histoplasmosis should be treated. For patients with severe life-threatening disease, immunocompromised hosts such as organ transplant recipients or corticosteroid-treated patients, and the rare patients with CNS or cardiac histoplasmosis, amphotericin B total dose (2.0 to 2.5 grams) is the drug of choice. Itraconazole, 200 to 400 mg daily for 6 to 12 months, is an effective alternative in immunocompetent patients with mild to moderate disease. Experience over the past decade with disseminated histoplasmosis in AIDS patients indicates that an aggressive approach to treatment is necessary in an attempt to prevent relapse. For AIDS patients with moderate to severe or life-threatening disease, intensive "induction" primary therapy with intravenous amphotericin B (total dose 1.0 to 2.0 grams) should be used to gain control of disease and reduce the organism load. For AIDS patients with milder disease, itraconazole (200 mg twice daily for 10 to 12 weeks) is highly effective primary therapy; fluconazole (400 to 800 mg daily) may be an effective alternative. Regardless of which primary therapy regimen is used, lifelong maintenance or suppressive therapy is required to prevent histoplasmosis relapse in patients with AIDS. At present, itraconazole (200 mg twice daily) is the drug of choice. In patients who cannot take itraconazole because of intolerance or drug interaction, fluconazole (200 to 400 mg daily) can be used. Ketoconazole is an inadequate primary or maintenance therapy in patients with AIDS. The approach of initiating therapy with intravenous amphotericin B and completing it with an oral agent may prove applicable to selected other patients with either chronic pulmonary or disseminated histoplasmosis.

The management of mediastinal fibrosis presumed secondary to *H. capsulatum* infection is largely unsatisfactory, as evidenced by progressive morbidity in many patients and a mortality rate of at least 30%. Antifungal chemotherapy is generally not recommended. In selected cases, surgical extirpation may be beneficial in alleviating entrapment or obstructive syndromes.

PROGNOSIS. Although primary pulmonary histoplasmosis may be associated with acute or chronic intrathoracic complications, this form of disease is usually self-limited. In contrast, chronic cavitary pulmonary histoplasmosis is usually progressive, resulting in respiratory insufficiency and death. Disseminated histoplasmosis is variable in its severity and course, depending on the immune status of the host. Although a single course of therapy may be curative in some patients, long-term maintenance therapy to prevent relapse is required in others, especially patients with AIDS.

Dismukes WE, Bradsher RW Jr, Cloud GC, et al.: Itraconazole therapy for blastomycosis and histoplasmosis. Am J Med 93:489, 1992. *In a prospective, nonrandomized open trial among 35 patients with non–life-threatening, nonmeningeal histoplasmosis treated for 2 or more months with itraconazole, the success rate was 86%.*

Wheat LJ: Diagnosis and management of histoplasmosis. Eur J Clin Microbiol Infect Dis 8:480, 1989. *A comprehensive review that includes an excellent perspective on the currently available serologic tests used to detect either antibody or antigen; includes 78 references.*

Wheat LJ, Connolly-Stringfield PA, Baker RL, et al.: Disseminated histoplasmosis in the acquired immune deficiency syndrome: Clinical findings, diagnosis and treatment, and review of the literature. Medicine (Baltimore) 69:361, 1990. *An informative review of disseminated histoplasmosis, a common opportunistic disease among AIDS patients living in or with history of exposure to the endemic area.*

Wheat LJ, Hafner R, Wulfsohn M, et al.: Prevention of relapse of histoplasmosis with itraconazole in patients with the acquired immunodeficiency syndrome. Ann Intern Med 118:610, 1993. *Results of this prospective, multicenter, open-label clinical trial indicate that itraconazole is safe and effective in preventing relapse of disseminated histoplasmosis in patients with AIDS.*

349 COCCIDIOIDOMYCOSIS

John N. Galgiani

DEFINITION. Coccidioidomycosis is a systemic infection due to the fungus, *Coccidioides immitis*, endemic to some deserts of the Western Hemisphere.

COCCIDIOIDOMYCOSIS

Causative fungus	*Coccidioides immitis*
Primary geographic distribution	Lower Sonoran deserts of the Western Hemisphere, including parts of Arizona, California, New Mexico, west Texas, and parts of Central and South America
Primary route of acquisition	Respiratory (inhalation of arthroconidia)
Principal site of disease	Lungs most common; spread to skin, bones, meninges, and other viscera uncommon but serious
Opportunistic infection in compromised hosts	Diffuse pneumonia and widespread infections common in patients with T lymphocyte defects or during high-dose corticosteroid therapy
Drug of choice for most patients	Usually no treatment required for primary pneumonia; usually fluconazole or itraconazole for extrapulmonary disease
Alternative therapy	Amphotericin B (especially with diffuse pneumonia); ketoconazole

ETIOLOGY. *C. immitis* is a dimorphic fungus that is classified as an ascomycete by ribosomal gene homology. In its vegetative state, mycelia with true septations mature to produce arthroconidia, single cells approximately 2 to 5 μm in size. After infection, an arthroconidium enlarges to as much as 75 μm in diameter as a spherule, undergoing internal septation to produce scores of endospores. When spherules rupture, packets of endospores are released, and these produce more spherules in infected tissue or revert to mycelia if removed from the body.

EPIDEMIOLOGY. *C. immitis* can be recovered from the soil of the low deserts of Arizona; the Central Valley of California; parts of other states, including New Mexico and Texas; and parts of Central and South America. Endemic regions follow the climatologic Sonoran life zone, which is characterized by modest rainfall, mild winters, and low humidity. *C. immitis* grows in a soil layer a few centimeters below the surface, and disruption of the dirt by windstorms

or construction equipment increases the release of fungal particles into the air. The risk of exposure increases during dry months that follow rainy seasons. Primary infection outside the endemic regions occurs rarely from exposure to contaminated bales of cotton or other fomites. Person-to-person transmission of pulmonary infection has not been reported, and isolation precautions are unnecessary.

INCIDENCE AND PREVALENCE. Using dermal hypersensitivity to coccidioidal antigens as an indicator of prior infection, the annual conversion rate within strongly endemic areas is normally 3%, representing 50,000 to 100,000 new infections and producing an incidence of approximately 60% within the general population. However, in the years 1990 to 1994, the number of clinically diagnosed infections was manyfold larger than in past years; in situations where exposure is unusually intense, such as at archeology sites or during military maneuvers within endemic regions, infections can develop in the majority of persons exposed for only a matter of days.

PATHOGENESIS AND PATHOLOGY. Virtually all coccidioidal infections are the result of inhaling arthroconidia into the lung. Within the small airways, proliferation engenders both acute inflammation, including eosinophils, associated with spherule rupture, and granulomatous inflammation, associated with mature, intact spherules. Focal pneumonia is often associated with ipsilateral hilar adenopathy, and less frequently, infection enlarges peritracheal, supraclavicular, and cervical nodes. Lesions occurring elsewhere are the result of hematogenous dissemination and usually develop within months of the initial infection. Although progressive dissemination results from <1% of infections, as many as 8% of persons with self-limited infection develop chorioretinal scars, suggesting that subclinical hematogenous spread may be frequent. Within weeks after infection, durable T-cell immunity normally arrests fungal proliferation, allowing inflammation to resolve and preventing reinfection in the future. However, control of the infection may not completely sterilize lesions, and reactivation of dormant infection or second infections is possible in patients whose cell-mediated immunity becomes deficient.

CLINICAL MANIFESTATIONS. At least two of every three infections are detected only by finding dermal hypersensitivity to coccidioidal antigens. Those who become ill usually experience a self-limited pulmonary syndrome. However, a minority of patients develop complications or progressive forms of infection that display a broad variety of manifestations and pose difficult problems for the clinician.

Primary Pulmonary Infections. Five to 21 days after exposure, symptoms develop; these may include fever, weight loss, fatigue, a dry cough, or pleuritic chest pain, and they are difficult to differentiate from those caused by other respiratory pathogens. Arthralgia without associated joint effusions is also frequent. Skin manifestations may also occur as a short-lived nonpuritic maculopapular rash, erythema multiforme, or erythema nodosum. The arthritic and dermatologic manifestations are thought to be mediated by circulating immune complexes or other immunologic phenomena and are referred to as "desert rheumatism." Radiographs of the chest may show no abnormalities or may demonstrate pulmonary infiltrates, either segmental or lobar. Hilar adenopathy is often a distinctive finding. Peripneumonic pleural effusions may occur and usually resolve without intervention, even though *C. immitis* is usually recoverable from the pleura. Eosinophilia is frequently a prominent finding in differential leukocyte counts of peripheral blood, and the erythrocyte sedimentation rate is usually elevated. Symptoms may persist for several weeks before improvement is clearly under way, and the illness, especially lassitude, may persist for months.

The primary pulmonary process produces a variety of sequelae. The most frequent is the development of a pulmonary nodule (Fig. 349–1), typically measuring 1 to 4 cm and lying within 5 cm of the hilus. Despite their harmless nature, coccidioidal nodules may engender concern because of their similarity to a malignant mass. For this reason, management usually requires percutaneous needle aspiration or resection. Another consequence of pulmonary coccidioidomycosis is cavitation of the infiltrate, which occurs in approximately 5% of pneumonias. Cavities are usually single, thin walled, in an upper lobe, and close to the pleura; they may cause pain, produce hemoptysis, or develop associated infiltrates. Infrequently a

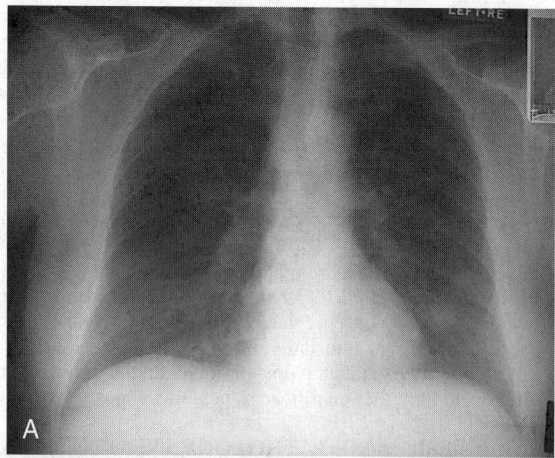

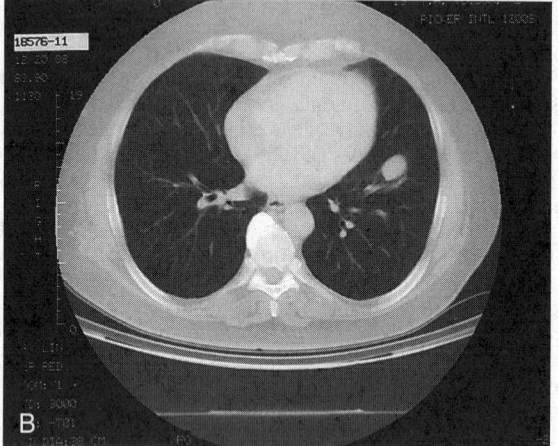

FIGURE 349–1. *A,* Benign nodule due to coccidioidomycosis. *B,* Computed tomographic image of the nodule in *A.*

cavity ruptures, forming a pyopneumothorax. This usually is the first symptom of coccidioidal infection and commonly occurs in otherwise healthy young males. An air-fluid level, detectable by roentgenography in the pleural space, often helps differentiate this problem from a spontaneous pneumothorax. Surgical resection of the cavity with closure of the bronchopleural fistula is the preferred treatment for this complication. The least common pulmonary complication is persistent fibrocavitary infection that progresses from involvement of lobes to involvement of both lungs.

Extrapulmonary Dissemination. Coccidioidomycosis usually results in dissemination beyond the lungs in immunosuppressed patients, such as organ recipients or those with AIDS or lymphoma. However, some patients have no underlying disease and do not manifest heightened susceptibility to other infections. The most common locations for disseminated lesions are skin (cutaneous papules or subcutaneous nodules); joints (especially the knee); bones, including vertebrae; and the basilar meninges. Such infections may produce one or many lesions and frequently are subacute or chronic in their presentation. When infections are more fulminant, they are usually in broadly immunosuppressed patients and produce fungemia detectable with blood cultures and diffuse reticulonodular embolic pulmonary infiltrates. Although the kidneys and the urinary bladder are rarely involved, *C. immitis* may be recovered from concentrated specimens of urine, because of either transient fungemia or focal dissemination to the prostate. In contrast to histoplasmosis, the gastrointestinal tract is rarely involved in coccidioidomycosis.

DIAGNOSIS. The diagnosis is firmly established by recovering *C. immitis* from clinical specimens. On direct examination of respi-

ratory specimens or tissue, spherules can be seen as large structures with refractile walls and internal organization and also on hematoxylin-eosin, silver, or periodic acid–Schiff stains of histologic preparations. The Gram stain does not detect spherules. In culture, mycelial growth is often evident within the first week of incubation. Except in the case of coccidioidal meningitis, in which cerebrospinal fluid (CSF) cultures are usually negative, isolation of the fungus is nearly always possible in patients with infections sufficiently severe to warrant therapy. In contrast, recovery of *C. immitis* may be difficult in patients who have only scant respiratory secretions associated with the initial pneumonia.

A presumptive diagnosis of coccidioidal infection is often based on detecting specific antibodies in serum. Within the first weeks of initial infections, a precipitin-type antibody is detected, usually by immunodiffusion techniques. Later, complement fixing (CF)-type antibodies usually appear. When reported quantitatively, CF antibodies generally are found to be highest in the most extensive infections and to decrease in concentration in patients whose infections are controlled. An important means of diagnosing coccidioidal meningitis is by detection of CF antibodies in the CSF, along with other abnormalities, such as leukocytosis, elevated protein concentration, or low glucose concentration.

TREATMENT. Because the primary infection is usually self-limited, treatment has been limited to patients with progressive illness. This was typical when amphotericin B was the only effective therapy and still remains a rational approach despite the advent of other agents, since none has been shown to either hasten the resolution of initial symptoms or prevent subsequent complications. Amphotericin B has been used successfully in cumulative doses of 1.0 to 3.0 grams for treating all types of coccidioidomycosis. However, it has not been uniformly effective and frequently has produced treatment-limiting morbidity and toxicity. Binding amphotericin B in liposomes or lipid complexes is being explored as a means of improving the therapeutic to toxic profile. Treatment of coccidioidal meningitis has necessitated intrathecal administration, which imposes additional toxicity and risks.

Azole antifungals have expanded the alternatives for treating coccidioidomycosis. Ketoconazole is orally effective and less toxic therapy than amphotericin B, but absorption is variable, gastrointestinal intolerance is frequent, and signs of dose-dependent suppression of steroidogenesis occur in some patients. More recently, two triazoles, fluconazole and itraconazole, have demonstrated efficacy without hormonal suppression. Fluconazole is also efficacious in the treatment of meningitis. Unfortunately, cessation of therapy often is followed by recurrence of lesions and therefore protracted, and in some patients continuous courses of therapy are needed to maintain control.

PROGNOSIS. After resolution of the initial infection, most patients maintain lifelong immunity, and second infections are very infrequent. Similarly, late recurrence is unlikely in the absence of intercurrent profound immunosuppression. In those in whom the initial infection cannot be resolved, the disease frequently follows a protracted course. Although infection is more debilitating than fatal, fulminant respiratory failure can occur, and if untreated, coccidioidal meningitis is nearly always fatal within 2 years.

Ampel NM, Dols CL, Galgiani JN: Coccidioidomycosis during human immunodeficiency virus infection. Results of a prospective study in a coccidioidal endemic area. Am J Med 94:235, 1993. *Estimates that the risk of active infection within southern Arizona during a 41-month-period was between 8.2 and 41.1%. Risk factors for coccidioidal disease were low CD4 counts or other AIDS-defining illnesses but not a history of prior coccidioidomycosis or a positive skin test.*

Catanzaro A, Galgiani JN, Levine BE, et al.: Fluconazole in the treatment of chronic pulmonary and nonmeningeal disseminated Coccidioidomycosis. Am J Med 98:249, 1995. *Of 75 evaluable patients, 50 improved with 200 mg or 400 mg per day of fluconazole therapy. A comparison of fluconazole and itraconazole should be completed in 1996 by the Mycoses Study Group.*

Galgiani JN, Catanzaro A, Cloud GA, et al.: Fluconazole therapy for coccidioidal meningitis. Ann Intern Med 119:28, 1993. *In 50 patients treated with 400 mg per day of fluconazole as sole therapy for coccidioidal meningitis, overall response was 79%, which compares favorably with a response of 57% to intrathecal amphotericin B in earlier studies. However, even in patients who respond well to this therapy, the risk of relapse if fluconazole is stopped is probably greater than 60%.*

Pappagianis D, Zimmer BL: Serology of coccidioidomycosis. Clin Microbiol Rev 3:247, 1990. *Comprehensive review of diagnostic tests for coccidioidomycosis.*

350 BLASTOMYCOSIS

William E. Dismukes

DEFINITION. Blastomycosis (North American blastomycosis, Gilchrist's disease) is an endemic systemic mycosis that occurs primarily in noncompromised hosts. As with the other important endemic mycoses, such as coccidioidomycosis and histoplasmosis, infection follows inhalation of the aerosolized spore form of the fungus. Clinical disease most commonly involves the lungs, skin, skeletal system, and male genitourinary tract.

BLASTOMYCOSIS

Causative fungus	*Blastomyces dermatitidis*
Primary geographic distribution	Endemic in North and South Central United States
Primary route of acquisition	Respiratory (inhalation of spores)
Principal sites of disease	Lungs, skin, bone, joints, prostate gland
Opportunistic infection in compromised hosts	Infrequent
Drug of choice for most patients	Itraconazole
Alternative therapy	Amphotericin B, ketoconazole, or fluconazole

---

ETIOLOGY. *Blastomyces dermatitidis,* the imperfect or asexual state of *Ajellomyces dermatitidis,* is a dimorphic fungus, growing as a mycelial form in the environment and in the laboratory at room temperature and as a yeast form in mammalian tissue and in the laboratory at 37°C. The yeast cells, which are identical *in vitro* and *in vivo* in tissue and fluid specimens, vary from 8 to 15 μm in diameter, have a thick, highly refractile cell wall, and reproduce by single broad-based buds. In the laboratory, growth of *B. dermatitidis* is somewhat slow; mold colonies may not appear for 1 to 3 weeks.

EPIDEMIOLOGY. Because no sensitive and specific skin test exists, the epidemiology of blastomycosis is less well understood than that of coccidioidomycosis and histoplasmosis. The incidence of clinical disease as a manifestation of blastomycosis appears to be lower than the incidence of clinical disease associated with the two other endemic mycoses. The prevalence of subclinical blastomycosis is largely unknown. Isolated cases of blastomycosis have been reported worldwide, including Africa and Central and South America; however, the disease is concentrated or endemic in the South and North Central United States, especially in areas bordering the Mississippi and Ohio River basins, and the Great Lakes. In these endemic areas, small point-source outbreaks of blastomycosis have been associated with recreational or occupational activities in wooded areas along waterways. Current evidence indicates that *B. dermatitidis* exists in warm, moist soil enriched by organic debris, including decaying vegetation or wood. It is not surprising, therefore, that persons with occupational or avocational exposure to soil and the outdoors appear to be at highest risk of acquiring infection. Data from point-source outbreaks indicate that the median incubation period from exposure to infection is about 43 days. Animals, especially dogs and horses, are also susceptible to infection, which may progress to clinical disease. Among humans, clinical illness is most common among middle-aged men. Although *B. dermatitidis,* in contrast to the other dimorphic fungi, is a relatively uncommon opportunistic pathogen, studies over the past decade indicate that blastomycosis is being increasingly observed in immunocompromised hosts, e.g., corticosteroid- and cytotoxic drug-treated patients, organ transplant recipients, and AIDS patients. This observation suggests that reactivation blastomycosis may be more common than previously suspected.

PATHOGENESIS AND PATHOLOGY. Humans and animals, for the most part, acquire infection by inhaling aerosolized conidia that convert to the yeast form in the lungs at body temperature. Percutaneous inoculation of *B. dermatitidis* has been documented rarely, as a result of either a laboratory accident or a dog bite. The clinical manifestations of disease at body sites other than lung (and rarely skin) result from the hematogenous spread of organisms.

Cell-mediated immunity appears to be the most important arm of host defense against *B. dermatitidis.* Recent *in vivo* and *in vitro* studies indicate that macrophages, stimulated by lymphokines, are more effective in inhibiting or killing the organism than are granulocytes. A growth-inhibiting or protective role of humoral immunity in blastomycosis has not been established. The typical histopathologic picture of pulmonary blastomycosis and other nonmucocutaneous sites of disease consists of noncaseating granulomas as well as clusters of neutrophils. By contrast, cutaneous and mucous membrane lesions are characterized by pseudoepitheliomatous hyperplasia with microabscesses.

CLINICAL MANIFESTATIONS. In general, blastomycosis is a chronic indolent systemic fungal disease associated with a variety of pulmonary and extrapulmonary manifestations. Among the latter, cutaneous disease predominates, occurring in about 40 to 80% of cases. Multiple organ involvement occurs in approximately 50 to 60% of cases. Extrapulmonary disease may occur in the absence of clinical or radiologic evidence of lung disease.

Pulmonary. Although precise data are not available, most primary infections are believed to be either asymptomatic or unrecognized as being due to *B. dermatitidis* on the basis of nonspecific flulike symptoms. In patients with proven acute pulmonary blastomycosis, the radiologic findings usually consist of infiltrative or nodular air space opacities, most often in the lower lobes. Pulmonary blastomycosis usually manifests as a chronic pneumonia syndrome, characterized by productive cough, pleuritic chest pain, dyspnea, weight loss, and low-grade fever. Although there are no distinguishing radiologic characteristics, consolidation, one or more fibronodular infiltrates or mass lesions with or without cavitation, is common, often mimicking the findings in other granulomatous diseases or bronchogenic carcinoma. Although hilar adenopathy and pleural effusions occur, they are uncommon. Patients with overwhelming pulmonary blastomycosis may develop diffuse, bilateral, interstitial alveolar infiltrates on the chest radiograph and clinical evidence of acute respiratory distress syndrome.

Skin. The cutaneous lesions, which often prompt the patient with blastomycosis to seek medical evaluation initially, are of two general types, verrucous and ulcerative; both types tend to occur more commonly on exposed parts. The verrucous lesions, which begin as papulopustules, are more characteristic; these progress slowly over weeks to months to become crusted, heaped-up, and warty in appearance, often with a reddish-black or violaceous hue, an area of central healing and scarring, and a well-circumscribed outer border. Microabscesses, manifested by black dots on the surface, are typically located at the periphery of verrucous lesions; removing the crusted eschar often reveals purulent material in which the yeast form of the organism can be demonstrated by wet preparation. Ulcerative lesions overlying a bed of friable red granulation tissue are less common. Occasionally, mucosal ulcerations may be found in the mouth, nose, or larynx, mimicking the mucocutaneous lesions of histoplasmosis. Lymphadenopathy in the region corresponding to the skin lesion or lesions is distinctly uncommon in patients whose cutaneous disease is secondary to hematogenous spread of organisms from a primary pulmonary focus.

Other. After lung and skin disease, bone and joint involvement is next most common and is seen in 10 to 50% of cases. Osteolytic lesions, with or without sclerotic margins, are typically located in long bones and vertebrae. Often, patients with bone disease present as a result of overlying chronic draining sinuses or contiguous soft tissue lesions rather than bone pain. Septic arthritis, which is much less common than osteomyelitis, is frequently secondary to contiguous extension. Up to one third of men with blastomycosis have genitourinary tract disease, manifested most commonly by prostatic enlargement with obstructive symptoms and less frequently by epididymitis. Central nervous system (CNS) disease in the form of either granulomatous meningitis or a mass lesion (intracerebral blastomycoma) occurs in about 5% of cases. Clinically apparent blastomycotic involvement of other organs, e.g., gastrointestinal tract, liver, spleen, adrenals, and kidneys, is unusual, except in patients with fulminant disseminated disease.

DIAGNOSIS. As is true for all systemic mycotic diseases, the definitive diagnosis of blastomycosis requires a positive fungal culture from clinical specimens. A presumptive diagnosis may be based on the finding of characteristic yeast forms in a wet preparation of sputum, pus, or other body fluid or in a histopathologic section of tissue, e.g., skin, lung, bone, or prostate. *B. dermatitidis* in wet preparations of fluid specimens mixed with 10% KOH appears as a broad-based single budding yeast and in fixed-tissue specimens stained with hematoxylin-eosin or periodic acid–Schiff (PAS) reagents as single or budding yeast cells with a doubly refractile cell wall. Because a presumptive clinical diagnosis based on "characteristic" skin lesions or radiologic findings is associated with an unacceptably high error rate, obtaining fluids or tissue from involved sites for culture and histopathologic study is mandatory in the evaluation of all patients with suspected blastomycosis. Moreover, documented cutaneous and/or pulmonary disease should signal the possibility of bone or genitourinary disease and lead to appropriate diagnostic studies, such as bone scan and prostate examination and massage. As a diagnostic test, the blastomycin skin test lacks sensitivity and specificity and should not be used. Similarly, the complement fixation assay for serum antibody is highly cross-reactive and of no diagnostic value. Recent studies suggest that immunodiffusion, enzyme immunoassay, or radioimmunoassay tests for antibody to the A antigen of *B. dermatitidis* or antibody to other more purified antigens, e.g., 120 kD, are better serologic markers of disease.

TREATMENT. At present, three drugs, amphotericin B, ketoconazole, and itraconazole, are approved for the treatment of blastomycosis. Although intravenous amphotericin B has been traditionally considered the drug of choice for all forms of disease, studies and experience gained over recent years indicate that the oral azoles, ketoconazole and itraconazole, are highly effective, especially in patients with chronic indolent disease and noninvolvement of the CNS. Ketoconazole should be initiated at a dosage of 400 mg per day, advanced by 200-mg increments at monthly intervals, up to a maximum of 800 mg per day in patients with progressive disease, and continued for a minimum of 6 months. Itraconazole in a dose of 200 to 400 mg per day for 6 months or longer is even more effective than ketoconazole (90 to 95% success rate versus 80%) and associated with less toxicity. Accordingly, itraconazole is considered the drug of choice for most patients with blastomycosis. However, itraconazole is more expensive than ketoconazole. Fluconazole, at usual therapeutic doses of 200 to 400 mg per day, is not as effective as ketoconazole or itraconazole. Higher doses of fluconazole, which are associated with higher costs and increased potential for toxicity, appear necessary for cure. Amphotericin B, a total dose of 1.5 to 2.5 grams, should be reserved for patients with overwhelming life-threatening or CNS disease, those rare patients who are immunocompromised, and those in whom oral azole therapy has failed. In selected situations, some investigators advocate an induction course of amphotericin B (total dose of approximately 500 mg) for a rapid fungicidal effect to gain control of disease, followed by maintenance or "consolidation" therapy with ketoconazole or itraconazole for 3 to 6 months. Although controversy exists about whether or not to treat patients with acute pulmonary blastomycosis who are identified as part of point-source outbreaks, available data suggest that most such patients do not require therapy. However, careful long-term follow-up of untreated patients is important to monitor for evidence of disease activity.

PROGNOSIS. In contrast to the past, now most patients with blastomycosis are identified and treated before the development of overwhelming or fatal disease. Antifungal therapy with either amphotericin B or an oral azole drug is associated with cure rates of ≥80% and relapse rates of <10%.

Brown LR, Swensen SJ, Van Scoy RE, et al.: Roentgenologic features of pulmonary blastomycosis. Mayo Clin Proc 66:29, 1991. *A well-illustrated description of the varied radiographic findings in pulmonary blastomycosis. Consolidation and mass patterns are most common, whereas hilar adenopathy and pleural effusion are rare.*

Dismukes WE, Bradsher RW Jr, Cloud GC, et al.: Itraconazole therapy for blastomycosis and histoplasmosis. Am J Med 93:489, 1992. *In a prospective, nonrandomized open trial, the success rate for 40 patients with non–life-threatening, non-meningeal blastomycosis treated with itraconazole for more than 2 months was*

95%.

Klein BS, Vergeront JM, Davis JP: Epidemiologic aspects of blastomycosis, the enigmatic systemic mycosis. Semin Respir Infect 1:29, 1986. *A valuable review that focuses on seven point-source epidemics and the ecologic niche of the organism.*

Meyer KC, McManus EJ, Maki DG: Overwhelming pulmonary blastomycosis associated with the adult respiratory distress syndrome. N Engl J Med 329:1231, 1993. *Overwhelming infection with* B. dermatitidis *can cause diffuse pneumonitis and the adult respiratory distress syndrome, even in immunocompetent hosts.*

Pappas PG, Threlkeld MG, Bedsole GD, et al.: Blastomycosis in immunocompromised patients. Medicine (Baltimore) 72:311, 1993. *This review documents the increasing occurrence of blastomycosis in compromised hosts, including corticosteroid-treated and oncologic patients, organ transplant recipients, pregnant patients, or those with AIDS, and describes the clinical manifestations and treatment approaches in these high-risk groups.*

351 PARACOCCIDIOIDOMYCOSIS
William E. Dismukes

DEFINITION. Paracoccidioidomycosis is a chronic granulomatous disease typically involving the lungs, skin, mucous membranes, and lymph nodes and limited to an endemic area extending from Mexico south to Argentina.

PARACOCCIDIOIDOMYCOSIS	
Causative fungus	*Paracoccidioides brasiliensis*
Primary geographic distribution	Endemic in Central America and parts of South America
Primary route of acquisition	Respiratory (inhalation of spores)
Principal sites of disease	Lungs, mucous membranes, skin, lymph nodes, liver, and spleen
Opportunistic infection in compromised hosts	Infrequent
Drug of choice for most patients	Itraconazole
Alternative therapy	Sulfonamide, amphotericin B, or ketoconazole

ETIOLOGY. The causative agent, *Paracoccidioides brasiliensis*, is a dimorphic fungus that grows as a mycelial form in nature and as an oval or round yeast form in tissues or at 37°C. Identifying characteristic multiple budding or "pilot wheel," thick-walled yeast cells, 10 to 40 μm in diameter, in tissue provides presumptive evidence of disease. Because the organism grows slowly on primary isolation, fungal cultures should be held for at least 4 weeks before discarding.

EPIDEMIOLOGY. Most cases occur in persons living in or with a history of prior exposure to southern Mexico, Central America, or South America; in selected countries such as Brazil, paracoccidioidomycosis is the most common systemic mycosis. Owing to the long period of latency, overt disease may develop in persons many years after they have left the endemic region. Infection is acquired by inhaling spores. Neither human-to-human transmission nor common-source outbreaks have been documented. The majority of cases occur in adult males, especially those who labor in the outdoors. The preponderance of cases in men may also be related to the observation that estrogens inhibit the mycelium-to-yeast transformation of the organism. Although cases have been reported in compromised hosts, in general, paracoccidioidomycosis is not considered an opportunistic fungal disease.

PATHOGENESIS AND PATHOLOGY. After inhaling spores, infection may remain confined to the lungs or may spread by lymphohematogenous dissemination to multiple organs. The host pathologic response caused by *P. brasiliensis* is similar to that caused by tissue invasion with *Blastomyces dermatitidis* and *Coccidioides immitis*, i.e., both granulomas and suppuration may develop. The type of tissue pathology and the spectrum of clinical disease are in large part dictated by the integrity of the cell-mediated defenses of the host.

CLINICAL MANIFESTATIONS. Pulmonary paracocciioidomycosis may be asymptomatic or result in symptomatic acute or chronic disease. Whereas the acute form of pulmonary paracoccidioidomycosis is usually nonspecific and indistinguishable from other influenza-like illnesses, the clinical and radiographic features of the chronic form often resemble those of chronic pulmonary coccidioidomycosis. Any or all lobes may be infected, but the upper lobes tend to be less frequently involved. In addition, cavities, if present, are usually small (so-called microcavities). Extrapulmonary disease, especially in persons younger than 30, may be acute in onset, is often manifested by lymphadenopathy and hepatosplenomegaly, and carries a poor prognosis. More typically, extrapulmonary disease in older adults is an indolent illness, manifested by oropharyngeal and laryngeal mucous membrane ulcers; verrucous, ulcerative, or nodular skin lesions, often on the face or mucocutaneous borders; and enlarged or necrotic, draining lymph nodes, especially in the cervical region. Other sites of less frequent involvement are the gastrointestinal tract, adrenal glands, testes, epididymis, and skeletal system. Central nervous system and eye disease secondary to *P. brasiliensis* are rare. A few cases of paracoccidioidomycosis have been observed in human immunodeficiency virus (HIV)–infected persons.

DIAGNOSIS. Demonstration of the characteristic "pilot wheel," multiple-budding *P. brasiliensis* yeast cells by wet mounts or KOH preparations of sputum, pus, or other body fluids or by special fungal stains of biopsy or cell-block specimens provides presumptive evidence of paracoccidioidomycosis. A positive culture of body fluid or tissue specimens is diagnostic. Two different serologic tests (agar gel immunodiffusion and complement fixation) are available through the Centers for Disease Control and Prevention in Atlanta. Precipitin bands appear early in the course of active infection and may persist for years, even after successful therapy. Complement-fixing antibodies appear later and are more useful in evaluating response to treatment. Both tests have high specificity. Alternative serologic tests, including enzyme-linked immunosorbent assay (ELISA) and counterimmunoelectrophoresis (CIE) as well as newer ones for detecting a 43-kD glycoprotein antigen and for antibodies to this antigen, are under investigation. Skin tests have no role in diagnosis.

TREATMENT. In the past, oral sulfonamides were the mainstay of therapy; however, these have two major drawbacks, namely, a high rate of relapse even after prolonged suppression therapy and a high frequency of adverse reactions, especially skin rashes. Intravenous amphotericin B is effective therapy and is usually used for more severe forms of paracoccidioidomycosis, such as pulmonary or disseminated multiorgan disease, and for more refractory cases. Follow-up chronic suppression therapy with sulfonamides is recommended. Oral antifungal azole drugs represent a significant advance in the treatment of this disease. Ketoconazole, an imidazole, is highly effective in both *in vivo* animal models and humans. Cure is usually achieved with dosages of 200 to 400 mg per day, given for at least 1 year. Itraconazole, a triazole, in a dose of 100 mg per day for 6 to 12 months, is as effective as ketoconazole, is better tolerated, and is associated with a lower relapse rate. As a result, many authorities now consider itraconazole the drug of choice for paracoccidioidomycosis. To date, experience in this disease with fluconazole, the other available oral triazole, has been limited. Because of the tropism of *P. brasiliensis* for the adrenal glands and the possibility of adrenal insufficiency during active disease or even after therapy is discontinued, periodic tests of adrenal function are recommended.

PROGNOSIS. Untreated disseminated paracoccidioidomycosis is generally fatal. As a rule, the more common indolent forms of adult disease, usually associated with reactivation, are amenable to prolonged therapy, given over months to years. Unfortunately, clinically significant fibrotic sequelae often persist despite therapy.

Brummer E, Castaneda E, Restrepo A: Paracoccidioidomycosis: An update. Clin Microbiol Rev 6:89, 1993. *A comprehensive review of the disease, focusing on the causative agent, epidemiology, pathogenesis, diagnosis, and therapy, with 329 references.*

Naranjo MS, Trujillo M, Munera MI, et al.: Treatment of paracoccidioidomycosis with itraconazole. J Med Vet Mycol 28:67, 1990. *Forty-five of 47 patients had the chronic form of disease. Itraconazole, 100 mg per day, given for a mean duration of 6 months, was highly effective, as measured by radiographic and cultural responses, falling serologic titers, and improvement in clinical severity scores.*

352 CRYPTOCOCCOSIS
William E. Dismukes

DEFINITION. Cryptococcosis is a systemic mycosis that most often involves the lungs and central nervous system (CNS) and, less frequently, the skin, skeletal system, and prostate gland. *Cryptococcus neoformans,* the causative organism, is the most common agent of fungal meningitis, and since the onset of the AIDS epidemic in the early 1980's, it has been increasingly recognized as an opportunistic fungal pathogen.

CRYPTOCOCCOSIS	
Causative fungus	*Cryptococcus neoformans*
Primary geographic distribution	Worldwide
Primary route of acquisition	Respiratory (inhalation of spores)
Principal sites of disease	Lungs, CNS, blood, skin, bone, joints, prostate gland
Opportunistic infection in compromised hosts	Frequent, especially in corticosteroid-treated and AIDS patients
Drug of choice in most patients	Amphotericin B (with or without flucytosine) or fluconazole
Alternative therapy	Itraconazole

ETIOLOGY. *C. neoformans* is a yeastlike round or oval fungus, 4 to 6 μm in diameter, which is surrounded by a polysaccharide capsule and which reproduces by budding. Characteristics used to distinguish genus *Cryptococcus* from other yeasts include a lack of pseudohyphae, carbohydrate, and nitrate assimilation and production of phenyloxidase, melanin, and urease. There are two varieties of *C. neoformans:* var. *neoformans* and var. *gattii,* and four different serotypes, A, B, C, and D (based on the antigenic specificity of the capsule). In the laboratory, *C. neoformans* var. *neoformans* (serotypes A and D) grows at 37°C on niger seed agar as smooth brown colonies within a few days after inoculation. By contrast, *C. neoformans* var. *gattii* (serotypes B and C) grows more slowly, and nonpathogenic *Cryptococcus* species grow poorly or not at all at 37°C. Color reactions on canavanine-glycine-bromthymol blue (CGB) agar are also used to determine varietal status. Nomenclature of the perfect or sexual states is based on mating properties. For example, strains of serotypes A and D, which include the majority of clinical isolates, can be mated to produce the perfect state (*Filobasidiella neoformans* var. *neoformans*).

EPIDEMIOLOGY. Cryptococcosis is worldwide in distribution. *C. neoformans* var. *neoformans* is found in soil and other environmental areas, especially those contaminated by pigeon droppings; pigeons themselves are not infected. Although less is known about the ecologic niche of *C. neoformans* var. *gattii,* this organism has been isolated recently from bark, wood, and leaves of river red gum (*Eucalyptus calmaldulensis*) trees in tropical and subtropical regions, the areas of the world in which this variety of *C. neoformans* is endemic. Although humans and animals acquire infection after inhaling aerosolized spores, clusters of cases or mini-outbreaks of cryptococcosis rarely occur. Only two unusual cases of presumed person-to-person transmission of cryptococcosis have been observed. There is no obvious age, gender, or occupational predilection. Immunosuppression related to altered T-cell function is the most common predisposing factor: Examples include corticosteroid therapy, lymphoreticular malignancies (especially Hodgkin's disease), sarcoidosis (even in the absence of corticosteroid therapy), HIV infection, organ transplantation, and perhaps diabetes mellitus. The association of cryptococcosis and organ transplantation probably relates in large part to immunosuppression with corticosteroids.

Cyclosporine, at least in a murine model, inhibits growth of *C. neoformans*. Among patients with AIDS in the United States, the incidence of cryptococcosis ranges from 5 to 10%; by contrast, in Africa and other developing areas, the incidence of cryptococcosis in AIDS patients is much higher. Although cryptococcosis occurs most frequently in immunosuppressed hosts, about 20 to 30% of patients with the disease have no apparent underlying condition or predisposing factor (except for unexplained CD4 cytopenia in some).

PATHOGENESIS AND PATHOLOGY. After aerosolized spores are inhaled, most infections begin with an asymptomatic pulmonary focus. In individuals with normal host defense, cryptococci remain localized in the lungs and are eventually eliminated. By contrast, in immunocompromised individuals, there is hematogenous spread to extrapulmonary organs. Neutrophils and later monocytes clear cryptococci from inflammatory sites. Phagocytosis by neutrophils and macrophages appears to be mediated in part by complement and several cytokines including interferon-γ, tissue necrosis factor, and GM-CSF. Cryptococcal polysaccharide is a major virulence factor and may be immunosuppressive, inhibit phagocytosis, and impair migration of leukocytes. Paradoxically, cryptococcal polysaccharide has also been shown to activate the alternative complement pathway. In general, immunity depends on functioning, sensitized T cells and an intact cell-mediated arm of host defense. Consequently, patients with defective or altered T-cell immunity, such as those with HIV infection, are highly susceptible to infection with *C. neoformans* and progressive disease. The incidence of cryptococcosis in AIDS patients is highly associated with CD4 counts < 100 cells per cubic millimeter. The preferential involvement of *C. neoformans* for the CNS is explained by the absence of complement and soluble anticryptococcal factors (present in normal serum) in normal cerebrospinal fluid (CSF), as well as a decreased to absent inflammatory response to cryptococci in brain tissue. As a result, well-formed granulomas are generally absent in histopathologic sections of infected tissue. The characteristic lesion in cryptococcal meningoencephalitis consists of cystic clusters of fungi; the basal ganglia and the cortical gray matter are the sites of heaviest involvement. In other organs such as the lung, the inflammatory response varies in intensity from minimal to heavy and consists of an array of cells, including organism-containing macrophages, giant cells, plasma cells, and lymphocytes. No necrosis is present, and tissue is usually displaced by multiplying organisms. Yeastlike cryptococci with characteristic narrow-based buds stain poorly with hematoxylin-eosin but are easily visualized with Gomori methenamine silver (GMS) or periodic acid–Schiff (PAS) stains. Mucicarmine stain further aids identification by giving a rose color to the polysaccharide capsule.

CLINICAL MANIFESTATIONS. Pulmonary Cryptococcosis. The pattern of pulmonary cryptococcal infection is highly variable, ranging from the extremes of saprophytic airway colonization without clinical or radiographic evidence of disease to full-blown acute respiratory distress syndrome in compromised hosts, such as AIDS patients. More typically, radiographic findings include either patchy pneumonitis or solitary or multiple small nodules in asymptomatic persons or those with mild to moderate symptoms, e.g., fever, malaise, cough, scant sputum, pleuritic pain, or rarely hemoptysis. Although tumor-like masses mimicking carcinoma are not uncommon, cavitation and pleural effusions are less likely. The course of pulmonary cryptococcosis is also variable. In patients with normal host defenses, spontaneous regression of both clinical and radiographic manifestations is the rule, although chronic stable infection is known to occur. In contrast, pulmonary cryptococcosis in immunocompromised patients is more likely to progress and therefore requires antifungal therapy. Pulmonary disease may occur in the absence of extrapulmonary cryptococcosis, and conversely, extrapulmonary disease, such as meningitis, may develop in the absence of apparent lung involvement.

Central Nervous System Cryptococcosis. Meningitis, usually subacute or chronic in nature, is the most common manifestation of CNS cryptococcosis. Complications include hydrocephalus, encephalitis, involvement of the optic pathways, brain stem vasculitis, and mass lesions (cryptococcomas) of the brain parenchyma or spinal cord. The clinical presentation and course of cryptococcal meningitis vary greatly, related in part to the underlying condition

and immune status of the host. In "normal" hosts, the onset is often insidious, whereas in compromised hosts, such as HIV-infected or corticosteroid-treated patients, the onset tends to be more acute and the course more rapidly progressive. The most common symptoms are headache and alteration in mental status, e.g., confusion, lethargy, obtundation or coma, and personality change. Nausea and vomiting are frequent; fever and stiff neck are less common. Ocular symptoms, such as blurred vision, photophobia, vision loss, and diplopia, secondary to perineuritic adhesive arachnoiditis, papilledema, optic nerve neuritis, chorioretinitis, or retinovitreal abscess, are present in about 25% of patients. Other findings include hearing deficits, seizures, ataxia, aphasia, and choreoathetoid movements. Dementia is important to recognize as a potential sequela because it may be curable. Cryptococcomas, which accompany cryptococcal meningitis in 5 to 20% of cases, are less common in patients with AIDS. Rarely, CNS cryptococcomas can be seen in the absence of meningeal disease. The mortality rate varies from 15 to 25%; most deaths occur in the first few weeks of illness.

Miscellaneous. After the lungs and CNS, the next most commonly involved organs in patients with disseminated cryptococcosis are the skin and skeletal system. Cutaneous manifestations occur in 10 to 15% of cases and usually take the form of papules, pustules, nodules, ulcers, or draining sinuses. Typically, cellulitis with prominent erythema and induration is seen in corticosteroid-treated transplant recipients, and umbilicated papules resembling molluscum contagiosum are observed in AIDS patients. Oral mucosal chancres have been reported rarely. Osteomyelitis is more common than septic arthritis. Less commonly involved sites of cryptococcal disease include pericardium, myocardium, muscle, liver, peritoneum, adrenal glands, kidneys, and prostate gland. Infections of these organs are being increasingly identified in AIDS patients. For example, the prostate has been reported to be a sanctuary of residual infection in this population group.

DIAGNOSIS. As with other systemic mycoses, the definitive diagnosis of cryptococcosis depends on demonstrating the characteristic yeastlike organism with its surrounding capsule in tissue or fluid obtained from involved sites, together with cultural confirmation. In addition, in patients with suspected cryptococcosis, the latex agglutination test to detect cryptococcal polysaccharide antigen in serum and CSF is an extremely important adjunct to diagnosis, unlike the situation for most other fungal disease, in which serologic tests lack specificity and sensitivity. Cryptococcal antigen is found in CSF in > 90% and in serum in about 75% of patients with meningitis, especially if serial specimens are examined over time. Titers are particularly high in patients with AIDS. In patients with extraneural cryptococcal disease, antigen is detected in only 25 to 50% of cases. Proper controls are necessary to eliminate rheumatoid factor, which may give rise to a false-positive result. Serum of patients with disseminated infection caused by *Trichosporon beigelii* may also test positive for cryptococcal antigen. False-negative tests for cryptococcal antigen may be due to low numbers of cryptococcal organisms invading tissue or in CSF, unencapsulated or poorly encapsulated strains, or a prozone phenomenon. Tests for cryptococcal antibody are not useful for diagnosis.

Pulmonary cryptococcosis is difficult to diagnose in most cases without obtaining lung tissue via bronchoscopy, open lung biopsy, or thorascopy. Wet preparations of sputum are only occasionally helpful, and sputum cultures are positive for *C. neoformans* in only 20% of cases. In patients with pleural effusions, fluid tested for cryptococcal antigen may be positive, thereby obviating a more invasive procedure. In every patient with established pulmonary cryptococcosis, a lumbar puncture should be performed, whether or not CNS disease is apparent. Blood cultures and tissue for culture and histopathologic study of any other suspected sites of involvement, e.g., skin or bone, should also be obtained.

The diagnosis of cryptococcal meningitis is easier to establish than the diagnosis of cryptococcal pulmonary disease. Once the diagnosis of meningitis is considered, a lumbar puncture should be performed. Most patients, except for those with AIDS, have significant CSF abnormalities, including elevated opening pressure, depressed glucose levels (hypoglycorrhachia) in half the cases, elevated protein levels, and a lymphocytic pleocytosis. The India ink preparation of centrifuged CSF to detect budding yeast cells and surrounding capsule is positive in 50 to 75% of cases; because the incidence of false-positive smears is high, confirmation of findings by culture is imperative. Culturing of centrifuged sediment of large volumes (5 to 10 ml) of CSF obtained by repeated lumbar punctures is associated with a positive culture rate of 90 to 95%. In AIDS patients, the CSF formula is often normal or only minimally abnormal, owing to a diminished or absent inflammatory response. Yet in most cases, cultures are positive, cryptococcal antigen titers are high, and India ink preparations reveal organisms. The chest roentgenogram may or may not be abnormal. Blood should be cultured and tested for antigen in all patients; these tests are positive more commonly in AIDS patients than in patients without AIDS. In addition, computed tomographic scans (CT) or magnetic resonance imaging (MRI) of the head is indicated in most patients, especially those with coma, suspected hydrocephalus, focal neurologic findings, seizures, or clinical deterioration after initial improvement.

TREATMENT. Approaches to therapy of cryptococcosis vary according to site(s) of involvement and underlying host status. Whereas all patients with CNS cryptococcosis or other forms of extrapulmonary disease require treatment, the majority of cases of pulmonary cryptococcosis alone, especially in the "normal" host, resolve without antifungal therapy. By contrast, other patients with pulmonary cryptococcosis, including patients with AIDS and other immunocompromising conditions, those with accompanying extrapulmonary disease, and those with progressive disease, require antifungal therapy. Although specific guidelines are poorly defined, the two commonly used drugs are amphotericin B (total dose 1.0 to 2.0 grams) and fluconazole (200 to 400 mg daily for 3 to 6 months). Fluconazole should be reserved for patients with mild to moderate forms of cryptococcal lung disease. As a rule, therapy should be continued until clinical, radiographic, and mycologic resolution of disease is evident. Surgical resection may be an important adjunct to drug therapy in patients with extensive lobar consolidation and large mass lesions.

The therapy of cryptococcal meningitis has been more extensively studied than the therapy of any other systemic fungal disease. Data indicate that (1) all patients require treatment; (2) several treatment regimens, including oral azole drugs, may be used; (3) a combination of amphotericin B and flucytosine is the regimen of choice, especially for patients with moderate to severe disease including complications such as obtundation, coma, blindness, cranial nerve palsies, and hydrocephalus; (4) regardless of regimen, 15 to 25% of patients die of this disease; and (5) treatment considerations are somewhat different for AIDS patients with cryptococcal meningitis (see below). Although the standard regimen is combination amphotericin B (0.5 to 1.0 mg per kilogram per day) and flucytosine (100 mg per kilogram per day) for 4 to 6 weeks, both the daily dose and total dose should be individualized, balancing the risks of toxicities of the drugs and the potential benefits of synergy and increased efficacy. Both renal function and serum flucytosine levels should be closely monitored, and flucytosine doses should be regulated to maintain serum concentrations in the range of 50 to 100 μg per milliliter. Potential toxic effects of flucytosine include bone marrow suppression, hepatitis, diarrhea, and rash. Although experience with fluconazole in non-AIDS cryptococcal meningitis is limited, this drug may be an effective alternative therapy. Intrathecal therapy with amphotericin B is usually reserved for patients who relapse or whose disease is refractory to prolonged courses of high-dose intravenous amphotericin B.

Because cryptococcal meningitis in AIDS patients may be highly refractory and associated with a relapse rate of 50% if therapy is stopped, both aggressive primary therapy and long-term maintenance therapy are required. For primary therapy, several alternative treatment regimens may be used. First, combination amphotericin and flucytosine may be given for the entire period of primary therapy. However, some AIDS patients may not tolerate flucytosine because of a high incidence of drug-induced cytopenias, often superimposed upon pre-existing bone-marrow suppression secondary to zidovudine, cytotoxic chemotherapy, and opportunistic infectious diseases. In addition, flucytosine should not be used unless serum levels can be monitored. In such situations, amphotericin B may be used alone. Second, azole therapy alone is effective in selected patients, e.g., those with mild disease and normal mental status at time of diagnosis. Fluconazole is favored over itraconazole, another triazole, in cryptococcal meningitis because of fluconazole's water solubility, minimal protein binding, and good to excellent penetration into CSF (60 to 80% of serum concentration). In addition, an intravenous formulation of fluconazole is available. A major disadvantage of fluconazole and itraconazole is their less rapid steriliza-

tion of CSF than with amphotericin B. As a result, amphotericin B with or without flucytosine should be preferentially used as primary therapy in more seriously ill AIDS patients such as those who are obtunded or comatose or who have widespread disseminated cryptococcosis. Third, therapy with amphotericin B and flucytosine or amphotericin B alone may be given for an initial 2 weeks as induction primary therapy, followed by an oral azole for 8 additional weeks as consolidation therapy. This unique approach, currently being evaluated, represents an attempt to sterilize the CSF more rapidly, reduce the number of early deaths, and avoid the potential for prolonged toxicity of the drugs used in initial treatment. Fourth, the combination of two oral drugs, flucytosine and fluconazole, has been studied in both animal models and to a lesser extent in patients with AIDS-associated cryptococcal meningitis. Until more data are available about the efficacy of this novel regimen, it cannot be recommended routinely over more established treatments. Finally, recent data indicate that passive antibody in the form of murine or humanized monoclonal antibodies has the potential to enhance cellular immunity; trials are ongoing.

Chemotherapy alone is not adequate treatment for all patients. Ventricular shunting of CSF should be performed in obtunded or comatose patients with hydrocephalus demonstrated by imaging studies. Among patients with no overt hydrocephalus but abnormal mental status and elevated intracranial pressure, treatment approaches include frequent lumbar punctures to cautiously lower CSF pressure, high-dose dexamethasone therapy, and temporary ventricular drainage.

Once primary therapy has sterilized the CSF, i.e., converted the fungal culture from positive to negative, maintenance therapy in AIDS patients should be initiated. Fluconazole (200 mg daily) is more effective in preventing relapse than amphotericin (1 mg per kilogram weekly) and much better tolerated, resulting in better patient compliance. Fluconazole is also more effective than itraconazole. Chronic suppressive therapy must be continued for life.

PROGNOSIS. The outcome of cryptococcosis is significantly worse in AIDS patients than in the non-AIDS population, as evidenced by higher mortality and relapse rates. Pretreatment prognostic factors, in addition to HIV infection, which adversely affect outcome in patients with cryptococcal meningitis, include an underlying condition predisposing to T-cell dysfunction; absence of headache as a presenting symptom; altered mental status as evidenced by obtundation, stupor, or coma; positive extraneural cultures for *C. neoformans*, CSF white cell count ≤ 20 per cubic millimeter; and high cryptococcal serum and CSF antigen titers. Among these factors, HIV infection and abnormal mental status appear to be most important. A rise in CSF antigen during suppressive therapy is associated with relapse; by contrast, other abnormalities of CSF such as hypoglycorrhachia, elevated protein, or positive India ink preparation may persist for months after therapy has been discontinued and do not appear to correlate with relapse.

PREVENTION. Because an environmental source of infection cannot be determined in the vast majority of patients who develop cryptococcal disease, attempts at eliminating *C. neoformans* from soil or other habitats are not feasible or practical. With the availability of effective, safe, oral antifungal drugs such as fluconazole and itraconazole, use of these as prophylactic agents in high-risk groups such as HIV-infected persons has been evaluated. Preliminary data indicate that oral fluconazole, 200 mg daily, in patients with CD4 counts < 200 cells per cubic millimeter, is more effective than clotrimazole troches in reducing the frequency of systemic fungal disease, especially cryptococcosis, but not in prolonging survival.

Levitz SM: The ecology of *Cryptococcus neoformans* and the epidemiology of cryptococcosis. Rev Infect Dis 13:1163, 1991. *Reviews of the two varieties of* C. neoformans *(var.* neoformans *and var.* gattii*) with emphasis on their distribution in nature and epidemiologic characteristics of patients infected.*

Powderly WG: Cryptococcal meningitis and AIDS. Clin Infect Dis 17:837, 1993. *Focuses on clinical and laboratory features as well as different treatment options, including primary therapy for acute disease and maintenance therapy to prevent relapse.*

Powderly WG, Saag MS, Cloud GA, et al.: A controlled trial of fluconazole or amphotericin B to prevent relapse of cryptococcal meningitis in patients with the acquired immunodeficiency syndrome. N Engl J Med 326:793, 1992. *The definitive trial showing that daily fluconazole is superior to weekly intravenous amphotericin B as maintenance preventive therapy in AIDS-associated cryptococcosis.*

Rex JH, Larsen RA, Dismukes WE, et al.: Catastrophic visual loss due to *Cryptococ-*

cus neoformans meningitis. Medicine (Baltimore) 72:207, 1993. *A thorough review of 49 cases with emphasis on pathogenesis, natural history, and management of this devastating complication of cryptococcal meningitis.*

Saag MS, Powderly WG, Cloud GA, et al.: Comparison of amphotericin B with fluconazole in the treatment of acute AIDS-associated cryptococcal meningitis. N Engl J Med 326:83, 1992. *A large clinical trial indicating that fluconazole is an effective alternative to amphotericin B as primary treatment of cryptococcal meningitis in AIDS.*

353 SPOROTRICHOSIS
William E. Dismukes

DEFINITION. Sporotrichosis is a chronic mycotic disease that typically involves skin, subcutaneous tissue, and regional lymphatics as a result of cutaneous inoculation of *Sporothrix schenckii.* Extracutaneous disease secondary to either lymphohematogenous dissemination or inhalation of organisms is rare.

SPOROTRICHOSIS

Causative fungus	*Sporothrix schenckii.*
Primary geographic distribution	Worldwide, mainly in temperate and tropical areas
Primary route of acquisition	Cutaneous inoculation
Principal sites of disease	Skin, lymphatics; less commonly, lungs and joints
Opportunistic infection in compromised hosts	Infrequent
Drug of choice for most patients	Itraconazole
Alternative therapy	Cutaneous disease: saturated solution potassium iodide, fluconazole, or surgery
	Excutaneous disease: amphotericin B

ETIOLOGY. *S. schenckii* is a dimorphic fungus that grows in nature and in the laboratory on Sabouraud's agar as a white mold, which, with time, becomes brownish black. In tissue and at 37°C, the organism exists as yeastlike cells, which appear as round, spherical, or cigar-shaped budding forms, 2 to 6 μm in size.

EPIDEMIOLOGY. Sporotrichosis is worldwide in distribution. *S. schenckii* appears to be ubiquitous in soil and in both living and decaying vegetation. Although the organism does not appear to infect plants, it may infect animals, especially cats and dogs, as well as humans, especially those who frequently handle or come in contact with mulch, sphagnum moss, hay, timber, and thorny bushes. Consequently, sporotrichosis is considered an occupational disease of certain groups, including farmers, nursery or forestry workers, gardeners, florists, landscapers, and carpenters. In 1988, the largest known epidemic of sporotrichosis in the United States occurred among 84 forestry workers exposed to sphagnum moss obtained from a single source. Transmission almost always results from the percutaneous introduction of organisms. In the majority of patients with extracutaneous disease, the route of acquisition is unclear. Rarely, pulmonary sporotrichosis may result from inhalation of aerosolized conidia. Although person-to-person transmission is not known to occur, transmission from animals, especially cats, to humans has been documented. The number of cases of cutaneous disease in males and females is similar; gender and age appear to play less of a role than does environmental exposure. By contrast, extracutaneous sporotrichosis is more common in males. *S. schenckii* is not considered an opportunistic fungal pathogen, although sporotrichosis in compromised hosts is being increasingly recognized. For example, cases have been observed in HIV-infected persons.

PATHOGENESIS AND PATHOLOGY. Cutaneous inoculation may follow either inapparent or obvious penetrating trauma. In the majority of patients, clinical disease does not extend beyond the site of inoculation or the draining lymphatics. Localized disease may persist for years, and cell-mediated immunity appears to be responsible for preventing or limiting the spread to extracutaneous sites. Conversely, multiorgan disease involving skin and distant sites, such as lungs, bones, and joints, is more common in immunosuppressed hosts.

The basic histopathologic pattern in cutaneous sporotrichosis is a combination of suppuration and granulomas, often accompanied by pseudoepitheliomatous hyperplasia. This pattern is not diagnostic, as it may also be seen in malignancy as well as other fungal diseases, such as blastomycosis, coccidioidomycosis, and chromomycosis. Because the yeastlike cells, typical of *S. schenckii,* are uncommonly identified in tissue sections, cultural confirmation is usually necessary for diagnosis. The finding of large asteroid bodies (radiate eosinophilic material surrounding fungal yeast cells) provides presumptive evidence of sporotrichosis.

CLINICAL MANIFESTATIONS. Two distinctive clinical forms of cutaneous and extracutaneous disease, which differ in management and prognosis, are seen.

Cutaneous. This form of sporotrichosis can be further divided into two types: plaque (or fixed) and lymphocutaneous. Plaque sporotrichosis, which is less common, consists of a single ulcerative or nodular lesion at the site of primary inoculation, usually on an exposed extremity or the face. The lesion begins as a small painless red papule, which gradually enlarges and finally ulcerates (sporotrichotic chancre). A violaceous hue and intermittent serosanguineous drainage are characteristic. Lymphocutaneous sporotrichosis, which is the more typical type and is found in about 75% of cases, represents an extension of the primary lesion. Subcutaneous nontender nodular lesions appear proximally along thickened lymphatics over days to weeks and occasionally ulcerate. Lymph nodes are rarely enlarged. Similarly, constitutional symptoms, such as fever and chills, are usually absent. This type of sporotrichosis, which usually remains confined to the primary site and its regional lymphatics, may wax and wane over years if untreated. Lymphohematogenous spread to distant organs is uncommon.

Extracutaneous. The pathogenesis of the majority of cases of extracutaneous sporotrichosis is uncertain because most cases are not accompanied by clinically apparent cutaneous disease. The skeletal system is the most commonly involved extracutaneous organ. Although indolent monarticular arthritis of the knees, ankles, wrists, and elbows is most frequent, osteomyelitis (especially of the tibia), tenosynovitis, and carpal tunnel syndrome have been reported. Multiarticular arthritis is more likely in compromised hosts with widespread hematogenous spread to multiple organs. Pulmonary sporotrichosis is far less common than osteoarticular disease. Fewer than 100 cases of pulmonary disease have been reported. This form of insidious infection occurs primarily in older male alcoholics and mimics reactivation tuberculosis. Thin-walled cavitary lesions in a single upper lobe are characteristic; bilateral fibrocavitary disease may be seen occasionally. Extrapulmonary spread of disease is uncommon. Ocular sporotrichosis results from traumatic inoculation of the conjunctiva or cornea; endophthalmitis is unusual. Chronic lymphocytic meningitis may be a complication of sporotrichosis, even in the absence of obvious extraneural disease. In any patient with chronic meningitis of unknown origin, cerebrospinal fluid (CSF) should be tested for antibody to *S. schenckii.*

DIAGNOSIS. As a rule, the diagnosis of sporotrichosis must be based on cultural demonstration of the organism in tissue or fluid obtained from involved sites, e.g., skin, subcutaneous nodule, joint, or lung. Histopathologic findings are usually nonspecific, and the characteristic yeastlike cells are often not identified by special stains such as Gomori methenamine silver or periodic acid–Schiff. Direct immunofluorescence, if available, may be helpful. Although testing of serum or CSF by latex agglutination or enzyme immunoassay for antibody to *S. schenckii* may be useful, especially in patients suspected of having extracutaneous disease, positive low-level antibody titers may be observed in normal persons. No skin test is commercially available.

TREATMENT. Conventional therapy for cutaneous sporotrichosis is saturated solution of potassium iodide, which is begun at a dosage of 5 drops three times a day and increased dropwise (3 to 5 drops per day) up to a maximum of 120 drops per day or until the development of iodine toxicity (manifested by rash, lacrimation, parotid swelling, or nonspecific gastrointestinal symptoms). Iodide therapy should be continued for at least 1 month after clinical resolution of the disease. Itraconazole in a dosage of 100 to 400 mg per day is an attractive alternative to iodide therapy for cutaneous sporotrichosis. Itraconazole is more effective than the other two oral azoles, ketoconazole and fluconazole, and better tolerated than potassium iodide. In addition, itraconazole (200 to 400 mg per day) is moderately effective in treating extracutaneous sporotrichosis. Amphotericin B should be reserved for patients with cutaneous or extracutaneous disease in whom iodide or azole therapy fails, and as therapy for immunocompromised patients with severe, life-threatening, widely disseminated sporotrichosis. In the latter group of patients, consideration may be given to switching to itraconazole after a successful induction course of amphotericin B. Cure rates may be improved in selected patients with bone and joint disease or single-cavity pulmonary disease by surgical resection of synovial tissue, bone, or lung, as an adjunct to antifungal therapy. Intra-articular amphotericin B may also be useful.

PROGNOSIS. Although untreated cutaneous sporotrichosis may remit and relapse for years, and rarely disseminate, the likelihood of cure with iodide or itraconazole therapy is high. In contrast, extracutaneous disease is more refractory, even to therapy including itraconazole, amphotericin B, and surgery; significant morbidity and mortality are frequent sequelae.

Calhoun DL, Waskin H, White MP, et al.: Treatment of systemic sporotrichosis with ketoconazole. Rev Infect Dis 13:47, 1991. *Oral ketoconazole was moderately effective in 11 patients with deep-seated sporotrichosis; durable responses were associated with prolonged treatment.*

Dixon DM, Salkin IF, Duncan RA, et al.: Isolation and characterization of *Sporothrix schenckii* from clinical and environmental sources associated with the largest U.S. epidemic of sporotrichosis. J Clin Microbiol 29:6, 1991. *A detailed microbiologic analysis of 21 clinical and 69 environmental isolates of* S. schenckii *associated with this sporotrichosis outbreak (84 cases).*

Sharkey-Mathis PK, Kauffman CA, Graybill JR, et al.: Treatment of sporotrichosis with itraconazole. Am J Med 95:279, 1993. *Results of this multicenter study in 27 patients show that itraconazole is effective and well-tolerated for lymphocutaneous and extracutaneous sporotrichosis.*

354 CANDIDIASIS
William E. Dismukes

DEFINITION. *Candida* species can cause a variety of clinical syndromes that are generically termed candidiasis and are usually categorized by site of involvement. Broadly speaking, the two most common syndromes are mucocutaneous candidiasis (e.g., stomatitis or thrush, esophagitis, and vaginitis) and invasive or deep organ candidiasis (e.g., fungemia, endocarditis, and endophthalmitis). In most patients, candidiasis is an opportunistic disease.

CANDIDIASIS

Causative fungus	*Candida* species (*C. albicans* most common)
Primary geographic distribution	Worldwide; part of normal flora of humans and in environment
Primary route of acquisition	Endogenous; person-to-person
Principal sites of disease	Mucous membranes (oropharynx, vagina), skin, esophagus, blood, liver, spleen, kidneys, eyes, heart
Opportunistic infection in compromised hosts	Frequent; e.g., mucosal disease in AIDS patients and deep organ disease in granulocytopenic patients
Drug(s) of choice for most patients	Mucosal disease: topical or oral azole drug (clotrimazole or fluconazole)
	Deep organ disease: amphotericin B or fluconazole
Alternative therapy for deep organ disease	Amphotericin B plus flucytosine

ETIOLOGY. Among more than 150 recognized species of *Candida, C. albicans* is the most commonly identified pathogen in humans. Other clinically important species include *C. tropicalis, C. parapsilosis, C. krusei, C. pseudotropicalis,* and *C. guilliermondi. Candida* organisms share two morphologic features: small, spherical yeast forms (4 to 6 μm), which reproduce by budding; and pseudohyphae (pseudomycelia), which are chains of elongated yeasts separated by constrictions. In body fluids or tissue, both budding cells and fragments of pseudohyphae may be visualized. Identification and speciation in the microbiology laboratory are based on both morphologic characteristics and results of metabolic tests. The ability of *C. albicans* to produce germ tubes in serum allows presumptive identification. *Torulopsis glabrata,* the most commonly encountered pathogenic species in the genus *Torulopsis,* resembles the yeast forms of other *Candida* species; because it does not produce a pseudomycelial form, *T. glabrata* is generally not considered a member of the genus *Candida.*

EPIDEMIOLOGY. Candidiasis occurs worldwide. *C. albicans* is part of the normal human flora of the mouth, gastrointestinal tract, and vagina; normally lives in balance with other microorganisms in the body; and, in most individuals, exists as a saprophytic colonizer or commensal. When various drugs or conditions, such as broad-spectrum antibiotics, corticosteroids, diabetes mellitus, or human immunodeficiency virus (HIV) infection, upset this balance, endogenous *C. albicans* may become a pathogen and cause either mucocutaneous or deep disease. *C. albicans* may also be recovered from soil, hospital environments, food, and other substrates. In contrast to *C. albicans,* the other *Candida* species that are pathogenic for humans less frequently colonize the skin, gastrointestinal tract, or vagina of normal individuals. These species more often reside in the environment and on inanimate objects and thus reach the body from exogenous sources; consequently, they are generally regarded as opportunistic fungal pathogens. Unlike other fungi, *Candida* species may be transmitted from person to person, e.g., between sexual partners, by hands of medical personnel, and during birth from colonized vagina to neonatal oropharynx.

Candidiasis, both mucocutaneous and deep forms, has emerged as the most common opportunistic fungal disease, owing to the progressively increasing use of antibiotics (both prophylactic and therapeutic); immunosuppressive and cytotoxic drugs; indwelling foreign bodies, including prosthetic heart valves, prosthetic joints, and intravascular monitoring devices; venous, arterial, urinary, and peritoneal catheters; and organ transplantation. In addition, the AIDS epidemic has been highly contributory.

PATHOGENESIS AND PATHOLOGY. Several components of the host defense system are important in protecting against infection with *Candida* species. An intact integumentary barrier, including skin and mucous membranes, prevents invasion of normally colonizing organisms, which possess adherence properties as yet not fully understood. *C. albicans* and *C. tropicalis* appear to be more adherent than other species, accounting in part for the frequency of these organisms as pathogens. Disruption or loss of normal barriers as a consequence of percutaneous catheters, endotracheal tubes, severe burns, or abdominal surgery is a common predisposing factor, especially to deep invasive or disseminated disease. Polymorphonuclear leukocytes and monocytes are the major cellular defenses against *Candida* species; intracellular killing largely depends on the myeloperoxidase, hydrogen peroxide, and superoxide anion systems. Although the role of tissue macrophages is unclear, lymphocytes and cell-mediated immunity appear to play a role. Abnormalities of host defense include T-cell dysfunction, which predisposes to mucocutaneous disease (oropharyngeal or esophageal candidiasis in HIV-infected persons as well as chronic mucocutaneous candidiasis), and granulocytopenia secondary to underlying disease or therapy, which predisposes to deep disease (candidemia or invasive candidiasis). In cutaneous candidiasis, histopathologic evidence of chronic dermatitis with yeasts confined to the stratum corneum is characteristic. By contrast, microabscesses interspersed in normal tissue are the characteristic pathologic finding in visceral candidiasis. Neutrophils appear initially, followed by histiocytes and giant cells and, in some cases, a readily apparent granulomatous response. In severely immunocompromised patients, the inflammatory response may be minimal or absent. Both yeasts and pseudohyphae can usually be visualized by special stains, such as periodic acid–Schiff or Gomori-methenamine-silver.

CLINICAL MANIFESTATIONS. Mucocutaneous Infections.

Thrush or oropharyngeal candidiasis is manifested by creamy white curdlike exudative patches on the tongue, buccal mucosa, palate, or other oral mucosal surfaces. These patches are actually pseudomembranes, which, upon removal, may leave a raw, bleeding, painful surface. Poorly fitting dentures may be a predisposing factor, and areas of erythema may be the only marker of disease. Cheilosis, an inflammatory reaction at the corners of the mouth, and atrophic changes, either acute or chronic, are less common presentations of oropharyngeal disease. Esophagitis, which may occur as an extension of thrush or may occur in the absence of thrush in up to one third of patients, is manifested typically by odynophagia, dysphagia, or substernal chest pain and uncommonly by bleeding. Thrush or esophagitis, occurring in the absence of any known predisposing condition, should raise the suspicion of HIV infection. Gastrointestinal candidiasis involving the mucosa of the stomach and small and large bowel is most common in patients with cancer and is an important source of disseminated infection.

Intertrigo, a cutaneous *Candida* infection involving warm, moist surfaces, such as the axillae, gluteal and inframammary folds, and groin, may be variable in appearance but is usually manifested as well-marginated, erythematous, exudative patches surrounded by satellite vesicles or pustules. Paronychia, a painful, tense, reddened swelling at the base of the nail or along the sides, is commonly caused by *Candida* species, especially in diabetics and persons whose hands are chronically immersed in water. Although *Candida* species may cause onychomycosis, this chronic deforming infection of the nails is most frequently due to one of the genera of superficial dermatophytes, such as *Trichophyton* or *Epidermophyton*. Vulvovaginitis, probably the most common *Candida* mucocutaneous infection in women, especially in association with pregnancy, oral contraceptives, antibiotic therapy, diabetes, and HIV infection, is characterized by thick, creamy vaginal discharge, erythematous labia, and intense pruritus. Balanitis in males, often acquired through sexual intercourse, is manifested by superficial vesicles and exudative patches, usually on the glans penis. *Candida* cystitis, which at cystoscopy resembles oral thrush, is most often a complication of an indwelling bladder catheter. Chronic mucocutaneous candidiasis, a rare condition manifested by a heterogeneous group of persistent, often disfiguring *Candida* infections involving skin, mucous membranes, hair, and nails, occurs primarily in persons with altered T-cell function or an endocrinopathy such as hypoparathyroidism or hypoadrenalism.

Deep Organ Candidiasis.

Numerous diagnostic categories or labels for serious or deep *Candida* infection exist, including candidemia, disseminated candidiasis, systemic candidiasis, invasive candidiasis, visceral candidiasis, and terms indicating involvement of specific organs, such as hepatosplenic candidiasis and ocular candidiasis. Here, discussion focuses on two major categories: candidemia, which may or may not be associated with visceral organ involvement; and disseminated candidiasis, which implies systemic multiorgan disease and encompasses other subgroups, such as visceral, invasive, and hepatosplenic disease.

Candidemia. Candidemia, which is usually defined as one or more positive blood cultures for *Candida* species, may occur in the presence or absence of clinical manifestations, e.g., fever or skin lesions. The incidence of candidemia has risen dramatically over recent years in association with the increased number of compromised hosts (e.g., those with AIDS, cancer, or burns, those in the postsurgical intensive care unit, and organ transplant recipients) managed by aggressive interventions, including empiric antibiotics, cytotoxic chemotherapy, hemodialysis, intravenous and intra-arterial catheters, other intravascular devices, and parenteral alimentation. In many hospitals, *Candida* has become one of the three to five most common microorganisms isolated from blood cultures. Previously, "transient candidemia" was used to imply short duration (< 24 hours) of fungemia and indicate either clearing of the candidemia upon removal of an infected intravascular catheter or a benign condition not requiring antifungal therapy. Recent data argue against this concept and suggest that catheter removal alone is in-

sufficient, even in the noncompromised patient, to prevent metastatic hematogenous dissemination to visceral organs. Accordingly, most investigators now believe that all patients with candidemia, regardless of duration or circumstances, deserve some form of antifungal treatment. Controversy at present centers on which drug, at what dose, and for how long (see Treatment below).

C. albicans is the most common species identified in blood. Studies from multiple medical centers indicate that *C. tropicalis* is a likely pathogen in the leukemic population, while *C. parapsilosis* fungemia occurs frequently in patients with solid tumor or nononcologic diseases, especially in association with cannula-related sepsis and hyperalimentation. *T. glabrata* resembles *C. parapsilosis* in its predilection for patients with solid tumors or nononcologic disorders.

Cannulas of various types are the most important portals of entry, accounting for more than one half of the episodes of candidemia. In almost all cases, removing cannulas, either peripheral or central, is necessary to eradicate candidemia. Other common sites of infection are the gastrointestinal tract, especially in granulocytopenic patients, and surgical wounds. The urinary and respiratory tracts, although frequently colonized by *Candida* species, are less common sources of bloodstream infection. The mortality rate of candidemia caused by all species is high, ranging from 40 to 80%. Mortality is significantly associated with a high APACHE II score, a rapidly fatal underlying disease, and sustained candidemia. The mortality rate in cannula-associated candidemia is lower than in candidemia related to other sources.

The frequency with which candidemia results in localized single-organ disease (e.g., ocular candidiasis) or widespread disseminated multiorgan disease is 20 to 40%. Premortem diagnosis of invasive or disseminated candidiasis must be based on histopathologic demonstration of *Candida* organisms invading tissue. Because blood cultures are negative in at least 50% of patients with disseminated candidiasis and there are no other reliable markers, such as serologic tests, disseminated *Candida* disease may not be suspected and appropriate invasive diagnostic procedures may not be performed. Autopsy series indicate that disseminated disease involving kidneys, liver, spleen, brain, myocardium, and eyes is most likely in patients with some rapidly fatal underlying disease, such as leukemia complicated by neutropenia, and is least likely in patients with candidemia in the setting of nononcologic disease, especially cannula-related sepsis. In addition, patients whose candidemia is treated are less likely to develop disseminated disease.

Cutaneous Lesions of Disseminated Candidiasis. Papulopustules or macronodules on an erythematous base, usually widely distributed over the trunk and extremities, are the hallmark lesions associated with persistent candidemia. Hemorrhagic bullae have also been reported.

Ocular Candidiasis. This form of localized candidiasis may result from either hematogenous spread or direct inoculation, e.g., after cataract extraction or intraocular lens implantation. Any eye structure may be infected; endophthalmitis is the most fulminant manifestation and may result in blindness. Single or multiple fluffy white cotton ball–like chorioretinal lesions, often extending into the vitreous, are characteristic. These lesions can be easily recognized on funduscopic examination and should be serially looked for in all patients with known candidemia.

Renal Candidiasis. Infection of the kidneys may be secondary to ascending extension from the bladder (*Candida* cystitis), resulting in papillary necrosis, caliceal invasion, or formation of a fungus ball in the ureter or renal pelvis. More commonly, renal candidiasis is secondary to hematogenous spread, in patients with either documented or undocumented candidemia, resulting in pyelonephritis with diffuse cortical and medullary abscesses. The triad of candidemia, candiduria, and *Candida* organisms within casts in urinary sediment provides presumptive evidence of upper urinary tract involvement.

Hepatosplenic Candidiasis. This visceral form of deep infection occurs most commonly in patients with hematologic malignancies, especially leukemia, who are in remission after prolonged chemotherapy-induced neutropenia. Gastrointestinal candidiasis complicated by portal fungemia is the source in most patients; documented candidemia or evidence of disease in other organs is usually absent. Persistent unexplained fever, right upper quadrant tenderness and pain, elevated alkaline phosphatase levels and multiple, scattered "bull's eye" lesions in the liver and spleen, demonstrated by abdominal ultrasonographic examination or computed tomography (CT), are features. Diagnosis is established by characteristic histopathology on liver biopsy.

Pulmonary Candidiasis. Whereas colonization by yeasts of the tracheobronchial tree is common in seriously ill, debilitated intensive care unit patients on ventilators, *bona fide* pneumonia caused by *Candida* species is rare. Diagnosis should be based on histopathologic evidence of yeast invasion.

Cardiac Candidiasis. Disseminated candidiasis is complicated frequently by *Candida* myocarditis (>50% of cases) and occasionally by *Candida* pericarditis. *Candida* is the most common cause of fungal endocarditis and should be suspected in the setting of indwelling cardiac prostheses, intravenous drug abuse, and prolonged use of central intravenous catheters for chemotherapy, hyperalimentation, or hemodynamic monitoring. Because fungal valvular vegetations are large and friable, major embolic events involving the central nervous system (CNS), coronary arteries, and large peripheral arteries are common.

Central Nervous System Candidiasis. Meningitis and intracerebral microabscesses as well as macroabscesses frequently complicate disseminated candidiasis. Cerebrospinal fluid pleocytosis, most often lymphocytic, hypoglycorrhachia, and elevated protein levels are typical; yeast organisms can be identified by wet preparation, Gram stain, or culture, in fewer than one half of cases. *Candida* meningitis may be a complication of ventricular shunt infection.

Musculoskeletal Candidiasis. Manifestations include myositis (abscess) in neutropenic patients and costochondritis, arthritis, and osteomyelitis (special predilection for vertebrae and intervertebral discs) in intravenous drug users. All of these complications may develop in any patient with disseminated candidiasis, whatever the setting or source.

DIAGNOSIS. Mucocutaneous lesions are diagnosed on the basis of clinical appearance and by examination of potassium hydroxide wet mounts or Gram-stained smears of lesion material obtained by scraping or swabbing. Masses of spherical budding yeast forms and pseudohyphae are characteristic. Patients suspected of having *Candida* esophagitis should undergo not only endoscopy and brushing but also biopsy in an attempt to histopathologically demonstrate mucosal invasion of *Candida* organisms. Esophagitis caused by either herpes simplex virus or cytomegalovirus may mimic the symptoms and appearance of *Candida* esophagitis; infection in a single patient caused by more than one microorganism is not unusual. Fungal blood cultures in patients with suspected candidemia or disseminated candidiasis should be performed using the highly sensitive lysis centrifugation method; this technique also allows more rapid detection of growth. Multiple serial cultures should be obtained. Data gathered over the past decade indicate that a single positive blood culture for *Candida* species should be assumed to represent clinically significant candidemia that merits antifungal therapy. The finding of heavy growth of *Candida* species in cultures of sputum, tracheal aspirate, wounds, or urine may increase the likelihood of bloodstream invasion but does not prove that dissemination has occurred. Because blood cultures may be negative in as many as 50% of patients with disseminated candidiasis, diagnosis must often depend on the results of histopathologic study and fungal cultures of tissue obtained by biopsy. Diagnostic procedures that should be considered include CT of the head, thorax, and abdomen; echocardiography; thoracentesis; arthrocentesis; lumbar puncture; and biopsy of skin, liver, kidney, myocardium, bone, muscle, or lung. Although quantitative or semiquantitative cultures of selected tissue specimens have been advocated as useful predictors of disseminated disease, no correlative data support this concept. Skin testing with *Candida* antigen may be useful in assessing for anergy but has no role in diagnosing candidiasis. Although much effort has been devoted to the development of reliable, simple, sensitive, and specific serologic assays for detecting serum antibodies to *Candida,* circulating *Candida* antigen (e.g., cell wall mannan or cytoplasmic enolase), or a metabolite, controversy persists about the value of these serodiagnostic procedures. Because false-positive and false-negative results are common, the decision to initiate treatment cannot be based on results of serologic tests alone. Over the past decade, numerous strain-typing methods have been developed to assist in the epidemiologic investigation and control of *Candida* species as nosocomial pathogens. Examples of older phenotypic methods include biochemical markers, isoenzyme patterns, sensitivity toward killer yeasts, and serotyping; newer genotypic methods include electrophoretic karyotyping, DNA probes, restriction endonuclease analysis of genomic DNA, restriction fragment length polymorphism, and random amplified polymorphic DNA. At present, the genotypic typing methods appear to be the most practical and sensitive means of discriminating strains of *Candida* species.

TREATMENT. In most patients with mucocutaneous infections, any one of several topical preparations, including nystatin, clotrimazole, miconazole, econazole, and ketoconazole, provides effective therapy. Nystatin suspension and clotrimazole troches appear to be equal in efficacy as therapy for oral thrush, but clotrimazole is better tolerated. Although the clinical manifestations of *Candida* vulvovaginitis are usually eliminated by local topical therapy with nystatin, clotrimazole, butoconazole, terconazole, or miconazole administered for 3 to 7 days, the disease tends to recur frequently in some patients. Newer approaches to acute vulvovaginitis use single-dose therapy, e.g., clotrimazole, 500-mg vaginal pessary; miconazole, 1200-mg ovule; or fluconazole, 150-mg oral tablet. In refractory cases, prolonged therapy with a topical agent or an orally absorbed azole, such as ketoconazole or fluconazole, provided that pregnancy has been excluded, may be beneficial. Oral ketoconazole, 200 to 400 mg daily, is the treatment of choice for chronic mucocutaneous candidiasis and must be continued indefinitely to avoid relapse. HIV-infected patients with mucocutaneous forms of candidiasis respond less rapidly than other patient groups and often with incomplete clearance of exudative patches. Nystatin suspension appears to be less effective than either clotrimazole troches or an oral drug, e.g., ketoconazole or fluconazole, in AIDS patients with oropharyngeal or esophageal candidiasis. Fluconazole appears to be more effective than ketoconazole. However, recent clinical microbiologic and epidemiologic data indicate an emerging problem of resistance to fluconazole among AIDS patients with oral thrush who are exposed either to repeated short courses of low-dose fluconazole therapy (50 to 100 mg daily) or prolonged prophylactic therapy. Although cross-resistance may develop to itraconazole, this triazole has been an effective therapeutic alternative in many patients with fluconazole-resistant disease. In refractory cases associated with severe disease and/or fluconazole-resistance, low-dose amphotericin B can be used.

Recent studies have established important guidelines regarding therapy of serious *Candida* disease, e.g., candidemia or disseminated candidiasis. First, in most patients with catheter-related candidemia, the catheter, if still present, should be removed. Second, in patients with suppurative peripheral thrombophlebitis, surgical segmental venous resection is necessary. Third, because of the high risk of metastatic complications of candidemia, such as endophthalmitis, osteomyelitis, arthritis, nephritis, myocarditis, and endocarditis, all patients with candidemia, even non-neutropenic hosts, deserve a course of antifungal chemotherapy. For patients with candidemia, both amphotericin B and fluconazole are effective in selected populations. Fluconazole, 400 mg daily for 14 days (initial intravenous therapy followed by oral therapy), should be reserved primarily for non-neutropenic patients with catheter-associated candidemia. Amphotericin B, 0.5 to 0.8 mg per kilogram per day for 7 to 14 days, should usually be given to compromised hosts, especially those who are granulocytopenic, patients with persistent candidemia (whatever the cause), and patients with septic shock syndrome due to *Candida* species. Until additional guidelines are forthcoming from ongoing prospective studies, the decisions regarding which drug to use and at what dosage must be based on the host defense status of the patient, underlying conditions, predisposing factors, and results of serial blood cultures and physical examinations for complications of candidemia.

Patients with documented disseminated disease, manifested as either localized deep disease (e.g., hepatosplenic candidiasis, CNS candidiasis, renal candidiasis, or *Candida* endocarditis) or multiorgan disease, should be treated with amphotericin B (total dose 2.0 to 3.0 grams), often in combination with flucytosine (75 to 125 mg per kilogram per day). Fluconazole may have a role in the therapy of hepatosplenic candidiasis, either as primary therapy or consolidation therapy after an initial course of amphotericin B, with or without flucytosine. Valve replacement is a necessary adjunct to chemotherapy in patients with *Candida* endocarditis.

Candida cystitis, in contrast to renal candidiasis, can be cured by removing the bladder catheter in the majority of cases. Therapeutic options available for managing candiduria that is persistent after catheter removal or in diabetic patients include oral flucytosine, 75 to 100 mg per kilogram per day for 7 to 10 days, or oral fluconazole, 100 to 200 mg per day for 7 to 10 days. Although both of these antifungal agents are excreted by the kidneys, fluconazole is preferred because it is less toxic. Eradicating candiduria in patients whose condition justifies a persistent indwelling catheter can be attempted with amphotericin B (50 μg per milliliter) or miconazole (50 μg per milliliter) bladder rinses.

Therapy for *Candida* peritonitis, which most often is a complication of continuous ambulatory peritoneal dialysis, is less straightforward. Ideally, the peritoneal catheter should be discontinued, and either intravenous amphotericin B or oral fluconazole should be administered until clinical symptoms and signs resolve and cultures become negative. For patients in whom the catheter must be maintained, instilling either amphotericin B or fluconazole in the dialysate fluid, has been successful.

Managing ocular candidiasis requires close cooperation with an ophthalmologist experienced in eye infections. For most cases of endophthalmitis, systemic amphotericin B with or without flucytosine plus vitrectomy to remove vitreous abscesses is required. Findings at vitrectomy may also be used to confirm the diagnosis. Data, largely from animal models, provide conflicting results about the efficacy of azole drugs as therapy of *Candida* endophthalmitis.

PREVENTION. Given the increasing incidence of nosocomial candidemia and its potential severity, awareness of the problem and measures aimed at prevention assume increasing importance. The frequency and duration of use of intravascular catheters and monitoring devices should be reduced, and subclavian central catheters should be changed at least weekly. Special attention should be paid to long-term access devices for chemotherapy such as Hickman or Broviac catheters. Similarly, the frequency, breadth, and duration of courses of antibiotics should be reduced. Antifungal drugs are commonly used in seriously ill hospitalized patients, especially those with granulocytopenia, to prevent *Candida* infection. Although fluconazole, the drug most commonly used, appears to be more beneficial in bone marrow transplant recipients than in patients with acute leukemia (see references), several concerns persist. Widespread injudicious use of oral azoles in prophylaxis does not offer protection against natively resistant pathogenic fungi (*Aspergillus* species, *Mucorales*, *Fusarium* species, *C. krusei*, and *T. glabrata*), and it may increase the likelihood of emergence of resistant organisms and may not be cost-effective.

Edwards JE Jr, Filler SG: Current strategies for treating invasive candidiasis: Emphasis on infections in nonneutropenic patients. Clin Infect Dis 14(suppl 1):S106, 1992. *A thoughtful perspective on the various approaches to serious* Candida *disease, including data to support each approach.*

Fraser VJ, Jones M, Dunkel J, et al.: Candidemia in a tertiary care hospital: Epidemiology, risk factors, and predictors of mortality. Clin Infect Dis 15:414, 1992. *Detailed univariate and multivariate analyses of the risk factors and predictors of mortality among 106 patients with candidemia over a one-year period. Of 30 patients who did not receive antifungal therapy, 19 (63%) died.*

Goodman JL, Winston DJ, Greenfield RA, et al.: A controlled trial of fluconazole to prevent fungal infections in patients undergoing bone marrow transplantation. N Engl J Med 326:845, 1992; Winston DJ, Chandrasekar PH, Lazarus HM, et al.: Fluconazole prophylaxis of fungal infection in patients with acute leukemia: Results of a randomized placebo-controlled, double-blind, multicenter trial. Ann Intern Med 118:495, 1993. *The first trial in bone marrow transplant recipients showed that fluconazole (400 mg per day) was more effective than placebo in preventing both superficial and systemic fungal infections, but overall mortality between the two treatment groups was not significantly different. By contrast, in the second trial in patients with acute leukemia, the same dose of fluconazole did not decrease the frequency of invasive fungal disease, reduce the empirical use of amphotericin B, or decrease the mortality rate.*

Lecciones JA, Lee JW, Navarro EE, et al.: Vascular catheter-associated fungemia in patients with cancer: Analysis of 155 episodes. Clin Infect Dis 14:875, 1992. *A retrospective review of central venous catheter–associated fungemia, primarily candidemia, over a 10-year period; results argue strongly for catheter removal.*

Sobel JD: Candidal vulvovaginitis. Clin Obstet Gynecol 36:153, 1993. *A practical overview of the pathogenesis, clinical manifestations, and treatment of this common mucosal infection in women.*

355 ASPERGILLOSIS
David A. Stevens

DEFINITION. Aspergillosis refers to infection with any of the species of the genus *Aspergillus*. These are in mold form in the environment, on artificial media, and when invading tissues.

ASPERGILLOSIS	
Causative fungus	*Aspergillus* species: *A. fumigatus, A. flavus, A. niger, A. terreus*
Primary geographic distribution	Ubiquitous: human habitat, soil, water, air
Primary route of acquisition	Inhaling spores
Principal site of disease	Lung
Opportunistic infection in compromised hosts	Invasive form, pulmonary
Drug of choice for most patients	Amphotericin, itraconazole
Alternative therapy	None

ETIOLOGY AND EPIDEMIOLOGY. Aspergilli are ubiquitous in the environment and have been isolated with ease from soil and air, and even swimming pools and saunas. They are associated with decaying matter and may grow in temperatures of 40 to 50°C, e.g., self-heating organic compost. The ease with which they are isolated from composting materials, silos, and the cooling canals of nuclear power plants has been an environmental and industrial concern. They are easily isolated from houses, particularly from basements, crawl spaces, bedding, humidifiers, ventilation ducts, potted plants, wicker or straw material, and house dust; in surveys they have been found in, for example, condiments, pasta, and marijuana samples. This pervasiveness should not make it surprising that they are sometimes found in normal expectorated sputa. They are important pathogens of insects (of economic importance to beekeepers) and birds, both domesticated and wild, and cause abortion in cattle. As they grow, they produce toxins, such as aflatoxin—one of the most potent carcinogens known—which contaminates the food chain, posing a risk to animals and humans. Their threat to hospitalized patients has been revealed in outbreaks of infection, particularly pulmonary infection in compromised hosts, associated with renovation and new construction. The suspected vector has been unfiltered air, as from inlets contaminated with bird excreta and fireproofing materials.

The most common species infecting humans are *A. fumigatus, A. flavus, A. niger,* and *A. terreus.* Some are speciated by the clinical laboratory only with difficulty, and they may be reported only as "*Aspergillus* species." In tissues they may be seen as septate hyphae, dichotomously branched (resembling the divergence of fingers from one another), and they may produce their characteristic conidia in tissues or artificial media, which is one way to differentiate them. If the septation can be seen, they can be differentiated from the zygomycetes; they may be confused with *Pseudallescheria boydii*, however, unless the characteristic terminal spores of the latter are seen.

Aspergillosis generally results from airborne conidia and is not contagious.

SYNDROMES. The main forms of clinical aspergillosis are shown in Table 355–1.

The *invasive* form of the disease is generally a problem of im-

TABLE 355–1. ASPERGILLOSIS SYNDROMES

Invasive disease	Asthma
Aspergilloma (fungus ball)	Invasive airways disease
Superficial bronchial disease	Bronchocentric granulomatosis
Extrinsic allergic alveolitis	Pleural disease
Mixed forms	Local disease
Allergic bronchopulmonary disease	Endocarditis

munocompromised hosts (see Ch. 266), and more aggressive immunosuppression and anticancer therapy are the most important factors contributing to the rise of *Aspergillus* infections. Series have reported an incidence as high as 41% in those with acute leukemia at autopsy, and in 89% of these cases it played a significant role in the death of the patient. In 97%, pulmonary involvement was present, and in 25%, the infection was disseminated widely to various organs. Similarly, in a group of heart transplant patients, the incidence of infection was 28%. This is also a problem in diabetics and patients with the neutrophil defect of chronic granulomatous disease. Diagnosis is difficult because aspergilli are frequently contaminants in sputum and even in other cultures when handled in the laboratory. In patients with leukemia, there is particularly an association with relapses of the malignancy, and usually three or four of the following factors are present: leukopenia, glucocorticoid therapy, cytotoxic chemotherapy, and broad-spectrum antibacterials. The classic picture is that of fever and pulmonary infiltrates or nodules, especially progressing to a cavity (usually when granulocytopenia is reversed), or wedge-shaped densities resembling infarcts. The pulmonary pathology in all these entities is that of hemorrhagic infarction and pneumonia. Pulmonary emboli are common because of the organism's tendency to invade blood vessel walls. These processes often combine to produce a "target lesion" pathologically, consisting of a necrotic center surrounded by a ring of hemorrhage. The sputum culture is positive in only 8 to 34% of cases, and obtaining tissue is necessary to make the diagnosis. Prospective culturing of the nose of granulocytopenic patients has been of some value, because a positive nasal culture (and particularly the presence of nasal *Aspergillus* lesions) has led to the early diagnosis of concurrent pulmonary or sinus disease. However, negative nasal cultures are common in pulmonary aspergillosis.

Targets of *disseminated disease* include the central nervous system, where abscesses are characteristic. The cerebrospinal fluid (CSF) glucose level is normal, and cultures of the CSF are negative. Mycelia invading blood vessels may produce a microangiopathic hemolytic anemia. Dissemination can result in Budd-Chiari syndrome, myocardial infarction, gastrointestinal disease, or skin lesions. Esophageal ulcers may produce gastrointestinal bleeding. Abscesses are common in the kidney, liver, and myocardium.

Endocarditis is associated with cardiac surgery, particularly prostheses, or intravenous drug abuse. Major arterial emboli occur in 83% of patients, and neurologic presentations are common. Only 8% have positive blood cultures, and this positivity is usually delayed 14 to 20 days, contributing to the poor record of diagnosis ante mortem, which is usually made on histologic examination of an embolus. Overall survival is about 5%, and these individuals have had valve replacement. The disease should be suspected in any post-cardiac surgery patient who presents with endocarditis or emboli and negative blood cultures.

The typical picture of an aspergilloma is a fungus ball (matted hyphae and debris) in a cavity in an upper lobe (Fig. 355–1). This has been reported as a complication in as many as 11% of old tuberculous cavities. The patients present with cough (87%), hemoptysis (81%), dyspnea (61%), weight loss (61%), fatigue (61%), chest pain (31%), or fever (25%). The sputum culture is positive in most. Total immunoglobulin G (IgG) and immunoglobulin A (IgA) levels are elevated. Invasion of the parenchyma is rare.

Pleural disease is associated with tuberculosis and bronchopleural fistulas. It may occur after surgery or spontaneously.

Allergic bronchopulmonary aspergillosis is usually seen superimposed on a background of chronic asthma (see Ch. 51) or cystic fibrosis. It is characterized by episodic airway obstruction, fever, eosinophilia, mucous plugs, positive sputum cultures, and the presence of grossly visible brown flecks in the sputum (hyphae), transient infiltrates and parallel "tram-line" or ring markings on chest radiographs, proximal bronchiectasis, upper lobe contraction, and elevated levels of total IgA and immunoglobulin E (IgE) especially when the patient is symptomatic. It is more common in agricultural areas and in the winter, presumably representing an association with stored agricultural products (especially moldy hay) and spore production. The eosinophilia is present in blood, sputum, and the lung on biopsy. The mucous plugs contain mycelia, and the plugs may be the cause of the infiltrates, with collapse and inflammation occurring peripherally, or inflammatory edema may be responsible. The parallel or ring markings are caused by thickened ectatic bronchi, and the upper lobe changes are a result of progressive apical fibrosis. The infiltrates may be nonsegmental and transient, with a clinical presentation of "eosinophilic pneumonia" and asthma, with eosinophils in blood and sputum; alternatively, they may be segmental, associated with the blocking of bronchi by plugs, and asthma and eosinophilia may be absent. A biphasic skin test response may assist in the diagnosis. A scratch test with *Aspergillus* antigens produces an immediate type I wheal and flare reaction, mediated by IgE and blocked by antihistamines, but not by corticosteroids. An intracutaneous test with the antigens produces a later (6 to 8 hours) Arthus-type reaction, mediated by IgG antibody and complement and blocked by steroids. Similarly, bronchial challenge with the antigens can produce a biphasic response. Immediate, short-lived wheezing may result, reproducing the asthmatic symptoms and associated with increased airways resistance; this can be blocked by β-blockers, antihistamines, and cromolyn, but not by steroids. There may be a later (2 to 6 hours) reaction, of two types. One is increased airways resistance, as described. The other is a restrictive defect occurring peripherally, which may be associated with influenza-like symptoms, fever, leukocytosis, and infiltrates. These reactions are associated with IgG precipitins and are believed to account for some transient infiltrates.

Extrinsic allergic alveolitis is an unusual form of *Aspergillus* lung disease and has been most associated with *A. clavatus* in malt workers. The patients develop a hypersensitivity pneumonitis with dyspnea and fever 4 hours after exposure. Diffuse micronodular infiltrates may be present at the time of symptoms. The patients have IgG precipitins and cell-mediated immune reactions against *Aspergillus* antigens, and granulomas are present on biopsy. Eosinophilia is not a feature. The scratch test is negative, although an intradermal test produces a reaction in 4 hours, with immunoglobulins and complement present on biopsy. Bronchial challenge produces a reaction in 4 hours, with systemic symptoms and a restrictive defect but without airways resistance. The entity can progress to irreversible fibrosis. The same pathophysiology may be involved in episodes following massive inhalation of spores, usually in farm environments. Symptoms are present within 24 hours, and granulomas are found on biopsy.

Superficial bronchial disease, an acute or chronic bronchitis with brown-flecked sputum, *extrinsic asthma* due to airborne conidia, and *bronchocentric granulomatosis,* a peribronchial destructive disease with wheezing or fever and weight loss, are other important pulmonary diseases. The aspergilloma, allergic, alveolitis, and superficial forms rarely progress to invasive disease. However, more *invasive airways disease* with ulcerative, pseudomembranous, or plaquelike tracheobronchitis has been recently described, particularly in immunocompromised hosts, and may presage parenchymal invasion. *Chronic necrotizing pulmonary aspergillosis* is a poorly defined entity that usually occurs in patients with underlying lung disease, often with features of invasive disease and aspergilloma.

Examples of *locally invasive disease* abound and are usually severe. These include invasion of burn wounds, keratitis, external otitis (particularly in the tropics), focal rhinitis (particularly in immunosuppressed and/or granulocytopenic hosts), sinusitis (in these hosts or following dental procedures) and osteomyelitis or endophthalmitis (after fungemia, trauma, or surgery). Cutaneous ulcers have been associated with the use of adhesive tape. Bloodborne dis-

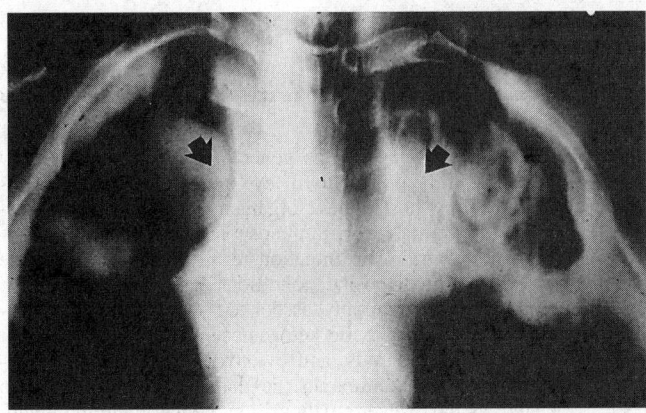

FIGURE 355–1. Tomogram of pulmonary aspergillomas.

ease in addicts can produce foci of dissemination that are similar to those associated with the invasive pulmonary form of the disease. A noninvasive form of sinus disease has a predominantly allergic component and eosinophilia. It is responsive to drainage and corticosteroids.

DIAGNOSIS. Some of the modalities of diagnosis have been mentioned in connection with specific syndromes. Antibody to *Aspergillus* has been detected by a variety of techniques and with a variety of antigen preparations. Data from the more commonly reported techniques suggest a high degree of sensitivity in allergic disease or aspergillomas, but generally a low sensitivity in invasive disease. As the frequency of false-positive reactions, even in the presence of other mycoses, is low, a positive test in invasive disease may be useful. IgE and IgG antibody specific to *Aspergillus* antigens is another serodiagnostic adjunct in allergic disease. Detection of antigenemia and of antigen in bronchoalveolar lavage fluid is also promising in diagnosis of invasive disease. The problem with all serodiagnostic modalities is the lack of a generally available, standardized technique. The physician should know the background data for the laboratory to which the specimens may be sent, i.e., the sensitivity and specificity of the assay in the various syndromes. Serial antibody testing in groups of patients predisposed to aspergillomas (i.e., those with lung cavities), to endocarditis (cardiac surgery patients), or to invasive disease may increase the utility of otherwise problematic serodiagnostic methods.

In severe disease, an aggressive, invasive approach, as well as making a tissue diagnosis early in the illness, appears to be a key to survival. In the appropriate clinical setting, such as an immunocompromised host with fever and a pulmonary infiltrate, repeated isolation of the same species in culture, and particularly a bronchial lavage or other endobronchial culture, correlates with invasive disease; sometimes even a single sputum culture (especially with heavy growth) may have to be the stimulus for therapy if invasive procedures cannot be done. Negative cultures do not rule out invasive disease.

THERAPY AND PREVENTION. In invasive disease, prompt, aggressive chemotherapy has produced superior survival statistics at some institutions, although recovery from neutropenia is a necessary accompaniment of recovery in almost every success. The role of granulocyte transfusions or colony-stimulating factors is unclear. In endocarditis, in addition to prompt, aggressive chemotherapy, valve replacement appears necessary. Locally invasive disease in other sites also requires systemic or local chemotherapy, particularly intravitreal therapy or nephrostomy irrigation in renal disease. Surgical excision has an important role in the invasion of bone, burn wounds, epidural abscesses, vitreal disease, sinus disease of noncompromised hosts, and removal of catheters for peritonitis and of silk sutures in bronchial stump (postpneumonectomy) aspergillosis. It may have a function in invasive pulmonary disease for which chemotherapy has failed.

In cases involving aspergilloma, there is evidence that patients with fever, cough, weight loss, malaise, and hemoptysis have an element of allergy, which can be demonstrated by bronchial challenge or the presence of specific IgG and IgE. These patients symptomatically improve if given glucocorticoids. Intravenous amphotericin B therapy of patients with aspergilloma produces results no better than those with routine pulmonary toilet. Intracavitary amphotericin, instilled through a catheter, is a heroic form of therapy that has been attempted in some patients. The role of surgery in this entity is controversial. Seven to 15% of mycetomas undergo spontaneous lysis. The overall operative mortality aggregated from several series is 7% but may be as high as 14% in some large series. The frequency of various operative complications is 22%, aggregated from several series, with a range of 7 to 60%. Furthermore, new aspergillomas have later developed after surgical successes. On the other hand, in various series, 18 to 26% of patients with adequate follow-up treated without surgery died of disease complications, usually hemoptysis, whereas 50% have shown significant improvement symptomatically and radiographically. If any consensus exists, it is that surgical resection has a role in recurrent, significant hemoptysis. An alternative therapy, particularly for the nonsurgical patient, is selective bronchial arterial embolization to the bleeding vessel.

In pleural disease, locally instilling nystatin, amphotericin, or miconazole has succeeded. In allergic disease, measures that have *not* worked include hyposensitization, avoidance of sites in the environment, and aerosolized corticosteroids. Cromolyn is inadequate in most patients. Aerosolized antifungals have produced remissions but do not prevent recurrences. Treating the clinical disease is more complicated than the effects of drug blockade demonstrable in challenge tests. The continuous use of systemic glucocorticoids can prevent the infiltrates and some accompanying symptoms. Intermittent use of glucocorticoids or raising the dose in patients on chronic therapy can produce rapid resolution of marked symptomatic episodes. The long-term beneficial effects of glucocorticoids are less clear; they are not so useful in arresting dyspnea or wheezing in the long term, and they do not prevent the development of the accompanying bronchiectasis. The proper approach to extrinsic alveolitis is to avoid the stimulus.

For those entities in which systemic chemotherapy is indicated, most clinical experience has been with amphotericin B. Its track record is generally poor in invasive or disseminated disease in compromised hosts (especially so in those with cerebral or hepatic disease or in bone marrow transplant patients). In the compromised host, it should be used aggressively, with prompt progression to a full therapeutic dose, which should be ≥ 1 mg per kilogram per day, if tolerated. Prophylactic therapy may have a role in patients who have survived invasive disease and will become neutropenic again. Rifampin almost always potentiates the activity of amphotericin *in vitro* against aspergilli, whereas results with flucytosine are unpredictable. Moreover, animal models have shown an enhanced effect of combinations of these drugs over that with amphotericin alone. Clinical data to support combination therapy are limited, but given the poor record of amphotericin alone in invasive disease, combination therapy appears a logical avenue to explore, particularly if synergy can be demonstrated. A few cures have been reported in invasive disease with flucytosine (which may have a role in cerebral or renal disease) or miconazole alone. Of the new azole drugs, itraconazole is clearly the most promising and as sole therapy has produced responses in invasive disease. Lipid-complexed amphotericin B and other drugs have demonstrated anti-*Aspergillus* activity *in vitro*, in models, and in some patients and may represent future avenues of exploration. Comparative clinical trials are needed to assess all alternative forms of systemic therapy.

In some centers, prophylaxis of susceptible patients, such as immunocompromised hosts, using intranasal, inhaled, or systemic antifungals, or allergic patients, using inhaled or systemic antifungals, has appeared to be a promising way to avoid disease and the need for therapy. Reducing airborne spores, such as by filtering hospital air and restricting contaminated materials (e.g., potted plants), is believed to be a worthwhile effort for patients who will be transiently immunosuppressed or neutropenic.

Denning DW, Stevens DA: The treatment of invasive aspergillosis. Rev Infect Dis 12:1147, 1990. *Reviews and tabulates data from more than 2000 published cases in 497 articles to give a current picture of therapeutic results.*

Vanden Bossche H, MacKenzie DWR, Cauwenbergh G (eds.): Aspergillus and Aspergillosis. New York, Plenum Press, 1988. *Contains 26 papers by experts on various clinical and microbiologic aspects of aspergillosis.*

356 MUCORMYCOSIS

Sandy F. S. Chun and David A. Stevens

DEFINITION. Mucormycosis is generally an acute and rapidly developing fungal infection caused by fungi of the class Zygomycetes. In healthy hosts, these organisms seldom cause infection. However, in debilitated or immunosuppressed hosts, they produce a fulminant opportunistic infection resulting in marked tissue destruction. Several predisposing conditions have been identified. The infection is most commonly associated with the acidotic patient, especially those in diabetic ketoacidosis. Prolonged treatment with antibiotics, corticosteroids, and cytotoxic drugs and, most recently, the use of deferoxamine in the dialysis patient have also been associated, as have severe malnutrition, hematologic malignancies, and extensive burns.

MUCORMYCOSIS

Causative fungus	The order Mucorales; *Rhizopus, Mucor* species most common
Primary geographic distribution	Ubiquitous: air, bread, fruit, vegetables, soil, manure
Primary route of acquisition	Inhaling spores
Principal sites of disease	Rhinocerebral, pulmonary, cutaneous, gastrointestinal, disseminated, central nervous system (CNS)
Opportunistic infection in compromised hosts	Pulmonary, rhinocerebral
Drug of choice for most patients	Amphotericin B
Alternative therapy	Amphotericin combined with rifampin, azoles, flucytosine

TABLE 356–1. CLINICAL MANIFESTATIONS OF MUCORMYCOSIS

Rhinocerebral	Gastrointestinal
Pulmonary	Widely disseminated
Cutaneous	Central nervous system

THE PATHOGENS. The pathogenic zygomycetes are largely in the order Mucorales, which is related to the term for this infection, mucormycosis. Zygomycosis has also been used to refer to the disease caused by organisms of the class, but that term would include diseases due to fungi of the order Entomophthorales. The latter diseases are different from those caused by the Mucorales (largely superficial infections) and are rare in North America. Phycomycosis is another older term in the literature describing the same infections. The Mucorales are morphologically distinct. Their hyphae are nonseptated, broad, and variable in size and shape. Furthermore, the branching of the hyphae is usually irregular and at right angles. Species of the genera *Rhizopus* and *Mucor* are the common pathogens of this group. Other genera, including *Absidia, Cunninghamella, Rhizomucor, Mortierella, Saksenaea, Syncephalastrum,* and *Apophysomyces,* have also been reported to cause disease. These fungi cannot be differentiated histopathologically. Further speciation requires culturing the pathogen and characterizing the isolates by their morphologic and physiologic features.

EPIDEMIOLOGY. The Mucorales are ubiquitous saprophytic fungi and are abundant in nature. They have been recovered from bread, fruits, vegetables, soil, and manure. These fungi have been isolated from the nose, stool, and sputum of healthy individuals. Despite their widespread distribution, they cause disease infrequently. Fortunately, even in the severely immunocompromised hosts, mucormycosis remains a rare opportunistic infection. The disease is not contagious.

PATHOGENESIS AND PATHOLOGY. Currently, there is no unifying concept of the pathogenesis of mucormycosis. In diseases of the airways (sinus, lung), the infection is presumed to originate from inhaled spores, although the lung may also be involved secondary to bloodstream invasion. Diabetic patients appear to be more frequently colonized. Whereas normal human serum can inhibit their growth, serum obtained from patients with diabetic ketoacidosis is not inhibitory and may even promote fungal growth. Undefined defects of macrophages and neutrophils contribute to the loss of immunity against this infection in the susceptible host. Corticosteroids weaken normal inhibitors of spore germination in tissue. Unlike most pathogenic fungi, these can grow in the absence of oxygen.

Invasion, thrombosis, and necrosis are the characteristic findings in this disease. Once the fungal spores have germinated at the site of infection, the hyphal elements are very aggressive and tend to invade blood vessels, nerves, lymphatics, and tissues. The infarction leads to further tissue hypoxia and acidosis, resulting in a vicious circle enhancing rapid growth and infection. The paucity of a granulomatous reaction is quite characteristic. The fungal hyphae sometimes have little or no inflammation around them.

CLINICAL MANIFESTATIONS. Mucormycosis can be manifested as at least six distinct clinical entities, dependent on the types of predisposing factors of the patient and the portal of entry of the organism (Table 356–1).

Rhinocerebral mucormycosis is the most frequent form of presentation, accounting for more than 75% of the cases in the literature. It commonly affects the poorly controlled diabetic patient who is also in ketoacidosis. It has also been reported in patients with hematologic malignancies who have been neutropenic for an ex-

tended period and who have received broad-spectrum antibacterial drugs or immunosuppressive therapy, in other acidotic patients, and in those with azotemia. This is one of the most rapidly fatal fungal diseases if left undiagnosed. Hyphae invade the paranasal sinuses and palate from the oronasal cavity. From the sinuses, especially the ethmoid sinus, the infection spreads to involve the retro-orbital region or the CNS. Epistaxis, severe unilateral headache, alteration in mental status, and eye symptoms such as lacrimation, irritation, or periorbital anesthesia are common symptoms. Examination of the nose may reveal the classic black necrotic turbinates (too often mistaken for dried blood) or even nasal septum perforation. However, at the early stage of infection, the nasal mucosa may appear only inflamed and friable. Facial cellulitis and palatal necrosis may be seen. The early eye findings include mild proptosis, periorbital edema, decreased visual acuity, or lid swelling. In more advanced orbital involvement, exophthalmos, complete ophthalmoplegia, conjunctival hemorrhage, blindness, fixed and dilated pupil, and corneal anesthesia may be found. These conditions result from fungal invasion of the roof of the orbit, affecting the nerves (third, fourth, and sixth cranial nerves and the ophthalmic branch of the fifth cranial nerve), muscles, and orbital vessels, a condition also known as the "orbital apex syndrome." The infection can spread through the superior orbital fissure or the cribriform plate to involve the brain. Cavernous sinus thrombosis is a frequent complication usually resulting from hematogenous spread from the ophthalmic veins.

This spread leads to additional cranial nerve involvement outside the orbital apex, specifically the trigeminal nerve ganglion and the root of the facial nerve, leading to ipsilateral paresthesia of the face or peripheral facial palsy. Internal carotid artery thrombosis, from retrograde spread from the ophthalmic artery or invasion from the cavernous sinus, is another late complication, leading to cerebral infarction. The middle ear may be involved via the blood, cerebrospinal fluid (CSF), or eustachian tube.

The radiographic manifestations are nonspecific. Plain roentgenograms of the sinuses and orbits may reveal nodular thickening of the mucosa of multiple sinuses, usually without air-fluid levels, or spotty destruction of the bone through the walls of the sinuses or into the orbit. Computed tomography or magnetic resonance imaging is useful in better defining the bone destruction and soft tissue involvement, which could be important in guiding subsequent surgical intervention. The CSF findings are usually nonspecific and often normal even in the presence of CNS involvement. The common findings are pleocytosis, with about 50% polymorphonuclear cells and slight protein elevation; hypoglycorrhachia is rare. Smear and culture of CSF are usually negative for fungus even in cases with documented meningeal involvement. Several infectious diseases can present a similar picture. Black necrotic lesions may also be seen with invasive aspergillosis and with infections by *Pseudomonas aeruginosa* or *Pseudallescheria boydii*. The only definitive method of differentiating between these possibilities is by examination of tissue. Cavernous sinus thrombosis due to *Staphylococcus aureus*, as well as rhinoscleroma, aggressive orbital tumor, midline granuloma, and other fungal infections, can mimic the disease as well.

Pulmonary mucormycosis occurs most frequently in patients with hematologic malignancies being treated with antibacterial drugs or immunosuppressive therapy. The presentation is usually acute, and the patients are often profoundly ill, with variable complaints of cough, fever, and sputum production. There is no specific lobar predilection. Pulmonary vascular thrombosis and infarction are universal findings. No pathognomonic clinical or radiographic findings exist. Sputum culture is usually negative. In fact, ante mortem diagnosis is seldom made because of the acuteness of the illness, the lack of consideration of the diagnosis, and the need for tissue to establish the diagnosis.

Invasive pulmonary aspergillosis or other mycoses, or nocardiosis, other bacterial infections, such as *Pseudomonas* infection, malignant invasion, hemorrhage, or pulmonary embolism and infarction may mimic the presentation of pulmonary mucormycosis.

Cutaneous mucormycosis is rare and is primarily a nosocomial infection in burn and blunt trauma victims. Local infection has also resulted from using contaminated elastic bandages. The involved area is erythematous and painful, with varying degrees of central necrosis that can progress to gangrenous cellulitis. This form of infection can also occur as a result of dissemination from another site of involvement. Skin and subcutaneous infection in diabetics can occur.

Gastrointestinal mucormycosis is the rarest form of infection. It is seen primarily in patients suffering from intrinsic abnormalities of the gastrointestinal tract or severe malnutrition. The infection is thought to arise from fungi entering the body with food. Any part of the gastrointestinal tract is susceptible to infection, with the stomach, terminal ileum, and colon being the most common sites. Wall invasion, ischemic infarction, and ulceration are characteristic. The diagnosis is frequently made at autopsy.

Disseminated mucormycosis is defined as infection occurring in two or more noncontiguous organ systems. The distant sites are infected by bloodstream invasion from a local site. Although any organ can be affected, the lungs and CNS are the two common sites. The outcome of this infection is almost invariably fatal.

Isolated CNS mucormycosis results from hematogenous spread and is seen primarily in intravenous drug addicts.

DIAGNOSIS. The diagnosis of any form of mucormycosis is dependent on direct and histologic examinations of scrapings and biopsies of necrotic material. In contrast to most fungi, these organisms are readily seen in hematoxylin and eosin-stained tissue. The Gomori methenamine silver stain is usually adequate, but some special fungus stains, such as periodic acid–Schiff, do not demonstrate the organism well. However, a more rapid but preliminary diagnosis can sometimes be made by demonstrating hyphal elements after potassium hydroxide digestion of fresh tissue scraping. The alkali digests some of the tissue debris, but not the fungus, and makes identifying the fungi easier. Swabs of discharge or abnormal tissue are not adequate and can give erroneous information. Fungal cultures are occasionally positive, but a negative culture result does not exclude the diagnosis nor make it less likely. The media used for culturing these fungi should not contain cycloheximide. At present, no skin tests or serologic methods are adequate for diagnosing mucormycosis. Blood cultures are not helpful.

THERAPY. The hallmarks of successful outcome in this aggressive infection rely on early diagnosis by invasive procedures, immediate correction of the underlying predisposing condition, aggressive surgical debridement, and early systemic amphotericin therapy. Amphotericin B is the only drug with proven clinical efficacy, and a high therapeutic dosage (such as 1.0 to 1.5 mg per kilogram per day, if tolerated) should be achieved as soon as possible. This may be reduced to alternate-day dosing once the patient is stabilized. Typically, a cumulative dose of 2 to 5 grams may be needed to achieve cure. Although local irrigation of infected sites with amphotericin is an unproven adjunct, given the difficulties in perfusion of infected areas because of the tendency to thrombosis, this measure seems logical. Similarly, potentiation of amphotericin with other drugs (such as rifampin, azoles, flucytosine) is of unproven benefit, but given the poor results with conventional therapy, this should be considered if susceptibility testing can be done *in vitro* with the patient's isolate to show synergy and exclude antagonism. The newer orally administered azole derivates have no proven activity alone against these fungi. Improvement of survival may necessitate repeated major surgical debridement of necrotic tissue, resulting in significant disfiguring. If the patient survives, major reconstructive surgery may be needed.

PROGNOSIS. Mucormycosis remains a disease with guarded prognosis. It is difficult to ascertain accurately the effectiveness of any therapeutic approach because the disease is relatively rare and there is a general bias toward reporting cases only if therapy is effective. With the introduction of amphotericin B in 1961, it is generally accepted that the survival rate significantly improved. Rhinocerebral mucormycosis is the most common form of infection and is thought to have an overall mortality rate of about 50%. Patients who develop hemiplegia, facial necrosis, or nasal deformity have a higher mortality. Pulmonary or disseminated mucormycosis frequently escapes ante mortem diagnosis, and only a handful of patients have been reported to recover from these. Superficial infec-

tions, particularly in immunocompetent patients, can be successfully treated with debridement and antifungal therapy. Deeper cutaneous infections of the extremities usually require amputation, and when the head or trunk is involved, the condition is commonly fatal.

At this time, the most aggressive approach we can take toward this lethal disease is rapid diagnosis and immediate institution of surgical debridement plus systemic and local chemotherapy.

Bigby TD, Serota ML, Tierney LM, et al.: Clinical spectrum of pulmonary mucormycosis. Chest 89:435, 1986. *This review emphasizes the pulmonary form and includes discussion of the microbiology, pathology, predisposing factors, clinical presentation, diagnosis, and treatment.*

Ingram CN, Sennesh J, Cooper JN, et al.: Disseminated zygomycosis: Report of four cases and review. Rev Infect Dis 11:741, 1989. *A presentation of four cases of disseminated disease and a comprehensive review of 181 cases reported in the English language literature. Hematologic malignancy is the major predisposing factor for dissemination. More than 90% of disseminated infections were diagnosed at autopsy.*

Sugar AM: Mucormycosis. Clin Infect Dis 14(Suppl. 1):S126, 1992. *A review of all forms of the disease.*

357 MYCETOMA

Michael S. Saag

DEFINITION. Mycetoma is a chronic, localized, subcutaneous infection characterized by draining sinus tracts that frequently discharge purulent material containing granules. The disease most often affects the lower extremities, with the majority of cases involving the foot. Originally described in the mid-1800's, the disease was initially referred to as "Madura foot," named after the region in India where it was first identified. Although still referred to as maduromycosis, the preferred name and the term used most often to describe the disorder is mycetoma.

EUMYCETOMA	
Primary geographic distribution	*P. boydii* (U.S.; N. America)
	L. senegalensis (W. Africa)
	M. grisea (S. America)
	M. mycetomatis (Worldwide; Saudi Arabia)
Primary sites of disease	Lower extremities; hands (direct inoculation)
Drug of choice	Itraconazole (as an adjunct to surgical debridement)
Alternative therapy	Ketoconazole Amphotericin B (resistant cases)

ACTINOMYCETOMA	
Primary geographic distribution	*A. madurae* (U.S.)
	S. somaliensis (Africa)
	A. pelletieri (S. America)
	N. brasiliensis (Mexico)
Primary sites of disease	Lower extremities; hands (direct inoculation)
Drug of choice	Trimethoprim/ sulfamethoxazole (as adjunct to surgery)
Alternative therapy	Dapsone Streptomycin

ETIOLOGY. More than 20 species of fungi and bacteria have been implicated as etiologic agents of mycetoma. Approximately 40% of cases are due to true fungi (eumycetoma), and 60% are caused by aerobic actinomycetes (actinomycetoma). The organisms are distributed throughout the world, and the predominant organisms responsible for disease are subject to regional variation. Etiologic agents of eumycetoma and actinomycetoma may be presumptively identified based on the characteristic pigment of their granules. A listing of the predominant causative organisms is given in Table 357–1.

EPIDEMIOLOGY. Mycetomas have been reported from all over the world but are endemic in tropical regions of Africa, India, Central and South America, and the Far East. The geographic distribution of the disease is more related to rainfall than any other climatic factor. Most of the etiologic agents have been cultured from the soil in endemic areas, and occasionally organisms have been identified on plant thorns, which may be responsible for intradermal inoculation. *Pseudallescheria boydii* is the most common cause of mycetoma in the United States and is readily isolated from the soil in the United States and Canada. *Nocardia brasiliensis* and *Actinomadura madurae* are the most frequently isolated organisms in Central America, South America, and the Caribbean.

The majority of cases occur in males, many of whom are field laborers or herdsmen who have long-term trauma to their feet while in wet or swampy soil. Although the disease afflicts people of all ages, most cases are reported in young adults. Person-to-person transmission is not believed to occur, and the disease is unrelated to animal contact.

PATHOGENESIS AND PATHOLOGY. In contrast to systemic mycoses, which are usually established via the respiratory route, mycetomas are initiated through direct inoculation of the organism into the skin or mucosal surface, frequently as a consequence of trauma. Although the foot is the most common site of infection, direct inoculation of organisms into the hand, back, neck, and back of the head can occur in individuals who carry loads contaminated with soil.

The precise mechanism of pathogenesis remains unknown. Once inoculated, the organism induces a subacute to chronic suppurative inflammatory response that is primarily neutrophilic in nature but that may be associated with a granulomatous reaction. Over time, localized necrosis, fibrosis, abscess formation, and, frequently, bone and joint disease ensue. Deep sinuses with fistulas commonly develop and present as draining sinus tracts on the skin surface. The purulent drainage from those tracts often contains grains or granules, which consist of the causative organism embedded in a host-derived, proteinaceous matrix. The size, character, and color of the granules suggest the underlying etiologic agent (see Table 357–1).

The inflammatory process usually extends along fascial planes and may result in substantial regional destruction of deep tissues and bone. Distal spread of disease via the lymphatics or the bloodstream may occur but is distinctly uncommon.

CLINICAL MANIFESTATIONS. Most cases of mycetoma present late in the course of a longstanding, chronic inflammatory disease. The initial lesion appears as a small, painless nodule several weeks to months after primary inoculation. The patient generally cannot recall a precipitating event or specific traumatic incident. The lesions slowly extend into deep tissues, and the resultant

lymphatic obstruction, fibrosis, and tissue thickening give the foot a shortened, raised appearance. Skin nodules may break down, yielding granulomatous tissue with serosanguineous to purulent discharge. Later in the course of disease, sinus tracts begin to appear through which the characteristic fungal granules are expelled onto the skin surface. The sinus tracts spontaneously heal, only to be replaced by new tracts at nearby sites. Eumycetomas tend to be more circumscribed, remain localized, and progress more slowly than actinomycetomas, which have less well defined margins, merge with surrounding tissue, and progress more rapidly. The lesions tend to remain painless until deep bone involvement occurs, although many patients may complain of a deep itching sensation during active disease progression. Systemic involvement is rare, and patients feel remarkably well even in the presence of advanced localized disease.

DIAGNOSIS. The definitive diagnosis of mycetoma depends on culture of the causative organism from tissue specimens. The disease is suspected in the appropriate clinical setting, especially when grains are identified in the purulent discharge. Examination of the grains can establish a differential diagnosis of eumycetoma or actinomycetoma based on the presence of characteristic broad (fungal) or narrow (actinomycete) filaments. The characteristics of the granules, when combined with geographic and epidemiologic information, can yield a presumptive identification of the specific organism. However, cultural data are required for confirmation. Serologic tests are not routinely available.

TREATMENT. The response to therapy is dependent on the underlying etiologic agent. Eumycetomas are unresponsive to antimicrobial therapy, although partial responses to amphotericin B, liposomal amphotericin B, miconazole, ketoconazole, itraconazole, and thiabendazole have been reported. Fortunately, eumycetomas tend to be well circumscribed, yielding ready access to surgical approaches. If the lesion is not removed in its entirety and residual disease is present, relapse is inevitable.

Actinomycetomas are more responsive to antimicrobial therapy. Regimens consisting of high-dose penicillin (10 to 12 million units per day), sulfadiazine (3 to 10 grams per day), or minocycline (150 mg twice daily) have been reported to have some effect. The most successful regimens consist of trimethoprim-sulfamethoxazole (160 mg of trimethoprim and 800 mg of sulfamethoxazole given twice daily), combined with either streptomycin (1 to 3 grams per day for 3 weeks) or rifampin (600 mg per day for 3 to 4 months); or dapsone (100 mg twice daily) combined with streptomycin (1 gram per day for 1 month, given intramuscularly). The dapsone regimen is often preferred owing to its low cost. Amoxicillin-clavulanic acid therapy has been successful in some cases which were unresponsive to conventional therapy. The duration of therapy with either the trimethoprim-sulfamethoxazole or the dapsone regimen is usually 9 months, depending on response.

PROGNOSIS. If the disease is diagnosed early, the prognosis for mycetoma is good. Unfortunately, many cases are not identified until late in the course of disease, when response to therapy is limited, and amputation may be required. When disease is located on the back, neck, trunk, or abdomen, very little therapeutic intervention can be offered. The prognosis for survival is quite good; however, the quality of life may be dramatically lessened.

Fincher RM, Fisher JF, Lovell RD, et al.: Infection due to the fungus acremonium (cephalosporium). Medicine 70:398, 1991. *Case report and review of the literature of this saprophytic organism that may cause disease in humans, especially immunocompromised hosts.*

Hay RJ, Mahgoub ES, Leon G, et al.: Mycetoma. J Med Vet Mycology 30(suppl. 1):41, 1992. *Overview of the epidemiology, immunodiagnosis, and treatment of eumycetoma and actinomycetoma.*

Magana M: Mycetoma. Int J Dermatol 23:221, 1984. *A thorough review of clinical aspects of mycetoma and therapeutic approaches.*

Mahgoub ES: Medical management of mycetoma. Bull WHO 54:303, 1976. *Summarizes general principles of diagnosis and management.*

Smego RA Jr, Gallis HA: The clinical spectrum of *Nocardia brasiliensis* infection in the United States. Rev Infect Dis 6:164, 1984. *An important review of the pathogenesis, diagnosis, and therapy of the most common cause of mycetoma worldwide.*

TABLE 357–1. CAUSATIVE ORGANISMS OF MYCETOMA AND THE CHARACTERISTIC PIGMENT OF THEIR ASSOCIATED GRANULES

Eumycetoma	Actinomycetoma
White to yellow grains	
Pseudallescheria boydii	*Nocardia brasiliensis*
Acremonium species	*Nocardia asteroides*
Trichophyton species	*Nocardia cavae* (tiny grains)
Microsporum species	*Actinomadura madurae* (large grains)
Fusarium species	
Aspergillus nidulans	
Yellow to brown grains	
Neotestudina (Zophia) rosatii	*Streptomyces somaliensis*
Black grains	
Madurella mycetomatis	*Streptomyces paraguayensis*
Madurella grisea	
Exophiala jeanselmei	
Leptosphaeria senegalensis	
Leptosphaeria thompkinsii	
Red to pink grains	
	Actinomadura pelletieri

358 DEMATIACEOUS FUNGAL INFECTIONS

Michael S. Saag

DEFINITION. The term "dematiaceous" is applied to fungi that produce an intrinsic characteristic pigment. Diseases caused by dematiaceous fungi are divided into two groups: chromomycosis (chromoblastomycosis) and phaeohyphomycosis.

ETIOLOGY. Chromomycosis is caused by several species of related fungi, most notably *Fonsecaea, Phialophora, Cladosporium*, and *Acrotheca* species. These agents are brown-pigmented saprophytes commonly found in soil and wood. The microscopic appearance, which is virtually identical for all of the causative agents, consists of thick-walled, dark brown bodies ("sclerotic cells" or "copper pennies"), single or clustered. Sclerotic cells represent an intermediate form between yeasts and hyphae and multiply by horizontal and vertical separation, not by budding.

Phaeohyphomycosis may be caused by several organisms, frequently referred to as "black" fungi. They differ from the agents of chromomycosis in their clinical appearance and the absence of sclerotic cells. The black fungi usually exist in tissues as yeast-like cells (solitary or in small chains), as septated hyphae (branched or unbranched), or as a combination of yeast and hyphae. The hyphal forms are frequently confused with *Aspergillus* species but may be distinguished by using the Fontana-Masson staining procedure (a melanin-specific stain) or via *in vitro* culture. The most common agents of phaeohyphomycosis identified in humans include species in the following genera: *Curvularia, Bipolaris, Exserohilum, Alternaria, Mycocentrospora, Pyrenochaeta, Trichomaris, Wangiella, Xylohypha,* and *Exophiala*.

EPIDEMIOLOGY AND PATHOGENESIS. The organisms causing chromomycosis and phaeohyphomycosis are worldwide in distribution. Chromomycosis occurs predominantly in young males and is usually inoculated into the skin via thorns, splinters, and other penetrating wounds. The disease is more prevalent in rural populations, especially among those with suboptimal nutritional status and personal hygiene. Chromomycosis appears to be endemic in certain areas, such as Madagascar and Costa Rica.

Phaeohyphomycosis is becoming an important disease among immunocompromised hosts. Despite the ubiquity of black fungi in the environment, disease due to these organisms had in the past been sporadic. More recently, however, clusters of cases have been reported from major medical centers as opportunistic infections in transplant recipients, especially bone marrow transplant patients.

CLINICAL MANIFESTATIONS. Chromomycosis initially manifests as a wart-like papule that slowly enlarges into a verruciform plaque. The lesions may progress to ulceration with or without an exudate. Over time, the lesions become dry and crusted with a raised border, which may be serpiginous. Large plaques frequently develop central scarring. Occasionally, the lesions become pedunculated and acquire a cauliflower-like appearance. Systemic spread to distal sites is distinctly uncommon, although spread through autoinoculation or via lymphatic drainage may occur. Rarely, widespread disseminated disease to the pancreas, liver, bowel, lymph nodes, meninges, and brain is noted.

Phaeohyphomycosis may occur as a wide spectrum of clinical disease. Superficial phaeohyphomycosis is the most benign and is found in the stratum corneum or around the hair shaft. Tinea nigra and black piedra are examples of this disorder. More invasive skin disease involving nonliving layers of keratinized epithelium include the dermatomycoses and onychomycoses. Mycotic keratitis may result in extensive corneal damage and subsequent blindness. Subcutaneous disease usually results from direct inoculation of fungi through intact skin. Cystic lesions with well-defined walls and central abscess formation, occasionally surrounding a foreign body such as a splinter, are characteristic.

Invasive phaeohyphomycosis is a potentially life-threatening disease that occurs predominantly in immunocompromised hosts. Localized invasive disease frequently occurs in the paranasal sinuses, lower respiratory tract, and bone. Disease due to *Cladosporium, Curvularia, Bipolaris, Xylohypha,* and *Exserohilum* species is especially prone to invade the central nervous system.

DIAGNOSIS. The diagnosis of chromomycosis and phaeohyphomycosis is made by histopathologic examination of tissue biopsy specimens or KOH (10%) preparations. The brown sclerotic cells of chromomycosis are readily identified, and special stains are not usually required. Phaeohyphomycosis is best diagnosed using the Fontana-Masson technique, which distinguishes organisms producing melanin from *Aspergillus* species. Cultures are required to identify the specific genera causing chromomycosis and phaeohyphomycosis. All cultures should be held for at least 8 weeks, since some of the organisms grow slowly. No serologic or skin tests are available.

TREATMENT. Surgical excision, when feasible, is the most effective mode of therapy for subcutaneous or deeply invasive disease. Unfortunately, unless lesions are diagnosed and treated early, the rate of relapse is high. Systemic antifungal therapy with amphotericin B is often used; however, the results are generally disappointing. Flucytosine (5-FC; 150 mg per kilogram per day) has been used on an investigational basis in patients with chromomycosis, with some success (16 of 23 patients cured); however, resistance developed in several treated patients. The response to therapy of phaeohyphomycosis is highly dependent on the causative organism. Many black fungi are resistant to 5-FC, and amphotericin B therapy yields variable results. Newer triazole antifungal agents, such as fluconazole and itraconazole, show some promise as effective agents.

Adam RD, Paquin ML, Petersen EA, et al.: Phaeohyphomycosis caused by the fungal genera *Bipolaris* and *Exserohilum*. Medicine 65:203, 1986. *These fungi have been previously misclassified as* Helminthosporium *or* Drechslera *species, but the latter fungi appear not to produce human disease. This paper serves as an excellent review.*

Bennett JE, Bonner H, Jennings AE, et al.: Chronic meningitis caused by *Cladosporium trichoides*. Am J Clin Pathol 59:398, 1973. *Comprehensive review of cerebral infection with dematiaceous fungi.*

McGinnis MR: Chromoblastomycosis and phaeohyphomycosis: New concepts, diagnosis and mycology. J Am Acad Dermatol 8:1, 1983. *Clear-cut exposition of clinical and mycologic criteria for these diagnoses. A very important review.*

Sudduth EJ, Crumbley AJ III, Farrar WE: Phaeohyphomycosis due to *Exophiala* species: Clinical spectrum of disease in humans. Clin Inf Dis 15:639, 1992. *An indepth review of infections due to* Exophiala. *Case report and review of the literature.*

359 INTRODUCTION TO HIV AND ASSOCIATED DISORDERS
Gerald L. Mandell

Disease, including the acquired immunodeficiency syndrome (AIDS), caused by the diabolically unique human immunodeficiency virus (HIV-1), has profoundly changed contemporary society and medical practice. The chapters in this part enable the physician to understand the virus and its effects on humans. In addition, there is an extensive discussion of involvement of various organ systems, both by the virus itself and by opportunistic infections. The management of patients with HIV infection is presented in detail.

In 1981, the first cluster of cases that we now call AIDS was recognized and reported. Nearly all of the early identified cases were in young homosexual men, but it was quickly learned that HIV infection could be transmitted by heterosexual contact and by blood transfer from infected to noninfected individuals.

After an initial flurry of fearful reactions by health care workers who believed that they were at a very significant risk for acquiring HIV infection, the facts are somewhat reassuring and protective procedures have been established. It is clear that the greatest risk to health care workers is needle stick (or other sharp) transmittal of blood from infected patients to health care workers, with an infection rate of about 3 per 1000. Universal precautions were established and appear to be a sensible and practical means for reducing nosocomial transmission of the virus. The premise is that blood and body fluids from all patients should be considered potentially infectious and appropriate precautions should be emphasized. Medical students and house officers training in many of our large medical centers are now just as likely to see patients with *Pneumocystis carinii* pneumonia as patients with pneumococcal pneumonia. The possibility of HIV infection must be considered in patients with a broad array of presenting symptoms because of the protean manifestations of this disease and its accompanying opportunistic infections and malignancies.

In the United States and other countries, governmental agencies are now reacting to the HIV infection pandemic. New civil rights and public health legislation has been passed. The potential penalty for acquiring a sexually transmitted disease has now escalated to death. Despite this, countries around the world have been relatively slow to realize that the rules of the game for sexual contact have changed. We can't wait for a magic vaccine to wipe out HIV infection. Educational efforts to reduce the spread of this disease have been supported by nearly all medical and public health groups but opposed by others on religious or moral grounds. The process for drug testing, development, and approval has been altered. Activist groups have caused re-examination of some of the processes and regulations regarding approval of new therapies. This has resulted in "fast tracks" for certain agents. The concept of "surrogate mark-

ers" for disease progression has emerged. In a disease where time from infection to death is close to 10 years, the use of survival measurements to determine efficacy of therapy would be impossibly slow. Therefore, surrogate markers such as CD4+ counts and number and severity of opportunistic infections are widely considered appropriate.

It is difficult to end this introduction on an optimistic note because, despite more than a decade of progress related to understanding the molecular biology of the virus and details of pathogenesis of the disease, neither a cure nor an effective vaccine is in sight. Despite intriguing observations and small gains, the big breakthrough has eluded us.

All practicing physicians must know the basics of AIDS pathogenesis, clinical disease presentation, and principles of management in order to effectively care for patients in the 1990's. A study of the following chapters will help to accomplish that.

360 IMMUNOLOGY RELATED TO AIDS
Bruce D. Walker

The clinical consequences of human immunodeficiency virus (HIV) infection are due to the ability of this virus to disarm the host immune system, a process that occurs by virtue of the fact that the primary target for the virus is the helper-inducer subset of lymphocytes. This lymphocyte subset, defined by its surface expression of the CD4 molecule, acts as the pivotal orchestrator of a myriad of immune functions. HIV infection can therefore be considered a disease of the immune system, characterized by the progressive loss of CD4-positive (CD4+) lymphocytes, (Table 360–1) with ultimately fatal consequences for the infected host.

Despite this immunosuppression induced by HIV, a number of specific immunologic defenses against the virus are generated in infected individuals and may contribute to the long asymptomatic phase following infection by keeping the virus at least partially contained. The potential significance of such responses is also underscored by the recent demonstration in animal AIDS models that

TABLE 360–1. POTENTIAL CAUSES OF CD4+ CELL DEPLETION

1. Direct toxic consequences of infection
2. Syncytia formation
3. Innocent bystander destruction of cells with adsorbed gp120
4. Impaired regeneration of the peripheral T cell compartment
5. Autoimmune destruction
6. Superantigens
7. Apoptosis

a state of vaccine-induced protective immunity can be achieved against retroviruses related to HIV. An understanding of the immunology related to HIV provides insight not only into the clinical sequelae of infection, but also into the prospects for development of an effective vaccine against HIV.

HIV-INDUCED IMMUNOSUPPRESSION

An understanding of HIV life cycle (see Ch. 361 and Fig. 360–1) is necessary to appreciate the induction of immunosuppresion.

The hallmark of HIV infection is progressive depletion of the CD4 helper-inducer subset of lymphocytes. Because of the central role of these cells in immunologic functioning, the clinical disease manifestations of immunosuppression and susceptibility to opportunistic infections and neoplasms are not surprising. The immunologic deficits associated with HIV infection are widespread and involve numerous interdependent effector arms of the immune system, including both cellular and humoral elements.

DIRECT IMMUNOSUPPRESSIVE PROPERTIES OF VIRAL PRODUCTS. Protein products of a number of retroviruses have been shown to have direct immunosuppressive properties independent of viral infection. A synthetic peptide corresponding to a highly conserved region in the HIV-1 gp41 transmembrane (TM) protein has been demonstrated *in vitro* to inhibit lymphocyte proliferative responses to mitogenic or antigenic stimuli. This region is analogous to a highly conserved immunosuppressive protein of human T-lymphotrophic virus I HTLV-I, and similar inhibitory TM proteins have been identified in other animal retroviral infections such as feline leukemia virus (FeLV). Whether such a phenomenon contributes to the global immunosuppression seen in HIV-infected individuals has not been determined, but the possibility that HIV proteins may be immunosuppressive has raised concerns about inclusion of such sequences in potential HIV vaccine candidates.

T LYMPHOCYTE ABNORMALITIES. Lymphocyte abnormalities associated with HIV infection can be classified as both quantitative and qualitative. Qualitative deficiencies become apparent soon after infection and before CD4 depletion is evident, and are largely related to intrinsic functional defects in the helper-inducer subset of lymphocytes. Studies using purified subpopulations of lymphocytes from AIDS patients have demonstrated a selective defect in soluble antigen (e.g., tetanus toxoid) recognition, although these cells are still able to undergo a normal degree of blast transformation and lymphokine production after exposure to mitogen (e.g., phytohemagglutinin). In other words, the weapon is loaded, but only mitogens and not antigens cause the trigger to be pulled. These studies also indicate that the central defect is lack of helper cell function rather than overabundance of suppressor cell activity. Other lymphocyte abnormalities observed with HIV infection include decreased lymphokine production, decreased expression of interleukin-2 (IL-2) receptors, decreased alloreactivity, and decreased ability to provide help to B cells. The functional T lymphocyte ab-

normalities also likely contribute to the loss of delayed type hypersensitivity reactions that become more prevalent as disease progresses.

The quantitative abnormality of T lymphocytes is the result of progressive depletion of the CD4+ helper T lymphocyte population (Table 360–1), which begins soon after primary infection. This downhill trend continues until the normal levels of 800 to 1200 CD4 cells per cubic millimeter drop below 50 cells per cubic millimeter and sometimes < 10 cells per cubic millimeter in the later stages of disease. CD4 cell depletion cannot be attributed solely to direct cytotoxic effects of virus infection, as only a minority of helper cells are actually infected, even in later stages of illness. Other factors potentially contributing CD4 depletion include (1) syncytia formation, in which a single infected cell fuses via its surface gp120 with the CD4 molecule on uninfected cells, forming multinucleated giant cells; (2) "innocent bystander" destruction of uninfected CD4 cells that have bound free gp120 to the CD4 molecule, rendering them susceptible to immune attack; (3) HIV infection of stem cells or HIV-induced thymic depletion, resulting in decreased helper cell production; (4) autoimmune mechanisms, whereby cross-reactive antibodies or cellular immune responses to the virus result in killing of uninfected CD4 cells; (5) superantigen effect, in which a viral protein would be hypothesized to lead to stimulation and ultimately depletion of CD4 lymphocytes bearing a specific T cell receptor; and (6) apoptosis, whereby virus or viral products would induce programmed cell death (PCD). Whatever the mechanisms of the CD4 cell depletion, the resultant consequence on immune function is so profound that total CD4 number is currently the best prognosticator of disease progression. The risk of certain opportunistic infections increases significantly when the total CD4 cell number is < 200 per cubic millimeter, which is why routine prophylaxis against *Pneumocystis carinii* pneumonic (PCP) is instituted at this stage. At levels below 50 to 100 cells per cubic millimeter the risk for other complications, such as disseminated mycobacterium avium or cytomegalovirus (CMV) infections, increases dramatically.

B LYMPHOCYTE ABNORMALITIES. As with T lymphocyte abnormalities in HIV infection, the B lymphocyte abnormalities are both quantitative and qualitative. Most characteristic, particularly in the early stages of infection, is intense polyclonal activation of B cells, evidenced clinically by elevated levels of immunoglobulins G and A, the presence of circulating immune complexes, and an increased number of peripheral blood B lymphocytes that secrete immunoglobulin spontaneously. These B cell abnormalities are unlikely to be a direct consequence of HIV infection of B cells. Whereas B cells can express low levels of CD4 and have been infected *in vitro*, there are no conclusive data indicating these cells became infected *in vivo*. Rather, the virus itself or viral proteins appear to directly interact with and stimulate uninfected cells. Other potential contributors to this polyclonal activation include concurrent viral infections. For example, CMV and Epstein-Barr virus (EBV) infection occur with greatly increased frequency in HIV-infected individuals and can lead to B cell hyperactivity.

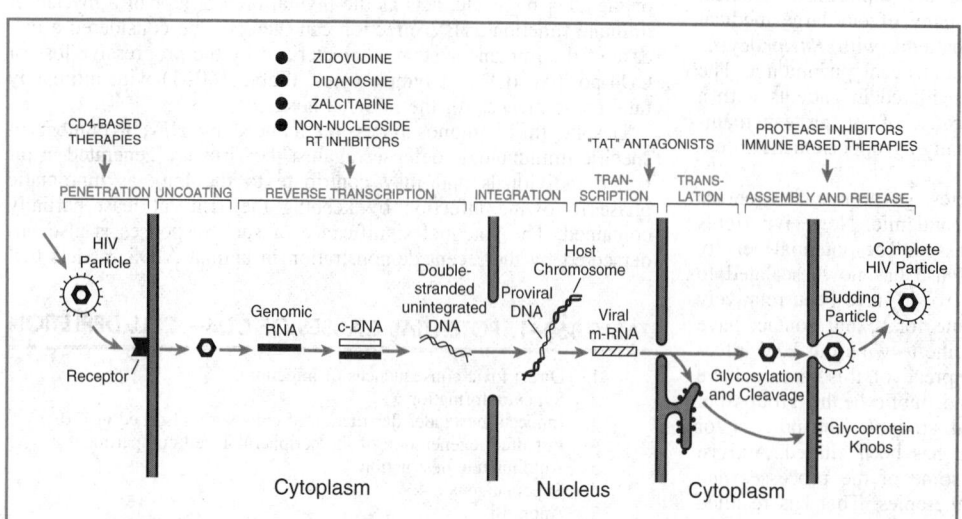

FIGURE 360–1. The life cycle of HIV. The target sites for antiretroviral agents are shown. (Reprinted with permission from Johnson VA, Hirsch MS: *In* AIDS Clinical Review. New York, Marcel Dekker, 1990, p 238.)

Functional abnormalities of B cells consist particularly of impaired antibody responses to antigenic stimuli, and impaired T cell helper function may also contribute to this problem. These impaired antibody responses may account for the increase in pyogenic infections seen in advanced HIV infection. In addition, decreased antibody responsiveness to vaccination against viruses such as influenza A and hepatitis B is also characteristic of late-stage HIV infection.

MONOCYTE/MACROPHAGE ABNORMALITIES. It has been clearly demonstrated that HIV also infects cells of the monocyte/macrophage lineage, probably by attaching to surface CD4 molecules on these cells. Infection and high-level replication of HIV have also been demonstrated in monocyte/macrophage progenitor cells of normal bone marrow and may contribute to the pancytopenia seen with HIV infection. Unlike CD4 lymphocytes, however, macrophages appear to be relatively resistant to the cytopathic effects of HIV infection and may therefore constitute a reservoir of infection. Macrophages may also play an important role in viral dissemination within the infected individual, in particular carrying virus across the blood-brain barrier to the central nervous system (CNS).

At least in part as a consequence of HIV infection, a number of monocyte/macrophage abnormalities have been detected in HIV-seropositive persons. The ability of monocyte/macrophages to act as antigen-presenting cells is impaired, particularly in later stages of illness. Some defects in these cells in AIDS patients may be a consequence of chronic *in vivo* activation, such as increased IL-2 receptor expression, IL-1 secretion, and increased chemotactic ligand receptor expression. The reasons for this chronic activation are likely multifactorial and may relate to exposure to viral proteins or lymphokines or to direct effects of HIV infection. These abnormalities may have immunopathogenic consequences, since defects in the ability to present antigens could ultimately impair the ability to sustain an immune response against HIV or other pathogens.

In the brain, cells of the macrophage lineage appear to be the major cell type infected with HIV and directly or indirectly may contribute to the CNS dysfunction observed in this disease. In the lung, infected alveolar macrophages may stimulate HIV-specific immune responses, the byproducts of which have been postulated to contribute to the observed alveolitis. Deficient T4 helper cell function may also indirectly contribute to the observed defects in monocyte/macrophages, since a minority of monocyte/macrophages appear to be actually productively infected *in vivo*.

NATURAL KILLER CELL ABNORMALITIES. Natural killer (NK) cells are thought to be an important component of immunosurveillance against virus-infected cells, allogeneic cells, and tumor cells. NK cells are typically large granular lymphocytes that recognize foreign antigens on cells, resulting in activation of lytic machinery. NK cells are phenotypically and numerically normal in AIDS patients, but they are functionally defective. This may relate in part to an observed defect in the trigger mechanism necessary to deliver the lethal blow to a target cell. In addition, defective lymphokine production in HIV-infected persons may also contribute to NK cell dysfunction. However, adding IL-2 to these cells *in vitro* only partially restores NK function.

AUTOIMMUNE ABNORMALITIES. Autoimmune phenomena are also part of the immunologic derangement in HIV infection and may also contribute to the disease manifestations seen clinically. When sensitive assays are used, circulating immune complexes can be detected in the majority of HIV-infected individuals. These may help to explain the occurrence of HIV-related arthralgias, myalgias, renal disease, and vasculitis.

Autoimmune mechanisms may also directly contribute to the immune suppression seen in AIDS. Sequence similarities exist between the HIV envelope transmembrane protein and human leukocyte antigen (HLA) class II proteins, and antibodies that cross-react with these two proteins have been detected in HIV-infected persons. Such autoantibodies could impair functioning of cells bearing class II antigens, either by directly eliminating these cells through antibody-dependent cellular cytotoxicity or by inhibiting their ability to interact with other cells.

VIRUS-SPECIFIC HOST IMMUNE RESPONSES (Table 360–2)

The initial phase of HIV infection is characterized by high-level viremia, associated with the ability to detect the viral core protein p24 in the serum. However, soon after infection the level of viremia and p24 antigenemia rapidly decreases (see Fig. 361–6). A long period of relatively asymptomatic infection ensues, suggesting that virus-specific immune responses may play a role in limiting viral replication and thereby disease progression. With the AIDS epidemic now entering its second decade, identification of the precise protective components of anti-HIV immunity remains an elusive goal, although significant progress continues to be made in characterizing HIV-specific humoral and cellular immune responses.

NEUTRALIZING ANTIBODIES. HIV infection induces B lymphocytes to produce antibodies directed against viral proteins, and some of these antibodies are capable of neutralizing the virus. Antibody responses are typically observed 1 to 3 months after primary infection, although longer periods before antibody responses develop have been documented in rare instances. Neutralizing antibodies directly neutralize free virus at a stage before the virus has entered the cell and become uncoated. In a number of viral infections, neutralizing antibody induced by immunization correlates with protection from subsequent viral infection. HIV-1 infection results in the production of HIV-specific antibodies directed at a number of viral proteins, and some of these antibodies demonstrate neutralizing activity. The primary target of neutralizing antibodies is the envelope glycoprotein, in particular a loop structure within a relatively hypervariable region of the gp120 glycoprotein termed the principal neutralizing domain or V3 loop, as well as epitopes in the region involved in CD4 binding that recognize conformationally determined regions that are composed of discontinuous segments brought together in the tertiary structure of the envelope protein.

Neutralizing antibodies have been demonstrated to be present at all stages of HIV infection, and although titers are generally lower in later stages of illness, attempts to correlate neutralizing antibody titers with disease progression have yielded conflicting results. Detailed studies in primary HIV-1 infection have demonstrated that antibodies capable of neutralizing the infecting strain of virus first appear after the clearance of the primary viremia, suggesting that other immune mechanisms may be important in the early control of viremia. In addition, it has been demonstrated that antibodies from infected persons at a given point in time tend to be poorly able to neutralize the infecting strain of virus, but much better at neutralizing isolates from other individuals or laboratory strains of virus. Although a number of animal studies have shown that neutralizing antibodies can confer protection against viral challenge, this protection has been largely in highly idealized situations in which maximal titers were induced just prior to challenge and a low inoculum of virus was given intravenously. Concern persists whether neutralizing antibodies alone would be able to confer protection against naturally acquired infection.

The ability of HIV-specific neutralizing antibodies to confer protection may be impaired in part by the high degree of antigenic variation exhibited by HIV. This antigenic variation is particularly pronounced in the envelope region of the virus, and virus variants may emerge within an infected individual that are neutralization resistant. This antigenic variation also has significant implications for vaccine design, since neutralizing antibodies generated in response to a single immunizing strain of virus are likely to neutralize only very closely related viruses, a phenomenon known as type specificity.

Antibodies also constitute the first line of defense at mucosal surfaces, in the form of secretory IgA. Such secretory antibodies have been found in blood, saliva, and other body fluids of persons infected with HIV, but their potential role as a protective immune response in HIV infection remains undetermined.

In sharp contrast to proposed protective attributes, HIV-specific antibodies have also been shown to promote HIV infection under certain experimental situations. Antibody binds to virions, and this complex appears to be taken up by some cells by binding of antibody through the cellular Fc receptor. This *in vitro* evidence for an-

TABLE 360–2. HIV-SPECIFIC IMMUNE RESPONSES

1. Neutralizing antibodies
2. Antibody-dependent cellular cytotoxicity
3. Natural killer cells
4. Cytotoxic T cells
5. Cellular proliferative responses

tibody-dependent enhancement is orders of magnitude less than that observed, for example, in dengue virus infection, and the clinical significance of this phenomenon is not known.

ANTIBODY-DEPENDENT CELLULAR CYTOTOXICITY (ADCC). Another mechanism the immune system can use to limit the spread of infection is ADCC, which involves both cellular and humoral components. ADCC is a process whereby virus-specific antibodies bind directly to viral proteins expressed on the surface of infected cells, thereby sensitizing these cells for lysis by cells that bind to the exposed Fc portion of the antibody. The cells mediating this response are typically NK cells, which express the CD16 Fc receptor for IgG. Antibodies that can mediate ADCC have been identified in the majority of HIV-infected individuals; these are present soon after seroconversion and are maintained throughout the disease course. The major ADCC target antigens are the envelope glycoproteins gp120 and gp41; *gag* proteins may also be involved. It has been postulated that ADCC may limit cell-cell spread of virus by providing an early cytotoxic host defense. ADCC may correlate with better clinical stage in children born to infected mothers, and ADCC titers have been shown to be higher in early stages of infection in some studies. However, the contribution of this immune response to protection from disease protection remains unclear.

NATURAL KILLER CELLS. *In vitro* evidence suggests that NK-type cells are not only important in ADCC, but also may bind free HIV-specific antibodies through their Fc receptors, arming them for attack against HIV-infected cells.

CYTOTOXIC T LYMPHOCYTES (CTL). Cytotoxic T lymphocytes have been demonstrated to be one of the protective host defenses generated in response to a number of viral infections. CTL can kill virus-infected cells by recognizing viral protein fragments on the infected cell surface, where these proteins form a binary complex with a surface HLA molecule. CTL recognition of this complex leads to lysis and elimination of the infected cell.

Although the hallmark of HIV infection is the development of profound immunosuppression, extremely vigorous HIV-specific CTL responses have been detected in the peripheral blood of infected individuals. These responses are directed not only against the major viral structural proteins, but also against the reverse transcriptase protein and regulatory proteins such as *vif* and *nef*. These responses appear to be mediated predominantly by CD8+ lymphocytes, which recognize processed HIV proteins on the surface of infected cells in conjunction with HLA class I (A,B,C) molecules. In addition to this so-called HLA-restricted CTL population, other cells appear to exist that can recognize HIV envelope protein on infected cells in an HLA-unrestricted fashion. These cells may be T cells or cells of the NK phenotype. Some studies have also suggested the existence of HIV-specific, CD4+ CTL restricted by HLA class II molecules.

Although a protective role for CTL has been demonstrated in numerous experimental models of viral infection, the question remains unresolved as to the possible protective role of CTL in HIV infection. Recent data demonstrate high levels of HIV-1–specific CTL in primary infection, and their appearance correlates with initial control of viremia. There is at least indirect evidence to suggest that the CTL response might indeed retard disease progression. For example, CD8+ lymphocytes from HIV-infected individuals can inhibit HIV replication in autologous CD4 lymphocytes *in vitro*. Similar inhibitory CD8 cells have also been identified in the SIV-infected macaque monkeys, and since cell contact is necessary for this inhibition to occur, it suggests that the cell mediating this response may be a classic CTL. Other indirect evidence that CTL may be important in retarding disease progression stems from studies quantifying HIV-specific CTL in infected persons. As clinical disease progresses, CTL numbers decline, which could help to explain the observed increase in viremia observed in later stages of illness.

Conversely, HIV-specific CTL have also been postulated to be deleterious to the host. These cells have been recovered from the lungs of subjects with lymphocytic alveolitis, suggesting that they may be inducing the alveolitis by attacking HIV-infected alveolar macrophages. In addition, CTL have been detected in the cerebrospinal fluid of HIV-infected individuals with neurologic disorders, prompting the hypothesis that CTL-mediated inflammatory reactions may contribute to the observed neurologic dysfunction. A possible mechanism may relate to the release of inflammatory cytokines by activated HIV-1–specific CTL. CTL could also contribute to the progressive decline in CD4 cells by eliminating those cells that become HIV infected.

CELLULAR PROLIFERATIVE RESPONSES. T cell immunity to viral pathogens consists not only of cytotoxic T lymphocytes, but also helper T cell proliferation and cytokine production in specific response to viral antigens. This CD4+ proliferative response is generally triggered by recognition of viral antigen in association with class II (HLA-D) molecules on the surface of antigen-presenting cells or B cells to be helped. Although HIV-specific proliferative responses are characteristically depressed in HIV-infected individuals, a number of epitopes eliciting these responses have been identified, particularly in the envelope glycoprotein gp120. Unfortunately, as with other HIV-specific immune responses, the precise contribution as a protective mechanism remains unclear. Recently it has been hypothesized that progression of HIV infection is associated with specific defects in T helper (Th) cell function. A switch from a predominantly Th1-type cytokine response, associated with the production of IL-2 and IFN-g following antigen or mitogen stimulation of peripheral blood mononuclear cells, to a predominantly Th2-type cytokine response, associated with the production of IL-4, IL-5, IL-6 and IL-10, has been observed by some investigators. Although this hypothesis remains quite controversial, it is perhaps intriguing that Th1-type responses to the HIV envelope protein have been detected in some exposed uninfected individuals.

IMMUNOTHERAPY FOR HIV INFECTION (Table 360–3)

Because the immune response elicited by HIV infection is ultimately incapable of protecting the host from disease progression, and because infection is associated with progressive deterioration of immune function, a number of approaches for immune-based therapy are being investigated. Passive immunotherapy with immunoglobulins as well as HIV-1–specific gamma globulins and monoclonal antibodies may have direct antiviral effects. Thymic hormones may influence the development of T cells, but clinical efficacy data are lacking. Cytokines may serve to regulate immune responses as well as HIV expression. Trials of intermittent IL-2 infusion are under way, with trials of IL-12 therapy planned. Preliminary *in vitro* studies have shown that IL-12 can restore some HIV-1–specific cell-mediated immune responses. Adoptive cellular therapy with autologous cloned HIV-1–specific CTL as well as polyclonal populations of CD8 cells are under way, and although efficacy has not yet been determined, the early data indicate that this approach seems to be safe. Trials of adoptive therapy with autologous uninfected CD4 cells to correct the CD4 cell deficit are being planned.

PROSPECTS FOR VACCINE DEVELOPMENT (Table 360–4)

Ultimate global control of the HIV epidemic will likely require a vaccine that can elicit protective immunity. Although efforts to define the components of protective immunity in infected persons have been unsuccessful thus far, recent data from animal models of retrovirus infection indicate that a state of protective immunity may be an attainable goal. When immunized with an attenuated, *nef*-deleted SIV, rhesus macaques were found to be protected when subsequently challenged with wild-type pathogenic SIV. Not only were the animals protected from low-dose challenge, but they were also protected from high-dose challenge. Although the precise mechanism whereby these animals were protected has not been deter-

TABLE 360–3. IMMUNE-BASED INTERVENTIONS FOR HIV INFECTION

Passive immunity
   Immunoglobulins
   Monoclonal antibodies
Thymic hormones
Cytokine treatment
   Interleukin-2
   Tumor necrosis factor
   Interferons
   Interleukin-12
Adoptive cellular therapy
Therapeutic vaccination

TABLE 360-4. POTENTIAL HIV-1 VACCINES IN CLINICAL TRIALS

1. Soluble protein/peptides
    gp160
    p24
    p17
    gp120
    V3 loop peptides
2. Recombinant live vaccines
    Vaccinia-HIV-1 gp160
    Canarypox gp160
3. Retroviral vectors
4. Pseudovirion vaccines
5. Whole inactivated HIV

mined, these results indicate that protective immunity may be an achievable goal for HIV infection.

Despite these promising results in the SIV model of HIV infection, a number of potential obstacles exist to the development of an effective AIDS vaccine (Table 360–5). Foremost among these is the genomic diversity of the viral genome. Most of this diversity occurs in the envelope gene, with as much as 20% divergence in nucleotide sequence among field isolates. Even within a single individual, multiple divergent strains of virus have been identified, reflecting an extremely high intrinsic mutation rate for the virus. The implications of such diversity for vaccine development are profound, since the virus acts as a moving target for any immune response that is generated. Another obstacle to be overcome is the type specificity of immune responses generated to candidate vaccines, since immune responses generated by an immunogen representing a single field isolate are unlikely to cross-react with all field isolates. In addition, although some of the protein-based HIV vaccine candidates have induced reasonably strong neutralizing antibodies when tested against laboratory strains of virus, these antibodies have been much less effective in neutralizing field isolates of HIV-1. The issue of antibody-dependent enhancement of HIV infection remains controversial and needs to be resolved so that high-risk individuals are not immunized and thereby potentially rendered more susceptible to infection. Once candidate immunogens are identified, animal testing for efficacy would be ideal, but may not be possible for a number of reasons. Unfortunately there is no good animal model of HIV infection. Although chimpanzees become infected with HIV, they do not develop disease. Rhesus macaques develop an immunodeficiency disease similar to AIDS when infected with SIV, but cannot be infected with HIV, are expensive to maintain, and are in limited supply. The potential utility of immunodeficient mice reconstituted with human fetal tissues, providing them with a "human" immune system, remains to be demonstrated. Perhaps the biggest obstacle will be demonstration of efficacy, which will require large field trials in populations showing a high enough incidence of new infection that statistically significant data can be generated in a reasonable period. Demonstration of efficacy in one population may not translate to other populations. For example, protection of persons infected by sexual exposure will not necessarily imply that such a vaccine would protect intravenous drug abusers as well, who may be exposed to a higher initial inoculum of virus. As with HIV-infected persons, the potential for discrimination against vaccines due to positive serology will have to be addressed.

Although these obstacles exist, a number of clinical trials are already under way with a variety of vaccine candidates. These include soluble *gag* or envelope proteins; recombinant vaccinia virus containing the HIV-1 envelope gene; pseudovirion vaccines that re-

TABLE 360-5. POTENTIAL OBSTACLES TO HIV VACCINE DEVELOPMENT

1. Genomic diversity of the viral genome
2. Type specificity of immune responses
3. Potential generation of enhancing antibodies
4. Lack of animal models of HIV infection and AIDS
5. Field trials to demonstrate efficacy
6. Indemnification of vaccinees from discrimination

semble whole HIV particles but are modified to exclude the viral genome or render it harmless; retroviral vectors; and whole killed virus vaccines. A number of these approaches are also being evaluated as potential therapeutic vaccines in an attempt to improve the host immune response to the virus. Combinations of some of these approaches are also under investigation. In subjects immunized with vaccinia-HIV-1 gp160, dramatic increases in HIV-1 envelope antibodies were observed when vaccinees were boosted with recombinant gp160 protein. Other approaches in various stages of preclinical development include use of recombinant BCG-HIV vectors as well as attenuated salmonella-HIV recombinants, which may be more effective at inducing mucosal immunity.

Cao Y, Qin L, Zhang L, et al.: Virologic and immunologic characterization of long-term survivors of human immunodeficiency virus type 1 infection. N Engl J Med 332:201, 1995. *Studies in seropositive subjects who have remained asymptomatic with normal and stable CD4 counts after 12 to 15 years of infection indicate low levels of plasma viremia, vigorous virus inhibitory CD8 lymphocyte responses, and strong neutralizing antibodies responses, as well as some degree of attenuation of the virus in a minority of subjects.*

Graham BS, Wright PF: AIDS vaccines. N Engl J Med 1995; submitted for publication. *Updated review on vaccines in Phase 1 and 2 trials.*

Koup RA, Safrit JT, Cao Y, et al.: Temporal association of cellular immune responses with the initial control of viremia in primary human immunodeficiency virus type 1 syndrome. J Virology 68:4650, 1994. *Characterization of the immune responses during primary infection.*

Levy JA: Pathogenesis of human immunodeficiency virus infection. Microbiol Revs 57:183, 1993. *Extensive review of HIV pathogenesis.*

Pantaleo G, Graziosi C, Fauci AS: The immunopathogenesis of human immunodeficiency virus infection. N Engl J Med 328:327, 1993. *A detailed review of the immunopathogenic mechanisms involved in HIV infection.*

Wei X, Ghosh SK, Taylor ME, et al.: Viral dynamics in human immunodeficiency type 1 infection. Nature, 373:117, 1995. *This study demonstrates that the life span of plasma virus and virus producing cells comprises a half-life of approximately 2 days, indicating that viremia is sustained by constant and rapid turnover of both free virus and infected cells.*

361 BIOLOGY OF HUMAN IMMUNODEFICIENCY VIRUSES

George M. Shaw

DISCOVERY OF HUMAN IMMUNODEFICIENCY VIRUSES

The identification of HIV-1 as the causative agent of acquired immunodeficiency syndrome (AIDS) just 3 years after the clinical syndrome was initially described represents a remarkable scientific achievement that had its roots in earlier discoveries of animal and human retroviruses (see Ch. 342). The selective loss of CD4+ helper T lymphocytes in patients with the disease implicated an agent with T-lymphocyte cell tropism. As expected for an etiologic agent, HIV-1 was shown to be uniformly present in subjects with AIDS and to reproduce the hallmark of disease, destruction of T lymphocytes, in tissue culture.

GENERAL BIOLOGIC PROPERTIES OF HIV-1

Soon after its discovery, HIV-1 was shown to be biologically, structurally, and genetically distinct from human T-lymphotrophic virus I (HTLV-I) and HTLV-II and more like members of the lentivirus subfamily of retroviruses (see Ch. 342). Unlike the leukemia viruses, which lead to immortalization of lymphocytes *in vitro* and *in vivo,* HIV-1 exhibits pronounced cytopathic properties for lymphocytes, causing syncytia formation and cell death. Morphologically, HIV-1 differs from HTLV-I and other type C oncogenic retroviruses in exhibiting a dense, cylindrical core surrounded by a lipid envelope typical of lentiviruses (Fig. 361–1).

The structural organization of HIV-1 is shown diagrammatically in Figure 361–2. Like all retroviruses, HIV-1 is a single-stranded plus-sense RNA virus. The RNA-dependent DNA polymerase, or reverse transcriptase, is packaged within the virion core and is responsible for replicating the single-stranded RNA genome through a double-stranded DNA intermediate, which in turn serves as the

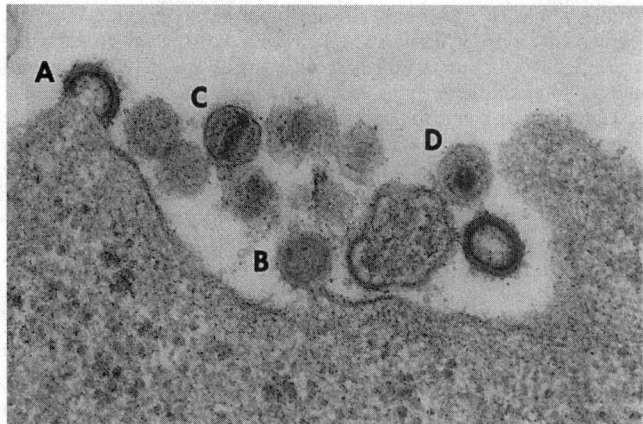

FIGURE 361–1. Transmission electron micrograph of HIV-1. Virions are shown at all stages of morphogenesis: early (A) and late (B) budding forms and cell-free mature virions (C and D) with condensed central cores. The diameter of virions is approximately 110 nm.

precursor molecule for proviral integration within the host cell genome. The major structural core proteins of HIV-1 are the p24 capsid protein and the p18 matrix protein, as shown. Surrounding the viral core protein structures is a bilayered lipid envelope that is derived from the outer limiting membrane of the host cell as the virus buds from the cell surface during replication. Studding this outer viral membrane are the envelope glycoproteins, gp120 and gp41, which are encoded by viral-specific genes and are responsible for cell attachment and entry.

The life cycle of HIV-1 is shown diagrammatically in Figure 361–3. Features of this life cycle distinguish retroviruses from all other viruses. The cell-free virion first attaches to the target cell through a specific interaction between the viral envelope and the host cell membrane. The specificity of this interaction between virus and cell has been shown to be due to a high-affinity specific interaction between the viral gp120 envelope glycoprotein and the target cell-associated CD4 molecule. Following virus adsorption, the viral and cellular membranes fuse, resulting in internalization of

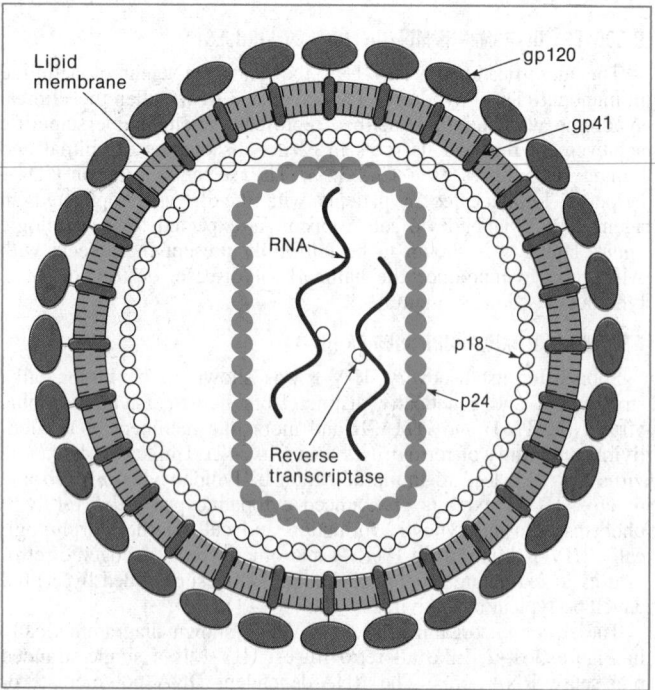

FIGURE 361–2. Structure of HIV-1. (Adapted from RC Gallo. Copyright © 1987 by Scientific American, Inc., and George V. Kelvin. All rights reserved.)

the nucleoprotein viral complex. Reverse transcription catalyzed by the viral reverse transcriptase generates a double-stranded DNA copy of the viral RNA within the nucleoprotein complex, and this migrates to the nucleus where covalent integration of viral DNA into the host chromosomes leads to formation of the provirus. Subsequent expression of viral DNA is controlled by a combination of viral and host cellular proteins that interact with viral DNA and RNA regulatory elements. Transcribed viral mRNA is translated into viral proteins, and new virions are assembled at the cell surface where genomic-length viral RNA, reverse transcriptase, structural and regulatory proteins, and envelope glycoproteins are assembled. Because the HIV-1 provirus is covalently integrated within the host cell chromosome, it represents a stable component of the host genome and is replicated and transmitted to daughter cells in synchrony with cellular DNA. Relevant to subsequent discussions of viral pathogenesis, the integrated provirus is thus permanently incorporated into the host cell genome and may remain transcriptionally latent or may exhibit high levels of gene expression with explosive production of progeny virus.

MOLECULAR STRUCTURE AND FUNCTION OF HIV-1

The genomic organization of HIV-1 is shown diagrammatically in Figure 361–4. The HIV-1 genome, like other retroviral genomes, is diploid, consisting of two identical viral RNA molecules assembled in a hydrogen-bonded 70S complex. These genomic subunits are plus strands of viral RNA in that they have the same chemical polarity as the mRNA from which viral products are translated. Like eukaryotic mRNA's, the genomic viral RNA contains a 5′ methylated-G nucleotide, a poly(A) tract of 100 to 200 nucleotides at its 3′ end, and a number of methylated(A) residues. Host cell–derived tRNA incorporated within the virion is base paired over a stretch of 18 nucleotides to the primer binding site of the genomic viral RNA near its 5′ terminus and serves to prime the synthesis of minus-strand DNA during the initial stages of viral replication following infection.

The HIV-1 genome is bounded by long terminal repeat (LTR) elements and contains genes encoding structural and enzymatic proteins (*gag, pol,* and *env*) found in all other replication-competent retroviruses. In addition to these, however, HIV-1 contains genes encoding other viral functions unique to this family of viruses that are responsible for their biologic behavior. The LTR sequences of HIV-1 direct and regulate expression of the viral genome (Fig. 361–5).

The *gag* gene encodes a precursor protein of 55 kilodaltons (p 55) which is cleaved into four smaller products with the linear order NH$_2$-p18-p24-p9-p7-COOH. These proteins constitute the core protein structure of the virus and also subserve nucleic acid and lipid membrane binding functions. The *gag* proteins of HIV-1, like those of other retroviruses, are synthesized as a polyprotein precursor that is subsequently cleaved during the viral maturation process. This facilitates the assembly of the different components of the virus core structure into a three-dimensional configuration that, when cleaved by a specific virus-derived protease, acquires the specialized functions characteristic of the mature virion. The polymerase gene products are translated from the same genomic RNA message as the *gag* proteins but in a different, overlapping reading frame as a result of ribosomal frame shifting. The *pol* gene encodes three proteins that are cleaved from a larger precursor polypeptide. These genes include NH$_2$-protease(p13)-reverse transcriptase (p66/p51)-integrase(p31)-COOH. The HIV-1 protease plays a critical role in virus biology, acting specifically to cleave *gag* and *pol* precursor polypeptides into functionally active proteins. The reverse transcriptase of HIV-1 is a magnesium-requiring RNA-dependent DNA polymerase responsible for replicating the RNA viral genome. The integrase protein is required for proviral integration into the host cell genome. The envelope gene *(env)* encodes a glycosolated polypeptide precursor (gp160) that is processed to form the exterior envelope glycoprotein (gp120) and the transmembrane glycoprotein (gp41), which anchors the envelope complex to the virus surface. It is the viral envelope that is responsible for CD4 binding, fusion, and virus entry.

Within the HIV-1 genome, there are additional genes that serve important viral functions and that distinguish HIV-1 from oncogenic retroviruses. These include the *vif, vpr,* and *vpu* genes located between *pol* and *env;* the *nef* gene located 3′ to the *env* and extending into the U3 region of the viral LTR; and the *tat* and *rev* genes, both

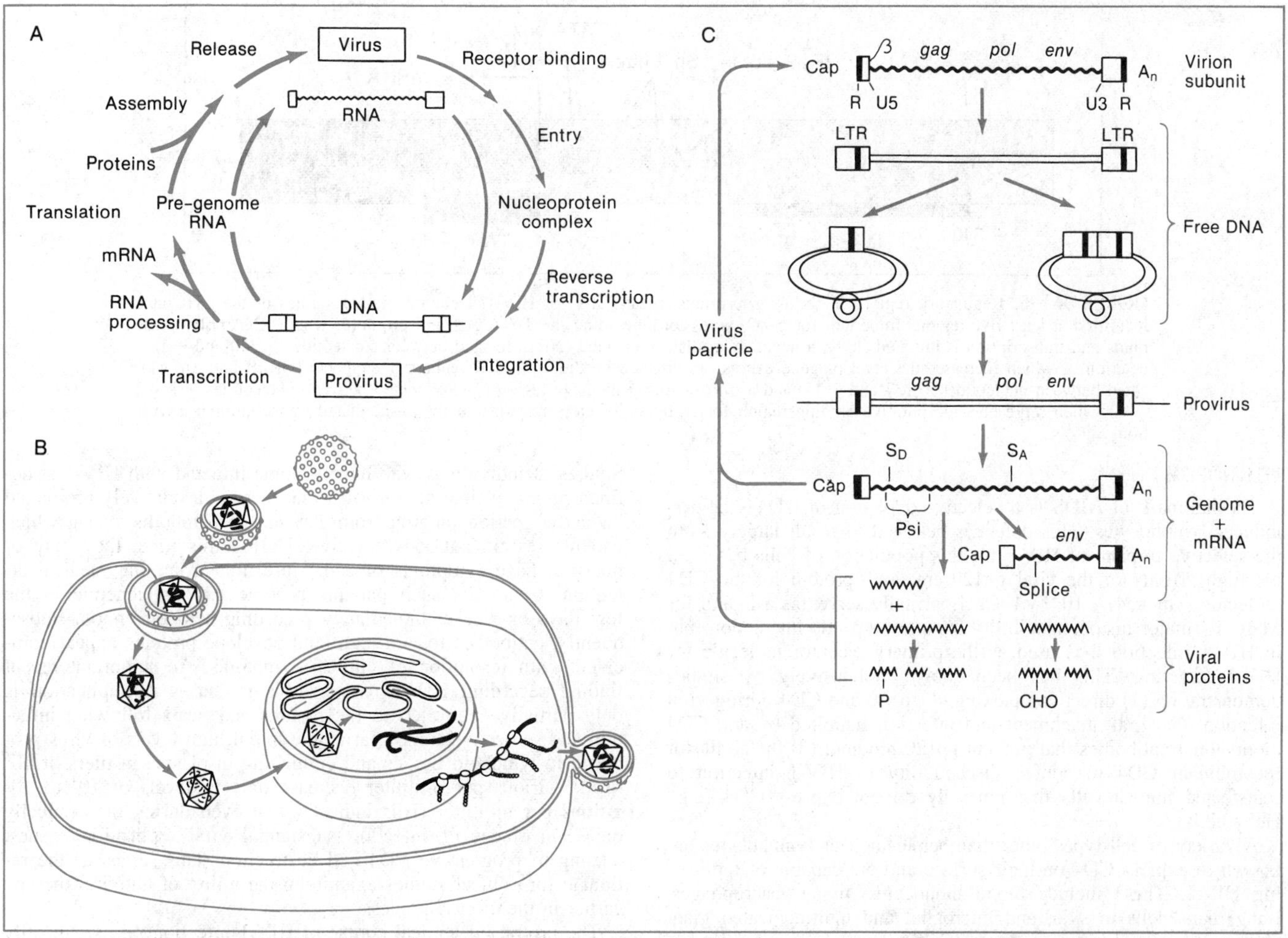

FIGURE 361–3. Different representations of the HIV-1 life cycle. *A,* An outline of the virus life cycle is shown, with thick arrows denoting amplification of viral products that may occur in the latter half of the replication cycle as a result of stimulation of virus expression. *B,* A pictorial overview of the virus life cycle outlined in *A,* beginning at the upper left and ending at the lower right. *C,* A detailed illustration of the major transformations of retroviral genetic information during the life cycle of HIV-1. Cap denotes the 5′ methyl-G-nucleotide, A_n the poly (A) tract, and S_D and S_A the splice donor and acceptor sites. Psi denotes the viral packaging signal sequence, P a phosphorylation site, and CHO a glycosylation site. (See text for discussion.) (Reprinted with permission from Varmus H, Brown P: Retroviruses. *In* Berg DE, Howe MM [eds.]: Mobile DNA. Washington, DC, American Society for Microbiology, 1989, p 53.)

of which exist as bipartite coding exons in the central and 3′ end of the virus. The *tat* gene encodes a 14-kDa protein that is essential for HIV-1 replication, upregulating HIV-1 expression at both transcriptional and post-transcriptional levels. The target sequence for *tat*-mediated upregulation of HIV-1 expression is the *trans*-acting responsive region (TAR) of the LTR, which apparently interacts with cellular factors induced by *tat* because the *tat* protein itself has not been shown to bind and activate TAR directly. The *rev* gene is also absolutely required for HIV-1 replication, facilitating transport of unspliced viral mRNA from the nucleus to cytoplasm. In the absence of *rev* genes, *gag* and *env* mRNA, transcripts are multiply spliced such that *gag* and *env* proteins are not made. The *vif* gene encodes a protein product of 23 kDa, which is required for the production of virions that are

fully infectious. The mechanisms of *vif* action are currently unknown. The *vpr* gene encodes a protein of 15 kDa which is involved in transport of the viral preintegration complex (see Fig. 361–3) to the nucleus. The *vpu* gene encodes a 16-kDa protein that is involved in virus assembly and release. The *nef* gene encodes a 27-kDa protein that decreases CD4 expression in virally infected cells, and by this or other means, accentuates viral pathogenesis *in vivo.*

In summary, HIV-1 encodes the usual structural and enzymatic proteins typical of other replication-competent retroviruses, including *gag, pol,* and *env,* but in addition it encodes a group of at least six regulatory or auxiliary proteins (*vif, vpr, vpu, tat, rev,* and *nef*) whose activities are critically important in regulating the life cycle and pathogenesis of the virus.

FIGURE 361–4. Genomic organization of HIV-1.

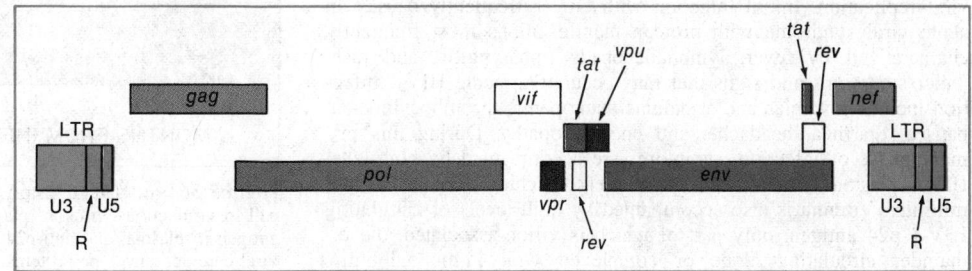

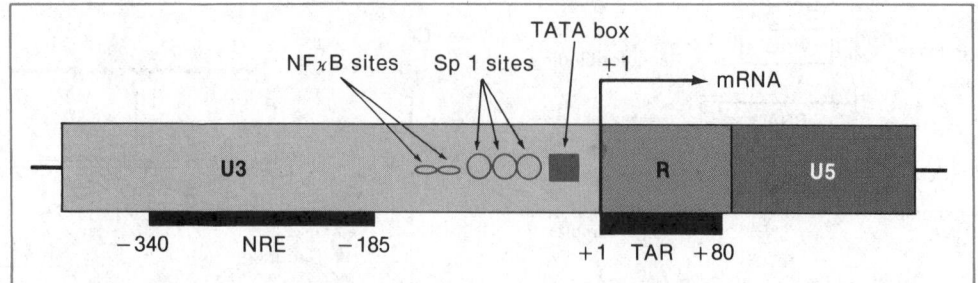

FIGURE 361–5. Regulatory regions in the long terminal repeat (LTR) of HIV-1. Deletion mutant studies of the LTR have identified at least five regions important for gene expression, including the TATA box and promotor where RNA polymerase binds and transcription is initiated (+1); a negative regulatory element (NRE) located between nucleotides −340 and −185, deletion of which increases the level of gene expression directed by the viral LTR; enhancer elements (NRκB and Sp1) located between nucleotides −137 and −17; and a *trans*-acting responsive region (TAR) located between nucleotides +1 and +80 which represents the putative binding region for regulatory factors responsible for *tat*-mediated transcriptional activation.

CELL TROPISM

The hallmark of AIDS is a selective depletion of CD4+ helper-inducer lymphocytes. This defect is believed to result largely from the selective tropism of HIV-1 for this population of cells based on the high affinity of the viral gp120 envelope protein for the CD4 molecule (km = 4×10^{-9}M). CD4 normally serves as a ligand for MHC II (major histocompatibility complex type II) interaction, but in HIV-1 infection it is used as the primary receptor molecule for HIV-1 targeting. This has been shown conclusively by studies demonstrating (1) direct complexing of gp120 and CD4 during viral infection; (2) viral attachment and infection inhibited by anti-CD4 monoclonal antibodies that prevent gp120 binding; (3) the ability of recombinant CD4 to confer susceptibility to HIV-1 infection to transfected human cells that normally do not express CD4 (e.g., HeLa cells).

A variety of cell types other than helper-inducer lymphocytes are known to express CD4 on their surface and are capable of replicating HIV-1. These include blood monocytes, tissue macrophages, Langerhans cells in skin, and microglial and multinucleated giant cells in the central nervous system (CNS). These cells generally express smaller amounts of CD4 on their cell surface but nonetheless have been shown to represent important reservoirs for HIV-1 *in vivo*. Infection of such cells, in fact, may play an important role in the pathogenesis of AIDS by sequestering the virus as described for other lentiviruses such as visna. Other cell types, including neurons, glial cells, B lymphocytes, colorectal epithelial cells, and myeloid precursors, which may or may not express small amounts of CD4 or CD4-related mRNA, have occasionally been shown to support HIV-1 replication, but the pathophysiologic significance of such findings in regard to viral pathogenesis *in vivo* is uncertain.

VIRAL PATHOGENESIS

Retroviral diseases are typically characterized by restricted viral gene expression, latency, and lifelong persistence of virus in the face of substantial host immune responses. From cohort studies of individuals infected with HIV-1 at known points in time, it is estimated that between 26 and 36% of infected individuals develop AIDS within 7 years of infection and that an additional 40% develop lesser signs of immune dysfunction. This protracted clinical course suggests that expression of the HIV-1 genome *in vivo* is downregulated as compared to *in vitro* infection of lymphocytes by HIV-1, which is characterized by explosive lytic viral infection.

Figure 361–6 depicts the natural history of HIV-1 infection of humans in relationship to clinical symptoms, immune function, and viral replication. Initial infection with HIV-1 frequently causes an acute viral syndrome with protean manifestations most frequently characterized by fever, lymphadenopathy, pharyngitis, and rash. Other symptoms and signs that may occur with acute HIV-1 infection include myalgias and arthralgias, leukopenia, thrombocytopenia, nausea, diarrhea, headache, and encephalopathy. During this primary phase of infection, symptoms are accompanied by high-level HIV-1 plasma viremia, with peak titers reaching 10^7 virions per milliliter. Viremia is also accompanied by high levels of circulating HIV-1 p24 antigen, only part of which is virion-associated, the remainder circulating alone or complexed with immunoglobulin.

Studies of individuals who have become infected with HIV-1 at defined points in time have shown that there is a relatively prolonged "window" period ranging from 2 weeks to 6 months during which patients remain antibody-negative. During this time, they may or may not have symptoms of acute infection prompting medical attention. Generally, such patients become p24 antigenemic in the few days or weeks immediately preceding seroconversion. Subsequently, antibodies to viral core and envelope proteins appear coincident with resolution of clinical symptoms. An important recent finding regarding HIV-1 pathogenesis is that viral replication is only partially controlled in the months and years following infection and seroconversion. That is, the initial high levels of virus produced in lymphoid tissues and circulating in plasma in titers of 10^6 to 10^7 virions per milliliter decrease only to levels of 10^3 to 10^5 virions per milliliter. This indicates that even during the clinically quiescent stages of infection substantial viral replication ensues, leading to progressive CD4 cell destruction. This serves as the rationale for clinical studies examining the utility of antiviral therapy earlier in the disease process.

The protracted clinical course of HIV-1 infection raises clinically relevant questions regarding viral pathogenesis: What are the mechanisms responsible for CD4+ cell loss *in vivo*? What are the viral and host interactions that underlie the chronicity of HIV-1 infection? The precise biologic mechanisms responsible for the cytopathic effects of HIV-1 *in vivo* are not known. Molecularly cloned HIV-1 proviral DNA, transfected into human cells, has been shown in cell culture experiments to contain all necessary information to generate infectious and cytopathic virus. Thus, there is no question that HIV-1 alone has the potential for direct cytopathic activity against CD4+ lymphocytes *in vitro* and *in vivo*. Expression of only the HIV-1 envelope on lymphocytes is sufficient for inducing fusion

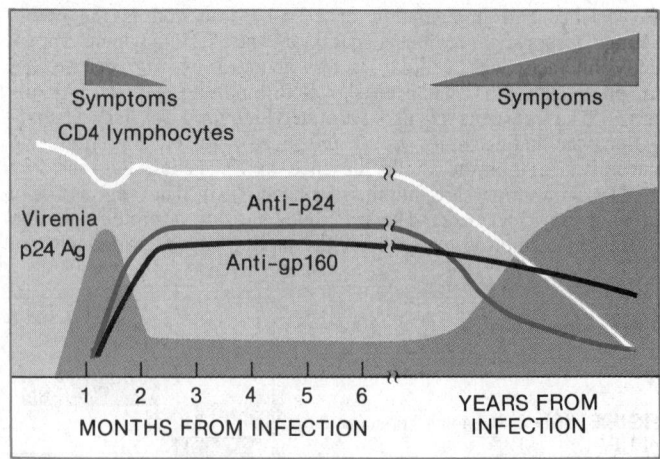

FIGURE 361–6. Natural history model for HIV-1 infection. Viremia denotes cell-free infectious virus in plasma, p24 Ag denotes circulating viral p24 antigen in plasma, and anti-p24 and anti-gp160 correspond to antibodies to viral core and envelope proteins.

of cells with normal uninfected CD4+ bystander cells, suggesting that syncytium formation mediated by gp120-CD4 interaction may also contribute to cell loss *in vivo*. However, other mechanisms of CD4 cell loss may also be operative. Cell-free HIV-1 gp120 envelope protein has been shown to adsorb to CD4+ cells and could serve as an effective antigen for mediating antibody-dependent cell-mediated cytotoxicity, and when processed by antigen-presenting cells, to constitute a target for direct T-cell cytotoxicity. The relative importance of these processes to CD4 cell loss *in vivo* remains to be determined. Similarly, in the CNS of infected individuals, wherein the predominant cell types infected with HIV-1 are cells of the monocyte/macrophage lineage, additional mechanisms of cytopathology are likely involved. Possibilities include the elaboration of cytotoxic factors from infected cells and interference with neurotropic factors, both leading to the clinically recognized AIDS dementia complex.

Viral and host factors responsible for the partial downregulation of HIV-1 replication following initial infection are also largely unknown. A strong humoral and cellular immune response to HIV-1 has been documented on the basis of ELISA, immunoblot, and radioimmunoprecipitation assays of patient sera and cell-mediated cytotoxicity to target cells displaying viral antigens. Neutralizing antibodies, antibody-dependent cell-mediated cytotoxicity, antibody-dependent complement-mediated cytotoxicity, MHC-restricted virus-specific cytotoxic T-lymphocyte-mediated cytotoxicity, and NK cell–mediated cytotoxicity have all been found to have activity against HIV-1 *in vitro* and may play an important role in the down-modulation of viral replication. However, the relative efficacy of the various immune effector arms and the changes that occur with time which eventually allow uncontrolled viral replication are unknown.

An additional component of the viral-host interaction of potentially great clinical importance is the regeneration capacity of the immune system. Recent studies of the clinical effects of novel, potent inhibitors of HIV-1 reverse transcriptase and protease genes indicate that patients with even severely depressed CD4 lymphocyte counts can experience substantial increases in such cells. Such responses have been of limited duration, however, owing to the development of viral resistance to these drugs. Yet they illustrate the potential benefits that may accrue if more effective antivirals are developed.

Genetic variability is a hallmark of HIV-1. The variability of the HIV-1 genome is characteristic of retroviruses in general because reverse transcription of viral RNA into proviral DNA and transcription of proviral DNA into genomic viral RNA are not subject to cellular proofreading mechanisms. The rate of nucleotide misincorporation by the viral reverse transcriptase is of the order of 10^{-4} per nucleotide per replication cycle. Because the HIV-1 genome is 10^4 nucleotides in length, this high rate of nucleotide misincorporation means that virtually no two viruses are identical and that HIV-1 isolates must, by definition, be described in terms of a "quasispecies" composed of populations of highly related but distinct viral genomes. Direct nucleotide sequence analysis of uncultured, virally infected human tissues using polymerase chain reaction amplification has confirmed these findings. The clinical importance of HIV-1 variability is still not fully understood. However, it is clear that viral resistance to reverse transcription inhibitors and protease inhibitors commonly develops and limits the effectiveness of these agents. Antigenic properties of the virus may also vary, thereby limiting the effectiveness of the immune response. Moreover, genetic variability leads to biologic changes in the virus over time, frequently resulting in the accumulation of virus strains with pronounced syncytium-inducing (SI) phenotypes in late stages of infection. Such a switch from non-SI to SI virus strains *in vivo* carries a worsened clinical prognosis.

HUMAN IMMUNODEFICIENCY VIRUS TYPE 2

Following the discovery of HIV-1 as the cause of epidemic AIDS in the United States, Europe, and Asia, patients in West Africa with AIDS-like symptoms were identified whose sera reacted more strongly with an immunodeficiency virus (SIV$_{MAC}$) isolated from captive rhesus macaques in US primate centers than with HIV-1. The identification of patients with serologic reactivity for SIV$_{MAC}$ raised the possibility that certain African human and simian populations could be infected with immunodeficiency viruses related to but distinct from HIV-1. An extensive survey of African primate species for such viruses led to the identification of distinct

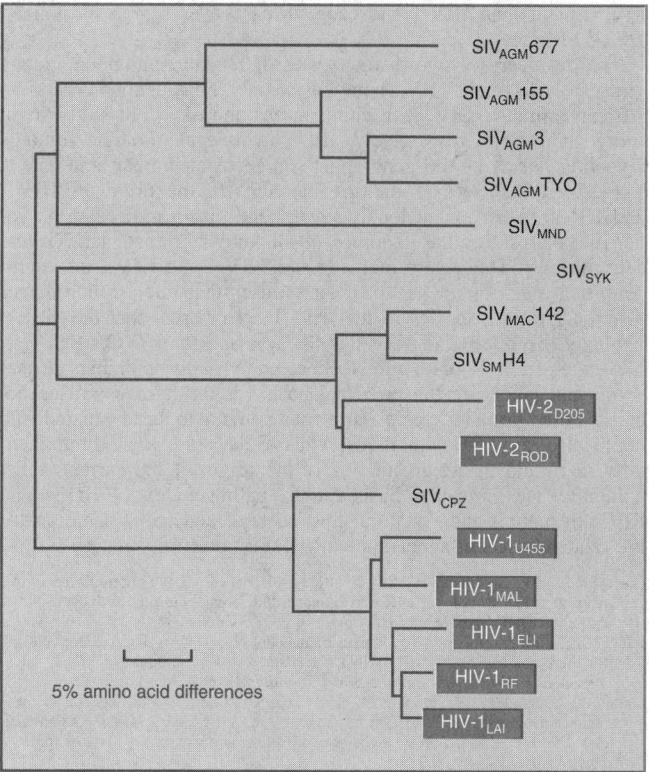

FIGURE 361-7. Phylogenetic relationships among primate lentiviruses, inferred from *pol* protein sequences. Independent isolates of SIV obtained from African green monkeys (AGM), mandrill (MND), Sykes' (SYK), rhesus macaque (MAC), sooty mangabey (SM), and chimpanzee (CPZ) are depicted along with representative isolates of HIV-1 and HIV-2 (boxed). The horizontal branch lengths are drawn to scale and can be used to determine the percentage difference in *pol* protein sequences between the different virus strains. The figure shows five major and roughly equidistant phylogenetic lineages of viruses (SIV$_{AGM}$; SIV$_{MND}$; SIV$_{SYK}$; SIV$_{MAC}$/SIV$_{SM}$/HIV-2; and SIV$_{CPZ}$/HIV-1). HIV-1 and HIV-2 appear as members of larger viral lineages composed of both simian and human derived viruses. Such relationships are indicative of cross-species transmission. (Adapted with permission from Hahn BH: Viral genes and their products. *In* Broder S, Merigan TC, Bolognesi D (eds.): Textbook of AIDS Medicine. Baltimore, Williams & Wilkins, 1994, p 21.)

SIV viruses present in African green monkeys (SIV$_{AGM}$), mandrills (SIV$_{MND}$), sooty mangabeys (SIV$_{SM}$), and chimpanzees (SIV$_{CPZ}$) (Fig. 361-7). West African patients with AIDS-like symptoms and healthy individuals at risk for AIDS were identified who were infected with a virus closely related to SIV$_{SM}$. This virus was isolated, molecularly cloned and characterized, and shown to represent a second major class of human immunodeficiency viruses termed HIV-2. Although originally limited geographically to West Africa, HIV-2 has now been identified in patients in Europe, the United States, South America, and India. HIV-2 is approximately 40 to 50% similar to HIV-1 in overall nucleotide sequence homology. There are two major differences in the genomic organization of HIV-1 and HIV-2. The *vpu* gene of HIV-1 is not present in HIV-2, and HIV-2 contains an additional gene, *vpx*, in its central region that is not present in HIV-1. Although the function of *vpx* is not entirely clear, it is packaged in the viral particle, like *vpr*, and it may have a similar function related to nuclear transport or processing of the viral preintegration complex. Antigenically, HIV-2 and HIV-1 are distinct, with greatest cross-reactivity in structural proteins and least in envelope proteins. Currently licensed ELISA tests to detect HIV-1 infection generally include HIV-2 antigens. However, confirmation requires specific testing by Western immunoblot using HIV-2–specific proteins as antigen. Like HIV-1, HIV-2 selectively infects CD4+ cells. Although HIV-2 can cause profound immunodeficiency and an AIDS syndrome indistinguishable from that caused by HIV-1, evidence suggests that HIV-2 may in general be less virulent than HIV-1 and cause disease over a more prolonged period of time.

The discovery of two distinct types of human immunodeficiency viruses (HIV-1 and HIV-2) having closely related counterparts in African primates (SIV$_{CPZ}$ in chimpanzees and SIV$_{SM}$ in wild-caught sooty mangabeys, respectively), along with epidemiologic findings revealing Africa as the geographic source of all human and SIV's, suggest cross-species (zoonotic) infection for the origin of HIV-1 and HIV-2. This conclusion is strengthened by a molecular phylogenetic analysis of the genomes of all known primate lentiviruses (Fig. 361–7). This figure indicates that HIV-1 and HIV-2 are members of a much larger group of lentiviruses that infect a number of different primate species in the wild. It is apparent that the closest phylogenetic relative of HIV-1 is SIV$_{CPZ}$, and for HIV-2, is SIV$_{SM}$. Nevertheless, it is premature to conclude that the chimpanzee and sooty mangabey are the proximal hosts for the human viruses because other primate species in Africa remain to be evaluated and could also serve as natural reservoirs. Such studies are fundamentally important to the elucidation of the origin of the current AIDS epidemic, the molecular basis for the pathogenicity of HIV's and SIV's in natural and unnatural host species, and an explanation for the relatively recent appearance of AIDS as an epidemic.

Barre-Sinoussi F, Chermann JC, Rey F, et al.: Isolation of a T-lymphotropic retrovirus from a patient at risk for acquired immune deficiency syndrome (AIDS). Science 220:868, 1983. *Discovery of HIV-1.*

Fauci AS: Multifactorial nature of human immunodeficiency virus disease: Implications for therapy. Science 262:1011, 1993. *Excellent review of immunopathologic mechanisms in HIV-1 disease and the scientific rationale for early treatment.*

Gallo RC, Salahuddin SZ, Popovic M, et al.: Frequent detection and isolation of cytopathic retroviruses (HTLV-III) from patients with AIDS and at risk for AIDS. Science 224:500, 1984. *Initial report conclusively identifying HIV-1 as the etiologic agent responsible for AIDS.*

Hahn BH: Viral genes and their products. *In* Broder S, Merigan TC, Bolognesi D (eds.): Textbook of AIDS Medicine. Baltimore, Williams & Wilkins, 1994, p 21. *Comprehensive up-to-date review of the molecular biology of HIV-1.*

Piatak M Jr, Saag MS, Yang LC, et al.: High levels of HIV-1 in plasma during all stages of infection determined by competitive PCR. Science 259:1749, 1993. *First study to accurately and systematically quantify HIV-1 in plasma throughout the entire course of infection, demonstrating the persistent nature of viral replication in vivo.*

Sharp PM, Robertson DL, Gao F, et al.: Origins and diversity of human immunodeficiency viruses. AIDS93/94: A Year in Review, in press. *Excellent review of the phylogenetic origins and evolutionary relationships among all known human and simian immunodeficiency viruses.*

Shaw GM, Hahn BH, Arya SK, et al.: Molecular characterization of human T-cell leukemia (lymphotropic) virus type III in the acquired immunodeficiency syndrome. Science 226:1165, 1984. *First description of the molecular cloning and analysis of the HIV-1 provirus.*

Weiss R, Teich N, Varmus H, Coffin J (eds.): RNA Tumor Viruses. Cold Spring Harbor, NY, Cold Spring Harbor Laboratory, 1982; Weiss R, Teich N, Varmus H, et al. (eds.): RNA Tumor Viruses 2/Supplements and Appendixes. Cold Spring Harbor, NY, Cold Spring Harbor Laboratory, 1985. *Textbooks on current knowledge of all retroviruses, including the three major groups of onco-, lenti- and spumaviruses.*

Xiping W, Sajal KG, Taylor ME, et al.: Viral dynamics in human immunodeficiency virus type 1 infection. Nature 373:117, 1995. *First description of viral and cellular kinetics underlying HIV-1 pathogenesis.*

362 EPIDEMIOLOGY OF HIV INFECTION AND AIDS

James W. Curran

The first cases of what has become known as the acquired immunodeficiency syndrome (AIDS) were reported in mid-1981 from Los Angeles, California. One month following these five reports of *Pneumocystis carinii* pneumonia (PCP) in young homosexual men, 26 cases of Kaposi's sarcoma (KS) in homosexual men in New York and California and additional cases of PCP and other opportunistic infections were reported. Reports of cases in the United States continued to rise, and soon the occurrence of PCP, KS, or other serious opportunistic infections in a person with unexplained immune dysfunction became known as AIDS. In retrospect, sporadic cases may have occurred in the United States, Europe, or Africa as much as three decades earlier, but the worldwide epidemic was not apparent until the 1980's.

TABLE 362–1. 1993 REVISED CLASSIFICATION SYSTEM FOR HIV INFECTION AND EXPANDED AIDS SURVEILLANCE CASE DEFINITION FOR ADOLESCENTS AND ADULTS*

	Clinical Categories		
CD4+ T-cell categories	(A) Asymptomatic, acute (primary) HIV or PGL†	(B) Symptomatic, not (A) or (C) conditions	(C) AIDS-indicator conditions
(1) ≥ 500/µL	A1	B1	C1
(2) 200–449/µL	A2	B2	C2
(3) < 200/µL AIDS-indicator T-cell count	A3	B3	C3

* Shaded areas indicate conditions included in the 1993 AIDS surveillance case definition for adolescents and adults. Clinical conditions in C are listed in Table 362–2.
† PGL = persistent generalized lymphadenopathy.

The initial occurrence of AIDS in homosexual men and injecting drug users (IDU's) suggested by 1982 that a transmissible agent was the likely cause. The transmissible agent hypothesis gained credence by early 1983 with the documented occurrence of AIDS in persons with hemophilia and in recipients of blood transfusions. Within a year, the retrovirus, now termed human immunodeficiency virus (HIV), was isolated and shown to be the cause of AIDS.

HIV INFECTION AND AIDS IN THE UNITED STATES

Since 1981, more than 985,000 cases of AIDS have been reported from 190 countries. More than 40% of these were reported from the United States, reflecting the relatively high incidence of the syndrome here and a well-established national active surveillance system. All 50 states require that AIDS be reported to state health departments and subsequently without names to the Centers for Disease Control and Prevention (CDC). The surveillance case definition for AIDS was initially developed before its cause was known but was revised following the development of diagnostic tests for HIV infection and the widespread use of CD4 lymphocyte monitoring in clinical management of persons with HIV disease. The current definition provides a consistent method to monitor trends of serious HIV-associated morbidity and mortality (Tables 362–1 and 362–2). Patients infected with HIV exhibit a spectrum

TABLE 362–2. CONDITIONS INCLUDED IN THE 1993 AIDS SURVEILLANCE CASE DEFINITION

Bacterial infections, multiple or recurrent*
Candidiasis of bronchi, trachea, or lungs
Candidiasis, esophageal
Cervical cancer, invasive†
Coccidioidomycosis, disseminated or extrapulmonary
Cryptococcosis, extrapulmonary
Cryptosporidiosis, chronic intestinal (> 1 month's duration)
Cytomegalovirus disease (other than liver, spleen, or nodes)
Cytomegalovirus retinitis (with loss of vision)
Encephalopathy, HIV-related
Herpes simplex, chronic ulcer(s) (> 1 month's duration); or bronchitis, pneumonitis, or esophagitis
Histoplasmosis, disseminated or extrapulmonary
Isosporiasis, chronic intestinal (> 1 month's duration)
Kaposi's sarcoma
Lymphoid interstitial pneumonia and/or pulmonary lymphoid hyperplasia*
Lymphoma, Burkitt's (or equivalent term)
Lymphoma, immunoblastic (or equivalent term)
Lymphoma, primary, of brain
Mycobacterium avium complex or *M. kansasii,* disseminated or extrapulmonary
Mycobacterium tuberculosis, any site (pulmonary† or extrapulmonary)
Mycobacterium, other species or unidentified species, disseminated or extrapulmonary
Pneumocystis carinii pneumonia
Pneumonia, recurrent†
Progressive multifocal leukoencephalopathy
Salmonella septicemia, recurrent
Toxoplasmosis of brain
Wasting syndrome due to HIV

* Children < 13 years old.
† Added in the 1993 expansion of the AIDS surveillance case definition for adolescents and adults.

of manifestations ranging from no symptoms to AIDS. Systems have been developed to classify these manifestations in children and adults. In states that require reporting of all HIV infections, a standard classification system is used.

INCIDENCE AND TRENDS OF AIDS IN THE UNITED STATES

By December 1993, 361,164 cases of AIDS in adults and children had been reported to the CDC; >220,000 were reported to have died, including >80% of those diagnosed before 1990. Among cases reported in 1993, 47% of cases in adults were homosexual or bisexual men without a history of intravenous drug use, and 6% were homosexual or bisexual IDU's. More than 60% of the reported cases in heterosexual men and women had a history of IDU, including half of the cases in women. One per cent of adults with AIDS had hemophilia or other coagulation disorders; 2% of cases were associated with transfusions, the vast majority of which had been received before 1985, when HIV antibody screening of all blood and plasma donations was instituted. In 1993, 9% of all cases of AIDS, including 37% of cases in women, were attributed to heterosexual contact with a person with documented HIV infection or in one of the other main transmission categories.

By December 1993, 5228 cases of AIDS had been reported in children younger than age 13, with >54% reported to have died. In 1993, >93% of pediatric AIDS cases resulted from perinatal transmission of HIV infection, 3% were attributed to transfusions, and 2% occurred in children with hemophilia. In 1993, rates of reported AIDS varied substantially by age, gender, race-ethnicity, and geographic area, emphasizing that overall HIV/AIDS occurrence in the United States was a product of "hundreds of epidemics" of varying intensity. Figure 362–1 depicts 1993 case rates by gender throughout the United States, highlighting these substantial geographic disparities.

AIDS has disproportionately affected black and Hispanic minority populations in the United States. In 1993, 55% of reported cases were in these minority populations; 36% of adult and 55% of pediatric cases were black and 18% of adult and 27% of pediatric cases were Hispanic. In contrast, blacks and Hispanics are estimated to account for 11.6% and 6.5% of the US population, respectively.

In 1993, AIDS rates were approximately 15 and 6 times higher for black and Hispanic women than for white women. The rates for black and Hispanic men were five and three times higher than for white men. Racial disparities in pediatric AIDS rates reflect those in women (Table 362–3). During the 1980's and early 1990's, AIDS cases increased more rapidly in those racial and ethnic minority

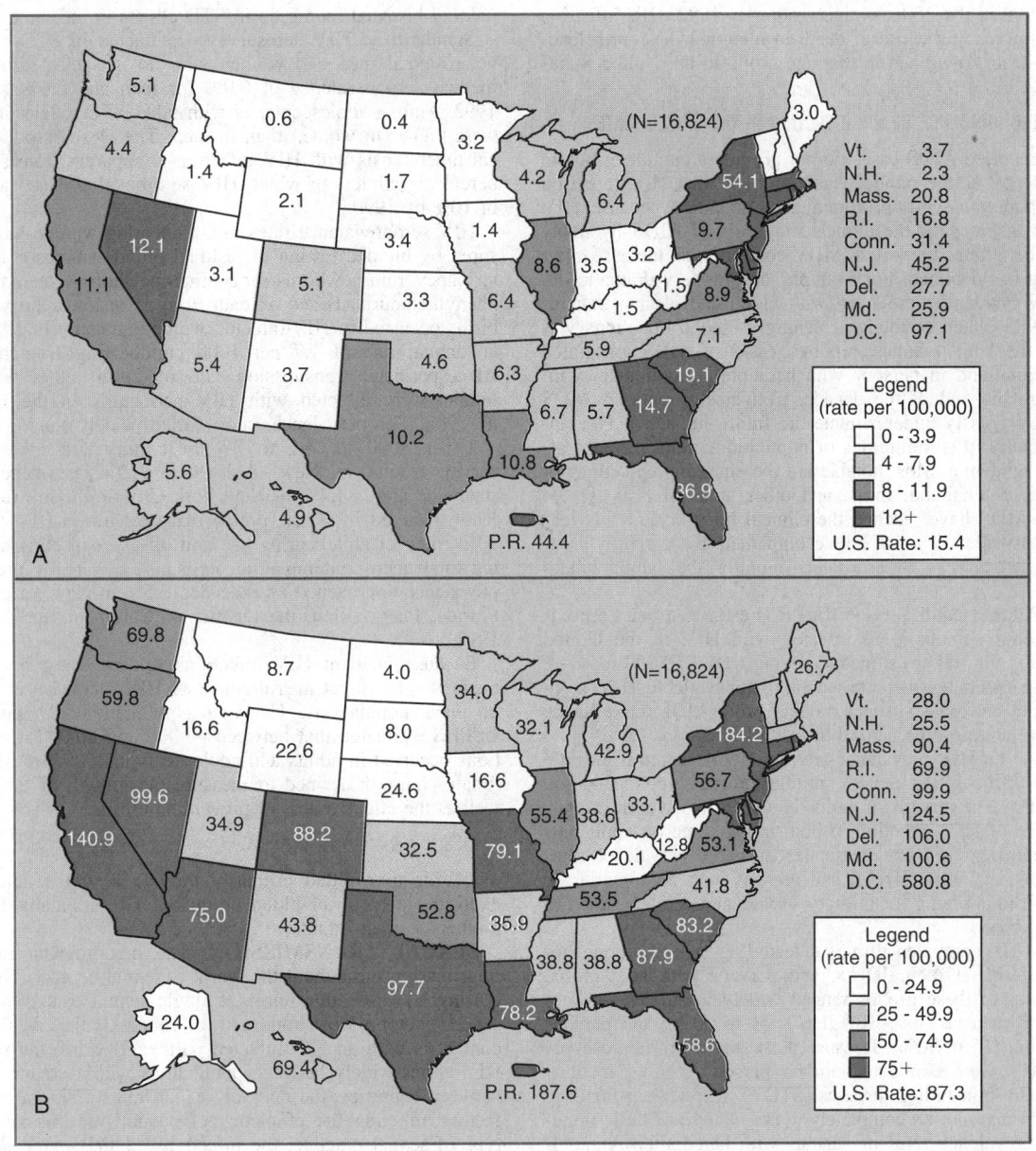

FIGURE 362–1. Adult/adolescent AIDS annual rates per 100,000 population, for cases reported in 1993 in the United States for *(A)* females and *(B)* males. (Source: Centers for Disease Control and Prevention: *HIV/AIDS Surveillance Report,* 5 (No.4):1, 1994.)

TABLE 362–3. NUMBER, PERCENTAGE, AND RATES* OF AIDS CASES, BY RACE/ETHNICITY—UNITED STATES, REPORTED IN 1993

| | Adult/Adolescent† | | | | | | | | | Children‡ | | |
| | Male | | | Female | | | Total | | | | | |
Race/Ethnicity	No.	%	Rate	No.	%	Rate	No.	%	Rate	No.	%	Rate
White, non-Hispanic	43,987	49	57	4,103	24	5	48,090	45	30	150	16	0.4
Black, non-Hispanic	28,792	32	266	9,220	55	73	38,012	36	162	532	55	7.2
Hispanic	15,301	17	146	3,324	20	32	18,625	18	90	263	27	3.6
Asian/Pacific Islander	665	1	21	97	1	3	762	1	12	5	1	0.3
American Indian/ Alaskan Native	281	<1	41	55	<1	8	336	<1	24	3	<1	0.6
Total minorities	45,039	51	179	12,696	75	47	57,735	54	111	803	84	4.8
Total¶	89,165	100	88	16,824	100	15	105,990	100	50	959	100	1.9

* Per 100,000 population. Population counts for 1993 were estimated from 1990 U.S. census data.
† Age ≥ 13 years.
‡ Age < 13 years.
¶ Includes 171 persons for whom race/ethnicity was unknown and one person for whom sex was unknown.

populations, particularly cases associated with injecting drug use or heterosexual HIV transmission.

HIV infection has a large impact on mortality in young adults in the United States, with three quarters of the nearly 37,000 deaths reported in 1992 in the 25 to 44 age group. By 1992, HIV infection had become the leading cause of death in men and the fourth leading cause of death in women in that age group in the United States (Fig. 362–2).

PREVALENCE AND INCIDENCE OF HIV INFECTION IN THE UNITED STATES

Trends in reported AIDS cases do not provide a complete picture of the prevalence of the public health problem that HIV infection poses for a population group, community, or nation because HIV infection *per se* precedes the clinical diagnosis of AIDS by many years. In some groups, reported AIDS continues to increase after HIV infection has declined. For example, despite very dramatic declines in HIV incidence associated with blood and plasma transfusions after 1985, when antibody screening of blood donations was instituted in the United States, reported cases of AIDS associated with transfusions and in persons with hemophilia continued to increase through the end of the decade. Conversely, reported AIDS case rates may grossly underestimate the future impact of HIV infection, especially in communities or populations more recently affected by the epidemic. Most notable are the emerging epidemics of HIV infection in Thailand, India, and other areas of Asia, where few cases of AIDS have reached the clinical horizon. For this reason, AIDS surveillance must be accompanied by carefully conducted HIV serosurveys to accurately monitor the public health problem.

The U.S. Public Health Service (USPHS) estimated that approximately 1 million persons were infected with HIV in the United States by 1990, with other estimates ranging from 750,000 to >1.2 million. These estimates were based on both available HIV seroprevalence data and on statistical models using AIDS surveillance data and information on the natural history of infection.

National data on HIV prevalence are directly measured from HIV testing of first-time blood donors, military recruit applicants, job corps applicants, and surveys of antibody status of newborn infants. The prevalence of HIV infection in both military recruit applicants and blood donors grossly underestimates true HIV prevalence rates because homosexual men, IDU's, and persons with hemophilia are discouraged from applying for military service and actively deferred from donating blood.

The highest HIV prevalence rates detected have been among homosexual or bisexual men, IDU's, and persons with hemophilia. Prevalence rates in these groups ranged widely in studies—homosexual/bisexual men (10 to 70%), IDU's, (1 to 50%), and persons with hemophilia (15 to 90%). Because most surveys in homosexual men and IDU's were conducted among persons seeking medical care for sexually transmitted diseases (STD's) or treatment for drug abuse, the data may not be completely representative of these populations. HIV prevalence rates in persons with hemophilia A and B were directly related to the amount of clotting factor received prior to 1985. HIV seroprevalence rates among female prostitutes varied

widely from 0 to >50%, with the differences largely attributed to the extent of injecting drug use in the population surveyed and the HIV prevalence among IDU's in the community at that time. HIV prevalence rates among male prostitutes parallel rates in homosexual and bisexual men seen in STD clinics in the same communities.

Standardized HIV serosurveys conducted in STD clinics among heterosexual men and women who do not inject drugs showed a median seroprevalence of 0.9% for men and 0.6% for women in 1992. Among adolescents, as with other STD's, HIV infection rates were higher in women than in men. The close association of clinical tuberculosis with HIV infection is apparent from surveys in tuberculosis clinics, in which HIV seroprevalence had a median rate of 10% by 1990.

HIV seroprevalence rates in childbearing women have been measured by blinded testing of residual blood samples collected on filter paper from newborns for routine metabolic screening such as for phenylketonuria. Based on data from 35 states, approximately 7000 births occurred in HIV-infected women annually in 1991–1992, for an annual rate of 1.7 per 1000 childbearing women nationwide. At a perinatal transmission rate of 20 to 30%, 1400 to 2100 infants were infected with HIV perinatally in the United States in 1992. Seroprevalence rates varied widely among states, from <1 per 1000 to >1 to 3% in northeastern urban areas. The survey results in New York State (HIV prevalence of 0.67% statewide and >1.4% in New York City in childbearing women in 1989) resulted in a state policy that encourages HIV counseling of all women of childbearing age and offers counseling and HIV testing to women contemplating pregnancy or already pregnant. Seroprevalence approached or exceeded 0.5% in New Jersey, Maryland, Florida, Puerto Rico, the District of Columbia, and New York by 1992.

Because incident HIV infections seldom cause persons to seek medical care, direct measurement of HIV incidence is very difficult in most populations. Using a combination of approaches, the USPHS estimated that between 40,000 and 80,000 new HIV infections occurred in adults and adolescents in 1989. HIV incidence estimates must be refined to measure the growth of the epidemic as well as the effectiveness of prevention efforts.

MODES OF TRANSMISSION OF HIV

HIV is transmitted primarily through sexual contact, parenteral exposure to blood or blood products, and perinatally from infected mothers to their infants.

SEXUAL TRANSMISSION. The predominant mode of HIV transmission throughout the world is sexual contact. The risk of acquiring HIV infection during a single sexual contact depends upon several factors. Most important, of course, is the likelihood that the contact is with an HIV-infected partner. Because the prevalence of HIV varies widely between populations within countries as well as between countries, the rates of sexual transmission also vary. Other factors affecting the efficiency of sexual transmission include the type of sexual practice; the infectivity of the source partner; coexisting genital infections in either partner, particularly those causing genital ulceration; and consistency of condom use. HIV transmis-

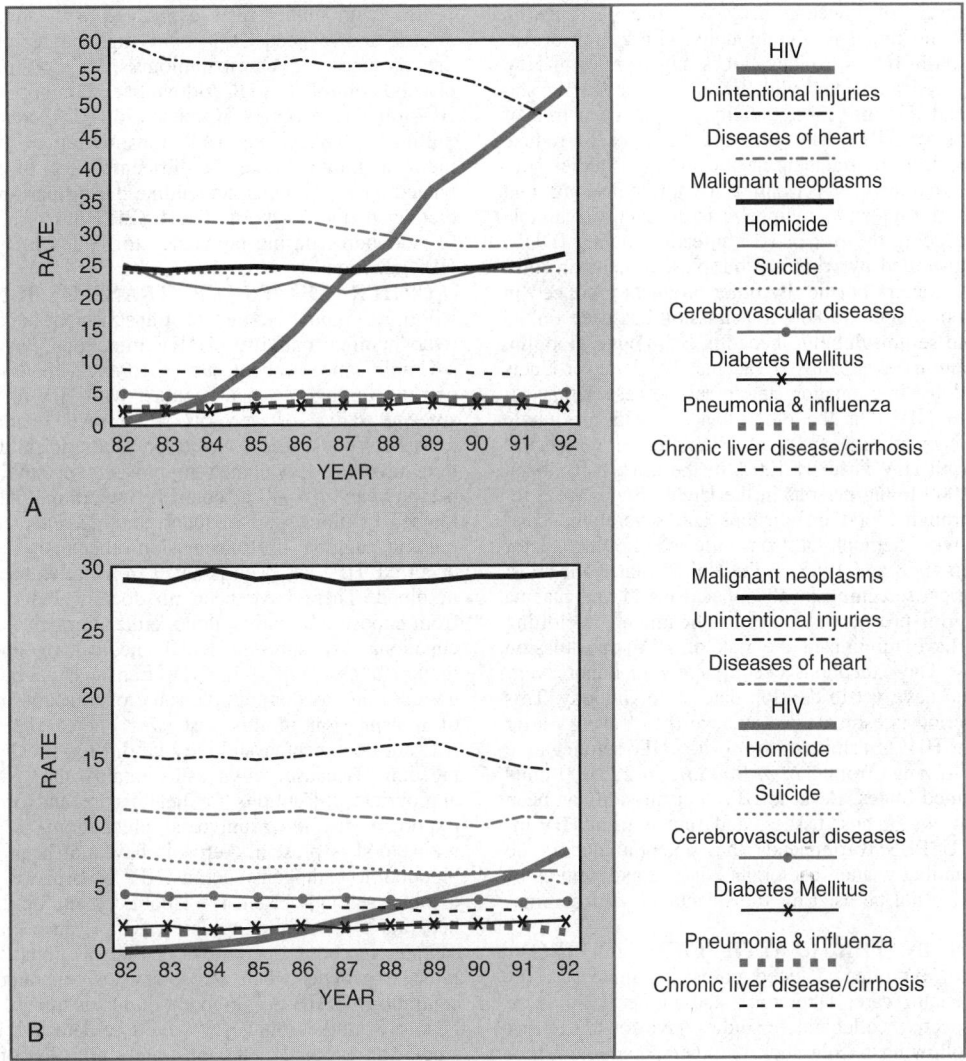

FIGURE 362–2. Death rates for leading causes of death among men *(A)* and women *(B)* aged 25 to 44, by year per 100,000 population in the United States, 1982–1992. (National vital statistics based on underlying cause of death, using final data for 1982 to 1991 and provisional data for 1992. Data for liver disease in 1992 were unavailable.)

sion has been attributed to vaginal, anal, and, less frequently, oral intercourse.

In epidemiologic studies among homosexual men, the risk of HIV acquisition increases with the number of sexual partners and the frequency of receptive anal intercourse, and practices associated with rectal trauma such as receptive "fisting" and anal douching. No sexual activity potentially involving the exchange of semen or blood, however, should be considered without risk. The relative efficiency of HIV transmission through various sexual practices was difficult to estimate precisely because most HIV-infected homosexual men in epidemiologic studies had engaged in multiple practices. Although the frequency of female-to-female transmission would seem to be quite low, such HIV infections associated with traumatic sexual practices have been reported. Most cases of HIV infection reported among bisexual women and lesbians are attributed to injecting drug use or heterosexual contact.

Most heterosexual transmission of HIV occurs during vaginal intercourse, although some studies suggest that receptive anal intercourse increases the risk of HIV transmission from an infected man to a woman. Some infected persons may be more efficient transmitters than others, perhaps owing to differences in viral strains or other factors. Transmission efficiency is inversely related to the immunologic status of the infected partner. In studies conducted among spouses and other steady sexual partners of HIV-infected persons, male-to-female, female-to-male, and male-to-male sexual transmission of HIV increased as the index partner's T-helper lymphocyte numbers declined. These findings are not surprising be-

cause the quantity of HIV in blood and semen increases as the disease progresses and the immune system weakens. Several studies have documented that infections such as *Haemophilus ducreyi,* *Treponema pallidum,* herpes simplex virus, and other pathogens causing genital or anal ulcers facilitate acquisition or transmission of HIV through sexual contact, most likely by disrupting the genital or anal skin and mucous membranes. Undoubtedly, the higher rates of untreated genital ulcer disease contribute to the high rates of sexual transmission of HIV observed in some areas of the developing world. Several investigators have reported increased risks of HIV acquisition for women with cervical infections with *Neisseria gonorrhoeae* or *Chlamydia trachomatis* or with cervical ectopy. To the extent that coexisting sexually transmitted infections increase the rate of HIV transmission, populations throughout the world with higher rates of these infections are at higher risk of HIV infection. Conversely, preventing and treating other sexually transmitted infections should have a beneficial effect on preventing HIV transmission. Cohort studies of couples discordant for HIV infection clearly indicate that consistent condom use reduces heterosexual as well as homosexual HIV transmission by ≥90% compared with inconsistent use or nonuse of condoms. Finally, preliminary studies suggest that antiretrovirals may reduce but not eliminate the risk of HIV transmission through sexual contact.

TRANSMISSION THROUGH PARENTERAL EXPOSURE TO BLOOD OR BLOOD PRODUCTS. HIV is transmitted to IDU's by parenteral exposure to contaminated injection equipment, including needles. Risk factors for infection include frequency of needle sharing, duration of injecting drug use, use of drugs in "shooting galleries," and living in a community with a high prevalence of HIV infection in IDU's. Among IDU's, higher rates of HIV infection have also been associated with lower socioeconomic status, homelessness, and minority race/ethnicity. As has been true of homosexual men, many IDU's have changed behavior to reduce their HIV risk, particularly by reducing needle sharing. Studies suggest that drug abuse treatment, street outreach with counseling, and measures to make sterile injection equipment more readily available all have a role in reducing the risk of HIV infection among IDU's.

HIV has been transmitted by whole blood, plasma, cellular components, and clotting factors but not by other products produced in the United States from blood. No HIV transmission has been linked to receipt of immune serum globulin, hepatitis B immune globulin, $Rh_o(O)$ immune globulin, or hepatitis B vaccine. The latter products have been produced by fractionation and other processes that remove and inactivate HIV. On the other hand, receipt of whole blood, packed cells, or plasma from an HIV-infected donor has been shown to transmit HIV virtually 100% of the time. It has been estimated that > 12,000 living persons in the United States were infected with HIV through blood transfusions and several thousand additional persons with hemophilia from infected clotting factor concentrates between 1978 and 1985. In the United States and most industrialized countries, screening of all donated blood and plasma for HIV, donor deferral procedures, and heat treatment of clotting factor concentrates have minimized the risk of HIV transmission through transfusions. The exceptions occur largely in donors very recently infected who have yet to develop detectable antibody. This so-called window period is estimated to average 6 to 8 weeks after infection. The rate of HIV transmission from such HIV-seronegative donors is estimated to range from 1 in 36,000 to 1 in 225,000 units transfused in the United States. Because HIV transmission has been reported in recipients of organs, tissues, and semen from HIV-infected donors, the USPHS recommends that potential donors be screened for HIV antibody and that organ, tissue, and semen of those who test positive not be used for transplantation or insemination.

TRANSMISSION IN THE HEALTH CARE ENVIRONMENT. Exposure to HIV-infected blood poses a definite risk for HIV infection for health care, laboratory, and home health care workers. Large prospective collaborative studies have found the risk of seroconversion following needle stick or other parenteral exposures to the blood of HIV-infected persons to be approximately 0.3%. In addition, there are a few well-documented published reports of infections in health care workers following mucous membrane or extensive skin exposures. Such transmission can occur, but the risk is much lower than following parenteral exposures.

Transmission of HIV infection from an infected dentist to six patients remains the only documented transmission of HIV to patients from a health care worker. These patients had no other confirmed exposure to HIV and each was infected with an HIV strain nearly identical genetically to that of the dentist and dissimilar to that of other HIV-infected persons in the area. Rarely, HIV infection transmission has been reported through inadvertent intravenous injection of blood from HIV-infected patients in home health care or hospital settings. Major nosocomial HIV outbreaks resulted from improper sterilization or reuse of contaminated injection equipment in Romania and in the former Soviet Union.

The risk of transmission of HIV, hepatitis B and C viruses, and other bloodborne pathogens to and from health care workers and patients can be minimized by close adherence to recommendations, which include universal precautions when caring for all patients.

PERINATAL TRANSMISSION. HIV is transmitted from an infected woman to her fetus or newborn during pregnancy or delivery or through breast-feeding. HIV detected in fetal tissues and HIV isolated in cord blood provide suggestive evidence that transmission can occur *in utero,* but recent studies suggest much if not most transmission occurs during the intrapartum period. HIV can be detected at birth by culture or polymerase chain reaction in only 30 to 50% of infants ultimately found to be infected. There are several reports of mothers who were infected through postpartum transfusions and subsequently transmitted HIV to their infants through breast-feeding. For that reason, the USPHS strongly recommends that HIV-positive mothers avoid breast-feeding in the United States,

where nutritionally adequate and safe substitutes are available. The rate of perinatal transmission in published studies varies from 13 to > 40% with higher rates associated with advanced maternal HIV disease and reduced CD4 count, higher rates of breast-feeding, and the presence of chorioamnionitis. In an important randomized placebo-controlled trial, zidovudine administered to asymptomatic HIV-infected pregnant women with CD4 counts > 200 per cubic millimeter reduced perinatal transmission by two thirds. The regimen was initiated after the thirteenth week of gestation and accompanied by intravenous zidovudine during parturition and 6 weeks of therapy to the newborn. The USPHS has issued guidelines on use of zidovudine during pregnancy to reduce perinatal transmission of HIV infection.

OTHER MODES OF TRANSMISSION. Throughout the world, the above routes of transmission have accounted for the overwhelming majority of HIV infections, but there has been considerable concern about other theoretical modes of transmission, especially through "casual" contact with HIV-infected persons, exposure to saliva or aerosols, or insect vectors. More than 700 nonsexual household contacts of adults or children with HIV infection have been evaluated in prospective studies. In thousands of person-years of close contact, including sharing bathroom and kitchen facilities, and frequent personal interactions including kissing and hugging, no transmission other than sexual or perinatal has occurred. HIV has been isolated from saliva but less frequently than in blood. There have been no documented transmissions of HIV from exposure to saliva alone, either through kissing or through occupational exposures in dental, medical, or laboratory settings. Although a case report of HIV transmission between siblings suggested a bite as the possible route of transmission, the precise mode of transmission in this case was unclear because seroconversion was not documented and the bite did not break the skin or result in bleeding. Because saliva can contain other pathogenic organisms, appropriate precautions for health care and dental workers remain important, including universal precautions if gross contamination with blood is present. Aerosols have not been reported to transmit bloodborne pathogens such as HIV or hepatitis B in the health care or other settings. Extensive laboratory and epidemiologic studies of hepatitis B have failed to detect HBsAg in respirable particles in air samples in dental operatories or dialysis units during procedures on infected patients when aerosols were generated. Because the concentration of HBsAg in body fluids is much higher than that of HIV, it is unlikely that HIV would be detected. Extensive laboratory studies have failed to demonstrate replication of HIV in insects that were fed high concentrations of HIV or injected with HIV-contaminated blood. Epidemiologic studies in the United States, Haiti, and Central Africa show no evidence of insect-borne HIV transmission.

The possibility of previously unrecognized modes of HIV transmission cannot be entirely excluded, but they are likely to be rare, if found.

AIDS AND HIV INFECTION OUTSIDE THE UNITED STATES

Within 3 years after the syndrome was recognized in the United States, cases of AIDS were reported from every continent. By June 1994, nearly 1 million cases had been reported from 190 countries to the World Health Organization (WHO) (Table 362–4). WHO estimated that > 40 million people would be infected with HIV by the end of the century. AIDS case reporting from developing countries is much less complete than in industrialized countries. Extensive HIV serosurveys in Africa, South and Central America, and parts of Asia provide evidence that AIDS case reports greatly un-

TABLE 362–4. CASES OF AIDS REPORTED TO WHO AS OF JUNE 30, 1994

Continent	Number of Cases	Number of Countries Reporting Cases
Africa	331,376	54
Americas	523,777	45
Asia	8,968	39
Europe	115,668	38
Oceania	5,330	14
Total	**985,119**	**190**

derestimate the magnitude of the HIV problem in many countries in these regions.

Modes of transmission of HIV are similar throughout the world, but the relative frequency varies considerably between countries and regions. In North America, Europe, Australia, New Zealand, and some areas of South America, the majority of HIV infections first occurred in homosexual men and IDU's; heterosexual and perinatal transmission initially resulted mostly from transmission from IDU's and their partners. In most countries in Africa and some in the Caribbean and South America, most HIV infections have occurred through heterosexual transmission. HIV seroprevalence rates are highest in urban prostitutes and sexually active young adults. High rates of infection in young women translate into a substantial amount of perinatal transmission. In some areas of Africa, pediatric HIV infection has significantly increased already high infant mortality rates. In many developing countries, transfusion of HIV-infected blood remains a substantial problem owing to inadequate blood banking and serologic testing capacity. Reuse of nonsterile needles and syringes and other medical practices have caused major HIV outbreaks in the former Soviet Union and Romania. In Asian countries such as Thailand and India, emergence of HIV infection as a major public health problem began in IDU's and prostitutes but rapidly spread more widely through heterosexual transmission to other young adult populations. In yet other countries, primarily in Eastern Europe, the Middle East, Asia, and the Pacific region, HIV has not yet been recognized as an important public health problem. The future course of HIV in these countries may depend upon their ability to anticipate and respond to the problem; it can be approximately predicted by the extent and pattern of sexually transmitted and transfusion-associated infections and the extent of injecting drug use which currently exists in each country.

A second human immunodeficiency virus, HIV type 2 (HIV-2), was first described in asymptomatic West Africans with AIDS in 1986. HIV-2 infection remains most prevalent in West Africa, although well-documented cases have been reported from Western Europe, Canada, Brazil, the United States, and Central Africa. HIV-2 is generally less virulent than HIV-1. The average viral titer is usually lower, perhaps explaining the lower rates of sexual and perinatal transmission and the slower rate of disease progression in persons infected with HIV-2 than HIV-1. HIV-1 and HIV-2 are closely related; tests for antibody for one virus often cross-react with those for the other. For example, licensed enzyme immunoassays for detecting HIV-1 find HIV-2 antibody in 60 to 90% of infected patients. In the United States combined HIV-1/HIV-2 assays are used to test donated blood. As of 1994, HIV-2 infection remained rare in the United States, with nearly all cases detected in persons from West Africa.

Recently additional HIV variants, classified together as subtype O, were reported from Cameroon. Although certain HIV antibody tests fail to detect these infections, these infections had not been detected in the United States by 1994 and were uncommon even in Cameroon. This situation reinforces the need for strong international collaboration in maintaining surveillance for variants of HIV and other emerging infections.

AIDS and human immunodeficiency virus infection in the United States: 1988 update. MMWR 38(S-4):1, 1989. HIV infection in the United States: A review of current knowledge. MMWR 36(S-6):1, 1987. The sentinel HIV seroprevalence surveys—special section. Pub Health Rep 105:113, 1990. National serosurveillance summary, Volume 3—Centers for Disease Control and Prevention, HIV/NCID/11-913/036; Gwinn M, Pappaioanou M, George JR, et al.: Prevalence of HIV infection in childbearing women in the United States. JAMA 265:1704, 1991. St. Louis ME, Connaugh A, Hayman CR, et al.: HIV infection in disadvantaged adolescents. JAMA 266:2387, 1991. These articles summarize recent methods and data on HIV seroprevalence in the United States.

1993 Revised classification system for HIV infection and expanded surveillance, case definition for AIDS among adolescents and adults. MMWR 41 (RR-17):1, 1992. Redfield RR, Wright DC, Tramont EA: The Walter Reed staging classification for HTLV-III/LAV infection. N Engl J Med 314:131, 1986. These are the most widely used classification systems in the United States.

Goedert JJ, Eyster EE, Biggar RJ, et al.: Heterosexual transmission of HIV: Association with severe depletion of T-helper lymphocytes in men with hemophilia. AIDS Res Hum Retroviruses 3:355, 1988. Holmberg SD, Horsburgh CR, Ward JW, et al.: Biologic factors in the sexual transmission of human immunodeficiency virus. J Infect Dis 160:116, 1989. Ellerbrock TV, Lieb S, Harrington PE, et al.: Heterosexual transmitted human immunodeficiency virus infection among pregnant women in a rural Florida community. N Engl J Med 327:1704, 1992. De Vincenzi I, et al.: A longitudinal study of human immunodeficiency virus transmission by heterosexual partners. N Engl J Med 331:341, 1994. Connor EM, Sperling RS, Gelber R, et al.: Reduction of maternal-infant transmission of human immunodeficiency virus type 1 with zidovudine treatment. N Engl J Med 331:1173, 1994. Recommendations of the U.S. Public Health Service Task Force on the use of zidovudine to re-

duce perinatal transmission of human immunodeficiency virus. MMWR 43(RR-1):1, 1994. These summarize available information on factors related to heterosexual transmission of HIV and prevention of perinatal transmission.

Mann JM, Tarantola DJM, Netter TW (eds.): AIDS in the World: A Global Report. Cambridge, Harvard University Press, 1992. This volume summarizes what is known about HIV infection and prevention activities throughout the world.

Update: Universal precautions for prevention of transmission of HIV, hepatitis B virus, and other bloodborne pathogens in health care setting. MMWR 37:337, 1988. Public Health Service statement on management of occupational exposure to HIV including considerations regarding zidovudine postexposure use. MMWR 39(RR-1):1, 1990. Recommendations for preventing transmission of human immunodeficiency virus and hepatitis B virus to patients during exposure-prone invasive procedures. MMWR 40(RR-8):1, 1991. These documents summarize data on transmission of HIV in the health care setting and list recommended precautions.

363 PREVENTION OF HIV INFECTION

Michael S. Saag

Prevention of HIV infection requires a thorough understanding of the modes of viral transmission, the populations at risk, and the established guidelines to avoid high-risk exposures. HIV has been identified in virtually every body fluid and tissue, including blood, semen, vaginal secretions, saliva, tears, breast milk, cerebrospinal fluid, amniotic fluid, urine, and fluid obtained from bronchoalveolar lavage. In most instances, the virus resides in lymphocytes present within body fluids; therefore, any fluid that contains lymphocytes could be implicated theoretically in the spread of the virus. Nonetheless, no cases of HIV transmission have been documented through any body fluids except blood and fluids grossly contaminated with blood, semen, vaginal secretions, and, rarely, breast milk. HIV has been transmitted through transplanted organs, including kidney, liver, heart, pancreas, and bone.

MODES OF HIV TRANSMISSION AND PREVENTION

SEXUAL TRANSMISSION. HIV infection is a sexually transmitted disease (STD). Like other STD's, HIV spreads bidirectionally and appears to be transmitted from male to female and female to male, with approximately equal efficiency. Although the majority of sexually transmitted cases reported in the United States occur via male homosexual activity, heterosexual transmission is one of the fastest growing modes of transmission reported in the United States and is the primary mode of disease acquisition in many African countries, where male-to-female prevalence ratios are approximately 1.1:1.

Certain cofactors are associated with an increased risk of acquiring HIV infection. Among homosexual men, receptive anal intercourse and contact with a large number of different sexual partners are the most important risk factors. Activities that may lead to damage of the rectal mucosa, such as rectal douching, manual penetration of the rectum ("fisting"), and concomitant ulcerative STD's, increase the likelihood of disease acquisition. Insertive rectal intercourse, fellatio, and ingestion of semen are associated with HIV transmission to a lesser degree. The likelihood of heterosexual acquired disease increases with a higher number of sexual partners, contact with intravenous drug users (IVDU's), prostitution, sexual practices that damage vaginal or rectal mucosa, and a previous history of other STD's. Female-to-female transmission has been reported via orogenital contact.

Prevention. Abstinence is the only absolute way of preventing sexual acquisition of HIV infection. Persons who have been engaged in a mutually monogamous relationship since the mid-1970's are at extremely low risk of acquiring disease; however, the assurance that both partners have remained "faithful" is sometimes difficult to confirm. For the majority of sexually active individuals it should be assumed that their partner is seropositive until demonstrated otherwise. Verbal claims of seronegativity should be viewed with skepticism. When a couple, heterosexual or homosexual, is establishing a long-term relationship, it may be recommended that they undergo serologic testing to determine their HIV status. However, the decision to be tested should be of mutual consent and viewed in the context that exposures outside the relationship may lead to seropositivity in the future.

In situations in which a decision to engage in sexual activity has been made and the HIV status of the partner is unknown or in doubt, safe sexual practices ("safe sex") should be implemented (Table 363–1). Mutual masturbation is considered "safe," assuming it is nontraumatic and not followed by ingestion of body fluids such as semen or vaginal secretions. Transmission of HIV has never been documented to occur through saliva; however, no group of patients has ever been studied who engage in deep "French" kissing as their sole means of sexual activity. Because HIV exists in saliva, albeit in very low titers, deep French kissing cannot be considered absolutely safe even though the likelihood of HIV transmission is extremely low. Condom use is the most effective means of preventing HIV infection among individuals who engage in vaginal or anal intercourse. To be effective, however, the condom should be made of latex and must be used properly. Natural skin condoms have been shown to leak in laboratory studies, whereas latex condoms maintain their integrity and are more durable. Nonoxynol-9, a spermicide with some antiviral activity, enhances the protective effects of condoms and should be used in conjunction with condoms either as a spermicidal jelly or impregnated into the latex condom itself. Petroleum-based lubricants enhance the likelihood of latex condom rupture and should be avoided. If needed, water-based lubricants such as K-Y Jelly should be used.

Both partners should be knowledgeable about the correct use of condoms. Discussions regarding condom use should occur before the need arises, and ideally, condom placement should be practiced in advance. A new condom should be used for each act of intercourse and each condom should be used only one time. Even under the best of circumstances, a 5 to 15% failure rate has been noted among couples using condoms as their sole means of contraception, and HIV transmission has been reported in discordant couples using condoms. Condom ineffectiveness is most often due to improper placement, falling off during intercourse, and rupture. Therefore, although condom use during intercourse is considered "safer" sex, it is not absolutely safe.

HIV TRANSMISSION IN INTRAVENOUS DRUG USERS. The primary mode of HIV transmission in IVDU's is sharing of contaminated needles and syringes. Sharing of injection paraphernalia ("works") is commonplace among IVDU's and is reinforced by the cultural, economic, and legal environment in the IVDU community. The risk of HIV transmission is highest among IVDU's who share needles and use drugs that are injected more often, such as cocaine. HIV is frequently transmitted from IVDU's to their sexual partners through both heterosexual and homosexual activity, and ultimately, the virus may be transmitted to their children via perinatal exposure. Many cases of heterosexual transmission, including transmission from prostitutes, are associated with intravenous drug use.

Prevention. The primary mode of preventing HIV transmission in IVDU's is to prevent the use of intravenous drugs in the first place. Education programs that are culturally sensitive and geared to young audiences have the best chance of preventing drug use. Access to treatment centers is the best approach for those individuals already using IV drugs. For those IVDU's who do not wish to seek treatment or who are unable to gain access to treatment, the

most effective way to prevent HIV infection is to avoid sharing needles and works. Where works are in short supply, needles and syringes should be cleaned after each use, preferably with readily accessible virucidal cleansers such as chlorine bleach (diluted 1:100). Some communities have adopted programs that provide free needles and syringes for IVDU's. Voluntary HIV testing and outreach programs that rigorously maintain confidentiality can be effective in reducing transmission to sexual partners of IVDU's. In order to be effective, antibody testing should be combined with intensive pretest and post-test counseling.

The efficacy of many community programs is limited, however, by cultural barriers, including lack of trust, fear of prosecution, misconceptions regarding the prevalence of HIV infection within the local drug-using population, and the use of ineffective language in delivering anti-HIV messages by program staff. When combined with the relative paucity of IV drug treatment resources, HIV education among IVDU's which ultimately results in behavioral changes represents the most challenging HIV prevention goal.

TRANSMISSION OF HIV THROUGH BLOOD PRODUCTS. HIV has been transmitted via transfusion of single-donor blood and blood products, including whole blood, fresh frozen plasma, packed red blood cells, cryoprecipitate, clotting factors, and platelets. Prior to May 1985, when the Red Cross began testing the blood supply for evidence of HIV antibodies, an estimated 10,000 to 12,000 individuals received blood products from HIV-infected donors. Most recipients develop infection after transfusion with HIV-tainted blood products, and recent data suggest that the time to development of advanced disease is shorter among transfusion recipients than among those who acquired their disease via sexual contact.

Since 1985, the rate of HIV transmission through transfusion has dropped precipitously. The current estimated rate of transmission is 1 in 40,000 to 1 in 200,000 units of blood, depending on the prevalence of HIV infection in the community where the blood was collected. Pooled plasma components often require 2000 to 30,000 donors per lot and represent a higher potential risk of transmission than single-donor blood products if the pooled product is not treated to eliminate infectious virus.

Prevention. Aggressive efforts by the American Red Cross have greatly reduced the risk of HIV transmission via transfusion in the United States. Voluntary self-deferral of donors at risk for HIV acquisition in the community was initiated in 1983. The effectiveness of self-deferral is limited, however, by social pressures. Some high-risk individuals view blood donation as a means of being tested for HIV and provide erroneous screening information in order to receive free, confidential evaluation of their HIV status. Other at-risk individuals may be coerced to participate in blood donation drives at work. Potentially infected donors may feel uncomfortable excusing themselves from donation and provide false information on screening in order to avoid possible disclosure of a high-risk lifestyle to their co-workers. Self-deferral programs are most effective when free, voluntary testing centers are readily available elsewhere in the community and when blood drives encourage potential donors to come to donation centers by themselves and not in groups.

The institution of HIV antibody testing of donated blood and blood products in 1985 has had the most dramatic effect on lowering the incidence of transfusion-related transmission. When combined with voluntary self-deferral, the blood supply has become relatively free of HIV. Heat inactivation processes for cryoprecipitate and clotting factor concentrates have virtually eliminated transmission of HIV through use of these products. Other products, such as immune globulin preparations and hepatitis B vaccines, are produced via methods that inactivate HIV and have never been associated with transmission of HIV.

TRANSMISSION OF HIV TO HEALTH CARE WORKERS. Transmission of HIV in the health care delivery setting has been the subject of intense investigation throughout the course of the epidemic. The percentage of health care workers with AIDS who have "no identified risk" for HIV infection has remained low ($<10\%$) and has not increased over time, despite the dramatic increase in the number of AIDS cases and concomitant exposure of health care workers to patients with HIV disease. More importantly, detailed studies examining the risk of specific exposures, such as needle stick injuries and mucous membrane exposures, have demonstrated very low risk of disease acquisition in the workplace. More than

TABLE 363–1. SAFE AND UNSAFE SEXUAL PRACTICES IN ORDER OF "SURENESS" OF SAFETY

Safe
   Abstinence
   Monogamous relationship with confirmed seronegative partner
   Manual sex (mutual masturbation)
   Kissing
   Intercourse with latex condom (used in combination with nonoxynol-9)
Unsafe
   Intercourse with "natural skin" condom
   Intercourse with latex condom lubricated with petroleum-based lubricants
   Unprotected orogenital sex
   Unprotected vaginal intercourse
   Unprotected anal intercourse

3628 health care workers have been examined prospectively in carefully designed surveillance studies at 10 high-incidence medical centers. The overall risk of seroconversion after a percutaneous needle stick from a known HIV-positive source is 0.25% per exposure. Although mucous membrane exposures to HIV-positive blood have resulted in seroconversion in at least three health care workers, prospective studies of over 900 splash exposures have failed to identify any seroconverters, implying that the risk of infection is even lower after mucous membrane exposure than through percutaneous needle stick. To date, no transmission has occurred after exposure to body fluids other than blood or fluids heavily contaminated with blood. Therefore, although the potential for HIV transmission to health care providers clearly exists, the risk of infection is inherently low and can be further minimized by following routine precautions to prevent transmission.

Prevention. In August 1987, the Centers for Disease Control and Prevention (CDC) published guidelines designed to minimize health care worker exposure to blood and body fluids which may be infected with blood-borne pathogens, such as HIV. These so-called universal precautions are based on the premise that any patient may be infected with bloodborne infectious agents and it may be difficult, if not impossible, to differentiate those with infection from their uninfected counterparts. Thus, all specimens containing blood or blood-tinged fluids obtained from *any* patient should be considered hazardous and handled as such (Table 363–2).

Handwashing is the cornerstone of universal precautions, as it is with all infection-control practices. Gloves should be worn when spillage of blood or body fluids is likely. Gloves should *never* be washed and should be changed after soiling or after gross contamination, with handwashing immediately after the gloves are removed. Gowns, protective eyewear, and masks are usually not needed except in circumstances in which splattering or splashing of blood-containing fluids is likely to occur. Masks should always be worn in situations in which eyewear is required. Reusable equipment should be cleansed of visible organic material, placed in an impervious bag, and returned to central supply for decontamination. Although heat is the single best decontamination method, chemical agents that possess mycobactericidal activity are effective against both hepatitis B and HIV and are acceptable alternatives when heat inactivation is impractical. Blood spills should be cleaned with appropriate caution. After placing gloves and other appropriate barrier precautions, excess blood should be removed with absorbent materials (e.g., paper towels), the area then cleaned with soap and water, and the area disinfected with a 1:10 solution of sodium hypochlorite (household bleach) and water. Health care workers with denuded skin, open lesions, or active dermatitis should avoid direct patient contact and should not process contaminated equipment or materials. Private rooms are generally not required for patients

TABLE 363–2. SUMMARY OF UNIVERSAL PRECAUTIONS

Specimens, including blood, blood products, and body fluids, obtained from *all* patients should be considered hazardous and potentially infected with transmissible agents.

Handwashing should be performed before and after patient contact; after removing gloves; and immediately if hands are grossly contaminated with blood.

Gloves should be worn when hands are *likely* to come in contact with blood or body fluids.

Gowns, protective eyewear, and masks should be worn when splashing, splattering, or aerosolization of blood or body fluids is *likely* to occur.

Sharp objects ("sharps") should be handled with great care and disposed of in impervious receptacles.

Needles should never be manipulated, bent, broken, or recapped.

Blood spills should be handled via initial absorption of spill with disposable towels, cleaning area with soap and water, followed by disinfecting area with 1:10 solution of household bleach.

Contaminated reusable equipment should be decontaminated using heat sterilization, or when heat is impractical, using a mycobactericidal cleanser.

Pocket masks or mechanical ventilation devices should be available in areas where cardiopulmonary resuscitation procedures are likely.

Health care workers with open lesions or weeping dermatitis should avoid direct patient contact and should not handle contaminated equipment.

Private rooms are not required for routine care; select circumstances, however, such as the presence of concomitant transmissible opportunistic diseases, may warrant respiratory, enteric, or contact isolation.

known to be HIV infected unless a concomitant opportunistic disease is present which requires respiratory, enteric, or contact isolation. Food service should be provided as usual on reusable dishware.

Because *all* blood and body fluids should be handled as potentially hazardous and *all* patients presumed to be infected, it makes little sense to identify infected patients or their specimens with "blood and body fluid" labels. The use of such labels on *known* infected patients implies that unlabeled specimens or specimens from patients of unknown status are less hazardous and may be handled with less care. Indeed, studies have shown that more than half of the specimens containing antibodies to either HbsAg or HIV went to the laboratory unlabeled. The handling of sharp instruments ("sharps") represents the greatest risk of HIV transmission to health care workers. Although sharp injuries cannot be entirely eliminated, the number of exposures can be reduced substantially by adhering to guidelines put forth in universal precautions. Before a sharp instrument is used, thought should be given regarding where the instrument will be disposed after use. Impervious containers should be readily available in all patient care areas and identified by the health care worker *prior to* "sharp" utilization. The containers should be checked frequently and should not be allowed to overfill. Used needles should never be manipulated, bent, broken, or recapped. Recapping of needles is the single most common activity that results in needle stick injuries.

Despite their logical basis and relative ease of implementation, universal precautions have not been accepted by many medical centers and health care providers. Recent studies have shown that > 50% of health care workers engage in inadequate infection control practices, even in high-impact AIDS centers, and up to 40% of the needle stick exposures were judged to be preventable. Although lack of adequate education may partly explain these findings, implementation of infection control practices has been generally poor historically. Between 200 and 400 health care workers die each year as a result of hepatitis B infection acquired on the job. The use of universal precautions helps minimize the transmission of many transmissible diseases in addition to HIV.

Even in the best of circumstances, accidental mucous membrane and percutaneous exposures to blood from HIV-infected patients do occur. Each institution and health care facility should adopt procedures for managing these exposures based on guidelines published by the CDC. The essential elements of management following needle stick or mucous membrane exposure include defining the type of exposure, appropriately evaluating the donor (patient) and recipient (health care worker) at the time of exposure, and follow-up of the health care worker for at least 1 year after exposure.

Proposed definitions of the types of exposure are summarized in Table 363–3. Health care workers with any kind of parenteral exposure should be counseled and evaluated for possible acquisition of HIV and receive routine prophylaxis against hepatitis B. The source patient (donor) should be evaluated for HIV infection; if the donor's HIV status is unknown, the donor should be informed about the incident and encouraged to allow voluntary, confidential screening of his/her blood for HIV and hepatitis B antibody. If the patient refuses or cannot give consent, he/she should be considered to be infected. In cases where exposure to HIV is documented or presumed to have occurred, the health care worker should be evaluated serologically for the presence of HIV as soon as possible after the exposure (baseline) and again at 6 weeks, 12 weeks, 24 weeks, and 1 year after the exposure to determine whether HIV transmission has occurred. The health care worker should report any acute illnesses that occur during the follow-up period, especially during the first 6 to 12 weeks after exposure. Exposed workers should follow the recommended guidelines for preventing HIV transmission, including using safe sexual practices, refraining from blood, semen, and organ donation, and avoiding breast feeding. If the source patient is seronegative for HIV and has no clinical manifestations of HIV disease, no further follow-up of the exposed health care workers is necessary, although some workers prefer follow-up for their own peace of mind. Serologic testing should be made available to all health care workers who are concerned about potential on-the-job exposure.

The use of zidovudine (AZT) prophylaxis following parenteral exposure to HIV remains controversial. Many clinicians favor using

TABLE 363–3. DEFINITIONS OF EXPOSURES TO BLOOD AND BODY FLUIDS FROM HIV-INFECTED PATIENTS

	Zidovudine Prophylaxis*
Massive parenteral exposure	Recommended
Transfusion of blood	
High-inoculum injection of blood (>1 ml) or laboratory materials containing high viral titers	
Definite parenteral exposure	Encouraged
Deep intramuscular injury with a needle contaminated with blood or a body fluid	
Small volume injection of blood or body fluid (<1 ml)	
Laceration caused by instrument contaminated with blood or body fluids	
Laceration inoculated with blood, body fluids, or virus samples (research materials)	
Possible parenteral exposure	Available
Subcutaneous or superficial injury with an instrument or needle contaminated with blood or body fluids	
Injury with a contaminated instrument or needle which does not cause visible bleeding	
Previous wound or skin lesion contaminated with blood or body fluids	
Mucous membrane exposure to blood or body fluids	
Doubtful parenteral exposure	Discouraged
Subcutaneous injury by instrument or needle contaminated with noninfectious fluids†	
Contamination of a wound, previous skin lesion, or mucous membrane with noninfectious fluids	
Intact skin visibly contaminated with blood	

  * Zidovudine 200 mg orally every 4 hours for 6 weeks; see text.
  † Body fluids considered to be potentially infectious include blood, blood products, cerebrospinal fluid, amniotic fluid, menstrual discharge, inflammatory exudates, pleural fluid, peritoneal fluid, pericardial fluid, and any fluid visibly contaminated with blood. All other fluids are considered noninfectious.

prophylactic AZT after massive or definite exposures based on the proven antiviral effect of AZT, the relatively infrequent and apparently reversible nature of serious adverse drug effects, and the demonstration in some animal models of retroviral infection that AZT, when given early after inoculation, modifies the course of disease. Others believe that AZT should not be administered based on the absence of postexposure prophylaxis data, the lack of information regarding toxicity in uninfected individuals, and the unknown long-term carcinogenic potential of AZT use. Although it is unlikely that any clinical trials will be able to resolve the issue owing to the large number of participants required (based on low rates of seroconversion) and the difficulty of enrolling exposed health care workers into placebo-controlled studies, very recent reports from the CDC indicate a 30% reduction in anticipated transmission rates of HIV to parenterally exposed health care workers who had received AZT prophylaxis. In many medical centers AZT prophylaxis has become a standard of practice. In those centers the option of AZT prophylaxis is offered to all health care workers with massive or definite exposures and discussed with those encountering possible parenteral exposures. Health care workers with doubtful parenteral or nonparenteral exposures generally should not take AZT prophylaxis. Those workers with massive or definite exposures who elect to take AZT prophylaxis should sign an informed consent that outlines the risks and benefits of AZT prophylaxis prior to starting therapy. The optimal timing and dosage of AZT prophylaxis are unknown; however, animal studies suggest that higher doses given as soon as possible after exposure have the best chance of being effective. Therefore, most centers that offer AZT prophylaxis to their employees have established mechanisms whereby the health care worker can be evaluated and the drug administered within 2 to 4 hours after the exposure. Dosing regimens vary from center to center but usually consist of 200 mg of AZT every 4 hours, with or without a 4 A.M. dose, for 4 to 6 weeks.

TRANSMISSION FROM INFECTED HEALTH CARE WORKERS TO THEIR PATIENTS. In July 1990, the first case of possible transmission of HIV from an infected health care worker (dentist) to his patients was reported. Six patients are believed to have acquired infection from the dentist based on the absence of other risk factors among the patients and the high degree of homology between the viruses isolated from the dentist and those isolated from the patients. Although each patient underwent an invasive procedure in the dental office, the precise mode of transmission remains unknown.

Based on the known transmission of other blood-borne pathogens from health care providers to their patients (e.g., hepatitis B), it was anticipated that HIV may also be transmitted in this fashion. Remarkably, despite the prolonged duration of the epidemic, the dentist described above remains the only documented case of transmission to patients in the health care setting. Several "look-back" studies of over 4000 patients who underwent invasive surgical procedures performed by HIV-infected physicians have failed to identify any additional cases of nosocomial transmission. Therefore, the risk of transmission from infected health care workers to patients is thought to be very low (between 1 in 42,000 and 1 in 420,000). Routine use of universal precautions should minimize the risk of transmission from HIV-infected patients to health care providers and vice versa.

VACCINE DEVELOPMENT

Education is the only means of HIV prevention currently available. Over the past few years significant efforts have been directed toward the development of an effective vaccine against HIV. Although substantial progress has been achieved, several obstacles still remain. Despite enormous advances in understanding the immunopathogenesis of HIV infection, the precise mechanism of protective immunity remains unknown. Without such knowledge, it is difficult to develop vaccines that are assured of targeting the appropriate arm of the immune system that confers long-term protective immunity. Another obstacle is the lack of correlation of data from animal models to the potential protective effects of vaccines in humans. Therefore, even if an effective vaccine were available, it would take years of human testing to demonstrate its effectiveness. Moreover, once a candidate vaccine is in human trials, the relatively low rate of HIV transmission and, in some cases, the difficulty in determining whether HIV infection has actually occurred will complicate the evaluation process. Despite the enormous progress made in vaccine development over the last few years, it will take several more years before protective efficacy can be established. Even if an effective vaccine is established, education will remain the primary mode of HIV prevention, owing to the difficulty in knowing how long the protective immune effect will last. Never before has so much been known about an epidemic during the time it was occurring. The challenge is to disseminate the knowledge to populations at risk in language they can understand and, ultimately, to modify activities so that the risk of transmission is minimized.

Blood spills should be handled via initial absorption of spill with disposable towels, cleaning area with soap and water, followed by disinfecting area with 1:10 of household bleach.

Centers for Disease Control: Recommendations for prevention of HIV transmission in health-care settings. MMWR 36(Suppl 2):1S, 1987. *Original description of universal precautions. Critical reading for all health care providers.*

Centers for Disease Control: Update: Investigations of persons treated by HIV-infected health-care workers—United States. MMWR 42:329, 1993. *Summary of look-back studies that examine the status of patients who received care from HIV-infected health care workers.*

Gerberding JL: Is antiretroviral treatment after percutaneous HIV exposure justified? Ann Intern Med 118:979, 1993. *Succinct overview of current thinking on postexposure prophylaxis. Cites key references.*

Lo B, Steinbrook R: Health care workers infected with the human immunodeficiency virus: The next steps. JAMA 267:1100, 1992. *Thoughtful review of the medical, epidemiologic, and ethical issues surrounding the practice of HIV-infected health care providers.*

364 NEUROLOGIC COMPLICATIONS OF HIV-1 INFECTION

Richard W. Price

The neurologic complications of HIV-1 infection are both common and varied. Indeed, only rarely do the central and peripheral nervous systems of HIV-infected patients remain unaffected through the course of their disease. Because each of the individual neurologic disorders is discussed in more detail elsewhere in this volume, the major purpose of this chapter is to provide an overview and a general guide to diagnosis and management. It is important to emphasize that differential diagnosis in these patients is far from an "academic exercise," because many of these conditions can be reversed, stabilized, or even cured with specific therapy.

Although the major susceptibility to neurologic complications occurs in the late phase of HIV-1 infection, at the time when immunosuppression leads to a marked increase in vulnerability to a host of conditions, patients may also manifest certain neurologic afflictions early in infection. Because the neurologic complications of early and late HIV-1 infection differ, they are considered separately. Indeed, because of these stage-related differences in susceptibility, when approaching diagnosis in HIV-infected patients it is important to characterize their "background" systemic HIV-1 infection, either clinically with respect to the presence or absence of previous opportunistic infections indicating compromised immunity or by assessment of surrogate markers, particularly the blood CD4+ lymphocyte count.

EARLY HIV-1 INFECTION

Although less common than in the late stages of HIV-1 infection, the nervous system may also be afflicted earlier, indeed as early as the stage of primary infection and seroconversion. Thus, individual reports have described examples of focal or diffuse encephalopathy, ataxia, myelopathy, and meningitis presenting either within the context of the mononucleosis-like HIV-1 seroconversion reaction or with minimal associated systemic symptoms. These conditions appear to evolve acutely or subacutely, to pursue a monophasic course, and to be followed by good, although not always complete, recovery. Peripheral nervous system disorders, including mononeuropathy involving cranial or segmental nerves, brachial plexopathy, and polyneuropathy, have also been reported during this phase. At times these peripheral and central nervous system (CNS) disorders occur together.

Subsequently, during the "clinically latent" phase of infection, several neurologic conditions have been reported. Among these is the Guillain-Barré syndrome and its more protracted counterpart, chronic idiopathic demyelinating polyneuropathy (CIDP), both of which are clinically indistinguishable from demyelinating polyneuropathies affecting non-HIV-1-infected individuals, except for higher cerebrospinal fluid (CSF) cell counts and perhaps a poorer prognosis. Response to treatment with corticosteroids, plasma exchange, and intravenous immunoglobulin has been noted, supporting presumption of an autoimmune pathogenesis. Because of the potential hazards of corticosteroids, plasma exchange and immunoglobulin are the preferred therapies. Isolated cases of a multi-

ple sclerosis–like demyelinating CNS disease have also been reported in this stage of HIV-1 infection, but this appears to be rare.

An additional important aspect of HIV-1 infection, with both diagnostic and pathogenetic implications, is the early development of CSF abnormalities, which presumably relate to early *asymptomatic HIV-1 infection of the CNS* soon after initial systemic infection. Prospective studies have reported that the majority of asymptomatic HIV-1-infected individuals exhibit mild CSF changes, including elevations in the cell count and protein and immunoglobulin levels as well as evidence of local "intra-blood-brain barrier" synthesis of anti-HIV-1 antibody. Additionally, in a substantial number of asymptomatic patients HIV-1 can be isolated from the CSF using culture techniques. These findings have not been shown to have an adverse prognostic significance for the subject; indeed, it is clear that patients with such abnormalities can continue to function without symptoms or signs of neurologic impairment. These "background" abnormalities may confound CSF analysis.

LATE HIV-1 INFECTION

The evolving, and eventually severe, impairment of immune defenses caused by HIV-1 renders the nervous system highly vulnerable to a broad spectrum of disorders. The following overview emphasizes general principles of pathogenesis and approach to diagnosis.

Pathophysiology

A number of pathophysiologic processes may lead to neurologic dysfunction in the late phase of HIV-1 infection (Table 364–1). These include conditions that distinguish the AIDS patient from other groups, such as *opportunistic infections, opportunistic neoplasms,* and several conditions that appear to relate to more *direct effects of HIV-1* itself. AIDS patients are also susceptible to the neurologic conditions that affect other acute and chronically ill populations, including metabolic brain disease resulting from systemic organ dysfunction, stroke related to nonbacterial thrombotic endocarditis or coagulopathies, toxic effects of medications, and primary psychiatric disturbances. Here we focus on those disorders that particularly distinguish AIDS patients.

OPPORTUNISTIC NERVOUS SYSTEM INFECTIONS. As with other organ systems, the spectrum of opportunistic infections of the nervous system results from the intrinsic vulnerabilities of the tissue (fertile soil) and the pattern of immunosuppression, in this case circumscribed impairment of T-cell/macrophage defenses. The patient's long-term history of exposure to particular organisms is also important because most of the opportunistic infections result from reactivation of latent infections rather than from new encoun-

TABLE 364–1. PATHOPHYSIOLOGIC CLASSIFICATION OF THE NEUROLOGIC COMPLICATIONS OF LATE HIV-1 INFECTION

Underlying Process	Examples
Opportunistic infections	Cerebral toxoplasmosis
	Cryptococcal meningitis
	Progressive multifocal leukoencephalopathy
	Cytomegalovirus encephalitis, polyradiculitis
Opportunistic neoplasms	Primary central nervous system lymphoma
	Metastatic lymphoma
Conditions possibly related to HIV-1 itself	AIDS dementia complex
	Aseptic meningitis
	Predominantly sensory polyneuropathy
Metabolic and vascular complications of systemic disease	Hypoxic, sepsis-related encephalopathies
	Stroke (nonbacterial thrombotic endocarditis, coagulopathies)
Toxic reactions	Dideoxyinosine, dideoxycytidine neuropathies
	AZT myopathy
Functional (psychiatric) disorders	Anxiety disorders
	Psychotic depression

ters with pathogens. An important implication of the pre-eminence of reactivated infection relates to serologic testing. Serology is most useful for assessing prior exposure to an organism and hence susceptibility to clinically important reactivation, but not for defining active infection. For example, patients with cerebral toxoplasmosis nearly always exhibit antecedent positive *Toxoplasma gondii* blood serology, and therefore a negative serum IgG antibody titer militates against this diagnosis. On the other hand, these serum antibody titers most often do not rise before or during the course of disease, and therefore a fourfold increase cannot be relied upon to establish disease activity. Moreover, as long as immunosuppression persists and therapy still cannot eliminate latent infection, suppressive antibiotic therapy must be maintained for the remainder of the patient's life.

The reason for the intrinsic vulnerability of the nervous system to certain infections (e.g., *T. gondii*) and not others (e.g., *Pneumocystis carinii*) in many cases remains uncertain. However, in some instances susceptibility relates to the capacity of local cells to support intracellular replication. Thus, the virus causing progressive multifocal leukoencephalopathy (PML), JC virus, causes a productive and lytic infection of oligodendrocytes and hence leads to spreading infection and demyelination as the processes of these myelin-producing cells disappear. In the case of HIV-1, productive infection appears to involve monocyte-derived macrophages and local microglial cells.

The circumscribed nature of the immunologic defect in AIDS determines the range of opportunistic infections, which therefore differs somewhat from that of other immunosuppressed states. For example, AIDS patients are particularly susceptible to cerebral toxoplasmosis but, unlike patients with organ transplants, are very unlikely to develop cerebral *Candida* or *Aspergillus* infections. For this reason, AIDS patients present a unique set of disease probabilities.

OPPORTUNISTIC NEOPLASMS. The major consideration in this category is primary brain lymphoma. These B-cell lymphomas arise in the CNS, usually are multicentric (at least microscopically), and only rarely metastasize systemically. Characteristically, they develop late in HIV-1 infection when blood CD4+ lymphocytes are low, i.e., in the same setting as major opportunistic infections. Indeed, the tumor cells are nearly always positive for Epstein-Barr virus (EBV), which likely plays an important role in their genesis. Radiation therapy usually results in tumor regression, but overall prognosis is poor, principally because other complications develop; the role of chemotherapy is uncertain, but aggressive treatment is often not possible because of reduced bone marrow reserves. Systemic lymphoma can also spread to the CNS, although usually to the leptomeninges rather than brain parenchyma. Although Kaposi's sarcoma has been reported to metastasize to brain, this is exceedingly rare.

EFFECTS OF HIV-1 ON THE NERVOUS SYSTEM. Several disorders have been suggested to relate in a more direct or fundamental way to HIV-1 infection. These include the AIDS dementia complex, aseptic meningitis, and perhaps predominantly sensory neuropathy. Although considerable uncertainty still exists regarding their cause and pathogenesis, the seeming uniqueness of these conditions in HIV-1-infected compared with other immunosuppressed patients, as well as more direct evidence of virus infection in some patients with the AIDS dementia complex, lends support to this contention.

Diagnosis: Neuroanatomic Approach

As with other neurologic disease, diagnosis in AIDS patients begins with localization of symptoms and signs and hence involves neuroanatomic classification (Table 364–2).

MENINGITIS AND HEADACHE. Several disorders may involve the leptomeninges in patients with advanced HIV-1 disease. The most important of these is infection by *Cryptococcus neoformans* (see Ch. 352). This condition usually presents subacutely with headache, nausea, vomiting, and confusion, just as in non-AIDS patients. However, importantly, in some patients initial symptoms can be remarkably benign, with only mild headache or fever. Likewise, the CSF findings may be bland, with few or no cells and little or no perturbation in either glucose or protein levels. For this reason the clinician should have a low threshold for lumbar puncture and

should routinely examine CSF for *Cryptococcus* (India ink stain, cryptococcal antigen determination, culture). Initial treatment is usually gratifying, although sterilizing the CSF is difficult and continued chronic therapy is required.

The syndrome of aseptic meningitis, presumably relating to direct HIV-1 infection of the leptomeninges, may complicate advanced HIV-1 infection but most often develops in the period of transition to AIDS. Both acute and chronic forms are accompanied by headache and meningeal symptoms, whereas signs of meningeal irritation are more characteristic of the acute group. Cranial nerve palsies affecting the seventh and, less often, the fifth and eighth nerves may complicate the course. The CSF shows a modest mononuclear pleocytosis, usually with normal glucose and mildly elevated protein. The presumption that this condition is due to direct HIV-1 infection of the meninges derives from the fact that the virus can be readily isolated from the CSF and no other cause has been identified. The syndrome itself is characteristically benign but may imply a poor prognosis in relation to impending progression to AIDS. The efficacy of antiretroviral or other therapies in this disorder has not been studied.

Other, less common meningeal disorders (including meningeal lymphoma, tuberculous meningitis, meningovascular syphilis) resemble their counterparts in the non-AIDS patient. A number of other conditions may present with symptoms resembling meningitis;

TABLE 364–2. NEUROANATOMIC CLASSIFICATION OF THE LATE COMPLICATIONS OF HIV-1 INFECTION

Meningitis and headache
  Cryptococcal meningitis
  Aseptic meningitis (HIV-1)
  Idiopathic, "HIV-1–related" headache
  Tuberculous meningitis (*Mycobacterium tuberculosis*)
  Syphilitic meningitis
  Lymphomatous meningitis (metastatic)
Diffuse brain diseases
  With preservation of consciousness
    AIDS dementia complex
  With concomitant depression of arousal
    Metabolic encephalopathies (alone or as an exacerbating influence)
    Toxoplasmosis ("encephalitic" form)
    Cytomegalovirus encephalitis
    Herpes encephalitis
Focal brain diseases
  Subacute
    Cerebral toxoplasmosis
    Primary CNS lymphoma
    Progressive multifocal leukoencephalopathy
    Tuberculous brain abscess (*M. tuberculosis*)
    Cryptococcoma
    Varicella-zoster virus encephalitis
    Herpes encephalitis
  Acute
    Vascular disorders
Myelopathies
  Subacute/chronic, progressive
    Vacuolar myelopathy
    HTLV-I–associated myelopathy
  Acute/subacute
    Transverse myelitis
      Varicella-zoster virus (herpes zoster)
      Spinal epidural or intradural lymphoma
    With polyradiculopathy
      Cytomegalovirus
Peripheral neuropathies
  Predominantly sensory polyneuropathy
  Toxic neuropathies (dideoxycytidine, dideoxyinosine)
  Autonomic neuropathy
  Cytomegalovirus polyradiculopathy
  Mononeuritis multiplex
  Herpes zoster
  Mononeuropathies associated with aseptic meningitis
  Mononeuropathies secondary to lymphomatous meningitis
Myopathies
  Polymyositis
  Noninflammatory myopathy
  AZT myopathy

for example, parenchymal brain diseases such as toxoplasmosis and primary CNS lymphoma may initially manifest with headache as an important symptom. More common, however, is the development of headache of uncertain cause. Although not well understood, this headache is not rare in late HIV-1 infection and at times can be a severe, debilitating problem. Whereas in some patients this headache may relate to systemic infection such as *P. carinii* pneumonia, in others the explanation is elusive and for this reason has been referred to as *HIV headache.*

PREDOMINANTLY FOCAL BRAIN DISORDERS. In approaching diagnosis of parenchymal brain disease, it is useful to separate the conditions that cause predominantly focal symptoms and signs from those producing more generalized brain dysfunction. Patients in the former group present with hemiparesis, aphasia, apraxia, hemisensory abnormalities, visual field loss, and the like, as a result of focal macroscopic lesions in cortical or subcortical brain regions. The most important of these are cerebral toxoplasmosis, which complicates the course of AIDS in 7 to 15% of patients, primary cerebral lymphoma developing in up to 5%, and PML, which occurs in perhaps 3%. Less common are a miscellany of other infections and cerebrovascular disorders.

Although the three major focal disorders all characteristically have a subacute onset and may be clinically indistinguishable, they tend to have somewhat different temporal profiles (Table 364–3). Thus, cerebral toxoplasmosis typically progresses most rapidly (over a few days) and PML evolves most slowly (over a few weeks), with primary CNS lymphoma somewhere in between. Each may cause similar neurologic deficits, but there are often differences in the associated findings. Thus, toxoplasmosis commonly presents with a combination of focal deficit and generalized encephalopathy with confusion or clouding of consciousness; fever and headache may also be present. This contrasts with PML, at least at onset, in which focal neurologic deficits are unaccompanied by either diffuse brain dysfunction or evidence of a systemic toxic state. CNS lymphoma, when accompanied by significant mass effect or when deep in the frontal or periventricular region, may cause more global mental dysfunction, but, again, these patients are usually afebrile without constitutional symptoms or signs.

Once the focal nature of the patient's symptoms and signs is recognized, use of neuroimaging techniques, including computed tomography (CT) or preferably magnetic resonance imaging (MRI), is critical both to confirm the presence of macroscopic focal disease and to determine the nature of the abnormalities (Table 364–3). Multiple lesions involving the cortex or deep brain nuclei (thalamus, basal ganglia) surrounded by edema strongly favor cerebral toxoplasmosis. In most cases *Toxoplasma* abscesses exhibit ringlike contrast enhancement on CT scan. Cerebral lymphoma may produce a similar neuroimaging appearance, although the lesions of lymphoma are usually less numerous (one or two definable lesions), commonly exhibit more diffuse or less clear-cut contrast enhancement, and are more often located in the white matter adjacent to the ventricles. PML characteristically involves the white matter, most often adjacent to the cortex, and is without mass effect or contrast enhancement.

After neuroimaging, the next step in diagnosing focal mass lesions often involves a trial of anti-*Toxoplasma* therapy. Pyrimethamine and sulfa therapy characteristically results in clinical improvement within a few days and distinct reduction of lesions on neuroimaging by 1 or 2 weeks. This rapid and consistent improvement allows treatment response to serve as a basis for diagnosis

and thereby obviates the need for brain biopsy in virtually all patients with toxoplasmosis. Biopsy is then reserved for cases with atypical clinical or laboratory features (including atypical neuroimaging appearance or negative *Toxoplasma* blood serology) along with those who fail to improve with treatment. It is important in the context of such therapeutic trial that, if possible, corticosteroids be avoided. Because the signs and symptoms, and even the neuroimaging abnormalities, of cerebral lymphoma may improve with corticosteroids, such treatment can confuse interpretation of the anti-*Toxoplasma* therapeutic trial. However, if cerebral edema threatens brain herniation, judicious short-term corticosteroids may be instituted along with appropriate specific therapy and subsequently tapered rapidly once the patient improves.

Other focal CNS disorders are uncommon but include some treatable lesions. This includes cryptococcoma, nearly always developing in the setting of meningitis. Varicella-zoster virus (VZV) can cause a demyelinating focal disease resembling PML, and cytomegalovirus (CMV) may rarely cause macroscopic lesions, sometimes with mineralization and contrast enhancement on neuroimaging, accompanied by focal clinical deficit. Herpes simplex viruses have also been reported to cause focal deficits. All of these evolve subacutely, as do the more common opportunistic problems. Acutely evolving neurologic deficits may follow seizures (Todd's palsy) or relate to poorly understood transient vascular syndromes resembling migraine clinically and pathogenetically. MRI and other studies are usually warranted in these patients to rule out other underlying disorders.

PREDOMINANTLY NONFOCAL BRAIN DISORDERS. The disorders presenting with more general or diffuse brain dysfunction and without focal features can be further divided into those in which consciousness remains fully preserved and those accompanied by a concomitant decrease in alertness. Most important among the former is the *AIDS dementia complex,* a clinical syndrome characterized by cognitive, motor, and, at times, behavioral dysfunction.

Both the incidence and severity of the AIDS dementia complex increase with advancing immunosuppression. The clinical syndrome is somewhat variable, and its pathologic substrate is heterogeneous. It appears to relate to effects of HIV-1 infection on the CNS rather than involving secondary opportunistic infection. Its early, mild form is usually characterized by impaired concentration and attention along with reduced mental agility, resulting in complaints of forgetfulness and slowness in performing complex mental tasks. In those who progress to more severe involvement, cognitive dysfunction worsens and involves other domains, and motor dysfunction becomes clinically manifest with gait unsteadiness and difficulty with rapid, fine movements of the hands. Personality change with apathy, lack of initiative, or, at times, hyperactivity and agitation may be part of the syndrome. In its most severe form, global dementia, paraplegia, and virtual mutism may evolve with resultant incapacity. Although it is in part a diagnosis of exclusion, the symptoms and signs of the AIDS dementia complex are sufficiently distinct to allow bedside diagnosis in most patients on the basis of their stereotypy. Neuroimaging characteristically reveals cerebral atrophy, and MRI may additionally demonstrate increased signal in white matter or basal ganglia. Several studies now suggest that zidovudine (AZT) can prevent and partially reverse the symptoms and signs of the AIDS dementia complex. Whether newer antiretro-

TABLE 364–3. COMPARATIVE CLINICAL AND RADIOLOGIC FEATURES OF CEREBRAL TOXOPLASMOSIS, PRIMARY CNS LYMPHOMA, AND PROGRESSIVE MULTIFOCAL LEUKOENCEPHALOPATHY

	Clinical Onset			Neuroradiologic Features		
	Temporal Profile	*Level of Alertness*	*Fever*	*Number of Lesions*	*Type of Lesions*	*Location of Lesions*
Cerebral toxoplasmosis	Days	Reduced	Common	Multiple	Spherical, ring-enhancing	Basal ganglia, cortex
Primary CNS lymphoma	Days to weeks	Variable	Absent	One or few	Irregular, weakly enhancing	Periventricular
Progressive multifocal leukoencephalopathy	Weeks	Preserved	Absent	Multiple	Nonenhancing	White matter

viral drugs have a similar therapeutic effect remains to be evaluated.

In the AIDS dementia complex there is relative preservation of alertness in relation to cognitive loss. This contrasts with most metabolic encephalopathies developing as sequelae of the systemic diseases suffered by AIDS patients; for example, hypoxia and sepsis are characteristically accompanied by a degree of lethargy and confusion which parallels the decline in cognition. Likewise, CNS-active drugs often cloud mentation and alertness together. Although such metabolic and toxic disorders may present alone, they may also have an exacerbating or unmasking influence on the AIDS dementia complex, resulting in a mixture of the two conditions. HIV-1-infected patients may also be more sensitive to neuroleptics and thereby manifest parkinsonian or other movement disorders as side effects at seemingly low doses.

Brain infections may also produce diffuse brain dysfunction. Although CNS toxoplasmosis characteristically causes focal neurologic symptoms and signs, in some patients generalized encephalopathy predominates. Similarly, CNS lymphoma may infiltrate deep structures and impair cognition and motor function without prominent focal symptoms or signs. The clinical importance of CNS CMV infection in this regard remains imprecisely defined. Scattered CMV infection of the brain is common at autopsy, but the clinical correlate of this finding is not clear, and likely it is often silent or mild. On the other hand, in a small number of patients CMV encephalitis may be severe with subacute clouding of consciousness and, at times, seizures. Herpes simplex virus types 1 and 2 may also cause subacute nonfocal encephalitis.

MYELOPATHIES. The most common spinal cord affliction in AIDS patients is the pathologically defined vacuolar myelopathy, which has been included within the broader clinical designation of the AIDS dementia complex because it is usually accompanied by evidence of concomitant brain dysfunction. The disorder is generally of subacute or gradual onset and progression with painless gait disturbance characterized by ataxia and spasticity. Bladder and bowel difficulty usually follow deterioration of gait, and sensory symptoms and signs are less prominent than gait dysfunction unless there is concomitant neuropathy. Patients do not manifest a distinct sensory or motor "level" as in transverse myelopathies but rather distal loss of large-fiber modalities accompanied by increased deep tendon reflexes (again, in the absence of neuropathy) and Babinski signs. The efficacy of AZT or other antiretrovirals in this subgroup of AIDS dementia complex patients is uncertain.

An additional, emerging cause of clinically similar myelopathy in HIV-1-infected patients relates to coinfection with a second retrovirus, human T-lymphotropic virus I (HTLV-I). Double infection results from the convergent epidemiologies of these infections related to intravenous drug abuse. Although pathologically distinct, clinical differentiation of vacuolar myelopathy and HTLV-I-associated myelopathy (HAM) may be very difficult. Diagnosis begins with suspicion based on risk and is supported by serologic documentation of HTLV-I infection, but the relative clinical contributions of the two viruses is problematic antemortem. In AIDS patients with myelopathy, laboratory diagnostic studies are principally directed at ruling out spinal cord disease other than vacuolar myelopathy because neither myelography nor spinal MRI usually detects vacuolar myelopathy or HAM.

PERIPHERAL NEUROPATHIES. The most common neuropathy in the late stages of HIV-1 infection is a distal, predominantly sensory, axonal neuropathy. Characteristically, sensory symptoms exceed both sensory and motor dysfunction. Although its prevalence has not been well defined, likely a mild form of this type of neuropathy is very common. In some patients these sensory symptoms become severe, and painful paresthesias and "burning feet" are disabling. Although suspected to relate to direct HIV-1 infection of nerve or dorsal root ganglia, this has not been directly confirmed, and the pathogenesis of this neuropathy is uncertain. Anecdotal experience suggests that it does not generally respond to AZT, and treatment therefore relies on symptom management with tricyclics and analgesics. Autonomic neuropathy has also been reported in AIDS patients, with presentation ranging from postural hypotension to cardiovascular collapse in the setting of surgery.

Of increasing importance in patient management are the toxic neuropathies caused by some of the newer antiretroviral nucleoside

drugs, including dideoxyinosine, dideoxycytidine, and d4T. These drugs cause dose-dependent axonal neuropathies with clinical features very similar to the AIDS-related sensory polyneuropathy discussed above, often heralded by distal extremity pain.

CMV causes an uncommon but therapeutically important infection of nerve roots. This polyradiculopathy is usually of subacute but fulminant onset, with pain and sacral sensory loss followed by ascending progression to flaccid paralysis. The CSF reveals a characteristic pleocytosis with polymorphonuclear cell predominance. Early diagnosis and prompt institution of ganciclovir or foscarnet treatment can lead to arrest and clinical improvement.

Less common than these polyneuropathies are two forms of mononeuritis multiplex. A relatively benign form may be seen earlier in infection during "clinical latency" and is self-limiting. A later, severe form may be caused by CMV and can be fatal if not treated.

MYOPATHIES. Several types of myopathy may complicate HIV-1 infection. Although classification and characterization of these conditions remain imprecise, both inflammatory and noninflammatory myopathies have been described, ranging in severity from asymptomatic creatine kinase elevation to severe proximal weakness. Patients with inflammatory, polymyositis-like illnesses have improved with steroid therapy.

AZT can also cause proximal weakness and loss of muscle mass. This toxic myopathy appears to develop only after prolonged use of the antiretroviral and perhaps relates to the drug's effect on mitochondria; muscle biopsy may reveal excessive or abnormal mitochondria. Discontinuing the drug usually results in clinical improvement.

Baumbartner JE, Rachlin JR, Beckstead JH, et al.: Primary central nervous system lymphomas: Natural history and response to radiation therapy in 55 patients with acquired immunodeficiency syndrome. J Neurosurg 73:206, 1990. *Describes an extensive experience with primary CNS lymphoma in AIDS.*

Berger JR, Kaszovitz B, Post JD, et al.: Progressive multifocal leukoencephalopathy associated with human immunodeficiency virus infection. Ann Intern Med 107:78, 1987. *A review of experience with PML in AIDS.*

Navia BA, Cho ES, Petito CK, et al.: Cerebral toxoplasmosis complicating the acquired immune deficiency syndrome: Clinical and neuropathological findings in 27 patients. Ann Neurol 19:224, 1986. *Describes clinical features of cerebral toxoplasmosis in AIDS.*

Navia BA, Jordon BD, Price RW: The AIDS dementia complex. I. Clinical features. Ann Neurol 19517, 1986. *Report characterizing the clinical features of the AIDS dementia complex.*

Porter SB, Sande M: Toxoplasmosis of the central nervous system in the acquired immunodeficiency syndrome. N Engl J Med 327:1643, 1992. *A review of experience with cerebral toxoplasmosis in AIDS.*

Price RWP, Perry SW (eds.): HIV, AIDS, and the Brain. New York, Raven Press, 1994. *A volume devoted to the effects of HIV-1 on the CNS, particularly the AIDS dementia complex.*

Price RW, Worley JM: Management of the neurologic complications of HIV-1 infection and AIDS. *In* Sande MA, Volberding PA (eds.): The Medical Management of AIDS. 4th ed. Philadelphia, WB Saunders, 1994, p 261. *A general review with updated full bibliography.*

Simpson DM, Wolfe DE: Neuromuscular complications of HIV infection and its treatment. AIDS 5:917, 1991. *A general review of the neuropathies and myopathies complicating HIV-1 infection.*

Zuger A, Louie E, Holzman RS, et al.: Cryptococcal disease in patients with the acquired immunodeficiency syndrome: Diagnostic features and outcome of treatment. Ann Intern Med 104:234, 1986. *Describes the clinical features of cryptococcal meningitis in AIDS.*

365 PULMONARY MANIFESTATIONS OF HIV INFECTION

Philip C. Hopewell

Lung disease, specifically *Pneumocystis carinii* pneumonia (PCP), was the first recognized mode of expression of infection with the human immunodeficiency virus (HIV). Since the original clusters of cases of PCP were reported in 1981, the respiratory system has continued to be a common site of involvement in persons infected with HIV. Although pulmonary disorders are more frequent among persons who have advanced immunosuppression, meeting the current surveillance definitions for the acquired immunodeficiency syndrome (AIDS), lung diseases also occur with an increased frequency in individuals with HIV infection who have lesser degrees of immunosuppression. This chapter describes the relative frequency and spectrum of lung diseases that occur among persons infected with HIV and focuses on the approach to evaluating symptoms that originate from the respiratory tract in this unique group of patients.

EFFECTS OF HIV ON RESPIRATORY TRACT DEFENSES

The hallmark of the effect of HIV infection on host immune response is a progressive reduction in the number of circulating CD4+ lymphocytes or "T-helper" cells (see Ch. 360 and 361). The CD4+ lymphocyte plays a central role in orchestrating both cellular and humoral immune responses. Consequently, as HIV disease becomes progressively more severe, the ability of the host to ward off or contain infecting organisms becomes more and more limited. Many of the immune defects that have been described in HIV-infected persons can be attributed simply to a reduction in numbers of CD4+ lymphocytes. However, HIV infection also induces functional defects in these cells: Circulating CD4+ lymphocytes fail to proliferate in response to antigens that have been encountered previously. This loss of memory may account for failure to continue to contain infections, such as with *Mycobacterium tuberculosis* or *P. carinii,* and for the inability to prevent reinfection, as may occur with *M. tuberculosis.* Reductions in production of interleukin-2 (IL-2) and interferon-γ by CD4+ lymphocytes from HIV-infected persons have also been demonstrated. These cytokines are responsible for stimulating clonal proliferation of specifically activated alveolar macrophages and lymphocytes. Defects in production of IL-2 and interferon-γ are detectable early in the course of HIV infection and account for a functional decrease in immune response out of proportion to reduced numbers of circulating CD4+ lymphocytes (see Ch. 360).

Alveolar macrophages from persons with HIV infection have reduced chemotactic ability, but the ability to phagocytose and kill ingested organisms is thought to be normal. Alveolar macrophages express CD4 surface antigens and thus can be infected with HIV, yet they remain viable. It has been postulated that these cells can serve as reservoirs in which HIV may be sequestered. The protected virions may then infect other cells. It has also been demonstrated that cytokines, especially tumor necrosis factor-α and IL-3, stimulated by opportunistic infections such as tuberculosis, result in upregulation of HIV production within macrophages. Given these findings, the alveolar macrophage may play roles in protecting both the host and the virus and may contribute to accelerated HIV disease in the presence of opportunistic infections.

CORRELATION OF RESPIRATORY TRACT DISORDERS WITH STAGE OF HIV DISEASE

The conceptual relationship between the frequency and spectrum of lung diseases and CD4+ lymphocyte count is shown in Figure 365–1. The data that support this concept have been derived from a large, national, multicenter investigation, The Pulmonary Complications of HIV Infection Study (PCHIS). The cohort that formed the basis for this study generally mirrored the characteristics of the known HIV-infected persons in the United States (that is, reported AIDS cases), had a broad range of severity of immune compromise (47% of the cohort had CD4+ lymphocyte counts >400 cells per microliter at the time of enrollment), and were followed for a median of 53 months.

Table 365–1 shows the diseases and their rates per 100 person-years of observation in the PCHIS. Because an HIV-negative control group made up of subjects from the two largest HIV transmission categories (homosexual/bisexual men and injecting drug users [IDU's]) was included, it was demonstrated that acute bronchitis, a disorder not usually regarded as opportunistic, is significantly more common among HIV-infected persons. It should be noted that because there were no study centers in areas in which histoplasmosis and coccidioidomycosis are endemic, there were few instances of these relatively common fungal infections of the lung noted in the cohort. This observation raises an important point: the spectrum of HIV-associated lung diseases varies with geographic location as well as with severity of immune compromise and the demographic (including transmission category) make-up of the HIV-infected population in any given medical center or geographic area.

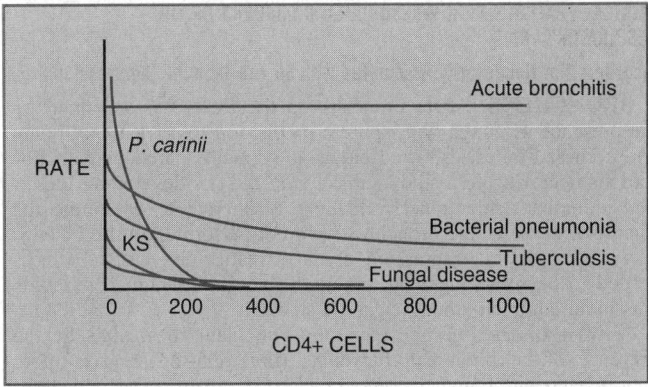

FIGURE 365–1. The relative frequency and spectrum of lung diseases change as the CD4+ lymphocyte count declines. This graph presents a conceptual depiction of these changes. The x-axis could also be equated with time following acquisition of HIV infection.

RELATIONSHIP OF RESPIRATORY TRACT DISEASES TO CD4+ LYMPHOCYTE COUNT, DEMOGRAPHIC CHARACTERISTICS, AND TRANSMISSION CATEGORY

PCP is the most common lung disease in persons with CD4+ counts <200 cells per microliter. However, in the PCHIS, 11 (6%) cases of PCP occurred in persons with CD4+ lymphocyte counts >200 cells per microliter. The patients with higher counts were marked by having other HIV-associated symptoms or findings such as fever, unintentional weight loss, oral thrush, and lymphadenopathy. Other lung diseases that usually occur only in persons with advanced HIV infection include fungal infections, pulmonary Kaposi's sarcoma (KS), lymphoma, and nontuberculous mycobacterial infections. In the case of *Mycobacterium avium* complex, it is difficult to determine if the organism is actually causing lung disease or is simply colonizing the airways. Thus, the frequency of *M. avium* complex lung disease is difficult to establish. The same difficulty applies to determining the frequency of cytomegalovirus (CMV) pulmonary disease.

Both demographic characteristics and HIV transmission category bear some relationship to the frequency of various lung diseases. Bacterial pneumonia tends to be more common among IDU's (with or without HIV infection) than in the other HIV transmission categories. Presumably, this relates, at least in part, to the effects of opiates on ventilation, cough, and ability to protect the airway. Tuberculosis is also more common in IDU's. Injection drug use had been shown to be a risk factor for tuberculosis prior to the HIV epidemic, so the finding of an increased amount of tuberculosis among drug users with HIV infection is not surprising.

Data from the PCHIS have shown that whites have a higher rate of PCP than blacks. Although the basis for this is unknown, the finding is consistent with the observation that PCP is rare in Africa. It has generally been assumed that the rarity of *P. carinii* in Africa is related to the organism being less common in the environment. However, the finding of a racial difference in risk suggests that genetic factors may play a role in predisposing whites to or protecting blacks from the disease.

TABLE 365–1. CUMULATIVE FREQUENCY OF DISEASES WITH RESPIRATORY TRACT INVOLVEMENT IN A COHORT OF PERSONS WITH HIV INFECTION (INCLUDES MULTIPLE EPISODES PER PERSON)

Diagnosis	Episodes per 100 Person-Years
Acute bronchitis	9.72
Pneumocystis carinii pneumonia	5.65
Bacterial pneumonia	5.63
Nontuberculous mycobacterial diseases	0.74
Interstitial lung disease	0.60
Pulmonary tuberculosis	0.58
Cytomegalovirus	0.42
Kaposi's sarcoma	0.33
Lymphoma	0.19
Cryptococcosis	0.16

CLINICAL FEATURES OF HIV-ASSOCIATED DISORDERS OF THE RESPIRATORY TRACT

Disorders Not Necessarily Associated with Severe Immune Suppression

BRONCHITIS. Acute bronchitis in the PCHIS was defined by the presence of cough with sputum production for at least 48 hours and a chest film that showed either no or stable parenchymal infiltrations occurring in a study subject who did not develop an identified pulmonary infection. Evaluations to attempt to determine the microbial cause of the bronchitis were not performed in the PCHIS. It was the general impression of the investigators that the illness tended to be self-limited but recurrent. Not surprisingly, bronchitis was more common among cigarette smokers.

Airways disease may be recognized on plain chest films by the presence of peribronchial thickening (Fig. 365–2A) and is more clearly seen on computed tomographic (CT) scans, especially thin-section scans (Fig. 365–2B). In addition, bronchiectasis may also occur without a recognized antecedent lung infection (Fig. 365–3). Bronchiectasis may also be a sequela of bacterial lung infection or, occasionally, PCP.

Although in the PCHIS cohort the episodes of acute bronchitis were neither associated with nor portended any other significant pulmonary diseases, the disorder may be problematic in that the symptoms may be mistaken as an indication for further, often invasive, evaluations. In general, however, bronchitis is recognizable by the absence of parenchymal infiltrations on chest films and, thus,

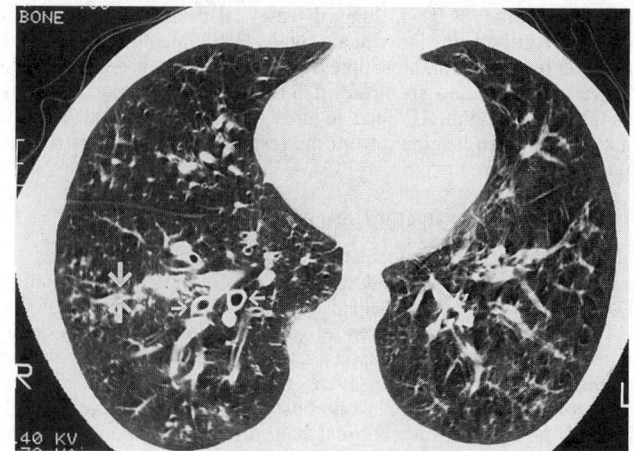

FIGURE 365–3. High-resolution CT scan of the chest of the patient whose films are shown in Figure 365–2. The scan is at a lower level and shows dilated airways with thickened walls indicative of bronchiectasis (*horizontal arrows*) and areas of mucus plugging and infiltration (*vertical arrows*). (Courtesy of Dr. James Gruden, Department of Radiology, San Francisco General Hospital.)

when the constellation of symptoms and findings described previously is noted, one should, generally, simply observe the patient, with or without antimicrobial therapy, and not undertake further evaluations.

BACTERIAL PNEUMONIA (see related chapter for each infection in Part XXI). As shown in Table 365–1, bacterial pneumonia occurred at a rate of 5.63 episodes per 100 person-years of observation in the PCHIS cohort. Bacterial pneumonia was defined as the presence of cough that was productive of purulent sputum, an area of parenchymal infiltration on chest film, and a response to antimicrobial therapy. A specific causative agent was identified in 35% of cases, a proportion that is consistent with the results of studies of the etiology of community-acquired pneumonia in persons without HIV infection.

Of the episodes for which the cause was established, *Streptococcus pneumoniae* accounted for 67% and *Haemophilus influenzae* 15%. These two agents have been generally ranked first and second in most reports of bacterial pneumonia in persons with HIV infection. In most reports, *Staphylococcus aureus* has been the third most common agent and seems to be especially common among persons with pulmonary KS. A long list of other bacterial pathogens has also been described as causing pneumonia in the setting of HIV infection (Table 365–2).

Bacterial pneumonia, especially pneumococcal pneumonia, commonly tends to be associated with bacteremia and, occasionally, sepsis syndrome. Other than the high frequency of bacteremia, the mode of clinical presentation of bacterial pneumonia does not differ in persons with and without HIV infection. Pneumonias caused by *S. pneumoniae* and *H. influenzae* tend to present as an acute illness of short duration characterized by fever, chills, and productive cough. Lobar consolidation is the most common finding on chest radiographs, and pleural fluid may be present.

The diagnostic evaluation should include sputum Gram stain and culture, Gram stain and culture of pleural fluid if present, and blood

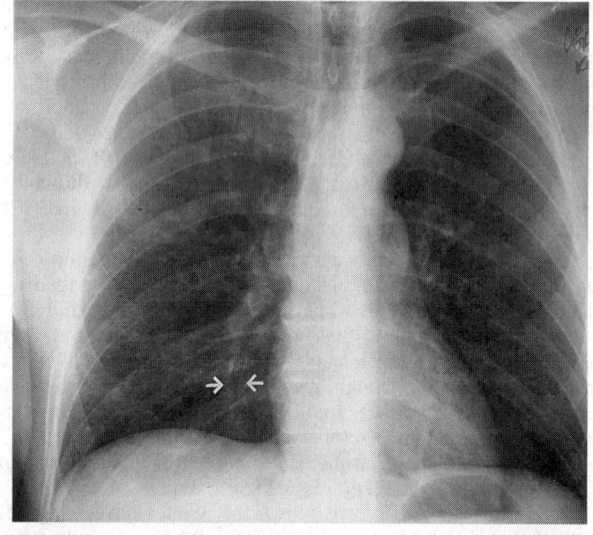

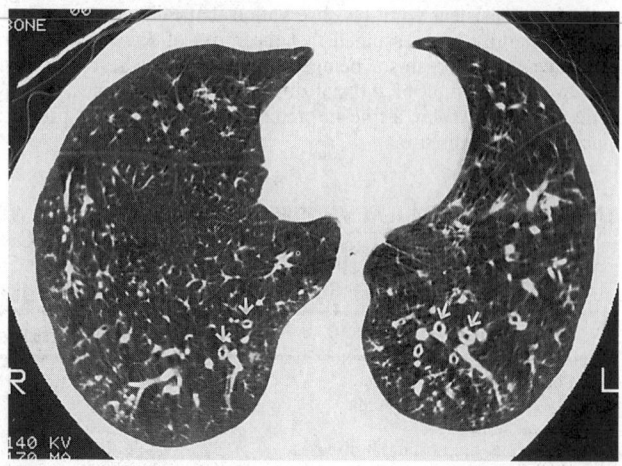

FIGURE 365–2. Bronchitis in HIV infection. *A,* A frontal view chest radiograph showing peribronchial thickening, right lower lung zone (*arrows*) consistent with bronchitis. *B,* A high-resolution CT scan of the chest showing bilateral peribronchial thickening (*arrows*) consistent with bronchitis. (Courtesy of Dr. James Gruden, Department of Radiology, San Francisco General Hospital.)

TABLE 365–2. REPORTED CAUSES OF BACTERIAL PNEUMONIA IN PERSONS WITH HIV INFECTION

Streptococcus pneumoniae
Haemophilus influenzae
Staphylococcus aureus
Nonpneumococcal streptococci
Pseudomonas aeruginosa
Moraxella catarrhalis
Rhodococcus equi
Neisseria meningitidis
Legionella species
Nocardia species
Actinomyces species

TABLE 365-3. FEATURES OF TUBERCULOSIS IN PATIENTS WITH HIV INFECTION

	Early in HIV Disease	Late in HIV Disease
Clinical course	More indolent Fewer systemic symptoms/signs	More acute Systemic symptoms/signs may predominate
Sites of disease	Predominantly pulmonary	Predominantly extrapulmonary and disseminated
Chest film	Upper lobe cavitary lesions	Diffuse or lower lobe infiltration Adenopathy Occasionally normal when lungs involved
Tuberculin test	Usually positive	Usually negative
Sputum smear/culture	Usually positive	Usually positive in patients with pulmonary disease
Infectiousness	Infectious when lungs are involved	Infectious when lungs are involved
Response to therapy	Excellent	Excellent

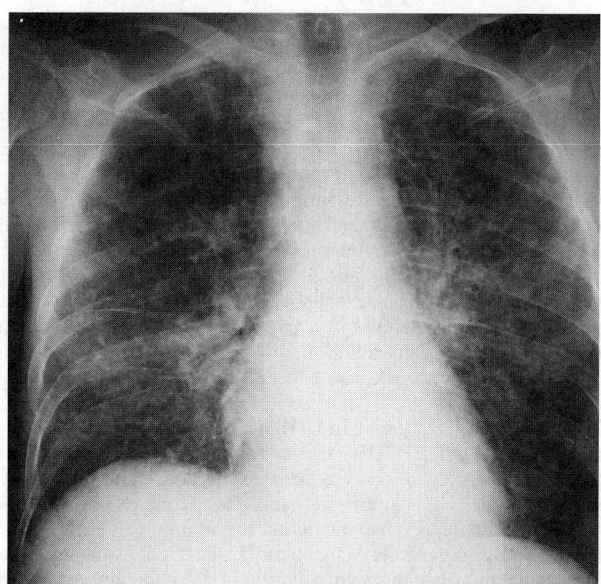

FIGURE 365-4. Frontal view chest radiograph showing diffuse pulmonary parenchymal infiltration and bilateral hilar and right paratracheal adenopathy. The patient had acid-fast bacilli seen on microscopic examination of his sputum, and *Mycobacterium tuberculosis* was isolated from sputum and blood. (Courtesy of Dr. James Gruden, Department of Radiology, San Francisco Hospital.)

cultures. Antimicrobial therapy should be guided by the usual principles for treating infectious disorders. The response to therapy should be prompt and comparable to the response of nonimmunocompromised patients. Clinicians should have a low threshold for initiating further diagnostic evaluations if the response is not prompt or is incomplete or there is worsening after an initial response. In a retrospective review of pneumococcal pneumonia in patients with HIV infection, all patients who failed to respond to usual antimicrobial therapy had superimposed PCP.

Another feature of HIV-associated bacterial pneumonia is the tendency for recurrence. This may be related to the failure to generate protective antibodies to the infecting organism or to bronchiectasis.

TUBERCULOSIS. Because *M. tuberculosis* is a very pathogenic organism, little or no immune compromise is needed for tuberculosis to develop. For this reason, tuberculosis tends to occur earlier in the course of HIV disease than diseases caused by less pathogenic organisms. The degree of immunosuppression present in a given patient has an important influence on the clinical features of tuberculosis in the presence of HIV infection, as described in Table 365-3. Persons with HIV infection and relatively well-preserved immune function tend to have "typical" features of tuberculosis, whereas tuberculosis that occurs among persons with advanced HIV disease commonly involves extrapulmonary sites and has diffuse lung infiltration with no cavitation and hilar and mediastinal adenopathy (Fig. 365-4). In terms of symptoms, tuberculosis may present as an acute illness or as a more indolent progressive process. When the lungs are involved, sputum smears and cultures are as likely to be positive in persons with HIV infection as in non–HIV-infected patients. However, because extrapulmonary sites are involved commonly, other diagnostic specimens are often necessary (Table 365-4).

Several studies have shown that persons with HIV infection and tuberculosis respond well to antituberculous therapy. In a series of patients, those who failed to respond to standard antituberculous therapy or who responded and then worsened had another superimposed disease, often PCP.

NONSPECIFIC AND LYMPHOID INTERSTITIAL PNEUMONITIS. In the PCHIS cohort, undiagnosed "interstitial disease" occurred at a rate of 0.33 cases per 100 person-years. It is not known, however, if these cases met the diagnostic criteria for either nonspecific interstitial pneumonitis (NIP) or lymphoid interstitial pneumonitis (LIP). LIP, although common in children with HIV infection, is thought to be rare in adults; thus, most of the cases in the PCHIS cohort were probably NIP. The cause of these conditions is not known, but it is speculated that they represent a response to the HIV itself. NIP tends to be self-limited in most instances and to resolve without therapy. LIP is more persistent and/or progressive but in some instances has seemed to respond to corticosteroids.

The diagnosis of both NIP and LIP can be made only by biopsy. Although transbronchial biopsy tissue is usually not sufficient to

provide a definitive diagnosis, findings that are consistent with NIP in the absence of any other identified diagnosis is sufficient to infer a diagnosis of NIP. Because of the apparent benign course of the disease and the lack of any therapeutic modalities, invasive tests to establish a diagnosis of NIP are not warranted.

Disorders Associated with Severe Immune Suppression

***PNEUMOCYSTIS CARINII* PNEUMONIA** (see Ch. 383). PCP is the most common lung disease in persons with advanced HIV infection. The presentation tends to be indolent, characterized by slowly progressive shortness of breath and nonproductive cough, usually accompanied by fever. In the PCHIS cohort, it was noted that virtually all episodes of PCP were marked by cough or shortness of breath, or both. If at least one of these symptoms was not present, PCP was not found. This study also examined the utility of screening for *P. carinii* by performing chest radiographs, pulmonary function tests, and examination of induced sputum on asymptomatic subjects. No cases of PCP were found. Based on these data, an evaluation for *P. carinii* should not be undertaken unless an HIV-infected person complains of cough and/or shortness of breath.

The radiographic findings of PCP are extremely varied. Most frequently there is diffuse "interstitial" infiltration, but there may be

TABLE 365-4. RESULTS OF MICROSCOPIC EXAMINATION AND MYCOBACTERIAL CULTURES IN PATIENTS WITH ADVANCED HIV INFECTION AND TUBERCULOSIS

Specimen	No. Positive/No. Tested (%)	
	Acid-fast Smear	*Culture*
Sputum	43/69 (62)	64/69 (93)
Bronchoalveolar lavage	9/44 (20)	39/44 (89)
Transbronchial lung biopsy	1/10 (10)	7/10 (70)
Blood	—	15/46 (33)
Lymph node	21/44 (48)	39/43 (91)
Bone marrow	4/22 (18)	13/21 (62)
Cerebrospinal fluid	—	4/21 (19)
Urine	—	12/17 (71)
Other*	5/31 (16)	24/32 (75)

* Includes pleural fluid/biopsy, pericardial fluid/biopsy, stool, liver biopsy, abscess drainage, peritoneal fluid, bone biopsy.

Data from Small PM, Schecter GF, Goodman PC, et al.: Treatment of tuberculosis in patients with advanced human immunodeficiency virus infection. N Engl J Med 324:289, 1991.

any manner of focal infiltrations, nodules or cavitary lesions, pneumatoceles, or miliary infiltration (Fig. 365–5). Focal upper lobe involvement that mimics tuberculosis is more common in persons who have been given aerosol pentamidine as prophylaxis against PCP. Pneumatoceles and spontaneous pneumothorax may occur with first episodes of PCP but are more common with subsequent episodes.

Commonly, the response to antipneumocystis therapy is slow, and radiographic abnormalities and gas exchange may worsen during the first 4 to 6 days of treatment. Co-administration of corticosteroids may minimize this initial worsening. Generally, particularly if the diagnosis has been established by bronchoscopy, most clinicians who repeat bronchoscopy early in the course of therapy find that it does not yield any additional diagnoses. However, worsening later in the course may be associated with a second, superimposed disease.

NONTUBERCULOUS MYCOBACTERIAL DISEASES (see Ch. 312). Soon after AIDS was initially described, it was recognized that a group of closely related mycobacteria collectively named *Mycobacterium avium* complex was a common cause of disseminated infection in patients with the syndrome. Although *M. avium* complex organisms are commonly isolated from respiratory tract specimens in persons with advanced HIV infection, actual lung disease is unusual. Occasionally, however, the organism may cause focal lung disease. Endobronchial lesions may be seen on bronchoscopy, and on biopsy these lesions may contain granulomas, a histologic feature that is unusual in other organs involved in disseminated *M. avium* disease. Colonization of the lungs may precede

and be a marker for subsequent disseminated *M. avium* infection. Disseminated *M. avium* complex disease occurs late in the course of HIV disease, usually when the CD4+ lymphocyte count is < 50 cells per microliter. Fever, weight loss, diarrhea, and abdominal pain are common symptoms. Pulmonary involvement is usually indicated by cough. Because it is difficult to distinguish between colonization and infection, the radiographic features of *M. avium* pulmonary disease are not well-defined. As noted above, focal infiltration may occur. Rarely, there may be diffuse lung involvement with an interstitial pattern on chest films. However, in the presence of a diffusely abnormal chest film, *M. avium* complex should not be accepted as the cause until other diseases have been excluded.

Among the nontuberculous mycobacteria, *M. kansasii* is a distant second to *M. avium* complex as a cause of disease in HIV-infected persons. As with *M. avium* complex, *M. kansasii* infections tend to be disseminated in persons with HIV infection. However, when *M. kansasii* is isolated from a respiratory tract specimen, it is more likely to be a cause of lung disease than is *M. avium* complex. As with most lung infections, *M. kansasii* usually presents with fever, cough, and, subsequently, shortness of breath. *M. kansasii* is probably more likely to cause diffuse infiltration on chest film than *M. avium* complex (see Ch. 312).

FUNGAL INFECTIONS (see Ch. 347 to 358). Both histoplasmosis and coccidioidomycosis are common HIV-associated infections in the areas in which the causative organisms are endemic and are seen sporadically outside of the endemic regions. The presenting clinical features of both histoplasmosis and coccidioidomycosis are nonspecific and variable. Histoplasmosis is commonly a protracted, febrile, wasting illness. Both infections are usually dissemi-

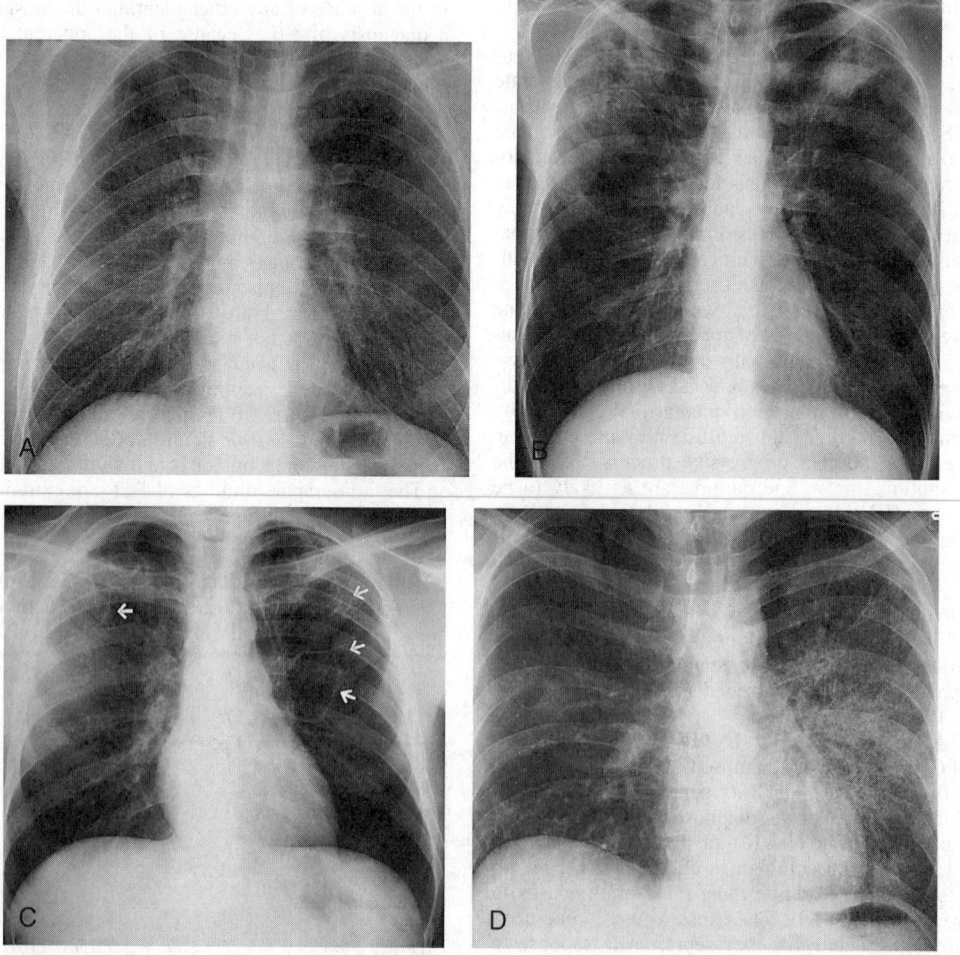

FIGURE 365–5. Radiographic findings of *Pneumocystis carinii* pneumonia (PCP). *A,* A frontal view chest radiograph showing diffuse hazy infiltration caused by early PCP. *B,* A frontal view chest radiograph with bilateral upper lobe infiltrations. *C,* A frontal view chest radiograph showing multiple bilateral thin-walled pneumatoceles *(arrows). D,* A frontal view chest radiograph with unilateral left-sided infiltration. (Courtesy of Dr. James Gruden, Department of Radiology, San Francisco General Hospital.)

nated, with respiratory symptoms and abnormal chest films reported in varying proportions. Both histoplasmosis and coccidioidomycosis can present with an acute sepsis syndrome including acute respiratory failure.

Chest radiographs are abnormal in the majority of patients, especially those who have respiratory symptoms. With histoplasmosis, the most common pattern is diffuse infiltration that is either reticulonodular or "alveolar." Coccidioidomycosis is associated with either localized or scattered nodular lesions or diffuse infiltration. For histoplasmosis, the diagnosis is commonly established by stain and culture of bone marrow, buffy coat, or blood. With coccidioidomycosis involving the lungs, specimens from the respiratory tract usually serve to establish the diagnosis.

Cryptococcosis is not limited to an endemic area. The presenting complaints are nonspecific and include fever, weight loss, fatigue, and headache, often present for a long period prior to diagnosis. Most often pulmonary involvement is silent, although in one large retrospective review, 31% of patients had respiratory complaints at the time of presentation. The findings on chest radiographs have been varied. Focal and diffuse infiltration, localized or scattered nodules, some of which may be cavitary, pleural effusions, and hilar adenopathy all have been described.

Aspergillosis has been diagnosed in a small number of patients with HIV infection. There are two patterns of *Aspergillus* pulmonary disease, one characterized by tissue invasion and the second largely an airway disease, obstructive bronchial aspergillosis. Reported risks in the setting of HIV infection have been neutropenia, use of corticosteroids, marijuana smoking, and use of broad-spectrum antimicrobial agents. Fever and cough that is sometimes productive of bronchial casts are the usual presenting complaints. The radiographic findings include focal infiltration, cavitary lesions, and pleura-based densities (Fig. 365–6). Atelectasis and airway filling patterns may be seen with obstructive bronchial aspergillosis.

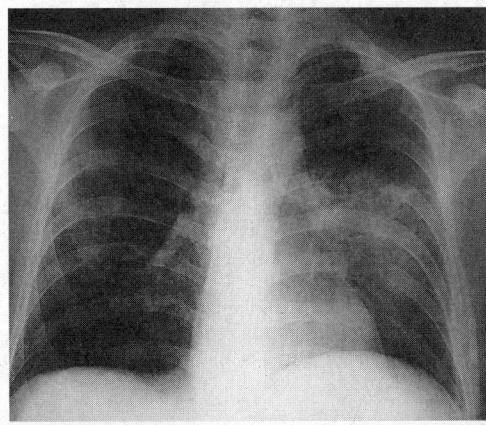

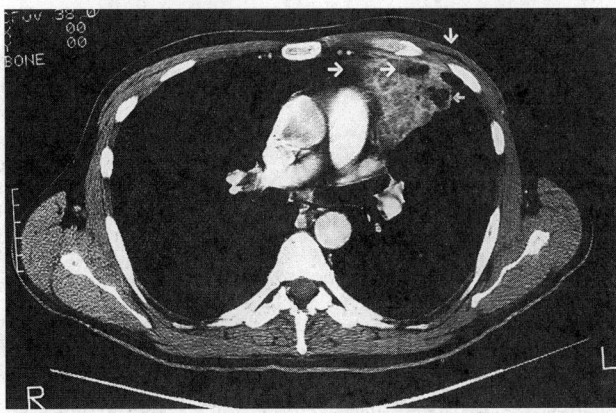

FIGURE 365–6. Invasive aspergillosis in an HIV-infected man. *A,* A frontal view chest radiograph showing infiltration in the right mid-lung zone. *B,* A CT scan of the chest at the level of the infiltration. The scan shows areas of necrosis *(horizontal arrows)* and probable chest wall invasion *(vertical arrow).* (Courtesy of Dr. James Gruden, Department of Radiology, San Francisco General Hospital.)

CYTOMEGALOVIRUS. CMV is commonly isolated from respiratory tract specimens in HIV-infected patients. However, it is unusual for lung disease to be attributable to this agent even when specific cytomegalic cells are seen on biopsy specimens. Thus, the diagnosis of CMV pneumonia can be made only when the virus is isolated in culture, specific histopathologic changes are seen on biopsy, and no other diagnosis is established. Because it is difficult to determine if CMV is the cause of lung disease in a given patient, the radiographic features of CMV pneumonia are not well-defined. In general, however, it is thought to cause diffuse infiltration that is not distinguishable from the pattern caused by many other organisms and by nonspecific interstitial pneumonitis.

NEOPLASTIC DISEASES. In the PCHIS cohort, KS involving the lungs occurred at a rate of 0.33 cases per 100 person-years of observation (14 [13%] pulmonary cases of 105 total cases), and pulmonary involvement with lymphoma occurred at a rate of 0.19 cases per 100 person-years. However, among persons with advanced HIV disease, pulmonary KS has been diagnosed in 8 to 14% of patients being evaluated for respiratory symptoms, in 21 to 49% of patients with respiratory symptoms and mucocutaneous lesions, and in 47 to 75% of patients with known KS undergoing autopsy. It is likely that the reported frequency of KS is less than actually occurs because the lung involvement may be clinically silent.

The diagnosis of pulmonary KS is nearly always established by the appearance of lesions on bronchoscopy. Typically, endobronchial KS is seen as flat, red or purple submucosal lesions that are similar in appearance to submucosal hemorrhages induced by bronchoscope trauma (see Color Plate 11*G*). The lesions may be found in any location, from vocal cords to peripheral airways, and tend to favor airway bifurcations. Because of their submucosal location, the lesions are difficult to biopsy; however, the findings are sufficiently characteristic in appearance to enable a high degree of diagnostic certainty. In a few instances, pulmonary parenchymal KS has been diagnosed by transbronchial or open biopsy in persons with no endobronchial lesions seen.

The chest radiographs of patients who had pulmonary KS without coexisting infection showed lesions that were predominantly central and consisted mainly of bronchial wall thickening and nodules (Fig. 365–7). Kerley B lines and pleural effusions were noted in 71 and 52%, respectively. Hilar or mediastinal adenopathy was present in 15%.

Non-Hodgkin's lymphoma is the second most frequent malignancy involving the lungs in patients with HIV infection. The frequency of pulmonary involvement in reported series is 0 to 25%. The presentation, even in patients who have pulmonary involvement, is generally dominated by systemic symptoms. The most common chest radiographic findings are patchy parenchymal infiltrates, nodules, and solitary masses. Intrathoracic adenopathy has been reported in a minority of cases. The diagnosis can be established by transbronchial biopsy, needle aspiration biopsy, or thoracoscopic or open biopsy.

AN INTEGRATED APPROACH TO DIAGNOSIS

Although the differential diagnosis of lung disease in a person with HIV infection is quite broad, the probabilities of the various diagnoses can be reduced in a given patient by knowing the patient's symptoms, HIV transmission category, and CD4+ lymphocyte count and further refined by the findings on the chest film. A general approach to the diagnostic evaluation in patients with a CD4+ lymphocyte count of ≤300 cells per microliter is shown in Figure 365–8.

First define the patient's symptoms, especially whether or not the patient has cough and/or shortness of breath. If cough is present, it is important to ascertain if it is productive of purulent sputum. It is very uncommon for patients with PCP to have purulent sputum. Moreover, depending on the stain used, the presence of purulent debris in respiratory tract specimens makes it difficult to detect *P. carinii* in smears of sputum or bronchoalveolar lavage (BAL) fluid. As noted previously, acute bronchitis and bacterial pneumonia are relatively more frequent among persons with higher CD4+ lymphocyte cell counts. Additionally, IDU's have higher rates of bacterial pneumonia and tuberculosis than persons in other HIV transmission categories. Also as noted, the differential diagnosis varies somewhat with the geographic area, with histoplasmosis and

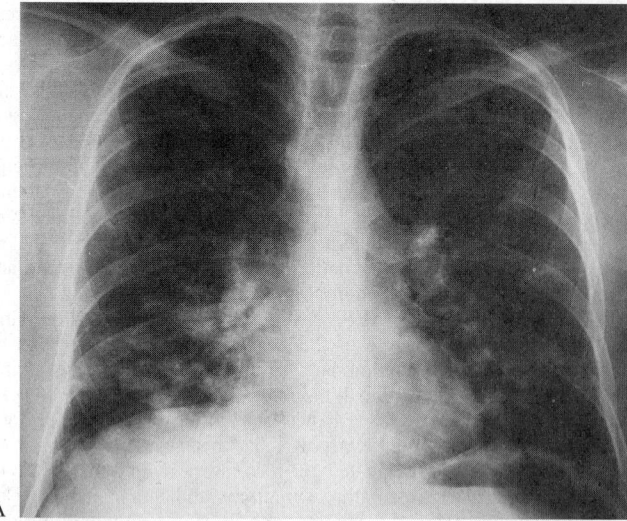

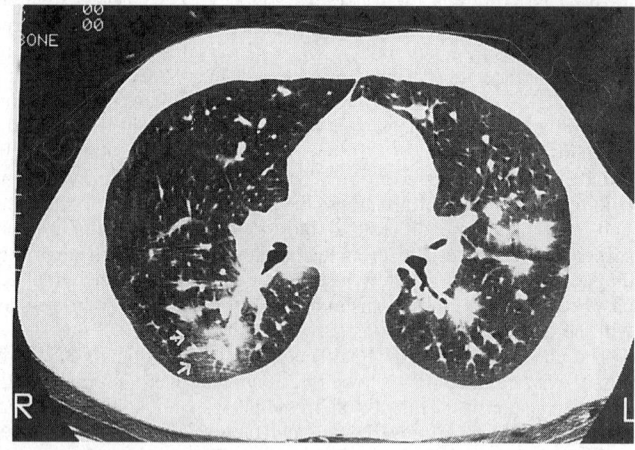

FIGURE 365–7. Kaposi's sarcoma (KS). *A,* A frontal view chest radiograph with typical findings of pulmonary KS. *B,* A high-resolution CT scan of the lower chest. Masslike peribronchovascular lesions typical of KS are seen. The lesions on the right side are surrounded by areas of fainter infiltration *(arrows),* a so-called halo sign that is highly suggestive of KS. (Courtesy of Dr. James Gruden, Department of Radiology, San Francisco General Hospital.)

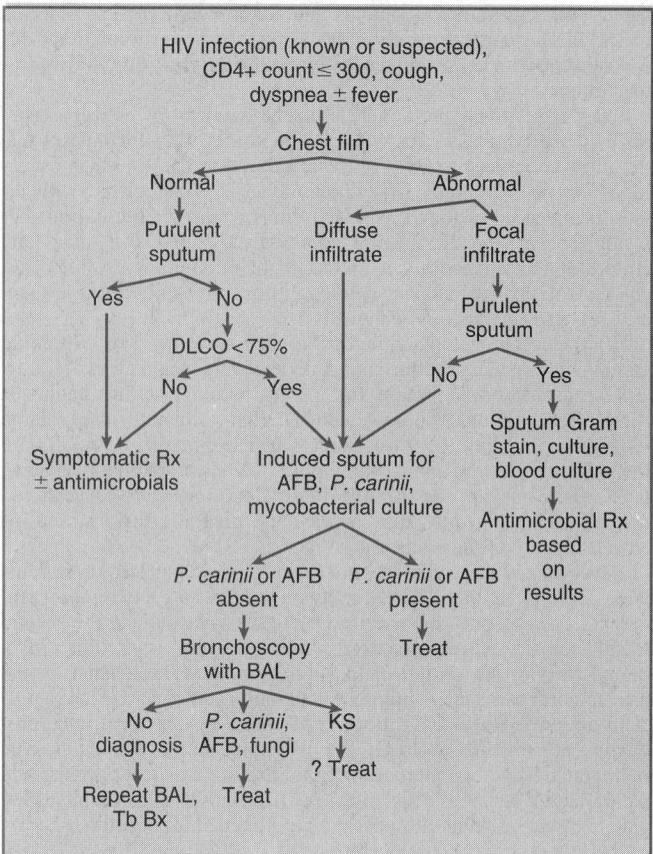

FIGURE 365–8. Algorithm of the diagnostic approach to patients who are known or suspected of having HIV infection resulting in significant immunocompromise, < 300 CD4+ lymphocytes per microliter. DLco = Pulmonary diffusing capacity for carbon monoxide; AFB = acid-fast bacilli; BAL = bronchoalveolar lavage; Tb Bx = transbronchial lung biopsy.

coccidioidomycosis being common in their respective endemic areas.

As in all patients with significant respiratory symptoms, radiographic examination of the chest is usually the first test. If the chest film shows no abnormalities in a patient with purulent sputum, the likely diagnosis is bronchitis. Patients with a diagnosis of bronchitis should be followed to be certain that the symptoms resolve and, if there is no resolution or worsening, further evaluation should be undertaken. It must be kept in mind that both tuberculosis and PCP may present with normal chest films.

Patients who have normal chest films and a nonproductive cough may also have bronchitis, but if the CD4+ lymphocyte count is < 300 cells per microliter, *P. carinii* should be considered. In this circumstance, pulmonary function testing with measurement of the diffusing capacity for carbon monoxide (DLco) should be performed. If the DLco is < 75% of the predicted normal value, further evaluation directed toward detecting *P. carinii* should be undertaken. A promising alternative approach that has not yet been fully evaluated is to replace measurement of the DLco with thin-section CT scanning using a limited number of images to reduce cost. This approach has the potential advantage of being able to distinguish among PCP, emphysema, and vascular obliteration caused by foreign particle embolization from intravenous drug use (Fig. 365–9).

If the chest film is abnormal, the next step depends on the type of abnormality. Focal infiltration, especially consolidation, in a pa-

tient with purulent sputum is most consistent with a diagnosis of bacterial pneumonia or tuberculosis (see Fig. 365–8). Sputum should be obtained for Gram stain, acid-fast stain, and cultures for pyogenic organisms and mycobacteria. If there is a poor response or worsening, further evaluation, especially for *P. carinii,* should be performed.

To this point much of the diagnostic approach is applicable for evaluating respiratory symptoms regardless of the HIV status of the patient. In the group of patients thought likely to have an HIV-re-

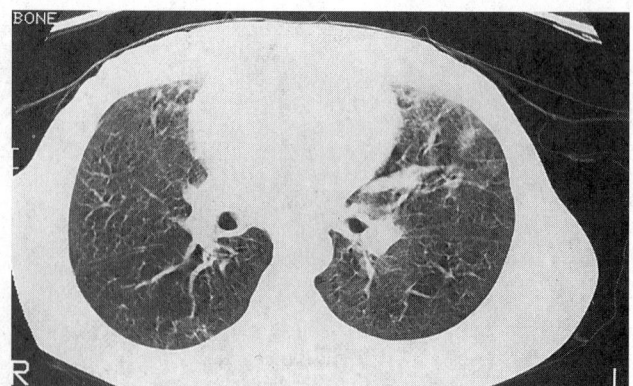

FIGURE 365–9. High-resolution CT scan of the chest of a patient who complained of shortness of breath but whose plain chest film was normal. The scan shows patchy "ground-glass" infiltration in the anterior portions of both lungs. The patient was found to have *P. carinii* in an induced sputum sample. The findings noted in the scan are typical of early *P. carinii* pneumonia. (Courtesy of Dr. James Gruden, Department of Radiology, San Francisco General Hospital.)

TABLE 365–5. EXAMINATION OF RESPIRATORY TRACT SPECIMENS

Specimen	Test
Spontaneous sputum	Gram stain, AFB stain, cultures for mycobacteria and pyogenic bacteria
Induced sputum	*P. carinii* stain, AFB stain, mycobacterial culture
Bronchoalveolar lavage fluid	*P. carinii* stain, AFB stain, mycobacterial and fungal cultures
Transbronchial biopsy tissue	Touch preparations and tissue stains for *P. carinii*, AFB stain, hematoxylin and eosin tissue stain, culture for mycobacteria and fungi
Needle aspiration biopsy tissue	*P. carinii* stain, AFB stain, cytologic examination, cultures for mycobacteria and fungi

AFB = Acid-fast bacilli.

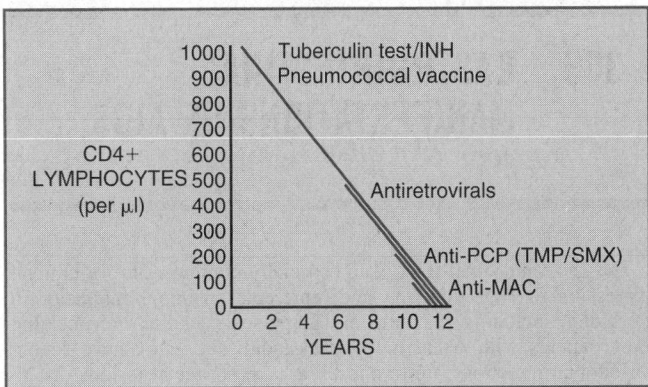

FIGURE 365–10. Schematic representation of the use of preventive interventions in persons with HIV infection. The timing of the interventions is based on the CD4+ lymphocyte count and the risk of the common HIV-associated lung infections. INH = Isoniazid; PCP = *P. carinii* pneumonia; TMP-SMX = trimethoprim-sulfamethoxazole; MAC = *Mycobacterium avium* complex.

lated opportunistic infection, however, there is considerable variation both in philosophy and in specific diagnostic tests used. Cogent arguments have been made for empiric treatment with antipneumocystis agents for patients thought highly likely to have PCP, with specific tests for the organism being reserved for patients who fail to respond. With or without an empiric therapeutic trial, when it is decided to seek a specific diagnosis, the approach used varies. In some institutions, as described subsequently, the first step is to examine induced sputum, with bronchoscopy being performed only in those patients with negative sputum examinations. In other institutions, bronchoscopy is the first procedure used to obtain respiratory tract specimens. Also, based on experience and preference, there are variations in the bronchoscopic procedure. Usually, BAL is performed with all procedures. Many clinicians also routinely perform a transbronchial biopsy at the time of initial bronchoscopy, whereas others perform biopsies on a case-by-case basis, and others do so only if the BAL does not provide a diagnosis (and perhaps not even then).

If there is diffuse or focal infiltration in a person with a nonproductive cough, generally the evaluation should be directed toward opportunistic organisms. In many institutions the next diagnostic step is to induce sputum by having the patient inhale a hypertonic (3%) saline mist generated by an ultrasonic nebulizer. Careful attention to the details of selecting patients and inducing, processing, and examining the sputum specimens is essential to obtain good results.

Diagnosis of mycobacterial disease and fungal infections can also be established by examining induced sputum. However, in HIV-infected patients, because of the high frequency of oral candidiasis, fungal cultures are frequently overgrown with *Candida* species.

Because the negative predictive value of a negative examination of induced sputum is in the range of 60%, patients having a negative sputum examination generally should undergo bronchoscopy with BAL unless another diagnosis has been established or the procedure is contraindicated. At San Francisco General Hospital, *P. carinii* infection, either alone or with another diagnosis, was found in 32% of bronchoscopic examinations in patients who had a negative sputum examination. KS was found in 15%, nontuberculous mycobacteria in 25%, *M. tuberculosis* in 5%, and fungal pathogens in 4%. In addition, nearly all of the pathogens were found by BAL, and only rarely did transbronchial biopsy provide additional information.

In patients whose chest films show focal or isolated nodular or mass lesions, needle aspiration biopsy, if the lesion is accessible, is an efficient diagnostic approach, and in some instances fluoroscopically guided transbronchial biopsy should be attempted. Enlarged intrathoracic lymph nodes may also be approached via needle aspiration biopsy, either through the bronchoscope (Wang needle) or via a transthoracic approach. The tests that should be performed on the various sorts of specimens described above are listed in Table 365–5.

PREVENTING LUNG DISEASES IN PERSONS WITH HIV INFECTION

Much of the improved survival for patients with HIV infection in recent years owes to the prevention of PCP. Hence, the use of antipneumocystis agents such as trimethoprim-sulfamethoxazole, dap-

sone, and pentamidine aerosol for persons with HIV infection and CD4+ lymphocyte counts < 200 cells per microliter is a high-priority intervention. This is described in more detail in Ch. 383.

Preventive interventions for tuberculosis also should be accorded a high priority. All HIV-infected persons should receive a tuberculin skin test, and, if the test is positive (≥ 5 mm induration), isoniazid preventive therapy should be given regardless of the CD4+ lymphocyte count. Isoniazid should also be given to all HIV-infected persons who have been exposed to a person with infectious tuberculosis regardless of the tuberculin test result. The use of isoniazid preventive therapy for nonexposed persons who are defined as anergic is not of proven benefit.

It is not established whether pneumococcal vaccine reduces the rate of pneumococcal disease in persons with HIV infection. However, because of the low likelihood of adverse reactions to the vaccine, any benefit would not be offset by risk. Data from the PCHIS cohort suggest that trimethoprim-sulfamethoxazole as antipneumocystis prophylaxis decreases the frequency of pneumococcal disease, thus providing an additional benefit for this preventive intervention.

Finally, it has been shown that prophylactic rifabutin reduces the frequency of *M. avium* complex disease by approximately 50%. Current recommendations are that rifabutin prophylaxis be given to persons with HIV infection and CD4+ counts of < 100 cells per microliter. Persons who are candidates for rifabutin should be carefully evaluated for tuberculosis. Rifabutin administered to a person who has undiagnosed tuberculosis would quickly result in resistance of *M. tuberculosis* to rifabutin *and* rifampin, a major antituberculosis drug. The relationship of preventive interventions to CD4+ lymphocyte count is summarized in Figure 365–10.

Chin DP: *Mycobacterium avium* complex and other nontuberculous mycobacteria in patients with HIV. Semin Respir Infect 8:124, 1993. *Describes the epidemiology, clinical presentation, diagnosis, and management of the nontuberculous mycobacterial diseases with a focus on M. avium complex.*

Hopewell PC: Tuberculosis and infection with the human immunodeficiency virus. *In* Reichman LB, Hershfield ES (eds.): Tuberculosis: A Comprehensive International Approach. New York, Marcell Dekker, 1993, p 369. *Describes the overall impact of HIV infection on all aspects of tuberculosis.*

Hopewell PC, Mazur H: *Pneumocystis carinii* pneumonia: Current concepts. *In* Sande MA, Volberding PA (eds.): The Medical Management of AIDS, 4th ed. Philadelphia, WB Saunders, 1994, p 367. *A comprehensive review of the epidemiology, pathogenesis, clinical features, diagnosis, and treatment of PCP.*

Irwin DH, Kaplan LD: Pulmonary manifestations of acquired immunodeficiency syndrome malignancies. Semin Respir Infect 8:139, 1993. *Describes the clinical features and management of pulmonary Kaposi's sarcoma and non-Hodgkin's lymphoma.*

Stansell JD: Pulmonary fungal infections in HIV infected persons. Semin Respir Infect 8:116, 1993. *Reviews the epidemiology, clinical features, diagnosis, and management of the fungal infections that involve the lungs in patients with HIV infection.*

Wallace JM, Rao V, Glassroth J, et al.: Respiratory illnesses in persons with human immunodeficiency virus infection. Am Rev Respir Dis 148:1523, 1993. *Describes the frequency and spectrum of lung diseases after 18 months of follow-up in a cohort of HIV-infected persons from the major transmission categories. Included are subjects who have little apparent immunosuppression.*

366 GASTROINTESTINAL MANIFESTATIONS OF AIDS

John G. Bartlett

The gastrointestinal tract is an especially common site for clinical expression of HIV infection and represents an important factor in morbidity, including malnutrition. Large-scale studies indicate that most patients with AIDS have oral candidiasis, many have severe periodontal infections, up to one third have perirectal lesions due to herpes simplex, 30 to 60% complain of chronic or intermittent diarrhea, and the average weight loss following an AIDS-defining diagnosis is 12 to 15 kg. Most of these complications represent opportunistic infections that occur only with advanced stages of immunosuppression when the T4 lymphocyte count is < 200 per cubic millimeter.

ORAL LESIONS. Oral candidiasis ("thrush") is encountered at some time in 80 to 90% of all patients with advanced stages of HIV infection. The usual finding is white patches that show yeast forms and pseudohyphae on KOH preparation. The diagnosis is usually made by visual appearance. The lesions usually respond to nystatin, clotrimazole troches, ketoconazole, or fluconazole, but relapse rates are high so that continuous therapy is often necessary. Oral hairy leukoplakia (OHL) is a newly recognized condition found exclusively in persons with HIV infection. *In situ* hybridization implicates Epstein-Barr virus. Typical lesions are patches of white fibrillar projections that are usually located on the tongue and often confused with thrush. OHL is usually asymptomatic, but occasional patients complain of pain or voice changes and respond to treatment with acyclovir. Herpes simplex virus (HSV) often causes painful oral lesions that have the typical appearance of vesicles on an erythematous base and break down to form ulcers. Herpetic lesions tend to be more severe and prolonged in patients with HIV infection. The usual treatment is acyclovir given orally or parenterally. The major source of confusion is aphthous ulcers of unknown origin that seem to respond best to topical or systemic corticosteroids. In patients with Kaposi's sarcoma, the oral cavity is often involved, most frequently with typical erythematous purplish raised lesions on the palate, although any site in the oral cavity may be involved. Most are asymptomatic; symptomatic lesions generally respond to radiation treatment. Periodontal disease is relatively common with either gingivitis or periodontitis. Treatment consists of topical chlorhexidine (Peridex) or systemically administered metronidazole.

ESOPHAGITIS. Odynophagia generally indicates an esophageal lesion. The most common cause is candidiasis, and most patients also have thrush. Alternative causes include HSV, cytomegalovirus (CMV), or aphthous ulcers. The diagnosis is optimally made with endoscopy showing grayish white plaques and smears or biopsy to demonstrate the causative agent. A presumptive diagnosis of *Candida* esophagitis is made in patients with thrush combined with odynophagia. Preferred drugs for *C. albicans* esophagitis are ketoconazole or fluconazole by mouth, or a brief course of amphotericin B by vein. HSV may be treated with acyclovir, CMV often responds to ganciclovir, and aphthous ulcers are optimally treated with systemic corticosteroids.

GASTRIC LESIONS. Patients with AIDS often have gastric achlorhydria; less common gastric lesions are Kaposi's sarcoma and opportunistic infections.

SMALL BOWEL AND COLON LESIONS. Acute and/or chronic diarrhea is a frequent complication, usually in the relatively late stages of HIV infection. In many instances, diarrhea is accompanied by severe weight loss, a combination referred to as "diarrhea-wasting syndrome" that is now included as an AIDS-defining diagnosis according to World Health Organization and Centers for Disease Control and Prevention definitions. The frequency of chronic diarrhea is usually reported at 30 to 60% for patients with AIDS, many have intermittent symptoms, and the small bowel is the most common site of pathologic changes. The most common

opportunistic pathogens responsible for chronic diarrhea (intermittent or continuous loose or watery stools for > 1 month) are *Cryptosporidium,* Microsporida, *Mycobacterium avium,* and CMV; each of these account for 15 to 40% of cases in large series.

Cryptosporidia tend to cause intermittent diarrhea that persists for months and may be responsible for severe fluid losses, dehydration, and electrolyte abnormalities. Small bowel biopsies show villous atrophy, crypt hyperplasia, and intraepithelial lymphocytes with typical schizonts that appear adherent to the brush border, but are actually just inside the basement membrane of the enterocyte. Functional tests show D-xylose malabsorption, and stools show no fecal leukocytes. The usual diagnostic test is a stool examination for oocysts that appear like yeast but are easily detected using modified acid-fast stains. Complications include papillary stenosis and obstruction of the common bile duct. No antimicrobial therapy has proven effective.

Microsporida are a group of extremely small unicellular parasites, with the most frequent species in AIDS patients being *Enterocytozoon bieneusi.* The organism cannot be easily detected in stool, so small intestinal biopsy with electron microscopy is often required. Histopathologic changes are similar to those noted with cryptosporidiosis except for the unique morphologic features and location of the organism within the cytoplasm of the enterocyte. No antimicrobial therapy has proven effective.

M. avium may cause pathologic changes in the small bowel which appear identical to those of Whipple's disease, but with large numbers of acid-fast bacilli. Most patients have *M. avium* bacteremia. The usual treatment is a combination of clarithromycin with ethambutol, clarithromycin with clofazimine, or all three drugs (see Ch. 312).

CMV commonly causes disseminated infection in the late stages of HIV infection at any level of the gastrointestinal tract including the mouth, esophagus, stomach, small bowel, colon, and perirectal region. The most common is a diffuse colitis with superficial ulcerations seen with computed tomographic (CT) scan or endoscopy. Symptoms ascribed to this infection include diarrhea, abdominal pain, and bloody stools. Less common are a solitary ulcer, toxic megacolon, or intestinal perforation. The diagnosis is generally established by demonstrating typical viral inclusions in intestinal biopsies. Ganciclovir and foscarnet are sometimes effective, although many patients do not respond.

Isospora belli is a protozoan parasite that accounts for about 1 to 3% of cases of chronic diarrhea in patients with advanced HIV infection. Large acid-fast oocysts (20 to 30 × 10 to 20 μm) are seen in the stool and trimethoprim-sulfamethoxazole (TMP-SMX) is effective therapy. *Entamoeba histolytica* and *Giardia lamblia* are occasionally encountered, but their frequency is no greater than in immunocompetent persons. *Blastocystis hominis* is found in stools of 10 to 15% of healthy heterosexual persons and 35 to 50% of asymptomatic homosexual men; its role as an enteric pathogen is unclear. Nonpathogenic ameba (*E. hartmani, E. coli, E. nana,* and *Iodamoeba butchii*) play no established role in diarrhea in persons with or without HIV infection.

Among bacterial pathogens, *Salmonella,* especially *S. typhimurium,* is found at least 20-fold more frequently in patients with AIDS than in the general population. Unusual features include the lack of an identifiable source of infection in most, a high rate of bacteremia (enteric fever), and the propensity of the infection to recur when treatment is discontinued. The favored drugs include ampicillin or amoxicillin, TMP-SMX, third-generation cephalosporins, and quinolones. Antibiotic-associated diarrhea or colitis due to *Clostridium difficile* is also relatively common in patients with HIV infection owing to their high rate of antibiotic consumption. Additional microbial pathogens to consider in acute diarrhea are *Shigella, Campylobacter jejuni,* and enteric viruses.

Tumors of the gastrointestinal tract associated with HIV infection include Kaposi's sarcoma, non-Hodgkin's lymphoma, cloacogenic carcinoma of the rectum, and squamous cell carcinoma of the rectum and anus. The most common of these is Kaposi's sarcoma, which has been found in gut tissue at autopsy in 40 to 50% of persons with typical cutaneous lesions. Endoscopy typically shows raised red nodules, but histologic confirmation is difficult owing to the depth of pathologic changes. The great majority are asymptomatic; less common presentations include diarrhea, subacute intestinal obstruction, protein-losing enteropathy, and rectal ulcer. The lymphomas associated with HIV infection are usually high-grade B-cell lymphomas that are extranodal in origin. The gastrointestinal tract is affected in up to 20%, and there may be involvement of any site from the oral cavity to the rectum.

AIDS ENTEROPATHY. Endoscopy in patients with advanced AIDS often shows morphologic changes in the small bowel in the absence of evidence for a superimposed opportunistic infection. Characteristic features are villous blunting, a reduced villus-crypt ratio, and an inappropriately low number of mitotic figures. In the absence of an enteric pathogen the findings are sometimes referred to as "AIDS enteropathy." Studies of gastrointestinal function in the presence of AIDS enteropathy usually show malabsorption with abnormal D-xylose and ^{14}C-glycerol-tripalmitin absorption tests. The cause of these changes is not known, but the major considerations include direct invasion by HIV, an opportunistic infection that has not been detected, small bowel overgrowth, autonomic nervous dysfunction, or immune dysfunction (reflecting the fact that 25% of lymphatic tissue is in the gut).

MANAGEMENT GUIDELINES FOR PATIENTS WITH DIARRHEA. Recommended tests should be tailored to the specific clinical findings and likely etiologic agents. For most patients with HIV infection and diarrhea that is severe or prolonged, the initial evaluation should include cultures for bacterial pathogens (*Salmonella, Shigella,* and *Campylobacter jejuni*), direct examination for ova and parasites, and a *Clostridium difficile* toxin assay. Previous studies indicate that a likely etiologic agent will be detected in 30 to 50% of patients, the most common in chronic diarrhea being *Cryptosporidium*. Those with persistent and unexplained diarrhea or disabling abdominal pain may undergo additional testing, including radiography with contrast, abdominal CT, and/or endoscopy. Extensive use of upper or lower endoscopy in this setting is controversial because the conditions often cannot be readily treated, giving a poor cost-benefit ratio. These conditions include AIDS enteropathy and infections with Cryptosporidia and Microsporida. The treatment of diarrhea in the patient with advanced infection should include appropriate antimicrobial agents directed against identified pathogens (Table 366–1). Nonspecific agents such as imodium or loperamide, indomethacin, somatostatin, or bismuth salts are sometimes useful. Nutritional consequences of chronic diarrhea need to be addressed as described below.

NUTRITIONAL SUPPORT. The average patient with AIDS loses 15 to 20% of his/her baseline weight during the course of the infection. Protein-calorie malnutrition is a common and serious sequela to late disease that may accelerate progressive immunosuppression. Contributing factors to malnutrition include a hypermetabolic state associated with chronic infection (especially with fever), oral lesions causing pain, esophageal lesions resulting in odynophagia, reduced taste sensation, depression, HIV-associated subcortical dementia, gastrointestinal side effects of medications, AIDS enteropathy, and opportunistic infections causing malabsorption. Therapeutic approaches are optimally based on the cause. Patients with chronic diarrhea should receive small, frequent meals that are low in fiber, residue, lactose, fat, and caffeine. These patients often require additional nutritional support, preferably using the oral route. Supplementary enteral nutritional feedings may include polymeric formulas or, for patients with severe enteropathy, elemental formulas.

"GAY BOWEL SYNDROME." This term is used in reference to the enteric and perirectal infections that are commonly encountered in homosexual men. Relevant in the context of HIV infection is the fact that the homosexual lifestyle is a risk category for both. However, the pathogens observed with gastrointestinal lesions in immunocompetent homosexual men and immunosuppressed patients with HIV infection are very different (Table 366–2). The former includes a number of sexually transmitted diseases combined with several conventional enteric pathogens. By contrast, the listing for patients with HIV infection is largely restricted to opportunistic infections and opportunistic tumors, reflecting immunosuppression. The single pathogen encountered in both lists is HSV, although this infection is distinctive in the two groups; HSV infections in patients with AIDS are usually more extensive, more severe, more prolonged, and more likely to involve acyclovir-resistant strains.

HEPATOBILIARY DISEASE. Prevalence rates of hepatitis B and hepatitis C viruses are high in AIDS patients, reflecting their prevalence among homosexual men, intravenous drug abusers, and hemophiliacs. Other causes of hepatocellular injury are CMV, HSV, and drugs (e.g., nucleoside analogues, TMP-SMX, isoniazid, rifampin). Cholestatic changes in liver function tests suggest *M. avium*, tuberculosis, histoplasmosis, and lymphoma. Cholangiopathy with biliary obstruction is usually caused by cryptosporidia or CMV; less common causes are microsporidiosis, lymphoma, and Kaposi's sarcoma.

ABDOMINAL SURGERY. The most common clinical syndromes in persons with HIV infection that require abdominal surgery are peritonitis associated with perforation due to CMV infection; lymphoma of the gut (most frequently with involvement of the terminal ileum with obstruction or bleeding); Kaposi's sarcoma; and *M. avium* infection involving retroperitoneal lymph nodes or spleen. Patients with cholangiopathy due to CMV or cryptosporidio-

TABLE 366–2. GASTROINTESTINAL LESIONS IN HOMOSEXUAL MEN AND PATIENTS WITH HIV INFECTION

Site	Immunocompetent Homosexual Men	Immune Deficiency with HIV Infection
Oral cavity	*Neisseria gonorrhoeae* Herpes simplex	*Candida albicans* Oral hairy leukoplakia Herpes simplex Aphthous ulcers Necrotizing gingivitis Kaposi's sarcoma
Esophagus		*Candida albicans* Cytomegalovirus Herpes simplex Aphthous ulcers
Small bowel	*Giardia*	*Cryptosporidium* *Isospora* Microsporidia *Mycobacterium avium* Cytomegalovirus *Salmonella typhimurium* "AIDS enteropathy" Lymphoma, B cell
Colon	*Chlamydia trachomatis* LGV serovars *Campylobacter* species *Shigella* *Etamoeba histolytica*	Cytomegalovirus
Anus, rectum	*Neisseria gonorrhoeae* *Treponema pallidum* Condyloma accuminatum Herpes simplex	Herpes simplex Cytomegalovirus

TABLE 366–1. TREATMENT OF ENTERIC PATHOGENS IN AIDS

Pathogen	Treatment
Candida albicans	
Thrush	Nystatin, clotrimazole, ketoconazole, or fluconazole
Esophagitis	Ketoconazole, fluconazole, or amphotericin B
Herpes simplex	Acyclovir
Cytomegalovirus	
Esophagitis	Ganciclovir
Enteritis/colitis	Ganciclovir (?) or foscarnet (?)*
Oral hairy leukoplakia	Acyclovir (symptomatic only)
Mycobacterium avium	Clarithromycin, clofazimine, ethambutol ± rifampin, ciprofloxacin or amikacin
Salmonella species	Ampicillin/amoxicillin, quinolone, trimethoprim-sulfamethoxazole, or third-generation cephalosporin
Clostridium difficile	Metronidazole or vancomycin
Campylobacter species	Erythromycin or quinolone
Entamoeba histolytica	Metronidazole + diloxanide
Giardia lamblia	Quinacrine or metronidazole
Isospora	Trimethoprim-sulfamethoxazole
Cryptosporidium	Paromomycin (?)*
Microsporidia	Albendazole (?)*

* (?) indicates that efficacy is not established.

sis often respond to endoscopic retrograde cholangiopancreatography, but recurrence rates are high. The experience to date indicates that patients with HIV infection tolerate surgical procedures well and do not have an unusually high incidence of postoperative complications.

Bartlett JG, Belitsos P, Sears C: AIDS enteropathy. Clin Infect Dis 16:726, 1992. *This is a review of AIDS enteropathy with a literature review, suggested diagnostic evaluation, and possible causes of "idiopathic AIDS enteropathy."*

Kotler DP, Clayton F, Scholes JV, Orenstein JM: Small intestinal injury and parasitic diseases in AIDS. Ann Intern Med 113:444, 1990. *The authors review histopathologic findings including electron microscopy in AIDS patients with cryptosporidiosis and microsporidiosis.*

Laughon BE, Druckman DA, Vernon A, et al.: Prevalence of enteric pathogens in homosexual men with and without acquired immunodeficiency syndrome. Gastroenterology 94:984, 1988. *This is an exhaustive study of stool to detect bacterial, viral, fungal, and parasitic pathogens in homosexual men without AIDS, with AIDS, and with proctitis or diarrhea.*

Nelson MR, Shanson DC, Hawkins DA, et al.: *Salmonella, Campylobacter* and *Shigella* in HIV-seropositive patients. AIDS 6:1495, 1992. *Analysis of stool cultures from 654 AIDS patients with diarrhea.*

Smith PD, Quinn TC, Strober W, et al.: Gastrointestinal manifestations in AIDS. Ann Intern Med 116:63, 1992. *Reviews the spectrum of enteric pathogens by organism; also addresses issues of immunopathogenesis, diagnosis, and therapy.*

367 CUTANEOUS SIGNS OF AIDS
Neal S. Penneys

Cutaneous signs and symptoms associated with AIDS increase in frequency and severity as the disease advances. However, infection by human immunodeficiency virus (HIV) may produce a transient macular roseola–like eruption. As HIV infection progresses, infectious processes and neoplastic disease are most often seen. Patients also may have symptoms such as pruritus without visible skin lesions.

Cutaneous infections are a common feature of AIDS. Superficial infections such as dermatophytosis, candidiasis, and scabies may be extensive and have altered appearances. Superficial fungal infections may coexist with other pathogens such as herpesvirus or cytomegalovirus to produce unusual complex cutaneous infections.

Cutaneous viral infections also may have unpredictable presentations. Molluscum contagiosum occurs commonly, is persistent, and lesions may become quite large. Human papillomavirus–induced lesions may occur, ranging from persistent verrucae to severe anogenital condyloma (see Color Plate 12A). Molluscum contagiosum and human papillomavirus lesions frequently occur in cosmetically sensitive areas. Locally destructive treatments such as curettage and cryotherapy are effective, but lesions almost always recur or new lesions develop, particularly as CD4 counts decrease.

Herpes zoster may be a reliable sign of the presence or progression of HIV infection in an otherwise asymptomatic person. With the diminishing immune response, the usually self-limited herpetic infections become chronic and fail to heal (see Color Plate 12B). Chronic herpetic lesions may not have the characteristic morphology of acute lesions in immunocompetent individuals. Both herpes simplex and herpes zoster viruses may produce disseminated skin lesions in HIV-infected individuals. The diagnosis of herpetic infections can be made by morphology of the clinical lesion, examination of a Tzanck preparation (Wright stain of a scraping taken from the base of a lesion), skin biopsy, viral culture, and/or molecular diagnostic methods. For chronic or recurrent herpetic infection and for long-term suppression, oral acyclovir therapy is helpful.

Unusual primary and disseminated infections occur in the skin in the context of HIV infection. Mucosal and cutaneous lesions of histoplasmosis, cryptococcosis, and other systemic fungal disorders can be signs of disseminated infection in AIDS patients. Mycobacterial infections produced by *M. tuberculosis, M. avium–intracellulare, M. haemophilum,* and others affect the skin in patients with AIDS. A long list of unusual or unique infections has been observed, including disseminated amebiasis, *Trichosporon beigelei,* sporotrichosis, *Strongyloides* infection, alternariosis, and superficial pheohyphomycosis. A new entity, bacillary angiomatosis caused by

Rochalimaea henselae/quintana, produces vascular proliferations in the skin as well as in other sites. Reiter's syndrome, with typical cutaneous findings, is found with increased frequency in patients with AIDS (see Color Plate 12C). It is safe to predict that unusual presentations of disseminated infectious diseases will continue to be described in the skin of AIDS patients.

Mucous membranes are commonly affected by infectious processes in patients with HIV infection. Oral candidiasis may be present and is one harbinger of the progression of HIV infection. Human papillomavirus and herpesvirus can produce lesions in the oral cavity. Oral hairy leukoplakia, a mixed infectious process, produces a characteristic "hairy" appearance to the sides of the tongue. Severe necrotizing gingivitis and recurrent oral ulcers are common. Lastly, disseminated infectious disease and malignant lymphoma can affect the mucous membranes.

The most common neoplasm in the context of AIDS is Kaposi's sarcoma (see Color Plate 12D). In AIDS, however, Kaposi's lesions may be solitary or disseminated, vary in color from light tan to deep purple, vary in appearance from macules to tumor nodules, arranged in a follicular, zosteriform, or linear pattern, and are generally atypical when compared with the lesions of Kaposi's sarcoma occurring in non–HIV-infected individuals. Kaposi's sarcoma found in AIDS patients frequently affects the mucosae. Other malignant tumors have an increased incidence in the setting of HIV infection, including squamous cell carcinoma and a variety of lymphomas, and all may have cutaneous involvement.

A number of poorly classified eruptions occur in AIDS patients. Best known is seborrheic dermatitis, which occurs in the usual locations but can be persistent and difficult to treat. Patients with AIDS also may have persistent pruritic eruptions, annular eruptions that resemble granuloma annulare, folliculitis, vasculitis, alopecia areata, vitiligo, porphyria cutanea tarda, eosinophilic folliculitis, and others. Certain well-characterized dermatoses such as psoriasis and atopic dermatitis appear to be worsened by the presence of HIV infection. Many AIDS patients receive a panoply of therapeutic agents that in turn produce a spectrum of cutaneous reactions including certain recognizable reactions, such as discolored nails from azidothymidine therapy (see Color Plate 12E).

Koehler JE, Quinn FD, Berger TG, et al.: Isolation of *Rochalimaea* species from cutaneous and osseous lesions of bacillary angiomatosis. N Engl J Med 327:1625, 1992. *Describes the entity bacillary angiomatosis and the organisms associated with its development in HIV-infected individuals.*

Penneys NS: Skin Manifestations of AIDS, 2nd ed. London, Martin Dunitz, 1995. *This reference is the easiest way to see the most common skin changes associated with HIV infection; has primary references.*

368 OPHTHALMOLOGIC MANIFESTATIONS OF AIDS
Mark A. Jacobson

Infectious or noninfectious ocular disorders, some of which may lead to severe visual impairment, have been reported in 40 to 90% of patients with AIDS referred for formal ophthalmoscopy. The true incidence of ophthalmic complications of AIDS can best be estimated from prospective observational cohort studies in which the incidence of cytomegalovirus (CMV) retinitis (the most common ophthalmologic complication of AIDS) has been reported. In several such studies, a range of 20 to 40% of AIDS patients have been diagnosed with CMV retinitis.

The differential diagnosis of HIV-associated ocular disease is best considered by its anatomic location.

DISEASES OF THE CHOROID, RETINA, AND VITREOUS

RETINAL MICROVASCULAR DISEASE (Table 368–1). The most common ophthalmologic complication observed in patients with HIV infection is retinal microvascular disease, which usually manifests as asymptomatic cotton-wool spots or small retinal hemorrhages. Cotton-wool spots have been reported in at least half of patients with AIDS and in up to 40% of patients with symptomatic HIV disease. Histopathologically, these lesions represent areas of

TABLE 368-1. DIAGNOSTIC FEATURES OF IMPORTANT CAUSES OF HIV-ASSOCIATED RETINITIS*

Feature	Cytomegalovirus	Retinal Necrosis (VZV, HSV)	Toxoplasmosis	Syphilis
Ocular symptoms	Floaters, visual field defect, or decreased visual acuity; painless	Floaters, visual field defect, or decreased visual acuity; pain common	Floaters, visual field defect, or decreased acuity; ± photophobia	Floaters, visual field defect, or decreased acuity; ± photophobia
Associated clinical findings	AIDS	Orolabial herpes, trigeminal herpes zoster	AIDS, encephalitis	Rash, hearing loss
Typical retinal lesion	Cottage-cheese exudate with hemorrhage	Confluent, gray or pale retina	White or yellow exudate	Variable
Typical retinal location	Adjacent to major vessel	Peripheral	Multifocal	Focal or posterior retina
Risk of retinal detachment	+++	++++	++	+
Serology, culture	Not helpful	Viral culture of skin lesion	*Toxoplasma gondii* IgG titer	VDRL, FTA-ABS

* Modified from Culbertson WW: Infection of the retina in AIDS. Int Ophthalmol Clin 29:108, 1989.

retinal ischemia. Both immune complex deposition and direct HIV retinal infection have been implicated in the pathogenesis of cotton-wool lesions. On funduscopic examination, they typically appear as white spots with feathered edges on the surface of the retina. A common location is near major posterior retinal vessels, and these lesions can have small associated retinal hemorrhages. It may be difficult to differentiate between cotton-wool spots and early lesions of CMV retinitis, which can have a very similar appearance. Sometimes the distinction can be made only by serial ophthalmoscopic examination. Cotton-wool spots remain stationary or resolve, whereas the lesion of CMV retinitis increases in size. Because cotton-wool spots virtually never cause symptomatic loss of vision and often spontaneously resolve, no treatment is indicated.

Small retinal hemorrhages and other microvascular abnormalities have been reported in up to 40% of patients with AIDS. These lesions also are asymptomatic, except in the rare case in which perifoveal involvement may result in visual blurring.

CYTOMEGALOVIRUS RETINITIS. CMV retinitis is the most common sight-threatening ocular opportunistic infection in patients with AIDS. It usually occurs only in patients with < 50 CD4+ (T helper) lymphocytes per microliter. The typical appearance is a white, cottage cheese–like retinal exudate often associated with hemorrhage and frequently located adjacent to major retinal vessels. In tissue sections, full-thickness retinal necrosis and swollen retinal cells containing intranuclear and intracytoplasmic inclusions are observed.

Patients with CMV retinitis typically present with complaints of painless visual impairment—either blurred vision, decreased visual acuity, or visual field defects—almost always affecting one eye more than the other. Several studies of untreated CMV retinitis have demonstrated a natural history of progressive retinal destruction caused by new retinal lesions or increasing size of previous lesions, which is usually evident within 1 month of initial diagnosis.

CMV retinitis is diagnosed primarily by its typical clinical appearance. The differential diagnosis includes cotton-wool spots, retinal hemorrhages, choroidal granulomas, acute and progressive outer retinal necrosis syndromes, and toxoplasmic and syphilitic retinitis. Differentiating between these entities may be difficult and the therapy of CMV retinitis is expensive, time-consuming, and toxic; therefore, the diagnosis retinitis must be confirmed by an experienced ophthalmologist. Because CMV can be isolated from approximately one quarter of patients with advanced AIDS but not more than three quarters of those AIDS patients who have CMV retinitis, viral cultures are neither sensitive nor specific diagnostic tests and are of value only as research tools.

The current standard therapy for CMV retinitis involves chronic intravenous treatment with either ganciclovir or foscarnet (Table 368-2). Ganciclovir is a nucleoside analogue prodrug that is preferentially phosphorylated within CMV-infected cells to an active drug, ganciclovir triphosphate, which inhibits CMV replication. Foscarnet is a pyrophosphate analogue that does not require phosphorylation for its anti-CMV activity. Although ganciclovir and foscarnet equally halt retinitis progression in 90% of cases, most AIDS patients have progressive retinal necrosis occur within 1 month after discontinuing therapy. Hence, therapy must be given indefinitely to minimize further, irreversible visual impairment. Both ganciclovir- and foscarnet-resistant strains of CMV have emerged and have been associated with therapeutic failure. In such cases, higher doses of these agents or using these agents in combination may be effective in controlling retinitis progression. Of note, foscarnet therapy has been associated with increased survival compared with ganciclovir therapy.

Because atrophy occurs in areas of active CMV retinitis, patients are susceptible to rhegmatogenous retinal detachment (resulting from a scar in a thinned portion of the retina). This complication often occurs during the healing stage, even in patients whose active retinitis has been controlled with antiviral therapy. For such patients, surgical reattachment by removing the vitreous and injecting silicone oil can be effective in restoring functional vision.

TOXOPLASMIC CHORIORETINITIS. Toxoplasmic chorioretinitis is rare compared to CMV retinitis but may complicate up to 20% of cases of AIDS-associated toxoplasmic encephalitis. Unlike toxoplasmic retinitis in immunocompetent individuals, which typically results from reactivation of congenitally acquired cysts latent in the retina, the AIDS-associated version does not appear to originate in pre-existing retinochoroidal scars but from organisms disseminating from nonocular sites of disease. Necrotizing retinal lesions are often bilateral and multifocal, and (as in CMV retinitis) may result in rhegmatogenous retinal detachment. Vitreous inflammation and anterior uveitis are more common and associated hemorrhage less common than in CMV retinitis. Because nearly all cases of toxoplasmic chorioretinitis are associated with toxoplasmic encephalitis, a computed tomographic or magnetic resonance scan of the brain should be done whenever this diagnosis is considered. Specific antiparasitic therapy (pyrimethamine and sulfadiazine, or pyrimethamine and clindamycin, in the same doses used to treat toxoplasmic encephalitis) is usually effective in preventing further retinal necrosis, but chronic maintenance therapy must be continued indefinitely to prevent relapse.

ACUTE RETINAL NECROSIS SYNDROME. Widespread, often bilateral, necrotizing retinitis caused by herpes simplex (HSV) or varicella-zoster virus (VZV) is now a well-characterized, although rare, AIDS-associated condition. Unlike CMV retinitis, this disease is often associated with ocular pain and concomitant keratitis or iritis. Many individuals have had recent or concurrent trigemi-

TABLE 368-2. THERAPY FOR CYTOMEGALOVIRUS RETINITIS

Standard dosing regimen for CMV retinitis
Ganciclovir
    Induction therapy: 5 mg/kg IV q12h × 14 days
    Chronic maintenance therapy: 5–6 mg/kg qd or 5 days/wk
Foscarnet
    Induction therapy: 90 mg/kg IV q12h × 14 days
    Chronic maintenance therapy: 90–120 mg/kg qd
Adverse effects
Ganciclovir
    Granulocytopenia
    Thrombocytopenia
    Azoospermia
Foscarnet
    Nephrotoxicity
    Ionized hypocalcemia (seizure or arrhythmia with overdose)
    Hypomagnesemia, hypophosphatemia, hypocalcemia, hypokalemia
    Genital ulcers
    Nephrogenic diabetes insipidus

nal zoster or orolabial HSV infection, and evidence of concurrent viral meningoencephalitis may be present. On funduscopic examination, widespread, pale or gray, peripheral retinal lesions are noted. Although intravenous acyclovir is effective in preventing further retinal necrosis, subsequent retinal detachment is a frequent, sight-threatening complication.

PROGRESSIVE OUTER RETINAL NECROSIS SYNDROME. Progressive outer retinal necrosis is a recently described clinical variant of VZV retinitis occurring in patients with CD4+ lymphocyte counts < 100 cells per microliter and characterized by multifocal, deep retinal lesions that rapidly progress to confluence. Less inflammatory cell response is observed in this condition than in acute retinal necrosis. The clinical response to available antiviral therapies is poor.

OTHER CAUSES OF CHORIORETINITIS AND VITRITIS. Cases of syphilitic retinitis have been reported in individuals with AIDS, symptomatic HIV disease, and asymptomatic HIV infection. There is no characteristic ophthalmologic appearance, but nearly all reported cases have had markedly positive serologic tests for active syphilis and dermatologic or central nervous system manifestations of secondary syphilis. Generally, response to intravenous penicillin therapy has been good. Disseminated pneumocystosis, *Mycobacterium tuberculosis,* and *Mycobacterium avium* complex infection with choroidal infiltrates have been described, but these lesions generally have not been sight-threatening. *Pneumocystis* choroiditis has been associated with use of inhaled pentamidine prophylaxis against *Pneumocystis carinii* pneumonia. Several cases of indolently progressive retinitis have been attributed to endogenous bacterial infection on the basis of retinal histopathology and response to broad-spectrum antibiotics. Also, vitritis (i.e., endophthalmitis) due to disseminated candidiasis may occur in parenteral drug users who are HIV infected or AIDS patients with indwelling central venous catheters.

OPTIC NEUROPATHY

Opportunistic infectious diseases affecting the optic nerve of patients with symptomatic HIV disease or AIDS may result in visual impairment or blindness. The most common cause of optic neuropathy is CMV infection. When CMV retinitis involves the optic disc, swelling of the optic nerve head (papillitis) leads to decreased visual acuity. This may occur in the presence or absence of other areas of retinitis and alternatively may affect the intraorbital optic nerve (optic neuritis) or retrobulbar nerve (retrobulbar neuritis). The retinal necrosis syndrome caused by herpes simplex or VZV infection may cause papillitis, and syphilis may cause papillitis, optic neuritis, or retrobulbar neuritis in patients at any stage of HIV disease. The most serious ocular complication of crytococcal meningitis is an arachnoiditis compressing the retrobulbar optic nerve and occasionally causing blindness. The cause of optic neuropathy can usually be established by seeking the other characteristic features of the specific infection. However, specific antimicrobial therapy for the cause of optic neuropathy often fails to improve vision once significant visual loss has occurred.

ANTERIOR UVEITIS

Severe anterior uveitis is uncommon in patients with HIV disease, but when such cases occur, syphilis or VZV infection is the most common cause. Mild, asymptomatic anterior uveitis commonly is observed in patients with CMV retinitis, but inflammation severe enough to cause symptoms is extremely rare. Occasional cases of toxoplasmic anterior uveitis have also been reported.

KERATITIS

Inflammatory disease of the cornea (keratitis) is most frequently caused by VZV or HSV, and the clinical features usually make diagnosis relatively simple. Patients with advanced HIV disease who develop this complication may require intravenous acyclovir therapy in addition to topical trifluridine. Microsporida infection has also been reported to cause keratitis in HIV-infected patients.

DISEASES OF THE CONJUNCTIVA AND ADNEXA

Kaposi's sarcoma has a predilection to involve ocular structures. Twenty of 100 patients with Kaposi's sarcoma examined at UCLA had ophthalmic lesions, 16 involving the eyelid and 7 the conjunctiva. In four of these patients, the ophthalmic lesion was the first and only clinically identified manifestation of Kaposi's sarcoma. Conjunctival Kaposi's lesions appear as bright red subepithelial nodules, and small lesions may be mistaken for subconjunctival hemorrhages. Periorbital edema may be caused by lymphangitic Kaposi's sarcoma, even in the absence of apparent ocular or cutaneous lesions. Most ocular lesions respond to local irradiation.

Nonspecific, nonpurulent conjunctivitis that often is self-limited has been reported in up to 10% of AIDS patients. Topical steroid and sulfa therapy may be beneficial for this condition. Other rare causes of conjunctivitis include syphilis, CMV, and molluscum contagiosum infection. Orbital Kaposi's sarcoma or Burkitt's lymphoma may present with ptosis and diplopia.

de Smet MD, Nussenblatt RB: Ocular manifestations of AIDS. JAMA 266:3019, 1991. *A practical clinical review that organizes ophthalmic complications of AIDS by anatomic structures.*

Gallant JE, Moore RD, Richman DD, et al.: Incidence and natural history of cytomegalovirus disease in patients with advanced human immunodeficiency virus disease treated with zidovudine. J Infect Dis 166:1223, 1992. *The largest prospective cohort study to evaluate the incidence of CMV retinitis in patients with HIV disease.*

Jacobson MA: Foscarnet therapy for AIDS-related opportunistic herpesvirus infections. *In* Volberding PA, Jacobson MA (eds.): AIDS Clinical Review 1992. New York, Marcel Dekker, 1992, p 173. *Reviews clinical pharmacology and rational therapeutic use of foscarnet.*

Studies of Ocular Complications of AIDS Research Group: Mortality in patients with the acquired immunodeficiency syndrome treated with either foscarnet or ganciclovir for cytomegalovirus retinitis. N Engl J Med 326:213, 1992. *The largest randomized trial to compare ganciclovir and foscarnet therapy for CMV retinitis.*

Winward KE, Hamed LM, Glaser JS: The spectrum of optic nerve disease in human immunodeficiency virus infection. Am J Ophthalmol 107:373, 1989. *A series of four patients with HIV-associated optic neuropathies (syphilitic, CMV, varicella-zoster virus, and cryptococcal).*

369 HEMATOLOGY/ONCOLOGY IN AIDS

*David T. Scadden and
Jerome E. Groopman*

HEMATOLOGIC ASPECTS OF HIV INFECTION

Hematologic abnormalities are frequent in HIV infection, and their pathogenesis is often multifactorial. Cytopenias are often the limiting factors in anti-infective and antineoplastic therapy for patients with HIV disease. Recombinant hematopoietic growth factors have been used to ameliorate anemia and neutropenia and can be important in treating such patients.

CYTOPENIA. HIV infection is associated most prominently with a decline in the number of CD4 lymphocytes over time. However, other cytopenias are also frequent, with anemia reported in 60%, thrombocytopenia in 40%, and neutropenia in 50% of patients with AIDS. These cytopenias occur in conjunction with progressive deterioration of immune function and are less common in the earlier stages of HIV infection. Thrombocytopenia is the exception and may constitute a manifestation of HIV infection during the asymptomatic phases. Many causes are frequently operative in the cytopenia in advanced HIV infection. Direct and indirect effects of HIV, opportunistic infections, neoplasms, and toxic antiretroviral, antimicrobial, or antitumor chemotherapy are the major factors to be considered. The differential diagnosis of cytopenia in HIV infection should primarily consider these causes. Evaluation of patients with low blood counts should focus on infectious processes and attendant myelotoxic effects of therapy. In addition to the usual laboratory approaches to cytopenia diagnosis based on impaired production, excess consumption, and/or sequestration, blood and marrow cultures and stains for fungi and mycobacteria should be performed. *Mycobacterium avium-intracellulare* (MAI), *Mycobacterium tuberculosis, Cryptococcus neoformans,* and *Histoplasma capsulatum* are often found within the marrow and lead to hematologic abnormalities. Cytomegalovirus (CMV) does not generally cause specific histopathologic changes of the bone marrow but may suppress hematopoiesis and is best cultured from the circulating buffy coat. Parvovirus infection may result in cytopenia (particularly anemia) and is often accompanied by characteristic giant pronormoblasts in the bone marrow. Neoplastic involvement of the marrow by B-cell lymphoma is frequent in AIDS patients with this malignancy, whereas Kaposi's sarcoma has only rarely been found in the bone marrow.

Bone marrow aspirate and biopsy in an HIV-infected patient with low blood counts is recommended, particularly in cases of fever of otherwise unknown cause and in staging of patients with non-Hodgkin's lymphoma.

Morphologic abnormalities of myeloid and erythroid lineages are often present in the bone marrow of patients with HIV disease in the absence of infection or neoplasm. These changes are nonspecific and include hypercellularity, dysplasia with frequent megaloblastosis, lymphoid aggregates, and increased eosinophils, plasma cells, and reticulin. The pathogenetic mechanisms for these morphologic abnormalities and the associated impaired hematopoiesis are not well defined. Laboratory studies of hematopoiesis in HIV infection have yielded variable and differing results. The bulk of evidence suggests that HIV does not directly infect early progenitors but may alter the proliferative capacity of progenitors by two possible mechanisms: (1) induction of inhibitory factors in the marrow microenvironment, or (2) interaction with the progenitor cell surface and induction of cell death (apoptosis) without infecting the cells.

THROMBOCYTOPENIA (see Ch. 152). Thrombocytopenia may be a presenting laboratory finding in an otherwise asymptomatic HIV-infected person. HIV infection should be considered in the differential diagnosis of thrombocytopenia, and the history should include questions regarding risk factors for this retrovirus. Clinically asymptomatic but thrombocytopenic HIV-infected patients have a similar rate of progression to AIDS as asymptomatic HIV-seropositive persons without thrombocytopenia. Thrombocytopenia is not a criterion for more advanced HIV disease according to the staging system developed by the Centers for Disease Control and Prevention (CDC). Multiple causes need to be considered in evaluating thrombocytopenia in HIV infection. Immune-mediated destruction and ineffective hematopoiesis are generally both operative. In addition, cases of AIDS with apparent hemolytic-uremic syndrome or thrombotic thrombocytopenic purpura have been described but are rare. Isolated thrombocytopenia is most often clinically similar to classic autoimmune thrombocytopenic purpura (ITP). Bone marrow examination reveals an increased number of megakaryocytes, and there are elevated levels of bound immunoglobulin on the platelet surface. However, the immunoglobulin is generally immune complexes often involving anti-HIV antibodies. Detection of antibody on platelet surfaces does not correlate with thrombocytopenia, possibly because reliculoendothelial cell dysfunction often occurs in AIDS and may reduce clearance of platelets. In addition to peripheral destruction of platelets, reduced production appears to be common in HIV disease. Even in patients with an ITP-like presentation, production is reduced. This mechanism predominates in patients with thrombocytopenia in the setting of AIDS.

The thrombocytopenia in HIV-infected patients has similar sequelae to classic immune thrombocytopenia, yet special attention to the issue of thrombocytopenia should be given in HIV-infected hemophiliacs. Complications from thrombocytopenia may be more severe in hemophiliacs, so therapy should be considered at a higher platelet count than in HIV-infected patients without other coagulation defects. An important observation has been the improvement in platelet count due to treatment with zidovudine (AZT) in HIV-infected patients with significant thrombocytopenia, regardless of risk group. Nearly two thirds of such patients may respond to AZT therapy and increase their platelet counts (mean of threefold increase) within 12 weeks of initiating treatment. If there is no response to AZT, then several treatment modalities may be considered, including interferon-α, splenectomy, corticosteroids, danazol, intravenous gamma globulin, anti-RhD preparations, or vincristine. Many of these have been successful in classic immune thrombocytopenia, particularly corticosteroids. Theoretical risk of steroid use exists in an HIV-infected individual including exacerbation of fungal infection, Kaposi's sarcoma, and activity of HIV itself. Nonetheless, most patients have tolerated corticosteroids for short intervals. Their long-term use in HIV-associated thrombocytopenia cannot be recommended.

ANEMIA. Anemia increases in incidence in HIV-infected patients as their degree of immune dysfunction worsens. The anemia is usually characterized as normochromic and normocytic, and iron studies are either normal or indicative of chronic disease. Occasionally the vitamin B_{12} level is decreased, but true vitamin B_{12} deficiency is uncommon; rather, transcobalamin transport may be altered and therapy with the vitamin does not lead to improved erythropoiesis. Should a low vitamin B_{12} level be found, then a true deficiency needs to be ruled out by a Schilling test and other studies (see Ch. 129).

The Coombs' test (antiglobulin) may be positive in the majority of patients with AIDS and in about a third of asymptomatic HIV-infected individuals. Although anti-i or other specific antibodies may occur, nonspecific binding of antiphospholipid antibodies or immune complexes to erythrocytes is more common. True hemolysis is unusual in HIV-infected patients as a cause of anemia.

Impaired erythropoiesis accounts for anemia in most HIV-infected individuals. Serum erythropoietin levels are often low for the degree of anemia in the patient without renal abnormalities and is of unclear origin. Parvovirus infection has been reported in HIV-infected patients and may result in red cell aplasia. Gamma globulin therapy has been reported to reverse this unusual cause of severe anemia.

The impairment in erythropoiesis due to HIV infection *per se* may be due to release of inhibitors and/or impaired production of trophic cytokines, as discussed above. Drug-induced anemia is frequent in HIV-infected patients. AZT is associated with both dose-related and idiosyncratic suppression of erythropoiesis. In the AZT Collaborative Working Group Study, anemia occurred in one third of AIDS patients following 6 weeks of treatment. This occurred at relatively high doses, and patients with severe immunosuppression were least tolerant of the drug. In other studies of AZT at doses of 300 to 600 mg per day, the decline in hemoglobin levels was less severe and the need for transfusion less frequent. The reductions in the recommended dosing have reduced the frequency and severity of anemia, but this toxicity remains a significant cause of anemia in AIDS patients. Of note, other antiretroviral drugs, dideoxyinosine (ddI) and dideoxycytidine (ddC), are not associated with anemia.

Macrocytic changes occur in the erythrocytes with AZT therapy. The mechanism of impaired erythropoiesis due to the drug appears to be impairment of DNA synthesis in developing progenitors. Recombinant erythropoietin therapy may decrease the transfusion requirement and increase the hemoglobin in anemic AIDS patients on AZT. The response to recombinant erythropoietin treatment is most clearly seen in patients with pretreatment serum erythropoietin levels below 500 mU per milliliter. Some anemic AIDS patients receiving AZT have developed red cell aplasia that does not improve with recombinant erythropoietin therapy.

NEUTROPENIA. Neutropenia occurs in the HIV-infected patient in concert with decreases in other cell counts with progressive deterioration of the immune system. As with the other cytopenias, neutropenia may be caused by impaired production and/or increased destruction of leukocytes. Antibody bound to granulocyte membrane structures has been observed in nearly one third of HIV-infected individuals. The presence of neutrophil-associated antibodies has not predicted the development of neutropenia. Impaired hematopoiesis is presumed to be the major cause of neutropenia due to HIV. In addition to neutropenia, neutrophil dysfunction has been reported in AIDS. The extent to which neutrophil defects, particularly in microbial killing, contribute to host immune impairment is unknown.

Neutropenia is most commonly caused by myelosuppressive therapy in AIDS patients. AZT treatment is at times limited by neutropenia, although neither ddI nor ddC seems to cause this problem. Other important therapies including trimethoprim-sulfamethoxazole for *Pneumocystis carinii* pneumonia, pyrimethamine-sulfadiazine for central nervous system (CNS) toxoplasmosis, acyclovir for disseminated herpes simplex or herpes zoster, and most prominently ganciclovir for CMV retinitis may be myelotoxic and result in neutropenia.

HEMATOPOIETIC GROWTH FACTORS. Suppression of leukocyte, as well as erythrocyte, production is a major issue in treating both HIV infection and its complicating infectious or neoplastic diseases. This problem may become less limiting as new antiretroviral therapies are developed and hematopoietic growth factors are used to over-ride myelotoxicity. The activity and safety of hematopoietic growth factors used to increase blood cell number in cytopenic HIV-infected individuals have been studied. The results have been quite encouraging with respect to the erythroid growth factor, erythropoietin, and the myeloid growth factors, granulocyte colony stimulating factor (G-CSF) and granulocyte macrophage colony stimulating factor (GM-CSF). It is clear that in most patients with anemia due to HIV infection and/or concomitant AZT therapy, with baseline serum erythropoietin concentrations <500 mU per milliliter, recombinant erythropoietin increases the hemoglobin and reduces the transfusion requirement. Use of the myeloid growth factors, G-CSF or GM-CSF, to ameliorate leukopenia due to HIV infection and/or therapy with AZT, interferon-α, or ganciclovir, has also been relatively successful. The myelotoxicity of these agents can be overcome using relatively low doses of G-CSF or GM-CSF. It is clear that with the myeloid growth factors as well as with erythropoietin, there is no sustained increase in blood cell production, so that therapy with the growth factor must be continued so long as the myelotoxic agent is administered.

The side effects of growth factor therapy seen in patients with HIV disease have been similar to those in other patients treated with these recombinant proteins. The major issue in the safety profile of the myeloid growth factors relates to their potential effects on replication of HIV. The preponderance of data indicate that HIV replication is stimulated *in vitro* by GM-CSF but not G-CSF. This is most clearly seen when isolates of HIV that are tropic for monocytes are studied. The data conflict as to whether this phenomenon occurs *in vivo*. There is also laboratory evidence that the antiretroviral effects of AZT in monocytes can be significantly augmented by the presence of GM-CSF. It appears that the growth factor increases the uptake and phosphorylation of AZT, resulting in higher intracellular concentrations of active drug. It is believed that GM-CSF should be considered for therapy only in combination with AZT based on these *in vitro* studies. G-CSF and erythropoietin do not appear to alter HIV expression and have been successfully combined with AZT, as stated above. Further clinical trials are required to demonstrate that adding the erythroid or myeloid growth factor not only allows for concomitant therapy with myelotoxic agents but significantly alters the natural history of patients with HIV disease.

ONCOLOGIC MANIFESTATIONS OF AIDS

Neoplasms, particularly Kaposi's sarcoma and B-cell lymphoma, are frequent in HIV-infected persons. Their development demonstrates the relationship of immune function to suppression of certain oncogenic events and provides a model to study the pathogenesis of these tumors. Clinical management of AIDS-associated neoplasia is complex because therapy should optimally address HIV and concurrent opportunistic infections as well as the tumors.

KAPOSI'S SARCOMA (see Ch. 110, 152, 367, and 475). Kaposi's sarcoma is the most frequent neoplastic manifestation of HIV infection. Indeed, it forms one of the CDC criteria that define an HIV-infected individual as having AIDS. Kaposi's sarcoma has been recognized in a number of other clinical and epidemiologic settings. The "classic" form of the neoplasm was described over a century ago in predominantly elderly men of Mediterranean and Jewish extraction. It generally involves lower extremities and is an indolent neoplasm. This form of Kaposi's sarcoma was also recognized in association with other malignancies, particularly lymphoma. This latter observation led to the hypothesis that immune surveillance was important in restricting the development of Kaposi's sarcoma. Another form of Kaposi's sarcoma was recognized in areas of Central Africa and has been termed the "endemic" form of the neoplasm. This occurrence in Africa was not related to infection with HIV. Again, the neoplasm was more frequently seen in men than in women but was generally more aggressive and involved lymph nodes and viscera.

Patients receiving immunosuppressive therapy, particularly for renal and hepatic transplants, were recognized to have a markedly increased incidence of Kaposi's sarcoma. This further supported the hypothesis that immunocompetence is important with respect to pathogenesis of this neoplasm. Of particular note has been well-documented resolution of Kaposi's sarcoma upon discontinuation of immunosuppressive therapy in these patients. Other disorders of the immune system, including systemic lupus erythematosus and pemphigus vulgaris, have also been associated with Kaposi's sarcoma.

The incidence of Kaposi's sarcoma has been estimated to be 20,000 times greater among HIV-infected individuals than in the general population. Although the neoplasm was originally diagnosed in 40% of AIDS patients when first reported in 1981, the incidence may be declining and is believed to now constitute approximately 15% of all AIDS patients in the United States. AIDS-associated Kaposi's sarcoma is more frequently seen among homosexual or bisexual men with HIV than in other risk groups with the virus. This suggests that HIV infection itself is not sufficient to account for the increased incidence of the disease; other factors may be important in the pathogenesis of the neoplasm. Early in the AIDS epidemic, it was suggested that CMV infection or the use of volatile nitrites could potentiate Kaposi's sarcoma. However, careful studies have not verified the importance of such candidate cofactors in the development of the neoplasm. Another hypothesis is that other cofactors of an infectious nature may be transmitted in tandem with HIV during intercourse and possibly during use of intravenous drugs. Molecular studies have recently identified a novel herpes virus genome in Kaposi's sarcoma lesions. A model of a neoplasm that distantly resembles Kaposi's sarcoma has been established in transgenic mice using the *tat* gene of HIV, but the significance of this to clinical Kaposi's sarcoma in AIDS is still unclear. It has been speculated that certain cytokines, such as interleukin-6, may be elaborated by the Kaposi's sarcoma cells and lead to autocrine proliferation. Reports of Kaposi's sarcoma in homosexual men not infected with HIV have provided further support to the hypothesis of an independent sexually transmitted infectious agent as an important cofactor in this neoplasm.

Histopathologically, these lesions are a mixture of different cell types. Endothelial cells are quite prominent within the Kaposi's sarcoma lesions, as is a prominent spindle cell proliferation surrounded by extravasated erythrocytes and macrophages. The cell of origin of the neoplasm is still debated, but permanent cell lines derived from the lesions suggest that the spindle cell is the primary neoplastic cell and is of mesenchymal origin.

Kaposi's sarcoma often is a cutaneous nonblanching red macule. As lesions increase in size, they often have surrounding ecchymoses and become more of a violet hue than red. At times, the lesions may become nodular and with advanced disease, the lesions may become confluent with large plaques developing, particularly on the legs. There is no orderly pattern of tumor progression, and presentation may be with lesions at multiple sites. The subsequent appearance of lesions is not affected if the primary lesion is excised. The rate of growth of the primary lesions, as well as the appearance of new lesions, can be quite variable. The lesions may occur on any cutaneous site and on mucous membranes. Lymphatic involvement is not unusual, and Kaposi's sarcoma may present as lymphadenopathy. Visceral involvement, particularly of trachea, lungs, and gastrointestinal tract, occurs commonly and may be seen in the absence of cutaneous disease. The most striking morbidity associated with Kaposi's sarcoma is that of lymph node involvement and consequent lymphedema involving the lower extremities, groin, and head and neck. Extensive parenchymal or pleural involvement of the lung may result in life-threatening respiratory compromise.

The diagnosis of Kaposi's sarcoma is relatively straightforward in HIV-infected individuals presenting with an erythematous or violaceous cutaneous or mucosal lesion. However, bacillary angiomatosis caused by *Rochalimaea* species may involve similar lesions. This process, which is treatable with antibiotics, should be excluded by Warthin-Starry staining of biopsy material. Following diagnosis, an assessment should be made of the rate of growth and distribution of the lesions. The presence of visceral disease does not necessarily correlate with poor response of lesions to therapy, so that an extensive evaluation for gastrointestinal or lymphadenopathic Kaposi's sarcoma is not indicated unless there are specific symptoms referable to such involvement. It should be pointed out that AIDS patients in general do not die of Kaposi's sarcoma, except for pulmonary Kaposi's sarcoma, but usually succumb to infectious complications. Thus, staging systems of the neoplasm have emphasized immunologic status and systemic symptoms in addition to the extent of the neoplasm. Recently, a classification system has been proposed which appears particularly useful for evaluating such patients. This system proposes a tumor (T), immunologic status (I), and systemic symptoms (S) staging (Table 369–1).

TABLE 369-1. KAPOSI'S SARCOMA (KS): RECOMMENDED STAGING CLASSIFICATION

	Good Risk (0) (All of the Following)	Poor Risk (1) (Any of the Following)
Tumor (T)	Confined to skin and/or lymph nodes and/or minimal oral disease*	Tumor-associated edema or ulceration Extensive oral KS Gastrointestinal KS KS in other non-nodal viscera
Immune system (I)	CD4 cells ≥ 200/μl	CD4 cells < 200/μl
Systemic illness (S)	No history of OI† or thrush No "B" symptoms‡ Performance status ≥ 70 (Karnofsky)	History of OI and/or thrush "B" symptoms present Performance status < 70 Other HIV-related illness (e.g., neurologic disease, lymphoma)

* Minimal oral disease is non-nodular KS confined to the palate.
† OI = Opportunistic infection.
‡ "B" symptoms are unexplained fever, night sweats, > 10% involuntary weight loss, or diarrhea persisting more than 2 weeks.
Modified from Krown SE, Metroka C, Wernz J: Kaposi's sarcoma in the acquired immune deficiency syndrome: A proposal for uniform evaluation, response, and staging criteria. J Clin Oncol 7:1201–1207, 1989.

The clinician should pursue therapy of Kaposi's sarcoma in patients with symptomatic visceral disease, lesions associated with edema, or rapidly evolving extensive cutaneous disease. Such patients usually require chemotherapy. The most active chemotherapeutic drugs appear to be doxorubicin, etoposide, vinblastine, bleomycin, and vincristine. Combinations of these agents, particularly doxorubicin, bleomycin, and vincristine, have been associated with a response rate of ≥50%. The combination of bleomycin and vincristine has been recommended for patients with borderline marrow function because the drugs are minimally myelotoxic and may be given in conjunction with AZT. Recent experience with liposomal formulations of anthracycline agents suggests that these may be particularly active in Kaposi's sarcoma. Response to chemotherapy usually occurs within the first few weeks of treatment. Unfortunately, the lesions regrow when the chemotherapy is stopped so that treatment needs to be chronic.

Patients with Kaposi's sarcoma who do not have rapidly progressive disease and therefore do not require immediate intervention may be treated with several other approaches. These include observation, single-agent interferon-α, local radiation, intralesional chemotherapy, local cryotherapy, or combinations of these. Antiretroviral therapy alone is not effective as an antineoplastic therapy for Kaposi's sarcoma. Selecting the optimal therapeutic approach involves determining the clinical status of the patient, particularly utilizing the staging classification (Table 369-1), as well as lifestyle issues. Patients who are categorized as "good risk" by the TIS staging system are also good candidates for response to interferon-α. Interferon-α may have not only antineoplastic but also anti-HIV effects. Therapy of Kaposi's sarcoma with single-agent interferon-α requires relatively high doses of the agent (18 to 36 million units daily). Recently, it has been recognized that similar benefit may be obtained using lower doses of interferon-α in combination with AZT, although with limiting hematologic toxicity. Such hematologic side effects may be overcome by using myeloid and erythroid growth factors. Interferon-α is associated with flulike side effects, and many patients were not able to tolerate prolonged therapy. It is unclear whether the antiviral as well as the antitumor properties of interferon-α make it a superior agent in the therapy of AIDS-associated Kaposi's sarcoma compared with chemotherapy alone or AZT in combination with chemotherapy (Table 369-2).

"Poor risk" patients by TIS staging should be given antiretroviral therapy because their major life-threatening complication of AIDS is related to immune suppression and opportunistic infection. Local treatment of disfiguring Kaposi's sarcoma lesions may be achieved using radiation therapy, chemotherapy, or cryotherapy in these patients. Radiation therapy is often avoided for mucosal Kaposi's sarcoma lesions because severe mucositis may result.

NON-HODGKIN'S LYMPHOMA. B-cell lymphoma frequently occurs in immunosuppressed individuals. Genetic disorders of the immune system such as Wiskott-Aldrich syndrome, as well as immunosuppressive therapy used in organ transplantation, are associated with malignant transformation of B cells and an oligoclonal or monoclonal lymphoma. Non-Hodgkin's B-cell lymphoma is emerging as a frequent manifestation of HIV infection as individuals with the retrovirus live longer as a result of better control of opportunistic infections. The initial relative risk of lymphoma in HIV-infected individuals compared with matched uninfected controls was 60 times; it is likely that this is an underestimate of the current risk. Thus, we expect to see an increasing incidence of B-cell lymphoma in this population.

Causative factors operative in the development of lymphoma in AIDS are likely to be multiple (see Ch. 145). HIV itself appears not be play a direct role but rather provides a permissive environment in which lymphoma develops. Lymphoma in this setting may be regarded as an opportunistic neoplasm and is considered an AIDS-defining illness. Proliferative signals to B cells, whether from dysfunctional T cells, aberrant cytokine production, or infections (such as Epstein-Barr virus), may induce polyclonal expansion of the B-cell population (see Ch. 341). This expanded population may provide targets for genetic abnormalities that lead to malignant transformation and emergence of several dominant clones. The oligoclonal populations of malignant B cells seen in some HIV-infected individuals with lymphoma support such a model. Ultimately, a single malignant clone may emerge, leading to a monoclonal neoplasm. The chromosomal abnormalities frequently seen in B-cell lymphoma involve translocation of loci encoding the immunoglobulin genes with the c-myc oncogene. Genetic evidence of Epstein-Barr virus is found in about one half of B-cell lymphomas in AIDS patients and virtually all primary CNS lymphomas in AIDS. A number of interacting factors are likely to be important in the pathogenesis of lymphoma in those patients with HIV infection united by the disorganization of immune function induced by HIV.

Clinically, B-cell lymphoma in AIDS patients tends to be of high-grade histologic pattern and follows an aggressive clinical course. Small, noncleaved or immunoblastic histologies are most frequent and account for nearly three fourths of all lymphomas in this setting. The remaining are usually a diffuse, large-cell type. The lower-grade lymphomas reported among HIV-infected individuals may represent background rather than neoplasm directly associ-

TABLE 369-2. TREATMENT OF KAPOSI'S SARCOMA

Interferon-α
Single agent	Alpha-2a (Roche)	18–36 mU SC daily for 8 weeks, then three times weekly
	Alpha-2b (Schering)	30 mU SC three times weekly
Combined therapy	Zidovudine	Zidovudine 100 mg PO every 4 hours while awake, interferon-α 5–10 mU SC three times weekly

Chemotherapy
Single agent	Doxorubicin	20–40 mg/m^2 IV every 3 weeks
	VP-16	100 mg/m^2 IV every 3 weeks or 50 mg PO daily as tolerated
	Vinblastine	4–8 mg IV weekly
Combined therapy	Vincristine/vinblastine	2 mg IV vincristine every 2 weeks 4–8 mg IV vinblastine on alternate weeks
	Doxorubicin/bleomycin/vincristine	Doxorubicin 20 mg/m^2 IV every 3 weeks Bleomycin 15 U/m^2 IV every 3 weeks Vincristine 2 mg IV every 3 weeks
	Bleomycin/vincristine	Bleomycin 15 U IV every 2–3 weeks Vincristine 2 mg IV every 2–3 weeks

ated with immunosuppression. Rarely, B-cell acute lymphoblastic leukemia or T-cell neoplasms have been reported.

Most patients have extranodular disease involving the gastrointestinal tract, CNS, liver, soft tissues, or bone marrow. In one large series, nearly 80% of all patients diagnosed with B-cell lymphoma in AIDS had non-nodular involvement. Lymphoma strictly confined to lymph nodes is uncommon. Gastrointestinal lymphoma may occur anywhere from the esophagus to the anus. Primary CNS lymphoma is usually immunoblastic in histologic type (see Ch. 364). Such patients generally have solitary mass lesions in the parenchyma of the brain, whereas CNS involvement in conjunction with systemic lymphoma is more often meningeal in location. All AIDS patients diagnosed with systemic non-Hodgkin's lymphoma should undergo careful CNS assessment with computed tomographic (CT) scan or magnetic resonance imaging (MRI) scan as well as lumbar puncture with cytology.

Most AIDS patients with B-cell lymphoma are classified as having stage III (involving both sides of the diaphragm without visceral involvement) or stage IV (visceral involvement). Systemic "B" symptoms are frequent, but fever should not be immediately ascribed to lymphoma in AIDS patients and secondary infectious causes need to be ruled out. Staging of patients should follow the approach used in other settings of non-Hodgkin's lymphoma, with particular attention to the gastrointestinal tract, bone marrow, and CNS. It is not clear that prognosis of lymphoma in AIDS is affected by stage, however.

The major differential diagnosis to be considered with primary CNS lymphoma is *Toxoplasma gondii* infection or progressive multifocal leukoencephalopathy (PML) (see Ch. 364). PML can usually be distinguished from CNS lymphoma by its lack of enhancement with gadolinium on MRI. CNS lesions due to lymphoma may be isodense or hypodense and contrast-enhancing on CT scan, and enhance on MRI, thereby resembling toxoplasmosis. Nonetheless, toxoplasmosis usually presents with multiple lesions throughout the neuraxis, whereas primary CNS lymphoma tends to be a single lesion located in a paraventricular site. Accessible lesions should be biopsied to distinguish between lymphoma and toxoplasmosis; lesions difficult to approach surgically may be empirically treated with antitoxoplasmal therapy for a limited time, generally 1 to 2 weeks. If no response is seen, lymphoma becomes more likely.

The treatment of AIDS-related B-cell lymphoma is controversial owing to the poor prognosis of the neoplasm and the limited tolerance of aggressive chemotherapy in this patient population. Both opportunistic infection and bone marrow suppression often limit the delivery of adequate dosage of chemotherapy on schedule. Patients with prior AIDS-defining illness, particularly a history of opportunistic infection, have a poor prognosis compared with patients who present with lymphoma as their initial manifestation of AIDS. Similarly, more severely immunocompromised patients with low CD4 cell numbers have a poor outcome and are less tolerant of chemotherapy than are those patients with more intact immune function.

Among "good prognosis" patients with relatively intact immune function and/or those presenting with lymphoma as their AIDS manifestation, aggressive therapy with combination regimens is indicated. For those patients who do not have CNS involvement at the time of presentation, prophylactic therapy to the CNS is often given to prevent CNS relapse. The response rate in these good-prognosis patients is similar to that of non-Hodgkin's lymphoma patients of stage IIIB or IVB without HIV (see Ch. 371), but the long-term survival rate is still poor owing to frequent relapse and intervening infections. Nonetheless, some patients have survived 12 months or longer disease-free following complete remission.

Patients with poor prognosis based on severe immune suppression and/or complicating opportunistic infections pose a particularly complex treatment dilemma. Some patients have opted for palliative therapy with corticosteroids because intensive chemotherapy may lead to further immune compromise and infection. Yet lymphoma is generally rapidly growing and fatal in patients who are not aggressively treated. Thus, the clinician needs to pursue therapy in such patients only with an informed discussion of the risks and benefits of treatment, honestly emphasizing the poor prognosis with or without chemotherapy.

Addition of antiretroviral therapy to chemotherapeutic regimens is now possible with nonmyelosuppressive anti-HIV drugs. However, the benefit of such therapy remains unknown.

The outlook is generally poor for patients with lymphoma, and the majority die within 9 months. No chemotherapeutic regimen has been identified as superior to others for AIDS patients with this neoplasm. The survival is even poorer for those with primary CNS lymphoma, on the order of 2 to 4 months. Although radiation therapy may result in a tumor response in the majority of these patients, the advanced stage of immunosuppression in which primary CNS lymphoma tends to occur generally limits the prognosis.

OTHER MALIGNANCIES. There is active clinical surveillance to determine whether neoplasms other than Kaposi's sarcoma and B-cell lymphoma may ultimately arise at an increased incidence in immunocompromised patients with HIV infection. It now appears that the incidence of Hodgkin's disease may be increased among HIV-infected individuals. In addition, there may be important differences in the course of Hodgkin's lymphoma in such patients, including a higher incidence of advanced disease, mixed cellularity histology, and extranodular disease. Furthermore, HIV-infected individuals with Hodgkin's disease appear to tolerate chemotherapy less well and have a higher incidence of tumor relapse than do those without HIV infection. This is likely due to their impaired hematopoiesis and the potential for opportunistic infections in such patients. In general, patients with HIV infection and Hodgkin's disease have a survival of <12 months. Further work is needed to better understand the altered pattern of Hodgkin's disease in the setting of HIV infection.

Hodgkin's disease therapy among HIV-infected patients should be according to guidelines for non–HIV-positive individuals (see Ch. 146). The major difference is to incorporate prophylaxis against opportunistic infections, particularly *P. carinii* pneumonia, and to be particularly alert to infectious complications during therapy.

Anal cancer and cervical cancer, neoplasms associated with papillomavirus infection, may occur with higher incidence in HIV-infected patients. This is due to the high prevalence of papillomavirus infection in groups at risk for HIV (see Ch. 314) and the high frequency of the premalignant condition, intraepithelial neoplasia in HIV-infected women. Frequent careful cervical examinations including colposcopy are indicated in HIV-infected women to detect early malignant change. Ongoing surveillance programs of HIV-infected individuals using Papanicolaou smears on cells from the transitional zone of the anus and cervix should provide important data as to the increased incidence and optimal surveillance programs for these cancers in this population. Invasive cancer of the uterine cervix has recently been added as an AIDS-defining illness in women infected with HIV.

Although anecdotal reports abound of other malignancies in HIV-infected individuals, it is unclear whether these occur above that of the background prevalence in the general population. Nonetheless, consideration should be given to the significance of the HIV infection in clinical management. These patients have a propensity to develop opportunistic infections when starting chemotherapy or radiation therapy and, in general, have fared poorly because of these infectious complications.

Ballem PJ, Belzberg A, Devine DV, et al.: Kinetic studies of the mechanism of thrombocytopenia in patients with human immunodeficiency virus infection. N Engl J Med 327:1779, 1992. *A study on thrombocytopenia in HIV disease.*

Henry DH, Beall GN, Benson CA, et al.: Recombinant human erythropoietin in the treatment of anemia associated with human immunodeficiency virus (HIV) infection and zidovudine therapy. Overview of four clinical trials. Ann Intern Med 117:739, 1992. *A summary of controlled trials using recombinant erythropoietin in HIV infection.*

Koehler JE, Quinn FD, Berger TG, et al.: Isolation of *Rochalimaea* species from cutaneous and osseous lesions of bacillary angiomatosis. N Engl J Med 327:1625, 1992. *Report of bacillary angiomatosis that may be confused with Kaposi's sarcoma.*

Levine AM: Acquired immunodeficiency syndrome–related lymphoma. Blood 80:8, 1992. *A review of AIDS-related lymphoma with an excellent bibliography.*

Lilenbaum RC, Ratner L: Systemic treatment of Kaposi's sarcoma: Current status and future directions. AIDS 8:141, 1994.

Luft BJ, Hafner R, Korzun AH, et al.: Toxoplasmic encephalitis in patients with the acquired immunodeficiency syndrome. N Engl J Med 329:995, 1993. *A discussion of outcomes from anti-toxoplasmosis treatment of CNS lesions in patients with AIDS.*

Palefsky JM: Anal human papilloma virus infection and anal cancer in HIV-positive individuals: An emerging problem. AIDS 8:283, 1994.

Pluda JM, Mitsuya H, Yarchoan R: Hematologic effects of AIDS therapies. Hematol Oncol Clin North Am 5:229, 1991. *A review of myelosuppression caused by drugs used in AIDS care.*

Roizman B: New viral footprints in Kaposi's sarcoma (editorial). N Engl J Med 332:1227, 1995. *Discusses the discovery of herpesvirus 8 by a novel technique and that the virus' footprints were found in cells affected by Kaposi's sarcoma.*

Tirelli A, Serraino D, Carbone A: Hodgkin disease and AIDS. Ann Int Med 118:313, 1993.

Zauli G, Vitale M, Carla Re M, et al.: *In vitro* exposure to human immunodeficiency virus type 1 induces apoptotic cell death of the factor-dependent TF-1 hematopoietic cell line. Blood 83:167, 1994. *A report of a possible mechanism of myelosuppression by HIV.*

370 RENAL, CARDIAC, ENDOCRINE, AND RHEUMATOLOGIC MANIFESTATIONS OF HIV INFECTION

Michael S. Saag

Infection with the human immunodeficiency virus type I (HIV) is a multisystem disease. Manifestations of pulmonary, gastrointestinal, neurologic, hematologic, and oncologic disease are well described in the literature, owing mainly to their high prevalence and often dramatic modes of presentation. In contrast, HIV-related renal, cardiac, endocrine, and rheumatologic diseases are more insidious in presentation. As overall survival of HIV-infected individuals continues to improve and therapeutic regimens become more sophisticated, clinicians will undoubtedly encounter disorders of the latter organ systems with increasing frequency.

RENAL DISEASE

Renal disease associated with HIV infection may present as fluid-electrolyte and acid-base abnormalities, acute renal failure, coincidental renal disorders, or a glomerulopathy directly related to underlying HIV infection, the so-called HIV-associated nephropathy (HIVAN). Originally observed in patients with AIDS and referred to as AIDS-associated nephropathy, recent studies have described the characteristic renal changes of HIVAN in both asymptomatic HIV-infected individuals and those with early symptomatic HIV disease, thereby broadening the definition to include all HIV-infected patients.

FLUID, ELECTROLYTE, AND ACID-BASE DISORDERS. Fluid-electrolyte disorders are common in patients with advanced HIV infection. Hyponatremia is noted in up to 40% of hospitalized AIDS patients and occurs in the setting of both hypovolemia and euvolemia. Hypovolemia, most often due to gastrointestinal fluid losses, is the most common cause of hyponatremia among this group of patients. The syndrome of inappropriate antidiuretic hormone release (SIADH) is responsible for the majority of cases of euvolemic hyponatremia and is most often due to underlying *Pneumocystis carinii* infection, malignancy, or central nervous system (CNS) disease. The presence of hyponatremia is associated with increased morbidity and mortality, especially in conjunction with certain opportunistic infections, such as cryptococcosis.

Adrenal insufficiency is a less frequent cause of hyponatremia. Although abnormalities of the adrenal glands are frequently reported at autopsy, overt adrenal insufficiency occurs in < 5% of patients. The typical findings of hyponatremia, hyperkalemia, non–anion gap metabolic acidosis, hypovolemia, renal salt wasting, and mild renal insufficiency are usually present in some combination.

Drugs are an important cause of fluid and electrolyte disorders in HIV-infected patients and can mimic the abnormalities associated with adrenal dysfunction. Hyperkalemia and non–anion gap metabolic acidosis have been noted in patients receiving parenteral pentamidine. Amphotericin B is associated with hypokalemia, hypomagnesia, renal tubular acidosis, and renal insufficiency. Foscarnet therapy is associated with decreased levels of ionized calcium and, on occasion, renal insufficiency. Chemotherapeutic agents used to treat AIDS-associated malignancies may lead to fluid and electrolyte disturbances through direct nephrotoxicity or gastrointestinal losses associated with prolonged vomiting or diarrhea.

ACUTE RENAL FAILURE. As with most chronic illnesses, acute renal dysfunction may develop as a complication in the management of HIV-infected patients. Prerenal azotemia often results from hypovolemia secondary to poor fluid intake, increased gastrointestinal losses, or both. Acute tubular necrosis can be ischemic in origin, usually secondary to hypotension or sepsis, or due to nephrotoxic agents. Acute interstitial nephritis is another complication associated with drugs used to treat HIV-related diseases. A listing of agents with nephrotoxic potential commonly used in HIV-infected patients is presented in Table 370–1.

Opportunistic infections, invasion of renal parenchyma with lymphoma or Kaposi's sarcoma, and amyloidosis, which occurs as a complication of subcutaneous narcotic abuse, all may result in interstitial nephritis. Other renal lesions, such as hepatitis B–induced membranous glomerulonephritis, IgA nephropathy, acute glomerulonephritis secondary to bacterial infection, direct infection of the renal parenchyma with cytomegalovirus (CMV), fungi, or mycobacteria, and the hemolytic-uremic syndrome have all been associated with renal dysfunction in HIV-infected individuals. The diagnosis and management of acute renal failure are no different in HIV-infected patients than in their uninfected counterparts.

HIV-ASSOCIATED NEPHROPATHY. *Definition.* HIVAN was first established as a unique clinical entity in 1984. Originally called AIDS-associated nephropathy (AAN), many investigators questioned whether AAN was indeed a unique manifestation of AIDS or simply represented heroin-associated nephropathy (HAN) occurring in intravenous drug users (IVDU's) who also happened to be infected with HIV. Although the lesions and clinical manifestations of HAN are similar to those of AAN, further studies have established clear distinctions between the two entities. Of note, AAN occurs in individuals, including children, who have never used intravenous drugs. Indeed, nearly half of the cases presenting with the manifestations of AAN have early (asymptomatic or minimally symptomatic) HIV disease. Therefore, HIVAN has replaced AAN as the most appropriate name for this entity.

Epidemiology. The first cases of HIVAN were described in major urban centers, such as New York and Miami, which also had many IVDU's among their HIV patient population. In contrast, centers whose HIV population consisted primarily of Caucasian homosexual and bisexual men, such as San Francisco and the National Institutes of Health, were not observing the renal changes of HIVAN in their patients, thereby implying that HIVAN was a manifestation of HAN. More recent epidemiologic data indicate that 50% of patients with HIVAN are IVDU's, with the remaining cases occurring in homosexual and bisexual men, immigrants from Haiti, women who have acquired HIV from heterosexual contacts, and children born to infected mothers, many of whom did not use intravenous drugs.

Over 90% of patients with HIVAN are black. No explanation regarding the high prevalence of cases among blacks has been established, although many investigators have speculated that cofactors such as superimposed infection(s) or specific immune response genes may be responsible.

Pathology and Pathogenesis. Focal and segmental glomerulosclerosis (FSGS) is the characteristic renal lesion identified in patients with HIVAN, occurring in 80 to 90% of patients. On gross inspection, the kidneys are usually enlarged and the cortical surface

TABLE 370–1. DRUGS WITH NEPHROTOXIC POTENTIAL COMMONLY USED IN THE TREATMENT OF HIV-RELATED DISEASE

Acyclovir	Nonsteroidal anti-inflammatory agents
Aminoglycosides	Penicillins
Amphotericin B	Pentamidine
Aspirin	Phenytoin
Cephalosporins	Rifabutin
Cimetidine	Rifampin
Cis-platinum	Spiramycin
Dapsone	Sulfonamides
Ethambutol	Tetracyclines
Foscarnet	Thiazides
Ganciclovir	Trimethoprim

is smooth, even in advanced uremia. Microscopic examination of early lesions reveals diffuse mesangial hyperplasia with minimal glomerular sclerosis over time. A variable number of glomeruli develop segmental sclerosis characterized by hyperplastic visceral epithelial cells with coarse cytoplasmic vacuoles, collapsed capillary walls or capillaries obliterated by protein deposits (hyalinosis), and foam cells (lipid-filled monocytes) in the lumina (Fig. 370–1). Bowman spaces are usually dilated and tubular damage is universal. Microcystic dilation of tubules is a unique feature of HIVAN not reported in the FSGS of HAN (Fig. 370–2). Interstitial changes consisting of mild edema with scattered mononuclear cells are usually evident in HIVAN kidneys but not nearly to the degree noted in HAN. Similarly, although interstitial fibrosis may be present in advanced HIVAN disease, it is not nearly as prominent as the marked interstitial fibrosis noted in HAN disease.

The etiology of HIVAN remains unknown; however, many investigators suspect that an infectious agent is responsible. Ultrastructural studies have demonstrated tubuloreticular structures in vascular endothelium as well as in circulating and tissue lymphocytes. Other findings, such as a large number of nuclear bodies existing as budding forms in renal and lymphoid tissues, have been interpreted by some investigators to suggest a viral etiology. *In situ* hybridization studies have demonstrated proviral HIV DNA in renal tubular and glomerular epithelial cells, implicating HIV as the causative agent. However, the predominance of HIVAN in blacks and the relative paucity of cases among Caucasian homosexual men suggest that other factors not yet identified must play a role in the pathogenesis of HIVAN.

Clinical Manifestations. HIVAN is characterized by the development of proteinuria, nephrotic syndrome, and rapidly progressive irreversible azotemia. The proteinuria is typically heavy and presents as an early manifestation. The time to the development of end-stage renal disease (ESRD) from the initial diagnosis of proteinuria is 4 to 16 weeks in patients with HIVAN, compared to 20 to 40 months among patients with HAN. Another clinical distinction between HIVAN and HAN is the relative absence of significant hypertension among patients with HIVAN. Accelerated hypertension is a hallmark of HAN. Peripheral edema and anasarca are conspicuously absent in a large number of HIVAN patients with high-grade proteinuria and hypoalbuminemia.

Nephropathy has been documented in patients months to years before the onset of clinical symptoms of early symptomatic HIV disease or AIDS. HIVAN is being reported with increasing frequency among HIV-infected children and appears to be independent of the risk factors for HIV infection in their mothers. It is anticipated that the incidence of HIVAN will continue to grow and should be considered as a diagnostic possibility in any HIV-infected patient who presents with unexplained proteinuria regardless of the stage of disease.

Diagnosis. Quantitative measurement of the amount of protein

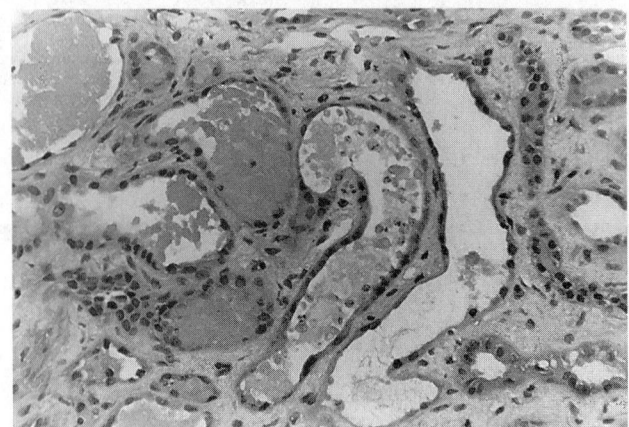

FIGURE 370–2. Dilated degenerated tubules demonstrating flattened epithelium and loss of nuclei and containing proteinaceous casts from a patient with HIV-associated nephropathy. (Hematoxylin-eosin; magnification × 200. Courtesy of Dr. William L. Clapp.)

excreted in the urine along with estimation of the creatinine clearance via a 24-hour urine collection should be performed early in the course of evaluation. Other reversible causes of renal insufficiency such as bacterial infection, crystalluria, and obstructive uropathy should be ruled out using urine culture, urinalysis, and ultrasonography. The kidneys are enlarged early in HIVAN and remain enlarged throughout the course of disease. The decision to perform renal biopsy should be made on a case-by-case basis depending on the clinical presentation, the likelihood of other diagnoses, and the therapeutic options available. Since a variety of other renal lesions, such as membranous nephropathy related to hepatitis B, membranoproliferative disease, and immune complex–related glomerular damage, may also present as nephrotic syndrome in HIV-infected patients, renal biopsy should be encouraged. The presence of the typical features of FSGS with tubular involvement as described above establishes the diagnosis of HIVAN when renal tissue is obtained.

Treatment. The lesions of HIVAN respond poorly if at all to currently available treatment regimens. In a few small studies, zidovudine has been shown to slow the progression of azotemia. Corticosteroids (60 mg prednisone daily over 2 to 6 weeks) recently have been shown to partially reverse the progressive azotemia and prevent the need for dialysis in a subgroup of patients. Until the use of corticosteroids is confirmed in larger studies, the treatment of HIVAN remains largely supportive. Nutritional support in the form of high-protein, high-calorie diets along with appropriate dosage adjustments of nephrotoxic drugs is crucial. Hemodialysis is of marginal benefit in prolonging survival of patients with advanced HIV disease once they have reached end-stage renal disease. Among patients with AIDS, hemodialysis provides short-term prolongation of life for 3 to 11 months. Patients who are asymptomatic or have early symptomatic HIV disease survive longer, with some patients living >4 years on chronic hemodialysis. Peritoneal dialysis should be considered in patients who are suitable candidates. Chronic ambulatory peritoneal dialysis (CAPD) may offer several advantages over hemodialysis, including avoiding leukopenia caused by the hemodialysis membranes, fewer problems with anemia, and theoretical advantages of less stimulation of HIV-infected T lymphocytes via membrane-induced cytokine release. A potential disadvantage of CAPD is the higher incidence of peritonitis. Renal transplantation is not considered a viable option in HIV-infected patients owing to the intensive immunosuppressive regimens required to prevent rejection. In some patients with advanced HIV infection or AIDS who develop HIVAN it may be appropriate to withhold dialysis support because of the generally poor prognosis. As always, such decisions should be individualized, taking into account the wishes of the patient, the family, and significant others.

CARDIAC DISEASE

A wide variety of cardiac abnormalities have been reported in HIV-infected patients, including ventricular dysfunction, myocarditis, pericarditis, endocarditis, and arrhythmias. Most often, cardiac involvement is clinically silent and is noted as an incidental finding

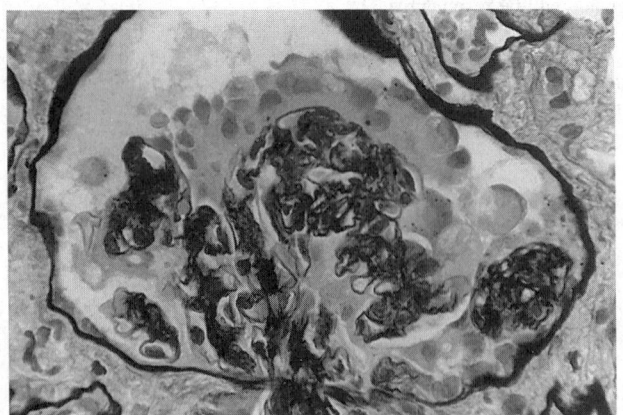

FIGURE 370–1. Glomerulus from a patient with HIV-associated nephropathy demonstrating global collapse of the glomerular capillaries, increased mesangial sclerosis, and a proliferative "cap" of visceral epithelial cells. (Silver methenamine; magnification × 400. Courtesy of Dr. William L. Clapp.)

at autopsy. When clinical symptoms are present, however, disease manifestations can be debilitating, and, in many cases, life threatening. Unlike HIV-associated renal disease, no specific cardiac syndrome or disease state has been described.

EPIDEMIOLOGY. Cardiac abnormalities have been observed in 25 to 75% of HIV-infected patients studied at autopsy. Myocardial disease is noted most frequently, occurring in >90% of subjects with cardiac findings. Pericardial disease, often with adjacent myocardial involvement, is observed in >20% of cases with cardiac abnormalities. Endocarditis is evident histologically in 3 to 5% of cases reported in autopsy series. No characteristic epidemiologic factor, such as age, gender, race, or means of acquiring HIV infection, has been identified which predisposes patients to cardiac disease. Although cardiac abnormalities are observed more frequently in AIDS patients, up to 30% of patients with early symptomatic HIV disease are noted to have abnormal findings on echocardiograms and electrocardiograms.

PATHOLOGY AND PATHOGENESIS. HIV-related heart disease may result from metastatic extension of a concomitant opportunistic infection or malignancy but most often is seen as lymphocytic infiltration of the myocardium or as an unspecified myocarditis. The mechanism responsible for the myocarditis remains unknown, although many investigators believe that HIV itself may be directly responsible. Other viruses, such as CMV, may be responsible for the development of myocarditis, although the typical "owl's eye" inclusion bodies are rarely seen in patients with HIV-associated cardiomyopathy. Additional mechanisms, such as postviral myocarditis or catecholamine-induced myocarditis, have been postulated, but little evidence exists to support their role.

A broad range of opportunistic infections and malignant diseases has been described in cardiac tissue examined at autopsy. Among the infectious disorders, fungal and viral pathogens are identified most often, followed by bacterial and protozoal infections (Table 370-2). Although the invading pathogen is frequently diagnosed at another primary site antemortem, cardiac involvement is rarely (<2%) identified before autopsy. This is largely due to the clinically silent nature of cardiac disease in HIV infection and a low index of suspicion by clinicians. Kaposi's sarcoma and metastatic lymphoma are the most common neoplastic diseases reported that invade the heart. Primary cardiac lymphoma has been reported rarely.

Pericardial disease is almost invariably associated with adjacent myocardial involvement. Pericarditis is usually nonspecific in origin, but when an etiologic process is identified, Kaposi's sarcoma or a pathogen such as *Mycobacterium tuberculosis* or *Cryptococcus neoformans* is responsible most often. Drugs used to treat HIV-associated disorders, such as doxorubicin for Kaposi's sarcoma, may cause myocardial damage. Other toxins, vitamin deficiencies, or metabolic abnormalities (e.g., hypothyroidism) may also result in myocardial dysfunction or pericardial disease.

Endocardial disease has been described in up to 3% of cases studied at autopsy and usually presents as either nonbacterial thrombotic (marantic) endocarditis or healed bacterial endocarditis.

TABLE 370-2. INFECTIOUS CAUSES OF CARDIAC DISEASE IN HIV-INFECTED PATIENTS

Bacteria
  Bacteria (endocarditis)
  Mycobacterium tuberculosis
  Mycobacterium avium-intracellulare
  Nocardia asteroides
  Actinomyces
Fungi
  Cryptococcus neoformans
  Histoplasma capsulatum
  Coccidioides immitis
  Candida species
  Aspergillus species
Viruses
  Cytomegalovirus
  Herpes simplex virus
  Human immunodeficiency virus
Protozoa
  Toxoplasma gondii
  Pneumocystis carinii

The precise etiology of marantic endocarditis is unknown, but it has been reported in other long-term wasting illnesses and malignant diseases. Vegetations are usually located on the mitral valve, although lesions on the tricuspid valve have been noted in up to 29% of AIDS patients with this disorder. Significant embolization to the spleen and brain was noted in >50% of patients with marantic endocarditis studied at autopsy. Bacterial endocarditis is reported rarely in AIDS patients. Healed lesions from previous bouts of bacterial endocarditis have been reported in autopsy series but are of little clinical significance.

CLINICAL FINDINGS. Most cardiac disease in HIV-infected patients is clinically silent. When symptoms are present they usually consist of the ordinary findings noted in non–HIV-infected patients with myocarditis or pericarditis, such as fever, dyspnea, chest pain, fatigue, cough, and orthopnea. Hepatomegaly and jugular venous distention are the most common signs noted on physical examination, followed by rales, systolic murmurs, and the presence of an S3 gallop. Signs of advanced pericardial disease with impending tamponade are among the most common clinical manifestations observed in patients who present with clinical symptoms of cardiac disease.

DIAGNOSIS. Demonstrated cardiomegaly on a chest roentgenogram is an important marker of underlying cardiac disease in HIV-infected patients. Right ventricular enlargement is usually the result of pulmonary artery hypertension, which in AIDS patients is often due to severe or recurrent opportunistic pneumonia. Left ventricular or biventricular enlargement is a characteristic finding of congestive cardiomyopathy due to any cause. Echocardiography is a more sensitive and specific noninvasive test that is used to assess the degree of ventricular dysfunction and to characterize the extent of pericardial effusion, if present. Several series have demonstrated echocardiographic abnormalities in up to 50% of HIV-infected patients who had no cardiac symptoms at the time of study. Ventricular enlargement, pericardial effusion, and ventricular hypokinesis were the abnormalities noted most frequently. In view of the overall silent nature of cardiac disease, the high likelihood that infiltrative processes will be evident and diagnosed at another site, and the often limited therapeutic options available for treating cardiac disease in HIV-infected patients, routine echocardiography should be discouraged in those without cardiac symptoms. The experience with endomyocardial biopsies in HIV-infected patients is quite limited; however, in those individuals who show signs of cardiac disease and have not had a specific diagnosis established, endomyocardial biopsy is a viable option for a definitive diagnosis.

Treatment. Supportive treatment consisting of diuretic therapy, reducing preload and afterload when appropriate, and correcting cardiac arrhythmias is the obvious initial approach to treating myocardial disease. Pericardial disease requires careful volume management with avoidance of aggressive diuresis or preload reduction. In the case of pericardial tamponade, surgical intervention is warranted. When the underlying etiology of the cardiac disease is known, appropriate therapy directed at the specific infectious agent or malignancy is indicated.

ENDOCRINE DISORDERS

Endocrine dysfunction has not been prominent in HIV infection. Nonetheless, all glands of the endocrine system may be infiltrated with opportunistic infections or malignancies or may be affected by drugs used to treat HIV-related disorders. The subtle presentations of endocrine diseases create difficult diagnostic challenges.

ADRENAL GLAND DYSFUNCTION. The adrenal gland is the endocrine gland most commonly affected in AIDS patients examined at autopsy, although clinical evidence of adrenal insufficiency is observed in <8% of AIDS patients. Widespread lipid depletion and varying degrees of adrenal necrosis are the most prevalent pathologic findings in postmortem examinations. Adrenal invasion by CMV is noted in up to 50% of patients with adrenal pathology. *Mycobacterium avium* complex, Kaposi's sarcoma, *C. neoformans,* and *Histoplasma capsulatum* involve the adrenal glands in 5 to 12% of cases. Drug therapy, with agents such as ketoconazole (adrenal dysfunction) or rifampin (increased clearance of cortisol) may also result in adrenal insufficiency. Fatigue, anorexia, nausea, vomiting, orthostatic hypotension, and hyponatremia are symptoms frequently noted in many HIV-infected patients; however, only a few with these symptoms are actually adrenal insufficient when evaluated using standard laboratory criteria.

Basal 8 A.M. plasma cortisol levels are usually higher in patients with advanced HIV disease than in asymptomatic patients and uninfected healthy controls. However, other ACTH-dependent steroids, such as desoxycorticosterone (DOC), compound B, and 18-hydroxy-DOC, are not elevated and show a blunted response to corticotropin (ACTH) stimulation, implying subnormal adrenal reserves. Patients who fail to achieve plasma cortisol levels >20 μg per deciliter 60 minutes after ACTH stimulation should be considered to have, or be at high risk of developing, adrenal insufficiency. Plasma ACTH levels are frequently normal or subnormal even when plasma cortisol levels are depressed, suggesting that adrenal insufficiency in some HIV-infected patients is due to a primary pituitary or CNS disorder. Treatment of adrenal insufficiency in HIV-infected patients is the same as in other individuals with abnormal adrenal function.

HYPOGONADISM. The most common abnormality of endocrine function noted clinically is hypogonadism. Decreased libido occurs in over one half of male patients with AIDS, and impotence, usually associated with low serum testosterone levels, is reported in up to 30% of AIDS patients. Serum gonadotropin levels may be below normal or inappropriately within normal limits in hypogonadal men with AIDS. When pituitary responsiveness to gonadotropin-releasing hormone is assessed in these hypogonadotropic males, normal release of luteinizing hormone (LH) and follicle-stimulating hormone (FSH) has been observed, suggesting a hypothalamic basis for the central hypogonadotropism. Other studies have demonstrated appropriately elevated levels of LH and FSH in hypogonadal men, implying primary testicular dysfunction. Drugs, such as ketoconazole, ganciclovir, and acyclovir have been associated with low testosterone levels or decreased spermatogenesis. Studies of gonadal function in women are limited, although menstrual irregularities are common in women with advanced HIV disease.

THYROID DISEASE. Thyroid function remains remarkably normal throughout the course of HIV disease. Low levels of thyroxine (T_4), triiodothyronine (T_3), and free-thyroxine index (FTI) in the setting of low concentrations of thyrotropin (TSH), the so-called euthyroid sick syndrome, is remarkably uncommon among ambulatory HIV-infected patients. Decreased levels of T_3 resin uptake and elevated levels of T_4-binding globulin are frequently noted in ambulatory patients with advanced disease; however, concentration of T_3 and T_4 are most often within normal limits. Invasive disease due to CMV, *P. carinii, C. neoformans,* Kaposi's sarcoma, and lymphoma have all been described in the thyroid. Remarkably, even patients with infiltrating opportunistic diseases of the thyroid gland usually remain euthyroid throughout the course of their disease. Nonetheless, despite the relative infrequency of clinical disease, hypothyroidism represents a potentially reversible cause of fatigue, malaise, altered mental status, and "failure to thrive" in HIV-infected individuals and should be routinely evaluated.

Less common causes of hypothyroidism in HIV-infected patients include adverse effects of medications. Ketoconazole has been associated with primary hypothyroidism on rare occasions. In addition, drugs that are strong inducers of hepatic microsomal enzymes, such as rifampin, may lead to increased clearance of T_4.

METABOLIC ABNORMALITIES. Hyponatremia is the most common electrolyte disturbance noted in HIV-infected individuals (see discussion in renal section). Disorders of carbohydrate metabolism have been reported in association with direct pancreatic invasion by opportunistic processes and with drug therapy. Pancreatic lesions caused by CMV, toxoplasmosis, Kaposi's sarcoma, and lymphoma are noted in up to 35% of cases at autopsy. Yet the development of type I diabetes mellitus has been reported in only a few instances. Hypoglycemia is the most common alteration in glucose metabolism. Direct toxic effects of drugs may induce premature release of insulin by β cells, resulting in hypoglycemic episodes that may be severe and prolonged. Pentamidine isothionate is the most common cause of hypoglycemia, occurring in 4 to 33% of treated patients. Renal insufficiency is a predisposing factor in the development of pentamidine-induced hypoglycemia. Although most hypoglycemic episodes result from parenteral administration of pentamidine, several cases have been reported in patients receiving aerosolized drug.

Disorders of calcium metabolism are relatively uncommon but do occur. Hypercalcemia is associated with HIV-related leukemia and lymphoma. Hypocalcemia usually is the result of drug therapy with agents, such as amphotericin B and foscarnet, which induce magnesium wasting and decrease levels of ionized calcium, respectively. CMV has been observed in parathyroid tissue; however, CMV-induced hypoparathyroidism is extremely rare.

Hyperlipidemia is noted commonly in HIV-infected patients. Isolated elevation of triglycerides is reported in up to 50% of patients with either asymptomatic HIV disease or AIDS. Although hypertriglyceridemia is routinely noted among patients with HIV wasting syndrome, no relationship has been noted between the serum triglyceride level and the degree of wasting. Elevation of cachectin (tumor necrosis factor), inhibition of lipoprotein lipase, and decreased clearance of circulating lipoproteins have all been proposed as potential mechanisms of hypertriglyceridemia, but no clear association of any of these factors has been established.

RHEUMATOLOGIC DISEASE

Rheumatologic manifestations of HIV disease are being recognized with increased frequency. Musculoskeletal complaints are reported in 33 to 75% of HIV-infected patients and may present as a variety of rheumatologic disorders (Table 370–3). The severity of disease ranges from intermittent arthralgias to debilitating arthritis and vasculitis. An array of autoimmune antibodies, including antinuclear, antiplatelet, antilymphocyte, antigranulocyte, and antiphospholipid (anticardiolipin and lupus anticoagulant) antibodies are associated with HIV infection along with circulating immune complexes, rheumatoid factor, and cryoglobulins. Despite the presence of these antibodies in some patients, the precise mechanisms by which the rheumatologic abnormalities develop have not been elucidated and most likely are different for each particular disorder.

TABLE 370–3. RHEUMATOLOGIC DISEASES ASSOCIATED WITH HIV INFECTION

Autoimmune phenomena
  Anticardiolipin antibodies
  Antigranulocyte antibodies
  Antilymphocyte antibodies
  Antinuclear antibodies
  Antiplatelet antibodies
  Circulating immune complexes
  Cryoglobulins
  Rheumatoid factor
Dermatologic
  Dermatomyositis
  Malar flush
  Psoriasis
Joint disease
  Arthralgias
  Arthritis
  Enthesopathies
  HIV-associated arthritis
  "Painful articular syndrome"
  Psoriatic arthritis
  Reactive arthropathy
  Reiter's disease
  Septic arthritis
  Systemic lupus erythematosus (lupus-like syndrome)
Myopathies
  Infectious (septic) myositis
  Myalgias
    Idiopathic
    Zidovudine-associated
  Necrotizing, noninflammatory myopathy
  Nemaline rod polymyositis
  Polymyositis
  Pyomyositis
Sjögren's syndrome
  Sicca complex
Vasculitis
  Central nervous system angiitis
  Eosinophilic vasculitis
  Henoch-Schönlein purpura
  Hypersensitivity (drug-induced)
  Leukocytoclastic vasculitis
  Polyarteritis nodosa
  Unspecified vasculitis

ARTHRALGIAS. Arthralgia is a common manifestation of acute HIV seroconversion, in addition to fever, myalgia, headache, sore throat, abdominal cramps, and lymphadenopathy. Generalized arthralgias are reported in up to one third of HIV-infected patients with minimally symptomatic disease. Some patients develop arthralgias and myalgias when zidovudine therapy is initiated; however, these symptoms are usually self-limited and abate within 4 to 6 weeks after starting treatment. The "painful articular syndrome" is characterized by severe articular pain of 2 to 24 hours' duration. Although uncommon, this disorder is quite incapacitating and usually unresponsive to oral nonsteroidal anti-inflammatory agents (NSAID's) or narcotic analgesics. Its etiology remains unknown. With the exception of the painful articular syndrome, most of the arthralgias associated with HIV disease are treated with nonsteroidal agents.

MYOPATHIES. Polymyositis-like illnesses, characterized by myalgias, proximal muscle weakness, and wasting, have been reported in several HIV-infected patients and have been the initial HIV-defining presentation in a few. The findings of creatinine phosphokinase (CPK) elevation (>5 times normal) and abnormal electromyography are indistinguishable from idiopathic polymyositis. Muscle biopsies reveal necrosis, fibrosis, and inflammation, but usually to a lesser extent than is noted in non–HIV-infected individuals. The presence of nemaline rods, often noted in muscle biopsies of older adults with myositis, suggests the likelihood of underlying HIV infection when noted in biopsy specimens obtained from younger adults, especially in the absence of inflammation.

Although virus-like particles have been demonstrated rarely in synovial tissue and HIV p24 antigen has been noted in the cytoplasm of degenerating muscle cells, no specific viral etiology has been determined. All attempts to culture HIV-1 from muscle tissue of patients with myositis have been unsuccessful.

Patients receiving long-term zidovudine therapy may develop myositis characterized by muscle weakness, elevated CPK levels, myalgias, and evidence of myopathy with a paucity of inflammatory cells on biopsy. Zidovudine-associated myositis usually responds to drug discontinuation and may recur on rechallenge. No definitive therapy exists for HIV-associated polymyositis, although corticosteroid therapy has been successful in reversing symptoms in some patients. If corticosteroid therapy is contemplated, the potential risks of superimposing immunosuppressive therapy on an immunocompromised host must be considered.

REITER'S SYNDROME. Reiter's syndrome is noted in up to 10% of HIV-infected patients who develop arthritis, and an additional 10 to 20% of patients are classified as having "reactive arthritis" because they lack the nonarticular features of Reiter's. Severe, persistent oligoarticular arthritis associated with urethritis, conjunctivitis, painless oral ulcerations, keratoderma blennorrhagicum, or circinate balanitis are the hallmarks of Reiter's disease in both HIV-infected and noninfected individuals. Clinical manifestations of Reiter's syndrome may precede or occur at the time of the initial diagnosis of HIV infection but most often follow the onset of immunodeficiency. HLA-B27 positivity is noted in 65 to 75% of HIV-infected patients with Reiter's syndrome. However, studies of African HIV patients with Reiter's disease or reactive arthritis revealed no increased incidence of HLA-B27, suggesting involvement of other gene markers in this group. *Shigella, Campylobacter, Ureaplasma,* and other bacterial species associated with the development of reactive arthropathies are rarely described in HIV patients with Reiter's syndrome. However, underlying concomitant sexually transmitted disease(s) may prove to be an important etiologic factor.

Treatment options for HIV patients with Reiter's disease are quite limited. Responses to NSAID's are minimal, and more potent immunosuppressive agents, such as methotrexate and azathioprine, frequently lead to opportunistic diseases and Kaposi's sarcoma shortly after initiation of therapy.

SJÖGREN'S SYNDROME. Xerophthalmia and xerostomia, the characteristic symptoms of Sjögren's syndrome (SS), have been reported with increasing frequency in AIDS patients. Features that closely resemble idiopathic SS, including sicca symptoms, a positive Schirmer test, abnormal salivary gland emptying, and abnormal salivary gland biopsies, have been reported in HIV-infected patients. As a result, it has been suggested that AIDS be an exclusionary disease for the diagnosis of idiopathic SS. The predominance of male patients, the absence of anti-Ro/SS-A and anti-La/SS-B antibodies, the absence of a well-defined connective tissue disease, the presence of HLA-DR52 and DR5 alleles instead of the characteristic A1, B8, DR3, DR2, and DQ1/DQ2 antigens, and a predominance of CD8+ lymphocytes instead of CD4+ cells infiltrating salivary tissue are the characteristic features of AIDS-associated SS, which differs from classic idiopathic SS. Treatment is primarily symptomatic.

SEPTIC ARTHRITIS. Joint space infection is remarkably uncommon in HIV-infected patients. Sporadic case reports have been published of septic arthritis due to fungal pathogens, such as *C. neoformans, H. capsulatum,* and *S. schenkii,* mycobacteria, and routine pyogenic organisms. The approach to diagnosis and treatment of septic arthritis is the same for HIV-infected patients as non–HIV-infected individuals.

HIV-ASSOCIATED ARTHROPATHY. A relatively uncommon arthritis has been described in patients with moderately advanced HIV disease who demonstrate no other signs of any recognizable rheumatologic disease. The so-called HIV-associated arthropathy (HIVAA) presents as a mono- or pauciarticular arthritis. The arthritis is usually severe, affects primarily the knees and ankles, and lasts from 1 week to 6 months. No extra-articular manifestations have been noted. The synovial fluid is noninflammatory in nature, although a mild synovitis consisting of a chronic mononuclear cell infiltrate is noted on biopsy. Rheumatoid factor, antinuclear antibodies, anti-DNA antibodies, and antibodies against RNP, Sm, Ro/SS-A, and La/SS-B are negative. No predominant HLA pattern has been described. NSAID's are of some benefit, but some patients require intra-articular steroid injections.

VASCULITIS. Several varieties of vasculitis have been reported in association with HIV infection. Necrotizing vasculitis of the polyarteritis nodosa type is reported most commonly and presents as a peripheral sensory or sensorimotor neuropathy. The vasculitis involves the medium-sized vessels of the nerves, skin, and muscle. None of the reported patients with HIV-related PAN were hepatitis B surface antigen positive. Primary angiitis of the CNS has been noted in two patients, one of whom had persistent varicella-zoster virus infection. Lymphomatoid granulomatosis has also been reported in HIV-infected patients. Henoch-Schönlein purpura has been reported rarely; however, no distinct etiology has been elucidated. Drug-induced hypersensitivity vasculitis, usually presenting as cutaneous disease, has been reported associated with penicillin, trimethoprim-sulfamethoxazole, amitriptyline, and griseofulvin. Recently, several cases of uveitis have been reported with rifabutin therapy, especially when this drug is administered with fluconazole and clarithromycin.

It is unclear whether HIV-associated vasculitis is the result of direct HIV invasion of the vessels, an immunologic reaction to an underlying viral infection, or a response to an opportunistic viral pathogen that invades vascular tissue. As with other serious rheumatologic manifestations of HIV disease, treatment options are limited by the underlying immunodeficiency of the host.

Buskila D, Gladman D: Musculoskeletal manifestations of infection with human immunodeficiency virus. Rev Infect Dis 12:223, 1990. *Extensively referenced review of the musculoskeletal complaints associated with HIV disease.*

Etzel JV, Brocavich JM, Torre M: Endocrine complications associated with human immunodeficiency virus infection. Clin Pharm 11:705, 1992. *A practical, easy-to-read overview of the endocrine abnormality seen in HIV-infected patients.*

Fernández SM, Cardenal A, Balsa A: Rheumatic manifestations in 556 patients with human immunodeficiency virus infection. Semin Arthritis Rheum 21:30, 1991. *One of the largest published reports on the rheumatological manifestations of HIV infection. Numerous tables, charts, and figures.*

Gherardi R, Belec L, Mhiri C, et al.: The spectrum of vasculitis in human immunodeficiency virus-infected patients. Arthritis Rheum 36:1164, 1993. *An up-to-date review of an uncommon yet diverse complication of HIV disease.*

Herskowitz A, Vlahov D, Willoughby S, et al.: Prevalence and incidence of left ventricular dysfunction in patients with human immunodeficiency virus infection. Am J Cardiol 71:955, 1993. *A study of 98 patients followed at Johns Hopkins Hospital Clinics who were evaluated for left ventricular dysfunction. Includes patients referred to the cardiology service as well as asymptomatic "controls."*

Kaul S, Fishbein MC, Siegel RJ: Cardiac manifestations of acquired immune deficiency syndrome: A 1991 update. Am Heart J 122:535, 1991. *Overview of the cardiac manifestations of HIV disease. Special focus on cardiomyopathy.*

Marks JB: Endocrine manifestations of human immunodeficiency virus (HIV) infection. Am J Med Sci 302:110, 1991. *A review of the pathologic and clinical reports in the literature regarding endocrinopathies in AIDS patients.*

Rao TKS: Human immunodeficiency virus (HIV) associated nephropathy. Annu Rev Med 42:391, 1991. *Succinct review of the renal complications of HIV disease, with special focus on the HIV-associated nephropathy.*

Smith MC, Pawar R, Carey JT, et al.: Effect of corticosteroid therapy on human immunodeficiency virus-associated nephropathy. Am J Med 97:145, 1994. *A recent study of a few patients successfully treated with corticosteroids for HIV-associated nephropathy.*

371 TREATMENT OF HIV INFECTION AND AIDS

Robert Yarchoan and Samuel Broder

Since the identification of AIDS as a new entity in 1981, dramatic changes have occurred in therapy for this disease and its related disorders. In 1984, therapy was either entirely supportive or directed at a bewildering array of infectious and oncologic complications. Identification of human immunodeficiency virus (HIV) as the causative agent of AIDS and elucidation of its life cycle have enabled the development of specific antiretroviral therapy. Such therapy is now recognized to be important in the treatment of AIDS. The available drugs, however, are not curative, and intense efforts to evaluate new therapeutic approaches to HIV infection and its associated conditions continue. In this chapter, we review some of the current approaches for treating AIDS patients. In addition, we discuss certain experimental approaches now being developed. In AIDS, as perhaps in no other disease, the line between approved and experimental therapy is difficult to draw.

The immunodeficiency in AIDS results, either directly or indirectly, from the progressive destruction of the immune system by HIV. In addition, HIV infection affects other organ systems (such as the central nervous system). T lymphocytes bearing CD4 antigen on their surface (CD4 cells or T4 cells), monocyte/macrophages, and monocyte-derived cells such as microglial cells are now recognized as the principal cellular targets for HIV. Although other cells are also susceptible to infection in certain settings, the clinical significance of this phenomenon is unclear. In infected individuals, the development and progression of disease require at least some level of ongoing infection of new cells by HIV. Thus, one could reason that interfering with HIV replication *in vivo* could halt (or even reverse) the progression of disease to AIDS. Indeed, the successful development of antiretroviral therapy has provided proof for this concept.

AZIDOTHYMIDINE (ZIDOVUDINE) AND OTHER DIDEOXYNUCLEOSIDES

The first three antiretroviral drugs to be developed and approved for the therapy of HIV infection are members of the class of compounds called dideoxynucleosides, special analogues of nucleosides that have a sugar and a purine or pyrimidine base. 3'-Azido-2',3'-dideoxythymidine, also called azidothymidine, zidovudine, or AZT (Fig. 371–1), was the first to enter clinical testing. Although this drug was initially synthesized as an anticancer agent, it was found to inhibit HIV replication in human T cells *in vitro* and was later found to have anti-HIV activity in monocytes and macrophages. In dideoxynucleosides, the 3'-hydroxy (—OH) group in the sugar is replaced by another group that does not form phosphodiester linkages. A number of dideoxynucleosides have been found to be potent inhibitors of HIV replication *in vitro,* and several, including AZT, have been shown to have clinical activity in patients with HIV infection.

Upon entering human cells, AZT and other dideoxynucleosides are activated (phosphorylated) to form a 5'-triphosphate moiety. This activation process, called anabolic phosphorylation, uses a series of enzymes (kinases) that usually serve to phosphorylate deoxynucleosides (Fig. 371–2). For many purposes, each drug in this broad family is unique. Even a one-atom shift in the sugar or the base of the parent compound can radically change activity and toxicity. There are substantial differences in the rates at which human cells phosphorylate these compounds and in their enzymatic pathways, and these differences may be important in their antiretroviral activity and differing toxicity profiles. For example, thymidine kinase, the enzyme responsible for the initial step in the phosphorylation of thymidine analogues such as AZT and 2',3'-didehydro-2',3'-dideoxythymidine (stavudine, d4T), is a cell cycle–dependent enzyme. As a result, the activity of this type of drug is relatively greater in replicating lymphocytes or cytokine-stimulated monocytes than in resting cells of the same lineage. By contrast, the activity of 2',3'-dideoxyinosine (ddI, didanosine) and 2',3'-dideoxycytidine

(ddC, zalcitabine) is not substantially affected by the state of activation of the cells. Therefore, these two classes of drugs may target different cell populations, and, as described below, this insight may be useful in guiding the development of combination regimens.

As triphosphates, dideoxynucleosides act as inhibitors at the level of HIV DNA polymerase (reverse transcriptase) (see Ch. 361). This unique viral enzyme catalyzes the conversion of HIV genetic information from RNA to DNA and subsequently catalyzes the formation of a second viral DNA strand, i.e., a copy complementary to the first. As 5'-triphosphates, dideoxynucleosides are believed to inhibit reverse transcriptase in two ways; as DNA chain terminators and as competitive inhibitors for binding deoxynucleoside 5'-triphosphates to relevant sites within reverse transcriptase. Reverse transcriptase, but not mammalian DNA polymerase alpha, preferentially uses dideoxynucleoside-5'-triphosphates in place of the respective physiologic 5'-triphosphates, and this is most likely one basis for their selective antiretroviral activity. Human mitochondrial DNA polymerase (gamma) is also relatively sensitive to inhibition by certain of these drugs, and, as discussed below, this may be a basis for clinical toxicities, including cases of hepatic steatosis and myopathy observed in patients receiving dideoxynucleoside therapy.

CLINICAL ACTIVITY OF ZIDOVUDINE. Phase I and II clinical trials of AZT conducted during 1985 and 1986 convincingly showed that the drug was effective at reducing morbidity and mortality in patients with advanced HIV infection (Fig. 371–3). The patients receiving AZT had increased numbers of CD4 cells, improved immunologic function, and a decreased viral load (as assessed by HIV p24 antigenemia). In addition, they had increased appetite, weight gain, and often reported feeling better, at least temporarily. In a 6-month multicenter double-blind randomized trial in which AZT was compared with placebo, patients who had severe early symptomatic HIV disease or who had had *Pneumocystis carinii* pneumonia were found to have a markedly reduced mortality and incidence of opportunistic infections upon receiving AZT compared with patients on placebo. Based on these studies, AZT was initially approved for patients with severe HIV infection at a recommended dose of 200 mg every 4 hours (1200 mg per day) around the clock. Since that time, it has been found that a maintenance regimen of 100 mg every 4 hours (600 mg per day), initiated after a month's therapy with 200 mg every 4 hours, is as effective as the initially recommended regimen and is less toxic. This is now the currently recommended dose schedule for patients with AIDS or advanced HIV infection. Many physicians do not use the higher dose during the first month of therapy and suggest that their patients omit the night-time dose, for a total of 500 mg per day. Also, many physicians believe that a regimen of 200 mg every 8 hours has equivalent activity and leads to increased patient compliance. Physicians should be alert for possible future modifications of the recommended dose of this drug. Of the dideoxynucleosides now available, AZT is generally recommended as the first-line drug for people with advanced HIV infection.

The pharmacokinetic profile of AZT is one of the factors that guide its usage. AZT is well absorbed by mouth; the average oral bioavailability is 63%. The circulating half-life is approximately 1.1 hours. Because of this relatively short half-life, a dosing schedule of every 4 hours was initially recommended. However, the active 5'-triphosphate moiety has an intracellular half-life of 1 to 3 hours, and as noted above, many physicians now use a regimen of 200 mg every 8 hours. Fifteen to 20% of an administered dose of zidovudine is excreted unchanged in the urine, whereas approximately 75% undergoes glucuronidation to an inactive form in the liver. AZT glucuronidation can be inhibited by certain other drugs, such as probenecid, which share this pathway, and these drugs can prolong the half-life of zidovudine. However, other drugs that undergo hepatic glucuronidation (e.g., acetaminophen) have no such effect. Studies are under way to evaluate the interactions of other drugs with AZT. Finally, AZT penetrates relatively well into the cerebrospinal fluid (CSF).

At the beginning of the epidemic, the expected survival of patients with fulminant AIDS was approximately 10 months. The expected survival of such patients has nearly doubled since that time. It is likely that a number of advances in diagnosis, prevention, and treatment of AIDS complications (particularly chemoprophylaxis for opportunistic infections such as *P. carinii* pneumonia) have contributed to this. However, when this specific factor has been looked at, the effect of AZT on survival has been observed over and above any contribution from chemoprophylaxis.

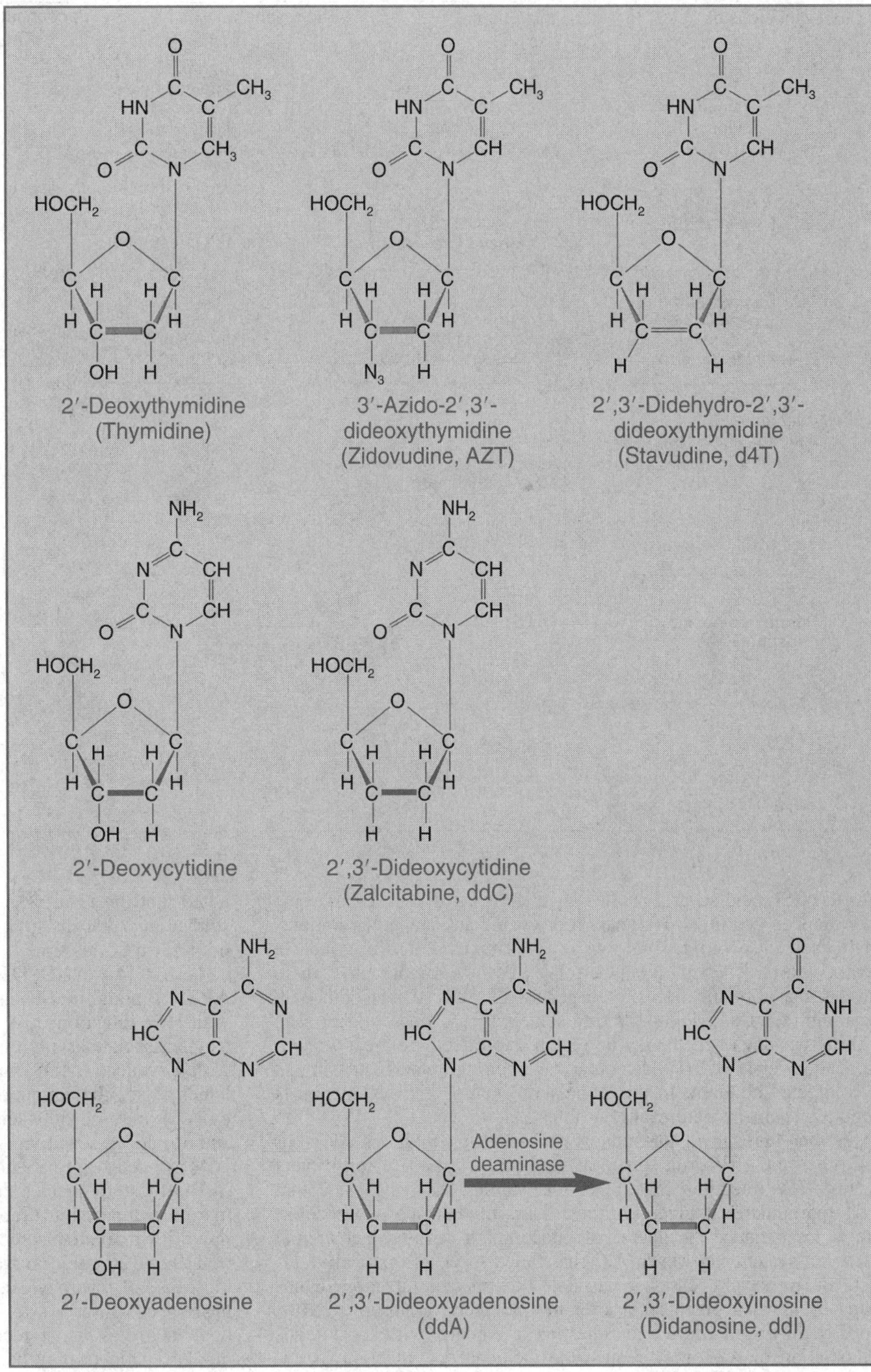

FIGURE 371-1. Structures of zidovudine (AZT), stavudine (d4T), zalcitabine (ddC), dideoxyadenosine (ddA), and didanosine (ddI), and their related physiologic deoxynucleosides. In each row, the physiologic deoxynucleoside is shown on the left and the related antiretroviral drug or drugs are shown to their right. In each case, a replacement of the 3′ hydroxy (—OH) group of the physiologic deoxynucleoside by an azido (—N₃) group or a hydrogen atom (—H) results in the formation of a potent antiretroviral drug. ddA is rapidly converted to ddI by the ubiquitous enzyme adenosine deaminase, and these can be considered alternate forms of the same drug for many purposes.

An unresolved issue is the optimal time to initiate AZT therapy. Five major double-blinded randomized trials of early AZT therapy have now been completed. Overall, these studies showed that AZT given to either asymptomatic or symptomatic patients with 200 to 500 CD4 cells per cubic millimeter resulted in a somewhat reduced progression of disease over 1 to 2 years. As a result of these observations, AZT was approved for HIV-infected patients with 500 CD4 cells per cubic millimeter or less. However, one study showed that the reduction in quality of life from the side effects of AZT was about equal to the increase associated with the effect on disease progression. Moreover, two of the studies specifically looked for an effect on survival, and in each case, no overall survival advantage was seen in patients given AZT early as opposed to those in whom the drug was withheld until symptoms developed. The consensus from these trials is that in regard to overall survival as an endpoint, administering AZT early is not proven to be better than later admin-

istration. It should be stressed that these results in no way refute the earlier findings that AZT initiated at the time of advanced HIV infection improves survival. Also, it should be remembered that these trials all involved AZT as a single agent, and the results do not necessarily apply to combination regimens.

Based on an informed discussion, some physicians and patients may elect to use AZT early whereas others may not. In either case, the physician should explain the results from the available clinical trials to the patient. Physicians should keep informed of changes in these recommendations as new trials are completed and analyzed.

In considering initiating therapy with AZT, physicians may weigh two factors: the presence of HIV-related thrombocytopenia and HIV-related dementia. HIV-infected patients sometimes develop thrombocytopenia, which can be rather severe. Several studies have now shown that AZT can reverse this process and is better tolerated in this population than are corticosteroids. Also, AZT can penetrate

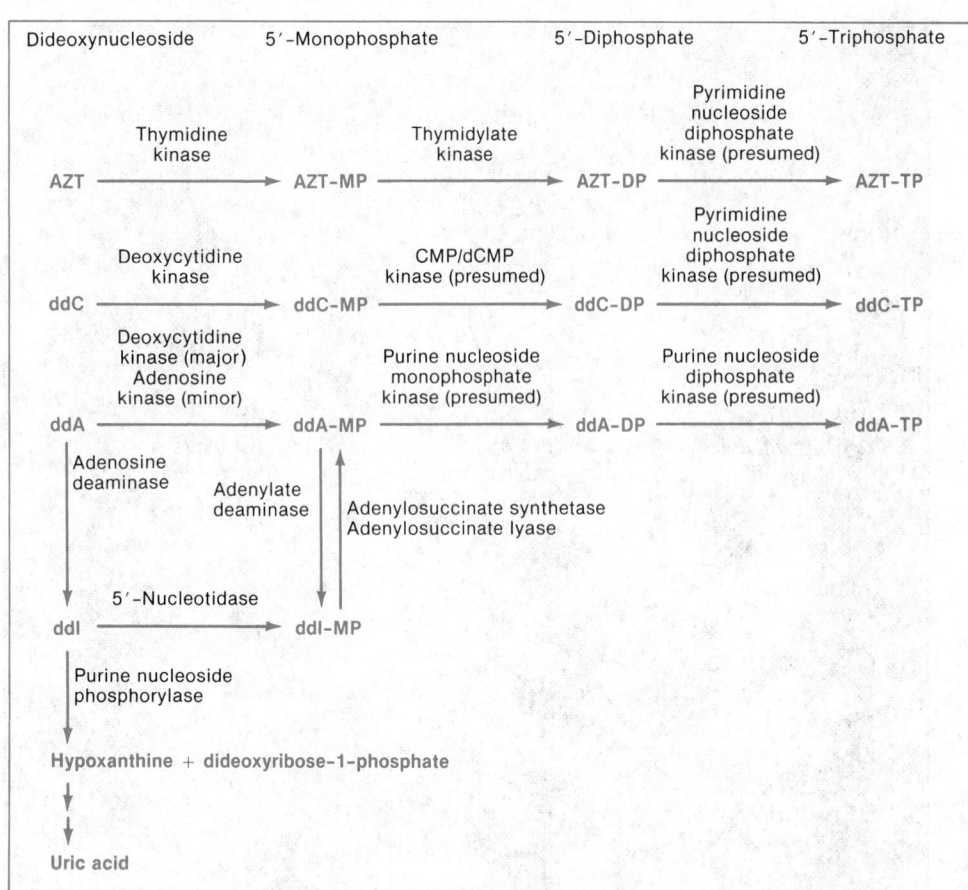

FIGURE 371–2. Activation pathways for zidovudine (AZT), zalcitabine (ddC), dideoxyadenosine (ddA), and didanosine (ddI) to the active triphosphate moieties in human cells. MP = 5′-monophosphate; DP = 5′-diphosphate; TP = 5′-triphosphate.

into the CSF, and several studies have shown that AZT can reverse HIV-induced cognitive dysfunction or even frank dementia. Patients have been observed to improve on psychometric testing, and, in several cases studied by positron emission tomography, there has been a normalization of the pattern of glucose metabolism in the brain (see Color Plate 12*F*). In some patients, doses higher than 500 mg per day of AZT may be required to effectively treat dementia. The reversal of HIV dementia has been particularly striking in HIV-infected children. In this population, neurologic dysfunction is often a prominent feature of HIV infection.

Another unresolved question is under what conditions AZT (or any other anti-HIV drug) given at the time of exposure can protect against HIV infection. Several animal studies have suggested that AZT (particularly if given within 2 hours of the time of infection) can at least reduce the degree of infection. In certain other animal retroviral systems, however, AZT has failed to yield a protective effect, and in several cases it has failed to prevent infection in humans even when given soon after the parenteral exposure to HIV. No data, however, address the question of whether postexposure administration of AZT may reduce the incidence of infection in humans. Many hospitals now offer a 4- to 6-week course of AZT to employees who have a substantial exposure to HIV, e.g., a needle stick with HIV-infected blood or a laboratory accident. In considering such therapy, physicians should weigh the risk of HIV infection occurring (about 1 in 200 for a needle stick), the short-term side-effects of AZT, and the unknown long-term sequelae of this drug.

Recent evidence from a recently conducted placebo-controlled trial, ACTG 076, indicates that AZT can reduce the transmission of HIV from the infected mother to her infant. In this study, the treatment consisted of a regimen of AZT administered to the mother during pregnancy (100 mg five times daily by mouth starting between weeks 14 and 34) and during labor and delivery (by the intravenous route), as well as to the infant during the first 6 weeks of life. Transmission of HIV infection was found to be reduced from 25.5% in the placebo control group to 8.3% in the treated group. The mothers in this study all had >200 CD4 cells per cubic millimeter and had never received anti-HIV therapy. No increase in congenital defects was seen in the AZT-treated infants. It should be

noted that the results cannot be extrapolated beyond the population studied and that the long-term effects of AZT exposure *in utero* are not known at this time.

TOXICITY AND OTHER LIMITATIONS OF AZT THERAPY. Although AZT has clearly been shown to benefit patients with HIV infection, it is by no means a perfect drug. Its long-term use is associated with a number of toxicities, particularly in patients with advanced AIDS, and on occasion the side effects may be lethal. Also, the immunologic and virologic improvement induced by AZT may be only temporary, especially in patients with AIDS, and a reduced sensitivity to the drug has been observed in strains of HIV isolated from patients on long-term therapy.

The most frequent toxicity associated with AZT therapy is bone marrow suppression (Table 371–1). The earliest sign is often anemia with marked macrocytic changes; a mean corpuscular volume of 110 to 120 cubic microns is not uncommon. AZT is now a leading cause of macrocytosis in several medical centers. Some patients have been observed to develop hypocellular or (rarely) aplastic bone marrows while receiving AZT. Later in the course of AZT therapy, patients may become neutropenic or thrombocytopenic. In some patients, the platelet count remains stable or paradoxically increases for some time, perhaps reflecting an effect against underlying HIV-induced thrombocytopenia. AZT-induced bone marrow suppression is most common in patients with advanced AIDS, low CD4 cell counts, pretherapy anemia, and pretherapy neutropenia. It is less problematic with the recently recommended dosage of 600 mg per day; however, even with this dosing schedule, it can occur in 30% or so of patients with advanced disease during the first year of therapy. HIV-infected patients often have vitamin deficiencies, particularly of vitamin B_{12}, and megaloblastic anemia from folic acid or vitamin B_{12} deficiency bears a certain similarity to AZT toxicity. It may thus be prudent to measure serum levels of folic acid and vitamin B_{12} and give replacement therapy if they are low; however, this intervention has not been shown to prevent or reverse AZT toxicity. It has been shown that genetically engineered erythropoietin (epoetin alfa) can partially ameliorate AZT-induced anemia, particularly in patients who do not have markedly elevated erythropoietin levels (see Ch. 369). For patients who develop severe

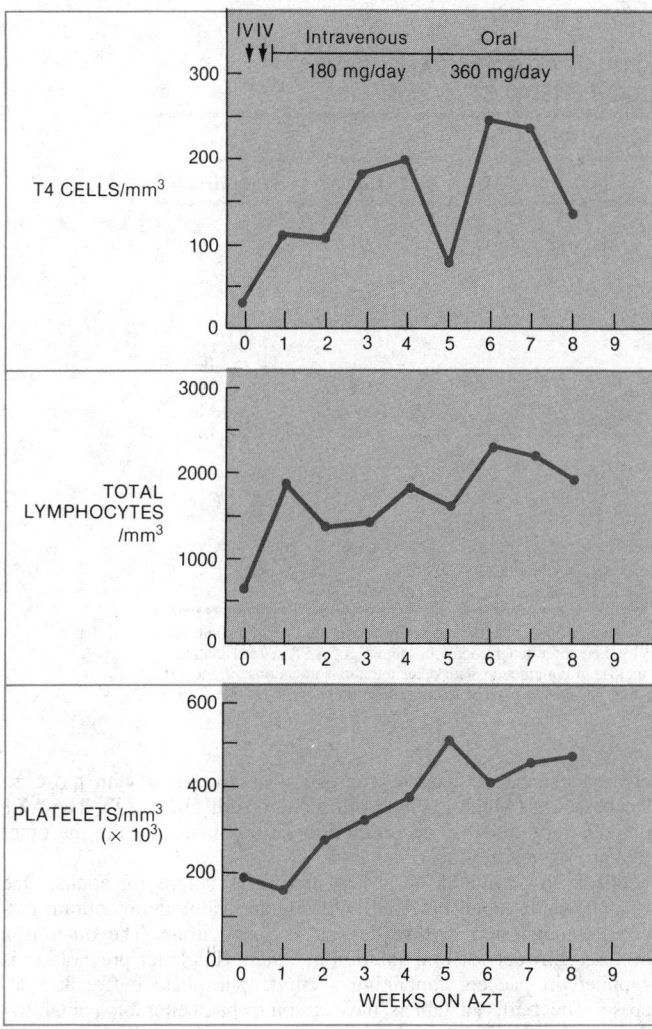

FIGURE 371–3. Course of the first patient to ever receive AZT. This patient, who had recently recovered from *Pneumocystis carinii* pneumonia, was treated on the National Cancer Institute service of the National Institutes of Health Clinical Center with 180 mg per day of AZT intravenously for 4 weeks, followed by 360 mg per day orally for 4 weeks.

anemia or neutropenia while receiving AZT, many physicians now favor switching to an alternative antiretroviral regimen (see below).

Myalgias are also common in patients receiving AZT. In addition, after long-term therapy (e.g., a year or more), a subset of patients may develop frank myopathy with muscle wasting and sometimes (but not always) elevations of creatine kinase. In rare cases, this side effect can lead to a catastrophic failure of systemic muscles. AZT-induced myositis can usually be distinguished from myositis caused by HIV by the presence of "ragged-red" fibers on biopsy, indicative of abnormal mitochondria (see Color Plate 12*G*). Paracrystalline inclusions in the mitochondria can be seen on electron microscopy. It is believed that this toxicity results from the inhibitory effect of AZT-5′-triphosphate on mammalian γ DNA polymerase, an enzyme found in the mitochondrial matrix. Some patients with this toxicity respond to a nonsteroidal anti-inflammatory drug, with or without a reduced dosage of AZT. In other cases, it may be necessary to discontinue the AZT. Certain patients who do not respond to the above interventions have been reported to respond to therapy with prednisone (40 to 60 mg daily). This potentially dangerous immunosuppressive drug should be used only in severe cases when other alternatives have failed.

Some HIV-infected patients receiving AZT, alone or in combination with other dideoxynucleosides, have been reported to develop a poorly understood syndrome involving severe macrovesicular hepatic steatosis (a condition related to Reye's syndrome) and lactic acidosis (see Color Plate 11*H*). A high proportion of these patients have died of this complication. Many had relatively early HIV infection and were well nourished or even obese. Also, a disproportionate percentage of such patients were female. It has been sug-

gested that, like zidovudine-induced myositis, this condition may be caused by mitochondrial toxicity.

Seizures, which can be fatal, have been reported as side effects of AZT, as has Stevens-Johnson syndrome on very rare occasions. Patients receiving AZT frequently complain of malaise, fatigue, nausea, or headaches. These often become less severe after several weeks on the drug. One approach to these symptoms is to start with a relatively low dose of AZT and work up to the full dose over a couple of weeks or so. Even with this approach, these symptoms are intolerable in a small percentage of patients. Some patients, particularly those of African-American ancestry, develop bluish fingernail discoloration as a result of AZT therapy (Color Plate 12*E*).

Improved survival from antiretroviral therapy may permit AIDS patients to live long enough to develop certain HIV-related complications. In particular, an unexpectedly high incidence of non-Hodgkin's lymphoma, in some instances approaching 10% of patients per year, has been observed in AIDS patients who have been closely followed for several years on AZT-containing regimens. These are probably not caused by AZT but rather represent the development of opportunistic tumors in drastically immunosuppressed patients.

The elevations in CD4 cell counts and declines in the load of HIV in patients receiving AZT generally last for only weeks or months, particularly in patients with advanced disease, and a growing body of data supports the notion that this is because viral resistance developed. AZT resistance, often 100-fold or more, is found in HIV isolated from the majority of patients with advanced disease who have received AZT for a year or more. Development of resistance is slower in patients with earlier HIV infection. Strains resistant to AZT generally have two or more mutations in the HIV *pol* gene (Table 371–2). Of these, the substitution of tyrosine (or phenylalanine) for threonine at codon 215 appears to be the most

TABLE 371–1. PRINCIPAL TOXICITIES OF DRUGS WITH ANTIRETROVIRAL ACTIVITY USED IN AIDS

Zidovudine (AZT)
1. Bone marrow suppression
   Red cells usually affected more than white cells or platelets
   Prominent increase in red cell mean corpuscular volume
   Marrow may become hypocellular
2. Malaise, fever, fatigue (especially during first few weeks)
3. Headaches (especially during first few weeks)
4. Myalgias
5. Myositis (in approximately 10% of patients after long-term use)
6. Hepatic steatosis, lactic acidosis (can be fatal)
7. Seizures (can be fatal)
8. Nausea, vomiting
9. Confusion, tremulousness (especially with high doses)
10. Bluish pigmentation of nails (especially in blacks)
11. Stevens-Johnson syndrome (very rare)

Didanosine (ddI)
1. Sporadic pancreatitis (can be fatal)
2. Painful peripheral neuropathy (involving feet)
3. Sporadic hepatitis (can be fatal)
4. Insomnia, irritability, anxiety
5. Macular erythematous skin rash (sporadic)
6. Retinal depigmentation (especially in children)
7. Increases in uric acid (from ddI metabolism)
8. Hyperamylasemia, hypertriglyceridemia
9. Diarrhea, hypokalemia (from citrate/phosphate/sucrose vehicle)
10. Neutropenia, thrombocytopenia (rare, relationship to drug unclear)
11. Seizures
12. Dry mouth
13. Diabetes mellitus (rare)

Zalcitabine (ddC)
1. Painful peripheral neuropathy (involving feet)
2. Aphthous stomatitis
3. Esophageal ulcerations
4. Pancreatitis (reported but rare)
5. Cardiomyopathy
6. Skin rash (may subside with continued treatment)
7. Fever (especially with high doses)
8. Thrombocytopenia (especially with high doses)
9. Hepatic steatosis or lactic acidosis (rare)

Stavudine (d4T)
1. Painful peripheral neuropathy
2. Elevations of hepatic transaminases
3. Bone marrow suppression, especially anemia

TABLE 371–2. SELECTED MUTATIONS IN HIV-1 REVERSE TRANSCRIPTASE ASSOCIATED WITH DRUG RESISTANCE

Codon	Wild Type	Drug						
		AZT	ddI	ddC	d4T	3TC	Pyridione	Nevirapine
41	Met	Leu						
50	Ile				Thr			
67	Asp	Asn						
69	Thr			Asp				
70	Lys	Arg						
74	Leu		Val					
100	Leu						Ile	Ile
103	Lys						Asn	Asn
106	Val							Ala
108	Val						Ile	Ile
135	Ile		Val					
151	Gln	Met	Met	Met	Met			
181	Tyr						Cys	Cys
184	Met		Val			Val		
188	Tyr						Cys	Cys
215	Thr	Tyr, Phe						
219	Lys	Gln, Glu						

Shown here are some of the principal mutations in the codons of reverse transcriptase of HIV conferring resistance to various anti-HIV drugs. The amino acids in the wild-type and mutated viruses are depicted by their three-letter codes. In the case of AZT, several mutations are generally required to yield high-level resistance. The mutation at codon 151, in conjunction with other mutations at codons 77 and 116, can confer resistance to multiple dideoxynucleosides. In the case of the non-nucleoside reverse transcriptase inhibitors pyridione (L-697, 661) or nevirapine, one mutation is sufficient to confer high-level resistance.

important. AZT-resistant strains generally preserve their sensitivity to most other dideoxynucleosides (including ddC and ddI), and this is one rationale for combination therapy with these agents.

DIDANOSINE. Several other dideoxynucleosides (see Fig. 371–2) and related nucleoside analogues have been found to be active against HIV in the laboratory. Of these, ddI, ddC, and d4T are currently approved in the United States, and others including the negative enantiomer of 2′,3′-dideoxy-3′-thiacytidine (3TC) are currently being tested in experimental protocols (Table 371–3). Upon being phosphorylated in target cells to their active moieties, all of these drugs are believed to work by the same general mechanism. However, because of differences in their intracellular or extracellular metabolism and effects on cellular DNA polymerases and normal nucleotides, various dideoxynucleosides may have fundamentally different activity and toxicity profiles. Each must be considered a different drug, and their mechanisms of action remain a matter for basic research.

The second such drug to be approved for the treatment of HIV infection was ddI. This drug is well absorbed by the oral route when given with appropriate buffers (oral bioavailability 40%). Although it has a relatively rapid serum half-life (average 1.6 hours), its active moiety, 2′,3′-dideoxyadenosine-5′-triphosphate, has an intracellular half-life of >12 hours, and it can thus be administered on a twice-daily regimen. Early clinical trials showed that ddI elevated CD4 cell counts and decreased the HIV viral load. Several large randomized trials comparing the relative efficacy of ddI and AZT in patients with AIDS or advanced HIV infection have shown that AZT was more effective than ddI in patients with AIDS or advanced HIV infection who had never before received AZT therapy. However, in patients who received as little as 8 weeks of prior AZT therapy, ddI was found to be more effective in preventing disease progression and to increase survival in some subsets (Fig. 371–4). Largely as a result of these studies, ddI is now approved for use in patients with advanced HIV infection who have received prolonged prior AZT therapy or who cannot tolerate AZT or who show disease progression during such therapy.

Certain subsets of patients may experience comparatively long actuarial survivals. Thus, for patients who entered a phase I study of ddI with CD4 counts between 100 and 300 cells per cubic millimeter, the estimated survival after 4 years was 80%.

There is recent evidence that a ddI-containing regimen is superior to AZT monotherapy in children with HIV infection. ACTG study 152 was designed to compare AZT, ddI, and a combination regimen of AZT and ddI in children with up to 6 weeks of prior anti-HIV therapy. An interim look at the data in February 1995 revealed that patients on the AZT monotherapy regimen had a significantly in-

creased chance of disease progression as compared with those on the best arm (which is either ddI alone or ddI plus AZT). The AZT monotherapy arm has accordingly been terminated, while the other two arms remain blinded.

ddI is now available in at least two formulations for adults. One is a chewable tablet buffered with dihydroxyaluminum sodium carbonate, magnesium hydroxide, and sodium citrate. The other is a buffered powder for oral solution in water. This latter preparation is supplied in packets containing a citrate phosphate buffer and sucrose. The buffered tablets have a somewhat better bioavailability than the buffered powder, and the dosages must be adjusted accordingly. For patients weighing at least 60 kg, the recommended dose is 400 mg of the tablets daily or 500 mg of the buffered powder daily, divided into two doses and taken on an empty stomach. For patients weighing <60 kg, the doses are 250 mg daily of the tablets or 334 mg of the buffered powder daily, again divided into two doses.

The principal toxicity of ddI is its potential for causing severe or even lethal pancreatitis (see Table 371–1). In the trials discussed above, the annual rate of pancreatitis in patients receiving ddI was about 7%, compared with a 3 to 4% annual rate in patients receiving AZT. As can be seen by the rates in AZT recipients, patients with HIV infection have an underlying high incidence of pancreatitis, and it is often difficult to distinguish ddI-induced pancreatitis from that caused by HIV infection, its complications, or other drugs. The incidence of pancreatitis is higher in patients with more advanced disease or with higher doses of ddI, and this is one of the factors that led to the current dosing recommendation. Some patients receiving ddI have asymptomatic hyperamylasemia, which may be of either salivary or pancreatic origin. Although it is prudent to temporarily discontinue ddI in patients with elevated levels of pancreatic amylase, the drug may be cautiously continued in patients who have only elevated salivary amylase levels. ddI should also be withheld in patients with hyperlipasemia or substantially elevated triglyceride levels, as these may reflect present or incipient pancreatic damage.

Patients receiving ddI should be counseled to avoid alcohol. A previous history of pancreatic disease should generally serve as a contraindication to ddI use. Also, other drugs that can cause pancreatitis, such as systemic pentamidine, high-dose sulfonamides, furosemide, and thiazide diuretics, should be avoided whenever possible in patients receiving ddI. In particular, ddI should be temporarily stopped when patients are treated for P. carinii pneumonia with intravenous pentamidine or sulfonamide-containing regimens (including trimethoprim-sulfamethoxazole). If appropriate, ddI can then be restarted after the completion of therapy. In the case of pentami-

TABLE 371-3. SELECTED ANTIRETROVIRAL DRUGS (EXPERIMENTAL AND APPROVED) FOR THE THERAPY TREATMENT FOR AIDS

Site of Effect	Name	Status (Fall 1994)	Comment
Viral binding	CD4-IgG chimera	Experimental	Blocks viral entry
	CD4-toxin hybrids	Experimental	May selectively kill HIV-producing cells
	Anti-HIV antibodies	Experimental	May block HIV fusion and entry
Reverse transcriptase	Zidovudine (AZT)	Approved	Principal toxicity is bone marrow suppression
	Didanosine (ddI)	Approved	Can cause pancreatitis or peripheral neuropathy
	Zalcitabine (ddC)	Approved	Peripheral neuropathy is dose-limiting toxicity
	Stavudine (d4T)	Approved	Can cause peripheral neuropathy
	Lamivudine (3TC)	Experimental	Resistance develops rapidly; especially active in combination with AZT
	Non-nucleoside reverse transcriptase inhibitors	Experimental	Resistance a problem with this class of drugs
	Phosphonoformate (Foscarnet)	Approved for cytomegalovirus	Also has some activity against HIV
Replicative efficiency	Genetic therapy approaches	Experimental	Inhibitions of *rev* and *tat* activity being studied
	Antisense oligonucleosides	Experimental	May have both sequence specific and nonspecific activities
Protein modification	Saquinavir	Experimental	Little toxicity. Being studied in combination trials. Resistance can develop.
	Other protease inhibitors	Experimental	Several now in clinical trial
			Clinical activity has been observed with some, but resistance can develop.
	Zinc finger inhibitors	Preclinical	Affect nucleocapsid protein; may also affect infectivity
Viral assembly and budding	Interferon-α	Approved for Kaposi's sarcoma	Antitumor activity against Kaposi's sarcoma. May also have anti-HIV activity

dine, which has a long serum half-life, it is probably prudent to wait at least 1 week before resuming ddI. Sulfonamides (including trimethoprim-sulfamethoxazole) at the doses used as prophylaxis for *P. carinii* pneumonia can be co-administered with ddI. Patients receiving ddI who develop abdominal pain should be advised to stop the drug immediately and be evaluated for pancreatitis. Physicians should probably avoid prescribing cimetidine or ranitidine along with ddI, as those drugs have the potential of increasing the absorption of ddI and can cause pancreatitis in their own right.

Some patients receiving ddI develop a painful peripheral neuropathy, primarily involving the feet. This is generally reversible upon discontinuing the drug, but the resolution may take weeks. Some patients with this condition have a decrease in their vibratory sense or ability to discriminate temperatures, but these objective findings are generally more subtle in relationship to the symptoms than in patients with HIV-induced peripheral neuropathy. Other reported side effects of ddI include seizures, headache, insomnia, irritability, vomiting, diabetes mellitus, hyperuricemia, and skin rash. Depigmentation of the retinal pigment epithelium, not associated with changes in visual acuity, has been reported, especially in children. Also, patients receiving the citrate/phosphate buffered form of

ddI may develop diarrhea, sometimes accompanied by life-threatening hypokalemia. This is generally attributed to the buffer/vehicle rather than to the ddI itself, and it may subside upon a change to the buffered tablets. Because ddI is given with buffers of gastric acidity, it should be given at least 2 hours after drugs such as ketoconazole or dapsone, whose absorption actually depends on gastric acidity.

HIV resistance had been reported to occur with ddI, but it is generally of a lesser degree than that observed with AZT. The most frequently observed mutation is a substitution of valine for leucine in codon 74 of the *pol* gene (see Table 371–2). Interestingly, this change can make AZT-resistant HIV with a mutation at codon 215 become more sensitive to AZT, and this has provided a rationale for using these drugs together in combination. Several pilot studies have shown that patients started on the combination of AZT and ddI often have elevated CD4 cells above baseline lasting for over a year, and some physicians use this combination in patients who progress on AZT therapy. While this regimen has not yet been approved, two large clinical trials have recently confirmed its clinical utility.

ZALCITABINE. ddC was the third drug to be approved for treating HIV infection. This drug was found to reduce the load of HIV in patients at even very low doses. On a weight basis, it is the most potent of the available antiretroviral nucleosides. It is well absorbed when given by mouth and is excreted by the renal route. In patients with advanced HIV infection who have not received prior antiretroviral therapy, ddC does not appear to be as clinically active as AZT. However, in patients who have had extensive prior AZT therapy, ddC appears to be as effective as continued AZT. Some investigators believe that a combination of AZT and ddC provides more durable elevations in CD4 counts than either agent used alone, particularly in patients with a CD4 count of > 150 cells per cubic millimeter.

The principal toxicity of ddC is a painful peripheral neuropathy, somewhat similar to that caused by ddI (see Table 371–3). Other toxicities include aphthous stomatitis, esophageal ulceration, cardiomyopathy, and a few reported cases of pancreatitis. Cases of lactic acidosis, hepatic steatosis, or fatal hepatic failure have also been reported. The differential toxicity profiles of AZT and ddC have led to their study in combination regimens. In a study of patients with advanced HIV infection who had had extensive pretreatment with AZT, however, the combination of AZT and ddC was overall no better than continued AZT therapy. Interestingly, however, patients who entered this study with 100 to 300 CD4 cells per cubic millimeter appeared to do better on the combination therapy. ddC as a single drug is currently approved at a dose of 0.75 mg three times daily for patients with advanced HIV infection who are intolerant of AZT or who have had disease progression while re-

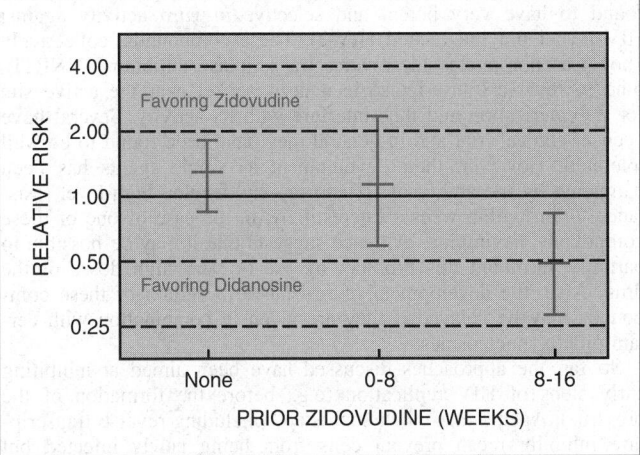

FIGURE 371–4. Comparative effectiveness of AZT and ddI in patients with advanced HIV-1 infection as assessed in ACTG Trial 116A. Shown are the relative risks of either a new AIDS-defining event or death in patients with varying prior experience with AZT. (Data from Abstract WS-B24-1 in the IXth International Conference on AIDS, Berlin, 1993 and from R. Dolin and the ACTG 116A team.)

ceiving AZT. In addition, it is indicated in combination with AZT for selected patients with advanced HIV infection (≤ 300 CD4 cells per cubic millimeter).

OTHER DIDEOXYNUCLEOSIDES. Stavudine (d4T) has recently been approved in the United States for patients who are intolerant of or deteriorating while receiving other approved therapies. The recommended dose is 40 mg twice daily for patients weighing at least 60 kg, and 30 mg twice daily for patients < 60 kg. Like AZT, this drug is a thymidine analogue. However, it is more efficiently phosphorylated in target cells, and it is active in patients at doses of 0.5 to 1.0 mg per kilogram per day. Its principal toxicities are painful peripheral neuropathy, anemia, and hepatitis. Some evidence exists that the phosphorylation of d4T in cells to its active moiety is inhibited by co-administering AZT, thus possibly interfering with its action. Their simultaneous use is not recommended outside the clinical trial setting. Another dideoxynucleoside, the negative enantiomer of 2',3'-dideoxy-3'-thiacytidine (lamivudine, 3TC), has been found to induce very little toxicity, whereas the development of high-level resistance may be a problem in its use as a single agent, it induces relatively prolonged effects on surrogate markers (viral load and CD4 count) when administered in combination with AZT.

OTHER ANTI-HIV THERAPIES

Many clinical trials of anti-AIDS drugs are currently under way, and physicians treating AIDS patients may need to counsel them about the advisability of entering a particular experimental protocol. As such, a basic knowledge of the strategies being considered to inhibit HIV replication at various steps in its life cycle may be of use (see Table 371–3).

As described in Ch. 361, the first step in the infection of a cell by HIV is its binding to a cellular receptor. The principal receptor for HIV binding is the first domain of CD4 glycoprotein, an important molecule found on helper T cells and certain other cells. Some experimental evidence indicates that under certain circumstances CD4-independent entry mechanisms may exist, although the clinical significance of this finding is unknown. Several groups have shown that various forms of genetically engineered soluble recombinant CD4 (containing the extracellular domains) can prevent the binding and infection of cells by HIV *in vitro*. However, these preparations were subsequently found to have less activity against fresh isolates of HIV than against laboratory strains, and they did not appear to have activity in patients.

As discussed above, much of the effort in developing anti-AIDS drugs has focused on reverse transcription. All of the dideoxynucleosides (as triphosphates) are thought to act at this step. In addition, trisodium phosphonoformate (foscarnet), a drug used to treat cytomegalovirus, has some activity against HIV at the level of reverse transcription. More recently, a diverse group of compounds, some of which are structurally related to the benzodiazepines, have been found to have very potent and selective *in vitro* activity against HIV-1 (but not the related HIV-2). These compounds, collectively known as non-nucleoside reverse transcriptase inhibitors (NNRTI), bind to reverse transcriptase in a deep pocket near the active site for polymerization and thus interfere with its activity. Several have been in clinical trial and in general they have been found to be well tolerated. However, their development as single agents has been hampered by the ability of HIV to rapidly develop high-level resistance, often within weeks. Interestingly, in the case of one of these compounds, nevirapine, evidence suggests that it may be possible to partially surmount this problem by use of very high doses of the drug. Also, the development of resistance to certain of these compounds may be delayed if they are given in combination with certain dideoxynucleosides.

So far, the approaches discussed have been aimed at inhibiting early steps of HIV replication (e.g., before the formation of the provirus). Agents that block such steps (including reverse transcriptase inhibitors) can prevent cells from being newly infected but have little or no effect on those that are already infected and producing virus. There is now a substantial interest in inhibiting late steps in HIV replication, in part because such agents are likely to be synergistic with inhibitors of early steps and in part because certain cells, such as macrophages, can produce HIV for long periods of time. One late target that has been the focus of a substantial re-

search effort is HIV protease. Certain proteins of HIV are first produced as large, relatively inactive polyproteins and later undergo a variety of modifications to form active proteins or glycoproteins. Proteolytic cleavage of the Gag-Pol fusion protein may occur very late, even within budding virions. Without a functional protease, the infectivity of the virus is severely diminished. The structure of this enzyme has recently been determined by radiographic crystallography, and a number of selective inhibitors have been identified. The principal problems initially encountered in developing this class of compounds have related to poor oral bioavailability, poor solubility, and complexity of synthesis. However, these have not been insurmountable, and several drugs have now entered clinical testing. One of the most extensively tested, saquinavir, was found in early clinical studies to have oral bioavailability of about 5%, to be well tolerated, to induce increases in CD4 counts, and to reduce the HIV viral load. It is an interesting agent; its use in combination with other anti-HIV agents is now being explored. Several other compounds, including L-735,524, ABT-538, and U-75875, are also undergoing clinical testing, and some of the preliminary clinical results have also been favorable. Some of these compounds may have better oral bioavailability than saquinavir. It is likely that within the next few years, one or more of these compounds will enter general clinical practice. However, the emergence of resistance has been observed with certain protease inhibitors as single drugs, and the potential of combination regimens to address this issue is a major topic for clinical research.

HIV replication is regulated by certain genetic elements (long terminal repeats) on the end of the viral genome and by several small viral-encoded proteins. Efficient viral replication requires the proper function of these regulatory elements, and as such they may also be targets for therapy. Specific inhibitors of these proteins are now being sought. Also, a number of cytokines and cellular factors have been identified that interact with the long terminal repeats and regulate HIV replication, and these may be targets for therapy. For example, tumor necrosis factor-α stimulates HIV replication, and HIV-infected patients have elevated levels of this factor. Certain drugs such as pentoxifylline inhibit its production, and this approach is now being tested in HIV-infected patients.

Another approach to inhibiting HIV replication has been the construction of "antisense" segments of modified DNA (e.g., phosphorothioate oligodeoxynucleotides). These are strands of DNA—modified to prevent degradation by cellular nucleases—with sequences complementary to that of HIV RNA. Such constructs may stop viral replication by bringing about a hybridization arrest at the level of the ribosome. A related approach being explored in the laboratory are ribozymes, RNA's that may cleave sequences in HIV RNA. Finally, a number of gene therapy approaches are being explored with the aim of rendering cells resistant to HIV replication. For example, cells may be protected against HIV by insertion of genes encoding for elements that block the activity of Tat or Rev, two regulatory elements of HIV. Clinical trials of such approaches are now under way. However, it is unlikely that any such approach will be widely used to treat AIDS over the next several years.

The last steps in the replication of HIV are viral assembly and budding. There is evidence that interferon-α can prevent HIV replication *in vitro*, in part by affecting viral budding. Interferons may have other sites of activity as well. Interferon-α has been found to have antitumor activity against Kaposi's sarcoma (see Ch. 369), particularly in patients with > 100 T4 cells per cubic millimeter who have disease limited to the skin, and it is approved for this indication.

A final word should be said about strategies to boost the immune system of individuals with HIV infection. The progression of HIV infection to fulminant AIDS represents an interplay between the infective potential of the virus and the ability of the immune system to interfere with this process. In most if not all patients, the virus eventually prevails in the absence of specific therapy and fulminant AIDS develops. Moreover, evidence indicates that abnormal cytokine stimulation in HIV-infected patients and imbalances in immune responses are an integral part of the disease process. At the same time, certain elements of the specific immune response against HIV slow down the progression to AIDS, and a judicious boosting of the immune system (or of the specific response to HIV) might prove to be advantageous to HIV-infected patients. A variety of experimental approaches to immunorestoration in AIDS are being explored, including cytokines (such as interleukin-2 [IL-2] or -12), immunostimulatory drugs, and extracorporeal expansion of immune elements. Recent evidence shows that periodic administration of IL-2, in combination with antiretroviral therapy, may induce increases in CD4 counts in certain patients. This experimental approach and others to enhance immune response are still under study.

As noted above, combinations of drugs may potentially offer several advantages over a given single agent. Indeed, it is likely that as individual drugs are developed, combination regimens become the mainstay of therapy for HIV infection. The use of several agents may help delay the development of HIV resistance. Also, certain combinations may have synergistic anti-HIV activity and preferentially affect different target cells. Moreover, combinations of drugs with different clinical toxicity profiles, for example AZT and ddC, may permit a sustained anti-HIV effect with reduced toxicity from either drug. Also, there is evidence that sustained elevations of CD4 cells may be attained with AZT plus ddI or AZT plus 3TC, in part because AZT resistance is partially reversed by mutations conferring resistance to ddI or 3TC. The potential number of permutations of drug combinations is large, and clinical studies are needed to sort out the relative merits of these approaches. Some drugs may be useful in suppressing certain opportunistic infections and thus have a secondary effect on HIV infection. For example, acyclovir can suppress herpes viruses and might thus indirectly reduce HIV infection (a nuclear regulatory protein of herpes viruses can activate HIV replication). The combination of AZT and acyclovir is usually tolerated by patients and is used by some physicians, particularly for patients who are troubled by recurrent herpes infection. Physicians should be cautioned against *ad hoc* patient experimentation with combination therapy, as unexpected drug interactions may occur.

GENERAL RECOMMENDATIONS

At present, four drugs are approved for the treatment of HIV infection. Results of a number of clinical trials have provided some guidance for using these agents. At the same time, however, different trials have sometimes provided conflicting results, and many questions remain about the optimal therapy of patients at different stages of their disease. In June of 1993, a panel convened by the National Institute of Allergy and Infectious Diseases sifted through the available data and made recommendations for the antiretroviral treatment of HIV infection (Table 371–4).

The panel recommended that symptomatic patients with < 500 CD4 cells per cubic millimeter or asymptomatic patients with < 200 CD4 cells per cubic millimeter start on antiretroviral therapy. The starting therapy of choice is AZT as a single agent, although the panel noted that combination therapy of AZT and ddI or AZT and ddC could also be considered. In a departure from previous recommendations, however, antiretroviral therapy is now considered optional for asymptomatic patients with 200 to 500 CD4 cells per cubic millimeter. Finally, antiretroviral therapy is not generally recommended for patients with > 500 CD4 cells per cubic millimeter outside of the setting of an experimental protocol. As noted in Table 371–4, a change to alternate antiretroviral drugs or combination therapy may be considered in patients who have disease progression on single-agent AZT therapy, and a change to alternate drugs should be considered in patients who cannot tolerate AZT. Finally, the panel recommended that no antiretroviral therapy coupled with supportive care be considered as a legitimate option in patients whose CD4 cell count drifts below 50 cells per cubic millimeter, if they cannot tolerate AZT.

In deciding on the appropriate therapy to use in an individual patient, physicians should consider the toxicity profiles of the various drugs, the specific disease symptoms, and the wishes of the patient. Physicians are advised to institute chemoprophylaxis for *P. carinii* pneumonia when the CD4 count falls below 200 cells per cubic millimeter (see Ch. 365 and 383). Also, chemoprophylaxis for *Mycobacterium avium* infection (see Ch. 312) with rifabutin is recommended for patients whose CD4 count has fallen below 100 cells per cubic millimeter. Yearly vaccinations with killed influenza virus are advisable; however, vaccinations with attenuated viruses should generally be avoided in this population.

Since the recommendations for anti-HIV therapy were made in 1993, results of two large clinical trials (ACTG 175 and Delta) have suggested that it may be worthwhile to begin treatment with a combination regimen. In both trials, one of which included patients with up to 500 cells/mm^3, initial therapy with either AZT and ddI or with AZT and ddC was found to be superior to that with AZT alone. In ACTG 175, monotherapy with ddI was found to be superior to AZT and equivalent to the combination regimens. The recommendations for anti-HIV therapy may be modified in the near future in light of these results. Also, 3TC (lamivudine) and some of the protease inhibitors are now available for compassionate use. Physicians should watch for ongoing developments that may profoundly affect accepted medical practice.

TABLE 371–4. RECOMMENDATIONS FOR ANTIRETROVIRAL THERAPY OF HIV-INFECTED ADULTS FROM A 1993 STATE-OF-THE-ART CONFERENCE

Clinical Status	CD4 Cell Count Range (cells/mm^3)	Recommendation
No previous antiretroviral therapy		
Asymptomatic	> 500	No therapy
Asymptomatic	200–500	Zidovudine or no therapy
Symptomatic	200–500	Zidovudine
Asymptomatic	< 200	Zidovudine
Symptomatic	< 200	Zidovudine*
Previous antiretroviral therapy		
Stable	≥ 300	Continue zidovudine
Stable	< 300	Continue zidovudine or change to didanosine
Progressing	50–500	Change to didanosine or zalcitabine*
Progressing	< 50	Change to didanosine or zalcitabine
Intolerant to zidovudine		
Stable or progressing	> 500	Discontinue antiretroviral therapy
Stable or progressing	50–500	Change to didanosine or zalcitabine
Stable or progressing	< 50	Change to didanosine or zalcitabine†

Recommendations are from a state-of-the-art panel convened by the National Institute of Allergy and Infectious Diseases in June 1993. Modified from Sande MA, Carpenter CCJ, Cobbs G, et al.: Antiretroviral therapy for adult HIV-infected patients. Recommendations from a state-of-the-art conference. JAMA 270: 2583, 1993.

* Some panel members would consider combination therapy with zidovudine plus didanosine or zidovudine plus zalcitabine.

† The option of discontinuing all nucleoside therapy can be considered in this population.

General Review

Johnston MI, Hoth DF: Present status and future prospects for HIV therapies. Science 260:1286, 1993. *Excellent overview of the current status of AIDS therapy. Extensive bibliography.*

Yarchoan R, Pluda JM, Perno CF, et al.: Anti-retroviral therapy of HIV infection: Current strategies and challenges for the future. Blood 78:859, 1991. *Clinical overview of therapeutic approaches now in use.*

Zidovudine

Concorde Coordinating Committee: Concorde: MRC/ANRS randomised double-blind controlled trial of immediate and deferred zidovudine in symptom-free HIV infection. Lancet 343:871, 1994. *Large placebo-controlled trial comparing early and late administration of zidovudine.*

Other Dideoxynucleosides

Abrams DI, Goldman AI, Launer C, et al.: A comparative trial of didanosine or zalcitabine after treatment with zidovudine in patients with human immunodeficiency virus infection. N Engl J Med 330:657, 1994. *Study comparing ddI and ddC as therapy for patients who progressed during AZT treatment or who could not tolerate it.*

Collier AC, Coombs RW, Fischl MA, et al.: Combination therapy with zidovudine and didanosine compared with zidovudine alone in HIV-1 infection. Ann Intern Med 119:786, 1993. *Article describing the combination therapy of AZT and ddI.*

Fischl MA, Stanley K, Collier AC, et al.: Combination and monotherapy with zidovudine and zalcitabine in patients with advanced HIV disease. Ann Intern Med 122:24, 1995. *Comparative trial of combination therapy with AZT and ddC versus monotherapy.*

Kahn JO, Lagakos SW, Richman DD, et al.: A controlled trial comparing continued zidovudine with didanosine in human immunodeficiency virus infection. N Engl J Med 327:581, 1992. *A comparative study of AZT and ddI in patients with at least 16 weeks of prior AZT therapy.*

Spruance SL, Pavia AT, Peterson D, et al.: Didanosine compared with continuation of zidovudine in HIV-infected patients with signs of clinical deterioration while receiving zidovudine. A randomized, double-blind clinical trial. Ann Intern Med 120:360, 1994. *Results of a trial comparing AZT and ddI and extensive prior AZT therapy in patients with AIDS or AIDS-related complex.*

Yarchoan R, Lietzau JA, Nguyen B-Y, et al.: A randomized pilot study of alternating or simultaneous zidovudine and didanosine therapy in patients with symptomatic immunodeficiency virus infection. J Infect Dis 169:9, 1994. *Article comparing alternating and simultaneous regimens of AZT and ddI.*

Resistance

Richman DD: Resistance of clinical isolates of human immunodeficiency virus to antiretroviral agents. Antimicrob Agents Chemother 37:1207, 1993. *Overview of HIV resistance.*

Recommendations for Therapy

Sande MA, Carpenter CCJ, Cobbs G, et al.: Antiretroviral therapy for adult HIV-infected patients. Recommendations from a state-of-the-art conference. JAMA 270:2583, 1993. *Provides an algorithm for antiretroviral therapy.*

372 MANAGEMENT AND COUNSELING FOR PERSONS WITH HIV INFECTION

John A. Bartlett

Physicians caring for persons with HIV infection must make crucial decisions in chronic management and counseling. The advances of the past 5 years, especially in the prevention and treatment of opportunistic infections, have led to an improved prognosis for patients with symptomatic HIV disease. The median survival for persons after their initial AIDS-defining illness has been extended to 2.5 years. Clinicians may evaluate their patients against a timeline of predictable complications (Fig. 372–1), and they are aided by improved diagnostic examinations and treatment options. The use of *Pneumocystis carinii* pneumonia (PCP) prophylaxis has led to fewer episodes of PCP as a complication of HIV infection, and other manifestations such as disseminated *Mycobacterium avium* complex (MAC) infection, cytomegalovirus (CMV) disease, and unexplained wasting have become more common. These decisions regarding the use of PCP prophylaxis and diligent attention to the early diagnosis and treatment of opportunistic infections have become incorporated into standards for clinical practice. However, some clinical decisions remain controversial, such as the optimal point for starting antiretroviral therapy, the use of combinations of antiretroviral therapy, and the use of prophylaxis against MAC. The clinician must practice HIV medicine in the context of an evolving knowledge base in which the results of clinical trials may not be absolute. Patients may be well informed about their illness and wish to participate in the decision-making process, to which they may make important contributions. In this environment the clinician has the opportunity to practice both the science and art of medicine, and the successful chronic management and counseling of HIV-infected persons offers the potential for dramatic rewards.

HIV PATHOGENESIS

The optimal choice of treatment(s) for HIV-infected persons must be guided by an understanding of viral pathogenesis (see Ch. 361). Advances in the past 5 years have resulted in an improved understanding of HIV pathogenesis, but many basic pathophysiologic questions remain unanswered. The relatively modest clinical impact of antiretroviral therapy is at least partially a reflection of this incomplete understanding, further complicated by repeated frustrations in the development of antiretroviral drugs (see Ch. 371).

Soon after the acquisition of HIV, the virus may achieve high levels, as assessed by quantitative virus culture, viral (p24) antigen detection, or polymerase chain reaction (PCR) for viral nucleic acids. After 2 to 4 weeks of this initial highly viremic phase, the amount of virus in the peripheral bloodstream significantly decreases, perhaps coincident with the generation of HIV-specific cellular immune responses. Despite the decreases in peripheral bloodstream viremia, HIV RNA can be detected by PCR in peripheral

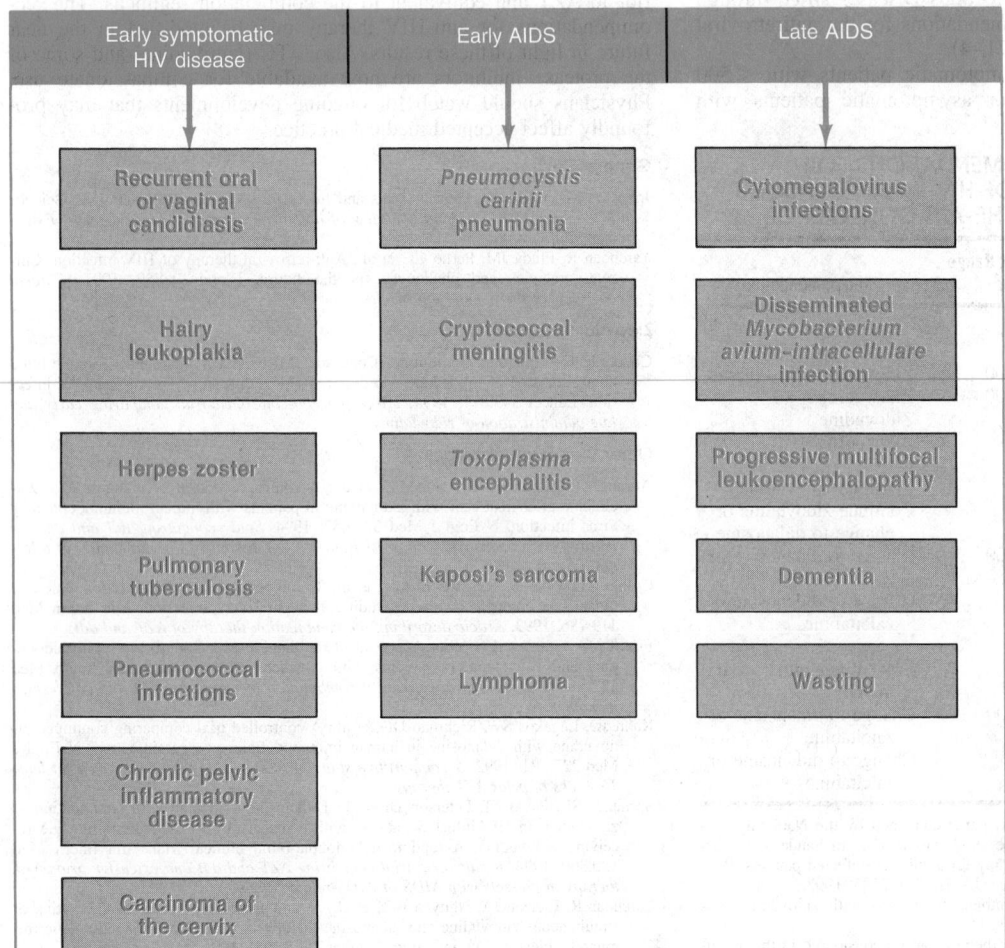

Early symptomatic HIV disease	Early AIDS	Late AIDS
Recurrent oral or vaginal candidiasis	*Pneumocystis carinii* pneumonia	Cytomegalovirus infections
Hairy leukoplakia	Cryptococcal meningitis	Disseminated *Mycobacterium avium-intracellulare* infection
Herpes zoster	*Toxoplasma* encephalitis	Progressive multifocal leukoencephalopathy
Pulmonary tuberculosis	Kaposi's sarcoma	Dementia
Pneumococcal infections	Lymphoma	Wasting
Chronic pelvic inflammatory disease		
Carcinoma of the cervix		

FIGURE 372–1. Time line of AIDS-related complications.

blood, even during asymptomatic HIV infection. The detection of HIV RNA suggests active HIV replication. New evidence indicates that HIV becomes predominately localized in lymphoid tissues during this period, especially lymph nodes, thymus, gastrointestinal lymphoid tissue such as Peyer's patches, and tissue macrophages in bone marrow, liver, spleen, and skin. HIV is concentrated in the germinal centers of lymph nodes during early HIV infection, and viral particles are frequently found there immediately adjacent to the processes of follicular dendritic cells, an area where activated T lymphocytes migrate for antigen recognition. In this microenvironment, uninfected activated CD4+ T lymphocytes may become HIV infected. This process may be further accelerated by the local production of tumor necrosis factor and interleukins-1 and -6 from B lymphocytes. These cytokines activate CD4+ T lymphocytes and macrophages, thus further increasing their susceptibility to and production of HIV. Thus, lymphoid tissue constitutes an important reservoir of ongoing viral replication, even during the asymptomatic period when less virus can be recovered from the peripheral bloodstream. As HIV infection progresses, normal lymph node architecture is destroyed and replaced with even larger amounts of virus, and in peripheral blood, increasing amounts of viral nucleic acid, p24 antigen, and culturable virus can be detected. These observations reinforce the need for effective antiretroviral therapy to control HIV replication.

However, direct viral infection and subsequent destruction of CD4+ T lymphocytes does not explain the entirety of HIV pathogenesis. Only 0.01 to 10% of circulating CD4+ lymphocytes contain viral nucleic acids, and this observation suggests that additional processes may contribute to CD4+ lymphocyte depletion. Experimental evidence suggests that autoimmune processes and the chronic immunologic activation of HIV infection may also participate in the destruction of CD4+ lymphocytes. Finally, little is known about important elements in the reconstitution of immunologic responses in an HIV-infected person. Current antiretroviral therapy provides only modest and transient rises in circulating CD4+ lymphocytes. Improved antiretroviral therapies may provide larger and more sustained increases, but given the alterations in lymphoid tissue including the thymus, lymph nodes, and bone marrow, the goal of immunologic reconstitution must consider abnormalities in these microenvironments.

CLINICAL EVALUATION OF THE PATIENT

The clinical approach to the HIV-infected patient should be guided by several important principles. First, it is important to establish the degree of immunosuppression in every patient through the history and physical examination and the measurement of absolute CD4+ lymphocyte count. Second, past histories of sexually transmitted diseases (STD's), positive PPD testing or exposure to tuberculosis, and places of residence may be very useful in predicting complications of HIV infection. Third, the sharing of pertinent medical information with patients may improve the quality of personal observations that they report to the physician in subsequent visits, and may also improve the physician's ability to establish early diagnoses, provide effective outpatient treatment, and communicate regarding treatment options and risk reduction. Information regarding the stage of HIV disease, and thus the degree of immunosuppression, provides important insight into predicting clinical complications and guiding therapeutic decisions. Such a clinical approach allows the physician to optimize the chronic management and counseling of HIV-infected persons.

THE INITIAL EVALUATION. The initial evaluation of an HIV-infected person should begin with a careful history of past evaluations for HIV infection. Previous history of risk behaviors, mononucleosis-like symptoms that could represent acute HIV infection, and previous HIV testing may all offer insight into the duration of HIV infection. Previous CD4+ lymphocyte counts, history of AIDS indicator conditions, or other clinical manifestations of HIV infection assist in establishing the patient's CDC (Centers for Disease Control and Prevention) classification of HIV infection (Fig. 372–2). The physician must also elicit a medical history, especially a history of STD's (syphilis, herpes simplex, hepatitis B, genital or perianal warts, and cervical dysplasia as important examples), past PPD testing or exposure to tuberculosis, substance abuse, and medication allergies. On physical examination, particular attention should be focused on the skin (severe seborrhea, molluscum contagiosum, chronic herpetic ulcerations, and Kaposi's sarcoma all suggest progressive HIV infection), lymph nodes (generalized lymphadenopathy usually correlates with earlier HIV infection and involution may signal progression of disease), oropharynx (candidiasis, oral hairy leukoplakia, and Kaposi's sarcoma indicate progression), genitalia (severe warts, recurrent vaginal candidiasis, frequently recurrent or severe herpetic ulcerations, cervical dysplasia, and Kaposi's sarcoma suggest progression), and central nervous system (neurocognitive and memory deficits suggest progression to AIDS dementia). The initial laboratory examination should include a complete blood count with differential, routine chemistries including liver enzymes and serum creatinine, absolute CD4+ lymphocyte count and CD4+ lymphocyte percentage, and syphilis and toxoplasma serologies. Patients should also undergo 5 TU PPD testing, and a positive response in an HIV-infected patient is defined as ≥ 5 mm induration. All HIV-infected patients should receive the pneumococcal pneumonia vaccine because of their increased risk of pneumococcal infections, and the influenza vaccine yearly. The hepatitis B vaccine may be given to previously uninfected patients.

Once the initial evaluation is complete (Table 372–1), the physician should be able to establish a CDC classification and use it to design a therapeutic plan. In addition, potential coinfections with *Treponema pallidum* or *Mycobacterium tuberculosis* should be recognized and treated for personal and public health benefits. Finally, counseling may result in the reduction of risk behaviors through education and the identification and treatment of substance abuse.

SUBSEQUENT EVALUATIONS. The intensity and frequency of follow-up examinations depend upon individual patient characteristics and progression of HIV disease. Absolute CD4+ lymphocyte counts should be followed at least every 6 months when ≥ 200 cells per cubic millimeter and should be followed more closely if they are rapidly changing or nearing a therapeutic landmark.

EVALUATING THE FEBRILE PATIENT. Fever is a common physical finding among patients with HIV infection, and the potential causes are many. Fever may indicate a self-limited viral upper respiratory tract infection in a patient with early HIV infection or the presence of PCP in a patient with progressive HIV infection. Differentiating the clinical manifestations of the two infections may be difficult for the physician; therefore, the physician should use any available information on HIV staging for the patient. In this context, the absolute CD4 lymphocyte count may be an extremely useful guide in assessing the likelihood of opportunistic infections. If the absolute CD4 lymphocyte count is > 200 cells per cubic mil-

FIGURE 372–2. CDC Classification System for HIV Infection. The shaded areas (classes A3, B3, C1-3) meet the CDC definition of AIDS. PGL = Progressive generalized lymphadenopathy.

	A Asymptomatic or PGL	B Early symptomatic HIV disease	C AIDS Indicator Conditions
1 CD4 > 500/mm³	A1	B1	C1
2 CD4 200-499/mm³	A2	B2	C2
3 CD4 < 200/mm³	A3	B3	C3

TABLE 372–1. INITIAL EVALUATION OF HIV-INFECTED PATIENTS

History
  How long have they been infected with HIV?
  What complications of HIV have occurred?
  What past evaluations have they undergone?
  What past treatments have they received?
  Any past history of STD's?
  Past history of positive PPD or exposure to tuberculosis?
  Medications and allergies?
  Substance abuse?
  Residential history?

Physical examination

Laboratory evaluation
  CBC with differential
  Chemistries including liver enzymes and serum creatinine
  Absolute CD4+ lymphocyte count and CD4+ lymphocyte percentage
  Syphilis and toxoplasma serologies

PPD testing

Immunizations
  Pneumococcal vaccine
  Influenza vaccine
  Hepatitis B vaccine if nonimmune

limeter, the likelihood of PCP or other opportunistic infections is significantly decreased. Thus, the absolute CD4 lymphocyte count may guide the most appropriate diagnostic considerations. Of note, the uncommon patient may present with an opportunistic infection at absolute CD4+ lymphocyte counts >200 cells per cubic millimeter; therefore, it is imperative to reconsider such diagnoses if the fever persists.

The source of fever is most frequently identified by a patient's history and physical examination; a directed diagnostic evaluation may then be undertaken. If no immediate source is apparent, patients with progressive HIV infection should have a blood culture for MAC and a serum cryptococcal antigen performed. Patients with persistent unexplained fevers may require repeated clinical and laboratory evaluations to elucidate its cause.

See Ch. 371 for discussion of specific antiretroviral therapies.

COMPLICATIONS OF HIV INFECTION

As HIV infection progresses, it creates increasing immunosuppression resulting in a predisposition to complicating opportunistic infections and neoplasms (Figs. 372–1 and 372–3). The pattern of these complications can be predicted by following a patient's absolute CD4+ lymphocyte count. On the basis of these correlations between absolute CD4+ lymphocytes and the predicted complications of HIV infection, clinicians can anticipate an increased risk of certain opportunistic infections in an individual patient, which may lead to an earlier diagnosis or the use of antimicrobial prophylaxis to prevent specific opportunistic infections. Successful prophylaxis has been identified against PCP, toxoplasmic encephalitis, disseminated MAC infection, and cryptococcal meningitis (Table 372–2).

Persons at highest risk for PCP include those recovering from their first episode (secondary prophylaxis, 1-year risk of recurrence without prophylaxis 60%), those with absolute CD4+ lymphocytes ≤200 cells per cubic millimeter (primary prophylaxis, 1-year risk of PCP ≥ 18%), those with CD4+ lymphocyte percentages <20%, and those with a non-PCP AIDS indicator condition (both primary prophylaxis). Sulfamethoxazole-trimethoprim (SMX-TMP) is the most successful prophylaxis against PCP, and dapsone or aerosolized pentamidine may be used as alternative prophylactic regimens in patients intolerant of SMX-TMP. SMX-TMP probably can also prevent toxoplasmic encephalitis among patients who are seropositive for previous infection with *Toxoplasma gondii*.

Recent clinical trials have demonstrated that rifabutin can delay disseminated MAC infection. Rifabutin is FDA-approved for patients at highest risk, usually those with absolute CD4+ lymphocytes < 100 cells per cubic millimeter. Fluconazole has also demonstrated efficacy in delaying cryptococcal meningitis in patients with absolute CD4+ lymphocytes <200 cells per cubic millimeter. Important longer-term issues that still need to be resolved with the use of rifabutin and fluconazole as prophylaxes include their effectiveness over prolonged periods, the possible evolution of resistance among MAC and cryptococcal isolates, pharmacokinetic interactions with other drugs commonly prescribed for patients with AIDS, and uncertain cost effectiveness.

PCP was once the most common AIDS indicator condition, but HIV-associated wasting, disseminated MAC infection, and CMV disease are now more common clinical manifestations. Undoubtedly the future complications of progressive HIV infection will continue to evolve as improved prophylactic strategies against additional opportunistic infections are identified and survival lengthens for persons with AIDS.

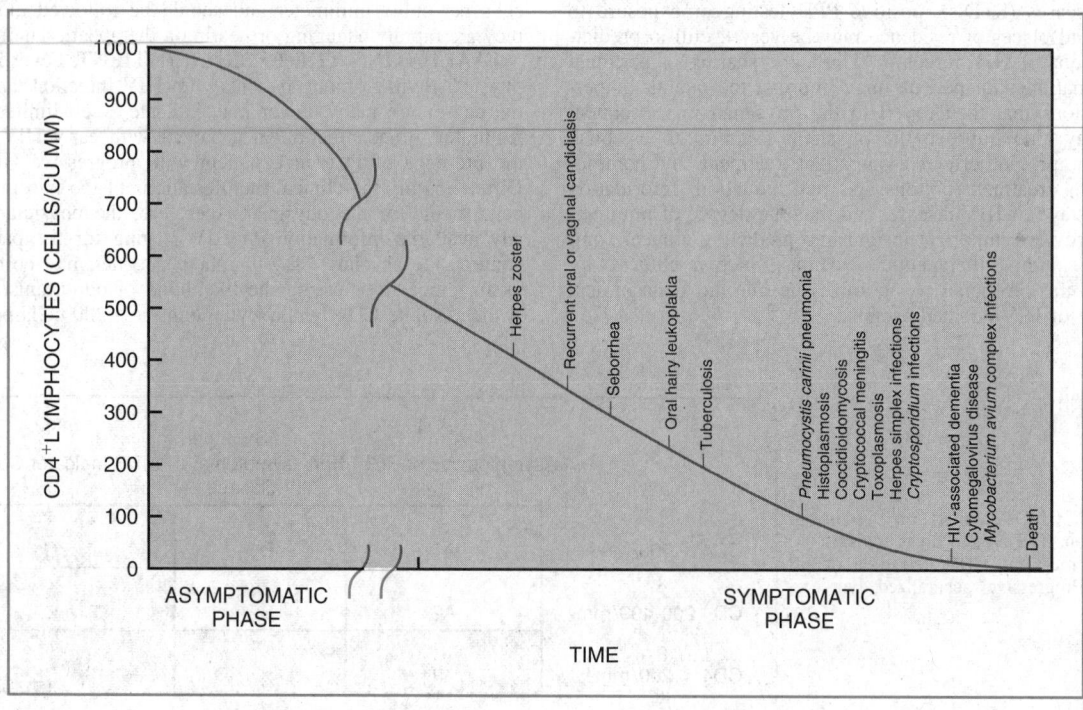

FIGURE 372–3. Complications of HIV disease as related to lymphocyte count.

TABLE 372-2. PROPHYLAXIS OF OPPORTUNISTIC INFECTIONS

Infection	Available Agents	Comments
Pneumocystis carinii pneumonia	SMX-TMP	SMX-TMP most effective and least expensive but potentially toxic
	Dapsone Aerosolized pentamidine	
Mycobacterium avium complex (MAC)	Rifabutin	Delay in disseminated MAC infection; costly; pharmacokinetic interaction with zidovudine; emergence of resistance unknown
Toxoplasmic encephalitis	SMX-TMP?	Preliminary data encouraging
Cryptococcal meningitis	Fluconazole	Delay in cryptococcal meningitis but costly; emergence of fungal resistance reported but of uncertain significance

SMX-TMP = sulfamethoxazole-trimethoprim.

When patients do develop opportunistic infections, clinicians should attempt to establish a diagnosis and initiate treatment as soon as possible. Early diagnosis results in an improved prognosis for most opportunistic infections, and with early diagnosis many patients may receive outpatient therapy. Successful outpatient therapy frequently results in greater patient satisfaction and lower health care costs.

Wasting is also a common complication of progressive HIV infection, either associated primarily with HIV itself or as a secondary manifestation of an opportunistic infection or neoplasm. The pathogenesis of HIV-associated wasting involves multiple potential processes: anorexia with decreased caloric intake, nausea and vomiting, intestinal malabsorption due to HIV enteropathy or an opportunistic infection in the gut, and the ineffective use of nutrients. The metabolic disarray induced in wasted patients with HIV infection results in profound catabolism, perhaps mediated by cytokines such as tumor necrosis factor, and interleukin-1 and -6. Reversing the wasting process may be extremely difficult; attempts to treat opportunistic infections, neoplasms, and the underlying HIV infection can improve nutritional status. Megestrol acetate and dronabinol have been used with modest success to stimulate appetite. Nutritional support may provide improvement in some patients, but in many the catabolism of late-stage HIV infection and its complications cannot be overcome.

COUNSELING

Counseling HIV-infected patients can present great challenges to their physicians. Many HIV-infected persons enter the physician-patient relationship with significant emotional distress and numerous complicating circumstances. These complicating circumstances can include issues of sexual orientation and sexuality, the need for risk reduction, substance abuse, societal discrimination, and increasing poverty as the epidemic evolves in the United States. The physician must enter this relationship prepared to address these issues with knowledge and compassion and without becoming judgmental about their content.

A crucial component involved in counseling HIV-infected persons is education concerning HIV disease, its transmission, and its potential treatments. This process should continue for the duration of the physician-patient relationship, and given the extensive knowledge base of many persons with HIV infection, there may be a mutual exchange of important information. The best medical interventions will not succeed unless HIV-infected persons have been carefully counseled regarding their potential benefits, costs, and acquisition. A well-informed patient can be a strong ally in tackling difficult therapeutic decisions, and many therapeutic decisions are currently not straightforward, such as the optimal time to initiate antiretroviral therapy. A well-informed patient may better recognize the early manifestations of HIV-related clinical complications and potential drug toxicities. Finally, a well-informed patient can constructively guide decisions regarding advance directives for his/her care if HIV disease progresses.

Education regarding the transmission of HIV and alterations in risk behavior is another important goal of counseling. Efforts to encourage behavioral changes resulting in temporarily decreased HIV transmission have succeeded in homosexual men in San Francisco, although recent evidence suggests an increasing number of new infections, especially among young individuals. Intensive efforts to decrease HIV transmission have also succeeded in smaller populations of injecting drug users and high-risk heterosexuals. All patients should be well informed regarding safer sex precautions and the avoidance of needle sharing. This information must be presented in language appropriate to the culture of the patient. Significant behavioral changes are frequently not accomplished during a single visit, and enduring change requires ongoing re-education and support from the physician.

Treating substance abuse (see Ch. 12) is crucial in decreasing the risk of HIV transmission through needle sharing and sexual contact and in avoiding the medical and psychological consequences of continued substance abuse. Physicians must advocate for their patients in seeking access to frequently inadequate and overwhelmed drug treatment programs. Physicians must acknowledge the high recidivism rates associated with substance abuse and continue to treat their recidivous patients firmly and without judgment. Finally, physicians should reinforce positively those recovering addicts who have succeeded in treatment and struggle to avoid relapse on a daily basis.

The clinical course of persons with HIV infection is frequently complicated by significant anxiety and depression. Pharmacologic measures may prove useful in their management, although anxiolytics should be used cautiously, given the prevalence of substance abuse in this population. In the circumstance of late-stage HIV infection complicated by HIV encephalopathy and depression, ritalin may prove useful. Physicians should identify AIDS service organizations in their community that may provide support services such as patient education, case management, transportation, shelter, food, medications, or support groups to their clients. Formal psychiatric referral may also be necessary in individual patients.

Complications

Hoover D, Saah A, Bacellar H, et al.: Clinical manifestations of AIDS in the era of pneumocystis prophylaxis. N Engl J Med 329:1922, 1993. *Reviews the changing clinical complications of AIDS.*

Nightingale S, Cameron W, Gordin F, et al.: Two controlled trials of rifabutin prophylaxis against *Mycobacterium avium* complex infection in AIDS. N Engl J Med 329:828, 1993. *The reports of two pivotal trials evaluating rifabutin prophylaxis against MAC infection.*

Counseling

Bartlett JG: Medical Management of HIV Infection. Glenview, IL, Physicians and Scientists Publishing Co., 1994. *A review for health care professionals describing the medical management of HIV-infected persons.*

Cates W, Hinman A: AIDS and absolutism—the demand for perfection in prevention. N Engl J Med 327:492, 1992. *Describes preventive measures for HIV infection and their role in public health.*

Hellinger F: The lifetime cost of treating a person with HIV. JAMA 270:474, 1993. *An informative review of the costs associated with treating HIV-infected persons.*

373 INTRODUCTION TO PROTOZOAN AND HELMINTHIC DISEASES

Adel A. F. Mahmoud

Human infections with parasitic protozoa and helminths account for a major proportion of the diseases caused by infectious agents. The magnitude of these infections is staggering; malaria infects 600 million, and ascariasis and trichuriasis 1 billion each, and 600 million are estimated to be infected with either schistosomiasis or filariasis. In spite of some worldwide efforts to control the spread and consequences of these infections, the associated morbidity and mortality have not been appreciably reduced. Furthermore, in the developed countries, infection with protozoa and helminths is being seen with increasing frequency in immigrants and is also among the more important causes of disease in the growing number of patients with depressed immune responses.

BIOLOGY OF PARASITIC PROTOZOA AND HELMINTHS

The host-parasite relationship in protozoan and helminthic infections is complex because of the distinctive biologic features of the organisms. Although protozoa are unicellular pathogens and are mainly microscopic in size, they are far larger than viruses and bacteria. Protozoa multiply within mammalian hosts, as do viruses, bacteria, and fungi. Infection, therefore, can be initiated by a relatively small inoculum of organisms, which then multiply within the host and reach the numbers that cause disease.

By contrast, helminths are multicellular organisms with well-developed organ structures. They vary in size from 1 cm to approximately 10 meters. Unlike other infectious agents, helminths do not multiply within mammalian hosts. Re-exposure is, therefore, necessary to increase the number of helminths in a host. This distinguishing feature has important clinical significance, as disease in most helminthiasis is closely related to intensity of infection. For example, anemia results from hookworm infection only if the individual is harboring a significant worm load or there are other reasons for nutritional deficiencies. In rare circumstances, such as strongyloidiasis in the immunosuppressed, the worm can increase population of its larval stage in humans through the autoinfection cycle.

Eosinophilia, when present, is a useful clinical manifestation of worm infections that migrate in host tissues. Worms that reside exclusively in body cavities, such as adult cestodes in the lumen of small intestine, are not associated with eosinophilia. Specific chemotherapy is usually followed by an increase in eosinophil count before it subsides to normal levels. Eosinophilia in helminthic infections may be related to the cell's ability to kill multicellular organisms. Because of the large size of most invading worms, these targets are killed by eosinophils extracellulary and killing is mediated by a combination of oxidative and nonoxidative mechanisms.

Parasitic protozoa and helminths have developed elaborate mechanisms for evading host protective responses. One of the best studied is antigenic variation noted in African trypanosomiasis. Parasitemia in infected individuals appears in waves, each representing a new parasite variable antigen. The trypanosomes are capable of expressing at least 100 different variable antigens, allowing a long chronic course of infection. The organisms contain individual genes for all the different variable glycoproteins, but only one is expressed at a time. The multiplicity of trypanosome variable glycoprotein genes and of mechanisms for introducing mutations into them illustrates the complexity and sophistication of the evasion techniques used by these pathogens.

The constantly changing nature of infectious disease is best illustrated in parasitic protozoan and helminthic infections. For example, new human pathogens such as *Isospora* and *Cryptosporidium* species have been appreciated only recently as causes of diarrheal illness, particularly in the immunosuppressed. These new developments add to difficulties in treating and controlling parasitic protozoa and helminths. Recently, new chemotherapeutic agents have been developed, such as praziquantel and ivermectin, which are safe and effective broad-spectrum antihelminthics. However, the ever-spreading resistance of the parasites causing malaria and their mosquito vectors to most available compounds is imposing a considerable challenge to clinicians and public health specialists.

APPROACH TO THE PATIENT WITH PROTOZOAN OR HELMINTHIC INFECTION

Because most of the clinical manifestations of protozoan and helminthic diseases are not specific or pathognomonic, a high degree of suspicion is essential. The simple question "Where have you been?" and knowledge of the general geographic distribution of parasitic protozoa and helminths often save exhaustive and costly diagnostic workups and may spare human lives. Furthermore, inquiry into the immune status of individual patients, other drug therapies, or other diseases may be helpful in establishing the diagnosis of an opportunistic protozoan or helminthic infection.

The next phase in attempting to reach correct diagnosis involves interpreting the presenting symptoms and signs. Peripheral blood eosinophilia remains an important and early indication of infections with tissue-invading worms. Definitive diagnosis in most cases requires isolation and identification of the specific pathogen. Because the number of cases seen by any single laboratory in North America is limited, expertise is required for correct identification that may not be available to many practicing physicians. Serologic testing for evidence of exposure to specific protozoa or helminths is currently available in many clinical or state laboratories or by consultation with the Centers for Disease Control and Prevention.

Centers for Disease Control: HHS Publication No. (CDC) 94-8280. Health Information for International Travel, Atlanta, Georgia, 1994, 188 pp. *A review of the geographic distribution of worldwide infections, updated yearly. It also contains the most recent recommendations for prophylaxis.*

Drugs for parasitic infections. Med Lett Drugs 35:111, 1993. *A review of antiparasitic drugs published and updated annually. It includes dose, availability, and alternative choices.*

Mahmoud AAF: Parasitic protozoa and helminths: Biological and immunological challenges. Science 246:1015, 1989. *A selected review of some of the unique biologic, immunologic, and molecular aspects of malaria and schistosomes that accounts for the ability of these organisms to invade and establish themselves as parasites in humans.*

Mahmoud AAF (ed.): Tropical and Geographical Medicine. 2nd ed. Companion Handbook. New York, McGraw-Hill, 1993. *Clinical, epidemiologic, and management principles for dealing with infectious diseases seen in North America and worldwide.*

Warren KS, Mahmoud AAF (eds.): Tropical and Geographical Medicine. 2nd ed. New York, McGraw-Hill, 1990. *Detailed description of the biology and molecular understanding of protozoa and helminths and the diseases they cause in individuals and in populations.*

Protozoan Diseases

374 MALARIA
Donald J. Krogstad

Malaria is a disease characterized by recurrent fever and chills associated with the synchronous lysis of parasitized red blood cells. Its name is derived from the belief of the ancient Romans that malaria was due to the bad air of the marshes surrounding Rome.

ETIOLOGY. Malaria is produced by intraerythrocytic parasites of the genus *Plasmodium*. Four plasmodia produce malaria in humans: *Plasmodium falciparum, P. vivax, P. ovale,* and *P. malariae.* The severity and characteristic manifestations of the disease are governed by the infecting species, the magnitude of the parasitemia, the metabolic effects of the parasite, and the cytokines released as a result of the infection.

INCIDENCE, PREVALENCE, AND RESURGENCE. *Incidence.* Although precise data are difficult to obtain, malaria is unquestionably one of the most common infectious diseases. At least 200 to 300 million cases of malaria occur each year, with 1 to 2 million deaths. Most deaths are due to *P. falciparum* infection and occur among children less than 5 years old in sub-Saharan Africa. One of the major unanswered questions about malaria is how plasmodia produce repetitive infections without stimulating an effective (protective) immune response.

Prevalence. The prevalence of malaria varies widely; it may reach 70 to 80% or more among children in hyperendemic areas during the transmission season. Thus its impact on the health of the developing world is enormous.

Resurgence. The major factors responsible for the resurgence of malaria are drug resistances: (1) the widespread resistance of the anopheline vector to economical insecticides such as chlorophenothane (DDT), and (2) the increasing prevalence of chloroquine resistance in *P. falciparum,* which is now endemic in South America, Southeast Asia, and Africa.

LIFE CYCLE AND EPIDEMIOLOGY. *Life Cycle.* The life cycle can be viewed as beginning with synchronous asexual replication of the erythrocytic stage of the parasite (Fig. 374–1). During the asexual erythrocytic cycle, the parasites mature from rings to trophozoites to schizonts, which ultimately rupture the red cell and release merozoites that enter uninfected red cells via receptors such as Duffy factor in *P. vivax;* the cycle is then repeated. By contrast, some erythrocytic parasites mature to sexual forms (gametocytes) that are ingested by the female anopheline mosquito. Within the mosquito intermediate host, male and female gametocytes mature to gametes, fuse to form an ookinete that matures to a zygote and ultimately produces the sporozoites that are infectious for humans. When an infected mosquito bites a human, sporozoites travel via the bloodstream to the liver, where they enter hepatocytes and mature to tissue schizonts, which release merozoites that are infectious for red cells and produce the asexual erythrocytic cycle. Two of the four species that infect humans (*P. vivax* and *P. ovale*) produce dormant (hypnozoite) forms in the liver, which mature 6 to 11 months or more after the initial infection and thus produce relapsing malaria.

Two characteristics of the life cycle are essential for the long-term survival of the parasite: multiplicity of replication and antigenic variability. *Multiplicity of replication* is apparent at each stage of the life cycle. The mature asexual erythrocytic schizont releases 8 to 32 merozoites when it ruptures its host red cell; up to 10,000 sporozoites result from one zygote; and 10,000 to 30,000 merozoites are released from one tissue (exoerythrocytic) schizont in the liver. This multiplicity of replication provides a redundancy that protects the parasite against losses from both immune and nonimmune host factors. *Antigenic variability* is associated with the morphologic changes that occur during the parasite's life cycle and similarly protects the parasite against the host immune response. For example, antibodies against sporozoites are ineffective against the asexual erythrocytic stages of the parasite. Similarly, immune responses directed against asexual erythrocytic stages have no effect against the sexual (gametocyte) stages of the parasite. In addition, antigenic variation exists among strains of the same species. These

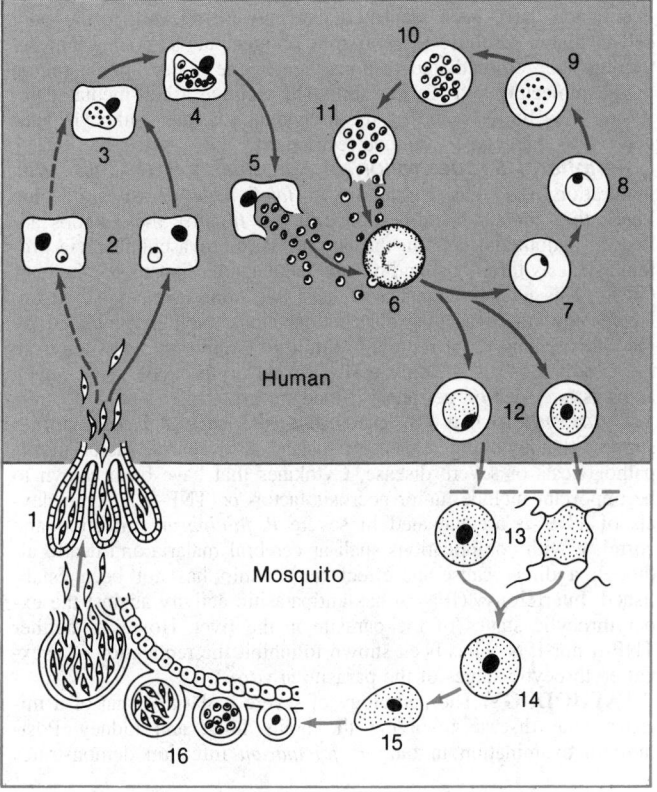

FIGURE 374–1. Life cycle of the malaria parasite. The lower and upper halves of the diagram indicate the anopheline mosquito and human parts of the cycle, respectively. Sporozoites from the salivary gland of a female *Anopheles* mosquito are injected under the skin (1). They then travel through the bloodstream to the liver (2) and mature within hepatocytes to tissue *schizonts* (4). Up to 30,000 parasites are then released into the bloodstream as *merozoites* (5) and produce symptomatic infection as they invade and destroy red blood cells. However, some parasites remain dormant in the liver as *hypnozoites* (*2, dashed lines from 1 to 3*). These are the parasites that cause relapsing malaria (in *P. vivax* or *P. ovale* infection). Once within the bloodstream, merozoites (5) invade red cells (6) and mature to the *ring* (7,8), *trophozoite* (9), and *schizont* (10) asexual stages. Schizonts lyse their host red cells as they mature and release the next generation of merozoites (11), which invade previously uninfected red cells. Within the red cell some parasites differentiate to sexual forms (male and female *gametocytes*) (12). When taken up by a female *Anopheles* mosquito, the gametocytes mature to *male* and *female gametes,* which produce *zygotes* (14). The zygote invades the gut of the mosquito (15) and develops into an *oocyst* (16). Mature oocysts produce *sporozoites,* which migrate to the salivary gland of the mosquito (1) and repeat the cycle. The dashed line between 12 and 13 indicates that absence of the mosquito vector prevents natural transmission via this cycle. Infection by the injection of contaminated blood bypasses this constraint and permits transmission among intravenous drug addicts or to recipients of blood transfusions. (Reproduced with permission from Krogstad DJ: Blood and tissue protozoa. *In* Schaechter M, Medoff G, Eisenstein BI [eds.]: Mechanisms of Microbial Diseases. 2nd ed © 1993, p 600, the Williams & Wilkins Company, Baltimore.)

observations are critically relevant to the development of a malaria vaccine (see below).

Epidemiology. The epidemiology of malaria is determined by the distributions of the anopheline mosquito vectors required for natural transmission and of the infected human reservoir. Both factors are present in endemic areas throughout the tropics. Important determinants of transmission include the vector population (vectors such as *Anopheles gambiae* in Africa are thought to be more efficient), temperature (elevated temperatures shorten the life of the vector and hasten the maturation of the parasite within the vector), and control programs (which reduce both the vector population and the prevalence of human infection).

Competent mosquito vectors are present in the United States (*A. albimanus* in the east and *A. freeborni* in the west). Although transmission in the United States is limited by the absence of infected humans, natural mosquito-borne transmission can and does occur with the importation of infected humans (e.g., the return of soldiers after their exposure in endemic areas). Mosquito-borne transmission (*introduced malaria*) occurred in the United States after World War II, the Korean War, the Vietnam War, and the arrival of refugees from Southeast Asia.

PATHOGENESIS. *Species-Dependent Factors.* Malaria is a multifactorial disease that can be explained in part, but not completely, by the magnitude of the parasitemia. *P. falciparum* is the most lethal parasite because it can invade red cells of any age and can thus produce unrestricted parasitemias involving 10^6 or more parasitized red cells per cubic millimeter of blood ($\geq 20\%$ of circulating red cells). Conversely, *P. vivax* and *P. ovale,* which invade only young red cells, are limited to parasitemias $\leq 25,000$ per cubic millimeter, and *P. malariae,* which invades only older red cells, is limited to parasitemias $\leq 10,000$ per cubic millimeter.

The Host Immune Response. Because millions of people experience repetitive episodes of malaria throughout their lives in the tropics, the immune response to natural infection is inadequate by definition. Thus the term *semi-immune* is used for residents of endemic areas who are at reduced risk of severe or complicated malaria but are reinfected regularly. The reasons for the inadequate host immune response are only partially clear and are likely to be central to developing a successful vaccine. For example, most exposed persons make antibodies directed against the repetitive epitope or epitopes on the surface of the sporozoite, and antibodies to asexual stages have been shown to reduce the magnitude of the parasitemia in children. However, cell-mediated immune responses are less frequent and may be essential for effective immunity. At least two factors have been identified that may be relevant to the poor cell-mediated response to sporozoite antigen: (1) The sites that determine the cell-mediated response are in the hypervariable region of the molecule, and (2) the ability to produce a cell-mediated response may be restricted by the individual's human leukocyte antigen (HLA) haplotype (immune restriction).

Peripheral Sequestration of Parasitized Red Cells. With maturation, red cells containing *P. falciparum* parasites develop knobs that contain histidine-rich proteins. *In vivo,* these knobs adhere to endothelial cells in the peripheral microvasculature via proteins such as thrombospondin, intercellular adhesion molecule 1, or CD36. This phenomenon has at least two consequences: (1) It enhances the microvascular obstruction and pathology produced by the parasite, and (2) it removes mature *P. falciparum* parasites from the circulation, so that only early asexual erythrocytic stages, such as rings, are seen on peripheral blood smears.

Cytokines in the Pathogenesis of Malaria. Recent studies suggest that cytokine release in malaria is a central factor in the pathogenesis of severe disease. Cytokines that have been shown to be important include tumor necrosis factor–α (TNF–α). Serum levels of TNF–α are elevated in severe *P. falciparum* infection and correlate with complications such as cerebral malaria and death, although a direct cause-and-effect relationship has not been established. Interferon-γ (IFN-γ) has antiparasitic activity against the exoerythrocytic stages of the parasite in the liver. However, neither TNF-α nor IFN-γ has been shown to inhibit the replication of asexual erythrocytic stages of the parasite *in vitro*.

PATHOLOGY. The pathology of severe malaria is that of a microvascular disease involving the brain, lung, and kidney. Postmortem examination in fatal *P. falciparum* infection demonstrates parasitized red cells in the capillaries of the brain and other affected organs. In severe cases, acute tubular necrosis may be present, and the liver, spleen, and other sites in the reticuloendothelial system may be filled with dark malarial pigment from the phagocytosis of parasitized red cells. This predominantly microvascular pathology is consistent with the importance of sequestration and cytokine release in the pathogenesis of severe *P. falciparum* malaria (see above). By contrast, the other malarias that infect humans produce lower parasitemias, do not sequester, and are rarely fatal.

CLINICAL MANIFESTATIONS. *Fever and Chills.* Most patients with malaria have recurrent fever and chills (at 48-hour intervals for *P. vivax* and *P. ovale* and at 72-hour intervals for *P. malariae*). By contrast, patients with *P. falciparum* infection typically have irregular fever and chills and rarely present with a regular 48-hour cycle of symptoms despite the 48-hour cycle of the parasite.

Coma. Coma (cerebral malaria) is the most feared complication of *P. falciparum* infection and has a substantial fatality rate. Although it has been attributed to the blockage of capillaries with parasitized red cells, both hypoglycemia and the effects of cytokines such as TNF-α are important factors. Hypoglycemia in *P. falciparum* malaria may have at least three causes: (1) insulin released from the pancreatic β cell by quinine or quinidine during treatment, (2) glucose consumption by the massive numbers of parasites present in the patient, and (3) liver glycogen depletion in persons who have not eaten for several days before seeking medical care because they were ill with malaria. Hypoglycemia is particularly important to consider because it is treatable. Although the effects of TNF-α undoubtedly contribute to cerebral malaria, it is difficult to separate them from the magnitude of the parasitemia because the concentration of TNF-α and the magnitude of the parasitemia correlate with each other.

Renal Failure. Patients with massive parasitemias may have dark urine from the free hemoglobin produced by hemolysis (blackwater fever) and may later develop renal failure. Although hemolysis alone should not produce renal failure, some degree of renal impairment is typical in such patients. In most instances, the patients recover uneventfully; however, acute renal failure may occur with a time course similar to that of other causes of acute tubular necrosis.

Pulmonary Edema. This complication also occurs in patients with high *P. falciparum* parasitemias ($\geq 5\%$ of circulating red cells). Hemodynamic measurements indicate that this is a noncardiogenic form of pulmonary edema with normal pulmonary arterial and capillary pressures. These findings and the association with high TNF-α levels suggest that the pathogenesis of pulmonary edema may be similar in malaria and bacterial septicemia.

Gastrointestinal Manifestations. Diarrhea is common among children with *P. falciparum* infection. Although the pathogenesis of this complication is unclear, postmortem studies of children with diarrhea demonstrate parasitized red cells in the microvasculature of the intestine.

DIAGNOSIS. *Giemsa-Stained Thick and Thin Smears.* The most direct way to diagnose malaria is to prepare and examine Giemsa-stained thick or thin smears using oil immersion magnification ($\times 1000$). Giemsa stain is preferable to Wright's stain, especially for persons with *P. vivax* or *P. ovale* infection, because the Schüffner's dots characteristic of those infections are often not visible with Wright's stain. Thick smears are more sensitive than thin smears because the red cells have been lysed. As a result, approximately 10 times as much blood can be examined per field and thus per unit of time. However, because the red cells have been lysed, it is not possible to determine the effect of the parasite on red cell size or the position of the parasite within the red cell on a thick smear (Table 374–1). Therefore, persons without previous experience in reading thick smears should consider using thin smears to identify the infecting parasite or parasites. A common mistake is to require characteristic gametocytes for a diagnosis of *P. falciparum* infection. Because gametocytes require longer to develop than asexual parasites (7 to 10 versus 2 days), they are usually not present in the peripheral blood when nonimmune tourists or expatriates first become symptomatic. Conversely, gametocytes are frequently present in the blood of semi-immune residents of endemic areas with few or no symptoms or asexual parasites. A second common mistake is to assume that the patient can have only one parasite species: Approximately 5% of persons with malaria have infections due to more than one parasite species.

TABLE 374-1. MALARIA PARASITES THAT INFECT HUMANS

	Parasitemia (per μl blood)	Complications
P. falciparum	$\geq 10^6$	Coma (cerebral malaria) Hypoglycemia Pulmonary edema, renal failure Anemia
P. vivax	$\leq 25,000$	Late (2–3 mo) splenic rupture
P. ovale	$\leq 25,000$	–
P. malariae	$\leq 10,000$	Immune complex nephrotic syndrome

	Morphology		
	Red Blood Cell Size	Schüffner's Dots	Stages
P. falciparum	No RBC enlargement	Absent	Rings, occasionally gametocytes
P. vivax	Enlarged host RBC	Present	All forms
P. ovale	Enlarged host RBC	Absent	All forms
P. malariae	No RBC enlargement	Present	All forms

	Relapse from Hypnozoites	Antimalarial Resistance
P. falciparum	No	Chloroquine and pyrimethamine-sulfadoxine
P. vivax	Yes	Possibly chloroquine
P. ovale	Yes	None known
P. malariae	No	None known

RBC = red blood cell

Fluorescent Staining with Acridine Orange.
Fluorescence microscopy is one of two new techniques for detecting malaria parasites in peripheral blood specimens. This technique takes advantage of the fact that parasitized red cells are less dense than unparasitized red cells. A finger stick specimen is taken into a capillary tube prepared with acridine orange (to stain the nucleic acid of the parasite) and an anticoagulant. After centrifugation, parasitized red cells are found at the top of the red cell layer just below the buffy coat. Experienced investigators can examine a blood specimen in 30 to 40 seconds (less time than necessary to examine a thick or thin smear).

DNA Probes.
Several investigators have developed *Plasmodium* and species-specific (e.g., *P. falciparum*-specific) DNA probes that can detect 40 to 100 parasites per microliter of blood (similar to the 1 to 10 parasites per microliter threshold of the thick smear). Problems that have recently been solved in the application of this technology include the use of signal systems as effective as ^{32}P that are not radioactive and the role of the polymerase chain reaction in enhancing sensitivity under field conditions.

Serology (Antigen Detection).
Recent studies suggest that testing for specific parasite antigens may be an alternative to microscopy. A commercial kit is now available for the diagnosis of *P. falciparum* infection based on detection of histidine-rich protein II.

Serology (Antibody Testing).
Testing for antibodies to plasmodia is of limited value. In endemic areas, most persons have antibody titers from previous infections whether or not they were infected recently. In addition, 3 to 4 weeks may be required to develop a diagnostic rise in antibody titer, whereas the decision to treat must be made in the first few hours of evaluation. However, serology may be of value retrospectively in nonimmune persons (expatriate tourists) who have been treated empirically for malaria without a microscopic diagnosis. For example, a high titer of antibodies against *P. vivax* suggests that the patient has had a recent *P. vivax* infection and should receive primaquine if it has not been given previously (see the section on treatment, below).

PREVENTION. Exposed nonimmune persons may prevent malaria by taking antimalarials prospectively (chemoprophylaxis); by using insect repellents and otherwise reducing contact with the anopheline vector; and possibly, in the future, by a malaria vaccine (immunoprophylaxis).

Chemoprophylaxis.
Drugs used for chemoprophylaxis must be safe because they are given to healthy persons for long periods. They should also have long serum half-lives so that they can be given infrequently. On the basis of these criteria, chloroquine is an excellent drug for chemoprophylaxis in areas without chloroquine-resistant *P. falciparum* (Table 374-2). It is the only chemoprophy-

TABLE 374-2. CHEMOPROPHYLAXIS OF MALARIA*

For Areas without Chloroquine-Resistant *Plasmodium falciparum*:

Chloroquine phosphate (Aralen)	500 mg/wk (300 mg chloroquine base) during exposure and for 4 wk after leaving the endemic area

For Areas with Chloroquine-Resistant *Plasmodium falciparum*:

Mefloquine (Lariam)	250 mg/wk during exposure and for 4 wk after leaving the endemic area
Doxycycline	100 mg/d during exposure and for 4 wk after leaving the endemic area

* Updated recommendations on malaria chemoprophylaxis may be obtained 24 hours a day, 7 days a week, through the Centers for Disease Control and Prevention (CDC) Hot Line at (404) 332-4555.

lactic agent known to be safe for pregnant women and does not produce retinal toxicity at the doses used for antimalarial chemoprophylaxis. Unfortunately, chloroquine-resistant strains of *P. falciparum* are now established in Southeast Asia, South America, and Africa. For areas with chloroquine-resistant *P. falciparum,* mefloquine is now the recommended chemoprophylactic agent, although resistance to mefloquine is developing in Southeast Asia. Doxycycline is an alternative, with the advantage that it also reduces the frequency of traveler's diarrhea. The disadvantages of doxycycline include the need to take it daily, photosensitivity reactions, and vaginitis. Because of hypersensitivity reactions to pyrimethamine-sulfadoxine (Fansidar) and both agranulocytosis and hepatitis with amodiaquine, neither of these agents is recommended for chemoprophylaxis.

Vector Control.
Because of widespread drug resistance in *P. falciparum,* increasing emphasis is placed on reducing exposure to the anopheline vector, especially in hyperendemic areas such as Africa. Strategies that are successful and should be considered include DEET-containing insect repellents and pyrethrin (insecticide)–impregnated bed nets. DDT is no longer effective in most regions of the world because of widespread resistance.

Immunoprophylaxis—Development of a Malaria Vaccine.
Although a malaria vaccine is not available, it is hoped that this goal will ultimately be achievable. Because the three major parasite stages in humans are antigenically distinct, a successful vaccine will likely need to contain at least three parasite antigens (sporozoite, merozoite, and gametocyte). However, a vaccine need not be 100% effective to be valuable. For example, a vaccine that would require boosting could be quite effective because of repetitive exposure to natural infection in endemic areas. In addition, a vaccine that limited the magnitude of the parasitemia could have a marked effect on survival even if it had no effect on the incidence of infection, because severe morbidity and death are associated with high parasitemias.

TREATMENT. Successful treatment of patients with malaria depends primarily on effective antimalarial drugs. However, it also depends on ancillary measures as diverse as the infusion of glucose and exchange transfusion. Monitoring of the blood glucose level is important because hypoglycemia is a common cause of coma and because both quinine and quinidine stimulate the release of insulin directly from the pancreatic β cell. Steroids are contraindicated in cerebral malaria because they prolong the duration of coma.

The treatment of chloroquine-susceptible malaria (*P. vivax, P. ovale,* or *P. malariae* malaria and chloroquine-susceptible *P. falciparum* malaria) is satisfactory (Table 374-3) because chloroquine is a safe and effective antimalarial. Some patients with chloroquine-resistant *P. vivax* have been treated successfully with 1500 mg chloroquine base (25 mg base per kilogram) orally after failing to respond to 600 mg base, whereas others have required treatment with mefloquine. However, the treatment of chloroquine-resistant *P. falciparum* malaria is unsatisfactory. Potential choices include quinidine, quinine, and mefloquine. For comatose patients, intravenous quinidine may be the safest treatment. The risk of quinidine cardiovascular toxicity is low with the measurement of serum quinidine levels (2.0 to 5.0 μg per milliliter is usually adequate; ≥ 6 μg per milliliter is potentially toxic) and cardiac monitoring (for a QT interval >0.6 second or QRS widening beyond 25% of baseline) during intravenous infusion. Although pyrimethamine-sulfadoxine (Fansidar) has been used for treatment, it is now controversial because of the

TABLE 374-3. TREATMENT OF MALARIA

P. vivax, P. ovale, P. malariae, and Chloroquine-Susceptible P. falciparum:

For patients unable to take oral medications:

IM chloroquine:	2.5 mg/kg IM q 4 hr or 3.5 mg/kg q 6 hr (total dose not to exceed 25 mg/kg base)
IV chloroquine:	10 mg/kg base over 4 hr, followed by 5 mg/kg base q 12 hr (given in a 2-hr infusion; total dose not to exceed 25 mg/kg base)

For patients able to take oral medications:

PO chloroquine:	10 mg/kg = 600-mg base, followed by an additional 300-mg base after 6 hr and 300-mg base again on days 2 and 3

Chloroquine-Resistant P. falciparum:

For patients unable to take oral medications:

IV quinidine:	6.25 mg/kg quinidine base (10 mg/kg quinidine gluconate) IV over 1 to 2 hr, followed by a constant infusion of 0.0125 mg/kg quinidine base (0.02 mg/kg quinidine gluconate) IV per minute until the parasitemia is < 1% or oral treatment is tolerated

For patients able to take oral medications:

PO quinine:*	650 mg quinine sulfate (540 mg quinine base) q 8 hr until significant improvement, or for 10 day

or

PO mefloquine:	750 mg as a single oral dose followed by 500 mg in 6–8 hr

or

PO halofantrine†	(500 mg q 6 hr × 3 doses, and repeat in 1 week) is an alternative, but is not effective against mefloquine-resistant parasite

or

PO pyrimethamine + sulfadoxine:	3 tablets (75 mg pyrimethamine plus 1500 mg sulfadoxine) as a single dose

To Prevent Relapse in P. vivax or P. ovale Infection:

PO primaquine:‡	15 mg primaquine base (26.3 mg primaquine phosphate) daily × 14 day

* In addition to oral quinine a number of investigators recommend tetracycline (250 mg PO q 6 hr for 7 to 10 days), pyrimethamine plus sulfadiazine or sulfisoxazole (25 mg twice daily plus 500 mg q 6 hr PO for 5 days), or 3 tablets of pyrimethamine-sulfadoxine (total of 75 plus 1500 mg PO once).
† Not yet available in the United States.
‡ To prevent potentially severe hemolysis, patients should be tested for glucose-6-phosphate dehydrogenase deficiency prior to treatment with primaquine.

increasing prevalence of resistance in areas of chloroquine resistance.

Patients with *P. vivax* or *P. ovale* infection should be tested for glucose-6-phosphate dehydrogenase deficiency before treatment with primaquine, which is used to eradicate persistent hypnozoites in the liver to prevent relapse.

PROGNOSIS. Virtually all patients with *P. vivax*, *P. ovale*, or *P. malariae* infection respond well to chloroquine and make an uneventful recovery. The chloroquine-resistant strains of *P. vivax* reported from Indonesia have thus far responded to treatment with either mefloquine or full-dose chloroquine (1.5 grams base). For patients with *P. falciparum* infection, the quantitative parasite count is the best predictor of the outcome. Patients with ≥5% parasitemia (≥ 250,000 parasites per microliter of blood) are at increased risk of severe and complicated malaria, including death. In addition to standard antimalarial treatment (outlined above), such patients should be considered for more heroic measures, such as exchange transfusion, if they do not improve within the first 12 to 24 hours of treatment.

Canfield CJ, Chongsuphajaisiddhi T, Danis M, et al.: Severe and complicated malaria. Trans R Soc Trop Med Hyg 89 (Suppl 2):1, 1990. *A comprehensive review of the pathogenesis and treatment of severe falciparum malaria.*

Good MF, Pombo D, Quakyi IA, et al.: Human T-cell recognition of the circumsporozoite protein of *Plasmodium falciparum:* Immunodominant T-cell domains map to the polymorphic regions of the molecule. Proc Natl Acad Sci USA 85:1199, 1988. *Evidence that the determinants of T-cell reactivity are in hypervariable regions of the circumsporozoite protein.*

Grau GE, Taylor TE, Molyneux ME, et al.: Tumor necrosis factor and disease severity in children with falciparum malaria. N Engl J Med 320:1586, 1989. *Serum levels of TNF are increased in children with severe falciparum malaria.*

Krogstad DJ, Gluzman IY, Klye DE, et al.: Efflux of chloroquine from *Plasmodium falciparum:* Mechanism of chloroquine resistance. Science 238:1283, 1987. *The*

basis of chloroquine resistance is rapid efflux of the drug from the resistant parasite.

Kwiatkowski D, Molyneux ME, Stephens S, et al.: Anti-TNF therapy inhibits fever in cerebral malaria. Q J Med 86:91, 1993. *Monoclonal antibodies against TNF-α do not reduce morbidity or mortality, although they do reduce fever in children with severe malaria.*

Miller LH, Good MF, Milon G: Malaria pathogenesis. Science 264:1878, 1994. *Major unresolved issues highlighted include the lack of protective immunity after natural infection and the role of factors such as cytokines and host receptor molecules in the cytoadherence associated with cerebral malaria.*

Udeinya IJ, Schmidt JA, Aikawa M, et al.: Falciparum malaria-infected erythrocytes specifically bind to cultured human endothelial cells. Science 213:555, 1981. *Knobs on falciparum-infected cells bind to endothelial cells and thus explain the sequestration of red cells with mature falciparum parasites.*

White NJ, Warrell DA, Chanthavanich P, et al.: Severe hypoglycemia and hyperinsulinemia in falciparum malaria. N Engl J Med 309:61, 1983. *Hypoglycemia results from utilization of liver glycogen stores while not eating in the early stages of the illness, from parasite consumption of glucose, and from the release of insulin from pancreatic β-cells by quinine (or quinidine).*

375 AFRICAN TRYPANOSOMIASIS (Sleeping Sickness)

Thomas C. Quinn

DEFINITION. Known widely as sleeping sickness, African trypanosomiasis is an acute and chronic disease caused by *Trypanosoma brucei*. The parasites are transmitted to humans through the bite of tsetse flies located in regions of Africa between 15 degrees north and 15 degrees south latitude. In humans, there are two distinct forms of the disease, East African trypanosomiasis caused by *T. brucei rhodesiense* and West African trypanosomiasis caused by *T. brucei gambiense*. Although there is some clinical overlap, East African trypanosomiasis primarily causes an acute febrile illness with myocarditis and meningoencephalitis that is rapidly fatal if not treated, whereas West African trypanosomiasis is characterized as a chronic debilitating disease with mental deterioration and physical wasting (Table 375–1). A closely related variant, *T. brucei brucei*, is noninfectious for humans, but causes a chronic wasting illness in cattle, called nagana, which has a considerable indirect effect on human nutrition in sub-Saharan Africa.

ETIOLOGY AND LIFE CYCLE. Trypanosomes are motile hemoflagellates with a single undulating membrane that passes along the length of the parasite, terminating in an anterior flagellum (see Color Plate 10*E*). Located anteriorly is a kinetoplast, an organelle containing topologically interlocked circular DNA molecules and mitochondria. In the peripheral blood of humans, trypanosomes vary in length from 10 to 40 μm. Both short stumpy and long slen-

TABLE 375-1. A COMPARISON OF GAMBIAN AND RHODESIAN SLEEPING SICKNESS

	Gambian (West African)	Rhodesian (East African)
Etiologic agent	*Trypanosoma brucei gambiense*	*Trypanosoma brucei rhodesiense*
Vector	*Glossina palpalis* or *tachinoides* (riverine tsetse)	*Glossina morsitans* (savanna tsetse)
Distribution	West and Central Africa	East Africa
Reservoir	Humans (domestic animals)	Wild game
Course of infection	Slow (months–years)	Rapid (< 1 yr)
Clinical features		
Lymphadenopathy	+ + (Winterbottom's sign)	±
Myocarditis, heart failure	−	+ +
Neurologic symptoms	+ +	+
Disseminated intravascular coagulation	−	+
Parasitemia	Low	High

der forms can be present in a patient at the same time. The different variants of *T. brucei* cannot be distinguished morphologically but can be identified by differences in pathogenicity for certain animals, as well as in biochemical requirements, electrophoretic pattern of component enzymes, and DNA hybridization.

T. brucei is transmitted by the tsetse fly *Glossina*, within which it undergoes several developmental changes. When biting an infected host, trypanosomes are ingested and within the insect midgut rapidly differentiate into procyclic forms with loss of their dense surface coat, composed of variant surface glycoprotein. After 2 to 3 weeks of multiplication within the midgut the procyclic trypanosomes migrate to the insect's salivary glands, where they change morphologically into epimastigotes. These forms further undergo multiplication and ultimately differentiate into metacyclic trypanosomes that are coated with characteristic variant surface glycoprotein and are infectious to mammalian hosts. When a new host is bitten by the tsetse fly, the trypanosomes present in the salivary glands are injected into the connective tissue and blood. Within the human host they divide by binary fission and undergo antigen variation, a process by which they continually change their variable surface glycoproteins (VSG) and evade the immune system of the host. With the bite of another tsetse fly, ingestion of the parasite occurs, and the life cycle of the organism is completed (Fig. 375–1). Mechanical transmission can theoretically also occur via blood transfusion or by interrupted biting of a tsetse fly feeding on an infectious person and directly thereafter biting an uninfected individual.

EPIDEMIOLOGY. It is estimated that African trypanosomiasis infects more than 20,000 Africans annually and that approximately 50 million people live at risk of acquiring trypanosomiasis because of the presence of the disease and its vector. Approximately 4 million square miles in Africa remain unpopulated because of the presence of *T. brucei brucei* infection, which results in the loss of domestic and wild animals, including cattle, waterbuck, bushbuck, and buffalo.

T. b. gambiense occurs primarily in the west and central regions of sub-Saharan Africa. Although it primarily infects humans, there may be animal reservoirs, such as pigs, dogs, and sheep. Gambian sleeping sickness is spread mainly by three species of tsetse fly, *Glossina palpalis, G. tachinoides,* and *G. fuscipes.* Distribution of these flies includes shaded areas along rivers and streams, where the conditions of temperature, darkness, and moisture are optimum.

T. b. rhodesiense differs from *T. b. gambiense* in that it is primar-

ily a parasite of wild game, with humans serving only as occasional hosts. The geographic distribution of *T. b. rhodesiense* is primarily East Africa from Ethiopia and eastern Uganda south to Zambia and Botswana. Rhodesian sleeping sickness is spread by tsetse flies of the *G. morsitans* group, including *G. pallidipes* and *G. swynnertoni.* These flies can survive in the open savanna, and Rhodesian sleeping sickness usually occurs among individuals visiting or traveling through an endemic area. Consequently, hunters, fishermen, and tourists are at risk, exposing themselves to vectors that usually feed on wild animals.

Imported African trypanosomiasis is a rare disease. Most cases were due to *T. b. rhodesiense* acquired by Americans who had been on safari in East Africa for a very brief period. Nearly all of these cases were initially misdiagnosed because of the unfamiliarity of United States physicians with this disease. With an increase in international travel, 20,000 Americans are now estimated to visit endemic areas yearly, and approximately 10,000 aliens enter the United States each year from countries in Africa where the infection is endemic.

PATHOGENESIS AND PATHOLOGY. Following the bite of the tsetse fly, trypanosomes accumulate in the connective tissue, where they multiply to produce a local chancre (trypanoma). The organisms subsequently spread through the lymphatics, resulting in enlargement of lymph nodes secondary to reactive plasma cell and macrophage infiltration. The trypanosomes eventually disseminate to the circulatory system, where the parasitemia usually remains at low intensity and the organisms multiply by binary fission. Systemic African trypanosomiasis without central nervous system (CNS) involvement is generally referred to as stage I disease.

The host immune response plays an integral role in the pathogenesis of African sleeping sickness, although the exact nature of the immunopathogenic reactions has not been clearly defined. Trypanosomes survive by periodically altering their surface antigenic coat, avoiding successful eradication by the host. Any single parasite may contain some 1000 genes for VSG which can be activated in a variety of ways and selected by the host-antibody response. Consequently trypanosomes occur in the peripheral blood of infected individuals in waves, with each parasite wave consisting of a serologically distinct organism.

Tissue damage is induced by either toxin production or immune complex reaction with release of proteolytic enzymes. Immune complexes consisting of variant antigens of the organism and complement-fixing antibodies have been demonstrated in both the circulation and the target organs of infected patients. The production of autoantibodies is a prominent feature, and they are frequently directed against antigen components of red cells, brain, and heart. Anemia secondary to autoimmune hemolysis can be severe, resulting in anoxia and further tissue destruction. Thus the host-parasite interaction can result in generalized febrile episodes, lymphadenopathy, and myocardial and pericardial inflammation, along with anemia, thrombocytopenia, disseminated intravascular coagulation, and renal disease primarily during the acute stage of the disease.

Stage II of human African trypanosomiasis involves invasion of the CNS, which occurs during the period of circulatory dissemination when trypanosomes localize in the small vessels of the CNS. Pathologic changes in the CNS are most prominent in chronic cases of Gambian sleeping sickness. The meninges are thickened and infiltrated with lymphocytes, plasma cells, and morular cells. Morular cells are modified plasma cells (up to 20 mm in diameter) with large granular inclusions that have been shown to consist of immunoglobulin. These cells may play an important role in the local production of immunoglobulin M (IgM) in the cerebrospinal fluid (CSF). Edema, hemorrhages, and granulomatous lesions are frequently present, along with thrombosis as a result of endarteritis and with neuronal degeneration.

African trypanosomes appear to induce a state of B cell polyclonal activation caused either by interference with host T cell control of antibody production or by a B cell mitogen released by the parasite. Polyclonal hypergammaglobulinemia, with very high levels of IgM, is commonly seen. High levels of nonspecific heterophile antibody, rheumatoid factor, and autoantibodies are also produced.

CLINICAL FEATURES. The signs and symptoms of sleeping sickness differ according to the infecting organism (Table 375–1).

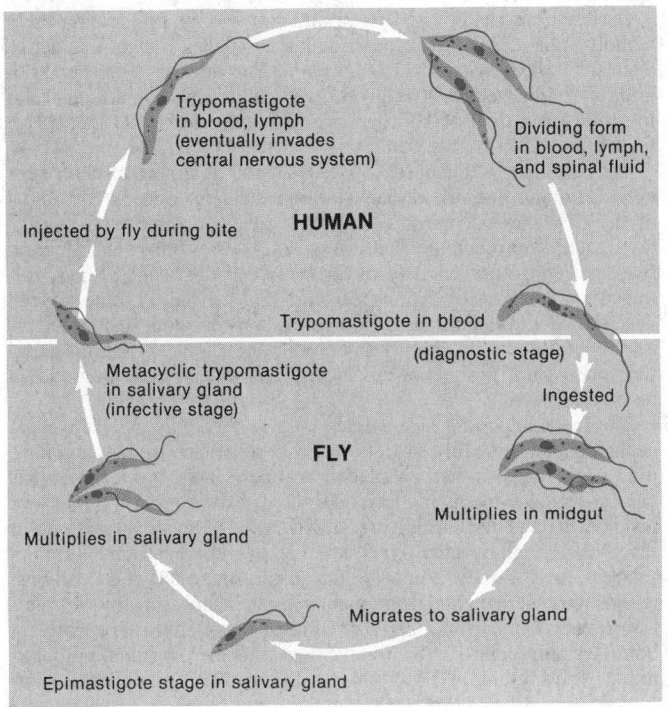

FIGURE 375–1. Life cycle of *Trypanosoma (Trypanozoon) brucei, T. (T.) b. gambiense,* and *T. (T.) b. rhodesiense.*

Rhodesian sleeping sickness, due to *T. b. rhodesiense,* causes a rapid progressive disease often resulting in cardiac failure and acute neurologic manifestations. Gambian sleeping sickness, caused by *T. b. gambiense,* is typically a more chronic illness with primarily neurologic features. However, this difference is not absolute; in some cases Gambian sleeping sickness can progress rapidly, and occasionally Rhodesian sleeping sickness may follow a more chronic course.

Gambian Sleeping Sickness. Within several days following the bite by an infected tsetse fly, a trypanosomal nodule or chancre develops, typically on the exposed parts of the body. Within a week the lesion becomes a hard, painful nodule surrounded by erythema and swelling, which persists for 1 to 2 weeks. After this incubation period, clinical features develop after systemic, lymphatic, and circulatory invasion of the trypanosomes. Fever, headache, dizziness, and weakness occur in the majority of these patients. Febrile episodes may last 1 to 6 days, alternating with afebrile periods. Lymphadenopathy with prominent supraclavicular and posterior cervical enlargement is seen in > 80% of infected individuals. Known as Winterbottom's sign, these enlarged lymph nodes are usually discrete, rubbery, and painless. Moderate splenomegaly may occur, and urticaria and erythematous rashes have also been observed. Electrocardiograms are often abnormal, but clinical signs of heart disease are unusual.

Six months to several years after symptoms first appear, the clinical features of this early hemolymphatic stage progress to a late meningoencephalitic stage. Behavioral and personality changes are often the first signs of CNS involvement. Later, more florid psychological changes may occur, with hallucinations and delusions. Reversion of sleep rhythm is characteristic, with drowsiness during the day, a feature from which the disease derives its name. Other nervous symptoms include tremor, most characteristically of the face and lips, and hyperesthesia, causing some patients to avoid common practices such as closing (Kerandel's sign) or locking doors (key sign). Without treatment, the patient's level of consciousness progressively deteriorates until there is lapse into stupor. Alterations in thermoregulation may lead to hypothermia or hyperthermia, and progressive neurologic alterations lead to convulsions, chorea, and athetosis. The CSF shows an increase in cells and protein, much of which is IgM. Free immunoglobulin light chains may be present. Most of the cells are lymphocytes, but a few are plasma cells and morula cells. Trypanosomes may also be evident within the CSF.

Rhodesian Sleeping Sickness. This disease is more acute than Gambian sleeping sickness, and symptoms usually occur a few days after the victim has been bitten by the tsetse fly. Alternating periods of high fever, malaise, and headache, followed by several days of well-being, are often misinterpreted as acute malaria infection. Lymphadenopathy is not prominent in this variety of the disease, and Winterbottom's sign is usually absent. Tachycardia with arrhythmias and extrasystoles is common. Anemia, thrombocytopenia, and disseminated intravascular coagulation are usually evident within the first several weeks of infection. Liver enzyme values are often elevated, and electrocardiograms are abnormal, usually reflecting underlying myocarditis. Neurologic features are similar to those described for Gambian sleeping sickness, but they occur much earlier and with more rapid deterioration. Without treatment the disease may result in death within a matter of weeks to months, without clear distinction into an early and late phase, as described for Gambian trypanosomiasis.

DIAGNOSIS. Although a presumptive diagnosis of trypanosomiasis is based on clinical suspicion, history of travel to areas where this disease is endemic, and tsetse fly exposure, confirmation of the diagnosis is based solely on the demonstration of trypanosomes. These organisms may be found in the blood (see Color Plate 10*E*), bone marrow, centrifuged CSF, lymph node aspirates, and scrapings from the chancre. Giemsa or Wright's stain of the buffy coat of centrifuged heparinized blood makes identification easier because the trypanosomes are often concentrated in the buffy coat. In one technique, referred to as the quantitative buffy coat (QBC), 60 μl of blood obtained by a fingerprick is drawn up in a glass hematocrit tube precoated with acridine orange and anticoagulate. Following centrifugation, the buffy coat can be examined and trypanosomes fluoresce greenish yellow, remain motile, and are easily identified. In patients with Gambian sleeping sickness, in which trypanosomes

are found less frequently in the blood, concentration methods such as ion exchange chromatography, diethylaminoethyl (DEAE) filtration, culture, or animal inoculation should be used.

All patients should have a lumbar puncture prior to and following therapy to determine whether CNS involvement is present. Documentation of CNS involvement is imperative because suramin, a drug effective against the hemolymphatic stage of *T. brucei,* does not penetrate the spinal fluid. CNS disease is manifested by pleocytosis and elevation of spinal fluid total protein and IgM levels. Trypanosomes can be found in most patients, provided that the CSF is examined immediately after collection and that clean glassware is used. For those patients in whom trypanosomes cannot be found, measuring the CSF IgM is often of great diagnostic help. A high CSF IgM value and a modest increase in total protein are almost pathognomonic of sleeping sickness.

Several immunodiagnostic tests have been developed for African trypanosomiasis, including an indirect hemagglutination test, indirect fluorescent antibody test, and enzyme-linked immunosorbent assay (ELISA), which are useful for epidemiologic surveys. A card agglutination trypanosome test (CATT) with prefixed trypanosomes is frequently used for rapid serodiagnosis. Although very sensitive, CATT may remain positive for several years after successful treatment, thereby decreasing its ability to differentiate between acute infection and a previous, treated infection.

TREATMENT. Suramin* is the drug of choice for the early hemolymphatic stage of both *T. b. gambiense* and *T. b. rhodesiense* infections before CNS invasion has occurred. Suramin does not cross the blood-brain barrier in increased amounts, and it does not cure the disease once CNS invasion has occurred. The dose is 20 mg per kilogram of body weight given intravenously up to a maximum single dose of 1 gram. Suramin is freshly prepared as a 10% aqueous solution. Intramuscular injection is not advised because of local irritation and pain. Suramin binds to plasma proteins and may persist in the circulation at low concentrations for as long as 3 months. A test dose of 200 mg is given initially; if no adverse side effects are noted, then full doses of the drug may be given on days 1, 3, 7, 14, and 21. A single course for an adult is usually 5 grams; it should not exceed 7 grams.

Suramin is a toxic drug that may result in idiosyncratic reactions in some individuals (1 in 20,000). The drug is excreted entirely by the kidneys; renal damage may result because the drug is deposited in the renal tubules. The urine should be examined before administering each dose of suramin, and if proteinuria or casts are present, treatment should be stopped. Other side effects include a papular eruption, photophobia, arthralgias, peripheral neuritis, fever, and agranulocytosis.

Pentamidine isethionate* is an alternative drug for treating early hemolymphatic African trypanosomiasis, but it is much less active against *T. rhodesiense* than is suramin. The dose is 4 mg per kilogram of body weight; it is given every other day by intramuscular injection for a total of 10 injections. Pentamidine is also ineffective for treating CNS trypanosomiasis.

The arsenical melarsoprol* (Mel B) is the treatment of choice for both Gambian and Rhodesian sleeping sickness once involvement of the CNS has occurred. The drug is given in three courses of 3 days each. The recommended dosage is 2.0 to 3.6 mg per kilogram per day given intravenously in three divided doses for 3 days, followed 1 week later by 3.6 mg per kilogram per day in three divided doses for 3 days. This latter course is then repeated 10 to 21 days later. Melarsoprol is a highly toxic drug and should be administered with great care. If signs of arsenical toxicity occur, the drug should be discontinued.

The most important side effects involve the CNS. A reactive encephalopathy, probably due to release of trypanosomal antigens, may occur early in the course of treatment, and its incidence has been reported to be as high as 18%. It may develop very rapidly or insidiously, and its mortality is about 50%. Clinical indications of reactive encephalopathy include high fever, headache, tremor, seizures, and finally coma. It has been suggested that corticosteroids protect patients from melarsoprol encephalopathy, but this assertion has not been clearly documented. An alternative drug for both systemic and CNS involvement includes difluoromethylornithine (eflornithine, DFMO), a specific, irreversible inhibitor of or-

---

* Available from the Centers for Disease Control and Prevention, Atlanta, GA.

boxylase. In one large trial of 207 patients with late-stage *T. b. gambiense* sleeping sickness, eflornithine was highly effective in successful treatment of both hemolymphatic and CNS stages of infection. Eflornithine dramatically reduced symptoms and rapidly cleared parasites from blood and CSF, even in those patients who had relapsed after melarsoprol therapy. The recommended dosage is 400 mg per kilogram per day given intravenously in four divided doses for 2 weeks, followed by 300 mg per kilogram per day given orally in four doses for 30 days. Frequent side effects include diarrhea and anemia. Unfortunately, its efficacy in *T. b. rhodesiense* has been quite variable, and its cost and long duration of therapy have limited its usefulness in the field. In addition, immunocompromised patients such as those with HIV infection do not respond to treatment as effectively with any of the above agents because a normal immune response is necessary for a cure. Regular follow-up with clinical examination of a lumbar puncture is necessary for all patients for at least 1 year after treatment.

PROGNOSIS. Untreated African sleeping sickness is almost invariably fatal. Many patients with early Gambian sleeping sickness may remain relatively well for months to years without treatment, but once CNS involvement has occurred, death is inevitable unless treatment is given. Death frequently results from pneumonia in Gambian sleeping sickness and from heart failure in Rhodesian sleeping sickness. Treatment with suramin in the early phase of sleeping sickness results in a cure rate of >90%. A few patients may subsequently develop CNS involvement and require further treatment. Mel B achieves a parasitologic cure in at least 90% of cases of advanced disease, and many patients may recover completely. Unfortunately, some patients are left with irreversible neurologic damage. Approximately 5% of patients may die during the course of Mel B therapy.

CONTROL AND PROPHYLAXIS. Measures to prevent and control African trypanosomiasis can be instituted at three different levels: surveillance and treatment, chemoprophylaxis, and vector control. Surveillance with treatment is necessary to reduce the human reservoir of infection, particularly in areas where epidemics have occurred in the past. Pentamidine has been successfully used as a chemoprophylactic in Gambian sleeping sickness when given as a single intramuscular injection of 4 mg per kilogram every 3 to 6 months. However, the drug is generally not recommended for mass use, and it appears to be ineffective against Rhodesian trypanosomiasis.

Vector control requires destruction of tsetse fly habitats by selective clearing of vegetation and spraying with insecticides, which are effective only temporarily. Because of the wide range of the tsetse fly, these vector control measures are not economically feasible except when it is necessary to break transmission in epidemics. For individual protection, avoidance of contact with infected tsetse flies is best achieved by the use of repellents and protective clothing.

A vaccine is not currently available because of the occurrence of antigenic variation. However, the potential for development of a vaccine has increased with the progress in cultivation of *T. brucei in vitro* and analysis of the chemical structure of its variant antigens.

Anonymous: Drugs for parasitic infections. *In* Abramowicz M (ed.): Med Lett Drugs Ther 35:111, 1993. *A listing of current recommendations for the treatment of all parasitic infections including trypanosomiasis.*

Cattand P, de Raadt P: Laboratory diagnosis of trypanosomiasis. Clin Lab Med 11:899, 1991. *A review of the various laboratory tests available for accurately diagnosing African trypanosomiasis.*

Hadjuk S, Adler B, Bertrand K, et al.: Molecular biology of African trypanosomes: Development of new strategies to combat an old disease. Am J Med Sci 303:258, 1992. *An excellent description of the mechanisms of antigenic variation which allow the parasite to avoid the host-immune response.*

Hunter CA, Kennedy PGE: Immunopathology in central nervous system human African trypanosomiasis. J Neuroimmunol 36:91, 1992. *A minireview of the different mechanisms potentially involved in the immunopathogenesis of CNS disease in human African trypanosomiasis.*

Jennings FW: Future prospects for the chemotherapy of human trypanosomiasis. Combination chemotherapy and African trypanosomiasis. Trans R Soc Trop Med Hyg 84:618, 1990. *A review of the different drug regimens for treating trypanosomiasis and discussion of their advantages and toxicities.*

Milord F, Pepin J, Loko L, et al.: Efficacy and toxicity of eflornithine for treatment of *Trypanosoma brucei gambiense* sleeping sickness. Lancet 340:652, 1992. *Clinical trial of eflornithine (DFMO) of 207 patients with late-stage* T.b. gambiense *sleeping sickness which demonstrated that eflornithine is as active and possibly less toxic than melarsoprol and is active for both stage I and stage II disease.*

376 AMERICAN TRYPANOSOMIASIS (Chagas' Disease)

Franklin A. Neva

DEFINITION. Chagas' disease, resulting from infection with the protozoan parasite *Trypanosoma cruzi,* is named after the Brazilian physician Carlos Chagas, who discovered the parasite. Distinction should be made between infection caused by the parasite, as manifested by positive serologic findings, and clinical disease. Chronic disease manifestations develop years after initial infection in the form of chronic cardiomyopathy with conduction defects or with dysfunction of the esophagus or colon (mega syndromes).

LIFE CYCLE OF THE ETIOLOGIC AGENT. The causative agent, *T. cruzi,* is usually transmitted as a zoonosis. Various species of blood-sucking reduviid bugs become infected when they take a blood meal from animals or humans who have circulating parasites, trypomastigotes, in the blood. The ingested parasites transform into epimastigotes and multiply in the midgut of the insect vector, where they later transform once again into metacyclic trypomastigotes in the hindgut of the bug. When the infected bug takes a subsequent blood meal, it frequently defecates during or after feeding, so that the infective metacyclic forms are deposited on the skin. Transmission to a second vertebrate host occurs when the feeding puncture site or a mucous membrane is inadvertently contaminated with infective bug feces. The parasites can penetrate a variety of host cell types, within which they transform into intracellular amastigote forms. In contrast to certain other intracellular organisms, amastigotes of *T. cruzi* are not enclosed in phagolysosomes. They multiply in the cytoplasm, elongate, transform into motile trypomastigotes, and rupture out of the cells. Liberated organisms penetrate new cells or are carried into the bloodstream to initiate further cycles of multiplication, preferentially in muscle cells, or are ingested by new vectors to maintain the cycle (Fig. 376–1).

Asymptomatic infected individuals with low-level parasitemia can transmit *T. cruzi* via blood transfusion. Another route of transmission of the parasite is congenital infection.

EPIDEMIOLOGY. *T. cruzi* and its arthropod vectors are widely distributed from the southern United States through Mexico and Central America into South America down to central Argentina and Chile. The parasite is restricted to the Western Hemisphere. In most countries where it occurs, the parasite cycle is sylvatic, i.e., it takes place in wild animals and their associated vector bugs. A peridomestic cycle occurs under conditions in which infected animals, such as opossums and rats, live close to human habitations, and vector bugs may invade houses to seek a blood meal. Certain species of triatomine bugs, such as *Triatoma infestans* and *Rhodnius prolixus,* have a great propensity to invade and breed in houses if suitable microenvironments are present. Cracks and holes in adobe mud huts or in crude wooden walls, thatched roofs, and household rubble provide hiding and breeding places for the bugs, which venture out at night to feed upon sleeping inhabitants. Under these conditions *T. cruzi* is transmitted from person to person—a domiciliary cycle—and Chagas' disease becomes a public health problem. Thus, human trypanosomiasis in Latin America is primarily an infection of rural poor people living in substandard housing.

The prevalence of antibodies to the parasite in human populations varies widely in different countries, as well as within regions of a country. A recent nationwide survey in Brazil found about 10% of the rural population to be infected. It is not unusual for up to half of all inhabitants in selected villages to be antibody positive. Countries with the highest incidence of both infection and disease due to *T. cruzi* include Brazil, Argentina, Chile, Bolivia, and Venezuela. It is estimated that in all of the Americas a total of 15 million people are infected. In many Latin American countries, positive serologic findings for *T. cruzi* constitute a social stigma; a lower socioeconomic background is implied, and employers are re-

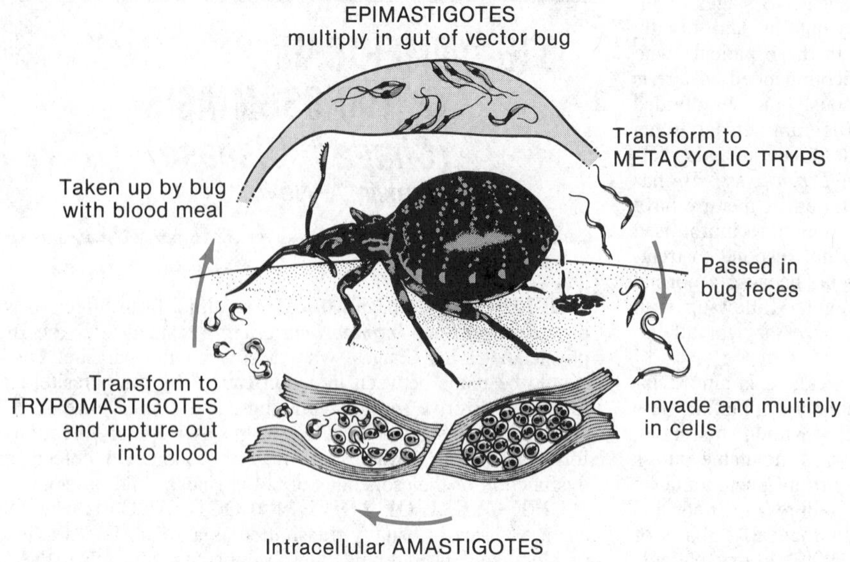

FIGURE 376-1. Life cycle of *Trypanosoma cruzi.*

luctant to hire someone who may later develop chronic Chagas' disease.

Considerable geographic variation exists in both the prevalence and the type of chronic disease manifestations. In Brazil, for example, cardiomyopathy and megadisease are common, and often a patient has both types of involvement. However, chagasic megaesophagus and megacolon are virtually unknown in Venezuela, Colombia, and Panama, whereas cardiomyopathy is relatively high, moderate, and low in prevalence, respectively. In general, the frequency of cardiac disease in Central America and Mexico in seropositive persons is low, even though rates of seropositivity may be substantial. Also in these countries heart disease tends to develop later in life than in Brazil.

The situation regarding Chagas' disease in the United States is interesting because only four autochthonous acute cases have been recognized despite the presence of *T. cruzi* in vector bugs as well as in animal reservoirs. The lack of transmission of *T. cruzi* to humans in this country is probably due to preference of the vectors for sylvatic habitats and their tendency to defecate late after feeding. Yet in some areas of the West, bites from aggressive and abundant reduviid bugs can be a source of annoyance to, and allergic reactions in, suburbanites and outdoorspeople. Because of increased Hispanic immigration in recent years, sporadic cases of chronic Chagas' disease will probably be encountered in the United States.

PATHOLOGY AND PATHOGENESIS. In *acute Chagas' disease,* a local inflammatory lesion called a chagoma may develop at the site of entry of the parasite. Histologically, the chagoma shows mononuclear cell infiltration, interstitial edema, and intracellular aggregates of amastigotes in cells of the subcutaneous tissue and muscle. Biopsy specimens from enlarged lymph nodes show hyperplasia, and amastigotes may be present in reticular cells. Skeletal muscle tissue from muscle biopsies have shown organisms and focal inflammation. In acute cases that have a fatal outcome there is invariably myocarditis with an enlarged heart. Microscopically, there is degeneration of cardiac muscle fibers and prominent but patchy areas of inflammation with nests of amastigotes in the muscles. The brain and meninges may also be parasitized in acute Chagas' disease. Virtually all organs and cell types can be invaded by *T. cruzi.*

The organs primarily affected in *chronic Chagas' disease* are the heart and certain hollow viscera, such as the esophagus and colon. Surprisingly, the intracellular *T. cruzi* usually cannot be found in the affected organs, or a few may be demonstrable after protracted search of many tissue sections. The heart in those patients with chronic disease who die suddenly, presumably of ventricular arrhythmias or heart block, may be normal in size or only moderately enlarged. Other patients with chronic chagasic cardiomyopathy develop cardiomegaly and die of intractable failure. The hearts are both hypertrophied and dilated, with thinning, especially at the apex to form a characteristic apical aneurysm. Mural thrombi, with subsequent embolization of the lungs and peripheral organs, are frequently seen. The coronary arteries are generally normal.

Microscopic findings in the heart are not specific, consisting of focal mononuclear cell infiltrates, hypertrophy of cardiac fibers with patchy areas of necrosis, variable fibrosis, and edema. The components of the conduction system of the heart most often involved by inflammatory changes are the sinoatrial and atrioventricular nodes, as well as the right branch and left anterior branches of the bundle of His. Andrade's detailed studies of these pathologic changes indicated that they correlated well with electrocardiographic (ECG) changes during life, but were diffusely scattered without specific localization to the conducting system.

When either the esophagus or the colon is affected in chronic Chagas' disease, the gross appearance is of dilatation and hypertrophy of the affected organ. The microscopic pathologic changes are disappointingly similar to those in the heart, again with no or very few organisms. However, myenteric ganglion cells are strikingly reduced in number. This type of parasympathetic denervation may also be found in other hollow viscera, such as duodenum, ureters, or biliary tree.

The significant pathology of *congenital Chagas' disease* is chronic placentitis, with inflammatory changes and focal necrosis in the chorionic villi. Amastigotes of *T. cruzi* are present in the lesions. The presence of lesions and organisms in the placenta may be associated with abortion, stillbirth, or acute disease in the fetus. However, pregnancy may result in a normal fetus, even though placental lesions are present.

The extent and clinical significance of pathologic changes in those individuals with antibodies to *T. cruzi* but without evidence of disease, i.e., the *indeterminate form,* are not yet clear. Such indeterminate cases may involve significantly reduced numbers of esophageal or colonic ganglion cells. It has been claimed that endocardial biopsy specimens from indeterminate cases have recognizable pathologic changes. In addition, in some indeterminate cases there is a chronic low level of parasitemia. Therefore, one point of view is that everyone with positive serologic findings has a continuing subclinical disease process that will become manifested with time. On the other hand, even in those areas where chronic Chagas' disease is common, one half or more of those with a positive serology will die of causes other than Chagas' disease. In most Latin American countries, where endemicity is much lower, a positive serologic finding constitutes a relatively small risk factor for later chronic disease.

The pathogenesis of acute Chagas' disease is straightforward, but the sequence of events leading to the late manifestations of chronic cardiomyopathy or megadisease is still poorly understood. Key features of the chronic disease that must be explained include the following: (1) a latent period of up to 20 years from presumed initial infection with *T. cruzi* before manifestations of cardiomyopathy or megadisease appear; (2) no or very few intracellular parasites in the affected organs, in contrast to abundant parasites in tissues in acute cases; (3) destruction of autonomic parasympathetic ganglia (Auerbach's plexus) of the esophagus and colon; and (4) great geographic variation in the frequency and type of chronic Chagas' disease. Genetic diversity in parasite strains, including variation in animal virulence, may explain geographic differences in disease. Exaggerated immune responses to *T. cruzi* are not present in patients with chronic Chagas' disease, at least as judged by humoral antibody levels and lymphocyte proliferative responses. The autoimmunity concept of pathogenesis lost favor when the tissue reactive antibody in patients was found to be heterophile in nature. Direct cell-mediated cytotoxicity to heart muscle has also been proposed as a mechanism for the chronic disease. An even more complicated type of autoimmune response involving anti-idiotypic antibodies as T cell antigens, as well as differential responses in antigen presentation, has also been proposed to explain chronic Chagas' disease. But a unifying concept of pathogenesis for chronic Chagas' disease is still lacking.

The indeterminate latent stage of infection with *T. cruzi* may be activated into a state of acute disease under conditions of severe immunosuppression. This can occur in seropositive recipients of organ transplants. Also, reports of activation of disease are increasing, especially with brain involvement similar to that produced by *Toxoplasma,* in patients with AIDS who also have latent *T. cruzi* infection.

CLINICAL PRESENTATION. In endemic areas, first exposure to *T. cruzi* generally is subclinical and goes unnoticed. When those initially exposed do develop clinical manifestations, the disease is an acute systemic infection. Chronic Chagas' disease, in contrast, evolves as a later sequela with specific organ involvement and no systemic features.

Acute Chagas' Disease. Although acute Chagas' disease is most commonly seen in children, it can occur at any age, depending on the nature of exposure to the causative organism. The incubation period under natural conditions cannot be established accurately but is probably at least a week. A local area of erythema and induration (chagoma) may develop in the skin at the site of parasite entry. When infection takes place via the conjunctival route, as it frequently does, the local periorbital swelling is referred to as Romaña's sign. The chagoma is often accompanied by regional adenopathy and persists for several weeks. Other signs of acute Chagas' disease include fever, generalized lymphadenopathy, hepatosplenomegaly, and transient skin rashes.

Myocarditis, accompanied by tachycardia and nonspecific ECG changes, can occur in the acute stage. Meningoencephalitis is another serious complication, particularly in very young patients. Fatal outcome in acute Chagas' disease is rare, but when it does occur, it is due to myocarditis and congestive failure or to meningoencephalitis.

Signs and symptoms of acute disease gradually subside within a few weeks to several months even without treatment. Trypanosomes, which have been demonstrable by direct microscopy in the peripheral blood during the acute phase, become more difficult to find and then disappear. The patient then enters the *indeterminate phase,* which is characterized by the presence of antibodies to *T. cruzi* and often also by the presence of low-level parasitemia in the blood demonstrable only by special sensitive methods. This state of apparent complete recovery with positive serologic findings may continue indefinitely without further evidence of disease or sequelae. However, a variable proportion of indeterminate cases, years to a decade or more later, will develop signs and symptoms of chronic Chagas' disease. Except for epidemiologic experience from a particular geographic region, there are no laboratory or clinical indicators to predict the likelihood of future chronic disease.

Chronic Chagas' Disease. Cardiac signs and symptoms are the most common manifestations of chronic disease and are apt to begin with palpitations, dizziness, precordial discomfort, and even syncope. These reflect a variety of arrhythmias, including ventricular extrasystoles, bouts of tachycardia, and various degrees of heart block. Sudden death due to ventricular tachycardia in an otherwise healthy young adult is not unusual. Symptoms due to arrhythmias may be present for a long time before cardiomegaly or evidence of cardiac failure appears. When congestive failure develops, it is predominantly right sided and is likely to lead to a fatal outcome

within a few years. Peripheral emboli to the brain or other organs are frequent.

Physical examination reveals only an irregular pulse, distant heart sounds, and perhaps a gallop rhythm. With failure, the heart can be very large, functional regurgitant murmurs may be heard, and there is often congestive hepatomegaly and peripheral edema.

The second most common chronic manifestation is megadisease of the esophagus or colon, most frequently the former. The symptoms are indistinguishable from idiopathic achalasia and include dysphagia, feeling of fullness after eating or drinking only small amounts, chest pain, and regurgitation. Aspiration with secondary pneumonia is a common complication in advanced cases, as are weight loss and cachexia. Salivary gland hypertrophy secondary to hypersalivation is sometimes seen. Esophageal cancer is reported to be more frequent in patients with chagasic megaesophagus, as with idiopathic achalasia.

Patients with chagasic megacolon suffer from chronic constipation and abdominal pain. Volvulus, obstruction, and perforation of the bowel may occur. An astonishing history of going several weeks between bowel movements has been obtained from some patients with severe megacolon. Megaesophagus and megacolon may both be present in the same patient, and cardiomyopathy can occur with either form of megadisease.

DIAGNOSIS. For both acute and chronic Chagas' disease, a history of possible exposure to *T. cruzi* should be sought. Usual tourist travel to endemic areas is not likely to provide sufficient exposure to infected vectors. Blood transfusion from a chronically infected donor can be a source of infection.

For *acute Chagas' disease* direct microscopic examination of anticoagulated blood or a buffy coat preparation for motile trypanosomes is the most important procedure. Organisms are more difficult to find on stained thin or thick blood films, but the morphology of organisms seen on direct microscopy should be confirmed in a stained preparation. Red cells may be lysed, using 0.083% NH_4Cl to concentrate parasites by centrifugation. If parasites cannot be found in the peripheral blood and acute disease is still suspected, blood can be cultured on NNN (Novy, MacNeal, and Nicolle's medium) or other suitable media. Inoculation of mice with the patient's blood may sometimes result in recovery of the parasite. Biopsy of an enlarged lymph node or of skeletal muscle for culture and/or histologic examination is another possibility.

The most sensitive technique for recovering trypanosomes from the blood is a procedure referred to as xenodiagnosis. It is basically a form of blood culture using the insect vector, by allowing up to 40 normal, laboratory-reared reduviid bugs to feed directly upon the patient or on the patient's blood through a membrane. Circulating parasites ingested by the bugs multiply in the gut and can be detected when the intestinal contents are examined 30 days later. Under experimental conditions, polymerase chain reaction techniques to demonstrate low levels of parasitemia appear promising, but no simple and specific methods are yet available for routine use.

Serologic testing is generally not needed to diagnose acute disease. Parasite-specific immunoglobulin M (IgM) antibodies detected by immunofluorescence or direct agglutination do not become positive until 20 to 40 days after the onset of symptoms. In certain situations this delayed antibody response permits the demonstration of seroconversion. Other laboratory tests often show nonspecific changes, such as a lymphocytic leukocytosis, elevated sedimentation rate, or transient ECG abnormalities. Reversible cardiomegaly and even pericardial effusion may occur.

The diagnosis of *chronic Chagas' disease* requires demonstration of antibodies to *T. cruzi* in the presence of the characteristic cardiac abnormalities and/or megadisease. Thus, except for the positive serologic findings, the diagnosis relies heavily upon clinical judgment in excluding other causes of heart disease or gastrointestinal dysfunction. A positive xenodiagnosis is strongly supportive, but not in itself diagnostic of chronic disease, since patients in the indeterminate phase may have low-level parasitemia. A variety of assays for specific antibody are available, and generally the results of different tests are comparable. However, there are cross-reactions in some tests with sera from patients with leishmaniasis or syphilis, for example. Therefore, in individual cases it may be helpful to confirm the presence of antibody to specific antigens of *T. cruzi* with more sophisticated tests, such as immunoblots.

Symptomatic heart involvement in the chronic disease is manifested by characteristic ECG abnormalities, often without cardiomegaly. The most common of these is complete right bundle branch block. Other frequent ECG findings are left anterior hemiblock, ventricular extrasystoles, and even complete heart block. If heart failure is present, radiographs and echocardiograms will show generalized cardiomegaly with a reduced ejection fraction (Fig. 376–2).

Chagasic megaesophagus in the early stages shows only delayed emptying and minimal dilatation on studies after a barium swallow. With more advanced disease, retention of swallowed material and esophageal dilatation are progressively increased. Manometric studies show spasm of the esophageal sphincter and uncoordinated peristaltic movements. Endoscopy should be performed to rule out malignant disease. However, all of these findings are indistinguishable from idiopathic achalasia. Barium enema with air contrast shows the dilated colon with impaired peristalsis, but other causes of colonic obstruction must be ruled out.

DIFFERENTIAL DIAGNOSIS. When acute Chagas' disease is symptomatic and severe, it can resemble a variety of acute systemic infections. Romaña's sign must be distinguished from other causes of unilateral orbital edema, such as the reaction to an insect bite, trauma, or orbital cellulitis.

Congenital infections are virtually indistinguishable from congenital toxoplasmosis, cytomegalic inclusion disease, and syphilis.

Various cardiomyopathies, such as postpartum, alcoholic, and endomyocardial fibrosis, can resemble chronic Chagas' heart disease. Endocardial biopsy is of dubious diagnostic value because of the nonspecific pathologic changes in chagasic cardiomyopathy; it might, however, identify other causes of heart disease. The characteristic heart murmurs of rheumatic valvular disease are helpful in differentiating this entity from chagasic cardiomyopathy. The value of positive serologic findings for *T. cruzi* in the differential diagnosis of both heart and megadisease will depend upon the background prevalence of antibodies in the general population.

TREATMENT. Two drugs with reasonable antitrypanosomal activity are currently in use for treating Chagas' disease. One of these is a nitrofuran derivative, nifurtimox*, which has been extensively evaluated. Nifurtimox is the only drug available in the United States for treating Chagas' disease; it is used in a dose of 8 to 12 mg per kilogram per day. The second drug, benznidazole, is a nitroimidazole derivative that appears to be equal to nifurtimox in efficacy, although there is less experience with its use. The exact mechanism of antitrypanosomal action of both of these drugs is not known.

There is now considerable evidence that if patients with acute Chagas' disease are treated with either nifurtimox or benznidazole,

---

* An investigational drug that must be obtained from the Centers for Disease and Prevention Control Drug Service (404-329-3670).

the extent of disease and parasitemia usually are reduced. But more important, many patients treated in the acute phase never develop antibodies to *T. cruzi*, or do so only transiently. From this observation, plus the fact that xenodiagnosis in such treated patients often is negative, it is assumed that parasites can be eliminated and the patient cured if treated in the acute stage. However, nifurtimox is not uniformly effective in producing these results, and parasite strains from certain geographic areas (Brazil) appear to be less responsive to treatment than do strains from other countries (Argentina and Chile).

The frequency of side effects from both nifurtimox and benznidazole is high; because they are administered for 60 to 90 days, drug toxicity is a serious problem. The most common adverse effect with nifurtimox is gastrointestinal intolerance, with anorexia, nausea, vomiting, and abdominal pain. Neurologic symptoms include restlessness, insomnia, disorientation, paresthesias, polyneuritis, and even seizures. Skin rashes can also occur. Peripheral neuropathy and bone marrow suppression have been reported with benznidazole. These side effects subside when the dosage of the drugs is reduced or treatment is stopped.

Since these drugs have shown effectiveness in treatment of acute Chagas' disease, some Latin American physicians are also treating chronic and indeterminate cases. There is no evidence that the established pathologic changes of chronic Chagas' disease can be reversed by nifurtimox or benznidazole therapy. The question of whether drug treatment in the indeterminate case, i.e., the asymptomatic patient with positive serologic findings, would prevent development of later chronic disease is controversial. Some data suggest that low-level parasitemia, as assessed by xenodiagnosis, can be reduced or eliminated after treatment with antitrypanosomal drugs, including allopurinol. But such studies require critical confirmation to establish their ultimate influence on the development of chronic disease, as well as risk versus benefit evaluation.

The treatment of patients with established chronic heart disease is supportive. Patients with frequent ventricular premature beats can benefit from antiarrhythmic drugs such as amiodarone. Cardiac pacemakers will prolong survival of those with complete heart block. The congestive failure of chagasic cardiomyopathy is disappointingly refractory to the usual cardiotropic drugs.

More options are open for managing and treating megadisease. In the early stages of megaesophagus, pneumatic dilatation of the sphincter is probably more effective than bougienage. For more advanced cases, various surgical procedures involving myotomy of the sphincter or partial resection are necessary. Early stages of megacolon can be managed by manipulating diet and using laxatives and occasional enemas. Sometimes an aperistaltic section of the colon can be resected in more severe cases.

PREVENTION. Chagas' disease could be eliminated as a serious health problem for the rural poor of Latin America by adequate housing and education. But stark socioeconomic realities dictate another approach to control. This consists mainly of the use of residual insecticides directed at domiciliary vectors. The use of benzene

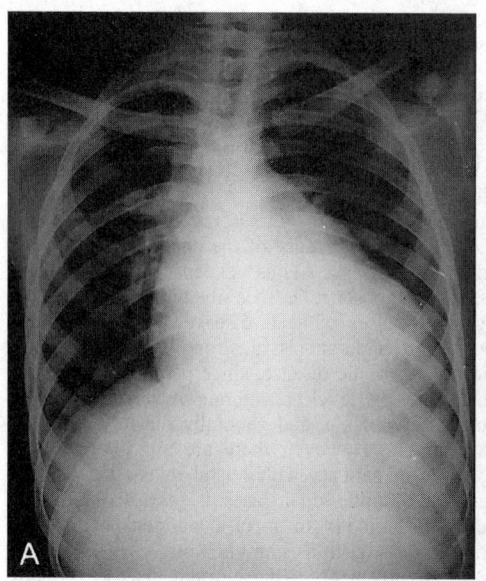
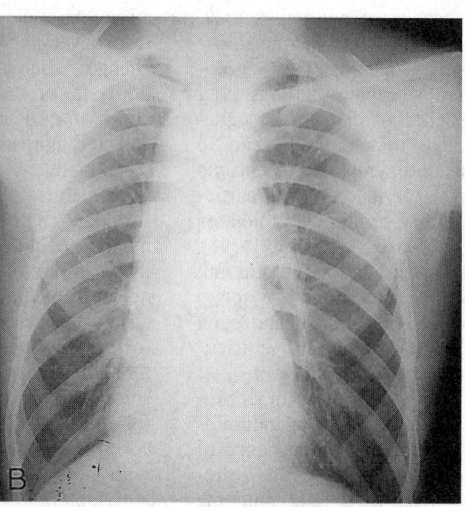

FIGURE 376–2. *A*, Cardiac silhouette in a patient with chronic chagasic cardiomyopathy and heart failure. *B*, Chest radiograph showing a widened mediastinum due to a greatly dilated megaesophagus of chronic Chagas' disease.

hexachloride (BHC), sprayed once or twice a year, has been very effective when used systematically.

Serologic testing in blood banks to avoid use of seropositive donors is carried out in endemic areas. Another precaution is to add 1:4000 gentian violet to blood 24 hours before use to kill trypanosomes that may be present. With the recent occurrence of several transfusion-associated cases of acute Chagas' disease in North America, the question of serologic screening of blood donors has been raised for areas of the country with large Latin American populations. The development of vaccines is still in the research stage.

Dias JCP: The indeterminate form of human chronic Chagas' disease. A clinical epidemiological review. Rev Soc Bras Med Trop 22:147, 1989. *A well-balanced review in English by a Brazilian expert. It documents the important point that infection with* T. cruzi *does not invariably progress to chronic disease.*

Kirchhoff LV: American trypanosomiasis (Chagas' disease)—A tropical disease now in the United States. N Engl J Med 329:639, 1993. *A concise "Current Concepts" review of the subject, including potential problems for blood banks and health care providers dealing with immigrant populations.*

Maguire JH, Hoff R, Sherlock I, et al.: Cardiac morbidity and mortality due to Chagas' disease: Prospective electrocardiographic study of a Brazilian community. Circulation 75:1140, 1987. *Antibodies to* T. cruzi *were present in 42% of the population. Excess mortality and development of abnormal ECGs were clearly related to positive serology.*

Rocha A, deMeneses ACO, daSilva AM, et al.: Pathology of patients with Chagas' disease and acquired immunodeficiency syndrome. Am J Trop Med & Hyg 50:261, 1994. *A review of 23 patients, 20 of whom had severe, multifocal meningoencephalitis; Chagas' disease was activated by AIDS.*

377 LEISHMANIASIS

Richard D. Pearson and Anastacio de Queiroz Sousa

Leishmaniasis is the name given to the spectrum of disease caused by *Leishmania* species, protozoa of the order Kinetoplastidia. It is endemic in widely scattered areas on every continent except Australia and Antarctica. The leishmania assume two distinct morphologic forms. They reside solely within mononuclear phagocytes as intracellular amastigotes in humans and other mammals, and they live as extracellular, flagellated promastigotes in the gut of their insect vectors, phlebotomine sandflies. With a few important exceptions such as visceral leishmaniasis in India, leishmaniasis is a zoonosis. Depending on the location, rodents, dogs, other animals, or humans are reservoirs. Transmission of the parasite requires a susceptible host, a sandfly vector, and an infected reservoir.

The clinical manifestations of leishmaniasis vary as a function of the parasite's pathogenicity, which differs among *Leishmania* species, and the host's immune responses. Some infections are asymptomatic and self-resolving, whereas others result in one or more of the three major forms of disease: cutaneous, mucosal (also termed mucocutaneous), and visceral leishmaniasis.

CLASSIFICATION AND LIFE CYCLE

The *Leishmania* species, their geographic locations, and the clinical syndromes that they produce are summarized in Table 377–1. The classification of *Leishmania* was originally based on their geographic location, clinical manifestations, vectors, and biochemical attributes. Speciation of isolates at World Health Organization reference laboratories is currently done by isoenzyme analysis. Species-specific monoclonal antibodies and kinetoplast-DNA (kDNA) probes are available in research laboratories. Recent experimental work suggests that polymerase chain reaction (PCR) methodology using *Leishmania* species-specific primers may emerge as the method of choice for speciation and diagnosis.

The leishmania live as intracellular amastigotes in parasitophorous vacuoles within mononuclear phagocytes in humans and other mammals (Fig. 377–1). Amastigotes are oval or round and approximately 2 to 3 microns in diameter. They have a relatively large eccentrically placed nucleus and a rod-shaped specialized mitochondrial structure, the kinetoplast. Promastigotes, which are found in the gut of the sandfly, are flagellated and extracellular.

Female sandflies, *Lutzomyia* species in Latin America and *Phlebotomus* species in the rest of the world, are responsible for transmitting leishmania. Some are peridomestic and live in rubble and debris near houses or farm buildings; others thrive in thick vegetation in forest areas. Sandflies are modified pool feeders. They ingest

TABLE 377–1. GEOGRAPHIC DISTRIBUTION AND CLINICAL DISEASE CAUSED BY *LEISHMANIA* SPECIES

Clinical Syndromes	Leishmania Species	Location
Visceral leishmaniasis		
Kala-azar: generalized involvement of the reticuloendothelial system (spleen, bone marrow, liver, etc.)	*L. donovani*	Indian subcontinent, North and East China, Pakistan, Nepal
	L. infantum	Middle East, Mediterranean littoral, Balkans, Central and Southwest Asia, North and Northwestern China, North and sub-Saharan Africa
	L. donovani (archibaldi)	Sudan, Kenya, Ethiopia
	Leishmania species	Kenya, Ethiopia, Somalia
	L. chagasi	Latin America
	L. amazonensis	Brazil (Bahia State)
	L. tropica	Israel, India, and "viscerotropic" disease in Saudi Arabia (U.S. troops)
Post–kala-azar dermal leishmaniasis	*L. donovani*	Indian subcontinent
	Leishmania species	Kenya, Ethiopia, Somalia
Old World cutaneous leishmaniasis		
Single or limited number of skin lesions	*L. major*	Middle East, Northwest China, Northwest India, Pakistan, Africa
	L. tropica	Mediterranean littoral, Middle East, west Asiatic area, Indian subcontinent
	L. aethiopica	Ethiopian highlands, Kenya, Yemen
	L. infantum	Mediterranean basin
	L. donovani (archibaldi)	Sudan, East Africa
	Leishmania species	Kenya, Ethiopia, Somalia
Diffuse cutaneous leishmaniasis	*L. aethiopica*	Ethiopian highlands, Kenya, Yemen
New World cutaneous leishmaniasis		
Single or limited number of skin lesions	*L. mexicana* (chiclero ulcer)	Central America, Mexico, Texas
	L. amazonensis	Amazon basin including Brazil and neighboring countries
	L. braziliensis	Multiple areas of Central and South America
	L. guyanensis (forest yaws)	Guyana, Surinam, northern Amazon basin
	L. peruviana (uta)	Peru (western Andes), Argentinean highlands
	L. panamensis	Panama, Costa Rica, Columbia
	L. pifanoi	Venezuela
	L. garnhami	Venezuela
	L. venezuelensis	Venezuela
	L. chagasi	Central and South America
Diffuse cutaneous leishmaniasis	*L. amazonensis*	Amazon basin including Brazil and neighboring countries
	L. pifanoi	Venezuela
	L. mexicana	Mexico, Central America
	Leishmania species	Dominican Republic
Mucosal leishmaniasis	*L. braziliensis* (Espundia)	Multiple areas in Latin America

Adapted from Pearson RD, Sousa AQ: Leishmania species: Visceral (kala-azar), cutaneous and mucosal leishmaniasis. *In* Mandell GL, Bennett JE, Dolin R (eds.): Principles and Practice of Infectious Diseases. 4th ed., New York, Churchill Livingstone, 1994, p 2428. Data from Lainson R, Shaw JJ: Evolution, classification and geographic distribution. *In* Peters W, Killick-Kendrick R (eds.): The Leishmaniases in Biology and Medicine, vol. 1. London, Academic Press, 1987, p 1.

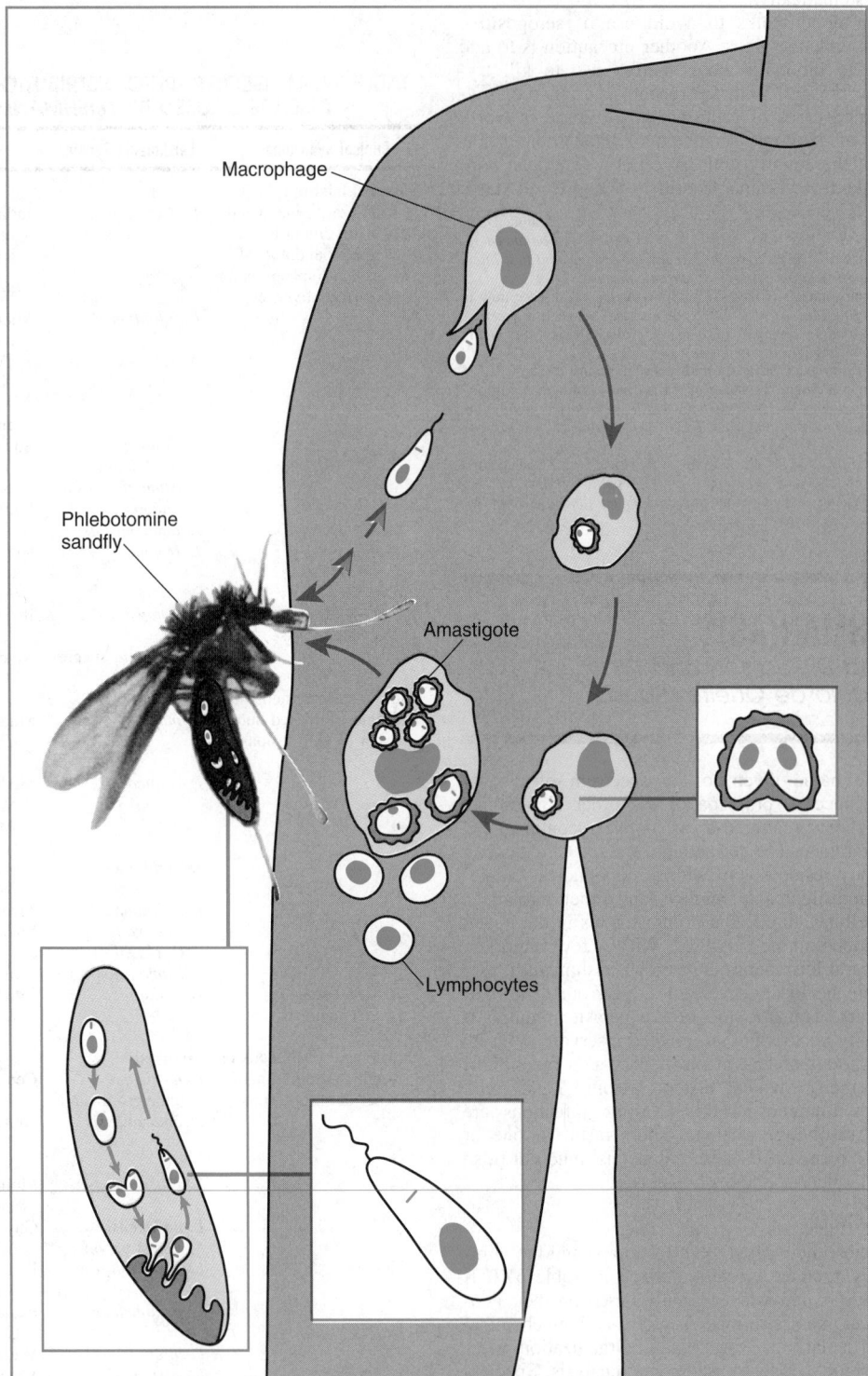

FIGURE 377-1. Life cycle of leishmania. Humans serve as the reservoir for *L. donovani* in India as depicted here. In most settings leishmaniasis is a zoonosis with rodents or canines as reservoirs.

amastigote-containing macrophages when they take a blood meal. Amastigotes transform to promastigotes, which then multiply and differentiate in the sandfly gut. The life cycle is completed approximately 1 week later when metacyclic promastigotes are deposited as the sandfly attempts to take its next blood meal. Sandfly saliva contains a factor(s) that enhances the promastigote's infectivity for macrophages.

IMMUNOLOGY

The control of leishmanial infections depends on T cell–mediated immune responses. Antileishmanial antibodies are produced, but they are not protective. Resolution of infection and protection

against reinfection correlate with the proliferation of CD4 cells of the Th1 type (see Ch. 221) that secrete interferon-γ and interleukin-2 (IL-2) in response to leishmanial antigens. Interferon-γ activates macrophages to kill intracellular amastigotes. Data from the murine system indicate that L-arginine–dependent nitric oxide production is the dominant effector mechanism. IL-12 appears to play an important role in the development of Th1 responses.

Potentially protective Th1 responses are suppressed in persons with progressive infections. Leishmania-specific CD4 cells of the Th2 type that produce IL-4 are responsible for suppressing the development of Th1 responses in mice. In humans with visceral leishmaniasis, IL-10 appears to mediate suppression. The early events that follow parasite inoculation seem to be crucial in determining whether protective or nonprotective T4 cell responses dominate, but they have not been fully defined.

VISCERAL LEISHMANIASIS

EPIDEMIOLOGY (Table 377–1). Visceral leishmaniasis is typically caused by *L. donovani* in India and Africa, and two closely related species—*L. infantum* in the Mediterranean littoral and *L. chagasi* in Latin America. The disease occurs sporadically or in epidemics. On occasion *Leishmania* species that are predominantly associated with cutaneous disease, e.g., *L. mexicana* and *L. major,* are isolated from patients with classic visceral leishmaniasis. In addition, a small group of American soldiers infected with *L. tropica* in Saudi Arabia during Operation Desert Storm (Persian Gulf War, 1991) developed a "viscerotropic" syndrome, with dissemination of amastigotes to the bone marrow, but without many of the manifestations of classic progressive visceral leishmaniasis.

Visceral leishmaniasis due to *L. donovani* is a major problem in eastern India and Bangladesh (Table 377–1). The disease is most common in young adults. Major epidemics followed the cessation of DDT spraying for malaria there. Humans appear to be the only reservoir of infection, and leishmania are transmitted by anthropophilic sandflies. *L. donovani,* which is also endemic in Kenya and Ethiopia, has been responsible for a large epidemic of visceral leishmaniasis among refugees in the Sudan. The reservoirs are rodents and small carnivores. Humans may serve as a reservoir during epidemics. Visceral leishmaniasis due to *L. infantum* occurs sporadically among children and persons with HIV and other immunocompromising conditions in southern Europe, the Middle East, and North Africa. In Brazil, Venezuela, Colombia, and other areas of Latin America, visceral leishmaniasis due to *L. chagasi* is typically found in scattered, rural areas, although large urban outbreaks have occurred in northeast Brazil. The majority of cases are in children younger than age 10.

IMMUNOPATHOLOGY. Infection with *L. donovani* and related organisms is acquired when promastigotes are inoculated by sandflies into an exposed area of skin. The parasites convert to amastigotes and multiply within mononuclear phagocytes. Although a cutaneous nodule or ulcer may develop, most patients are unaware of the site of primary inoculation. Amastigotes subsequently disseminate via regional lymphatics and the vascular system to mononuclear phagocytes throughout the reticuloendothelial system. The majority of infections with *L. donovani, L. chagasi,* and *L. infantum* are asymptomatic and resolve spontaneously. A minority progress to classic, full-blown visceral leishmaniasis, known in many areas as kala-azar. In Brazil, a subset of children infected with *L. chagasi* has a prolonged course with minimal symptoms; in some the infection eventually resolves spontaneously, whereas in others it progresses to classic visceral leishmaniasis.

In patients with progressive visceral leishmaniasis, increased numbers of mononuclear phagocytes are found in the liver and spleen, resulting in hypertrophy. In the liver there is a dramatic increase in the number and size of Kupffer cells, many filled with amastigotes. The spleen often is massively enlarged, and splenic lymphoid follicles are replaced by parasitized mononuclear cells. Amastigote-containing mononuclear phagocytes are found in the bone marrow, lymph nodes, skin, intestinal tract, and other organs. Circulating immune complexes are common, and there is histologic evidence of deposition in the kidney, but renal failure is rare.

CLINICAL MANIFESTATIONS. The incubation period with symptomatic infection is quite variable but usually ranges from 3 to 8 months. The onset of visceral leishmaniasis is often insidious and difficult to date, and the disease usually has a subacute or chronic course. In some cases, however, there is an abrupt onset of fever and chills suggestive of malaria. Symptoms include fever, malaise, anorexia, weight loss, and enlargement of the abdomen. Fever may be intermittent, remittent with twice-daily temperature spikes to 38 to 40°C, or less commonly, continuous. It is usually well tolerated.

Hepatomegaly and splenomegaly are hallmarks of visceral leishmaniasis; the spleen is firm and nontender and frequently becomes massively enlarged (Fig. 377–2). Patients in India may develop hyperpigmentation, which led to the name kala-azar, meaning black fever in Hindi. Jaundice is occasionally present. Late in visceral leishmaniasis patients may develop epistaxis, gingival bleeding, and petechiae on their extremities. They may have edema and ascites due to hypoalbuminemia. The majority of patients with visceral

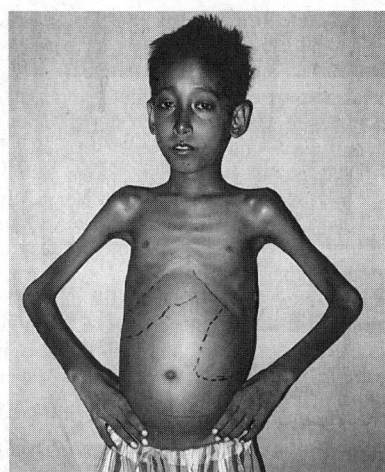

FIGURE 377–2. Indian patient with kala-azar. Note wasting of thorax and shoulder girdle and hepatosplenomegaly as outlined.

leishmaniasis and concurrent HIV present in the classic manner, but splenomegaly may be absent, and atypical presentations with involvement of the lungs, pleura, oral mucosa, esophagus, stomach, small intestine, or skin have been reported.

On laboratory examination, anemia, thrombocytopenia, neutropenia, and hypergammaglobulinemia are common. The anemia is usually normocytic and normochromic unless complicated by blood loss. The white blood count may be as low as 1000 per cubic millimeter; eosinopenia is common. Platelets are also decreased. The erythrocyte sedimentation rate is elevated. The levels of gamma globulin are markedly increased, at times in the range of 9 to 10 grams per deciliter. This is a result of polyclonal B cell activation. Circulating immune complexes and rheumatoid factors are also present in the majority of patients. Liver enzymes and bilirubin are elevated in some.

Untreated persons with visceral leishmaniasis have a progressive, downhill course over several months or more. Severe cachexia may develop. Patients with advanced visceral leishmaniasis evidence neutropenia as well as anergy to multiple T cell antigens. Bacterial pneumonia, measles, dysentery, tuberculosis, gangrenous stomatitis, and other secondary infections are common and frequently contribute to death.

Viscerotropic Leishmaniasis. In the *L. tropica*–related "viscerotropic" syndrome observed in American military personnel who served in Operation Desert Storm, symptoms included chronic low-grade fever, malaise, fatigue, and in some instances, diarrhea. The troops did not develop splenomegaly or the progressive wasting associated with classic visceral leishmaniasis.

Post–Kala-azar Leishmaniasis. A small percentage of persons in India and Africa who are treated for visceral leishmaniasis develop post–kala-azar dermal leishmaniasis after the other manifestations of disease have resolved. In Africa the lesions develop shortly after treatment and persist for several months. In India they appear up to 2 years after treatment and persist for as long as 20 years. The skin lesions vary from hyperpigmented macules to frank nodules and contain *L. donovani* amastigotes. They are frequently found on the face, trunk, and extremities.

DIAGNOSIS. A presumptive diagnosis of visceral leishmaniasis is easily made by the classic clinical presentation in an endemic area. The diagnosis may be delayed or missed in an immigrant or traveler returning to a nonendemic country, particularly if the person has concurrent HIV infection and lacks splenomegaly. The diagnosis is confirmed by identifying *Leishmania* species amastigotes in tissue or by growing promastigotes in culture. Splenic aspiration results in a diagnosis in 96 to 98% of cases. It is relatively safe when performed by an experienced physician, but significant hemorrhage occurs on occasion, particularly in patients with clotting abnormalities. Bone marrow aspiration results in a diagnosis in more than half of the cases. Alternative sites for aspiration and/or biopsy include the liver and lymph nodes if they are enlarged, or culture of the buffy coat. In patients with concurrent HIV infections amastigotes are frequently identified in unexpected sites such as bronchoalveolar lavage fluid, pleural effusions, or biopsies of lesions in the oral pharynx, larynx, stomach, or intestine.

Antileishmanial antibodies are present in high titer in immunocompetent patients with visceral leishmaniasis. They can be measured by enzyme-linked immunosorbent assay (ELISA), indirect immunofluorescence assay, direct agglutination tests, or several alternative assays. Persons with advanced HIV and those with viscerotropic *L. tropica* infections frequently have low or undetectable antileishmanial antibodies. The leishmanin skin test, also known as the Montenegro test, is negative in persons with visceral leishmaniasis, but it becomes positive in the majority of those who undergo successful chemotherapy and in those with self-resolving infections. The antigen preparation is not approved for use in the United States.

CUTANEOUS AND MUCOSAL LEISHMANIASIS

EPIDEMIOLOGY (see Table 377–1). *Leishmania* species produce a spectrum of cutaneous and mucosal lesions. Most common are chronic, localized, ulcerative lesions, often referred to as "oriental sores" (see Color Plate 9*F*). They are seen periodically among Western travelers who visit or work in endemic areas. Cutaneous leishmaniasis in Latin America is caused by *L. mexicana, L. braziliensis,* and several related species, and on occasion, by *L. chagasi.* It is a zoonosis. The reservoirs are usually forest rodents. Humans become infected when they settle or work in or near forested areas. *L. braziliensis* is also responsible for mucosal leishmaniasis.

Most cases of cutaneous leishmaniasis outside of Latin America are caused by three *Leishmania* species. *L. major* is an important problem among settlers, visitors, and troops in endemic rural areas of the Middle East, Central Asia, and North Africa. Rodents are the principal reservoir. *L. tropica* is usually found in urban areas of the Middle East, the Mediterranean littoral, India, Pakistan, and Central Asia. The reservoirs are dogs and humans. *L. aethiopica* is endemic in Ethiopia, Kenya, and southwest Africa, where hyrax are reservoirs. On occasion *L. donovani* or *L. infantum* is isolated from cutaneous lesions.

IMMUNOPATHOLOGY. The peripheral blood mononuclear cells from patients with classic cutaneous leishmaniasis proliferate and produce interferon-γ and IL-2 in response to leishmanial antigens *in vitro,* and patients evidence delayed-type hypersensitivity responses to leishmanial antigens *in vivo.* The chronic course of the disease appears to be due to the dominance of Th2-like responses and other suppressive factors at the site of the lesion.

The spectrum of cutaneous leishmaniasis includes several variants. On one extreme is the anergic variant diffuse cutaneous leishmaniasis, a rare syndrome in which parasites disseminate in the skin, producing multiple nodular lesions composed primarily of histiocytes filled with amastigotes. These lesions do not ulcerate. No evidence of a Th1 response is seen in patients with diffuse cutaneous leishmaniasis. Peripheral blood mononuclear cells do not proliferate or produce interferon-γ or IL-2 in response to leishmanial antigens, and there are no delayed-type hypersensitivity responses to intradermally injected antigens. Clinically this is somewhat analogous to lepromatous leprosy.

In contrast to mucosal leishmaniasis there is a chronic, destructive, granulomatous inflammatory response. Amastigotes are often scant. There is evidence of a vigorous Th1-like response. Peripheral blood mononuclear cells proliferate and secrete interferon-γ in response to leishmanial antigens, and there are pronounced delayed-type hypersensitivity responses to intradermally inoculated antigens. Clinically, this hyperergic variant is somewhat analogous to tuberculoid leprosy.

CLINICAL MANIFESTATIONS. *Cutaneous Leishmaniasis.* Cutaneous leishmaniasis may involve single or multiple lesions. They are relatively heterogeneous and vary as a function of the infecting *Leishmania* species and the host's immune response. A typical lesion starts as an erythematous papule at the site where promastigotes are inoculated by a sandfly, slowly increases in size, becomes a nodule, and eventually ulcerates. "Wet" lesions are covered with exudate, and have raised borders (see Color Plate 9*F*). They are frequently associated with superficial, secondary bacterial or fungal infections. Other lesions are "dry" with a central crust.

Satellite lesions may be found at or near the edges of the primary site of infection. On occasion cutaneous leishmaniasis may appear nodular, suggesting skin cancer. Rarely, cutaneous leishmaniasis involves local lymphatics, mimicking sporotrichosis. Cutaneous lesions persist for months and in some cases years before they spontaneously heal, leaving flat, hypopigmented, atrophic scars.

It was once thought that cutaneous leishmaniasis was confined to the skin, but recent observations in Brazil indicate that *L. braziliensis* can cause regional lymphadenopathy, fever, and other constitutional symptoms before the primary cutaneous lesion becomes apparent. These symptoms and findings resolve as the skin ulcer develops. Splenomegaly occurs in some patients. It is thought that *L. braziliensis* may disseminate to distant mucosal sites during this early phase of infection.

Diffuse Cutaneous Leishmaniasis. Diffuse cutaneous leishmaniasis is a rare anergic variant. It starts as a localized papule that does not ulcerate, and satellite lesions develop as amastigotes disseminate in the skin (Fig. 377–3). Eventually multiple cutaneous nodules develop on the face and extremities. The disease progresses slowly and often persists for decades.

Leishmaniasis Recidiva. Leishmaniasis recidiva, typically associated with *L. tropica* infection in the Middle East, is a chronic syndrome with skin lesions on the face or exposed extremities that enlarge slowly, tend to heal in the center, and persist for many years. Biopsies of the lesions reveal chronic inflammatory changes; amastigotes are sparse.

Mucosal Leishmaniasis (Espundia). A small percentage of persons with *L. braziliensis* infection in Latin America develop mucosal lesions of the nose, mouth, pharynx, or larynx months to years after the primary skin ulcer heals (see Color Plate 9*G*). The disease typically begins with nasal inflammation and stuffiness, followed by ulceration of the mucosa. The lesions are characterized by a chronic granulomatous response. There is destruction of the mucosa and eventually of the underlying cartilage of the nasal septum or palate. Patients evidence brisk Th1 responses to leishmanial antigens, and the tissue destruction appears to be due to a hyperergic immune response. The differential diagnosis of American mucosal leishmaniasis includes paracoccidioidomycosis, histoplasmosis, tertiary syphilis, tertiary yaws, sarcoidosis, Wegener's granulomatosis, midline granuloma, rhinoscleroma, and basal cell carcinoma.

DIAGNOSIS. The diagnosis of cutaneous leishmaniasis should be considered in any person with a chronic, localized skin lesion who has been exposed in an endemic area. It is confirmed by identifying amastigotes in touch preparations, by histopathology, or by growing promastigotes in culture. A punch biopsy and aspirate should be obtained from the margin of the lesion after it has been meticulously cleaned. Touch preparations are stained with a Wright-Giemsa preparation. The remaining tissue should be divided and used for culture and histopathology. Antileishmanial antibodies are

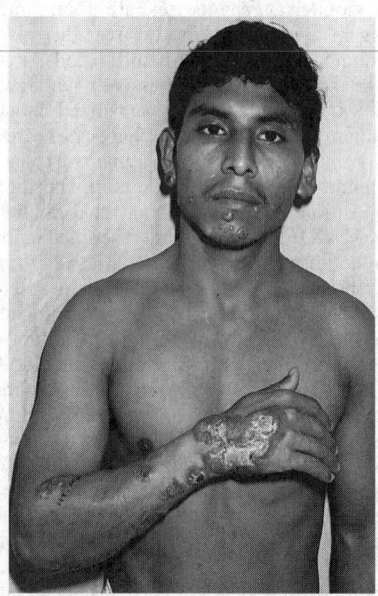

FIGURE 377–3. Patient with diffuse cutaneous leishmaniasis of 5 years' duration. Note nonulcerative lesions of chin, ear lobes, right arm, and hand.

often detectable in the serum of patients with cutaneous leishmaniasis, but the titers are usually low. The leishmanin skin test is positive in persons with simple cutaneous leishmaniasis, leishmaniasis recidiva, and mucosal leishmaniasis, but nonreactive in patients with diffuse cutaneous leishmaniasis.

Parasites are often scant in mucosal lesions due to *L. braziliensis*. A positive leishmanin skin test, the presence of antileishmanial antibodies, exposure in an endemic area, and evidence of a healed cutaneous lesion allow for a presumptive diagnosis.

TREATMENT

VISCERAL LEISHMANIASIS. Pentavalent antimonials, stibogluconate sodium (Pentostam), and meglumine antimonate (Glucantime) remain the treatment of choice for visceral leishmaniasis, but clinical failures are becoming increasingly prevalent in many areas, and these drugs are associated with important untoward effects. Stibogluconate sodium is available in the United States through the CDC Drug Service.* It is also used in Europe, Africa, and India. Meglumine antimoniate is available in Latin America, France, and in Francophone countries in Africa.

Stibogluconate sodium and meglumine antimoniate are administered on the basis of their pentavalent antimony content. When properly manufactured and stored, they appear to be of comparable efficacy and toxicity. The recommended treatment course is 20 mg of pentavalent antimony per kilogram body weight per day for 20 to 28 days. A prolonged course is frequently used in patients who do not respond completely to the initial course of therapy.

Recent reports suggest that chemical pancreatitis is common in patients receiving pentavalent antimonials. Other side effects include pain at the injection site when the drug is given intramuscularly, arthralgias, myalgias, nausea, vomiting, liver enzyme abnormalities, and ST-T wave changes by electrocardiography. Cardiac toxicity and sudden death have occurred in patients who received more than the recommended dose.

Amphotericin B and pentamidine are alternative drugs, but both have important side effects (see Ch. 347). Amphotericin B (0.5 to 1.0 mg per kilogram every other day for up to 8 weeks or for a total dose of 1.5 to 2.0 grams) has been used successfully to treat patients who fail antimony therapy. Recombinant interferon-γ plus a pentavalent antimonial have proven to be effective in patients with visceral leishmaniasis who fail pentavalent antimonial therapy alone. Unfortunately, recombinant interferon-γ is expensive and available only for patients on experimental protocols.

CUTANEOUS LEISHMANIASIS. Cutaneous lesions that are large or located in cosmetically important sites and those that are caused by *L. braziliensis* or other *Leishmania* species associated with mucosal disease should be treated. Small, inconspicuous, or healing lesions caused by *Leishmania* species that are not associated with mucosal disease can be followed expectantly. Pentavalent antimonials, stibogluconate sodium and meglumine antimoniate, effectively treat cutaneous leishmaniasis in many situations, but, as described above, they are frequently associated with toxicity, and clinical failures are becoming increasingly prevalent. Full doses of 20 mg per kilogram body weight per day are recommended for 20 to 28 days; lower doses may favor the development of antimony resistance. Cutaneous lesions heal slowly during antimony therapy. A number of other drugs and therapeutic approaches, including local treatment and immunotherapy, are under study and have their proponents, but the data are insufficient to recommend their general use.

Therapeutic failures with pentavalent antimonials are common in persons with diffuse cutaneous leishmaniasis, leishmaniasis recidiva, and mucosal leishmaniasis. Amphotericin B is an alternative. Preliminary data suggest that recombinant interferon-γ administered with a pentavalent antimonial can be used to effectively treat patients with diffuse cutaneous leishmaniasis.

PROPHYLAXIS

Personal protection with insect repellents containing DEET applied to skin and permethrin-treated clothing can reduce the frequency of sandfly bites in visitors to endemic areas. Fine mesh netting can be used for protection at night. Unfortunately, these measures are seldom practical for residents of endemic areas.

---

* Centers for Disease Control and Prevention, Atlanta, Georgia 30333; telephone 404-639-3670 (evenings, weekends, and holidays 404-639-2888).

Addy M, Nandy A: Ten years of kala-azar in West Bengal, Part I. Did post–kala-azar dermal leishmaniasis initiate the outbreak in 24-Parganas? Bull WHO 70:341, 1992. *An experience with visceral leishmaniasis in India discussing the potential role of humans with post–kala-azar dermal leishmaniasis as a reservoir of infection.*

Badaró R, Johnson WD Jr: The role of interferon-γ in the treatment of visceral and diffuse cutaneous leishmaniasis. J Infect Dis 167(Suppl 1):S13, 1993. *Recombinant interferon-γ plus a pentavalent antimonial appear promising for treating visceral or diffuse cutaneous leishmaniasis refractory to antimony therapy.*

Grogl M, Thomason TN, Franke ED: Drug resistance in leishmaniasis: Its implications in systemic chemotherapy of cutaneous and mucocutaneous disease. Am J Trop Med Hyg 47:117, 1992. *Pentavalent antimonial resistance is becoming increasingly common; recommends 20 mg per kilogram body weight of pentavalent antimony daily for 20 to 28 days, depending on the leishmanial syndrome being treated.*

Herwaldt BL, Berman JD: Recommendations for treating leishmaniasis with sodium stibogluconate (Pentostam) and review of pertinent clinical studies. Am J Trop Med Hyg 46:296, 1992. *Discusses the use of pentavalent antimonials in treating leishmaniasis.*

Locksley RM, Louis JA: Immunology of leishmaniasis. Curr Opin Immunol 4:413, 1992. *Excellent review of immunology of leishmanial infections and the role of cytokines in controlling cell-mediated immune responses.*

Magill AJ, Grögl M, Gasser RA Jr, et al.: Visceral infection caused by *Leishmania tropica* in veterans of Operation Desert Storm. N Engl J Med 328:1383, 1993. *Some Operation Desert Storm soldiers developed a viscerotropic syndrome with L. tropica, resulting in a temporary ban on blood and organ donations from all those involved in the operation.*

Reed SG, Scott P: T-cell and cytokine responses in leishmaniasis. Curr Opin Immunol 5:524, 1993. *Excellent review of the immunology of leishmaniasis.*

Wilson ME, Donnelson JE, Pearson RD, et al.: Macrophage receptors and *Leishmania*. In Korkonen TK, Hovi T, Makela PH (eds.): Molecular Recognition in Host-Parasite Interactions. New York, Plenum Publishing, 1992, p 17. *The receptors and ligands that mediate leishmania-macrophage interactions are discussed.*

378 TOXOPLASMOSIS

Carlos S. Subauste and Jack S. Remington

DEFINITION. *Toxoplasma gondii* is a protozoan that commonly infects mammals and birds throughout the world. *T. gondii* infection in humans is usually asymptomatic. However, clinical and/or pathologic evidence of disease (toxoplasmosis) occurs in some cases, particularly in the immunodeficient patient and fetus. Infection is characterized by two stages: acute (recently acquired) and chronic (latent). For information on congenital toxoplasmosis, the reader is referred to the Remington and Klein text (see end of this chapter).

LIFE CYCLE. *T. gondii* exists in three forms: the tachyzoite, which is the asexual invasive form; the tissue cyst (containing bradyzoites), which persists in tissues of infected hosts during the chronic phase of the infection; and the oocyst (containing sporozoites), which is produced during the sexual cycle in the intestine of cats (the definitive host). The extraintestinal asexual cycle is present in all incidental hosts and in cats. After ingestion of tissue cysts or oocysts, bradyzoites or sporozoites, respectively, are released into the intestinal lumen, where they invade surrounding cells, become tachyzoites, and disseminate throughout the body via the blood and lymphatics. The *tachyzoite* has a crescent shape, measures approximately 3 by 7 μm, requires an intracellular habitat for survival, and can infect all mammalian cells. Continued multiplication ultimately results in destruction of the host cell and release of tachyzoites, which can then infect other cells. Tachyzoites are found in tissues during the acute stage of the infection or during reactivation of the chronic infection. Freezing and thawing, desiccation, and gastric secretions kill tachyzoites. Development of immunity is associated with disappearance of tachyzoites and formation of tissue cysts. *Tissue cysts* measure from 10 to 200 μm in diameter, may contain up to several thousand bradyzoites, can be found in all organs, and are most readily observed in myocardial, skeletal, and smooth muscle and the central nervous system (CNS). In humans, they appear to persist for life. Unlike tachyzoites, bradyzoites released from tissue cysts are relatively resistant to the digestive process of the gastrointestinal tract. The enteroepithelial sexual cycle results in the formation of oocysts in the cat's intestine. *Oocysts* measure 10 to 12 μm in diameter, are excreted in the feces 3 to 34 days after the cat becomes infected, and continue to be excreted for 7 to 20 days, after which excretion rarely recurs. They become infectious only after they are excreted and sporulation occurs; the duration of this process depends on environmental conditions but usually takes 2 to 3 days. They may remain infectious in the environment for more than 1 year.

EPIDEMIOLOGY. *T. gondii* infects humans throughout the world. In the United States, depending on geographic locale and population group, 3 to 67% of adults have serologic evidence of infection. In other parts of the world, including tropical countries and some areas of western Europe, up to 90% of adults are seropositive. Transmission to humans occurs by ingesting tissue cysts or oocysts, the transplacental route, blood product transfusion, organ transplantation (kidney, heart, liver), and laboratory accident. Epidemics of toxoplasmosis due to eating undercooked meat or exposure to infected cat feces have occurred. In the United States, transmission by eating undercooked or raw meat containing tissue cysts or of vegetables or other food products contaminated with oocysts appears more common than transmission by contact with cat feces. Commercial cuts of pork and lamb (but rarely beef) may contain tissue cysts that remain infectious unless the meat is frozen to −20° C or heated to 66° C.

The incidence of congenital toxoplasmosis in the United States ranges from 1 in 1000 to 1 in 8000 live births. Transplacental infection resulting in congenital infection can occur in immunocompetent pregnant women with acute *T. gondii* infection and in immunocompromised pregnant women with reactivation of a chronic infection. If the acute infection in the mother goes untreated, congenital infection occurs in approximately 15% of fetuses when maternal infection is acquired during the first trimester, 30% when acquired in the second trimester, and 60% when acquired in the third trimester. The earlier the transmission to the fetus, the more severe the outcome. Toxoplasmic encephalitis (TE) in AIDS patients (and in Hodgkin's disease and bone marrow transplant recipients) in the United States is almost always due to reactivation of a chronic infection. Therefore, the incidence of this disease is proportional to the prevalence of *T. gondii* antibodies (latent infection) in a given population and the stage of HIV infection in these patients (usually CD4 count <200 per cubic millimeter). In the United States, *T. gondii* seroprevalence in HIV-infected individuals varies from 10 to 45%. It is estimated that 20 to 47% of HIV-infected, *T. gondii*–seropositive patients ultimately develop TE.

PATHOGENESIS. Following infection by the oral route, tachyzoites disseminate from the gastrointestinal tract and can invade virtually any cell or tissue, where they proliferate and produce necrotic foci surrounded by inflammation. In immunocompromised individuals, acute infection may result in severe damage to multiple organs. Both cell-mediated immunity and humoral immunity play a crucial role in resistance against *T. gondii*. Despite a normal immune response, tissue cysts form in multiple organs. Although disruption of cysts or "leakage" of bradyzoites from cysts appears to occur in normal hosts without causing disease, this can result in life-threatening disease in immunocompromised patients. Immunocompetent children or adults with congenital *T. gondii* infection can develop a localized reactivation that usually manifests clinically as recurrent retinochoroiditis.

CLINICAL MANIFESTATIONS. *Acute Infection in Immunocompetent Patients.* *T. gondii* infection is symptomatic in only approximately 10 to 20% of immunocompetent individuals. In these patients, toxoplasmosis most often presents as lymphadenopathy. Although any or all lymph node groups may be involved, cervical lymphadenopathy is most common; nodes are usually discrete, nontender, nonsuppurative, and asymptomatic. However, some patients may present with fever, myalgias, arthralgias, fatigue, headache, sore throat, maculopapular rash, urticaria, hepatosplenomegaly, small numbers (<10%) of atypical lymphocytes, and rarely myocarditis. Involvement of retroperitoneal or mesenteric nodes may be associated with abdominal pain. Toxoplasmic lymphadenopathy is a self-limited disease, although fatigue and/or lymphadenopathy may persist or recur for months. Clinical illness due to reinfection from an exogenous source has not been reported.

Ocular Toxoplasmosis in Immunocompetent Patients. *T. gondii* infection has been reported to be responsible for approxi-

mately 35% of retinochoroiditis in older children and adults in the United States. Individuals with recently acquired infection uncommonly develop ocular involvement. *T. gondii* retinochoroiditis usually presents as a late manifestation of congenital infection. These latter patients are usually asymptomatic until adolescence or adulthood. Reactivation is uncommon after age 40. Patients may present with blurred vision, scotoma, pain, photophobia, or epiphora. Macular involvement may impair central vision. Systemic symptoms usually do not accompany ocular involvement. Ophthalmologic examination reveals multiple yellow-white, cotton-like patches with indistinct margins, located in small clusters in the posterior pole. Retinochoroiditis in the context of congenital infection is often bilateral, whereas retinochoroiditis in patients with recently acquired infection is typically unilateral. Retinochoroiditis may be part of a syndrome of panuveitis; isolated anterior uveitis has not been associated with *T. gondii*. Lesions may heal spontaneously, in which case they become atrophic with whitish gray plaques with distinct margins surrounded by areas of black choroidal pigment. Lesions at different stages of development may occur simultaneously. Multiple relapses may occur and may result in glaucoma and loss of vision.

Toxoplasmosis in Immunocompromised Patients. Numerous conditions that compromise the immune system have been associated with toxoplasmosis, including AIDS, Hodgkin's disease, and the use of corticosteroids or other immunosuppressive agents for treating malignancies, collagen-vascular disorders, or prevention of organ transplant rejection. In patients with these conditions, toxoplasmosis may be due to exogenous acquisition of infection or, more commonly, to reactivation of a latent infection. It is often rapidly progressive and fatal if untreated. Clinical manifestations are most commonly secondary to involvement of the CNS, lungs, eyes, and heart. TE is the most common manifestation and is also the most frequent cause of intracerebral mass lesions in patients with AIDS (see Ch. 364). TE typically presents with focal neurologic abnormalities of subacute onset, frequently accompanied by nonfocal signs and symptoms such as headache, altered mental status, and fever. The most common focal neurologic sign is motor weakness, but patients may also present with cranial nerve abnormalities, speech disturbances, visual field defects, sensory disturbances, cerebellar signs, focal seizures, and movement disorders. Meningeal signs may be present. Cerebrospinal fluid (CSF) may show slight mononuclear pleocytosis, increased protein, and normal glucose levels. Although radiologic findings are not pathognomonic, the presence of multiple lesions in AIDS patients strongly favors the diagnosis of TE, whereas the presence of a single lesion makes TE less likely. Computed tomographic (CT) scans usually show multiple bilateral cerebral lesions, which tend to be located at the corticomedullary junction and the basal ganglia. These lesions are generally hypodense and show ring enhancement after intravenous contrast. CT scans tend to underestimate the number of lesions and may show a single lesion when magnetic resonance imaging (MRI) reveals two or more lesions. MRI is more sensitive and should be performed in patients with suspected TE whenever feasible, but especially if only a single lesion is seen on CT. MRI scans show TE lesions as high signal abnormalities on T2-weighted imaging. The differential diagnosis of TE includes CNS lymphoma, progressive multifocal leukoencephalopathy, and infections due to other opportunistic pathogens.

Toxoplasmic pneumonitis may develop in the absence of extrapulmonary disease. Its clinical and radiologic features are nonspecific and may mimic *Pneumocystis carinii* pneumonia. Patients present with fever, dyspnea, and nonproductive cough, and their chest radiographs usually show bilateral interstitial infiltrates. Although ocular toxoplasmosis is infrequent in AIDS patients, it is still the second most common cause of retinal infection in these patients. It should be distinguished from ocular involvement due to cytomegalovirus, syphilis, herpes simplex, varicella zoster, *P. carinii*, lymphoma, and fungi. Clinical manifestations secondary to cardiac involvement occur but are unusual. In non-AIDS immunocompromised patients, congestive heart failure, arrhythmias, and pericarditis have been noted. Toxoplasmic myocarditis can mimic heart transplant rejection.

DIAGNOSIS. Toxoplasmosis can be diagnosed by isolating the organism; serology; polymerase chain reaction (PCR); demonstrating tachyzoites in tissues or body fluids by histology or cytology; and demonstrating characteristic lymph node histology. Isolation of

T. gondii is accomplished by inoculating blood, CSF, bronchoalveolar lavage (BAL) fluid, amniotic fluid, or tissue specimens into mice or cell culture. Mouse inoculation is more sensitive than cell culture. Many commercial serology kits to detect *T. gondii* antibodies are not adequate and give unacceptable numbers of false-positive and/or false-negative results. Only the most commonly used tests are discussed here. IgG antibodies can be detected with the Sabin-Feldman dye test (considered the gold standard), indirect fluorescent antibody (IFA), agglutination, or enzyme-linked immunosorbent assay (ELISA) tests. IgG antibodies measured by the dye test and IFA test usually appear 1 to 2 weeks after infection, peak (usually ≥ 1:1000) in 6 to 8 weeks, and gradually decline thereafter; low titers (1:4 to 1:64) usually persist for life. The agglutination test is a sensitive and inexpensive method to screen for IgG antibodies.

Detecting IgM antibodies is frequently useful to diagnose the acute infection. Their absence virtually excludes this diagnosis in immunocompetent patients. IgM antibodies appear as early as 5 days after infection and usually disappear after a few weeks or months; low levels can, however, persist for more than 1 year.

Diagnosis of acute *T. gondii* infection often requires performing and evaluating a panel of tests in a reference laboratory. This is critical in pregnant women, who may choose abortion when informed of a positive IgM test. Recent infection is likely when serial specimens obtained at least 3 weeks apart and tested in parallel show significant rise in IgG antibody titers, and/or by the presence of IgM, IgA, or IgE titers in conjunction with an "acute profile" in the differential agglutination test. The usefulness of serology in HIV-infected patients is mainly to identify those at risk for developing toxoplasmosis. Therefore, all HIV-positive patients should be tested for the presence of IgG antibodies. In addition, serologic tests may be misleading in chronically infected patients who receive heart or other organ transplants because these patients can show rising titers of IgG and IgM antibodies without clinical evidence of active *T. gondii* infection. Definitive diagnosis of toxoplasmosis in immunodeficient patients ultimately relies on histologic studies, isolating the parasite, and/or identifying *T. gondii* DNA from appropriate sites. However, a presumptive diagnosis of TE in AIDS patients can be made in the presence of a compatible clinical presentation, the presence of multiple ring-enhancing lesions on CT or MRI scans, and the presence of IgG antibodies. HIV-infected patients who present with a single lesion on MRI scan or who are seronegative for *T. gondii* antibodies should be considered for brain biopsy.

PCR has been used successfully on CSF, amniotic fluid, samples from BAL, and blood to diagnose toxoplasmosis. Routine histologic and cytologic staining may not allow tachyzoites to be identified in tissue sections. An immunohistochemical method should be used to confirm their presence. The presence of multiple cysts in tissue sections near an area of inflammation and necrosis is highly suggestive of active infection. The histologic features of toxoplasmic lymphadenopathy are considered diagnostic.

TREATMENT. The need for and duration of therapy depend on the clinical manifestations of toxoplasmosis and the immune status of the patient.

Acute Infection in Immunocompetent Patients. Patients with toxoplasmic lymphadenitis do not require antimicrobial therapy unless symptoms are severe and persistent. Pyrimethamine plus sulfadiazine is considered the regimen of choice and is synergistic against tachyzoites. It is not active against the tissue cyst form. In adults, a loading dose of 200 mg of pyrimethamine is administered orally in two divided doses on the first day. Thereafter, patients receive 25 to 50 mg per day orally. Owing to the prolonged half-life of pyrimethamine (4 to 5 days), administration every 2 to 4 days has been suggested. Sulfadiazine is administered as a loading dose of 75 mg per kilogram (up to 4 grams) orally followed by a daily dose of 100 mg per kilogram (up to 6 grams) divided in two doses. Other sulfonamides have less activity against *T. gondii*. Treatment is usually continued for 2 to 4 weeks followed by reassessing the patient's condition. Because pyrimethamine is a folate antagonist, the most common side effect is dose-related bone marrow suppression. Patients receiving pyrimethamine should thus be placed on a daily oral dose of 5 to 10 mg of folinic acid (*not* folic acid) and have complete blood cell and platelet counts measured twice weekly. Patients receiving sulfonamides should maintain high urinary flow to prevent crystal-induced nephrotoxicity. Other important side effects of sulfonamides are fever, rash, leukopenia, and hepatitis. Infections acquired after a blood transfusion or laboratory accident may be severe and therefore should be treated.

Ocular Toxoplasmosis in Immunocompetent Patients. Patients with toxoplasmic retinochoroiditis may be treated with pyrimethamine plus sulfadiazine (P + S). Clindamycin, either alone or in combination with pyrimethamine or sulfadiazine, has also been effective. Systemic corticosteroids are added to the regimen when retinochoroiditis involves the macula, optic nerve head, or papillomacular bundle.

Acute Infection in Pregnant Women. Spiramycin at a dose of 3 grams daily* appears to reduce the incidence of fetal infection by about 60%. If prenatal diagnosis reveals infection in the fetus, the pregnant patient should receive pyrimethamine and sulfadiazine in order to treat the fetus. Owing to potential teratogenicity, pyrimethamine should not be administered in the first 16 weeks of pregnancy.

Toxoplasmosis in Immunocompromised Patients. Immunodeficient patients with toxoplasmosis or with serologic evidence of an acute *T. gondii* infection should be treated. Chronic asymptomatic infection does not require treatment. In non-AIDS immunodeficient patients, therapy is usually administered until 4 to 6 weeks after all clinical evidence of toxoplasmosis resolves. Treatment is usually based on the presumptive diagnosis of TE (see section on diagnosis). Treatment of toxoplasmosis in AIDS patients has two phases: acute stage therapy and maintenance treatment. Acute therapy should be administered for at least 3 weeks; 6 weeks is recommended in patients with severe illness or when significant clinical and/or neuroradiologic response has not been achieved. P + S and pyrimethamine plus clindamycin (P + C) have been used with comparable results (Table 378–1). Most patients respond to these regimens, and neurologic improvement usually occurs within the first 7 days. Brain biopsy should be considered if clinical improvement does not occur during the first 2 weeks of treatment or if deterioration occurs during the first 3 days. Many AIDS patients do not tolerate one or the other regimen because of rash (P + S), rash and diarrhea (P + C), or bone marrow suppression (P + S, P + C). Short courses of corticosteroids can be administered to treat cerebral edema and intracranial hypertension. The mortality rate in treated patients ranges from approximately 1 to 25%. Because most AIDS patients relapse when treatment is discontinued, maintenance therapy is necessary. The optimal regimen has not been identified. Usually the same drugs used for acute therapy are continued but at lower doses (Table 378–1). For patients who do not tolerate any of these regimens for acute stage or maintenance therapy, alternatives listed in Table 378–1 can be tried in combination with pyrimethamine.

PREVENTION. Preventing the infection is particularly important for seronegative immunocompromised patients and pregnant women. Patients should be instructed to eat meat only if it is well cooked, to wash their hands after touching undercooked meat, and to wash fruits and vegetables. In addition, patients should avoid contact with cat feces. It seems prudent to avoid transfusions of blood products from a seropositive donor to a seronegative immunocompromised patient when feasible. If possible, seronegative recipients should receive transplanted organs from seronegative donors. If not feasible, seronegative patients who receive organs from seropositive donors should be treated with pyrimethamine, 25 mg daily for 6 weeks.

For primary prophylaxis in *T. gondii* seropositive HIV-infected patients with a CD4 count < 200 cells per cubic millimeter, administering either trimethoprim-sulfamethoxazole, pyrimethamine-dapsone, or pyrimethamine-sulfadoxine (Fansidar) is indicated to prevent development of toxoplasmosis (Table 378–2). To attempt to prevent congenital toxoplasmosis, routine serologic screening of pregnant women has been recommended so that fetuses at risk can be detected. Serologic status of pregnant women should be evaluated no later than the 10th or 12th week of gestation. Those who are seronegative should be retested at the 20th to 22nd week and then again near term. Administering spiramycin to acutely infected

---

* Obtained from the Food and Drug Administration: phone 301-443-4280.

TABLE 378–1. GUIDELINES FOR ACUTE AND MAINTENANCE THERAPY OF TOXOPLASMIC ENCEPHALITIS IN AIDS PATIENTS

	Acute Therapy	Maintenance Therapy*
Suggested regimens		
Pyrimethamine	Oral 200 mg loading dose, then 50 to 75 mg qd	25 to 50 mg qd
plus		
Folinic acid (leucovorin)	Oral, IV, or IM 10 to 20 mg qd (up to 50 mg qd)	10 to 20 mg qd
plus one of the following		
Sulfadiazine or	Oral 1 to 1.5 g q 6 hr	1 g q 12 hr
Clindamycin	Oral or IV 600 mg q 6 hr (up to IV 1200 mg q 6 hr)	300 mg q 6 hr
Pyrimethamine-sulfadoxine (Fansidar)	No adequate data	1 tablet t.i.w.
Alternative regimens†		
Trimethoprim-sulfamethoxazole	Oral or IV, 5 mg (trimethoprim component)/kg q 6 hr	No adequate data
Pyrimethamine	No adequate data	50 mg qd
plus		
Folinic acid		10 to 20 mg qd
Pyrimethamine and folinic acid	As in suggested regimens	As in suggested regimens
plus one of the following		
Clarithromycin or	Oral 1 g q 12 hr	1 mg q 12 hr
Azithromycin or	Oral 1200 to 1500 mg qd	1200 to 1500 mg qd
Atovaquone or	Oral 750 mg q 6 hr	750 mg q 6 hr
Dapsone	Oral 100 mg qd	100 mg b.i.w.

* Drugs administered orally.
† Data inadequate for definitive recommendation.
Adapted from Wong SY, Remington JS: Toxoplasmosis in the setting of AIDS. *In* Broder S, Merigan TC Jr, Bolognesi D (eds.): Textbook of AIDS Medicine. Baltimore, Williams & Wilkins, 1994.

TABLE 378–2. PRIMARY PROPHYLAXIS FOR TOXOPLASMOSIS IN AIDS PATIENTS*

For the *T. gondii*–seropositive HIV-infected individual†

Trimethoprim-sulfamethoxazole	1 DS tab qd
	2 DS tab b.i.w.
Pyrimethamine-dapsone	Pyrimethamine, 50 mg once a week, plus dapsone, 50 mg qd
	Pyrimethamine, 25 mg b.i.w., plus dapsone, 100 mg b.i.w.
	Pyrimethamine, 75 mg once a week, plus dapsone, 200 mg once a week
Pyrimethamine-sulfadoxine (Fansidar)	3 tablets every two weeks
	1 tablet b.i.w.

For prevention of congenital transmission of *T. gondii* in seropositive, HIV-infected pregnant women‡

Spiramycin	1 g q 8 hr

DS = double strength.
* Drugs are administered orally.
† These regimens have been reported to be effective for primary prophylaxis of toxoplasmic encephalitis in AIDS patients.
‡ Although at present no data are available on the efficacy of prophylaxis against congenital transmission in this group of patients, we consider it prudent to recommend spiramycin because preliminary studies by Mitchell and colleagues suggest that the transmission rate for congenital toxoplasmosis in these women is remarkably and significantly higher than in non–HIV-infected, *T. gondii*–seropositive women.
Adapted from Wong SY, Remington JS: Toxoplasmosis in the setting of AIDS. *In* Broder S, Merigan TC Jr, Bolognesi D (eds.): Textbook of AIDS Medicine. Baltimore, Williams & Wilkins, 1994.

pregnant women (see section on treatment) appears to reduce the incidence of congenital infection by approximately 60%.

Dubey JP: Toxoplasma, neospora, sarcocystis, and other tissue cyst-forming coccidia of humans and animals. *In* Kreier JP (ed.): Parasitic Protozoa, vol. 6. San Diego, Academic Press, 1993, p 1. *Comprehensive review of the biology of* T. gondii.

Israelski DM, Remington JS: Toxoplasmosis in the non-AIDS immunocompromised host. *In* Remington JS, Schwartz MN (eds.): Current Clinical Topics in Infectious Diseases, vol. 13. Boston, Blackwell Scientific, 1993, p 322. *A review of the association of toxoplasmosis with disorders, other than AIDS, that compromise the immune system.*

Luft BJ, Hafner R, Korzun AH, et al.: Toxoplasmic encephalitis in patients with the acquired immunodeficiency syndrome. N Engl J Med 329:995, 1993. *A critically evaluated prospective study on the clinical/radiologic course of patients treated with pyrimethamine plus clindamycin for toxoplasmic encephalitis.*

Remington JS, McLeod R, Desmonts G: Toxoplasmosis. *In* Remington JS, Klein KO (eds.): Infectious Diseases of the Fetus and Newborn Infant. 4th ed. Philadelphia, WB Saunders, 1995, p 140. *A comprehensive discussion of congenital toxoplasmosis and the diagnosis and management of acute* T. gondii *infection during pregnancy.*

Wong SY, Remington JS: Toxoplasmosis in the setting of AIDS. *In* Broder S, Merigan TC, Bolognesi D (eds.): Textbook of AIDS Medicine. Baltimore, Williams & Wilkins, 1994, p 223. *A comprehensive overview of the clinical presentation, diagnosis, management, and prevention of toxoplasmosis in AIDS patients.*

379 CRYPTOSPORIDIOSIS
Rosemary Soave

Cryptosporidiosis is a gastrointestinal infection characterized by watery diarrhea, abdominal cramps, malabsorption, and weight loss. It is usually a severe, unrelenting illness in immunocompromised patients, particularly those with the acquired immunodeficiency syndrome (AIDS), and a self-limited disease in the immunologically normal host. It is caused by the coccidian protozoan *Cryptosporidium*, long associated with disease in animals. In 1981–1982, identification of *Cryptosporidium* in 47 AIDS patients with severe enteritis brought the protozoan to the attention of the medical community. As more physicians have looked for this parasite, the number of reported cases of cryptosporidiosis has continued to rise, and it has come to be recognized as an emerging threat to domestic and global health. There is currently no known effective therapy.

THE PROTOZOAN. *Cryptosporidium* (which means "hidden spore") belongs to the class Sporozoa and the suborder Eimeriorina, or true coccidia. Other pathogens of humans in this group include *Toxoplasma gondii, Isospora belli,* and the recently recognized *Cyclospora* species. Although 20 species within the genus *Cryptosporidium* have been described, cross-transmission experiments suggest that little or no host specificity exists. *C. parvum* is the species responsible for disease in humans and mammals.

The 4- to 5-μm, spherical, acid-fast *Cryptosporidium* oocyst is the environmentally resistant form of the parasite that is identified in fecal specimens (Fig. 379–1). Sporulated (mature) oocysts contain four elliptical (2 to 4 × 6 to 8 μm), flat, aflagellar but motile sporozoites that are released (excystation) in the host intestinal tract upon dissolution of the oocyst's outer wall. Sporozoites implant on the host mucosal epithelium and undergo asexual and sexual development within a parasitophorous vacuole. The parasite–host cell relationship is unique in that the parasite is intracellular, i.e., en-

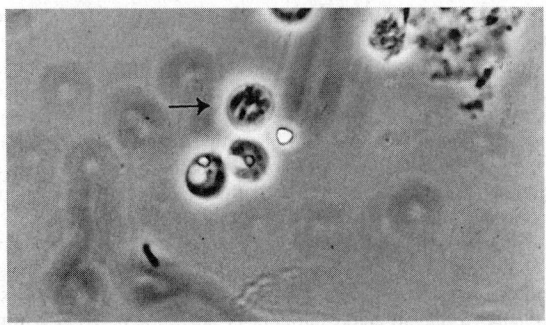

FIGURE 379-1. Wet mount of human stool showing three cryptosporidial oocysts and sporozoites *(arrow)* (×630).

veloped by a host cell membrane, but extracytoplasmic. Sporozoites develop into trophozoites and subsequently undergo asexual multiplication (merogony), formation of macrogametes and microgametes (gametogony), fertilization, and oocyst formation. Newly formed oocysts that are expelled in the feces are immediately infective. The ability of *Cryptosporidium* to develop completely within one host (monoxenous life cycle) imparts a tremendous potential for reinfection and may contribute to the refractory nature of the illness that is seen in *Cryptosporidium*-infected AIDS patients.

EPIDEMIOLOGY. Although more than 100 reports of cryptosporidial infection have emanated from at least 60 countries spanning 6 continents, the true prevalence of cryptosporidiosis in either immunocompetent or immunocompromised hosts is unknown. These surveys of selected populations have revealed infection rates ranging from 0.6 to 20% in the developed world and 4 to 32% in the developing world. Available reports indicate that *Cryptosporidium* is ubiquitous and a major cause of diarrhea worldwide. They also suggest that higher infection rates are associated with young age (< 2 years); warm, wet weather; and overcrowding. In addition, several studies have revealed higher than expected rates of seropositivity, suggesting that active or recent cryptosporidial infection may be common in the general population. As of 1986, the Centers for Disease Control and Prevention estimated that 3 to 4% of AIDS patients had cryptosporidiosis. In recent studies, approximately 16% of AIDS patients with diarrhea were found to be infected. By contrast, more than 30% of AIDS patients in Haiti and parts of Africa have cryptosporidiosis. Asymptomatic carriage of the parasite has been documented in immunocompetent and immunocompromised subjects, but the frequency with which it occurs and its significance have yet to be determined.

Transmission of *Cryptosporidium* between humans and domestic animals has been well documented, and it is likely that both serve as reservoirs of the disease. For humans, however, spread from person to person and via contaminated water is more common than zoonotic transmission. Person-to-person transmission has been implicated in day care center outbreaks, clusters of infection among contacts of index cases, spread between sexual partners, and nosocomial spread of infection among patients and health care workers. Contaminated water is responsible for infection in travelers and swimmers, and for a number of major community outbreaks in the United States and the United Kingdom. In the spring of 1993, an outbreak of waterborne cryptosporidiosis in Milwaukee, Wisconsin, caused diarrheal illness in approximately 403,000, 4,400 of whom required hospitalization. This was the largest waterborne outbreak ever recorded in the United States. *Cryptosporidium* oocysts are often detected in pristine and sewage-contaminated surface waters, treated and untreated sewage effluent, and municipal water supplies. The public health impact of low levels of *Cryptosporidium* oocysts in drinking water is unknown and currently under study. The infectious dose of *Cryptosporidium* appears to be very low but has not yet been defined. The *Cryptosporidium* oocyst is very resistant to common disinfectants; it is unaffected by chlorine concentrations in drinking water or swimming pools. Boiling water for 1 minute eliminates the risk of acquiring *Cryptosporidium* from contaminated drinking water. *Cryptosporidium* infectivity may also be destroyed by freeze-drying or by treatment with 5 to 10% ammonia, 70% to full-strength bleach, or 10% formaldehyde.

PATHOLOGY AND PATHOGENESIS. *Cryptosporidium* has

been found in the pharynx, esophagus, stomach, duodenum, jejunum, ileum, appendix, colon, rectum, gallbladder, pancreas, bile, and pancreatic ducts, as well as within colonic submucosal vessels of infected immunocompromised (primarily AIDS) patients. The parasite has also been detected in sputum, tracheal aspirates, bronchoalveolar lavage, and lung tissue of a small number of immunocompromised patients with gastrointestinal cryptosporidiosis. Light microscopic evaluation of Giemsa-stained or hematoxylin-eosin–stained *Cryptosporidium*-infected tissue reveals small, spherical, basophilic structures along the epithelial cell brush border. Ultrastructural studies reveal the entire spectrum of endogenous stages of the organism adherent to the enterocyte surface and enveloped by a membrane, believed to be derived from the host cell. Histologic changes are nonspecific and minimal, resembling those described for giardiasis, i.e., villous atrophy, crypt elongation, and minimal subjacent inflammatory infiltrates of the lamina propria. By contrast, marked histologic changes ranging from acute inflammation to gangrenous necrosis of the gallbladder and biliary duct epithelium have been described for patients with cryptosporidial cholangitis or cholecystitis.

The pathogenic mechanisms by which *Cryptosporidium* causes enteritis are unknown. The secretory nature of the diarrhea and the presence of malabsorption suggest that an enterotoxin-mediated mechanism and/or physical destruction of the brush border may be operative.

CLINICAL MANIFESTATIONS. The spectrum of cryptosporidial infection ranges from asymptomatic infection to fulminant diarrhea. Cryptosporidiosis is characterized by watery diarrhea, cramping abdominal pain (often exacerbated by food ingestion), weight loss, and flatulence. Nausea, vomiting, anorexia, myalgias, and malaise may also be present. Fever, leukocytosis, and eosinophilia are not common. Fecal examination reveals cryptosporidial oocysts and mucus, but no leukocytes or blood. Vitamin B_{12}, xylose, and fat malabsorption have been documented. Radiographic abnormalities are nonspecific and include prominent mucosal folds, intestinal wall thickening, small bowel dilatation, and disordered motility.

The incubation period for human cryptosporidiosis appears to be between 2 and 14 days. The severity and course of the illness are determined by host immunocompetence. In the immunologically normal host, infection is often explosive in onset and lasts an average of 10 to 14 days. Clearance of the parasite from stool lags behind clinical resolution by 2 to 3 weeks, thus creating problems for infection control. Although self-limited, symptoms are often severe enough to justify therapeutic intervention, were it available. Infection in AIDS patients often begins insidiously and escalates in severity as the underlying immune defect becomes more profound. Frequent (6 to 25), voluminous (1 to 25 liters) daily bowel movements, profound weight loss, and stool oocyst shedding often persist for months.

Biliary cryptosporidiosis has been documented only in immunocompromised patients. Because invasive procedures that may not be justified in the absence of treatment options are a prerequisite for definitive diagnosis, the incidence of this complication is not known. Most patients with biliary cryptosporidiosis have classic signs of cholangitis, including severe right upper quadrant pain, nausea, and vomiting. Serum levels of alkaline phosphatase and γ-glutamyl transpeptidase are elevated, but serum bilirubin and transaminase levels are usually normal. Radiographic evaluation may reveal a dilated gallbladder, thickened gallbladder wall, and dilated bile ducts with luminal irregularities. Patients undergoing endoscopic retrograde cholangiopancreatography (ERCP) are often found to have cryptosporidia studding the surface epithelium and in the bile. In certain instances, cholecystectomy or endoscopic papillotomy has resulted in transient improvement of both symptoms and laboratory abnormalities.

DIAGNOSIS. The diagnosis of cryptosporidial enteritis is based on identifying the oocyst form of the parasite in fecal specimens. Since 1981, various staining techniques for detecting oocysts have been popularized, including several modifications of the acid-fast stain (Kinyoun, Ziehl-Neelsen), the fluorescent auramine-rhodamine stain, and the periodic acid-Schiff (PAS) and carbol fuchsin–negative stains. With the acid-fast stain, acid-fast (red) oocysts may be easily distinguished from yeast that are similar in size and shape but are not acid fast (they stain green). Although the acid-fast stain is commonly used because it is quick and inexpensive, recent studies suggest that it is quite insensitive. Concentration of stool, such as by centrifugation, enhances sensitivity. A fluorescein-labeled monoclonal antibody directed at the oocyst wall and an enzyme-linked immunosorbent assay (ELISA) antigen-capture microtiter assay are now commercially available. The sensitivity, specificity, and relative merits of the various methods for fecal diagnosis of cryptosporidiosis have not been fully defined, but the latter two techniques appear to be more sensitive than staining methods, and their role in the clinical laboratory is currently being investigated. Because the pattern of fecal oocyst shedding in human cryptosporidiosis has not been determined, and the sensitivity of the various methodologies is also not known, the optimal number of negative stool specimens required to confirm the absence of cryptosporidia has yet to be defined. If the acid-fast stain is used to detect *Cryptosporidium*, it is important to note that *Cyclospora*, a newly recognized acid-fast coccidian parasite that causes a clinical syndrome indistinguishable from cryptosporidiosis, may be mistaken for *Cryptosporidium*. Precise measurement of oocyst size is used to differentiate *Cryptosporidium* (4 to 5 μm) from *Cyclospora* (8 to 10 μm). Accurate identification is crucial because *Cyclospora* appears to be sensitive to trimethoprim-sulfamethoxazole.

Although the sensitivity and specificity of stool examination compared with small intestinal biopsy have not been determined, stool examination appears to be more sensitive. In addition to being invasive and costly, intestinal biopsies may be falsely negative owing to autolysis during processing and sampling difficulties related to the parasite's patchy distribution and the paucity of inflammatory changes to guide the endoscopist.

Anticryptosporidial IgG and IgM have been detected in both immunocompetent persons and patients with AIDS by immunofluorescent assay (IFA) and ELISA. Antibody titers rise within 6 to 8 weeks after the onset of infection and decline within 1 year. Immunocompetent hosts generally have higher titers. The IgM response is often absent or minimal in patients with AIDS. Serologic studies are not useful in diagnosing acute cryptosporidiosis but do have a role in defining the epidemiology of the disease.

TREATMENT. There is currently no known effective therapy for cryptosporidiosis. Identification of potentially active agents has been severely hampered by the absence of an asymptomatic, small-animal model of the chronic disease and by an inability to cultivate the organism *in vitro*. Investigational therapy has not been given to the immunocompetent host with cryptosporidial enteritis because illness in these patients is usually self-limited. Persons receiving corticosteroids or cytotoxic agents may be successfully managed by discontinuing the immunosuppressive drugs.

Because of the severe nature of the illness in AIDS patients with cryptosporidiosis, a vast array of antidiarrheal, antimicrobial, and immunomodulating agents have been administered in an unprecedented manner with little preclinical data to support their use. Early anecdotal reports of success using the antitoxoplasma macrolide spiramycin led to two controlled studies with this agent. A placebo-controlled clinical trial of oral spiramycin in 54 AIDS patients with cryptosporidiosis failed to show any difference between placebo and drug. Subsequent pharmacokinetic studies suggested that this may have been due to suboptimal drug absorption. In a single-blind, placebo-controlled study of intravenous spiramycin, 5 of 31 patients had clinical and parasitologic improvement, but the results were not statistically significant and there was unacceptable toxicity. The veterinary agents diclazuril and letrazuril also failed to demonstrate efficacy in placebo-controlled trials. Preliminary results from a recently concluded placebo-controlled study of the lactose-free form of oral azithromycin reveal a statistically significant correlation between parasitologic response and higher serum azithromycin levels. Further studies with both oral and intravenous azithromycin are about to begin. Paromomycin, a poorly absorbed, oral antiamebic aminoglycoside, has been associated with symptomatic relief in a subset of AIDS patients when given at a dose of 2 grams per day. However, parasitologic response is rare, and relapses are common in spite of continued therapy. Paromomycin is currently being studied in an AIDS Clinical Trials Group (ACTG)–sponsored placebo-controlled trial.

The mechanisms by which the immunocompetent host success-

fully deals with cryptosporidial infection are poorly understood but appear to include both intact T cell- and B cell-mediated immunity. Novel attempts at modulating immune function in *Cryptosporidium*-infected patients centered on using immune bovine colostrum, bovine milk globulins, and bovine transfer factor have provided interesting and conflicting results that require further investigation.

In the absence of any proven effective therapy for cryptosporidiosis, careful management of fluid and electrolyte balance is of paramount importance. All classes of nonspecific antidiarrheal agents, including the long-acting, parenterally administered somatostatin analogue octreotide acetate, may be useful, when used in trial-and-error fashion, for individual patients. However, their safety in *Cryptosporidium*-infected patients is not known. Total parenteral nutrition often provides major benefits, but its use is controversial owing to the need for an invasive procedure and its high cost.

Current WL, Garcia LS: Cryptosporidiosis. Clin Microbiol Rev 4:325, 1991. *A well-written epidemiologic, parasitologic, and clinical review.*
Mac Kenzie WR, Hoxie NJ, Proctor ME, et al.: A massive waterborne outbreak of *Cryptosporidium* infection associated with a filtered public water supply in Milwaukee, Wisconsin, March and April, 1993. N Engl J Med 331:161, 1994. *This article describes the largest waterborne outbreak recorded in the United States.*
Mannheimer SB, Soave R: Protozoal infections in patients with AIDS: Cryptosporidiosis, isoporiasis, cyclosporiasis and microsporidiosis. Infect Dis Clin North Am 8:483, 1994. *A comprehensive, fully referenced review of the clinical aspects of infection with* Cryptosporidium *and other enteritis-producing protozoans.*

380 GIARDIASIS
David P. Stevens

DEFINITION. Giardiasis is an infection of the small intestine caused by the flagellated protozoan *Giardia lamblia*. Its hallmarks are diarrhea, malabsorption, and weight loss.

ETIOLOGY. The organism exists in two forms: the motile, flagellated, pear-shaped trophozoite, 12 to 15 μm in length; and the smaller, tough-walled oval cyst. Trophozoites either attach to the microvilli of the intestinal epithelium with the characteristic attaching disc or they move about by means of flagellae in the unstirred layer of mucus just above the epithelial surface. The trophozoites, carried caudally by peristalsis, eventually encyst and pass into the environment. The cyst is resistant to many environmental stresses, including concentrations of chlorine normally found in treated municipal water supplies. Infection of a subsequent host occurs with ingestion of as few as 10 to 25 cysts. Excystation occurs in the acid environment of the stomach, and infection proceeds in the small intestine of the new host.

EPIDEMIOLOGY. Giardiasis is found in all climates and spreads by a variety of routes. Well-documented epidemics have demonstrated person-to-person spread in day care centers for children and nursing homes. Food contaminated after cooking is an infrequent cause of *Giardia* epidemics. A common source of spread is contaminated water. Dozens of epidemics have been described consequent to the breakdown of community water filtration systems. Indeed, *Giardia* is the most frequent cause of waterborne diarrhea in the United States. Animal reservoirs of infection probably contribute to surface water contamination. Campers and backpackers must be particularly mindful of the risk of drinking untreated water.

Giardia is a frequent source of diarrhea in travelers returning from endemic areas (western United States, Rocky Mountain areas). The incubation period is 7 to 21 days, so it is common for infected travelers to visit their physician several weeks after returning home. This longer incubation period serves to distinguish giardiasis from more explosive diarrhea caused by toxigenic *Escherichia coli* and other forms of infectious traveler's diarrhea that have shorter incubation periods (see Ch. 298).

PATHOGENICITY. Jejunal mucosal biopsies from infected persons range in appearance from normal to marked subtotal mucosal atrophy with submucosal inflammatory cell infiltration, reduced villus height, and elongated crypts. Electron microscopic observation of epithelial cells beneath overlying adherent trophozoites shows deformation and blunting of the individual microvilli. In spite of morphologic clues, the pathogenic mechanism for these changes remains speculative. Host humoral and cellular immune responses occur, but their roles in protection as well as pathogenesis are unclear. The increased prevalence of giardiasis in persons with immune deficiency syndromes argues for the role of immunity in host defense.

CLINICAL MANIFESTATIONS. Infection can be asymptomatic. Clinical illness, however, is associated with some or all of the following: diarrhea, cramps, flatulence, nausea, excessive tiredness, bloating, anorexia, and chills. Reversible lactase deficiency and malabsorption of fat and vitamin B_{12} have been documented. The infection is frequently self-limited, but a prolonged, indolent illness with progressive weight loss is possible.

DIAGNOSIS. Symptoms typically associated with giardiasis are nonspecific, and diagnostic tests are of low sensitivity. The diagnosis is established by observing cysts or trophozoites in stools or trophozites in small bowel contents. Because the organism may be excreted in stool intermittently and its demonstration is elusive, at least three stool specimens should be examined before a negative conclusion is drawn. Immunologic tests for *Giardia* antigens in stool are commercially available but expensive. If no organisms are detected, the small bowel contents may be sampled. This can be achieved by tube aspiration or by passing a string that will absorb sufficient jejunal fluid for examination. Microscopic examination of a wet preparation of jejunal contents usually reveals motile organisms when infection is present. Small bowel biopsy may be performed in situations in which these measures are unsuccessful. The small bowel roentgenogram usually shows an edematous mucosa, but this finding is nonspecific. Hematologic values are normal.

There is occasional justification for a trial of therapy in the patient who has the typical signs and symptoms of giardiasis but negative tests for the organism.

TREATMENT. Therapy is with quinacrine hydrochloride, 100 mg three times per day for 7 days. When this drug is contraindicated, metronidazole,* 250 mg three times per day for 7 days, is an alternative. Therapy with either drug is unsuccessful in approximately 10% of patients, requiring a second course. Treatment of infected persons in highly endemic areas is of questionable value because reinfection occurs readily when water supplies are contaminated. All infected persons in nonendemic regions should be treated.

Flanagan PA: *Giardia*—diagnosis, clinical course and epidemiology. Epidemiol Infect 109:1, 1992. *An excellent discussion of the epidemiology of giardiasis.*

Hopkins RS, Juranek DD: Acute giardiasis: An improved clinical case definition for epidemiologic studies. Am J Epidemiol 133:402, 1991. *The sensitivity and specificity of diagnostic approaches are examined.*

Sullivan PS, DuPont HL, Arafat RR, et al.: Illness and reservoirs associated with *Giardia lamblia* infection in rural Egypt: The case against treatment in developing world environments of high endemicity. Am J Epidemiol 127:1272, 1988. *Treatment issues for highly endemic regions are considered.*

381 AMEBIASIS
Jonathan I. Ravdin

Human amebiasis is due to infection with the enteric protozoan *Entamoeba histolytica*. This parasite infects 1% of the world's population, with the disease burden highest in poor, developing areas. To manage patients with amebiasis appropriately, physicians must know the biology of the organism, risk factors for infection, mechanisms of disease, pathogenesis and host immunity, the presenting manifestations of the invasive syndrome, the correct diagnostic approach, alternative therapeutic drug regimens, and strategies for preventing infection.

BIOLOGY OF *E. HISTOLYTICA* AND EPIDEMIOLOGY. Infection results from ingestion of the fecally excreted acid-resistant cyst form. Excystation occurs in the small bowel, leading to colonization of the colon with trophozoites. Transmission of infection results from fecal contamination of water or food or direct fecal-oral contact because of poor hygiene or anal-oral sexual practices. Epidemiologic and molecular biology studies indicate that there are distinct strains, the pathogenic *E. histolytica* and the nonpathogenic *Entamoeba dispar.* Infection with the latter is more common but does not result in systemic invasive disease or antigenic exposure. Approximately 10% of those with pathogenic *Entamoeba* infection present clinically with invasive amebiasis, although all manifest a serum antibody response. The relative frequency of histolytica and dispar infection varies, depending on geographic area. Regions of the world with a high incidence of invasive amebiasis include Mexico, parts of South America, western and South Africa, the Indian subcontinent, the Middle East, and Southeast Asia. High-risk groups in the United States include sexually promiscuous male homosexuals, the institutionalized mentally retarded population, and travelers or emigrants (especially Mexican-Americans) from areas of high prevalence. Groups that, when infected, can experience an increased severity of invasive amebiasis are the very young (under age 2 years), pregnant women, malnourished individuals, and patients on corticosteroids.

PATHOGENESIS AND HOST IMMUNITY. *E. histolytica* trophozoites cause disease by sequentially adhering to colonic mucins, disrupting mucosal barriers with proteolytic enzymes, and contact-dependent lysis of host cells, including responding inflammatory cells. Trophozoite adherence to colonic mucins is mediated by a galactose-binding surface protein; attachment by this protein is the first step in the amebic lysis of human cells. Intestinal infection with *E. dispar* usually clears within 8 to 12 months without evidence of a specific immune response. Cure of invasive amebiasis is associated with resistance to recurrent disease, but not necessarily immunity to asymptomatic intestinal infection. Protective immunity is apparently mediated by development of a serum antibody and an amebicidal cell-mediated immune response with lymphokine-activated macrophages and a CD8 subset of cytotoxic lymphocytes serving as effector cells. Acute amebiasis is associated with the occurrence of antigen-specific suppression of cell-mediated responses to *E. histolytica*, facilitating parasite survival in tissues. It is unclear whether the mucosal secretory IgA antiamebic antibody response that develops after pathogenic infection has any protective role.

CLINICAL DISEASE SYNDROMES. The disease syndromes caused by *E. histolytica* are summarized in Table 381–1. It is unknown whether health is impaired by asymptomatic infection with *E. dispar* or *E. histolytica*. Occasionally, infected patients present with nonspecific gastrointestinal complaints, such as bloating and cramps, without evidence of invasive colitis. Amebic rectocolitis is characterized by the subacute onset of bloody diarrhea over days, abdominal tenderness, weight loss, and fever in only one third of cases. Fulminant colitis with perforation is uncommon; patients are in a toxic state, are acutely ill, and have a rigid, tender abdomen. Toxic megacolon is an unusual complication that is associated with the inappropriate use of corticosteroids when amebic colitis is mistaken for idiopathic inflammatory bowel disease. Chronic nondysenteric amebic colitis can manifest with years of intermittent bloody diarrhea, a syndrome symptomatically indistinguishable from ulcer-

---

TABLE 381–1. CLINICAL SYNDROMES ASSOCIATED WITH *E. HISTOLYTICA* INFECTION

Intestinal Disease
Asymptomatic infection
Acute rectocolitis (dysentery)
Fulminant colitis with perforation
Toxic megacolon
Chronic nondysenteric colitis
Ameboma
Extraintestinal Disease
Liver abscess
Liver abscess complicated by:
  Peritonitis
  Empyema
  Pericarditis
Lung abscess
Brain abscess
Genitourinary disease

Reproduced with permission from Mandell GL, Douglas RG Jr, Bennett JE (eds.): Principles and Practices of Infectious Diseases. 3rd ed. New York, Churchill Livingstone, 1989.

---

* This use is not listed in the manufacturer's directive but is recommended by the Centers for Disease Control and Prevention.

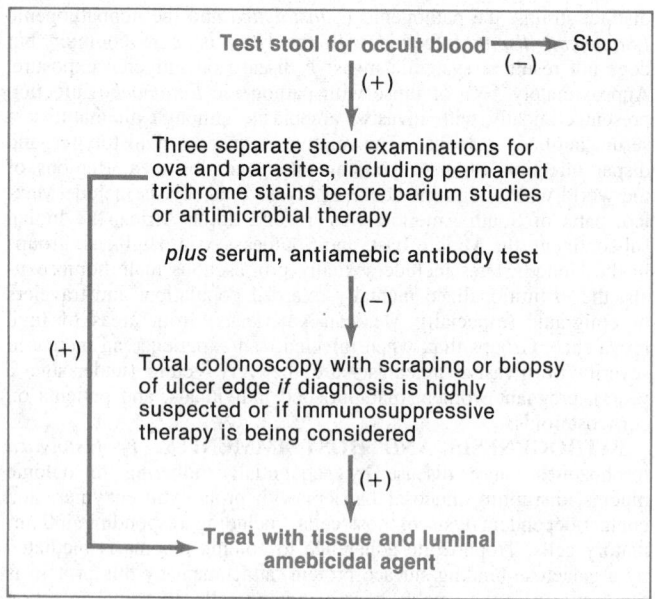

FIGURE 381-1. Diagnostic evaluation for acute amebic rectocolitis in a patient with suggestive epidemiology and clinical manifestations. (Reproduced with permission from Kass EH, Platt R [eds.]: Current Therapy in Infectious Disease-3. Philadelphia, BC Decker, 1990.)

ative colitis. Ameboma is a rare segmental form of chronic amebic colitis that is more common in the cecum and ascending colon and presents as a tender abdominal mass that can be confused with colonic carcinoma.

Extraintestinal disease consists mainly of amebic liver abscess, which can occur up to 5 months after the onset of intestinal infection. The presentation may be acute with fewer than 10 days of high fever and marked right upper quadrant tenderness. Alternatively, with more than 10 days of symptoms, fever is less frequent and pain and weight loss predominate. Fewer than a third of patients have concurrent diarrhea. Extension of an amebic liver abscess into the peritoneum or pericardium is a very acute clinical presentation that is more likely with a left lobe abscess. Disease can extend to the pleura, causing empyema, or, less likely, disseminate hematogenously to the lung and brain.

DIFFERENTIAL DIAGNOSIS AND WORKUP. Algorithms for the diagnosis of amebic colitis and liver abscess are provided in Figures 381-1 and 381-2, respectively. The differential diagnosis of acute amebic colitis includes infection due to *Shigella, Campylobacter, Salmonella, Yersinia,* and invasive *E. coli* species or *Clostridium difficile* toxin–mediated disease. Amebiasis is one

cause of inflammatory colitis in which fecal leukocytes may be absent, owing to the ability of trophozoites to lyse human neutrophils. Recently, several research groups succeeded in correctly diagnosing *E. histolytica* and *E. dispar* intestinal infections by directly detecting amebic antigen in feces and serum. Although these diagnostic tests may soon be available, in current clinical practice, the diagnosis of intestinal amebiasis still rests upon the morphologic identification of trophozoites in fecal specimens. At least three stool samples are necessary to reach a 90% yield; samples should be refrigerated or placed in fixative if they cannot be processed immediately. Laboratories in the United States frequently falsely identify fecal leukocytes as trophozoites; careful study with skilled microscopy is necessary. Serology for antiamebic antibodies is positive in >90% of patients with amebic colitis longer than 1 week in duration and is very helpful in making a correct diagnosis. Interpretation of results can be difficult in highly endemic areas, where up to 25% of the population is seropositive owing to the persistence of serum antibodies for years after asymptomatic *E. histolytica* infection. Endoscopy with biopsies of the ulcer edge is diagnostic in 90% of cases; this is helpful for a rapid diagnosis and to differentiate amebiasis from idiopathic inflammatory bowel disease.

The key study for diagnosing amebic liver abscess is abdominal ultrasonography, a rapid, noninvasive procedure that differentiates biliary tract disease from a nonhomogeneous cavitary defect in the liver. The differential diagnosis can then be narrowed to amebic liver abscess, pyogenic bacterial abscess, echinococcal cyst, and hepatoma. Attention to epidemiologic risk factors and detecting serum antiamebic antibodies are usually sufficient to establish the diagnosis, with the caveat that serology may be negative in patients with fewer than 7 days of symptoms. However, if there is sufficient risk for a bacterial abscess and a serologic study is not immediately available, then a "skinny-needle" aspiration, guided by ultrasonography or computed tomography, can be performed. This procedure with culture will diagnose and assist in therapy of a bacterial abscess; aspiration of an amebic abscess yields a yellow proteinaceous fluid often without white blood cells or amebas. The trophozoites are found in tissue at the periphery of the liver lesion.

THERAPY. Regimens for treating amebiasis are summarized in Table 381-2. Therapy of invasive amebiasis requires a tissue-active agent followed by a drug effective in the bowel lumen. In pregnant women, the use of nonabsorbable agents (paromomycin) or the judicious use of metronidazole is advisable. It is controversial whether therapy is necessary for asymptomatic intestinal infection without evidence of tissue invasion; however, this may be advisable in areas where pathogenic *E. histolytica* infection is likely or reinfection is not expected. Careful follow-up stool examinations are necessary, as all available agents are not always effective in eradicating intestinal infection. Patients with amebic liver abscess respond gradually to therapy with decreased pain and fever over 3 to 5 days. A small minority do not respond at all within 3 days or have a very large abscess that appears close to rupture; needle aspiration is indicated in such patients. After aspiration, continued therapy with metronidazole should be adequate. Recent studies revealed

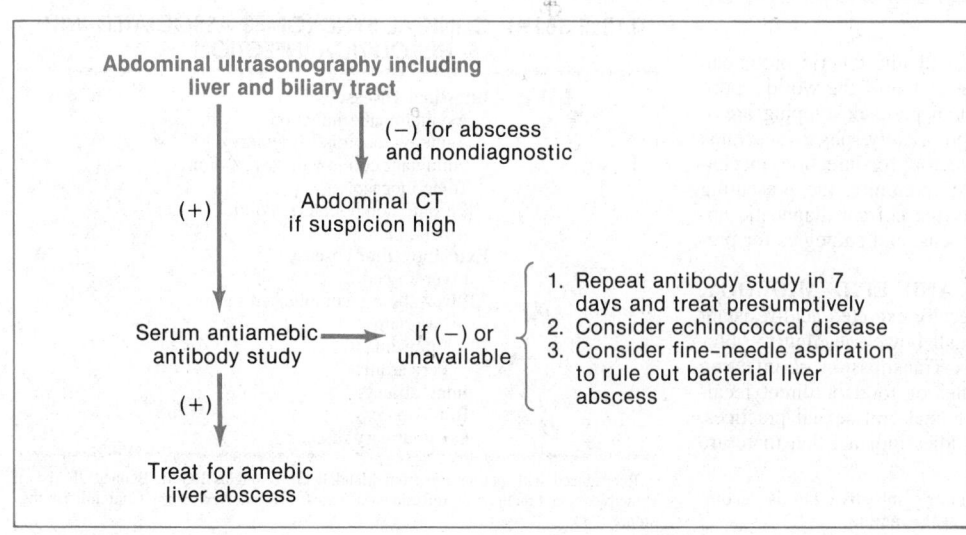

FIGURE 381-2. Diagnostic evaluation for amebic liver abscess in a patient with suggestive epidemiology and clinical manifestations. (Reproduced with permission from Kass EH, Platt R [eds.]: Current Therapy in Infectious Disease-3. Philadelphia, BC Decker, 1990.)

TABLE 381–2. THERAPEUTIC REGIMENS FOR TREATMENT OF AMEBIASIS*

Cyst Passers
Diloxanide furoate, 500 mg t.i.d. × 10 days, or
Paromomycin, 30 mg/kg/day in 3 divided doses × 5–10 days, or
Tetracycline, 250 mg q.i.d. × 10 days, then diiodohydroxyquin, 650 mg t.i.d. × 20 days

Invasive Rectocolitis
Metronidazole, 750 mg t.i.d. × 5–10 days
   or 2.4 grams qd × 2–3 days
   or 50 mg/kg × 1 dose
   plus diloxanide furoate or paromomycin or if metronidazole not tolerated
Dehydroemetine, 1–1.5 mg/kg/day × 5 days plus diloxanide furoate or paromomycin

Liver Abscess
Metronidazole, 750 t.i.d. × 5–10 days or 2.4 mg qd × 1–2 days plus diloxanide furoate or paromomycin or if metronidazole not tolerated
Dehydroemetine, 1–1.5 mg/kg/day × 5 days plus diloxanide furoate or paromomycin

* All dosages are for oral administration except dehydroemetine, which is given intramuscularly; metronidazole can be used intravenously.
Adapted with permission from Mandell GL, Douglas RG Jr, Bennett JE (eds.): Principles and Practices of Infectious Diseases. 3rd ed. New York, Churchill Livingstone, 1989.

a high incidence of intestinal infection in patients with amebic liver abscess. To avoid a recurrence of disease, therapy must include a luminal cysticidal agent.

PREVENTION. *E. histolytica* infection can be prevented by the availability of clean water, adequate sanitation, and avoidance of sexual practices or living conditions that facilitate direct fecal-oral contamination. Boiling is the only reliable way of killing cysts; halide solutions are not reliable. In endemic areas, uncooked foods such as salads and vegetables should be avoided. No vaccine or acceptable form of chemoprophylaxis is available; however, current research on the pathogenesis of amebiasis and the host immune response has led to the identification of multiple *E. histolytica* antigens that are effective as subunit vaccines in experimental models of amebic liver abscess.

AMEBIC MENINGOENCEPHALITIS

Amebic meningoencephalitis is a rare clinical syndrome caused by the free-living amebas *Naegleria fowleri* and *Acanthamoeba* species. *N. fowleri* causes a primary amebic meningoencephalitis (PAM), whereas *Acanthamoeba* produces a subacute granulomatous amebic encephalitis (GAE).

N. fowleri in trophozoite or flagellate form grows best at high temperatures (46° C); encystment occurs at low temperatures. *Acanthamoeba* species, which have a trophozoite and cyst form, grow at normal ambient temperatures (25 to 35°C). PAM is a highly infrequent disease despite the massive exposure of populations to warm fresh water. GAE is usually restricted to immunosuppressed populations, such as those with AIDS or those with organ transplants. *N. fowleri* enters the central nervous system (CNS) by penetrating the nasal mucosa and cribriform plate and is highly cytolytic. GAE probably results from hematogenous dissemination and can be distinguished from PAM by the presence of cysts in tissue.

PAM is characterized by the abrupt onset of headache, fever, and meningismus, with rapid development of focal neurologic findings, including olfactory loss. A neutrophilic cerebrospinal fluid (CSF) pleocytosis is frequently associated with increased CSF protein and hypoglycorrhachia. A negative CSF Gram stain result, India ink preparation, culture for bacteria, and cryptococcal antigen study in a patient with acute meningitis who has a history of exposure to fresh water suggests the need to examine the CSF for motile trophozoites (10 to 30 μm), a finding that is diagnostic. In contrast, GAE manifests subacutely over weeks with focal CNS signs, headache, fever, and depressed mental status and is often complicated by seizures. The presence of *Acanthamoeba* organisms in a nodular or ulcerative skin lesion is helpful; study of the CSF usually reveals a nonspecific lymphocytosis with abnormally elevated protein levels. A brain biopsy is necessary to differentiate GAE from toxoplasmosis, pyogenic brain abscess, and other causes of focal CNS disease.

There is no treatment known to be efficacious for PAM or GAE. Treatment with systemic and intrathecal amphotericin B was associated with survival in two patients with PAM. *Acanthamoeba* organ-

isms are usually susceptible *in vitro* to ketoconazole, micronazole, 5-flucytosine, and pentamidine. After determination of susceptibility of the patient's isolate *in vitro,* the above agents and amphotericin B can be considered. These are rare disorders, and the risk of PAM from diving or waterskiing in warm fresh water cannot be quantified. Other opportunistic infections are much more frequent than those caused by *Acanthamoeba* in immunosuppressed patients.

Katzenstein D, Rickerson V, Braude A: New concepts of amebic liver abscess derived from hepatic imaging, serodiagnosis, and hepatic enzymes in 67 consecutive cases in San Diego. Medicine (Baltimore) 61:237, 1982. *Excellent clinical study of amebic liver abscess.*
Martinez AJ: Infection of the central nervous system due to Acanthamoeba. Rev Infect Dis 5:S399, 1991. *An up-to-date review of* Acanthamoeba *infections, including epidemiology, clinical course, diagnosis, and treatment.*
Ravdin JI: Diagnosis of invasive amoebiasis—time to end the morphology era. Gut 35:1018, 1994. *The most recent authoritative review of the approach to diagnosis of amebic infection.*
Ravdin JI, Petri WA: Entamoeba histolytica. In Mandell GL, Bennett JE (eds.): Principles and Practices of Infectious Disease, 4th ed. New York, Churchill Livingstone, 1994. *This detailed review of clinical amebiasis is well referenced and the most recent available.*
Ravdin JI, Schain DC, Kelsall B: Antigenicity, immunogenicity and vaccine efficacy of the galactose-specific adherence protein of Entamoeba histolytica. Vaccine 11:241, 1993. *Latest update on research relevant to vaccine development.*

382 OTHER PROTOZOAN DISEASES
Richard D. Pearson

OTHER ENTERIC PROTOZOANS

A number of enteric protozoa in addition to *Entamoeba histolytica, Giardia lamblia,* and *Cryptosporidium parvum,* which are discussed in other chapters, can cause disease (Table 382–1). They are acquired by ingesting cysts or oocysts in contaminated water or food. The parasites excyst and multiply in the lumen of the bowel, or in some cases within intestinal epithelial cells. Enteric protozoal pathogens should be considered in patients with persistent diarrhea, abdominal pain, and related symptoms, particularly if they have AIDS or a history of international travel.

The diagnosis is made by identifying cysts, oocytes, or trophozoites in the stool. Microscopic examinations should be performed by experts because fecal debris may be confused with parasites, and, conversely, pathogenic protozoa may be scant or difficult to differentiate from nonpathogens such as *Entamoeba coli, Endolimax nana, Iodamoeba bütschlii, Trichomonas hominis,* or *Chilomastix mesnili.* Therapy includes rehydration and administration of antiprotozoal drugs (Table 382–1).

Drugs for parasitic infections. Med Lett Drugs Ther 35:111, 1993. *Consensus recommendations for treating parasitic diseases are provided in tables. Key articles are referenced.*
Jernigan J, Guerrant RL, Pearson RD: Parasitic infections of the small intestine. Gut 35:289, 1994. *A good starting point for a review of recent literature on enteric protozoal pathogens.*

BABESIOSIS

Babesiosis is a tick-borne, malaria-like illness caused by *Babesia* species that infect erythrocytes of mammals. Most infections in the United States are due to *B. microti,* which is endemic on the chain of islands off the coast of New England and New York that includes Nantucket, Martha's Vineyard, Long Island, Block Island, and Shelter Island, and in Connecticut. The major reservoir in those areas is the white-footed mouse, *Peromyscus leucopus.* The vector is the deer tick, *Ixodes scapularis,* the same tick that transmits *Borrelia burgdorferi,* the cause of Lyme disease (see Ch. 321). The cycle begins when larvae feed on infected mice and acquire *Babesia.* Infection is transmitted to humans when nymphs, the next stage, feed on them. Blood transfusions have been implicated in a few cases. Sporadic cases of babesiosis have been reported from other areas of the United States, including California, Georgia, Washington, and Wisconsin. Some have been caused by different *Babesia*

TABLE 382–1. OTHER ENTERIC PROTOZOA

Organism	Epidemiology	Manifestations	Therapy*
Balantidium coli	Primarily an infection of animals, especially pigs, but also affects humans	Asymptomatic, or mild and self-resolving; a few cases are more severe with abdominal pain, blood, and mucus in the stool	Tetracycline (500 mg q.i.d. for 10 days) *Alternative:* Metronidazole (750 mg t.i.d. for 5 days) *or* Iodoquinol (650 mg t.i.d. for 20 days)
Blastocystis hominis	Probably worldwide, including North America; often found concomitantly with *Giardia lamblia*	Pathogenicity is debated	The need for treatment is debated, but efficacy has been reported with: Metronidazole (750 mg t.i.d. for 10 days) *or* Iodoquinol (650 mg t.i.d. for 20 days)
Cyclospora species (previously known as cyanobacterium-like bodies [CLB])	Distribution appears to be world-wide	May produce severe, watery diarrhea and fatigue lasting for weeks	Trimethoprim, 160 mg and Sulfamethoxazole, 800 mg b.i.d. for 3 days
Dientamoeba fragilis	Worldwide distribution; frequently found concomitantly with the pinworm, *Enterobius vermicularis*	Most asymptomatic; diarrhea reported	Iodoquinol (650 mg t.i.d. for 20 days) *or* Paromomycin (25–30 mg/kg body weight/day in 3 doses for 7 days) *or* Tetracycline (500 mg q.i.d. for 10 days)
Entamoeba polecki	Most cases reported from Papua New Guinea, but probably worldwide distribution; primarily found in pigs and monkeys; human infections are rare	Most asymptomatic; some have symptoms similar to *Entamoeba histolytica* colitis	Metronidazole (750 mg t.i.d. for 10 days)
Isospora belli	Worldwide distribution, most prevalent in Latin America and Africa	Self-limited diarrhea in immuno-competent residents and travelers, but persistent, severe diarrhea in patients with AIDS	Trimethoprim 160 mg plus sulfamethoxazole 800 mg q.i.d. for 10 days then b.i.d. for 3 weeks
Microspordia (*Enterocytozoon bieneusi* and *Septata intestinalis*)	Apparent worldwide distribution	Pathogenicity debated; frequently found in the stool of AIDS patients with persistent diarrhea	Uncertain; Abendazole 400 mg b.i.d. may be helpful for *E. bieneusi* and may cure *S. intestinalis*
Sarcocystis species	Common pathogens of animals; rare in humans; acquired by ingesting contaminated beef or pork	Nausea, vomiting, abdominal pain, and diarrhea. Eosinophilic necrotizing enteritis has been observed in the small intestine	No specific therapy

* Recommendations based on Drugs for parasitic infections. Med Lett Drugs Ther 35:111, 1993. The dosages and durations are for adults.

species. In Europe, *B. divergens* and *B. bovis* are transmitted by *Ixodes ricinus.*

B. microti infections are often asymptomatic or mild and self-resolving, but they can cause severe, malaria-like disease, particularly in the elderly, splenectomized patients, and the immunocompromised. The incubation period varies from 1 to 6 weeks; most patients are unaware of a tick bite. Symptomatic patients typically experience irregular fever, sweats, chills, myalgia, fatigue, and other constitutional symptoms. Unlike malaria, there is no periodicity to the disease. Fever is frequently the only finding on physical examination, but hepatomegaly and splenomegaly are present on occasion. There is evidence of hemolytic anemia of varying severity and often thrombocytopenia. The white count is normal or slightly depressed, and there may be elevations of liver enzymes and bilirubin. Untreated, symptomatic babesiosis may last from a few weeks to several months.

Babesiosis is diagnosed by identifying intraerythrocytic *Babesia* in blood smears. On rare occasions dividing parasites make up four daughter cells that appear as the characteristic tetrad (Maltese cross) in an infected erythrocyte.

The majority of cases of babesiosis in immunocompetent patients are asymptomatic or mild and resolve spontaneously without treatment. In adults with serious *Babesia* infections the treatment of choice is clindamycin, 1.2 grams twice a day parenterally or 600 mg three times a day orally, plus quinine, 650 mg three times a day orally for 7 days.

Telford SR 3d, Gorenflot A, Brasseur P, et al.: Babesial infections of humans and wildlife. *In* Kreier JP, Baker JR (eds.): Parasitic Protozoa. 2nd ed. New York, Academic Press, 1993, p 1. *The epidemiology, clinical manifestations, and therapy of human and animal babesiosis are reviewed in detail.*

TRICHOMONIASIS

Trichomonas vaginalis is among the most prevalent of all pathogenic protozoa. As many as 3 million women are infected each year in the United States alone. The organism is oval, approximately 10

by 15 μ wide, and has four free flagella at its anterior pole and a fifth in an undulating membrane that runs along the cell. *Trichomonas vaginalis* is usually spread by sexual contact. The highest incidences of disease are among women with multiple sexual partners and those who present with other sexually transmitted diseases (see Ch. 314). It can also be passed from infected mothers to their newborn daughters, but it is seldom symptomatic in girls before menarche. *T. vaginalis* is able to survive for some time in moist environments, and nonvenereal transmission can occur.

As many as half of the *T. vaginalis* infections in women are asymptomatic. The remainder are associated with vaginal discharge, vulvovaginal irritation, dyspareunia, or dysuria. The discharge tends to be watery and copious, but in some cases it is thick and may be yellow or green. Patients may notice an odor, but that is more common with bacterial vaginosis. On pelvic examination there is usually inflammation of the vaginal walls. Punctate hemorrhages on the exocervix, causing the classic "strawberry cervix," are uncommon on gross inspection, but they are observed in approximately half of infected women if colposcopy is performed. The pH of the vaginal contents is typically elevated above the normal level of 4.5, as it is in bacterial vaginosis. In contrast, the pH remains low in women with *Candida* vaginitis.

Most men with *T. vaginalis* are asymptomatic, but the organism is isolated on occasion from men with symptoms of urethritis who are negative for *Neisseria gonorrhoeae* and *Chlamydia trachomatis* (see Ch. 315). Urethral discharge is usually scant in such cases. On rare occasions *T. vaginalis* can cause epididymitis, produce superficial penile ulcerations which are usually located under the prepuce, or involve the prostate.

Diagnosis of trichomonas vaginitis is usually made by identifying the parasite in vaginal discharge. The trophozoites have a twitching movement with active flagella. They are seen in wet mounts of vaginal secretions in approximately 60% of infected women. Polymorphonuclear leukocytes are usually present. Culture is the most sensitive method of diagnosis, and commercial kits are now available. In men a wet mount of material from a platinum loop scraping of the anterior urethra reveals the organism in approximately half of the cases. Prostatic massage prior to collecting urine for trichomonas culture is the most sensitive diagnostic approach. Serodiagnostic studies lack sensitivity and specificity.

Metronidazole is the treatment of choice; a single dose of 2 grams is effective. All sexual partners must be treated concurrently to prevent reinfection. Metronidazole, 250 mg three times a day for 7 days, is an alternative. Single-dose therapy ensures patient compliance, but the higher dose can produce nausea and a metallic taste. Metronidazole also has a disulfiram-like effect, and patients consuming it with alcohol may develop severe nausea, vomiting, and flushing. The use of metronidazole is relatively contraindicated during pregnancy. Treatment failures with metronidazole are encountered. Some are due to reinfection, others to poor compliance, but a subset is apparently due to metronidazole resistance. In such cases high doses of metronidazole have been administered for longer periods of time. Tinidazole, which is not licensed for use in the United States, is also effective for trichomoniasis when administered as a single 2-gram dose.

Krieger JN, Jenny C, Verdon M, et al.: Clinical manifestations of trichomoniasis in men. Ann Intern Med 118:844, 1993. *Summarizes the clinical manifestations of trichomoniasis in men.*

Lossick JG, Kent HL: Trichomoniasis: Trends in diagnosis and management. Am J Obstet Gynecol 165:1217, 1991. *An excellent review of the diagnosis and treatment of women with trichomoniasis.*

Rein MF: *Trichomonas vaginalis. In* Mandell GL, Bennett JE, Dolin R: Principles and Practice of Infectious Diseases, 4th ed. New York, Churchill Livingstone, 1995, p 2493. *The epidemiology, diagnosis, and treatment of trichomoniasis are reviewed.*

383 *PNEUMOCYSTIS CARINII* PNEUMONIA
Fred R. Sattler

Pneumocystis pneumonia remains the most frequent case-defining infection in AIDS (see Ch. 365). Nearly 20,000 first episodes of pneumocystis continue to be reported to the Centers for Disease Control and Prevention (CDC) each year. A large number of second or third episodes also occur annually in AIDS patients but do not require reporting to the CDC.

Moderate to severe episodes cause appreciable morbidity, and even with effective therapies, 20 to 25% are fatal. For mild episodes, the fatality rate is <3%, but the diagnosis is often difficult, as signs and symptoms may mimic community-acquired infections and the presentation is often atypical in patients receiving prophylaxis for pneumocystis. It is, therefore, imperative that episodes be detected when alteration of gas exchange is mild and lung damage is minimal if hospitalization and mortality are to be minimized. Thus, clinicians caring for HIV patients must be aware of various manifestations of pneumocystis so that therapy can be initiated early.

ETIOLOGY. *Pneumocystis carinii* is a eukaryotic microbe with morphologic features similar to those of protozoa. Lack of growth on fungal culture media and response to therapies used to treat protozoan infections have supported the notion that it is a protozoan. However, *P. carinii* has an affinity for fungal stains, its ultrastructure is more similar to fungi, and molecular analysis of its 16S ribosomal RNA and mitochondrial DNA indicates that it is phylogenetically closely related to the *Ascomycetes* yeasts. Moreover, the base pair sequence of its mitochondrial DNA contains genes of NDH dehydrogenase subunits and cytochrome oxidase subunits, which show 60% similarity with fungi but only 20% homology with protozoa. Finally, the dihydrofolate reductase (DHFR) of *P. carinii,* as with fungi, is a single enzyme with lower molecular weight than the dual thymidylate synthetase–DHFR activity present in protozoa.

Establishing whether *P. carinii* is a fungus is not moot. Although pneumocystis does not respond to antifungal drugs such as amphotericin or fluconazole, β-glucan synthesis in the cyst wall is inhibited by antifungal agents such as echinocandins and papulocandins.

These agents are active against both the cyst and trophozoite forms of *P. carinii* in experimental infections. By contrast, traditional antipneumocystis therapies affect only the trophozoites. Novel therapeutic approaches that affect both stages of the life cycle are therefore being developed in an attempt to improve treatment response rates.

EPIDEMIOLOGY AND TRANSMISSION. Within the first few years of life, nearly all children have serologic evidence of exposure to *P. carinii.* Thus, the most accepted hypothesis for pathogenesis has been that *P. carinii* remains latent in the lung and reactivation occurs during severe immune depression. Yet, there is little to support chronic carriage because the organism is not detected in lung sections at autopsy of previously healthy individuals or by polymerase chain reaction (PCR) in bronchoalveolar lavage fluid of immunocompetent adults.

P. carinii is found incidentally in lungs of immunocompromised patients, and genetic sequences of the organisms have been detected in the absence of histologic evidence of infection in immunocompromised patients. Case clusters and familial spread have been reported, and in one natural history study of HIV patients, upper respiratory infections peaked in winter months followed by pneumocystis pneumonia 4 months later, indicating that *P. carinii* was acquired by exposure to persons coughing during earlier months when community respiratory infections were common. These data suggest that *P. carinii* may be acquired by person-to-person spread.

PATHOGENESIS AND PATHOPHYSIOLOGY. In cortisone-treated rats, inhaled *P. carinii* adheres to type 1 alveolar cells through fibrinonectin. After several weeks, small clusters of *P. carinii* can be detected in alveolar spaces. Later, air sacs become filled with organisms, indicating that replication is slow but proliferation is extensive. Two morphologic forms of the organism are readily detected. The majority are small pleomorphic trophozoites. A more mature, larger, thick-walled cyst containing up to eight intracystic bodies is less prevalent. Histology typically shows foamy alveolar exudates consisting of degenerative *P. carinii* cell membranes, surfactant, host proteins, and a modest number of alveolar macrophages. As infection progresses, septal hypertrophy occurs and interstitial edema and mononuclear cells accumulate. Similar abnormalities occur in humans.

In patients, these abnormalities result in increased alveolar-capillary permeability, which is associated with impaired gas exchange and decreased membrane diffusing capacity, compliance, total lung capacity, and vital capacity. Soon after antipneumocystis therapy begins, lung function is further impaired by the inflammatory response, as evidenced by a rapid decline in oxygenation. This inflammatory reaction appears to be mediated by tumor necrosis factor-α (TNF-α) and interleukin-1, -6, and -8 released by alveolar macrophages. TNF-α is modulated by the β-glucan component of the cell wall of the organism, providing further evidence that *P. carinii* is a fungus.

RISK FOR INFECTION. In laboratory rodents, depletion of T lymphocytes is the critical determinant in producing pneumocystis pneumonia. In humans, pneumocystis occurs in association with lymphoreticular malignancy, certain congenital disorders, and therapy with cyclosporine or corticosteroids which have in common variable defects in T-cell function. In patients with HIV, the risk of developing pneumocystis is related to deficiency of T-lymphocytes with CD4 surface phenotype. The median CD4 count is 50 to 70 at the time of first episodes. That pneumocystis may occur with transient declines in CD4 counts to <100 during primary HIV infection suggests that the level of CD4 immunity and not the stage of HIV infection is important in determining risk for infection. Although >90% of episodes occur with <200 CD4 cells, pneumocystis may occur at higher CD4 counts in individuals whose CD4 cells are declining rapidly and those with thrush and fever.

HISTOPATHOLOGY. Microscopy of lung tissue from AIDS patients with pneumocystis shows prominent eosinophilic, foamy intra-alveolar exudate, proliferation of type II pneumocytes, but only mild interstitial inflammation. Detection of *P. carinii* requires special stains for identification. The cysts are uniformly 5 to 7 μm and easily collapse to appear as helmet or banana shapes. Trophozoites are smaller, measuring 1 to 4 μm, and unlike the cysts are pleomorphic.

Diffuse alveolar damage is commonly found on biopsy sections.

Interstitial fibrosis is present in approximately 6% and intraluminal fibrosis in almost 40% of cases and appear to be related to the severity of the inflammatory response and duration of therapy. By contrast, acute exudative alveolar damage is unusual and hyaline membranes have been detected in <5% of lung biopsies but occasionally may be so prominent that they obscure the eosinophilic alveolar material typical of most cases. Other less common histologic abnormalities include cysts and cavities, granulomas, lymphocytic interstitial infiltrates, microcalcifications, vasculitis, and alveolar proteinosis. In patients with cavitation and pneumothorax, there is tissue invasion with *P. carinii* in the interstitium, and unlike the typical findings, greater proportions of trophozoite than cysts are present.

CLINICAL MANIFESTATIONS. Early recognition and treatment are imperative. Figure 383–1 shows that the risk of a fatal outcome increases progressively for patients whose room air PaO_2 are ≤ 75 mm Hg and alveolar-arterial oxygen differences ([A − a]DO_2) are ≥ 35 at presentation. Clinicians must therefore be familiar with both the typical manifestations and the less common presentations of pneumocystis.

Typical Presentations. The onset of pneumocystis pneumonia in AIDS patients is usually insidious. The cardinal manifestation is a hacking, usually nonproductive cough that may have been present for weeks. Retrosternal chest tightness, intensified by coughing and inspiration, is also common. Fever occurs in 80 to 90%. Dyspnea occurs later when oxygenation is moderately to severely impaired.

Physical findings are often limited and nonspecific. There is usually no tachypnea with mild episodes, whereas respiratory distress and use of accessory respiratory muscles may be present with severe episodes. Auscultation of the lungs is frequently normal because rales occur in only 30 to 40% of cases and are usually a late finding in severe episodes. Occasionally patients have wheezing or overt bronchospasm. In one report 84% of patients had peak expiratory flow rates (PEFR) <80% of predicted, with 54% of these responding to bronchodilator therapy. By contrast, in HIV patients without pneumocystis, only 23% had low PEFR and only 3% of these exhibited bronchodilator responses.

Physical findings outside the lung may assist in the clinical assessment. In patients not receiving antifungal drugs, oral thrush is a nearly universal finding. Facial seborrheic dermatitis is also common. Generalized adenopathy with lymph nodes >1 cm is rare because patients with pneumocystis generally have severe immunodeficiency with hypoplastic lymph nodes.

Some gender differences exist in the clinical presentation and course. In one study of 2526 men and 544 women, women were more likely to be hospitalized for their first episode of pneumocystis, were less likely to be white, and were more likely to die in the hospital. These findings suggest that pneumocystis is less likely to be diagnosed early in the course of infection in women.

Atypical Presentations. **Pneumothorax and Cavitation.** Pneumothoraces that may be associated with refractory bronchopleural fistulas and chronic lung cavitation are an increasingly frequent presentation and may occur in up to 10% of episodes. Pneumothoraces occurred spontaneously in 20 (2%) of 1030 patients with AIDS at one medical center; 50 to 95% of episodes are associated with active pneumocystis pneumonia. Thus, HIV patients with spontaneous pneumothorax should undergo workup and treatment for pneumocystis along with management of the pneumothorax.

Lung destruction and cavitation are manifested by solitary, thin-walled cavities, regional honeycombing, blebs, or bullae formation; these findings are often bilateral, usually occurring in the upper lobes and preceding pneumothraces.

Although cavitation and pneumothorax were initially associated with aerosol pentamidine prophylaxis, these complications may occur without aerosol therapy, in nonsmokers, at presentation of first episodes of pneumocystis, and before bronchoscopy or mechanical ventilation and barotrauma.

Extrapulmonary Pneumocystis. Infection with *P. carinii* may occur outside the lung in 0.5 to 3.0% of patients with pneumocystis pneumonia. At the time extrapulmonary pneumocystis is diagnosed, >50% have active pulmonary infection with *P. carinii*. Nucleotide sequences of the *P. carinii* DHFR gene have been detected by PCR in blood of 5 of 11 patients with pneumocystis pneumonia, which suggests that hematogenous dissemination occurs during acute pneumonia.

Clinical presentations have included external auditory polyps, mastoiditis, choroiditis, cutaneous lesions or digital necrosis secondary to vasculitis, small bowel obstruction, ascites with gross nodules in the stomach and duodenum, hepatic or splenic infiltration, hilar or mediastinal lymphadenopathy, thyroiditis, thymic involvement, and hematologic cytopenias due to involvement of the bone marrow. At autopsy disseminated infection has been documented in other organs, including abdominal lymph nodes, pancreas, gastric mucosa, adrenal glands, myocardium, kidneys, and central nervous system. Lymph nodes, liver, spleen, and bone marrow have been the most commonly affected organs.

Histology of affected organs show foci of eosinophilic frothy exudates, and special stains reveal *P. carinii*. Unlike in the lung, these lesions are often calcified (punctate or rimlike) and show vasculitis with invasion of vessel walls by *P. carinii*.

Clinical manifestations of extrapulmonary pneumocystosis are generally nonspecific (e.g., fever and sweats). Two infections are associated with specific symptoms or signs. *P. carinii* involving the thyroid may present with neck pain, hyperthyroidism or hypothyroidism, and goiter, which may be a multinodular or solitary neck mass. The thyroid is usually "cold" on ^{125}I scanning. The diagnosis is made by fine-needle aspiration. The other infection is choroiditis. Lesions consist of slightly elevated, yellow-white plaques, generally limited to the choroid without involvement of retinal vessels (unlike cytomegalovirus [CMV] retinitis) and without evidence of intraocular inflammation (see Color Plate 11*F*). Identifying typical choroidal lesions may provide the first clue of *P. carinii* infection.

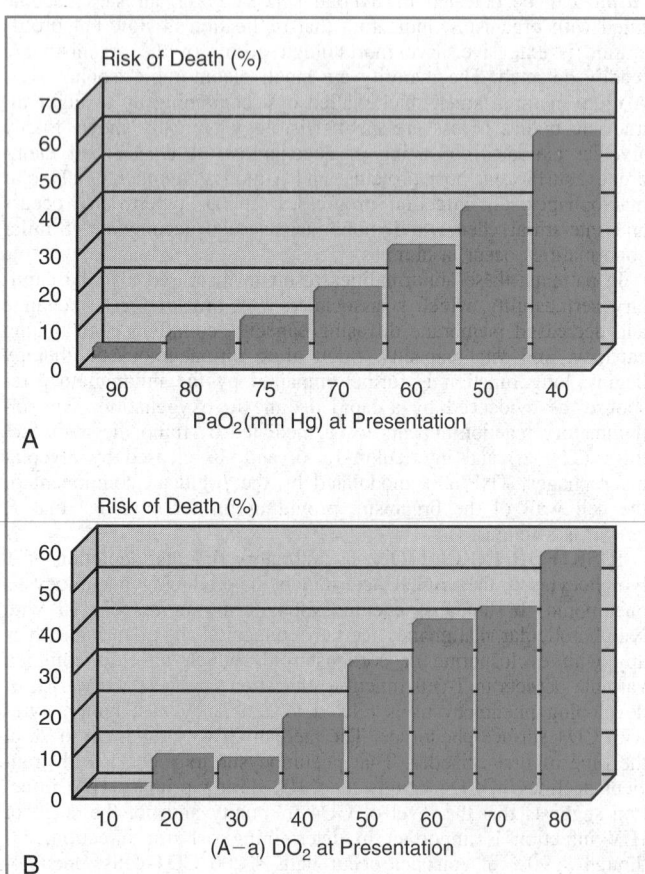

FIGURE 383–1. *A*, Risk of death, according to the partial pressure (Pao$_2$) of oxygen on room air at time of admission to the hospital for patients receiving conventional therapies without adjunctive corticosteroids. *B*, Risk of death, according to alveolar-arterial oxygen difference [(A − a)Do$_2$] on room air at time of admission to the hospital for patients receiving conventional therapies without adjunctive corticosteroids. (Adapted from the United States Public Health Service Consensus Statement on the Use of Corticosteroids as Adjunctive Therapy for Pneumocystis Pneumonia in the Acquired Immunodeficiency Syndrome.)

The lungs are involved in nearly 90% of cases, but eye involvement may be the only evidence of extrapulmonary infection.

Extensive and widespread extrapulmonary infection portends a poor prognosis, with organ failure and death occurring frequently, whereas involvement of a single extrapulmonary site is often associated with a favorable response to therapy for *P. carinii.*

LABORATORY ABNORMALITIES. *Pulmonary Function Tests.* Hypoxemia is the most useful marker of pneumocystis and is highly predictive of outcome. At presentation, $PaO_2 < 80$ mm Hg or an $(A - a)DO_2$ of > 15 on room air occurs in $> 80\%$ of episodes.

In patients with pneumocystis who have normal or nearly normal PaO_2, $(A - a)DO_2$, and chest radiographs, graded exercise testing results in increases in the $(A - a)DO_2$ and oxygen desaturation can be demonstrated with pulse oximetry. The carbon monoxide (CO)-diffusing capacity, DL_{CO}, is also a sensitive marker but nonspecific. Despite the lack of specificity, DL_{CO} values $> 80\%$ make pneumocystis unlikely (i.e., negative predictive values are $> 98\%$). In AIDS patients with asthma who have cough and hypoxemia, results of DL_{CO} should be normal when hypoxemia is due solely to bronchospasm.

Radiographic Procedures. **Routine Radiology.** Routine chest radiographs typically show interstitial infiltrates, beginning in perihilar areas and spreading to the lower and finally upper lung fields. The apices are usually spared. Alveolar patterns with air bronchograms may be superimposed on the interstitial process in more advanced infection, although alveolar infiltrates may be the initial presentation in up to 10% of cases. In 10 to 30% of cases the radiographic presentation is atypical with asymmetric or predominantly upper lobe infiltration—especially for patients who received prophylaxis with inhaled pentamidine. Other atypical abnormalities include nodules, cysts, pneumatoceles, cavitation with "honeycombing," pneumothorax, thoracic adenopathy with or without calcifications, pleural effusions, abscesses, lobar or segmental consolidation, solitary parenchymal nodules, or postobstructive infiltration secondary to endobronchial nodules of *P. carinii.* In one series of 100 patients with pneumocystis, cysts were documented in 34% and of these, 32 had multiple cysts measuring 1.0 to 5.0 cm that occurred predominantly in upper lobes. Cysts resolved partially or completely in most cases with specific therapy for pneumocystis, but 12 (35%) of the 34 patients developed pneumothoraces compared with only 2 of 30 patients without cysts. These cystic/cavitary lesions may mimic tuberculosis (Fig. 383–2). By contrast, 10 to 20% of patients with documented pneumocystis have had normal chest radiographs at presentation.

Computed Tomography (CT). Scans typically show fine, diffuse alveolar consolidation with bronchial wall thickening even when chest radiographs are normal and less often show regional consolidation or cystic airspaces. Low attenuation lesions and calcifications of lymph nodes, spleen, liver, and kidneys may be present in patients with extrapulmonary involvement. The value of CT is primarily for patients with normal chest radiographs or unexpected extrapulmonary pneumocystis.

Nuclear Imaging. Nuclear imaging may be of ancillary value in some cases. Gallium-67 accumulates in activated macrophages through transferrin receptors in areas of lung inflammation, but pulmonary uptake is not specific for *P. carinii* pneumonia. Specificity is improved when scans are reported as positive only if gallium uptake in lung equals or exceeds uptake in liver. Although images are not read until 48 to 72 hours after injection, gallium imaging may be useful for patients with chronic lung disease who have worsening respiratory symptoms.

Lactate Dehydrogenase. Serum lactate dehydrogenase (LDH) is more elevated in pneumocystis than in matched patients with other pulmonary complications of HIV. Although serum levels of LDH are not highly specific, the sensitivity was $> 90\%$ in one study of patients with dyspnea and pneumocystis when values were > 220 IU per liter. Moreover, at presentation, LDH values > 500 IU per liter are associated with an increased risk for a fatal outcome. Equally important, serial tests gradually improve in survivors.

CD4 Counts. Typically counts are < 100 cells per cubic millimeter and $> 90\%$ of patients have values < 200 when first diagnosed with pneumocystis.

DIAGNOSIS. *Bronchoalveolar Lavage.* Bronchoalveolar lavage (BAL) is the cornerstone of diagnosis of pneumocystis and consistently has a sensitivity of 86 to 96%. The diagnostic yield was reported to be only 62% for patients with acute pneumocystis

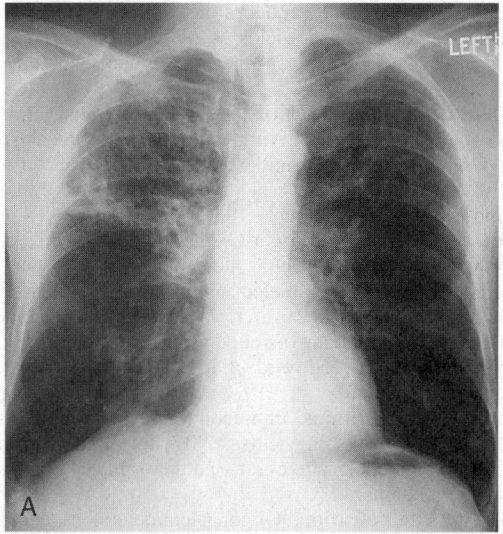

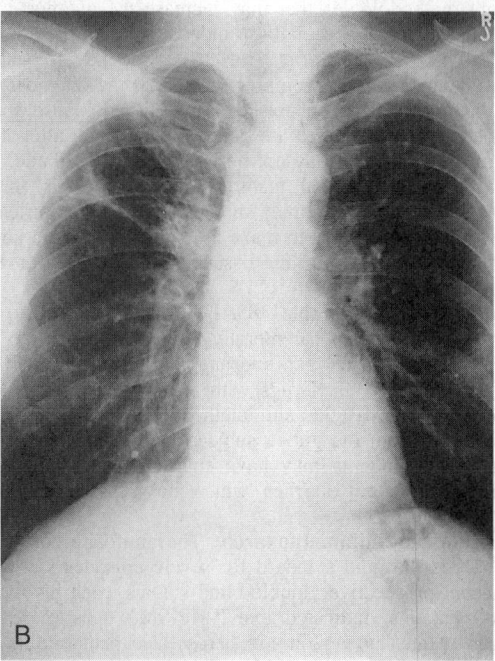

FIGURE 383–2. *A,* This chest radiograph was obtained from a 42-year-old homosexual man who presented with a 14-month history of chronic cough, dyspnea with minimal exertion, and 25-pound weight loss. He was treated for 8 weeks with four standard antituberculous drugs plus intravenous amikacin, but cultures for *Mycobacterium tuberculosis* remained negative. A repeat induced sputum at that time showed large numbers of *P. carinii. B,* Chest radiographs from the same patient after a 3-week course of therapy with oral trimethoprim-sulfamethoxazole (15 mg per kilogram per day of the trimethoprim component). At the completion of the therapy, his cough and dyspnea had completely subsided.

who had received inhaled pentamidine and who had disease predominantly in upper lobes. Several approaches may increase the yield for such patients. Bilateral BAL resulted in a diagnosis in 94%, compared with 84% in patients previously undergoing BAL on one side. Because there may be severalfold more organisms recovered from upper than from lower lobes, sampling involved sites is likely to increase the yield.

Transbronchial Biopsy. The yield from transbronchial biopsy approaches BAL if tissue is obtained without crush artifact and contains at least 25 alveoli. If both BAL and transbronchial biopsies are obtained, the diagnostic sensitivity approaches 100%.

Sputum Induction. Pulmonary secretions may be obtained by ultrasonic nebulization of hypertonic saline. If these specimens are treated with mucolytic agents to solubilize oral debris prior to centrifugation, cytostaining procedures have resulted in diagnostic yields of 15 to 90%. Fluorescent staining with monoclonal antibodies for *P. carinii* generally produces the highest yields. Because the sensitivity is variable and yields $>80\%$ have been consistently achieved in only a few centers, a negative induced sputum does not exclude the diagnosis.

Identification of P. carinii. Cyst Wall Stains. The standard staining procedure for identifying *P. carinii* in clinical specimens has used Gomori's methenamine silver because the sensitivity is generally $>95\%$. Toluidine blue O also stains the cyst, is more rapid, and is comparably reliable.

Noncyst Wall Stains. Wright-Giemsa and Diff-Quik stains are commonly used and stain trophozoites, nuclei of cysts, and intermediate forms and can be completed within 30 minutes. However, organisms may be missed in 10 to 15% of cases. Papanicolaou silver stains the nonspecific foam surrounding large clusters of *P. carinii*, but organisms are not readily identified. The methodology is quick and useful for screening.

Immunochemical Stains. Immunofluorescent staining with monoclonal antibody results in yields $>90\%$ for BAL specimens and appears to be more sensitive for sputum samples than silver or Wright-Giemsa stains.

Molecular Identification. Oligonucleotide probes and PCR are promising methodologies that may increase the diagnostic yield in identifying *P. carinii*, especially in induced sputum specimens.

TREATMENT. *Initiating Therapy.* The key to successfully treating pneumocystis is prompt suspicion of the diagnosis and initiating therapy early when episodes are mild. Because sputum induction and bronchoscopies are generally not done after hours and results of special stains may not be immediately available, most patients with typical clinical features of pneumocystis (if there is moderate-to-severe hypoxemia) should be treated empirically. This does not impair the ability to make a diagnosis, as large numbers of *P. carinii* are detectable in lung tissues and secretions for weeks after the onset of therapy.

Severe Episodes (Table 383–1). **Parenteral Therapy.** Initial therapy should be given parenterally for patients with moderate-to-severe impairment in oxygen exchange, namely $Pao_2 <70$ mm Hg or an $(A - a)Do_2 >35$. Drugs with high oral bioavailability such as trimethoprim (TMP) and sulfamethoxazole (SMX) may be erratically absorbed from the gut in subjects with severe hypoxemia. In addition, AIDS patients may have enteropathy and malabsorption even in the absence of diarrhea, which may result in subtherapeutic drug concentrations.

Trimethoprim-Sulfamethoxazole. The antifolate combination of TMP-SMX is the gold standard for severe episodes (see Ch. 371). Three recent prospective, double-blind studies, each involving more than 300 patients, indicated that TMP-SMX was more effective than trimetrexate, atovaquone, or aerosolized pentamidine in AIDS patients with pneumocystis. Although there are no comparably rigorous studies comparing TMP-SMX with parenteral pentamidine, TMP-SMX is associated with less serious toxicities.

The most frequent potentially serious toxicity with TMP-SMX is neutropenia (Table 383–2). Because this reaction is dose-dependent, many clinicians choose a lower dose TMP-SMX (15 mg per kilogram per day of TMP). Several controlled trials have indicated that the lower dose results in survival rates $\geq 88\%$ for severe episodes, suggesting that the lower dose does not compromise effectiveness.

Parenteral Pentamidine. Parenteral pentamidine is also highly effective. As with TMP-SMX, toxic reactions are common with parenteral pentamidine (Table 383–2). In one study in which patients received a minimum of 14 days of therapy, nephrotoxicity (>1 mg per deciliter rise in serum creatinine) occurred in 64% of patients, hypotension in 27%, and hypoglycemia in 21% (serum glucose <60 gm per deciliter). Impaired renal function and hypoglycemia are dose-dependent and more likely to be seen after 2 weeks of therapy or a total dosage of >4 grams. Hypotension generally occurs during or shortly after intravenous infusions and may last several hours, although low blood pressures may persist for several months.

Hypoglycemia is the most treacherous reaction and occurs in 10 to 20% of AIDS patients treated with pentamidine and results from sudden increases in serum insulin caused by lysis of pancreatic beta cells. Because of the prolonged binding of pentamidine to tissues, precipitous hypoglycemia may occur after pentamidine is discontinued, and fatal reactions have occurred up to 2 weeks after the last dose. When hypoglycemia is detected, pentamidine should be discontinued and patients should be monitored closely with daily capillary glucose measurements for several weeks.

Trimetrexate. Trimetrexate (NeuTrexin) is a powerful antifolate drug that binds to the DHFR of *P. carinii* nearly 1500 times more avidly than TMP and is concentrated in *P. carinii*. In a pivotal licensure study, trimetrexate was effective but inferior to TMP-SMX for moderate-to-severe episodes. Treatment-terminating toxicity, particularly critical neutropenia, thrombocytopenia, and anemia, occurs significantly less often with trimetrexate than with TMP-SMX.

Adjunctive Corticosteroids (Table 383–3). The major breakthrough in the search for more effective therapies for pneumocystis has been the irrefutable evidence that mortality for severe episodes can be reduced nearly twofold by use of corticosteroids within 72 hours after beginning conventional therapy. In addition, oxygen desaturation occurs less often and fewer patients need mechanical ventilation with adjunctive corticosteroids. The only adverse consequence of steroids has been an increased incidence of mucocutaneous herpes infections in one trial.

Adjunctive corticosteroids could be deleterious if prescribed with empiric antipneumocystis therapy for patients who actually have pulmonary fungal infection or tuberculosis, because these patients may initially improve, thereby delaying diagnosis and specific therapy. Moreover, corticosteroids can aggravate and accelerate the progression of cutaneous and pulmonary Kaposi's sarcoma.

Salvage Therapy. Once patients have developed respiratory failure during treatment for pneumocystis, prognosis is poor. Parenteral TMP-SMX, pentamidine, trimetrexate, eflornithine, and clindamycin-primaquine have all been evaluated for salvage in uncontrolled studies and appear to provide limited success in rescuing overtly failing patients. There is little reason to favor any of these therapies, but parenteral drugs are preferable.

Mild Episodes (see Table 383–1). For mild episodes ($Pao_2 >70$ mm Hg or an $[A - a]Do_2 <35$), treatments should be nontoxic and suited for home therapy because mortality rates are $<5\%$ with standard therapies. TMP-SMX is inexpensive and conveniently given orally but results in a high frequency of side effects.

Atovaquone. Atovaquone (Mepron) is an oral hydroxynapthoquinone developed as an antimalarial compound and has an excellent safety profile. The drug inhibits mitochondrial electron transport necessary for the biosynthesis of pyrimidines in protozoa, but its mode of action for *P. carinii* is unknown.

In the pivotal licensure study of atovaquone for 322 patients with mild to moderately severe ($[A - a]Do_2 <45$) pneumocystis pneumonia, failures due to inadequate therapeutic response occurred in 31% of patients receiving atovaquone and 16% with TMP-SMX ($P = 0.002$). Patients in whom treatment failed were more likely to have low plasma concentrations of atovaquone ($<15 \mu g$ per millimeter) and diarrhea. Atovaquone must be given with food because blood levels are two- to threefold lower when the drug is taken on an empty stomach.

Trimethoprim-Dapsone. Trimethoprim-dapsone, like TMP-

TABLE 383–1. ESTABLISHED THERAPIES FOR INITIAL TREATMENT OF *PNEUMOCYSTIS CARINII* PNEUMONIA

Intravenous therapies
1. Trimethoprim-sulfamethoxazole — 5/25 mg/kg every 6–8 hours
2. Pentamidine* — 4 mg/kg once daily
3. Trimetrexate plus — 45 mg/M² once daily
   leucovorin — 20 mg/M² every 6 hours
4. Clindamycin plus — 900 mg every 8 hours
   primaquine base (oral)† — 15–30 mg once daily

Oral therapies
1. Trimethoprim-sulfamethoxazole — 2 double-strength tablets t.i.d.
2. Trimethoprim plus — 4–5 mg/kg t.i.d.
   dapsone — 100 mg once daily
3. Clindamycin plus — 456–600 mg t.i.d. or q.i.d.
   primaquine base — 15–30 mg once daily
4. Atovaquone‡ — 750 mg t.i.d.

Aerosol therapy
1. Pentamidine — 600 mg daily via Respirgard II§

* Intramuscular therapy may cause sterile abscesses and should be avoided.

† The combination is not advisable in situations in which absorption may be impaired (severe hypoxemia, vomiting, diarrhea, ileus, malabsorption) because clindamycin alone has no activity against *P. carinii*.

‡ Must be given with food because serum concentrations are 2- or 3-fold lower when drug is administered on an empty stomach.

§ Administered at 50 psi and 8 liters per minute of oxygen.

TABLE 383-2. TOXICITIES ASSOCIATED WITH STANDARD THERAPIES FOR
***PNEUMOCYSTIS* PNEUMONIA**

Drug	Frequent Causes of Morbidity	Infrequent Causes of Morbidity
Trimethoprim-sulfamethoxazole	Fever Morbilliform rash Nausea and vomiting Neutropenia* Thrombocytopenia† Anemia‡	Stevens-Johnson syndrome Exfoliative dermatitis Diarrhea Liver test abnormalities Elevated serum creatinine Hyperkalemia Hyponatremia Renal impairment Hallucinations or agitation
Parenteral pentamidine	Fever Morbilliform rash Nausea and vomiting Renal impairment Hypoglycemia Hypotension Pancreatitis	Hypocalcemia Ventricular tachycardia/fibrillation Torsades de pointes Neutropenia Thrombocytopenia Liver test abnormalities Ketoacidosis and diabetes Hypomagnesemia Myoglobinuria Hematuria
Trimetrexate plus leucovorin	Fever Morbilliform rash	Liver test abnormalities Neutropenia Thrombocytopenia Mucositis
Dapsone	Fever Morbilliform rash Nausea and vomiting	Methemoglobinemia Hemolytic anemia Sulfone syndrome
Clindamycin	Fever Morbilliform rash Diarrhea	Liver test abnormalities *C. difficile* colitis
Primaquine	Nausea Abdominal distress Neutropenia	Methemoglobinemia Hemolytic anemia Hypertension Arrhythmias
Atovaquone	Rash	Fever Nausea and vomiting Liver test abnormalities
Inhaled pentamidine	Cough Bronchospasm Metallic taste	Contact dermatitis Morbilliform rash Hypoglycemia Pancreatitis Renal impairment

* Reduce to < 1000 per deciliter
† Reduce to < 50,000 per deciliter
‡ > 2 gram per deciliter decline

SMX, results in sequential folate blockade in *P. carinii*. Dapsone (a sulfone) binds to the *P. carinii* dihydropteroate synthetase twofold more avidly than SMX. Treatment-terminating neutropenia and elevation of liver tests occur less frequently than with TMP-SMX.

Clindamycin-Primaquine. Clindamycin and the antimalarial drug primaquine together have excellent activity against *P. carinii* in a cell culture system and in cortisone-treated rats, but neither agent alone is highly effective. The combination has been effective for pneumocystis both as initial therapy and for patients intolerant of or failing conventional therapies, with response rates in the range of 90% regardless of whether clindamycin is given intravenously or orally and whether the dose of primaquine base is 15 or 30 mg daily. This combination may be somewhat better tolerated than TMP-SMX, but controlled trials have not established whether it is as effective as TMP-SMX.

Adjunctive Corticosteroids (Table 383-3). The U.S. Public Health Service has not recommended adjunctive corticosteroids for mild episodes because mortality with conventional therapies is very low if there is minimal impairment of oxygenation at baseline. However, a recent study indicated that desaturation is less, exercise tolerance is better, and LDH returns to baseline more quickly with adjunctive corticosteroids in episodes of mild to moderate severity.

OUTCOME AND PROGNOSIS. Clinical parameters associated with an increased risk for fatal outcome have included at presentation an elevated serum LDH of > 500 IU per deciliter, $Pao_2 < 70$ mm Hg or $(A - a)Do_2 > 35$, BAL neutrophils > 5%, and low T3 and reverse T3 hormone concentrations.

Changing Therapy. It is often difficult to know when a pa-

tient is failing a specific therapy. Persistence of fever or lack of improvement on chest radiographs is common, and persistence or progression of infiltrates frequently occurs even in patients who ultimately are cured. A sustained respiratory rate > 35 per minute or absolute increase in room air $(A - a)Do_2 > 20$ above baseline have proven reproducible endpoints for failure and objective justification for changing therapy and searching for other infectious complications in the lung.

Supportive Care. Evidence suggests that the degree of alveolar damage is the most important determinant of outcome. Thus, as with ARDS, which has similar histologic features to severe pneu-

TABLE 383-3. ADJUNCTIVE CORTICOSTEROIDS* FOR PATIENTS WITH PNEUMOCYSTIS AND
$(A-a)Do_2 \geq 35$ mm Hg OR $Pao_2 \leq 70$ mm Hg

	Dose	Treatment Days
Oral		
Prednisone	40 mg b.i.d.	1–5
	40 mg once daily	6–10
	20 mg once daily	11–end of therapy
Intravenous		
Methyl-prednisolone	30 mg b.i.d.	1–5
	30 mg once daily	6–10
	15 mg once daily	11–end of therapy

* Efficacy established only when adjunctive corticosteroids are initiated within 72 hours of starting specific treatment for *P. carinii*.

TABLE 383–4. PROPHYLACTIC THERAPIES FOR PREVENTION OF *PNEUMOCYSTIS* PNEUMONIA

Drug	Dose or Regimen	Alternate Dose or Regimen
Antifolate regimens		
Trimethoprim-sulfamethoxazole	1 DS tablet daily	1 DS tablet three times weekly
	(160 mg trimethoprim, 800 mg sulfamethoxazole)	1 SS tablet daily
Dapsone	100 mg tablet daily	50-mg tablet once or twice daily
Dapsone-pyrimethamine	50 mg tablet dapsone daily	None
	50 mg tablet pyrimethamine	Weekly
Sulfadoxine-pyrimethamine	1 tablet weekly (sulfadoxine 500 mg, pyrimethamine 25 mg)	None
Pyrimethamine-sulfadiazine or pyrimethamine-clindamycin	Induction or maintenance doses for toxoplasmic encephalitis*	None
Aerosolized pentamidine		
Respirgard II jet nebulizer	300 mg monthly	None established
Fisons' ultrasonic nebulizer	60 mg every 2 weeks†	None
Other regimens		
Atovaquone	Unknown	None
Primaquine-clindamycin	Unknown	None

* Patients receiving therapy for toxoplasmosis are unlikely to need additional prophylaxis for pneumocystis because pyrimethamine-sulfadiazine has been used successfully to treat pneumocystis pneumonia, and the combination of pyrimethamine-clindamycin is similar to the regimen of primaquine-clindamycin, which is also effective treatment for pneumocystis.
† Five 60 mg doses within the first 14 days for "loading," one dose on day 21, and then every 2 weeks thereafter.
DS = double strength; SS = single strength.

mocystis, good supportive care is crucial for severely ill patients with pneumocystis. Continuous positive airway pressure by face mask improves oxygenation in patients with tachypnea and desaturation refractory with standard masks and may mitigate the need for mechanical ventilation.

Mechanical Ventilation and Intensive Care Unit Care. For AIDS patients on mechanical ventilators in intensive care units (ICU), mortality has ranged from 30 to 50% in recent reports, supporting the value of aggressive measures in selected patients with severe episodes. Low albumin, arterial pH < 7.35, or need for positive end expiratory pressure > 10 cm H_2O after 96 hours in the ICU portend a severalfold greater risk for a fatal outcome. Thus, patients with better nutritional status and who are not acidotic or have less severe alveolar damage may benefit most from ICU care.

PROPHYLAXIS (Table 383–4). The U.S. Public Health Service has advised that patients at high risk for pneumocystis receive prophylactic therapies. Those at highest risk include (1) patients with prior pneumocystis and (2) those with < 200 CD4+ cells. TMP-SMX is currently the most effective therapy for prophylaxis of pneumocystis. In several studies, the relative hazard of developing pneumocystis was approximately three to four times less with TMP-SMX than with aerosolized pentamidine.

In controlled trials, dapsone has been comparable to aerosolized pentamidine but somewhat inferior to TMP-SMX. When combined with pyrimethamine (usually 50 mg once weekly), the two drugs are also highly effective in preventing toxoplasmosis.

Bozzette SA, Sattler FR, Chui J, et al.: A controlled trial of early adjunctive treatment with corticosteroids for *Pneumocystis carinii* pneumonia in the acquired immunodeficiency syndrome. N Engl J Med 323:1451, 1990. *A pivotal study demonstrating that adjunctive corticosteroids reduce mortality for patients with severe pneumocystis.*
Hardy DW, Feinberg J, Finkelstein DM, et al.: A controlled trial of trimethoprim-sulfamethoxazole or aerosolized pentamidine for secondary prophylaxis of *Pneumocystis carinii* pneumonia in patients with the acquired immunodeficiency syndrome. AIDS Clinical Trials Group Protocol 021. N Engl J Med 327:1842, 1992. *Results demonstrate the superiority of TMP-SMX compared with aerosolized pentamidine for preventing pneumocystis in AIDS patients with prior pneumocystis.*
Hughes W, Leoung G, Kramer F, et al.: Comparison of atovaquone (566C80) with trimethoprim-sulfamethoxazole for the treatment of *Pneumocystis carinii* pneumonia in patients with the acquired immunodeficiency syndrome (AIDS). N Engl J Med 328:1521, 1993. *Results established the relative effectiveness and tolerability of atovaquone for therapy of mild to moderately severe pneumocystis.*
Sattler FR, Frame P, Davis R, et al.: Trimetrexate with leucovorin versus trimethoprim-sulfamethoxazole for moderate to severe episodes of *Pneumocystis carinii* pneumonia in patients with AIDS: A prospective, controlled multicenter investigation of the AIDS Clinical Trials Protocol 029/031. J Infect Dis 170:165, 1994. *Results established the relative effectiveness and tolerability of trimetrexate for moderate to severe pneumocystis pneumonia.*
Toma E, Fournier S, Dumont M, et al.: Clindamycin/primaquine versus trimethoprim-sulfamethoxazole as primary therapy for *Pneumocystis carinii* pneumonia in AIDS: A randomized, double blind pilot trial. Clin Infect Dis 17:178, 1993. *Results confirm prior reports of the incidence of adverse effects with two treatment regimens and suggest that clindamycin-primaquine is highly effective as initial therapy for pneumocystis.*
Travis WD, Pittaluga S, Lipschik GY, et al.: Atypical pathologic manifestations of *Pneumocystis carinii* pneumonia in the acquired immunodeficiency syndrome. Review of 123 lung biopsies from 76 patients with emphasis on cysts, vascular invasion, vasculitis, and granulomas. Am J Surg Pathol 14:615, 1990. *Report describes the pathologic findings of* pneumocystis *in patients with AIDS.*

Helminthic Diseases

384 CESTODE INFECTIONS
Charles H. King

The eight cestode species that most commonly cause human infection are listed in Table 384–1. Although this class of parasites is often referred to, collectively, as "tapeworms," it is important to note that not all cestode parasites develop into tapeworms in the human host. The key to understanding the rather broad spectrum of cestode-associated illness is to recall that these parasites divide their life cycle between two or more different animal hosts, termed *intermediate* and *definitive* hosts. The intermediate host harbors the immature parasite as a tissue cyst, whereas the subsequent definitive host harbors the mature parasite as a tapeworm. For a given cestode species, humans may serve as *either* intermediate or definitive hosts.

The *intermediate* host is typically an insect or herbivorous (omnivorous) vertebrate that ingests parasite eggs in fecally contaminated food or water. The cestode eggs hatch into invasive oncospheres in this primary host's intestinal tract, then migrate into the host viscera or muscles to develop into immature cystic forms, called cysticerci or cysticercoids (for Cyclophyllidea cestodes such

TABLE 384-1. COMMON HUMAN CESTODE INFECTIONS

Species	Stage Found in Humans	Common Name	Pathology	Therapy
Diphyllobotrium latum	Adult	Fish tapeworm	Pernicious anemia	Niclosamide Praziquantel
Hymenolepis nana	Adult	Dwarf tapeworm	Rarely symptomatic	Niclosamide Praziquantel
Taenia saginata	Adult	Beef tapeworm	Rarely symptomatic	
Taenia solium	Adult	Pork tapeworm	Rarely symptomatic	Niclosamide Praziquantel
	Larva	Cysticercosis	Brain and tissue cysts	Albendazole* Praziquantel Surgery
Echinococcus granulosus	Larva	Hydatid cyst disease	Solitary tissue cysts	Surgery Albendazole*
Echinococcus multilocularis	Larva	Alveolar cyst disease	Multilocular cysts	Surgery Albendazole*
Taenia multiceps	Larva	Bladderworm, coenurosis	Brain and eye cysts	Surgery
Spirometra mansonoides	Larva	Sparganosis	Subcutaneous larvae	Surgery

* This drug has not been approved by the Food and Drug Adminstration at the time of publication.

as *Taenia* and *Hymenolepis*), or procercoid and plerocercoid larvae (for Pseudophyllidea cestodes such as *Diphyllobothrium*). Humans become intermediate hosts for cestode species by ingesting parasite eggs in food or water, as in echinococcosis, or rarely by direct transfer of plerocercoid larvae from animal tissues, as in sparganosis.

The *definitive* host for a cestode species is a carnivorous or omnivorous mammal that acquires infection by consuming larval cysts in the uncooked tissues of an intermediate host. Upon exposure to stomach acid and bile salts in the digestive tract, the larvae excyst and develop into mature tapeworms within the intestinal lumen. Adult tapeworms contain two sections: a *scolex* (or head) used to adhere to the wall of the intestine, and a *strobila*, or tapelike chain of developing segments called proglottides. The hermaphroditic proglottides produce large numbers of fertile, infectious parasite eggs that reach the environment either free or enclosed within parasite segments in the host's feces. Carnivorous humans become definitive hosts by ingesting cyst-infested meat of intermediate hosts (e.g., fish, pork, or beef), after which the cysts develop into intraluminal, intestinal tapeworms.

We are strictly definitive hosts for the cestodes *Diphyllobothrium latum* (the "fish" tapeworm) and *Taenia saginata* (the "beef" tapeworm). These adult tapeworms do not enter the tissues of the human body and cause only minimal clinical symptoms. In contrast, we are solely intermediate hosts for *Echinococcus granulosus* (hydatid cyst disease), *E. multilocularis* (alveolar cyst disease), *Taenia multiceps* (coenurosis), and *Spirometra* species. In the human body, these parasites develop as larval cysts and cause significant symptomatic tissue damage.

There are two exceptions to this rule. First, patients with *T. solium* infection may be infected with larval cysts (cysticercosis), adult tapeworms ("pork" tapeworm), or both. Second, in the case of the dwarf tapeworm, *Hymenolepis nana*, complete egg-to-tapeworm development can take place within a single human host. *H. nana* can thus be transmitted directly from person to person, and internal autoinfection may substantially increase the tapeworm burden of an infected individual. For all other cestode infections, increases in parasite burden occur only by means of continued exposure to egg-contaminated or larvae-infested foods and water.

INTESTINAL CESTODE (TAPEWORM) INFECTIONS

Diphyllobothrium latum

D. latum tapeworms are the largest parasites that infect humans, ranging up to 10 meters in length. Infection is acquired by ingestion of parasite cysts in the tissues of smoked or uncooked fresh water fish (e.g., as sushi, sashimi, or ceviche). Tapeworms develop to maturity within 3 to 6 weeks after exposure and may survive for up to 20 years. Infection is prevalent (up to 2% of local residents) in many parts of the world; endemic foci are found in lake or delta regions of Scandinavia, the former Soviet Union, Japan, Europe, Chile, and North America. Contamination of fresh water bodies by raw sewage increases the risk for *D. latum* infection, but stable

transmission may also occur owing to local infection of alternate definitive hosts, such as foxes, wolves, minks, and bears.

CLINICAL MANIFESTATIONS. For most patients, *D. latum* infection produces few, if any, symptoms. These are typically limited to nonspecific complaints of weakness, dizziness, craving for salt, diarrhea, and intermittent abdominal discomfort. Occasional patients may experience vomiting, severe abdominal pain, and weight loss. In cases of multiple infection, biliary or intestinal obstruction may occur. One to 2% of patients with *D. latum* infection develop significant vitamin B_{12} deficiency, resulting in megaloblastic anemia and/or neurologic disease. Folate deficiency may also occur. Vitamin B_{12} deficiency is a product of extensive vitamin uptake by the worm as well as worm-induced interference with gastrointestinal uptake by the host (despite normal gastric acidity and intrinsic factor production). Vitamin B_{12} deficiency is most common among older patients and is more likely to occur in patients with low dietary intake of vitamins, multiple tapeworms, or a tapeworm in the proximal jejunum. In the debilitated host, nervous system complications can be quite extensive and can range from peripheral neuropathy to the syndrome of severe combined degeneration (see Ch. 223).

DIAGNOSIS. The diagnosis of *D. latum* infection is made by stool examination for characteristic operculated eggs that are 65 by 45 μm. Recovery of proglottides is infrequent owing to segment degeneration during intestinal transit.

TREATMENT. Treatment is with niclosamide or praziquantel, as summarized in Table 384-2. Severe vitamin B_{12} deficiency can be rapidly treated by parenteral vitamin injections.

PREVENTION. Fish tapeworm infection is prevented by avoiding consumption of raw, smoked, or salted fish from endemic areas. Parasite cysts may be killed by cooking (above 56°C for 5 minutes) or by freezing (−20°C for 24 hours).

Hymenolepis nana

H. nana, or dwarf tapeworm, is found frequently in warm, dry climates and is prevalent in Southern and Eastern Europe, Asia, Africa, Central and South America, and Australia. It is the only human tapeworm that does not require an intermediate host. In the small intestine, hatching eggs release oncospheres that penetrate the villi of the mucosa. Four to 5 days later, the developed cysticercoid ruptures out of the villus and a parasite scolex attaches to the lining of the ileum, maturing in 10 to 12 days. Mature worms are small, measuring 25 to 40 mm long by 1 mm wide. Autoinfection can occur internally, i.e., within the small bowel, or externally, via the fecal-oral route, resulting in heavy infection. With time, however, a regulatory immunity to infection may develop, so that *H. nana* infection can be spontaneously cleared. Intensive infection is more common in institutionalized, malnourished, or immunodeficient individuals.

CLINICAL MANIFESTATIONS. The clinical manifestations of *H. nana* vary with intensity and may include diarrhea, anorexia, abdominal pain, and pallor. A statistical association with phlyctenular

TABLE 384–2. THERAPY FOR INTESTINAL CESTODE (TAPEWORM) INFECTION

	Niclosamide	Praziquantel
Dosage		
Adults	2 grams (4 tablets)	10–12 mg/kg for all age groups
Children >34 kg	1.5 grams (3 tablets)	(25 mg/kg for *H. nana*)
Children 11–34 kg	1 gram (2 tablets)	
Administration	For most tapeworm species, taken as a single dose; tablets must be thoroughly chewed before swallowing to obtain complete therapeutic effect; a 7-day course of drugs used for *H. nana,* with reduced pediatric doses on days 2–7	Taken as a single dose for all species; may repeat after 7 days for heavy *H. nana* infections
Side effects	Nausea, vomiting, abdominal pain, diarrhea, drowsiness, dizziness, headache, pruritus	Mild but frequent, including dizziness, myalgias, nausea, vomiting, diarrhea, abdominal pain
Pregnancy	No known mutagenic effects; considered safe if indicated; because of risk of cysticercosis by autoinfection in *T. solium* tapeworm infection, therapy should not be delayed	

keratoconjunctivitis has been observed and has been tentatively ascribed to the immune response to infection.

DIAGNOSIS. The diagnosis of *H. nana* infection is made by examining stool for eggs 30 to 47 μm that have a characteristic double membrane. Proglottides are usually not seen in the stool.

TREATMENT. Treatment is with niclosamide or praziquantel, as outlined in Table 384–2. Compared with the treatment of other tapeworm infections, longer courses of niclosamide and higher doses of praziquantel are recommended for the therapy of *H. nana* infection because of the relative resistance of larval cysticercoids to drug therapy. Because of the potential for late emergence of worms from viable cysticercoids remaining in the ileum, heavily infected individuals should be retested for infection and retreated 10 to 14 days after initial therapy.

PREVENTION. Because *H. nana* is easily transmitted from person to person, sanitation and hand washing are essential to control this parasite. Mass chemotherapy may also be used to suppress endemic transmission, particularly within closed institutions.

Taenia saginata

T. saginata, or beef tapeworm infection, is widespread in cattle-breeding areas of the world. Endemic foci (defined as prevalence >10%) are found in the southern Russian republics, in the Near East, and in central and eastern Africa. Infection is less common in other parts of the world but is found at prevalence rates of 0.1 to 5% in Europe, Southeast Asia, and South America. Infection is acquired by consuming cysticerci in the muscle tissue of infected cattle. The consumption of dishes such as steak tartare, "bleu" or rare steak, and undercooked shish kebabs is associated with infection in North American travelers to endemic areas.

CLINICAL MANIFESTATIONS. *T. saginata* infection may cause nonspecific complaints of weakness and mild abdominal discomfort in a minority (one third) of patients. Because *T. saginata* proglottides are motile, they may cause acute abdominal symptoms by migrating into and obstructing the appendix or the pancreatic and biliary ducts. A psychologically distressing feature of infection (and often the first symptom reported by the patient) occurs when motile proglottides migrate out of the anus onto skin or clothing or when they are observed moving in the feces.

DIAGNOSIS. The diagnosis of taeniasis is most readily established by stool examination and perianal inspection for parasite proglottides and eggs. It is not possible, however, to distinguish *T. saginata* eggs from those of *T. solium* morphologically, and the definitive diagnosis of *T. saginata* infection requires pathologic examination of proglottid features or DNA hybridization studies. In practice, because patients with *T. solium* are at risk for self-infection with cysticercosis (see below), and because medical therapy for taeniasis is both safe and highly effective, treatment of an undetermined *Taenia* species infection should not be delayed pending speciation of the infecting tapeworm.

TREATMENT. Treatment of beef tapeworm infection is with praziquantel or niclosamide, as outlined in Table 384–2. Both medications are highly effective in eliminating infection, and no special preparation or purgation is required. After therapy, the parasite scolex is digested within the gastrointestinal tract before it is passed in the feces. Although with the highly effective medications currently in use one no longer needs to collect the scolex to be assured that the parasite head has been expelled, digestive destruction of the

head limits our ability to establish a species-specific clinical diagnosis for individual *Taenia* infections.

PREVENTION. *T. saginata* infection is prevented by avoiding foods containing undercooked or raw beef. As for the fish tapeworm, cooking to 56°C for 5 minutes or freezing at −20°C for 7 to 10 days destroys the infective larvae.

Taenia solium

T. solium, also known as pork tapeworm, causes human infection in two different forms. Individuals who consume undercooked pork containing intermediate parasite cysts develop intestinal *T. solium* tapeworms. Individuals who consume parasite eggs may develop intermediate parasite cysts within the tissues of the body. (This condition, called *cysticercosis,* is described in more detail in the section on tissue cestode infections.) Autoinfection, most likely via the fecal-oral route, is possible, and a single patient may harbor both adult tapeworm and tissue cysticerci. *T. solium* infection is prevalent in Mexico, Central and South America, Africa, the Cape Verde Islands, southern Europe, Southeast Asia, and the Philippines. Most infections seen in the United States and Canada are found in immigrants from these endemic foci.

CLINICAL MANIFESTATIONS. *T. solium* tapeworms are relatively short (3 meters) but may survive for several decades once established in the human jejunum. Generally, tapeworm infections with *T. solium* produce minimal or no symptoms, being limited to mild, nonspecific abdominal complaints. Unlike *T. saginata* proglottides, the segments of *T. solium* are nonmotile and are unlikely to cause obstruction.

DIAGNOSIS. The diagnosis of intestinal infection with *T. solium* tapeworm is made by examining the stool for eggs and proglottides. Because the eggs are morphologically indistinguishable from those of *T. saginata,* study of the proglottid or head of the tapeworms is required for species identification. Stool samples and proglottides should be handled with care because of the risk of acquiring cysticercosis by accidental ingestion of *T. solium* eggs.

TREATMENT. *T. solium* tapeworm infection is treated with either niclosamide or praziquantel, as outlined in Table 384–2. Once diagnosis is established, therapy should be instituted as soon as possible because of the risk of autoinfection with cysticercosis. Therapy of concurrent cysticercosis is substantially longer and more intensive than that for intestinal infection and is described in detail in the section on tissue cestode infections.

Other Intestinal Cestodes

Other tapeworms that occasionally infect humans include the dog tapeworm *Dipylidium caninum* and the rodent tapeworm *Hymenolepis diminuta.* These are most common in children and are acquired by inadvertently ingesting the intermediate larval forms of these parasites in the bodies of fleas or other insects. Usually, *D. caninum* and *H. diminuta* infections produce minimal symptoms. Diagnosis is established by stool examination, and infections are readily treated with standard doses of niclosamide or praziquantel.

TISSUE CESTODE (CYST) INFECTION

Echinococcosis

Human echinococcosis causes significant morbidity and mortality in livestock-raising regions in all parts of the world. The causative agents of "hydatid" and "alveolar" cyst disease in humans are the intermediate larval forms of the tapeworms *Echinococcus granulosus* and *E. multilocularis,* respectively.

Like other cestodes, *Echinococcus* tapeworms have both intermediate and definitive hosts. For *Echinococcus* species, dogs and other canines are the definitive hosts. Tapeworm-infected animals pass eggs in their feces, which contaminate the local environment. Contamination of grazing areas and foodstuffs results in egg ingestion by intermediate hosts, e.g., humans, sheep, goats, camels, and horses for *E. granulosus* and mice or other small rodents for *E. multilocularis.* Life cycle transmission is completed when the definitive carnivore host consumes meat or offal of the intermediate host that contains hydatid or alveolar cysts. Protoscolices within the cysts mature in the lumen of the canine gut to become adult, egg-bearing tapeworms. Because the cysts of *Echinococcus* contain a germinal layer that can produce multiple internal "daughter" cysts by asexual budding, an individual dog may develop infection with dozens of tapeworms after consuming a single large cyst. Once the tapeworms mature, a heavily infected dog may contaminate 10 or more hectares of ground with infectious eggs in the space of a week.

In most areas of the world, burial practices make humans a "dead-end" host for *Echinococcus;* i.e., human infection does not perpetuate transmission in the local ecosystem. Nevertheless, the "inadvertent" hydatid cyst disease caused by *E. granulosus* and the more aggressive alveolar cyst disease caused by *E. multilocularis* are severe or even fatal illnesses for a significant minority of infected individuals.

EPIDEMIOLOGY. *E. granulosus* is common in livestock-raising areas of both developed and developing countries. Sheep- and goat-herding populations that keep dogs as pets or work animals are at highest risk for hydatid cyst disease. Until recently, hydatid disease was common in Australia, New Zealand, Argentina, Chile, Ireland, Scotland, the Basque country, the Mediterranean basin, and throughout middle Europe. Currently, the area with the highest prevalence in the world is the Turkana and Samburu regions of northwestern Kenya, where domestic and feral transmission of *E. granulosus* is perpetuated among nomadic farmers by poor hygienic practices. Occasional hydatid disease transmission is also found in central Asia, Mexico, the United States, and South America.

Alveolar cyst disease due to *E. multilocularis* is usually transmitted by wild animals, e.g., foxes and bush dogs, and is found in the arctic regions of the United States, Canada, and the former Soviet Union, as well as in rural areas of Europe and Turkey.

CLINICAL MANIFESTATIONS. Human disease caused by *Echinococcus* species results from bloodborne invasion of the liver (50 to 70% of patients), lungs (20 to 30%), or other organs by developing parasite oncospheres. As these mature, they grow within tissues by concentric enlargement *(E. granulosus)* or by extension through adjacent host tissues *(E. multilocularis).* At any given time, most infected individuals are asymptomatic, and it may take 5 to 20 years for a cyst to grow to sufficient size (3 to 15 cm) to cause symptoms. When present, symptoms and findings refer to the anatomic site of involvement and derive from local inflammation, secondary bacterial infection, obstruction, or local mass effect. In hydatid cyst disease, the growing cyst becomes surrounded by a fibrous capsule formed by host immune reaction. Within this primary unilocular cyst, multiple daughter cysts, each containing an infective protoscolex, develop by asexual budding of the germinal layer. In alveolar cyst disease, the parasite cyst is not well separated from surrounding tissues, and lateral budding and malignancy-like growth (including distant metastasis of daughter cysts) may occur.

Patients with symptomatic hydatid liver cysts may complain of abdominal discomfort or mass in the right upper quadrant. Cyst leakage into the peritoneal cavity or pleural space may be associated with fever, urticaria, or a severe anaphylactoid reaction. Invasion of the biliary system often leads to the passage of daughter cysts into the common bile duct, with clinical and chemical evidence of intermittent obstruction resembling cholerdocholithiasis. Individuals with symptomatic hydatid involvement of the lungs present with cough, hemoptysis, and pleurisy. Spontaneous rupture of the cyst may lead to intrathoracic spread or to evacuation of daughter cysts via the bronchus. At either lung or liver sites, bacterial superinfection may cause an acute presentation with symptoms of sepsis. Hydatid involvement of the brain is marked by slow-onset mass effect, hydrocephalus, and often seizures. Cysts of the bone frequently fail to form a discrete capsule but rather cause local erosion of the cortex, resulting in pathologic fracture.

Symptomatic alveolar cyst disease most frequently refers to liver involvement and manifests as vague, mild upper quadrant and epigastric pain. Signs of hepatomegaly or obstructive jaundice may be present. Occasionally, metastatic lesions in the lung or brain are the first to cause symptoms by local inflammation or mass effect.

DIAGNOSIS. Laboratory evaluation may show marked eosinophilia, but this finding is inconstant (30% prevalence). In hydatid cyst disease, radiographic and ultrasonographic studies typically show characteristic large, avascular cysts containing internal structures consistent with daughter cysts. Detection of mural calcification strongly favors the diagnosis of hydatid cyst. The differential diagnosis includes hemangioma, metastatic carcinoma, and remote bacterial or amebic liver abscess. Confirmatory evidence of infection may be obtained by serology (sensitivity of 60 to 90%, depending on the test used). Serologic testing is available commercially or from the Centers for Disease Control and Prevention (CDC), Atlanta, GA (through local state health departments). Until recently, it has not been recommended to perform closed aspiration on the cyst for diagnosis, as cyst leakage has the potential to initiate a severe allergic reaction and may result in the metastatic spread of daughter cysts. However, a recent clinical series has reported successful computed tomography (CT)–guided thin-needle aspiration of hydatid cysts for diagnosis. This procedure, when followed by immediate instillation of ethanol to kill viable protoscoleces, was associated with minimal side effects and was followed by apparent regression of cysts on CT scans. Further trials of this simplified approach to diagnosis and therapy appear warranted.

With alveolar cyst disease due to *E. multilocularis,* the organism's appearance on radiographic and sonographic imaging often mimics that of hepatic carcinoma. A definitive diagnosis may require either angiography or open biopsy at surgery. Precautions must be taken to prevent metastatic dissemination of daughter cysts at the time of surgery.

TREATMENT. Stable, asymptomatic, calcified cysts do not require specific therapy but should be monitored by serial imaging over several years to ensure a benign resolution. When technically feasible, expanding, symptomatic, or infected cysts are best removed *in toto* at surgery, with care taken to isolate and kill the cyst (with hypertonic saline (25 to 30 grams per deciliter) or other cidal agents (such as iodophor or ethanol) prior to excision, to avoid secondary spread or parasite cysts. Surgical resection should include careful closure of biliary and enteric fistulas and extensive postoperative drainage of the cyst bed to prevent fluid accumulation and secondary bacterial infection. Alveolar cyst disease may require wide resection, i.e., total lobectomy of liver or lung, to remove all cyst material.

In many cases, symptomatic echinococcal cysts are not amenable to resection. In such cases, oral drug therapy with the anthelminthics, either long-term mebendazole (40 mg per kilogram of body weight per day in three divided doses for 6 to 12 months) or albendazole* (400 mg twice a day for one to eight periods of 28 days each, separated by drug-free rest intervals of 14 to 28 days), has been recommended for cure or palliation. Cure rates, particularly for difficult cases with recurrent or extrahepatic/extrapulmonary cysts, have been low (< 33%), although a majority of patients show some improvement. Because the efficacy of drug therapy is limited, a combined medical-surgical approach should be formulated for each patient.

Cysticercosis

Cysticercosis represents human tissue infection with the intermediate cyst forms of the pork tapeworm *T. solium.* Cysticercosis is acquired by ingestion of *T. solium* eggs in contaminated foods. Infection prevalence is approximately 1 to 10% in endemic areas of Latin America, India, Asia, Indonesia, and parts of Africa. Because of its potentially life-threatening complications, cysticercosis has greater clinical significance than does intestinal *T. solium* tapeworm

---

* This drug has not been approved by the Food and Drug Administration at the time of publication. In the United States, compassionate use may be available through SmithKline Beecham Pharmaceuticals, Philadelphia, PA.

infection, particularly if cyst disease involves the CNS, the eyes, the heart, or other vital organs.

CLINICAL MANIFESTATIONS. Clinical manifestations depend on the location and number of infecting cysts. Cysticerci are bladder-like, fluid-filled cysts containing an invaginated protoscolex. They are often surrounded by a dense fibrous capsule of host origin. In infected humans, cysticerci are usually multiple, 0.5 to 2 cm in size, and distributed widely throughout the body. Many patients have minimal, if any, symptoms of infection. However, symptomatic *neurocysticercosis* (i.e., cerebral cysticercosis, eye or spinal cord involvement) requires medical attention. This syndrome has an estimated mortality of up to 50%, and any neurologic, cognitive, or personality disorder in an individual from an endemic area should be considered a possible manifestation of undiagnosed neurocysticercosis. In the past decade, diagnosis of this condition has been facilitated by CT scanning and magnetic resonance imaging (MRI), both of which are highly sensitive in detecting CNS cysticerci. Patients with CNS involvement have an average of 10 cysts distributed throughout the brain and spinal cord. These cysts may be in different stages of development, with symptoms commonly arising when older cysts begin to die, lose osmoregulation, and release antigenic material to provoke significant host inflammatory response.

In practice, neurocysticercosis may be divided into six discrete syndromes for management. In the *acute invasive* stage of cysticercosis, immediately after infection, the patient may experience fevers, headache, and myalgias associated with significant peripheral eosinophilia. Heavy infection at this stage may result in a clinical picture of "cysticercal encephalitis" associated with coma and rapid deterioration. This presentation should be treated aggressively with antiparasitic agents and anti-inflammatory drugs. After cysticerci become established, *parenchymal CNS cysticercosis* (50% of cases) is associated with seizures, intellectual impairment, and personality changes. Compression due to swelling or inflammation around the cysts may result in focal deficits, signs of cerebral edema, and/or hydrocephalus. Seizures may be focal (jacksonian), referring to the specific cortical locus of involvement, or may be generalized. *Subarachnoid cysticercosis* (30% of cases) is frequently associated with obstruction of cerebrospinal fluid (CSF) flow. Intracranial hypertension may manifest as vomiting, headache, and visual disturbances. Sensorial changes may include apathy, amnesia, dementia, hallucination, and emotional disturbance. Like other forms of basilar meningitis, pericysticercal inflammation at the base of the brain may cause obstruction or vasculitis of the cerebral arteries, leading to intermittent ischemia or stroke. *Intraventricular cysticercosis* (15% of cases) is, because of its location, the most difficult to diagnose and treat. Symptomatic cysts are most frequent in the fourth ventricle, where they cause outflow obstruction and increased intracranial pressure without localizing signs. An aggressive variant of ventricular neurocysticercosis, called racemose cysticercosis, frequently involves the basal cisterns. This form of cysticercosis has been noted most often in young women and involves multiple, rapidly spreading cysts in the cerebrum and around the base of the brain. Whereas symptoms due to isolated cysts may remit, racemose cysticercosis usually has a progressive, deteriorating course if therapy is not given. Those with *spinal cysticercosis* may present with cord compression, radiculopathy, transverse myelitis, or signs of meningitis, depending on the location of involvement. *Ocular cysticercosis* is a distinct syndrome that manifests as eye pain, scotomata, and decreasing vision due to iridocyclitis, clouding of the vitreous, and retinal inflammation or detachment.

DIAGNOSIS. A definitive diagnosis of cysticercosis requires examination of biopsy material obtained from a tissue cyst. However, a presumptive diagnosis may be made on the basis of a history of residence in an endemic area, the presence of characteristic radiographic findings on plain films (calcified cysts in soft tissues) or scans (multiple, low-density, enhanced, and unenhanced lesions on CT or MRI), and suggestive laboratory findings. Infection with *T. solium* tapeworm is present in about 25% of neurocysticercosis cases. In neurocysticercosis, examining the CSF may show hypoglycorrhachia, elevated total protein levels, and lymphocytic and eosinophilic pleocytosis (5 to 500 cells per microliter). Serum and CSF enzyme-linked immunosorbent assay (ELISA) and Western

blot testing for specific immunoglobulin M (IgM) and immunoglobulin G (IgG) anticysticercal antibodies has a sensitivity of 75 to 100%. These tests are available through commercial laboratories or from the CDC (samples should be sent through state health departments). It should be noted, however, that antiparasite antibodies may persist long after infection, and a positive IgG serology merely indicates prior *Taenia* exposure, not necessarily active disease. The differential diagnosis of neurocysticercosis includes tumor, hydatid cyst disease, vasculitis, and chronic fungal and mycobacterial infection.

TREATMENT. Given the high prevalence of cysticercosis in some areas of the world, it is evident that most cysticerci do not cause significant symptoms. For *symptomatic* cysts outside the CNS, the optimal therapy is surgical removal, as this ensures complete elimination of the cyst. In the case of symptomatic neurocysticercosis, which carries an associated mortality of up to 50%, therapy is definitely indicated, but surgery may be risky or technically unfeasible. An alternative approach to controlling some forms of neurocysticercosis has been demonstrated in recent clinical studies: Drug therapy with either praziquantel (50 mg per kilogram per day in three divided doses for 14 to 30 days) or albendazole* (15 mg per kilogram per day for 30 days) has been associated with alleviation of symptoms and regression of cyst size and number in patients with viable (nonenhancing) cysts in the cerebral parenchyma. However, drug therapy has provided only limited improvement in patients with arachnoiditis and no improvement in patients with intraventricular cysts. For these latter presentations, the treatment of choice remains surgery and/or palliation with shunting, anticonvulsants, and anti-inflammatory agents. It should be noted that in about 20% of treated cases, starting drug therapy is associated with a severely symptomatic, increased inflammatory response at the site of the cyst. This inflammation may be controlled with corticosteroids, but corticosteroids are not recommended for routine use in all patients, as they may significantly alter the pharmacokinetics of the anthelminthics used to treat infection. Follow-up tomographic scanning should be repeated 3 months after therapy is stopped to ensure adequate response. If necessary, a repeat course of drug therapy with the alternate agent may be given to improve response. Because parasite-induced ocular inflammation does not respond well to systemic anti-inflammatory agents, patients with cysticercosis of the eye (20% of cases of neurocysticercosis) should not receive drug therapy until the eye disease has been controlled surgically.

Coenurosis

A different, but more rare, form of tissue cysticercosis may be caused by larval stages of the dog tapeworms *T. multiceps* and *T. serialis*. Lesions tend to be solitary and are distinguished pathologically from *T. solium* cysticerci on biopsy. Ocular involvement is common, and surgical resection is currently the only effective mode of therapy.

Sparganosis

Sparganosis is a tissue cestode infection caused by the plerocercoid larval stages of *Spirometra* species tapeworms of cats and other carnivores. Humans may become infected by ingesting infected water fleas *(Cyclops),* by ingesting uncooked meat from infected animals (reptiles, birds, or mammals), or by cutaneous exposure (e.g., via traditional skin or eye poultices) to uncooked, infected meat. Usually, the larva encysts within the intestinal submucosa or skin. In some cases, however, parasites may invade the eye or CNS and cause significant inflammatory pathology at the site of encystment. Occasionally, proliferation into surrounding tissues occurs by lateral budding of the parasite (termed *sparganum proliferum*). The treatment of choice for sparganosis is ethanol injection and/or surgical removal, as limited experience with medical anthelminthic therapy has shown no beneficial effect.

Davis A, Dixon H, Pawlowski Z: Multicentre clinical trials of benzimidazole carbamates in human cystic echinococcosis (phase 2). Bull WHO 67:503, 1989. *Review of experience in multicenter trials of medical therapy for hydatid and alveolar cyst disease.*

Del Brutto OH, Sotelo J: Neurocysticercosis: An update. Rev Infect Dis 10:1075, 1988. *Extensive review of the diagnosis and treatment of this varied and complex disease. Contains a useful flow diagram on therapy for neurocysticercosis.*

Filice C, Di Perri G, Strosselli M, et al.: Parasitologic findings in percutaneous

---

* This drug has not been approved by the Food and Drug Administration at the time of publication.

drainage of human hydatid liver cysts. J Infect Dis 161:1290, 1990. *Description of a small series of patients undergoing CT-guided diagnosis and treatment of hydatid cyst disease.*

King CH, Mahmoud AAF: Drugs five years later: Praziquantel. Ann Intern Med 110:290, 1989. *A summary of data on the anthelminthic agent praziquantel since its release in the United States. Includes a listing of doses recommended for cestode therapy: with references.*

Pawlowski ZS: Cestodiases: Taeniasis, cysticercosis, diphyllobothriasis, hymenolepiasis and others. *In* Warren KS, Mahmoud AAF (eds.): Tropical and Geographical Medicine. 2nd ed. New York, McGraw-Hill, 1990, p 490. *A detailed review of cestode infections (excluding Echinococcus species).*

Schantz PM, Okelo GBA: Echinococcosis (hydatidosis). *In* Warren KS, Mahmoud AAF (eds.): Tropical and Geographical Medicine. 2nd ed. New York, McGraw-Hill, 1990, p 505. *Review of human infection with* Echinococcus *species. Useful for hydatid disease as well as less common E. multilocularis and E. vogeli infections.*

385 SCHISTOSOMIASIS
(Bilharziasis)
Adel A.F. Mahmoud

DEFINITION. Schistosomiasis, a chronic worm infection, affects more than 200 million people in the world; several hundred million more live in endemic areas and are at risk of exposure to the parasites. The schistosomes are blood flukes that parasitize the venous channels of the definitive human host; infection is transmitted via fresh water snails. Humans may be infected by one of five species: *Schistosoma haematobium, S. mansoni, S. japonicum, S. intercalatum,* or *S. mekongi.* Each species is endemic in specific geographic areas of the world; infection in humans may result in defined clinical syndromes. Other species that occasionally infect humans include *S. bovis, S. matthei,* and some avian schistosomes. Currently, schistosomiasis is endemic in various areas of Africa, Asia, South America, and the Caribbean islands. In the United States, there are approximately 400,000 infected individuals; these include Puerto Ricans, and immigrants or travelers exposed while in endemic areas. Because of the absence of susceptible snails, the life cycle of the schistosomes cannot be established in this country.

ETIOLOGY. The schistosomes differ from other trematodes that infect humans in that they have separate sexes. The species of schistosomes that infect humans share some common features, although they are morphologically distinctive. Each worm has two suckers (anterior and ventral), and the bifurcate intestinal ceca unite posteriorly. The larger male (0.6 to 2.2 cm × 2 to 4 mm) has a ventral gynecophoral canal in which the female is held during copulation. The slender female worm (1.2 to 2.6 cm × 1 to 2 mm) has a rounded body with pointed ends.

Adult schistosome worms parasitize defined sites of the venous vasculature of humans. *S. haematobium* worms inhabit the venous plexus around the lower end of the ureters and the urinary bladder, whereas *S. mansoni, S. japonicum, S. intercalatum,* and *S. mekongi* are located in the mesenteric veins. Sexual maturity of female worms requires the presence of living mature males; when ready to deposit eggs, the worms move against the bloodstream toward the small venous radicles. The female schistosomes deposit ova singly or in bunches, depending on the species of the parasite, and retreat in the direction of blood flow. Egg deposition has been estimated at 300 per day for female *S. haematobium* and *S. mansoni* worms and 3000 per day for *S. japonicum.* The ova of each species have characteristic morphologic features, which are of diagnostic importance. Once deposited in the host, eggs attempt to penetrate the venous capillaries and escape to the bladder or intestinal lumen; enzymatic secretions are thought to aid egg migration. The proportion of ova escaping from infected individuals varies in each species and also may depend on the extent of pathology and state of resistance in the host. Eggs that fail to reach the lumen of urinary tract or gut are trapped in these organs or may be carried to other organs such as the liver; these ova cause inflammatory and immunopathologic changes that are a major cause of disease in schistosomiasis. The schistosome eggs, when deposited by female worms, contain immature miracidia; they take approximately 10 to 12 days to develop while migrating through the host tissues. Once mature, miracidia have a mean lifespan of 11 to 12 days.

Indiscriminate urination and defecation by infected individuals result in dissemination of the parasite eggs in the environment. In fresh water the schistosome ova hatch within a few hours. Miracidia escape head first and swim, usually near the surface of water; they remain infective to the snail intermediate host for approximately 8 hours. On encountering the specific snail, the miracidia penetrate its tissues and undergo tremendous asexual multiplication and transformation into hundreds of cercariae. Schistosome infection of snails causes varying degrees of pathology in their liver and sexual organs and reduces their lifespan. Development of schistosomes inside the snail takes approximately 4 to 6 weeks, but it varies with the species of the parasite and mollusc and with changes in environmental conditions. Cercariae, the infective forms to humans, emerge from the snails under specific conditions of light and temperature; they are elongate with a pear-shaped body and a long forked tail and measure approximately 400 to 600 μm in length. They can survive in fresh water for almost 72 hours but lose their infectivity considerably within the first 24 hours. Cercariae attach to skin of mammalian hosts by their oral or ventral suckers. Burrowing of the skin is helped by vertical vibratory movements of their bodies and secretions of the cephalic penetration glands; the process is usually completed within a few minutes. During penetration, the cercariae shake off their tails and change into the next stage of the life cycle, the schistosomula, which lie in tunnels in the stratum corneum parallel to the skin surface. Schistosomula are covered by a heptalaminar membrane (instead of the trilaminar cercarial membrane) and can no longer survive in fresh water. They are thought to remain in the skin for 1 to 3 days before migrating to the lungs, finally reaching the liver in 2 to 4 weeks. In the intrahepatic portal system, the worms complete the major digestive and sexual stages of their development. Adult worms start their migration to their final habitat in 2 weeks and mate; viable eggs can be seen in the excreta 5 to 9 weeks after cercarial penetration. Figure 385–1 shows the stages of the life cycle of schistosomes.

The mean lifespan of adult schistosome worms inside the human host is not known exactly. Several individual case reports indicate that worms may live 20 to 30 years. This, however, represents extreme cases, as examination of infected individuals who migrate to nonendemic areas indicates that the mean lifespan of the worms is in the range of 3 to 10 years.

EPIDEMIOLOGY. The endemicity of schistosomiasis in any specific area depends on the unsanitary disposal of urine and feces, the presence of suitable snail hosts, and human exposure to cercaria-infected bodies of water. Furthermore, the epidemiology of schistosomiasis is complex because of the existence of several stages of the life cycle of the parasite and the multitude of factors affecting each. Since adult schistosomes, like many parasitic

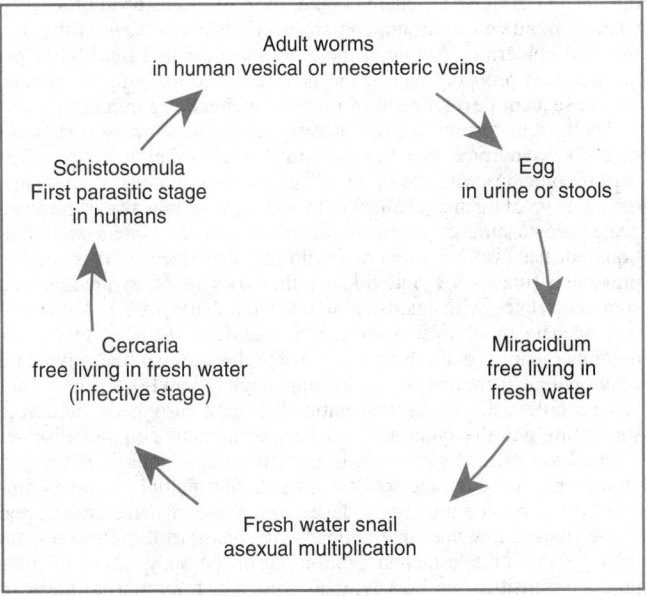

FIGURE 385–1. Schistosome life cycle.

worms, do not multiply in the human body, a close correlation exists between worm load and fecal or urinary egg counts; estimates of intensity of infection can therefore be obtained by ova-enumerating procedures. Quantifying worm loads is important epidemiologically as well as for the individual patient, as it determines the potential of participation in transmission of schistosomiasis and predicts, to a large extent, the risk of morbidity and pathologic outcome.

In endemic areas, schistosomiasis prevalence and intensity show characteristic association with age. Schistosomiasis is acquired early in childhood; prevalence and intensity gradually increase to a peak in the second decade of life. In older individuals, a modest reduction of prevalence may be seen along with a sharp fall in intensity of infection. The marked drop in intensity in adults may be due to a decrease in their water-related activities. Development of immunity may also explain the age-related decrease in intensity. Intensity of infection in endemic communities shows another characteristic feature: Most infected individuals harbor low worm loads, and only a small proportion acquire heavy infection. The underlying mechanism of this clustering of heavy infection in schistosomiasis is not known but may be due to varying degrees of susceptibility and/or response of humans to the parasites.

In some areas, the endemicity of schistosomiasis may be maintained by animal reservoirs; this is especially the case with *S. japonicum,* which infects dogs and cows. Although both *S. haematobium* and *S. mansoni* can infect primates and rodents, the role of these animals as reservoirs does not seem to be epidemiologically important.

PATHOGENESIS. Schistosomiasis is initiated by cercarial penetration of skin; inside the host three maturational forms of the parasite evolve: schistosomula, adults, and eggs. These stages are associated with morphologic, biochemical, and antigenic changes of the worm, which add to the complexity of the host-parasite relationship. Disease caused by schistosomiasis occurs mainly in those with high eggs counts. This relationship, however, is not exact, as the roles of other factors such as genetic background and immunologic modulatory mechanisms are now being elucidated.

Three distinct disease syndromes caused by schistosomiasis have been described; each corresponds roughly to a stage in the parasite development in the host. Cercarial dermatitis, or swimmer's itch, may be seen in infections with human schistosomes but is more common when avian or other nonhuman cercariae penetrate the skin. Swimmer's itch caused by nonhuman schistosomes is commonly seen in the north-central United States, where some lakes are infected. The condition has also been reported in subjects exposed to *S. mansoni* or *S. haematobium* but rarely after exposure to *S. japonicum.* Primary exposure to these larvae results in either no reaction or immediate pruritic macular rash. On repeated exposures, sensitization occurs, and a more pronounced papular eruption develops with erythema, edema, and pruritus. Histopathologically, edema, round cell infiltrate, and eosinophilia can be seen in the dermis and epidermis. Although the mechanism of this reaction is not known, it is probably due to the host response to dying larvae and the subsequent development of humoral and cellular immunity.

Acute schistosomiasis, or Katayama fever, is a serum sickness–like syndrome that occurs 3 to 9 weeks after infection. This period coincides with the onset of egg production and its associated increase in antigenic challenge to the host. Clinically significant acute schistosomiasis occurs more often with *S. japonicum* infections but has also been reported with the other species. It is seen in previously unexposed individuals; the severity of symptoms and signs correlates with intensity of infection. Very little is known of the mechanism of this syndrome; it manifests itself as fever, abdominal pain, and headache with hepatosplenomegaly and eosinophilia. Increases of serum immunoglobulin (Ig) G, IgM, IgE, and specific antischistosomal antibodies have also been observed, suggesting that the syndrome is a form of immune complex disease.

The basic pathologic lesion in chronic schistosomiasis is the egg granuloma. Although the schistosomes do not multiply in the definitive host, they continually produce eggs; some of these are trapped in the tissues. Enzymes and antigens are subsequently released from the eggs to facilitate their migration out of the body. These parasite products sensitize the host lymphocytes, which migrate to areas of egg deposition and recruit other cells, and a compact cellular infiltrate "granuloma" is formed. Several cell types are prominent in the schistosome egg granuloma: lymphocytes, macrophages, eosinophils, and fibroblasts. The size of these granulomas and the resulting fibrosis lead to most of the chronic fibro-obstructive lesions in schistosomiasis. In *S. haematobium* infection, granulomas at the lower end of the ureters impede urine flow and cause hydroureter and hydronephrosis. In infections with other schistosome species, granulomas in the intestinal wall are associated with the abdominal manifestations of the disease, and those in the liver result in presinusoidal obstruction of portal blood flow, portal hypertension, splenomegaly, and esophageal varices. Less commonly, eggs may be carried to almost any organ or tissue in the body, eliciting granuloma formation and its pathologic sequelae. The size of the granulomatous response represents a delicate balance between sensitizing and modulating mechanisms. In chronic schistosomiasis, granulomas spontaneously modulate—i.e., their size decreases significantly—and may result in slowing the progression of disease manifestations. Modulation has been shown to be mediated by several arms of the host's immune system, including serum antibodies, anti-idiotypic antibodies, immune complexes, suppressor lymphocytes, and macrophages. Functionally, granulomas serve to destroy the parasite eggs.

The immune response of individuals with schistosomiasis includes humoral as well as cellular components. The degree and extent of these responses provide the balance between asymptomatic infection and disease manifestations. Furthermore, mechanisms that control the host immune response, such as genetic background, have been demonstrated to influence the extent of granuloma formation and consequently disease. The host immune response to schistosome antigens also is inversely related to intensity of infection; impaired responses are seen only in those with heavy worm loads. Whether the defect in immunity is a cause or consequence of infection is not yet clear. Another aspect of the host's immune response in schistosomiasis relates to the development of peripheral blood as well as tissue eosinophilia. Schistosomiasis, similar to other worm infections with tissue phases, results in a significant increase in eosinophils, especially during the acute phase of infection. Later, in the chronic stage, the eosinophil count may not be significantly elevated. Eosinophils are seen in subcutaneous tissues around the entry points of cercariae, and they constitute approximately 50% of the cells in egg granulomas. Eosinophils have been shown to play a central role in host defenses against the invading stage of the parasite (schistosomula) and the phase (ova) retained in the tissues.

MANAGEMENT. Diagnosis of schistosomiasis must be based on the clinical presentation, positive geographic history, and finding the parasite eggs in the excreta or biopsy material. Quantification of infection and assessment of viability of the eggs are important procedures not only for planning therapy but also for prognostic evaluation. For physicians practicing in nonendemic areas, e.g., North America, most infected individuals have the early acute and nonspecific features of the infection. Eosinophilia and serologic evidence of exposure to schistosome infection are two particularly helpful laboratory findings. Appropriate management of individuals with schistosomiasis must take into consideration the extent of disease and intensity of infection. Antischistosomal therapy, if given early during the course of disease, may lead to reversal of pathologic lesions. In late cases, chemotherapeutic measures may be useful only in preventing further damage from the presence of the parasite.

CONTROL. The intimate relationship between humans and bodies of fresh water in their environment leads to schistosomiasis endemicity. In addition, the lack of precise knowledge of the epidemiology of infection and disease has hampered efforts to control it. Several developments, such as single-dose oral chemotherapeutic agents and better appreciation of transmission dynamics, have led to a clearer definition of strategies for control of schistosomiasis. Ideally, eradication of infection should be the target, but this is impossible to achieve with the currently available tools and the economic and social structure of the endemic areas. Research toward antischistosome vaccine is progressing, but its practical use lies in the future. A more realistic approach is based on control of disease and reduction of transmission. The measure currently advocated is targeted chemotherapy, combined with focal eradication of the organism if needed. In addition, health education, attempts at raising socioeconomic standards, providing privies, and abandoning obsolete agricultural practices offer means for achieving progress in containing this infection.

Those traveling to endemic areas should be given proper advice. There are virtually no safe fresh water bodies in most of the areas endemic for schistosomiasis. Avoiding contact with these water sources is strongly recommended.

SCHISTOSOMIASIS HAEMATOBIA (Urinary Bilharziasis)

S. haematobium infection is endemic in Africa and some parts of the Middle East; it is highly prevalent in the Nile Valley and extends along the Mediterranean coast of the continent. In West Africa it is more widely disseminated than *S. mansoni;* its distribution in East and South Africa is patchy. In Southwest Asia the endemic area includes most countries of the Middle East and Arabian peninsula. Clinically, infection with *S. haematobium* is the most significant of the human schistosome infections because symptoms such as hematuria and dysuria occur early and affect approximately two thirds of infected individuals. In endemic areas, extensive hydroureters and hydronephrosis can be demonstrated in a considerable proportion of infected children; the natural history of these lesions and the course of disease in adults have not been clearly defined.

Adult male *S. haematobium* worms are distinguished by their finely tuberculate surface and by the presence of four to five large testes. The ovaries are found in the posterior half of the female body and contain 20 to 30 eggs (Table 385–1). The main intermediate hosts of *S. haematobium* in North Africa and the Middle East are fresh water snails of the genus *Bulinus;* in Africa south of the Sahara they belong to the subgenus *Physopsis.*

PATHOLOGY AND CLINICAL MANIFESTATIONS. In the urinary bladder, the formation of egg granulomas leads to hyperemia, tubercles, ulcers, and polyps; as healing proceeds, sandy patches and scarring may be seen. Obstructive uropathy is the main functional disturbance caused by schistosomiasis haematobia. Other urinary tract disorders, such as bacteriuria, calculi, and bladder cancer, have been epidemiologically associated with *S. haematobium* infection. Ova of *S. haematobium* have occasionally been found in the lungs with subsequent focal pulmonary arteritis and diffuse hypertensive arteriolar changes; chronic cor pulmonale may occur in these patients.

Swimmer's itch and acute schistosomiasis have rarely been described in *S. haematobium* infection. By contrast, symptoms related to the urinary tract, including dysuria, hematuria, or frequency, occur in a large proportion of infected individuals. Hematuria is characteristically terminal, but with extensive ulceration the whole stream of urine may be bloody, along with passage of clots. In late cases, symptoms related to secondary infection of the urinary tract, severe obstructive uropathy, or neoplasia may appear. Urine examination reveals proteinuria and hematuria; both signs are closely related to intensity of infection. An association between *S. haematobium* infection and bacteremia, mainly caused by *Salmonella* organisms, has been reported. Renal function may be compromised in patients with obstructive uropathy. Cytoscopic examination shows some degree of pathology in almost all infected individuals, the most common being hyperemia near the ureteral openings and the bladder trigone. Sandy patches, tubercles, ulcers, and polyps may also be seen. Imaging studies show bladder calcification in approximately 50 to 80% of infected individuals. Other pathologic lesions are also frequently seen in 40 to 60% of patients, including obstructive uropathy, hydroureters, hydronephrosis, and filling defects in the bladder and ureters.

DIAGNOSIS. Urine examination for *S. haematobium* eggs can be performed by direct or concentration methods (Table 385–1). Once *S. haematobium* infection is diagnosed, urinary tract pathology should be assessed by ultrasonography. In addition, care must be taken in some endemic areas for early detection of bladder cancer by appropriate cytologic and histologic examinations.

TREATMENT. See Management of Schistosomiasis, below.

SCHISTOSOMIASIS MANSONI (Intestinal or Hepatosplenic Bilharziasis)

Infection with *S. mansoni* is endemic in Africa, the Middle East, South America, and some Caribbean islands. The distribution of schistosomiasis mansoni in Africa overlaps with that of schistosomiasis haematobia. In Southwest Asia, it occurs in Yemen and Saudi Arabia. *S. mansoni* is sporadically distributed all over the northern part of South America and is endemic in several Caribbean countries and islands and in many parts of Puerto Rico.

Adult male *S. mansoni* worms have a grossly tuberculate surface and usually contain seven small testes. In the female, the ovary occupies the anterior half of its body, with a short uterus containing one to four ova (Table 385–1). The intermediate snail hosts of *S. mansoni* are species of the genus *Biomphalaria* in Africa and *Australorbis tropicorbis* in the Americas.

PATHOLOGY AND CLINICAL MANIFESTATIONS. Acute schistosomiasis mansoni is the most common early presentation encountered by physicians in North America. Symptoms appear between 3 and 7 weeks after exposure and include fever, anorexia, abdominal pain, and headache. Less often, diarrhea, nausea, and

TABLE 385–1. DIAGNOSIS OF SCHISTOSOMIASIS

Schistosome	Eggs	Diagnosis
S. haematobium	Mainly found in urine but may be found in stools or rectal biopsy Eggs: 143×50 μm; spindle shaped: rounded anterior, conical posterior, tapering to a terminal delicate spine	Obtain urine sample at midday (when eggs are excreted); more than one sample may be needed Examine urine directly or by filtering 10 ml urine through Nuclepore membrane Rectal biopsy in suspected cases with normal urine Serologic testing to diagnose early or light infection
S. mansoni	Eggs: 155×66 μm; oval with lateral, long spine	Examine stool for eggs Use Kato thick smear method for quantification purposes Rectal biopsy or serologic testing to diagnose stool-negative cases, particularly in lightly infected patients
S. japonicum	Found in stool; eggs: 89×67 μm; oval or rounded with lateral, short, sometimes curved spine	Examine stool for eggs Kato thick smear (for quantitative assessment) Rectal biopsy for those with light infections, especially with less common manifestation (i.e., cerebral schistosomiasis)
S. mekongi	Found in stool; eggs: 60×32 μm; smaller than eggs of *S. japonicum*	Examine stool for eggs
S. intercalatum	Found in stool; eggs: 180×65 μm; terminal spine	Examine stool for eggs

vomiting may occur. Hepatosplenomegaly, eosinophilia, and increased serum immunoglobulins are the main clinical signs. Most of these manifestations correlate significantly with intensity of infection as evaluated by stool egg counts.

Schistosoma mansoni eggs are primarily deposited in the small veins around the large intestine; some of the eggs may be trapped in the gut wall or break loose into the portal circulation to be carried to the small intrahepatic portal venules. On examination, the intestinal mucosa appears red and granular with pinpoint elevations surrounded by hyperemic zones. There may be minute hemorrhages and ulcerations. Sessile and pedunculated polyps, mainly in the rectosigmoid area, have been reported in Egyptians infected with *S. mansoni,* but not in persons from other endemic areas. Pathologic examination of the liver in lightly infected individuals shows schistosome eggs with and without granulomas and mild portal inflammation. In advanced cases, the typical picture of Symmers' fibrosis is seen; the eggs are concentrated in and around large portal tracts with marked fibrosis and obstructive portal venous lesions. The lobular arrangement of liver parenchyma and its function are usually maintained. However, these structural changes lead to marked alteration of hepatic hemodynamics, such as obstruction of portal blood flow through the liver and increase in number and size of intrahepatic arterial branches, thus shifting the blood flow through the liver from mainly portal to arterial sources. Portal hypertension leads to congestive splenomegaly and formation of portosystemic venous shunts at the lower end of the esophagus and other sites. In these patients, schistosome eggs may find their way to the pulmonary circulation, bypassing the obstructed portal blood flow. In the lungs, granulomas form around the trapped eggs, leading to arteriolar fibrosis and pulmonary hypertension.

Nervous system involvement in schistosomiasis mansoni is rare; the main clinical presentation, as in schistosomiasis haematobia, is transverse myelitis. The preferential involvement of the spinal cord may be due to the anatomic location of adult worms. The underlying pathologic lesions are usually granulomas forming around eggs in the spinal cord.

Infection with *S. mansoni* does not have characteristic or specific symptomatology. Early symptoms are those of acute schistosomiasis and are all nonspecific. These include fever, weakness, headache, and abdominal pain. This is particularly the case in travelers who are accidentally exposed to infection in endemic areas. In chronic schistosomiasis mansoni, infected individuals have a slightly higher incidence of crampy abdominal pain (21 to 48%) and bloody diarrhea (4 to 28%) than do matched uninfected controls from the same endemic area. Other frequently mentioned nonspecific symptoms, such as weakness, inability to work, or diarrhea, have not been convincingly demonstrated in any controlled studies. Significant enlargement of the liver is seen in 4 to 11% of infected subjects, and splenomegaly occurs in 3 to 7%. Patients with schistosomal hepatosplenomegaly have a unique form of liver disease. The pathophysiologic changes are based on alteration of hemodynamics, fibrosis of large portal tracts, and very little derangement of liver function. Enlargement of the liver usually occurs in the left lobe, but later, in the course of infection and particularly in adults, uniform hepatomegaly may be seen. Ultrasonographic examination of the liver shows evidence of specific patterns of fibrosis, which distinguishes this syndrome from other causes of hepatomegaly. Simultaneously, gross enlargement of the spleen may occur; the organ is characteristically rubbery hard. Laboratory examination may show indications of anemia and a low degree of eosinophilia but little changes in liver function are seen until late in the course of disease. Total serum proteins are usually normal, but gamma globulin increases are common. An association between schistosomal hepatosplenomegaly and hepatitis B antigen and antibody presence has been described, but its pathophysiologic significance is not clear. Although hepatosplenomegaly usually occurs in heavily infected individuals, other underlying mechanisms may be involved. An association between human leukocyte antigen (HLA) haplotypes and schistosomal hepatosplenomegaly has been demonstrated. In patients with pure schistosomal fibrosis uncomplicated by cirrhosis or viral hepatitis, liver function is preserved for a long time. The presenting feature often is an episode of hematemesis caused by rupture of esophageal varices without prior complaints. Bleeding may recur several times while the liver parenchyma maintains its normal

functions. Finally, however, symptoms and signs of liver cell failure ensue, along with the development of stigmas of chronic liver disease and ascites.

Several less-defined clinical syndromes have been associated with schistosomiasis mansoni. In infected laboratory animals as well as in individuals with chronic schistosomiasis mansoni, antigen-antibody complexes have formed and deposited in the kidney glomeruli. However, the prevalence of this syndrome and the rate at which it occurs in schistosomiasis are unknown. Cor pulmonale in schistosomiasis is a better defined disease entity, although its incidence is not known. It usually occurs in patients with advanced hepatosplenic schistosomiasis mansoni or japonica because of the development of collateral circulation. In *S. haematobium*–infected individuals, the anatomic location of adult worms may help eggs reach the systemic circulation directly and become trapped in the pulmonary arterioles. Patients with schistosomal pulmonary hypertension present clinically with symptoms and signs similar to those in cor pulmonale of other causes. Aneurysmal dilatation of the pulmonary artery and its branches, along with right ventricular hypertrophy, may occur.

DIAGNOSIS. See Table 385–1.

TREATMENT. See Management of Schistosomiasis, below.

SCHISTOSOMIASIS JAPONICA

On the main Asian continent, schistosomiasis japonica is prevalent in some parts of China, Thailand, Laos, Cambodia, and Malaysia. It is also endemic in the Philippines and Celebes. This schistosome species characteristically infects humans and domestic animals such as cats, dogs, and cattle, thus providing reservoir hosts that may contribute to its endemicity in certain areas of the Far East. The intermediate hosts for *S. japonicum* are snails of the genus *Onchomelania*.

Adult *S. japonicum* male worms have a nontuberculate surface and seven medium-sized testes. The ovary occupies the middle part of the body of female worms and contains 50 to 100 ova (Table 385–1).

PATHOLOGY AND CLINICAL MANIFESTATIONS. Cercarial dermatitis is not a prominent feature of schistosomiasis japonica. Katayama fever, or acute schistosomiasis, was named after the district in Japan previously endemic for *S. japonicum* infection. Symptoms usually begin 5 to 7 weeks after infection and are similar to those associated with schistosomiasis mansoni. The clinical features usually subside in a few days but may last for several months, and fatalities have been reported. The chronic manifestations of schistosomiasis japonica are related to ova deposited in the intestines and liver; adult worms produce 10 times more eggs than those of *S. mansoni*. These ova are laid in aggregates and remain so in the intestinal wall or when carried to the liver by the portal blood flow. In addition, *S. japonicum* eggs differ from those of *S. mansoni* in their tendency to calcify in tissues. Schistosomiasis japonica granulomas vary in size tremendously and tend to show signs of necrosis.

Individuals with chronic schistosomiasis japonica may have no symptoms or several nonspecific complaints. Controlled surveys in endemic areas have shown no particular increase in complaints of weakness, abdominal pain, or diarrhea in infected individuals. Clinical signs of hepatosplenomegaly are more frequently seen in infected than in uninfected individuals, but they were not uniformly correlated with intensity of infection. Severe hepatosplenic disease caused by schistosomiasis japonica may be seen in endemic areas, but its prevalence and relationship to intensity of infection and other complicating factors are unknown.

Cerebral schistosomiasis japonica is a unique syndrome reportedly occurring in 2 to 4% of infected individuals in the endemic countries. *S. japonicum* infection of the central nervous system preferentially affects the brain. The lesions consist of large aggregates of eggs in the cerebral venous system, but adult worms have never been found in the brain. Cerebral schistosomiasis japonica occurs clinically early in the course of the infection; the most frequent manifestation is focal jacksonian epilepsy; less commonly, generalized encephalitis may be the presenting feature.

DIAGNOSIS. See Table 385–1.

TREATMENT. See Management of Schistosomiasis, below.

OTHER HUMAN SCHISTOSOMES

Endemic foci for *S. intercalatum* are found in Central and West Africa. Adult worms inhabit the mesenteric blood vessels, and terminal spine eggs are seen in stools of infected individuals. Symptoms usually ascribed to this species of schistosome include abdominal pain, diarrhea, and blood in stools. Diagnosis is based on positive geographic history and finding parasite ova upon fecal examination (see Table 385–1).

S. mekongi is the most recent schistosome species to be described as a cause of infection and disease in humans. The parasite is endemic in some parts of the mainland of Southeast Asia. Adult worm and eggs are similar to those of *S. japonicum;* ova of *S. mekongi* are, however, smaller. In symptomatic patients, a syndrome not unlike that due to *S. japonicum* has been observed. It includes abdominal pain, diarrhea, and heptosplenomegaly. Diagnosis is established by fecal examination for parasite ova (see Table 385–1).

MANAGEMENT OF SCHISTOSOMIASIS

Chemotherapy is the major antischistosome strategy for eradication of parasites in infected individuals and for reducing incidence, intensity, and morbidity in populations of endemic areas. The current drug of choice is praziquantel, a pyrazinoisoquinoline derivative that is effective against all species of schistosomes that infect humans. Praziquantel has several advantages as the chemotherapeutic agent of choice, including oral administration, low incidence of toxicity and side effects, and marked antiparasitic activity. The recommended dose of praziquantel for treatment of infections with *S. haematobium*, *S. intercalatum*, or *S. mansoni* is 40 mg per kilogram of body weight administered once. For *S. japonicum* infection, administration of 30 mg per kilogram twice in 1 day is recommended, and for *S. mekongi,* 20 mg per kilogram three times in 1 day. These dosages have been shown to result in parasitologic cure in approximately 80% of treated individuals and in a highly significant reduction of intensity of infection. Side effects of praziquantel are rare, usually mild, and self-limiting. These include abdominal pain, headache, dizziness, and skin rashes.

The effect of antischistosome chemotherapeutic agents on disease manifestations is variable. It is dependent on the duration of infection and extent of disease. Treatment is expected to result in reversal of pathology, e.g., hematuria and hepatosplenomegaly, in infected children. By contrast, adults with established fibro-obstructive disease in the liver and urinary tract may not show significant clinical improvement following chemotherapy. Other therapeutic or surgical methods may therefore be necessary to correct the anatomic lesions. Furthermore, medical management of the chronic sequelae of schistosomiasis, such as liver fibrosis, portal hypertension, and esophageal varices, should be conducted according to established practices and taking into consideration the unique pathophysiologic characteristics of disease due to schistosomiasis.

Abdel-Salam E, Abdel Khalik A, Abdel-Meguid A, et al.: Association of HLA class I antigens (A1, B5, B8, and CW2) with disease manifestations and infection in human schistosomiasis mansoni in Egypt. Tissue Antigens 27:142, 1986. *A large-scale, population-based study of association between certain HLA haplotypes and hepatosplenomegaly due to schistosomiasis mansoni.*

Hofstetter M, Nash TE, Cheever AW, et al.: Infection with *Schistosoma mekongi* in Southeast Asian refugees. J Infect Dis 144:420, 1981. *Description of clinical and parasitologic features of schistosomiasis mekongi.*

King CH, Lombardi G, Lombardi C, et al.: Chemotherapy based-control of schistosomiasis haematobia. II. Metrifonate vs. praziquantel in control of infection associated morbidity. Am J Trop Med Hyg 42:587, 1990. *Presents data on long-term effects of metrifonate and praziquantel on the clinical and ultrasonographic manifestations of* S. haematobium *infection in school-aged children.*

Lukas NW, Boros DL: Lymphokine regulation of granuloma formation in murine schistosomiasis mansoni. Clin Immunol Immunopath 68:57, 1993. *Up-to-date review of the regulatory immunologic mechanisms in schistosome granulomas.*

Mahmoud AAF: Strategies for vaccine development: Schistosomiasis. Ann NY Acad Sci 589:136, 1989. *Summary of available protective monoclonal antibodies and purified schistosome antigens with promise as vaccines.*

Mahmoud AAF, Abdel Wahab MF: Schistosomiasis. *In* Warren KS, Mahmoud AAF (eds.): Tropical and Geographical Medicine, 2nd ed. New York, McGraw-Hill, 1990, pp. 458–473. *Detailed description of the parasitologic, immunologic, molecular, and clinical aspects of infection and disease.*

Mott KE, Dixon H, Osei-Tutu E, et al.: Relation between intensity of *Schistosoma haematobium* infection and clinical hematuria and proteinuria. Lancet 1:1005, 1983. *Correlation of proteinuria and hematuria with counts of* S. haematobium *eggs in urine.*

World Health Organization: The Control of Schistosomiasis. Technical Report Series 728, pp. 1–86. World Health Organization, Geneva, Switzerland, 1993. *Up-to-date examination of the epidemiology, morbidity, and methods of control of schistosomiasis. Also includes summary of control programs in endemic areas and outline for strategy of morbidity control.*

386 LIVER, INTESTINAL, AND LUNG FLUKE INFECTIONS
Adel A.F. Mahmoud

Flukes are parasitic worms of the phylum Platyhelminthes. These organisms are dorsoventrally flattened and are typically bilaterally symmetric. With the exception of the schistosomes, all flat worms of clinical significance are hermaphroditic. Morphologically the body of adult worms is leaf shaped and possesses two prominent suckers, one located anteriorly and the other ventrally. These are attachment organs that help anchor adult worms in their habitat within the organs of the definitive host. During the typical life cycle of a flat worm, the organism utilizes two, three, or more hosts; one is the definitive host and the others are intermediate hosts. The parasite undergoes developmental and multiplicative cycles within these hosts, the exception being sexual reproduction, which occurs only in the adult stage of the parasite, usually within the definitive host. All adult parasitic trematodes are obligate parasites. They challenge the protective mechanisms of the definitive hosts because of their size, complex anatomic and antigenic structure, and remarkable abilities to evade expulsion. Clinically relevant flukes are usually grouped according to the main location of adult worms in the definitive host.

Approximately 50 million individuals are infected worldwide; the liver flukes *Clonorchis sinensis, Opisthorchis felineus*, and *O. viverrini* are the most prevalent. Liver, intestinal, and lung flukes are similar morphologically, but vary in size from 1 mm to 7 cm. The pattern of life cycle of these flukes is similar. Eggs are passed in the feces or sputum of infected individuals. These ova are usually oval with an operculum and vary in size by species. Eggs hatch in the aquatic outside environment, releasing miracidia that seek specific snail intermediate hosts where they undergo several asexual multiplication steps, resulting finally in the release of cercariae. This stage is free living but of limited lifespan; it has to encyst on vegetation or in the tissues of fish or crabs where it changes into the metacercarial stage, which is infective to humans. Human acquisition of infection depends on ingestion of metacercaria in raw or improperly cooked aquatic plants or animals. Diagnosis of a specific tissue fluke is a significant clinical challenge: Knowing the geographic distribution of infection, the specific symptoms and signs, and the proper identification of eggs in feces or sputum samples is a necessary step. Recently the specificity and sensitivity of serologic tests have progressed to being helpful in diagnosis with a certain degree of confidence. The most important parasitologic, clinical, and diagnostic features of liver, intestinal, and lung flukes are summarized in Table 386–1.

LIVER FLUKES

Several species of liver flukes are capable of inducing significant morbidity and mortality in humans. Opisthorchiasis and clonorchiasis are the most common of these infections.

Opisthorchiasis

Human infection is caused by *O. viverrini* or *O. felineus,* parasitic flukes of cats, dogs, and other fish-eating mammals. Human infection is acquired by ingestion of metacercariae found in the second intermediate host (cyprinoid fish, carp). The metacercariae excyst in the duodenum and migrate through the ampulla of Vater to reach their final habitat in the bile ducts. The incidence of *O. viverrini* in northeastern Thailand (Table 386–2) has recently been increasing, reaching 90% of the population in specific foci.

PATHOGENESIS AND CLINICAL FEATURES. Adult flukes inhabit the distal bile ducts and may occasionally be seen in the gallbladder. The majority of infected individuals are asymptomatic. Lesions have been demonstrated in the biliary system, varying from hyperplasia of ductal epithelium to obstruction and bile retention. There is significant correlation between intensity of infection and severity of observed lesions. The association of *O. viverrini* and

TABLE 386-1. MAJOR LIVER, INTESTINAL, AND LUNG FLUKE INFECTIONS IN HUMANS

Infection	Causative Organisms	Second Intermediate Host	Size of Adult Fluke (mm)	Final Habitat in Humans	Size of Eggs (μm)
Opisthorchiasis	O. viverrini O. felineus	Cyprinoid fish	5–10 × 1–2	Distal bile ducts, gallbladder	28 × 16 Operculated
Clonorchiasis	C. sinensis	Carp fish	10–24 × 3–5	Bile and pancreatic ducts	29 × 16 Operculated
Fascioliasis	F. hepatica F. gigantica	Aquatic vegetation or water	20–30 × 13 75 × 20	Large biliary ducts	140 × 75 Inconspicuous operculum 175 × 80
Fasciolopsiasis	F. buski	Aquatic plants	50–75 × 8–20	Small intestine	135 × 35 Small operculum
Paragonimiasis	P. westermani	Fresh and brackish water crabs	7–16 × 4–8	Lungs, brain, or abdominal organs	100 × 60 Operculated

cholangiocarcinoma, known for many years, has recently been examined by the International Agency for Research on Cancer. The consensus is that enough evidence exists to classify O. viverrini as a human carcinogen.

Most infected individuals are asymptomatic; infection is diagnosed when the characteristic eggs are found during routine fecal examination. Since very few controlled studies have been performed on infected and uninfected populations of endemic areas, the specificity of symptoms and signs is questionable. Symptomatic infections are associated with right upper quadrant discomfort, dyspepsia, and change in bowel habits. Generalized symptoms such as decrease of appetite and weight loss have also been observed. In severe cases, relapsing cholangitis and cholecystitis may occur. An association between O. viverrini and cholangiocarcinoma, gallstones, and obstructive jaundice has been reported. Liver enlargement is demonstrated in most symptomatic individuals along with imaging evidence for biliary tree disease.

Infection with O. felineus has a characteristic clinical course. In its acute phase (2 to 3 weeks after infection), the clinical features include irregular fever, lymphadenopathy, myalgia, and eosinophilia. In chronic infections, symptoms and signs of biliary disease resemble those of O. viverrini infection; however, the worms may also be found in the pancreatic duct, causing manifestations related to this organ.

Clonorchiasis

C. sinensis is also frequently referred to as the Chinese or oriental liver fluke. Carnivorous animals such as dogs, cats, and rats are probably the reservoir hosts in nature. Human infection is acquired by ingestion of the second intermediate host, a fresh water carp of the family Cyprinidae. In endemic areas (Table 386–2), many species of this family have been found to be parasitized with C. sinensis metacercariae. Clonorchiasis is also seen in many coun-

tries, including the United States among immigrants from endemic areas. Importation of C. sinensis is a risk in the international food trade.

PATHOGENESIS AND CLINICAL FEATURES. The life cycle, pathology, and clinical manifestations of clonorchiasis are similar to those of opisthorchiasis. Adult flukes reside in the medium-sized and small bile ducts. They may also be found in the gallbladder, common bile duct, and the pancreatic duct. In early infection the pathologic features consist of edema and epithelial desquamation in bile ducts associated with an inflammatory response. Later, metaplasia and glandular proliferation occur with dilatation and thickening of bile ducts. The final pathologic insult is related to marked periductal fibrosis. The specificity of symptoms due to clonorchiasis such as anorexia, epigastric pain, or diarrhea has been questioned in studies performed on immigrants to the United States from the Far East. In chronic infection as seen in endemic areas, the association with cholangitis, gallstones, and cholangiocarinoma has been reported repeatedly. Sonography or computed tomography (CT) demonstrates the pathologic changes in the liver: flukes within dilated bile ducts and periductal changes.

Fascioliasis

Human infection with the zoonotic flukes Fasciola hepatica and F. gigantica is acquired by ingestion of parasitic metacercariae that are attracted to various aquatic plants or through drinking water contaminated with the infective stage of the organisms. The natural hosts of fascioliasis include sheep, goats, cattle, and horses; endemic regions are listed in Table 386–2. Once the infective metacercariae are consumed they excyst in the duodenum, penetrate its wall, and travel via the peritoneal cavity to enter the liver through its capsule. The organisms migrate into the liver parenchyma to reach their final habitat in large bile ducts.

PATHOGENESIS AND CLINICAL FEATURES. Human fascioliasis is usually associated with mild clinical features. The resulting syndromes may conveniently be divided into the *acute migratory phase*, while the organisms are finding their way through the peritoneal cavity to the hepatic liver capsule and parenchyma, and the *established phase*, which is associated with the mature flukes taking residence in the bile ducts. The acute phase is marked with fever, right upper quadrant or epigastric pain, and eosinophilia. The clinical presentation may last 4 to 8 weeks after ingestion of metacercariae and is usually self-limited. It has to be noted that stool examination during this phase is usually negative for parasite eggs. During the established phase, most infected individuals are asymptomatic. Some may complain of abdominal pain and dyspepsia. Hepatomegaly and jaundice may be noted, as well as significant peripheral blood eosinophilia. Borderline changes in liver function tests have also been reported. CT of the liver may help in demonstrating hepatic lesions, including the nodular or the more characteristic linear hypodense tracks, particularly if they are located subcapsularly. In the *biliary stage*, ultrasonography may demonstrate the adult flukes in the bile ducts or gallbladder.

Dicroceliasis

Human infection with Dicrocoelium dendriticum or D. hospes is rare (Table 386–2). Dicroceliasis is a zoonosis in sheep, goats, deer,

TABLE 386-2. GEOGRAPHIC DISTRIBUTION OF FLUKES

Fluke	Distribution
Liver	
Opisthorchis viverrini	Thailand, Laos, Cambodia
O. felineus	Russia, Eastern and Central Europe
Clonorchis sinesis	China, Japan, Korea, Taiwan, Vietnam Hong Kong (imported fish from China)
Fasciola hepatica	United States, Europe, Africa, Asia
F. gigantica	less common; Africa, Asia, Hawaii
Dicrocoelium sp.	Europe, Africa, Asia, North America
Intestinal	
Fasciolopsis sp.	Taiwan, Thailand, Bangladesh, India, plus other Asian and Western countries
Echinostoma sp.	Indonesia, Philippines, Thailand, Taiwan
Heterophyes heterophyes	Egypt, Iran, the Far East, Southeast Asia
Metagonimus yokogawai	China, Japan, Korea, Taiwan
Gastrodiscoides hominis	India, Southeast Asia, Russia
Lung	
Paragonimus sp.	Asia, West Africa, Central and South America

and other herbivores. Its life cycle is similar to that of other liver flukes except that metacercariae encyst in ants, the second intermediate host. Humans are infected via eating metacercariae-containing ants. Most cases of dicroceliasis are asymptomatic. In those with heavy infection, vague abdominal complaints—vomiting, diarrhea or constipation, and biliary colic—have been observed.

INTESTINAL FLUKES

Human infection with one of more than 50 species of intestinal trematodes has been reported from the Far East, Middle East, and North Africa. Clinically significant disease may be encountered in infection with only few species, as outlined below.

Fasciolopsiasis

The giant intestinal fluke *Fasciolopsis buski* inhabits the small intestine of pigs. The life cycle of the helminth is similar to that of *Fasciola hepatica*. Humans are infected by ingestion of raw stems, leaves, and pods of aquatic plants with encysted metacercariae. The geographic distribution is listed in Table 386–2. Endemicity depends on close contact among water plants, pigs, and populations that consume raw aquatic plants.

F. buski attach to the mucosa of small intestine, particularly the duodenum and jejunum. Most infected individuals are asymptomatic. The site of attachment, however, becomes ulcerated, following which there is a local inflammatory response. In heavy infection, intestinal obstruction and protein-losing enteropathy have been reported. With heavy infection, abdominal pain and diarrhea may be observed along with edema and anasarca because of hypoalbuminemia.

Echinostomiasis

Humans can be infected with any of several genera of the family Echinostomatidae (Table 386–2). The common species are *Echinostoma ilocanum, E. malayanum,* and *E. revolutum.* Adult flukes are parasites of the small intestine of birds and mammals. Humans are occasionally infected after eating undercooked *Pila,* other fish, and tadpoles. Mature adult worms attach to intestinal mucosa causing ulceration and subsequent inflammatory response. Little morbidity has been reported in association with echinostomiasis. High-intensity infection may be associated with abdominal pain and diarrhea.

Heterophyiasis

Heterophyes heterophyes infects not only humans (Table 386–2) but also cats, dogs, and other fish-eating mammals. Infection is acquired by ingestion of the fish second intermediate host, which contains the fluke metacercariae. The common fish hosts include mullet and minnow and the brackish water fish *Mugil capito.* They are usually consumed either raw or salted. Metacercariae can live in salted fish for approximately 1 week. Adult *H. heterophyes* attach to the mucosa of jejunum and upper ileum, producing shallow ulcers and mild inflammatory response. Symptomatic patients complain of gastroenterocolitis with diarrhea and tenesmus. Stools characteristically contain abundant mucus and occasionally blood.

OTHER INTESTINAL FLUKES

Several other species may cause disease limited to defined geographic areas (Table 386–2). *Metagonimus yokogawai* life cycle and the associated disease syndromes are similar to *H. heterophyes* infection, but *M. okogawai* may invade the mucosa of small intestine, resulting in ulceration and granuloma formation. Another intestinal fluke, *Gastrodiscoides hominis* (Table 386–2), has its final habitat in humans in the cecum. Clinically it is believed to produce mucous diarrhea.

Lung Flukes: "Paragonimiasis"

Human infection by species of *Paragonimus* may cause considerable pulmonary or extrapulmonary morbidity. *Paragonimus* infection exists in nature in humans and carnivores. There are at least 10 species of *Paragonimus* known to cause human disease; of these *P. westermani* is most common (Table 386–2). Infection is acquired by ingestion of metacercariae encysted in fresh water and brackish water crabs or crayfish (raw or undercooked). Infection may also be transmitted to humans through contaminated utensils used to prepare crabs or crayfish. Rarely, consumption of wild boar meat may result in transmission of immature flukes to humans where they complete their development into adult worms.

PATHOGENESIS AND CLINICAL FEATURES. Disease in infected humans is related to migration of young flukes from the gastrointestinal tract to their final habitat (early or acute stage) and more characteristically results from adult worms becoming established in the lungs or at extrapulmonary sites (late or chronic stage).

Acute paragonimiasis occurs during the 3-week period following infection. It passes unnoticed in most infected individuals. Symptoms include diarrhea, abdominal pain, fever, and malaise associated with cough, dyspnea, and night sweats. Pulmonary paragonimiasis results from invasion of the host lungs and establishment of adult worms in cysts or abscess cavities. The lung parenchyma demonstrates hemorrhage and an inflammatory response of predominantly eosinophils. Worm cysts are 1 to 2 cm in diameter and usually contain one or two worms. Pathologic changes in the remaining lung tissues may result in bronchopneumonia, bronchiectasis, fibrosis, and pleural thickening. The established pulmonary stage of paragonimiasis results usually in mild chronic cough with production of mucoid rusty-brown sputum. Hemoptysis that may be severe and life threatening occurs rarely. Microscopic examination of sputum demonstrates necrotic tissue and parasite eggs. Physical examination of patients with pulmonary paragonimiasis is usually within normal limits. Chest radiography may be normal in 10 to 20% of cases. Typical changes in the lungs include pathway infiltrate and ring shadow with a crescent-shaped "corona." Cystic and nodular lesions are also commonly seen. Furthermore, pleural lesions, including effusion, pneumothorax, and thickening, may be encountered in approximately two thirds of infected individuals. Other imaging methods, e.g., CT, may define better the pulmonary abnormalities, including worm migration tracks.

Extrapulmonary paragonimiasis occurs either because maturing flukes migrate to tissues other than the lungs, or adult flukes migrate from the lungs to other tissues. It is believed that extrapulmonary paragonimiasis may be mainly due to *Paragonimus* flukes other than *P. westermani.* The tissues most commonly affected are the brain, abdominal organs, and skin. In cerebral paragonimiasis, the clinical presentation may be acute or chronic. Acute cerebral paragonimiasis presents as fever, headache, visual disturbances, paralysis, and generalized or focal convulsions. Evidence for an intracranial inflammatory process may be demonstrated as papilledema, high cerebrospinal fluid pressure, and eosinophilic pleocytosis. Chronic cerebral paragonimiasis is characterized by space-occupying lesions that cause epilepsy or paralysis. Abdominal or cutaneous paragonimiasis results from invasion of liver, spleen, or skin by maturing or adult flukes. This results in space-occupying lesions, abscesses, or migratory swellings.

MANAGEMENT OF LIVER, INTESTINAL, AND LUNG FLUKE INFECTIONS

Diagnosis of human infection with liver, intestinal, or lung flukes requires knowledge of the geographic distribution of these infections, a high degree of clinical correlations of mainly nonspecific symptoms and signs with history of possible exposure, and peripheral blood eosinophilia. Definitive diagnosis is established by finding the characteristically shaped fluke eggs in fecal samples (liver, intestinal, and lung worms) or in sputum paragonimiasis. Occasionally eggs are obtained in samples of other tissue fluid, e.g., bile or in biopsy tissue. In general, the sensitivity of fecal or sputum examination is enhanced by examining two or three separate specimens. Seroimmunodiagnostic tests are available for fascioliasis and paragonimiasis. They are particularly helpful in early infection in which parasitologic diagnosis is usually negative. Serodiagnosis is an essential step in the work-up in an unusual clinical presentation.

Chemotherapy for fluke infections has become a more effective management strategy with the introduction of praziquantel. This orally administered 1-day antihelminth results in cure rates of 70 to 90% and an even more remarkable decrease in egg counts. Its administration is associated with few side effects. The recommended dose of praziquantel is 75 mg per kilogram body weight divided into three doses and given in 1 day. For fascioliasis the drug of choice is bithionol given orally as 30 to 50 mg per kilogram every other day for 10 to 15 doses.

Prevention of infection with any of the above parasitic trematodes depends on proper medical advice given to individuals traveling or planning to reside in endemic areas (see Ch. 268). Avoidance of ingestion of suspect intermediate hosts and the proper washing, cooking, or preservation methods of such food items is the most effective strategy. Engaging in some of the local dietary habits in endemic areas is to be discouraged. Water for drinking must be properly purified to avoid the possible transmission of *F. hepatica*. Control of parasitic trematodes in endemic areas is a much more complex challenge. It involves changing long-established cultural, dietary, and sanitary habits. With the availability of a safe broad-spectrum antihelminth (praziquantel), chemotherapy may play a significant role in controlling infection and disease. As a long-term strategy, vaccines and socioeconomic development will be needed.

Drugs for Parasitic Infections: The Medical Letter on Drugs and Therapeutics. 35:111, 1993. *Yearly update of drugs of choice and alternatives.*

Harinasuta T, Bunnag D: Liver, Lung and Intestinal Trematodiasis. *In* Warren KS, Mahmoud AAF (eds.): Tropical and Geographical Medicine, 2nd ed. New York, McGraw-Hill, 1990, pp. 473–489. *An authoritative description of the causing agents, clinical syndromes, and management strategies.*

Im JG, Whang HY, Kim WS, et al.: Pleuropulmonary paragonimiasis: Radiologic findings in 71 patients. AJR 159:39, 1992. *Retrospective evaluation of 71 individuals with evidence of pleuropulmonary paragonimiasis. Report details frequency of specific radiographic and CT findings.*

King CH: Liver, lung and intestinal trematodiasis. *In* Mahmoud AAF (ed.): Tropical and Geographical Medicine, 2nd ed. Companion Handbook. New York, McGraw-Hill, 1993, pp. 149–154. *Summary of the salient clinical features, diagnostic and therapeutic approaches to tissue fluke infection.*

Lim JH: Radiologic findings of clonorchiasis. AJR 155:1001, 1990. *Detailed description of the epidemiology and parasitology of clonorchiasis as well as the sonographic and CT findings based on examining a large group of infected individuals.*

387 NEMATODE INFECTIONS
James W. Kazura

Nematodes (phylum Nematoda), or roundworms, include a vast number of species of free-living and parasitic helminths. These multicellular organisms differ from unicellular bacteria and protozoa in that they have organ systems with specialized nervous, muscular, gastrointestinal, and reproductive functions. Parasitic nematodes vary in length from several millimeters to approximately 2 meters and four larval stages and adult worms of both sexes. With the exception of *Strongyloides* and a few other helminths of medical importance, larvae are produced after mating of sexually mature adult worms, which by themselves are incapable of multiplying in the mammalian host. The inability of adult worms to replicate has important implications for the propensity of this class of organism to establish an infection and cause disease. Unlike the situation pertaining to bacterial, viral, or protozoan infections, casual or a low degree of exposure to infective stages of parasitic helminths generally does not result in patient infection or pathologic manifestations. Repeated or intense exposure to a large number of infective larvae is required for infection to be established and disease to develop.

Nematode infections are endemic in both temperate and tropical climates. They are transmitted either by the fecal-oral route or by inoculation of infective larvae into the skin, primarily by blood-feeding intermediate insect vectors. The prevalence of infection is greatest in circumstances conducive to the development and transmission of infective forms of the parasites, i.e., overcrowded, perennially warm geographic areas with poor sanitation, such as in many developing countries of Africa, Asia, and Latin America and economically poor areas of North America and Europe.

The epidemiology of human nematode (as well as trematode and cestode) infections has several unique features. The infection in an endemic area has a negative binomial distribution; i.e., the majority of individuals have low parasite burdens and a small number harbor relatively high burdens. Persons in the latter group are important from an epidemiologic perspective in that they contribute most substantially to transmission and are most likely to develop pathologic

manifestations. This characteristic implies that transmission in an endemic area may be decreased or interrupted by reduction of the parasite burden in a small proportion of the population. In addition, because total worm load correlates directly with the propensity to develop disease, treatment of lightly infected persons may not be indicated or may be unnecessary, especially if the available chemotherapy has major side effects.

Nematode infections of medical importance may be broadly classified into those in which the route of infection, larval migration, and disease manifestations are primarily gastrointestinal and those that affect other tissues. The former group includes hookworms (*Ancylostoma duodenale, Necator americanus*), the roundworm *Ascaris lumbricoides*, the pinworm *Enterobius vermicularis*, and the whipworm *Trichuris trichiuria*. Animal intestinal nematodes such as *Trichostrongylus* and *Anisakis* species also occasionally infect and cause disease in humans. *Trichinella spiralis, Strongyloides stercoralis*, and *Angiostrongylus cantonensis* infect humans by the oral route, but disease manifestations are due primarily to migration in other tissues. Tissue-invasive nematodes include lymphatic filariae (*Wuchereria bancrofti, Brugia malayi*, and *B. timori*), skin-dwelling *Onchocerca volvulus* and *Loa loa*, and the guinea worm, *Dracunculus medinensis*.

Anderson RM, May RM: Helminthic infections of humans: Mathematical models, population dynamics, and control. Adv Parasitol 24:1, 1985. *An excellent discussion of the relationship of the biology of parasitic helminthic infections to their epidemiology and control strategies.*

INTESTINAL NEMATODES

These infections include hookworm disease, ascariasis, enterobiasis, trichuriasis, and rarely animal nematodiases. They are prevalent in temperate and tropical areas of the world, especially those with overcrowding and poor sanitation. Intestinal nematode infections have little morbidity in most cases and are easily treated with mebendazole.

Hookworm Disease

ETIOLOGY AND EPIDEMIOLOGY. The major hookworms that infect humans are *Ancylostoma duodenale* and *Necator americanus*. *A. ceylanicum* infection is less common and occurs primarily in the South Pacific. Animal hookworms such as *A. braziliense* and *Uncinaria stenocephala* do not undergo full development in incidentally exposed humans. Infection occurs when exposed skin maintains contact for several minutes with soil contaminated with parasite eggs containing viable larvae. Larvae penetrate the skin and subsequently migrate to and mature in the lungs. The parasites then break into the air spaces, ascend the trachea, and are swallowed. Adult worms mature in the upper small intestine and attach to the mucosa. Female worms release more than 10,000 eggs per day, which are passed in the stools and deposited in the soil. The prepatent period (duration of time between infection and passing of eggs in the feces) is 40 to 105 days. Adult hookworms have a lifespan of 2 to 5 years.

Hookworms infect over 1 billion persons worldwide. The highest prevalences of infection (80 to 100%) occur in tropical and less developed countries, where environmental and socioeconomic conditions are especially favorable to transmission. These include warm, moist soil; lack of public sewage disposal systems; and the habit of walking barefoot. The higher prevalence of hookworm infection in children than adults results from more frequent exposure of skin to larvae in soil. Acquired resistance is minimal or does not appear to develop as a consequence of previous infection.

PATHOGENESIS AND CLINICAL MANIFESTATIONS. Hookworm disease is due primarily to gastrointestinal blood loss and attendant iron deficiency anemia. The latter correlates directly with the total worm burden. Adult worms attached to the mucosa of the upper small intestine digest ingested blood as well as cause focal bleeding. *A. duodenale* is estimated to cause a blood loss of 0.3 ml per day per worm; *N. americanus* induces loss of approximately 0.03 ml per day. Light infections (feces with < 400 eggs per gram) do not cause blood loss sufficient to induce iron deficiency. Nutritional deficiencies secondary to coexisting conditions that result in low iron stores (e.g., malabsorption or insufficient dietary intake in children and multiparous women) contribute significantly to morbidity. Hypoproteinemia has been reported in children with hookworm disease in less developed countries. This complication is most likely due to coexisting malnutrition rather than gastrointestinal disease caused by hookworm infestation *per se*. Abdominal signs or symptoms are not caused by hookworm infection.

Pruritus at the site of larval skin penetration ("ground itch") occurs occasionally. In the case of primary exposure, local itching and erythematous papules lasting 1 week develop. More intense pruritus, vesiculation, and edema of 2 to 3 weeks' duration may occur after repeated exposure to infective larvae. Hookworm larvae migrating through the lungs rarely cause pulmonary symptoms.

DIAGNOSIS. Hookworm infection is diagnosed by identification of the characteristic round eggs containing convoluted larvae. Direct smears of freshly passed stool using the Kato or other techniques are satisfactory for the diagnosis of moderately to heavily infected cases (> 400 eggs per gram).

TREATMENT AND PREVENTION. Mebendazole is the treatment of choice (Table 387–1). The ideal method for preventing hookworm infection is improvement of hygienic conditions. Use of footwear, especially by children, is currently the only practical means of avoiding infection.

Ascariasis

ETIOLOGY AND EPIDEMIOLOGY. *Ascaris lumbricoides* are roundworms 2 to 3 cm in length that reside in the lumen of the jejunum and in the mid-ileum. Infection occurs by the oral route when soil containing embryonated eggs is ingested. Larvae are released from eggs in the small intestine, penetrate the gut, and migrate to the liver and then lungs via the blood or lymphatic circulation. Following maturation in the lungs over a 4-week period, the parasites ascend the respiratory tract and are swallowed. Adult worms reach sexual maturity (i.e., female worms release eggs that are detectable in feces) approximately 60 days after infection.

Ascariasis affects approximately one quarter of the world's population and is likely the most prevalent helminthiasis of humans. Infection is common in Africa, Asia, and Latin America, especially in areas of high population density and unhygienic conditions. The use of human feces as fertilizer, defecation in soil, and hand-to-mouth contact with contaminated soil are major factors that contribute to the spread of *Ascaris*. The ability of *Ascaris* eggs to remain viable in harsh environmental conditions (embryonated eggs remain infectious after exposure to freezing temperatures and desiccation for several weeks) also facilitates transmission.

PATHOGENESIS AND CLINICAL MANIFESTATIONS. Disease caused by *A. lumbricoides* is infrequent and generally correlates with the intensity of infection. The majority of infected individuals are asymptomatic.

Symptomatic cases can be divided into two broad categories based on the phase of infection and site of pathology, i.e., pulmonary or gastrointestinal tract. Pulmonary disease is caused by the migration of larvae in the small vessels of the lung and their subsequent rupture into alveoli. Tissue damage is thought to be due to the host immune response, which includes production of immunoglobulin E (IgE) and eosinophilia. Transient pulmonary infiltrates, fever, cough, dyspnea, and eosinophilia lasting 1 to several weeks are the major clinical manifestations. This complex of symptoms and signs is frequently seasonal and coincidental with environmental changes that favor development of infective-stage larvae in eggs (e.g., spring rains that follow cold and dry periods). Intestinal signs and symptoms are due either to obstruction caused by the presence of an exceptionally large number of parasites in the small intestine or to migration of adult worms to unusual sites, such as the biliary tree or pancreatic duct. Intestinal obstruction almost always occurs in children < 6 years old. The onset is sudden and characterized by colicky abdominal pain and vomiting. Heavily infected children are also prone to biliary disease or pancreatitis secondary to *Ascaris* lodging in the ducts draining these organs. A malabsorption syndrome characterized by steatorrhea and low vitamin A levels has been reported in Latin American children with ascariasis.

DIAGNOSIS. Intestinal infection is diagnosed by the presence of the typical oval, thick-shelled *Ascaris* eggs in thick smears of fecal specimens. The existence of adult worms in pancreatic or biliary ducts should be suspected in children who have high egg outputs in conjunction with jaundice or pancreatitis. Pulmonary ascariasis cannot be diagnosed on the basis of identification of ova in feces because adult worms have not yet matured and reached the intestinal tract. Biopsy of the lung is unlikely to demonstrate larvae and is not recommended.

TREATMENT AND PREVENTION. Treatment for uncomplicated intestinal ascariasis is listed in Table 387–1. Treatment causes neuromuscular paralysis of the worms and expulsion of intact helminths. No specific treatment is recommended for pulmonary ascariasis because the condition is self-limited.

The major means of preventing *Ascaris* infection is improvement of hygienic and socioeconomic conditions. Mass chemotherapy successfully reduces worm loads but requires frequent treatment.

Enterobiasis

Enterobius vermicularis or pinworm infection is cosmopolitan in its distribution. It is common in overcrowded settings and spreads rapidly in conditions in which person-to-person contact is frequent, such as in institutions for children.

Infection occurs by the fecal-oral route. Embryonated eggs carried on the fingernails, bed clothing, or bedding are ingested and hatch in the upper small intestine. Larvae develop in the large bowel into adult worms 2 to 5 mm long. Female worms migrate nightly out of the rectum and deposit large numbers of ova (11,000 per worm) in the perianal and perineal areas. Larvae in the deposited eggs become infective within several hours of exposure to ambient oxygen. Infectivity is usually maintained for 1 to 2 days.

The vast majority of pinworm infections are asymptomatic or associated with perianal pruritus and consequent sleep deprivation. *E. vermicularis* is a rare cause of appendicitis and, when the adult worms follow an aberrant path of migration, vulvovaginitis, urethritis, or peritonitis.

The diagnosis of pinworm infection is easily made by identifying ova on a piece of cellophane tape applied to the perirectal area in the morning. *E. vermicularis* eggs are oval and slightly flattened on one side. It is unusual to find eggs in feces or adult worms in the perianal area. Repeated examinations may be necessary.

Treatment (Table 387–1) is mebendazole given to affected individuals as well as close associates, such as family members. Although personal cleanliness is recommended as a means of limiting transmission, there is no clear-cut demonstration that it prevents infection.

Trichuriasis

Trichuris trichiuria or whipworm infection is similar to pinworm infection in that it is limited to the gastrointestinal tract and does not have a tissue migratory phase. Eggs containing infective larvae mature in warm, moist soil over a 2-week period. Ingested eggs

TABLE 387–1. TREATMENT FOR INTESTINAL NEMATODES

Nematode	Treatment
Hookworm	Mebendazole, 100 mg orally b.i.d. for 3 days. Do not give to pregnant women; iron supplementation (if warranted by anemia and complicating illnesses)
Ascaris	Mebendazole, 100 mg orally b.i.d. for 3 days. Children with heavy infections, biliary tract obstruction: piperazine, 50–75 mg/kg body weight for 2 days
Enterobius	Pyrantel pamoate, 11 mg/kg once, with a repeated dose 2 weeks later; maximum single dose, 1 gram. Several treatments may be required (every 3–4 months) if exposure continues (i.e., in institutional setting)
Trichuris	Mebendazole, at same dosage as for ascariasis
Other animal nematodes	
Trichostrongylus	Pyrantel pamoate, 11 mg/kg once; maximum dose of 1 gram
Anisakis	Thiabendazole, 25 mg/kg b.i.d. for 3 days if surgery is not required
Capillaria	Mebendazole, 200 mg b.i.d. for 20 days. Alternative: thiabendazole, 25 mg/kg q.d. for 30 days. Supportive care: replace fluid and electrolytes, high-protein diet
Gnathostoma	For subcutaneous lesions: surgical removal. For CNS infection: mebendazole, 200 mg q3h for 6 days OR albendazole, 400–800 mg q.d. for 21 days

hatch in the small bowel and subsequently develop in epithelial cells of the cecum and ascending colon into adult worms that are 40 mm in length. The body of the parasite protrudes into the colonic lumen. Its anterior portion has a whiplike shape.

As is the case with most intestinal nematode infections, trichuriasis is most common in overcrowded areas with poor sanitation. The estimated prevalence worldwide is 800 million, with approximately 2 million cases in the southern United States. Children are more frequently infected than adults and also more likely to have higher worm burdens.

Adults with trichuriasis are usually asymptomatic. In children with heavy infections (> 10,000 eggs per gram of feces), a syndrome of dysentery, growth retardation, and rectal prolapse has been described. The pathologic manifestations include infiltrates of eosinophils and neutrophils accompanied by epithelial denudation. Complicating diseases such as shigellosis and amebiasis may contribute to this condition in children.

Whipworm infection is diagnosed by identification of football-shaped eggs in direct smears of fecal specimens. Mebendazole at the same dosage indicated for ascariasis is satisfactory treatment is listed in Table 387–1.

Other Animal Nematodiases

Humans may serve as paratenic hosts for several nematodes that ordinarily parasitize the intestine of other mammals. These helminths are incapable of completing their life cycle in humans and display aberrant migration patterns in both intestinal and nonintestinal tissues.

Several species of the genus *Trichostrongylus* infect both humans and domestic ruminants. The infection is found widely in the Middle and Far East and Australia. Ova are passed in the stool of ruminants and hatch in the soil. Humans are incidentally infected when larvae are ingested with leafy vegetables. The adult worms live in the intestines and suck small amounts of blood; heavy infections result in anemia. Diagnosis is made by identifying ova, which resemble those of hookworm, in the stool. Treatment is listed in Table 387–1.

Anisakis is an intestinal nematode of marine mammals. Several species of saltwater fish are intermediate hosts. Human infection occurs when raw fish is eaten. The larvae of both *Anisakis* and *Phocanemia decipiens* have been implicated. Most cases have been reported in Japan or Western Europe, particularly Scandinavia. The larvae invade the wall of the small intestine or stomach, causing pain and, rarely, intestinal obstruction or perforation. Gastric anisakiasis can be diagnosed endoscopically and treated by removal of the worms. Intestinal anisakiasis often resembles an acute abdomen, leading to laparotomy. Thiabendazole treatment is listed in Table 387–1. Infection is prevented by cooking or freezing fish prior to eating.

Capillaria philippinensis infection has been reported from the Philippines and Thailand. This nematode is thought to parasitize birds, with fish and crustaceans serving as intermediate hosts. Humans are infected by eating the raw intermediate hosts. The ingested larvae mature and live in the crypts of the small intestine, where they reproduce. The result is often a heavy infection; up to 40,000 adult worms have been recovered at one autopsy. The clinical syndrome includes severe malabsorption and protein-losing enteropathy. The diagnosis is made by finding eggs or larvae in the stool; an intradermal test is also available. The treatment of choice is mebendazole (Table 387–1).

Gnathostoma spinigerum is an intestinal nematode of dogs and cats; fish are intermediate hosts. The infection is endemic in rodents in the Far East and Thailand. Human infection has also been reported in South America. Infective larvae are ingested by humans in raw or undercooked fish. The larvae do not complete their life cycle in humans but migrate through the body. The most frequent site is subcutaneous tissues, where larvae are found in eosinophilic granulomas. A few weeks after infection, pruritic or painful subcutaneous nodules and swellings appear. These may be migratory and develop into abscesses. In CNS gnathostomiasis, hemorrhagic tracts may be found in the brain. Fever, vomiting, and abdominal pain occur a few days after larvae are ingested. Paralysis of the extremities, encephalitis, and subarachnoid hemorrhage have been reported. Eye

involvement with uveitis and orbital cellulitis represents a third variety.

Peripheral eosinophilia is usual in cutaneous gnathostomiasis; the diagnosis may be established by biopsy. In CNS infection, blood eosinophilia is an inconstant feature, but eosinophils are present in the cerebrospinal fluid (CSF), as in the case of angiostrongyliasis. Treatments are listed in Table 387–1. The infection may be prevented by thorough cooking of fish.

Several nematodes that ordinarily parasitize the intestine of monkeys occasionally infect humans. *Oesophagostomum* has been reported from Africa, Asia, and Brazil; it is responsible for the formation of granulomas in the intestinal wall. *Ternides deminutus* is sometimes found in the human colon in Africa and Asia; a heavy infection may cause anemia. *Physaloptera mordens,* also reported from Africa, may attach itself to the esophagus, stomach, or small intestine of humans. The definitive host of *Lagochilascaris minor* is unknown. About 30 human cases have been reported from Central and South America, usually with worms invading the soft tissues of the neck, throat, and sinuses.

Drugs for Parasitic Infections. Med Lett 35:111, 1993.
Khuroo MS, Zargar SA, Mahajan R: Sonographic appearances in biliary ascariasis. Gastroenterology 93:267, 1987. *A discussion of the ultrasound appearance of this unusual but clinically important aspect of ascariasis.*
Schad GH, Banwell JG: Hookworms. *In* Warren KS, Mahmoud AAF (eds.): Tropical and Geographical Medicine. New York, McGraw-Hill, 1990. *A general review of biology, clinical aspects, and epidemiology of hookworm infection. Synthesizes a large amount of confusing literature.*
Smith JW, Wootten R: Anisakis and anisakiasis. Adv Parasitol 16:93, 1978. *An exceptionally complete review.*

TOXOCARIASIS

DEFINITION. Visceral larva migrans (VLM) and ocular larva migrans (OLM) are caused by ingestion and subsequent development and migration of embryonated eggs of the canine roundworm *Toxocara canis.* Roundworms of cats *(T. cati)* and raccoons *(Baylisascaris procyonis)* also rarely cause VLM.

ETIOLOGY. In its normal canine host, *T. canis* follow a route of migration similar to that described for *Ascaris;* i.e., ingested larvae penetrate the small intestine, migrate to the lungs, are reswallowed, and develop into adult worms in the small intestine; the adult worms lodge there and release eggs that are passed in the feces. When embryonated *T. canis* eggs are ingested by humans, larvae also migrate throughout the body (lung, liver, brain, muscles, and occasionally eyes) but fail to complete development to the adult stage. Tissue necrosis secondary to penetrating larvae and associated host inflammatory reactions, such as eosinophil-rich granulomas, are the underlying cause of disease.

EPIDEMIOLOGY. Toxocariasis is endemic in both temperate and tropical areas of the world. The vast majority of symptomatic cases occur in young children. This age group is most likely to be infected by virtue of frequent and intimate handling of dogs (especially newborn puppies that may be hyperinfected), playing in areas where dogs and cats defecate (e.g., public sandboxes), and the habit of geophagia. The potential of exposure to embryonated eggs is high in that *T. canis* infection is common in dogs (a 20% infection rate in dogs in the United States).

CLINICAL MANIFESTATIONS. The vast majority of children who ingest *T. canis* eggs are asymptomatic. VLM is the most common clinically defined entity attributable to *T. canis.* It is most frequent in children younger than 5 (there are no published series of adults with VLM) and is characterized by fever < 39°C; pulmonary symptoms, including wheezing and cough; and, less frequently, pain in the right upper quadrant. These symptoms have a gradual onset and resolve over 4 to 8 weeks. Physical signs include wheezing and hepatomegaly in about one quarter of cases. Larvae less commonly migrate to the brain and heart and cause focal neurologic defects and heart failure.

OLM has an incidence approximately one tenth that of VLM and affects children older than 8 to 10 years. Visual disturbances due to VLM are not distinguishable from other causes of focal intraretinal granulomas or space-occupying lesions, such as tuberculosis and retinoblastoma. *T. canis* larvae may migrate intraretinally and produce transient and recurrent impairment of vision.

DIAGNOSIS AND TREATMENT. VLM is diagnosed on the basis of suspicion of ingestion of *T. canis* eggs in a child with the symptoms described above. Eosinophilia, elevated erythrocyte sedimentation rate, and generalized hypergammaglobulinemia are also consistent with the diagnosis. Biopsy to document the presence of larvae is insensitive and not recommended. An enzyme-linked immunosorbent assay (ELISA) for measuring anti-*Toxocara* antibodies is helpful if elevated immunoglobulin M (IgM) antibodies and a rise in titer between acute and convalescent phases are documented. Most cases of VLM are not life threatening and are self-limited. Treatment is therefore not required. In persons with severe pulmonary, cardiac, or neurologic involvement and high-grade eosinophilia ($> 10,000$ per cubic millimeter of blood), diethylcarbamazine, 6 mg per kilogram per day in three doses for 7 to 10 days, and corticosteroids may be used to reduce symptoms and shorten the course of the illness. No controlled studies, however, demonstrate the efficacy of chemotherapy.

OLM represents a diagnostic dilemma in that it must be distinguished from intraretinal neoplasms and infections. Expert ophthalmologic consultation is necessary. Computerized tomography and fluorescein angiography are helpful in diagnosis. Elevated anti-*Toxocara* antibody titers in aqueous fluid relative to serum values are consistent with OLM. It is unclear if anthelminthics are useful for the treatment of OLM.

VLM and OLM may be prevented by periodic deworming of dogs, especially puppies, and limiting their defecation in public places.

Glickman LT, Schantz PM, Cypess RH: Epidemiologic characteristics and clinical findings in patients with serologically proven toxocariasis. Trans R Soc Trop Med Hyg 73:254, 1979. *An excellent description of the major clinical manifestations of toxocariasis.*

CUTANEOUS LARVA MIGRANS

Animal hookworms, most frequently the dog parasite *Ancylostoma braziliense* and less commonly *Uncinaria stenocephala* and *Bunostomum phlebotomum*, are the major causative agents of cutaneous larva migrans, or creeping eruption. *Ancylostoma duodenale, Necator americanus,* and *Strongyloides stercoralis* may produce a similar syndrome during the phase of infection that involves penetration of the skin.

The disease occurs when skin comes into direct and prolonged contact with hookworm larvae contained in the feces of dogs, cats, or humans. Moist areas visited by animals, such as vegetation near beaches and exposed soil covered by porches, are common sites in which humans may be infected. Cutaneous larva migrans in the United States is most prevalent in southern coastal regions.

Clinical manifestations result from penetration and migration of larvae in the epidermal-dermal junction of the skin. Within several hours of contact with exposed skin, the patient notes pruritus and raised erythematous serpiginous lesions. The lesions migrate approximately 1 cm per day and evolve into bullae. Multiple lesions may appear if large areas of the body have been exposed, as in sunbathing.

Creeping eruption may be treated by topical application of thiabendazole oral suspension. This may be prepared by trituration of a 500-mg tablet in 5 grams of petroleum jelly. If untreated, cutaneous larva migrans is self-limited; signs and symptoms resolve in several weeks to 2 months.

ANGIOSTRONGYLIASIS

Angiostrongylus cantonensis is a cause of eosinophilic meningitis in Asia and the South Pacific. Small numbers of cases have also been reported in Cuba and Africa. *Angiostrongylus costaricensis* is a rare cause of gastrointestinal bleeding. The nematode is limited in its distribution to Central and South America. Humans are infected with these rodent (primarily rat) nematodes after ingesting poorly cooked or raw intermediate mollusc hosts, such as snails, slugs, and prawns. Fresh vegetables may also be contaminated with infective larvae and serve as a vehicle of infection.

In the case of *A. cantonensis* infection, ingested infective larvae penetrate the gut wall and migrate to small vessels of the meninges and, less commonly, the spinal cord and eye. An intense local inflammatory reaction ensues within 1 week. Fever, meningismus, and headache develop in association with eosinophilic pleocytosis of the CSF. Strabismus, paresthesias, and vomiting have been observed in a minority of cases. Diagnosis is based on a history of ingesting potentially contaminated foodstuffs and the presence of eosinophils in CSF. Larvae are usually not found in CSF. Other in-

fectious causes of eosinophilic meningitis include *Trichinella spiralis, Taenia solium, Toxocara canis, Gnathostoma spinigerum,* and *Paragonimus westermani*. Symptomatic *A. cantonensis* infection resolves over a 2-week period. The value of anthelminthic therapy or corticosteroids has not been established.

A. costaricensis larvae penetrate the mucosa of the terminal ileum, appendix, and ascending colon. The larvae subsequently develop into adult worms in the local lymphatics and mesenteric arterioles. Eggs released by the female worms elicit multiple eosinophil-rich granulomatous reactions that cause edematous, thickened bowel and necrosis (secondary to mesenteric blood vessel obstruction). Clinical presentations typically include right-sided abdominal pain, vomiting, and fever. Abnormal laboratory findings include leukocytosis with eosinophilia. Parasite larvae and eggs are not present in stools. A palpable mass secondary to granulomatous lesions may be present and cause intestinal obstruction. Less frequently, gastrointestinal bleeding is the principal manifestation. Treatment is surgical. There is no demonstrated benefit of specific anthelminthic chemotherapy.

Koo J, Pien F, Kliks M: Angiostrongylus (Parastrongylus) eosinophilic meningitis. Rev Infect Dis 10:1155, 1988. *An excellent discussion of the biology of the helminth and the clinical manifestations of human infection.*

TRICHINOSIS

DEFINITION. Infection by *Trichinella spiralis* occurs when infective larvae are eaten in undercooked pork or other meats. The majority of infected individuals are asymptomatic. Clinical manifestations in heavily infected persons include diarrhea, myalgias, fever, and, less commonly, myocarditis and neurologic disease. Trichinosis occurs in all areas of the world, including the Arctic and temperate regions. The incidence of trichinosis in the United States has decreased markedly over the past several decades.

ETIOLOGY. Infection is initiated by ingesting infective larvae encysted in striated muscle. Excystment occurs in the acid-pepsin environment of the stomach, and parasites develop into sexually mature adult worms in the upper to middle small intestine of the human host. Completion of the enteric phase of the parasite life cycle takes about 1 week, with adult worms remaining viable and productive of larval offspring for an additional 3 to 5 weeks. The systemic phase commences 1 week after infection, when larvae released by female worms migrate through blood vessels and lymphatics and invade multiple organ systems. Mature third-stage larvae develop in host-derived nurse cells in striated skeletal and cardiac muscle, where they become encysted and remain viable for years. As is the case with most helminthiases, the severity of symptoms is related to the total parasite load. Because adult worms are incapable of reproducing themselves, the number of infective larvae ingested is the most important determinant of worm load (i.e., number of larvae that invade muscle and other tissues).

EPIDEMIOLOGY. *T. spiralis* infection is enzootic in omnivorous and carnivorous animal populations, including rats, bears, and aquatic mammals of the Arctic. The nematode is introduced into domestic animals such as pigs and horses by feeding them garbage containing carcasses of these animals, most commonly rats. Human infection usually occurs in two settings: first, when undercooked or smoked pork products or beef contaminated with nematodes is eaten, and second, when flesh of poorly cooked wild game, such as bear or boar meat, is ingested. An important source of infection in Alaskan and Canadian Arctic native populations is uncooked walrus meat.

The annual incidence of human trichinosis in the United States has decreased from more than 450 in 1947-1949 to fewer than 56 between 1982 and 1986. This decline is primarily due to fewer cases related to ingestion of commercial pork products. Recent cases in the United States occur in point-source outbreaks associated with eating game or noncommercial pork products.

PATHOGENESIS AND CLINICAL MANIFESTATIONS. Tissue-invasive *T. spiralis* larvae elicit an eosinophilic granulomatous reaction that may result in significant end-organ tissue damage and dysfunction. Skeletal muscle is the most frequent site involved. Myocardial damage, pulmonary infiltration, and focal neurologic damage secondary to invasion by larvae are seen in only the most heavily infected persons. The systemic phase of infection usually occurs

2 to 3 weeks after ingestion of infective larvae and may last for 2 months. Clinical manifestations typically include myalgias (especially of the gastrocnemius and masseter), periorbital edema, and fever. Myocardial damage may manifest as heart failure or dysrhythmias.

The enteric phase of infection may cause gastrointestinal signs and symptoms, such as diarrhea and abdominal cramps. These typically occur within 1 week of eating contaminated meat and last less than 2 weeks. Reports from the Canadian Arctic suggest that the *T. spiralis* larvae that infect walrus meat may cause diarrhea of 1 to 3 months' duration.

DIAGNOSIS. A diagnosis of trichinosis should be considered in individuals with generalized myalgias and eosinophilia (>600 eosinophils per cubic millimeter). Serologic testing for *T. spiralis* antibodies is available at the Centers for Disease Control and Prevention. Elevation of IgM antibodies or a more than fourfold rise in titer between acute and convalescent phases of infection is helpful in diagnosis. The levels of creatine phosphate kinase and of serum immunoglobulins and the erythrocyte sedimentation rate are also increased for several weeks after infection. Muscle biopsy (e.g., of the gastrocnemius) may demonstrate larvae, although their absence does not exclude the diagnosis.

TREATMENT AND PREVENTION. If patients present at a time when adult parasites are in the intestine (i.e., during the initial 1 to 2 weeks after infection, when gastrointestinal symptoms are prominent), mebendazole is recommended at a dosage of 200 to 400 mg three times per day for 3 days, followed by 400 to 500 mg three times per day for 10 days. It is not clear if larvae in muscle are killed by this drug, and treatment is primarily symptomatic with antipyretics and analgesics. Although there are too few recent cases to establish a possible beneficial effect of corticosteroids, they may be useful to diminish the severity of inflammation when signs of myocarditis, neurologic disease (e.g., seizures, focal weakness), or pulmonary insufficiency develop. *T. spiralis* infection is prevented by killing larvae in meat products. This is achieved by heating until no trace of pink flesh remains. Freezing, smoking, or exposure to microwaves does not reliably kill the helminth.

Bailey TM, Schantz PM: Trends in the incidence and transmission patterns of trichinosis in humans in the United States. Comparisons of the periods 1975-1981 and 1982-1986. Rev Infect Dis 12:5, 1990. *A comprehensive review of the epidemiology of trichinosis.*
MacLean JD, Viallet J, Law C, et al.: Trichinosis in the Canadian Arctic: Report of five outbreaks and a new clinical syndrome. J Infect Dis 160:513, 1989. *Excellent description of severe gastrointestinal manifestations of* T. spiralis *in a population in which the prevalence of trichinosis is among the highest in the world.*

STRONGYLOIDIASIS

DEFINITION. *Strongyloides stercoralis* infection is endemic in warm climates worldwide, including the southern United States. In immunologically normal individuals, infection is usually asymptomatic or causes gastrointestinal dysfunction, manifest as abdominal pain, bloating, or bleeding. Persons who have deficient cell-mediated immunity can develop an autoinfective and hyperinfective life cycle of the nematode that markedly increases the total worm load. Life-threatening acute pulmonary disease and organ dysfunction due to dissemination of larvae to aberrant sites such as the brain, pancreas, and kidneys may result in immunocompromised hosts.

ETIOLOGY. *S. stercoralis* infection occurs when skin contacts free-living filariform larvae in the soil. After penetrating the skin, the parasite embolizes to the small vessels of the lungs via the venous circulation. Rhabditiform larvae then break into the alveolar spaces, ascend the respiratory tree, and are swallowed. Further development to adult worms occurs in the duodenum and upper jejunum, where egg-laying parasites live in the mucosa and submucosa. Rhabditiform larvae are released from eggs and are passed from the body in stools. Infective filariform larvae develop in the soil by two alternative means, either by direct transformation from rhabditiform larvae or indirectly from free-living intermediate forms.

Several unusual features of the life cycle of *S. stercoralis* are crucial to understanding how this parasitic nematode causes life-threatening disease. First, unlike the vast majority of human helminthic parasites, adult worms reproduce parthogenetically in the gastrointestinal tract. The total worm burden in the host may therefore be greatly increased in the absence of repeated exposure to infective larvae in the environment. Second, rhabditiform larvae may develop into infective filariform larvae in the gastrointestinal tract as well as after passage in feces. Occurrence of the former process in immunocompromised hosts allows autoinfection, whereby larvae pass directly through the bowel (internal autoinfection) or perianal skin (external autoinfection) to reinitiate migration and development in the lungs. When this event is frequent, a hyperinfection syndrome ensues. Disseminated strongyloidiasis refers to a situation of hyperinfection in which the organisms also migrate to and cause pathology in organs not usually traversed by larvae, such as the CNS.

EPIDEMIOLOGY. *S. stercoralis* infection is endemic in Africa, Asia, Latin America, and areas of Eastern and Southern Europe. Prevalence rates based on stools examined for rhabditiform larvae vary from more than 40% in areas of sub-Saharan Africa to 1 to 7% in rural Eastern Europe. In the United States, the infection is endemic in rural Appalachia and other parts of the South. Prevalences range from 0.4 to 3% in the United States. Refugees from Asia have a higher prevalence of infection than do indigenous Americans. Surveys of homosexual men indicate a frequency of infection of 3.9%. It is likely that most studies of prevalence underestimate infection because they are based on examination of a single stool specimen, which is less sensitive than multiple examinations performed over days or weeks.

Strongyloidiasis is especially common in overcrowded situations in which sanitation and personal hygiene are poor, such as in institutions for retarded children and POW camps. An unusually high frequency of *S. stercoralis* infection has also been reported in persons with asymptomatic human T cell lymphotropic virus (HTLV) type I infection.

PATHOGENESIS. Adult worms and larvae penetrating the upper small bowel cause an enteritis characterized histopathologically by eosinophil and mononuclear cell infiltration of the lamina propria. Edema and mucosal atrophy are present on gross examination. Ulcerative lesions with hemorrhages are present in the most severe cases. Filariform larvae in the lungs elicit an inflammatory response in the alveoli consisting of mononuclear cells and eosinophils. In hyperinfection syndrome, these may coalesce and result in alveolar hemorrhage.

Autoinfection leading to exceptionally high worm loads (hyperinfection) and disseminated strongyloidiasis occur in persons with deficient cell-mediated immunity. Groups at risk include persons who are chronically taking corticosteroids, renal transplant recipients, patients with Hodgkin's disease and other lymphomas, and leukemic patients. Because *S. stercoralis* may persist and remain asymptomatic for decades after exposure, it is important to keep in mind that a change in immune status may convert a previously asymptomatic infection to hyperinfection. In this regard, there is a suspected association between acquired immunodeficiency syndrome (AIDS) and disseminated strongyloidiasis.

CLINICAL MANIFESTATIONS. More than 50% of immunocompetent infected persons are asymptomatic. The frequency of clinical manifestations among infected immunocompromised subjects is not known.

Signs and symptoms of *S. stercoralis* infection are attributable to the presence of adult worms in the upper gastrointestinal tract and larval invasion and attendant host pathologic responses in the lung, skin, and aberrant sites of migration, such as the brain, eyes, pancreas, and kidney. Immunocompetent individuals rarely develop signs or symptoms attributable to larval migration outside the gut.

Gastrointestinal disease usually manifests as abdominal bloating, vague epigastric pain, and diarrhea with nausea. Symptoms are exacerbated by eating. Hematochezia and melena occur in <20% of subjects with intestinal strongyloidiasis. Major causes of morbidity related to *S. stercoralis* infection of the intestine are paralytic ileus, small bowel obstruction, and a malabsorption syndrome.

Pulmonary signs and symptoms in immunocompromised persons with hyperinfection syndrome are similar to those seen in the adult respiratory distress syndrome, i.e., acute onset of dyspnea, productive cough, and hemoptysis. These are accompanied by fever, tachypnea, hypoxemia, and respiratory alkalosis. *Strongyloides* larvae may also invade the CNS, pancreas, and eye and cause signs and symptoms attributable to tissue destruction in these sites.

Dermatologic manifestations include self-limited creeping eruption and, more commonly, larva currens. The latter is due to migration of filariform larvae produced by a process of external autoinfection as described above. The larvae elicit serpiginous erythematous papules and occasionally urticaria around the buttocks, upper thigh, and lower abdomen. Larva currens has been noted among former prisoners of war in the South Pacific.

DIAGNOSIS. The unequivocal diagnosis of *S. stercoralis* infection depends on identifying larvae in host tissues or gastrointestinal and pulmonary secretions. The existence of filariform larvae in stools implies an active autoinfection.

Intestinal strongyloidiasis is most easily diagnosed by identification of parasites in direct smears of freshly passed stools. Rhabditiform larvae are 225 to 380 μm in length. Repeated examinations and concentration of stools increase the sensitivity of this method from approximately 25 to 80%. Examination of fluid obtained by duodenal aspiration or passage of a swallowed string into the upper small bowel may also be used if stool examinations are negative. Serologic tests are sensitive but not generally available. The differential diagnosis of intestinal *S. stercoralis* infection includes sprue, peptic ulcer, regional enteritis, and ulcerative colitis.

Hyperinfection syndrome and disseminated strongyloidiasis are diagnosed by identification of filariform larvae (500 to 600 μm long) in gastrointestinal secretions, as described above, or in pulmonary tissues, secretions, or washings, such as those obtained by bronchoalveolar lavage or in sputum. Larvae have also been recovered from CSF, peritoneal washings, kidneys, urine, skin, and brains of immunocompromised persons.

Accompanying laboratory abnormalities frequently include eosinophilia. However, eosinophilia may not develop in immunocompromised hosts. Lack of eosinophilia is therefore not helpful in excluding strongyloidiasis in the differential diagnosis. The differential diagnosis of hyperinfection and disseminated strongyloidiasis includes overwhelming bacterial or fungal sepsis.

COMPLICATIONS. Disseminated strongyloidiasis is frequently accompanied by fungal or bacterial sepsis. Gram-negative enterococcal and polymicrobial septicemia has been observed. These infections likely result from translocation of gut organisms by migrating larvae.

TREATMENT. Uncomplicated intestinal strongyloidiasis should be treated with thiabendazole (25 mg per kilogram of body weight twice daily for 2 days with a maximum of 3 grams per day). Parasitologic cure rates are >90%. Thiabendazole at the same daily dosage should be given to immunocompromised patients with hyperinfection syndrome (i.e., pulmonary disease) or disseminated disease. The drug should be continued for a minimum of 5 to 7 days, although 1 to 2 weeks may be required if organ dysfunction and larval recovery persist. Symptomatic improvement and failure to detect larvae in gastrointestinal secretions or other sites is indicative of cure. Corticosteroids and other immunosuppressive agents should be discontinued when possible.

PREVENTION. Infection is preventable by avoiding skin contact with contaminated soil. Immunocompromised patients in endemic areas should be advised to avoid walking barefoot. Persons residing in endemic areas who are to become immunosuppressed (e.g., for renal transplantation) should have their stools examined three times for the presence of larvae, and they should be treated if the examination is positive. Because infected individuals may be incorrectly categorized as uninfected by this test, it is suggested by some authorities that prophylactic thiabendazole (25 mg per kilogram of body weight daily for 2 days) be given in the month preceding iatrogenic immunosuppression. Positive serology for *S. stercoralis* is also an indication for thiabendazole administration prior to immunosuppression.

Cook GC: *Strongyloides stercoralis* hyperinfection syndrome: How often is it missed? Q J Med 64:625, 1987. *Discusses in detail the differential diagnosis and pitfalls in diagnosis of strongyloidiasis in the immunocompromised host.*

Robinson PD, Lindo JF, Neva FA, et al.: Immunoepidemiologic studies of *Strongyloides stercoralis* and human T lymphotropic virus type I infection in Jamaica. J Infect Dis 169:692, 1994. *Describes the association between HTLV-I infection and strongyloidiasis.*

DeVault GA Jr, King JW, Rohr MS, et al.: Opportunistic infection with *Strongyloides stercoralis* in renal transplantation. Rev Infect Dis 12:653, 1990. *Excellent discussion of clinical presentation and management of hyperinfection in immunocompromised hosts.*

Lessnav K-D, Can S, Talavera W: Disseminated *Strongyloides stercoralis* in human immunodeficiency virus–infected patients. Treatment failure and a review of the literature. Chest 104:119. *A discussion of the difficulties in diagnosis in AIDS patients.*

388 FILARIASIS
*Eric A. Ottesen**

388.1 Introduction

Eight filarial parasites commonly infect humans (Table 388–1), but three are responsible for most of the pathology associated with these infections. These are the lymphatic dwelling filariae *Wuchereria bancrofti* and *Brugia malayi* and the subcutaneous filarid *Onchocerca volvulus*.

All eight species are transmitted by biting arthropods (Table 388–1) and go through complex life cycles that include a slow maturation phase of 3 to 18 months from the time infective larvae are introduced by the vector until the adult worms mature and reside in the lymph nodes, subcutaneous tissue, or body cavities. The offspring of these adults (microfilariae) are 200 to 300 μm long and 5 to 9 μm wide. They either circulate in the blood or migrate through the skin, awaiting ingestion by the appropriate arthropod in which they develop over 1 to 2 weeks to infective forms capable of initiating this life cycle again. Adult worms are long lived (5 to 20 years), while microfilariae live probably 6 to 15 months. Patent infection is generally not established unless exposure to infective larvae is intense and prolonged, and manifestations of disease usually develop slowly.

Diagnosis can be extremely difficult because in endemic populations it relies almost exclusively on parasitologic techniques to demonstrate microfilariae in the blood or tissue, and at present there are no completely satisfactory methods for making a definitive diagnosis in states of "amicrofilaremic" or "amicrofiladermic" filariasis (i.e., infections without demonstrable microfilariae). When microfilariae circulate in the blood, they do so with or without a distinct periodicity (Table 388–1). Some are garbed in sheaths whereas others are sheathless. These two features, as well as other more subtle morphologic distinctions, are helpful diagnostically. Microfilariae in the blood can be identified either by direct observation of Giemsa-stained blood smears or, more sensitively, by concentration techniques using Knott's method (examination of centrifuged sediment after mixing 1 ml of blood with 9 ml of 2% formalin) or membrane filtration of 1 ml or more of blood through a 3-μm or 5-μm pore Nuclepore membrane filter. Skin microfilariae are best sought by performing skin snips as described in Ch. 388.4. Antibody detection, although helpful in certain situations, is generally nondiagnostic because it cannot differentiate current from past infection or exposure and because of antigenic cross-reactivity between the filariae and other helminth parasites. Newer diagnostic methods based on detecting circulating antigen in blood or parasite DNA from skin snips or blood are more sensitive and currently are being readied for general use.

Diethylcarbamazine (DEC)† had been the single mainstay of treatment for all filarial infections since the late 1940's; however, it shows variable effectiveness for the different infections. The new drug ivermectin,‡ because of greater efficacy and safety, has replaced DEC as the drug of choice for onchocerciasis; it is currently under evaluation for use in lymphatic and other filariases. Suramin,‡ although extremely toxic, can also be used for onchocerciasis.

Ottesen EA: Filarial Infections. Infect Dis Clin North Am 7:619, 1993. *A practical approach to the clinical management of each of the filarial infections of humans.*
World Health Organization: Lymphatic filariasis: The disease and its control. Fifth report of the WHO Expert Committee on Filariasis. WHO Tech Rep Ser 821:1,

* The author wishes to acknowledge the previous contributions of Bruce Greene, M.D., (onchocerciasis) and Donald Hopkins, M.D., (dracunculiasis).
† Not commercially available in the United States but may be obtained in special circumstances from Lederle Laboratories, Pearl River, NY.
‡ Available from the Centers for Disease Control and Prevention, Parasitic Disease Drug Service, Atlanta, GA.

TABLE 388–1. THE COMMON FILARIAL PARASITES OF HUMANS

Species	Distribution	Vector	Primary Pathology	Microfilariae Primary Location	Periodicity	Presence of Sheath
Wuchereria bancrofti	Tropics worldwide	Mosquitoes	Lymphatic, pulmonary	Blood, hydrocele fluid	Nocturnal, subperiodic	+
Brugia malayi	Southeast Asia, West Pacific	Mosquitoes	Lymphatic, pulmonary	Blood	Nocturnal, subperiodic	+
Brugia timori	Indonesia	Mosquitoes	Lymphatic	Blood	Nocturnal	+
Onchocerca volvulus	Africa; Central and South America	Black fly	Skin, eye, lymphatic	Skin, eye	None or minimal	−
Loa loa	Africa	Deer fly	Allergic	Blood	Diurnal	+
Mansonella perstans	Africa; South America	Midge	? Allergic	Blood	None	−
Mansonella streptocerca	Africa	Midge	Skin	Skin	None	−
Mansonella ozzardi	Central and South America	Midge	Vague	Blood	None	−

1992. A broad review of lymphatic filariasis and directions that research and control efforts should take in the future.

World Health Organization: Onchocerciasis: The infection and its control. Report of the WHO Expert Committee on Onchocerciasis. WHO Tech Rep Ser, 1995, in press. A broad review of onchocerciasis and the directions that research and control efforts should take in the future.

388.2 Lymphatic Filariasis

ETIOLOGY. There are three lymphatic-dwelling filarial parasites of humans, *Wuchereria bancrofti, Brugia malayi,* and *Brugia timori.* Adult worms are threadlike in form (2 to 10 cm long by < 0.4 cm wide) and usually reside in the lymph nodes or afferent lymphatic channels. The female worms produce large numbers of microfilariae (200 to 300 μm long), which circulate in the peripheral blood awaiting ingestion by mosquito intermediate hosts, which are necessary to continue the parasite's life cycle. After about 2 weeks the microfilariae develop into infective third-stage larvae (L_3's). When infected mosquitoes feed, these L_3's leave the mosquito mouth parts and come to rest on the surface of the host's skin. Only if they manage to penetrate the skin through the puncture at the site of the bite can transmission be successful; after a further developmental period lasting as long as 4 to 12 months, adult worms can again be found in the lymphatic tissues, where they mate and produce another generation of microfilariae. The adult parasites may remain viable in the human host for decades.

EPIDEMIOLOGY. Almost 120 million people have lymphatic filariasis—105 million with bancroftian and 13 million with brugian filariasis. For *W. bancrofti,* humans are the only definitive host and thus the only reservoir for infection. *W. bancrofti* is found throughout the tropics and subtropics, including areas of South America and the Caribbean, Africa, Asia, and the Pacific. Two forms of the parasite are distinguished by the periodicity of their circulating microfilariae. Nocturnally periodic forms have microfilariae detectable in peripheral blood primarily at night, whereas in the subperiodic forms the microfilariae are usually present in the blood at all hours but with maximal levels often in the late afternoon. Generally, subperiodic bancroftian filariasis is found only in the Pacific islands east of 160 degrees E longitude (including New Caledonia, Fiji, Samoa, Ellis Island, Cook Islands, Society Islands, and the Marquesas); elsewhere *W. bancrofti* is generally nocturnally periodic. The natural vectors are *Culex quinquefasciatus* in urban settings and usually anopheline or aedean mosquitoes in rural areas.

The distribution of brugian filariasis is much more restricted, being limited primarily to parts of Malaysia, Indonesia, India, China, Korea, the Philippines, and Japan. Again, there are both nocturnally periodic and subperiodic forms of the parasite. The former is more common and is transmitted in coastal rice fields primarily by mansonian and anopheline mosquitoes; mansonian mosquitoes, found in swamp forests, are the major vectors of the subperiodic form. Un-

like *W. bancrofti, B. malayi* can be a natural infection of cats and can be established in a number of laboratory animals. *B. timori* has been described from only two Indonesian islands.

PATHOLOGY. Most of the pathology of bancroftian and brugian filariasis is associated with the lymphatics. Although details of the pathogenesis are lacking, the progression of pathologic changes is becoming clearer. Even in entirely asymptomatic individuals with microfilaremia but no overt clinical manifestations of infection, lymphatic structural and functional abnormalities are often severe. Compromised function ultimately leads to lymphedema that is at first reversible. With continued assault on this compromised lymphatic system by persistent parasites and by complicating localized bacterial and fungal superinfections, the lymphedema becomes irreversible and leads to chronic elephantiasis of the limbs, breasts, or genitalia, or to chyluria. The location of lymphatic damage determines the site and type of pathology expressed.

Adult worms, residing in the afferent approaches or cortical sinuses of the lymph nodes, induce local reactions by undefined mechanisms that result in dilatation of the lymphatics and hypertrophy of the vessel walls. Endothelial and connective tissue proliferation leads to polypoid growths that protrude into the lymphatic lumen, and even while the vessels remain patent, normal lymphatic function is not ensured. Both earlier lymphangiography studies and more recent lymphoscintigraphy studies have clearly documented the development of a characteristic tortuosity of the lymph vessels with loss of valvular function and backflow of lymph leading to lymph stasis and lymphedema even during this "preobliterative phase."

Because of a still undefined interplay between the host immune system and the parasite, local inflammatory and granulomatous reactions subsequently develop around dying or dead adult worms, with infiltration of plasma cells, eosinophils, and giant cells. Fibrosis occurs, and the fragmented parasites are either completely resorbed or partially calcified. Lymphatic obstruction develops, and associated bacterial-induced inflammation or superinfection may further complicate the lymphatic damage. Although there is subsequent formation of collateral lymphatics and some recanalization of obstructed vessels, lymphatic function remains compromised. Repeated infection and increasing host response to the parasite leads to the chronic changes of advanced elephantiasis.

CLINICAL MANIFESTATIONS. Although previously not much emphasized, a major distinction exists between the clinical presentation of lymphatic filariasis in individuals native to the endemic regions (whose exposures have been lifelong) and that of those entering such areas and meeting the infection for the first time. In these latter (e.g., long-term visitors, military personnel, settlers) the most common presentations are localized inflammatory reactions, especially adenolymphangitis, and evidence of immediate hypersensitivity responses to the parasites (i.e., urticaria, eosinophilia, and immunoglobulin E [IgE] elevations). Only rarely do such individuals present with the contrasting set of findings characteristic of the infection in those native to the endemic areas, particularly asymptomatic microfilaremia.

Patients manifesting *asymptomatic microfilaremia* rarely come to the physician's attention except through an incidental finding of microfilariae in the peripheral blood smear during mass surveys in endemic regions, or when blood eosinophilia leads to a diagnostic evaluation for filariasis. Such asymptomatic persons appear to be clinically unaffected by the parasites. However, recent studies have shown dramatically that this asymptomatic state belies severe underlying pathology, both lymphatic functional abnormalities seen on lymphoscintigraphy and renal pathology manifested as hematuria and proteinuria. It is likely that some but not all of these individuals become symptomatic, but factors determining such clinical changes are unknown.

"Filarial fever" is the term given to acute febrile episodes (often with shaking chills), accompanied by painful lymphatic inflammation (lymphadenitis and lymphangitis) and transient local edema that occur up to 6 to 10 times per year and usually last 3 to 7 days before subsiding spontaneously. Although appreciated only recently, "filarial fevers" appear to be really two different clinical syndromes, one initiated by host immunologic responses to lymphatic-dwelling parasites and the other, seemingly more common, induced by bacterial superinfection of limbs with already compromised lymphatic function. The former is characterized by a *retrograde* lymphangitis and "cold" edema of the affected limb and the latter by a cellulitis-type of presentation with a warm edematous extremity. Such inflammatory reactions occur in the upper and lower extremities with both bancroftian and brugian filariasis, but involvement of the genital lymphatics is almost exclusively a feature of *W. bancrofti* infection. Thus, acute *W. bancrofti* episodes may also involve funiculitis, epididymitis, scrotal pain, and tenderness. Patients with filarial fevers may be microfilaremic but more often are not.

As lymphatic damage progresses, the edema and anatomic distortion that were initially transient develop into the permanent changes of elephantiasis. Pitting edema yields to brawny edema, and both thickening of subcutaneous tissue and hyperkeratosis develop. Fissuring of the skin develops along with nodular and papillomatous hyperplastic changes. Superinfection (with skin bacteria and dermatophytes) becomes an increasing problem. In addition, in bancroftian filariasis affected genital lymphatics may lead to scrotal lymphedema or hydrocele, whereas involvement of the retroperitoneal lymphatics can increase hydrostatic pressure in the renal lymphatics, causing their rupture into the renal pelvis or tubules and leading to chyluria. Characteristically, such chyluria is intermittent, sometimes lasting for days or weeks before abating spontaneously and then recurring; often it is most prominent in the morning after the patient first arises.

DIAGNOSIS. Diagnosis is most certainly made by identifying the parasites themselves, usually microfilariae in the blood, hydrocele fluid, or chylous urine. These fluids can be examined directly (20 cubic millimeters on a slide with or without red blood cell lysis), after concentration of the parasites by centrifugation in 2% formalin (Knott's technique), or after filtration through a membrane (3- to 5-μm Nuclepore) filter. The time of blood collection should take into account the parasite's possible nocturnal periodicity. More recently, ultrasound techniques have been successfully and simply used to visualize rapidly moving ("dancing") adult worms in the dilated scrotal lymphatics of infected men; such findings are absolutely pathognomonic of filarial parasites.

Because many persons with filariasis (especially those with chronic pathology) are not microfilaremic, diagnosis must often be made clinically. The differential diagnosis is broad but in the acute episodes primarily includes thrombophlebitis, infection, and trauma. The edema and other lymphatic obstructive changes associated with chronic filariasis must be distinguished from the manifestations of congestive heart failure, malignant disease, trauma, postsurgical scarring, and a number of less common congenital and idiopathic abnormalities of the lymphatic system. The many disorders associated with serum IgE and blood eosinophil elevations must be considered in evaluating asymptomatic filarial infections. Several specific points may help in this differential diagnosis: (1) Exposure to filariae must be prolonged or intense (for at least several months) before persons become infected; (2) the physical finding or history of *retrograde* lymphangitis can often aid in distinguishing filarial from bacterial lymphangitis; (3) although lymphadenopathy is characteristic of filariasis, alone it is never diagnostic; (4) lymphangiographic and lymphoscintigraphic patterns of elephantiasis and chyluria are well defined, so that even though not always diagnostic,

these tests can sometimes be useful in distinguishing filarial from congenital or neoplastic lymphatic abnormalities; (5) although total serum IgE and blood eosinophil levels are often elevated in filarial infections, they cannot distinguish filarial from other helminth infections except in the case of the tropical eosinophilia syndrome (see Ch. 388.3).

Until recently, serologic and skin tests have not generally been helpful in diagnosing filariasis *except* in those individuals not native to the endemic regions. The primary reason is that residents of endemic areas with their lifelong exposures to mosquito-borne filarial larvae develop high levels of antifilarial antibodies, regardless of whether they actually acquire infection. The recent development of assays to detect circulating antigens liberated by adult worms (and present in the blood both day and night) promises to revolutionize the serologic approach to diagnosing filariasis.

TREATMENT. The approach to treating lymphatic filariasis is currently undergoing dramatic changes. Although DEC† (6 mg per kilogram per day) remains the only drug registered for use in lymphatic filariasis, ivermectin‡ (400 μg per kilogram per day) is an equally potent microfilaricide. DEC is also effective in killing some, although not all, adult worms, but for ivermectin there is still uncertainty about its potential adulticidal activity. Most surprising has been the recent finding that a single dose of DEC has essentially the same long-term effectiveness in decreasing microfilaremia and apparent killing of adult worms as the 1- to 3-week courses previously recommended. For control programs, this finding has enormous implications; for individual clinic patients, however, it is not certain that earlier recommendations for the longer courses of DEC should be scaled back to single-day dosing; specific clinical studies still need to address this issue.

The side effects of DEC treatment, whether single-dose or multiple doses, can be troublesome, especially in brugian filariasis. These include fever, chills, headache, dizziness, nausea, vomiting, and arthralgias, all usually occurring in the first 24 to 36 hours. Both the likelihood of developing such reactions and the degree of their severity are directly related to the number of circulating microfilariae. Thus, the side effects of DEC at the recommended (6 mg/kg) dosage are due not to direct drug toxicity but to inflammatory responses of the host to dying parasites. To avoid these reactions in highly parasitemic persons, one can initiate treatment with very small doses of DEC or premedicate the patients with steroids, as suggested for loiasis (see Ch. 388.5). A very few patients may also develop filarial fever episodes with lymphangitis and lymphadenitis in the first days after DEC treatment. All of these side effects occur early in treatment and generally subside even when the drug is continued.

Chronic lymphedema and elephantiasis have recently been shown to have a surprising degree of reversibility. All such affected patients should receive long-term low-dose DEC (to eradicate persistent or new filarial infections) and diligent attention to local care of the lymphedematous extremity through limb elevation, use of special massage techniques and elastic stockings, and especially prevention of superficial bacterial and fungal infection. More severely affected patients may benefit remarkably from surgical decompression of the lymphatic system through "nodovenous shunt" surgery followed by excision of redundant tissue. Hydroceles can be repeatedly drained or managed surgically. Chyluria also can sometimes be corrected surgically, but, interestingly, many cases have been reported in which diagnostic lymphangiography itself appears to have terminated the leak of chyle into the urine, probably as a result of its sclerosing effects.

PREVENTION. DEC kills developing preadult forms of many filarial species, and its value as a prophylactic agent in humans (10 mg per kilogram on 2 consecutive days each month) has recently been established. In addition, for public health programs to control lymphatic filariasis, a single dose of DEC given yearly to an entire community dramatically reduces the prevalence of infection. Similarly, small doses administered intermittently (or even as an additive to common table salt) to all residents of an endemic region (e.g., 3 mg per kilogram monthly) reduce the number of bloodborne microfilariae in the community to levels so low that successful transmission of the infection by mosquitoes cannot occur. Other approaches to filariasis control designed to eradicate the mosquito vectors have also proved effective for the short term but have been difficult to sustain.

Amaral F, Dreyer G, Figueredo-Silva J, et al.: Live adult worms detected by ultra-sonography in human bancroftian filariasis. Am J Trop Med Hyg 50:753, 1994. *The first description of a successful new technique for noninvasive localization and visualization of living adult-stage* W. bancrofti *worms. Such adult worms could be identified in more than half of all asymptomatic microfilaraemic men evaluated.*

Chodakewitz JA: Ivermectin and lymphatic filariasis: Clinical update. Parasitol Today, 1995. *A thorough review of the most recent trials comparing single-dose DEC, single-dose ivermectin, and the combination of these single-dose regimens to effect microfilarial clearance from the blood of patients with* W. bancrofti *or* B. malayi *infections.*

Ottesen EA: The human filariases: New understandings, new therapeutic strategies. Curr Opinion Infect Dis 7:550, 1994. *A look at the dramatic advances of the past 2 to 3 years that are transforming the way filariasis is both understood and managed.*

Witte MH, Jamal S, Williams WH, et al.: Lymphatic abnormalities in human filariasis as depicted by lymphoangioscintigraphy. Arch Intern Med 153:737, 1993. *Thirty-three patients with symptomatic (acute or chronic) lymphatic filariasis from South India were evaluated by lymphoscintigraphy, which was shown to be a simple, safe, reliable, noninvasive method for examining the peripheral lymphatic system. The abnormalities noted in these patients included delayed or absent tracer transport, tortuosity of the deep lymphatics, dermal diffusion, retrograde tracer flow, and faint or absent regional node visualization.*

388.3 Tropical Eosinophilia

Tropical eosinophilia is a syndrome of acute and chronic lung disease first defined in the 1940's but not generally recognized as being of filarial origin until the 1960's. Its main clinical features are a history of residence in a filaria-endemic region; paroxysmal cough and wheezing, which generally occur at night; scanty sputum production; occasional weight loss, low-grade fever, and adenopathy; and extreme blood eosinophilia (>3000 per microliter). It is more common in men than in women. Chest roentgenograms can be normal but generally show increased bronchovascular markings, diffuse interstitial lesions, or mottled opacities primarily involving the mid and lower lung fields. Tests of pulmonary function almost always indicate restrictive abnormalities and often obstructive defects as well. The association of the syndrome with filarial infection was first recognized by finding very high levels of antifilarial antibody in these patients and by noting the favorable response to treatment with antifilarial drugs (now diethylcarbamazine† [DEC], 6 to 10 mg per kilogram per day for 3 to 4 weeks). Later, several reports described microfilariae or their degenerating remnants in lung biopsy specimens. Most recently, extremely high levels of total serum IgE (usually 10,000 to 100,000 ng per milliliter) have been found in these patients, and an appreciable fraction of this IgE has been shown to be directed against filarial antigens.

Because of these and other findings, tropical eosinophilia is now considered a form of "occult filariasis" in which host immunologic hyperresponsiveness to the parasite results in such rapid clearance of microfilariae from the blood that this stage of the parasite is essentially never detectable. Generally, this microfilarial clearance takes place in the lungs, and the clinical symptoms appear to result largely from the allergic and inflammatory reactions elicited by the cleared parasites. In some subjects, however, trapping of the microfilariae occurs predominantly in other organs of the reticuloendothelial system (liver, spleen, lymph nodes), and in these persons the major clinical manifestations are those resulting from hepatomegaly, splenomegaly, or lymphadenopathy. It had been postulated that infection with nonhuman filarial parasites is the major cause of tropical eosinophilia. Almost certainly, however, the syndrome is caused not by an "abnormal parasite" but rather by an abnormal host response to those same parasites (*Wuchereria bancrofti* and *Brugia malayi*) that commonly cause lymphatic filariasis (see Ch. 388.2). In this respect, tropical eosinophilia may be similar to another pulmonary eosinophilic disorder, allergic bronchopulmonary aspergillosis, both in its clinical expression and in its pathogenesis (see Ch. 355).

Diagnosis depends primarily on distinguishing tropical eosinophilia from the other important eosinophilic syndromes with pulmonary involvement, namely, Löffler's syndrome, chronic eosinophilic pneumonia, allergic aspergillosis, certain vasculitis syndromes, the idiopathic hypereosinophilia syndrome, drug allergies, and some helminth infections. Although there is no one clinical or laboratory criterion that will distinguish tropical eosinophilia from these other conditions, a history of residence in the tropics, high levels of specific filarial antibodies, and a response to DEC therapy are the most helpful differential points. Within 3 to 7 days after DEC is begun, symptoms improve markedly or disappear. Resolution may not be complete, however, and relapse may occur months to years later and require retreatment. DEC will not, of course, reverse permanent pulmonary damage (primarily an interstitial fibrosis), which frequently develops prior to successful diagnosis and treatment of the disorder.

Ottesen EA, Nutman TB: Tropical pulmonary eosinophilia. Ann Rev Med 43:417, 1992. *A brief overview of the newer clinical and pathogenetic aspects of the TPE syndrome, with references to the appropriate primary sources.*

388.4 Onchocerciasis (River Blindness)

ETIOLOGY. Onchocerciasis, most commonly causing skin and eye disease, results from infection with the filarial parasite *Onchocerca volvulus*. Transmission is via the bites of black files (*Simulium* species) that ingest microfilariae from the skin of an infected person while taking a blood meal. After 6 to 8 days of development in the vector, the larvae are infective and can be transmitted to another person when the fly bites again. Over a period of several months, the larvae develop into adult worms that coil into spherical bundles surrounded by host fibrotic and granulomatous tissue located in the subcutaneous tissues and deeper fascial planes. After a prepatent period of 9 to 18 months, the adult male and female worms reproduce sexually to yield millions of microfilariae that migrate primarily through the skin and ocular tissues.

Microfilariae are highly motile, unsheathed and approximately 200 to 300 μm long and 6 to 9 μm wide. Adult female worms are 23 to 70 cm in length, while the males are 3 to 6 cm long and weigh only 1% as much as the female. The average life span of the adult worm is estimated to be 8 to 10 years and that of the microfilariae, 13 to 14 months.

PREVALENCE AND EPIDEMIOLOGY. *O. volvulus* infects an estimated 17 million persons, principally in 27 countries of equatorial Africa in a broad belt extending from the Atlantic coast on the west to the Red Sea and Indian Ocean on the east. More limited foci are also found in Yemen and in six countries of the Americas (Guatemala, Mexico, Venezuela, Brazil, Colombia, and Ecuador).

Endemicity of *O. volvulus* in human populations is dependent upon habitation of fly-infested areas by sufficient numbers of people who are exposed to human-biting flies during daily activities such as farming, fishing, bathing, washing and water collection. Because the flies depend on waterways for egg-laying and reproduction, they concentrate around streams and rivers. As a result, infection and disease in human populations tend to be similarly distributed; hence the term *river blindness*. Generally, the vectors fly a few kilometers from waterways, but they may be carried by winds for hundreds of kilometers.

The incidence of blindness varies in different regions (thought to be related to parasite strain), but until recently onchocerciasis has been the fourth leading cause of blindness; in some hyperendemic areas more than half the adults became blind. A much higher percentage of persons develops skin disease, and because both of these severe disabilities typically occur during the third and fourth decades of life, the impact of the disease on the community is particularly devastating, frequently incapacitating the heads of households.

PATHOLOGY AND PATHOGENESIS. The disease affects primarily the skin, lymph nodes, and ocular tissues. In the skin, histopathology reflects a low-grade chronic inflammatory process, the end stage of which is loss of elastic fibers, atrophy, and fibrosis.

Onchocercomata, which are fibrous subcutaneous nodules containing adult worms, show a rim of chronic inflammation with fibrosis and extensive capillary infiltration surrounding the worms themselves. Lymph nodes show chronic inflammatory changes and, in some cases, fibrosis and atrophy. In the eye, neovascularization and scarring of the cornea lead to loss of transparency and blindness. The rest of the eye is frequently involved by a chronic nongranulomatous inflammatory process that leads to anterior uveitis and associated chronic complications, chorioretinitis with damage to the retinal pigment epithelium, and optic atrophy.

The basis for the pathologic changes of onchocerciasis is believed to be the host reaction to chronic infection with microfilariae. Numerous factors appear to contribute to the pathologic changes, including toxic or tissue-altering products of host granulocytes and lymphoid cells that are involved either in killing microfilariae or in responding to their spontaneous or natural death, and toxic products of the microfilariae themselves.

CLINICAL MANIFESTATIONS. The earliest signs of infection include pruritus, intermittent papular rash sometimes with thickening of the skin which may be localized to one area of the body, and conjunctivitis. In expatriate visitors to endemic areas, who are usually lightly infected, these are frequently the only manifestations. The onchocercomata are 0.5- to 3-cm subcutaneous nodules that are firm, nontender and freely movable if not attached to periosteum. They frequently occur in clusters overlying bony prominences, including the superior iliac crests, the coccyx, the greater trochanter of the femur, the bony thorax, and the head. With chronic infection, permanent skin changes occur, including loss of elasticity, a chronic, scaling hyperkeratotic maculopapular pruritic rash with mottled hypopigmentation or hyperpigmentation, and, finally, atrophy, leading in some cases to areas of skin breakdown and superinfection. The chronic skin manifestations are intermittently punctuated by transient episodes of localized rash, erythema, and edema. In Central America the dermal manifestations are most prominent around the head and neck, whereas in Africa they more commonly involve the trunk, buttocks, and lower extremities. Lymph node involvement is usually manifested by enlargement, particularly in the inguinal and femoral regions, and in some cases by secondary obstructive changes in the groin region or in an extremity. Also seen when massively enlarged inguinal nodes develop in the presence of appreciable dermal atrophy is the characteristic clinical picture of "hanging groin."

In the eye the earliest manifestations are punctate keratitis and anterior uveitis. Chronic changes include sclerosing keratitis, chorioretinitis (which leads to progressive constriction of visual fields), optic atrophy, and complications due to persistent anterior uveitis, including miosis, pupillary distortion, and glaucoma. In general, the severity of the eye disease correlates with intensity and duration of infection.

DIAGNOSIS. The diagnosis can be made clinically by the presence of onchocercomata, typical skin changes, or eye findings of onchocerciasis, especially microfilariae visualized by slit-lamp examination of the cornea or anterior chamber in otherwise normal-appearing eyes. Diagnosis is most frequently made by finding microfilariae of *O. volvulus* in the patient's skin. "Skin snips" are taken using either a corneoscleral biopsy instrument or a razor blade, to yield approximately 1 to 2 mg of skin, including superficial dermis. The skin is placed in saline or water, and the microfilariae that emerge are counted after a 3-hour or overnight incubation. Alternatively, the snips can be processed for polymerase chain reaction (PCR) amplification of parasite DNA, a technique more sensitive than direct visualization. Because distribution of microfilariae is not uniform, four to six snips should be done in different areas, including the hips, calves, and shoulders. Instruments used for skin snipping should be disposable or thoroughly sterilized between patients. Although elevated titers of antifilarial antibodies may support the diagnosis of onchocerciasis, a definitive immunodiagnostic technique has not yet been developed.

TREATMENT. Invermectin‡ is now the drug of choice to treat onchocerciasis. The dosage is 150 μg per kilogram, given every 6 or 12 months. Because it kills microfilariae but not adult worms, retreatment is necessary over a period of years. Expatriate visitors to endemic countries often require more than once-a-year treatment because of rapid recurrence of pruritus in these hyperreactive individuals. Ivermectin is not approved for use in pregnant

women, nursing mothers within 1 week of delivery, or children under age 5.

DEC† should *not* be used to treat patients with onchocerciasis because the severe inflammatory reaction ("Mazzotti reaction") induced by the rapid killing of microfilariae can actually cause pathology (especially in the eye) worse than the infection itself. Although qualitatively similar posttreatment reactions can occur after ivermectin (including fever, pruritus, lymphadenitis, arthralgia, and postural hypotension), their incidence and severity are much less, and essentially no exacerbation of ocular lesions occurs. Suramin, although it does kill adult worms, has appreciable toxicity (especially renal) and must be given intravenously at approximately weekly intervals over 2 to 3 months, so it should be used with caution and only where there can be careful monitoring.

Surgical removal of nodules containing adult worms is appropriate for cosmetic reasons but cannot be expected to cure infection because for every palpable nodule there are four to nine nonpalpable ones.

PROGNOSIS. With treatment, the early ocular and cutaneous changes are reversible, but for persons living in an endemic area, therapy must be given repeatedly because ivermectin does not kill the adult parasites and, thus, does not eliminate the infection. The atrophic skin changes, sclerosing keratitis, and established lesions in the posterior segment of the eye are not helped by therapy.

PREVENTION. Protective clothing, insect repellents, and avoiding areas harboring the vector are useful measures for visitors to endemic areas, but there is no available chemoprophylaxis. Vector control is difficult and expensive but has achieved excellent success in the 11-country Onchocerciasis Control Program in West Africa. The remarkable Mectizan Donation Program, in which the manufacturer of ivermectin (Merck & Co., Inc.) has pledged to donate, without cost, all the drugs needed to treat all patients in all endemic areas for as long as necessary, has spurred the organization of massive control programs throughout the endemic regions of Africa and the Americas, supported by governmental and nongovernmental development organizations, the World Bank, and the Inter American Bank. The effect of these efforts promises to be a dramatic decline in the incidence and prevalence of onchocerciasis and, most importantly, in the disease it inflicts on affected individuals.

Duke BOL: The population dynamics of *Onchocerca volvulus* in the human host. Trop Med Parasitol 44:61, 1993. *Data from disparate sources are cleverly compiled to allow interpretation and extrapolation leading to astounding conclusions about the number of adult worms and microfilariae in* O. volvulus–*infected patients.*

Dull B: Mectizan Donation and the Mectizan Expert Committee. Acta Leidensia 59:399, 1990. *Describes organization of a program that provided over 30 million once-yearly doses of ivermectin to 8 million individuals in onchocerciasis-endemic regions of Africa and the Americas (end, 1994).*

Ottesen EA: Immune responsiveness and the pathogenesis of human onchocerciasis. J Infect Dis, in press. *Reviews a confusing array of studies dealing with the immune responses of onchocerciasis patients. Proposes that it is not so much the proinflammatory response to O. volvulus microfilariae that is responsible for the skin and eye pathology as it is the "bystander" damage by host immune and phagocytic cells attempting to contain or prevent inflammatory responses to the vast number of microfilariae dying "naturally" each day.*

World Health Organization: Onchocerciasis: The infection and its control. Report of the WHO Expert Committee on Onchocerciasis. WHO Tech Rep Ser 1995, in press. *A broad review of onchocerciasis and the directions that research and control efforts should take in the future.*

388.5 Loiasis

Loa loa is indigenous only to the rain forest belt of western and central Africa. Mature female parasites, about twice the size of the males, are 50 to 70 mm long and 0.5 mm wide. They live for many years in the subcutaneous tissue in humans, usually attracting attention only when they cross the eye subconjunctivally. The sheathed microfilariae produced by these females circulate in the blood with a diurnal periodicity that peaks at about noon.

Clinical loiasis presents in two primary forms, one more common among individuals native to endemic regions and the other more common in visitors to these areas who acquire infection. Among the natives, loiasis is often entirely asymptomatic until an adult worm appears moving across the eye or blood examination reveals microfilaremia. Such individuals may also have occasional episodes of "Calabar swellings." These are characteristic localized areas of erythema and angioedema (up to 5 to 10 cm in diameter) that occur primarily on the extremities and last 1 to 3 days before regressing spontaneously. These swellings appear to be a hypersensitivity reaction to the adult worm, whose presence can also be detected in some patients by either a subcutaneous crawling sensation or the appearance of a fine vermiform hive in the skin. When the inflammation extends to nearby joints or peripheral nerves, corresponding symptoms may develop. Nephropathy (probably immune complex mediated) and, more rarely, encephalopathy have also been reported.

The major difference between this presentation and that seen in visitors who acquire infection is the greater predominance of allergic or hyperreactive symptoms in the latter. Episodes of angioedema are likely to be more frequent and debilitating, and patients are much less likely to have microfilariae in the blood. In addition, they often present with extensive blood eosinophilia (30 to 60% of an elevated total leukocyte count), much like patients with tropical eosinophilia (Ch. 388.3). Diagnosis in these patients often cannot be made parasitologically and must be based on the characteristic history, clinical presentation, blood eosinophilia, and elevated filarial antibody titers. If untreated, a small (but undefined) percentage of such patients develops severe cardiomyopathy, presumably secondary to the hypereosinophilia elicited by the infection.

Treatment is with DEC, 6 to 10 mg per kilogram per day for 2 to 3 weeks. The drug is extremely effective against microfilariae, but less so against adult worms, so that multiple courses of treatment are often necessary before signs and symptoms completely resolve. In cases of heavy microfilaremia (greater than several hundred microfilariae per milliliter of blood), inflammatory reactions may be so severe as to include coma and death. Thus, treatment of such persons must be done cautiously, using one or more of the following options: very low initial DEC doses, pretreatment with steroids, pheresis to remove circulating microfilariae, or albendazole, instead of DEC, which appears to kill adult worms but not the microfilariae. DEC is effective in preventing loiasis when taken in prophylactic doses of 300 mg weekly.

Carme B, Boulesteix J, Boutes H, et al.: Five cases of encephalitis during treatment of loiasis with diethylcarbamazine. Am J Trop Med Hyg 44:684, 1991. *An excellent critical review of the past experiences and implications of the likelihood of encephalitis developing following treatment of loiasis patients with diethylcarbamazine.*

Klion AD, Ottesen EA, Nutman TB: Effectiveness of diethylcarbamazine in treating loiasis acquired by expatriate visitors to endemic regions: Long-term follow up. J Infect Dis 169:604, 1994. *Thirty-two expatriates with loiasis contracted in endemic areas were treated one or more times with 3-week courses of DEC and were followed 2 to 15 years after treatment. Only 38% were cured after one course of treatment, and no clinical or laboratory parameters (including eosinophilia and specific filarial serology) were found either to predict a successful outcome posttreatment or to define when a patient was completely cured.*

Nutman TB, Miller KD, Mulligan M, et al.: Diethylcarbamazine prophylaxis for human loiasis: Results of a double-blinded study. N Engl J Med 319:752, 1988. *A placebo-controlled study in Peace Corps volunteers showing clearly that clinical loiasis can be prevented by weekly DEC in long-term visitors to endemic countries.*

388.6 Dracunculiasis

Dracunculiasis, or guinea worm disease, is caused by infection with the parasite *Dracunculus medinensis*. It occurs in the Indian subcontinent and Africa, where up to 1 million persons living in rural areas are affected annually; more than 100 million persons remain at risk of infection.

Diagnosis of patent infections is easy. The thin adult female worms, each up to 1 meter long, emerge directly through the skin, usually of the lower leg, ankle, or foot. The worms emerge 10 to 14 months after victims have drunk water containing infected *Cyclops,* a barely visible crustacean that serves as the parasite's intermediate host. When persons harboring such emerging worms enter a stag-

nant source of drinking water, such as a step well or pond, larvae are released into the water, where some are ingested by *Cyclops.* When humans drink water containing *Cyclops* with infective larvae, the larvae penetrate the intestinal or stomach wall, mature, and mate, after which the male worms die.

The adult worms emerge slowly, over a period of weeks or months. Emergence may be preceded by generalized allergic symptoms and is usually accompanied by a blister that ruptures to form an ulcer at the site of emergence. Some worms present first as a serpentine cord just beneath the skin or at the center of an abscess. No immunity develops, so persons in endemic areas are infected year after year.

The great social and economic significance of dracunculiasis, which rarely is fatal, derives from the fact that emergence of the worm is very painful and is often associated with swelling, local arthritis, and secondary infection. Thus, victims are often unable to farm or sometimes even walk for weeks or months. Over half of the adults in a village may be crippled at the same time, and the seasonal infection tends to occur precisely when villagers need to harvest or plant their crops. School attendance is also affected.

Treatment is difficult because anthelminthics such as thiabendazole or metronidazole only marginally reduce the duration of emergence and associated pain. Aspirin can help relieve the pain. Emerging worms are best rolled around a small stick as their predecessors have been for centuries, care being taken not to break the worm (which would exacerbate the inflammation). Some worms can be removed surgically. Victims should be immunized against tetanus, which is sometimes caused by secondary infection of the ulcer around the emerging worm. Persons at risk should be taught to boil their drinking water or filter it through a cloth and to avoid entering sources of drinking water when the infection is patent.

Because the most effective intervention against this infection is to provide safe drinking water, efforts began during the International Drinking Water Supply and Sanitation Decade (1981–1990) to provide safe water to dracunculiasis-endemic areas as a priority and thereby eliminate the disease. By the end of 1993 all endemic countries were working to eradicate the disease by 1995. The annual number of cases of dracunculiasis reported to WHO was reduced by 75% between 1989 and 1993.

Hopkins DR, Ruiz-Tiben E, Kaiser RL, et al.: Dracunculiasis eradication: Beginning of the end. Am J Trop Med Hyg 49:281, 1993. *A recent review of all aspects pertaining to control and eradication of dracunculiasis.*

388.7 Other Filarial Infections

PERSTANS FILARIASIS

Mansonella perstans (formerly *Dipetalonema perstans, Acanthocheilonema perstans*) is distributed in a broad belt across the center of Africa and in northeast South America. Adult worms, up to 70 to 80 mm long, reside in the body cavities (pleural, peritoneal, and pericardial) and in the mesentery, perirenal, and retroperitoneal tissues. Microfilariae are liberated *unsheathed* from the females and circulate in the blood without regular periodicity.

M. perstans infection was long thought to be asymptomatic, because up to 90% of individuals with the parasite appeared to have no difficulty with it. Subsequent studies, however, indicate clearly that *M. perstans* is capable of inducing a variety of symptoms, including angioedematous swellings much like the "Calabar swellings" of loiasis; fever; headache; pain in bursae and/or joint synovia, in serous cavities, or over the liver; neurologic or psychological symptoms; and extreme exhaustion. There is some evidence that symptoms are more prominent in outsiders coming to endemic regions, but in all series at least a quarter of such patients were asymptomatic despite persistent microfilaremia.

Treatment with DEC,† 5 to 6 mg per kilogram per day for 2 to 3 weeks is often ineffective, and although other drugs have been tried (e.g., mebendazole, albendazole, ivermectin), none has proven to be reliably effective. When the parasites are eliminated, however, patients characteristically lose their symptoms (no matter how vague), lose their eosinophilia, and regain a sense of well-being.

Adolph PE, Kagan IG, McQuay RM: Diagnosis and treatment of *Acanthocheilonema perstans* filariasis. Am J Trop Med Hyg 11:76, 1962. *Results from a series of patients observed in the United States after returning from missionary work in Africa.*

Clarke V deV, Harwin RM, MacDonald DF, et al.: Filariasis: *Dipetalonema perstans* infections in Rhodesia. Cent Afr J Med 17:1, 1971. *Discussion of the clinical expression of M. perstans filariasis in Africans and Europeans living in East Africa.*

STREPTOCERCIASIS

Mansonella streptocerca is transmitted by midges, especially *Culicoides grahami*. It occurs in the tropical forest belt of Africa from Ghana to Zaire. The adult worms are subcutaneous, especially over the torso; and the microfilariae, which have characteristic shepherd's-crook tails, are found in the skin (see Ch. 388.4 for skin-snipping technique).

Infection is usually symptomless, but the adult worms may produce hypopigmented macules (to be distinguished from leprosy), and the microfilariae occasionally cause pruritic papular rashes similar to those of onchocerciasis. Both adult worms and microfilariae are killed by DEC† (e.g., 7 to 10 days of treatment at 6 mg per kilogram per day).

Meyers WM, Connor DH, et al.: Human streptocerciasis: A clinicopathologic study of 40 Africans (Zairians) including identification of the adult filaria. Am J Trop Med Hyg 21:528, 1972. *Covers the clinical aspects and gives references to other aspects.*

MANSONELLA OZZARDI INFECTION

M. ozzardi is restricted in distribution to Central and South America and certain islands of the Caribbean. Adult worms have been recovered in humans only twice, both times from the peritoneal cavity. *Unsheathed* microfilariae circulate in the blood with little or no periodicity.

Many investigators consider these parasites to be nonpathogenic, but one of the fullest clinical studies of an affected population found that the major clinical presentation is severe articular pain or dysfunction, especially in the arms and shoulders. Headache, fever, pulmonary symptoms, adenopathy, hepatomegaly, and pruritic skin eruptions also occurred in a small number of patients with a frequency greater than that in nonparasitized individuals in the same population. DEC† has little or no effect on this infection, but ivermectin‡ appears to be effective therapy.

Marinkelle CJ, German E: Mansonelliasis in the comisaria del Vaupes of Colombia. Trop Geogr Med 22:101, 1970. *A very complete and interesting account of clinical manifestations ascribed to M. ozzardi infections in South American Indians.*

Nutman TB, Nash TE, Ottesen EA: Ivermectin in the successful treatment of a patient with *Mansonella ozzardi* infection. J Infect Dis 156:662, 1987. *A single case report presenting clinical and immunologic evidence for the effectiveness of ivermectin (140 µg per kilogram given once) in an M. ozzardi infection.*

HUMAN DIROFILARIASIS

Dirofilaria species are filarial parasites mostly of dogs, cats, and raccoons that sometimes infect humans but almost never fully develop to complete their life cycles in this abnormal host. The distribution of cases is worldwide and reflects the distribution of the parasites in animals.

Two general types of clinical presentation predominate. Pulmonary dirofilariasis, caused by the dog heartworm *D. immitis*, usually presents as an asymptomatic solitary pulmonary nodule but occasionally with chest pain, cough, or hemoptysis. Microscopically there is local eosinophilia and granuloma formation accompanied by infarction and thrombosis around an impacted, immature worm. The second common clinical presentation is that of a subcutaneous nodule found anywhere on the body (or within the eye) that results usually from infection with the subcutaneous dwelling filarids of dogs *(D. repens)* or raccoons *(D. tenuis)* but occasionally from infection with *D. immitis.* Local lesions again are granulomatous and eosinophilic and are sometimes accompanied by bacterial superinfection.

Definitive diagnosis and treatment most often result from the same surgical (excisional) procedure. Blood eosinophilia is not a *regular* finding in these patients nor are detectable antifilarial antibodies. Furthermore, because the worms are usually incompletely developed, microfilaremia occurs only in the rarest of circumstances. These "abnormal" parasite infections do not respond to DEC, and their treatment is primarily surgical.

Dissanaike AS: Zoonotic aspects of filarial infections in man. Bull WHO 57:349, 1979. *A scholarly, readable discussion of the human's interaction with zoonotic filarial infections.*

389   ARTHROPODS AND LEECHES
William L. Krinsky

ARTHROPODS AS AGENTS OF DISEASE

Disease associated directly with arthropods results from toxins, or allergic responses to the organisms or their products when humans are exposed by bites or stings, simple contact, or invasion through the skin or natural orifices. Arthropods most often involved in these types of exposure are listed in Table 389–1.

Physicians usually become aware of insects and their relatives (spiders, mites, ticks, scorpions, millipedes, and centipedes) when patients present with skin lesions caused by arthropods, when infestations of the creatures themselves are seen, when foreign bodies extracted from skin or sense organs are identified as arthropods, or when respiratory symptoms develop in response to arthropods or their products. Dermatoses associated with arthropods and human infestations with arthropods (e.g., lice, mites, fly larvae) are discussed in detail in this chapter. Arthropods as vectors are mentioned here; detailed discussions of arthropod-borne pathogens may be found elsewhere in this book.

Biting Arthropods

LOUSE INFESTATIONS (Pediculosis)

Pediculosis is infestation of the body with lice. The observation of louse eggs (nits) cemented to hairs of the scalp or lice themselves confirms the diagnosis of head louse *(Pediculus capitis)* infestation. Nits (or lice) attached to the seams of clothing (often in undergarments) indicate the presence of body lice *(P. humanus)*, and nits or lice attached to pubic hairs indicate a pubic (crab) louse *(Phthirus pubis)* infestation.

The eggs are pearly yellow-white and opaque, elongate-oval, about 0.8 mm long and 0.3 mm wide, and are attached singly to each hair or clothing fiber. After hatching, the nits appear translucent and opalescent. Although nits may be numerous, usually not more than 10 to 20 lice are associated with infested persons. The head louse egg is cemented on a hair about 1 mm above the scalp surface.

Head and body lice are very similar in appearance. Adult head lice are 2.5 to 3.5 mm long, and adult body lice are 3.0 to 4.5 mm

TABLE 389–1. ARTHROPODS CAUSING HUMAN PATHOLOGY

Human Exposure	Arthropod	Antigens or Toxins
Bites	Insects (lice, bedbugs, and other true bugs; fleas; flies including mosquitoes, black flies, biting midges, sandflies, horse and deer flies, stable flies, tsetse flies, keds; ants)	Salivary secretions, venoms
	Arachnids (chigger and other rodent and bird mites; ticks, spiders)	
	Centipedes	
Stings	Insects (some ants, wasps, and bees)	Venoms
	Arachnids (scorpions)	
Invasion	Insects (fly larvae, *Tunga* fleas)	Salivary secretions, excretions
	Arachnids (scabies mites)	
Simple contact	Insects (caterpillars, pupae, or adults of moths and butterflies; blister and some rove beetles)	Setae, spines, secretions (venoms) and excretions
	Arachnids (stored product mites)	
	Millipedes	

long. Each immature and adult head and body louse has three pairs of about equal-sized legs bearing claws for gripping hairs or fibers. Adult pubic lice, somewhat crablike in appearance, are 1 to 2 mm long, about as broad, grayish white or yellowish brown, and they have forelegs narrower than the other pairs. All immature lice (three stages in each species) resemble their respective adults except in size, and all immature lice and adults are obligate bloodsucking ectoparasites. The body louse is the only known natural vector of the pathogens of louse-borne typhus, trench fever, and louse-borne relapsing fever.

Head lice and their nits are found most frequently in the hair over the postauricular and occipital regions. Body lice are usually not found on the body but are seen in clothing, with nits in the seams and creases in areas that contact the body. Crab lice and nits are found on hairs in the pubic and perianal regions, sometimes on hairs on the thighs and abdomen, less commonly on axillary hairs, beard, mustache, eyebrows, eyelashes, and rarely on the scalp. Pubic infestations are found only in postpubertal individuals.

The skin lesions produced by the bites of lice are erythematous papules that may be accompanied by urticaria or lymphadenopathy. Extensive erythema and pruritus result from hypersensitivity to louse saliva. Crab lice typically induce nonpruritic small gray-blue macules (0.3 to 1.0 cm in diameter) with irregular borders (maculae ceruleae) that may persist for months. The lesions produced by any of the species may be covered with hair matted with eggs, dried serous secretions, and dark louse excrement. The latter, seen on the body or in underclothing, should trigger a search for lice. Excoriations from scratching disguise bite lesions and may lead to impetigo or to furuncular or eczematous lesions. The possibility of louse infestation should be considered when pyoderma is seen. The combination of lichenification and pigmentation in chronically infested individuals is called vagabond's disease (morbus vagabondus). A nondescript macular or papular erythematous rash on the trunk may be the presenting sign for an undiscovered head louse infestation. Postauricular and posterior cervical lymphadenopathy in the absence of other node enlargement should suggest head lice. Body louse infestation may be differentiated from scabies by the absence of lesions on the hands and feet and the common occurrence of lesions in the intrascapular region. The differential diagnosis of louse-induced dermatitis from various mite-induced lesions or non–arthropod-associated dermatoses is made by finding nits or lice.

Treatment includes shampoos, creams, and lotions containing insecticides. The most often used preparations contain lindane (γ benzene hexachloride) or pyrethrins. Malathion and permethrin, a synthetic pyrethrin, are being used more frequently because of their ovicidal effect. One effective treatment for head lice is a shampoo with permethrin (1%) creme rinse. Pubic louse infestations in nonocular regions are effectively treated with a 5-minute application of lindane (1%) shampoo to the infested areas. Lindane should be used with caution on infants, children, and pregnant women. Infested clothing and linen should be washed in hot water (60°C) for 20 minutes or dry cleaned.

After treatment, lice and nits can be removed using a metal comb with teeth 0.1 mm apart. Moisture or oil rinses may make this easier. Mechanical removal is recommended for facial pubic louse infestations.

Preventing recurrence involves treatment of infested human contacts and materials (fomites). Pillow cases, hats, scarves, and other items should be washed or cleaned. Infested combs and brushes should be cleaned and boiled or soaked for 1 hour in lindane shampoo or Lysol (2%). Head and body lice survive only about 3 days (10 days maximum) away from the body. Sexual partners of persons with pubic lice should be treated, and bedding, towels, and clothing should be washed or dry cleaned. Pubic lice do not survive longer than 24 hours away from a body. Transmission via toilet seats is unlikely. Fumigation after any louse infestation is unnecessary, but vacuuming is helpful to remove stray lice and shed hairs with affixed nits.

FLEA BITES

Most fleas, unlike lice, do not infest the body. The common flea species that suck blood from humans visit the body for a few minutes to hours, when feeding occurs. As in louse infestations, flea bites generally cause pruritus. Each bite lesion is an erythematous papule with a hemorrhagic punctum. Sensitization of an individual to flea saliva may result in papular urticaria (common in affected children), bullous eruptions, or erythema multiforme-type lesions. Bites are usually multiple and irregularly grouped. Bites in adults appear as widespread papules that become lichenified or as grouped papules overlying erythema or edema. Persons entering a previously infested room that has been vacant for weeks or months often suffer from multiple bites on the ankles and legs as hungry fleas emerge from pupal cocoons in floor crevices, debris, or carpeting. As with louse bites, excoriated lesions may become infected and furuncular.

Flea eggs are usually laid off the host, and larvae live off the host, feeding on organic debris. Adults reach their hosts by jumping. Flea species that most often bite humans are the cat flea (Ctenocephalides felis), the dog flea (C. canis), and the human flea (Pulex irritans). Occasionally, household infestations with fleas may arise from abandoned wild animal nests built near houses.

Treatment of flea bites is symptomatic and involves using antipruritic and anti-inflammatory creams or lotions or oral antihistamines. Secondary infections may require antibiotic therapy. Infested pets should be treated with specific insecticides. Floors, carpets, upholstered furnishings, and pets' sleeping quarters should be sprayed or dusted with insecticides to kill larval, pupal, and adult fleas. A thorough cleaning, including vacuuming, of infested premises should eliminate the insects. Because fleas at all stages can live for weeks or months, a repeat insecticide application may be necessary.

Persons may protect themselves from fleas with repellents containing diethyl metatoluamide. Wild animal (especially rodent) fleas that feed on humans may transmit the bacilli of plague or tularemia, as well as the less virulent rickettsia of murine (flea-borne) typhus. Less common pathogens transmitted by accidental ingestion of fleas (mostly by children) are the dwarf tapeworm Hymenolepis diminuta and the dog tapeworm Dipylidium caninum.

BEDBUGS AND KISSING BUGS

Bedbugs (Cimicidae) are flat, mahogany-brown, wingless insects (5 to 7 mm long). Most species are bloodsucking ectoparasites of birds and bats. Two species (Cimex lectularius and C. hemipterus) feed almost exclusively on humans; the former is cosmopolitan; the latter has a tropical distribution. Both species cause irritating, pruritic bite lesions in sensitized individuals. The bugs become engorged with blood in 3 to 15 minutes and feed only at night or in subdued light. They hide in crevices of bedding, beds, floors, and furnishings and in wood and paper trash accumulations during the day. The bites are often seen in short linear groups and vary from small urticarial lesions to large erythematous papules or bullae. The lesions are often excoriated, and eczematous reactions and pyoderma may be seen. Hypersensitivity reactions may include asthma, generalized urticaria, and arthralgia. Although some affected persons complain of being awakened at night, most are troubled by the lesions on arising in the morning. Treatment is symptomatic. Prevention includes removing debris that harbors the bugs, using insecticides in crevices, and cleaning infested furnishings.

Triatomine kissing bugs (Reduviidae) that suck blood from a diversity of hosts are found in the New World subtropics and tropics and in Asia. Most of these cone-nosed bugs (8 to 38 mm long) are tan, brown, or black, with yellow or red spots around the dorsal edge of the abdomen. The bugs feed rapidly at night. Sensitive individuals may develop papular lesions, small vesicles, or, in the extreme, large urticarial or hemorrhagic nodular to bullous lesions. Generalized anaphylactoid reactions, including shock and angioneurotic and laryngeal edema, have occurred. Kissing bugs may feed anywhere on the body. Domesticated species in the tropics are found most often in thatched houses or those with mud floors. In the southwestern United States, a species (Triatoma protracta) living in wood rat nests in desert areas occasionally invades homes. Treatment of bites or allergic reactions is symptomatic. In Central and South America, these insects are vectors of Chagas' disease trypanosomes.

MOSQUITOES AND OTHER BLOODSUCKING FLIES

Mosquitoes (Culicidae) are found worldwide, breeding wherever there is stagnant water. While biting, a female mosquito (3 to 6 mm long) induces a pruritic wheal that becomes an erythematous papule. In sensitive persons, bullous lesions, cellulitis, or hemorrhagic necrotic reactions may follow the bites. Systemic anaphylactic reactions are rare. The most serious medical problems associated with mosquitoes relate to their transmission of the agents of yellow fever, dengue, arboviral encephalitides, malaria, and filariasis.

Biting midges (Ceratopogonidae), also called "punkies" or "no-see-ums" because of their minute size (most are 0.6 to 2 mm long), give a painful bite. The resulting erythematous punctiform lesions may become papular and pruritic. Vesicles may develop that ooze fluid for days. These midges, especially *Culicoides* species, bite mostly on exposed parts of the body and may be pestiferous in sandy seashore or marshy breeding areas. Biting occurs mostly at dawn or dusk.

Black flies (Simuliidae), also called buffalo gnats, are small (1 to 5 mm long), humpbacked, tan to black insects that breed only in running water. They are troublesome bloodsuckers in northern temperate regions. The bites may become hemorrhagic papules that ooze blood for hours. These lesions may be painful and cause recurrent pruritus. Lymphadenopathy is common in sensitive individuals, who may develop localized edema. Cephalalgia, fever, and nausea may occur following large numbers of bites. Black fly species found at high elevations in Central and South America and along rivers in Africa transmit *Onchocerca volvulus,* the etiologic agent of river blindness.

Phlebotomine sandflies (Psychodidae) are delicate, small (2 to 3 mm long), hairy flies found mainly in subtropical and tropical areas. Various species are abundant in rain forests in the New World and in arid areas in the Mediterranean region and Asia. Biting occurs at night or in subdued light. The bites may be painful, occur usually on the extremities, and cause pruritus and elevated pale urticarial lesions that become papular. Vesicular or bullous lesions may occur. Phlebotomine flies are vectors of sandfly (pappataci) fever, bartonellosis, and leishmaniasis.

Other flies that may attack humans and cause painful bites are horse and deer flies (Tabanidae), stable flies, and tsetse flies. Tsetse flies, found only in Africa, transmit the trypanosomes of African sleeping sickness.

Treatment of any of these fly bites is symptomatic and includes topical corticosteroids and oral antihistamines to reduce itching. Personal protection from biting flies involves using screen enclosures, headnets, and insect repellents. Protective clothing and open mesh jackets impregnated with repellents are effective.

CHIGGERS AND OTHER BITING MITES

Chiggers are the larvae (six-legged stage) of trombiculid (itch or harvest) mites. These larvae (0.15 to 0.40 mm long) are white to yellow or orange-red and are found on many vertebrates. Human infestation occurs following contact with grassy or shrubby vegetation inhabited by the mites. First exposure may not produce dermatitis or may produce only slightly irritating, transient erythematous macules or papules (1 to 2 mm). The more commonly seen skin reactions to chigger feeding are extremely pruritic, papular, papulovesicular, or papulourticarial lesions (4 to 20 mm) that persist with burning and itching for days to weeks. The lesions may fade and flatten or become hemorrhagic, purpuric, or vesicular. Diagnosis depends on morphology and distribution of lesions, exposure history, and observation of the mites. Engorging chiggers may be apparent as minute reddish blebs embedded in hair follicles. The mites most often attach to skin covered by clothing, especially near belts, straps, or elastic bindings. Scrub itch mites of Asia and South Pacific Islands usually do not cause dermatitis, but they are vectors of scrub typhus rickettsiae.

Other biting mites that are rarely recovered from the lesions they cause are pyemotid (straw, hay, or grain itch) mites, cheyletoid (cat or dog fur and predatory) mites, and dermanyssid (chicken, red, house mouse, tropical rat, fowl, and rodent) mites. All of these mites are extremely small (about 0.4 to 1 mm long), and depending on the species, the six-legged larvae or eight-legged nymphs and adults may attack humans. The resulting skin lesions may be extremely variable.

The differential diagnosis of mite-induced dermatitis depends on associating the patient with a source of mites. Sources include wild and domestic animals, agricultural commodities, dried floral arrangements, infested furniture, and, in chigger-associated cases, particular outdoor habitats.

Treatment of dermatitis is symptomatic. Antipruritic lotions and creams or oral antihistamines are useful. Secondary infections may

require antibiotic therapy. Rare allergic reactions, including edema and asthma, require emergency treatment. Prevention of recurrences depends on destroying or fumigating the mite source. Personal repellents (containing sulfur or diethyltoluamide) are helpful in preventing chigger infestation, although avoiding infested areas is the best prevention. *Rickettsia tsutsugamushi* is the only pathogen of major medical importance specifically associated with mite transmission. *R. akari*, the causative agent of rickettsialpox, is transmitted by the house mouse mite.

TICK BITES AND TICK PARALYSIS

Ticks, like mites, are arachnids that have six-legged larvae and eight-legged nymphs and adults. Ticks, found worldwide, are grouped in two major families, soft ticks (Argasidae) and hard ticks (Ixodidae). The former, which have rugose integuments, are associated with restricted habitats, such as rodent burrows and bird nests, and rarely feed on humans. When they do, most attach for only a matter of minutes and produce maculate, erythematous lesions (6 to 30 mm in diameter). Some species in Africa cause extensive ecchymosis; pain, pruritus, edema, ulceration, and necrotic lesions have also been observed. The pajoroello (talaja) tick (*Ornithodoros coriaceus),* found in Mexico, California, and Oregon, is known to produce hemorrhagic, painful lesions. Soft ticks are of primary medical importance as vectors of the borreliae of relapsing fevers.

Hard ticks have smooth, hard, shiny integuments and are found on a diversity of animals and in grass and forests. Ticks carried on dogs, cats, or other animals sometimes drop off and attach to humans. Hard ticks remain embedded in the skin for days while becoming engorged with blood and usually do not cause pain or discomfort. Engorging ticks, mistakenly identified as pedunculated moles or warts, are usually noticed only by chance observation. Typical tick bite lesions are small indurations with peripheral erythema. Unusual manifestations of hard tick bites include various forms of nonspecific dermatitis, acrodermatitis chronica atrophicans, necrotic ulcers, and alopecia. Most hard ticks attach, feed, drop off, and are never noticed. Nodular lesions that may persist for years at the sites of bites must be differentiated from malignant conditions, such as lymphomas. Hard ticks are vectors of the causative agents of various arboviral hemorrhagic fevers and encephalitides, several kinds of tickborne typhus (including Rocky Mountain spotted fever), tularemia, babesiosis, erhlichiosis, and Lyme disease. An engorging tick itself may induce tick paralysis (discussed below).

Attached soft ticks may be easily removed by gentle traction with a forceps. Hard ticks require strong constant traction. Use of heat, flames, or caustic substances may cause unnecessary harm to the patient. Hard ticks, embedded in sensitive sites, such as the ear canal or genitals, may be covered with petrolatum. The ticks then detach within about 2 hours and can be gently removed. Complete extraction of the mouthparts lessens the chance of secondary infection. Persistent nodules that cause discomfort should be surgically excised.

Tick paralysis is an unusual form of ascending flaccid paralysis that occurs while a tick is attached to the body. Mostly children (especially girls) are affected. Tick paralysis in humans has been associated with only a small number of hard tick species in North America, Europe, South Africa, and Australia. Most cases have been caused by the Rocky Mountain wood tick (*Dermacentor andersoni*) in western North America and the common dog tick (*D. variabilis)* in eastern North America. Although nonspecific numbness or irritability may occur before the onset of paralysis, the initial consistent sign is *weakness in the legs*. Leg tendon reflexes are reduced or absent, and Romberg's sign is often present. Sensory changes are rarely noted. Blood counts and lumbar puncture usually give no indication of the disease. Complete paralysis of the extremities may occur within a few days after a tick attaches. If the cause is unrecognized, paralysis usually progresses, causing speech dysfunction, dysphagia, and ultimately death from aspiration or respiratory paralysis. If a tick is found, removal usually results in reversal of paralysis with a return to normal function in hours to weeks, depending on the severity of the neurologic deficit. The patient should be examined for other ticks, with special attention to concealed areas, such as the scalp, ear canals, axillae, popliteal fossae, anus, and genitals. Even after all ticks are removed, death may occur from bulbar or respiratory paralysis.

The clinical presentation of tick paralysis may suggest poliomyelitis, Guillain-Barré syndrome, diphtheritic polyneuropathy, transverse myelitis, botulism, or other acutely developing neuropathies. The specific agent of *Dermacentor* tick paralysis is unknown. Prevention of tick bites and tick paralysis includes avoiding tick-infested habitats. Individuals and their pets who enter such habitats should be thoroughly examined for ticks. Personal measures that may prevent ticks from reaching the skin include wearing long-sleeved shirts and long pants, tucking pants legs into socks, and using chemical repellents.

SPIDER BITES

All spiders are eight-legged arachnids that use venom to immobilize their prey. Relatively few species have mouthparts (chelicerae) large and strong enough to inject venom into human skin. Among the better known spiders that cause moderate to severe reactions in humans are the widows (*Latrodectus* species) of the Old and New World, brown spiders (*Loxosceles* species) of the Americas and southern Africa, wandering spiders (*Phoneutria* species) in South America, species of *Chiracanthium* in both hemispheres, and funnel web spiders (*Atrax* species) in Australia.

The black widow (shoe button) spider *(Latrodectus mactans)* female may bite if it or its web is disturbed. Its abdomen is 6 mm wide and 9 to 13 mm long and is shiny black with a reddish hourglass marking or less well defined markings on the underside. The spider lives in sheltered, dark, dry places, such as in garages and in old stone walls and outhouses. The bite, which may not be felt, may become slightly swollen and appear as two erythematous puncture marks. Within a few hours, a bitten person develops intense muscle pains and commonly a tightening feeling in the chest. Abdominal (boardlike) rigidity and waves of excruciating cramping pain are characteristic. Respiratory distress, nausea, vomiting, profuse perspiration, headache, vertigo, paresthesias of the extremities, hyperactive reflexes, speech difficulty or visual dysfunction may occur. In untreated adults, the pathologic effects of the venom usually disappear within 2 to 3 days. Death from cardiac or respiratory arrest occurs mostly in very young children and elderly or hypertensive persons.

The differential diagnosis requires consideration of various abdominal and vascular crises, such as perforated ulcer, acute appendicitis or pancreatitis, cholelithiasis, nephrolithiasis, splenic, renal, or mesenteric embolism, volvulus, porphyria, tetanus, and strychnine and lead poisoning. The generalized muscle pain, the lack of abdominal tenderness, and the peripheral sensory changes help to differentiate the widow spider bite.

A specific antivenin is effective against all *Latrodectus* venom and neutralizes the effects of the venom. Because the antivenin is derived from horses, horse serum sensitivity testing is required before the antivenin is administered. Parenteral opioids and benzodiazepines relieve pain in patients who cannot take antivenin.

The brown (violin or fiddleback) spiders, including *Loxosceles reclusa* (brown recluse) and *L. laeta* of the western hemisphere, are also secretive, living in secluded places in houses and nesting in clothing, and they may bite when disturbed. They are 10 to 15 mm long and have a dark violin-shaped mark on the brown to gray cephalothorax. Their bites are most often recognized when a serious condition, *necrotic arachnidism,* is the result. The sometimes painful lesion that develops 2 to 6 hours after a bite is a bulla or pustule surrounded by concentric rings of ischemia and erythema. Within 24 to 48 hours, the lesion becomes cyanotic, and a central necrotic area begins to form. This area may slowly expand (up to 20 cm) over days to weeks. The resulting ulcer may not heal for weeks or months. Systemic reactions to the bite include fever, chills, edema, nausea, vomiting, dizziness, myalgias, and arthralgias; morbilliform and petechial eruptions may occur within 48 hours of the bite. A fatal complication, most often seen in children, is *intravascular hemolysis,* followed by hemoglobinuria and acute renal failure.

Treatment of necrotizing lesions is mainly symptomatic and may include antibiotic therapy for secondary infection. Curettage of bite wounds under local anesthesia as well as dapsone therapy promotes healing.

CENTIPEDE BITES

Centipedes are multilegged, elongated (up to 30 cm) arthropods with one pair of legs on each body segment. The first pair of legs is modified as poison claws that are used to inject venom into prey. Centipedes, which shun the light and are found under rocks and forest litter, rarely bite. The characteristic bite lesion has two punctate hemorrhages in the center of an erythematous swelling. Centipede bites may cause severe (fiery) local pain that may be followed by inflammation, edema, and superficial necrosis. Systemic reactions may include headache, dizziness, and vomiting. The transient effects of a bite may be accompanied by irregular pulse, muscle spasm, or lymphadenopathy. In general, centipede bites cause no long-term pathologic effects.

Stinging Arthropods
BEE, WASP, AND ANT STINGS

Bees, wasps, and ants (order Hymenoptera) include solitary and social species. Females have an egg-laying tube (ovipositor) that has been modified as a sting that secretes venom from abdominal glands. Social bees include honeybees and bumblebees, which all have two pairs of membranous wings and are stocky, hairy, and often yellow and black or brown. The honeybee *(Apis mellifera)* and its close relatives are found worldwide and often are responsible for human sting reactions. The honeybee has a barbed sting that becomes embedded in skin, and as the bee tries to escape, it leaves its venom apparatus and other abdominal organs and soon perishes. Vespid wasps (yellow jackets, hornets, paper wasps) are smooth insects, sleeker than bees and often yellow and black or with combinations of yellow, red, brown, or black. These wasps make the paper nests found in trees, under eaves of houses, or underground. Honeybees and bumblebees may sting when disturbed while seeking nectar or pollen at flowers. Vespid wasps may become pestiferous around food. Mutillid wasps (velvet ants, cow killers), which are hairy and wingless, sometimes sting in sandy, arid environments.

Human reactions to stings usually include intense local pain, followed by the appearance of a red punctum surrounded by a blanched area and erythema. A wheal forms and the swelling and erythema, accompanied by pruritus, may last for a few hours. Multiple stings, especially on the face, may cause extensive edema, multiple vesicles, bullae, or purpura. Treatment includes gentle removal of the sting by scraping with a sharp blade (in cases of honeybee envenomation), and use of ice and topical hydrocortisone or oral antihistamines. Severe and sometimes fatal allergic reactions to stings of bees and wasps in sensitized individuals are discussed in Ch. 227.

Ants (Formicidae) of some species can sting, causing severe pain. Two groups of New World stinging ants are the fire ants (*Solenopsis* species) and harvester ants (*Pogonomyrmex* species). These ants build ground nests that protrude as large mounds. An ant may grip the skin with its mandibles and then insert its sting. The ant may pivot and sting many times. This behavior, compounded by the common occurrence of mass attacks, leads to a clustering of lesions. The usual reaction to the sting is fiery, sharp pain, followed by a wheal and flare response. A clear vesicle appears that becomes pustular after about 24 hours. This sterile pustule may persist for 3 to 10 days and dry as a crust that sloughs, leaving a macule, scar, or fibrous nodule. Systemic reactions such as dizziness, nausea, vomiting, profuse perspiration, cyanosis, and asthma occur in allergic individuals but may also be seen in cases of multiple stings. Symptomatic treatment of local reactions is similar to that for bee and wasp stings.

SCORPION STINGS

Scorpions are mostly subtropical and tropical arachnids that have a pair of lobster-like claws (pedipalps) anteriorly and a curved spine posteriorly that is an outlet for the proteinaceous venom produced by a pair of venom glands. Scorpions are nocturnal predators that sting quickly and repeatedly when disturbed in their hiding places under rocks, lumber, and vegetation or in shoes, bedding, or clothing left on the ground. In the United States, one scorpion species, *Centruroides exilicauda,* of about 40 native species causes severe pathologic effects. This small (about 6 cm long), straw-colored species is found in Arizona. The arid regions that extend from

North Africa to India are inhabited by the most abundant and dangerous scorpions.

The nature and severity of human reactions to scorpion stings are not consistent with the size, appearance, or aggressiveness of different species. Intense and immediate pain at the site of a sting is common to all cases. When a mildly toxic scorpion is involved, the pain may be followed by local swelling and perhaps skin discoloration, regional lymphadenopathy, pruritus, or paresthesias, and less commonly by nausea and vomiting. These reactions are transient, lasting for minutes to as long as 24 hours. The more toxic species cause local pain but little or no skin response, and systemic effects are usually noted within a few minutes to 24 hours after the sting. Symptoms may include anxiety, drowsiness, syncope, increased salivation, lacrimation, perspiration, diminished vision, photophobia, numbness and sluggishness of the tongue, vomiting, diarrhea or involuntary defecation and micturition, priapism, muscular fibrillations or spasms, and convulsions. Clinical signs may include hypotension or hypertension, irregular pulse, tachycardia and arrhythmias, irregular respiration, rapid shifts in body temperature, oliguria or polyuria, and hemiplegia. Laboratory tests may reveal hyperglycemia, glycosuria, aspartate transaminase (AST) increase, hematuria, and melena. Pathologic changes that may lead to death include myocarditis, pulmonary edema, and shock. Respiratory paralysis is the usual immediate cause of death. In the most toxic cases, death may occur within minutes of the sting or not for over 40 hours later, but most deaths occur in 2 to 20 hours after the sting. The mortality is highest in children. It is important to closely monitor affected patients because sudden relapses, often involving acute respiratory distress, may occur after a patient's condition seems to have stabilized.

The most important treatment for moderate to very toxic stings is an antivenin. Antivenin to *C. exilicauda* is available in Arizona from the Antivenom Production Laboratory, Arizona State University, Tempe, Arizona 85281 (602-965-6443 or 602-965-1457) and Poison Control in Phoenix (602-253-3334). Antivenins against other species are available from laboratories in Mexico, Brazil, Europe, Africa, and Asia. In India, where antivenin is not available, acute pulmonary edema and hypertension have been successfully treated with vasodilators, such as prazosin hydrochloride.

Early treatment of stings may include cooling the sting site for up to 2 hours and using a local anesthetic. Oxygen administration or artificial respiration, sodium phenobarbital injection, and parenteral solutions, including blood plasma, may be needed to treat respiratory distress, convulsions, and shock, respectively. Calcium gluconate (10 ml of 10% solution) given as a slow intravenous injection reduces muscle spasms. In the United States, morphine and meperidine are contraindicated because they enhance the toxic effects of *C. exilicauda* venom. Morphine and barbiturates are not recommended for treating scorpion stings because these drugs inhibit the bulbar respiratory centers.

Personal protection includes wearing heavy gloves and boots when reaching into hidden areas in which scorpions may hide. Shaking out shoes and other materials left on the ground before using them is essential. Removing litter from around houses, sealing cracks in foundations, and selective use of pesticides are helpful means of preventing scorpions from inhabiting houses and gardens.

Invasive Arthropods

SCABIES

The scabies mite *(Sarcoptes scabiei)*, unlike the other mites discussed, burrows into the skin and, because it reproduces on humans, can maintain a continuous infestation. Fertile female mites burrow into the skin and lay their eggs as they tunnel. Immature stages (larvae and nymphs) move out to the surface and enter hair follicles. Further development and mating take place near the skin surface. The mite burrows are slightly raised, curved, or tortuous gray lines, 5 to 15 mm long, and at the end of each is a female, a minute pearly bleb. The burrows are restricted to the horny layer of the skin and occur most often in the sides of the fingers, the interdigital webs, flexor surfaces of the wrists, elbows, skin around the nipples, and penis. Other lesions, including erythematous papules, lichenified patches, and pustules, which occur in sites other than the burrows, may be seen on the abdomen, thighs, and buttocks. In infants and young children, burrows may occur in the palms and soles, and papular lesions may be seen on the scalp, face, and neck.

Intense pruritus begins from 2 to 6 weeks after first exposure to the mite. Definitive diagnosis of the lesions is often difficult because of excoriations. In very clean individuals, few lesions may be present, and burrows may not be clearly visible. Generalized urticarial papules may result from previous treatment with fluorinated corticosteroids. Some patients have pruritic inflammatory nodules (≤ 12 mm in diameter) that occur on covered skin, especially the axillae, abdomen, scrotum, and penis. A severe form of scabies most often seen in immunologically compromised persons is called *crusted scabies.* As the name implies, warty plaques occur frequently on the hands and feet, and extensive scaling covers the scalp to the trunk or below. Horny debris collects under the fingernails, which are usually distorted and thickened. Pruritus, erythema, and lymphadenopathy may occur.

Diagnosis of any scabies infestation depends on observing a mite in skin scrapings of a burrow or *in situ,* by gently raising the top of a burrow with a sterile needle and looking with a magnifier. In most scabies cases, only 10 to 15 mites are present on the body. In crusted scabies, large numbers of mites are present. To obtain a scraping of a burrow, an area suspected of infestation is scraped with a scalpel blade. The scraped material is examined at 50 to 100 times magnification. The movements of a living mite may be observed if the material is placed on a slide without any mounting media. Otherwise, the scraping may be cleared in potassium hydroxide (20%) or suspended in mineral oil under a coverslip on the slide. The adult female mite is about 300 to 400 μm long, oval, with the dorsum convex and venter flattened. It has four pairs of legs, two pairs directed anteriorly and two posteriorly. Each anterior leg ends in an unjointed stalk with a distensible thin-walled sac at its tip; each posterior leg ends in a long, thick bristle. The size of the mite egg is about 100×150 μm.

Scabies lesions initially may be diagnosed as those of other skin conditions, e.g., neurodermatitis, dermatitis herpetiformis, lichen planus, and various other kinds of mite-associated dermatitis, such as that caused by *Cheyletiella* fur mites. The distribution of lesions and observation of the mite rule out these other diagnoses. Secondary infections appearing as pyoderma are common, and nephrogenic strains of streptococci infecting the lesions may cause acute glomerulonephritis.

Treatment of uncomplicated scabies is with one of various acaricides. Permethrin (5% in dermal cream) in a single-dose regimen of 8 to 14 hours has recently been used with success. Lindane (1%) cream or lotion is often used in an 8- to 12-hour treatment for adults, followed by thorough washing. Use of lindane on infants and pregnant women is discouraged. Pruritus and dermatitis may persist for days after adequate treatment. Antipruritic medications are often prescribed.

Transmission occurs during contact with infested persons or with clothing recently worn by such persons. Transmission between bed partners is common and does not require body contact. All household and intimate contacts should be treated to prevent recurrence or continued transmission. The female mite survives for only 2 to 3 days away from a host; therefore, as with louse infestations, fumigation is unnecessary. Clothing, especially undergarments, bedding, and towels, should be laundered in hot water.

Scabies mites infesting domestic animals, including dogs and cats, occasionally cause dermatitis in humans, but the lesions are usually limited to the areas that contact the animals. These mites are usually not recovered from humans.

MYIASIS AND TUNGIASIS

Myiasis is the infestation of living vertebrate tissue by fly larvae. Many flies (order Diptera) that normally deposit eggs or larvae on carrion, manure, or decaying organic matter sometimes deposit their immature stages in open wounds or infected human tissues. These include blow flies, also called greenbottle or bluebottle flies (Calliphoridae), flesh flies (Sarcophagidae), and house flies (Muscidae). The larvae of some of these flies are attracted to draining infections or to clothing stained with urine or feces. The larvae crawl into lesions or natural orifices when an infected person sleeps on the ground or is otherwise exposed to flies. Individuals immobilized because of physical illness or old age who have such open lesions or infections, and especially those who are living in poor sanitary conditions, are particularly susceptible. Urogenital myiasis may cause dysuria, hematuria, and pyuria.

Some fly larvae invade intact skin of domestic animals or humans; species in this group include the human bot fly (*Dermatobia hominis*) found in Central and South America, the African tumbu fly *Cordylobia anthropophaga,* and some species of *Wohlfahrtia* that have a predilection for the tender skin of infants.

Fly larvae that live in food, e.g., vinegar flies (Drosophilidae) and cheese skippers (Piophilidae), are sometimes accidentally ingested and may cause gastrointestinal discomfort.

Wound or dermal myiasis often results in furuncular lesions, and an infested individual notices a swelling and feels pain or movement under the skin where the larvae are feeding on tissue fluids. On top of a lesion can be seen two dark respiratory openings (spiracles) through which the larva breathes. Treatment consists of gently compressing the swelling and removing the larva with a forceps. A local anesthetic may be helpful because recurved spines may hold the larva tightly under the skin. Topical antibiotics are used to control or prevent secondary infections. Removal of larvae that crawl into sensory openings or urogenital and anal orifices may require irrigation or surgical intervention. Intestinal myiasis is usually self-limited, ceasing when the larvae are passed in the stool. Dermal myiasis of most kinds, if untreated, progresses until the mature larvae back out of the skin and drop to the ground to pupate. The physical and emotional distress caused by the presence of living larvae can be prevented if a physician considers the possibility of such an infestation and removes the larvae early in the infestation. Prevention requires frequent wound dressing changes and use of window and door screens.

Tungiasis is the infestation of vertebrate, including human, skin by the female flea *Tunga penetrans* (chigoe, jigger, or sand flea). This flea occurs in sandy soil in subtropical and tropical regions of the Americas, the West Indies, and Africa. It usually feeds between the toes, under a toenail, or in the sole of the foot and becomes embedded as it gorges on blood. The flea, which remains embedded permanently, may cause irritation, pain, or pruritus, and the resulting swelling is often pustular. Secondary skin infections and tetanus are complications of infestations, and autoamputation of digits in Africans is apparently caused by inflammatory reactions to the flea.

Treatment of tungiasis includes removing the flea with a sterile needle or blade, tetanus vaccination, and use of topical antibiotics. Personal protection against *T. penetrans* includes wearing footwear and using insect repellent. Sleeping above the ground surface usually prevents the flea from reaching the body.

Arthropods and Contact Dermatitis

Various species of nonbiting mites found in stored products may cause dermatitis when they contact human skin. These microscopic foodstuff mites (Acaridae, Glycyphagidae) are found in commodities, including grains, cereals, seeds, bulbs, dried herbs, copra, dried vegetables, cured meats, mushrooms, humus, cheese, and animal and plant material used for stuffing furniture, pillows, and mattresses. Dried fruit mites (Carpoglyphidae) are found not only in dried fruits but also in jams, jellies, spoiled fruit, wine, caramel, flour, and dried milk products. The skin reactions to these mites vary, but pruritic diffuse erythema with urticarial wheals or erythematous papular eruptions is common. Laborers in granaries, food-processing plants, and commercial kitchens and dockworkers are most susceptible.

Another form of pruritic dermatitis is caused by contact with various caterpillars, pupae, adults, and some egg masses of moths and butterflies (order Lepidoptera). Urticating setae and spines on these life forms may cause mechanical irritation of the skin or may have toxic effects. Contact with setae, spines, or hairs may cause intense stinging or fiery pain, followed by the formation of wheals, local edema, erythema, and pruritus. Less common reactions include lymphadenopathy, cephalalgia, shocklike symptoms, or convulsions.

Treatment of dermatitis caused by foodstuff and dried fruit mites or lepidopteran spines or setae is symptomatic. Antipruritic substances, including antihistamines, corticosteroids, and anesthetics, have been used. Commodities containing mites must be fumigated or destroyed. Spines or setae of lepidopterans may be removed

from the skin with fine forceps. Protective clothing and thorough washing of exposed materials help prevent continuation of these forms of dermatitis.

A third form of contact dermatitis results from vesicants produced by blister beetles (Meloidae) and some rove beetles (Staphylinidae). Cantharidin, first isolated from the meloid called the Spanish fly, is found in all species of blister beetles. Contact with this substance causes mild to severe vesicular dermatitis.

Similar lesions, which usually follow a burning sensation and tanning of the skin, result from contact with millipedes. Some species of these herbivorous myriapods exude a fluid from pores along the length of the body. Secretions from the aforementioned beetles or millipedes cause burning pain and conjunctivitis if they are rubbed into the eyes.

Treatment of toxic dermatitis associated with beetles or millipedes includes rapid washing of the skin or eyes, if affected, and use of local anesthetics. The dermal reactions caused by contact with mites, lepidopterans, beetles, and millipedes are usually transitory and do not have long-lasting effects.

PENTASTOMIASIS (Linguatuliasis)

Pentastomiasis is infestation with pentastomids, little-known arthropods called tongue worms. These bloodsucking endoparasites are found as adults in the lungs of reptiles and birds or in the nasal cavity of carnivores, especially cats and dogs. Herbivores are normal intermediate hosts, but humans and other mammals can be dead-end aberrant hosts for the larvae. Ingested eggs hatch, and the larvae burrow through the intestine and migrate to diverse tissues, where they molt several times and become encysted as third-stage larvae.

Human infestations have occurred in Europe, Africa, Asia, and North, Central, and South America. Two species account for most cases, *Armillifer armillatus,* found in pythons and other vipers in tropical Africa, and *Linguatula serrata,* found in canids in Europe and the Near and Middle East.

Infection occurs by accidental ingestion of tongue worm eggs, contaminating food or drink, picked up on fingers from handling infected snakes or lizards, or from improperly cooked or raw reptiles. The third-stage larvae (20 to 25 mm long) encysted in fibrous capsules occur most often in the liver and are rarely noted except incidentally at autopsy or as calcified cysts (3 to 6 mm in diameter) on radiographs. Rarely, a mass of cysts in the intestinal wall may cause obstruction. Cysts compressing vital structures such as bile ducts or bronchi may lead to infections or obstructions.

Linguatuliasis, the direct infection of humans with third-stage larvae of *Linguatula* species, occurs most often in Lebanese people who eat raw or inadequately cooked liver or lymph nodes of goats and sheep. The ingested larvae migrate to the nasopharynx from the stomach. These larvae (5 to 10 mm long) cause Halzoun's syndrome, characterized by paroxysmal coughing, sneezing, and nasal and lacrimal discharge, accompanied by pain and itching in the throat. Other symptoms may include hoarseness, dyspnea, dysphagia, and vomiting. Submaxillary and cervical lymph nodes may be enlarged. Recovery in most cases is spontaneous in 7 to 10 days; however, death from asphyxiation due to tonsillar edema has been reported. A similar syndrome seen in Sudan, Turkey, and Greece is called Marrara's syndrome.

Prevention of pentastomiasis includes proper cooking of exotic foods such as herbivore organs and reptiles, improved hygiene of persons handling reptiles, and ingestion only of clean water and thoroughly washed raw vegetables.

LEECHES AS AGENTS OF DISEASE (Hirudiniasis)

Leeches of medical importance are bloodsucking annelid worms. Each has a ventral anterior or posterior sucker. The former encloses teeth that cut through the skin after the leech attaches. Feeding occurs within a half hour or more.

The leeches most often feeding on humans are aquatic (freshwater) species of *Hirudo,* the cosmopolitan medicinal leeches; *Limnatis,* the nasal leeches found from the Canary Islands east through Europe, Africa, and Asia; *Dinobdella,* found in Asia; and terrestrial species of *Haemadipsa,* found in Asia, Indonesia, Australia, Pacific Islands, and Central and South America. Humans are subject to attack by large leeches in tropical rain forests or to infestation with aquatic species while wading or swimming.

Wounds produced by leeches often go unnoticed, except for the oozing blood or prolonged bleeding caused by an anticoagulant, hirudin. Pruritus is common at bite sites, and although leeches are not known to transmit any human pathogens, secondary infections may occur. Immature aquatic leeches may be ingested with water and infest the upper respiratory and digestive tracts or may invade the mouth, nose, eyes, vagina, urethra, or anus of swimmers.

Attachment of leeches to the nasal passages may cause epistaxis. Attachment to the larynx may cause hoarseness, dyspnea, and hemoptysis, and attachment to the pharynx or esophagus may cause dysphagia and hematemesis. Hemorrhaging from leech infestations may be so severe, especially in children, that anemia occurs, leading to death.

Techniques used for removing leeches from the respiratory and digestive tracts include a steady pull on the specimen with a forceps or hemostat or narcotizing the leech with a spray of 5% cocaine hydrochloride before removal. In genitourinary infestations, irrigation with a strong salt solution may cause the leeches to detach. A leech attached to skin or respiratory or digestive tract surfaces may be induced to release its grip by holding it in a hemostat and touching the exposed part of the worm with a small flame or other cauterant.

Preventing attack by aquatic and land leeches includes use of protective clothing and insect repellents. Repellents applied to boots, trouser legs, and exposed skin are quite effective, but, because they are water soluble, must be reapplied every few hours in wet tropical regions where leeches are commonly found.

Alexander JO: Arthropods and Human Skin. Berlin, Springer-Verlag, 1984. *This is the first and best comprehensive text devoted to dermatologic problems associated with arthropods.*

Clark RF, Wethern-Kestner S, Vance MV, et al.: Clinical presentation and treatment of black widow spider envenomation: A review of 163 cases. Ann Emerg Med 21:782, 1992. *This is the largest reported series of* Latrodectus *envenomations and the largest series to receive antivenin.*

Drabick JJ: Pentastomiasis. Rev Infect Dis 9:1087, 1987. *This review discusses biology, parasitology, clinical manifestations, pathology, diagnosis, treatment, and epidemiology.*

Hurwitz S: Clinical Pediatric Dermatology. Philadelphia, WB Saunders, 1993, p 405. *Has excellent photographs of lice and scabies and associated skin lesions, as well as a review of flea, bedbug, mosquito, and other arthropod bites and stings.*

Southcott RV: Injuries from Coleoptera. Med J Austral 151:654, 1989. *Discusses the nature of chemical irritants produced by beetles and reviews clinical cases.*

390 SNAKE BITES
Jay P. Sanford

EPIDEMIOLOGY. Of the nearly 3500 species of snakes, fewer than one tenth are venomous. The poisonous varieties belong to five families (Table 390–1). Throughout the world, snake bites are estimated to account for 30,000 to 40,000 deaths annually. The largest number occur in Burma (Russell's viper) and Brazil (*Bothrops* species, lance-headed vipers). In the United States, the number of snake bites is estimated at 8000 per year. Twenty to 60% of the bites by venomous snakes in the United States result in little or no envenomation (poisoning). The states with the highest bite rates are North Carolina, Arkansas, Texas, Georgia, West Virginia, Mississippi, and Louisiana. Despite the large number of bites with enven-

TABLE 390–1. VENOMOUS SNAKES OF THE WORLD

Family	Common Varieties	Geographic Distribution
Crotalidae	Pit vipers (rattlesnakes, water moccasins, copperheads), fer-de-lance, bushmaster	Americas, Asia
Elapidae	Cobras, kraits, mambas, coral snakes, death adder	Worldwide except Europe
Columbridae	Boomslangs, bird snakes	Africa
Hydrophidae	Sea snakes	Indo-Pacific waters
Viperidae	True vipers (Russell's viper), puff adder	Worldwide except Americas

omation, fewer than 15 deaths occur annually, and almost all these are due to rattlesnake bites.

Coral snakes, eastern and western varieties, are found in southern and western states (North Carolina, South Carolina, Georgia, Florida, Alabama, Mississippi, Louisiana, Arkansas, Texas, New Mexico, and Arizona). Their fangs are short and permanently erect. They envenomate through chewing movements. Since they are nocturnal and shy, they rarely bite humans.

The pit vipers (Crotalidae) are identified by a small depression between the eyes and nostrils. Their fangs are long and hinged, folding back when the mouth is closed and erect when open. Upon contact, venom is expressed by muscular contraction. The pit vipers are generally aggressive. The eastern (*Crotalus adamanteus*) and western (*C. atrox*) diamondback rattlesnakes are the largest and most dangerous in the United States. Their distribution includes the aforementioned states plus California, Nevada, and Oklahoma. Cottonmouths *(Agkistrodon piscivorus),* or water moccasins, are found along streams in the southern and southeastern states. They may inflict facial bites when disturbed while resting on tree branches. Contrary to lore, they can bite under water. Copperheads *(A. contortrix),* or highland moccasins, have a geographic distribution similar to the cottonmouths. Their bite is painful but rarely fatal.

PATHOGENESIS. Because of the heterogeneous composition and multiplicity of effects, snake venoms cannot be classified simply as neurotoxic, cardiotoxic, myotoxic, or hematotoxic on the basis of the snake family (Table 390–2).

Venoms from Elapidae and Hydrophiodae snakes contain basic polypeptides that produce presynaptic and/or postsynaptic neuromuscular block with resultant flaccid paralysis, including respiratory paralysis. Cobra cardiotoxin, an additional basic polypeptide, depolarizes cell membranes of skeletal, cardiac, and smooth muscles, thus contributing to paralysis. Venom of the South American rattlesnake (*Crotalus durissus*) contains an acidic protein with nondepolarizing curare-like neuromuscular blocking effects. Viperatoxin isolated from the Palestine viper causes a peripheral nerve conduction block. A variety of enzymes, mostly hydrolases and phospholipase A, are present in most venoms. Bradykinin is released from bradykininogen by most crotalid and viperid venoms but not by Elapidae except the king cobra (*Ophiophagus hannah*). The venom of a single snake seldom contains all of the toxins. The composition and potency of venom are highly variable and differ not only among species but even among individual snakes.

SYMPTOMS AND SIGNS. *Pit Viper Envenomation.* In the United States, most victims reach a physician within 15 minutes to 3 hours. At that time, it is essential to determine whether or not en-

TABLE 390–2. BIOCHEMISTRY OF SNAKE VENOMS

Toxins	Family	Mechanism of Injury/Death
Neurotoxin (basic polypeptide)	Elapidae, Hydrophidae, South American rattlesnake (*Crotalus durissus terrificus*), Palestine viper (*Vipera palestinae*)	Respiratory paralysis
Cardiotoxin	Elapidae	Cardiovascular depression
Enzymes	Elapidae, Hydrophidae, Crotalidae, Viperidae	Hemolysis
Phospholipase A		
5-Nucleotidase		
Phosphodiesterase		
Deoxyribonuclease II		
Ribonuclease		
Adenosine-triphosphatase		
Nucleotide pyrophosphatase		
Exopeptidase		
Hyaluronidase	(Absent in spitting cobra)	
L-Amino acid oxidase		
Acetylcholinesterase	Elapidae (absent in spitting cobra, mamba, coral snake)	
Alkaline phosphatase		
Acid phosphatase		

venomation has occurred and, if it has occurred, to determine the severity; this has important therapeutic implications. The clinical effects are summarized in Table 390–3. The most important early findings are swelling at the bite, usually occurring within 10 minutes, and pain, although pain may be absent. Mild envenomation is characterized by local edema (1 to 5 inches in diameter) and pain without systemic symptoms or signs. With moderate envenomation, local findings are more extensive—edema of 6 to 12 inches in diameter. Systemic findings occur: weakness, sweating, nausea, faintness, dizziness, ecchymoses, and tender regional lymph nodes. With severe envenomation, systemic involvement includes tachycardia, tachypnea, hypothermia, hypotension, ecchymoses, paresthesias of the scalp and finger and toe tips, and muscle fasciculations. With very severe envenomation, gingival bleeding, hematemesis, hematuria, melena, oliguria, and coma occur.

Over the first 12 hours, the skin develops a tense, discolored appearance and bullae, which may be either serous or hemorrhagic.

Coral Snake Envenomation. The bite wound usually resembles scratch marks and is somewhat painful, but there is little or no edema. The onset of systemic manifestations is usually delayed 1 to 6 hours. Paresthesias around the bite may occur within several hours. Systemic symptoms may include weakness, apprehension, giddiness, nausea, vomiting, excess salivation, and even a sense of euphoria. Bulbar and cranial nerve paralysis may develop with ptosis, diplopia, papillary dilation, excess salivation, dysphagia, dysphonia, and respiratory failure. Paralysis may last 6 to 14 days, and muscular strength may not be fully regained for 6 to 8 weeks.

LABORATORY FINDINGS. Proteolytic enzymes in venoms not only damage tissue but also have a marked effect on coagulation, thrombin-like activity being most prominent. Within the first few hours, there is a drop in platelets owing to local consumption (occasionally to < 10,000 per milliliter), a decrease in fibrinogen, and an increase in fibrin degradation products. Striking increases in prothrombin time and partial thromboplastin time occur with severe envenomation. Erythrocytes show a peculiar "burring," indicating membrane damage, and drops in hematocrit and hemoglobin concentration occur.

With pit viper envenomation, baseline laboratory tests should include complete blood count, platelet count, prothrombin time, partial thromboplastin time, bleeding time, urinalysis, and serum electrolytes. Blood should be obtained for typing and crossmatching. In patients with moderate or more severe envenomation, arterial blood gas determinations and an electrocardiogram are indicated. Hematologic studies should be repeated every 4 to 6 hours for the first day or until the coagulopathy has stabilized. With coral snake envenomation, repetitive coagulation studies are not indicated.

TREATMENT. **First Aid** (Table 390–4). The initial goal of first aid is to minimize systemic absorption of the toxin. This is accomplished by restraining the patient to minimize muscular activity, applying compressive dressings, and transporting to the hospital with as little effort exerted by the patient as circumstances permit. With neurotoxic venoms, absorption may result in respiratory arrest, for which resuscitation is essential. Respiratory paralysis may develop within 15 minutes following cobra bites. The snake should be killed if this can be done quickly and safely and taken with the patient to allow accurate identification; this may obviate unnecessary therapy. The dead snake must be handled with care, since the head of an ap-

TABLE 390–4. FIRST AID: GOAL: MINIMIZE SYSTEMIC ABSORPTION OF TOXIN UNTIL ANTIVENIN CAN BE ADMINISTERED

Do's	Don'ts
Minimize muscular activity and immobilize affected part (splint the limb, carry the patient).	
Wipe bite site.	Perform incision and suction of bite wound.
Kill snake and take with patient to enable accurate identification.	Allow "dead" snake to bite care givers or patient.
Apply absorption, delaying compressive bandage over bite site and up entire limb.	Apply tourniquet or occlude arterial blood supply.
Transport to nearest medical treatment facility.	Place affected part in ice.
Observe for respiratory arrest; pulmonary resuscitation may be required.	Give patient alcohol.

parently dead snake can deliver a venomous bite for up to an hour after being severed. The potential value of incision and suction is less than the risks, which include delay in antivenin (antivenom) administration. The site of the bite should be wiped but not incised. Incisions can aggravate bleeding, damage nerves and tendons, introduce infection (especially with mouth suction), and delay healing. An absorption-delaying compressive bandage, preferably crepe (not a tourniquet), should immediately be applied firmly, as for a sprain, over the bite site and up the entire limb. The affected part should be immobilized (splinted) promptly. If available, an inflatable splint provides both compression and immobilization. The patient should be promptly transported to the nearest medical treatment facility. The compressive bandage should not be released during transit. The affected area should not be placed in ice. Cryotherapy results in greater tissue damage with the potential for necessitating amputation.

Hospital Care. On admission it is important to determine, if possible, if the bite was inflicted by a pit viper—specifically, rattlesnake, moccasin, or copperhead—or a coral snake and whether envenomation has occurred. The mainstay of therapy is physiologic monitoring in an intensive care unit and, for rattlesnake bites with envenomation, antivenin, which is a horse serum product; hence it has a high potential of causing serum sickness later. There are two antivenins: one polyvalent for North American pit vipers and another for eastern coral snakes. Water moccasion and copperhead bites can be managed without antivenin, avoiding immediate anaphylactic reactions and later serum sickness. With rattlesnake bites, for minor envenomation, antivenin is not indicated. For more serious rattlesnake envenomation, antivenin should be administered. For mild envenomation, 3 to 5 ampules of antivenin should be diluted (10 ml each) and then added to 500 ml of intravenous fluid and infused over 30 minutes to 2 hours. Antivenin should not be given as one-ampule increments. Skin or conjunctival sensitivity tests are unreliable in predicting early reactions to antivenin. All patients given antivenin should be regarded as likely to have a reaction; the incidence ranges from 3 to 54%. Epinephrine should be available in a syringe before the infusion is started. At the first sign

TABLE 390–3. PIT VIPER ENVENOMATION: SYMPTOMS AND SIGNS (PERCENTAGE)

Local		Systemic							
		Generalized		Hematologic		Neuromuscular			
Fang marks	100	Weakness	70	Thrombocytopenia	42	Paresthesia of scalp, fingertips	63
Edema	74	Tachycardia	60	Increased clotting time	37	Faintness, dizziness	57
Pain	65	Hypotension	54	Decreased hemoglobin	37	Paresthesias of affected part	57
Vesicles	40	Sweating	43	Burring of RBC	18	Fasciculations	41
Necrosis	27	Nausea/vomiting	42	Thrombocytosis	16		
		Hypothermia	42	Bleeding	15		
		Tachypnea	40				
		Regional adenopathy	40				

Adapted from Russell FE: Snake venom poisoning in the United States. Annu Rev Med 31:247, 1980.

of anaphylactoid reaction, bronchospasm, hypotension, or angio-edema, the infusion should be stopped and 0.5 ml of 1:1000 epinephrine injected intramuscularly. This is almost always effective, and the antivenin infusion can be restarted. A history of allergy to horse serum contraindicates antivenin unless the risk of death from envenomation is high and the patient is pretreated with epinephrine. If the amount of antivenin is adequate, swelling will not progress and paresthesias will decrease. If progression occurs, the dose should be repeated. For moderate envenomation 5 to 10 vials, for severe envenomation 10 to 20 vials, and for very severe envenomation up to 40 vials (400 ml) may be required. In one series, the average dose required for adults with severe bites was 16 vials. Larger doses are required for bites in children and for those involving the fingers. Antivenin neutralizes both the local and the systemic effects of the venom.

In coral snake bites, if any symptoms or signs develop within the first several hours, 3 to 5 vials of antivenin (*Micrurus fulvius*) should be given intravenously. Even in the absence of symptoms, patients should be observed in the hospital for approximately 48 hours because onset of symptoms may be delayed and insidious. If neurotoxic signs appear (Table 390–3) an edrophonium test should be done: atropine sulfate (0.6 mg) given by slow intravenous infusion, followed by edrophonium chloride (10 mg) given intravenously over 2 minutes. If improvement occurs, neostigmine methylsulfate should be administered (beginning with 25 μg per kilogram of body weight per hour) by continuous infusion.

Antibiotics are usually recommended. Bacteriologic cultures of rattlesnake venom and fangs show growth from over 90% of specimens (venom or fangs) cultured. Aerobic gram-negative bacilli (*Enterobacter* sp., *Pseudomonas* sp.) and histotoxic clostridia (*Clostridum perfringens*) are the predominant isolates. On the basis of the microbiologic results, one of the newer β-lactam antibiotics—piperacillin, ceftazidime, ticarcillin clavulanate, or piperacillin tazobactam—is most appropriate. While clinical experience has not been reported, ciprofloxacin plus metronidazole orally should be an effective regimen. A tetanus toxoid booster is recommended.

In the severely envenomated patient, concurrent supportive measures include the management of shock and of respiratory and renal failure. Glucocorticoids have been recommended, but a controlled trial of prednisone therapy helped neither local nor systemic effects of viperine poisoning. Despite the hypofibrinogenemia and increase in fibrin degradation products, heparin is not of benefit.

Decompressive fasciotomy is indicated only if edema within closed muscular compartments is inadequately controlled, compartmental pressures are 30 mm Hg or higher, and arterial blood supply is compromised. From the end of the first to the third week, the majority of patients will develop serum sickness, the prevalence approximating 1% per milliliter of horse serum administered. Steroids are useful for treatment of serum sickness reactions.

PROGNOSIS. If adequate antivenin has been administered intravenously, mortality is virtually nil. If cryotherapy has been avoided, amputation or serious resultant deformities are uncommon. Only a few cases of snake bite poisoning in pregnancy have been reported. However, with envenomation by pit vipers, fetal loss has been 43% and maternal mortality 10%.

BITES CAUSED BY SNAKES NOT FOUND IN THE UNITED STATES

VIPER (VIPERIDAE) BITES. Bites by Russell's viper are the leading cause of fatal snake bite in Pakistan, India, Bangladesh, Sri Lanka, Burma, and Thailand. They are an occupational hazard of rice farmers. Up to 70% of the protein content of the venom is phospholipase A2, which can induce hemolysis, rhabdomyolysis, presynaptic neurotoxicity, and shock. Geographic variation in clinical manifestations is striking. The most common systemic signs are those of neurotoxicity; external ophthalmoplegia, ptosis, difficulty in opening the mouth ("pseudotrismus"), and inability to protrude the tongue. Symptoms include drowsiness, headache, vomiting, and abdominal pain. Incoagulable blood commonly leads to spontaneous hemorrhage, often massive. Generalized muscle tenderness, myoglobinuria, and oliguria also are common. In some countries, viper bite envenomation is the most common cause of acute renal failure. Management requires intensive supportive therapy and specific antivenin. Antivenin is most effective when administered within 4 hours, 400 to 500 ml often being required. Adequate doses restore blood coagulability but do not reverse shock, nephrotoxicity, or my-

otoxic signs. Causes of death include shock; pituitary, intracranial, and gastrointestinal hemorrhage; and tubular or renal cortical necrosis. Individuals who recover often show clinical or laboratory evidence of hypopituitarism.

COBRA (ELAPIDAE) BITES. Bites are almost invariably painful. Local necrosis is often preceded by bullae, which may not develop for 2 to 4 days after the bite. Neurotoxic symptoms may appear as early as 3 minutes after a bite, with onset rare after 6 hours. Respiratory paralysis may occur within 15 minutes. Responses to intravenous edrophonium chloride (administered as above) usually occur. The effectiveness of cobra antivenin is inconsistent. Maintaining adequate ventilation is essential. In survivors, neurotoxic manifestations usually resolve within a week.

Burch JM, Agarwal R, Mattox KL, et al.: The treatment of crotalid envenomation without antivenin. J Trauma 28:35, 1988. *A report of 81 patients managed by close physiologic monitoring in an intensive care unit without antivenin or surgical therapy. Excellent results were obtained.*

Curry SC, Kraner JC, Kunkel DB, et al.: Noninvasive vascular studies in management of rattlesnake envenomations to extremities. Ann Emerg Med 14:1081, 1985. *Provides details for monitoring, using noninvasive arterial studies. All but 1 of 25 patients received antivenin, and none underwent early surgical decompression.*

Dunnihoo DR, Rush BM, Wise RB, et al.: Snake bite poisoning in pregnancy. J Reprod Med 37:653, 1992. *A good review of snake bites in general as well as in pregnancy.*

Gold BS, Barish RA: Venomous snake bites. Emerg Med Clin North Am 10:249, 1992. *An excellent recent review.*

Malasit P, Warrell DA, Chanthavanich P, et al.: Prediction, prevention and mechanism of early (anaphylactic) antivenom reactions in victims of snake bites. Br Med J 292:17, 1986. *A study demonstrating the futility of intradermal and conjunctival tests for hypersensitivity.*

Tun-Pe, Phillips RE, Warrell DA, et al.: Acute and chronic pituitary failure resembling Sheehan's syndrome following bites by Russell's viper in Burma. Lancet 2:763, 1987. *A study of 33 patients; of 24 survivors, 46% had evidence of pituitary insufficiency.*

Watt G, Meade BD, Theakston RDG, et al.: Comparison of tensilon and antivenom for the treatment of cobra-bite paralysis. Trans R Soc Trop Med Hyg 83:570, 1989. *Results of a double-blind study of edrophonium versus placebo and a study of antivenin.*

391 VENOMS AND POISONS FROM MARINE ORGANISMS
Jay W. Fox

It is generally accepted that the term *envenomation* implies penetration by an organism for delivery of a venom containing one or more toxins. In contrast, poisons are toxins that are acquired from the environment by mechanisms such as absorption, inhalation, and ingestion. In the marine environment, both forms of intoxication occur, with effects ranging from mild irritation and discomfort to death. Previously, most clinically relevant intoxications were envenomations from marine organisms primarily found in tropical and subtropical waters. In recent times, however, severe outbreaks of poisoning from ingesting marine organisms containing toxins have occurred. This is likely due to increased microorganism growth in coastal waters as a result of eutrophication. Encroachment on the marine environment for recreation, living space, and food sources may be expected to increase the frequency of adverse encounters with venomous and poisonous marine organisms. This chapter discusses the marine organisms responsible for the majority of clinically significant intoxications, with emphasis on the pharmacologic and symptomatic properties of the toxins. Table 391–1 lists names of venomous and poisonous marine organisms that can produce severe intoxication or death and whether antivenin is available. The sites of action of some marine neurotoxins are depicted in Figure 391–1.

VENOMOUS MARINE ORGANISMS

Venomous marine organisms deliver their venoms by biting and stinging (Table 391–1). Envenomation involves penetration of the skin. Thus, consideration must be given to the potential of infection by microorganisms, especially in situations involving deep puncture

TABLE 391-1. SIGNIFICANT VENOMOUS AND POISONOUS MARINE ORGANISMS

Organism	Type of Envenomation (poisoning)	Primary Toxins	Antivenom Available
Sea snakes (Hydrophiidae)	Bite	Post-synaptic neurotoxin	Yes
Blue-ringed octopus (Octopodidae)	Bite	Post-synaptic neurotoxin (tetrodotoxin)	No
Cone shell (Conidae)	Bite	Pre- and post-synaptic neurotoxins	No
Box jellyfish (*Chironex fleekeri, Chiropsolmus quadrigatus*)	Sting	Hemolysins, proteinases, cardiotoxin necrotoxins	Yes
Portuguese man-o-war (*Physalia physalis*)	Sting	Hemolysins, proteinases, cardiotoxin necrotoxins	No; may be a need
Sea nettles (*Chrysaora quinquecirrha; Cyanea capillata*)	Sting	Hemolysins, proteinases, cardiotoxin necrotoxins	No; generally no need
Sea anemone (*Anemonia sulcata*)	Sting	Neurotoxins	No; generally no need
Scorpionfish (Scorpaenidae)	Sting/puncture	Hemolysins, necrotoxins ?	Yes
Lionfish (Scorpaenidae)	Sting/puncture	Hemolysins, necrotoxins ?	No
Stonefish (Scorpaenidae)	Sting/puncture	Hemolysins, necrotoxins ?	Yes
Weeverfish (Trachinidae)	Sting/puncture	Hemolysins, necrotoxins ?	No
Stingrays (Rajiformes)	Sting/puncture	?	No
Dinoflagellates			
Gambierdiscus toxicus	Poisonous (found in fish)	Ciguatera poisoning, ciguatoxins, maitotoxin (neurotoxins)	
Ptychodiscus brevis	Poisonous (found in shellfish)	Neurotoxic shellfish poisoning (NSP), neurotoxins	
Gonyaulax spp.	Poisonous (found in shellfish)	Paralytic shellfish poisoning (PSP)	
Pyrodinium spp.	Poisonous (found in shellfish)	Saxitoxin, neosaxitoxin and gonyautoxin	
Jania spp.	Poisonous (found in shellfish)	Okadaic acid (phosphatase inhibitors)	
Pufferfish (Tetraodontiformes)	Poisonous	Tetrodotoxin (neurotoxin)	No
Porcupinefish (Tetraodontiformes)	Poisonous	Tetrodotoxin (neurotoxin)	
Sunfish (*Mola* spp.)	Poisonous	Tetrodotoxin (neurotoxin)	

wounds and bites, as well as to the treatment of the toxicologic effects of the venom.

SEA SNAKES. Sea snakes are members of the family Hydrophiidae and are generally found in tropical and subtropical waters. Sea snakes are very common in the coastal waters of Thailand, Indonesia, the Persian Gulf, Australia, and India. With regard to the Americas, one species of sea snake, *Pelaramis platurus,* the yellow-bellied sea snake, is found in the Pacific coastal waters of Central America. These snakes are very capable swimmers but do not come ashore and are relatively immobile on land. They inject their venom with two small maxillary fangs (2 to 4 mm) containing ducts con-

nected to venom glands located posterior and ventral to the maxillary bone. The relatively short aspect of the fangs prevents effective envenomation through most protective clothing such as dive suits. In the case of human envenomation, if the subject reacts by violent retraction the fangs are often dislodged from the maxillary bone of the snake and may remain in the site.

Because of the nature of the venom and the size of the fangs, the sea snake bite itself is generally not painful. One or two small prick marks are present at the envenomation site, as occasionally are additional marks from the other teeth in the snake's mouth. The primary toxin in sea snake venom is a postsynaptic peptide neurotoxin

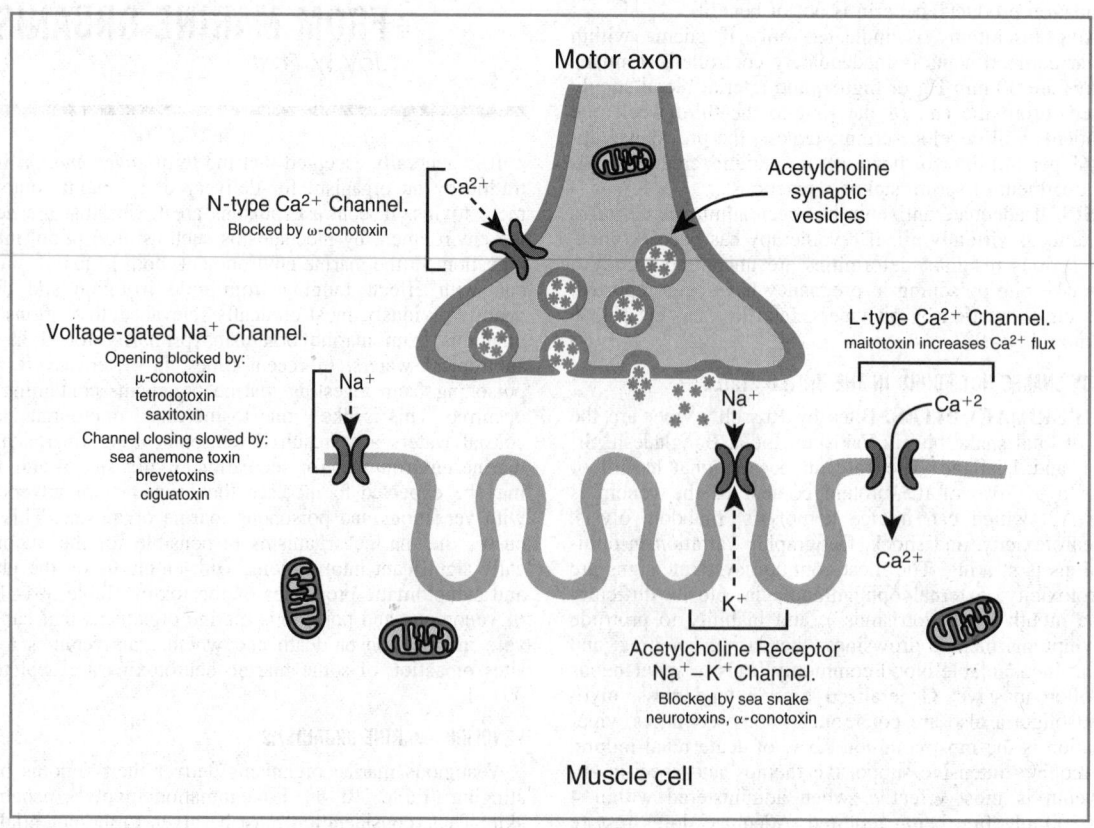

FIGURE 391-1. Schematic representation of a motor axon synapse and the sites of action of various marine neurotoxins.

that functions by blocking the acetylcholine receptor at neuromuscular junctions (Fig. 391–1). The symptoms of sea snake envenomation are mainly neurologic and typically appear within 30 minutes to 2 hours after the bite. Ptosis, dysphagia, and nonrigid paralysis occur and in severe cases respiratory failure may occur. In severe cases respiratory intervention may be necessary.

MOLLUSKS. Blue-Ringed Octopus. The blue-ringed and spotted octopuses (*Hapalochlaena maculosa* and *H. lunulata*), found in Australian waters, inject their venom by a relatively painless bite producing two small puncture wounds. Hemorrhage at the site may occur. The major toxic component in the venom is tetrodotoxin, a postsynaptic neurotoxin that causes perioral and intraoral paresthesias, dysphagia, nausea, ataxia, aphonia, flaccid muscular paralysis, and respiratory distress or failure. Fatal envenomations have occurred.

Cone Shells. Cone shell venoms are injected into victims through a hollow, harpoon-like tooth. The venom is primarily neurotoxic, causing paresthesias, hypotension and respiratory impairment/failure. Three types of neurotoxins have been identified in cone shell venoms: ω-conotoxin, α-conotoxin, and μ-conotoxins, all of which are short polypeptides. The ω-conotoxins block depolarization-induced Ca^{2+} uptake through N-type pre-synaptic channels (Fig. 391–1). The bite is very painful and may be followed by such systemic symptoms as dysphagia, aphonia, pruritus, blurred vision, syncope, muscular paralysis, and respiratory and cardiac failure. In cases of severe envenomation, preparation for cardiovascular and respiratory support should be made. Rare cases of coagulopathies have been noted. Fatal envenomations have occurred.

Weeverfish/Scorpionfish/Stonefish/Lionfish. Weeverfish are of the Trachinidae family while the scorpionfish, stonefish, and lionfish all belong to the family Scorpaenidae. Members of the Scopraenidae family are mostly found in tropic and subtropic waters. Weeverfish occur in European and African waters. All of these fish sting by using dorsal spines. Additionally, anal spines of the Scorpaenidae fish and opercular spines of the Trachinidae fish can also deliver venom. The spines are encased in an integumentary sheath that is torn when the spine punctures the victim's skin. Venom glands are located at the base of the spine.

Few details are known regarding the biochemistry and pharmacology of the toxins in weeverfish venom. The sting of the weeverfish is extremely painful and may produce systemic effects such as aphonia, fever, chills, dyspnea, cyanosis, nausea, syncope, hypotension, and arrhythmias. The wound is edematous, erythematous, and ecchymotic. Bacterial infection is typical and gangrene has been known to develop in severe cases of infection. The venom may be somewhat heat-labile, and soaking in tolerably hot water may relieve some pain as well as attenuate the effects of the venom. Death from weeverfish sting is rare.

Scorpionfish (*Scorpanena*) are primarily found in tropical and subtropical waters and the Mediterranean. The stings of these fishes have been described to be very similar to those of the weevers. Lionfish (*Pterois*) dwell in tropical waters; their stings generally are the most severe of all of the fish stings and occasionally cause death. Because the venom is heat-labile, soaking in hot water is recommended. The stonefish (*Synanceja*) group is found throughout the India-Pacific area, China, Australia, and the Indian Ocean, and is considered to be the most venomous fish. Symptoms are similar to those from the stings of members of the other groups. Hot water soaking of the wound site is recommended. As with all fish stings, care should be taken to ensure that no broken portions of the spines remain in the wound; vigilance against bacterial infections should be observed.

COELENTERATES. Jellyfish and Anemones. These organisms belong to the Cnidaria phylum, thus named because of their venomous organelles, cnidae. The cnidae found in jellyfish and anemones (termed nematocysts and spirocysts respectively) are located on exposed tentacles. On tactile stimulation the tentacles send forth a tethered projectile to deliver venom through the dermis. As the victim's surrounding musculature contracts, the venom is disseminated. The toxins contained in the venom from these organisms have not been fully documented. Hemolysins, DNAses, and histamine releasers have been identified in some venoms. Several peptide toxins have been characterized from the sea anemone, *Anemonia sulcata,* which act similarly to α-scorpion toxins by inactivating the Na^+ channel. Stings by jellyfish and anemones typically produce immediate pain at the site of envenomation, followed by ery-

thematous, urticarial lesions. Anaphylaxis is not common in most situations unless previous sensitization has occurred. Depending on the severity of the sting, wheals and whip-like patterns at the sites of envenomation may appear within a few minutes or be delayed by several hours, followed in some cases by dermal necrosis. Recurrence of eruptions days after the envenomation have been reported. Systemic reactions may include muscle spasms and cramps, vomiting, nausea, diarrhea, diaphoresis, and in rare cases cardiorespiratory failure. Verapamil will eliminate cardiac arrhythmia but will not ameliorate respiratory depression. Unfired nematocysts on tentacles adhering to the skin may be neutralized by either vinegar or baking soda depending on the species of jellyfish. Vinegar seems to be most useful for the Portuguese man-of-war (*Physalia physalis*) and Australian blue bottle (*P. utriculus*) stings while baking soda appears more efficacious for sea nettle (*Chrysaora quinquecirrha*) stings. Box jellyfish (*Chironex fleckeri*) found in Australian waters are perhaps the most venomous jellyfish, producing very severe stings that may cause death due to hypotension, muscular and respiratory paralysis, and ultimately cardiac arrest. Treatment of box jellyfish stings must include consideration of the option of respiratory support and administration of an antivenin.

Sponges. Some sponges colonized by coelenterates elaborate toxins that can produce either a pruritic allergenic dermatitis or an irritant dermatitis. These toxins are delivered by the sharp spicules present in the sponges, which when handled penetrate the dermis. The toxins can cause the typical sponge diver's disease characterized by local burning and itching, which in severe cases may be accompanied by soft tissue edema and purulent vesiculation. Serious illness is rare.

Corals. Fire coral (*Millepora alcicornis*) is found in shallow tropical waters. Stings are a common consequence of brushing or rubbing against the coral. Envenomation produces a burning or stinging sensation followed by severe pruritus. Edematous wheals may occur but generally dissipate over the course of several days. The site of envenomation should be soaked in dilute acetic acid or isopropanol to relieve pain.

BRISTLEWORMS. Bristleworms (Annelida) are segmented invertebrates found in tropical Pacific waters and the Gulf of Mexico. The bristles present on the segments of the organism are capable of penetrating the skin and producing a severely painful envenomation with pruritus and burning that may persist for several days. Local paresthesia is likely and may linger for weeks. Treatment is symptomatic, with consideration of possible tetanus infection. Little is known regarding the chemistry of bristleworm venoms.

SEA URCHINS. Of the echinoderms, sea urchins and sea stars are responsible for most stings to humans. The venom is delivered by the long spines and pedicellariae protruding from the sea urchin body. The spines are covered at the tips with a venom sac that is broken when it penetrates the skin. The pedicellariae, present on some species of sea urchins, are pincer-like appendages carrying venom glands. The toxins of sea urchin venoms are not well-characterized. Stings can produce pain, hemorrhage, aphonia, paresthesias, paralysis, hypotension, nausea, syncope, and respiratory distress. Immersion in hot water helps inactivate heat-labile toxins in the venoms. Attached pedicellariae and embedded spines must be removed to prevent additional envenomation.

STINGRAYS. Stingrays (order Rajiformes) are found in most seas but are predominant in the Indo-Pacific area. Venom is delivered by stings from spines (one or more) present on the tail of the stingray. Stingray spines are retroserrated on the margins and are covered by an integumentary sheath. Venomous glandular tissue is located at the base of the spines. On puncture of the skin, the sheath is torn by the serrated spine and venom flows along the two ventrolateral grooves of the spine into the surrounding tissue. One of the identified toxins in the venom is serotonin. The spines are often deeply embedded in the tissue and difficult to extract due to the retroserration. Care must be taken to remove all spine and sheath fragments. A sting produces severe pain and edema, which in extreme cases is accompanied by hemorrhage, syncope, vomiting, hypotension, and cardiac arrhymia. In rare cases death can occur, especially if the pericardial, peritoneal, or pleural cavities are penetrated. Soaking the wound in hot water inactivates some of the heat-labile toxins in the venom.

POISONOUS MARINE ORGANISMS

Marine poisoning nearly always results from consumption of a fish or shellfish harboring various toxins. The causes of three types of marine poisoning are fish or shellfish containing toxins produced by dinoflagellates (Ciguatera, neurotoxic shellfish, paralytic shellfish, and diarrhetic shellfish poisoning); fish that produce their own toxin (Tetraodontiformes fish); and fish containing significant levels of bacteria that have metabolized histidine to histamine resulting in pseudoallergenic reactions.

CIGUATERA POISONING. Ciguatera toxins have been identified in over 400 species of fish. During blooms of the dinoflagellate *Gambierdiscus toxicus,* toxins produced by these organisms concentrate in the fish to levels that are toxic to humans when ingested. The primary toxins responsible for ciguatera poisoning are ciguatoxin(s), which are cyclic polyethers, and act as excitatory agents by binding to Na^+ channels. Maitotoxin, from the same dinoflagellate, is a water-soluble polyether, and acts by enhancing Ca^{2+} entry through L-type Ca^{2+} channels. Symptoms of ciguatera poisoning generally appear within 2 to 12 hours following ingestion of contaminated fish. Gastrointestinal symptoms including diarrhea, abdominal pain, nausea, and vomiting appear first, followed by neurologic and cardiovascular symptoms. Neurologic symptoms include aphonia, dental dysesthesias, fatigue, tremor, ataxia, pruritus, extremity and perioral dysesthesia, vertigo, headache, myalgias, arthralgias, temperature reversal, and hyporeflexia. Cardiovascular symptoms, such as bradycardia and hypotension, occur least often. There is no specific treatment for ciguatera poisoning; supportive, symptom-based therapy is indicated. Death from ciguatera poisoning has occurred but is rare.

NEUROTOXIC SHELLFISH POISONING (NSP). NSP is caused by eating shellfish that contain brevetoxins produced by the dinoflagellate *Ptychodiscus brevis.* Brevetoxins are cyclic polyethers that function similarly to the ciguatoxins. Gastrointestinal and neurologic symptoms of intoxication appear within 3 hours toxic shellfish is eaten and are similar to those of ciguatera poisoning. Treatment is supportive. No deaths have been reported for NSP.

PARALYTIC SHELLFISH POISONING (PSP). PSP is significantly more severe than NSP and predominantly involves neurologic symptoms with less pronounced gastrointestinal symptoms such as nausea, vomiting, and diarrhea. The toxins responsible for PSP are from the dinoflagellate genera *Gonyaulax, Pyrodinium,* and *Jania* and are harbored in a variety of shellfish. The primary PSP toxins—saxitoxin, neosaxitoxin, and gonyautoxin—are heterocyclic compounds that block nerve and muscle action potentials by binding to Na^+ channels. The site of binding overlaps with tetrodotoxin, resulting in paralysis. Symptoms appear soon after consumption of contaminated shellfish (minutes to hours) beginning with circumoral and extremity paresthesias. Additional neurologic symptoms, such as ataxia, arthria, dysphagia, dysmetria, diaphoresis, and tachycardia, soon follow the initial paresthesias. Respiratory depression or failure can occur and may result in death, usually within 12 hours of the onset of symptoms. As with other shellfish poisoning, therapy is supportive, with close attention given to potential respiratory distress or failure.

DIARRHETIC SHELLFISH POISONING (DSP). DSP is also caused by eating shellfish that are contaminated by dinoflagellate toxins. The two primary toxins associated with DSP are okadaic acid(s) and pectenotoxins. Okadaic acid is a polyether derivative of a 38 carbon fatty acid. It functions as an inhibitor of protein phosphatase-1 and -2A and causes smooth and cardiac muscle contraction. Symptoms of DSP begin with abdominal cramps and nausea and progress to diarrhea. Additional, delayed symptoms occurring approximately 35 hours after ingestion may appear and include vomiting, vertigo, diarrhea, cramps, and headache. Treatment is supportive.

TETRAODONTIFORMES (PUFFERFISH, PORCUPINEFISH, AND SUNFISH) POISONING. Pufferfish (also called blowfish, balloonfish, and toadfish), porcupinefish and sunfish (*Mola* spp.) have a very potent toxin, tetrodotoxin, present in their liver, gonads, intestines, and skin. The flesh of the fish (fugu) is a delicacy in Japan and prepared by specially trained chefs to avoid serving significant amounts of toxins. Tetrodotoxin is a heterocyclic compound that binds at voltage-sensitive Na^+ channels (at an overlapping site with saxitoxin) to block Na^+ passage, preventing nerve and muscle action potentials, thus resulting in paralysis. Symptoms occur rapidly (several minutes to several hours) beginning with circumoral paresthesias and progressing to widespread paresthesias. Following the initial paresthesias, additional symptoms soon follow including ataxia, weakness, aphonia, diaphoresis, excess salivation, dyspnea, dysphagia, weakness, and respiratory distress or failure. Gastrointestinal symptoms include nausea, vomiting, and diarrhea. Coagulopathologies have been reported in association with tetrodotoxin intoxication. Respiratory intervention is crucial in light of the potential for complete flaccid paralysis. Without respiratory assistance, death is not unusual in cases of severe intoxication.

SCOMBROID FISH POISONING. Scombroid poisoning is a pseudoallergic fish poisoning caused by consumption of certain types of fish that have been improperly stored, including the scombroid fish (tuna, mackerel, wahoo, bonito, albacore, skipjack) and nonscombroid fish (mahi-mahi, amberjack, sardines, and herring). The poisoning results from high levels of histamine and saurine present in the fish because of bacterial catabolism of histidine. Presentation of symptoms from intoxication is rapid (within minutes to hours), beginning with a flushing of the skin, oral paresthesias, pruritus, urticaria, nausea, vomiting, diarrhea, vertigo, headache, bronchospasm, dysphagia, tachycardia, and hypotension. Therapy should follow a course for allergenic reaction and anaphylaxis. Symptoms usually resolve in several hours.

Adams ME: Neurotoxins. Trends Neurosci 17(4)(Suppl) 1994. *This issue is a concise tabulation of neurotoxins, their biological sources and pharmacological activities.*
Auerbach PS: Marine envenomations. N Engl J Med 325:486, 1991. *A thorough guide to the types of marine envenomations and symptoms that they cause.*
Burnett JW: Human injuries following jellyfish stings. Maryland Med J 41:509, 1992. *This article describes the mechanism of jellyfish stings and therapy.*
Hall S, Strichartz G (eds.): Marine Toxins: Origin, Structure and Molecular Pharmacology. American Chemical Society, Washington, DC, 1990. *This is a collection of papers on marine toxins with particular emphasis on experimental pharmacology.*
Miller DM (ed.): Ciguatera Seafood Toxins. CRC Press, Boca Raton, Fl. 1991. *A compilation of information on the toxicology of ciguatoxin poisoning.*
Tu AT (ed.): Marine Toxins and Venoms, Handbook of Natural Toxins, Vol. 3. New York, Marcel Dekker Inc., 1988. *This volume discusses many types of marine toxins as well as a section on treatment.*

Section One—Principles of Clinical Neurologic Diagnosis

392 CLINICAL STUDY OF THE PATIENT

392.1 Approach to the Patient

Fred Plum and Jerome B. Posner

The continuing triumphs of genetic, cellular, and molecular biology that have marked the past 20 years have added greatly to our understanding of neurologic-neuromuscular function and the causes and mechanisms of neurologic diseases. At last count, more than 115 distinct genetic disorders of the nervous system have been assigned to specific chromosomal loci. In more than 50 of these, the particular gene or abnormal gene product has been delineated, and hardly a month passes without new discoveries in this realm. Efforts to transfer missing genes to deficient hosts have been started, and functionally effective nerve cell transplants have been placed successfully in the human brain in efforts to correct parkinsonism. The identification and results of experimental applications of a variety of neurotrophic factors hold promise that effective new treatments for certain neurodegenerative disorders may be close at hand. These triumphs presage entirely new and potentially remarkable approaches to future neurologic therapy.

Despite these advances, the fundamental challenge in successfully diagnosing and treating patients with neurologic symptoms or disease remains in (1) understanding the genesis of their complaints, (2) parsimoniously but effectively using laboratory aids to rule in or out the presence of specific structural-chemical disease, and (3) managing them with full recognition that the individual physician represents the most important component in improving the health and spirits of another, suffering human being.

The evaluation of patients whose complaints potentially implicate the nervous system challenges the physician on several levels. New neurologic symptoms often frighten patients. They are afraid of pain, and often disturbed by the threat of becoming crippled and terrified of having chronic disorders such as Alzheimer's and other degenerative diseases. They may use misleading or incorrect terminology to describe their symptoms, and some repress crucial information because they fear its implications. Another issue is the ambiguity of many neurologic complaints. Ultimately, all symptoms of whatever origin are neurologic, because they necessarily require abnormal stimulation of either peripheral or central neuroreceptor systems to make themselves felt. Separating primary neurologic symptoms from those reflecting trouble in other bodily organs represents only a first small step down the diagnostic trail. Even seemingly direct neurologic complaints such as headache, nausea, dizziness, tinnitus, fatigue, and generalized weakness are as likely to signal the presence of an emotional disorder as a somatic neurologic abnormality, and the distinction often evades laboratory investigation. To assign the basis of such complaints accurately requires that the physician know why *this* symptom occurred in *this* patient at *this* particular time. To reach such answers often takes time and repeated questioning, but until these matters are understood, the physician can neither treat present disability nor anticipate future developments.

Even more important than separating emotional from somatic neurologic complaints is recognizing the urgency for prompt diagnosis and treatment of serious neurologic disorders. If nerve cells die they cannot regenerate or be repaired. Furthermore, the older the patient, the less likely the brain is able to substitute new, learned functions for those damaged or destroyed by disease. The guiding principle in treating neurologic illness is that the more rapidly the doctor can reach an accurate diagnosis, the easier it becomes to prevent progression and reduce future disability. The mandate is clear: In seriously and acutely ill patients with neurologic abnormalities, life- or brain-threatening complications must be treated immediately even while proceeding with diagnostic procedures that may take much longer to complete. By contrast, patients whose diseases lack quick and specific remedies (e.g., most psychosomatic disorders, degenerative diseases, or residua of severe trauma) usually need far more from the doctor than mere drugs or operations can supply.

Several important maxims apply to all treatment situations. When emergencies occur, protect the brain first, no matter what successive steps must follow. Relieve pain even while proceeding with diagnosis. Give reassurance, hope, and explanation at every step along the way. In order to plan long-term management effectively and economically, try to construct an accurate prognosis as early as possible. In acute, self-limited illnesses, such as meningococcal meningitis or most cases of acute inflammatory polyneuritis, for example, one usually can predict the probable outcome within a few days of onset. For most such patients one can even predict the convalescent time required before they return to their former occupations. With diseases with intermediate outcomes, such as multiple sclerosis, full recovery is less certain and the risk of relapse or chronic disability requires the physician to appraise all aspects of the patient's life in order to give proper guidance. At the worst extreme are patients who suffer severe head trauma, or become severely crippled from stroke or demented from Alzheimer's disease. They may never recover independence, and their proper early management often requires the doctor to advise families about major social and financial readjustments that will be required in the future. How doctors manage such complexities determines their effectiveness as physicians.

392.2   Clinical Diagnosis
Fred Plum and Jerome B. Posner

A logical approach to neurologic problems yields high clinical dividends in accuracy of diagnosis and selection of appropriate therapy. The following imperatives outline a widely used strategy.

Focus strongly on the relevant history, weighing the biologic implications of the patient's symptoms in relation to known neuroanatomic and physiologic perturbations. Vague symptoms can sometimes reflect educational problems or mental decline in the patient. Alternatively, they may hint more at a distressed psyche than a diseased soma. By contrast, perturbations of specific sensory, motor, or language pathways often produce symptoms that almost immediately point to the general anatomic region and pathophysiology of the patient's neurologic abnormality.

Heed chronology. Remote, temporary sensorimotor or visual symptoms affecting a 35 year old who several years later develops an "acute" paraparesis suggests an exacerbating and remitting disorder such as multiple sclerosis rather than a new spinal neoplasm. Conversely, a several-year history of sharply episodic, brief experiences of depersonalization accompanied by automatic behavioral activity in a patient with a recently developing unilateral headache suggests temporal lobe seizures accompanying an enlarging intracranial mass lesion rather than the onset of a migraine late in life.

Try to place the origin of symptoms and signs on at least a crude neuroanatomic map. Do they suggest disease in a single anatomic locus or do they reflect dysfunction affecting several different anatomic areas? Do they suggest a system disorder (e.g., motor neuron disease or neuromuscular disease) rather than a focal structural lesion, e.g., a single spinal neoplasm producing focal lower motor neuron changes at one level with upper motor neuron abnormalities extending below that level?

Are the symptoms and signs consistent with known physical disorders? For example, chronic weakness and fatigue lasting more than 6 months unaccompanied by physical or laboratory abnormalities suggest chronic anxiety-depression rather than structural disease or systemic metabolic dysfunction. Beware, however; some diseases affecting the nervous system move so slowly that their early symptoms and signs may not be readily localizable. A corollary to not overdiagnosing somatic disorders is that it is equally important not to entertain psychiatric diagnoses unless other findings or projective tests support such conclusions. For example, low-grade astrocytomas of the frontal lobe may produce new-onset behavioral abnormalities long before they cause focal abnormalities on the neurologic examination or unequivocal abnormalities in magnetic resonance images.

Form etiologic hypotheses logically, apply common sense, and consider the common before the rare. Age, previous symptoms, epidemiologic frequency, gender in X-linked diseases (e.g., muscular dystrophy or adult-onset optic atrophy) as well as personal changes in the home and workplace all can contribute important elements that must be weighed in the evaluation.

Reach ultimate diagnosis only on strong evidence, known principles of anatomy, the presence of objectively perturbed neurologic function, and knowledge of disease mechanisms. Avoid undue efforts to fit signs and symbols into inexact syndromes. Physicians who too rapidly try to match symptoms and signs into an iteratively constructed diagnosis often prematurely make conclusions that they later find difficult to surrender. Keeping an open mind in making preliminary hypotheses and awareness that early working diagnoses are necessarily subject to change makes one capable of meeting changes that may emerge from the clinical course or laboratory findings. Lastly and importantly, order tests sparingly, armed with knowledge of what each procedure can or cannot provide and how it specifically may help to diagnose or confirm the particular patient's problem.

392.3   The Neurologic History
Jerome B. Posner

When a patient presents with a neurologic complaint, the clinical history usually supplies a greater proportion of the diagnostically relevant information than does either the neurologic examination or the nervous system images. Many neurologic diseases (e.g., migraine and, often, epilepsy) are not accompanied by abnormal physical or laboratory findings, and in these instances the physician must depend solely on the history to reach an appropriate diagnosis. Even when the patient suffers from a neurologic disease marked by physical signs and/or laboratory abnormalities, the history usually supplies about 80% of the total diagnostic information. Furthermore, because neurologic abnormalities affect such important functions as thinking, moving, and feeling, it is unusual to have significant abnormal signs that have not been reflected in symptoms. (Exceptions occur in demented patients and those with lesions of the nondominant parietal lobe, characterized by denial of disability. In these instances, abnormal behavior may be recognized by family and friends.) Thus, findings on examination not recognized by the patient or family are likely to be irrelevant or even misleading. By contrast, symptoms complained of by the patient, such as mild weakness or alterations of sensation, are probably significant even if too subtle to be detected by the examination. Because patients so keenly appreciate neurologic symptoms, a meticulous history often allows a physician to localize the disease anatomically and to understand its pathophysiology even before the physical examination.

Taking the neurologic history usually occupies the majority of time spent in an initial visit with a patient suffering a neurologic disorder. At the completion of the history, the physician should be able either to make a definite diagnosis or to formulate three or four hypotheses that can be tested by the physical and laboratory examinations. To reach this goal, the experienced physician gradually develops a targeted approach, similar to that which follows.

BE INTERESTED AND SUPPORTIVE. Try not only to gain diagnostic information but also to learn enough about the patient's psychologic and social background to establish a satisfactory doctor-patient relationship. Diagnostic information is often lost when patients do not volunteer symptoms that they believe would not interest the physician or that are too intimate to tell to an "unsympathetic stranger." The patient is usually more readily forthcoming if the physician demonstrates interest, reassurance, and support.

BE ALERT TO NONVERBAL CUES. What the patient does is often as important as what he or she says. The patient's overall appearance and demeanor, tone of voice, or a sigh or a tear in discussing what appear to be relatively trivial symptoms may be important clues to an underlying depression or severe anxiety over those symptoms.

REQUIRE PRECISION. Do not accept jargon or names of diseases from the patient. Jargon terms such as "dizziness" or diagnostic appellations such as "sinus headache" require an exact definition.

MAINTAIN A BALANCE BETWEEN LISTENING AND ASKING. Elicit the history in the patient's own words and, whenever possible, allow the patient to tell the story without interruption. Excessive interruptions imply impatience or disinterest and may lead to the exclusion of vital information. However, the physician must ask direct questions to encourage relevance, achieve precision, and place each symptom in its correct context. If the information is not volunteered, the physician must ask about the intensity and frequency of the complained symptoms, their duration, events and factors that precipitate or relieve them, and any other symptoms associated in time with the patient's major complaint.

FORM HYPOTHESES. Do not be a passive recipient of the patient's story. While taking the history, one must sift and distill the information in order to retain the relevant and discard the irrelevant. Concurrently, one must form hypotheses about the nature of symptoms as they are presented and test those hypotheses by asking pertinent questions. Hypotheses are tested and refined during the course of taking the history, so that by the end the physician has a few potential diagnoses to guide the physical and laboratory examinations. The best hypotheses are broad explanations of the patient's symptoms in anatomic and/or pathophysiologic terms, which are gradually refined into etiologic terms as the history develops. Hypotheses should give preference to illnesses that are probable (i.e., common diseases are more likely than rare diseases), serious (e.g., brain tumors should be considered before tension-type headache), treatable (e.g., spinal cord meningioma and vitamin B_{12} deficiency should be ruled out before making a diagnosis of multiple sclerosis), and novel (some patients have rare diseases, and these should not be forgotten).

ALWAYS TAKE A COMPLETE HISTORY. Even if the diagnosis seems clear from the chief complaint and the present illness, elicit other aspects of the patient's history in order to confirm or repute other physical or psychologic disabilities that could contribute to the patient's discomfort. In particular, inquire about the patient's mood (e.g., depressed or suicidal?), usual daily activities (and whether the illness interferes with them), sexual activities, the nature of psychologic and physical support at home, and the patient's view of the illness and its effects.

END BY SUMMARIZING. At the end of the history, summarize the history as you understand it, asking the patient if the summary is correct and if anything has been overlooked.

OBTAIN FURTHER HISTORY FROM THE PATIENT'S FAMILY AND FRIENDS. If the history appears incomplete, and particularly if part of the illness involves changes in mental state or episodic unconsciousness, ask family, friends, and colleagues to supply missing elements, giving their views on how the signs and symptoms affect the patient's daily life.

392.4 The Neurologic Examination
Fred Plum

Several texts contain detailed techniques of bedside neurologic examinations. In most clinical circumstances, however, an understanding of a few fundamental principles about the nervous system plus mastery of a brief but systematically thorough approach to the examination can give reliable and effective answers. The secret is to learn well an approach that covers the main elements of nervous system function and to be familiar with ways to seek out more exhaustive evaluations if and when the history or examination suggests special abnormalities. Under all circumstances, however, the details of how one examines the patient should be geared to evaluating clinical hypotheses derived from the history.

An effective neurologic examination proceeds from general to specific in its principles and rostral to caudal in its anatomy. The examination checks on the integrity of major functions but avoids details that do not relate to the complaints of most patients. Evaluate the level of arousal (see Ch. 393). In awake and talking patients, begin to evaluate mental status and language as they give their histories. Apply at least a brief mental examination on everyone, but be gentle and understanding: "How has your memory been? Can I just check a couple of points with you?" Check orientation. Examine memory for recent events, for public figures, and for three unrelated words after a 5-minute interval. Review the capacity to handle abstractions (boy—dwarf, small tree—bush, proverbs). Provide a problem in simple arithmetic (the number of nickels in $1.35). Check serial sevens. Have the patient repeat five numbers or spell "world" backward. Be patient and remember that anxiety can compromise the performance of even a normal mind. If in doubt, perform a minimental status evaluation (see Table 400–3). Have the patient stand and walk; bear in mind that the nervous system is the organ of communication and behavior, and that one learns most about humans by watching them attempt natural tasks. To detect apraxia (see Ch. 399) watch the patient at least partially dress and undress; remark on alertness-dullness; hyperactivity-apathy; adventitious movement–akinesia; visible deformities, asymmetries, or weaknesses in functional tasks; hypertrophies-atrophies; cutaneous abnormalities (pox, birthmarks, café au lait spots, pigmented or hair spots over spinal defects); a straight, flat, or crooked spine. Learn to observe constantly and closely, comparing what you see with what you already have encountered in thousands of people

living normal lives. Wise physicians gain experience not only from their patients but from the everyday world in which they live.

Examine cranial functions. Palpate the skull and test the neck gently for suppleness and length. Then examine the following in every patient: vision, the optic fundi, pupillary activity, ocular movements, corneal reflexes, jaw movement, facial movement, hearing, swallowing, speaking, and breathing. One can omit examinations of smell, taste, facial sensation, labyrinthine-vestibular activity, sternocleidomastoid function, or detailed tongue movements unless symptoms suggest an abnormality of these areas. Examine in everyone the extremities and trunk for hypertrophy or atrophy, size, gross strength, muscle tonus, adventitious movements (e.g., tremors, fasciculations, tics), coordination (rhythmic movements and point-to-point tests), and reflexes. If the patient has no sensory symptoms, he/she is unlikely to have significantly abnormal sensory signs. Nevertheless, check the distal extremities briefly for the threshold perception of vibration and pin prick. Examine the plantar responses. Evaluate autonomic and sphincter functions only if the history has suggested dysfunction involving these areas. Get in the habit of examining the neck over the carotid arteries for bruits that may herald partial stenoses. Above all, be systematic and consistent in the approach and *do not jump at diagnosis until all the evidence is in*. Doctors tend to make diagnoses quickly and surrender wrong ones reluctantly. By contrast, they view even partial unknowns as challenging problems. Try to choose the latter approach until matters become certain.

USE OF LABORATORY TESTS. Advances in laboratory methods during recent years have remarkably increased the accuracy of diagnosis and physiologic evaluations. At the same time, the excess of technology raises the costs of medical care unnecessarily. More than anything else, the physician's ordering practices influence this aspect of health care costs. Doctors must recognize the precise advantages for both positive and negative knowledge that derive from each test, then gear their ordering to hypotheses gained from the history and whatever additional clues come from the neurologic examination. For example, when managing an adult with recent onset of headache, the results of a computed tomographic scan, whether normal or abnormal, commonly help management and may provide the patient with great reassurance. However, to repeat scans or irrelevant tests just for the sake of "a complete workup" wastes the time and resources of all concerned.

Glick TH: Neurologic Skills. Examination and Diagnosis. Boston, Blackwell Scientific Publications, 1993. *Provides a detailed approach to the neurologic history, examination, and formulation of diagnoses.*
Guarantors of Brain. Aids to the Examination of the Peripheral Nervous System. London, Bailliere and Tindall, 1986. *An indispensable pictorial guide to the motor and sensory distribution of the dermatomes and peripheral nerves.*

392.5 Neurologic Diagnostic Procedures
Jonathan D. Victor

LUMBAR PUNCTURE

Sampling the cerebrospinal fluid (CSF) is indispensable for the diagnosis of central nervous system infections and needs to be performed on an emergency basis when bacterial meningitis is suspected. Table 392–1 lists other indications for lumbar puncture, as well as major contraindications.

ELECTRODIAGNOSTIC STUDIES

Examinations performed in the clinical neurophysiology laboratory are best viewed as extensions of the bedside neurologic examination. The neurologic examination, fundamentally, is a series of observations of the patient's response to a traditional set of standard stimuli. The techniques of clinical neurophysiology allow one to detail the responses with a greater temporal resolution, to demonstrate the activity of single cells and cell populations that underlie the responses, and to quantify the observations.

TABLE 392-1. COMMON INDICATIONS AND CONTRAINDICATIONS FOR LUMBAR PUNCTURE

Diagnostic indications
  Known or suspected meningitis and encephalitis
    Acute: bacterial, viral
    Subacute: tuberculous, syphilitic, fungal, neoplastic
    Chronic: syphilitic, granulomatous, neoplastic
  Intracranial or intraspinal hemorrhage, if CT or MRI is not available
  Multiple sclerosis
  Acute polyneuropathy
  Suspected benign intracranial hypertension (pseudotumor), if CT or MRI is negative
Therapeutic indications
  Intrathecal administration of antimicrobial or chemotherapeutic agents
  CSF drainage in benign intracranial hypertension or communicating hydrocephalus
Contraindications
  Intracranial hypertension due to mass lesion or obstructive hydrocephalus
  Bleeding diathesis
  Local skin or epidural infections

Neurophysiologic tests are not etiologic tests. They do not replace the basic neurologic paradigm of reasoning from localization to possible causes but rather add to the precision and sensitivity with which functional pathology can be defined.

Electroencephalography

The electroencephalogram (EEG) is a record of the spontaneous electrical activity of the brain as recorded on the scalp. The clinical EEG is typically recorded from 8 to 16 pairs of electrodes (called "derivations"). The "international 10-20" system of electrode placement provides coverage of the scalp at standard locations denoted by the letters F (frontal), C (central), P (parietal), T (temporal), and O (occipital) with subscripts (odd for left-sided placements, even for right-sided placements, and "z" for midline placements).

EEG signals have a typical amplitude of 30 to 100 μV and an irregular wavelike variation in time (Fig. 392-1A). The main generators of the EEG are thought to be postsynaptic potentials, with the largest contribution arising from pyramidal cells. The minute amplitude of the EEG compared to the ECG is a consequence of two facts: The normal ECG is generated by cells that are synchronously activated and geometrically aligned; the normal EEG is generated by cells that are asynchronously activated and, in general, not geometrically aligned. Thus, the EEG is a composite record of fluctuating correlations between the activities of many populations of cells.

Ongoing EEG activity, called the *background,* is described in terms of frequency ranges: less than 3.5 Hz (delta), 4 to 7.5 Hz (theta), 8 to 13 Hz (alpha), and greater than 13.5 Hz (beta). In awake but relaxed normal adults, the background consists primarily of alpha activity in occipital and parietal areas and beta activity in central and frontal areas. Variations in this pattern occur as a function of age (particularly in the first years of life) and behavioral state (e.g., vigilant versus relaxed versus drowsy versus asleep; eyes open versus eyes closed).

EEG ABNORMALITIES. EEG abnormalities can be divided into two categories: alterations in the background activity and paroxysmal activity. Global *background abnormalities* accompany diffuse brain dysfunction associated with developmental delay, metabolic disturbances, infections, and degenerative diseases. EEG background abnormalities are never specific enough to establish a diagnosis. For example, the *burst-suppression* pattern illustrated in Figure 392-1B may be seen in severe anoxic brain injury as well as in coma due to barbiturates. Several encephalopathies, however, have characteristic EEG features that suggest a diagnosis. For example, an excess of beta activity suggests intoxication with barbiturates, benzodiazepines, and related drugs. *Triphasic slow waves* (Fig. 392-1C) are typical of metabolic encephalopathies, particularly those due to hepatic and renal dysfunction. Creutzfeldt-Jakob disease and subacute sclerosing panencephalitis have characteristic EEG signatures, consisting of background alterations associated with periodic paroxysmal discharges (see below).

Psychiatric illness is not associated with prominent changes in the EEG. Thus, a normal EEG helps to distinguish pseudodementia

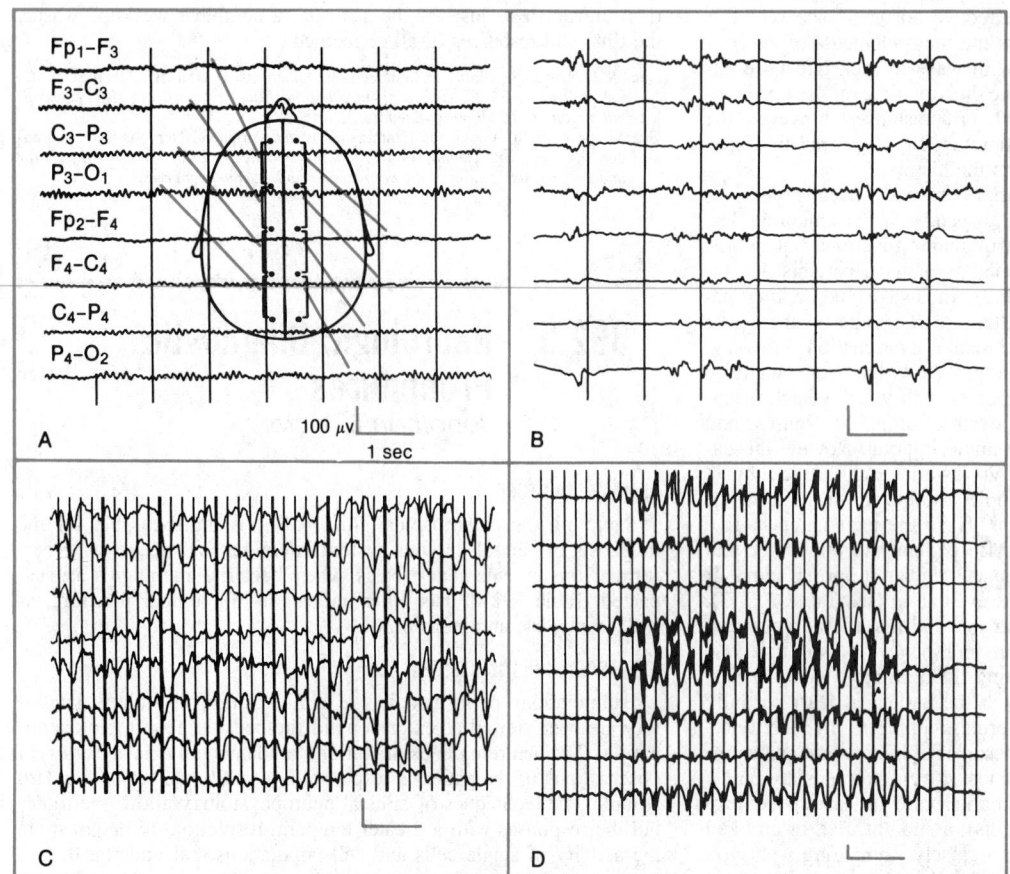

FIGURE 392-1. Normal and abnormal EEG's. *A,* The EEG of a normal alert adult. *B,* Burst-suppression, a pattern seen in severe cerebral dysfunction. *C,* Triphasic slow waves, seen in metabolic encephalopathies. *D,* A brief spike-and-wave seizure. In each record, the top four tracings are from parasagittal left-sided bipolar electrode placements (Fp$_1$-F$_3$, F$_3$-C$_3$, C$_3$-P$_3$, P$_3$-O$_1$); the lower four tracings are from the corresponding right-sided placements (Fp$_2$-F$_4$, F$_4$-C$_4$, C$_4$-P$_4$, P$_4$-O$_2$). The scale represents 1 sec and 100 μV. Note the reduced vertical scale in D.

from dementia and psychogenic unresponsiveness from neurologic disease.

Thalamocortical connections play a major role in establishing the normal EEG background. Thus, although brain stem and diencephalic activity is not directly registered in the EEG, structural lesions of the brain stem may cause diffuse changes in background activity via their effect on thalamocortical relays.

The EEG is an adjunctive test in the determination of brain death. An active EEG readily distinguishes de-efferented or locked-in states (such as severe Guillain-Barré syndrome and basal pontine infarction) from cortical inactivity (see Ch. 394). Electrocerebral silence, however, does not necessarily imply brain death, because it may be produced by reversible conditions such as barbiturate intoxication and hypothermia.

Focal or lateralized background abnormalities in the EEG imply similarly localized disturbances in brain function and thus suggest the presence of underlying structural lesions. CT and MRI have largely supplanted the EEG for anatomic localization. An important exception is herpes simplex encephalitis, which may produce focal abnormalities in temporal leads before imaging techniques demonstrate structural changes.

Paroxysmal EEG activity ("spikes" and "sharp waves") reflects pathologic synchronization of neurons. As such, this finding identifies a brain region with epileptogenic potential. Spikes and sharp waves commonly appear in the EEG records of epilepsy patients during interictal periods. The location and character of EEG paroxysms and their relationship to the background help to classify the epileptic disorder, guide rational anticonvulsant therapy, and assist prognosis. (See also Ch. 433.) Some patients with epilepsy may not show paroxysmal activity on a routine EEG, either because the focus is infrequently active or because it is too small or too deep to be evident in scalp recordings. The diagnostic yield of the EEG can be increased by *activation procedures,* such as hyperventilation and photic stimulation, by prolonged ambulatory monitoring, or through the use of special recording sites, including nasopharyngeal leads, anterior temporal leads, and surgically placed subdural and depth electrodes.

During a seizure, paroxysmal EEG activity becomes continuous and rhythmic and replaces normal background activity (see Ch. 433). In partial seizures with secondary generalization, paroxysmal activity begins in one brain region and spreads to uninvolved regions. The EEG identifies a focal onset of seizures more accurately than clinical observation alone. In primary generalized seizures, paroxysmal EEG activity is bilateral at onset. An example is shown in Figure 392–1*D.*

Whether focal or generalized, seizures with motor manifestations are unlikely to be subtle clinical events. However, sensory seizures, psychomotor seizures, and other forms of seizures without major motor manifestations may require an EEG for identification and diagnosis.

Evoked Potentials

External stimuli evoke changes in the ongoing electrical activity of the brain that may be extracted from scalp recordings by signal-averaging techniques. The three modality-specific evoked potentials discussed below form the bulk of clinical practice.

VISUAL EVOKED POTENTIALS (VEP). The VEP is commonly elicited by stimulation of the retina with repetitive reversals of black-and-white checkerboard patterns. The most robust component is an occiput-positive wave several microvolts in amplitude, occurring approximately 100 msec after pattern reversal. Termed the P-100, its cellular origins include a mixture of excitatory and inhibitory synaptic signals. The VEP is recorded separately for each eye. Interocular differences in P-100 latency imply prechiasmal conduction abnormalities, and bilateral delay in the P-100 latency implies bilateral conduction defects in the visual system. Since VEP's measure central response time rather than visual resolution, they may be abnormal in patients with normal visual acuity and visual fields. VEP's are particularly useful in identifying unsuspected optic nerve or cerebral abnormalities in patients whose clinical signs point to disease affecting the brain stem or spinal cord. Demonstration of such multifocal lesions in the appropriate setting fortifies the clinical diagnosis of multiple sclerosis. Delayed optic nerve conduction may also be due to compressive lesions (e.g., pituitary tumor), metabolic disorders (e.g., vitamin B_{12} deficiency), and other neurodegenerative diseases (e.g., olivopontocerebellar atrophy). In patients who cannot or will not cooperate with behavioral tests, VEP's elicited by a graded series of stimuli provide a measure of visual resolution and contrast sensitivity.

BRAIN STEM AUDITORY EVOKED POTENTIALS (BAEP). The BAEP is commonly elicited by brief clicks presented to one ear, while random noise is presented to the other ear. The normal response, recorded by an electrode at the ear referenced to the vertex, consists of a series of submicrovolt waves at approximately 1-msec intervals. Wave I is generated at the distal end of the eighth nerve; wave III is generated along auditory pathways at the level of the superior olive, and wave V is generated at the level of the inferior colliculus. BAEP abnormalities commonly accompany mass lesions in the cerebellopontine angle and intraparenchymal brain stem lesions affecting the auditory pathways. Because the BAEP shows a stereotyped maturational pattern in the first 2 years of life, it is a valuable means of assessing the developmentally delayed or at-risk neonate. BAEP's elicited by a sequence of increasingly intense click stimuli provide a measure of auditory threshold in infants and patients who cannot cooperate with behavioral tests. In the appropriate clinical setting, absence of BAEP potentials rostral to wave II accompanied by still-remaining peripherally generated potentials supports the diagnosis of brain death.

SOMATOSENSORY EVOKED POTENTIALS (SEP). A SEP may be elicited by brief electrical stimulation delivered to any of several sensory nerves and dermatomes, but median, peroneal, and posterior tibial nerves are most commonly used. Scalp electrodes placed over somatosensory areas record submicrovolt potentials, and the spinal cord volley and peripheral nerve action potential often can be recorded by appropriately placed electrodes. With median nerve stimulation, potentials generated at medullary and midbrain-thalamic levels can be identified. Compressive, demyelinating, or metabolic disturbances affecting central sensory pathways delay centrally generated potentials but not potentials generated prior to entry to the spinal cord. Upper- and lower-extremity SEP's, in conjunction with nerve conduction studies and EMG, can help to identify radiculopathies and plexopathies.

OTHER PHYSIOLOGIC MEASURES OF BRAIN ACTIVITY. The limited anatomic information provided by the EEG has motivated new approaches to provide measures of brain function with better spatial resolution. *Magnetoencephalography (MEG),* the recording of magnetic fields generated by intracranial current loops, achieves a higher spatial resolution than the EEG because magnetic fields are virtually unaffected by the volume-conduction effects that distort the brain's electrostatic fields. Because MEG retains millisecond temporal resolution, it adds to the ability of electrical recordings to localize the generators of evoked potentials and epileptic spikes. Unfortunately, the minute size of the brain's magnetic fields and the costly and cumbersome nature of present-day detectors limit the application of MEG.

Imaging techniques identify activity-induced changes in cerebral blood flow and metabolism and thus sacrifice temporal resolution to achieve better spatial resolution. *Positron emission tomography (PET)* achieves a spatial resolution of < 1 cm and can exploit specific ligands and metabolites to probe transmitter systems or metabolic pathways, but it is very costly and requires the injection of significant amounts of a radioisotope. PET has demonstrated characteristic global patterns of metabolic derangements that distinguish the vegetative state and several forms of dementia, and has characterized the metabolic abnormalities in a variety of extrapyramidal disorders.

Functional magnetic resonance imaging (fMRI), which can be performed either with or without administration of a paramagnetic contrast agent, has an ultimate spatial resolution of about 1 mm and can be used to make multiple measurements in the same subject. In normal subjects and in patients, PET and fMRI have identified local brain regions activated by specific sensory, motor, and cognitive tasks. These techniques have the potential to demonstrate localized functional abnormalities of the brain even in the absence of structural changes.

Nerve Conduction Studies and Electromyography

NERVE CONDUCTION STUDIES. Most peripheral nerves can be stimulated percutaneously at one or more points along their length. The induced electrical activity of muscles can be recorded with surface electrodes or with appropriately inserted needle electrodes. The *conduction velocity* of motor nerves can be calculated from the difference in latency of the motor response evoked by stimulation at two or more points along their length. Conduction velocity in sensory nerves can be determined by recording sensory nerve action potentials elicited by electrical stimulation at proximal or distal sites.

Nerve roots and segments of peripheral nerves that lie too close to the spinal cord to be studied directly may be examined by the F-response and H-reflex. The *F-response* is the compound muscle action potential that results from antidromic conduction of a volley along a motor nerve to the anterior horn cell body and back again to muscle. The *H-reflex*, a muscle response that represents the electrical equivalent of the monosynaptic stretch reflex, is elicited by stimulating sensory fibers in the corresponding peripheral afferent nerve. Usually, it is readily recorded only in the soleus after stimulation of the tibial nerve and thus serves to test the S1 root only.

Compound nerve action potentials are elicited by electrical stimulation of a peripheral nerve and are recorded by electrodes placed at a second site along the nerve. The response is dominated by the larger and more rapidly conducting myelinated nerve fibers. Accordingly, demyelinating neuropathies characteristically slow the conduction velocities. By contrast, axonal neuropathies, in which individual cell bodies or axons fail, decrease the amplitude of evoked motor and sensory responses but preserve normal conduction velocities until all of the largest myelinated fibers are affected.

Routine clinical tests cannot readily assess the function of unmyelinated fibers. Percutaneous microneurographic recording from single nerve fibers in the intact peripheral nerve represents an investigational approach to study unmyelinated and small myelinated fibers.

Electromyography (EMG) is performed by inserting a needle electrode into the muscle. At rest, a normal muscle with normal innervation remains electrically silent. With denervation, spontaneous activity occurs, consisting predominantly of fibrillation potentials and positive sharp waves. *Fasciculation potentials*, representing synchronous firing of entire motor units, occur mainly in anterior horn cell disorders and mechanical disturbances affecting motor nerve roots and may result in fasciculations that visibly dimple the overlying skin. *Fibrillation potentials* and *positive sharp waves*, which represent electrical activity of single muscle fibers, occur predominantly in neurogenic lesions but can also be seen in dystrophies and inflammatory myopathies.

Electromyographic recording during voluntary muscle contraction permits observation of individual motor units and their pattern of *recruitment*. In myopathies, degeneration of muscle fibers leads to a decrease in the size of motor units: Voluntary contraction recruits a normal number of units but with small amplitude and short duration. In denervated muscle, voluntary activity recruits a decreased number of units. With chronic denervation, collateral sprouting by remaining motoneurons leads to residual motor units of abnormally large amplitude and duration. *Myotonic discharges*, abnormal repetitive discharges that vary in amplitude and frequency, are seen in a variety of specific myopathies.

Table 392–2 summarizes how nerve conduction studies and EMG distinguish myopathies from neuropathies and indicate whether a neuropathy is demyelinating or axonal. Note that radiculopathies are distinguished from polyneuropathies on the basis of the distribution of the affected nerves and muscles rather than the findings in the affected areas. Detailed analysis of EMG activity may also help analyze central disturbances of motor control.

NEUROMUSCULAR TRANSMISSION STUDIES. Diseases of the neuromuscular junction are identified by the presence of abnormal neuromuscular transmission in the setting of otherwise normal nerve conduction studies. At the normal neuromuscular junction, the amount of acetylcholine released exceeds severalfold the requirements for activating the muscle. Repetitive action potentials cause a mild decrement in acetylcholine release, but the safety factor prevents a decrement in the postsynaptic response. In myasthenia gravis, immunologic blockade reduces the safety factor of the postsynaptic receptors. As a result, repetitive stimulation of a motor nerve elicits a rapid diminution of the evoked muscle action potential paralleling the decreasing amounts of acetylcholine released. In botulism and Eaton-Lambert syndrome, repetitive stimulation overcomes a presynaptic blockade and produces a gradual increase in the size of the evoked muscle action potential.

Pathologic reductions in the safety factor magnify the normal variability of the time interval between nerve action potential and depolarization of the postsynaptic fiber. This increased variability, or "jitter," can be assayed by simultaneously recording two muscle fibers in the same motor unit with single-fiber EMG electrodes. The jitter study is a more sensitive test of defective neuromuscular transmission than repetitive stimulation.

Aminoff MJ (ed.): Electrodiagnosis in Clinical Neurology, 3rd ed. New York, Churchill Livingstone, 1992. *Comprehensive introduction to EEG, EP, EMG, and other modalities.*

Chiappa KH: Evoked Potentials in Clinical Medicine, 2nd ed. New York, Raven Press, 1990. *Emphasis on practical matters and interpretation.*

Fisch BJ: Spehlmann's EEG Primer, 2nd ed. New York, Elsevier, 1991.

Kimura J: Electrodiagnosis in Diseases of Nerve and Muscle: Principles and Practice, 2nd ed. Philadelphia, FA Davis, 1989. *A standard reference.*

Niedermeyer E, Lopes da Silva F: Electroencephalography: Basic Principles, Clinical Applications, and Related Fields, 2nd ed. Baltimore, Urban and Schwartzenberg, 1987. *Encyclopedic, authoritative.*

Regan D: Human Brain Electrophysiology. New York, Elsevier, 1989. *Encyclopedic, emphasis on fundamentals and evoked potentials.*

TABLE 392–2. TYPICAL ELECTROPHYSIOLOGIC FEATURES OF NEUROPATHIES AND MYOPATHIES

	Nerve Conduction Velocity	F-response	H-reflex	Electromyography
Inflammatory myopathy or dystrophy	Normal	Normal	Normal	Fibrillations; positive sharp waves; small motor units
Metabolic myopathy	Normal	Normal	Normal	Small motor units
Axonal neuropathy	Normal	Normal	Normal	Fibrillations; positive sharp waves; fasciculations; large motor units with distal predominance
Demyelinating neuropathy	Slowed diffusely	Delayed or absent diffusely	Delayed or absent	Normal motor units
Radiculopathy	Normal	Delayed or absent in damaged root	Delayed or absent if S1 is involved	Fibrillations; positive sharp waves; fasciculations; large motor units if chronic
Motoneuron disease	Normal	Normal	Normal	Fibrillations; positive sharp waves; fasciculations; large motor units diffusely

392.6 Radiologic Imaging Procedures
Michael Deck

Management of neurologic disorders has improved dramatically over the last 20 years because of revolutionary developments in imaging techniques such as computed tomography (CT), magnetic resonance imaging (MRI), positron emission tomography (PET), and single photon emission computed tomography (SPECT). During the last 5 years these methods have improved spatial resolution, and fast spin echo and echo planar imaging by MRI have made possible physiologic studies of blood flow. At the same time, cerebrospinal fluid (CSF) flow and even activation studies of the cerebral cortex have become available.

Magnetic resonance spectroscopy (MRS) uses hydrogen and phosphorus to measure the concentrations of metabolites in brain volumes as small as 1 cm^3 and has been useful in tumors, ischemia, and various metabolic disorders.

Magnetic resonance angiography (MRA) uses various complicated pulse sequences to image cervical cerebral arteries. The technique has been applied to diagnosing carotid artery stenosis, aneurysms of the circle of Willis, and thrombosis of the intracranial venous sinuses.

Interventional therapeutic approaches to intracranial aneurysms, arteriovenous malformations, vascular spasm, and vascular tumors such as meningiomas and chemodectomas are now available at most tertiary-level hospitals. Selective or superselective intra-arterial and intravenous administration of thrombolytic agents for the treatment of acute stroke and superselective chemotherapeutic agents for malignant brain tumors are currently under evaluation and appear promising.

THE SKULL AND BRAIN

PLAIN RADIOGRAPHY. Plain radiographs of the skull are routinely taken in frontal, lateral, and half-axial projections. Such films are useful principally in the initial evaluation of head trauma in which fractures of the vault and base may influence subsequent management. *Most skull radiographs, however, are taken for medicolegal reasons. Their value is limited because of poor correlation with injury of the underlying brain.* Depressed bone fragments may require elevation. Involvement of the paranasal sinuses or mastoid air cells may result in meningitis and indicate a use for prophylactic antibiotics. CT and MRI have supplanted plain radiographs in evaluating intracranial trauma and mass lesions such as tumors, hematomas, and infarcts, in detecting optic foramen enlargement due to tumors, and in identifying bony sclerosis due to meningiomas. CT and MRI also demonstrate tumors and inflammatory lesions of the paranasal sinuses as well as the craniovertebral junction better than do plain radiographs.

COMPUTED TOMOGRAPHY. CT uses an x-ray tube with a tightly collimated beam passing through the anatomic area under study. An array of 520 to 4800 x-ray detectors measures the radiation absorbed by the organs targeted by the beam during a 360-degree rotation lasting 1 to 6 seconds. Computers now formulate the analogue output from each detector to calculate a coefficient of absorption for each "pixel" in the field, using a mathematical process called filtered back projection. The resulting image is displayed on a cathode-ray tube monitor that may be viewed directly or photographed onto transparent film. CT images from current equipment demonstrate anatomic structures in the skull and brain with high spatial resolution. Fresh hemorrhages within either the brain or the subarachnoid, subdural, or epidural spaces can be identified because of the greater x-ray attenuation of clotted blood. Areas of calcification may have similar appearances but are usually more irregular and have a higher attenuation value. Many CT examinations use contrast enhancement with intravenous iodinated material to demonstrate normal vascular structures as well as the abnormal endothelial permeability that accompanies certain types of tumors and inflammatory processes.

Although contrast enhancement can add critical information in many CT examinations of the brain, the material also carries a small risk of adverse anaphylactic reactions. The general population has about a 1 in 10,000 chance of serious anaphylactic reaction and a 1 in 40,000 to 100,000 chance of death. These dangers increase fourfold in patients with previous allergic history to iodinated contrast material, iodine, or shellfish. The risk may be reduced by administering an antihistamine drug immediately before or 50 mg of prednisone orally 24, 12, and 6 hours before the injection. Special techniques can improve the resolution of CT and generate physiologic data. These include the following:

1. Coronal projections image the floor of the skull, the sella turcica, and the petrous bones.

2. Image reformatting generates coronal or sagittal images from multiple axial images. The technique depends on absolute immobilization of the patient and produces good resolution. It increases, however, the amount of radiation to the brain and potentially the eye. Three-dimensional reformatting may be useful for displaying surfaces and contours and is increasingly used by craniofacial surgeons to evaluate facial trauma and congenital anomalies, including craniosynostosis.

3. Ultrathin sections of 1.5 mm or less examine areas requiring high detail, such as the sella turcica, orbits, and petrous bones.

4. Bone targeting uses a special reconstruction algorithm to define fine anatomy such as the ossicles and osseous labyrinth of the petrous bone.

5. Dynamic scanning consists of performing rapid sequence scans after rapidly injecting a bolus of contrast agent. The subsequent contrast enhancement and washout can help to differentiate an aneurysm or arteriovenous malformation from a vascular tumor.

6. CT cisternography and myelography are performed by injecting water-soluble nonionic contrast material (iohexol or iopamidol) into the subarachnoid space and running the contrast material to scan the area of suspected abnormality. The technique may help to delineate tumors of the sella region, foramen magnum, and spinal canal. It may also be used to investigate CSF rhinorrhea and CSF dynamics in hydrocephalic patients.

MAGNETIC RESONANCE IMAGING. MRI, a rapidly evolving technology, has replaced CT as the examination of choice for most neurologic conditions (Table 392–3). Nuclear magnetic resonance occurs when hydrogen atoms or certain other elements with an odd number of nuclear particles such as sodium or phosphorus are placed in an intense magnetic field of between 3000 and 15,000 gauss (0.3 to 1.5 tesla). The nuclei behave like small magnets and align themselves in the field. When stimulated by a pulse of radio energy of a specific frequency (the Larmor frequency) determined by the intensity of the main magnetic field, the nuclei flip off axis. While in this energized state, the nuclei spin in phase as they subsequently relax into their original alignment with the main magnetic field, emitting a small radiofrequency signal. The MR image is gen-

TABLE 392–3. IMAGING MODALITY OF CHOICE IN DISEASES OF THE CNS

	CT	CT + C	MRI	MRI + Gd
Brain				
Gliomas	+	++	+++	++++
Metastases	+	+++	+++	++++
Meningiomas	+	+++	++	++++
Lymphoma	+	++	+++	++++
Postoperative and radiation therapy	+	++	++	++++
Hematomas	+++	0	++++	0
Subarachnoid hemorrhage	+++	0	+	0
Aneurysm and arteriovenous malformation	+	++	+++	0
Head trauma	+++	0	+++	0
Infarcts	++	+	+++	++
Abscess	+	++	+++	++++
AIDS	+	+++	+++	++++
Multiple sclerosis	0	+	++++	++++
Hydrocephalus/atrophy	++	++	++++	0
Congenital anomalies	+	+	++++	0
Sellar tumors	+	++	++++	+++
Posterior fossa				
Acoustic neurinoma	+	++	++++	+++
Meningioma	+	+++	+++	++++
Epidermoids	+	+	++++	0
Cholesterol granuloma	+	+	++++	0
Basilar artery aneurysm	+	++	++++	0
Craniovertebral junction	+	+	++++	0
Intra-axial gliomas	+	++	++++	+++
Spine				
Trauma	+++	0	+++	0
Degenerative disc disease	+++	0	++++	0
Postoperative disc disease	++	+++	+++	++++
Metastatic bone disease	++	0	++++	+++
Arteriovenous malformation of the cord	0	+	+++	+++

CT = Computed tomography; C = contrast enhancement; MRI = magnetic resonance imaging; Gd = gadolinium enhancement.

erated by many such magnetic resonance signals, transformed by a computer using techniques similar to those employed in CT. The resulting images demonstrate a high contrast between various tissues owing largely to differences in the rate at which magnetized nuclei in tissues of different chemical composition resume their original state (T1 and T2). The intensity of the MR image may be measured on the viewing console using a movable cursor similar to that on a CT scanner. Using standard "spin-echo" imaging sequences, a short T1 relaxation time of tissues such as fat results in high intensity (bright), whereas a long T1 relaxation time (CSF) results in CSF producing low signal intensity. Conversely, a short T2 relaxation time in tissues such as fat results in a low signal intensity, and a long T2 relaxation time in CSF results in a high signal intensity.

Accordingly, the contrast of fat, brain, and CSF on a T1-weighted spin echo (TE 30, TR 500) reverses itself on a T2-weighted spin echo (TE 80, TR 2000). The concentration of protons also affects intensity, as it is their signal that is being measured. Other factors affecting signal intensity include flow, magnetic susceptibility, paramagnetic effects, and the static field strength of the device.

MR images may be obtained in axial, coronal, sagittal, or oblique planes by changing the switching of the instrument's several magnetizing coils. Paramagnetic contrast agents developed for use with MRI contain elements such as gadolinium that, because of the large number of unpaired electrons in their outer shells, have a marked effect on the T1, or spin-lattice relaxation time, of protons. Gadolinium chelated to DTPA (Gd-DTPA) is used to define areas of increased vascularity and/or capillary permeability.

MRI is contraindicated for patients who harbor cardiac pacemakers or ferrous foreign bodies such as shrapnel. Intracranial aneurysm clips provide an absolute contraindication unless it is known for certain that they are made from nonmagnetic titanium or stainless steel. The presence of metal prostheses, spinal rods, certain metallic dental implants, and metallic cranioplastic prostheses may produce interfering artifacts but carry no risk of injury to the patient.

CEREBRAL ANGIOGRAPHY. Most cerebral angiograms are performed with an intra-arterial catheter inserted over a guide wire into the femoral artery and passed upward to the aortic arch or into the carotid or vertebral artery. Although cerebral angiography is a relatively safe procedure in experienced hands, complications, such as arterial damage, emboli to the brain, and contrast neurotoxicity, occur in 1 to 2% of procedures. New, less toxic, but more expensive non-ionic contrast agents are now replacing traditional ionic contrast materials. The use of smaller catheters facilitates examination of outpatients.

Arterial digital subtraction angiography (DSA) uses computerized imaging enhancement to improve the contrast of the injected contrast agent and to lower the dose required. Recently developed equipment with a 1k × 1k matrix produces such superb images that all arteriograms may be performed without using x-ray film. Instantaneous viewing of the subtracted images and software techniques such as road-mapping, rotational sequences, and density analysis have resulted in shorter examination times and improved studies.

Intravenous DSA uses similar equipment and rapid injections of contrast material into a peripheral vein or the right atrium. Imaging commences after a suitable delay to allow the contrast to pass through the pulmonary circulation into the systemic arteries. The procedure may be performed as an outpatient procedure for demonstrating the aortic arch and great vessels in the neck, as well as the intracranial cerebral arteries and veins. Intravenous DSA is not satisfactory for demonstrating small aneurysms of the circle of Willis or intracranial arterial abnormalities such as occlusions from emboli or vasculitis. Its rate of complications is similar to that of arterial angiography.

THE SPINE

RADIOGRAPHY (PLAIN FILMS). Conventional radiography of the spine demonstrates bony abnormalities such as degenerative disc disease, primary and metastatic tumors, and fractures of the vertebral bodies. Plain radiographs are the best method for demonstrating osteophytes in the neural foramina in the cervical, thoracic, and lumbar spine. Plains films should be obtained prior to myelography, CT, or MRI to identify segmentation anomalies at the thoracolumbar and lumbosacral junctions.

COMPUTED TOMOGRAPHY. CT of the spine demonstrates abnormalities of the spinal cord, meninges, vertebral bodies, and intervertebral articulations as well as those affecting paravertebral and prevertebral soft tissues. CT supplemented with intravenous contrast enhancement may be used to demonstrate vascular tumors of the spinal cord and meninges and can be valuable in distinguishing recurrent herniation of lumbar intervertebral discs from postsurgical scarring.

Postmyelogram CT or CT with intrathecal contrast improves delineation of subtle nerve root displacement due to posterolateral herniation of the intervertebral discs and associated osteophytes. It is also useful in demonstrating cysts and hydromyelia of the spinal cord, conditions in which CT may detect entry of contrast agent into the cavity 12 to 24 hours after intrathecal injection.

MAGNETIC RESONANCE IMAGING. MRI of the spine has replaced CT as the examination of choice because it gives better resolution of the spinal cord, subarachnoid space, and vertebral anatomy. It clearly depicts the intervertebral discs, showing the state of hydration of the nucleus pulposus and the condition of the annulus, usually with clear and unequivocal demonstration of any rupture of the annulus.

MRI of the spine with enhancement by Gd-DTPA defines spinal cord tumors and inflammatory processes of the meninges and differentiates recurrent disc herniation from postoperative scar tissue.

MYELOGRAPHY. Myelography is the most sensitive examination for demonstrating intradural mass lesions and can be helpful when an MRI is equivocal or shows multilevel disc disease without a predominant level of pathology. Iodinated water-soluble non-ionic contrast agent (iohexol, iopamidol) is introduced by lumbar puncture or, if indicated, by lateral cervical puncture (C1–C2). The contrast is hyperbaric and flows by gravity. By tilting the patient on a radiographic table, the contrast may be manipulated under fluoroscopic control from the lumbosacral region to the base of the skull.

Complications of myelography are rare, and the study is often performed as an outpatient procedure. Nevertheless, neurotoxic and other complications occasionally can occur. They include injury to nerve roots by the lumbar puncture needle as well as subarachnoid, subdural, or epidural bleeding. Much rarer events include infections or compression by mass lesions due to changes of pressure in the subarachnoid space.

IMAGING TECHNIQUES IN SPECIFIC DISEASE CATEGORIES

Tumors of the Cerebral Hemispheres

GLIOMAS (Fig. 392–2). Gliomas are demonstrated best with MRI because of sensitivity to slight changes in water content producing an area of hyperintensity on T2-weighted images. Tumors adjacent to the skull are seen best on MRI because of the absence of bone artifact. Differentiation of tumor from peritumoral edema may be obvious or difficult depending on the tumor margin but is improved with Gd-DTPA enhancement, which may demonstrate the areas of blood-brain barrier disruption or hypervascularity. Pre-gadolinium T1-weighted images may demonstrate hyperintensity due to hemorrhage into the tumor. Careful comparison of MRI images with multiple biopsies at the time of surgery has shown that tumor cells may extend well beyond the areas of contrast enhancement and may even be found in the opposite cerebral hemisphere.

METASTASES. MRI usually reveals metastases better than contrast-enhanced CT. Occasionally metastases may be overlooked on a regular MRI or contrast-enhanced CT but are clearly demonstrated on a postcontrast MRI. Because gadolinium-enhanced MRI is the superior examination, it should be performed when metastases are suspected or when evaluating "extent of disease."

Multiple metastases may resemble other disease processes such as *Toxoplasma* abscesses or even the active stage of multiple sclerosis. An accurate history is always required and sometimes even a biopsy. *A solitary metastasis may often resemble a glioma or a primary lymphoma and if it is located close to the skull, it may be difficult to distinguish from a meningioma. Metastases, whether solitary or multiple, usually are well circumscribed. Surrounding edema may be minimal or extensive, depending on the cell type and steroid therapy.*

MENINGIOMAS (Fig. 392–3). Meningiomas are usually well demonstrated on contrast-enhanced CT or MRI, but if small they may be difficult to identify on MRI without contrast. Almost all meningiomas exhibit intense homogeneous gadolinium enhancement; visualization, particularly of the components adjacent to the inner table of the skull, may be superior. MRI scans in multiple

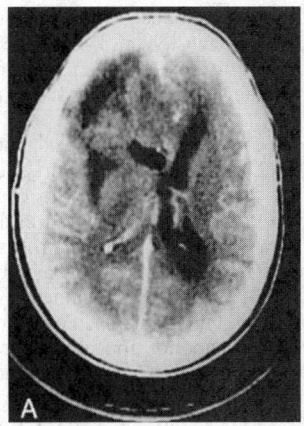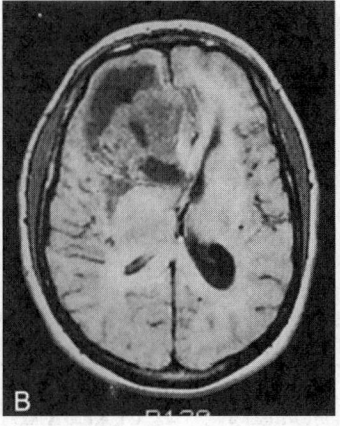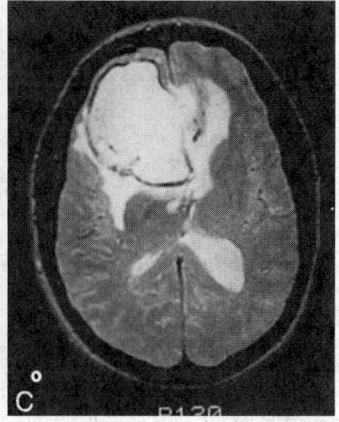

FIGURE 392–2. Right frontal glioblastoma multiforme. *A,* CT axial section with iodinated contrast enhancement. *B,* MRI axial section, 500/30 SE (T1-weighted). *C,* MRI axial section, 2000/80 SE (T2-weighted).

planes increase the examiner's confidence about the extracerebral location of these tumors.

Postoperatively, enhanced MRI is superior to enhanced CT for demonstrating residual tumor, invasion of the venous sinuses, and surgical scar formation.

LYMPHOMAS. MRI detects primary and secondary lymphoma of brain better than CT. The changes may sometimes resemble meningiomas or gliomas, thus requiring a biopsy for ultimate diagnosis. Patients with AIDS may simultaneously harbor lymphoma and *Toxoplasma* granulomas that cannot be differentiated by MRI except by evaluating the response to anti-*Toxoplasma* therapy.

TUMOR STATUS. Postoperative evaluation of tumor recurrence and radiation necrosis may be difficult with either CT or MRI if only a single examination is available. Contrast enhancement on CT and MRI may persist for several months after surgery, and radiation therapy may open the blood-brain barrier to contrast agents so as to resemble a deteriorating process on follow-up examinations. Chronic postradiation changes with demyelination of white matter are detected better on MRI than CT. Radiation necrosis may be indistinguishable from recurrent tumor by either enhanced MRI or CT. PET using fluorodeoxyglucose to measure regional cerebral metabolic rate typically demonstrates hypoactivity in areas of radionecrosis and hyperactivity in recurrent tumor. Some gliomas, however, may have low metabolic activity due to cystic components or a low grade of malignancy, sometimes making differentiation uncertain.

Other Brain Lesions

HEMATOMAS AND HEMORRHAGE. CT contributes importantly to the diagnosis of parenchymatous intracranial hemorrhage and is routinely performed as an emergency procedure following recent severe head injury or stroke. Acute hemorrhages appear as areas of increased density depending on the anatomic location (spherical or irregular for intracerebral, lentiform if chronic subdural, and concavo-convex if acute subdural or epidural). The CT-recorded increased density of clot fades so that by 10 to 14 days after bleeding occurs, the area may become isodense relative to brain, leaving a thin rim of contrast enhancement. Subacute subdural hematomas are frequently visualized better after contrast because of enhancement of the adjacent brain surface. Subsequently the aging clot, although unchanged in size, becomes hypodense, approaching the density of the CSF.

Intracranial hemorrhages cause rapid and complex changes in MRI scans during the first 4 days. Accordingly, the appearance of bleeding depends upon time of onset, source (arterial or venous), location (subarachnoid, subdural, intraparenchymal), and whether or not rehemorrhage has occurred. Other factors affecting reliability include the pulse sequences used and the field strength of the magnet.

An acute hemorrhage in any location appears isointense or slightly hyperintense on T1-weighted spin-echo images, but is hyperintense or heterogeneous on T2-weighted spin-echo techniques. At this stage hemorrhages resemble an acute infarct, tumor, or abscess/granuloma. The presence of blood, however, may be inferred from a gradient-echo scan that accentuates the magnetic susceptibility effect of the iron in hemoglobin and results in a zone of marked hypointensity.

During the first 24 hours after clot formation, oxyhemoglobin red cells change to deoxyhemoglobin and methemoglobin, resulting in a decreased signal intensity on the T2-weighted spin-echo images. Between 3 and 6 days after clot formation, lysis affects red cells with accumulation of extracellular deoxyhemoglobin and methemoglobin that results in a shortening of the T1 relaxation time, leading to increased signal intensity on T1-weighted spin-echo images.

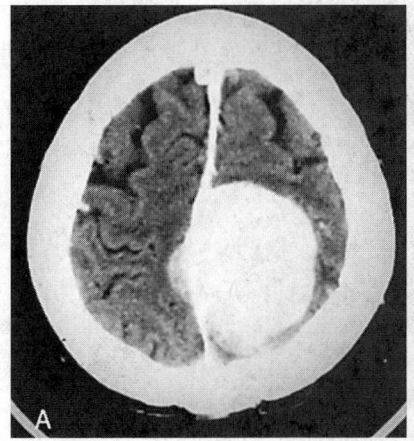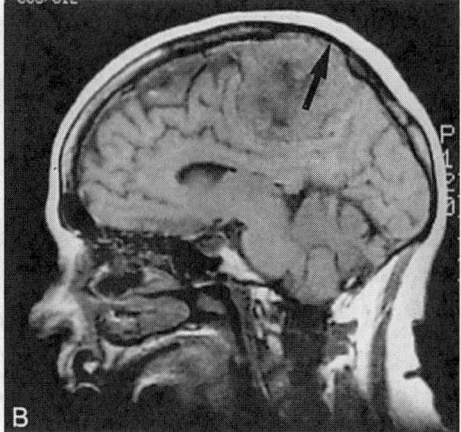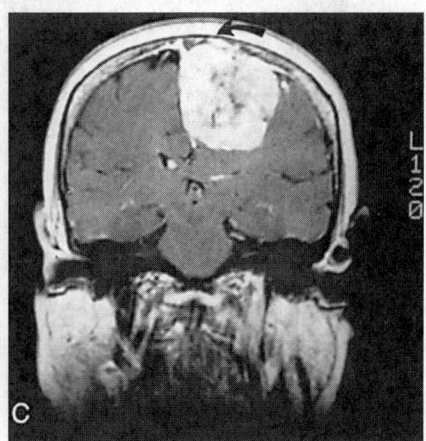

FIGURE 392–3. Left parietal parasagittal meningioma. *A,* CT axial section with iodinated contrast enhancement. *B,* MRI sagittal 500/30 SE section demonstrates invasion of the superior sagittal sinus *(arrow). C,* MRI coronal 500/30 SE section after intravenous administration of gadopentetate dimeglumine demonstrates intense enhancement of the tumor, dural extension, and invasion of the superior sagittal sinus *(arrow).*

After about 5 days, when red cell lysis is complete, deoxyhemoglobin converts to methemoglobin, resulting in a marked decrease in T1 relaxation time and an increase in the T2 relaxation time. This produces high signal intensity on T1- and T2-weighted spinecho images, the unmistakable hallmark of hemorrhage. This appearance remains for 30 to 40 days, after which the T1 hyperintensity gradually decreases. Finally, the aging hemorrhage approaches the signal intensity of CSF, but the margin may remain hypointense (dark) owing to the paramagnetic effect of hemosiderin in surrounding macrophages.

Because of these complex changes, CT often detects hemorrhage more easily during the first 48 hours. If gradient-echo techniques are used, MRI may be more sensitive than CT during this time, although fresh hemorrhage may be indistinguishable from old hemorrhage or areas of abnormal brain mineralization.

ANEURYSMS AND ARTERIOVENOUS MALFORMATIONS (Fig. 392–4).

Aneurysms and arteriovenous malformations may be diagnosed by CT because of curvilinear calcifications, contrast enhancement of the lumen, and mass effect. MRI is superior to CT because the rapidly flowing blood in the lumen of the aneurysm or the nidus of a malformation results in a "signal void." Aneurysms as small as 3 mm may be detected, and surrounding hemorrhage in the brain is readily identified. Giant aneurysms >1 cm in diameter may have turbulent flow leading to heterogeneous signal intensity, similar in appearance to mural thrombosis. Magnetic resonance angiography (MRA) shows promise in detecting aneurysms and arteriovenous malformations, but detection depends upon the imaging factors and the velocity of flow within the lesions. The accuracy of MRA has not yet reached that of cerebral angiography.

Subarachnoid hemorrhage, usually due to rupture of an aneurysm, is better shown on CT than on MRI because of the effects of CSF on clot formation, deoxyhemoglobin accumulation, and resolution of the hemorrhage. *In suspicious cases, however, subarachnoid hemorrhage should never be excluded unless a lumbar puncture is normal.* Cerebral arteriography remains essential to demonstrate the anatomy of the aneurysm neck, exclude multiple aneurysms, and identify blood flow patterns. Angiography also detects anatomic anomalies of the circle of Willis prior to surgical or endovascular intervention.

Arteriovenous and venous malformations may be differentiated on MRI, but cerebral arteriography is required to differentiate a venous malformation from a small, "high-flow" arteriovenous malformation. Angiography is similarly necessary to demonstrate the dural component of an arteriovenous malformation, which may not be visible on MRI or MRA.

Cavernous hemangiomas, small benign tumors that arise in the cerebral hemispheres, cerebellum, or brain stem, cause gradual neurologic deterioration due to small, recurrent hemorrhages. On CT they appear as hyperdense masses with variable contrast enhancement. On MRI they produce a pathognomonic appearance with heterogeneous hyperintensity on T1-weighted spin-echo and a dark rim on T2-weighted technique. A cerebral arteriogram may be normal except for a faint homogeneous stain, usually without a mass effect.

HEAD TRAUMA. Following serious head trauma, conventional radiographs of the skull detect fractures of the skull vault and associated fractures of the facial bones and cervical spine. Particular attention to the upper cervical spine is required in the elderly because of the possibility of a fractured odontoid process or a "bamboo" fracture of the spine affected by ankylosing spondylitis.

Computed tomography is the best examination for demonstrating acute brain contusions or intracranial hemorrhages during the first 48 hours. Later, MRI is superior for imaging small hemorrhagic collections and revealing cerebral contusions and axonal shearing injuries.

CEREBRAL INFARCTS (Fig. 392–5). CT is currently the most frequently used imaging modality in acute stroke. Any degree of significant hemorrhage can be detected, permitting an early decision about use of anticoagulants.

MRI, however, demonstrates changes in the brain parenchyma earlier and, with gradient-echo techniques, is extremely sensitive for the presence of hemorrhage. With the addition of MRA, it is also superior for detecting thrombosis of the carotid or intracerebral arteries and venous sinus occlusions.

An acute infarct appears as an area of hyperintensity on T2-weighted spin-echo images within 4 hours after onset of the stroke; CT images may remain normal for the first 12 to 24 hours. After 4 days, areas of contrast enhancement may be detected with CT or even earlier with MRI owing to the development of pial and subpial collateral arteries and capillaries. MRI and CT equally well demonstrate old infarcts with areas of focal brain atrophy or encephalomalacia, but MRI using T2 spin-echo or gradient-echo techniques better shows areas of old hemorrhage.

In elderly patients with hypertension or arteriosclerosis and in patients with vasculitis such as lupus erythematosus, foci of hyperintensities on T2-weighted MRI images often appear in the cerebral hemispheres or cerebellum, even though the CT remains normal.

INFLAMMATORY BRAIN LESIONS. CT and MRI demonstrate inflammatory changes due to herpes simplex encephalitis, progressive multifocal leukoencephalopathy, and cytomegalovirus infection because of brain edema, mass effect, and occasionally contrast enhancement. MRI is superior to CT for demonstrating multiple granulomas such as those that complicate AIDS; gadolinium enhancement increases their detectability. Sometimes neither CT nor MRI differentiates concurrent inflammatory lesions, such as *Toxoplasma* granulomas from tuberculomas or neoplasm such as primary lymphomas.

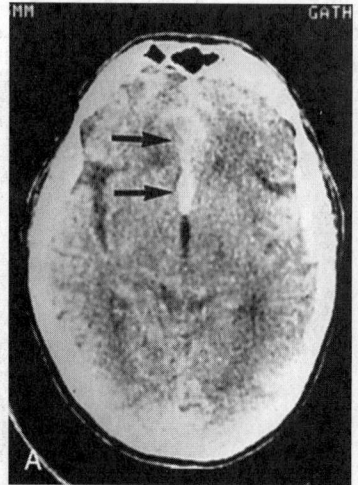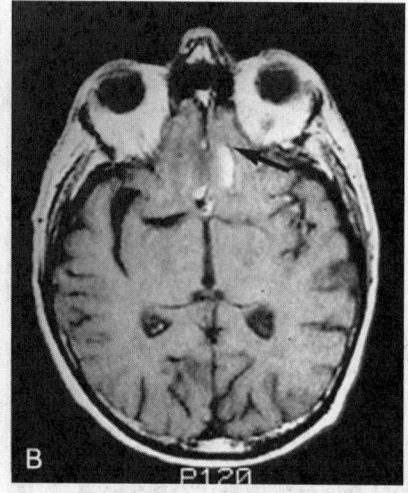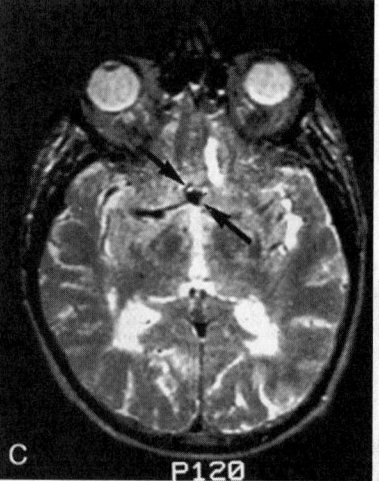

FIGURE 392–4. Subarachnoid hemorrhage due to rupture of anterior communicating artery aneurysm. *A,* CT axial section demonstrates hyperdense blood in the interhemispheric fissure *(arrows). B,* MRI axial 500/30 SE section demonstrates hyperintense blood along the olfactory groove *(arrow). C,* MRI axial 2000/80 SE section (T2-weighted) scan demonstrates the aneurysm of the anterior communicating artery *(arrows).*

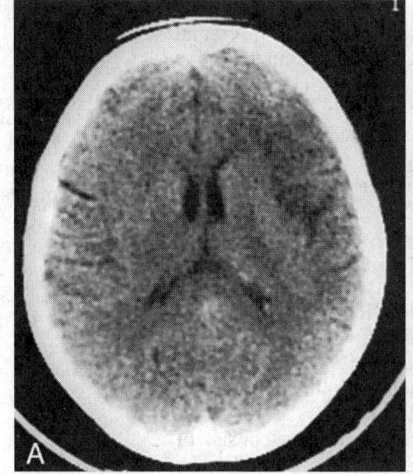
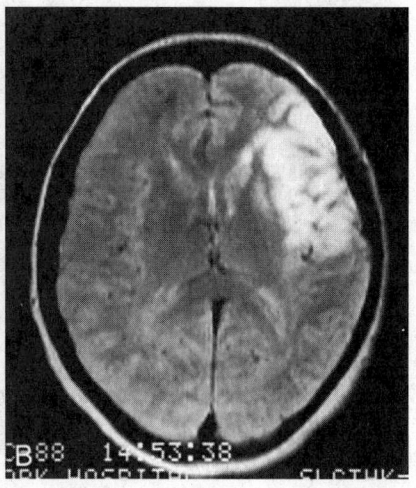

FIGURE 392–5. Acute left frontal infarct. *A,* CT axial section at 24 hours demonstrates a vague area of decreased attenuation of the left frontal lobe. *B,* MRI axial 2000/30 SE section reveals a very hyperintense area of the left frontal lobe with involvement of the cerebral cortex and adjacent basal ganglia due to a partial occlusion of the middle cerebral artery.

MRI with gadolinium enhancement is superior to CT for demonstrating acute and chronic meningitis, including sarcoid, as well as subdural and epidural empyemas. Contrast-enhanced MRI and CT detect intracerebral abscesses equally well; MRI with contrast enhancement best detects abscesses adjacent to the ethmoid sinuses and petrous temporal bones.

MULTIPLE SCLEROSIS (MS) AND WHITE MATTER DISEASES (Fig. 392–6). MRI identifies brain lesions in about 80% of patients with known MS, compared with 25% found by CT scans. Contrast enhancement after Gd-DTPA differentiates active plaques from old, healed lesions.

Focal hyperintensities resembling those of MS occur frequently in elderly patients and are usually due to ischemic demyelination or to multiple small infarcts. Similar lesions also can follow radiation therapy, Lyme disease, and severe recurrent migraine attacks; they also may be caused by generalized vascular inflammatory diseases such as lupus erythematosus. Small, disseminated metastases may have a similar appearance.

HYDROCEPHALUS AND ATROPHY. Both hydrocephalus and cerebral atrophy are associated with loss of brain volume and increased volume of CSF (see Ch. 436). MRI is the examination of choice for differentiating hydrocephalus from cerebral atrophy and for localizing the site of obstruction. MRI with gadolinium enhancement may detect small, infiltrating tumors or chronic meningitis.

In the presence of chronic aqueduct stenosis or colloid cysts obstructing the third ventricle, asymptomatic caudal herniation of the brain stem through the tentorium may be demonstrated on sagittal MR images.

CONGENITAL ANOMALIES. MRI is the best imaging modality for demonstrating and understanding most developmental anomalies of the brain. Multiplanar coronal, sagittal, and axial images make structural changes more apparent, and MRI better distinguishes areas of brain damaged by perinatal anoxia, injury, and infections.

SELLAR TUMORS. MRI is superior to CT in delineating tumors of the pituitary gland, the suprasellar region, and the optic chiasm. Contrast enhancement is essential in CT studies of this region and is increasingly used with MRI examination.

MR images in the sagittal and coronal planes demonstrate the normal pituitary gland, including the hyperintense posterior pituitary. Microadenomas are detected reliably using thin-section T1-weighted spin-echo sequences in the coronal plane. Following Gd-DTPA administration, microadenomas exhibit delayed enhancement relative to the surrounding normal tissue and therefore appear hypointense early and hyperintense late.

Analysis of the signal intensity (on T2-weighted images) separates solid fibrous adenomas from soft or cystic ones. Craniopharyngiomas and meningiomas differ from each other by their suprasellar location, tissue characteristics, and post–Gd-DTPA enhancement pattern. The precise location of adjacent cranial nerves and cerebral arteries may be identified, aiding the preoperative planning and surgical removal of the tumor.

POSTERIOR FOSSA LESIONS. MRI is the examination of choice for posterior fossa lesions because of its multiplanar capabilities, absence of bone artifacts, and superior contrast detection between gray and white matter and CSF. Tumors arising outside the cerebellum and brain stem can be differentiated from primary intra-axial tumors. Tumors arising in the skull base and clivus are detected because of replacement of the normal high signal intensity of fat-containing bone marrow. The MRI examination should be modified for the posterior fossa to include high-resolution coronal and axial images with T1-weighted spin echo. Enhancement with Gd-DTPA is increasingly used to demonstrate the total extent of meningiomas and to rule out additional tumors.

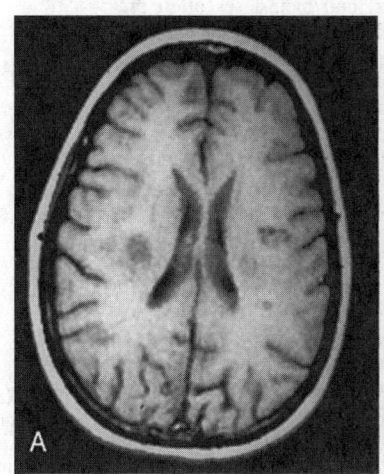
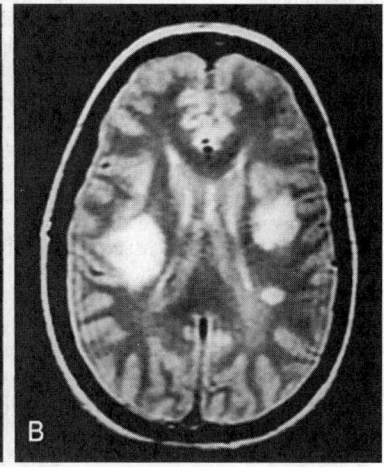

FIGURE 392–6. Multiple sclerosis. *A,* MRI axial 500/30 SE section reveals several areas of low signal intensity due to plaques of demyelination. *B,* MRI axial 2000/40 SE (proton-density) section demonstrates that the areas of demyelination are more numerous and larger.

ACOUSTIC NEURINOMAS. These benign tumors usually originate from the superior vestibular division of the eighth cranial nerve in the internal auditory canal of the petrous temporal bone (see Ch. 435).

MRI demonstrates acoustic neurinomas as slightly hypointense or isointense masses in the internal auditory canal, with extension into the adjacent cerebellopontine angle cistern (see Ch. 435). On T2-weighted images the tumor becomes hyperintense but may be obscured by the hyperintensity of the surrounding CSF. The separate divisions of the seventh and eighth cranial nerves are visible on the contralateral side. Such tumors enhance after gadolinium administration.

MENINGIOMAS OF THE POSTERIOR FOSSA. Meningiomas can grow anywhere in the posterior fossa. Those in the cerebellopontine angle appear similar to acoustic neurinomas but rarely extend into the internal auditory canal. Gadolinium enhancement is necessary to visualize the tumor's dural beak.

EPIDERMOID TUMORS. These interesting tumors consist of glittering white folds of epidermal tissue surrounded by CSF. The tumors produce a mass effect and insinuate themselves into the adjacent cisterns, wrapping around blood vessels and cranial nerves. On CT the lesions appear as fluid densities, sometimes resembling an arachnoid cyst. Epidermoid tumors show no contrast enhancement.

MRI demonstrates the full extent of the tumor, and subtle changes in signal intensity on T2-weighted spin-echo images usually differentiate the growth from surrounding CSF. Considerable deformity of the brain stem can precede abnormal neurologic signs.

CHOLESTEROL GRANULOMAS OF THE PETROUS APEX. These unusual lesions often contain brown fluid with cholesterol crystals thought to result from an inflammatory response to hemorrhage into infected petrous apical air cells. Compression of adjacent cranial nerves V, VI, VII, or VIII often results.

BASILAR ARTERY ANEURYSMS. Both saccular and fusiform aneurysms may be difficult to diagnose on CT in the axial plane. Diagnosis is straightforward on MRI because of the characteristic signal void of the lumen and the clear anatomic localization. MRA may demonstrate the lumen well, depending on the velocity of flow within it.

ARACHNOID CYSTS. Primary arachnoid cysts of the posterior fossa occur in the prepontine cistern, cerebellopontine angle, and cisterna magna. On MRI they demonstrate a signal intensity identical to that of CSF. The associated mass effect of the cyst usually differentiates it from an enlarged cisterna magna.

CRANIOVERTEBRAL JUNCTION. MRI is superior to CT for demonstrating basilar impression, whether due to congenital anomalies at the craniovertebral junction or to soft bones such as in Paget's disease or osteogenesis imperfecta. Brain stem compression caused by atlantoaxial subluxation due to rheumatoid arthritis or trauma is also well shown. Abnormally low cerebellar tonsils due to Chiari I malformation or the Arnold-Chiari malformation are easily detected.

INTRA-AXIAL POSTERIOR FOSSA TUMORS. *Brain Stem.* Intracranial tumors of the brain stem such as gliomas, ependymomas, cavernous hemangiomas, and metastases often present with progressive unilateral or bilateral cranial nerve palsies similar to extracranial tumors. Imaging techniques are crucial for the diagnosis and usually determine treatment. Surgical biopsy may have an unacceptably high complication rate.

MRI examination with multiple planes, multiple sequences, and contrast enhancement demonstrates the intra-axial location and extent of the mass with a high degree of confidence. Differentiation between a glioma and an ependymoma may be possible based on the sharply defined edge of an ependymoma and its location near the ventricular surface. Metastases of the brain stem vary in appearance, depending upon the site of origin, and may be mistaken for granulomas, lymphomas, and gliomas.

Cerebellar Tumors. Medulloblastomas as well as solid and cystic astrocytomas are usually well demonstrated with CT or MRI with contrast enhancement. Hemangioblastomas, often cystic, are better shown on MRI with contrast enhancement. The upper spinal cord should be included in the study because the area may contain additional tumor nodules.

TRAUMA. Conventional radiographs are obtained initially to demonstrate fracture and dislocations. After mid-position views with a collar have revealed normal alignment and an intact odontoid process, radiographs of the cervical spine are usually taken in flexion and extension to detect instability due to ligamentous injury. CT is helpful in demonstrating fractures of the neural arch and articular facets as well as transverse fractures of the vertebral body and post-traumatic disc herniations that may result in cord or nerve root compression. If spinal cord injury is evident clinically, MRI examination is useful to identify hematomyelia or epidural hematoma and may assist in the decision for conservative or surgical management.

DEGENERATIVE DISC DISEASE. Plain radiographs should be taken to demonstrate the vertebrae; disc space views in flexion and extension often help to show instability at the intervertebral articulations.

MRI is the study of choice in all areas of the spine for demonstrating degeneration or prolapse of the discs (Fig. 392-7). Images are obtained in the sagittal plane, the oblique axial planes, and through the intervertebral discs using various T1- or T2-weighted spin-echo sequences or gradient-echo techniques. Disc prolapse is identified and the annular deficit is usually clearly seen. Spinal stenosis, if present, is readily identified, and spinal cord or cauda equina compression may be detected.

In postoperative patients with recurrent symptoms, MRI with gadolinium enhancement can differentiate recurrent disc prolapse from postoperative scarring in the epidural space.

If MR images are degraded from metallic clips, rods, or other fixation devices or by patient motion, a CT examination of the area may substitute. Intravenous iodinated contrast is used to differentiate enhancing epidural scans from recurrent disc disease.

PRIMARY TUMORS, HYDROMYELIA, AND DEMYELINATING DISORDERS OF THE SPINAL CORD. MRI is the study of choice (Fig. 392-8). Gadolinium enhancement is required to demonstrate areas of increased vascularity in the spinal cord due to inflammatory and neoplastic processes. Intramedullary cysts due to small gliomas and ependymomas may be mistaken for hydromyelia on nonenhanced studies, but the tumor is readily detected on the post–Gd-DTPA images. Meningeal metastases either from systemic cancer or from CNS tumors show nodular enhancement after Gd-DTPA administration.

METASTATIC BONE DISEASE. MRI is the most accurate technique for detecting osseous metastases and epidural masses that may cause a cord or cauda equina compression. Such examinations are replacing emergency myelography and are usually sufficient to

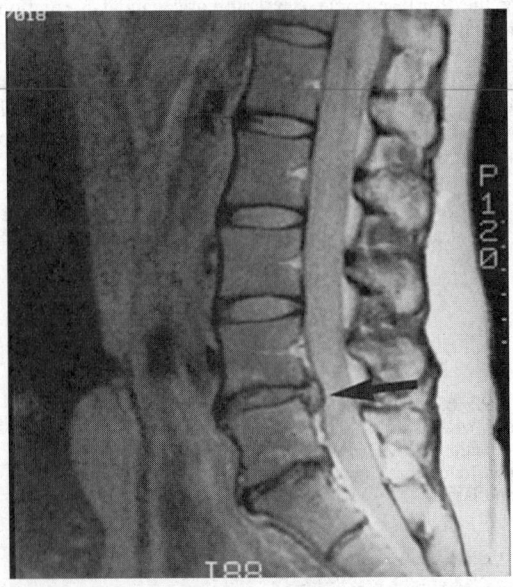

FIGURE 392-7. Herniation of a lumbar intervertebral disc. MRI 1500/30 SE sagittal section reveals a midline posterior prolapse of the nucleus pulposus of the L4/5 intervertebral disc (*arrow*) with an obvious dehiscence of the annulus fibrosis.

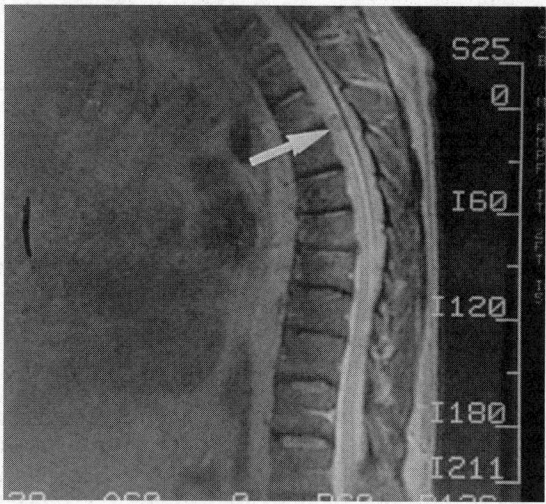

FIGURE 392–8. Thoracic neurofibroma. MRI 2000/80 SE sagittal section demonstrates an ovoid tumor *(arrow)* overlying the thoracic spinal cord.

direct appropriate radiation therapy. MRI or CT may be used to direct needle biopsies of suspected metastases of the vertebrae.

ARTERIOVENOUS MALFORMATIONS OF THE SPINAL CORD. Although large arteriovenous malformations may be identified on MRI or MRA, myelography is necessary to identify small malformations. Selective spinal arteriography with injections of contrast material directly into multiple intercostal and lumbar arteries is required to identify the precise feeding arteries, the nidus of the malformation, and the draining veins.

Brant-Zawadski M, Norman D (eds.): Magnetic Resonance Imaging of the Central Nervous System. New York, Raven Press, 1987. *An atlas of MRI demonstrating the classic appearances of a variety of brain lesions.*
Huk WJ, Gademann G, Friedmann G: Magnetic Resonance Imaging of Central Nervous System Diseases. Berlin, Springer-Verlag, 1990.
Newton TH, Potts DG (eds.): Advanced Imaging Techniques: Modern Neuroradiology. Vol. 2. San Anselmo, Calif., Clavedel Press, 1983. *Contains, among other useful information, an excellent description of the physics and techniques of various imaging modalities written for nonphysicians.*
Stark DD, Bradley WG (eds.): Magnetic Resonance Imaging. St. Louis, CV Mosby, 1988. *A comprehensive text containing detailed technical and clinical descriptions of MRI.*

Section Two—Disorders of Cerebral Function

393 DISTURBANCES OF CONSCIOUSNESS AND AROUSAL
Fred Plum

DEFINITIONS AND MECHANISMS OF ALTERED CONSCIOUSNESS

Consciousness is a brain-generated psychological state expressed in two dimensions: wakefulness and the self-aware cognition of past events and future anticipations which accompany the normal wakeful state. Disease or dysfunction that impairs either aspect of this combination causes the conditions defined in Table 393–1. Occasionally, however, either certain forms of neurologic damage or the presence of a severe psychiatric disorder can mimic an unconscious state. A later section discusses these potentially deceptive conditions.

Impaired consciousness can be *sustained,* i.e., prolonged for periods lasting for hours or more, or *brief,* with the lapse enduring for no more than a few seconds to an hour or so. The longer an abnormal state of consciousness lasts, the more likely it is to reflect structural damage to the brain rather than a transient alteration in its function. Sustained alterations of consciousness are discussed in Ch. 394. Brief loss of consciousness is considered in Ch. 396.

The normal capacity to awaken and direct attention depends upon ontogenetically primitive arousal mechanisms lodged within or in close association with the ascending reticular activating system (ARAS). The ARAS consists of a loosely organized, fairly dense column of neurons which extends forward along the brain's central core from approximately the upper third of the pons to the deep midline reaches of the hypothalamus and the thalamus. The system includes cholinergic, adrenergic, and serotoninergic fibers as well as others employing still undefined neurotransmitters. The self-aware, cognitive aspects of consciousness depend largely on the interconnected neural networks of the cerebral hemispheres and their extensive interconnections with the thalamus, basal ganglia, and cerebellum. Normal conscious states depend on the continuous, effective interaction between these cerebral systems and the subcortical activating mechanisms.

Impairments of consciousness can be partial or complete, acute or chronic. By definition, acute disturbances of consciousness always include at least some reduction in alertness and attention. These reductions often are accompanied by diffuse impairments of normal cognitive activity, reflecting a close interdependence between cortical cognitive mechanisms and the ascending activating systems. Accordingly, acute lesions that affect either the ascending system or diffusely impair large amounts of the cortex reduce the level of consciousness. Acute damage to or depression of the ARAS carries a high risk of blocking cortical arousal because its anatomic subcortical cross-sectional area is small, yet the system projects diffusely to the cortex and subcortical structures. By contrast, any given region of cortex feeds back to only a limited subcortical area

TABLE 393–1. STATES OF ALTERED CONSCIOUSNESS OR UNRESPONSIVENESS

Coma: A state of unarousable unresponsiveness; even strong exteroceptive stimuli fail to elicit recognizable psychological responses.

Stupor: Spontaneous unarousability interruptable only by vigorous, direct external stimulation.

Hypersomnia, pathologic drowsiness, obtundation: Terms applied to an increase above the patient's normal sleep/wake ratio, often accompanied during wakefulness by reduced attention and interest in the environment.

Delirium: An acute or subacute reduction in awareness, attention, orientation, and perception ("clouding of consciousness"), usually fluctuating and accompanied by abnormal sleep/wake patterns and often psychomotor disturbances.

Syncope: A brief loss of consciousness due to global failure of cerebrovascular perfusion.

Dementia: A sustained or permanent multidimensional or global decline in cognitive functions, usually without impaired arousal.

Vegetative state: A sustained, complete loss of cognition. Wake/sleep cycles and other autonomic functions remain relatively intact. The condition can either follow acute, severe bilateral cerebral damage or develop gradually as the end stage of a progressive dementia.

Locked-in state: A condition in which intellectual activity is preserved but cannot be expressed because of total incapacity to express voluntary responses due to impaired junction of descending motor pathways in the brain or peripheral motor nerves. Most such patients can use vertical eye movements to signal by code; some can grunt by code.

so that disease or dysfunction at the cerebral level usually must be widespread to cause stupor or coma. The tempo of the damage also is important. With disease that gradually affects either the cortex or the ascending activating mechanisms alone, arousal mechanisms tend to adapt so rapidly that wakefulness never is altogether lost. Accordingly, slowly progressive, severe cerebral disease causes a multifaceted dementia rather than the reduced arousal that results from acute disturbances. Among subcortical reticular structures, the posterior hypothalamus is essentially the only locus in which a chronic lesion produces a prolonged loss or reduction of the capacity to reawaken.

394 SUSTAINED IMPAIRMENTS OF CONSCIOUSNESS
Fred Plum

Three kinds of neurologic disorders may produce sustained impairment of consciousness. These include (1) focal supratentorial mass or destructive lesions that either secondarily compress or directly destroy deep midline thalamic-hypothalamic activating structures, (2) posterior fossa mass or destructive lesions that compress or destroy the brain stem's upper pontine–mesencephalic reticular formation, and (3) metabolic-diffuse abnormalities that acutely or subacutely impair the functions of the two cerebral hemispheres, the brain stem, or both. Metabolic abnormalities especially tend to affect both cerebral and subcortical arousal mechanisms concurrently. Table 394–1 enumerates the more common specific causes of stupor and coma according to these mechanisms.

PATHOPHYSIOLOGY AND CATEGORICAL DIAGNOSES OF DELIRIUM, STUPOR, AND COMA

INTRACRANIAL MASS LESIONS. Intracranial mass and destructive lesions that immediately or eventually impair consciousness can arise either above or below the tentorium, the fibrous structure that divides the diencephalon and forebrain from the brain stem. Whether such lesions lie in the supra- or subtentorial compartments, their effects and outcome depend on (1) the geographic anatomy of the abnormality, (2) its size and rate of enlargement, and (3) any reactive changes it causes in surrounding brain. These

TABLE 394–1. THE COMMON CAUSES OF STUPOR AND COMA

Supratentorial lesions (causing secondary upper brain stem dysfunction)
  Cerebral hemorrhage
  Large cerebral infarction
  Subdural hematoma
  Epidural hematoma
  Brain tumor
  Brain abscess (rare)
Subtentorial lesions (compressing or destroying the rostral reticular formation)
  Pontine or cerebellar hemorrhage
  Brain stem infarction
  Brain stem or cerebellar tumor
  Cerebellar abscess
Metabolic and diffuse lesions (see also Table 394–5)
  Exogenous poison
  Infections
    Meningitis
    Encephalitis
  Concussion and postictal states
  Anoxia or ischemia
  Hypoglycemia
  Ionic and electrolyte disorders
  Endogenous toxin due to organ failure or deficiency
  Nutritional deficiency
Psychogenic unresponsiveness

TABLE 394–2. CHARACTERISTICS OF SUPRATENTORIAL LESIONS LEADING TO COMA

Initiating symptoms usually cerebral-focal: aphasia; focal seizures; contralateral hemiparesis, sensory change, or neglect; frontal lobe behavioral changes; headache.
Dysfunction moves rostral to caudal: e.g., focal motor → bilateral motor → altered level of arousal.
Abnormal signs usually confined to a single or adjacent anatomic level (not diffuse).
Brain stem functions spared unless herniation develops.

changes include tissue edema and vasodilatation as well as proliferative inflammatory and glial responses. Their volume and effect can be as dangerous as the primary lesion itself because they can triple the size of the primary lesion. Such severe reactions are especially prominent in and around malignant neoplasms, acute infarctions, hemorrhages, or abscesses. Because the skull is inexpansible, all enlarging masses eventually cause intracranial shifts and compressions that endanger the vitality of adjacent and remote brain areas.

As mass lesions form and enlarge within the cranial cavity, local intracranial compliance declines, cerebrospinal fluid flow and absorption are impeded, and the intracranial pressure rises. If the process is not interrupted, intracranial distortion and pressure eventually increase sufficiently to impede the blood supply in areas of compressed tissue. When this occurs, arteriolar resistance intermittently fails, leading to temporary, recurrent increases in intracranial blood volume which produce brief but dangerous episodes of greatly increased intracranial pressure, called *pressure waves*.

As could be expected, functional neurologic abnormalities accompanying the above pathophysiologic changes occur earliest in regions in and adjacent to the primary lesion, then gradually extend to affect more remote brain areas made vulnerable by being compressed against unyielding edges of bone or dura. Particularly at risk of this complication are structures that become squeezed against the falx cerebri or herniate into the restricted apertures of the tentorial notch or foramen magnum, thereby impacting areas critical to consciousness and even survival (Fig. 394–1).

SUPRATENTORIAL MASS LESIONS CAUSING COMA. Enlarging supratentorial lesions most often produce stupor or coma by shifting brain tissue either horizontally across the midline or caudally toward the tentorium. The process compresses and displaces the diencephalon, impairing arousal mechanisms and producing distinctive clinical features (Table 394–2). Localizing symptoms almost always appear first, followed, as the lesion enlarges, by the development of altered consciousness. In keeping with this sequence, most patients demonstrate a combination of *focal* hemispheric signs, e.g., sensorimotor abnormalities, aphasia, or visual field defects, followed by signs of *diffuse* supratentorial dysfunction, consisting of nonfocal headache, reduced attention, confusion, and somnolence. Sometimes supratentorial masses arise and enlarge in neurologically silent areas such as the frontal lobes or the subdural space. In such instances, signs and symptoms of diffuse cerebral dysfunction and increased intracranial pressure may predominate, producing papilledema, confusion, apathy, or hypersomnolence. In either event, brain imaging discloses a large, space-occupying lesion, characteristically displacing adjacent tissues either caudally, across the midline, or both. Unless the brain already has begun to herniate into the tentorial notch, pupillary and oculovestibular reflexes remain intact. Decerebrate motor responses develop only as a late sign.

Transtentorial herniation complicating supratentorial mass lesions begins either with downward displacement of the diencephalon (central herniation) or with the uncus of the temporal lobe squeezing against the midbrain in the tentorial notch (uncal herniation) (Table 394–3). With impending *central* herniation, stupor becomes gradually deeper, and patients sigh, yawn, or develop periodic breathing. The pupils shrink to 1 to 2 mm in diameter, reflecting hypothalamic dysfunction, but retain their light reflexes. Later, one or both pupils may ominously dilate. Loss of forebrain inhibition on the brain stem results in the development of brisk oculomotor reflexes (see Ch. 403). Until mesencephalic insufficiency develops, oculovestibular reflex responses (cold caloric test) are marked by tonic deviation of the eyes toward the stimulated side. Bilateral upper motor neuron signs develop, eventually leading to decerebrate

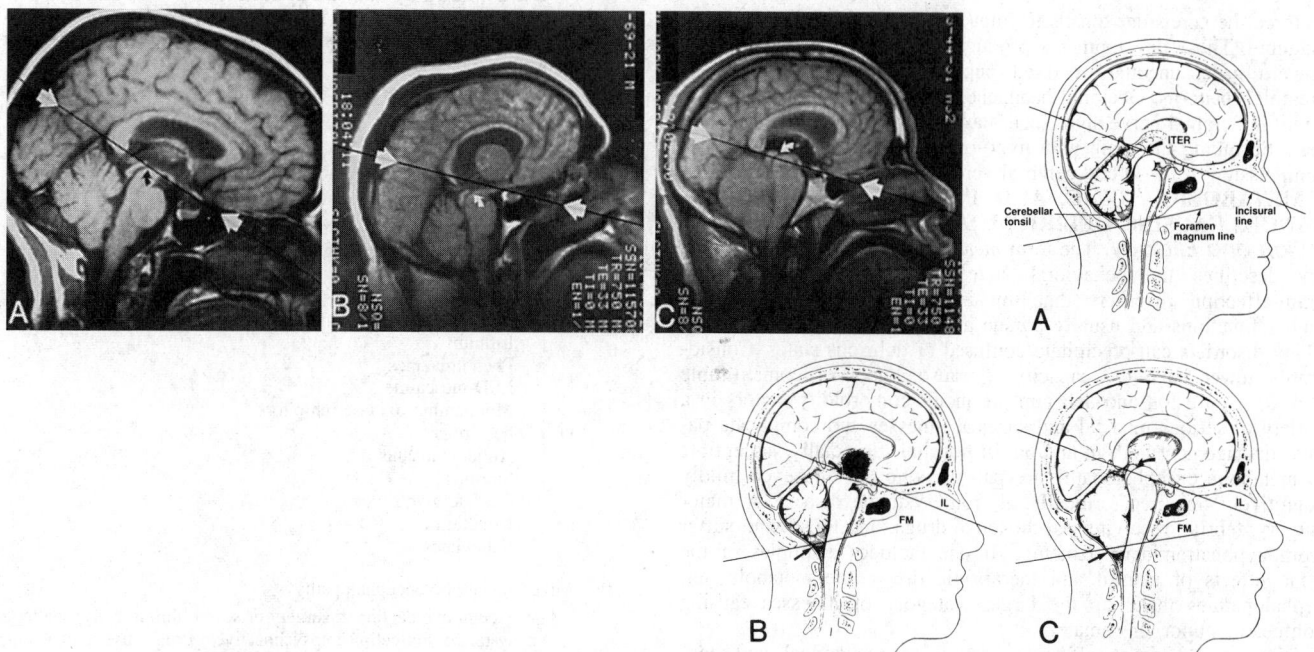

FIGURE 394–1. Midsagittal diagrams and magnetic resonance images of a normal adult brain compared with downward and upward transtentorial herniation as well as foramen magnum herniation. *A,* Normal 45-year-old male brain. The incisural line (IL) defines the plane of the tentorial opening, which extends from the junction between the vein of Galen and the cerebral venous straight sinus posteriorly to the anterior clinoid process. The iter, i.e., the rostral opening of the aqueduct of Sylvius *(black curved arrow)* lies on or within 2 mm of the IL. The cerebellar tonsils remain well above the foramen magnum. *B,* Downward transtentorial herniation due to a chronic colloid cyst lying in the third ventricle of a 52-year-old man (dark round shadow on diagram). The curved white arrow on the MRI scan points to the aqueduct, posterior thalamus, and mesencephalon, which are displaced 8 mm caudally of the IL. The cerebellar tonsils are visible at the level of the foramen magnum. *C,* Upward tentorial plus foramen magnum herniation has occurred secondary to a cerebellar lymphoma in a 32-year-old man with HIV-I infection. The cerebellum is enlarged. The iter *(black curved arrow)* and the rostral mesencephalon have herniated 6 mm above the IL, and the brain stem is flattened against the base of the skull. The cerebellar tonsils have herniated into the foramen magnum.

or decorticate reflex posturing, worse on the body side contralateral to the brain mass.

A similar progression of abnormal signs accompanies *uncal* herniation, except that as the uncus slides over the tentorial edge, it may compress the third nerve before it squeezes the diencephalon (Table 394–3). Shortly afterward, third nerve paralysis usually develops and the involved eye turns outward. If the herniating process continues, it paralyzes the opposite third nerve and other mesencephalic functions begin to fail. To be effective, treatment must be initiated before these late signs of deterioration appear.

SUBTENTORIAL MASS OR DESTRUCTIVE LESIONS CAUSING COMA. Subtentorial mass or destructive lesions cause stupor or coma if they directly damage or compress the ascending activating systems that arise from the paramedian rostral pontine tegmentum and mesencephalon. Such coma-causing abnormalities always affect adjacent neuro-ophthalmologic centers, causing telltale signs that pinpoint the anatomy of damage (Table 394–4).

Most subtentorial lesions that cause coma by directly injuring the upper brain stem (e.g., infarcts or hemorrhages) cause coma from the outset. The pupils are always abnormal, owing to dysfunction or destruction of pontine sympathetic pathways, third nerve nuclei, or their internuclear fibers. Dysconjugate eye movements are common, as are nystagmus, bizarrely or independently moving eyes, ocular bobbing, or ocular deviation. Unilateral facial anesthesia involving both the brow and lower face, absent caloric responses to either side, and conjugate eye deviation toward the paralyzed arm and leg all suggest a subtentorial lesion. The combination of flaccidity in the arms and flexor responses in the legs signifies pontine-midbrain damage. Brain imaging identifies cerebellar or pontine hemorrhage as well as expanding cerebellar hematomas, neoplasms, or most infarctions. MR produces better images of the cerebellum and brain stem than CT scans.

Compressive lesions of the posterior fossa, such as hemorrhages, abscesses, or tumors of the cerebellum or fourth ventricle, rarely cause coma until late in their course, at which time they may cause the mesencephalon to herniate upward through the tentorial notch

TABLE 394–3. SIGNS OF INCIPIENT DOWNWARD HERNIATION

	Central	Uncal
Arousal	Impaired early, before other signs	Impaired late, usually with other signs
Breathing	Sighs, yawns, sometimes Cheyne-Stokes respirations	No early change
Pupils	First small reactive (hypothalamus), then one or both approach midposition	Ipsilateral pupil dilates, followed by somatic third nerve paralysis
Oculocephalic responses	Initially sluggish, later tonic conjugate	Unilateral third nerve paralysis
Motor signs	Early hemiparesis opposite to hemispheric lesion followed late by ipsilateral motor paresis and extensor plantar response	Motor signs late, sometimes ipsilateral to lesion

TABLE 394–4. TELLTALE SIGNS OF PRIMARY SUBTENTORIAL LESIONS CAUSING COMA

Onset of coma often sudden
Symptoms of brain stem dysfunction may precede coma
Localizing brain stem signs always exist
  Caloric responses disconjugate or absent
  Pupil(s) abnormal: pinpoint (pons), fixed (midbrain), irregular and/or unequal (midbrain-pontine)
  Often "bizarre" signs: ocular bobbing, ataxic breathing, etc.
  Often signs of cerebellar or bilateral motor dysfunction

or force the cerebellar tonsils to impact downward into the foramen magnum. These developments produce deepening stupor, failure of upward gaze, unequal or fixed pupils, and irregularly irregular breathing patterns. Occipital headache, nystagmus, diplopia, nausea, vomiting, cranial nerve signs, and ataxia often precede unconsciousness. Shrinking the brain with hypo-osmotic fluids and surgical decompression of the lateral cerebral ventricles can be life-saving.

METABOLIC, TOXIC, AND DIFFUSE BRAIN DISTURBANCES CAUSING DELIRIUM, STUPOR, AND COMA. *Definition and Etiology.* The term *metabolic* or *diffuse encephalopathy* describes the behavioral state produced by a group of brain-affecting disorders that impair predominantly the organ's higher functions and usually pursue a temporary, reversible course. Many disorders can precipitate confused or delirious states. Considerably fewer have the capacity to cause stupor or coma (Table 394–5). Confusion and delirium are major comorbidity factors in a variety of serious medical and surgical illnesses and complicate patient management both in and out of hospital. Especially susceptible to metabolic encephalopathy are patients who are old, even mildly cognitively impaired, critically ill from systemic disease or major surgery, febrile, receiving psychoactive drugs, and those who suffer from hyponatremia or azotemia. If one includes examples of the toxic effects of abused and therapeutic drugs, the metabolic encephalopathies make up the largest category of illnesses causing confusion, stupor, or coma.

Disorders or drugs affecting several neurochemical and neuropharmacologic systems can cause a metabolic encephalopathy. Prominent examples are drugs with either anticholinergic or sedative effects. Other common causes include a number of inflammatory or infectious illnesses, physiologic disturbances such as epilepsy or complicated migraine, diffuse brain trauma, and disseminated structural lesions such as certain forms of cancer or cerebral thromboembolism. Diffuse, acute or subacute, bilateral, multi-level cerebral and subcerebral dysfunction that almost always spares pupillary reactivity is the hallmark of metabolic encephalopathy and is only rarely produced by structural brain disease.

Terminology. Classic neurologic thinking has employed the terms *delirium* and *acute toxic psychosis* for the more blatantly agitated and severely disoriented, hallucinatory-delusional forms of metabolic encephalopathy. Quieter, less severe disturbances have been termed *acute* or *subacute confusional states.* This chapter often uses these terms because they are more descriptively informative than the usage adopted by the American Psychiatric Association's Diagnostic Manual, which applies the term *delirium* to all examples of acquired confusion, agitation, disorientation, or hallucinations occurring in the setting of structural or known neurochemical brain disease.

Clinical Features. Table 394–6 lists the most consistent and specific symptoms of acute confused-delirious states. Frequent premorbid features include fractures, age over 80 years, and at least mild cognitive impairment. The clinical evaluation of these conditions attempts first to determine whether the observed changes are due to metabolic rather than structural brain disease or psychiatric dysfunction. One then proceeds to define the particular metabolic or structural defects and treat them. Evaluations of the history, the pattern of impaired consciousness, motor activity, and autonomic activity help answer the first question, whereas the general physical examination, evaluation of pulmonary ventilation, and laboratory tests assist with the second (Table 394–7). The history is especially important and should inquire into previous systemic medical illnesses, psychiatric history, access to potentially intoxicating drugs or alcohol, and recent changes in behavior.

State of Consciousness and Mental Content. Disorders of attention are the earliest sign and the hallmark of metabolic brain disease. Some patients act quietly perplexed, preoccupied, and unable to concentrate. Others appear hypervigilant and distractible, picking at the bedclothes and attending briefly to each new environmental stimulus no matter how trivial or irrelevant. Still others lose contact with the environment, becoming completely preoccupied and often frightened by vivid fragmentary hallucinations or delusions. Early attentional deficits may be subtle and easily mistaken for normal, slightly odd behavior. Soon, however, other symptoms emerge, including emotional lability, insomnia or drowsiness, and often vivid nightmares. As delirium worsens, some patients express the fear of

TABLE 394–5. POTENTIAL CAUSES OF TOXIC, METABOLIC, OR DIFFUSE BRAIN DYSFUNCTION CAUSING DELIRIUM OR COMA

I. Exogenous poisons
  A. Alcohol–sedative drug abuse, acute or chronic, immediate or withdrawal
  B. Acid poisons or poisons with acidic breakdown products:
      Paraldehyde
      Methyl alcohol
      Ethylene glycol
  C. Psychotropic drugs, acute or chronic:
      Opiates and their congeners
      Cocaine
      Amphetamines
      Tricyclic antidepressants and anticholinergic drugs
      Lithium
      Phenothiazines
      LSD-mescaline
      Monoamine oxidase inhibitors
  D. Other drugs:
      Anticonvulsants
      Steroids
      Cardiac glycosides
      Cimetidine
      Salicylates

II. Mixed metabolic encephalopathy
    Age + cognitive decline ± surgery or severe illness ± hyponatremia ± systemic infection ± psychoactive drug use ± azotemia ± darkened environment.

III. Deprivation of oxygen, substrate, or metabolic cofactors
  A. Hypoxia (interference with oxygen supply to the entire brain; cerebral blood flow normal)
      1. Decreased oxygen tension (usually $Pao_2 < 35$ mm Hg) and content of blood: pulmonary disease, alveolar hypoventilation, decreased atmospheric oxygen tension (e.g., high altitude)
      2. Decreased oxygen content of blood—normal tension:
          Anemia (Hb < 40% normal)
          Carbon monoxide poisoning
          Methemoglobinemia
  B. Ischemia (diffuse or widespread multifocal interference with blood supply to brain; often with accompanying hypoxia)
      1. Decreased cerebral blood flow resulting from decreased cardiac output:
          Hemorrhagic or septic shock
          Stokes-Adams syndrome, cardiac arrest, cardiac arrhythmias
          Myocardial infarction
          Aortic stenosis
          Pulmonary embolism
      2. Decreased cerebral blood flow resulting from decreased systemic peripheral resistance:
          Syncope: orthostatic, vasovagal
          Carotid sinus hypersensitivity
          Hypovolemia
      3. Decreased cerebral blood flow due to generalized or multifocal increase in cerebrovascular resistance:
          Hyperventilation syndrome
          Increased blood viscosity (polycythemia, cryo- and macroglobulinemia, sickle cell anemia)
          Subarachnoid hemorrhage (both hemotoxic and vasospasm)
      4. Decreased local cerebral blood flow due to widespread small vessel occlusion or tissue necrosis:
          Disseminated intravascular coagulation
          Systemic lupus erythematosus
          Endocarditis, bacterial or nonbacterial
          Cardiopulmonary bypass
          Small emboli (fat, fibrin, platelets)
      5. Alterations of blood flow due to failure of autoregulation:
          Hypertensive encephalopathy
  C. Hypoglycemia:
      Hyperinsulinism: exogenous; endogenous
  D. Cofactor deficiency:
      Thiamine (Wernicke's encephalopathy)
      Pyridoxine
      Vitamin B_{12}

IV. Diseases of organs other than brain
  A. Nonendocrine organs:
      Liver (hepatic coma)
      Kidney (uremic coma)
      Lung (CO_2 narcosis)

TABLE 394–5. POTENTIAL CAUSES OF TOXIC, METABOLIC, OR DIFFUSE BRAIN DYSFUNCTION CAUSING DELIRIUM OR COMA *Continued*

    B. Hyper- and/or hypofunction of endocrine organs:
        Panhypopituitarism
        Thyroid (myxedema-thyrotoxicosis)
        Parathyroid (hyper- and hypocalcemia)
        Adrenal (Addison's disease, Cushing's disease)
    C. Other systemic diseases:
        Diabetes
        Cancer and its treatments
        Porphyria
        Sepsis

  V. Abnormalities of fluid, ionic, or acid-base environment of CNS
    A. Water and sodium (hyper- and hyponatremia; hypo- and hyperosmolality
    B. Acidosis (metabolic and respiratory)
    C. Calcium (hyper- and hypocalcemia)

  VI. Disordered temperature regulation
    A. Hypothermia
    B. Heat stroke, fever, malignant neuroleptic syndrome

  VII. Infections or inflammation of CNS
    A. Leptomeningitis
    B. Encephalitis
    C. Acute "toxic" encephalopathy
    D. Parainfectious encephalomyelitis
    E. Cerebral vasculitis
    F. Subarachnoid hemorrhage

  VIII. Miscellaneous diseases of uncertain pathophysiology
    A. Seizures and postictal states
    B. Concussion
    C. Right middle cerebral or left posterior cerebral infarctions
    D. Migraine

"going crazy." Others lie quietly or sleep when left alone. None reads for substance or attends to the surrounding world with any interest. With more severe metabolic disturbances, patients become drowsy and some become stuporous or comatose. The prevailing affect depends partly on the nature of the illness and partly on how rapidly it develops. Previous personality often has surprisingly little influence on delirious behavior. Rapidly developing metabolic abnormalities are more likely to produce agitation or stupor than are those that evolve more slowly.

Disturbances in cognition accompany altered alertness and awareness, causing difficulties with immediate recall and the ability to abstract. Normal subjects readily recall and repeat six or seven digits forward and five or six backward and can identify the common denominator between such pairs as an apple and an orange or a fly and a tree; confused patients cannot. But the examiner must be cautious; innate intelligence and education also determine cognitive abilities. Unless the physician already knows the patient, it may be difficult to attribute mild mental changes to a metabolic defect. Loss of memory for recent events and disorientation for time are hallmarks of organic brain disease. Orientation to place and time should be specifically tested by asking the date and year, the day of the week, and the present location.

Perceptual errors, e.g., mistaking the physician for someone else, as well as illusions and hallucinations, are more serious symptoms. Hallucinations are common and usually animate. They frighten and agitate some patients, but others tolerate them quietly and must be asked about their presence. Delirious hallucinations or delusions may be visual, auditory, or tactile, alone or in combination; rarely are they systematic. By contrast, schizophrenic delusions or halluci-

TABLE 394–6. PRINCIPAL SYMPTOMS OF ACUTE CONFUSED-DELIRIOUS STATES

Acute onset and fluctuating course
Inattention
Disorganized thinking
Memory impairment
Disorientation
Altered sleep-wake cycle

TABLE 394–7. PHYSICAL SIGNS OF METABOLIC ENCEPHALOPATHY

Confusion, lethargy, delirium often precede or replace coma
Motor signs, if present, usually symmetric
Bilateral asterixis, myoclonus appear
Pupillary reactions usually preserved
Sensory abnormalities usually absent
Hypothermia common
Abnormal signs reflect incomplete brain dysfunction at multiple anatomic levels

nations are usually systematic in pattern and consist almost exclusively of endogenous auditory perceptions.

Characteristically, the mental status examination fluctuates in metabolic encephalopathy. Delirious patients typically become more disoriented at night and in unfamiliar surroundings. The presence of restraints, intermittent background noise, and unfamiliar activity accentuates their confusion.

Motor Activity. Bilateral tremor, asterixis, and multifocal myoclonus are hallmarks of metabolic brain disease. The *tremor* ranges from fine to coarse, is irregular at a rate of about eight to ten per second, and involves the distal more than proximal parts of the extremities. Coarse tremor such as accompanies certain drug withdrawals or intoxications may be so heavy that it shakes the bed.

Asterixis describes an abnormal, irregular, distal involuntary jerking movement, best elicited with arms outstretched, hands pronated, and fingers extended. Severe examples border on myoclonus. Asterixis is encountered rarely, and then unilaterally, in patients with structural brain disease.

Multifocal myoclonus consists of sudden nonrhythmic, nonpatterned coarse jerks affecting resting groups of muscles. Multifocal myoclonus occurs most frequently in uremia, in hypercarbic-anoxic encephalopathy, with penicillin or lithium overdose, and in association with the progressive dementia of Creutzfeldt-Jakob disease (see Ch. 428.6).

Psychomotor activity in delirium can range from extremes of picking at the bedcovers, sustained restlessness, and thrashing about to total immobility. Increased psychomotor activity is typical of acute deliria such as delirium tremens. More commonly, toxic confusional states are marked by lethargy, drowsiness, and general bradykinesia. Other patients may be unwilling or unable to stay in bed. They pace the halls, move constantly, and often shout vulgarities or aggressive threats. Unless restrained, many confused patients fall in trying to walk or during efforts to climb out of bed.

Speech is often abnormal. Patients with increased psychomotor behavior often speak rapidly, muttering or slurring speech into an incomprehensible jumble. Bradykinetic patients may speak slowly, monotonously, and so softly as to be barely heard.

Seizures, hyperactive stretch reflexes, and *signs of mild focal brain dysfunction* frequently accompany severe metabolic brain disease, especially after alcohol-sedative withdrawal. The seizures are usually generalized and the motor abnormalities usually symmetric. Nevertheless, focal paresis and focal seizures occasionally occur, especially with hypoglycemia, hepatic encephalopathy, or postanoxic encephalopathy.

Autonomic Activity. *Pupillary light reactions are preserved in metabolic coma with rare exceptions, and their absence requires a specific search for a pre-existing or acute structural lesion.* Nevertheless, a few exceptions exist; the ingestion of drugs possessing an anticholinergic action can paralyze the pupils transiently in either mid-position or dilation. Also, exposure to severe anoxia or asphyxia can produce fixed mid-position or dilated pupils. If sustained, these imply irreversible brain stem damage. In general, the pupils usually remain symmetric in metabolic brain disease, but are often asymmetric and sometimes fixed in patients comatose from structural brain disease.

Hypothermia is common in sedative intoxication as well as with hypoglycemia and myxedema. *Hyperthermia* with profuse perspiration and tachycardia accompanies most agitated deliria and is especially common with delirium tremens. Hyperthermia without perspiration suggests anticholinergic drug ingestion, infection, heat stroke, or the malignant neuroleptic syndrome. Less severe, unexplained

TABLE 394-8. LABORATORY EVALUATION OF METABOLIC BRAIN DISEASE

Test	Reason for Test
Immediately Reported	
Glucose	Hypoglycemia, hyperosmolar coma
Na$^+$	Osmolar abnormalities
Ca^{2+}	Hyper- or hypocalcemia
BUN	Uremia
Arterial blood pH, PCO_2, PO_2	Acidosis, alkalosis, hypoxia
Lumbar puncture	Infection, hemorrhage, meningeal carcinomatosis
Later Reported	
Liver function tests	Hepatic coma
Sedative drug levels	Overdose
Blood and CSF culture	Sepsis, encephalitis, meningitis
Full electrolytes, including Mg^{2+}	Electrolyte imbalance
Coagulation profile	Intravascular coagulation
EEG	Seizure disorder

hyperthermia can reflect idiosyncrasy to a variety of widely used drugs, including salicylates.

Laboratory Tests. The causes of metabolic coma are legion. In many instances the history (e.g., of drug abuse, systemic disease, exposure to toxins) immediately suggests the cause. When this is uncertain, tests listed in Table 394-8 should be performed immediately to establish or rule out the presence of life-threatening metabolic defects. Unless strong evidence indicates a specific metabolic or infectious process causing the delirium, diagnostic brain imaging is desirable. Imaging shows no immediately pertinent abnormalities in metabolic encephalopathy but may reveal pre-existing abnormalities such as chronic subdural hematoma or previous brain damage, the effects of which can mimic or accentuate metabolic delirium.

PSYCHIATRIC DISORDERS. Psychiatric disorders capable of producing the behavioral appearance of impaired consciousness include delirious stages of acute schizophrenic or manic attacks, the nearly total withdrawal of severe depression or certain forms of catatonia, and the pseudocoma of hysteria and malingering (Table 394-9). Especially in the early stages of such disorders, distinction from physiologic alterations of consciousness sometimes can be difficult. Psychiatric amnesia is the most common pseudo-organic symptom and the most readily diagnosed. One should suspect psychiatric amnesia when the experience covers sharply delineated periods of time, has an abrupt onset and offset with total amnesia in the middle, is nonprogressive in nature, and relates either to experiences that provoked severe anxiety or to potentially punishable behavior. Catatonic withdrawal states or psychotic deliria in psychiatric illness sometimes can be difficult to differentiate from those of

TABLE 394-9. PSYCHIATRIC STATES RESEMBLING ACUTE IMPAIRMENT OF CONSCIOUSNESS

1. **Catatonic states.** Uncommon conditions occurring in either schizophrenic or severe depressive illness which may resemble organic stupor. Mutism, bilateral motor resistance, hypokinesia, and even rigidity are common. Absent are pathologic reflexes, as well as abnormal brain images, EEG's, and laboratory chemical tests.
2. **Acute psychotic deliria.** Uncommon. Involves adult patients of any age, more frequently those older than 50 years. The state can arise with either affective or schizophrenic disorders. Agitation, fear, and hypermobility are prominent. Auditory or visual hallucinations occur, not necessarily paranoid but usually systematized. Fast, coarse tremor can be present and tends to last longer than drug-alcohol withdrawal tremors. Verbal responses, when elicitable, usually reflect orientation for time and place, but distractibility or muteness often limits mental testing. Pathologic reflexes are lacking. EEG and laboratory chemical tests remain normal in the absence of medical complications. The condition can be difficult to diagnose, but an agitated delirium that lasts longer than 2 weeks almost always reflects psychiatric disease. Some end in catatonia or death unless treated with neuroleptics,
3. **Hysteria-malingering.** Unarousable unresponsiveness, usually of brief duration, unaccompanied by physiologic abnormalities and often associated with obviously factitious responses to stimulation.

metabolic origin, but applying the guidelines given in Table 394-10 usually provides the answers. As a general rule, however, if the patient's cooperation can be elicited to obtain satisfactory answers, recent memory and cognitive functions usually turn out to be preserved in the functional psychoses. Patients with extreme anxiety may hyperventilate, producing respiratory alkalosis, a diffusely slow electroencephalogram, and sometimes tetany. Otherwise, physical and laboratory evaluations in psychogenically altered consciousness remain normal.

Patients with hysterical pseudocoma have normal somatic neurologic examinations. Breathing is eupneic or voluntarily hyperpneic. Most such patients lie supine and quietly unresponsive, with limbs remaining either flaccid or resisting movement in unpredictable patterns. Eyelids usually are closed, actively resist opening, and may spontaneously flutter. Furthermore, the eyelids are incapable of the slow closure that follows passive raising of the lids of patients with physiologic coma. The pupils in psychiatric unresponsiveness are briskly responsive or, if cycloplegics have been self-instilled, widely dilated. Oculocephalic responses are unpredictable, but if the diagnosis is doubtful, irrigating the tympanum with 50 ml of cold water produces physiologic nystagmus rather than the tonic eye deviation or absent responses shown by comatose patients with structural or metabolic disease. Sometimes, the eyes may deviate toward the bed when the patient is turned to one side.

Occasionally, psychiatric pseudodelirium or unresponsiveness can be superimposed on underlying physical illness. An example is the patient hospitalized with a severe medical or neurologic illness who becomes so anxious that he or she is unable to cope and withdraws psychologically to the point of unresponsiveness. In such doubtful instances, slow infusions of small amounts of sodium amobarbital (Amytal interview) may allow the physician to establish contact and rapport with the patient. Because the drug may similarly awaken patients rendered unconscious by continuous focal seizures, close clinical observation and, if possible, an EEG are best done before the test.

ACUTE CENTRAL NERVOUS SYSTEM POISONING. Table 394-11 lists the most frequent acute neurotoxic poisonings in the United States, gives their principal signs of toxicity, and outlines their treatment. To find descriptions of poisons not included in

TABLE 394-10. ORGANIC AND FUNCTIONAL PSYCHOSES COMPARED

Variable	Organic	Functional
Onset	Usually > 30 years	Usually < 40 years
Family history	Usually negative	Often psychiatrically abnormal
Immediate history	Drugs, alcohol, acute medical or neurologic illness	No established medical or neurologic features
Psychology of history	Psychologically coherent	Psychologically incoherent
Major (psychotic) symptoms	Agitation, tremor, noisiness, inattention	Same
Orientation and memory	Abnormal	Normal if answers obtained
Delusions or hallucinations	Visual, sometimes olfactory or auditory; nonsystematic (chaotic)	Mainly auditory; systematic: tell a story
Mood	Fearful or apathetic; delusions often regarded as unwanted	Consistent with psychotic symptoms
Coma or akinetic (catatonic) state	Systemic and/or neurologic signs present; EEG abnormal	Neurologic signs absent; EEG normal
Fever, leukocytosis	Signs of medical illness often present	Absent (except malignant hyperthermia or catatonia)
Alcohol-drug intoxication or withdrawal	Often present	Absent
Clinical or EEG seizures	Often present	Absent

TABLE 394–11. COMMON DRUG POISONINGS, SIGNS OF TOXICITY, AND TREATMENT

Drug	Signs and Symptoms		Diagnostic Test	Treatment
	Mild	*Severe*		
Opiates Heroin Morphine Meperidine Methadone Hydromorphone Oxycodone Levorphanol	"Nodding" drowsiness, small pupils, urinary reention, slow and shallow breathing; skin scars and subcutaneous abscesses; duration 4–6 hours; with methadone, duration to 24 hours	Coma; pinpoint pupils, slow irregular respiration or apnea, hypotension, hypothermia, pulmonary edema	Response to naloxone Urine	Naloxone, 0.4 mg intravenously or intramuscularly; repeat at 15-minute intervals if patient responds and gradually increase intervals; repeat in 3 hours if necessary; if no response by second dose, suspect another cause; treat shock; find and detect infection
Sedatives–hypnotics syndromes Alcohol Barbiturates Chloral hydrate Glutethimide (Doriden) Meprobamate (Equanil)	Confusion, rousable drowsiness, delirium, ataxia, nystagmus, dysarthria, analgesia to stimuli	Stupor to coma; pupils reactive, usually constricted; oculovestibular response absent; motor tonus initially briefly hyperactive, then flaccid; respiration and blood pressure depressed; hypothermia.	Blood, urine, breath Blood Blood Blood	Intubate, ventilate, lavage; drainage position; antimicrobials; keep mean blood pressure > 90 mm Hg and urine output > 300 ml per hour; avoid analeptics; hemodialyze severe phenobarbital poisoning
Benzodiazepines (Librium, Valium, Tranxene, Ativan, Dalmane, etc.)	Usually taken with another sedative if poisoning is attempted	Coma seldom severe if drug taken alone	Blood	As above; diuresis of little help
Toxic-hyperactive syndromes Amphetamines Methylphenidate	Euphoria, sometimes paranoid, repetitive behavior, dilated pupils, tremor, hyperactive reflexes; hyperthermia, tachycardia, arrhythmia	Agitated, assaultive and paranoid excitement; occasionally convulsions; hyperthermia; circulatory collapse.	Blood	Chlorpromazine
Cocaine	Similar but less prominent than above; less paranoid, often euphoric	Twitching; irregular breathing, tachycardia, arrhythmia, occasionally convulsions; myocardial infarction; acute stroke; vasculitis; chronic paranoid psychosis or depression	Blood, urine	Diazepam plus labetalol for cardiovascular crisis
MAO inhibitors (Parnate, Nardil, Eutonyl, etc.)	Hypertensive crises, agitation, drowsiness, ataxia	Hypotension; headache; chest pain; agitation; coma, seizures and shock	Clinical	Symptomatic; gastric lavage
Neuroleptics (phenothiazines, butyrophenones, etc.)	Acute dystonia, somnolence, hypotension	Coma; convulsions (rare); arrhythmias; hypotension	Blood	Anticholinergics; diphenhydramine; symptomatic; gastric lavage
Psychedelics (LSD, mescaline, psilocybin, phencyclidine)	Confused, disoriented, perceptual distortions, distractable, withdrawn or eruptive, leading to accidents or violence; wide-eyed, dilated pupils; restless, hyperreflexic; less often, hypertension or tachycardia	Panic		Reassure; diazepam satisfactory; avoid phenothiazines
Scopolamine-atropine (knockout drops, Transderm delirium)	Agitated or confused, visual hallucinations, dilated pupils, flushed and dry skin	Florid toxic disoriented delirium, visual hallucinations; later, amnesia, fever, dilated fixed pupils, hot flushed dry skin, urinary retention		Reassure; sedate lightly, (1) avoid phenothiazines; (2) do not leave alone
Antidepressants Tricyclics (Tofranil, Elavil, Desipramine, etc.)	Restless, drowsiness, tachycardia, ataxia, sweating	Agitation, vomiting, hyperpyrexia, sweating, muscle dystonia, convulsions, tachycardia or arrhythmia	Blood	Symptomatic; gastric lavage Intensive care, anticonvulsants, and antiarrhythmics for severe cases
Lithium	Mild lethargy	Sustention-intention tremor, lethargy; muteness with appearance of distraction; coma; multifocal seizures; slow or fluctuating course	Blood	Hydrate if mild; hemodialyze for delirium, coma, or convulsions
Acid-forming intoxicants Methanol (formic); ethylene glycol (oxalic and hippuric); other organic alcohols	Inebriation with hyperpnea	All produce progressive hyperventilation, drunkenness, stupor, eventually convulsions and death. Early blindness with methanol	Blood shows increasingly severe anion gap acidosis	Inhibit hepatic alcohol dehydrogenase by giving alcohol until acidosis controlled; treat acidosis vigorously
Salicylate Aspirin	Tinnitus, dyspnea	Older persons: confusional state or toxic delirium leading to stupor, convulsions, coma	Blood salicylate > 60 mg/dl	Alkaline diuresis

this section, especially chronic neurotoxic agents, the reader should consult the textbooks listed in the references. Almost all drugs in overdose amounts are likely to be mixed with intoxicating amounts of alcohol, thereby making their clinical signs more difficult to appraise. Nevertheless, clinical evaluation must be used to diagnose the specific agent causing several of these reaction patterns because chemical tests are in many instances either unavailable or impractically slow. When any doubt exists, one should keep admission serum samples for possible later analysis. With most of the drugs, tolerance develops to chronic ingestion and individuals may react differently to similar doses. Accordingly, blood levels and size of the dose are unreliable guides to the potential depth of coma or other complications. The mixing of agents adds to the unreliability. Only the opiates and some of the sedatives create an immediate risk of death; concurrent alcohol ingestion enhances both these risks. Opiate poisoning is discussed in greater detail in Ch. 12.

Pathogenesis. All sedative drugs depress the central nervous system, although not equally on a gram-molecular weight basis, and often produce different degrees of inhibition on individual central structures. The duration of action varies widely and depends largely on how the particular drug is detoxified or eliminated. The benzodiazepines, short-acting barbiturates, pentobarbital, secobarbital, and amobarbital are detoxified by the liver, as is methaqualone. They exert their maximal effects promptly after being absorbed and, even in huge doses, seldom cause neurologic depression lasting longer than 3 to 5 days. The benzodiazepine group especially possesses a wide margin of safety between their hypnotic effects and any serious depression of breathing and circulatory control. Barbital and phenobarbital are partially detoxified by the liver and partially excreted in the urine. Severe poisoning with the latter agent can cause coma lasting 10 to 14 days. Furthermore, as a class, the barbiturates have a relatively high capacity to halt breathing control and produce hypotension.

A withdrawal syndrome consisting of tremulousness, agitation, and sometimes delirium and convulsions can develop after prompt withdrawal from chronic exposure to any of the hypnotic sedatives. Convulsions are a particular problem after withdrawal from barbiturates, methaqualone, and, to a lesser extent, benzodiazepines.

Clinical Manifestations. Stupor or coma caused by depressant drug poisoning usually presents the characteristic picture of acute general anesthesia. The depression of the central nervous system tends to be bilateral and symmetric and the drug usually simultaneously depresses junction at many levels, including the spinal cord. Respiratory and circulatory controlling mechanisms in the lower brain stem are affected only with very high doses or not at all. Except with the now obsolete sedative glutethimide and with extremely large doses of barbiturates, the pupillary light reflexes are preserved. Within the first half hour or so after suddenly taking a sedative in potentially anesthetic doses, patients can demonstrate muscular hypertonus or even spasticity as the result of uneven depression of different neurologic levels. Within a short time, usually less than an hour, flaccidity supervenes, and the stretch reflexes disappear. Even moderate degrees of drug depression can depress or block the oculovestibular reflexes.

Despite their lack of exact correlation, blood levels of short-acting barbiturates of more than 2.5 mg per deciliter and phenobarbital levels of more than 12 mg per deciliter are associated with very deep coma to the level at which apnea and hypotension become management problems. Apnea rarely supervenes with the benzodiazepines, even at very high doses.

Diagnosis. The combination of acutely occurring unresponsiveness, with preserved or sluggish pupillary reactions, absent oculovestibular reactions, motor areflexia, hypothermia, and relative depression of respiration and circulation is clinically diagnostic of sedative-anesthetic drug poisoning. Only infarction or hemorrhage of the pons resembles this clinical state, and with lesions of the pons the pupils are usually small or pinpoint, the stretch reflexes are generally preserved or hyperactive, and the plantar responses become extensor. Specific chemical tests detect barbiturates, glutethimide, meprobamate, methaqualone, and bromides in blood or urine, and can be done as emergency measures.

CLINICAL EVALUATION OF DELIRIUM, STUPOR, OR COMA

The immediate step consists of assuring vital cardiorespiratory systems and protecting against further damage to the central nervous system. Once these measures are taken, the keys to diagnosis, specific treatment, and prognosis lie in carefully examining the patient, systematically seeking the answers to a few central questions:

Is the process neurogenic or psychogenic in origin?

If neurogenic, is (are) the lesion(s) supratentorial, subtentorial, focal, or multifocal-diffuse?

Once the immediate cause of loss of consciousness is under control, is the appropriate treatment medical or surgical?

If the illness is nonstructural, is it exogenously toxic or endogenously metabolic, already maximal (e.g., postanoxic, postintoxicant), or progressive; is it worsening or improving?

Which immediate treatment best halts the pathologic process and sustains the patient?

DIFFERENTIAL HISTORY. If sudden unconsciousness is not an expected consequence of an already known illness, witnesses to the onset provide the most helpful immediate information. Was the onset gradual or abrupt? Was it preceded by headache and, if so, of what location and duration? Was paralysis or seizure activity observed? Were antecedent or prodromal symptoms noted? Did the onset occur in a circumstance or geographic area in which drugs, trauma, or foul play could be suspected? What medications might the patient have taken? Beyond these immediacies, what has been the patient's physical and mental health for the past few days, weeks, or months?

PHYSICAL AND NEUROLOGIC EXAMINATION. In cases of deep unresponsiveness, one first carries out steps 1 to 5 described below under Emergency Management, then proceeds with the physical examination. Under urgent circumstances, the physician should be able to conduct a highly focused, pertinent physical and neurologic examination on patients in coma in less than 5 minutes. This includes appraising cardiopulmonary status as indicated above and systematically carrying out the main features of the examination outlined in Table 394–12. In the course of the above, trauma or seizures make themselves evident. In patients with coma of unknown cause, clues should be sought to drug exposure, as well as to past serious medical or psychiatric problems. Companions should be asked about recent neurologic function and dysfunction.

For patients presenting with less severe impairments, i.e., acute-subacute confusion, delirium, or hypersomnolence, the examiner can take a more deliberate approach. Usually, a detailed history can precede the exigencies of stabilizing vital functions and a thorough organ-by-organ physical examination can be conducted. Either way, by the end of the initial examination, the findings should begin to indicate which of the four major causes of coma, as listed in Table 394–1, is responsible for the patient's acute problem. At that juncture, one can move toward obtaining supplementary or reinforcing laboratory tests as indicated below.

LABORATORY STUDIES. Unless the acutely obtained clinical findings make the diagnosis and appropriate treatment immediately obvious, blood should be drawn for laboratory tests listed in Table 394–8. Lumbar puncture is best deferred until after a contrast-enhanced brain CT or an MRI is obtained, so long as the images can be obtained promptly as an emergency procedure. If imaging is not available and the findings suggest acute, treatable meningitis or encephalitis, the physician has no choice but to proceed cautiously with lumbar puncture, using a No. 20 or 22 needle. The EEG (see Ch. 392) is diagnostically indispensable for detecting delirious states caused by continuously recurring partial complex seizures. A normal EEG rules out organic causes of acute unresponsiveness.

EMERGENCY MANAGEMENT OF COMA. Faced with acute coma of uncertain origin, one must treat the patient first, even as the history and initial diagnostic tests are being applied. Certain measures apply to the care of all patients:

1. *Assure an adequate airway and oxygenation.* Immediately check and clean out the upper airway. If the patient is deeply unresponsive, insert an endotracheal airway, but first give 1 mg of atropine intravenously to guard against hypoxigenic vagally induced asystole. Be sure that no neck fracture exists before extending the head for intubation. Auscultate both lung bases to ensure that the lower airway is open. Ventilate if necessary and keep arterial Pao_2 greater than 80 mm Hg and $Paco_2$ 30 to 35 mm Hg. To empty the stomach in comatose patients suspected of acute orally ingested drug poisoning, initiate lavage only *after* the cuffed airway tube is in place.

2. *Maintain circulation.* Insert venous line(s) and start Ringer's

TABLE 394-12. THE NEUROLOGIC EXAMINATION IN COMA

1. Guarantee vital functions as indicated in text.
2. Feel the scalp for hematomas: they overlie fracture lines; be sure the neck is not fractured; test *gently* for stiff neck.
3. Test language. Test arousability by words, loud sounds, noxious stimuli. If vocalizations occur, check quickly for appropriate phrases, actual words, and presence or absence of aphasia.
4. Do a neuro-ophthalmologic examination.
   Funduscopy (if difficult, defer until patient is stabilized)
   Papilledema? (increased intracranial or venous sinus pressure)
   Hemorrhages (subarachnoid hemorrhage; hypertensive encephalopathy; diabetes; hypoxic-hypercarbic encephalopathy)
   Pupils
   Light reaction. Use bright flashlight and, if necessary, a magnifying glass if uncertain. Absence means potentially fatally deep sedative poisoning or acute or chronic structural brain stem damage (e.g., tabetic pupils).
   Equality. 15% of normals have mild anisocoria but new or >2 mm dilation means parasympathetic (third nerve) palsy.
   Extraocular movements. Absence acutely means deep drug poisoning, severe brain stem damage, Wernicke's encephalopathy, polyneuropathy, or botulism.
   Dysconjugate at rest means an acute third, fourth, or sixth nerve palsy or internuclear ophthalmoplegia. Tonic conjugate deviation toward a paralytic arm and leg means forebrain seizures or a contralateral pontine destructive lesion; away from the paralytic arm and leg means forebrain gaze paralysis.
   Spontaneous eye movements. In coma patients, nystagmus, bobbing, or independently moving eyes all mean brain stem damage.
   Oculocephalic (away from direction of head turning) or oculovestibular (toward cold caloric irrigation) responses. Absence of responses means drugs or severe brain stem disease; dysconjugate responses with equal pupils mean internuclear ophthalmoplegia, with unequal pupils mean third nerve disease.
5. Examine the motor systems.
   Strength
   Unilateral weakness or motionlessness of arm and leg means contralateral supraspinal upper motor neuron lesion, most often cerebral; if of arm, leg, and face, contralateral cerebral lesion. Occasionally arm and leg weakness can reflect contralateral brain stem lesion.
   All four extremities weak or motionless implies metabolic disease; less likely is brain stem disease (tone and reflexes increased) or peripheral disease (tone and reflexes decreased).
   Attempt to elicit reflex posturing
   Arm flexed, leg extended—contralateral deep cerebral-thalamic dysfunction
   Arm and leg extended—thalamic or mesencephalic lesion
   Arms extended and legs flexed or flaccid—pontine lesion
   Legs flexed, arms flaccid—pontomedullary or spinal lesion
   Compare side-to-side reflexes and examine plantar responses.
6. Seek seizure activity or abnormal movements. (1) Generalized? (2) Focal? (3) Multifocal? (4) Myoclonic?
   Control 1 immediately, 2 and 3 deliberately; if 4, treat underlying disease.
   Acute tremor, asterixis, multifocal myoclonus—seek metabolic cause.
7. Inspect breathing.
   Regular hyperpnea: metabolic acidosis; pulmonary infarction; congestive failure or aveolar infiltration; sepsis; salicylism; hepatic coma
   Cyclically irregular (Cheyne-Stokes): low cardiac output plus bilateral cerebral or upper brain stem dysfunction
   Irregularly irregular gasping, slow or weak: lower brain stem dysfunction (including hypoglycemia, drug effects), less often peripheral ventilatory paralysis
8. Proceed with laboratory tests and emergency management as described in text.

lactate solution. Determine and maintain a satisfactory cardiac rate and rhythm. Avoid overhydration but keep mean blood pressure at 80 to 90 mm Hg, using dopamine if necessary. In poisoning cases maintain urine flow at 300 ml or more per hour. In any patient during the early stages of coma, check electrolytes initially and at 12-hour intervals thereafter.

3. *Draw blood for emergency laboratory analysis.* Give IV Narcan to protect against opiate intoxication and 50 mg thiamine to prevent accentuation of Wernicke's encephalopathy.

4. *Give glucose.* If hypoglycemia is a possible diagnosis, give 50 ml of 50% glucose. Draw blood first in order not to lose evidence for the diagnosis. The glucose does not appreciably intensify serum hyperosmolality.

5. *Stop generalized motor seizures.* Repetitive convulsions can result from either cerebral structural lesions, pre-existing epileptic disorders, or acquired metabolic-diffuse encephalopathies. Status epilepticus can cause coma and within a short period of time produces irreversible brain damage as well. Follow the protocol for treatment provided in Table 433-7. Start treatment with intravenous diazepam.

6. *Restore blood acid-base and osmolar balance.* Extremes of either acidosis or alkalosis usually reflect profound metabolic problems, severe circulatory insufficiency, the postictal state (muscular lactic acidosis), or hyperadrenocorticism. Because severe metabolic acidosis can precipitate cardiovascular irregularity and alkalosis depresses breathing, they should be corrected. Extreme hypo- and hyperosmolality are equally dangerous to brain and should be corrected, the first by withholding fluids (except water by mouth) and stopping diuretics and the second by administering fluids (and insulin for hyperglycemia). Beware of too rapid reversal. Osmotic delays across the blood-brain barrier during treatment can lead to large fluid shifts in or out of the brain. Also, too rapid correction of hyponatremia can produce central pontine myelinolysis (see Ch. 406). A reasonable goal in treating osmolal shifts is to correct blood by about 0.5 mOsm per hour.

7. *Treat infection.* Several kinds of infection can cause or intensify delirium and coma. Obtain nose, throat, blood, and wound cultures, and perform lumbar puncture if indicated. With any sign of infection, begin antimicrobial treatment after obtaining the cultures cited above, based on either the results of smears or the most probable clinically suggested organism.

8. *Treat extreme body temperatures.* Hyperthermia above 40° C or hypothermia below 34° C should be brought to within 3° C of normal.

9. *Consider specific antidotes.* Many, if not most, patients admitted to emergency rooms in coma have taken an overdose of drugs, often in combination. For narcotic overdose, give 0.4 mg of naloxone intravenously every 5 minutes until the subject awakens. If the subject might be an addict, dilute the dose in 10 ml of saline and give slowly, trying to minimize withdrawal phenomena. Remember that naloxone's duration of action of 2 to 3 hours is shorter than that of several narcotics, and repeated dosing may be required. Analeptics of any kind are contraindicated.

Recently, flumazenil, a benzodiazepine antagonist, has been found useful in treating patients with benzodiazepine overdose, with or without concurrent ingestion of other depressant drugs. Length of unresponsiveness was shortened, and complications were reduced. The agent has not yet been released for use in the United States.

10. *Control agitation,* employing diazepam or haloperidol as necessary.

11. *Prevent complications.* If possible, keep unconscious patients semiprone in the drainage position and change their position from side to side, but never place them fully supine. In most instances, treat potential pulmonary infection with a broad-spectrum antibiotic. Poisoned patients and many with head injuries are unconscious for only a few days, and the risk of emergence of drug-resistant bacterial infections is of less concern than is pneumonia caused by already aspirated material. It is wise to protect the corneas against abrasions, using ophthalmic ointment and, if necessary, taping the lids shut.

RECOVERY AND PROGNOSIS. Patients recovering from coma require close medical supervision. Severe pneumonitis can develop as late as 3 to 4 days after recovery. If antimicrobial drugs were started during coma, they are best continued for at least 48 hours after it ends. Permanent physical sequelae are rare. Among 356 of our own cases of sedative drug overdose, residual brain injury was observed only once (in a patient who suffered an acute cardiac arrest). Peripheral nerve injuries from pressure developed in 6 subjects, and 14 subjects had pressure skin lesions leaving scars. There were no other physical residua.

Convalescent management varies according to the patient's underlying psychiatric disorder and attitudes. Suicide attempts are never accidents, and reports of near-fatal ingestion caused by misunderstanding the dose or forgetting previous doses carry little validity. The expert opinion of a psychiatrist should be sought before deciding whether to release or to institutionalize a patient. The immediate prognosis is good, but many patients try again over the years.

PROGNOSIS IN SEVERE BRAIN DAMAGE

Accurately forecasting the patient's outcome is central to appropriate patient care and consideration. Modern medical advances currently save many lives that only a few years ago would have been lost to severe disease or trauma. Unfortunately, however, when severe brain dysfunction accompanies acute illness, these advances create the risk that vigorous treatment may be followed by an unwanted outcome. According to Harris polls, most persons in the United States prefer death to a life of severe, permanent neurologic disability and they often express this view in the form of an advanced declaration. Several empirically based guidelines can help the physician predict with a high degree of certainty neurologic outcomes following illnesses causing severe brain damage or coma.

Nontraumatic Coma

The outcome from medical coma depends on (1) its cause, and (2) excepting only depressant drug poisoning, the initial severity and extent of neurologic damage as revealed by clinical neurologic signs obtained within the first few days of illness.

Depressant drug poisoning, no matter how deep the coma, reflects a state of general anesthesia. Barring severe complications, almost all patients with drug intoxication who reach medical attention recover completely. This favorable prognosis applies even when coma is so profound that normal brain stem reflexes and the EEG temporarily disappear. Because most comas of unknown origin that precipitate emergency house calls or emergency room visits are due to drug ingestion, such initially undiagnosed patients should receive maximal treatment unless direct evidence points to severe structural brain damage and the use of drugs by ingestion or for therapy has been ruled out.

Aside from drug poisoning, coma occurring during the course of medical illness and lasting more than a few hours carries a poor prognosis, with only about 15% of patients returning to close to their pre-illness state of health. The major problem in making early treatment decisions lies in discriminating between patients who have a chance of reaching a good outcome and those whose chances of neurologic recovery are extremely small. In making such early decisions, the presence or absence of certain clinical signs of abnormal forebrain and/or upper brain stem function have been found to be powerful predictors of eventual outcome. The nature of the underlying illness and age have less of an influence and only slightly modify the predictive accuracy of early signs.

The clinical tests most valuable for estimating the capacity for recovery after medical coma are identical to those used in diagnosing and following the later course of the patient in coma. In most instances, early functional changes evolve so rapidly that one cannot reliably estimate the outcome of coma within the first minutes to hours, a time when improvement often occurs. After about 6 hours, however, so long as the patient has not received heavy doses of sedative drugs or alcohol, certain neurologic findings begin to correlate increasingly with the potential for neurologic recovery or otherwise. By the end of the first day, clinical signs accurately predict about two thirds of the patients who actually will do well. With each successive day, the signs develop greater predictive power. When considered appropriate to the patient's expressed wishes, treatment can be adjusted accordingly.

Some patients in coma due to a medical disease die from their initial illness within a short time. Ignoring that premise, Table 394–13 lists clinical signs found in a prospective study to predict either a good or a poor outcome from coma due to nonsurgical disease. Good outcome means a possible return to the level of health that pre-existed the coma-causing illness. Poor outcome means that the patient will be permanently, severely disabled either cognitively, physically, or both. The table emphasizes that signs of brain stem dysfunction (absent pupillary or corneal responses, imperfect or absent oculocephalic responses, or abnormal motor responses to stimulation) worsen prognosis and, in combination, indicate a nearly hopeless outlook when they persist beyond the third day.

Following an acute diffuse brain injury such as follows cardiac arrest, a few patients become immediately vegetative following the ictus and remain so as the days pass into weeks. Most who fail to speak until after the end of the second week are left with prominent intellectual defects, especially in recent and anterograde memory, even if sensorimotor activities return to normal. Persistence of coma or the vegetative state in an adult for >4 weeks almost never is associated with later complete recovery and the longer the mindless state lasts, the greater the chance of permanent disability. Care must be taken in such instances to rule out a locked-in state (see Table 393–1).

Traumatic Coma

Coma following head injury has a statistically better outcome than that associated with medical illness. About 50% of patients in coma from head injury die, many instantly. Acute treatment may somewhat improve the outcome of those who reach hospital. Recovery in traumatic cases is closely linked to age: the younger the better. As with medical coma, severely abnormal neuro-ophthalmologic signs reflecting brain stem dysfunction imply a poor prognosis, with approximately 90% of such patients either dying or remaining in near-vegetative states.

TABLE 394–13. CLINICAL SIGNS OF GOOD OR POOR OUTCOME FROM COMA

Good Prognosis	Poor Prognosis
1 day: Awake. No neuro-ophthalmologic abnormalities; speaking at least words. Possibility of poor outcome = 30%	Not awake. Pupils and oculocephalic reflexes absent and flaccid motor system. Possibility of good outcome = 2%
3 days: Corneal responses present, speaks words, moves. Possibility of poor outcome = 26%	No words; corneal responses and appropriate motor responses absent. Possibility of good outcome = 0%
1 week: Eyes open, says words, makes localized motor responses. Possibility of poor outcome = 1%	No wakefulness, motor system flaccid. Possibility of good outcome = 0%

Data derived from best outcome studies of 500 optimally treated patients in coma from nontraumatic, non–drug poisoning causes. From Levy DE, Bates D, Caronna JJ, et al.: Prognosis in non-traumatic coma. Ann Intern Med 94:293, 1981.

Dreisbach RH, Robinson WO: Handbook of Poisoning, 11th ed. Norwalk, CT, Appleton and Lange, 1987. *Succinct and handy, an excellent quick source to consult in emergencies, especially for poisoning in children.*

Francis J, Martin D, Kapoor WN: A prospective study of delirium in hospitalized elderly. JAMA 263:1097, 1990. *Among 229 elderly patients, 50 suffered delirium. Abnormal sodium levels, illness severity, previous dementia, fever or hypothermia, and neuroleptic drug use were major risk factors.*

Gilman AG, Rall TW, Nies AS, Taylor P (eds.): Goodman and Gilman's The Pharmacological Basis of Therapeutics, 8th ed. New York, Pergamon, 1990. *The "bible" of pharmacology and associated toxicology addresses major drug poisonings in authoritative chapters.*

Haddad LM, Winchester JF: Clinical Management of Poisoning and Drug Overdose. Philadelphia, WB Saunders, 1990.

Levy DE, Caronna JJ, Singer BH, et al.: Predicting outcome from hypoxic-ischemic coma. JAMA 253:1420, 1985. *Prospective correlations were obtained between early neurologic signs and eventual course in 210 patients, mostly with cardiac arrest. By 72 hours, signs accurately selected between good or poor eventual outcome in >75% of patients.*

Plum F: Coma and related global disturbances of the human conscious state. *In* Jones EG, Peters A (eds.): Cerebral Cortex. Vol. 9, Altered Cortical States. New York, Plenum Press, 1991. *A recent chapter describing current advances in pathophysiology.*

Plum F, Posner JB: Diagnosis of Stupor and Coma, 3rd ed., rev. Philadelphia, FA Davis, 1982. *Provides more discussion of the material described in this chapter.*

Reich JB, Sierra J, Camp W, et al.: Magnetic resonance imaging measurements and clinical changes accompanying transtentorial and foramen magnum herniation. Ann Neurol 33:159, 1993. *Readily interpreted sagittal images of the brain demonstrate the physical existence of pathologic brain herniations and their relationship to clinical findings.*

395 BRAIN DEATH
Fred Plum

Modern resuscitative devices can maintain the functions of the heart, lungs, and visceral organs for hours or days after the life-maintaining centers of the brain stem tissue have stopped functioning. The economic waste of this hopeless process, as well as the increasing success of organ transplant programs, has led countries worldwide to adopt the principle that death of the person occurs when either the brain or the heart irreversibly fails in its functions. In the United States the time of brain death has been accepted as

TABLE 395-1. CRITERIA FOR DIAGNOSIS OF BRAIN DEATH

1. Nature and duration of coma must be known
   a. Known structural disease or irreversible systemic metabolic cause
   b. No chance of drug intoxication or hypothermia; no paralyzing or potentially anesthetizing drugs recently given for treatment
   c. Body temperature must be above 34°C
   d. Six-hour observation of no brain function is sufficient in cases of known structural cause when no drug or alcohol is involved in causation or treatment; otherwise, 12 hours plus negative drug screen required
2. Absence of cerebral and brain stem function
   a. No behavioral or reflex responses can be elicited by noxious stimuli applied above foramen magnum level
   b. Fixed pupils
   c. No oculovestibular response to 50 ml ice water calories
   d. Apneic off ventilator with oxygenation for 10 minutes
   e. Systemic circulation may be intact
   f. Purely spinal reflexes may be retained
3. Supplementary (optional) criteria (any one is diagnostic)
   a. EEG must be largely isoelectric for 30 minutes at maximal gain
   b. Brain stem-evoked responses must reflect absent function in vital brain stem structures
   c. No cerebral circulation present on angiographic examination

the time of the person's death in legal terms. Many states accept the brain death concept by statute, and in no state has the principle failed to meet legal challenge. The Presidential Commission set as the criterion for brain death the "irreversible cessation of all functions of the entire brain, including the brain stem." Guidelines for the practical application of these principles are listed in Table 395-1. One of the supplementary criteria often is particularly desirable when making decisions at 6 hours to facilitate organ transplant.

Certain points in the diagnosis of brain death must be emphasized. *Recoverable drug depressant poisoning can in all ways except stopping the cerebral circulation resemble brain death and must be explicitly ruled out.* In any doubtful case, any evidence of EEG activity or of reflex activity of the brain stem means that the brain is not dead and contravenes immediate discontinuation of life support. Purely spinal reflex activity, however, can persist after brain death, including reflexes of the limbs and even some remarkably complex movements, including flexion of the trunk and raising of outstretched arms.

It is recommended that physicians faced with applying and acting upon the diagnosis of brain death familiarize themselves with the additional pertinent material listed in the references and whenever possible obtain confirmation with an experienced consultant.

Abrams MB, et al.: Deciding to Forego Life-Sustaining Treatment. A Report on the Ethical, Medical, and Legal Issues in Treatment Decisions. President's Commission for the Study of Ethical Problems in Medicine and Biomedical and Behavioral Research. Washington, DC, United States Government Printing Office, March, 1983. *A long and thoughtful report on the problems associated with the terminally ill and the neurologically hopelessly damaged patient.*

Barber J, et al.: Guidelines for the determination of death: Report of the medical consultants on the diagnosis of death to the President's Commission for the Study of Ethical Problems in Medicine and Biomedical and Behavioral Research. Neurology 32:395, 1982. *The detailed report describing that cardiac death and brain death are equivalent and giving criteria for each.*

Council on Scientific Affairs and Council on Ethical and Judicial Affairs: Persistent vegetative state and the decision to withdraw or withhold life support. JAMA 263:426, 1990. *The article provides criteria for the diagnosis of permanent unconsciousness and summarizes the data that support their reliability.*

396   BRIEF LOSS OF CONSCIOUSNESS
Fred Plum

Brief loss of consciousness (BLOC), defined as loss of self-awareness lasting from a few minutes to as much as an hour, is a relatively common symptom. If one excludes conditions readily diagnosed by circumstances or history such as acute traumatic concussion, a known recurrent minor seizure disorder, or accidental insulin-induced hypoglycemia, most such cases are due to causes

TABLE 396-1. PRINCIPAL CAUSES AND APPROXIMATE FREQUENCIES OF BRIEF LOSS OF CONSCIOUSNESS OF UNKNOWN ORIGIN

Syncope	
Primarily neurogenic-vasodepressor	55%
Primarily cardiogenic	10%
Central nervous system	<10%
First seizure	
Cerebrovascular insufficiency	
Subarachnoid hemorrhage	
Intracranial pressure waves	
Drugs-metabolic	<10%
Alcohol-sedative blackouts	
Narcotic overdose	
Hypoglycemia—exogenous or endogenous	
Antihypertensive drugs	
Diagnosis unknown	15–20%

listed in Table 396-1. As the table indicates, *syncope,* defined as brief unconsciousness due to a temporary, critical reduction of cerebral blood flow, is by far the most common cause of BLOC. With any of the conditions, however, reliable observations of the attack itself often are unavailable. Under such circumstances, a careful history and physical examination, including any possible information gained from witnesses, generally give more diagnostic information than any other approach.

Certain immediate guidelines aid in differential diagnosis. Patients under age 50 years with no previous history of cardiac disease, seizures, antihypoglycemic medication, or drug-alcohol abuse almost all turn out to have either benign, neurally mediated reflex syncope or a disorder undiagnosable from available evidence. Such patients rarely require an evaluation more elaborate than a careful history and physical examination plus standard blood counts and blood chemistry determinations. Tilt table studies are said to induce autonomically generated hypotension in neurally mediated reflex syncope, but specificity often is low. For those over age 40, an electrocardiogram (ECG) should be obtained. Computed tomography and electroencephalographic examinations are not cost-effective in the absence of additional abnormal neurologic symptoms or signs.

396.1   Syncope

ETIOLOGY AND INITIAL CONSIDERATIONS. A brief dysfunction of vasodepressor cardiovascular reflexes causes most syncope. Less frequent causes include primary cardiovascular disease or the drugs used to treat it, primary or secondary orthostatic hypotension, and, rarely, cerebral arterial vascular disease. Seizure disorders or psychiatric episodes represent possibly confusing conditions when only a retrospective history can be obtained. Acute, severe vertiginous attacks sometimes can induce secondary, reflex syncope. Hysterical unresponsiveness, although not uncommon, cannot be diagnosed reliably in retrospect. Diagnostic signs of such attacks are given in Table 396-2.

Among patients over age 50 with no historical or physical features suggesting cardiac, neurologic, or systemic illness, benign syncope remains the most common cause of unexplained BLOC.

TABLE 396-2. SIGNS OF PSYCHOGENIC PSEUDOSYNCOPE

Lids close actively, may flutter, and often resist examiner's attempt to open them.
Breathing: eupnea or acute hyperventilation.
Pupils responsive or dilated (self-administered cycloplegic).
Oculocephalic responses unpredictable; calorics produce quick nystagmus.
Motor responses unpredictable, often bizarre and self-protecting.
No pathologic reflexes. EEG normal in awake patient.

Nevertheless, most authorities recommend at least 24 hours of prolonged ECG monitoring in such instances. In Kapoor's study of 433 mostly older patients (mean age, 56 years) with presumed syncope, prolonged ECG recording independently provided important diagnostic information in approximately 20%. In the event of any evidence suggesting cardiac disease, invasive electrophysiologic testing may be useful.

MECHANISMS OF SYNCOPE. Unconsciousness results when generalized cerebral blood flow declines to approximately 40% of normal. Such a drop usually reflects a fall in cardiac output by half or more, and a fall in mean erect arterial blood pressure to below 40 to 50 mm Hg. Given this principle, it comes as no surprise that posture contributes importantly to the event. Syncope of any cause is far more common in the sitting or standing position than during recumbency. Indeed, recumbent syncope must be regarded as reflecting either serious cardiovascular disease or neurologic disease until proved otherwise.

Pathophysiologic changes in several bodily systems can cause these changes. These include (1) temporarily abnormal neural reflexes acting on an otherwise normal cardiovascular system (this category includes the most common causes of fainting in persons who have no history of serious cardiovascular disease); (2) abnormal intrinsic cardiovascular function, including especially disease of the conduction system predisposing to malignant arrhythmias; (3) impaired right heart filling secondary to functionally increased resistance to venous return; (4) acute or subacute blood loss; (5) increased resistance of cervical or intracranial arterial vascular beds; (6) subacute or chronic autonomic insufficiency. Table 396–3 lists subcategories of these disorders which are discussed more fully in the following paragraphs.

Neurogenic Mechanisms in Normal and Abnormal Cardiovascular Control. Sympathetic and parasympathetic influences on the cardiovascular system normally act in a finely tuned manner to slow the heart (vagal) and regulate the degree of constriction of the large venous capacitance vessels of the trunk and extremities (sympathetic outflow). Imbalance, be it a reflection of paralysis or excessive activity in either system, can perturb heart rhythm and rate, slacken venomotor tone, and lead to either reduced left ventricle output, reduced right heart filling, or the two combined. Hypoperfusion sufficient to produce vagal reflex syncope can require as much as 30 seconds or more to evolve or can occur so abruptly as to produce immediate unconsciousness. To produce primary cardiac syncope, sinus bradycardia in most healthy persons must fall below about 30 to 35 beats per minute. Asystole for longer than 3 to 5 seconds usually causes fainting in the erect position at any age. Higher rate and shorter duration thresholds apply to older patients and those with diseased hearts. Atrioventricular arrest,

TABLE 396–3. PRINCIPAL MECHANISMS OF SYNCOPE

I. Mainly impaired right heart filling
   A. Reflex abnormalities
      1. Vasodepressor ("vasovagal"): capacitance veins dilated, cardiac rate normal or slow
      2. Primary or secondary autonomic insufficiency (Ch. 402)
   B. Hypovolemia: hemorrhage, acute salt-water loss, protein loss, enteropathy, burns
   C. Mechanically impaired right heart return: Valsalva maneuver, tussive excess, abrupt chest compression; term pregnancy; pulmonary embolism; pericardial tamponade
II. Globally impaired cardiac output
   A. Reflex abnormalities
      1. Vagal sinus arrest
         a. Psychophysiologic (rare)
         b. Visceral stimulation: glossopharyngeal neuralgia, swallow syncope, direct tracheal stimulation, dilatation of hollow viscus
         c. Carotid baroreceptor sensitivity
   B. Intrinsic cardiac disease (with or without reflex enhancement) (Table 396–4).
III. Primary cerebral ischemia (uncommon)
   A. Multivessel cervical arterial obstructive disease
   B. Transient acute increase in intracranial pressure (plateau waves)
   C. Basilar migraine (rare in adults)
   D. Vertebral-basilar TIA's (rare)

however, is extremely uncommon in persons with healthy hearts, possible exceptions being overtrained athletes, persons taking cocaine, and rare "hypervagal" subjects undergoing severe psychophysiologic threats.

PHYSIOLOGIC REFLEX (VASOVAGAL) SYNCOPE. *Acute vasodepressor syncope* is the most common cause of fainting and typically is marked by a diphasic course. During an initial brief period of apprehension and anxiety, heart rate, blood pressure, total systemic resistance, and cardiac output inconsistently may increase. The vasodepressor phase follows, during which blood pressure falls and cardiac output declines. Both sympathetic and parasympathetic abnormalities are involved, because atropine prevents the bradycardia but not the depressor response. Progressive sensations of lightheadedness, giddiness, abdominal sinking sensations, nausea, urinary urgency, and finally "gray-out" or faintness accompany the vasodepressor component.

During vasodepressor syncope, subjects appear pale and the accompanying parasympathetic hyperactivity characteristically induces piloerection and sweating. Because cardiac action continues, awareness and normal cardiovascular reflexes usually return promptly once the subject becomes supine. Vomiting or explosive diarrhea may follow. Occasionally, emotionally generated dysautonomic influences on the heart can be so profound as to induce arrhythmia. Investigators have speculated that this mechanism can cause sudden death associated with sudden grief or fright.

Fainting is more likely in circumstances of emotional perturbation, in hungry subjects, after a heavy, alcohol-supplemented meal, in a warm, moist environment, and after prolonged standing. A few individuals give a history of lifelong susceptibility to fainting attacks. Rarely, one gets a history suggesting predisposition to vasodepressor syncope based on an autosomal dominant trait, with family members in several generations having been susceptible to recurrent vasodepressor attacks.

Visceral reflex syncope acts via the same medullospinal pathways as the examples cited above. A sense of faintness or even complete syncope can follow immediately after any of the following: emptying a full bladder from the standing position *(micturition syncope)*, acute visceral pain (as occurs with a suddenly distended gut or an abrupt joint or ligament injury), an attack of severe vertigo (as occurs with Ménière's disease), or a migraine attack.

The diagnosis of vasodepressor syncope is made largely by history; rarely are the events medically witnessed. Among young persons who lack histories or physical findings of neurologic or cardiovascular disease, treatment is symptomatic. Furthermore, when consulting on such cases we have never found either brain imaging or EEG useful. When impending sensations of faintness threaten, persons should be promptly placed supine. Placing the head far forward in a sitting position is usually ineffective. Subjects who have fainted should be mobilized slowly, because the reflex abnormality occasionally can persist for as long as 2 hours. Prophylactic treatment has little value except when fainting occurs in response to a disease or injury that requires attention. Occasionally, overtrained athletes with chronically slow hearts and a history of syncope during exertion are helped by a regimen of reduced training combined with oral anticholinergic agents.

SYNCOPE DUE PRIMARILY TO CARDIAC CAUSES. Pathologic reflex (vagovagal) attacks result primarily from failure of left heart output associated with reflexly induced changes in the cardiac rhythm, including nodal or sinus arrest, atrioventricular asystole, atrioventricular block, sinoatrial block, and ventricular arrhythmias. Usually these are accompanied by relatively minor vasodepressor changes in the peripheral vasculature, implying a lesser sympathetic abnormality. Most patients with vagovagal attacks belong to the older population and have associated heart disease, resulting in abnormally intense cardiac responses to a relatively normal degree of increased parasympathetic stimulation or sympathetic inhibition. Vagal bradycardia or arrest occasionally is induced by sudden emotional stimuli but more commonly follows acute noxious or abnormal visceral stimulation. Severe bradycardia or arrest especially accompanies glossopharyngeal neuralgia, swallowing in patients with mechanical esophageal lesions, sudden painful dilatations of a hollow viscus, prostatic manipulation, tracheal stimulation, or visceral wounds.

Cardiac syncope almost always reflects serious heart disease. Given a normal heart, neither bradycardia above 30 beats per minute nor tachycardia up to 200 beats per minute causes syncope in the supine or seated position so long as functioning vasomotor reflexes remain. Analyses of large series of patients show serious associated cardiac risk factors, including those listed in Table 396–4. In the case of patients over 40 years of age or those showing such risk factors, prolonged (Holter) monitoring of cardiac activity is indicated. In the absence of specific predisposing abnormalities discovered by history, physical examination, and such ECG monitoring, however, additional studies such as direct electrophysiologic studies of the heart, cardiac catheterization or coronary angiography may add helpful information. Management of cardiac syncope depends upon the nature of the underlying heart disease. Affected persons should be considered for pacemaker insertion.

OTHER CAUSES OF FAINTING. *Orthostatic Hypotension.* Acute orthostatic hypotension occasionally occurs in normal persons after acute blood loss, e.g., cryptic gastrointestinal hemorrhage, or following prolonged standing as with soldiers at parade rest in a hot sun; affected subjects undergo a sudden collapse of sympathetic reflex tone. Recurrent symptoms of syncope or faintness accompanying the erect position usually can be traced to the presence of the chronic use of diuretics, vasodepressor drugs β-adrenergic blockers, or neurologic disorders involving the peripheral or central nervous system. Chronic hypovolemia, such as occurs in elderly cardiac or systemically ill patients, also predisposes to syncope, especially following periods of bed rest or prolonged sitting. Increased age as well as many drugs accentuate tendencies to orthostatic hypotension. The latter include most antihypertensive agents and many of the antidepressants, phenothiazines, and sedatives. Neurogenic causes of autonomic insufficiency are discussed in Ch. 402.

Orthostatic hypotension sufficient to cause cerebral symptoms can occur either rapidly upon standing or develop insidiously over seconds or minutes. Although symptoms of faintness and giddiness predominate, some patients lack such prodromal warnings, presumably because of the absence of strong efferent parasympathetic activity. Sometimes when chronically ill patients sit for long periods or stand, they become confused or tremulous without the usual sensations of faintness or collapse. Diagnosis comes from observing an acute or progressive decline in the mean blood pressure of more than 10 to 15 mm Hg in the erect position. Autonomic insufficiency can be inferred by observing an unchanging pulse rate despite the hypotension, and confirmed by tilt-table tests or by identifying other autonomic impairment. The simplest way to evaluate sympathetic tone at the bedside is to take the pulse while the supine patient performs a vigorous Valsalva maneuver for a matter of 30 seconds or so. The normal response consists of a palpable post-Valsalva slowing of pulse and a 10 to 30 mm Hg rise in mean blood pressure.

Treatment of orthostatic hypotension depends upon the cause. Symptomatic treatment requires eliminating drugs that cause hypotension, correcting causes of blood volume depletion, and applying elastic stockings to the lower extremities. When other measures fail, an increased salt intake and, subsequently, administering the salt-retaining steroid fludrocortisone, 0.3 to 0.8 mg per day in divided doses, can be cautiously initiated. The chronic use of vasopressor agents seldom helps. Patients can be at least partially reconditioned by erect activity. Every effort should be made to keep them up and walking.

Mechanically Impaired Right Heart Filling. In patients with congestive heart disease or cardiopulmonary failure, a strong *Valsalva maneuver* or sustained coughing (*tussive syncope*) raises intrathoracic pressure sufficiently to impede venous return and induce syncope. *Term pregnancy* causing compression of abdominal veins can occasionally induce a similar, posturally related effect. *Pulmonary embolism* and *acute cardiac tamponade,* due most often

to subpericardial aortic dissection, act similarly to reduce the right heart filling and critically reduce cardiac output.

Recurrent symptoms of chronic hypovolemia are common in the chronically ill, especially in cardiac patients, the elderly, and those kept at bed rest for sustained periods (in whom baroceptor reflexes also become blunted). Syncope is a risk in all these groups, especially with prolonged motionless sitting.

Cerebral Vascular Disease. Intrinsic cerebral vascular diseases only rarely cause episodes of brief loss of consciousness. Although syncopal episodes might be expected on anatomic grounds as part of the symptom complex associated with vertebral-basilar insufficiency, such is seldom the case. Several reports describing large series of patients with vertebral-basilar insufficiency make no mention of such events. I have observed only two well-documented cases over the years. By contrast, brief periods of confusion or even unconsciousness occasionally mark the course of patients with severe stenosis or occlusion of one or both internal carotid arteries; they may or may not show concurrent narrowing of the vertebrobasilar system. In a few such patients, pulse and blood pressure have been monitored through the attacks, which are marked by brief unresponsiveness associated with transient amnesia but no seizures or EEG changes. Surgical removal of carotid stenoses have helped some, but not all, affected patients. Presumably the spells reflect transient, global blood flow reductions to the cerebral hemispheres associated with hemodynamic insufficiency in cervical arterial circulations.

396.2 Nonsyncopal Causes of Brief Alterations of Consciousness

HYPERVENTILATION. The disorder is mechanistically closely related to syncope in that a globally reduced cerebral blood flow gives rise to sensations of giddiness, faintness, and other distress. Full unconsciousness rarely occurs without some additional abnormal maneuver. The abnormal state is most often part of an anxiety response and often is accompanied by sensations of suffocation, pressure on the chest, and a sense of being unable to obtain the satisfaction of a lung-filling deep breath. Extreme or prolonged hyperventilation can produce feelings of unreality with anxiety bordering on panic.

Symptoms and signs include feelings of unreality, difficulty in concentrating, and several hard-to-explain sensory complaints, such as unilateral or bilateral chest pain or paresthesias involving the body and extremities. Symptoms of facial twitching, carpal spasm, and perioral paresthesias are more easily understood as part of alkalotic tetany.

Hyperventilation occasionally precipitates syncope under special circumstances. Children sometimes voluntarily hyperventilate, then perform a vigorous Valsalva maneuver to induce syncope (fainting lark). Athletes may repeat a similar sequence in contests such as weight lifting or squat jumps. More dangerous is a pattern wherein underwater swimmers hyperventilate before diving, then exhaust their oxygen reserves before producing sufficient carbon dioxide to produce dyspnea. The ensuing cerebral hypoxia can induce fatal submersion syncope.

SEIZURE DISORDERS. Seizure disorders (see Ch. 433) may be confused with syncope under four principal circumstances:

1. *Rapid, profound syncope* may induce a single brief tonic seizure or series of clonic twitches as a result of abrupt cerebral ischemia (*convulsive syncope*). The response is more likely when the subject has made maximal efforts to stand or sit despite premonitory symptoms. Features that are more consistent with syncope than epilepsy include the psychologic circumstances and physical appearance, the associated medical conditions and body position, the brief quality of the seizure, its rapid recovery, and the presence of a normal neurologic examination and interictal EEG.

2. *Akinetic seizures* consist of attacks of suddenly falling or

TABLE 396–4. CARDIOVASCULAR ABNORMALITIES FREQUENTLY ASSOCIATED WITH SYNCOPAL ATTACKS

Myocardial infarction	Pacemaker malfunction
Aortic stenosis	Ventricular tachycardia
Severe cardiomyopathy	Sick sinus syndrome
Severe hypertension	Complete heart block
Pulmonary embolism	Asystole ($> \pm 3$ sec erect, ± 8 sec supine)
Pulmonary hypertension	Bradycardia < 44/min
Dissecting aortic aneurysm	Tachycardia > 160–180/min

pitching to the ground, starting in early childhood. Similar episodes occur in the supine position and are marked by unresponsiveness accompanied by generalized muscular hypotonia or brief body spasm. Diagnosis rests on the typical history, the age of onset, and the presence of an abnormal EEG. *Absence (petit mal) seizures* rarely provide a diagnostic problem because children with petit mal, although out of contact, neither fall nor turn pale and usually have no memory of the episode. The EEG is abnormal and frequently diagnostic.

3. *Partial complex (psychomotor) seizures* sometimes include brief behavioral automatisms in which the subject recalls only being out of contact and may retrospectively consider himself to have suffered a state of unconsciousness. Usually the presence of a characteristic, self-recognized aura or set of incipient symptoms indicates the diagnosis. Falling to the ground rarely occurs unless a generalized seizure develops. Witnessed attacks and the abnormal EEG usually are typical.

4. *Postictal unresponsiveness* from grand mal attacks produces unconsciousness lasting minutes, the duration usually depending on the severity of the preceding convulsion. Diagnosis is a problem only if the seizure was unwitnessed, in which case the state may look like concussion or profound fainting. Even so, the postictal state is marked initially by flushing (cyanosis), giving way to pallor, hyperpnea, and deep unresponsiveness, none of which occurs in syncope.

HYPOGLYCEMIA (see Ch. 206). Hypoglycemia, usually caused by excess exogenous rather than endogenous insulin, can produce a variety of relatively brief episodes of neurologic dysfunction. These can consist, variably, of brief confusional episodes, seizures of a variety of types, narcolepsy-like syndromes, and focal or tetraparetic weakness with or without coma but not resembling syncope. Diagnosis depends on suspicion plus the detection of blood sugars of less than 30 to 40 mg per deciliter during an attack.

DRUG OR ALCOHOL BLACKOUTS. Drug or alcohol blackouts consist of episodes of such severe intoxication that they anesthetize memory for the event, leaving the subject with an episode of focal amnesia. Many are accompanied by "passing out," consisting of deep, barely arousable sleep.

CONCUSSION-POSTCONCUSSION AMNESIA. Variable periods of memory loss for immediate subsequent events can follow brief periods of concussive unconsciousness. The usual question is whether an intrinsic malady caused the fall or the fall represented the whole illness. Only diagnostic diligence can solve the issue.

ACUTE INTRACRANIAL HYPERTENSION. Plateau waves, associated with this condition, can produce brief episodes of loss of consciousness that resemble syncope. Occasionally, brief unconsciousness may accompany the onset of acute subarachnoid hemorrhage. The episode, which is syncopal in its abruptness and often accompanied by either a tonic extensor spasm or brief clonic jerks, is most often due to an acute cardiac arrhythmia or asystole accompanying the onset of bleeding. Cerebral hemorrhage with intraventricular rupture can produce similar events.

DROP SPELLS. As discussed in Chapter 404, these are poorly understood attacks affecting older persons. The legs suddenly and unexplainedly give way, and the women fall, often injuring themselves but experiencing no observed interruption of consciousness. The cause is unknown.

CONVERSION REACTIONS OR MALINGERING (PSEUDOSYNCOPE). Hysterical or other forms of psychogenic unresponsiveness are almost impossible to diagnose in retrospect. If such a condition occurs during the physical examination, the diagnosis can be concluded by the absence of physiologic abnormality and the presence of additional, often bizarre features (see Table 396–2). Most subjects awaken with gentle but firm confrontation. A few do so only when advised that psychiatric admission lies in store. Mutilating stimuli are neither justified nor often successful in proving the diagnosis.

Aminoff MJ, Scheinman MM, Griffin JC, et al.: Electrocerebral accompaniments of syncope associated with malignant ventricular arrhythmias. Ann Intern Med 108:791, 1988. *Ten of 17 episodes of syncope caused by electrically induced ventricular tachycardia or arrhythmia had accompanying tonic seizures or irregular muscular twitching. The results illustrate the high incidence of convulsive syncope.*

Benditt DG, Remole S, Milstein S, et al.: Syncope: Causes, clinical evaluation and current therapy. Annu Rev Med 43:283, 1992. *A comprehensive review.*

Kapoor WN: Evaluation and management of syncope. JAMA 268:2553, 1992. *A well-*

balanced review of the author's large personal series plus others in the recent literature.

Mandis AS, Linzer M, Salem D, et al.: Syncope. Current diagnostic evaluation and management. Ann Intern Med 112:850, 1990. *A comprehensive review of the problem identifying rare as well as common causes and emphasizing laboratory evaluations, especially of cardiovascular mechanisms.*

397 DISORDERS OF SLEEP AND AROUSAL

Fred Plum

BIOLOGY OF NORMAL SLEEP. Of all normal visceral functions, the fundamental value of sleep remains the least well understood. Its restorative rewards are self-evident, as is the fact that severe degrees of sleep deprivation impair cognitive and systemic functions alike. Yet the cell-molecular bases for these elementary experiences remain unknown, just as do the signals that induce sensations of drowsiness or the biochemical tissue changes that accompany refreshing sleep. Brain-regulating mechanisms that generate normal sleep cycles and the underlying macrophysiology of sleep states are better understood and are discussed in subsequent paragraphs.

Normal adult sleep-wake patterns repeat themselves on an approximately 24-hour cycle, of which wakefulness occupies approximately two thirds. The suprachiasmatic nucleus of the hypothalamus sets the overall circadian rhythm, and the environmental light-dark cycle as well as the individual's personal activities establish the specific clock hours of the pattern. Suprachiasmatic outputs similarly induce circadian patterns of function in other hypothalamic regulatory nuclei and influence arousal and sleep-related nuclei located in the upper brain stem as well. Perturbations in this normal system occur readily. The abrupt changing of environmental clock time by three or more hours such as occurs with shift changes of working hours or transmeridian air travel induces jet lag, characterized by several days of fractionated sleep patterns poorly coordinated with practical requirements. Similarly, psychologically induced hyperarousal, depression, or severe illness all can disrupt the comforting nurtures of normal circadian sleep.

Needs for sleep among normal individuals vary widely and tend to decline with age. Adults sleep less than children and men less than women, with most normal adults sleeping regularly between about 7 and 9 hours per day, but with extremes of 4 and 11. Tropical inhabitants typically displace part of their total sleep time to afternoon hours in keeping with a hemicircadian intrinsic cycle of alertness and sleepiness. Normal sleep evolves in non-REM stages graded 1 to 4 [on the basis of electroencephalographic (EEG) changes and depth of unarousability] and REM sleep, which alternate through the night in approximately 90-minute cycles. REM is a cortically active sleep stage, consisting of rapid, wakeful-like EEG patterns, rapid eye movements, and markedly reduced voluntary muscle activity. The biologic importance of these phase shifts is little understood but much debated. Whatever their explanation, an abnormal regulation of the timing of REM sleep is a central feature of narcolepsy, discussed below. In the absence of a sleep disorder, the subjective experience of sleep is uninterrupted in most persons under about age 40. Stages 3 and 4 sleep, as defined by standard EEG criteria, decline gradually throughout adulthood. Awakenings at the transition of REM to non–REM sleep tend increasingly to interrupt the sleep pattern, especially over about age 60.

INSOMNIA. A recent, abrupt onset of insomnia in an adult most often relates to the advent of systemic illness, grief, newly appearing personal or financial preoccupations, dietary indiscretions, or jet lag. A more gradual development marks the sleeplessness that often follows drug or alcohol use, aging, a new-onset or recurrent depressive disorder, a major change in personal relationships, or rarely, the development of a neurologic disorder. The insomniac who snores may have obstructive sleep apnea, and the insomniac with restless legs syndrome may have periodic limb movements (discussed below). Syphilitic general paresis, Huntington's disease, and Parkinson's disease all occasionally produce insomnia early in their course. Similar problems accompany certain of the cerebellar degenerations, brain stem injuries, or strokes, as well as very rare cases of prion disease called fatal familial insomnia (see Ch. 428.6). Chronic insomnia of many years' duration unaccompanied by pain, aging, or debilitating illnesses such as chronic cardiopulmonary diseases, cancer, or severe arthritis generally has physically benign implications. It may represent either a normal individual variation of sleep requirements or a chronic psychiatric disorder associated with symptoms of anxiety and depression.

Given the multiple circumstances that may interfere with sleep, management not only becomes difficult but often must be individualized (Table 397–1). Hypnotic drugs find their ideal use in patients with recent-onset insomnia, with short-acting benzodiazepines being the agents of choice. All drugs of this class induce tolerance more slowly than their predecessors (e.g., barbiturates) but still lose their effectiveness if used uninterruptedly for more than a few weeks. Also, all are habituating and predispose to withdrawal symptoms after more than a few days of continuous use. Accordingly, all should be prescribed at a minimum dose for naive subjects, particularly elderly ones. Of the group, triazolam (Halcion) and zolpidem (Ambien) are favored for inducing sleep, whereas flurazepam (Dalmane) and quazepam (Doral) are effective in sustaining the duration of sleep. Triazolam at doses >0.25 mg sometimes impairs recent memory or leaves unpleasant hangovers. Flurazepam and quazepam have desalkyl metabolites with long half-lives, which may accumulate to produce side effects after 10 to 14 days of use. With all these drugs, the best approach is to administer them for two or three nights prior to retiring and then halt their intake so as to compare the results and resume, if necessary, with similarly interrupted patterns for not longer than 5 weeks. Tapered doses should be scheduled over a several-day period to avoid withdrawal symptoms.

For patients with more sustained and refractory insomnia, the following guidelines may be helpful.

1. Encourage the insomniac to maintain a regular bedtime and arising time and not to spend excessive time in bed. This regularity needs to include weekends.

2. Reassure the insomniac that although his/her feelings of fatigue, heavy limbs, fuzzy thinking, and giddy sensations may relate to the ostensible sleep lack, no evidence indicates that even long-term insomnia injures health.

3. Emphasize that insomniacs only know when they are awake. Direct observations usually show that they sleep more than they think.

4. Strongly recommend that the insomniac give up alcohol and all kinds of psychoactive drugs not being prescribed for psychiatric illness. All these agents, with time, risk enhancing the sleep loss because of tolerance or withdrawal effects.

5. Take simple steps first. Have patients reduce tea or coffee to morning hours. Prescribe specific effective daily exercise. Eliminate long midday naps. Give enough analgesics to relieve pain. Reduce the size of evening meals and avoid red meat. Try taking hot baths in the evening. Replace noisy atmospheres with earphones playing music or a white noise generator.

6. If depression or chronic pain persists, try tricyclic or other relevant antidepressants in appropriate doses given at bedtime.

7. If other approaches fail, consider a combination of appropriate antidepressants such as a tricyclic in modest doses, combined with behavioral therapy.

8. Reassure elderly insomniacs that their sleeplessness is probably physiologic, not psychological. Urge them to read or listen to music or other tapes when awake. Install steady noise backgrounds

TABLE 397–1. SIMPLE MEASURES TO HELP CHRONIC INSOMNIACS

Maintain a regular schedule with reduced time in bed.
Reassure them that insomnia rarely impairs physical health.
Emphasize that insomnics know only awakening, not sleep time.
Urge avoidance of alcohol, cigarettes, stimulants, polypharmacy, red meat, heavy evening meals. Urge daily exercise.
Treat pain, counteract random nighttime noise. Urge evening hot baths, serene atmospheres.
Avoid hypnotics. Consider, if appropriate, antidepressants or behavioral therapy.

TABLE 397–2. THE PARASOMNIAS

Largely in Children	Adults
Headbanging	Bruxism
Sleepwalking	Restless legs
Night terrors	Periodic limb movements
Bedwetting	Sleep apnea
Nightmares (mostly children but any age)	REM behavior disorder

(e.g., by electric fan or the like) to dampen sudden environmental noises.

9. Use sedatives seldom, in small doses, and for periods of 3 weeks or less. Short- to middle-acting benzodiazepines probably are best, but prescribe them for elderly persons at no more than half the size of the usual adult dose.

10. For severe problems, combine antidepressants and behavioral therapy. Consider expert consultation with a sleep specialist.

SPECIAL CASES. *Parasomnias.* The parasomnias consist of a group of motor or autonomic disorders that can delay or disrupt the course of normal sleep (Table 397–2). Most of these conditions affect children, but a few interfere with the sleep patterns of adults and are described here.

Bruxism (teeth grinding) can occur at any age beyond puberty. A few examples are familial, but most become clinically apparent in a setting of tension and anxiety. Wearing a teeth shield while asleep may ameliorate the noisy grinding and the morning headaches that go with it but may not substitute adequately for needed psychiatric attention aimed toward reduction of stress and anxiety.

Restless legs syndrome usually affects selected adults in their elder years. The symptoms consist of unpleasant sensations in the calves and an urge to move the legs, leading to uncontrolled movement, pacing, or rubbing to temporarily alleviate the discomfort. About half of cases are familial. The subjective symptoms may delay sleep onset and/or interrupt or shorten its duration. Annoying periodic limb movements occur during sleep in the vast majority of patients with this condition. These movements also can be found in almost any other sleep disorder (e.g., sleep apnea, narcolepsy) and in up to 40% of asymptomatic elderly persons. In most such cases, there are far fewer movements per night than in restless legs syndrome. Current treatment includes carbamazepine (Tegretol), carbidopa-levadopa (Sinemet), or a low-potency narcotic such as oxycodone or propoxyphene (Darvon). None have dramatic effects.

Night terrors rarely affect adults. When so, they usually reflect a recent personal crisis or, when recurrent, drug-alcohol excess, structural lesions of the brain, or serious psychiatric disorders.

Somnambulism may extend into midlife after late childhood onset. Severe cases in which the behavior poses a threat to the patient should be treated with intermediate half-life benzodiazepines such as lorazepam (Ativan) at 0.5 to 2 mg at bedtime. The principal differential diagnosis is nocturnal partial complex seizures. A recently identified parasomnia is the *REM behavior disorder,* which typically affects older males. These patients act out their dreams and frequently sustain injuries as a result. Treatment consists of clonazepam (Klonopin) at 0.5 to 3 mg at bedtime.

Narcolepsy and Daytime Hypersomnolence. Narcolepsy is a specific neurologic syndrome consisting of excessive daytime drowsiness, cataplexy (85 to 90% of patients), and less often, the additional phenomena of sleep paralysis and intense dreamlike hallucinations at sleep-wake transitions (50 to 60% of patients). More than 90% of cases possess the DQB1-0602 haplotype, possibly related to a gene mutation on chromosome 6. Since less than 10% of cases are immediately familial, autoimmune mechanisms or additional genetic influences have been postulated. The exact disease mechanism remains unknown, and most persons with similar haplotypes do not develop the illness.

Clinically, chronic excessive daytime sleepiness without an increase in 24-hour sleep identifies the illness. Other features are listed in Table 397–3. Narcolepsy equally affects men and women, has its onset mostly before age 25, and lasts a lifetime. Chronic daytime sleepiness accompanied by intermittent, minutes-long sleep

TABLE 397–3. CLINICAL FEATURES OF NARCOLEPSY

Chief symptoms: Near-constant sleepiness, boredom-related immediate sleep, cataplexy, signs or history of other diseases lacking
Associated symptoms: Sleep paralysis, presleep hallucinations-dreams, disrupted nocturnal sleep
Onset: During young adulthood or before
Differential diagnosis: Sleep apnea syndromes, acute or chronic sleep deprivation, metabolic encephalopathy; rarely, structural brain disease, psychiatric disease

episodes that are most often associated with boring sedentary circumstances provide the hallmarks. Although nighttime sleep tends to be repeatedly spontaneously interrupted and slightly shortened, total sleep time remains within a normal range. The intensity and frequency of daytime attacks vary from sufferer to sufferer; when severe, the disease interferes with memory, affects employment, and may lead to traffic and other accidents.

Diagnosis of narcolepsy depends on the typical, unremitting chronic history, a young age of onset, and the exclusion of other hypersomnia-inducing disorders. Moderate to severe sleep apnea and chronic sleep deprivation are far more frequent causes of daytime hypersomnolence than narcolepsy. Also, structural lesions of the brain or idiopathic hypersomnia rarely are causes of daytime hypersomnolence. A careful history and physical examination will eliminate most of these disorders. Because narcolepsy is a lifelong condition which often requires the chronic use of controlled substance stimulants, diagnosis should be confirmed by the laboratory multiple sleep latency test before starting treatment.

Cataplectic attacks consist of brief, jelly-like bodily weakness accompanying laughter or other strong emotion. *Sleep paralysis* describes a usually brief experience of feeling unable to move after awakening from a period of sustained sleep. As a phenomenon, it overlaps similar experiences of adolescence and usually ends abruptly, apparently by self-will or by mild sensory stimulation. Presleep (hypnogogic) or postsleep (hypnopompic) hallucinations are intense and sometimes bizarre; they strongly resemble the experiences of some normal persons following severe sleep deprivation.

Narcolepsy is best treated with stimulants to counteract daytime drowsiness and tricyclic antidepressants to reduce cataplectic attacks. Methylphenidate or dextroamphetamine in divided doses up to 60 mg daily are most effective. Pemoline (Cylert) in divided doses up to 112.5 mg daily is also effective and produces less irritability and tension. The incidence of unwanted side effects mounts above these levels, and the drugs should be started at low, spaced doses, because some narcoleptics require only moderate stimulation. Scheduled short naps can be very effective at reducing daytime drowsiness and the dose of medication. Cataplexy requires separate treatment and often can be completely controlled with imipramine or desipramine (50 to 150 mg daily), given in gradually increasing doses. Abstaining from all drugs one day each week helps to maintain beneficial drug effects for most patients. Usually, the stimulant drugs retain their beneficial effects for many months or even years.

Sleep Apnea. Sleep apnea occurs relatively frequently and occasionally can become sufficiently severe to interfere with health or even cause unexpected death. Clinically important sleep apnea occurs as a result of three disease categories: (1) cardiopulmonary obstructive disorders, (2) anatomic changes in the airways associated with development, aging, and supplementary medical problems (Table 397–4) and (3) neurologic or neuromuscular disorders. The neurologic causes have the least frequency; interaction often occurs between either of the first two causes and the third.

Airway obstruction with or without partial cardiopulmonary decompensation produces the largest group of medically important obstructive apneas. Age and maleness carry intrinsic risks, reflected in the high rates of snoring and temporary choking (obstructive apnea) that affect older men during otherwise uncomplicated sleep. When one adds to partial obstruction the burdens of obesity, which both narrows the upper (supraglottic) airway and increases resistance against diaphragmatic contraction, nocturnal breathing becomes commensurately more obstructed at the pharyngeal level and more of an effort. Any additional upper airway obstruction, whether from the swellings of allergy, the increased secretions of tobacco-dam-

aged mucous membranes, or the pre-existence of developmentally narrowed canals, threatens to produce nocturnal respiratory decompensation. The recurrent obstructive apneas, each ending in a brief and insensible arousal, eventually produce daytime fatigue and sleepiness, with resultant deterioration of the personality, decline in work habits, and intellectual slowness. In the morbidly obese, daytime blood gases begin to deteriorate due to restrictive lung disease. If the problem proceeds uncorrected, heart failure, arrhythmias, hypertension, and premature death may ensue.

Nonobstructive sleep apnea also may occur during the course of acute severe congestive heart failure or with acute exacerbations of chronic obstructive pulmonary diseases. With either event, hypoxic-hypercarbic central respiratory depression plus peripheral fatigue, depressant drugs, and sleep may seriously elevate the breathing threshold. The result produces a cardiopulmonary emergency.

Central sleep apnea, sometimes called "secondary sleep apnea," when it results from progressive peripheral or central neurological abnormalities, has a relatively low incidence (Table 397–4). Peripheral or central-peripheral neurologic diseases act by gradually reducing ventilatory capacity to the point of physiologic insufficiency, reflected either by progressive dyspnea or the presence of an insidiously gradual decompensation of arterial blood gases. Whether because of inherent insensitivity or by adaptation, central brain stem respiratory sensitivity to hypercarbia-hypoxia becomes blunted, and sleep may further elevate the breathing threshold leading to episodic apnea of varying severity. Most of the potential causes listed in Table 397–4 can be recognized easily from historical and physical evidence. Two that are sometimes overlooked consist of adult acid maltase deficiency, which sometimes produces selective diaphragmatic failure, and acute-subacute bilateral brachial neuropathy, which can silently interrupt phrenic nerve conduction.

Treatment of sleep apnea depends on accurate diagnosis as to the severity of the problem and application of mechanical techniques of proved worth. Evaluation by an experienced sleep disorders center usually can help in such steps and in suggesting a program of treatment. The usual first approach is to apply continuous positive airway pressure (CPAP) during the night via the nasal route. Nasal CPAP induces remarkable improvement in as many as 90% of patients with obstructive sleep and in some patients with central sleep apnea. Weight loss by exercise and a reasonable diet can be very effective at reducing or eliminating obstructive sleep apnea, if accomplished and maintained. Concomitant use of nasal CPAP during weight loss can relieve the condition entirely. Any amount of alcohol increases the severity of obstructive sleep apnea, which nevertheless can be overcome with an appropriate CPAP level. Heavy al-

TABLE 397–4. CLINICALLY IMPORTANT SLEEP APNEAS

Neurologic Mechanisms	Systemic Abnormalities
Peripheral Neuromuscular Disorders	
Uncommon; all reflect gradually progressive weakness in respiratory muscles combined with desensitization of brain stem respiratory centers	Severe, acute congestive heart failure
	Obstructive pulmonary disease with chronic hypercarbia-hypoxemia
Gradually progressive muscular dystrophies, especially myotonic and acid maltase deficiency	
Chronic severe myasthenia gravis	
Severe postpolio syndrome with marginal respiratory reserve	
Progressive amyotrophic lateral sclerosis, progressive bulbar palsy	
Central Disorders	
Lower brain stem structural disease	*Airway Obstructive Disorders*
Respiratory center desensitization secondary to recurrent hypoxia-hypercarbia	Predominantly males
	Obesity
	Mostly ages 40–70
	Congenital or developmental upper airway narrowing
	Secondary narrowing: Allergic rhinitis, hypertrophied tonsils, tongue, or pharyngeal tumors, hypothyroidism, acromegaly

cohol users often have difficulty complying with any treatment, including CPAP. Unless clearly abnormal and substantial airway obstruction exists, surgery on the upper airway seldom offers sustained improvement. Nasal CPAP may help clear the right-sided heart failure associated with obstructive sleep apnea in the context of obesity-hyperventilation or chronic obstructive pulmonary disease.

Other patients with central or sleep apnea require artificial ventilation by other means, for which several kinds of instruments are available. The need for tracheostomy or other surgical procedures has almost completely disappeared during recent years.

Culebras A (ed.): The neurology of sleep. Neurology 42(suppl 6):94, 1992. *Eleven authorities provide well-written, comprehensive reviews and discussion of the subject. Articles on narcolepsy and sleep apneas offer especially useful information.*
Kryger MH, Roth T, Dement WC (eds.): Principles and Practice of Sleep Medicine. 2d ed. Philadelphia, WB Saunders, 1994. *A detailed, comprehensive textbook addresses all aspects of the subject.*
Mignot E, Lin X, Kalil J, George C, et al.: DQB1-0602 (DQw1) is not present in most non-DR2 Caucasian narcoleptics. Sleep 15(5):415, 1992. *This and the following paper informatively discuss haplotypes in narcolepsy.*
Mignot E, Lin X, Hesla P-E, Dement WC, et al.: A novel HLA DR 17, DQ1 (DQA1-0102/DQB1-0602 Positive) haplotype predisposing to narcolepsy in Caucasians (Letter to the Editor). Sleep 16:764, 1993.

398 DIAGNOSIS OF REGIONAL CEREBRAL DYSFUNCTION

Antonio R. Damasio

Localizing the site of neurologic dysfunction based on clinical signs and symptoms is crucial to the assessment of neurologic diseases. Although noninvasive neuroimaging techniques localize many brain lesions, the abnormalities associated with some diseases often elude all but research-level imaging procedures. For instance, in most degenerative diseases, the regional anatomic defect can be defined only on the basis of clinical signs. Another example is the diagnosis of most epileptogenic foci, a key element in the therapeutic management of epileptic patients.

Figure 398–1 diagrams the regional neuroanatomy of the adult human brain. The accuracy of regional clinical diagnosis depends on numerous factors. First, elementary motor and sensory disorders relate to dysfunction in motor and sensory pathways and can be detected earlier than disorders of thinking or language, which result from dysfunction in association cortices. The localization of the underlying lesions is generally more precise in the former than in the latter. This difference reflects the fine anatomic and functional modularity of the primary sensory and motor systems and the fact that cognitive processes depend on distributed anatomic systems beyond the primary areas. Furthermore, the neural substrate for integrative processes varies individually, different individuals having different endowments for specific abilities. For instance, language or visuospatial skills are linked to a variety of genetic and epigenetic factors and are influenced by age, educational background, and even gender. Second, the type of pathologic lesion and its rate of development influence the rate of appearance and the extent of symptoms. Most infarcts damage the brain and lead to an abrupt onset of signs followed by at least some improvement. By contrast, most intracranial tumors generate symptoms gradually and the brain adapts to the tumor enlargement. Some slow-growing meningiomas can reach the size of a plum before they cause detectable dysfunction, whereas small brain metastases from a carcinoma elsewhere in the body may cause major symptoms rapidly. Third, the mass effect and the edema that accompany large infarcts and some tumors may cause a shift of brain structures and thereby compress remote and otherwise intact areas of the brain against the rigid frame of the dural meninges and skull. Such compression can generate false localizing signs, lead to impaired attention, and interfere with wakefulness (see Ch. 396).

OCCIPITAL LOBES

The occipital cortices are solely dedicated to visual processing. Signals from both lateral geniculate nuclei arrive in each primary visual cortex (Brodmann's area 17), which occupies the superior and inferior banks of the calcarine fissure (see also Ch. 404.2). This region contains a retinotopic projection of visual information. The inferior visual field maps onto the superior calcarine fissure and vice versa; the right visual field maps into the left calcarine region and conversely for the left visual field; the central part of the retina projects onto the caudal part of the calcarine region, at the occipital pole, while progressively more peripheral sectors of the retina project to more anterior sectors of the calcarine region. Beyond area 17, visual information is widely distributed by a large number of functionally distinct regions, located within the association cortices of Brodmann's areas 18 and 19. The main goals of these parallel processing units are (1) to generate representations of the form, volumetric shape, texture, movement, color, and spatial location of stimuli in the external world, and (2) to serve as distributed storage sites for the records of visual perception that become committed to memory and are later used in the processes of visual recall, recognition, imagetic thinking, and dreaming.

Damage to the calcarine cortices (Table 398–1) or to the optic radiations as they approach the calcarine region causes varied field defects for form vision (hemianopias or quadrantanopias) depending on the region affected (e.g., damage to the left superior calcarine region causes a right inferior quadrantanopia; damage to an entire calcarine region leads to a hemianopia). When damage is confined to inferior occipital cortices but spares the calcarine regions, patients may develop *achromatopsia,* a disturbance of color perception without compromise of form vision (damage to the left side causes right hemiachromatopsia and vice versa). Damage to left occipital cortices and underlying periventricular white matter combined with destruction of the interhemispheric visual pathways often causes a disorder of reading without concomitant impairment of writing *(alexia without agraphia).* This may be accompanied by an impairment of color naming without impairment of color perception *(color anomia).* Bilateral damage to inferior visual association cortices causes *agnosia,* a selective impairment of visual recognition (see Ch. 399). Lesions that extensively involve the right occipital cortices (inferior *and* superior) can cause agnosia for unique faces and places, and lesions that involve left occipital cortices (inferior *and* superior) can cause agnosia for manipulable objects. Bilateral damage to superior visual association cortices leads to disturbances of visual attention *(visual disorientation or simultanagnosia)* and stereo vision *(astereopsis).* Visual disorientation can also result from bilateral superior parietal lesions, as a component of Balint syndrome (see Parietal Lobe, below). Lesions that involve the lateral occipital cortices about their middle tier can cause defects of motion perception. Infarctions in the territory of one or both posterior cerebral arteries are the most common cause of pathology in the occipital lobes.

TEMPORAL LOBE

The temporal lobes contain structures necessary for visual and auditory perception, language, memory, and affect. The most characteristic signs of temporal lobe damage are impairments of memory, which can be caused by lesions of either side, and impairments of language, usually related to dominant hemisphere lesions (see Ch. 399). The cortical structures related to vision are located in the inferior and lateral aspects of the lobe (part of area 37, areas 20 and 21). They are higher-order association cortices that receive information from the occipital association cortices. The inferior component of the geniculocalcarine pathway (Meyer's loop) courses in the depth of the temporal lobe (see Ch. 403).

The primary auditory cortices (areas 41 and 42) are located in the first temporal gyrus at the end of the most complex chain of subcortical processing stations of any sensory portal of the brain. They represent acoustic frequencies and intensities for a large range of pitched and unpitched sounds (speech, music, environmental noises) so as to permit their recognition and spatial localization. The record of those representations is contained in the auditory association cortices that surround the primary cortices bilaterally, in the superior temporal gyrus (largely area 22). Although the auditory input from the contralateral ear prevails functionally over the ipsilateral input, each cortex receives information from both ears; unilateral temporal lesions never cause deafness.

The medial temporal lobes contain cortical and subcortical struc-

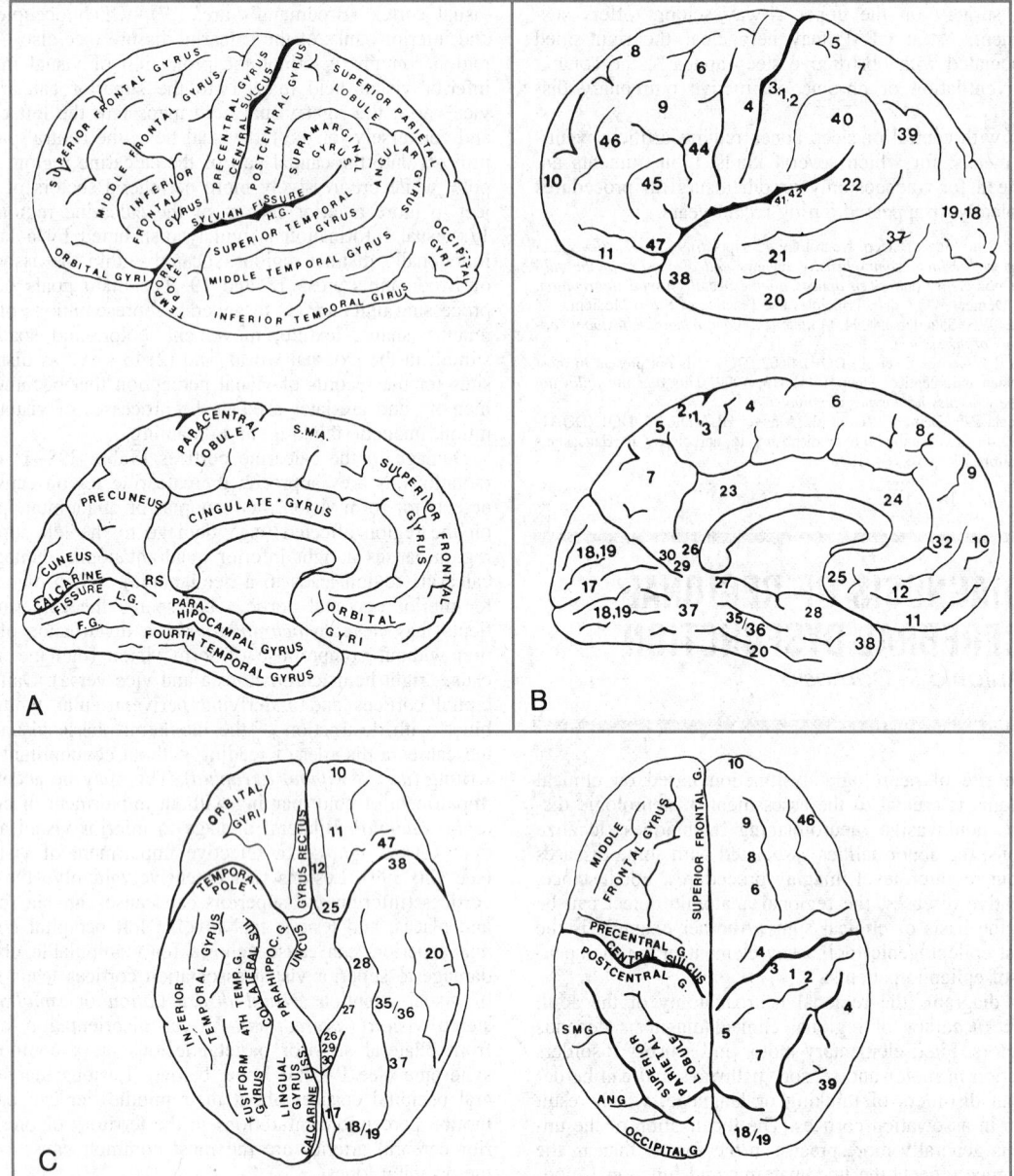

FIGURE 398-1. The principal gyri, sulci, and Brodmann's cytoarchitectonic areas of the human brain. *A,* Gyri and sulci in lateral *(top)* and mesial *(bottom)* views. *B,* Brodmann's areas in lateral *(top)* and mesial *(bottom)* views. *C,* Gyri, sulci, and Brodmann's areas in orbital *(left)* and superior *(right)* views.

tures of the limbic system, e.g., the entorhinal cortex (area 28) located in the anterior part of the parahippocampal gyrus; the hippocampal formation; and the amygdala. These highly interconnected structures correlate perceptual inputs, ongoing verbal and nonverbal thought operations, and the status of the internal milieu. This correlation is indispensable for emotional expression, affective experience, and memory. Lesions of this region severely impair those functions.

The temporal lobes can be compromised by numerous pathologic processes (Table 398-2). Epileptogenic scars and intracranial tumors are common; head injury often damages anterior temporal structures; herpes simplex encephalitis has a predilection for the region; the highest and earliest concentration of cytoskeletal pathology in Alzheimer's disease is in entorhinal cortex and hippocampus; and the hippocampus is selectively vulnerable to anoxia. Patients with temporal epileptogenic lesions experience a variety of abnormalities of visceral sensation, thought process, and even sense of self. They exhibit emotional and motor disturbances that can appear before or during a seizure. In some patients, more subtle but longer-lasting behavioral changes develop between seizures. Tables 398-3 and 398-4 list major ictal and interictal symptoms. Bilateral removal of this region in animals causes the Kluver-Bucy syn-

drome, a disorder characterized by indiscriminate sexual behavior, excessive orality, and placidity. The full syndrome rarely develops in humans, but some components can occur in patients with extensive bilateral temporal damage caused by herpes simplex encephalitis and in patients with dementias of degenerative or post-traumatic origins.

PARIETAL LOBE

The anterior aspect of the parietal lobe contains the postcentral gyrus where Brodmann's areas 3, 1, and 2 receive somatosensory information hailing from nerve terminals in the contralateral half of the body (the projections are somatotopically organized, with the largest share given to the phonatory apparatus and hand). These cortices interlock with the primary motor cortex in the precentral gyrus (area 4) and project to the superior parietal lobules (areas 5 and 7) and inferior parietal lobules (areas 39 and 40, respectively, the angular and supramarginal gyri). Another target of somatic sensation is area S2, located in the upper bank of Sylvian fissure, and yet another is the insula, the latter being especially related to visceral information. These cortices generate dynamic representations of the perceiver's body and of three-dimensional stimuli as apprehended by somatosensory processing. They interweave such repre-

TABLE 398-1. CHARACTERISTIC MANIFESTATIONS OF OCCIPITAL LOBE DAMAGE

Sign	Qualification	Lesion
Hemiachromatopsia	Right or left field	Left or right inferior mesial cortex and white matter
Pure alexia	Noted anywhere in intact field	Left inferior cortex and white matter (including outflow of calosum)
Color anomia	Seen only in left visual field in combination with right hemianopia	Left inferior and mesial
Visual agnosia	Noted anywhere in intact field	Usually bilateral inferior (but right occipital may involve faces and places and left occipital may involve manipulable objects)
Visual disorientation	Noted anywhere in intact field	Bilateral superior
Astereopsis	Noted anywhere in intact field	Bilateral superior
Impaired movement detection	Noted anywhere in intact field	Bilateral superior

TABLE 398-3. ICTAL MANIFESTATIONS OF TEMPORAL LOBE EPILEPTIC FOCI

Medial Basal Structures	Lateral Structures
Olfactory hallucinations	Language impairment; hissing, roaring, or clicking; vertigo
Memory disturbances (dejà vu or jamais vu); forced thinking, dreamy state	

Epigastric distress
Blank staring
Repetitive automatisms

sentations with appropriate motor programs as well as pertinent visual and auditory information.

Damage to the sector of the postcentral somatosensory cortex to which signals from the hand usually project in either hemisphere impairs the ability to recognize form (astereognosia), scale, texture, and weight of objects in the contralateral hand. (The thresholds for touch, pain, vibration, and temperature are generally not disturbed.)

Damage to the dominant or nondominant inferior parietal lobule causes diverse manifestations. The dominant somatosensory cortex develops dynamic representations of (a) the body and its movements (especially those of the hand and phonatory apparatus) and (b) the shapes of objects located within arm's reach (in so-called intrapersonal space). Dysfunction in the area of the dominant angular gyrus disrupts reading and writing, planning and execution of representational hand movements in specific contexts (apraxia), arithmetic skills (acalculia), finger recognition (finger agnosia), right-left orientation, and the ability to copy drawings and diagrams and to execute three-dimensional constructions (constructional apraxia). Dysfunction in the dominant supramarginal gyrus is mainly associated with aphasia (Table 398–5).

The nondominant parietal cortices hold a dynamic representation of extrapersonal space (the space beyond arm's reach) based on somatosensory, visual, and auditory cues. *Both* hemispaces are represented in this region. The attentional survey of external sensory events and projected movements in both hemispaces also depend on this nondominant region, damage to which leads to complex defects in spatial processing. The defects are especially pronounced in the hemispace opposite the lesion and cause the commonly encountered *neglect syndrome*. Not only is the left hemispace inappropriately at-

TABLE 398-2. MANIFESTATIONS OF TEMPORAL LOBE DAMAGE

	Unilateral	Bilateral
Posterolateral	Aphasia* Pure-word deafness* Amusia†	Global auditory agnosia (includes aphasia, amusia, and agnosia for environmental sounds)
Medial	Verbal* or nonverbal memory impairment Complex seizures	Amnesia
Anterolateral and inferior	Anomia* Nonverbal memory impairment Visual agnosia Complex seizures	Amnesia

* Usually left hemisphere
† Right hemisphere only

tended but the left side of the body itself may be neglected and left hemiplegia or hemisensory loss may be ignored or actively denied (anosognosia). The ability to negotiate a route without hitting obstacles placed to the left side of the body, the skill to follow a previously known and automated route (in a house or town), and the capacity to learn a new route are all compromised by nondominant inferior parietal lesions. Unlike their counterparts with left-sided lesions, patients with such nondominant injuries show little concern for their condition and often have an indifferent affect. An adequate rehabilitation program must take into account this reduced motivation. Patients may become confused when these structures are affected on the right side together with the nearby auditory cortices.

Bilateral damage confined to superior parietal lobules causes ocular apraxia (the inability to direct gaze voluntarily toward new visual stimuli appearing in the periphery of the visual field), bilateral optic ataxia (the inability to generate precise contralateral hand movements toward an outbound target under visual guidance), and an impairment of visual attention, a breakdown in the ability to apprehend the visual panorama in a cogent, seamless manner (this is known as visual disorientation or simultanognosia). The combination of ocular apraxia, optic ataxia, and visual disorientation constitutes the Balint syndrome. Common causes are bilateral infarctions in the border zone between the posterior and middle cerebral artery territories and bilateral metastases. Unilateral damage to the superior parietal lobule causes optic ataxia and defective pursuit eye movements.

FRONTAL LOBES

The human frontal cortices encompass nearly half of the entire cortical mantle and include a large number of diverse anatomic fields. Their operations assist with movement control (Table 398–6); general problem solving; planning; decision making; generation of willful responses; regulation of social behaviors, emotion, and autonomic function; and regulation of thought and language. Understanding of structural and junctional relationships is less advanced for frontal cortices than for other cerebral regions. Furthermore, such impairments are less easy to detect in clinical and laboratory settings than in real life.

The motor sector of the frontal lobe (the precentral and premotor cortices) is located mainly in the lateral frontal surface but spills into the mesial surface as well. The precentral cortex (area 4 or M1) contains a somatotopic representation of contralateral body movements in which the phonatory apparatus and hand are accorded the largest share. It is the principal target of re-entrant projections from cerebellum and motor thalamus. The premotor region (area 6) is part of a network for motor programming, and it receives re-entrant projections from basal ganglia as well as projections from the posterior sensory cortices. It integrates incoming movement-related information for final relay to the corticospinal

TABLE 398-4. INTERICTAL TRAITS OF PATIENTS WITH TEMPORAL LOBE EPILEPTIC FOCI

Lack of humor
Sadness
Obsessiveness
Metaphysical preoccupation
Hyposexuality
Dependence

TABLE 398–5. MANIFESTATIONS OF PARIETAL LOBE DAMAGE

Superior parietal lobule		Bilateral damage causes Balint syndrome. Unilateral damage causes mainly optic ataxia and transient abnormalities of pursuit eye movements.
Inferior parietal lobule	left	Aphasia; alexia; agraphia; acalculia; constructional apraxia; right/left disorientation; finger agnosia
	right	Neglect; anosognosia; inappropriate affect
Post-rolandic cortices		Subjective alterations in somatic sensation. Astereognosia

tract. Part of the nearby area 8, known as the frontal eye field, relates to voluntary eye movements (seizures originating in this area cause the eyes to deviate *away* from the lesion; damage by an infarction makes the eyes deviate *toward* the lesion). The mesial aspect of area 6 contains the supplementary motor area (SMA or M2). The SMA is anatomically contiguous with the rest of the premotor cortex but constitutes a functionally separate region. (It contains a whole body map in its relatively small cortical surface.) Damage to area 4 causes varied degrees of focal paralysis in the contralateral side of the body or face (involvement of corticospinal projections in corona radiata or internal capsule causes less focal paralyses). Damage to the lateral aspect of area 6 causes impairments of motor learning and execution as well as transient forms of neglect, whereas involvement of the SMA leads to mutism and contralateral akinesia. Infarctions and parasagittal tumors in this region often compromise part of both the SMA and the nearby cingulate gyrus (area 24) located immediately beneath the cingulate sulcus. The cingulate is a limbic cortex and its acute damage also causes akinesia, mutism, transient neglect, and an impairment of motivation. Tumors impinging in this region may cause speech arrest and seizures characterized by vocalization and may trigger involuntary movement synergies involving contralateral limbs and trunk.

Involvement of the posterior orbital surface is associated with disturbances of social behavior. These include inability to recognize the social significance of real-life situations and an inability to plan appropriate actions with a personal and social consequence. On occasion, especially with large lesions, patients may exhibit inappropriate demeanor (facetiousness). During the acute phase of medial frontal damage patients are generally akinetic and inattentive and some may urinate or defecate in public although sphincter function per se is preserved.

Areas 44 and 45 on the dominant side are known as Broca's

TABLE 398–6. MOTOR SYMPTOMS OF FRONTAL LOBE DISEASE*

	Structural Damage	Seizure
Precentral gyrus	Focal distal weakness, maximal in lower face, hand, less often foot; increased reflexes, mild spasticity, Babinski sign	Jacksonian: focal onset on face, thumb, foot. "March" toward trunk.
Corona radiata or internal capsule	Hemiplegia; increased spasticity	
Premotor (lateral)	Ocular ipsiversion; paratonic resistance to passive motion; grasping; hypokinesia; optic ataxia, aphasia	Adversive: ocular contraversion
Premotor (mesial)	Mutism	Involuntary synergies (elevated arm and leg, body turning); speech arrest and/or vocalization

* All arise contralateral to the brain lesion.

area. Their damage causes aphasia (see Ch. 399). Damage to the nondominant side of this area alters the prosodic qualities of speech. The most anterior regions of the frontal lobe accommodate the prefrontal cortices (areas 46, 47, 9, 10, 11, 12), damage to which impairs decision making and planning, reduces creativity, and alters the regulation of affect and emotion. With permanent damage, the magnitude of the deficit relates directly to the bilaterality or unilaterality of the lesion, the size of the lesion, and the previous intellectual caliber and occupation of the patient. Relatively small unilateral lesions produce minor impairments that are difficult to detect and tend to resolve. Large bilateral prefrontal lesions, however, although they leave motor, perceptual, and language functions intact, are incompatible with maintaining a socially adapted, fully self-conscious, and creative personality. The defects are most noticeable in patients who undergo bilateral prefrontal ablations for the treatment of large midline brain tumors. Even then, however, the impairments can be better sensed by appraising social and occupational behavior than by neuropsychologic tests, most of which may be passed flawlessly.

The frontal lobes are especially vulnerable to closed head injury, resulting in many of the signs described above as well as in the formation of cortical scar tissue and the appearance of seizures. The lateral sectors are frequently compromised by infarctions secondary to middle cerebral artery occlusions and meningiomas. The mesial sector often suffers infarctions or hemorrhages, secondary to ruptured aneurysms of the anterior communicating or anterior cerebral arteries. Meningiomas arising in the falx are another common cause of damage. The posterior orbital sector is often involved by herpes simplex encephalitis, by hemorrhages from ruptured anterior circulation aneurysms, and by meningiomas arising in the sphenoid and ethmoid regions. The brunt of the effects of normal-pressure hydrocephalus is seen in damage to the frontal white matter. Finally, prefrontal cortices can be markedly involved in Pick's disease, and both prefrontal and frontal limbic cortices are involved to some extent in Alzheimer's disease. When large tumors involve frontal lobe structures, especially malignant gliomas which may arise in one frontal lobe and traverse the corpus callosum to involve the other, patients exhibit many of the disturbances outlined above, impairments of attention and balance (see Ch. 404), and the release of primitive reflexes (grasp reflex, Gegenhalten or paratonia, echopraxia).

Damasio AR, Damasio H: Cortical systems for retrieval of concrete knowledge: The convergence zone framework. *In* Koch C (ed.): Large-Scale Neuronal Theories of the Brain. Boston, MIT Press, 1994, p 61. *A framework for the understanding of cognition at the level of systems.*

Damasio H, Damasio AR: Lesion Analysis in Neuropsychology. New York, Oxford University Press, 1989. *A method to study the anatomic location of cerebral lesions, and a review of advances in neuropsychology.*

Damasio AR, Tranel D, Damasio H: Somatic markers and the guidance of behavior: Theory and preliminary testing. *In* Levin HS, Eisenberg HM, Benton AL (eds.): Frontal Lobe Function and Dysfunction. New York, Oxford University Press, 1991, p. 217. *Examples of the extreme dissociation of behavior caused by frontal lobe damage. The lesions prompt a variety of socially unacceptable behaviors but do not interfere with language or memory. The intelligence quotient is unaltered.*

Heilman K, Valenstein E (eds.): Clinical Neuropsychology, 3rd ed. Oxford, Oxford University Press, 1993. *A multiauthored collection of essays on major aspects of neuropsychology.*

Mesulam M-M (ed.): Principles of Behavioral Neurology. Philadelphia, FA Davis, 1985, p. 125. *Another collection of comprehensive reviews on neuropsychology.*

Penfield W, Jasper W: Epilepsy and the Functional Anatomy of the Human Brain. Boston, Little, Brown and Company, 1954. *The classic monograph on what epilepsy and the electrical stimulation of the cerebral cortex tell us about the neural substrates of higher brain function.*

399 DISTURBANCES OF MEMORY AND LANGUAGE

Antonio R. Damasio

The concerted operation of multiple but relatively specific neural systems is the basis for the most complex human abilities: the acquisition and categorization of knowledge (learning and memory), the translation of knowledge in a verbal or signed code (language), the manipulation of nonverbal and verbal knowledge in thought processes, the ability to select responses and solve problems (planning, decision making, creativity), and the reflection upon ongoing cognitive activities in the perspective of one's autobiography (self-consciousness). These functions presume the normal operations of emotion (the impetus to sustain a given mental activity or action) as well as attention (the ability to concentrate willfully on a specific mental content to the exclusion of others).

MEMORY AND ITS IMPAIRMENTS

Memory is the ability to (1) make a record of interactions between the brain and the body proper or between the entire organism and the external world; (2) to store concepts derived from the categorization of those records; and (3) to manipulate the records internally for recall and recognition. The terms "learning" and "memory" are used almost interchangeably, although learning should be used only to denote "memory acquisition."

Unless the process of consolidation takes over, the memory of objects or events that we perceive or imagine is retained only briefly (< 60 seconds). The material held during that period is said to be in *short-term memory* or *immediate memory* (Table 399–1). This brief memory is preserved in most amnesias. If those materials are to be recorded into *long-term memory,* an active physiologic process must start promptly. The process of consolidation takes time, and recently acquired memories are more vulnerable to decay than those that have been held long and internally rehearsed. Newer memories are known as *recent* memories, and older memories as *remote.*

Memory for unique faces, objects, or events is usually known as *episodic* (e.g., the memory of a personal friend or a favorite landscape). Memory for classes of objects or events is known as *generic* or *semantic* (e.g., the knowledge that allows us to categorize a car as a transport vehicle, a dog as an animal, or a given locale as urban or rural). Episodic and semantic memories constitute factual knowledge and are known as *declarative.* Declarative memory contrasts with *procedural* memory, which is based on skills rather than facts and refers to actions rather than to the knowledge necessary to acquire those actions. The playing of an instrument, typing, and swimming are examples of *procedural* memory. Procedural memory is spared in most amnesias.

MEMORY MECHANISMS. The thesaurus of facts and rules acquired in a lifetime is largely stored in the association cortices of every lobe of both hemispheres. Several subcortical nuclei assist the process of learning and recall. Memories are dynamically and flexibly distributed in neuron ensembles linked by patterned and hierarchically organized corticocortical and commissural connections. Access to single-modality memories depends on association cortices near the primary sensory cortex that conveyed the information in the first place (the impaired access or partial destruction of those cortices causes an *agnosia*—Table 399–2). Access to memories of polymodal events depends on cortices farther away from sensory sources. Finally, access to unique and complex polymodal episodes depends on inferior and anterolateral temporal cortices as well as some prefrontal cortices (impaired access or partial damage to such cortices causes *amnesia*).

The ability to form a permanent record depends on the normal operation of the hippocampal system, the basal forebrain, and the diencephalon, as well as several brain stem nuclei. The elucidation of the respective roles of these components is imperfect, but it appears that the hippocampus, which is informed about relationships between components of an event via connections from the higher-order association cortices, binds and stabilizes information according to its appropriate temporal and spatial links. The stabilization

TABLE 399–1. TYPES OF MEMORY

Factual (declarative)
Skill (procedural)

Short-term (immediate)—less than 60 seconds
Long-term—more than 60 seconds

Recent
Remote

Episodic (unique entities and events)
Generic (same as semantic; pertains to nonunique entities, as members of a conceptual category)

TABLE 399–2. TYPES OF MEMORY IMPAIRMENT

Agnosia	Impaired recognition of stimuli presented in one sensory channel (e.g., object, face, voice, melody) that cannot be explained by defective perception.
Anomia	Impaired retrieval of the name for a stimulus (e.g., object or face) that is otherwise properly perceived and properly recognized.
Amnesia	A pervasive impairment of the ability to recall and recognize unique events and unique stimuli. The defect is independent of the sensory channel used to probe memory (e.g., given a unique person, *neither* the face *nor* the voice is recognizable).
Aphasia	A pervasive impairment of linguistic processing (e.g., structure of sentences; assembly of phonemes in a word; retrieval of words from the lexicon).
Dysarthria	Defective articulation of speech sounds without compromise of linguistic processing. When the articulation breakdown is complete, the term *anarthria* applies.

appears to involve molecular and cellular changes during long-term potentiation. Through the interconnected amygdala the hippocampus also influences basal forebrain, diencephalon, and brain stem nuclei. The basal forebrain and brain stem, in turn, provide the cerebral cortex with neurochemical inputs that probably contribute to stabilize records at the cellular level (acetylcholine, noradrenaline, dopamine, serotonin, and probably other, still ill-defined mediators and modulators). The hippocampal interconnections with the diencephalon sample the status of the internal milieu at the time of a given sensory experience, informing on the value of a particular stimulus or event in the context of instinctual goals. Finally, the ascending brain stem reticular formation contributes importantly because most learning presumes attention and arousal.

The neural structures and systems involving the acquisition of procedural memories are different: After bilateral destruction of hippocampus and basal forebrain, perceptuomotor skills remain intact and new motor skills can be learned. The motor and sensory cortices, the cerebellum, the neostriatum, and the motor nuclei of the thalamus are the key structures in this circuitry. A discussion of the molecular and cellular changes related to memory is outside the scope of this chapter.

MEMORY DISORDERS. Table 399–3 lists several terms that are helpful in describing and classifying the amnesias. The terms *anterograde* and *retrograde* are especially important. Anterograde designates the time compartment operating *since* the amnesia began and refers to the partial or complete inability to remember events during that period. Retrograde refers to information gained *prior* to the onset of amnesia that may not be retrievable in recall or recognition. Retrograde amnesia can be as short as hours or days, as is often the case in post-traumatic situations, or may extend back years or even decades, as in Korsakoff's amnesia or the amnesias that follow herpes simplex encephalitis.

Some middle-aged and elderly persons have an increasing but isolated difficulty in recalling proper names and recent events of limited importance. This "benign forgetfulness" is not a predictor of the progressive dementias and is best treated with prompt and vigorous reassurance. The most frequent causes of incapacitating mem-

TABLE 399–3. TYPES OF AMNESIA

Retrograde	Amnesia for information learned before the onset of illness
Anterograde	Amnesia for information that presented itself after onset of illness
Global	Information cannot be retrieved through *any* sensory channel
Modality-specific	Same as associative agnosia; information cannot be retrieved through the affected channel, e.g., vision
Permanent	
Stable	Example: postencephalitic
Progressive	Example: Alzheimer's disease
Transient	Examples: transient global amnesia, post-traumatic amnesia

TABLE 399–4. CAUSES OF AMNESIA

Alzheimer's disease and other degenerative dementias
Head injury
Herpes simplex encephalitis
Ruptured anterior circulation aneurysms with infarction in basal forebrain
Infarctions in other memory-related systems, e.g., medial thalamic nuclei; temporal cortices
Anoxic/ischemic encephalopathy
Wernicke-Korsakoff encephalopathy
Psychogenic amnesia

ory loss are the degenerative dementias, head injury, cerebrovascular disease, encephalitis, brain anoxia and ischemia, and nutritional impairment (Table 399–4).

Part of our knowledge about the critical contribution of the hippocampal formation to memory came from a patient who underwent *bilateral medial temporal lobe resection* to treat epilepsy. He became severely amnesic postoperatively and has remained unable to learn factual memories to this day. His severe anterograde amnesia contrasts with a largely spared retrograde memory and with preserved generic memories and procedural learning. The amnesias caused by *postanoxic encephalopathy,* in which anterograde memory is heavily compromised, also are caused by hippocampal damage in which the CA1 sector is selectively damaged. Together with the evidence that specific areas of the entorhinal cortex and subiculum are damaged in amnesic patients with *Alzheimer's disease,* these findings underscore the importance of hippocampus in memory (see Ch. 400). *Herpes simplex encephalitis* commonly damages the hippocampal region but also involves other anterolateral and inferior regions of the temporal cortices. Such patients suffer not only an anterograde memory defect but also a severe retrograde amnesia. Bilateral damage to hippocampus can also be caused by infarctions in the territory of the posterior cerebral arteries. Infarctions in the area of the basal forebrain (septal nuclei, nucleus accumbens, nucleus basalis of Meynert) due to ruptured aneurysms in the anterior circulation are also associated with amnesia. Both anterograde and retrograde memory are compromised, but unlike with temporal lobe amnesia, the defect is mild and tends to improve, and appropriate cueing helps recall. *Head injury* is another major cause of amnesia. *Korsakoff's syndrome* is a severe amnesia that compromises both anterograde and retrograde memories and is accompanied by confabulation and lack of insight. It is caused by severe thiamine deficiency, generally in the setting of alcoholism, and often accompanies or follows acute Wernicke encephalopathy (see Ch. 406) or delirium tremens (see Ch. 11).

Transient global amnesia (TGA) is a self-limited memory impairment during which the patient can identify himself but is unable to recall events preceding the episode and generally cannot recognize places. Patients with TGA remain attentive, have normal language and reasoning, and are generally distressed by their disorientation. They tend to ask repeatedly where they are, what they have been up to, and what is going on. Most TGA episodes last about 4 or 5 hours (but may be shorter or longer) and gradually clear. The attacks leave no residual impairment and are generally nonrecurrent. Status epilepticus with complex partial or petit mal seizures may mimic TGA but can be distinguished because patients with seizures are generally noninquisitive and inattentive. Most TGA attacks occur in middle-aged or older persons and may reflect transient ischemia or local neurochemical changes in memory-related areas of the temporal lobe or thalamus.

Psychogenic amnesia is generally greatest for emotionally important events and may erase circumscribed epochs of the past while leaving intact epochs immediately preceding or following the amnesic period. It may include disorientation to self. Questions such as "Who am I?" or "What is my name?", unless uttered during delirium or a seizure, raise the possibility of a psychogenic process. Psychogenic amnesia must be distinguished from emotional upheaval (which often impairs attention and produces inconsistent performance in psychological testing), from depression (which slows mentation and reduces communication), and from organic amnesias (in which emotionally reinforced material tends to be recalled better than neutral events, and disorientation is worst for time, less for place and persons, but never for self).

Treatment. Patients with acute post-traumatic amnesia tend to recover spontaneously. The same is true of amnesia caused by overmedication or delirium. Memory loss caused by depression (pseudodementia) has a good prognosis when effectively treated. A less fortunate prognosis accompanies amnesia following prolonged post-traumatic coma. When coma lasts more than 2 or 3 weeks, most patients over 25 years old tend not to recover from the memory loss. Patients with amnesia due to herpes encephalitis recover only when the lesions are mostly or solely unilateral and even then retain substantial impairments. In most amnesias the recovery is inversely proportional to the initial severity and depends on the extent and placement of lesions. The bulk of improvement usually takes place within the first year after onset. Neuroactive peptides, neurotransmitter precursors, neurotransmitters, and special dietary agents have no proven usefulness in chronic organic amnesia.

AGNOSIA. Agnosia is the inability to recognize a previously familiar sensory stimulus despite the integrity of elementary perception of the stimulus and the absence of defects of intelligence, motivation, or attention. It is a percept stripped of its meaning. The disorder is a form of monomodal amnesia, a disability that prevents a sensory stimulus from triggering previously acquired information that would reveal its identity. Agnosia results from dysfunction of association cortices of the affected sensory modality, which contain records of purely modal processing. *Visual agnosia* is the most frequent example. It consists of the selective failure to recognize familiar faces (prosopagnosia) or objects (visual object agnosia). The phenomenon is generally associated with bilateral occipitotemporal lesions.

LANGUAGE AND ITS DISORDERS

Verbal languages are arbitrary symbolic codes in which words stand for external stimuli, actions, and relationships, as well as for the intellectual and emotional reactions that such stimuli evoke in the perceiver. The normal brain acquires and stores a dictionary of such words in at least one language, a lexicon, and develops a highly automated process of two-way translation between the mechanism to reconstruct word representations and the mechanism to reconstruct nonverbal representations of objects, actions, or concepts. The process of language comprehension is the translation of sentences (structured sequences of words) into sequences of approximate nonverbal counterparts whose ongoing manipulation is known as thought. Nouns, verbs, or adjectives have fairly direct referential nonverbal equivalents. On the contrary, functor words (conjunctions, prepositions and adverbs, verb endings) refer to relationships. Functors, together with word order, are the key to the grammatical organization of sentences (syntax). The formulation of speech or writing is the rendering of a nonverbal thought process into a syntactic frame filled with appropriate lexical elements. The lexical and syntactic operations of language depend on phonemic and graphemic devices, which can enact correspondences between sounds, their visual representations, and the articulatory patterns that permit their sensorimotor implementation in phonetic utterances or writing. Oral verbal expression also depends on word stress and the intonational contour of sentences, i.e., the fundamental frequency of the sounds in an utterance as well as the durational elements of speech. The term *prosody* subsumes the latter qualities of verbal expression.

NEURAL SUBSTRATES OF LANGUAGE. Verbal language is characteristically human, and its experimental study is restricted to human beings. Considerable knowledge has been gathered about the neural substrates of language from the cognitive and neuroanatomic study of patients with acquired impairments caused by focal brain lesions (aphasias). Most such studies have relied largely on postmortem, computed tomography, and magnetic resonance imaging analysis, although more recent evaluations have used positron emission tomography (PET). Electrical stimulation of different regions of the cerebrum during surgery for seizures or motor disorders also has provided information on the neural representation of language. A salient finding, first noted more than a century ago and since confirmed, is that the left hemisphere of about 95% of individuals is especially adroit at language processing. In left language-dominant persons all aspects of language depend largely on left-hemisphere processing, with the partial exception of some aspects of prosody. Handedness is an imperfect but clinically useful indicator of language dominance. In almost all right-handed persons the left hemisphere is dominant for language, and its damage in key areas leads to severe aphasia. Most left-handed and ambidextrous persons (about 70%) are also left language-dominant, although they may have additional language representation in the right hemisphere. About one third of left-handers have either bilateral language representation or right-hemisphere language representation. Such persons are at a disadvantage in that lesions of either side can cause aphasia, although the disability tends to be less severe and to improve. Even extremely right-handed individuals with full language dominance in the left hemisphere possess some language representation in the opposite hemisphere (especially for nouns and verbs; adjectives are poorly represented and functor words probably not at all). The right hemisphere of such a person has little access to speech output and little syntactic capability. It has been suggested that gender is an important variable in language representation, but the available data are not conclusive. Language representation is different in children. Most children who suffer severe brain lesions up to age 5 or 6 years can recover from aphasia and continue to develop language to nearly normal levels. Left-hemisphere lesions sustained later, especially after puberty, have the same consequences as for adults.

Some asymmetric functional abilities have been related to neuroanatomic cerebral asymmetries. The left planum temporale, the area of association cortex located immediately behind the transverse gyrus (the primary auditory cortex), is measurably larger than the right in about 70% of individuals. The difference is visible on gross inspection and in the microscopic cytoarchitectonic structure of the area. Such persons possess a longer sylvian fissure on the left than on the right, reflecting the larger extent of the posterior temporal region, and more horizontally placed so as to accommodate a more voluminous left lower parietal lobule (supramarginal gyrus and angular gyrus).

Language depends on a wide network of cortical and subcortical processing units, and its knowledge and operations are distributed within key cortical regions (see Fig. 398–1). The principal set of language areas is located around the left sylvian fissure (the perisylvian language region). In its posterior aspect lies Wernicke's area (the posterior auditory association cortex, or Brodmann's area 22; it includes the planum temporale and the posterior portion of the first temporal gyrus. Immediately below and behind lies area 37, the lateral aspect of which, in the posterior sector of the second and third temporal gyri, is committed to language. Above and behind the sylvian fissure lie the supramarginal gyrus (area 40) and the angular gyrus (area 39). In the anterior aspect of the perisylvian region in the inferior and posterior aspects of the frontal operculum lie areas 44 and 45, also known as Broca's area. Between sit the motor and sensory regions associated with sensory motor phonatory representations. Also contributing to the language network are components of the basal ganglia (especially in the head of the caudate nucleus and parts of the putamen), some thalamic nuclei, the supplementary motor areas (especially the one on the left), and the anterior cingulate gyri.

THE APHASIAS. Aphasia (or dysphasia) is a disturbance of the comprehension or formulation of verbal messages caused by newly acquired brain disease. Although developments in cognitive science have led to a linguistic-based approach to aphasia, Geschwind's diagnosis of aphasic disorders in terms of the comprehension of language, the fluency of output, and the ability to repeat sentences remains clinically useful because of the strong relationship between these traits and the anatomic sites of the underlying lesions. Table 399–5 summarizes the important clinical clues.

Damage to the posterior sector of the left superior temporal gyrus and its surround causes *Wernicke aphasia*. Patients speak fluently, with normal melodic contour, and even a normal syntactic frame. However, they select wrong words (semantic paraphasias), so the intelligibility of their otherwise well-formed verbal messages may be low (jargon aphasia). Likewise, their comprehension of verbal message is poor because of their inability to translate words into nonverbal meanings. Wernicke aphasics with severe comprehension defects may develop paranoid reactions and become homicidal or suicidal. Wernicke aphasia must be distinguished from *auditory agnosia,* the inability to recognize objects or actions by the characteristic sounds they make (due to bilateral lesions in auditory cortex), and *pure word deafness,* an agnosia restricted to words (due to dominant lesions undercutting the auditory cortex) that allows patients to recognize nonspeech sounds and to produce normal speech. It is also different from the logorrhea of manic states, the logical thought derailment of schizophrenia, and the verbal salads of chronic schizophrenics.

Posterior lesions outside the Wernicke area produce more restricted disturbances. Lesions of the supramarginal gyrus give rise to *conduction aphasia,* a disorder in which the patient speaks fluently, has relatively preserved comprehension, but makes sound substitution errors (phonemic paraphasias). The major impairment of repetition stands out among these comparatively milder defects. Other strategically placed lesions of the posterior dominant hemisphere selectively compromise reading or writing. Alexia (inability to comprehend written language while retaining relatively normal vision) without concomitant writing impairment results when a lesion destroys the left visual cortex and, in addition, involves the outflow of the splenium of the corpus callosum. This placement cuts off projections that otherwise connect the unaffected right visual cortex to language areas of the left. Despite their inability to

TABLE 399–5. DIAGNOSTIC POINTERS TO THE MOST FREQUENT APHASIA TYPES

Type of Aphasia	Speech	Comprehension	Repetition	Other Signs	Localization
Broca	Nonfluent; effortful	+	−	Right hemiparesis worse in arm; aware of defect; frustrated	Lower posterior frontal
Wernicke	Abundant; fluent; well articulated	−	−	Often none; may be euphoric and/or paranoid	Posterior and superior temporal
Conduction	Fluent with some articulatory defects	+	−	Often none; cortical sensory loss in right arm	Usually supramarginal gyrus; may extend to insula and primary auditory cortex
Global	Scant; nonfluent	−	−	Right hemiparesis worse in arm; may present *without* hemiparesis	With hemiparesis: massive perisylvian lesion; without hemiparesis: separate Broca and Wernicke area damage
Transcortical motor	Nonfluent; explosive	+	+		Anterior or superior to Broca area
Transcortical sensory	Scant; fluent	−	+		Surrounding Wernicke area, posteriorly or inferiorly
Atypical ("basal ganglia")	Fluent dysarthric	−	−/+	Right hemiparesis worse in arm	Head of caudate; anterior limb of capsule
Atypical ("thalamus")	Fluent	−	+	Attentional and memory defects in acute phase	Anterolateral thalamus

+ = Intact or largely preserved
− = Impaired

comprehend the written word, patients with "pure" alexia can speak and write normally, in contrast to those with a combination of *alexia with agraphia* (impairment of writing despite normal motor function of the hand), in whom both reading and writing are compromised. In its pure form the abnormality is rare and follows lesions of the left angular gyrus. More frequently alexia and agraphia are accompaniments of Wernicke aphasia.

Broca aphasia is characterized by nonfluent, effortful, melodically flat speech, often shorn of functor words and marred by poor word order. The syntactic defect far outweighs the lexical impairment. Comprehension is well preserved in conversation. Broca aphasia must be distinguished from dysarthria, a disorder of speech articulation that does not impair the linguistic structure of communication. Many Broca aphasics are mute in the first hours or days after the onset of the disorder and only gradually develop the characteristic verbal signs. The intent to communicate, however poorly, is rarely in question. The lesion compromises Broca's area and adjacent cortical and subcortical territories. Because of patterns of vascular supply, many such patients also suffer a contralateral hemiplegia. Apraxia is added when the lesion involves the adjacent premotor cortex. Aphasia caused by lesions confined to Broca's area has a comparatively good prognosis.

Global aphasia consists of a severe loss of all aspects of language operation. Acutely, patients are often mute and have a right hemiplegia. The paucity of speech may become chronic, the patient being able neither to comprehend nor to produce language (except in the form of expletives or brief phrases). Despite rehabilitation efforts, the prognosis is poor, and patients often become depressed and listless, more so than Wernicke aphasics. As indicated in Table 399–5, two possible localizations can be associated with global aphasia.

With all the aphasias described above, patients are unable to repeat long sentences after the examiner. With some language defects, however, repetition is preserved. The dissociation between intact repetition and disturbed comprehension or speech output implies that Wernicke and Broca regions, as well as their interconnections, must be intact and that the causative lesions may lie near but outside those areas. There are two frequently encountered aphasias of this type: *transcortical motor* and *transcortical sensory* (Table 399–5).

Mutism accompanies a variety of conditions. It may describe the initial state of patients who evolve into Broca or global aphasics but produce no speech at all acutely. It may describe patients with bilateral premotor lesions who often remain chronically mute. Mutism has been applied to the paroxysmal speech arrest caused by seizures arising out of the supplementary motor or Broca areas, generally as an irritative response to an overlying tumor, and to the absence of speech in acute psychoses. Prominent mutism affects patients with lesions of the dominant-sided supplementary motor area and/or nearby cingulate, who not only do not speak but show no inclination to communicate through facial expression or gestures. Those patients also are generally motionless and when they recover do not exhibit aphasic symptoms. Mutism is not *anarthria,* a severe impairment of articulation that prevents speech but allows both the vivid expression of the intent to communicate and the frustration of not being able to do so (anarthria is caused by bulbar or pseudobulbar defects and can be confirmed by the presence of other signs of nuclear and supranuclear paralysis of lingual–vocal cord functions). Nor is mutism the same as *aphonia,* in which the phonatory apparatus is locally inoperative for mechanical or psychogenic reasons.

Some aphasias can be caused by infarcts in the dominant basal ganglia, especially when they involve the head of the caudate and the anterior limb of the internal capsule, and by infarcts in anterolateral nuclei of the dominant thalamus. Their occurence indicates that subcortical structures contribute to language processing, probably by assisting cortical units. The basal ganglia aphasias most often show a combination of fluent, dysarthric speech accompanied by impaired auditory comprehension and a right hemiparesis. The thalamic aphasias resemble transcortical sensory aphasia.

Although seizures or transient vascular insufficiency can cause brief language disturbances, the development of a selective disturbance in language that lasts more than a few hours always reflects a structural and focal lesion. The most common causes are infarction and hemorrhage in the distribution of a major cortical artery branch. Less frequent causes are head trauma and space-occupying lesions.

Damasio AR: Aphasia. N Engl J Med 326:531, 1992. *A description of different aphasia types and their localization.*
Damasio AR, Tranel D, Damasio H: Face agnosia and the neural substrates of memory. Annu Rev Neurosci 13:89, 1990. *A discussion of the cognitive and neuropsychological aspects of this intriguing phenomenon, with information applicable to the understanding of memory.*
Dudai Y: The Neurobiology of Memory: Concepts, Findings, Trends. Oxford, Oxford University Press, 1989. *A comprehensive review of the neuroscience of memory.*
Ojemann GA, Creutzfeldt OD: Language in humans and animals: Contribution of brain stimulation and recording. *In* Plum F, Mountcastle VB, et al. (eds.): Handbook of Physiology, Section 1: The Nervous System. Vol. V, Higher Functions of the Brain, Part 2. Bethesda, MD, American Physiological Society, 1987, p. 675. *Electrical stimulation and recording from the cerebral cortex provide clues to the neural basis of language.*
Victor M, Adams RD, Collins GH: The Wernicke-Korsakoff Syndrome and Related Neurologic Disorders Due to Alcoholism and Malnutrition, 2nd ed. Philadelphia, FA Davis, 1989. *The classic monograph on the subject provides evidence for the role of the diencephalon in memory.*

400 ALZHEIMER'S DISEASE AND RELATED DEMENTIAS

Antonio R. Damasio

The term *dementia* describes a pervasive decline in a number of mental functions resulting in the loss of personal and social independence in a previously competent individual. Although a defect in memory is often the core impairment in dementia, the term applies only to patients who have additional impairments in intellect as reflected by defective reasoning, decision making, and judgment. Those impairments are usually accompanied by disturbances in language and spatial orientation. Isolated defects in memory (amnesia) or in language (aphasia) do not qualify for the diagnosis of dementia even when their severity curtails normal behavior. The term *dementia* also does not apply to mentally retarded individuals who have never become intellectually competent and should not be applied to disturbances of attention, regardless of how profound they may be. The terms *confusional state* and *delirium* refer to the latter conditions.

From a physiopathologic standpoint, dementia occurs when several of the cerebral systems that support learning, memory, language, emotion, and reason are rendered dysfunctional by *any* neurologic disease process. Dementia can remain stable when the disease is self-limited (such as may follow brain damage from cardiac arrest or head trauma). In most instances, however, the dementia develops insidiously, as a result of diseases such as Alzheimer's or communicating hydrocephalus. Although the term *dementia* is equally appropriate for either stable or evolving mental decline, in practice it denotes a gradual, progressive condition.

Table 400–1 lists the most frequent causes of progressive dementia. Dementia has never been a rare occurrence but of late its frequency has been rising steeply. In part, this may reflect public and physician awareness of the condition, but the remarkable rise of longevity in the industrialized world is probably the key factor. Progress in medicine and living standards has extended life expectancy by about 15 years, dramatically increasing the incidence

TABLE 400–1. THE MOST FREQUENT CAUSES OF PROGRESSIVE DEMENTIA

Alzheimer's disease
Other degenerative diseases, e.g., Pick's, Parkinson's, Huntington's; Lewy body disease; progressive supranuclear palsy
Multiple cerebral infarcts
Chronic drug use
Depression
Intracranial mass lesions
Communicating hydrocephalus
Endocrine and metabolic disorders
CNS infections, e.g., HIV, opportunistic, syphilis, Creutzfeldt-Jakob disease

TABLE 400–2. TREATABLE CAUSES OF DEMENTIA

Inappropriate or excessive use of medications or alcohol
Resectable intracranial tumors
Subdural hematomas
Depression
Communicating hydrocephalus
Endocrine and metabolic disorders, e.g., hypothyroidism, vitamin B_{12}
   deficiency
CNS infections

TABLE 400–3. OUTLINE OF MINI–MENTAL STATUS EXAMINATION*

Test	Score
What is the year, season, date, day, month?	5
Where are you: state, county, town, place, floor?	5
Name three objects: State slowly and have patient repeat (repeat until patient learns all three)	3
Do reversal serial 7's (five steps) or spell "WORLD" backwards	5
Ask for the three unrelated objects above	3
Name from inspection a pencil, a watch	2
Have patient repeat "No if's, and's, or but's"	1
Follow a three-stage command (1 pt each) ("Take a paper in your hand, fold it, and put it on the floor.")	3
Read and obey, "Close your eyes."	1
Write a simple sentence	1
Copy intersecting pentagons	1

* From Folstein MF, Folstein SE, McHugh PR: Minimental state. A practical method for grading the cognitive state for the clinician. J Psychiatr Res 12:189, 1975. The authors found that out of a possible total score of 30, mean score for dementia was 9.7, depression with cognitive impairment was 19.0, and uncomplicated affective depression was 27.6.

of late-life neurologic diseases, with degenerative diseases and especially Alzheimer's disease topping the list. Some recent studies have claimed that as many as 50% of individuals over the age of 80 develop Alzheimer's disease. Even assuming some exaggeration in those predictions, the impact of this disease in medicine and society cannot be overemphasized. Furthermore, not all dementia is of the Alzheimer type: Many patients so affected have conditions that are partially or completely reversible (Table 400–2).

Diagnosing Dementia

The diagnosis of dementia must be rigorously made and be followed by an attempt to uncover its probable cause. The imperative first step lies in establishing that a decline in cognitive and behavioral capacities exists. Many normal older individuals inappropriately sense that their mental abilities are diminishing. It is as important to reassure such persons about the benign nature of their complaints as to make a diagnosis of dementia in those who suffer it. Forgetfulness, especially of proper names, is common at any age and is accentuated by anxiety, fatigue, and depression. Benign forgetting, however, is accompanied neither by amnesia for recent social and personal events nor by impaired judgment (although depression may severely impair planning and decision making). A probing history and interview, together with a normal neurologic examination, can rapidly exclude the possibility of dementia. In addition, brief tests such as those listed in the Whitehouse reference offer simple measures of psychological ability that can be used to reassure the concerned patient.

If the brief examinations and detection tests suggest that dementia exists, the next step is to establish a premorbid baseline, something that the patient may be unable to provide and may depend on testimony from a reliable relative or escort. What is the patient's education and cultural background? What have been his or her professional and social achievements? Whenever possible, specific information should be sought about years of education, degrees achieved, professional positions, personality, and the judgment of colleagues, friends, and relatives.

The examination should evaluate the following: (1) orientation, (2) attention, (3) social appropriateness, (4) affect, (5) memory, and (6) language. Most of these emerge almost automatically as the evaluation proceeds. What is the patient's attitude toward the examiner? Is he or she cooperative? socially appropriate? attentive and able to communicate verbally? oriented to time and place? Can the patient relate recent public and personal events (the accuracy of the latter corroborated by an escort)? Patients with early Alzheimer's disease tend to be cooperative, socially appropriate, and attentive, but their recent memory clearly shows a decline. Patients with dementia due to brain tumors, central nervous system (CNS) infections, or hydrocephalus are more often distractible, less appropriate, and careless of appearances.

Some traditional mental status tests, such as the recall of three unrelated words at 5 minutes, the reverse spelling of "WORLD," or the backwards subtraction of serial 7's, can give helpful hints but are not reliable. Many nondemented patients with aphasia, amnesia, parietal lobe dysfunction, or mere distraction can fail such tests; conversely some patients with early dementia can pass them. The popular Mini–Mental Status Examination fares better (Table 400–3).

In doubtful cases, a formal evaluation conducted by a trained neuropsychologist offers the most reliable means to diagnose the presence and severity of dementia. Such evaluations quantify intellectual and problem-solving ability, memory, speech and language, perception, attention, concentration, and personality. Many standardized tests, such as the Wechsler Adult Intelligence Scale—Revised, the Wechsler Memory Scale—Revised, and the Benton Visual Re-

tention Test, permit a diagnostic precision that cannot be approximated by bedside evaluations or screening batteries. Formal neuropsychological examination is especially useful in distinguishing dementia from depression.

Differential Diagnosis

There are more than 50 possible causes of dementia, but many are rare and the most frequent, Alzheimer's disease, has a fairly distinctive profile. Nonetheless, only histologic analysis of brain tissue at autopsy offers an absolute confirmation of Alzheimer's disease, and the clinical diagnosis remains one of exclusion. Because some of the less frequent causes of dementia can be treated and occasionally may mimic Alzheimer's disease, it is important to identify them or rule them out. The distinction depends largely on the results of a small group of critical tests (Table 400–4).

ALZHEIMER'S DISEASE

PATHOGENESIS AND MANIFESTATIONS. Alzheimer's disease is caused by a progressive and selective degeneration of neuron populations in the entorhinal cortex, the hippocampus, the high-order association cortices of the temporal, frontal, and parietal regions, and some subcortical nuclei in the basal forebrain, thalamus, and brain stem. The neuronal damage and the attending loss of synaptic density disable several neural systems essential to learning and retrieval of memories. By itself, the cortical component of the damage would explain the prominent memory defects of Alzheimer patients. In addition, however, damage to cholinergic neurons in the basal forebrain results in a loss of delivery of acetylcholine to the cerebral cortex, whereas damage to the brain stem's locus coeruleus precludes the delivery of norepinephrine to the cerebral cortex. Those neurochemical defects are likely to worsen, if not independently explain, many of the behavioral changes seen in Alzheimer patients. At autopsy, the brains of Alzheimer patients are atrophied, especially in the regions where most neurons die. Characteristically, the motor and primary sensory cortices remain unaffected, as do the basal ganglia and cerebellum. Histologically, the diseased neurons are seen to contain cytoplasmic neurofibrillary

TABLE 400–4. USEFUL TESTS IN THE EVALUATION OF DEMENTIA

Brain computed tomography or magnetic resonance imaging
Neuropsychologic evaluation
Complete blood count and erythrocyte sedimentation rate, serologic test for syphilis
Metabolic screen (SMA 12–16)
Serum TSH, vitamin B_{12} level
Chest radiograph
Cerebrospinal fluid analysis: cells, protein
Electroencephalography

tangles composed of paired helical filaments visible with special stains. The most prominent anatomic change, however, consists of amyloid plaques containing degenerated neuronal fragments surrounding a small, dense core of amyloid material.

The neuropathologic diagnosis of Alzheimer's disease depends not only on the presence of neurofibrillary tangles and neuritic plaques but also on their anatomic distribution and quantity. Neurofibrillary tangles are present in other diseases, including the dementia that follows repeated boxing injuries. Neuritic plaques are present in the brains of normal aged persons, although less abundantly than in the Alzheimer brain. Such findings lead some investigators to believe that Alzheimer's dementia may represent an accelerated form of brain aging rather than a conventional disease.

In about 25% of cases of Alzheimer's disease, the history reveals a relative affected by the disease, and in some rare families the disease can start early (fifth or sixth decade) and affect the offspring in an autosomal dominant pattern. Also, patients with trisomy 21 (Down syndrome) develop the neuropathologic changes of Alzheimer's disease in their third or fourth decade. Current research studies indicate a linkage of Alzheimer's disease to chromosomes 14, 19, and 21. Recent investigations also reveal that the genotype for ApoE, a protein known for its role in cholesterol transport, is a risk factor in Alzheimer's disease. Homozygotes for ApoE$_4$ have high risk for the disease compared with E$_3$ or E$_2$ homozygotes. E$_4$ heterozygotes have an intermediate risk. The search for toxins, infectious agents, and nutritional or environmental factors has been disappointing.

Clinically, Alzheimer's disease is characterized by a relentless impairment of memory and reasoning that generally begins insidiously and can progress for a decade or longer. In most cases, Alzheimer's disease starts after age 60, and the incidence increases with each decade thereafter. Analyses show a greater incidence in women, which may reflect in part their increased longevity compared with men. A high level of education may be a protective factor. In most patients the gradual impairment of memory dominates the early clinical picture. They fail to learn new recent events, both public and personal. A defect in recognition of previously known familiar places or situations often inaugurates the symptoms. The impairments worsen with time. Despite preserving their speech, motor performances, and social graces, patients are not able to retain employment and become unable to cope with the activities of daily living. A loss of affective resonance is common, which relatives may describe as shallowness or lack of interest. Unwise decisions regarding property or investments are often made during these early stages of the disease. Signs of poor judgment and a deterioration of social relationships commonly ensue.

Alzheimer's disease may take other forms of onset. Some patients become suspicious of friends, employers, or spouse, and exhibit paranoid behavior, especially during the evening hours. They may awaken in the night disoriented to place and time and behaving in acute psychotic fashion. In another variant, language may be especially compromised. In those instances memory for words suffers the most and disturbs naming of specific objects and people. Finally, the disease may begin by compromising visual attention. Patients report an inability to perceive simultaneously more than one object in the visual field and become unable to orient themselves along previously familiar routes. Whatever the variant of onset, a pervasive impairment of memory eventually sets in. In striking contrast to the intellectual decay, motor performance (strength, coordination) remains preserved in most cases during the first years of the disease. Some patients with Alzheimer's disease can even learn *new* motor skills despite their ravaged ability to retain new factual information. Nevertheless, exceptions exist. A patient has been described with left hemiplegia and dementia whose autopsy revealed neuropathologic changes entirely characteristic of Alzheimer's disease. Also, some patients may exhibit extrapyramidal signs, in which case the course is usually more rapid. It is possible that some of the latter patients have a pathologic entity known as Lewy body dementia, hallmarked by a coexistence of Alzheimer changes and an abundance of Lewy bodies in cortical neurons.

No reliable antemortem marker exists for Alzheimer's disease. Accordingly, diagnosis must be formulated in terms of probability, based on the identification of a typical profile and the exclusion of similar conditions. In order to diagnose probable Alzheimer's disease, one must (1) document the dementia by careful bedside examination or neuropsychological tests revealing scores significantly below the range commensurate with the patient's age, educational level, and past performance; (2) verify impairment of memory; and (3) verify that the onset of dementia was not sudden or rapidly progressive. A diagnosis of Alzheimer's disease should *not* be entertained if early in the presentation (1) there are motor signs such as hemiparesis or gait disorder (but see exceptions above); (2) there is loss of somatic sensation; (3) there is a visual field defect; and (4) seizures have occurred. The electroencephalogram (EEG) should be normal early in the course of the disease, although as the disease progresses it may reveal a nonspecific pattern of slowing. The cerebrospinal fluid should also be normal, containing no cells and either a normal or mildly elevated protein level. Computed Tomography (CT), or Magnetic Resonance Imaging (MRI) scans may be normal early in the course or reveal enlargement of sulci. The enlargement can become quite pronounced in late stages but is generally more symmetric and severe than in Pick's disease (see below). Positron emission tomography has revealed a consistent pattern of diminished metabolic activity in the temporoparietal regions.

MANAGEMENT. There is no cure for Alzheimer's disease, and no drug tried so far can alter the progress of the disease. Although tacrine may rarely ameliorate symptoms in some patients, its results are usually disappointing and its side effects include severe hepatotoxicity. There are ways, however, in which caregivers can ameliorate the manifestations of the disease. During early stages, when patients can remain at home, strategically placed cue cards around the house can help their orientation so as to carry on tasks relating to their self-care. Variations of such a strategy also can help patients cope with nondemanding social activities. An emphasis on tasks that require motor skills (music playing, dancing, card playing, typing, drawing) can help to make the days more pleasurable to the patient and less frustrating to caretakers. Appropriate drugs help to cope with bouts of anxiety, depression, or paranoid ideation that some patients show. Drugs also can be used to regulate the sleep cycle and avoid nighttime waking and "sundowning." Reduction of environmental stresses and random sensory stimuli can yield surprisingly good results in this regard. Eventually a decision is needed regarding nursing home placement and the securing of appropriate medical care in such a setting. The Alzheimer's Disease and Related Disorders Association has chapters in every state which can guide physicians and patients to dedicated services. A valuable guide to management is referenced at the end of this chapter.

DISTINGUISHING ALZHEIMER'S DISEASE FROM OTHER DEMENTIAS

Treatable Dementias

INAPPROPRIATE OR EXCESSIVE USE OF MEDICATIONS. This is perhaps the most frequent and treatable dementia. It can coexist with Alzheimer's disease, and excessive drug use must be ruled out before the diagnosis of Alzheimer's disease is entertained. Cough suppressants, barbiturates, benzodiazepines, tricyclic antidepressants, monoamine oxidase inhibitors, anticholinergics, and digitalis are the common offenders. The combination of some of these drugs with alcohol in an elderly and frail individual can mimic Alzheimer's disease.

DEPRESSION. This should always be considered in the differential diagnosis because it can present as mental decline, in which case it is known as masked depression or pseudodementia. Expert psychological testing is the key to diagnosis. A number of neuropsychological tests are capable of specifically discriminating depression from Alzheimer's disease. The Benton Visual Retention Test, for example, is passed by nearly all patients who are eventually diagnosed as having pseudodementia, whereas patients with Alzheimer-type dementia fail or perform at the borderline level.

BRAIN TUMORS AND SUBDURAL HEMATOMAS. Tumors that involve structures of the limbic system, e.g., meningiomas that compress frontal lobe structures or gliomas that infiltrate the white matter of frontal and temporal cortices, often present as dementia. Distractibility, bradykinesia, and apathy dominate the clinical picture and a CT or MRI scan easily confirms the suspicion. In most instances, meningiomas can be resected with success. The elderly are prone to develop subdural hematomas after relatively minor, and thus easily forgettable, head injuries. Such hematomas, especially when bilateral, can lead to dementia, often with little in the way of a telltale history. CT or MRI is diagnostic.

COMMUNICATING HYDROCEPHALUS. Communicating hydrocephalus of the so-called normal-pressure variety is another late-life condition easily detected by brain imaging. The lateral ventricles and the third ventricle are enlarged, the sulci may be effaced, and the sampling of cerebrospinal fluid pressure in a routine lumbar puncture may fail to reveal an elevation because the pressure waves that pound the ventricular walls are intermittent. Not uncommonly the past history reveals a significant neurologic antecedent such as bacterial meningitis, subarachnoid hemorrhage, or severe head injury. The dementia is probably due to pervasive dysfunction in white matter pathways surrounding the ventricles. The clinical picture is dominated by impaired attention and flatness of emotional expression and always includes a gait disorder and urinary incontinence, neither of which affects early Alzheimer's patients. The gait disorder consists of a loss of the automatic motor patterns that are normally engaged in walking (apraxia) combined with a broad-based ataxia. An intraventricular shunt may reverse the symptoms in selected patients.

OTHER CAUSES. Endocrine and metabolic disorders, especially hypothyroidism and vitamin B_{12} deficiency, also can cause dementia. They are easily detectable and largely correctable. Syphilis and fungal infections can cause reversible dementias. In the appropriate setting, syphilis is an especially important diagnostic consideration. Many other dementias exist that can be reversed upon correcting the conditions to which they are secondary. Chronic liver disease, chronic lung disease, and uremia are obvious examples.

Nontreatable Forms of Dementia

PICK'S DISEASE. In spite of its rarity, the number of Pick's disease cases appears to be rising. This is a degenerative condition characterized by a markedly asymmetric loss of neurons in the frontal and anterior temporal regions. In some cases, the involvement is virtually unilateral and may be largely confined to either the temporal or frontal lobe (hence the term *lobar atrophy*). An intriguing preponderance for involvement of the left hemisphere has been noted. Histologic analysis reveals loss of cortical neurons in the atrophied areas. Two signs that assist with the microscopic diagnosis are the presence of Pick's neurons (pale, swollen neurons that fail to take conventional stains and are thus achromatic) and Pick's bodies (silver-staining cytoplasmic inclusions easily distinguishable from neurofibrillary tangles). Pick's neurons are most commonly found in the frontal region, whereas Pick's bodies are found predominantly in the temporal region. Neurofibrillary tangles and neuritic plaques are not histologic features of the disease.

Pick's disease has two prevalent profiles. Both usually begin in the sixth or seventh decade and affect women more frequently than men. In one profile, the patient has a gradual mental decline not unlike that seen in Alzheimer's disease but in which impairments of judgment, social appropriateness, and affect predominate over the memory defect. Not uncommonly, these patients make unwise business decisions and if they live alone they may care little about their appearance. Eventually, memory impairment sets in. This profile correlates with preponderant involvement of the frontal lobe. In the other prevalent profile, patients begin by complaining of a problem with name finding. Few specific names for objects or people can be produced, although speech articulation, syntactic processing, memory, and judgment may be intact. In most instances, within 2 to 5 years, memory and judgment begin to decline. The anatomic correlate is involvement of the *left* temporal lobe. Incidentally, Pick's original description was of the latter profile, although the former has become the textbook standard.

The left temporal form of Pick's disease brings into the discussion an elusive entity known as *progressive aphasia without dementia*. The pattern observed in some of the patients resembles that of Pick's disease, but the language disorder has remained the most prominent or sole symptom. It is possible that these cases are examples of Pick's disease in which involvement beyond the left temporal cortices is minimal or delayed. Other evidence suggests that the condition reflects either a variant of Alzheimer's disease or a nonspecific spongiform degeneration. The diagnosis of Pick's disease in the early stages is hazardous, although after about 2 years of evolution the clinical profile becomes suggestive. By then, state-of-the-art CT or MRI should provide evidence of asymmetric lobar atrophy.

PARKINSON'S DISEASE. Dementia complicates a sizable number of cases of idiopathic parkinsonism. From a clinical stand-point it is important to ensure that the mental decline is not due to the effects of anticholinergic medication or to the multifarious cognitive changes induced by levodopa. Histologic study of brain tissue of demented patients with Parkinson's disease has shown in many but not all instances abundant neurofibrillary tangles and neuritic plaques identical to those encountered in Alzheimer's disease.

HUNTINGTON'S DISEASE. Patients with Huntington's disease are prone to a host of cognitive and behavioral changes (see Ch. 411). Depression and psychotic states are part of the clinical picture. They may precede chorea and dystonia and persist into the later stages, producing a high suicide rate. Measurable mental decline is often found as the disease progresses. Distractibility and slowness of cognitive processing hallmark the presentation. The dementia is best explained by extensive cortical dysfunction secondary to neuron loss in the basal ganglia, especially in the caudate.

MULTIPLE VASCULAR LESIONS. A variety of conditions resulting in multiple strokes, large and small, can cause dementia. The following should be considered:

1. Multiple small infarcts (multiple-infarct dementia), occurring at different points in the history and involving cortical or subcortical gray matter, especially in the territories of middle cerebral and anterior cerebral arteries. The history and physical examination of such patients invariably reveal systemic hypertension, diabetes, signs of widespread vascular disease, or a combination of the above. The age range is similar to that during which degenerative diseases strike, but a careful history and neurologic examination disclose distinctive clues. For instance, the development of the dementia is stepwise, punctuated by specific events during which disturbances of speech, orientation, or motor impairment developed, often followed by some recovery. In short, the mental decline is cumulative but not gradual. (But note that the patient may lack memory and insight and thus smooth out the history profile and mislead the examiner. Helpful additional clues include focal motor defects, especially weakness, ataxia, or urinary incontinence. Alzheimer's disease shows neither of these abnormalities during its early clinical course.)

2. Multiple demyelinating lesions occurring in the surround of a blood vessel are revealed by MRI in the subcortical white matter. This puzzling condition, sometimes called Binswanger's disease or subcortical arteriosclerotic encephalopathy, can have a dementia profile indistinguishable from that of Alzheimer's disease. Most affected patients are hypertensive, however, although the condition has been described in normotensive individuals. Both CT and MRI reveal enlargement of the lateral ventricles disproportionate to the enlargement of the cortical sulci. MRI also reveals an abundance of periventricular lucencies, which show up as white on T2-weighted images. It should be noted that similar lucencies can be seen in normal older individuals but generally without ventricular enlargement of the same magnitude.

3. Multiple infarcts caused by vasculitis such as congophilic angiopathy, isolated angiitis of the central nervous system, and systemic lupus erythematosus. These are all rare conditions that present in a far more severe and dramatic way than degenerative diseases, multiple-infarct dementia, or Binswanger's disease. Such patients usually become acutely ill and are more likely to be admitted to an inpatient service than to remain ambulatory. The severity of the condition usually is paralleled by a relatively rapid course compared to the longer time scale of most of the other dementias discussed above. Other clues help the diagnosis. For instance, congophilic angiopathy causes medium to large *hemorrhagic* infarctions. Congophilic angiopathy often coexists with Alzheimer's disease for reasons that are not clear. Lupus is rare in the elderly, and the signs of systemic involvement are diagnostic. Isolated angiitis is more elusive, but the severity and rapidity of the course help the diagnosis.

CENTRAL NERVOUS SYSTEM INFECTIONS. Until recently, the most frequent form of nontreatable infectious dementia was the transmissible form of Creutzfeldt-Jakob disease, a spongiform encephalopathy discussed in Ch. 428.6. Over the past decade, immune suppression in the setting of HIV infection has become the most common infectious cause of dementia. In some cases the dementia is due to direct HIV involvement of the cerebral parenchyma; in others it is caused by opportunistic infections.

Folstein MF, Folstein SE, McHugh PR: Minimental state. A practical method for grading the cognitive state for the clinician. J Psychiatr Res 12:189, 1975. *The authors found that out of a possible total score of 30, mean score for dementia was 9.7, depression with cognitive impairment was 19.0, and uncomplicated affective depression was 27.6.*

Lippa CF, Smith TW, Swearer JM: Alzheimer's disease and Lewy body disease: A comparative clinicopathological study. Ann Neurol 35:81, 1994. *An attempt to establish Lewy body disease as a pathologic entity.*

Mace NL, Rabin PV: The 36-hour Day. A Family Guide to Caring for Persons with Alzheimer's Disease, Related Dementing Illnesses, and Memory Loss in Later Life. Baltimore, Johns Hopkins University Press, 1981. *An invaluable book for families and friends of the affected.*

Plum F, Gandy S: The dementias. Research Proceedings of the Association of Nervous and Mental Diseases, Vol. 73. American Psychiatric Assn Press, 1995.

Selkoe DJ: Aging brain, aging mind. Sci Am, September, 1992, p. 135. *An overview of current research on aging and dementia.*

Van Hoesen GW, Damasio AR: Neural correlates of cognitive impairment in Alzheimer's disease. *In* Plum F (ed.): Handbook of Physiology: Higher Functions of the Nervous System. Bethesda, MD, American Physiological Society, 1987, p. 871. *A review of the neuropsychological and neurobiologic characteristics of the disease.*

Whitehouse PJ (ed.): Dementia. Philadelphia, FA Davis, 1993. *A comprehensive monograph as many aspects of the dementias, with multiple authorities describing epidemiologic, neurobiologic, and clinical aspects of the problem. Sections also address management, legal issues, and current drug trials.*

401 PSYCHIATRIC DISORDERS IN MEDICAL PRACTICE

Gary J. Tucker

At various times most people experience anxiety, depression, sleep disturbance, and/or somatic preoccupation. In most cases such symptoms are transient, and their precipitants are often evident—an upcoming examination, a new job, marriage, divorce, work or family problems. In these instances the physician has no difficulty in reassuring the patient that the symptoms are transient and situational. However, when these symptoms persist and/or when they occur in situations that have no clear precipitants, they should arouse the physician's concern. In order to determine whether someone has a psychiatric illness, the following questions must be considered: (1) Do the signs and symptoms fit a psychiatric diagnosis? For example, when patients say they are sad or depressed, do their symptoms meet the diagnostic criteria for a diagnosis of depression? (2) Is there a family history of similar symptoms? Many psychiatric illnesses tend to have a genetic or familial basis. (3) Is the longitudinal pattern of the symptoms consistent with the natural history of a psychiatric disorder? Emotional symptoms associated with specific situations are usually classified as reactions to the situation (see Grief Reactions); they do not usually become psychiatric disorders. (4) Are the symptoms incapacitating? All persons have enduring patterns of relating, perceiving, and reacting to others. These constitute a person's personality and may take the form of such patterns as obsessive, passive, or antisocial personality traits. When such characteristics interfere with the individual's ability to function, however, the condition is regarded as a disorder, named for the predominant personality characteristic. (5) Do delusions and hallucinations exist? Delusions and hallucinations in the absence of other medical causes always indicate major psychiatric illness. Although illusory phenomena can often occur at times of tiredness, intoxication, or fever, their occurrence in clear states of consciousness should alert the physician to the presence of major psychiatric illness.

The proper delineation of psychiatric disorders from normal emotional reactions rests on a careful history, a mental status evaluation, and a knowledge of psychiatric syndromes. If the findings of the history and mental status evaluation do not fit into any of the known psychiatric syndromes, the physician should reserve judgment and follow the patient. In many cases, the symptoms neither persist nor return and all can be reassured. If the symptoms con-

TABLE 401–1. CLUES TO NONPSYCHIATRIC DISORDERS AFFECTING BEHAVIOR

1. The signs and symptoms do not fit into an established psychiatric diagnostic category.
2. There is no prior psychiatric history or symptoms.
3. The patient demonstrates an abrupt change in behavior or personality.
4. Signs and symptoms fluctuate rapidly.
5. The condition does not respond to treatment.

tinue, the physician may recognize a clear psychiatric syndrome. With all persistent emotional and behavioral symptoms, however, the physician must first rule out systemic medical disorders.

DIFFERENTIATING PSYCHIATRIC DISORDERS FROM MEDICAL DISORDERS

As biologic studies of psychiatric patients progress and specific psychopharmacologic agents are found to affect behavior, it becomes increasingly evident that psychiatric disorders are disorders of central nervous system (CNS) functioning. This awareness includes recognition that the CNS has a limited number of ways of responding to stress. For example, hallucinations can arise from psychologic causes, from toxins in the blood, from head trauma, from seizure disorders, from acute strokes, and from fever. With such potentially diverse causes, it is imperative that the physician seek clues to differentiate the causes of the behavior change (Table 401–1).

Many clues in the history can suggest something other than an intrinsic psychiatric illness as a cause of abnormal behavior. Most patients with psychiatric illnesses have had psychiatric symptoms or reveal seeds of the current disturbance in their histories. When a patient presents with a good premorbid social history, a good work history, a warm and supportive family, and well-preserved personality, the physician should seek nonpsychiatric factors to explain the behavior change. Many physicians tend erroneously to view behavior changes only in a psychological framework. Abrupt changes in behavior, personality, mood, or ability to function should be evaluated for possible organic causes. As indicated, most decompensating patients with psychiatric illness report having had similar, albeit less severe, symptoms in the past. To give an example: A 60-year-old man who has been formal and proper his entire life but abruptly becomes bawdy and flirtatious is probably not experiencing the onset of a major psychiatric illness but rather is showing personality changes associated with a new, structural disorder of the brain or of body metabolism. Rapid fluctuations in mental status also suggest a new organic disturbance rather than a psychiatric disorder. Patients with psychiatric disease seldom are delusional and hallucinating in the morning but free of these symptoms the same evening (or vice versa). By contrast, the resolution of the delusions and hallucinations associated with schizophrenia typically requires days to weeks. Similarly, motor behavior does not change rapidly in psychiatric illness. Patients with encephalopathies, by contrast, often have a "motor drivenness" with episodic desires to move about, to get up and walk. This restlessness is particularly prominent in delirious states (see Ch. 393). Lastly, and perhaps most subtly, when a patient does not respond to the usual interventions one should suspect the possibility of an incorrect diagnosis. For example, when a patient with hallucinations and delusions has been treated unsuccessfully with adequate doses of neuroleptic medications for an appropriate period of time with no change in the symptoms, the physician should consider the possibility of a disorder other than schizophrenia. These simple guidelines often alert the clinician to multiple diagnostic possibilities.

Diagnostic and Statistical Manual of Mental Disorders, 4th ed. Washington, DC, American Psychiatric Association, 1994. *A useful, widely accepted outline of diagnostic features of the gamut of psychiatric disorders.*

Goodwin D, Guze S: Psychiatric Diagnosis, 4th ed. New York, Oxford University Press, 1989. *An excellent overall text on descriptive psychiatry and the basis for diagnostic groupings.*

Lishman W: Organic Psychiatry, 2nd ed. Oxford, Blackwell, 1987. *A comprehensive description of neurologic and medical complications of behavioral disorders.*

Pincus J, Tucker G: Behavioral Neurology, 3rd ed. New York, Oxford University Press, 1985. *This monograph discusses differential diagnosis and behavioral aspects of neurologic disease as well as neurologic aspects of psychiatric disorders.*

Schiffer RB, Klein RF, Sider RC: The Medical Evaluation of Psychiatric Patients, New York, Plenum Press, 1989. *A detailed explication of the comorbidity of medical illnesses and behavioral symptoms.*

Schizophrenia and some forms of affective disorders constitute the major psychotic illnesses. (Psychosis is defined as the presence of hallucinations and/or delusions.) In 1911 Eugene Bleuler, a Swiss psychiatrist, described the central features of schizophrenia as a psychotic process manifested by disturbed thinking, changes in the emotional responsiveness of the patients, and a preoccupation with their own inner life, or autism. By schizophrenia he did not mean a "split personality" but more a splitting of psychologic functions. While some functions, such as the ability to communicate, were often impaired, others, such as memory and mathematical abilities, were sustained. In essence, this early concept remains a good clinical definition of the schizophrenic process.

Schizophrenia most often starts in late adolescence. The course is usually marked by a decline in psychosocial functioning, with a tendency for the patient to become downwardly mobile in social function. The introduction of neuroleptics in 1954 brought about some improvement in the treatment of these patients. Current treatment aims toward shorter hospitalizations for schizophrenics with more vigorous attempts to retain the patient in a community setting. Physicians encounter two principal groups of schizophrenic patients, one with an acute florid psychotic illness and the other suffering chronic illness with less florid symptoms. The care of these two groups differs in that the acute management is simple, whereas the care and rehabilitation of the chronic patient can be extremely difficult. The nationally pursued process of "deinstitutionalization" of the mentally ill has thrust this latter patient population into our everyday world.

DIAGNOSTIC CRITERIA AND CLINICAL SIGNS AND SYMPTOMS. Table 401–2 lists the diagnostic criteria for schizophrenia. Hallucinations and delusions can occur in affective disor-

TABLE 401–3. USUAL SYMPTOMATIC PATTERNS OF PSYCHOTIC DISORDERS

	Acute Schizophrenia	Mania	Major Depression	Delirium
Delusions	++++	++++	+++	++
Hallucinations	++++	++	++	+++
Disorientation/ confusion	0	0	0	++++
Incoherent speech	++++	+++	0	++++
Depressed mood	+	0	++++	+
Grandiosity	++	++++	0	0

ders and organic conditions; however, the course of these latter illnesses is different. With schizophrenia, the greater the number of delusions and hallucinations present, particularly persecutory delusions, delusions of control, firmly fixed mood-incongruent delusions, and auditory hallucinations, the more likely is the person to progress to a chronic psychotic condition (Table 401–3). Other prominent symptoms of schizophrenia are the presence of incoherence and the inability of patients to communicate in a logical and goal-directed fashion. As an example of the speech of a schizophrenic, the patient may respond as follows when asked why he was brought to the hospital: "You are a Nazi; God sent me to save the world; I have a lovely apartment; your eyes are blue."

The stipulation that these criteria must last for a 6-month period (demonstrating a deterioration from a previous level of functioning) defines a more chronic population. When the duration of symptoms is shorter than 6 months, it is inadvisable to use the diagnosis of schizophrenia. This allows the clinician to withhold judgment and encourages a search for other disorders. This is particularly important with the first episode of psychotic illness, in that it is difficult to differentiate an acute manic episode from an acute schizophrenic episode. Psychotic episodes due to toxic drug reactions, sleep deprivation, and medical causes invariably last less than 6 months.

In the past many subtypes of schizophrenia have been described, but their predictive validity has been poor except for catatonia and paranoia. Catatonic symptoms include either markedly retarded motor behavior (often to the point of no voluntary movement, the patient retaining any posture into which he is passively placed) or markedly agitated motor behavior. The importance of a catatonic diagnosis, in either the retarded or the agitated form, has retained some validity in conferring a better prognosis, but there is also evidence that catatonia may be more related to affective disorders than to schizophrenia. The paranoid forms of schizophrenia also show some unique features in that the paranoid delusions are often the only major symptoms and they tend to remain stable over time.

EPIDEMIOLOGY. The prevalence of schizophrenia in the general population is about 1% for lifetime risk, or about an 0.5 in 1000 incidence of recorded or treated cases per year in the United States. The schizophrenic syndrome has a similar worldwide incidence, the only cultural difference being that prognosis for recovery seems better in rural than in urban settings. The prevalence rate is eight times higher in the lower than in the higher socioeconomic environments. Because the parents of schizophrenics have a social class distribution similar to that of the general population, the lower position of the patients appears to be a result of the illness rather than the cause of it.

Seventy per cent of schizophrenics become ill between ages 15 and 35, and the illness affects males slightly more than females. Peak onset in males lies between 15 and 24 years and in females between 25 and 34 years. There are slight ethnic differences, with a higher incidence in Scandinavian countries and in nonwhites. The chronicity of the illness presents an enormous cost. A recent study notes that although schizophrenia affects only one-twelfth as many persons as does myocardial infarction, the cost is six times as great.

PATHOPHYSIOLOGY. The pathophysiology of schizophrenia is unknown, nor has an anatomic origin of the symptoms been determined. Nevertheless, a number of conditions (including trauma, seizure disorders, and Huntington's disease) can produce schizo-

TABLE 401–2. SCHIZOPHRENIA AND OTHER PSYCHOTIC DISORDERS

A. **Characteristic symptoms:**
   At least two of the following, each present for a significant portion of time during a 1-month period (or less if successfully treated):
   1. Delusions
   2. Hallucinations
   3. Disorganized speech (e.g., frequent derailment or incoherence)
   4. Grossly disorganized or catatonic behavior
   5. Negative symptoms, i.e., affective flattening, alogia, or avolition
   [Note: Only one A symptom is required if delusions are bizarre or hallucinations consist of a voice keeping up a running commentary on the person's behavior or thoughts, or two or more voices conversing with each other.]

B. **Social/ occupational dysfunction:**
   For a significant portion of the time since the onset of the disturbance, one or more major areas of functioning such as work, interpersonal relations, or self-care are markedly below the level achieved prior to the onset (or when the onset is in childhood or adolescence, failure to achieve expected level of interpersonal, academic, or occupational achievement).

C. **Duration:**
   Continuous signs of the disturbance persist for at least 6 months. This 6-month period must include at least 1 month of symptoms that meet criterion A (i.e., active phase symptoms) and may include periods of prodromal or residual symptoms. During these prodromal or residual periods, the signs of the disturbance may be manifested by only negative symptoms or two or more symptoms listed in criterion A present in an attenuated form (e.g., odd beliefs, unusual perceptual experiences).

D. **Schizoaffective and mood disorder exclusion:**
   Schizoaffective disorder and mood disorder with psychotic features have been ruled out because either (1) no major depressive or manic episodes have occurred concurrently with the active phase symptoms or (2) if mood episodes have occurred during active phase symptoms, their total duration has been brief relative to the duration of the active and residual periods.

E. **Substance/ general medical condition exclusion:**
   The disturbance is not due to the direct effects of a substance (e.g., drugs of abuse, medication) or a general medical condition.

Modified from Diagnostic and Statistical Manual of Mental Disorders, 4th ed. Washington, DC, American Psychiatric Association, 1994.

phrenia-like hallucinations and delusions. Many authors have reported a higher than normal incidence of nonlocalizing neurologic abnormalities in schizophrenia, changes that are not present in other psychiatric conditions. These include defects in stereognosis, graphesthesia, and various skilled motor activities. Minor vestibular system defects, usually consisting of a reduction in the nystagmus response unrelated to medication use, have been noted in schizophrenic patients. Deficits in smooth-pursuit eye movements during pendulum tracking have been reported in schizophrenia as well as in other psychoses. Other evidence of CNS damage, including electroencephalographic (EEG) abnormalities, is tantalizingly frequent.

Twenty-five per cent of hospitalized schizophrenic patients show abnormally slow EEG tracings using standard recording techniques. Computed tomographic and magnetic resonance imaging studies have both shown lateral ventricle and third ventricle enlargement, widened cortical sulci, cerebellar atrophy, cerebral asymmetry, and decreased brain density consistently in many, but not all, studies in subgroups of schizophrenic patients. Not all of these changes occur in the same subgroups. Although the implications of these findings are unclear, the findings correlate with increased cognitive disturbance, poorer premorbid adjustment, and longer duration of illness. Many of the neurologic findings are consistent with changes found in other types of neurodevelopmental disorders. As more standardization of the techniques and diagnostic criteria occurs, there should be greater consistency of findings. Using the more dynamic measures, changes have been reported in the cerebral blood flow in the anterior frontal regions, the temporal cortex, and the globus pallidus, as well as decreased D_2 receptor sites in schizophrenics. Neuropsychologic testing shows a great deal of overlap between the findings in patients with clear-cut organic disease and those with schizophrenia to the point that the tests often fail to distinguish between the two conditions.

Strong evidence implicates a genetic factor in schizophrenia to a degree that 10 to 15% of the offspring of a schizophrenic parent are at risk for the disease. Furthermore, the coincidence of schizophrenia in monozygotic twins is roughly 60%. Additional evidence for a genetic factor comes from studies of children of schizophrenic parents who are raised by either their natural or adoptive, nonschizophrenic parents: The chances of developing the disease are identical in both instances, regardless of the environment. Despite these findings, family factors have been implicated in other ways. In families with much highly charged emotional interaction, schizophrenic patients seem to do very poorly. Less emotionally stimulating environments appear to allow the schizophrenic to function better.

Additional indirect evidence for biologic mechanisms in schizophrenia derives from pharmacologic studies: (1) Most of the neuroleptic drugs effective in controlling schizophrenic symptoms act as dopamine blockers in the CNS. (2) Many psychoactive drugs such as mescaline and amphetamines are dopaminergic and also have the potential for creating psychotic reactions. Further suggestions of altered dopamine metabolism in schizophrenic patients come from the inconsistent findings of both elevated and reduced levels of homovanillic acid, its major metabolite in the CSF and urine. As yet, most of these biologic findings, as well as the results of parallel animal studies, are too inconsistent or incomplete to permit unifying hypotheses.

PROGNOSIS AND TREATMENT. Prognosis in schizophrenia is poor and specific therapy lacking. Over a 25- to 30-year period, approximately one third of patients show some recovery or remission, and the remainder either have major residual symptoms or are still hospitalized. The major treatment is neuroleptic medication.

Table 401–4 lists the drugs most commonly used in the treatment of schizophrenia. The goal of treatment is to decrease as many of the symptoms as possible. As long as hallucinations, delusions, and disorganized thinking persist, the accepted practice is to increase the dose of medication until reaching a maximum decrease in symptoms. The response is usually achieved in a period of 2 to 3 weeks, with decreases in hallucination and thought disorder and a variable response of delusions. The most frequent limiting factor is the appearance of extrapyramidal side effects, the most common of which are dystonia, akathisia (restlessness), and parkinsonism. These occur most commonly in the first 2 to 4 months of drug use.

There is little difference in efficacy in the neuroleptics (Table

TABLE 401–4. DRUGS COMMONLY USED FOR TREATMENT OF SCHIZOPHRENIA*

Drug	Daily Dosage Range (mg)
Phenothiazines	
Chlorpromazine (Thorazine)	300–1500
Thioridazine (Mellaril)	150–800
Perphenazine (Trilafon)	8–64
Trifluoperazine (Stelazine)	4–60
Fluphenazine (Prolixin)†	2–20
Butyrophenones	
Haloperidol (Haldol)†	2–40
Thioxanthenes	
Thiothixene (Navane)	6–60
Atypical neuroleptics	
Clozapine (Clozaril)	50–900
Risperidone (Risperdal)	2–6

* Owing to untoward extrapyramidal reactions, one often needs to administer these drugs along with such drugs as benztropine mesylate (Cogentin), trihexyphenidyl HCl (Artane), diphenhydramine HCl (Benadryl).

† Comes in two injectable slow-release forms that can be given every 10 days to 3 weeks.

401–4), and lack of efficacy usually reflects too low a dose. If, however, no response occurs to a phenothiazine-type drug (e.g., chlorpromazine), one usually changes to another class of neuroleptics, such as a butyrophenone (haloperidol) or a thioxanthene. Two new neuroleptics have recently become available. Clozapine is the best studied and is clinically effective in 30% of cases that have been refractory to other neuroleptics. Clozapine is of interest for several other reasons in that it does not seem to cause either extrapyramidal symptoms or tardive dyskinesia. It has a tendency to cause agranulocytosis (1 to 2% incidence) and has very little effect on D_2 receptors. Risperidone has also been recently released and shows promise as a novel neuroleptic with few reports of tardive dyskinesia. It also has little effect on D_2 receptors. The physician should become familiar with one drug from each of these classes of neuroleptics for acute and maintenance use. The major long-term hazard in the use of most of these medications is tardive dyskinesia.

Tardive dyskinesia is a syndrome of involuntary movements, usually choreoathetoid, that may affect the mouth, lips, tongue, extremities, or trunk. Although usually associated with use of neuroleptics for 6 months or more, tardive dyskinesia can occur with shorter administration. Patients on neuroleptics should be periodically evaluated for these abnormal movements. A frequent early sign consists of vermicular movements of the tongue. Anticholinergic drugs do not help this condition. The symptoms may decrease with an increase of the medication, but such improvement usually is only temporary and may lead to a vicious circle of worsening chorea and increased drug dosages. The cause of tardive dyskinesia is not known, but it is believed to represent the development of dopaminergic hypersensitivity. In many instances gradually decreasing the dose of neuroleptics induces a slow remission of the symptoms (see also Ch. 411).

Despite the above conditions, the use of neuroleptics is effective, and the drugs should be used to help the patient function with as few symptoms as possible despite the potential side effects. Removing schizophrenic patients from medication greatly increases the chances of hospitalization within the following 6 months. This lag represents a major problem in that most patients immediately feel and do better without the medications. As a result, families and patients often fail to associate the cessation of medication with the subsequent relapse.

In spite of the fact that typical neuroleptics are the treatment of choice for schizophrenia, they are not a panacea and there are alternative or adjunctive agents that the clinician may consider. At this stage these agents should be regarded as novel. They include medications such as anticonvulsants, benzodiazepines, calcium channel blockers, and monoamine agonists and antagonists.

Most criteria for judging prognosis in schizophrenia are related to short-term outcome and can be summarized by saying that the more acute and florid the early symptoms or, as some have phrased it, the more the patient has "positive" symptoms (delusions, hallucinations, agitation, and depressive symptoms), the more likely he is to recover from the acute episode. The more insidious the onset and the

Drug	Dose*	24-hr Maximum
Haloperidol (Haldol)	5–10 mg every 1–2 hr IM or PO	50 mg
Thiothixene (Navane)	5–10 mg every 2–4 hr IM or PO	40 mg
Lorazepam (Ativan)	0.5–1.0 mg every 1–2 hr IM or PO	10 mg

* Doses should be 50 to 75% reduced in the elderly or medically ill.

more lacking in emotional display (negative symptoms), the worse the short- and long-term prognoses. The natural history of the illness (even in treated patients) seems to be of two major types: (1) an episodic, relapsing course with each episode resulting in a lower level of psychosocial functioning; and (2) a gradual, slow decline in functional ability. Both courses eventually result in a progressive loss of psychosocial capacities. Treatment efforts in schizophrenia have taken a rehabilitative, or psychoeducational, approach in which the family is educated about the problems of schizophrenia and issues of living are openly dealt with.

ACUTE USE OF NEUROLEPTIC MEDICATION. Neuroleptic drugs are useful for nearly all patients who are markedly agitated with or without delusions and hallucinations and irrespective of diagnosis (Table 401–5). They help to control agitated states associated with delirium and dementia. In elderly patients and in those with delirium and/or dementia, however, the doses should be much lower until the patient's reaction is ascertained. Because acutely agitated psychotic patients respond to lorazepam as well as to neuroleptics, the initial use of benzodiazepines is probably safer in cases in which the source of the agitation is not known and in manic states for which long-term neuroleptic medication is not planned.

Andreasen N: Schizophrenia. Washington, DC, American Psychiatric Press, 1994. *A comprehensive review of current knowledge about schizophrenia.*

Hogarty GE, McEvoy JP, Muntez M, et al.: Dose of fluphenazine, familial expressed emotion and outcome in schizophrenia: Results of a two-year controlled study. Arch Gen Psychiatry 45:797, 1988. *An excellent study on the role of psychosocial factors.*

Lyon M, Barr CE, Cannon TD, et al.: Fetal neural development and schizophrenia. Schizophrenia Bull 15:149, 1989. *Excellent discussion of the neurodevelopmental findings in schizophrenia.*

Pickar D, Owen RR, Litman RE, et al.: Clinical and biologic response to clozapine in patients with schizophrenia: Crossover comparison with fluphenazine. Arch Gen Psychiatry 49:345, 1992. *Good discussion of novel neuroleptic use.*

Shore D: Schizophrenia 1993. Schizophrenia Bull 19:1, 1993. *An excellent review of all aspects of schizophrenia.*

Suddath RL, Christison GW, Torrey EF, et al.: Anatomical abnormalities in the brains of monozygotic twins discordant for schizophrenia. N Engl J Med 322:789, 1990. *Discussion of new brain imaging findings in schizophrenia.*

AFFECTIVE DISORDERS

A difficulty in clinical diagnosis is that similar terms are used to describe feeling states that differ greatly in degree and sometimes in kind. Such is the case with the term *depression*. In common use the meaning may extend from a description of a brief pang of regret to profound feelings of futility and suicidal despair. At what point along this spectrum does one label the condition "illness"? When does normal grief become pathologic? This section discusses these questions.

The most recent characterization of depressive illness has been simplified into *bipolar disorders* (manic-depressive), identifying wide swings of mood; *major depressive illness,* marked by severe depressive symptoms but without manic swings; and two milder forms, *cyclothymic disorder* and *dysthymic disorder* (formerly called depressive neurosis). These last two terms describe milder forms of bipolar disorders and depression that fall short of the specific diagnostic criteria for the more serious disorders.

Symptoms of depression also are classified by the company they keep. A psychiatric condition alone would be classified as an affective disorder, but when symptoms of affective disorders accompany medical conditions, they are defined as being due to a specific medical condition. Marked depressive symptoms have been noted with various endocrine disorders, brain tumors, seizure disorders, vitamin deficiencies, and particular neurologic disorders such as multiple sclerosis, Parkinson's disease, and stroke. Depressive symptoms also can be associated with drugs used to treat medical conditions.

In at least some instances, the consistency of the symptoms may reflect the fact that similar neurotransmitter systems are altered in both the primary and secondary affective disturbances.

Major Depression

The symptomatology and diagnostic criteria for major depression are listed in Table 401–6. Although many patients have single episodes of major depressive illness, the condition also can be repetitive, and this recurrent condition is frequently called unipolar depressive illness. Fifty percent of patients with a single episode of major depression eventually will have another depressive episode.

The key features of major depression are a markedly gloomy mood in which there is a loss of interest in life, a lack of pleasure in almost all activities, and a general feeling of hopelessness and worthlessness. The illness takes the form of a cognitive change in which the patient seemingly looks at the world with "black glasses," and everything thought about or accomplished is minimized or negated: The wealthy and successful career person talks about his or her impending financial doom and general lack of accomplishment in life; the gifted artist dismisses his creations as trivial. When vegetative functions (sleep, appetite, psychomotor activity) are markedly impaired and a complete loss of pleasure accompanies almost all activities with no reactions to pleasurable stimuli, we often add the term *melancholia*. Some severe depressions can present in a highly anxious, agitated state. The history of previous episodes (either manic or depressive) aids in the diagnosis.

Affective Disorders in the Elderly

At the two ends of life, childhood and aging, the psychopathology of affective disorders is less distinct than during the years between. Elderly patients may have many dysphoric symptoms but not meet the precise diagnostic criteria for major affective disorder. Diagnosis in the elderly is also complicated by two factors: (1) the behavioral and cognitive changes caused by the aging of the CNS (although, other than minor memory impairments, the presence of cognitive impairments should make the clinician consider a more

TABLE 401-6. MAJOR DEPRESSIVE EPISODE

A. At least five of the following symptoms have been present during the same 2-week period and represent a change from previous functioning; at least one of the symptoms in either (1) depressed mood or (2) loss of interest or pleasure.
  1. Depressed mood most of the day, nearly every day, as indicated by either subjective report (e.g., feels sad or empty) or observation made by others (e.g., appears tearful). Note: in children and adolescents, can be irritable mood.
  2. Markedly diminished interest or pleasure in all, or almost all, activities most of the day, nearly every day (as indicated by either subjective account or observation made by others).
  3. Significant weight loss or weight gain when not dieting (e.g., more than 5% of body weight in a month), or decrease or increase in appetite nearly every day. Note: in children, consider failure to make expected weight gain.
  4. Insomnia or hypersomnia nearly every day.
  5. Psychomotor agitation or retardation nearly every day (observable by others, not merely subjective feelings of restlessness or being slowed down).
  6. Fatigue or loss of energy nearly every day.
  7. Feelings of worthlessness or excessive or inappropriate guilt (which may be delusional) nearly every day (not merely self-reproach or guilt about being sick).
  8. Diminished ability to think or concentrate, or indecisiveness, nearly every day (either by subjective account or as observed by others).
  9. Recurrent thoughts of death (not just fear of dying), recurrent suicidal ideation without a specific plan, or a suicide attempt or a specific plan for committing suicide.
B. The symptoms cause clinically significant distress or impairment in social, occupational, or other important areas of functioning.
C. The symptoms are not due to the direct effects of a substance (e.g., drugs of abuse, medication) or a general medical condition (e.g., hypothyroidism).

Modified from Diagnostic and Statistical Manual of Mental Disorders, 4th ed. Washington, DC, American Psychiatric Association, 1994.

comprehensive workup for dementia), and (2) the presence of other medical illnesses with their attendant medications.

The most common psychiatric symptoms in community populations of older adults are those of depression (15%), hypochondriasis (14%), suspiciousness (17%), and persecutory ideation (4%). As many as one third complain of difficulty in falling asleep, awakening during the night, or being sleepy during the day. All these symptom rates increase for the institutionalized elderly. By contrast, cases fulfilling the specific diagnoses of major depression, dysthymia, and schizophrenia occur at a much lower rate than in younger populations.

Although the aged patient may not meet full diagnostic criteria for affective disturbance, persistent symptomatology nevertheless deserves a trial of cautious pharmacologic intervention. This is particularly true of elderly patients who have cognitive impairments. Community samples of aged populations show about a 4 to 5% prevalence of severe cognitive impairment. The figure may not entirely reflect degenerative brain disease, however, because the biologic changes that occur with affective illness also can cause cognitive impairments detected by both neuropsychological testing and clinical neurologic examination. This is true in younger populations as well. The abnormalities can include not only problems with memory and orientation but signs of minor neurologic impairment as well; all may clear after a trial of antidepressive medication. The term "pseudodementia" has been used for these potentially treatable cognitive changes in elderly affectively disordered patients.

DIAGNOSIS. The diagnosis of affective disorders is made on clinical grounds as discussed above. Many tests to aid the diagnosis of depression have been introduced, including the dexamethasone suppression test (DST), the thyroid-stimulating hormone (TSH) response (see below), and many measures of disturbed sleep function such as rapid eye movement (REM) latency. Unfortunately, none has proved to be diagnostically reliable or specific for affective disorder. In diagnosing depression, the interview is central.

EPIDEMIOLOGY. The gender distribution of major depression is almost two-to-one female to male. The peak age incidence for women is 35 to 45 years, whereas the age pattern is less clear for men. There may also be an increased incidence in women in their early 50's. The prevalence is about 3.2 per 100 males and about 4.5 to 9.3 per 100 females. Incidence is 82 to 201 new cases per 100,000 for men and 247 to 598 new cases per 100,000 for women. The mean duration of first attack of an untreated depressive illness is about 13 months. The episodes, if they recur, are likely to be similar in nature and respond to treatment in a similar fashion. As with bipolar illness, alcoholism is a frequent complication of depressive illness, particularly when it has a recurring course.

Patients in primary care clinics (5 to 10%) and on medical inpatient services (15%) show an increased prevalence of depression.

PATHOPHYSIOLOGY. Pathophysiologic theories of affective disorders have developed along three major lines: (1) endocrine studies; (2) neurotransmitters; and (3) electrophysiologic studies. Depressed patients frequently have elevated levels of cortical steroids in the blood and urine and at least half fail to suppress cortisol secretion after dexamethasone administration. TSH response to thyrotropin-releasing hormone also has been found to be aberrant in many depressed patients, even though their blood T_3 and T_4 levels are normal. Growth hormone, prolactin, gonadal hormones, corticotropin-releasing factor, and melatonin have all been shown to have diminished responses in subgroups of affective disorders. Although none of these findings is specific for any type of depressive illness or consistent in all depressive illnesses, they nevertheless suggest the presence of pituitary-hypothalamic dysfunction in affective disorders.

Studies of neurotransmitters in depression have been stimulated largely by the success of antidepressant pharmacologic agents. Many of the tricyclic compounds and the monoamine oxidase inhibitors (MAOI) effective in the treatment of depression increase the availability of catecholamines and indolamines in the CNS. L-Dopa, used to treat Parkinson's disease, is a major catecholamine (dopamine) precursor and may in itself induce mania. These and other observations have given rise to the catecholamine-indolamine hypothesis of depression. The theory postulates that a certain level of amines and/or receptor sensitivity to catecholamines functions to generate a normal mood. Receptor insensitivity or a depletion of

amines, or a decrease in their synthesis or storage, leads to depression. Conversely, if the amines are in excess or the receptors are hypersensitive, mania may develop. Recently, the acetylcholine system has also been implicated in affective disorders, a "balance" between adrenergic and cholinergic function being postulated as necessary for the stabilization of mood. Neither theory is entirely satisfactory because the tricyclic drugs affect many receptor systems and their main action may be one of changing or regulating the sensitivity of the receptor rather than acting directly as neurotransmitters. Furthermore, newer drugs that have antidepressant effects do not affect these transmitter systems. One study, for example, has found that the anticonvulsant carbamazepine favorably influences the course of certain patients with bipolar illness.

Electrophysiologic studies on affective illness have concentrated on changes in sleep functions, especially the presence of changes in the REM sleep pattern during episodes of active illness. A subgroup of patients with affective disorder shows a shortened REM latency. Furthermore, analyses of circadian rhythms provide increasing evidence for autumn and winter precipitation of some bipolar disorders, with depressive illnesses apparently related to diminished ambient light in winter climates. The change has been correlated with alterations of melatonin metabolism.

TREATMENT. Mild depression usually manifests itself as feelings of sadness and self-deprecation, coupled with slight sleep and appetite disturbances. In such patients an attempt at counseling about the events in their lives and helping delineate appropriate priorities and activities, along with prescriptions for adequate exercise, diet, rest, and general health measures, may suffice. When symptoms become more marked, particularly when they disturb sleep and appetite, and the person becomes unable to perform work, school, or household tasks, one should consider adding antidepressant medication to the above regimen (Table 401–7). If the symptoms have been present for a number of years, a trial of medication may be in order. With prominent depressive symptomatology hospitalization may be necessary, the major indication being to prevent suicide (the risk among persons with major affective disorders is 15%). To ask all patients with depression of mood, apathetic fatigue, or ill-defined somatic symptoms if they have ever considered suicide not only is wise but can elicit an important signal to intensify treatment.

The approach and response to drug therapy in depression vary considerably among both physicians and patients. Perhaps the best prediction of a favorable response is if a blood relative has responded well to a similar agent. In patients who present primarily with insomnia and marked vegetative disturbances as well as some agitation, amitriptyline (or nortryptyline) is somewhat more sedat-

TABLE 401–7. ANTIDEPRESSANT DRUGS

Drug	Daily Dosage Range (mg)*	Anticholinergic Effects
Tricyclics		
Imipramine (Tofranil)	50–150	++
Amitriptyline (Elavil)	50–150	+++
Nortriptyline (Aventyl)	50–150	++
Desipramine (Norpramin, Pertofrane)	50–150	+
Doxepin (Sinequan)	150	++
Tetracyclic		
Maprotiline (Ludiomil)	50–225	+
Serotonin reuptake inhibitors		
Fluoxetine (Prozac)	10–80	0
Sertraline (Zoloft)	50–200	0
Paroxetine (Paxil)	20–40	0
Other		
Bupropion (Wellbutrin)	300–450	0
Trazodone (Desyrel)	150–600	0
Venlafaxine (Effexor)	75–350	±
MAOI's†		
Phenelzine (Nardil)	15–90	++
Tranylcypromine (Parnate)	20–30	++

* In most cases the dose should be reduced 30 to 50% in the elderly and medically ill.
† Monoamine oxidase inhibitors.

ing, particularly if given at bedtime. Imipramine (or desipramine) is less sedating and often avoids the drowsiness that amitriptyline causes. After initial complete blood count, liver profiles and, in older patients, an ECG, it is best to start these medications in single doses at bedtime. An initial starting dose of 50 mg may be rapidly increased every several days until a total dosage of 150 mg per night is reached. As stated earlier, with elderly patients all psychotropic drugs should be used cautiously, and doses of antidepressants should be decreased by 30 to 50% from the above. For example, one would start an elderly patient on 10 or 25 mg of an antidepressant such as nortriptyline at bedtime or even every other night. For prolonged treatment the elderly often respond to smaller doses (10 to 75 mg). If after 6 weeks the elderly patient has not responded to doses as high as 75 mg and there are no marked side effects, doses can be slowly increased. Similarly, in otherwise healthy adults, if no response to 150 mg per day appears within 6 weeks, the dosage can often be increased to as much as 200 to 300 mg (beyond manufacturers' guidelines). It is wise, however, to obtain the counsel of a specialist prior to using these doses. If there is still no response one could switch to another tricyclic or immediately to an MAOI.

The new serotonin reuptake inhibitors such as fluoxetine, paroxetine, and sertraline have all been shown to be as effective as the tricyclics but have the advantage of fewer side effects. However, there are side effects with these new medications, and increased agitation can be a significant problem. The agitation responds to decreasing the dose. Weight gain and sexual dysfunction also have been noted. Blood level measurements are available for most of the tricyclic antidepressants, although their main usefulness is to indicate that the person is taking and absorbing the drug. Only nortriptyline has a known therapeutic window (50 to 140 ng per milliliter).

It is useful to caution patients that the antidepressants do not produce an immediate response, although if given at bedtime they may improve sleeping immediately. Also, the prominent anticholinergic side effects and hypotension are often a bother, and patients should be forewarned. Some of the supposed side effects of the medication are also accompaniments of the depressive illness, and patients, if questioned, may reveal that they have had many of the symptoms prior to taking the medication. Several of the newer antidepressants, such as fluoxetine and bupropion, have different actions. One must recognize that the tricyclics have a quinidine-like effect and have been used to treat some cardiac arrhythmias.

For patients who fail to respond to antidepressants, psychiatric consultation is critical. However, some have found it useful to add 0.25 μg per day of triiodothyronine (T_3) to the tricyclic dosage, particularly in women. Also, the addition of lithium to tricyclic regimens has been found to have an augmenting effect on the response to antidepressant tricyclics (neither of the above is an FDA-approved use).

The MAOI's returned to usage recently with the introduction of fluoxetine and bupropion. They had been underutilized in the United States owing to their tendency to cause hypertensive crises following the ingestion of foods containing tyramine. However, for patients not responding to tricyclic medications or those with atypical depressions marked predominantly by anxiety symptoms, they are quite effective. Patients can be started on MAOI drugs immediately following tricyclic cessation. The reverse, however, does not hold, and patients stopping an MAOI drug must wait 7 to 14 days before starting a tricyclic antidepressant. If dietary restrictions are followed and sympathetic amine medications are avoided, MAOI's are usually safe, their major side effects being hypotension and insomnia. They have milder anticholinergic effects and often are easier to tolerate than the tricyclic antidepressants, but the specific side effects and indications for use are still being delineated.

In older patients who fail to respond to pharmacotherapeutic interventions, as well as in others with complicated medical conditions which the drugs might adversely affect, electroconvulsive therapy (ECT) is probably the safest treatment. Whereas 60% of most affective disturbances respond to pharmacotherapy, close to 80% improve after ECT. There are few contraindications: When ECT is administered in association with modern anesthetic techniques, the morbidity is reduced to that of the anesthesia alone. With careful monitoring, even patients with recent cerebral or myocardial insults can be treated with ECT.

PROGNOSIS. Antidepressant drugs should be continued for 6 to 20 weeks after patients become free of symptoms. More prolonged treatment is desirable for those who have had recurrent episodes. Many patients have been maintained for years on tricyclic antidepressants and MAOI's without major impairment. Nevertheless, in spite of the best treatment, between 15 and 20% of depressives go on to a chronic course. Most patients with a single episode resume normal function. Some use the depressive episode as a chance to reorganize their lives and proceed to function better than they had previously.

Dysthymic Disorder (Depressive Neurosis)

The symptoms consist of a depressed mood of longstanding duration with a severity less intense than in a major depressive disorder. These patients often seem to have situational reasons for their illness. Many present primarily with physical complaints to physicians. Substance and drug abuse, as well as personality profiles that involve dependency and obsessional symptomatology, are often part of the clinical picture. The diagnostic criteria are outlined in Table 401–8.

As this condition is treated in many settings, the epidemiologic distribution is difficult to determine. One estimate of prevalence is 60 per 1000. Women predominate. Familial patterns have not been established. There is evidence that various personality conflicts and situational precipitants are related to these conditions more than to the other affective disorders.

Many types of short-term psychotherapy have been effective in treating these conditions. Patients who respond poorly to psychotherapy often benefit from antidepressant medication.

GRIEF REACTIONS

Physicians often find it emotionally difficult to deal with the loved ones of patients who have died or been seriously injured, yet such contacts provide important preventive medicine. Grief should be looked upon as a biologic process with psychological roots. Issues of loss and attachment are prominent in bereavement. In normal bereavement 50% of persons experience depressed mood, sleep disturbances, and crying lasting anywhere from 2 to 6 months. Furthermore, many grief reactions resolve only slowly over a number of years. This is particularly true in older persons.

During bereaved states general health deteriorates, and serious illnesses often increase. Some persons lose contact with reality and blame themselves, constantly asking, "Why did this happen?" Others even have difficulty in accepting that the person is dead. Anger and withdrawal can prevail. Some survivors, particularly when the death was violent, experience stress responses similar to those of combat veterans, who in addition to the symptoms related above may have frequent and often violent intrusive mental images.

These normal reactions can blur into a more serious state with intense and prolonged symptoms lasting 6 months or more. Some survivors undergo a delayed response, functioning well immediately after the event but experiencing later symptoms of bereavement, often precipitated by the death of another person or the anniversary of the death of the loved one. Others can develop hypochondriacal symptoms resembling those of the deceased. Panic attacks and depressive illness may develop also in prolonged grief reactions.

The management of grief reactions can often be undertaken by the physician in his/her normal contact with the bereaved survivor. Lindeman has outlined several valid principles: (1) Allow the patient to share his feelings about the death of the relative. The physician can be extremely helpful in discussing the normal process of

---

TABLE 401–8. DYSTHYMIC DISORDER

A. Depressed mood (or can be irritable mood in children and adolescents) for most of the day, for more days than not, as indicated either by subjective account or by observation made by others, for at least 2 years (1 year for children and adolescents).

B. Presence, while depressed, of at least three of the following:
1. Low self-esteem or self-confidence, or feelings of inadequacy
2. Feelings of pessimism, despair, or hopelessness
3. Generalized loss of interest or pleasure
4. Social withdrawal

Modified from Diagnostic and Statistical Manual of Mental Disorders, 4th ed. Washington, DC, American Psychiatric Association, 1994.

grief and the reactions that people experience. (2) Review the relationships of the deceased with the important people in their lives. (3) Help grieving persons to accept their feelings and fears about things such as their ability to cope, their fears about "going crazy," and anger. (4) Discuss with the bereaved how they are adapting to the stress and what modes they are using to cope. (5) Attempt to formulate the future relationships between the bereaved and others in their lives. (6) Find new persons with whom the bereaved can develop relationships.

Although the above matters can only be touched on in the acute situation, they often can be dealt with over time. Even the gathering of information about these areas helps many patients. If the condition progresses to an abnormal degree, the use of appropriate medications is indicated, e.g., for affective disturbance or panic disorder. Mild sedation and hypnotics at the acute stage are also useful. Support groups have been organized to deal with both the normal and excessive processes of grieving and appear to help.

SUICIDAL BEHAVIOR

About 75% of patients who commit suicide have seen a physician within the previous 6 months. Most practicing physicians encounter half a dozen potentially suicidal patients per year, among whom 10 to 12 actually commit the act over the ensuing years. The figures illustrate how important it is for the physician to detect various clues. Suicide rates are higher in patients with psychiatric problems, with the highest incidence occurring in those with affective disorders or alcoholism or those who are in the early post-hospital phase of schizophrenic disorders. Suicidal behavior is not specific to any single psychiatric disturbance. Suicidal behavior occurs across a spectrum of mental illness, and it should be treated as a problem distinct from the major psychiatric disorders. Effective pharmacologic treatments for depression and schizophrenia have been available since the 1950's, yet there is no evidence that these treatments have reduced the suicide rate of either population. Therapy that may help in avoiding suicide include enhancing the patient's social supports, improving his or her problem-solving and other coping skills, and initiating treatments designed to reduce drug and alcohol use, especially during periods of stress.

The typical victim of attempted suicide is a white female, 20 to 40 years of age, who ingests pills, usually after an interpersonal conflict. By contrast, the typical successful suicide victim is a white male, 45 years of age or older, often separated, widowed, or divorced, who lives alone and may be unemployed or retired. Patients who commit suicide suffer a high incidence of recently poor physical health and evidence of psychiatric disturbance. Many have a previous history of suicide attempts or threats.

Patients often wish to discuss their suicidal fears, but many physicians are made uncomfortable by discussing the matter. Such a reaction is more than a lack of compassion: It represents bad medicine. The question must be approached understandingly, but almost all seriously ill adults should be asked gently if they have had thoughts about death or suicide. Comments patients make about feeling they would be "better off dead" or "people would be better off without me" should be taken seriously. Preoccupations with funerals, cemetery lots, and the buying of weapons should make the clinician suspicious. Any patient who presents with vague complaints should be asked about his or her emotional state. If any indication of suicidal intent is forthcoming, one must immediately evaluate its seriousness, inquiring gently about the following: (1) Has the person considered actual suicide? If so, what plans have been made and how specifically? The more specific, the more worrisome. (2) What other psychopathology exists? Is the patient agitated, seriously depressed, etc.? (3) What precipitating stresses exist? (4) Are there persons whom the patient trusts and who could help? (5) Will the person agree to work with you and contact you if his suicidal feelings intensify? (6) If no reassurance comes from the patient or relatives that the situation can be managed at home, hospitalization may be necessary. Physicians who find themselves unable to provide such a supporting role should consider requesting psychiatric consultation for the patient.

An even more difficult evaluation is how to treat those who have made a recent unsuccessful suicide attempt. After a suicide attempt there often is a brief period of days to weeks of lightening of the depressive mood, after which strong self-destructive feelings reappear. The more lethal the risk (i.e., the higher was the potential risk of death in the initial suicide attempt), the more determined should be the effort to provide psychiatric treatment, preferably in a hospital. If patients express an explicit intent to die, often stated with determination and conviction, there is no question about the necessity for hospitalization.

Most patients after suicide attempts should have a psychiatric consultation. When this is impossible, the nonpsychiatric physician must assess the suicidal potential. Part of the evaluation can also serve as the initial formation of a doctor-patient relationship. If they have a supportive environment and will keep contact, some of these patients can be managed as outpatients. Physicians should beware of writing potentially lethal prescriptions for patients who may have suicidal tendencies. For example, for a routine dosage schedule of tricyclic antidepressants (150 mg per day), even a week's supply provides a potentially lethal overdose.

SUICIDE IN ADOLESCENTS. Somewhere between 9 and 18% of children and adolescents have made suicide attempts. This astoundingly high figure correlates with turmoil in the family as well as disturbed parent/child interactions. There are also significant correlations with substance abuse, depressive illness, and conduct disorders in children and adolescents as well as histories of physical and sexual abuse. Many of these children and adolescents had threatened suicide previously. Many have done poorly in school and have records of chronically aggressive behavior. One of the most difficult questions is whether to hospitalize an adolescent at risk for suicide. The answer relates primarily to the severity of the suicidal behavior and the patient's intent to "be dead." Interestingly, in adolescents, it also relates to the presence of assaultive behavior in that the hostility toward others can also be directed against the self. The environmental supports available to see someone through a depressive episode also mitigate the need for hospitalization. It is extremely important in treating the adolescent to provide some form of individual counseling, usually centered on coping skills and cognitive therapy, as well to work with the environmental support system or the patient's family. Pharmacologic treatment is effective for affective illness in adolescents.

SUICIDE AND AGING. Persons older than 70 years have a higher suicide rate, with single males at the peak. Risk factors include unemployment, isolation, poor health, pain, feelings of being rejected, history of mental illness, and previous suicide attempts. A history of alcoholism is a high comorbid factor. Many elderly indirectly pursue suicide by stopping eating or necessary medications. Electroconvulsive therapy is often the most effective form of treatment.

Bipolar Disorders

Bipolar disorders (previously called manic-depressive disorders) probably make up the most homogeneous diagnostic grouping in psychiatry, as they consist of a marked change in mood that varies from major depressive episodes (as discussed) (see Table 401–6) to significant manic episodes as defined below. There is usually a return to normal behavior between episodes. There is little difficulty in recognizing the illness if one looks at the longitudinal course. However, if patients are examined only briefly, at a particular moment in time, manic excitement can be confused with schizophrenic psychosis. The depressive phase of bipolar illness can also be misconstrued as a catatonic state.

DIAGNOSTIC CRITERIA AND CLINICAL SIGNS AND SYMPTOMS. The manic phase of the illness is characterized by an expansive euphoric mood in which grandiose plans and ideas predominate. It is important to be aware that despite this expansiveness and grandiosity, patients who are frustrated or disagreed with often become irritable and sometimes aggressive. The major diagnostic criteria are listed in Table 401–9. The patient can be psychotic in the manic phase, with delusions and hallucinations consistent with the grandiosity; persecutory delusions, feelings of being controlled, can also be present. At times it is difficult to distinguish an excited schizophrenic patient from a manic one. As already stated, one must examine the longitudinal course of the illness, until either a depressive episode occurs or the course deteriorates after remission of the acute symptom, in order to diagnose a schizophrenic process. In all instances, it is crucial to rule out organic factors.

The average age at onset of bipolar disorder is about 30 years, but about 20% of patients have an onset below the age of 20. In fe-

TABLE 401-9. MANIC EPISODE

A. A distinct period of abnormally and persistently elevated, expansive, or irritable mood, lasting at least 1 week (or any duration if hospitalization is necessary).

B. During the period of mood disturbance, at least three of the following symptoms have persisted (four if the mood is only irritable) and have been present to a significant degree:

1. Inflated self-esteem or grandiosity
2. Decreased need for sleep (e.g., feels rested after only 3 hours of sleep)
3. More talkative than usual or pressure to keep talking
4. Flight of ideas or subjective experiences that thoughts are racing
5. Distractibility (i.e., attention too easily drawn to unimportant or irrelevant external stimuli)
6. Increase in goal-directed activity (either socially, at work or school, or sexually) or psychomotor agitation
7. Excessive involvement in pleasurable activities that have a high potential for painful consequences (e.g., the person engages in unrestrained buying sprees, sexual indiscretions, or foolish business investments).

C. The mood disturbance is sufficiently severe to cause marked impairment in occupational functioning or in usual social activities or relationships with others to necessitate hospitalization to prevent harm to self or others.

D. The symptoms are not due to the direct effects of a substance (e.g., drugs of abuse, medication) or a general medical condition (e.g., hypothyroidism).

Modified from Diagnostic and Statistical Manual of Mental Disorders, 4th ed. Washington, DC, American Psychiatric Association, 1994.

males, the onset of the condition seems to have a bimodal distribution, with one peak falling between 20 and 30 years and the other between 40 and 50 years. The peak age at onset of schizophrenia is much younger, but the age at onset of bipolar illness overlaps enough so that the differential diagnosis of a psychotic illness in a young person is difficult and may change as the clinical picture evolves over time. Almost half the patients with bipolar disorders have at least two to three episodes of illness, and as many as a third experience seven or more episodes of illness once the pattern has started. Each episode of illness, whether manic or depressive, can last from 4 to 13 months; some go on to chronicity and some cease much sooner. The course of the illness has been modified significantly with the advent of lithium therapy, especially with respect to diminishing both the severity and the frequency of the episodes. The shorter durations are usually related to the effectiveness of the treatment. Although some patients rapidly alternate between extremes over 2 to 4 days, most episodes have a longer duration and, frequently, after a manic phase a depressive phase follows. Chronicity, again as opposed to schizophrenia, is not a major problem with manic-depressive illness, being cited as low as 1% in some studies. Mortality with bipolar illness averages between two and two and one-half times the expected rate for that age; suicide occurs in about 8 to 10%.

EPIDEMIOLOGY. The lifetime risk for developing bipolar illness ranges from 0.6 to 0.9% of the population. The new-case incidence per hundred thousand per year is from 9 to 15 in men and from 7.4 to 32 in women. The risk increases with a family history of bipolar illness. The genetic pattern in bipolar illness is uncertain but suggests autosomal dominance with incomplete penetration. There is a 72% concordance in monozygotic twins and a 19% concordance in same-sex dizygotic twins. Both the course of illness and the response to treatment are similar among blood relatives. In one well-studied Amish family, the abnormal gene has been identified on chromosome 11. Other families with equally strong genetic patterns have not possessed this particular chromosomal alteration.

PATHOPHYSIOLOGY. Most of what is known about the pathophysiology of bipolar illness is similar to what is known about the biology of the major depressive disorders.

DIAGNOSIS AND TREATMENT. The treatment of bipolar disorders has three distinct aspects: the manic episode, the major depressive episode, and long-term maintenance therapy. Prior to any specific therapy, an adequate medical workup is necessary in order to be certain that the patient suffers from a primary affective illness. The patient in an acute manic state is delusional, grandiose, and hyperactive and in this condition looks similar to any patient with

psychosis. If this is the first episode, one cannot differentiate this state phenomenologically from the first episode of schizophrenia or a psychosis due to physical illness. The differential diagnosis with the first episode rests on a careful history, family history, and physical and laboratory examination. The past history and the nature of onset of the illness are important, as noted previously. Furthermore, most psychiatric disorders have a familial pattern. A psychiatrist should be involved in the evaluation of patients who present with their first psychotic episode.

The treatment of the acute manic phase is usually undertaken in the hospital, as it is imperative to protect the patient from his own misdeeds, e.g., spending inordinate amounts of money, making embarrassing speeches. If the family is supportive, however, and feels it can control the situation, treatment can be started outside of the hospital. Lithium is not useful for the acute management of mania and if the patient is severely agitated, sedation is necessary. Neuroleptics are not used in the long-term treatment of bipolar illness, but benzodiazepines, particularly lorazepam, can effectively control most acute manic states (see Table 401-5). If the agitation cannot be controlled with medication, the clinician should obtain psychiatric consultation to consider using ECT to control the manic excitement. Manic excitement creates a medical emergency in which patients can die from exhaustion.

Although most general physicians treat acute mania rarely, they may more often encounter the use of lithium. Lithium effectively prevents relapses in >60% of bipolar illnesses. The drug is slightly more effective in preventing manic than depressive episodes. Nevertheless, its use should be considered with any repetitive affective disturbance.

Prior to the beginning of lithium therapy, a CBC, urinalysis, electrolytes, creatinine, BUN, thyroid studies, and a baseline ECG and EEG should be obtained. Chronic medical illnesses, especially renal insufficiency, can contraindicate use of the agent. Lithium has a half-life of 24 to 36 hours, and it takes at least 4 days to achieve a steady state. The specific therapeutic effectiveness is not evident until at least 4 to 10 days after institution of therapy. Consequently, lithium is not a good medication for the acutely agitated or manic patient but should be started early in anticipation of maintenance use. It is necessary to monitor the serum level of lithium, adequate levels for acute illness being in the range of 0.8 to 1.4 mEq per liter. For maintenance therapy, satisfactory responses accompany blood levels of 0.4 mEq per liter. Dose and blood level, however, should be titrated against clinical effectiveness for each patient. Once maintenance levels are reached, patients usually can be maintained for long periods with minimal contact. Doses usually are given twice daily, as absorption from the gastrointestinal tract is rapid and the drug peaks in the serum within 1 to 2 hours. *Serum lithium levels of more than 2 mEq per liter are highly dangerous and represent a medical emergency requiring immediate hospitalization and, sometimes, hemodialysis.* Of most concern with regard to side effects in the long-term use of lithium is the development of mild leukocytosis, hypothyroidism, diabetes insipidus, and, occasionally, renal tubular damage. Although these long-term side effects are not trivial, they are uncommon and must be weighed against the propensity of untreated patients to be recurrently hospitalized. For patients who do not respond to lithium therapy or cannot tolerate it, increasingly encouraging reports describe the effective use of carbamazepine and valproic acid in treating bipolar conditions.

The depressive phase of bipolar illness is treated the same as for any major depressive disorder, as outlined previously.

Patients with bipolar disorders are often reluctant to continue with their medications, particularly lithium, because they feel it inhibits them, decreases their energy, or affects their creativity. Consequently, a good deal of discussion about these issues is pertinent for the patient and especially for the family. The enlistment and assistance of the family of the patient with bipolar disorder are important. During either acute mania or severe depressive reactions, verbal interventions with patients often are difficult, and it is useful simply to repeat some major reassuring statements—that they are patients, that they are going to get better, and that this is not their normal state. Although the role of precipitants is not clear in the onset of bipolar illness, it is important for patients to remain in treatment. This often can be accomplished by helping them understand stressful situations in their lives. Family and marital counseling often is useful.

PROGNOSIS. The more episodes a patient has, the more likely he or she is to have another. Nevertheless, if one takes as indices of outcome successful marital and occupational adjustment, approximately two thirds of patients do well. About 15% have some improvement, and the remainder do poorly. Although manic or depressive episodes may cause much acute social disruption, including job loss and marital strife, the wide spacing of episodes often prevents long-term social decay. Patients with bipolar disease usually function normally between episodes. Accordingly, a major goal of treatment is to protect the patient during episodes so as to minimize social disruption. Nevertheless, although the prognosis is not as devastating as in schizophrenia, it is still fraught with a significant amount of periodic and, sometimes, long-term functional disability.

Goodwin FK, Jamison KR: Manic Depressive Illness. New York, Oxford University Press, 1990. *An excellent review of all aspects of affective disorders.*
Parkes CM, Weise RS: Recovery from Bereavement. New York, Basic Books, 1983. *Excellent summary of treatment of grief.*
Pfeffer CR: Clinical perspectives on treatment of suicidal behavior among children and adolescents. Psychiatr Ann 20:143, 1990. *An excellent general article on the management of suicidal behavior in children and adolescents, applicable to adults as well.*
Sadovay J, Lazarus L, Jarvick L: Review of geriatric psychiatry. Washington, DC, American Psychiatric Press, 1991. *An excellent and comprehensive review of geriatric psychiatry.*
Shucter S, Zisook S: Treatment of spousal bereavement. Psychiatr Ann 16:295, 1986. *An excellent discussion of treatment of bereavement.*

ANXIETY DISORDERS

Anxiety is the most ubiquitous psychiatric symptom and one of the most common of all disorders that present to the general physician. It occurs as part of most major psychiatric syndromes, particularly depressive ones. Anxiety accompanies at least some aspects of most normal lives, and it can be an effective stimulus to improved performance. The performance curve follows an inverted U: A little anxiety can improve performance, performance then plateaus as the anxiety increases, and eventually too much anxiety causes a decrease in the ability to function. Currently, anxiety disorders are divided into two major categories: (1) panic disorders, which are episodic, "attack-like" symptoms; and (2) generalized anxiety disorder, which is a persistent state of anxiety, commonly associated with somatic complaints and labeled somatization disorder.

Patients with anxiety symptoms are extremely high users of medical services, usually complaining vaguely that "something is wrong." A retrospective study of 55 patients with panic disorder referred from primary care physicians for psychiatric consultation revealed that 89% initially presented with one or two somatic complaints. In most, somatic misdiagnoses had continued for months or years. The most frequent symptom patterns were (1) cardiac (chest pains, tachycardia, irregular heartbeat); (2) gastrointestinal (epigastric distress); (3) neurologic (headache, dizziness/vertigo, syncope, or paresthesias): and (4) chronic fatigue or fibromyalgia. In a random survey of 195 patients in a primary care practice screened with structured interviews, 13% met DSM-III criteria for panic disorder.

DIAGNOSTIC CRITERIA AND CLINICAL SIGNS AND SYMPTOMS. A panic attack produces a distinct symptomatic event. There is a precipitous sensation of feelings of fear, impending doom, or imminent death, accompanied by a potential host of physical symptoms (Table 401–10). In fact, when a patient presents with somatic symptoms as listed above and shows no abnormal physical signs or laboratory findings, one should strongly consider panic disorder.

Affected patients often complain of the physical symptoms in an agitated state. These circumstances differ markedly from chronic anxiety states, in which symptoms are more gradual and do not create life-threatening fears. Generalized anxiety disorder is a pervasive feeling of anxiety or "nervousness" that lacks the attack-like characteristics of panic disorder. The symptoms of generalized anxiety disorders are mainly muscle tension, autonomic hyperactivity, and apprehensive hypervigilant behavior.

A strong association links *agoraphobia* and panic attacks. Agoraphobia is defined as a morbid fear and avoidance of being alone or

TABLE 401–10. PANIC DISORDER WITHOUT AGORAPHOBIA

A. Both of the following symptoms:
  1. Recurrent unexpected panic attacks, defined as a discrete period of intense fear or discomfort, in which at least four of the following symptoms developed abruptly and reached a peak within 10 minutes: (1) palpitations, pounding heart, or accelerated heart rate; (2) sweating; (3) trembling or shaking; (4) sensations of shortness of breath or smothering; (5) feeling of choking; (6) chest pain or discomfort; (7) nausea or abdominal distress; (8) feeling dizzy, unsteady, lightheaded, or faint; (9) derealization (feelings of unreality) or depersonalization (being detached from oneself); (10) fear of losing control or going crazy; (11) fear of dying; (12) paresthesias (numbness or tingling sensations); (13) chills or hot flushes.
  2. At least one of the attacks has been followed by a month (or more) of (a) persistent concern about having additional attacks; (b) worry about the implications of the attack or its consequences (e.g., losing control, having a heart attack, "going crazy"); or (c) a significant change in behavior related to the attacks.
B. Absence of agoraphobia
C. The panic attacks are not due to the direct effects of a substance (e.g., drugs of abuse, medication) or a general medical condition (e.g., hypothyroidism).
D. The anxiety is not better accounted for by another mental disorder, such as obsessive-compulsive disorder (e.g., fear of contamination), post-traumatic stress disorder (e.g., in response to stimuli associated with a severe stressor), separation anxiety disorder, or social phobia (e.g., fear of embarrassment in social situations).

Modified from Diagnostic and Statistical Manual of Mental Disorders, 4th ed. Washington, DC, American Psychiatric Association, 1994.

being in public places, resulting in a marked restriction of travel, often to the point of becoming housebound. In many cases the agoraphobia is secondary to panic attacks: The patient restricts activities for fear of having a panic attack and thereby develops an agoraphobic profile. Consequently, one looks for the presence of panic attacks or panic attack–like symptoms in patients with agoraphobia, as they often respond to the same treatment given for panic attacks. Simple phobias, e.g., fear of flying, heights, snakes, respond better to behavioral management than to drug treatment and are usually associated with generalized anxiety rather than panic-like episodes.

EPIDEMIOLOGY. Recent epidemiologic studies of panic disorder have noted a prevalence rate of 0.4 to 1.2 per 100. The rates are highest in persons aged 25 to 44 years and in the separated and divorced. The rates are lowest in persons over the age of 64 and bear no relationship to race or education. For agoraphobia the prevalence rates are between 2.5 and 5.8 per 100. There is a marked prevalence for women (two to four times that of men), with an age range of 18 to 64 years. The rates for generalized anxiety disorder range from 2.5 to 6.4 per 100, again slightly more common in young women. Genetic studies have shown that monozygotic twins have higher concordance for anxiety disorders than do dizygotic twins when the proband has panic disorder but not when he/she has a generalized anxiety disorder.

PATHOPHYSIOLOGY. Panic attacks can be precipitated in susceptible patients by sodium lactate infusions, caffeine (PO), CO_2 inhalation, yohimbine (PO), isoproterenol (IV), and benzodiazepine receptor antagonists. All of these agents interact with the noradrenergic system and particularly the locus coeruleus system, which contains most of the brain's noradrenergic cell bodies.

TREATMENT. Two major treatments are available for panic attacks, one pharmacologic, the other psychological. The key to treatment is the establishment of a supportive relationship with the patient. Affected patients are often frightened, concerned about "going crazy" and/or dying, and somewhat ashamed of their symptoms. It is useful for the physician immediately to reassure the patient by clarifying that what he/she experiences is part of a well-known illness that causes these feelings. It is often useful to educate patients with appropriate reading material.

Well-controlled studies have demonstrated the effective treatment of panic attacks with tricyclic antidepressants (particularly imipramine), MAOI's (particularly phenelzine), and the benzodiazepines (particularly alprazolam). The doses and treatment pattern of the tricyclics and the MAOI's are similar to those used for affective disorders, and the dose of alprazolam is usually between 4 and

6 mg per day. At times β-blocking agents offer relief, but not so dramatically as the antidepressants and alprazolam. The doses of the antidepressants may need to be somewhat higher for these conditions than for affective disorders (tricyclics are usually used in the range of 150 to 300 mg*; the MAOI's in the range of 60 mg* or more per day). The new serotonin reuptake inhibitors are also effective in anxious patients but should be given in very small doses owing to their tendency to cause increased agitation. Pharmacologic treatment should last for 6 months to 1 year after response, with the drugs then gradually tapered. β-Blocking agents can be useful for treating the tachycardia and palpitations associated with panic attacks. β Blockers can also be used to decrease the cardiac symptoms associated with tricyclic use, which is often reassuring to the patient.

The treatment of generalized anxiety disorders has less clear guidelines. Although benzodiazepines and psychologic interventions are commonly emphasized, their benefit is more difficult to evaluate. A patient on benzodiazepines for 6 to 12 months may experience withdrawal symptoms on cessation of medication. Furthermore, one must be concerned and cautious about the addicting potential of the benzodiazepines and to some extent the tricyclics. Consequently, the treatment of generalized anxiety disorders should rely heavily on counseling, relaxation techniques, behavioral modification, exercise, and similar modalities rather than on prolonged pharmacologic interventions.

Certain medical conditions can simulate panic attacks and must be excluded. These include arrhythmias, angina, respiratory illnesses, asthma, obstructive pulmonary disease, various endocrine disturbances (hyperthyroidism, pheochromocytoma), seizure disorders, vertiginous conditions, pharmacologic stimulants and caffeine, and withdrawal syndromes, particularly from CNS depressants, e.g., alcohol, barbiturates, or occasionally, benzodiazepines. Medical conditions that are often noted in patients with severe panic attacks include episodic hypertension, peptic ulcer disorder, and mitral valve prolapse.

Sequelae of the Vietnam conflict brought attention to *post-traumatic stress disorders*. The basic differentiation of post-traumatic stress disorder from generalized anxiety disorder is the presence of a clear antecedent that could potentially cause distress in almost anyone. Another major characteristic of post-traumatic stress disorder is the re-experiencing of the trauma, through either recurring or intrusive recollections, dreams, or sudden feelings that the event is about to recur. Affected persons often exhibit a lack of emotional responsiveness or involvement with the world after the trauma. Other symptoms may include hyperalertness, heightened "startle responses," sleep disturbance, guilt, and memory and concentration difficulties. Affected persons may avoid activities that could evoke recollections of the traumatic event. Although medications are sometimes useful for acute symptoms (especially if accompanied by panic attacks or depressive symptoms), the major treatment of post-traumatic stress is psychotherapeutic, particularly group sessions. At times narcosynthesis has been used successfully.

PROGNOSIS IN ANXIETY DISORDERS. The ubiquity of anxiety symptoms and the blurring of panic disorder into generalized anxiety or chronic anxiety and phobic states, as well as a strong association with depressive illness, make a prognosis difficult to establish. In general, panic disorder may run a limited course with episodic patterns; long periods of remission can intervene with no symptomatology at all. Only about one quarter of patients with panic disorder are treated, implying a high incidence of spontaneous remission in cases that do not come to medical attention. Nevertheless, many patients become housebound for a significant part of their lives. Follow-up studies of 5 to 20 years' duration show that about 50 to 60% of the patients recovered or were much improved. Drug abuse and alcoholism are potentially serious complications.

Katon W: Panic Disorder in the Medical Setting. Washington, DC, American Psychiatric Press, 1991. *An excellent overview of the relation between anxiety and somatic symptoms.*

Roy-Byrne P: Anxiety: New Findings for the Clinician. Washington, DC, American Psychiatric Press, 1988. *A comprehensive summary of diagnostic and treatment studies of anxiety disorders.*

Sonnenberg S, Blank A, Talbott J: The Trauma of War. Washington, DC, American Psychiatric Press, 1985. *A good review of current knowledge on post-traumatic stress disorder.*

---

* Exceeds manufacturer's recommended dosage.

SOMATIZATION DISORDERS

Somatization disorders consist of psychologically engendered symptoms suggesting organ dysfunction for which associated physical or laboratory evidence of dysfunction is either absent or trivial in relation to the degree of complaint. If physicians can find no clear biologic mechanism for a set of symptoms because they are too vague, diffuse, or disparate (or even anatomically impossible) and the symptoms could fulfill some purpose in the patient's life (e.g., would help to avoid some area of responsibility, deny failure, or evoke increased attention by the family or others), they should suspect a purely psychologic disorder. However, these patients should not be treated lightly. Many vague symptoms arise early in organic disease, and patients must be examined carefully, supported, and followed. Similarly, patients with unfounded symptoms should also be evaluated for major depression and panic disorder, as persons with these conditions can present primarily with somatic complaints. Patients who tend toward somatization often have histories that are characterized by disturbed interpersonal relations and emotional disruptions (Table 401–11).

Diverse disorders can present as medically unfounded somatic symptoms, including hypochondriasis, conversion disorder (hysteria), psychogenic pain disorders, factitious disorders, and malingering. What ties these conditions together are the following characteristics: (1) symptoms that suggest a physical disorder; (2) no demonstrable clinical signs or evident physiologic abnormality; (3) evidence that the symptoms may be associated with psychological factors; (4) symptoms that do not seem to be under voluntary control (except in malingering and factitious disorder).

DIAGNOSTIC CRITERIA AND CLINICAL SIGNS AND SYMPTOMS. Somatization disorders include a wide variety and number of symptoms (Table 401–12). The remarkable phenomenon is the lack of accompanying physical or important laboratory abnormalities. The syndrome occurs mostly in females, with a population incidence of about 1%. The condition runs in families; in men it correlates with the occurrence of sociopathy and alcoholism rather than somatic symptoms.

PATHOPHYSIOLOGY. The condition is marked by an empiric collection of symptoms, the exact cause and pathophysiology of which are not understood. Most patients have limited education and lack sophistication; however, there are many exceptions to this characterization. Most explanations have been sociologic and psychological and center on the somatization as a signal of personal distress. Consequently the behavior is often interpreted as a way to obtain help from caregivers or as a mechanism of obtaining social supports and, perhaps, manipulating relationships. It has also been postulated to represent a cognitive style whereby somatic symptoms are used in place of emotional expression.

TREATMENT. These patients are difficult to treat effectively. Perhaps the most important factor should be an attempt to rule out depressive and panic disorders. Patients with somatization disorders can persuade physicians that there is an urgent need to intervene; however, this temptation should be resisted. Careful evaluation of the history is extremely important for, as is evident, most of them do not respond to treatment. It is not that they enjoy their pain but that they are seeking other things, e.g., attention, relief from other problems. Perhaps the most important thing the physician can con-

TABLE 401–11. COMMON FEATURES IN THE HISTORIES OF PATIENTS WITH SOMATIZATION SYMPTOMS

1. Developmental histories of gross neglect, child abuse, and/or sexual abuse
2. Unstable adult relationships characterized by multiple divorces and often physical violence
3. Past family histories of alcoholism
4. A past history of alcohol abuse prior to the start of somatization
5. Past history of substance abuse
6. A positive review of systems on medical history
7. A polysurgery history
8. A history of litigious relationships with authority figures
9. Past history of psychiatric illness
10. Modeling of pain behavior in their families as way of solving problems and coping with intimate relationships

TABLE 401-12. SOMATIZATION DISORDER

A. A history of many physical complaints beginning before the age of 30, occurring over a period of several years, and resulting in treatment being sought or significant impairment in social or occupational functioning.

B. Each of the following criteria must have been met at some time during the course of the disorder. To count a symptom as significant, it must not be fully explained by a known general medical condition, or the resulting complaint or impairment is in excess of what would be expected from the history, physical examination, or laboratory findings.
1. *Four pain symptoms:* A history of pain related to at least four different sites or functions (such as head, abdomen, back, joints, extremities, chest, rectum, during sexual intercourse, during menstruation, or during urination).
2. *Two gastrointestinal symptoms:* A history of at least two gastrointestinal symptoms other than pain (such as nausea, diarrhea, bloating, vomiting other than during pregnancy, or intolerance of several different foods).
3. *One sexual symptom:* A history of at least one sexual or reproductive symptom other than pain (such as sexual indifference, erectile or ejaculatory dysfunction, irregular menses, excessive menstrual bleeding, vomiting throughout pregnancy).
4. *One pseudoneurologic symptom:* A history of at least one symptom or deficit suggesting a neurologic disorder not limited to pain (conversion symptoms such as blindness, double vision, deafness, loss of touch or pain sensation, hallucinations, aphonia, impaired coordination or balance, paralysis or localized weakness, difficulty swallowing, difficulty breathing, urinary retention, seizures, dissociative symptoms such as amnesia, or loss of consciousness other than fainting).

Modified from Diagnostic and Statistical Manual of Mental Disorders, 4th ed. Washington, DC, American Psychiatric Association, 1994.

vey to patients is that they will neither seriously worsen nor die, and although the physician may not know the cause of the complaint he is willing to support them through the illness episode. In fact, it is almost paradoxic that by scheduling these patients for frequent regular visits the doctor often not only saves time but may decrease the patient's need to develop symptoms in order to be seen. After the clinician becomes certain of the diagnosis and of the absence of a pathologic process, laboratory studies should be kept to a minimum, as the more tests that are ordered, the more the patient becomes convinced that something is wrong. The tendency to dispense medications to these patients not only invites addiction but produces such a confusion and plethora of drugs that they become a cause of untoward symptoms. The major goal of treatment should be to keep to a minimum the medical and surgical interventions. A general attempt should be made to substitute inquiry into the patient's life as opposed to procedures. The most helpful attitude for the doctor to adopt is to be more interested in maintaining the relationship than in curing the symptoms and to emphasize that a successful outcome is to reduce the number of doctors the patient sees and the number and amount of medicines he/she takes. The scheduling of visits can be based on the frequency of visits over the past 2- to 3-month period.

PROGNOSIS. Somatization disorders are more a way of life than a discrete episodic illness. The patient maintains a propensity for expression of emotional need or distress with somatic symptoms. Although the episodes may wax and wane, it is clear that these patients are wedded to the medical establishment.

Other Conditions Associated with Somatic Symptoms

Although the term *hysteria* has been dropped from official use and such conditions are now termed *conversion reactions,* such patients make up about 1% of a neurologist's practice. The predominant disturbance in conversion disorder is a loss or alteration in physical functioning suggesting a physical disorder. As a rule, the loss or distortion of neurologic function is not fully explained by any known disease detectable by physical and laboratory examination. Much of what has been covered with regard to somatization disorder is true of hysterical conditions. These patients do not necessarily have histrionic personalities. They do have physical complaints, but when examined closely their symptoms fail to indicate anatomic-physiologic patterns; rather, they conform more to a psychological reaction.

Hypochondriasis is often simple to recognize in that the patient presents with a belief that a disease is present for which diagnosis and treatment are necessary. The complaints are more circumscribed, with often minute examination and description of bodily functions to the physician. As the physician talks to the patient he becomes increasingly aware that the patient is more concerned about the belief of illness than the discomfort from symptoms. In fact, the symptoms are not especially distressing or painful. This is in marked contrast to the patient with chronic pain whose pain is often out of proportion to the physical findings.

In patients with chronic pain, the continuation of the pain often allows the avoidance of activities in the patient's life or the obtaining of emotional or financial support from others. Affected patients frequently have histories of addiction, seeing many physicians, and undergoing multiple surgical procedures.

The genesis of many of the above conditions lies at an involuntary level in that the symptoms and the motivation for them lie outside the conscious control of the patient. Two conditions, factitious disorder and malingering, are voluntarily controlled by the patient. These patients, often described as having *Münchausen's syndrome,* induce illnesses in themselves, e.g., fevers (by injection), dermatitis, blood disease (anemia), or seizures. Affected patients are often associated with the health professions, and one can discern no clear goal or gain from their behavior. They frequently are peripatetic, traveling from hospital to hospital. When a factitious disorder is diagnosed, these patients should be confronted openly as to their behavior and what treatment (as some may be necessary) will or will not be provided. In true malingering, the goal of the illness behavior is often evident (or evident after extensive inquiry), and the condition is usually less a chronic than a factitious disorder. Most cases consist of partial malingering, in which an individual exaggerates symptoms of a real disease or attributes a voluntarily induced disability to an accident or injury. In these conditions the physician tends to be angry with the patient, but it is better to confront him or her about the situation in a nonjudgmental manner. Particularly when compensation issues surround the case, treatment is pointless until legal questions or damage awards are settled.

Katon W, Egan K, Miller D: Chronic pain: Lifetime psychiatric diagnosis and family history. Am J Psychiatry 142:1156, 1985. *An interesting study of the relationship between pain syndromes and psychiatric problems.*

Marsden CD: Hysteria—A neurologist's view. Psychol Med 16:277, 1986. *An excellent review of hysteria.*

Quill T: Somatization disorder. JAMA 254:3075, 1985. *A good discussion of the physician's role in the treatment of patients with somatic disorder.*

Smith R: Somatization Disorder in the Medical Setting. Washington, DC, American Psychiatric Press, 1991. *Emphasizes importance of the ability to diagnose somatization disorder in the primary care setting.*

Section Three—
Pathophysiology and
Management of Major
Neurologic Symptoms

402 AUTONOMIC DISORDERS AND THEIR MANAGEMENT

Clifford B. Saper

Disorders of the autonomic nervous system are of great importance to internal medicine, as they can present as disorders of virtually any organ system in the body. Furthermore, the central regulation of autonomic response is closely tied to neuroendocrine control, and both are often involved by central disorders. Aspects of neuroendocrine disease are discussed in Chapters 200 to 202 and 204. This chapter focuses on disorders of the autonomic nervous system (Table 402–1) and discusses them in the overall context of diseases affecting basic integrative functions of the nervous system.

DISORDERS OF PERIPHERAL AUTONOMIC FUNCTION

The peripheral autonomic nervous system consists of three main divisions: the *parasympathetic* division, which includes the outflow from the cranial nerves and the low lumbar and sacral spinal cord; the *sympathetic* division, which comprises the autonomic outflow from the thoracic and high lumbar segments of the spinal cord; and the *enteric* nervous system, which includes neurons that are intrinsic to the wall of the gut. The details of the organization of the peripheral autonomic nervous system are covered in basic anatomy and physiology texts.

Knowledge about the different neurotransmitter and receptor types associated with the peripheral autonomic nervous system has resulted in the availability of a wide range of drugs to modify autonomic responses. Some key autonomic drugs and their clinical uses are listed in Table 402–2. These are covered in detail in clinical pharmacology texts.

Pandysautonomias

ACUTE PANDYSAUTONOMIA. Widespread failure of the autonomic nervous system may evolve acutely or subacutely as part of a parainfectious inflammatory polyneuropathy (of the Guillain-Barré type). In rare cases, the autonomic neuropathy predominates and, when severe, may be life threatening. Wide swings in blood pressure and heart rate occur but usually reverse themselves in a few minutes. Generally, putting the patient into the Trendelenberg position is sufficient to maintain cerebral perfusion during hypotensive periods. Cardiac arrhythmias of all types may occur, presumably as a result of the instability of autonomic innervation of the cardiac conducting system. These must be treated gingerly, as the underlying conduction abnormality may change very rapidly.

TETANUS. A similar subacute pandysautonomia is also seen in severe cases of tetanus. Tetanus toxin, elaborated by *Clostridium tetani* organisms in an infected wound, is transported by autonomic as well as motor axons back to the spinal cord, where it is taken up by and inactivates the terminals of inhibitory interneurons. Treatment of the motor manifestations of tetanus by paralyzing and sedating the patient does little to abate the autonomic storm. Up to 40% of patients with tetanus in an intensive care environment may suffer cardiac arrest as a result of arrhythmias. They are generally easily resuscitated with standard measures.

CHRONIC AUTONOMIC NEUROPATHY. The axons of the peripheral autonomic nervous system generally are of small caliber and poorly myelinated or unmyelinated. Certain polyneuropathies that have a predilection for small-diameter axons can result in autonomic changes. *Amyloid neuropathy* often includes a major autonomic component that may present as a gastrointestinal motility disorder or orthostatic hypotension. Similarly, *diabetic neuropathy*, although it is often dominated by sensory or motor complaints, may cause widespread autonomic failure. The neuropathy of *acute inter-*

TABLE 402–1. DISORDERS OF THE AUTONOMIC NERVOUS SYSTEM

Peripheral Autonomic Disorders
  Pandysautonomias
    Acute pandysautonomia
    Tetanus
    Chronic autonomic neuropathy
    Familial dysautonomia
    Idiopathic autonomic insufficiency (Shy-Drager syndrome)
  Regional dysautonomia
    Horner's syndrome
    Paraspinal tumors
    Somatosympathetic dysreflexia
    Reflex sympathetic dystrophy (causalgia)
  Disorders of specific autonomic functions
    Pupillary disorders
      Horner's syndrome
      Oculomotor paresis
    Cardiovascular disorders
      Glossopharyngeal neuralgia
      Carotid sinus hypersensitivity
    Sweating disorders
      Hyperhidrosis
      Anhydrosis
    Gastrointestinal disorders
      Disorders of motility
      Vomiting
    Genitourinary disorders
      Incontinence
      Urinary retention
      Spastic bladder
      Impotence

Disorders of Central Autonomic Integration
  Emotional disorders
    Panic disorder
    Psychosomatic illness
    Cardiac arrhythmias
  Thermoregulatory disorders
    Poikilothermia
    Paroxysmal hypothermia
    Hyperthermia and fever
    Neuroleptic malignant syndrome
  Feeding disorders
    Hyperphagia and obesity
    Hypophagia and inanition
  Disorders of fluid and electrolyte regulation
    Hypernatremia, hyperosmolality, and absence of thirst
    Hyperdipsia, hyponatremia, and water intoxication
    Paroxysmal hyponatremia
  Central reproductive disorders
  Arousal disorders
    Hypersomnolence
    Insomnia

TABLE 402-2. SYSTEMIC EFFECTS OF SOME COMMONLY USED AUTONOMIC DRUGS

Receptor Type	Drug Type (example)	Tissue	Effect
Muscarinic cholinergic	Antagonist (atropine)	Pupil	Mydriasis
		Salivary gland	Dry mouth
		Bronchi	Dilation
		Heart	Tachycardia
		Gut	Decreased motility and secretion
α-Adrenergic	Antagonist (phenoxybenzamine)	Blood vessels	Vasodilation
α$_1$-Adrenergic	Agonist (phenylephrine)	Blood vessels	Vasoconstriction
	Antagonist (prazosin)	Blood vessels	Vasodilation
β-Adrenergic	Agonist (isoproterenol)	Heart	Increased rate and contractility
β$_1$-Adrenergic	Antagonist (metoprolol)	Blood vessels	Decreased rate and contractility
β$_2$-Adrenergic	Agonist (terbutaline)	Bronchi	Dilation

mittent porphyria or certain toxic agents, such as *Vacar* (a rat poison), may have a prominent autonomic component. Acute poisoning with *organophosphate insecticides* that block acetylcholinesterase results in a hypercholinergic state, including miosis and cardiac slowing, that lasts for several days. The neuropathy that follows several weeks later usually does not have a strong autonomic component. Other peripheral neuropathies that may have an autonomic component are listed in Table 402–3.

CHRONIC DYSAUTONOMIA. Recessively inherited *familial dysautonomia* of the Riley-Day type is most commonly seen in Ashkenazi Jewish children. Symptoms referable to the autonomic nervous system and relative indifference to pain are present from birth.

Idiopathic autonomic insufficiency of the *Shy-Drager* type may develop as a chronic degenerative condition in middle age or late adult life owing to loss of neurons in the autonomic ganglia as well as in the preganglionic cell groups in the medulla and spinal cord. The presenting complaint is often orthostatic hypotension, but signs or symptoms of pupillary, gastrointestinal, genitourinary, sweating, or other autonomic abnormalities are elicited on history and physical examination.

Idiopathic autonomic insufficiency is distinguished from non-neurologic causes of orthostatic hypotension by the lack of compensatory tachycardia, indicating impairment of either the peripheral or central components of the baroreceptor reflex. Severe autonomic neuropathy affecting the glossopharyngeal or vagus nerves may also impair the baroreceptor response but is typically associated with other evidence of sensory or motor neuropathy. Other cardiovascular signs include loss of sinus arrhythmia and absence of normal overshoot in the diastolic blood pressure during phase IV of the Valsalva maneuver. An abnormally accentuated blood pressure re-

sponse to intravenous infusion of norepinephrine is consistent with widespread denervation supersensitivity. A detailed list of tests of autonomic insufficiency is provided in Table 402–4.

Idiopathic autonomic insufficiency is part of a spectrum of disorders, ranging from isolated orthostatic hypotension, with or without parkinsonian features, to *multisystem atrophy* with evidence of cerebellar and extrapyramidal involvement. When idiopathic autonomic insufficiency is associated with a multisystem neurologic degenerative disease, it may be accompanied by ataxia, rigidity, bradykinesia, tremors, weakness, or other neurologic disturbances. Additional cell loss is seen in other affected areas in multisystem atrophy.

Orthostatic hypotension is generally the most disabling aspect of autonomic degeneration. Indomethacin may be effective in selected patients. Other patients require elastic stockings or even entire lower body suits to reduce blood pooling in the lower extremities during standing. Treatment with mineralocorticoids, such as fludrocortisone, can expand intravascular blood volume and cause elevation of blood pressure in all positions. In such patients, the head of the bed should be elevated in recumbency to minimize hypertensive effects on the brain. Occasionally, oral sympathomimetic agents, such as ephedrine, or monoamine oxidase inhibitors are employed. The latter must be used with caution, as the ingestion of vasoactive amines present in many common foods, including certain wines, cheeses, pickled foods, and smoked meats, can cause severe hypertension.

Regional Dysautonomia

The segmental organization of the sympathetic nervous system can result in regional disturbances of function. The most common of these is caused by injury to the cranial sympathetic innervation arising from the superior cervical ganglion, or *Horner's syndrome*. Miosis, ptosis, and anhydrosis may occur if the ascending sympathetic fibers are injured below the level at which they enter the skull with the internal carotid artery. Damage to sympathetic fibers along the course of the intracranial carotid artery produces only oculosympathetic paresis (Raeder's syndrome). Unfortunately, this difference is only of marginal value clinically, as the Horner's syndrome produced by extracranial lesions is often incomplete. Lesions of the central descending sympathoexcitatory pathway, running through the lateral portions of the brain stem from the hypothalamus to the spinal cord, may produce a central Horner's syndrome, in which there is miosis and ptosis as well as loss of sweating over the entire ipsilateral body. Postganglionic Horner's syndrome can be differentiated from preganglionic or central lesions by pharmacologic testing (Table 402–4). The most common cause of Horner's syndrome is atherosclerotic disease affecting the vasa nervorum originating in the carotid artery. However, Horner's syndrome may also be seen when an intrathoracic or cervical tumor involves the sympathetic chain. Hence, evaluation of Horner's syndrome should include radiographic or magnetic resonance examination of the pulmonary apices and paracervical area.

Paraspinal tumors at lower levels along the sympathetic chain may cause loss of sweating over the involved dermatomes. This deficit can be appreciated by running the handle of a tuning fork down the skin in the paraspinal region. The smooth movement is interrupted by the dry skin at the level of the lesion. Occasionally, compression of a midthoracic spinal root, which carries visceral sensory fibers, by a disc or tumor may present as abdominal pain.

TABLE 402-3. PERIPHERAL NEUROPATHIES THAT MAY HAVE AN AUTONOMIC COMPONENT

Autonomic symptoms often prominent
  Guillain-Barré syndrome
  Amyloid neuropathy
  Diabetic neuropathy
  Acute intermittent porphyria
  Vacar (rat poison)
Autonomic symptoms may occur
  Renal failure
  Toxic neuropathies
    Vinca alkaloids
    Perhexiline maleate
    Thallium
    Arsenic
    Mercury
    Organic solvents
    Acrylamide
  Vasculitis
    Systemic lupus erythematosus
    Rheumatoid arthritis
    Mixed connective tissue disease
  Thiamine deficiency
  Leprosy
  Charcot-Marie-Tooth disease
  Fabry's disease

TABLE 402–4. TESTS OF AUTONOMIC FUNCTION*

Test	Interpretation
Pupillary responses	
4% cocaine	Pupillodilatation indicates release of normal catecholamine stores.
1% hydroxyamphetamine	Pupillodilatation indicates denervation supersensitivity.
1% phenylephrine	
0.1% epinephrine	
0.1% pilocarpine	Pupilloconstriction indicates denervation supersensitivity.
2.5% methacholine	
Sweating responses	
Thermal sweating	Regional absence of sweating indicates sympathetic cholinergic denervation.
Galvanic skin response	Increased conductivity under mild stress indicates normal adrenergic innervation.
1:1000 pilocarpine	Intradermal injection causes axon reflex sweating.
1:10,000 acetylcholine	
Axon reflex	
1:1000 histamine	Intradermal injection normally causes wheal and flare.
Cardiovascular responses	
Orthostatic challenge	Pulse normally increases and diastolic blood pressure falls < 15 mm Hg.
Carotid sinus massage	Normally causes fall in blood pressure and heart rate.
R-R interval	Normally increases during inspiration (sinus arrhythmia).
Valsalva maneuver	Longest to shortest R-R interval ratio normally is ≥ 1.4.
Cold pressor test	Immersing hand in ice water normally increases blood pressure and heart rate.
Plasma catecholamines	Normally increase response to standing or stress.
Norepinephrine infusion 0.05 μg/kg/min	Diastolic blood pressure increase ≥ 20 mm Hg indicates supersensitivity.
Genitourinary, rectal responses	
Cremasteric reflex	Stroking skin of thigh normally causes testicular retraction.
Anal wink reflex	Scratching perianal skin normally causes anal sphincter contraction.
Bulbocavernosus reflex	Squeezing glans penis or clitoris normally causes anal sphincter contraction.

* For details see McLeod and Tuck, 1987.

Stimulation of pain fibers at any level results in both local (spino-spinal) and generalized (spino-bulbo-spinal) *somatosympathetic reflex responses,* including sweating, vasoconstriction, and pupillodilatation. In patients with a pre-existing spinal cord transection, a noxious stimulus below the level of the transection may produce only local sympathetic reflex responses. Hence it is important in the paraplegic patient to investigate asymmetric sympathetic responses for a local lesion that might cause pain in an intact individual.

Following injury to peripheral nerves, aberrant regeneration may result in *reflex sympathetic dystrophy.* It is believed that the sympathetic efferent fibers form excitatory synapses along the course of damaged peripheral sensory nerves. Normally innocuous sensory stimulation, such as covering the affected limb with a sheet or with clothing, may cause excruciating burning pain, associated with variable autonomic changes. Atrophic changes in the skin and bone may reflect abnormal sympathetic innervation or disuse. Relief can sometimes be obtained with guanethidine or phenoxybenzamine. If regional sympathetic block alleviates pain, removal of the affected ganglion can produce permanent relief.

Disorders of Specific Autonomic Functions

PUPILS. Anisocoria, asymmetry of pupillary size, may reflect a deficit of sympathetic innervation of the smaller pupil (causing miosis) or parasympathetic innervation of the larger one (causing mydriasis). Because both the oculosympathetic and oculomotor (parasympathetic) innervations participate in lid elevation, ptosis if present generally indicates the abnormal eye. Anisocoria may be longstanding and of little clinical significance, but pupillary asymmetry of recent onset should be evaluated by a neurologist. Impairment of sympathetic innervation of the iris (pupillodilator) muscle is not always accompanied by ptosis or a sweating deficit (Horner's syndrome). The pupilloconstrictor fibers travel in the dorsomedial part of the oculomotor nerve, where they may be selectively affected by temporal lobe herniation or by an aneurysm of the posterior communicating artery. Pharmacologic testing may aid in the identification of the pupillary abnormality (Table 402–4). The most common cause of a large pupil is instillation of atropinic eye drops or application of a scopolamine patch near the face (to prevent motion sickness); the pharmacologically dilated pupil does not respond even to strong solutions of pilocarpine. Another common cause of a large, poorly reactive pupil is *Adie's syndrome,* an idiopathic condition involving degeneration of the ciliary ganglion. The pupil usually shows sector paralysis and constriction with accommodation, and it dilates and responds to light after a period in complete darkness. The abnormal pupil responds briskly to 0.1% pilocarpine (Table 402–4), and there is concomitant loss of tendon reflexes in most cases.

CARDIOVASCULAR. The baroreceptor reflex is an important protective response, causing bradycardia and peripheral vasodilatation to counteract an acute increase in blood pressure, or the reverse response during hypotension. The afferent fibers for the response run in the glossopharyngeal (carotid sinus) and vagus (aortic depressor) nerves, whereas the efferent response includes both parasympathetic and sympathetic components. Injury to the glossopharyngeal or carotid sinus nerves in the neck (often by a tumor) can cause episodic attacks of hypotension and bradycardia, which often present as syncope. In most cases, there is an associated pain or paresthesia in the cutaneous distribution of the glossopharyngeal nerve (in the external auditory meatus or the pharynx), known as *glossopharyngeal neuralgia.* The situation is analogous to tic doloreaux, in which there are intermittent volleys of firing in the affected nerve. Atropine or a transvenous pacemaker may prevent the bradycardia associated with the attacks, but loss of vasoconstrictor tone sometimes results in symptomatic hypotension despite these maneuvers. Anticonvulsants, particularly phenytoin and carbamazepine, may prevent the attacks.

Carotid sinus syncope (see Ch. 396) is a condition seen most commonly in elderly individuals with carotid atherosclerosis. Even mild pressure over the carotid bulb, such as a tight shirt collar, can produce a full-blown carotid sinus response, resulting in syncope. The diagnosis is made by gently compressing the carotid artery below the angle of the jaw while the electrocardiogram (ECG) is monitored. Facilities for cardiac resuscitation must be immediately available, as the compression may result in sinus arrest. Vigorous massage should be avoided, as it may dislodge an embolus, resulting in a transient or even permanent neurologic deficit. Treatment of carotid sinus hypersensitivity is the same as that for glossopharyngeal neuralgia.

SWEATING. Human sweat glands are innervated by both noradrenergic sympathetic fibers (mediating emotional responses) and cholinergic sympathetic fibers (thermal sweating). Certain somatosympathetic reflexes can produce generalized or regional sweating, in response to innocuous or noxious somatosensory stimuli. *Paroxysmal localized hyperhidrosis* is a rare condition that probably represents an exaggeration of normal somatosympathetic reflexes. Generalized hyperhidrosis, particularly involving the hands and the soles of the feet, is most likely a normal variant. Drugs directed at interrupting α-adrenergic transmission (phenoxybenzamine, clonidine) have been useful in some cases of localized hyperhidrosis. In extreme cases, regional sympathectomy has been performed.

Idiopathic anhydrosis may be segmental or generalized. This rare condition is sometimes associated with Adie's syndrome (Ross syndrome), but in other cases there are no other signs of autonomic impairment. In some cases the impairment is preganglionic and in others postganglionic, as judged by the axon reflex sweating response (Table 402–4). In most recorded patients, the deficits have been stable and did not go on to involve other autonomic functions.

GASTROINTESTINAL. Disorders of intestinal motility, which may be due to damage to the parasympathetic innervation of the gut or to dysfunction of the enteric nervous system itself, are discussed in Chapter 101. Specific abnormalities of esophageal contraction and colonic tone have been noted in patients suffering from depression and may predict response to antidepressant medication.

Vomiting is a neurally mediated gastrointestinal reflex that is coordinated by neurons in the medullary reticular formation. Chemical emetic agents such as certain narcotics or dopaminergic agonists act at the area postrema, a chemosensory zone on the fourth ventricular surface of the medulla, to elicit the vomiting reflex. Local dopaminergic connections are thought to mediate the response, and antidopaminergic drugs such as prochlorperazine may act at the level of the area postrema to suppress vomiting. Intractable vomiting without any gastrointestinal abnormalities has been reported in certain patients with tumors involving the medullary cell groups controlling vomiting or their connections. Treatment of the tumor with steroids and radiation therapy generally results in improvement.

GENITOURINARY. The urinary bladder is composed of interlacing smooth muscle fibers of the detrusor covered by an internal mucous membrane and an outer serosa. The detrusor is innervated by parasympathetic neurons located in the intermediolateral column at the second through fourth sacral segments. Additional motor neurons located in the ventral horn at the same levels constitute Onuf's nucleus. Their axons run through the pelvic nerve to innervate striated accessory muscles of micturition (including the external urethral sphincter) in the pelvic floor. Neurons of Onuf's nucleus are strikingly preserved in motor neuron disease but are lost along with autonomic preganglionic cells in idiopathic autonomic insufficiency. The internal sphincter at the bladder neck is innervated via the hypogastric nerve by sympathetic prevertebral pelvic ganglia whose preganglionic innervation arises from the intermediolateral column at the T12–L1 level.

Bladder relaxation during filling and subsequent coordination of micturition are under the control of Barrington's nucleus, located in the floor of the fourth ventricle at the pontine level. Brain stem control of micturition is, in turn, under voluntary regulation by areas within the cerebral sensory and motor cortex. When bladder fullness is sensed and the environmental conditions are appropriate, micturition is initiated by Barrington's nucleus, under forebrain control. There is a fall in external sphincter pressure, resulting in reflex relaxation of the internal sphincter and contraction of the bladder.

Forebrain impairment results in loss of voluntary control of micturition but does not otherwise affect the complex sensory and motor program that results in normal voiding. Incontinence in such patients can be managed by using adult diapers or external urinary collection devices without risk of frequent urinary tract infections or damage to the upper urinary tract. Injury to the bulbospinal pathway from Barrington's nucleus to the sacral intermediolateral column, however, causes major disruption of coordinated bladder function. Acutely following spinal cord injury there is a period of spinal shock, during which the bladder does not undergo reflex contraction as it fills. Such patients require urinary catheterization to prevent vesical and renal damage.

One to 2 weeks following injury, spinal reflex control of the bladder returns. Some patients can induce reflex bladder emptying by somatosensory stimulation, such as stroking the skin over the thigh. The spastic bladder reflexively contracts at a lower volume

TABLE 402–5. SOME COMMONLY PRESCRIBED DRUGS THAT MAY IMPAIR URINARY FUNCTION

Antiarrhythmics	Antiparkinsonian agents
Atropine	Amantadine
Disopyramide	Dopa/carbidopa
Antihistamines	Bromocriptine
Diphenhydramine	Benztropine
Neuroleptics	Trihexyphenidyl
Haloperidol	Antispasmodics
Chlorpromazine	Baclofen
Antidepressants	
Amitriptyline	
Imipramine	

and, because detrusor action is not coordinated with sphincter opening, rarely empties completely. Injury to sensory nerves supplying the bladder also may cause overfilling and incomplete emptying, indicating the importance of sensory feedback in bladder control. Patients with significant postvoid residual urine are at increased risk for urinary tract infections, but bladder overfilling with elevated pressures above 40 mm H_2O may ultimately be a greater problem. Elevations in pressure above 40 mm H_2O may require continuous or intermittent catheterization to prevent damage to the upper urinary tract.

Pharmacologic intervention, aimed at augmenting or suppressing autonomic motor responses of the bladder or internal sphincter, has only limited value. Bethanacol, a cholinergic agonist, is used to augment bladder contraction to improve emptying. It is most effective in combination with an α-adrenergic blocker, such as phenoxybenzamine or prazocin, that simultaneously reduces pressure of the internal sphincter. Baclofen may be used to decrease spastic contraction of the external sphincter. Drugs that have atropinic properties, including a surprising variety of antiarrhythmic, antihistamine, neuroleptic, and antidepressant medications, may inhibit bladder contraction, resulting in overfilling and urinary retention (Table 402–5).

Erectile function in males is under parasympathetic control by the same sacral levels as the urinary system. Sensory afferent fibers travel via the pudendal nerve, while parasympathetic motor fibers run in the pelvic nerve. Sympathetic innervation via the hypogastric nerve contracts the seminal vesicles during ejaculation and closes the bladder neck to prevent retrograde emission. Although supraspinal influences are of great importance, reflex erection and ejaculation can occur in patients after spinal injury. Neurogenic impotence can result either from damage to descending pathways relaying forebrain influence from the hypothalamus to the sacral preganglionic neurons or from injury to the sensory or parasympathetic motor innervation of the penis. A variety of drugs that block either parasympathetic or sympathetic function can interfere with erectile function (Table 402–6). As erections normally occur several times nightly during periods of rapid eye movement sleep, it is possible to document organic disorders of erection by measuring penile tumescence overnight. Disorders of male sexual function are considered in Ch. 209.

TABLE 402–6. SOME COMMONLY PRESCRIBED DRUGS THAT MAY IMPAIR ERECTILE FUNCTION

Drugs causing impotence	Drugs causing priapism
Parasympatholytics	Chlorpromazine
Atropine	Thioridazine
Amitriptyline	Trazodone
Sympatholytics	Prazosin
Methyldopa	Dopa/carbidopa
Guanethidine	
Clonidine	
Propranolol	
Prazosin	
Vasodilators	
Hydralazine	
Diuretics	
Hydrochlorothiazide	
Antihistaminergic	
Cimetidine	

ORGANIZATION OF CENTRAL AUTONOMIC AND ENDOCRINE REGULATION. The autonomic nervous system is under three levels of central control. The *preganglionic* neurons located in the medulla and the spinal cord provide the final common pathway for central autonomic control. Each of these neurons integrates the inputs from many sources, including afferents from higher levels of the nervous system and local reflex responses. A series of *brain stem and spinal* cell groups coordinates *reflex control* of the autonomic nervous system. These nuclei receive cranial (parasympathetic) and spinal (sympathetic) afferent information and control a variety of important reflexes (e.g., swallowing, maintaining blood pressure, initiation of voiding). Both the preganglionic neurons and the brain stem reflex neurons are under the control of *forebrain integrative* cell groups that coordinate autonomic function with behavior and with endocrine control.

The hypothalamus is the most important area for integration of behavior with autonomic responses and with neuroendocrine control of the anterior and posterior pituitary glands (Fig. 402–1). Because the hypothalamus consists of tightly packed, interwoven pathways and cell groups, it is unusual for an injury to involve selectively a single functional system. Nevertheless, considerable progress has been made in determining the anatomic substrates for specific integrative functions, and disorders of these systems are occasionally encountered (Table 402–7). In addition, autonomic dysfunction is a frequent concomitant of emotional disorders.

Emotional Disorders

Portions of the insular and cingulate areas of the cerebral cortex and the amygdala are believed to regulate autonomic responses to emotional stress. In healthy individuals, stress can induce sympathetic responses, such as pupillodilatation, dry mouth, and increases in blood pressure. In patients with *panic disorder* (see Ch. 401), such autonomic responses can become overwhelming and convince the patient that there is a serious organic problem. PET studies show increased metabolism in the structures of the medial temporal lobe and the insular cortex during panic attacks. After eliminating the possibility of pheochromocytoma (see Ch. 204.2), anxiolytic or antidepressant drugs are usually found helpful. Clomipramine is likely to become the drug of choice for this disorder.

In some individuals under chronic emotional stress, a variety of syndromes are seen implicating autonomic control of the internal organs. Although *psychosomatic illness* is often thought to be nonorganic and may respond to psychotherapeutic drugs, there is considerable evidence that some organic disorders seen in anxious

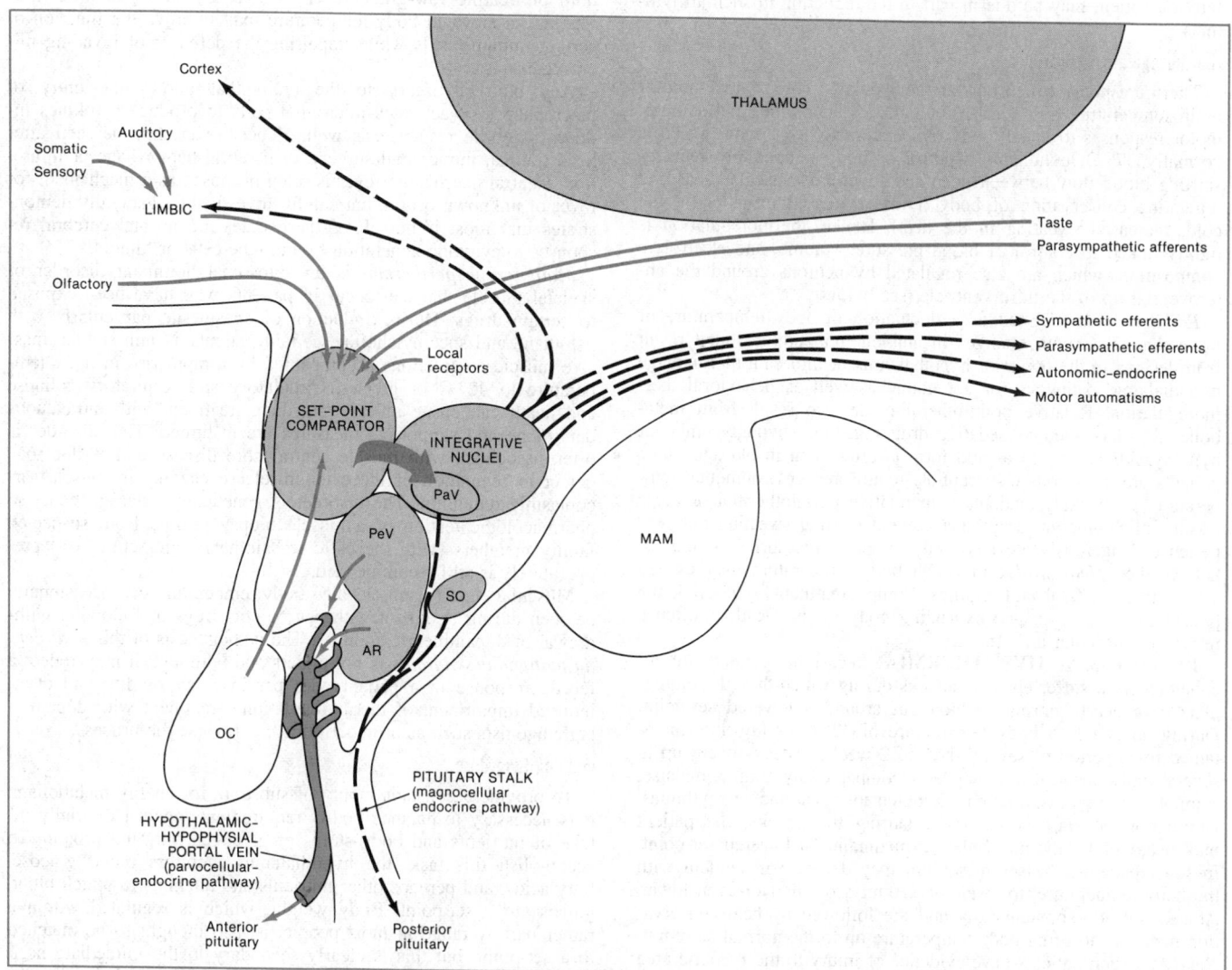

FIGURE 402–1. Schematic illustration of the functional organization of the hypothalamus. General and visceral sensory, limbic, and local interoceptive (e.g., osmolality and temperature) information is compared against a homeostatic set-point by integrative cell groups in the preoptic area and tuberal hypothalamus. Efferent autonomic responses from the paraventricular nucleus (PaV) and lateral hypothalamic area are then integrated with anterior pituitary control via the periventricular (PeV) and arcuate (AR) nuclei and posterior pituitary control via the supraoptic (SO) and paraventricular nuclei, and with behavioral regulation exercised mainly by the lateral hypothalamic area. MAM = mamillary body; OC = optic chiasm. (Amended from Saper CB: Hypothalamus. *In* Pearlman AL, Collins RC (eds): Neurobiology of Disease. New York, Oxford University Press, 1989, p 197.)

TABLE 402–7. REGIONAL HYPOTHALAMIC SYNDROMES

Region	Normally Regulates	Disorders
Preoptic	Blood volume, pressure, and electrolytes	Paroxysmal hyponatremia
		Essential hypernatremia
	Thermoregulation	Paroxysmal hypothermia
Tuberal	Gastrointestinal tract and feeding	Hyperphagia (ventromedial lesions)
		Hypophagia (lateral lesions)
	Reproduction	Hypogonadism
	Emotions	Rage responses
Posterior	Arousal	Hypersomnolence
	Descending autonomic and motor pathways	Poikilothermia

patients also may be caused by autonomic dysregulation. For example, swallowing disorders often represent abnormal control of peristalsis. Erosive gastritis and even frank ulceration may occur as a result of autonomic dysfunction. Perhaps the most serious problems are encountered in patients with pre-existing cardiac abnormalities, who may have cardiac arrhythmias under stressful conditions. Retrospective studies of victims of sudden death due to lethal ventricular arrhythmias indicate a much higher incidence of behavioral stress in the period preceding the attack. The protective affect of β-adrenergic blockers against sudden death in the post-myocardial infarction patient may be due in part to the reduction in such arrhythmias.

Thermoregulatory Disorders

Thermoresponsive neurons in the medial preoptic area monitor brain temperature and activate autonomic, endocrine, and somatomotor responses to match body temperature to a set-point, which is normally 37° C in humans. Control of body temperature requires shifting blood flow between deep and superficial vascular beds and regulating conservation of body fluids (increased urination in the cold, increased sweating in the heat). Hence, thermoregulation is tightly linked to control of blood pressure, volume, and electrolyte composition, which are also regulated by neurons around the anteroventral tip of the third ventricle (see below).

Poikilothermia, defined as a fluctuation in body temperature of more than 2° C with changes in ambient temperature, may result from lesions in the posterior hypothalamus or midbrain that damage hypothalamic pathways for autonomic as well as behavioral thermoregulation. Relative poikilothermia can also result from metabolic disorders such as sedative drug ingestion, hypoglycemia, or hypothyroidism, and in a mild form is often seen in old age. Such patients are dangerously susceptible to lowered environmental temperature. Conversely, patients with relative poikilothermia or those taking anticholinergic drugs that prevent thermal sweating may experience dangerously elevated body temperatures during periods of hot weather. *Heat stroke,* in which body temperature may exceed 42° C, is often fatal and requires prompt treatment by cooling the patient in an ice bath and expanding body fluids. Death is often a result of ventricular arrhythmia.

PAROXYSMAL HYPOTHERMIA. Occasional patients are encountered who suffer episodic attacks during which they thermoregulate in a nearly normal fashion but around a lowered set-point. During an attack, a body temperature of 32° C or lower is maintained for a period of several days to 2 weeks. Attacks occur up to several times per year and may be accompanied by fatigue, malaise, somnolence, hypoventilation, hypotension, cardiac arrhythmias, lacrimation, ataxia, and asterixis. During the attacks, the patient may behaviorally thermoregulate to maintain the lowered set-point. In some patients, the serum sodium may decrease in tandem with the body temperature, to levels of 110 mEq per liter or even lower. Attacks subside spontaneously and are followed by heat conservation measures to bring body temperature up to the normal set-point. Nearly all such patients have evidence of injury to the preoptic area of the hypothalamus. Paroxysmal hypothermia is sometimes seen in patients with agenesis of the corpus callosum, most likely because the corpus callosum and the preoptic area are both embryologic derivatives of the lamina terminalis, which fails to form normally. Anticonvulsants have been prescribed to alleviate attacks but have rarely been effective.

FEVER AND HYPERTHERMIA. During an immune response, macrophages release cytokines, such as interleukin-1 and tumor necrosis factor, that act on neurons or glial cells at the organum vasculosum of the lamina terminalis, a vascular structure outside the blood-brain barrier that sits in the anteroventral tip of the third ventricle, to cause a febrile response. Prostaglandins are a critical mediator for producing fever and some of the endocrine and metabolic changes that accompany it. Fever, an upward resetting of the thermoregulatory set-point, is achieved by normal heat conservation mechanisms, including shivering and behavioral thermoregulation. Drugs that inhibit the generation of prostaglandins are the mainstay of treatment of fever, but there is considerable debate on the wisdom of treating low-grade fever ($< 38.5°$ C) during an infectious illness. An elevated body temperature may improve the function of certain immune cells while impairing the defenses of invading microorganisms.

Any physical injury to the brain that allows the entry of macrophages or activates microglial cells to produce cytokines induces a febrile response as well. Hence, fever may be seen after head trauma, intracranial surgery, or cerebral hemorrhage or infarction. Central neurogenic fever is often proposed as a mechanism for fever of unknown origin, but careful investigation generally demonstrates that most if not all of these cases are normal cerebral responses to cytokine generation by immune cells or tumors.

Malignant hyperthermia is an autosomal dominant disorder of skeletal muscle that can occur in patients who have been exposed to certain drugs. During induction of anesthesia, particularly with halothane and succinylcholine, certain patients sustain sudden massive muscle contractions accompanied by a rapid rise in body temperature to 42° C or greater. Circulatory and respiratory collapse and death can ensue unless immediate treatment with intravenous dantrolene and supportive measures are instituted. This disorder is often associated with muscle central core disease and is due to a defect in regulation of the calcium-release channel in muscle sarcoplasmic reticulum. The disorder is genetically heterogeneous, so pharmacologic testing of a muscle biopsy sample from suspected family members (with the caffeine-halothane contracture test) preoperatively is still recommended.

Muscular rigidity and elevated body temperature can occasionally be seen during treatment with neuroleptic drugs or following withdrawal of dopaminergic agonists. The pathogenesis of this *neuroleptic malignant syndrome* is not understood, although it may reflect a febrile response in a patient with parkinsonian rigidity and drug-induced impairment of thermoregulation. Treatment with dopaminergic agonists such as bromocriptine can reverse the process.

Feeding Disorders

To provide a constant supply of substrate for energy metabolism, it is necessary to balance bodily requirements against the daily intake of nutrients and body stores of glycogen, fat, and protein. To accomplish this task, the hypothalamus monitors blood glucose, fatty acids, and perhaps other nutrients and attempts to match blood glucose to a set-point. Body weight, which is regulated within a rather narrow range in most people, is also thought to be matched to a set-point, but this is clearly secondary to the immediate need for metabolic substrate. The neural mechanisms regulating energy metabolism and feeding are mainly coordinated in the region of the ventromedial nucleus of the hypothalamus and the nearby paraventricular nucleus. The control of feeding is closely related to autonomic control of the gastrointestinal system.

HYPERPHAGIA AND OBESITY. Lesions in the region of the ventromedial nucleus of the hypothalamus can result in massive overeating and obesity. Experimental studies indicate that overeating is largely in response to parasympathetically mediated hyperinsulinemia, causing a chronically lowered blood glucose. Transection of the vagus nerve below the diaphragm corrects insulin secretion and overeating. Hence, hypothalamic hyperphagia is mainly a disorder of autonomic control of the pancreas, with a resultant attempt to defend the blood glucose set-point.

The *Klein-Levin syndrome* is a poorly understood disorder in which patients, typically adolescent boys, have episodic attacks of somnolence, often sleeping up to 20 hours per day. When awake, they appear dull and often confused and consume enormous quantities of food. Attacks may last up to 2 weeks and can recur several times per year. Pathologic verification of the site of the lesion in typical cases is lacking, but a similar syndrome may be seen acutely in encephalitis involving the hypothalamus.

The *Prader-Willi syndrome* is a congenital disorder due to a deletion in chromosome 15, which includes mental retardation, hypogonadism, and hyperphagia, often with massive obesity. The cause of the overeating is not known.

HYPOPHAGIA AND INANITION. Large lesions in the region of the lateral hypothalamic area, at the level of the ventromedial nucleus, result in aphagia, which may recover to hypophagia and regulation around a new, lower body weight set-point. Such lesions, which must be bilateral, are usually devastating, and selective impairment of eating on this basis has rarely been reported in adults. More often, patients with hypothalamic damage and inanition are somnolent and show a variety of endocrine abnormalities. There is no evidence for injury to the hypothalamus in anorexia nervosa.

Children may demonstrate a quite different response to congenital hypothalamic tumors or malformations. In the diencephalic syndrome of infancy, there is profound emaciation, despite good feeding and linear growth. The affected children are often exceptionally good-natured. The difference from adults with similarly placed tumors probably reflects the capacity for plasticity and formation of new neuronal connections during development.

Central Disorders of Fluid and Electrolyte Regulation

The medial preoptic area, around the anteroventral tip of the third ventricle, plays a critical role in regulating blood pressure, volume, and electrolyte composition. Endocrine control (mineralocorticoids and especially vasopressin), autonomic regulation (control of blood flow in different vascular beds, innervation of sweat glands and kidney, especially the juxtaglomerular apparatus controlling renin release), and behavioral response (drinking) all play important roles in this process. Disorders of the release of vasopressin, by neurons whose cell bodies are located in the supraoptic and paraventricular nuclei, are discussed in Ch. 75 and 202.2. Coordinated central disorders of fluid regulation are rare.

HYPERNATREMIA, HYPEROSMOLALITY, ABSENCE OF THIRST. Neurogenic hypernatremia is a rare disorder marked by impairment of the normal responses to osmolar stimuli. Hence, there is a deficit in vasopressin response to increased sodium and osmolality and an absence or relative deficiency of thirst. Vasopressin response to hypovolemia may be maintained, and there is preservation of habitual drinking of water (often related to meals) which may be sufficient to maintain serum osmolality under normal conditions. During hot weather, when there is increased loss of water through evaporation of sweat, patients often fail to increase their water consumption adequately and may suffer attacks of fatigue, fever, muscle cramps and tenderness, and even myoglobinuria (associated with hypokalemia). With serum sodium in excess of 180 mEq per liter, patients may experience confusion or even become stuporous, and some may die.

The hypothalamic injury giving rise to essential hypernatremia has been accurately localized in only a few cases but in all of these seems to involve the preoptic area in the region of the anteroventral third ventricle. Treatment consists of training the patient to drink adequate amounts of fluids, particularly during hot weather. Spironolactone, chlorpropamide, and thiazide diuretics have been used to reduce serum sodium and increase potassium. During an attack of severe hypernatremia, when it becomes necessary to provide intravenous fluid and potassium supplementation, it is important not to reduce serum sodium by more than 20 mEq per liter per day. More rapid correction has been associated with central pontine myelinolysis, which may leave the patient quadriplegic.

HYPERDIPSIA, HYPONATREMIA, AND WATER INTOXICATION. Excessive water drinking in the absence of either hypovolemia or serum hyperosmolality is termed primary hyperdipsia and must be distinguished from the compensatory hyperdipsias of diabetes insipidus, diabetes mellitus, and polyuric renal failure. In the absence of inappropriate vasopressin secretion, symptoms of water intoxication, such as stupor, delirium, or convulsions, are infrequent. Most severe hyperdipsia occurs in persons who have psychiatric disturbances. We have seen only one case of primary hyperdipsia, in a patient who had suffered an attack of encephalitis involving the hypothalamus during childhood.

PAROXYSMAL HYPONATREMIA. Many of the patients with paroxysmal hypothermia (see above) suffer simultaneous hyponatremia, which may be sufficiently severe (serum sodium < 110 mEq per liter) to cause symptoms of confusion or even convulsions. The serum sodium is regulated around the reduced set-point but may respond to fluid restriction.

Central Reproductive Disorders

Reproductive hormonal control, behavior, and the associated autonomic responses are controlled by poorly defined mechanisms in the medial basal hypothalamus overlying the pituitary stalk. To the extent that it relies upon control of blood flow in specific vascular beds, the autonomic regulation of sexual function must be coordinated with control of body temperature and fluid balance. The change in body temperature that accompanies ovulation and the fluid shifts seen in the perimenstrual period in women are examples of this integration.

Reproductive endocrine disorders are covered in Ch. 202.1 and 208.1. Male erectile function, which is dependent upon sacral parasympathetic innervation of the penis, may be affected by diseases of the peripheral autonomic nervous system (see above) as well as psychogenic factors acting at the level of the forebrain. Diagnosis and treatment of male sexual dysfunction is discussed in Ch. 209.

Arousal Disorders

The function of the autonomic nervous system is to augment the activity of various organ systems to deal with perturbations of internal homeostasis. Of all the body's organs, the single most important one to activate during an external threat is the brain. The ascending activating system, running from the brain stem reticular formation to the diencephalon, increases the responsiveness of the forebrain to external stimuli and may be considered a cerebral component of the autonomic system. Ch. 393, 394, and 396 describe the details of altered states of consciousness. We discuss here briefly disorders associated with lesions of the ascending arousal system. Sleep disorders are discussed in Ch. 397.

HYPERSOMNOLENCE. Following lesions of the ascending activating system at the level of the rostral brain stem, there is typically impairment of level of consciousness acutely. After a few weeks, the forebrain recovers spontaneous wake-sleep cycles. Prolonged sleeplike stupor lasting longer than a few weeks is seen only when lesions involve the posterior diencephalon. It is not clear whether this continued somnolence results from injury to the thalamus, to the hypothalamus, or to the connections of these structures. Methylphenidate, amphetamine, and bromocriptine have been used in these patients, with some anecdotal reports of success.

INSOMNIA. Sleep is an active process, requiring the participation of hypnogenic influences arising from the lower brain stem and serotoninergic neurons in the midbrain raphe. We have seen one patient in whom destruction of the medulla, below the level of the ascending activating system, resulted in a chronically wakeful state. Lesions of the preoptic area may also cause a decrease in sleep, which is closely related to a deficit in thermoregulation.

Peripheral Autonomic Disorders

Lefkowitz RL, Hoffman BB, Taylor P: Neurohumoral transmission: The autonomic and somatic motor neuron systems. *In* Gilman AG, Rall TW, Nies AS, Taylor P: The Pharmacological Basis of Therapeutics. New York, Pergamon, 1990, p 84. *A thorough review of peripheral autonomic organization and neurotransmission.*
McGuire EJ: The innervation and function of the lower urinary tract. J Neurosurg 65:278, 1986. *A thoughtful review of the physiology and pathophysiology of micturition.*
McLeod JG, Tuck RR: Disorders of the autonomic nervous system: Part 1. Pathophysiology and clinical features. Ann Neurol 21:419, 1987. *A recent review of autonomic physiology and pathophysiology.*

McLeod JG, Tuck RR: Disorders of the autonomic nervous system: Part 2. Investigation and treatment. Ann Neurol 21:519, 1987. *A guide to pharmacologic testing and treatment of autonomic dysfunction.*

Schwartzman RJ: Reflex sympathetic dystrophy. Curr Opin Neurol Neurosurg 6:531, 1993. *A review of the pathophysiology and clinical aspects of reflex sympathetic dystrophy.*

Central Autonomic Disorders

Loewy AD, Spyer KM: Central Regulation of Autonomic Functions. New York, Oxford Press, 1990. *A comprehensive series of reviews on the central components of the autonomic nervous system.*

Plum F, van Uitert R: Non-endocrine diseases and disorders of the hypothalamus. Res Publ Assoc Res Nerv Ment Dis 56:415, 1977. *A comprehensive review of the integrative disorders of autonomic function.*

Quane KA: Mutations in the ryanodine receptor gene in central core disease and malignant hyperthermia. Nature Genetics 5:51, 1993. *An analysis of the genetics of malignant hyperthermia.*

Saper CB: Hypothalamus. *In* Pearlman AL, Collins RC: Neurobiology of Disease. New York, Oxford Press, 1990, p 197. *A review of hypothalamic regulation of integrated functions and their disorders.*

Saper CB, Breder CD: The neurologic basis of fever. N Engl J Med, 330:1880, 1994. *A review of the mechanisms of fever and hyperthermia.*

Talman WT: Cardiovascular regulation and lesions of the central nervous system. Ann Neurol 18:1, 1985. *A review of central control of the circulation and the effects of nervous system lesions on cardiac arrhythmias and blood pressure control.*

403   THE SPECIAL SENSES
Robert W. Baloh

403.1   Smell and Taste

Approximately 2 million American adults suffer from disorders of taste and smell, yet there is relatively little information available on how to evaluate or treat these patients. These disorders have been neglected because they are seldom fatal and, unlike abnormalities of vision and hearing, are not considered serious handicaps. Chemosensory disorders, however, often reduce the enjoyment and quality of life and are important to patients who suffer from them. Disorders of taste interfere with digestion because taste stimulants alter salivary and pancreatic flow, gastric contractions, and intestinal motility. Smell also contributes to the anticipation and ingestion of food because much of what we taste derives from olfactory stimulation during ingestion and chewing. The inability to detect noxious tastes and odors can result in food- or gas poisoning, particularly in elderly subjects. In the extreme, chemosensory disorders can lead to overwhelming stress, anorexia, and depression.

ANATOMY. The sensory receptor for taste, the taste bud, is made up of approximately 50 cells arranged to form a pear-shaped organ. The life span of these cells is about 10 days, and they are constantly being renewed from dividing epithelial cells surrounding the bud. Taste buds are located on the tongue, soft palate, pharynx, larynx, epiglottis, uvula, and the upper one third of the esophagus. The taste buds located on the anterior two thirds of the tongue and on the palate are innervated by the seventh cranial nerve. The ninth cranial nerve innervates the posterior one third of the tongue and the folds or clefts on the lateral border of the tongue. The ninth and tenth nerves innervate taste buds in the pharynx. Afferent signals from the taste buds project to the nucleus of the solitary tract in the medulla and then via a series of relays to the thalamus and postcentral somatosensory cerebral cortex. Free nerve endings of the fifth cranial nerve are found on the tongue and in the oral cavity, and lesions involving these pathways also can alter taste perception.

Olfactory receptors lie in a roughly dime-sized area of specialized pigmented epithelium that arches along the superior aspect of each side of the nasal mucosa. Specialized bipolar sensory cells in this region thrust short receptor hairs into the overlying mucosa to detect aromatic molecules as they dissolve. As with taste buds, the specialized receptor portion of the bipolar neuron undergoes continuous renewal, turning over approximately every 30 days. Thin axons of the bipolar neurons course through small holes in the cribri-

form plate of the ethmoid bone to form connections in the overlying olfactory bulb on the ventral surface of the frontal lobe. From here second- and third-order neurons project directly and indirectly to the prepiriform cortex and parts of the amygdaloid complex of both sides of the brain, representing the primary olfactory cortex.

PATHOPHYSIOLOGY OF CHEMOSENSORY DISORDERS. Disorders of taste and smell can be divided into local, systemic, and neurologic (Table 403–1). The taste buds and the specialized receptor portion of the bipolar olfactory cells are constantly being renewed, and the process of renewal can be affected by nutritional, metabolic, and hormonal states, therapeutic radiation, drugs, and age. For example, with interruption of mitosis by antiproliferative agents, a return of normal taste function takes a minimum of 10 days, while a return to normal olfactory function takes more than 30 days. Numerous local conditions such as colds and allergies, chronic sinusitis, and nasal polyposis can influence the sense of smell by restricting airway patency. Accidental blows to the head can shear the fine axons of the bipolar olfactory neurons, resulting in loss of smell. Lesions of the fifth, seventh *(chorda tympani),* and ninth nerves can lead to disordered taste sensation. Olfactory and gustatory disturbances can serve as important diagnostic signs for focal neurologic lesions (e.g., frontal lobe tumors). Hallucinations of smell and taste occur with epileptogenic lesions affecting the mesial temporal lobe and insular region, respectively. Finally, olfactory disturbances and hallucinations occur with a number of psychiatric illnesses (particularly depressive illness and schizophrenia).

EXAMINATION OF TASTE AND SMELL. Olfaction can be tested grossly at the bedside with a few easily recognized odors such as coffee, chocolate, and the roselike aroma of the compound phenylethyl alcohol. (Avoid nasal irritants.) Each nostril is tested separately to determine whether the problem is unilateral or bilateral. Gustatory sensation is typically tested with weak solutions of sugar, salt, and acetic acid, or vinegar. The patient must keep his tongue protruded and respond to questions either by nodding the head or pointing to names of the tastes written on cards. The anterior two thirds and posterior one third of the tongue should be tested separately.

COMMON CAUSES OF LOSS OF SMELL AND TASTE. The most frequently encountered causes of loss of smell are local obstructive disease, viral infections, head injuries that sever the neurons crossing through the cribriform plate, and normal aging. Patients can lose their sense of smell not only from chronic allergies and sinusitis but also from the nasal sprays and drops that they use to treat these conditions. The most common cause of loss of the sense of taste is drug ingestion, particularly antirheumatic and antiproliferative drugs and drugs containing sulfhydryl groups in their molecular structure, such as penicillamine and captopril. Patients with poor dental hygiene commonly complain of distortions of taste. Many of the systemic disorders listed in Table 403–1 probably have their effect by decreasing the rate of turnover of sensory receptors on the tongue and olfactory epithelia. Disturbances of smell and taste in malnourished patients have been attributed to specific deficiencies in vitamins and minerals, such as zinc. However, it is possible that the loss of protein and calorie intake impairs the functioning of taste buds and olfactory cells in the same manner that it impairs the regeneration of intestinal epithelia. Viral illnesses such as influenza and viral hepatitis produce disorders of both taste and smell. The loss of olfactory sensation after viral illnesses may be due to scarring of the subepithelial tissue and the replacement of

TABLE 403–1. COMMON CAUSES OF LOSS OF TASTE AND SMELL

	Taste	Smell
Local	Radiation therapy	Allergic rhinitis, sinusitis, nasal polyposis, bronchial asthma
Systemic	Cancer, renal failure, hepatic failure, nutritional deficiency (B_3, zinc), Cushing syndrome, hypothyroidism, diabetes mellitus, infection (influenza), drugs (antirheumatic and antiproliferative)	Renal failure, hepatic failure, nutritional deficiency (B_{12}), Cushing syndrome, hypothyroidism, diabetes mellitus, infection (viral hepatitis, influenza), drugs (nasal sprays, antibiotics)
Neurologic	Bell's palsy, familial dysautonomia, multiple sclerosis	Head trauma, multiple sclerosis, Parkinson's disease, frontal tumor

olfactory epithelium with respiratory epithelium. Multifocal neurologic disorders such as multiple sclerosis can affect the central olfactory and gustatory pathways at multiple levels, and therefore abnormalities of taste and smell are common in such patients. Treatment, other than avoiding drugs known to affect taste or smell, is unsatisfactory.

Estrem SA, Renner G: Disorders of smell and taste. Otolaryngol Clin North Am 20:133, 1987. *Concise clinical review.*
Schiffman SS: Taste and smell in disease. N Engl J Med 308:1275, 1337, 1983. *A well-referenced two-part short review.*
Taste and smell disorders: parts 1 and 2. Ear Nose Throat J 68:286, 291, 297, 316, 331, 352, 354, 362, 373, 386, 393, 398, 1989. *Two issues devoted to diagnosis and management.*

403.2 Neuro-ophthalmology

The mechanistic understanding of vision impairment along with disturbances of pupillary and oculomotor control lies close to the heart of diagnosing neurologic disorders. Diseases of the eye itself are further considered in Part XXV.

VISION

One of the most difficult diagnostic problems is vision loss that cannot be explained by obvious abnormalities of the eye. In order to properly evaluate such a patient the examining physician must be familiar with the anatomy and physiology of the afferent visual system. The afferent visual pathways cross at right angles to the major ascending sensory and descending motor systems of the cerebral hemispheres and in their anterior portion are intimately related to the vascular and bony structures at the base of the brain. Not surprisingly, localization of lesions within the afferent visual pathways has great localizing value in neurologic diagnosis.

ANATOMY OF THE VISUAL PATHWAYS. Light entering the eye falls on the retinal rods and cones, which transduce the stimulus into neural impulses to be transmitted to the brain. The distribution of visual function across the retina takes a pattern of concentric zones increasing in sensitivity toward the center, the fovea. The fovea consists of a "rod-free" central grouping of approximately 100,000 slender cones. The ganglion cells subserving these cones send their axons directly to the temporal aspect of the optic disk, forming the papillomacular bundle. Axons originating from ganglion cells in the temporal retina must curve above and below the papillomacular bundle, forming dense arcuate bands.

The arteries supplying the optic nerve and retina both derive from branches of the ophthalmic artery. The central retinal artery approaches the eye along each optic nerve and pierces the inferior aspect of the dural sheath about 1 cm behind the globe to enter the center of the nerve. The artery emerges in the fundus at the center of the nerve head, from which it nourishes most of the retina by superior, medial, inferior, and lateral branches. Anastomotic branches derived from the choroidal and posterior ciliary arteries supply the nerve head itself and the macular region. Venous drainage from the retina and nerve head flows primarily via the central retinal vein, whose course of exit from the eye parallels that of the entry of the artery. The venous anatomy explains why inflammatory lesions of or adjacent to the optic nerve head cause venous distention and ipsilateral papilledema (optic neuritis), whereas inflammation lying posterior to the point where the vein leaves the nerve produces only visual loss without swelling of the nerve head (retrobulbar neuritis).

What each eye "sees" is termed its visual field (Fig. 403–1). The nasal side of the left eye and the temporal side of the right eye see the left side of the world, and the upper half of each retina sees the lower half of the world. Behind the eye, the optic nerve passes through the optic foramen and sphenoid bone to reach the optic chiasm. In the chiasm, nerves from the nasal half of each retina decussate and join the fibers from the temporal half of the contralateral retina. From the chiasm, the optic tracts pass around the cerebral peduncles to reach the lateral geniculate ganglia of either side. At the level of the geniculus, fibers serving corresponding points in each retinal half visual field lie adjacent to each other, and this proximity is maintained in the subsequent relay to the calcarine cortex. The geniculocalcarine radiation initially fans out into superolat-

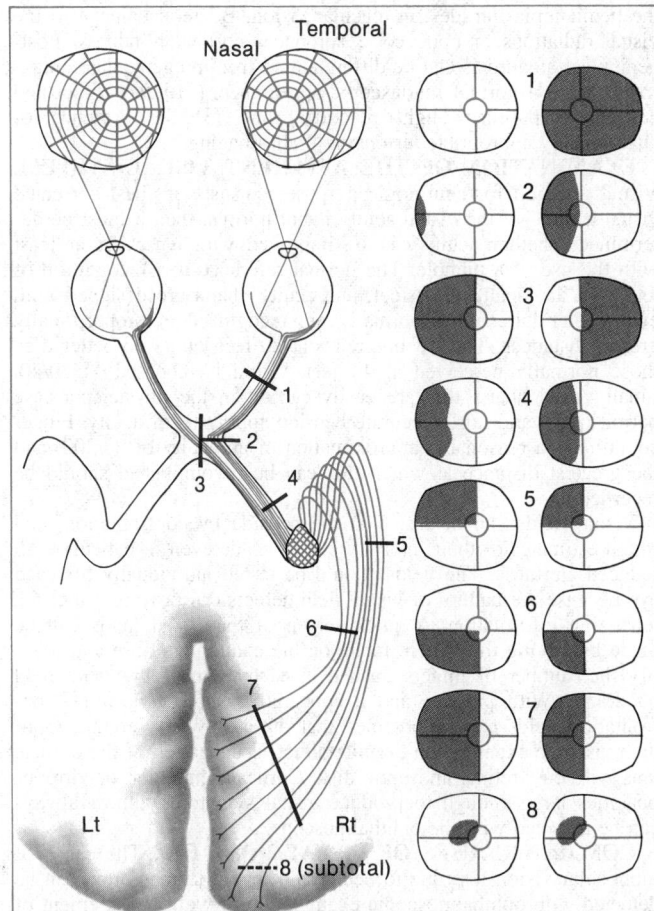

FIGURE 403–1. Visual fields that accompany damage to the visual pathways. 1. Optic nerve: Unilateral amaurosis. 2. Lateral optic chiasm: Grossly incongruous, incomplete (contralateral) homonymous hemianopia. 3. Central optic chiasm: Bitemporal hemianopia. 4. Optic tract: Incongruous, incomplete homonymous hemianopia. 5. Temporal (Meyer's) loop of optic radiation: Congruous partial or complete (contralateral) homonymous superior quadrantanopia. 6. Parietal (superior) projection of the optic radiation: Congruous partial or complete homonymous inferior quadrantanopia. 7. Complete parieto-occipital interruption of optic radiation: Complete congruous homonymous hemianopia with psychophysical shift of foveal point often sparing central vision, giving "macular sparing." 8. Incomplete damage to visual cortex: Congruous homonymous scotomas, usually encroaching at least acutely on central vision.

eral and inferolateral projections, the latter passing around the lateral ventricle and for a short distance into the temporal lobe (Meyer's loop) before turning posteriorly to head for the striate cortex of the occipital lobe. At the occipital pole, the striate cortex (Area 17) lies along the superior and inferior bands of the calcarine fissure, with macular fibers projecting most posteriorly to the occipital pole and more peripheral retinal projections lying more anteriorly.

LOCALIZATION OF LESIONS WITHIN THE VISUAL PATHWAYS. Monocular vision loss is due to a lesion of one eye or its retina or optic nerve. Binocular visual loss, on the other hand, can result from disease located anywhere in the visual pathways from the retinae to the occipital poles. Lesions involving or compressing the optic chiasm produce nonhomonymous visual abnormalities that affect the unilateral visual fields incongruously (e.g., the bitemporal hemianopia illustrated by Lesion 3 in Fig. 403–1). Optic tract abnormalities are comparatively rare but produce characteristic visual changes. The fibers serving identical points in the homonymous half fields do not fully commingle in the anterior optic tract, so lesions encroaching on this structure produce incongruous and usually incomplete homonymous hemianopias. Lesions on the geniculate ganglia, visual radiations, or visual cortex produce congruent hemianopic field defects that may go unrecognized unless the hemianopia intrudes on macular vision. Bilateral damage to the visual radiations or optic cortex produces cortical blindness. Postgeniculate amaurosis can be differentiated from pregeniculate amaurosis by (1) a normal funduscopic appearance, (2) intact direct and consensual pupillary light reactions, and (3) the presence of anatomically appropriate lesions by brain imaging.

EXAMINATION OF THE AFFERENT VISUAL SYSTEM. Visual function for neurologic purposes consists of "best corrected visual acuity." If the visual acuity is not normal, then it must be determined whether acuity can be improved with lenses or at least with the use of a pinhole. The normal reference is a recognition of letters at an idealized 20 feet, and acuity charts are designed with even larger letters that normally are recognized at proportionally greater distances. Thus, if one reads at 20 feet letters no better than those normally perceived at 40 feet, vision is recorded as 20/40. Small visual charts that are easily carried in the physician's case permit quick and fairly accurate bedside appraisals of acuity. Finger counting is a reasonable approximation of an acuity of 20/200, and the greatest distance at which this can be accomplished should be recorded.

Visual fields can be tested at the bedside by confrontation, and rough estimates of their integrity can be made even in patients with reduced alertness. The fields should be tested individually for each eye because the pattern of visual field defects can provide important localizing information. A quick screen of the visual fields can be made by having the patient fixate on the examiner's nose and identify the number of fingers flashed in each of the four visual field quadrants. With practice and a cooperative subject, accurate confrontation fields can be obtained that outline even scotomas. Ophthalmoscopic examination permits direct visualization of the cornea, lens, vitreous, retina, and optic disk. Corneal, lenticular, or vitreous opacities large enough to produce visual symptoms almost always can be detected with the ophthalmoscope.

COMMON CAUSES OF VISUAL LOSS. *Eye.* The cause of monocular vision loss due to ocular and retinal lesions often can be detected with ophthalmoscopic examination or with measurement of intraocular pressure. *Glaucoma* caused by impaired absorption of the aqueous humor results in a high intraocular pressure that usually produces gradual visual loss, "halos" seen around illuminated lamps, and, often, pain and redness in the affected eye. Infrequently, rapid vision loss can occur with few premonitory symptoms. Diagnosis comes from the tonometric measurement of a high intraocular pressure and may be suspected by palpating an abnormally firm globe and observing a deep, pale optic cup and attenuated blood vessels. *Retinal tears and detachments* give rise to unilateral distortions of the visual image seen as sudden angulations or curves of objects containing straight lines (metamorphopsia). *Hemorrhages* into the vitreous humor or unilateral *infections* or *inflammatory lesions* of the retina can produce scotomas that in all ways resemble those resulting from primary disease of the central visual pathway.

Binocular vision loss due to retinal disease in younger subjects is usually due to *heredodegenerative conditions.* Vascular diseases, diabetes, idiopathic (senile) macular degeneration, and bilateral retinal detachments are causes in older age groups. In the *pigmentary retinal degenerations* visual loss begins peripherally and proceeds centrally, and often very slowly, before acuity (central vision) is impaired. By contrast, *macular degenerations* impair central vision early in their course. Most of the retinal degenerations produce characteristic and recognizable ophthalmoscopic appearances. With pigmentary degenerations the visual fields shrink progressively in size. With macular degenerations, on the other hand, the fields show noncongruent central scotomas.

Optic Nerve. Acute or subacute monocular vision loss due to optic nerve disease is most commonly produced by demyelinating disorders, vascular obstruction, or neoplasm. Demyelinating disease of the nerve head (*optic neuritis* or *papillitis*) produces papilledema along with loss of central vision in the affected eye only; subjectively unrecognized scotomas sometimes may be found in the other eye. Demyelination in the optic nerve behind where the retinal vein emerges (*retrobulbar neuritis*) initially leaves a normal-looking disk but a central or paracentral scotoma. With chronic demyelinating disorders the optic disk becomes pale and atrophic. More than 50% of patients who initially present with optic neuritis or retrobulbar

TABLE 403-2. COMMON CAUSES OF TRANSIENT MONOCULAR VISION LOSS

Category/ (Typical Duration)	Causes	Differential Features
Thromboembolism (1–5 min)	Atherosclerosis	Other atherosclerotic vascular disease, associated crossed hemiparesis, angiography (carotid atheromata)
	Cardiac	Valvular disease, mural thrombi, atrial fibrillation, recent MI
	Blood dyserasia	Blood tests + for sickle cell anemia, macroglobulinemia, multiple myeloma, polycythemia, etc.
Vasospasm (5–30 min)	Migraine	Ipsilateral headache, other classic aura, and family history
Vascular compression (few sec)	Papilledema	Precipitated by position change, Valsalva maneuver, or pressure waves
	Tumor	Associated slowly progressive monocular visual loss
Vasculitis (1–5 min)	Temporal arteritis	Associated headache, polymyalgia rheumatica, palpable temporal artery, elevated sed rate

neuritis go on to develop typical symptoms and signs of multiple sclerosis. Vascular lesions produce either total amaurosis or a sector field defect consistent with an intraocular arterial occlusion *(ischemic optic neuropathy).* The common causes of transient monocular vision loss and their differential features are listed in Table 403–2. *Tumors* invading the optic nerve or space-occupying lesions compressing it anywhere between the orbit and the chiasm cause gradually decreasing central vision (intrinsic or far advanced lesions) or a sector defect of the peripheral visual field. With such chronic lesions the affected optic nerve becomes visibly atrophic.

Acute binocular vision loss due to bilateral optic nerve disease is most often caused by demyelinating disease and less frequently by optic nerve or retinal vascular disease or by toxic or nutritional optic neuropathies. In younger persons and those lacking a clear history of toxic exposures demyelinating lesions overwhelmingly predominate (optic neuritis). Symptoms are of abrupt or subacute onset with visual blurring or loss of acuity, which may progress rapidly to blindness within hours or days. There may be pain about the eyes, particularly on eye movement.

Papilledema resulting from increased intracranial pressure occasionally causes vision loss under one of three circumstances: (1) acute transient episodes of amaurosis lasting a few seconds and attributable to acute increases in intracranial pressure (plateau waves) that interfere with retinal venous drainage into the cavernous sinus or with vascular irrigation of the occipital lobe; (2) acute bilateral sustained amaurosis following abrupt surgical relief of longstanding, severely increased, intracranial pressure (a rare cause); and (3) progressive loss of peripheral vision with longstanding, severe papilledema, presumably owing to pressure atrophy of the most peripherally lying fibers in the tightly sheathed optic nerve. Table 403–3 gives the main differential points between papilledema and optic neuritis. Subacute or chronic binocular vision loss due to optic nerve disease results mainly from *toxic nutritional* causes and the *inherited optic atrophies.* The latter sometimes accompany spinocerebellar degeneration or selectively affect the optic nerves in

TABLE 403-3. DIFFERENTIATION OF OPTIC NEURITIS FROM PAPILLEDEMA

	Optic Neuritis	Papilledema
Central-cecocentral vision loss	Present	Absent
Distribution	Usually unilateral	Usually bilateral
Ocular pain on movement	Present	Absent
Direct light reflex	± Reduced	Intact
CT and MRI scan of head	Normal	Often abnormal
Visual evoked responses	Abnormal	Normal
Lumbar puncture pressure	Normal	Elevated

both juveniles and adults (Leber's forms). With either cause, visual loss is moderate or severe and primarily or initially affects central vision; ophthalmoscopy shows mild to moderate primary optic atrophy.

Chiasm and Optic Tract. Patients with lesions of the optic chiasm and optic tract are often unaware of visual impairment until the deficit encroaches on central vision in one or both eyes. Intrinsic or extrinsic neoplasms and parachiasmal arterial aneurysms are the most common lesions in this location. *Gliomas* that arise in the chiasm are rare in adulthood but, when they occur, impair central vision early. Extrinsic space-occupying lesions compressing the chiasm can arise from the superior, lateral, or inferior aspect and include *dysgerminomas, craniopharyngiomas, pituitary adenomas, meningiomas* arising from the sphenoid bones, and large *aneurysms* of the carotid artery. The diagnosis rests on finding the characteristic visual field abnormalities (bitemporal hemianopsia for chiasm and incongruous homonymous hemianopsia for optic tract lesions) and identifying the specific lesion with computed tomography (CT) or magnetic resonance imaging (MRI). Pituitary apoplexy (due to acute hemorrhage into the gland, occurring most frequently in patients with unrecognized pituitary adenomas) can result in sudden vision loss. Prompt neurosurgical intervention under steroid coverage is required for most patients.

Visual Radiations and Occipital Cortex. Lesions involving the postgeniculate visual pathways most often result from *vascular damage, traumatic injuries, neoplasms* or, rarely, *inflammatory* or *degenerative disorders* involving the cerebral white matter. Their localization can be deduced by the resulting visual field defects. Vascular disease of the occipital lobes is the most common cause of homonymous visual field defects in the middle-aged and elderly population. Typically, the onset of such field defects is associated with other signs and symptoms of transient ischemic episodes in the vertebrobasilar distribution. Bilateral damage to the visual radiations or occipital cortex produces *cortical blindness.* Most often, there are other signs of vascular disease including focal neurologic findings. *Anton's syndrome* refers to cortical blindness with denial of visual defect. Affected patients not only deny the fact that they are blind but confabulate details of their visual environment from memory. Autopsy studies reveal lesions of the medial, temporal, and parietal lobes as well as the calcarine cortex. *Tumors* are rarely confined to the limits of the occipital lobes; therefore neurologic deficits with occipital tumors are rarely only visual.

PUPILLARY CONTROL

The neuromechanisms that control pupil size and reactivity are complex, yet they can be evaluated by simple clinical procedures. The diameter of the pupil is determined by the antagonistic actions of the iris sphincter and dilator muscles with the latter playing a minor role. If the sphincter muscle is severed or ruptured it does not retract toward one quadrant but rather continues to function except in the altered segment. Therefore, the pupillary response can be evaluated even in the presence of significant damage to the iris.

ANATOMY AND LOCALIZATION OF LESIONS WITHIN PUPILLARY PATHWAYS. The size of the pupil is governed by tonic balance between sympathetic and parasympathetic innervation of the muscles of the iris. Sympathetic stimulation dilates the pupil, and parasympathetic stimulation constricts it. In the normal resting state, light entering the eye provides the major stimulus governing the size of the pupil (Fig. 403–2). Light activates the retinal rods and cones with maximal sensitivity in the macular area. The optic nerve fibers follow the crossed and uncrossed visual pathways to the pregeniculate portion of the optic tracts, where the receptor fibers for light diverge to the pretectal nucleus located at the midbrain diencephalic junction. Interneurons project from this nucleus to the Edinger-Westphal nuclei atop the midbrain third nerve complex of either side. From that point paired parasympathetic efferents leave the midbrain with the third nerves to travel in the interpeduncular space across the petroclinoid ligament and edge of the tentorium, where, after traversing the cavernous sinus, they enter the superior orbital fissure. In the orbit the parasympathetic efferents synapse in the ciliary ganglion from which short ciliary nerves enter the eye to reach the pupillary muscles.

The principal sympathetic control of the pupil originates in the ventral lateral hypothalamus (first-order neuron) from which fibers descend ipsilaterally to the lower brain stem tegmentum and thence to the cervical cord, where they lie superficially and synapse with the preganglionic neurons in the intermedial lateral column of the upper three thoracic segments. Preganglionic fibers (second-order neurons) emerge with the ventral roots of C8, T1, and T2, and ascend in the neck to synapse in the superior cervical ganglion adjacent to the base of the skull. Postganglionic (third-order neurons) pupillary fibers accompany the internal carotid artery through the

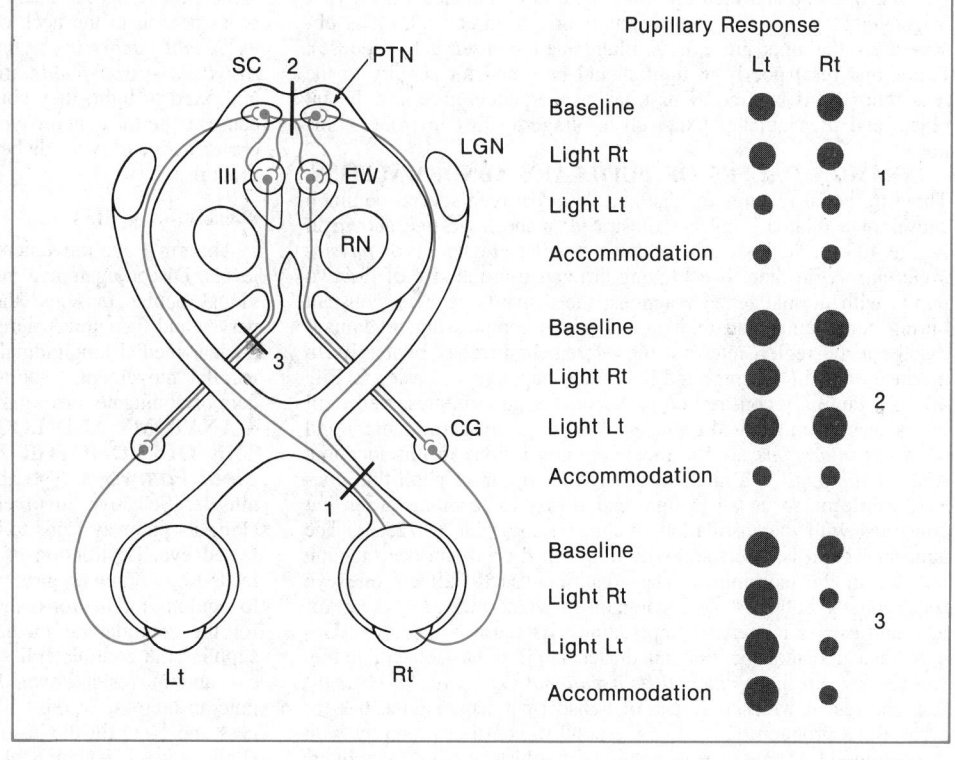

FIGURE 403–2. Pupillary responses associated with lesions of the (1) optic nerve, (2) pretectum, and (3) oculomotor nerve. SC = Superior colliculus; PTN = pretectal nucleus; EW = Edinger-Westphal nucleus; LGN = lateral geniculate nucleus; RN = red nucleus; CG = ciliary ganglion.

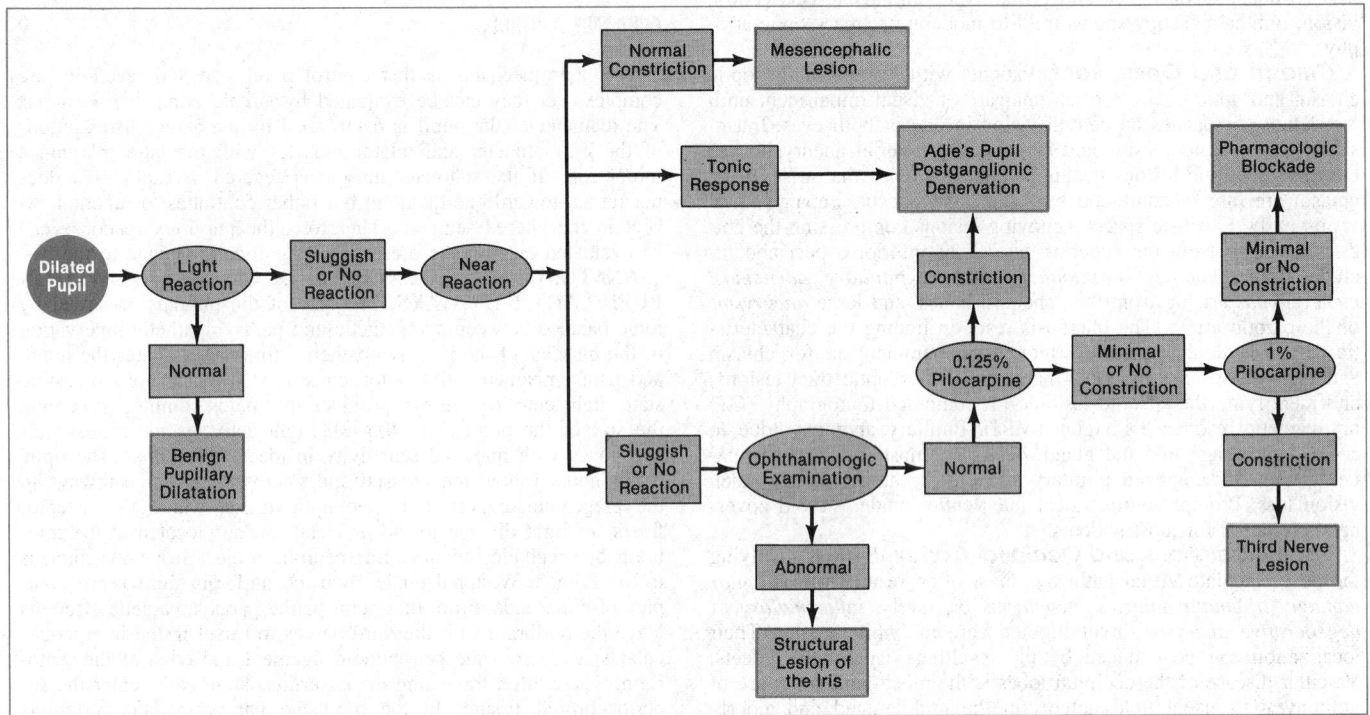

FIGURE 403–3. Evaluation of a dilated pupil.

skull, leaving it to follow the ophthalmic branch of the trigeminal nerve to reach the pupillodilator muscle of the eye.

Sympathetic paralysis of the eye with ptosis and miosis (Horner's syndrome) can result from lesions anywhere along the course of the pathway described above. Topical diagnosis is made best by identifying associated signs in the brain stem or neck or along the carotid artery.

EXAMINATION OF THE PUPIL. The pupillary response to light should be examined in a dimly lighted room, in which case the pupils are in a semidilated state. First, the size and symmetry of the pupils are assessed by shining a dim light onto the face from below so that both pupils are seen simultaneously in the indirect illumination. To test light reactivity, gaze is directed at a distant object and first one and then the other pupil is illuminated with a very bright light source. If a pupil reacts poorly to direct light, it is observed as the opposite eye is illuminated (consensual response). Pupils that react poorly to light should be tested for activity to the near reflex. This is done by first having the patient gaze at a distant object and then quickly fixate on his fingertip just in front of his nose.

COMMON CAUSES OF PUPILLARY ABNORMALITIES. The differential features for distinguishing between several common causes of a dilated pupil are illustrated in the logic tree shown in Figure 403–3. With so-called benign pupillary dilatation or *physiologic anisocoria* there is a lifelong difference in the size of the two pupils with normal reflex reactions; the disparity remains constant during constriction and dilatation. Lesions compressing or damaging the tectal region interrupt the afferent light reflex bilaterally to produce dilated (> 5 mm) and light-fixed pupils (e.g., Lesion 2, Fig. 403–2). Pupillary constriction on accommodation is preserved until late stages. Tumors of the pineal gland (e.g., dysgerminomas) and *localized infarctions* are the most common lesions in this location. *Adie's tonic pupil* is a medium-to-large (3 to 6 mm) pupil that constricts little or not at all to light and slowly to accommodation but constricts with the instillation of dilute pilocarpine (0.125%). The abnormal pupil is associated with diminished or absent deep tendon reflexes in the extremities. The condition usually affects one eye (occasionally both), is more common in women 25 to 45 years of age, and carries no serious implications. Its cause is unknown. Unexplained unilateral or bilateral dilated pupil as an isolated finding can result from the *accidental or intentional instillation of mydriatics.* The recent widespread use of transdermal scopolamine has increased the problem. Failure of the pupil to constrict promptly with pilocarpine (1%) gives the diagnosis if the history is unclear. Inter-

ruption of the emerging third nerve in the ventral midbrain or along the proximal part of its course produces a mid-dilated pupil 6 to 7 mm in diameter. Important causes of compression of the third nerve in this region are *aneurysms, neoplasia,* and *brain herniation* due to increased intracranial pressure. In nearly all cases the pupillary involvement is associated with other signs of third nerve involvement (see below). Rarely, compressive lesions such as a posterior communicating artery aneurysm can present with an isolated dilated pupil.

As noted above, the causes of *Horner syndrome* are numerous because of the long course of sympathetic innervation to the eye. It is unlikely that a patient with a central nervous system lesion will present with an isolated Horner syndrome. The most common lesions producing Horner syndrome involve the ascending second-order neuron in the neck or the extracranial postganglionic neuron; *malignant tumors in the apex of the lung* are by far most common. *Argyll-Robertson pupils* are small (1 to 2 mm), unequal, irregular, and fixed to light; they constrict to accommodation. Their principal cause is tertiary neurosyphilis, although partial Argyll-Robertson changes occur with diabetes and certain of the autonomic neuropathies.

OCULOMOTOR CONTROL

Abnormal eye movements can result from disturbances at several levels. Disconjugate eye movements result from lesions of the individual ocular muscles, the myoneural junctions, the oculomotor nerves and their three paired nuclei in the brain stem, and the internuclear medial longitudinal fasciculus (MLF) that yokes the eyes in parallel movements. Supranuclear lesions typically produce disorders of conjugate gaze (gaze palsies).

ANATOMY AND LOCALIZATION OF LESIONS WITHIN THE OCULOMOTOR PATHWAYS. *Nuclear and Internuclear Pathways.* The abducens nerve supplies the lateral rectus muscle. Selective involvement of the abducens nerve anywhere along its pathway leads to isolated weakness of abduction of the affected eye. Destruction of the abducens nucleus in the brain stem leads to a conjugate gaze paralysis (ipsilateral) because, in addition to oculomotor neurons, the nucleus contains interneurons destined for the contralateral medial rectus nucleus. The trochlear nucleus supplies the contralateral superior oblique muscle which intorts the eye and moves it down. Patients with superior oblique weakness note an increase in diplopia with head tilt toward the side of weakness and often tilt the head in the opposite direction. At rest there is slight upward deviation of the involved eye, and downward movement is impaired when the affected eye is turned in. The third cranial nerve supplies the remaining ocular muscles. Involvement of the third nerve nucleus in the midbrain always produces at least some bilateral oculomotor weakness; the superior rectus division of the nucleus supplies the contralateral superior rectus muscle (all other divisions supply ipsilateral muscles). Peripheral third nerve paralysis can result from lesions damaging the structure anywhere from its origin from the ventral midbrain to where it enters the orbit via the superior orbital fissure. Depending on its completeness, a third nerve palsy produces a widely dilated pupil, severe ptosis, and an externally deviated eye held in position by the unopposed contraction of the lateral rectus muscle. In such conditions, the continued trochlear action reveals itself by intorsion of the eye when the subject attempts to look down and in.

The MLF interconnects the abducens nucleus in the pons with the contralateral oculomotor nuclear complex in the midbrain. It terminates cephalad in the interstitial nucleus in the rostral midbrain and can be traced as far caudad as the thoracocervical region of the spinal cord (coordinating nuchal-ocular control). Lesions involving the MLF characteristically produce an internuclear ophthalmoplegia (INO) with which the eyes are conjugate in the primary position but disconjugate on lateral gaze. With a fully developed INO on lateral gaze away from the side of the lesion the contralateral eye abducts and shows nystagmus, whereas the ipsilateral adducting eye partially or completely fails to move nasally because of failure of ascending impulses to reach the third nerve nucleus. Adduction for convergence is usually relatively maintained. Upbeat gaze-evoked nystagmus typically occurs with INO.

Supranuclear Pathways. The pathway descending from the frontal eye fields in the frontal lobe regulates rapid voluntary eye movements *(saccades).* A signal from the frontal eye field activates a burst of firing in the contralateral horizontal gaze center in the paramedian pontine reticular formation. This high frequency burst (or pulse) of neuronal firing is transmitted directly to the nearby sixth nerve nucleus and via MLF to the contralateral third nerve nucleus. For voluntary vertical gaze both frontal eye fields send signals to the vertical gaze center in the pretectum (probably the interstitial nucleus of the MLF). Acute lesions involving a frontal eye field (e.g., hemorrhage or infarction) result in transient (24 to 72 hours) inability to direct the eyes contralaterally. Vertical eye movements are not affected by unilateral frontal lobe lesions. Bilateral damage to the frontal eye fields or their descending pathways may produce the inability to move the eyes voluntarily (horizontal or vertical) despite preserved reflex eye movements, a condition called *oculomotor apraxia.* Lesions involving the horizontal gaze center in the pons produce an ipsilateral paralysis of conjugate gaze and tonic deviation of the eyes to the contralateral hemiorbit. Lesions of the pretectum selectively impair vertical gaze with the vertical upgaze center being slightly rostral and dorsal to the vertical downgaze center.

Pathways descending from the parieto-occipital region of the two hemispheres subserve slow visual tracking or *smooth pursuit movements.* The exact location of these descending pursuit pathways is not completely known, but there are strong projections to the ipsilateral superior colliculus and ipsilateral pons. The cerebellar flocculus is also a critical relay station for smooth pursuit pathways. Lesions of the parieto-occipital region, pons, and cerebellum impair smooth pursuit and optokinetic slow phases when the target moves ipsilateral to the lesion. The *convergence* center is located in the rostral-dorsal midbrain near the vertical gaze center. Lesions in this region typically impair convergence and voluntary vertical gaze (particularly up-gaze). Pathways for cortical control of vergence have not been identified. The fourth supranuclear oculomotor control system, the *vestibulo-ocular reflex,* and its examination are discussed below.

EXAMINATION OF EYE MOVEMENTS. Fixation and gaze holding are tested by having the patient look center, right, left, up, and down. Each position should be held steady and unwavering with the observer documenting carefully abnormal movements or ocular disconjugacies. Each supranuclear oculomotor control system is examined separately. *Saccades* are tested by having the patient fixate alternately on two targets such as the examiner's finger and nose; the speed and accuracy are noted. *Smooth pursuit* is tested by slowly moving a target back and forth and up and down and observing the patient's ability to produce smooth tracking movements. It the target velocity is low (less than 30 degrees per second) normal subjects should be able to pursue without requiring catch-up saccades. *Convergence* is tested by having the patient follow a target moving from far to near. The degree of normal convergence varies considerably and depends on the cooperation of the patient. A clear sign that the patient is attempting to converge is simultaneous pupillary constriction.

COMMON CAUSES OF ABNORMAL OCULOMOTOR CONTROL. *Strabismus.* The flow chart in Figure 403–4 outlines the logic for determining the common causes of strabismus. A comitant strabismus present since childhood is usually a benign *congenital disorder.* As noted earlier, latent congenital strabismus can become manifest in adulthood in association with a systemic illness. An acquired skew deviation (vertical displacement of the ocular axes) can result from any number of lesions involving the brain stem and has little localizing value. Noncomitant strabismus can result from restrictive disease of the orbit or from abnormal muscle or oculomotor nerve function. The presence of mechanical restriction is confirmed by the use of forced duction testing. (After a topical anesthetic is applied to the eye, the ophthalmologist grasps the muscle insertion with a large blunt-toothed forceps and identifies mechanical restriction.) Common causes of *orbital restrictive disease* include dysthyroid ophthalmopathy, orbital pseudotumor, trauma, and orbital mass lesions. Variable strabismus that increases with fatigue suggests the likelihood of *myasthenia gravis* (see Ch. 459). A Tensilon test can usually confirm the diagnosis. If both restrictive disease and myasthenia gravis have been excluded, most patients with noncomitant strabismus have processes affecting the oculomotor nuclei, their fascicles, or the cranial nerves themselves. Common causes of an *isolated third nerve palsy* in an adult include aneurysm, vascular occlusive disease (including diabetes mellitus), trauma, and neoplasm. Typically, but not always, third nerve lesions due to vascular disease spare the pupil. Vascular disease and trauma are by far the most common causes of *isolated trochlear nerve palsies.* The abducens nerve is particularly vulnerable to isolated traumatic involvement because of its long pathway outside the brain stem. Lesions at distant sites that produce increased intracranial pressure can lead to abducens nerve dysfunction producing a "false localizing sign." Other common causes of *isolated sixth nerve palsies* are vascular disease, trauma, and neoplasm. About one fourth of cases with cranial nerve palsies (third, fourth, or sixth nerves) remain undiagnosed.

Internuclear Ophthalmoplegia (INO). INO may be unilateral or bilateral, partial or complete, depending on the location of the lesion and the degree of damage to the MLF. *Demyelinating* and small *vascular lesions* are the most common cause of unilateral INO unaccompanied by other ocular palsies or brain-stem signs. Larger brain-stem lesions that damage one or more oculomotor nuclei plus the MLF often produce bizarre combinations of disconjugate eye movements coupled with nuclear oculomotor palsies. Myasthenia gravis can produce an ophthalmoparesis resembling INO owing to the greater involvement of the medial rectus compared to the lateral rectus. Demyelinating diseases are by far the most common causes of bilateral INO involvement.

Disorders of Conjugate Gaze. As noted earlier, infarction of the frontal cortex results in transient contralateral gaze paresis. Tumors and infarction of the paramedian pontine reticular formation produce ipsilateral horizontal gaze paralysis. With the so-called locked-in syndrome (secondary to basilar artery thrombosis) voluntary horizontal eye movements are absent; the patient's only remaining motor functions are vertical eye and lid movements. Lesions of the pretectum typically affect only vertical eye movements, although the descending pathways from the frontal eye fields to the horizontal gaze centers in the pons can also be affected. With the *dorsal midbrain syndrome* (Parinaud syndrome) patients present with a conjugate up-gaze paresis. When they attempt to make upward saccades they develop convergence retraction nystagmus. As noted earlier, impaired convergence and light–near dissociation of the pupillary reflexes are also part of the syndrome. The most common causes of the dorsal midbrain syndrome include tumors of the pineal gland (dysgerminomas), aqueductal stenosis, and localized infarction.

Nystagmus. Spontaneous nystagmus can be congenital or acquired. *Congenital nystagmus* typically has a high frequency and variable wave form (occasionally pendular) and is highly fixation-dependent. It is usually not associated with a structural brain lesion. The lifelong history confirms the diagnosis. Spontaneous nystagmus

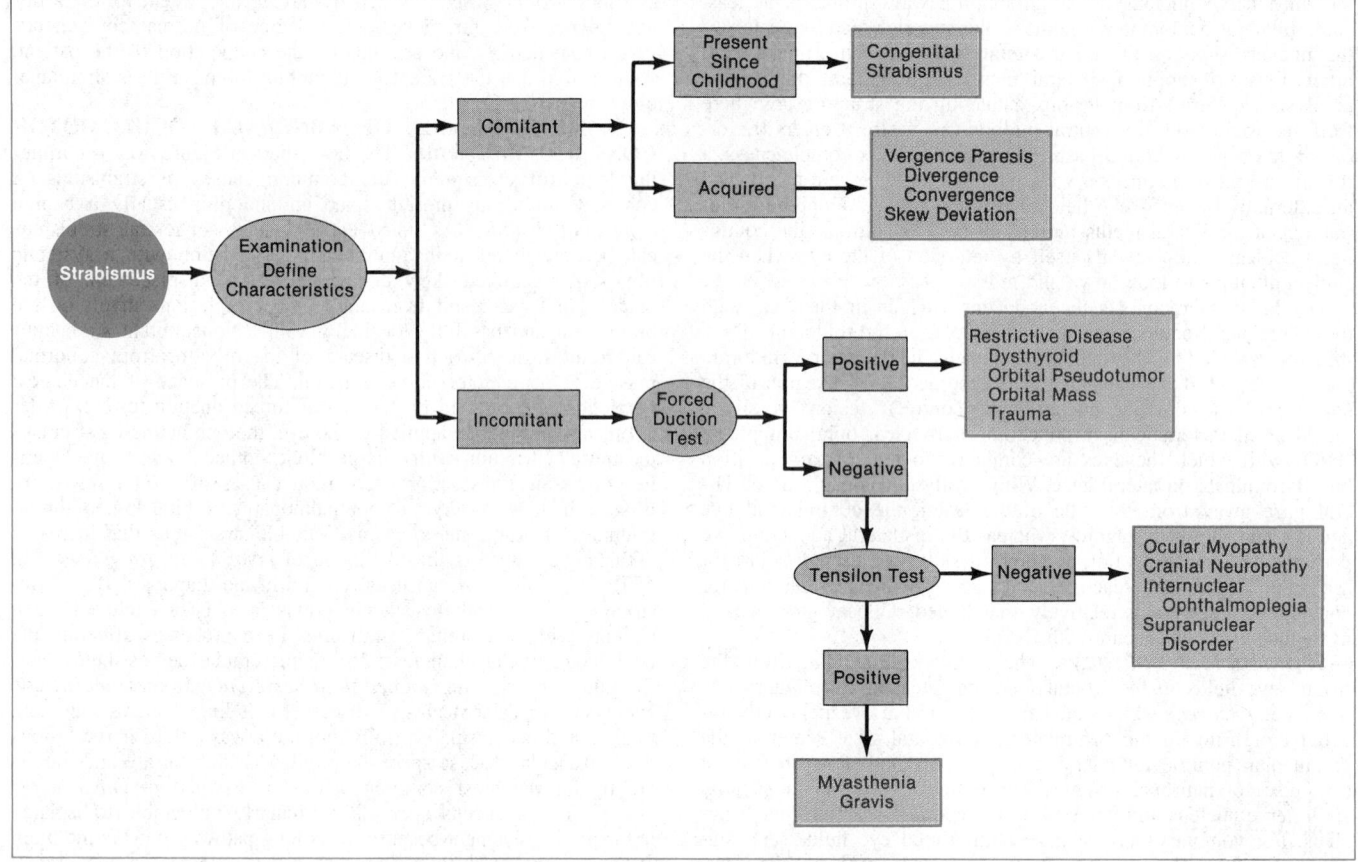

FIGURE 403–4. Diagnostic approach to strabismus.

due to a *peripheral vestibular* lesion (i.e., in the labyrinth or vestibular nerve) usually has combined horizontal and torsional components and is strongly inhibited with fixation (Table 403–4). Acquired persistent spontaneous nystagmus that is not inhibited by fixation indicates a lesion in the brain stem and/or cerebellum *(central vestibular)*. The latter is often purely vertical or horizontal because the vertical and horizontal vestibulo-ocular pathways separate beginning at the vestibular nuclei. Spontaneous *downbeat nystagmus* is commonly seen with lesions of the medulla or cervicomedullary junction (e.g., Arnold-Chiari malformation).

Gaze-evoked nystagmus is always in the direction of gaze and is usually present with and without fixation. It is most commonly produced by ingestion of *drugs* such as phenobarbital, phenytoin, alcohol, and diazepam. It can also occur in patients with such varied conditions as myasthenia gravis, multiple sclerosis, and cerebellar atrophy. Asymmetric horizontal gaze-evoked nystagmus indicates a structural brain-stem or cerebellar lesion (particularly at the cerebellopontine angle) with the lesion usually being on the side of the

larger amplitude nystagmus. *Rebound nystagmus* is a type of gaze-evoked nystagmus that either disappears or reverses direction as the eccentric gaze position is held. When the eyes are returned to the primary position nystagmus occurs in the direction of the return saccade. Rebound nystagmus occurs in patients with cerebellar atrophy and focal structural lesions of the cerebellum; it is the only variety of nystagmus thought to be specific for cerebellar involvement. *Disconjugate gaze-evoked nystagmus* most commonly results from lesions of the MLF (see above), but it can also occur with other lesions of the brain stem involving the oculomotor nuclei. Positional nystagmus is discussed below.

Other Ocular Oscillations. *Ocular bobbing* consists of a fast conjugate downward eye movement followed by a slow return to the primary position. The phenomenon accompanies severe displacement or destruction of the pons or, much less often, metabolic CNS depression. *Ocular myoclonus* consists of continuous rhythmic pendular oscillations, most often vertical, with a rate of 2 to 5 beats per second. Often it accompanies palatal myoclonus and has a similar pathogenesis. *Square wave jerks* and *ocular flutter* consist of brief, intermittent, horizontal oscillations (saccades) arising from the primary gaze position. These types of ocular oscillation are most commonly seen with cerebellar disease but can also accompany more diffuse central nervous system disorders. *Opsoclonus* consists of rapid, chaotic, conjugate, repetitive, saccadic eye movements (dancing eyes). One type of opsoclonus accompanies cerebellar dysfunction, but the most chaotic varieties are associated with brain-stem encephalitis or the remote effects of systemic neoplasm, especially neuroblastoma in children. *Ocular dysmetria* refers to over- and undershooting of saccadic eye movements often followed by multiple attempts at refixation. It reflects cerebellar dysfunction.

TABLE 403–4. KEY DISTINGUISHING FEATURES OF PERIPHERAL AND CENTRAL TYPES OF SPONTANEOUS AND POSITIONAL NYSTAGMUS

Type of Nystagmus	Peripheral (End Organ and Nerve)	Central (Brain Stem and Cerebellum)
Spontaneous	Unidirectional, fast phase away from lesion, combined horizontal torsional, inhibited with fixation	Bidirectional or undirectional; often pure horizontal, vertical, or torsional; *not* inhibited with fixation
Static positional	Direction-fixed or direction-changing, inhibited with fixation	Direction fixed or direction-changing, *not* inhibited with fixation
Paroxysmal positional	Vertical-torsional occasionally horizontal-torsional, vertigo prominent, fatigability, latency	Often pure vertical, vertigo less prominent, no latency, nonfatigable

Burde RM, Savino PJ, Trobe JD: Clinical Decisions in Neuro-ophthalmology. St. Louis, CV Mosby, 1985. *Liberal use of flow charts to help the clinician answer the question, "Given the symptom and signs, what is the disease?"*

Glaser JS: Neuro-ophthalmology, 2nd ed. Hagerstown, MD, Harper & Row, 1990. *An excellent one-volume didactic introductory text.*

Leigh RJ, Zee DS: The Neurology of Eye Movement, 2nd ed. Philadelphia, F. A. Davis Company, 1991. *An up-to-date monograph that gives the clinical and physiologic details of modern investigations on ocular control.*

403.3 Hearing and Equilibrium

The neural pathways subserving hearing and those most important for equilibrium and spatial orientation are anatomically proximate in much of their course from their end organs in the inner ear to their termination in the superior portion of the temporal lobe. Because of the close anatomic linkage, disorders that affect hearing often affect equilibrium, and vice versa. For this reason they are considered together here. Despite their anatomic propinquity, however, substantial pathophysiologic differences make clinical examination of the two systems quite different. The auditory system is physiologically relatively isolated, so that its function and dysfunction can be tested independently of other neural systems. The vestibular system, in contrast, has many close physiologic links with the motor system (particularly the cerebellum, oculomotor system, and autonomic nervous system) and can be tested only indirectly by noting secondary effects on oculomotor and cerebellar functions. Abnormalities of the auditory system lead to only a few well-defined and unique symptoms (i.e., hearing loss or tinnitus). Abnormalities of the vestibular system can cause symptoms that mimic disorders of the other neural structures. Such symptoms include dizziness, ocular abnormalities (nystagmus), motor abnormalities (including ataxia or sudden falls), and autonomic abnormalities (including nausea, vomiting, and even syncope).

HEARING

ANATOMY AND PHYSIOLOGY OF HEARING. In normal hearing, sound waves are transmitted from the tympanic membrane via the three ossicles of the air-filled middle ear (air conduction) to the oval window and the basilar membrane of the fluid-sealed cochlea. The ossicles serve to increase the gain from the tympanum to oval window about 18-fold, compensating for the loss that sound waves moving from air to fluid would otherwise suffer. In the absence of this system, sound may reach the cochlea by vibration of the temporal bone (bone conduction) but with much less efficiency (approximately 60 dB loss). Hair cells lying along the cochlear basilar membrane detect the vibratory movement of that membrane and transduce vibration into nerve impulses. The nerve impulses are relayed via nerve cells that synapse at the base of hair cells and have their bodies in the spiral ganglion to the cochlear nucleus of the ipsilateral pontine tegmentum. The spiral cochlea mechanically analyzes the frequency content of sound. For high-frequency tones only sensory cells in the basilar region are activated, whereas for low-frequency tones all or nearly all sensory cells are activated. Therefore, with lesions of the cochlea and its afferent nerve the hearing levels for different frequencies are usually unequal, typically resulting in better hearing sensitivity for low-frequency than for high-frequency tones. Within the brain stem, auditory signals ascend from the ventral and dorsal cochlear nuclei to reach the superior olivary nuclei of both sides. Thus nervous system lesions central to the cochlear nucleus do not cause monaural hearing loss, and, conversely, unilateral central lesions do not cause deafness. From these structures the pathway projects by way of the lateral lemnisci to the inferior colliculi. Each inferior colliculus transmits to the other and to its ipsilateral medial geniculate body, which in turn sends the final projection to the transverse auditory gyrus lying in the superior portion of the ipsilateral temporal lobe.

The normal ear can detect sound frequencies ranging between 20 and 20,000 Hertz (Hz); the upper range drops off fairly rapidly with advancing age. The ear is most sensitive between 500 and 4000 Hz, which roughly corresponds to the frequency range most important for understanding speech. The hearing level in this range has several practical implications in terms of the degree of handicap and the potential for useful correction with amplification. A 30- to 40-dB hearing level in the speech range would impair normal conversation, whereas an 80-dB hearing level would make everyday auditory communication almost impossible (the social definition of deafness).

LOCALIZATION OF LESIONS WITHIN THE AUDITORY PATHWAYS. *Conductive hearing loss* results from lesions involving the external or middle ear. It is typically characterized by an approximately equal loss of hearing at all frequencies and by well-preserved speech discrimination once the threshold for hearing is exceeded. Patients with conductive hearing loss can hear speech in a noisy background better than in a quiet background because they can understand loud speech as well as anyone.

Sensorineural hearing loss results from lesions of the cochlea and/or auditory division of the eighth cranial nerve. With sensorineural hearing loss the hearing levels for different frequencies are usually unequal, typically resulting in better hearing for lower- than for high-frequency tones. Patients with sensorineural hearing loss often have difficulty hearing speech that is mixed with background noise and may be annoyed by loud speech. Three important manifestations of sensorineural lesions are diplacusis, recruitment, and tone decay. Diplacusis and recruitment are common with cochlear lesions; tone decay usually accompanies eighth nerve involvement.

Central hearing disorders result from lesions of the central auditory pathways. As a rule patients with central lesions do not have impaired hearing for pure tones, and they can understand speech as long as it is clearly spoken in a quiet environment. If the listener's task is made more difficult with the introduction of background noise or competing messages, performance deteriorates more markedly in patients with central lesions than in normal subjects.

EXAMINATION OF HEARING. *Bedside Test.* A quick test for hearing loss in the speech range is to observe the response to spoken commands at different intensities (whisper, conversation, shouting). Tuning fork tests permit a rough assessment of the hearing level for pure tones of known frequency. The clinician can use his own hearing level as a reference standard. In the Rinne test nerve conduction is compared to bone conduction by holding a tuning fork (preferably 512 Hz) against the mastoid process until the sound can no longer be heard. It is then placed 1 inch from the ear and in normal subjects can be heard about twice as long by air as by bone. If bone conduction is better than air conduction, the hearing loss is conductive, but care must be taken to assure that the bone conduction is not heard in the normal ear. In the Weber test, the tuning fork is placed on the patient's forehead or upper teeth. Normally this sound is referred to the center of the head. If it is referred to the side of unilateral hearing loss, the hearing loss is conductive; if it is referred away from the side of unilateral hearing loss, the loss is sensorineural.

Audiometry. *Pure tone testing* is the nucleus of most auditory examinations. Pure tones at selected frequencies are presented via either earphones (air conduction) or a vibrator pressed against the mastoid portion of the temporal bone (bone conduction), and the minimal level that the subject can hear is determined for each frequency. Two speech tests are routinely used. The *speech reception threshold* (SRT) is the intensity at which the patient can correctly repeat 50% of the words presented. The SRT is a test of hearing sensitivity for speech and should reflect the hearing level for pure tones in the speech range. The *speech discrimination test* is a measure of the patient's ability to understand speech when it is presented at a level that is easily heard. In patients with eighth nerve lesions speech discriminations can be severely reduced, even when pure tone thresholds are normal or nearly normal, whereas in patients with cochlear lesions discrimination tends to be proportional to the magnitude of hearing loss.

Brain stem auditory evoked responses (BAER) can be recorded from scalp electrodes at 0 to 10 msec (early), 10 to 50 msec (middle), and 50 to 500 msec (late) following a click stimulus. The early potentials reflect electrical activity at the cochlea, eighth cranial nerve, and brain stem; the later potentials reflect cortical activity. Computer averaging of the responses to 1000 to 2000 clicks separates the evoked potential from background noise. Early evoked responses may be used to estimate the magnitude of hearing loss and to differentiate among cochlea, eighth nerve, and brainstem lesions.

CAUSES OF HEARING LOSS. *Conductive Hearing Loss.*
The logic for identifying common causes of hearing loss is shown in Figure 403–5. The history, examination, and audiometry usually provide the key differential features. The most common cause of conductive hearing loss is *impacted cerumen* in the external canal. This benign condition is usually first noticed after bathing or swimming when a droplet of water closes the remaining tiny passageway. The most common serious cause of conductive hearing loss is inflammation of the middle ear, *otitis media,* either infected (suppu-

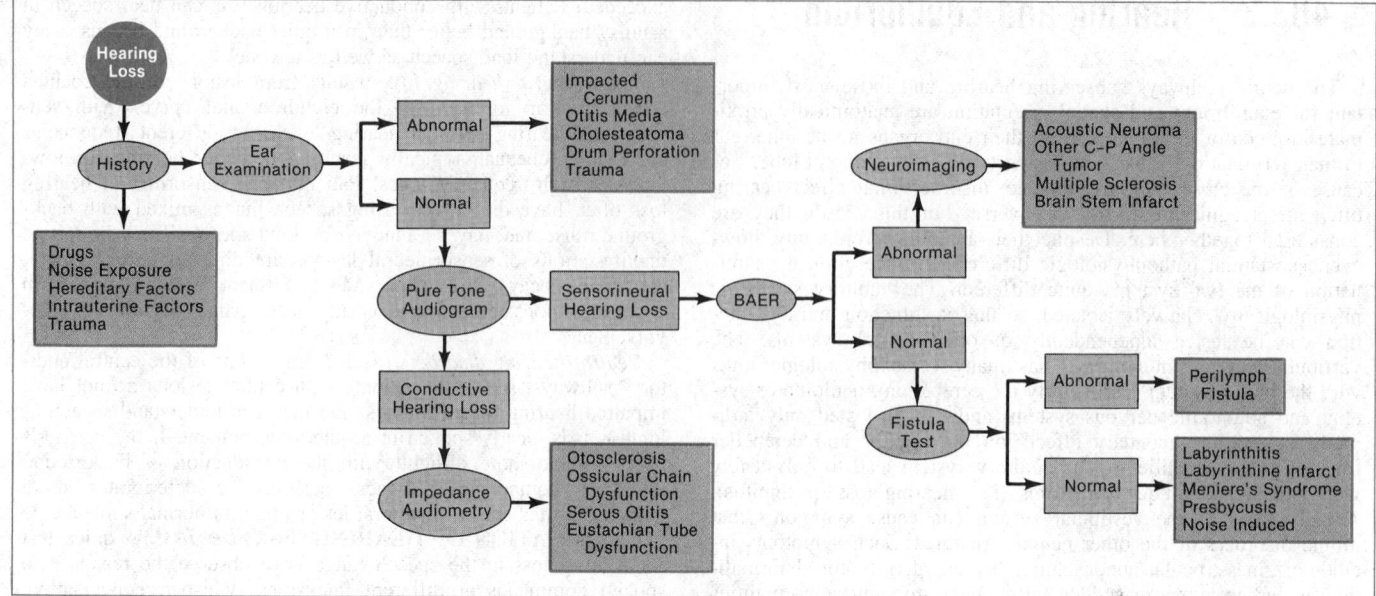

FIGURE 403–5. Evaluation of hearing loss.

rative) or noninfective (serous). Fluid accumulates in the middle ear, impairing the conduction of airborne sound. Since the air cavity of the middle ear is in direct connection with the mastoid air cells, infection can spread through the mastoid bone and, occasionally, into the intracranial cavity. Chronic otitis media with perforation of the tympanic membrane can result in an invasion of the middle ear and other pneumatized areas of the temporal bone by keratinizing squamous epithelium *(cholesteatoma).* Cholesteatomas can produce erosion of the ossicles and bony labyrinth, resulting in a mixed conductive sensorineural hearing loss. *Otosclerosis* commonly produces progressive conductive hearing loss by immobilizing the stapes with new bone growth in front of and below the oval window. The hearing loss is typically conductive, although in some persons the cochlea may be invaded by foci of otosclerotic bone, producing an additional sensorineural hearing loss. Otosclerosis usually stabilizes when the hearing level reaches 50 to 60 dB and rarely progresses to deafness. Other common causes of conductive hearing loss include trauma, congenital malformations of the external and middle ear, and glomus body tumors.

Sensorineural Hearing Loss. Genetically determined deafness, usually from hair cell aplasia or deterioration, may be present at birth or may develop in adulthood. The diagnosis of *hereditary deafness* rests on the finding of a positive family history. In many instances the inheritance is through a recessive gene or a dominant gene with low penetrance, making it difficult to determine the genetic nature of the disorder. *Intrauterine factors* resulting in congenital hearing loss include infection (especially rubella); toxic, metabolic, and endocrine disorders; and anoxia associated with Rh incompatibility and difficult deliveries.

Acute unilateral deafness usually has a cochlear basis. *Bacterial or viral infections* of the labyrinth, *head trauma* with fracture or hemorrhage into the cochlea, or *vascular occlusion* of a terminal branch of the anterior inferior cerebellar artery all can damage extensively the cochlea and its hair cells. An acute idiopathic, often reversible, unilateral hearing loss strikes young adults and is presumed to reflect an isolated viral infection of the cochlea and auditory nerve terminals. Sudden unilateral hearing loss often associated with vertigo and tinnitus can result from a *perilymphatic fistula.* Such fistulae may be congenital or may follow stapes surgery or head trauma. *Drugs* cause acute and subacute bilateral hearing impairment. Salicylates, furosemide, and ethacrynic acid have the potential to produce transient deafness when taken in high doses. More toxic to the cochlea are aminoglycoside antibiotics (gentamicin, tobramycin, amikacin, kanamycin, streptomycin, and neomycin). These agents can destroy cochlear hair cells in direct relation to their serum concentrations. Some antineoplastic chemotherapeutic agents, particularly cisplatin, cause severe ototoxicity.

Subacute relapsing cochlear deafness occurs with *Ménière syndrome,* a condition associated with fluctuating hearing loss and tinnitus, recurrent episodes of abrupt and often severe vertigo, and a sensation of fullness or pressure in the ear. Recurrent endolymphatic hypertension (hydrops) is believed to cause the episodes. Pathologically, the endolymphatic sac is dilated, and the hair cells become atrophic. The resulting deafness is subtle and reversible in the early stages but subsequently becomes permanent and is characterized by diplacusis and loudness recruitment. The disorder is usually unilateral, but in about 20 to 40% of patients bilateral involvement occurs.

The gradual, progressive, bilateral hearing loss commonly associated with advancing age is called *presbycusis.* Presbycusis is not a distinct disease entity but rather represents multiple effects of aging on the auditory system. It may include conductive and central dysfunction, although the most consistent effect of aging is on the sensory cells and neurons of the cochlea. The typical audiogram of presbycusis is a symmetric high-frequency hearing loss gradually sloping downward with increasing frequency. The most consistent pathology associated with presbycusis is degeneration of sensory cells and nerve fibers at the base of the cochlea. The recurrent trauma of *noise-induced hearing loss* affects approximately the same cochlear region and is almost as common, particularly among those with exposure to loud explosive or industrial noises. Loud, blaring, modern music has become a recent offender. The loss almost always begins at 4000 Hz and does not affect speech discrimination until late in the disease process. With only brief exposure to loud noise (hours to days) there may be only a temporary threshold shift, but with continued exposure permanent injury begins. The duration and intensity of exposure determine the degree of permanent injury.

Hearing loss from direct damage to the acoustic nerve in the petrous canal occasionally results from infection within or trauma to the surrounding bone; severe deafness of abrupt onset marks the event and is usually associated with acute vertigo due to concurrent vestibular nerve injury. Progressive unilateral hearing loss that arises insidiously and worsens by almost imperceptible degrees is characteristic of benign neoplasms of the cerebellopontine angle, such as *acoustic neuromas.* In about 10% of cases the hearing loss can be acute, apparently owing to either hemorrhage into the tumor or compression of the labyrinthine vasculature.

Central Hearing Loss. Central hearing loss is unilateral only if it results from damage to the pontine cochlear nuclei on one side of the brain stem. Such can occur with *ischemic infarction* of the lateral brain stem (e.g., occlusion of the anterior inferior cerbellar artery), a plaque of *multiple sclerosis,* or, rarely, invasion or compression of the lateral pons by a *neoplasm* or *hematoma.* Bilateral *degeneration* of the cochlear nuclei accompanies some of the rare recessive inherited disorders of childhood. As noted, clinically important unilateral hearing loss never results from neurologic disease arising rostrad to the cochlear nucleus. Although bilateral hearing loss could, in theory, result from bilat-eral destruction of central hearing pathways, in practice this is rare because involvement of neighboring structures in brain stem or hemisphere would usually produce overwhelming neurologic disability.

TREATMENT OF HEARING LOSS. If an underlying disorder has not yet destroyed the auditory system and can be ameliorated medically or surgically, hearing may be improved or preserved. Most patients with otosclerosis respond to stapedectomy. Closure of a perilymph fistula may improve hearing. Antibiotic and decongestive treatment of otitis media should prevent permanent hearing loss. A low-salt diet and diuretics are effective in selective cases of Meniere syndrome, particularly if episodes are precipitated by premenstrual water retention. Hearing aids amplify sound, usually with the goal of making speech intelligible. Patients with conductive hearing loss require simple amplification, but those with sensorineural hearing loss often need frequency-selective amplification in order to make hearing aids useful. Recent advances in acoustic technology have markedly improved the outlook for the latter. Monitoring audiograms in patients with noise- or ototoxic drug exposure are critical for prevention of permanent hearing loss.

TINNITUS. The flow chart in Figure 403–6 outlines the logic for determining the common causes of tinnitus. A careful history should be taken to identify common offending drugs (Table 403–5). With *objective tinnitus* the patient hears a sound arising external to the auditory system, a sound that can usually be heard by the examiner with a stethoscope. Objective tinnitus usually has benign causes such as noise from temporomandibular joints, opening of eustachian tubes, or repetitive muscle contractions. Sometimes, in a quiet room, the patient can hear the pulsatile flow in the carotid artery or a continuous hum of normal venous outflow through the jugular vein. The latter can be obliterated by compression of the jugular vein or extreme lateral rotation of the neck. Pathologic objective tinnitus occurs when patients hear turbulent flow in vascular anomalies or tumors (e.g., glomus jugulare tumor). Objective tinnitus may also be an early sign of increased intracranial pressure. Such tinnitus, which is usually overshadowed by other neurologic abnormalities, can be obliterated by pressure over the jugular vein. It probably arises from turbulent flow through compressed venous structures at the base of the brain.

TABLE 403–5. DRUGS COMMONLY ASSOCIATED WITH TINNITUS

Quinidine	Propranolol
Salicylates	Levodopa
Indomethacin	Aminophylline
Carbamazepine	Caffeine

Subjective tinnitus can arise from sites anywhere in the auditory system. The sounds most frequently complained of are metallic ringing, buzzing, blowing, roaring, or, less often, bizarre clanging, popping, or nonrhythmic beating. Tinnitus heard as a faint, moderately high-pitched, metallic ring can be observed by almost anyone who concentrates attention on auditory events in a quiet room. Sustained louder tinnitus accompanied by audiometric evidence of deafness occurs in association with both conductive and sensorineural hearing loss. Tinnitus observed with otosclerosis tends to have a roaring or hissing quality, while that associated with Meniere syndrome often produces sounds that vary widely in intensity with time and quality, sometimes including roaring or clanging. Tinnitus with other cochlear or auditory nerve lesions tends to be higher pitched and ringing in quality. Audiometric and brain stem–evoked response testing can help distinguish between lesions involving the conducting apparatus, the cochlea, and the auditory nerve.

Tinnitus without observable deafness appears sporadically and for variable lengths of time in many persons without other evidence of an ongoing pathologic process. In many instances one suspects that the auditory experience is no more than an anxious preoccupation with normal auditory physiology.

TREATMENT OF TINNITUS. Most patients with tinnitus can be helped by detailed interview together with the relevant examination and laboratory investigations followed by reassurance where this can be given. Often exacerbating factors such as chronic anxiety and depression can be identified. In patients with hearing loss and tinnitus a hearing aid may improve communication in two ways, as amplification of ambient sound may effectively mask the tinnitus. This mechanism probably explains the frequent observation that removal of cerumen from the external auditory canal to im-

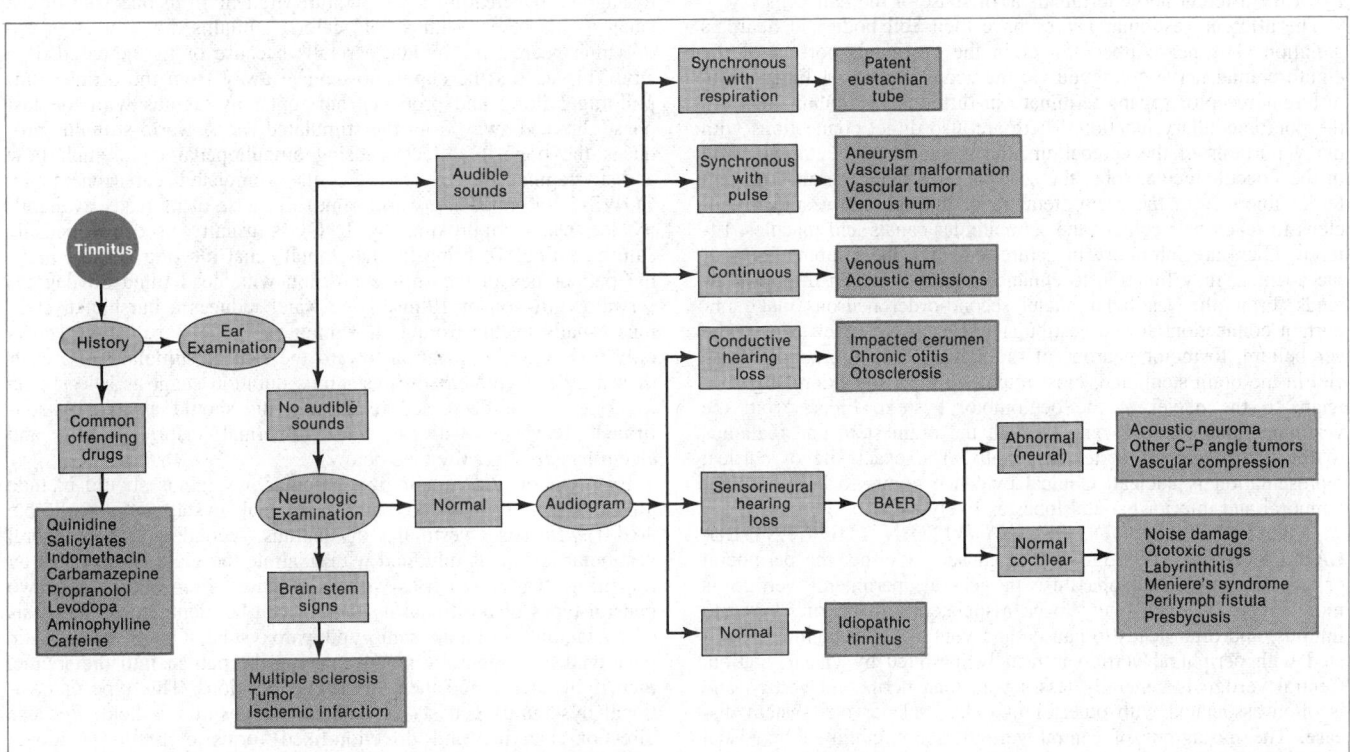

FIGURE 403–6. Evaluation of tinnitus.

prove ambient hearing also improves tinnitus. Also, when cerumen is attached to the tympanic membrane, tinnitus may result from local mechanical effects on the conductive system. For patients who find their tinnitus most obtrusive when trying to sleep, a bedside FM clock radio tuned between stations can provide an effective masking sound that will switch itself off after the patient falls asleep. A careful drug history should be taken, and a drug-free trial period should be considered when possible. Some patients who notice that caffeine, alcohol, or nicotine exacerbates their tinnitus experience significant relief when these drugs are discontinued.

EQUILIBRIUM—VESTIBULAR SYSTEM

ANATOMY AND PHYSIOLOGY OF THE VESTIBULAR SYSTEM. The paired vestibular end organs lie within the temporal bones next to the cochlea. Each organ consists of three semicircular canals that detect angular acceleration and two otolith structures, the utricle and saccule, that detect linear acceleration (including gravitational). Like the cochlea, these organs possess hair cells that act as force transducers, converting the forces associated with head acceleration into afferent nerve impulses. The hair cells of the three semicircular canals, each of which is oriented at right angles to the others, are concentrated in the crista, where they are embedded in a gelatinous mass called the cupula. Movement of the head causes the endolymph to flow either toward or away from the cupula, bending the hair cells and, depending on the direction of endolymphatic movements, either exciting or inhibiting the afferent nerve firing. Because the afferent nerves arising from the semicircular canals are tonically active, the baseline activity can be increased or decreased depending on the direction of hair cell bending. Furthermore, the two sets of semicircular canals are approximately mirror images of each other, so that rotational movement of the head that excites one canal inhibits the analogous canal on the opposite side. The hair cells of the utricle and saccule are concentrated in an area called the macule. The macule of the utricle lies approximately in the plane of the horizontal canal and the macule of the saccule is approximately in the plane of the anterior canal. The hair cells are embedded in a membrane that contains calcium carbonate crystals or otoliths; the density of otoliths is considerably greater than that of the endolymph. Linear accelerations of the head combine with the linear acceleration of gravity to distort the otolith membrane, thereby bending the underlying hair cells and modulating the activity of the afferent nerve terminals at the base of the hair cells.

The afferent vestibular nerves have their cell bodies in Scarpa's ganglion. The nerve fibers travel in the vestibular portion of the eighth cranial nerve contiguous to the acoustic portion. Fibers from different receptor organs terminate in different vestibular nuclei at the pontomedullary junction. There are also direct connections with many portions of the cerebellum, the greatest representation being in the flocculonocular lobe, the so-called vestibular cerebellum. Efferent fibers from the brain stem travel through the vestibular nucleus to reach hair cells of the semicircular canals and macules. Efferent fibers are inhibitory in nature and, like the efferent fibers of the cochlea, may function to enhance inputs to which the brain attends. From the vestibular nuclei second-order neurons make important connections to the vestibular nuclei of the other side, to the cerebellum, to motor neurons of the spinal cord, to autonomic nuclei in the brain stem, and, most importantly for the examining clinician, to the nuclei of the oculomotor system. Fibers from the vestibular nuclei also ascend through the brain stem and thalamus to reach the cerebral cortex bilaterally. The exact site of cortical representation is unclear. Clinical evidence points to both superior temporal and inferior parietal lobes as likely sites.

LOCALIZATION OF LESIONS WITHIN THE VESTIBULAR PATHWAYS. Vertigo can be caused by either the peripheral or central vestibular apparatus. In general, peripheral vertigo is more severe, is more likely to be associated with hearing loss and tinnitus, and often leads to nausea and vomiting. Nystagmus associated with peripheral vertigo is usually inhibited by visual fixation. Central vertigo is generally less severe than peripheral vertigo and is often associated with other signs of central nervous system disease. The nystagmus of central vertigo is not inhibited by visual fixation and frequently is prominent when vertigo is mild or absent.

EXAMINATION OF THE VESTIBULAR SYSTEM. Most vestibular problems presenting to the physician are episodic, and often there are neither symptoms nor signs when the physician examines the patient. The history, therefore, can become paramount for identifying vestibular dysfunction. The history should attempt to distinguish vertigo (the illusion of movement in space) from light-headedness (presyncope), ataxia (disequilibrium of the body without true movement in space), and psychogenic symptoms (the feeling of dissociation or, sometimes, dysequilibrium). If the history is not clear, bedside provocative tests to mimic the symptom may assist in making a pathophysiologic diagnosis. Hyperventilation, which lowers the $Paco_2$ and decreases cerebral blood flow, causes a light-headed sensation associated with syncope. Ask the patient to hyperventilate maximally for 1 to 3 minutes to cause light-headedness. If the episode mimics the patient's symptoms it suggests that anxiety and hyperventilation may be playing an important role. In addition, during the course of hyperventilation the patient may suffer dry mouth, chest tightness, and paresthesias, which may be recognized as part of the spontaneous attacks, thus helping in diagnosis.

Bedside tests of vestibulospinal function are often insensitive because most patients can use vision and proprioceptive signals to compensate for any vestibular loss. Patients with acute unilateral peripheral vestibular lesions may past point or fall toward the side of the lesion, but within a few days balance returns to normal. Patients with bilateral peripheral vestibular loss have more difficulty compensating and usually show some imbalance on the Romberg and tandem walking tests, particularly with eyes closed.

The vestibulo-ocular reflex can be tested at the bedside by inducing physiologic nystagmus and searching for pathologic nystagmus. In an alert human, rotating the head back and forth in the horizontal plane induces compensatory horizontal eye movements that are dependent on both the visual and vestibular systems. The doll's-eye test is a test of vestibular function in a comatose patient, since such patients cannot generate pursuit or corrective fast components. In this setting conjugate compensatory eye movements indicate normally functioning vestibulo-ocular pathways. Because the vestibulo-ocular reflex has a much higher frequency range than the smooth pursuit system, a qualitative bedside test of vestibular function can be made by having the patient shake his head back and forth at frequencies above 1 Hz while reading a standard visual acuity chart. A decrease in visual acuity of more than one line compared with testing with the patient's head kept still indicates an abnormal vestibulo-ocular reflex.

The caloric test uses a nonphysiologic stimulus to induce endolymphatic flow in the horizontal semicircular canal and horizontal nystagmus by creating a temperature gradient from one side of the canal to the other. With a cold caloric stimulus the column of endolymph nearest the middle ear falls because of its increased density. This causes the cupula to deviate away from the utricle (ampullofugal flow) and produces horizontal nystagmus with the fast phase directed away from the stimulated ear. A warm stimulus produces the opposite effect, causing ampullopedal endolymph flow and nystagmus directed toward the stimulated ear (mnemonic: COWS—cold opposite, warm same). Because of its ready availability ice water (approximately 0° C) is usually used for bedside caloric testing. To bring the horizontal canal into the vertical plane the patient lies in the supine position with head tilted 30 degrees forward. Infusion of 10 ml of ice water induces a burst of nystagmus usually lasting from 1 to 3 minutes. A comatose patient shows only a slow tonic deviation toward the side of stimulation. Greater than a 20% asymmetry in nystagmus duration suggests a lesion on the side of the decreased response. This should always be confirmed, however, with standard bithermal caloric testing and electronystagmography (see below).

Examination for pathologic vestibular nystagmus should include a search for spontaneous and positional nystagmus (see Table 403–4). Because vestibular nystagmus secondary to peripheral vestibular lesions is inhibited with fixation, the yield is increased by impairing fixation (such as with +30 lenses, Frenzel glasses). Two general types of positional nystagmus can be identified on the basis of nystagmus duration: static and paroxysmal. One induces static positional nystagmus by slowly placing the patient into the supine, then right lateral, and then left lateral positions. This type of positional nystagmus persists as long as the position is held. Because direction-changing and direction-fixed forms of static positional nystagmus occur with both peripheral and central vestibular lesions, their presence indicates only a dysfunction somewhere in the

TABLE 403–6. DISTINGUISHING BETWEEN VESTIBULAR AND NONVESTIBULAR TYPES OF DIZZINESS

	Vestibular	Nonvestibular
Common descriptive terms	Spinning (environment moves), merry-go-round, drunkenness, tilting, motion sickness, off-balance	Light-headed, floating, dissociated from body, swimming, giddy, spinning inside (environment stationary)
Course	Episodic	Constant
Common precipitating factors	Head movements, position change	Stress, hyperventilation, cardiac arrhythmia, situations
Common associated symptoms	Nausea, vomiting, unsteadiness, tinnitus, hearing loss, impaired vision, oscillopsia	Perspiration, pallor, paresthesias, palpitations, syncope, difficulty concentrating, tension headache

From Baloh RW, Honrubia V: Clinical Neurophysiology of the Vestibular System. 2nd ed. Philadelphia, FA Davis, 1990.

vestibular system. As with spontaneous nystagmus, however, lack of suppression with fixation and signs of associated brain-stem dysfunction suggest a central lesion.

Paroxysmal positional nystagmus is induced, after a brief delay, by a rapid change from erect sitting to supine head-hanging left, center, or right position (the so-called Hallpike maneuver). It is initially high in frequency but dissipates rapidly (within 30 seconds to 1 minute). The most common variety of paroxysmal positional nystagmus, benign positional nystagmus, usually has a 3- to 10-second latency before onset and rarely lasts longer than 30 seconds. The nystagmus is always torsional with fast phase directed upward (i.e., toward the forehead). It is usually prominent in only one head-hanging position, and a burst of nystagmus in the reverse direction occurs when the patient reassumes the sitting position. Another key feature is the severe vertigo and nystagmus that the patient experiences with the initial positioning which, with repeated positioning, rapidly disappear (fatigability). Benign positional nystagmus is a sign of vestibular end-organ disease (see below).

Electronystagmography (ENG) is a technique for recording eye movements that allows precise quantification of both physiologic and pathologic nystagmus. A standard ENG test battery includes (1) tests of visual ocular control (saccades, smooth pursuit, and optokinetic nystagmus); (2) a careful search for pathologic nystagmus with fixation and with eyes open in darkness, and (3) measurement of induced physiologic nystagmus (caloric and rotational). ENG can be helpful in identifying a vestibular lesion and localizing it within the peripheral and central pathways.

EVALUATING THE "DIZZY" PATIENT. The history is key because it determines the type of dizziness (vertigo, light-headed, feeling of dissociation, disequilibrium), associated symptoms (neurologic, audiologic, cardiac, psychiatric), precipitating factors (position change, trauma, stress, drug ingestion), and predisposing illness (systemic viral infection, cardiac disease, cerebrovascular disease). Features that distinguish between vestibular and nonvestibular types of dizziness are summarized in Table 403–6. The examination should include complete neurologic, head and neck, and cardiac assessments. When focal neurologic signs are found, neuroimaging usually leads to specific diagnosis. When vertigo is present without focal neurologic symptoms or signs, audiometry and electronystagmography aid in localizing the lesion to the labyrinth or eighth nerve. Patients with hyperventilation syndrome and/or acute anxiety should be identified after the history and examination so that needless tests are not obtained. A detailed cardiac evaluation (including Holter monitoring) often identifies the cause of episodic presyncopal light-headedness.

COMMON CAUSES OF VERTIGO. The logic for identifying common causes of vertigo is shown in Figure 403–7.

Physiologic Vertigo. Physiologic vertigo includes common disorders such as *motion sickness, space sickness,* and *height vertigo.* In these conditions vertigo (defined as an illusion of movement) is minimal or absent while autonomic symptoms predominate. With height vertigo, patients often experience acute anxiety and panic reaction. Individuals with motion sickness and space sickness typically develop perspiration, nausea, vomiting, increased salivation, yawning, and generalized malaise. Gastric motility is reduced and digestion impaired. Even the sight or smell of food is distressing. Hyperventilation is a common sign, and the resulting hypocapnia leads to changes in blood volume, with pooling in the lower parts of the body predisposing to postural hypotension and syncope. An unusual variant of motion sickness continues when the subject returns to stationary conditions after prolonged exposure to motion. Typically, affected patients report that they feel the persistent rocking sensation of a boat long after returning to solid ground. Rarely, the syndrome can last for months to years after exposure to motion and can even be incapacitating. The cause is unknown.

Physiologic vertigo can often be suppressed by supplying sensory cues that help to match the signals originating from different sensory systems. Thus, motion sickness, which is exacerbated by sitting in a closed space or reading (giving the visual system the miscue that the environment is stationary), may be improved by looking out at the environment and watching it move. Height vertigo, caused by a mismatch between sensation of normal body sway and lack of its visual detection, can often be relieved either by sitting or by visually fixating a nearby stationary object.

Benign Positional Vertigo (BPV). BPV is by far the most common cause of pathologic vertigo. Patients with this condition

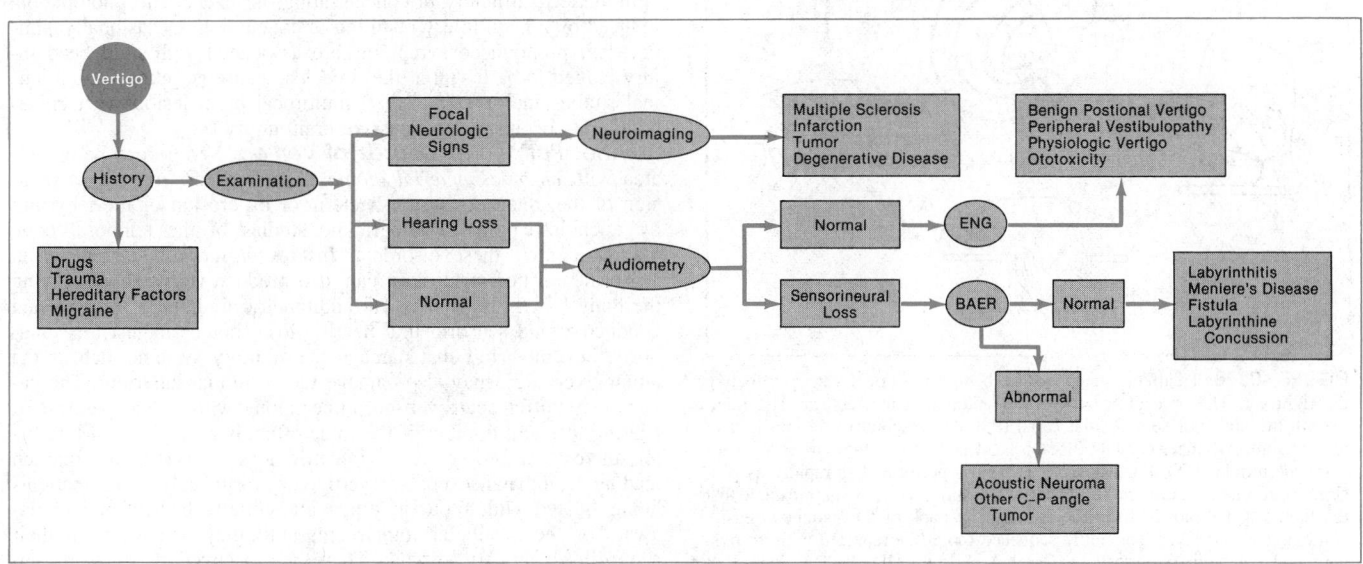

FIGURE 403–7. Evaluation of vertigo.

develop brief episodes of vertigo (less than 1 min) with position change, typically when turning over in bed, getting in and out of bed, bending over and straightening up, or extending the neck to look up. BPV can result from *head injury, viral labyrinthitis,* and *vascular occlusion,* or it may occur as an isolated symptom of unknown cause (in about 50% of cases). The latter is particularly common in the elderly. This syndrome is important to recognize because in the vast majority of patients, the symptoms spontaneously remit. It does commonly recur, however. The diagnosis rests on finding characteristic fatigable paroxysmal positional nystagmus after a rapid change from the sitting to the head-hanging position (see above). BPV is thought to result from free-floating calcium carbonate crystals (normally attached to the utricular macule) that inadvertently enter the long arm of the posterior semicircular canal. The crystals move within the endolymph and artificially displace the cupula. Consistent with this theory, the burst of paroxysmal positional nystagmus is in the plane of the posterior canal of the "down ear," and the positional nystagmus disappears after the ampullary nerve has been surgically resected from the posterior canal on the diseased side. If the history and physical findings are typical, a simple bedside positioning maneuver can remove the debris from the posterior semicircular canal in most patients (Fig. 403–8). If the history or findings are atypical, the condition must be distinguished from other causes of positional vertigo that may occur with tumors or infarcts of the posterior fossa.

Acute Peripheral Vestibulopathy ("Acute Labyrinthitis").

One of the most common clinical neurologic syndromes at any age is the acute onset of vertigo, nausea, and vomiting lasting for several days and not associated with auditory or neurologic symptoms. Most affected patients gradually improve over 1 to 2 weeks, but some develop recurrent episodes. A large percentage report an upper respiratory tract illness 1 to 2 weeks prior to the onset of vertigo. This syndrome occasionally occurs in epidemics (epidemic

vertigo), may affect several members of the same family, and more often erupts in the spring and early summer. All of these factors suggest a viral origin, but attempts to isolate an agent have been unsuccessful, except for occasional findings of a herpes zoster infection. Pathologic studies showing atrophy of one or more vestibular nerve trunks, with or without atrophy of their associated sense organs, are evidence of a vestibular nerve site and, probably, viral cause for many patients with this syndrome *(viral neurolabyrinthitis).* In some patients attacks of acute vestibulopathy (usually less severe) recur over many months or years. There is no way of predicting whether a person who suffers a first attack will have repetitive attacks.

Meniere Syndrome.

The typical clinical features of Ménière syndrome are described earlier (see p. 2022). This disorder accounts for about 10% of all patients with vertigo. The diagnosis is based on documenting episodic severe attacks accompanied by more or less continuous tinnitus and fluctuating hearing levels on audiometric testing.

Migraine.

Vertigo is a common symptom with migraine. It can occur with headaches or in separate isolated episodes, and it can predate the onset of headache. So-called benign paroxysmal vertigo of childhood is often the first symptom of migraine. The mechanism of vertigo with migraine is not clear, but damage to the inner ear occurs in about one third of patients. A few develop typical features of Ménière syndrome.

Post-traumatic Vertigo.

Vertigo, hearing loss, and tinnitus often follow a blow to the head that does not result in temporal bone fracture, the so-called *labyrinthine concussion.* Although they are protected by a bony capsule, the delicate labyrinthine membranes are susceptible to blunt trauma. Blows to the occipital or mastoid region are particularly likely to produce labyrinthine damage. *Transverse fractures* of the temporal bone typically pass through the vestibule of the inner ear, tearing the membranous labyrinth and lacerating the vestibular and cochlear nerves. Complete loss of vestibular and cochlear function is the usual sequela, and the facial nerve is interrupted in approximately 50% of cases. Examination of the ear often reveals hemotympanum, but bleeding from the ear seldom occurs because the tympanic membrane usually remains intact. As noted above, *benign positional vertigo* is also a common sequela of head trauma. *Fistulae* of the oval and round windows can result from impact noise, deep-water diving, severe physical exertion, or blunt head injury without skull fracture. The mechanism of the rupture is a sudden negative or positive pressure change in the middle ear or a sudden increase in cerebrospinal fluid pressure transmitted to the inner ear via the cochlear aqueduct and internal auditory canal. Clinically, the rupture leads to the sudden onset of vertigo or hearing loss, or both. Surgical exploration of the middle ear is warranted when there is a clear relationship between the onset of vertigo or hearing loss, or both, and the onset of severe exertion, barometric change, head injury, or impact noise.

Postconcussion Syndrome.

The so-called postconcussion syndrome refers to a vague dizziness (rarely vertigo) associated with anxiety, difficulty in concentrating, headache, and photophobia induced by a head injury resulting in concussion. Occasionally, similar, less pronounced symptoms are associated with mild head injury judged to be trivial at the time. The cause is unknown, but animal studies indicate that small multifocal brain lesions (petechiae) commonly occur after concussive brain injury.

Other Peripheral Causes of Vertigo.

Vertigo can be associated with *chronic bacterial otomastoiditis,* either from direct invasion of the inner ear by the bacteria or by erosion of the labyrinth by a cholesteatoma. Radiographic studies of the temporal bone readily identify these disorders. Just as *otosclerosis* can result in sensorineural hearing loss, it can also produce vertigo by involving the bony labyrinth. The typical audiometric findings of a combined conductive and sensorineural hearing loss should suggest this diagnosis. Several *drugs* that damage the auditory system, such as the aminoglycosides, may also damage the vestibular labyrinth. The patient may suffer acute vertigo, either along with or independent of hearing loss and tinnitus, if the toxic effect is asymmetric. More often there is a progressive symmetric loss of vestibular function leading to imbalance but not vertigo. Unfortunately, many patients being treated with ototoxic drugs are initially bedridden and unaware of the vestibular impairment until they recover from their acute illness and try to walk. Then they discover that they are unsteady on their feet and that the environment tends to jiggle in front

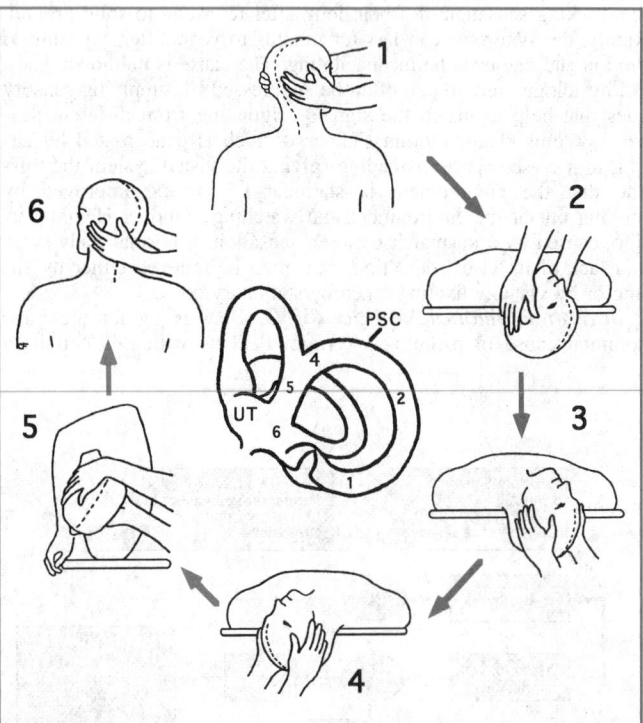

FIGURE 403–8. Treatment maneuver for benign positional vertigo affecting the right ear. The procedure is reversed for treating the left ear. The numbers in the posterior semicircular canal (PSC) correspond to the position of the calcium carbonate crystals in each head position as they are moved toward the utricle (UT). Each position change is performed as rapidly as possible to accelerate the particles. Positions 2 and 3 are the same except that the therapist has moved from the front to the back of the patient to easily continue the maneuver. The entire sequence should be repeated until no nystagmus is elicited. (Courtesy of Carol A. Foster, MD, UCLA School of Medicine.)

of their eyes (*oscillopsia*). Younger patients adapt after weeks to the labyrinthine failure; older ones may be left permanently disabled. Usually there is no nystagmus (because of the symmetric involvement), but the patient is ataxic. Caloric and rotational tests during electronystagmography can document impairment or absence of vestibular function. The best treatment is prevention. If the drug is discontinued early during the course of symptoms the disorder may stabilize or improve.

Vascular Insufficiency. Vertebrobasilar insufficiency is a common cause of vertigo in the elderly (see also Ch. 419). Whether the vertigo originates from ischemia of the labyrinth, brain stem, or both structures is not always clear because the blood supply to the labyrinth, eighth cranial nerve, and vestibular nuclei originate from the same source, the basilar vertebral circulation. Vertigo with *vertebrobasilar insufficiency* is abrupt in onset, usually lasting several minutes, and is frequently associated with nausea and vomiting. Associated symptoms resulting from ischemia in the remaining territory supplied by the posterior circulation include visual illusions and hallucinations, drop attack and weakness, visceral sensations, visual field defects, diplopia, and headache. These symptoms occur in episodes either in combination with the vertigo or alone. Vertigo may be an isolated initial symptom of vertebrobasilar ischemia, but repeated episodes of vertigo without other symptoms should suggest another diagnosis. Vertebrobasilar insufficiency usually is caused by atherosclerosis of the subclavian, vertebral, and basilar arteries. Occasionally, episodes of vertebrobasilar insufficiency are precipitated by postural hypotension, Stokes-Adams attacks, or mechanical compression from cervical spondylosis. Diagnostic studies including CT scans are usually normal because the vascular insufficiency is transient and function returns to normal between episodes. Angiography can be helpful in confirming the diagnosis but carries a risk and rarely leads to definitive therapy.

Vertigo is a common symptom associated with *infarction of the lateral brain stem or cerebellum,* or both. The diagnosis usually is clear, based on the characteristic acute history and pattern of associated symptoms and neurologic findings. Occasionally cerebellar infarction or hemorrhage presents with severe vertigo, vomiting, and ataxia without associated brain-stem symptoms and signs that might suggest the erroneous diagnosis of an acute peripheral vestibular disorder. The key differential point is the finding of clear cerebellar signs (extremity- and gait ataxia) and gaze-evoked nystagmus. Such patients must be watched carefully for several days because they may develop progressive brain-stem dysfunction owing to compression by a swollen cerebellum.

Cerebellopontine-Angle Tumors. Most tumors growing in the cerebellopontine angle (e.g., *acoustic neuroma, meningioma, epidermal cyst*) grow slowly, allowing the vestibular system to accommodate so that they produce a vague sensation of disequilibrium rather than acute vertigo. Occasionally, however, episodic vertigo or positional vertigo heralds the presence of a cerebellopontine-angle tumor. In virtually all patients, retrocochlear hearing loss is present, best identified by an abnormal brain-stem auditory evoked response. Magnetic resonance imaging (MRI) of the cerebellopontine angles is the most sensitive diagnostic study for identifying a cerebellopontine-angle tumor.

Other Central Causes of Vertigo. Acute vertigo may be the first symptom of *multiple sclerosis,* although only a small percentage of young patients with acute vertigo eventually develop multiple sclerosis. Vertigo in multiple sclerosis is usually transient and often associated with other neurologic signs of brain-stem disease, in particular, internuclear ophthalmoplegia or cerebellar dysfunction. Vertigo may also be a symptom of *parainfectious encephalomyelitis* or, rarely, *parainfectious cranial polyneuritis.* In this instance the accompanying neurologic signs establish the diagnosis. The *Ramsay-Hunt syndrome* (geniculate ganglion herpes) is characterized by vertigo and hearing loss associated with facial paralysis and, sometimes, pain in the ear. The typical lesions of herpes zoster, which may follow the appearance of neurologic signs, are found in the external auditory canal and over the palate in some patients. Rarely is herpes zoster responsible for vertigo in the absence of the full-blown syndrome. *Granulomatous meningitis* or *leptomeningeal metastasis* and cerebral or systemic *vasculitis* may involve the eighth nerve, producing vertigo as an early symptom. In these disorders cerebrospinal fluid analysis usually suggests the diagnosis. Patients suffering from *temporal lobe epilepsy* occasionally experience vertigo as the aura. Vertigo in the absence of other neu-

rologic signs or symptoms is never caused by epilepsy or other diseases of the cerebral hemispheres.

TREATMENT OF VERTIGO. Treatment of vertigo can be divided into three general categories: specific, symptomatic, and rehabilitative. Specific therapies include antibiotics for bacterial or syphilitic labyrinthitis, anticoagulants for vertebrobasilar insufficiency, and surgery for acoustic neuroma. When possible, treatment should be directed at the underlying disorder. In most cases, however, symptomatic treatment is either combined with specific therapy or is the only one available (e.g., with acute peripheral vestibulopathy). Many different classes of drugs have been found to have antivertiginous properties, and in most instances the exact mechanism of action is uncertain. All of these agents produce potentially unpleasant side effects, and the decision on which drug or combination to use is based on their known complications and on the severity and duration of the vertigo. An episode of prolonged, severe vertigo is one of the most distressing symptoms that one can experience. Affected patients prefer to lie still with eyes closed in a quiet, dark room. Antivertiginous drugs with sedation such as phenergan (25 mg four times daily [q.i.d.]) or diazepam (5 mg q.i.d.) may be helpful. Prochlorperazine suppositories (25 mg) may stop vomiting. In more chronic vertiginous disorders, when the patient is trying to carry on normal activity, less sedating antivertiginous medications such as meclizine (25 mg q.i.d.) or transdermal scopolamine (0.5 mg every 3 days) may provide relief. Vestibular rehabilitation exercises are designed to help the patient compensate for permanent loss of vestibular function.

Baloh RW, Honrubia V: Clinical Neurophysiology of the Vestibular System, 2nd ed. Philadelphia, FA Davis, 1990. *Monograph reviewing basic and clinical aspects of vestibular function.*

Brandt T, Steddin S: Current view of the mechanism of benign paroxysmal positioning vertigo: Cupulolithiasis or canalolithiasis? J Vest Res 3:373, 1993. *Why the positioning maneuver works.*

Hazell JWP: Tinnitus I, II and III. J Otolaryngol 19:1, 6, 11, 1990. *Up-to-date clinical review.*

Nadol JB: Hearing loss. N Engl J Med 329:1092, 1993. *Timely review.*

404 DISORDERS OF MOTOR FUNCTION

404.1 Weakness, Asthenia, and Fatigue
Fred Plum

The terms *weakness, asthenia,* and *fatigue* imprecisely overlap. *Weakness* most often refers specifically to reduced motor capacity, either regional or general in distribution. Table 404–1 lists specific disorders and mechanisms producing weakness. Rowland's textbook chapter well describes the clinical findings. *Asthenia* carries the mixed definition of loss of strength, energy, or vitality—hardly unambiguous synonyms. Long usage reflects the double meaning, the term *asthenia* having been applied equally to the poorly understood state of psychic weakness (neurasthenia) and to the biologically well-established muscle weakness of myasthenia gravis. Medically, *weakness* is best used to describe demonstrably reduced muscle strength in specific area(s) of the body. *Asthenia* is too ambiguous to be useful.

Table 404–2 defines several particular acute or subacute disorders that may cause generalized weakness. Beyond these classes of specifically identifiable disorders, however, most chronic weakness unaccompanied by diagnosable neurologic or appropriate medical conditions is more likely to have a psychiatric than a neurologic genesis.

Fatigue, as employed in medical terms, describes a reduction in performance due to excessive effort or an experienced deterioration

TABLE 404–1. CAUSES OF ACUTE OR SUBACUTE WEAKNESS

Condition	Examples or Mechanisms
Joint or muscle injury-inflammation	Movement of the part induces pain.
Primary muscle disease	Genetically transmitted muscle or mitochondrial disorders; inflammatory or granulomatous myopathies; corticosteroid administration
Neuromuscular junction	Myasthenia gravis; Lambert-Eaton myasthenic syndrome
Peripheral motor or sensorimotor pathways (lower motor neuron)	Damage to peripheral motor nerves, spinal motor roots, anterior horn cells
	N.B.: Dysfunction of proprioceptive sensory pathways can produce the illusion of weakness secondary to impaired position sense.
Corticospinal pathways (upper motor neuron)	Disease or injury to the system anywhere from above the anterior horn cell to frontal lobe motor areas
Basal ganglia	Hypokinesia, slow starting, and weakness in parkinsonism
Cerebellum	Sense of incomplete strength with neocerebellar damage
Hysterical or pretended weakness	Signs inconsistent with specific physiologic failure

in capacity. Fatigue lasting weeks or months can accompany or follow several serious illnesses listed in Table 404–2. Fatigue can be local or general, acute or chronic, and, depending on circumstance, the sense of exhaustion may follow, accompany, or precede attempts at either motor or intellectual effort. Most short-term fatigue lasting for minutes to as much as a few weeks in duration can be traced to recognized antecedents, such as acute systemic illness, severe emotional perturbation, or intense effort of either a physical or intellectual nature. Recurrent, rapidly developing fatigue involving local or generalized striated muscle is typical of myasthenia gravis or, less often, the metabolic myopathies (see Ch. 457). Multiple sclerosis and Parkinson's disease characteristically are accompanied by chronic feelings of fatigue, usually worse at the end than at the beginning of the day. Processes such as tuberculosis, systemic cancer, subacute endocarditis, collagen vascular disease, and certain endocrinopathies represent less frequent causes. Subacute, disabling fatigue also can accompany early HIV involvement of the brain, but that condition also causes recognizable abnormalities in cognitive capacities.

Medical records going back a number of years indicate that many otherwise healthy adults experience continuous fatigue either chronically or in restricted epidemics to a degree sufficient to interfere with employment or domestic responsibilities. Recently identified as having *chronic fatigue syndrome,* such subacutely or chronically fatigued patients compared with nonexhausted controls have not shown higher long-term antibody titers against Epstein-Barr virus,

TABLE 404–2. MEDICAL-NEUROLOGIC ILLNESSES COMMONLY ASSOCIATED WITH ACUTE-SUBACUTE GENERALIZED WEAKNESS OR FATIGUE

Systemic	Neurologic
Acute bacterial-viral infections	Myasthenia gravis
Thyrotoxicosis	Early polyneuropathy
Post–myocardial infarction	Multiple sclerosis
Addison's disease	Parkinsonism
Disseminated malignancy	Postconcussion syndrome
Anticancer chemotherapy	Sustained drug use
Acute hepatitis; acute Epstein-Barr virus or Lyme disease	
Severe anemia	

Lyme borreliosis, or other organisms. Studies to date find few relevant physical or laboratory abnormalities in most chronically fatigued patients.

All well-analyzed studies of patients with chronic debilitating fatigue emphasize the high incidence of the symptoms (up to 25% or more of primary care patients), the lack of identifiable medical abnormalities, and a high incidence of psychiatric disorder. Symptoms of chronic anxiety, personality disorders, or depression have been identified in as many as 80% of such cohorts. The condition frequently includes somatoform complaints unaccompanied by physical or laboratory abnormalities as well as expressions of autonomic dysfunction including breathlessness, palpitations, tachycardia, constipation-diarrhea, sexual impairment, inappropriate sweating, and unsatisfactory sleep patterns. Prospective and retrospective studies consistently have identified significantly more manifestations of depression, somatic anxiety, and emotional maladjustment than were expressed by nonfatigued controls chosen from patients with neuromuscular disease or recovering from known viral illnesses. No satisfactorily evaluated treatment program has been forthcoming for persons with chronic fatigue. Most patients with somatoform disorders of this kind have sustained better outcomes when "floated" by physicians providing repeated reassurances at short intervals than by psychiatrists attempting intense psychotherapy. Advisory psychiatric consultation, as well as modest doses of tricyclic antidepressants for some, have at times been found to reduce an otherwise high rate of incapacitating somatoform complaints.

As Wilson et al. conclude, "The lack of specificity in the treatment of chronic fatigue syndrome encourages pseudoscience and the proliferation of those willing to exploit patients' beliefs in simplistic pathophysiologic models. In this, little has changed since the 19th century when treatment by rest and reflexology were embraced by many physicians as a model for managing the neurasthenic patient."

Kroenke K, Wood DR, Mangelsdorff AD, et al.: Chronic fatigue in primary care. Prevalence, patient characteristics and outcome. JAMA 260:929, 1988. *Among 1159 consecutive outpatients in primary care clinics, 24% described chronic fatigue as a major problem. Screening psychometric instruments identified depression, somatic anxiety, or both among 80% of fatigued patients versus 12% of controls.*
Rowland LP: Weakness: The syndromes caused by weak muscles. *In* Rowland LP (ed.): Merritt's Textbook of Neurology, 8th ed. Philadelphia, Lea & Febiger, 1989, p 50. *A systematic explanation of patterns of weakness accompanying disease entities ranging from muscle to brain.*
Schlueberg A, Straus SE, Peterson P: Chronic fatigue syndrome research. Definition and medical outcome assessment. Ann Intern Med 117:325, 1992. *An NIH workshop found no consistency in patient physical findings or laboratory tests to confirm the diagnosis. Similarities to the fibromyalgia syndrome and necessity for psychiatric screening were emphasized.*
Wilson A, Hickie I, Lloyd A, et al.: The treatment of chronic fatigue syndrome: Science and speculation. Am J Med 96:544, 1994. *A team including specialists in psychiatry, infectious diseases, and immunopathology sets out sensible guidelines for evaluation and management.*

404.2 Ataxia and Related Gait Disorders
Fred Plum

The brain is the organ of behavior, and the perceptive physician can learn a great deal about patients by observing their natural behavior in everyday tasks such as talking, writing, taking a coat off or putting it on, and especially how they coordinate their movements in the everyday acts of walking and turning. Natural walking represents a well-coordinated continuum of a series of falls under the momentum of a forwardly pushed torso and head. Normal gaits vary widely but have certain features in common. Head and trunk are held generally erect with the face and eyes looking forward rather than consistently either skyward or earthward. The four extremities interact gracefully, easily, and reciprocally, with right arm and left leg moving in one direction and left arm and right leg taking the opposite direction. Normally, the legs stride along a nearly straight line with footprints spaced approximately 1 to 3 inches to either side, the spread depending somewhat on walking speed and terrain. Upon that background, the following abnormal gaits can be compared.

ATAXIA. Ataxia is a failure of muscular coordination expressed as irregularity or awkwardness of movement. Most often the analysis of ataxia as a diagnostic problem lies in distinguishing disturbances in proprioceptive control from those caused by weakness, cerebellar-vestibular abnormalities, or the influence of toxic drugs.

PROPRIOCEPTIVE (SENSORY) ATAXIA. Proprioceptive ataxia can result from abnormalities anywhere along the afferent pathway from peripheral nerve, dorsal root, dorsal spinal funiculus, or the sensory projection from the thalamus to the parietal lobe cortex. The functional defect results from an impaired perception of the location of the body part combined with relatively preserved strength in the member.

Bilateral peripheral nerve or root lesions cause a defect that characteristically (1) affects the lower more than the upper extremities, (2) involves position sense as much as or more than vibratory sensation, (3) shows absent or greatly reduced deep tendon reflexes, and (4) produces a broad-based, weaving gait that with severe sensory loss becomes lurching, sometimes leg flinging, or pounding, and is worse in the dark (rombergism). Spinal dorsal column lesions produce similar symptoms except that position loss may be more profound, the signs may be less equally symmetric, the tendon reflexes can be preserved, and pathologic reflexes may be present if the abnormality involves the corticospinal tract. Patients with peripheral or spinal sensory ataxia are subjectively well aware of their deficits. They are also aware that their lack of coordination is not due to "dizziness," which distinguishes them from patients with vestibular disorders. Parietal or thalamoparietal proprioceptive impairment produces an ataxia that is usually unilateral and (1) affects the contralateral upper extremity as severely as the lower, (2) impairs position sense disproportionately more than vibration, and (3) may go partially unrecognized or be denied by the patient (anosognosia).

CEREBELLAR ATAXIA. The motor abnormality depends on the localization of the cerebellar lesion and whether or not adjacent or related neural structures are involved. Thus midline, lateral-hemispheric, and cerebellar outflow lesions each tend to produce somewhat distinct syndromes. These differences become blurred when cerebellar tumors compress the adjacent brain stem to produce additional dysfunction or when diseases such as multiple sclerosis or spinocerebellar degeneration affect remote neurologic structures.

Spinocerebellar disorders produce a predominantly sensory ataxia superimposed on which is a variable degree of cerebellar dyssynergia. Specific cerebellar inflow and outflow pathways are commonly affected. The disorders involve predominantly the lower extremities.

Midline cerebellar dysfunction results principally from degenerative (nutritional-alcoholic) or neoplastic (e.g., medulloblastoma, hemangioblastoma, metastasis) disease. The gait is characteristic with legs thrust widely apart and extended, the arms extended in compensatory balance, and walking accomplished by short steps. Affected patients usually look at the ground for additional sensory stabilization and turn *en bloc*. With extension into the anterior midline cerebellum, stretch reflexes become hyperactive. As the disorder advances, rhythmic truncal titubation appears, often associated with abnormal rhythmic movements of the upper extremities and, eventually, nystagmus. Posterior midline space-occupying lesions may add retropulsion (see below) to this symptom complex.

Lateral cerebellar hemispheric abnormalities produce ipsilateral hypotonia and incoordination of the limbs, an irregular swaying gait and a tendency to drift toward the side of the lesion. The feet are spread apart, although not so broadly as with midline lesions, and patients characteristically cannot manage close-footed tandem walking. Rombergism is absent, but, as with all ataxias, distorted vision or closing the eyes accentuates the patient's unsteadiness. Rhythmic movements and point-to-point tests are impaired in both the upper and lower extremities. If classic intention tremor appears, it indicates a lesion involving the dentate nucleus or the superior cerebellar peduncle.

DRUNKENNESS. Drunkenness, whether due to alcohol or drugs, results mainly from bilateral labyrinthine-vestibular dysfunction and is accompanied by sensations of both vertigo and dizziness. Few patients with cerebellar disease suffer as much incapacity as the reeling, lurching, twisting, and falling inebriate. Lesser degrees of intoxication produce unsteadiness, a tottering, cautious gait with the feet placed moderately widely apart, clumsiness, dysarthria, and nystagmus in all directions.

VESTIBULAR ATAXIA. Lesions anywhere along the peripheral eighth nerve pathway from labyrinth to brain stem can cause vestibular ataxia. Affected patients tend to drift toward the side of impairment and then quickly correct the deviation in the opposite direction. Turning accentuates their unsteadiness and induces missteps. Bilateral damage or degeneration of the vestibular nuclei in the brain stem results in a narrow-based ataxia with poor compensating movements in the limbs. Patients may drift or fall to either side, and some show a tendency to retropulsion and falling backward. Closing the eyes accentuates the gait disorder.

SPASTIC ATAXIA. Combined bilateral abnormalities of the spinal dorsal columns and cortical spinal tracts produce a characteristic broad-based tottering and sometimes pounding gait with the knees held high but the legs moving stiffly. The condition occurs with demyelinating diseases and other intrinsic spinal disorders such as vascular malformations, cobalamin deficiency, arachnoiditis, and, occasionally, neoplasms.

FRONTAL LOBE GAIT DISORDERS. Patients with frontal lobe disease can suffer any of several gait disorders, depending upon the anatomic distribution of the lesions. Unilateral injury to the foot-leg area of the somatosensory cortex produces a focal monoparesis, whereas bilateral motor-premotor damage results in a relatively narrow-based, stiff-legged impairment, sometimes with scissoring of the legs. More anteriorly placed premotor and prefrontal abnormalities arise in association with deep bilateral tumors, multiple cerebral infarctions, or communicating, "low pressure" hydrocephalus. The ensuing ataxia consists of a severe difficulty in initiating walking or otherwise using the lower extremities so long as the patient is in the erect position. The feet appear glued to the floor (magnet reaction), and efforts to walk often consist of short shuffles or even hops before the legs get moving. Walking, once (or if) it begins, proceeds as a halting and broad-based movement made easier by guidance or support. At least some dementia almost always accompanies the gait disorder.

Patients with frontal ataxia of this type show a considerably greater ability to move their legs when lying supine than when standing. Examination of the lower extremities discloses an increased paratonic resistance to passive movements coupled with bilateral plantar grasp responses, extensor thrust responses and, usually, accentuated tendon reflexes. These reflex abnormalities and physiologic dysfunctions best explain the difficulty in movement.

HEMIPARESIS. Both pyramidal-corticospinal and extrapyramidal motor disorders may have a hemiparetic pattern, potentially confusing their early differentiation. Severe spastic hemiplegia from damage to the corticospinal tract or the full-blown stooped, festinating, semishuffling gait of parkinsonism is so well known and readily recognized as to require no discussion. In their initial stages, both pyramidal and extrapyramidal disorders produce mild or inconstant weakness, a susceptibility to easy fatigue in the affected member, and a sense of stiffness. Both corticospinal hemiparesis and parkinsonian hemiparesis incipiently produce a gait disorder marked by a slack arm and a reduction of automatic accessory movements on the affected side, a tendency to scuff the toe, and a degree of bodily akinesia. Both may result in an increase in muscular resistance to passive stretch on the involved side. The following points help in differential diagnosis. Patients with early pyramidal tract dysfunction tend to have unilaterally increased reflexes on the affected side. When walking, they flex the wrist and fingers, circumduct the lower extremity, and hold the foot in an equinovarus position. Patients with early hemiparetic parkinsonism, by contrast, tend to have greater facial and bodily hypokinesia, to stoop, to have difficulty in performing two independent motor acts simultaneously, and show mild cogwheel resistance on rotary movements of the elbow or wrist. They extend the affected wrist and step the weak foot forward rather than circumducting it. The foot itself is held in simple varus position. The deep tendon reflexes may or may not be slightly asymmetric.

ELDERLY GAIT DISTURBANCES. Any of several specific visual, somatosensory, or motor diseases may impair walking in elderly persons. Typical difficulties include a tendency to take slow, short, mincing, and unsteady steps. A stooped position coupled with a moderately broad-based, unsteady gait, sometimes results from a chronic communicating hydrocephalus (see Ch 436).

RETROPULSION. A tendency to step backward from the standing position or to fall backward while sitting can be a symptom of several serious, acquired midline abnormalities of the brain. Occasionally, the abnormality is associated with large, unilateral frontal lobe neoplasms that produce an increase in intracranial pressure and intracranial shift. Retropulsion of posterior fossa origin is especially dangerous, as it often comes on suddenly and is accompanied by a loss of the normal postural protective mechanisms that guard against injury during falling.

ANTALGIC GAIT. Posture and walking abnormalities developed to minimize back, hip, and other leg pain can sometimes mimic neurologic abnormalities. They can be differentiated by finding the painful lesion and an absence of abnormal neurologic signs.

HYSTERICAL GAIT. Hysteria can mimic a variety of hemiparetic, steppage, or ataxic gait disorders. With a hemiparetic type, the pattern usually reveals its genesis by an atypical dragging behind of the affected leg during a series of hops or supported steps. The most obviously factitious hysterical disorder is a lurching, irregularly based, sometimes bent-forward walk in which the patient grasps any object in reach for support and reels inconsistently from side to side. Such patients may sink to the floor but almost never endure an unsupported, self-injuring fall. Other than the gait abnormality, the neurologic examination is normal in these patients.

Keane JR: Hysterical gait disorders: 60 cases. Neurology 39:586, 1989. *A lively and perceptive evaluation of the problem finds that dystonia and chorea are most likely to be overlooked, and that prompt diagnosis leads to the best outcomes.*

Nutt JG, Marsden CD, Thompson PD: Human walking and higher level gait disorders, particularly in the elderly. Neurology 43:268, 1993. *A clinical and neurophysiologic analysis of a large number of cases.*

405 DISORDERS OF SENSATION
Jerome B. Posner

405.1 Major Sensory Symptoms

An organism perceives its environment through its sensory systems. When a sensory system is disordered, sensation may be diminished, increased, or distorted. Table 405–1 lists definitions for major sensory abnormalities.

THE NEUROBIOLOGY OF SENSORY PATHWAYS

Two major sensory pathways subserve cutaneous sensation and conscious perception. The first subserves the sensations of pain, temperature, and crude touch. The receptors are naked nerve endings connected either to small (5 μ), thinly myelinated, "A delta" fibers, which conduct at about 35 meters per second, or to unmyelinated "C" fibers (1 to 2 μ), which conduct at about 0.5 meter per second. Those sensory fibers, all of which have their cell borders in the dorsal root ganglia, enter the spinal cord and synapse in the dorsal horn. Most ascending (second order) pain fibers cross the spinal cord and divide into two groups: the neospinothalamic tract, which is believed to subserve the perception of intensity and localization of pain, temperature, and crude touch, and the paleospinothalamic tract, which is believed to subserve the arousal and emotional components of pain. The axons of the neospinothalamic tract ascend in the anterolateral quadrant of the spinal cord. The axons terminate in the thalamus, principally within the ventral posterolateral nucleus (VPL) ipsilateral to the side of their ascent. Third-order neurons from the thalamus project to somatosensory area 1 (sensorimotor cortex), with the same somatotopic localization as other sensory modalities. Lesions of pain pathways sometimes lead to chronic "neuropathic pain"; one type is called thalamic pain. The paleospinothalamic tract, whose cells of origin in the dorsal horn receive C-fiber input, consists of crossed and uncrossed fibers. Most fibers cross in the anterior commissure and ascend in the spinal cord more ventral than the neospinothalamic tract. Many of the fibers of the paleospinothalamic tract send collaterals to the reticular formation of the brain stem.

The second system subserving the functions of light touch, position sense, and tactile localization begins as cutaneous mechanoreceptors connected to larger myelinated fibers. These large fibers also enter the spinal cord via the dorsal root ganglion and ascend without synapsing in the posterior and to a lesser extent lateral columns of the cord to reach the gracile and cuneate nuclei in the low brain stem. Second-order neuron fibers then decussate and ascend in the medial lemniscus to reach the contralateral ventral posterolateral thalamus. Third-order neurons projected from the thalamus terminate in the cerebral cortex, predominantly in the sensorimotor strip surrounding the Rolandic fissure. Lesions of this system lead to loss of position sense of the limbs and body in space, inability to localize tactile stimuli or to distinguish between one and two closely placed stimuli, and inability to describe accurately the size, shape, and texture of objects (stereoanesthesia). Subcortical lesions of the system also cause loss of the ability to recognize vibratory sensation (pallesthesia).

LOCALIZATION OF SENSORY DISORDERS

PERIPHERAL NERVES. Many diseases of peripheral nerves affect both large and small fibers, leading to a diminution of all sensory modalities to approximately equal degree. In some disorders of peripheral nerves, either small or large fibers can be involved preferentially, leading to a "dissociated sensory loss." When small fibers are predominantly affected, pain and temperature sensation are involved out of proportion to light touch, vibration, and position sense. Spontaneous pain and burning dysesthetic sensations are common and often provide the presenting complaints. Because autonomic fibers are also small, trophic changes in skin and joints may accompany such a small-fiber peripheral neuropathy, but because motor fibers and the afferent portion of the stretch reflex are subserved by large fibers, these functions are relatively preserved. Such selective small fiber damage is sometimes encountered in diabetes and is common in some of the hereditary neuropathies as well as in toxic-nutritional neuropathies (see Ch. 449 and 450).

Large fiber damage, more common in demyelinating neuropathies, is characterized by profound loss of localizing touch and proprioception, with relative preservation of crude touch, pain, and temperature sensation. Paresthesias are common. The deep tendon reflexes are lost because of damage to large afferent fibers and there is usually weakness as well.

The diagnosis of a peripheral neuropathy (see Ch. 445 to 452) involving sensory fibers is established by the distribution of the sensory loss, which may be in the distribution of a single nerve, multiple individual nerves, or a symmetric distal stocking-and-glove distribution. Polyneuropathies are distributed distally because longer axons are more vulnerable to disease than shorter ones. In general, mononeuropathies are caused by local disease (e.g., compression entrapment), or vascular disorders (e.g., polyarteritis) and polyneuropathies by immunologic or metabolic disorders (e.g., demyelination-inflammatory neuropathy, diabetes, uremia, nutritional neuropathy).

SPINAL CORD. Dissociation of sensory loss is more common in spinal cord disorders than in those originating in peripheral nerves or roots. Lesions of the posterolateral columns produce profound loss of position and vibration sense with normal crude touch pain, and temperature sensation. Usually corticospinal tracts are involved as well, causing hyperactive reflexes and extensor plantar responses. Lesions of the spinothalamic tract or of crossing fibers from the posterior horn to the spinothalamic tract cause loss of pain and temperature sense with preservation of vibration, position, and localizing touch. Such dissociated sensory loss is common in syringomyelia and may occur with infarction of the anterior portion of the spinal cord from occlusion of the anterior spinal artery. In both of these disorders, motor function may be relatively well preserved. When only one side of the spinal cord is involved, proprioceptive sensation is lost on the ipsilateral side and pain and temperature sensation on the contralateral side, both below the level of the lesion. A small band of decreased sensation to all modalities resulting from damage to the posterior horn marks the level of the lesion. This so-called Brown-Séquard syndrome is sometimes seen with tumors compressing or invading the spinal cord and is common in radiation myelopathy. Lesions of the spinal cord are rarely confused with those of peripheral nerves because the sensory loss in spinal

TABLE 405–1. MAJOR SENSORY SYMPTOMS DEFINED

Hypesthesia, anesthesia: reduction or loss of cutaneous touch sensation
Hypalgesia, analgesia: reduction or loss of cutaneous pain sensation
Hyperesthesia: lowered sensory threshold to cutaneous touch
Hyperalgesia: lowered cutaneous threshold to noxious stimuli
Hyperpathia: elevated threshold to noxious stimuli with accentuated discomfort above the threshold
Paresthesias: spontaneously arising exteroceptive sensation (e.g., pins and needles sensations, burning sensations)
Dysesthesias: unpleasant distortion of innocuous afferent stimuli
Allodynia: the perception of an ordinarily nonpainful stimulus as painful or excruciating

cord lesions is usually proximal as well as distal and restricted to those segments damaged below the spinal cord level. Furthermore, motor signs of upper motor neuron disease, particularly extensor plantar responses, usually correctly identify the central nature of a spinal cord disorder rather than point to a peripheral disturbance.

BRAIN STEM. In the lower brain stem, spinothalamic and proprioceptive pathways remain separated, lateral lesions of the medulla causing loss of pain and temperature sensation on the ipsilateral side of the face (a result of damage to the descending root of the trigeminal nerve) and the contralateral side of the body. This sensory abnormality is usually accompanied by other signs of lateral medullary damage (Wallenberg's syndrome) and spares proprioceptive pathways. Higher in the brain stem, as the two pathways converge in their route toward the thalamus, damage causes contralateral sensory loss to all modalities, usually accompanied by cranial nerve palsies, ataxia (from the cerebellar outflow), and motor weakness.

CEREBRUM. In the thalamus, damage to the ventral posterolateral nucleus causes decreased sensation of all modalities on the contralateral side of the body and face. Sensory loss is often accompanied by dysesthesias and sometimes pain.

Lindblom U, Ochoa JL: Somatosensory function and dysfunction. *In* Asbury AK, McKhann GM, McDonald WI (eds.): Diseases of the Nervous System, 2nd ed. Philadelphia, WB Saunders, 1992, p 213. *A concise but comprehensive discussion.*

405.2 Headache and Other Head Pain

Headache ranks ninth among the causes of visits to physicians and is a major source both of time lost from work and of medical diagnostic procedures. The frequency of disabling headache is explained in part by the rich nerve supply to the head (including afferent nerve fibers from trigeminal, glossopharyngeal, vagus, and upper three cervical nerves). Head pain can result from distortion, stretching, inflammation, or destruction of pain-sensitive nerve endings as a result of intra- or extracranial disease in the distribution of any of the aforementioned nerves. Most head pain carries a benign prognosis. The physician's twofold task is first to distinguish more common, benign head pain from rarer but more serious causes and then to administer appropriate treatment. The diagnosis can usually be established by history and physical findings alone; skull radiographs, computed tomographic (CT) and magnetic resonance (MR) images, and other diagnostic tests are seldom required. Table 405–2 is a simplified classification of the pathogenesis of head pain. The overwhelming majority of headaches are either migraine or so-called tension headaches, with both abnormalities frequently playing a role in a given individual.

MIGRAINE AND OTHER VASCULAR HEADACHES

The term *vascular headache* applies to a group of clinical syndromes of unknown origin in which the final step in pathogenesis of the pain appears to be dilatation of one or more branches of the carotid artery, leading to stimulation of sensitized periarterial nociceptors by noxious substances released by the artery or nerve. Such substances as serotonin, substance P, bradykinin, histamine, prostaglandins, and calcitonin gene–related peptides alone or in combination have all been implicated in the pathogenesis of vascu-

TABLE 405–2. PATHOPHYSIOLOGIC CLASSIFICATION OF HEADACHE

Vascular Headache
  Migraine headache
    Classic migraine
    Common migraine
    Complicated migraine
    Variant migraine
  Cluster headache
    Episodic cluster
    "Chronic" cluster
    Chronic paroxysmal hemicrania
  Miscellaneous vascular headaches
    Carotidynia
    Hypertension
    Orgasmic, exertional, and cough headache
    Hangover
    Toxins and drugs
    Occlusive vascular disease

Tension Headache
  Common tension headache

Depressive equivalent
Conversion reaction
Temporomandibular joint dysfunction
Atypical facial pain

Traction-Inflammation Headache
  Cranial arteritis
  Increased or decreased intracranial pressure
  Extracranial structural lesions
  Pituitary tumors

Extracranial Structural Lesions
  Parnasal sinusitis and tumors
  Dental infections
  Otitis
  Ocular lesions
  Pituitary tumors
  Cervical osteoarthritis

Cranial Neuralgias

lar headache. Most vascular headaches are unilateral, often but not always throbbing, and recurrent over months or years. Individual headaches are precipitated in some by identifiable environmental, dietary, or psychological factors. During the course of a vascular headache, the involved arteries may be tender to the touch. Most vascular headaches can be relieved by prompt administration of ergotamine or sumatriptan; recurrent headaches can often be prevented by one of several prophylactic drugs (see below). So-called common migraine may affect as many as 25% of the population. Other vascular headache syndromes are less common, but each has distinctive clinical findings.

Classic Migraine

Classic migraine is distinguished by an onset that includes well-defined symptoms of neurologic dysfunction that precede or, less often, accompany the headache. Neurologic symptoms are usually visual, consisting of bright flashing lights (scintillation or fortification scotomata) beginning in the center of a visual half-field and radiating over 10 to 30 minutes outward toward the periphery. Less commonly, the visual abnormalities are monocular (retinal) or consist of hemianoptic loss of vision in place of or following the scintillating scotomata. Other neurologic disturbances that can occur in classic migraine include unilateral paresthesias, usually involving the hand and perioral area, aphasia, hemiparesis, and hemisensory defects. An uncommon variant named *basilar artery migraine* occurs predominantly in children and adolescents and is characterized by vertigo, ataxia, and diplopia, along with hemiparesis or hemisensory changes. Rarely, confusion, stupor, or even coma may develop. Neurologic symptoms of classic migraine usually last no longer than 30 minutes and generally clear before the headache phase begins. Rarely, such signs may persist for hours or even days.

The pathogenesis of the neurologic dysfunction is not fully understood. Measurements of regional cerebral blood flow during episodes of classic migraine have shown a wave of focal hyperemia followed by abnormally low flow spreading from posterior to anterior over the cerebral cortex. The flow reduction may be sufficient to cause the neurologic symptoms and, rarely, cerebral infarction. In most cases, however, the changes are insufficient to explain the neurologic symptoms. One explanation is that a wave of physiologic "spreading" depression spreads across the cortex, accounting for both the neurologic symptoms and the changes in blood flow. Changes in brain blood flow do not accompany common migraine, even though the headache phase of the illness is similar. Thus, it is likely that if "spreading depression" is the cause of the neurologic symptoms of migraine, it is only one of several precipitating factors that may produce the headache.

The syndrome of classic migraine has four parts: (1) A *prodromal phase* occurs in a minority of patients and consists of an alteration of mood, often occurring for 24 or more hours before the headache. In some patients, known precipitants such as red wine commonly induce an attack. (2) The second phase consists of the *neurologic symptoms* described above. These may occur without subsequent headache (termed migraine equivalent), particularly in older people. (3) The third phase usually begins as the neurologic symptoms clear and characteristically consists of a unilateral throbbing frontotemporal *headache* on the side opposite the neurologic symptoms. The headache is frequently accompanied by nausea, photophobia, vomiting, diarrhea, phonophobia (noise intolerance), and a general feeling of being unwell. The headache commonly lasts 4 to 6 hours but may persist for 1 or more days. Prolonged headaches may change into a dull, aching, bilateral pain extending back into the neck and shoulders. The headache phase is often terminated either by vomiting or by a period of sleep. (4) The *post-headache* phase is characterized by a feeling of exhaustion, tenderness of the scalp and recurrence of head pain on sudden head movement.

The diagnosis of classic migraine is made by history; physical findings are absent, and laboratory evaluation is not helpful. When the attacks are atypical, particularly when neurologic disability is severe or prolonged, CT or MR imaging may be required to rule out structural lesions of the brain. Such instances are rare. The treatment of classic migraine is similar to that of common migraine (see below), except that classic migraine attacks usually occur no more than four or five times a year and rarely more than once a month.

Common Migraine

Common migraine is similar to classic migraine but lacks the neurologic symptoms. Many persons with classic migraine also have episodes of common migraine. Common migraine is characterized by recurrent headaches, often severe, frequently beginning unilaterally, and usually associated with malaise, nausea and/or vomiting, and photophobia. The disorder often begins in childhood, affects women more often than men, and runs in families (70% of patients give a family history). Identifiable factors that often precipitate individual headaches are holidays and weekends, menstrual periods, foods (especially red wine, chocolate, nuts, and aged cheese), environmental stimuli (such as bright sunlight, too much sleep, and undue emotional stress or resentment). Medical conditions and their treatment may also precipitate attacks. Vasodilators such as nitroglycerin and antihypertensives and serotonin releasers such as reserpine, as well as estrogens and oral contraceptives, have been reported to cause migraine attacks in susceptible individuals. The diagnosis is usually made by the history. Important historical points that help distinguish migraine from tension-type headaches (see below) include their unilaterality, their association with nausea or vomiting, the tendency of migraine to awaken one from sleep, a positive family history, and a positive response to sumatriptan or ergotamine. When the diagnosis is in doubt, treatment of the patient for common migraine often clarifies the issue.

TREATMENT. The best treatment for migraine is prevention. The patient should avoid known precipitating factors. Medications known to cause migraine should be withdrawn if others can be substituted. Foods commonly implicated may also be withdrawn and, if withdrawal is effective, replaced one at a time to determine the specific precipitant. The patient should attempt to avoid undue stress or fatigue and not to sleep excessively on weekends. If these methods fail and severe headaches occur frequently (once a week or more), pharmacologic prophylaxis is indicated. Several agents have been reported effective in the prophylaxis of migraine, but not every patient responds to each agent. Effective drugs include β-adrenergic, serotonin, and calcium channel blockers, antidepressants, nonsteroidal anti-inflammatory agents, valproic acid, and others.

Acute attacks, if mild, often respond to analgesic agents and bedrest. More severe attacks are best treated by ergotamine or sumatriptan. Either drug, given parenterally, is sufficiently effective (85 to 90%) to be useful as a diagnostic test. Oral ergot 1 to 2 mg given at the onset of a headache is effective in fewer patients. Better results can be achieved with sublingual or rectal preparations, preferably one half of a 2-mg ergotamine rectal suppository. The side effects of *ergotism* (muscle pain, vasoconstriction, mottled

skin, peripheral gangrene, multifocal encephalopathy) make it unwise to treat frequent migraine headaches in this way, and one should switch to prophylaxis if the headaches occur more than once a week. For patients who present to emergency departments with severe headaches sumatriptan by injection is the drug of choice.

Migraine Variants

Several migraine syndromes differ sufficiently from classic and common migraine to earn separate names. *Ophthalmoplegic migraine* describes an ocular motor palsy occurring during the course of a severe migraine attack. Ophthalmoplegic migraine usually begins in childhood and is characterized by unilateral pupillary dilatation, ptosis, and paralysis of ocular muscles occurring 12 to 24 hours *after* the beginning of an attack of severe migraine. The ophthalmoplegia usually clears within hours to days but frequently recurs. Angiography may be required to rule out a carotid aneurysm. *Hemiplegic migraine* is a familial syndrome in which aphasia, confusion, and hemiparesis or hemiplegia precede or more often accompany the migraine attack. Repetitive episodes alternating from side to side may occur over many years. *Complicated migraine* defines attacks of migraine prodromes in which the focal neurologic defects may last for the entire headache attack and even leave permanent residua. The few available anatomic studies of such patients have shown ischemic brain infarction involving the functionally impaired region.

Cluster Headache

Cluster headaches are short-lived attacks of severe, acute, and intense unilateral head pain that recurrently occur in clusters lasting several weeks, only to disappear for months or years. It is only about one twenty-fifth as common as migraine. The disorder affects men much more than women and usually begins between the third and sixth decades. Clusters characteristically occur in the spring and fall and last 3 to 8 weeks. The individual headaches occur one to several times a day, particularly at night, awakening the victim from sleep. Each attack, which lasts 30 minutes to 2 hours, is characterized by rapid onset of a knife-like pain in the nostril or behind the eye which spreads to involve the forehead. During the attack, the ipsilateral nostril may water and the eye tear. In about 20% of instances, a Horner syndrome develops. The headache pain may be so severe that these patients restlessly pace the floor, bang their head against the wall, and may threaten suicide. The headache disappears as abruptly as it arises, usually without residua. Unlike migraine, cluster headaches do not make persons systemically ill. No nausea, vomiting, or exhaustion appear when the headache ceases. When clusters are occurring (but not between) alcohol invariably induces attack. When the headaches occur frequently, the Horner syndrome may outlast the head pain.

The pathogenesis of cluster headache is unknown, although it is believed to relate to migraine. The diagnosis is established by the characteristic history. Treatment of an acute attack is usually not worthwhile, since by the time the patient absorbs the analgesic agents the attack is over. In some patients the headache rapidly responds to oxygen inhalation. Several drugs prevent attacks of cluster headache. Ergotamine tartrate given prophylactically in a dose of 1 mg four times a day, or 2 mg at bedtime if the attacks are all nocturnal, is often effective. The drug should be withdrawn every seventh day to prevent the symptoms of ergotism and to see if the cluster has ceased. Other drugs reported to be effective in some patients include those listed for migraine prophylaxis.

Cluster Variants

Several variants of cluster headache require different treatment. *Chronic paroxysmal hemicrania* is a rare disorder consisting of cluster headaches that appear many times a day and recur unremittingly for years. There may be as many as 10 to 20 headaches daily, each lasting 10 to 30 minutes. Indomethacin* orally in doses of 75 to 150 mg daily has relieved all subjects. A cluster variant characterized by daily cluster headache without remission, multiple brief jabs of pain in the head, and a background of continuous unilateral headache of variable severity exacerbated by exertion has recently been described and is said to respond to indomethacin in

---

* This use is not listed in the manufacturer's directive.

most instances. Patients who did not respond to indomethacin did so to tricyclic antidepressants.

Other Vascular Headaches

Orgasmic headaches are short-lived bilateral throbbing headaches that occur in either sex and appear abruptly at orgasm. The headache usually disappears within minutes to an hour or more and may recur repetitively. Usually the illness is self-limited, but if not it may respond to 1 mg of ergot given an hour before sexual activity. *Exertional headache* occurs, as the name implies, during active exercise. It is usually bilateral and throbbing and may last several hours, responding well to indomethacin. Vascular headaches have been reported to follow minor *trauma* to the carotid artery in the neck and *carotid endarterectomy.* The headaches are unilateral, recurrent, and severe and usually respond to prophylaxis with propranolol. *Carotidynia* is the name given to spontaneous vascular headaches associated with unilateral anterior neck pain and/or carotid tenderness. They usually respond to the same treatment as migraines. When attacks of carotid pain and/or headache recur, the diagnosis is not difficult, but the first attack must be distinguished from a spontaneous dissection of the carotid artery and may require angiography for diagnosis.

Hangover headache is part of a larger syndrome, usually including premature awakening from an evening of overindulgence and often accompanied by a fine tremor of the extremities, mild gastric distress or nausea, mental dulling, and mild incoordination. The pathogenesis relates to alcohol withdrawal, dehydration, and the toxic effect of various congeners found with different intoxicants. *Nitrites* can induce pulsating headache and, occasionally, facial flushing, most often after the ingestion of processed foods ("hot dog" headache). *Monosodium glutamate* has been blamed for the "Chinese restaurant syndrome," characterized by postprandial headache, tight sensations about the face and head, and, less often, giddiness and diarrhea.

Cough headache is, as the name implies, sudden and often severe headache related to cough. The headache may last only seconds or may persist minutes to hours after a single cough or a coughing paroxysm. In some patients, cough headache is a symptom of an intracranial mass lesion. Most patients, however, do not have underlying structural disease; in these patients the disorder is probably similar to exertional and orgasmic headaches and has a vascular origin. *"Ice pick"* headaches are brief (1 to 2 seconds), sharp focal head pains occurring at unpredictable intervals and at different areas of the head. They do not indicate intracranial disease. *Thunderclap* headaches are sudden, severe, "exploding" pains that involve the entire head and resolve slowly over hours. Although such headaches occasionally reflect a small subarachnoid hemorrhage, most are without pathologic significance. A severe thunderclap headache probably deserves evaluation by lumbar puncture to look for subarachnoid blood. If found angiography may be indicated to seek an intracranial aneurysm.

Hypertensive headaches occur only in patients with very severe or episodic hypertension. They are characterized by early-morning, usually throbbing, occipital headache that responds to the treatment of the hypertension.

TENSION-TYPE HEADACHES

Tension-type headache is the term applied to a form of benign head pain that occasionally affects most persons. The disorder is characterized by pain of mild to moderate intensity, usually bilateral in location, and typically pressing or "tight" in quality. The pain may be chronic or episodic; if episodic, it may last minutes to days. The feeling of being unwell—with nausea, photophobia, and phonophobia so common with migraine—is usually absent. Tension-type headaches are uncommon, but associated symptoms can include dizziness, blurring of vision, and tinnitus.

The pathogenesis of the disorder is unknown. The term *tension-type headache* describes both the pericranial muscle tightening and tenderness found in some patients and the emotional anxiety and psychological tension present in others. The role of these two factors in pathogenesis is not clearly established. Tension headaches affect some persons daily. They usually begin in early afternoon or evening, with a dull occipital or frontal pain that may spread to grip the entire head "in a vise." Unique among headaches, the pain may remain constant for days, weeks, or months and is often associated with tenderness in the posterior cervical, temporalis, or masseter muscles. Tension-type headaches are more frequent in women, in individuals who are tense and anxious, and in those whose work or posture requires sustained contraction of posterior cervical, frontal, or temporal muscles. The symptoms of common migraine and tension headaches overlap, and many persons suffer from both. The distinguishing features favoring tension-type headaches include pressure or tightness, which is worst at the back of the neck, increased severity of pain as the day progresses, and pain that is preceded by or associated with anxiety-producing situations. Tension-type headaches seldom awaken the patient from sleep. They do not respond to ergot preparations.

In many respects muscle pain and tenderness in tension headaches resemble the fibromyalgia syndrome, whatever that disorder may be.

TREATMENT. The first step in treating tension-type headache lies in identifying causal factors, if any. Many such patients are depressed and respond to treatment with antidepressant agents such as amitriptyline. Others are tense and anxious and respond to anti-anxiety agents such as diazepam. This drug, in a dose of 15 to 20 mg a day for 2 to 3 weeks, is often effective as a diagnostic test. The relief of chronic headache establishes the diagnosis for the physician and helps to convince the patient that tension and anxiety are playing a major role. Also, these drugs frequently break up a cycle of anxiety–muscle tension–anxiety, so that a short course may give prolonged relief. Physical dependence at doses <30 mg a day is rare.

An individual headache may be treated with aspirin. This drug is probably more useful for tension headaches than acetaminophen because of its anti-prostaglandin properties. Vasoactive agents used for the treatment of migraine have no role although sumatriptan should be tried at least once. Some clinics report that biofeedback treatments effectively relieve muscle contraction and thus the headache. For sharply localized, painful areas present at the site of headache, injection with local anesthetics may transiently relieve the headaches. Sometimes massage has a similar effect. Chronic ingestion of analgesic agents may cause tension-type headaches. Withdrawal of the medication usually relieves the headaches.

Tension-Type Headache Variants

Several rather characteristic headache syndromes of unknown cause may be variants of tension-type headache. One is the so-called temporomandibular joint syndrome. Patients complain of unilateral or bilateral head pain, usually in the temporal region and in the jaw, often radiating into the ear. The pain is often associated with tenderness of the masseter and temporalis muscles and may be exacerbated by chewing. Accompanying symptoms often include limitation of full movement at the temporomandibular joint when opening the jaw, bruxism, and malocclusion. The disorder sometimes responds to dental manipulation, particularly use of a mouth guard during sleep that prevents bruxism. However, for most patients analgesics and anxiolytic agents effectively treat such muscle-contraction head pains. *Post-traumatic headaches* are dull, generalized, aching head pains that follow head injury. The injury is often mild. Patients suffering the "post-traumatic syndrome" complain of headache often coupled with unsteadiness, giddiness, difficulty concentrating, insomnia, and fatigue. Compensation issues seem to have no effect. The headache often persists for months or years. Treatment, like that of tension-type headaches, consists of psychological support, reassurance, and the use of mild analgesics or anxiolytic agents. Patients should be encouraged to return to work as soon as possible and to try to live a normal life despite the symptoms. The disorder can blend into *depressive headache,* a chronic generalized headache, usually vaguely described, sometimes associated with giddiness and unsteadiness, that occurs as a frequent and sometimes predominant manifestation of depression. The treatment of choice is an antidepressant drug.

Atypical Facial Pain

Atypical facial pain or *atypical facial neuralgia* describes a syndrome characterized by steady aching facial pain, usually unilateral, localized to the lower part of the orbit, maxillary area, and sometimes the jaw. The pain begins without a known precipitating episode and may last for hours, days, or indefinitely. It may spread to involve the head or neck, and muscles of the jaw and neck are often tender. Sometimes autonomic symptoms including sweating, flushing, rhinorrhea, and pallor are present. The disorder usually affects women, often in early middle age. Patients are tense, anxious, and often chronically depressed. The pathogenesis of the illness is unknown. The autonomic changes have led some to suggest that the syndrome is a migraine variant, and the muscle tenderness and depression have led others to suggest that it be classified with tension-type headache. Patients suffering from atypical facial pain should be examined carefully for pathology of the eyes, nose, teeth, sinuses, and pharynx, but such is rarely found. Careful psychological evaluation often reveals a masked depression. Treatment is usually unsatisfactory. Analgesic agents are usually not helpful, and patients respond poorly to psychotherapy. Antidepressants sometimes help. It is important to recognize that the syndrome is not caused by structural disease and that patients require no invasive diagnostic or therapeutic procedures. Above all, surgical "treatment," including dental extraction, does more harm than good. This disorder should not be confused with trigeminal neuralgia, discussed below; carbamazepine is ineffective.

HEAD PAIN DUE TO TRACTION OR INFLAMMATION

Cranial Arteritis

This condition receives detailed consideration in Ch. 246 but deserves mention here as an important cause of headache in the elderly. The illness almost always appears after age 60 and usually later. It begins with unilateral or bilateral temporal, occipital, or fronto-occipital head pain of variable intensity, often coupled with tenderness of the painful areas. Many patients have pain in the jaw muscles, making chewing uncomfortable. Nodules occasionally are palpable on affected vessels. The great risk is occlusion of retinal arteries secondary to untreated inflammation. Diagnosis depends on suspicion and usually on the presence of an elevated erythrocyte sedimentation rate. Diagnosis should be confirmed by arterial biopsy because definitive steroid treatment, once started, often must be maintained for many months. Because migraine-vascular headaches and depressive headaches also can have their onset in the elderly, a confirmed diagnosis is essential.

Alterations of Intracranial Pressure

Headache from altered intracranial pressure is caused by compression or traction of pain-sensitive vascular and neural structures over the apex and base of the brain. In the instance of *intracranial hypotension,* the loss of spinal fluid decreases the buoyancy of the brain so that the organ descends when the upright position is assumed, exerting traction on structures at its apex and compression on structures at its base. Compensatory vasodilation may also contribute to the pain. (In rare instances, the small bridging veins that enter the sagittal sinus may rupture and cause subdural hematomas.) In *intracranial hypertension,* the source of pain is probably compression of vascular and neural structures at the base of the brain by tumor or edematous brain.

INTRACRANIAL HYPERTENSION. Increased intracranial pressure per se does not lead to headache unless pain-sensitive structures are distorted. Many patients with high intracranial pressure from brain tumors, jugular venous obstruction, hydrocephalus, or pseudotumor cerebri do not suffer headache. If headache is present, it may be mild or severe, throbbing or steady, localized or generalized. When localized, it usually overlies the site of the lesion, but posterior fossa lesions may cause bifrontal headache. The headache is characteristically at its worst early in the morning, although, unlike cluster headache, it usually does not awaken the patient from sleep. It is exacerbated by stooping, coughing, moving the head suddenly, or straining at stool. Many patients prefer to sleep in the sitting position. The headache is rarely continuously intense. Transient rises of intracranial pressure called plateau waves (see Ch. 436) sometimes cause 5 to 20 minutes of severe headache accompanied by nausea, vomiting, or other neurologic signs. These episodes are commonly precipitated by assuming the upright posture but can also be precipitated by coughing, sneezing, or straining.

The treatment of headache related to increased intracranial pressure is the treatment of the underlying disease. Mild analgesics give temporary relief; narcotic analgesics should not be used because of their tendency to produce respiratory depression and further raise the pressure in neurologically compromised individuals.

INTRACRANIAL HYPOTENSION (see Ch. 436) **AND LUMBAR PUNCTURE HEADACHE.** Intracranial hypotension usually follows a lumbar puncture and is due to continued leakage of cerebrospinal fluid (CSF) through a rent in the dural sheath. The syndrome develops 12 hours to several days after the lumbar puncture and is characterized by headache on assuming the upright position. There is no evidence that a period of recumbency after a lumbar puncture prevents subsequent development of the headache. The headache usually begins as a dull ache in the posterior cervical area, radiating laterally toward the shoulders and cephalad toward the frontal area. It persists, often growing more severe, as long as the patient remains upright. When most severe it may be associated with diaphoresis, nausea, and vomiting. Persistent headache of intracranial hypotension can lead to diplopia, probably a result of traction on the abducens nerves. The diagnosis is made by history; spontaneous intracranial hypotension is suspected by the history of positional headache and confirmed by low (< 30 mm H_2O) or even negative CSF pressure on attempted lumbar puncture. The fluid is usually normal, but there may be an elevated protein concentration if the needle has entered a subdural or epidural fluid collection. Analgesics relieve the mildest headaches; the most severe ones can be controlled only by assuming the recumbent position.

EXTRACRANIAL STRUCTURAL CAUSES OF HEADACHE

Nasal and Sinus Headache

Although acute or chronic inflammation and neoplasms of the paranasal sinuses can cause headache, most patients who have been diagnosed as having sinus headaches are in fact suffering from either vascular or tension-type headache. True paranasal sinus headaches result from acute inflammation causing pain localized over the involved sinus and associated with stigmata of acute infection, including fever, swelling, and tenderness over the sinus and engorgement of the turbinates, ostia, nasofrontal ducts, and superior nasal spaces. Most of the discomfort comes from the ostia, which are many times more sensitive than the poorly innervated walls of the sinuses. True sinus headache is dull and aching, made worse by changing head position, and seldom associated with nausea and vomiting. Sinus headache is treated with decongestants and analgesics. Persistent purulent discharges should be cultured and appropriate antimicrobial drugs employed. Chronic suppurative disease in the frontal, ethmoid, and sphenoid sinuses, or in the mastoid air cells, may result in osteomyelitis and inflammation of adjacent cranial tissues. Headache persisting after surgical drainage of a diseased sinus suggests extradural and possibly subdural infection. More chronic inflammation and neoplasms, particularly when they occur in the sphenoid sinus, may not be accompanied by the usual physical signs of sinusitis. In such instances, CT or MR scan may be required to establish the diagnosis.

Dental Pain

Noxious stimuli in a tooth usually evoke local toothache, but severe dental pain can be difficult to localize. Afferent fibers from the teeth are contained in the second and third divisions of the trigeminal nerve, and tooth pain can be referred to areas of the head supplied by these nerves. More commonly, in association with toothache, tooth extraction, or a tender, diseased tooth, distant tissues exhibit surface hyperalgesia, tenderness, and vasomotor reactions, such as tender eyeballs, reddening of the conjunctivae, and tenderness of the auricular and temporal tissues. Because of secondary muscle contraction, other sites of tenderness and pain may be noted behind the ears, behind the lower border of the mastoid process, and in the muscles of the occiput, neck, and shoulders. The upper teeth frequently hurt in association with disease of the nasal and paranasal structures. Occasionally, in coronary insufficiency, pain is experienced in the lower jaw. One should beware of ascribing bizarre pains in and around the jaws to a dental origin unless unequivocal acute inflammatory dental lesions are present. Dental extraction rarely ameliorates neuralgias or atypical facial pain. Headache should not be attributed to a diseased tooth unless the injection of procaine into the tissues about the suspected tooth greatly reduces the intensity of, or eliminates, such headache.

Severe pain in the vicinity of the ear can be caused by disease of the teeth, acute tonsillitis, inflammatory and neoplastic disease of the larynx and nasopharynx, temporomandibular joint disorders, tumors, inflammation in the posterior fossa, and disease of the cervical spine and its soft tissues. Pain in the ear is also associated with vascular headaches, atypical facial pain, and herpes zoster of the fifth and seventh cranial nerves and, rarely, the glossopharyngeal nerve. True glossopharyngeal neuralgia causes severe pain radiating from the tonsil into the ear. It has the usual timing feature of "tic" (see Cranial Neuralgias below).

Headaches due to primary ear disease almost always indicates inflammation or destructive disease. Acute otitis media (purulent or nonpurulent), furunculosis of the ear canal, traumatic rupture of the tympanum, and fracture of the anterior wall of the bony canal all cause pain in the ear associated with tenderness of adjacent skeletal muscles. Osteomyelitis of the mastoid bone may be associated with inflammation of the nearby periosteum as well as of dura and adjacent tissues (epidural abscess)—both sources of pain in or behind the ear. Pain in this region also accompanies tumors of the acoustic nerve and inflammation and thrombosis of the lateral sinus.

Eye Pain and Headache

Many minor eye disorders are blamed for headache, which actually turns out to be tension-type head pain. The pain of *glaucoma* at first remains localized in the eyeball, then extends along the rim of the orbit and, finally, throughout most of the area supplied by the ophthalmic division of the trigeminal nerve. Nausea and vomiting sometimes accompany such headaches, which can become prostratingly severe if not treated promptly.

With inflammation of the iris and ciliary body, light may cause intense pain in the eye and adjacent areas because of movement of the inflamed iris. When the iris is immobilized, pain is allayed.

Pituitary Pain

Headache caused by pituitary tumors is the result of compression and distortion of pain-sensitive structures at the base of the skull, particularly the diaphragma sella. Pain is generally referred to the frontal or temporal regions bilaterally and may on occasion be referred to the vertex or occipital regions. The pain can occur at any time and is frequently chronic and unremitting. The diagnosis can be established by MRI of the pituitary fossa. Acute headache occurring with known pituitary lesions *(pituitary apoplexy)* usually results from infarction or hemorrhage into the tumor. Sudden expansion of the tumor may compromise the overlying optic chiasm, leading to visual loss, or invade the laterally lying cavernous sinus, causing ocular palsies. Pituitary apoplexy is usually treated surgically by drainage of the hemorrhagic or infarcted material.

Neck Pain

Osteoarthritis of the zygapophyseal joints of the upper cervical spine is an occasional cause of perplexing headache. The pain is generally constant and aching and perceived in the upper cervical and occipital areas. It may radiate to the vertex of the head or even the orbit. At times, vertex or orbital pain is more severe than occipital and neck pain, leading to confusion in diagnosis. The pain probably results from entrapment of the C3 root by overgrowth of the C2 zygapophyseal joint. A syndrome of unilateral upper nuchal and occipital pain accompanied by ipsilateral numbness of the tongue occurring on sudden turning of the head is probably explained by compression of the second cervical root in the atlanto-occipital space. Such acute pain can be prevented by restricting neck movement with a cervical collar. Upper cervical nerve blocks relieve more chronic pain and are useful diagnostically as well as therapeutically.

CRANIAL NEURALGIAS

The term *cranial neuralgias* refers to several distinctive head pains that appear to result from sudden and excessive discharge from the involved nerve. The best-known cranial neuralgia is trigeminal neuralgia. The concept of cranial neuralgias has been expanded to include the chronic burning pain that frequently follows herpes zoster infection of the nerve.

TRIGEMINAL NEURALGIA. Trigeminal neuralgia (tic douloureux) is characterized by sudden, lightning-like paroxysms of pain in the distribution of one or more divisions of the trigeminal nerve. Most trigeminal neuralgia is caused by compression of the trigeminal nerve by normal but aging arteries or veins of the posterior fossa. In some patients there is no identifiable structural disease. Occasionally trigeminal neuralgia may be a symptom of a gasserian ganglion tumor, multiple sclerosis, or a brain-stem infarct involving the descending root of the trigeminal nerve.

The history is diagnostic. The pain occurs as brief, lightning-like stabs, frequently precipitated by touching a trigger zone around the lips or the buccal cavity. At times, talking, eating, or brushing the teeth serves as a trigger. The pains rarely last longer than seconds, and each burst is followed by a refractory period of several seconds to a minute in which no further pain can be precipitated. The pains, however, often occur in clusters so that the patient may report somewhat erroneously that each pain lasts for hours. The pain is limited to one or more divisions of the trigeminal nerve, usually the second, or third, or both. Spontaneous remissions and exacerbations are common, the exacerbations tending to occur in spring and fall. Between paroxysms of pain, the patient is asymptomatic. Tic pain rarely occurs at night. In idiopathic trigeminal neuralgia, the neurologic examination is entirely normal. In symptomatic trigeminal neuralgia, there may be sensory changes in the distribution of the trigeminal nerve, and such a finding should prompt a careful search for structural disease of the nervous system.

Carbamazepine usually is effective in doses varying from 400 to 800 mg a day, but because of its sedative properties the initial dose is 100 mg twice daily, gradually increased to the required maintenance dose. The drug is primarily an anticonvulsive, not an analgesic, and is effective only for specific kinds of pain such as trigeminal neuralgia, glossopharyngeal neuralgia, and the lightning pains of tabes dorsalis. Baclofen, phenytoin, and pimozide are also usually effective. Other occasionally effective drugs include valproate, lorazepam, and mexiletine.

The most popular operations consist of lesioning of the gasserian ganglion (either by radiofrequency or glycerol injections) and posterior fossa craniotomy to relieve the compression of the trigeminal nerve by vascular structures. Gasserian ganglion lesions can be made under local anesthesia, are generally effective initially, but have a high relapse rate. Posterior fossa craniotomy is as effective as gasserian ganglion lesions and appears to have a lower relapse rate. The purpose of both operations is to relieve pain with little or no loss of sensation, thus preventing the dreaded complications of anesthesia dolorosa.

GLOSSOPHARYNGEAL NEURALGIA. Glossopharyngeal neuralgia is characterized by pain similar to that of trigeminal neuralgia but in the distribution of the glossopharyngeal and vagus nerves. The trigger zone is usually in the tonsil or posterior pharynx, and the pain spreads toward the angle of the jaw and the ear. Occasional patients suffer cardiac slowing or arrest during these attacks as a result of the intense afferent discharge over the glossopharyngeal nerve. Carbamazepine is often effective, and if it fails, the other drugs used for trigeminal neuralgia therapy may help. If drug therapy is unsuccessful, glossopharyngeal nerve roots are sectioned in the posterior fossa. Symptomatic glossopharyngeal neuralgia is occasionally the presenting complaint of a tonsillar tumor, and careful examination of the pharynx and tonsillar fossa must be carried out.

OTHER NEURALGIAS. Similar but much rarer disorders than trigeminal or glossopharyngeal neuralgia have been reported to involve the greater occipital nerve and the nervus intermedius portion of the facial nerve. The clinical features and treatment of these rare disorders are similar to those for trigeminal neuralgia.

DIAGNOSTIC EVALUATION

Headache is extremely common and the excessive application of expensive and highly technical laboratory procedures to its diagnosis and management has been a substantial cause of unnecessary medical costs. Set against this truism is the fact that in some instances a timely MRI or lumbar puncture can give life-saving information about an otherwise undiagnosable problem. Given these antitheses, the following principles may help in management.

1. Patients with chronic classic or common migraine or with chronic tension-type headache rarely require more than a careful history and examination. Even when the unilateral prodromes and headache of longstanding, classic migraine consistently affect the same side, the incidence of associated intracranial lesions remains so low that scans are unnecessary and arteriography unjustified.

2. Headaches that have begun or worsened recently deserve investigation. This principle especially applies to headaches that have a consistently focal distribution, follow trauma, or begin after the age of 30 years. MRI is more sensitive than CT.

3. The EEG is almost never useful in the diagnosis of diseases causing headache and can be omitted. Skull radiographs are so rarely useful that they should be omitted. Even for trauma, CT scans have discriminating capacities far superior to those of plain films and make radiographs unnecessary.

4. Diagnostic lumbar puncture should be performed with any acute headache that (a) is accompanied by fever or (b) is explosive or the most severe headache ever suffered (a history typical of acute subarachnoid hemorrhage—but see thunderclap headache, p. 2033). Lumbar puncture should, if possible, be deferred until after CT scanning with other forms of acute headache, especially if stiff neck but no fever is present. (This combination may indicate partial herniation of cerebellar tonsils into the foramen magnum secondary to an intracranial mass lesion.)

5. Now that CT and MRI are widely available, radioisotopic brain scanning rarely if ever adds useful information and is expensively superfluous.

Lance JW: Mechanism and Management of Headache. Oxford, Butterworth Heinemann, 1993. *A monograph describing pathophysiology, diagnosis, and management of headaches and other head pain in a clear and concise style.*

Lauritzen M: Pathophysiology of the migraine aura. The spreading depression theory. Review article. Brain 117:199, 1994. *A comprehensive description of the pathophysiology of the migraine aura.*

Olesen J, Tfelt-Hansen P, Welch KMA (eds.): The Headaches. New York, Raven Press, 1993. *A multi-authored comprehensive text covering the basic and clinical aspects of all headache syndromes.*

405.3 Some Specific Pain Syndromes

Some chronic painful disorders are associated with a specific constellation of signs and symptoms which establishes them as identifiable pain syndromes. Those most commonly encountered in clinical practice include the *neuropathic pain* disorders of diabetic polyneuropathy (see Ch. 449), sympathetically maintained pain, postherpetic neuralgia, phantom limb pain, and the *non-neuropathic pain* syndromes, fibromyalgia and myofascial pain. Taken together, these syndromes cause chronic, usually unremitting pain that is often disabling and difficult and frustrating to treat.

SYMPATHETICALLY MAINTAINED PAIN. This term applies to severe pain, usually burning in quality and associated with autonomic changes including swelling, vasomotor instability, and abnormalities of sweating. The pain syndrome usually follows an injury, often minor, to an extremity. If the injury has involved a peripheral nerve, particularly the sciatic or median nerve, the syndrome is called *causalgia*. If the injury does not involve the peripheral nerve, if there has been no trauma, or if the syndrome follows a visceral illness (e.g., myocardial infarction), the term applied is *reflex sympathetic dystrophy*. (Older and outmoded terms include post-traumatic painful osteoporosis, Sudek's atrophy, post-traumatic spreading neuralgia, minor causalgia, and shoulder-hand syndrome.) The exact pathophysiology of the disorder is unknown, but, as the name implies, efferent activity of the sympathetic nervous system plays an important role in both the pain and the autonomic symptoms.

The disorder is characterized by severe and continuous pain exacerbated by emotional stress and usually associated with severe hyperpathia so that moving or touching the limb is often intolerable. At first the pain is localized to the site of injury or the distribu-

tion of an injured nerve, but with time it spreads to involve the entire extremity. Spread to other areas of the body sometimes occurs. Along with the pain go vasomotor changes including vasodilatation (warm and dry skin) or vasoconstriction (cyanosis, cool skin). Other autonomic changes may include edema and either hypo- or hyperhidrosis; trophic changes of the skin, subcutaneous tissues, muscles, and bone (osteoporosis) also occur. The entire symptom complex rarely affects any one patient, and one sign or symptom usually predominates. Untreated, the disorder can lead to muscle atrophy, fixation of joints, and a useless extremity. The diagnosis is largely clinical but can be supported by tests showing autonomic instability or trophic changes including increased bone uptake on radionuclide scans, bone atrophy on plain radiographs, and temperature abnormalities on thermography.

The earlier the treatment, the more effective it is likely to be. Treatment is directed at repeatedly blocking sympathetic outflow to the involved site while stimulating and mobilizing the painful area. Some physicians endorse sympatholytic agents (e.g., phenoxybenzamine up to 120 mg in divided doses) and short courses of corticosteroids. Nevertheless, many patients fail to respond. In refractory patients pharmacologic agents directed at neuropathic pain, including tricyclic antidepressants (e.g., amitriptyline, 50 to 150 mg at bedtime), anticonvulsants (e.g., carbamazepine, 600 to 800 mg a day in divided doses), and oral local anesthetics (e.g., mexiletine, up to 300 mg three times a day) can be tried. Refractory cases should be referred to a multidisciplinary pain clinic.

POSTHERPETIC NEURALGIA. Postherpetic neuralgia refers to severe and prolonged burning pain with occasional lightning-like stabs in the involved dermatome after an attack of herpes zoster. Severe postherpetic neuralgia is usually a disease of elderly patients and, like most chronic pain, is exacerbated by emotional upset and relieved to some degree by distraction. Touching the involved area may exacerbate the pain. Treatment is not satisfactory. Initial treatment should be directed toward stimulating the painful area. In some patients brisk rubbing applied repeatedly with a terrycloth towel or stimulation of the dermatome with a cutaneous electrical stimulator may bring relief which outlasts the stimulus, occasionally permanently.

Most patients require multimodality therapy, which includes stimulation of the area, physical therapy, psychological support, and pharmacologic treatment. The application of topical pharmacologic agents, such as lidocaine, sometimes gives temporary relief, and anecdotal evidence claims that topical application of capsaicin is useful. Lancinating pains, which are usually a minor component, usually respond to anticonvulsants (e.g., carbamazepine, 400 to 600 mg a day in divided doses), but anticonvulsants do not affect the continuous pain. The latter may be treated by tricyclic antidepressants or mexiletine (see above). Neuroleptics (e.g., fluphenazine 1 to 3 mg daily) may also be helpful. When conservative approaches fail, one should consider either anesthetic approaches with subcutaneous local injection or sympathetic blockade. The only surgical approach that has proved at all useful is to lesion the dorsal root entry zone, and even that remains controversial. Adrenocorticosteroids and acyclovir, both of which may diminish pain in the acute stage, have no effect on the development of postherpetic neuralgia. In many patients, the disease runs its course and, after a year or two, disappears spontaneously.

The pharmacologic approach includes tricyclic antidepressants, anticonvulsants, neuroleptics, and sometimes sympathetic blockade. Referral to a multidisciplinary pain center may be helpful.

PHANTOM LIMB PAIN. Phantom limb pain is a chronic and severe pain appearing to be localized in an amputated or totally denervated limb. All patients suffer phantom sensations after amputation and as many as 60 to 70% suffer pain, especially if they had severe preambulation pain. The pain may resemble that suffered before amputation or may seem like muscle pain with the phantom in a cramped or uncomfortable position. Usually the pain lessens and disappears with time, but sometimes it becomes chronic and severe. Therapy is difficult. Painful neuromas should be ruled out but are uncommon; even when these are removed, the pain is not usually relieved. Surgery to the CNS is seldom helpful. The pain may be triggered by touching the amputation stump or even healthy areas. Sometimes phantom pain can be permanently abolished by cutaneous stimulation, either rubbing or electrical stimulation, or by repeated anesthetic blocks of peripheral nerves proximal to the stump. The pharmacologic approach is the same as that described for the neuropathic pains above, including referral to a multidisciplinary pain center.

FIBROMYALGIA AND MYOFASCIAL PAIN. Fibromyalgia (also called fibrositis) is characterized by widespread or generalized musculoskeletal pain associated with morning stiffness, disturbed sleep and fatigue (nonrestorative sleep), and at times by vague complaints of a feeling of swelling or paresthesias. On examination, *tender points* can be found at multiple sites over muscles and ligaments, particularly at the upper borders of the trapezius, supraspinatus, and upper gluteal area and below the lateral epicondyle of the elbow and the medial epicondyle of the femur. The disorder usually occurs in middle-aged women and is often associated with fatigue, anxiety, and depression. Tension headaches and irritable bowel syndrome are common.

The myofascial pain syndrome refers to chronic pain in a regional distribution associated with trigger point(s). *Trigger points* are tender, sometimes hardened areas in a muscle which, when palpated, reproduce the distribution of the spontaneous pain. When injected with a local anesthetic, both the local and referred pain are temporarily relieved.

The pathophysiology of these syndromes is poorly understood. Some observers have reported microscopic changes at trigger points (so-called fibrous nodules), suggesting that a tonic contraction of muscle has led to structural changes. Others have suggested that release of noxious substances, such as lactic acid, potassium, or kinins from chronically contracted muscles, may be responsible for the pain and tenderness associated with the syndromes. No theory has stood the test of time.

Treatment is often difficult and frustrating. Some patients may benefit from mild analgesic drugs, heat, and massage. In others with trigger points (myofascial pain), massage or injection of trigger points with local anesthetics may give relief. Biofeedback, with the patient trying consciously to relax contracted muscle recorded by surface EMG, has been reported to be useful. Antidepressants are modestly effective and produce at least a short-term remission in about 20% of patients. For most patients, a combination of physical methods with investigation and treatment of associated psychological disorders is necessary if long-term relief is to be achieved.

Fields HL, Leibeskind JC (eds.): Progress in Pain Research and Management. Volume 1. Pharmacological Approaches to the Treatment of Chronic Pain: New Concepts and Critical Issues. Seattle, IASP Press, 1994. *A recent monograph describing pain syndromes and their pharmacologic management.*

Schott GD: Visceral afferents: Their contribution to "sympathetic dependent" pain. Brain 117:397, 1994. *A review of the physiology of causalgia and related painful disorders.*

Wall PD, Melzack R (eds.): Textbook of Pain. London, Churchill Livingstone, 1994. *A compendium of basic, clinical, and therapeutic aspects of most pain syndromes.*

405.4 The Painful Back
David S. Howell

The back is a complex structure serving weight-bearing and locomotor functions. It provides for major support of body structures and transmission of loading forces through the sacroiliac joints to the lower limbs. The fundamental functioning unit is an articular triad composed of two zygoapophyseal joints posteriorly and the intervertebral disc anteriorly. The disc is composed of a nucleus pulposus encompassed by the annulus fibrosus. These structures are arranged in a series and stabilized throughout the spine by ligaments. The spinal bones also encase the spinal cord and the cauda equina and through successive foramina rootlets connect the spinal cord with peripheral neural pathways (See Ch. 444 for discussion of cervical spine, Ch. 238 for spondylarthropathies, Ch. 440 for intervertebral disc disease.)

ETIOLOGY. In Table 405–3, the numerous causes of back pain are displayed according to disease subgroups. Although all vertebral levels can be affected, pain in the low back is most prevalent. The majority of patients have problems relating to functional or mechanical disturbances, and these must be distinguished from a wide variety of diseases either of focal origin or referred from multiple organ systems. Among degenerative diseases, low back pain is a leading cause of industrial absenteeism and chronic disablement.

MEDICAL HISTORY. Sex. Compression vertebral fractures

TABLE 405–3. ETIOLOGY OF BACK PAIN

Mechanical or traumatic
  Paraspinal ligaments and musculature
    Myofascial syndrome, sacroiliac strain
  Spondylogenic
    Osteoarthritis-related lesions—zygoapophyseal joints
    Degenerative lesions—intervertebral discs
    Mechanical insufficiency, congenital and acquired, of ligaments and bones
    Spondylolisthesis
    Spinal stenosis
    Fractures
Metabolic
  Vertebral bodies, partial collapse and distortion—osteoporosis; osteomalacia—Paget's disease—often with secondary osteoarthritis
Tumors
  Neural tumors, osteosarcoma, metastatic tumors, e.g., from breast, thyroid, kidney
  Myeloma, lymphoma, leukemia
Systemic inflammatory disease
  Spondylitis (ankylosing)—Reiter's disease; psoriatic or enteropathic arthropathy
  Disseminated ankylosing skeletal hyperostosis
Infections
  Pyogenic, fungal, tuberculous disc infection, herpes zoster infection, paraspinal abscesses
Referred pain
  Vascular—aneurysms, sclerosis of aorta and branches
  Tumors or inflammation of pleural, pulmonary, pericardial, cardiac, or neck origin
  Viscerogenic disease of gallbladder, pancreas, stomach, intestines, kidneys, ureters, bladder, prostate, uterus
  Pelvic or retroperitoneal tumors or inflammation
Nonorganic components
  Hysterical conversion
  Learned painful behavior
  Psychosis
  Litigation neurosis, malingering
  Chronic pain syndrome
  Substance abuse

from osteoporosis have their highest prevalence in postmenopausal women. Gynecologic pathology, such as endometriosis, is the basis for some referred patterns of back pain. Reiter's disease, ankylosing spondylitis, and back injuries are found more commonly in males.

Age. Young people with back pain most commonly suffer from muscle or ligament strains, congenital abnormalities, injury, spondyloarthropathies, and herniated disc syndromes. In middle and old age, osteoporosis, vertebral collapse, degenerative states, including spinal stenosis, and malignant lesions are common.

Family History. Familial patterns of segregation are often detected in respect to spondyloarthropathies and uncommonly in respect to spinal degenerative conditions.

Nature of Pain. Events or conditions that accelerate or retard symptoms should be explored. The chronic inflammatory diseases (spondyloarthropathies) are associated with increased pain and stiffness on inactivity. Patients with lumbar disc protrusion and radicular pain generally are relieved by lying flat with the knees flexed and are uncomfortable sitting. Sudden or acute onset of symptoms is suggestive of a mechanical or infectious origin of symptoms, respectively. Constitutional symptoms such as fever, weight loss, and fatigue are important clues to infectious, inflammatory, or neoplastic disorders.

In regard to localization, the dorsal segment suggests osteoarthritis, vertebral fracture, neoplasm, herpetic radiculitis, or referred pain from the viscera (see later paragraph). Localization of pain in the low back is usually of little help in regard to differential diagnosis. Claudication-type pain, with onset after sustained walking, suggests either spinal stenosis or arterial insufficiency. The former condition often refers pain to the thigh and is poorly relieved by standing still. Usually neurogenic claudication is relieved by sitting, whereas vascular claudication is reduced by standing.

Referred Pain. A deep aching pain referred to various sites in the upper and midback may be engendered by lesions in the upper gastrointestinal tract. Pain of malignant disease (whether local or referred) is typically severe and unrelieved by change of position or mild analgesics.

In respect to neuropathic symptoms, alteration of the structure of the vertebral foramina may lead to radicular dissemination of pain. In such instances, compression or traction of nerve rootlets or extension of inflammation to them can lead to sensory and motor nerve symptoms and signs, i.e., paresthesias, hypoesthesias, and muscle weakness.

Symptomatology. Discogenic pain is characteristically aggravated by cough or sneeze. Rarely, loss of bowel or urinary sphincter function can result from cord compression or bilateral involvement of sacral nerve roots from spinal stenosis, tumors, or infectious lesions.

PHYSICAL EXAMINATION. General examination of the back is discussed in Ch. 233. Descriptions here are confined to vertebral compression fractures, degenerative disc disease, and lumbosacral strains and sprains.

Lumbosacral Strain. This and related myofascial syndromes are the most common ailments seen in the office practice of rheumatology. A history of injury is often followed by prompt or delayed low back pain. Transient disc prolapse, subluxation of facet joints, and injury to muscles or ligaments are diagnostic considerations. Physical signs are usually limited to paravertebral muscle spasm, tenderness, and restricted lower back motion without evidence of nerve root involvement.

Vertebral Compression Fractures. These are the most common complication of osteoporosis, with the resultant traction or compression of rootlets adjacent to collapsed vertebrae. Severe pain may begin suddenly, associated with the postural strain of lifting heavy objects or hyperflexing the trunk. Major physical findings consist of localized tenderness and muscle spasm related to the level of the nerve roots affected. Poorly localized back pain may be associated with osteoporosis in the absence of vertebral collapse. Metastatic tumor, myeloma, and metabolic bone disease, especially osteopenia of aging, are common underlying conditions.

Discogenic Disease. The most common form of low back pain with radiculitis is associated with prolapse, protrusion, or extrusion of intervertebral disc substance. Usually the onset of acute symptoms is preceded by chronic intermittent low back pain, although a discrete injury may precipitate an attack. Ninety percent of disc herniations are localized at L4–L5 or L5–S1 levels. Discs involving the L4 nerve root may cause pain referred along the course of the femoral nerve upon hip extension and knee flexion. Knee extension may be weak and the patellar reflex reduced or absent. Patients with L5 nerve root disturbance complain of classic sciatic distribution of pain, i.e., radiating to the posterior thigh and anteromedial leg and foot, in association with weakness of the toe extensors. First sacral radiculopathy is associated with pain over the posterior thigh, calf, and heel, weakness of the ankle and toe flexors, and reduced or absent Achilles tendon reflex. Frequently, loss of neurologic function is subtle and requires repeated testing to document. A positive response to straight-leg raising is most frequently indicative of L4–L5 or L5–S1 disc protrusion. Usually there is pain on hip flexion with the knee extended and absence of pain on repetition of hip flexion with the knee flexed (Lasègue's sign). The cauda equina syndrome is a form of spinal stenosis and is an uncommon but important complication of massive disc prolapse. In the cauda equina syndrome, central midline disc displacement causes paralysis of the sacral root with bladder and bowel dysfunction. It is characterized by severe bilateral leg pain, urinary retention, weakness of the anal sphincter, and bilateral nerve root abnormalities. Once complete neurologic block has occurred, pain is often alleviated, and the patient requires a neurologic examination to verify the need for emergency surgery.

Spondylolisthesis. This condition, which refers to forward displacement of one vertebra on another, commonly involves the L4–L5 and L5–S1 levels. Bursts of segmental severe girdle pain are typical, often worse on activity and relieved by rest.

LABORATORY PROCEDURES. These are dictated by the results of medical history and physical examination. Simple radiographs of the back may suffice if a traumatic injury is causative. In instances of suspected metabolic disturbance, appropriate screening tests, such as serum calcium, phosphorus, and alkaline phosphatase measurements, should be obtained. Complete blood counts, sedimentation rate, urinalysis, and automated serum chemical profiles are sometimes justified to clarify the diagnosis. Anemia and an elevated sedimentation rate should prompt a more extensive search for infectious, inflammatory, and neoplastic diseases.

RADIOGRAPHIC STUDIES. *Routine Radiographic Studies.* These include frontal, lateral, and oblique films of the lumbosacral spine, which can demonstrate foraminal encroachment, compression fractures, degenerative changes, and subluxation of zygoapophyseal joints, as well as internarrowing. There may be severe degenerative changes on the radiographs, with few or no relevant symptoms, and severe back pain may occur in the absence of significant radiographic signs and be of discogenic origin.

Additional Imaging Procedures. When surgical intervention is planned or a diagnosis remains questionable and requires an imperative answer and high resolution, computed tomography (CT) and magnetic resonance imaging (MRI) (noninvasive) are increasingly preferred to myelography. It is not usually necessary to perform discography (injection of radiopaque dye directly into the disc). When osteomyelitis or neoplastic involvement is likely, radionuclide bone scans are helpful. A percutaneous vertebral biopsy under fluoroscopic guidance may be performed to establish histopathologic diagnosis or bacteriologic diagnosis at highly suspicious sites obvious from scans or radiographs. Electromyography can confirm the presence of nerve root deficits.

Management. Conservative therapy for mechanical disorders of the spine and disc herniation focuses on bed rest, analgesics, and anti-inflammatory medication. Long-term use of anti-inflammatory agents should be accompanied by prophylactic protection against peptic ulceration. Application of moist heat, e.g., hydrocollator packs wrapped with a wet towel, may relieve pain and muscle spasm. The amount of bed rest is dependent on the severity of symptoms. After bed rest, gradual ambulation and a program of exercises, together with back protection including a lumbosacral support, are recommended. Most cases of disc herniation respond to conservative therapy; those unresponsive require further measures, including epidural steroids and nerve root or sleeve infiltrations with steroids. Before surgery is indicated, a psychological assessment and exercises emphasizing back stretching and abdominal strengthening should be attempted.

Progressive muscular weakness and progressive neurologic deficit despite bed rest and other aforementioned measures, as well as the cauda equina syndrome, are indications for surgery. Relative indications for laminectomy are severe pain unrelieved by bed rest and recurrent episodes of incapacitating pain; 90 to 95% improvement is anticipated following surgery, although 70% of patients experience relief of pain whether or not the disc is removed.

Following either conservative therapy or surgery, a program of prophylactic management includes postural education, performance of a daily exercise program to strengthen the lumbar and abdominal muscles, and avoidance of lower spine stress. Besides laminectomy, joint fusion for spondylolisthesis and discogenic disease or unroofing procedures for spinal stenosis are sometimes necessary. Myelography, CT, or MRI is indicated preoperatively to establish definitively the nature and extent of disease as well as the level of vertebral involvement.

Acute symptoms from compression fractures require appropriate rest and relief of pain with analgesics. Activities must be selected to avoid additional compression fractures. (See Ch. 217 for management of osteoporosis.)

Brown MD, Ray CD, et al.: In Weinstein JN (ed.): Clinical Efficacy in the Diagnosis and Treatment of Low Back Pain. New York, Raven Press, 1992, pp 279–280. *A flow scheme of diagnostic steps and alternative modes of treatment as well as assessment of their value.*

Brown MD, Rydevik B: Advances in the understanding and treatment of low back pain and sciatica. Orthop Clin North Am 22: April, 1991. *An overview of the present management of low back pain, with emphasis on controlled trials and newer diagnostic techniques.*

Manmiche C, Hessels EG, Bentzen L, et al.: Clinical trials of intensive muscle training for chronic low back pain. Lancet 2:862, 1988. *An appropriate program is described for motivated patients with pain refractory to conventional measures.*

Weber H: Lumbar disc herniation: A controlled prospective study with 10 years of observation. Spine 8:131, 1983. *A classic set of observations on the natural history of the disease and discussion of management.*

406 NUTRITIONAL DISORDERS OF THE NERVOUS SYSTEM
Robert Messing

Characteristic neurologic syndromes result from deficiency of certain nutrients (Table 406–1). In developing countries, nutritional disorders usually result from starvation or from limited diets. In developed countries of North America and Europe, acquired nutritional disorders are found most often in chronic alcoholics (Table 406–2). They also occur with food faddism, starvation due to cancer or malabsorption syndromes, psychiatric illness, or infantile malnutrition. Genetic factors may contribute to vulnerability in some disorders such as the Wernicke-Korsakoff syndrome and two rare vitamin E deficiency syndromes. Part XVI discusses the metabolism of most of the medically important vitamins as well as many details of their deficiencies. This chapter emphasizes the major neurologic syndromes seen in developing countries and briefly describes their management.

VITAMIN B₁ (THIAMINE) AND THE WERNICKE-KORSAKOFF SYNDROME

CLINICAL MANIFESTATIONS. This acute neurologic disorder most often results from the malnutrition of alcoholism but can also accompany other conditions (Table 406–3). The triad of ophthalmoplegia, gait ataxia, and a confusional state is characteristic, but the condition should be suspected in any confused alcoholic. The most common ocular abnormality is nystagmus, usually horizontal, less often vertical. Ocular palsies are also common, particularly affecting lateral rectus function, unilaterally or bilaterally. Complete external ophthalmoplegia and ptosis are unusual, and pupillary light responses are rarely impaired. Gait ataxia results from cerebellar involvement and is usually not associated with limb ataxia or dysarthria. The most common mental disturbance is a quiet confusional state with profound disorientation, apathy, drowsiness, and impaired memory. Acutely, some patients suffer a severe delirium, most likely reflecting alcohol withdrawal. Stupor and coma occur rarely. About 80% of patients have a distal symmetric sensorimotor polyneuropathy, which is symptomatic in two thirds of cases. Associated autonomic disturbances include tachycardia, hypertension, hypotension, and hypothermia. Beriberi heart disease, another thiamine deficiency disorder, is also associated with neuropathy. Although CNS deficits may occur in nutritionally deprived infants with beriberi, adults with Wernicke's encephalopathy do not develop beriberi heart disease.

PATHOLOGY. Demyelination, necrosis, gliosis, and vascular proliferation are found within the mamillary bodies, periventricular regions of the diencephalon and midbrain, the floor of the fourth ventricle, the superior and inferior colliculi, and the superior cerebellar vermis.

TREATMENT. Treatment with thiamine corrects some or all of the abnormalities. Because intestinal absorption is impaired in alcoholics, thiamine (100 mg per day) should be administered parenterally for several days. Glucose increases thiamine utilization, and if

TABLE 406–2. NEUROLOGIC DISORDERS ASSOCIATED WITH ALCOHOLISM

Disorders due directly to alcohol
  Intoxication
  Withdrawal seizures
  Delirium tremens
  Fetal alcohol syndrome
Nutritional deficiency disorders
  Wernicke-Korsakoff syndrome
  Pellagra
  Amblyopia
Disorders that may involve alcohol and poor nutrition
  Cerebellar degeneration
  Alcoholic myopathy
  Alcoholic polyneuropathy
  Alcoholic dementia
Disorders associated with electrolyte abnormalities
  Central pontine myelinolysis
Disorders of unknown cause
  Marchiafava-Bignami syndrome

given prior to administration of thiamine, can precipitate or worsen the encephalopathy. Outpatient therapy should provide 50 mg of oral thiamine a day for at least 6 weeks and weekly thereafter. Ophthalmoplegia and gaze palsies usually begin to resolve during the first day of treatment. Nystagmus, ataxia, and confusion improve over days to weeks. Many patients are left with nystagmus, some with gait ataxia, and some with amnesia.

Many patients with the acute Wernicke-Korsakoff syndrome retain a residual disorder of memory—Korsakoff's amnestic syndrome. They are unable to learn new information (anterograde amnesia) and have difficulty recalling established recent memories (retrograde amnesia). Some confabulate to fill gaps in memory. In contrast to the deficit in memory, other intellectual skills and language are better preserved. Lesions involving the midline diencephalon and the dorsal medial nuclei of the thalamus may account for the memory disturbance. Treatment is the same as for Wernicke's encephalopathy. About 20% recover completely from Wernicke-Korsakoff psychosis over several months, but a quarter do not and require long-term care.

ALCOHOLIC DEMENTIA

Many alcoholics develop enlarged cerebral ventricles and other signs of brain shrinkage which can be visualized on computed tomographic and magnetic resonance scans of the brain. Many such patients also show impairments on psychometric examination. Pathologically, the brain shows white matter pallor and loss of neurons mainly in premotor cortex. In their early stages, such changes may relate to reduced water content of brain, and during this time radiologic and cognitive abnormalities may lessen if drinking stops. With continued alcoholism, however, the process continues and

TABLE 406–1. MAJOR NEUROLOGIC SYNDROMES DUE TO ACQUIRED NUTRITIONAL DEFICIENCY

Protein-calorie malnutrition	Developmental neurologic defects
Vitamin A	Night blindness
Vitamin B₁ (thiamine)	Polyneuropathy, Wernicke-Korsakoff syndrome
Niacin, L-tryptophan	Pellagra, polyneuropathy
Pyridoxine	Polyneuropathy, seizures
Multiple B vitamins	Amblyopia, polyneuropathy
Folate	? Polyneuropathy, ? myelopathy, ? dementia
Vitamin B₁₂	Combined systems disease, polyneuropathy, dementia
Vitamin D	Myopathy
Vitamin E	Spinocerebellar degeneration
Iodine	Cretinism

TABLE 406–3. CONDITIONS PREDISPOSING TO WERNICKE'S ENCEPHALOPATHY

Chronic alcoholism
Starvation
Persistent vomiting
  Hyperemesis of pregnancy
  Gastric cancer
  Gastritis
  Intestinal obstruction
  Digitalis intoxication
Systemic diseases
  Malignancy
  Hepatic failure
  Disseminated tuberculosis
  Uremia
Iatrogenic
  Gastrointestinal surgery with malabsorption
  Hemodialysis or peritoneal dialysis
  Prolonged intravenous feeding
  Refeeding after starvation
Anorexia nervosa

sooner or later becomes permanent. The cerebral abnormalities may partly result from nutritional deficiency, although animal studies indicate that alcohol can cause direct neuronal damage in spite of adequate nutrition.

ALCOHOLIC-NUTRITIONAL NEUROPATHY

CLINICAL MANIFESTATIONS. Alcoholics and other nutritionally deprived persons commonly develop a mixed axonal-demyelinating polyneuropathy (see Ch. 450) with pain and paresthesias in the feet. More severe cases develop leg weakness and symptoms involving the hands. The pain is often burning in character and can be so severe as to make light touch and deep pressure intensely uncomfortable and to inhibit walking.

Muscle weakness and wasting, when present, affect the legs more than the arms and are most prominent distally. Sensory abnormalities usually involve all modalities, but pain and temperature sensation are involved early. Sensory abnormalities are more severe distally, and the legs are more involved than the arms. The deep tendon reflexes are diminished or absent, especially at the ankles. Depression of the ankle deep tendon reflexes is common in asymptomatic patients. In rare cases the condition involves the vagus nerve and the thoracoabdominal sympathetic chain, resulting in hoarseness, dysphagia, vocal cord paralysis, and hypotension. The cerebrospinal fluid protein levels most often are normal. The diagnosis usually is evident on clinical grounds. Electrodiagnostic studies seldom are needed but, if obtained, show signs of denervation with reduced amplitude of sensory and motor action potentials but relatively preserved nerve conduction velocities.

PATHOLOGY AND TREATMENT. The pathologic findings are mainly those of axonal degeneration with secondary demyelination. A specific vitamin deficiency has not been identified in alcoholic neuropathy; similar polyneuropathies occur with deficiencies of thiamine, niacin, or pyridoxine. Possibly, alcohol may have a direct toxic effect on peripheral nerves. Treatment consists of a balanced diet of supplemental B vitamins and abstinence from alcohol. Several weeks may elapse before motor improvement begins. Recovery is generally slow and incomplete.

ALCOHOLIC MYOPATHY

Some alcoholic patients suffer from an acute syndrome of focal or generalized muscle pain, tenderness, swelling, and weakness, beginning abruptly during a drinking binge. Affected muscles are swollen, tender, and indurated with the edematous overlying skin taking on a dusky color. Affected patients may have associated cardiac failure, an arrhythmia, or an impaired swallowing capacity due to pharyngeal weakness. The serum creatine kinase (CK) level is moderately or markedly elevated and, in severe cases, myoglobinuria may cause acute renal failure, hyperkalemia, and death. The diagnosis is readily made clinically, but if doubt prevails, electromyography usually shows evidence of a myopathy (see Ch. 392.5) and muscle biopsy reveals necrosis of muscle fibers. Recovery follows days to weeks of abstinence and adequate nutrition, occasionally leaving residual proximal muscle weakness. Animal experiments indicate that both nutritional deprivation and prolonged alcohol intoxication contribute to the acute muscle necrosis.

In contrast to acute myopathy, proximal muscle weakness and atrophy develop in some alcoholics over a period of weeks or months with little or no muscle pain. The symptoms of chronic alcoholic myopathy reflect the proximal muscular distribution, with the lower extremities usually being affected more than the upper ones. The serum CK is usually normal but may be elevated in some cases, especially after recent drinking. Electromyography usually shows myopathic changes in proximal muscles, and muscle biopsies show mild degenerative abnormalities without widespread necrosis. Alcoholic myopathy and cardiomyopathy (see Ch. 43) often develop concurrently. Improvement usually occurs with 2 to 3 months of abstinence from alcohol and restored nutrition; in some muscle power never returns completely to normal.

ALCOHOLIC CEREBELLAR DEGENERATION

Degeneration of the cerebellum occurs frequently in chronic alcoholics and has also been documented after severe nutritional depletion unrelated to alcohol abuse. Most patients give a history of episodic binge drinking superimposed on heavy consumption of alcohol for many years. Symptoms usually begin insidiously with progressive unsteadiness and difficulty in walking. Sometimes the

disorder evolves rapidly, especially after a binge or severe systemic illness. Affected patients have striking gait ataxia, walking with hesitant, wide-based steps. More severe examples include truncal ataxia as well. Some patients may demonstrate impaired heel to shin tests, but nystagmus, dysarthria, and ataxia of the upper extremities are rare. The features of a distal polyneuropathy are present in about half of the patients. The most prominent pathologic abnormality is degeneration of neurons in the anterior and superior cerebellar vermis. Within these areas all neuronal elements are affected, but the Purkinje cells appear to be especially vulnerable. Similar lesions often accompany cases of Wernicke's encephalopathy, suggesting that the two conditions are closely linked. It is not certain, however, that cerebellar degeneration is due solely to thiamine deficiency. A direct toxic effect of alcohol and an underlying genetic susceptibility to cerebellar damage may contribute. Cerebellar dysfunction stabilizes and sometimes improves with abstinence, adequate nutrition, and supplemental B vitamins.

NUTRITIONAL AMBLYOPIA

This disorder appears most commonly in malnourished alcoholics and appears to be due to deficiency of several B vitamins. It is characterized by insidious and progressive loss of visual acuity and the ability to distinguish colors. Examination discloses bilateral and symmetric central or paracentral scotomas, and, in advanced stages, optic atrophy. Polyneuropathy or a history of the Wernicke-Korsakoff syndrome may coexist. Substantial improvement in vision with complete return of acuity and visual fields can follow early treatment with group B vitamins. In advanced cases, visual impairment may be permanent.

MARCHIAFAVA-BIGNAMI DISEASE

This rare disorder, diagnosed only at autopsy, seldom is described nowadays. The pathology consists of bilateral, symmetric demyelination of the corpus callosum and adjacent white matter, supplemented in some instances with demyelination of the middle cerebellar peduncles. Early symptoms include irritability, aggressiveness, and confusion, often followed by apathy and bilateral spasticity or rigidity. Some case reports describe acute seizure disorders, stupor, or coma. The cause is not well understood, but most or all established cases have been associated with chronic alcoholism and the histologic features closely resemble those found in central pontine myelinolysis (see Ch. 432). Circumstances suggest that the two conditions may be variations of the same process.

PELLAGRA

Pellagra is an uncommon disorder resulting specifically from a deficiency of nicotinic acid (niacin) or its amino acid precursor tryptophan but often incorporating deficiency symptoms of other B vitamins including pyridoxine. Pellagra is uncommon in developed countries because of fortification of processed foods with niacin but is occasionally encountered in chronic alcoholics or institutionalized patients. Manifestations include diarrhea, glossitis, anemia, and erythematous skin lesions in sun-exposed areas. Neurologically, affected persons are irritable and depressed, suffer from insomnia, and have difficulty concentrating. Later, confusion, hallucinations, or paranoid thoughts appear, usually accompanied by spastic weakness. Physical signs include cerebellar deficits, optic neuropathy, and often, a sensorimotor polyneuropathy. Pathologic changes are found throughout the neuraxis and many neurons, particularly the large Betz cells of the motor cortex, show chromatolytic changes. Pellagra responds to administration of niacin along with other B vitamins, although the cerebral symptoms may not resolve completely.

PYRIDOXINE (VITAMIN B₆) DEFICIENCY

A deficiency of dietary pyridoxine in adults causes a sensorimotor polyneuropathy. Pyridoxine is converted by pyridoxal kinase and pyridoxine phosphate oxidase to its active form, pyridoxal phosphate. Pyridoxal phosphate is a cofactor for several enzymes, including glutamic acid decarboxylase, which generates the major inhibitory neurotransmitter γ-aminobutyric acid (GABA) from glutamic acid. Patients taking isonicotinic acid hydrazide (INH) for tuberculosis are at risk for pyridoxine deficiency because INH complexes with pyridoxal phosphate. In addition to polyneuropathy, typical central nervous system, skin, and gastrointestinal manifestations of pellagra may appear in some patients receiving INH. All may be prevented by concomitant administration of pyridoxine.

Persons who ingest an overdose of INH also may develop convulsions, which respond to pyridoxine.

COBALAMIN AND FOLIC ACID DEFICIENCY

The normal and abnormal metabolism of vitamin B_{12} and folic acid is discussed in Ch. 133 in relation to megaloblastic anemias. The following sections describe the principal neurologic abnormalities.

VITAMIN B_{12} DEFICIENCY. Severe vitamin B_{12} deficiency leads to subacute degeneration of peripheral nerve axons plus subacute degeneration of white matter in the dorsal and lateral columns of the spinal cord. Spongy changes as well as foci of myelin and axonal loss affect these areas, with the posterior columns showing maximal involvement at the cervical and upper thoracic levels. Eventually, optic nerve and cerebral white matter can become similarly damaged.

Patients with vitamin B_{12} deficiency first complain of paresthesias, most commonly described as tingling "pins and needles" sensations or numbness, typically affecting the feet bilaterally and sometimes the hands. If the disease goes untreated, gait ataxia sooner or later develops, producing symptoms that intensify with walking in the dark. Further neurologic deterioration in untreated patients progresses relentlessly but at individually varying rates of speed. Ataxia is commonly followed by leg weakness and by bowel and bladder dysfunction. Neuropsychiatric symptoms include apathy, depression, irritability, paranoia, nocturnal confusion, and dementia. Intellectual deterioration rarely develops in the absence of other neurologic signs. Failing vision with central scotomas occurs rarely.

Initially, there may be few objective findings aside from minimal, distal impairment of vibratory sensation involving the legs and sometimes the hands. Subsequently, position sense becomes impaired and sensory changes eventually reach the trunk and arms. Flexion of the neck may elicit tingling paresthesias in the back and legs (Lhermitte's sign). Patellar and ankle deep tendon reflexes are usually diminished or absent, and in the late stages there may be decreased perception of touch, pain, and temperature in the distal lower extremities. Eventually, spinal cord involvement leads to symmetric spastic weakness in the legs and extensor plantar responses.

Diagnosis and Pathophysiology. Most patients with neurologic disease have serum vitamin B_{12} concentrations of less than 100 pg per milliliter. However, approximately 5% of patients have levels between 100 and 200 pg per milliliter. Serum methylmalonic acid and total homocysteine levels are usually elevated and can be used to demonstrate cobalamin deficiency in such patients with slightly depressed vitamin B_{12} levels. As emphasized in Chapter 133, most vitamin B_{12}–induced neurologic disorders have an associated macrocytic anemia. Often, however, such persons are taking folic acid in vitamin pills, which prevents the tell-tale anemia. Direct diagnostic measures are discussed in Chapter 133. Neurologic disorders that can be confused with cobalamin deficiency include peripheral neuritis and, in late cases, multiple sclerosis, cervical spondylosis, spinal cord tumors, and syphilitic meningomyelitis. A virtually identical syndrome has been reported after chronic abuse of nitrous oxide. The importance of this observation is that both nitrous oxide abuse and vitamin B_{12} deficiency result in elevated levels of homocysteine and methylmalonic acid. Nitrous oxide oxidizes the cobalt ion of cobalamin from an active monovalent state to an inactive trivalent state and selectively inhibits methionine synthase. Nitrous oxide causes myelopathy in humans and animals and can be prevented in animals by supplementation with methionine. Therefore, inhibition of methionine synthase may be crucial for the development of neurologic disease in vitamin B_{12} deficiency.

Treatment. Intramuscular administration of cobalamin is the only effective treatment for vitamin B_{12} deficiency, whether due to pernicious anemia or to other malabsorptive states. Most symptomatic improvement occurs during the first 6 months of therapy, although it may not be complete for a year or more. Treatment is discussed in detail in Ch. 133.

FOLATE DEFICIENCY. Only a small proportion of patients with low serum folate levels develop nervous system manifestations, and it is not certain whether or not the two are causally related. Methyltetrahydrofolate, a folic acid derivative, is a cofactor for vitamin B_{12}–dependent methionine synthase. Folate deficiency should be considered in patients suffering from nutritional failure plus a combination of neuropathy, dementia, or symptoms of suba-

cute combined degeneration of the spinal cord with normal vitamin B_{12} levels. Chronic alcoholism is the most important cause of folate deficiency, which also complicates malabsorption due to gastrointestinal diseases. Trimethoprim, methotrexate, oral contraceptives, and the anticonvulsants phenytoin and phenobarbital may intensify folate deficiency by interfering with folate absorption, storage, or metabolism but are not consistently associated with a neurologic disorder. Deficient patients may develop megaloblastic anemia that appears identical to that seen in vitamin B_{12} deficiency (see Ch. 133). Treatment with 1 mg of folate several times a day followed by maintenance with 1 mg daily is usually sufficient to control anemia but if the latter is due to vitamin B_{12} deficiency folate does not prevent neurologic deterioration.

VITAMIN D DEFICIENCY

The radiographic, biochemical, and treatment considerations in vitamin D deficiency are discussed in Ch. 212 and 213. Proximal limb weakness may occur in patients with malabsorption or dietary deficiency of vitamin D. Symptoms may also develop with prolonged use of phenytoin or phenobarbital, which appear to increase target organ resistance to vitamin D. In addition to limb weakness, neck muscles may be weak and there may be a waddling gait. Bulbar and ocular muscles are spared. Osteoporotic bone pain often affects the pelvic girdle and spine and may be associated with multiple fractures and vertebral collapse. The serum CK level is usually normal or slightly elevated, and biopsies show minor, nonspecific muscle fiber atrophy. Myopathic changes are present on electromyography. Serum alkaline phosphatase is elevated, and serum calcium and phosphorus may be decreased. Laboratory abnormalities, bone pain, and weakness usually respond to vitamin D therapy.

VITAMIN E (TOCOPHEROL) DEFICIENCY

This rare condition occurs in the setting of severe malabsorption of lipids (see Ch. 103) plus two rare disorders affecting the nervous system: abetalipoproteinemia and isolated vitamin E deficiency. The clinical syndrome consists of a spinocerebellar degeneration resembling Friedreich's ataxia (see Ch. 413). Weakness and gait unsteadiness are common complaints. Neurologic signs include loss of deep tendon reflexes and reduced vibratory sensation in the feet. Position sensation is less affected and pain and temperature sensations may be normal. Limb and gait ataxia are common, as are mild to moderate proximal weakness, although weakness can be diffuse or predominantly distal. Babinski's sign develops in fewer than half of the cases. About half of the patients have nystagmus, ptosis, or partial external ophthalmoplegia.

Vitamin E is an antioxidant that appears to protect unsaturated fatty acids of membrane phospholipids from oxidative degradation. Deficiency of vitamin E causes loss of large-caliber myelinated axons of peripheral nerves and degeneration of posterior columns and spinocerebellar tracts in the spinal cord. Degenerative changes are also present in the cerebellar cortex, and there is accumulation of lipid pigment in nerve cell bodies in dorsal root ganglia, anterior horn cells, and brain stem motor nuclei. Plate- or disc-like swellings in axons are noted in the posterior columns.

Oral preparations of vitamin E, 200 to 600 mg a day, or intramuscular injections of 50 to 100 mg every 3 to 7 days may prevent progression of neurologic disease. The clinical picture and serum level should be followed and dose adjusted accordingly. Supplementation with bile salts may enhance intestinal absorption.

Blass JP: Vitamin and nutritional deficiencies. *In* Siegel GJ, Agranoff BW, Albers RW, et al. (eds.): Basic Neurochemistry, 5th ed. New York, Raven Press, 1994. *A clear discussion of the neurochemistry of vitamins.*

Charness ME, Simon RP, Greenberg DA: Ethanol and the nervous system. N Engl J Med 321:442, 1989. *A scholarly review with many references.*

Harper CG, Giles M, Finaly-Jones R: Clinical signs in the Wernicke-Korsakoff complex: A retrospective analysis of 131 cases diagnosed at necropsy. J Neurol Neurosurg Psychiatry 49:341, 1986. *Correct antemortem diagnosis was reached in only 20% of cases; most overlooked examples lacked ophthalmoplegia.*

Healton EB, Savage DG, Brust JCM, et al.: Neurologic aspects of cobalamin deficiency. Medicine 70:229, 1991. *A comprehensive review of 189 patients suggests that neurologic symptoms may occur without anemia and in fact are worse in those without anemia.*

Layzer RB: Neurologic Manifestations of Systemic Disease. Philadelphia, FA Davis, 1985. *Excellent discussions of neuropathies and myopathies associated with nutritional deficiencies.*

Satya-Murti S, Howard L, Krohel G, et al.: The spectrum of neurologic disorders from vitamin E deficiency. Neurology 36:917, 1986. *A study of nine patients and a helpful bibliography.*

Section Four—The Extrapyramidal Disorders

Joseph Jankovic

407 INTRODUCTION

The term *extrapyramidal* refers to the anatomic and functional characteristics that distinguish the basal ganglia–regulated motor system from the pyramidal (corticospinal) and cerebellar systems. Extrapyramidal movement disorders are divided descriptively into *hypokinesias,* characterized by poverty and slowness of movement; *hyperkinesias,* manifested by abnormal involuntary movements; and miscellaneous motor disturbances (Table 407–1). Before discussing the clinical, pathophysiologic, and therapeutic aspects of the different movement disorders, it is important to review the anatomic and functional organization of the basal ganglia.

FUNCTIONAL AND NEUROCHEMICAL ANATOMY OF THE BASAL GANGLIA

The six paired nuclei that constitute the basal ganglia include the caudate nucleus, putamen, globus pallidus (or pallidum), nucleus accumbens, subthalamic nucleus, and substantia nigra (Fig. 407–1). The caudate nucleus and putamen, although separated by the internal capsule, share cytoarchitechtonic, chemical, and physiologic properties; they are often referred to as the *corpus striatum,* neostriatum, or simply striatum. The striatum is a highly inhomogeneous structure composed of subregions termed striosomes and matrix. The limbic system provides major input to the striosomes, whereas neocortical areas primarily project to the matrix. Although the internal capsule separates the internal segment of the globus pallidus (GPi) and the pars reticulata of the substantia nigra (SNr), evidence suggests that these nuclei should also be regarded as a single functional structure. The term *lenticular nucleus* refers to the putamen and globus pallidus combined because of their lenslike shape.

Recent anatomic and physiologic data suggest a complex organization of the basal ganglia and related structures (Fig. 407–1). According to this schema, the sensorimotor, association, and limbic cortical areas provide anatomically and functionally segregated inputs to the dorsal (the caudate and putamen) and ventral (nucleus accumbens, not shown) striatum. The somatosensory, motor, and premotor cortical areas project mainly to the putamen, and the posterior parietal and temporal and frontal association cortical areas project largely to the caudate and nucleus accumbens. The anatomy is consistent with the concept that the putamen is primarily concerned with motor function and the caudate is more involved with emotional and cognitive processes. The corticostriatal afferents are mediated by the excitatory neurotransmitter glutamic acid. The other major striatal afferents originate in the substantia nigra pars

TABLE 407–1. MOVEMENT DISORDERS

Hypokinesias	Hyperkinesias	Miscellaneous
Parkinsonism	Tremor	Ataxia
Hypomimia	Dystonia	Gait disorders
Dysarthria	Chorea	Hyperreflexia
Sialorrhea	Athetosis	Hemifacial spasm
Micrographia	Ballism	Myokymia
Shuffling gait	Tics	Stiff-person syndrome
Other signs of	Myoclonus	Psychogenic
bradykinesia	Stereotypy	
and rigidity	Akathisia	
	Restless legs	
	Paroxysmal	
	dyskinesias	

compacta (SNc), which provides major dopaminergic inhibitory input to the basal ganglia via the nigrostriatal pathway. Other inhibitory inputs to the striatum arise from the brain stem raphe nuclei (serotonergic) and from the locus ceruleus neurons (noradrenergic). The striatum is composed largely of cholinergic neurons, and some excitatory cholinergic projections to the striatum originate in the midline intralaminar thalamic nuclei.

The striatal nuclei project somatotopically to the external segment of the globus pallidus (GPe) and the GPi and SNr complex. The striatal efferents utilize the inhibitory neurotransmitter γ-aminobutyric acid (GABA). The subthalamic nucleus (STN) regulates the output of the basal ganglia to the thalamus by modulating the inhibitory GABAergic afferents from the GPe and the excitatory glutamatergic efferent projections to the GPi-SNr complex. The efferent inhibitory GABAergic projections from the GPi terminate in the thalamus. The thalamic nuclei in turn project to the supplementary motor area of the cortex and the primary motor cortex.

MOVEMENT DISORDERS

Single-cell recordings in behaving animals and other studies have demonstrated that one of the primary roles of the basal ganglia is to scale the movement amplitude and velocity rather than to initiate movements. Besides their crucial role in the execution of movement, the basal ganglia also seem to be involved in the preparation for movement.

In addition to impaired voluntary movements, dysfunction in the basal ganglia can also cause a variety of abnormal involuntary movements. Correlations between the various types of abnormal movements and sites of experimental and pathologic lesions have provided helpful insights into and better understanding of the function of the basal ganglia. The remainder of this section is organized according to the major categories of movement disorders into hypokinetic (parkinsonian), hyperkinetic, and miscellaneous movement disorders (see Table 407–1).

HYPOKINESIAS (PARKINSONIAN DISORDERS)

Bradykinesia is manifested clinically by slowness of automatic and spontaneous movements and impaired ability to initiate voluntary movements (akinesia). This typical parkinsonian symptom presumably results from loss of the inhibitory dopamine input to the striatum and hypoactivity of the GPe neurons. This, in turn, causes functional disinhibition (excitation) of the STN, inducing an increase of neuronal activity in the GPi, thereby raising the tonic inhibitory output from the basal ganglia (GPi) to the thalamus and to the cortical projection areas (Fig. 407–2). The altered activity in the "motor" circuit is manifested by increased movement time, which becomes particularly prolonged when a parkinsonian patient performs sequential movements.

Rigidity, another cardinal sign of parkinsonism, is demonstrated clinically by increased resistance against passive movement of a body part, usually associated with the "cogwheel" phenomenon. A parkinsonian patient perceives rigidity as a feeling of joint stiffness and muscle tightness. The pathophysiologic mechanisms of rigidity have been attributed to pallidal disinhibition resulting in increased suprasegmental activation of normal spinal reflex mechanisms.

Postural instability due to loss of righting reflexes can cause propulsion (tendency to fall forward) and retropulsion (tendency to fall backward). It is one of the most disabling symptoms of Parkinson's disease. The mechanism of postural instability is unknown, but it has been attributed primarily to involvement of the pallidum. Other hypokinetic manifestations are listed in Table 407–1.

HYPERKINESIAS (ABNORMAL INVOLUNTARY MOVEMENTS)

Tremor is a rhythmic oscillatory movement produced by alternating or synchronous contractions of opposing muscle groups.

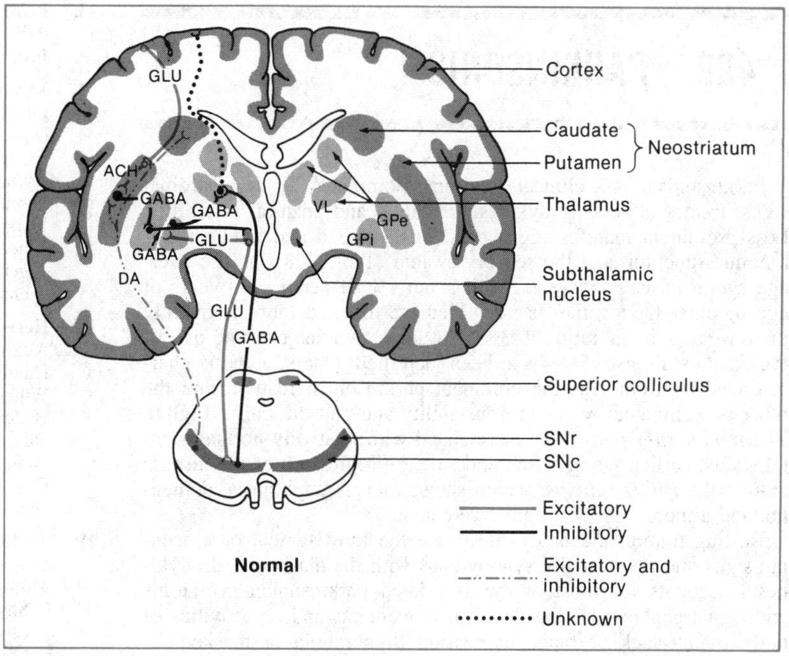

FIGURE 407-1. Anatomy of the basal ganglia and their connections. ACH = acetylcholine; GABA = γ-aminobutyric acid; GLU = glutamate; GP = globus pallidum (e = external, i = internal); DA = dopamine; SN = substantia nigra (c = compacta, r = reticulata); VL = ventrolateral.

Tremors are divided into rest or action tremors; the latter are further subdivided into postural or contraction tremors (e.g., arms outstretched in front of the body or in a "wing-beating" position) and kinetic or intention tremors (e.g., during target-directed movement, such as the finger-to-nose maneuver). *Rest tremor,* usually asymmetric at onset, is the typical tremor of Parkinson's disease. When it involves the hands, it causes a supinating-pronating oscillatory (pill-rolling) movement at approximately 4- to 6-Hz frequency. Parkinsonian tremor also often involves the legs, feet, lips, tongue, chin, and voice but almost never affects the head or neck. *Postural tremor,* with frequency ranging between 4 and 12 Hz, is most typically seen in patients with essential tremor. *Kinetic (intention) tremors* are slow and more irregular movements with a rate of 1.5 to 3 Hz. Kinetic tremors usually indicate an abnormality of the cerebellum or its outflow pathways (the dentate nucleus, the superior cerebellar peduncle, and contralateral red nucleus).

Dystonia is produced by involuntary, sustained (tonic) or spasmodic (rapid or clonic), patterned, and repetitive muscle contractions, frequently causing twisting (e.g., torticollis), flexing or extending (e.g., writer's cramp, retrocollis), and squeezing (e.g., blepharospasm, writer's cramp) movements or abnormal postures. Dystonia is usually constant but occurs in some cases only during particular activities. Examples of task-specific dystonias include writer's or typist's cramp and inversion of a foot while running. As dystonia progresses, the involuntary contractions also appear at rest. A characteristic feature of dystonia is that the spasms lessen in intensity with "sensory tricks," such as touching one side of the face to maintain a primary position, thus counteracting involuntary torticollis. Dystonia can fluctuate in intensity and is exacerbated by stress, fatigue, activity, or a change in posture. It subsides during sleep, relaxation, and hypnosis. These features and the bizarre nature of dystonic patterns sometimes are wrongly attributed to psychogenic causes. About half of patients with dystonia have a coexistent postural tremor, identical to essential tremor. The anatomic substrate for dystonia is unknown. Clinicopathologic studies of patients with secondary dystonias most often implicate the putamen and the rostral brain stem in their genesis.

Chorea consists of continuous, abrupt, rapid, brief, flowing, unsustained, irregular, and random jerklike movements. Choreic patients frequently mask the abnormal movements by voluntary semipurposeful activities. A characteristic feature of chorea is the inability to maintain voluntary sustained contraction. Examples include an inability to sustain manual grip or tongue protrusion and the dropping of objects. Muscle stretch reflexes are usually "hung up" and "pendular." Affected patients typically have a peculiar irregular and dancelike gait. The pathogenesis of chorea is unknown. Some findings point to abnormalities in caudate function. A selective loss of the GABA-enkephalin striatal neurons projecting to the GPe, found in Huntington's disease, results in excessive inhibition of STN neurons.

The movement disorders of athetosis (Ch. 411), ballism (Ch. 411), myoclonus (Ch. 412), tics (Ch. 412), and stereotypies (Ch. 412) are discussed in later chapters of this section.

DeLong MR: Primate models of movement disorders of basal ganglia origin. TINS 13:281, 1990. *A review of the MPTP model of parkinsonism used in the study of basal ganglia circuitry. Hyperactivity of the STN is associated with bradykinesia, and a chemical lesion in the STN ameliorates this cardinal sign.*

Hallett M: Physiology of basal ganglia disorders: An overview. Can J Neurol Sci 20:177, 1993. *An excellent review of current understanding of the basal ganglia connections in the normal and diseased brain.*

Jankovic J, Tolosa E (eds.): Parkinson's Disease and Movement Disorders. Baltimore, Williams & Wilkins, 1993. *A comprehensive review of hypokinetic, hyperkinetic, and miscellaneous movement disorders.*

Marsden CD, Fahn S (eds.): Movement Disorders 3. London, Butterworths Heinemann, 1994. *A comprehensive review of different movement disorders by recognized experts.*

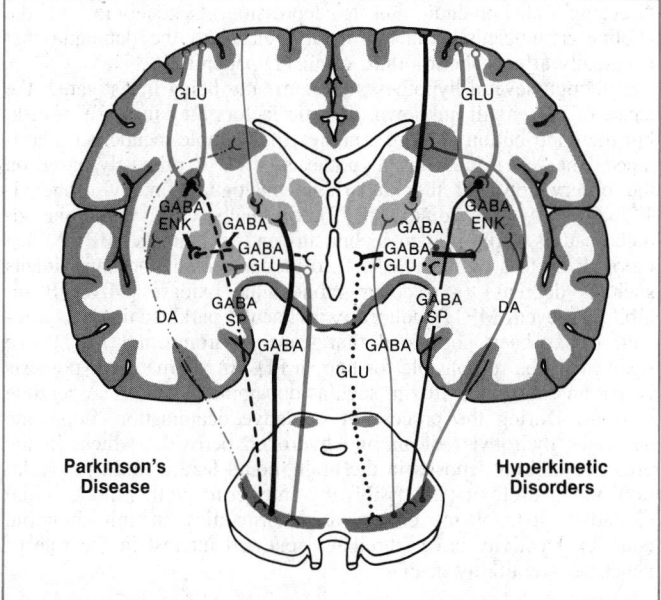

FIGURE 407-2. Functional organization of the basal ganglia in parkinsonian disorders and hyperkinetic movement disorders. ACH = acetylcholine; GABA = γ-aminobutyric acid; GLU = glutamate; DA = dopamine; ENK = enkephalin; SP = substance P.

408 PARKINSONISM

Parkinsonism is a clinical syndrome dominated by four cardinal signs: tremor at rest, bradykinesia, rigidity, and postural instability. Less prominent manifestations concern the mood and intellect, autonomic function, and the sensory system (Table 408–1). The average age at onset is 55 years, with about 1% of persons 60 years of age or older having the disease. Men are affected more frequently than women by a ratio of 3:2. At least two major subtypes of Parkinson's disease (PD) have been identified: One subtype is characterized by tremor as the dominant parkinsonian feature, and the other is dominated by postural instability and gait difficulty (PIGD). The *tremor subtype* of PD is associated with relatively normal mental status, earlier age at onset, and slower progression of the disease than is the *PIGD subtype,* which shows more bradykinesia, dementia, and a more rapidly progressive course.

Resting tremor and bradykinesia are the most typical parkinsonian signs and are virtually synonymous with the diagnosis. Bradykinesia accounts for most of the associated parkinsonian symptoms and signs: general slowing down of movements and of activities of daily living; lack of facial expression (hypomimia or masked facies); staring expression due to decreased frequency of blinking; impaired swallowing, which causes drooling; hypokinetic and hypophonic dysarthria; monotonous speech; small handwriting (micrographia); difficulties with repetitive and simultaneous movements; difficulty in arising from chair and turning over in bed; shuffling gait with short steps; decreased arm swing and other automatic movements; and start hesitation and freezing. Freezing, manifested by sudden and often unpredictable inability to move, is one of the most disabling of all parkinsonian symptoms.

Several disorders other than PD can cause at least part of the parkinsonian syndrome (Table 408–2). Non-PD parkinsonian disorders can be distinguished clinically from PD by the presence of atypical findings, absence or paucity of tremor, and poor response to levodopa. The last feature may be partly explained by the fact that postsynaptic dopamine receptors are preserved in PD, but they are decreased in the other parkinsonian syndromes.

PARKINSON'S DISEASE

Pathogenesis

The most typical pathologic hallmarks of PD are (1) neuronal loss with depigmentation of the substantia nigra (SN) and (2) Lewy bodies, which are eosinophilic cytoplasmic inclusions in neurons consisting of aggregates of normal filaments. These abnormalities are most prominent in the ventrolateral region of the SN that pro-

TABLE 408–1. NONMOTOR DISTURBANCE IN PARKINSON'S DISEASE

Neurobehavioral Abnormalities in Parkinson's Disease

Personality changes (apathy, lack of confidence, fearfulness, anxiety, emotional lability and inflexibility, social withdrawal, dependency)

Dementia (tip-of-the-tongue phenomenon [partial anomia], spatial disorientation, paranoia, psychosis, hallucinations)

Bradyphrenia (slow thought processes, loss of concentration, difficulty with concept formation)

Depression

Sleep disturbance

Sexual dysfunction

Psychiatric side effects of therapy

Other Nonmotor Manifestations of Parkinson's Disease

Autonomic dysfunction (orthostatic hypotension, respiratory dysregulation, flushing, "drenching sweats," constipation, sphincter and sexual dysfunction)

Sensory symptoms (paresthesias, pains, akathisia; visual, olfactory, and vestibular dysfunction)

Seborrhea, pedal edema, fatigue, weight loss

TABLE 408–2. CAUSES OF THE PARKINSON SYNDROME

I. Primary (Idiopathic) Parkinsonism
Parkinson's disease
Juvenile parkinsonism

II. Secondary (Acquired, Symptomatic) Parkinsonism
Infectious: postencephalitic, slow virus
Drugs: neuroleptics (antipsychotic, antiemetic drugs), reserpine, tetrabenazine, α-methyldopa, lithium, flunarizine, cinnarizine
Toxins: MPTP, CO, Mn, Hg, CS_2, methanol, ethanol
Vascular: multi-infarct, hypotensive shock
Trauma: pugilistic encephalopathy
Other: parathyroid abnormalities, hypothyroidism, hepatocerebral degeneration, brain tumor, normal-pressure hydrocephalus, syringomesencephalia

III. Heredodegenerative Parkinsonism
Autosomal dominant Lewy body disease
Huntington's disease
Wilson's disease
Hallervorden-Spatz disease
Olivopontocerebellar and spinocerebellar degenerations
Familial basal ganglia calcification
Familial parkinsonism with peripheral neuropathy
Neuroacanthocytosis

IV. Multiple-System Degeneration (Parkinsonism-Plus)
Progressive supranuclear palsy
Multiple-system atrophy
  Shy-Drager syndrome
  Striatonigral degeneration
  Olivopontocerebellar atrophy
Parkinsonism-dementia-ALS complex
Corticobasal ganglionic degeneration
Alzheimer's disease
Hemiatrophy-parkinsonism

jects to the putamen. At least an 80% loss of dopaminergic neurons in the substantia nigra and the same degree of dopamine depletion in the striatum must appear before clinical symptoms of PD become evident.

Motor symptoms of PD result chiefly from degeneration of the nigrostriatal pathway, causing a deficiency of dopamine in the putamen and, to a lesser degree, the caudate nucleus. The cognitive deficits and some neurobehavioral symptoms have been attributed to degeneration of the dopaminergic mesocortical and mesolimbic pathways, and the associated autonomic dysfunction may be partly caused by dopamine depletion in the hypothalamus. Besides dopamine deficiency, impairment of the other neurotransmitters may be responsible for some of the associated findings. For example, degeneration of the noradrenergic locus ceruleus may contribute to the "freezing" phenomenon and to depression. Degeneration of the cholinergic nucleus basalis probably relates to the dementia that eventually affects about a third of all PD patients.

Although several hypotheses are currently being investigated, the cause of PD is still unknown. Genetic factors may increase its risk, but the contribution is more complex than simple mendelian inheritance. The "environmental" hypothesis of PD is primarily based on the observation that the meperidine analogue 1-methyl-4-phenyl-1,2,3,6-tetrahydropyridine (MPTP), originally used by heroin addicts, causes parkinsonism in humans and in animals. MPTP must be oxidized to a pyridine MPP+ to be neurotoxic, and antioxidants such as deprenyl (a selective monoamine oxidase [MAO]-B inhibitor) prevent MPTP-induced experimental parkinsonism. As a result, it has been postulated that some environmental MPTP-like toxin might be responsible for human PD. An alternative hypothesis is that an endogenous toxin, such as dopamine, damages susceptible neurons. During the process of oxidative deamination, dopamine generates hydroxyl radicals and hydrogen peroxide, which, in the presence of iron deposits in the brain, could lead to lipid peroxidation and neurotoxicity, possibly by interfering with mitochondrial oxidative metabolism. Observed abnormalities in mitochondrial complex I activity have stimulated renewed interest in the role of genetic susceptibility in PD.

Treatment

The finding that deprenyl prevents MPTP-induced parkinsonism stimulated interest in antioxidative therapy as a means of retarding the progression of PD. Some but by no means all studies have found that deprenyl slows the development of motor disability and the rate of disease progression when used in the early stages of PD. Deprenyl also may provide moderate symptomatic relief. After starting deprenyl, many patients report improvement in their energy level and bradykinetic symptoms. The effect may be due to deprenyl's ability to increase striatal concentrations of dopamine by blocking its metabolism by MAO. The addition of one of the anticholinergic drugs, such as trihexyphenidyl, may provide additional symptomatic relief, particularly in younger patients and patients in whom tremor predominates. Associated depression, present in many parkinsonian patients, can be treated with tricyclic antidepressants, such as amitriptyline or nortriptyline. Because the anticholinergics, including the tricyclics, can produce undesirable psychological symptoms as well as side effects, such as dry mouth, blurring of vision, and urinary hesitancy, amantadine may offer a useful alternative, particularly in elderly patients. Amantadine, however, although helpful in controlling both tremor and bradykinesia, can also cause adverse effects, including livedo reticularis, ankle edema, exacerbation of congestive heart failure, and mild anticholinergic side effects. Its beneficial effects seldom last more than a few months.

Many neurologists favor employing combinations of deprenyl, the anticholinergics, and amantadine until they no longer provide a satisfactory control of parkinsonian symptoms. At that point levodopa combined with carbidopa, a peripheral dopa decarboxylase inhibitor, is added to the antiparkinsonian regimen. The starting dosage of carbidopa/levodopa is 25 mg/100 mg twice daily, to be gradually increased over 3 weeks to three times per day. The dosage is then adjusted, depending on the severity of symptoms and occupational demands. Some patients require as much as 25 mg/250 mg four or five times daily; others tolerate only smaller doses. Although levodopa can suppress tremor, it is most useful in controlling bradykinesia and rigidity. Postural instability may be ameliorated by levodopa in early stages. Levodopa is contraindicated in patients with diagnosed melanoma and should be used with caution in those with prominent psychosis or dementia, peptic ulcer disease, and cardiac arrhythmias.

About 15% of parkinsonian patients fail to improve with levodopa from onset of therapy. Most of these nonresponders probably suffer from a form of postsynaptic parkinsonism rather than PD. A failure to respond to levodopa should also suggest the possibility of a wrong diagnosis, a drug interaction (concomitant use of dopamine receptor blocking agents, such as antipsychotic and antiemetic drugs), and pharmacokinetic reasons, such as insufficient dosage, slow stomach emptying, and competition for absorption in the small intestine and at the blood-brain barrier by amino acids in protein meals. Almost all patients who initially improve lose their response to levodopa some time between 3 and 8 years after onset.

PD patients lose their response to levodopa because of (1) natural progression of the disease and (2) development of complications as a result of chronic levodopa therapy. Although nonneuronal elements may participate in the conversion of levodopa to dopamine, the surviving striatal dopaminergic terminals progressively lose their capacity for conversion of levodopa to dopamine, and the patient develops motor fluctuations and symptomatic deterioration.

The most challenging problem in managing PD is treating levodopa complications. Thanks to carbidopa and similar agents, systemic side effects are seldom prominent. The most common central side effects of levodopa therapy include psychiatric problems, dyskinesias (seen in about 80% of patients after 3 years of therapy), and clinical fluctuations (seen in about 50% of patients after 5 years of therapy). The most common form of clinical fluctuation is the wearing-off effect, characterized by end-of-dose deterioration and recurrence of parkinsonian symptoms due to shorter (sometimes only 1 to 2 hours) duration of benefit after a given dose of levodopa. Slow-release preparations of levodopa (e.g., Sinemet CR, Madopar CR) prolong the plasma (and presumably brain) levels and may be useful in treating or preventing motor fluctuations. Deprenyl may prolong the duration of benefit from each levodopa dose.

Because the onset of levodopa-induced complications seems to be related to the duration of levodopa therapy, some authorities delay initiating levodopa therapy until the patient's symptoms begin to interfere with normal activities. Once levodopa treatment is initiated, the dose should be maintained as low as possible (Fig. 408–1). Some authorities believe that instead of increasing the dosage of levodopa, dopamine agonists such as bromocriptine pergolide should be introduced early in the course of anti-PD therapy. In experimental studies, pergolide has been shown to exert its dopaminergic effects without presynaptic dopamine, and it may improve parkinsonian symptoms even before levodopa is given. Some authorities, therefore, give pergolide as the first dopaminergic drug. However, as symptoms increase, dopamine agonists must be com-

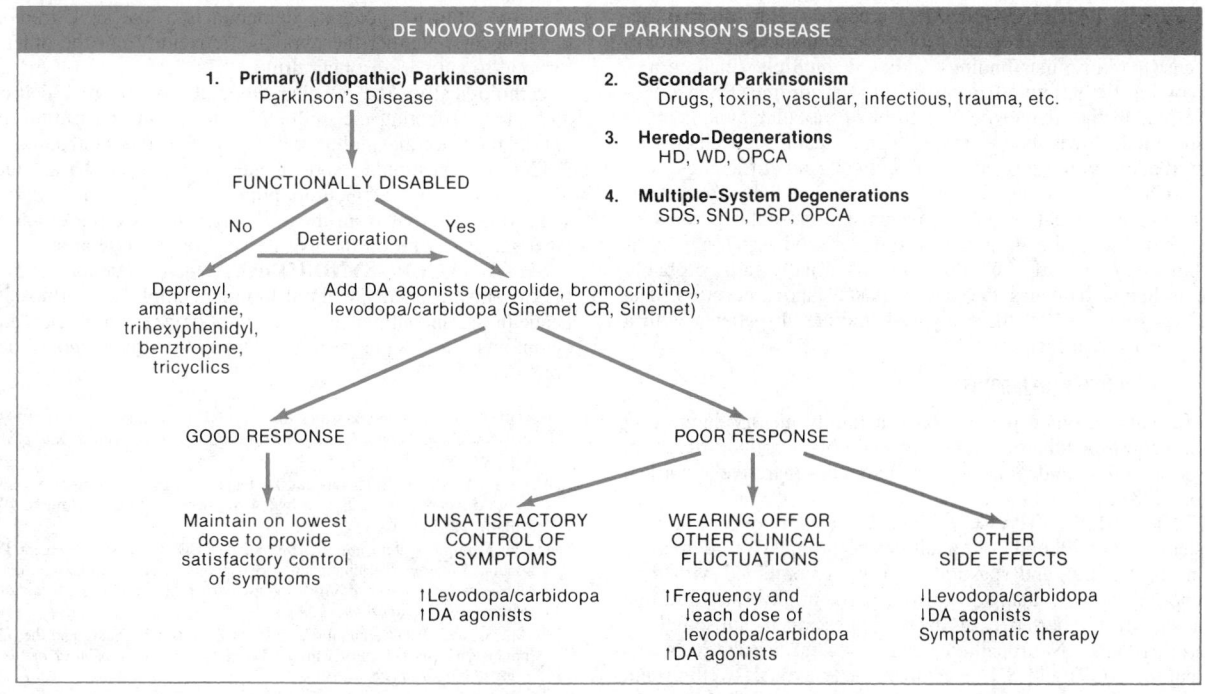

FIGURE 408–1. Diagrammatic representation of therapeutic approach to patients with parkinsonism. DA = dopamine; HD = Huntington's disease; OPCA = olivopontocerebellar atrophy; PSP = progressive supranuclear palsy; SDS = Shy-Drager syndrome; Sinemet CR = controlled-release levodopa/carbidopa; SND = striatonigral degeneration; WD = Wilson's disease.

bined with levodopa. The starting dosage for bromocriptine is 1.25 mg twice a day and for pergolide, 0.05 mg twice a day. The dosage should be increased slowly to prevent gastrointestinal, psychiatric, autonomic, and other side effects. The side effects of dopamine agonists are similar to those of levodopa, although dopamine agonists may produce hallucinations, delusions, and other psychiatric symptoms more often than does levodopa. They also can cause erythromelalgia, a painful erythema of the legs not usually seen with levodopa. Other motor and nonmotor symptoms of PD may require more specific therapy.

Surgical treatment of PD remains of uncertain value. Stereotaxic thalamotomy is occasionally employed in an attempt to ameliorate disabling tremor. In addition, pallidotomy and thalamic stimulation sometimes may provide relief of parkinsonian symptoms. Surgical transplantation of fetal substantia nigra into the striatum remains under investigation.

As with all progressive, disabling diseases, psychological support of patients and family offers important help. Patients should be encouraged to learn about their disease (by reading educational material provided by the national and local support organizations) and, above all, to remain physically and socially active.

SECONDARY PARKINSONISM

POSTENCEPHALITIC PARKINSONISM. Many individuals who survived the acute febrile illness and encephalopathy during the pandemics of encephalitis lethargica (von Economo's encephalitis) between 1919 and 1926 later developed a variety of movement disorders, including parkinsonism. Although the virus or viruses responsible for encephalitis lethargica were never isolated, infections caused by coxsackie, Japanese B, and western equine encephalitis viruses have since been identified as being complicated by parkinsonism. In general, postencephalitic parkinsonism has a slower progression and is more sensitive to levodopa therapy.

DRUG-INDUCED PARKINSONISM. Drugs that deplete the presynaptic stores of dopamine, such as reserpine and tetrabenazine (an investigational drug not available for general use in North America), and drugs that block the dopamine receptors, such as antipsychotic and antiemetic agents, can cause a parkinsonian syndrome clinically indistinguishable from idiopathic parkinsonism (PD). The same drugs can also cause a variety of other movement disorders, such as akathisia, dystonic reactions, and various tardive syndromes (e.g., tardive stereotypy, tardive dystonia, and tardive akathisia).

VASCULAR PARKINSONISM. Cerebrovascular disease accounts for only a small proportion of parkinsonism. Single strokes rarely cause parkinsonian findings, although multiple small infarctions involving the striatum can produce the syndrome. Brain imaging is helpful in the diagnosis. One form of vascular parkinsonism is the so-called "lower body parkinsonism," manifested chiefly by gait disturbance with short steps, "freezing," and difficulties with turning. (Chronic communicating, "low-pressure" hydrocephalus causes a similar clinical picture.) Patients with vascular parkinsonism may have dementia, hyperactive reflexes, and urinary incontinence, but tremor is rare. Levodopa therapy usually fails, probably because ischemia damages the striatal postsynaptic receptors. The diagnosis is suggested by these atypical findings in patients with a history of stroke risk factors.

HEREDODEGENERATIVE PARKINSONISM

Very few parkinsonian patients have a family history suggesting a specific pattern of inheritance. With such a history, the differential diagnosis should include one of the heredodegenerative disorders (see Table 408-2).

HALLERVORDEN-SPATZ DISEASE. This rare condition is manifested by childhood or adult-onset progressive dementia, bradykinesia, rigidity, and spasticity, variously combined with dystonia, choreoathetosis, ataxia, seizures, amyotrophy, and retinitis pigmentosa. Most reported cases have suggested an autosomal recessive inheritance. Neuropathologically, iron accumulates in the globus pallidus (GP) and SN, accompanied by axonal swelling and

neuronal degeneration in the basal ganglia, corticospinal tract, and cerebellum. Cysteine, found to be increased in the GP, possibly chelates iron, causing generation of free radicals and subsequent neuronal degeneration.

FAMILIAL BASAL GANGLIA CALCIFICATIONS. Calcium may accumulate in the basal ganglia in association with hypoparathyroidism or as a result of a familial disorder, sometimes referred to as Fahr's disease. Affected patients exhibit parkinsonism, chorea, dementia, and palilalia. Brain imaging may detect basal ganglia calcification in clinically unaffected relatives.

OLIVOPONTOCEREBELLAR AND SPINOCEREBELLAR DEGENERATIONS. The combination of parkinsonism and cerebellar ataxia characterizes olivopontocerebellar degeneration or atrophy (OPCA), a heterogeneous group of neurodegenerative disorders most often inherited in an autosomal dominant pattern, but occasionally occurring sporadically. In addition to the parkinsonism-ataxia complex, patients with OPCA often exhibit marked dysarthria, neuro-ophthalmologic signs, and a variable degree of upper and lower motor neuron signs (see Ch. 413).

MULTIPLE-SYSTEM DEGENERATION (PARKINSONISM-PLUS)

Approximately 10 to 15% of all patients with parkinsonian findings have a more widespread disorder classified clinically as "parkinsonism-plus syndrome" and pathologically as a "multiple-system degeneration." In addition to parkinsonism, such patients suffer from additional findings that may include supranuclear ophthalmoparesis (progressive supranuclear palsy), dysautonomia (Shy-Drager syndrome), ataxia (OPCA), laryngeal stridor (striatonigral degeneration), apraxia and alien hand (corticobasal degeneration), dementia (Alzheimer's disease with parkinsonism and diffuse Lewy body disease), and a combination of dementia and motor neuron disease (parkinsonism-dementia-amyotrophic lateral sclerosis [ALS] complex). The cause of all forms of this syndrome is unknown.

PROGRESSIVE SUPRANUCLEAR PALSY. Progressive supranuclear palsy (PSP) accounts for about 8% of all parkinsonian patients evaluated in a PD clinic. PSP has its onset in the seventh decade, about 10 years after the usual onset of PD. Initial symptoms consist of a gradual onset of postural instability, unsteady gait, and supranuclear vertical ophthalmoparesis, first expressed by impairment of downward gaze. Later, upward and then lateral conjugate gaze also become impaired, but until the advanced stage, the external ophthalmoparesis can be overcome by labyrinthine stimulation via the oculocephalic maneuver. Patients with PSP often exhibit axial rigidity, nuchal dystonia, and a rigid-dystonic facial expression. Mild to moderate dementia is a late sign; tremor almost never occurs. Neither the hypokinetic rigidity nor the other changes respond to antiparkinsonian drugs.

Pathologically, PSP is characterized by selective neuronal loss and gliosis affecting the midbrain tegmentum and tectum, the internal segment of the globus pallidus (GPi), the subthalamic nucleus (STN), the vestibular and dentate nuclei, the basal nucleus of Meynert, and the pedunculopontine nucleus. Neurofibrillary tangles, somewhat different from those in Alzheimer's disease, and granulovacuolar degeneration involve nerve cells in these areas.

SHY-DRAGER SYNDROME. When patients with atypical parkinsonism (usually without tremor) complain of orthostatic lightheadedness, incontinence, sexual impotence, and other autonomic symptoms, the diagnosis of Shy-Drager syndrome should be considered (see Ch. 402).

Calne DB: Treatment of Parkinson's disease. N Engl J Med 329:1021, 1993. *A review of the pharmacology of levodopa, deprenyl, dopamine agonists and of other therapeutic strategies.*

Jankovic J, Marsden CD: Therapeutic strategies in Parkinson's disease. *In* Jankovic J, Tolosa E: Parkinson's Disease and Movement Diseases. Baltimore, Williams & Wilkins, 1993, p 115.

Quinn N: Multiple system atrophy. *In* Marsden CD, Fahn S: Movement Diseases-3-London, Butterworth-Heinemann, 1994, p 262. *A clinicopathologic correlation of a large series of cases of Shy-Drager syndrome, olivopontocerebellar atrophy, and striatonigral degeneration.*

Stacy M, Jankovic J: Differential diagnosis of Parkinson's disease and the other parkinsonian syndromes. Neurol Clin 10:341, 1992. *A survey of most of the secondary forms of parkinsonism.*

409 TREMORS

ESSENTIAL TREMORS

Essential tremor is the most common type of tremor encountered in developed countries. The tremor is inherited in an autosomal dominant pattern with high penetrance. Affected patients lack the hypokinetic features and rigidity of Parkinson's disease (PD), discussed in the preceding chapter. Essential tremor typically produces flexion-extension oscillation of the hands at the wrists or adduction-abduction movements of the fingers when arms are outstretched in front of the body. Although frequently referred to as "benign essential tremor," it may be partially disabling, often causing spilling of liquids and interfering with handwriting. Essential tremor also frequently involves the head and voice, which helps to differentiate it from parkinsonian tremor. Another useful distinguishing feature is the occurrence of essential tremor during maintenance of posture; parkinsonian tremor is usually present when the affected body part is at relative rest. Parkinsonian patients, however, often exhibit postural tremor, and patients with essential tremor may have tremor at rest, suggesting an overlap between PD and essential tremor.

The frequency of essential tremor ranges from 4 to 12 Hz, and the oscillation may be produced by either alternating or synchronous contractions of antagonistic muscles. Some forms occur only during a specific activity, such as writing or holding an object in a particular position. Such *focal task-specific tremors* may be associated with task-specific dystonias ("occupational cramps") or with generalized essential tremor and dystonia. Nearly half of all patients with essential tremor show evidence of an associated dystonia. The nature of the link is unknown.

Essential tremor has many variants, including isolated head, voice, tongue, facial, and chin tremors and orthostatic tremor. Although considered a variant of essential tremor, orthostatic tremor usually does not respond to propranolol; clonazepam, however, provides satisfactory control in most patients. Focal tremor may be rarely induced by trauma to the affected body part. This peripherally induced tremor is often associated with focal dystonia and reflex sympathetic dystrophy.

β-Adrenergic blocking drugs (e.g., propranolol at 80 to 240 mg per day) are the most effective agents in the treatment of essential tremor. Modest doses of alcohol also reduce the tremor in most instances, but this is an impractical approach to treatment. Other occasionally useful drugs include primidone (starting dosage is 25 mg at bedtime; the daily dosage can be gradually increased to 750 mg per day), lorazepam, and alprazolam. Patients with a disabling essential tremor that does not respond satisfactorily to medications sometimes improve with local injections of botulinum. Thalamotomy is used as a last resort but high-frequency thalamic stimulation is gaining wider acceptance as a treatment of disabling tremors unresponsive to pharmacologic therapy.

Blond S, Caparros-Lefebvre D, Parker F, et al.: Control of tremor and involuntary movement disorders by chronic stereotactic stimulation of the ventral intermediate thalamic nucleus. J Neurosurg 77:62, 1992. *A review of experience with thalamic stimulation in treatment of severe tremors.*

Lou J-S, Jankovic J: Essential tremor: Clinical correlates in 350 patients. Neurology 41:234, 1991. *A comprehensive analysis of clinical features of a large cohort of patients with essential tremor.*

410 DYSTONIAS

DEFINITION. Dystonia is a syndrome dominated by involuntary, sustained (tonic) or spasmodic (rapid or clonic), patterned, and repetitive muscle contractions, frequently causing twisting (e.g., torticollis), flexing or extending (e.g., writer's cramp, retrocollis), and squeezing (e.g., blepharospasm) movements or abnormal postures. Dystonia is frequently associated with other movement disorders, particularly tremor, myoclonus, and parkinsonism. About 1 of 3000

people are diagnosed as having dystonia, but the true prevalence is probably much higher.

CLASSIFICATION. Dystonia may vary in severity, and it may progress as follows: task-specific (occurring only during a specific activity, such as writing or typing) → action (present only during, not necessarily specific, activity) → overflow (involving adjacent muscles) → at rest (present even during rest) → fixed postures (joint contractures). Dystonia is exacerbated by stress, fatigue, activity, or a change in posture and is relieved by sleep, relaxation, hypnosis, and a variety of sensory tricks. Whereas most dystonias are continual, some occur paroxysmally and some have marked diurnal variations (Fig. 410–1). Partly because of fluctuations in severity, sometimes influenced by the emotional state of the patient, dystonia is often mistakenly attributed to psychogenic causes.

Dystonia can be classified according to its *distribution* as focal, segmental, multifocal, generalized, or unilateral (hemidystonia). Most childhood-onset dystonias begin focally, usually in one foot; other body parts become involved later, eventually resulting in generalized dystonia. In contrast, adult-onset dystonias tend to remain focal or segmental. Examples of focal dystonia include blepharospasm, oromandibular dystonia, torticollis, spasmodic dysphonia, and occupational (e.g., writer's, typist's, pianist's) cramps (Fig. 410–1). Blepharospasm is categorized as a *focal* dystonia when it occurs alone (essential blepharospasm). Also, blepharospasm is often associated with dystonic movements in the adjacent facial, oromandibular, laryngeal, and neck muscles. This *segmental dystonia* is sometimes referred to as Meige's syndrome, but the term *"cranial-cervical dystonia"* is more descriptive.

The most common form of dystonia is *cervical dystonia*. According to the position of the head, cervical dystonia can be categorized as torticollis, laterocollis, anterocollis, retrocollis, or a combination of these abnormal postures. There is a 3:2 female preponderance, and the onset is usually in the fifth decade. Local pain is reported by about half the patients, and radiculopathy complicates cervical dystonia in about 20%. Half of all patients with cervical dystonia have an associated head-neck tremor. The tremor can be dystonic, seen only when the patient attempts to keep the head straight; essential, in which case the tremor persists irrespective of the position of the head; or a combination of dystonic and essential. About half the patients report a movement disorder such as tremor or dystonia in family members. The cause of most cervical dystonias is unknown. In 15% of cases, however, cervical dystonia can be attributed to either local trauma or an exposure to neuroleptic drugs.

PATHOGENESIS. The pathoanatomy of dystonia is unknown, but studies suggest a functional involvement of the basal ganglia,

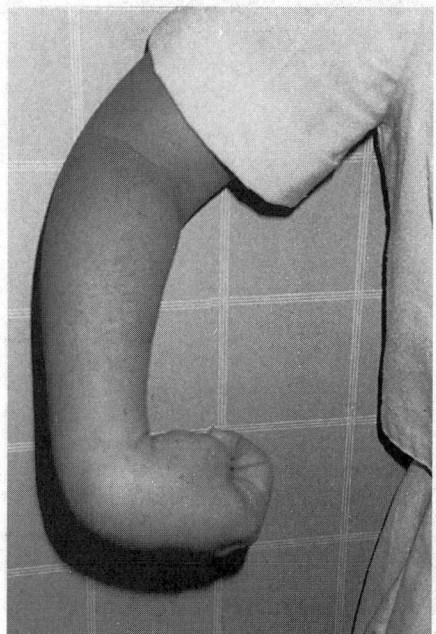

FIGURE 410–1. Focal dystonia of the distal right arm.

particularly the putamen, and the brain stem. Brain imaging and autopsy examinations usually yield normal findings. Postmortem biochemical analyses have found evidence of enhanced noradrenergic transmission in the rostral brain stem.

PRIMARY DYSTONIA

This category accounts for 90% of cases. Primary dystonias with onset in childhood have been previously termed *dystonia musculorum deformans.* Childhood-onset dystonias are often inherited, usually in an autosomal dominant pattern; about half of adult-onset cases seem to have a genetic basis. Other members of the family may have only partial manifestations, such as club foot, scoliosis, torticollis, writer's cramp, bruxism, or essential tremor. Genetic dystonia seems to have a higher prevalence among Ashkenazi Jews, but both Jewish and non-Jewish dystonias have been linked to a marker in the q32–q34 region of chromosome 9. An X-linked dystonia has been recently described in Filipino families. A dopa-responsive dystonia has been linked to a marker on chromosome 14.

SECONDARY DYSTONIA

Occasionally, a specific, and potentially treatable, cause of dystonia can be identified (see Fig. 410–1). One of the most important examples is *Wilson's disease,* described in detail in Ch. 188. Neurologic symptoms represent the first manifestations in about 50% of patients with this autosomal recessive disorder, appearing during their second or third decade.

Tardive dystonia is a persistent form of dystonia caused by exposure to dopamine receptor blocking drugs, such as major tranquilizers (e.g., chlorpromazine, thioridazine, fluphenazine, thiothixene, haloperidol, loxapine, amoxapine) and certain antiemetics (e.g., prochlorperazine, metoclopramide) (Fig. 410–2). Levodopa can also cause intermittent dystonia (and focal dystonia may be the presenting symptom of Parkinson's disease). In all drug-induced dystonias, the offending drug should be withdrawn or the dosage reduced whenever possible. In contrast to focal, segmental, or generalized dystonia, hemidystonia is associated with an identifiable cause in most cases. These include subcortical infarction, arteriovenous malformation, abscess, tumor, and other lesions, some of which can be treated surgically. There are many other causes of secondary dystonia, but only a few are amenable to therapy.

TREATMENT. Treatment consists of supportive therapy (e.g., relaxation techniques, prostheses), medications, botulinum toxin injections, and surgery. The anticholinergic drugs are sometimes beneficial. Trihexyphenidyl, the most frequently used anticholinergic, must be started in low doses and slowly increased to tolerance, perhaps up to 60 mg per day. Some children can tolerate such high doses, but anticholinergic side effects usually limit adult tolerance to 20 to 25 mg daily or less. In advanced cases, dopamine-depleting and dopamine receptor blocking drugs may be added. Muscle relaxants (e.g., diazepam or lorazepam), baclofen, and carbamazepine sometimes provide benefit. About 10% of patients with childhood or adolescent dystonia improve with levodopa. Diurnal fluctuations with exacerbation of the movement disorder toward the end of the day are typical in this form of dystonia. In patients with refractory focal dystonia and, less often, segmental dystonia, injection of the paralysis-inducing botulinum toxin into the contracting muscles provides effective, albeit temporary, relief. Such approaches are best left to those with experience in this treatment.

Patients who are socially and occupationally disabled by dystonia despite optimal medical therapy, including botulinum toxin, sometimes can be helped surgically. Surgical procedures include orbicularis myectomy for blepharospasm, cervical rhizotomy for neck dystonia, and thalamotomy for hemidystonia or generalized (predominantly distal) dystonia. Such procedures are effective in a majority of patients but have both potentially serious complications and high rates of symptom recurrence, making them a last resort.

Fletcher NA, Harding AE, Marsden CD: A genetic study of idiopathic torsion dystonia in the United Kingdom. Brain 113:379, 1990. *A review of inheritance in dystonic families in England suggests that 85% are inherited in an autosomal dominant pattern with 40% penetrance.*

Jankovic J, Brin M: Therapeutic applications of botulinum toxin. N Engl J Med 324:1186, 1991. *A critical review of studies using botulinum toxin in different dystonic and other disorders.*

Jankovic J, Fahn S: Dystonic disorders. *In* Jankovic J, Tolosa E (eds.): Parkinson's Disease and Movement Disorders. Baltimore, William & Wilkins, 1993, p 337. *Comprehensive review of clinical aspects and treatment of dystonia.*

411 CHOREAS, ATHETOSIS, AND BALLISM

HUNTINGTON'S DISEASE

Huntington's disease (HD), an autosomal dominant disorder with complete penetrance, is the phenotype of an expanded triple repeat sequence of a novel gene located at chromosome 4p16.3. Dementia and various emotional and psychiatric disturbances are prominent. The estimated prevalence of HD in the United States is 4 to 8 per 100,000 people. Although about 10% of HD cases begin before age 20, the peak age at onset is in the fourth and fifth decades. Juvenile HD often first manifests with progressive parkinsonism, dementia, and seizures. In contrast, adult HD often starts with the insidious onset of clumsiness and adventitious, fidgety, random, brief movements. Initially, these purposeless movements may be incorporated into and masked by normal intentional acts, delaying the recognition of chorea. Chorea often begins distally, but as the disease progresses, it becomes generalized and can interrupt voluntary movements. Characteristically, patients with HD have difficulty in maintaining tongue protrusion or a steady grip, and their gait is often irregular, hesitant, unsteady, and dancelike. Other motor symptoms include dysarthria, dysphagia, and postural instability.

Neuropsychological symptoms may precede motor changes. They may consist of personality changes, apathy, social withdrawal, agitation, impulsiveness, depression, mania, paranoia, delusions, hostility, hallucinations, or psychosis. Cognitive changes are manifested chiefly by loss of recent memory and impaired judgment. Progressive motor dysfunction, dementia, and incontinence eventually lead to institutionalization and death. The duration of illness from onset to death is about 15 years for adult HD and 8 to 10 years for the juvenile variant.

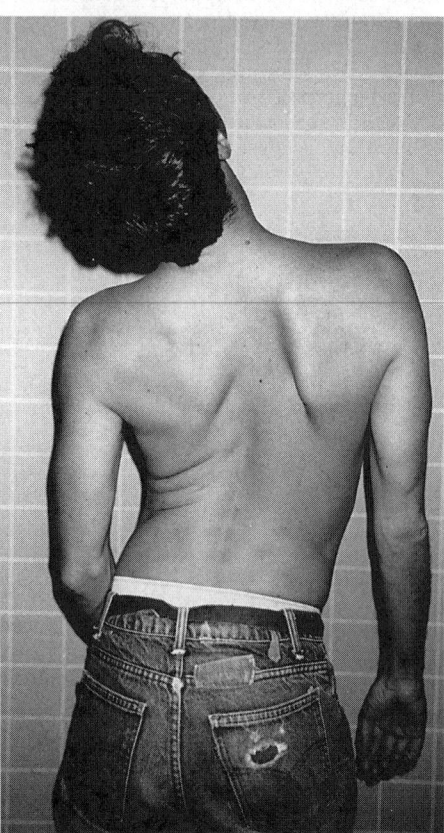

FIGURE 410–2. Truncal dystonia in a manic-depressive patient with tardive dystonia secondary to a variety of antipsychotic drugs.

Postmortem changes in HD brains include neuronal loss and gliosis in the cortex and the striatum, particularly the caudate nucleus. Chorea seems to be primarily related to the loss of striatal neurons projecting to the lateral globus pallidus (GPe), whereas rigid-akinetic symptoms correlate with the additional loss of striatal neurons projecting to the medial globus pallidus (GPi). Loss of medium-sized spiny neurons, which normally constitute 80% of all striatal neurons, is associated with a marked decrease in γ-aminobutyric acid (GABA) synthesis. Acetylcholine activity declines, presumably reflecting a degeneration of cholinergic striatal interneurons. Neuropeptides are markedly altered in HD: Levels of substance P, cholecystokinin, and metenkephalin decrease, but somatostatin, thyrotropin-releasing hormone, neurotensin, and neuropeptide Y levels increase. The number of dopamine, acetylcholine, and serotonin receptors is lowered in the striatum.

Reliable clinical diagnosis depends on the combination of chorea, emotional disturbances, progressive dementia, and a family history suggestive of autosomal dominant inheritance. Because spontaneous mutations are rare, lack of family history raises questions of paternity or misdiagnosis. As noted, the mutated Huntington gene consists of unstable expanded CAG repeats. When the repeat number exceeds 42, the diagnosis of HD is certain. The test is now used to confirm the clinical diagnosis of HD and to identify presymptomatic patients.

Treatment is symptomatic. The psychosis may improve with neuroleptics, such as haloperidol, pimozide, fluphenazine, and thioridazine, but these drugs can induce tardive dyskinesia and other adverse effects and should be used only if absolutely necessary. Monoamine-depleting drugs, such as reserpine (0.25 mg to 8 mg per day) and tetrabenazine (an investigational drug not available for general use in North America), may relieve chorea, do not cause tardive dyskinesia, and may be as effective as the dopamine-blocking drugs. Unfortunately, these drugs can cause or exacerbate depression, sedation, akathisia, and parkinsonism. Anxiolytics and antidepressants may be useful in some patients. Genetic aspects of HD should be discussed openly with the patients to provide them and their relatives with nondirective counseling.

OTHER CHOREIC DISORDERS

Besides HD, other rare, genetically transmitted choreas include *benign hereditary chorea,* a nonprogressive chorea with childhood onset, and *paroxysmal choreoathetoses. Senile chorea* is a rare symptom complex in which chorea begins after age 60 and is unaccompanied by the neurobehavioral symptoms or family history of HD. Some patients have been reported to have pathologic changes identical to those of HD; others have had predominant degeneration of the putamen rather than the caudate. *Neuroacanthocytosis,* also referred to as "chorea-acanthocytosis," usually presents in the third or fourth decade of life with a combination of self-mutilation manifested by lip and tongue biting, generalized chorea, lingual dystonia, and motor and phonic tics. Other features include seizures, amyotrophy, areflexia, and elevated levels of serum creatine phosphokinase. Wet blood or Wright-stained fast-dry smears reveal more than 15% of red blood cells as acanthocytes. Neuroimaging usually demonstrates caudate atrophy. The condition most often has a pattern of autosomal recessive inheritance. *Sydenham's chorea,* now uncommon, has an autoimmune basis, most often appearing as a consequence of infection with group A streptococcus. Unlike arthritis and carditis, which occur soon after such infection, chorea and various neurobehavioral symptoms may be delayed for 6 months or longer. Chorea appearing during pregnancy (chorea gravidarum), with use of birth control pills, or during the course of systemic lupus erythematosus probably has a similar pathogenesis.

ATHETOSIS

Athetosis is a slow form of chorea characterized by twisting, writhing movements. It most often accompanies static encephalopathy due to cerebral palsy, kernicterus, prematurity, glutaric aciduria, poststroke hemiplegia, and other causes of early life brain damage. In some cases, the movement disorder becomes progressive after decades of no apparent change. Athetosis usually does not respond to pharmacologic therapy.

BALLISM

Ballism is a form of forceful, flinging, high-amplitude, coarse chorea. Because the involuntary movement usually affects only one side of the body, the term hemiballism is used. The condition is often preceded by hemiparesis associated with a hemorrhagic or ischemic stroke involving the contralateral subthalamic nucleus (STN) or adjacent structures. Less common causes of hemiballism include abscess, arteriovenous malformation, cerebral trauma, hyperosmotic hyperglycemia, tumor, and multiple sclerosis. Most of these lesions involve the STN, but hemiballism has been described occasionally in patients with lesions outside the STN. Dopamine-blocking and -depleting drugs, used in the treatment of chorea, benefit most patients with hemiballism, but the disorder usually subsides spontaneously within several weeks. Occasional examples of prolonged disabling and medically intractable hemiballism can be treated with contralateral thalamotomy or pallidectomy.

Albin RL, Reiner A, Anderson KD, et al.: Striatal and nigral neuron subpopulations in rigid Huntington's disease: Implications for the functional anatomy of chorea and rigidity-akinesia. Ann Neurol 27:357, 1990. *Using neuropeptide immunochemistry, the investigators conclude that chorea correlates with damage to the striatal projections to GPe, whereas parkinsonian signs observed in some HD patients result from additional damage in the projections to the GPi.*

Albin RL, Tagle DA: Genetics and molecular biology of Huntington's disease. Trends Neurosci 18:11, 1995. *Summarizes the recent literature and emphasizes the role of "triple-repeats" in neurogenetics.*

Fahn S: Paroxysmal dyskinesias. *In* Movement Disorders 3. London, Butterworth-Heinemann, 1994, p 310. *A comprehensive survey of hyperkinetic movement disorders occurring intermittently.*

412   TICS, MYOCLONUS, AND STEREOTYPIES

TICS

Tics are involuntary, abrupt, sudden, isolated, brief movements *(motor tics);* sounds produced by nose, mouth, or throat *(vocal/phonic tics);* or sensations *(sensory tics).* Motor tics may be simple (e.g., eye blinking, nose twitching, head jerking) or complex (e.g., repetitive touching, jumping, kicking, pelvic gyrations). Similarly, vocal/phonic tics may be simple (e.g., throat clearing, grunting, sniffing) or complex (e.g., echolalia, palilalia, coprolalia). Characteristics of tics include suppressibility, increase with stress and excitement, decrease with distraction and concentration, suggestibility, waxing and waning, and possible persistence during sleep.

The most common cause of tics is the *Gilles de la Tourette syndrome,* a genetic disorder dominated by tics and a variety of behavioral manifestations. Transient tics of childhood and persistent simple tics probably represent fragmentary forms of Tourette's syndrome. The following criteria are diagnostic: (1) Both multiple motor and one or more phonic tics must be present, although not necessarily concurrently; (2) the tics occur many times, nearly every day or intermittently through a period of more than a year; (3) the anatomic location, number, frequency, complexity, type, and severity of tics change over time; (4) onset is before age 21; and (5) involuntary movements and noises cannot be explained by other medical conditions. Because of the fluctuating, heterogeneous, and often bizarre manifestations, affected patients frequently have their illness misdiagnosed by physicians and are mistreated by schoolmates, teachers, co-workers, and strangers.

Epidemiologic studies suggest that most cases of Tourette's syndrome are genetic, occurring commonly and with penetrance approaching 100%, particularly in males. A few cases may be nongenetic, triggered or caused by neuroleptics, carbon monoxide poisoning, head trauma, viral encephalitis, cocaine abuse, or opiate withdrawal. Many affected patients suffer from obsessive-compulsive disorder and have problems with attention and learning. Sleep disorders include parasomnias, bedwetting, and interruption by tics.

Therapy varies. Because most patients experience waxing and waning of symptoms and a generally favorable natural course, reassurance and behavioral therapy may be sufficient in mild cases. Drugs are indicated when tics cause physical discomfort or social embarrassment. Judicious use of dopamine receptor blocking drugs, such as fluphenazine, pimozide, and haloperidol, may reduce the

TABLE 412–1. NEUROLEPTIC-INDUCED MOVEMENT DISORDERS

Acute Disorders	Chronic Disorders
Dystonic reaction	Tardive dyskinesia
Parkinsonism	Stereotypic: oral-facial-lingual-masticatory
Akathisia	Trunk-pelvic
Neuroleptic malignant	Respiratory
syndrome	Choreic: limbs
	Tardive dystonia; tics; myoclonus;
	tremor; akathisia; parkinsonism

frequency and severity of tics and ameliorate impulsive and aggressive behavior. These drugs, however, cause sedation, depression, and weight gain. Furthermore, tardive dyskinesia is a potentially serious complication of chronic neuroleptic therapy. Clonazepam, clonidine, fluoxetine, and clomipramine seem to be particularly helpful in the treatment of obsessive-compulsive disorder and other behavioral problems frequently associated with Tourette's syndrome.

MYOCLONUS

Myoclonus is a jerklike movement produced by a sudden, rapid, and brief contraction (positive myoclonus) or a muscle inhibition (negative myoclonus). *Segmental myoclonus* usually involves either the branchial structures, innervated by the lower cranial nerves and upper cervical nerve roots, or other body parts innervated by the spinal roots and nerves; it consists of rhythmic (1 to 3 Hz) contractions caused by a lesion of the brain stem or spinal cord. *Palatal myoclonus* results from acute or chronic lesions involving the anatomic triangle linking dentate, red, and inferior olivary nuclei. *Generalized myoclonus* is believed to reflect discharges arising from the brain stem reticular formation and is categorized as physiologic, essential, epileptic, or symptomatic. Two forms of myoclonus are associated with sleep: physiologic sleep myoclonus, occurring normally during initial phases of sleep, and nocturnal myoclonus, now called *"periodic movements of sleep,"* often associated with *"restless legs syndrome"* as well as with abnormal involuntary movements while the person is awake.

Causes of generalized myoclonus include acute and prolonged hypoxia and ischemia; various metabolic, infectious, and toxic factors; and exposure to neuroleptic drugs (tardive myoclonus). Myoclonus can be associated with familial chorea and dystonia and with many neurodegenerative disorders, including parkinsonism, progressive myoclonus epilepsy, and a variety of rare heredodegenerative disorders. Multifocal myoclonus often develops in the late stages of Creutzfeldt-Jakob disease and, less frequently, Alzheimer's disease.

The specific pathogeneses of myoclonus are unknown. Clonazepam, lorazepam, valproate, carbamazepine, and 5-hydroxytryptophan have been reported to have antimyoclonic activity. Clonazepam, at a dosage of 1 to 9 mg per day, is the drug of first choice, but the development of adverse effects, such as drowsiness, ataxia, and sexual dysfunction, often limits its usefulness.

STEREOTYPIES

The term "stereotypy" denotes a continuous or intermittent, involuntary, coordinated, patterned, repetitive, rhythmic, purposeless, but seemingly purposeful and ritualistic movement. Stereotypies may be simple (e.g., chewing movement, foot tapping, body rocking) or complex (e.g., complicated rituals, sitting down and arising from a chair). They can be volitionally suppressed. Stereotypies can accompany a variety of human behavioral disorders, such as anxiety, obsessive-compulsive disorders, Tourette's syndrome, schizophrenia, akathisia, autism, and mental retardation. Stereotypies and self-stimulatory or self-injurious behavior constitute the most recognizable symptoms in mentally retarded and autistic patients.

Tardive dyskinesia, a persistent movement disorder caused by exposure to dopamine receptor blocking drugs, is a frequently encountered stereotypy. Many other tardive movement disorders can result from the use of dopamine receptor blocking drugs (neuroleptics) (Table 412–1). The term "akathisia" describes the combination of stereotypy and a sensory component, such as an inner feeling of restlessness. The disorder particularly affects the lower extremities ("restless legs") and often is worse at night, causing insomnia, and it may be associated with periodic movements of sleep (see Ch. 397). Elderly women appear to be at particularly high risk for tardive dyskinesia. The mechanism of the disorder is poorly understood but is believed to result from the development of supersensitive dopamine receptors caused by chronic neuroleptic blockade. Prevention is the best treatment for the drug-induced movement disorders. Whenever possible, drugs other than the neuroleptics should be used for psychiatric or gastrointestinal problems. When no alternative exists, the dosage and duration of exposure should be kept at a minimum. Spontaneous remissions of tardive dyskinesia occasionally follow withdrawal of the offending agent. Dopamine-depleting drugs, such as tetrabenazine or reserpine, are the most effective drugs in its symptomatic treatment.

Jankovic J: Tardive myoclonus and other drug-induced movement diseases. Clin Neuropharmacol, in press. *A comprehensive review of clinical and pharmacological features of tardive dyskinesias and other movement disorders produced by dopaminergic or antidopaminergic drugs.*

Jankovic J: Tourette's syndrome: Phenomenology, pathophysiology, genetics, epidemiology and treatment. *In* Appel SH (ed.): Current Neurology, Vol 13. Chicago, Mosby-Year Book, 1993, p 209. *A critical review of current knowledge about the motor and behavioral aspects of Tourette's syndrome.*

Marsden CD, Fahn S (eds.): Movement Disorders 3. London, Butterworth-Heinemann, 1994, p 503. *A comprehensive review of movement disorders, including tics, myoclonus, and stereotypies.*

Section Five—
Degenerative Diseases of
the Nervous System

Robert B. Layzer

The term "degenerative diseases" refers to a varied assortment of central nervous system disorders characterized by gradual and progressive loss of neural tissue. This section deals with several degenerative diseases of unknown cause: the hereditary ataxias, paraplegias, and amyotrophies; the phakomatoses; syringomyelia; and amyotrophic lateral sclerosis. Several important diseases are discussed in other chapters concerned with dementia, extrapyramidal diseases, and autonomic disorders. Some degenerative diseases are difficult to classify because they involve multiple anatomic locations; these *multisystem atrophies* have arbitrarily been assigned to the chapters that deal with their principal symptom (see Table 413–1).

413 HEREDITARY CEREBELLAR ATAXIAS AND RELATED DISORDERS

The symptoms of hereditary ataxia may be intermittent or progressive. *Intermittent or periodic ataxia* occurs in children with a variety of recessively inherited biochemical disorders, such as aminoacidurias and disorders of pyruvate metabolism. A rare, autosomal dominant disease known as hereditary periodic ataxia is characterized by attacks of vertigo, nystagmus, ataxia, and dysarthria, lasting several hours; it responds to prophylactic treatment with acetazolamide.

Progressive ataxia occurs in children with known biochemical disorders such as abetalipoproteinemia and some of the lipidoses, but most diseases in this category are of unknown origin. Those that begin before age 20, including Friedreich's ataxia and ataxia-telangiectasia, are usually inherited in an autosomal recessive fashion, whereas most adult-onset types are autosomal dominant.

FRIEDREICH'S ATAXIA

This autosomal recessive disease, with a carrier frequency of nearly 1 in 100 and a prevalence of 2 in 100,000, is probably the most common type of hereditary ataxia. The biochemical mechanism is unknown, but the abnormal gene has been mapped to the long arm of chromosome 9.

PATHOLOGY. At autopsy the spinal cord is atrophic. There is loss of nerve cells in the dorsal root ganglia and Clarke's columns and "dying-back" degeneration of nerve fibers in the dorsal columns, pyramidal tracts, spinocerebellar tracts, and peripheral nerves. Minor changes are present in the brain stem and cerebellum. The heart shows chronic interstitial fibrosis and ventricular hypertrophy.

CLINICAL MANIFESTATIONS. Progressive ataxia of gait usually begins in childhood or adolescence and within a few years is accompanied by loss of deep reflexes, limb ataxia, Babinski signs, and cerebellar dysarthria. The ability to walk is lost about 15 years after onset. Most patients eventually exhibit scoliosis, pronounced impairment of vibration and position sense in the lower extremities, and pes cavus. Some develop wasting of distal limb muscles, a stocking-glove deficit of superficial sensation, nystagmus, deafness, or optic atrophy. Intellect remains normal. A hypertrophic cardiomyopathy is present in most patients and often leads to supraventricular arrhythmias; heart failure is probably the major cause of death. Insulin-dependent diabetes mellitus develops in 10 to 20% of patients. The mean age at death is 37 years.

DIAGNOSIS. Sensory nerve action potentials are small or absent. Electromyography may show signs of denervation in distal limb muscles, but motor nerve conduction velocities are normal. The cerebrospinal fluid is normal except for mild elevation of the protein content in a few cases. Magnetic resonance (MR) imaging often shows atrophy of the cervical spinal cord; the medulla may also be small, but the cerebellum is spared. Electrocardiography often shows inverted T waves, right- or left-axis deviation, and right

or left ventricular hypertrophy; conduction disturbances are uncommon.

DIFFERENTIAL DIAGNOSIS. The constellation of progressive ataxia, areflexia, Babinski signs, and onset before age 25 is usually diagnostic. However, a similar picture can occur in vitamin B_{12} deficiency and in two hereditary autosomal recessive disorders, abetalipoproteinemia and selective vitamin E deficiency. True Friedreich's ataxia is sometimes confused with a less common autosomal recessive type of early-onset progressive ataxia, in which the tendon reflexes are preserved; in the latter syndrome, optic atrophy, scoliosis, and electrocardiographic abnormalities are rare.

ATAXIA-TELANGIECTASIA

Ataxia-telangiectasia is an autosomal recessive, multisystem disease affecting the skin, nervous system, and immune system. Its prevalence has been estimated at 1 to 2 per 100,000. The condition is described further in Ch. 223.

ADULT-ONSET CEREBELLAR ATAXIA

Hereditary ataxia starting in adult life is nearly always an autosomal dominant disorder with multiple neurologic manifestations, among which cerebellar signs are prominent. In Europe the prevalence is 1 to 10 per 100,000 population. The syndrome is genetically heterogeneous; one type is caused by expansion of an unstable trinucleotide repeat on chromosome 6p, another is linked to chromosome 12q, and the Azorean form (Machado-Joseph disease) is linked to chromosome 14q.

PATHOLOGY. Many cases have the pathologic features of olivopontocerebellar atrophy, with loss of neurons in the inferior olives and pontine nuclei (which provide major afferent pathways to the cerebellum), as well as degeneration of the spinocerebellar tracts, corticospinal tracts, and posterior columns. Neuronal degeneration is sometimes found in the cerebellar cortex, dentate nucleus, basal ganglia, midbrain, cerebral cortex, and spinal cord, including the anterior horns. The pathology, however, is as variable as the clinical findings, even within a given family. In Machado-Joseph disease, the cerebellar cortex and olives are spared.

CLINICAL MANIFESTATIONS. The age of onset, although variable, is usually between 20 and 50. Cerebellar ataxia of gait, dysarthria, and incoordination of the limbs usually dominate the clinical picture, so that the ability to walk is lost within 15 years. The other manifestations are extremely variable. Babinski signs and increased reflexes are commonly present, and some patients have spastic weakness in the legs. Vibration and position sense are sometimes lost as the disease advances, and the reflexes may disappear as the primary sensory neurons degenerate. Extrapyramidal findings may include impassive facies, cogwheel rigidity, chorea, athetosis, dystonia, and facial dyskinesia. Many patients have supranuclear oculomotor disorders such as lid retraction, ptosis, nystagmus, slow eye movements, and gaze paresis, especially upgaze. Optic atrophy, with pale discs, is common. Pigmentary degeneration of the retina, beginning in the macula, is an early and constant feature in some families, suggesting that these cases may be genetically distinct. Personality change or dementia, muscle wasting and fasciculation in the tongue and distal extremities, and bulbar symptoms of dysphagia or hoarseness are other common manifestations. Death occurs approximately 20 years after onset, at an average age of 57.

TABLE 413-1. THE MULTISYSTEM ATROPHIES

Disease	Heredity	Principal Feature	Associated Features	Chapter
Shy-Drager syndrome	Sporadic	Autonomic insufficiency	Parkinsonism, cerebellar ataxia, dysphagia, laryngeal stridor, amyotrophy	402
Progressive supranuclear palsy	Sporadic	Ophthalmoplegia, especially vertical	Gait ataxia, axial dystonia, parkinsonism, pseudobulbar palsy, dementia	410
Kearns-Sayre syndrome	Sporadic	Ptosis and ophthalmoplegia	Short stature, cerebellar ataxia, retinal degeneration, heart block, deafness, mitochondrial myopathy, mental deficiency, Babinski signs	454
Hereditary ataxias, adult type	Autosomal dominant	Cerebellar ataxia	Ophthalmoplegia, dementia, parkinsonism, dystonia, optic atrophy, retinal degeneration, dysphagia, amyotrophy	413

A few families seem to have a "pure" cerebellar syndrome beginning in the seventh decade of life. These cases (cerebellar cortical atrophy) tend to have a more benign prognosis.

DIAGNOSIS. In the olivopontocerebellar atrophy syndrome, MRI may show atrophy of the cerebellar folia and pons, with enlargement of the fourth ventricle and pontine cisterns. In pure cerebellar cortical atrophy, only the cerebellum is shrunken. The cerebrospinal fluid is usually normal. Sensory nerve action potentials are small or absent in patients with absent reflexes; in patients with preserved reflexes, somatosensory evoked potentials may be abnormal.

DIFFERENTIAL DIAGNOSIS. Nonhereditary cases of late-onset cerebellar degeneration are at least as common as the hereditary kind. Some are associated with alcoholism or a visceral malignancy, but in many, no apparent cause can be established. These patients' cerebellar symptoms tend to begin between the ages of 40 and 60 and may be accompanied by dementia, extrapyramidal signs, or Babinski signs. Some cases of this kind have the pathologic features of olivopontocerebellar atrophy, but whether there is any genetic link to the autosomal dominant ataxias is unclear. It should be noted that patients presenting with ataxia may later develop the typical signs of progressive supranuclear palsy or one of the other multisystem atrophies listed in Table 413–1.

Harding AE: The Hereditary Ataxias and Related Disorders. Edinburgh. Churchill Livingstone, 1984. *A detailed review of the hereditary cerebellar ataxias and spastic paraplegias, including the author's own study of several hundred patients and family members. A modern classic.*

Orr HT, Chung M, Banfi S, et al.: Expansion of an unstable trinucleotide repeat in spinocerebellar ataxia type 1. Nature Genetics 4:221, 1993. *Reports the first specific gene defect to be found in a hereditary ataxia.*

414 HEREDITARY SPASTIC PARAPLEGIAS

This is a diverse group of uncommon diseases whose main symptom is an insidiously beginning, progressive spasticity of the lower extremities. Families with "pure" hereditary spastic paraplegia (Strümpell's disease) are the most numerous, but many rare variants have been reported in which spasticity is associated with other neurologic, ocular, or cutaneous manifestations, overlapping with the spinocerebellar degenerations. The prevalence of these diseases is not well established. Rare examples of *primary lateral sclerosis,* although sporadic in incidence, may belong to this class.

PATHOLOGY. In the pure form, the spinal cord shows degeneration of the lateral corticospinal tracts and posterior columns, most severe in the thoracic region. Less often there is minor degeneration of the spinocerebellar tracts, anterior corticospinal tracts, anterior horn cells, and cortical Betz cells.

CLINICAL MANIFESTATIONS. Most patients with pure hereditary spastic paraplegia continue to walk for many years and have a normal lifespan. Many cases begin in infancy with delayed walking, but the onset can be as late as the seventh decade. Spasticity of the legs and a stiff, slow gait are the main symptoms. Affected persons walk on their toes, trip easily, and are unable to run. About one fourth have pes cavus. The legs show hyperactive reflexes, clonus, and Babinski signs, whereas the arms are usually normal. Later the legs may become weak, the arms may show increased reflexes, and distal muscle wasting may develop, especially in the hands. Vibration and position sense may become impaired in the legs, and many patients develop urinary frequency, urgency, and precipitancy, although sexual function remains normal. Most patients become unable to walk sometime in the sixth or seventh decade.

DIAGNOSIS. The cerebrospinal fluid is normal. Electromyography may show denervation in the distal limb muscles, but the sensory nerve action potentials are preserved, even in patients showing decreased vibration and position sense. Somatosensory evoked po-

tentials, however, are consistently small or unobtainable, reflecting a degeneration of dorsal column fibers.

DIFFERENTIAL DIAGNOSIS. Hereditary spastic paraplegia must be distinguished from nonhereditary causes of slowly progressive myelopathy such as cervical spondylosis, intraspinal tumor, arteriovenous malformation or fistula of the spinal cord, multiple sclerosis, amyotrophic lateral sclerosis, and myelopathy associated with human T cell lymphotropic virus 1 (HTLV-1 tropical spastic paraparesis, Ch. 428.3). MRI has simplified diagnosis of many of these conditions.

415 HEREDITARY AND ACQUIRED INTRINSIC MOTOR NEURON DISEASES

Degenerative diseases of several kinds can attack the large motor neurons of the spinal cord or the brain to produce selective impairment of muscle strength or motor skill. Those of childhood are largely hereditary, whereas the major adult disorder, amyotrophic lateral sclerosis, is nearly always sporadic, with few clues illuminating either its cause or molecular pathogenesis. Table 415–1 lists the major disorders in this category, and the references provide greater detail on the many subtypes.

HEREDITARY AMYOTROPHIES

Hereditary spinal muscular atrophy is a syndrome of progressive muscular weakness and atrophy resulting from selective degeneration of the motor neurons of the spinal cord. A comparable disorder of the lower brain stem nuclei produces progressive bulbar palsy. Many different clinical syndromes have been delineated based on the age of onset, the pattern of muscular weakness, the rate of progression, and the mode of inheritance. Using this approach, at least 15 separate genetic disorders can be recognized. It has been estimated that 1 in 40 Caucasians carries a gene for spinal muscular atrophy. No consistent biochemical defect is known, although hexosaminidase deficiency has been identified in a few cases.

PATHOLOGY. At the time of postmortem examination in the spinal cases, the anterior horns show gliosis and loss of large neurons, and many of the remaining motor neurons are undergoing degeneration. The ventral roots are atrophic owing to loss of myelinated nerve fibers. Similar changes are observed in the motor nuclei of the brain stem in bulbar cases.

In the well-developed infantile and childhood types, microscopic examination of the skeletal muscles using histochemical techniques shows large groups of round, atrophic muscle fibers and large groups of hypertrophied fibers staining uniformly as either type 1 or type 2. These features reflect the continuing process of denervation and reinnervation. However, at an early stage of infantile spinal muscular atrophy the only finding may be uniform atrophy of all

TABLE 415–1. THE MAJOR INTRINSIC MOTOR NEURON DISEASES

Hereditary
  Spinal muscular atrophy
    Type I. Acute, infantile (Werdnig-Hoffmann disease)
    Type II. Late infantile and childhood type
    Type III. Juvenile and adult types
  Familial amyotrophic lateral sclerosis (ALS)
Acquired
  Acute: anterior poliomyelitis
  Chronic:
    ALS alone
    Anterior horn cell degeneration associated with spinocerebellar degeneration, Shy-Drager syndrome, parkinsonism, Creutzfeldt-Jakob disease
    Remote neoplasms, other
  Primary lateral sclerosis (rare)

muscle fibers, with preservation of the normal "checkerboard" fiber-type pattern. In slowly progressive cases of juvenile or adult onset, atrophic muscle fibers are found mainly in small groups; most muscle fibers are of normal size but are arranged in groups of uniform fiber type. After many years some muscle fibers show secondary myopathic changes, such as internal nuclei, splitting, or degeneration.

ACUTE INFANTILE SPINAL MUSCULAR ATROPHY

Werdnig-Hoffmann disease is a fatal, early infantile form of spinal and bulbar muscular atrophy that appears to be a single genetic entity. Inherited as an autosomal recessive abnormality on chromosome 5q, it is one of the most common fatal hereditary diseases of childhood, with an annual incidence of 1 in 20,000 live births and a carrier frequency in the general population of about 1 in 80. The abnormal gene is located on the long arm of chromosome 5.

In at least one third of the cases, there is a prenatal onset, with reduced fetal movements, weakness at birth, or congenital joint deformities. In the remainder of cases, the disease becomes apparent in the first 2 or 3 months of life. There is progressive, flaccid weakness of the trunk and limbs, with severe hypotonia, poor head control, and diminished movements of the limbs, more severe in the proximal muscles. Weakness of the intercostal muscles causes retraction of the chest during inspiration; the cry is weak, and coughing is ineffective. Bulbar weakness causes difficulty in sucking and swallowing. The tendon reflexes are usually absent. Death occurs before 3 years of age; 50% of the patients die in the first 7 months of life and 95% in the first 18 months.

The serum creatine kinase activity and the cerebrospinal fluid are normal. Electromyography shows reduced activation of motor unit potentials, many of which are of increased size, duration, and complexity. Fibrillations and fasciculations are rarely observed. It is important to distinguish this disease from treatable disorders such as infant botulism and chronic inflammatory polyneuropathy. The former is identified by repetitive nerve stimulation tests showing abnormal neuromuscular transmission and the latter, by abnormalities of nerve conduction and increased protein levels in the cerebrospinal fluid.

PROGRESSIVE MUSCULAR ATROPHY IN CHILDREN

PROXIMAL TYPE. Clinically, this is a rather diverse disorder, but most cases are now thought to be caused by a single autosomal recessive gene, located on the long arm of chromosome 5, near or at the locus for Werdnig-Hoffmann disease. The incidence of this syndrome is 1 in 24,000 live births, and the carrier rate is approximately 1 in 90. A milder, autosomal dominant form is also known.

Weakness starts anytime from birth to 8 years of age, usually before 1 year of age. The weakness affects the trunk and limbs and initially is more severe in proximal muscles. The limb muscles become atrophic, the tendon reflexes are lost, and joint contractures may develop. Fasciculations are not prominent but may be apparent in the fingers, producing a fine, irregular tremor. The face and jaws may be weak, and the tongue may be atrophic and show fasciculation.

Children with early onset may never be able to walk and often develop severe scoliosis, limb deformities, and respiratory insufficiency. Many eventually die of pulmonary infection, but some very weak patients survive into adult life, the progress of the disease apparently having arrested early in childhood. Children with a later onset of weakness tend to have a milder course, with slowly progressive proximal weakness, increased lumbar lordosis, and a waddling gait. Those with autosomal recessive inheritance rarely walk after age 20, whereas those with the rare autosomal dominant form may still be walking in middle age.

Serum creatine kinase activity may be mildly or moderately increased in patients with slowly progressive weakness, apparently because of secondary myopathic changes in muscle. The cerebrospinal fluid is normal. Electromyography shows the typical changes of chronic denervation and reinnervation as well as fibrillations and fasciculations, serving to distinguish these patients from similar patients with muscular dystrophy.

Many of these children benefit from active and passive physical therapy and the judicious use of lightweight braces. Special attention should be given to spinal support to counteract scoliosis. Later in childhood, surgical immobilization of the spine may be indicated.

DISTAL TYPE. This category includes both dominant and recessive disorders and accounts for about 10% of all cases of spinal muscular atrophy. Distal limb weakness and muscle wasting, more severe in the lower extremities, usually begins in early childhood and tends to be mild and slowly progressive. Three quarters of the patients have pes cavus, and, except for the absence of sensory deficits, the disorder is often clinically indistinguishable from Charcot-Marie-Tooth disease. However, patients with spinal muscular atrophy have normal conduction in motor and sensory nerves. A rare scapuloperoneal type, with autosomal recessive inheritance, is characterized by distal leg weakness and scapular winging, starting in infancy; there may also be bulbar symptoms such as laryngeal stridor.

SPINAL MUSCULAR ATROPHY OF ADOLESCENT OR ADULT ONSET

Patients with late-onset spinal muscular atrophy have slowly progressive muscular weakness and usually continue to walk for two or three decades or more. Although much less common than the infantile and childhood types, the adult types include at least four clinical and eight genetic categories.

PROXIMAL TYPE. These patients resemble those with muscular dystrophy, and clinical examination may offer few clues to the neurogenic character of the proximal weakness. Fasciculations and muscle cramps are usually not prominent, and the serum creatine kinase activity may be substantially increased. To add to the confusion, males with onset of symptoms in their teens may have large calves. Some patients eventually develop mild bulbar symptoms, such as dysphagia. Electromyography serves to establish the neurogenic nature of the disorder, and muscle biopsy is rarely needed. Families with autosomal dominant and autosomal recessive inheritance have been described. A distinctive X-linked recessive variety, known as bulbospinal neuronopathy, is associated with gynecomastia and dysphagia. It is caused by expansion of a trinucleotide repeat within the gene coding for the androgen receptor.

SCAPULOPERONEAL AND FACIOSCAPULOHUMERAL TYPES. Both myopathic and neurogenic scapuloperoneal syndromes are known, and several varieties begin in the second or third decade of life. Autosomal dominant, autosomal recessive, and X-linked recessive forms have been described. The common feature of these disorders is progressive atrophy and weakness of the shoulder girdle and lower leg muscles, although weakness eventually may spread to the other limb muscles. Electromyography and muscle biopsy can distinguish the anterior horn cell diseases from the muscular dystrophies, but the prognosis is similar in both groups. A few families have an autosomal dominant form of spinal muscular atrophy resembling facioscapulohumeral muscular dystrophy.

DISTAL TYPE. This is usually a childhood disorder, but there are a few families with distal amyotrophy beginning in the third or fourth decade of life, inherited as an autosomal dominant trait. Some familial as well as adult cases exhibit onset in middle age and such a slow progression as never to be incapacitating, even in old age.

AMYOTROPHIC LATERAL SCLEROSIS

Amyotrophic lateral sclerosis (ALS) is a fatal degenerative disease of the central nervous system characterized by slowly progressive paralysis of the voluntary muscles.

INCIDENCE. The annual incidence is about 1 case per 100,000 population, the prevalence being 4 to 6 cases per 100,000. Geographical pockets of much higher incidence in Guam, the Kii peninsula of Japan, and western New Guinea suggest possible, still unknown, exogenous causes. Ninety-five percent of cases in the United States are sporadic, but a few families have several members with the typical clinical picture of sporadic ALS arising in an autosomal dominant pattern. Males are affected slightly more often than females. Although the disease can appear as early as the third decade of life, most cases begin after age 40, and the incidence increases into the eighth decade.

PATHOLOGY. Degeneration of the motor neurons of the spinal cord and lower brain stem is marked by extensive cell loss and astrocytic gliosis. Swellings containing neurofilaments are often found on axons close to their cell bodies. As the Betz cells and large pyramidal neurons of the motor cortex disappear, the corticospinal tracts degenerate, leaving gliosis of the lateral columns of the spinal cord. The ventral spinal roots are depleted of large myelinated nerve fibers, but surviving axons develop distal sprouts that reinnervate some muscle fibers, so that skeletal muscle histopathology shows both muscle fiber atrophy and fiber-type grouping.

ETIOLOGY. Few clues exist to the cause of ALS. Some authors regard the disease as a manifestation of premature aging or a deficiency of a neurotrophic factor. Other speculations include toxic exposure to minerals such as lead or aluminum, deficiency of calcium or magnesium, infection by an unidentified virus, and autoimmunity. Benign paraproteinemia has been encountered in a small proportion of patients, and antiganglioside antibodies have been found in the serum in a majority of the cases, but the significance of these findings is unclear. Recently, some familial cases were linked to a gene coding for the enzyme superoxide dismutase, located on chromosome 21q. This finding has stimulated research into a possible role of free radical toxicity in the pathogenesis of ALS.

CLINICAL MANIFESTATIONS. The major symptom consists of slowly progressive muscle weakness involving the limbs, trunk, breathing muscles, throat, and tongue. Most patients have a mixture of lower and upper motor neuron symptoms, although either may predominate. The former include muscle weakness, wasting, fasciculations, and cramps; the latter include stiffness and slowness of movement, slow and clumsy speech, and explosive release of laughter and crying (pseudobulbar palsy). The ocular muscles are not affected except in patients who survive long times after bulbar paralysis has begun. No impairment affects bladder, bowel, or sexual function. The stretch reflexes are diminished in severely denervated muscles, but more often signs of lower motor neuron weakness are combined with brisk reflexes, a finding nearly specific to ALS. Babinski signs are often present. Sensation is normal except for an expected diminution of vibration sense in the feet in older patients. Occasional cases develop a progressive dementia.

The onset is insidious, and initial symptoms may be confined to a single limb (especially the distal muscles), both limbs on one side, or to lower cranial nerves. Gradually the patchy and asymmetric weakness becomes widespread, and patients become unable to walk, dress, or feed themselves. There is loss of weight because of muscle atrophy and impaired swallowing; the speech becomes unintelligible; choking interferes with eating and sleeping; and breathing becomes difficult even at rest. Death occurs from pulmonary infection and insufficiency. The average survival is 3 years after onset of symptoms, but a few severely debilitated patients live for 10 years or longer.

DIAGNOSIS. Because there are no specific laboratory tests, the diagnosis is based principally on clinical criteria. The disease to be diagnosed as ALS should have a relentlessly progressive, gradual course; lower motor neuron signs should exist at widely separate levels of the nervous system, or upper motor neuron signs should be found well above the level of the lower motor neuron signs; and no conflicting findings such as sensory loss, incontinence, or ocular weakness should be present. The cerebrospinal fluid is normal except for a mild elevation of protein concentration in some cases. Brain and spinal cord imaging is unrevealing. Electromyography shows active and chronic denervation in multiple muscles of the brain stem, upper and lower extremities, and trunk; motor nerve conduction velocity is normal or slightly reduced, and sensory nerve conduction is normal. Serum creatine kinase activity is normal or moderately increased.

DIFFERENTIAL DIAGNOSIS. Although ALS is nearly always fatal, a few patients stop deteriorating or even recover normal strength, but such cases are extremely rare. Other motor neuron disorders, treatable myelopathies and neuropathies, and even thyrotoxic myopathy must be distinguished from ALS (Table 415–2).

TREATMENT. With a disease as grim as ALS, the physician must be careful to avoid premature misdiagnosis. Once the diagnosis is certain, however, some explanation must be given to the patient and the family. This requires considerable tact and gentleness; often it is best to convey the information gradually on successive visits, allowing the relentless progression of weakness to speak for itself.

No medication has been shown to be beneficial, and physical therapy does not delay the neuromuscular deterioration. Quack remedies surface periodically; for their own protection, patients

TABLE 415–2. DIFFERENTIAL DIAGNOSIS OF AMYOTROPHIC LATERAL SCLEROSIS

Disease	Distinguishing Features
Benign fasciculations	No weakness, atrophy, or electromyographic (EMG) abnormality
Motor neuron diseases	
*Lead or mercury toxicity	Increased lead or mercury levels
Benign focal amyotrophy	Onset in youth, strictly focal, no upper motor neuron signs
Postpolio progressive muscular atrophy	Slow course, no upper motor neuron signs
Subacute motor neuronopathy in lymphoma	Plateau in few months, later improvement
*ALS in lung cancer or B cell dyscrasia	Improves on treatment of tumor
Hereditary spinal muscular atrophy	Symmetric, slow course, no upper motor neuron signs
*Thyrotoxic myopathy with fasciculations	Myopathic EMG
*Compressive myelopathy due to cervical spondylosis or extramedullary tumor	Sensory symptoms, no lower motor neuron signs in legs, cord compression on MRI or myelography
*Immune-mediated multifocal motor neuropathy	Multifocal nerve conduction block, very high antiganglioside antibody titers

* Treatable conditions

who wish to try experimental forms of treatment should be referred to a reputable academic center.

Patients with impaired gait may benefit from using a cane or a walker, and patients who suffer from severe dysphagia without other disabling symptoms can be offered nasogastric tube feeding or a gastrostomy. The most difficult medical question, however, involves the therapeutic role of artificial ventilation. Most patients, understanding the hopeless prognosis, prefer not to be kept alive artificially in a state of total paralysis, unable to communicate except with eye movements. Nevertheless, some of these patients have survived for several years, living at home with the help of a devoted and intelligent family. It is important to discuss these issues when patients are in the early stages of respiratory involvement, so that they can make decisions in advance about whether or not to accept emergency resuscitation during a respiratory crisis.

PRIMARY LATERAL SCLEROSIS

Primary lateral sclerosis (PLS) denotes a rare condition characterized by painless, gradually progressing spastic weakness that involves the lower limbs and may ascend to involve the arms and bulbar muscles. In most instances, the disease begins in middle or late life and usually lasts more than a decade before intercurrent illness causes death. Typically, neurologic examinations show a relatively symmetric spastic paraparesis or quadriparesis with heightened deep tendon reflexes and extensor plantar responses but no hint of sensory abnormality. Neither clinical nor electrical studies detect evidence of skeletal muscular denervation. Similarly, imaging procedures disclose no relevant abnormalities involving either brain or spinal cord. The cerebrospinal fluid remains unremarkable, and appropriate tests fail to disclose HIV, HTLV, or other inflammatory processes. Autopsy examinations, performed in a number of cases, have revealed ascending bilateral demyelination of the thoracolumbar corticospinal tracts extending anywhere from the lower cord up to the cerebral peduncles. Cerebral degeneration has not been noted. The cause of PLS is not known, but sporadically arising familial spastic paraplegia cannot be excluded in cases selectively involving the lower extremities. No specific treatment exists, although baclofen may bring modest relief of stiffness.

Brzustowicz LM, Lehner T, Castilla LH, et al.: Genetic mapping of chronic childhood onset spinal muscular atrophy to chromosome 5q 11.2–13.3. Nature 344:540, 1990. *Evidence that the infantile and childhood types of spinal muscular atrophy are allelic disorders of a single gene.*

Deng H-X, Hentati A, Tainer JA, et al.: Amyotrophic lateral sclerosis and structural defects in Cu, Zn superoxide dismutase. Science 261:1047, 1993. *Mutations of the gene for superoxide dismutase, important for scavenging of toxic free radicals, cause reduced red cell enzyme activity in familial ALS.*

Martin JB: Molecular genetics in neurology. Ann Neurol 34:757, 1993. *Provides an informative table.*

Pringle CE, Hudson AJ, Munoz DG, et al.: Primary lateral sclerosis: Clinical features, neuropathology, and diagnostic criteria. Brain 115:495, 1992. *The most comprehensive article about an uncommon disease, carefully reported.*

Williams AC (ed.): Motor Neuron Disease. London, Chapman and Hall, 1994. 776 pp. *In addition to offering full clinical accounts of motor neuron disorders, this book reviews current research on pathogenesis of ALS and gives helpful advice about medical management.*

416 SYRINGOMYELIA

Syringomyelia is a disorder of the spinal cord and, often, the lower brain stem, characterized by slowly progressive enlargement of a fluid-filled cyst (syrinx) within the cord or medulla. Most cases are congenital in origin, related to maldevelopment of the cervicomedullary junction; others are caused by arachnoiditis, intraspinal tumor, or trauma.

PATHOLOGY. In congenital cases, the cyst is thought to represent an enormously dilated remnant of the fetal central canal, which usually does not communicate with the fourth ventricle. It is lined by glial tissue, and in places by remnants of ependyma, and contains clear fluid identical to cerebrospinal fluid. Extending from the high cervical level or medulla to the thoracic or lumbar cord, the cavities vary in shape and size at different levels. Most patients have a Chiari type of congenital cerebellar malformation, in which flattened ectopic tonsils descend caudally so as to obstruct both the exit foramina of the fourth ventricle and the subarachnoid space at the foramen magnum.

Acquired syringomyelia may result from basal arachnoiditis, obstructing the cerebrospinal fluid pathways around the foramen magnum, or may develop in a segment of the cord rendered abnormal by an intramedullary tumor, spinal arachnoiditis, or severe traumatic injury. In nontumor cases the cavity is lined only by glia, whereas in tumor cases the cyst wall may contain both tumor and glial cells.

PATHOGENESIS. The mechanism of cyst formation and expansion is poorly understood. In congenital syringomyelia the cavity probably originates before birth as a dilatation of the primitive central canal. Enlargement of the cyst is somehow related to obstruction of the subarachnoid space at the cervicomedullary junction by the ectopic cerebellar tonsils, causing a pressure gradient between the cyst and the subarachnoid space, especially during straining, coughing, or sneezing. The mechanism may be similar in cases of basal arachnoiditis. In patients with spinal arachnoiditis, the cyst may originate in an area of ischemic myelomalacia, and in cases associated with tumor or severe injury there is cystic degeneration of the spinal cord before the syrinx starts to expand. Why the cyst continues to enlarge in these noncommunicating cases is hard to understand, because there is no apparent pressure gradient between the cyst and the subarachnoid space. Obstruction of cerebrospinal fluid circulation due to spinal arachnoiditis may be an important factor.

CLINICAL MANIFESTATIONS. The classic clinical picture of congenital syringomyelia is of a slowly progressive, asymmetric, destructive process in the central portion of the cervical and thoracic spinal cord, damaging the anterior horn cells, the crossing spinothalamic tract fibers, and the lateral corticospinal tracts. This causes muscle weakness and wasting in the hands and arms; scoliosis owing to denervation of paraspinal muscles; loss of arm reflexes; spastic weakness of the lower extremities; and a *dissociated sensory loss* with impaired perception of pain and temperature in the neck, arms, and upper trunk and preserved light touch perception and proprioception. Some patients experience a deep, aching pain in the neck or arms. Symptoms usually begin between 25 and 40 years of age and advance relentlessly for decades, although one third of the patients have long periods of stability. The deficits may worsen suddenly after a fall or after coughing or sneezing. Ten percent of patients develop a painless arthropathy of the shoulder, elbow, or hand. Extension into the medulla may cause nystagmus, dysphagia, or wasting of the tongue, and some patients have hydro-

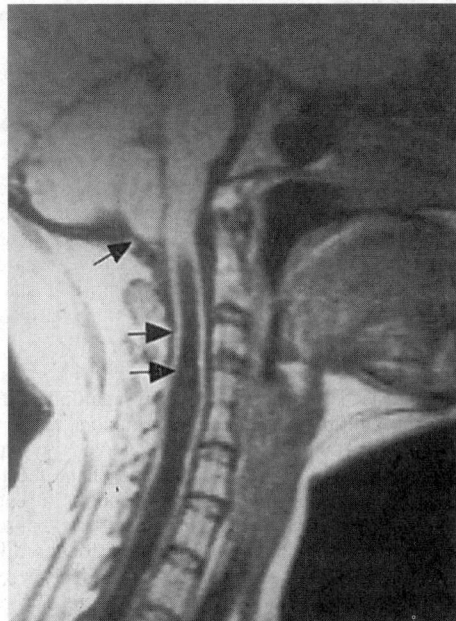

FIGURE 416-1. Magnetic resonance image of upper spine and foramen magnum in a patient with syringomyelia and a small Chiari I malformation *(single arrow)*. The syrinx appears as a dark central area in the cervical and thoracic spinal cord *(double arrows)*.

cephalus or cerebellar signs related to an associated Chiari malformation.

The manifestations of acquired syringomyelia depend on the segment of the spinal cord affected. Posttraumatic syringomyelia, developing in paraplegic or quadriplegic patients months or years after the injury, is revealed by weakness and sensory impairment rising craniad from the transected level. The cases associated with arachnoiditis following previous purulent meningitis, subarachnoid hemorrhage, surgery, trauma, or spinal anesthesia tend to involve the thoracic and lower cervical segments. Syringes associated with intramedullary spinal cord tumor extend for variable distances rostrad or caudad to the tumor.

DIAGNOSIS. Magnetic resonance (MR) imaging, outlines the size and extent of the cavity as well as the presence of cerebellar ectopia, arachnoiditis, or an intraspinal tumor (Fig. 416-1). Electromyography reveals active and chronic denervation in wasted upper extremity muscles, but sensory nerve conduction is normal in the analgesic hand because the lesion is located proximal to the dorsal root ganglia. The cerebrospinal fluid is normal except for a raised protein content in cases associated with tumor or arachnoiditis.

TREATMENT. Various surgical procedures have been devised in the hope of arresting the neurologic deterioration. None has been reliably successful. If hydrocephalus is present, placement of a ventriculoperitoneal shunt may be sufficient to cause the syrinx to collapse, but seldom halts its progression. For congenital syringomyelia associated with cerebellar ectopia, it is customary to perform a posterior decompression of the foramen magnum, ensuring that the fourth ventricle communicates with the subarachnoid space. Acquired syringomyelia is usually treated by decompressing the cyst via a syringoarachnoid, syringopleural, or syringoperitoneal shunt. It has not been established that the outcome of any of these procedures is superior to the natural history of the disease. Some neurosurgical reports suggest that these operations often reduce chronic pain and arrest the progression of neurologic symptoms but long-term follow-up is lacking.

Anderson NE, Willoughby EW, Wrightson P: The natural history and the influence of surgical treatment in syringomyelia. Acta Neurol Scand 71:472, 1985. *A thoughtful critique of the uncertain role of surgical treatment for syringomyelia.*

Oldfield EH, Muraszko K, Shawker TH, Patronas NJ: Pathophysiology of syringomyelia associated with Chiari I malformation of the cerebellar tonsils. Implications for diagnosis and treatment. J Neurosurg 80:3, 1994. *Uses light-tech imaging to analyze fluid dynamics in the syrinx and advocates a new approach to treatment.*

417 THE PHAKOMATOSES

The phakomatoses, or neurocutaneous syndromes, are congenital disorders characterized by disordered growth of ectodermal tissues, producing distinctive skin lesions and malformations or tumors of the nervous system. More than 20 syndromes have been described, the most important of which are neurofibromatosis 1 and 2, tuberous sclerosis, and Sturge-Weber disease.

NEUROFIBROMATOSIS 1 (von Recklinghausen's Disease)

Neurofibromatosis 1 is characterized by multiple café au lait spots on the skin, multiple peripheral nerve tumors, and a variety of other dysplastic abnormalities of the skin, nervous system, bones, endocrine organs, and blood vessels. It is one of the most common genetic diseases, occurring approximately once in every 3000 births. It is inherited as an autosomal dominant trait, but 40 to 60% of cases are clinically sporadic. Even allowing for the difficulty of detecting the trait in mild cases, there seems to be a remarkably high mutation rate, on the order of 10^{-4} per locus per generation. The responsible gene, which occupies a 300-kilobase region of chromosome 17q, codes for a GTPase-activating protein (neurofibromin), which functions as a tumor suppressor.

PATHOLOGY. The peripheral nerve tumors are of two types, schwannomas and neurofibromas, the latter derived from both Schwann cells and perineural fibroblasts. Neurofibromas of sensory nerve twigs produce the distinctive subcutaneous nodules; in peripheral nerve trunks the tumor appears as a fusiform enlargement or plexiform neuroma. Schwannomas arise in cranial and spinal nerve roots and also in peripheral nerve trunks. Both types of tumor occasionally become malignant. The brain may show disordered architecture, hamartomas, gliomas, and meningiomas.

CLINICAL MANIFESTATIONS. Some manifestations are congenital, but most appear during childhood and adult life. Café au lait spots become larger and more numerous with age; most patients eventually have more than six spots greater than 1.5 cm in diameter. Other skin lesions include freckles (axillary freckles being specific to this disease); soft pedunculated cutaneous neurofibromas, and firm subcutaneous neurofibromas.

Plexiform neurofibromas may grow to enormous size, leading to grotesque overgrowth of soft tissues and bone in a limb or around the orbit. Enlarging nerve trunk tumors may cause pain and impair sensory-motor function; intraspinal nerve root tumors do the same and also compress the spinal cord. Gliomas of the optic nerve and chiasm are the most frequent intracranial tumor; they usually behave indolently as hamartomas do. A hamartoma of the hypothalamus may cause precocious puberty.

About 10% of children are mentally deficient, and about 10% develop seizures, half in association with an intracranial tumor. Kyphoscoliosis, dysplasia of the skull, bowed legs, and other bone abnormalities are common. Pheochromocytoma occurs in about 5% of patients, usually in adult life. Hypertension may result from renal artery dysplasia.

DIAGNOSIS. The diagnosis is usually clinically evident, but biopsy of a neurofibroma can be diagnostic in cryptic cases. Spinal nerve root tumors often have a dumbbell shape, with intraspinal and extraspinal components; these are most readily identified on MRI. For diagnosis of intracranial tumors and hamartomas either CT or MRI is suitable.

TREATMENT. Most patients live a normal life with few or no symptoms. Small cutaneous or subcutaneous neurofibromas can be removed if they are painful or frequently irritated, but large plexiform neurofibromas usually should be left alone. A few become malignant with continued invasion and fatal outcome. Symptomatic peripheral nerve trunk schwannomas can sometimes be removed safely by an experienced surgeon. Intraspinal and intracranial schwannomas are approached in the usual surgical fashion. Optic nerve gliomas are generally treated with radiation, but it is not clear whether this improves the outcome.

NEUROFIBROMATOSIS 2

This rare disease is characterized by the occurrence of bilateral acoustic neuromas and often other intracranial tumors, such as meningiomas and ependymomas. A few café au lait spots are present in 42% of cases. The disease is inherited as an autosomal dominant trait, but 50% of cases are new mutations. The responsible gene, located on chromosome 22q, codes for a cytoskeletal protein (merlin) which is presumed to function as a tumor suppressor. Family members at risk for the disease should be screened regularly with hearing tests and brain stem auditory evoked responses.

TUBEROUS SCLEROSIS

The phenotype of tuberous sclerosis consists of mental deficiency, epilepsy, and a characteristic facial eruption known as adenoma sebaceum. The disease is inherited as an autosomal dominant trait, but about 80% of the cases are sporadic, owing to new mutations. Two separate gene loci have been linked to the syndrome, one on chromosome 9q and the other on chromosome 16p.

PATHOLOGY. The facial papules of adenoma sebaceum are angiofibromas. The cerebral hemispheres contain multiple hamartomas characterized by disordered architecture, proliferating and abnormal astrocytes, and deposits of calcium. The common retinal hamartomas are also probably of glial origin. Visceral lesions include multiple rhabdomyomas of the heart, multiple angiomyolipomas of the kidneys, and cystic transformation of the lungs by proliferating fibrous, muscular, and vascular tissue.

CLINICAL MANIFESTATIONS. Mental deficiency may be mild or severe, but one third of affected individuals have normal or even superior intelligence. Seizures occur in 80% of cases, usually starting before the age of 5, and are often difficult to control with medication. In infants the seizures often take the form of infantile spasms; these children tend to be more severely impaired mentally. Occasionally, diagnosis escapes attention until late adolescence or adult life, when investigation of a seizure disorder of new onset discloses subtle skin lesions or multiple retinal or intracranial hamartomas.

Nearly all patients have distinctive skin lesions. Hypopigmented spots are present from the time of birth in nearly 100% of patients; they are more numerous on the trunk and are easier to see with a Wood's lamp. The next most common is adenoma sebaceum, a papular, salmon-colored eruption about the center of the face and in the nasolabial folds. It usually becomes more prominent after puberty. Leathery "shagreen" patches over the lower back and fibromas of the nailbeds affect perhaps 40% of patients.

Retinal hamartomas affect about half the patients. About 30% of patients have cardiac rhabdomyomas, which sometimes cause arrhythmia or congestive heart failure. Renal tumors occur in two thirds of patients and are usually asymptomatic, although pain and bleeding can occur. Cystic disease of the lungs, an uncommon complication, mainly affects women over the age of 20; the symptoms include pneumothorax, dyspnea, cyanosis, and cor pulmonale.

DIAGNOSIS. Clinical diagnosis often is obvious. MRI is the procedure of choice and identifies both calcified and uncalcified tubers and nodules. Adenoma sebaceum, ungual fibromas, and hypopigmented spots are diagnostically specific, but retinal hamartomas also occur in neurofibromatosis.

Treatment is confined to symptomatic control of the epilepsy and to surgical therapy of the occasional hamartoma that undergoes gliomatous changes and enlarges to produce symptoms.

STURGE-WEBER SYNDROME

The Sturge-Weber syndrome is a nonhereditary, congenital disorder of facial and cerebral blood vessels characterized by a facial angioma (port-wine stain), seizures, and mental deficiency. The condition involves a defect of embryonic development, with persistence of a vascular plexus in the cephalic portion of the neural tube. The incidence is about 5 in 100,000 births.

The facial angioma is usually unilateral but may extend to the other side and conforms largely but not strictly to trigeminal nerve subdivisions. There may be cavernous angiomas of the tongue, gums, or mouth, and choroidal angiomas may cause congenital glaucoma. An angioma of the occipital and parietal leptomeninges accompanies the facial nevus on the same side, and the underlying cerebral hemisphere is atrophic, with degenerative changes and deposits of iron and calcium in the superficial layers of the cerebral cortex. The cortical calcifications and atrophy are easily seen on brain CT. Neurologic symptoms develop in infancy or early childhood, consisting of focal or generalized seizures. Half of the children become mentally impaired, and one third develop a hemiparesis. When seizures are difficult to control with medication, early surgical removal of the affected part of the brain may improve control and prevent intellectual deterioration.

Gomez MR (ed.): Tuberous Sclerosis, 2nd ed. New York, Raven Press, 1988. *Gives detailed information about multiple organ involvement in tuberous sclerosis, with excellent illustrations of the skin and retinal lesions.*

Gutmann DH, Wood DL, Collins FS: Identification of the neurofibromatosis type 1 gene product. Proc Natl Acad Sci 88:9658, 1991. *The title identifies the content.*

Mulvihill JJ (moderator): Neurofibromatosis 1 (Recklinghausen disease) and neurofibromatosis 2 (bilateral acoustic neurofibromatosis): An update. Ann Intern Med 113:39, 1990. *A succinct review of clinical and genetic features of both syndromes.*

Trofatter JA, MacCollin MM, Rutter JL, et al.: A novel moesin-, ezrin-, radixin-like gene is a candidate for the neurofibromatosis 2 tumor suppressor. Cell 72:791, 1993. *Characterizes the probable structure of the causative gene abnormality.*

Section Six—
Cerebrovascular Diseases

William A. Pulsinelli

418 CEREBROVASCULAR DISEASES—PRINCIPLES

The family of cerebrovascular diseases can be classified according to whether they affect the brain's vascular supply either focally or diffusely (Fig. 418–1). The generic term "stroke" signifies the abrupt impairment of brain function caused by a variety of pathologic changes involving one (focal) or several (multifocal) intracranial or extracranial blood vessels. Approximately 80% of all strokes are caused by too little blood flow (ischemic stroke), and the remaining 20% are nearly equally divided between hemorrhage into brain tissue (parenchymatous hemorrhage) or the surrounding subarachnoid space (subarachnoid hemorrhage). In contrast, diseases that affect the heart or the systemic circulation cause generalized hypoperfusion and diffuse brain dysfunction or injury. Ischemic stroke and the hypoperfusion syndromes affecting the brain share much pathophysiology, and both processes are considered together in Ch. 419; hemorrhagic stroke is addressed in Ch. 420.

EPIDEMIOLOGY

The annual incidence and death rate for stroke have declined steadily in the United States throughout the twentieth century and for most European countries and Japan since approximately 1960. In the United States, a 1% per year decrease in the annual mortality

rate from stroke recorded since 1915 accelerated in the early 1970's to approximately 5% per year. A recent analysis indicates that the stroke incidence has stabilized at approximately 0.5 to 1.0 per 1000 population. Incidence rates in western European countries are slightly higher (1.5 per 1000), but several eastern European countries and Japan have rates of 3 per 1000 based at least partly on environmental, dietary, and smoking habits. At these current rates, stroke remains the third leading cause of medically related deaths and the second most frequent cause of neurologic morbidity in developed countries.

Several other important facts about stroke incidence have emerged: incidence and death rate for stroke are higher among blacks than whites in the United States; approximately similar rates affect men and women, in contrast to the male predominance for myocardial infarction; and there is a strikingly higher incidence (20 to 30 per 1000) for those over age 75.

CEREBROVASCULAR ANATOMY

Since most strokes are caused by abnormalities within the cerebral circulation, an understanding of cerebrovascular anatomy helps in arriving at the correct diagnosis and determining the underlying pathogenesis and prognosis.

The brain is supplied by four major arteries: the left and right internal carotid and vertebral arteries (Fig. 418–2). The left common carotid artery arises from the aortic arch, but the other vessels originate from branches of the aorta; the right common carotid artery stems from the innominate artery, and the left and right vertebral arteries take off from their respective subclavian arteries.

INTERNAL CAROTID ARTERIES. Each common carotid artery bifurcates into an internal and external carotid artery in most

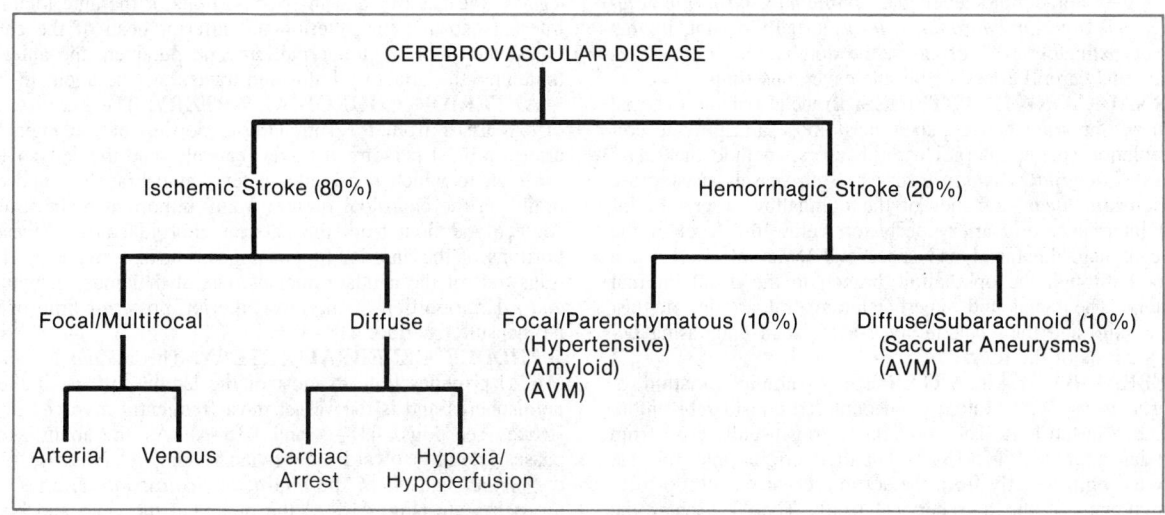

FIGURE 418–1. Classification of cerebrovascular disease.

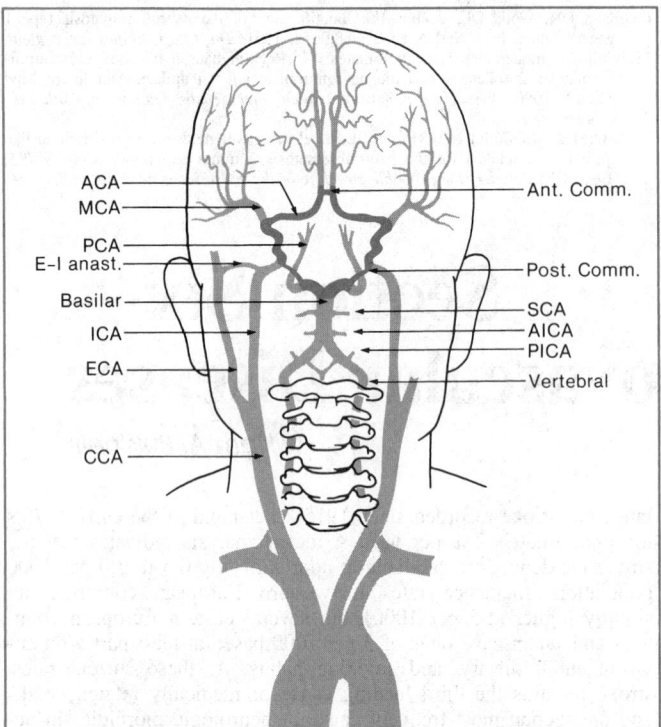

FIGURE 418–2. Extracranial and intracranial arterial supply to the brain. Vessels forming the circle of Willis are highlighted in dark red. Abbreviations for intracranial and extracranial arteries are as follows: ACA = anterior cerebral artery; MCA = middle cerebral artery; PCA = posterior cerebral artery; E-I anast = extracranial-intracranial anastomosis; ICA = internal carotid artery; ECA = external carotid artery; CCA = common carotid artery; Ant. Comm. = anterior communicating artery; Post. Comm. = posterior communicating artery; SCA = superior cerebellar artery; AICA = anterior inferior cerebellar artery; PICA = posterior inferior cerebellar artery. (Modified from Lord R: Surgery of Occlusive Cerebrovascular Disease. St. Louis, C.V. Mosby Company, 1986; with permission.)

individuals just below the angle of the jaw and approximately at the level of the thyroid cartilage (Fig. 418–2). The *internal carotid artery (ICA)* enters the skull through the foramen lacerum and travels a short distance within the petrous portion of the temporal bone. It then enters the cavernous sinus before penetrating the dura and ascends above the clinoid processes to divide into the *anterior* and *middle cerebral arteries.* The portion of the internal carotid artery that lies between the cavernous sinus and the supraclinoid process forms an S shape and is sometimes referred to as the "carotid siphon." The internal carotid artery gives off its first important branches at the supraclinoid level, the *ophthalmic, posterior communicating,* and *anterior choroidal arteries* usually arising in that order. In approximately 10% of cases, the ophthalmic artery arises from the internal carotid artery within the cavernous sinus.

EXTERNAL CAROTID ARTERIES. Branches of the external carotid artery, important because they anastomose and provide collateral circulation to the internal carotid artery, include the *facial artery* and the *superficial temporal artery.* Both vessels anastomose with the *supratrochlear* branches of the ophthalmic artery. In instances of internal carotid artery occlusion below the level of the ophthalmic branch, the facial and superficial temporal arteries can supply blood through the ophthalmic branch to the distal internal carotid artery. The facial and superficial temporal arteries lie just beneath the skin, and their palpability can assist in diagnosing occlusion or stenosis of the ICA.

VERTEBRAL-BASILAR ARTERIES. Anatomic variation of the *vertebral artery* (VA) system is encountered considerably more frequently than in the ICA. The vertebral arteries usually arise from the subclavian arteries (Fig. 418–2), but their origins may migrate proximally to begin directly from the aortic arch or distally to form a common branch of the thyrocervical trunk. The VA's enter the foramen of the sixth cervical vertebra or, much less commonly, the

fourth, fifth, or seventh vertebral level. The VA's ascend through the transverse foramina and exit at C1, where they turn 90 degrees posteriorly to pass behind the atlantoaxial joint before penetrating the dura and entering the cranial cavity through the foramen magnum. The portion of the vertebral artery that loops behind the atlantoaxial joint is prone to mechanical trauma, and rotation of the head to approximately 60 degrees may cause arterial narrowing and reduce blood flow to the ipsilateral vertebral artery.

Intracranially, the vertebral arteries lie lateral to the medulla oblongata and then course ventrally and medially, where they unite at the medullopontine junction to form the *basilar artery (BA).* The BA bifurcates at the pontomesencephalic junction into the *posterior cerebral arteries (PCA's).*

In as many as 20% of all individuals, the right or left VA's terminate before reaching the BA, leaving the latter to be supplied inferiorly by a single vessel. Intracranial branches of the VA's include medial branches, which unite to form the *anterior spinal artery,* and lateral branches to the dorsolateral medulla and posterior cerebellum, called the *posterior inferior cerebellar arteries.*

CIRCLE OF WILLIS. The *circle of Willis* (Fig. 418–2) is formed by the union at the base of the brain of both anterior cerebral arteries via the *anterior communicating artery* and the middle cerebral arteries with the posterior cerebral arteries on each side via the *posterior communicating arteries* (Fig. 418–2). Anomalies of the circle of Willis occur frequently; in large autopsy series of normal individuals, more than half showed an incomplete circle of Willis. The most common sites for such abnormalities, which usually present as hypoplasia or atresia, are the posterior communicating arteries (22%) and the anterior cerebral arteries (10%).

ANTERIOR CEREBRAL ARTERIES. The *anterior cerebral arteries* (ACA's) pass medially above the optic chiasm and head rostrally toward the interhemispheric fissure, where they arch caudally to lie just dorsal to the corpus callosum (Fig. 418–3). In approximately 10% of normal individuals, the A1 segment of the ACA (the portion between the middle cerebral and anterior communicating arteries) is atretic or absent, leaving its distal portion to be supplied by the opposite ACA via the anterior communicating artery. Branches of the ACA supply the frontal poles, the superior surfaces of the cerebral hemispheres where their distal branches anastomose with those of the middle cerebral artery, and all of the medial surfaces of both cerebral hemispheres with the exception of the calcarine cortex. Cortical areas served by the ACA include the motor and sensory cortex of the legs and feet, the supplementary motor cortex, and the presumed cortical micturition center lying in the paracentral lobule (Figs. 418–3 and 418–4).

The A1 and A2 segments (the portion between the anterior communicating artery and the genu of the corpus callosum) give off many small branches that penetrate the anterior perforated substance of the brain. These small penetrating branches include all of the *anterior* and some of the *medial lenticulostriate* arteries. Usually, there is a dominant medial striate vessel called the *recurrent artery of Heubner,* which arises in most instances from the A1 segment of the ACA. This artery penetrates the perforated substance of the brain and, along with the other small perforators, supplies (Fig. 418–4) the anterior and inferior portions of the anterior limb of the internal capsule, the anterior and inferior head of the caudate nucleus, the anterior globus pallidus and putamen, the anterior hypothalamus, the olfactory bulbs and tracts, and the uncinate fasciculus.

ANTERIOR CHOROIDAL ARTERY. The *anterior choroidal artery* arises from the supraclinoid portion of the internal carotid artery in most persons. It travels caudally and medially over the optic tract, to which it provides a few small branches, and enters the brain via the choroidal fissure. Many important brain structures receive blood flow from the anterior choroidal artery; these include portions of the anterior hippocampus, uncus, amygdala, globus pallidus, tail of the caudate nucleus, lateral thalamus, geniculate body, and a large portion of the most inferior, posterior limb of the internal capsule (see Fig. 418–4).

MIDDLE CEREBRAL ARTERY. The *middle cerebral artery (MCA)* provides flow to most of the lateral surface of the cerebral hemispheres and is the vessel most frequently involved in ischemic stroke (see Figs. 418–3 and 418–4). As the main MCA trunk passes laterally toward the sylvian fissure, it gives rise to some of the *medial* and all of the *lateral lenticulostriate* arteries. These arteries irrigate (Fig. 418–4) the putamen, the head and body of the caudate nucleus, the lateral globus pallidus, the full vertical extent

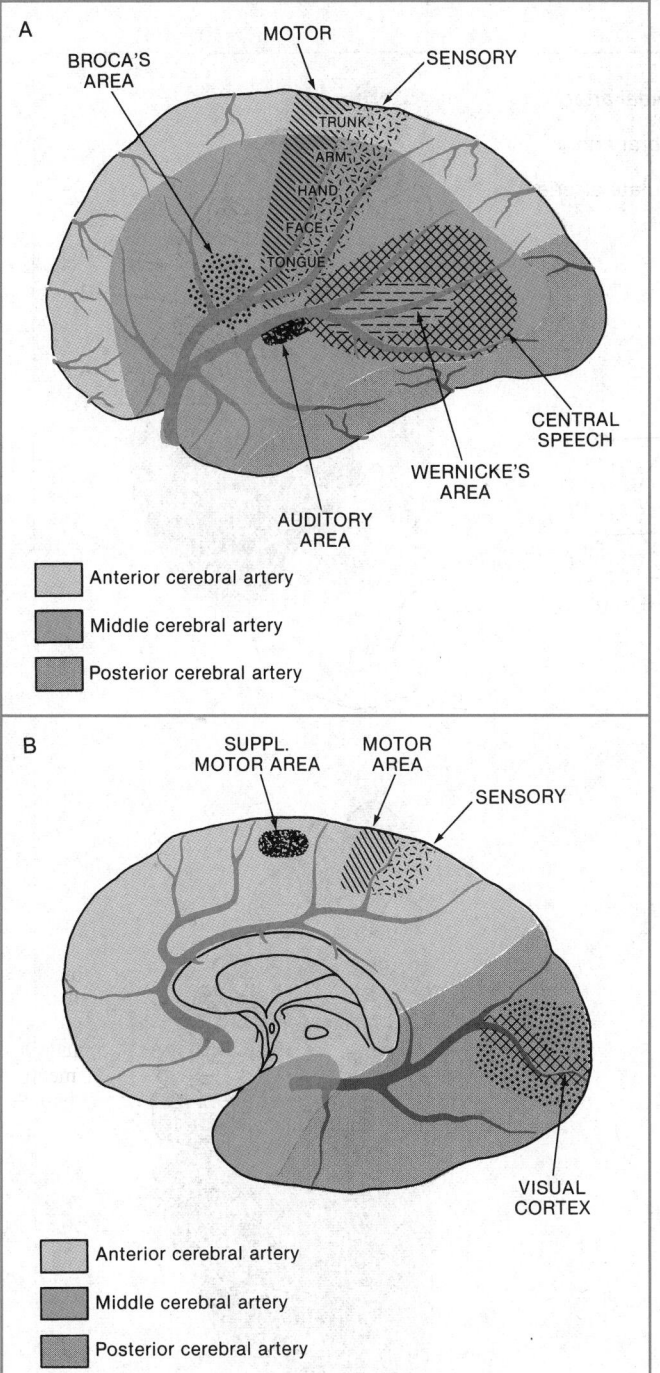

FIGURE 418–3. Lateral *(A)* and medial *(B)* views of the cerebral hemisphere showing the surface distributions of the anterior, middle, and posterior cerebral arteries.

of the anterior limb of the internal capsule, and a superior portion of the posterior limb of the internal capsule. The MCA then extends into the sylvian fissure, where it branches into several smaller arteries grouped into a superior division, which feeds the cortical surface above the fissure, and an inferior division, which supplies the cortical surface of the temporal lobe. The territory of the MCA includes the major motor and sensory areas of the cortex, the areas for contraversive eye and head movement, the optic radiations, auditory sensory cortex, and, in the dominant hemisphere, the motor and sensory areas for language.

POSTERIOR CEREBRAL ARTERIES. Blood flow to both *posterior cerebral arteries (PCA's)* derives primarily from the BA (70% of the time) and from the ICA (10% of the time). In the remaining 20%, one PCA is supplied by the internal carotid artery and the other by the basilar artery. The PCA's pass dorsal to the third cranial nerves and across the cerebral peduncles and then as-

cend upward along the medial edge of the tentorium, where they branch into anterior and posterior divisions. The anterior division (Figs. 418–3 and 418–4) supplies the inferior surface of the temporal lobe, where its terminal branches anastomose with branches of the MCA. The posterior division supplies the occipital lobe, where its terminal branches anastomose with both the ACA and the MCA. In its most proximal course along the base of the brain, the PCA gives off several groups of penetrating arteries commonly referred to as the thalamogeniculate, the thalamoperforating, and the posterior choroidal arteries. The red nucleus, the substantia nigra, medial parts of the cerebral peduncles, the nuclei of the thalamus, the hippocampus, and the posterior hypothalamus receive blood from these penetrating branches (Fig. 418–4).

BRAIN-STEM BLOOD FLOW. At all rostrocaudal levels of the brain stem, the ventral medial portion is supplied by short paramedian vessels; the ventrolateral portion by short circumferential branches from the vertebral or basilar arteries; and the dorsolateral portion and cerebellum by long circumferential branches, which include the *posterior inferior cerebellar* arteries, which arise from the vertebral arteries, and the *anterior inferior* and *superior cerebellar* arteries, which arise from the basilar artery (Fig. 418–5A and B).

The pyramids, the inferior olives and medial lemnisci, the medial longitudinal fasciculi, and the emerging fibers of the hypoglossal nerve (Fig. 418–5A) derive blood from the vertebral arteries. Longer branches from the vertebral arteries and posterior inferior cerebellar arteries supply the spinothalamic tracts, the vestibular nuclei, the sensory nuclei of the fifth cranial nerve, the descending fibers of the sympathetic nervous system, the restiform body, and the emerging fibers of the vagus and glossopharyngeal nerves. The most cephalad and dorsal segment of the medulla includes the vestibular and cochlear nuclei, which, along with the posterior portion of the cerebellum, receive flow from the posterior inferior cerebellar artery.

The basilar artery gives rise to perforating branches as it spans the ventral midline pons and midbrain (Fig. 418–5B). These short perpendicular branches distribute blood to the paramedian structures, including the corticospinal tracts, the pontine reticular nuclei, the medial lemnisci, the medial longitudinal fasciculi, and the pontine reticular nuclei. The *anterior inferior cerebellar artery* feeds blood to the lateral pons, including the emerging seventh and eighth cranial nerves, the trigeminal nerve root, the vestibular and cochlear nuclei, and the spinothalamic tracts. It also branches to the most dorsal and lateral of these structures on its dorsal course toward the cerebellum.

At the midbrain level, the basilar artery lies in the midline in the peduncular fossa. Short branches pass laterally and dorsally to both sides to supply the cerebral peduncles, the emerging fibers of the third nerve, medial portions of the red nuclei, the medial longitudinal fasciculus, the oculomotor nuclei, and the midbrain reticulum. The superior cerebellar arteries contribute to the dorsal midbrain supply, including that of the colliculi and the superior portion of the cerebellum on each side.

VENOUS DRAINAGE. The veins in the brain, unlike those in many other parts of the body, do not accompany the arteries (Fig. 418–6). Cortical veins drain into the superior sagittal sinus, which runs posteriorly between the cerebral hemispheres. Deeper structures drain into the inferior sagittal sinus and great cerebral vein (of Galen), which join at the straight sinus. The straight sinus runs posteriorly along the attachment of the falx cerebri and tentorium and joins the superior sagittal sinus at the torcular Herophili, from which the two transverse sinuses arise. Each transverse sinus passes laterally toward the petrosal bone to become the sigmoid sinus, which exits the skull into the internal jugular vein. Each cavernous sinus communicates with its contralateral twin and surrounds the ipsilateral carotid artery; both drain posteriorly into the petrosal sinuses, which in turn drain into the sigmoid sinus.

NORMAL PHYSIOLOGY

CEREBRAL METABOLISM AND BLOOD FLOW. The brain performs no mechanical work; nevertheless, the energy demands to support normal electrophysiologic brain activity in conscious humans equal, on a per weight basis, those of metabolically active tissues like the heart and kidney. Aerobic glucose metabolism provides the energy necessary to drive membrane ion pumps,

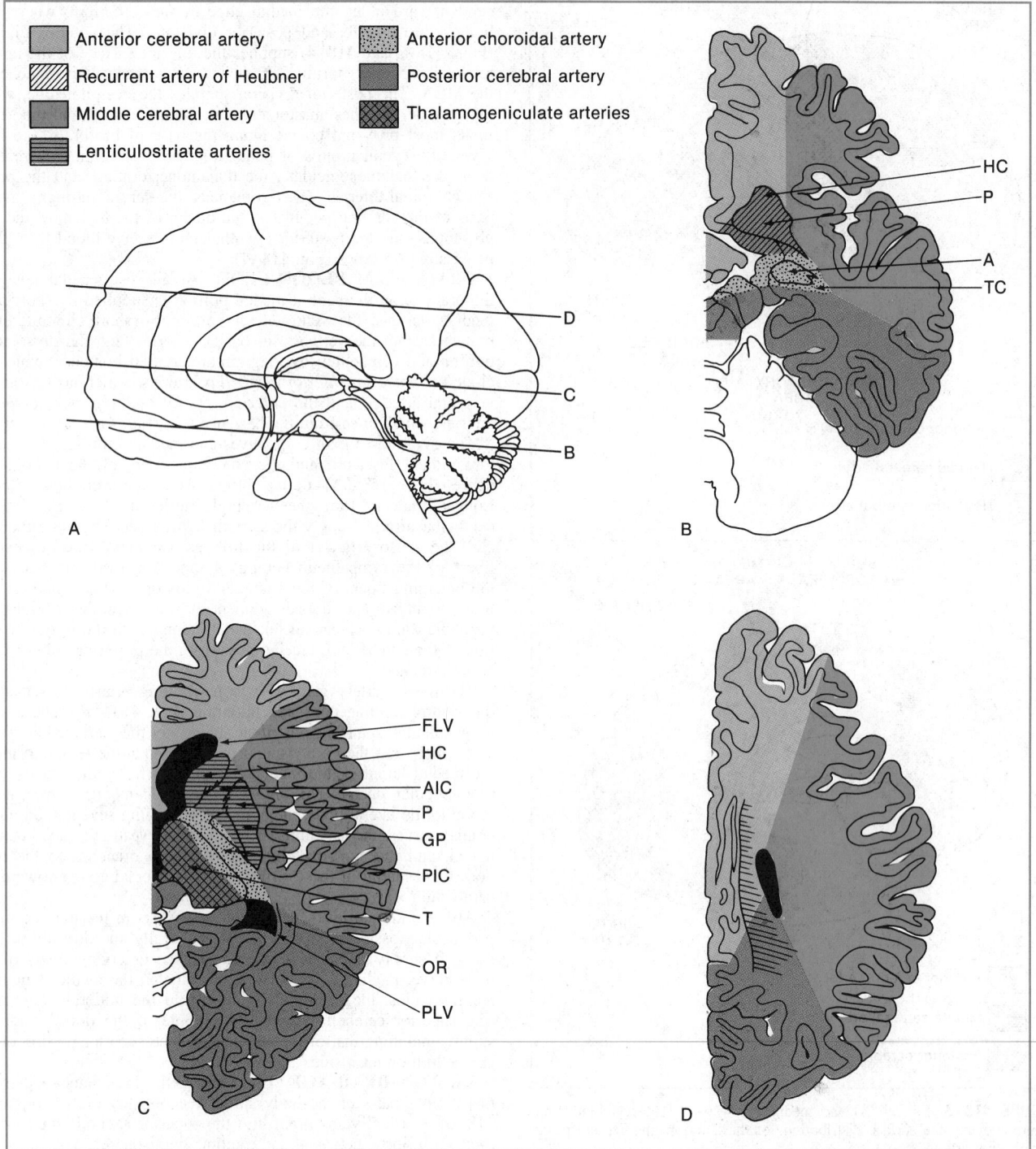

FIGURE 418–4. Arterial supply of deep brain structures. *A,* Sagittal view of the brain showing the computed tomographic (CT) planes through which views B, C, and D were taken. *B,* CT plane through the head of the caudate nucleus (HC), putamen (P), amygdala (A), tail of the caudate nucleus (TC), hypothalamus, temporal lobe, midbrain, and cerebellum. *C,* CT plane through the frontal horn of the lateral ventricle (FLV), head of the caudate nucleus (HC), anterior and posterior limbs of the internal capsule (AIC, PIC), putamen (P), globus pallidus (GP), thalamus (T), optic radiations (OR), and posterior horn of the lateral ventricle (PLV). *D,* CT plane through the centrum semiovale. (Modified from De Armond S, et al: Structure of the Human Brain, A Photographic Atlas, 3rd ed. New York, Oxford University Press, 1989; with permission.)

synthesize, store, and release neurotransmitters, and maintain tissue structure. The normal, conscious human consumes approximately 160 μmol O$_2$ and 30 μmol glucose per 100 grams of brain each minute (Table 418–1).

Approximately 10% of available blood glucose is extracted and phosphorylated by the brain in a single pass, yet only 80% of this glucose is used to generate energy. The 5:1 ratio of O$_2$ versus glucose consumption (Table 418–1) indicates that approximately 20% of glucose carbons are not oxidized. Approximately 10 to 15% of glucose is metabolized to lactate, which may be lost to the circula-

tion; the remainder is used for the synthesis of neurotransmitters, fats, and, to a small degree, proteins. Each mole of glucose metabolized by the brain through glycolysis and the mitochondrial respiratory chain therefore yields approximately 30 mol ATP instead of the expected 38.

Unlike muscle or other tissues, the brain stores few glucose, glycogen, or other high-energy phosphate (ATP, phosphocreatine) reserves but instead relies on a sizable and well-regulated blood flow to satisfy its immediate needs for energy. Cerebral blood flow (CBF) averages 60 ml per 100 grams of brain per minute in the

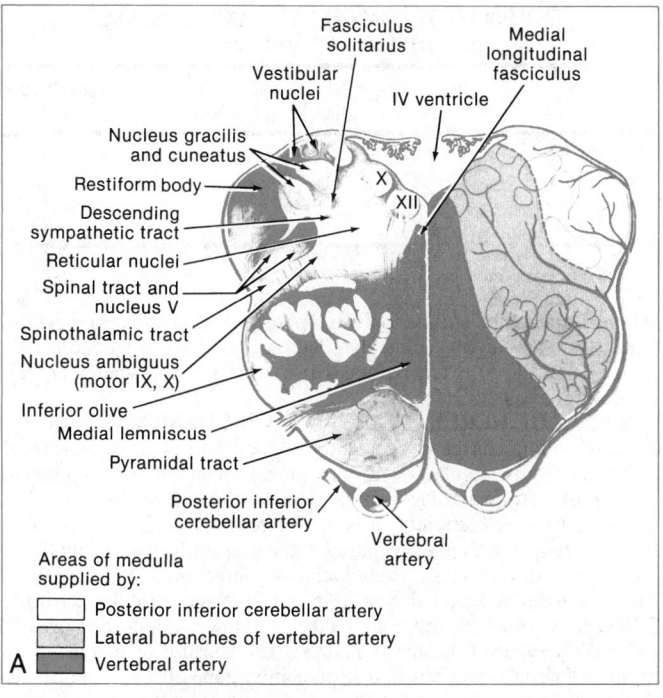

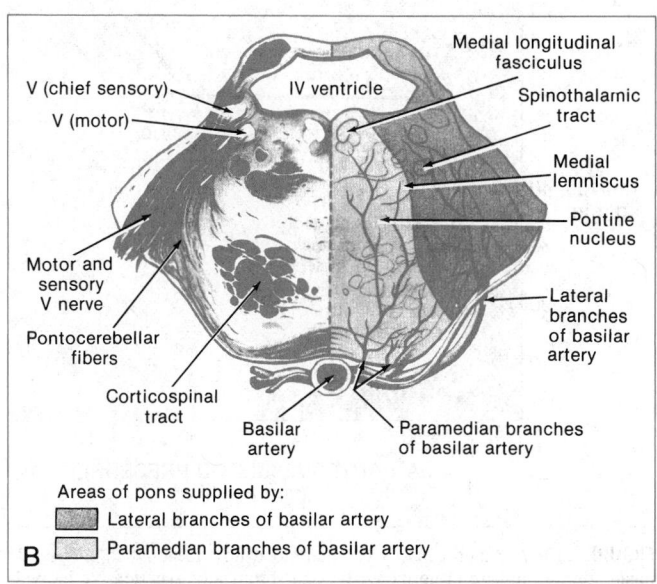

FIGURE 418–5. *A,* Cross-section of the medulla oblongata at the level of the hypoglossal nuclei (XII). Short branches of the vertebral and anterior spinal arteries supply the medial medulla. Longer circumferential branches, including the posterior inferior cerebellar artery, supply the lateral portions of the medulla. *B,* Cross section of the midpons. The medial portion receives the blood supply from short, perforating basilar artery branches. More laterally, the blood supply comes from lateral basilar artery branches.

normal, conscious human; in the absence of such flow, the brain has sufficient high-energy stores to support normal metabolic needs for only a few minutes. At normal arterial O_2 tensions and blood glucose concentrations, CBF delivers 350 mmol O_2 and 260 mmol glucose to 100 grams of brain each minute (see Table 418–1).

These values exceed the brain's normal consumption rates of O_2 and glucose by factors of approximately 2 and 9, respectively. The blood vascular reserves for both O_2 and glucose must be small, as is illustrated by the fact that all changes of synaptic activity, whether related to thinking, talking, or directing muscular activity, are tightly *coupled,* both temporally and anatomically, to an almost instantaneous, proportional increase in CBF. The anatomic segregation of the brain's functional activities results in an ever-changing mosaic of regional metabolic/blood flow values that reflect moment-to-moment changes in electrophysiologic activity.

The coupling of CBF to regional synaptic activity and metabolic activity represents only one of several important mechanisms regulating normal CBF. Changes in the respiratory rate or volume, which lead to even mild hyper- or hypocapnia, respectively dilate or constrict cerebral resistance vessels, so that CBF shows a linear relationship to Pa_{CO_2}. This normal physiologic response to Pa_{CO_2} is exploited clinically to treat cerebral herniation syndromes. Mechanical hyperventilation to a Pa_{CO_2} of 20 to 25 mm Hg reduces CBF by approximately 40 to 45% and normal adult cerebral blood volume from 50 ml to approximately 35 ml. While seemingly small, this 15-ml reduction often suffices to retard the progression of cerebral herniation. The response is short-lived, however, and brain and blood HCO_3^- and H^+ ions control blood vessel tone re-equilibrate within 30 to 60 minutes.

A complex system of neural pathways regulates CBF in response to normal and abnormal circumstances. Some of these neural pathways participate in *autoregulation,* a process which maintains CBF at a constant level despite wide fluctuations in cerebral perfusion pressure.

Because cerebral venous pressures closely approximate the intracranial pressure, autoregulation values usually are expressed in terms of mean arterial pressure.

FIGURE 418–6. Venous drainage of intracranial structures. SSS = superior sagittal sinus; CV = cortical veins; ISS = inferior sagittal sinus; ICV = internal cerebral vein; GV = great vein of Galen; *SS = straight sinus; TH = torcular herophili; PS = petrosal sinus; CS = cavernous sinus; TS = transverse sinus; SS = sigmoid sinus; LS = lateral sinus; IJ = internal jugular vein. (Reproduced with permission from Gates P, Barnett HJ, Mohr JP, et al. [eds.]: Stroke: Pathophysiology, Diagnosis and Management. New York, Churchill Livingstone, 1986.)

TABLE 418–1. METABOLIC ACTIVITY (NORMAL CONSCIOUS MAN)

	Consumed	Supplied
	(100 grams brain/min)	
CBF	60 ml	—
O_2	156 μmol	350 μmol
Glucose	33 μmol	260 μmol

CBF = cerebral blood flow.

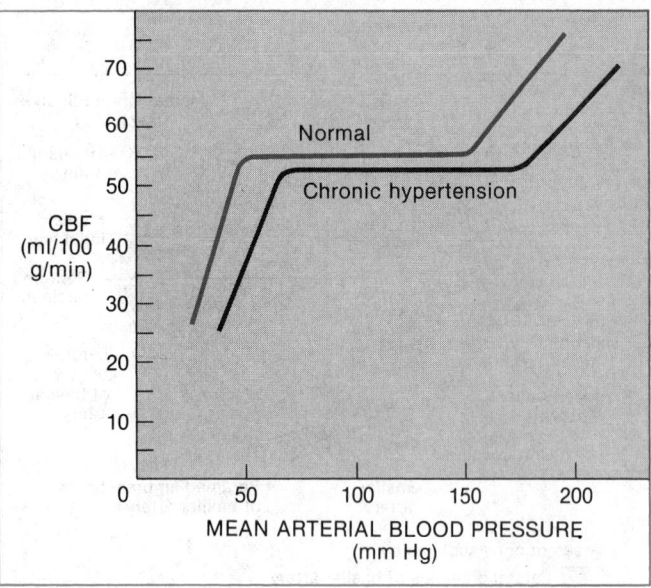

FIGURE 418-7. Autoregulatory cerebral blood flow response to changes in mean arterial pressure in normotensive and chronically hypertensive individuals. Note the shift of the curve toward higher mean pressures with chronic hypertension.

Normal autoregulation has both upper and lower limits (Fig. 418-7); at mean arterial pressures above 150 mm Hg, blood flow increases and capillary pressure rises, while at mean arterial pressures below 50 mm Hg, CBF falls. Increased capillary pressure in hypertensive patients may be a factor in intracerebral hemorrhage and hypertensive encephalopathy. In patients with chronic hypertension, the upper and lower autoregulatory limits are shifted toward higher systemic pressures (Fig. 418-7). Consequently, too rapid therapeutic reduction of blood pressure to apparently normal levels carries the risk of further lowering of cerebral blood flow in hypertensive patients with ongoing cerebral ischemia. Chronic treatment with antihypertensive agents readjusts the autoregulatory curve toward more normal values.

BLOOD-BRAIN BARRIER. Regulation within narrow limits of the extracellular ionic and molecular composition is more important for the normal function of the brain than for any other organ. Small changes in the extracellular concentrations of, for example, Na^+ ions or the neurotransmitters glutamate or norepinephrine greatly alter neuronal function. The blood-brain barrier, is composed anatomically of unique endothelial cells that lack the usual transendothelial channels and that seamlessly abut one another (tight junctions). This anatomy protects the brain against the fluctuating composition of blood and minimizes the entry of potentially toxic compounds.

The entry of nutrients and egress of metabolic products cross the blood-brain barrier via simple diffusion, facilitated transport, or active transport. Lipid-soluble compounds rapidly diffuse across endothelial cell membranes, while polar compounds must be transported on special carrier molecules that are driven either by concentration gradients (facilitated transport) or through the expenditure of energy (active transport). Gas molecules such as O_2 and CO_2 freely diffuse across plasma membranes and rapidly equilibrate between blood and brain. Glucose, a highly polar molecule, enters the brain on a special carrier with a Km (7 to 8 mM) just slightly higher than the normal blood glucose concentration. The rate of brain glucose transport is normally two to three times faster than the metabolism of glucose, but since glucose uptake depends so highly on its concentration, a reduction of blood sugar to one-third the normal amount, caused by either ischemia or hypoglycemia, may compromise normal metabolism (Table 418-2).

PATHOPHYSIOLOGY/PATHOLOGY OF CEREBRAL ISCHEMIA

A failed delivery of O_2 and glucose to the brain generates a cascade of events that vary qualitatively and quantitatively with the severity of the insult. The severity of cerebral ischemia, defined as the degree and duration of blood flow loss, largely determines

TABLE 418-2. HUMAN HYPOXIC-ISCHEMIC THRESHOLD VALUES

	PaO$_2$ (torr)	CBF (ml/100 grams/min)	Blood Glucose (mg/dl)
Normal	90	60	80
Stupor	30-40	20-30	25-30
Coma	20-30	15-20	20-25
Brain Injury	< 20	< 15	< 20

whether the brain suffers only temporary dysfunction, irreversible injury to a few highly vulnerable neurons (selective ischemic necrosis), or damage to extensive areas involving all cell types (cerebral infarction).

TYPES OF CEREBRAL HYPOXIA-ISCHEMIA. Cerebral hypoxia-ischemia can be conveniently divided into focal or multifocal ischemia from vascular occlusion, global ischemia from complete failure of cardiovascular pumping, and diffuse hypoperfusion-hypoxia caused by respiratory disease or reduced perfusion pressure. *Focal cerebral ischemia,* resulting most frequently from embolic or thrombotic occlusion of extracranial or intracranial blood vessels, variably reduces blood flow within the involved vascular territory. Blood flow to the central zone of the ischemic vascular bed usually is severely reduced but rarely reaches zero because of partial filling from collateral blood vessels. In transition zones between normally perfused tissue and the severely ischemic central core, blood flow is moderately reduced. This rim of moderately ischemic tissue has been called the "ischemic penumbra," and although brain cells in this region remain viable longer than do those in the ischemic core, they too will die if left deprived of adequate blood flow.

Focal cerebral ischemia sufficient to cause clinical signs or symptoms and lasting only 15 to 30 minutes causes irreversible injury to specific, highly vulnerable neurons. If the ischemia lasts an hour or longer, infarction of part or all of the involved vascular territory is inevitable. Clinical evidence of permanent brain injury from such ischemia may or may not be detectable, depending upon the region and the amount of brain tissue involved (see Ch. 419).

Global cerebral ischemia, typically caused by cardiac asystole or ventricular fibrillation, reduces blood flow to zero throughout all of the brain. Global ischemia lasting more than 5 to 10 minutes is usually incompatible with recovery of consciousness in normothermic humans. Brain damage from more transient global ischemia, uncomplicated by periods of prolonged hypotension or hyperglycemia, is limited to specific populations of highly vulnerable neurons. This "selective ischemic necrosis" of neurons involves, for example, the CA1 pyramidal neurons of hippocampus, the cerebellar Purkinje cells, and the pyramidal neurons in neocortical layers 3, 5, and 6 (Table 418-3). While selective ischemic necrosis of neurons typifies transient global ischemia, such injury may also accompany prolonged hypoxemia, carbon monoxide poisoning, and focal cerebral ischemia of brief duration. Cardiac resuscitation complicated by prolonged hypotension or hyperglycemia may cause cerebral infarction, particularly in border zones that lie between the terminal branches of major arterial supplies.

Diffuse cerebral hypoxia, uncomplicated by cerebral ischemia, is limited to conditions of mild to moderate hypoxemia, since myocardial contractility and blood pressure fall with severe hypoxemia. As a consequence, pure cerebral hypoxia causes cerebral dysfunction but not irreversible brain injury. Individuals with pure cerebral hypoxia from altitude sickness, pulmonary disease, or severe anemia present with confusion, cognitive impairment, and lethargy. The on-

TABLE 418-3. ORDER OF DECREASING NEURONAL VULNERABILITY TO ANOXIA

Hippocampus
    CA1, CA4 > CA3 > granule cells
Cerebellum
    Purkinje > stellate and basket > granule > Golgi cells
Striatum
    Small and medium-sized > large neurons
Neocortex
    Layers 3,5,6 > layers 2,4

set of coma signals cardiovascular compromise and imminent brain damage. With relatively *acute* changes in arterial oxygen tension from normal to a Pa$_{O_2}$ of 40 mm Hg (see Table 418–2) or with a fall in the hemoglobin concentration below 7 grams per deciliter, compensatory increases of cerebral blood flow become inadequate, and clinical signs and symptoms of cerebral hypoxia develop.

NEUROPATHOLOGY OF CEREBRAL ISCHEMIA. Ischemic injury to the brain can be classified on the basis of cytopathologic criteria into four types. Cerebral *autolysis,* observed most frequently in brain-dead patients preserved on mechanical ventilators for several days, reflects enzymatic autodigestion of the tissue.

Cerebral *infarction,* usually caused by focal vascular occlusion, is characterized histopathologically by necrosis of neurons, glia, and, in some areas, endothelial cells. Cerebral infarcts are frequently described grossly as pale (anemic) or "hemorrhagic," (showing gross petechial bleeding). Most often, the hemorrhagic areas lie along border zones of partially perfused tissue and occur most frequently with transient embolic occlusion followed by reperfusion of the infarcted vascular bed.

Transient arrest of the cerebral circulation (global ischemia) for periods of a few minutes causes *selective ischemic necrosis of highly vulnerable neurons* (see Table 418–3).

The time required for histologic changes to reach their maximum in areas of cerebral infarction differs markedly from the time course of injury encountered in selective ischemic necrosis. Infarction usually requires only a few hours before histologic stains sharply outline the distinct margins between living and dying neurons and glia. By contrast, selective ischemic necrosis of neurons evolves more slowly and sometimes requires several days or more to reach its full extent.

Another distinctive neuropathologic lesion due to ischemia is *demyelination* of the central hemispheric white matter. Such injury is usually the consequence of carbon monoxide poisoning or other prolonged periods of moderately severe hypoxemia or cerebral hypoperfusion. Within these lesions, nerve cell axons are demyelinated, and oligodendroglial cells die off.

MOLECULAR MECHANISMS. In severely ischemic brain tissue, energy-rich compounds become depleted within seconds to a few minutes (see Table 418–2). Soon thereafter, the tissue begins to lose structural integrity. As energy-dependent membrane pumps fail, neuronal and glial cell membranes depolarize and allow the influx of Na$^+$ and Ca^{2+} ions and the efflux of K$^+$ ions. Elevated intracellular Ca^{2+} and other second messengers activate lipases and proteases, which in turn release membrane-bound free fatty acids and denature proteins. Depolarization of presynaptic terminals releases abnormally high concentrations of excitatory and inhibitory neurotransmitters, which may further exacerbate injury. If blood flow is restored in 15 to 30 minutes and no other complicating variables, such as hyperglycemia, are involved, most of these events are reversible, and only selectively vulnerable neurons will die. If ischemia lasts hours or more, cerebral infarction develops.

In contrast to the rapid cascade of events caused by severe ischemia, moderate ischemia triggers poorly defined mechanisms that sacrifice electrophysiologic activity to preserve brain structure, at least temporarily. Acute reduction of blood flow below one-half that of normal exceeds the capacity of compensatory mechanisms, such as an increased extraction of O$_2$ and glucose extraction by the tissue. The electroencephalogram (EEG) slows, and if ischemia is diffuse, the patient becomes confused, lethargic, or stuporous. The molecular mechanisms that induce this "anoxic anesthesia" are unknown. Depletion of whole tissue energy reserves is not an explanation, since these remain normal, partly as a consequence of the decreased energy demand normally used to maintain membrane ion pumps and EEG activity. With slightly greater ischemia, all synaptic activity ceases and the EEG becomes isoelectric. This too occurs before high-energy stores are depleted, indicating that generalized energy failure cannot explain the early loss of synaptic activity. Prompt recovery of blood flow restores full function and structural integrity to the tissue. If moderate ischemia persists for several hours, however, irreversible injury begins to develop, possibly as a consequence of compromised calcium homeostasis. Tissues with partial depletion of ATP and impaired calcium homeostasis may benefit from pharmacologic therapies that reduce calcium movement through voltage-dependent and neurotransmitter-dependent ion channels.

CEREBRAL EDEMA. Pathologic increases in the water content of the brain (edema) accompany all types of ischemic and hemorrhagic stroke. Brain swelling and raised intracranial pressure relate proportionally to the volume of the accumulated water; in some instances, they can cause neurologic deterioration and death by transtentorial herniation. Cerebral edema and herniation represent the immediate cause of death in one-third of all ischemic and three-quarters of all hemorrhagic fatal strokes.

Brain edema is categorized on the basis of pathophysiologic and anatomic criteria as intracellular or interstitial. Intracellular edema, also called cytotoxic edema, represents an accumulation of intracellular osmoles and water causing cell swelling at the expense of the interstitial brain volume. Intracellular edema develops rapidly in ischemic brain tissue as energy-dependent membrane ion pumps fail and Na$^+$ and other osmoles enter the cell from the interstitial and vascular compartments. Cell swelling occurs predominantly in astrocytes, but neurons, oligodendroglial cells, and endothelial cells also are involved to a lesser degree. The osmolality of ischemic brain increases acutely from 310 mOsm to approximately 350 mOsm. The intracellular accumulation of water increases from a normal value of approximately 79 to 81% of brain weight, an addition insufficient in most instances to cause cerebral herniation. If cerebral circulation is re-established before permanent brain injury develops, intracellular brain edema resolves within a matter of hours without permanent sequelae.

Interstitial brain edema, also called "vasogenic edema," occurs later than the intracellular form. Damage to blood-brain barrier endothelial cells allows macromolecules such as plasma proteins to enter the interstitial space, carrying with them osmotically bound water. Interstitial brain edema following cerebral infarction progressively worsens for 3 to 4 days after a stroke. Fluid accumulation within the vicinity of damaged endothelial cells and the zone of infarction can raise the local water content of brain by as much as 10%. Such large volume increases can lead to transtentorial herniation and similarly fatal consequences.

Barnett HJ, Mohr JP, Stein BM, et al. (eds.): Stroke: Pathophysiology, Diagnosis and Management. New York, Churchill Livingstone, 1992. *A comprehensive two-volume overview of all aspects of ischemic and hemorrhagic stroke.*

Caplan LR, Stein RW: Stroke: A Clinical Approach. Boston, Butterworth, 1986. *A pragmatic description of the diagnosis and treatment of stroke.*

Plum F, Pulsinelli WA: Cerebral metabolism in hypoxic-ischemic brain injury. *In* Asbury AK, McKann GM, McDonald IW (eds.): Disease of the Nervous System. Philadelphia, W.B. Saunders Company, 1992. *A contemporary review of the pathogenesis of ischemic injury to brain.*

419 ISCHEMIC CEREBROVASCULAR DISEASE

419.1 Focal Ischemia

CLASSIFICATION

The clinical manifestations of focal ischemic stroke result from interference with blood circulation to the brain; the precise signs and symptoms depend on the region deprived of flow. For any brain region, however, focal ischemia can be classified into categories that have important clinical implications.

STROKE VERSUS TRANSIENT ISCHEMIC ATTACK (TIA). *Stroke* is defined as a neurologic deficit lasting more than 24 hours caused by reduced blood flow in a particular artery supplying the brain. The usual pathologic outcome is infarction. A *transient ischemic attack,* or *TIA,* by contrast, is defined arbitrarily as a similar neurologic deficit lasting less than 24 hours. Originally, the defined time limit for TIA's was less than 1 hour, but this was subsequently expanded to the longer interval for practical purposes. Nevertheless, most TIA's resolve within an hour. Once a deficit has lasted longer than an hour, it is likely to be classified as a presump-

acute phase of the ischemic stroke only to seek out a mass lesion and only after a noncontrast scan has been obtained.

CT scans immediately delineate primary cerebral hemorrhage, but hemorrhagic conversions of an ischemic infarct usually develop only after 1 to 2 days. A few continue to appear for up to 4 weeks.

Magnetic resonance imaging (MRI) is more sensitive than CT to changes in tissue structure and may provide a more accurate and earlier measure of cerebral infarction (Fig. 441–7). MRI, however, is more costly, and, with the present equipment, requires more time to perform than CT; in addition, the need to exclude ferromagnetic materials from the MRI suite, as well as the difficulty in monitoring patients in the scanner, makes MRI unsuitable for many acutely ill patients. If the diagnosis remains in doubt, MRI may be used after the acute phase to verify infarction.

Lumbar Puncture. Lumbar puncture (LP) is no longer widely used to diagnose routine stroke because, (1) noninvasive CT or MRI detects cerebral hemorrhage and, (2) anticoagulation begun within 6 hours after a lumbar puncture risks causing a spinal epidural hematoma. An LP is important, however, in diagnosing neurosyphilis or meningitis, as, for example, in patients with acute stiff neck who show no blood on brain imaging. If an LP is to be done in suspected stroke, it should be preceded by brain imaging and funduscopic examination to rule out raised intracranial pressure.

Noninvasive Cerebrovascular Examination. Several noninvasive techniques help to evaluate the cerebrovascular supply. Indirect tests that examine blood flow in the periorbital or orbital circulation include *Doppler sonography* and *quantitative oculopneumoplethysmography* (OPG).

Direct examination of the common, internal, and external carotid arteries is best achieved with *duplex ultrasonography.* Duplex ultrasonography consists of B-mode ultrasonography, which produces a real-time image of the carotid vessels and a range-gaited pulsed Doppler that is visually guided by the B-mode image to measure the frequency shift associated with increased blood velocity through a stenotic lumen. The combination of the precise location of the Doppler frequency signal and the B-mode image provides the most accurate noninvasive method for analyzing disease of the extracranial circulation. Limitations of the technique include (1) access to only the portion of the carotid circulation that lies between the clavicles and the mandible (in approximately 10% of patients, the carotid bifurcation lies above the angle of the jaw, making ultrasonography difficult or impossible), (2) absorption of sound waves by calcium within a mural plaque, which may "shadow" and obscure a plaque on a distal vessel wall, and (3) echolucency of acute thrombi, which can be indistinguishable from flowing blood.

The direction and velocity of blood flow in the intracranial blood vessels originating from the circle of Willis may be examined with low-frequency *pulsed transcranial Doppler,* a technique still being evaluated for its usefulness as a diagnostic tool. The intracranial blood vessels also can be examined on reconstructed CT or MRI images. An evolving technique involves the imaging of flowing blood using *magnetic resonance angiography.* The procedure produces images of the extracranial and intracranial blood vessels, as well as atherosclerotic abnormalities of the carotid bifurcation; some aneurysms can also be detected.

Cerebral Angiography. Intracranial and extracranial *cerebral angiography* of elderly patients prone to ischemic stroke carries a 2 to 4% risk of producing a reversible neurologic deficit and a 0.5 to 1.0% risk of permanent neurologic deficits or death. Accordingly, angiography should be reserved for specific indications in which it may reveal abnormalities amenable to therapy. Examples include a search for fibromuscular dysplasia, arterial dissection, cranial arteritis, or as a preparation for cerebrovascular surgery. *Digital subtraction arteriography* permits use of smaller amounts of intravascular contrast material and may thus be of lower risk, especially in patients with marginal renal or cardiac function. *Digital subtraction venous angiography* is no longer widely used because of its unreliability in detecting plaque ulcerations and in differentiating carotid stenosis from complete occlusion.

Other Techniques. Methods for measuring cerebral blood flow in the clinical arena are still largely investigational; they include *positron emission tomographic (PET)* methods, usually using radiolabeled water or carbon dioxide; *single-photon emission computed*

tomography (SPECT); and radiolabeled and stable *xenon* inhalation techniques.

DIFFERENTIAL DIAGNOSIS OF ISCHEMIC STROKES AND TIA'S

The clinical diagnosis of ischemic or hemorrhagic stroke relies primarily on the clinician's understanding of brain function and pathology. Deficits that evolve over weeks are usually caused by a brain mass, either *primary or metastatic brain tumor* or *brain abscess. Subdural hematoma* should be distinguishable from stroke by the hematoma's more prolonged course and its combination of diffuse and focal dysfunction.

TIA's may be confused with classic or complicated *migraine,* the former being associated with scintillating scotomata and the latter with hemiparesis or other focal deficits; some of the underlying pathophysiology may be ischemic for both TIA's and migraine, but evidence is accumulating that nonischemic electrical disturbances (spreading depression) may be involved in the pathophysiology of migraine.

Seizures can be confused with TIA's. Most seizures produce motor activity or positive sensory phenomena, whereas most strokes and TIA's produce weakness and sensory loss. Nevertheless, seizures can sometimes produce these "negative" symptoms. The postictal state following (unobserved) seizures is even more likely to imitate an ischemic deficit. Serial observations usually permit the differentiation of stroke from seizure, but rapid differentiation may be difficult and may interfere with early stroke treatment. As with migraine, strokes and seizures can coexist: A small proportion of strokes (about 10%), especially embolic strokes, are associated at onset with seizures.

Hemorrhagic stroke often enters the differential diagnosis for ischemic stroke. Although the anatomic locations of the two may differ, with hemorrhage seldom involving a discrete vascular territory, clinical differentiation can be uncertain, making CT scan necessary. Other illnesses included in the differential diagnosis of vertebrobasilar ischemia include, as mentioned above, nonspecific dizziness, Meniere's disease, or peripheral vestibulopathy.

CAUSES AND PATHOGENESIS (Table 419-2)

ATHEROSCLEROSIS. Atherosclerosis of extracranial and intracranial arteries accounts for approximately two thirds of all ischemic strokes and an even greater proportion of those affecting patients over the age of 60. Atherosclerosis causes strokes either by *in situ stenosis or occlusion* or by *embolization* of plaque material to distal cerebral vessels. In either case, the clinical and pathologic effects depend on the adequacy of collateral circulation to the affected vascular territory. It is not uncommon for unilateral or, more rarely, bilateral occlusion of the internal carotid artery to develop without neurologic symptoms, especially if the stenosis or occlusion develops slowly. In instances of marked stenosis or occlusion of extracranial arteries that is combined with intracranial atherosclerosis, cerebral perfusion sometimes can relate closely to small changes in blood pressure. One effect can be a worsening stroke deficit associated with orthostatic blood pressure changes that would otherwise be considered normal.

The more common effect of atherosclerosis is that a platelet-fibrin embolus detaches from a plaque and floats distally, where it occludes a smaller branch. Such emboli are likely to produce symptoms, since the more distal the occlusion, the less likely can collateral filling prevent damage. In cases of artery-to-artery embolization, the embolus usually emanates from a plaque at the base of the aorta, the bifurcation of the common carotid artery, or at the point where the vertebral arteries originate from the subclavian arteries.

EMBOLI OF CARDIAC ORIGIN. Cerebral emboli of a cardiac source may account for up to one third of all ischemic strokes. Thrombus formation and the release of thromboemboli from the heart are promoted by arrhythmias and structural abnormalities of the valves and chambers.

Mural Thrombi. Mural thrombi typically form under areas of dyskinetic myocardium damaged by *myocardial infarction.* As many as 35% of patients with recent anterior wall infarction harbor mural thrombi, and if not anticoagulated, nearly 40% of these will embolize systemically within 4 months after the myocardial infarction. *Cardiomyopathies* can also predispose to mural thrombi and embolization. In one study, systemic emboli were found in approximately 15% of patients with congestive or dilated cardiomyopathy,

TABLE 419-2. CAUSES OF ISCHEMIC STROKE

Atherosclerosis

Emboli of Cardiac Origin

Mural thrombus
  Myocardial infarction (anterior wall sputum, akinetic segment)
  Cardiomyopathy (infectious, idiopathic, Chagas' disease)
Valvular heart disease
  Rheumatic heart disease
  Bacterial endocarditis
  Nonbacterial endocarditis (carcinoma, Libman-Sacks)
  Mitral valve prolapse
  Prosthetic valve
Arrhythmia (atrial fibrillation)
Cardiac myxoma
Paradoxical emboli

Vasculitides

Primary CNS vasculitis
Systemic necrotizing vasculitis (polyarteritis nodosa, allergic angitis)
Hypersensitivity vasculitis (serum sickness, drug-induced, cutaneous vasculitis)
Collagen vascular diseases (rheumatoid arthritis, scleroderma, Sjögren's disease)
Giant cell (temporal arteritis, Takayasu's arteritis)
Wegener's granulomatosis
Lymphomatoid granulomatosis
Behçet's disease
Infectious vasculitis (neurovascular syphilis, Lyme disease, bacterial and fungal meningitis, tuberculosis, acquired immunodeficiency syndrome [AIDS], ophthalmic zoster, hepatitis B)

Hematologic Disorders

Hemoglobinopathies (sickle cell, HbSC)
Hyperviscosity syndromes (polycythemia, thrombocytosis, leukocytosis, macroglobulinemia, multiple myeloma)
Hypercoagulable states (carcinoma, pregnancy, puerperium)
Protein C or S deficiency
Antiphospholipid antibodies (lupus anticoagulant, anticardiolipin antibody)

Drug Related

"Street drugs" (cocaine, "crack," amphetamines, lysergic acid, phencyclidine, methylphenidate, sympathomimetics, heroin, pentazocine)
Alcohol
Oral contraceptives

Other

Fibromuscular dysplasia
Arterial dissection (trauma, spontaneous, Marfan's syndrome)
Homocystinuria
Migraine
Subarachnoid hemorrhage/vasospasm
Other emboli (fat, bone marrow, air emboli)
Moyamoya

a subgroup of the condition that is usually caused by alcohol abuse or viral infections. Patients who also had atrial fibrillation had a higher incidence of embolism (33%) than did those without (14%). None of the cardiomyopathy patients on anticoagulation, however, experienced systemic emboli.

Valvular Heart Disease. Although less common than previously, *rheumatic heart disease* often gives rise to systemic embolization. In one series, 20 to 25% of patients with mitral stenosis developed systemic emboli, although most had coexisting atrial fibrillation.

Acute or subacute *infective endocarditis* produces vegetations on heart valves, and debris that can embolize into the cerebral circulation. Many emboli are relatively small, but those associated with endocarditis caused by staphylococci, fungi, or yeast often are large enough to occlude proximal intracranial arteries. Systemic emboli are found in as many as 30% of patients dying from infective endocarditis. Prompt recognition of the heart lesion plus the presence of fever, a murmur, petechiae, and other characteristics, in patients with underlying valvular disease or intravenous drug use should prompt blood cultures and treatment with antibiotics to reduce the risk of embolism. Anticoagulation is not effective and may increase the risk of parenchymal bleeding. Infective endocarditis is associated with other forms of cerebrovascular disease, including cerebral hemorrhage, subarachnoid hemorrhage, and mycotic aneurysm, as well as cerebral abscess.

Embolization from heart valves also occurs in *nonbacterial endocarditis (NBTE),* in which predominantly platelet-fibrin vegetations form on the heart valves and then embolize into the systemic circulation. NBTE occurs commonly in association with cancer of the stomach, prostate, ovary, pancreas, and lung. In one autopsy series of patients with NBTE, cerebral emboli were found in one third. Clinically, diffuse encephalopathy as well as focal stroke is observed; associated disseminated intravascular coagulation accompanies about 20% of cases.

Libman-Sacks (atypical verrucous) endocarditis is associated with systemic lupus erythematosus. Soft, friable vegetations form on the leaflets of any of the heart valves, not just the tricuspid valve, as believed earlier. Systemic (and cerebral) emboli are rare.

Mitral valve prolapse describes a billowing of the mitral leaflets into the left atrium during systole. Although usually asymptomatic, some patients experience palpitations or chest pain. The diagnosis is suggested by auscultatory and echocardiographic criteria, but normal standards are uncertain, making the true incidence unknown; it is estimated to be 6 to 10% in healthy young women. In part because of different diagnostic criteria, the role of mitral valve prolapse in cerebral embolism remains controversial: Several analyses of strokes in young adults suggest a disproportionately high representation of patients with mitral valve prolapse, but others indexed on patients with mitral valve prolapse suggest that systemic embolism is infrequent. Coexisting infective endocarditis or arrhythmia contributes to cerebral embolism.

Prosthetic heart valves carry a high risk of systemic (including cerebral) embolism; mechanical heart valves have a higher risk than biologic valves (e.g., porcine). The overall risk of embolism is roughly equivalent in anticoagulated patients with mechanical valves and in nonanticoagulated patients with biologic valves: 1 to 3% per year for aortic prostheses, and 3 to 5% per year for mitral substitutions.

Arrhythmias. *Atrial fibrillation,* with or without valvular disease, strongly increases the risk of embolic ischemic stroke, especially in patients over the age of 60. In one large series, the risk of ischemic stroke was 6 to 7% per year in nonanticoagulated patients. The risk is highest shortly after development of atrial fibrillation: Up to one third of emboli occur in the first month. Embolism can also accompany therapeutic cardioversion. About 35% of patients with nonvalvular atrial fibrillation sooner or later will have an ischemic stroke. In some, embolism underlies the stroke; in others, the fault lies in coexisting intrinsic cerebrovascular disease associated with coronary artery disease. Even thyrotoxic, nonvalvular atrial fibrillation is associated with a 10 to 12% risk of stroke. The one group without a strikingly increased risk is patients with isolated atrial fibrillation, associated with other clinical evidence of cardiopulmonary disease.

Cardiac Myxoma. Cardiac tumors are uncommon, occurring in about 0.05% of autopsies. *Myxomas* account for about 35% of all intracardiac tumors but are the ones most likely to embolize, from either overlying thrombus or the tumor itself. In one series, about one-quarter of patients with autopsy-proven cardiac myxomas had clinical evidence of strokes. Aneurysms and intracranial hemorrhage were also reported. The coexistence of hemolytic anemia due to red blood cell trauma and lysis sometimes suggests a cardiac tumor, but firm diagnosis requires echocardiography or angiography.

Paradoxical Emboli. Emboli of venous origin have long been known to cross a patent foramen ovale into the systemic circulation. Studies using bubble echocardiography found that 40% of stroke patients under age 55 with a normal cardiac evaluation by history, examination, and ECG had a patent foramen ovale detected by bubble echocardiography.

VASCULITIDES. A group of disorders classified as vasculitides cause focal or multifocal cerebral ischemia through inflammation and necrosis of extracranial and/or intracranial blood vessels. The pathogenesis of vascular inflammation differs among these disorders, but all involve some deposition of humoral and cellular immune complexes and infiltration of polymorphonuclear and mononuclear cells in blood vessel walls. In most cases, the cause of the inflammatory response is unknown, but in others, infection, a postinfectious or neoplastic process, or a hypersensitivity immune reaction triggers the inflammation.

Segmental inflammation of cerebral blood vessels causes cerebral ischemia acutely at the site of involvement through platelet aggregation and/or clot formation or chronically through fibrinoid necrosis, which narrows the vessel lumen. Central nervous system (CNS) vasculitis, although a rare cause of stroke, is itself not uncommon and should enter the differential diagnosis whenever a young patient presents with a stroke or a patient of any age presents with a diffuse unexplained encephalopathy.

Symptoms of CNS vasculitis include cognitive disturbances, headache, and seizures (encephalopathy), which occur more frequently than with focal neurologic dysfunction. The diagnosis depends on the angiographic appearance of a "beadlike" segmental narrowing of cerebral blood vessels and/or the finding of characteristic inflammatory histopathology in leptomeningeal and cortical biopsy specimens. Cerebral angiograms may appear normal in 20 to 30% of histologically positive cases. In addition, because of the segmental or "skip" nature of the inflammatory response, the histopathology may go undetected in the presence of a positive angiogram.

The diagnosis of CNS vasculitis is aided by the presence or absence of peripheral nervous system or systemic organ involvement and by identifying the underlying cause of the inflammation. Primary CNS vasculitis, Behçet's disease, Takayasu's arteritis, and temporal arteritis are notable for their infrequent involvement or noninvolvement of the peripheral nervous system. By contrast, the hypersensitivity and systemic necrotizing vasculitides frequently produce polyneuropathies.

Primary CNS arteritis, giant cell arteritis, and vasculitis associated with certain CNS infections deserve specific attention, since these may present initially or solely with neurologic signs and symptoms.

Primary CNS Arteritis. Primary arteritis of the CNS, also called granulomatous arteritis of the CNS, causes headache and other encephalopathic-like symptoms in young or middle-aged individuals. The course is usually insidiously progressive but may wax and wane for periods of several months. It is a diagnosis of exclusion.

Giant Cell Vasculitis. Temporal arteritis and Takayasu's arteritis are characterized by a granulomatous vasculitis of medium-sized and large arteries. Temporal arteritis affects predominantly patients over the age of 60, causing constitutional symptoms such as fever, malaise, weight loss, and headache. In half the patients, symptoms consistent with polymyalgia rheumatica may coexist, including jaw, neck, and facial pain, as well as morning stiffness. Tenderness and pain over the temporal arteries and an elevated erythrocyte sedimentation rate are frequently, but not always, present. Biopsy of the superficial temporal artery provides the definitive diagnosis. Because of the segmental nature of the vasculitis, serial sections should be examined. Even then, typical features of fever, malaise, tender scalp vessels, and a grossly elevated sedimentation rate dictate the early initiation of corticosteroid therapy because of the high risk of acute ischemic blindness. A *dramatic* improvement in constitutional symptoms is semidiagnostic.

Takayasu's arteritis affects primarily young women and involves mainly the aortic arch, the large brachiocephalic arteries derived from the arch, and the abdominal aorta. Mononuclear infiltrates and fibrous proliferation produce progressive narrowing of the lumen of these vessels, causing reduced flow into the upper extremities (hence the name "pulseless disease") and cerebral ischemia. Although initially diagnosed in Japanese women, it has been recognized in Western countries.

Infectious Vasculitis. Bacterial, fungal, and viral infections can induce CNS vasculitis and cerebral ischemia (Table 419–2). Neurosyphilis and its meningovascular complications have increased considerably in recent years (see Ch. 422) and should be considered in patients with atypical or unexplained cerebrovascular disease.

HEMATOLOGIC ABNORMALITIES. Hemoglobinopathy. Among the hemoglobinopathies, *sickle cell disease* is by far the most common cause of stroke. In sickle cell disease, a single substitution of the amino acid valine for glutamate at the sixth position of the β-globin molecule causes the mutant molecule HbSS to become highly insoluble and polymerize under deoxygenated conditions. The polymerization alters the erythrocyte's shape ("sickling") and decreases the cell's deformability, leading to increased blood viscosity, microvascular sludging, and microvascular infarction. Sickle cell disease also causes hyperplasia of fibrous tissue and muscle cells of the vascular intima, leading to stenosis and occlusion of some medium to large cerebral arteries.

Ischemic stroke occurs in approximately 15% of patients with HbSS and in a much smaller percentage of those with sickle cell trait (HbSA) or HbSC. At normal arterial oxygen saturations of 95 to 100% in HbSS, some sickling is present, and at 65%, i.e., just slightly lower than normal venous oxygen saturation, approximately 75% of erythrocytes sickle. Ischemic stroke arises most frequently in children, whereas hemorrhagic stroke is more common in adults with HbSS; subarachnoid hemorrhage in patients with sickle cell disease is frequently the result of a ruptured saccular aneurysm.

Small changes in oxygen tension, dehydration, acidosis, or infection can precipitate sickle cell crisis and stroke. Cerebral angiography causes an increased risk for patients with sickle cell disease. In instances when such angiography is necessary to evaluate the source of intracerebral hemorrhage, the level of HbSS should be reduced to less than 20% through transfusions.

Hyperviscosity Syndrome. Cerebral blood flow relates inversely to blood viscosity. The latter is directly proportional to the number of circulating red and white blood cells, the aggregation state, the number of platelets, and the plasma protein concentration. Blood flow (BF) is inversely proportional to the deformability of erythrocytes and blood velocity (shear rate). Patients with the hyperviscosity syndrome can either have focal neurologic dysfunction or, more frequently, diffuse or multifocal signs or symptoms, including headache, visual disturbances, cognitive impairment, and seizures.

Cellular hyperviscosity, associated with *polycythemia, thrombocytosis,* or *leukocytosis* of any cause, can reduce BF below threshold levels for cerebral dysfunction and injury. Hematocrits above 50%, white cell counts $> 150,000$ per μl, and platelet counts in excess of 1 million per μl increase the risk of stroke.

Elevated plasma protein concentrations caused by *macroglobulinemia* or *multiple myeloma* elevate plasma viscosity and increase stroke risk. Approximately 25% of patients with macroglobulinemia experience some form of cerebral ischemia, and a lesser number of patients with multiple myeloma experience the hyperviscosity syndrome. Of the various forms of multiple myeloma, those with a predominance of immunoglobulin A (IgA) most frequently develop a hyperviscosity syndrome because this particular molecule is likely to form high molecular weight polymers.

Hypercoagulable States. Cancer, particularly the adenocarcinomas, pregnancy, and the puerperium have all been associated with a "hypercoagulable state" that predisposes to arterial and venous thrombosis. Despite the fact that any one of several abnormalities, including elevations of fibrinogen levels, alterations of partial thromboplastin or prothrombin times, and platelet aggregation, occurs in the hypercoagulable state, no tests have been devised to diagnose it specifically.

Protein C or S Deficiency. Proteins C and S are two naturally occurring anticoagulants synthesized in the liver via vitamin K–dependent mechanisms. Deficiencies of either are rare, dominantly inherited, and expressed phenotypically by incomplete penetrance. Homozygotes develop serious and frequently fatal clotting abnormalities at birth, while heterozygotes may show no signs of hypercoagulability. Proteins C and S act in concert to inactivate the activated coagulating Factors V and VIII; protein C also triggers the endogenous fibrinolytic pathways. Deficiencies in either are associated with ischemic vascular disease. Because of incomplete penetrance, the occurrence of thrombosis and stroke in the adult is extremely rare.

Antiphospholipid Antibodies. A strong epidemiologic association links a group of antiphospholipid antibodies to cerebral ischemia manifested clinically as atypical migraine, TIA, recurrent strokes, or ischemic encephalopathy. These antibodies bind to membrane phospholipids and include anticardiolipin antibody, the lupus anticoagulant, and antibodies causing a false-positive VDRL. The pathogenetic relationship between the antibodies and enhanced cerebral thrombosis is unknown. The syndrome may manifest at any age but usually affects patients younger than 50. Antiphospholipid antibodies often accompany collagen vascular disease, especially systemic lupus erythematosus, as well as valvular heart disease.

Circulating titers of phospholipid antibodies correlate poorly with either the incidence or the severity of cerebral ischemia.

DRUG-RELATED CAUSES OF STROKE. An extensive list of "street" drugs (see Table 419–2) has been associated with stroke, reflecting as much the social patterns of drug abuse as the unique properties of the drugs themselves. The sharing of nonsterile needles to inject many of these drugs intravenously (e.g., heroin, cocaine) may precipitate infectious processes (bacterial endocarditis, hepatitis B, mycotic aneurysms) that lead to strokes. Several of the drugs are potent vasoconstrictors and may initiate cerebral vasospasm. Others have been associated with cerebral vasculitis caused either by immune responses to the primary drug or by hypersensitivity to contaminating adulterants. The intravenous injection of oral medications (pentazocine [Talwin], methylphenidate [Ritalin]) that have been crushed and suspended in water can cause cerebral microemboli owing to particles of talc and cellulose used as ingredients in the pills. The particles are thought to be trapped by pulmonary arterioles, causing local arteritis and later arteriovenous shunts that allow the microemboli to reach the CNS.

Over-the-counter cold remedies and nasal decongestants containing sympathomimetics such as ephedrine, phenylpropanolamine, and phenoxazoline have been associated with ischemic stroke. Cases have been reported following the prolonged use of oral cold medications as well as in patients who chronically overuse nasal decongestants.

The risk of ischemic and hemorrhagic stroke is increased from 4- to 13-fold among users of high-dose estrogen contraceptives. The coexistence of hypertension, prolonged use of the pill, smoking, a previous history of migraine, and age exceeding 35 years seems to enhance the risk of contraceptive-related stroke. A clear association between stroke and the newer low-dose estrogen contraceptives has not been established.

OTHER CAUSES OF STROKE. *Fibromuscular dysplasia* (or hyperplasia) describes areas of segmental nonatherosclerotic arterial narrowing, usually caused by fibroplasia and smooth muscle proliferation, that alternate with rings of medial thinning. The uncommon condition affects the carotid and vertebral arteries, usually at the level of the second cervical vertebra rather than at the origin of the vessels; it also affects the renal arteries and is associated with hypertension. Fibromuscular dysplasia predominates in women and occurs, on the average, in the sixth decade of life. It produces ischemic stroke both by the hemodynamic effects of stenosis and by thromboembolism. The condition is also associated with aneurysm formation and with arterial dissection. Angiography usually makes the diagnosis, although flow studies with MRI may prove useful. Because of its rarity, there is little information about treatment.

A *dissecting aortic aneurysm,* although uncommon, can occlude major branches of the aorta supplying the cranial circulation and produce ischemic strokes. Chest, back, or abdominal pain accompanying the stroke and differences in palpable pulses or in blood pressure in the limbs suggest the diagnosis. Emergency angiography is needed to confirm it.

Extracranial *dissections of the carotid artery* are increasingly recognized. Many follow relatively trivial trauma (e.g., pharyngeal injury with blunt objects in children, and neck torsion, sometimes from chiropractic manipulation, in adults). Some are associated with fibromuscular dysplasia, others with a variety of childhood conditions, including Ehler-Danlos and Marfan's syndromes as well as tuberous sclerosis. Pathologically, intraluminal blood enters the subintimal or medial vascular planes, and the lumen becomes progressively narrowed and thrombosed. Carotid artery dissections can sometimes be recognized clinically by intense ipsilateral pain. Angiography may be needed for diagnosis, but MRI is sometimes sufficient.

Homocystinuria is characterized by dislocated ocular lenses, bone deformities, a marfanoid appearance, mental retardation, accelerated atherosclerosis, and arterial or venous thromboses. Several different genetic defects can cause homocystinuria, but the most frequent is a deficiency of the enzyme cystathionine β-synthase. Approximately one third of affected individuals have one or more strokes by the age of 15 years. In some studies, heterozygous homocystinuria has been reported in as many as one quarter of young persons who have suffered strokes. Treatment with pyridoxine or folic acid may limit disease progression.

Reactive vascular narrowing *(vasospasm)* causes ischemic strokes in two settings. One causes substantial disability in *subarachnoid*

hemorrhage (Ch. 420.1). Vasospasm also presumably explains ischemic strokes seen in a small number of patients with *migraine* headaches. Migraineurs develop ischemic strokes, either in conjunction with migraine (in which case they appear to result from a prolonged migraine attack) or remote from the attack (in which case more traditional stroke mechanisms, such as atherosclerosis, are likely to be responsible).

Fat emboli typically occur several days after trauma that includes fracture of the long bones. Although focal ischemic strokes may occur, more typically the condition manifests with seizures and a diffuse encephalopathy consistent with disseminated embolization. Associated findings include petechiae and fat emboli visible on funduscopic examination. Fat globules may be identified in urine or CSF.

Air emboli can occur with open heart surgery, in patients with pneumothorax, or in divers who ascend too rapidly to the surface. Air emboli cause altered mental status and seizures, but the changes are maximal immediately after the embolization. Segmental areas of pallor may be observed on the tongue, and there may be marbling of the skin and air emboli seen on funduscopic examination. When caused by sudden decompression, the condition is treated in a decompression chamber.

Moyamoya is a rare condition that is most common among the Japanese, in whom it has been reported to affect fewer than 0.1 per 100,000 of the general population. Diagnosis requires demonstration of bilateral terminal internal carotid artery occlusion that involves the origins of the MCA and ACA. An abnormal vascular network develops at the base of the brain that is believed to provide collateral circulation. The abnormal collateral channels appear on angiograms as a "smoky haze," hence the Japanese term "moyamoya." The cause of the vascular occlusion is unknown, but it occurs most commonly in children (peak incidence at age 6 years), in whom it may be associated with ischemic stroke; in adults, it more commonly causes hemorrhage. A similar angiographic picture occasionally accompanies acute tonsillitis, atherosclerosis, meningitis, cancer, trauma, and radiotherapy.

A condition in which the walls of small arteries are thickened and disorganized, referred to by some as lipohyalinosis, was originally believed to underlie small, subcortical brain infarcts called *lacunes.* Traditional causes of stroke, including diabetes and hyperlipidemia, have appeared in these patients with almost the same frequency as in those with nonlacunar, ischemic stroke. Perhaps as a result, treatment recommendations, which initially differed for lacunar strokes, now parallel those for nonlacunar strokes.

PREVENTION AND TREATMENT OF STROKE

Currently, there are several promising but no proven therapies for acute ischemic stroke. Even when effective treatments become available, the physician's opportunity to treat and the utility of a particular pharmacotherapy will be hampered by time constraints; the evolution of irreversible brain damage occurs within 2 to 3 hours of focal vascular occlusion (see Ch. 418). Such considerations place a premium on preventing stroke.

The reduction of stroke risk factors, through therapy for hypertension, diabetes mellitus, smoking, atherosclerosis, and cardiac arrhythmias (Table 419–3) is largely responsible for the marked decline in the incidence of stroke over the past 30 to 40 years.

RISK FACTORS AND PRIMARY PREVENTION THERAPIES

Stroke risk factors have been determined on the basis of mathematical abstractions of epidemiologic data that imply an association or a cause-effect relationship. This section categorizes such risk

TABLE 419–3. PREVENTION OF STROKE

Treat hypertension and diabetes mellitus
Stop smoking
Limit alcohol intake
Control diet and obesity
Thoughtful use of oral contraceptives
Anticoagulants for atrial fibrillation and selected acute myocardial
 infarctions
Antiplatelet agents for carotid/vertebrobasilar atherosclerosis
Endarterectomy for symptomatic carotid artery atherosclerosis of 70–99%

factors as *definite* or *presumed* and indicates whether they are related to *genetic* and *lifestyle* factors or to *disease processes*. Treatable risk factors are emphasized, and the expected outcome of such prophylactic therapy is presented.

DEFINITE GENETIC AND LIFESTYLE RISK FACTORS. *Hypertension.* This is the most powerful risk factor for stroke. Even within relatively "normal" ranges of blood pressure, the risk of stroke increases by approximately 50% for every 5 mm Hg increase in diastolic pressure throughout the range of 70 to 110 mm Hg. All components of blood pressure (systolic, diastolic, mean) correlate with the incidence of stroke, and the elevation of the systolic pressure is probably a direct cause of stroke that is independent of the secondary complications of hypertension, such as atherosclerosis or arterial rigidity. The risk of stroke is approximately four times greater in patients with definite hypertension (160/95 mm Hg) than in normotensive individuals and is twofold higher in so-called borderline hypertensive individuals. Antihypertensive therapy that lowers the diastolic pressure by as little as 6 mm Hg reduces stroke risk by nearly one quarter in as little as 2 to 3 years. Data from the Framingham Study indicate that the control of hypertension is as beneficial in reducing stroke risk in persons over 70 as it is at earlier ages.

Smoking. Smoking increases stroke risk twofold to fourfold. Those who stop smoking substantially reduce their risk of stroke over a period of 2 to 5 years, but their level of risk may not return completely to that of nonsmokers.

Age, Gender, and Race. Age, gender, and race are all unalterable risk factors for stroke, but they may signal treatable disease processes. The incidence of stroke approximately doubles with each decade between ages 45 and 85. Unlike cardiovascular ischemia, in which the incidence in men is approximately three times that in women, stroke occurs only 1.3 times more often in men than in women. The stroke risk in U.S. blacks is approximately 1.3 times that of whites. Some of the differences may be related to environmental or lifestyle factors, since southeastern blacks have a higher stroke rate than do northern ones. Similarly, the high incidence of stroke in the Japanese is not seen in their kindred living in Hawaii.

POSSIBLE GENETIC AND LIFESTYLE RISK FACTORS. *Cholesterol, Lipids, Diet, and Obesity.* Several dietary factors and obesity may play a role in stroke incidence, but the evidence is inconclusive. Diet and obesity may predispose toward diabetes mellitus and cardiovascular disease, and such patients have a higher chance of dying of stroke than do age-matched controls. Despite the incontrovertible relationship between elevated blood cholesterol and lipids and coronary artery disease, no conclusive evidence currently links lipid abnormalities to stroke. Nevertheless, most authorities strongly advise stroke-prone patients to lower elevated cholesterol and triglyceride levels. Because of the relationships that link obesity with diabetes mellitus, elevated blood pressure, and lipid abnormalities, weight control also is recommended for stroke-prone patients.

Alcohol. Moderate alcohol consumption relates inversely to the incidence of atherosclerosis and coronary artery disease, and a similar reduction of stroke risk with moderate alcohol consumption has also been suggested but not proved. By contrast, binge drinking increases the incidence of both hemorrhagic and ischemic stroke, especially when combined with cigarette smoking. Much of the latter risk may be attributable to a combination of hemoconcentration and hypertension associated with heavy alcohol consumption.

Oral Contraceptives. Although formerly available high-dose estrogen oral contraceptives were related to stroke, the association is less clear for current preparations. Nevertheless, the combination of oral contraceptives with other risk factors, such as migraine, smoking, hypertension, and age greater than 35 years, may act in combination to raise stroke risk, and many recommend against oral contraceptives in such circumstances.

DEFINITE DISEASE-RELATED RISK FACTORS. *Heart Disease.* Rheumatic valvular disease plus atrial fibrillation increases the risk of stroke 17-fold. Chronic or paroxysmal atrial fibrillation without lesions of the heart valves is associated with a fivefold increase in the risk of stroke. Chronic anticoagulation with warfarin is recommended for most fibrillators, especially those with a history of prior embolism, the presence of a left atrial thrombus on two-dimensional echocardiography, the coexistence of dilated or hypertrophic cardiomyopathy or of thyrotoxic heart disease, and

prior to direct-current (DC) conversion. Asymptomatic individuals over age 60 may be considered for anticoagulation on an individual basis. Preliminary data from a U.S. study indicated that treatment of chronic atrial fibrillation with warfarin or aspirin reduced the risk of embolic stroke by approximately 80%; other studies indicate that only warfarin confers such benefits. Furthermore, low-dose warfarin with a target prothrombin time ratio that is 1.2 to 1.5 times the control value conferred protection similar to that conferred by conventional warfarin therapy. Valvular disease related to bacterial or nonbacterial endocarditis, myxomatous degeneration of the mitral valve or other diseases causing mitral valve prolapse, mitroannular calcification, and prosthetic heart valve replacements all predispose toward cerebral emboli.

Myocardial infarction involving the anterior wall or septum is associated with a mural thrombus in up to one third of patients, and of these, approximately 15% will suffer a cerebral embolus within a 2-year interval. Acute anticoagulation therapy with heparin, with later conversion to warfarin therapy, is recommended for patients with myocardial infarction involving the anterior or septal wall or in patients with an intramural thrombus detected by two-dimensional echocardiography. Anticoagulation should continue until the two-dimensional echocardiogram indicates resolution of the thrombus. Such therapy reduces the incidence of stroke by approximately one half.

Stroke and TIA. The occurrence of an initial stroke is a powerful predictor of recurrent stroke. Patients between the ages of 45 and 65 years have a 10- to 20-fold increased risk of having a recurrent versus an initial stroke. The comparative risk drops to eightfold for those over the age of 65. The apparent decrease in the incidence of recurrent stroke with age reflects the marked increase in the incidence of an initial stroke in patients over the age of 65. The annual stroke risk following a TIA is 5% per year, which declines to 3% after 3 years. After the occurrence of amaurosis fugax, the annual risk of stroke is 1 to 2%.

Strong evidence derived from meta-analyses supports the use of prophylactic aspirin to protect against strokes in patients with prior strokes or TIA's. Similarly prophylactic antiplatelet therapy with ticlopidine has also been shown to protect against such secondary events. A decision to use antiplatelet or anticoagulant therapy in patients with prior strokes must take into account both the individual patient's risk of further functional loss and the risks of treatment.

Asymptomatic Carotid Stenosis. Individuals with asymptomatic carotid stenosis or carotid bruits have approximately a 1.5- to 2-fold increase in the risk of stroke compared with the general population. Cerebral infarction in this population, however, occurs as frequently in a vascular territory different from the stenotic artery as in the involved one. Asymptomatic carotid stenosis or bruit is a marker of cerebrovascular disease and signals an increased risk of stroke, but not necessarily one in the territory of the involved vessel. No large, randomized placebo-controlled trials have shown any efficacy of prophylactic antiplatelet therapy in patients with asymptomatic carotid stenosis or bruits.

Although prophylactic aspirin therapy in a healthy population of U.S. physicians reduced the incidence of myocardial infarction, no change occurred in the incidence of ischemic stroke, and a slight increase was detected in the incidence of hemorrhagic stroke. Antiplatelet agents cannot be recommended for stroke prophylaxis in healthy individuals.

Other Diseases. Diabetes mellitus is a risk factor independent of hypertension and is associated with an approximate threefold increase in the risk of stroke. No present data indicate that normalization of the blood sugar level reduces the incidence of stroke. Polycythemia, sickle cell disease, migraine, CNS vasculitis, and several infectious diseases all somewhat increase the risk of stroke.

SURGICAL TREATMENT FOR THE PREVENTION OF STROKE. The role of *prophylactic surgery* in the prevention of ischemic stroke is only partly resolved. A multi-institutional, randomized trial of an external carotid artery–middle cerebral artery anastomosis showed no benefit, and the procedure has been largely abandoned. *Carotid endarterectomy*, designed to remove stenotic plaques from diseased carotid arteries, was developed in the mid-1960's, and from 1971 until about 1984 the number of such operations steadily increased, despite controversy concerning its efficacy. Several multicenter trials in North America and Europe are currently examining the indications and efficacy of carotid endarterectomy versus medical therapy in symptomatic and asymptomatic

TABLE 419-4. GUIDELINES FOR CAROTID ENDARTERECTOMY

1. Recent ischemic symptoms (TIA, minor stroke)
2. Angiographically proven ipsilateral stenosis (70–99%)
3. Surgical risk ≤ 5%
4. Five-year cardiovascular life expectancy > 50%

carotid stenosis. Initial results from two studies indicate that endarterectomy significantly reduces ipsilateral stroke in patients with recent symptoms of ischemia and angiographically proven 70 to 99% ipsilateral carotid artery stenosis. Only patients with a 50% or greater 5-year life expectancy were entered in the study. The procedure is not appropriate for vertebrobasilar disease (Table 419–4). Patients with less than 30% stenosis were best treated medically. The best therapy for patients with 30 to 69% stenosis remains under examination. Likewise, we await the results of ongoing randomized trials to determine the comparative efficacy of medical therapy versus endarterectomy in patients with asymptomatic carotid stenosis. Although *angioplasty* is used widely for coronary artery disease, its utility for cerebrovascular atherosclerosis has not been established.

Surgery for *subclavian steal* is almost never indicated. This steal is a radiographic finding associated with occlusion or severe stenosis of a proximal subclavian artery, resulting in retrograde flow in the ipsilateral vertebral artery. The finding is only rarely associated with symptoms of vertebrobasilar ischemia when the ipsilateral arm is exercised. In most cases, it is merely a radiographic curiosity.

MANAGEMENT AND TREATMENT OF ACUTE TIA STROKE

Patients clinically diagnosed as having *acute cerebral ischemia* should be admitted to the hospital unless the deficit has existed for several days and is stable. The initial history and physical examination emphasize the rapid diagnosis of ischemic cerebral ischemia (TIA or stroke) and the exclusion of seizures, hypoglycemia, tumor, and other alternative diagnoses (Table 419–5). As already noted, a normal CT scan within the first several hours is consistent with an ischemic stroke. Admission is also advised for patients with *new-onset TIA's* or those in whom TIA's are occurring with markedly increasing frequency or severity (*crescendo TIA's*).

GENERAL MANAGEMENT. Once admitted, stroke patients should be maintained for at least 24 hours at bed rest to avoid postural hypotension. Since autoregulation (see Ch. 418) is usually ineffective in areas of ischemic brain, CBF will decline if systemic blood pressure falls because of postural changes or volume restriction. Hypertension, if present, should be treated, but with limited, stepwise reductions in blood pressure, for the same reason (Table 419–5). If patients have bulbar dysfunction affecting chewing or swallowing, mouth feedings should be avoided to reduce the chance of aspiration. Virtually all patients should have intravenous catheters placed to facilitate urgent treatments. If oral feedings are restricted for prolonged periods, supplementation with intravenous thiamine becomes important to prevent Wernicke's disease; eventually, hyperalimentation or feeding by nasogastric or gastrostomy tube may be needed.

In the early days of an ischemic stroke, passive range-of-motion exercises to the affected limbs can help retain mobility and prevent contractures. Later, more intensive rehabilitation individualized to improve gait, speech, dexterity, and ability to manage activities of daily living become important. Patients often benefit from brief, intensive rehabilitation in specialized hospitals before being sent home. All patients at bed rest should be encouraged to flex and extend their ankles periodically to reduce the chances of deep venous thrombosis, and all should also take occasional deep breaths to combat atelectasis.

PHARMACOTHERAPY (Table 419–6). No pharmacologic therapy has been proved effective for acute ischemic stroke. Nonetheless, several agents are used, depending on the underlying pathophysiology. Intravenous *heparin* is frequently begun on an acute basis for progressing or incomplete stroke, but as already noted, results are difficult to determine. An important point is that none of the studies of heparin have examined the effect of beginning within the first hours after stroke onset, so that poor study design may have masked detection of any benefit. A current multicen-

ter trial in North America of heparinoid therapy in acute stroke may provide better guidelines.

Despite underlying bleeding into the blood vessel wall, patients with vascular dissections are often treated with heparin in an effort to maintain patency of the vascular lumen and limit the likelihood of embolism; no proof of benefit exists. Patients with lacunar strokes were previously considered not to be helped by heparin, but some authorities have modified that view in recent years.

Patients whose strokes are attributed to emboli of cardiac origin are frequently treated acutely with heparin. Chronic oral anticoagulation is usually started concurrently, but debate surrounds the use of heparin until oral anticoagulation takes effect. Some advocate heparin because of concern about early re-embolization and the possibility that warfarin (Coumadin) sometimes enhances coagulability during the first 6 to 8 hours of therapy; others worry about the risks of hemorrhage into the initial stroke. It seems clear that the risk of bleeding is greater for larger infarcts. A reasonable course is to begin heparin and then begin warfarin after a CT scan at 48 hours reveals a small nonhemorrhagic infarct or at 5 to 7 days for a large nonhemorrhagic infarct (Table 419–6). Evidence of a hemorrhagic infarct should delay anticoagulation by 4 to 6 weeks.

TABLE 419-5. EVALUATION OF ACUTE FOCAL NEUROLOGIC DYSFUNCTION

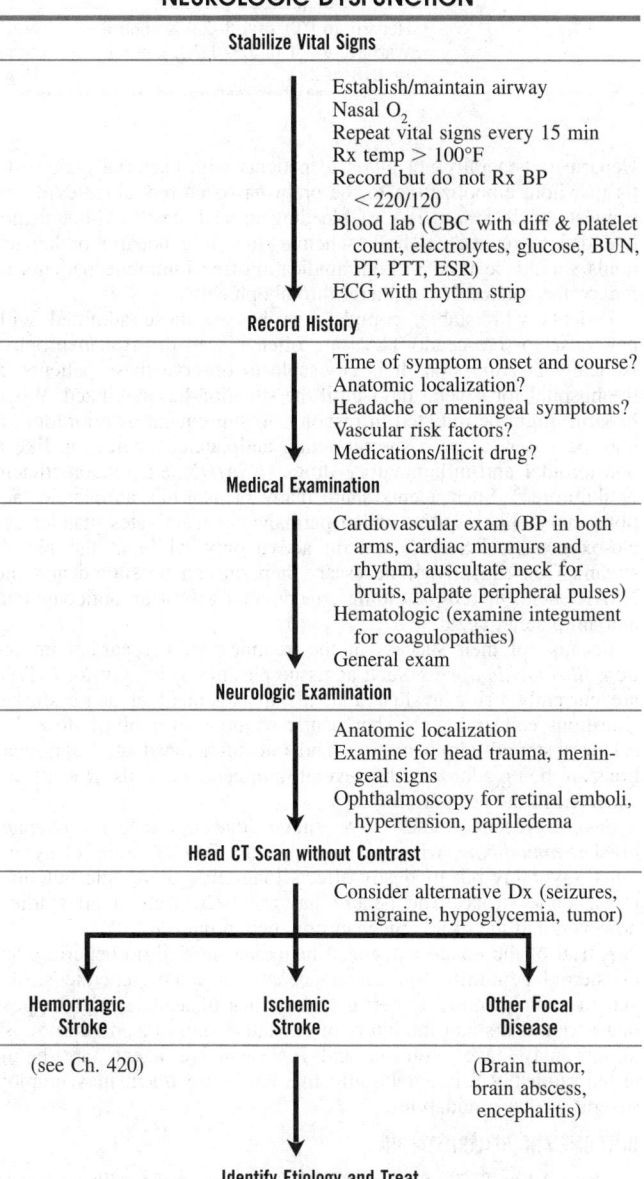

Stabilize Vital Signs

Establish/maintain airway
Nasal O$_2$
Repeat vital signs every 15 min
Rx temp > 100°F
Record but do not Rx BP
< 220/120
Blood lab (CBC with diff & platelet count, electrolytes, glucose, BUN, PT, PTT, ESR)
ECG with rhythm strip

Record History

Time of symptom onset and course?
Anatomic localization?
Headache or meningeal symptoms?
Vascular risk factors?
Medications/illicit drug?

Medical Examination

Cardiovascular exam (BP in both arms, cardiac murmurs and rhythm, auscultate neck for bruits, palpate peripheral pulses)
Hematologic (examine integument for coagulopathies)
General exam

Neurologic Examination

Anatomic localization
Examine for head trauma, meningeal signs
Ophthalmoscopy for retinal emboli, hypertension, papilledema

Head CT Scan without Contrast

Consider alternative Dx (seizures, migraine, hypoglycemia, tumor)

Hemorrhagic Stroke — (see Ch. 420)

Ischemic Stroke

Other Focal Disease — (Brain tumor, brain abscess, encephalitis)

Identify Etiology and Treat

(see TABLE 419–6)

TABLE 419–6. MANAGEMENT OF ACUTE FOCAL BRAIN ISCHEMIA

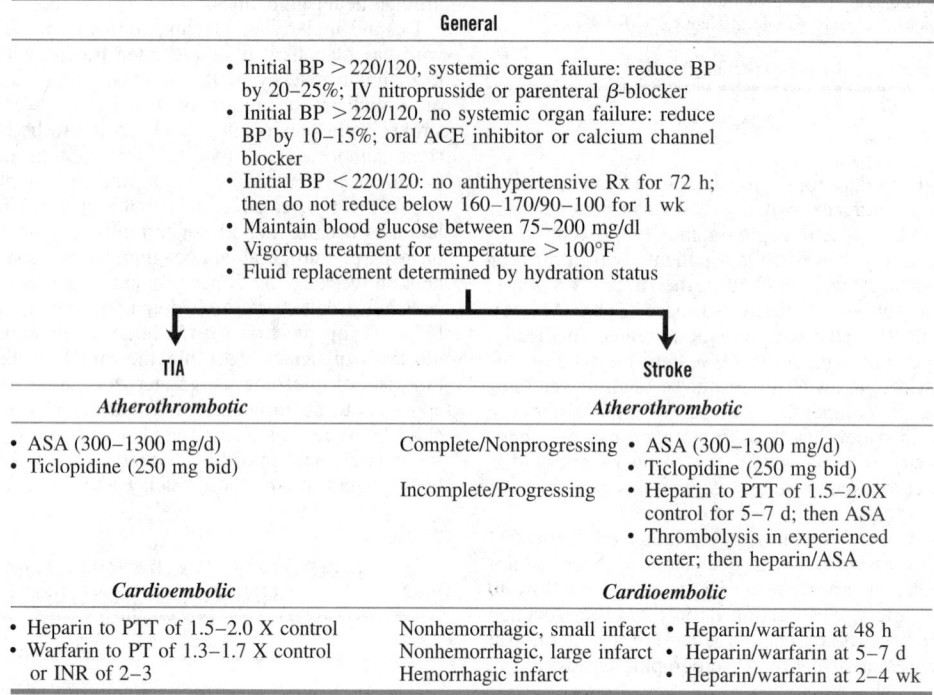

General

- Initial BP > 220/120, systemic organ failure: reduce BP by 20–25%; IV nitroprusside or parenteral β-blocker
- Initial BP > 220/120, no systemic organ failure: reduce BP by 10–15%; oral ACE inhibitor or calcium channel blocker
- Initial BP < 220/120: no antihypertensive Rx for 72 h; then do not reduce below 160–170/90–100 for 1 wk
- Maintain blood glucose between 75–200 mg/dl
- Vigorous treatment for temperature > 100°F
- Fluid replacement determined by hydration status

TIA	Stroke
Atherothrombotic	*Atherothrombotic*
• ASA (300–1300 mg/d) • Ticlopidine (250 mg bid)	Complete/Nonprogressing • ASA (300–1300 mg/d) • Ticlopidine (250 mg bid) Incomplete/Progressing • Heparin to PTT of 1.5–2.0X control for 5–7 d; then ASA • Thrombolysis in experienced center; then heparin/ASA
Cardioembolic	*Cardioembolic*
• Heparin to PTT of 1.5–2.0 X control • Warfarin to PT of 1.3–1.7 X control or INR of 2–3	Nonhemorrhagic, small infarct • Heparin/warfarin at 48 h Nonhemorrhagic, large infarct • Heparin/warfarin at 5–7 d Hemorrhagic infarct • Heparin/warfarin at 2–4 wk

Heparin is generally not given to patients with bacterial endocarditis in whom embolization to the brain has occurred, since evidence suggests an increased risk of bleeding in such cases. Although not intended to reduce cerebral ischemia, low-dose heparin or heparinoids should be used in contraindication-free immobile patients to reduce the chance of peripheral thrombophlebitis.

Patients with stable, complete strokes or those admitted with new-onset or crescendo TIA's are often placed on *aspirin* prophylactically at admission. It is advisable to observe these patients in the hospital for several days until the situation has stabilized. When heparin might be initiated in response to subsequent deterioration, it may be wiser to use a shorter-acting antiplatelet medication like a nonsteroidal anti-inflammatory drugs (*NSAID's,* e.g., indomethacin or ibuprofen). Such agents share many of aspirin's antiplatelet actions, but unlike aspirin, which permanently inactivates platelet cyclo-oxygenase, NSAID's remain active only while in the bloodstream. Consequently, if necessary, heparin can be started and the NSAID held, thereby avoiding concomitant use of an anticoagulant and antiplatelet agent.

Because of their success in the treatment of myocardial infarction, *fibrinolytic agents,* such as tissue plasminogen activator (t-PA), are currently being evaluated in the management of acute stroke. Questions concerning the therapeutic window, fibrinolytic dose, local or systemic administration, and rate of hemorrhagic complications are being addressed by several multicentered trials. Results are expected in the near future.

Several recent studies have shown that the calcium channel blocker *nimodipine,* when given within the first 12 hours of symptoms, favorably but modestly affects long-term neurologic outcome in ischemic stroke. The benefit has not been seen in all studies, however, and the drug's mechanisms remain unclear.

A trial of the opiate antagonist naloxone showed no benefit. Corticosteroid administration has no benefit in acute ischemic stroke and may be harmful. Experimental studies of acute stroke suggest that antioxidants and inhibitors of excitatory amino acid neurotransmitters may have promise, and representative agents are being tested clinically. Ultimately, effective stroke treatment may employ several of these modalities.

OUTCOME AND REHABILITATION

About 10 to 15% of patients with ischemic stroke will die, some because of brain swelling or neurologic dysfunction directly related to the stroke (e.g., impaired respiration with medullary infarctions), but most because of systemic complications, such as myocardial in-

farction, pulmonary embolism, and pneumonia. Several studies show an association of stroke with subendocardial necrosis. Most large population studies report that about one fifth of patients surviving stroke require long-term institutionalization and one third to one half of the remaining are left with various disabilities. Most functional recovery takes place during the first 3 months, but some continued slow improvement is possible.

Probably because of overlapping risk factors, the leading cause of death in patients who survive the initial stroke is myocardial infarction, underscoring the importance of cardiac evaluation. Patients who have had one stroke are at increased risk of having additional ones, particularly when the first stroke is attributed to emboli of cardiac origin.

VENOUS STROKE

Although considerably less common than arterial cerebrovascular disease, venous occlusions can cause massive damage and death. As with ischemic strokes from arterial disease, the primary mechanism of brain damage is reduction in capillary blood flow, in this instance because of increased outflow resistance. Back-transmission of high pressure into the capillary bed usually results in early brain swelling from edema and superimposes a potentially severe degree of hemorrhagic infarction in subcortical white matter.

The most dangerous form of venous disease arises when the superior sagittal sinus is occluded, but obstruction of a transverse sinus or one of the major veins over the cerebral convexity (e.g., vein of Labbé) also can produce significant damage. Venous occlusions occur most commonly in association with coagulopathies, often in the puerperal period or in patients with disseminated cancer, and sometimes as a result of contiguous disease, such as infection or cancer. The transverse sinus can be occluded as a consequence of inner ear infections, producing a once common condition called otitic hydrocephalus.

With *superior sagittal sinus obstruction,* veins draining into the sinus from the superior and medial surfaces of both cerebral convexities are commonly obstructed, and thus in its early stages, the condition can result in bilateral weakness and sensory changes in the legs. This bilaterality should alert the clinician to the possibility of sinus thrombosis. Brain swelling and bilateral involvement can produce lethargy or stupor early in the course. Seizures occur more often with venous than with arterial occlusion, possibly because of the irritating effect of parenchymal blood on the cortex.

The differential diagnosis of venous obstruction can include traditional arterial strokes but more often extends to diffuse processes such as herpes simplex encephalitis and meningitis. Diagnosis depends on the recognition of impaired venous flow. Increasingly, this is detected by loss of flow artifact on MRI. On contrast CT scans, a nonenhanced triangular area surrounded by contrast in the posterior sinus (the empty "delta" sign) should suggest the diagnosis. Since MRI is not infallible, angiography is still the definitive diagnostic procedure, but attention must be directed to films showing the venous phase.

The management of venous sinus thrombosis increasingly relies on the use of heparin anticoagulation, even in the presence of superimposed parenchymal hemorrhage. Venous occlusions are serious and often fatal, but acute anticoagulation started as soon as the diagnosis is recognized appears to lessen substantially the morbidity and mortality of the condition. Anticonvulsants should be used as needed to control seizures and limit concomitant increases in CBF that might otherwise aggravate brain swelling and bleeding. Nonanticoagulated superior sagittal sinus occlusion that is not complicated by infection carries a mortality rate of 25 to 40%. Uncontrolled series suggest that early heparin therapy can reduce the mortality and morbidity by more than half.

419.2   Diffuse Ischemia

Brief diffuse cerebral ischemia causes syncope without any permanent sequelae (see Ch. 396). Prolonged diffuse ischemia, by contrast, has devastating consequences. The most common cause is cardiac asystole or other forms of overwhelming cardiopulmonary failure. Aortic dissection and global hypoxia or carbon monoxide poisoning can cause a similar picture.

Diffuse hypoxia-ischemia typically kills neurons in the hippocampus, cerebellar Purkinje cells, the striatum, and cortical layers 3, 4, and 6. Clinically, it results in unconsciousness: coma followed often by the eyes-open vegetative state. If patients do not regain consciousness within 2 to 3 days, the prognosis for return of independent function becomes very poor. Early absence of pupillary light reflexes, corneal reflexes, and reflex eye movements predict a poor outcome. Patients lacking all of these responses even within the first day of hypoxic-ischemic coma have less than a 5% chance of resuming independent activities within 1 year (see Ch. 394). Even if consciousness is regained, such patients often suffer long-term impairment of memory and sometimes a variety of sensorimotor syndromes consistent with lesions located in a boundary zone distribution.

Other than prompt and aggressive efforts to restore cardiovascular circulation, no treatments have been found to help patients who are comatose after cardiac arrest. A randomized, multi-institutional trial of barbiturates was without benefit, and corticosteroids may even be harmful. In young patients hypoxic because of drowning, evidence suggests that hypothermia may prolong resistance to ischemic damage, but therapeutic hypothermia in adults can induce cardiac arrhythmias and has not yet been tested. Chronically unconscious patients have not been shown to benefit from either physical or electrical stimulation programs.

Antiplatelet Trialists' Collaboration: Secondary prevention of vascular disease by prolonged antiplatelet treatment. Br Med J 296:320, 1988. *A meta-analysis of 31 randomized trials concluded that aspirin reduces stroke risk by 22%.*

Barnett HJ, Mohr JP, Stein BM, et al. (eds.): Stroke: Pathophysiology, Diagnosis and Management. New York, Churchill Livingstone. 1992. *A comprehensive review of the diagnosis and management of ischemic and hemorrhagic stroke.*

Brott T, Broderick J, Kothari R: Thrombolytic therapy for stroke. Curr Opinion Neurol 7:25, 1994.

Collins R, Peto R, MacMahon S, et al.: Blood pressure, stroke, and coronary heart disease, Part 2. Short-term reductions in blood pressure: Overview of randomised drug trials in their epidemiological context. Lancet 335:827, 1990. *A meta-analysis showing a strong association between even modest hypertension and stroke and striking benefits from blood pressure management.*

Easton JD, Wilterdink JL: Carotid endarterectomy: Trials and tribulations. Ann Neurol 35:5, 1994. *Review of published and ongoing trials of carotid endarterectomy for symptomatic and asymptomatic patients.*

Editorial: Left ventricular thrombosis and stroke following myocardial infarction. Lancet 335:759, 1990. *A brief summary of recommended anticoagulation therapy to reduce embolic stroke after myocardial infarction.*

Pulsinelli WA, Jacewicz M, Buchan AM: Hypoxic-ischemic disorders in stroke. *In* Johnston MD, McDonald R, Young AB (eds.): Scientific Basis of Neurologic Drug Therapy. Philadelphia, FA Davis, 1992. *Contemporary review of the pharmacologic treatment of ischemic stroke.*

Sandercock P: Recent developments in the diagnosis and management of patients with transient ischemic attacks and minor ischemic strokes. Q J Med 78:101, 1991. *A review of current diagnosis and management of transient ischemic attacks and stroke.*

Stroke Prevention in Atrial Fibrillation Study: Preliminary report of the Stroke Prevention in Atrial Fibrillation Study. N Engl J Med 322:863, 1990. *Preliminary report of a multi-institutional study emphasizing the importance of warfarin or, at least in the nonelderly, aspirin to prevent stroke in atrial fibrillation.*

420   HEMORRHAGIC CEREBROVASCULAR DISEASE

Approximately 20% of all strokes consist of intracranial hemorrhages, half into the subarachnoid space and the remainder within the brain itself. The acute rise in intracranial pressure from arterial rupture causes loss of consciousness in approximately half the patients, and many of these die of cerebral herniation (see Ch. 443). However, since hemorrhage into the subarachnoid space or brain parenchyma causes less tissue injury than does ischemia, patients who survive often show a remarkable recovery.

Like ischemic stroke, hemorrhagic stroke can be thought of as diffuse (subarachnoid and/or intraventricular) or focal (intraparenchymal). Subarachnoid hemorrhage (SAH) is caused by rupture of surface arteries (aneurysms, vascular malformations, head trauma), with blood usually limited to the cerebrospinal fluid (CSF) space between the pial and arachnoid membranes (Table 420–1). Intracerebral hemorrhage is most frequently caused by the rupture of arteries lying deeply within the brain substance (hypertensive hemorrhage, vascular malformations, head trauma), but in some instances the force of blood from ruptured surface arteries may penetrate the brain parenchyma. Blood within the cerebral ventricles results either from reflux of subarachnoid blood through the fourth ventricular foramina or by extension from a site of intraparenchymal hemorrhage.

420.1   Aneurysmal Subarachnoid Hemorrhage

EPIDEMIOLOGY

Rupture of a saccular or "berry" aneurysm causes approximately 80% of all SAH's, 5% are caused by mycotic aneurysm rupture, and an even smaller percentage reflects bleeding from atherosclerotic, neoplastic, or dissecting cerebral aneurysms. The incidence of aneurysmal SAH is approximately 10 per 100,000 population, with 80% of these occurring in persons 40 to 65 years old, 15% in those 20 to 40 years old, and 5% in those below 20 years of age. Women are slightly more likely than men (3:2) to suffer rupture of a cerebral aneurysm, especially during pregnancy.

TABLE 420–1. CAUSES OF SPONTANEOUS INTRACRANIAL HEMORRHAGE

1. Arterial aneurysms
   a. "Berry" aneurysm
   b. Fusiform aneurysm
   c. Mycotic aneurysm
   d. Aneurysm with vasculitis
2. Cerebrovascular malformations
3. Hypertensive-atherosclerotic hemorrhage
4. Hemorrhage into brain tumor
5. Systemic bleeding diatheses
6. Hemorrhage with vasculopathies
7. Hemorrhage with intracranial venous infarction

ETIOLOGY AND PATHOGENESIS

SACCULAR ANEURYSMS. The pathogenesis of saccular aneurysms reflects a combination of congenital, acquired, and hereditary factors. Congenital defects in the muscle and elastic tissue of the arterial media, seen at autopsy in 80% of normal vessels of the circle of Willis, gradually deteriorate as they are exposed over time to the hemodynamic stresses of pulsatile blood flow. These defects lead to microaneurysmal dilatations (<2 mm) of the circle of Willis arteries in 15 to 20% of the population. Larger (>5 mm) aneurysms are found in 5% of the population, characteristically distributed at the arterial bifurcations. Eighty percent are located in the anterior, carotid artery–derived, arterial circulation; the rest lie along the bifurcations of vertebrobasilar arteries (Fig. 420–1).

The remarkably high incidence of wall defects in the media of normal vessels, the high frequency of incidental microaneurysms, and the tendency for aneurysms to enlarge with time and rupture imply that both congenital and acquired factors influence the pathogenesis of rupture. On the other hand, the relative rarity of SAH (10 per 100,000 population) suggests that other factors, possibly genetic, may predispose to aneurysm formation. A modest incidence of familial saccular aneurysms as well as their association with polycystic kidney disease, Ehlers-Danlos syndrome, and other connective tissue disorders implicates hereditary factors. Although hypertension per se is not a significant risk factor for aneurysmal SAH, aneurysms have been known to rupture under conditions associated with a sudden rise in blood pressure, including extremes of emotional excitement and physical exertion such as coitus and athletic events.

FUSIFORM ANEURYSMS. Fusiform or ectatic aneurysms acquire their name from the spindle-shaped dilatation and elongation that occur in large arteries at the site of arteriosclerotic narrowing. These aneurysms develop most frequently in the basilar artery but also may affect the internal, middle, and anterior cerebral arteries of individuals with widespread arteriosclerosis and hypertension. They rarely rupture and are difficult to treat when they do because their shape and stiff walls preclude easy surgical clipping. Progressive dilatation and the tortuous elongation of the vessel cause neurologic dysfunction most frequently by compressing surrounding structures. Typically, ectatic aneurysms of the basilar artery compress cranial nerves V, VII, and VIII, causing facial pain, hemifacial spasm, and hearing loss with vertigo, respectively. Fusiform aneurysms may initiate the features of cerebellopontine angle tumors, or they may mimic pituitary and suprasellar mass lesions.

MYCOTIC ANEURYSMS. Mycotic cerebral aneurysms are caused by septic degeneration of arterial wall muscle and elastic tissue. They form in distal cerebral arteries at the point where small septic cardiogenic emboli lodge. They are frequently multiple and can be found in either the anterior or the posterior cerebral circulation.

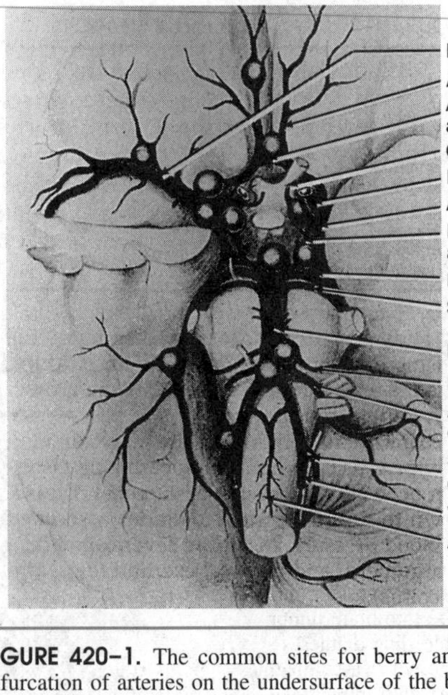

CLINICAL PRESENTATION

Prodromal signs and symptoms frequently precede the catastrophic rupture of saccular aneurysms. Focal headaches occasionally may signal compression of pain-sensitive structures from an expanding aneurysm, in which case the headache is usually progressive. They also may generate "sentinel" leaks of sudden, focal head pain. Such sentinel headaches are frequently severe and may be accompanied by nausea or vomiting or may cause meningeal irritation. Despite the similarity of these headaches to common migraine, most patients can distinguish between the two. Patients with suspected sentinel headache should have computed tomographic (CT) scans and, if these are negative, lumbar punctures to exclude active bleeding.

Compression of the oculomotor nerve by an expanding aneurysm of the posterior communicating artery at its junction with either the internal carotid or the posterior cerebral artery and, less frequently, of the superior cerebellar artery, can cause ipsilateral ophthalmoparesis, ptosis, and later pupillary dilatation with loss of the pupillary light reflex. Orbital pain frequently, but not always, accompanies these signs. The clinical picture may resemble diabetic involvement of cranial nerve III, but the latter usually spares the pupil. Other compression syndromes from cerebral aneurysms include amnesia combined with varying degrees of cranial nerve III paresis and quadriparesis from large strategically placed, basilar-tip aneurysms. Giant (>2.5 cm) aneurysms of the internal carotid artery lying within the cavernous sinus can cause unilateral ophthalmoplegia and orbital pain by compressing cranial nerves III, IV, VI, and the first division of V. Giant aneurysms of the supraclinoid portion of the internal carotid artery can produce unilateral vision loss or field defects through compression of the optic nerve or tracts.

Rupture of saccular aneurysms into the subarachnoid space seldom is associated with focal signs or symptoms. Nearly half of patients so affected lose consciousness, at least transiently, as intracranial pressure exceeds cerebral perfusion pressure. Approximately 10% of patients remain in coma for several days, depending upon the location of the aneurysm and the amount of bleeding. Patients who remain conscious and those who awaken from coma commonly recall the sudden onset as producing the "most excruciating headache" of their life. Rupture of an intracranial aneurysm in the absence of headache is rare, and some reported cases probably reflect amnesia for the event.

In addition to the frequent change in the level of consciousness, acute SAH causes meningeal irritation, nuchal rigidity, and photophobia, symptoms that may require several hours to develop. Subhyaloid retinal hemorrhages occur in 20 to 30% of patients as a result of increased intracranial pressure, raised retinal venous pressure, and dissection of blood along the optic nerve sheath. Blood pressure is frequently elevated, and body temperature usually rises, particularly during the early days after bleeding as subarachnoid blood products produce a chemical meningitis. Focal neurologic dysfunction is not a prominent feature of SAH unless there is associated compression by the aneurysm of surrounding brain structures, the jet of blood dissects directly into a clinically relevant brain region, or vasospasm occurs as a complication (see below).

LABORATORY EXAMINATION

Serum electrolytes should be measured at the time of hospital admission to serve as a baseline for detecting later complications. A complete blood count, including platelets and clotting times, should be obtained to evaluate possible infection or hematologic or clotting abnormalities. The electrocardiogram (ECG) may show various abnormalities, including heightened T waves, shortened PR intervals, peaked or inverted T waves, and increased U waves. These ECG abnormalities and subsequent arrhythmias have been attributed to multifocal myocardial necrosis caused by elevated levels of circulating catecholamines.

CT scans reveal subarachnoid blood within the basal cisterns in about three quarters of patients within 48 hours of bleeding. Magnetic resonance (MR) images have a lower index of accuracy. Detection of intracranial blood on the CT scan, however, becomes more difficult with time as blood and its breakdown products be-

Middle cerebral artery
Anterior cerebral artery
Anterior communicating artery
Ophthalmic artery
Internal carotid artery
Anterior choroidal artery
Posterior communicating artery
Posterior cerebral artery
Superior cerebellar artery

Basilar artery
Internal auditory artery
Anterior inferior cerebellar artery
Posterior inferior cerebellar artery
Vertebral artery
Anterior spinal artery

FIGURE 420–1. The common sites for berry aneurysms to develop at the bifurcation of arteries on the undersurface of the brain.

come isodense. Blood localized to the basal cisterns, the sylvian fissure, or the intrahemispheric fissure more frequently indicates rupture of a saccular aneurysm, while blood lying over the convexities or within the superficial parenchyma of the brain is more consistent with either the rupture of an arteriovenous malformation or a mycotic aneurysm. The amount and location of blood within the subarachnoid space relate directly to an aneurysm's location and the likelihood of subsequent vasospasm (see below). Importantly, an early CT scan also allows a baseline evaluation of ventricular size to compare against possible later hydrocephalus. A contrast-enhanced CT scan may aid in the identification of an arteriovenous malformation and some large (> 1.0 cm) aneurysms but should be obtained only after a noncontrast study has been completed, since contrast agents may obscure detection of subarachnoid blood.

If the CT scan fails to show blood, a lumbar puncture is diagnostic. To avoid puncture of the venous plexus lying on the anterior wall of the spinal canal, the spinal needle should be advanced slowly, with frequent removal of the trocar to detect first entry of the subarachnoid space. A traumatic lumbar puncture usually can be distinguished from SAH by the failure of the latter to show a decrease in the red blood cell (RBC) count between the first and last tubes of CSF (Table 420–2). In addition, in the presence of bloody fluid, one of the CSF samples should be centrifuged immediately and the supernate examined for the presence of hematin or xanthochromia by visual inspection and testing the fluid with a benzidene (Hemoccult) stick. Red blood cells in the spinal canal begin to lyse within 2 to 3 hours, and the centrifuged supernate will then appear pink. Later (10 hours) as the hemoglobin is converted to bilirubin, the fluid develops a yellow tinge. The CSF pressure is usually elevated and may remain so for many days. Spinal fluid samples taken within the first 24 hours often show a white blood cell (WBC) count consistent with the normal circulating WBC-RBC ratio (ca. 1:1000); later samples contain increased polymorphonuclear and mononuclear cells secondary to chemical meningitis caused by breakdown products of subarachnoid blood. The CSF blood glucose level is usually normal early, but as chemical meningitis develops, the level may decline, but rarely to less than 40 mg per dl. The protein content of the CSF is usually elevated, consistent with contamination by blood (1 mg per dl fluid for every 1000 RBC's).

Cerebral angiography remains the definitive study to detect the source of SAH. In instances in which the diagnosis of aneurysmal SAH is certain, the timing and need for a cerebral angiogram should be determined by surgical considerations (see below). When diagnostic doubt exists, the angiogram should be performed immediately. Since as many as one third of patients with aneurysmal SAH harbor multiple cerebral aneurysms, both carotid and vertebral arteries should be examined. (Among patients with multiple cerebral aneurysms, almost half have identically placed aneurysms in the left and right circulation, so-called mirror aneurysms.) Cerebral angiography fails to detect the source of bleeding in 10 to 20% of cases. Such patients are thought to have a better prognosis, with only a 1 to 2% annual chance of recurrent SAH. Failure to detect the source of bleeding may result from obliteration of an aneurysm through clotting; because bleeding was caused by rupture of a small, superficial venous angioma; or when hemorrhage has occurred from a spinal cord aneurysm or arteriovenous malformation (AVM). The presence of back pain or spinal cord symptoms at onset should prompt a search for a spinal source of hemorrhage. Repeat cerebral angiography is indicated 3 to 4 weeks later when the initial angiogram is negative and no other clues to the bleeding site can be found.

Cerebral angiography is recommended immediately in patients who have septic endocarditis and SAH to search for possible my-

TABLE 420–2. "TRAUMATIC TAP" OR SUBARACHNOID HEMORRHAGE?

	"Traumatic Tap"	Spontaneous Subarachnoid Bleed
Xanthochromia	Absent	Onset: 4–6 hr Duration: approximately 6 wk
Red cell count (serial tubes)	Decreasing	Constant
Blood clot formation	Rapid	Slower

cotic aneurysms. Since 25% of patients with subacute bacterial endocarditis and evidence of systemic embolism harbor one or more cerebral mycotic aneurysms, they should also undergo cerebral angiography.

LATE MEDICAL AND NEUROLOGIC COMPLICATIONS

The medical complications of SAH include cardiac myonecrosis and arrhythmias attributed to abnormal levels of circulating epinephrine. Symptomatic hyponatremia may also develop from the inappropriate secretion of antidiuretic hormone.

Late neurologic complications include *rebleeding* from the same aneurysm, cerebral *vasospasm* and its ischemic consequences, *hydrocephalus* caused by blockage of CSF outflow pathways, and occasionally *seizures*. Aneurysmal rerupture is suggested by new headache or neurologic worsening but can be diagnosed firmly only if a repeat CT scan or lumbar puncture shows the presence of new blood in the subarachnoid space. Approximately one third of patients with aneurysmal SAH rebleed during the first month, the incidence being highest during the first 2 weeks after the initial bleed. Patients with an unclipped aneurysm who survive their initial bleed for more than 1 month have a 2 to 3% yearly risk of rebleeding.

Cerebral vasospasm as diagnosed by cerebral angiography is defined as an abnormal narrowing of cerebral arteries. Vasospasm has been reported in up to 75% of patients with SAH, half of whom develop strokelike neurologic signs and symptoms. The peak onset for vasospasm is between days 3 and 14, but the complication can develop as late as 3 weeks after SAH. Arteries forming the circle of Willis and their major branches are the initial site of involvement, with more distal arteries becoming involved later. The amount and location of blood detected within the basal cisterns on CT scans correlate with the incidence and location of vasospasm.

The molecular mechanisms causing cerebral vasospasm are unknown but probably involve release of vasoactive amines and polypeptides, which pathologically influence vascular smooth muscle contraction. Vasospastic vessels show medial necrosis within the first few weeks, and later medial atrophy, subendothelial fibrosis, and intimal thickening.

Communicating hydrocephalus may develop as early as the first or second week after SAH. Patients with more extensive bleeding are more likely to develop the complication, but its incidence correlates with the amount of blood on CT images less clearly than does the development of vasospasm. Red blood cells and their breakdown products cause hydrocephalus by obstructing CSF outflow pathways at the level of the fourth ventricle and through the pacchionian granulations lining the venous sinuses. Seldom does communicating hydrocephalus require surgical treatment early after SAH.

Seizures are infrequent but occasionally complicate SAH. Seizures usually signal cortical damage either from bleeding into the neocortex or from ischemic necrosis.

TREATMENT

SACCULAR ANEURYSMS. The definitive therapy for a ruptured saccular aneurysm consists of surgical clipping of the aneurysm to prevent rebleeding. Medical therapy aims to reduce the risk of rebleeding and cerebral vasospasm and to prevent other medical complications before and after surgical intervention. Patients should be kept quiet at bed rest, with the administration of appropriate analgesics for the treatment of headache and gentle sedation. Stool softeners minimize straining with subsequently increased intracranial pressure. Hypertension should be treated, but not aggressively, since some of the elevated pressure may represent a normal compensatory mechanism to maintain cerebral perfusion pressure in the face of increased intracranial pressure or cerebral arterial narrowing. Systolic pressures in the range of 160 to 170 mm Hg and diastolic pressures in the range of 90 to 100 mm Hg are acceptable. The voltage-regulated calcium channel antagonist nimodipine should be given orally in a dosage of 60 mg every 4 hours for 21 days. Although it does not reduce the frequency of vasospasm, nimodipine lowers by one third the incidence of cerebral infarction in patients suffering SAH and cerebral vasospasm.

The effects of cerebral vasospasm can also be partly overcome by raising cerebral perfusion pressure through plasma volume expansion and pressor agents, usually phenylephrine or dopamine.

TABLE 420-3. HUNT CLASSIFICATION OF PATIENT'S CONDITION

Grade	Condition
0	Unruptured aneurysm
1	Asymptomatic or minimal headache and slight nuchal rigidity
1A	No acute meningeal or brain reaction but with fixed neurologic deficit
2	Moderate to severe headache, nuchal rigidity; no neurologic deficit other than cranial nerve palsy
3	Drowsiness, confusion, or mild focal deficit
4	Stupor, moderate to severe hemiparesis, possible early decerebrate rigidity and vegetative disturbances
5	Deep coma, decerebrate rigidity, and moribund appearance

Such measures, however, may raise the risk of rebleeding and should be undertaken only in patients with surgically clipped saccular aneurysms.

The optimal time to clip a ruptured saccular aneurysm remains controversial. Several studies show that patients with a Hunt grade (Table 420-3) of 1 to 3 do best if the aneurysm is clipped within 24 to 36 hours of the onset of bleeding. Otherwise, an increasingly accepted approach is to operate either within the first 3 days or after days 10 to 14. The logic relates to the timing of intrinsic rebleeding and the onset of cerebral vasospasm. Since the incidence of aneurysmal rebleeding is highest during the first 2 weeks after SAH and the mortality associated with each bleed approaches 40 to 50%, the aneurysm should be clipped as soon as possible. Nevertheless, undertaking aneurysmal surgery in the presence of active vasospasm has been associated consistently with poor neurologic outcomes. As a result, most surgeons avoid operating during days 3 to 10, when maximal cerebral vasospasm is likely. In patients whose aneurysm is clipped early, preliminary studies suggest that lysing blood clots in the basal cisterns with fibrinolytic drugs, followed by washing the blood out, may reduce subsequent vasospasm. Aneurysmal clipping should be delayed until 10 to 14 days after the last documented SAH in patients who present to hospital later than 3 days, who have active vasospasm on early cerebral angiograms, or who fall initially into a poor clinical grade (Hunt 4 and 5). In instances of delayed surgical intervention, most authorities recommend repeating the cerebral angiogram prior to surgery to rule out the continued presence of vasospasm. Some neurosurgeons also recommend postoperative angiograms to verify proper clip placement and obliteration of the aneurysm.

MYCOTIC ANEURYSMS. Unruptured mycotic aneurysms should be treated with antibiotics appropriate for the infecting organism and followed angiographically. Single aneurysms and those in surgically accessible areas should be considered for prompt surgical clipping.

PROGNOSIS

The mortality rate from aneurysmal SAH amounts to a daunting 50 to 60% after 1 year. Almost half such patients die before reaching the hospital, and most of the remaining die during the first month. An equally high mortality accompanies each episode of rebleeding. Approximately 25% of survivors have persistent neurologic deficits.

Unruptured cerebral aneurysms detected incidentally during cerebral angiography bleed at a yearly rate of 1 to 3%. Aneurysm size is strongly associated with the likelihood of rupture, so that saccular aneurysms less than 5 mm should be followed carefully, aneurysms between 5 and 10 mm may be considered for surgical clipping, and those greater than 10 mm should be clipped at the earliest convenience. The experience of the surgical team critically affects decisions and outcome concerning such treatment.

420.2 Hemorrhage from Vascular Malformations

CLASSIFICATION AND EPIDEMIOLOGY

Congenital vascular malformations of the brain and spinal cord fall into five categories according to vessel size and type. *Venous angiomas,* the most common cerebrovascular malformations, are composed entirely of veins and usually lie close to the brain's surface. Hemorrhage from a venous angioma is uncommon and rarely fatal. Nevertheless, these lesions have gained considerable attention, since they are readily detected by CT scans. They seldom produce seizures or headaches. A cerebral *varix* is a single dilated vein and very rarely causes clinical symptoms.

Telangiectasias are uncommon vascular anomalies composed of tangles of small, capillary-like vessels. They are usually located deep in the brain (diencephalon, brain stem, cerebellum) and rarely produce symptoms. Because of their strategic location, hemorrhage from these small vessels can occasionally be fatal.

Cavernous angiomas are large sinusoidal channels served by large feeding arteries and veins. Many of the channels thrombose, and the remainder have very low blood flow, which makes their visualization on angiograms difficult. They are readily detected by CT scan and rarely bleed, but they may cause headaches and seizures.

The most common symptomatic vascular anomaly is the *arteriovenous malformation* (AVM). AVM's are composed of tangles of arteries connected directly to veins without intervening capillaries. The resulting vessels are thin walled owing to poorly developed elastic and muscle tissue within the media. The large arteries, which feed the AVM, usually show hypertrophy of the media and thickening of the endothelium. Brain tissue is usually absent from the AVM but when present is nonfunctional. AVM's can be located anywhere in the brain and can produce headaches, seizures, focal neurologic deficits, or intracranial hemorrhage. Intracranial hemorrhage from vascular malformations accounts for 1% of all strokes and 10% of all SAH's. The prevalence of AVM's among the general population is uncertain, but autopsy studies of unselected patients indicate that 4 to 5% harbor some form of vascular malformation, of which only 10 to 15% produce symptoms. Familial cases of AVM's are rare, indicating that the problem reflects sporadic abnormalities in embryologic development.

CLINICAL PRESENTATION

Most AVM's manifest with intracranial hemorrhage, a lower proportion causing seizures or progressive neurologic disability as first symptoms. The initial hemorrhage tends to occur during the second through fourth decades, with the risk of rebleeding averaging approximately 6 to 7% the first year, 2% after 5 years, and 1 to 2% thereafter. The decline in the incidence of rebleeding with time may reflect the spontaneous thrombosis of arterial feeders. The initial and subsequent hemorrhages are associated with a 10% chance of death. If the rebleed rate of 1 to 2% is maintained for life, the young individual who presents with a hemorrhagic AVM faces a 50 to 60% chance of an incapacitating or fatal repeat hemorrhage during a normal lifespan.

AVM's may bleed into the subarachnoid space, into the brain parenchyma, or into the ventricular system. Focal neurologic signs and symptoms depend upon the severity of the bleed and the extent to which brain parenchyma has been destroyed. Bleeding into the subarachnoid space is usually less severe than with saccular aneurysms, and blood tends to localize over the cerebral convexities rather than in the basal cisterns. The incidence of cerebral vasospasm with AVM hemorrhage appears less than for aneurysm SAH, perhaps because less blood accumulates around the large arteries at the base of the brain. No explanation has been provided for the observation that small AVM's (<2.5 cm) tend to bleed more frequently than do large AVM's (>5 cm).

Approximately one third of patients who harbor an AVM present with seizures, of which about half have a focal onset. Focal neurologic deficits independent of seizures also develop, resulting from vascular thrombosis and brain tissue hypoperfusion caused by either vascular compression or a "steal" syndrome. Shunting of blood through arteriovenous fistulas may draw blood away from normal brain tissue, causing hypoperfusion and dysfunction of the brain proximal to the AVM. With treatment of the AVM, either through surgical resection or by embolization of the feeding arteries, some of these focal neurologic signs may improve or disappear. Approximately 10% of patients with AVM's have a history of headache, the location of which seldom coincides with the site of the AVM. Some AVM-associated headaches closely resemble migraine, but unlike migraine, most AVM-associated headaches rarely alternate between the two sides of the head.

LABORATORY EXAMINATION

The laboratory evaluation for intracranial hemorrhage from an AVM is similar to that described for aneurysmal SAH. A CT scan with contrast is diagnostic in approximately 85% of patients. MR images are equally, if not more, effective in diagnosis. Angiography remains the definitive test to identify the AVM and delineate its feeding arteries and draining veins. Since approximately 10% of AVM's are associated with saccular aneurysms, four-vessel angiography is indicated even if the AVM is defined by unilateral carotid injection. In addition, extracranial or contralateral arteries occasionally supply intracranial AVM's and should be considered in the angiographic evaluation.

TREATMENT

Uncertainties concerning the natural history of unruptured AVM's, as well as the efficacy and complications associated with newer forms of interventional therapy, make it difficult to define a simple set of guiding therapeutic principles. Generally speaking, unruptured AVM's that manifest with either seizures or headache may be treated conservatively, especially in patients older than 55 to 60 years. In such patients, hypertension should be controlled, platelet antiaggregating agents and anticoagulants avoided, and anticonvulsants given to control the seizures.

Interventional therapeutic options include surgical resection of the AVM, embolization of the feeding arteries, or radiation-induced thrombosis. Various considerations, including age, degree of neurologic dysfunction, and location of the AVM, must be considered when choosing treatment. The present custom is to treat younger patients (<55 years) more aggressively, resecting surgically accessible AVM's, since removal of the AVM and *all* its arterial feeders is curative. In older patients or if the AVM lies in language-vulnerable areas or deep in the brain, use of focused gamma x-rays or proton beam radiation is safer but only effective in lesions less than 3 cm in diameter. Embolization of the feeding arteries is rarely recommended as the sole interventional therapy, since such an approach totally obliterates the arterial feeders in only about 40% of cases. Arterial embolization is frequently used in conjunction with either surgery or focused radiation therapy.

420.3 Focal Cerebral Hemorrhage

Focal hemorrhage occurs spontaneously in three common settings: hypertension, ruptured AVM's, and amyloid (or congophilic) angiopathy. Additional contributing causes are excessive anticoagulation, systemic bleeding diatheses, and trauma.

EPIDEMIOLOGY

In the United States, primary intracerebral hemorrhage occurs with an incidence of about 12 per 100,000 population, a rate similar to that for SAH but only 10% that for ischemic stroke. Age-adjusted rates for men are about 50% higher than for women, and rates for blacks are over twice those for whites. As with ischemic stroke, the incidence appears to be declining; excluding hemorrhage associated with anticoagulation, the rate in Rochester, Minnesota, fell from about 15 per 100,000 in 1945 to 5 per 100,000 in the early 1970's. The incidence of hypertension also declined in frequency during the same period, but no conclusive data link the two trends.

PATHOLOGY

The pathologic picture of primary intracerebral hemorrhage typically consists of a large confluent area of blood that clots and then weeks later begins slowly to be phagocytosed; after several months, the only residuum may be a small, collapsed cavity lined by hemosiderin-containing macrophages. Although hemorrhages may destroy brain tissue locally, histologic examination suggests that displacement of normal brain tissue and dissection along fiber tracts account for much of the pathology.

PATHOGENESIS

Hypertension can produce hemorrhages throughout the brain, but usually they occur in four central locations: external capsule–putamen, internal capsule–thalamus, central pons, and cerebellum (Fig. 420–2). A smaller number arise in the subcortical white matter, especially in the polar regions of the frontal, temporal, and occipital lobes. Bleeding producing central hemorrhages is believed to result from rupture of microaneurysms in small, intracerebral arteries (50 to 150 μm in diameter). The pathology of the microaneurysms includes replacement of normal lining endothelium, media, and elastic tissue with fibrous tissue and fat. Similar changes can lead to necrotic vascular degeneration, which, along with microaneurysms, predisposes to hemorrhage. A strong relationship links microaneurysms to hypertension; in one autopsy series, microaneurysms were found in 46 of 100 hypertensive brains and in 85% of hypertensive persons with hemorrhages, but in only 7 of 100 normotensive brains.

Amyloid (or congophilic) angiopathy is a pathologic diagnosis, increasingly encountered in the elderly. Unrelated to generalized amyloidosis and occasionally hereditary, the condition often appears in the brains of patients with Alzheimer's disease and has been associated with nonhypertensive hemorrhages in the cerebral polar and white matter areas (Fig. 420–2). It is rare in patients under age 55. Amyloid deposits, chemically related to those in Alzheimer plaques, are seen in the media and adventitia of medium- and small-sized arteries. Multiple small hemorrhages may be associated with the condition.

Anticoagulation, fibrinolysis, and other hematologic abnormalities can be associated with intracerebral hemorrhages. Warfarin anticoagulation has been implicated in about 10% of primary intracerebral hemorrhages. With the less aggressive programs of low-dose warfarin anticoagulation (target prothrombin time ratio of 1.2 to 1.5) now used for peripheral venous disease and to prevent arterial embolism, the rate of intracranial bleeding in one recent study had fallen to under 1% with 2 years of treatment. Data from large-scale studies of fibrinolysis (e.g., tissue plasminogen activator,

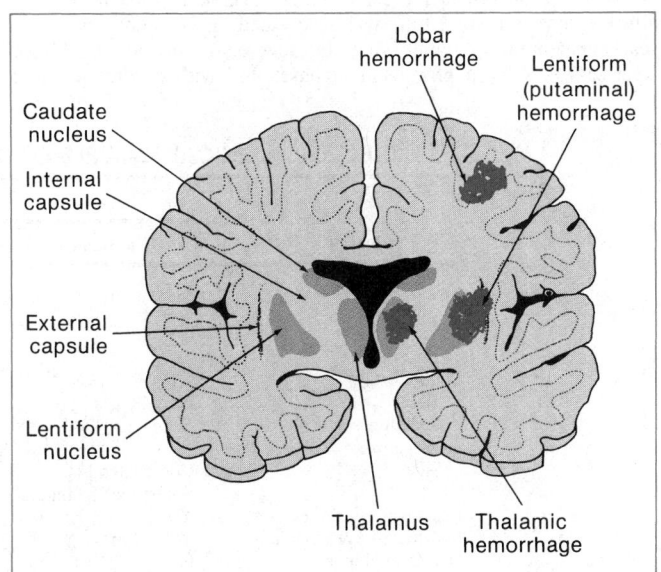

FIGURE 420–2. A coronal section through the cerebral hemispheres illustrating thalamic, putaminal, and lobar subcortical hemorrhages.

t-PA) in acute myocardial infarction indicate that at a total t-PA dose no greater than 100 mg, the rate of symptomatic intracerebral hemorrhage is only about 0.5% (although in one small series, it was 5%); at higher doses of 150 mg, the rate rises to about 1.5%. Cerebral hemorrhages occur in *leukemia, polycythemia, hemophilia,* and other clotting abnormalities, and they also occur in patients using *amphetamines* and *cocaine.*

Although *trauma* causes intracerebral (as well as subarachnoid) hemorrhage, the diagnosis is usually aided by the history as well as by coexistent external signs of trauma, SAH, and, on CT scan, multifocal, inhomogeneous hemorrhages and areas of decreased density (see Ch. 487).

CLINICAL PRESENTATION

Large cerebral hemorrhages usually produce catastrophic, acute syndromes. The onset is often associated with physical (or emotional) activity; onset during sleep is rare. Common early features include alterations in consciousness, headache, nausea, and vomiting. Although uncommon, seizures occur, possibly reflecting cortical irritation by blood. With the increasing ability to recognize less dramatic hemorrhages by using CT and MRI, neurologists now realize that hemorrhages also can produce less severe dysfunction that may be indistinguishable clinically from ischemic stroke. Clinical evolution over hours is common and usually attributed to secondary brain swelling.

The clinician should be able to recognize common hemorrhagic syndromes (Table 420–4) to anticipate dangerous brain swelling and provide appropriate medical and supportive management.

PUTAMINAL HEMORRHAGE (35 TO 50%). Patients with massive putaminal hemorrhages (Fig. 420–3) become lethargic or comatose within minutes to hours of onset and concurrently develop contralateral weakness (including face) and a contralateral hemianopsia and gaze paresis (with eyes deviated toward the hemorrhage).

THALAMIC HEMORRHAGE (10 TO 15%). Some patients with thalamic hemorrhages lose consciousness early in the clinical course, but those who are awake often experience contralateral hemiparesis, sensory changes, and homonymous hemianopsia (the last often clearing quickly).

PONTINE HEMORRHAGE (10 TO 15%). Traditional teaching held that coma always accompanied the onset of pontine hemorrhage, but refined imaging shows that this is not always the case with smaller hemorrhages. In the comatose patient, small, reactive pupils are common, oculovestibular responses are lost early, and vomiting often occurs at onset. Patients usually have quadriplegia and bilateral extensor posturing.

CEREBELLAR HEMORRHAGE (10 TO 30%). Because cerebellar hemorrhage initially spares the brain stem, consciousness is usually preserved in the early stages. Occipital headache is usually the first symptom, followed by unsteady gait, clumsiness, nausea, and vomiting, which may be severe and repetitive. Motor weakness is seldom prominent at onset, but with progression and

brain stem compression, contralateral hemiparesis and caloric-resistant ipsilateral gaze paresis help to localize the lesion to the posterior fossa. Pupillary reactions are usually preserved. Further deterioration in arousal can result from several sources: extension into or compression of the brain stem, herniation of cerebellar tissue downward through the foramen magnum or upward across the tentorium, or hydrocephalus caused by obstruction of CSF flow into or out of the fourth ventricle. Prompt recognition and treatment of cerebellar hemorrhage by this stage can be life saving.

LOBAR CEREBRAL HEMORRHAGE. Lobar hemorrhages typically occur with amyloid angiopathy. The clinical presentation depends on the actual location of the hemorrhage, but there are some common features. Most patients are elderly; headache, nausea, and vomiting probably occur with about the same frequency but less intensity as in deep, hypertensive hemorrhages. Coma and seizures are less common, possibly because the bulk of the hemorrhage is comparatively small and located in subcortical white matter.

LABORATORY EXAMINATION

Noncontrast CT scans demonstrate areas of hemorrhage as zones of increased density and rule out infarction (Fig. 420–3). Spontaneous hemorrhages typically display homogeneous areas of increased density and a mass effect, whereas hemorrhagic infarctions are characterized by areas of increased density (blood) interspersed with areas of decreased density (infarction). CT does not always distinguish reliably between a primary intraparenchymal hemorrhage and a hematoma resulting from a ruptured aneurysm. Similarly, some primary intracerebral hemorrhages dissect into the ventricular or subarachnoid system, inducing secondary intraventricular hemorrhage or SAH.

The MRI picture of hemorrhage depends on the precise sequence used and the age of the hemorrhage. At present, the advantages and disadvantages of MRI in this condition remain incompletely described, particularly in the early hours after onset. One advantage of MRI is its ability to detect small hemorrhages, especially in the brain stem. Cerebral angiography is seldom used to evaluate acute hemorrhages, except those attributed to mycotic aneurysms being evaluated for surgical intervention.

TREATMENT

The management of acute parenchymal hemorrhage is supportive, but vigilance for transtentorial or foramen magnum herniation must be exercised, particularly with cerebellar hemorrhages. Incipient herniation is initially treated with hyperventilation (which takes advantage of the vasoconstricting effect of hypocapnia; see Ch. 394) and osmotic agents (e.g., mannitol), but both of these interventions lose effectiveness with time. Corticosteroids have not been effective in treating brain edema from cerebral hemorrhage, and since they carry added risks (e.g., immunologic compromise, gastrointestinal hemorrhage), they are not advocated.

Direct surgical evacuation of acute spontaneous cerebral hemorrhage seldom is justified, occasional cerebellar hemorrhages providing a possible exception. What few comparative studies are available suggest that acute surgical evacuation of hematomas from the

TABLE 420–4. CLINICAL FEATURES OF COMMON HYPERTENSIVE HEMORRHAGES

Clinical	Site of Hemorrhage			
	Putaminal	*Thalamic*	*Pontine*	*Cerebellar*
Unconsciousness	Later	Later	Early	Late
Hemiparesis	Yes	Yes	Quadriparesis	Late
Sensory change	Yes	Yes	Yes	Late
Hemianopic	Yes	Yes	No	No
Pupils:				
Size	Normal	Small	Small	Normal
Reaction	Yes	Yes or no	Yes or no	Yes
Gaze paresis:				
Side	Contralateral Sometimes ipsilateral	Contralateral	Ipsilateral	Ipsilateral
Response to calories	Yes	Yes	No	Yes or no
Downward eye deviation	Yes	No	No	
Ocular bobbing	No	No	Sometimes	Sometimes
Gait lost	No	No	Yes	Yes
Vomiting	Occasional	Occasional	Often	Severe

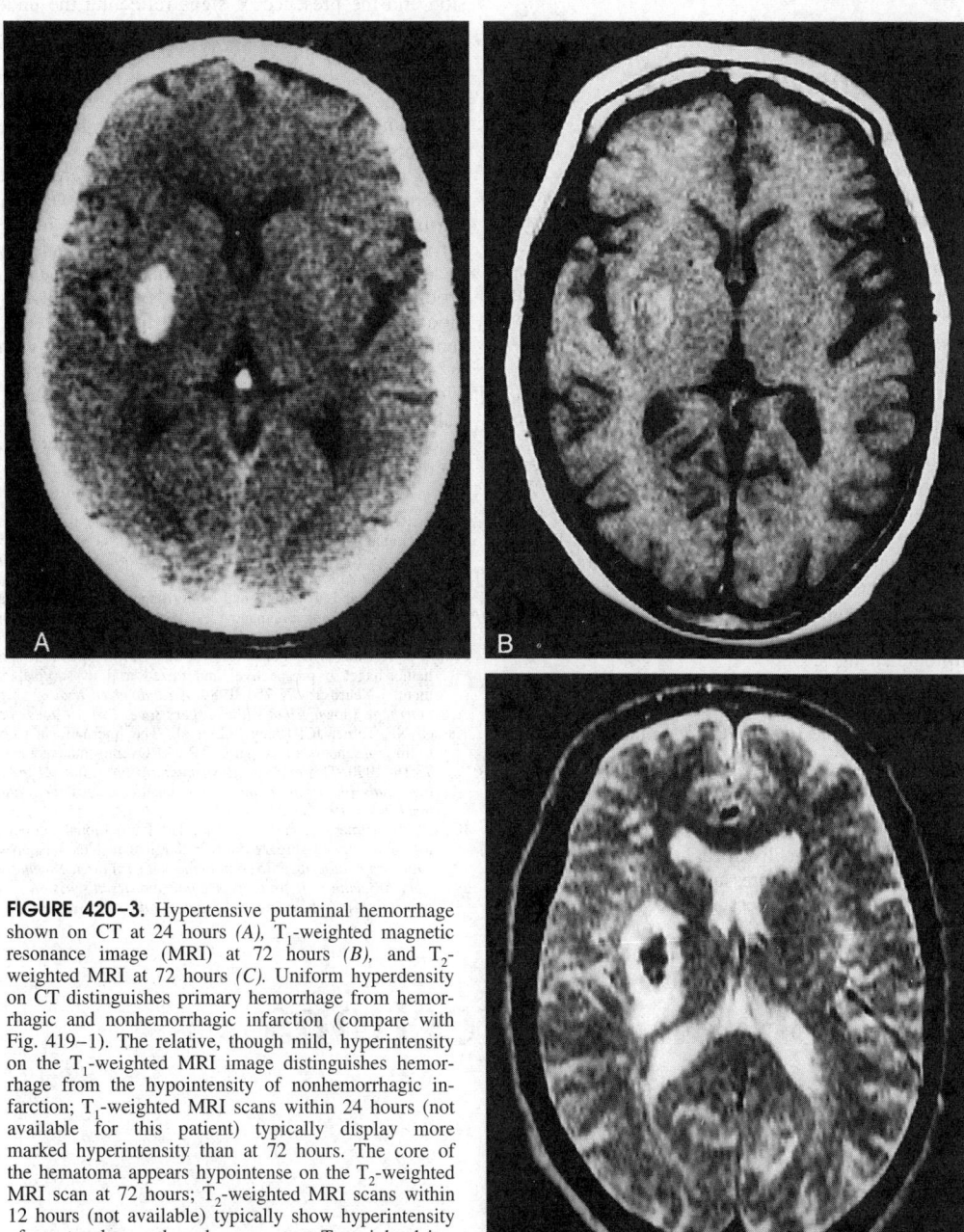

FIGURE 420–3. Hypertensive putaminal hemorrhage shown on CT at 24 hours *(A)*, T$_1$-weighted magnetic resonance image (MRI) at 72 hours *(B)*, and T$_2$-weighted MRI at 72 hours *(C)*. Uniform hyperdensity on CT distinguishes primary hemorrhage from hemorrhagic and nonhemorrhagic infarction (compare with Fig. 419–1). The relative, though mild, hyperintensity on the T$_1$-weighted MRI image distinguishes hemorrhage from the hypointensity of nonhemorrhagic infarction; T$_1$-weighted MRI scans within 24 hours (not available for this patient) typically display more marked hyperintensity than at 72 hours. The core of the hematoma appears hypointense on the T$_2$-weighted MRI scan at 72 hours; T$_2$-weighted MRI scans within 12 hours (not available) typically show hyperintensity of greater degree than do concurrent T$_1$-weighted images. The rim of hyperintensity in C probably represents edema fluid. (Reproduced with permission from Zimmerman RD, et al.: AJNR 9:47–57, 1988.)

cerebral hemispheres do not substantially improve mortality and considerably increase the risk of severe residual neurologic disability if the patient survives. With the cerebellum, lateral ventricular shunting appears to produce results as good as or better (fewer neurologic residua) than surgical removal of hematomas, although lesions greater than 3 cm in diameter that continue to compress the brain stem after the shunt is placed occasionally benefit from evacuation.

As with ischemic strokes, blood pressure should not be lowered precipitously in patients with acute cerebral hemorrhage, since parenchymal blood and edema formation are likely to compress the tissue vascular bed and increase vascular resistance; an abrupt and steep reduction in systemic blood pressure could lower perfusion pressure below the critical threshold, thereby superimposing ischemic on hemorrhagic damage.

PROGNOSIS

The prognosis with intraparenchymal hemorrhage is surprisingly good in patients who survive the acute illness, but mortality is higher (30 to 40%) than in ischemic stroke (10 to 20%). As with ischemic stroke, recent studies show that about one fifth of patients surviving hemorrhage require institutionalization; in contrast to ischemic stroke, however, most of the remaining survivors of hemorrhage achieve a good status or complete recovery. Age and large hemorrhage size are associated with a worse prognosis, and prognosis after extensive brain stem hemorrhage is guarded. In contrast to SAH, the risk of recurrent hemorrhage is relatively low, the exception being that AVM's can rebleed at rates approaching 2% per year within the first several years of the initial bleed.

PROPHYLAXIS

Epidemiologic data strongly suggest that control of hypertension reduces the risk of hypertensive intraparenchymal hemorrhage. Careful control of anticoagulation and avoidance of other agents known to be associated with hemorrhage (e.g., amphetamines) should reduce the risk of hemorrhage. At present, there is no way to control the risk of bleeding from amyloid angiopathy.

420.4 Hypertensive Encephalopathy

Hypertensive encephalopathy is a syndrome that accompanies markedly elevated blood pressures. Clinically, the disorder is characterized by symptoms of increased intracranial pressure (headache, nausea, vomiting, visual blurring) and of focal neurologic dysfunction, along with seizures and progressive stupor and coma. Retinal changes characteristic of severe hypertension are common and often include hemorrhages or papilledema, but arteriolar narrowing may be the only abnormality.

The cause of neurologic dysfunction is not clearly established. One theory, largely discounted, was based on observed retinal vasospasm and suggested that similar intracerebral vasospasm caused focal ischemia and resultant neurologic dysfunction. More recent evidence rests on the observation that with severe hypertension the upper limit of cerebral arterial autoregulation is exceeded, and blood flow rises passively with further increases in systemic blood pressure. Coincidentally, progressively higher pressures are transmitted into the capillary system, causing movement of plasma and even some cellular elements from blood into surrounding brain tissue. Resulting local and diffuse edema is postulated to cause the focal and diffuse neurologic changes.

Uremia uncomplicated by hypertension can produce a similar clinical picture, but this is easily excluded by determining the blood urea nitrogen (BUN) or creatinine values. Other complications of hypertension to be considered in the differential diagnosis include hemorrhagic and ischemic stroke, but in these conditions, focal signs predominate, whereas in hypertensive encephalopathy they are accompanied by prominent signs of diffuse dysfunction. Increased intracranial pressure from obstructive hydrocephalus, brain tumor, or subdural hematoma, particularly if pressure is transmitted into the fourth ventricle, can elevate blood pressure and slow the pulse.

Usually, the absence of retinal changes suggesting chronic hypertension and the presence of signs reflecting the underlying neurologic diagnosis differentiate such neurogenic hypertension from hypertensive encephalopathy.

Hypertensive encephalopathy is a medical emergency. Treatment should be directed to acute, deliberate lowering of blood pressure (e.g., with intravenous nitroprusside), but avoiding hypotensive or even normal levels. In most patients with chronic hypertension, the upper and lower limits of autoregulation are shifted upward, and if systemic pressure is lowered below the lower limit of the patient's intrinsic autoregulation (which can rise as high as 120 mm Hg), cerebral ischemia can result. When associated with pregnancy (eclampsia), hypertensive encephalopathy usually responds well to prompt delivery of the fetus. Hypercapnia, by dilating cerebral blood vessels, can exacerbate the effects of hypertensive encephalopathy, and seizures also are associated with further increases in cerebral blood flow and capillary pressure. Both should be avoided by controlled ventilation, when required, with anticonvulsants such as intravenous diazepam, 10 to 20 mg given slowly in repeated doses as needed to control seizures, and followed by phenytoin or carbamazepine.

Brown RD Jr, Wießbers DO, Forbes G, et al.: The natural history of unruptured intracranial arteriovenous malformations. J Neurosurg 68:352, 1988. *A follow-up study of 168 patients to define the natural history of clinically unruptured intracranial AVM's.*

Dias MS, Sekhar LN: Intracranial hemorrhage from aneurysms and arteriovenous malformations during pregnancy and the puerperium. Neurosurgery 27:855, 1991. *A review article discussing risks and medical and surgical management.*

Juvela S, Heiskanen O, Potanen A, et al.: The treatment of spontaneous intracerebral hemorrhage: A prospective randomized trial of surgical and conservative treatment. J Neurosurg 70:755, 1989. *A randomized trial of 52 patients with brain hemorrhage showing that while surgery saves lives, it does not improve function.*

Kassell NF, Torner JC, Haley EC, et al.: The International Cooperative Study on the timing of aneurysm surgery. Part 1: Overall management results. J Neurosurg 73:18, 1990. *This manuscript summarizes the results of the International Cooperative Study on saccular aneurysms and documents the status of medical management in the 1980's.*

Kassell NF, Torner JC, Jane JA, et al.: The International Cooperative Study on the timing of aneurysm surgery. Part 2: Surgical results. J Neurosurg 73:37, 1990. *This manuscript describes 3521 patients with ruptured saccular aneurysms who came from 68 centers. It presents a contemporary discussion of the diagnosis of SAH, prevention of rebleeding, vasospasm, and early versus late surgical intervention.*

Section Seven—Infections and Inflammatory Disorders of the Nervous System

Roger P. Simon

421 PARAMENINGEAL INFECTIONS

Parameningeal central nervous system (CNS) infections include those that affect brain parenchyma directly (brain abscess), those that produce suppuration in potential spaces covering the brain and spinal cord (epidural abscess and subdural empyema), those that produce occlusion of the contiguous venous sinuses and cerebral veins (cerebral venous sinus thrombosis), and remote infectious processes (bacterial endocarditis and sepsis) that result in diffuse, multifactorial involvement of the CNS.

BRAIN ABSCESS

Brain abscess is an uncommon disorder accounting for only 2% of intracranial mass lesions. Abscesses produce localized, circumscribed, enlarging CNS infections that produce symptoms and findings similar to those of other space-occupying lesions, such as brain tumors. Brain abscesses, however, often progress more rapidly than tumors and more frequently affect meningeal structures.

ETIOLOGY. Infections resulting in brain abscess originate or extend from extracerebral locations. Although the most frequent predisposing factors have changed over the past decades and vary with a hospital's population and referral base, the most common (Table 421–1) are bloodborne metastases from unknown sources and from lung or heart, direct extension from parameningeal sites (otitis, cranial osteomyelitis, sinusitis), recent or remote head trauma or neurosurgical procedures, and infections associated with cyanotic congenital heart disease. Bloodborne infections seed the brain via hematogenous spread and produce abscesses in brain re-

TABLE 421–1. SUMMARY OF UCSF CASES ACCORDING TO TIME PERIODS

	1970–1974	1975–1980	1981–1986	Total
Number of Cases	22	33	47	102
Etiology				
Local infection	2(9)	4(12)	13(28)	19(19)
Cardiac	6(27)	6(18)	5(11)	17(17)
Surgery	1(4)	7(2)	8(17)	16(16)
Trauma	2(9)	1(3)	6(13)	9(9)
Pulmonary	4(18)	4(12)	1(2)	9(9)
Immunocom-promise	2(9)	2(6)	2(4)	6(6)
Other	1(4)	4(12)	0(0)	5(5)
Unknown	4(18)	4(12)	13(28)	21(21)
Organisms				
Aerobic	16(73)	27(82)	34(72)	77(75)
Anaerobic	5(23)	8(24)	7(15)	20(20)
Multiple	5(23)	8(24)	7(15)	20(20)
None cultured	6(27)	6(18)	14(30)	26(25)
Deaths	9(41)	3(9)	2(4)	14(14)

Figures in parentheses indicate percentages.
Adapted with permission from Mampalam TJ, Rosenblum ML: Trends in the management of bacterial brain abscesses: A review of 102 cases over 17 years. Neurosurgery 23:451, 1988.

gions in proportion to the blood flow; accordingly, parietal lobe abscesses predominate. Extension of infection from otitis and mastoiditis involves contiguous brain regions of the temporal lobe and cerebellum, whereas abscesses resulting from sinusitis affect the frontal and temporal lobes. Currently, the most common cause of brain abscess in many urban hospitals is toxoplasmosis occurring in immunodeficiency states due to co-infection with the human immunodeficiency virus (HIV).

PATHOLOGY. On the basis of findings of clinical and experimental research, most brain abscesses evolve over a number of stages, beginning with vascular seeding of brain parenchyma, producing early cerebritis during the first 1 to 3 days. Inflammatory infiltrates of polymorphonuclear cells, lymphocytes, and plasma cells follow within 24 hours. By 3 days, the surrounding area shows a marked increase in perivascular inflammation. The late cerebritis phase develops approximately 4 to 9 days after infection, during which time the center becomes necrotic, containing a mixture of debris and inflammatory cells. Neovascularity is maximal at this time. Early reactive astrocytes surround the zone of infection and proceed to early capsule formation between approximately 10 and 13 days. At this time, the necrotic center shrinks slightly, and a well-developed peripheral fibroblast layer evolves. The late capsule stage continues to evolve between 14 days and 5 weeks, with continual shrinking of the necrotic center and a *relative decrease* in the inflammatory cells. The capsule thickens as reactive astrocytes proliferate.

BACTERIOLOGY. The pathogenic organisms vary considerably, depending on the clinical circumstances. *Staphylococcus aureus* is the most common isolate in trauma-related cases. In patients with HIV-associated disease, *Toxoplasma* is the most common organism and bacterial abscesses are rare. Among other abscesses, the most commonly isolated pathogens are anaerobic organisms, but aerobic and microaerobic streptococci, *Staphylococcus aureus*, *Bacteroides, Proteus,* and other gram-negative bacilli may also be found (Table 421–1). *Actinomyces, Nocardia,* and *Candida* are less frequent offenders. Infection is often polymicrobial. Culture-negative abscesses from surgical specimens occur in 30% of antibiotic-treated patients and in 5% of patients operated on before antibiotic administration.

CLINICAL PRESENTATION. Signs of infection may be minimal or absent. Almost half of affected patients maintain a normal body temperature, and fewer than a third show a peripheral white cell count above 11,000 per microliter. Neck stiffness is rare in the absence of increased intracranial pressure.

Otherwise, the presenting features resemble those of any expanding intracranial mass (Table 421–2). A headache of recent onset is the most common symptom, representing distortion or irritation of pain-sensitive structures within the cranial vault, especially those of the great venous sinuses and the dura about the base of the brain. If the process continues untreated, isolated headache will increase in

TABLE 421–2. BRAIN ABSCESS: PRESENTING FEATURES IN 43 CASES

Headache	72%
Lethargy	71%
Fever	60%
Nuchal rigidity	49%
Nausea, vomiting	35%
Seizures	35%
Ocular palsy	27%
Confusion	26%
Visual disturbance	21%
Weakness	21%
Dysarthria	12%
Stupor	12%
Papilledema	10%
Dysphasia	9%
Hemiparesis	9%
Dizziness	7%

Reproduced with permission from Chan CH, Johnson JD, Hofstetter M, et al.: Brain abscess: A study of 45 consecutive cases. Medicine 65:415, 1986.

severity and become accompanied by focal signs such as hemiparesis or aphasia, followed by obtundation and coma. The period of evolution may be as brief as many hours or as long as many days to weeks with more indolent organisms. Seizures may occur with abscesses involving the cortical gray matter.

CEREBROSPINAL FLUID EXAMINATION. Cerebrospinal fluid (CSF) examination is not useful in diagnosis because the findings range from normal to those of purulent meningitis, depending on the walling off of the brain abscess or its closeness to CSF compartments (Table 421–3). More important, because abscesses often expand rapidly, lumbar puncture may aggravate impending transtentorial herniation. If possible, the procedure should be deferred until after brain images are obtained, which may eliminate the need for CSF analysis.

NEUROIMAGING. CT and MR are the imaging studies of choice for brain abscesses and monitoring their response to therapy. MRI is especially useful for posterior fossa abscesses, as it provides an artifact-free view of the brain stem and cerebellum. In addition, MRI with intravenous gadolinium contrast is superior in demonstrating cerebritis surrounding edema, the extent of mass effect, or associated venous thrombosis. MRI with or without gadolinium is preferable to CT for demonstrating multiple lesions.

The evolution of the abscess can be followed radiologically. In the early cerebritis stage, CT images reveal a low-density lesion

TABLE 421–3. SUMMARY OF LUMBAR FLUID CHANGES ASSOCIATED WITH BRAIN ABSCESS*

		Number of Patients	Per Cent
Pressure			
<200 mm		38	38
200–300 mm		35	35
>300 mm		26	26
	Total	99	
White cells per mm³			
<5		61	29
5–100		81	38
>100		71	33
	Total	213	
Protein (mg per dl)			
<50		26	24
50–100		38	35
>100		44	41
	Total	108	
Glucose (mg per dl)			
>40		89	79
<40		23	21
	Total	112	

* Most of these data were obtained before brain imaging was widely available.
Reproduced with permission from Fishman RA: Cerebrospinal Fluid in Diseases of the Nervous System. Philadelphia, WB Saunders, 1980, p 264.

with partial ring enhancement. In the late cerebritis and early capsule stage, well-formed ring-enhancing lesions are seen. The ring enhancement is typically thin walled and uniform, with subtle medial thinning adjacent to the ventricular system. Thick, nonuniform, or nodular enhancement should raise suspicion of an alternative cause. Delayed contrast scans show diffusion of contrast material into the lucent center. In the late capsule stage, well-formed ring enhancement may be seen with no delayed diffusion of contrast. Other ring-enhancing lesions that may mimic the image of brain abscess include primary and metastatic tumor, a resolving infarct or hematoma, and, rarely, demyelinating disease.

TREATMENT. Pyogenic brain abscesses are treated with antibiotics combined with surgical aspiration or excision. Aspiration offers the advantage of identifying the infecting organism and may be performed stereotactically with CT guidance while the patient is under local anesthesia; excision requires craniotomy. Surgical therapy is required when significant mass effect is present, when the abscess adjoins the ventricular surface (raising the possibility of catastrophic rupture into the ventricular system), when abscesses arise in the posterior fossa (with the potential of brain stem compression), or when abscesses reach a large size (>cm diameter) or become refractory to medical therapy. In selected cases antibiotics alone are appropriate, as in the case of surgically inaccessible, multiple abscesses (seen in 10% of patients) or abscesses in the early cerebritis stage. If the causal organism is not identified, antibiotic coverage should be directed toward the most likely organisms (streptococci and anaerobes). A suggested regimen includes penicillin G, 4 million units given intravenously (IV) every 4 hours, and metronidazole, 15 mg per kilogram IV over 1 hour, followed by 7.5 mg per kilogram given IV or orally every 6 hours. If staphylococcal infection is suspected (e.g., because of a history of trauma or intravenous drug abuse), vancomycin should be added. Concomitant corticosteroid therapy may attenuate edema surrounding abscesses.

The resolution of abscesses can be followed by serial CT or MRI. Antibiotics must be continued until the abscess cavity resolves completely, usually 6 to 8 weeks, although in surgically treated patients it may be 4 weeks. A failure to demonstrate abscess shrinkage in 4 weeks constitutes an antibiotic failure; a surgical procedure should then be performed. Of note is that the ring enhancement may persist after clinical and CSF normalization.

Abscesses associated with HIV infection are assumed to be due to *Toxoplasma gondii*. The diagnosis is confirmed by response to empiric treatment with daily doses of sulfadiazine, 12 to 15 mg per kilogram, given orally, and pyrimethamine, 25 to 50 mg, given orally. An alternative regimen is pyrimethamine given orally and clindamycin, 900 to 1200 mg IV every 6 hours (or 600 mg orally every 6 hours) for patients allergic to sulfa drugs.

PROGNOSIS. The current mortality rate is 5 to 15%, depending on locale and the nature of pre-existing illness. Outcome correlates inversely with the abscess size and the degree of neurologic dysfunction at presentation, but less well with age, cause, number of abscesses, or corticosteroid use.

SPINAL EPIDURAL ABSCESS

Infection within the epidural space about the spinal cord is an uncommon but readily diagnosable and treatable potential cause of paralysis and death. Its incidence is 0.5 to 1.0 per 10,000 hospital admissions in the United States, but the frequency is substantially increased in the intravenous drug-using population.

CLINICAL PRESENTATION. Patients are usually systemically ill with fever (to 38° to 39° C) in virtually all acutely evolving cases and in the majority of those with a subacute evolution. The initial feature is acute or subacute neck or back pain, with focal percussion tenderness being a prominent feature in the great majority; stiff neck and headache are common. As the infection progresses, over hours, days, or weeks, radicular pain occurs, the site varying with the location of the abscess. The pain can be mistaken for sciatica, a visceral abdominal process, chest wall pain, or cervical disc disease. If the condition goes unrecognized at this stage, the symptoms can rapidly evolve, over a few hours to a few days, to produce weakness and finally paralysis occurring distal to the spinal level of the infection. In this clinical setting, spinal epidural

abscess should be assumed, systemic antibiotics begun, and urgent neuroradiologic confirmatory diagnostic procedures pursued.

The differential diagnosis includes compressive and inflammatory processes involving the spinal cord (transverse myelitis, intervertebral disc herniation, metastatic tumor), which can usually be differentiated clinically by the absence of systemic infection. Transverse myelitis, however, may be associated with fever; the most useful differential feature is its rapid evolution to maximum deficit within 24 hours or less. Other infectious processes that may produce back or neck pain or tenderness must be excluded (bacterial meningitis, perinephric abscess, disc space infection, bacterial endocarditis). *Spinal subdural empyema* can cause a similar syndrome but is much less frequent.

ETIOLOGY. Infections of the epidural space originate from contiguous spread or via hematogenous routes from a distant source. Cutaneous sites of infection are the most common remote sources, especially in intravenous drug users. Abdominal, respiratory tract, and urinary sources are also common. Osteomyelitis may be a cause by either direct extension or hematogenous spread, especially when associated with sepsis. Contiguous spread of infection occurs, most commonly from psoas abscesses, decubitus ulceration, perinephric and retropharyngeal abscesses, surgical sites, or epidurally placed catheters. Whether or not spread can occur from pelvic infections via spinal veins remains unsettled. Minor back trauma has been implicated in producing a hematoma near the spine, which is subsequently seeded via hematogenous sources.

PATHOPHYSIOLOGY. The anatomy of the epidural space dictates the location of the abscess, the frequency of epidural infections being proportional to the volume of the epidural space. Because the size of the intravertebral canal remains relatively constant while the circumference of the spinal cord changes, this is maximal in the thoracic region and least at the cervical spine enlargement. Further, as the dura about the cord is adherent to the vertebral column anteriorly, more epidural abscesses lie posteriorly and because no anatomic barriers separate spinal segments in the posterior epidural space, such abscesses usually extend over three to five or more vertebral segments.

As the epidural space is not confined rostrocaudally, there is no clear abscess cavity or focal mass to provide a situation of simple compression for spinal cord compromise in epidural abscess. Clinical signs often are substantially greater than would have been predicted from the anatomic extent of pus or granulation tissue found at surgical exploration. Further, in many instances, no frank compression is found on postmortem examination. The spinal cord dysfunction is likely to reflect toxic processes secondary to inflammation, as well as venous thrombosis, thrombophlebitis, ischemia, and edema.

BACTERIOLOGY. Causative organisms can be identified by culture or Gram stain from pus obtained at exploration (90% of cases), blood cultures (60 to 90% of cases), or CSF (20% of cases). *Staphylococcus aureus* accounts for most infections, followed by streptococci and gram-negative anaerobes. Tuberculous abscesses remain common, representing as many as 25% of cases in high-risk populations.

DIAGNOSIS. CSF examination is often performed because of associated fever and meningeal signs. The fluid usually is nonspecifically abnormal, containing normal or decreased glucose levels, a moderately elevated protein content (400 to 500 mg per milliliter), and a lymphocytic pleocytosis (22 to 150 per cubic millimeter). Spinal fluid cultures yield organisms in about 25% of cases and Gram stains are rarely positive. Almost 90% of patients show a peripheral blood leukocytosis.

Plain spine radiographs, with attention to the area of percussion tenderness, may show osteomyelitis/discitis, a compression fracture, or a paravertebral mass. Gadolinium-enhanced MRI is the study of choice for the evaluation of a suspected epidural abscess because of its superior ability to demonstrate the craniocaudal extent of the extradural soft tissue mass, associated mass effect upon the cord or cauda equina, and potential signal abnormalities within the discs, vertebral bone marrow, and spinal cord. The addition of an intravenous gadolinium contrast agent better defines central necrosis suggestive of abscess rather than cellulitis. If MRI is unavailable or technically impossible, CT with myelography usually provides adequate information. A normal plain CT alone does not exclude the diagnosis.

TREATMENT. The disease is fatal in the absence of antibiotic therapy. Unless culture and sensitivities dictate otherwise, penicillinase-resistant penicillin (nafcillin, 12 grams per day, or oxacillin, 12 grams per day) with an aminoglycoside (gentamicin, 5 mg per kilogram per day) should be started empirically as antistaphylococcal treatment for presumed bacterial infection. For confirmed *Staphlyococcus aureus* abscesses, penicillinase-resistant penicillin can be used alone, but many authorities add rifampin (300 mg every 12 hours) because of its ability to penetrate the abscess cavity. Therapy should be continued intravenously for 3 to 4 weeks in the absence of osteomyelitis and 6 to 8 weeks with associated osteomyelitis. Surgical decompression was once thought to be mandatory in all cases; now early diagnosis by CT or MRI scans allows for effective medical therapy prior to occurrence of neurologic complications. Medical management of cervical epidural abscess requires close neurologic monitoring because of the small space available for abscess expansion and the high potential for quadriparesis. If blood cultures are negative, needle aspiration or laminectomy may be necessary to determine the causative organism.

PROGNOSIS. The chances of partial or complete recovery relate inversely to the amount of neurologic dysfunction at the time of diagnosis. Patients with abnormalities limited to pain recover without deficit. Approximately half the patients with some weakness have complete resolution, and nearly half the patients with paralysis of less than 36 hours' duration show some recovery of motor function. In tuberculous epidural abscess, recovery of motor function has been reported even after paralysis lasting for weeks.

VENOUS SINUS THROMBOSIS SECONDARY TO INFECTION

Thrombosis of cerebral veins or sinuses may be of idiopathic origin (see Ch. 419), may occur in the setting of hematologic disorders or coagulation abnormalities (see Ch. 153), or may result from local or contiguous infectious processes. The last-named syndromes are dealt with here.

Venous drainage from the brain begins with venules and veins that drain into the great venous sinuses. The venous sinus system itself lacks valves, permitting retrograde propagation of clots or infections emanating from structures such as those located in the central portion of the face or the middle ear.

Septic Cavernous Sinus Thrombosis

The cavernous sinuses comprise the most caudal dural venous chambers at the skull base. The paired structures lie on either side of the pituitary fossa, immediately above the midline sphenoid sinus. The cavernous sinus encloses the "cavernous portion" of the internal carotid artery; the third, fourth, and sixth cranial nerves en route to the apex of the orbit; and the ophthalmic and maxillary branches of the trigeminal nerve, which supply sensation to the forehead, periocular regions, cornea, and malar area of the face. Septic cavernous sinus thrombosis most commonly results from extension of infections involving the neighboring sphenoid and ethmoid sinuses, the central portion of the face, or the pharynx or tonsils.

Presenting symptoms are headache and/or lateralized facial pain, followed in a few days to weeks by fever, and involvement of the orbit, producing proptosis and chemosis secondary to obstruction of the ophthalmic vein. Paralysis of oculomotor nerves follows rapidly. Sensory dysfunction in the first and second divisions of the trigeminal nerve and a decrease in the corneal reflex are less obvious. Further involvement of the contiguous orbital contents follows, with mild papilledema and decreased visual acuity, sometimes progressing to blindness. Extension to the opposite cavernous sinus or to other intracranial sinuses with cerebral infarction, or increased intracranial pressure secondary to impaired venous drainage can result in stupor, coma, and death.

The differential diagnosis includes carotid cavernous sinus fistula (diagnosed by ocular bruit and an afebrile state); idiopathic granulomatous involvement of the cavernous sinus (the Tolosa-Hunt syndrome) or orbit (orbital pseudotumor, diagnosed by relative sparing of the orbital contents); and orbital cellulitis (infection localized to the orbit but sparing the structures of the cavernous sinus). Some overlap often occurs between involvement of these contiguous structures of the orbit and involvement of the cavernous sinus.

The CSF is abnormal in almost all cases, sometimes with a profile resembling that of purulent meningitis or parameningeal infection.

The most common causative organism is *Staphylococcus aureus*, with streptococci and pneumococci being less common; anerobic infection has been reported. Radiologic evaluation includes sinus imaging, with attention to the sphenoid and ethmoid sinuses. MRI (with and without intravenous gadolinium contrast) can often demonstrate venous thrombosis by illustrating the lack of the normal "flow void" within vascular structures. Cranial CT scans, employed with or without intravenous contrast material, are less helpful but may show a subtle increase in size and enhancement on the thrombosed sinus. MR angiography may demonstrate extrinsic narrowing of the intracavernous portion of the internal carotid artery.

Treatment relies on early diagnosis and consists of the prompt drainage of infected paranasal sinuses as well as specific antistaphylococcal agents, such as nafcillin or oxacillin, given intravenously. Heparin anticoagulation may reduce morbidity from associated brain ischemia, but this treatment remains controversial in cases involving infection.

Lateral Sinus Thrombosis

Septic thrombosis of the lateral sinus results from acute or chronic infections of the middle ear. The symptoms consist of ear pain followed by headache, nausea, vomiting, and vertigo, evolving over several weeks. On examination, most patients are febrile. An abnormality on otologic examination is nearly invariable; mastoid swelling may be seen. Sixth cranial nerve palsies can occur, but other focal neurologic signs are rare. Papilledema occurs in half the cases, and elevated CSF pressure is present in most, especially with occlusion of the right lateral sinus (which is the major venous conduit from the superior sagittal sinus). CSF contents are usually normal, although a perimeningeal inflammatory profile may be seen.

Treatment includes intravenous antibiotics to cover staphylococci and anerobes (nafcillin or oxacillin with penicillin or metronidazole). Surgical drainage (mastoidectomy) may be required. Increased intracranial pressure seldom needs direct treatment unless visual fields show progressive constriction. The outcome is usually favorable.

Septic Sagittal Sinus Thrombosis

This uncommon condition occurs as a consequence of purulent meningitis, infections of the ethmoid or maxillary sinuses spreading via venous channels, compound infected skull fractures, or, rarely, neurosurgical wound infections. Symptoms include manifestations of elevated intracranial pressure (headache, nausea, and vomiting) that evolve rapidly to stupor and coma. Seizures and hemiparesis may result from cortical infarction. The rate of progression, severity of symptoms, and prognosis are all related to the location of thrombosis involving the sinus. When only the anterior third of the sinus is obstructed, symptoms are less intense and evolve more slowly. If or when the thrombosis progresses to involve the middle and posterior thirds of the sinus, deterioration progresses more rapidly and outlook for recovery declines.

CSF abnormalities accompany well over half the cases. The opening pressure is increased in proportion to the extent of the sagittal sinus involvement, and a pleocytosis usually reflects the association of a meningeal or parameningeal process.

Radiologically, septic sagittal sinus thrombosis may be excluded by visualization of the normal sagittal sinus during the venous phase of cerebral angiography; the diagnosis can usually also be made by MRI, which demonstrates an abnormal increase in signal intensity (absent flow void) within the affected venous sinus. Contrast-enhanced CT scanning may reveal a contrast void lying at the junction of the transverse and sagittal sinuses (the region of the torcula); this so-called delta sign represents an intraluminal clot surrounded by contrast material.

Intravenous antibiotics should be directed at organisms recovered from the meningeal process or the meningeal site. *Staphylococcus aureus* (including the methicillin-resistant strains), β-hemolytic streptococci, pneumococci, and gram-negative aerobes such as *Klebsiella* are the most common organisms. Initial antibiotic treatment should include vancomycin and a third-generation cephalosporin. Associated paranasal sinusitis should be drained surgically. Heparin use has been little tested in septic venous thrombosis, but experience with noninfected sinus thrombosis has shown it to reduce both morbidity and mortality appreciably (see Ch. 419).

Neurologic Complications of Infectious Endocarditis

Neurologic complications occur in one third of patients with bacterial endocarditis and triple the general mortality rate of the disease. Most of these complications derive from valvular vegetations. Cerebral (but not systemic) emboli are more common from mitral valve endocarditis, for reasons unknown. The time of embolization during the course of endocarditis depends upon the virulence of the organism and whether it produces acute or subacute disease. With acute endocarditis (predominantly staphylococci or enterococci), embolization occurs early, often during the first week, while in subacute disease (predominantly viridans group streptococci or enterococci) emboli occur over the full course of treatment and occasionally after treatment is completed. Emboli lodge in the peripheral branches of the middle cerebral artery, in most cases with resultant hemiparesis. Focal seizures may result.

Whether or not warfarin anticoagulation decreases the risk of embolization remains a controversial issue. This therapy was administered in an earlier period to decrease platelet fibrin vegetations that sequestered the bacteria away from the body's defenses. Current evidence suggests a high rate of hemorrhagic intracerebral complications from warfarin anticoagulation in native valve endocarditis, but not in prosthetic valve endocarditis. Mechanisms to explain the difference remain unknown. Nevertheless, most authorities believe that patients already receiving chronic anticoagulation at the time of diagnosis of endocarditis should be maintained on such therapy.

Mycotic aneurysms complicate endocarditis in 2 to 10% of cases and are more common in acute than subacute disease. The middle cerebral artery is most commonly involved, with the aneurysms being located distally in the vessel, differentiating them from congenital berry aneurysms. The process by which the aneurysmal dilatation occurs remains in dispute, although embolization of infectious vegetations is accepted as the inciting event. Aneurysmal rupture results in 80% mortality, and early diagnosis is therefore important. Whom to subject to angiography is uncertain. However, clinical or radiologic evidence of cerebral or other embolization defines the high-risk group. Other suggested indications for angiography include severe headache (presumably the result of aneurysmal leakage). When an unruptured aneurysm is identified by angiography, it may resolve with antibiotic therapy alone. Such patients need a follow-up angiogram to document an interval decrease in aneurysm size. Otherwise, surgical therapy requires excision of the infected portion of the artery. Patients with proximal mycotic aneurysms have a greater risk of perioperative stroke than do those with distal involvement.

Small brain abscesses may complicate the course of endocarditis, but macroscopic abscesses are rare, most occurring in the setting of acute, rather than subacute, endocarditis. Multiple microabscesses, however, can result in a diffuse encephalopathy similar to that seen in sepsis. Such lesions may escape detection on CT scanning and are not amenable to surgical drainage. Antibiotic treatment of the primary disease is indicated.

A CSF pleocytosis occurs in 70% of patients with neurologic complications, but in an unknown number of patients in whom the CNS is clinically spared. The CSF profile may be that of a purulent meningitis (polymorphonuclear predominance, elevated protein level, and low glucose level) or that of a perimeningeal infection (lymphocytic predominance, modest protein elevation, and normal glucose level). A hemorrhagic component may be seen. Purulent CSF is associated with signs of meningeal irritation and infection with a virulent organism.

SUBDURAL EMPYEMA

Empyema refers to infection in a preformed space, in this case that separating the dura and arachnoid. Subdural empyema is responsible for one fifth of localized intracranial infections and results from direct or indirect extension from infected paranasal sinuses via a retrograde thrombophlebitis or, less frequently, untreated chronic otitis. Unilateral empyema is most common, as the falx prevents passage across the midline, but bilateral and/or multiple concurrent empyemas occur. Cortical venous thrombosis or brain abscess develops in approximately one fourth of cases; purulent meningitis is a less common accompaniment.

Symptoms initially reflect those of chronic otitis or sinusitis, upon which lateralized headache (a universal feature), fever, and obtundation become superimposed. Vomiting, meningeal signs, and focal neurologic abnormalities (hemiparesis or seizures) usually follow. If the disease remains untreated, obtundation progresses, and the septic mass and swollen underlying brain soon lead to venous thrombosis or death from herniation. The major differential diagnosis is that of meningitis. Nuchal rigidity and obtundation occur in both, but papilledema and lateralizing deficits are more common in empyema. Lumbar puncture, if obtained because of the suspicion of meningitis, reveals an elevated intracranial pressure accompanied by an increased protein content and a polymorphonuclear pleocytosis with usually a normal glucose concentration in the CSF. Either CT or MRI can be diagnostic of empyema, showing an extra-axial, crescent-shaped mass with an enhancing rim lying just below the inner table of the skull over the cerebral convexities or the interhemispheric fissures. MRI better detects underlying parenchymal edema as well as the infection itself.

Treatment requires both prompt surgical drainage of the empyema cavity and high-dose intravenous antibiotics directed toward organisms found at the time of craniotomy. The bacteriology of subdural empyemas is similar to that of sinusitis and cerebral abscess, discussed above. Anticonvulsants should be administered prophylactically, as seizures are common.

If cortical infarction from venous thrombosis does not occur, the prognosis is surprisingly favorable, although chronic epilepsy results in one third of patients.

CRANIAL EPIDURAL ABSCESS

Infections of the epidural space coexist most often with subdural empyema and less frequently with chronic sinusitis or otitis alone. Symptoms and signs are headache and fever with focal neurologic abnormalities due to the coexistent subdural empyema or brain abscess. The diagnosis is made with MRI or contrast-enhanced CT scan (which demonstrate a peripherally enhancing lenticular-shaped lesion in the epidural space), and the abscess is treated by surgical drainage followed by systemic antibiotics. In uncomplicated cases, the prognosis is excellent.

MALIGNANT EXTERNAL OTITIS

This necrotizing osteitis occurs in elderly patients with diabetes. The associated organism, *Pseudomonas aeruginosa,* is part of the normal flora of the external ear. In this case, it produces an external otitis that fails to respect normal anatomic boundaries. The result consists of a rapidly evolving syndrome of ear pain, facial swelling, osteomyelitis of the base of the skull, and purulent meningitis accompanied by multiple cranial nerve palsies. Urgent treatment with antipseudomonal penicillin or a third-generation cephalosporin combined with an aminoglycoside, as well as surgical debridement and drainage, is essential. The mortality rate is high.

Brain Abscess

Haimes AB, Zimmerman RD, Morgello S, et al.: MR imaging of brain abscesses. AJR 152:1073, 1989. *Reviews MRI of brain abscesses and its differential diagnosis.*

Maniglia AJ, Goodwin WJ, Arnold JE, et al.: Intracranial abscesses secondary to nasal, sinus, and orbital infections in adults and children. Arch Otolaryngol Head Neck Surg 115:1424, 1989. *Association of sinus disease with brain abscesses is reviewed.*

Patel KS, Marks PV: Management of focal intracranial infections: Is medical treatment better than surgery? J Neurol Neurosurg Psychiatry 53:472, 1990. *Discussion of the issue of nonsurgical management.*

Yang SY, Zhao CS: Review of 140 patients with brain abscess. Surg Neurol 39:290, 1993. *Clinical features, bacteriology, imaging, and treatment discussed.*

Spinal Epidural Abscess

Darouiche RO, Hamill RJ, Greenberg SB, et al.: Bacterial spinal epidural abscess. Review of 43 cases and literature survey. Medicine (Baltimore) 71:369, 1992. *A large recent series. Issue of medical versus surgical treatment addressed.*

Del-Curling O Jr, Gower DJ, McWhorter JM: Changing concepts in spinal epidural abscess: A report of 29 cases. Neurosurgery 27:185, 1990. *A recent neurosurgical series.*

Redekop GJ, Del MR: Diagnosis and management of spinal epidural abscess. Can J Neurol Sci 19:180, 1992. *Reviews 25 recent cases; presentations, treatment, outcome.*

Teman AJ: Spinal epidural abscess. Early detection with gadolinium magnetic resonance imaging. Arch Neurol 49:743, 1992. *Early imaging addressed.*

Venous Sinus Thrombosis Secondary to Infection

DiNubile MJ, Boom WH, Southwick FS: Septic cortical thrombophlebitis. J Infect Dis 161:1216, 1990. *Fourteen-year experience from a single center.*

Neurologic Complications of Infectious Endocarditis

Davenport J, Hart RG: Prosthetic valve endocarditis 1976–1987. Antibiotics, anticoagulation, and stroke. Stroke 21:993, 1990. *Anticoagulation in prosthetic valve endocarditis is readdressed.*

Jones HJ, Siekert RG: Neurological manifestations of infective endocarditis. Review of clinical and therapeutic challenges. Brain 112:1295, 1989. *Two decade experience. Central and peripheral nervous systems reviewed in addition to imaging and treatment.*

Subdural Empyema

Bok AP, Peter JC: Subdural empyema: Burr holes or craniotomy? A retrospective computerized tomography–era analysis of treatment in 90 cases. J Neurosurg 78:574, 1993. *Surgical treatment is reviewed.*

Pathak A, Sharma BS, Mathuriya SN, et al.: Controversies in the management of subdural empyema. A study of 41 cases with review of literature. Acta Neurochir 102:25, 1990. *A recent large series and literature review.*

Weingarten K, Zimmerman RD, Becker RD, et al.: Subdural and epidural empyemas: MR imaging. AJR 152:615, 1989. *MRI is described.*

Cranial Epidural Abscess

Krauss WE, McCormick PC: Infections of the dural spaces. Neurosurg Clin North Am 3:421, 1992. *Epidural and subdural infections and treatment reviewed.*

Malignant External Otitis

Johnson MP, Ramphal R: Malignant external otitis: Report on therapy with ceftazidime and review of therapy and prognosis. Rev Infect Dis 12:173, 1990. *A recent review of clinical and therapeutic aspects.*

422 NEUROSYPHILIS

The resurgence of primary and secondary syphilis (now estimated to be 14.7 cases per 100,000) first occurred in the promiscuous homosexual male population but has more recently spread to the heterosexual community via prostitutes. If untreated, approximately 7% of patients with primary syphilis infection develop some form of symptomatic neurosyphilis.

PATHOPHYSIOLOGY. Each of the neurologic manifestations of syphilis results from a chronic, insidious meningeal inflammatory process caused by treponemal invasion of the central nervous system (CNS). An inflammatory response in the cerebrospinal fluid (CSF) occurs in 34% of asymptomatic persons with syphilis, with the CSF abnormalities peaking at 13 to 18 months after the primary infection. This CNS invasion dictates the risk of future symptomatic and asymptomatic neurosyphilis, which amounts to approximately

30% following a primary infection but falls to 1% or less if CSF examination is normal 5 years after the primary infection (Merritt, 1946).

CLINICAL SYNDROMES. The clinical manifestations of neurosyphilis are divided into acute syphilitic meningitis, cerebrovascular syphilis, syphilitic dementia (general paresis), and tabes dorsalis. These entities, however, overlap clinically. For instance, paresis and tabes may coexist (taboparesis). After primary infection, these clinical subtypes of neurosyphilis follow a predictable time course (Fig. 422–1) based on the evolution of the meningeal inflammatory process. Symptomatic syphilitic meningitis is the earliest manifestation of nervous system syphilis. The meningeal inflammation later extends to involve the cerebral blood vessels and, when symptomatic, results in cerebrovascular neurosyphilis (usually seen within the first 5 years following primary infection). The so-called parenchymal forms of neurosyphilis (paresis and tabes) develop after a more protracted interval.

Acute Syphilitic Meningitis. Symptomatic meningeal syphilis occurs during the first months to a year or two after the primary infection, with 10% of cases occurring coincident with a secondary rash. The course is subacute. Headache is common, and asymmetric cranial nerve abnormalities are prominent (especially those involving auditory function, facial strength, eye movements, and unilateral or bilateral papilledema due to involvement of the optic nerve). Patients are afebrile; meningeal signs are often present, and some experience at least a degree of confusion. The CSF usually contains syphilitic antibodies and shows a lymphocytic pleocytosis. Accurate diagnosis is important, as mild symptoms may resolve without treatment and leave the patient at risk for progression to the fixed deficits associated with the later forms of neurosyphilis.

Cerebrovascular Syphilis. As the meningeal inflammatory process progresses, a diffuse vasculitis evolves, compromising the cerebral arteries traversing the subarachnoid space and producing a subacute encephalopathy with ischemia-caused focal features. Associated symptoms include confusion, personality change, and intellectual decline, usually followed by the emergence of focal deficits resulting from occlusion of specific vessels. Branches of the middle cerebral artery are most often involved, but any cerebral or spinal vascular bed may be affected alone or in combination, with ischemic lesions evolving over a period of several hours or days. The resulting syndrome differs from thromboembolic stroke because of the associated encephalopathy, the multifocal pattern, and the subacute time course.

Diagnosis is confirmed by finding an inflammatory spinal fluid

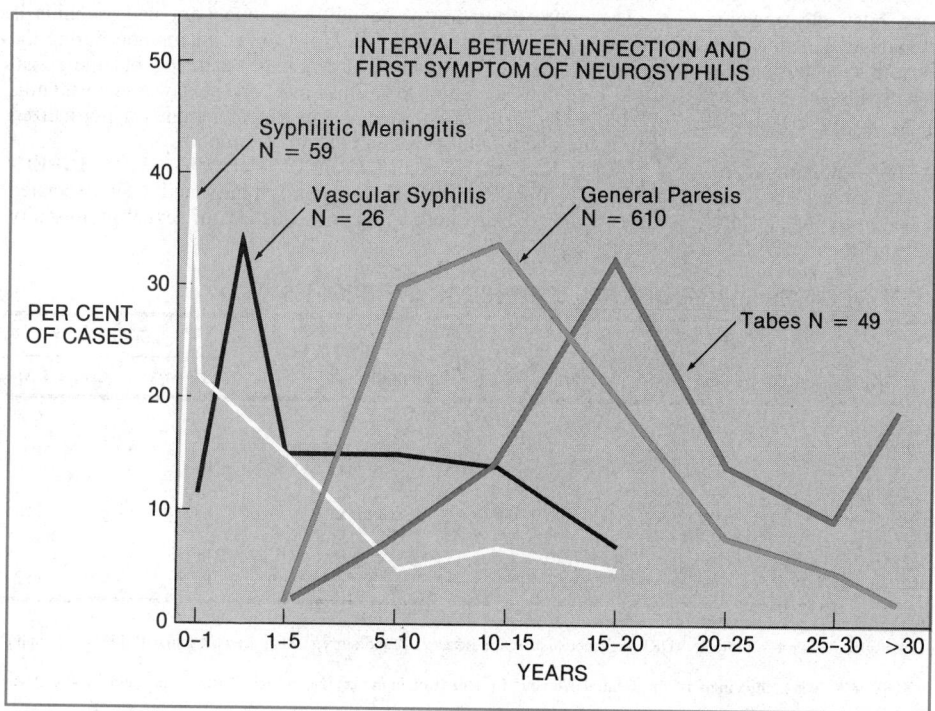

FIGURE 422–1. Interval between primary and symptomatic neurosyphilis by type (meningeal, vascular, paresis, tabes), abstracted from the literature and presented as per cent of total cases within type. (Reproduced with permission from Simon RP: Neurosyphilis. Arch Neurol 42:606, 1985. Copyright 1985, American Medical Association.)

positive serology; angiography is unnecessary, but if per-demonstrates vasculitis of medium-sized arteries. Areas of ischemia imaged by CT or MRI in association with the characteristic CSF suggest the diagnosis.

Syphilitic Dementia. Dementia paralytica, or general paresis of the insane, is caused by the diffuse meningoencephalitic form of neurosyphilis. Affected patients usually present 5 to 15 years or more after the primary infection. General paresis affects men four to seven times more frequently than women, perhaps because the infectivity of *Treponema pallidum* declines during pregnancy.

The clinical pattern of syphilitic dementia can mimic almost any organic brain syndrome. The colorful descriptions of grandiose delusional states and psychosis are well known, but these conditions were uncommon even in the prepenicillin era. Then, as now, a simple dementing illness predominated. In advanced cases, tremors of the hands, tongue, and lips resulted, producing a striking dysgraphia and dysarthria. Few untreated cases reach such an advanced stage.

Several features differentiate paresis from other causes of dementia. Syphilitic dementia has a relatively early onset, most commonly beginning between ages 30 and 50, and it progresses rapidly if untreated, being fatal within months to a few years. An inflammatory CSF is always found, and the blood and CSF serologies always contain syphilitic antibodies in diagnostic amounts.

Tabes Dorsalis. The term denotes a myeloneuropathy that characteristically follows the primary infection by 10 to 20 years. The primary lesions affect either the proximal dorsal root entry zones or the dorsal root ganglia. As with paresis, a marked male predominance (7:1) was noted in the prepenicillin era.

The classic triad of symptoms includes lightning pains, sensory ataxia, and urinary disturbance. The most common and earliest signs include pupillary abnormalities, lower extremity areflexia, and the Romberg sign. Lightning pains are transient, agonizing, shooting pains affecting the legs most commonly but potentially arising in any region of the body. Characteristic is an early loss of vibration and position sense attributed to secondary degeneration of the posterior columns of the spinal cord. The proprioceptive impairment engenders a wide-based, unsteady gait that is exacerbated by elimination of visual input (eye closure): the Romberg sign. Bladder hypotonia with overflow incontinence results from deafferentation of the lower sacral sensory nerve roots. Rectal incontinence is uncommon; genital sensory and autonomic impairment eventually results in impotence. Peripheral autonomic impairment, along with loss of peripheral nociceptive afferent fibers, is responsible for the development of trophic (Charcot) joint deformities and distal extremity ulcers.

Of the pupillary abnormalities, half have the classic Argyll Robertson pattern, being small, irregular, and bilaterally reacting poorly to light but constricting briskly to accommodation (the phenomenon of light–near dissociation). Other pupillary abnormalities in tabes include unilateral mydriatic pupils with loss of pupillary light reflex. The sensory impairment is responsible for the loss of deep tendon reflexes.

CEREBROSPINAL FLUID EXAMINATION. A chronic, insidious, inflammatory response within the CSF (Table 422–1) accompanies each of the clinical syndromes of neurosyphilis and pro-vides the ultimate diagnostic test establishing the presence of active neurosyphilis and/or its response to therapy. The absence of a CSF inflammatory response excludes a diagnosis of active neurosyphilis and therefore precludes a clinical response to antibiotic therapy. As with any chronic meningitis, the γ globulin portion of the protein content is commonly elevated, and oligoclonal bands may be present.

Active neurosyphilis produces an abnormal CSF. The possibility of a negative serology in neurosyphilis is difficult to ascertain from the classic literature because of using the relatively insensitive Wasserman test and the unrecognized inclusion of nonsyphilitic syndromes of cerebrovascular disease and viral meningitis. When the clinical diagnosis was characteristic, however, only rare cases showed a negative CSF serology (even with the Wasserman reaction): In 100 paretic patients reported by Merritt (1946), the CSF Wasserman test was positive in every case. Wilson also reported universal CSF positivity in 77 cases of paresis. Theoretically, a negative CSF VDRL might occur in the presence of severe immunosuppression, as a prozone phenomenon, or, in an early case, as a manifestation of the CSF inflammatory response preceding seropositivity. This last situation may explain occasional recent reports of false-negative results or delayed conversions in early meningeal syndromes.

The role of the more sensitive treponemal test (fluorescent treponemal antibody [FTA]) in diagnosing CNS syphilis remains uncertain because of a high false-positive response and decreased sensitivity (75%); without supporting clinical or laboratory data, the diagnostic value of a reactive CSF FTA is unknown. An additional confirmatory test is to inject CSF into rabbit testes; a reactive testicular swelling and recovery of spirochetes prove treponemal infectivity.

TREATMENT. Because neurosyphilis of all clinical types is associated with a CSF inflammatory response, the CSF cell count provides the ultimate monitor of the effectiveness of therapy. Normalization of the spinal fluid is the required endpoint of antibiotic therapy. Once the CSF remains normal, clinical relapses fail to occur.

Penicillin is the drug of choice. Various regimens from 12 to 24 mU per day have been suggested, but it is not clear that the higher doses alter the clinical outcome. Intramuscular benzathine penicillin usually results in undetectable levels in CSF and accordingly should not be used for treatment of neurosyphilis. Spirocheticidal levels (0.03 IU per milliliter, 0.018 μg per milliliter) in CSF occur with 12 million units of IV penicillin daily in four divided doses. Some regimens include probenecid to increase concentrations in CSF by decreasing reabsorption of penicillin through the choroid plexus. Probenecid, however, also decreases parenchymal penicillin concentrations by competing for uptake at membrane transport sites.

The optimal duration of penicillin treatment for neurosyphilis is uncertain. Complete normalization of CSF is uncommon during the usual 2- to 3-week course of intravenous treatment, but the spinal fluid continues to return to normal over the next weeks to months (Table 422–2). Proof of adequate treatment requires a normalized cell count and a falling protein content at 6 months.

HUMAN IMMUNODEFICIENCY VIRUS (HIV) INFECTION IN NEUROSYPHILIS. Neurosyphilis and HIV-associated disease may coexist, both being consequences of sexual promiscuity

TABLE 422–1. CSF FINDINGS IN VARIOUS NEUROSYPHILITIC SYNDROMES

Syndrome	OP	WBC	Glu	Prot	Gamma Globulin*	VDRL	
						Blood	*CSF*
Meningitis	170	154 (94% L)	29	95		1:64	1:4
Cerebrovascular	192	58 (87% L)	41	119	IgG index .93	1:512	1:16
Paresis		220	49	305	IgG index 1.99	1:128	1:8
Tabes (active)		62		140		1:16	1:28
Tabes (inactive)		2	76	43		1:16	1:2

* Normal IgG index = 0.23 to 0.64.

OP = Opening pressure; WBC = white blood cells; Glu = glucose; Prot = protein; VDRL = Venereal Disease Research Laboratory; CSF = cerebrospinal fluid; L = lymphocytes; IgG = immunoglobulin G.

From Simon RP, Bayne LL: Neurosyphilis. *In* Martin J, Tyler K (eds.): Infections of the Central Nervous System (Contemporary Neurology Series). Philadelphia, FA Davis, 1993, p 237.

TABLE 422-2. CEREBROSPINAL FLUID (CSF) RESPONSE TO PENICILLIN TREATMENT*

	Admission	Day 7	Day 21	6 Mo
Opening pressure, mm CSF	120	–	–	Normal
Cells/cu mm	207 (94% L)	100 (100% L)	24 (100% L)	0
Glucose, mg/dl	51	66	54	66
Protein, mg/dl	50 (14.4% gamma globulin)	38	48	34
Serology (VDRL)				
CSF	1:2	1:1	–	–
Blood	1:64	1:64	1:64	1:64

* Meningovascular syphilis treated with aqueous penicillin G, 24 million units daily for 21 days; data from Holmes MD, Brant-Zawadski MM, Simon RP: Clinical manifestations of meningovascular syphilis. Neurology 34:553, 1984.

or intravenous drug abuse. Syphilitic syndromes in these patients do not differ in either time course or clinical presentation from those in the pre-AIDS era. Cases identified as "penicillin resistant" may merely have coexistent HIV-induced CSF pleocytosis that is not altered by penicillin therapy. In addition, the occasional recovery of treponemes following penicillin treatment for syphilis in HIV-coinfected patients was similarly observed in the pre-AIDS era. A recent comparison of syphilitics with or without HIV coinfection found no difference from the classically reported illness in clinical presentations, course of disease, serologic expression, or effect of treatment.

The principles of treating neurosyphilis in HIV-coinfected patients are similar to those used in patients without the retrovirus disease; intravenous penicillin should be used in spirocheticidal doses, and the spinal fluid should be monitored as an index of therapy. As noted, when the inflammatory response is due partly to syphilis and partly to HIV infection, only a portion of the pleocytosis will disappear, leaving a new plateau of CSF cellularity. The Centers for Disease Control and Prevention (CDC) recommends that patients coinfected with HIV and syphilis for more than 1 year have an examination of their CSF, whether or not they have neurologic symptoms.

Gourevitch MN, Selwyn PA, Davenny K, et al.: Effects of HIV infection on the serologic manifestations and response to treatment of syphilis in intravenous drug users. Ann Intern Med 118:350, 1993. *No difference was found in presentation, course, response to treatment, and serology with or without HIV coinfection.*
Hook EW III: Management of syphilis in human immunodeficiency virus-infected patients. Am J Med 93:477, 1992. *Reviews management issues in the HIV coinfected.*
Merritt HH, Adams RD, Solomon HC: Neurosyphilis. 2nd ed. New York, Oxford University Press, 1946. *The classic descriptive work of the prepenicillin era.*
Musher DM, Hamill RJ, Baughn RE: Syphilis in the presence of human immunodeficiency virus infection. Ann Intern Med 113:872, 1990. *A critique of the association between syphilis and HIV infection.*
Simon RP: Neurosyphilis. Arch Neurol 42:606, 1985. *A review of the clinical syndromes, CSF, and serologic diagnostic criteria.*

Section Eight—Viral Infections of the Nervous System

423 INTRODUCTION

Richard W. Price

Agents belonging to nearly all the major groups of animal viruses can infect the central nervous system (CNS). The spectrum ranges from the large, complex DNA herpesviruses to small, relatively simple viruses with DNA or RNA genomes, such as the papovaviruses and retroviruses. Also included are prions, unique transmissable agents that cause the spongiform encephalopathies. As a result, neurologic manifestations of viral infections can be almost equally diverse, extending from the typical acute febrile encephalitides to chronic progressive disorders that clinically resemble degenerative neurologic diseases.

In most cases, particularly in those infections presenting as acute encephalitis, nervous system involvement is an uncommon complication of a relatively common systemic infection. In adaptive terms, extension of infection to the CNS is "accidental" and may even preclude survival of the virus and its transmission to a new host. For example, the polioviruses cause enteric infections in which replication in the gut and fecal-oral transmission determine the essential survival and transmission of the organism; extension of infection to anterior horn cells of the spinal cord devastates the host but does not contribute to the "life cycle" of the virus. By contrast, the neurotropic herpesviruses, including herpes simplex virus type 1, are exquisitely adapted to cause latent and reactivated infection within the peripheral nervous system; in this case, the sensory neuron is the reservoir for latent virus, and reactivated virus exploits axoplasmic transport to reinfect the epithelium and consequently induce local shedding of virus. However, even in the case of the herpesviruses, CNS complications, such as acute herpes encephalitis, are "acci-dental" and not essential in the organism's adaptive strategy. By contrast, rabies is an illness in which CNS infection plays a central role in the life cycle of the virus: Involvement of the brain produces "rabid," biting behavior that actually contributes to virus transmission.

Viruses can enter the nervous system along a number of avenues. Transport up peripheral nerves can allow direct passage from epithelium or viscera to the CNS; once virus enters the brain, similar intraneural passage by axoplasmic transport can facilitate further spread. A number of viruses are transported along nerve processes by both orthograde and retrograde axoplasmic transport systems. This mode allows rapid passage over long distances and also provides an avenue protected from immunologic interference. Most viruses, however, enter the brain by hematogenous dissemination with passage across the vascular endothelium. As a general rule, agents that travel over neural routes tend to produce initially focal neurologic symptoms and signs, whereas those that disseminate hematogenously cause more diffuse clinical changes. Numerous exceptions exist, however. One reason for this lies in the selective vulnerability to infection of particular nervous system structures or cells. Focal or multifocal disease can also follow general hematogenous dissemination in a random seeding of brain regions. Many viruses preferably infect the meninges rather than the brain, gaining access via the fenestrated capillary endothelium of the choroid plexus.

Within the nervous system some viruses do not discriminate among neurons and glial or endothelial cells, whereas others choose selective targets. Such selectivity is often determined by cell-surface molecules, principally glycoproteins, that serve as receptors for viruses underlying their specific attachment and subsequent entry into cells. Different cell types may vary in their capacity to support virus-directed metabolism and replication.

Virus-cell interactions can assume a number of courses: *abortive infection* results in little or no change in the cell and no virus replication; *acute productive/lytic infection* is characterized by a full replication cycle with production of progeny and subsequent cell death; *chronic productive infection* may allow prolonged release of progeny virus without cell death; in *latent infection,* the viral genome resides quiescently in the cell, but retains the capacity to reactivate subsequently; *transforming infection* results in increased and characteristically abnormal cell proliferation, usually in the absence of virus replication; *defective infection* may result in nonproductive infection or production of incomplete particles yet causes varying degrees of cell alteration and viral antigen expression.

As with other types of organisms, neural injury and dysfunction accompanying viral infections relate to varying contributions of the *direct* effects of the virus and its genome (e.g., neuronal death caused by herpes simplex virus or oligodendroglial cell death caused by JC virus), the *indirect* effects mediated by antigen-specific host responses (e.g., lysis of infected cells by cytotoxic T lymphocytes), and less specific cell-coded neurotoxic gene products (e.g., nitric oxide and quinolinic acid) released in association with cytokine reactions. The relative importance of these factors in individual infections depends both upon the interactions of the invading organism with the cells it infects and the profile of host cell responses that it elicits. This balance is highly variable from one virus to the next and importantly influences the time course, morbidity, and degree of recovery from each infection.

Diagnostic approaches to viral diseases depend on the clinical setting and specific agents involved. The arsenal of available diagnostic methods is steadily growing. For many acute infections the time-honored serologic techniques assessing host antibody responses in serum and, at times, cerebrospinal fluid remain the most useful and cost effective. Although some infections elicit diagnostic tissue reactions (e.g., Negri body in rabies), for most infections newer techniques have displaced simple histopathology in identifying infection in tissue; these include detection of viral antigens using specific antibodies and of viral nucleic acids using *in situ* hybridization. Although more direct identification of viruses in blood or other clinical specimens by culture isolation generally remains difficult and costly, the introduction of the polymerase chain reaction (PCR) gene amplification technique to clinical virology is now rapidly expanding the diagnostic capability of the laboratory.

In the past, limitations of treatment made specific virologic diagnosis either largely an "academic exercise" or important principally for epidemiologic purposes. Efforts to combat viral disease consisted exclusively of prevention through active, or at times passive, immunization. In the past two decades, however, antiviral chemotherapy has become a practical reality. Effective therapy is now available for neurotropic herpesviruses and antiviral treatment can temporarily retard progression of HIV-1 infection. The promise thus exists for more effective treatments for infection by these viruses as well as for the development of chemotherapeutic agents that will act selectively against other important viruses causing neurologic diseases.

Johnson RT: Viral Infections of the Nervous System. New York, Raven Press, 1982. *Although now outdated in certain details, this remains an excellent introduction to the general principles of viral infection of the nervous system.*

Johnson RT, Burke DS, Elwell M, et al.: Japanese encephalitis: Immunocytochemical studies of viral antigen and inflammatory cells in fatal cases. Ann Neurol 18:567, 1985. *An exemplary contribution describing viral and immunologic pathology of Japanese encephalitis.*

Tsai T: Arboviral infections in the United States. Infect Dis Clin North Am 5:73, 1991. *A general review of arboviral infections, including clinical and epidemiologic aspects.*

424 ACUTE VIRAL MENINGITIS AND ENCEPHALITIS

Richard W. Price

DEFINITIONS. The terms *viral meningitis* and *viral encephalitis* refer to infections of the leptomeninges and brain parenchyma, respectively. When the spinal cord is involved along with the brain, the term *viral encephalomyelitis* may be used. When both meninges and brain parenchyma appear to be infected, *viral meningoencephalitis* sometimes is employed, although viral encephalitis is almost always accompanied by meningeal inflammation. The nonspecific term *aseptic meningitis* refers to an inflammatory process of the meninges accompanied by a predominantly mononuclear cell pleocytosis and not caused by pyogenic bacterial infection. Although viral infections are the most common cause of aseptic meningitis, infections by other types of organisms, as well as chemical irritation of the meninges and reactions to certain medications, can cause a similar clinical picture and cerebrospinal fluid profile. Most viral meningitides are benign and self-limiting with a low acute morbidity and only rare long-term sequelae. Although viral encephalitides are also often benign, they more frequently result in morbidity and mortality.

Acute central nervous system (CNS) infections caused by a variety of viruses are appropriately considered together because of their largely indistinguishable clinical aspects. Viral infections causing more distinct neurologic symptoms and signs are considered separately in subsequent sections.

ETIOLOGIES. Many viruses can cause acute encephalitis or meningitis (Table 424–1). Table 424–2 indicates the most common virus groups and the syndromes they produce.

Enteroviruses are small, nonenveloped RNA viruses of the picornavirus family with numerous serotypes. Over 50 have been associ-

TABLE 424–1. VIRUSES ASSOCIATED WITH ACUTE CENTRAL NERVOUS SYSTEM INFECTIONS IN THE UNITED STATES

RNA Viruses
  Picornaviruses (enteroviruses)
    Polioviruses
    Coxsackieviruses, groups A and B
    Echoviruses
    Enteroviruses
  Togaviruses
    Eastern equine encephalitis*
    Western equine encephalitis*
    St. Louis encephalitis*
    Powassan*
    Tick-borne encephalitis
    Rubella
  Bunyavirus
    California encephalitis* (includes LaCross subtype)
  Orbivirus
    Colorado tick fever*
  Arenavirus
    Lymphocytic choriomeningitis
  Rhabdovirus
    Rabies
  Orthomyxoviruses and paramyxoviruses
    Influenza
    Parainfluenza
    Mumps
    Measles
  Retroviruses
    Human immunodeficiency virus type 1
DNA Viruses
  Herpesviruses
    Herpes simplex, types 1 and 2
    Varicella-zoster
    Epstein-Barr
    Cytomegalovirus
    Adenoviruses

* Arthropod-borne viruses (arboviruses).

TABLE 424-2. RELATIVE FREQUENCY OF MENINGITIS AND ENCEPHALITIS OF KNOWN VIRAL ETOLOGY

Viral Agent	Viral Meningitis (%)	Viral Encephalitis (%)
Enteroviruses	83	23
Arboviruses	2	30
Mumps	7	2
Herpes simplex	4	27
Varicella	1	8
Measles	1	<1

Reproduced with permission from Jubelt B: Enterovirus and mumps virus infections of the nervous system. Neuro Clin 2:187, 1984.

ated with meningitis or encephalitis. The family includes members of the coxsackie A and B, echovirus and newer enterovirus groups, as well as the three poliovirus subtypes (see Ch. 425).

Arboviruses include agents of several families that are transmitted by mosquitoes or ticks. More than 15 different arboviruses have been associated with encephalitis in varied areas of the world. In the United States, the five most important are eastern and western equine encephalitis, St. Louis encephalitis, California encephalitis (with most cases involving the LaCross subtype), and Colorado tick fever. Less common within the continental states are Venezuelan equine encephalitis and Powassan encephalitis.

Herpes simplex virus type 1 causes severe encephalitis, but usually with characteristic focal features, whereas herpes simplex virus type 2 causes aseptic meningitis in association with primary or secondary genital herpes (see Ch. 426). Lymphocytic choriomeningitis (LCM) virus, an arenavirus, is a sporadic cause of meningitis and occasionally encephalitis. Aseptic meningitis has now been recognized as a complication of acute infection by the retrovirus causing the acquired immunodeficiency syndrome (AIDS; see Part XXII). Adenoviruses are respiratory viruses that only rarely cause meningitis or severe childhood encephalitis.

The acute neurologic disease associated with measles, vaccinia, and rubella infections in most cases represents postinfectious encephalomyelitis (see Ch. 429). This may also be true of the encephalitis that has occasionally been reported with influenza and parainfluenza virus infections.

EPIDEMIOLOGY. Viral meningitis and encephalitis are relatively common disorders. In one study in Rochester, Minnesota, for example, the incidence of aseptic meningitis was nearly 11 per 100,000 person-years, and that of viral encephalitis was more than 7 per 100,000 person-years. This finding was compared with a rate of 8.6 episodes of bacterial meningitis. A relatively low mortality rate in this study (3.8%) may have reflected the inclusion of milder cases and the predominance of the LaCross type of viral encephalitis. In other epidemiologic settings, the mortality may be considerably greater. In general, a specific cause is identified in only about 10 to 15% of cases of meningitis and encephalitis in the United States.

Each virus causing CNS infection has its own epidemiologic pattern. Because of the predominance of enteroviruses and arboviruses, the overall incidence of viral meningitis and encephalitis peaks in the late summer. Enterovirus epidemics in temperate climates characteristically take place with transmission occurring by the fecal-hand-oral route. They often involve young children, with rapid spread in family or social groups. The geographic and seasonal incidence of arbovirus infection relates to the life cycle of arthropod vectors and animal reservoirs (see Ch. 346) and their contact with humans. Eastern equine encephalitis virus is limited largely to the Atlantic and Gulf coasts, while western equine encephalitis virus is confined to the western two thirds of the country, with the highest incidence in the middle states. The latter virus causes many more human infections than does the eastern virus, but only 1 in 100 infected persons develops encephalitis. St. Louis encephalitis virus causes disease in both rural and urban areas over a large part of the United States. In the rural areas, the virus has the same pattern as western encephalitis virus, but in urban areas more explosive outbreaks can occur. In recent years, the LaCross subtype of the California encephalitis virus has been related every year to cases spread widely over the United States, particularly in the east and midwest, mostly in children. Colorado tick fever occurs in the Rocky Mountain area; about 18% of infected patients develop meningitis, but encephalitis is rare. Venezuelan encephalitis has spread into Florida and the southwestern states and, in most of those infected, produces an influenza-like illness, but about 3% develop acute meningitis or encephalitis. Powassan virus is a rare cause of encephalitis in Canada and along the northern border of the United States.

Lymphocytic choriomeningitis virus is the major zoonotic virus causing meningitis and encephalitis. Humans acquire the infection by contact with dust or food contaminated by excreta of the common house mouse. Human disease is more common in winter, when the natural host tends to move indoors. Lymphocytic choriomeningitis virus has also been found in hamsters, and human infections have been traced to laboratory and pet hamsters.

Mumps virus spreads by the respiratory route, with infection occurring throughout the year but increasing in incidence during the spring. Although mumps virus infects the two genders equally, males develop meningitis three times more frequently than females.

PATHOGENESIS. Events leading up to the development of the acute viral encephalitides and meningitides can be divided into three stages. The first involves exposure of an external body surface to the virus, usually with local replication of the "inoculum." In the case of enteroviruses, the infecting virus is contained in body fluids or excreta from infected persons and transferred by direct contact or within contaminated environmental materials. The arboviruses, by contrast, are introduced by an arthropod bite. The next stage involves systemic viremia and amplification of virus in visceral organs; a secondary viremia may lead to invasion of and replication within the nervous system or meninges. With the exception of rabies virus, the neurotropic herpesviruses, and perhaps the polioviruses, agents that cause acute viral encephalitis or meningitis reach the nervous system hematogenously. This factor accounts for the widespread distribution of cerebral dysfunction associated with most of the encephalitides.

In viral encephalitis, infection of neurons, glial cells, and even vascular endothelium leads to cell dysfunction and sometimes cell death. Inflammatory responses follow. Clinical symptoms and signs depend on the distribution of infection and on both the direct effect of the virus and the secondary inflammatory reactions in the tissue. The relative contribution of each to brain dysfunction depends on the particular infecting virus. The remarkable degree of recovery in many patients suggests that secondary inflammatory and immune responses often predominate.

CLINICAL MANIFESTATIONS. Most acute viral encephalitides and meningitides produce similar symptoms with variations depending on the particular virus. Often CNS manifestations are preceded or accompanied by fever, malaise or myalgia, gastrointestinal disturbance, respiratory symptoms, or rash. These are followed by headache, photophobia, stiff neck, and other signs of meningeal irritation, usually with an intensity milder than that of bacterial meningitis.

When encephalitis exists, evidence of diffuse or, less commonly, focal brain dysfunction accompanies or overshadows signs of meningeal irritation. Patients characteristically exhibit altered attention and consciousness, ranging from confusion to lethargy or coma. Motor function may be abnormal, with weakness, altered tone, or incoordination, reflecting dysfunction of the cortex, basal ganglia, or cerebellum. Severe cases may cause difficult-to-control generalized or focal seizures. Some patients exhibit myoclonus or tremor. Hypothalamic involvement may lead to hyperthermia or hypothermia, autonomic dysfunction with vasomotor instability, or diabetes insipidus. Abnormalities of ocular motility, swallowing, or other cranial nerve functions are uncommon. Spinal cord infection is usually inconspicuous but can result in flaccid weakness, with acute loss of reflexes in the most severe cases. Focal symptoms other than seizures are usually minor and overshadowed by generalized brain dysfunction; some patients may show hemiparesis, visual disturbance, or sensory loss. Focal involvement of limbic structures is particularly characteristic of herpes encephalitis (see Ch. 426).

The time course of acute viral meningitis and encephalitis varies. The onset may occur within a matter of hours or evolve more slowly over a few days. Usually, maximum deficit appears within 1 to 4 days.

LABORATORY FINDINGS. Examination of the cerebrospinal fluid is essential. The presence of 10 to 1000 mononuclear cells per cubic millimeter is characteristic. On occasion, early examination may show acellular fluid or predominance of polymorphonuclear leukocytes, but the typical mononuclear pleocytosis soon evolves. The pressure may be elevated, while the glucose level is characteristically normal or only modestly reduced. The protein content is usually elevated (50 to 100 mg per deciliter) and may exhibit increased immunoglobulin concentration and the presence of oligoclonal bands. An increased protein content and number of cells may persist for weeks or months after convalescence, and oligoclonal bands can be detected for an even longer period.

Systemic laboratory findings may vary, depending on the etiologic agent. Generally, the white blood cell count is not elevated, but either elevations or depressions can be seen, usually with a lymphocytic predominance. Involvement of salivary glands or pancreas in mumps may elevate the serum amylase level.

Neurodiagnostic tests usually reveal nonspecific abnormalities, with notable exception in the case of herpes simplex encephalitis (see Ch. 426). Computed tomography (CT) and magnetic resonance imaging (MRI) are usually normal early in the course of the nonherpetic viral encephalitides, but focal edema and contrast enhancement may appear in the more severe cases. The greatest value of these neuroimaging procedures lies in excluding alternative diagnoses.

DIAGNOSIS. With a few exceptions, the neurologic and laboratory findings accompanying the acute viral meningoencephalitides are insufficiently distinct to allow an etiologic diagnosis, and it may even be difficult to distinguish these disorders from a number of nonviral diseases. The epidemiologic setting (e.g., time of year, exposure to insects, the local community) and accompanying systemic manifestations may be helpful in presumptive diagnoses. Thus, involvement of the nervous system by mumps virus is usually suspected from associated clinical parotitis or pancreatitis, although the neurologic disease can be the sole or presenting clinical manifestation; conversely, a certain history of previous mumps eliminates this diagnostic possibility. Several enterovirus infections produce a rash, which usually accompanies the onset of fever and persists for 4 to 10 days. In infections by coxsackievirus A5, 9, and 16, and echovirus 4, 6, 9, 16, and 30, the rash is typically maculopapular and nonpruritic and may be confined to the face and trunk or may involve extremities, including the palms and soles. Echovirus 9 infections can cause a petechial rash resembling meningococcemia. Herpangina, characterized by gray vesicular lesions on the tonsillar fossae, soft palate, and uvula, can accompany group A coxsackie infection. In coxsackievirus A16 and, rarely, other group A serotype infections, a vesicular rash may involve hands, feet, and oropharynx. As discussed below, the encephalitis related to Epstein-Barr virus occurs in the setting of acute mononucleosis. The principally postinfectious encephalitides related to measles and varicella follow overt systemic diseases with characteristic rashes.

Because no specific treatment exists for acute viral meningitis and encephalitis (except herpes), and their signs and symptoms are often nonspecific, exclusion of other diagnoses becomes important. Potentially confusing are partially treated bacterial meningitis; rickettsial infections; Lyme disease; meningitis caused by a variety of nonpyogenic organisms, including *Mycobacterium tuberculosis* and *Cryptococcus neoformans* and other fungi; meningeal or parameningeal bacterial infections; brain abscess; subacute bacterial endocarditis; and the cerebral vasculitides. Among noninfectious causes, trimethoprim-sulfamethoxazole, nonsteroidal analgesics, OKT3 antibody given to enhance immunosuppression, intravenous immunoglobulin, and certain other drugs may occasionally cause a sterile meningeal reaction. Without a cerebrospinal fluid examination, the differential diagnosis becomes even broader, encompassing additional toxic and vascular diseases. Most alternative diagnoses can be suspected or eliminated by the history, the cerebrospinal fluid profile, or brain imaging.

Despite the absence of effective treatment, specific virologic diagnosis is useful both for prognosis in the individual patient and for epidemiologic implications for the populations at risk. Diagnosis usually relies on serology, although direct detection of the organism in the cerebrospinal fluid, blood, or stool may sometimes be achieved. Selection of tests and their interpretation depend upon the particular organism. Almost all acute viral syndromes occur in the setting of a first encounter with the agent, which then results in

lasting immunity. In these cases, seroconversion documented by a fourfold or greater rise in antibody titers between acute and convalescent sera is a principal means of diagnosis. A notable exception is herpes simplex encephalitis, in which antibody titers must be more cautiously interpreted (see Ch. 426). Attempts at direct viral isolation are of limited value in clinical management and must be tailored to the suspected agent. Arboviruses and enteroviruses can be isolated from the blood but are seldom recoverable at the time of clinically evident meningitis or encephalitis. During the acute disease, coxsackieviruses and echoviruses are most readily isolated from stool or cerebrospinal fluid and, in some cases, throat washings. Lymphocytic choriomeningitis virus can be isolated from blood or cerebrospinal fluid. Mumps virus may be isolated from saliva, throat washings, or cerebrospinal fluid. Type 2 herpes simplex virus may be cultured from the cerebrospinal fluid or identified in genital lesions. Polymerase chain reaction (PCR) screening of cerebrospinal fluid undoubtedly will improve specific diagnosis in the future.

TREATMENT. Treatment of acute viral encephalitis and meningitis (except herpes) is directed at symptom relief, supportive care, and preventing and managing complications. Strict isolation is not essential, although when enteroviral infection is suspected, precautions in handling of stools and the practice of careful hand washing should be instituted. Persons with measles, chickenpox, rubella, or mumps virus infections should observe the usual precautions of isolation from susceptible individuals. Arboviruses are not characteristically spread from person to person because they require an intermediate insect vector.

The headache and fever of meningitis can usually be managed with judicious doses of acetaminophen. Severe hyperthermia ($> 40°C$) may require vigorous therapy, but mild temperature elevations may serve as a natural defense mechanism and are best left untreated.

Patients with severe encephalitis often become comatose. Because, however, some may achieve remarkable recovery, vigorous support and avoidance of complications are essential. Meticulous care in an intensive care unit setting with respiratory and nutritional support is usually justified.

Although seizures sometimes complicate encephalitis, prophylactic anticonvulsants are not routinely recommended. If seizures develop, they can usually be managed with phenytoin and phenobarbital. If status epilepticus ensues, appropriate vigorous therapy should be instituted to prevent secondary brain injury and attendant hypoxia (see Ch. 433). Similarly, secondary bacterial infections should be sought and promptly treated.

Steroids should probably generally be avoided in the treatment of encephalitis because of their inhibitory effects on host immune responses.

PROGNOSIS. Full recovery from viral meningitis usually occurs within 1 to 2 weeks of onset, although some patients describe fatigue, light-headedness, and asthenia persisting for months.

The prognosis of encephalitis depends on its cause. Arbovirus encephalitides have variable mortality rates; that with eastern equine encephalitis is approximately 30%; with St. Louis, 10%; with western equine, 10%; with Venezuelan equine, 1%; and with California, less than 0.5%. The mortality rates for western equine encephalitis are greater in children under 1 year of age; for St. Louis encephalitis they are greater in the elderly. Nonfatal encephalitis caused by eastern, western, and St. Louis viruses leaves a relatively high rate of neurologic sequelae. Encephalitis associated with mumps or LCM virus is rarely associated with death, and sequelae are infrequent. Hydrocephalus has been reported as a late sequela of mumps meningitis and encephalitis in children.

Chonmaitree T, Baldwin CD, Lucia HL: Role of the virology laboratory in diagnosis and management of patients with central nervous system disease. Clin Microbiol Rev 2:1, 1989. *A review of laboratory procedures used in the diagnosis of acute viral diseases of the CNS.*

Evans AS: Viral Infections of Humans: Epidemiology and Control, 3rd ed. New York, Plenum Publishing Corporation, 1989. *A useful text dealing with the epidemiology of viral infections; contains individual chapters dealing with the major groups, including the arboviruses, enteroviruses, and herpesviruses.*

Nicolosi A, Hauser WA, Beghi E, et al.: Epidemiology of central nervous system infections in Olmstead County, Minnesota, 1950–1981. J Infect Dis 154:399, 1986. *Provides incidence figures for viral meningitis and encephalitis.*

Whitley RJ: Viral encephalitis. N Engl J Med 323:242, 1990. *A recent review that emphasizes herpes encephalitis management and differential diagnosis.*

425 POLIOMYELITIS

Richard W. Price

DEFINITIONS. Poliomyelitis (acute anterior poliomyelitis, infantile paralysis) is an acute illness caused by the three strains of poliovirus. The disease selectively destroys the motor neurons of the spinal cord and brain stem to cause flaccid asymmetric weakness. Until recently one of the most feared of all human infectious diseases, poliomyelitis is now almost entirely preventable by vaccination.

ETIOLOGY. The three antigenically different strains of poliovirus (types 1, 2, and 3) are classified in the genus *Enterovirus* within the family Picornaviridae. These are small (approximately 270 nm), roughly spherical particles with icosahedral symmetry containing a single-stranded RNA core and are surrounded by a protein capsid. Lacking a lipid envelope, the polioviruses are resistant to lipid solvents and stable at low pH.

INCIDENCE, PREVALENCE, AND EPIDEMIOLOGY. In the United States, the number of cases of paralytic poliomyelitis, has fallen to just a few cases yearly, thanks to the widespread use of an effective vaccine. In less advanced regions of the world, paralytic polio continues to occur, with a seasonal incidence in temperate zones but a more even distribution throughout the year in tropical areas. Poliovirus is acquired by the oral route and subsequently replicates in the oropharynx and lower gastrointestinal tract. It may be secreted for a week or two in saliva and for more prolonged periods in feces, which provides the major avenue of host-to-host transmission. Spread of polioviruses is greatly influenced by standards of hygiene, and greatest dissemination occurs within families or other crowded circumstances.

Paralysis is an unusual complication of poliovirus infection. During an epidemic, only 1 to 2% of infections result in neurologic symptoms and signs with another 4 to 8% suffering nonspecific (minor) illness. A number of factors increase the incidence of paralytic disease, including advancing age, recent hard exercise, tonsillectomy, pregnancy and impairment of B lymphocyte (antibody) defenses. Immunity to each of the three types of poliovirus is lifelong, but infection with one strain does not necessarily protect against subsequent infection by another. In the United States, poliomyelitis due to live-attenuated strains is as common as disease related to wild-type virus.

PATHOGENESIS AND PATHOLOGY. Polioviruses selectively infect certain neuronal populations, inducing highly stereotyped pathology, and in this manner contrast with most of the viruses causing acute encephalitis or meningitis.

The poliovirus invades the nervous system only after prior systemic replication. An initial alimentary phase with local replication in the intestinal mucosa and spread to the local lymphatics is followed by a viremia which seeds the nervous system. Once within the central nervous system, poliovirus may disseminate along neural pathways, attacking principally motor neurons of the spinal cord and lower brain stem, the brain stem reticular formation, and, to a lesser extent, the precentral gyrus. Convalescent poliomyelitis is characterized by loss of motor neurons and denervation atrophy of their associated skeletal muscles.

CLINICAL MANIFESTATIONS. The incubation period from virus exposure to the neurologic phase characteristically lasts between 4 and 10 days but may be prolonged to 4 to 5 weeks. The major illness usually begins with fever and malaise, followed within hours by generalized headache, vomiting, and within another day by the development of neck and back stiffness. Patients often are drowsy but on arousal are irritable and apprehensive. Progression may stop at this point. When paralysis develops, it usually begins on the second to fifth day after the onset of headache. Weakness, however, may be among the initial symptoms or, rarely, may be delayed for 7 to 10 days. Children generally exhibit less intense systemic symptoms than do adults, who characteristically appear acutely ill and are tremulous, flushed, and agitated. Their muscles are often sensitive and stiff.

Poliomyelitis preferentially damages the larger somatic motor neurons. In most cases, the involvement tends to include the lumbar segments more than the cervical and the spinal cord more than the brain stem. The consequent paralyses are usually asymmetric, weakness characteristically being more proximal than distal. In mild cases paralysis affects only parts of muscles rather than selective peripheral nerve or nerve root distributions. Sensory changes are lacking. The paralysis may render one member useless yet entirely spare the contralateral arm or leg. About 50% develop acute urinary retention. The trunk musculature is least commonly affected. The affected muscles are flaccid, and the deep tendon reflexes may be absent. Atrophy develops rapidly, usually beginning within a week in paralyzed muscles and progressing over the ensuing weeks. The motor deficit rarely progresses for more than 3 to 5 days.

About 10 to 15% of cases affect the lower brain stem motor nuclei. Involvement of the ninth and tenth cranial nerve nuclei leads to paralysis of pharyngeal and laryngeal musculature. Parts of the facial muscles can be involved, either unilaterally or bilaterally. Less often, the tongue and muscles of mastication become paralyzed. External oculomotor weakness occurs rarely. The pupils are spared. Direct involvement of the brain stem reticular formation can disrupt breathing and swallowing and can produce serious disturbances in cardiovascular control. Poliomyelitis seldom causes permanent functional paralysis of the bulbar muscles, probably because of the relatively small size of the motor units served by brain stem nuclei and because overwhelming disease in these critical segments usually kills the patient.

DIAGNOSIS AND DIFFERENTIAL DIAGNOSIS. Because of its rarity in the United States, poliomyelitis may present diagnostic difficulties. Its early phases must be differentiated from other acute meningitides, and when paralysis ensues, a major differential diagnosis is with the Guillain-Barré syndrome and other predominantly motor polyneuropathies. However, no other acute disease produces headaches, stiff neck, fever, and asymmetric flaccid paralysis without sensory loss coupled with an increase in white blood cells in the cerebrospinal fluid (CSF). Rarely, the CSF shows a persistence of significant pleocytosis in polyneuritis, and CSF protein levels above 100 mg per milliliter are frequent. Acute intermittent porphyria may cause a motor polyneuropathy somewhat similar to postinfectious polyneuropathy. At times, acute transverse myelitis may be confused with poliomyelitis, but findings of a sensory-motor spinal level at the appropriate spinal cord segment usually serves to separate an inflammatory cord transection from diffuse anterior horn cell involvement (see Ch. 428.1). Rarely, coxsackievirus and echoviruses have been reported to cause encephalitides with prominent (but not extensive) motor neuron symptoms and signs. Diagnosis can be established by isolation of virus from blood or CSF or by serologic evidence of acute poliovirus infection. In cases related to vaccine strains, viral isolates can be distinguished in the laboratory.

TREATMENT. There is no specific treatment, but supportive care is important in reducing suffering during the acute attack, in maintaining vital functions to ensure survival, and perhaps in modifying the overall outcome and disability. Important measures include preventing contractures, maintaining airway and cardiovascular stability, and preventing excessive calcium mobilization and bed sores.

PROGNOSIS. Death in poliomyelitis is usually the result of bulbar involvement and is attributable to respiratory and cardiovascular impairments. Mortality has been considerably reduced with modern management of respiratory insufficiency. Patients who survive an episode of acute paralytic poliomyelitis usually recover considerable motor function. Generally, motor improvement begins within the first weeks after onset, and 60% of eventual recovery is achieved by 3 months.

The Postpolio Syndrome. A number of patients with previous poliomyelitis develop further motor deterioration later in life. In some this relates simply to musculoskeletal decompensation or other factors but does not involve new weakness. However, other persons suffer a true loss of strength termed the postpolio syndrome. This disorder is characterized by an insidiously slow but gradually progressive weakness beginning 30 or more years after an attack of poliomyelitis. Most commonly it adds to the weakness of already affected muscles; less often, weakness develops in muscles previously thought to be normal. This weakness is often accompanied by fasciculations, and there may be additional atrophy. Muscle biopsy shows type grouping consistent with active denervation-reinnervation. Overall, the prognosis is good, with only slow progression of further weakness, which rarely leads to a severe increase in disability or to death. The most likely pathogenesis consists of senescence of surviving, expanded motor units. This development must be distinguished from motor neuron disease of a more malignant variety (see Ch. 415), which has also been described many years after acute poliomyelitis but appears to be much less common than the more gradual and benign postpolio syndrome.

PREVENTION. Poliomyelitis can be prevented by either live-attenuated or killed polio vaccines. These are now given routinely in Western cultures, although the practice of immunization has relaxed as the threat of developing paralytic poliomyelitis has become less conspicuous. If this trend is not reversed, a resurgence of the disease can be expected. An important consequence of accurate diagnosis of poliomyelitis is the prompt institution of local vaccination programs for communities at risk, including subcultures in which vaccination is avoided for religious or other reasons.

Price RW, Plum F: Poliomyelitis. *In* Vinken PJ, Bruyn GW (eds.): Handbook of Clinical Neurology, Vol. 32, Part I. Amsterdam, Elsevier-North Holland, 1978. *A general review of clinical and biologic aspects of poliomyelitis.*

Windebank AJ, Litchy WJ, Daube JR, et al.: Late effects of paralytic poliomyelitis in Olmsted County, Minnesota. Neurology 41:501, 1991. *A study characterizing the long-term clinical sequelae of a population sample with previous poliomyelitis.*

426 HERPESVIRUS INFECTIONS OF THE NERVOUS SYSTEM

Richard W. Price

Three of the six human herpesviruses (see also Ch. 339 through 341) share an essential "neurotropism" in their adaptation for survival and transmission. Herpes simplex virus types 1 and 2 (HSV-1 and HSV-2) and varicella-zoster virus (VZV) all establish in sensory ganglia a latent infection that can subsequently reactivate to release progeny virus into the territory of the ganglion's epithelial innervation. The major neurologic complications of these infections in adults include adult-type herpes simplex encephalitis caused by HSV-1; aseptic meningitis, radiculitis, and sacral autonomic insufficiency caused by HSV-2; and encephalitis, myelitis, radiculopathy, and vasculitis complicating herpes zoster. Prompt diagnosis of infections by these viruses is important because they are now amenable to selective antiviral drug therapy. Two of the remaining human herpesviruses, Epstein-Barr virus and cytomegalovirus, although largely lymphotropic, can also cause neurologic disease in the setting of systemic illness. Recent reports also suggest that human herpesvirus-6 can cause encephalitis in immunosuppressed patients.

426.1 Herpes Simplex Encephalitis (HSE)

Adult-type HSE is a sporadic disease with a severe morbidity and high mortality. Both HSV-1 and HSV-2 are capable of causing encephalitis, but type 1 by far predominates. In contrast, HSV-2 accounts for the great majority of neonatal herpetic encephalitis, which is not considered here.

EPIDEMIOLOGY AND PATHOGENESIS. Although the most common identified cause of severe, sporadic viral encephalitis in the United States, HSE is nonetheless uncommon. The disease afflicts persons of all postneonatal ages, with peaks of incidence in late childhood and middle age. It occurs with approximately equal frequency throughout the year, and case-to-case transmission does not occur. Curiously, immunosuppression plays no apparent role.

HSV-1 is a ubiquitous organism; more than 90% of adults exhibit serologic evidence of exposure and likely harbor latent ganglionic infection. Recurrent cold sores resulting from viral reactivation occur in perhaps one fourth of adults. Although HSE may occur as a primary infection, it likely more often results from reactivated virus or perhaps from reinfection by a new strain of virus.

The characteristic gross and microscopic pathology of herpetic infection, particularly its anatomic localization, distinguishes HSE from other encephalitides. Although often asymmetric, the disease is usually bilateral and afflicts the medial temporal and inferior frontal lobes and related "limbic" structures, including the hippocampus, amygdaloid nuclei, olfactory cortex, insula, and cingulate gyrus. Necrosis with petechial hemorrhage is so intense that the disease was once called *acute necrotizing encephalitis*. Microscopically, hemorrhagic necrosis with mononuclear inflammation characterizes involved areas, with neurons and glia often containing Cowdry type A intranuclear inclusions during the acute phase of infection. The gray matter is affected predominantly, but infection extends into the white matter as well.

CLINICAL MANIFESTATIONS. HSE most commonly presents as a subacute or acute illness causing local and diffuse cerebral dysfunction. Typically, patients are febrile, although in as many as 10% fever may be absent, and thus herpes encephalitis warrants consideration even in afebrile patients who present with an altered mental status. Severe headache, focal or generalized convulsions, and alterations in behavior and consciousness are the most prominent symptoms. Common symptoms including disorientation, delusions, agitation, personality changes, or dysphasia sometimes lead erroneously to psychiatric referral. Motor paralyses are present in fewer than half of affected individuals.

DIAGNOSIS. Evaluation of suspected HSE has been an area of controversy, principally related to the issue of diagnostic brain biopsy. Among the arguments for brain biopsy are that (1) it is the most sensitive and accurate diagnostic method, contrasting with the insensitivity and difficulty in early interpretation of serologic studies and neurodiagnostic procedures; and (2) this procedure results in identification of alternative diagnoses, some of which respond to specific treatment. Arguments against brain biopsy relate to its potential short- and long-term sequelae, the benignity of empiric therapy, and the improved sensitivity and accuracy of magnetic resonance imaging (MRI) compared with earlier diagnostic methods. Broad application of DNA detection is likely to further obviate the need for biopsy. Important issues regarding management also relate to the facilities, expertise, and experience available to the patient at the admitting hospital. Nevertheless, we recommend that most patients be managed without biopsy and that the combination of clinical and laboratory features warrants an approach utilizing empiric therapy.

The most important step in management involves prompt recognition of HSE as a diagnostic possibility and rapid institution of acyclovir therapy. Among the important neurodiagnostic evaluations in patients suspected of having HSE are MRI, cerebrospinal fluid (CSF) analysis, and electroencephalography. Whereas computed tomographic (CT) scanning is surprisingly insensitive in detecting early HSE, with two fifths or more patients having normal scans, MRI more often detects characteristic abnormalities. The latter include virtually pathognomonic increased signal, particularly on T2-weighted sequences, in the same regions showing pathology at autopsy: the medial temporal and insular cortical regions as well as the inferior frontal cingulate gyri, often bilateral (Fig. 426–1). The MRI also allows more sensitive detection of alternative diagnoses, such as brain abscess, vasculitis, or demyelination. Some patients are so ill or agitated that MRI may require general anesthesia. In some, biopsy might be needed.

CSF examination is also important in detecting evidence of virus infection. Most patients exhibit a mononuclear pleocytosis with 50 or more leukocytes per cubic millimeter, although fewer or even a normal number of cells may be noted. The protein content is usually mildly elevated, and the glucose level is normal or only mildly reduced. Like MRI, CSF analysis may also be useful in establishing alternative diagnoses, such as bacterial or fungal infection. In more than three fourths of patients, the electroencephalogram exhibits focal abnormalities, most often showing spike and slow-wave or sharp-wave patterns over the involved temporal lobes.

Attempts at isolating HSV-1 from CSF rarely succeed. New methods of diagnosis seek detection of viral antigens (by enzyme-

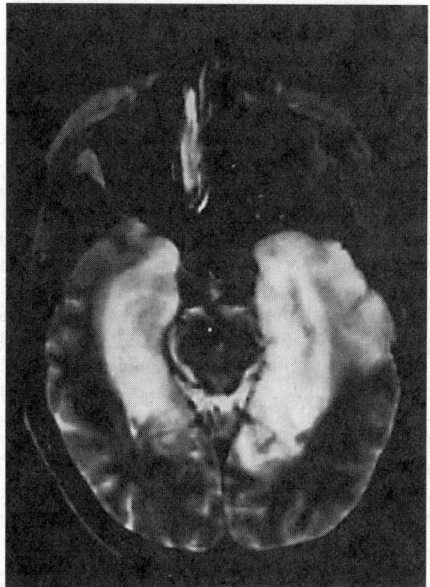

FIGURE 426-1. MRI scan of a 54-year-old woman with herpes simplex encephalitis who presented with fever, dysphasia, and confusion. The T2-weighted image shows increased signal in both medial temporal lobes, with more extensive involvement on the left (right side of figure).

linked immunosorbent assay) or nucleic acid by polymerase chain reaction (PCR) gene amplification show great promise. In the research laboratory PCR has been shown to be sensitive and specific in detecting HSV-1 DNA sequences in CSF. Isolation of the virus from the oropharynx is useless because no relationship exists between symptomatic or asymptomatic viral shedding at such peripheral sites and brain infection. HSV-1 is often reactivated by other neurologic diseases eliciting fever, creating a source of false-positive serologic responses.

In contrast to the epidemic encephalitides, in which documentation of seroconversion provides a major method of diagnosis, in HSE serologic testing is often inconclusive. This is particularly true at the onset, when prompt diagnosis is critical. During convalescence analyses of blood, antibody titers can give false-negative or false-positive results. Assessment of intrathecal anti–HSV-1 antibody production appears to be quite useful, however.

TREATMENT. The introduction of antiviral therapy has greatly improved the outcome of HSE. This was first demonstrated with vidarabine, and even greater benefit has been shown with acyclovir, which has become the treatment of choice. HSE is treated by an intravenous infusion of 10 mg per kilogram given over a 1-hour period every 8 hours for 10 days. The therapeutic efficacy of acyclovir is restricted to the herpesviruses by virtue of the drug's selective interaction with two virus-coded enzymes, thymidine kinase and DNA polymerase; acyclovir is thus not a broad-spectrum antiviral. Because acyclovir is excreted principally by the kidney, caution must be exercised in patients with renal impairment. Side effects of acyclovir are generally few, although neurotoxicity rarely occurs, manifested as altered consciousness, tremors, hallucinations, and seizures. Other aspects of care also require meticulous attention. Optimally, patients with HSE should be managed in the intensive care setting of a tertiary referral center.

PROGNOSIS. Both age and initial neurologic status significantly influence the prognosis in HSE. Even with antiviral therapy, patients who are comatose when first treated often fare poorly. Extensive infection and brain damage are present in most of these patients as a result of a more fulminant illness and, sometimes, a delay in beginning therapy. Many patients, however, particularly those younger than 30 years old who are neurologically intact when treatment begins, recover normal or nearly normal function. Patients with minor neurologic deficits may survive without severe long-term sequelae and return to normal function if diagnosis is made and specific treatment is instituted early in the course. In a few patients, and despite antiviral treatment, HSE can relapse within a few weeks after the acute disease, resulting in severe sequelae. The pathogenesis of such relapses is unknown.

426.2 Neurologic Complications of Genital Herpes

Genital herpes, most often caused by HSV-2, may be complicated by local or radicular pain, aseptic meningitis, autonomic (bowel, bladder, and sexual) dysfunction, and, rarely, myelitis. These complications are more common in association with primary genital herpes but may occur with recurrent disease as well. Prodromal neuritic symptoms commonly precede recurrences and may involve the buttock, the groin, or, less commonly, the lower extremities.

Aseptic meningitis and autonomic dysfunction may occur either independently or together. Meningitic symptoms are associated with primary genital herpes in about one fourth of patients, but only a minority require hospitalization. Its course is benign, usually clearing in 4 to 10 days without residua. The CSF profile is typical of an aseptic meningitis, with a mononuclear pleocytosis, mild protein elevation, and normal, or occasionally reduced, glucose level. When the history clearly implicates an epidemiologic and temporal relationship with genital herpes and the CSF findings are those of a typical mononuclear profile, a clinical diagnosis can usually be made. Specific diagnosis can often be established by isolation of HSV-2 at lumbar puncture.

Urinary retention, constipation, and sexual impotence in association with genital herpes are less common than meningitis. Symptoms and signs of a sacral sensory radiculopathy sometimes accompany the autonomic changes. The pathophysiology of this disorder is uncertain, but direct herpetic infection of nervous system structures is likely. Fortunately, autonomic dysfunction is reversible, and patients can be assured that their symptoms will probably clear. Although unusual, these autonomic symptoms can recur. It is important to consider and pursue the diagnosis of HSV-2 infection in patients who present with isolated bladder, bowel, or sexual dysfunction. It is critical not to make an inappropriate diagnosis of spinal neoplasm or, especially, early multiple sclerosis. When there is a clear history of genital herpes, the cause of autonomic dysfunction is usually readily established clinically. Inspection and viral culture of genital lesions, plus accompanying antibody titers, which may appear and rise slowly only in primary HSV-2 infection, provide additional help.

In adults, HSV-2 only rarely produces adult-type herpes encephalitis indistinguishable from that caused by HSV-1. Transverse myelopathy due to HSV-2 is very rare.

Epithelial HSV-2 primary infections and recurrences can be treated with acyclovir, but the effect on the neurologic complications of genital herpes is uncertain. In the absence of adequate data, it appears appropriate to give acyclovir for neurologic complications of primary genital herpes.

In patients with frequent recurrent attacks of genital herpes, early, self-initiated treatment of recurrent lesions with oral acyclovir has been advocated, beginning therapy at the onset of prodromal symptoms. This approach is probably appropriate for the rare patient with recurrent herpetic meningitis.

426.3 Neurologic Complications of Varicella-Zoster Virus Infections

Herpes zoster (HZ) (shingles, zona) is a dermatomal cutaneous infection caused by reactivation of the VZV that normally lies latent in sensory ganglia following an early attack of varicella. In addition to its cutaneous manifestations, zoster is accompanied by neuritic symptoms and may be complicated by an array of neurologic sequelae. The VZV is distantly related to HSV, sharing only minor antigen cross-reactivity.

INCIDENCE AND EPIDEMIOLOGY. HZ is a common disorder, with an annual incidence estimated at 3.4 cases per 1000 persons. Unlike varicella, HZ occurs throughout the year, with neither significant clustering of cases nor seasonal or yearly preponderance. Case exposure in HZ is rarely identified. Two factors, age and immunosuppression, significantly influence its incidence. The disease is uncommon in childhood, relatively constant in those between 20 and 50 years of age (approximately 2.5 cases per 1000 annually), and thereafter doubles its incidence in those between the ages of 50 and 60 and redoubles it in those between age 80 and 90. Immunosuppression due to systemic disease (in particular, Hodgkin's disease and other lymphoreticular malignancies), cytotoxic drugs, corticosteroids, radiation therapy, or infection by human immunodeficiency virus (HIV) predisposes. In some cases, a history of neoplasm, radiation exposure, or physical injury in the proximity of the dorsal root ganglion or nerve is elicited.

Age is an important factor also in the development of postherpetic neuralgia, which develops almost exclusively in persons older than 50 years of age. The incidence of postherpetic pain varies, ranging between 15 and 75%, depending on clinical definition of the syndrome and selection of patients. Immunosuppression predisposes to spread of virus beyond the ganglion-nerve-dermatome unit into the central nervous system or systemically.

PATHOGENESIS AND PATHOLOGY. Although controversial, evidence suggests that VZV is latent in ganglionic satellite cells rather than neurons. Once latent virus reactivates, it can spread within the sensory ganglion and travel centrifugally over the peripheral nerve processes, eventually seeding the skin with the dermatomal vesicular rash.

Cell-mediated defenses rather than humoral immunity are critically involved in protecting the host during HZ. Pathologically, acutely infected dorsal root ganglia and nerve show the presence of a mononuclear inflammatory response, neuronal degeneration with intranuclear Cowdry type A inclusion bodies, and similar infection of surrounding satellite cells. The peripheral nerve may contain parallel changes. In more severe cases, dorsal root ganglia above and below the primarily affected ganglion also show active herpetic infection.

CLINICAL MANIFESTATIONS. Prodromal sensory symptoms include dermatomal pain, itching, or paresthesias, which often precede by several days the eruption of the segmental rash. The early pain of zoster may be confused with other types of neuropathic or visceral pain. Rarely, no rash appears but the role of VZV is suggested by a rise in antibody titers (*zoster sine herpete*). The most frequently involved dermatomes are those extending from the third thoracic to the second lumbar segments and the first (ophthalmic) division of the trigeminal nerve. The rash itself initially consists of erythematous macules that vesiculate over 12 to 24 hours. Normally the vesicular fluid pustulates within 72 hours; in a week the pustules begin to dry, and crusting takes place by 10 to 12 days. The crusts, in turn, fall off in 2 to 3 weeks. In the immunocompromised host, this time course may be protracted. In uncomplicated cases, the rash heals with a variable degree of superficial scarring, at times leaving areas of hyperpigmentation or depigmentation, which may be anesthetic. More severe cases may leave denervation of a large segment of the dermatome.

Zoster can affect any of several of the cranial nerves. The ophthalmic division of the trigeminal nerve is the most commonly affected, and the condition may be complicated by spread to orbital structures, resulting in acute and long-term ocular sequelae. Spread of cutaneous rash along the bridge of the nose to its tip should be taken as a signal of impending ocular infection, prompting early ophthalmologic consultation. Facial palsy, with or without accompanying loss of taste on the anterior two thirds of the tongue, may accompany either otic zoster (Ramsay Hunt syndrome), with rash confined to a segment of the auricle, or the second and third cervical dermatomes (cervical collar zoster). Occasionally, infection of the ninth and tenth or fifth cranial nerve may precede facial weakness. As with other motor syndromes (see below), weakness is often delayed for a variable period after the rash. Eighth nerve dysfunction with sensorineural hearing loss or vertigo occurs in the same setting as facial palsy but with less frequency. HZ may rarely cause facial palsy in the absence of rash (*sine herpete*). Zoster of the ninth and tenth cranial nerves is unusual and may be overlooked without a careful search for the pharyngeal rash or ipsilateral laryngeal or pharyngeal palsy.

HZ of the extremities or trunk can also be complicated by segmental motor weakness, the motor loss usually corresponding to the involved cutaneous dermatome. Weakness characteristically develops from a few days to 2 weeks after the onset of the rash, and longer delays are rare. Its onset is characteristically abrupt, occurring over hours or 1 or 2 days, with little or no subsequent deterioration. Weakness abates or disappears in about 85% of cases.

Myelitis of variable extent is a less common complication of HZ and results from direct viral invasion of the spinal cord, perhaps augmented by local inflammatory responses. It occurs most commonly in the immunosuppressed person and, like motor paresis, is characteristically delayed after the onset of the rash. The most common manifestation is bladder dysfunction. Other signs include mild or transient asymmetric reflexes, lower extremity weakness, and sensory disturbance. Severe myelopathy can produce a partial Brown-Séquard syndrome or total cord transection. Characteristically, involvement lies at the same spinal cord segment as the rash but may ascend to a higher level. Spinal MRI or myelography may be needed to rule out coexisting epidural tumor.

At least three types of brain involvement may complicate zoster: diffuse encephalitis, focal parenchymal infection, and vasculitis. Headache, stiff neck, and mild diffuse encephalitis often accompany acute HZ but are difficult to distinguish from the effects of fever, sepsis, narcotic analgesics, and other underlying medical problems. Most such patients recover fully. In more severe diffuse encephalitis, chances for recovery may also be good if other complications of the disease do not intervene. The clinical picture is that of acute or subacute lethargy or delirium accompanied by CSF pleocytosis with few focal features.

Focal VZV encephalitis is a rare complication in immunosuppressed patients that can resemble progressive multifocal leukoencephalopathy. The onset may be temporally remote from the cutaneous rash. The cerebral lesions involve principally the white matter. Brain biopsy is required for diagnosis, allowing identification of Cowdry type A inclusions or of VZV antigens or nuclei acids.

Cerebral vasculitis is probably the most common serious postzoster central nervous system complication. Affected patients usually develop delayed contralateral hemiplegic strokes following trigeminal ophthalmic division zoster owing to inflammation or occlusion of the internal carotid artery and its major branches ipsilateral to the rash. The delay between the rash and the onset of cerebral dysfunction varies from none to as long as 6 months, with a mean interval of 7 weeks. A more widespread cerebral vasculitis following zoster in other locations has also been reported. The pathogenesis is still incompletely understood, but the characteristic involvement of local vessels innervated by the infected ganglion, in conjunction with reports suggesting the presence of viral nucleocapsids and viral antigens within vessels, suggests that the arteries are directly infected. Additional contributions may be made by secondary local inflammatory responses and thrombosis, leading to vascular occlusion or distal embolization. Arteriographic evidence of vasculitis or occlusions in the involved vessels and the clinical setting usually allow diagnosis.

DIAGNOSIS. The clinical diagnosis of HZ is seldom difficult. The dermatomal distribution and the evolution of the vesicular rash are characteristic, and only rarely does herpes simplex infection assume a similar pattern and confuse the diagnosis. Difficulty, however, may occur early in the disease, when pain or other sensory symptoms precede the rash. The rare case of zoster sine herpete may require additional methods of diagnosis, and, in cases with an occult rash, a careful search is necessary. When there is a question of the diagnosis, a Tzanck test examining lesion scrapings, a direct culture, or immunohistochemical identification of infected cells can provide specific identification of VZV. Serology may also be helpful, although the commonly used complement fixation test can cross-react between HSV and VZV.

THERAPY. The goals are to relieve the acute segmental infection, to curtail spread of infection either systemically or to other areas of the nervous system, and to prevent postherpetic neuralgia. The means available consist of using antiviral drugs to interrupt viral replication and perhaps corticosteroids to modify local inflammatory responses. Treatment of individual patients must take into account their background risk for particular complications.

Because involvement of the ophthalmic division of the trigeminal nerve risks spreading to orbital structures, such infections should receive early antiviral treatment. Systemic antiviral therapy should also be used for immunosuppressed patients, who are more susceptible to severe disseminated infection. In young patients with normal immune function, there is usually no requirement for specific therapy because zoster is usually mild with swift recovery and no residua. Older nonimmunosuppressed persons are susceptible to postherpetic neuralgia. A recent large clinical study showed that prednisone had no protective effect against the neuralgia.

The antiviral treatment of choice for HZ is acyclovir. The nucleoside can abort the rash and prevent systemic spread when administered promptly by the intravenous route. The recommended intravenous dosages vary from 5 to 10* mg per kilogram infused every 8 hours for 5 days. More recently, the use of oral acyclovir has been suggested at a dosage of 800 mg* every 4 hours with omission of the nighttime dose, particularly in individuals who are not at marked risk of developing viral complications.

Intravenous acyclovir is indicated for patients in whom VZV infection progresses to cause myelitis or encephalitis, although delay in institution reduces its overall effect. No satisfactory data indicate whether either acyclovir or steroids improve the outcome of HZ-associated motor weakness. Similarly, there is no proven effective treatment for zoster-associated cerebral vasculitis. Postherpetic neuralgia is discussed in Ch. 405.3.

426.4 Neurologic Complications of Cytomegalovirus and Epstein-Barr Virus Infections

Both human cytomegalovirus (CMV) and Epstein-Barr virus (EBV) infections can cause neurologic disease. In children CMV is an important and relatively common cause of congenital neurologic deficit, but central and peripheral nervous system infections in adults occur almost exclusively in the setting of immunosuppression. Central nervous system (CNS) complications of EBV infections occur in the setting of acute mononucleosis. Both CMV and EBV have been implicated in triggering the Guillain-Barré syndrome.

CMV encephalitis and, less commonly, meningoencephalitis or myelitis have been reported as opportunistic infections in adults suffering from impaired cell-mediated immunity. Earlier these complications were reported most commonly in patients undergoing organ transplantation. Recently their occurrence has been noted principally in association with acquired immunodeficiency syndrome (AIDS). The clinical features of CMV brain infection have been imprecisely characterized, but they generally resemble the physical and cognitive impairments of a metabolic encephalopathy (see Ch. 394). At times, focal deficits (e.g., hemiparesis) or seizures are superimposed. Pathologically, infection of the brain is marked by scattered microglial nodules, some of which contain typical cytomegalovirus intranuclear inclusions. As many as one fourth of autopsied AIDS patients have neuropathologic evidence of CNS cytomegalovirus infection, although in most the infection appears to be mild, and its contribution to symptoms uncertain. Some patients may exhibit ventricular subependymal abnormalities or small abscess-like lesions on MRI. Hyponatremia is a common feature.

Recently, CMV has been found to cause severe ascending polyradiculopathy. This syndrome is usually characterized by the subacute evolution of severe, painful polyradiculopathy that begins with sacral or lumbar sensory, motor, and autonomic dysfunction.

The diagnosis of CMV encephalitis is difficult. Most AIDS patients, particularly homosexual men, have circulating antibody to

the virus which can be isolated from urine or blood, yet they do not suffer nervous system infection. For this reason, serologic evaluation and systemic virus isolation are not particularly helpful in diagnosis; rather, one must rely principally on clinical suspicion. More recently, use of polymerase chain reaction (PCR) to amplify CMV DNA in CSF has been shown to be diagnostic. CMV polyradiculopathy can be diagnosed by the CSF findings, including the prominence of neutrophils, isolation of virus, and PCR amplification. The antiviral drugs ganciclovir and foscarnet have been reported effective in treating certain manifestations of CMV infection, including particularly the retinopathy that sometimes complicates AIDS but also CMV polyradiculopathy.

The neurologic complications of EBV infection range from symptoms of headache, photophobia, weakness, and fatigue to more serious, but uncommon, complications. The latter have been described principally in the context of individual case reports. They include encephalitis, meningoencephalitis, Guillain-Barré syndrome, Bell's palsy, acute cerebellar ataxia, and transverse myelitis. It is likely that most of these neurologic complications result from immune-mediated injury rather than direct viral infection. EBV is also implicated in the primary CNS lymphoma complicating AIDS and the immunosuppression of organ transplantation.

Aurelius E, Johansson B, Skoldenborg B, et al.: Rapid diagnosis of herpes simplex encephalitis by nested polymerase chain reaction assay of cerebrospinal fluid. Lancet 337:189, 1991. *A series demonstrating high sensitivity and specificity of polymerase chain reaction detection of HSV-1 DNA in CSF of patients with encephalitis.*

Bashir R, Luka J, Cheloha K, et al.: Expression of Epstein-Barr virus proteins in primary CNS lymphoma in AIDS patients. Neurology 43:2358, 1993. *Describes expression of EBV RNA and protein in primary CNS lymphomas.*

Devinsky O, Cho E-S, Petito CK, Price RW: Herpes zoster myelitis. Brain 114:1181, 1991. *A case series characterizing myelitis complicating HZ.*

Drobyski WR, Knox KK, Majewski BS, Carrigan DR: Brief report: Fatal encephalitis due to variant B human herpesvirus-6 infection in a bone marrow-transplant recipient. N Engl J Med 330:1356, 1994. *A detailed case report of a virologically well-studied patient with fatal encephalitis associated with HHV-6 infection.*

Holland NR, Power C, Matthews VP, et al.: Cytomegalovirus encephalitis in acquired immunodeficiency syndrome (AIDS). Neurology 44:507, 1994. *A case series analyzing the clinical and laboratory features of a group of autopsy-proven patients with CMV encephalitis.*

Miller RG, Storey JR, Greco CM: Ganciclovir in the treatment of progressive AIDS-related polyradiculopathy. Neurology 40:569, 1990. *Describes the clinical and therapeutic aspects of cytomegalovirus polyradiculopathy in AIDS patients.*

Straus SE: Overview: The biology of varicella-zoster virus infection. Ann Neurol 35:S4, 1994. *A general review of VZV introducing a symposium on VZV and postherpetic neuralgia containing several other useful brief reviews.*

Whitley RJ, Gnann JW: Acyclovir: A decade later. N Engl J Med 327:782, 1992. *A review of the clinical uses of acyclovir.*

Wood MJ, Johnson RW, McKendrick MW, et al.: A randomized trial of acyclovir for 7 days or 21 days with and without prednisolone for treatment of herpes zoster. N Engl J Med 330:897, 1994. *A clinical trial showing no additional effect of prolonging acyclovir treatment and only a modest short-term effect of prednisolone on healing of the acute zoster rash; neither longer antiviral treatment nor the corticosteroid influenced the incidence of postherpetic pain.*

---

427 RABIES
Richard W. Price

DEFINITION. Rabies is a viral infection with nearly worldwide distribution that affects principally wild and domestic animals but also involves humans, resulting in a devastating, almost invariably fatal encephalitis.

ETIOLOGY, PATHOGENESIS, AND PATHOLOGY. Rabies virus is a bullet-shaped, enveloped, single-strand RNA virus classified in the rhabdovirus family and *Lyssavirus* genus. It has particular neurotropic properties, and unlike many of the other viruses causing acute encephalitis, it appears to require central nervous system (CNS) infection as an essential part of its "life cycle."

Viral transmission to both animals and humans characteristically results from the bite of a rabid animal, although cases of transmission by aerosol in the laboratory or in a bat cave and by transplanted infected corneal tissue have also been recorded. Once the

---

* Exceeds manufacturer's recommended dosage.

virus breaches the protective epithelium, it reaches the CNS via peripheral nerves, exploiting retrograde axoplasmic transport. The interval between the bite and the onset of disease ranges from days to a year or more, but in most cases lasts 1 to 2 months. This delay may relate to amplification of the virus in peripheral tissues, particularly skeletal muscle, before it gains access to the CNS over motor and sensory nerves. During this delay, the virus can be eliminated by host immune mechanisms; indeed, it is this delay that affords an opportunity for prophylactic postexposure immunization after the rabid bite. Once virus enters peripheral and central nervous system pathways, immune defenses are unable to suppress further replication and spread of infection, which includes axoplasmic transport and perhaps transsynaptic transmission.

The CNS is involved in the subsequent transmission of the virus by infected animals in two essential ways: (1) Infection of certain brain regions underlies the characteristic behavioral changes in the rabid animal, leading to increased biting activity; and (2) antegrade transport of the virus to salivary glands leads to virus shedding. In concert, these two aspects of infection ensure transmission and survival of the virus in the wild. They also have practical diagnostic implications for the human disease. The characteristic altered behavior in humans often results in a distinct clinical picture distinguishing rabies from other viral encephalitides. Antegrade virus transport also affords a means of diagnosing rabies by isolation from saliva or immunohistochemical staining of infected cutaneous nerves innervating hair follicles.

Pathologic findings include both nonspecific and specific abnormalities. A considerable discrepancy often occurs between the degree of pathologic change, particularly neuronal loss, and the severe antemortem clinical state. Nonspecific changes include perivascular mononuclear infiltrates and microglial response, although inflammation may be scant in relation to the widespread distribution of infected cells detected immunohistochemically. Similarly, neuronal destruction is less prominent than the abundance of viral antigen, which is located principally in neurons but also in astrocytes. More specific changes include the presence of Negri bodies, eosinophilic neuronal intracytoplasmic inclusion composed of viral nucleoprotein. At autopsy, infection is usually widespread in the brain, but with prominent involvement of the brain stem and spinal cord and also involvement of the hippocampus, basal ganglia, cortex, and other structures. The relation of virus infection of neurons and the attendant inflammatory reaction to the clinical manifestations remains incompletely understood. Rabies infection of neurons may alter their membrane properties or synaptic transmission. Whatever the means, patients eventually manifest widespread brain dysfunction that terminally impairs respiratory and autonomic control.

EPIDEMIOLOGY. The epidemiology of rabies varies in different parts of the world, falling into two patterns. In *sylvatic rabies,* infection is maintained in wildlife reservoirs. Thus, in the United States, rabies is endemic in the striped skunk in the midwestern states and California, in the raccoon in the southeastern and mid-Atlantic states, in the red fox in northern New York and adjacent regions of Canada and in the gray fox in parts of the southwestern states; bat rabies has a wide geographic range. A similar pattern holds in other developed nations, where human rabies is rare and more often results from direct contact with wildlife than from secondary transmission to the domestic dog or cat and then to humans. This pattern contrasts with that in much of Asia, Africa, and Latin America, where *urban rabies* is maintained as an epizootic infection in the domestic dog and human disease is far more common. Viral strains differ among various animal hosts.

CLINICAL MANIFESTATIONS. After the silent incubation period, clinical rabies frequently begins with a prodromal phase, which may include nonspecific symptoms of malaise, fever, and headache but also more specific local symptoms related to the site of the original bite. These include itching, paresthesias, or other sensations beginning in the area of the healed wound and then spreading to a wider region and eventually involving the whole limb or side of the body.

Within a few days, the full-blown illness begins, taking one of two forms—encephalitic *(furious)* or paralytic *(dumb)* rabies—perhaps depending on the source and strain of the infecting virus. In its initial phase, encephalitic rabies is often distinguished from other viral infections by irritability of the patient and hyperactivity of a

number of automatic reflexes. Periods of calm lucidity may alternate with confusion and seeming intense anxiety precipitated by internal or external stimuli. Hydrophobia, with reflexive intense contraction of the diaphragm and accessory respiratory and other muscles, is induced upon attempts to drink or even at the sight of water. Similarly, blowing or fanning air on the chest may induce intense laryngeal, pharyngeal, or other muscle spasms (aerophobia). High fever persists throughout the illness.

Paralytic rabies is less common and more readily misdiagnosed. Patients present with weakness, usually beginning in the bitten extremity and spreading to involve all four limbs and the facial muscles. Early in the course, both consciousness and sensory function are spared. Helpful signs include myoedema and piloerection, and fever is also present. As the diseases progresses, it may converge with the encephalitic form, accompanied by some of the same irritative phenomena. Both forms evolve into lethargy and coma, with prominent alterations of respiratory and cardiovascular function. Tachycardia may precede bradycardia with ectopic rhythms, and the breathing pattern becomes irregular with cluster or periodic respirations. Patients succumb to respiratory failure or cardiovascular collapse within a mean interval of 4 days from onset, although a few may survive as long as 3 weeks or more. Intensive supportive care may extend survival longer; rare cases with partial vaccine-induced immunity have been reported to survive with intensive care.

DIAGNOSIS. Rabies is usually suspected on the basis of a history of animal bite or other exposure, although in as many as one third of cases no such history is obtained. Definitive antemortem diagnosis is established by immunohistochemical identification of rabies virus antigen in hair follicle nerve endings of biopsied skin, usually obtained from the nape of the neck. Isolation of virus from saliva or the presence of antirabies antibodies in blood in the absence of vaccination or in the cerebrospinal fluid may also be used to establish diagnosis. Postmortem diagnosis is usually made by histologic or immunohistochemical examination of the brain.

The differential diagnosis depends on the clinical presentation and the epidemiologic setting. In the case of paralytic rabies, diagnosis is most often confused with the Guillain-Barré syndrome, poliomyelitis, or other neuropathies or myelopathies, while the encephalitic form must be differentiated from other viral and infectious encephalitides, tetanus, and toxic encephalopathies. In regions where vaccine is prepared using neural tissue (still the practice in many regions of the world with the highest rates of rabies), allergic encephalomyelitis remains a principal differential diagnosis.

TREATMENT AND PREVENTION. Established CNS disease remains essentially untreatable. Disease prevention relies on public health measures to reduce animal reservoirs and on postexposure immune prophylaxis to abort viral penetration of the CNS after a rabid bite or other contact. Although clinical rabies is a rare disease in most developed countries such as the United States, the decision to administer active prophylaxis remains a relatively common clinical issue. The physician first determines the type of possible exposure; an open wound or disrupted mucous membrane exposed to saliva may warrant postexposure prophylaxis, whereas contact of saliva with intact skin may not. The first step in management is to administer prompt local wound care, thoroughly washing with soap or iodine. The epidemiologic setting is important in determining the likelihood that the biting animal might be rabid and often requires consultation with local health authorities to ascertain which animals carry rabies in the geographic setting. In the absence of previous vaccination, both passive (rabies immune globulin of human origin) and active (diploid cell vaccines) immunizations are administered. Presently, tissue culture–derived vaccines are safe, with a low incidence of major adverse reactions, in contrast to earlier nerve tissue–derived vaccines.

Baer GM, Bridbord K, Hui FW, et al. (eds.): Research towards rabies prevention. Rev Infect Dis (Suppl)10:S5773, 1988. *A compendium of brief papers presented at a symposium dealing with various aspects of rabies, particularly strategies for prevention, but covering a broad range of related tissues.*

Centers for Disease Control: Rabies Prevention—United States, 1991: Recommendations of the Immunization Practices Advisory Committee (ACIP). MMWR 40 (RR-3):1, 1991. *Outlines US guidelines for rabies prophylaxis.*

Fishbein DB, Robinson LE: Rabies. N Engl J Med 329:1632, 1993. *An outstanding and succinct review of the epidemiology and management of rabies and rabies exposure.*

Hemachudha T: Rabies. *In* McKendall RR (ed.): Handbook of Clinical Neurology, vol 12: Viral Diseases. Amsterdam, Elsevier Science Publishers, 1989, p 383. *A particularly valuable review of the clinical neurologic aspects of rabies.*

428 SLOW VIRUS INFECTIONS OF THE NERVOUS SYSTEM

Richard W. Price

428.1 Introduction

The term *slow infections* was first applied by Bjorn Sigurdsson to a group of transmissible diseases of sheep characterized by an incubation period and course measured in months or years rather than hours or days, as in typical acute viral or bacterial infections. Subsequently, several human diseases sharing these characteristics have been described. Although often considered together because of their chronic nature, these disorders are in fact heterogeneous with respect to their clinical manifestations, neuropathology, etiology, and pathogenesis. Although in some instances the infections are accompanied by inflammatory pathology, others clinically and pathologically more closely resemble degenerative or hereditary diseases of the nervous system. Two of the sheep diseases upon which Sigurdsson based his concept of slow infections, *visna* and *scrapie,* have subsequently proved to have human counterparts. Visna is caused by a retrovirus and somewhat resembles the nervous system infections caused by the human immunodeficiency virus type 1 (HIV-1) responsible for acquired immunodeficiency syndrome (AIDS) and tropical spastic paraparesis caused by human T cell lymphotropic virus type I (HTLV-I), while scrapie closely parallels Creutzfeldt-Jakob disease and kuru.

The agents causing the slow infections are taxonomically diverse, as are the mechanisms by which they maintain chronic progressive infection and cause clinical symptomatology (Table 428–1). Thus, HIV-1 is an RNA-containing retrovirus that codes for a DNA intermediary that can integrate into the host genome and persist for the life of the cell; progressive multifocal leukoencephalopathy is caused by a small, nonenveloped DNA-containing papovavirus; subacute sclerosing panencephalitis is due to the enveloped RNA measles virus; and Creutzfeldt-Jakob disease is caused by an agent that has not yet been definitively identified but may consist of a modified cell protein only (see Ch. 428.6). Contributions of host immune responses to the development and symptomatology of these diseases are varied. In the case of progressive multifocal leukoencephalopathy, a conventional virus that circulates commonly in the human community and is ordinarily associated with little, if any, disease causes devastating central nervous system (CNS) infection in the presence of depressed host cell-mediated immunity. HIV-1 causes profound systemic disease by virtue of its predilection for infecting the helper-inducer (CD4+) subset of T lymphocytes, with the resultant systemic immunosuppression perhaps playing a role in

the subsequent development of progressive brain disease by this same virus. In this setting of perturbed immunity, CNS injury results from "indirect" mechanisms whereby uninfected cells are damaged by toxic products released from infected and reactive macrophages. The pathogenesis of myelopathy caused by HTLV-I also most likely significantly involves immunopathologic mechanisms. Subacute sclerosing panencephalitis appears to result from defective replication in the brain of a once-common conventional virus and is accompanied by an exuberant but ineffective antibody response. In the case of Creutzfeldt-Jakob disease, immunosuppression plays no role in the development or progression of the disease, and indeed there is little evidence that the host recognizes the infectious agent as foreign.

The diversity of the agents causing these slow infections, along with their variable cell and tissue tropism, host susceptibility, and pathologic reactions, has led to speculation that viruses may play a role in several of the common neurodegenerative disorders, including multiple sclerosis, amyotrophic lateral sclerosis, parkinsonism, and Alzheimer's disease. To date, however, no direct evidence for such an infectious cause of any of these disorders has been identified.

Tyler KL, Martin JB: Infectious Diseases of the Central Nervous System. Philadelphia, FA Davis, 1993. *Contains a detailed and informative section on viral diseases of the nervous system.*

428.2 Human Immunodeficiency Virus Infection and the AIDS Dementia Complex

DEFINITION. Among the common neurologic complications of human immunodeficiency virus type 1 (HIV-1) infection (see Ch. 364) is the *AIDS dementia complex,* which appears to relate pathogenetically in an elemental way to the AIDS virus itself rather than to secondary opportunistic infection. The nomenclature for this "subcortical" dementing syndrome is still in a state of flux, and several alternative terms have been used, including AIDS dementia and *HIV-1-associated cognitive/motor complex.* This section continues to use the earlier AIDS dementia complex terminology and the functional staging categories outlined in Table 428–2. Neither peripheral neuropathy nor psychological reactive states are intrinsic parts of the AIDS dementia complex.

CLINICAL MANIFESTATIONS. The AIDS dementia complex is characterized by a triad of cognitive, motor, and behavioral dysfunction. Patients' earliest symptoms usually consist of difficulties with concentration and memory. They complain of losing their train of thought or conversations and find that they need to keep lists to maintain their daily schedules. Many complain of "slowness" in thinking. Complex tasks at work or in the home, such as balancing the checkbook or reconciling other personal financial affairs, become increasingly difficult and take longer to complete.

Despite these early complaints, in stage 0.5 to 1, bedside screening or mental status testing may yield results within the normal range, although characteristically patients are slower and less facile than previously. With advancing disease (stages 2 to 3), patients perform poorly on tasks requiring concentration and attention, such as word and digit reversals and serial subtraction. Eventually, a larger array of mental status tests becomes abnormal, accompanied by psychomotor slowing.

Symptoms of motor dysfunction usually are less prominent than those of intellectual impairment. However, motor abnormalities, including, particularly, slowing of rapid successive and alternating movements of the extremities and eyes, are almost always noted on examination. Abnormal reflexes are common, with generalized hyperreflexia (in the absence of concomitant neuropathy) along with release signs such as snout or glabellar responses. With disease progression, symptomatic difficulty with balance or incoordination may be evident; patients may inadvertently drop things or become

TABLE 428–1. HUMAN SLOW VIRUS INFECTIONS OF THE CENTRAL NERVOUS SYSTEM

Disease	Etiologic Agent	
	Name	*Classification*
AIDS dementia complex	Human immunodeficiency virus type 1	Retrovirus (RNA)
Tropical spastic paraparesis	Human T cell lymphotropic virus type 1	Retrovirus (RNA)
Progressive multifocal leukoencephalopathy	JC virus	Papovavirus (DNA)
Subacute sclerosing panencephalitis	Measles virus	Paramyxovirus (RNA)
Progressive rubella panencephalitis	Rubella virus	Togavirus (RNA)
Creutzfeldt-Jakob syndrome, Gerstmann-Sträussler disease, kuru	–	Spongiform encephalopathy agents, prions

TABLE 428-2. AIDS DEMENTIA COMPLEX (ADC) STAGING

ADC Stage	Characteristics
Stage 0 (normal)	Normal mental and motor function.
Stage 0.5 (equivocal/ subclinical)	Either minimal or equivocal *symptoms* of cognitive or motor dysfunction characteristics of ADC or mild signs (snout response, slowed extremity movements), but *without impairment of work or capacity to perform activities of daily living* (ADL). Gait and strength are normal.
Stage 1 (mild)	Unequivocal evidence (symptoms, signs, neuropsychological test performance) of functional intellectual or motor impairment characteristic of ADC, but able to perform *all but the more demanding aspects of work or ADL.* Can walk without assistance.
Stage 2 (moderate)	Cannot work or maintain the more demanding aspects of daily life, but able to perform *basic activities of self care.* Ambulatory, but may require a single prop.
Stage 3 (severe)	*Major intellectual incapacity* (cannot follow news or personal events, cannot sustain complex conversation, considerable slowing of all output), *or motor disability* (cannot walk unassisted, requiring walker or personal support, usually with slowing and clumsiness of arms as well).
Stage 4 (end stage)	*Nearly vegetative.* Intellectual and social comprehension and responses are at a rudimentary level. Nearly or absolutely mute. Paraparetic or paraplegic with double incontinence.

slower and less precise with hand activities, including writing. Gait incoordination may result in frequent tripping or falling or in a perceived need to exercise new care in walking. In more advanced disease, ataxia and, subsequently, leg weakness limit ambulation. Patients with early or predominating spastic-ataxic gait are usually shown to have vacuolar myelopathy pathologically (see below). Bladder and bowel incontinence is common in the late stages of the disease.

Psychological depression appears to be surprisingly infrequent in these patients, despite the prominence of psychomotor slowing. Patients appear uninterested and lack initiative but are not dysphoric. A minority develop a more agitated organic psychosis with manic features.

Patients with a severe progressive course who reach stage 4 characteristically lie quadriparetically in bed with a vacant stare and incontinence. They may be mute or exhibit an extraordinary delay in making brief verbal responses. Unless intercurrent illness develops, the level of arousal is usually preserved.

DIAGNOSIS AND DIFFERENTIAL DIAGNOSIS. Diagnosis relies on identifying the characteristic clinical features of the AIDS dementia complex and excluding other conditions. No single laboratory test establishes the presence of the syndrome. In those with milder forms, perhaps the major difficulty is in distinguishing true cognitive impairment from the effects of fatigue and systemic illness or from psychiatric conditions, including anxiety, depression, or hypochondriasis. The history is critical in establishing functional decline, and an observant friend or family member may provide particularly helpful information. Neuropsychological testing can define impairment of attention and motor speed but must be interpreted appropriately, taking into account the patient's background, including age and education, as well as confounding conditions such as substance abuse, previous head trauma, and the effects of various medications. Such studies are also useful for quantifying the patient's progression or response to treatment.

In those with more severe disease, the differential diagnosis most commonly centers on distinction from the other neurologic complications noted in HIV-1-infected patients (see Ch. 364) or, less commonly, from dementing or myelopathic neurologic disease observed in the normal population. Both neuroimaging procedures and cerebrospinal fluid (CSF) examination are diagnostically essential,

principally to eliminate other conditions rather than to establish a diagnosis of the AIDS dementia complex. Computed tomography (CT) and magnetic resonance imaging (MRI) almost always detect cerebral atrophy with widened cortical sulci and enlarged ventricles. In some patients, MRI also shows patchy or diffuse signal changes in the hemispheric white matter and, less commonly, the basal ganglia or thalamus (Fig. 428-1).

Routine CSF analysis is not specifically diagnostic, and findings may be indistinguishable from those in asymptomatic HIV-1-infected patients, with variable elevation of protein content or mononuclear cells. Elevations of CSF neopterin and β_2-microglobulin levels have been reported to correlate with the presence and severity of the AIDS dementia complex, but these markers of immune activation are also increased in CNS opportunistic infections and are not specific. HIV-1 isolation from the CSF is not diagnostically helpful because the virus can also be cultured from asymptomatic seropositive subjects. The p24 core protein is seldom detected by immunoassay in the CSF of patients with milder clinical disease and therefore generally is not useful.

EPIDEMIOLOGY. The frequency of the AIDS dementia complex increases as the systemic effects of HIV-1 infection and resultant immunosuppression worsen. This complication is rare in patients who are otherwise asymptomatic but begins to become more frequent in those manifesting constitutional symptoms (fever, weight loss, malaise). Its prevalence increases further as the CD4+ blood T lymphocyte counts fall and opportunistic infections develop. Preterminally this neurologic syndrome is common. However, precise prevalence figures are not available, and, indeed, with the introduction of antiviral treatment, the epidemiologic pattern of neurologic AIDS may be changing. Milder forms of the AIDS dementia complex, with a static or indolently progressive course, are more common in patients with preserved immune function (CD4+ lymphocyte counts above 200 per cubic millimeter), whereas the progressive and more severe forms characteristically develop in patients with more advanced immunosuppression. In addition, although there is a general parallel between the onset and severity of the AIDS dementia complex and the onset and severity of systemic complications, wide individual variability exists; at one extreme are patients with little or no systemic disease but with severe AIDS dementia complex, while at the other end some patients with repeated episodes of opportunistic infection may remain neurologically preserved.

PATHOLOGY AND PATHOGENESIS. The neuropathologic findings in patients with the AIDS dementia complex include at least three "subsets" of major abnormalities: (1) central gliosis and white matter pallor, (2) multinucleated cell encephalitis, and (3)

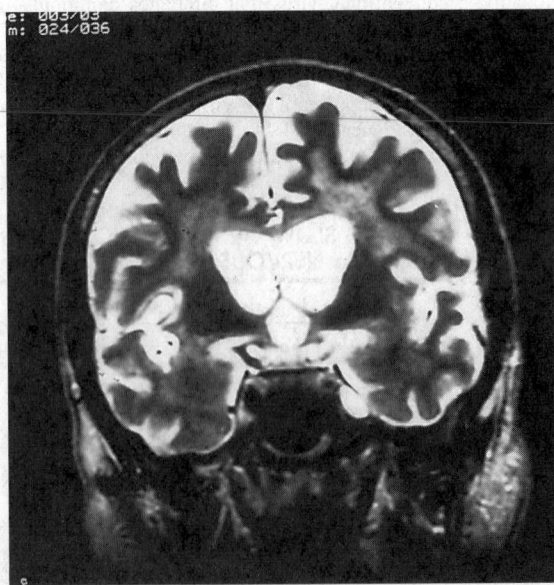

FIGURE 428-1. A coronal T2-weighted MRI of the brain of a patient with AIDS dementia complex showing typical atrophy with enlarged lateral and third ventricles and subarachnoid space along with "patchy" increased signal in the central white matter.

vacuolar myelopathy. In general, these findings correlate with the clinical severity. Central gliosis and white matter pallor are almost universal findings and, in isolation, are the major abnormality in patients with milder AIDS dementia complex. Rarely, they are the only abnormalities in patients with even more severe clinical symptoms and signs. Virologic studies to date have little or no viral burden in brains of this subgroup of patients.

Multinucleated cell encephalitis is characterized by the presence of perivascular and, at times, parenchymal cell reactions that include macrophages and microglial cells along with multinucleated cells derived from fusion of these two cell types. These multinucleated cells are infected by HIV-1, and, indeed, the cell fusion likely results from interaction of the viral glycoproteins gp120 and gp41 with the CD4 cell receptor. Multinucleated cell encephalitis is thus properly referred to as *HIV-1 encephalitis* and is noted in patients with more severe and progressive AIDS dementia complex.

Vacuolar myelopathy, while defined pathologically, can also often be distinguished clinically on the basis of the predominant myelopathic symptoms and signs. Patients with this condition usually present with spastic-ataxic gait difficulty but with proportionally little sensory disturbance and usually no definable sensory "level." Histologically, the disorder closely resembles subacute combined spinal cord degeneration accompanying vitamin B_{12} deficiency. Its pathogenesis is uncertain, but clearly independent of the type of productive infection that produces multinucleated giant cells.

The pathogenesis of the neurologic injury underlying the AIDS dementia complex has been difficult to unravel from a number of aspects. Because the major "functional elements" of the brain, i.e., the neurons, oligodendrocytes, and astrocytes, do not appear to be productively infected, it remains uncertain how these cells are damaged. In both the gliosis-pallor and the vacuolar myelopathy subsets, overt HIV-1 brain infection is absent or undetectable, and even in multinucleated cell encephalitis the magnitude of neurologic dysfunction often appears to exceed the distribution and extent of productive infection. Speculation has centered on possible indirect mechanisms of injury involving toxic molecules of either viral (e.g., gp120) or cellular (e.g., cytokines elaborated by uninfected cells responding to infection) origin. It is also possible that nonproductive infection of glia might lead to cell dysfunction without virus replication as a result of restricted viral genome transcription or translation. Whatever the mechanisms, however, HIV-1 infection, either of brain or of systemic organs, appears to be the *prime mover* in the pathogenesis of the AIDS dementia complex and thus the major target of therapy.

TREATMENT AND PROGNOSIS. Several reports now suggest that zidovudine (also azidothymidine, or AZT) relieves, at least partially, the symptoms and signs of the AIDS dementia complex. Therapeutic effect has been documented by improvement in neuropsychological test performance in several studies. Dose recommendations remain uncertain, but in the absence of precise information, conventional dosage (100 mg every 4 hours during wakefulness) is advised. Limitations of treatment relate to toxicity, (bone marrow suppression and, less often, myopathy), but, eventually, probable drug resistance. In patients whose neurologic condition deteriorates on these doses, the clinician may attempt to increase the dose, although toxicity is more likely. Additional antiretroviral drugs are currently being assessed with respect to their effect on this condition.

Symptomatic management is important. In the subset of patients who present with mania, lithium or neuroleptics may be helpful. However, these patients may be unusually susceptible to the side effects of neuroleptics and other psychotropic drugs, and thus treatment should be cautious and begin with low doses.

Navia BA, Jordan BD, Price RW: The AIDS dementia complex: I. Clinical features. Ann Neurol 19:517, 1986. Navia BA, Cho ES, Petito CK, et al.: The AIDS dementia complex: II. Neuropathology. Ann Neurol 19:525, 1986. *Companion articles describing the clinical and pathologic features of the AIDS dementia complex.*

Price RW, Perry S: HIV, AIDS, and the Brain. New York, Raven Press, 1994. *A collection of papers dealing with clinical and pathogenetic aspects of the AIDS dementia complex and brain HIV infection.*

Sidtis JJ, Gatsonis C, Price RW, et al.: Zidovudine treatment of the AIDS dementia complex: Results of a placebo-controlled trial. Ann Neurol 33:343, 1993. *A report of a clinical trial assessing zidovudine therapy for the AIDS dementia complex.*

Sidtis JJ, Price RW: Early HIV-1 infection and the AIDS dementia complex. Neurology 40:323, 1990. *A review of the issue of the AIDS dementia complex in asymptomatic HIV-1 seropositive individuals. Provides staging scheme given in this chapter.*

428.3 Human T Cell Lymphotropic Virus Type I– Associated Myelopathy and Tropical Spastic Paraparesis

DEFINITION. Human T cell lymphotropic virus type I (HTLV-I) was the first human retrovirus to be identified in the laboratory and the second, after human immunodeficiency virus type 1 (HIV-1), to be implicated in neurologic disease. This connection was made when a survey in Martinique discovered that nearly 60% of patients with tropical spastic paraparesis (TSP) were seropositive for HTLV-I. A similar serologic association was soon established in other tropical areas, and, concomitantly, Japanese workers implicated this virus in the myelopathy occurring principally in the Kyushu district; they proposed the name HTLV-I–associated myelopathy (HAM). Subsequent comparison of the clinical and laboratory features indicated that the tropical and Japanese conditions are, in fact, the same disease.

ETIOLOGY AND EPIDEMIOLOGY. HTLV-I is a genomically complex virus classified among the oncogenic retroviruses. Although infection is most often asymptomatic, the virus has been implicated in acute T cell lymphoma/leukemia (ATLL) as well as HAM/TSP. In Japan it is estimated that myelopathy develops in about 1 in every 2000 infected carriers and ATLL in perhaps 1 in 10,000 carriers; the two conditions rarely coexist. Infection is widely prevalent in much of the Caribbean, in certain parts of South Africa, South India, Colombia, Peru, and the Seychelles Islands, as well as Japan. In the United States, endemic infection is found principally in certain parts of the Southeast, chiefly among blacks; however, the influx of Caribbean and other migrants, as well as perhaps transfusion-related transmission, has resulted in more widespread sporadic dispersion. Infection is thought to be transmitted sexually from males to females, in breast milk, and by transfusion, the last factor having led to serologic blood donor screening. Although some preliminary observations suggested that multiple sclerosis might be associated with this retrovirus, numerous subsequent studies have failed to substantiate such a connection.

HTLV-I–associated myelopathy usually afflicts individuals between 20 and 65 years old and most commonly begins between ages 35 and 45 years. For those infected early in life, this implies a very prolonged incubation period. In patients infected by transfused blood, however, the incubation period is as short as 5 or 6 months. Otherwise, most cases are sporadic, although there is an occasional familial incidence. The variability in disease expression among those infected has led to the suggestion that host factors, including histocompatibility immune response genes, might be cofactors in the disorder's development.

CLINICAL MANIFESTATIONS. The salient feature of HTLV-I myelopathy is spastic paraparesis or paraplegia. Typically, the onset is gradual, with steady disease progression over months to years and a tendency in many instances to stabilize later on. Occasionally, the disorder begins more abruptly and has a more irregular course. Patients almost universally exhibit spastic legs; bladder and bowel disturbance is present in more than three quarters, while only about half have position or vibratory sensory impairment. Low back stiffness and pain are common. The gait may at times appear ataxic, and probably fewer than one tenth of affected persons have symptoms of neurologic dysfunction outside the spinal cord. Optic atrophy, nerve deafness, peripheral neuropathy, a clinical picture of pseudo-amyotrophic lateral sclerosis with anterior horn cell disease, and polymyositis have all been noted. Patients may also have systemic findings involving the lung (lymphocytic alveolitis), skin, and eyes (cotton-wool spots).

Characteristic CSF findings include oligoclonal immunoglobulin bands and intrathecal synthesis of anti-HTLV-I antibodies. The CSF cell count may be normal or show a mild lymphocytic pleocytosis; lymphocytes with flower-like nuclear changes similar to those seen in ATLL may be present. About half of patients have abnormal signal in the cerebral white matter detected by magnetic resonance imaging (MRI), indicating subclinical involvement.

The diagnosis of TSP/HAM relies principally on the identification of the clinical manifestations and documentation of viral infection; CSF abnormalities, including the high level of antibodies to the virus, are also helpful. Because of the high rate of asymptomatic HTLV-I infection, other neurologic conditions are likely to develop in seropositive patients, and thus the diagnosis requires more than simply ascertaining the presence of antibodies in a patient with spinal cord or other neurologic abnormalities. In addition, current serologic screening methods do not discriminate between HTLV-I and the related retrovirus, human T cell lymphotropic virus type II (HTLV-II), which also may be associated with a similar myelopathy. Additional testing with Western blot or more direct characterization of the viral genome by polymerase chain reaction can discriminate between the two viruses.

PATHOLOGY AND PATHOGENESIS. The spinal cord corticospinal tracts are most severely affected, although abnormalities are usually more widely distributed. Perivascular inflammation involving lymphocytes, macrophages, and plasma cells, along with fibrosis, is notable. Gliosis is prominent, with loss of myelin and, frequently, axons as well. Although the brain also contains scattered perivascular inflammation, parenchymal changes are usually minimal or absent. Immunologic studies show activation of major histocompatibility class I antigens in association with the inflammatory and gliotic responses.

Although HTLV-I antigens have been noted in some cases, most other attempts to identify infected cells have been negative, indicating that productive infection is minimal. This observation, along with the prominence of inflammation and the therapeutic response to immunosuppressive measures, suggests that immunopathologic processes are involved in the genesis of spinal cord injury. HTLV-I infection is associated with a state of immune activation with circulating activated T cells. Whether the neurologic injury relates to immune reactions to HTLV-I antigens and consequent "innocent bystander" injury of adjacent neural tissue or to true autoimmunity with activation of immune responses against self-antigens is uncertain.

TREATMENT AND PROGNOSIS. Immunosuppression using corticosteroids, plasma exchange, or other measures has been reported, principally by the Japanese, to alleviate HTLV-I myelopathy, although remission may not be well sustained. Antiviral therapy (with zidovudine or newer antiretroviral drugs used for AIDS) has not yet been clearly assessed in TSP/HAM. As noted above, the course and outcome are variable. Usually the disease becomes disabling, but not directly life limiting; thus supportive measures are of paramount importance, as in other spinal cord diseases.

Lehky TJ, Fox CH, Koenig S, et al.: Detection of human T-lymphocyte virus type I (HTLV-I) tax RNA in the central nervous system of HTLV-I-associated myelopathy/tropical spastic paraparesis patients by in situ hybridization. Ann Neurol 37:167, 1995. *HTLV-I RNA was found in the spinal cords of three HAM/TSP patients, including in astrocytes; contains an up-to-date reference list related to pathogenesis.*

Roman GC, Vernant J-C, Osame M (eds.): HTLV-I and the Nervous System. Proceedings of an international meeting organized by the Departments of Neurology of Texas Tech University and La Meynard Hospital, April 15–16, 1988, Fort-de-France, Martinique, French Antilles. New York, Alan R. Liss, 1989. *Contains reviews of the clinical, epidemiologic, and biologic aspects of TSP/HAM.*

428.4 Subacute Sclerosing Panencephalitis and Progressive Rubella Panencephalitis

Subacute sclerosing panencephalitis (SSPE), a "slow" infection caused by measles virus, usually affects children, but its onset can extend into young adulthood. Patients usually have a history of measles within the first 2 years of life, and it is speculated that such early host exposure allows emergence of persistent defective virus replication. Fortunately, its incidence has markedly decreased in recent years.

Clinically, SSPE usually begins with cognitive and behavioral changes; progresses to include motor dysfunction with prominent myoclonus choreoathetosis, dystonia, and rigidity; and usually pursues a progressive course with steady deterioration over 1 to 3 years to eventual rigid quadriparesis and a vegetative state. The condition is more common in a rural setting and affects males more often than females. The electroencephalogram (EEG) reveals periodic complexes with synchronous bursts at two or three slow waves per second, recurring at 5- to 8-second intervals. The CSF is characterized by a high immunoglobulin concentration, oligoclonal bands, and abundant intrathecal synthesis of antibody to measles virus antigens. Serum measles antibody titers are also high. These findings are usually sufficiently characteristic for diagnosis, but brain biopsy may be needed for definitive diagnosis in some cases. The distinct pathology of SSPE includes gliosis, loss of myelin, and perivascular infiltrates of lymphocytes and plasma cells in white and gray matter. Intranuclear inclusions containing viral nucleocapsids are noted in both neurons and glia.

Measles virus may also cause a subacute encephalitis in the immunocompromised host. The prominence of cognitive and motor dysfunction in these patients resembles SSPE, but the clinical setting, its subacute onset and more rapid evolution, and the presence of seizures rather than myoclonus are distinctive. Brain pathology includes abundant intranuclear inclusions, but inflammation is minimal, and neither serum nor CSF antibody titers against measles virus are high. For this reason, brain biopsy is usually needed for diagnosis.

Progressive rubella panencephalitis is a rare disorder resembling SSPE but caused by rubella virus and developing as a complication of either the congenital rubella syndrome or, more typically, childhood rubella. A hiatus of years separates early infection from the onset of neurologic deterioration, which is characterized by behavioral changes, intellectual decline, ataxia, spasticity, and sometimes seizures. Myoclonus is not a prominent feature, as it is in SSPE. Serology or viral isolation from brain or peripheral blood lymphocytes confirms the cause.

With the advent of widespread measles and rubella immunization, these disorders have been all but eliminated in the United States, although SSPE still occurs in less developed parts of the world. There is no known treatment.

Graves M: Subacute sclerosing panencephalitis. Neurol Clin 2:267, 1984. *A thorough general review of SSPE.*

Wolinsky JS: Subacute sclerosing panencephalitis, progressive rubella panencephalitis, and multifocal leukoencephalopathy. *In* Waksman B (ed.): Immunologic Mechanisms in Neurologic and Psychiatric Disease. New York, Raven Press, 1990, p 259. *An excellent review of the pathogenesis of SSPE and subacute rubella encephalitis.*

428.5 Progressive Multifocal Leukoencephalopathy

DEFINITION. Progressive multifocal leukoencephalopathy (PML) is an opportunistic viral infection of the CNS caused by a papovavirus, JC virus. Initially described in patients with a variety of underlying disorders accompanied by impaired T lymphocyte/macrophage-mediated immune defenses, it now most frequently occurs in patients with advanced human immunodeficiency virus type 1 (HIV-1) infection. It is one of the clinical AIDS-defining opportunistic complications. As the name implies, clinical PML affects principally the white matter of the brain, often with more than one lesion and characteristically pursuing an inexorably progressive course.

ETIOLOGY AND EPIDEMIOLOGY. Two factors are important in the development of PML: exposure to JC virus in the past and suppression of T cell-related immune defenses against the virus. With respect to the former, JC virus has a virtually worldwide distribution, and the majority of the population exhibits serologic evidence of exposure by the teenage years. Primary infection is benign, and, indeed, disease accompanying initial exposure has not been clearly defined. PML appears to result almost always from reactivation of latent JC virus infection rather than from recent exposure. The virus is thus innocent, except under circumstances in which the host's T lymphocyte-directed immunity is impaired and rendered unable to suppress JC virus reactivation and subsequent continued replication and spread. Recent studies indicate that JC virus infection in PML patients is not confined to the brain but also involves peripheral blood mononuclear cells, probably chiefly B lymphocytes.

Whereas the incidence of PML has increased with the AIDS epidemic to complicate perhaps 2 to 5% of cases, it may also complicate organ transplantation, lymphoreticular and hematologic malignancies (particularly in the context of cytoreductive chemotherapy), autoimmune disorders, and other immunosuppressed states associated with T lymphocyte dysfunction.

CLINICAL MANIFESTATIONS AND DIAGNOSIS. PML is characterized by the gradual onset and steady progression of focal neurologic dysfunction, usually involving the cerebral hemispheres. Thus, patients may present with homonymous visual field disturbance, hemiparesis, hemisensory disturbance, aphasia, apraxia, or other "cortical" dysfunction, depending on the location of the demyelinating focus. Posterior fossa abnormalities with cerebellar dysfunction or signs of brain stem involvement are less common. Most often the patient is otherwise well, without constitutional symptoms (e.g., fever, malaise), and consciousness is preserved. Headache or seizures are unusual, occurring in 10% or fewer of patients.

Diagnosis is often suspected on the basis of the underlying condition (e.g., AIDS) and the clinical presentation of focal neurologic deficit. Neuroimaging is helpful in demonstrating loss of white matter rather than an expanding mass (as, for example, in toxoplasmosis or primary CNS lymphoma). Computed tomographic (CT) scanning is less sensitive than magnetic resonance imaging (MRI), both with respect to detecting multiple lesions and in distinguishing white matter localization, most commonly adjacent to the cerebral cortex (Fig. 428–2). Characteristically, contrast enhancement is absent. Although MRI in the AIDS dementia complex may show multifocal abnormalities in the white matter that superficially resemble those of PML, patients with AIDS dementia complex usually do not have focal neurologic symptoms and signs and MRI lesions do not show on T1 MRI sequences as they do with PML.

CSF is usually acellular, with normal or only mild elevation of protein content. Serologic studies usually document the presence of serum antibodies against JC virus, but this is of limited diagnostic utility because antibody titers are indistinguishable from those of

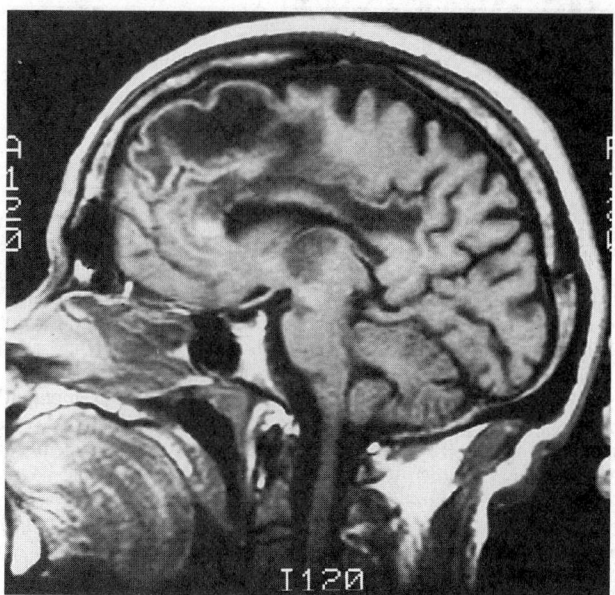

FIGURE 428–2. A sagittal T1-weighted MRI of a patient with advanced progressive multifocal leukoencephalopathy showing marked loss of white matter in the frontal lobe and cingulate gyrus with preservation of the cortical gray matter.

the normal population and do not rise with the onset or progression of the disease. CSF antibodies are usually not detected. Culture of the virus from CSF or blood is difficult, and not useful for diagnosis. Identification of viral nucleic acid in the CSF, blood, or urine using PCR appears promising, but the sensitivity and specificity have yet to be fully defined. Accordingly, brain biopsy is necessary for definitive diagnosis. The distinct histologic abnormalities usually permit diagnosis on routinely processed and stained tissue, but immunohistochemical identification of JC antigens or *in situ* hybridization to identify viral nucleic acid may be useful.

PATHOLOGY AND PATHOGENESIS. The pathology of PML provides an example of the selective effects of a virus on different cell populations within the brain. Thus, the major macroscopic finding of demyelination results from the progressive productive-lytic infection of oligodendrocytes. Lesions begin as microscopic centers of infection, which then spread concentrically outward; oligodendrocytes are lost in the center, and their nuclei are swollen, with inclusions at the periphery. Because myelin is composed of the elaborated cytoplasmic membranes of these cells, their lysis results in the characteristic demyelination; in mild lesions, axons are relatively spared, while in more severe coalescent foci, frank cavitation results. Macroscopic pathology consists of multiple foci of enlarging demyelinating "plaques." Astrocytes undergo marked alteration, with formation of bizarre nuclei resembling transformed cells, but without true malignant potential. Neurons are spared. Inflammation is usually minimal.

TREATMENT AND PROGNOSIS. There is no established treatment for PML. Case reports of response to cytosine arabinoside administered intravenously or intravenously are now being followed up by a controlled clinical trial. Of note, spontaneous remissions have been reported, including several in patients with AIDS.

Berger JR, Kaszovitz B, Post MJD, et al.: Progressive multifocal leukoencephalopathy associated with human immunodeficiency virus infection: A review of the literature with a report of sixteen cases. Ann Intern Med 107:78, 1987. *A review of AIDS-associated PML.*
Houff SA, Major EO, Katz DA, et al.: Involvement of JC virus-infected mononuclear cells from the bone marrow and spleen in the pathogenesis of progressive multifocal leukoencephalopathy. N Engl J Med 318:301, 1988. *A report emphasizing the presence of systemic JC virus infection in PML.*

428.6 Creutzfeldt-Jakob Disease

Paul E. Bendheim

DEFINITION. Creutzfeldt-Jakob disease (CJD) is a subacute central nervous system (CNS) disorder characterized by a progressive dementia, myoclonus, and distinctive electroencephalographic (EEG) and neuropathologic findings. Although uncommon, it is the most prevalent of the human subacute spongiform encephalopathies—fatal diseases that can arise either by dominant genetic inheritance, transmission of a unique pathogen, or sporadically.

ETIOLOGY. CJD is a unique disease in that it can apparently arise by two separate mechanisms, genetic and infectious. Most cases, however, are sporadic and in these the pathogenetic mechanism remains unknown. CJD is closely related to kuru and several rare, inherited human diseases termed the *Gerstmann-Straüssler-Scheinker syndrome* (GSS) and *fatal familial insomnia* (FFI). *Scrapie* is an analogous spongiform encephalopathy of sheep and goats experimentally transmissible to other animal species. As proposed in a remarkable insight by Parry 35 years ago, natural scrapie in sheep is genetic in origin, but the protein encoded by this mutated gene can behave as an infectious particle and transmit the disease to susceptible hosts. The scrapie agent is not known to cause disease in humans. The transmissible CJD, GSS, kuru, and animal spongiform encephalopathy agents are unlike any known virus or other well-characterized transmissible pathogen. This has resulted in the terms *slow virus, virion,* and *prion* being used interchangeably with "agent" to refer to them. These agents probably consist of protein only, and no nucleic acid component is needed to transmit the disease to susceptible hosts.

Kuru is a disease previously endemic among the Fore people inhabiting an area in the eastern highlands of Papua New Guinea. Cerebellar dysfunction, dementia, and progression to death within 2 years were typical. Women and children were affected much more frequently than men. Circumstantial evidence indicates that the kuru agent was transmitted through the ritual handling of affected tissues, especially brain, from deceased relatives. This cultural practice was discontinued, and the incidence of kuru has decreased dramatically since 1959. Brain tissues from patients dying of kuru were inoculated into the brains of chimpanzees, which, after a prolonged incubation period, developed a similar disease. Subsequently, the neuropathology of kuru and that of CJD as well as GSS were noted to be similar, and experimental transmission studies using CJD-affected or GSS-affected brain were undertaken successfully, eventually in a wide range of laboratory animals.

Progress in characterizing the transmissible agents of scrapie and CJD has partially clarified the distinct yet related mechanisms by which human CJD arises. The pivotal elements in the molecular pathogenesis are the PrP gene located on the short arm of human chromosome 20, and its product, the cellular protein PrP. PrP is normally expressed in neurons and other cells; its function is not known, but its concentration is critically controlled. The transmissible CJD agent is composed of degradation-resistant aggregates of PrP. It is postulated that when exogenous PrP "infects" a susceptible individual, it "replicates" by incorporating normal PrP into new aggregates in a process that resembles crystallization. These abnormal aggregates of PrP increase in concentration and size until they interfere with normal neuronal function. Genetic cases of CJD arise when disease-initiating mutations occur in the PrP gene and result in an intrinsically degradation-resistant form of PrP. The aggregation of these proteins occurs spontaneously, without the exogenous "seeding" crystal needed in transmissible cases. Nearly a score of PrP gene mutations have been identified in more than 100 families affected with various clinical types of CJD. Certain other allelic variations in the PrP gene, although insufficient to produce disease solely on a genetic basis, may predispose to developing CJD from an exogenous "infection" with the CJD agent. The molecular mechanisms by which sporadic cases occur are not yet delineated. Possibilities include somatic mutations in the PrP gene, post-translational changes in PrP itself which promote its abnormal accumulation, or other metabolic events that affect the processing of PrP. The unifying concept underlying the various causes of CJD is that aggregated PrP behaves as an *endogenous neurotoxin*. When PrP derived from either a normal gene (e.g., infectious cases) or a mutated gene (e.g., genetic cases) is not adequately degraded, it accumulates to toxic levels in the CNS.

The CJD agent provokes no inflammatory response or specific antibody production. It is resistant to chemical and physical treatments that inactivate most viruses, including heat, formaldehyde, nuclease digestion, and ultraviolet and ionizing radiation. This agent can be inactivated by procedures that denature proteins. Unique fibrillar structures are observed in electron micrographs of samples prepared from brain tissue of individuals with CJD. They resemble the abnormal fibrils that accumulate in scrapie-affected animals and represent an aggregated form of the CJD protein.

INCIDENCE AND EPIDEMIOLOGY. On a worldwide basis, the incidence of CJD is between one and two cases per million population. This incidence peaks in the fifth through seventh decades, although cases have been documented as early as the second decade. The genders are equally affected. Approximately 300 deaths occur in the United States each year. Higher rates have been noted in Israel among Libyan-born Jews and in circumscribed areas of the former Czechoslovakia and Chile.

CJD usually occurs sporadically in middle-aged adults without known exposure. A family history is evident in 8 to 15% of patients, and these patients are usually found to have a mutation in the PrP gene. Several reports document iatrogenic human-to-human transmission by cornea transplants and via the reuse of stereotaxic EEG electrodes that had unknowingly been previously implanted in a patient with CJD. Several cases have resulted from the use of dura mater allografts. Additional clusters of cases suggesting neurosurgical transmission have been reported. In the past decade, CJD has been diagnosed in individuals in both the United States and Europe who had received human pituitary gland growth hormone replacement therapy. It seems apparent that certain lots of the cadaveric hormone preparation were contaminated with the CJD agent. Incubation periods were between 4 and 21 years, emphasizing the astonishingly long incubation times of the spongiform encephalopathies. Additional cases may yet appear because more than 10,000 patients worldwide received this form of human growth hormone prior to its discontinuation in 1985. Also, four cases of CJD developed in Australian women who had been treated with pituitary gonadotropin for infertility.

Worldwide, the incidence of CJD is the same in countries with endemic sheep scrapie as it is in those without scrapie, indicating that there is no apparent transmission to humans from this animal reservoir. During the past decade a major outbreak of a new veterinary disease, bovine spongiform encephalopathy (BSE) or mad cow disease, has appeared in Great Britain. A few cases of BSE have been reported in other European countries. BSE has not occurred in the United States. BSE appears to have had its origin in the use of food supplements contaminated with the sheep scrapie agent. Although unlikely, it is too early in the BSE epidemic in Great Britain to determine if the passage of the scrapie agent through cattle poses any increased risk to humans. Nevertheless, British authorities have taken measures to prevent human consumption of contaminated beef.

PATHOLOGY. The pathologic findings in CJD are limited to the CNS, although the transmissible agent can be detected in many organs. Cortical neuronal depletion, marked reactive astrocytosis, intracellular vacuolar or spongiform change, and the absence of inflammation are the major features. Amyloid fibrils and plaques composed of the CJD protein occur in virtually all cases. The immunochemical detection of the protease-resistant protein PrP, *in situ* or after extraction, allows rapid confirmation of the diagnosis.

CLINICAL MANIFESTATIONS. Vague psychiatric or behavioral symptoms suggesting a personality change often herald the onset of CJD, but within a few weeks or months a relentlessly progressive dementia becomes evident. Myoclonus is usually present and often prominent at some time during the course. Deterioration is usually rapid, and 90% of victims die within 1 year. CJD patients are afebrile and have normal blood and cerebrospinal fluid profiles. The EEG in at least 75% of cases at late clinical stages shows a diffusely slow background with superimposed complexes, which may or may not be associated with myoclonus.

The dementia can be accompanied by signs of involvement of any part of the CNS. Most patients develop signs of cerebellar and pyramidal tract dysfunction as the disease advances. Visual disturbances, extrapyramidal signs, and various dysphasias often occur. The terminal stage is marked by decorticate and decerebrate postures, stupor, and coma. Massive myoclonic responses to auditory or other sensory stimuli may create the false impression that the patient is alert and responsive.

Subtypes of CJD based on distinctive clinical presentations have been delineated. The optic type features visual disturbances, usually cortical blindness. The dyskinetic form has prominent extrapyramidal signs, whereas the ataxic variant resembles kuru with its marked cerebellar involvement. *Gerstmann-Straüssler-Scheinker syndrome* is an autosomal dominant, genetically transmitted form of CJD with slower progression and signs of spinocerebellar ataxia. A specific mutation in the gene that codes for the CJD precursor protein has been found in some patients with this familial form of CJD. This mutation results in a protein with leucine substituted for proline at PrP codon 102, a step that promotes its aggregation into the characteristic brain amyloid. *Fatal familial insomnia* patients have a subacute course with untreatable insomnia, motor disturbances, dysautonomia, another specific PrP gene mutation, and marked atrophy of thalamic nuclei.

DIAGNOSIS. The diagnosis of CJD should be considered when a relatively rapidly progressive dementia develops in an adolescent or adult patient with normal spinal fluid. The presence of myoclonus or the characteristic EEG recording is strongly supportive, but often either or both are absent in early stages. All treatable diseases that can cause dementia need to be specifically tested for before a presumptive diagnosis of CJD or another untreatable dementia is made. Neither brain imaging nor laboratory evaluations are useful in diagnosis. Brain biopsy has been the usual method to establish definitive diagnosis. Research level, two-dimensional electrophoresis, however, has also provided accurate diagnosis in an increasing number of cases. In early cases, psychological depression, the AIDS dementia complex, and a number of rare dementias, including collagen vascular diseases and paraneoplastic limbic encephalitis, must be considered. Rarely, lithium toxicity can present with a clinical picture and EEG pattern resembling those of CJD. Discontinuation of the drug results in improvement within a few weeks.

Alzheimer's disease (see Ch. 400), the most common neurodegenerative dementia, usually has a more protracted course, without either the myoclonus or the typical EEG of CJD. Amyloid deposi-

tion in the brain is a pathologic hallmark of both ease and CJD, but the amyloid proteins deposited i eases are structurally unrelated. The development o bodies for both these amyloid proteins allows rapid differentiation between CJD and Alzheimer's diseas biopsy or postmortem examination is done.

TREATMENT AND PROGNOSIS. No effective available, and CJD appears to be uniformly fatal.

PREVENTION. Although CJD can be transmitted, health care workers and others having contact with patie higher than that to the general population. Isolation of pa not indicated, but certain guidelines should be followed. I workers should wear gloves when handling tissues, bloo spinal fluid. Accidental skin contact with possibly contaminate ids or materials should be followed by washing with 1 N so hydroxide or a 1:10 dilution of 5% household chlorine bl (sodium hypochlorite). All laboratory samples should be clea marked and needles disposed of properly. The agent can be inac vated on contaminated surfaces using a 1:10 dilution of bleach fo 1 hour. Surgical and pathologic instruments should be steam autoclaved for 1 hour at 132°C. No organs, tissues, or tissue products from patients with CJD or with any ill-defined neurologic disease should be used for transplantation or replacement therapy.

Chesebro BW (ed.): Transmissible spongiform encephalopathies: Scrapie, BSE and related human disorders. Curr Topics Microbiol Immunol 172:1, 1991. *A multiauthored monograph with reviews on clinical, etiologic, genetic, epidemiologic, pathologic, and research aspects of CJD, kuru, scrapie, and BSE.*

Brown P, Gibbs CJ Jr, Rodgers-Johnson P, et al.: Human spongiform encephalopathy: The National Institutes of Health series of 300 cases of experimentally transmitted disease. Ann Neurol 35:513, 1994. *Clinical features are detailed in this large series of documented cases.*

Brown P, Goldfarb LG, Gajdusek DC: The new biology of spongiform encephalopathy: Infectious amyloidoses with a genetic twist. Lancet 337:1019, 1991. *A thoughtful summary of several disease-associated mutations and an insightful discussion on the seeming paradox of a disease that is both genetic and infectious.*

Prusiner SB, Hsiao KK: Human prion diseases. Ann Neurol 35:385, 1994. *A detailed review of the genetics of CJD.*

Rosenberg RN, White CL III, Brown P, et al.: Precautions in handling tissues, fluids, and other contaminated materials from patients with documented or suspected Creutzfeldt-Jakob disease. Ann Neurol 19:75, 1986. *Safety guidelines for health care workers and specific decontamination protocols for surgical and pathologic instruments.*

Section Nine—Neurologic Disorders Associated with Altered Immunity or Unexplained Host-Parasite Alterations

Richard A. Rudick

429 CENTRAL NERVOUS SYSTEM COMPLICATIONS OF VIRAL INFECTIONS AND VACCINES

Central nervous system (CNS) signs arising during the course of systemic infection usually reflects CNS invasion by the inciting organism. Less frequently, systemic infections or use of certain vaccines gives rise to CNS abnormalities that do not reflect direct in-

fection of nervous tissue, but rather result from presumed autoimmune or toxic mechanisms. Several reasonably distinct patterns of involvement have been delineated. Two of these, *acute disseminated encephalomyelitis* (ADEM) and *acute necrotizing hemorrhagic encephalopathy* (ANHE), appear to be mediated by immune mechanisms and have a peripheral nervous system counterpart, acute inflammatory polyneuropathy, or the Guillain-Barré syndrome. The remainder, Reye syndrome, acute toxic encephalopathy, and acute cerebellar ataxia of childhood, are likely to be toxic in origin.

ACUTE DISSEMINATED ENCEPHALOMYELITIS

DEFINITION AND NOMENCLATURE. Acute disseminated encephalomyelitis is an uncommon acute inflammatory disease of the CNS which occurs following viral infections or vaccination.

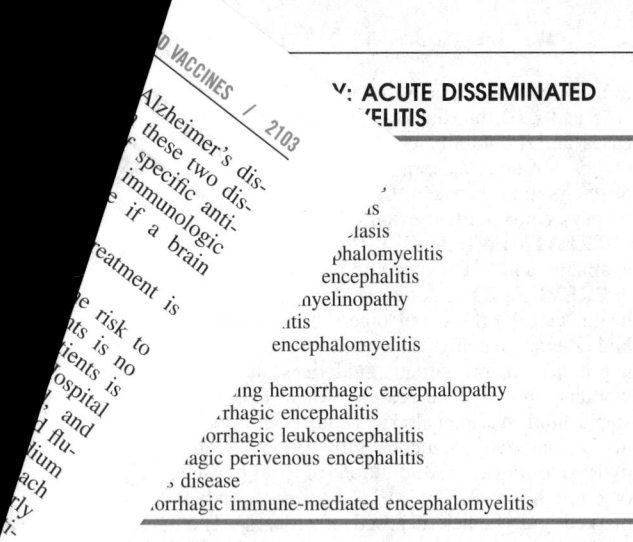

TABLE 429–1. ...Y: ACUTE DISSEMINATED ...ELITIS

...s
...lasis
...phalomyelitis
encephalitis
...nyelinopathy
...itis
encephalomyelitis
...ng hemorrhagic encephalopathy
...rhagic encephalitis
...orrhagic leukoencephalitis
...agic perivenous encephalitis
... disease
...orrhagic immune-mediated encephalomyelitis

... thought to be immune mediated. Brain and spinal cord ...nent is usually widespread but may at times be limited to ...e areas such as the optic nerves or a single spinal cord level. ...ous names have been used to describe this syndrome (Table ...9–1), but the term ADEM is appropriately descriptive. The classic features of ADEM (Table 429–2) include an antecedent event, commonly a viral illness, followed after a latent period by acute onset of multifocal or diffuse CNS signs, the potential for extensive or even complete recovery, and pathologic evidence of perivascular inflammation and demyelination.

ETIOLOGY AND PATHOGENESIS. Table 429–3 lists the principal events preceding ADEM, although many cases occur without a known precipitant. Of the various viral infections, ADEM occurs more frequently with RNA viruses that bud from infected cells. Viral infections associated with exanthems, such as measles, rubella, and varicella, are particularly common antecedents, but the disease also follows mumps, influenza, herpes simplex, or viruses causing banal nonspecific upper respiratory infections. The syndrome has been observed after vaccination for rabies, rubella, pertussis, influenza, or vaccinia, or in association with various medications. Neurologic manifestations usually occur 6 to 10 days after the exanthem, viral symptoms, or vaccination.

A compelling analogy links the ADEM complicating rabies vaccination with the animal disorder *experimental allergic encephalomyelitis* (EAE). Inoculation of susceptible animals with brain homogenates, highly purified myelin components, or peptides containing the encephalogenic sequences of myelin basic protein (MBP) or proteolipid protein (PLP) can induce acute CNS perivascular inflammatory and demyelination histologically identical to the pathology observed in ADEM. In animals with EAE, neurologic signs appear 10 to 14 days after sensitization to myelin antigens in association with humoral and cellular immune responses to the inciting CNS antigen. Furthermore, EAE can be transferred to naive animals by injecting T lymphocytes from the immunized animals, suggesting that this cell type is of primary importance in the pathogenesis. ADEM complicating rabies vaccination is considered a human form of EAE. ADEM was observed in as many as one of every 600 individuals following rabies vaccination using inactivated inoculum of fixed rabies virus propagated in animal brain. The complication of rabies vaccination called "neuroparalytic accident" was caused by vaccine contamination with CNS antigens. Both complement-fixing antibody and specific lymphocyte proliferative responses to crude and purified CNS antigens have been measured in blood of patients receiving rabies vaccine, with the most abnormal responses in patients with neuroparalytic accidents. Current rabies vaccines derived from virus grown in human diploid cells appear to be essentially free of neural complications (see Ch. 427).

TABLE 429–2. CARDINAL FEATURES OF ACUTE DISSEMINATED ENCEPHALOMYELITIS

Preceding event—usually viral illness
Latent period followed by acute onset of multifocal or diffuse CNS signs
Potential for extensive recovery
Pathologic features of perivascular inflammation and demyelination; vessel damage and hemorrhage variable

TABLE 429–3. PRINCIPAL CONDITIONS PREDISPOSING TO ACUTE DISSEMINATED ENCEPHALOMYELITIS

Infections
Measles
Varicella-zoster
Influenza
Rubella
Mycoplasma pneumoniae
Respiratory agents
Epstein-Barr
Vaccines: smallpox, measles, rabies (Semple vaccine)

ADEM following viral infection may also be immune mediated. Lymphocytes that proliferate in the presence of MBP, complement-fixing antibodies to neural tissue, and humoral factors with demyelinating activity have been described. Encephalitis is relatively frequent following measles (1:1000 cases), but there is little evidence to implicate invasion of the CNS by measles virus as an obligate prerequisite. Theoretical data support the possible importance of sequence similarities between measles virus or other viral antigens and CNS proteins such as MBP and PLP. Very early in the course of measles ADEM, specific proliferative responses to MBP are apparent in the lymphocytes of children, and measurable quantities of MBP are released into CSF. These findings support the hypothesis that acute measles transiently alters the immune system, which in some persons results in a breakdown of tolerance to CNS antigens. Despite the usual absence of CNS symptoms, this process appears to occur frequently, as reflected by a high incidence of abnormal-appearing electroencephalograms (EEG's). Both EEG abnormalities and clinical ADEM can occur after vaccination with live-attenuated measles virus but at a markedly lower frequency, with ADE arising in about one in 1 million vaccinated persons.

INCIDENCE. Valid incidence figures for ADE are difficult to derive. Encephalitis complicates about one in 1000 cases of measles. ADEM following vaccination for smallpox is of only historical interest but occurred in the United States with a reported incidence of 2.9 per million primary vaccinations. ADEM following other childhood viral illnesses or vaccinations is uncommon. Most adult cases of ADEM have no identifiable antecedents.

PATHOLOGY. Characteristic lesions typically occur around venules within the white matter of brain and spinal cord. Leptomeninges contain lymphocytes, plasma cells, and occasional polymorphonuclear cells early in the course. Shortly thereafter, there is a perivenular mononuclear inflammatory infiltration. Myelin in this distribution becomes fragmented and eventually entirely absent. There is relative axonal sparing. This primary lesion can occur throughout the neuraxis but tends to be most prominent in the centrum semiovale of the cerebrum and in the pontine white matter. Repair occurs through remyelination. In certain cases, large, confluent demyelination can take on a superficial resemblance to the plaques of multiple sclerosis, differing primarily in that all lesions reflect a similar time of onset.

CLINICAL MANIFESTATIONS. In adults, neurologic symptoms often first suggest the illness. With the childhood exanthems, CNS symptoms usually begin about 5 days after the onset of the rash. The clinical disorder can resemble any of the acute encephalitides. Typically, nonspecific symptoms of fever, headache, anorexia, and vomiting are rapidly followed by meningeal signs, altered consciousness, and focal signs referable to brain, spinal cord, optic nerves, or spinal roots. About half the patients experience one or more generalized seizures. Neurologic signs consist of some combination of pyramidal tract dysfunction, cranial nerve signs, movement disorders, sensory system dysfunction, cerebellar signs, and loss of muscle stretch reflexes. Stupor, delirium, or coma develops in severe cases. The EEG is abnormal, with widespread slowing of background rhythms. The cerebrospinal fluid in children almost invariably shows a modest mononuclear pleocytosis of 20 to 200 cells per cubic millimeter and occasionally higher. The fluid contains a slight elevation of protein content, a normal glucose level, and a raised MBP. Tests for oligoclonal bands are usually negative. After several days, magnetic resonance imaging (MRI) characteristically demonstrates scattered white matter lesions, at least some of which enhance with paramagnetic agents during the acute phases of the disease.

The duration of active CNS disease varies from days to weeks, often with a protracted convalescence. The overall mortality is about 20%. About 90% of survivors recover completely or nearly completely, although severe residual deficits can occur.

DIAGNOSIS. Diagnosis in ADEM is by exclusion. The most important consideration is CNS infection. In pathologic series of clinically diagnosed ADEM occurring during the course of mass vaccination programs, postmortem examination showed that the majority of patients had other illnesses, including potentially treatable CNS infections. In the setting of a recent exanthem, viral illness, or vaccination, ADEM may be suggested. Differentiation from an initial severe episode of MS (see Ch. 432) can be difficult, particularly because relapsing forms of ADEM have been reported.

TREATMENT. Treatment consists of supportive care, including the use of anticonvulsants and, when necessary, intensive care monitoring. Although sometimes used clinically, neither corticosteroids nor other immunosuppressive drugs have established efficacy.

ACUTE NECROTIZING HEMORRHAGIC ENCEPHALOPATHY

Acute necrotizing hemorrhagic encephalopathy (ANHE) is considered the hyperacute form of ADEM. As with ADEM, many names have been applied to this syndrome (see Table 429–1). ANHE is thought to have a similar immunopathogenesis to ADEM. Typically, the illness arises spontaneously or following an uneventful upper respiratory illness. Sudden headache precedes the neurologic symptoms, which include seizures and rapid progression from lethargy to coma in a matter of a few hours to several days. Major focal neurologic abnormalities are common and may suggest lateralized cerebral involvement. Systemic signs and symptoms include fever and marked peripheral leukocytosis. The accompanying CSF pleocytosis usually shows a preponderance of polymorphonuclear cells and sometimes evidence of hemorrhage. More than 80% of all recognized cases of ANHE are fatal, although these findings may be biased by selective reports of postmortem studies. The brain is usually swollen, and examination shows bilateral but asymmetric abnormalities, with petechial hemorrhages scattered throughout the white matter. Microscopic lesions consist of features reminiscent of hyperacute forms of EAE. The clinical differential diagnosis includes ADEM and acute viral encephalitis, especially herpes simplex encephalitis (see Ch. 426). Computed tomography (CT) or MRI may be diagnostically helpful in selected cases. Therapy is supportive.

Griffin DE: Monophasic autoimmune inflammatory diseases of the CNS and PNS. Res Publ Assoc Res Nerv Ment Dis 68:91, 1990. *A review of recent advances in unraveling parainfectious nervous system disease.*

Kesselring J, Miller DH, Robb SA, et al.: Acute disseminated encephalomyelitis—MRI findings and the distinction from multiple sclerosis. Brain 113:291, 1990. *Multifocal white matter lesions indistinguishable from those seen in MS in most patients with ADEM.*

430   REYE SYNDROME

DEFINITION. Reye syndrome is a form of hepatic encephalopathy with fatty infiltration of the liver, markedly raised intracranial pressure, and brain edema. The illness follows one of several common viruses or hepatotoxicity from commonly used drugs.

ETIOLOGY AND PATHOGENESIS. Reye syndrome appears to be due to an abnormality of mitochondrial fatty acid metabolism. Entry of fatty acids into mitochondria or beta-oxidation itself may be impaired. Biochemical manifestations of Reye syndrome, regardless of the precipitant, include hypoglycemia, accumulation of fatty acids, fatty acyl CoA's, and acyl carnitines. Accumulated products further injure mitochondria, further impairing beta-oxidation. Reye syndrome almost always follows a viral infection, and epidemiologic studies strongly support a link between the use of aspirin and Reye syndrome. The syndrome most commonly follows influenza A, influenza B, herpes varicella zoster, and to a lesser extent several other common virus infections. Little evidence links the precipitating viral infection directly to either the central nervous system (CNS) or hepatic involvement. A toxic origin is proposed for both types of involvement. Hepatic dysfunction results in various meta-

bolic derangements including hyperammonemia, lactic acidemia, and elevated levels of serum free fatty acids. These metabolic derangements have been implicated in the pathogenesis of the brain swelling and increased intracranial pressure that dominate the clinical course of severe cases. The precise mechanism of mitochondrial impairment remains to be clarified.

INCIDENCE. Reye syndrome occurs most commonly among children between 1 and 15 years of age but has been reported in adolescents and is increasingly recognized in adults. Inner city black infants may be especially at risk for the disease. Prospectively derived incidence figures for the most susceptible age groups are as high as 6.2 per 100,000 children.

PATHOLOGY. The liver shows a noninflammatory, panlobular, hepatocellular accumulation of lipid droplets and both histochemical and ultrastructural evidence of inflammation. At postmortem examination, swelling of astrocytic foot processes and ultrastructural changes in mitochondria similar to those seen in hepatic mitochondria may be found in the greatly swollen brain.

CLINICAL MANIFESTATIONS AND COURSE. Reye syndrome is a biphasic disorder. As symptoms of the initial viral illness begin to wane or clear, intractable vomiting appears in association with lethargy or delirium. Early diagnosis is confirmed by the findings of nonicteric hepatic dysfunction, an elevated arterial blood ammonia level, and serum transaminase levels that exceed three times normal levels. Hepatic enlargement is present in about one half of the cases. Children under 1 year of age often show hypoglycemia. Signs of CNS deterioration include the development of generalized seizures, deepening obtundation, and transtentorial herniation. The cerebrospinal fluid is under increased pressure but is acellular, with otherwise normal constituents.

DIAGNOSIS. Diagnosis rests on the clinical findings and appropriate biochemical abnormalities. Liver biopsy usually is not necessary. CNS infection, inborn errors of metabolism, such as ornithine transcarbamoylase deficiency and systemic carnitine deficiency, and the presence of known hepatotoxins, including valproate, salicylates, and paracetamol, must be actively excluded. A childhood syndrome, distinguishable from Reye syndrome only by the absence of hepatic involvement and a high incidence of acute convulsions, can follow both banal viral infections and vaccination.

TREATMENT. Affected patients require intensive care monitoring until the course of the disease is well established. Hypoglycemia and electrolyte abnormalities must be corrected. Many authorities suggest hydration with solutions of high glucose content. Appropriate measures should be taken to monitor intracranial pressure continuously in the more severely affected cases, as judicious control of intracranial hypertension contributes to a favorable outcome. Mortality is about 10%.

Ede RJ, Williams R: Reye's syndrome in adults. Br Med J 296:517, 1988. *Although uncommon, such cases do occur and need management different from that for children.*

Pranzatelli MR, DeVivo DC: Pharmacology of Reye syndrome. Clin Neuropharmacol 10:96, 1987. *A comprehensive review including detailed recommendations for medical management.*

431   NEUROLOGIC COMPLICATIONS IN THE IMMUNOLOGICALLY COMPROMISED HOST

Immunodeficient states induced by a variety of intrinsic or exogenous mechanisms greatly reduce the central nervous system's (CNS) natural resistance to infection (for mechanisms, see Ch. 266). Many well-known and a few uncommon causes of immune compromise exist, some examples being genetically related immune deficiency disorders (see Ch. 223); splenectomy; the giving of active immune suppressants to facilitate renal, bone marrow or other organ transplants or protect against severe autoimmune disorders; applying chemotherapy or radiation therapy for cancer or allied disorders; and the intrinsic capacity of HIV-1 to destroy CD4 lymphocytes. Each of these conditions predisposes to serious infections of the CNS, and some can foster primary or secondary lymphoma production in the brain or, rarely, the spinal cord.

In transplant recipients, hospital-acquired bacterial species provide the major early risk (see Ch. 266 and 267). Early on, severe immunosuppression of any kind also commonly reactivates herpes viruses, most frequently herpes simplex, then herpes varicella virus, and, least often, cytomegalovirus (see Ch. 426). Sooner or later, with continued immunosuppression nosocomial bacterial and mycotic infections may arise (see Ch. 267).

Among cancer patients (e.g., Hodgkin's disease or hairy cell leukemia) as well as in certain hematologic disorders or other less common conditions, splenectomy may be indicated. It increases the risk of bacterial meningitis (see Ch. 151). Other immunosuppressed patients are similarly at risk for either bacterial or fungal infections of the brain-meninges. Progressive multifocal encephalopathy (see Ch. 428.5) nowadays most often appears as a complication of AIDS, but the condition also may arise in patients suffering from other forms of severe immunosuppression as well as sporadically. Potential CNS immunologic complications of AIDS, among which differentiation between toxoplasmosis and lymphoma may be difficult, are discussed in Ch. 364 and 428.2.

Section Ten—The Demyelinating Diseases

432 MULTIPLE SCLEROSIS AND RELATED CONDITIONS
Richard A. Rudick

This section discusses diseases primarily affecting central nervous system (CNS) myelin; demyelinating peripheral neuropathies are discussed in Ch. 447. CNS myelin is an elaborate extension of the oligodendrocyte cell membrane. A single oligodendrocyte myelinates as many as 20 or 30 different CNS axonal segments, each over a length of 1 mm or less. Oligodendrocyte membrane extensions wrap around the axons in a concentric fashion to form the

TABLE 432–1. DISEASES OF MYELIN

Idiopathic, presumably autoimmune (this chapter)
  Recurrent or chronically progressive demyelination (multiple sclerosis and its variants)
  Monophasic demyelination (may be first clinical episode of multiple sclerosis)
    Optic neuritis
    Acute transverse myelitis
  Acute disseminated encephalomyelitis; acute hemorrhagic leukoencephalopathy
    Following infection, with or without exanthem
    Following vaccination
Viral infections (see Ch. 423–428)
  Progressive multifocal leukoencephalopathy
  Subacute sclerosing panencephalitis
Nutritional disorders (see Ch. 406)
  Combined systems disease (vitamin B_{12} deficiency)
  Demyelination of the corpus callosum (Marchiafava-Bignami disease)
  Central pontine myelinolysis
Anoxic-ischemic sequelae (see Ch. 394)
  Delayed postanoxic cerebral demyelination
  Progressive subcortical ischemic encephalopathy
Leukodystrophies (this chapter)
  Primarily affecting CNS myelin
    Adrenoleukodystrophy (Schilder's disease)
    Pelizaeus-Merzbacher disease
    Spongy degeneration
    Others (Alexander's disease, Canavan's disease)
  Central peripheral nervous system
    Metachromatic leukodystrophy
    Globoid cell (Krabbe's disease)

myelin sheath. Tightly compacted mature myelin consists of parallel layers of bimolecular lipids apposed to layers of hydrated protein. Lipids, including cerebroside, phospholipids, and cholesterol, constitute 75% of myelin's dry weight. Myelin proteins include proteolipid protein, myelin basic protein, myelin-associated glycoprotein, and a number of less abundant proteins detectable by electrophoretic separation. Active myelin synthesis starts *in utero* and continues for the first 2 years of life; slower synthesis continues during childhood and adolescence. Turnover of mature myelin continues at a slower rate throughout life. Both developing and mature forms of myelin are readily susceptible to injury by the disease described in this section.

Table 432–1 classifies the several forms of myelin diseases. Acquired disorders are separated from developmental abnormalities. Multiple sclerosis (MS) and its variants are by far the most common diseases in this group. Viral infections, nutritional disorders, and anoxic-ischemic sequelae are discussed in Ch. 423 through 428, 406, and 394. The leukodystrophies are uncommon disorders but instructive because recent genetic and biochemical advances have elucidated the mechanisms causing many of these conditions.

MULTIPLE SCLEROSIS

DEFINITION. MS is a disorder of unknown cause, defined clinically by characteristic symptoms, signs, and progression and pathologically by scattered areas of inflammation and demyelination affecting the brain, optic nerves, and spinal cord. The first symptoms of MS most commonly occur between the ages of 15 and 50. Most MS patients recover to some degree from individual bouts of inflammatory demyelination, producing the classic exacerbating-remitting course seen early in the disease. Diagnosis requires intermittent or progressive CNS symptoms buttressed by evidence for two or more CNS white matter lesions and occurring in an appropriately aged patient who lacks an alternative explanation such as recurrent strokes or systemic lupus erythematosus. The diagnosis is based on clinical features; currently available laboratory tests support the diagnosis but are not directly diagnostic.

ETIOLOGY. The cause of MS is unknown, but it is now widely believed that the pathogenesis involves immune-mediated inflammatory demyelination. Pathologic examination of MS brain shows the hallmarks of an immunopathologic process—perivascular infiltration by lymphocytes and monocytes, class II MHC antigen expression by cells in the lesions, lymphokines and monokines secreted by activated immune cells, and the absence of overt evidence for infection. Additional evidence for an autoimmune pathogenesis includes (1) immunologic abnormalities in blood and cerebrospinal fluid (CSF) of MS patients, notably selective intrathecal humoral immune activation, lymphocyte subset abnormalities, and a high frequency of activated lymphocytes in blood and CSF; (2) an association between MS and certain MHC class II allotypes; (3) the clinical response of MS patients to immunomodulation—patients tend to improve with immunosuppressive drugs and worsen with interferon-gamma (IFN-γ) treatment, which stimulates the immune response; and (4) striking similarities between MS and experimental allergic encephalomyelitis (EAE)—an animal model in which recurrent episodes of inflammatory demyelination can be induced by inoculating susceptible animals with myelin basic protein or proteolipid protein.

Epidemiologic studies suggest environmental and genetic factors in the etiopathogenesis of MS. The uneven geographic distribution of the disease and the occurrence of several point-source epidemics have suggested environmental factors; however, intense study over the past 30 years has failed to establish an infectious cause. Migration studies have shown that exposure to undefined environmental factors prior to adolescence is required for subsequent development of MS. A genetic influence is well-established by excess concordance in monozygotic compared with dizygotic twins, clustering of MS in families, racial variability in risk, and association with class II MHC allotypes. In Caucasians, the HLA class II haplotype DR15,DQ6,Dw2 appears strongly and consistently associated with an increased risk of MS.

The evidence—immunologic, epidemiologic, and genetic—supports the concept that exposure of a genetically susceptible individual to an environmental factor(s) during childhood (perhaps any one of many common viruses) leads eventually to immune-mediated inflammatory demyelination. The precise interplay between genetic, environmental, and immunologic factors and the nature of the environmental trigger(s) remains to be elucidated.

INCIDENCE, PREVALENCE, AND EPIDEMIOLOGY. The annual *incidence* rate for MS ranges in different populations from 1.5 to 11 per 100,000. Several studies suggest that the incidence rate has increased over time. For example, data from Olmsted County, Minnesota, suggested a gradual increase in annual incidence during the past century from about 1.2 per 100,000 between 1905 and 1914 to about 6.2 per 100,000 between 1975 and 1984. In all studies, the highest age- and gender-specific rates occur in women between 20 and 40 years of age.

Worldwide prevalence differs according to geography. Distribution of MS has been well studied in North America, Northern Europe, Australia, and New Zealand. In both hemispheres, MS is more common in the temperate zones, decreasing toward the equator. The *prevalence* of MS in the northern United States, Canada, and northern Europe is at least 100 per 100,000 population; in certain regions, the prevalence of MS exceeds 300 per 100,000 people, compared with less than 5 per 100,000 people in the tropics. Regional heterogeneity has been reported within high prevalence zones, and several reports describe MS clusters in small areas. In the Faroe Islands, for example, a well-reported outbreak of MS occurred during the 20 years following the start of World War II, suggesting the effects of an unidentified environmental factor.

PATHOLOGY. Brain, optic nerves, and spinal cord from MS patients contain scattered areas of myelin loss ranging in size from 1 mm to several centimeters in diameter with relatively intact axons. The borders between histologically normal tissue and demyelinated zones are usually well-demarcated but may shade from normal to thinning before bare axons occur. Some areas show diffuse partial myelin loss. Although plaques may occur in any myelinated area of the CNS, the most commonly affected regions include optic nerves, periventricular cerebral white matter, and cervical spinal cord.

The earliest event in development of the MS lesion is breakdown of the blood-brain barrier, followed by perivenular mononuclear infiltrates, and quickly thereafter by circumscribed areas of myelin breakdown. Macrophages invariably occupy sites of active demyelination and appear necessary for myelin loss. B lymphocytes and plasma cells surround small CNS blood vessels, and T lymphocytes and monocytes infiltrate CNS parenchyma. Products of the immune response, including immunoglobulins, interleukins, interferons, and tumor necrosis factor, accompany the acute MS lesion. Tissue edema reaches a maximum after about 1 month, following which lesions evolve over several months into permanently demyelinated gliotic scars depleted of oligodendrocytes. After the initial events, immature oligodendrocytes appear and presumably participate in remyelination. As a rule, however, oligodendrocytes and remyelination regenerate insufficiently to explain the remarkable clinical recovery observed in many patients.

LABORATORY ABNORMALITIES. *Cerebrospinal Fluid.* Immune activation within the CNS is a cardinal feature of MS. Increased CSF immunoglobulin levels, reflecting the presence of intrathecal humoral immune activation, appear in 80 to 90% of MS patients. CSF gamma globulin normally represents less than 13% of total CSF protein, but in MS patients the proportion often rises much higher. After separating CSF gamma globulin fractions by agarose or polyacrylamide gel electrophoresis, separate discrete "oligoclonal" bands (OCB) can be detected in 70 to 80% of patients. The sensitivity for detecting OCB can be increased by separating CSF by isoelectric focusing or by staining the gels or nitrocellulose blots with anti-immunoglobulin antibodies. As with most diagnostic tests, however, as the sensitivity of the method increases, the specificity decreases; CSF OCB also can be observed in patients with CNS infections or inflammatory diseases and have been reported with tumors or strokes. Increased CSF levels of free kappa light chains develop less frequently than OCB but are more specific for MS than IgG abnormalities. The amount of antibody synthesis within the CNS can be quantified by measuring the CSF and serum IgG and albumin levels and calculating a CSF IgG synthesis rate. CSF protein is normal or only slightly elevated in MS; levels above 75 mg per deciliter require an alternative explanation. CSF cell count is nearly always < 50 mononuclear cells per microliter; cell counts > 100 cells per microliter require a search for an infectious cause. Myelin destruction releases myelin basic protein (MBP) into CSF, which can be detected by radioimmunoassay. The MBP level correlates to some extent with disease activity and lesion location; none is detectable in normal individuals or during quiescent periods in MS patients. MBP levels rise in association with acute attacks or rapid disease progression. This serves as an index of disease activity but is not specific to MS; myelin injury from any other cause, such as acute brain infarction, increases CSF MBP.

In the presence of a slight mononuclear pleocytosis and normal protein, the presence of oligoclonal bands, selectively increased IgG levels, and free kappa light chains provide strong support for the diagnosis of MS when CNS syphilis, subacute sclerosing panencephalitis, chronic meningitis, CNS Lyme disease, HTLV-I myelopathy, or other infectious diseases have been excluded.

Sensory Evoked Potentials

Myelin allows rapid propagation of the nerve action potential. Myelin loss from any cause slows conduction velocity or causes conduction block. Conduction along sensory pathways can be measured by inducing a response to a visual, auditory, or somatosensory stimulus. Measurement of the latency after stimulus of the visual evoked potential (VEP) is used most widely (see Ch. 392.5). In most laboratories, the normal VEP latency is less than approximately 105 msec. Increased latency indicates an abnormality in the optic nerve on that side. Evoked potentials are considered extensions of the clinical examination, allowing for objective measurement of lesions within specific pathways. They have not proved useful for monitoring progression of disease or response to therapy.

Imaging Procedures

Computed tomographic (CT) brain scans sometimes reveal hypodense regions in white matter, but the imaging modality is relatively insensitive and usually shows no abnormalities. For these reasons, magnetic resonance imaging (MRI) has largely supplanted CT scanning. Abnormal head MRI scans show abnormalities in more than 85% of clinically definite MS patients. Typical lesions (Fig. 432–1) are multifocal, appear hyperintense on intermediate and T2-weighted MR images, and occur predominantly in the periventricular white matter, corpus callosum, cerebellum, cerebellar peduncles, brain stem, and spinal cord. Usually MRI reveals many more hyperintense lesions than clinically anticipated. Intravenous paramagnetic agents, such as gadolinium, demonstrate acute lesions, which appear hyperintense on T1-weighted images. Serial studies have demonstrated that gadolinium enhancement appears and disappears in a given lesion in about 4 weeks. MRI is used widely to confirm a diagnosis of suspected MS and to rule out other conditions. MRI abnormalities are not specific for MS, particularly in patients older than 50, who commonly develop nonspecific MRI signal changes of uncertain significance. The specificity of MRI lesions for MS increases with lesions ≥ 6 mm in diameter that are adjacent to the

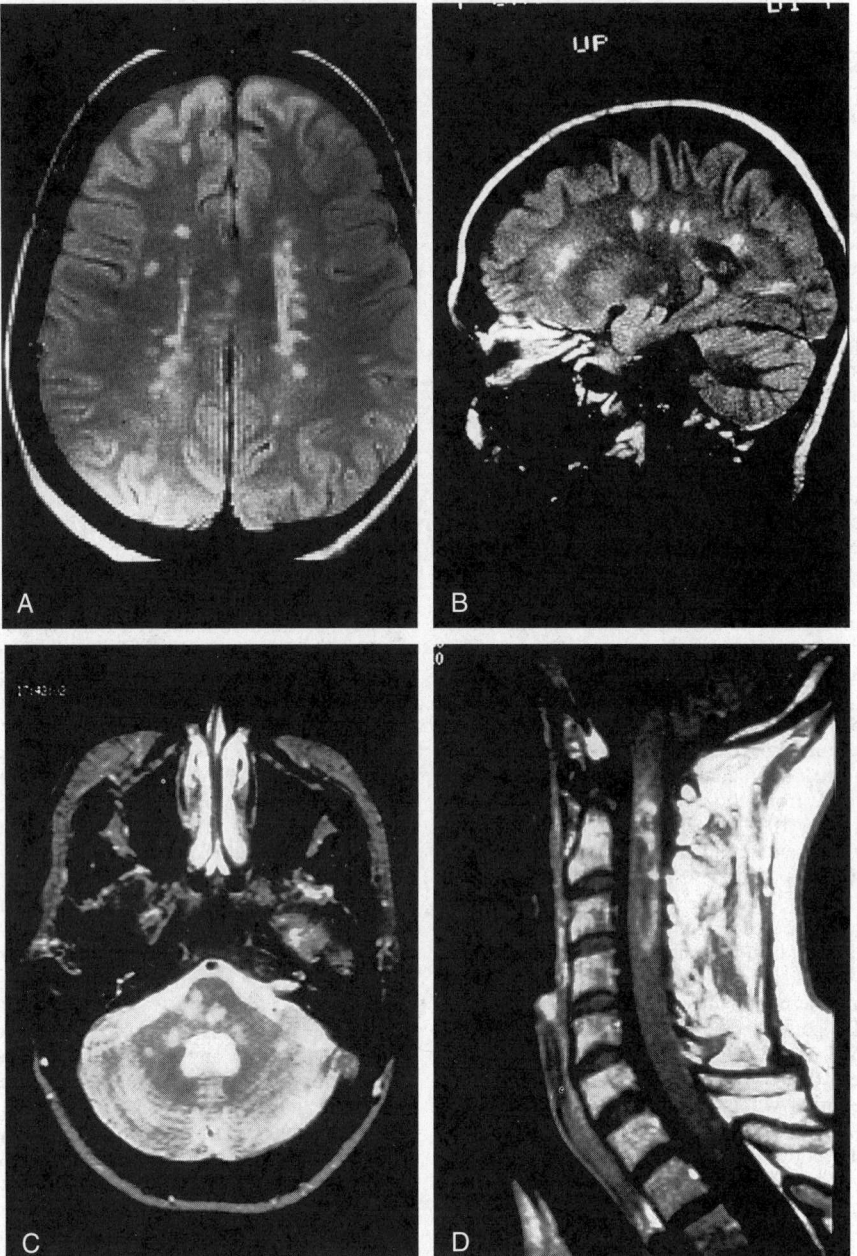

FIGURE 432–1. Magnetic resonance imaging of brain and spinal cord from a patient with clinically definite multiple sclerosis. *A,* Transverse section just above the bodies of the lateral ventricles. Note the numerous high-signal lesions adjacent to the bodies of the lateral ventricles in the deep cerebral white matter. *B,* Sagittal proton-density image showing ovoid lesions extending from the lateral ventricles into the deep cerebral white matter. *C,* T2-weighted section through the brain stem and cerebellum at the level of the middle cerebellar peduncles showing numerous high-signal lesions in the pons, cerebellar peduncles, and cerebellum. *D,* T1-weighted sagittal image through the cervical spinal cord following administration of gadolinium. Note the elongated intrinsic cervical spinal cord lesion with gadolinium enhancement as signified by high signal around the periphery of the lesion. (Courtesy of Barbara Banger, M.D., Cleveland Clinic Foundation Department of Neuroradiology.)

lateral ventricles, particularly when accompanied by brain stem, cerebellar, and spinal cord lesions. Use of MRI as a research tool to measure treatment effect or disease progression is rapidly evolving. Whether or not such studies are cost-effective for measuring clinical progress is debatable. Newer magnetic resonance–based techniques such as magnetization transfer imaging may allow differentiation between inflammation and demyelination. Such a distinction may become important as future therapies evolve.

CLINICAL MANIFESTATIONS. *Onset, Common Clinical Manifestations, and Course.* Women are affected more frequently than men—with a 3:2 ratio. Symptom onset occurs between ages 20 and 50 and peaks at approximately age 30. Nevertheless, children younger than 12 and adults over 50 occasionally present with their first symptom. MS produces myriad neurologic symptoms and signs, depending on the anatomic sites of involve-

ment. In younger patients, the disease usually starts with a subacute or acute onset of focal neurologic symptoms and signs, most often reflecting disease in optic nerves, pyramidal tracts, posterior columns, cerebellum, central vestibular system, or medial longitudinal fasciculus. Older individuals commonly present with insidiously progressive myelopathy, manifest as some combination of progressive spastic leg weakness, axial instability, and bladder impairment. In a large group of MS patients studied at the University of Western Ontario in the 1970's (Table 432–2), approximately 30% of patients presented with visual symptoms, 30% with sensory symptoms, 20% with gait or balance disturbance, and the remaining 20% with various other symptoms. In general, as the disease progresses, new symptoms and signs appear, old symptoms and signs recur, and residual symptoms and impairments increase.

Visual symptoms include monocular visual loss, oscileopsia, or

TABLE 432-2. INITIAL SYMPTOMS IN MS PATIENTS*

Symptom	Percentage of Cases
Sensory disturbance in one or more limbs	33
Disturbance of balance and gait	18
Visual loss in one eye	17
Diplopia	13
Progressive weakness	10
Acute myelitis	6
Lhermitte's sign	3
Sensory disturbance in face	3
Pain	2

* From Paty DW, Poser CM: Clinical symptoms and signs of multiple sclerosis. *In* Poser CM (ed.): The Diagnosis of Multiple Sclerosis. New York, Thieme and Stratton, 1984, p 27.

diplopia. Gait disorder results from spastic leg weakness, axial instability, and lower extremity sensory loss. Spasticity consists of increased muscle tone, hyperreflexia, and limb spasms, accompanied by weakness and loss of dexterity. Spasticity in MS patients almost always affects the lower more than the upper extremities. Upper extremity impairment includes sensory loss resulting in a clumsy hand, cerebellar ataxia, or less commonly spastic weakness. Bladder dysfunction includes urinary urgency with urge incontinence or hesitancy and incomplete emptying. Neuropsychological problems are common and include depression, emotional lability, and cognitive impairment.

Increased body temperature by as little as 0.5° C transiently reduces neurologic function in some patients. In the setting of increased ambient temperature, strenuous physical activity, or fever, patients may experience transient worsening of symptoms. This results from slowed axonal conduction induced by heating, and the new symptoms disappear within hours of regaining normal body temperature.

At least 70% of patients improve in the days to months following their initial bout, with the degree of improvement ranging from slight to virtual disappearance of the neurologic dysfunction. Although most patients experience exacerbations and remissions early in the course of their illness, as time goes by, recovery from individual bouts decreases, fixed impairment and disability remain, and the course becomes chronically progressive. About 30% of patients experience chronically progressive problems from the onset of disease, especially those aged more than 45 years. Ten years after onset, about half of all patients are still able to carry out their household and/or employment responsibilities. Fifteen years after onset about half require a cane to walk. Approximately 25 years after onset, at least half are unable to walk, even with assistance. By contrast, some individuals, perhaps as many as a third, occupy the extremes of either avoiding disability altogether or having unusually severe limitations, becoming bedridden within months after onset. The average interval from clinical onset to death is 35 years, with terminal factors due to sepsis from urinary tract infection, decubiti, aspiration pneumonia, or suicide.

Factors Affecting the Clinical Course. The only predictable factor in MS is its unpredictability in the individual patient. *It has become clear, however, that certain features carry a relatively poor prognosis. These include progressive disease from onset, preponderance of motor and cerebellar signs, and a near diagnostically abnormal head MRI at first presentation. Conversely, favorable indicators include a high degree of recovery after the first attack, predominance of sensory symptoms, and benign condition 5 years after symptom onset.*

Several studies have found that infections of almost any type increase the risk for exacerbation. This is thought to result from immune system activation, with an associated increase in MS disease activity. As with numerous autoimmune diseases, MS disease activity decreases during pregnancy but increases somewhat in the postpartum period. The overall progression of MS, however, is not affected by one or more pregnancies.

DIAGNOSIS. Despite increasing reliance on sophisticated brain imaging, CSF, and electrophysiologic tests, the diagnosis of MS is based on *clinical* features *supplemented* by laboratory tests, rather than the other way around. The Schumacher criteria have been widely used for diagnosis of MS. Clinically definite MS exists when an appropriate clinical history is supported by (1) objective abnormalities of CNS function in the neurologic examination; (2)

TABLE 432-3. WASHINGTON COMMITTEE CRITERIA FOR DIAGNOSIS OF MULTIPLE SCLEROSIS*

Category	Attacks	Clinical Evidence		Para-clinical Evidence†	CSF OB/IgG
Clinically definite MS					
1	2	2			
2	2	1	and	1	
Laboratory-supported definite MS					
1	2	1	or	1	+
2	1	2			+
3	1	1	and	1	+
Clinically probable MS					
1	2	1			
2	1	2			
3	1	1	and	1	
Laboratory-supported probable MS					
1	2				+

* From Poser CM, et al.: New diagnostic criteria for multiple sclerosis: Guidelines for research protocols. Ann Neurol 13:227, 1983.
† MRI or evoked potential studies.

examination or history indicating involvement of two or more areas of the CNS; (3) CNS disease predominantly reflecting white matter involvement; (4) involvement of the CNS following either a pattern of two or more episodes, each lasting > 24 hours and a month or more apart, or a slow or stepwise progression of signs and symptoms over at least 6 months; (5) patient age between 10 and 50; and (6) signs and symptoms that cannot be better explained by another disease process. These criteria are based entirely on clinical features. Laboratory testing plays an increasingly important role in documenting multicentric CNS lesions and eliminating alternative diagnoses. This is reflected in diagnostic criteria developed more recently that incorporate sensory evoked potentials and MRI to identify disseminated lesions, and CSF IgG abnormalities to support the diagnosis (Table 432–3).

Two common errors confound the diagnosis of MS. The first occurs in a patient with clear neurologic disease who has an alternative diagnosis (Table 432–4). Certain clinical or laboratory "red flags" are useful in alerting the clinician about a possible diagnostic error in this situation (Table 432–5). The two most useful red flags include disease that could be explained by a single lesion in the nervous system and the absence of a clinical remission. In a patient with localized disease, the working assumption must be that a definable, non-demyelinating, structural lesion exists. Depending on the clinical features, diagnostic testing should be used to rule out brain or spinal cord tumor, arteriovenous malformation, cervical spondylosis with cord compression, cervical or thoracic disc herniation, Chiari malformation, brain abscess, or a parenchymal mass

TABLE 432-4. CONDITIONS COMMONLY MISTAKEN FOR MULTIPLE SCLEROSIS

Vascular diseases
  Small-vessel cerebrovascular disease
  Vasculitis
Structural lesions
  Craniocervical junction tumor, malformation of base of skull
  Anomaly
  Posterior fossa tumor or arteriovenous malformation
  Spinal cord tumor or cervical spondylosis
Degenerative diseases
  Motor system disease
  Spinocerebellar degeneration
Infections
  HTLV-I infection
  HIV myelopathy or HIV-related cerebritis
  Lyme disease
Other conditions
  Cobalamin deficiency
  Sjögren's syndrome
  Sarcoidosis
  Nonspecific MRI abnormalities

TABLE 432-5. RED FLAGS IN THE DIAGNOSIS OF MULTIPLE SCLEROSIS*

Syndrome that could be explained by localized disease
Steadily progressive disease, absence of clinical remission
Absence of oculomotor, optic nerve, sensory, or bladder involvement
Normal cerebrospinal fluid

* Modified from Rudick RA, Schiffer RB, Schwetz K, et al.: Multiple sclerosis: The problem of incorrect diagnosis. Arch Neurol 43:578, 1986.

from sarcoidosis. MRI is the most sensitive differential screening procedure and currently eliminates the need for CT scanning or myelography in almost all cases.

Degenerative, infectious, or neoplastic diseases must be considered in patients with a steadily progressive course. Disorders that can be incorrectly diagnosed as MS include spinocerebellar degeneration, cervicomedullary syringomyelia, basilar invagination, motor neuron disease, HTLV-1 myelopathy, HIV-related myelopathy or brain infection, and neoplasms such as parenchymal lymphoma. Spinocerebellar degeneration and motor neuron disease are suspected by symmetric neurologic impairment restricted to characteristic neural systems and by the absence of CSF inflammatory change or response to corticosteroids.

Progressive myelopathy should prompt testing for HTLV-1, HIV, and very long chain fatty acids to rule out adrenoleukodystrophy (ALD). On rare occasion, CNS lupus or vitamin B_{12} deficiency may be clinically indistinguishable from MS. These disorders should be ruled out by determining antinuclear antibodies and vitamin B_{12} levels at the time of diagnosis.

Small vessel cerebrovascular disease should be considered in the hypertensive patient, particularly in those lacking CSF abnormalities typical of MS. MRI may help distinguish MS from small-vessel cerebrovascular disease; MS patients more commonly have lesions adjacent to the brain ventricles and involvement of the corpus callosum.

The second common type of diagnostic error occurs in patients with no definable neurologic disease. Patients commonly acquire an MS diagnosis because of nonspecific neurologic symptoms such as weakness, fatigue, or tingling, at times supplemented by minimal nonspecific signal changes on brain MRI. The absence of objective neurologic signs at any time, patterns of weakness or sensory loss that fail to conform to known neuroanatomic systems, and disability out of proportion to objective clinical findings raise the suspicion of psychogenic illness. One must be open-minded, however, because MS can begin with sensory symptoms, fatigue, or other nonspecific symptoms. In many cases, it is necessary to follow the patient over time before an accurate diagnosis can be made.

TREATMENT. Education. MS patients and their families need information about MS after a diagnosis has been made. Typical questions include the following: (1) *"What will happen to me?"* One of the major psychological burdens for an MS patient is uncertainty about the future course of his or her illness. The physician should acknowledge the unpredictable course but emphasize the spectrum of severity and the significant proportion of patients who remain neurologically intact for many years. (2) *"How can I control my illness?"* Most patients have beliefs about what will improve or worsen their MS. The patient's need for control over the disease can often be focused on healthy life styles like fitness programs or appropriate diet. (3) *"When should I call you?"* Patients should be advised to call when necessary but should be routinely seen at 6- or 12-month intervals. This allows ongoing assessment of neurologic impairment and results in a gradual decline in the need for telephone calls. (4) *"Will my children get this?"* The lifetime risk to a child of a mother with MS is 3 to 5%; this is a 30- to 50-fold increase over that for the general population, but still a small risk. (5) *"Can I have a baby?"* Pregnancy has a predictable effect on the pattern of MS, as discussed above. It appears that breast feeding has little if any effect on the frequency, timing, or severity of postpartum exacerbations, and the bulk of evidence suggests that the overall course of MS, including the eventual degree of disability, is unaffected by one or more pregnancies. Women with mild to moderate disability should plan pregnancies primarily on the basis of issues other than MS.

Symptom Pharmacotherapy. *Spasticity* may be reduced by a combination of physical measures and antispastic drugs. The GABA-agonist baclofen is the drug of choice but should be individualized because it is effective over a wide dose range. Baclofen should be instituted slowly to avoid sedation or weakness and withdrawn slowly to avoid confusional states or seizures. Diazepam may be used as an adjunct to baclofen, particularly for patients with nocturnal spasms causing sleep disturbance. Even a small dose of diazepam may potentiate the benefits of baclofen. Dantrolene is an alternative antispastic drug for patients who do not respond well to baclofen or diazepam or cannot tolerate the sedation that sometimes complicates the use of these drugs. Dantrolene exerts its effects at the muscle; consequently, motor weakness almost always accompanies dantrolene's antispastic effect. Dantrolene should be used cautiously in patients with myocardial disease, and it occasionally causes toxic hepatitis. Patients with severe spasticity not effectively managed with the above measures may benefit from intrathecal baclofen administered continuously at a rate of 200 to 800 μg per day via a fully implantable infusion pump.

Dystonic spasms consist of brief, recurrent, painful posturing of one or more extremities, not associated with altered consciousness or urinary incontinence. Dystonic spasms are easily controlled with carbamazepine or phenytoin. *Ataxia* is difficult to treat pharmacologically. Intention tremor may respond to clonazepam, which should be instituted slowly to avoid sedation. Clonazepam should be initiated at 0.5 mg at bedtime and increased gradually to an endpoint of sedation or effective control of tremor. One or more tonic-clonic seizures occur in about 5% of MS patients. A single motor seizure predicts a subsequent seizure in an MS patient and should be treated with an adequate dose of phenytoin. *Bladder symptoms* require at a minimum urinalysis, culture, and postvoid residual volume. In the absence of a urinary tract infection or urinary retention > 100 ml, anticholinergic agents such as oxybutynin or propantheline are effective. Urinary tract infection or significant urinary retention in an MS patient requires urologic evaluation. *Fatigue* in MS, when disabling and not caused by depression, can be treated effectively with amantadine, 100 mg twice a day. Pemoline is effective for some individuals who have not responded to amantadine.

Heat sensitivity results from conduction failure in partially demyelinated CNS fibers. Patients may benefit from cool showers or air conditioning. Dramatic deterioration can accompany fever in patients with advanced MS, and elevated body temperatures should be aggressively treated, with specific infections being managed with appropriate antibiotics.

Pain syndromes consist of trigeminal neuralgia or more atypical facial pain, paroxysmal limb paresthesias presenting as brief tic-like pain, burning dysesthesias, Lhermitte's phenomenon, and chronic back pain due in most cases to mechanical stress caused by ataxia and weakness. Trigeminal neuralgia or disagreeable paresthesias may respond to carbamazepine or alternatively to amitriptyline, phenytoin, or baclofen. If medical therapy fails, trigeminal rhyzotomy is an alternative. Chronic low back and leg pain are usually alleviated with nonsteroidal anti-inflammatory drugs and physical therapy. A proper walking aid, ankle foot orthosis, or proper seating is critical. Coexistent herniated discs should be ruled out in the MS patient with radicular pain, particularly when an ankle or knee tendon reflex is absent.

Depression or *emotional distress* is often underrecognized and inadequately treated. Depression is particularly common when the illness is first diagnosed or when it worsens significantly. Depression has a significant negative impact on quality of life, social relationships, and job performance and should be treated aggressively with psychiatric referral or antidepressant drugs. For depressed MS patients with anxiety and insomnia, amitriptyline is effective and inexpensive. For patients with coexisting bladder symptoms, imipramine is useful because its α-adrenergic properties may improve bladder dysfunction. For older patients or patients with memory impairment, a tricyclic with less anticholinergic activity, such as desipramine or nortriptyline, or a serotonin reuptake inhibitor may be better tolerated. *Emotional lability,* which may be distressing and socially disabling for some MS patients, may improve with low doses of amitriptyline.

Cognitive dysfunction may be difficult to recognize clinically but should be suspected in any MS patient with poor work performance, family disintegration, or noncompliance with medical or rehabilitative therapies, particularly when the explanation for the problem is unclear. Neuropsychological tests should include sensitive measurements of complex attention and information processing, learning and recent memory, concept formation, and problem solving. There is no known effective drug therapy, although patients often can learn compensatory strategies and may benefit from cognitive rehabilitation.

Disease Pharmacotherapy. Numerous trials of drugs have been directed at improving the long-term course of MS or shortening the course of acute exacerbations. Nearly all current experimental therapy trials include MRI measures of outcome, and measures of clinical outcome have improved.

Corticosteroid Therapy. Recent evidence suggests that intravenous methylprednisolone (MP) has a more rapid onset of action and better efficacy than corticotrophin or other steroid preparations in limiting acute exacerbations. No evidence exists that chronic corticosteroid therapy slows or halts progression of MS. Furthermore, excessive or injudicious use of steroids gradually lessens their value, and most patients eventually become steroid-unresponsive. For major clinical exacerbations, intravenous MP, 500 or 1000 mg per day for 3 days, can be administered safely in an outpatient setting, followed by prednisone, 60 mg in a single morning dose for 3 days, tapering off over 12 days.

Immunomodulatory Therapy. Betaseron (interferon β-1b), a human recombinant interferon-β preparation, has been shown to reduce the frequency of MS exacerbations and the progression of MRI lesions in ambulatory patients with exacerbating-remitting MS. The drug is FDA approved for MS patients in this category, being administered at a dose of 8 million IU every other day by subcutaneous injection. Adverse effects include flulike symptoms, injection site inflammatory reactions, and occasional blood transaminase elevations. Avonex (interferon β-1a), a different form of recombinant human β interferon, at a dose of 6 MIU administered by weekly IM injections also has been shown to decrease MRI disease activity. The principal observed side effects were flulike symptoms. Various drugs that suppress the immune system have been reported to show partial efficacy. These include cyclophosphamide, cyclosporine, azathioprine, and methotrexate. Methotrexate, administered orally at a dose of 7.5 mg weekly, was found to reduce the proportion of patients with chronic progressive MS who worsened during a 2-year treatment period compared with placebo-treated patients. This dose results in minimal apparent toxicity. Cyclophosphamide and cyclosporine have some reported benefit but are limited by toxicity. Evidence indicates that azathioprine reduces the rate of exacerbations, but the relative and ultimate benefits of azathioprine and interferon-β have not been determined. Currently, it is safest to restrict immunosuppressive drugs to centers operating within the context of controlled protocols.

MULTIPLE SCLEROSIS VARIANTS

NEUROMYELITIS OPTICA (*DEVIC'S DISEASE*). Neuromyelitis optica is a syndrome characterized by partial or complete transverse myelopathy and optic neuritis. Loss of vision and paraplegia may occur in either order, and the two major components of the disease may be widely separated in time. The syndrome of neuromyelitis optica may occur as the result of acute disseminated encephalomyelitis, systemic lupus erythematosus, or sarcoidosis as well as during the course of typical MS or in isolation without apparent cause. In the latter case, it is considered a variant of MS.

CONCENTRIC SCLEROSIS. Concentric sclerosis is a rare form of demyelinating disease characterized by rapidly progressive demyelination. It appears to be a variant of rapidly progressive MS. Clinically, the disease begins with the acute or subacute onset of altered behavior, difficulty in communication, mutism, apathy, and headache. CSF is usually normal. Imaging shows extensive lesions in cerebral white matter. Concentric sclerosis may be suspected clinically but can be diagnosed only by its characteristic histopathology. Alternating bands containing demyelinated and partially demyelinated axons radiate concentrically. Oligodendrocyte loss characterizes the bands of demyelination.

MONOPHASIC DISORDERS RELATED TO MULTIPLE SCLEROSIS

OPTIC NEURITIS. Optic neuritis denotes acute or subacute partial or complete loss of vision in one or both eyes due to inflammation. Almost all patients with inflammatory optic neuritis experience pain in, around, or behind the affected eye, followed within a day or two by visual loss. Visual loss of varying intensity progresses for as long as 1 week. Optic neuritis is classified as *retrobulbar neuritis* when the lesion is in the posterior two thirds of the optic nerve and *papillitis* when the lesion is in the anterior portion of the optic nerve. The latter leads to an ophthalmoscopic appearance similar to that of acute papilledema resulting from increased intracranial pressure but differing from the latter by the association of markedly reduced visual acuity. Visual fields in optic neuritis reveal a central or ceco-central scotoma of varying degree. Color vision is impaired, and a deafferented, Marcus-Gunn pupil may exist. Unless the patient has papillitis, ophthalmoscopic examination remains normal for the first 2 to 3 weeks, after which the disc pales, with loss of small vessels on the disc, or more severe atrophy may develop. Visual function almost always recovers to some degree, usually within weeks. Blindness as the result of optic nerve demyelination of MS seldom occurs.

The syndrome of optic neuritis can be caused by several diseases, of which MS is by far the most common. Tobacco-nutritional amblyopia, Leber's disease, vasculitis, optic nerve compression on any basis, neurosyphilis, ischemic optic neuropathy, pernicious anemia, or sarcoidosis produce most cases not caused by MS. Optic neuritis is usually easily differentiated from optic nerve ischemia, which has an abrupt onset, affects older individuals, and results in field cuts consistent with retinal artery occlusions. Compressive optic neuropathy causes slowly progressive visual loss. Vasculitis or sarcoidosis can usually be distinguished by characteristic funduscopic features and by the presence of uveitis.

Many patients with idiopathic isolated optic neuritis eventually develop MS, the reported frequency in several series varying from 13 to 85% according to the length of follow-up. The presence of CSF oligoclonal bands or brain MRI abnormalities significantly increases the risk of early conversion to MS. Patients with idiopathic monosymptomatic optic neuritis who have periventricular MRI abnormalities have about a 35% chance of developing MS within 2 years and an 85% chance of developing MS within 5 years.

More rapid but not necessarily greater total visual recovery occurs by treating optic neuritis with intravenous methylprednisolone. A 3-day course of intravenous MP followed by a prednisone taper within 8 days of the onset appears to reduce by about 50% the likelihood of conversion from idiopathic optic neuritis to MS during 2 years of follow-up.

ACUTE TRANSVERSE MYELITIS. Acute transverse myelitis denotes rapidly developing paraparesis or paraplegia as the result of spinal cord dysfunction. Abrupt or rapidly developing back or radicular pain may be followed by ascending paresthesias and weakness beginning in the feet. Urinary and fecal retention or incontinence is common. Progression varies from minutes, as with infarction, to steady or stepwise progression over several days. Progression over days may occur with both spinal cord compression due to a tumor and MS. It is also common to observe patients with sensory symptoms below a particular dermatome corresponding to the spinal cord level of involvement, with or without ataxia and variable degrees of leg weakness. It may be difficult to distinguish idiopathic transverse myelitis from compressive myelopathy. Therefore, the syndrome of acute transverse myelitis demands immediate diagnostic evaluation.

Several disorders can produce an acute transverse myelopathy (Table 432–6). The most important to rule in or out immediately are compressive lesions, including spinal or epidural abscess, tumor, herniated intervertebral disc, or injury; vascular occlusion due to arteritis, aortic dissection, aortic surgery, or arteriovenous malformation; varicella-zoster infection; and autoimmune disease including MS. In many instances, a careful history suggests the cause and the appropriate approach. Nevertheless, the evaluation must include an *immediate* imaging procedure such as MRI with attention to the level of involvement to rule out spinal cord compression. Cord compression from metastatic tumor may present acutely even though the tumor has been present for weeks or longer. Central herniated intervertebral discs may cause acute cord compression without producing local pain. Rapidly progressing myelopathy in a previously healthy person should always raise the question of spontaneous epidural, subdural, or intraparenchymal abscess or bleeding, the latter occurring from an arteriovenous malformation or as a complication of anticoagulation or blood dyscrasia. About one third of patients with idiopathic transverse myelitis give a history of an antecedent upper respiratory or flulike illness. Transverse

TABLE 432-6. ACUTE OR SUBACUTE TRANSVERSE MYELOPATHY

Associated with infection
  Bacterial
    Spinal epidural abscess
    Intramedullary abscess
  Viral, e.g., varicella-zoster
  Postviral, e.g., rubella with disseminated encephalomyelitis
Compression
  Tumor, especially metastatic
  Trauma
  Herniated intervertebral disc
Vascular
  Acute extradural, subdural, or parenchymal hemorrhage
  Dissecting aortic aneurysm
  Arteritis
  Lupus erythematosus
Idiopathic

myelitis may also follow several other infectious illnesses such as mycoplasma or measles with virus infection.

Transverse myelitis and slowly progressive myelopathy are common manifestations of MS, either as a first clinical manifestation or a late development. A syndrome suggesting complete cord transection rarely occurs. As with optic neuritis, CSF oligoclonal bands or an abnormal brain MRI suggesting MS makes clinically definite MS likely.

Proper treatment requires an expeditious diagnosis. When cord compression is present, surgical decompression and treatment with antibiotics or with corticosteroids are needed immediately. Treatment may halt progression but may not restore lost function. In idiopathic transverse myelopathy, MS, or cord compression, corticosteroids may reduce edema and lead to earlier restitution of function, although the effect on long-term outcome is uncertain. The treatment of choice for neoplastic cord compression is dexamethasone; for idiopathic transverse myelitis, intravenous methylprednisolone is preferable. Patients must be supported by bladder catheterization, ventilatory support, and proper protection from compression neuropathies as necessary. Prognosis varies widely, recovery ranging from almost none at all to complete, depending on the degree of acute necrosis.

LEUKODYSTROPHIES

The leukodystrophies (see Table 432–1) are dysmyelinating diseases in that myelin formation or maintenance is impaired by a genetically determined biochemical defect. A biochemical defect is known for several, but they remain relatively rare, incurable disorders, affecting individuals from the first months of life to the 20's.

ADRENOLEUKODYSTROPHY. Adrenoleukodystrophy (ALD) includes two genetically determined disorders that cause dysfunction of adrenal glands and nervous system myelin. There are two distinct types of ALD—the X-linked form and a recessive form, termed neonatal ALD. Neonatal ALD is a rare disorder characterized by early and severe psychomotor retardation, seizures, retinopathy, hepatomegaly, and dysmorphic features occurring in infants of either gender.

The X-linked form of ALD is phenotypically heterogeneous, even though the disease is associated with a common biochemical defect. The two common patterns of X-linked ALD are the childhood form and adrenomyeloneuropathy. In the childhood form, boys develop normally until age 4 to 8, when they manifest behavioral changes with progressive cognitive decline leading over years to a chronic vegetative state. Young men with adrenomyeloneuropathy experience progressive paraparesis and bladder dysfunction. Almost all such ALD patients have adrenal insufficiency, although the degree varies considerably. Less common phenotypes of X-linked ALD include adrenal insufficiency without nervous system involvement, progressive dementia in adults, and asymptomatic males with the same metabolic deficiency as affected relatives. Occasionally, female heterozygotes develop neurologic disturbances that resemble MS. The basis for clinical heterogeneity despite a common metabolic defect is unknown. Tissues and body fluids of patients with X-linked ALD contain high levels of unbranched saturated very

long chain fatty acids. Fatty acids accumulate because of deficient peroxisomal catabolism, although the precise nature of the enzyme defect is not clear. The gene for X-linked ALD has been mapped to Xq28.

The diagnosis of X-linked ALD may be suspected in males with the clinical features described above. CSF shows inflammatory changes that may be identical to those seen in MS, although the CSF protein is usually higher in ALD. MRI shows symmetric lesions in the posterior parietal and occipital white matter. Endocrine testing reveals primary adrenal insufficiency. The diagnosis is confirmed by demonstrating increased levels of very long chain fatty acids in blood, tissue, or cultured fibroblasts. Most female heterozygotes can be identified using these methods as well. A DNA probe is available for gene screening, and prenatal diagnosis is possible through biochemical and genetic screening of amniocytes.

Pathologic examination shows widespread demyelination in CNS and peripheral myelin, with numerous lipid lamellar inclusions throughout the tissue. Many lesions exhibit cellular infiltration with lymphocytes and macrophages, suggesting an inflammatory component to pathogenesis.

Treatment of X-linked ALD consists of adrenal hormone replacement and dietary restriction of long chain fatty acids. Preliminary evidence suggests that bone marrow transplantation may slow progression of the disease, but there is no specific treatment at present.

PELIZAEUS-MERZBACHER DISEASE. Pelizaeus-Merzbacher disease represents a group of a poorly characterized and heterogeneous disorders with extensive CSF myelin destruction associated with myelin breakdown products staining bright red with the usual fat stains. The so-called sudanophilic leukodystrophies are thus distinguishable pathologically from the metachromatic leukodystrophies. The sudanophilic staining characteristic results from high levels of cholesterol esters; it is observed in the aminoacidurias, adrenoleukodystrophy, and Pelizaeus-Merzbacher disease. The latter is a rare leukodystrophy inherited as an X-linked recessive trait and primarily affecting males. The condition begins in infancy and progresses slowly to produce extensive, diffuse, symmetric disturbances of myelin associated with gliosis within the cerebrum and cerebellum. The peripheral nervous system is not affected. The underlying biochemical defect is unknown, and no treatment is available.

SPONGY DEGENERATION OF WHITE MATTER. Many disorders can produce the pathologic changes leading spongiform degeneration of myelin. These include various metabolic derangements, exposure to hexachlorophene, carbon monoxide, cyanide, isoniazid, actinomycin D, amphotericin B, methyl ester, and methotrexate.

METACHROMATIC LEUKODYSTROPHY. Metachromatic leukodystrophy (MLD) is the most common leukodystrophy. MLD is a lysosomal storage disease caused by deficiency of arylsulfatase A. Patients develop diffuse dysmyelination, usually starting in the first 10 years of life. The process leads to dementia, convulsions, cranial nerve abnormalities, and finally severe spasticity or rigidity. Death usually occurs after 2 to 4 years. Juvenile and adult-onset cases have been reported. In the adult form of MLD, patients develop mental deterioration that evolves progressively to severe dementia, pyramidal tract, and cerebellar signs. The diagnosis is suspected in an infant or child with progressive dementia, convulsions, and spasticity and in a young adult with progressive dementia, particularly in the face of absent tendon reflexes and elevated CSF protein.

The arylsulfatase A gene has been cloned and characterized. Nearly all patients have deficient arylsulfatase A enzyme activity, resulting in accumulation of sulfatides in lysosomes within central and peripheral nervous system tissue. Occasionally, arylsulfatase A activity is low, but the individual remains unaffected. This is termed pseudodeficiency. An increased urinary excretion of sulfatide and reduced arylsulfatase A activity in venous blood or cultured fibroblasts is diagnostic. Pathologically, sulfatides (which stain metachromatically) accumulate in oligodendrocytes and Schwann cells and within myelin lamellae. Sulfatides also collect within neurons, liver, gallbladder, kidneys, and spleen. Some evidence suggests that bone marrow transplantation may slow or halt progression of MLD.

GLOBOID CELL LEUKODYSTROPHY (KRABBE'S DISEASE). Globoid cell leukodystrophy is characterized biochemically as deficient galactocerebroside β-galactosidase activity. The disease affects infants in the first 2 to 3 months of life and is transmitted as an autosomal recessive trait. Rare instances occur in late infancy or in adulthood. The activity of galactocerebroside β-galactosidase can be determined in serum, peripheral leukocytes, or fibroblasts. Neuropathologic examination reveals marked loss of myelin throughout the brain, with the presence of round or oval mononuclear cells the size of large glia or as large, irregular multinucleated cells, termed globoid cells, containing galactocerebroside. Infants with the disorder usually progress to a vegetative state within their second year. Late onset cases present with progressive motor impairment and less frequently visual failure. No treatment is known.

Multiple Sclerosis

Anderson DW, Ellenberg JH, Leventhal CM, et al.: Revised estimate of the prevalence of multiple sclerosis in the United States. Ann Neurol 31:333, 1992. *Increased the estimated number of United States MS cases to 350,000.*

Ebers GC, Sadovnick AD: The geographic distribution of multiple sclerosis: A review. Neuroepidemiology 12:1, 1993. *Provides a synthesis of available epidemiologic information. A combination of both genetic and environmental factors appears to explain the available data on MS and geography.*

Goodkin DE, Rudick RA, Ross JS: The use of brain magnetic resonance imaging in multiple sclerosis. Arch Neurol 51:505, 1994. *Provides an overview of the use of MRI in MS patients.*

Prineas J, Kwon E, Goldenberg P, et al.: Multiple sclerosis. Oligodendrocyte proliferation and differentiation in fresh lesions. Lab Invest 61:489, 1989. *Elegantly describes and illustrates the tissue alterations produced by MS.*

Ransohoff RM, Tuohy VK, Lehmann PV: The immunology of multiple sclerosis: New intricacies and new insights. Curr Opin Neurol Neurosurg 7:242, 1994. *Reviews recent advances in our understanding of immunopathogenesis.*

Rudick RA: Helping patients live with multiple sclerosis. What primary care physicians can do. Postgrad Med 88:197, 1990. *Provides practical management strategies for primary physicians caring for MS patients and their families.*

Rudick RA, Birk KA: Multiple sclerosis and pregnancy. *In* Goldstein PJ, Stern BJ (eds.): Neurological Disorders of Pregnancy, 2nd ed rev. Mount Kisco, NY, Futura Publishing, 1992, p 165. *Reviews the relationship between pregnancy and MS, with emphasis on reproductive and pregnancy counseling.*

Rudick RA, Goodkin DE (eds.): Treatment of Multiple Sclerosis. Trial Design, Results and Future Perspectives. London, Springer-Verlag, 1992. *The first monograph with a comprehensive summary of the state of MS experimental therapeutics.*

Runmarker B, Andersen O: Prognostic factors in a multiple sclerosis incidence cohort with twenty-five years of follow-up. Brain 116:117, 1993. *Describes favorable prognostic indicators, including a high degree of recovery after first exacerbation, predominance of sensory symptoms, and benign condition 5 years after symptom onset.*

Schumacher G, Beebe G, Kibler R, et al.: Problems of experimental trials of therapy in multiple sclerosis: Report by the panel on the evaluation of experimental trials of therapy in multiple sclerosis. Ann NY Acad Sci 122:552, 1965. *Defined clinical criteria that are still valid for the diagnosis of MS.*

Optic Neuritis

Beck RW, Cleary PA, Anderson MM, et al.: A randomized, controlled trial of corticosteroids in the treatment of acute optic neuritis. N Engl J Med 326:581, 1992. *Reported that treatment of optic neuritis with intravenous MP improved the rate of visual recovery but not the extent of eventual return of vision.*

Beck RW, Cleary PA, Trobe JD, et al.: The effect of corticosteroids for acute optic neuritis on the subsequent development of multiple sclerosis. N Engl J Med 329:1764, 1993. *Found that treatment with intravenous MP reduced the likelihood of progression from optic neuritis to clinically definite MS within 2 years by 50%.*

Optic Neuritis Study Group: The clinical profile of optic neuritis. Experience of the optic neuritis treatment trial. Arch Ophthalmol 109:1673, 1991. *Provides definitive clinical and laboratory features of 448 patients with acute optic neuritis studied according to a comprehensive standardized protocol.*

Transverse Myelitis

Ropper AH, Poskanzer DC: The prognosis of acute and subacute transverse myelopathy based on early signs and symptoms. Ann Neurol 4:51, 1978. *Reviews the experience of a large general hospital with an excellent description of the clinical findings and follow-up.*

Tippett DS, Fishman PS, Panitch HS: Relapsing transverse myelitis. Neurology 41:703, 1991. *Describes patients with recurrent episodes of transverse myelitis, no evidence for brain stem or forebrain lesions, and absence of CSF oligoclonal bands. This is probably a variant of MS.*

Leukodystrophies

Aubourg P, Blanche S, Jambaque I, et al.: Reversal of early neurologic and neuroradiologic manifestations of X-linked adrenoleukodystrophy by bone marrow transplantation. N Engl J Med 322:1860, 1990. *Suggests a benefit from bone marrow transplantation.*

Gieselmann V, von Figura K: Advances in molecular genetics of metachromatic leukodystrophy. J Inherited Metab Dis 13:560, 1990. *Reviews the genetics of MLD.*

Krivit W, Shapiro E, Kennedy W, et al.: Treatment of late infantile metachromatic leukodystrophy by bone marrow transplantation. N Engl J Med 322:28, 1990. *Suggests a benefit from bone marrow transplantation.*

Moser HW, Bergin A, Cornblath D: Peroxisomal disorders. Biochem Cell Biol 69:463, 1991. *Provides a comprehensive overview of the biochemical abnormalities underlying ALD.*

Moser HW, Moser AB, Naidu S, Bergin A: Clinical aspects of adrenoleukodystrophy and adrenomyeloneuropathy. Devel Neurosci 13:254, 1991. *Provides an authoritative overview of clinical features.*

Moser HW, Moser AB, Smith KD, et al.: Adrenoleukodystrophy: Phenotypic variability and implications for therapy. J Inherited Metab Dis 15:645, 1992. *Provides the largest experience with bone marrow transplants and suggests that results are encouraging.*

Seitelberger F: Pelizaeus-Merzbacher's disease. *In* Vinken P, Bruyn G (eds.): Handbook of Clinical Neurology, vol 10. Amsterdam, North-Holland, 1970, p 150. *An excellent review of this and related degenerative diseases of myelin.*

Wanders RJ, Tager JM: Peroxisomal fatty acid beta-oxidation in relation to adrenoleukodystrophy. Devel Neurosci 13:262, 1991. *Provides the present state of knowledge regarding the organization of peroxisomal fatty acid oxidation with emphasis on X-linked adrenoleukodystrophy.*

Section Eleven—
The Epilepsies

433 THE EPILEPSIES
Timothy A. Pedley

DEFINITION

Epilepsy is a term applied to a group of chronic conditions whose major clinical manifestation is the occurrence of *epileptic seizures:* sudden and usually unprovoked attacks of subjective experiential phenomena, altered awareness, involuntary movements, or convulsions.

Although a diagnosis of epilepsy requires the presence of seizures, not all seizures imply epilepsy. Seizures are a relatively common symptom of brain dysfunction, and they may occur during the course of many acute medical or neurologic illnesses in which brain function is temporarily deranged *(acute symptomatic seizures)* (Table 433–1). Such seizures are most often self-limited and do not persist after the underlying disorder has resolved. Seizures can also occur as a reaction of the brain to physiologic stress, sleep deprivation, fever, and alcohol or sedative drug withdrawal. Occurrence of seizures in such everyday settings is exceptional and implies an increased seizure susceptibility (lowered seizure threshold). The latter may reflect poorly understood genetic factors that determine an individual's intrinsic resistance to minor physiologic, metabolic, or toxic insults. Finally, isolated seizures also sometimes occur for no discoverable reason as unprovoked events in presumably healthy people. None of these kinds of seizures represent epilepsy.

ETIOLOGY

Epilepsy can arise from a variety of conditions and pathophysiologic mechanisms. About 70% of adults and 40% of children with new-onset epilepsy have partial (focal) seizures (Fig. 433–1A). In most of these, it is not possible to identify a specific cause, although the focal nature of the seizures generally implies a cerebral injury or lesion (so-called *cryptogenic* epilepsy) (Fig. 433–1B). The most common specific lesions are hippocampal sclerosis, gangliogliomas and glial tumors, cavernous malformations, neuronal mi-

TABLE 433–1. POTENTIAL CAUSES OF ACUTE SYMPTOMATIC SEIZURES

Medical conditions
  Metabolic disarray
    Hyponatremia (< 120 mEq/L)
    Hypernatremia (> 145 mEq/L)
    Hypoglycemia (< 40 mg/dl)
    Hyperglycemia (> 400 mg/dl)
    Hyperosmolality (> 300 mOsm/L)
    Hypocalcemia (< 7 mg/dl)
  Drug-induced seizures
    Isoniazid, imipenem
    Theophylline, aminophylline
    Lidocaine
    Meperidine
    Ketamine, halothane, enflurane, methohexital
    Amitriptyline, maprotiline, imipramine, doxepin, fluoxetine
    Haloperidol, trifluoperazine, chlorpromazine
    Ephedrine, phenylpropanolamine, terbutaline
    Methotrexate, BCNU, asparaginase
    Cyclosporine
    Cocaine (crack), phencyclidine, amphetamines
    Alcohol (especially withdrawal)
  Illnesses
    Behçet's disease
    Eclampsia
    Hypertensive encephalopathy
    Liver failure
    Polyarteritis nodosa
    Porphyria
    Renal failure
    Sickle cell disease
    Syphilis
    Systemic lupus erythematosus
    Thrombotic thrombocytopenic purpura
    Whipple's disease
Neurologic conditions
  Angiitis of the nervous system
  Meningitis
  Encephalitis
  Acute head trauma (impact seizures)
  Stroke
  Brain abscess
  Brain tumor

grational defects (cortical dysplasia) and hamartomas, encephalitis, cerebral trauma, and hemorrhage. Not all patients with cerebral pathology develop epilepsy; how a particular lesion or injury causes a region of brain to become epileptogenic is poorly understood at this time.

Although specific mendelian (e.g., tuberous sclerosis, hyperglycinemia, Lafora's disease), chromosomal (Down syndrome), or mitochondrial (MELAS) genetic diseases account for only about 1% of epilepsy cases, heritable factors are important in a much higher percentage, especially in children. Forms of epilepsy that are demonstrably more heritable than others (e.g., childhood absence epilepsy, juvenile myoclonic epilepsy) are increasingly referred to as *idiopathic* or *primary* epilepsies. Common features include a variable family history, generalized spike-wave abnormality on EEG, and onset in childhood or adolescence.

Family history, cerebral injury, and neurologic disease are all risk factors for epilepsy, and the magnitude of the increased risk relative to the population at large can be specified for a number of different conditions that predispose to seizures. In many patients, several factors coexist, and the development of epilepsy reflects the interaction of acquired brain pathology and genetic predisposition.

CLASSIFICATION AND CLINICAL MANIFESTATIONS

Although a number of different classification schemes have been proposed to describe seizures and the various types of epilepsy, the most widely used today are those of the International League Against Epilepsy.

Classification of Epileptic Seizures

Seizures are classified by their clinical manifestations supplemented by EEG data (Table 433–2). There are many different kinds of seizures, each with characteristic behavioral changes and electro-

physiologic alterations that usually can be detected by EEG recordings. The particular manifestations of any single seizure depend on several factors: (1) whether most or only a part of the cerebral cortex is involved at the beginning; (2) the functions of the cortical areas where the seizure originates; and (3) the subsequent pattern of spread within the brain. The International Classification reflects these considerations in two important ways. First, it divides seizures into two fundamental types: those with onset limited to part of one cerebral hemisphere (*partial* or *focal* seizures), and those that involve the cerebral cortex diffusely from the beginning (*generalized* seizures). Second, the International Classification recognizes that seizures are dynamic and evolving and that patients show variations in seizure pattern depending on the extent and manner of spread of the electrical discharge. Thus, simple partial seizures may evolve into complex partial seizures, and either simple or complex partial seizures can evolve into secondarily generalized tonic-clonic convulsions.

PARTIAL SEIZURES. The initial events of a seizure, described either by the patient or by an observer, are usually the most reliable indication to determine if a seizure begins focally. *Simple* partial seizures result when the ictal discharge occurs in, and remains limited to, a circumscribed area of cortex. This is often referred to as the *epileptogenic focus*. Consciousness is not depressed, and patients can interact normally with their environment except for limitations imposed by the seizure on specific localized brain functions. Many symptoms or phenomena can be the expressions of simple partial seizures. Subjective sensory and psychoillusory phenomena are referred to collectively as *auras* and affect about 60% of patients with focal epilepsy. Sensory symptoms such as localized paresthesias, numbness, vertigo, auditory hallucinations, and unformed visual hallucinations occur with seizures beginning in the corresponding primary sensory areas. Psychoillusory symptoms arise from ictal discharges in limbic and association cortex and include dysmnesic symptoms, such as feelings of familiarity (*deja vu*) and unfamiliarity (*jamais vu*); dreamy states, feelings of unreality and depersonalization; time distortion; emotional symptoms such as fear or depression; visual illusions such as multiple images (polyopsia) or distortions of size (micropsia and macropsia); and hallucinatory phenomena, such as unpleasant smells, stereotyped visions, or familiar voices. Autonomic symptoms reflect ictal involvement of limbic structures that lie in the mesial temporal or frontal lobe and project to the hypothalamus and brain stem. Examples of autonomic phenomena include an epigastric rising sensation (especially common with seizures beginning in the mesial temporal lobe), nausea, lightheadedness, pallor or flushing, pupillary dilation, piloerection, salivation, and urinary incontinence.

Simple partial seizures with motor signs begin with *clonic* (rhythmic jerking) or *tonic* (stiffening) movements of a discrete body part. Because of their large cortical representation, muscles of the face and hand are involved often. When the seizure discharge begins in the primary motor cortex and spreads to involve the rest of the precentral gyrus, clonic movements progress in an orderly sequence (*"jacksonian march"*) that reflects the homunculus representation (e.g., thumb to fingers to face to leg). More often, however, ictal discharges involve supplementary or other secondary motor areas of the frontal lobe and produce contralateral flexion and elevation of the arm, contralateral turning of the head and eyes, and tonic extension of the ipsilateral arm (the so-called fencer's posture). Other simple partial motor signs include speech arrest, vocalizations, and eye blinking.

Simple partial seizures may be followed by a transient neurologic abnormality reflecting postictal depression of the epileptogenic cortical area. Thus, focal weakness may follow a simple partial motor seizure, numbness a sensory seizure, and blindness or amblyopia an occipital lobe seizure. These reversible neurologic deficits are collectively referred to as *Todd's paralysis* and rarely last for more than 48 hours. Similarly, prompt examination of a patient after a seizure may reveal transient focal abnormalities that provide useful clues to the site of seizure origin.

Complex partial seizures impair consciousness and produce unresponsiveness. In temporal lobe seizures, loss of consciousness results when the ictal discharge spreads bilaterally to involve both hippocampal and amygdala areas, the parahippocampal gyri and, to some extent, the entorhinal cortex and subfrontal, especially septal, regions. About 70 to 80% of complex partial seizures arise from the temporal lobe, and more than two thirds of these originate in mesial temporal lobe structures, especially hippocampus, amygdala, and

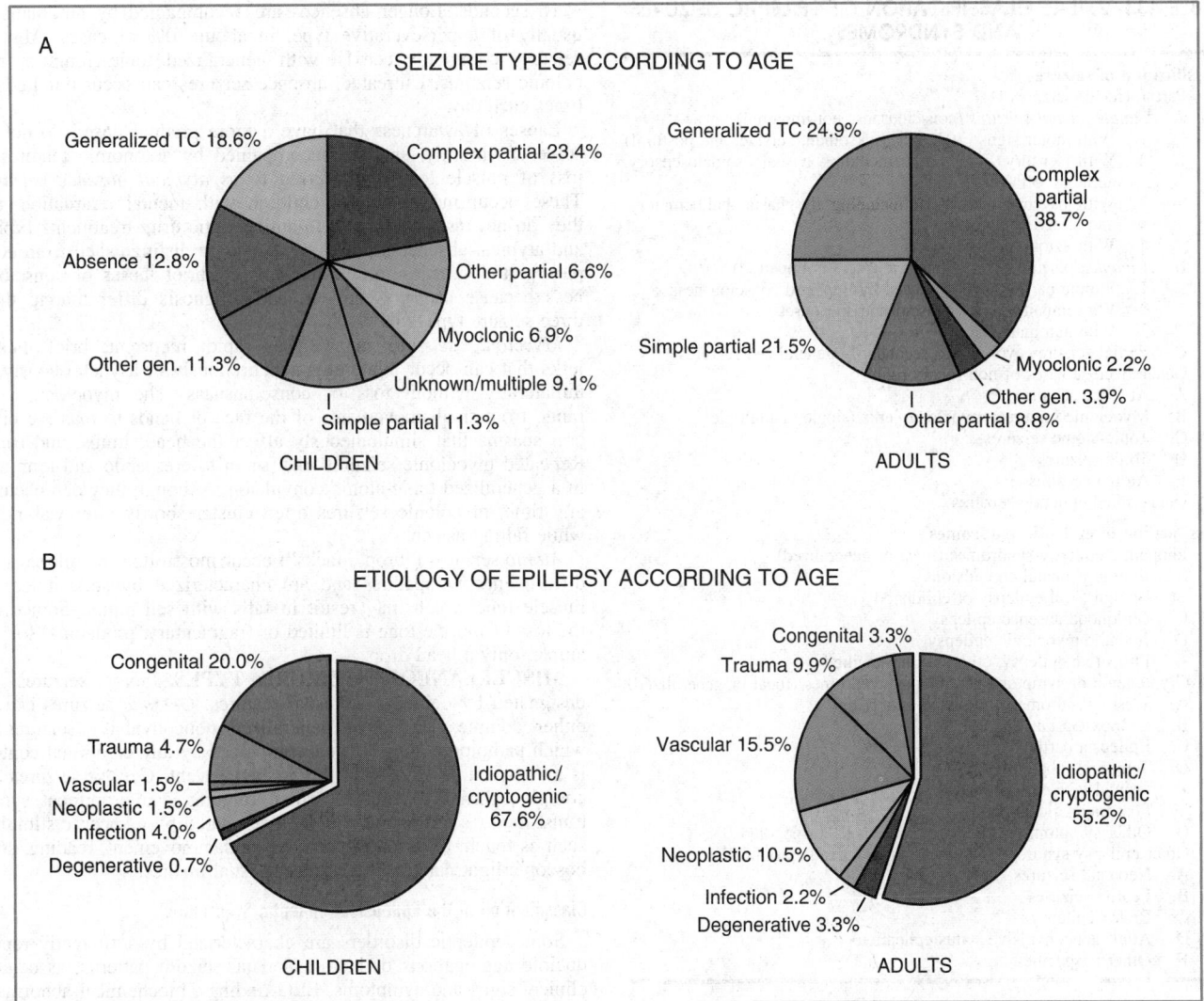

FIGURE 433–1. *A,* Proportion of seizure types as a function of age for newly diagnosed cases of epilepsy in Rochester, Minnesota, 1935–1984. *B,* Etiology of epilepsy in all newly diagnosed cases in Rochester, Minnesota, 1935–1984. TC = tonic-clonic. (Modified from Hauser et al, Epilepsia 34:453–468, 1993.)

parahippocampal gyrus. Remaining cases of complex partial seizures arise mainly from the frontal lobe, with smaller percentages originating in parietal and occipital lobes. Many complex partial seizures evolve from simple partial seizures; consciousness becomes impaired as the seizure progresses. Complex partial seizures preceded by an olfactory aura are referred to as *uncinate fits* because of their origin in or near the uncus of the medial temporal lobe. Clinical tradition teaches that uncinate fits have a higher association with brain tumors than other types of complex partial seizures.

The typical complex partial seizure of temporal lobe origin consists of a motionless stare accompanied by alteration of consciousness followed by *automatisms* (repetitive purposeless complex movements) and, often, dystonic positioning of the arm or hand *contralateral* to one seizure discharge. Oroalimentary automatisms are most common and include lip smacking, swallowing, and sucking and chewing movements. Gestural automatisms, such as fumbling, picking at clothes or objects, hand wringing, and patting movements, are also frequently encountered and are typically expressed maximally in the lines *ipsilateral* to the epileptogenic temporal lobe. There may be clumsy perseveration of ongoing motor tasks, such as eating, drawing, walking, or washing dishes. Some patients show a degree of residual ability to react to their environment during the seizure, although their behavior is typically inappropriate. Complex partial seizures usually last 45 to 90 seconds and are followed by a period of confusion and disorientation lasting several more minutes. Without EEG recording, it is difficult to de-

termine where the ictal state ends and postictal behavior begins. Characteristically, patients are amnesic for details of the seizure that occurred after the aura. There may be transient postictal aphasia when the seizure involves the dominant temporal lobe.

Complex partial seizures of frontal lobe origin are atypical and often differ dramatically from those originating in the temporal lobe. Although there are many variations, frontal lobe complex partial seizures tend to (1) begin and end abruptly; (2) be brief with few, if any, postictal symptoms; (3) express prominent, but often bizzare, motor manifestations such as asynchronous thrashing or flailing of arms and legs, pelvic thrusting, pedalling leg movements, and loud vocalizations, all of which can at first suggest psychogenic attacks; and (4) show minimal or nonlocalizing changes with scalp EEG recordings.

Psychomotor, temporal lobe, and *limbic* seizures are all terms that have been used in the past to describe many of the ictal behaviors now classified as complex partial seizures, but they are not synonymous. Not all complex partial seizures arise from the temporal lobe, nor do all involve the limbic system. Some temporal lobe and limbic phenomena reflect unilateral ictal discharges and may not be associated with significant alteration of awareness, the *sine qua non* of complex partial seizures. Finally, automatisms (the "psychomotor" element) are not invariably present in complex partial seizures.

GENERALIZED SEIZURES. Generalized seizures begin diffusely and involve both cerebral hemispheres simultaneously from the outset. They lack clinical and EEG features that indicate a lo-

TABLE 433-2. ILAE CLASSIFICATION OF EPILEPTIC SEIZURES AND SYNDROMES

Classification of seizures
I. Partial (focal) seizures
   A. *Simple partial seizures* (consciousness not impaired)
      1. With motor signs (including jacksonian, versive, and postural)
      2. With sensory symptoms (including visual, somatosensory, auditory, olfactory)
      3. With psychic symptoms (including dysphasia, hallucinatory, and affective changes)
      4. With autonomic symptoms
   B. *Complex partial seizures* (consciousness is impaired)
      1. Simple partial onset followed by impaired consciousness
      2. With impairment of consciousness at onset
      3. With automatisms
   C. Partial seizures evolving to secondarily generalized seizures
II. Generalized seizures of non-focal origin
   A. Absence seizures
   B. Myoclonic seizures; myoclonic jerks (single or multiple)
   C. Tonic-clonic seizures
   D. Tonic seizures
   E. Atonic seizures
III. Unclassified epileptic seizures

Classification of epileptic syndromes
I. Idiopathic epilepsy syndromes (focal or generalized)
   A. Benign neonatal convulsions
   B. Benign focal epilepsy of childhood
   C. Childhood absence epilepsy
   D. Juvenile myoclonic epilepsy
   E. Idiopathic epilepsy, otherwise unspecified
II. Cryptogenic or symptomatic epilepsy syndromes (focal or generalized)
   A. West's syndrome (infantile spasms)
   B. Lennox-Gastaut syndrome
   C. Epilepsia partialis continua
   D. Temporal lobe epilepsy
   E. Frontal lobe epilepsy
   F. Post-traumatic epilepsy
   G. Other symptomatic epilepsies, otherwise unspecified
III. Other epilepsy syndromes of uncertain or mixed classification
   A. Neonatal seizures
   B. Febrile seizures
   C. Reflex epilepsy
   D. Adult nonconvulsive status epilepticus
   E. Other unspecified

calized cerebral origin. Generalized seizures are subdivided mainly on the basis of the presence or absence and character of ictal motor manifestations. These features, in turn, depend on the extent to which subcortical and brain stem structures are engaged in elaboration of the ictal discharge.

Generalized tonic-clonic seizures (*grand mal convulsions*) are characterized by abrupt loss of consciousness with bilateral tonic extension of the trunk and limbs (*tonic phase*), often accompanied by a loud vocalization as air is forcefully expelled across tightly contracted vocal cords (the *"epileptic cry"*), followed by bilaterally synchronous muscle jerking (*clonic phase*). In some patients, a few clonic jerks precede the tonic-clonic sequence; in others, only a tonic or a clonic phase is seen. Urinary incontinence is common, fecal incontinence rare. The actual ictus does not usually last more than 90 seconds. The postictal phase is marked by transient deep stupor followed in 15 to 30 minutes by a lethargic, confused state with automatic behavior. As recovery progresses, many patients complain of headache, muscle soreness, mental dulling, lack of energy, or mood changes lasting as long as 24 hours.

Generalized tonic-clonic seizures result in a number of striking but transient physiologic changes, including blood hypoxia and lactic acidosis, elevated plasma catecholamine levels, and increased concentrations of creatine kinase, prolactin, corticotropin, cortisol, beta-endorphin, and growth hormone. Complications include oral trauma, vertebral compression fractures, shoulder dislocation, aspiration pneumonia, and sudden death, which may be related to acute pulmonary edema, cardiac arrhythmia, or suffocation.

Absence seizures (*petit mal seizures*) occur mainly in children and are characterized by sudden, momentary lapses in awareness (the absence attack), staring, rhythmic blinking, and, often, a few small clonic jerks of arms or hands. Behavior and awareness return

immediately to normal. There is no postictal period and usually no recollection that a seizure has occurred. Most absence seizures last < 10 seconds. Longer absences are accompanied by automatisms, usually of a perseverative type, in about 70% of cases. Absence seizures commonly coexist with generalized tonic-clonic or myoclonic seizures. Untreated, absence seizures can occur hundreds of times each day.

Lapses of awareness that have a more gradual onset, do not resolve as abruptly, and are accompanied by autonomic features or loss of muscle tone are referred to as *atypical absence seizures.* These occur most often in children with mental retardation, and they do not respond as well to antiepileptic drug treatment. Typical and atypical absence seizures must also be distinguished from complex partial seizures manifested only by brief lapses of consciousness because cause, treatment, and prognosis differ among these three seizure types.

Myoclonic seizures manifest as rapid, recurrent, brief muscle jerks that can occur bilaterally, synchronously or asynchronously, or unilaterally without loss of consciousness. The myoclonic jerks range from small movements of the face or hands to massive bilateral spasms that simultaneously affect the head, limbs, and trunk. Repeated myoclonic seizures may seem to crescendo and terminate in a generalized tonic-clonic convulsion. Although they can occur at any time, myoclonic seizures often cluster shortly after waking or while falling asleep.

Atonic seizures ("drop attacks") occur most often in children with diffuse encephalopathies and are characterized by sudden loss of muscle tone which may result in falls with self-injury. Sometimes the loss of muscle tone is limited or fragmentary, producing, for example, only a head drop.

MISCELLANEOUS SEIZURE TYPES. Some seizures are designated by unique or unusual features. *Gelastic* seizures can be either complex partial or generalized nonconvulsive seizures in which pathologic laughter unaccompanied by any emotional content is a conspicuous feature of the epileptic event. *Cursive* seizures are complex partial seizures in which running is a prominent symptoms. *Reflex* seizures are attacks precipitated by a specific stimulus, such as touch, a musical tune, a particular movement, reading, stroboscopic light patterns, or complex visual images.

Classification of the Epilepsies (Epileptic Syndromes)

Some epileptic disorders are characterized by sufficiently reproducible aggregations of historical data, seizure patterns, associated clinical signs and symptoms, EEG findings, biochemical abnormalities, and imaging results that distinct *epileptic syndromes* can be defined. Furthermore, classifying the kind of epilepsy a patient has, or identifying a person's specific epileptic syndrome, is more important than describing seizures. This is because such a diagnosis has implications for diagnostic evaluation, treatment, genetic counseling, and prognosis. The most widely used classification scheme today is the 1989 revision of the International League Against Epilepsy's Commission on Classification and Terminology (Table 433–2).

The ILAE classification separates major groups of epilepsy first on the basis of whether seizures are partial (*localization-related [focal] epilepsies*) or generalized (*generalized epilepsies*), and second, by cause (*idiopathic, symptomatic,* or *cryptogenic epilepsy*). Idiopathic epilepsies and syndromes are those that have no demonstrable underlying cause other than a probable hereditary predisposition. Symptomatic epilepsies and syndromes are those resulting from a known or assumed brain disorder. Cryptogenic epilepsies and syndromes are those in which the cause is unknown, although a symptomatic basis is assumed because of circumstantial evidence or similarities to cases in which the cause is known. Subtypes of epilepsy are grouped by age and, in the case of focal epilepsies, by the anatomic location of the presumed site of seizure onset.

A fundamental problem with the ILAE classification is that it is entirely empirical, with clinical and EEG data emphasized over specific etiologic information (e.g., gene abnormalities, biochemical or metabolic defects). Nonetheless, this realistically reflects current knowledge about most epilepsies today. Furthermore, defining common epilepsy syndromes has great practical value.

FEBRILE SEIZURES. Febrile seizures are the most common cause of convulsions in children: They affect between 3 and 5% of all children in the United States and Europe under the age of 5 years. Most febrile seizures occur between the ages of 6 months and 4 years, although sometimes they occur in children as old as 6 or 7 years. About 30% of children have more than one attack; chance of recurrence is greatest if the first seizure occurs before 1 year of age or there is a family history of febrile seizures. Although the vast majority of affected children have no long-term consequences, febrile seizures increase the risk of developing epilepsy later. This risk is low for most children, about 2 to 3%, but it approximates 10 to 13% in those who have had prolonged or focal seizures, who have a family history of afebrile seizures, or who were neurologically abnormal before the first febrile seizure. Febrile seizures are not associated with, nor do they cause, mental retardation, below average IQ, poor school performance, or behavior problems. Prophylactic treatment is generally not indicated because of the benign prognosis. If treatment is considered at all, rectal administration of diazepam only during febrile illnesses is effective, safe, and preferable to chronic therapy using phenobarbital.

BENIGN PARTIAL EPILEPSY OF CHILDHOOD WITH CENTRAL-MIDTEMPORAL SPIKES. This is one of the most common epileptic syndromes of childhood, representing about 15% of all pediatric epilepsies. Seizures usually begin between the ages of 4 and 13 years; affected children are otherwise normal. Most have seizures principally or only at night. Because sleep promotes secondary generalization, parents report only tonic-clonic convulsions; any focal signature is usually missed. In contrast, seizures occurring during the day are typically focal and express themselves with twitching of one side of the face, speech arrest, drooling, and paresthesias of the face, gums, tongue, and inner cheeks. Seizures may progress to include hemiclonic movements or hemitonic posturing. EEG's show a distinctive pattern of stereotyped epileptiform discharges over the central and midtemporal regions. Prognosis is invariably good, and seizures disappear by mid to late adolescence. Outcome is not affected by treatment, but carbamazepine prevents recurrent attacks.

CHILDHOOD ABSENCE (PETIT MAL) EPILEPSY. This disorder begins most often between the ages of 4 and 12 years in children who are neurologically and intellectually normal. Absence attacks can often be precipitated by hyperventilation. The EEG is diagnostic, showing stereotyped 3-Hz spike-wave discharges in association with a typical spell (Fig. 433–2). Generalized tonic-clonic seizures occur in 30 to 50% of cases. Ethosuximide (10 mg per kilogram per day or, in older children, 250 mg two or three times daily) and valproate (15 to 30 mg per kilogram per day) are equally effective against absence seizures; valproate is preferable if generalized tonic-clonic seizures coexist.

JUVENILE MYOCLONIC EPILEPSY. This is one of the most frequently encountered types of idiopathic generalized epilepsy. It begins most often between the ages of 8 and 20 years in otherwise healthy individuals. When fully developed, the syndrome is characterized by morning myoclonic jerks, generalized tonic-clonic seizures that occur just after awakening, normal intelligence, a family history of similar seizures, and an EEG that shows generalized 4- to 6-Hz spike-wave and polyspike-wave discharges. Valproate controls attacks in > 80% of cases, but indefinite treatment is required in most cases because of the high rate of seizure relapse following attempted drug withdrawal.

LENNOX-GASTAUT SYNDROME. This term is used for a heterogeneous group of early childhood epileptic encephalopathies that have in common physical brain abnormalities, mental retardation, uncontrolled seizures, and an EEG pattern that shows generalized 1.5- to 2.5-Hz sharp-slow wave discharges ("slow spike-and-wave pattern"). No treatment is consistently effective; management is best directed by specialists in the field.

TEMPORAL LOBE EPILEPSY. This is the most common epileptic syndrome of adults, accounting for at least 40% of epilepsy cases. Seizures begin in late childhood or adolescence, and there is often a history of febrile seizures. Virtually all patients have complex partial seizures, some of which secondarily generalize. Epigastric or visceral auras are frequent. Interictal EEG's usually show epileptiform discharges over the anterior temporal region (Fig. 433–3). Most patients with temporal lobe epilepsy have impaired memory, and some show a decrease in either verbal or visuospatial skills, depending on whether the epileptogenic temporal lobe is dominant or nondominant.

Temporal lobe epilepsy arises most often from mesial temporal limbic structures, typically in association with a characteristic lesion known as *hippocampal sclerosis.* Hippocampal sclerosis refers to variable but selective neuronal loss, especially in the CA1 (Sommer's sector), CA3, and dentate gyrus regions of the hippocampus (Fig. 433–4). Secondary gliosis occurs, and corresponding atrophy of the hippocampal formation can be recognized on magnetic resonance brain scans (see below). Neurons in the hippocampal CA2 region (resistant zone) and granule cell layer are relatively spared. In 20% of cases, temporal lobe epilepsy is caused by other structural lesions such as cavernous malformations, hamartomas, cortical dysplasia, glial tumors, and scars related to previous head injuries or encephalitis. Some temporal lobe seizures are symptoms of frontal or occipital lesions which initiate ictal discharges that propagate into mesial temporal lobe structures.

Antiepileptic drugs are usually successful in suppressing secondarily generalized seizures, but > 50% of patients continue to have partial seizures. In drug-resistant cases, temporal lobectomy is the treatment of choice.

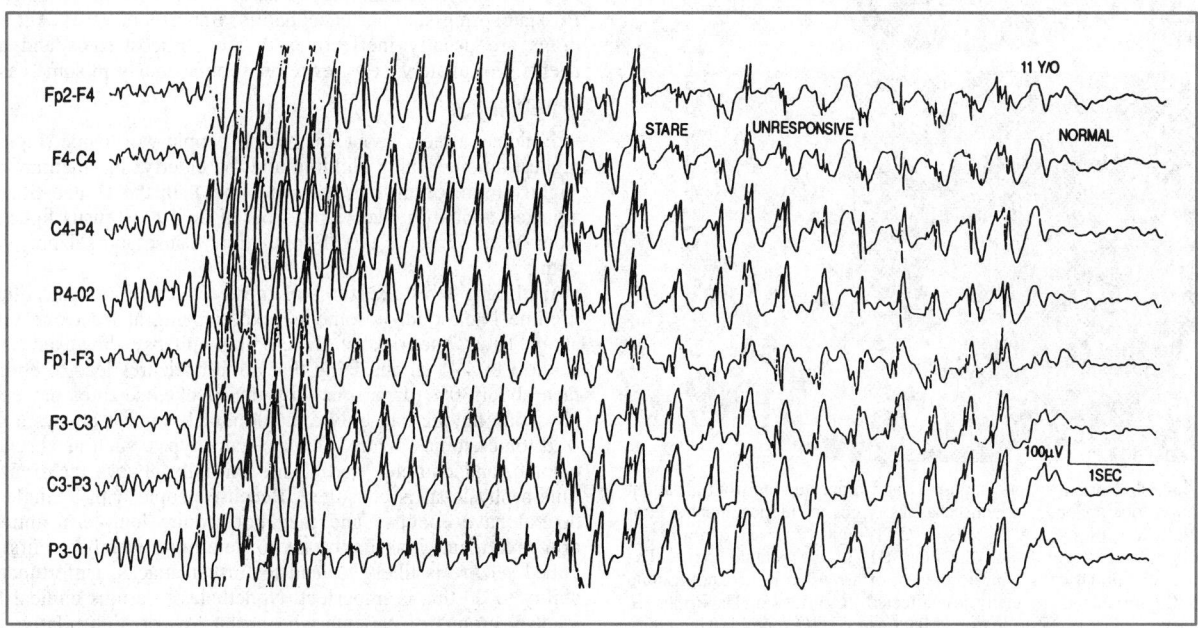

FIGURE 433–2. Childhood absence epilepsy. The EEG shows the typical pattern of generalized 3-Hz spike-wave complexes associated with a clinical absence seizure.

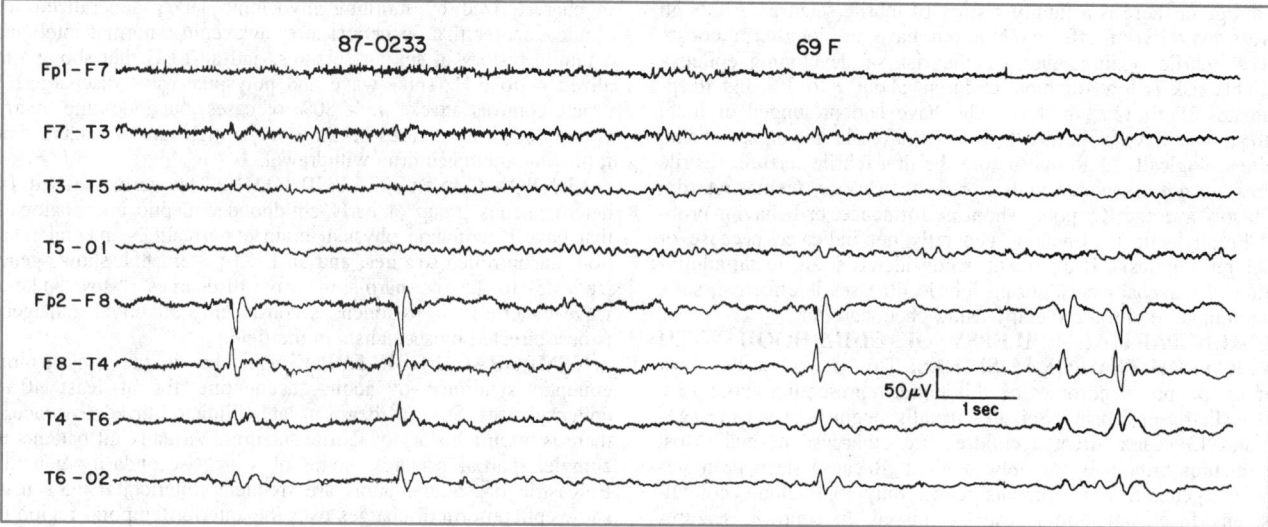

FIGURE 433-3. Temporal lobe epilepsy. Epileptiform discharges are seen focally over the right temporal lobe (bottom four lines), and there is intermixed irregular slow-wave activity not seen on the other side.

POST-TRAUMATIC EPILEPSY. The chance of developing post-traumatic epilepsy relates directly to the severity of the head injury. Following penetrating wounds and other severe head injuries, for example, about one third of patients develop seizures within 1 year. Severe head injuries are defined by the presence of a cerebral contusion, intracerebral or intracranial hematoma, unconsciousness or amnesia lasting more than 24 hours, or persistent abnormalities on neurologic examination, such as hemiparesis or aphasia. Although the majority of patients develop seizures within 1

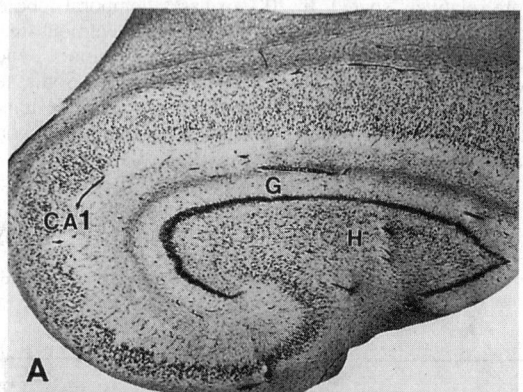

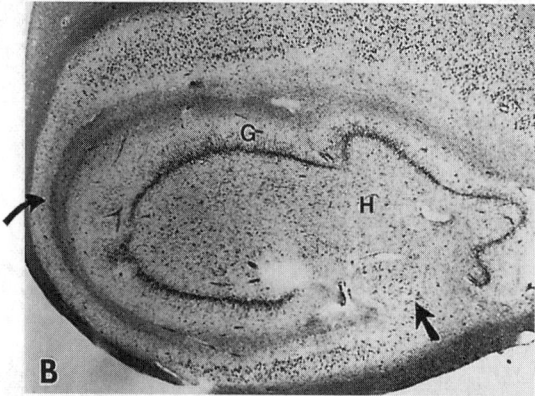

FIGURE 433-4. Normal hippocampus *(A)* and hippocampus from a patient with temporal lobe epilepsy showing changes typical of hippocampal sclerosis *(B)*. Note loss of pyramidal cells in CA1 region *(curved arrow, left)*, CA4 *(straight arrow, right)*, and the hilus (H) of the dentate gyrus. The CA2 region (pyramidal cells lying to the left of arrow on right) and granule cell layer (G) are characteristically less affected. (Courtesy of Dr. Robert S. Sloviter, Departments of Neurology and Pharmacology, Columbia University and Helen Hayes Hospital, New York, New York.)

to 2 years of injury, new-onset seizures may still appear 5 or more years later. Two thirds of patients with post-traumatic epilepsy have partial or secondarily generalized seizures. Mild head injuries (uncomplicated brief loss of consciousness, no skull fracture, absence of focal neurologic signs, no contusion or hematoma) do not increase the risk of seizures.

Impact seizures (a generalized convulsion occurring at the time of, or immediately after, the injury) and *early seizures* (those occurring within the first 1 to 2 weeks) represent acute reactions of the brain to the trauma. Seizures beginning after 10 to 14 days reflect an increased risk of developing post-traumatic epilepsy.

Early seizures should be treated with phenytoin. Phenytoin should also be given prophylactically for 1 to 2 weeks to patients who have sustained severe head injuries in order to minimize complications from seizures occurring during acute management. In the absence of overt attacks, phenytoin should be discontinued after 2 weeks because no data indicate that antiepileptic drugs prevent the development of later epilepsy.

EPILEPSIA PARTIALIS CONTINUA (EPC). This term refers to continuous focal seizures involving part or all of one side of the body. In adults, EPC occurs with severe strokes, primary or metastatic brain tumors, metabolic encephalopathies (especially hyperosmolar nonketotic hyperglycemia), encephalitis, and subacute or rare chronic inflammatory diseases of the brain (Kozhevnikov's Russian spring-summer encephalitis; Behçet's disease). Antiepileptic drugs are usually ineffective, as are corticosteroids and antiviral agents. Fortunately, seizures remit spontaneously in some cases.

EPIDEMIOLOGY

Epilepsy affects about 45 million people worldwide. Incidence is highest among young children and the elderly, and men are affected slightly more often than women (1.5:1). In the United States, age-adjusted annual incidence rates based on 1990 census figures range from 31 to 57 per 100,000 population. Cause and seizure type vary with age.

Excluding febrile seizures or those related to an acute illness, the lifetime likelihood of someone experiencing at least one seizure is about 10%. The risk of developing epilepsy, however, is lower, about 3 to 4%, emphasizing that not all seizures lead to epilepsy. In fact, about 30% of persons with unprovoked seizures present to the physician having had only a single attack, almost always a generalized tonic-clonic seizure. Other seizure types, such as absence, myoclonic, and complex partial, are virtually always recurrent by the time a physician is consulted. Because people with a single seizure do not have epilepsy and may not require long-term antiepileptic drug treatment, it is important to determine whether a first unprovoked seizure is likely to lead to further attacks. Unfortunately, the ability to do this is imperfect. Nonetheless, various clinical features identify groups of patients who are at low or high relative risk for further seizures, and this helps in making treatment decisions and advising patients. The high-risk group consists of individuals with a history of significant brain injury and an abnormal EEG. For these patients, recurrence risk at 2 years is about 65%. By contrast, recurrence risk is only 24% in persons with an idiopathic generalized seizure, a normal EEG, and a negative family history for seizures or epilepsy. Following a second seizure, risk of further seizures rises to >80%. A second seizure, therefore, is a reliable indication of epilepsy.

Persons with epilepsy have increased mortality rates compared with the general population. Most of this increased risk occurs in patients with symptomatic epilepsy in whom mortality relates to the underlying condition. In patients with idiopathic or cryptogenic epilepsy, the increased risk of death is related mainly to accidents, especially drowning. Autopsy and clinical series have reported an increased risk of sudden unexplained death, presumably due to cardiac arrhythmia, pulmonary edema, or myocardial infarction, but the actual incidence has not been documented.

PATHOGENESIS

Seizures result from the synchronous interactions of large populations of neurons that intermittently discharge in abnormal patterns. Because of the large number of processes that regulate cortical excitability, it is unlikely that there is a single epileptogenic mechanism. Nonetheless, neurophysiologic studies in a variety of experimental preparations have shown that "epileptic" neurons share a number of properties, although the total expression of these varies according to the particular model.

Intracellular recordings from neurons in an epileptogenic focus show recurring high-voltage, long-duration depolarizations with superimposed high-frequency bursts of action potentials. The extracellular current flow generated by these *paroxysmal depolarizing shifts* (PDS's) results in the interictal EEG spike or sharp wave, the characteristic epileptiform discharge that signifies susceptibility to seizures. PDS generation involves several mechanisms, including increased excitability resulting from changes in intrinsic voltage-dependent membrane currents, newly active excitatory circuits, attenuation or loss of effective postsynaptic inhibition and other inhibitory processes, as well as increased effectiveness of excitatory synapses. In neurons showing "epileptic" patterns of behavior, ordinary synaptic inputs may elicit exaggerated or pathologically amplified responses. Activation of the N-methyl-D-aspartate (NMDA) type of glutamate receptors potentiates cellular excitability and leads to sustained neuronal depolarization and calcium influx. Prolonged NMDA receptor activation and excessive accumulation of intracellular calcium also result in neuronal toxicity and may lead to cell death ("epileptic brain damage") following severe repetitive seizures or status epilepticus. In some areas of cortex, hippocampus for example, subsets of neurons which normally fire in bursts may serve as pacemaker cells for other groups of neurons during epileptogenic activities.

Although it is not known in detail what causes the transition from an interictal to an ictal state, development of sustained experimental seizures reflects decreasing effectiveness of inhibitory mechanisms accompanied by increasing evidence of excitation. PDS's become more frequent and involve ever larger numbers of neurons and more distant areas of cortex, a situation that results in progressive depolarization of neurons both within and outside the original focus. During frequent interictal epileptiform discharges and especially during seizures, extracellular potassium and intracellular calcium concentrations increase and contribute to the overall excitability of the epileptic neuronal aggregate. During the seizure itself, neurons are tonically depolarized and fire continuously in a sustained, high-frequency discharge (corresponding to the tonic phase of the seizure). The seizure ends as phasic repolarizations interrupt the continuous firing pattern (the correlate of the clonic phase) and gradually restore membrane potentials to normal or to a temporary hyperpolarized state (postictal depression). Phenytoin and carbamazepine are effective anticonvulsants because they produce a use-dependent block of sodium channels, thus limiting the capability of neurons to fire at high-frequency rates. The benzodiazepines and barbiturates exert their anticonvulsant effect by enhancing postsynaptic GABA-mediated inhibition through an effect on the chloride ionophore.

In the focal epilepsies, abnormal neuronal behavior originates in and may remain confined to a restricted area of the cortex. The brain possesses powerful mechanisms to suppress and restrain abnormal electrical behavior. Typically during focal interictal discharges or focal seizures, areas surrounding the epileptogenic cortex are inhibited (surround inhibition), as is the homotopic contralateral cortex and areas of the thalamus and brain stem. Only when these restraining influences are overcome does a seizure spread and become secondarily generalized.

In temporal lobe epilepsy, certain neurons within the dentate gyrus of the hippocampus have been identified as being especially vulnerable to injury. Selective loss of mossy cells and of neurons containing somatostatin and neuropeptide Y results in deafferentation of the normally powerful GABA inhibitory neurons within the dentate gyrus, rendering them nonfunctional. As a result, the granule cells of the dentate gyrus become disinhibited and respond with abnormal synchronous bursts to cortical stimuli. Subclinical electrographic seizures develop and further damage vulnerable cell populations, creating a self-enhancing cycle of cell loss, impaired control of hippocampal excitability, and, eventually, clinical seizures associated with the pathologic picture of hippocampal sclerosis. How other lesions (e.g., tumors or cavernous malformations) cause focal epilepsy is less well understood.

The thalamus plays a critical role in generating generalized seizures and the generalized spike-wave EEG patterns that accompany them. The bilateral synchrony of generalized seizures and the rhythmicity of spike-wave discharges appear to depend on two main factors—a unique set of ionic conductances, including a T-type calcium current, which enable neurons in the thalamic nucleus reticularis to function as pacemaker control cells, and the special anatomy and pharmacology of the thalamocortical system. The substantia nigra also is critical to the expression of generalized convulsions, especially the tonic phase; GABA-ergic inhibitory transmission in the substantia nigra plays a regulatory role in the propagation of both primary and secondarily generalized seizure discharges. Because there are no consistent, demonstrable pathologic changes in the brains of patients with idiopathic generalized epilepsy, susceptibility to these seizures likely results from inherited biochemical membrane or neurotransmitter defects that result in abnormal excitability within the involved circuits.

DIAGNOSIS

Accurate diagnosis is the cornerstone of rational management. The diagnostic evaluation has three objectives: (1) to determine if the patient has epilepsy; (2) to classify the seizures and type of epilepsy accurately and determine if the clinical data fit a particular epilepsy syndrome; and (3) to identify, if possible, a specific underlying cause.

History

A detailed and accurate history is imperative and the single most important factor in diagnosis. Because patients usually have only limited awareness of their behavior during a seizure, additional information usually must be obtained from family members or other close observers. The historical summary should provide a clear description of the patient's seizures, including details of any aura; the neurologic status between attacks; any reproducible precipitants; and relevant risk factors for epilepsy such as a family history of seizures or a history of severe head trauma, encephalitis or meningitis, and febrile seizures (Table 433–3). In children and young adults, one should inquire about gestation, birth, postnatal course, and early development. If a patient has been treated previously, it is

TABLE 433–3. ESSENTIAL FEATURES OF THE SEIZURE HISTORY

Date and circumstances of first attack
First consistent event in the seizure (Is there an aura? Are initial symptoms/signs focal or lateralizing?)
Subsequent evolution of the seizure, in sequence
Postictal manifestations (Todd's paralysis)
Is there more than one seizure type?
Average rate of occurrence; longest seizure-free interval since onset
Seizure precipitants (alcohol, sleep deprivation, particular stimuli, stress)
Is there a pattern to seizure occurrence (circadian, catamenial)?
Has there been a change in characteristics of the seizure?
Symptoms of neurologic or systemic disease between seizures. Are these static, intermittent, or progressive?
Risk factors for epilepsy (family history, cerebral injury)

important to learn what drugs were used, the doses and blood levels that were achieved, and therapeutic or adverse effects.

Physical Examination

Although the physical examination is normal in most patients with epilepsy, abnormal findings, when present, can be helpful in two ways. First, physical signs may point to an underlying neurologic or systemic disorder of which the seizures are a part. Phakomatoses, for example, are commonly associated with seizures and may be suggested by café-au-lait spots, a facial angioma, hypopigmented macules, axillary freckling, and shagreen patches. Second, focal neurologic signs indicate localized cerebral pathology. Asymmetry in the size of the hands, feet, or face signifies a longstanding abnormality of the cerebral hemisphere contralateral to the smaller side. Third, absence seizures can be triggered in untreated patients by having them hyperventilate for 2 to 3 minutes.

Laboratory Tests

ELECTROENCEPHALOGRAPHY. EEG is the most important diagnostic test for epilepsy. EEG findings are useful and sometimes essential for establishing the diagnosis, classifying seizures correctly, identifying epileptic syndromes, and making therapeutic decisions. In combination with appropriate clinical findings, *epileptiform* EEG patterns termed "spikes" or "sharp waves" strongly support a diagnosis of epilepsy. In patients with seizures, focal epileptiform discharges indicate focal epilepsy, whereas generalized epileptiform activity indicates a generalized form of epilepsy. The particular pattern of epileptiform activity, defined by the morphology, spatial distribution, repetition rate, and other characteristics of the discharges, assists in identifying a particular type of epilepsy or epileptic syndrome. A note of caution is warranted, however. Most EEG's are obtained between seizures, and interictal abnormalities alone can never prove or refute a diagnosis of epilepsy. Epilepsy can be definitively established only by recording a characteristic ictal discharge during a clinical attack. Unfortunately, this is uncommon during routine EEG recordings. A further factor that can confound interpretation of interictal EEG's is the occurrence of similar epileptiform abnormalities in about 2% of normal people; many of these, especially in children, are asymptomatic markers of a genetic trait. Finally, epileptiform-like waveforms or artifacts can be misinterpreted and erroneously considered to be evidence of seizure susceptibility.

About 40 to 50% of patients with epilepsy show epileptiform abnormalities on their initial EEG. The chance of capturing epileptiform activity is enhanced by sleep deprivation for 24 hours before the test and having the patient sleep during a portion of the EEG recording. Serial EEG's also increase the yield of positive tracings. A small number of persons with epilepsy, however, continue to have normal interictal EEG's despite all efforts to record an abnormality.

Specialized epilepsy centers in tertiary referral hospitals include monitoring units equipped with simultaneous EEG and closed-circuit television capability as well as computer-assisted detection and analysis systems. These facilities have greatly improved management of selected patients by giving physicians the means to distinguish epileptic from nonepileptic paroxysmal events, to make precise electrical-clinical correlations, and to localize epileptogenic foci for resective surgery.

NEUROIMAGING STUDIES. Anatomic imaging using computed tomography (CT) or magnetic resonance imaging (MRI) complements EEG data by identifying structural brain pathology that may be causally related to the development of epilepsy. MRI is substantially more sensitive than CT in detecting epileptogenic cerebral lesions. Hippocampal sclerosis, defects of neuronal migration, gangliogliomas and some gliomas, and cavernous malformations are readily seen with MRI but may be missed using CT. It is important to obtain a complete imaging study that includes both T1- and T2-weighted images in coronal and axial planes. Imaging in the coronal plane perpendicular to the long axis of the hippocampus has improved detection of hippocampal atrophy and gliosis (Fig. 433–5), findings that correlate with the pathologic picture of mesial temporal sclerosis and an epileptogenic temporal lobe. An even more sensitive measure of hippocampal atrophy compares volume measurements of a patient's hippocampus with similar quanti-

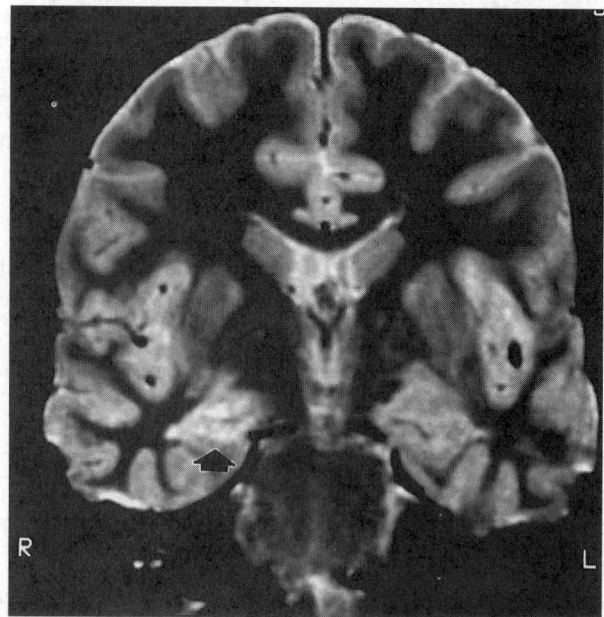

FIGURE 433–5. Coronal MRI scan at the level of the anterior temporal lobe showing changes consistent with right-sided hippocampal sclerosis. The right hippocampal formation *(arrow)* is atrophic compared with the left and shows signal changes (white areas) indicating gliosis. (Courtesy of Dr. Stephen Chan, Division of Neuroradiology, Columbia-Presbyterian Medical Center, New York, New York.)

tative data obtained in normal controls. Gadolinium infusion does not improve detection of cerebral lesions associated with epilepsy, although it often aids in differentiating among types of cerebral pathology.

A CT or, preferably, MRI scan should be obtained in all patients suspected of epilepsy over the age of 18 years and in all children with partial seizures (except those with benign focal epilepsy of childhood), abnormal neurologic findings, or focal slow-wave abnormalities on EEG. All patients with refractory seizures should have an MRI scan even if earlier CT scans were normal.

In contrast to these structural imaging methods, positron emission tomography (PET) and single photon emission computed tomography (SPECT) offer functional views of the brain. These techniques use physiologically active, radiolabeled tracers to image the brain's metabolic activity (PET) or blood flow (SPECT). For example, about 70% of patients with temporal lobe epilepsy show focal hypometabolic areas on interictal PET scans that correspond to the epileptogenic focus. Abnormalities using PET or SPECT are often demonstrated even when MRI or CT is normal. By and large, these specialized procedures are reserved for research-level studies rather than diagnosis.

BLOOD TESTS. Routine blood tests rarely offer diagnostic assistance in otherwise healthy patients with epilepsy. Serum electrolytes, liver function tests, and an automated blood count may be useful, however, as baseline studies before starting antiepileptic drug therapy. Blood tests are necessary and frequently informative in older patients with acute or chronic systemic disease. Consideration should be given to obtaining blood or urine samples from adolescents and young adults with unexplained generalized seizures to screen for substance abuse, especially cocaine.

LUMBAR PUNCTURE. Lumbar puncture is mandatory if there is any suspicion of meningitis or encephalitis. It is otherwise unnecessary and need not be performed routinely. Repeated generalized seizures and convulsive status epilepticus can increase cerebrospinal fluid protein content slightly and produce a pleocytosis of up to 100 WBC's per cubic millimeter for 24 to 48 hours. CSF pleocytosis should be attributed to seizures only in retrospect; infection or intracranial inflammatory processes should always be assumed first.

ELECTROCARDIOGRAM (ECG). An ECG should be obtained in any young person with a first generalized seizure if there is a family history of arrhythmia, sudden unexplained death, or episodic unconsciousness. An ECG should also be obtained in any patient with a history of cardiac arrhythmia or valvular disease.

Not every paroxysmal event is a seizure, and misidentification of other conditions as epilepsy leads to ineffective, unnecessary, and potentially harmful treatment. In addition, misdiagnosis accounts for a substantial portion of patients whose spells have not responded to antiepileptic drug treatment.

A variety of conditions can be confused with epilepsy, depending on the age of the patient and the nature and circumstances of the attacks (Table 433–4). It is not always possible to distinguish among various diagnostic possibilities on clinical grounds alone, and admission to a specialized monitoring unit is frequently necessary.

Nonepileptic paroxysmal disorders have in common the occurrence of sudden, discrete events characterized by abnormal or inappropriate behavior, variable responsiveness, changes in muscle tone, and various postures or movements. These conditions are far more common and variable in their presentation in children than in adults. Many of the disorders simulating epilepsy in childhood can be viewed as transient "developmental" conditions that require no treatment other than reassurance.

Syncope (see Ch. 396.1) refers to the symptom complex that results when there is a transient, global reduction in cerebral perfusion with associated hypoxia. Loss of consciousness lasts only a few seconds, uncommonly a minute or more, and recovery is rapid. If the cerebral hypoxia is sufficiently severe, the syncopal episode may include brief tonic posturing of the trunk or a few clonic jerks of the arms and legs (convulsive syncope). Similarly, some forms of *migraine* can be mistaken for seizures, especially if headache is atypical or mild. Basilar artery migraine, a rare variant seen most often in adolescents and young adults, can include lethargy, mood changes, confusion and disorientation, vertigo, bilateral visual disturbances, and alteration or loss of consciousness.

Psychogenic seizures frequently cause intractable "epilepsy" in adults and may represent 20% or more of cases referred to an epilepsy monitoring unit. Definitive diagnosis requires video/EEG documentation, although a history of atypical and nonstereotyped attacks, emotional or psychological precipitants, psychiatric illness, complete lack of response to antiepileptic drugs, and repeatedly normal interictal EEG's suggests the possibility of psychogenic seizures. *Panic attacks* and anxiety attacks with hyperventilation can superficially resemble partial seizures with affective, autonomic, or special sensory symptoms. Prolonged hyperventilation results in muscle twitching or spasms (tetany), and affected patients may faint.

Episodic dyscontrol is a poorly defined entity consisting of intermittent periods of inappropriately violent and destructive behavior that is out of character for the patient. Abnormal EEG's have been reported in children with the episodic dyscontrol syndrome, but most affected adults have little evidence of a structural brain disorder.

TABLE 433–4. NONEPILEPTIC EPISODIC DISORDERS IN ADOLESCENTS AND ADULTS

Movement disorders
    Myoclonus
    Paroxysmal choreoathetosis
    Hyperexplexia (startle disease)
Migraine
    Confusional
    Vertebrobasilar
*Syncope and cardiac arrhythmias
Behavioral/psychiatric disorders
    *Psychogenic seizures
    *Hyperventilation syndrome
    *Panic disorder
    Dissociative states ("fugue states")
    Episodic dyscontrol
Narcolepsy and sleep apnea
    Automatic behavior syndrome
    Partial cataplexy
Transient ischemic attacks
*Transient global amnesia
    Acute confusional states
*Alcoholic blackouts
    Hypoglycemia attacks

* Most commonly encountered

MEDICAL TREATMENT

The First Seizure

Patients with their first epileptic seizure should be screened for symptoms and signs of an acute medical or neurologic illness. Brain imaging with MR or CT need not be done emergently unless there is a high likelihood of an acute cerebral lesion or the patient remains obtunded. Most patients recover rapidly following an isolated seizure, so several hours of observation are usually sufficient to assess the clinical progress, obtain additional relevant information, and review the results of laboratory tests. Hospitalization is not necessary provided that there is no suspicion of an underlying illness and a responsible family member or friend can observe the patient closely at home. If these criteria cannot be met, or if there is uncertainty about them, hospitalization is indicated. If the patient is sent home, there should be a clear plan for follow-up and re-evaluation.

Whether an antiepileptic drug should be prescribed following a first seizure is a matter of controversy. Although a large multicenter randomized study from Italy has recently demonstrated that antiepileptic drugs reduce the risk of relapse following a first unprovoked generalized tonic-clonic seizure, no information exists regarding the effect of early treatment on long-term prognosis, especially with regard to such important issues as whether early treatment reduces the severity of epilepsy or increases the chance of entering a prolonged remission. As indicated earlier in this chapter, chronic treatment of all first seizures would expensively overtreat three quarters of the patients. We believe that the decision to treat should be based on the physician's estimate of the risk of further seizures; the consequence to the patient of recurrent seizures; a reasonable expectation that the patient will comply with the treatment regimen; and the risk of adverse effects from antiepileptic drug therapy (10 to 30%). Patients are classified as being at low risk for further seizures if they have a normal EEG, normal physical examination, no history of significant cerebral injury, a normal brain imaging study, and absence of a family history of epilepsy. We recommend treating patients after a first seizure only if they have two or more of these risk factors. Nevertheless, the final decision regarding treatment must always be individualized, considering the potential psychological, vocational, and physical consequences of further seizures for each patient.

Selection of Antiepileptic Drugs

The treatment of epilepsy has three main objectives: (1) to eliminate seizures or reduce their frequency to the maximum extent possible; (2) to avoid chronic drug-related adverse effects; and (3) to assist the patient in maintaining or restoring normal vocational and psychosocial adjustment. Although each of these goals is possible, unfortunately no medical treatment currently available can permanently eliminate ("cure") epilepsy. Furthermore, fewer than 50% of adults treated for chronic partial and secondarily generalized seizures become seizure free for more than 12 months with currently available drugs.

Drugs used to treat different kinds of seizures are listed in Table 433–5. Well-controlled prospective studies have shown that carbamazepine, phenytoin, primidone, and phenobarbital are equally effective in suppressing partial and secondarily generalized seizures. In individual patients, however, failure to respond to one drug does not preclude a good response to another. Valproate is somewhat less effective against complex partial seizures than either carbamazepine or phenytoin but it is of comparable efficacy against secondarily generalized seizures. Despite similar pharmacologic potency, these drugs differ substantially in terms of side effects and pharmacokinetic properties. Thus, tolerability and ease of dosing schedule determine the particular choice of drug for an individual patient. Cost may be another consideration. Phenytoin has a long half-life and may be given once or twice daily after midadolescence. In contrast, carbamazepine must be administered more often, which increases problems with compliance for some patients. On the other hand, concern about phenytoin's occasional undesirable cosmetic effects (gingival hypertrophy, hirsutism, and coarsening of the facial features) makes carbamazepine the drug of choice for other patients, especially younger ones. Primidone and phenobarbital have a high incidence of sedative and cognitive side effects and are rarely recommended as initial therapy.

TABLE 433-5. DRUGS USED IN TREATING DIFFERENT TYPES OF SEIZURES

Type of Seizure	Drugs
Simple and complex partial	Carbamazepine, phenytoin; valproate; gabapentin, lamotrigine as add-on; primidone, phenobarbital
Secondarily generalized	Carbamazepine, phenytoin, valproate; gabapentin, lamotrigine as add-on; phenobarbital, primidone
Primary generalized seizures	
Tonic-clonic	Valproate; carbamazepine, phenytoin; lamotrigine
Absence	Ethosuximide, valproate; lamotrigine
Myoclonic	Valproate; clonazepam
Tonic	Valproate, felbamate; clonazepam

Note: The utility and clinical spectrum of lamotrigine, felbamate, and gabapentin have not yet been established, and the position of these drugs in the table should be viewed only as tentative.

Valproate is the drug of first choice for generalized-onset seizures. It can be used effectively as monotherapy in 80% of patients even when several types of generalized seizures coexist. Phenytoin and carbamazepine are only slightly less effective against generalized tonic-clonic seizures, but they may exacerbate absence and myoclonic seizures which frequently accompany generalized tonic-clonic seizures. Ethosuximide is as effective as valproate in treating typical absence seizures and, because of fewer side effects, is the drug of choice when no other seizure type exists. Clonazepam has some utility in treating myoclonic seizures, but tolerance tends to develop.

Drug Dosage and Pharmacokinetic Principles

Table 433-6 gives the usual dose and relevant pharmacokinetic data for each of the most commonly used antiepileptic drugs. Following absorption, a drug is distributed between the plasma and various tissue compartments. Because most antiepileptic drugs are fractionally bound to serum proteins, an equilibrium exists between the plasma concentrations of protein-bound and free (unbound) drug. Only unbound drug is capable of crossing the various lipoprotein membranes that surround brain receptor sites, making only this portion of the total drug concentration available to produce the desired effect. Antiepileptic drug blood levels that are routinely determined by laboratories reflect total plasma drug concentrations (bound plus unbound fractions). When protein binding is altered by disease (e.g., uremia), physiologic state (e.g., pregnancy), or other drugs (e.g., valproate), determining the unbound fraction provides a more accurate reflection of the drug's concentration in the brain's extracellular space. Measuring free levels can be helpful whenever there is a discrepancy between the total plasma concentration and the expected clinical effect.

A drug's *half-life* is a measure of the rate at which a drug is eliminated, mainly through metabolism or excretion. Drug half-life determines the dosing interval for antiepileptic drugs; this should amount to less than one third to one half the drug's half-life at steady state in order to minimize fluctuations in plasma concentrations. *Steady state* refers to the equilibrium that is established between drug intake and clearance. The time it takes for a drug to achieve steady-state conditions is determined by its half-life. For practical purposes, steady state is reached at an interval equal to five times the drug's half-life. Because a drug continues to accumulate in the body until steady state is reached, plasma drug levels are reliable only when they are measured under steady-state conditions. Similarly, time to steady state determines how rapidly the dose of any antiepileptic drug can be increased. Phenytoin is an exception because of its nonlinear kinetics. Phenytoin's half-life is dose-dependent, which means that steady-state concentration at one dose cannot be used to predict directly the steady-state concentration at a higher dose. For example, phenytoin's half-life is about 24 hours at plasma concentrations of 10 to 20 μg per milliliter. However, its half-life increases to 36 hours (or more) at concentrations of 25 μg per milliliter.

The care of patients with epilepsy has been greatly improved by the widespread availability of reliable data on therapeutic plasma concentrations of antiepileptic drugs. Most published therapeutic ranges for the various antiepileptic drugs have been derived from relatively small numbers of patients and reflect average blood levels that were empirically effective in controlling seizures with minimal or no adverse effects. As a result, optimal blood levels for some patients fall either above or below the recommended levels. Some patients, for example, consistently have side effects at low or "therapeutic" concentrations, whereas others benefit from "toxic" levels without experiencing side effects. Blood levels, therefore, are useful guidelines that assist in achieving optimal therapy but they should never be the goal of treatment. A level in the low to mid-therapeutic range is a reasonable target when initiating treatment, but subsequent dose adjustments should be based on the patient's clinical progress, seizure frequency, and appearance of drug-related side effects. As a guide to future management, blood levels can be re-

TABLE 433-6. ANTIEPILEPTIC DRUGS—DOSAGE AND PHARMACOKINETIC DATA

	Usual Dosage (per 24 hr)	Oral Availability (%)	Protein Bound (%)	Clearance (ml/min/kg)	Urinary Excretion (unchanged %)	Volume of Distribution (liters/kg)	Half-life (hours)	"Therapeutic" Concentrations (μg/ml)
Carbamazepine*	Adult: 800–1600 mg Child: 10–40 mg/kg/day	75–85	74	1.3 (post-induction) (very variable)	<1	0.8–2.0	11–22†	6–12
Ethosuximide	Adult: 750–1500 mg Child: 10–75 mg/kg/day	>90	0	0.19 (higher in children)	18	0.62–0.69	45–60 (children mean: 36)	40–100
Felbamate	Adult: 2400–3600 mg Child: 15–45 mg/kg/day		25–35		50	0.70	18–24	20–60
Gabapentin	Adult: 900–3600 mg	51–59	<3		77–80		5–8	>2
Lamotrigine	Adult: 75–200 mg	>70	55		10		30 (14–50)	1–5
Phenobarbital	Adult: 90–180 mg Child: 2–6 mg/kg/day	100	45–50	0.062 (higher in children)	25	0.54–0.70	99 (shorter in children)	15–40
Phenytoin	Adult: 300–500 mg Child: 4–12 mg/kg/day	90	90	Capacity limited V_{max} = 5.9 mg/kg/day K_M = 5.7 μg/ml	2	0.78	6–42 (concentration dependent)	10–20
Primidone‡	Adult: 750–1250 mg Child: 6–12 mg/kg/day	92	19	0.59–0.94	42	0.64–0.72	8–15	5–12
Valproate	Adult: 1000–3000 mg Child: 10–70 mg/kg/day	100	93 (concentration dependent)	0.11	2	0.19	14–20	50–120

* The carbamazepine metabolite carbamazepine-10,11-epoxide is also pharmacologically active: values given are for the parent compound.
† The half-life of carbamazepine is considerably longer when the drug is first introduced, prior to autoinduction of hepatic microsomal enzymes.
‡ Primidone's primary metabolites, phenobarbital and phenylethylmalonamide, are also pharmacologically active; values given are for the parent compound.
From Pedley TA, Scheuer ML, Walczak TS: In Rowland LP (ed.): Merritt's Textbook of Neurology, 9th ed. Malvern, PA, Lea & Febiger, 1994.
Blood levels for lamotrigine, felbamate, and gabapentin have not been firmly established. These values are only estimates based on initial clinical trials.

peated when control of seizures is achieved or when toxic side effects appear. Noncompliance is the most common reason that a therapeutic drug level is not achieved using recommended dosing schedules. Therapeutic drug monitoring helps to minimize unpredictable drug interactions in patients taking two or more drugs and to compensate for hepatic or renal effects on drug elimination.

Initiating Antiepileptic Drug Therapy

Treatment should start with a single drug chosen according to the patient's type of seizure, considering adverse effects, required dosing schedule, and cost. With the exception of phenobarbital and phenytoin, antiepileptic drugs should be started in low doses to minimize acute toxicity and then increased to a maintenance schedule according to the patient's tolerance and the drug's pharmacokinetics. Most common side effects are temporary, and these are minimized if the dose is built up slowly. Nausea can be minimized by taking the medication with meals. Sedation may be less likely if a higher dose is given at bedtime.

If therapeutic blood levels need to be achieved rapidly, one should consider starting with drugs for which loading doses are practical, such as phenytoin or phenobarbital. Other drugs can gradually be substituted once seizures are controlled.

All antiepileptic drugs are capable of producing adverse effects, and the prescribing physician must be familiar with these. The most common side effects are *dose-related* and typically occur when the drug is first given or when the dose is increased. Dose-related side effects usually correlate with plasma concentrations of the drug or its major metabolites. *Idiosyncratic* reactions create the most serious and life-threatening side effects of antiepileptic drugs. All antiepileptic drugs can cause similar idiosyncratic reactions, including rash, Stevens-Johnson syndrome, agranulocytosis, thrombocytopenia, aplastic anemia, and hepatic failure. Idiosyncratic reactions are not dose-related, and no laboratory test can identify individuals specifically at risk for them. Routine blood monitoring at set intervals is costly and ineffective. Minor elevations in liver SGOT and SGPT occur in about 25 to 30% of patients with epilepsy, and these neither correlate with clinical symptoms nor predict development of hepatitis or liver failure. Isolated elevations in GTT levels seem to have little use as an indication of clinically significant liver dysfunction in persons with epilepsy. Nearly 20% of patients taking carbamazepine develop a benign leukopenia with WBC counts below 4000 per millimeter. A few patients have WBC counts that drop transiently below 2500 per millimeter. The risk of developing aplastic anemia is not increased in this group, nor is there an increased rate of infections or other possible complications that might be attributed to leukopenia.

When Initial Treatment Fails

Monotherapy results in satisfactory control of seizures (>90% reduction) in about 60% of patients. Of patients in whom the first drug was ineffective, about half respond to an alternative drug used alone. Of the remaining, fewer than half have improved control by addition of a second drug. Felbamate, gabapentin, and lamotrigine have recently been approved as adjunctive therapy in patients with partial and secondarily generalized seizures. They are useful additions to phenytoin, carbamazepine, and valproate when these drugs fail as monotherapy. Although the new drugs have a number of desirable features and generally better therapeutic indices compared with more familiar agents, it is too soon to predict what their ultimate place will be in the treatment of epilepsy. Felbamate, for example, has already proved to be too toxic (aplastic anemia, liver failure) for routine use.

Pregnancy Concerns

Epilepsy should not discourage a woman from becoming pregnant: Well over 90% of women taking antiepileptic drugs have healthy babies. Nonetheless, epilepsy affects the pregnancy in many ways, and it is important that women be informed before conception about possible problems and the steps that can be taken to minimize these. Overall, women with epilepsy demonstrate 1.5 to 3 times higher rates of complications of pregnancy regardless of treatment. These include increased risks of intrapartum bleeding, toxemia, abruptio placentae, premature labor, and stillborn births. About one third of women with epilepsy experience increased seizures during pregnancy. This is mostly due to falling antiepilep-

tic drug levels associated with a variety of physiologic changes that promote increased volume of distribution and clearance. Thus, antiepileptic drug levels should be followed closely during pregnancy, especially after the first trimester.

In the general population, *major fetal malformations* (cardiac defects, cleft lip or palate, neural tube defects, including spina bifida and anencephaly) occur in about 2% of pregnancies. This risk is increased to 5 to 6% in infants born to women with epilepsy who have taken a single antiepileptic drug during pregnancy. Valproate increases the chance of neural tube defects by 1.5%, and carbamazepine polytherapy may also raise this specific risk by 0.5%, especially if there is a family history of neural tube defects. Use of two or more drugs carries a 10% risk of major fetal malformations.

Minor anomalies (nail hypoplasia, hypertelorism, low-set ears, prominent lips, broad-based nose) are also increased in infants of mothers with epilepsy, but this seems to reflect both genetic and drug-related factors. Such anomalies occur at increased rates independent of treatment status, although antiepileptic drug therapy increases the risk further to a slight degree. It was formerly thought that particular profiles of these anomalies could be attributed to specific drugs (e.g., fetal hydantoin syndrome or fetal valproate syndrome), but recent data indicate that all antiepileptic drugs can produce similar anomalies.

Virtually all antiepileptic drugs promote a hemorrhagic diathesis in the newborn. Intramuscular vitamin K, which is given routinely to babies, is occasionally inadequate to prevent hemorrhage. Therefore, oral vitamin K, 20 mg per day, should be prescribed for the mother during the last month of pregnancy.

The risk of neural tube defects is reduced, perhaps eliminated, by preconceptive use of folic acid, 1 mg per day. Ultrasonography and amniocentesis done at 18 to 19 weeks of gestation have a nearly 95% accuracy rate in experienced hands of identifying neural tube defects and other major malformations. Serum α-fetoprotein determinations have a 25% false-negative rate.

SURGICAL TREATMENT

Surgical intervention should be considered when seizures fail to respond to antiepileptic drugs and when they continue to disrupt patients' quality of life. Advances in surgical techniques and improved methods of identifying epileptogenic brain areas have made surgical treatment an option for more patients with uncontrolled seizures today than ever before. In 1985, for example, there were about 500 operations for epilepsy in the United States; in 1990, there were over 1500.

In the past, there was considerable disagreement about when to refer patients for surgery, and many physicians viewed it as a therapy of last resort. As a result, until very recently the average time from epilepsy diagnosis to operation was about 20 years. Currently, increasing numbers of neurologists believe that it is possible to identify patients who are likely to benefit from surgery earlier in the course of their illness, and that minimizing the delay between onset of seizures and successful intervention provides better seizure control, psychosocial outcome, and quality of life.

Few patients benefit from further attempts at medical treatment if seizures are not controlled following two trials of high-dose monotherapy using appropriate drugs and one trial of rational combination therapy. These steps can be accomplished within 1 to 2 years. At that point, the detrimental effects of continued seizures, often exacerbated by drug toxicity, warrant referral to a specialized epilepsy center.

The most common type of epilepsy surgery, and the one with which there is the greatest experience, is *focal cortical resection.* Surgery should be considered for any patient with focal seizures whose attacks remain disabling despite optimal medical therapy. Three criteria identify the ideal patient for resective surgery: (1) the seizures begin in an identifiable and localized area of cortex; (2) the surgical excision can encompass the epileptogenic region; and (3) the required resection does not impair neurologic function. These requirements are met most often by patients with temporal lobe epilepsy or other focal epilepsies associated with a demonstrable cerebral lesion (e.g., cavernous malformation, ganglioglioma). Over two thirds of such patients become seizure free, and approximately 90% have sufficiently fewer seizures to improve substantially their quality of life. The outcome is less favorable for patients undergoing nonlesional extratemporal resections: About 45% of patients become seizure free; another 35% have worthwhile improvement.

Two other surgical procedures are used much less often and only for highly selected cases of persons with longstanding, uncontrolled seizures, usually beginning in childhood. *Corpus callosotomy* is indicated for intractable atonic and secondarily generalized tonic-clonic seizures such as occur in severe epileptic encephalopathies like the Lennox-Gastaut syndrome. *Hemispherectomy* is an effective operation for children with severely incapacitating unilateral seizures associated with hemiatrophy, hemiparesis, and a useless hand (infantile hemiplegia syndrome).

PROGNOSIS OF EPILEPSY

About 60 to 70% of people with epilepsy achieve a 5-year remission of seizures within 10 years of diagnosis. About half of these patients eventually become seizure free without anticonvulsant drugs. Factors favoring remission include an idiopathic form of epilepsy, a normal neurologic examination, and an onset in early to middle childhood (excluding neonatal seizures).

Thirty percent of patients, usually with severe epilepsy starting in early childhood, continue to have seizures and never achieve a remission. In the United States, the prevalence of intractable epilepsy cases approximates 1 to 2 per 1000 population.

Discontinuing Antiepileptic Drugs

Because epidemiologic studies have shown that many patients with epilepsy become seizure free for an extended period, a number of investigators have attempted to identify which patients can discontinue antiepileptic drugs without a high risk of relapse. Successful drug withdrawal is most likely if initial seizure control was readily achieved using monotherapy; there were relatively few seizures before remission; and the EEG and neurologic examination are normal just before drugs are discontinued. In addition, longer seizure-free intervals (4 years rather than 2) reduce the likelihood of relapse. Conversely, risk of relapse is high if seizure control was difficult to establish and required polytherapy; if there were frequent generalized tonic-clonic seizures before control was achieved; and if the EEG demonstrates moderate or severe disturbances of background activity or active epileptiform activity at the time drug withdrawal is considered.

STATUS EPILEPTICUS

Various types of status epilepticus take either convulsive or nonconvulsive forms. *Convulsive status epilepticus* is a medical emergency that requires timely and appropriate treatment in order to minimize serious systemic and neurologic morbidity. Like self-limited seizures, convulsive status may be either idiopathic and of generalized onset or secondary to bilateral spread from a focal epileptogenic brain area. *Nonconvulsive status* presents as a new-onset sustained confusional state.

Convulsive status epilepticus is the first manifestation of epilepsy in about 10% of cases; more than 50% of patients with status epilepticus do not have a history of epilepsy. An acute precipitating factor or specific cause, such as metabolic abnormalities, drug abuse, hypoxia, infection, stroke, or tumor, can be identified in 50 to 65% of patients with status epilepticus. The mortality rate approaches 30% in adults, but death usually relates to the underlying condition. Status epilepticus itself accounts for death in about 10% of cases.

Treatment protocols are designed to eliminate seizure activity and to identify and treat any underlying medical or neurologic disorder. Initial management focuses on ensuring adequate oxygenation and maintaining blood pressure (Table 433–7). There must be unimpeded access to the circulation, and cardiac function must be monitored continuously. Diagnostic studies should be initiated concurrently with blood obtained for antiepileptic drug levels, blood count, and routine chemistries. Brain imaging is necessary, but control of seizures must be the first priority. Lumbar puncture must be performed if meningitis is strongly suspected. If, however, focal neurologic signs point to a mass lesion, antibiotics should be given and a CT scan obtained first. In adults, thiamine followed by glucose should be administered to counteract hypoglycemia unless an adequate glucose concentration has been demonstrated.

Table 433–7 presents the recommendations of the Epilepsy Foundation of America for treating status epilepticus. A benzodiazepine, either diazepam (10 mg, repeated once) or lorazepam should be given, followed immediately by intravenous phenytoin, 20 mg per kilogram, at a rate not exceeding 50 mg per minute. If seizures continue, an additional 5 mg per kilogram of phenytoin should be given. About 80% of patients respond to this protocol. If status is refractory, the patient should be admitted to an intensive care unit and anesthetized with intravenous pentobarbital, 5 mg per kilogram, followed by 25 to 50 mg every 25 to 50 minutes as necessary to produce a burst-suppression pattern on continuously monitored EEG. Maintenance doses are 1 to 3 mg per kilogram per hour. Ventilatory assistance and vasopressors are invariably required.

Nonconvulsive status epilepticus is difficult to diagnose and is frequently unrecognized. It presents most often in middle-aged or elderly persons without a history of seizures. Onset is generally abrupt, with a fluctuating confusional state that can last for days to weeks. Although clouding of consciousness occurs to a varying degree, the absence of stupor or coma contributes to misdiagnosis. Nonconvulsive status epilepticus may be mistaken for psychosis because of the abrupt development of bizarre behavior, inappropriate affect, paranoia, delusions, and catatonia. Alternatively, memory loss, confusion, and mood changes may predominate and suggest a metabolic/toxic encephalopathy or dementia. Some patients have recurrent episodes.

TABLE 433–7. PROTOCOL FOR TREATING STATUS EPILEPTICUS

Time (min)	Action*
0–5	Diagnose status epilepticus by observing continued seizure activity or one additional seizure
	Give oxygen by nasal cannula or mask; position patient's head for optimal airway patency; consider intubation if respiratory assistance is needed
	Obtain and record vital signs at onset and periodically thereafter; control any abnormalities as necessary; initiate ECG monitoring
	Establish an IV in one or both arms using catheter; draw venous blood samples for glucose level, serum chemistries, hematology studies, toxicology screens, and determinations of antiepileptic drug levels
	Assess oxygenation with oximetry or periodic arterial blood gas determinations
6–9	If hypoglycemia is established or a blood glucose determination is unavailable, administer glucose; in adults, give 100 mg of thiamine first, followed by 50 ml of 50% glucose by direct push into the IV; in children, the dose of glucose is 2 ml/kg of 25% glucose
10–20	Administer either 0.1 mg/kg of lorazepam at 2 mg/min or 0.2 mg/kg of diazepam at 5 mg/min by IV; if diazepam is given, it can be repeated if seizures do not stop after 5 min; if diazepam is used to stop the status, phenytoin should be administered immediately to prevent recurrent status
21–60	If status persists, administer 15–20 mg/kg of phenytoin by IV no faster than 50 mg/min in adults and 1 mg/kg per min in children; monitor ECG and blood pressure during the infusion; phenytoin is incompatible with glucose-containing solutions—the IV should be purged with normal saline before the phenytoin infusion
>60	If status does not stop after 20 mg/kg of phenytoin, give additional doses of 5 mg/kg to a maximal dose of 30 mg/kg
	If status persists, give 20 mg/kg of phenobarbital by IV at 100 mg/min; when phenobarbital is given after a benzodiazepine, the risk of apnea or hypopnea is great, and assisted ventilation is usually required
	If status persists, give anesthetic doses of drugs such as pentobarbital; ventilatory assistance and vasopressors are virtually always necessary

* Time starts at seizure onset. ECG = electrocardiogram; IV = intravenous line.

From Dodson WE, DeLorenzo RJ, Pedley TA, et al: Treatment of convulsive status epilepticus: Recommendations of the Epilepsy Foundation of America's working group on status epilepticus. JAMA 270:854, 1993.

Diagnosis depends on demonstrating seizure discharges in the EEG accompanying symptoms. Most patients show continuous or nearly continuous 1- to 2.5-Hz generalized spike-wave activity similar to generalized absence status ("spike-wave stupor") that occurs in children. Rarely, however, the EEG ictal activity is localized, usually to the frontal or temporal lobes, indicating that in these patients the nonconvulsive status is a form of continuous partial seizure activity. Intravenous diazepam (5 to 10 mg) or lorazepam (1 to 2 mg) suppresses epileptiform EEG abnormalities and produces dramatic improvement in the patient's mental state. Long-term seizure control is achieved using valproate, phenytoin, or carbamazepine.

A specific cause cannot be identified in most cases. Sometimes, however, nonconvulsive status results from electrolyte imbalance, drug toxicity (e.g., lithium), or a focal cerebral lesion (e.g., frontal lobe infarction).

PSYCHOSOCIAL ISSUES

Epilepsy and its personal effects result from multiple interacting factors, of which seizures are only a part. The extent of a patient's disability or quality of life may relate more to physical limitations caused by neurologic abnormalities, psychological factors, or adverse drug effects than to the seizures themselves. This observation is underscored by patients who become seizure free following surgery but who remain disabled and unable to find employment, establish relationships, or become independent in other ways. Not the least of epilepsy's disabling aspects is the episodic nature of the condition: Periods of relative well-being are punctuated by unpredictably occurring attacks that impose their own limitations, create embarrassment, and reinforce negative stereotypes. Recurrent seizures, despite treatment, are graphic reminders of medicine's failure. Adults experience discrimination at work and loss of mobility because they cannot drive.

The treatment of epilepsy can be effective only when interacting medical, psychological, and environmental factors are addressed successfully. Areas of psychosocial difficulty should be identified early in the course of treatment and an appropriate plan of management developed. This often requires a multidisciplinary approach to disabilities that have social, educational, vocational, and psychological dimensions. The physician must be sensitive to these issues, even if they are not voiced explicitly. In fact, psychosocial concerns may be the major focus of the majority of follow-up visits. The physician has a special responsibility to educate society as well as the patient and family in order to counter the many misperceptions, myths, and prejudices that are ascribed to epilepsy.

Berg AT, Shinnar S: The risk of seizure recurrence following a first unprovoked seizure: A quantitative review. Neurology 41:965, 1991. *A meta-analysis of the most important papers to evaluate the development of and risks for epilepsy following a first unprovoked seizure.*

Delgado-Escueta AV, Janz D: Consensus guidelines: Preconception counseling, management, and care of the pregnant woman with epilepsy. Neurology 42(suppl 5):149, 1992. *An essential and current summary of the risks and management options for women with epilepsy who desire to become pregnant. Practical recommendations are included.*

Dodson WE, DeLorenzo RJ, Pedley TA, et al.: Treatment of convulsive status epilepticus: Recommendations of the Epilepsy Foundation of America's working group on status epilepticus. JAMA 270:854, 1993. *A consensus report describing the epidemiology, pathogenesis, morbidity and mortality, treatment, and prognosis of status epilepticus.*

Engel J Jr (ed.): Surgical Treatment of the Epilepsies, 2nd ed. New York, Raven Press, 1993. *A comprehensive volume covering all aspects of the surgical treatment of epilepsy and emphasizing advances between 1986 and 1992.*

First Seizure Trial Group. Randomized clinical trial on the efficacy of antiepileptic drugs in reducing the risk of relapse after a first unprovoked tonic-clonic seizure. Neurology 43:478, 1993. *The first prospective study to compare the effect of treatment versus no treatment on risk of further seizures following a first convulsion.*

Freeman JM, Vining EPG, Pillas DJ: Seizures and Epilepsy in Childhood: A Guide for Parents. Baltimore, Johns Hopkins Press, 1990. *Despite the title, this sensitive and thorough review of epilepsy and its impact on quality of life is suitable for patients of all ages and their families.*

Hauser WA, Hesdorffer DC. Epilepsy: Frequency, Causes and Consequences. New York, Demos, 1990. *An encyclopedia of facts regarding all aspects of epilepsy.*

Hauser WA, Annegers JF, Kurland LT: Incidence of epilepsy and unprovoked seizures in Rochester, Minnesota: 1935–1984. Epilepsia 34:453, 1993. *This ambitious study provides the best available data regarding seizure incidence and complements an earlier prevalence study by the same investigators.*

Sloviter RS: The functional organization of the hippocampal dentate gyrus and its relevance to the pathogenesis of temporal lobe epilepsy. Ann Neurol 35:640, 1994. *The most coherent hypothesis and review of supporting experimental and clinical data linking the development of mesial to temporal sclerosis.*

Section Twelve— Intracranial Tumors and States of Altered Intracranial Pressure

Nicholas A. Vick

434 INTRACRANIAL TUMORS

Approximately 17,000 new cases of primary brain tumors are treated each year in the United States. Metastases are even more frequent and contribute considerably to suffering and death from systemic cancer. The diversity of brain tumors makes it important to attend to what is characteristic about each histologic type because attention to biologic specificity guides therapy and certainly will advance future understanding.

The classification of brain tumors is a subject with confusing terminology. This text employs a simpler approach, classifying brain tumors into *metastatic, primary extra-axial,* and *primary intra-axial* (Table 434–1). These categories include all of the primary brain tumors listed in the World Health Organization classification (Table 434–2), adds pituitary and metastatic tumors, and is obviously simple. Moreover, it follows practical clinical thinking. This chapter deals with the general biology, clinical features, and treatment of brain tumors as an overall problem. The following chapter describes the particular behavior of the most important subtypes in accordance with the outline of Table 434–1.

GENERAL CONSIDERATIONS

"Is it benign or malignant?" is invariably the first question patients, families, and physicians ask when confronted with a diagnosis of brain tumor. About a third of primary brain tumors can be called benign. Meningiomas and acoustic neuromas are good examples, they grow slowly, often can be removed completely, and rarely recur.

The concept of malignancy in the central nervous system (CNS) has a different meaning from that which applies to systemic cancers. The term "malignant" has nothing to do with metastasis out of the CNS, which is extraordinarily rare. It has everything to do with

TABLE 434–1. COMMON BRAIN TUMORS IN ADULTS WITH PERCENTAGE INCIDENCE BY CATEGORY*

Metastatic	Primary Extra-axial	Primary Intra-axial
Lung (37)	Meningioma (80)	Gioblastoma (47)
Breast (19)	Acoustic neuroma (10)	Anaplastic astrocytoma (24)
Melanoma (16)	Pituitary adenoma (7)	Astrocytoma (15)
Colorectum (9)	Other (3)	Oligodendroglioma (5)
Kidney (8)		Lymphoma (2)
Other (11)		Other (7)

* These figures, given in parentheses, can be extremely variable from one center to another, depending on referral pattern. They are given here as general estimates based upon many published series.

anatomic location and the possibility of complete surgical removal. Unless a tumor can be completely excised to the last cell, all intracranial neoplasms are potentially malignant in that they may recur, and often do.

INITIAL EVALUATION

SYMPTOMS AND SIGNS. Brain tumors present in two patterns, not necessarily mutually exclusive. One consists of nonfocal symptoms of *increased intracranial pressure,* such as headaches, nausea, vomiting, confusion, and lethargy. The other consists of symptoms or signs of *focal brain dysfunction,* such as hemianopia, hemiparesis, cranial nerve palsies, or focal seizures (Table 434–3). Such signs of focal brain dysfunction may have convincing localizing value even before an image of the brain is made by computed tomography (CT) or magnetic resonance imaging (MRI). Some tumors that arise in neurologically "silent" areas, such as the parietal or frontal association cortices, may produce only nonfocal generalized symptoms of headache, confusion, behavioral change, or, eventually, a seizure, despite growing to a considerable size. Although the capacity to reach early diagnosis by CT or MRI has greatly reduced the numbers of patients in whom symptoms of increased intracranial pressure represent initial complaints, examples still remain, especially in association with fast-growing tumors and in children. The latter are particularly likely to have tumors in the posterior fossa that tend to obstruct spinal fluid pathways earlier than do supratentorial tumors. As implied, the tempo with which a brain tumor grows also influences the presenting symptoms. Despite the fixed space of the skull (once infantile sutures have closed), the human brain possesses a remarkable capacity to make room for a slowly growing tumor (Fig. 434–1). Because of this, and even allowing for the relative rapidity of growth of aggressive brain tumors such as glioblastomas, the rule is that the patient usually appears better clinically than might be expected from the degree of abnormality seen on CT or MRI scan.

DIFFERENTIAL DIAGNOSIS. Patients who present with symptoms and signs of increased intracranial pressure or a first convulsive seizure need to be hospitalized. Diagnosis and treatment

TABLE 434–2. WORLD HEALTH ORGANIZATION CLASSIFICATION OF BRAIN TUMORS*

A. Astrocytic tumors
  1. Astrocytoma
    a. Fibrillary
    b. Protoplasmic
    c. Gemistocytic
  2. Pilocytic astrocytoma
  3. Subependymal giant cell astrocytoma (ventricular tumor or tuberous sclerosis)
  4. Astroblastoma
  5. Anaplastic (malignant) astrocytoma
B. Oligodendroglial tumors
  1. Oligodendroglioma
  2. Mixed oligoastrocytoma
  3. Anaplastic (malignant) oligodendroglioma
C. Ependymal and choroid plexus tumors
  1. Ependymoma
    Variants:
    a. Myxopapillary ependymoma
    b. Papillary ependymoma
    c. Subependymoma
  2. Anaplastic (malignant) ependymoma
  3. Choroid plexus papilloma
  4. Anaplastic (malignant) choroid plexus papilloma
D. Pineal cell tumor
  1. Pineocytoma (pinealcytoma)
  2. Pineoblastoma (pinealoblastoma)
E. Neuronal tumors
  1. Gangliocytoma
  2. Ganglioglioma
  3. Ganglioneuroblastoma
  4. Anaplastic (malignant) gangliocytoma and ganglioglioma
  5. Neuroblastoma
F. Poorly differentiated and embryonal tumors
  1. Glioblastoma
    Variants:
    a. Glioblastoma with sarcomatous component (mixed glioblastoma and sarcoma)
    b. Giant cell glioblastoma
  2. Medulloblastoma
    Variants:
    a. Desmoplastic medulloblastoma
    b. Medullomyoblastoma
  3. Medulloepithelioma
  4. Primitive polar spongioblastoma
  5. Gliomatosis cerebri

* This is one of several formal schemes that are based on neuropathologic criteria. Metastasis is not considered, and one can get no sense of a given tumor as a *clinical* problem, as suggested by the simple classification in Table 434–1.

measures must be started at once; it may be unsafe to wait. Those who present with focal neurologic impairment and who do not have symptoms of increased intracranial pressure may reasonably be evaluated in the outpatient setting for other conditions that are often considerations in the differential diagnosis of brain tumor (Table 434–4). The tempo of evolution of symptoms and signs of focal

TABLE 434–3. FOCAL CLINICAL MANIFESTATIONS OF BRAIN TUMORS

Frontal lobe	**Temporal lobe**	**Sella/optic nerve/pituitary**
Generalized seizures	Complex partial (psychomotor) seizures	Endocrinopathy
Focal motor seizures (contralateral)	Generalized seizures	Bitemporal hemianopia
Expressive aphasia (dominant side)	Behavioral changes	Monocular visual defects
Behavioral changes	Olfactory and complex visual auras	**Pons/medulla**
Dementia	**Corpus callosum**	Cranial nerve dysfunction
Gait disorders, incontinence	Dementia (anterior)	Ataxia, nystagmus
Basal ganglia	Behavioral changes (posterior)	Weakness, sensory loss
Hemiparesis (contralateral)	Asymptomatic (mid)	Spasticity
Movement disorders rare	**Thalamus**	**Cerebellopontine angle**
Parietal lobe	Sensory loss (contralateral)	Deafness (ipsilateral)
Receptive aphasia (dominant side)	Behavioral changes	Loss of facial sensation (ipsilateral)
Spatial disorientation (nondominant side)	Language disorder (dominant side)	Facial weakness (ipsilateral)
Cortical sensory dysfunction (contralateral)	**Midbrain/pineal**	Ataxia
Hemianopia (contralateral)	Paresis of vertical eye movements	**Cerebellum**
Occipital lobe	Pupillary abnormalities	Ataxia (ipsilateral)
Hemianopia (contralateral)	Precocious puberty (boys)	Nystagmus
Visual disturbances (unformed)		

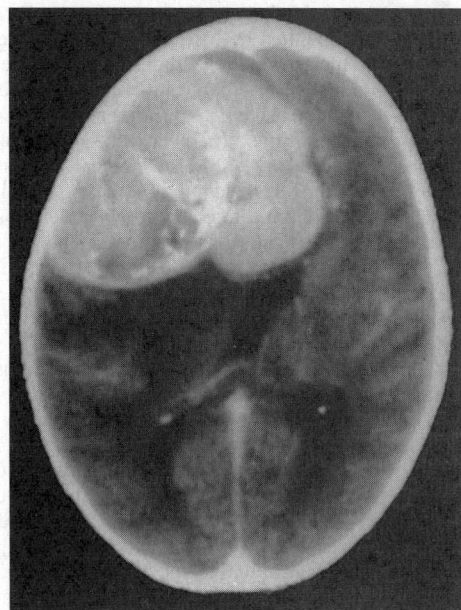

FIGURE 434-1. CT scan with contrast of a meningioma in a patient who presented with mild cognitive deficits, illustrative of the size a slow-growing tumor can attain in the brain. The tumor was completely resected.

TABLE 434-4. THE MAIN DIFFERENTIAL DIAGNOSES OF BRAIN TUMORS

Hematomas, especially in tumors that have a tendency to bleed, such as melanoma
Abscesses, including fungal
Granulomas
Parasitic infections, such as cysticercosis
Vascular malformations, especially those without arteriovenous shunts
Solitary large plaques of multiple sclerosis
Seldom, progressive strokes

neurologic impairment, much more than their severity, governs urgency of evaluation. The tempo also strongly influences diagnostic considerations. Although an occasional brain tumor may manifest with such rapid onset of hemiparesis or aphasia that a stroke is mimicked, most do not. Associated aspects of the history, such as recent head trauma, previous episodes of reversible neurologic impairment, or recent infection and fever, should direct attention to diagnostic alternatives such as subdural hematoma, multiple sclerosis, or cerebral abscess. Simply stated, it is the careful history, not the neurologic examination, that usually points to the alternative diagnoses.

IMAGING AND OTHER DIAGNOSTIC PROCEDURES

Brain imaging by MRI or CT scans is an indispensable component of the modern diagnosis of the presence but not the type of brain tumors. One type of tumor can look like another or even resemble nonneoplastic mass lesions, such as brain abscesses, fungal infections, parasitic invasions, demyelinating diseases, or strokes. For definitive diagnosis and adequate treatment planning, one must obtain a tissue diagnosis whenever possible. This can be made either by direct surgical biopsy or, in the case of some nonneoplastic conditions, by judging CT or MRI responses to particular therapies.

MRI is almost always superior to CT scanning in diagnosing intracranial mass lesions. MRI outlines posterior fossa structures and tumors with a clarity that CT cannot achieve because of x-ray distortions due to the bony structure of that region. In several types of tumor, particularly the low-grade gliomas, MRI may show extensive brain infiltration in cases that fail to produce any image abnormality on CT or, at most, a vague low density. Although either MRI or CT should be used with contrast enhancement in cases of suspected brain tumor, the passage of such contrast agents beyond the blood-brain barrier into the tissue does not necessarily imply the presence of a histologically malignant tumor. For example, although malignant gliomas almost always show contrast enhancement, so do meningiomas, which are entirely benign if they can be fully removed surgically.

CT scans done without contrast enhancement are of little value in the diagnosis of brain tumors or other mass lesions. Although it is true that hemorrhage, calcifications, hydrocephalus, and shift can be well seen on a noncontrast CT scan, the interpretation of even these conditions is tentative because each can have an underlying causative structural abnormality such as a brain tumor, which may fail to appear on a noncontrast CT study. Allergy to CT dye is rare and readily manageable. Currently available nonionic CT dyes have an extremely low incidence of side effects. There is little risk that currently used CT dyes will cause renal dysfunction in normally hydrated patients who are not known to have kidney disease.

MRI initially provided two types of images, designated T1 and T2. For brain tumors, the former generally showed a well-demarcated area of low density and the latter, bright whiteness that encompassed a more extensive region owing to the signal of the surrounding brain edema (Fig. 434-2). With the availability for general usage in 1988 of *gadolinium contrast for MRI*, a new set of criteria of usage and differential diagnostic considerations in brain imaging have quickly evolved (Table 434-5). T1 gadolinium imaging is the most precise way to image a brain tumor, and often patients can be followed during and after treatment with that type of study alone. Such an approach is easier for patients because it reduces the length of time otherwise spent on T2 scanning. Now and

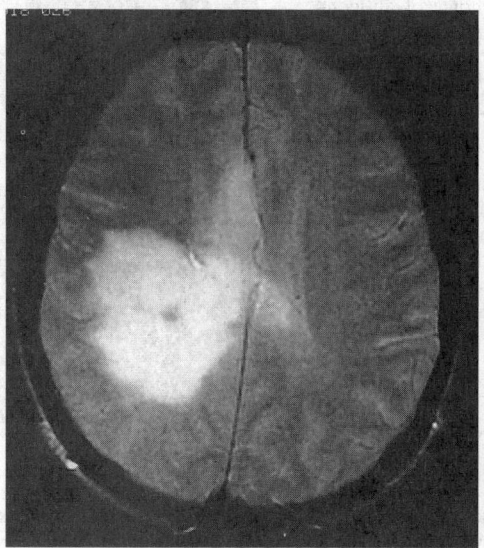 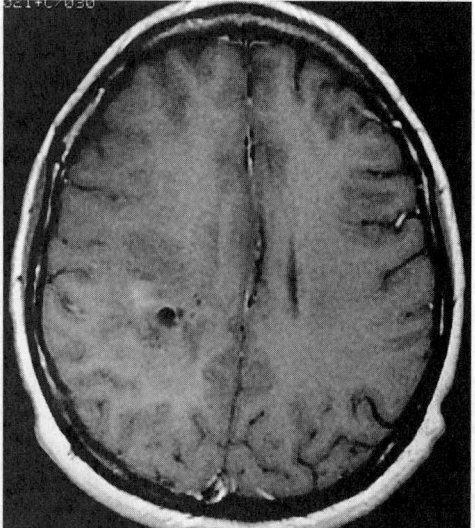

FIGURE 434-2. Low-grade astrocytoma as imaged by MRI. On the left, T2-weighted image; on the right, T1-weighted image, gadolinium contrast with minimal enhancement. The images are typical of this tumor, which is being detected with increasing frequency in seizure patients by MRI. Many are invisible on CT scans.

TABLE 434–5. T1 GADOLINIUM MRI CHARACTERISTICS OF BRAIN TUMORS

Metastases	These are remarkably variable (Fig. 434–3). Some enhance brightly and solidly with gadolonium. Others are in ring configuration. Many are invisible with contrast CT.
Acoustic neuromas	These are invariably intensely contrasted by gadolinium, even more reliably than by CT.
Meningiomas	Same as for acoustic neuromas.
Pituitary adenomas	These always enhance less than the normal pituitary gland. MRI is superior in every way to CT, especially when thin slices and magnified views are ordered.
Glioblastoma	These are almost always in ring configuration.
Anaplastic astrocytomas	These are sometimes solidly bright; they are often patchy, may be noncontrasting, and may look like low-grade astrocytoma.
Low-grade astrocytomas	These do not enhance. They are often invisible by CT or are imaged only as vague low density.
Oligodendrogliomas	These generally do not enhance unless anaplastic and are often invisible on CT unless they are calcified.
Primary brain lymphomas	These usually exhibit homogeneous enhancement and are smoothly rounded. Periventricular location is common. They are multiple in about a fourth of cases. This lesion does not often look like glioblastoma but is easily mistaken for metastases if multiple.

then, T2 images are useful. For example, T2 images, besides showing the extent of edema, also delineate the demyelinating effects of radiation upon white matter.

Cerebral angiography seldom is used in the diagnosis of brain tumors. In a few circumstances, neurosurgeons, in preparation for surgery, require a more precise knowledge of the pattern and position of blood vessels that can be obtained only by angiography. The procedure is also used to embolize highly vascular meningiomas, or to study cerebral dominance by injection of sodium amytal into the carotid artery (the Wada test) in left-handed individuals who are to have surgery near language areas. Preoperative determination of cerebral localization helps surgeons to plan the extent of surgery and avoid postoperative language deficits.

Examination of the *spinal fluid* has limited indication in the diagnosis of brain tumors. One is to rule in or out an inflammatory disorder mimicking a brain tumor. Another is to establish the diagnosis of benign intracranial hypertension in patients with uninformative MR images (see Ch. 436). In addition, spinal fluid cytology may be useful for determining instances of malignant meningitis secondary to metastatic neoplasms, in association with spinal spread of medulloblastoma in some children and in identifying primary lymphomas of the brain in cases in which MRI changes are ambiguous.

The routine electroencephalogram (EEG) has no role in the diagnosis of brain tumors and does not assist in the choice of anticonvulsant drugs for brain tumor patients. However, specialized intraoperative neurophysiologic techniques such as depth electrode studies and intraoperative monitoring may be useful in identifying and removing epileptogenic areas adjacent to brain tumors or to avoid resection of critical brain regions adjacent to tumors.

Positron emission tomography (PET) is able to quantify biochemical functions, such as oxygen and glucose utilization, within tumors as well as normal brain tissue. PET scanning is a powerful research tool of limited availability for routine clinical purposes. Its spatial resolution is inferior to that of both CT and MR. In patients with brain tumors who develop recurrent symptoms after radiation therapy, PET can differentiate with about 70% accuracy radiation-induced injury from tumor recurrences. These disorders appear identical on MRI.

TREATMENT

PREOPERATIVE CONSIDERATIONS AND MEDICAL MANAGEMENT. In almost every instance when a brain tumor is suspected on the basis of the combined results of history, physical findings, and imaging studies, the *first consideration is its surgical resectability.* There are exceptions, such as cases of multiple brain

metastases in a patient with known systemic cancer. Patients with single brain metastases, defined by MRI, may be candidates for surgical resection of the metastasis, depending on their systemic medical status. It is unproductive to embark upon an extensive systemic evaluation in the search for an unknown primary cancer in patients with a single resectable presumed brain metastasis. If a primary tumor is not quickly revealed by a careful medical evaluation, with special attention to skin (for melanoma), breasts, and lungs, the pathologic diagnosis of the brain tumor needs to be disclosed by resection or, if unresectable owing to its position, by biopsy.

Although small meningiomas or acoustic neuromas usually do not require treatment to reduce intracranial pressure, in the majority of brain tumor patients it is appropriate to start *dexamethasone* promptly. The purpose is to reduce intracranial pressure, which accompanies the majority of brain tumors, and to relieve neurologic symptoms caused by peritumoral brain edema (Fig. 434–3). Dexamethasone's long biologic half-life and steady action upon the brain have made it the steroid of choice for treating patients with brain tumors. It should be started with an oral dose of 16 mg, followed with 8 mg twice daily. It is well absorbed by mouth, and its action by that route is almost as rapid as when given intravenously. Antacids are seldom necessary. If focal neurologic symptoms are due to peritumoral vasogenic edema, dexamethasone induces improvement within 48 hours and usually sooner. If there is no benefit, the neurologic symptoms are likely to be due to damage of the brain tissue by the tumor and not to edema.

Edema associated with brain tumors is due chiefly to abnormally fenestrated endothelium in the tumor, which permits excess flow of fluid from capillaries into the growth. Normally, solutes are transported through capillaries into brain by dissolving in and diffusing through the cerebral endothelium, a phenomenon dependent on lipid solubility and molecular size. Endothelial cells also possess some facilitated or carrier-mediated processes that are stereospecific, saturable, and independent of lipid solubility and molecular size. In brain tumors, these selective properties of the blood-brain barrier are overwhelmed by increased bulk flow and hydraulic conductivity through the defective endothelium. The result is vasogenic edema, and it is this reaction that dexamethasone so greatly reduces.

In instances of extreme intracranial pressure, the speed and action of dexamethasone are not sufficient to reduce the brain swelling quickly enough to prevent complications. In such instances, hyperosmotic solutions of *mannitol* must be given. The usual dosage is 0.5 to 2.0 grams per kilogram given intravenously over 15 minutes, followed by additional boluses of 25 grams as needed. The osmotic action of mannitol occurs within minutes. Clinical improvement may be dramatic. It is unusual for brain tumor patients preoperatively to decompensate so severely from increased intracranial pressure that intubation becomes necessary. Nevertheless, this does occur. In such cases the $Paco_2$ must be decreased by passive hyperventilation to approximately 25 mm Hg. The effect constricts

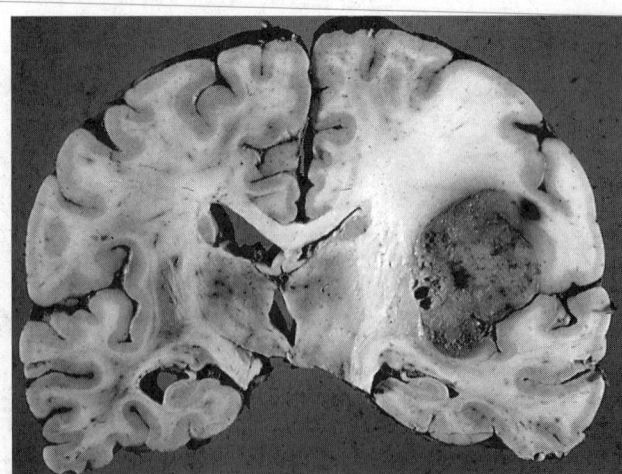

FIGURE 434–3. Gross coronal pathologic specimen of a solitary metastasis from a non–small cell lung carcinoma to the right cerebral hemisphere. The tumor is well circumscribed. It causes marked edema that greatly expands the cerebral white matter. Metastatic tumors such as this can often be surgically resected.

the cerebral vasculature and promptly induces a major reduction of intracranial pressure, which can be life saving.

About 20% of brain tumor patients develop *seizures* some time in their lives, even if they do not have seizures at the time of diagnosis. It is conventional and probably effective to treat all patients with supratentorial tumors with anticonvulsants before surgery. Most patients with acoustic neuromas or other posterior fossa tumors have a low probability of convulsive seizures and do not need such drugs. Phenytoin is the best initial drug because it can be administered either intravenously or orally, unlike either carbamazepine or valproic acid, which can be used only orally. An intravenous drug is especially useful for continuation during the perioperative period. If required, patients may be switched easily to alternative oral drugs later. Phenytoin should be started orally, giving 1000 mg over 12 hours, or intravenously, with 1000 mg given over 1 hour. Thereafter, the usual dosage is 300 to 400 mg daily, administered in one dose or split between breakfast and dinner, along with dexamethasone. Periodic blood levels need to be checked to adjust the dosage to ensure concentrations of 10 to 20 μg per milliliter.

SURGERY. Although complete excision of a brain tumor is the ultimate goal in every case, this is not always possible. Even potentially curable tumors, such as meningiomas or acoustic neuromas, may reside in positions that make complete resection technically impossible. Malignant gliomas lack microscopic boundaries, even though they may appear by imaging studies to have well-defined limits. How much surgical success can be achieved with these tumors depends on several factors, including the tumor's proximity to indispensable areas, the skill and experience of the neurosurgeon and the preoperative level of neurologic function. The combination of current standards of neurosurgical anesthesia, the capacity to control intracranial pressure, and the recent addition of lasers to other operative tools such as the operating microscope have greatly increased the surgeon's capacity for well-chosen radical resection. Correspondingly, the relative risks of surgery have become less age dependent than was previously the case. The greatest surgical risk is to neurologic function and the fear of unacceptable postoperative neurologic deficits. For this reason, radical operations upon tumors involving language areas, sensorimotor regions, the basal ganglia, corpus callosum, and brain stem are generally avoided. However, partial removal in these areas by stereotaxic methods may be surprisingly effective. MR images facilitate such surgery by showing that the tumor has pushed aside critical brain structures and that a macroscopic tumor edge can be delineated. It has been repeatedly shown that resection of the maximal amount of tumor consistent with functional preservation provides patients with better and longer lives.

A number of tumors cannot be even partially resected because they invade indispensable areas of the brain. Most are intra-axial tumors, such as the gliomas. Although imaging techniques may produce a characteristic picture suggestive of a particular histologic diagnosis, treatment planning demands a tissue diagnosis. All brain regions may be approached by MR-guided stereotaxic biopsy. The tissue specimens are small, but they are almost invariably adequate to establish a diagnosis. Morbidity, chiefly hemorrhage, occurs in about 2% of cases. Patients usually need to remain in the hospital for less than 48 hours. Open biopsies of brain tumors are not justifiable. If the skull and dura are to be opened, the surgeon should be prepared to do a gross total resection or, at least, a major removal of as much tumor as is consonant with preservation of neurologic function.

Deep leg vein thrombophlebitis leading to pulmonary embolism is a recurrent postoperative problem only partially helped by prophylactic application of compression boots. Early passive exercises and mobilization are imperative. The staff must monitor and maintain anticonvulsant levels to prevent postoperative seizures. Dexamethasone should be administered at adequate levels for at least 5 days to minimize surgically induced brain edema.

RADIATION THERAPY. All forms of external beam radiation, whether γ photons emitted from ^{60}Co sources or x-rays generated from linear accelerators, act similarly. They produce fast-moving electrons and free radicals in biologic tissue that interrupt chemical bonds between DNA base pairs. Affected cells either die or become so altered that their mitotic rate is greatly diminished. Radiation therapy is given in small daily fractions to build to a total dose. It appears safer and more effective to do this than to give larger frac-

tions over shorter periods. Hyperfractionation, defined as two (or more) doses during a day, does not seem to be worthwhile. Therapeutic brain irradiation with particulate radiation such as neutrons has been attempted experimentally at facilities with cyclotrons. Such densely ionizing radiation has shown no therapeutic advantage over x-rays. Interstitial (implanted) radiation therapy (brachytherapy) is usually given in the form of $^{125}I_3$ or $^{192}Ir_4$ in "seeds" placed by stereotaxic techniques. This method permits localized high-dosage radiation with sharp edges and sparing of the adjacent brain. Considerable controversy exists about the utility of interstitial radiation therapy, but it can be effective in well-selected patients. Other nonoperative radiosurgical techniques include the "gamma knife" and linear accelerators adapted to provide focused therapeutic beams. Efficacy has been shown for metastases but not for gliomas.

The *complications of radiation therapy* are often reported as infrequent, perhaps 2 to 5% of cases. These figures, are unrealistically low if one includes effects on long-term survivors. They reflect the fact that most irradiated patients with brain tumor die before brain injury appears. A high percentage of patients receiving whole-brain radiation develop dementia or impaired mobility. Often, postradiation neurologic damage may not become fully developed for several years. Local field rather than whole-brain radiation has reduced the incidence of dementia in long-term survivors. Dementia is a considerable problem in children who survive radiation therapy for medulloblastoma. The incidence may reach 50% or more in those who survive treatment for 5 years.

External beam radiation therapy has value in controlling the growth of malignant gliomas and metastatic brain tumors. It doubles median survival time for both types of tumors. Radiation therapy, however, has little, if any, value for recurrent meningiomas and acoustic neuromas. These are almost invariably better handled by reoperation. Primary brain lymphomas are so responsive to radiation therapy that many neurologists and radiation therapists continue to use it alone despite the fact that chemotherapy may prove to provide superior initial treatment. It has already been mentioned that solitary brain metastases are best managed by surgical resection before radiation therapy.

CHEMOTHERAPY. Chemotherapy for brain tumors has had a disappointing record. The reasons are many, but inadequacy of drug delivery, tumor cell heterogeneity, and inherent resistance are among the important ones. Almost all efforts have been directed toward the primary brain tumors, especially the gliomas. Established brain metastases, however, respond about as well as systemic metastases do in many cancers, especially breast and small cell lung cancer. BCNU (biscloroethylnitrosurea), the most frequently used drug, remains the most effective single agent available to treat the malignant astrocytomas. The combination of procarbazine, CCNU (cyclohexylchloroethylnitrosourea), and vincristine is the most effective multidrug regimen for the malignant astrocytomas, and it is probably superior to BCNU. It has an unusually beneficial effect against oligodendrogliomas. No more than 10% of patients with malignant gliomas have meaningful and durable responses to chemotherapy, whether it is given immediately after radiation therapy (when its effect is especially hard to assess) or at the time of recurrence. Efforts to improve response to chemotherapy by delivering drugs through the carotid artery have not been successful. BCNU has intolerable toxicity when given by the intra-arterial route. Cisplatin is being studied for possible utility as an intra-arterial drug in highly selected patients.

The pharmacokinetics of drugs used in brain tumor chemotherapy are not well understood. Knowledge about their ability to gain adequate concentration within the tumors is minimal, and almost nothing is known about chemosensitivity. Nonetheless, occasional remarkable responses to chemotherapy do occur in patients with gliomas. Among other primary intra-axial brain tumors, primary brain lymphoma has a reasonably good response rate. The drugs used are those given regularly for systemic lymphoma. Patients with primary brain lymphoma do better with chemotherapy added than with radiation therapy alone. On average, 3- to 4-year survivals can now be expected.

Several additional forms of medical treatment for brain tumors have been attempted experimentally. These include slow release of BCNU from implanted biodegradable polymers and the administration of interferons, other biologic response modifiers, and radionuclides coupled with monoclonal antibodies. None has met with appreciable success to date. In all probability, much new biologic knowledge, such as the sequential genetic events that influence the malignant transformation and progression of brain tumors, will be required before new medical treatments become practical realities.

Hildebrand J (ed.): Management in Neuro-Oncology. EOS Monographs. Berlin, Springer-Verlag, 1992. *A short review of management of brain tumors.*

Morantz RA, Walsh JW (eds.): Brain Tumors. A Comprehensive Text. New York, Marcel Dekker, 1994. *A comprehensive text written by experienced physicians.*

Twijnstra A, Keyser A, Ongerboer de Visser BW: Neuro-Oncology. Primary Tumors and Neurological Complications of Cancer. Amsterdam, Elsevier, 1993. *A summary of current concepts in diagnosis and management.*

435 SPECIFIC TYPES OF BRAIN TUMORS AND THEIR MANAGEMENT

METASTATIC TUMORS

All systemic cancers are capable of metastasizing to the intracranial contents and skull, although some do so more readily than others. The most frequent are lung, breast, and melanoma. This is not surprising because they are among the most common cancers. In many instances, brain metastases produce symptoms before the primary tumor is suspected. Furthermore, the primary cancer may not be found without considerable effort.

Patterns of metastasis to the nervous system have some variability, but none is truly characteristic. Non–small cell carcinoma of the lung and renal carcinoma tend to be associated with single metastases, whereas small cell carcinoma of the lung, breast carcinoma, and melanoma often generate multiple secondary deposits. The metastases may be miliary in melanoma. T1 gadolinium magnetic resonance imaging (MRI) scans are critical in the imaging of brain metastases (Fig. 435–1). *Multiple metastases* may be revealed with this method, whereas T2 MRI and contrast computed tomography (CT) may show only one or, in rare instances, none. For multiple metastases, whole-brain irradiation is the best form of treatment as long as the patient's systemic condition indicates a potential for high-quality survival. Patients with widespread systemic metastasis

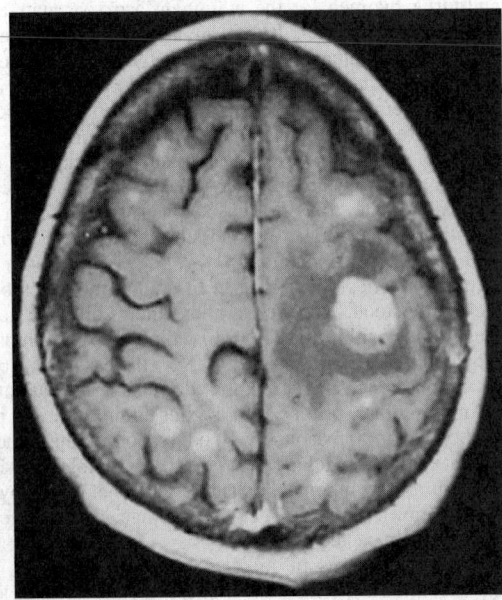

FIGURE 435–1. MRI scan, T1 gadolinium, of multiple metastases from breast carcinoma. The tumors were not visible on CT, even after giving a contrast agent.

TABLE 435–1. METASTATIC BRAIN TUMORS

These tumors affect 10% of cancer patients (and still another 20% have dural meningeal involvement).

At least 50% are multiple.

If solitary (the only metastatic lesion in the body), surgery clearly provides best results in most cases. Surgery may be the best approach even if other metastases are present in patients in good condition.

Radiation therapy is useful palliation but not curative. Long-term survivors may have consequential side effects such as dementia.

who are unlikely to survive more than a few months are best treated with dexamethasone alone.

The major benefit of aggressive surgery in patients with a *single brain metastasis* is for the quality of life that remains. Studies of evaluation of performance are compelling. Some of the best outcomes are in patients with a non–small cell lung carcinoma and a single metastasis to the brain. Surgical removal of both tumors sometimes leads to a protracted remission from the disease. With most brain metastases, however, 2-year mortality is similar between surgical patients and those who receive radiation therapy alone. Most patients with systemic metastases die of their systemic illness and not their brain metastasis.

Metastases to the dura and meninges are relatively common. Meningeal carcinomatosis produces headache, cranial nerve palsies, and stiff neck. These symptoms are due to the presence of tumor cells within the spinal fluid and to small deposits on the meninges around cranial nerves, at the base of the brain, and upon spinal roots. The diagnosis is made by cytologic examination of large-volume spinal fluid specimens. As many as three or more spinal taps may be needed to find cancer cells in some cases. The spinal fluid protein level is generally elevated, and the glucose concentration may be low. The latter changes are sufficiently characteristic, in the absence of evidence of infection, to suggest the diagnosis. T1 gadolinium MRI scanning may image the small deposits in the meninges. They are especially evident in the cauda equina even in the absence of clinical symptoms referable to lumbosacral nerve roots. The treatment of meningeal carcinomatosis includes irradiation of the brain and spinal cord, which usually provides benefit but rarely long remission. In patients with limited systemic metastases, intrathecal chemotherapy with methotrexate through an Ommaya reservoir is appropriate; occasional patients respond impressively. Most do not, however, and the effective treatment of meningeal carcinomatosis remains a difficult problem. In the future, the still experimental treatment of meningeal carcinomatosis with isotope-emitting radionuclides coupled to monoclonal antibodies may replace intrathecal chemotherapy.

Table 435–1 lists some key features of metastatic brain tumors.

PRIMARY EXTRA-AXIAL TUMORS

Meningiomas, acoustic neuromas, and pituitary adenomas are the most frequent in this group, which, by definition, are tumors that are not of the brain itself but of its coverings, the cranial nerves, and the adjacent structures. These primary "extra-axial" tumors differ from brain tumors in many ways. They are not of neuroectodermal origin, they are histologically unrelated, and most are truly benign because they can be cured by excision. They exert effects upon the brain by pressure and only occasionally by actual invasion.

Meningiomas, which are growths of the fibroblast-like cells of the dura and arachnoid villi, account for about 15% of all primary brain tumors. They occur more often in women. The biologic explanation is unknown, but the finding has stimulated interest in the presence of progesterone receptors in the tumors. Meningiomas may occur many years after radiation delivered to the head, in which setting they may be multiple. A relationship to head trauma has never been convincingly documented. A few are familial. Such cases, as well as most apparently sporadic examples, are associated with a loss of a portion of chromosome 22, similar to that which characterizes neurofibromatosis type 2.

Most meningiomas arise as solitary tumors in characteristic sites, such as over the cerebral convexities, attached to the sagittal sinus or at the base of the brain attached to the dura of the sphenoid sinus, the olfactory grooves, or the region of the sella. In some of these areas, they may be difficult to remove completely without excessive risk and may recur slowly but repeatedly. Many grow so slowly that serial CT or MR images suggest no enlargement over many years. This slow growth sometimes permits the brain to accommodate them with modest symptoms even when they reach a large size (see Fig. 434–1). Many are detected incidentally. Small, asymptomatic meningiomas are often best watched by imaging studies at intervals; in the elderly, even large, asymptomatic ones may not require surgery.

Acoustic neuromas consist of distinctive growths of Schwann cells (schwannoma) of the eighth cranial nerve. Almost all are unilateral and not apparently familial. Bilateral acoustic neuromas are rare, familial, and diagnostic of neurofibromatosis type 2. This autosomal dominant condition occurs with nearly 100% penetrance in successive generations and derives from a gene deletion on chromosome 22.

Acoustic neuromas grow on the nerve into a round mass just as it emerges from the acoustic canal into the cerebellopontine angle. Some produce symptoms when they are small and confined within the canal. Others may go unsuspected until they grow to rather large size, filling the cerebellopontine angle and compressing the brain stem. Acoustic neuromas greatly surpass in frequency any other tumor of cranial nerves. Partial or complete nerve deafness is characteristic and usually the first symptom. As acoustic neuromas grow, they sequentially affect the fifth and then the seventh cranial nerves on the same side. When large, they cause cerebellar ataxia on the same side and, ultimately, symptoms of brain stem dysfunction. MRI scans accurately detect even very small acoustic neuromas. All patients who develop hearing loss in the middle years of life should be considered to have an acoustic neuroma until proved otherwise. Audiometry alone is suggestive but not diagnostic; caloric tests of labyrinthine function almost always show abnormalities, but the most efficient physiologic study is the auditory evoked response. Current microsurgical techniques yield remarkably good results, usually preserving the seventh nerve and, occasionally, hearing as well.

Pituitary Adenomas

These tumors may cause endocrine symptoms, such as hypothyroidism, amenorrhea, galactorrhea, infertility, acromegaly, or Cushing's syndrome (Ch. 159). With the exception of these hormonal impairments, early symptoms, if any, are usually limited to nonspecific headaches. As pituitary adenomas enlarge, they erode the sella turcica and extend above it to compress the optic nerves, eventually causing bitemporal visual field defects. Rare hemorrhages into large pituitary tumors can cause *pituitary apoplexy,* producing a characteristic syndrome of sudden-onset headache, partial ophthalmoplegia, and blindness in one or the other eye. Emergency surgical decompression must be applied to preserve vision.

Current endocrinologic and MRI techniques facilitate the diagnosis of pituitary tumors, especially if 1-mm cuts and magnified views through the sella are obtained. Medical treatment with bromocriptine may be effective but is slow in yielding results. The drug must be continued indefinitely. Only surgical removal can produce a cure. The safety and efficiency of transsphenoidal pituitary surgery warrant its consideration in all patients, including those with microadenomas that are confined to the sella and larger tumors that, in the past, could be approached only by a subfrontal craniotomy. Radiation therapy may be required in occasional patients who have large and incompletely removed macroadenomas.

Less common primary extra-axial tumors include *craniopharyngiomas,* related *suprasellar epidermoid cysts,* and *Rathke cleft cysts.* Although they reflect congenital abnormalities of the brain and most frequently become symptomatic in childhood, as many as one third of these tumors can first appear in adult life, some as late as the sixth decade. In adults, craniopharyngiomas may compress the frontal lobes and occasionally cause dementia. Such tumors are almost always benign and surgically curable if they can be separated from adjacent parasellar structures, optic nerves, and hypothalamus. Pineal region tumors include *pineocytomas* and *pineoblastomas* derived from pineal parenchymal cells, as well as *teratomas* and *germinomas.* These two groups appear with about equal frequency, have the capacity to be biologically aggressive, and are difficult to manage surgically. Characteristic symptoms and signs include increased intracranial pressure, paresis of upward gaze, pupillary dysfunction, convergence nystagmus, and hydrocephalus due to obstruction of cerebrospinal fluid outflow pathways. Precocious puberty occurs in young males, the result of destruction of the pineal by germinomas. The true pineal tumors may cause delayed puberty. Intracranial *chordomas,* tumors of residual notochordal tissue, are rare and usually arise within the skull at the base of the brain, on the clivus. They are regionally invasive and rarely can be controlled even with aggressive surgery and radiation therapy. *Lipomas* occur chiefly in midline structures, especially over the corpus callosum. *Arachnoid cysts* can arise anywhere on the surface of the brain; some grow to remarkable size. Most arachnoid cysts are incidental, cause no symptoms, and are best left alone. Their infrequency, as well as that of the other extra-axial tumors mentioned, stands in contrast to the frequency and clinical importance of meningiomas and acoustic neuromas (see Table 434–1).

PRIMARY INTRA-AXIAL TUMORS

This group includes astrocytomas, oligodendrogliomas, ependymomas, medulloblastomas, less common neuroectodermal tumors, and primary brain lymphoma. They share the quality of direct, invasive involvement of the substance of the brain, making them rarely curable by surgical excision. Accordingly, gliomas are fundamentally malignant, although some may behave in an indolent manner.

Astrocytomas are the most common gliomas. Their cause is unknown, familial examples constituting only 1% of cases. Astrocytomas have occurred as a late consequence of radiation to the head or skull. The most aggressive variant, *glioblastoma multiforme,* accounts for more than 50% of all primary brain tumors. Glioblastoma (astrocytoma IV) is distinguished pathologically from the less aggressive *anaplastic astrocytoma* (astrocytoma III) on histopathologic grounds, and the two have important clinical differences. Glioblastoma is more common, is more characteristic of older age groups, and has a median survival time of less than 1 year even with aggressive treatment with surgery, radiation therapy, and chemotherapy. By contrast, patients with anaplastic astrocytoma have a median survival time of slightly more than 2 years. Age is an important variable for both of these tumors: The younger the patient, the better the prognosis. Glioblastoma in children, for example, has a median survival of more than 2 years. In adults, men are affected more often than women. Anaplastic astrocytomas and glioblastoma occur in multicentric locations in about 5% of cases. In these instances, they may be mistaken for multiple cerebral metastases or for primary brain lymphoma on imaging studies.

Glioblastomas and anaplastic astrocytomas produce a similar clinical picture, and CT or MR images may be somewhat alike (Fig. 435–2). In most instances, the onset is relatively rapid and heralded by seizures, headaches, and focal neurologic deficits. A minority of patients with these tumors have relevant histories of seizures with onset years before; one assumes that such malignant growths evolve from long-existing, low-grade astrocytomas. Sequential genetic alterations occur in astrocytomas as they become more aggressive. Loss of chromosome 10 is characteristic of

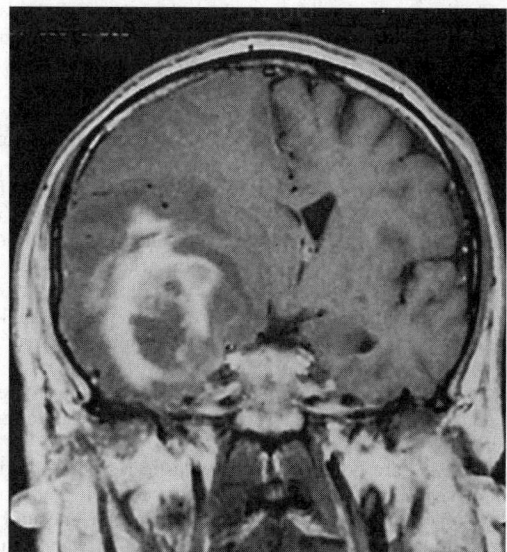

FIGURE 435–2. MRI scan, T1 gadolinium enhanced, of a temporal lobe glioblastoma, showing typical ring configuration of contrast with central necrosis and marked mass effect.

glioblastoma cells and may occur subsequent to loss of chromosome 17, which is common in lower-grade astrocytomas. The latter is likely related to a mutation of a tumor suppressor gene, p53, on this chromosome.

Low-grade astrocytomas can pursue a highly variable course, and many of them do not progress to malignancy. Indeed, some are extremely indolent in their growth, so that the median survival time of patients with low-grade astrocytomas is 7 years from the time of diagnosis. This prognosis means little in individual cases, however, because the course of these tumors is, as noted before, highly variable. In some patients, low-grade astrocytomas transform to glioblastoma within a few years, whereas other astrocytomas can remain indolent for 10 years or more. Many low-grade astrocytomas spread too extensively before diagnosis can be made to allow surgical resection (see Fig. 434–2). By contrast, smaller, favorably situated ones sometimes can be totally removed and the patient apparently cured. Paradoxically, astrocytomas associated with large cysts have a much better prognosis. This favorable circumstance occurs most often in the cerebellum in children and young adults but also in the cerebral hemispheres. Brain stem astrocytomas cannot be operated upon except in rare instances when they are exophytic. Most infiltrate the brain stem and enlarge it. In a similar way, optic nerve astrocytomas, an uncommon cause of vision loss that affects chiefly children, enlarge the optic nerves and may erode the optic foramina. They grow slowly, are sometimes associated with neurofibromatosis, and are often best left untreated until MRI scanning documents unequivocal tumor growth or vision declines. What to do at that point is controversial. Many authorities withhold radiation treatment for low-grade astrocytomas, at least until all other approaches fail and for as long as the quality of life can be maintained. Two important reasons support this position. One is that little well-controlled evidence indicates that radiation greatly shrinks these tumors, eradicates them, slows their growth, or prevents their conversion into malignant astrocytomas. The other, as already remarked upon, is that radiation damages the normal brain, producing selective neuronal injury, areas of radiation necrosis, or both.

Oligodendrogliomas are the most "benign" of the gliomas, although some develop anaplastic features. Their clinical manifestations usually are indistinguishable from those of low-grade astrocytomas. Seizures are an important early symptom. Oligodendrogliomas occur chiefly in the cerebral hemispheres and especially in the frontal lobes. Many contain flecks of calcium, demonstrable by brain imaging. Complete surgical resection is the therapeutic goal but often cannot be realized because of the size and location of the tumors. Despite their slow growth, most oligodendrogliomas respond well to chemotherapy. As many as 80% improve with a regimen that combines procarbazine, CCNU, and vincristine. This response to chemotherapy seems to be superior to that observed with radiation therapy alone. Oligodendroglioma is the primary intra-axial tumor most likely to bleed spontaneously. In addition, anaplastic oligodendrogliomas tend to spread through the spinal fluid to the meninges. A few of these tumors eventually become so anaplastic that they histologically and clinically resemble glioblastomas.

Medulloblastomas occur chiefly in the region of the fourth ventricle and affect principally children and young adults. They cause characteristic symptoms of cerebellar and brain stem dysfunction. In children, aggressive surgery and radiation therapy yield a 5-year survival of 50%, but many children treated in this manner suffer serious, permanent postradiation intellectual deficits. Several reports indicate that chemotherapy with cyclophosphamide and vincristine improves survival, and other drugs are being tried.

Medulloblastoma is characterized by an amplification of the *c-myc* oncogene and abnormalities of chromosome 17. Medulloblastomas arising in the cerebral hemispheres resemble, or may be the same as, *primitive neuroectodermal tumors* (PNET). These tumors are radiosensitive, like medulloblastomas of the fourth ventricle and cerebellum, and at times respond temporarily to aggressive chemotherapy.

Gangliogliomas are composed of neoplastic astrocytes and abundant dysmorphic neoplastic neurons. They occur chiefly in the temporal lobes of children and young adults, have an unusually slow growth rate, and may have a good prognosis even when untreated. Some are associated with tuberous sclerosis.

Primary brain lymphoma is increasing in frequency among both the acquired immunodeficiency syndrome (AIDS) and, for unknown reasons, the non-AIDS populations. These growths involve the brain diffusely, producing infiltrating and often multicentric tumors that tend to lie deep in the brain and adjacent to ventricular surfaces. Almost all of these tumors are B cell derived; the eye is the only other extranodal site that is regularly involved concomitantly. Only rare patients go on to develop systemic lymphoma, and that occurs late in the disease. Primary brain lymphoma is fundamentally unresectable. Steroids are an important component of treatment; dexamethasone is uniquely chemotherapeutic for this tumor. Median survivals of 3 years can now be expected with the addition of multidrug chemotherapy to radiation therapy.

Rare intra-axial brain tumors include *choroid plexus papillomas* and *carcinomas,* which are even less common than the benign but troublesome *colloid cysts* of the third ventricle. The last-mentioned lesion may cause hydrocephalus by blocking the outflow of cerebrospinal fluid from the lateral ventricle. *Capillary hemangioblastomas* arise in the cerebellum and elsewhere. They are sometimes associated with an autosomal dominant inherited disorder that includes retinal angiomatosis as well as cysts and tumors of the pancreas, kidneys, and adrenals (von Hippel syndrome). Some of these cerebellar capillary hemangioblastomas secrete erythropoietin and cause polycythemia.

Vascular malformations of the brain often can be mistaken for gliomas. They frequently manifest with nonhemorrhagic symptoms such as seizures. They sometimes resemble brain tumors in appearance on CT or MRI, and some, especially of the capillary variety (which lack large arteriovenous shunts), cannot be imaged by cerebral angiography. Many of these abnormalities lie in the brain stem and thalamus; because they are indistinguishable from brain tumors on even the best imaging studies, they may undergo biopsy as a diagnostic step, with devastating results. Vascular malformations of the brain involving large-caliber vessels are readily diagnosed by CT or MR images even without cerebral angiography.

Abscesses and *granulomas* of the brain cannot usually be distinguished from tumors by CT or MRI alone. If systemic evaluations fail to suggest a proper diagnosis, reliable management demands that biopsy be used. Even in the non-AIDS population, surprising alternatives to the clinical and radiologic diagnosis of a brain tumor are regularly revealed by biopsy. In many instances, potentially tragic errors of management can be avoided by taking as a direct approach and studying the tissue of the intracranial lesion.

Fadul C, Wood J, Thaler H, et al.: Morbidity and mortality of craniotomy for excision of supratentorial gliomas. Neurology 38:1374, 1988. *Documents convincingly the safety and efficacy of aggressive surgery for gliomas.*

Kyritsis AP, Levin VA: Chemotherapeutic approaches to the treatment of malignant gliomas. Adv Oncol 8:9, 1992. *A short but authoritative and useful review.*

Loeffler JS: Radiotherapy in managing malignant gliomas: Current role and future directions. Adv Oncol 8:14, 1992. *Covers the field well, including newer approaches and techniques.*

Patchell RA, Tibbs PA, Walsh JW, et al.: A randomized trial of surgery in the treatment of single metastasis to the brain. N Engl J Med 322:494, 1990. *An important paper, not only for its conclusion, which clearly supports surgery for a single metastasis, but also because it is an example of what careful clinical trials in neuro-oncology can achieve. Jerome Posner's editorial comments on this paper, and on metastasis in general, are in the same issue and are masterful.*

Posner JB: Neurological Complications of Cancer. Philadelphia, FA Davis, 1995. *A discussion of diagnosis and management of metastatic brain tumors.*

Russell DS, Rubinstein LJ: Pathology of Tumours of the Nervous System. 5th ed. Baltimore, Williams & Wilkins, 1989. *The definitive text, indispensable, scholarly, complete, and beautifully redone by Professor Rubinstein just before his death in 1989.*

436 DISORDERS OF INTRACRANIAL PRESSURE

INTRACRANIAL HYPERTENSION

GENERAL PRINCIPLES. Cerebrospinal fluid (CSF) pressure in excess of 250 mm CSF is usually a manifestation of serious neurologic disease. Intracranial hypertension is most often associated with rapidly expanding mass lesions, CSF outflow obstruction, or cerebral venous congestion; however, a variety of systemic and central nervous system disorders may be accompanied by an increase in intracranial pressure (ICP) (Table 436–1). Lumbar CSF pressure

TABLE 436-1. PATHOGENESIS OF INCREASED INTRACRANIAL PRESSURE

Perturbation	Proximate Cause	Clinical Example
Increased dural sinus venous pressure	Sinus compression or occlusion	Sagittal sinus thrombosis Otitic hydrocephalus Brain tumors
	Increased sinus blood flow	OC$_2$ retention Arteriovenous malformation
	Increased peripheral venous pressure	Internal jugular vein occlusion Superior vena cava syndrome Congestive heart failure
Increased CSF outflow resistance	Ventricular outflow obstruction Obliteration of the cisternal and/or convexity subarachnoid space Plugging of the arachnoid villi	Brain tumors Aqueductal stenosis Meningitis Extradural or subdural masses Cerebral masses or edema Subarachnoid hemorrhage Infectious polyneuritis Spinal cord tumors
Increased rate of CSF formation	Increased choroidal CSF formation Increased extrachoroidal CSF formation	Choroid plexus papilloma Hypo-osmolality Cerebral edema
Unknown	Increased cerebral volume Increased sagittal sinus pressure Increased CSF outflow resistance	Benign intracranial hypertension

may not accurately reflect ICP. In patients with intracranial mass lesions and brain herniation, lumbar CSF pressure may be normal or even low despite grossly elevated supratentorial CSF pressure. Kinking of the aqueduct of Sylvius by adjacent mass lesions, diencephalic–temporal lobe transtentorial herniation, or cerebellar compression of the fourth ventricle, with or without accompanying descent of the cerebellar tonsils into the foramen magnum, can impede the free transmission of CSF into the lumbar subarachnoid space.

Table 436-2 lists the principal symptoms and signs associated with intracranial hypertension. Headache is produced by traction on pain-sensitive cerebral blood vessels or dura mater at the base or, less often, the vertex of the brain. Signs reflect the presence of impending herniation with intermittent vascular compression, midline shift, or axial distortion of the brain stem (see Ch. 393). In the absence of such shifts, increased ICP alone may be asymptomatic. *Papilledema* is the most reliable sign of ICP; but in many patients with increased ICP, it fails to develop. This is particularly true in the elderly. Retinal venous pulsations, when present, imply that CSF pressure is normal or not significantly elevated, but their absence is not helpful diagnostically. Patients with increased ICP often complain of worsening symptoms, particularly headache, in the morning, perhaps because plateau waves (spontaneous elevations of ICP) occur more commonly during sleep.

The initial treatment of any patient with increased ICP whose neurologic status is deteriorating is aimed at reducing the volume of the intracranial contents in an attempt to prevent brain damage (Table 436-3). If ICP approaches the systolic blood pressure, the cerebral perfusion pressure decreases and irreversible ischemia may develop. The definitive treatment of intracranial hypertension is ulti-

mately determined by the nature of the underlying pathologic process.

Benign Intracranial Hypertension

Benign intracranial hypertension is a syndrome of increased ICP unaccompanied by localizing neurologic signs, intracranial mass lesion, or CSF outflow obstruction in an alert, otherwise healthy-looking patient. Such patients are almost always obese and more often women. Benign intracranial hypertension (also called pseudotumor cerebri, or idiopathic intracranial hypertension) may be associated with a variety of systemic and iatrogenic disorders (Table 436-4). The cause is usually unknown. Chronically increased ICP may give rise to the "empty sella syndrome," which refers to a radiographically globular enlargement of the sella turcica, an incompetent diaphragma sellae, and a compressed but functioning pituitary.

The diagnosis of benign intracranial hypertension is one of exclusion. Intracranial masses (tumors, hematomas, infections) and CSF outflow obstruction must be excluded by computed tomography (CT) or magnetic resonance imaging (MRI). Magnetic resonance angiography (MRA) is necessary to rule out dural venous sinus thrombosis. Lumbar puncture, which is usually deferred until CT or MR has revealed a normal or small ventricular system, is required to confirm the diagnosis. Lumbar spinal fluid pressure is elevated, frequently above 300 mm CSF, but the composition of the fluid is normal; the protein content is usually in the low normal range, below 20 mg per deciliter.

PATHOPHYSIOLOGY. In most cases, the cause is unknown. Chronically elevated ICP implies an increase in dural sinus venous pressure, an increase in CSF outflow resistance, an increase in the rate of CSF formation (if it ever really occurs), or some combination of these factors. One or more of these mechanisms must elevate the CSF pressure. Pathogenetic hypotheses that postulate an in-

TABLE 436-2. SYMPTOMS AND SIGNS OF INTRACRANIAL HYPERTENSION

Common	Less Common
Headache	Hearing distortion or loss
Tinnitus	Vertigo
Vomiting (with or without nausea)	Facial weakness
Visual obscurations, visual loss, photopsias	Shoulder/arm pain
Papilledema	Neck pain or rigidity
Diplopia	Ataxia
Lethargy and increased sleep	Paresthesias of extremities
Psychomotor retardation	Anosmia
Pain on eye movement	Trigeminal neuralgia

TABLE 436-3. EMERGENCY TREATMENT OF IMPENDING HERNIATION IN ACUTELY DECOMPENSATING PATIENTS

Therapy	Dosage or Procedure	Onset (Duration) of Action
Hyperventilation	Lower Paco$_2$ to 25 to 30 mm Hg	Seconds (minutes)
Osmotherapy	Mannitol, 0.5 to 2.0 gm/kg intravenously over 15 minutes, followed by 25 gm as needed	Minutes (hours)
Corticosteroids	Dexamethasone, 50 mg intravenous push, followed by 50 mg daily in divided doses	Hours (days)

TABLE 436–4. SYSTEMIC AND IATROGENIC DISORDERS ASSOCIATED WITH BENIGN INTRACRANIAL HYPERTENSION

Commonly Prescribed Drugs
Nalidixic acid
Nitrofurantoin
Phenytoin
Sulfonamides
Tetracycline
Vitamin A
Endocrine and Metabolic Disorders
Addison's disease
Cushing's syndrome
Hypoparathyroidism
Levothyroxine therapy
Menarche, pregnancy, oral contraceptives
Obesity and irregular menses
Steroid therapy/withdrawal
Hematologic Disorders
Cryoglobulinemia
Iron deficiency anemia
Miscellaneous Disorders
Dural venous sinus obstruction/thrombosis
Head trauma
Internal jugular vein ligation
Lupus erythematosus
Middle ear disease

crease in brain bulk consequent to an increase in cerebral blood volume or in brain water content (interstitial brain edema) do not provide an adequate explanation. The constancy of obesity, often extreme, has suggested the possibility of a disorder of the hypothalamus. But no data have emerged to support this idea. Despite decades of knowledge of the association with obesity, the link remains completely obscure. The strikingly greater incidence in women than in men (4:1) is also unexplained but surely important in some way.

CLINICAL MANIFESTATIONS. Most patients complain of headache. Other common early symptoms include nausea and vomiting, visual disturbances, retro-ocular pain, diplopia, tinnitus, and vertigo. Bilateral papilledema, the cardinal feature, is almost always present and may be associated with peripapillary retinal hemorrhages, exudates, or both. Vision loss, the only serious complication of idiopathic intracranial hypertension, may occur either early or late in the course of the disease but is seen less than feared. Transient obscurations of vision do not predict subsequent failure of vision. Characteristically, visual field testing reveals enlarged blind spots. Quantitative visual field testing should be performed at monthly intervals early in the disease. Diplopia, caused by unilateral or bilateral abducens palsy, may develop as a false localizing sign. The remainder of the neurologic examination is almost always normal. It is important to distinguish pseudopapilledema—an anomalous elevation of the optic disc—from true papilledema, which is prima facie evidence of increased ICP. Anomalous elevation of the disc, which may be associated with identifiable hyaline bodies (drusen), should suggest the diagnosis of retinitis pigmentosa.

In some instances, benign intracranial hypertension is a self-limited disease in which CSF pressure returns to normal as clinical symptoms remit over several months. However, clinical improvement is not always accompanied by a reduction in CSF pressure, and there is a vexing subgroup of patients whose pressure remains persistently elevated after neurologic signs and symptoms have resolved. The course of such cases implies that clinical symptoms may be independent of the absolute magnitude of CSF pressure and that chronically raised ICP may be totally asymptomatic. In addition, despite persistently elevated CSF pressure, patients do not become hydrocephalic. The ventricular system remains small, or no larger than normal. This finding suggests that whatever mechanism "resets" CSF pressure above normal does not predispose to the development of communicating hydrocephalus and that the two conditions are biologically unrelated.

TREATMENT. Unfortunately, no convincing evidence exists that any of the frequently recommended treatment modalities are regularly efficacious. The high rate of spontaneous remission com-

plicates the evaluation of various therapies. At present, four general approaches to symptomatic treatment are used: (1) repeated lumbar puncture, (2) pharmacologic treatment, (3) ventriculosystemic or lumboperitoneal shunting, and (4) incision of the optic nerve sheath.

Frequent (such as alternate day), large-volume lumbar punctures may provide relief of symptoms and document the occurrence of remission. Either it is beneficial, or remission occurs independently during the period of treatment. Corticosteroids and diuretics have been the mainstay of medical treatment, and both are effective; or, again, the disease remits during the period of treatment. Dexamethasone, furosemide, and acetazolamide are often tried. CSF shunting procedures are not without risk, and their long-term efficacy remains to be established. Incision of the optic nerve sheath for the relief of papilledema is the treatment of choice for patients whose visual fields are deteriorating. Surprisingly, in some patients, headache and papilledema on the contralateral side are relieved as well as the ipsilateral papilledema.

HYDROCEPHALUS

Hydrocephalus refers to the net accumulation of CSF within the cerebral ventricles and their consequent enlargement. Although acute obstructive hydrocephalus usually produces a sudden increase in intraventricular pressure, CSF pressure is frequently normal (or low) in patients with chronic hydrocephalus. It is customary to distinguish between "noncommunicating" and "communicating" hydrocephalus; the former is produced by lesions that obstruct the intracerebral CSF circulation at or proximal to the foramina of Luschka and Magendie, the latter by obstruction of the basal cisterns or convexity subarachnoid space in such a way that the ventricular system communicates with the spinal subarachnoid space but CSF cannot drain through the arachnoid villi into the superior sagittal sinus. Because both "noncommunicating" and "communicating" types of hydrocephalus are obstructive and both are treated by shunts, the distinction really has less meaning than that usually ascribed to it. Perhaps the important distinction should be between obstructive and nonobstructive hydrocephalus. Ventricular dilatation associated with severe cerebral atrophy, sometimes called "hydrocephalus ex vacuo," is the best example of nonobstructive hydrocephalus.

DIAGNOSIS. Hydrocephalus is easily diagnosed by MRI. The diagnosis must take into account the increase in ventricular volume that accompanies normal aging and the presence or absence of cerebral atrophy. Enlargement of the temporal horns and an inability to visualize the sylvian and interhemispheric fissures or cerebral sulci, plus the presence of periventricular lucencies (CT) or periventricular hyperintensity (MR), favor the diagnosis of hydrocephalus. A normal or small fourth ventricle in the presence of enlarged lateral and third ventricles suggests aqueductal stenosis.

ACUTE VERSUS CHRONIC HYDROCEPHALUS. Sudden, complete ventricular outflow obstruction leads to acute hydrocephalus, coma, and, if untreated, death; partial obstruction is more common and only moderately less dangerous (Table 436–5). Chronic hydrocephalus in the adult is most often caused by aqueductal stenosis or the complications of subarachnoid hemorrhage. Other reported causes and associations are listed in Table 436–5. In

TABLE 436–5. CAUSES OF HYDROCEPHALUS

Acute
Cerebellar hemorrhage/infarction
Colloid cyst of the third ventricle
Exudative meningitis
Head trauma
Intracranial tumor/hematoma
Spontaneous subarachnoid hemorrhage
Viral encephalitis
Chronic
Aqueductal stenosis
Ectasia and elongation of the basilar artery (rare)
Granulomatous meningitis
Head trauma
Hindbrain malformations
Meningeal carcinomatosis
Brain and spinal cord tumors
Spontaneous subarachnoid hemorrhage
Syringomyelia

many instances, the cause of symptomatic chronic hydrocephalus ("normal-pressure hydrocephalus") cannot be determined. Unequivocally asymptomatic hydrocephalus may be found in approximately 4% of patients over the age of 60 who consult neurologists.

CLINICAL MANIFESTATIONS. The patient with acute obstructive hydrocephalus may have severe headache, lethargy, signs of increased ICP, papilledema, abducens palsy, and signs of the causative lesion. Hyperactive reflex and bilateral extensor plantar responses are almost invariably present. Ventricular CSF pressure is markedly increased, but if CSF pathways are blocked, this increase may not be transmitted to the lumbar subarachnoid space. Patients with chronic communicating hydrocephalus, including normal-pressure hydrocephalus, have a progressive dementia characterized by forgetfulness and psychomotor retardation, an unsteady gait, and urinary incontinence. Bilateral pyramidal and extrapyramidal signs may be present. Some patients have a parkinsonian appearance. The lumbar CSF pressure is usually normal or nearly normal in range, although overnight recording of ventricular CSF pressure may reveal intermittent waves of elevated pressure.

TREATMENT. Acute hydrocephalus responds dramatically to ventricular drainage and CSF diversion. Treatment of the primary lesion is the treatment of choice, although temporary ventricular decompression or ventriculosystemic shunt may be necessary in some cases. Ventricular shunting has also been used for patients with chronic communicating hydrocephalus. Unfortunately, not all patients respond, or response may be delayed for weeks or months; moreover, there are no reliable clinical or neuroradiologic predictors of shunt response. Recent onset and mild dementia remain better predictors than does isotope cisternography. Absence of cerebral atrophy and temporary improvement after lumbar puncture seem to correlate with benefit from a shunt operation.

INTRACRANIAL HYPOTENSION

CSF pressure measured at a lumbar puncture site, with the patient in the lateral decubitus position, normally ranges from 70 to 200 mm CSF (5 to 15 mm Hg). Low or zero lumbar CSF pressure can be recorded under several circumstances, as indicated in Table 436–6. Symptoms of the first two or three circumstances on that list are likely to be dominated by the underlying illnesses. The remainder of the circumstances tend to cause a consistent syndrome characterized by severe, throbbing frontal and occipital headache, which usually appears within 30 seconds after the patient assumes an erect posture and subsides completely upon the patient's lying flat. Associated complaints may include dizziness, nausea, stiff neck, photophobia, and, rarely, diplopia due to an associated abducens nerve palsy. The disorder often arises 1 to 21 days after lumbar puncture. The pathogenesis is as for lumbar puncture headache (Ch. 405.2).

Rare cases of CSF hypotension may occur spontaneously, producing, in previously healthy persons, symptoms similar to those already described. The onset can be acute or subacute and is occasionally precipitated by mild trauma, such as a fall on the buttocks or a casual bump to the head. The cause usually remains unknown, although isotope cisternography sometimes reveals spontaneous rupture of a dural nerve sheath. Diagnosis can be difficult because zero spontaneous pressures in the lumbar subarachnoid space can give the false impression of missing the thecal sac. Treatment is symptomatic; spontaneous recovery usually requires days to a few weeks. When post–lumbar puncture symptoms are persistent, disabling, or both, an epidural "blood patch" is indicated. The actual need for blood patches is far less than the frequency with which the procedure is done by worried physicians for impatient sufferers of post–lumbar puncture headache. The procedure involves the injection of 10 ml of the patient's own blood into the epidural space to seal a presumed dural leak. Rarely, in long-lasting cases, surgical exploration has exposed the dural leak, which must be sutured. In patients suffering from either lumbar puncture–induced or spontaneous intracranial hypotension, an MRI of the brain may reveal intense enhancement of the meninges. Occasionally, subdural effusions develop. The process is benign and clears when the intracranial hypotension resolves.

Lyons HK, Meyer FB: Cerebrospinal fluid physiology and the management of increased intracranial pressure. Mayo Clin Proc 65:684, 1990. *A superb review with excellent references.*

Pannullo S, Reich JB, Krol G, et al.: MRI changes in intracranial hypotension. Neurology 43:919, 1993. *A description of patients with intracranial hypotension and meningeal enhancement on MRI.*

Petersen RC, Bahram M, Laws ER Jr: Surgical treatment of idiopathic hydrocephalus in elderly patients. Neurology 35:307, 1985. *A clinically oriented review of the indications for, risks of, and benefits to be expected from the surgical treatment of normal-pressure hydrocephalus.*

Radhadkrishnan K, Ahlskog JE, Garrity JA, et al.: Idiopathic intracranial hypertension. Mayo Clin Proc 69:169, 1994.

Ropper AH, Kennedy SK: Neurological and Neurosurgical Intensive Care. 3rd ed. Rockville, MD, Aspen Publishers 1993. *Chapter 3 is a brief but excellent resource, with 129 well-chosen references, on all aspects of the treatment of intracranial hypertension.*

TABLE 436–6. CAUSES OF ABNORMALLY LOW (0–50 mm) CSF PRESSURE

Dehydration-hypovolemia
Cranial-intraspinal CSF block
Post–CNS surgery
CSF fistula
Post–lumbar puncture drainage
Spontaneous-idiopathic; dural nerve sheath tear

Section Thirteen—Injury to the Head and Spinal Cord

Lawrence F. Marshall

437 HEAD INJURY

GENERAL CONSIDERATIONS

Head injury is a major public health problem. Nonpenetrating traumatic brain injury is responsible for more than 50,000 deaths a year in the United States, and many people have long-term intellectual and behavioral residua. Severe head injury mainly affects young people between 15 and 30 years, but spares no age or socioeconomic group. Missile injury, particularly gunshot wounds to the skull and brain, are far from confined to urban areas of socioeconomic decay.

MECHANISM OF BRAIN DAMAGE

The pathology of head injury includes a spectrum of changes. Underlying almost all nonpenetrating brain trauma is diffuse axonal injury, a condition in which axons are either sheared at the time of impact or degenerate soon after because of irreversible traumatic or ischemic damage to the fibers. Superimposed upon such white matter changes are contusions, which represent hemorrhage mixed into the tissue, and hematomas, more focal collections of blood. Hematomas can occur on the external surface of the dura (extradural hematoma), under the dura and over the underlying brain (subdural hematoma), or within the substance of the brain (intraparenchymal hematoma). In mild and moderate head injury the frequency of surgical hematomas is low. As the degree of neurologic injury increases, however, the severity of diffuse axonal injury rises in almost direct proportion, as does the frequency of intracranial hematomas.

Cell-molecular abnormalities due to regional anoxia plus direct trauma add to the above changes. Trauma releases an excess of excitatory amino acids as well as inflammatory mediators and free radicals, all in the bruised or ischemic areas. Blood-brain barrier breakdown follows, inducing tissue edema and increased intracranial pressure due to brain enlargement.

Damage to the brain as a result of traumatic injury occurs through a variety of dynamic processes. The impact, in addition to causing immediately variable degrees of abnormality, sets into motion a series of events which, if left uninterrupted, may result in much more severe changes in the tissues and even death. The last 15 years have made it increasingly apparent that primary damage to the brain that at first seems moderate and compatible with a good recovery in many cases may give way to the later development of intracranial hematoma or ischemic brain damage as a result of shock and/or hypoxia.

PRIMARY DAMAGE

Primary traumatic damage to the brain can be separated into three basic processes: (1) diffuse axonal injury (DAI), (2) brain contusion, and (3) intracranial hematoma. DAI always occurs in severe head injury and has a predilection for the brain stem, corpus callosum, and deep white matter. Experimental studies suggest that minor degrees of DAI probably occur in patients who suffer only a *concussion,* i.e., a transient loss of consciousness usually associated with no or minimal residua. With more severe head trauma, the number of areas and the severity of DAI increase proportionately. Some patients with near-fatal injury suffer white matter injuries that completely interrupt long sensorimotor pathways at the cervicomedullary junction.

Brain contusions as shown in Figure 437–1 are common. Traumatic contusions can occur throughout the brain but are more frequent on the cortical surface and in the superficial white matter. Contusions vary in size from <2 to 3 ml to much larger. Such ar-

eas of tissue injury are important for several reasons. First, they represent areas of damage to the brain. Second, contusions may act as mass lesions because of the development of secondary edema in the surrounding tissues. Such mixtures of edema and hemorrhagic tissue may enlarge, progressively causing brain displacement and distortion. Third is intracranial hemorrhage which can result in epidural, subdural, or intraparenchymal hematomas.

Epidural hematomas usually result from moderate impact injuries. A baseball striking the head, an assault producing only a transient loss of consciousness, or a fall from a horse are typical precipitating events. Extradural hematomas characteristically follow fractures of the temporal bone associated with laceration of the middle meningeal artery. In some instances, the hemorrhage may follow a fracture tearing one of the major draining venous sinuses of the brain. The clinical course is classically described as a transient loss of consciousness, followed by a period of lucidity and then a rather abrupt deterioration. Actually, this sequence occurs in only a minority of patients: Some lose consciousness immediately following impact, whereas others deteriorate abruptly without a history of initial loss of consciousness.

In the apparently minimally injured patient brought to an emergency room following an ostensibly minor head injury CT scans are the procedure of choice because they detect both skull and major parenchymal injuries. If CT is unavailable, a skull x-ray to detect fractures should be obtained before sending the patient home. Elderly patients should always have CT scans before being discharged. Trauma patients should be hospitalized for close observation if the neurologic examination is abnormal or if consciousness is altered in any way. The early detection of extradural hemorrhages is of utmost importance because most affected patients do not initially have irreversible brain damage.

Subdural hematomas are divided into three subgroups: acute, subacute, and chronic. An *acute subdural hematoma* almost always signifies severe brain injury and is associated with significant DAI and contusions. Most such patients are unconscious from impact, and half die. Recent studies have demonstrated that early surgery for acute subdural hematomas somewhat improves outcome, particularly in patients who show little other associated injury to the brain. The frequency of subdural hematomas increases with age, presumably because age-associated brain atrophy more readily allows the expansion of such venous bleedings. Most subdural hematomas are caused by laceration of the bridging veins that drain blood from the surface of the brain into the major sinuses or by laceration of cortical veins in the region of the sylvian fissure. Acute subdural hematomas are especially likely following assaults, falls (particularly in the elderly or alcoholic), and motor vehicle accidents when the head is decelerated suddenly on impact.

Subacute subdural hematomas consist of blood clots that underlie the dura on the surface of the brain, developing from 48 hours to 1 week following injury. Some must arise within a few hours of impact but do not reach a sufficient size to cause either depression of consciousness or a focal neurologic deficit. Patients with subacute subdural hematomas are usually older than age 50, occasionally have been taking anticoagulants, and usually have less serious head injuries than those with acute subdural hematomas. Only a small percentage are in coma when first seen and, if the hematoma is diagnosed promptly following its onset, most enjoy a good outcome.

Chronic subdural hematomas have distinct qualities. They usually occur between 1 and 6 weeks following injury, often bilaterally. Many follow trivial injuries, such as striking the head on a door, with no associated loss of consciousness. Indeed, affected patients often forget the inciting event. Patients with chronic subdural hematomas characteristically come from older age groups and many suffer from chronic illnesses, including alcoholism and dementia. Headache, worse in the morning, hypersomnolence or confusion, mild focal weakness, difficulty writing, and unsteadiness are common complaints. Chronic subdural hematomas, because of age-related shrinkage of the brain, may reach a substantial size in excess of 100 cc before the patient seeks medical attention. The treatment is relatively straightforward. Some resolve spontaneously. For larger clots, a twist drill hole and puncture of the dura suffice for many patients. Many surgeons leave a drain in the subdural space to allow gravity drainage for 24 to 48 hours following evacuation of the clot. In some instances, particularly if CT scanning reveals an area of increased density, two burr holes are placed to allow irrigation of the subdural space. Craniotomy should be avoided if possible.

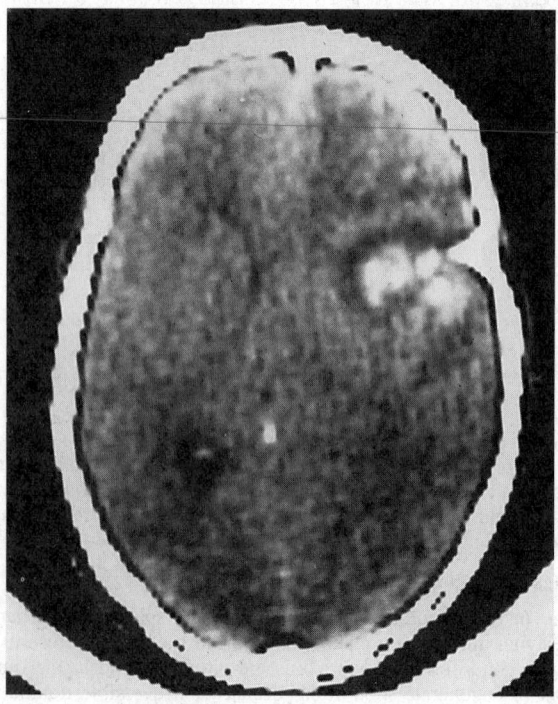

FIGURE 437–1. Brain contusion.

The third type of intracranial hematoma is the *intraparenchymal hemorrhage,* sometimes called intracerebral hemorrhage. These may vary in size from 1 to 100 ml, but they are usually considered for surgical drainage only when they exceed 15 to 20 ml. Long-term prognosis often is poor.

PREHOSPITAL CARE AND INITIAL RESUSCITATION

Head injuries often occur under circumstances that traumatize other organ systems as well. Fractures of the long bones and injuries to the chest and abdomen are common, particularly as a result of motor vehicle accidents or pedestrian-vehicle interactions. Until recently, concerns about secondary insults such as shock and hypoxia arose primarily among the more severely injured. Present evidence, however, indicates that even moderate levels of hypotension can convert a reversible brain injury to one with ischemic brain damage. Accordingly, immediate and adequate restitution of blood pressure and intravascular fluid volume, as well as early steps to prevent or treat hypoxia, represent essential preventive measures.

Utilization of the Glasgow Coma Scale (GCS) shown in Table 437–1 provides a simple and reproducible means for serially assessing the head-injured patient. This examination, which assesses the patient's ability to respond to pain, to speak, and to open his or her eyes, when performed in concert with examination of the pupils, serves as an excellent field guide to the severity of injury. All four limbs must be tested for responsiveness either to verbal command or to pain in order not to overlook focal neurologic deficits, such as hemiparesis, paraparesis, or quadriparesis. Changes in pupillary responsiveness suggest brain stem compression, which must be detected early and dealt with promptly if treatment is to be successful.

Patients who cannot follow commands, do not open their eyes to noxious stimuli, and fail to utter words or comprehensible sounds are considered in coma (GCS score of 8 or less) and require early assurance of a secured airway. The frequency of shock and hypoxia increases in proportion to the severity of injury. Hypoxia occurs in approximately one third of all severe head injuries, and pulmonary shunting affects more than half. Because of these changes, early controlled intubation, often at the scene of the injury, is highly recommended. Search for sources of hemorrhage is essential and should include the less obvious ones such as scalp lacerations and pelvic fractures. If such cannot be found, neurogenic hypotension should be suspected. Fluid resuscitation should begin at the scene, recognizing the difficulties in administering large amounts of fluid under these conditions. Current evidence suggests that even with modern paramedic systems shock often receives inadequate treatment in the field and that newer strategies, utilizing hypertonic saline or pressor agents, may be required. Studies show that the

presence of hypotension at outset almost doubles the mortality of head injury.

Once the airway has been secured and fluid resuscitation initiated, stabilization of the cervical spine and transport become the next priorities. In general, the neck should be placed in a neutral position. However, if the patient is awake and chooses to hold the neck in an unusual position, it should not be forced. Some patients with cervical spine fractures but no neurologic deficit have been made quadriplegic by ill-advised attempts to straighten the neck.

Upon arrival at the hospital the priorities of maintaining airway and circulation remain uppermost. Adequate oxygenation with a Pao_2 above 80 and moderate hyperventilation to $Paco_2$ of 35 mm Hg to control brain swelling are initial objectives. A mean blood pressure of at least 90 mm Hg is mandatory.

CT SCANNING

The availability of rapid-sequence CT scanning has revolutionized the care of the head injured. Patients with focal neurologic deficits and severe injuries, i.e., a GCS score of 8 or less, should be scanned as soon as airway and hemodynamic stability are ensured. To minimize the risks of transportation and movement, deteriorating patients should be accompanied by a physician, and even stable but seriously injured patients should have an experienced emergency room or trauma nurse present at all times. Supervised respiratory assistance should assure adequate ventilation during transport and during the scan.

The results of CT scans heavily influence subsequent management. If a surgical lesion is demonstrated, the patient should be taken to the operating room immediately. Otherwise severe traumatic injuries are best treated in intensive care units, with lesser injuries being handled in units that provide close observation.

Several findings on the CT scan, other than intracranial hematomas, merit close attention and warn of possible deterioration. Compression or absence of the mesencephalic cistern augurs a high degree of brain swelling and death, even in patients whose clinical examination at the time suggests only a moderately severe injury. Unilateral or bilateral hemispheric swelling almost always predicts the likelihood of dangerous intracranial hypertension.

SERIAL ASSESSMENT

Close observation, with particular attention to the development of tachypnea and bradycardia, is important. Table 437–2 lists signs that portend potential intracranial catastrophe. An increase in systolic blood pressure of 15 mm Hg or more or a decline in heart rate of 15 beats per minute often gives the first hints of the development of an intracranial mass lesion.

Tachypnea holds particular importance. Respiratory rates over 20 per minute are abnormal in patients over 15 years of age and may indicate an increase in intracranial pressure or the development of pulmonary failure or infection. Similarly, increasing headache is often present but overlooked; it may reflect a rising intracranial pressure. The use of continuous flow sheets in an intermediate care setting or in a neurologic observation unit assists in monitoring the course and detecting subtle changes in vital signs.

INTENSIVE CARE MANAGEMENT OF THE SEVERELY HEAD INJURED

The overriding objective in the care of the severely head injured is to prevent further insults to the traumatized brain. The situation requires meticulous attention to detail and continuous vigilance to detect and counteract deterioration in hemodynamic, pulmonary, and neurologic function. The brain's vulnerability to secondary injury extends beyond shock and hypoxia. Fever increases the metabolic rate of the tissue by approximately 13% for each degree Celsius, a demand that the already injured brain may not be able to meet. Seizures are a major threat—they increase tissue energy requirements and trigger a rise of up to 400% in cerebral blood flow, accentuating any existing increase in the intracranial pressure.

The objectives in the critical care of head injury shown in Table 437–3 illustrate an approach that includes both the avoidance of systemic insults to the brain and the treatment of intracranial hypertension. Elevations of intracranial pressure above the normal of 15 mm Hg accompany most severe head injuries, and some believe that they contribute directly to further tissue damage if left untreated. Compression of the mesencephalic cistern detected by CT

TABLE 437–1. GLASGOW COMA SCALE

The Glasgow Coma Scale is a practical means of monitoring changes in level of consciousness, based upon eye opening and verbal and motor responses. The responsiveness of the patient can be expressed by summation of the figures. The lowest score is 3, the highest is 15.

Eyes open	Spontaneously (eyes open does not imply awareness)	4
	To speech (any speech, not necessarily a command)	3
	To pain (should not use supraorbital pressure for pain stimulus)	2
	Never	1
Best verbal response	Oriented (to time, person, place)	5
	Confused speech (disoriented)	4
	Inappropriate (swearing, yelling)	3
	Incomprehensible sounds (moaning, groaning)	2
	None	1
Best motor response	Obeys commands	6
	Localizes pain (deliberate or purposeful movement)	5
	Withdrawal (moves away from stimulus)	4
	Abnormal flexion (decortication)	3
	Extension (decerebration)	2
	None (flaccidity)	1
	Total Score	

TABLE 437–2. SIGNS OF POTENTIAL INTRACRANIAL CATASTROPHE AND WHAT THEY MAY SIGNIFY

Signs	Changes	Potential Meaning
Respiration	Rate > 20	} Pulmonary edema or pneumonitis
Pulse	Change > 10/min and/or heart rate < 60	} Each may indicate elevated ICP with transtentorial herniation
Blood pressure	Change in systolic > 15 mm Hg and/or widening pulse pressure	
Headache*	Is it increasing?	Often indicates increased ICP
Pupils	Enlargement Asymmetry Irregular shape (oval) Decrease in reactivity Change from preresuscitation	}
Motor	Decrease of 1 point on GCS New focal deficit	} Increased mass effect New hemorrhage Recurrent hemorrhage
Level of consciousness		Increased ICP Seizures Hypotension
	Abrupt decrease	
	Transient	Seizures Hypoxia
	Progressive decrease	Rehemorrhage Brain stem involvement Septicemia Electrolyte imbalance Vasospasm Hydrocephalus

* All changes except headache may occur in both awake and unconscious patients. GCS = Glasgow coma scale; ICP = intracranial pressure.

scans and referred to as "diffuse swelling," is frequent in patients with even moderately severe injuries. Because mortality in such cases can be reduced from approximately 85 to 35% with early and rapid intervention for intracranial hypertension, most academic neurosurgical centers record the intracranial pressure (ICP) continuously so as to treat intracranial hypertension whenever it develops. Several available techniques are discussed in the references to this chapter.

ICP monitoring should not be initiated in patients with coagulation disturbances. Patients in whom multiple contusions can be detected by a first CT scan can be assumed to have a trauma-related coagulopathy that will correct itself within a few hours, after which a ventricular cannula can be inserted.

The treatment of *traumatic intracranial hypertension* is central to the intensive care of the critically brain injured patient. The cornerstone of management is to adjust baseline ventilation to maintain a Pco_2 in the 35 to 37 mm Hg range, permitting brief periods of greater hyperventilation to respond to sudden increases in intracranial pressures. Levels of extreme hyperventilation may produce excessive vasoconstriction. The head should be maintained in a neutral position because turning it to the right or left may introduce venous obstruction and a rise in ICP. Also, the head should be elevated to not more than 30 degrees. Intravascular volume must be

maintained using balanced salt solutions. Dextrose and water should be avoided. Head trauma often induces salt retention initially so that half normal saline may be most useful to meet fluid needs. Because hyperglycemia is known to exacerbate ischemic brain injury in experimental animals, it appears wise to avoid glucose infusions.

Sedation and pain relief are essential in the initial phases of treatment. Morphine sulfate by continuous infusion of 2 to 8 mg per hour is the least complicated and most effective regimen. Muscle relaxation with vecuronium or other short-acting agents is occasionally helpful in patients in whom ICP is difficult to control, but otherwise is not necessary. Muscle relaxants should be accompanied by adequate sedation.

Anticonvulsants have a limited but important use in acute traumatic head injury. Phenytoin given for the first 7 days after injury reduces the incidence of post-traumatic epilepsy during that period. No study has shown a protective effect when medication was continued beyond the first week.

LONG-TERM CONSEQUENCES OF SEVERE HEAD INJURY

Severe head injury causes serious long-term intellectual and behavioral impairment. Most such patients suffer difficulties in recent memory, abstract thinking, and rapid information processing. Depression, fatigue, and impetuosity accentuate these cognitive deficits. Long-term deficits of motor function are relatively uncommon and less socioeconomically important. Many rehabilitation programs have been developed to assist the severely head injured in the management of these problems. Counseling of the family is essential. Divorce, suicide, and spouse abuse can be reduced in frequency by early intervention.

MINOR HEAD INJURY

Minor head injury is defined as including a GCS score of 13 to 15 following emergency room or hospital admission combined with a return to a normal level of consciousness within 24 hours. Most but not all such patients have normal CT scans. Patients suffering minor head injuries characteristically experience early post-traumatic problems with recent memory, concentration, and abstract thinking. In most instances such problems subside within the first 1 to 3 months following minor injury. Approximately 15% are left with cognitive deficits that do not completely remit. Age is a specific risk factor, and many elderly persons develop chronic dizziness and disequilibrium after even minor trauma. Such symptoms

TABLE 437–3. ICU MANAGEMENT OF SEVERE HEAD INJURY AND INTRACRANIAL HYPERTENSION

1. Head elevated 30 degrees and in neutral plane
2. Intubation with controlled ventilation to an arterial $Paco_2$ of 30–35 mm Hg
3. Good pulmonary toilet
4. Maintain fluid balance with 0.5 normal saline
5. Maintain systolic arterial pressure between 100 and 160 mm Hg
6. Maintain cerebral perfusion pressure > 70 mm Hg (CPP = MAP − ICP)
7. Adequate sedation
8. Muscle relaxants prn (must use sedation concurrently)
9. Maintain normothermia
10. Adequate anticonvulsant therapy
11. Ventricular drainage for intracranial hypertension
12. Mannitol 0.25 mg/kg if No. 11 fails or is not available
13. Hypnotic for elevated ICP in patients with diffuse or hemispheric swelling

are classified as a *post-traumatic or postconcussive syndrome*. Recent evidence indicates that a small percentage of patients suffer modest but permanent residual cognitive impairment.

Many patients with minor head injuries suffer transiently from insomnia, depression, and headache. Early support and reassurance from the physician often improve these symptoms. If headache persists for more than 60 to 90 days, propranolol, 30 to 60 mg in three divided doses, may bring relief.

MODERATE HEAD INJURY

Patients who have not been rendered comatose but have a depressed level of consciousness for several hours or days following injury are classified as having suffered moderate head injuries. These patients have GCS scores of 9 to 12. Such patients almost always suffer measurable cognitive and behavioral difficulties over the long term. Nevertheless, many eventually return to gainful employment. Even so, the potential for social disruption is high, and traits of impetuousness and heightened irritability often create socioeconomic problems. Depression is frequent and may respond to tricylic antidepressants. Intervention, using a variety of psychological services including social workers and psychiatrists, has a more favorable impact if carried out early rather than after the problems have overwhelmed the patient and family.

Foulkes MA, Eisenberg HM, Jane JA, et al.: Report on the traumatic coma data bank. J Neurosurg (Suppl) 75:51, 1991. *Outcome data and much more are described in a cohort of 1030 head-injury victims treated from onset in a multicenter trial.*

Marshall SB, Marshall LF, Vos H, et al.: Neuroscience Critical Care: Pathophysiology and Patient Management. Philadelphia, WB Saunders, 1990. *Particular emphasis on assessment of the neurologically impaired patient, modern neuroradiology, and intensive care.*

Ropper AH (ed.): Neurological and Neurosurgical Intensive Care, 3rd ed. New York, Raven Press, 1993. *A well-edited volume that contains an excellent, detailed chapter on head injury by Chestnut and Marshall.*

Temkin NR, Dikmen SS, Wilensky AJ, et al.: A randomized, double-blind study of phenytoin for the prevention of post-traumatic seizures. N Engl J Med 323:497, 1990. *Four hundred and four patients with serious head trauma were randomly assigned treatment with phenytoin or placebo within 24 hours of injury; significant reduction in seizure incidence (P < 0.001) occurred only between drug loading time and day 7.*

438 SPINAL CORD INJURY

Most injuries to the spinal column do not traumatize the spinal cord, but there are still approximately 35 spinal cord injuries per million Americans each year. In addition to the neurologic deficit that such injuries can produce, they often result in persistent and severe pain and, if not treated properly, bony deformity. The mortality rate of spinal cord injury has fallen to less than 5% and long-term survival is now the rule. Associated with this, however, are tremendous costs stemming from medical treatment, lost occupations, and the need for life-long medical and emotional support systems.

NATURE OF THE INJURY

About half of all serious spinal injuries affect the cervical level, with nearly 50% of such patients becoming quadriplegic. Next most frequent is high thoracic cord damage, with the remainder distributed variously at lower spinal levels. Three major abnormalities damage the tissue: destruction from either direct trauma, e.g., gunshot wounds or secondary bone displacement; compression by displaced or broken bones; and ischemia due to compression or laceration of spinal arteries. Postinjury edema of spinal soft tissues and the cord itself accentuates these changes.

Spinal cord injuries can be categorized as complete or incomplete. Acute, complete injuries most often produce *spinal shock*, with loss of all sensorimotor functions including flaccidity and loss of reflexes at and below the level of injury. A few such cases may involve sustained priapism. Less severe injuries can produce a *central cord syndrome* resulting from ischemia or hematomas of the cervical cord (Fig. 438–1). These result in a syringomyelia-like clinical syndrome characterized by weakness in the distal upper extremities combined with impaired or lost pain and temperature sensations in the arms but sparing of touch and often of all functions below the cervical cord level. The upper extremity weakness generally improves in such cases. Other patterns of cord injury may produce an anterior spinal artery syndrome (see Ch. 443) or a partial hemisection, producing distal weakness and proprioceptive loss ipsilateral to the cord damage accompanied by contralateral pain and temperature impairment.

EMERGENCY MANAGEMENT

For the physician, crucial elements in treatment arise at the accident scene or within the first few hours at the hospital. After that time, experienced neurosurgeons or orthopedists provide care, supplemented if possible by resources of a tertiary care center.

At the site of injury three major concerns are paramount: maintenance of ventilation, protection against shock, and neck immobilization to prevent further spinal cord damage. Damage to high thoracic or cervical spinal levels creates the immediate risk of ventilatory failure due to acute paralysis of intercostal-abdominal muscles, the diaphragm, or both. Untoward movement of the neck risks converting a partial injury to a complete one, making nasotracheal intubation preferable to standard peroral intubation. Tracheostomy or cricothyroidotomy should be avoided if possible because these procedures often put pressure on the vertebral column.

Severe hypotension often follows cervical injury because the lesion interrupts the descending sympathetic pathways; bradycardia characteristically accompanies the low blood pressure. Such neurogenic hypotension can be distinguished from hypovolemic shock by the tachycardia of the latter. In either case, the legs should be elevated gently to improve venous return and fluids delivered in amounts sufficient to counter both the traumatic and neurogenic aspects of the problem. Severe hypotension during the early minutes

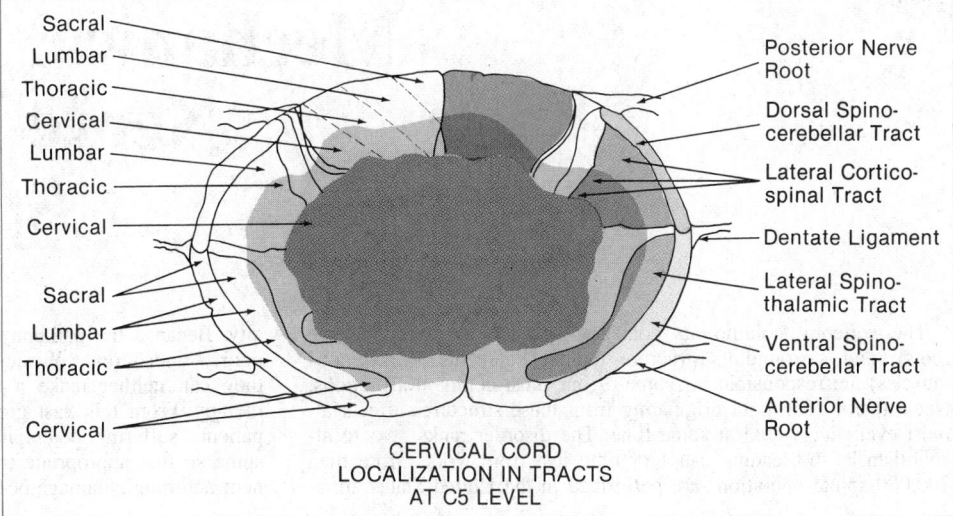

FIGURE 438–1. Diagrammatic description of the spinal pathways at the lower cervical level showing the usual distribution of the contusion-hemorrhage that causes a central cord syndrome.

Sacral
Lumbar
Thoracic
Cervical
Lumbar
Thoracic
Cervical
Sacral
Lumbar
Thoracic
Cervical

Posterior Nerve Root
Dorsal Spinocerebellar Tract
Lateral Corticospinal Tract
Dentate Ligament
Lateral Spinothalamic Tract
Ventral Spinocerebellar Tract
Anterior Nerve Root

CERVICAL CORD LOCALIZATION IN TRACTS AT C5 LEVEL

or hours after injury is itself a potential cause of spinal cord damage.

The neck and spine should be immobilized as gently as possible at the injury site, using a carrying board, sandbags and adhesive tape, or a Philadelphia collar. Soft collars are ineffective. The head is best maintained in a neutral position but should not be forced into such an attitude lest the maneuver induce further spinal cord damage.

Recent controlled studies indicate that giving large doses of methylprednisolone within 8 hours of the onset of trauma appears to reduce the degree of eventual neurologic dysfunction in acute traumatic paraplegia. Dose levels used in the study trial included immediate intravenous administrations of 30 mg per kilogram of body weight of the steroid followed by continuous infusion of 5.4 mg per kilogram per hour for the next 23 hours. Treatment begun more than 8 hours after injury was not helpful.

HOSPITAL CARE

The medical care of spinal cord injuries is a specialty unto itself. Such patients often are critically ill owing to a combination of systemic injuries, blood and fluid loss, various fractures, and infections. Considerable expertise is required for the accurate interpretation of spinal radiographs. The treating physician must not accept as normal plain radiographs that do not demonstrate all of the cervical vertebrae. An overlooked spine injury can be catastrophic if, for example, an odontoid fracture or an injury to C7 results later in sudden instability. Patients with cervical fracture-dislocations usually are placed in skeletal traction with skull fixation prior to administering definitive surgical repair. Injuries to the thoracic or lumbar level are the exception; because traction has little benefit, open surgery, when indicated, usually is carried out earlier.

Medical management emphasizes the guiding principles of trauma care. Rotating beds reduce the risk of decubitus erosions, meticulous chest physiotherapy and pulmonary toilet can minimize lung complications, and cardiovascular as well as fluid-electrolyte stability requires continuous attention. Pneumatic antiembolism stockings, vigorous fluid replacement, and early mobilization have reduced the frequency of deep venous thromboses in such patients by one third. Vena caval filters should be considered for severely immobilized patients who do not require early surgery. Nearly all patients with traumatic cord injury require prolonged urinary bladder catheterization. Meticulous effort to prevent infection should be applied from the start and, whenever staff experience permits, in-dwelling catheters should be replaced by intermittent catheterization at 4- to 6-hour intervals. Acidification of the urine with vitamin C or cranberry juice helps to reduce the incidence of infection.

Trauma patients require heavy nutrition to feed the demands of wound healing and the efforts of rehabilitation. For those who cannot eat, enteral solutions sufficient to meet caloric need can be started within 3 to 4 days after injury. Every effort should be given to supplying appetizing food and vitamins subsequently.

Autonomic dysfunction complicates the convalescence of more than half of patients who suffer severe spinal cord injuries above the midthoracic level. Disconnected distal autonomic pathways can induce a variety of troublesome phenomena, including systemic hypertension, reflex sweating, skin flushing, headache, and painful flexor spasms of the lower extremities. Bladder distention and infection frequently trigger such reflex dysautonomia and require urgent treatment. Diazepam, in small doses initially, and baclofen given chronically may be useful for the treatment of reflex spasms. Some centers have successfully used the continuous intrathecal administration of baclofen by an indwelling pump to prevent such disabling reflex spasms.

PHYSICAL AND OCCUPATIONAL THERAPY AND REHABILITATION

Almost all patients with spinal cord injury require prolonged postacute care. Those with complete transections have suffered a devastating injury with life-long functional and psychiatric consequences. Early physical and emotional therapy are crucial. Early range of motion prevents contractures, diminishes the risk of venous thrombosis, protects the skin, and boosts morale. A comprehensive and individualized management plan is essential. Patients and family members must be counseled in detail about probable changes in lifestyle. All of these features are best carried out in experienced rehabilitation centers that can provide assistance in home modification, driver retraining, and vocational rehabilitation. Depression following an initial period of denial occurs in almost all patients and may be masked by jocularity. If the rehabilitation team moves quickly to provide emotional as well as physical management, many patients with spinal cord injury can return to a competitive place in society. Most of the injured do best if a single physician organizes the long-term aspects of urinary tract management, skin care, sexual problems, and emotional-vocational needs.

Bracken MB, Shepard MJ, Hellenbrand KG, et al.: A randomized, controlled trial of methylprednisolone or naloxone in the treatment of acute spinal cord injury. N Engl J Med 322:1405, 1990. *The first study to clearly demonstrate the efficacy of pharmacologic treatment for spinal cord injury.*

Cooper PR: Management of Posttraumatic Spinal Instability. *In* Neurosurgical Topics. Park Ridge, IL, American Association of Neurological Surgeons, 1990.

Section Fourteen— Mechanical Lesions of Nerve Roots and Spinal Cord

Jerome B. Posner

The vertebral column, its contents (spinal cord, exiting nerve roots), and surrounding structure (spinal ligaments, paraspinous muscles) are responsible for some of our most common afflictions. Neck and/or back pain originating from these structures affects almost every individual at some time. The disorder ranks next to alcoholism as the leading cause of time lost from work. More than 200,000 spinal operations are performed in the United States annually. Because the pathophysiology of most neck and back pain is poorly understood, physicians often encounter patients in whom they can neither make a certain diagnosis nor prescribe rational therapy. From this vast group they must cull the small number of patients suffering potentially remediable structural disease of the spine so that appropriate treatment can be instituted before permanent neurologic damage occurs.

439 ANATOMY, PHYSIOLOGY, AND DIFFERENTIAL DIAGNOSIS

ANATOMY AND PHYSIOLOGY OF THE SPINE

The spine is composed of two functional segments. The *anterior segment* containing two adjacent vertebral bodies separated by an intervertebral disc bears weight and cushions the spine during such activities as walking and running. The posterior segment is composed of the vertebral arches, the transverse processes, the posterior spinous processes, and the paired articulations known as *facets* with the facet joint between them. It protects the contained spinal cord and nerve roots and allows the spine to move in extension and rotation. The midcervical and lower lumbar levels are particularly mobile, making them susceptible to mechanical disorders such as osteoarthritis and herniated discs (see Ch. 440). Several ligaments offer the spine passive support and paravertebral muscles support the spine actively by voluntary and reflex contraction.

The *periosteum* of the vertebral body is pain-sensitive so that compression fractures are at least initially painful (Fig. 439–1). The *intervertebral disc* is probably not pain-sensitive. However, if the disc bulges and compresses the outer layers of the anulus fibrosus or the posterior longitudinal ligament, pain may result. Posteriorly, the synovium-lined *facet joints* are pain-sensitive and may be a source of neck and back pain, although the intraspinal ligaments holding the posterior elements are not. Most of the pain-sensitive structures are innervated by the recurrent meningeal or sinuvertebral nerves, a branch of each spinal nerve that arises just distal to the dorsal root ganglion and re-enters the spinal canal through the intervertebral foramen. The *paravertebral muscles* surrounding and supporting the spine are also pain-sensitive, particularly when overstretched or in spasm. These muscles are probably the most common source of acute neck and back pain. The pain-sensitive *nerve root* usually occupies only a small portion of the intervertebral foramen through which it exits the spinal canal. When the spine is extended (i.e., hyperlordotic posture), the intervertebral foramen becomes smaller, potentially impinging on the nerve root and leading to overlap of the facet joints, giving potential irritation of pain-sensitive synovial membranes.

The spinal cord and its attached motor, sensory, and autonomic nerve roots are the primary occupants of the spinal canal. The spinal cord itself extends in the adult from the first cervical to the first lumbar vertebral body, and the spinal roots continue in the subarachnoid space to the second sacral vertebra. The caudal portion of the spinal cord is called the *conus medullaris,* and the bunched

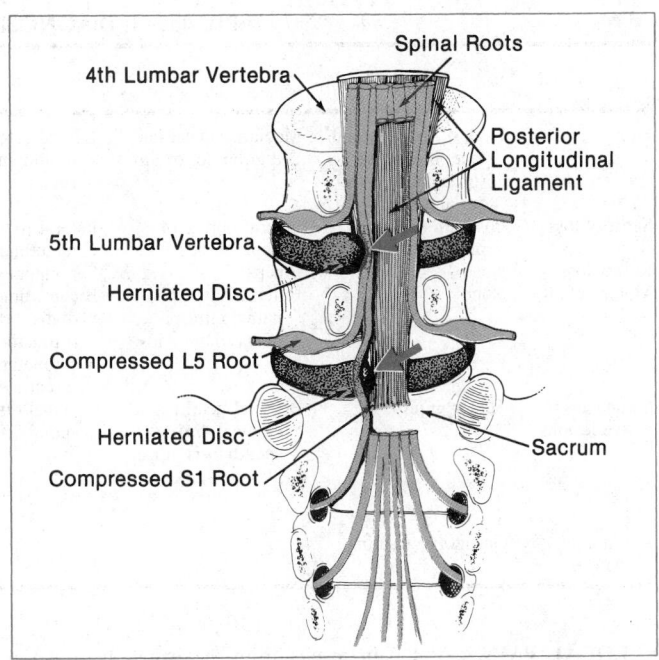

FIGURE 439–2. Nerve root compression by herniated disc. The figure illustrates that the posterior longitudinal ligament tapers as it reaches the lower lumbar area, leaving a weakened area laterally allowing disc herniation. An L4–L5 disc is shown lateral to the L5 root, displacing it medially; a herniated disc between L5 and S1 displaces the root laterally. (From Posner JB: Back pain and epidural spinal cord compression. Med Clin North Am 71:185, 1987.)

lumbar and sacral roots that exit below the cord are the *cauda equina.*

Within the canal several processes can compress or deform the spinal cord and its roots. In the cervical spine, the spinal cord and vertebral segments lie at approximately the same level; thus, the C5 vertebral body marks the C5 spinal segment and emerging nerve roots are virtually horizontal. The more caudad spinal cord segments and vertebral segments move out of alignment so that thoracic spinal cord segments gradually become two to three levels higher than the corresponding vertebral segments. Most of the lumbar and sacral cord is found between T10 and L1 lumbar segments. As a result, the nerve roots travel a descending pathway in the subarachnoid space before exiting via the vertebral foramen. In addition, because there is a C8 spinal segment and no C8 vertebral body, cervical spine nerve roots above C8 exit above the vertebral body with the same number (e.g., the C4 root exits between C3 and C4). Thus, a herniated C4–C5 disc may compress the C5 or C6 root but not the C4 root.

In the thoracic and lumbar spine, nerve roots leave the intervertebral foramen just below the pedicle arising from the vertebra of the same number so that a herniated disc between L4 and L5 vertebral bodies usually compresses the L5 nerve root; a herniated disc between L5 and S1 usually compresses the S1 root (Fig. 439–2). If the disc protrudes medially (less common than laterally protruding discs), an L4–L5 disc may compress sacral roots rather than the L5 lumbar root. Only if the disc completely extrudes into the vertebral canal does an L4–L5 disc compress the L4 root.

The size of the vertebral canal relative to the spinal cord varies from level to level and among individuals. There is generally more space in the lumbar and cervical areas than in the thoracic area. In some individuals the spinal canal is congenitally small (spinal stenosis). Disc herniation or osteoarthritis is more likely to cause myelopathy in these individuals than in those with capacious canals.

TYPES OF PAIN

The cardinal symptom of lesions of the spine or its contents is pain. The type and location of pain often help substantially in diagnosis.

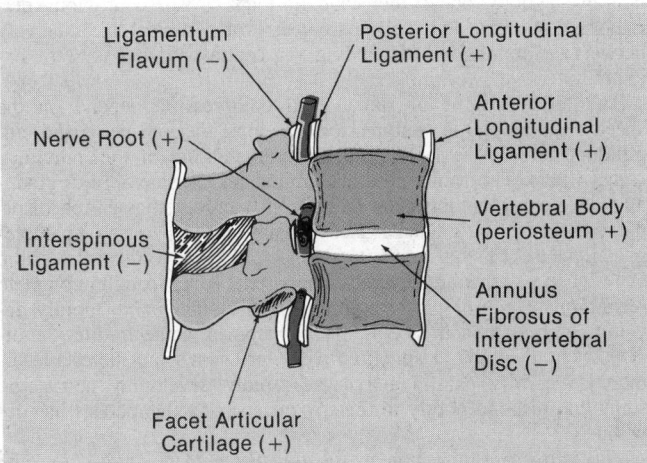

FIGURE 439–1. Pain-sensitive structures of the spine. This lateral view indicates the pain-sensitive structures with a plus sign (+) and those structures not pain-sensitive with a minus sign (−). (From Posner JB: Back pain and epidural spinal cord compression. Med Clin North Am 71:185, 1987.)

TABLE 439-1. DIAGNOSIS OF NERVE ROOT LESIONS

	C2–C3	C5	C6	C7	C8	Nerve T1
Pain	Back of head, lateral face, behind ear (occasionally vertex and orbit)	Medial scapula, lateral border of arm	Lateral forearm, thumb and index finger	Posterior arm, lateral hand, mid-forearm, and medial scapula	Medial forearm and hand	Deep aching in shoulder and axilla to olecranon
Sensory loss	Posterior scalp, pinna, lateral face	Lateral border of upper arm	Lateral forearm, including thumb	Mid-forearm and middle finger	Medial forearm and little finger	Axilla down to olecranon
Reflex loss	None	Biceps	Supinator	Triceps	Finger stretch	None
Motor deficit	None	Deltoid, supraspinatus, infraspinatus, rhomboids	Biceps, brachioradialis, brachialis, (pronators and supinators of forearm)	Latissimus dorsi, pectoralis major, triceps, wrist extensors, wrist flexors	Finger flexors, finger extensors, flexor carpi ulnaris (thenar muscles in some patients)	*All* small hand muscles (in some thenar muscles via C8)
Some causative lesions	Tumor, injury	Brachial neuritis, cervical disc or spondylosis, upper plexus injury	Cervical disc or spondylosis	Cervical disc or spondylosis	Pancoast tumor, rare in disc lesions or spondylosis, metastatic tumor, thoracic outlet syndrome	Pancoast tumor, cervical rib, outlet syndromes, metastatic carcinoma in deep cervical nodes
Autonomic changes	Gustatory sweating					Horner's syndrome

LOCAL PAIN. Local pain results from the irritation of nerve endings at the site of the pathologic process. Metastatic tumors and osteoporotic collapse of a vertebral body cause pain at the site of the lesion by irritation of nerve endings in the periosteum of the vertebral body. Metastatic tumors involving the vertebral body that do not distort the periosteum are usually painless. Intervertebral discs cause local pain when they compress nerve endings in the anulus fibrosus or posterior longitudinal ligament. Local pain is usually steady, aching, and associated with tenderness to palpation or percussion. Most spine pain from mechanical causes (e.g., herniated disc) occurs either in the neck or low back because these structures are most mobile and more subject to injury. Tumors often strike the thoracic area, and osteoporotic vertebral collapse often affects the structurally weaker thoracic vertebral bodies.

The *character* of the local pain is helpful diagnostically. Pain caused by lumbar muscle or ligamentous strain or by herniated disc usually disappears when the patient lies recumbent. The pain of spinal stenosis, on the contrary, is often absent when lying or sitting and occurs only when the patient walks. Vertebral metastases with or without epidural spinal cord compression cause pain that is often more prominent when lying and sometimes is relieved by sitting up; many patients with spinal cord compression elect to sleep in a sitting position. Even if pain is absent in the lying position, movement such as turning over in bed or arising may be particularly painful.

REFERRED PAIN. Referred pain arises from deep somatic or visceral structures and is perceived at a distant site within the same spinal segment but not necessarily in dermatomal distribution (radicular pain, see below). Referred pain, like local pain, has a deep aching quality and is often associated with tenderness of subcutaneous tissues and muscles at the site of referral. Maneuvers that affect local pain usually have the same effect on referred pain. Pain referred from pathologic abnormalities of the cervical spine often is either just medial to the scapula or over the lateral aspect of the arm; pain referred from the low back is usually appreciated in the buttocks and posterior thighs, although rarely below the knees. Pain from the upper lumbar spine is often referred to the flank, groin, and anterior thigh. Pain also can be referred to the spine from lesions of thoracic or abdominal viscera, a prominent example being the back pain from pancreatic carcinoma.

MUSCLE PAIN. Muscle pain occurs when an injury to or structural abnormality of the spine induces paravertebral muscle spasm. Sustained contraction of paravertebral muscles gives rise to chronic aching pain, usually felt lateral to the midline of the neck or back. Palpation may reveal evidence of spasm and tenderness. At times, when areas of extreme sensitivity (trigger points) are palpated, the pain may be felt not only locally in the muscle but also may be referred to distant structures. Trigger points define myofascial pain syndromes, common causes of neck and back pain without structural abnormalities of the spine (see Ch. 405).

RADICULAR PAIN. Radicular pain is the prominent symptom of nerve root compression. Nerve roots are not usually pain-sensitive. However, chronic compression leads to edema and, perhaps, inflammation and demyelination; the root then becomes sensitive to stretching or compression. When compressed, the pain may be experienced only in the cutaneous distribution (dermatome) of the involved root or may be felt locally and deep in muscles that it supplies. Root pain is usually exacerbated by increasing intraspinal pressure by coughing, sneezing, and straining.

FUNICULAR PAIN. Funicular pain is caused by compression of the long tracts of the spinal cord. It is less sharp than radicular pain and often described as a cold, unpleasant sensation in the extremity. It is more diffuse than radicular pain but is usually exacerbated by movements that stretch the cord (neck flexion, straight leg raising) or increase intraspinal pressure.

SIGNS OF NERVE ROOT AND SPINAL CORD DYSFUNCTION

In addition to pain, chronic compression of nerve roots can produce paresthesias, sensory loss, weakness, atrophy, and hyporeflexia in root-supplied areas, thus localizing the lesion. Knowing the myotomal and dermatomal distribution of spinal roots (Table 439–1) often allows one to localize the lesion and suggest its cause: Involvement of a single root is more likely to occur with intervertebral disc herniation (see Ch. 440), whereas multiple root dysfunction is likely to be caused by tumor or chronic inflammation. Myotomal and dermatomal localization must be used cautiously. Not every body obeys the standard maps. Also, contiguous dermatomes overlap, and the apparent size of a dermatome can vary between examinations, depending on central nervous system excitability.

The clinical signs of spinal cord compression depend on the speed with which the compression develops, the transverse and longitudinal site of the lesion, and the vulnerability of the individual spinal fibers. The spinal cord accommodates considerably to gradually developing compression (e.g., from meningiomas); such disorders can cause the gradual onset of painless paraparesis or paraplegia. Because of this accommodation, subsequent decompression, even when patients are severely paraparetic, often leads to complete resolution of neurologic symptoms. On the other hand, rapidly developing lesions such as epidural hematomas, acute midline herniated discs, or epidural spinal cord compression from metastatic tumor are usually painful and cause rapidly developing neurologic signs that respond poorly to therapy once severe paraparesis has developed.

The site of compression in the transverse plane may determine clinical signs. Laterally located lesions compressing one side of the spinal cord may cause the Brown-Séquard syndrome (ipsilateral hemiparesis, vibration and position sense loss, with contralateral pain and temperature loss); compression of the posterior portion of the cord may cause bilateral position and vibratory loss, with

TABLE 439–1. DIAGNOSIS OF NERVE ROOT LESIONS Continued

Roots T4	T10	L2	L3	L4	L5	S1	S2–S4
Anterior chest and/or upper back	Midback and/or anterior abdomen	Across thigh	Across thigh	Down to medial malleolus	Back of thigh, lateral calf, dorsum of foot	Back of thigh, back of calf, lateral foot	Buttocks, genitalia, back of thigh
Usually none (upper back and chest at nipple level)	Usually none (midback and abdomen at umbilicus level)	Often none	Often none	Medial leg	Dorsum of foot	Behind lateral malleolus	Buttocks, genitalia
None	Decreased abdominal reflex	None	Adductor reflex	Knee jerk	None	Ankle jerk	Bulbocavernosus
Not discernible	None	Hip flexion, adduction of thigh	Knee extension, adduction of thigh	Inversion of foot	Dorsiflexion of toes and foot (latter L4 also)	Plantar flexion and eversion of foot	Bladder and bowel
Intravertebral or paravertebral tumor, herpes zoster	Intravertebral and paravertebral tumor, herpes zoster	Neurofibroma, meningioma, neoplastic disease; disc lesions very rare except at L4 <5%			Disc lesions, metastatic malignancy, neurofibromas, meningioma		Tumor, midline disc
Chest wall, piloerection, hyperhidrosis, unilateral gynecomastia, galactorrhea	Chest wall, piloerection, hyperhidrosis, retrograde ejaculation	Alterations in temperature and color of all or parts of the leg or thigh					Incontinence, impotence, urinary retention

preservation of pain and temperature sensation and of motor power. However, most lesions twist the cord as they compress it and also interfere with the vascular supply to sites beyond the compression. Accordingly, one can depend only in a general way on the neurologic signs to evaluate the exact transverse site of compression. Cervical lesions cause quadriplegia; thoracic lesions, paraplegia; and upper lumbar lesions, normal motor function with bowel and bladder dysfunction and extensor plantar responses (conus medullaris syndrome). Lesions below the first lumbar vertebral body compress the cauda equina, causing loss of bowel and bladder function with lower motor neuron leg weakness and normal plantar reflexes.

The corticospinal tracts and posterior columns are more vulnerable to compression than others. As a result, weakness, spasticity, and reflex hyperactivity tend to be the earliest signs of spinal cord compression, with paresthesias, and vibratory and position sense loss occurring soon thereafter. Loss of pain and temperature sensation and of bladder and bowel function usually occur late.

APPROACH TO THE PATIENT

Most mechanical lesions of the spine and its contents begin with pain and only later cause other neurologic dysfunction. There are many causes of neck or back pain. One survey listed over 100 causes (Table 439–2). The task for the physician is to separate potentially serious disease from more common causes of back pain.

HISTORY. The diagnostic evaluation begins with the history. Most spine pain begins acutely or subacutely and often follows, by minutes to hours, some unaccustomed physical activity, particularly lifting or bending. Patients may awaken stiff and sore in the morning or may develop acute back pain on arising without any obvious precipitating event. Most neck pain begins as a stiff neck, often on awakening, without a history of unusual activity. In many patients, neck or low back pain recurs episodically over many years. Most neck or back pain is dull and aching in quality, exacerbated by movement and relieved by rest. Pain that is present when the patient is immobile and cannot be relieved by positional manipulation should lead the physician to consider a more serious disorder (e.g., tumor or extruded disc). *Radicular pain,* particularly if accompanied by paresthesias or loss of sensation, indicates mechanical compression of the nerve root supplying that dermatome and implies identifiable structural disease (e.g., herniated disc). *Referred pain* does not imply compression of a root.

EXAMINATION. Special attention should be paid to mobility of the spine and paravertebral structures. Most patients who complain of a stiff neck have some limitation of movement of the cervical spine, but if gradual movement of the cervical spine causes intense

pain, if pain on neck flexion is referred to the thoracic or lumbar area, or if neck flexion causes paresthesias radiating into the arms, legs, or back (Lhermitte's sign), spinal cord compression should be suspected. Most low back pain not caused by a herniated disc is exacerbated by flexion and relieved by lying down. The paravertebral muscles are often in spasm, and tender to palpation and straighten the normally lordotic lumbar spine. Almost any severe low back pain, particularly if it radiates into a lower extremity, can increase when the extended leg is raised from the bed (straight leg raising sign). However, pain referred to the contralateral back or leg when the nonpainful leg is raised (crossed straight leg raising) implies

TABLE 439–2. SOME CAUSES OF BACK PAIN

Common Causes
  Degenerative disorders
    Osteoarthritis, facet syndrome
    Herniated disc
    Spinal stenosis
    Nerve root entrapment
  Muscle dysfunction
    Spasms, fatigue, fibromyalgia, and myofascial pain
  Psychosomatic (e.g., stress, conversion reaction, tension states)
  Trauma
    Lumbar strain (acute or chronic)
Less Common Causes
  Congenital disorders
    Facet tropism (asymmetry)
    Transitional vertebra
    Spondylolysis and spondylolisthesis
  Infections (e.g., disc space infection, tuberculosis, epidural and subdural abscess, herpes zoster, meningitis, sacroiliac joint infection)
  Inflammatory diseases (e.g., ankylosing spondylitis, arachnoiditis, rheumatoid arthritis)
  Metabolic disorders (e.g., osteoporosis, gout, diabetic neuropathy, Paget's disease)
  Postoperative (e.g., sequelae of scar formation, arachnoiditis)
  Scoliosis (e.g., idiopathic, postparalytic, aging)
  Trauma
    Lumbosacral, sacroiliac strain
    Compression fracture (vertebral body or transverse process)
  Dislocation or subluxation
  Tumors
    Benign bone and neural tumors (e.g., neurinoma, ependymoma, meningioma, osteoid osteoma, hemangioma, osteoblastoma)
    Malignant bone and neural tumors
      Primary (e.g., multiple myeloma, osteosarcoma)
      Secondary (metastases)
  Visceral disease (e.g., visceral inflammation, female pelvic pathology, retroperitoneal pathology, aortic aneurysm, prostatic disease)

root compression. Forced extension of the hip (reverse straight leg raising) can elicit pain from upper lumbar root disease (L4 and above). Point tenderness over a spinous process raises the suspicion of involvement of the vertebra by either tumor or infection.

The neurologic examination is important. Sensory loss, reflex diminution, and weakness all suggest neurologic disease that requires further evaluation. The distribution of abnormalities localizes the lesion. Patients in severe pain may be reluctant to move the painful part, making normal muscles appear weak. Likewise, guarding can affect deep tendon reflexes, either increasing or decreasing them with respect to the normal side. Clear and reproducible neurologic signs, particularly sensory loss in a dermatomal distribution or a diminished stretch reflex, imply root compression.

Careful examination can reveal inconsistencies (e.g., leg pain on straight leg raising that appears when the patient is recumbent but not when sitting) that suggest a psychological rather than a physiologic basis.

LABORATORY AIDS TO INVESTIGATION. For most patients with back or neck pain, laboratory tests are neither required nor helpful. Plain radiographs of the spine rarely reveal clinically unsuspected findings. Radiographic examination of neck or back should be undertaken only when the history and examination suggest specific findings (e.g., fracture or dislocation). If the clinical examination points to other significant disease of the neck or back (e.g., herniated disc) and if pain does not respond to conservative measures in a few weeks, the physician should proceed directly to MRI, which can identify all elements of the spinal column and its contents in multiple planes. Patients suspected of harboring tumors, infection, or vascular disease should be imaged without delay.

The only abnormalities not easily identified by MRI are subluxations of vertebral bodies with movement. Flexion and extension plain radiographs of the neck or back settle that issue. Images of the neck and back must be interpreted with caution because degenerative disc changes are frequently found in asymptomatic patients and increase with age. MRI, even though more expensive than CT and *radionuclide bone scan,* is so much more sensitive that it will probably replace these tests. Invasive tests, such as *myelograms, spinal angiography,* and *discography,* should be reserved for specialists. Thermography has no value.

Electromyography and nerve conduction studies, particularly using H and F responses, can help identify the presence and site of proximal sensory and motor root damage and anterior horn cell dysfunction. *Somatosensory evoked potentials* can be recorded along the spinal cord or in the brain after a peripheral nerve is stimulated and can sometimes identify the approximate site of a spinal cord lesion (see Ch. 392.2).

MANAGEMENT OF THE PATIENT WITH NECK AND BACK PAIN. If no clinical findings suggest serious structural disease of the spine, nerve roots, or spinal cord, patients should be treated as if they suffered from an acute neck or back strain, without further diagnostic evaluation. For severe pain, the best treatment probably consists of 2 to 3 days bed rest on a firmly supported mattress in the position most comfortable. The best position for low back pain is usually semi-Fowler's position (head slightly elevated with pillows under the knees). For neck pain use a cervical pillow that maintains the normal lordotic curve rather than flexes the neck as regular pillows do. A soft cervical collar may be as effective in immobilizing the neck as bed rest. Bed rest may be combined with analgesic agents (usually aspirin or acetaminophen) and with local heat. Patients should be encouraged to stay recumbent except to go to the toilet until pain diminishes. As pain subsides, patients should gradually ambulate and begin gentle stretching and strengthening exercises. Other treatment modalities, including traction, procaine or saline injection into trigger points, transcutaneous stimulation, and spinal manipulation, are not more efficacious than the regimen described above. One recent study suggests that chiropractic manipulation of the back produces more rapid and prolonged relief of nonsciatic low back pain than does physical therapy with or without manipulation. Manipulation of the neck is potentially dangerous, however, because it can occlude the vertebral arteries as they enter the skull. A recent randomized study of patients with acute, nonspecific low back pain suggests that maintaining ordinary activity leads to faster recovery than either bed rest or back-mobilizing exercises.

Using standard therapy, 70 to 80% of patients become free of pain and able to return to full activity within a 4-week period. During the period of rest, repeated physical and neurologic examinations are unwise because vigorous movement can exacerbate pain and delay improvement. A small minority of patients continue to have chronic pain, and they, along with those whose initial examination has suggested more serious disease, need further evaluation.

Deyo RA, Rainville J, Kent DL: What can the history and physical examination tell us about low back pain? JAMA 268:760, 1992. *How to approach a patient with back pain.*
LaRocca H: A taxonomy of chronic pain syndromes: 1991 Presidential Address, Cervical Spine Research Society Annual Meeting, December 5, 1991. Spine 17(105):S344, 1992. *The entire supplement discusses diseases of the cervical spine.*
Malmivaara A, Häkkinen U, Aro T, et al.: The treatment of acute low back pain—Bed rest, exercises, or ordinary activity? N Engl J Med 332:351, 1995.
Nachemson AL (ed.): Newest knowledge of low back pain. Solutions in sight. *In* Clinical Orthopaedics and Related Research, #279. Philadelphia, JB Lippincott, 1992, p 2. *Extensive discussion of acute and chronic low back pain and its management.*
Shekelle PG, Adams AH, Chassin MR, et al.: Spinal manipulation for low-back pain. Ann Intern Med 117:590, 1992. *May help in acute low back pain.*

440 INTERVERTEBRAL DISC DISEASE

HERNIATED DISC. Herniated intervertebral discs are the most common cause of neck or low back pain associated with a clearly defined structural abnormality. Lumbar and cervical strain and myofascial pain syndromes (see Ch. 439) are more common but not marked by clear pathologic abnormalities. Between each two vertebral bodies is a fibrocartilaginous intervertebral disc. The disc consists of a soft inner nucleus pulposus (a remnant of the notochord) surrounded by thicker fibrous tissue (the anulus fibrosus). The gelatinous nucleus pulposus acts as a shock absorber between adjacent vertebral bodies. With advancing age, the nucleus loses fluid, volume, and resiliency, and the disc structure becomes more susceptible to trauma and compression. Tears develop in the anulus as a result of repeated minor trauma, and eventually, if they enlarge, a portion of the soft nucleus pulposus herniates. When disc material herniates into the vertebral canal, it can compress nerve endings and nerve roots, causing pain and other symptoms. Generally, the disc herniates lateral to the posterior longitudinal ligament, thus compressing spinal roots as they enter the intervertebral foramen. Occasionally the disc herniates more centrally, compressing either the spinal cord in the cervical or thoracic area or the cauda equina in the lumbar area. The term *herniated disc* refers to a disc that maintains continuity with the nucleus pulposus; extruded disc refers to a free fragment within the spinal canal. The signs and symptoms of herniated discs are caused by compression of either nerve roots or the spinal cord. The specific signs and symptoms depend in part on whether the predominant compression is spinal cord or nerve root, and in part on the level at which the neural structures are compressed (see Ch. 439). The most common sites of lumbar disc herniation are between L4 and L5 and L5 and S1, compressing the L5 and S1 roots, respectively. L3–L4 herniations are less common. In the cervical area, the common herniations occur between C5 and C6 (C6 root) and, especially, C6 and C7 (C7 root). Less commonly, herniations appear between C3 and C4, C4 and C5, and C7 and T1. Thoracic disc herniations are uncommon but can cause severe myelopathy because the thoracic area is the narrowest of the entire vertebral canal and the cord has a relatively poor vascular system. Although clinical localization in diagnosis of disc disease is usually quite accurate, an extruded disc fragment sometimes may be large enough to affect several roots or may migrate from the disc space in which it herniated, to cause signs at a distance.

The most common symptom of a herniated disc is pain. Local pain is felt as a dull aching in the neck or back, with an associated stiffness of those structures, frequently occurring episodically in response to minor trauma (or no discernible trauma at all) months or years prior to the development of radicular pain. Radicular pain may occasionally be the first sign of disc disease but is more likely to follow repeated bouts of local pain. Radicular pain is generally sudden in onset, often following minor trauma such as a twist, turn, or unusual bend. Radicular pain is perceived as sharp and well localized and may radiate from the back along the entire distribution of the involved root or affect only a portion of the dermatome. Both local and radicular pain have the characteristics of being exacerbated by activity and relieved by rest.

With cervical disc herniation, most patients hold their necks stiffly and resist passive movement. Lateral bending either to or away from the side of the herniated disc frequently exacerbates both the local and radicular pain. The patient may be more comfortable with the neck slightly flexed but usually prefers the recumbent position. Patients with lumbar disc disease are most comfortable lying, most uncomfortable sitting, and a little less uncomfortable standing. The back is held stiffly, so that the normal lumbar lordotic curve disappears; pain is usually exacerbated by extension of the back. Slow forward bending sometimes relieves the pain. Muscle spasm is prominent with both cervical and lumbar disc disease. Raising the intraspinal pressure, as by coughing, sneezing, or straining, increases the pain sharply. Stretching the compressed root also aggravates the pain. In the upper extremities, extending the arm and laterally flexing the neck to the opposite side sometimes reproduces radicular pain. In the lower extremities, raising the extended leg with the patient recumbent frequently reproduces the pain of an L5 or S1 radiculopathy and, if the pain is felt when the opposite leg is raised (crossed straight leg raising), the sign is highly reliable. Symptoms of L4 radiculopathy can often be reproduced by extending the hip (stretching the femoral nerve) when the patient is lying in the prone position. Often tenderness is present along the entire distribution of the nerve(s) supplied by the compressed root as well as in muscles supplied by the root. In patients with cervical disc disease, palpation or light percussion of the brachial plexus and the supraclavicular fossa or axilla often causes pain. In patients with lumbar disc disease, palpation over the femoral nerve (L4) in the groin or over the sciatic nerve (L5–S1) in the calf, thigh, or buttocks often causes severe pain. Occasionally tenderness in the calf (the posterior tibial nerve) is so striking as to suggest that the patient is suffering from thrombophlebitis rather than disc herniation. Other neurologic signs that commonly accompany disc disease include paresthesias and sensory loss in the distribution of the involved root and motor weakness in the myotome supplied by that root. The most important single sign is a diminished or absent reflex, giving objectively verifiable evidence of neurologic disease.

If an intervertebral disc herniates medially rather than laterally, it may spare the root and involve the spinal cord directly. When this occurs, there may be little or no pain or pain in a bilateral radicular distribution. Sometimes the pain is felt at a site far distant from the disc herniation as a result of compression of long sensory tracts in the spinal cord (funicular pain). The signs and symptoms of cord involvement are the same as those of compression of the spinal cord by other mass lesions. In contradistinction to diseases that arise within the spinal cord itself, compressive lesions tend to spare bladder and bowel function until late. (The exception is when the compression occurs either at the conus medullaris or in the cauda equina.)

The diagnosis of herniated disc is deduced from the characteristic clinical symptoms and findings. In many patients with radiculopathy, findings are minimal and the history must establish the diagnosis. When the patient complains of back pain, with or without a radicular component, but has no motor, sensory, or reflex changes to suggest the site of a radiculopathy, the differential diagnosis includes pain arising from pain-sensitive nerve endings in the muscles, ligaments, and joints of the vertebral bodies and the paravertebral structures. These structures must be examined carefully to determine which of them is responsible. MRI is helpful (see Ch. 439).

Controversy surrounds the management of herniated discs. Most physicians believe that the first step is bed rest. Some have reported that adrenocorticosteroids, either taken orally or injected into the epidural space, may hasten resolution of pain and other symptoms. No controlled studies support this recommendation. Steroids injected into the epidural or subarachnoid space are contraindicated and may produce severe inflammatory reactions. Surgery is indicated when (1) bed rest fails, and the patient is incapacitated by severe, intractable pain; (2) a centrally placed lumbar disc compresses the cauda equina, producing urinary dysfunction; (3) motor weakness (e.g., foot drop) is severe and gets worse on bed rest; or (4)

acute cervical or thoracic discs cause substantial myelopathy. The best operation removes the involved disc, leaving as much bone as possible intact. Fusion of the lumbar spine is rarely indicated. Lumbar disc operations are done posteriorly via a laminotomy. Cervical disc operations may be done either posteriorly to decompress the cord or anteriorly across the neck to remove the disc without disturbing posterior bony elements. The surgical approach for myelopathy should probably be anterior if the disc is in the cervical area and lateral if the disc is in the thoracic area.

SPONDYLOSIS. Spondylosis is a term applied to chronic degenerative disease of intervertebral discs associated with reactive changes in the adjacent vertebral bodies. Spondylotic changes in the neck and low back increase with age and are almost invariably present in the elderly. Spondylosis is usually asymptomatic except when the reactive tissue compresses a nerve root or the spinal cord. When this occurs, the signs and symptoms are similar to those of herniated disc disease, but the onset is less abrupt and the treatment often more difficult. In both the cervical and lumbar areas, spondylosis is more likely to cause spinal cord or cauda equina symptoms if the sagittal diameter of the spinal canal is congenitally narrow.

Cervical Spondylosis. Most patients suffer either radiculopathy or myelopathy, but not both. Pain is common but usually less acute and severe than with herniated discs. Even muscle spasm may be absent. However, the vertebral degenerative changes in the neck lead to limitation of movement in all directions. The classic picture of cervical spondylotic myelopathy is one of little or no pain but slowly developing weakness, atrophy, and fasciculations in the upper extremities, particularly the small muscles of the hand, accompanied by spastic paraparesis with decreased proprioception in the legs. At first the findings may suggest a diagnosis of amyotrophic lateral sclerosis. However, in cervical spondylosis there are sensory changes, particularly vibration loss in the lower extremities, and in amyotrophic lateral sclerosis fasciculations are found outside of cervical segments. The differential diagnosis also includes other compressive lesions of root and spinal cord as well as chronic multiple sclerosis.

The diagnosis of cervical spondylitic myelopathy is established with MRI, which accurately delineates the size of the cervical canal and the site of spinal cord and/or root compression.

The natural history of cervical myelopathy and radiculopathy varies. Many patients experience long periods of pain relief and remission or stabilization of neurologic symptoms, making it difficult to evaluate the effect of a particular treatment. Many physicians prefer, once having established the diagnosis, to begin conservative treatment with a brief period of bed rest accompanied by cervical traction and stabilization of the neck with a soft collar. If collar and traction are successful, they should be continued. However, if the patient develops progressive neurologic signs in the face of conservative treatment, surgical therapy is indicated. Most neurosurgeons believe that if the spinal cord compression occurs at one or two segments, anterior removal of the disc material with spinal fusion is the preferred course. If more than a few segments are involved, laminectomy with foraminotomy is preferred.

In some patients with cervical spondylosis (or with congenital narrowing of the cervical spinal canal, or both), neurologic symptoms are exacerbated by exercise, with pain, numbness, and weakness appearing when a particular extremity is exercised. The pathogenesis is thought to be compression of the spinal cord so severe that the blood supply to the area cannot increase during its activity, leading to ischemia of cord and root structures (pseudoclaudication).

Lumbar Spondylosis. Most of the considerations described above apply. The symptoms of lumbar spondylosis are similar to those of herniated disc, often occurring at multiple levels. One outstanding difference is the frequent presence of *pseudoclaudication* from cauda equina compression in patients with spinal stenosis due to either spondylosis or congenital narrowing. Typically, symptoms and signs are evoked or accentuated by walking and include pain, paresthesias, and weakness in the lower extremities. All of the symptoms may disappear when the patient ceases walking, even though he remains in the standing position. At times, however, the symptoms may be exacerbated by prolonged standing and relieved only by sitting or lying down. Pseudoclaudication of the cauda equina may be distinguished from intermittent vascular claudication in several ways: in vascular disease, the pulses in the lower extremities are usually absent or become absent as exercise begins. Also, the symptoms are usually reproducible and stereotypic; i.e., the patient can predict the exact distance he can walk at a given speed before symptoms develop. Symptoms of cauda equina pseudoclaudication are less stereotypic, so that on some days patients can walk much longer distances than on others. The reason for this variability is not known. In patients with pseudoclaudication, the narrowed lumbar canal is easily measured by MRI. With severe lumbar stenosis, conservative treatment usually fails, and decompressive laminectomy is the treatment of choice.

OTHER CAUSES OF BACK AND NECK PAIN. Several common pathophysiologically poorly understood disorders that cause pain in the back or neck can be confused with intravertebral disc disease or cervical or lumbar spondylosis. These include pain arising in lumbosacral, sacroiliac, or zygapophyseal joints or pain that arises in adjacent supporting structures, including muscle. These disorders usually cause chronic aching local pain that, when severe, may be referred to distant sites. Typical radicular pain never occurs. As a group, the diagnosis is usually suspected by finding tenderness at a specific muscle site or limitation of motion in a specific joint. The diagnosis is supported by a lidocaine block, which should completely relieve the pain if the presumptive diagnosis is correct.

The *facet syndrome* is believed to result from osteoarthritis or trauma of the zygapophyseal joints or their synovial membranes. In the low back it is characterized by pain in the back, buttocks, and thighs. It is often relieved by flexion and aggravated by extension of the spine and frequently accentuated by rest and relieved by movement. Characteristically the area is stiff and painful in the morning and improves somewhat as the day wears on. There is tenderness to palpation of the joint. Anesthetic blocks of the joint relieve both the local and referred pain. Similar chronic pain may have its origin in the lumbosacral or sacroiliac joints.

Musculoskeletal pain is also a common but poorly understood cause of low back and probably neck pain. In patients with painful muscle spasm the normal lordotic curve is usually straightened and tight, and tender muscles can be palpated by the examiner. Local anesthetic blocks, followed by gentle mobilization, usually relieve the spasm and the pain. Prolonged contraction of muscles, such as results from sustained posture or psychological stress, may produce similar pain and tenderness. Fibromyalgia and myofascial pain syndromes often affect the neck and back. They are discussed in Ch. 405.

Braakman R: Management of cervical spondylotic myelopathy and radiculopathy [editorial]. J Neurol Neurosurg Psychiatry 57:257, 1994. *A review of clinical findings and treatment.*

Kanner RM: Low back pain. Semin Neurol 14:272, 1994. *A nice description of management of patients with pain from disc disease and other causes of low back pain.*

Wall PD, Melzack R (eds.): Textbook of Pain. London, Churchill Livingstone, 1994. *A compendium of basic, clinical, and therapeutic aspects of most pain syndromes, including disc disease.*

441 NEOPLASMS OF THE SPINAL CANAL

Neoplastic growths that cause nerve root or spinal cord compression can be paravertebral, extradural, intradural, or intramedullary (Fig. 441–1). Most of those causing spinal cord compression are extradural and metastatic. Extradural neoplasms originate in the vertebral body surrounding the spinal cord and compress spinal roots or cord without invading them. Intradural neoplasms also cause symptoms by compressing spinal roots or cord without invading, but unlike extradural neoplasms the majority are benign and slow growing. Intramedullary neoplasms cause symptoms both by invading and by compressing spinal structures; the tumors may be either benign or malignant.

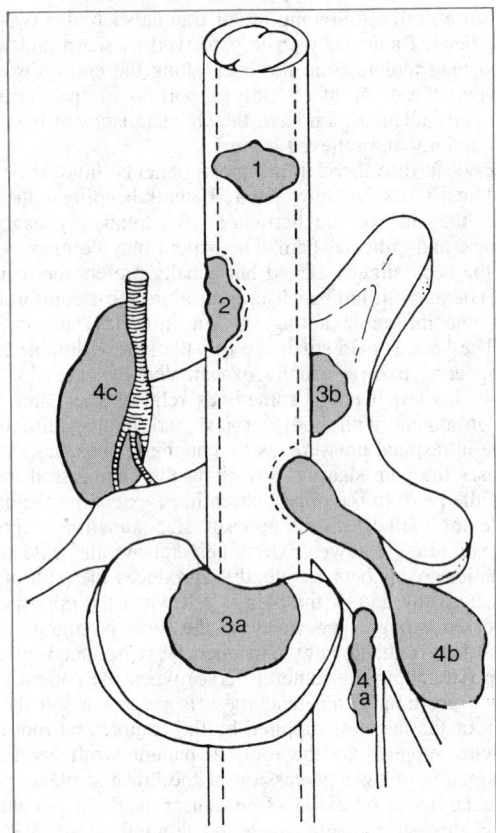

FIGURE 441–1. Pathophysiology of myelopathy caused by neoplasms. 1, The tumor may arise in or metastasize hematogenously to the substance of the spinal cord (intramedullary). 2, The tumor may be extraparenchymal but intradural. 3, The tumor may be extradural, extending either from the vertebral body (3a) or from a spinous process (3b), and cause symptoms by compressing the spinal cord. 4, The tumor may originate in or spread to the paravertebral space and produce its symptoms either by (4a) invading nerve roots, (4b) invading the epidural or subdural space through the intervertebral foramen, or (4c) compressing radicular arteries to cause spinal cord ischemia. (From Andreoli TE, Carpenter CCJ, Plum F, Smith LH Jr [eds.]: Cecil Essentials of Medicine. Philadelphia, WB Saunders, 1986.)

PARAVERTEBRAL TUMORS. Neoplastic lesions that begin in or metastasize to the paravertebral space often cause serious and perplexing neurologic problems. The tumor may extend longitudinally within the paravertebral space, progressively compressing or invading nerve roots. At times, such tumors grow through an intervertebral foramen and compress not only the nerve root but also the spinal cord. Rarely, spinal cord symptoms may be caused by paravertebral tumors compromising radicular arteries that supply the spinal cord. If the tumor is more lateral than the immediate paravertebral space, the brachial, lumbar, or sacral plexus may be compressed, causing symptoms similar to root compression but with a different pattern of sensory and motor loss. The symptoms of extravertebral tumor begin insidiously with severe, unremitting pain, often with a burning quality localized just lateral to the spine and radiating in a bandlike pattern in the distribution of the involved dermatome(s). If the lesion involves abdominal or thoracic roots, motor and sensory changes are usually not appreciated by either the patient or the examiner. Autonomic changes may be a prominent or the only neurologic sign. Hyperhidrosis occurring in a band coinciding with the site of the pain strongly suggests the diagnosis. When the tumor involves cervical or lumbar roots, the pain may be soon followed by numbness in fingertips or toes, with accompanying weakness and reflex diminution, depending on the roots involved. Autonomic changes, including anhidrosis or hyperhidrosis, may affect the arm or leg. Horner's syndrome or diaphragmatic paralysis often accompanies cervical or upper thoracic paravertebral tumors. The diagnosis is best established by MR scans of the level suggested by the clinical findings. The scans can also determine whether the lesion has grown through the intervertebral foramen or has eroded vertebral bodies.

The differential diagnosis of paravertebral tumor includes disorders that cause paravertebral pain with or without compression of nerve roots. *Myofascial pain syndromes* cause low back or neck paravertebral pain with referred pain into arms or legs. On examination one often finds an area of exquisite muscle tenderness on a taut band of muscle. Relief of pain often can be produced by injecting the trigger point with saline solution or a local anesthetic. Temporary relief of pain after such injection does not imply that structural disease is absent; the trigger points may be a reaction to spinal or nerve root disease. In myofascial syndromes, autonomic, sensory, or motor changes are not usually present. Disease of kidneys and other viscera lying in the retroperitoneal space may cause aching pain similar to that of paravertebral tumors, but usually not radiating or associated with autonomic, motor, or sensory changes. Percussion of the involved viscera reproduces the pain that is described as a dull ache rather than a neurogenic burning pain. Chronic pain after a thoracotomy *(post-thoracotomy pain)* probably results from entrapment of nerve roots at the time of surgery, perhaps with neuroma formation. Such pains can sometimes be relieved by paravertebral anesthetic blocks.

The management of paravertebral masses depends on the diagnosis. In patients known to have cancer, particularly lymphomas or carcinomas of the breast or lung, the tumor can be assumed to be metastatic and should be treated with radiation therapy and, if available, chemotherapy. If the patient has no history of cancer, a biopsy is required and, depending on the site of the lesion, resection may be attempted both to establish a diagnosis and to decompress the nerve roots. Once the diagnosis is established by biopsy, further therapy such as radiation or chemotherapy may be indicated.

EXTRADURAL TUMORS. Extradural neoplasms compress spinal roots and cord in one of three ways. Either they arise in vertebrae surrounding the spinal cord and grow into the epidural space or they arise in the paravertebral space and grow through the intervertebral foramen to compress the cord laterally. Rarely, tumors may arise in the epidural space itself, without involving either vertebral or paravertebral structures. Most extradural neoplasms are metastatic (e.g., carcinomas of the breast, lung, prostate, or kidney). Some extradural neoplasms arise *de novo* in the vertebral bodies (e.g., chordoma, osteogenic sarcoma, myeloma, chondrosarcoma). A minority of extradural neoplasms are benign (e.g., osteoma, osteoid osteoma, angioma). Because extradural neoplasms usually destroy bone before causing spinal cord compression, local pain is the first symptom and may precede either radicular pain or other symptoms of spinal cord compression by weeks or months. Rarely the first symptoms may be spinal cord dysfunction. As with other causes of spinal cord compression, extradural neoplasms cause symptoms first distally and later proximally. Thus, even thoracic and cervical neoplasms generally cause weakness and numbness in the legs before trunk and upper extremity muscles are involved. The diagnosis of extradural spinal cord compression must be suspected by the history of pain followed by signs and symptoms of spinal cord dysfunction and confirmed by radiographic study. About 85% of patients suffering from extradural spinal cord compression have bone lesions at the site of compression on plain radiographs. MRI establishes the site and degree of spinal cord compression.

The differential diagnosis of extradural neoplasms includes inflammatory disease of bone and epidural abscess (e.g., vertebral tuberculosis, bacterial osteomyelitis), acute or subacute epidural hematomas, herniated intervertebral discs, spondylosis, and, very rarely, extramedullary hematopoiesis (in patients with severe and chronic anemias) or epidural lipomatosis (in patients on chronic steroid therapy). MRI often distinguishes those from tumor, but sometimes definitive diagnosis requires biopsy of the lesion either via decompressive laminectomy or by percutaneous needle biopsy.

The treatment of extradural neoplasms depends on the cause. Most neoplasms that cause extradural spinal cord compression are malignant and progress rapidly. Once spinal cord symptoms begin, paraplegia may develop in hours to days. Paraplegia is usually irreversible, whereas treatment often can correct mild to moderate spinal cord dysfunction. Thus, early diagnosis and effective emergency treatment of extradural spinal cord compression are mandatory. The treatment of patients known to be suffering from cancer who develop signs and symptoms of spinal cord compression from extradural metastases is radiation therapy. Therapy should begin with corticosteroids (dexamethasone, 16 to 100 mg daily) to decrease spinal cord edema, followed immediately by radiation ther-

apy. If effective chemotherapeutic agents are available, they should be used in conjunction with steroids and radiation therapy. In patients not known to be suffering from a primary cancer, metastatic disease is the most common cause of extradural spinal cord compression, but definitive diagnosis must be made by biopsy. Such patients should begin corticosteroid therapy followed by surgery with removal of as much tumor as possible for diagnostic and therapeutic purposes. If a malignant neoplasm is encountered, radiation therapy should begin as soon after the surgery as is practical. In a few patients in whom radiation therapy and chemotherapy are ineffective, resection of the vertebral body involved by tumor may delay or prevent the development of paraplegia. Benign extradural tumors require surgery.

INTRADURAL EXTRAMEDULLARY TUMORS. Most intradural tumors are benign. Meningiomas and neurofibromas are the two most common types. Teratomas, arachnoid cysts, and lipomas are less common. *Meningiomas* occur in middle-aged and elderly women, predominantly in the thoracic region. Another common site is at the foramen magnum. Meningiomas are benign, slow growing, and usually located on the posterior aspect of the spinal cord. Pain is usually the first symptom, but in about 25% the meningioma is painless, the first symptoms being those of spinal cord compression. Paresthesias and sensory changes beginning distally in the lower extremities are a frequent early symptom and are often mistaken for peripheral neuropathy. As the disease progresses, however, corticospinal tract signs betray the spinal origin. Even when spinal cord signs and symptoms are obvious, the lack of pain may lead one to suspect a degenerative or demyelinating disease such as multiple sclerosis rather than a neoplasm. MRI with contrast enhancement usually is diagnostic. The treatment of spinal cord meningiomas is surgical removal.

The second common cause of intradural spinal cord compression is *neurofibroma*. Because these tumors usually arise from the dorsal root, radicular pain is often the first symptom, preceding signs of spinal cord compression by months or years. When spinal cord compression develops, it progresses slowly. Some patients with spinal neurofibroma suffer from neurofibromatosis. That diagnosis may be suspected either by a positive family history or by the cutaneous stigmata of the disease. A neurofibroma may extend on either side of the intervertebral foramen, involving the root both in the paravertebral space and within the spinal canal. The cerebrospinal fluid protein is almost always elevated. The diagnosis is established by MRI. Surgical extirpation of the lesion usually leads to complete recovery.

Occasionally *metastatic tumors* involving the leptomeninges present with intradural mass lesions. Pain is almost always prominent, and spinal cord compression develops more rapidly than with the more benign intradural tumors. In addition, malignant cells are frequently encountered in the spinal fluid. The spinal fluid glucose may be decreased, the protein elevated. The treatment of intradural malignant neoplasms is radiation therapy and chemotherapy because complete surgical extirpation is almost never possible. Because the tumor usually seeds the entire subarachnoid space, radiation therapy, if it is to have more than temporary effect, must either be delivered to the entire neuraxis or be supplemented by chemotherapy.

INTRAMEDULLARY TUMORS. The most common intramedullary spinal tumors are astrocytomas (usually low grade) and ependymomas. Other tumors that occasionally cause intramedullary spinal lesions are hemangioblastomas, lipomas, and hematogenous metastases. Pain is an early symptom of most intramedullary tumors, and signs of spinal cord dysfunction progress rapidly or slowly, depending on the growth characteristics of the tumor. Intramedullary tumors are often associated with syringomyelia, the syrinx sometimes being at a distance from the primary tumor and producing its own symptoms of spinal dysfunction. The so-called characteristic signs of intramedullary spinal cord lesions (dissociated sensory loss, sacral sparing, and early onset of bladder and bowel dysfunction) are not reliable enough clinically to distinguish intramedullary from extramedullary lesions; that diagnosis is established by MRI. In some patients with longstanding benign intramedullary lesions, plain radiographs of the spine may show widening of the spinal canal and erosion of the pedicles. The differential diagnosis of intramedullary tumors includes intramedullary abscesses and syringomyelia without tumor. A definitive diagnosis is established by biopsy. Successful surgical removal of intramedullary tumors is possible, particularly with ependymomas and hemangioblastomas and sometimes with gliomas as well. Highly skilled and experienced surgeons are necessary for tumors to be removed without increasing neurologic symptoms. If the tumor cannot be totally excised, postoperative radiation therapy often delays recurrence.

Ependymomas have a predilection to involve the lower end of the spinal cord and the filum terminale. An unusual syndrome sometimes produced by such tumors is hydrocephalus with headache, papilledema, and enlarged cerebral ventricles. The pathogenesis of the hydrocephalus is believed to be the plugging of pacchionian granulations by protein exuded from the tumor into the spinal fluid.

Byrne TN, Waxman SG (eds.): Spinal Cord Compression. Philadelphia, FA Davis, 1990. *Specific chapters cover non-neoplastic as well as neoplastic causes of spinal cord compression and noncompressive myelopathies simulating spinal cord compression.*
Posner JB: Neurologic Complications of Cancer. Philadelphia, FA Davis, 1995. *A current discussion of the diagnosis and management of metastatic disease of the spine.*

442 INFLAMMATORY DISEASES COMPRESSING THE SPINAL CORD

Inflammatory diseases that compress nerve roots and spinal cord can be extradural, intradural, or intramedullary. Extradural inflammatory lesions include vertebral tuberculosis or bacterial osteomyelitis with extradural extension and primary extradural bacterial abscesses. These entities are discussed in Ch. 421. Intradural but extramedullary inflammatory diseases include bacterial, fungal, and parasitic meningitis, inflammatory disease of the leptomeninges of unknown cause such as sarcoidosis or Behçet's syndrome, and reactions to foreign substances such as myelographic contrast material, spinal anesthetics, or steroids. Occasionally, leptomeningeal infiltration with tumor or subarachnoid hemorrhage causes an inflammatory response of the leptomeninges that mimics subacute or chronic infection. All of these inflammatory intradural lesions can lead to spinal arachnoiditis. *Spinal arachnoiditis* is characterized by neck and back pain and by radicular pain in the distribution of the roots involved in the inflammatory process. Dysfunction of multiple roots, particularly in the lumbosacral area, is common; occasional patients go on to develop signs of spinal cord dysfunction (often caused by syrinx formation), which may progress to paraplegia. The diagnosis of spinal arachnoiditis is established by myelography. A myelogram reveals spotty and irregular collections of contrast material with impairment of the flow through the subarachnoid space. Sometimes there is a complete block to the passage of the myelographic contrast material. The spinal fluid may contain an increased cellular response and a decreased glucose concentration. The protein concentration is usually elevated. Sometimes a specific infectious organism can be identified either by microscopic examination or by culture. There is no therapy for spinal arachnoiditis unless a specific treatment-sensitive infective agent is identified.

Intramedullary infectious processes include bacterial and parasitic abscesses and acute transverse myelitis. These entities are discussed under the appropriate chapter headings.

Byrne TN, Waxman SG (eds): Spinal Cord Compression. Philadelphia, FA Davis, 1990. *Chapters discuss vascular and inflammatory causes of spinal cord compression and noncompressive myelopathies mimicking spinal cord compression.*
Caplan LR, Norohna AB, Amico LL: Syringomyelia and arachnoiditis. J Neurol Neurosurg Psychiatry 53:106, 1990. *A well-referenced discussion of chronic arachnoiditis and its sequelae.*
Dolan RA: Spinal adhesive arachnoiditis. Surg Neurol 39:479, 1993. *A review of 41 cases.*

443 VASCULAR DISORDERS COMPRESSING THE SPINAL CORD

Extradural, intradural, and intramedullary vascular disorders all can cause spinal cord compression. The most common and serious extradural vascular disease is *spinal epidural hematoma*. Hemorrhage into the spinal epidural space may occur spontaneously or be associated with trauma, a bleeding diathesis, or a vascular malformation. It is particularly common in patients being treated with anticoagulants. It may occasionally follow lumbar puncture, particularly in patients with bleeding abnormalities. Hemorrhage usually arises from the epidural venous plexus and tends to collect over the dorsum of the spinal cord covering several segments. The clinical picture is characterized by the sudden onset of severe localized back pain and the rapid development of spinal cord dysfunction, often leading to complete paraplegia in several hours. If the patient has a known bleeding disorder, the clinical diagnosis is easily established. In patients without known bleeding or clotting disorders, the differential diagnosis includes acute epidural abscess and acute transverse myelopathy. Although occasional patients recover from paraparesis related to epidural spinal cord compression spontaneously, the majority require emergency surgical evacuation if neurologic function is to be preserved. The more rapidly the paralysis develops and the longer the delay in decompression, the less likely is the patient to recover.

Intradural but extramedullary vascular lesions are usually caused by hemorrhage from *vascular malformations* on the surface of the spinal cord. *Spinal subarachnoid hemorrhage* is characterized by the sudden onset of back pain, often with a radicular component with or without the development of signs of spinal cord compression. Lumbar puncture reveals evidence of subarachnoid hemorrhage with red cells, xanthochromic spinal fluid, and usually an elevated protein concentration. In the absence of spinal cord signs, the differential diagnosis includes spontaneous intracerebral subarachnoid hemorrhage.

Vascular malformations also may lie within the substance of the spinal cord where they can give rise to intramedullary hemorrhage (hematomyelia) as well as subarachnoid hemorrhage. The sudden development of partial or complete transverse myelopathy is the most common onset. If blood leaks into the subarachnoid space, pain in the neck and back and other signs of meningeal irritation occur.

Arteriovenous malformations may also compress the spinal cord or give rise to hemodynamic changes that result in spinal ischemia. In such cases, distortion and compression of the cord by enlarged, abnormal vessels occur only gradually, producing slowly progressive symptoms of spinal cord dysfunction. Exacerbation of symptoms may accompany menstrual periods or pregnancy.

Complete or partial recovery of function can follow episodes of spinal cord ischemia or even small hemorrhages. The unchanging localization of the attacks and the prominence of pain help differentiate arteriovenous malformations from other recurrent neurologic disorders such as multiple sclerosis. Rarely, a bruit may be heard by auscultation over the site of the malformation. MRI identifies most hemorrhages and vascular malformations, but angiography with regional catheterization of radicular vessels is necessary to identify feeding vessels as a preliminary step to surgical treatment. Advances in microsurgery have increased the chances for satisfactory removal of these lesions. Embolization of the malformation or ligation of feeding arteries has been performed when the abnormality cannot be removed surgically.

Amson JA, Spetzler RF: Surgical resection of intramedullary spinal cord cavernous malformations. J Neurosurg 78:446,1993. *Description of a clinical entity usually not diagnosed before the advent of MRI.*
Dawson DM, Potts F: Acute nontraumatic myelopathies. Neurol Clin 9:585, 1991. *Diagnosis and management of vascular myelopathies. Entire issue is devoted to spinal cord disorders.*

444 CONGENITAL ANOMALIES OF THE CRANIOVERTEBRAL JUNCTION, SPINE, AND SPINAL CORD

Congenital anomalies of the spine are common and are often encountered on radiographs of patients suffering from neck or low back pain. Some congenital anomalies such as *spina bifida occulta* can be considered variants of normal and are probably never responsible in and of themselves for low back pain. Others such as the *Klippel-Feil syndrome* (congenital fusion of two or more cervical vertebrae) are not responsible for neck pain or other neurologic symptoms except when associated with coexisting congenital anomalies of the central nervous system. Congenital abnormalities of the spine that are common and usually asymptomatic but that must be considered potential causes of neck or back pain include *facet tropism* (misalignment of the facets on the two sides of the corresponding vertebral body; several authorities believe that this increases rotational stress on the facet joints and may cause back pain); *transitional vertebrae,* such as in sacralization to a lumbar vertebra or lumbarization of a sacral vertebra (these alter spinal mechanics and result in instability and stress, sometimes producing back pain); and *spondylolisthesis* (forward slipping of one vertebral body onto another caused by a defect between the articular facets). A third group of congenital anomalies of the spine consists of those that are likely to cause not only neck or back pain but also neurologic disability. These include *basilar impression,* which is often associated with *Arnold-Chiari malformation* (see later discussion). Severe spinal *scoliosis* or *kyphosis,* congenital *stenosis* of the lumbar or cervical spinal canal, anterior and lateral spinal *meningoceles,* and *diastematomyelia* are other causes of back pain and neurologic disability. Diastematomyelia is a bony abnormality that divides the spinal canal, leading to duplication of the spinal cord. It is usually associated with evidence of spina bifida on plain radiographs, and sometimes the bony septum can be identified as well. Patients who become symptomatic in adulthood almost always have some cutaneous abnormality, especially hypertrichosis over the sacral area. The disorder may be associated with other congenital abnormalities of the central nervous system as well.

ARNOLD-CHIARI MALFORMATION

INFANTILE FORM. The Arnold-Chiari malformation is characterized by downward displacement of the cerebellum through the foramen magnum of the skull and by similar caudal elongation of the medulla. The infantile form is commonly associated with other midline defects such as spina bifida and meningocele, hydrocephalus caused by aqueductal or fourth ventricular obstruction, and other congenital malformations of the brain and cord. Therapy is directed toward surgical relief of the hydrocephalus with a ventricular shunting procedure and repair of the meningomyelocele. Prognosis is poor for patients with extensive defects.

ADULT FORM. The malformation may be asymptomatic until adult life, when the patient gradually develops symptoms and signs of dysfunction of the cerebellum, lower cranial nerves, pyramidal tracts, and posterior columns. Posterior cranial displacement may occur with coughing or straining. Downbeat nystagmus is characteristic. At times the initial signs may be those of hydrocephalus secondary to obstruction of the cerebrospinal fluid pathways or to coexisting syringomyelia of the cervical spinal cord and medulla (see Ch. 416). Commonly there is radiographic evidence of fusion of the cervical vertebrae, or basilar impression, but MR scan establishes the diagnosis even when there are no coexisting bony abnormalities. The Arnold-Chiari malformation in adults may simulate syndromes produced by tumors near the foramen magnum or by multiple sclerosis. Surgical enlargement of the foramen magnum and decompression of the cervicomedullary junction benefit selected cases.

BASILAR IMPRESSION AND PLATYBASIA

Basilar impression refers to abnormal invagination of the cervical spine into the base of the posterior fossa of the skull. The diagnosis is made from sagittal MR reconstructions that show excessive protrusion of the tip of the odontoid process of the axis into or above the foramen magnum. *Platybasia* refers to flattening of the base of the skull, wherein lateral roentgenograms of the skull reveal flattening of the angle between the orbital plates of the anterior fossa and the clivus, the sloping anterior floor of the posterior fossa. The abnormality by itself has no clinical significance.

These malformations are usually developmental in origin, and there may be hereditary transmission. Occasionally, basilar impression may result from metabolic bone diseases such as rickets, osteitis deformans, osteomalacia, osteogenesis imperfecta, or fibrous dysplasia. Minor degrees of deformity of the base of the skull give rise to no symptoms. The neck appears shortened, and its movements may be limited. More severe invagination may produce signs of impaired function of the cerebellum, lower cranial nerves, pyramidal tracts, and posterior columns. Syringomyelia and syringobulbia may be present. Increased intracranial pressure may develop owing to obstruction of the foramina of the fourth ventricle and the basal cisterns. The clinical manifestations must be differentiated from those caused by neoplasms in the region of the foramen magnum and multiple sclerosis. When neurologic signs are progressive, surgical decompression of the posterior fossa and upper cervical cord may be indicated.

Oldfield EH, Muraszko K, Shawker TH, Patronas NJ: Pathophysiology of syringomyelia associated with Chiari I malformation of the cerebellar tonsils. J Neurosurg 80:3, 1994. *New concepts of the pathophysiology of the disorder.*

Vinken PJ, Bruyn GW, Klawans HL, Myrianthopoulos NC (eds.): Handbook of Clinical Neurology. Volume 50, Malformations. New York, Elsevier Science Publishers, 1987. *A recent comprehensive review of congenital malformations of the brain and spine.*

Section Fifteen—Diseases of the Peripheral Nervous System

John W. Griffin

The peripheral nervous system, through its motor, sensory, and autonomic divisions, serves as a major interface between the central nervous system and the environment. Diseases of the peripheral nervous system, termed *peripheral neuropathies,* are among the most prevalent neurologic conditions. They range in severity from the mild sensory abnormalities found in up to 70% of patients with longstanding diabetes to fulminant, life-threatening paralytic disorders such as the Guillain-Barré syndrome. Differential diagnosis of peripheral nerve disease can be challenging because the catalogue of disorders that can produce neuropathies is extensive. Although a wide variety of symptoms and signs can result from diseases of the peripheral nervous system, the repertoire of underlying cellular pathology is limited, so that only a few clinical or pathologic features are specific to individual neuropathies. Nevertheless, the past 5 years have seen rapid advances in diagnosis and therapy. An increasing number of nerve diseases are now amenable to treatment, and the peripheral nervous system has a much greater capacity for regeneration and repair than the central nervous system, so that functional improvement is a realistic goal for a lengthening list of neuropathies.

Differential diagnosis in the peripheral nervous system begins with classification of the *clinical features* of the neuropathy, and uses elucidation of the *underlying pathophysiology*, primarily as reflected in electrodiagnostic tests, as a differential tool. On these bases, the specific laboratory tests that are likely to prove useful can be defined.

445   Anatomy and Basic Terminology

The peripheral nervous system (PNS) contains motor, sensory, and autonomic fibers. The motor, sensory, and autonomic fibers are anatomically discrete as they leave their nerve cell bodies (for example, in the ventral roots and the dorsal roots) and again as they approach their nerve terminals, but are admixed throughout most of the peripheral nerves. The lower motor neurons in the ventral horn of the spinal cord give rise to axons that pass through the ventral root before joining their sensory and autonomic counterparts in the mixed spinal nerves. In contrast, the primary sensory neuron is a unique cell type. The nerve cell body, located in the dorsal root ganglion, gives rise to a single axonal stem process that bifurcates into a peripheral branch, which extends down a peripheral nerve, and a central branch, which passes through the dorsal root and enters the spinal cord. In a subpopulation of these sensory neurons (the large neurons subserving joint position and vibratory sensibility), the axons of the central processes pass up the ipsilateral dorsal column of the spinal cord to synapse in the gracile and cuneate nuclei of the medulla oblongata. In the lumbar region of an adult, the dorsal and ventral spinal roots may be 12 inches or more in length; in contrast, in the cervical region the spinal roots are only about two inches long.

Injury to the spinal roots produces *radiculopathy*. The root at a single level may be injured by compression due to a herniated nucleus pulposus (intervertebral disc) or from metastatic cancer. The characteristic clinical features of an isolated root lesion are sensory symptoms with loss of cutaneous sensibility in the segmental or *dermatomal* distribution, as well as weakness in the muscles innervated by that root. If the affected nerve root subserves a tendon reflex, the tendon reflex is depressed or lost. Involvement of spinal roots at many levels *(polyradiculopathy)* can be produced by infiltrative processes, such as carcinomatous meningitis. The clinical picture reflects the specific root levels involved.

The term *peripheral neuropathy* connotes any disease of the peripheral nervous system (PNS). Involvement of a single peripheral nerve constitutes *mononeuropathy,* as seen, for example, following inadvertent intraneural injury to the sciatic nerve during intramuscular injections. *Multiple mononeuropathy* (mononeuropathy multiplex) describes focal involvement of more than one individual peripheral nerve. For example, diabetes and vasculitis, by damaging the small blood vessels supplying the peripheral nerves, can produce injury to several widely distributed individual nerves. *Polyneuropathy* designates a widespread and generally symmetric disorder of the PNS. Polyneuropathies usually produce distally predominant loss of sensation, strength, and tendon reflexes.

Gardner E, Bunge RP: Gross anatomy of the peripheral nervous system. *In* Dyck PJ, Thomas PK, Griffin JW, et al. (eds.): Peripheral Neuropathy, 3rd ed. Philadelphia, W.B. Saunders, 1993, pp. 8–27. *This is the major comprehensive monograph on this subject with well-written chapters, designated in subsequent subsections of this section, on both common and rare disorders.*

446   PATHOPHYSIOLOGY OF PERIPHERAL NEUROPATHIES

Normal function of myelinated nerve fibers depends on the integrity of both the axon and its myelin sheath. The simplest type of nerve injury is transection of the axon. The axon distal to the site of transection degenerates while that proximal to the injury survives and has the potential for regeneration. As the axon degenerates the myelin in the distal stump is also broken down and cleared. Axonal degeneration due to a focal nerve injury occurs, for example, in radiculopathies due to severe compression of the nerve root and in focal ischemic injury to roots and nerves. In the symmetric polyneuropathies, the underlying pathology is usually a slowly evolving type of axonal degeneration that involves the ends of long nerve fibers first and preferentially. With time, the degenerative process involves more proximal regions of long fibers, and shorter fibers are affected. This pattern of *distal axonal degeneration* or *"dying back"* of nerve fibers results from a wide variety of metabolic, toxic, and heritable causes. The resulting clinical picture includes early loss of the tendon reflex at the ankle, and weakness that initially involves the intrinsic muscles of the feet, the extensors of the toes, and the dorsiflexors at the ankle; the motor signs are accompanied by distally predominant loss of large-fiber sensory modalities such as vibratory sensibility in the toes. With progression, the hands are similarly involved, and the process may spread more proximally up the legs and arms. The resulting pattern of sensory loss is frequently termed a *stocking-and-glove* pattern. Recovery from axonal degeneration requires nerve regeneration, a notoriously slow process.

Demyelination of a peripheral nerve at even a single site can block conduction, resulting in a functional deficit identical to that seen after axonal degeneration. In contrast to repair by regeneration, however, repair by remyelination can be quite rapid. Autoimmune attack on the myelin sheath occurs in the *inflammatory demyelinating* neuropathies and some neuropathies associated with paraproteinemias. Inherited disorders of myelin are the other major category of demyelinating neuropathy. Uncommon causes include some toxic, mechanical, and physical injuries to nerve. Although these examples have nearly pure demyelination, and other neuropathies have axonal degeneration exclusively, many neuropathies have an admixture of both axonal degeneration and demyelination. This mixed pathology reflects the mutual interdependency of the axons and the myelin-forming Schwann cells.

On the basis of the clinical features alone, it is difficult to predict whether a patient has a predominantly axonal or demyelinating pattern of peripheral nerve injury. Electrodiagnostic tests—nerve conduction velocity and electromyography—provide a tool for assessing the relative contributions of axonal loss and demyelination. Nerve conduction studies are done by stimulating individual nerves with electrodes at two sites, one proximal to the other, and measuring the velocity of conduction of the action potential between those two sites. In addition, for both sensory and motor nerves, the amplitude of the evoked response can be determined. In general, axonal degeneration decreases the amplitude of the evoked action potential out of proportion to the degree of reduction in conduction velocity, whereas demyelination produces prominent reductions in conduction velocities.

Griffin JW, Hoffman PN: Degeneration and regeneration in the peripheral nervous system. *In* Dyck PJ, Thomas PK, Griffin JW, et al. (eds.): Peripheral Neuropathy, 3rd ed. Philadelphia, W.B. Saunders, 1993, pp. 361–376.

Schaumburg HH, Berger AR, Thomas PK: Disorders of Peripheral Nerve, 2nd ed. Philadelphia, F.A. Davis Co., 1992. *A highly readable succinct but informative monograph aimed especially at the general physician.*

447 IMMUNE-MEDIATED NEUROPATHIES

GUILLAIN-BARRÉ SYNDROME (Acute Inflammatory Demyelinating Polyneuropathy)

The Guillain-Barré syndrome (GBS) is characterized clinically by weakness or paralysis affecting more than one limb, usually symmetrically, associated with loss of tendon reflexes and with increased spinal fluid protein without pleocytosis. Since the advent of polio vaccination, GBS has become the most frequent cause of acute flaccid paralysis throughout the world. In the 1960's, the pathologic substrate of many cases of GBS was shown to be lymphocytic infiltration of the spinal roots and peripheral nerves, with macrophage-mediated demyelination and a variable degree of secondary axonal degeneration. On this basis, GBS became virtually synonymous with *acute inflammatory demyelinating polyneuropathy* (AIDP) (Table 447–1). At the present time it seems preferable to retain the clinical term *GBS,* because it is becoming increasingly clear that a small proportion of cases in North America and Europe, and a large proportion of cases in other regions, especially in the developing world, are characterized by noninflammatory acute axonal degeneration. These cases are clinically indistinguishable and have similar spinal fluid profiles. They are termed the axonal forms of GBS.

GBS is almost certainly an immune-mediated disorder. It follows some type of infectious disorder in approximately 60% of cases. The best documented antecedents include infection with *Campylobacter jejuni,* herpesviruses, and mycoplasma. *C. jejuni* is often associated with more severe "axonal" cases and most likely sensitizes the immune system to antigens shared between the organism and the peripheral nerve.

CLINICAL MANIFESTATIONS. The initial symptoms often consist of tingling and "pins-and-needles sensations" in the feet and may be associated with dull low-back pain. By the time of presentation, which usually occurs within hours or a very few days after first symptoms, weakness has usually supervened. The weakness is usually most prominent in the legs, but the arms or cranial musculature may be involved first. Tendon reflexes are lost early, even in regions where strength is retained. Because the spinal roots are usually prominently involved, GBS can involve short nerves (axial and intercostal as well as cranial nerves) as well as long ones. Weakness progresses, with the nadir reached within 30 days, and usually by 14 days. Progression can be alarmingly rapid, so that critical functions such as respiration can be lost within a few days or even a few hours.

The potential for respiratory insufficiency, as well as swallowing difficulty and autonomic dysregulation, underlies the life-threatening nature of GBS. In the past, mortality was as high as 15%. With modern critical care and the adjunctive therapies outlined below, mortality has fallen to about 2%. The first aspect of management is prompt and accurate initial diagnosis. At the time of presentation, a high index of clinical suspicion is necessary. No laboratory test is specific for GBS, but careful electrodiagnostic testing can usually identify at least mild abnormalities during the early stages. Although elevation of the spinal fluid protein level is characteristic, it usually rises only after the first week, not within the first few days when the diagnosis may be uncertain. At the earliest stages, the differential diagnosis includes non-neuropathic conditions such as spinal cord diseases (for example, transverse myelitis) and acute myopathies.

TREATMENT. Because of the potential for rapid deterioration, patients with a presumptive diagnosis of GBS usually require hospitalization for observation. Monitoring should include frequent measurement of the vital capacity and ability to swallow. Intensive-care observation and insertion of an airway should be initiated early, before declining ventilatory strength, autonomic dysregulation, or fatigue due to unproductive coughing erupts into an acute emergency. Such early intervention largely prevents life-threatening crises. Most of the reduction in mortality in GBS derives from modern intensive care.

Two adjunctive therapeutic techniques are of benefit. *Plasmapheresis*—the exchange of the patient's plasma for albumin—was the first treatment definitively shown to shorten the time to recovery. Infusion of high doses of *human immunoglobulin* intravenously also produces benefit. Both treatments are effective, and the choice should be individualized. In patients with limited venous access, gamma globulin is easier to administer. When the veins are sufficient for plasmapheresis, it may be the preferable treatment; experience with plasmapheresis is greater, and it may produce a lower incidence of relapse after initial improvement. The use of corticosteroids alone is not beneficial. Whether either plasmapheresis or intravenous immunoglobulin is useful in the axonal variants of GBS is undetermined.

Thorough education of the patient about the possibility of rapid deterioration and about the overall favorable prognosis is an important early step. While able to breathe and speak, patients should be instructed in a communication system with nurses and family so that they will be able to make themselves understood if intubation and respiratory support are required.

The prognosis for GBS varies with age, severity, and the extent to which axonal degeneration exceeds demyelination. A middle-aged patient who requires respiratory assistance, and who receives plasmapheresis early in the course, on the average resumes walking about 3 months later (6 months without plasmapheresis). Indeed,

TABLE 447–1. GUILLAIN-BARRÉ SYNDROME AND RELATED IMMUNE-MEDIATED NEUROPATHIES

Disorder	Type	Clinical Characteristics	Pathophysiology	Treatment
Guillain-Barré syndrome	Acute inflammatory demyelinating polyneuropathy	Prominent or predominant motor involvement of acute onset	Demyelination, lymphocytic infiltration	Plasmapheresis; intravenous immunoglobulin (IVIg); corticosteroids alone ineffective
	Acute inflammatory demyelinating polyneuropathy	Ataxia, ophthalmoparesis, and areflexia of acute onset	Antibodies against the ganglioside GQ1b	(Probably) plasmapheresis or IVIg
	Axonal GBS	Motorsensory or pure motor forms	Noninflammatory axonal degeneration predominates; strongly associated with antecedent *Campylobacter jejuni* infection	(Probably) plasmapheresis or IVIg
Chronic inflammatory demyelinating polyneuropathy		Slower onset; may be recurrent	Widespread demyelination with remyelination, secondary axonal loss; may occur in association with monoclonal gammopathy	Corticosteroids, plasmapheresis, IVIg
Multifocal motor neuropathy		Stepwise involvement of individual nerves; nearly pure motor involvement	Focal demyelination	IVIg or cytotoxic agents; corticosteroids and plasmapheresis ineffective

many recover much more promptly than that. Relapses, if they occur, should be re-treated with plasmapheresis or gamma globulin.

Arnason BGW, Soliven B: Acute inflammatory demyelinating polyradiculopathy. *In* Dyck PJ, Thomas PK, Griffin JW, et al. (eds.): Peripheral Neuropathy, 3rd ed. Philadelphia, W.B. Saunders, 1993, pp. 1437–1497.

Hartung H-P, Stoll G, Toyka KV: Immune reactions in the peripheral nervous system. *In* Dyck PJ, Thomas PK, Griffin JW, et al. (eds.): Peripheral Neuropathy, 3rd ed. Philadelphia, W.B. Saunders, 1993, pp. 418–444.

McKhann GM, Cornblath DR, Griffin JW, et al: Acute motor axonal neuropathy: A frequent cause of acute flaccid paralysis in China. Ann Neurol 33:333, 1993. *Describes a large epidemic of a GBS variant occurring in an underdeveloped country.*

Ropper AH, Wijdicks EFM, Trauax BT: Guillain-Barré Syndrome. Philadelphia, F.A. Davis, 1991. *A thorough analysis of all aspects of the disorder.*

van der Meche FGA, Schmitz PIM, Dutch Guillain-Barré Study Group: A randomized trial comparing intravenous immune globulin and plasma exchange in Guillain-Barré syndrome. N Engl J Med 326:1123, 1992.

Yuki N, Yoshino H, Sato S, et al.: Severe acute axonal form of Guillain-Barré syndrome associated with IgG anti-GD$_{1a}$ antibodies. Muscle Nerve 15:899, 1992.

CHRONIC INFLAMMATORY DEMYELINATING NEUROPATHY

Chronic inflammatory demyelinating neuropathy (CIDP), sometimes referred to as chronic GBS, bears similarities to the clinical, pathologic, and laboratory pictures seen in acute GBS. It differs primarily in the time course and in the absence of identifiable antecedent events. The differences in response to therapy, however, suggest that the precise immunopathogenetic mechanisms are likely to differ.

CLINICAL MANIFESTATIONS. CIDP can occur at any age. The usual picture is one of slowly evolving weakness beginning in the legs, with widespread areflexia and loss of large-fiber (vibratory) sensibility on examination. In the more rapidly evolving cases of CIDP, the distinction from GBS is arbitrary. In general, in patients with acute GBS the nadir is reached within 4 weeks, while in patients with CIDP more time is required. The diagnosis is supported by prominent demyelinating features on nerve conduction studies and by elevation of the protein level of the spinal fluid.

Blinded trials showed that, unlike GBS, most cases of CIDP respond to corticosteroids alone. CIDP also responds to plasmapheresis. Intravenous gamma globulin improves some cases. In most instances the first choice of therapy is with corticosteroids, using the lowest dosage required to achieve and maintain an adequate response. Plasmapheresis, while simple and safe, usually must be repeated every several weeks to maintain a response and entails substantial expense. Nevertheless, this form of therapy is valuable in patients who do not respond to corticosteroids or in whom unacceptable corticosteroid doses are required or side effects supervene.

Dyck PJ, O'Brien PC, Oviatt KF, et al.: Prednisone improves chronic inflammatory demyelinating polyradiculoneuropathy more than no treatment. Ann Neurol 11:136, 1982.

Dyck PJ, Prineas J, Pollard J: Chronic inflammatory demyelinating polyradiculoneuropathy. *In* Dyck PJ, Thomas PK, Griffin JW, et al. (eds.): Peripheral Neuropathy, 3rd ed. Philadelphia, W.B. Saunders, 1993, pp. 1498–1517.

MULTIFOCAL MOTOR NEUROPATHY

An uncommon related disorder, *multifocal motor neuropathy*, occurs as "pure motor" multiple mononeuropathy. A patient may describe, for example, development of unilateral wristdrop (radial nerve involvement) followed by footdrop on the other side (peroneal nerve involvement). In addition, tendon reflexes may be lost outside the distribution of weakness, but the sensory examination is normal even in weak limbs. The pathologic characteristic, inflammatory demyelination, resembles that seen in CIDP, but is highly focal and largely spares sensory nerve fibers. A characteristic electrodiagnostic feature is the presence of *conduction block,* a reflection of the focal demyelination. The spinal fluid protein is usually normal. A nonspecific but helpful laboratory finding, noted in about 70% of cases, is markedly increased anti-GM$_1$ ganglioside antibodies in the serum. Multifocal motor neuropathy is noteworthy because it can be confused with more ominous disorders such as amyotrophic lateral sclerosis, but responds favorably to intravenous immunoglobulin as well as to cytotoxic therapy. Neither corticosteroids nor plasmapheresis brings improvement.

Chaudhry V, Corse AM, Cornblath DR, et al.: Multifocal motor neuropathy: Response to human immune globulin. Ann Neurol 33:237, 1993.

Pestronk A, Cornblath DR, Ilyas AA, et al.: A treatable multifocal motor neuropathy with antibodies to GM$_1$ ganglioside. Ann Neurol 24:73, 1988.

NEUROPATHIES ASSOCIATED WITH MONOCLONAL GAMMOPATHIES

Peripheral neuropathy occurs in some monoclonal gammopathies, both the benign type and myeloma. Monoclonal proteins of IgM, IgG, and IgA types are all associated with neuropathy. In some instances the monoclonal protein has been shown to cause the neuropathy. For example, some IgM monoclonal proteins react with sugars found on a specific Schwann cell protein, the *myelin-associated glycoprotein* (MAG). The monoclonal protein intercalates into the myelin lamellae, producing a distinctive pathologic feature, abnormally wide spacing between adjacent myelin lamellae, and consequent demyelination. The neuropathy can be reproduced in experimental animals (chickens) by passive transfer of the monoclonal IgM from patients. A few other nerve epitopes have been defined with which specific paraproteins react. However, for most of the IgG and IgA monoclonal proteins the mechanism of nerve injury is not known.

CLINICAL MANIFESTATIONS. The clinical picture of the neuropathy varies. The IgM monoclonal antibodies with "anti-MAG" reactivity typically produce neuropathy with prominent large-fiber sensory loss and sensory ataxia, as well as milder weakness. The electrodiagnostic tests indicate demyelination, albeit admixed with nerve fiber loss. In other cases with IgM monoclonal proteins there is a distinctive picture that includes scleroderma-like skin changes, hepatomegaly, and endocrine abnormalities, as well as neuropathy (the POEMS syndrome described below). Other individuals with monoclonal proteins have a clinical picture identical to CIDP, and still others have distally predominant axonal degeneration.

Identification of a monoclonal protein does not necessarily mean that the protein is the cause of the neuropathy. Most of the monoclonal proteins found in patients with neuropathy are classed as monoclonal gammopathies of unknown significance, a group alternatively termed benign monoclonal gammopathies because there is no evidence of multiple myeloma at the time of presentation. The incidence of such monoclonal proteins increases with age. Especially in older patients, before the presumption is accepted that the paraprotein causes the neuropathy, it is important to exclude other causes of neuropathy, such as diabetes or alcoholism.

Three disorders should be specifically sought in individuals with paraproteins and neuropathy: (1) There is a special association of neuropathy with solitary plasmacytomas, often osteosclerotic. The POEMS syndrome—polyneuropathy, organomegaly, endocrinopathy (hirsutism, testicular atrophy), monoclonal IgM protein, and skin pigmentation—is highly associated with osteosclerotic myelomas. A skeletal radiographic survey is essential in patients with monoclonal proteins and neuropathy. (2) Cryoglobulinema, with or without monoclonal gammopathy, can produce neuropathy, and the possibility should be excluded. (3) The monoclonal proteins may result in amyloid deposition in nerve and thus produce neuropathy indirectly. Amyloid deposition is particularly associated with excretion of light chains in the urine. The distinctive neurologic picture of amyloidosis often suggests the possibility of amyloid neuropathy (see below). Unlike most other neuropathies, there is a predilection for involvement of small sensory and autonomic nerve fibers, so that the history may include painless injuries to the feet or hands and evidence of autonomic dysfunction, including impotence and orthostatic hypotension. Definitive diagnosis of immunoglobulin-associated amyloidosis is by histology. Fat pad aspiration and muscle biopsy may be useful before undertaking biopsy of rectal ganglia or peripheral nerve.

The one category of paraproteinemic neuropathies in which treatment is clearly beneficial is that of the solitary plasmacytomas. Excision and radiation of the plasmacytoma can be curative. In other paraproteinemic neuropathies, some reports suggest modest benefit from plasmapheresis or other forms of therapy in neuropathies associated with benign monoclonal gammopathies. In general, however, the degree of improvement is insufficient for the nuisance and expense of therapy. The effort is better focused on gait training and protection from falls. No therapy has been shown to slow progression of amyloid neuropathy.

Kyle RA, Dyck PJ: Osteosclerotic myeloma (POEMS syndrome). *In* Dyck PJ, Thomas PK, Griffin JW, et al. (eds.): Peripheral Neuropathy, 3rd ed. Philadelphia, W.B. Saunders, 1993, pp. 1288–1293.

Kyle RA, Dyck PJ: Amyloidosis and neuropathy. *In* Dyck PJ, Thomas PK, Griffin JW, et al. (eds.): Peripheral Neuropathy, 3rd ed. Philadelphia, W.B. Saunders, 1993, pp. 1294–1309.

Kyle RA, Dyck PJ: Neuropathy associated with the monoclonal gammopathies. *In* Dyck PJ, Thomas PK, Griffin JW, et al. (eds.): Peripheral Neuropathy, 3rd ed. Philadelphia, W.B. Saunders, 1993, pp. 1275–1287.

IMMUNE-MEDIATED ATAXIC NEUROPATHIES

In this category are three disorders: *carcinomatous sensory neuropathy, sensory ganglionitis associated with features of Sjögren's syndrome,* and *idiopathic sensory ganglionitis.* All three are characterized clinically by subacute or slowly developing proprioceptive sensory loss leading to gait ataxia and inability to localize arms and/or legs. Patients show rombergism: They can stand with feet together and eyes open, but fall when they close their eyes, reflecting loss of kinesthetic sensibility. Tendon reflexes usually disappear, but strength remains. Pathologic changes in all three disorders include lymphocytic infiltration of the dorsal root ganglia, with destruction of the primary sensory neurons and associated degeneration of their central and peripheral processes. Large sensory neurons are predominantly affected, leaving pain and thermal sensibilities relatively intact. Electrodiagnostic studies document the absence of sensory nerve action potentials and preservation of motor responses. Spinal fluid protein may be normal or contain increased protein. Modest pleocytosis often accompanies the carcinomatous disorder.

The possibility of occult carcinoma underlying an immunogenic (paraneoplastic) ataxic neuropathy adds urgency to differential diagnosis. The most frequent associations include small cell carcinoma of the lung, breast carcinoma, and ovarian carcinoma. In addition to clinical screening for these possibilities, a useful serologic test is the anti-Hu antibody, which reacts with a 37-kD neuronal nuclear protein. Although the presence of anti-Hu antibodies is neither perfectly sensitive nor specific, their association with ataxic neuropathy strongly suggests underlying carcinoma. It should be noted that carcinoma has also been associated with other types of neuropathy, including bland, slowly evolving, sensory motor neuropathy. However, this type of neuropathy is usually an accompaniment of advanced stages of cancer and is rarely a presenting manifestation. The evaluation for occult carcinoma is directed toward those uncommon patients with pure sensory ataxic neuropathy.

Another group of patients with a similar clinical and pathologic picture have features of Sjögren's syndrome, including keratoconjunctivitis sicca and elevated antinuclear antibody titers (Ch. 263). Surprisingly, these patients only occasionally have joint disease or other extraglandular manifestations of Sjögren's syndrome, and most will not have sought medical attention before neuropathy develops. Affected patients are likely to have associated autonomic insufficiency, including pupils that are large and are more reactive to accommodation than to light (Adie's pupils).

A third group of patients with idiopathic sensory ganglionitis have no associated systemic disease. Because this group of disorders often have a very acute onset, they may be misdiagnosed as Guillain-Barré syndrome. This group is referred to as *idiopathic sensory neuronopathy.*

Unfortunately, cytotoxic or corticosteroid therapy only rarely benefits any of these sensory ganglionitis disorders. The gait ataxia produces substantial early disability, but relearning through gait training, rehabilitation, and physical therapy allows a large proportion of affected individuals to resume daily activities.

Griffin JW, Cornblath DR, Alexander E, et al.: Ataxic sensory neuropathy and dorsal root ganglionitis associated with Sjogren's syndrome. Ann Neurol 27:304, 1990.
McLeod JG: Paraneoplastic neuropathies. *In* Dyck PJ, Thomas PK, Griffin JW, et al. (eds.): Peripheral Neuropathy, 3rd ed. Philadelphia, W.B. Saunders, 1993, pp. 1583–1590.
Windebank AJ, Blexrud MD, Dyck PJ, et al.: The syndrome of acute sensory neuropathy: Clinical features and electrophysiologic and pathologic changes. Neurology 40:584, 1990.

VASCULITIC NEUROPATHIES

Peripheral nerves have extensive collateral circulation and are relatively invulnerable to occlusion of large peripheral arteries. By contrast, they are susceptible to focal interruption of circulation within the individual nerve fascicles due to small blood vessel diseases. As a result, many types of systemic vasculitis affect the peripheral nerves. They are one of the most frequently damaged organ systems in polyarteritis nodosa and are frequently involved in rheumatoid arteritis, Sjögren's syndrome, and the vasculitides associated with infections such as hepatitis B, Lyme disease, and HIV. They are less frequently affected in Wegener's granulomatosis because of its restricted regional involvement. The peripheral nerves can be the predominant site of vasculitis, producing a syndrome referred to as vasculitis restricted to the peripheral nervous system. This disorder offers special diagnostic challenges, because the usual footprints of systemic inflammatory disease, including elevated sedimentation rate, are often absent.

CLINICAL MANIFESTATIONS. The clinical manifestations of all of these vasculitic neuropathies reflect the patchiness of the underlying disease. The characteristic picture consists of multiple mononeuropathy, often evolving in a stepwise fashion, so that wristdrop from radial nerve palsy may occur on one side followed by footdrop on the other, with patchy areas of subjective numbness or sensory loss appearing elsewhere on the extremities. The asymmetry and the length-independence of the nerves involved suggest small vessel disease of nerve. In the absence of diabetes mellitus, vasculitis becomes the prime diagnostic consideration. Evaluation of multiple mononeuropathy includes screening of patients to detect evidence of systemic vasculitis in the skin, kidneys, eyes, and other organs. Ultimately, vasculitis is a histologic diagnosis, and if no other organ involvement is identified, combined nerve and muscle biopsy is needed to establish diagnosis.

Treatment of vasculitic neuropathies consists of treatment of the underlying vasculitis. In a neuropathy apparently restricted to the peripheral nervous system, corticosteroids may be tried initially, but most patients require cytotoxic therapy comparable to that used for polyarteritis.

Said G, Lacroix-Ciaudo C, Fujimura H, et al: The peripheral neuropathy of necrotizing arteritis: A clinicopathological study. Ann Neurol 23:461, 1988.

448 HEREDITARY NEUROPATHIES

Heritable neuropathies rank among the most prevalent inherited neurologic diseases. Because many occur in midlife and because the family history is often previously unrecognized, the heritable disorders constitute an important aspect of differential diagnosis.

CHARCOT-MARIE-TOOTH DISEASE

DEFINITION. The eponymic designation, *Charcot-Marie-Tooth* (CMT) disease, identifies a group of heritable disorders of peripheral nerves that share clinical features, but differ in their pathology and the specific genetic abnormalities, as shown in Table 448–1. One group of disorders, classed together as CMT type I (CMT I), is characterized pathologically by abnormalities of peripheral myelination and, at a molecular level, by abnormalities of specific proteins found in the myelin sheaths or Schwann cells. The CMT II group is characterized by axonal degeneration.

PATHOGENESIS. Most forms of CMT disease reflect an autosomal dominant trait, but some similar clinical phenotypes overlap different genetic abnormalities. Several gene abnormalities can cause CMT I (Table 448–1). Three specific gene abnormalities have been identified. The most prevalent is duplication of a segment of chromosome 17 that encodes the peripheral myelin protein-22 (PMP-22) gene. A chromosome 1-linked form is due to an abnormality of another myelin protein, termed P_0. Recently a sex-linked form has been related to abnormalities of the connexin-32 gene. The gene defects in the axonal forms are not yet known.

PATHOLOGY. The pathology of the demyelinating forms of CMT is characterized by excessive numbers of Schwann cells forming concentric rings around nerve fibers. Termed *onion bulbs* because of their appearance on microscopic examination, the wrappings lead to a palpable and often visible increase in the size of certain nerves, such as the ulnar nerve at the elbow or the greater auricular nerve running from the posterior margin of the sternocleidomastoid muscle to the base of the ear. Because of the increase in the size of the nerves, the demyelinating forms of CMT disease are termed *hypertrophic neuropathies.*

CLINICAL MANIFESTATIONS. All forms of CMT disease tend to occur in the second to fourth decades with insidiously evolving footdrop. On examination, one finds distal wasting of the intrinsic muscles of the feet, the anterior tibial group, and the

TABLE 448–1. CHARCOT-MARIE-TOOTH (CMT) AND RELATED HERITABLE NEUROPATHIES

Disorder	Type	Clinical Features	Pathophysiology	Inheritance	Gene Defect
CMT I		Slowly evolving motor-sensory neuropathies with high arches, hammer toes, hypertrophic nerves	Demyelination and remyelination with onion bulbs		
	a			Dominant	Duplication of a segment of chromosome 17 encoding PMP-22
	b			Dominant	Point mutation in the myelin protein P_0
	x			Sex-linked	Mutation in connexin 32
CMT II		Similar, without hypertrophic nerves	Distally predominant axonal degeneration	Dominant	Unknown
CMT III (Dejerine-Sottas disease)		Early onset, severe motor-sensory neuropathy	Severe hypomyelination with onion bulbs	Recessive	Mutation in P_0

calves. A variable degree of impaired large-fiber sensory function is reflected in elevated vibratory thresholds in the toes. Tendon reflexes are lost, at least at the ankles. Typically a foot deformity exists, with high arches (pes cavus) and hammer toes, reflecting longstanding muscle imbalance in the feet. Upon specific questioning, affected individuals recall that they were never athletic, that they could not run, jump, or ice skate along with their peers. Often they report frequent ankle sprains. In general, these problems attract little concern on the part of patients or their families, reflecting the lifelong nature and slow evolution of the disease. Patients can frequently identify several other family members who have similar foot deformities. The most useful diagnostic test lies in the identification of the clinical features in other family members. Even mild or subclinical forms of the disease are usually identified readily on examination.

TREATMENT. Most patients with CMT disease enjoy a nearly full spectrum of occupational and daily activities, and they have a normal lifespan. The footdrop can be relieved by appropriate bracing of the ankle. Occasionally, however, the disease produces much greater deficits. Genetic counseling and education of affected individuals and their families is important, both for reassurance and to preclude unnecessary diagnostic evaluation of affected members in future generations.

AMYLOID NEUROPATHIES

All forms of amyloid neuropathy are due to extracellular deposition of the fibrillary protein, amyloid, in peripheral nerve and sensory and autonomic ganglia, as well as around blood vessels in nerves and other tissues. The nonhereditary type of amyloidosis associated with monoclonal immunoglobulins has been described above. The forms of heritable amyloidosis, at one time classified by geographic origin of the first families recognized, have been shown by molecular genetic techniques to represent a variety of point mutations in the transthyretin (prealbumin) gene. The most frequent variant transthyretin protein results from substitution of methionine for valine at position 30 in the molecule. In all forms of amyloidosis, the precise means by which amyloid deposition injures nerve remains unresolved. Mechanical distortion of neurons in the sensory and autonomic ganglia and of nerve fibers, as well as vascular involvement due to amyloid deposition around blood vessels, both may contribute.

CLINICAL MANIFESTATIONS. In all forms of amyloidosis the outstanding abnormalities affect the small sensory and autonomic fibers. Involvement of small fibers responsible for pain and thermal sensibilities leads to loss of the ability to perceive mechanical and thermal injury and tissue damage. As a result, painless injuries present a major hazard of this disorder; in advanced stages they can lead to chronic infections or osteomyelitis of the feet or hands, and the need for amputation. The autonomic dysfunction produces orthostatic hypotension, impotence, and, in late stages, bladder and bowel incontinence. Until the late stages, strength, touch-pressure sensibility, and vibratory sensation are usually preserved. In some of the heritable forms (as well as in immunoglobulin-associated amyloidosis), median nerve entrapment may occur because of amyloid deposition. Diagnosis of systemic amyloidosis is made by histologic demonstration of amyloid in biopsy of nerve, muscle, fat aspirate, or other tissue. The heritable forms are normally autosomal dominant, so that the diagnosis may be suggested

by family history. The specific genetic abnormality can be identified by molecular genetic analysis. No definitive treatment for any form of amyloid neuropathy is available, but education in prevention of injury to anesthetic limbs can preserve function.

449 METABOLIC NEUROPATHIES

DIABETIC NEUROPATHIES

Diabetes is the most frequent cause of peripheral neuropathy worldwide. Incidence figures depend on the employed definition; at least some peripheral nerve abnormalities can be detected in about 70% of patients with longstanding diabetes, and symptomatic neuropathy affects 5 to 10%. The diabetic neuropathies include a variety of clinical forms, including symmetric polyneuropathies, and a variety of forms of individual nerve injury (Table 449–1).

DIABETIC POLYNEUROPATHY

Diabetic polyneuropathy is symmetric and usually distally predominant, beginning with sensory loss in the feet. It is the most frequent of the diabetic neuropathies. It is uncommon at the time of diagnosis of diabetes, but its prevalence increases with duration of diabetes. The precise pathogenesis remains a matter of controversy, but a signal recent advance has been the demonstration that, like the ocular and renal complications, diabetic neuropathy can be reduced in incidence and in severity by maintaining blood sugar levels close to normal. This effect of "tight control" is consistent with the hypothesis that hyperglycemia itself contributes to nerve damage. The complications of hyperglycemia that injure nerves may include one or more of the following: abnormalities of nerve vasculature and blood flow, leading to angiopathic injury; metabolic effects of abnormalities in polyol pathways; and nonenzymatic glycosylation of nerve proteins.

CLINICAL MANIFESTATIONS. The neuropathy is usually asymptomatic at the onset, a stage during which abnormalities in sensation and reflexes may be detected on routine examination. The symptomatic phase usually begins insidiously, but some cases have an abrupt onset, and in a small percentage of patients this appears to be precipitated by the institution of insulin. Unlike most other

TABLE 449–1. DIABETIC NEUROPATHIES

Diabetic polyneuropathies
  Rapidly reversible physiologic dysfunction associated with hyperglycemia
  Symmetric polyneuropathy
    Sensorimotor neuropathy
    "Small-fiber" neuropathy, with autonomic dysfunction, reduced pain sensibility, spontaneous burning pain
Diabetic mononeuropathies and plexopathies
  Diabetic third nerve palsy
  Diabetic fourth nerve palsy
  Diabetic truncal neuropathy
  Diabetic lumbosacral plexopathy

neuropathies, in diabetes small-fiber sensibility as well as large-fiber sensation are typically reduced, resulting in elevated pin, thermal, and vibratory thresholds. The small-fiber dysfunction is often manifested by spontaneous neuropathic pain. This includes bothersome *dysesthesias*—unpleasant sensations evoked by normally innocuous stimuli, such as the bedsheets on the toes at night. There may be continuous burning or throbbing pain, and walking often is distressing ("It feels like I'm walking on coals."). In addition, sudden intense "lightning" pains may affect the feet and legs.

Some degree of autonomic insufficiency is frequent in diabetic neuropathy. Manifestations include loss of the normal sinus arrhythmia; failure of blood pressure restoration and cardiac acceleration on standing, sometimes producing orthostatic hypotension; impotence; constipation; and a particularly distressing symptom, diabetic diarrhea, with unpredictable loose stools and fecal incontinence. In some patients, these "small-fiber" abnormalities, including neuropathic pain, loss of pin and thermal sensibility, and autonomic dysfunction, dominate the clinical picture.

The diagnosis of diabetic polyneuropathy is straightforward in established diabetics with typical clinical pictures. Electrodiagnostic studies, usually unnecessary, document neuropathy, and spinal fluid protein is frequently moderately elevated. Conversely, diabetic neuropathy is the most *overdiagnosed* cause of peripheral nerve disease. In general, the diagnosis of diabetic neuropathy can comfortably be made only in the setting of longstanding diabetes, usually insulin-requiring. If only recent mild hyperglycemia is present, the diagnosis of diabetic polyneuropathy should be regarded as suspect.

TREATMENT. The approach to management of diabetic hyperglycemia is outside the scope of this chapter, but there is increasing reason to think that primary prevention as well as slowing of the progression of established diabetic neuropathy is abetted by correction of blood sugar to as nearly normal values as possible ("tight control"; see Ch. 218). Once the diagnosis of diabetic polyneuropathy is established, no other specific treatment for the neuropathy is currently available. Symptomatic management includes use of tricyclic antidepressants or carbamazepine for the spontaneous neuropathic pain. Full therapeutic doses are required, and the dosage must be slowly increased to minimize side effects such as dizziness. Opiates are contraindicated, but high doses of amitriptyline sometimes help. The major goal in management of diabetic polyneuropathy is prevention of the cycle of painless injury, ulceration, cellulitis, osteomyelitis, and osteolysis that underlies much of the functional disability produced by this disorder and that contributes to an ultimate requirement for amputation. The loss of pain sensibility on examination should trigger increased vigilance. Painless injuries can largely be prevented by education, avoidance of physical and thermal hazards to the feet, well-fitting shoes, and frequent inspections of the feet. Erythema or injury is treated promptly with removal of the aggravating factor, such as an ill-fitting shoe. Cessation of weight bearing until healing occurs can minimize ulceration. Meticulous skin and nail care is required.

One of the most distressing aspects of the autonomic neuropathy is impotence. A variety of methods, including intracavernous injection of yohimbine, have been advocated and are helpful to some patients. Other genitourinary disturbances include retrograde ejaculation and disordered micturition. Milder cases of diabetic diarrhea may respond to agents such as diphenoxylate.

MONONEUROPATHY AND MULTIPLE MONONEUROPATHIES

Diabetes also can cause a variety of mononeuropathies and multiple mononeuropathies. They represent vascular insufficiency or infarction in nerve, presumably caused by disease of the small blood vessels. Their onset is typically abrupt and often painful.

CLINICAL MANIFESTATIONS. Characteristic is *diabetic third nerve palsy,* characterized by sudden inability to adduct the eye or open the lid. Unlike third nerve compression from intracranial masses or carotid aneurysms, the pupil is typically spared. The sixth nerve, the femoral nerve, or other major nerves of the extremities, may be similarly involved.

In another characteristic syndrome, best termed *diabetic lumbosacral plexopathy,* affected persons develop pain in the hip with asymmetric weakness of the proximal leg muscles over days to a few weeks. The disorder often occurs in a setting of recent severe (>10%) loss of body weight and frequently appears to be a "femoral" neuropathy, with quadriceps weakness and loss of the tendon reflex at the knee. Careful examination, however, usually discloses more widespread involvement of muscles innervated by

the lumbosacral plexus, typically including the hamstring and gluteus muscles. Although the complaints may be referable to one side, mild abnormalities often affect the contralateral side. In addition, evidence of more symmetric polyneuropathy, with reduced tendon reflexes of the ankles, elevated sensory thresholds, and often weakness of toe extension and ankle dorsiflexion, may exist. The limited pathologic data available suggest that this is a consequence of small vessel disease in the lumbosacral plexus, perhaps amplified by associated atherosclerotic disease in the aortic bifurcation. In any event, the prognosis is surprisingly favorable; pain decreases within weeks, and strength returns to the affected muscles within weeks to months. At the onset this disorder can be confused with intraspinal disease or polyradiculopathy. Diabetic lumbosacral plexopathy is sometimes called diabetic amyotrophy, but this term is best avoided, because it has also been applied to a syndrome of widespread muscle wasting that occasionally develops in diabetics in association with a period of weight loss. A final noteworthy mononeuropathy is *diabetic truncal neuropathy*. Patients have pain in the distribution of one or more intercostal nerves, often associated with hypesthesia and numbness. Like the other diabetic mononeuropathies, recovery over months is the rule.

Dyck PJ, Karnes JL, Daube J, et al.: Clinical and neuropathological criteria for the diagnosis and staging of diabetic polyneuropathy. Brain 108:861, 1985.

Johnson PC, Doll SC, Cromey DW: Pathogenesis of diabetic neuropathy. Ann Neurol 19:450, 1986.

Max MB, Culnane M, Schafer SC, et al.: Amitriptyline relieves diabetic neuropathy pain in patients with normal or depressed mood. Neurology 37:589, 1987.

HEPATIC NEUROPATHY

Polyneuropathy is sufficiently uncommon in chronic liver disease that other underlying causes that can affect both liver and peripheral nerves (alcoholism, primary biliary cirrhosis) should be sought.

THYROID DISEASE

Myxedema neuropathy is usually a minor manifestation of myxedema, but areflexia and distal sensory loss can be seen. Cerebellar ataxia and behavioral changes usually predominate.

UREMIC NEUROPATHY

This peripheral neuropathy is associated with chronic renal insufficiency. Electrophysiologic abnormalities routinely occur when creatinine clearance is less than 10% of normal, but the severity and rate of progression of symptomatic uremic polyneuropathy vary widely. The syndrome usually consists of distally predominant, symmetric, motor-sensory polyneuropathy. In some patients, there is marked motor predominance, so that footdrop and leg weakness are major manifestations. In others, paresthesias and, occasionally, burning dysesthesias are early symptoms. In either event, loss of tendon reflexes, initially at the ankle, is characteristic. Electrophysiologic and pathologic studies indicate that both distal axonal degeneration and demyelination occur in uremic neuropathy, but the precise underlying mechanisms remain uncertain.

An important outcome of the past 30 years' experience with dialysis and renal transplantation is recognition that this peripheral neuropathy is both preventable and treatable by amelioration of the renal insufficiency. While both approaches are helpful, renal transplantation produces much better preservation of peripheral nerve function.

PORPHYRIC NEUROPATHY

The intermittent porphyrias, considered fully in Ch. 187, are important diagnostic considerations in acute neuropathies. The most prevalent of these disorders, acute intermittent porphyria (AIP), is associated with recurrent episodes of neuropathy, which are typically acute or subacute in onset. Paresthesias and dysesthesias of the extremities occur and in severe episodes are associated with rapidly evolving weakness or paralysis, mimicking the axonal form of Guillain-Barré syndrome, often associated with bladder dysfunction and constipation. The associated CNS effects may contribute to alterations in level of consciousness as well as hysteria-like or psychotic behavior, potentially delaying recognition of the emergent nature of the neuropathy. During acute attacks, most patients with AIP have increased excretion of porphobilinogen and delta-aminolevulinic acid in the urine. This simple diagnostic assay should be considered in any patient with acute paralytic neuropathy. The treatment of acute porphyric attacks is described in Ch. 187.

CRITICAL CARE NEUROPATHIES

An increasingly frequently recognized disorder, critical care neuropathy is encountered in patients following a severe medical illness, is often complicated by sepsis, and requires prolonged intensive care. Motor involvement predominates. Although it is usually most severe distally, it can impair the "weaning" of patients from ventilatory support. The underlying pathology appears to be axonal degeneration. The etiology is unclear, and no effective therapy other than time and adequate nutrition is known. Most affected persons recover completely.

450 TOXIC NEUROPATHIES

A wide array of environmental, occupational, recreational, and pharmaceutical agents can produce peripheral nerve disease. For agents in which the period of exposure is limited, the diagnosis is often suggested by subacute neuropathy. Most, although not all, neurotoxins produce distal axonal degeneration. The picture typically includes distally predominant sensory loss, loss of tendon reflexes at the ankles, and distal weakness. With continued exposure, the symptoms may progress more proximally; even after the offending agent is withdrawn, progression sometimes may continue, a phenomenon termed *coasting*. Nevertheless, withdrawal represents the optimal treatment. Tables 450–1 and 450–2 list important pharmaceutical and environmental toxins.

Persons with pre-existing nerve disease may be unusually susceptible to neurotoxins. For example, those with Charcot-Marie-Tooth disease can experience devastating toxic reactions to standard level chemotherapeutic doses of vincristine. In all toxic neuropathies the key to treatment lies in prompt recognition and withdrawal.

Schaumburg HH, Berger AR, Thomas PK: Disorders of Peripheral Nerve, 2nd ed. Philadelphia, F.A. Davis, 1992.

ALCOHOL-NUTRITIONAL NEUROPATHY

Polyneuropathy in persons with chronic alcoholism usually occurs in a setting of associated nutritional deficiency (see Ch. 456). The pathogenesis of alcohol-nutritional-deficiency neuropathy remains undefined. Most persons with alcoholic neuropathy have evidence of multifactorial nutritional deficiency, but in some, nutritional background seems adequate, and the direct contribution of alcohol cannot be excluded. The pathology of alcohol-nutritional neuropathy is that of a bland "dying back" disorder affecting both sensory and motor fibers. The initial symptoms are pain and paresthesias, beginning on the soles of the feet, sometimes evolving to

TABLE 450–1. PHARMACEUTIC NEUROTOXINS

Antiretrovirals (ddI, ddC)
Chloramphenicol
Cisplatin
Clioquinols
Dapsone
Disulfiram (Antabuse)
Ethambutol
Ethionamide
Gold
Hydralazine
Isoniazid
Metronidazole and misonidazole
Nitrofurantoin
Penicillamine
Perhexiline
Phenytoin (rare)
Pyridoxine
Stilbamidine
Suramin
Thalidomide
Vincristine/vinblastine

TABLE 450–2. INDUSTRIAL AND ENVIRONMENTAL NEUROTOXINS

Metals
  Arsenic
  Lead
  Mercury
  Thallium
Substance abuse
  Alcohol
  Glue (hexacarbons) inhalation
  Nitrous oxide inhalation
Industrial poisons
  Acrylamide
  Carbon disulfide
  Cyanide (chronic)
  Dichlorophenoxyacetic acid
  Dimethylaminopropionitrile
  Ethylene oxide
  Hexacarbon (n-hexane) (glue sniffer, occupational exposure to solvents, glues, or glue thinner)
  Organophosphorus esters (triorthocresyl phosphate, leptophos, mipafox, trichlorphon)
  Polychlorinated biphenyls
  Tetrachlorbiphenyl
  Trichloroethylene (trigeminal neuropathy)

burning feet and severe hyperpathia and often associated with aching and tenderness of the calves. Weakness is initially distal, and tendon reflexes are lost first at the ankles. Treatment with nutritional supplementation, including thiamine and multivitamins, and cessation of alcohol ingestion are highly beneficial in the early stages of the disease. In advanced cases the disease may continue to progress for a period after initiation of therapy, and recovery may be incomplete.

451 NEUROPATHIES ASSOCIATED WITH INFECTIOUS DISEASES

HUMAN IMMUNODEFICIENCY VIRUS (HIV) INFECTION

A variety of nerve diseases can accompany HIV infection (see also Ch. 428.2). The *Guillain-Barré syndrome* (GBS) and *chronic inflammatory peripheral neuropathy* (CIDP) tend to occur early in HIV infection, when CD4 counts are 250 to 500, and before development of AIDS. They presumably reflect early immune dysregulation. They are distinguished by the frequent presence of pleocytosis, an uncommon finding in seronegative GBS and CIDP. Their course and response to treatment are similar to those observed in seronegative patients.

Cytomegalovirus (CMV) infection of nerve occurs in the setting of clinically evident AIDS and in association with systemic CMV infection. CMV can produce multiple mononeuropathy associated with focal infection of endothelial cells of the nerve, macrophages, and Schwann cells. A dramatic and potentially treatable disorder is *CMV polyradiculopathy*. It develops in persons with AIDS and is characterized by abrupt pain in the back and legs with rapidly progressing paraparesis and areflexia. A distinctive finding is polymorphonuclear pleocytosis, usually associated with markedly increased spinal fluid protein. Cytologic examination sometimes can identify CMV inclusions in spinal fluid. The differential diagnosis includes herpesvirus-associated transverse myelopathies. Prompt diagnosis of CMV polyradiculopathy is important, because some patients respond well to antiviral therapy with ganciclovir and/or foscarnet.

The most prevalent neuropathic complication of HIV infection is *sensory neuropathy of AIDS*. In advanced AIDS, affected patients typically complain of pain on the soles of the feet and discomfort while walking. Neuropathic pain may be intense, associated with loss of small and large-fiber sensory modalities, with a variable, usually mild, degree of motor impairment. Typically the reflexes are lost at the ankle but exaggerated at the knees. This pattern reflects both neuropathy and a CNS disease such as vacuolar myelopathy. Pathologic studies of the sensory neuropathy have shown noninflammatory distally predominant axonal degeneration of sensory fibers. Both large and small fibers are lost. The pathogenesis is unknown, but the disease does not appear to be produced by local productive HIV infection within the nerves themselves. The treatment is symptomatic.

Griffin JW, Wesselingh SL, Griffin DE, et al.: Peripheral neuropathies in HIV infection: Similarities and contrasts with the central nervous system. In HIV, AIDS, and the Brain. Association in Research on Nervous and Mental Disease Proceedings, Vol 92. New York, Raven Press, 1994.

LYME DISEASE (BORRELIOSIS)

Neuropathic consequences can predominate in some patients with Lyme disease (see Ch. 343). The geographic area of the patient as well as history of the characteristic antecedent rash may suggest the diagnosis. The neuropathy is usually a multiple mononeuropathy, with a high predilection of facial nerve involvement, mimicking idiopathic Bell's palsy.

LEPROUS NEUROPATHY

The clinical manifestations of leprosy are virtually exclusively those of peripheral neuropathy and its sequelae. Although WHO has set a target for eradication of active leprosy by the year 2000, at least 5 million individuals with residual disease will remain worldwide. In all forms of leprosy, infection of the skin with *Mycobacterium leprae* and destruction of cutaneous nerve fibers are the primary events. The major classes, *lepromatous* and *tuberculoid,* differ in the extent of postimmune response to the organism.

In *lepromatous leprosy,* no effective cellular immune response is mounted, and large numbers of bacilli reside within the skin, where they infect predominantly the Schwann cells of intracutaneous nerves. With time, Schwann cells throughout the peripheral nervous system are affected, with a striking distribution of nerve fiber damage related to environmental temperatures. Organisms proliferate in the nerve fibers in the coolest regions of the skin, such as the ears, the lateral area of the face, and the digits, before they affect warmer areas covered with clothing. The resulting cutaneous sensory loss includes strikingly selective loss of pain sensibility.

The other major form of the disease, *tuberculoid leprosy,* is characterized by an active inflammatory response to the organism with much of the nerve damage probably resulting from the immune response. Tuberculoid disease and the intermediate form, *borderline disease,* produce a less stereotyped, more patchy and asymmetric neuropathy.

Painless injuries and painless traumatic joint diseases are the major sequelae of both forms of leprosy. Recent data have shown that chemotherapy for leprosy is associated with regeneration of nerve fibers. In general, however, nerve fibers do not successfully reinnervate the skin, so that cutaneous anesthesia and its complications persist. In addition to chemotherapy, education and protection from painless injuries, as described for diabetic polyneuropathies, can substantially modify the outcome.

Miko TL, Le Maitre C, Kinfu Y: Damage and regeneration of peripheral nerves in advanced treated leprosy. Lancet 342:521, 1993.
Sabin TD, Swift TR, Jacobson RR: Leprosy. In Dyck PJ, Thomas PK, Griffin JW, et al. (eds.): Peripheral Neuropathy, 3rd ed. Philadelphia, W.B. Saunders Company, 1993, pp. 1354–1379.

452 ENTRAPMENT AND COMPRESSIVE NEUROPATHIES

The peripheral nerves are vulnerable to chronic compression or entrapment in a variety of sites. The most frequently encountered are median nerve compression at the wrist within the carpal tunnel *(carpal tunnel syndrome);* median nerve compression in the upper

forearm; ulnar nerve compression in the hand *(cubital tunnel syndrome),* wrist, or at the elbow *(tardy ulnar nerve palsy);* tibial nerve compression behind the medial malleolus *(tarsal tunnel syndrome);* and peroneal nerve compression over the lateral fibular head. Because of its prevalence, carpal tunnel syndrome deserves specific comment.

CARPAL TUNNEL SYNDROME

Entrapment of the median nerve at the wrist reflects the limited available space for the median nerve because of the surrounding bone, joint, and ligaments, as well as the tendons and synovium passing through the canal. Repetitive motion of the fingers is a highly publicized exacerbating element, but other precipitating factors that should be considered include trauma, osteoarthritis, ganglionic cysts, myxedema, and rarely, amyloid deposition. Mild symptoms typically involve paresthesias of the first three digits, often occurring overnight and relieved by shaking or elevating the hands. In more severe disease, objective sensory loss in the median nerve distribution, weakness of median-innervated muscles such as the abductor pollicis brevis, and prolongation of nerve conduction across the carpal tunnel (prolonged distal latency) are characteristic. The diagnosis is supported by identification of *Tinel's sign,* in which tapping the carpal tunnel elicits paresthesias in the median nerve distribution, and by paresthesias produced by sustained flexion of the wrist.

The treatment of carpal tunnel syndrome requires consideration of the relationship between symptoms and occupational or recreational activities. Treatment begins with splinting of the wrist in slight dorsiflexion during sleep, thereby increasing the cross-sectional area of the carpal tunnel. Injection of corticosteroids into the carpal tunnel and use of potassium-sparing diuretics are helpful in some patients. More severe carpal tunnel syndrome is treated surgically by release of the carpal ligament.

BELL'S PALSY

Unilateral facial paralysis of acute onset frequently occurs on an idiopathic basis (Bell's palsy). The etiology and pathophysiology remain unknown. The diagnosis is one of exclusion: facial nerve palsies also occur in the setting of *herpes zoster oticus,* in which they are typically associated with otalgia and varicelliform lesions affecting the external ear, ear canal, or tympanic membrane. Facial paralysis of a lower motor neuron type can be caused by *infiltrative disease in the meninges,* such as carcinomatous meningitis, and by *inflammatory diseases* such as sarcoidosis and Lyme disease. *Primary tumors of the facial nerve* can occur with apparently rapidly developing facial paralysis, although often in retrospect more subtle facial asymmetry had developed over a longer period. Facial paralysis can also occur in primary *CNS disease* affecting the pontomedullary junction, such as multiple sclerosis. Facial palsy has been noted in individuals with HIV infection, particularly in the early stages shortly after initial infection.

These considerations excluded, most cases of facial paralysis reflect idiopathic Bell's palsy. Patients typically notice facial paralysis on inspection in the mirror in the morning, and the disorder appears to come on overnight in many instances. Onset of facial paralysis may be heralded or accompanied by pain behind the ear (in the region of the stylomastoid foramen). The severity of paralysis varies widely. The prognosis can to some extent be predicted by electrophysiologic examination of the facial nerve after the first several days. In most cases, prognosis is quite favorable. Some believe that a course of oral corticosteroids with rapid tapering may improve the prognosis and is widely used, but this has never been verified. In severe cases, protection of the cornea from drying and injury is essential.

TRIGEMINAL NEURALGIA (TIC DOULOUREUX)

Trigeminal neuralgia is a recurring pain syndrome in which episodes of abrupt stabbing pain involve the second or third divisions of the trigeminal nerve. This and other painful cranial neuralgias are discussed in Ch. 455.

Section Sixteen—Diseases of Muscle (Myopathies) and Neuromuscular Junction

Andrew G. Engel

453 GENERAL APPROACH TO MUSCLE DISEASES

Muscle diseases are caused by derangements in the structure or function of the muscle fiber or in the innervation, blood supply, or connective tissue elements of muscle. A myopathy is a muscle disease not related to a demonstrable alteration in the innervation of muscle. To facilitate the understanding of muscle diseases, this chapter begins with a brief overview of the structure and function of muscle.

BASIC STRUCTURE AND FUNCTION OF MUSCLE

Each voluntary muscle contains myriad muscle fibers. A small proportion of the fibers is confined to muscle spindles that function as mechanoreceptors and participate in regulating the motor tone. The remaining muscle fibers are innervated by α motor neurons. A *motor unit* consists of one α motor neuron and the muscle fibers it innervates. The number of motor units per muscle and the number of muscle fibers per motor unit vary from muscle to muscle. In general, motor units are smaller in small muscles subserving delicate movements than in large muscles maintaining posture or exerting strong force. Muscle fibers belonging to different motor units intermingle with each other, so that the territories of individual motor units overlap. All muscle fibers in a motor unit share similar properties or are of the same type. Three major muscle-fiber (and motor-unit) types can be recognized: Type I, slow-twitch, fatigue-resistant fibers are high in oxidative enzymes but low in glycolytic enzymes. Type IIB, fast-twitch fatigable fibers are high in glycolytic enzymes and low in oxidative enzymes. Type IIA, intermediate-twitch, fatigue-resistant fibers are high in glycolytic enzymes and have an intermediate content of oxidative enzymes. In most human muscles the three fiber types occur in about equal proportions. Because the motor unit territories overlap, the fiber types intermingle randomly.

Adult muscle fibers are about 50 μm in diameter. The myofibrils, which account for most of the fiber volume, are associated with mitochondria, glycogen granules, transverse (T) tubules, and sarcoplasmic reticulum (SR). The myofibrils, 0.5 to 1.0 μm wide, consist of repeating units, or sarcomeres, limited by Z disks. The latter anchor 1 μm-long thin filaments that extend from each Z disk toward the center of the sarcomere. The thin filaments interdigitate with 1.6 μm-long thick filaments in the central region (A-band) of the sarcomere. The sarcomeres of adjacent myofibrils lying in register give the striated appearance to the muscle fiber. The thin filaments are composed of actin, troponin, and tropomyosin. The thick filaments are made up nearly entirely of regularly arrayed myosin molecules. The head of each myosin molecule projects laterally from the thick filament and can serve as a cross-bridge between myosin and actin. The T tubules are inward extensions of the muscle fiber surface membrane and propagate the action potential into the depth of the fiber. The SR abuts on the T tubules and partially envelops individual myofibrils. In the resting state the SR sequesters calcium into its lumen by means of an ATPase and thereby maintains a very low calcium concentration (about 10^{-7} M) around the myofilaments.

When the T tubules are depolarized by an action potential, voltage sensors embedded in their wall open calcium release channels positioned on the abutting SR surfaces and calcium escapes from the SR into the myofilament space. The released calcium binds to troponin on the thin filaments which then act on tropomyosin to allow repeated binding of the myosin cross-bridges to actin. Each binding is associated with a conformational change in the cross-bridge that exerts a force on the thin filament toward the center of the sarcomere. The cross-bridge cycle requires adenosine triphosphate (ATP), which is split by an ATPase on the cross-bridge. If ATP is depleted, the cross-bridges remain attached to the thin filaments and the muscle becomes stiff, as in rigor mortis. When ATP is available, the unloaded fiber shortens, the thin filaments are propelled into the A band, and the Z disks are pulled closer together in every sarcomere. The active state subsides with calcium reuptake by the SR; interaction between actin and the cross-bridges ceases and relaxation sets in.

THE DIAGNOSIS OF MUSCLE DISEASES

The diagnosis of a muscle disease rests on the clinical data, the electromyogram (EMG), and the muscle biopsy. None of the three approaches is individually adequate, but their combined use yields the correct diagnosis in a very high proportion of cases. Examples of disorders that are similar by clinical criteria but require muscle biopsy and EMG for accurate diagnosis are polymyositis, limb-girdle dystrophy, and adult acid maltase deficiency; distal muscular dystrophies, progressive muscular atrophy, and the slow-channel myasthenic syndrome; and benign congenital myopathies, mitochondrial myopathies, and childhood or juvenile spinal muscular atrophies.

CLINICAL DATA. *The Genetic History.* This is relevant to diagnosis as well as counseling. A negative family history, however, does not exclude either autosomal recessive inheritance, an incompletely penetrant autosomal-dominant gene in one parent, or a new mutation. In autosomal dominant disorders (e.g., myotonic and facioscapulohumeral dystrophy or the familial periodic paralyses) a negative family history needs to be validated by examination of both parents. The clinical examination or biochemical tests may help in detecting heterozygotes in autosomal-recessive or X-linked-recessive diseases. In Duchenne and Becker dystrophy, carrier detection and prenatal diagnosis are facilitated by analyses of dystrophin and DNA.

The History of the Illness. **Age at Onset, Duration, and Rate of Progression of Symptoms.** Most benign congenital myopathies, congenital muscular dystrophy, congenital myasthenic syndromes, a number of inherited metabolic myopathies, and the acute form of spinal muscular atrophy present in infancy. Duchenne dystrophy usually presents in early childhood. Many inherited myopathies, inherited anterior horn cell diseases, and most hereditary peripheral neuropathies present in childhood or early adult life. Limb-girdle, Becker, and facioscapulohumeral dystrophy usually present in adolescence; myotonic, oculopharyngeal, limb-girdle, and distal dystrophies can present in adult life. Dermatomyositis and scleroderma can begin in childhood or adult life; pure polymyositis is unusual before adolescence; and sporadic inclusion-body myositis seldom presents before the fifth decade.

Muscle weakness evolving over a few hours suggests an exogenous intoxication (e.g., organophosphorus or barium poisoning), periodic paralysis, or rhabdomyolysis. An abrupt onset of symptoms also can occur in myasthenia gravis or with other defects of neuromuscular transmission. Acute muscle weakness appearing during or after recovery from a Reye syndrome–like metabolic crisis suggests an enzyme defect in organic acid metabolism associated with secondary carnitine deficiency. Weakness evolving over a few days to a few weeks can occur in acute postinfectious polyneuropathy (Guillain-Barré syndrome), toxic neuropathies, and acute dermatomyositis. A subacute evolution, over a period of weeks to months, is seen in motor neuron disease; some metabolic myopathies, such as corticosteroid-induced or thyrotoxic myopathy; late-onset nemaline myopathy; and most cases of dermatomyositis and idiopathic polymyositis. A slow evolution over a number of years is typical of most dystrophies but can also occur in the inflammatory myopathies, such as inclusion body myositis, and in some cases of motor neuron disease.

Effects of Exercise, Rest After Exercise, Diet, and Temperature. Weakness appearing or increasing during exercise suggests a defect of neuromuscular transmission or in muscle energy metabolism. Weakness that decreases with exercise but increases during rest after exercise is typical of the periodic paralyses. Fasting or a high-fat diet may provoke or worsen symptoms in patients with defects of fatty acid oxidation. Exposure to cold worsens myotonia and can provoke weakness in periodic paralysis and paramyotonia congenita. Exposure to heat can increase neuromuscular transmission defects.

Symptoms in Muscle Diseases. Relatively few symptoms are associated with diverse muscle diseases: weakness, decrease of muscle bulk, increased fatigability, muscle pain, cramps, stiffness, and discoloration of the urine caused by myoglobinuria. The cardinal symptom is muscle weakness, but patients often describe its consequences instead of speaking of weakness. Patients complaining of cramps sometimes suffer from contractures or tetany. The term *stiffness* is used to describe a variety of conditions, such as the stiff-man syndrome, neuromyotonia, and myotonia.

Muscle Weakness. Weakness of the cranial, cervical, torso, and limb muscles presents stereotypically. Weakness of muscles supplied by cranial nerves causes drooping of the eyelids (ptosis, third cranial nerve); double vision (diplopia, third, fourth, and sixth cranial nerves); failure of the eyelids to close at night, altered facial expression, difficulty in whistling or sucking from a straw (seventh cranial nerve); inability to close the jaw, difficulty in chewing hard food (fifth cranial nerve); and difficulty in pronouncing words (dysarthria), hypernasal voice, nasal regurgitation of liquids, and difficulty in swallowing (dysphagia) (tenth and twelfth cranial nerves). Weakness of the cervical muscles is shown by difficulty in lifting the head from a pillow or holding the head erect, and weakness of the truncal muscles by difficulty in rolling over in bed or sitting up from the supine position. Weakness of the arm muscles is related as difficulty in holding the arms overhead, lifting heavy objects, or using the hands for motor tasks. Weakness of the pelvic girdle and of the proximal lower extremity muscles is reflected by difficulty in rising from sitting or squatting, climbing stairs, or stepping in or out of the bathtub. Weakness of the distal lower extremity may cause flopping of the feet or difficulty in rising on the toes.

Other Symptoms. In evaluating *abnormal fatigability,* it is important to define the duration and intensity of exercise that provokes it. Even mild exercise can induce fatigue in patients with defects of neuromuscular transmission or with mitochondrial myopathies that involve an electron transport complex. Brief periods of intense, anaerobic exercise precipitate fatigue in patients with glycolytic enzyme defects, but sustained exercise is required to induce fatigue in carnitine palmityltransferase deficiency.

Muscle pain (myalgia) at rest can occur in some of the inflammatory myopathies (especially dermatomyositis and the eosinophilia-myalgia syndrome); during acute viral infections; in polymyalgia rheumatica, myxedema, myotonic disorders, and necrotizing vasculitis; during attacks of myoglobinuria; and in neuropathies associated with vitamin B_1 deficiency, arsenic intoxication, and alcoholism. *Muscle pain during and after exercise* is experienced when the energy supply to muscle is restricted, as with defects in glycolysis or fatty acid oxidation, AMP deaminase defi-

ciency, or ischemia (as in intermittent claudication, scleroderma, and amyloidosis involving muscle), or in normal persons after unusually strenuous exercise.

Muscle cramps last from seconds to minutes, are associated with high-frequency (up to 150 Hz) discharges of the motor units, and can be initiated by strong contractions and stopped by stretching the muscle. They occur with dehydration, azotemia, hyponatremia, and myxedema, in partially denervated muscles, and sometimes in normal individuals without known cause.

Muscle contractures are electrically silent, last from a few to more than 30 minutes, occur only in patients with glycolytic enzyme defects, are provoked only by exercise, and involve only those muscles that are exercised.

The facial and carpopedal spasms of *tetany* occur with hypocalcemia or hypomagnesemia and are associated with high-frequency (up to 300 Hz) axonal discharges. High-frequency electrical discharges also occur in muscle in the *stiff-man syndrome, neuromyotonia,* and *myotonia,* arising in the spinal cord, the peripheral nerves, and the muscle fiber surface membrane, respectively.

In *myotonic disorders* mechanical or electrical stimuli applied to any region of the muscle fiber surface membrane elicit repetitive spike discharges that wax and wane in amplitude and frequency. Mechanical deformation of the membrane during contraction acts as positive feedback, again depolarizing the membrane. The result is tetanic contraction of the individual fibers. The symptoms are stiffness, difficulty in relaxing muscles after a strong contraction, being muscle-bound at the beginning of exercise, and improvement with continued exercise.

Myoglobinuria follows the excessive release of myoglobin from muscle during a period of rapid muscle fiber destruction (rhabdomyolysis). Weakness, muscle pain, and malaise are associated features.

The Clinical Examination. Inspection. This can reveal muscle atrophy, hypertrophy, contractures, winging of the scapulas, fasciculations (twitching of portions of muscles at rest caused by single contractions of motor units), and myokymia (fine undulating movements of muscles associated with sustained abnormal motor-unit activity). The examiner also notes the patient's stance and gait, ability to walk on toes and heels, and hop on one foot, and rise from sitting, squatting, or lying supine.

Inspection provides information on the distribution of weakness, which is then confirmed by detailed manual muscle testing. For example, weakness of the pelvic girdle muscles causes a waddling gait; if there is also weakness of the back extensor muscles, the gait is also lordotic with hyperextension of the upper torso. Muscle atrophy consistently predicts muscle weakness, but not all weak muscles are atrophic, and muscle atrophy can be masked by obesity. Muscle hypertrophy not from voluntary exercise is common in myotonia congenita; it also occurs in the course of Duchenne and Becker and—less commonly—of limb-girdle dystrophy. Hypertrophy may appear with chronic partial denervation, acid maltase deficiency, the permanent myopathy of periodic paralysis, myxedema, sarcoidosis, amyloidosis, and cysticercosis. The nonspecific term *pseudohypertrophy* refers to enlargement of a weak muscle.

Manual Muscle Testing. The British Medical Research Council provides a commonly used rating scale for muscular weakness: 5, normal power; 4, active movement against gravity and resistance; 3, active movement against gravity; 2, active movement with gravity eliminated; 1, trace contraction; 0, no contraction.

The distribution of the weakness can help in formulating the clinical diagnosis. Weakness greater in proximal than distal muscles suggests a myopathy rather than a neuropathy. Predominantly distal muscle weakness suggests a neuropathy but can also occur in myotonic and other distal dystrophies and inclusion body myositis. Selective involvement of some muscles with sparing of others is more likely to occur in dystrophy than in inflammatory muscle disease, but it can also accompany such diverse entities as adult acid maltase deficiency, focal myositis, or the slow-channel myasthenic syndrome. The external-ocular and other cranial muscles can be affected by the Guillain-Barré syndrome, neuromuscular transmission defects, some mitochondrial myopathies, oculopharyngeal dystrophy, and myotubular myopathy. Diffuse, symmetric weakness of multiple cranial muscles with ptosis but with sparing of the ocular movements suggests myotonic dystrophy. Motor neuron disease can affect the bulbar muscles but spares the external ocular muscles ex-

TABLE 453-1. CLINICAL CLUES DIFFERENTIATING MUSCLE FROM NERVE DISEASE

	Myopathy	Neuropathy-Neuronopathy
Distribution	Mainly proximal and symmetric	Distal if symmetric; nerve or root distribution if mono- or multifocal
Atrophy	Late and mild	Early and prominent
Onset	Usually gradual	Often rapid
Fasciculations	Absent	Sometimes present
Reflexes	Lost late	Lost early
Tenderness	Diffuse in myositis	Focal in nerve or root disease
Cramps	Rare	Common
Sensory loss	Absent	Often present
Muscle enzymes	Usually elevated	Usually not or slightly elevated

cept rarely in terminal stages. Selective weakness of the triceps, wrist extensor, finger extensor, iliopsoas, hamstring, anterior tibial, and peroneal muscles, with relative sparing of other muscles, suggests upper motor neuron involvement.

Other Findings. *Action myotonia* is observed as an inability to open the fist or the eyes promptly after closing them tightly for a few seconds. *Percussion myotonia* appears as a local postpercussion contraction followed by abnormally slow relaxation. It can best be observed in the tongue, deltoid, thenar, and extensor digitorum communis muscles. A local swelling appearing for a few seconds at the site of percussion is not myotonia but *myoedema,* seen in myxedema and emaciation.

The *tendon reflexes* are diminished in proportion to the weakness in most myopathies; an early loss of tendon reflexes is observed in neurogenic diseases of muscle, inclusion body myositis, the Lambert-Eaton myasthenic syndrome, and a number of benign congenital myopathies. Slow relaxation of the reflexes is typical of myxedema.

A complete *examination of the nervous system* is also relevant to the evaluation of muscle weakness. Table 453–1 lists clinical guidelines that differentiate nerve from muscle disease. Peripheral neuropathy, ataxia, neurosensory hearing loss, myoclonus, fluctuating neurologic deficits, and mental deterioration can be associated with mitochondrial myopathies.

Recognition of the *signs or symptoms of an associated illness* can point to the cause of the myopathy. Examples are collagen-vascular diseases, sarcoidosis, amyloidosis, the endocrine myopathies, and the mitochondrial myopathies with multisystem involvement. *Involvement of organs or tissues other than muscle* provides further diagnostic clues. For example, cardiomyopathy can be associated with myotonic dystrophy, a dystrophinopathy, Emery-Dreifuss dystrophy, certain types of periodic paralysis, thymomatous myasthenia gravis, and late-onset nemaline myopathy. Cardiomyopathy and/or hepatic enlargement can occur in sarcoidosis and in the myopathies associated with deficiencies of acid maltase, debranching enzyme, carnitine, acyl-CoA dehydrogenase, and a mitochondrial electron transport complex.

Nonorganic Findings Simulating Muscle Disease. See Table 453–2.

Serum Enzymes of Muscle Origin. The serum creatine kinase (CK) level is elevated in many muscle diseases. The enzyme is released into serum from injured skeletal or cardiac muscle. CK is a dimer of muscle-specific (M) and brain-specific (B) monomers, and the different CK isoenzymes can be distinguished by electrophoretic analysis. Mature muscle contains predominantly the MM isoen-

TABLE 453-2. SYMPTOMS OR SIGNS OF FUNCTIONAL MUSCLE DISEASE

Vague complaints
Migrating or diffusely constant muscle pain without tenderness
Excessive, nonfocal tenderness
"Give-way" weakness during testing
Bizarre sensory deficits
Hysterical gait or postures

TABLE 453-3. MOLECULAR GENETIC FINDINGS IN MYOPATHIES

Disease	Gene Locus/Defect	Inheritance
Duchenne/Becker dystrophy	Xp21 Large deletions in 2/3; small rearrangements in 1/3	XLR
Emery-Dreifuss dystrophy	Xq28	XLR
Facioscapulohumeral dystrophy	4q35*	AD
Severe childhood limb-girdle dystrophy	13q12	AR
Limb-girdle dystrophy	15q	AR
Limb-girdle dystrophy	5q	AD
Myotonic dystrophy	19q13 Unstable DNA: excess trinucleotide repeats	AD
Hypokalemic periodic paralysis	1q31–q32; mutations in T tubule voltage sensor	AD
Hyperkalemic periodic paralysis/paramyotonia congenita	13q13.1–13.3; point mutations in muscle sodium channel gene	AD
Myotonia congenita	7q35; point mutations in muscle chloride channel gene	AR or AD
Central core disease/malignant hyperthermia	19q13.1	AD
Nemaline myopathy	1q21–1q23*	AD
Myotubular myopathy	Xq28*	XLR
Acid maltase deficiency	17q23	AR
Myophosphorylase deficiency	11q13	AR
Muscle phosphofructokinase deficiency	1cenq32	AR
Phosphoglycerate kinase deficiency	Xq13	XLR
Muscle phosphoglycerate mutase deficiency	7p12–p13	AR
Lactate dehydrogenase deficiency	11p15.4	AR
Carnitine palmitoyltransferase II deficiency	1p11–p13	AR
Kearns-Sayre syndrome	Mitochondrial DNA; deletions	Sporadic
MELAS	Mitochondrial DNA; tRNA-(lys) point mutation	Maternal
MERRF	Mitochondrial DNA; tRNA-(leu, ile) point mutations	Maternal
LHON	Mitochondrial DNA; point mutations in complex 1, or cyt *b*	Maternal
NARP	Mitochondrial DNA; point mutation in complex 6	Maternal

* Other gene loci may also exist.

XLR, X-linked recessive; AD, autosomal dominant; AR, autosomal recessive; MELAS, mitochondrial encephalomyopathy, lactic acidosis, and strokelike episodes; MERRF, myoclonic epilepsy with ragged-red fibers; LHON, Leber's hereditary optic neuroretinopathy; NARP, neurogenic muscle weakness, ataxia, and retinitis pigmentosa. (Data from table by Jean-Claude Kaplan and Bertrand Fontaine, Neuromuscular Disorders 1:89, 1994.)

zyme, whereas in mature cardiac muscle the MB form predominates. Accordingly, abnormal CK release from muscle increases mostly the MM isoenzyme, whereas CK release from heart increases the MB form in serum. Injured muscle releases other enzymes, such as aldolase, lactate dehydrogenase, and aspartate aminotransferase, but the increases are less marked and can derive from other tissues, such as the liver and erythrocytes. The serum CK level is a sensitive index of muscle fiber injury in a myopathy; it also can increase slightly or modestly in motor neuron disease, in chronic peripheral neuropathies, after severe voluntary exertion, or following a convulsion.

ELECTROMYOGRAPHY (EMG). This test consists of the analysis of spontaneous, evoked, and voluntarily generated potentials from nerve and muscle. The procedure is useful in distinguishing between broad categories of disease, such as myopathy versus neuropathy, or demyelinating versus axonal neuropathy. In some instances the types of electrical potentials and the pattern of abnormality suggest a disease category, such as an inflammatory myopathy, a myotonic disorder, or a storage myopathy. A progressive decrease of the amplitude of the compound muscle action potential evoked by low-frequency repetitive nerve stimulation (decremental response) is observed with defects of neuromuscular transmission.

Sequential assessment of an EMG abnormality can provide useful information on the distribution, degree of activity, and progression of a disease. For example, persistent fibrillation potentials in polymyositis reflect continuing disease activity; the decremental response can be used to monitor the course of myasthenia gravis; and alterations in nerve conduction velocities are a guide to the progression of peripheral neuropathies. Further details of the usefulness of EMG are given in Ch. 392.2, 446, and 459.

THE MUSCLE BIOPSY. Biopsy specimens are used for light microscopic, ultrastructural, and biochemical studies. In most instances, light microscopic observations with enzyme histochemical studies are sufficient and sometimes critical for diagnosis.

Muscles showing mild to moderate weakness are biopsied. Strong muscles may not show diagnostic pathologic change, and in more severely affected muscles excessive amounts of connective tissue may obscure the basic pathologic process. Muscles that have been injected (as is often the case for the deltoid) or recently examined by EMG are unsuitable for diagnosis. The reference provides details of light and electron microscopic findings as well as diagnostic biochemical studies that can be obtained on muscle biopsies.

Molecular Genetic Studies. These are important because they help in diagnosis and carrier detection. Thus far, molecular genetic studies have contributed more to diseases of muscle than to those of any other tissue (Table 453–3).

Engel AG, Franzini-Armstrong C (eds.): Myology, 2nd ed. New York, McGraw-Hill, 1994. *A multiauthored book on the anatomy, physiology, and biochemistry of skeletal muscle, the approach to muscle diseases, and the clinical aspects of muscle diseases.*

454 MUSCULAR DYSTROPHIES

Muscular dystrophies are inherited myopathies associated with progressive muscle weakness, destruction and regeneration of the muscle fibers, and eventual replacement of the muscle fibers by fibrous and fatty connective tissue. There is no accumulation of metabolic storage material in the muscle fibers. A current classification is shown in Table 454–1.

DYSTROPHINOPATHIES. The term includes X-linked allelic disorders resulting from mutations of the large dystrophin gene located at Xp21 (see Table 453–3). At least five different tissue-specific dystrophin transcripts exist. Dystrophin in skeletal muscle is a 420-kD subsarcolemmal cytoskeletal protein concentrated in transverse riblike rings over each sarcomere and interacting with other cytoskeletal proteins, and a dystrophin-associated protein (DAP) complex links the cytoskeleton of the sarcolemma to the extracellu-

TABLE 454–1. CLASSIFICATION OF THE MUSCULAR DYSTROPHIES

X-linked recessive dystrophies
  Duchenne/Becker dystrophies and other dystrophinopathies
  Emery-Dreifuss dystrophy
Autosomal recessive dystrophies
  Severe childhood limb-girdle dystrophy
  Chromosome 15q-linked limb-girdle dystrophy
  Autosomal recessive distal dystrophies
    With necrotizing features
    With rimmed vacuoles
  Congenital muscular dystrophies
    Without cerebral abnormalities
    With ocular and cerebral abnormalities
Autosomal dominant dystrophies
  Myotonic dystrophy
  Facioscapulohumeral dystrophy
  Oculopharyngeal dystrophy
  Chromosome 5q-linked limb-girdle dystrophy
  Autosomal dominant scapuloperoneal dystrophy
  Autosomal dominant distal dystrophies
    With onset in upper limbs (Welander type)
    With onset in lower limbs
    Tibial muscular dystrophy

lar matrix. Dystrophin deficiency results in a secondary DAP deficiency. Further, deficiency of a 50-kD DAP component in itself causes a severe autosomal recessive muscular dystrophy (see below). The severity of the resulting phenotype usually depends upon whether the dystrophin mutation shifts the translational reading frame. The two major dystrophinopathy phenotypes are Duchenne and Becker dystrophy.

Duchenne Dystrophy. Most patients have a frameshifting mutation and severe dystrophin deficiency that can be demonstrated by immunoblotting or immunostaining of muscle. The combined dystrophin and secondary DAP deficiency weaken the sarcolemma, resulting in ultrastructurally detectable sarcolemmal tears. The result permits the influx of calcium-rich extracellular fluid and complement into the muscle fiber. Activation of intracellular proteases and complement leads to fiber necrosis.

The incidence of Duchenne dystrophy is close to 1 in 3300 male births, the mutation rate being about 1 in 10,000. The disease is present at birth, produces symptoms during early childhood, leads to failure of ambulation near the end of the first decade, and causes death near the end of the second decade. The serum creatine kinase (CK) level is markedly elevated from birth and decreases gradually as muscle bulk is lost. Early symptoms are developmental delays, difficulty in running or climbing stairs, frequent falls, and enlargement of the calves. Initially the weakness is more proximal than distal. Except for the sternocleidomastoids, the cranial muscles and the external anal sphincter are spared. The proximal tendon reflexes disappear by the age of 10. Joint contractures commonly appear in most patients between 6 and 10 years of age. After ambulation is lost, all muscles atrophy and paraspinal muscle weakness leads to progressive kyphoscoliosis. Weakness of the respiratory muscles can be detected after the age of 10, but the diaphragm is relatively spared. Respiratory failure, with or without respiratory infections, occurs terminally. The heart is affected with scarring of the posterobasal portion of the left ventricle, producing tall right precordial R waves and deep left precordial Q waves in the electrocardiogram in 90% of the patients. Clinically significant cardiomyopathy is uncommon and in only 10% of cases is death related to cardiac dysfunction. Central nervous system involvement is indicated by lower than average intelligence and mild cerebral atrophy.

Infrequently, Duchenne dystrophy manifests in females who have Turner's (XO) or Turner's mosaic (X/XX or X/XX/XXX) syndrome, a structurally abnormal X chromosome, or an X-autosomal translocation. In a few female heterozygotes, the disease manifests because of incomplete inactivation of the maternal X chromosome.

Becker Dystrophy. Most patients have a non-frameshifting mutation, so that a reduced amount of an abnormal dystrophin is produced, resulting in a milder syndrome than Duchenne dystrophy. Immunoblots of muscle extracts distinguish between Becker and Duchenne dystrophy as well as between sporadic cases of Becker and limb-girdle dystrophy.

Becker dystrophy has an incidence of about 1 per 20,000 male births. The disorder begins later and evolves more slowly than Duchenne dystrophy: The mean age of onset of symptoms, becoming chair-bound, and death are 12, 30, and 42 years, respectively. Most patients show marked calf muscle enlargement until the terminal stage. Calf pain on exercise is a frequent and early symptom. The serum CK level is markedly elevated even in preclinical stages of the disease but begins to decline after the age of 20. Contractures develop at the wheelchair stage. Electrocardiographic abnormalities develop in about 40%. A small proportion of the patients have a dilated cardiomyopathy unrelated to the severity of the myopathy.

Other Dystrophinopathies. Other, milder dystrophinopathy phenotypes are represented by exercise intolerance associated with myalgias, muscle cramps, or myoglobinuria; minimal limb-girdle weakness or quadriceps myopathy; asymptomatic elevation of the serum CK level; cardiomyopathy with only mild muscle weakness; and fatal X-linked cardiomyopathy without muscle weakness. The different dystrophin phenotypes are determined by the site of the mutation in the dystrophin gene and whether the mutation affects the expression of the cardiac isoform of dystrophin.

DIAGNOSIS. In families in which a dystrophinopathy has been previously diagnosed, the clinical findings can define the diagnosis. Special studies are recommended for the diagnosis of new cases, but the approach to a given patient is likely to depend on the cost and availability of the various diagnostic procedures. In all the dystrophinopathies, immunoblotting of muscle is more reliable than immunostaining. Deletional analysis of genomic DNA obtained from leukocytes or muscle, using the polymerase chain reaction with multiple primers to amplify deletion-prone exons, identifies 65% of all mutations but may not distinguish between frameshifting and non-frameshifting mutations.

X-LINKED MUSCULAR DYSTROPHY WITH EARLY JOINT CONTRACTURES AND CARDIOMYOPATHY (EMERY-DREIFUSS DYSTROPHY). Recent genetic linkage studies have mapped this disease to band q28 of the X chromosome. The disease presents in childhood, progresses slowly, and involves distal or proximal muscles in the lower extremities and proximal muscles in the upper extremities. The serum CK is moderately elevated. Contractures of the knees, elbows, and cervical and dorsolumbar spine appear early. Atrial conduction defects and paralysis, requiring treatment by pacemaker, appear later. The disorder has been referred to as Emery-Dreifuss dystrophy and as X-linked scapuloperoneal myopathy, the distinction depending only on whether the proximal or distal muscles are affected in the lower limbs. The lack of muscle hypertrophy, early contractures, slow progression, relatively low serum CK, and overt cardiac involvement distinguish this disease from Duchenne dystrophy; all these features but the slow progression differentiate it from Becker dystrophy. When cardiomyopathy cannot be detected or the pedigree of X-linked inheritance is not established, the disease can be difficult to distinguish from the rigid-spine syndrome or other heterogeneous scapuloperoneal syndromes.

LIMB-GIRDLE SYNDROMES. *Definition and Classification.* The term applies to a clinically heterogeneous syndrome characterized by weakness of pectoral- or pelvic-girdle but not of facial muscles. The disorders can be separated into three major categories:

1. Genetically distinct limb-girdle dystrophies mapped to chromosomal loci. This category includes three entities (see Table 453–3).
2. Limb-girdle dystrophies observed in large kinships and with a well-defined pattern of inheritance but still not linked to a chromosomal locus. These disorders include autosomal dominant benign myopathies, or as yet uncharacterized autosomal recessive muscular dystrophies.
3. Other limb-girdle syndromes. This group identifies by default progressive myopathies involving the limb-girdle muscles that cannot be identified specifically by currently available criteria.

The Differential Diagnosis of Limb-Girdle Syndromes. All patients with limb-girdle syndromes need to be further investigated by EMG and muscle biopsy. In those with a positive family history, the differential diagnosis includes inherited metabolic myopathies (e.g., acid maltase deficiency or a lipid storage myopathy); morphologically distinct congenital myopathies or their late-onset variants (e.g., nemaline, central core, and myotubular myopathies); or progressive muscular atrophy. In sporadic cases of a limb-girdle syndrome the differential diagnosis includes the same diseases, and also inflammatory myopathies (polymyositis, inclusion body myositis, or sarcoidosis confined to muscle), endocrine myopathies, sporadic Duchenne dystrophy, Duchenne or Becker dystrophy manifesting in female carriers, other dystrophinopathies, and sporadic Emery-Dreifuss dystrophy before the appearance of joint contractures or cardiomyopathy.

FACIOSCAPULOHUMERAL DYSTROPHY. The inheritance is autosomal dominant with high penetrance and variable expression (see Table 453–3). The disease presents in childhood or adult life. It involves the facial muscles early and then descends to the scapular fixators, the muscles of the upper arm, and the anterior leg muscles. Early physical signs include failure to bury the eyelashes, an expressionless face, pouting lips, winging of the scapulas when the arms are raised, and an inward-sloping anterior axillary fold. The rate of progression and the extent to which pelvic girdle, forearm, and lower torso muscles are eventually affected vary considerably between and within different families. There is no muscle hypertrophy; joint contractures are uncommon; and the serum CK level is normal or shows mild elevation. In some families a conspicuous inflammatory reaction appears in affected muscles, but the course of the illness is unaltered by corticosteroid therapy. In others an asso-

ciated sensorineural hearing loss occurs, with or without retinal telangiectasis and progressive painless blindness (Coats syndrome). The differential diagnosis includes progressive muscular atrophy, congenital myopathies (e.g., nemaline, central core, and myotubular myopathy), mitochondrial myopathies, sporadic cases of Emery-Dreifuss dystrophy before the appearance of joint contractures or cardiomyopathy, the scapuloperoneal syndrome, the slow-channel myasthenic syndrome, and polymyositis.

MYOTONIC DYSTROPHY. Transmission of myotonic dystrophy is by dominant inheritance with high penetrance and variable expressivity. The gene locus and defect are now known (see Table 453–3). Part of the sequence predicts the gene product to be a member of the protein kinase family. The disease is associated with abnormal expansion of CTG repeats in the 3′ untranslated region of the gene. The age of onset, the expressivity of the disease, and the severity of the congenital myotonic dystrophy have been correlated with the number of repeats. How the gene defect causes tissue injury and myotonia is not yet understood. The incidence is about 1 in 7500 births. A typical distribution of the weakness, myotonia, and multisystem abnormalities characterizes the disease.

Myotonic dystrophy presents in childhood or adult life with a mean age at onset of 19 years. Myotonic symptoms either precede or accompany the muscle weakness. As the disease evolves, the myotonia diminishes in muscles severely affected by the dystrophic process. Distal limb, levator palpebrae, masticatory, facial, cervical, pharyngeal, laryngeal, and upper esophagus muscles are commonly affected. External ophthalmoplegia is rare. Weakness also can appear in proximal limb and respiratory muscles. The latter, when severe, results in alveolar hypoventilation, hypercapnia, arterial oxygen unsaturation, and increasing somnolence. Action myotonia is commonly observed in facial, lid elevator, and hand muscles; percussion myotonia is usually found in tongue, thenar, finger extensor, and selected proximal limb muscles.

Myotonic dystrophy produces systemic abnormalities including frontal baldness, subcapsular cataracts, testicular atrophy and ovarian dysfunction in adult life, extrathyroidal hypometabolism, endorgan unresponsiveness to insulin, mental changes, and hypercatabolism of IgG. Cardiac conduction defects are common and can cause sudden death. Gastrointestinal smooth muscle involvement results in reduced lower esophageal and gastric motility and dilatation of segments of the colon. Some patients have bouts of diarrhea alternating with constipation and colicky abdominal pain. Less frequent manifestations are pigmentary retinal degeneration and cranial anomalies (hyperostosis cranii, small sella turcica, large paranasal sinuses, and prognathism).

Muscle biopsies characteristically show very large muscle fibers with numerous central nuclei, sarcoplasmic masses, ring fibers, and variable type 1 fiber atrophy. Necrotic fibers are uncommon. The serum CK level is normal or only slightly elevated.

DISTAL DYSTROPHIES. A number of genetically distinct entities have been recognized. Different types of *autosomal dominant distal muscular dystrophies* have been described. That observed in a large Scandinavian kinship by Welander presents between the fourth and sixth decades with selective weakness and atrophy of the forearm extensor and intrinsic hand muscles and then involves the anterior leg and small foot muscles. In patients homozygous for the dominant gene, the onset is earlier and proximal muscles are also affected. Another form of distal dystrophy observed in some districts of Finland selectively involves the anterior tibial muscles; the upper extremities are never affected. In other non-Scandinavian kinships with late onset and dominant inheritance, the disease first involves the lower extremities. The serum CK level is normal or slightly increased. Two varieties of *autosomal recessive distal muscular dystrophies* have been described. In both there is a juvenile onset and the lower limbs are affected before the upper. In one type there is frequent fiber necrosis and regeneration and the serum CK level is markedly increased. In the other type the muscle fibers harbor rimmed vacuoles and the serum CK level is only slightly increased.

The differential diagnosis of the distal muscular dystrophies includes myotonic dystrophy, inclusion body myositis, debranching enzyme deficiency, distal mitochondrial myopathy, distal chronic spinal muscular atrophy, and the neuronal form of peroneal muscular atrophy.

OCULOPHARYNGEAL MUSCULAR DYSTROPHY. The disease, inherited as autosomal dominant, presents in the fifth or sixth decade with progressive ptosis and dysphagia. Later, all external ocular and other voluntary muscles may become affected. Death usually results from starvation or aspiration pneumonia. The serum CK level is normal or slightly increased. Muscle biopsy discloses intranuclear tubular filaments and rimmed vacuoles in the muscle fibers.

THE RIGID-SPINE SYNDROME. This is a heterogeneous disorder in which muscle contractures involve the spine as well as other joints. An autosomal dominant form presenting with proximal muscle weakness in the first decade is also recognized. In most cases the disease is sporadic, begins in the first decade, and results in widespread muscle weakness and atrophy during the second decade.

CONGENITAL DYSTROPHIES. See Table 454–1.

TREATMENT OF THE MUSCULAR DYSTROPHIES. There is no specific treatment of any of the muscular dystrophies. Physical therapy to prevent contractures, orthoses, and corrective orthopedic surgery can be used to improve the quality of life in some stages. The cardiac conduction defects in Emery-Dreifuss dystrophy and myotonic dystrophy may require treatment by pacemaker. The myotonia in myotonic dystrophy is rarely a clinical problem but can be treated with phenytoin (0.3 to 0.6 gram daily) or by quinine (0.3 to 1.5 grams daily).

Preventive treatment consists of prenatal diagnosis in families with known pedigrees, carrier detection, and genetic counseling. Some Duchenne carriers are recognized by immunostaining muscle for dystrophin, which may show scattered dystrophin-negative fibers. In some Becker carriers dystrophin of abnormal size or amount is detected by immunoblotting. Close to 65% of Duchenne or Becker carriers and fetuses at risk can be identified by DNA analysis using cDNA probes or the polymerase chain reaction; carriers not identified this way may still be detected in families with known carriers by linkage analysis. In myotonic dystrophy, the detection of an abnormal number of CTg repeats in the 3′ untranslated region of the gene allows prenatal diagnosis and detection of presymptomatic cases. However, this test may not detect all carriers.

Recent advances in molecular genetics have raised hopes for gene therapy of Duchenne dystrophy, but this approach is still in its infancy.

Ahn AH, Kunkel LM: The structural and functional diversity of dystrophin. Nature Genetics 3:283, 1993. *A concise and comprehensive account of what is currently known about the dystrophin gene and dystrophin.*

Barohn RJ, Miller RG, Griggs RC: Autosomal recessive distal dystrophy. Neurology 41:365, 1991. *A good review of the currently recognized forms of distal dystrophies.*

Clarke A: Report of the ENMC workshop on the limb-girdle muscular dystrophies. J Med Genet 29:753, 1992. *An informative survey of the genetically distinct forms of limb-girdle dystrophy.*

Engel AG, Franzini-Armstrong C (eds.): Myology, 2nd ed. New York, McGraw-Hill, 1994. *Excellent, comprehensive descriptions of the muscular dystrophies by multiple experts.*

Matsumura K, Campbell KP: Dystrophin-glycoprotein complex: Its role in the molecular pathogenesis of muscular dystrophies. Muscle Nerve 17:2, 1994. *A summary of recent developments that pave the way for a better understanding of muscular dystrophies.*

Nicholson LVB, Johnson MA, Bushby KMD, et al.: An integrated study of 100 patients with Xp21-linked muscular dystrophy using clinical, genetic, immunochemical and histopathological data. III. Differential diagnosis and prognosis. J Med Genet 30:475, 1993. *A clearly written guide to the use and interpretation of currently available tests for the dystrophinopathies.*

455 MORPHOLOGICALLY DISTINCT CONGENITAL MYOPATHIES

DEFINITIONS AND BASIC CONCEPTS. The diseases in this group are characterized by the following features:

The course is nonprogressive or relatively nonprogressive. The prognosis is generally benign except in reducing body myopathy and in the X-linked form of myotubular myopathy.
A distinct pattern of inheritance is observed in some diseases (e.g., central core disease, nemaline myopathy); others are genetically heterogeneous (e.g., myotubular myopathy).

TABLE 455–1. MORPHOLOGICALLY DISTINCT CONGENITAL MYOPATHIES

Central core disease
Nemaline (rod) myopathy
Myotubular (centronuclear) myopathy
    Severe X-linked recessive form
    Milder autosomal recessive and dominant forms
Multicore disease
Congenital fiber type disproportion
Fingerprint body myopathy
Sarcotubular myopathy
Reducing body myopathy
Trilaminar myopathy
Myopathy with focal lysis of type I fibers
Spheroid/cytoplasmic body myopathies

Muscle weakness is present at birth or appears in early childhood. It is proximal or diffuse and may or may not involve the cranial muscles.
The muscle bulk is normal or reduced. There is no muscle hypertrophy.
The deep tendon reflexes are reduced or absent in most cases.
Skeletal abnormalities related to the weakness, such as a high-arched palate, kyphoscoliosis, dislocated hips, and pes cavus, are common.
The serum CK level is normal, except in some older patients with myotubular or sarcotubular myopathy.
The EMG is normal or suggests a myopathy. Spontaneous electrical activity is absent in all cases, except for fibrillation potentials and myotonic discharges in some cases of myotubular myopathy.
Each disease has one or more distinguishing, but not specific, morphologic features. Type I fiber preponderance and small type I fibers occur in most disorders.

Table 455–1 lists the currently recognized morphologically distinct congenital myopathies.

Late-Onset Variants. Adult-onset cases of central core disease, nemaline myopathy, myotubular myopathy, and multicore disease exist. In some cases mild congenital disease becomes recognized only after additional progression in adult life or when discovery of an affected younger relative prompts investigation of other family members.

Two other forms of late-onset nemaline myopathy are noteworthy. One is sporadic, evolves subacutely or chronically, affects the proximal limb and torso but not the cranial muscles, and may cause death from respiratory failure. The CK level is normal. Some cases possess an associated monoclonal gammopathy. Histologically, there is progressive accumulation of nemaline rods and progressive atrophy of rod-containing fibers. Another late-onset form occurs in a familial setting, is associated with cardiomyopathy, and can result in sudden death.

Fardeau M, Tomé FMS: Congenital myopathies. *In* Engel AG, Franzini-Armstrong C (eds.): Myology, 2nd ed. New York, McGraw-Hill, 1994, p 1487. *A comprehensive, well-illustrated review. It raises numerous unanswered questions about etiology and nosology.*

456 INFLAMMATORY MYOPATHIES

DEFINITION AND CLASSIFICATION. Inflammatory myopathies represent a heterogeneous group of disorders (Table 456–1). Most are diffuse in distribution, but some are focal, affecting circumscribed regions in single or multiple muscles. Some are caused by or related to bacterial, parasitic, or viral infections. In most other inflammatory myopathies the cause is undetermined, but an autoimmune origin is suspected. This section focuses on selected aspects of the idiopathic inflammatory myopathies not covered in other chapters.

TABLE 456–1. CLASSIFICATION OF INFLAMMATORY MYOPATHIES

Infections
  Parasitic: toxoplasmosis, sarcosporidiosis, African trypanosomiasis, American trypanosomiasis, cysticercosis (*Taenia solium*), trichinellosis
  Bacterial: pyomyositis, septic myositis, gas gangrene (*Clostridium welchii*), leprous myositis
  Spirochetal: Lyme disease (*Borrelia burgdorferi*)
  Viral: acute myositis following influenza or other viral infections, retrovirus-related myopathies (HIV, HTLV-I)
Idiopathic, autoimmune origin suspected
  Pure polymyositis
  Dermatomyositis
  Inclusion body myositis
  Scleroderma involving muscle
  Inflammatory myopathy associated with another autoimmune disease (systemic lupus erythematosus, rheumatoid arthritis, Sjögren's syndrome, rheumatic fever, overlap syndromes, chronic graft-versus-host disease, polyarteritis nodosa)
  Sarcoidosis involving muscle
  Inflammatory myopathies with eosinophilia
    Eosinophilic polymyositis
    Localized eosinophilic myositis
    Eosinophilic perimyositis
    Diffuse fasciitis with eosinophilia
    Eosinophilia-myalgia induced by L-tryptophan preparations
  Focal myositis
    Focal proliferative myositis
    Localized nodular myositis
      Pseudothrombophlebitis of a calf muscle
    Orbital myositis
  Polymyalgia rheumatica*
Other inflammatory myopathies
  Localized myositis ossificans
  Generalized myositis ossificans

---

* There are no inflammatory changes in muscle.

Myopathies Related to Retrovirus Infections. These can appear early or late in the course of immunodeficiency virus (HIV) infections. The most common form is HIV-associated polymyositis, which presents early in the infection and is mediated by T cells. Necrotizing myopathy without inflammation, or myopathies with nemaline rods or giant cells, necrotizing vasculitis, focal myositis in the form of pseudothrombophlebitis, and recurrent myoglobinuria without other predisposing factors also can occur. Attempts to immunolocalize HIV antigens in muscle fibers have consistently failed, and the manner in which the HIV virus induces myopathies is unclear. Zidovudine, an agent for treatment of the HIV infection, may induce a toxic mitochondrial myopathy coexistent with the HIV-related myopathy.

Human T cell leukemia virus type I (HTLV-I), an agent associated with chronic spastic paraparesis, also can be associated with polymyositis, but the virus has not been shown to infect muscle fibers.

Autoimmunity in Idiopathic Inflammatory Myopathies. Authorities have inferred an autoimmune cause in inflammatory myopathies from one or more of the following observations: (1) The myopathy is associated with another identifiable autoimmune disease (e.g., systemic lupus erythematosus or rheumatoid arthritis). (2) Laboratory tests suggest an altered immune state (e.g., myositis-specific antibodies, increased serum gamma globulins, decreased total hemolytic complement in serum, and positive tests for antibodies against native DNA, other nuclear or cytoplasmic antigens, or rheumatoid factor). (3) Muscle contains a predominantly mononuclear inflammatory exudate. (4) Evidence exists of focal invasion and destruction of muscle fibers by antigen-specific cytotoxic T cells. (5) The diseases respond to corticosteroids or other immunosuppressants. The first criterion, if fulfilled, represents strong, but indirect, evidence. Laboratory tests suggesting an altered immune state are positive in a minority of patients with dermatomyositis and in polymyositis. A mononuclear inflammatory exudate, however, also can occur in some genetically determined muscle diseases (e.g., Duchenne or facioscapulohumeral dystrophy). Inclusion body myositis, in which an inflammatory exudate is often prominent, most cases of scleroderma, and some cases of pure polymyositis

and dermatomyositis do not respond to immunosuppressants. Further, neither the factors that initiate self-sensitization nor the sensitizing antigen has been defined in any of the major inflammatory myopathies (idiopathic polymyositis, inclusion body myositis, dermatomyositis, and scleroderma). None has been transferred to an experimental animal.

Sporadic Inclusion Body Myositis. This entity differs from other idiopathic inflammatory myopathies in several respects. It fails to respond to corticosteroids or other immunosuppressants. Most patients are older than 50, and there is male predominance. The disease evolves slowly, affecting the lower limbs first, involving both proximal and distal muscles, and resulting in selectively severe weakness and atrophy of the quadriceps. Facial, cervical, and pharyngeal muscles are usually spared. Deep tendon reflexes disappear early from the affected limbs. The serum CK level is mildly elevated or normal. The EMG indicates myopathic changes and abnormal electrical irritability, as in dermatomyositis or polymyositis, but there may be additional neurogenic features as well. Affected muscles show a typical pattern of histologic change: rimmed vacuoles in a significant proportion of the fibers; eosinophilic intranuclear and cytoplasmic inclusions in a few fibers that also are congophilic and react positively for ubiquitin and β-amyloid protein; small groups of atrophic fibers without type grouping; and an endomysial and a lesser perivascular inflammatory exudate. The exudate is enriched in cytotoxic T cells that focally surround, invade, and destroy non-necrotic fibers. Necrotic fibers occur but are less common than in polymyositis. Ultrastructural studies show that the rimmed vacuoles contain myeloid structures and other cytoplasmic degradation products and that the inclusions consist of microtubular filaments. The differential diagnosis includes motor neuron disease, distal muscular dystrophies, peripheral neuropathies, and pure polymyositis. The diagnosis is usually clarified by a careful study of the muscle biopsy.

Differences Between Dermatomyositis and Pure Polymyositis. Dermatomyositis and pure polymyositis resemble each other in the predominantly proximal distribution of the muscle weakness, a mononuclear inflammatory exudate in muscle, myopathic changes, spontaneous electrical activity in the EMG, and responsiveness to corticosteroid therapy. Consequently, they are often treated as a single entity in evaluating their cause, natural history, and therapy. Several aspects of dermatomyositis differentiate it from pure polymyositis, however: (1) The characteristic rash of dermatomyositis is lacking in pure polymyositis. (2) Capillary injury and necrosis are early and constant findings in dermatomyositis. Many of the injured capillaries react for the membrane attack complex of complement, whereas other vessels are found to be occluded by platelet thrombi or to harbor microtubular inclusions. (3) Muscle fibers at the periphery of the fascicles undergo selective degeneration and atrophy. (4) The inflammatory exudate is concentrated at perimysial and perivascular sites and is enriched in B cells and helper T cells. (5) There is no evidence for T cell–mediated cytotoxicity directed against the muscle fibers. These findings suggest that a humoral response against vascular elements plays an important role in the pathogenesis of dermatomyositis.

By contrast, no capillary necrosis or loss develops in pure polymyositis. The inflammatory exudate contains fewer B cells and helper T cells than in dermatomyositis, and B cells are virtually absent from the endomysium. Focal invasion and destruction of non-necrotic muscle fibers by antigen-specific cytotoxic T cells accompanied by macrophages indicate cell-mediated cytotoxicity directed against the muscle fiber. Necrosis of isolated fibers also occurs. These findings suggest that a component of the muscle fiber surface membrane is a target of the immune effector response.

Differences Between Scleroderma and the Other Major Inflammatory Myopathies. In scleroderma, the serum CK level is either normal or only slightly elevated, the resting EMG is often normal, and necrotic fibers are uncommon. The pathologic changes involve fibrosis and inflammation affecting the perimysium and the perimysial blood vessels. The inflammatory cells at these sites are predominantly T cells and macrophages. The findings suggest a cell-mediated immune response against a perimysial and/or vascular component in muscle.

Eosinophilia-Myalgia Related to L-Tryptophan Preparations. This syndrome appeared in 1989 in patients consuming L-tryptophan preparations. The features consisted of eosinophilia ($> 10^9$ per liter), marked myalgias, fasciitis, and often a peripheral neuropathy. Interstitial pneumonitis, myocarditis, and encephalopathy occurred in some subjects. An autoimmune pathogenesis was implicated by onset or progression of the syndrome after withdrawal of the L-tryptophan preparation, inflammatory cells in the affected tissues, and responsiveness to immunotherapy in some cases. The pathologic substrate is an interstitial inflammation associated with an occlusive microangiopathy and fibroplasia. The triggering factor appears to be 1,1'-ethylidenebis[tryptophan], a contaminant of L-tryptophan produced by a single manufacturer.

Myositis Ossificans. The *localized form* appears as a tender swelling after trauma to a muscle. After a few months this becomes hard and ossified. Therapy consists of excision. The *generalized form* represents an autosomal dominant disease with variable expressivity that begins in childhood, involves many muscles, and causes progressive rigidity of body parts. The initial lesions appear in fascia and dermis and are associated with inflammation, local hemorrhage, and connective tissue proliferation. Cartilage and bone formation occur at a later stage. Other congenital malformations (microdactyly of the great toe, exostoses, absence of upper incisors or of ear lobules, and hypogenitalism) are found in most patients. There is no effective therapy.

Engel AG, Franzini-Armstrong C (eds.): Myology, 2nd ed. New York, McGraw-Hill, 1994. *Comprehensive descriptions of the clinical and laboratory features and therapy of polymyositis, dermatomyositis, inclusion body myositis, and other inflammatory and HIV-associated myopathies by multiple authors.*

Mastaglia FL (ed.): Inflammatory myopathies. *In* Ballière's Clinical Neurology, vol 2, no 3. Philadelphia, Ballière Tindall, 1993. *A detailed survey by multiple authors of the clinical and pathologic aspects of the major subtypes of inflammatory myopathies.*

457 METABOLIC MYOPATHIES

GLYCOGEN STORAGE DISEASES. These are described in detail in Ch. 170. When muscle is involved, glycogen-filled vacuoles appear in the fibers; the glycogen excess can vary from slight to marked, and definitive diagnosis requires demonstration of a specific enzyme deficiency. Of the several glycogenoses, only glucose-6-phosphate dehydrogenase and liver phosphorylase deficiencies fail to affect muscle. All glycogenoses that affect muscle are transmitted as autosomal-recessive traits except phosphoglycerate kinase deficiency, which is X-linked recessive.

Acid Alpha-1,4-Glucosidase (Lysosomal Acid Maltase) Deficiency. The gene encoding the enzyme maps to chromosome 17q23. Various mutations affecting the synthesis, phosphorylation, maturation, and catalytic activity of the enzyme have been identified. Three major clinical variants exist. The *infantile type* presents in early infancy with generalized and rapidly progressive weakness and heart, tongue, and liver enlargement. There is widespread and marked glycogen excess in tissues, including lower motor neurons. Death occurs from cardiorespiratory failure before the age of 2 years. The *childhood type* presents in infancy or early childhood as a myopathy. Weakness is more proximal than distal, and there may be calf enlargement simulating muscular dystrophy. Glycogen excess is less marked and confined to muscle. Death occurs before age 20 of respiratory failure. The *adult type* presents between the second and seventh decade of life, either with slowly progressive limb muscle weakness that mimics limb-girdle dystrophy or polymyositis, or with insidiously developing ventilatory insufficiency leading to respiratory failure. In all three types the serum CK level is increased, but to less than 10 times normal. The EMG in affected muscles shows myopathic changes and excessive abnormal electrical irritability, including myotonic discharges (but there is no clinical myotonia). Muscle biopsy demonstrates a vacuolar myopathy with high glycogen content and acid-phosphatase reactivity in the vacuoles, an appearance that otherwise occurs only in chloroquine myopathy and a rare cardioskeletal lysosomal storage disorder without acid maltase deficiency.

Debranching Enzyme Deficiency. The gene for the enzyme maps to chromosome 1p21. A disabling myopathy affecting both proximal and distal muscles can appear in childhood or (more commonly) in adult life. Often there is a history of a protuberant abdomen and hypoglycemic episodes in childhood, along with muscle fatigue on exertion. Persistent hepatomegaly and biventricular cardiac hypertrophy are found in most cases. There is a diminished glycemic response to epinephrine and glucagon and an impaired rise of lactic acid after ischemic exercise. The EMG shows myopathic changes and abnormal electrical irritability in affected muscles.

Branching Enzyme Deficiency. The disease presents in infancy with progressive hepatosplenomegaly and failure to thrive. The abnormal starchlike glycogen, which resists diastase digestion, induces nodular cirrhosis and liver failure. Death occurs in early childhood from liver or heart failure. Muscle weakness is variable; if present, the tongue is severely affected.

Phosphorylase b Kinase (PBK) Deficiency. This syndrome shows marked clinical and genetic heterogeneity. Cardiac PBK deficiency is a fatal disease of infancy. An autosomal recessive form presents in childhood with weakness or hepatomegaly that improves with age; PBK is deficient in muscle, liver, and erythrocytes. An X-linked recessive disease presents in children with asymptomatic hepatomegaly or mild hypoglycemia; PBK is deficient in liver and erythrocytes. Another form of PBK deficiency which is restricted to muscle presents with exercise intolerance and myoglobinuria or a late-onset myopathy simulating muscular dystrophy.

Glycolytic Enzyme Defects: Myophosphorylase, Phosphofructokinase (PFK), Phosphoglycerate Kinase (PGK), Phosphoglycerate Mutase (PGM), and Lactate Dehydrogenase (LDH) Deficiencies. Table 453–3 lists the molecular genetic findings. The common clinical features are periodic myoglobinuria following strenuous exertion since childhood; easy fatigability; and a venous lactate level that fails to rise after ischemic exercise in myophosphorylase and PFK deficiencies, and fails to rise or rises by less than 100% in PGK, PGM, and LDH deficiencies. Muscle cramps are prominent. They are caused by electrically silent contractures and are not associated with ATP depletion; their mechanism is not understood. The muscle glycogen excess is slight to modest. Permanent muscle weakness and atrophy are initially slight, but may increase with age. Fatal infantile variants have been identified in myophosphorylase and PFK deficiency. In PFK deficiency hyperuricemia and gout occur in some cases, and there is mild hemolytic disease caused by a partial erythrocyte enzyme defect. PGK mutations result in either severe hemolytic anemia and neurologic deficits but no myopathy, or produce a myopathy with only the features described above.

DISORDERS OF FATTY ACID METABOLISM. Long-chain fatty acids taken up by muscle are utilized for energy metabolism or incorporated into triglycerides and stored as lipid droplets. Long-chain fatty acids entering the catabolic pathway are esterified with coenzyme A (CoA) to form acyl-CoA's. These react with carnitine to form acylcarnitines in a reaction catalyzed by carnitine palmitoyltransferase (CPT) I, an enzyme positioned on the inner surface of the inner mitochondrial membrane. The acylcarnitines are transported through the inner mitochondrial membrane by a carnitine-acylcarnitine translocase and then reconverted to acyl-CoA's by CPT II. The acyl-CoA's undergo repeated cycles of beta-oxidation, generating acetyl-CoA's that enter the citric acid cycle or form ketone bodies. The inner mitochondrial membrane is impermeable to long-chain fatty acids, CoA, and acyl-CoA's. Consequently, carnitine, carnitine-acyltransferases, and carnitine-acylcarnitine translocase jointly regulate the oxidation of fatty acids and modulate the intramitochondrial CoA/acyl-CoA ratio. Excessive intramitochondrial accumulation of an acyl-CoA compound leads to its conversion to a corresponding acylcarnitine. The acylcarnitine leaves the mitochondrion via the translocase, diffuses out from the cell, and is preferentially excreted by the kidney. If this process continues, muscle and body carnitine stores become depleted.

Derangements in fatty acid oxidation produce a variety of syndromes that affect muscle and other organs. The possible consequences include one or more of the following: intermittent energy shortage in muscle causing *rhabdomyolysis* and *myoglobinuria;* intramitochondrial acyl-CoA excess and CoA deficiency, secondary carnitine depletion, and inhibition of multiple mitochondrial enzyme systems (these events trigger a *Reye syndrome–like metabolic crisis,* see Ch. 429); and triglyceride accumulation in muscle producing a *lipid-storage myopathy.* Many carnitine-deficiency syndromes are secondary to another metabolic defect in fatty acid oxidation, branched-chain amino acid metabolism, or the respiratory chain. A lipid storage myopathy can be caused by primary carnitine deficiency or by another defect of fatty acid oxidation with or without secondary carnitine deficiency (Table 457–1).

Carnitine Palmitoyltransferase Deficiency. Infantile and adult forms of the disease exist. The most common cause of adult CPT deficiency is a homozygous Ser113Leu mutation in the CPT II gene (see Table 453–3). In affected patients who are heterozygous for this mutation, a second mutation in the CPT II gene is likely. The symptoms consist of muscle aching, fatigability, and periodic myoglobinuria on sustained exertion, especially if combined with fasting and exposure to cold. There are no symptoms between attacks, and the muscle lipid content is normal or only slightly increased.

Acyl-CoA Dehydrogenase Deficiencies. Deficiencies of the long-chain, medium-chain, and short-chain specific enzymes, and in the factors that transfer electrons from multiple acyl-CoA dehydrogenases to coenzyme Q (multiple acyl-CoA dehydrogenase deficiency), have been identified. Each syndrome causes secondary carnitine depletion, a lipid storage myopathy, and organic aciduria. The urinary organic acid and acylcarnitine profiles reflect the site of the metabolic block. *Short-chain acyl-CoA dehydrogenase deficiency* is associated with adult-onset lipid storage myopathy. Ketogenesis is not impaired and there are no metabolic crises. The other acyl-CoA dehydrogenase deficiencies produce intermittent metabolic crises resembling Reye syndrome. *Long-chain acyl-CoA dehydrogenase deficiency* usually has a neonatal onset and is associated with hepatomegaly and cardiomyopathy. *Medium-chain acyl-CoA dehydrogenase deficiency* usually presents in the first or second year of life with a metabolic crisis. Between attacks the patients are well or have mild weakness, easy fatigability, and mild hepatomegaly. *Multiple acyl-CoA dehydrogenase deficiencies* are genetically and biochemically heterogeneous. Severe neonatal forms with cardiomyopathy and milder late-onset cases have been described. Some cases respond to riboflavin therapy. The acyl-CoA dehydrogenase deficiencies are treated with a low-fat, high-carbohydrate diet and L-carnitine supplements (2 to 4 grams daily in adults and 100 mg per kilogram daily in infants and children). Crises can be prevented by avoiding fasting and maintaining alimentation at all times, especially during febrile illnesses. The crises are treated by intravenous therapy to correct the hypoglycemia and electrolyte abnormalities, and by L-carnitine, initially 100 mg per kilogram and then 25 mg per kilogram every 4 hours.

Primary Carnitine Deficiency Syndromes. Primary systemic carnitine deficiency is an autosomal recessive disease due to impaired carnitine transport in muscle, heart, renal and intestinal epithelia, and fibroblasts. Defective intestinal absorption and a renal

TABLE 457–1. DISORDERS OF LIPID METABOLISM AFFECTING MUSCLE

Primary muscle or systemic carnitine deficiency
Organic acidurias with acyl-CoA dehydrogenase deficiencies*
  Long-chain acyl-CoA dehydrogenase deficiency
  Medium-chain acyl-CoA dehydrogenase deficiency
  Short-chain acyl-CoA dehydrogenase deficiency
  Multiple acyl-CoA dehydrogenase deficiency
  Long-chain 3-hydroxyacyl-CoA dehydrogenase deficiency
  Short-chain 3-hydroxyacyl-CoA dehydrogenase deficiency
Organic acidurias with defects in branched-chain amino acid metabolism*
  Isovaleryl-CoA dehydrogenase deficiency†
  Propionyl-CoA carboxylase deficiency
  Methylmalonyl-CoA mutase deficiency
  β-hydroxy-β-methylglutaric-CoA lyase deficiency
Defects in mitochondrial respiratory chain or energy utilization‡
  Block at NADH-coenzyme Q reductase (Complex I deficiency)
  Mitochondrial ATPase deficiency (Complex V deficiency)
Miscellaneous disorders‡
  Idiopathic Reye syndrome
  Valproate therapy

* Associated with secondary carnitine deficiency.
† This enzyme is also an acyl-CoA dehydrogenase.
‡ Only some patients become carnitine deficient and accumulate lipid in muscle.

TABLE 457–2. CLASSIFICATION OF MITOCHONDRIAL MYOPATHIES

Nuclear DNA defects
  Hypermetabolic myopathy (Luft syndrome)
  Defects proximal to the mitochondrial respiratory chain
    Carnitine palmitoyltransferase deficiency
    Primary and secondary carnitine deficiency syndromes
    Acyl-CoA dehydrogenase deficiencies
    Defects in the pyruvate dehydrogenase complex
  Defects of the mitochondrial respiratory chain
    Coenzyme Q deficiency
    Complex I deficiency
    Complex II deficiency
    Complex III deficiency
    Complex IV deficiency
Mitochondrial DNA mutations
  Kearns-Sayre syndrome
  PEO due to mitochondrial myopathy
  MERRF
  MELAS
  Maternally transmitted mitochondrial myopathy and cardiomyopathy
  NARP
  LHON
Defective interaction of nuclear and mitochondrial DNA
  Multiple mitochondrial DNA deletions
  Myoneurogastrointestinal disorder and encephalopathy
  Mitochondrial DNA depletion*

* Affects infants. See chapter by Morgan-Hughes in Engel AG, Franzini-Armstrong C (eds.): Myology, 2nd ed. New York, McGraw-Hill, 1994.

PEO, Progressive external ophthalmoplegia; MERRF, myoclonic epilepsy with ragged red fibers; MELAS, mitochondrial encephalomyopathy with lactic acidosis and strokelike episodes; NARP, neurogenic muscle weakness, ataxia, and retinitis pigmentosa; LHON, Leber's hereditary optic neuroretinopathy.

carnitine leak caused by the transport defect result in further tissue carnitine depletion. The disease is associated with cardiomyopathy, weakness, and episodes of hypoketotic hypoglycemic encephalopathy; it responds to carnitine replacement therapy. A myopathic form of primary carnitine deficiency also exists and may respond to prednisone therapy.

Other Lipid Storage Myopathies. Autosomal recessive and dominant lipid storage myopathies associated with lifelong weakness, myalgias, and electrical myotonia, but without carnitine deficiency, have been described. *Chanarin's disease* is a rare autosomal recessive condition with congenital ichthyosis, steatorrhea, and lipid storage in muscle fibers, hepatocytes, gastrointestinal epithelial cells, epidermal cells, monocytes, myelocytes, and fibroblasts.

MITOCHONDRIAL MYOPATHIES. Mitochondrial diseases can arise from mutations in nuclear or mitochondrial DNA or stem from a defective interaction between nuclear and mitochondrial DNA. Some mitochondrial DNA mutations are transmitted by vertical maternal inheritance; others arise *de novo* in the maternal ovum or in early embryonic life. Table 457–2 shows a current classification of the mitochondrial myopathies.

In many mitochondrial myopathies a substantial proportion of the muscle fibers contains subsarcolemmal and intermyofibrillar accumulations of structurally and functionally abnormal mitochondria. These fibers appear "ragged red" in the trichrome stain and "ragged blue" when reacted for succinate dehydrogenase and may fail to react for cytochrome c oxidase (CCO). Some fiber segments are CCO-negative without containing an excess of mitochondria. A segmental distribution of the histologic abnormalities along the length of individual muscle fibers and CCO negativity of only a proportion of the fibers point to a mutation in mitochondrial DNA.

Many mitochondrial myopathies produce slowly progressive weakness of limb and/or external ocular and other cranial muscles, abnormal fatigability on sustained exertion, and lacticacidemia on exertion or even at rest. Some affect multiple organs or systems, and the myopathy is but one facet of a multisystem disease.

Defects Proximal to the Mitochondrial Respiratory Chain. These include the primary carnitine deficiencies, acyl-CoA dehydrogenase deficiencies, carnitine palmitoyltransferase deficiency (all dealt with above), and *defects in the pyruvate dehydrogenase complex*. The latter are associated with various neurologic syndromes that include movement disorders, ataxia, neuropathy, subacute necrotizing encephalomyelopathy (Leigh's syndrome), and fatal infantile lactic acidosis. Muscle biopsy shows ragged red fibers, lipid excess, or denervation atrophy.

Defects in the Mitochondrial Respiratory Chain. The mitochondrial respiratory chain includes four distinct enzyme complexes and also coenzyme Q and cytochrome c. The components are attached to the inner mitochondrial membrane and carry reducing equivalents from reduced nicotinamide adenine dinucleotide (NADH), flavin adenine dinucleotide ($FADH_2$), and electron-transferring flavoprotein (ETF) to molecular oxygen. A fifth complex, an ATPase, uses released energy to phosphorylate ADP to ATP in a tightly coupled process. Defects in the electron transport complexes are associated with marked clinical, biochemical, and genetic heterogeneity. The reasons for this are that each complex is composed of multiple subunits, different subunits of a given complex are encoded by different genes, some subunits of a given complex are encoded by mitochondrial rather than nuclear DNA, some subunits are tissue specific, and some subunits are developmentally regulated.

Coenzyme Q Deficiency. A deficiency of mitochondrial coenzyme Q is associated with a familial syndrome of marked lipid and mitochondrial excess in muscle, severe lactacidemia, intermittent myoglobinuria, progressive muscle weakness, cognitive deficits, cerebellar ataxia, and seizures. The activities of complex I, II, III, and IV and cellular cytochrome levels are normal.

Complex I (NADH-Coenzyme Q Oxidoreductase) Deficiency. Most of these begin in childhood and allow survival to adult life. Either muscular or central nervous system manifestations dominate the clinical picture. In the former group the findings include muscle weakness, exercise intolerance, exertional lactacidemia, and ragged red fibers in muscle. Headaches, progressive visual loss, hemiparesis, dysphasia, dementia, dystonia, and cerebral atrophy affect the latter group. A fatal infantile form exists.

Complex II (Succinate-Dehydrogenase) Deficiency. A deficiency of complex II together with decreased levels of the mitochondrial enzyme aconitase has been observed in patients with lifelong exercise intolerance and recurrent episodes of myoglobinuria. In other patients, a biochemical deficiency of succinate dehydrogenase in muscle is associated with severe infantile myopathy and lactic acidosis or syndromes that phenotypically resemble Leigh syndrome or the Kearns-Sayre syndrome (discussed below).

Complex III (Coenzyme Q–Cytochrome C Oxidoreductase) Deficiency. These begin in childhood or adult life. Muscle weakness, exercise intolerance, exertional lactacidemia, and ragged red fibers are constant findings. Some patients also have external ophthalmoplegia and/or dementia, myoclonus, ataxia, pyramidal signs, and loss of proprioception. The muscle symptoms in one patient were improved by treatment with menadione and vitamin C, agents that can function as electron transfer mediators instead of complex III.

Complex IV (Cytochrome C Oxidase) Deficiency. Several syndromes are associated with this defect, and are detailed in the references.

Mitochondrial DNA Mutations. Mitochondrial DNA (mtDNA) can undergo point, deletion, or duplication mutations. With homoplasmic mutations, a single population of mutant mtDNA appears in all cells and produces a single clinical syndrome. With heteroplasmic mutations, normal and mutant forms of mtDNA coexist in the same cell, and subsequent cell replication leads to uneven segregation of normal and mutant DNA. The phenotypic expression depends on the proportion of mutant to normal mtDNA in cells of a given tissue, as well as tissue dependence on oxidative metabolism and the severity of the oxidation-phosphorylation defect.

Kearns-Sayre Syndrome. The mutations in the major syndromes are listed in Table 453–3. Most cases are sporadic and stem from heteroplasmic DNA deletions in the maternal ovum or during early embryonic life. The syndrome presents under age 20, and is associated with progressive external ophthalmoplegia (PEO), retinitis pigmentosa, and ragged red fibers, plus at least one of the following: heart block, cerebellar syndrome, or a high spinal fluid protein content. More than half of the patients have hearing loss, mental defect, short stature, and lactic acidosis; less than half have cystic changes or calcification of the basal ganglia, pyramidal signs, seizures, peripheral neuropathy, endocrine disturbances (e.g., hypogonadism, diabetes, hypoparathyroidism), or renal Fanconi syndrome. The presence of heart block requires treatment by pacemaker.

Progressive External Ophthalmoplegia Due to a Mitochondrial Myopathy. Not only external ocular but also other cranial as well as cervical, truncal, and limb muscles can be affected. One or more elements of the Kearns-Sayre syndrome also occur in some patients. About half the patients have mitochondrial DNA deletions. The disease is sporadic, indicating that the deletions are found only in somatic cells.

Myoclonus, Generalized Seizures, Ragged Red Fibers (MERRF). The disease presents in children or adults and is associated with progressive myoclonus, seizures, cerebellar ataxia, and muscle weakness. Short stature, dementia, hearing loss, and optic atrophy are frequent; spasticity, central hypoventilation, endocrinopathies, and peripheral neuropathy occur less often.

Mitochondrial Encephalomyopathy with Lactic Acidosis and Strokelike Episodes (MELAS). The same mutations that cause MELAS can also be found in some patients with PEO or other encephalomyopathies without strokelike episodes. In 25% of MELAS patients the family history is consistent with maternal inheritance. More than 90% of MELAS patients have normal early development, experience strokelike episodes before age 40, and have focal or generalized seizures, lactic acidosis, and ragged red fibers in muscle. Brain imaging during strokelike episodes shows areas of encephalomalacia affecting areas lying outside of the territories of the main cerebral arteries. Other frequent features consist of dementia, hearing loss, short stature, and episodic vomiting. Less than half of the patients have calcification of the basal ganglia, ataxia, myoclonus, optic atrophy, episodic coma, increased spinal fluid protein content, or cardiomyopathy. The diagnosis is based on strokelike episodes before the age of 40, seizures or dementia or both, ragged red fibers in muscle or lactic acidosis or both, plus two of the other frequent features.

Maternally Transmitted Mitochondrial Myopathy and Cardiomyopathy. This disorder is caused by another heteroplasmic point mutation at nucleotide 3260 in the mitochondrial $tRNA^{Leu(UUR)}$ gene. It is associated with lactic acidosis and ragged red fibers in muscle. Other features of MELAS are absent.

Neuropathy, Ataxia, and Retinitis Pigmentosa (NARP). In addition to the features characterizing the syndrome, some patients also suffer from developmental delay, seizures, and proximal muscle weakness. Muscles lack ragged red fibers. In some families the same mutation results in Leigh syndrome.

Leber's Hereditary Optic Neuroretinopathy (LHON). The disease is more frequent in men than in women. It presents in young adults with optic neuritis and telangiectasia around the optic disk and results in central loss of vision. Cerebellar ataxia, spasticity, posterior column signs, peripheral neuropathy, and cardiac conduction defects also can occur. Morphologic and biochemical abnormalities affect muscle mitochondria.

Defective Interactions of Nuclear and Mitochondrial DNA. **Multiple Mitochondria DNA Deletions.** This disorder is clinically and genetically heterogeneous, transmitted as an autosomal dominant or recessive trait. The clinical features, which vary from family to family, comprise proximal muscle weakness, PEO, cataracts, hearing loss, ataxia, peripheral neuropathy, mental retardation, and hypoparathyroidism. In one family, two brothers suffered from recurrent myoglobinuria after exertion or fasting.

Myoneurogastrointestinal Disorder and Encephalopathy. This autosomal recessive disorder is associated with PEO, mitochondrial myopathy, neuropathy, abnormal intestinal motility with bouts of vomiting and diarrhea, leukoencephalopathy, and lactic acidosis. Multiple deletions in mitochondrial DNA and biochemical defects in complex IV or I have been observed.

ENDOCRINE MYOPATHIES. Muscle weakness can be a symptom of any endocrine disorder. The serum CK level is normal, except in myxedema and in uremic hyperparathyroidism. The EMG is normal or myopathic without spontaneous electrical activity. The histologic alterations in muscle are often nonspecific, such as type II fiber atrophy, focal increases and decreases in mitochondria, and focal myofibrillar degeneration. Fiber necrosis and regeneration and connective tissue proliferation are uncommon.

Glucocorticoid-Induced Myopathy. Muscle weakness commonly occurs in Cushing's syndrome and in patients receiving relatively high doses of glucocorticoids. Fluorinated drugs (dexamethasone, triamcinolone) are more pathogenic than nonfluorinated ones (prednisone). Considerable variation exists in the minimal dosage that induces myopathy. However, daily treatment for 3 months with 60 mg prednisone in divided doses induces some weakness in nearly all patients. Women are more susceptible than men, and divided daily doses are more pathogenic than single or alternate daily doses. The onset is usually insidious but occasionally sudden with diffuse myalgias. The weakness is more proximal than distal and affects the lower more than the upper limbs. Hip and ankle flexors are selectively severely affected. The cranial muscles are spared. The serum CK level remains normal. Therapy consists of reducing the steroid dosage to the lowest possible level. Muscle strength returns to normal within 1 to 4 months after therapy is stopped.

Adrenal Insufficiency. Weakness is a typical feature, closely related to derangements in fluid and electrolyte balance and possibly to the associated hypotension. Joint contractures, especially of the knees and not related to muscle weakness, may also occur. Hyperkalemia in chronic adrenal insufficiency can be a cause of secondary periodic paralysis (discussed below).

Thyrotoxic Myopathy. This appears in 80% of untreated cases of hyperthyroidism. The hyperthyroid state can be mild and of long duration or present for only a few weeks before the onset of the weakness. Weakness is predominantly proximal, less often both proximal and distal. The deep tendon reflexes are hyperactive or normal. The serum CK level remains normal. The EMG shows myopathic motor unit potentials but never fibrillation potentials.

Graves' ophthalmopathy is described in Ch. 203. Thyrotoxic periodic paralysis is considered below.

Hypothyroid Myopathy. Muscle aching, cramps, slow relaxation of the reflexes, ridging of the muscles on percussion (myoedema), and an increase of the serum CK level are common findings in myxedema. Muscle enlargement and limb-girdle weakness occur only occasionally.

Muscle Symptoms in Hyperparathyroidism and Osteomalacia. Proximal muscle weakness, fatigability, and muscle pain and tenderness, usually with bone pain and tenderness, can occur in primary and secondary hyperparathyroidism and in osteomalacia.

A more malignant syndrome can appear in uremic hyperparathyroidism. Here, metastatic calcification of the media and proliferation of the intima of small blood vessels produce skin and visceral infarcts and a necrotizing myopathy with marked elevation of serum enzymes and myoglobinuria.

Muscle Symptoms in Hypoparathyroidism. The typical neuromuscular symptom is tetany. This is considered in Ch. 214.

Acromegaly and Hypopituitarism. Acromegaly initially causes muscle hypertrophy, particularly if the disorder begins before growth ceases. Later, generalized weakness and atrophy develop. Muscle biopsies can show segmental muscle fiber degeneration, type I or type II fiber atrophy, or no pathologic change. The serum CK level remains normal. A hypertrophic distal neuropathy and nerve entrapment are common in acromegaly.

Pituitary failure in adults results in weakness and fatigability with little muscle atrophy. The weakness itself may reflect the combined influence of thyroid, adrenal, and growth hormone deficiencies.

THE PERIODIC PARALYSES (PP). These disorders occur as either inherited (primary) or acquired (secondary) illnesses and can be further classified according to measurable alterations in the serum potassium level during attacks (Table 457–3). The primary types are transmitted by autosomal dominant inheritance, but nearly a third of the cases arise sporadically. It is important to realize that in the primary forms the serum potassium decreases or increases but may still remain within the normal range during attacks and is normal or low-normal between attacks. By contrast, in secondary PP caused by potassium wastage or retention the serum potassium is always markedly reduced or elevated during and even between attacks. In each type of PP the propagation of the muscle fiber action potential fails during an attack.

The different types of periodic paralysis share several common features: (1) Paralytic attacks last from < 1 hour to as long as several days. (2) Weakness can be localized or generalized. (3) Tendon reflexes diminish and then disappear during attacks. (4) Muscle fibers become inexcitable to direct or indirect electrical stimulation during the attacks. (5) Generalized attacks begin proximally and spread distally. Respiratory and cranial muscles tend to be spared except in the most severe attacks. (6) Rest after exercise provokes weakness in the muscles that were exercised. Continued mild exercise aborts attacks. (7) Exercise followed by rest of a single muscle can induce weakness of that muscle without detectable change in

TABLE 457-3. CLASSIFICATION OF THE PERIODIC PARALYSES

Primary
  Hypokalemic
  Normokalemic
  Hyperkalemic
    without myotonia
    with myotonia
    with paramyotonia
  Paramyotonia congenita
  With cardiac arrhythmia (hyper-, hypo-, or normokalemic)
Secondary
  Hypokalemic
    Thyrotoxic
    Urinary potassium wastage
    Gastrointestinal potassium wastage
    Barium intoxication
  Hyperkalemic
    Renal insufficiency
    Adrenal insufficiency

the potassium level in the systemic circulation. (8) Exposure to cold can provoke weakness in the primary forms of the disease. (9) Complete recovery occurs after initial attacks. (10) In the primary disorders permanent weakness and a persistent vacuolar myopathy can develop with or without repeated attacks. Despite these similarities, the different forms of PP differ in their response to sodium, potassium, or carbohydrate loading, as well as their pattern of urinary electrolyte excretions during attacks, and in some of their clinical features.

Primary Hypokalemic Periodic Paralysis. The disease is caused by mutations in the voltage sensor of the T tubule. Attacks begin in the first or second decade and become less frequent or cease during the fourth or fifth decade. When attacks recur daily, the patient is weakest in the morning and becomes stronger as the day passes. High dietary sodium or carbohydrate intake as well as excitement provokes or exacerbates the episodes. Major attacks are associated with urinary retention of sodium, potassium, chloride, and water. The diagnosis is supported by a positive family history and a decrease in serum potassium during an attack. An abnormally low serum potassium level between attacks suggests secondary rather than primary PP. In diagnosing sporadic cases one must exclude potassium wastage and thyrotoxicosis. The oral or intravenous administration of glucose, 2 grams per kilogram of body weight, combined with 10 to 20 units of insulin given subcutaneously, may provoke an attack within 2 to 3 hours. Depression of the serum potassium during the attack and a favorable response to 2.5 to 7.5 grams of potassium chloride (KCl) given orally must be demonstrated. Provocative tests must never be done in patients already hypokalemic, and potassium chloride must not be given to patients unless they have adequate renal or adrenal reserve.

Thyrotoxic Periodic Paralysis. This disease resembles primary hypokalemic PP in the changes in serum and urinary electrolytes that accompany the attacks and in the response to glucose, insulin, potassium, and rest after exercise. However, 95% of the cases are sporadic, the male to female ratio is 6:1, most cases occur among Orientals, the onset is usually in adult life, and correction of the hyperthyroidism prevents further attacks.

Barium-Induced Periodic Paralysis. The accidental ingestion of absorbable barium salts such as barium carbonate induces hemorrhagic gastroenteritis, hypertension, cardiac arrhythmias, convulsions, hypokalemia, and muscle paralysis. Barium blocks potassium channels and thereby reduces potassium efflux from muscle; potassium uptake by muscle, mediated by the sodium-potassium pump, continues, and hypokalemia results.

Periodic Paralysis Secondary to Urinary or Gastrointestinal Potassium Loss. Paralytic attacks do not occur unless the serum potassium falls below 3 mEq per liter, and during the attacks the serum potassium decreases even further. Other neuromuscular complications of severe potassium depletion include a necrotizing myopathy, myoglobinuria, and latent or manifest tetany.

Primary Hyperkalemic Periodic Paralysis and Paramyotonia Congenita. These diseases are now known to be allelic, caused by mutations in the α-subunit of the adult muscle sodium channel gene. In primary hyperkalemic periodic paralysis, the attacks begin in the first or second decade. They are often brief but can last up to several days. Between attacks the serum potassium is normal or slightly lower than normal. During major attacks potassium moves out from muscle. The serum potassium increases but may not exceed the normal range, and the urinary potassium excretion increases. Myotonic, paramyotonic, and nonmyotonic forms of hyperkalemic PP can be distinguished. In *myotonic hyperkalemic PP* myotonia can be detected in facial, tongue, finger extensor, and thenar muscles between attacks. In *paramyotonic hyperkalemic PP,* exposure to cold causes widespread and severe myotonia. Exercise in the cold is followed by prolonged weakness not reversed by rewarming. Paralytic attacks are provoked by orally administered KCl, 50 to 100 mg per kilogram, given in an unsweetened solution in the fasting state. The test is contraindicated in subjects already hyperkalemic or those without adequate renal or adrenal reserve. In pure *paramyotonia congenita* potassium loading does not induce weakness. Unlike in myotonia congenita, the myotonia is worsened rather than improved by exercise. Exercise in the cold causes prolonged electrically silent stiffness and weakness not relieved by rewarming.

Secondary Hyperkalemic Periodic Paralysis.
This can occur when the serum potassium level exceeds 7 mEq per liter. The usual cause is renal or adrenal insufficiency, but hyperkalemia from exposure to spironolactone and during attacks of malaria also has caused paralytic attacks. The diagnosis is suggested by the presence of a very high serum potassium level during attacks, persistent hyperkalemia between attacks, and the associated primary disorder.

Primary Normokalemic Periodic Paralysis.
There are no consistent changes in the serum potassium during the attacks. The existence of the disease has been questioned because some patients are sensitive to potassium salts. The observations suggest that normokalemic PP is a heterogeneous entity.

Primary Periodic Paralysis with Cardiac Arrhythmia.
Affected patients suffer from PP and tachyarrhythmias that can cause sudden death. The cardiac symptoms are provoked or worsened by hypokalemia and digitalis and are refractory to disopyramide phosphate, propranolol, or phenytoin, but may respond to imipramine. Dysmorphic features, such as short stature, clinodactyly, and microcephaly can also occur. The PP has been clearly related to hyperkalemia in some patients, but hypokalemic and normokalemic PP were diagnosed in others.

Therapy of the Periodic Paralyses.
In all forms of primary PP acetazolamide, from 250 mg to 2 grams daily, can prevent attacks or decrease their frequency. The metabolic acidosis induced by the drug may prevent sodium channel inactivation by small depolarizations. Prolonged exposure to the drug promotes the formation of renal calculi.

The treatment of attacks of *primary hypokalemic PP* consists of giving 2 to 10 grams of oral KCl. Preventive therapy includes acetazolamide, a low-carbohydrate and relatively low-sodium (2.3 grams per day) diet, and 2.5 grams of KCl taken orally three times daily. *Thyrotoxic PP* is treated by antithyroid therapy, KCl supplements, and a low-carbohydrate, low-sodium diet. Acetazolamide is ineffective.

In *primary hyperkalemic PP* one treats the acute attacks with 2 grams per kilogram of glucose by mouth and 15 to 20 units of crystalline insulin subcutaneously. The inhalation of 1.3 mg metaproterenol every 15 minutes for three doses, or of 0.18 mg albuterol repeated once after 10 minutes, has aborted acute attacks. Preventive treatment consists of acetazolamide or thiazide diuretics and frequent high-carbohydrate meals. Tocainide, 300 to 400 mg three to four times daily, prevents cold-induced stiffness and weakness in paramyotonic hyperkalemic PP and paramyotonia congenita. The drug acts by blocking sodium channels in muscle.

The periodic paralyses caused by excessive wastage or retention of potassium are treated by correcting existing electrolyte abnormalities and, if possible, removing the existing cause. In acute barium poisoning, 10 ml of a 10% solution of sodium sulfate is administered intravenously every 30 minutes until symptoms subside.

NUTRITIONAL AND TOXIC MYOPATHIES.
Diffuse muscle atrophy and weakness associated with type II fiber atrophy are commonly observed in malnourished or cachectic patients. The muscle weakness in nutritional osteomalacia has been attributed partly to disuse and partly to malnutrition.

Vitamin E Deficiency.
This has now been implicated in progressive gait and limb ataxia, sensorimotor neuropathy, extraocular muscle paresis, and a myopathy in which giant abnormal lysosomes accumulate in muscle. The cause is a malabsorption syndrome, as detailed in Ch. 103 and 406. High doses of vitamin E may be of benefit.

Myopathy in Alcoholism.
An acute necrotizing myopathy associated with myoglobinuria occurs in chronic alcoholics after a bout of drinking. Hypokalemia caused by sweating, vomiting, diarrhea, and renal wastage may act as a precipitating factor. The hypokalemia may be followed by hyperkalemia as myoglobinuria and renal failure develop. A subacute alcoholic myopathy with proximal muscle weakness and elevation of the serum CK level may also exist. If so, it is usually associated with a chronic neuropathy.

Chloroquine Myopathy.
The side effects of the drug include macular and corneal degeneration, peripheral neuropathy, and myopathy. Muscle weakness appears when the daily dosage is 500 mg for a year or longer. Pathologically, the condition produces a vacuolar myopathy and constitutes a prototype for myopathies due to an excited autophagic mechanism.

Emetine Myopathy.
Emetine, an ipecac alkaloid, is used to treat amebiasis. Side effects include cardiotoxicity and muscle weakness. A reversible myopathy involving proximal limb muscles has been observed in patients with feeding disorders who abuse ipecac to induce vomiting and in alcoholics receiving emetine for aversion therapy. The pathologic findings include focal destruction of mitochondria and focal myofibrillar degeneration.

Other Toxic Myopathies.
Epsilon amino-caproic acid, an inhibitor of fibrinolyis and of clot dissolution, infrequently causes myalgias, myonecrosis, and myoglobinuria. *Colchicine* in customary doses induces a vacuolar myopathy in patients with gout and renal insufficiency who attain elevated plasma drug levels. The antiarrhythmic agent amiodarone can induce an autophagic myopathy and a peripheral neuropathy. *Lovastatin,* an inhibitor of mevalonic acid and cholesterol biosynthesis, causes a necrotizing myopathy with or without myoglobinuria in less than 0.5% of patients. Concomitant therapy with immunosuppressants increases the risk of myopathy. *Isoretinoic acid,* a vitamin A analogue for treating acne, infrequently causes myalgias, elevation of the serum creatine kinase, and reversible muscle damage. *Cocaine* abuse can result in a necrotizing myopathy and myoglobinuria. The myopathy induced by *zidovudine* is considered in Ch. 456.

MYOGLOBINURIA.
The clinical syndrome of myoglobinuria is associated with brown discoloration of urine by myoglobin and metmyoglobin. Myoglobin, a 17,000-molecular-weight protein with a prosthetic heme group, is present in muscle at a concentration of 1 gram per kilogram. It has a lower renal excretory threshold than hemoglobin. Small amounts of myoglobin not sufficient to discolor urine are excreted in various necrotizing myopathies. The visible discoloration of urine by myoglobin indicates both massive and acute muscle destruction (rhabdomyolysis) and warns of impending renal damage. The pigment has to be distinguished from hemoglobin and porphyrins. If there is no hemoglobinemia or hematuria, a positive benzidine test strongly suggests myoglobinuria. However, myoglobinuria itself can induce microhematuria, and certain identification of myoglobin must be made specifically. The immunoprecipitation assay has the virtue of being simple and quantitative but is so sensitive that it detects the pigment in the absence of overt myoglobinuria.

Muscle pain, swelling, and weakness precede overt myoglobinuria by a few hours. In addition to myoglobin, phosphate, potassium, creatine, and muscle enzymes are released into the circulation. The heme pigment in the glomerular filtrate and casts in the tubules cause proteinuria, hematuria, and tubular necrosis. Renal failure is more likely if hypotension, acidosis, and hypovolemia coexist. With increasing renal insufficiency, hyperphosphatemia, hypocalcemia, tetany, and life-threatening hyperkalemia appear. Death may result from renal or respiratory failure. Otherwise, the myoglobinuria and proteinuria disappear in 3 to 5 days. The marked hyperenzymemia decreases gradually, and muscle strength returns relatively slowly after major attacks. EMG abnormalities can persist for several months.

Myoglobinuria can have many causes: metabolic, infectious, toxic, ischemic and/or traumatic, secondary to another myopathy, and idiopathic. It is likely that many of the so-called idiopathic cases have a metabolic or infectious cause.

Myoglobinuria Caused by a Metabolic Disturbance.
The common denominator is impaired substrate utilization for energy metabolism or a critical substrate deficiency in the face of ex-

cessive demands for energy. Most diseases in this group were considered earlier in this chapter. Deficiencies of phosphorylase kinase, myophosphorylase, phosphofructokinase, phosphoglycerate mutase, phosphoglycerate kinase, and lactate dehydrogenase block anaerobic glycolysis; coenzyme Q and succinate dehydrogenase deficiencies interfere with oxidative phosphorylation; and carnitine palmitoyltransferase deficiency impairs fatty acid oxidation when it is most needed. Substrate deficiency in the face of excessive demands and derangements of muscle metabolism account for the myoglobinuria associated with malignant hyperthermia, the malignant neuroleptic syndrome, and the abrupt withdrawal of antiparkinson drugs. Substrate deficiency may also account for the myoglobinuria that occurs after severe exercise in untrained individuals, as in military recruits.

Almost any severe metabolic insult can cause myoglobinuria. These include carbon monoxide poisoning, extreme hypoglycemia, severe hypokalemia, hypernatremia, or water intoxication.

Myoglobinuria with Infections. This can occur after influenza A, herpes simplex, Epstein-Barr, and coxsackievirus infections and early in the course of HIV infection. The precise mechanism is not understood. Myoglobinuria also occurs with bacterial infections accompanied by high fever and sepsis, and with muscle gangrene caused by clostridial infection.

Toxic Myoglobinuria. The myoglobinuria associated with alcoholism was considered above. Intoxication with barbiturates, amphetamine, cocaine, and other narcotics, especially if associated with agitation or coma, can produce myoglobinuria. Myoglobinuria occurring with lovastatin, epsilon amino-caproic acid, or amiodarone was discussed earlier in this chapter. The toxin of the Malayan sea snake, *Enhydrina schistosa,* induces myalgias, trismus, flaccid paralysis, and myoglobinuria.

Ischemic and Traumatic Myoglobinuria. Massive ischemia of muscle from any cause (e.g., major vessel occlusions, angiopathy in uremic hyperparathyroidism), crush injuries, or prolonged pressure on dependent muscles in the immobile comatose patient can induce myoglobinuria. Localized ischemic necrosis of muscle and sometimes myoglobinuria occurs in severe forms of the anterior tibial syndrome.

Myoglobinuria Secondary to Other Myopathies. Myoglobinuria has been observed infrequently in acute dermatomyositis (where the cause is probably ischemia), systemic lupus erythematosus, and mild dystrophinopathies.

Treatment. The acute episode is treated by rest, maintenance of adequate urine flow by hydration and diuretics, and alkalinization of the urine with sodium bicarbonate. Other measures consist of treatment of the renal insufficiency as required and removal of the offending cause if possible.

DiMauro S, Wallace DC (eds.): Mitochondrial DNA in Human Pathology. New York, Raven Press, 1993. *A review of the current status of the mitochondrial DNA diseases by multiple authors.*

Engel AG, Franzini-Armstrong C (eds.): Myology, 2nd ed. New York, McGraw-Hill, 1994. *Chapters by DiMauro and Tsujino, Engel and Hirschhorn, Zierz, DiDonato, Morgan-Hughes, Penn, Victor and Sieb, Kaminski and Ruff, and Lehmann-Horn, Engel, Ricker, and Rüdel provide detailed and up-to-date reviews of the metabolic myopathies.*

Hirano M, Ricci E, Koenigsberger MR, et al.: MELAS: An original case and clinical criteria for diagnosis. Neuromusc Disord 2:125, 1992. *A careful analysis of 70 cases of MELAS and criteria for the clinical diagnosis of the disease.*

458 MISCELLANEOUS MYOPATHIES

INFILTRATIVE MYOPATHIES. *Systemic Amyloid Myopathy.* The most common neurologic complication in various types of amyloidosis is a predominantly sensory-autonomic neuropathy. Amyloid deposition in muscle is frequent, but the muscle involvement is usually subclinical. Occasionally amyloidosis presents or is associated with an overt myopathy characterized by muscle enlargement, macroglossia, stiffness, exertional muscle pain, and

proximal or diffuse weakness. Electromyography shows myopathic features in proximal muscles with or without changes of neuropathy distally. The amyloid deposits, identified by their metachromasia and affinity for Congo red stain, appear between and around the mural elements of the small vessels and extend into the interstitial spaces where they tightly surround individual muscle fibers.

Hypertrophic Branchial Myopathy. This sporadic illness presents between the second and fourth decades of life and is restricted to muscles that derive from the embryonic branchial cleft. The disease evolves with slowly progressive, asymmetric, bilateral enlargement of temporalis, masseter, and pterygoid muscles. Weakness is minimal or absent. The swelling itself is painless but may lead to pain with jaw opening. The EMG and muscle biopsy show nonspecific myopathic alterations in the affected muscles. There is no satisfactory treatment. When chewing is impaired, partial excision of the enlarged muscles has proved beneficial.

SYNDROMES ASSOCIATED WITH ABNORMAL MUSCLE ACTIVITY. These can be caused by (1) abnormal neural activity in the central nervous system (e.g., dystonia, tetanus, stiff-man syndrome); (2) abnormal excitability of the peripheral nervous system (neuromyotonia, tetany, cramps); (3) abnormal excitability of the muscle fiber surface membrane (myotonic disorders); (4) a defect within the muscle fiber resulting in abnormal mechanical activity (e.g., malignant hyperthermia, contractures without electrical activity, and slow relaxation of electrically silent muscle fibers). Dystonia, tetanus, and tetany are considered in Ch. 289, 410, and 412. The remaining entities were discussed earlier in this section or are discussed below.

Stiff-Man Syndrome. This is a disease of adult life affecting men more frequently than women. Initially intermittent spasms of axial and limb muscles are followed by continuous stiffness that immobilizes the patient. Agonist and antagonist muscles are affected simultaneously, preventing voluntary movement. The EMG shows constant firing of normal motor unit potentials in the stiff muscles. There are no signs of cerebral or spinal cord disease. Spinal anesthesia relieves the spasms. The disease is frequently associated with organ-specific autoimmune diseases, and especially insulin-dependent diabetes mellitus. In a series of 13 patients, 4 had circulating antiglutamic acid decarboxylase as well as anti–islet cell and other organ- and non–organ-specific autoantibodies; 4 had an associated solid tumor and antibodies recognizing a 125-kD antigen; and 5 had no evidence of any known autoantibody. As glutamic acid decarboxylase converts glutamic acid to the inhibitory neurotransmitter γ-aminobutyric acid (GABA), the findings suggest that at least in some patients the disease is caused by immune-mediated impairment of GABAergic inhibitory pathways. Relatively high doses of diazepam or baclofen, which increase GABA-mediated central inhibition, and clonidine, which prevents norepinephrine release from nerve terminals, may improve or relieve the symptoms.

Neuromyotonia. This can be generalized or focal. *Generalized neuromyotonia,* or Isaacs' syndrome, is sporadic or familial. Some of the familial cases are associated with a peripheral neuropathy; some of the sporadic cases have an intrathoracic malignancy. Abnormal impulses arising in peripheral motor axons produce continuous muscle fiber activity that persists even during sleep. Depending on the site of origin in the axon, the abnormal activity is abolished by proximal nerve block or block of neuromuscular transmission. The EMG shows very high frequency (150 to 300 Hz) recurring bursts of motor unit potentials. The involuntary activation of multiple motor units causes stiffness and delayed relaxation of the affected muscles and continuous, small, undulating movements of the overlying skin (*myokymia*). Phenytoin or carbamazepine may inhibit the abnormal discharges and relieve the symptoms. Evidence supports an autoimmune cause of this syndrome, possibly an immune response to peripheral nerve potassium channels. Some patients respond to plasmapheresis; some cases are associated with myasthenia gravis, thymoma, or anti-acetylcholine receptor antibodies; and some cases are induced by exposure to penicillamine. Further, some of the electrophysiologic features of the disease can be transferred from humans to mice with IgG.

Similar high-frequency and rhythmically recurring bursts of motor unit potentials occur in *facial myokymia* seen with demyelinating or other lesions of the brain stem.

Focal neuromyotonia can occur following peripheral nerve lesions, but here the firing rate is slower (30 to 60 Hz). The delayed relaxation of an affected muscle after a willed contraction mimics action myotonia.

A benign syndrome of *muscle cramps, fasciculations, and myokymia* associated with low-frequency bursts of motor unit potentials also occurs and may incorrectly suggest the diagnosis of early motor neuron disease.

A syndrome associated with *myokymia, hyperhydrosis, mental symptoms, thymoma,* and *anti-acetylcholine receptor antibodies* but without symptoms of myasthenia gravis has been recently described.

Schwartz-Jampel Syndrome. This autosomal recessive disease begins in early childhood. It is characterized by chondrodystrophy, bone and joint deformities, short stature, a doleful facial expression with blepharospasm, hypertrichosis, muscle stiffness, and muscle hypertrophy or atrophy. There is delayed muscle relaxation suggesting myotonia. The EMG, however, shows high-frequency repetitive discharges, not myotonic discharges. Muscle biopsy reveals neurogenic and myogenic features.

Myotonia Congenita. Autosomal dominant (Thomsen's disease) and autosomal recessive forms of paramyotonia congenita are recognized. The two types of myotonia are associated with different point mutations of the muscle chloride channel gene and are therefore allelic disorders. Both diseases are benign and associated with diffuse muscle hypertrophy and diffuse action, percussion, and electrical myotonia. Cold increases the myotonia, and sustained exercise improves it. The membrane defect consists of a markedly reduced chloride conductance. Quinine, 0.3 to 1.5 grams daily, or phenytoin, 0.3 to 0.6 gram daily, relieves the myotonia.

Slow Relaxation of Electrically Silent Muscle Fibers. This is a rare disease in which there is impaired muscle relaxation that is rapidly worsened by exercise. The slowly relaxing fibers are electrically silent. The defect lies within the calcium-pump ATPase of the sarcoplasmic reticulum.

Rippling Muscles. This is a benign and dominantly inherited disorder presenting in late childhood or adult life. Sporadic cases also occur. Local percussion of a muscle evokes myoedema. This is replaced by a longitudinal depression parallel to the long axis of the muscle which then moves to the periphery of the muscle in 10 to 20 seconds in a wave that resembles the plucking of a chromatic scale on a harp. The response to percussion superficially resembles myotonia, but the rippling muscles are electrically silent. Mild muscle pain, stiffness at the beginning of exercise, and mild elevation of the serum CK level are associated features.

Grimaldi LME, Martino G, Braghi S, et al.: Heterogeneity of autoantibodies in stiff man syndrome. Ann Neurol 34:57, 1993. *A timely review of the evidence for the autoimmune pathogenesis of the disease.*

Newsom-Davis J, Mills KR: Immunological association of acquired neuromyotonia (Isaacs' syndrome). Brain 116:453, 1993. *Provides a clear description of the neurophysiologic aspects and evidence for an autoimmune origin of the syndrome.*

Ricker K, Moxley RT, Rohkamm R: Rippling muscle disease. Arch Neurol 46:405, 1989. *A good description of an uncommon disease and a review of the literature.*

Rüdel R, Ricker K, Lehmann-Horn F: Nondystrophic myotonias. *In* Engel AG, Franzini-Armstrong C (eds.): Myology, 2nd ed. New York, McGraw-Hill, 1994, p 1291. *A detailed account of the clinical, electrophysiologic, and molecular genetic aspects of the nondystrophic myotonias.*

459   DISORDERS OF NEUROMUSCULAR TRANSMISSION

DEFINITION AND BASIC CONCEPTS. Disorders of neuromuscular transmission can be acquired or inherited and are associated with abnormal weakness and fatigability on exertion. In each disorder the safety margin of neuromuscular transmission is compromised by one or more specific mechanisms. These mechanisms involve acetylcholine (ACh) synthesis or packaging of ACh quanta (6,000 to 10,000 molecules) into synaptic vesicles, the exocytotic release of ACh quanta from the nerve terminal by nerve impulse, and the efficiency of the released quanta to generate a postsynaptic depolarization. The efficiency of the released quanta depends on the

geometry of the synaptic space, the density of postsynaptic ACh receptors (AChR's), and the conductance and open time of the AChR ion channel. The depolarization induced by a single quantum gives rise to a miniature end-plate potential (MEPP); that induced by a larger number of quanta released by nerve impulse generates an end-plate potential (EPP). The EPP amplitude must exceed a critical threshold to activate the voltage-sensitive sodium channels around the end-plate and thereby generate a muscle fiber action potential. Neuromuscular transmission fails when the EPP fails to reach this critical threshold.

Table 459–1 shows a classification of currently recognized defects of neuromuscular transmission. Botulism is described in Ch. 288, the others in this chapter. The congenital syndromes are discussed in the indicated references.

MYASTHENIA GRAVIS (MG). This is an acquired autoimmune disorder in which pathogenic autoantibodies induce AChR deficiency at the motor end-plate. The safety margin of neuromuscular transmission is compromised by the small amplitude of the MEPP and consequently of the EPP. Circulating AChR antibodies are present in 80 to 90% of the cases, and IgG and complement components are deposited on the postsynaptic membrane. AChR deficiency results from complement-mediated lysis of the junctional folds, accelerated internalization and destruction of AChR cross-linked by antibody (modulation), and, to a lesser extent, by antibodies blocking the binding of ACh to AChR.

Clinical Features. The incidence is two to five per year per million and the prevalence 13 to 64 per million. The female to male ratio is 6:4. The disease may present at any age, but the incidence in women peaks in the third decade and in men in the sixth or seventh decade.

MG can involve either the external ocular muscles selectively or the general voluntary muscle system. The symptoms may fluctuate from hour to hour, day to day, or over longer periods. They are provoked or worsened by exertion, exposure to extremes of temperature, viral or other infections, menses, and excitement. Ocular muscle involvement is usually bilateral, asymmetric, and typically associated with ptosis and diplopia. Weakness of other muscles innervated by cranial nerves results in loss of facial expression, everted lips, a smile that resembles a snarl, jaw drop, nasal regurgi-

TABLE 459–1. CLASSIFICATION OF DISORDERS OF NEUROMUSCULAR TRANSMISSION

Autoimmune
Myasthenia gravis
Lambert-Eaton myasthenic syndrome
Congenital
Presynaptic defects
Familial infantile myasthenia (defect in ACh resynthesis or packaging)*
Paucity of synaptic vesicles and reduced quantal release‡
End-plate AChE deficiency*
Kinetic abnormalities of AChR with AChR deficiency
Classic slow-channel syndrome§
Miscellaneous mutations causing prolonged open time of the AChR channel§
AChR deficiency and short channel open time‡
Kinetic abnormalities of AChR without AChR deficiency
High-conductance fast-channel syndrome*
Syndrome attributed to abnormal interaction of ACh with AChR*
Partially characterized syndromes
Congenital myasthenic syndrome resembling LEMS‡
AChR deficiency with paucity of secondary synaptic clefts*
Partially characterized AChR deficiencies‡
Familial limb-girdle myasthenia*
Benign CMS with facial malformations*
Toxic
Botulism
Drug-induced
Organophosphate intoxication

---

* Autosomal recessive inheritance
† Autosomal recessive inheritance in some cases
‡ Autosomal recessive inheritance suspected
§ Autosomal dominant inheritance
ACh, acetylcholine; AChE, acetylcholinesterase; AChR, acetylcholine receptor; CMS, congenital myasthenic syndrome

tation of liquids, choking on foods and secretions, and a slurred, hypernasal speech with a reduced volume. Abnormal fatigability of the limb muscles causes difficulty in combing the hair, lifting objects repeatedly, climbing stairs, walking, and running. Depending on the severity of the disease, dyspnea can appear on moderate or mild exertion or be present even at rest. The abnormal fatigability can be demonstrated by asking the patient to look up without closing the eyes for a minute, to count loudly from 1 to 100, to hold the arms abducted to the horizontal position for a minute, or to perform repeated deep knee-bends. The tendon reflexes remain normally active even in weak muscles. Atrophy of masseter, temporal, facial, or tongue muscles, and less often of other muscles, occurs in about 15% of patients.

Initially, the symptoms are purely ocular in 40%, generalized in 40%, and involve only the extremities in 10%, and only the bulbar or bulbar and eye muscles in another 10%. Subsequently, the weakness can spread from ocular to facial to lower bulbar muscles and then to torso and limb muscles, but the sequence may vary. Proximal limb muscles are affected more than distal ones. In the most advanced cases the weakness is universal. By the end of the first year, the ocular muscles are affected in nearly all patients. The symptoms remain ocular in only 16%. In nearly 90% of those in whom the disease becomes generalized, this occurs within the first year after the onset. Progression is most rapid within the first 3 years, and more than half of the deaths caused by MG occur in that period. Spontaneous remissions lasting from weeks to years can occur. Long remissions are uncommon, and most remissions occur during the first 3 years.

Two thirds of patients with MG have thymic hyperplasia and 10 to 15% have thymoma. A few with thymoma also develop myocarditis or giant cell myositis. In about 10% the MG is associated with another autoimmune disease, such as hyperthyroidism, polymyositis, systemic lupus erythematosus, Sjögren's syndrome, rheumatoid arthritis, ulcerative colitis, pemphigus, sarcoidosis, pernicious anemia, or Lambert-Eaton myasthenic syndrome.

A clinical classification of MG, originally proposed by Osserman, is based on the distribution and severity of symptoms: group 1, ocular; group 2A, mild generalized; group 2B, moderately severe generalized; group 3, acute fulminating; group 4, late severe. Another classification, proposed by Vincent and Newsom-Davis, is based on the age of onset and the presence or absence of thymoma: Type 1, MG with thymoma: The disease is usually severe and the AChR antibody level is high; there is no association either with sex or HLA antigen. Type 2, no thymoma, onset before age 40: The AChR antibody level is intermediate; there is female preponderance and an increased association with HLA-A1, HLA-B8, and HLA-DRw3 antigens (HLA-B12 in Japan). Type 3, no thymoma, onset after age 40: The AChR antibody level tends to be low; there is male preponderance and increased association with HLA-A3, HLA-B7, or HLA-DRw2 antigens (HLA-A10 in Japan). Striated muscle antibodies are found in 90%, 5%, and 45%, respectively, in the three types. The association with other autoimmune diseases is highest in Type 3 and lowest in Type 1.

Transient Neonatal MG. Circulating AChR antibodies can be detected in most infants born to myasthenic mothers, but only 12% of such children develop MG, usually during the first few hours of life. The findings are feeble cry, feeding and respiratory difficulty, general or facial weakness, and ptosis. The mean duration is 18 days. There is no relation between the severity of MG in mother and infant. The disease is caused by the transfer of AChR antibodies from mother to infant.

Diagnosis. This is based on the characteristic history, physical examination, anticholinesterase tests, and laboratory studies. The latter include EMG studies, tests for AChR antibodies, and in selected cases, microelectrode studies *in vitro* of neuromuscular transmission and ultrastructural and cytochemical studies of the endplate.

Anticholinesterase Tests. Edrophonium given intravenously acts within a few seconds, and its effects last for a few minutes. One to 2 mg of the drug is injected intravenously over 15 seconds. If no response occurs in 30 seconds, an additional 8 to 9 mg is injected. The evaluation of the response requires objective assessment of one or more signs, such as degree of ptosis, range of ocular movements, and the force of the hand grip. Possible cholinergic side effects of

the drug include fasciculations, flushing, lacrimation, abdominal cramps, nausea, vomiting, and diarrhea. The drug must be given cautiously to patients with cardiac disease, for it may cause sinus bradycardia, atrioventricular block, and, rarely, cardiac arrest. Atropine is used to reverse toxicity. Intramuscular neostigmine, 0.5 to 1.0 mg, acts maximally in about 30 minutes, and its effects last up to 2 hours, allowing a more leisurely evaluation of changes in clinical status.

Electromyography. Supramaximal stimulation of a motor nerve at 2 to 3 Hz results in a 10% or greater decrement of the amplitude of the evoked compound muscle action potential from the first to the fifth response. The test is positive in nearly all patients provided that two or more distal and two or more proximal muscles are examined. The decrement is caused by a normally occurring decrease in the number of quanta released from the nerve terminal, and hence in the amplitude of the EPP, at the beginning of low-frequency stimulation. In MG the EPP amplitude is already reduced by the AChR deficiency, and the additional decrease during stimulation blocks transmission at an increasing number of end-plates. Single-fiber EMG compares the timing of action potentials between pairs of closely adjacent muscle fibers in the same motor unit during a willed contraction. In MG the low amplitude and relatively long rise time of the EPP cause abnormally long interpotential intervals and intermittent blocking of action potential generation at some fibers.

Serologic Tests. The usual AChR antibody test measures the binding of antibody to AChR labeled with radioactive α-bungarotoxin. The toxin itself is attached irreversibly to the ACh binding site of AChR. The antibody binding test is positive in nearly all adults with moderately severe or severe MG, in 80% with mild generalized MG, and in 50% with ocular MG, but in only 25% of those in remission. The test is less reliable in juvenile than in adult MG. In a few patients only antibodies that block the binding of ACh to AChR can be detected. The antibody titer correlates only loosely with disease severity, but in individual patients a >50% decrease in titer for more than 12 months is nearly always associated with sustained clinical improvement. Striated muscle antibodies also occur in MG patients. Their role remains unknown, but they often are associated with thymoma.

Other Diagnostic Studies. Immune deposits can be localized at the MG end-plate in cryostat sections even when circulating AChR antibodies cannot be detected. C3 localization is technically the easiest and most convenient way to confirm the suspected diagnosis.

Differential Diagnosis. This includes neurasthenia, the Miller Fisher variant of inflammatory polyneuropathy, oculopharyngeal dystrophy, mitochondrial myopathies involving the external ocular and/or other cranial and limb muscles, intracranial mass lesions compressing cranial nerves, drug-induced myasthenic syndromes, and other disorders of neuromuscular transmission listed in Table 459–1. Neurasthenia is recognized by giving way on muscle testing and the lack of objective clinical and laboratory findings. In myopathies involving the ocular muscles, the weakness does not fluctuate, diplopia is seldom a symptom, the muscle biopsy may show distinct morphologic abnormalities, and pharmacologic and laboratory tests for MG are negative. Drug-induced and other myasthenic syndromes are considered below.

Therapy. Anticholinesterases, alternate-day prednisone treatment, azathioprine, thymectomy, and plasmapheresis are currently used to treat MG. Anticholinesterases are useful in all clinical forms of the disease. Pyridostigmine bromide (Mestinon) (60-mg tablets) acts for 3 to 4 hours, and neostigmine bromide (15-mg tablets) for 2 to 3 hours. The former drug has fewer muscarinic side effects and is therefore more widely used. One half to four tablets of pyridostigmine bromide are given every 4 hours in the daytime. This medication is also available in 180-mg "time-span" tablets for use at bedtime and as a syrup for children and patients requiring nasogastric feeding. If troublesome muscarinic side effects occur, these can be treated with 0.4 to 0.6 mg atropine given orally two or three times daily. Postoperatively or in critically ill patients intramuscularly injectable pyridostigmine bromide (the dose is one thirtieth of the oral dose) and neostigmine methylsulfate (the dose is one fifteenth of the oral dose) can be used.

Progressive weakness despite increasing amounts of anticholinesterases signals the onset of a cholinergic or myasthenic crisis. Cholinergic crises are associated with muscarinic effects, such as abdominal cramps, nausea, vomiting, diarrhea, miosis, lacrimation, increased bronchial secretions, diaphoresis, and bradycardia. In a myasthenic crisis the muscarinic effects are not conspicuous, and 2 mg edrophonium given intravenously improves rather than worsens the weakness. In practice, however, the two types of crises often are difficult to distinguish, and overmedication of a myasthenic crisis can convert it into a cholinergic crisis. Therefore, patients who have increasing difficulty with respiration, feeding, or handling secretions and who are not responding to relatively high doses of anticholinesterases are best treated by drug withdrawal, tracheal intubation or tracheostomy, support with respirator, and intravenous feeding. Refractoriness to drug therapy usually disappears after a few days.

In patients with generalized disease not responding adequately to modest doses of anticholinesterases, other forms of therapy must be employed. Thymectomy increases the remission rate and improves the clinical course of MG. Although controlled clinical studies of thymectomy according to age, gender, severity, and duration of disease have never been carried out, there is general agreement that the best response occurs in young women with hyperplastic thymus glands and high antibody titer. Thymoma represents an absolute indication for thymectomy because the tumor is often locally invasive. Computed tomography of the mediastinum is a sensitive screening test, but it can give false-positive results.

Alternate-day prednisone treatment induces remission or significantly improves the disease in more than half the patients. The treatment is relatively safe provided that one institutes the usual precautions for patients taking corticosteroid therapy. With an average dose of 70 mg on alternate days, the average time for significant improvement is 5 months. After the improvement reaches a plateau the dose must be lowered gradually over several months to establish the minimum maintenance dose.

Azathioprine in doses of 150 to 200 mg per day also induces remissions or measurable improvement in more than half the treated patients. The minimum time for improvement is 3 months. Surveillance to detect side effects (pancytopenia, leukopenia, serious infection, and hepatocellular injury) must be maintained during therapy.

Plasmapheresis is indicated in severe generalized or fulminating MG refractory to other forms of treatment. Daily exchanges of 2 liters of plasma result in objective improvement and lower the AChR antibody titer in a few days. Plasmapheresis, however, is highly expensive and does not confer greater long-term protection than immunosuppressants alone.

Intravenous immunoglobulin therapy at a dose of 400 mg per kilogram for 5 consecutive days or 1 gram per kilogram for 2 consecutive days may improve severe MG within 2 to 3 weeks of the start of therapy. The mean duration of the response is 9 weeks in patients also treated with corticosteroids and 5 weeks in those who are not.

LAMBERT-EATON MYASTHENIC SYNDROME. This is an acquired autoimmune disease in which pathogenic autoantibodies cause a deficiency of voltage-sensitive calcium channels at the motor nerve terminal. The deficiency restricts calcium ingress when the terminal is depolarized by nerve impulses and thereby reduces the probability of quantal release. Among patients over 40 years 70% of men and 30% of women have an associated carcinoma, usually a small-cell carcinoma of the lung. The syndrome may predate tumor detection by up to 3 years. Non-neoplastic cases have an association with other autoimmune disorders, HLA-B8 and DRw3 antigens, and organ-specific autoantibodies.

Patients have weakness and fatigability of proximal limb and torso muscles with relative sparing of extraocular and bulbar muscles. The lower limbs are more severely involved than the upper ones. On maximal voluntary contraction the force produced by a weak muscle increases for a few seconds and then again decreases. The tendon reflexes are hypoactive or absent in most patients. Autonomic manifestations (dry mouth, impotence, decreased sweating,

orthostatic hypotension, or altered pupillary reflexes) occur in one half of the patients.

On EMG, the amplitude of the compound muscle action potential evoked by a single nerve stimulus from rested muscle is abnormally small. Repetitive stimulation at 2 Hz induces a further decrement, but stimulation at frequencies higher than 10 Hz or voluntary exercise for a brief period markedly facilitates the response so that the evoked potential attains normal amplitude.

Anticholinesterases are only slightly effective. Guanidine hydrochloride (10 mg per kilogram per day) or 3,4-diaminopyridine (1 mg per kilogram per day) increases quantal release from the nerve terminal and relieves the symptoms. However, the former drug has severe toxic side effects, and the latter is not yet available in clinical practice. Optimal treatment of non-neoplastic cases consists of modest doses of alternate-day prednisone and 2 mg per kilogram per day of azathioprine.

DRUG-INDUCED MYASTHENIC SYNDROMES. These are uncommon in clinical practice. Tetracycline, polymyxin and aminoglycoside antibiotics, antiarrhythmic agents (procainamide, quinidine), β-adrenergic blockers (propranolol, timolol), phenothiazines, lithium, trimethaphan, methoxyflurane, and magnesium given parenterally or in cathartics reduce the safety margin of neuromuscular transmission. However, overt myasthenic symptoms do not usually appear unless an overdose of the drug is administered or the renal or hepatic elimination of the drug is impaired. The same drugs and inhalation anesthetic agents also can potentiate neuromuscular blocking agents used during surgical procedures and both may worsen or unmask pre-existing disorders of neuromuscular transmission. Calcium channel blocking drugs can worsen the transmission defect in the Lambert-Eaton myasthenic syndrome.

Succinylcholine, a depolarizing blocking drug, is used to induce muscle relaxation during anesthesia. A single dose of the drug sufficient to cause transient apnea is eliminated by plasma pseudocholinesterase in 2 to 10 minutes. In approximately 1 of 2500 patients receiving the drug, prolonged apnea occurs and persists up to several hours. Most of these patients have an autosomal recessive abnormality of the plasma pseudocholinesterase. In some genetic variants the plasma pseudocholinesterase activity is abnormally low; in others the enzyme shows increased sensitivity to inhibition by dibucaine.

ORGANOPHOSPHATE INTOXICATION. Organophosphate insecticides irreversibly inhibit cholinesterases. Poisoning occurs by accident or when the compounds are ingested with suicidal intent. The accumulation of ACh at central, muscarinic, and nicotinic cholinergic synapses is associated with alterations in sensorium, convulsions, coma, severe muscarinic side effects, cramps, fasciculations, and muscle weakness from a depolarization block as well as desensitization of AChR at the neuromuscular junction. Therapy consists of gastric lavage with more than 100 liters of water, followed by the use of activated charcoal and oral cathartics, respiratory support, and anticonvulsants as needed. Atropine, 1 to 2 mg intramuscularly every hour, can be used to control the excessive secretions. Pralidoxime (1 gram intravenously, repeated in 20 minutes if necessary) has been used with variable success.

Engel AG: Congenital myasthenic syndromes. Neurol Clin 12:401, 1994. *A thorough review of the current status of the congenital myasthenias and of the investigative approaches to these diseases.*

Engel AG, Franzini-Armstrong C (eds.): Myology, 2nd ed. New York, McGraw-Hill, 1994. *Chapters by Engel and Magleby ably discuss the detailed anatomy, physiology, and clinical dimensions of neuromuscular transmission.*

Gutmann L, Besser R: Organophosphate intoxication: Pharmacologic, neurophysiologic, clinical, and therapeutic considerations. Semin Neurol 10:46, 1990. *A lucid analysis of the pathophysiologic basis of the symptoms and a reliable guide to therapy.*

O'Neill JH, Murray MF, Newsom-Davis J: Lambert-Eaton myasthenic syndrome: A review of 50 cases. Brain 3:577, 1988. *A comprehensive review of the clinical and basic science aspects of the disease.*

PART XXV

EYE DISEASES

John W. Gittinger, Jr.

Because many systemic diseases affect the eyes, ophthalmoscopy is a necessary skill for the physician. The pupil of the eye is a window opening onto the arterioles and venules of the retina, the optic disc, and the pigmented tissues of the fundus. Ch. 403 describes the autonomic and somatic motor disorders of ocular control and reviews the clinically important anatomy of the visual pathways. The chapters that follow highlight the interrelationship between ocular and systemic disease, beginning with a discussion of visual loss, then providing a brief review of the two common ophthalmic disorders—cataract and glaucoma, before turning to ocular entities and ocular manifestations of medical disorders that nonophthalmic physicians are likely to encounter.

460 VISUAL LOSS

Visual loss may be either transient (see Ch. 403) or permanent, with most of the potential causes capable of producing either one. A major purpose of the ophthalmologic examination is to establish the cause of visual loss. The need for correction of vision with glasses is called *refractive error*. When evaluating a patient for reduced vision, only the best-corrected acuity should be considered. Uncorrected acuity is of little interest in assessing the pathophysiology of the eye. Refractive errors include myopia, hyperopia, and astigmatism; presbyopia (literally "aging eye") refers to the loss of accommodation as the lens hardens with age, making focusing at near difficult even in eyes without refractive error *(emetropia)* after about age 45.

In myopia the eye is too large for its refractive power, and the image of a distant object focuses in front of the retina. Diverging light rays from nearer objects focus on the retina; thus, the person is "nearsighted" in that near vision is clearer than distance vision. A moderate degree of myopia thus compensates for presbyopia, an important consideration as permanent surgical correction of myopia is becoming more common.

In hyperopia, the eye is too small, and the image has not yet come into focus when it reaches the retina. In young persons, accommodation compensates for low degrees of hyperopia, but such hyperopia accelerates the age of onset of symptoms of presbyopia. Astigmatism reflects different degrees of refractive error along two perpendicular corneal meridians. An eye often has both myopia or hyperopia and astigmatism. Except when it reflects a structural alteration, as in high myopia, the need for refractive correction is considered a variant of normal, not a disease process.

Many conditions can cause visual loss (Table 460–1). Normal visual development in an infant requires formed images on the retina and intact visual pathways in the rest of the brain. A neonatal eye with a dense opacity of the media such as a mature cataract (see below) cannot develop useful vision unless the opacity is removed soon after birth and any resulting large refractive error corrected promptly. Visual development proceeds through crucial states; any interruption of these stages during infancy or early childhood can permanently limit the normal capacity for processing visual information even if the causative condition is treated later on. If both eyes are involved, the development of nystagmus (rhythmic to-and-

TABLE 460–1. DIFFERENTIAL DIAGNOSIS OF VISUAL LOSS

Opacities of the media	Corneal opacities (leukomas, edema, dystrophy) or irregularity; anterior chamber blood or inflammation; cataract; vitreous opacities
Chorioretinal disease	Macular and other retinal degenerations; retinal detachment; toxic, vascular, and traumatic retinopathies; infectious and inflammatory chorioretinitis; retinal tumors
Optic nerve disease	Glaucoma, other optic neuropathies (inflammatory, toxic, traumatic, vascular, hereditary); compressive and infiltrative neuropathy; optic nerve tumors
Visual pathway disorders	Vascular, inflammatory, infectious, degenerative developmental, neoplastic
Amblyopia	Strabismic, nutritional deprivation, anisometropic, ametropic, idiopathic
Psychogenic	

fro movements of the eye) at about 3 or 4 months of age signifies that this crucial period has been exceeded.

Normal adult levels of visual acuity can be measured electrophysiologically by age 6 months, but the neural connections that permit fine visual processing become permanently established only later in childhood. During the first few years of life, strabismus—misalignment of the visual axes of the two eyes—may result in suppression of central vision in one eye. Such visual loss in an eye that appears anatomically normal is termed *amblyopia*—a term also sometimes applied to processes that reduce vision but produce only subtle ophthalmoscopic changes, e.g., toxic-nutritional amblyopia. A large, uncorrected refractive error—*ametropia*—or a major difference in the refractive error in the two eyes—*anisometropia*—may also lead to amblyopia. Strabismic amblyopia is potentially reversible until 6 to 10 years of age, when the neural processing networks for vision become fixed for life. With this final step in visual development, the visual system achieves adult inflexibility so that misalignment of the visual axes results in permanent diplopia rather than suppression. An adult with acquired misalignment of the visual axes who does not experience diplopia probably has either reduced vision or a history of childhood strabismus.

Careful ophthalmic examination and appropriate testing should allow classification of reduced vision into one of the categories listed in Table 460–1: opacities of the media, chorioretinal disease, optic nerve disease, visual pathway disorders, amblyopia, or psychogenic visual loss. Two or more processes may affect the same eye.

Albert DM, Jakobiec FA: Principles and Practice of Ophthalmology. Philadelphia, WB Saunders, 1994. *This multivolume, multiauthored text features many color illustrations.*

Miller NR: Walsh and Hoyt's Clinical Neuro-ophthalmology. 4th ed. Baltimore, Williams & Wilkins, 1982–1995. *This encyclopedic review by one individual details many ocular entities with systemic manifestations.*

Tasman W, Jaeger EA: Duane's Clinical Ophthalmology. Philadelphia, JB Lippincott, revised annually. *Another multivolume text bound in a loose-leaf format that facilitates yearly updates and additions of selected chapters.*

PSYCHOGENIC VISUAL LOSS

Visual loss not attributable to an organic process is termed *psychogenic*. Alternative designations are functional, nonorganic, nonphysiologic, hysterical, and malingering. The last two are best avoided. Hysteria suggests to some a sexual bias and must be considered a psychiatric rather than an ophthalmologic diagnosis; malingering imputes motives that are difficult to prove. Functional visual loss, the usage currently preferred by some authorities, is potentially confusing because *functional* is used in other senses in medicine; e.g., *functional amblyopia* refers to those forms of amblyopia in which the process is potentially reversible with treatment (strabismic, ametropic, and anisometropic). In these instances there is presumably an underlying physiologic alteration in the visual system itself.

Psychogenic visual loss is not necessarily a diagnosis of exclusion. Certain patterns of visual loss cannot be explained by organic disease. Concentric constriction of visual fields is a common finding in nonphysiologic visual loss but also occurs with advanced glaucoma and retinitis pigmentosa as well as after bilateral occipital infarctions. Failure of the visual field to expand to an appropriate stimulus with increased testing distance—tubular fields—is, however, diagnostic of psychogenic visual loss. Similarly, patients who claim to be completely blind in one eye but who have normal pupillary reactions, full stereopsis, or normal ipsilateral visual evoked responses must have a nonphysiologic component to their visual loss. Other testing techniques also may result in normal subjective responses from a supposedly blind eye.

Most cases of psychogenic visual loss occur in the setting of minor psychological reactions rather than major psychiatric disorders. Sometimes organic and nonorganic components coexist. Affected patients should be evaluated by a neurologist or ophthalmologist familiar with psychogenic visual loss. Unless the visual loss prevents the patient from working or attending school, simple reassurance and careful follow-up with treatment of intercurrent organic abnormalities constitute appropriate management, and in some cases spontaneous improvement occurs.

461 CATARACT

A cataract is any lens opacity; cataracts characteristically produce painless, gradual loss of vision. Cataracts are described according to their location, e.g., nuclear (deep in the lens), cortical (more superficial), and capsular or subcapsular (on or immediately beneath the capsule). Cataracts are further classified as immature, mature, or hypermature. An immature cataract has some clear cortex; a mature cataract is totally opaque—the pupil appears white *(leukokoria)*. A hypermature cataract has liquefied cortex that may leak through the capsule and excite destructive inflammation. Immature cataracts are usually removed for visual reasons. A mature or hypermature cataract in an eye with potentially useful vision should be removed to prevent irreversible damage from lens-induced inflammation.

ETIOLOGY. Congenital cataracts are a feature of rubella embryopathy and often are associated with other congenital malformations. Acquired cataracts may result from trauma, radiation, or metabolic disorder. Several examples of colorful cataracts have diagnostic but little visual significance. In Wilson's disease, orange copper deposits may appear on the anterior capsule ("sunflower cataract"). Chlorpromazine administration may result in a brown or white dusting on the anterior lens surface. Red, green, and blue opacities in the lenticular cortex ("Christmas tree cataract") characterize myotonic dystrophy, but are occasionally encountered in its absence.

Hypocalcemia may be cataractogenic. Cataracts occur in disorders of carbohydrate metabolism: hypoglycemia, galactosemia, and diabetes mellitus. Although diabetics do not necessarily have an increased incidence of cataracts, those that occur progress rapidly, perhaps because of varying lens hydration.

Systemic corticosteroids promote formation of central posterior subcapsular cataracts. Because of the path that light must take through the lens, such opacities reduce vision more than similar eccentric or anterior ones. Posterior subcapsular cataracts affect focusing especially when the pupil is small, as in bright light or with close work; difficulties with driving and reading are often their first symptoms.

Most cataracts have no known cause. The common nuclear scle-

rotic or senile cataract is often familial, but no specific factors have been proven to accelerate or retard its development.

TREATMENT. With the exception of mature and hypermature cataracts and of immature cataracts that have swollen sufficiently to threaten to precipitate angle-closure glaucoma (see below), most cataracts are removed for visual reasons. Considerations in planning cataract extraction are the patient's visual needs, the potential for improvement, and the risks of surgery. A person who drives requires surgery when the better eye falls below an acuity of 20/40, the legal minimum for a driver's license in most states. By contrast, an elderly patient with 20/200 acuity and limited visual needs may be content without surgical intervention. Care must be taken to identify intercurrent ocular disease; removal of the lens of an eye with advanced glaucoma or macular degeneration does not improve vision.

The risk of cataract surgery is relatively small. Despite the possibility of intraocular hemorrhage, postoperative infection, corneal decompensation, or problems with wound healing, the chances for a good visual outcome are excellent. Even successful cataract surgery, however, increases the likelihood of subsequent retinal detachment, and a small percentage of eyes postoperatively develop prolonged cystoid macular edema with reduced acuity.

General anesthesia constitutes a major portion of the risk of cataract surgery. Because cataract extraction can usually be performed under local or even topical anesthesia, general anesthesia should be avoided in medically fragile patients.

Jaffe NS, Jaffe MS, Jaffe GF: Cataract Surgery and Its Complications. 5th ed. St. Louis, CV Mosby, 1990. *This profusely illustrated monograph addresses most of the issues of modern cataract surgery; includes extensive references.*

462 GLAUCOMA

Glaucoma comprises a group of disorders in which elevated intraocular pressure damages the optic nerve. The major types of glaucoma are open-angle, angle-closure, congenital, and secondary. The dynamics of aqueous humor control intraocular pressure. The aqueous humor is derived from blood by a process of secretion and ultrafiltration in the ciliary body. Aqueous humor then passes from the posterior chamber through the pupil to fill the anterior chamber, the space between the back of the cornea and the plane of the iris and pupil. The aqueous humor is reabsorbed through the trabecular meshwork, located in the angle between the cornea and the iris, to enter Schlemm's canal, which connects with the venous system (Fig. 462–1).

OPEN-ANGLE GLAUCOMA

In chronic open-angle glaucoma, the most common type, a block at the level of the trabecular meshwork impairs aqueous humor reabsorption. Intraocular pressure rises above its normal maximum of 21 mm Hg, gradually destroying axons and supporting tissue at the optic disc. The prevalence of open-angle glaucoma varies with the population studied and the diagnostic criteria employed. A conservative estimate in United States and European adults is 0.5%. Patients with increased intraocular pressure without signs of optic nerve damage are considered to have *ocular hypertension.* Treatment of ocular hypertension may be initiated if the pressure exceeds 30 mm Hg or in certain other situations.

Open-angle glaucoma is ordinarily asymptomatic until well advanced. Only rarely does the elevated intraocular pressure cause corneal edema, with the attendant perception of halos around lights. Pain is not characteristic. Initially only the peripheral visual field is lost; visual acuity remains normal until late in the course of the disease. Diagnosis depends on measuring intraocular pressure, examining the optic disc, and testing the visual fields. Gonioscopy, the visualization of the angle structures under high magnifications with special contact lenses, distinguishes an angle-closure from an open-angle mechanism.

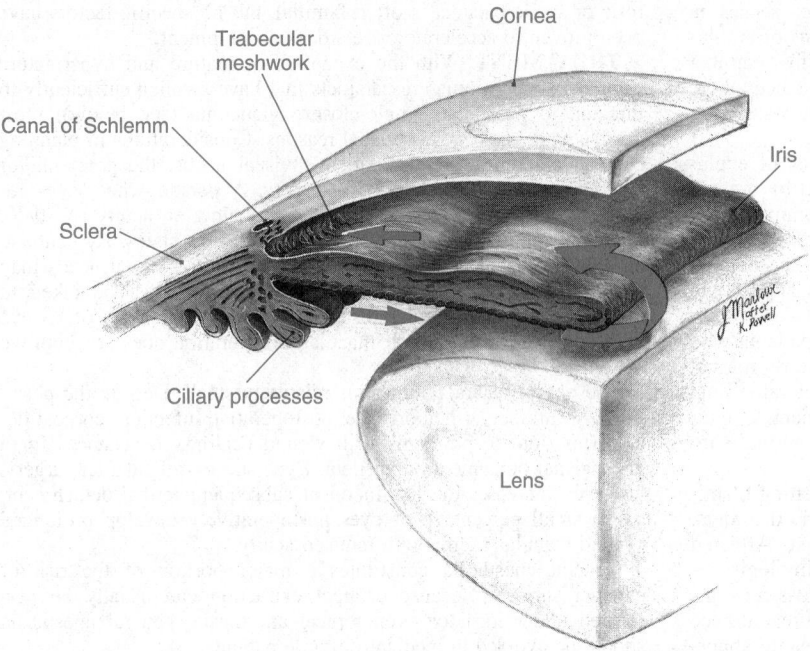

FIGURE 462-1. Circulation of aqueous humor in the normal eye. Aqueous is produced in the ciliary body and its processes, fills the posterior chamber (which also contains the lens), passes through the pupil *(large arrow)*, and is reabsorbed through the trabecular meshwork into the canal of Schlemm.

The treatment of open-angle glaucoma is primarily medical. Topical administration of parasympathomimetics (pilocarpine and carbachol), β-adrenergic blockers (e.g., timolol), and sympathomimetics (epinephrine and dipivefrin) decreases intraocular pressure. When these medications—individually and in combination—fail to arrest progressive disc damage producing visual field loss, topical indirect parasympathomimetics (echothiophate) and systemic carbonic anhydrase inhibitors (acetazolamide and methazolamide) may be useful.

If visual loss progresses with maximum tolerated medical therapy, surgery is indicated. *Laser trabeculoplasty* opens aqueous outflow channels by burning the surface of the trabecular meshwork. If all else fails, a surgical fistula can be created between the anterior chamber and the subconjunctival space. Such filtering procedures allow direct absorption of aqueous humor by subconjunctival and episcleral vessels.

The management of open-angle glaucoma involves early recognition, careful follow-up, and patient compliance with therapeutic regimens. Routine measurement of intraocular pressures (tonometry) at general physical examinations is often advocated; however, careful ophthalmoscopy with referral of patients whose central excavation ("cup") exceeds one third of the disc's area may be an equally effective screen.

ANGLE-CLOSURE GLAUCOMA

Angle-closure glaucoma develops when the normal path of aqueous flow is interrupted in an eye with a shallow anterior chamber, the consequence of a structurally anomalous anterior segment. Intraocular pressure remains normal until resistance to aqueous flow through the pupil—pupillary block—bows the iris forward to obstruct the resorptive surfaces in the angle. The pressure then rises precipitously, characteristically to above 50 mm Hg (Fig. 462-2).

Acute angle-closure glaucoma classically presents as a red, painful eye with decreased vision. The pupil is about 6 mm and fixed; the corneal light reflex is dulled. The patient is diaphoretic and nauseated and often vomits. Such typical angle-closure glaucoma is easy to recognize. The elderly, however, do not necessarily develop the full set of clinical signs and symptoms, and angle-closure glaucoma should be considered in all patients with a fixed, mid-dilated pupil and decreased vision even in the absence of a red eye or pain. The correct diagnosis can be made by slit-lamp examination with tonometry. Occasionally, chronic or subacute angle-closure glaucoma mimics open-angle glaucoma. Gonioscopy is then used to distinguish between the two mechanisms.

Dilating the pupils precipitates angle-closure in predisposed eyes. The risk of pharmacologic dilation is correlated with the depth of

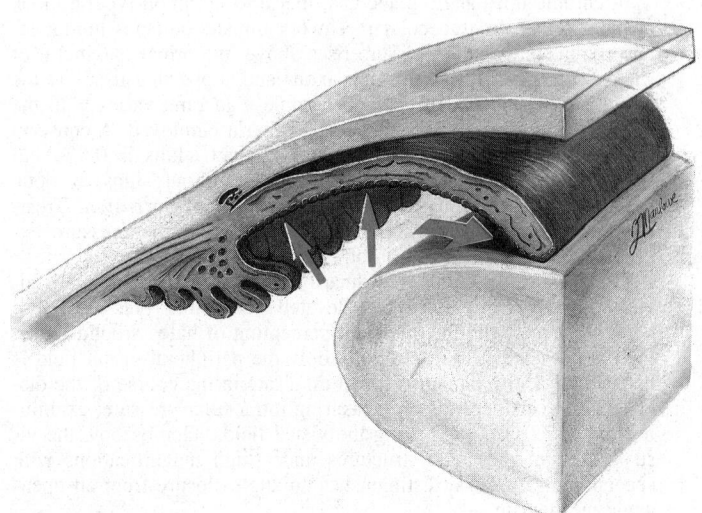

FIGURE 462-2. Angle-closure glaucoma. Owing to an anatomic anomaly in the anterior segment of the eye, the aqueous becomes trapped behind the pupil, bowing the iris forward (iris bombé) to cover the trabecular meshwork, which lies in the angle between the iris and the cornea.

the anterior chamber; eyes with shallow anterior chambers are at risk for angle-closure glaucoma. This distinction is not always easy to observe, and even experienced ophthalmologists sometimes cannot determine with certainty whether an angle will close with dilation. The likelihood of angle closure increases with age, and everyone over the age of 50 should be considered to have this potential. This does not mean that pupils of an older patient with a normal anterior chamber should not be dilated, but rather that dilation should be performed with a short-acting mydriatic agent such as tropicamide and the patient observed until the mydriatic wears off.

Nonophthalmologists should probably not routinely dilate pupils of adult outpatients. Children and inpatients may have dilation if there is no other contraindication such as recent head trauma, an iris-fixated intraocular lens, or impending general anesthesia. With these exceptions, the diagnostic benefits of dilation outweigh the risk of precipitating angle closure. Should angle-closure glaucoma develop, it can be recognized and promptly treated.

An acute angle-closure attack creates an emergency. Initial management consists of administration of parenteral acetazolamide, oral glycerol or (in diabetics) isosorbide, or intravenous mannitol, plus topical pilocarpine and a β-adrenergic antagonist. Once the attack has been broken, the anatomic predisposition can be circumvented by connecting the posterior and anterior chamber through the peripheral iris, usually with a *laser iridotomy*. The anterior segment abnormality that underlies angle-closure glaucoma is bilateral, and prophylactic surgery on the other eye is generally indicated.

CONGENITAL AND SECONDARY GLAUCOMA

Congenital glaucoma is an open-angle glaucoma that results from dysgenesis of the angle structures. Increased intraocular pressure enlarges the immature eye *(buphthalmos);* a corneal diameter greater than 12 mm in a child suggests congenital glaucoma. Secondary glaucoma develops as the consequence of another ocular disease. Examples of secondary glaucomas include angle-closure glaucoma precipitated by intumescence of the lens, glaucoma developing as a result of new vessels forming in the angle (as occurs with diabetes or other ocular vascular disease), and glaucoma in the chronically inflamed eye of a patient with juvenile rheumatoid arthritis. In addition, severe blunt trauma causing bleeding into the anterior chamber *(hyphema)* damages angle structures and predisposes to the subsequent development of open-angle glaucoma.

Secondary, lens-induced angle-closure glaucoma is treated by surgical removal of the lens. Most other secondary glaucomas are managed in much the same way as primary open-angle glaucoma. Neovascular glaucoma is difficult to treat. If ischemia is the stimulus, as occurs with diabetes or retinal vascular occlusion, ablation of ischemic tissues by photocoagulation may halt progression. If neovascularization continues, medical control becomes ineffective. Filtering procedures generally fail because tissue proliferation closes the surgical fistula, a problem that may be avoided by connecting the anterior chamber and the subconjunctival space with a plastic valve or by using antimetabolites to inhibit tissue growth. Destruction of the ciliary body by an externally applied energy source (thermal, laser, ultrasound) controls intraocular pressure but seldom preserves useful vision.

Glaucoma of any type in which all light perception has been lost is called *absolute glaucoma*. Enucleation (removal of the eye) is the definitive treatment for a blind, painful eye, although topical medications or retrobulbar injection of alcohol may relieve discomfort and allow the eye to be retained.

463 DISC SWELLING AND OPTIC ATROPHY

The optic disc marks the transition from retina to optic nerve. The central retinal artery and vein pass through the disc and bifurcate on its surface. There is considerable normal variation in the disc's ophthalmoscopic appearance. A central excavation or cup occupies a variable portion of its substance; vessels are often seen

TABLE 463–1. CAUSES OF DISC SWELLING

Increased intracranial pressure (papilledema)	Compressive optic neuropathy
Inflammatory optic neuropathy (papillitis)	Graves' disease
Infiltrative optic neuropathy	Sphenoid wing meningioma
Sarcoidosis	Vasculopathies
Leukemia and other malignancies	Anterior ischemic optic neuropathy
Optic nerve tumors	Central retinal vein occlusion
Angioma	Toxic-metabolic optic neuropathy
Optic nerve meningioma	Idiopathic
Childhood optic nerve glioma	Pseudopapilledema
Malignant optic nerve glioma	Optic disc drusen
Metastatic carcinoma	Hyperopia
	Other anomalies

curving over the edge of this cup. Over 1 million axons originate in the ganglion cells of the retina and pass through each optic disc. Although these axons are nearly transparent, a bright ophthalmoscope visualizes fine reflective striations on the disc's surface and the immediately surrounding retina. Disc swelling can be a consequence of ischemia, infarction, infiltration, or local changes in tissue pressures (Table 463–1).

PAPILLEDEMA (see Color Plate 13*B*)

The term *papilledema* literally describes disc swelling from any cause; some prefer to reserve this term for disc swelling from increased intracranial pressure. The swelling and elevation of the disc observed ophthalmoscopically primarily reflect accumulation of axoplasm and are most obvious just adjacent to the disc's normal borders.

Papilledema from increased intracranial pressure is usually bilateral but may be asymmetric. With rapid increases in intracranial pressure, the veins become engorged and hemorrhages appear on the disc and adjacent retina. With only rare exceptions, visual acuity remains normal in acute papilledema. Chronic papilledema may lead to secondary optic atrophy and permanent loss of vision (see below). Surgical fenestration of the optic nerve sheath in eyes with visual loss may halt progression.

PSEUDOPAPILLEDEMA

Certain normal disc appearances resemble papilledema. Hyperopic eyes are small, with consequent axonal crowding at the disc that may be confused with swelling. Optic disc drusen, depositions of hyaline material in the prelaminar optic nerve, sometimes present as disc elevation in young persons. If they cannot be recognized with careful ophthalmoscopy, these calcified optic disc drusen may be visualized on computed tomography or ultrasonography. In older persons, the previously buried drusen become visible ophthalmoscopically as refractile bodies that resemble rock crystals (see Color Plate 13*D*). Anomalous discs are often discovered incidentally. One clue to their nature is the frequent absence of the physiologic cup; in true papilledema the cup is preserved until the disc swelling is far advanced.

OPTIC NEURITIS

Papillitis indicates an inflammatory or demyelinating neuritis located in the anterior optic nerve. In approximately half of eyes with optic neuritis the disc appears normal initially; this is *retrobulbar optic neuritis*. In papillitis, the disc is swollen and may be hemorrhagic, an appearance ophthalmoscopically indistinguishable from the papilledema that results from increased intracranial pressure. Unlike disc swelling from increased intracranial pressure, however, acuity and visual field are characteristically affected, and the condition is usually unilateral (see also Tables 403–2 and 403–3).

The management of optic neuritis is controversial. Recent studies indicate that, although visual outcome is not affected by corticosteroid administration, the incidence of other episodes of demyelination may be decreased.

ANTERIOR ISCHEMIC OPTIC NEUROPATHY

Whereas papillitis is largely a disease of the young, acute disc swelling and loss of vision in older persons suggest infarction and are termed *anterior ischemic optic neuropathy*. Often only the superior or inferior half of the disc is involved, with consequent altitudinal loss of the inferior or superior visual field. Most ischemic optic neuropathy is idiopathic, but the disorder may be the initial manifestation of giant cell or temporal arteritis, a disease of the elderly described in Ch. 246. Nonarteritic anterior ischemic optic neuropathy tends to occur in discs with small cups, and the second eye eventually becomes involved in about two fifths of cases.

The treatment of arteritic anterior ischemic optic neuropathy is directed to the underlying giant cell arteritis (see Ch. 246). Surgical incision of the optic nerve sheath does not appear to be effective treatment for nonarteritic anterior ischemic optic neuropathy.

OTHER CAUSES OF DISC SWELLING

Bilateral disc swelling may accompany severe hypertension and constitutes a hypertensive crisis (see Ch. 37). Markedly decreased intraocular pressure, encountered after ocular surgery or injury, also produces disc swelling, and the disc may swell acutely during an attack of angle-closure glaucoma. Disc swelling is also a feature of some toxic and hereditary optic neuropathies. Compression causes disc swelling only when the optic nerve is constricted. This occurs in some patients with the orbitopathy of Graves' disease (see Ch. 466), pseudotumor of the orbit (see Ch. 466), and sphenoid wing meningioma. Intrinsic tumors of the optic nerve, the most common being glioma and meningioma, may present as disc swelling and visual loss. Infiltration and swelling of the optic nerve heads are also encountered in leukemia, metastatic carcinoma, and sarcoid.

OPTIC ATROPHY

Optic atrophy results from death of the axons in the retina and optic nerve. Disc pallor and optic atrophy are not synonymous; some temporal pallor is a feature of normal discs. A lesion anywhere from the retina through the optic tract can cause optic atrophy. Lesions behind the lateral geniculate in early life occasionally cause trans-synaptic degeneration and optic atrophy. Optic atrophy may be classified as primary, secondary, or glaucomatous. *Primary optic atrophy* refers to progressive pallor without loss of disc substance, a sign of retrograde or anterograde degeneration from compression, vascular injury, or toxic metabolic injury to the axons. *Secondary optic atrophy* develops after disc swelling, as in chronic papilledema. Vascular and glial changes may give the disc an irregular, milky gray appearance with ill-defined borders. The distinction is not always clinically evident. *Glaucomatous optic atrophy* denotes loss of disc substance, already referred to as increased cupping.

Optic atrophy is difficult to recognize in young children, in whom the discs may have a pale appearance normally. In adults with nuclear sclerotic cataracts, pallor may be masked by the lens acting as a yellow filter. The diagnosis of optic atrophy should not be made unless there is evidence of alteration in visual function: decreased acuity or field or, in infants, nystagmus.

Ultimately, optic atrophy is not a clinical finding but a pathologic entity. In retinitis pigmentosa there is a primary dystrophy of the rods and cones. The ganglion cells remain intact, but secondary vascular and gliotic changes produce a waxy pallor of the disc that is not a true optic atrophy because the axons are preserved.

LEBER'S HEREDITARY OPTIC NEURORETINOPATHY (LEBER'S DISEASE)

This disorder, often called Leber's optic atrophy, classically presents as acute or subacute visual loss in men around the age of 20 years. Women are much less often affected, with later onset. Initially the discs appear swollen because of opacification of the peripapillary nerve fiber layer (see Color Plate 13*F*), but the swelling does not represent edema, since fluorescein angiography demonstrates only telangiectatic vessels that do not leak dye.

With time central vision is lost in both eyes, and optic atrophy evolves. Although no effective treatment exists, vision occasionally improves spontaneously. The disorder is transmitted via an abnormality in maternal mitochondrial DNA, explaining the unusual heredity in which men cannot transmit the disease but all women in pedigrees are either affected or carriers. Most cases can be diagnosed by study of mitochondrial DNA from peripheral leukocytes. The availability of these molecular diagnostic tests has expanded the limits of the phenotype to include cases of optic neuropathy not having the characteristic clinical manifestations.

464   UVEITIS

Uveitis denotes inflammation of the uveal tract, which consists of the iris, ciliary body, and choroid. There are two major clinical types, anterior and posterior (Table 464–1). Anterior uveitis, also known as *iritis* or *iridocyclitis,* has as its hallmark cells in the anterior chamber; the iris itself seldom appears inflamed. Posterior uveitis may take the form of *chorioretinitis.* The choroid and retina are so intimately connected that it is difficult to have inflammation of one without the other.

Acute anterior uveitis causes congestion of the eye, often producing a halo of injection surrounding the cornea that is described as ciliary flush. Frequently, the eye is painful, vision reduced, and the pupil small and poorly reactive. The diagnosis is confirmed by the presence of free cells in the aqueous humor, visible as bright points of light as the slit-lamp beam passes through the normally optically empty anterior chamber. In more severe inflammation, *keratitic precipitates,* cellular aggregates on the back of the cornea, appear. When these are large and oily, the inflammation is called *granulomatous iritis,* a variant sometimes associated with systemic inflammatory disease such as sarcoid, syphilis, and tuberculosis. The cause of most anterior uveitis is unknown.

UVEITIS AND ARTHRITIS. Juvenile rheumatoid arthritis (see Ch. 237) and ankylosing spondylitis (see Ch. 238) are especially likely to be associated with uveitis. Young men with ankylosing spondylitis have recurrent acute iritis that responds to standard treatments (see below). Most are HLA-B27 positive. By contrast, the uveitis accompanying juvenile rheumatoid arthritis is chronic and may initially be subclinical. Young women with the pauciarticular form of juvenile rheumatoid arthritis who develop uveitis often have grossly normal-appearing eyes, with the cellular reaction apparent only by slit-lamp examination. With time, adhesions called posterior synechiae form between the iris and lens, potentially causing secondary pupillary block glaucoma or occlusion of the pupil. Chronic inflammation may lead to cataract formation and ectopic calcification in the corneal epithelium, called *band keratopathy.* Hypercalcemia alone also causes band keratopathy.

Physicians treating seronegative pauciarticular arthritis should consider scheduling slit-lamp and dilated examinations several times a year. Posterior synechiae are also detectable with a hand light after instillation of mydriatics, as the pupil does not fully dilate and develops an irregular, scalloped border.

REITER'S SYNDROME. The triad of arthritis, urethritis, and conjunctivitis suggests Reiter's syndrome (see Ch. 238). This develops most often in men between the ages of 20 and 40 as a nonbacterial urethritis followed by polyarthritis and ocular inflammation. The initial ocular manifestation is usually a mucopurulent conjunctivitis, followed in many cases by an anterior uveitis. Keratitis and episcleritis also occur. As in ankylosing spondylitis, with which it shares similarities, HLA-B27 is often positive.

BEHÇET'S SYNDROME. Uveitis or retinitis is a cardinal feature of Behçet's syndrome (see Ch. 249). In some cases a layer of white cells forms in the lower portion of the anterior chamber; such

TABLE 464–1. DISEASES ASSOCIATED WITH UVEITIS

	Infectious	Other
Anterior (iridocyclitis)	Herpes zoster Herpes simplex Hansen's disease	Ankylosing spondylitis Rheumatoid arthritis Reiter's syndrome
Posterior (chorioretinitis)	Toxoplasmosis Toxocariasis Histoplasmosis Measles	
Both anterior and posterior	Syphilis Coccidioidomycosis Onchocerciasis Brucellosis	Sarcoid Behçet's syndrome Vogt-Koyanagi-Harada syndrome Inflammatory bowel disease

hypopyon uveitis is considered characteristic. In other patients the primary ocular manifestation is a retinal vasculitis and vitritis. Rarer neuro-ophthalmic manifestations such as cranial nerve palsies or homonymous hemianopias are part of a wider central nervous system (CNS) involvement.

UVEOMENINGITIS. Another systemic disease with characteristic ocular inflammation is uveomeningitis (Vogt-Koyanagi-Harada syndrome). This disorder, more common in darkly pigmented people, affects the uvea, retina, meninges, and skin. Manifestations include meningeal signs, alopecia, poliosis, vitiligo, tinnitus, and dysacusis. There may be an anterior or posterior uveitis with exudative retinal detachment. The visual prognosis is guarded even with aggressive treatment with systemic steroids and other immunosuppressants.

MALIGNANCY MASQUERADING AS UVEITIS. A steroid-responsive exudative process simulating uveitis can be the presentation of a lymphoreticular neoplasia (variously called reticulum cell sarcoma, histiocytic sarcoma, or—when the brain is involved—primary CNS lymphoma) in persons over age 40. The cytology of a vitreous aspirate may be diagnostic. Radiation treatment has palliative value.

An apparent iritis developing during a course of treatment for leukemia may represent infiltration of the anterior segment. Diagnosis and therapy are similar to the above.

TREATMENT. Treatment consists largely of topical or, when the inflammation is prolonged or severe, systemic immunosuppression. Prednisolone or dexamethasone topically constitutes initial therapy. Topical administration of mydriatic-cycloplegics in anterior uveitis reduces discomfort and retards posterior synechiae formation. Severe and prolonged inflammation or posterior uveitis may require periocular corticosteroid injections or oral prednisone. Cytotoxic immunosuppressive agents are sometimes used.

---

465 OCULAR INFECTIONS

Ocular infections and inflammations are most sensibly grouped according to their locations. The most common superficial infection is *blepharoconjunctivitis,* or more simply, *conjunctivitis.* Infection of the lacrimal gland is *dacryoadenitis;* infection of the lacrimal drainage system, *dacryocystitis.* Corneal involvement is called *keratitis. Uveitis, scleritis,* and *episcleritis,* which are seldom infectious, are discussed elsewhere (see Ch. 464 and 468). Infection or inflammation inside the eye is *endophthalmitis.* An infectious *vitritis* is a form of endophthalmitis. Some *chorioretinitis* is infectious. *Panophthalmitis* refers to infections that extend through the sclera or cornea and involve adjacent orbital tissues.

CONJUNCTIVITIS

Causes include allergic, viral, bacterial, chlamydial, and chemical agents. Mild acute viral conjunctivitis, with a watery discharge and lids sealed closed upon awakening, usually requires only warm or cool compresses and a topical vasoconstrictor to whiten the eye. Topical antibiotics are sometimes prescribed to prevent superinfections but offer no clear advantages. Severe or chronic conjunctivitis should be managed by an ophthalmologist.

GONOCOCCAL CONJUNCTIVITIS. Purulent bacterial conjunctivitis usually responds to topical antibiotics. An important exception is hyperpurulent gonococcal conjunctivitis, a disease of the newborn *(gonococcal ophthalmia neonatorum)* and of sexually promiscuous adults. The eye is markedly inflamed with a copious discharge and swollen lids. The discharge should be Gram stained and cultured on appropriate media. Treatment consists of parenteral antibiotics and saline lavage of ocular secretions. Because of the emergence of penicillinase-producing strains, use of a β-lactamase–resistant cephalosporin such as ceftriaxone is warranted. Untreated gonococcal infection can penetrate the intact eye and destroy it; treatment should be started as soon as the diagnosis is suspected.

CHLAMYDIAL CONJUNCTIVITIS. In some parts of the world chronic chlamydial conjunctivitis leads to conjunctival scarring and corneal vascularization, a disease known as *trachoma* (see Ch. 323). The resulting blindness is an important international public health problem. In developed countries, chlamydial infection manifests as a subacute conjunctivitis, frequently with associated urethritis. Although a keratitis may be present, severe corneal damage does not ensue. Chlamydial conjunctivitis, also called *inclusion blennorrhea* because of the cytoplasmic inclusions found in Giemsa-stained conjunctival scrapings, is difficult to eradicate in adults by topical antibiotics alone and should be treated with systemic tetracycline or erythromycin.

HERPETIC KERATITIS (see Color Plate 13*A*). Viral keratitis is a common and potentially serious consequence of infection with herpes simplex. The corneal involvement may be recognized by the characteristic *dendrite,* a branching epithelial ulcer. Topical antiviral agents promote healing, but recurrence is frequent, with increasing risk of corneal stromal involvement and scarring. Topical steroids activate epithelial herpes infections and should not be used without ophthalmologic consultation in any patient with a red eye. Herpes zoster ophthalmicus also sometimes produces an acute dendritic keratitis, which usually requires no treatment.

CORNEAL ULCERS

Bacterial and fungal infections of the cornea are a serious threat to vision. Corneal ulcers tend to develop in the context of ocular trauma or contact lens wear, after surgery, or with pre-existing corneal disease. Corneal ulceration appears as an area of white, gray, or yellow infiltrate that stains with fluorescein. Affected patients should be referred promptly to an ophthalmologist for evaluation and treatment with topical antibiotics and other measures.

ENDOPHTHALMITIS

Infection inside the eye most often follows accidental or surgical perforation. Epidemics have occurred following the use of contaminated irrigating solutions in intraocular surgery. Less commonly, infections elsewhere metastasize to the eye. Bacterial endophthalmitis must be treated aggressively if there is to be any chance of preserving vision. When the infection is recognized, cultures and smears are taken from the anterior chamber and vitreous cavity by aspiration, and a course of intravitreal and sometimes systemic, topical, and periocular antibiotics is begun. The choice of antibiotics depends on what organisms, if any, are found on Gram stain. Surgical vitrectomy may be warranted.

CANDIDA ENDOPHTHALMITIS. *Candida albicans* is the most prevalent organism causing metastatic (endogenous) endophthalmitis. Fungemia after prolonged use of intravenous catheters or parenteral drug abuse results in colonization of the eye, with multiple white, fluffy chorioretinal infiltrates. These often involve the macula, reducing central vision. Careful direct ophthalmoscopy through a dilated pupil is indicated in patients at risk. Most *Candida* endophthalmitis requires systemic or intravitreal administration of antifungal agents, although spontaneous resolution has been observed.

INFECTIOUS CHORIORETINITIS

CONGENITAL TOXOPLASMOSIS (see Color Plate 13*H*). This is a common type of infectious chorioretinitis acquired *in utero.* This protozoan parasite can remain dormant in pigmented chorioretinal scars for many years and then become active, with white infiltration at the border of the scar and an overlying vitritis. If a previously uninvolved macula is threatened or the degree of inflammation is severe, antibiotic treatment may be indicated.

CYTOMEGALOVIRUS RETINITIS (see Color Plate 14*G*). Cytomegalovirus (CMV) retinitis appears in immunosuppressed hosts as a discrete area of white or yellow retinal opacification with associated hemorrhage and vascular sheathing. The ophthalmoscopic picture resembles that of a branch retinal vein occlusion (see Ch. 469), but in CMV retinitis one eye often has multiple foci, and there is a tendency for bilateral involvement.

Diagnosis can be made clinically in most cases. Dosages of immunosuppressive drugs should be reduced, if possible. Treatment with foscarnet or ganciclovir results in temporary regression of the process, which then breaks through the antiviral therapy and progresses to severe visual loss unless the underlying immunosuppression can be reversed.

OTHER INFECTIOUS CHORIORETINITIDES. Syphilis and tuberculosis may present as chorioretinitis or uveitis. Herpes simplex retinitis resembles that of cytomegalovirus. Cryptococcal meningitis may have an associated chorioretinitis. Focal chorioretinitis can accompany subacute sclerosing panencephalitis (see Ch. 428.4).

466 ORBITAL DISEASE AND TUMORS

GRAVES' ORBITOPATHY. Graves' orbitopathy consists of inflammation and infiltration of orbital tissues, with characteristic enlargement and scarring of the extraocular muscles. The varied clinical manifestations include lid retraction, exophthalmos, increased intraocular pressure, limitation of eye movement, and decreased vision from optic neuropathy or corneal drying *(exposure keratitis).* Graves' orbitopathy frequently develops in persons previously treated for hyperthyroidism. When the orbitopathy first manifests, the patient may be hyperthyroid, euthyroid, or hypothyroid. A clinical picture consistent with Graves' orbitopathy in the absence of a demonstrable thyroid abnormality, even to sophisticated testing, is referred to as *ophthalmic Graves' disease.* Coronal computed tomography (CT) or magnetic resonance imaging (MRI) demonstrating enlarged ocular muscles is a sensitive diagnostic maneuver.

Graves' orbitopathy is the most frequent cause of both unilateral and bilateral exophthalmos. Retraction of the upper lid to expose sclera above the cornea exaggerates the appearance of exophthalmos and predisposes to corneal drying. Tethering of the eye by fibrotic muscles produces a mechanical ophthalmoplegia and diplopia. Movement up and out is often restricted; pure loss of abduction mimicking sixth nerve palsy occurs. Ophthalmoplegia is not necessarily accompanied by exophthalmos.

Enlarged ocular muscles at the apex of the orbit may compress the optic nerve, producing disc swelling and visual loss. Severe exposure or progressive visual loss from compressive optic neuropathy is an indication for treatment. Systemic steroids reduce exophthalmos and temporarily relieve optic nerve compression. Surgical decompression of the orbit by one of several routes is one definitive therapy; orbital irradiation is also used. Once the orbitopathy has stabilized, surgical approaches to the extraocular muscles and lids may improve diplopia and correct persistent lid retraction.

INFLAMMATORY PSEUDOTUMOR OF THE ORBIT. Orbital pseudotumor is an idiopathic inflammation that falls within the spectrum of lymphoproliferative disorders. Its clinical manifestations are pain, exophthalmos, and limitation of eye movement. There may also be erythema and swelling of the lids. Orbital pseudotumors can mimic orbital infection, true tumors, or the orbitopathy of Graves' disease. The major sites of inflammation are muscle *(myositis),* nerve *(perineuritis),* sclera *(scleritis),* or lacrimal gland *(dacryoadenitis).*

If the inflammation is posterior to the orbital apex in the walls of the cavernous sinus, the painful ophthalmoplegia that results is called the *Tolosa-Hunt syndrome.* Orbital pseudotumor merges pathologically and clinically with orbital lymphoma, which in turn merges with systemic lymphoma.

Initial evaluation of a patient with clinical signs and symptoms of orbital pseudotumor includes orbital ultrasonography and CT or MRI. A trial of high-dose systemic corticosteroids is usually indicated prior to biopsy. Orbital biopsy is not a trivial undertaking and should be reserved for steroid-unresponsive or recurrent processes. Some histologically benign infiltrations do not respond to corticosteroids. Biopsy in such cases reveals fibrous tissue described as *sclerosing pseudotumor.* Occasionally, a patient with a histologically benign pseudotumor subsequently develops a systemic lymphoma.

A necrotizing vasculitis, Wegener's granulomatosis, must also be included in the differential diagnosis of orbital pseudotumor, especially when the inflammation is bilateral. Most cases of Wegener's granulomatosis involve contiguous sinus structures, but local ocular forms of the disease have been reported. The combination of progressive proptosis and sinus disease also suggests orbital aspergillosis, especially in persons who are immunosuppressed or reside in warmer climates.

RHABDOMYOSARCOMA. Rhabdomyosarcoma is the most common malignant tumor of the orbit during the first decade of life and also occurs during the second and third decades. The initial presentation is usually ptosis with lid infiltration and proptosis. Progression may be extremely rapid, the clinical picture mimicking trauma or cellulitis. Biopsy and prompt treatment with irradiation and chemotherapy result in a high percentage of survival, although vision in the eye on the side of the tumor is seldom preserved.

OTHER ORBITAL TUMORS. Many types of primary, secondary, and metastatic tumors involve the orbit. Most present with exophthalmos, visual loss, and limitation of eye movement. High degrees of malignancy are rare with meningiomas, gliomas, hemangiomas/lymphangiomas, and dermoids. Carcinomas of the lacrimal or meibomian glands represent a serious threat to life, and some cases require *exenteration*—the removal of the orbital contents. Carcinoma from contiguous sinuses invades the orbit, and breast carcinoma is especially likely to metastasize to the orbit.

467 INTRAOCULAR TUMORS

RETINOBLASTOMA. Retinoblastoma, a malignancy of the retina, is the most common intraocular tumor of childhood and one of the more common childhood tumors at any site. One third are bilateral. About 6% of retinoblastomas are inherited in an autosomal dominant pattern; half of these are bilateral. Ninety percent of retinoblastomas are discovered before the age of three. Adults who have survived retinoblastoma are at risk for the development of other malignancies, especially osteogenic sarcomas.

MALIGNANT MELANOMA. Primary melanomas develop in the conjunctiva, iris, ciliary body, or choroid; skin melanomas have a predilection for metastasis to the eye and orbit. Malignant melanomas of the choroid are the most common primary intraocular tumor of adulthood. Most occur in middle-aged whites. The prognosis of malignant melanoma of the choroid depends upon size, cytology, and the presence of extrascleral extension. Choroidal malignant melanomas often metastasize to the liver.

The differential diagnosis of a pigmented intraocular mass includes benign choroidal nevus, senile disciform macular degeneration (also known as central exudative hemorrhagic retinopathy), peripheral exudative hemorrhagic chorioretinopathy, choroidal hemangioma, and hypertrophy or hyperplasia of the retinal pigment epithelium. Many eyes removed because of the suspicion of malignant melanoma have been found to have unexpectedly benign pathologies.

Enucleation is the traditional treatment for malignant melanoma of the choroid. Other approaches include photocoagulation, radiation therapy, and local resection. Many pigmented choroidal tumors can be followed safely without intervention, especially when they are found incidentally in the seeing eyes of elderly patients.

METASTATIC CARCINOMA TO THE EYE. Once considered rare, metastatic cancer is now recognized as the most common ocular malignancy of adulthood, with an incidence exceeding that of choroidal melanoma. Most frequent are carcinomas invading the choroid (see Color Plate 13*E*), the most likely primary being breast, followed by carcinomas of the lung, then kidney, gastrointestinal tract, testis, and prostate. With lung or renal carcinoma, the primary site may be inapparent at the time the metastasis is detected. If tumor is identified elsewhere, removal of the eye is seldom indicated. Palliative radiation therapy or chemotherapy may preserve vision, and enucleation should be performed only if the eye is blind and painful.

Shields JA, Shields CL: Intraocular Tumors: A Text and Atlas. Philadelphia, WB Saunders, 1992. *An extensively illustrated and referenced overview by two experienced clinicians.*

468 EPISCLERITIS, SCLERITIS, AND THE DRY EYE

To a neurologist, the eye is anterior extension of the brain; to a rheumatologist, the eye is a joint. Medicine and ophthalmology come together in the diagnosis and management of rheumatoid and connective tissue disorders. Uveal manifestations are discussed in Ch. 464, the toxicity of drugs used in treatment in Ch. 470, and the retinal changes in Ch. 469.

EPISCLERITIS AND SCLERITIS

Inflammation of the collagenous shell of the eye can be either superficial *(episcleritis)* or deep *(scleritis)*. The transparent, avascular cornea is continuous with the opaque, vascular sclera and may be secondarily involved. Episcleritis resembles a localized conjunctivitis. The inflammation is deeper, however, and the dilated vessels do not always blanch with topically applied phenylephrine 2.5%, as they would in a pure conjunctivitis. Episcleritis usually is self-limited, although it may be recurrent, and it does not permanently damage the eye. Most episcleritis is idiopathic, but the disorder may be encountered in rheumatoid arthritis, polyarteritis nodosa, Wegener's granulomatosis, systemic lupus erythematosus, dermatomyositis, progressive systemic sclerosis, and relapsing polychondritis.

Scleritis is more likely than episcleritis to accompany a systemic disease, although the list of associations is about the same for the two disorders. Any portion of the sclera may be affected. The diagnosis is especially difficult with posterior scleritis, which may present as ocular pain or as an exudative retinal detachment. Anterior scleritis often becomes a prolonged, indolent inflammation with eventual permanent structural alteration of tissues. Pain may be prominent and severe. Inflammation in scleritis is initially localized and may be nodular or diffuse. With prolonged inflammation, scleral thinning results in a localized bluish discoloration as the underlying choroid becomes visible. Scleral necrosis with perforation is possible; this is especially frequent in association with rheumatoid arthritis. The adjacent cornea may melt away.

Management of scleritis is difficult. Local steroid injections may predispose to perforation. Systemic corticosteroids and other antirheumatic drugs are useful in some patients. The ocular process often closely parallels the activity of the underlying disease, which should guide systemic therapy.

KERATOCONJUNCTIVITIS SICCA. Corneal inflammation as the result of drying is referred to as *keratoconjunctivitis sicca*. Keratoconjunctivitis sicca, a dry mouth (xerostomia), and a connective tissue disorder constitute *Sjögren's syndrome.* The underlying pathophysiology appears to be an autoimmune reaction affecting the lacrimal and salivary glands. Sjögren's syndrome is common in patients with rheumatoid arthritis, especially middle-aged women. Complaints of burning, irritation, or excessive secretions suggest a dry eye but are notoriously nonspecific.

Diagnosis depends on demonstration of tear hyposecretion (usually by decreased wetting of a strip of litmus or filter paper placed between the lower lid and the eye in the inferior cul-de-sac—the Shirmer test) accompanied by corneal and conjunctival epithelial damage. Once epithelial cells start to slough, the corneal surface takes up fluorescein instilled into the conjunctival sac. Devitalized cells that have not yet been sloughed stain with rose bengal, making this dye an even more sensitive test for keratitis sicca.

Treatment consists of replacing tear volume and reducing tear turnover. Various preparations of artificial tears are available; those that do not contain preservatives are preferable if frequent administration is required. Other maneuvers include temporary or permanent occlusion of the lacrimal puncta to reduce tear outflow and placement of contact lenses, moisture chambers, or goggles over the eyes to decrease evaporation.

469 OCULAR VASCULAR DISEASE

SYSTEMIC HYPERTENSION AND ARTERIOSCLEROSIS

Although the retinal vascular abnormalities in hypertension are nonspecific and variable, they can be important diagnostically and therapeutically. The effects of blood pressure on the retinal vessels depend on both its absolute level and its duration. Although essential hypertension is a disease of arterioles, the retinal vascular bed lacks sympathetic innervation, and the fundus changes must be considered secondary.

Arteriolar narrowing is the most common hypertensive change and the most difficult to differentiate as abnormal. The normal ratio of the diameters of the arteriolar and venous blood columns is 2:3 or 3:4. A decrease in this ratio can best be appreciated in the smaller branches away from the disc. Other findings include microaneurysms, hemorrhages, lipid deposits, and edema. Retinal and disc edema usually follows a rapid increase in systemic blood pressure. Disc edema defines one type of malignant hypertension or hypertensive crisis and may be the presenting sign of markedly elevated blood pressure. By contrast, opacification (or sclerosis) of the vessel walls—described as copper or silver wiring—accompanies longstanding, uncontrolled hypertension and is rarely encountered now because of effective antihypertensive therapies.

Thickening of the arteriolar wall explains arteriovenous nicking and venous dilation distal to the crossing. Cotton-wool spots are signs of local ischemia; hemorrhages and hard exudates reflect vascular leakage. Microaneurysms result from irreversible structural alterations in the capillary walls. Retinal vascular occlusions (see below) and ischemic optic neuropathy (see Ch. 463) are potential consequences of hypertensive vascular changes.

Hypertension accelerates atherosclerosis, but atherosclerosis does not require hypertension. The only pure arteriosclerotic funduscopic change is atheroma of the retinal arterioles. These are seen as yellow-white plaques in the central retinal artery or its first branches, where the arteries still have an internal elastic lamina. These plaques should be differentiated from calcific or lipid emboli, which are usually smaller or more peripheral. Other retinal emboli include platelet-fibrin emboli that move through the arterioles and cause some cases of transient monocular blindness, talc emboli that appear as small white flecks in drug abusers using adulterated heroin, and septic emboli from subacute bacterial endocarditis that manifest as white-centered hemorrhages (Roth spots—Color Plate 14*B*). A rare but important cause of retinal embolism is cardiac myxoma (see Ch. 47).

DIABETIC RETINOPATHY (see Color Plate 14*B*, 14*E*, and 14*F*)

Diabetic retinopathy, the most common of the vascular retinopathies, shares many features with hypertensive retinopathy. The pathophysiologic defect appears to lie at the level of the retinal capillaries. Progressive degeneration of the capillary walls results in leakage (hemorrhages and exudates), diffuse and focal expansion (microaneurysms), and closure of small vessels. The ischemic retina in the focal areas of nonperfusion elaborates factors stimulating new vessel and fibrous ingrowth. Radiation therapy given as treatment for head and neck cancers may produce similar injury to the retinal capillary wall cells.

Diabetic retinopathy is classified as *background* or *proliferative.* Background retinopathy is further subdivided into *simple* background—with microaneurysms, dot/blot hemorrhages, and hard exudates—and a *preproliferative* form. In preproliferative retinopathy there is beading of veins, cotton-wool spots, and numerous intraretinal hemorrhages. Also characteristic is intraretinal new vessel pathology, so-called *intraretinal microvascular anomalies.*

In proliferative retinopathy, neovascularization appears on the disc and elsewhere, especially along the major vascular arcades. Fibrovascular proliferation and vitreous hemorrhages may follow. Proliferative diabetic retinopathy confers a poor visual prognosis.

Background retinopathy reduces visual acuity when there is edema or exudation in the macula. More new cases of blindness result from background retinopathy with macular edema than from proliferative retinopathy, because the former is much more prevalent. Background retinopathy with macular edema commonly presents in type 2 diabetics over age 50.

TREATMENT. Good diabetic control appears to retard the progression of retinopathy. Ablation of ischemic retina by panretinal photocoagulation helps preserve central vision in eyes with early proliferative retinopathy, making this the current treatment of choice. Advanced proliferative retinopathy may require removal of the vitreous and its contents through instruments inserted through the pars plana of the ciliary body. In such cases the prognosis is guarded, but an estimated 50 to 75% of patients undergoing pars plana vitrectomy experience some visual improvement.

OTHER VASCULAR RETINOPATHIES (see Color Plate 14)

SYSTEMIC LUPUS ERYTHEMATOSUS. Retinopathy is common but nonspecific; the most frequent findings are retinal hemorrhages and cotton-wool spots. Cotton-wool spots are not exudations, but represent localized areas of axoplasmic stasis caused by ischemia, which may indicate active vasculitis. Patients with lupus also may have hypertensive retinopathy. Central nervous system involvement may be associated with optic nerve and chiasmal neuropathy, papilledema, ocular motor cranial nerve palsies, hemianopias, and a migraine-like syndrome.

HEMATOLOGIC DISEASE. Anemia and thrombocytopenia predispose to retinal and subconjunctival hemorrhages. Retinal hemorrhages that result from leukemia often have a white center— the classic but nonspecific Roth spot mentioned above. Leukemia can cause *hyperviscosity retinopathy,* characterized by venous tortuosity and dilation, retinal hemorrhages, and vascular occlusions. A chronically elevated leukocyte count also predisposes to capillary drop-out and microaneurysm formation, but proliferative retinopathy is rare. Other causes of hyperviscosity retinopathy are Waldenström's macroglobulinemia, multiple myeloma, polycythemia, and sickle cell anemia. In extreme cases, sludging of blood in the veins is visible ophthalmoscopically.

PERIPHERAL RETINAL NEOVASCULARIZATION. Diabetic retinopathy affects largely the posterior pole of the eye. The retinopathy of prematurity (previously known as retrolental fibroplasia) and *sickle cell disease* have their major impact on the peripheral retina. The ocular and systemic manifestations of sickling hemoglobinopathies correlate poorly. In patients with sickle cell anemia, proliferative retinopathy is rare. Peripheral neovascularization is more common in sickle cell hemoglobin C disease (SC) and sickle cell thalassemia (S-thal). Patients with sickle cell trait usually have no ocular findings, although hypoxia encountered at high altitudes may precipitate hemorrhages and vascular occlusions.

The ocular findings in *sickle hemoglobinopathies* include small, dark red, comma-shaped conjunctival vascular segments, best observed on the inferior bulbar conjunctiva after instillation of a topical vasoconstrictor. Ischemic infarction of iris segments is also observed. In addition to peripheral neovascularization that often resembles the sea fan coral, other characteristic retinal findings include hemorrhages that have a salmon pink coloration from hemoglobin breakdown products and black chorioretinal scars with irregular borders in the equatorial periphery.

About one fifth of proliferative sickle retinopathy regresses spontaneously. The rest, if untreated, progress to retinal detachment and vitreous hemorrhage. Treatment consists of photocoagulation or transscleral cryotherapy or diathermy.

RETINAL VASCULAR OCCLUSIONS

CENTRAL RETINAL ARTERY OCCLUSION (CRAO) (see Color Plate 14*C*). The central retinal artery is a branch of the ophthalmic artery, in turn a branch of the internal carotid artery. Occlusion of the central retinal artery causes sudden, usually nearly complete visual loss in one eye. Ophthalmoscopy reveals arteriolar narrowing and vascular stasis which is recognizable ophthalmoscopically as segmentation of the venous blood column—"boxcar" pattern. Bilateral boxcarring is a useful sign of circulatory arrest and death.

Within hours the infarcted superficial layers of the retina lose their normal transparency and assume a milky white translucency. Because the thin retina of the fovea receives its nutrition from the underlying choroid, this region retains its normal color and contrasts with the surrounding infarcted retina to produce a cherry red spot. Bilateral cherry red spots are also encountered in children with congenital lipid storage diseases, the most common being Tay-Sachs, in which abnormal metabolic products partially opacify the ganglion cell layer that surrounds but does not extend across the fovea.

Eventually arterial flow is restored and the edema resolves. The disc, initially normal because it derives its blood supply from the surrounding choroid, gradually becomes pale and atrophic as its axons degenerate. After several weeks it is difficult to distinguish a central retinal artery occlusion from other causes of primary optic atrophy.

In some persons, portions of the retina are supplied by vessels arising from the choroidal circulation, and such areas may be spared if the central retinal artery alone is occluded. A CRAO deprives most eyes of useful vision. CRAOs are the result of emboli (atheromatous, myxomatous, and material from diseased or artificial heart valves), of local small vessel disease, or of carotid occlusion. A CRAO is sometimes the initial sign of giant cell arteritis or polyarteritis nodosa. CRAO has been reported in patients with sickle cell trait after trauma or other stress.

Acute central retinal artery occlusion is an emergency. In a few instances prompt action may dislodge an embolus and restore circulation in time to prevent retinal death and thus preserve vision. For a nonophthalmologist, intervention consists of firm, intermittent pressure on the globe with the heel of the hand, alternately raising and lowering intraocular pressure. A mixture of 95% oxygen and 5% carbon dioxide may also be administered by mask for several minutes at a time, monitoring respiratory status. Ophthalmologists use other measures: retrobulbar injection of local anesthetic to dilate the arteries and anterior chamber paracentesis to lower the pressure in the ocular vascular bed.

BRANCH RETINAL ARTERY OCCLUSION (BRAO) (see Color Plate 14*D*). Branch arterial occlusions present as sudden, partial loss of peripheral vision. On dilated fundus examination a wedge-shaped area of pale, infarcted retina is seen spreading outward from an arteriolar bifurcation. Branch retinal artery occlusions are almost always embolic in origin, the most common source of emboli in older adults being the ipsilateral carotid artery. In children and young adults, migraine, coagulation abnormalities, increased intraocular pressure, and oral contraceptives may predispose to vascular occlusions.

CENTRAL RETINAL VEIN OCCLUSION (CRVO) (see Color Plate 14*A*). The dramatic ophthalmoscopic findings of dilated, tortuous veins, extensive retinal hemorrhages, and disc swelling in one eye have classically been called a central retinal vein occlusion. Experimental evidence suggests that such hemorrhagic retinopathy requires both arterial ischemia and venous disease.

Visual prognosis varies. In the fully developed form usually encountered in older persons, vision is poor and generally remains so. Panretinal photocoagulation may decrease the risk of subsequent neovascular glaucoma in selected cases. A less severe ophthalmoscopic picture is encountered in younger patients. Acuity in such *nonischemic central retinal vein occlusion* or *venous stasis retinopathy* is only slightly reduced, and the visual prognosis is good. Ischemic oculopathy following carotid occlusion produces a similar retinopathy; the diagnosis is suggested by low retinal arterial pressure measured by ophthalmodynamometry or oculopneumoplethysmography.

A CRVO presents as unilateral visual loss in older adults but, unlike a CRAO, is not an emergency, as there is no accepted immediate therapy. There are also no specific accompanying diseases. Hypertension and diabetes are loosely associated, and hypercoagulable states must be considered, especially if there is bilateral retinopathy.

BRANCH RETINAL VEIN OCCLUSIONS. Patients with branch vein occlusions complain of blurred vision. In the fundus, hemorrhages and cotton-wool spots spread out in a wedge from an arteriovenous crossing. As in CRVO, there are few specific systemic associations. Neovascular glaucoma is rare, but vision persistently reduced by macular edema may respond to photocoagulation. Branch retinal vein occlusion must be distinguished from viral retinitis (see Ch. 465).

470   THE EYE AND MEDICATIONS

DRUGS WITH OCULAR SIDE EFFECTS

ANTICHOLINERGICS. A variety of systemic drugs have ocular side effects. Any medication with anticholinergic properties can dilate the pupil and diminish accommodation. This is the basis for the unhelpful caution against use in patients with glaucoma found in drug information inserts of medications that alter autonomic function such as antidepressants, tranquilizers, bronchodilators, and vasoconstrictors. Only when there is a potential for angle closure are such drugs contraindicated, and this is usually unrecognized. Patients on therapy for open-angle glaucoma are at little risk, as mydriasis usually does not affect their intraocular pressures. If the patient has a known angle-closure mechanism, previous iridectomy should have all but eliminated the danger of dilation. Of the systemic anticholinergic drugs, transdermal scopolamine is the most likely to dilate and fix pupils and paralyze accommodation, either by systemic absorption or through inadvertent instillation into the conjunctival sac by a contaminated finger.

CORTICOSTEROIDS. Prolonged administration of systemic corticosteroids often leads to the formation of posterior subcapsular cataracts. Topical corticosteroids increase intraocular pressure in genetically predisposed persons. Topical steroids also activate herpes simplex keratitis and should be prescribed only under the supervision of an ophthalmologist.

QUININE AND CHLOROQUINE. Quinine may cause acute blindness, with narrowing of the retinal arterioles. An overdose increases the probability of toxic effects, but rare persons are sensitive even to therapeutic doses. Other symptoms of quinine toxicity include dizziness, tinnitus, and hearing loss. Central vision may improve, with persistent constriction of peripheral field and evolution of optic atrophy.

The synthetic antimalarials chloroquine and hydroxychloroquine have a specific retinal toxicity. This usually appears only after prolonged administration in doses exceeding 250 mg per day for chloroquine and 400 mg per day for hydroxychloroquine. The parafoveal retina is most affected, and reduction in visual acuity may not develop until toxicity is moderately advanced. Chloroquine binds to pigmented tissues, exerting a toxic effect on the retinal epithelium with loss of pigmentation in a target-like or bull's-eye pattern around the fovea. Discontinuation of the drug may improve matters, but progressive visual loss may continue if the process is advanced.

AMIODARONE. Amiodarone represents a class of drugs having the property of cationic amphiphilia. Amiodarone binds to polar lipids and accumulates within lysosomes, producing whorl-like depositions of pigment in the corneal epithelium similar to the keratopathy of Fabry's disease (see Ch. 174.1). These seldom interfere with vision and resolve if the drug is discontinued. Instances of disc swelling and visual loss resembling anterior ischemic optic neuropathy (see Ch. 463) have been encountered in patients receiving amiodarone. The degree of visual loss from such amiodarone papillopathy must be balanced against the risk of cardiac arrhythmia in deciding whether to decrease the dosage.

THIORIDAZINE. Phenothiazines are potentially toxic to retina and retinal pigment epithelium, producing a coarse pigmentary degeneration. Of those now in common use, only thioridazine has clinically significant toxicity, and then only with dosages exceeding 1 gram per day for prolonged periods.

ETHAMBUTOL. Various drugs have been implicated in optic neuropathies. Only with ethambutol is the incidence of such side effects high enough that monitoring is considered mandatory. The physician administering ethambutol should perform monthly checks

TABLE 470–1. SYSTEMIC SIDE EFFECTS OF TOPICAL OCULAR HYPOTENSIVES

β-Blockers (timolol, betaxolol, levobunolol)
  Bronchospasm
  Bradycardia/hypotension
  Light-headedness/depression/fatigue
  Neuromuscular blockade in myasthenia gravis

Miotics
  Pilocarpine
    Brow ache (usually transient)
    Cholinergic overdose
  Echothiophate
    Prolonged action of succinylcholine or procaine

Sympathomimetics (epinephrine, dipivefrin)
  Tachycardia
  Atrial and ventricular arrhythmias
  Hypertension
  Headache

of acuity and color vision, especially when dosages exceed 15 mg per kilogram.

SYSTEMIC SIDE EFFECTS OF TOPICAL OCULAR MEDICATIONS
(Table 470–1)

Medications in solution are easily absorbed from the nasal mucosa, and systemic side effects are more likely with drops than ointments. Dilation of the pupil with 10% phenylephrine solution has been known to precipitate hypertension; topical epinephrine may increase ventricular extrasystoles. A single administration of timolol maleate to an asthmatic patient has induced bronchospasm and respiratory arrest.

Topical anticholinergics such as atropine, scopolamine, and cyclopentolate may contribute to confusional states in the elderly. Cyclopentolate is occasionally a cause of acute hallucinations and even psychosis in the young. Pilocarpine, used in large doses in the treatment of acute angle-closure glaucoma, has resulted in cholinergic overdose characterized by nausea, vomiting, salivation, and gastrointestinal cramps. As these are also symptoms of the angle-closure attack itself, such toxicity may not be immediately recognized, leading to continued administration and cardiovascular collapse.

Echothiophate iodide, an organophosphate used in the treatment of some forms of childhood strabismus and of open-angle glaucoma, predisposes to cholinergic crisis, which may mimic an acute surgical abdomen. Also, patients receiving echothiophate have impaired metabolism of succinylcholine. Use of succinylcholine during the induction of general anesthesia in a patient receiving echothiophate has caused death.

CARBONIC ANHYDRASE INHIBITORS

Acetazolamide and methazolamide inhibit aqueous production and are used systemically to reduce intraocular pressure when topical medications are inadequate. Most patients experience paresthesias; their absence is thought by some to indicate noncompliance. Carbonic anhydrase inhibitors rarely cause blood dyscrasias and also can induce a systemic acidosis, producing a syndrome of malaise and anorexia, depression, and weight loss that responds to concurrent administration of sodium bicarbonate. Acetazolamide also increases the incidence of urolithiasis. The combination of a carbonic anhydrase inhibitor and a thiazide diuretic may deplete body potassium. Carbonic anhydrase inhibitors should be administered with caution to people with known allergy to sulfonamides.

Grant WM, Schuman JS: Toxicology of the Eye. 4th ed. Springfield, IL, Charles C Thomas, 1993. *The latest update of a standard reference.*

PART XXVI

SKIN DISEASES

471 INTRODUCTION
Frank Parker

The skin is a dynamic organ containing many tissues, cell types, and specialized structures, which together serve multiple functions crucial to health and survival. One of the largest and most versatile of organs, it provides a number of unique functions. First it is the interface with our environment and serves many functions crucial to survival, including protection against the elements (including UV light, mechanical and chemical injury, invasion by infectious agents, and prevention of desiccation) and thermoregulation. Second, it functions as a sensory receptor, monitoring diverse environmental stimuli. Third, it plays an active role in immunologic surveillance. Last, in many instances it actively "mirrors" internal disease processes.

Skin problems are exceedingly common: 30% of Americans have dermatologic conditions requiring a physician's care (Table 471–1). Also, the skin and its appendages (the hair and nails) play a paramount role in our psychological makeup. Third the skin can be readily examined and biopsied and cared for under the eyes of the physician and patient.

TABLE 471–1. PREVALENCE OF COMMON DERMATOLOGIC DISEASES IN THE UNITED STATES*

	Rate per 1000	Numbers (in 1000's)
Fungus infections	81.1	15,733
Tinea pedis	38.7	7509
Tinea unguium	21.8	4232
Tinea versicolor	8.4	1623
Tinea cruris	6.7	1301
Acne vulgaris	68.1	13,217
Cystic acne	1.9	375
Acne scars	1.7	321
Seborrheic dermatitis	28.2	5476
Verruca vulgaris	8.5	1684
Folliculitis	8.0	1553
Atopic dermatitis	6.9	1332
Lichen simplex chronicus	4.5	882
Hand eczema	1.6	311
Dyshidrotic eczema	2.1	405
Psoriasis	5.5	1070
Vitiligo	4.9	957
Herpes simplex	4.2	824

* Persons 1 to 74 years of age—noninstitutionalized.
Reprinted from the chapter by Dr. Marie-Louise Johnson in the 17th edition of the *Cecil Textbook of Medicine,* with her permission.

Arnold HL, Odom RB, James WP: Andrew's Diseases of the Skin. Philadelphia, W.B. Saunders, 1990. *An up-to-date text covering cogent aspects of clinical dermatology.*

Fitzpatrick TB, Eisen AZ, Wolff K, et al.: Dermatology in General Medicine, 3rd ed. New York, McGraw-Hill, 1987. *A detailed and well-illustrated textbook covering all aspects of dermatology. Two volumes.*

Rook A, Wilkinson DS, Ebling FJG, et al.: Textbook of Dermatology. Oxford, Blackwell Scientific, 1986. *This three-volume multiauthored text covers every aspect of dermatology in great detail. It is well written and referenced.*

472 STRUCTURE AND FUNCTION OF SKIN
Frank Parker

The skin serves a variety of functions that can be correlated with specific properties of epidermal or dermal regions. The epidermis differentiates to form anucleate cornified cells that act as a relatively impermeable protective barrier to the outward loss of body fluids and the inward penetration of various substances and microorganisms. These lamellae of cornified surface cells together with the brown pigment melanin also play an important role in protecting against the carcinogenic effects of ultraviolet radiation. Two components of the dermis, its unique circulatory system and specialized cutaneous appendages, the sweat glands, play a vital role in the body's thermoregulation. Finally, the skin is important immunologically. Both the epidermis (Langerhans' cells) and dermis (epidermodermal junction structures) predispose to a number of immunologic reactions that generate inflammatory skin diseases.

ANATOMIC CONSIDERATIONS

The skin is composed of two mutually dependent layers: the outer *epidermis* and inner *dermis,* both cushioned on the fat-containing subcutaneous tissue, the *panniculus adiposus* (Figs. 472–1 and 472–2).

EPIDERMIS. The epidermis is a continuously renewing multi-layered organ that constantly differentiates. The stratified structure contains two main zones of cells (keratinocytes), an inner region of viable cells, the *stratum germinativum,* and an outer layer of anucleate cells known as the *stratum corneum,* or horny layer. Three strata of cells are recognized in the germinativum: the *basal, spinous,* and *granular* layers, each representing progressive stages of differentiation and keratinization of the epidermal cells as they evolve into the dead, tightly packed stratum corneum cells on the skin surface.

The epidermis is derived from the mitotic division of the basal cells resting on the basement membrane *(basal lamina),* with the daughter cells moving outward to the surface, where they become polyhedral as they synthesize increasing quantities of keratin. These *stratum spinosum cells* attach to one another mechanically by desmosomes, complex modifications of the cellular membranes that impart a spinous or quill-like appearance to the cells. Desmosomes play a crucial role in maintaining the adherence of the epidermal cells to one another. Desmosomes contain several intracellular proteins (i.e., desmoplakins, which are the paraneoplastic pemphigus autoantigens) and transmembrane proteins (desmogleins, which function as the pemphigus folaceous and pemphigus vulgaris autoantigens). With further outward displacement the differentiating cells of the spinous layer become flattened, and refractile keratohyalin granules appear in the cytoplasm, accounting for the designation of *granular layer* that rests just below the stratum corneum. These granules are the site of active synthesis of filaggrin, which causes keratin filaments to aggregate in parallel array, forming the tough, "chemically resistant" internal structure of the stratum corneum cells.

The transformation from viable granular cells to anucleate, non-

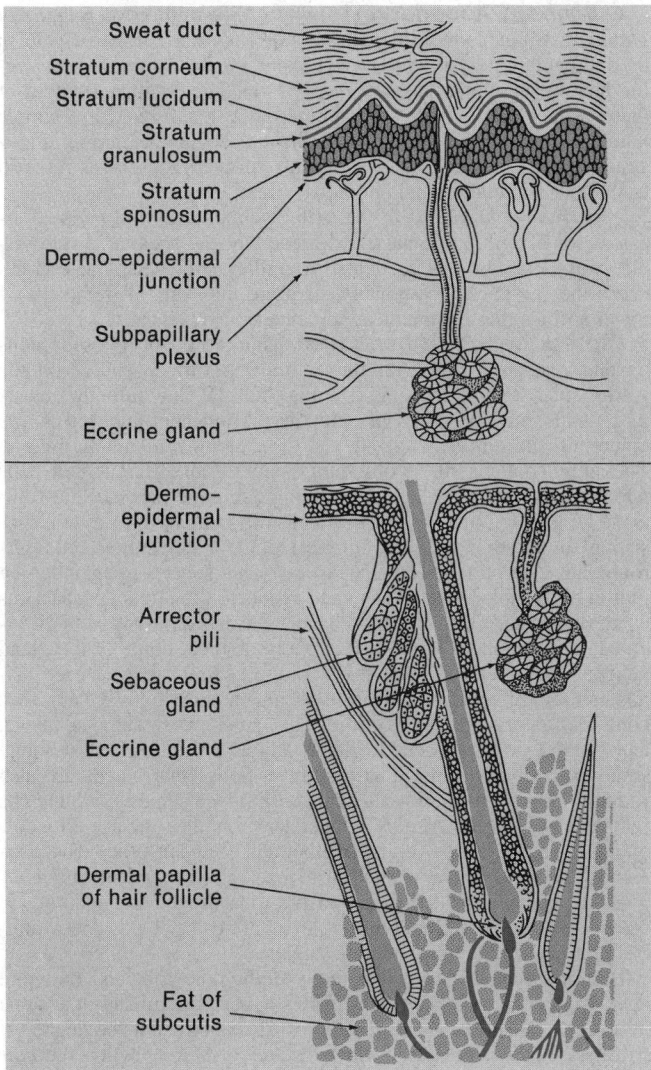

FIGURE 472-1. Structure of the skin. (Adapted from the 17th edition of the *Cecil Textbook of Medicine* with the permission of Dr. Marie-Louise Johnson.)

Two other cell types are found in the epidermis, the *melanocyte* and the *Langerhans' cell*. Both are dendritic cells with cytoplasmic arms that stretch out to contact the keratinocytes in their vicinity. The melanocytes are pigment (melanin)-producing cells that are arrayed in the basal epidermal layer and hair follicles, whereas the Langerhans' cells are usually found in the suprabasal layers of the epidermis, and at times in the dermis. Each dendritic cell has a different origin and function.

Melanocytes evolve in the neural crest of the embryo and migrate to the skin in early embryonic life. These cells synthesize brown, red, and yellow melanin pigments that give the skin its distinctive coloration. Melanocytes contain submicroscopic organelles (melanosomes) which synthesize melanin. A specific enzyme, tyrosinase, found within the melanosome, oxidizes tyrosine to dihydroxyphenylalanine (DOPA) and then to DOPA quinone. Additional nonenzymatic oxidation and polymerization occur to form the final product, melanin. Two kinds of melanin are recognized: eumelanin (brown-black biochrome) and phaeomelanin (yellow-red biochrome that contains large quantities of cysteine). The genetic make-up of the individual determines which melanin is produced, thus providing the various colors and hues of skin and hair. Once melanosomes are fully melanized, the resulting granules are transported out the dendritic processes of the melanocyte and transferred into the adjacent epidermal cells or hair.

Langerhans' cells, derived from bone marrow, contain a unique submicroscopic racket-shaped organelle (Birbeck granule) that plays a major immunologic role in the skin (Fig. 472–2). They contain surface receptors for immunoglobulins, and Ia-antigens, capturing

viable cornified cells is abrupt. The cornified layer consists of up to 25 layers of tightly packed, highly flattened horny cells.

The differentiation of the epidermal cells involves the formation of fibrous proteins known as *keratin*. The process of maturation of the epidermis (cornification) is complete in the stratum corneum yielding cells with mature keratin, namely, a system of filaments embedded in a continuous matrix (which is probably derived from the keratohyalin granules) within a thickened cell membrane. The stratum corneum limits the rate of passage of ions and molecules into and out of the skin. The insolubility and protective qualities of the stratum corneum is the result of (1) masses of keratin fibers embedded in keratohylin within the corneocytes, (2) the thickened cell membrane or cornified envelope, and (3) the deposition glucosylceramide and acylceramines in the intercellular s between the corneocytes by lamellated membrane bound organelles found in the upper spinous layer.

The basal layer of epidermis has a permanent population of germinal cells whose progeny undergo the specific pattern of differentiation just described. The new keratinocytes require about 14 days to evolve into stratum granulosum cells and another 14 days to reach the surface of the stratum corneum and be shed. Proper control of proliferation of basal cells and their subsequent orderly differentiation into keratinized stratum corneum cells produces the smooth, pliable surface of the skin. Alterations in the homeostatic state of cell division, defects in differentiation, or changes in exfoliation from the surface can lead to irregularities in the skin surface, characterized as roughening, scaling, and hyperkeratosis (accumulation of excessive layers of stratum corneum).

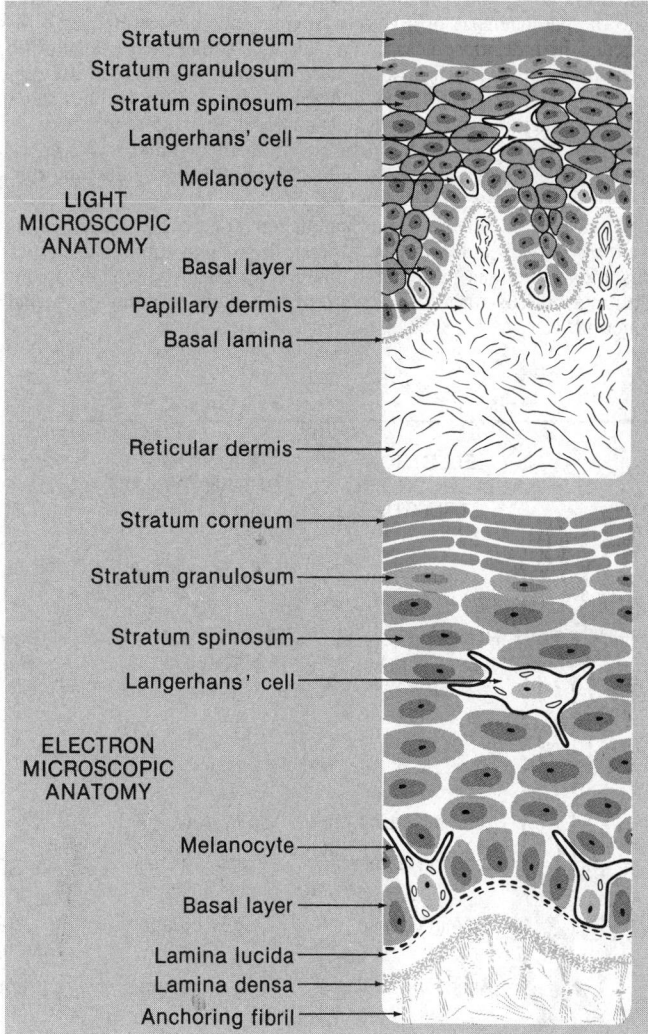

FIGURE 472-2. Diagrammatic representation of the light microscopic and electron microscopic anatomy of the skin.

external antigenic materials that contact the skin and circulating them to draining lymph nodes. Langerhans' cells thus play a central role in delayed hypersensitivity reactions of the skin (allergic contact dermatitis).

DERMIS. Beneath the epidermis lies the principal mass of the skin, the dermis, which is a tough, resilient tissue with viscoelastic properties. It consists of a three-dimensional matrix of loose connective tissue composed of fibrous proteins (collagen and elastin) embedded in an amorphous ground substance (glycosaminoglycans). At the microscopic level the collagen fibers resemble an irregular meshwork oriented somewhat parallel to the epidermis. Coarse elastic fibers are entwined in the collagenous fibers, being particularly abundant over the face and neck. This fibrous and elastic matrix serves as a scaffolding within which networks of blood vessels, nerves, and lymphatics intertwine and the epidermal appendages, sweat glands, and pilosebaceous units rest.

Dermoepidermal Junction. The structures situated at the interface between the epidermis and dermis constitute an anatomic functional unit of complex membranes and lamellae laced by divergent types of filaments that together serve to support the epidermis, weld the epidermis to the dermis, and act as a filter to the transfer of materials and inflammatory or neoplastic cells across the junction zone. At the level of light microscopy, this boundary zone is seen as an undulating pattern of rete ridges (downward finger-like or ridge-like extensions of the epidermis) and dermal papillae (upward projections of the dermis into the epidermis) (Fig. 472–2). Periodic acid-Schiff (PAS) staining discloses a thin uniform zone of intense reaction along this undulating junction which represents the basement membrane. Electron microscopic, immunoelectron microscopic, immunologic, biochemical, and genetic studies have elucidated the complexity of this region and are providing new insights into the pathogenesis of a variety of cutaneous diseases. Keratin filaments, hemidesmosomes, lamina lucida, lamina densa, anchoring filaments, and anchoring fibrils each function to maintain different levels of basement membrane adhesion. Figure 472–3 outlines these general structures, their molecular composition, and some diseases in which there is either a genetic defect in the synthesis of components of these structures or an autoantibody formed against the molecular components of the structure.

A variety of inherited mechanobullous diseases (epidermolysis bullosa) as well autoimmune bullous diseases (pemphigoid, herpes gestationis, bullous systemic lupus erythematosus) involve separation and bullous formation at various levels of the dermoepidermal junction.

Cutaneous Appendages. Two to three million *eccrine sweat glands* distributed over all parts of the body surface participate in thermoregulation by producing hypotonic sweat that evaporates during heat or emotional stress (Fig. 472–1). The combined output of these glands may exceed 1.5 liters per hour. Each gland is a simple tubule with a coiled secretory segment deep in the dermis and a straight duct extending up to the skin's surface. The glands respond to thermal stimulation and emotional stress.

Apocrine sweat glands in the axillae, circumanal and perineal areas, external auditory canals, and areolae of the breasts secrete viscid, milky material that accounts for axillary odor when bacteria degrade the secretion. Presumably, they are the vestigial remnants of lower species that communicate by cutaneous chemicals.

Pilosebaceous Appendages. Hair units, or pilosebaceous appendages, are found over the entire skin surface except on the palms, soles, and glans penis (see Fig. 472–1). Hair follicles consist of a shaft surrounded by an epithelial sheath continuous with the epidermis, the sebaceous gland, and the arrector pili smooth muscle. The bulb contains the proliferating pool of undifferentiated cells which gives rise to various layers comprising the hair and the follicle. The proliferating cells in the bulb differentiate into a hair consisting of keratinized, hard, imbricated, flattened cortex cells surrounding a central medullary space. The sebaceous glands are multilobular holocrine glands that connect into the pilosebaceous canal (hair canal) through the sebaceous duct. Germinative undifferentiated sebaceous cells at the periphery of each lobule of the gland generate daughter cells that move to the central areas of each acinus as they differentiate and form sebum (a complex oily substance composed of tri- and diglycerides, fatty acids, wax esters, squalene, and sterols). Most sebaceous glands adjoin a hair follicle, although some open directly on the skin surface. Sebaceous glands are also found normally in the buccal mucosa (Fordyce's spots), around the female areola (Montgomery's tubercles), on the prepuce (Tyson's glands), and in the eyelids (meibomian glands). The sebaceous glands and certain hair follicles are androgen-dependent target organs. Follicles particularly responsive to androgen stimulation are found over the frontal and vertex areas of scalp, beard, chest, axillae, and upper and lower pubic triangles.

Hair follicles are formed in early embryonic life, and no more develop after birth. Males and females have approximately the same number of hair follicles distributed over the body, but the degree of hairiness depends on two distinct features of hair growth—the *hair cycle* and the *hair pattern*. Hair growth consists of recurring cycles of growth, regression, and resting. The resting hair lies high in the follicle, where it forms a stubby hair bulb that is easily shed. Growth begins with a burst of mitotic activity and the follicle

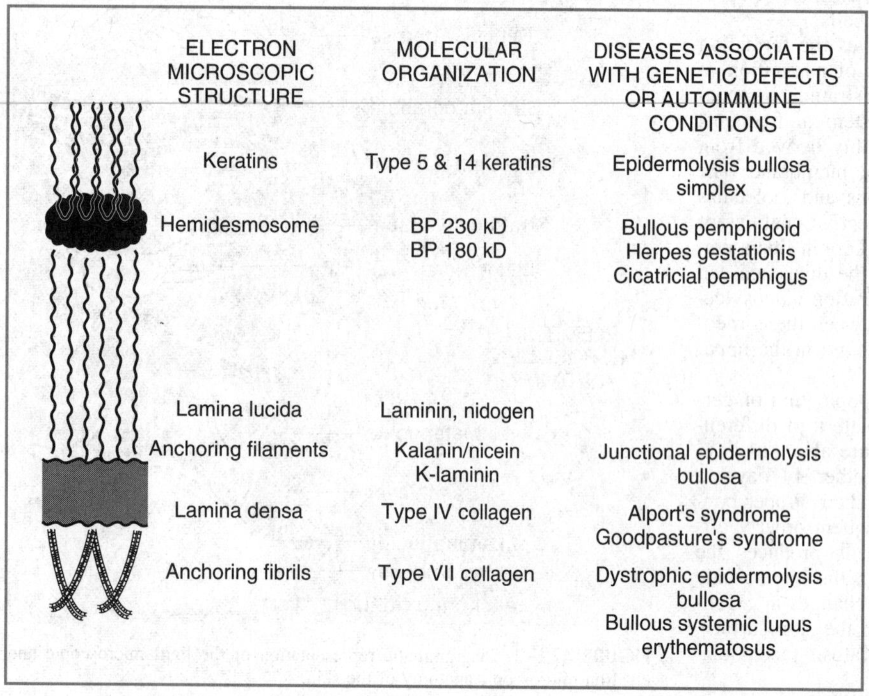

ELECTRON MICROSCOPIC STRUCTURE	MOLECULAR ORGANIZATION	DISEASES ASSOCIATED WITH GENETIC DEFECTS OR AUTOIMMUNE CONDITIONS
Keratins	Type 5 & 14 keratins	Epidermolysis bullosa simplex
Hemidesmosome	BP 230 kD BP 180 kD	Bullous pemphigoid Herpes gestationis Cicatricial pemphigus
Lamina lucida	Laminin, nidogen	
Anchoring filaments	Kalanin/nicein K-laminin	Junctional epidermolysis bullosa
Lamina densa	Type IV collagen	Alport's syndrome Goodpasture's syndrome
Anchoring fibrils	Type VII collagen	Dystrophic epidermolysis bullosa Bullous systemic lupus erythematosus

FIGURE 472–3. Structures and diseases of the dermoepidermal junction.

grows downward to reconstitute a new hair bulb. The hair bulb cells divide rapidly and keratinize to form a new hair shaft that dislodges the old resting club telogen hair. Regression provides a brief respite when mitosis ceases and the hair follicle pulls upward in the dermis as the hair shaft evolves into a resting club hair. In the adult scalp 85% of the hairs are in a growth state, 14% in a resting state, and 1% in regression. Considerable variation in timing of the hair cycle occurs from one region of the body to another, and the duration of growth determines the length of hairs.

Hair cycles also vary with the second important feature of hair growth, namely, hair pattern or the type of hair growing in each follicle. Two types of hairs are seen: vellus hair (fine, soft, short, non-pigmented, and common on "nonhairy" areas of the body) and terminal hair (coarse, long, pigmented, and found on hairy areas of the body).

Dramatic changes occur at puberty in both hair cycle and hair pattern mediated by either testosterone or dihydrotestosterone. The increased hairiness results from the conversion of vellus hair follicles to large terminal follicles. In the axillae and lower pubic triangle this conversion is mediated by testosterone and androstenedione. In other regions such as the beard, chest, upper pubic triangle, nostrils, and external ears, this conversion is mediated by dihydrotestosterone. Paradoxically, DHT also mediates the reverse process, namely, the miniaturization of large terminal follicles into vellus hairs. Such physiologic miniaturization occurs with the reshaping of the frontal hairline from a straight line to an M-shaped configuration at puberty. This occurs in all men and in the majority of women.

Maternal androgens ensure full development and function of sebaceous glands at birth. The vernix caseosa covering the neonate is mostly sebum. Normally sebaceous glands atrophy after birth, until puberty, when androgens again stimulate their activity. Acne is often one of the earliest signs of puberty. Disorders of androgen excess in adult women (e.g., polycystic ovary syndrome) are also associated with increased sebaceous activity and acne. Estrogens in large amounts decrease gland size and secretion.

FUNCTIONS OF THE SKIN

PROTECTION. Several structures in the skin, including the stratum corneum, melanin, cutaneous nerves, and the dermal connective tissue, provide important survival functions. The skin protects against the loss of essential fluids, the entrance of toxic agents and microorganisms, and damage from ultraviolet radiation, mechanical shearing forces, and extreme environmental temperatures.

The *stratum corneum* serves as a low-permeability barrier that retards water loss from the inner epidermal hydrated layers and also shields against environmental damage. The barrier properties of the horny layer are of practical importance from several points of view: Excessive drying or inflammatory reactions in the skin (e.g., eczema) lead to roughness, scaling, and disruption of the normally compact layers of horny cells. This leads to increased transepidermal water loss and, if severe (as in generalized exfoliative dermatitis, erythroderma, or burns), can contribute to fluid and electrolyte imbalance. With breaks in the horny layer, external substances more readily gain entrance to the underlying epidermis. Thus, various chemical substances, including medications placed on injured skin, have a greater opportunity to be absorbed or to act as haptens or antigens, increasing the possibility of allergic contact dermatitis. This becomes particularly common when topical antibiotics are applied to chronically inflamed skin, leading to superimposed allergic contact dermatitis. The disruption of the barrier also increases the chance of colonization of pathologic bacteria in the skin, especially in the presence of tissue fluid exudates, which serve as excellent culture media. Percutaneous absorption of various topical medications used in treating skin conditions, can be enhanced by hydrating the stratum corneum with the use of occlusive plastic wraps.

The stratum corneum normally harbors a number of aerobic and anaerobic resident organisms (i.e., *Staphylococcus epidermidis,* diphtheroids, *Proprionibacterium acnes,* and *Pityrosporon*). Breaks in the stratum corneum, poor hygiene, and excessive humidity (especially in intertriginous areas) all contribute to cutaneous infections such as impetigo, erysipelas, folliculitis, furunculosis, and ecthyma.

A second structural component that provides protection is the *melanocyte,* which produces melanin pigment. Melanin is a large polymer that has the unique capability of absorbing light over the broad range of 200 to 2400 nm wave lengths. It serves as an excellent screen against the untoward effects of solar ultraviolet radiation, such as aging and wrinkling of the skin and the development of cutaneous neoplasms. The importance of melanin is dramatically illustrated by the high incidence of skin cancers in sun-exposed areas of the body, particularly in light-skinned, blue-eyed, easily sunburned individuals and in albinos. Ultraviolet light exposure also causes aging and wrinkling of the skin. Neither sex nor race affects the number of melanocytes in the epidermis. Negroid skin contains the same number of melanocytes as Caucasian skin, but the pigmentation is more intense as a result of the synthesis of more melanin that is dispersed throughout the melanocytes and adjacent keratinocytes. Accordingly, black skin is much less likely to form skin cancers, and it ages more slowly than white skin.

Dermal nerves play an important role in bodily protection. Nerve endings are extensively distributed in the skin in two general morphologic types: free nerve endings and specialized endings (Pacini's and Meissner's corpuscles), which mediate many sensations including pain, pressure, and itch. Loss of sensation (e.g., diabetic neuropathy) may result in deep traumatic ulcers (trophic ulcers) without the patient's awareness. Damage to the dermatomal nerves (e.g., herpes zoster) may result in prolonged burning pain and hypesthesias (postherpetic neuralgia).

Itch is mediated by cutaneous nerves. It may occur in conjunction with a number of dermatologic diseases or without clinically evident skin disease (pruritus) (Tables 472–1 and 472–2). Itch and pain are carried on unmyelinated C fibers found in the upper portion of the dermis of the skin, mucous membranes, and cornea. The afferent C fibers enter the dorsal horn of the spinal cord, synapse, cross the midline, and ascend the spinothalamic tracts to the thalamus. Then the impulse proceeds to the sensory area of the postcentral gyrus of the cortex. Cutting the spinothalamic tract, as in an anterolateral hemichordotomy, abolishes pain and itch. A variety of peripheral mediators stimulate the C fibers and induce itching. These include histamine, trypsin, proteases, peptides (bradykinin, vasoactive intestine peptide, substance P—all potent histamine releasers), and bile salts. Prostaglandins are modulators of pruritus rather than primary mediators, lowering the threshold to itching evoked by both histamine and pain. Central modulators of pruritus, such as systemic morphine, cause itch while relieving pain by acting on central opiate receptors. Regrettably, no single pharmacologic agent effectively treats all kinds of pruritus.

Generalized itching in the absence of primary skin disease (pruritus) may be an important sign of internal disease (Table 472–2). An important cause of pruritus is psychic stress. Some patients with psychogenic pruritus believe the itching is caused by invisible parasites in the skin. Such patients scratch until excoriations and prurigo papules (thickened papular areas of skin due to constant rubbing) evolve in areas that the patient can readily reach (extremities, scalp, upper back). Dry skin (xerosis) is a common cause of itching in older individuals. Certain drugs (aspirin, opiates) can cause itching without a visible rash. Patients with polycythemia vera display a unique form of itching triggered by sudden changes in temperature, especially when they emerge from a warm bath. The itch is prickly in nature and lasts minutes to hours.

The tough, viscoelastic properties imparted to the skin by the fibrous proteins (collagen and elastin) and amorphous ground substance that make up the dermis protect the skin against shearing forces. The viscous and elastic properties of the ground substance allow it to resist compression and accept molding, thus reducing point pressure on sensitive skin structures.

TABLE 472–1. SKIN DISEASES ASSOCIATED WITH ITCHING

Xerosis (dry skin)
Insect infestations (scabies, pediculosis, insect bites)
Dermatitis (atopic, contact, nummular) including poison ivy contact
Drugs (opiates, aspirin, quinidine)
Lichen planus
Urticaria
Dermatitis herpetiformis (burning itch)
Sunburn
Fiberglass dermatitis
Seborrheic dermatitis

TABLE 472-2. PRURITUS ASSOCIATED WITH SYSTEMIC DISEASE

Systemic Disease	Postulated Cause
Uremia	Secondary hyperparathyroidism, high skin calcium concentration, proliferation of mast cells, xerosis
Obstructive biliary disease	High concentrations of bile salts in skin
Primary biliary cirrhosis	
Cholestatic hepatitis secondary to drugs (chlorpropamide)	
Intrahepatic cholestasis of pregnancy	
Extrahepatic biliary obstruction	
Hematologic and myeloproliferative disorders	Unknown
Lymphoma including Hodgkin's disease	
Mycosis fungoides	
Polycythemia vera	
Iron deficiency anemia	
Endocrine disorders	Unknown
Thyrotoxicosis	
Hypothyroidism	
Diabetes	
Carcinoid	Serotonin
Visceral malignancies	Unknown
Breast, stomach, lung	
Psychiatric disorders	Unknown
Stress	
Delusions of parasitosis	
Neurologic disorders	Unknown
Multiple sclerosis (paroxysmal itching)	
Notalgia paraesthetic—local itch of back, medial shaft scapula (local neuropathy)	
Brain abscess	
CNS infarct	

THERMOREGULATION. Thermoregulation is subserved concomitantly by the cutaneous vasculature and the sweat glands. A massive network of interconnecting musculocutaneous arteries and venules, as well as capillaries, arteriovenous shunts, and small venules, plays a crucial role in the maintenance of body temperature (see Fig. 472–1). Most of the skin's blood resides in the large venous plexus, through which blood slowly moves close to the surface, dissipating heat. Equally important in thermoregulation is the formation of eccrine sweat, which provides cooling by evaporation from the skin's surface. Every gram of water that evaporates from the skin loses 580 calories of heat.

Blood flow through the skin is 10 to 20 times that required to supply needed metabolites and oxygen. Under basal conditions about 8.5% of the total blood flow passes through the skin, controlled primarily by the sympathetic nervous system. Blood flow can increase up to 3.5 liters per minute with exercise in a warm environment thereby dissipating large amounts of heat. Both central (hypothalamic heating) and peripheral thermoreceptors stimulate sweating via the sympathetic nervous system, but in the case of sweat glands, acetylcholine is the postganglionic transmitter. Increase in body core temperature is the strongest stimulus for inducing sweating, whereas peripheral (cutaneous) thermoreceptors are only one tenth as effective in eliciting perspiration.

Response to cold begins when cool blood passes the hypothalamus, which elicits both heat conservation and production mechanisms. Sympathetic stimuli constrict cutaneous blood vessels and hypothalamic impulses activate shivering, which increases heat production by as much as 50%. Conversely, when warm blood irrigates the hypothalamus, central heat production ceases and cutaneous blood vessels dilate allowing heat loss from the skin surface. Vasodilatation also occurs reflexly through direct warming of the skin surface (in warm environments). In addition, stimulation of the hypothalamus produces sweating and increases evaporative heat loss. Periodic exposure to heat or to heat and work stresses (i.e., daily 1- or 2-hour exposures for 10 to 14 days) enhances the secretory capacity of the eccrine sweat glands (acclimatization).

The crucial role of cutaneous vasculature in thermoregulation and cardiovascular homeostasis can be reversed by widespread inflammatory conditions of the skin causing *erythroderma*. Diseases such as generalized dermatitis, psoriasis, drug reactions, and underlying lymphomas, can cause generalized, inflammatory-based cutaneous vasodilatation that can divert 10 to 20% of cardiac output through the skin. To maintain blood pressure, cardiac output must increase and older individuals with impaired cardiac reserve can develop high-output failure accompanied by tremendous loss of body heat with wide swings in temperature and shivering.

THE SKIN AS AN ENDOCRINE ORGAN. Many metabolic activities of the skin are under hormonal regulation. Not only do sebaceous glands and certain hair follicles respond readily to androgens, but they are capable of many diverse steroid transformations, as described above.

Dihydrotestosterone causes sebaceous glands to enlarge at puberty, stimulates the growth of certain hair (male sexual hair of the beard, chest, upper pubic triangle, nose, and ears), and generates the growth and development of the external genitalia. Drugs such as cimetidine and spironolactone have antiandrogenic activity and have been used to treat acne and hirsutism. In addition, thyroid hormones can regulate hair growth and alter the texture of the skin (fine, sparse hair and smooth, soft skin in hyperthyroidism; coarse hair and cool, rough, thick skin in hypothyroidism). Other hormones affect melanin pigment formation, melanocyte-stimulating hormone, and estrogen-stimulating skin pigmentation.

THE SKIN AS AN IMMUNOLOGIC ORGAN. The epidermis and the dermoepidermal junctional area participate actively in immunologic reactions. The skin includes immunologically important cells including keratinocytes, Langerhans' cells, and melanocytes as well as immunologic structures such as the lamina lucida and basal lamina that are involved in bullous reactions of the skin.

Epidermal Immunologically Important Cells. The most important immunologic cell in the epidermis is the Langerhans' cell, comprising 2 to 5% of the total epidermal cell population. Langerhans' cells contribute to a number of immunologic reactions, including macrophage–T cell interaction, T and B lymphocyte interactions, graft versus host (GVH) reactions, and skin graft rejection. The Langerhans' cell synthesizes and expresses Ia antigens (Class II antigens, immune response gene–associated antigens) that are crucial in processing and presenting allergens to sensitized T lymphocytes critical in the elicitation of delayed hypersensitivity contact dermatitis. Lymphokines, made by the Langerhans' cells during these immunologic reactions, augment and enhance these processes and also contribute to the accompanying inflammatory response.

Keratinocytes participate in immunologic responses by expressing Ia antigens on their surfaces in such conditions as GVH reaction, mycosis fungoides, allergic contact dermatitis, lichen planus, and tuberculoid leprosy. In these conditions the keratinocytes make lymphokines, particularly interleukin 1, which provides a second signal supplementing macrophages (Langerhans' cells) in mitogen- and antigen-induced T cell activation. In addition, epidermal cells make other cytokines such as prostaglandin-E2 and leukotrienes that participate in inflammatory reactions in the skin. Keratinocytes are the immunologic target in the pemphigus group of diseases in which circulating autoantibodies against intercellular antigen of the epidermis and mucous membrane epithelium initiate intraepidermal acantholytic bullae.

The Dermoepidermal Junction. A variety of inflammatory diseases often characterized by bullous reactions seem to be mediated by immunoreactants, including IgG, IgA, and IgM, and complement deposition along the dermoepidermal junctional area. The anatomic site of blister formation correlates with the position of deposition of these immunoreactants. The antigens in several diseases have been isolated and partially characterized. The use of immunofluorescent techniques at the light microscopic and especially the ultrastructural level has been helpful in more precisely diagnosing these bullous conditions. These are summarized in Table 472–3, along with immunofluorescent skin findings in connective tissue diseases.

INFLAMMATORY REACTIONS IN THE SKIN AND WOUND HEALING. Cutaneous inflammation reflects the sum of the effects of biologic products of cells (mast cells, infiltrating neutrophils, monocytes/macrophages, lymphocytes) as well as the effects of the products of the complement system, membrane-

TABLE 472–3. IMMUNOFLUORESCENT CUTANEOUS FINDINGS IN IMMUNOLOGICALLY MEDIATED SKIN DISEASE

Diseases	Biopsy Findings of Direct Immunofluorescence Immunoreactants (DIF)	Ultrastructural Localization of Immunoreactants	Site of Blister Formation on Routine Light Microscopic Pathology	Serum Findings: Indirect Immunofluorescence (IIF)
Bullous Diseases				
Pemphigus (all forms)	Deposits of IgG intercellular areas between keratinocytes	Between keratinocytes	Suprabasilar in pemphigus vulgaris; substratum corneum in pemphigus foliaceus	IgG antibodies to intracellular areas of keratinocytes in 95% of patients
Bullous pemphigoid	IgG and/or complement (C) in basement membrane zone (BMZ)	Lamina lucida and hemidesmosomes—upper part lucida and sub-basal cells	Subepidermal	IgG Ab to BMZ in 70%
Cicatrical pemphigoid	IgG and/or C in BMZ	Lamina lucida	Subepidermal	IgG antibodies BMZ in 10%
Herpes gestationis	Complement in BMZ—occasionally IgG	Lamina lucida—close to lamina densa	Subepidermal—sub-basal cell—above lamina densa	IgG antibodies BMZ in 20% (HG factor in 25%)
Dermatitis herpetiformis	IgA and C in dermal papillae (granular deposits)	Granular IgA associated with microfibril bundles in dermal papilla	Subepidermal in dermal papillae—papillar dermal microabscesses	No circulating antibodies
Epidermolysis bullosa acquisita	IgG, C3 in BMZ	Sublamina densa amorphous granular deposits	Subepidermal	Frequent IgG autoantibodies
Linear IgA bullous dermatosis in childhood	IgA and complement in linear deposition in BMZ	—	Subepidermal	No circulating antibodies
Connective Tissue Diseases				
Bullous SLE	IgG, IgM, and complement in BMZ in involved and normal skin—linear homogenous	Just beneath lamina densa (basal lamina)	Subepidermal	Circulating antibodies to BMZ; ANA found in 90%
Discoid LE	IgG, other Ig, and C in lesional skin at BMZ	—	—	No circulating antibodies to BMZ, ANA titers normal
Systemic LE	IgG band at BMZ in normal skin (over 90% in sun-exposed areas)	—	—	Elevated ANA titers
Systemic sclerosis	Nucleolar IgG	—	Epidermal thinning and increased dermal collagen	ANA, speckled, 85%, centromere + in CREST syndrome
MCTD	IgG/IgM in BMZ in some patients; nuclear IgG in epidermis	—	—	Speckled ANA and ENA (extractable nuclear antigens)
Dermatomyositis	Negative	—	—	ANA often normal range

derived arachidonic acid metabolic pathways (prostaglandins and leukotrienes) and the Hageman factor–dependent pathways of coagulation, fibrinolysis, and kinin generation. Early phases of wound healing also encompass many of these reactions.

Cutaneous Inflammation. Several pathophysiologic reactions initiate inflammation, including infectious, immunologic, and toxic processes that affect the epidermis or dermis, or both. Mast cells in the skin function not only as the sentinel cells in immediate-type hypersensitivity reactions but also as major effector cells in inflammatory reactions. They release (1) histamine, prostaglandin D2, and leukotrienes, which cause vascular dilatation and increased permeability, redness, swelling, pain, and itch; (2) chemotactic factors for eosinophils and neutrophils; (3) proteases that interact with the complement, kinin, and fibrinolytic pathways; and (4) heparin, which contributes to local angiogenesis. Degranulation of mast cells occurs in response to various antigens that cross-link IgE on the mast cell surface (immediate hypersensitivity reactions), to by-products of complement activation C3a and C5a (as occurs in leukocytoclastic vasculitides), and to radiocontrast media, aspirin, insect venom, and various physical stimuli. Circulating peripheral blood cells infiltrate local tissue sites in response to chemotactic factors released by mast cells and other infiltrating cells. Basophils release histamine and chemotactic substances, such as those involved in allergic contact reactions, bullous pemphigoid, erythema multiforme, and inflammatory responses. Neutrophils release myeloperoxidase, acid hydrolases, and neutral proteases that are active against microbes and cause tissue destruction (dermatitis herpetiformis, psoriasis, leukocytoclastic vasculitis, and bacterial infections of the skin). Eosinophils release major basic protein and peroxidase (allergic drug reactions in the skin, bullous pemphigoid). Lymphocytes release lymphokines that modulate immunologic and inflammatory responses (lichen planus, lupus erythematosus, allergic contact dermatitis, tuberculoid leprosy). Monocytes and macrophages engulf foreign proteins and microorganisms (granulomatous reactions in

the skin such as sarcoidosis, deep fungus and acid-fast bacilli infections, and cutaneous foreign body responses). Both classic and alternate complement pathways release products that induce mast cell degranulation and induce inflammation. (The activation of the system seems to contribute to inflammatory reactions in hereditary complement deficiencies causing lupus erythematosus–like syndromes or pyodermas, as well as necrotizing vasculitis.)

Wound Healing in the Skin. Healing proceeds temporally in three phases: substrate, proliferative, and remodeling. The initial substrate phase, encompassing the first 3 to 4 days after wounding, is so named because the cellular and other interactions lead to preparation for subsequent events. During this phase vascular and inflammatory components prevail (vascular clotting in the severed vessels; leukocyte and macrophage chemotaxis into the area to ingest bacteria, debride the wound, and degrade collagen). The proliferative phase (10 to 14 days after wounding) results in regeneration of epidermis, neoangiogenesis, and proliferation of fibroblasts with increased collagen synthesis and closure of the skin defect. The final remodeling takes place over 6 to 12 months, during which time a more stable form of collagen is laid down to form a scar of progressively increasing tensile strength. In some instances so much collagen is deposited in the healing wound that an elevated *hypertrophic scar* (red, raised scar within the boundaries of the original wound) or keloid (scar tissue extending beyond the boundaries of original injury into surrounding normal tissue) is produced. Keloids occur most commonly over the anterior chest, upper back, and deltoid regions. They rarely regress, and they recur after excision.

THE COSMETIC IMPORTANCE OF SKIN. Aging alters virtually all the structures and functions of the skin. Environmental insults, especially chronic sun exposure, cause far greater damage to the skin than time itself.

Changes with aging at the structural, physiologic, and biochemical level are as follows: Epidermal turnover rate decreases approximately 50% between the third and seventh decades. Concurrent loss of dermal elastic and collagen fibers accounts for the paper-thin, transparent quality of aged skin and the easy rupture of dermal vessels. An increasing cross-linkage of collagen and elastin accompanies aging, making the dermis more rigid and less able to withstand shearing forces. Aged skin, when "tented up," only slowly returns to its original form, whereas young skin readily snaps back. Sundamaged aged skin shows microscopic collagen damage. Dermal collagen is replaced by amorphous basophilic staining material. This condition, termed *elastosis*, results in deep wrinkling and furrowing, especially over the face and back of the neck, and yellow papules and nodules in a reticular pattern on the face. Decreases occur in the number of functioning sebaceous and sweat glands contributing to the dryness of aged skin and to impaired thermoregulation in aged persons. Reduction in the vascular network in the skin surrounding hair bulbs and eccrine and sebaceous glands may be responsible for the atrophy of these appendages with age. A 50% reduction in the number of Langerhans' cells may account in part for the age-associated decrease in immune responsiveness and allergic contact dermatitis reactions in the elderly. Loss of enzymatically active melanocytes (10 to 20% per decade) causes irregular pigmentation of the skin and graying of the hair. Gradual reduction occurs in the number of body hairs, especially in the scalp, axillary, and pubic regions (related in part to decreased androgen production). Linear growth of nails also decreases by 30 to 50% between early and late adulthood. Often nails become brittle and thickened. A number of proliferative growths are associated with aging skin, including skin tags (acrochordon), cherry angiomata, seborrheic keratosis, lentigenes, and sebaceous hyperplasia.

Orkin O, Maibach HI, Dahl MV: Dermatology. Norwalk, CT, Appleton & Lange, 1991. *A complete, well-written text covering the structure and function of the skin as well as clinical dermatology.*

Soter NA, Baden HP: Pathophysiology of Dermatologic Diseases, 2nd ed. New York, McGraw-Hill, 1991. *A well-written, concise text that explores the scientific basis of cutaneous diseases.*

473 EXAMINATION OF THE SKIN AND AN APPROACH TO DIAGNOSING SKIN DISEASES
Frank Parker

General considerations in history taking and physical examination:

THE DERMATOLOGIC HISTORY

A proper history includes the following: where the patient's skin condition first appeared; what it resembled and what symptoms, if any, were associated with it; how the skin disease progressed and changed and what has been done to treat it.

A careful review of the systemic medications (both proprietary and prescribed) that the patient is taking is in order. The relationship of the onset of the skin rash to the use of systemic internal medications is particularly crucial in evaluating the possibility of a drug reaction.

A history of atopic diseases or skin cancer and a careful family history of skin problems help to identify genetic and familial aspects of dermatosis.

If one suspects contact dermatitis, a detailed work and hobby history can identify exposure to allergens or irritants. Environmental exposure to the elements such as sun, cold, and heat may provoke skin reactions. When dealing with possible infectious and parasitic processes of the skin, it is useful to seek for similar problems among family members or sexual partners.

Psychologic stress, although seldom a sole cause of cutaneous conditions, can exacerbate many dermatoses (e.g., acne, psoriasis, seborrhea, atopic eczema).

THE PHYSICAL EXAMINATION

Dermatology is a visual specialty and the examiner's eye and a magnifying lens are its most important tools. Good lighting is essential, either daylight or fluorescent light simulating daylight. At times side lighting in a darkened room is useful for detecting minimally raised or depressed lesions.

The skin should be examined systematically from head to toe, so as to evaluate all regions of the integument, including the nails and mucous membranes. It is not unusual for the informed and observant physician to find some significant skin lesion, such as a basal cell carcinoma or even a melanoma, of which the patient is unaware. The general assessment of the entire skin allows the examiner to determine the pattern of the problem before focusing on specific lesions. Distribution may follow neural (as in a dermatome) or vascular patterns (as in livedo reticularis). In addition, factors related to the patient's general medical condition can also be discerned in the skin by noting signs of aging, pigmentation, trauma, nutrition, and hygiene. Color changes related to underlying systemic conditions (e.g., jaundice with hepatobiliary conditions, cyanosis with various cardiopulmonary diseases, diffuse hyperpigmentation with Addison's disease, paleness with anemia) all are important.

In each region of the body the physical examination includes three maneuvers: (1) *Observation* for color or surface changes. It is extremely important when observing skin lesions to use an alcohol sponge to wipe off existing cosmetics, oil, or foreign material. (2) *Touch or light stroking* to perceive texture changes, warmth, and moisture. Smoothness or roughness of the skin depends on such things as normal keratinization, proper hydration of the stratum corneum, and normal cutaneous blood flow. (3) *Palpation* to determine the consistency and pliability of the skin by stretching the integument between the fingers. Plasticity depends on the normal structure and function of dermal connective tissue and ground substance.

Because there are many hundreds of dermatoses, a logical process of elimination is required to narrow the possibilities, first to specific groups of diseases and finally to one condition. Such a diagnostic approach is based on specific morphologic descriptions of the skin lesions, together with an appropriate history and laboratory tests. Three steps are involved in this systematic approach. First, the entire skin is examined for primary and secondary skin lesions that allow the examiner to place the patient in one of nine diagnostic groups (the second step) (Table 473–1). Many skin conditions are found in each group, but all of the conditions in a given group express the same primary and secondary lesions. The third step involves singling out the patient's disease from the others in the group. This is done by looking for specific features, such as the distribution of skin lesions, any unusual shapes of the lesions or arrangement of several lesions (annular, serpiginous, dermatomal), color of the lesion including dominant hue and the color pattern, and the surface characteristics (particularly the appearance of scales or verrucous or vegetative changes).

STEP 1: DESCRIPTION OF PRIMARY AND SECONDARY SKIN LESIONS. Primary skin lesions are uncomplicated abnormalities that represent the initial pathologic change, uninfluenced by complications such as infection, trauma, or therapy. Secondary lesions reflect progression of the disease or scratching or infection of the primary lesions. Most of the primary changes can, at times, occur as secondary manifestations; for example, pustules may appear as primary lesions of folliculitis or as secondary lesions when scaling, itching lesions are scratched and infected. The trick is to recognize any single primary skin lesion as the initial change characteristic of the disease.

The terminology used to describe primary and secondary skin changes is the basic language of dermatology, the means by which one can accurately describe skin diseases to a colleague. If this terminology is not used correctly it is difficult to arrive at the precise diagnosis of skin diseases. Each descriptive word is not only a short account of what is seen on the surface of the skin but also relays specific information about processes within the skin. A diagrammatic representation and description of primary and secondary skin lesions are presented in Table 473–1.

STEP 2: ASSIGNMENT OF THE LESION TO A MAJOR GROUP OF DISEASES. Each disease within a given group shares the same primary and secondary skin lesions. Some diseases have overlapping traits so they may be assigned to more than one group.

TABLE 473–1. MAJOR GROUPS OF DERMATOLOGIC DISEASES BASED ON THE CLINICAL MORPHOLOGY OF THE SKIN CONDITION

Group	Clinical Morphology	Examples of Diseases in the Group
Eczema or dermatitis	Macules (erythema), papules, vesicles, lichenification, fine scaling, excoriations, tions, crusting	Contact dermatitis, atopic dermatitis, stasis dermatitis, photodermatitis, scabies, dermatophytoses, exfoliative dermatitis, candidiasis
Maculopapular eruptions	Macules, erythema, papules	Viral exanthems, drug reactions, verruca vulgaris, Kawasaki's disease, vasculitic and purpuric eruptions
Papulosquamous dermatoses	Papules, plaques, erythema with unique scales	Psoriasis, Reiter's syndrome, pityriasis rosea, lichen planus, seborrheic dermatitis, ichthyosis, secondary syphilis, mycosis fungoides, parapsoriasis
Vesiculobullous diseases	Vesicles, bullae, erythema	Herpes simplex and zoster, hand-foot-and-mouth disease, insect bites, bullous impetigo, scalded skin syndrome, pemphigus, pemphigoid, dermatitis herpetiformis, porphyria cutanea tarda, erythema multiforme
Pustular diseases	Pustules, cysts, erythema	Acne vulgaris and rosacea, pustular psoriasis, folliculitis, gonococcemia
Urticaria, persistent figurate erythemas, cellulitis	Wheals and figurate, raised erythema, scaling	Urticaria, erythema annulare centrifugum, erysipelas, necrotizing fasciitis
Nodular lesions	Nodules and tumors, some associated with erosions and ulceration	Benign and malignant tumors—basal cell cancer, squamous cell cancer, rheumatoid nodules, xanthomas
Telangiectasias, atrophic, scarring, ulcerative diseases	Atrophic, sclerotic telangiectasias and ulcerative changes	Connective tissue diseases, radiation dermatitis, lichen sclerosus et atrophicus, vascular insufficiency (arterial and venous), pyoderma gangrenosum
Hyper- and hypomelanosis	Increased and decreased melanin deposition in skin	Acanthosis nigricans, café au lait spots, vitiligo, tuberous sclerosis, xeroderma pigmentosum, chloasma, freckles

An arbitrary grouping that has proved to be of practical value is listed below and is used later in this chapter to discuss specific diseases within each group (Table 473–1).

STEP 3: NARROWING THE POSSIBILITIES TO THE EXACT DIAGNOSIS. Of great importance is the distribution of the skin disease, for many conditions have typical patterns or affect specific regions. For example, psoriasis commonly affects extensor surfaces and atopic eczema flexor areas of the extremities (Fig. 473–1). Photoreactions are confined to parts of the body exposed to sunlight. Involvement of the palms and soles is seen in erythema multiforme, secondary syphilis, psoriasis, and eczema. Contact dermatitis to exogenous allergens or irritants often presents with unusual patterns and distributions corresponding to the areas where the offending material came in contact with the skin. The best way to examine for distribution is to step away from the patient and view from a few feet away.

An important clue in differentiating diseases lies in the shape of the individual lesions and the arrangement of several lesions in relation to each other. A *linear* arrangement of lesions may indicate a contact reaction to an exogenous substance brushing across the skin, a pathologic process involving a vascular or lymphatic vessel, or a cutaneous nevus (Fig. 473–1). *Zosteriform* refers to lesions arranged along the cutaneous distribution of a spinal dermatome. They are unilateral and denote herpes zoster and, occasionally, metastatic carcinoma of the breast or the dermatomal hemangiomatous growths of Sturge-Weber syndrome. *Annular* lesions are circular with normal skin in the center. Annular macules are observed in drug eruptions, secondary syphilis, and lupus erythematosus. Resolving hives may leave annular configurations. Annular lesions with scale suggest dermatophytosis or pityriasis rosea. *Iris* lesions are a special type of annular lesion in which an erythematous annular macule or papule develops a second red ring or a purplish papule or vesicle in the center (target or bull's-eye lesion). Iris lesions are seen in erythema multiforme. *Arciform* lesions form par-

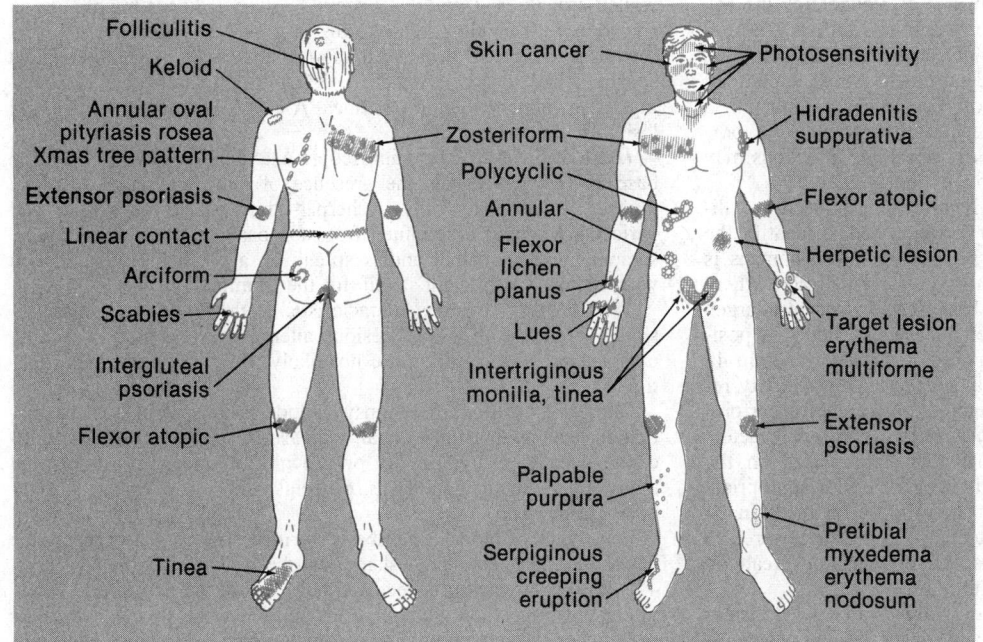

FIGURE 473–1. Configurational and regional diagnostic aids for the diagnosis of primary and secondary skin lesions.

tial circles or arcs and may be seen in dermatophyte infections. *Polycyclic* patterns evolve when numerous annular lesions enlarge and run together. Creeping eruptions and psoriasis produce *serpiginous* (snakelike, undulating, linear) patterns. *Herpetiform* refers to a grouping of lesions such as occurs in herpes simplex or dermatitis herpetiformis.

Other physical features influence diagnoses. Dry, lichenified lesions suggest a chronic state, whereas wet, weeping, macerated lesions suggest acute reactions. Abscesses are soft and fluctuant, whereas nodules are usually firm. Redness caused by dilatation of superficial blood vessels blanches with pressure, whereas erythema caused by extravasated blood as occurs in petechiae and purpuric lesions does not blanch. Hues of brown to black usually indicate melanin, although some drugs (e.g., tetracycline) cause brown-black pigmentation in the skin. The variation in color from melanin is related to the depth of the pigment in the skin—the deeper the pigment the more blue-black the color.

DIAGNOSTIC TESTS AND AIDS IN EXAMINATION OF THE SKIN

Certain aids and procedures, when combined with the history and physical examination assist accurate diagnosis.

VISUAL AIDS. *Magnification*. Magnification of skin lesions can detect the follicular plugging seen in discoid lupus erythematosus, or fine telangiectasias in the pearly, opalescent borders of basal cell cancers.

***Transillumination*.** Oblique lighting in a darkened room can help to detect slight degrees of elevation or depression of lesions as well as fine wrinkling or atrophy of the epidermis. The application of a penlight directly to nodular lesions in a dark room may give clues as to their density and make-up. Cystic lesions allow transmission of some light, whereas nodules composed of cellular infiltrates do not.

***Diascopy*.** Firm pressure with a microscope slide against skin lesions differentiates erythema of capillary dilatation from that of extravasated blood. Sarcoidosis, tuberculosis, and other granulomatous inflammatory reactions in the skin are suggested if diascopy of the lesions shows a characteristic "apple-jelly" or glassy, fawn-colored appearance.

***Long-wave Ultraviolet or Wood's Light Examination*.** Long-wave ultraviolet light (UVA) (360 nm) is useful in evaluating several conditions of the skin. Wood's light exaggerates the differences in the degree of pigmentation when the skin is examined with the lamp in a dark room. Melanin is a universal absorber of UV light, so decreased melanin shows more reflection (light color) and increased melanin less reflection (darker color). Pigment in the epidermis is exaggerated with UVA light, but that in the dermis is not, so a reasonable guess as to the site of melanin in the skin can be made. Wood's light may be the only means of recognizing the hypomelanotic ash leaf-shaped macules of tuberous sclerosis. The extent of vitiligo and melanotic nevi (which appear darker than surrounding normal skin) can also be determined. Some superficial fungal infections of the scalp fluoresce blue-green; erythrasma, a superficial intertriginous bacterial infection that produces a porphyrin, fluoresces a brilliant coral red; *Pseudomonas* infections may give off yellow-green color under a Wood's light.

CLINICAL TESTS. *Patch Tests*. Patch testing is used to validate a diagnosis of allergic contact sensitization and to identify the causative allergen. Because the entire skin of sensitized humans is allergic, the test reproduces the dermatitis in one small area where the allergen is applied, usually on the back. The suspected allergen is applied to the skin, occluded, and left in place 48 hours. A positive test reproduces an eczematous response at the test site from 48 hours up to a week later. The latter is a delayed hypersensitivity reaction. Considerable experience is required to accurately perform and interpret patch tests. *Photopatch testing* is performed to detect photocontact allergy. Suspected photoallergens are placed on the skin in two sets. One set of allergens is irradiated with appropriate wavelengths of light after the patches are in place on the skin 24 hours; the second set of the same photoallergens is kept covered to serve as controls. Photoallergens cause an erythematous reaction that is evident 24 hours after exposure to light.

***Physical Contact Testing*.** *Darier's sign* is the development of an urticarial and flare reaction after vigorously rubbing cutaneous mast cell (urticaria pigmentosa) lesions of the skin. The rubbing degranulates the mast cells, releasing histamine.

Nikolsky's sign demonstrates disadherence of the epidermal cells to one another. Pushing, rubbing, or rotating normal skin near bullous lesions causes the epidermis to be dislodged, leaving a moist, glistening defect. This sign is present in various forms of pemphigus and in toxic epidermal necrolysis.

The *Koebner phenomenon* occurs in certain skin diseases that tend to evolve new skin lesions after traumatic injury in areas of apparently normal skin. Thus, psoriasis may evolve within surgical scars and after sunburn or in the wake of a drug reaction involving the skin. Lichen planus may also exhibit this phenomenon.

Pathergy, the development of pustular and ulcerative lesions at the site of needle puncture, is suggestive of Behçet's syndrome and pyoderma gangrenosum.

Hair-pull examination is done to assess hair loss in the scalp. It is often useful to pull vigorously on scalp hairs to determine whether there is an increased number of falling hairs (normally only one or two can be removed with a tug of a group of hairs between the thumb and forefinger); ascertain the ratio of anagen to telogen hairs; and examine the hairs under a microscope for various congenital malformations of the shaft. Normally 10 to 15% of scalp hairs are in their resting phase. The percentage rises in naturally shed hair.

***Paring Hyperkeratotic Lesions to Differentiate Warts from Calluses*.** After the hyperkeratosis is pared away, the wart displaces and obliterates epidermal ridges and small bleeding points, and black and red dots become visible. In calluses the epidermal ridges are not interrupted, and no vessels are seen within the callus.

LABORATORY PROCEDURES. *Gram Stain and Cultures*. Gram stain for bacteria and bacteriologic cultures are important when the primary lesion is a pustule or furuncle or appears to be impetigo. When an unusual cutaneous infection is considered in an immunosuppressed patient, a skin biopsy specimen can be minced or ground in a sterile mortar and cultured for aerobic and anaerobic bacteria, including typical and atypical mycobacteria, deep fungi, and *Candida*. A more rapid method of screening for infectious agents in immunosuppressed patients (often the first sign of septicemia in such patients is pustules, nodules, or ulcerative lesions) is to perform frozen sections on a skin biopsy specimen taken from the lesion and to obtain Gram stains, acid-fast bacterial stains, and PAS stains (to identify fungal and yeast elements). This may provide a diagnosis within a few hours.

***Examination and Culture for Fungi and Candida*.** The presence of mycelia may be ascertained by applying 10% potassium hydroxide (KOH) to scale or exudative material scraped from suspected lesions and briefly heating the slide to dissolve the keratin. Hyphal elements can be observed by direct microscopic examination. Dermatophyte hyphae appear as long, branching, refractile, walled structures; *Candida* appears as shorter, linear hyphae in association with budding yeast forms (Fig. 473–1); tinea versicolor is seen as round yeast forms with short, club-shaped hyphae (so-called spaghetti and meatballs pattern). KOH examination of skin scrapings is mandatory to rule out tinea. A classic dictum is "if the skin lesion is scaly, scrape it."

***Tzanck Smear*.** The microscopic examination of cells from the base of vesicles reveals the presence of giant epithelial cells and multinucleated giant cells in herpes simplex, herpes zoster, and varicella. Material is obtained from the base of a vesicle by gentle scraping with a scalpel and is spread on a glass slide and stained with Giemsa's or Wright's stain for the examination.

***Skin Biopsy*.** Lesions characteristic of the eruption (primary lesions) should be biopsied. Lesions altered by scratching, infection, crusting, or lichenification are not likely to provide useful information.

Clinical indications for biopsy include lesions thought to be malignant; lesions that fail to heal, increase in size, bleed easily, or ulcerate spontaneously; tumors or growths of uncertain nature; and many inflammatory conditions, especially those for which the diagnosis is uncertain.

Four types of biopsies can be performed. The choice of technique determines the size and shape of the specimen obtained (Fig. 473–2). The procedure selected should secure the tissue most likely to contain the pathologic alterations and leave the smallest cosmetic defect. For the most complete histopathologic assessment an *ellipti-*

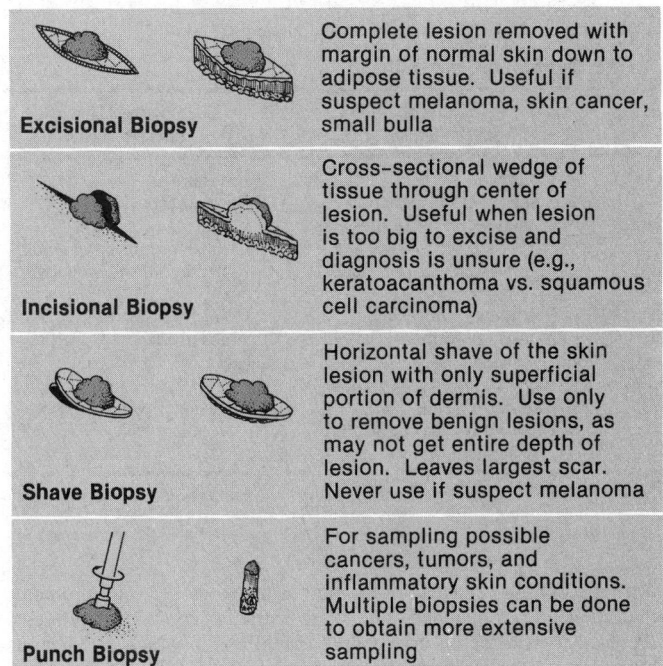

Excisional Biopsy	Complete lesion removed with margin of normal skin down to adipose tissue. Useful if suspect melanoma, skin cancer, small bulla
Incisional Biopsy	Cross-sectional wedge of tissue through center of lesion. Useful when lesion is too big to excise and diagnosis is unsure (e.g., keratoacanthoma vs. squamous cell carcinoma)
Shave Biopsy	Horizontal shave of the skin lesion with only superficial portion of dermis. Use only to remove benign lesions, as may not get entire depth of lesion. Leaves largest scar. Never use if suspect melanoma
Punch Biopsy	For sampling possible cancers, tumors, and inflammatory skin conditions. Multiple biopsies can be done to obtain more extensive sampling

FIGURE 473–2. Methods of skin biopsy.

cal, full-thickness excision is best because, in one procedure, the entire lesion is removed and secured for diagnosis and the remaining defect is easily sutured. The excisional biopsy technique is indicated when malignant melanoma is suspected or when a lesion is deep in skin or subcutaneous tissue and its orientation in surrounding tissue is relevant for diagnosis. A second procedure is the *paramedian incisional biopsy,* in which a thin but deep elliptical section is taken through the center of the lesion including normal skin at each end. This is especially useful in diagnosing large keratoacanthomas. A third biopsy method is the *shave,* or *parallel incision,* in which Xylocaine is injected locally under the lesion to lift it above the skin surface, and a scalpel (the knife horizontal to the skin surface) is used to "shave" off the protruding part of the skin and lesion. This technique is useful for diagnosing malignant and benign tumors when subsequent treatment by curettage and electrodesiccation is anticipated. It should never be used when melanoma is suspected, because the specimen obtained is too superficial for adequate histologic grading. Shave biopsy is convenient for removing superficial benign tumors such as seborrheic keratoses or skin tags. The fourth technique, *punch biopsy,* utilizes a tubular blade to cut out a circular plug of skin by slightly rotating and pushing the cutting edge deep into the dermis. The specimen is clipped off at its base with scissors, and the defect can be readily closed with sutures. Punch biopsies are used to diagnose inflammatory diseases and tumors.

If a first skin biopsy does not provide an answer, it is necessary and appropriate to rebiopsy. It is useful to give the pathologist an adequate clinical history to aid the interpretation.

474 PRINCIPLES OF THERAPY
Frank Parker

GENERAL CONSIDERATIONS

The goals of therapy are to define and remove the cause of a disorder, restore the structural and functional integrity of the skin, and relieve symptoms. Relief of such symptoms as itching, pain, or cosmetic disfigurement is an important goal. Damaged skin needs protection, as its barrier function is impaired. This can be assured with dressings and by minimizing scratching and avoiding abrasive

clothing and soaps or chemicals. Removal of debris, such as excessive scale, hyperkeratoses, crusts, and infection, is also a crucial goal of therapy if the skin is to heal. Topical and systemic medications, dressings, and other treatments can alter skin temperature and blood flow and thus favorably affect the metabolism of the skin.

TOPICAL MODES OF THERAPY

SOAKS AND WET DRESSINGS. Water, with or without various additives, can provide many benefits to the skin, including soothing comfort, antipruritic effects, and increased rate of epidermal healing with hydration and debridement of crusts, dead skin, and bacteria.

Baths. When the area of involvement is too large to apply compresses, a bath is useful. Baths with whirlpool action are favored for debridement of large or deep ulcers. Medicated baths can evenly distribute soothing antipruritic and anti-inflammatory agents to widespread lesions. Starch and oatmeal complexes are commercially available in forms suitable for tub baths. Bath oil prevents drying by leaving a thin film of emollient on the skin. The tub should be one-half full and the soak should last no longer than 20 to 30 minutes to avoid maceration. Warm baths cause vasodilation and may increase itching; cool baths constrict vessels and usually soothe pruritus. The best time to apply lubricants is immediately after the bath so that they may hold water in the hydrated stratum corneum.

Wet Dressings. Water and medication can be applied to the skin with dressings (finely woven cotton, linen, or gauze) soaked in solution. As water evaporates, the skin cools and pruritus lessens. For maximal benefit from evaporation, dressings should be no more than a few layers thick and dipped in the solution and reapplied to the area of treated skin every few minutes for 15 to 30 minutes several times a day. Wet compresses, especially with frequent changes, provide gentle debridement, the cleansing resulting from transfer of crusts, scales, and cutaneous debris to the compress. If the compresses are permitted to dry (wet to dry compresses) and become adherent, the debriding effect can further damage the skin. Dried-out dressings should be remoistened to facilitate removal. Wet compresses also leach water-binding proteins from the stratum corneum and epidermis, causing drying, a desirable effect for moist, oozing and weeping lesions. Therefore they are useful in treating acute vesicular, bullous, oozing or weeping conditions as well as crusty, swollen, and infected skin.

Open wet dressings are applied directly to the skin, leaving the dressing exposed to the air to evaporate. Frequent reapplication debrides exudate, crust, and bacterial contamination and dries out the skin, rapidly decreasing oozing and weeping.

Closed wet dressings, in which the moist fabric dressings are applied to the skin and covered with an impervious material such as plastic, oil cloth, or Saran wrap, may be useful when maceration and heat retention are required. For example, they may be appropriate if there is excessive keratin of the palms or soles or when an early abscess needs heat to localize the infection.

Dry dressings protect the skin, apply medications, keep clothing and sheets from rubbing, and keep dirt away. Such dressings also prevent scratching and rubbing. In cases of neurodermatitis or stasis dermatitis, they often are left in place for several days. Soft casts or castlike boots (e.g., Unna boot) serve the same purposes.

The medication most commonly added to baths and dressings is aluminum acetate, which serves to coagulate bacterial and serum protein. As a 5% preparation it is known as Burow's solution, and it must be further diluted for use. Burow's solution can be readily made by dissolving tablets or powder packets in appropriate amounts of water. (One tablet or packet in 500 ml = 1:20 concentration.) Potassium permanganate and silver nitrate stain the skin, may be absorbed if used over large raw areas of skin, and in high concentrations may burn the skin. They seldom are used nowadays.

Other means of cleansing and debridement of wounds, in addition to wet compresses, include such products and procedures as absorption beads or granules that suck debris and exudate out of wounds (Debrisan, Duoderm granules), hydrogen peroxide, whirlpool treatments, and various enzymatic products including trypsin/chymotrypsin, fibrinolysin, collagenase, and streptokinase. Antimicrobial agents are seldom applied by surface dressings be-

TABLE 474-1. GUIDELINES FOR SOME DRESSING MATERIALS

Dressing	Polyurethane Films	Hydrocolloid Wafers	Hydrogel Sheets, Granules	Hydrophilic Powders, Pastes
Examples	Opsite Tegaderm	Duoderm Restore	Vigilon Gelperm sheets Spenco second skin dressing	Envisan Bard absorption
Indications	Protect red wounds Autolysis of yellow or exudative wounds	Protect red wounds Autolysis of yellow wounds	Protect red wounds Autolysis of yellow wounds	Cleansing infected wounds Protection of red wounds
Advantages	Wound visible Waterproof, decreases pain Decreases friction Cost effective	Absorbent, good barrier, reduces pain, easy to store	Absorbent, reduces pain, good conformity	Good filler for deep wounds, absorbent
Disadvantages	Nonabsorbent Sticks to healthy tissue	Odor with removal Nontransparent	Poor barrier Need cover dressing to secure	Occasional pain on application, can leak

Also useful are the alginate materials (Kaltostate and Sorbsan) that absorb wound exudate. Alginates are fibers processed from brown seaweed into pads. Exudate transforms the fibers to a gel at the wound interface.

cause huge quantities would be required to reach therapeutic concentrations.

"Occlusive dressings" are being used with increasing frequency in the treatment of acute wounds and chronic venous, diabetic, and pressure ulcers. A variety of new dressing materials are available, including polyurethane films, hydrocolloidal wafers, hydrogel sheets, and hydrophilic powders and pastes. Table 474-1 lists examples of these dressing materials and some indications for use. In general, these materials provide good protection, help promote healing, and provide pain reduction of skin ulcerations.

TOPICAL MEDICATIONS. Most topical medications consist of two major agents, the active ingredient or specific medication and the vehicle or base in which the active material is dissolved.

Bases or Vehicles. Bases come in a variety of forms. *Powders* promote dryness by absorbing evaporative moisture. They reduce maceration and friction in intertriginous areas. Powders may be inert chemicals (corn starch, talcum), or may contain medications. *Lotions* are suspensions of insoluble powders in water. As water on the skin surface evaporates, it cools and leaves a uniform film of powder on the surface. The addition of alcohol increases the cooling effect. *Creams* are emulsions of oil in water (more water than oil). They vanish into the skin because water evaporates and the residual oil is spread thinly and imperceptibly over the skin. *Ointments* consist of oils with variably smaller amounts of water added in suspension. They have a pleasant lubricating effect on dry or diseased skin, but they give a greasy feeling to the skin and clothing. Oils in bases give a softening effect to the skin by forming an occlusive layer that traps water and retards evaporation. Thus, ointments with large amounts of oil give a more sustained, softening effect than creams or lotions. Some ointments containing large percentages of inert oil may be occlusive and retain heat, increase pruritus, and increase percutaneous absorption of active ingredients. The more occlusive ointments should not be used on oozing or infected areas, as the resulting occlusion and warmth may increase bacterial growth. *Pastes* are mixtures of powder and ointment (e.g., zinc oxide paste). *Sprays* are propelled aerosols.

Selection of a base or emollient depends on the condition being treated and the needs of the patient. Lotions are useful for pruritic, oozing reactions. Petrolatum, by contrast, retains heat and promotes hydration and even maceration of the stratum corneum. Ointments are used most often on dry, scaling conditions in which endogenous hydration of the stratum corneum is defective. Between these extremes is a spectrum of possibilities that permit some cooling but add lubrication.

Active Agents—Specific Agents. *Topical steroids* provide effective local anti-inflammatory and antipruritic effects. Topical steroids cause immediate and profound constriction of cutaneous blood vessels. This is believed to prevent mobilization of polymorphonuclear leukocytes and monocytes into the reaction site. They also interfere with the inflammatory activities of already present cells (e.g., mast cells). Corticosteroids used in topical preparations are intrinsically active without need for further metabolism; this accounts for their rapid effect on cutaneous blood vessels as manifested by blanching of the skin. Therapeutic action is also rapid. Topical steroids slow the mitotic rate of fibroblasts, decrease collagen synthesis and possibly enhance collagen catabolism. They further interfere with phagocytosis and the skin's ability to fight off bacterial, viral, and fungal infections. All effective topical corticosteroids have the basic hydrocortisone structure. A 1% concentration of hydrocortisone ointment or cream serves as a norm for comparing potency of subsequently modified topical steroids. By fluorinating hydrocortisone or adding acetonide, the potency of the steroid is greatly enhanced.

Topical corticosteroid preparations may be classified in a general way as of low, intermediate, or high potency (Table 474-2). The potency corresponds closely to the degree of anti-inflammatory effectiveness as well as to the incidence and severity of associated side effects. Although some corticosteroids (particularly fluorinated compounds) are more topically active than others, the potency of a preparation also relates to the concentration of active drug in the vehicle and the nature of the vehicle. Because corticosteroids are poorly soluble in most vehicles, many preparations deliver only a fraction of the drug to target cells. Of the various types of vehicles used in steroid preparations, ointments are the most efficient because they most effectively dissolve steroids, and the occlusive nature of ointments increases stratum corneum permeability. Second

TABLE 474-2. POTENCY RANKING OF SOME COMMONLY USED TOPICAL STEROIDS

Potency	Generic Name	Clinical Application
Most potent	Clobetasol propionate cream and ointment 0.5%, halobetasol propionate cream and ointment 0.5%, betamethasone dipropionate cream and ointment 0.5%, clobetasol propionate cream and ointment 0.5%, halcinonide cream and ointment 0.1%, fluocinonide ointment 0.5%	Recalcitrant psoriasis, discoid lupus, recalcitrant lichen planus, nummular eczema
Intermediate potency	Triamcinolone acetonide 0.1%, betamethasone nolerate cream 0.1%, amcinonide cream 0.17%	Dermatitis—allergic contact, atopic eczema, neurodermatitis
Low potency	Hydrocortisone cream and ointment 2.5% and 1.0%, desonide cream and ointment 0.5%, locoid ointment 0.1%, dexamethasone sodium phosphate cream 0.1%	Intertrigo, pruritus ani, seborrheic dermatitis

in order of efficiency is acetone-alcohol gel, whereas creams and lotions are less useful. Table 474–2 lists examples of topical steroids and their grouping according to potency.

The adverse effects of topical steroids relate almost exclusively to the intermediate and high-potency compounds. Epidermal and dermal atrophy can be pronounced; decreased collagen synthesis and reduced stromal support for dermal blood vessels lead to telangiectasia, purpura, and striae. These are especially likely to occur in intertriginous "occluded" areas of the skin and on the face. Fluorinated steroids can cause a perioral scaling, papular and pustular dermatitis, or facial redness, telangiectasia, and acne rosacea-like eruption. Potent topical steroids applied for prolonged periods around the eyes can occasionally cause glaucoma and even cataracts. Topical steroids can predispose to or worsen skin infections such as folliculitis, tinea, and candidiasis. Systemic absorption of potent topical steroids may lower plasma cortisol levels when they are used with occlusion over as little as 20% of the body, but this is unusual.

Intermediate-potency steroids are useful in most dermatologic conditions. Ointments are useful for thickened skin or for dry, exposed areas where creams or gel preparations rapidly evaporate. Low-potency steroids are used to treat the face and the thin and occluded skin of the groin and genital area. Lotions and gels are best for hairy areas. High-potency steroid preparations should not be used to treat most dermatologic conditions. Their use is primarily reserved for areas of skin that have been substantially thickened by disease, such as dense plaques of psoriasis or chronic dermatitis. Table 474–3 gives some guidelines for selecting the steroid potency and vehicle most useful in various areas of the body.

Topical steroids are usually applied once or twice a day. The stratum corneum acts as a reservoir and continues to release topical steroid into the skin after the initial application. Chronic dermatoses become less responsive after prolonged use of topical steroids. This phenomenon is referred to as *tachyphylaxis.* Changing to another topical steroid often overcomes this phenomenon.

Intralesional corticosteroids are used to shrink inflammatory acne cysts and hypertrophic scars and keloids. They are occasionally injected into unresponsive, localized dermatoses such as alopecia areata, granuloma annulare, discoid lupus erythematosus, psoriasis, and lichen simplex chronicus. Several types of steroids are used for this purpose, varying in their duration of action. Triamcinolone acetonide is the most widely used, and its maximal duration of action is 4 to 6 weeks. Triamcinolone hexacetonide is longer acting (6 to 8 weeks); injectables of shorter duration (2 to 4 weeks) include Celestone and Decadron. The steroids should be diluted to less than 5 mg per milliliter to avoid the risk of causing skin atrophy. Intralesional steroid preparations are crystalline and dissolve in the tissues slowly over weeks to months. To avoid disfiguring atrophy, great care is necessary in using low concentrations and shaking the diluted material just prior to injecting into the dermis.

Topical Antibiotics. These help suppress bacteria in erosions or superficial infections and occasionally in chronic leg ulcers. Silver sulfadiazine preparations are particularly useful as an adjunct to currently accepted principles of burn wound care. The commonly used topical antibiotics are bacitracin, neomycin, clindamycin phosphate, erythromycin, and tetracycline hydrochloride. The latter three are used to treat acne vulgaris. All topical antibiotics have the potential to sensitize, but neomycin is particularly prone to do so, especially after long-term use on chronic stasis dermatitis and leg ulcers. Mupirocin, a new topical antibiotic ointment, is particularly useful in treating staphylococcal and streptococcal infections of the skin; when used three times a day for a week it eliminates 87% of skin pathogens and may decrease nasal staphylococcus carriers.

Topical Antifungal Agents. Antifungals treat localized infections by superficial dermatophytes, *Candida,* and tinea versicolor. Topical broad-spectrum antifungal preparations effective against all of these organisms include clotrimazole, econazole, and miconazole creams and lotions used twice daily. Topical agents useful against dermatophytes but not *Candida* include haloprogin and Tinactin. Over-the-counter preparations, perhaps less effective against dermatophytes, are undecylenic acid and Verdefam. No topical preparations are useful against nail infections with these fungal organisms. Nystatin creams, oral suspensions, and vaginal tablets are effective against *Candida* infections in various areas of the body. Ketoconazole is a broad-spectrum imidazole antifungal agent highly effective against dermatophytes, *Candida,* and tinea versicolor. It is available in cream and oral forms.

Tars and Anthralin. Crude coal tar is often applied directly to the skin to treat psoriasis. Tars increase the effectiveness of ultraviolet light and reduce the accelerated mitotic rate of keratinocytes in psoriasis. Tars are often incorporated into shampoos for control of seborrheic dermatitis and in bath oils for use in psoriasis.

Anthralin is a synthetic coal tar derivative that is used in the treatment of psoriasis. Both tar and anthralin cause staining of clothing and skin. They can also be irritating. Anthralin must be started at the lowest concentrations (0.1%) and initially left on the skin for short periods of time (0.5 hour) to avoid irritation.

Antiparasitic Topical Medications. Antiparasitics are employed for the treatment of pediculosis capitis, pediculosis pubis, and scabies. The lice of pediculosis corporis live in the seams of clothes and bedding. These must be disinfected by washing or dry cleaning. One per cent gamma benzene hexachloride (lindane), cromatiton, and pyrethrin compounds (RID) all are useful in treating pediculosis and scabies. Lindane is not suggested for children less than 6 years of age or for pregnant or lactating women. Permethrin 5% (Elimite Cream), a synthetic pyrethroid used for the treatment of scabies, has been particularly effective with one application, especially as some scabies organisms appear to be developing resistance to lindane. Other, but less effective forms of therapy for scabies, include 10% crotamiton (Eurax) and topical sulfur ointments (5% in HEB cream). These require frequent applications.

Antiseptic Cleaners. These bacteriostatic or bactericidal agents are used as local or generalized skin cleansers and for wound irrigations. "Chlorhexidine" is active against gram-positive and negative bacteria and some fungi and yeasts. *Antiseptic* iodinated compounds slowly liberate iodine, which is effective against bacteria, fungi, yeasts, and viruses. One of the most frequently used preparations is povidone-iodine.

Sunscreens. Sunscreens help protect the skin from the acute and chronic effects of UV radiation. They are rated by their sun protective factor (SPF). The SPF, which ranges from 3 to 50, is the factor by which the product extends the period of exposure to reach the sunburn reaction that would have taken place without the sunscreen. The action of topical photoprotectives is to reduce penetration of photoactive nonionizing radiation. Such protection can be achieved by either absorbing or reflecting the radiation. No sunscreen enhances tanning. Rather, if partial block is achieved, it permits melanin production relative to the radiation transmitted and the inherent capacity of the partially protected skin to respond. Most sunscreens are less effective in blocking UVA (320 to 400 nm) than UVB (290 to 320 nm). Para-aminobenzoic acid and its esters protect the skin from UVB and allow UVA to pass. Other non-PABA chemical sunscreens such as benzophenones and cinnamates are also useful against UVB and, to some extent, UVA. If protection against UVA is required, a sunscreen containing benzophenones or anthranilate compounds should be sought. For complete protection

TABLE 474–3. GUIDELINES FOR SELECTING TOPICAL STEROIDS

Location or Type of Lesion	Suggested Potency of Steroid	Suggested Vehicle
Areas of Body		
Trunk, arms, legs	Intermediate or low	Ointment or cream
Palms, soles	Intermediate or high	Ointment
Scalp	Intermediate or low	Lotion, gel, aerosol
Intertriginous areas	Low	Cream, lotion
Face	Low	Cream, lotion
Area around eyes	Low	Cream or ophthalmic preparation
Ears	Intermediate or low	Cream, gel, or lotion
Types of Lesion		
Dry, scaling, fissuring, lichenified lesion	Intermediate	Ointment
Thickened, hyperkeratotic skin patches	High	Ointment
Oozing, weeping lesions	Intermediate	Lotion, cream
Ulcerative lesions	Do not use topical steroids	

or total blockade of UVB and UVA, physical sunscreens containing titanium dioxide, zinc oxide, or iron oxide are available as heavy creams or pastes that reflect ultraviolet light.

Topical Scar and Keloid Treatment. Silicone (Sialastic) gel sheeting has been found to prevent and treat chronic hypertrophic and keloid scars. Sialastic gel sheeting is a soft semiocclusive polymer that, when chronically bandaged to the scar for 12 to 24 hours per day for at least 2 months, makes hypertrophic and keloid scars flatter and more flexible. The mechanism is not known.

SYSTEMIC MODES OF THERAPY FOR DERMATOLOGIC CONDITIONS

ANTIHISTAMINES. The most specific use of antihistamines is to ameliorate or halt histamine-mediated disorders such as urticaria, angioedema, and allergic rhinitis. Antihistamines also suppress non-histamine-induced itching by soporific side effects. Antihistamines are of two major classes, the classic H_1 blockers and the newer H_2 blockers, which also decrease gastric acid secretion. H_1 blockers have three problems: (1) They don't block all the effects of histamine. (2) They provide only limited protection against anaphylaxis because mediators other than histamine are involved in this reaction. (3) They are not selective in their effects (i.e., they also have anticholinergic and sedative effects). Antihistamines (H_1 blockers) can be arranged into several groups depending on their molecular configurations (Table 474-4).

An effective agent for a given patient may be selected from one group or from a combination of groups, but its effects are unlikely to be enhanced by combining antihistamines within a given group. If response to one antihistamine is minimal, another from a different group should be added or substituted. Evidence that blood vessels in human skin have H_2 as well as H_1 receptors has led to the evaluation of H_2-receptor antagonists such as cimetidine in combination with an H_1 antagonist, and the combination has proved to be effective in the treatment of some cases of chronic urticaria otherwise unresponsive to H_1 antagonists.

Antihistamines should be started in moderate doses until sufficient improvement or troublesome side effects develop. Generally, they are administered three or four times a day. Low doses should be given to elderly patients, as they are unusually sensitive to central nervous system side effects such as confusion, dizziness, and syncope, as well as to urinary retention, dry mouth, and blurred vision. In children, paradoxically, antihistamines may induce hyperactivity.

SYSTEMIC STEROIDS. Systemic steroids are used for a number of dermatologic conditions, but they have several drawbacks: (1) Prolonged administration leads to adrenal suppression and susceptibility to infection. (2) Many diseases such as psoriasis and atopic dermatitis may worsen after steroid withdrawal. (3) Safer and simpler therapy is available for most common dermatoses. Systemic

TABLE 474-4. ANTIHISTAMINES ARRANGED ACCORDING TO THEIR MOLECULAR CONFIGURATION

Antihistamine Group	Generic Name (Proprietary Name)
H₁ receptor antagonist	
Ethanolamine	Diphenhydramine (Benadryl)
	Clemastine (Tavist)
Piperidines	Cyproheptadine (Periactin)
	Azatadine (Optimine)
Phenothiazines	Promethazine (Phenergan)
	Trimeperazine (Temaril)
Alkylamines	Chlorpheniramine (Chlortrimeton)
	Dexchlorpheniramine (Dimetane)
Ethylenediamines	Tripelannamine (Pyribenzamine)
	Pyrilamine (Neoantergan)
Piperazines	Hydroxyzine (Atarax)
	Meclizine (Bonamine)
Nonsedating antihistamine	Terfenadine (Seldane)
	Astemizole (Hismanil)
	Loratadine (Claritan)
Miscellaneous H₁ receptor antagonists	
Tricyclic compounds	Doxepin (Sineovan)
H₂ receptor antagonist	Cinetidine (Tagamet)
	Ranitidine (Zantac)

TABLE 474-5. THE ORAL AZOLE DRUGS

Agent	Tablet Strength	Absorption	Common Adverse Effects
Ketoconazole	200 mg	Acid in stomach Best on empty stomach	N, V, pruritus, rash, headache, hepatitis 2-10% patients, anaphylaxis in large doses, adrenal insufficiency, decreased libido, gynecomastia
Fluconazole	50, 100 200 mg	No effect of acid or food on absorption	N, V, rash, hepatitis is rare, headache, confusion, leukopenia, Stevens-Johnson syndrome especially in AIDS
Itraconazole	100 mg	Acid in stomach	N, V, pruritus, rash, hepatitis is rare, hypokalemia, hypertension

corticosteroids are used in three types of situations. First, patients severely ill with life-threatening diseases known to be responsive to corticosteroids (anaphylactic reactions, extensive erythema multiforme, acute exfoliative dermatitis, pemphigus vulgaris) should be started as high doses—80 to 100 mg daily. Second, patients with acute and severe but self-limited conditions are treated with steroids to control or suppress episodes. Examples include widespread poison ivy dermatitis, extensive sunburn, and acute generalized urticaria of known cause. Third, steroids are used for patients with chronic dermatologic conditions that, because of periodic exacerbations, intermittently require low doses (15 to 20 mg) of prednisone together with supportive topical therapy. Examples include flares of chronic atopic dermatitis, pemphigoid, and some connective tissue diseases.

SYSTEMIC ANTIFUNGAL AGENTS. Several systemic agents are available for treating not only systemic but superficial fungal infections. These can be considered as two types of medications: (1) griseofulvin and (2) oral azol drugs, including ketoconazole, fluconazole, and itraconazole.

Griseofulvin is active against dermatophytes but not against tinea versicolor or *Candida*. It is fungistatic, entering the horny layer of the skin via the sweat and the nails by incorporation into the keratinizing cells of the nail matrix. The entire nail must grow out with griseofulvin incorporated into it before the tinea at the distal end of the nail is affected. Accordingly, griseofulvin must be taken for many months before dermatophyte infections of the toenails disappear. Less time is required for infections of the fingernails and glabrous skin. Griseofulvin has rare side effects, including photosensitivity, urticaria, angioedema, headaches, gastrointestinal upset, and granulocytopenia. The drug may intensify underlying porphyria. Alleged, hepatotoxicity is not well documented. Griseofulvin also decreases the activity of warfarin-like drugs so that patients taking these agents may require dosage adjustments after griseofulvin therapy. Griseofulvin comes in several different packaging forms. Manufacturer's instructions for its use should be consulted before specifically ordering the drug. Griseofulvin also is effective in treating tinea capitus, onychomycosis, and tinea corporis too extensive for topical therapy and for superficial fungal infections in immunosuppressed patients.

Azol drugs are synthetic compounds that are classified as imidazoles (miconazole and ketoconazole) or triazoles (itraconazole and fluconazole) according to whether they contain two or three nitrogen atoms, respectively, in the five-membered azole ring. The antifungal effects of the azoles are due to their ability to inhibit ergosterol synthesis, critical for maintaining fungal membrane integrity. Ketoconazole and itraconazole are available only for oral use, requiring an acid environment for optimal absorption. Fluconazole is available in both oral and intravenous formulations.

Table 474-5 outlines some information regarding these azoles. Ketoconazole is effective against dermatophytes and, unlike griseofulvin, also against tinea versicolor and *Candida*. Several instances of fatal hepatocellular toxicity have been recorded, so ketoconazole should be used only for extensive cutaneous dermatophyte infections unresponsive to griseofulvin or for extensive cutaneous *Candida* infections. Liver enzyme levels should be determined before starting treatment and monitored at monthly intervals during treatment. Because most cases of azole-related hepatitis occur during the first few months of treatment, monitoring is especially important during this time. (Aminotransferase determinations are particularly sensitive in identifying early drug-induced hepatitis.)

It is not entirely clear what the role of itraconazole and fluconazole will be in treating superficial fungal infections. Several reports have noted favorable results of treating tinea corporis and cruris, onychomycosis, and cutaneous candidiasis with once-weekly doses of oral fluconazole for 2 to 4 months (150 to 200 mg once a week).

RETINOIDS. Retinoids are derivatives of natural vitamin A compounds. Two retinoids, isotretinoin and etretinate, are available for use in the treatment of dermatologic conditions. Retinoids decrease epidermal cell proliferation and keratinization and inhibit sebaceous gland activity. Etretinate has been found to be useful in severe psoriasis, especially the erythrodermic and pustular forms, as well as in several forms of ichthyosis. Isotretinoin has proved to be especially useful in severe cystic acne, often inducing prolonged remissions for several years after the drug is given for the usual 3- to 4-month course. The retinoids have many side effects, including cheilitis, conjunctivitis, dryness and fragility of skin, congenital malformations (heart defects, hydrocephalus, microtia), osteophytic growths on the vertebrae, epiphyseal closure in growing youngsters, corneal opacities, night blindness, and elevations of very low density and low density lipoproteins. 13-cis retinoic acid (Accetane) should be given for severe nodulacystic acne. When given in doses of 0.5 to 1.0 mg per kilogram for 4 to 5 months, clearing of the acne occurs in 85 to 95% of patients, and some 85% of these patients remain essentially clear of their acne indefinitely. Some 10 to 15% of patient's acne recurs and requires repeat courses of isotretinoin.

SYSTEMIC GOLD SALTS. Chrysotherapy has been useful in the treatment of autoimmune bullous disease, particularly pemphigus vulgaris. Intramuscular compounds have been used in the same manner as in rheumatoid arthritis. Remissions with a mean duration of 21 months or longer have been obtained in some patients with these bullous diseases. Generally a total dose of 400 to 600 mg of gold must be given before bullae respond. The experience with oral gold (Aurinotin) is limited in its use in dermatologic conditions.

SYSTEMIC ANTIBIOTICS. These are frequently used to treat cutaneous bacterial infections and conditions aggravated by bacterial overgrowth such as acne vulgaris, acne rosacea, and acute dermatitis. Most cutaneous bacterial infections involve *Staphylococcus aureus* or *Streptococcus pyogenes* (erysipelas, cellulitis, folliculitis, furunculosis, carbunculosis). Penicillins, cephalosporins, and erythromycins are commonly used to treat these conditions. Erythromycin and tetracyclines can control acne vulgaris and acne rosacea. Trimethoprim-sulfamethoxazole is used for pyodermas in patients allergic to penicillin or caused by methicillin-resistant *S. aureus,* as an alternative therapy for gonorrhea, and occasionally for the treatment of acne vulgaris. The sulfone antibiotic dapsone is occasionally used successfully to treat noninfectious diseases such as dermatitis herpetiformis, pyoderma gangrenosum, and leukocytoclastic cutaneous vasculitis.

ANTIMALARIALS. Chloroquine, hydroxychloroquine, and quinacrine benefit cutaneous lupus erythematosus, polymorphic light eruption, solar urticaria, and porphyria cutanea tarda. Antimalarials bind DNA, inhibit the LE cell phenomenon and antinuclear antibody reactions, block chemotaxis, and antagonize histaminic responses, all of which may be related to the therapeutic effects on the diseases mentioned above. Cutaneous and mucous membrane pigmentation, nausea, diarrhea, and cycloplegia are common toxic effects, but retinopathy is the adverse reaction of greatest concern. Quinacrine does not cause retinopathy.

SYSTEMIC ANTIVIRAL AGENTS. Acyclovir and vidarabine can treat herpes simplex and zoster skin and systemic infections. Ch. 339 details their usage.

SYSTEMIC CYTOSTATIC DRUGS. Cytotoxic drugs such as methotrexate, cyclophosphamide, azathioprine, and hydroxyurea are used in a number of skin conditions when they cannot be controlled by more conventional means. Thus, psoriasis, when it is generalized, severe, and life-ruining, may be treated with modest doses of methotrexate, azathioprine, or hydroxyurea; life-threatening bullous diseases such as pemphigus vulgaris are occasionally treated with these agents as an alternative to high doses of corticosteroids.

SULFONES AND SULFONAMIDES. Dapsone and sulfapuridine are the most commonly used sulfa preparations in dermatology. Dapsone is most commonly used to treat leprosy. Sulfone and sulfonamides are used most often to control dermatitis herpeti-

formis. Dapsone is also useful in treating cutaneous vasculitis, pyoderma gangrenosum, bullous forms of systemic erythematosus, and brown recluse spider bites.

A common side effect of dapsone is hemolysis and methemoglobinemia (especially in patients deficient in the enzyme glucose-6-phosphate dehydrogenase). Patients require frequent laboratory monitoring including a complete blood count differential, chemistry profile, reticulocyte count, and methemoglobin level.

ULTRAVIOLET LIGHT AS A THERAPEUTIC AGENT. UV phototherapy is used primarily in psoriasis and to treat vitiligo but may also help patients with nummular and atopic eczema, pityriasis rosea, the pruritus of uremia, and mycosis fungoides. UV light units are available in two wavelength ranges, UVB (the sunburn range of 280 to 320 nm) and UVA (long wavelength spectrum of 320 to 400 nm). The use of topical tar preparations, which "photosensitize" the skin to UVB wavelengths, adds to the effectiveness of treatment. Used over many weeks to months, the approach is highly effective in controlling psoriasis.

UVA light units are employed by dermatologists and commercial suntan centers to cause tanning rather than burning. The ability of UVA to evoke a sunburn is 1000 times less than that of UVB. The primary use of UVA is to treat severe, extensive psoriasis and vitiligo. It is used in combination with topical or oral psoralen, a drug that binds to DNA in the skin and sensitizes it to the effects of UVA. The long-term side effects of such therapy are unknown, although it may induce squamous and basal cell cutaneous carcinomas. The unprotected cornea and retina can be damaged by UV light. Stringent guidelines for protecting the eyes must be observed.

Shelley WB, Shelley GD: Advanced Dermatologic Therapy. Philadelphia, WB Saunders, 1987.

475 SKIN DISEASES OF GENERAL IMPORTANCE
Frank Parker

Chapter 473 discusses an approach to diagnosing skin diseases based on the specific morphologic descriptions of primary and secondary skin lesions. The nine ensuing groups, encompassing the majority of skin diseases, are listed in Table 473–1. This chapter discusses some of the diseases in each of these groups, providing the clinician with a differential diagnosis.

THE ECZEMAS (DERMATITIS)

Eczematous dermatitis is an inflammatory response of the skin to multiple exogenous and endogenous agents, although often the cause is not clear. Eczemas are defined by their clinical appearance and are subdivided either by their pattern of distribution or by etiologic factors (when known). Many eczematous processes are related to immunologic reactions (Table 475–1).

The term *eczema* or *eczematous dermatitis* is applied to eruptions characterized histologically by epidermal intercellular edema, termed *spongiosis*. Eczemas can be acute, with marked spongiosis causing red papules and vesicles and oozing, weeping, and crusting, or they may be chronic, with redness, scaling, fissuring, and especially lichenification. Both acute and chronic forms of eczema may affect the same patient, with the acute reaction progressing to oozing and crusting; with continued pruritus, the patient's rubbing and scratching converts the eczema to the chronic, dry, lichenified form. The hallmarks of all types of eczematous dermatitis are marked pruritus and varying degrees of erythema along with papules, vesicles, fine scaling, or lichenification. The histology of various types of eczemas is the same; skin biopsies identify a lesion as an eczematous reaction, but it does not differentiate among the various types of eczema.

CONTACT DERMATITIS. Contact dermatitis is the best understood and potentially the most correctable of eczematous reactions. For any such rash, the clinician should first determine

TABLE 475-1. ECZEMATOUS DERMATITIS SKIN ERUPTIONS NOT DISCUSSED IN TEXTS

Clinical Type	Etiology or Suspected Cause	Distinctive Diagnostic Findings
Eczematous drug-induced reaction	Drugs such as penicillin taken internally	Generalized eczema reaction evolves after taking medications (usually 10 or more days after first beginning drug; sooner if previously exposed) and clears with stopping drugs
Dermatophyte and *Candida* eczematous reactions	Dermatophytes and *Candida* induce eczematous inflammatory reaction	Dermatophyte or yeast found in scales or exudate
Infectious eczematoid dermatitis	Products from draining infected skin areas induce eczema reaction—linear infections, leg ulcers	Occurs near site of infection or other draining lesion; clears with treatment of infection
Dermatophytid	Hypersensitivity reaction occurring on distant areas of skin in response to products from fungal infection of other areas of skin	Often vesicular eruption of palms or fingers with dermatophyte infection of feet
Nonspecific eczematous dermatitis	No obvious cause—diagnosis of exclusion after above eczemas ruled out	Acute and chronic eczema patches anywhere on body; severe itching

whether it could be a contact reaction. If the cause can be identified, its avoidance cures it. There are two types of contact dermatitis, *irritant* and *allergic*. Irritant contact dermatitis is produced by substances that simply irritate or have a direct toxic effect on the skin, such as acids, alkalis, solvents, and detergents; no immunologic process is involved. Allergic contact dermatitis, on the other hand, is a delayed-type hypersensitivity reaction that occurs in response to a wide variety of allergens commonly found in the environment. The allergens consist of small molecular weight substances that act as haptens and bind to proteinaceous components of the skin to form the sensitizing antigen. Sensitization to the allergen requires 10 to 14 days to develop after the first encounter; subsequent exposure elicits the eczematous response in 1 to 7 days (delayed hypersensitivity).

The onset of irritant reactions after exposure to topical substance varies. Skin damage is evident within hours after contact with a strong irritant. Weaker irritants may require multiple applications and days or weeks before the development of the eczema (e.g., housewife's eczema of the hands due to chronic exposure to water and detergents). Contact dermatitis accounts for more than 50% of all occupational illnesses (excluding injury). In the industrial setting, approximately 70% is irritant and 30% allergic contact dermatitis.

Both irritant and allergic contact eczemas are initially confined to sites of contact, providing a diagnostic clue. Allergic reactions to plants, appear as linear, red, papular and vesicular streaks where the plant brushes across the skin. Allergies to metals (especially nickel) cause eczematous reactions under rings or watchbands or on the lobes of ears (earrings). Dermatitis under a ring may also stem from trapped water and irritating soap residues.

The most common allergens causing allergic contact dermatitis are pentadecylcatecol (allergen in poison oak, ivy, and sumac as well as in cashews, mangos, and ginko trees), paraphenylenediamine (a substance in hair dyes which cross-reacts with benzocaine and hydrochlorothiazide), nickel, mercaptobenzothiazol and thiuram (components in rubber), and ethylenediamine (a preservative in many medications and also found in industrial dyes and insecticides). Other common sources of contactants include topical medications (neomycin, anesthetics such as benzocaine, topical antihistamines), preservatives (ethylenediamine, merthiolate), vehicles (propylene glycol), and cosmetics (fragrances, preservatives, paraphenylenediamines). A detailed history of the patient's occupation, hobbies, habits, clothing, cosmetics, and topical medications is necessary to find the contactant.

Therapy of contact dermatitis is avoidance of the irritant or allergen if possible. Sometimes protective clothing is curative. Barrier creams are of little benefit. Acute, severe generalized contact dermatitis is treated with a short (10- to 14-day) course of systemic steroids and wet dressings or baths. Milder eczematous reactions respond to topical steroids and systemic antihistamines.

PHOTODERMATITIS. A variety of skin reactions, termed photosensitivity reactions, may occur in response to exposure to ultraviolet light. Some appear as eczematous reactions, so-called photoallergic dermatitis, which may occur in response to topical as well as systemic substances in the presence of UV light. The distribution of the eczematous eruption in light-exposed areas is an important feature in the differential diagnosis, with the cheeks, nose, forehead,

and tips of ears as sites of predilection. The backs of hands and forearms are also frequently involved and the history of exposure to UV light prior to the onset of the reaction is important in identifying light sensitivity (see Fig. 473–1).

Photoallergic dermatitis is immunologic. Absorption of a specific wavelength of ultraviolet light by a topical substance or a systemic drug (which is deposited in the skin from the vascular circulation) causes chemical conversion of the substance or drug to a hapten that binds cutaneous proteins to become a complete antigen capable of eliciting a type IV delayed hypersensitivity reaction similar to an allergic contact dermatitis reaction. Photoallergic reactions appear only where the UV light hits the skin, even though the systemic drug or topical photoallergen is present in the skin all over the body; i.e., the reaction depends on UV light hitting the skin with the allergen in it. Long wavelength UVA light usually generates these reactions. Because UVA light penetrates window glass, the reaction often occurs from indoor exposure. Such drugs as thiazides and phenothiazines can cause photoeczematous reactions, as can a number of topically applied substances, such as methylcoumarin, musk ambrette, halogenated salicylanilids, and topical sunscreening agents. Photopatch testing can identify substances in materials causing these reactions. Avoidance of the offending material is often curative. Oral or topical steroids relieve the inflammatory reaction.

ATOPIC DERMATITIS. This chronic, eczematous condition of the skin is often associated with a personal or family history of asthma, allergic rhinitis, and atopic eczema. Pruritus is prominent, and the consequent scratching and rubbing lead to lichenification, most typically in the antecubital and popliteal flexural areas. The eczema usually manifests itself after the first few months of life, appearing on the face and extensor areas of the extremities as acute and subacute, red, vesicular and oozing dermatitis. Many cases resolve spontaneously by puberty only to recur in adolescence and adulthood as a chronic dermatitis with scaling, dryness, and lichenification over the face, neck, upper chest, and characteristically the antecubital and popliteal fossae (flexural dermatitis). Atopics have a readily identifiable facies with diffuse erythema, perioral pallor, and a redundant crease or fold below the lower eyelids. The palms often have an increased number of skin markings, noticeable as fine cross-hatched lines. Stroking the skin in atopic dermatitis causes a white line, or dermatographism, probably due to dermal edema and vasoconstriction.

The cause of atopic dermatitis is not known, but a number of immunologic and pharmacologic abnormalities associate with the skin condition. For example, IgE reagenic antibodies are increased in 80% of atopic patients, especially those with extensive skin disease (such patients respond to many antigens applied by skin prick testing), but these antibodies seem not to *cause* atopic eczema. Avoiding antigens to which these patients react by scratch test does not improve the eczema. Patients with atopic eczema also have depressed cell-mediated immunity. This may account for the overproduction of IgE, resulting in unusual susceptibility to cutaneous herpes simplex, vaccina, molluscum contagiosum, and wart infections. Neutrophil and monocyte chemotaxis is reduced during exacerbations of eczema, explaining the frequent staphylococcal skin infections in these patients. Treatment with oral antibiotics to reduce staphylococcal flora (or overt staphylococcal infections such as fol-

PLATE 13   EYE DISEASES

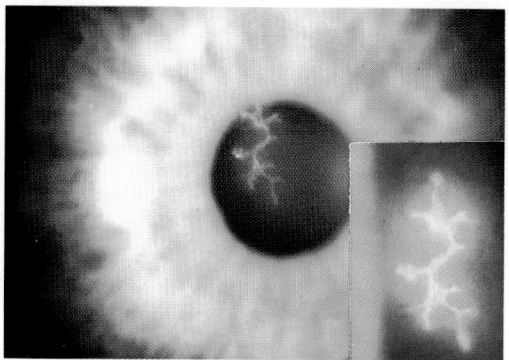

A, Herpes simplex corneal epithelial keratitis in diffuse light and *(inset)* in light passed through a cobalt blue filter after fluorescein staining.

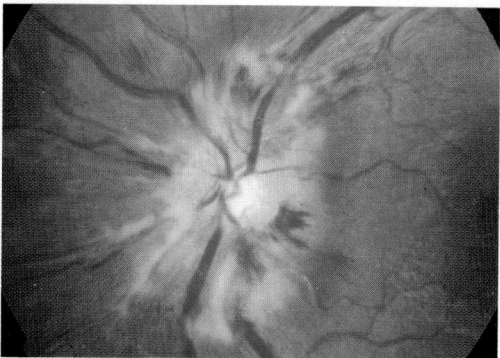

B, Papilledema in a young person. Note disc swelling, hemorrhages, and exudates, with preservation of the physiologic cup.

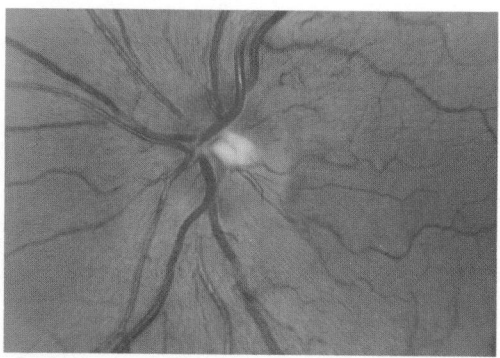

C, Disc in acute Leber's hereditary optic neuropathy. The disc tissue appears hyperemic, with peripapillary telangiectasia and opacification of the nerve fiber layer. Fluorescein angiography revealed no dye leakage.

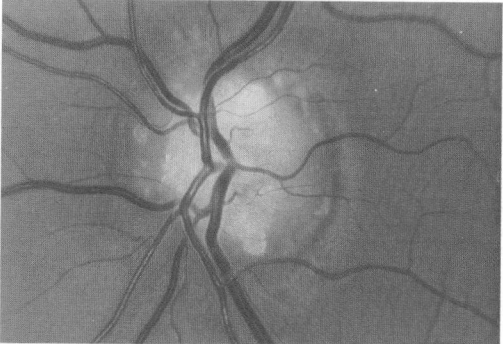

D, Optic disc drusen (also called hyaline bodies). Although obvious here, these calcified excrescences may be difficult to see in young persons, in whom the disc elevation they produce is mistaken for papilledema. (Also, they should be distinguished from retinal drusen—see *F* below.)

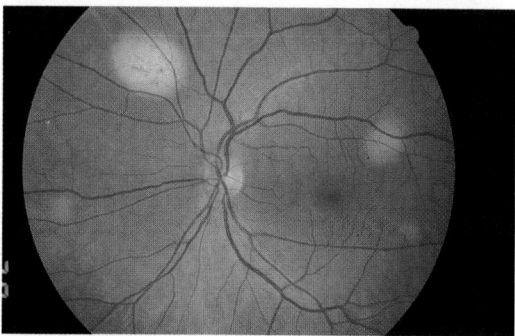

E, Multiple white choroidal metastases in a man with lung carcinoma.

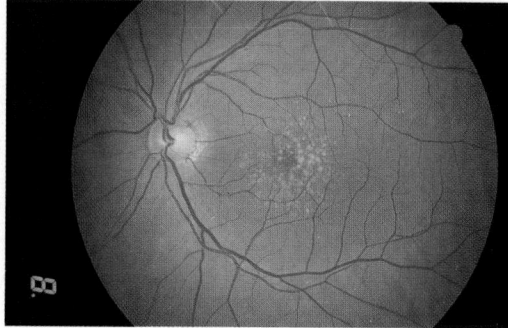

F, Retinal drusen. Multiple small white dots in the macula that represent abnormal accumulations in the retinal pigment epithelium basement (Bruch's) membrane. Such drusen are often precursors to visual loss from senile macular degeneration. (These should be distinguished from optic disc drusen—see *D* above.)

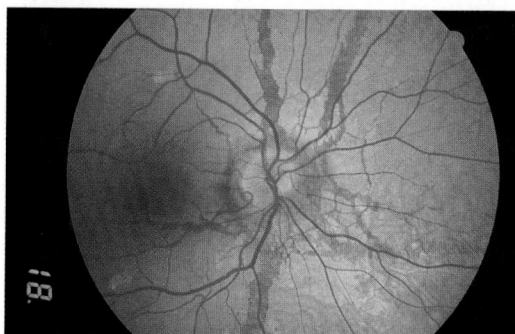

G, Angioid streaks in pseudoxanthoma elasticum. Breaks in the retinal pigment epithelium basement (Bruch's) membrane radial and circumferential to the disc indicate an underlying defect in elastic tissue formation.

Photographs taken by Mr. Harry Kachadoorian, C.R.A., University of Massachusetts Medical School, Worcester, Massachusetts.

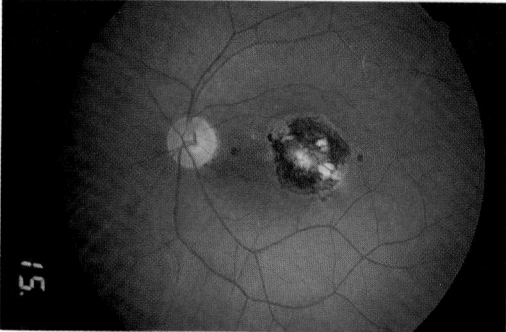

H, Macular chorioretinal scar. The appearance is typical of congenital toxoplasmosis, although other causes of chorioretinitis are included in the differential diagnosis.

PLATE 14 EYE DISEASES

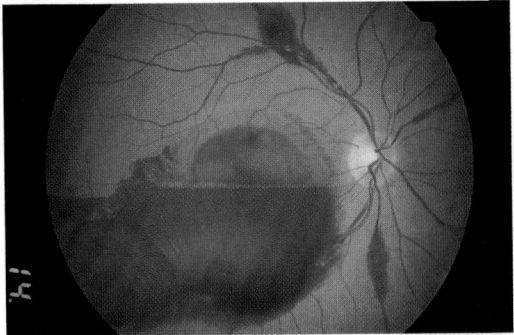

A, Preretinal (subhyaloid) hemorrhage. This occurred after a difficult intubation in an asthmatic woman with a previously normal eye examination. Similar findings are seen as a manifestation of diabetic retinopathy and in association with subarachnoid hemorrhage. The blood forms a meniscus with the patient in the upright position.

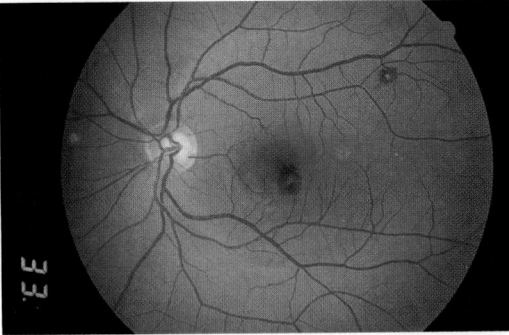

B, Roth's spots. Multiple white centered hemorrhages in a man with recurrent subacute bacterial endocarditis. White centered hemorrhages are also seen with leukemia and diabetes. The small white scars are probably the residua of previous episodes.

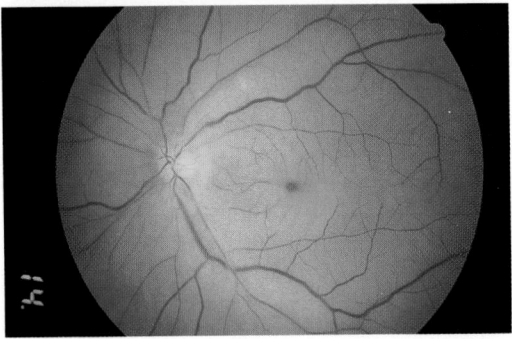

C, Central retinal artery occlusion. The retina is diffusely pale, lending a prominence to the normal coloration of the central fovea, often described as a cherry red spot.

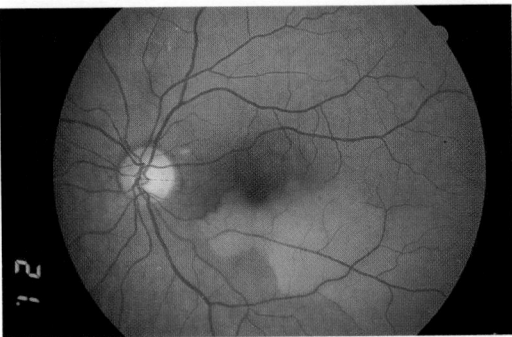

D, Inferior branch retinal artery occlusion. A pie-shaped sector of pale, infarcted retina extends from the embolic occlusion at the first branch of the arteriole of the inferior temporal arcade.

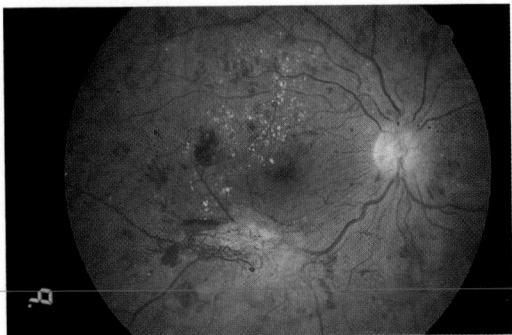

E, Proliferative diabetic retinopathy. Multiple hemorrhages, exudates, and new vessels are visible, with chorioretinal striae extending toward an area of fibrovascular proliferation along the inferior temporal arcade.

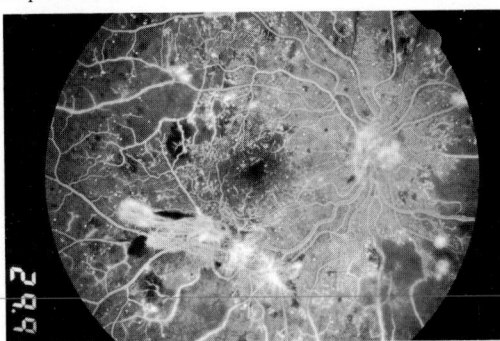

F, Fluorescein angiogram of the same fundus pictured in *E.* The new vessels, especially at the disc and the area of fibrovascular proliferation, are seen to leak fluorescein. Many of the "dot hemorrhages" are revealed as microaneurysms that fill with dye.

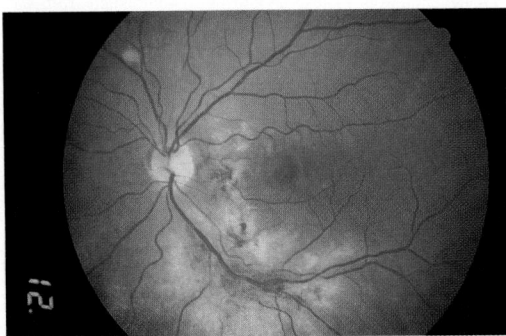

G, Cytomegalovirus retinitis in a patient with AIDS. There is a sector of retinal necrosis and hemorrhages along the inferior temporal arcade.

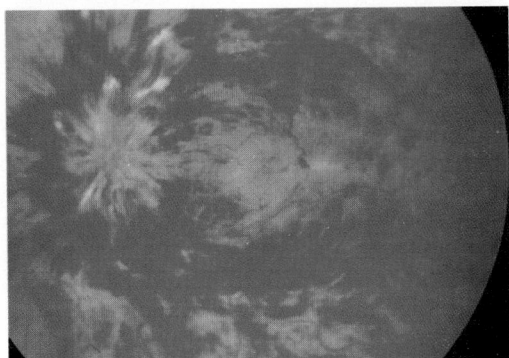

H, Central retinal vein occlusion. The disc is swollen with diffuse retinal hemorrhages and cotton-wool spots.

Photographs taken by Mr. Harry Kachadoorian, C.R.A., University of Massachusetts Medical School, Worcester, Massachusetts.

PLATE 15 SKIN DISEASES

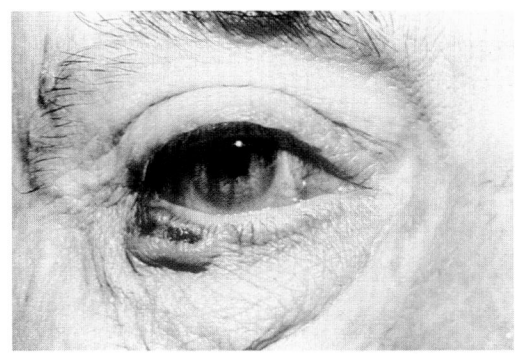

A, Basal cell cancer. Tumor with rolled, opalescent borders and central "rodent" ulcer.

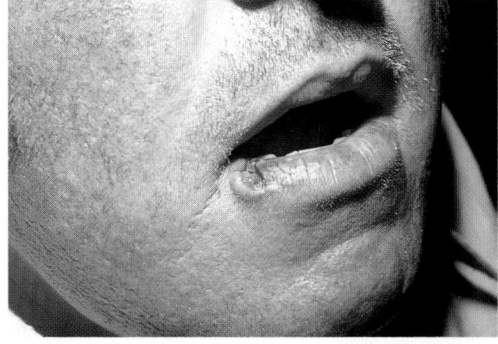

B, Squamous cell cancer. Firm nodule with eroded surface on the lower lip.

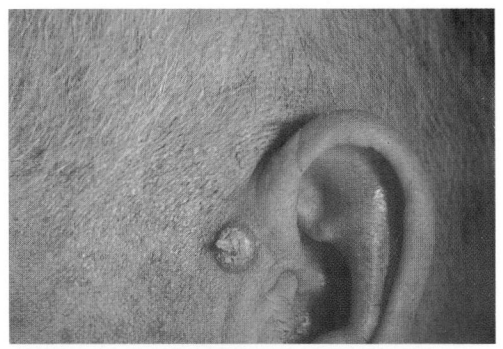

C, Cutaneous horn. Keratotic horn evolving from red nodule at base. These commonly are squamous cell cancers.

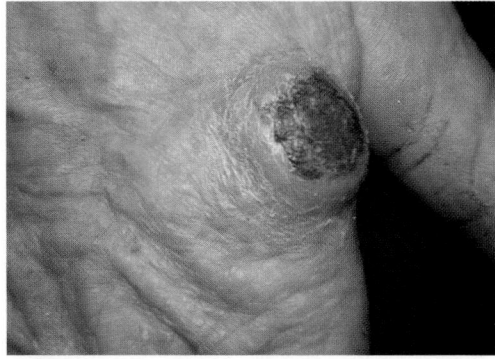

D, Keratoacanthoma. Large nodular lesion with central keratotic crater.

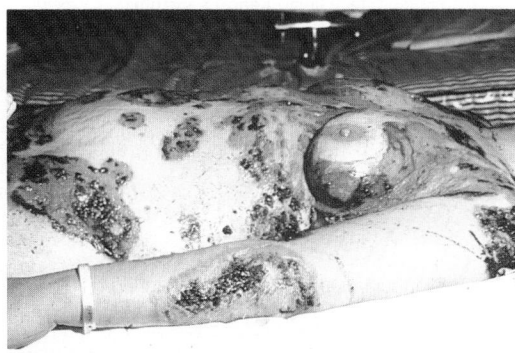

E, Pemphigus vulgaris. Intraepidermal bullae are easily ruptured, leaving superficial crusted erosions with thin shreds of blister roof along the edges. Careful examination reveals some intact blisters (primary lesions) below the breast.

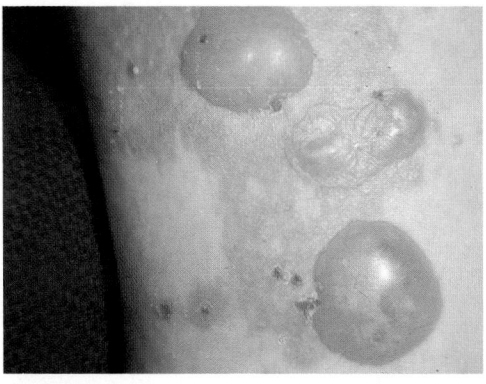

F, Bullous pemphigoid. Tense subepidermal bullae on an erythematous base.

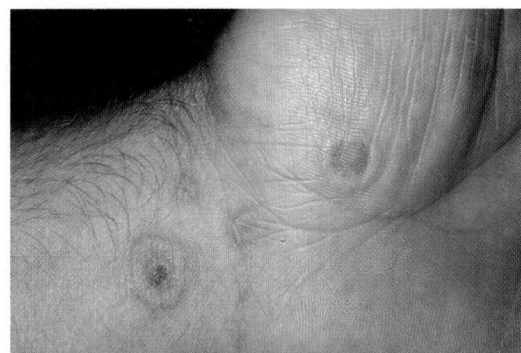

G, Erythema multiforme. Target or "bull's-eye" annular lesions with central vesicles and bullae.

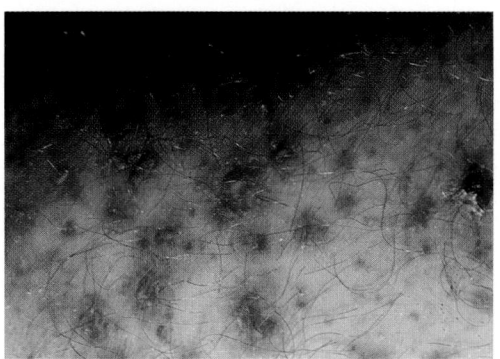

H, Palpable purpura. Leukocytoclastic vasculitis commonly causes raised purpuric and ulcerated lesions on legs.

PLATE 16 SKIN DISEASES

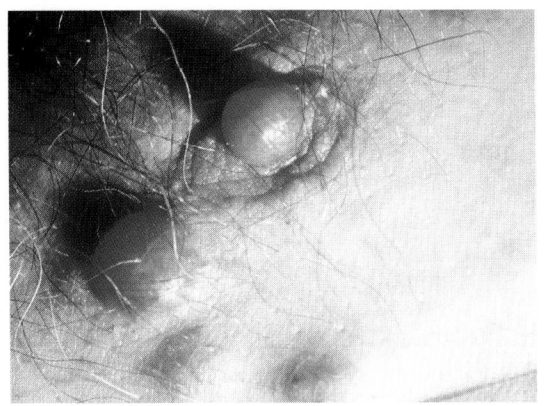

A, Skin metastases. Firm, hard, red nodules.

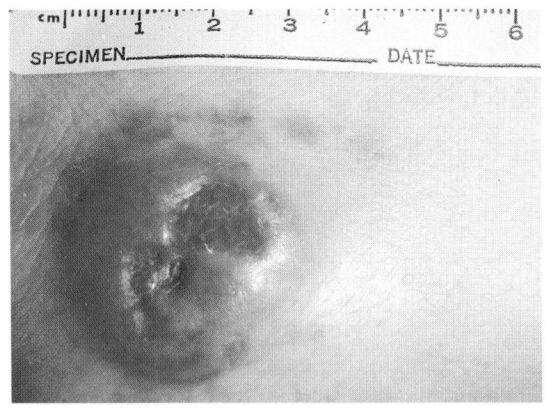

B, Mycosis fungoides, tumor stage.

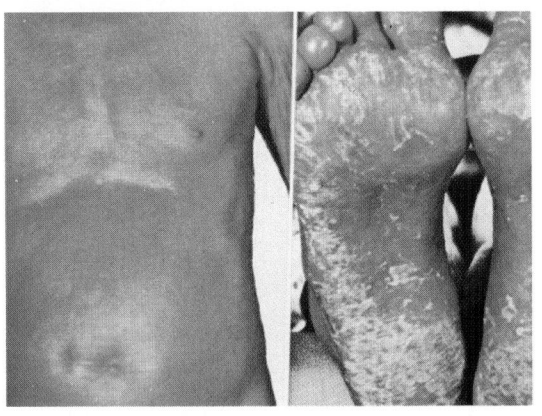

C, Sézary syndrome, exfoliative dermatitis stage.

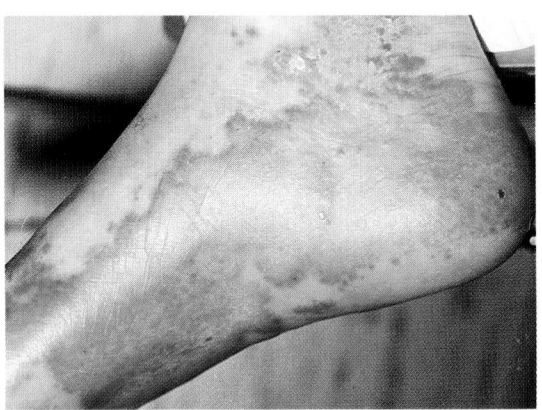

D, Classic Kaposi's sarcoma.

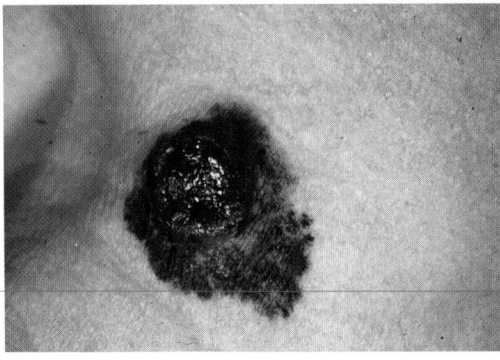

E, Malignant melanoma. Darkly pigmented, nodular lesion with irregular outline, irregular shades of dark pigmentation, and irregular surface configuration.

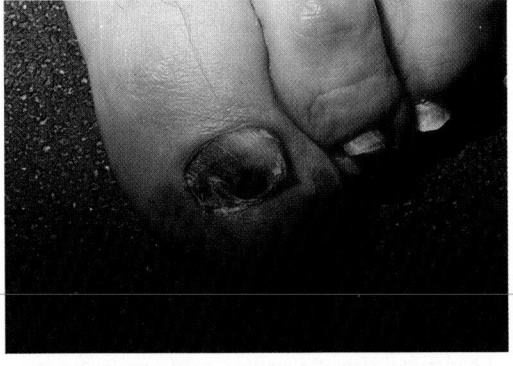

F, Subungual melanoma. Dark blue-black pigment within nail bed, with irregular dark pigment on the tip of the great toe.

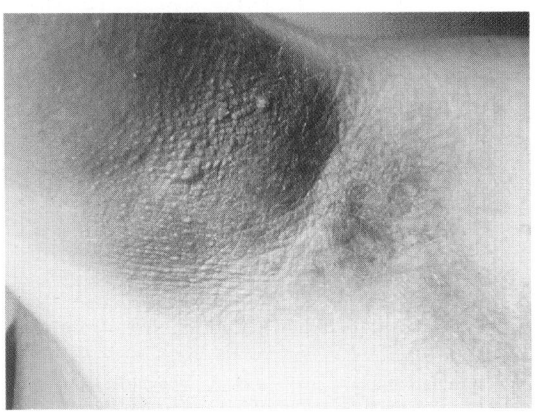

G, Acanthosis nigricans. Axillary lesion.

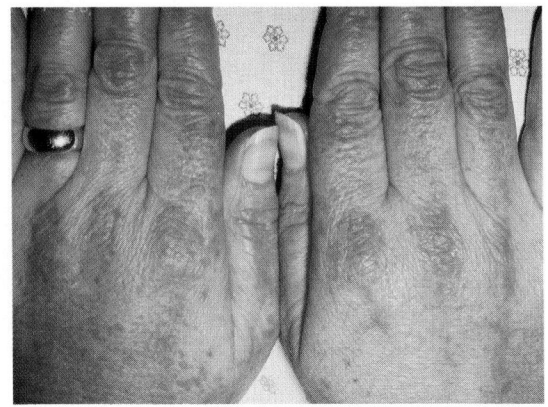

H, Dermatomyositis. Gottron's papules over the knuckles.

PLATE 17 SKIN DISEASES

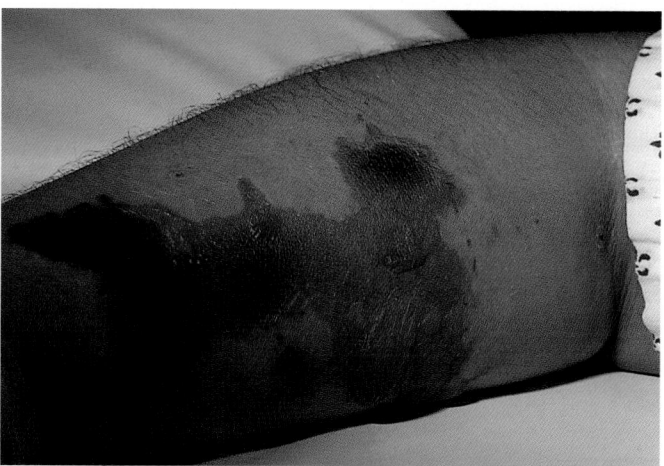

A, Macule—flat circumscribed color change. This is a purpuric area of skin in a patient with purpura fulminans.

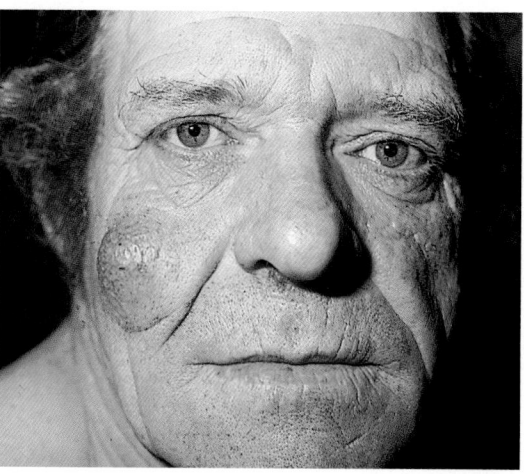

B, Cyst—large semisolid sac. An infundibular cyst on the right cheek. Note that this is a smooth, round, nodular lesion.

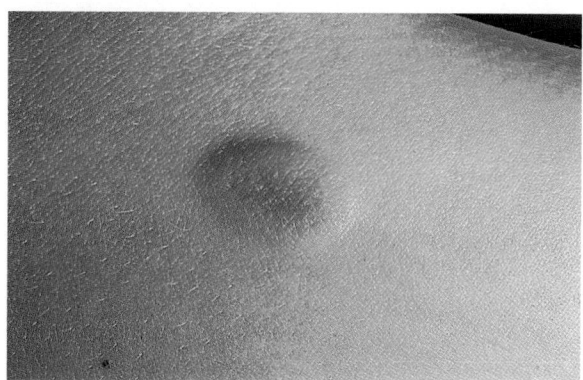

C, Papule—a solid elevation of 1 cm or less. This is a papule of granuloma annulare.

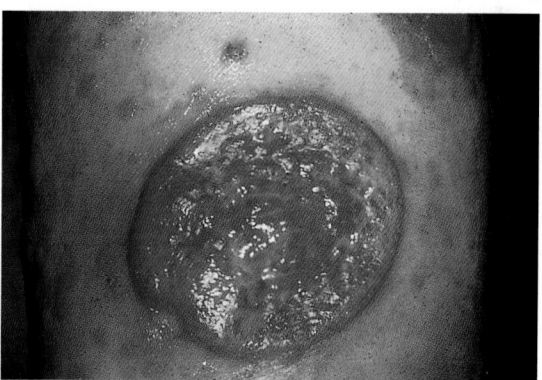

D, Plaque—a raised, circumscribed, flat-topped lesion. A typical mycosis fungoides–eroded plaque.

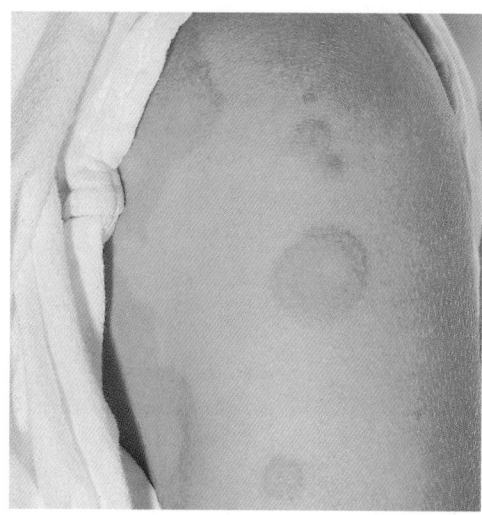

E, Wheal—erythematous edematous plaque that is evanescent. This is a urticarial lesion due to penicillin.

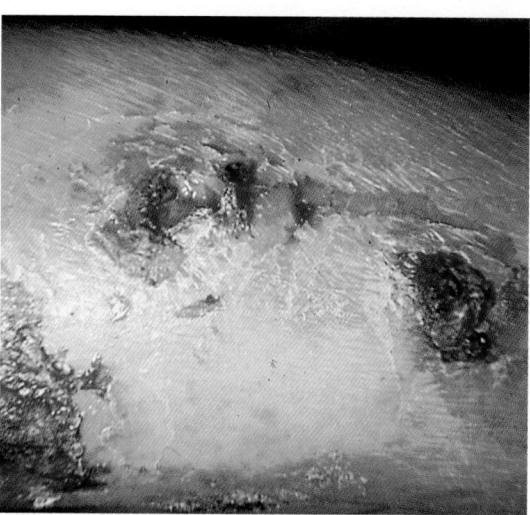

F, Erosion—superficial denudation of epidermis. Ecthyma—a superficial staphylococcal infection.

PLATE 18　SKIN DISEASES

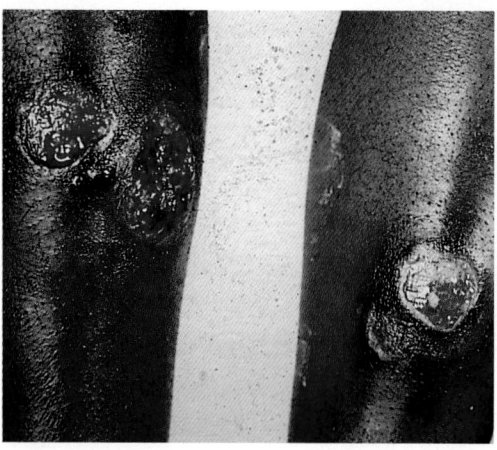

A, Ulcer—deep defect in the skin extending to the dermis. These ulcers are secondary to ischemia due to sickle cell anemia.

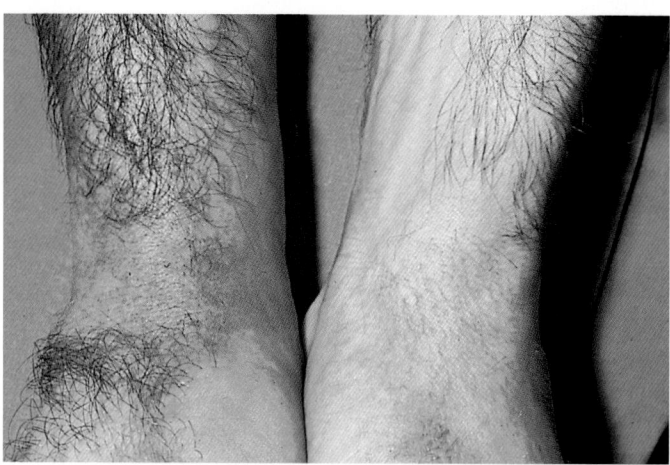

B, Atrophy—loss of epidermal or dermal substance with thinning of skin. Here the atrophy is due to scleroderma. Note loss of hair follicles and shiny atrophic areas of skin.

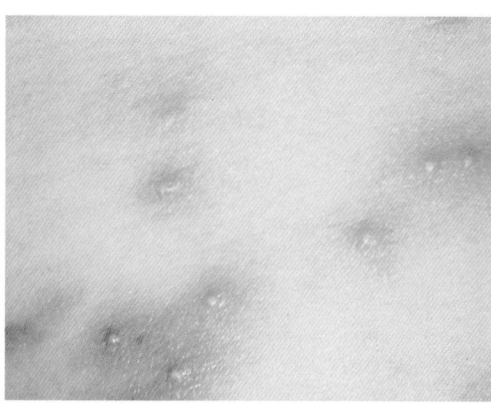

C, Pustule—fluid-filled sac filled with neutrophils. This patient had hot tub dermatitis due to *Pseudomonas* infection.

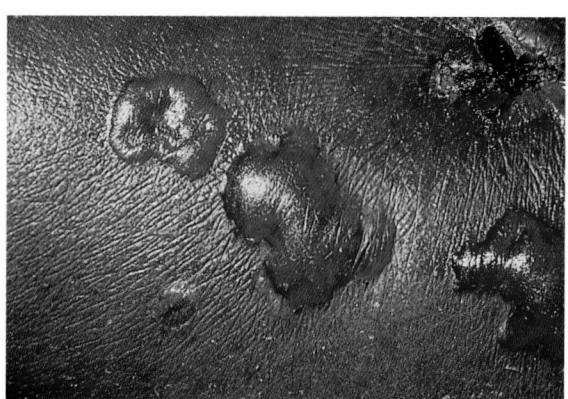

D, Bullae—fluid-filled lesions 0.5 cm or larger—bullous impetigo.

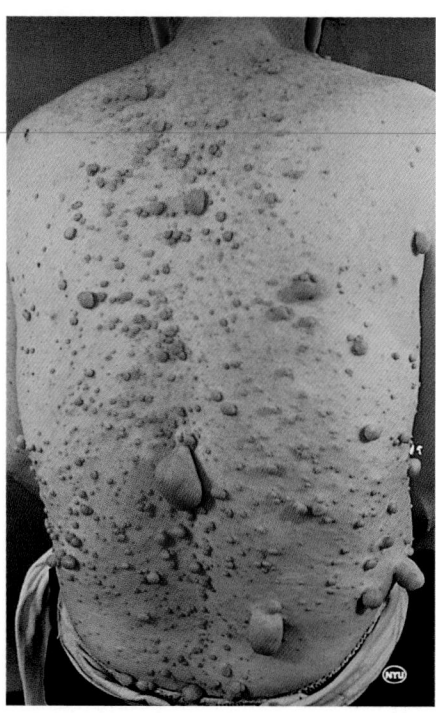

F, Scar—an area of replacement fibrosis of the dermis or subcutaneous tissue. These scars are healed diabetic ulcers.

E, Nodules—solid, large (>1 cm) deep-seated mass in dermal or subcutaneous tissues. These nodules are neurofibromas in a patient with neurofibromatosis.

PLATE 19 SKIN DISEASES

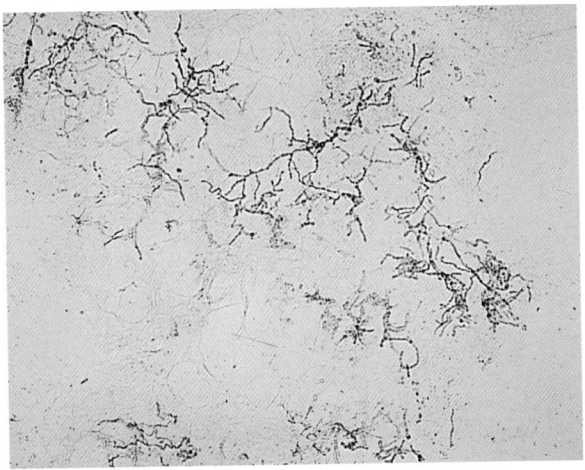

A, Tzanck smear of herpes simplex. Positive Tzanck smear is seen as multinucleated giant cell.

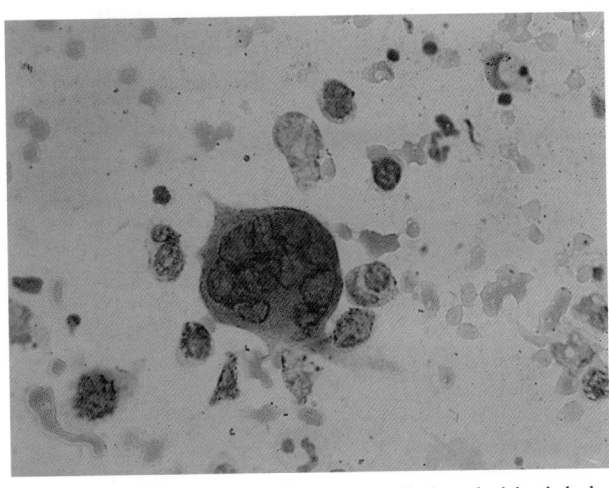

B, KOH preparation. Fungi appear as refractile branched hyphal elements after skin stratum corneum scrapings are incubated with 20% KOH for several minutes.

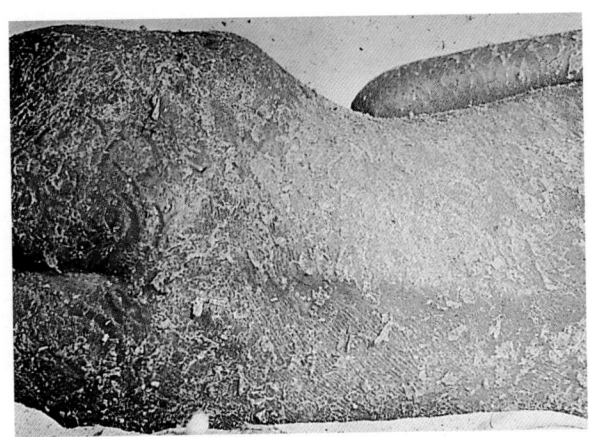

C, Exfoliative erythroderma. Diffuse inflammatory reaction of the entire skin with thickening, lichenification, redness, and scaling.

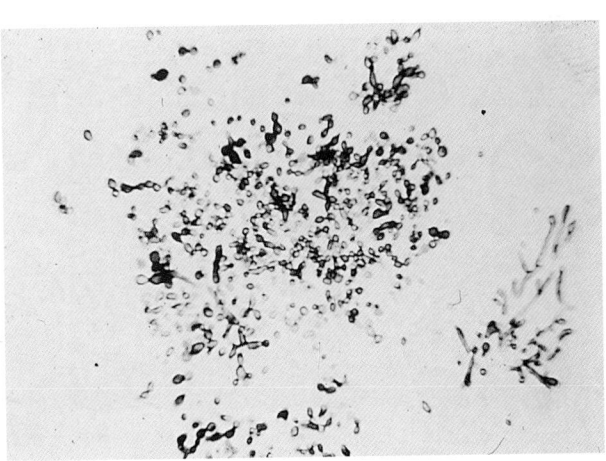

D, Candida albicans. KOH examination of candidal skin lesion. Short, stubby hyphae and budding yeast elements.

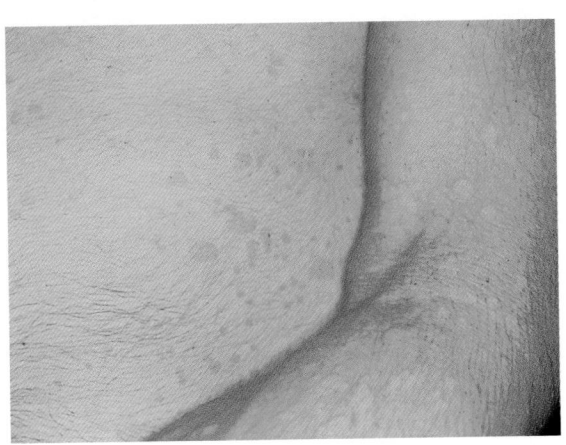

E, Tinea versicolor. Discrete areas of red-brown scaling lesions on the trunk.

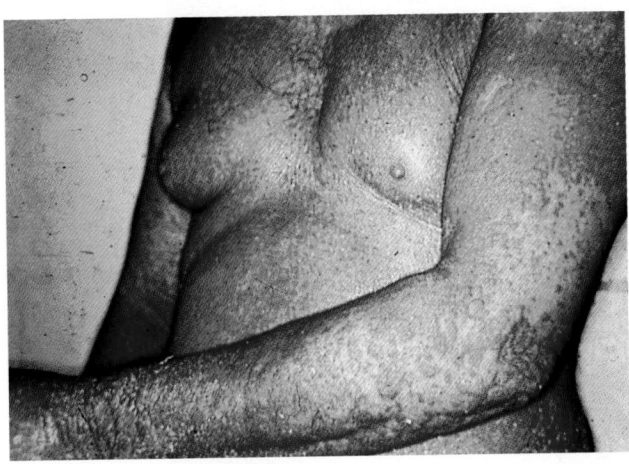

F, Drug eruption. Macular erythematous and somewhat scaling diffuse eruption. Penicillin drug rash.

PLATE 20   SKIN DISEASES

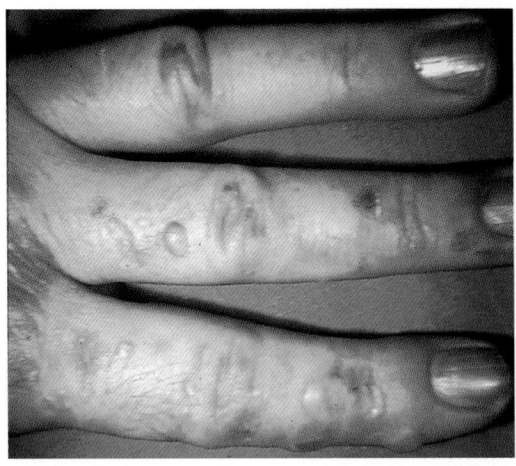

A, Porphyria cutanea tarda. Vesicular eroded and crusted lesions that leave scars. Lesions are precipitated by exposure to sun and trauma to the skin.

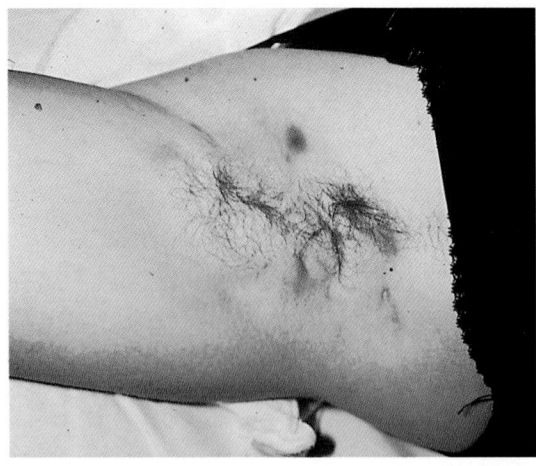

B, Hidradenitis suppurativa. Tender cystlike abscess in the axilla with retracted scars and sinus tracts.

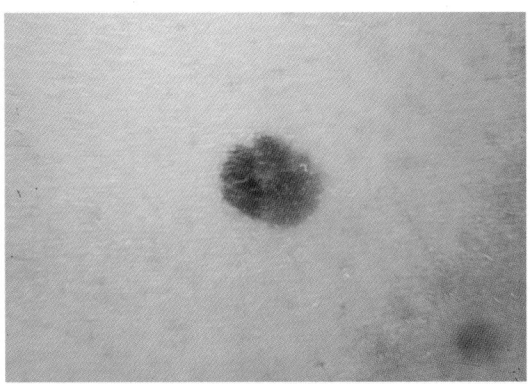

C, Junctional nevus. Uniformly pigmented, flat lesion. Note sharply demarcated borders and symmetry of the lesion.

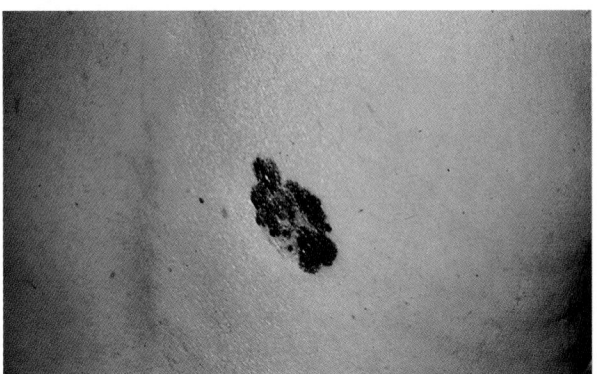

D, Superficial spreading melanoma. A darkly pigmented lesion with irregular outline and considerable scalloping of the borders and asymmetry.

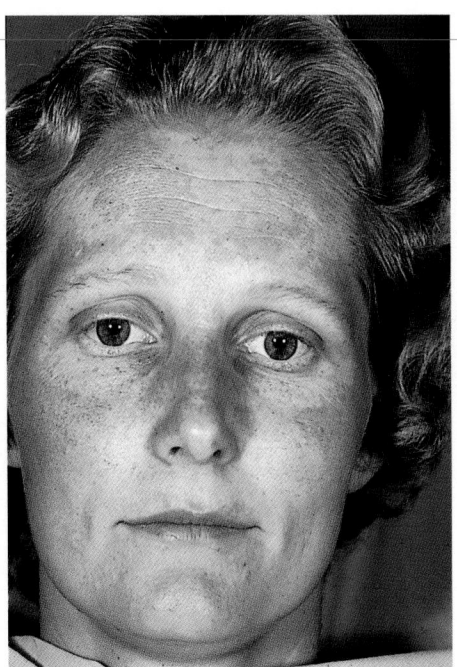

F, Tuberous sclerosis. Characteristic area of depigmentation with ash leaf configuration, on leg.

E, Melasma. Light brown hyperpigmentation of the cheeks and forehead.

liculitis, furuncles, or cellulitis) often results in marked improvement in the eczema.

Atopic individuals are often tense, resentful, aggressive, and restless, but whether this accompanies the diathesis or merely results from living with chronic, unremitting itching and skin inflammation is not certain. Either way, the physician must help the patient meet the stresses of life.

Keratoconjunctivitis and stellate anterior subcapsular cataracts are associated with atopic eczema, particularly in patients with extensive skin changes. The conjunctivitis and keratitis usually start in childhood. The cataracts may also begin at a young age and form rapidly, often by age 20. Keratoconus is seen in 25% of atopics.

The treatment of atopic dermatitis is the same as for other eczematous eruptions and includes topical steroids, emollients, and systemic antihistamines. In some children (less than 2 years of age) food allergy can cause atopic dermatitis, but dietary factors remain controversial. Skin tests or RAST tests help identify which foods may be responsible. Positive results must be confirmed with controlled food challenges and elimination diets. Allergic immediate skin testing and desensitization have been of little value.

Skin irritation must be avoided by wearing soft cotton clothing. Counseling, psychotherapy, and stress reduction sometimes help. Patients often worsen during the autumn and winter seasons when central heating and a dry environment dramatically decrease humidity. The frequent use of emollients is the best treatment for skin dryness, especially immediately after bathing when the skin is hydrated. Topical corticosteroids are the most important means of controlling the inflammatory response, and the least potent forms should be used, usually in an ointment base. Systemic steroids should be used only in short courses to overcome exacerbations not controlled by topical steroids.

STASIS DERMATITIS. This is an eczematous eruption of the lower legs secondary to peripheral venous insufficiency. Venous incompetence causes increased hydrostatic pressure and capillary damage with extravasation of red blood cells and serum. These conditions trigger an inflammatory, brawny, edematous, red, and hyperpigmented petechial scaling or weeping reaction, usually around the medial malleolus or distal one third of the lower leg. Secondary allergic contact dermatitis frequently complicates the problem when neomycin is used chronically to treat accompanying stasis ulcers. Management consists of preventing venous stasis and edema with supportive hose while the patient is ambulatory. Weight reduction helps obese patients. The eczema is treated with topical steroids and wet compresses when oozing and crusting are present. Occasionally chronic stasis dermatitis, when secondarily infected, can undergo exacerbation with spread of the acute inflammation to distant areas of the body, a condition known as *autosensitization dermatitis*. These secondary eczematous patches evolve on the face, neck, and extensor areas of the extremities. Topical steroids (occasionally oral ones for severe reactions) control the reactions; antibiotics may be needed to halt cutaneous infection.

NUMMULAR ECZEMATOUS DERMATITIS. This condition is defined by recurrent, coin-shaped patches predominantly on the extensor surfaces of the arms and legs, less often the trunk. Minute patches of vesicles and papules spread to become scaling and thickened, occasionally clearing in the center so that they may resemble superficial fungal infections. Mild to severe pruritus accompanies the patches. Although the cause is unknown, many factors acting alone or in combination may contribute. Dry skin is frequent, and the disease reaches a peak in winter months. Irritating substances such as wool, soap, and frequent bathing may contribute. The combination of topical steroids (usually of intermediate potency), 3% crude coal tar, and ultraviolet light treatments helps to control the persistent eczema.

LICHEN SIMPLEX CHRONICUS. Also known as neurodermatitis, this is a chronic, pruritic, lichenified eczematous eruption that results from constant scratching. Pruritus often precedes the scratching, and rubbing induces lichenification, initiating a vicious circle. In most patients it is a nervous habit. Patches of neurodermatitis commonly affect the nape of the neck, lower legs, groin, or other regions within easy reach of the hands. Occasionally constant scratching results in scaling, thickened, excoriated papules and nodules. Treatment consists of explaining the cause and the need to stop rubbing. Topical steroids and oral antihistamines may be helpful. Steroids injected into the lesion break the itching cycle more successfully than topical oils.

SEBORRHEIC DERMATITIS. Seborrheic dermatitis is characterized by erythematous, eczematous patches with yellow, greasy scales localized to hairy areas and regions of the skin with high concentrations of sebaceous glands, especially the middle of the face, nasolabial folds, eyebrows, ear canals, retroauricular folds, and presternal areas. Dandruff is scaling of the scalp without inflammation. Severe cases can involve the axillae and groin regions. Seborrheic dermatitis may appear in infants until about 6 months of age ("cradle cap"); after that it disappears until after puberty. Patients with neurologic disorders, such as Parkinson's disease or stroke, may have a dramatic flare of their seborrhea. Although the cause of seborrhea is unknown, the associations with emotional stress and neurologic disease suggest a central nervous system influence. Some studies suggest that the condition is related to excessive growth of yeast organisms *(Pityrosporum)* on the skin. It is sometimes difficult to differentiate seborrhea from psoriasis when the latter is localized to the scalp, ears, and face.

Antiseborrheic shampoos containing tar, sulfur, salicylic acid, selenium sulfide, or zinc pyrithione provide the most useful treatment. The shampoo should be used daily, rubbed into the scalp and left on for 5 minutes before rinsing. Inflammatory seborrhea that does not respond to shampoos alone may benefit from a topical steroid lotion or gel in hairy areas and hydrocortisone cream for facial glabrous skin. Continual use of shampoo and topical steroids is required for control. The use of topical or oral antiyeast medication, ketoconizole, helps in some patients.

XEROTIC ECZEMA AND ECZEMA CRAQUELE. These conditions are characterized by chapping and symptomatic dryness that may lead to visible fissuring through the stratum corneum, giving criss-crossing cracks that resemble dried mud. Such changes occur most commonly in winter, and they respond to emollients and/or hydrocortisone ointments.

HAND ECZEMA. Hand eczema is most common in housewives, cooks, food handlers, and medical personnel. The most common precipitators are constant exposure to mild primary irritants (soap, water), frequent hand washing, atopy, and nummular dermatitis. Allergic contact dermatitis may be another cause. *Dyshidrotic eczema* (pompholyx), a relatively noninflammatory, recurrent, pruritic, vesicular eruption of the palms and soles of unknown cause, differs from other hand eczemas in that the primary involvement is on the palm instead of the dorsum of the hands. The term *dyshidrotic eczema* suggests malfunction of the sweat ducts, but this is a misnomer. Pompholyx, from the Greek meaning bubble, is a more apt term. Emotional stress tends to be a trigger. Vesicles on the palms can also represent *dermatophytid*, an allergic reaction to a dermatophyte infection on the feet. If potassium hydroxide (KOH) examination of the feet is positive, treatment of the fungus clears up the palmar reaction as well.

Treatment of hand dermatitis involves avoidance of primary irritants such as soap, solvents, detergents, and frequent exposure to water. The use of cotton gloves with rubber gloves over them is useful in protecting the hands in water. Topical steroids and emollients may help, but topical steroids are often required.

EXFOLIATIVE DERMATITIS (ERYTHRODERMA). Total body cutaneous erythema, edema, scaling, and fissuring may occur as an idiopathic entity without preceding dermatologic or systemic disease, or it may result from a variety of cutaneous (atopic or contact dermatitis, psoriasis, seborrheic dermatitis, autosensitization, pityriasis rubra pilaris) or systemic disorders (mycosis fungoides, lymphomas, leukemias) as well as a reaction to drugs (antibiotics, barbiturates, antiepileptic agents, gold). Other organ systems are affected by the general erythroderma and changes in the stratum corneum barrier function. The diffuse redness and warmth of the skin reflect vasodilation and increased blood flow through the immense cutaneous vasculature. Five to 8% of the total cardiac output may be directed to the dilated, inflamed, cutaneous vasculature. In older individuals with underlying cardiac disease, high output heart failure may ensue. Also increased heat loss may lead to decreased core temperature, shivering, and swings in temperature. Oral steroids decrease the cutaneous inflammation and correct the abnormalities. In less acute situations total body applications of topical steroids with plastic sauna suit occlusion reverse the erythroderma.

FUNGAL INFECTIONS OF THE SKIN. Fungal infections may be confused with eczema. These infections include dermatophytosis, candidiasis, and tinea versicolor. *Dermatophytes* are a homogeneous group of fungi that live on the keratin of the stratum corneum, nails, and hair and frequently provoke a cutaneous inflammatory reaction with pruritus, redness, scaling, and vesiculation. Three genera of dermatophytes cause these infections: *Trichophyton, Microsporum,* and *Epidermophyton.* Dermatophytosis of the trunk (tinea corporis) can be caused by several species (*T. rubrum* and *T. mentagrophytes* are most common), resulting in annular inflamed patches with elevated scaling and, at times, vesicular borders with a tendency for central clearing. The eruption may be widespread and may mimic nummular eczema. Extensive, red, scaling lesions with elevated serpiginous borders may occur in diabetic and immunosuppressed patients. Ringworm of the scalp appears as scaling areas of hair loss with black dots indicating breakage of hair shafts. Most infections are now due to *T. tonsurans* or *M. canis.* The latter agent may fluoresce under Wood's light, but this should not be used for diagnosis. Rather, examination with KOH preparations and cultures for fungi should be performed (using plucked hairs and scales from the affected areas). Tinea cruris infection in the groin appears as red patches with elevated serpiginous and scaling borders. The scrotum is seldom involved. Erythrasma is still another type of intertriginous erythema caused by a *Corynebacterium* infection. It appears as velvety red patches with fine scale which, under Wood's light, fluoresce a diagnostic coral pink color. Erythromycin clears the infection. Tinea of the feet (pedis) and hands (manum) often present together. Infections of the feet appear in three forms: (1) interdigital maceration, scaling, and fissuring; (2) diffuse, dry, scaling and mild erythema of the plantar surface, often extending onto the sides of the feet in a "moccasin" distribution, occasionally associated with dry scaling of one palm; (3) vesiculopustular lesions on the insteps of the feet. Involvement of the nails—onychomycosis—often accompanies hand and foot dermatophytosis.

Candidiasis, particularly involvement by *C. albicans,* causes inflammatory skin reactions. Intertriginous moniliasis occurs in the groin, perineum, gluteal folds, inframammary areas, axillae, and digital webs. Typically, the folds become macerated and erythematous with small satellite papules and erosions around the periphery of the main lesion. Obesity, diabetes, and use of antibiotics may play a role in *Candida* infection. Chronic mucocutaneous candidiasis is a rare condition characterized by superficial *Candida* infection of the skin, nails, and oral and genital mucosal surfaces complicating a variety of systemic immunodeficiencies (see Ch. 354). *Tinea versicolor,* a common superficial fungus infection caused by *Pityrosporon orbiculare,* is identified by scaling, red to brown or white, oval patches over the neck, trunk, and upper arms. As the name versicolor implies, the lesions vary in color. During the summer months when the skin is exposed to ultraviolet light, the lesions appear hypopigmented, as the infection prevents the involved skin from forming pigment. Examination of the lesion with KOH reveals budding yeast forms and club-shaped hyphae.

Either topical or systemic agents can treat fungal infections of the skin. If the dermatophytic or candidal glabrous skin infection is localized, econazole, miconazole, clotrimazole, and ciclopirox creams, ointments, and lotions are effective when applied two to three times a day for 3 to 4 weeks. Tinea versicolor also responds to these agents, but selenium sulfide antidandruff shampoo is less expensive and also effective. Application of the shampoo to the involved areas of skin for 10 minutes each night for 3 to 4 weeks clears the disease, although the hypopigmentation does not resolve until the patient is exposed to the sun. Regular shampooing with selenium sulfide reduces reinfection rates. Widespread fungal lesions, or those resistant to topical therapy, may require systemic agents. Griseofulvin is an effective, safe agent and the treatment of choice for dermatophyte infections, but it is not effective for *Candida.* The drug must be given for varying periods of time, depending on the site of infection. The micronized form (Ultrafine, U/F) seems to be most consistently effective. Approximately 10 mg per kilogram per day is used in children and 1 gram per day in adults.

Ketoconazole is a second oral medication useful for dermatophytes, but it is also effective in *Candida* infections. Because ketoconazole occasionally causes severe liver damage, it should not be used initially for dermatophyte infections. It is useful in mucocutaneous candidiasis at a dose of 200 to 400 mg per day in adults. Because of its toxicity, liver function tests should be performed every 2 to 4 weeks.

MACULOPAPULAR SKIN DISEASES

The rashes included in this group represent diverse cutaneous and systemic conditions characterized by widespread erythematous macules and papules. Some of the conditions also have associated petechiae or purpura.

VIRAL EXANTHEMS. Because many *viral exanthems* are maculopapular, this group of skin diseases is often termed morbilliform, or measles-like. The clinical appearance of virus-induced erythema is not specific for a given etiologic agent; other signs and symptoms help to suggest a particular viral agent. Most viral exanthems are preceded by a prodrome of fever and constitutional symptoms. A history of previous exposure to infected individuals should be obtained. Incubation times vary from days to weeks depending on the virus. Drug history may also be important, especially with infectious mononucleosis, in which only 3% of patients have a maculopapular or petechial eruption, but with the administration of ampicillin the frequency approaches 100%. In measles (rubeola) and rubella, the erythematous macules and papules begin on the face and spread to the trunk and extremities, fading with desquamation in 6 days in rubeola and on the third day in rubella. The rashes associated with enterovirus infection are most commonly rubella-like but occasionally are purpuric. Exanthem subitum (roseola infantum) displays fleeting, discrete, red papules surrounded by a whitish halo that begins on the trunk and then evolves on the neck. Erythema infectiosum (fifth disease) is an alarming appearing red, "slapped cheek" rash over the face with reticulate maculopapular lesions on the extremities that clear in 3 to 6 days. Mucous membranes are sometimes involved. In rubella, red spots occur on the soft palate. In measles, Koplik's spots, tiny gray-white papules on an erythematous base, are found on the buccal mucosa opposite the molars. An erythematous, maculopapular rash that begins peripherally on the palms and soles and spreads to the trunk, often with a petechial component, is seen in *atypical measles.* This is a hypersensitivity reaction to wild measles virus in a partially immune, vaccinated host.

Verruca vulgaris and *molluscum contagiosum* are two examples of viral infections confined to the skin which elicit unique papular lesions. Wart papilloma virus induces various forms of warts: *common warts,* dome-shaped papules with corrugated, hyperkeratotic surfaces; *flat warts,* slightly raised, smooth, flat-topped papules often on the hands and face; *plantar warts,* painful papules on the soles of the feet covered by a thick callus with black puncta within the lesion; *condylomata acuminata,* or venereal warts, soft, moist, sessile, pedunculated and verrucous papules involving the perianal and genital areas. *Molluscum contagiosum* is caused by a DNA poxvirus that infects epidermal cells to induce smooth, dome-shaped, translucent papules with a central umbilication from which a cheesy core can be expressed. These lesions occur most commonly on the trunk, face, and genitals. The treatment of warts relies on a variety of nonspecific destructive techniques, including liquid nitrogen cryotherapy, salicylic and lactic acid combinations, cantharidin, and podophyllin. Molluscum contagiosum lesions are removed by curettage of the central core, liquid nitrogen freezing, or cantharidin application for short periods of time (30 to 60 minutes).

SCARLETINIFORM ERUPTIONS. Scarlet fever, *Kawasaki's syndrome,* and *toxic shock syndrome* also present with erythematous macular and papular eruptions. Group A streptococcal pharyngitis or tonsillitis with a strain producing erythrogenic toxin initiates a confluent, papular eruption with sandpaper texture that begins on the neck and upper chest and evolves over the abdomen and extremities. The face is flushed, and circumoral pallor is prominent. Extensive desquamation occurs in 4 to 5 days. Punctate redness of the palate and strawberry tongue coexist.

Kawasaki's syndrome, a condition of unknown cause, displays a morbilliform or scarletiniform eruption more prominent on the trunk than the face. Most distinctive are magenta red discolorations of the palms and soles associated with indurative edema of the hands and feet. The skin and extremity changes occur within 3 to 4 days of the onset of fever, along with mucous membrane inflammatory changes consisting of conjunctivitis and strawberry tongue. Palm, sole, and finger tip desquamation occurs 10 to 18 days after the onset of fever. Asymmetric lymphadenopathy, especially in the cervical area, is seen in 75% of patients—hence the name *mucocu-*

Toxic shock syndrome is a serious condition arising from toxins elaborated by *Staphylococcus aureus* infections, often in menstruating women using tampons but also in patients with postsurgical infections. The rash is an erythematous, macular, diffuse eruption that blanches readily with pressure followed by desquamation of the affected skin, in association with fever, strawberry tongue, hypotension, vomiting, and renal insufficiency. The rash often spares the skin where clothing fits tightly with pressure on the skin, e.g., waistline where underwear elastic and belt press tightly.

DRUG REACTIONS. Drug reactions can cause reactions that mimic nearly all forms of skin conditions. The most common eruptions, however, are hives and morbilliform rashes. The erythematous macules and papules that often become confluent usually begin within a week of initiating the drug. Unfortunately, no laboratory tests can identify a responsible drug, so reliance must be placed on the history. Often patients are taking several drugs. In trying to select the offending medication from the list, variables to consider are the temporal relationship between the initiation of the drug and the rash and the odds that a given drug is likely to cause an eruption. Drugs most likely to cause maculopapular eruptions include trimethoprim-sulfamethoxazole, penicillin G, semisynthetic penicillins, ampicillin, quinidine, gentamicin sulfate, and blood products. Itching is common with drug reactions, and fever may occur. It is difficult to differentiate the maculopapular drug rash from viral exanthems except that viral prodromata and viral mucous membrane lesions are lacking in drug rashes.

The mechanisms of most cutaneous drug reactions are not understood. Only 10% of drug reactions have a clearly identified immunologic basis. Specific mechanisms of immunologically mediated drug reaction can be due to immediate hypersensitivity (IgE or type I–mediated), cytotoxic antibody reactions (type II), circulating immune complexes (type III), and even type IV delayed hypersensitivity. The mechanisms of nonimmunologically mediated drug reactions include toxic overdose, idiosyncratic responses, drug interactions, and pharmacologic side effects.

Most cutaneous drug reactions remit within 2 to 3 weeks after the drug is stopped. Symptomatic therapy includes antihistamines, occasionally systemic steroids, and application of topical steroids.

PURPURIC MACULOPAPULAR SKIN LESIONS. These should cause the physician to consider a different group of conditions. Purpura, because it represents extravasation of red blood cells outside the cutaneous vessels, cannot be blanched as erythema can. Purpura can be classified as nonpalpable (macular) and palpable (papular). Nonpalpable purpura results from bleeding into the skin without associated inflammation of the vessels and indicates either a bleeding diathesis or blood vessel fragility. Nonpalpable purpura can be *petechial* (macules < 3 mm) or *ecchymotic* (macules > 3 mm). Thrombocytopenia causes petechiae, whereas abnormalities in the blood-clotting cascade commonly cause ecchymoses. Necrotic ecchymoses are found when thrombi form in dermal vessels, leading to infarction and hemorrhage as in disseminated intravascular

coagulation (DIC). Palpable purpura results from inflammatory damage to cutaneous blood vessels, the inflammation causing elevated lesions as in vasculitis.

Nonpalpable Purpuras. Nonpalpable purpuras include thrombocytopenic conditions, senile or actinic purpura, blood clotting abnormalities, Schamberg's disease, hypergammaglobulinemic conditions, and disseminated intravascular coagulation. *Actinic (senile) purpura* is a common problem in older individuals, the result of increased vessel fragility reflecting dermal connective tissue damage from chronic sun exposure and aging. Minor trauma induces ecchymoses, usually on the dorsum of the hands and forearms. The skin in these areas is thin and fragile. Topically or systemically administered steroids can induce similar purpura. Other causes of vascular fragility of the skin include *amyloidosis* and the *Ehlers-Danlos syndrome. Schamberg's disease,* or *pigmented purpuric dermatitis,* is an idiopathic capillaritis that causes petechial lesions of the lower legs (occasionally the arms and trunk) in association with hyperpigmentation. The lesions have the appearance of cayenne pepper. Occasionally Schamberg's disease is secondary to a drug reaction. Petechiae and purpura also occur in *hypergammaglobulinemic purpura,* a syndrome characterized by episodes of fever and arthralgias which appear to be the result of immune complex–mediated damage to small blood vessels. *Disseminated intravascular coagulation* (DIC) refers to uncontrolled clotting within blood vessels with the formation of diffuse thrombosis. The skin is frequently involved with hemorrhage, ecchymosis, and infarction. DIC occurs in association with bacterial sepsis (particularly meningococcemia), as a postviral or poststreptococcal infection phenomenon *(purpura fulminans),* or in conjunction with malignancies such as prostatic carcinoma and acute myelocytic leukemia. The most distinctive hemorrhagic skin lesions are stellate (star-shaped) purpuric ecchymoses with necrotic centers. The center of the lesion is dark gray, indicative of necrosis and impending slough. Petechiae are seen, and hemorrhagic bullae, acral cyanosis, mucosal bleeding, and prolonged bleeding from wound sites can occur. Patients may be systemically ill with fever, shock, and renal failure.

A variety of infectious diseases cause cutaneous petechiae, purpura, or ecchymoses. Already mentioned is *meningococcemia,* in which the organisms produce acute vasculitis or local Shwartzman-like reactions with erythematous macules, petechiae, purpura, and ecchymosis on the trunk and legs. These may become confluent, often with central necrosis. Patients with acute meningococcemia are ill with fever, malaise, headache, meningeal signs, and hypotension. The skin lesions of *disseminated gonococcemia* begin as tiny red papules and petechiae and then evolve into painful purpuric pustules and vesicles scattered on the distal extremities. Fever, polyarthritis, or monoarticular arthritis may be present. The rash of *Rocky Mountain spotted fever* appears between the second and sixth day of the illness, initially as small, erythematous macules that blanch on pressure but then evolving into petechiae, purpura, and ecchymoses. The rash first occurs on the acral areas and then spreads to the extremities and trunk. Small areas of necrosis may occur on the fingers, toes, and ear lobes. Fever, severe headache,

TABLE 475–2. TYPES OF VASCULITIS AND ASSOCIATED SKIN LESIONS

Type of Vasculitis	Blood Vessels Involved	Type of Skin Lesion
Leukocytoclastic or hypersensitivity angiitis: Henoch-Schönlein purpura, cryoglobulinemia, hypocomplementemic vasculitis	Dermal capillaries, venules, and occasional small muscular arteries in internal organs	Purpuric papules, hemorrhagic bullae, cutaneous infarcts
Rheumatic vasculitis: systemic lupus erythematosus; rheumatoid vasculitis	Dermal capillaries, venules, and small muscular arteries in internal organs	Purpuric papules; ulcerative nodules; splinter hemorrhages; periungual telangiectasia and infarcts
Granulomatous vasculitis Churg and Straus allergic granulomatous angiitis	Dermal small and larger muscular arteries and medium muscular arteries in subcutaneous tissue and other organs	Erythematous, purpuric, and ulcerated nodules, plaques, and purpura
Wegener's granulomatosis	Small venules, arterioles of dermis, and small muscular arteries	Ulcerative nodules; peripheral gangrene
Periarteritis: classic type limited to skin and muscle	Small and medium muscular arteries in deep dermis, subcutaneous tissue, and muscle	Deep subcutaneous nodules with ulceration; livedo reticularis; ecchymoses
Giant cell arteritis: temporal arteritis, polymyalgia rheumatica, Takayasu's disease	Medium muscular arteries and larger arteries	Skin necrosis over scalp

toxicity, confusion, and myalgias commonly occur. *Infective endocarditis* is associated with petechial and purpuric skin lesions. Petechiae appear in crops in the conjunctivae, buccal mucosa, upper chest, and extremities. Splinter hemorrhages (linear, red to brown streaks under the fingernails or toenails); Osler nodes (2- to 15-mm, tender, red nodules on the pads of the fingers and toes); and Janeway lesions (small, painless plaques and palpable, purpuric nodules on the palms or soles) may be seen. The skin lesions are related to immune complex vasculitis or septic emboli.

Palpable Purpuras. *Vasculitis* and *necrotizing angiitis* are terms used in disorders in which there is segmental inflammation in the blood vessel wall with accumulation of neutrophils and fibrinoid necrosis. The vascular reaction is mediated by immune complexes. Papules with purpura result from extravasation of blood from the damaged vessels. Although all sizes of blood vessels may be affected, the vasculitis in the skin involves venules. If the process is extensive or if large vessels are involved, skin necrosis and ulceration may occur. Depending upon the size of the blood vessels affected, at least five types of vasculitis may involve the skin. The size and type of vessels in the skin, in turn, determine the kind of morphologic lesion (Table 475–2).

In general, as the vasculitis involves progressively larger and more deeply situated vessels, the skin lesions become more nodular, with larger ulcerative or gangrenous processes. The term *granulomatous vasculitis* refers to angiitis associated with a histiocytic proliferation that also involves necrotizing granulomas in the connective tissue of multiple organs, causing rhinorrhea, sinusitis, cough, arthralgias, and ocular and neurologic symptoms (Churg-Strauss vasculitis).

Necrotizing leukocytoclastic vasculitis can occur in a variety of settings including (1) sepsis, (2) connective tissue disease—especially systemic lupus erythematosus and rheumatoid arthritis, (3) cryoglobulinemia, (4) drug reactions, and, occasionally (5) underlying carcinomas, lymphomas, or leukemias. In many instances no apparent cause is found.

Circulating immune complexes have been demonstrated in patients with necrotizing angiitis. Immunoglobulins and complement are found in the affected vessel wall by direct immunofluorescence. The immune complexes lodge in the small vessel walls and activate the complement system, forming the anaphylatoxins C3a and C5a, which recruit neutrophils that induce inflammatory and necrotic damage to the vessel with accompanying fragmented nuclei of the neutrophils (so-called nuclear dust).

Several syndromes are associated with leukocytoclastic vasculitis, depending on the organ systems affected. *Henoch-Schönlein syndrome* occurs most often in children, frequently preceded by an upper respiratory infection and accompanied by arthralgias, abdominal pain, and renal vasculitis. IgA is usually found along with complement in the involved vessels on direct immunofluorescence. *Hypocomplementemic vasculitis* is characterized by urticaria-like lesions, arthritis, and low serum complement. IgG and C3 are present in vessels taken from early skin lesions. Facial and laryngeal edema may also occur. A third form consists of purpura, arthralgia, weakness, and *mixed cryoglobulinemia* (mixed cryoglobulins contain IgG and IgM with anti-IgG or rheumatoid factor activity), which may be idiopathic or occasionally associated with systemic lupus erythematosus, infectious mononucleosis, lymphomas, or primary biliary cirrhosis.

If the vasculitis is idiopathic and cutaneous, the skin responds to prednisone (60 to 80 mg per day) or dapsone (100 to 150 mg per day). Systemic vasculitides may require prednisone and cyclophosphamide (2 mg per kilogram per day).

Necrotizing cutaneous vasculitis may occur in association with *hepatitis B* and in patients with *intestinal bypass surgery* for morbid obesity or in patients with jejunal diverticula or other gastrointestinal conditions characterized by bacterial overgrowth. An *arthritis-dermatitis syndrome* with intestinal bypass surgery may occur with polyarthritis and palpable purpura or purpuric nodules and pustules on the trunk, legs, feet, and arms. Antigenic components of the intestinal bacterial overgrowth lead to the formation of cryoprotein immune complexes that deposit in the skin and joints, causing a hypersensitivity vasculitis and nondeforming arthritis. Antibiotics such as chloramphenicol, sulfamethoxazole-trimethoprim, tetracycline, and metronidazole have been reported to improve the condition.

PAPULOSQUAMOUS SKIN DISEASES

Unique scales are the common characteristic of diseases in this group (Table 475–3). *Squamous* refers to scaling that represents thickened stratum corneum and thus implies an abnormal keratinization process. The lesions, in addition to being scaly, are characterized by sharply demarcated, red to violaceous papules and plaques that result from thickening of the epidermis and/or underlying dermal inflammation.

PSORIASIS. Psoriasis is a genetically determined, chronic epidermal proliferative disease of unpredictable course. Onset is most frequent in early adult life, but it may begin at any age. Once the disease becomes manifest, it may remain localized to a few areas or may cause intermittent or continuous generalized disease.

The lesions appear as erythematous papules and plaques surmounted by silvery, thick scales that resemble mica (micaceous) and that are easily removed and may accumulate in the patient's clothing or bed (Fig. 475–1). In intertriginous areas maceration pre-

TABLE 475–3. ADDITIONAL PAPULOSQUAMOUS SKIN DISEASES

Disease	Appearance of Lesion	Distribution	Mucous Membrane Involvement	Other Features
Secondary syphilis	Ham red or copper colored scaling papules and plaques, sometimes annular	Generalized: palms and soles often involved	Mucous patches, often white or red; condyloma warts of anal area	Condylomata in genital area; serologic test for syphilis positive
Pityriasis rubra pilaris	Red, scaling plaques and patches with follicular horny excretions, especially on dorsum of hands and fingers; diffuse, yellow hyperkeratoses of palms and soles	Often diffuse, rough scaling erythema involving entire body with islands of normal skin ("island sparing")	Occasionally lacy white plaques in mouth	Remits spontaneously in 2–4 years; nail changes as in psoriasis
Pityriasis lichenoides et varioliformis acuta (Mucha-Habermann disease)	Red, discrete, palpable papules that vesiculate and then become hemorrhagic, crust, scale, and leave a scar	Scattered lesions over trunk and extremities	May resemble leukocytoclastic vasculitis	May resolve in a few months or persist for years
Pityriasis lichenoides et varioliformis chronica (chronic parapsoriasis)	Guttate to larger, red slightly scaling papules and plaques; nonpruritic	Usually on trunk	Some forms may represent early stages of mycosis fungoides	Responds to UVB light treatments
Mycosis fungoides	Persistent, pruritic, red, thickened plaques with fine scales as seen in eczema, or thick mica-like scales suggestive of psoriasis; may ulcerate	Scattered asymmetrically over trunk, extremities; girdle area often first area involved	Neoplastic T-cell lymphoma	May show islands of normal skin within red areas

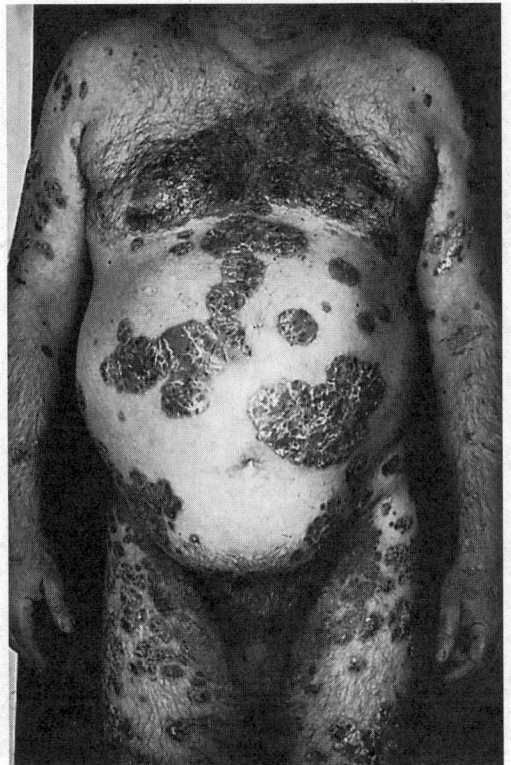

FIGURE 475-1. Psoriasis. (From the 17th edition of the Cecil Textbook of Medicine, with the permission of Dr. Marie-Louise Johnson.)

vents scales from accumulating, but the lesions remain red and sharply defined. Classically, lesions are distributed symmetrically over areas of bony prominence such as elbows and knees. They also commonly occur on the trunk and scalp and in the intergluteal cleft. These latter two areas are frequently overlooked. Palms and soles may be involved, with diffuse redness, scaling, and, at times, pustular lesions. Nail involvement occurs in up to 50% of patients. The nails may be pitted with small ice pick-like depressions on the surface of the nail plate. Onycholysis can also occur, in which a plaque of psoriasis in the distal nail bed causes a red-brown discoloration that is reminiscent of an oil stain under the nail. Another helpful diagnostic feature is the Koebner phenomenon, in which intense trauma to the skin induces new skin lesions. Thus, scratches or surgical incisions elicit linear papulosquamous lesions that should alert the physician to the diagnosis. This may also explain the high incidence of psoriasis on the elbows and knees. Other aggravating factors include streptococcal infections, emotional stress, overuse of alcohol, and drugs, including lithium and beta blockers. Several common variants of psoriasis may also be seen: (1) *guttate psoriasis,* in which numerous, small papular lesions with silvery scales evolve suddenly over the body, often 1 to 3 weeks following streptococcal pharyngitis; (2) *inverse psoriasis,* in which plaques evolve in intertriginous areas and thus lack the typical silver scale because of maceration and moisture; (3) *pustular psoriasis,* a form of the disease in which superficial pustules occur in one of three presentations—pustules studding typical plaques; pustules confined to the palms and soles; and a rare generalized eruption in which pustules evolve abruptly on large areas of erythematous skin accompanied by fever and leukocytosis; (4) *erythroderma*—occasionally the psoriasis can become generalized to involve erythema and scaling of the entire integument. This may occur secondary to a general Koebner phenomenon with overvigorous therapy, a drug reaction, or withdrawal of oral steroids; (5) *psoriatic arthritis*—arthritis may accompany psoriasis in 10 to 15% of cases.

At times Reiter's syndrome may be confused with psoriasis. The skin lesions of the two disorders are indistinguishable clinically and histologically. In Reiter's syndrome pustular and hyperkeratotic papules and plaques commonly occur on the palms and soles (keratoderma blenorrhagica) and scaling, red patches evolve encircling the glans penis and within the groin (balanitis circinata). The presence of asymptomatic erosions on the tongue and buccal mucosa,

urethritis, iritis or conjunctivitis, arthritis, and occasionally diarrhea should suggest the diagnosis.

The pathogenesis of psoriasis is unknown, but it appears to be a multifactorial disease in patients who are genetically predisposed. There is an increased prevalence of psoriasis in individuals with HLA antigens BW17, B13, and BW37. Thirty percent of patients have a family history of disease. The basic alteration represents an accelerated cell cycle in an increased number of dividing cells, culminating in rapid epidermal cell proliferation. Cellular turnover is increased seven-fold, and the transit time from the basal layer to the top of the stratum corneum is 3 or 4 days rather than the usual 28. This rapid turnover of keratinocytes alters keratinization, resulting in thickened epidermis (seen as papules and plaques) and parakeratotic stratum corneum (silvery scales). The mechanism underlying this benign proliferative reaction is unknown.

The goal of therapy is to decrease epidermal proliferation and underlying dermal inflammation. There is no curative agent for psoriasis, and treatment suppresses the condition only as long as it is administered. Three types of topical therapies are employed: (1) topical steroids, usually with intermediate and strong potency agents administered once or twice a day; (2) topical tars and anthralin preparations, often used once a day in combination with topical steroids; (3) ultraviolet light, either UVB with tar or UVA with oral psoralens (see Ch. 474). Recently a new medication, calcipotriene ointment (dovonex 0.005%), has been released for psoriasis treatment. This Vitamen D ointment restricts the hyperproliferative reaction. This topical preparation seems to be as effective as medium-potency topical steroids and so it has "steroid sparing effects" on the use of potent topical steroids. It is used twice a day and can irritate the skin, especially when used on the face and in body folds.

Two systemic types of therapy are available, but because of their side effects these should be reserved for severe widespread disease that is unresponsive to topical measures: (1) antimetabolites or antimitotic agents, including methotrexate, azathioprine, and hydroxyurea. The most commonly used is methotrexate in low doses, usually given on a weekly basis. Because these agents affect bone marrow and liver (in the case of methotrexate), complete blood counts and liver function tests should be performed regularly, together with intermittent liver biopsies. (2) Etretinate, a retinoid, is particularly useful in pustular and erythrodermic forms of psoriasis. Careful monitoring of blood counts, plasma triglycerides, and liver function is required, and avoidance of pregnancy during the use of this drug is mandatory. In fact, the drug should probably not be used in women of childbearing age.

PITYRIASIS ROSEA. Oval or round, tannish pink or salmon colored, scaling papules and plaques appear rapidly over the trunk, neck, upper arms, and legs (Fig. 475–2). Several features of this self-limited papulosquamous condition are unique. The generalized eruption is preceded by a single lesion, termed the "herald patch," that is commonly misdiagnosed as "ringworm." The patch can occur anywhere but often appears on the neck or lower trunk area and precedes the general rash by several days to a week. The oval

FIGURE 475–2. Pityriasis rosea. (From the 17th edition of the Cecil Textbook of Medicine, with the permission of Dr. Marie-Louise Johnson.)

patches have an unusual fine, white scale located near the border of the plaques, forming a collarette. The lesions follow skin cleavage lines, in a pattern likened to a Christmas tree. The condition spontaneously involutes in 1 to 2 months. Recurrences are rare. Itching can be prominent.

Pityriasis rosea occasionally is preceded by a mild upper respiratory infection, and its greatest incidence is in the winter months, suggesting a viral cause. However, the disease does not occur endemically and is not transmitted person to person.

Such conditions as tinea corporis and guttate psoriasis may be considered in the differential diagnosis, but two possibilities should always be entertained: drug eruption and secondary syphilis. If the rash persists longer than 2 or 3 months or generalizes to involve the trunk, extremities, and especially the face, a drug reaction should be considered. Such medications as gold compounds, barbiturates, captopril, clonidine, and tripelennamide can cause such a rash. Secondary syphilis should be suspected and a serologic test obtained if the rash involves palms and soles and if fever, coryza, or mucous membrane erosions (so-called mucous patches) are present.

Treatment of pityriasis rosea is usually not necessary, although topical corticosteroids and antihistamines may relieve itching and decrease erythema. Ultraviolet light (UVB), given as three to five treatments eliciting a mild erythema reaction, often clears the rash.

LICHEN PLANUS. This idiopathic, pruritic, inflammatory condition of the skin is included in the papulosquamous group of diseases because the primary lesion is a unique papule. The papules are flat topped (planus) and polygonal in configuration (i.e., the sides conform to normal fine skin folds) and have a lilac or purple hue. They may have visible scales on their surface, but more characteristic are subtle, fine white dots or white reticulated lines (Wickham's striae) surmounting the shiny, flat tops (resembling the appearance of a lichen). Wickham's striae are more visible under a hand lens after the application of a drop of mineral oil to the surface of the papule. The Koebner phenomenon occurs in lichen planus, so linear streaks of papules at the sites of skin trauma may be noted.

Although lichen planus can occur anywhere on the body, typical locations are the ankles, wrists, mouth, and genitalia. There may be only a few papules or innumerable ones in a generalized distribution. Mucous membranes are commonly involved, the lesions appearing most frequently as asymptomatic white streaks in a reticulated pattern on the buccal mucosa, tongue, gums, or lips. At times blisters and erosions are superimposed (erosive lichen planus), causing severe discomfort. Lichen planus involving the male genitalia may appear as violaceous annular lesions. Rarely, lichen planus may appear as violaceous annular and polycyclic lesions on the legs and arms, or as hyperkeratotic, follicular, scarring alopecia. All lichen planus lesions leave residual hyperpigmented macules in their wake.

The cause of lichen planus is not known, but two conditions may mimic lichen planus skin lesions and thus offer clues to an immune cause. Certain drugs such as thiazides, phenothiazines, gold, quinidine, and antimalarials can cause lichen planus-like, generalized eruptions. Also, some patients with graft-versus-host disease also develop a skin reaction that closely resembles lichen planus. The eruption can evolve into the usual chronic graft-versus-host sequelae of diffuse dermal sclerosis, cicatricial alopecia, reticulated pigmentation, and ulceration.

For other, mostly less frequent, papulosquamous skin diseases, see Table 475–3. Icthyoses are listed in Table 475–4 and illustrated in Figure 475–3.

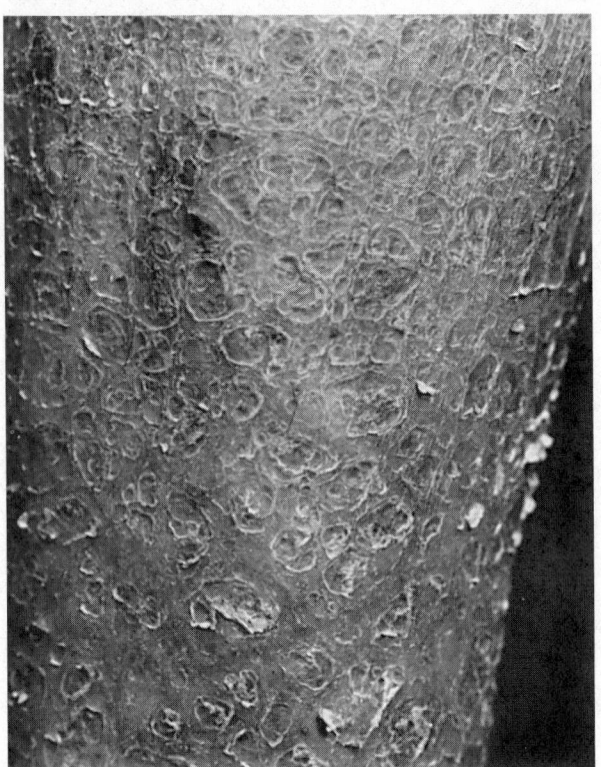

FIGURE 475–3. Ichthyosis. (From the 17th edition of the Cecil Textbook of Medicine, with the permission of Dr. Marie-Louise Johnson.)

VESICULOBULLOUS DISEASES

Vesicles and bullae, when intact, are readily recognized primary skin lesions. Crusts or superficial erosions are secondary lesions that lead one to suspect a preceding fluid-filled primary lesion. The cause of blistering disease includes bacterial and viral infections, contact dermatitis, and autoimmune and metabolic diseases. The pathogenesis of the blister formation is often helpful in understanding its anatomic location: Blisters occur either within the epidermis (intraepidermal) or at the dermoepidermal junction (subepidermal) (Table 475–5).

Intraepidermal vesicles or bullae usually contain clear fluid (but may become filled with purulent material secondarily) and have very thin roofs, so they are flaccid in appearance and are easily broken. At times the blisters are difficult to recognize, and only erosions, crusts, or the thin shreds of the epidermal blister roofs remain. Subepidermal blisters, on the other hand, have an epidermal roof and are tense and remain intact. Hemorrhagic fluid is common in subepidermal blisters because of their location close to dermal capillaries.

Biopsy of early vesicles or blisters is imperative in diagnosis. Immunofluorescence studies on biopsy material may differentiate certain immunologically mediated diseases. Pathologic studies are most informative when performed early, before therapy has been initiated.

INTRAEPIDERMAL VESICULOBULLOUS DISEASES. Pathologic processes involved in epidermal blister formation include spongiosis, primary cell damage, and acantholysis. Spongiosis, a common form of blister formation in eczematous processes, represents edema between cells of the prickle layer and liquefaction

TABLE 475–4. ICHTHYOSIFORM DERMATOSES

	Inheritance	Onset	Distribution	Clinical Associations	Kinetics
Lamellar ichthyosis	Autosomal recessive	Birth	Body, palms, soles	Ectropion	Increased
Epidermolytic hyperkeratosis	Autosomal dominant	Birth	Predominant flexural involvement	Blisters	Increased
X-linked ichthyosis (steroid sulfatase deficiency)	X-linked	Birth	Trunk	Corneal opacities	Normal
Ichthyosis vulgaris	Autosomal dominant	Childhood	Spares flexural areas	Atopy	Normal

Reprinted from the chapter by Dr. Marie-Louise Johnson in the 17th edition of the Cecil Textbook of Medicine, with her permission.

TABLE 475-5. LESS COMMON VESICULOBULLOUS DISEASES

Location of Blister in Skin	Cause If Known	Important Physical Findings	Other Facts of Note in History or Laboratory Results
Autoimmune			
Cicatricial pemphigoid	Subepidermal IgG linear in basement membrane zone	Scarring blisters in the mucous membrane; 25% have blisters on skin	Causes blindness; stenosis of urethra, anal areas
Dermatitis herpetiformis (vesicles in dermal papillae)	Immunologic deposition of IgA in dermal papillae	Grouped, symmetrically distributed vesicles and urticarial papules on scalp, scapulae, buttocks, elbows, knees	Intense burning, itch; high incidence of asymptomatic celiac sprue
Metabolic			
Porphyria cutanea tarda	Metabolic defect in porphyrin metabolism	Tense bullae that leave scars in sun-exposed areas; bullae induced by sun, trauma	May also see facial hirsutism and hyperpigmentation
Bullous disease of renal disease	Unknown	Bullae usually in extremities	
Bullous disease in diabetics	Unknown	Large bulla on acral areas	
Mechanicobullous diseases			
Epidermolysis bullosa (split above, below, and within dermal-epidermal zone)	Variety of inherited conditions	Tense blisters that erode and scar, especially in recessively inherited forms; can lead to severe scars covering digits	Severe forms may involve mouth, esophagus
Epidermolysis bullosa acquista (blister below lamina densa)	Linear IgG and C3 deposits below lamina densa	Tense blisters that lead to scars and millia in pressure and trauma sites on hands, feet; scarring mucous membrane lesions also occur	Circulating antibody to sublamina densa antigen found

of cells which gradually increases the size of the fluid spaces. Primary epidermal cell damage with fluid accumulation is seen in viral infections and friction damage. Blisters may also occur when cellular desmosomal attachments and intercellular cementing substances are immunologically or chemically altered, causing dyshesion referred to as acantholysis (pemphigus).

Bullous impetigo, a subcorneal infection of the skin with staphylococcal and/or streptococcal organisms, causes large, fragile, clear or cloudy bullae that form thin, honey-yellow crusts and a delicate collarette-like remnant of blister roof after the blisters rupture. Autoinoculation results in satellite lesions. The superficial epidermal blistering is caused by the toxic effects of an epidermal toxin elaborated by certain strains of these bacterial organisms.

A more serious variant of bullous impetigo is *staphylococcal scalded skin syndrome,* usually affecting infants and characterized by the formation of rapidly progressive, painful, erythematous patches in which large flaccid bullae evolve and shed as large sheets of skin, leaving a denuded, scalded-appearing surface. With only slight trauma the skin readily slides off, much like wet wallpaper slides off a wall (Nikolsky's sign—see Ch. 473). In contrast to localized bullous impetigo in which the *Staphylococcus aureus* may be recovered in the skin lesions, the bullae of scalded skin syndrome are sterile, although a staphylococcal infection may be found in the conjunctiva, nose, or pharynx. The widespread intraepidermal blistering results from an epidermal toxin elaborated by specific strains of *Staphylococcus* and hematogenously carried to the skin. These are penicillinase-resistant strains of *Staphylococcus* and therefore require methicillin-type antibiotics.

A somewhat similar condition, *toxic epidermal necrolysis* (TEN), occurs in adults, often secondary to drugs (e.g., ampicillin, allopurinol) and occasionally to *Staphylococcus* infections in an immunosuppressed patient. TEN is a reaction to a variety of antigenic materials that cause a suprabasilar split in the epidermis with necrosis of much of the overlying epidermis. Because of the more extensive destruction of epidermis and barrier stratum corneum layer (as opposed to staphylococcal scalded skin syndrome, in which the split is subcorneal), TEN is often fatal and, when extensive, should be treated as a widespread burn would be cared for. TEN also often involves the mucous membranes and therefore may be confused with Stevens-Johnson syndrome (see below).

Viral infections of the skin may cause vesicles and bullae by virtue of direct infection of the keratinocytes and the destructive effect on the cells. Vesicles caused by viruses often display two important characteristics: (1) they tend to occur in groups on an indurated erythematous base, and (2) they often take on an umbilicated appearance.

Herpes simplex infections are discussed in Ch. 339.

A complication of herpes simplex infection, *erythema multiforme,*

is a hypersensitivity skin and mucous membrane reaction that evolves 1 to 2 weeks following herpetic recurrences as a result of a herpesvirus–containing immune complex reaction to the herpes antigen. Herpes infection is only one etiologic stimulus leading to erythema multiforme (see below).

Diagnosis of herpes infections (including zoster and varicella) is made with a Tzanck preparation of material taken from the roof of vesicles. The contents are smeared onto a slide and stained with Wright or Giemsa stain to reveal multinucleated giant cells (see Ch. 473).

Acyclovir administered orally or intravenously is the most frequently used form of therapy for primary and recurrent forms of herpes (see Ch. 339).

Varicella infection, when initially encountered, causes chickenpox, a generalized pruritic eruption with widespread, delicate vesicles on an erythematous base which have been likened to a dew drop on a rose petal. They often become umbilicated, hemorrhagic, and pustular and may leave scars. Chickenpox lesions occur predominantly on the trunk but also involve the head, extremities, and mucous membranes of the mouth and conjunctiva. Successive crops of lesions evolve for a week. Ch. 336 discusses the systemic illness. *Herpes zoster* is a recrudescence of latent varicella virus in persons who previously had varicella. Zoster appears as grouped, umbilicated, and, at times, hemorrhagic vesicles and pustules on an erythematous base situated unilaterally along the distribution of cranial or spinal nerve roots. Frequently several immediately adjacent dermatomes are involved. Bilateral involvement is rare. Zoster is frequently associated with a prodrome of severe radicular pain in the involved areas. A common useful sign in making the diagnosis is hypesthesia of the dermatomal areas—the patient often bitterly complains that the rubbing of clothing on the area is intolerable. Most patients with herpes zoster are over 50 years of age, and cancer patients (especially those with lymphomas such as Hodgkin's disease) are particularly prone to this infection. In such patients or in immunocompromised individuals, cutaneous dissemination from the original dermatome may occur, as well as visceral involvement of liver, lung, and central nervous system. Treatment of herpes zoster is usually symptomatic with Burow's compresses, analgesics, and acyclovir, especially in immunocompromised patients (800 mg five times per day orally for 10 days). Postherpetic neuralgia is common in individuals over 50 (see Ch. 405). Systemic corticosteroids may reduce acute herpetic pain; whether they reduce the risk of postherpetic neuralgia is debatable. *Insect bites* including flea and fire ant bites may also induce vesicles or bullae, a response to injected toxins or foreign chemicals or proteins in the bite or an allergic reaction to them.

Pemphigus diseases cause blistering in the epidermis by virtue of the process of acantholysis. *Pemphigus vulgaris* and a variant, *pem-*

phigus vegetans, which heals with hypertrophic, "vegetative" surfaces, are acquired autoimmune diseases of the skin and mucous membrane. The superficial bullae, evolving just above the basal layer, readily rupture, leaving denuded, bleeding, weeping and crusted erosions over the body which do not heal. The oral mucosa is almost always involved and is frequently the presenting site. The painful erosions characteristically spill over the vermilion border of the lips and onto the skin. Lesions of the skin occur anywhere but often in pressure and friction areas. The blisters arise on normal-appearing skin. Untreated pemphigus vulgaris progresses slowly with extensive denudation, leading to fluid and electrolyte imbalance, sepsis, and death. Pain from mouth lesions prevents adequate food intake. Skin biopsy of early vesicles should be obtained for routine histologic examination. The edge of a bulla, including adjacent normal skin, should be examined by direct immunofluorescence to make the diagnosis. Immunofluorescence shows deposits of immunoglobulins (usually IgG) and/or C3 in the intercellular spaces around keratinocytes. Antibodies to the intercellular areas of the epidermis are found in the serum. Circulating antibodies to the epidermis are directed against several polypeptide components of the epidermal desmosomes. Their titers somewhat reflect disease activity, and they may contribute to the defective epidermal adhesion. High doses of systemic steroids (100 to 200 mg of prednisone per day) over prolonged periods usually control the disease. Methotrexate and other cytotoxic agents are useful as steroid-sparing agents. Treatment with intramuscular gold often is successful, occasionally inducing long-term remissions (see Ch. 474).

Pemphigus foliaceus is a less severe disease in which the acantholytic separation within the epidermis is in the upper portion of the prickle layer. *Pemphigus erythematosus* may be a localized variant of pemphigus foliaceus presenting with superficial blisters, erosions, and crusting and oozing over the scalp and face in a seborrheic dermatitis–like rash or often simulating the butterfly rash of systemic lupus erythematosus. Mucous membrane involvement in pemphigus foliaceus and pemphigus erythematosus is unusual, and lower doses of systemic steroids generally control these conditions. Immunofluorescent studies on skin from the edge of lesions reveal immunoglobulin and/or C3 in the intercellular areas of the upper portions of the epidermis.

Familial benign pemphigus, or Hailey-Hailey disease, is a dominantly inherited disorder with suprabasal cell acantholysis, the groups of bullae arising on erythematous skin in the flexural areas (neck, axillae, groin). Spreading erosions display vesicles and pustules at the borders with a moist, granular center. Warm weather and superficial bacterial infections seem to cause flares with spontaneous exacerbations and remissions continuing for years. Familial benign pemphigus differs from other forms of pemphigus in its genetic pattern, absence of mouth lesions, benign course, and absence of intercellular antibodies. Antibiotics, both topical and systemic, may improve acute flares of the disease. If *Candida* infection is superimposed, topical antifungal agents are often of benefit. When chronic vegetating lesions are present, surgical removal with skin grafting may be useful.

DERMAL-EPIDERMAL VESICULOBULLOUS DISEASES. Separation of the epidermis from the dermis occurs in a variety of bullous diseases resulting from autoimmune and immunologic reactions, metabolic disturbances, and a number of inherited mechanicobullous conditions (see Table 475–5).

Bullous pemphigoid is an autoimmune disorder of the elderly, in which tense, large blisters occur on normal or erythematous skin, often in the groin, axillae, and flexural areas. Only one third of patients have oral blisters. Healing usually occurs in some blisters without scarring while new lesions evolve. Itching may be severe or absent. Skin biopsies display a subepidermal blister through the lamina lucida (at the electron microscopic level), and direct immunofluorescence reveals deposition of the IgG immunoglobulin and complement directed against an antigen in the lamina lucida. The prognosis is good, and the disease usually subsides after months or years. Widespread bullae require therapy with 40 to 60 mg of oral prednisone per day and occasionally with immunosuppressive agents.

Another subepidermal blistering disease, *herpes gestationis,* is a rare autoimmune condition that occurs during pregnancy and the postpartum period. The name of the disease is misleading, for it is not associated with herpesvirus infection. The blisters develop at any time throughout the course of pregnancy, although they most often begin during the second and third trimesters and subside a few weeks post partum. Some patients may experience transient flares or recurrences with each menstrual period or following the use of oral contraceptives. There are recurrences with subsequent pregnancies. Herpes gestationis is a pruritic condition with numerous tense vesicles arising on both normal-appearing and erythematous areas of skin. Arcuate and polycyclic red plaques with peripheral blistering are seen. The lesions first appear on the abdomen and then spread to involve the entire integument. Skin biopsy findings are indistinguishable from those of bullous pemphigoid by light microscopy, and examination of perilesional skin by direct immunofluorescence reveals C3 and less often an IgG linear band just below the epidermis. There is associated fetal mortality as high as 30%, and there is also an increased rate of premature live births. Transient vesiculobullous lesions may infrequently occur in some otherwise healthy infants of affected mothers. Occasionally the patients' intractable pruritus and extensive bullae respond to high-potency topical steroid ointments and diphenhydramine, but most patients require oral prednisone (20 to 60 mg daily) throughout pregnancy with intermittent tapering.

Cicatricial pemphigoid (benign mucosal pemphigoid) and dermatitis herpetiformis are described in Table 475–5.

Erythema multiforme is an immunologic reaction in the skin and mucous membranes often mediated by circulating immune complexes that evolve in response to a number of antigenic stimulae (infections, drugs, connective tissue disease). As the name implies, the skin reaction is characterized by a variety of lesions, namely, erythematous plaques, blisters, and target or bull's-eye lesions. The mucous membranes of the mouth and eye may also be involved, and this is referred to as *Stevens-Johnson syndrome.* Typically the cutaneous lesions favor the extremities (often the palms) and are symmetric. Target lesions are diagnostic and are recognized by a central, dark purple area or a blister surrounded by a pale, edematous, round zone, surrounded in turn by a peripheral rim of erythema. In Stevens-Johnson syndrome the skin disease is more widespread, with blisters and painful erosions in the mouth and eyes. The patients look and feel ill with fever, prostration, and difficulty in eating. Histologically, subepidermal separation is found in the blistering center of the target lesion, and when early lesions are biopsied, immunofluorescence reveals immunoglobulin and complement in the walls of the small dermal blood vessels; the inflammation and bulla form in response to vascular damage and leaking. In one half of cases no cause is found for the reaction, but a cause should be sought in all cases, especially drugs (penicillins, barbiturates, phenytoin [Dilantin], and sulfonamides) and infections (herpes simplex, *Streptococcus, Mycoplasma pneumoniae*). Recurrent herpes simplex infection is the most common cause of recurrent erythema multiforme. It is not clear whether medical therapy favorably alters the course of idiopathic erythema multiforme, although treatment of a precipitating infection seems appropriate and acyclovir may prevent recurrences of herpes-associated erythema multiforme. Stopping suspected drugs is also imperative. The value of systemic steroids in erythema multiforme and Stevens-Johnson syndrome is controversial. In addition, IV fluids may be required in patients with severe oral involvement, and topical anesthetics (viscous Xylocaine) may help to decrease mouth discomfort.

An example of a bullous disease caused by a metabolic disorder is *porphyria* (see Table 475–5 and Ch. 187).

Other metabolic bullous diseases are those seen with chronic renal disease and diabetes mellitus. These also are briefly described in Table 475–5, as are mechanobullous conditions.

PUSTULAR DISEASES OF THE SKIN

Pustules usually bring to mind infection, but not all pustular dermatoses are caused by pathogenic microorganisms. Pustular conditions often occur in association with erythematous papules, cysts, and nodules and may open to form crusts (Table 475–6).

NONINFECTIOUS PUSTULAR SKIN DISEASES. *Acne* is the most common pustular condition of the skin. It is an inflammatory disorder affecting pilosebaceous units and is usually found over the face and upper trunk. Several pathogenic factors play a role as individuals enter puberty: (1) androgens stimulate the sebaceous glands and increase sebum production (see Ch. 472); (2) abnormal keratinization and impaction in the pilosebaceous canal

TABLE 475-6. ADDITIONAL NONINFECTIOUS PUSTULAR DISEASES OF THE SKIN

Name of Skin Condition	Cause	Important Physical Findings	Other Facts of Note in Histroy or Laboratory Results
Perioral dermatitis	May be caused by potent topical steroids; variant of acne	Perioral and periorbital red scaling patches, papules, and pustules	
Pustular psoriasis	Variant of psoriasis	Sterile pustules localized to palms and soles or generalized over body	Patient is toxic with fever, leukocytosis; can die of generalized form
Miliaria pustulosa	Occlusion of sweat glands in hot environment	Discrete red papules or pustules with red base over trunk, especially back	

(comedones) obstruct sebum flow; (3) proliferation of anaerobic bacteria, *Propionibacterium acnes,* predisposes to rupture of the pilosebaceous unit with extravasation into the surrounding dermis, resulting in sterile, inflammatory papules, pustules, and cysts. These later lead to disfiguring scarring. Therapy of acne is usually successful in controlling the disease until the patient "grows out" of this condition. Topical agents that remove comedones such as benzoyl peroxide and topical vitamin A preparations are particularly effective because their action allows sebum to flow freely onto the surface of the skin. Topical and oral antibiotics (tetracycline and erythromycin) are indicated in patients with inflammatory papules and pustules. Oral 13-*cis*-retinoic acid (Accutane) decreases sebaceous gland size and sebum production. This drug should be used primarily for severe cystic acne because in high daily doses it produces undesirable side effects and can be teratogenic. Spironolactone, the potassium-sparing diuretic, has antiandrogenic properties that have resulted in its increasing use in women with difficult-to-control acne. Used in doses of 100 to 200 mg per day along with routine forms of acne therapy, the condition frequently is brought under control. The clinician should recognize that other factors may play a role in exacerbating acne, including oil-based cosmetics and drugs (androgenic hormones, antiepileptics [phenytoin], high-progestin birth control pills, systemic corticosteroids when taken in high doses, and iodide- and bromide-containing agents). Occasionally endocrinologic conditions characterized by excess androgen secretion may cause acne, i.e., polycystic ovarian disease, adrenal or ovarian tumors.

Rosacea is a chronic inflammatory disorder affecting the blood vessels and pilosebaceous units of the face in middle-aged individuals. Patients with rosacea have papules and pustules superimposed on diffuse erythema and telangiectasia over the central portion of the face. An important component is easy flushing and blushing of the face often accentuated when alcohol, caffeine-containing, or hot spicy foods are ingested. Hyperplasia of the sebaceous glands, connective tissue, and vascular bed of the nose sometimes causes *rhinophyma* or a large, red, bulbous nose (see Fig. 475–4). Ocular complications occur in a small but significant number of rosacea patients; these include blepharitis, chalazion, conjunctivitis, and keratitis. Progressive keratitis can lead to scarring and blindness. Rosacea and the eye complications usually respond well to tetracycline, and/or metronidazole but the antibiotic must be continued for life (at the lowest dose that suppresses the condition) because rosacea recurs when therapy stops. High-potency topical corticosteroid preparations may induce or aggravate pre-existing rosacea and should not be used for long periods of time on the face.

INFECTIOUS CAUSES OF SKIN PUSTULES. *Folliculitis,* an *S. aureus* infection of the hair follicle, appears as pustules with a red rim with hair emanating from the center of the pustule. Folliculitis typically occurs in hairy regions where clothing rubs (buttocks, thighs) or on the face. The key to diagnosis is finding a central hair in the pustule. Occasionally the follicular infection can extend more deeply to form a larger, red, fluctuant nodule that "points" in order to drain pus from one (furuncle) or more follicles (carbuncle). Systemic antibiotics such as erythromycin or dicloxacillin usually clear extensive infections; topical antiseptic cleansers such as povidone-iodine or chlorhexidine can resolve mild folliculitis and may be useful in preventing recurrences.

Candidiasis appears as beefy red patches in intertriginous, moist areas characteristically surrounded by satellite pustules. Paronychia, a painful red swelling in the periungual regions of the finger, may also drain pus in which *Candida* can be found with a KOH prepa-

ration. Topical agents such as clotrimazole and miconazole are used two or three times a day. These must be used for many weeks before the infection clears.

Hot tub folliculitis is a generalized, pruritic folliculitis caused by *Pseudomonas aeruginosa* that is acquired in contaminated hot tubs, whirlpools, or swimming pools. It usually begins 6 hours to 5 days after hot tub soaking and affects many people using the facility. It appears as a vesicular and then pustular eruption over the trunk, buttocks, legs, and arms but spares the head and neck. *Pseudomonas* can often be cultured from fresh pustules. In most instances the folliculitis resolves within 7 to 10 days without specific treatment. Infected tubs and pools should be cultured for *Pseudomonas* and disinfected.

Dermatophytes can, at times, infect hair follicles and result in pustules, particularly in the beard (tinea barbae) and scalp (kerions). These are readily confused with a bacterial folliculitis. Kerions appear as indurated, boggy, inflammatory plaques studded with pustules. These intense inflammatory reactions to superficial dermatophytes (especially *T. verrucosum*) respond to griseofulvin therapy, although a short course of oral corticosteroids is also useful.

Deep fungal infections such as *blastomycosis, sporotrichosis,* and *coccidioidomycosis* may cause pustules, as well as verrucous, ulcerative papules and nodules. Sporotrichosis characteristically spreads up cutaneous lymphatics and appears as nodular, pustular lesions in a linear distribution.

SYSTEMIC INFECTIONS CAUSING PUSTULES ON THE SKIN. A variety of septicemias including gonococcemia, staphylococcal septicemia, and *Candida* septicemia (in immunosuppressed patients) cause pustular lesions associated with purpura.

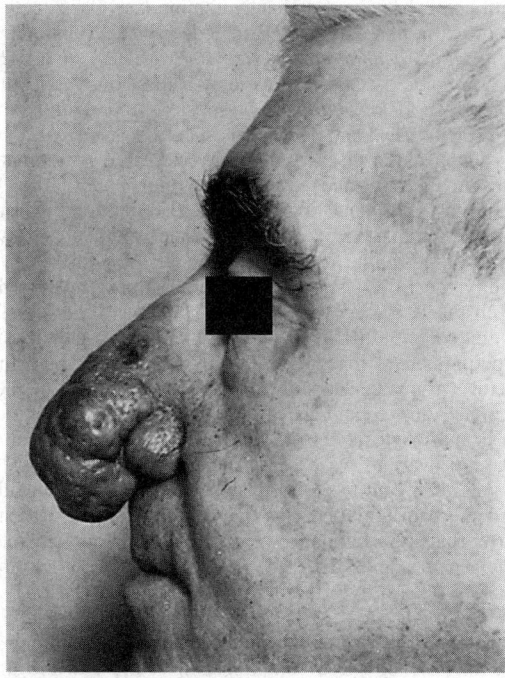

FIGURE 475–4. Rhinophyma. (From the 17th edition of the Cecil Textbook of Medicine, with the permission of Dr. Marie-Louise Johnson.)

URTICARIA, PERSISTENT FIGURATE ERYTHEMAS, CELLULITIS

This group of skin lesions is of disparate appearance and origin. The common feature is a raised edematous, red plaque with a sharply demarcated border.

URTICARIAL REACTIONS. Urticaria, the most common condition in this group, appears as wheals, transient erythematous and edematous swellings of the dermis caused by local increase in permeability of capillaries and small venules. This increased permeability results from histamine and other chemical substances released from cutaneous mast cells by Type I IgE hypersensitivity reactions, as well as by nonimmunologic mechanisms (see Ch. 224). Certain agents such as aspirin, opiates, and some foods degranulate mast cells directly without an allergic mechanism. Other urticarial reactions are immunologically mediated by such allergens as infections (viral, i.e., hepatitis, sinus and tooth infections), infestations (systemic parasites), drugs, pollens, and injections (blood products, vaccinations). Physical modalities—light (solar urticaria), cold (cold urticaria), heat or exercise (cholinergic urticaria), or pressure or rubbing of the skin (dermatographism)—cause other such "hives". Hives are transient, any given lesion lasting < 24 hours, although new ones may continuously evolve. Acute urticaria (i.e., lasting < 6 weeks) often results from drugs and the cause is frequently identified. The cause of chronic urticaria (lasting > 6 to 8 weeks) is more difficult to identify. Hives covering large areas and producing deep tissue swelling are termed *angioedema*. This condition can involve the tongue and throat and impinge upon the airway. In such patients a careful history about medications (including over-the-counter drugs, especially cold tablets or medications containing aspirin) should be elicited. Infections such as sinusitis or apical abscess of teeth must be looked for. In addition, physical types of urticaria should be considered: *cholinergic* urticaria is characterized by evanescent multiple, small wheals surrounded by a wide pink flare induced by heat and exercise; *solar* urticaria by large plaques in sun-exposed areas; *cold* urticaria by wheals that evolve with exposure to cold. Urticaria accompanied by fever and arthralgias occurs in serum sickness reactions and in the prodromata of viral hepatitis. Occasionally urticaria occurs in conjunction with internal conditions such as malignancies or connective tissue diseases. Hereditary angioedema, an autosomal dominant disorder, causes recurrent urticaria, angioedema, intestinal colic, and life-threatening laryngeal edema.

If the cause for the urticaria cannot be found or avoided, symptomatic control is achieved with antihistamines or oral steroids. Acute angioedema or laryngeal edema requires rapid systemic treatment with epinephrine and diphenhydramine (see Ch. 224).

Other urticaria-like skin lesions include *erythema multiforme* (see above); *juvenile rheumatoid arthritis skin lesions*—small, 2- to 3-mm, salmon-colored hives that last only a few hours appearing with fever spikes; *erythema margination*—lesions found in 10% of patients with acute rheumatic fever (see Ch. 277). *Urticaria pigmentosa* (mastocytosis), a disease caused by increased accumulations of mast cells in the skin and at times in lymph nodes, liver, spleen, bones, and gastrointestinal tract (see Ch. 231), presents with multiple tan to brown, papular spots that urticate when rubbed owing to the release of histamine from the mast cells. A skin biopsy specimen readily identifies increased numbers of mast cells in the dermis. When the lesions develop in early childhood, the condition is usually limited to skin and the lesions resolve by puberty, leaving only hyperpigmented macules. If the skin lesions evolve in adulthood there is a greater chance for mast cell infiltration of the organ systems noted above, and the skin lesions persist. Symptoms and findings in mastocytosis depend on the organ systems involved and the release of various vasoactive substances contained in the increased masses of mast cells. Hepatosplenomegaly, lymphadenopathy, and bone pain may occur secondary to infiltrates. Patients may experience flushing, palpitations, headache, syncope, hypotension, abdominal pain, and diarrhea, all related to histamine and prostaglandin release from the mast cells.

FIGURATE ERYTHEMAS. This is a group of uncommon conditions characterized by annular, polycyclic, and geographic erythematous skin lesions. These conditions, in contrast to the urticarial reactions, persist for many days or even years, moving slowly or rapidly over the skin surface (hence, the term sometimes used for these reactions—persistent figurate erythema). Usually no specific cause is found for these lesions, but some may be associated with underlying malignancies. Erythema repeus, characterized by a series of swirling woodgrain-like red lines, is found in association with adenocarcinomas of the breast, lung, or gastrointestinal tract or with other fungal infections. Erythema annulare centrifugum is a slowly enlarging annular lesion that clears in the center with collarette scaling on the inner edge of the red rings. It is found at times with cutaneous dermatophyte infections, systemic *Candida* infections, the ingestion of blue cheese, parasitic bowel diseases, and autoimmune disorders.

Erythema chronicum migrans is the unique annular skin lesion found in Lyme disease caused by a spirochete inoculated by infected tick bites (see Ch. 321 and Color Plate 10*B*).

CELLULITIS. Although superficially resembling urticaria, these inflammatory infections of the dermis are readily distinguished from hives by their persistent, slowly enlarging nature as well as their pain and warmth. Group A streptococci and *S. aureus* are most commonly responsible. *Erysipelas* is sometimes identified separately from cellulitis. It displays a sharply demarcated painful border and an "orange-peel" epidermal surface. Group A *Streptococcus* is the usual cause. Patients usually feel ill and are febrile. Cellulitis on the lower legs in adults may develop from fissures between the toes from tinea pedis. Systemic antibiotics, erythromycin, dicloxacillin, or the cephalosporins are the most commonly used drugs.

Necrotizing fasciitis is a special form of cellulitis involving the deep fascial structures underlying the skin. Rapidly evolving in enclosed fascial spaces, usually in diabetics or immunosuppressed patients, these infections are caused by a mixture of aerobic and anaerobic gram-negative organisms and must be diagnosed early by deep fascial biopsy and treated immediately with broad-spectrum antibiotics and surgical debridement.

NODULES AND TUMORS OF THE SKIN

Skin nodules and tumors may evolve within the epidermis or the dermis and subcutaneous tissue, arising in various skin appendages and structures, including melanocytes. Such lesions may represent benign or malignant growths, infiltrative or inflammatory reactions. In many instances the structures giving rise to the nodule reflect the colors of these structures. Vascular lesions appear red to purple, whereas lesions involving melanocytes appear pigmented.

Most epidermal nodules are recognized by localized thickening of the epidermis or corneum with hyperkeratosis or scale. Dermal or subcutaneous nodules appear as lumps, often with no alteration in the overlying epidermis.

Of primary concern is whether a nodule is benign or malignant. This is not always easy, and skin nodules and tumors often must be biopsied. Some clinical generalizations can be made in distinguishing benign from malignant tumors (Table 475–7).

NONPIGMENTED NODULES—BENIGN. *Warts* are benign epidermal growths caused by papilloma viruses (see above, under Maculopapular lesions).

Sebaceous hyperplasia occurs as papular and occasionally nodular lesions on the faces of individuals past 50 years of age. Proliferation of sebaceous glands surrounding a hair follicle appears as groups of yellow papules evolving in an annular configuration with a central pore. Sebaceous hyperplasia may be clinically difficult to differentiate from basal cell cancers, although the yellow discoloration and central pore may help. At times skin biopsy may be necessary. No treatment is generally required.

TABLE 475–7. CLINICAL FEATURES HELPFUL IN DISTINGUISHING BENIGN FROM MALIGNANT TUMORS

Clinical Feature	Benign	Malignant
Configuration	Symmetric, sharp borders	Asymmetric, irregular borders
Rate of growth	Slow	Slow or rapid
Friability	No friability	Often friable
Bleeding or ulceration	Seldom bleed or ulcerate	Often bleed and ulcerate
Consistency	Firm or soft	Usually firm to hard
Color	Uniform color and pigmentation	Irregularity of color and pigmentation

Keratoacanthomas, or self-healing epitheliomas, are rapidly growing, biologically benign neoplasms of epidermal keratinocytes. The lesions resolve spontaneously, leaving a scar. Keratoacanthomas are usually found on sun-exposed areas and begin as flesh-colored papules that rapidly grow over a period of 6 weeks, evolving a central keratin-filled crater. The lesions remain for 6 to 8 weeks and then subside. Such lesions are best excised because they leave unsightly scars and are difficult to differentiate from squamous cell cancer, even histologically.

Epidermal inclusion cysts appear as flesh-colored, firm nodules in the skin, particularly over the scalp and trunk. A helpful diagnostic sign is a central enlarged pore where the epidermis has invaginated to form the cyst. If the central pore is patent, slight squeezing will express white, cheesy, foul-smelling keratin and sebum. Bothersome cysts can be excised.

Lipomas are more deeply situated than epidermal inclusion cysts. Although they can feel firm and even rubbery, like a cyst, they usually are multilobulated and softer in consistency. If the diagnosis is in doubt and especially if the lesion is firm, a biopsy is indicated. Lipomas may be multiple. Familial multiple epidermal cysts and lipomas, fibromas, and osteomas associated with intestinal polyps are recognized as Gardner's syndrome.

Neurofibromas, focal proliferations of neural tissue within the dermis, may present in two forms: (1) soft, flesh-colored, protruding nodules that, on compression, can be invaginated into what feels like a defect in the skin (buttonhole sign), and (2) deep, firm, dermal or subcutaneous nodules. Neurofibromas may be solitary, but when they are multiple *von Recklinghausen's disease* should be considered, especially when café au lait spots (light brown macules) and axillary freckling are seen.

NONPIGMENTED NODULES—MALIGNANT. Malignant tumors of the epidermas—*basal cell* and *squamous cell carcinomas*—relate to the amount and intensity of electromagnetic radiation, including ultraviolet light and x-radiation, the skin has received over a lifetime. Accordingly, such cancers occupy sun-exposed areas, especially the face, neck, arms, and hands. The cancers are more common in patients living in southern latitudes of the northern hemisphere and in Australia, especially in persons with a light complexion whose occupations keep them outdoors. These epidermal cancers also are more common in immunosuppressed patients, attesting to the importance of the immune surveillance system in cancer. A personal or family history of skin cancer should sharpen attention to the possibility of cancer.

Basal cell carcinomas arise from the basal cells of the epidermis. They rarely metastasize, but they can cause extensive, local destruction. Four clinical forms should be recognized: (1) the *nodular* type, the most common, appears as a pearly or opalescent, irregularly shaped papule or nodule with a central depression or crater; telangiectasias and a rolled, waxy border are often in evidence. When ulceration and crusting occur, it is referred to as a rodent ulcer (Fig. 475–5). Often the raised, waxy border is subtle and is observed more readily by stretching the skin. (2) *Superficial* basal cell carcinoma is recognized as a red, slightly scaling, eczematous plaque that may be slightly eroded and crusted. Careful examination reveals a threadlike, pearly, rolled edge. This is an easily overlooked neoplasm, frequently confused with psoriasis or eczematous patches. A high index of suspicion, along with skin biopsy, is needed to make the diagnosis. (3) *Pigmented* basal cell carcinoma appears as a blue-black nodule or plaque with a pearly, opalescent sheen. Melanocytes are not histologically involved in these cancers, merely stimulated to make more pigment but not worsening the prognosis. (4) *Scarring* or *sclerosing* basal cell cancers present as atrophic, white, sometimes slightly eroded or crusted plaques with telangiectasia. This is the most difficult form to cure because of its indistinct borders. The diagnosis of basal cell carcinoma should be confirmed by biopsy. Treatment depends on the location of the lesion, the morphologic type, the size of the tumor, and whether it is primary or recurrent. Treatment modalities include curettage and electrodesiccation, scalpel excision, radiation therapy, and cryotherapy. Properly selected, each modality has a cure rate greater than 90%. A specialized form of excision is used for recurrent basal cell cancers, sclerosing basal cell cancers, and large primary basal cell cancers in regions in which recurrences are likely (particularly in the nasolabial folds and the periorbital and immediate preauricular areas). The Mohs surgical technique utilizes frozen section histologic mapping of the tumor to determine its extent.

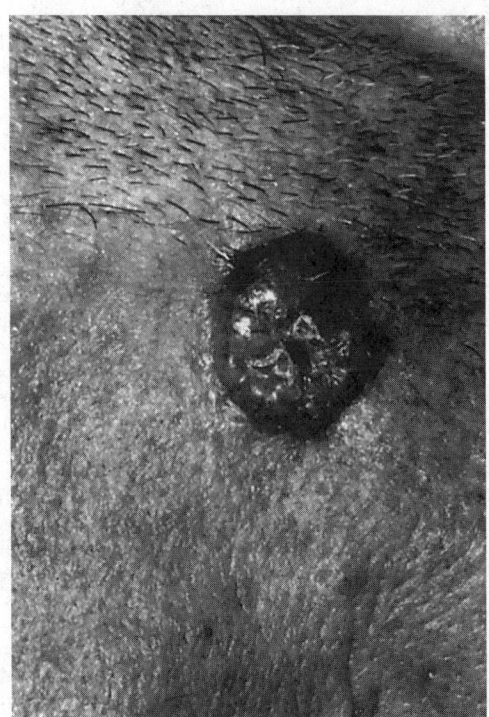

FIGURE 475–5. Basal cell epithelioma. (From the 17th edition of the Cecil Textbook of Medicine, with the permission of Dr. Marie-Louise Johnson.)

Squamous cell carcinoma, a malignant neoplasm of the keratinocytes, is a less common but more aggressive type of cancer. Squamous cell carcinoma is locally invasive and has the potential to metastasize. It occurs primarily on the head and neck, upper extremities, and trunk, presenting as firm, red, smooth or verrucous nodules. Hyperkeratoses may be prominent. The cancers also display increased friability, ulceration, and crusting (Fig. 475–6). *Bowen's disease* is a squamous cell cancer *in situ,* appearing as red, scaling, crusted, sharply demarcated plaques. Squamous cell cancer *in situ* on the penis in uncircumcised males evolves as velvety red patches on the glans and foreskin. Bowen's disease and erythroplasia are banal, easily overlooked conditions that can metastasize if

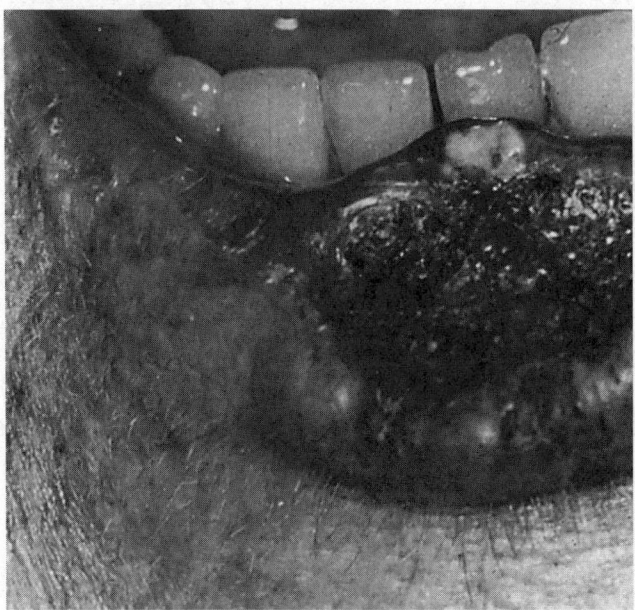

FIGURE 475–6. Squamous cell carcinoma. (From the 17th edition of the Cecil Textbook of Medicine, with the permission of Dr. Marie-Louise Johnson.)

not diagnosed early. *Actinic keratoses,* precancerous lesions of atypical keratinocytes, appear as red, ill-marginated macules and papules with yellow-brown, adherent scales in sun-damaged skin. They may evolve into squamous cell cancers. Any lesion suspected of being a squamous cell cancer should be biopsied. Excision is the treatment of choice. Actinic keratoses are treated with liquid nitrogen freezing or, if numerous, with topical 5-fluorouracil applied as 1 or 5% cream or solution over 2- to 4-week period.

PIGMENTED NODULES—BENIGN. *Seborrheic keratoses* are epidermal cell neoplasms that appear on the face and trunk in middle age. These 2-mm to 5-cm, elevated, tan to brown or occasionally black, round to oval lesions have a verrucous or crumbly, greasy surface and a stuck-on appearance. No therapy is necessary unless they are of cosmetic concern, and then liquid nitrogen cryotherapy or curettage is an effective means of removal.

Dermatofibromas are areas of focal dermal fibrosis accompanied by overlying epidermal thickening and hyperpigmentation. Clinically, they look like brown papules or nodules. A useful diagnostic test is the "dimple sign," in which pinching the lesion results in central dimpling of the overlying epidermis. Some dermatofibromas are dark brown in color and occasionally raise the concern of melanoma, but the fibromas are symmetric and uniform in color. The lesions occur frequently on the lower extremities and less often on the arms, and they may be multiple. Although therapy is usually not required, simple excision can be done.

Nevi, or *moles,* are benign accumulations of pigment-forming nevus cells. They may be congenital or acquired, and most nevi evolve before age 35. There are three forms, representing various stages of biologic evolution and growth: *Junctional nevi* are light to brown macular lesions. *Compound nevi* have flat, junctional portions along with brown papules with a smooth or rough surface; these evolve from junctional nevi in older children and young adults. Later, *intradermal nevi* evolve from the compound nevi as flesh-colored to brown papules or sessile growths (Fig. 475–7). Although nevi vary in appearance and color, individually they are uniform in color, symmetric in their growth and configuration, and usually <6 mm in diameter. Occasionally nevi darken in color or may itch, and new nevi may develop during pregnancy, but symptomatic nevi that change should be regarded suspiciously.

PIGMENTED NODULES—MALIGNANT. Malignant melanoma is the cutaneous neoplasm of melanocytes and nevus cells. Useful clinical features in their diagnosis are called the A-B-C-D's (Table 475–8).

Several clinical forms or presentations of melanoma can be identified, each demonstrating the characteristics described in Table

TABLE 475–8. THE A-B-C-D'S

A = Asymmetry of the lesion is due to irregular, random growth of the malignant cells associated with irregular surface topography and papules and nodules.
B = Borders of the tumors are irregular with notching and pigment "spilling" out beyond the edges.
C = Color variegation consists of browns, blacks, blues, and even shades of red and white. The variations in color represent different depths of invasion of pigment cells along with inflammatory reaction and immunologic response to the malignant cells.
D = Diameter or size of melanomas tends to be greater than 6 mm before they are recognized.

475–8. *Lentigo maligna melanoma* is a slowly evolving, multicolored lesion on the head and neck. It is preceded by lentigo maligna (*in situ* melanoma), which extends peripherally and is an unevenly pigmented, dark brown to black macule that can grow to a size of 5 to 7 cm over a period of many years before nodules develop dermal invasion. *Superficial spreading melanoma* may occur on any area of the body, appearing as irregularly pigmented lesions with papules, nodules, and notched borders. Invasion into the dermis occurs more rapidly than in lentigo maligna melanoma. *Nodular melanoma* appears as a rapidly growing, blue-black, smooth or eroded nodule (Fig. 475–8). It invades dermis early in its evolution, making premetastatic diagnosis difficult. *Acral lentiginous melanoma* occurs on the palms, soles, and digits. It evolves as an irregular, enlarging, variegate-colored, brown to black growth similar to lentigo maligna melanoma but more aggressive in dermal invasion early in its course. Only minor degrees of papular elevation may be associated with deep invasion.

One third of melanomas may arise from existing nevi, so that a change in size, shape, and color or itching of a pigmented lesion (a common symptom in melanomas) should be carefully investigated. Early diagnosis is the key to survival. The deeper the malignant cells invade the dermis, the more likely is metastasis. The depth of dermal invasion can be microscopically measured from the granular cell layer in the epidermis to the deepest penetration of melanoma cells into the dermis. Thin melanomas (<0.76 mm) enjoy a virtually 100% cure rate. If the depth is greater than 1.6 mm, only 20 to 30% survive for 5 years.

Any suspicious pigmented lesion must be biopsied, preferably by excision. Definitive surgical excision should be undertaken only after confirmation of melanoma is established histologically. In large lesions such as lentigo maligna, it is acceptable to do incisional biopsy prior to definitive therapy. Suspicious pigmented lesions should never be shave-biopsied or shave-excised, nor should they be electrocauterized. Full-thickness tissue through the entire lesion is required for diagnostic and prognostic evaluation.

The precise cause of melanoma is unknown, but sunlight and heredity have been suggested as risk factors. The occurrence of melanoma has been increasing during the past few decades. Famil-

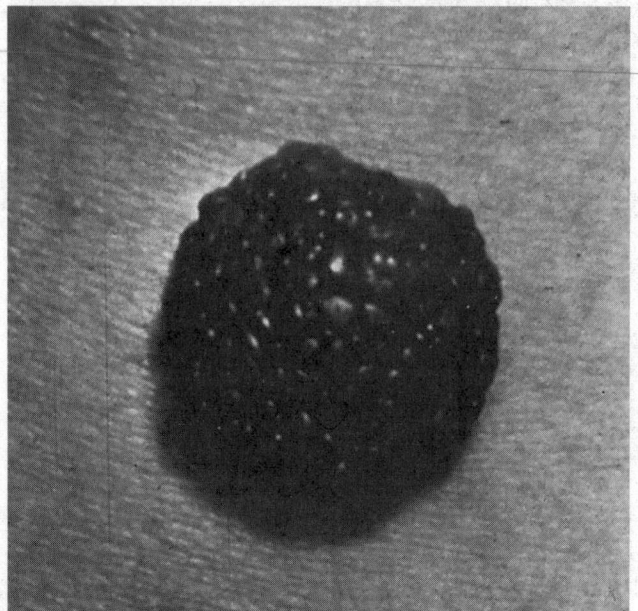

FIGURE 475–7. Intradermal nevus. (From the 17th edition of the Cecil Textbook of Medicine, with the permission of Dr. Marie-Louise Johnson.)

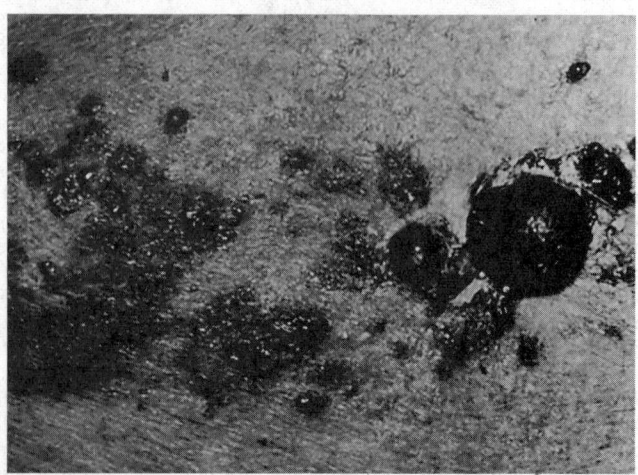

FIGURE 475–8. Nodular melanoma. (From the 17th edition of the Cecil Textbook of Medicine, with the permission of Dr. Marie-Louise Johnson.)

ial occurrence of malignant melanoma affects families with the *dysplastic nevus syndrome.* Numerous atypical, haphazardly colored, red-brown nevi with irregular borders appear over the trunk, extremities, and scalp. Biopsy of these atypical nevi reveals disordered melanocytic proliferation. The nevi may have an increased risk of developing melanoma, although the melanomas can also arise from normal skin in these persons. Close clinical follow-up and excision of suspicious nevi are important.

VASCULAR TUMORS OF THE SKIN. *Hemangiomas,* benign proliferations of dermal vessels, appear at or soon after birth as red, blue, or purple, flat, papular, or nodular lesions. Their appearance depends upon the number, size, and depth of the proliferating vessels. Thus, capillary angiomas are composed of small, superficial vessels causing *nevus flammeus* and *strawberry hemangiomas. Cavernous hemangiomas* are made up of larger and deeper vessels. Cavernous and strawberry angiomas often enlarge at an alarming rate over the first year or two and then usually involute by age nine or ten. Cavernous hemangiomas are less likely to resolve and sometimes may be deeply situated. Large lesions located in strategic locations (around the eye and mouth) may require systemic steroids in efforts to shrink these tumors. Platelet consumption by large cavernous hemangiomas may occur in the *Kasabach-Merritt syndrome.* Ordinarily hemangiomas require no therapy; watchful waiting allows them to resolve spontaneously, the cosmetic result usually being superior to that obtained by therapeutic intervention. When large hemangiomas ulcerate, bleed, or impinge on vital structures or functions (e.g., around the ears, eyes, nose, mouth), oral steroids given over short periods of time in the dose of 1 to 2 mg per kilogram body weight shrinks the tumor temporarily while awaiting the natural involution. Interferon α also has been used to shrink large hemangiomas that do not respond to steroids.

Pyogenic granuloma, a bright red, raspberry-like growth that can reach a centimeter in size, is friable and bleeds easily when traumatized. These lesions occur most often on arms, legs, fingers, and hands. They enlarge rapidly within weeks but have no malignant potential; they represent capillary hemangiomatous proliferation and follow injury or surgery. The term *pyogenic* is a misnomer, as no infectious process is involved. These lesions are treated with excision, curettage and electrocauterization, or cryotherapy. Occasionally amelanotic melanomas may present as a pyogenic granuloma, so pathologic examination of pyogenic granulomas should be performed.

Kaposi's sarcoma is a rare neoplasm of multifocal origin which presents as red-purple to blue-brown macules, plaques, and nodules of the skin and other organs. The cutaneous lesions may be firm or compressible, solitary or numerous, and may even appear initially as a dusky stain, especially about the toes.

These round-cell and spindle-cell sarcomas also can reside in viscera and until their association with AIDS seemed to occur predominantly in older men, leading to their demise. In Europe and North America, where Kaposi's sarcoma is more frequently seen among Jews and those of Mediterranean descent, the lesions commonly affect the lower extremities, are indolent, and often are associated with chronic lymphedema, indicating tumor infiltration of the lymphatics. Men are affected 10 to 15 times more often than women, are usually in their seventh decade, and have an average survival time of approximately 10 years. The incidence of such Kaposi's sarcoma reported for the United States is < 0.1 per 100,000 population and < 0.02% of all malignancies.

In tropical Africa, an endemic belt of Kaposi's sarcoma exists at an altitude of 1200 to 1500 meters where the disease accounts for 3 to 9% of all malignancies, afflicting blacks while sparing whites and Indians. It has a peak incidence in the first decade, with most patients less than 20 years of age, and with survival of less than 3 years. Visceral rather than cutaneous involvement and marked lymphadenopathy are the predominant, unique clinical signs in these African children.

The selective geographic distribution of the lymphadenopathic type of Kaposi's sarcoma resembles that of Burkitt's lymphoma. Electron microscopic studies that affirm an association between cytomegalovirus and Kaposi's sarcoma make another parallel with Burkitt's lymphoma, the malignancy so closely linked to the Epstein-Barr virus. In the acquiring of Kaposi's sarcoma, therefore, infectious agents and immune status seem to be significant, as well as genetic and environmental factors. Kaposi's sarcoma has been observed to complicate systemic lupus erythematosus being treated

with immunosuppression and to appear along with tumors of lymphoreticular origin in the immunosuppressed recipients of renal transplants. It is known to coexist with other primary malignancies. However, its appearance as an aggressive lethal tumor in the young male homosexual is a stunning observation of grave concern. Those affected have a mean age in the fourth decade. Their skin lesions are generalized in distribution and are smaller, softer, and lighter in color than the classic firm, indurated lesions of the legs. Mucous membrane tumors or symptomatic visceral or lung lesions may appear before cutaneous hemorrhagic sarcomas. Average survival time from onset is less than 2 years.

Such fulminant Kaposi's sarcoma appears alone or with *Pneumocystis carinii* pneumonia and other opportunistic infections in increasing numbers in male homosexuals and drug abusers. A small painless red nodule of the skin, easily overlooked, can signal a profoundly compromised immune state and grave prognosis (see Ch. 367 and Color Plate 16D).

INFLAMMATORY NODULES OF THE SKIN. *Erythema nodosum* is an inflammatory reaction in subcutaneous fat which represents a hypersensitivity response to a number of antigenic stimuli. Well-localized, multiple, tender, red, deep nodules, 1 to 5 cm in size, usually develop bilaterally over the pretibial areas. They eventually involute, leaving yellow-purple bruises. Ulceration does not occur. Immunoglobulin and complement deposition has been found in deep blood vessels in early lesions, and in some patients circulating immune complexes have been detected. The localization of the painful nodules to the lower legs may relate to hemodynamic factors. Although no cause can be found in many patients, the following factors have been identified: drugs (especially oral contraceptives), pregnancy, inflammatory bowel disease, sarcoidosis, streptococcal infection, *Yersinia* enterocolitis, deep fungus infections, and tuberculosis. If the cause cannot be identified and eliminated, symptomatic therapy with aspirin, nonsteroidal anti-inflammatory medications, potassium iodide, or short courses of systemic steroids may be useful.

Subcutaneous fat necrosis is a condition in which tender, red nodules occur on the lower legs and thighs in patients with pancreatitis or pancreatic carcinoma. The skin lesions may occur in the absence of signs associated with the internal carcinoma. Serum amylase and lipase values are elevated, and skin biopsy provides diagnostic findings.

Rheumatoid nodules are subcutaneous inflammatory lesions usually found over elbows, knees, and fingers in patients with severe rheumatoid arthritis and high rheumatoid factor titer (see Ch. 237).

NODULES ASSOCIATED WITH METABOLIC DISEASES AND MISCELLANEOUS CONDITIONS. *Xanthomas* are focal collections of lipid-containing histiocytes in the dermis and tendon sheaths. They appear as yellowish papules (eruptive xanthomas), plaques (xanthelasma), nodules (xanthoma tuberosum), and xanthomas in tendon and tendon sheaths (xanthoma tendinosum). Xanthomas often arise in association with inherited hyperlipoproteinemias (see Ch. 173) or in several underlying metabolic diseases that alter lipoprotein metabolism, such as diabetes, hypothyroidism, cholestatic liver disease, pancreatitis, renal disease, and certain drug reactions (e.g., 13-*cis*-retinoic acid). Xanthelasma usually develops in the absence of hyperlipidemia, although hypercholesterolemia (and increased low density lipoproteins) may be present.

Patients with gout occasionally deposit sodium urate in the skin, forming firm, hard papules and nodules (tophi) that may discharge whitish crystals in the pinnae of the ears and periarticular areas.

ATROPHIC SKIN CONDITIONS WITH SCARRING, INDURATION, ULCERATION, AND TELANGIECTASIAS

Connective tissue diseases are the most common conditions that lead to this spectrum of cutaneous changes.

SCARRING. *Lupus erythematosus* may be localized to the skin (discoid lupus) or present as a systemic condition (see Ch. 240). Discoid lupus skin lesions appear as red plaques with white, cohesive scales that often are accentuated in the follicular openings (follicular plugging). The plaques eventually atrophy, with depression and scarring along with hypopigmentation in the center of the lesions and a hyperpigmented rim. The lesions usually occur in sun-exposed areas and, when they involve the scalp, cause scarring alopecia. Systemic lupus erythematosus presents as an erythematous rash with a violaceous hue, accentuated in sun-exposed areas, especially the malar area, producing a butterfly configuration. Telangiectasias may also be prominent, and, at times, fine scaling is seen. Occasionally bullae, erosions, and ulcers also occur. Periungual telangiectasia is a prominent finding in systemic lupus as well as in other connective tissue diseases. Subacute lupus is a form in which psoriasiform skin patches are found on the face and trunk. Skin biopsy for both routine and direct immunofluorescence pathologic examination is useful in confirming the diagnosis.

Dermatomyositis findings include violaceous edema of eyelids (heliotrope), flat-topped papules over the knuckles (Gottron's papules), and reticulated patches of hyper- and hypopigmentation, erythema, and telangiectasia (poikiloderma) found on the V of the neck, face, elbows, and knees.

X-radiation can cause chronic skin changes of atrophy, telangiectasias, irregular pigmentation, and eventually ulceration. Within these areas malignant changes may later appear.

DERMAL INDURATIONS (SCLEROSIS). *Scleroderma* is a condition in which excessive collagen is found in the dermis (see Ch. 241). *Morphea* is localized scleroderma confined to the skin, whereas *systemic scleroderma,* or *progressive systemic sclerosis,* is a more extensive form in which fibrosis diffusely involves the skin as well as internal organs (see Ch. 241). Morphea lesions are asymptomatic, oval to irregular, whitish, firm, thickened patches with an erythematous border. The plaques are most often found on the trunk. The thickened skin in progressive systemic sclerosis is not sharply demarcated, but rather causes indurated, "hidebound" tight skin over the fingers, toes, and extremities (acrosclerosis). Thickening of the facial skin causes smoothness and loss of wrinkles except for furrowing around the mouth. Ulcerations followed by pitted scars occur on the finger tips. Telangiectasia may be prominent, appearing as periungual telangiectasias and multiple, small punctate macules on the face and hands (matlike telangiectasia). A variant of systemic scleroderma, the *CREST syndrome,* displays extensive telangiectasias over face and hands. Patients with *hereditary hemorrhagic telangiectasia* also display telangiectasia, particularly around the mouth and nose and on the fingers as well as vascular malformations in the gastrointestinal tract and, at times, the lung. No cutaneous induration is found in this condition.

Lichen sclerosus et atrophicus may be confused with morphea, presenting as porcelain white, atrophic, indurated plaques most commonly on the vulva or on the male genitalia (balanitis xerotica obliterans). At times it occurs as scattered patches on the trunk. Purpuric areas may also be seen within the lesions.

Myxedema may cause a doughy thickening of the skin from deposition of glycosaminoglycans in the dermis. This may be localized to the pretibial areas (pretibial myxedema) as firm, nonpitting plaques and nodules with accentuation of the follicular orifices giving a *peau d'orange* appearance.

CUTANEOUS ULCERS. Primary skin ulcers are caused by a wide variety of conditions. The location of the ulcers, the symptoms associated with them, and the rapidity of their appearance are important clues in diagnosing their various causes.

Ulcers of the extremities are frequently associated with vascular disease. Sudden pain associated with numbness of an extremity and ulceration suggest arterial occlusion. Ulceration of digits associated with a purplish red color with dependency and pallor when the extremity is elevated suggests arteriosclerotic peripheral vascular disease. Brawny edema, brown discoloration, and dermatitis over the lower legs in association with ulcers around the malleoli are seen with venous insufficiency. Sickle cell anemia causes ulcerations in the lower third of the leg. Areas of pressure and trauma, particularly on the foot, in patients with peripheral neuropathy, are susceptible to neurotrophic ulcers *(mal perforans),* as in diabetes and leprosy. The skin around the ulcer is anesthetic and callused. Pressure sores or decubitus ulcers occur in immobilized debilitated patients. Shearing forces, friction, moisture, and pressure contribute to the development of these sores. The sacral and coccygeal areas, ischial tuberosities, and greater trochanters are favored sites. The best treatment of pressure sores is prevention by frequently moving immobilized patients, keeping the skin clean, and using air mattresses.

An unusual and dramatic ulcerative condition, *pyoderma gangrenosum,* often begins as an inflammatory nodule or pustule resembling a furuncle which breaks down, ulcerates, and gradually enlarges peripherally. Fully developed, the lesions are moderately deep, red, necrotic ulcers with undermined, violaceous, edematous borders. These lesions, which typically evolve on the lower legs, are postulated to represent a Shwartzman-like hypersensitivity reaction to a number of underlying internal conditions, including chronic ulcerative colitis, regional ileitis, rheumatoid arthritis, dysproteinemias, and occasionally leukemia or lymphoma. In over one half of the cases no cause is identified.

Ecthyma gangrenosum is characterized by ulcerative lesions, often in the body folds (anogenital and axillary areas), in immunosuppressed patients with *Pseudomonas* septicemia. The painless lesions begin as hemorrhagic bullous patches that become necrotic and ulcerate and are surrounded by considerable erythema with a central gray to black eschar. *Pseudomonas* can be cultured from these skin lesions.

Genital ulcers suggest venereal disease, including herpes simplex (see above), syphilis (indurated, painless, round ulcer with a clean base), chancroid (single or multiple, soft, painful, purulent ulcers with undermined erythematous edges), lymphogranuloma venereum (transient, painless skin ulcer with associated inguinal adenopathy), and granuloma inguinale (small nodules on genitalia which erode and become filled with velvety red granulation).

Multiple genital ulcers also occur in *Behçet's syndrome* in association with oral ulcers and ocular disease (iridocyclitis). Erythema nodosum, arthritis, and neurologic and intestinal involvement may also occur. The oral and genital ulcers are small, painful aphthae. Occasionally sterile pustules and ulcers occur at the site of minor trauma such as blood sampling.

Geometric, bizarre-shaped, angular ulcers are characteristic of a self-inflicted, factitial cause.

HYPER- AND HYPOPIGMENTATION OF THE SKIN

Disorders of melanin pigmentation can be classified as hypomelanoses (decreased or absent epidermal melanin) or hypermelanoses (increased epidermal or dermal melanin). Hyper- and hypomelanosis can be further subdivided into localized or generalized (total body) alterations of pigmentation.

Hyperpigmentary Conditions

LOCALIZED PIGMENTARY CONDITIONS. *Freckles* (ephelides) are light brown-red macules found in sun-exposed areas which are caused by increased melanin production in normal numbers of melanocytes. These occur in fair-complexioned individuals with red or sandy hair. Ultraviolet radiation increases melanin production in these lesions.

Lentigines are also hyperpigmented macules, but they occur because of increased numbers of melanocytes in the basal layer of the epidermis. Two types are recognized: (1) *lentigo simplex,* which occurs in early life and is congenital, and (2) *actinic lentigines,* which are acquired in middle age and are related to sun damage over the face, arms, and dorsum of the hands. Actinic lentigines are sometimes difficult to distinguish from early lentigo maligna on the face, but actinic lentigines have no malignant potential. The *multiple lentigines syndrome* is a rare, dominantly inherited condition characterized by hundreds of lentigines on the trunk, head, extremities, palms, and soles, and it is associated with *E*lectrocardiographic abnormalities, *O*cular hypertelorism, *P*ulmonary stenosis, *A*bnormal genitalia, *R*etarded growth, and *D*eafness (thus the acronym LEOPARD syndrome). Another dominantly inherited condition is *Peutz-Jeghers syndrome,* distinctive for its numerous lentigines occurring around the mouth, eyes, hands, and feet in association with gastrointestinal polyps, gastrointestinal hemorrhage, and occasionally malignant degeneration of the polyps.

Melasma (chloasma) of the face usually affects women, and in this instance the melanocytes produce more melanin than normal in response to hormonal factors (occurs during pregnancy or while on birth control pills) in association with ultraviolet radiation. This type of pigmentation occurs symmetrically over the malar eminences, forehead, and upper lip. The lesions may fade with delivery but often persist and are accentuated when birth control pills are used. Hydroquinone, a bleaching agent (2 to 4% creams), may help reduce the pigmentation, but many authorities believe these are of no value and that they may worsen the problem. Sunscreens are also useful.

Postinflammatory hyperpigmentation is the term given to macular pigmentation following inflammatory skin diseases (lichen planus typically causes brown to blue pigmentation).

Café au lait spots are light brown (coffee-with-cream hue) macules that occur on the trunk and extremities in neurofibromatosis (Fig. 475–9). Six or more such lesions, each greater than 1.5 cm in diameter, are diagnostic for this dominantly inherited disease. Axillary freckling, discrete neurofibromas (Fig. 475–10), and large plexiform neurofibromas along with bony abnormalities combine to make this a disfiguring condition. Ten percent of the normal population have isolated café au lait spots. In *Albright's disease* (polyostotic fibrous dysplasia) three or four large, irregularly shaped (so-called coast-of-Maine configuration), hyperpigmented macules are usually found unilaterally distributed on the buttocks or cervical area.

Xeroderma pigmentosum is a rare, heterogeneous group of diseases with hereditary deficiencies of enzyme systems in the skin that repair ultraviolet-induced damage to keratinocyte and melanocyte DNA. This inability to maintain the integrity of DNA leads to extreme sun sensitivity and multiple freckles over the face, lips, conjunctivae, and extremities which evolve into variably sized pigmented patches interspersed with hypopigmented areas. Keratoses, keratoacanthomas, basal and squamous cell cancers, and malignant melanomas evolve and frequently lead to early death. This entity should be thought of whenever one finds otherwise unexplained extreme sensitivity to the sun or excessive freckling in youngsters. This disease can be subtle in its initial presentation, and total avoidance of the sun from early life may prevent subsequent fatal skin cancers.

GENERALIZED HYPERPIGMENTATION. Diffuse brown hyperpigmentation is a feature of *Addison's disease* with accentuation of the pigment in body folds (palmar creases), pressure points (knuckles, elbows), and gingival mucous membrane. A similar type of diffuse hyperpigmentation is seen following adrenalectomy in patients with Cushing's disease due to a pituitary tumor, as well as in patients with pancreatic and lung carcinomas. In all of these instances the generalized hypermelanosis results from overproduction of melanocyte-stimulating hormone (MSH) and adrenocorticotropic hormone (ACTH). These trophic hormones share common amino acid sequences. Both MSH and ACTH secretions are increased in Addison's disease as a result of diminished output of cortisol by the adrenals. Oat cell cancers of the lung and pancreatic carcinomas

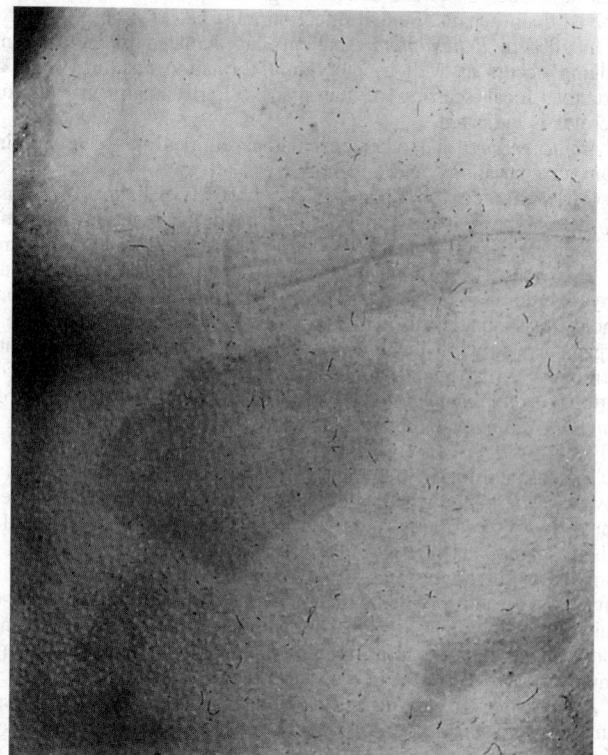

FIGURE 475–9. Café au lait spot. (From the 17th edition of the Cecil Textbook of Medicine, with the permission of Dr. Marie-Louise Johnson.)

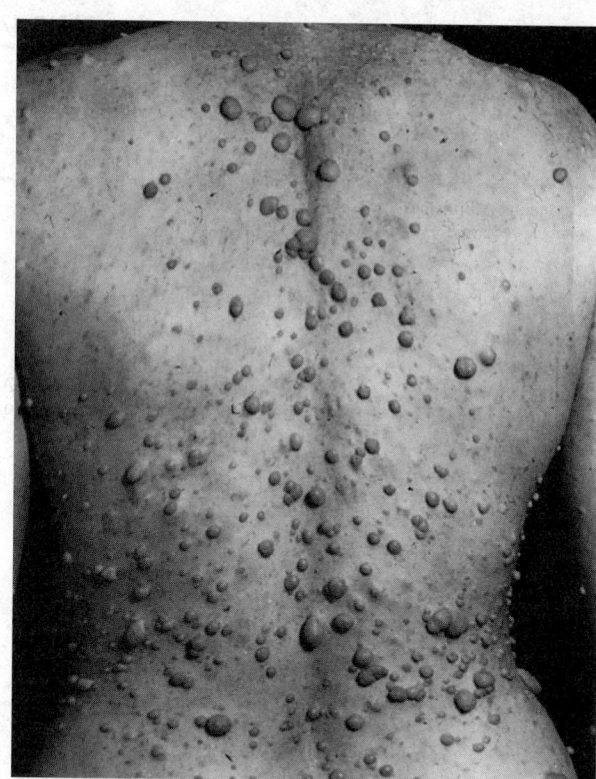

FIGURE 475–10. Neurofibromatosis—von Recklinghausen's disease. (From the 17th edition of the Cecil Textbook of Medicine, with the permission of Dr. Marie-Louise Johnson.)

have been found to excrete increased amounts of MSH, thus causing similar hyperpigmentation. Melanocyte MSH receptors bind MSH, which stimulates intracellular cyclic AMP, and this, in turn, increases tyrosinase activity and pigment formation in melanocytes.

A number of drugs can cause Addisonian-like hypermelanosis including busulfan, cyclophosphamide, and nitrogen mustard. Blue-gray pigmentation may occur either diffusely or in localized patches following use of chlorpromazine, minocycline, and antimalarial drugs. In addition, inorganic trivalent arsenicals (found in insecticides and contaminated water) may also produce a generalized brown pigmentation, but in this instance the hypermelanosis is studded with small, scattered, depigmented macules (likened to rain drops on a dusty road) and punctate keratoses on the palms and soles. *Hemochromatosis* causes a metallic gray-brown, generalized hyperpigmentation resulting from the combination of increased pigment formation in the skin and iron deposition.

Hypopigmentary Conditions

LOCALIZED PIGMENTARY CHANGES. *Vitiligo*, a circumscribed hypomelanosis of progressively enlarging amelanotic macules in a symmetric distribution around body orifices and over bony prominences (knees, elbows, hands), is familial in 36% of cases. In one third of cases some spontaneous repigmentation occurs, particularly in sun-exposed areas. White hairs are common in the vitiliginous areas. Although most patients with vitiligo are healthy, there is an increased association with certain autoimmune conditions such as thyroiditis, hyperthyroidism, Addison's disease, pernicious anemia, and diabetes mellitus. Melanocytes are absent from the vitiliginous macules. Circulating complement-binding antimelanocyte antibodies have been found in some vitiligo patients. The use of PUVA may give some repigmentation, but it may require 200 or more such treatments.

Piebaldism is a local hypopigmentary condition representing an autosomal dominant hypomelanosis on the extremities, anterior surface of the thorax, and especially over the midline of the forehead and central scalp. A white forelock is typical. The hypomelanosis stems from the lack of normal migration of the melanocytes to these regions during embryologic development.

TABLE 475–9. ALBINISM

	Inheritance	Frequency	Skin Color	Pigmented Nevi Freckles	Hair	Eyes Color	Red Reflex
Oculocutaneous Albinism Tyrosinase-negative	AR*	1 in 34,000	pink/white	none	white	gray-blue	present
Tyrosinase-positive	AR	blacks: 1 in 15,000 whites: 1 in 40,000	white-cream	present	white-yellow red; darkens	blue-yellow brown	present but may be absent in dark races
Yellow-mutant	AR	rare—Amish, Polish, German-American; blacks (American, Ceylonese, African)	white at birth, slightly tan possible	present	white-birth red/yellow 6 mos	blue at birth; darkens	present
Chédiak-Higashi syndrome	AR	rare in most countries; none in blacks	pink/white	present	blond-dark brown-steel gray	blue to brown	present but diminishes with time
Oculocutaneous Albinoidism	AD†		pink/white	?	white blond	blue	present
Ocular Albinism Vogt	X-linked	uncommon	normal	present	normal	blue	
Forsius-Eriksson	X-linked	less common	normal	present	normal	blue	
Autosomal recessive	AR	10 families	normal	present	normal	blue	present

A common localized form of hypopigmentation, *pityriasis alba,* appears as slightly pink and hypopigmented, oval to round patches with mild, fine scaling. These occur on the cheeks of children, but they may also be found on the trunk, mimicking the hypopigmented, scaling patches seen in tinea versicolor (a KOH examination of the scales may be necessary to differentiate these two conditions). Pityriasis alba is most frequently seen in atopic dermatitis patients.

Tuberous sclerosis, an autosomal dominant condition, displays white macules in almost all cases. The depigmented macules involve the trunk or buttocks in an oval or mountain ash-leaf configuration. The presence of three or more macules strongly suggests tuberous sclerosis, and because the hypomelanotic patches are present at birth, they represent one of the earliest signs of the condition. Examination with Wood's light is often useful in visualizing the lesions, which histologically contain melanocytes with decreased numbers of melanosomes. Newborns with unexplained seizures or mental retardation should be screened with a Wood's light for the presence of the white spots. Ch. 417 gives details of the systemic disorder. CT brain scans are also useful in defining the tumorous dysplasia.

Certain chemicals, particularly phenol derivatives, when applied to the skin, may cause permanent depigmentation. Hypomelanosis has been observed on the hands of black-skinned individuals wearing rubber gloves in which hydroquinone is used as an antioxidant.

GENERALIZED HYPOPIGMENTATION. (Albinism). Table 475–9 lists these hereditary disorders, all of which produce generalized hypomelanosis of the skin, hair, and eyes.

REGIONAL DIAGNOSIS OF SKIN DISEASES—COMMONLY ENCOUNTERED PROBLEMS BY ANATOMIC REGION

Many skin diseases have a predilection for certain areas or regions of the body, often related to variations in the structure and function of the integument (Table 475–10).

Disorders of the Nails

The nail is a plate of hard keratin synthesized from an invagination of the epidermis. The proximal nail fold houses the matrix of the nail where basal cells rapidly proliferate and differentiate into the nail plate, which grows over the nail bed. Nails grow continuously throughout life. The average fingernail grows 0.5 to 1.2 mm per week, whereas toenails grow at one half to one third this rate. It takes a fingernail about 5.5 months and the toenails 12 to 18 months to regrow from the matrix, although rate of growth slows as the individual gets older. Table 475–11 provides a terminology to describe defects in nail formation.

SKIN DISEASES INVOLVING NAILS. Nail changes in *psoriasis* have been described above. Fingernails are more frequently involved than toenails. Fungal infection must be ruled out.

In 10% of *lichen planus* patients, accentuated longitudinal nail ridging occurs as well as pterygium formation resulting from destructive focal scarring of the matrix. Early treatment with oral steroids is indicated.

Atopic eczema and other eczematous entities may cause pitting, transverse striations, and onycholysis.

Onychomycosis, or fungal infections of the nail, may be caused by dermatophyte (tinea unguium) or candidal infections. Infection of toenails is more frequent than fingernails, but all nails may be involved. The nail plate is discolored, thickened, crumbly, and onycholytic with accumulation of debris. White superficial onychomycosis appears as white patches in the toenail plate due to organisms growing on the surface barely penetrating the nail. Scrapings reveal hyphae upon KOH examination. An unusual condition, *chronic mucocutaneous candidiasis,* is caused by widespread *Candida albicans* infection leading to diffuse white thickening of all nails.

Topical antifungal therapy is ineffective. Oral griseofulvin is given for dermatophyte infection until the nails appear clear. Ketoconazole (200 mg daily) is an alternative should griseofulvin fail or when *Candida* is the causative agent. Oral therapy requires 4 to 6 months for fingernails and 12 to 16 months for toenails. In older individuals toenail problems may never be eradicated because the nails grow so slowly. Residual fungal spores in shoes and the environment no doubt cause frequent recurrences; topical antifungal powders may be helpful in long-term prophylaxis.

Paronychia, or painful, red swelling of the nail fold, is usually caused by *C. albicans.* At times a small abscess or purulent discharge is seen. This infection usually occurs in hands constantly exposed to a wet environment (bartenders, janitors). Therapy consists

TABLE 475–9. ALBINISM (Continued)

	Eyes				Hair Bulb Incubation (Tyrosine)	Defect	Melanosome Maturation by Stage	Complications or Associated Problems
Nystagmus	Photophobia	Visual Acuity	Pigment in Fundus	Other				
marked	severe	legally blind	none	–	negative	no tyrosinase	I-unmelan-ized II	skin malignancy basal cell ca squamous cell ca
present but less	present but variable	severe defect in children; may improve with age	none; some with age	pigment cart-wheel effect pupil, limbus	positive	no access of en-zyme to tyro-sine	I, II, some III, rare IV	skin malignancy basal cell ca squamous cell ca
present but variable	present but variable	marked defect; may improve with age	none; some with age	pigment cart-wheel effect	neg to pos?	unknown ? pheomelano-genesis	I, II, III	unknown
absent or slight	absent or slight	normal or slight decrease	some; increase with age	normal for cart-wheel effect	positive	giant melano-somes, lethal defect in leukocytes	I, II, III, IV	infections; hematologic and neuro-logic abnor-malities; lym-phoreticular malignancy
no	no	normal or slight decrease	punctate		positive	unknown	unknown	none
present	severe	marked decrease	reduced		positive			
latent	absent or slight	color blind			positive			
present	severe	marked decrease			positive			

* AR = Autosomal recessive.
† AD = Autosomal dominant.
Reprinted from the chapter by Dr. Marie-Louise Johnson in the 17th edition of the Cecil Textbook of Medicine, with her permission.

of avoidance of water and the use of antifungal solutions two or three times a day for a month or two.

NAIL DISTURBANCES IN SYSTEMIC DISEASES. *Splinter hemorrhages* result from the extravasation of blood from longitudinally oriented vessels of the nail bed. Although often thought to be associated with bacterial endocarditis, they are much more commonly associated with trauma. *Beau's lines* are nonspecific, appearing as transverse depressions across the nail plates following any severe disability that temporarily interferes with nail growth. *Longitudinal pigmented bands* occur most often in response to trauma or a nevus located in the matrix. *Yellow nail syndrome* exhibits yellow thickening of the nails with absence of the lunula and variable degrees of onycholysis accompanying pulmonary conditions such as bronchiectasis, pleural effusion, and chronic obstructive pulmonary disease. Lymphedema of the extremities may coexist. *Clubbing* of the nails (increased bilateral curvature of the nails with enlargement of the soft connective tissue of the distal phalanges resulting in the flattening of the obtuse angle formed by the proximal end of the nail and the digit) occurs most often with bronchiectasis, lung abscess, and pulmonary neoplasms. Cardiovascular disease and chronic gastrointestinal diseases (ulcerative colitis, sprue) are also associated with clubbing. Clubbing accompanied by bone pain and proliferative periostitis is termed *hypertrophic osteoarthropathy*. The condition is most often associated with bronchogenic squamous cell carcinoma.

TUMORS OF THE NAIL. A variety of benign tumors occur around the nail unit. These include *periungual fibromas, myxoid cysts,* and *subungual exostoses*. Surgical removal is the only certain means of cure.

The main malignant tumor involving the nails is *melanoma,* which appears as a pigmented area at the base of the nail or as a longitudinal pigmented streak in the nail. Nevi can give the same appearance, and biopsy of the lesion in the matrix is the only absolutely certain way of making a diagnosis.

Disorders of the Mucous Membranes

Any abnormality of color, texture, or appearance of the mucous membranes should be investigated. Malignant changes should be suspected in infiltrated or ulcerated lesions and a biopsy performed.

Ch. 96 discusses disorders of the oral mucous membranes, the tongue, and the salivary glands.

Alterations of Hair Growth

HAIR LOSS (ALOPECIA)

Physical, chemical, and emotional events cause fluctuations in hair growth and if severe enough may stop growth entirely. The physical examination is important in noting the pattern of hair loss and whether or not scarring is present. Nonscarring alopecia may be a temporary phenomenon, whereas scarring is indicative of permanent hair loss.

NONSCARRING ALOPECIA. Localized Alopecia. *Alopecia areata* is characterized by well-circumscribed, round or oval patches of nonscarring hair loss, usually over the scalp or in the beard, eyebrows, or eyelashes. Erythema may be present early in the course of the patches. Characteristically the periphery of patches of hair loss is studded with fractured hairs with tapered shafts. Histologic features include small dystrophic hair follicles and a lymphocytic infiltrate around the hair bulbs. Occasionally all the scalp hair is lost (alopecia totalis), and all the body hair may fall out (alopecia universalis). Alopecia areata has a variable, unpredictable course. Most patients regrow hair within a few months, but one fourth of them experience recurrences. The more extensive the alopecia, the poorer the prognosis. Alopecia involving the occipital region or eyebrows, lashes, and nasal hairs portends a poor prognosis. Alopecia areata may have an autoimmune pathogenesis, being occasionally associated with Hashimoto's thyroiditis and pernicious anemia. Topical, intralesional, and systemic steroids give variable benefits. Recent modes of therapy include induction of allergic or irritant contact dermatitis (1% anthralin, or topical dinitrochlorobenzene), photochemotherapy with PUVA, and topical minoxidil.

Tinea capitis is most likely to be confused with alopecia areata. Tinea infection appears as one or more patches of hair loss with mild scaling and erythema and broken hair shafts leaving residual black stumps (black dot ringworm). Nonfluorescing *Trichophyton tonsurans* is the usual cause. Griseofulvin is the drug of choice.

Trichotillomania refers to traumatic, self-induced alopecia and results from compulsive twisting and rubbing, which causes breaking

TABLE 475–10. REGIONAL DERMATOLOGY

Region of Skin	Type of Skin Group	Disease Process
Scalp	Papulosquamous and eczematous	Psoriasis, seborrheic dermatitis, tinea capitis, eczema (atopic, contact)
	Pustular	Folliculitis, kerion
	Nodular	Nevi, seborrheic keratosis, pilar cysts, verruca
	Atropic and telangiectatic	Connective tissue disease, scleroderma, discoid LE
Face	Pustular	Acne, rosacea, folliculitis, tinea
	Papulosquamous and eczematous	Psoriasis, seborrheic dermatitis, contact dermatitis (cosmetics), atopic dermatitis, impetigo, lupus erythematosus, photodermatitis
	Vesicular	Herpes zoster and herpes simplex, insect bites
	Nodular	Basal cell cancers, squamous cell cancers, melanomas, keratoacanthomas, nevi, actinic keratosis
Trunk	Papulosquamous and eczematous	Psoriasis, atopic and contact eczema, tinea versicolor, pityriasis rosacea, scabies
	Vesiculobullous	Pemphigus, bullous pemphigoid
	Maculopapular	Secondary syphilis, drug reaction, viral exanthems
	Nodular	Nevi, seborrheic keratosis, lipoma, basal cell cancer, keloid, neurofibroma, angiomas, melanoma
	Pustular	Acne
	Urticarial	Hives
Arms and forearms	Eczematous and papulosquamous	Contact dermatitis—plants; atopic dermatitis, lichen planus
	Nodular	Nevi, warts, seborrheic keratosis, actinic keratosis
	Atrophic telangiectasis	Scleroderma, dermatomyositis
Legs	Eczematous and papulosquamous	Contact dermatitis, stasis dermatitis, atopic dermatitis, psoriasis, lichen planus
	Nodular	Erythema nodosum, dermatofibromas, nevi, melanoma, Kaposi's sarcoma, lipoma
	Maculopapular	Vasculitis, Schamberg's disease, actinic purpura, pretibial myxedema
	Atrophic, telangiectatic, and ulcerative	Scleroderma, dermatostasis ulcers, arterial insufficiency
Genitalia and groin	Eczematous and papulosquamous	Contact dermatitis, seborrheic dermatitis, scabies, pediculosis pubis, psoriasis, Reiter's syndrome, erythrasma, tinea, candidiasis, lichen planus, intertrigo, lichen simplex chronicus
	Vesiculobullous	Herpes simplex, Stevens-Johnson syndrome
	Ulcerative and atrophic	Syphilis, chancroid, lymphopathia venereum, Behçet's syndrome
	Nodular	Verrucae vulgaris, erythroplasia of Queyrat, squamous cell cancer, sebaceous cyst, molluscum contagiosum
	Pustular	Hidradenitis suppurativa
Hands	Eczematous and papulosquamous	Allergic contact and irritant contact dermatitis, dyshidrosis, pyoderma, tinea, dermatophytids, scabies, atopic dermatitis, secondary syphilis
	Vesiculobullous, pustular	Erythema multiforme, hand-foot-and-mouth disease, porphyria cutanea tarda, psoriasis
	Nodular	Warts, squamous cell cancer, actinic keratosis, keratoacanthoma, pyogenic granuloma, granuloma annulare, synovial cysts
	Hypopigmented	Vitiligo
	Atrophic-telangiectatic	Scleroderma, dermatomyositis
Feet	Eczematous and papulosquamous	Contact dermatitis, atopic dermatitis, tinea, psoriasis, lichen planus
	Vesiculobullous	Tinea, epidermolysis bullosa, erythema multiforme
	Nodules	Verruca, corn, nevus
	Atrophic-telangiectatic	Scleroderma

and epilation of the hair shafts. The scalp is usually affected, less often the eyebrows and lashes. If the patient can be given insight, the condition it is self-limited. More severe emotional problems should be referred to a psychiatrist.

Women who develop hair thinning at the margins of the scalp may be using excessive traction or other traumatic hair styling techniques *(traction alopecia)*. Overtight hair curling such as corn rowing and the use of hot combs to straighten hair leads to progressive hair thinning and even scarring.

Hair loss is sometimes seen in the scalp of patients with *secondary syphilis*. The hair loss is spotty, often "moth-eaten" in appearance.

Androgenic alopecia, or male pattern baldness, involves the frontal, vertex, and upper occipital regions of the scalp while spar-

TABLE 475–11. POTENTIAL DEFECTS IN NAIL FORMATION

Brittleness—easy breaking of nail tips
Leukonychia—white discoloration of nails
Striations—longitudinal ridges running parallel or perpendicular to the length of the nail
Onycholysis—separation of the nail plate from the bed
Onychogryphosis—hypertrophy and thickening of the nail
Onychomycosis—dystrophy, destruction of the nail due to yeast and fungal infections
Pitting—discrete pitlike depressions in the nail surface
Koilonychia—spoon-shaped deformity of the nails (concave nail with everted edges)
Pterygium formation—growth of cuticle onto the nail plate

ing the posterior and lateral margins. The process may begin at any age after puberty, with temporal recession of hair usually noted first. There is no actual loss of hair but rather the conversion of thick terminal hairs to fine, unpigmented, poorly seen vellus hairs. Common baldness is genetically predetermined and androgen dependent. Males who are castrated prepubertally or men born with low testosterone production, as in Klinefelter's syndrome, do not become bald, regardless of their genetic predisposition to balding. Women may also show balding, but it is milder with only diffuse thinning. Women with elevated androgen levels, as occur in masculinizing disorders, have baldness in a pattern similar to that in men. Surgical techniques such as hair transplants (plugs of hair-bearing areas from the sides of the scalp placed in the thinned frontal and crown areas) or scalp reduction may be useful in some patients. Thinning of hair growth is characteristic of old age in both genders.

Diffuse or Generalized Alopecia. Stress alopecia, or *telogen effluvium,* is a transient, reversible, diffuse hair loss of scalp hair that results from alterations in the normal hair cycle (see Ch. 472). Severe emotional and physiologic stress (high fever, systemic illness, major surgery with general anesthesia, crash diet) and certain drugs (heparin, coumarin, allopurinol, amphetamines, β-blocking agents, lithium, probenecid, thiouracil) may cause growing hairs to convert to resting hairs, which are subsequently shed. Pregnancy and oral contraceptives cause hairs to grow continually, rather than cycling at programmed times. After childbirth or discontinuation of oral contraceptives, growing follicles "catch up" by simultaneously resting; shedding follows 2 to 4 months later. If the stress resolves, the hair regrows in 4 to 6 months. Diffuse hair loss may not be noticeable until there is greater than 50% scalp hair loss. Gentle pulling of the hair verifies the degree of shedding; if more than five hairs come out when a dozen are grasped, excessive shedding is present.

Toxic alopecia occurs if hair growth is disrupted. Newly synthesized hair shafts are weakened and the hair breaks readily. Thinning may be extreme, occurring within a few weeks of an insult, involving all 80% of actively growing follicles. Chemotherapeutic agents, especially doxorubicin and related agents, exert their effect on rapidly growing cells in the hair bulb and commonly cause hair damage in cancer patients receiving chemotherapy. Radiation therapy to the scalp area does the same thing. *Retinoids* and *hypervitaminosis A* cause hair loss owing to their interference with keratinization.

Diffuse hair loss over the scalp occurs in *hypothyroidism*, associated with hair that is dry and brittle, and severe malnutrition.

Seborrheic dermatitis, with erythema and yellow, greasy scales throughout the scalp, may be associated with mild, diffuse hair loss. Treatment with tar shampoos and topical steroids to control the inflammatory response reverses the condition.

Diffuse scalp hair loss can follow *hair shaft weakness*, either acquired (due to braiding, permanent wave solutions, or excessive heat when drying or straightening hair) or congenital. Patients with congenital hair weakness have sparse fine or wiry hair from early childhood.

SCARRING ALOPECIA. Scarring alopecias display atrophy of the scalp and absence of hair follicles. Cicatricial areas of hair loss can result from a variety of pathologic processes that permanently destroy the hair follicles.

Localized Scarring Alopecia. Systemic lupus erythematosus causes diffuse, nonscarring alopecia of the scalp in 20% of patients, along with short, broken (lupus) hairs in the frontal margin. *Discoid lupus erythematosus* causes oval scarring areas of alopecia. Typical plaques have an active erythematous margin, white atrophic center, and telangiectasias and keratin-filled follicles.

Morphea, when it involves the scalp, causes firm, hairless, ivory colored, indurated lesions. At times morphea takes on linear patterns that simulate saber wound (*en coup de sabre*).

A number of *physical injuries* such as mechanical trauma, burns, and radiation dermatitis may also cause local scarring alopecias.

Nonlocalized Scarring Alopecia. Lichen planus may cause diffuse, patchy scarring alopecia (*lichen planopilaris*). Typical lichen planus lesions are often found in other areas of the body. Biopsy may help in the diagnosis.

HIRSUTISM (EXCESSIVE HAIR GROWTH)

Excessive hair growth, usually a complaint of females, may be due to either endocrinologic or nonendocrinologic conditions. When women are affected in those areas of the body which normally develop hair as a secondary sex characteristic in males, their hirsutism generally reflects treatable endocrinopathy, as these follicles respond to high concentrations of testosterone and can convert various androgens to dihydrotestosterone (see Ch. 472).

NONENDOCRINE HIRSUTISM. *Ethnic* or *racial hirsutism* is characterized by excessive hair growth on the upper lip, beard area, chest, nipples, or lower abdomen in women without menstrual abnormalities or masculization. Type of hair, rate of hair growth, and distribution of hair over the body differ among the races, relating to variations in the sensitivity of follicles to circulating androgens. A male pattern of hirsutism is more common in females whose ancestors came from the southern parts of Europe. Asians and native Americans have less body hair. If serum testosterone, dehydroepiandrosterone, and androstenedione are normal, bleaching or shaving may make the hair less noticeable. Electrolysis permanently destroys hair follicles but is time consuming and costly. Spironolactone,* which has antiandrogenic properties (200 mg per day), used for a period of 12 months is also useful in decreasing hair growth.

Certain *drugs* may increase hair growth. Androgenic or steroidal medications, such as anabolic steroids, corticosteroids, and contraceptives may cause increased hair growth in the beard, chest, and groin areas. Drugs such as phenytoin, phenothiazines, cyclosporine, and minoxidil cause excess hair in both men and women anywhere on the body.

---

* This use is not listed in the manufacturer's directive.

ENDOCRINE HIRSUTISM. A distinction must be made between hirsutism caused by increased androgen production with and without virilization. In general, virilization is a sign of markedly elevated androgens derived from the adrenal glands or ovaries, especially adrenogenital syndrome, congenital adrenal hyperplasia, Cushing's disease or syndrome, Stein-Leventhal syndrome (polycystic ovarian syndrome), and occasionally malignant adrenal or ovarian tumors. Any woman with hirsutism and accompanying virilization should be tested for excess cortisol and androgen production.

Simple or *idiopathic hirsutism* denotes hirsute women in whom a specific diagnosis cannot be made and who have normal or slightly elevated adrenal or ovarian androgens. Such patients have been successfully treated with cyclically administered birth control pills or with spironolactone.

PHOTOSENSITIVITY AND OTHER REACTIONS TO LIGHT

Certain wavelengths of light can induce a number of undesirable cutaneous reactions, including sunburn, skin aging, carcinogenesis, and a variety of photosensitivity reactions (see Fig. 473–1).

The solar spectrum that commonly affects human skin is in the ultraviolet light range (290 to 400 nm), which is subdivided into three bands designated as UVC (shorter than 290 nm), UVB (290 to 320 nm), and UVA, or long-wave ultraviolet light (320 to 400 nm). UVC does not reach the earth, being absorbed by ozone; UVB, or the sunburn spectrum, causes burning, tanning, aging, and carcinogenic changes in the skin. UVA is melanogenic and erythrogenic, but the amount of energy required to produce these effects is 1000 times greater than UVB. UVA causes skin reactions through window glass, and these wavelengths are often responsible for photoreactions in which chemical photosensitizers and UV radiation interact to cause inflammatory skin reactions.

The incidence of photoreactions depends on a number of factors such as the amount of light reaching the earth's surface, season of the year, latitude and weather conditions, and thickness of the ozone layer, as well as topographic features of the environment. Certain climatologic and environmental factors influence the amount of sunlight hitting the skin. For example, 50% of the daily ultraviolet light is emitted between 11 A.M. and 2 P.M.: Avoiding exposure during this time may minimize photoreactions. Sitting in the shade does not protect against UV exposure, because 50% of the ambient ultraviolet light is received; 90% of ultraviolet light penetrates clouds, so one can get sunburns even in the shade and on cloudy days.

Direct Photo Effects on the Skin

ACUTE EFFECTS. Sunburning and tanning are attributed primarily to UVB light, although prolonged exposure to UVA can produce mild burn and marked hyperpigmentation. The sunburn reaction produces a complex inflammatory process causing dyskeratotic cells, spongiosis, vacuolation of keratinocytes, and edema from capillary leakage, 12 to 24 hours after exposure. Occasionally, in addition to redness and pain, blisters may evolve. Prostaglandins may play a role in the burn reaction, as they are found in increased quantities in sunburned skin. Aspirin, indomethacin, or prostaglandin synthesis inhibitors can reduce the burn.

Three to 4 days after a sunburn, new melanin pigment is formed. Several cellular and molecular changes occur in the skin after each sunburn reaction which, if repeated, may lead to the chronic effects of UV light. A few days after UV light burning, epidermal mitosis and hyperplasia occur and DNA, RNA, and proteins in the skin are damaged.

CHRONIC EFFECTS. Degenerative changes of the skin consisting of wrinkling, telangiectasias, and keratoses result from chronic exposure to UV light. The skin may become furrowed and leathery and develop yellow papules and plaques due to degeneration of the dermal collagen. These changes are caused by both UVB and UVA radiation. Such changes can be minimized by daily topical applications of effective sunscreens.

A number of malignant and premalignant skin lesions are associated with chronic sun exposure, including actinic keratoses, keratoacanthomas, basal cell and squamous cell carcinomas, and probably melanomas.

Indirect Photo Effects on the Skin

Photoreactions that occur when systemic or topical chemicals induce photosensitivity or when there is an underlying immunologic, biochemical, or genetic abnormality that predisposes to sun sensitivity are considered indirect reactions; that is, the sun alone does not cause photoreactions.

EXOGENOUS FACTORS CAUSING PHOTOSENSITIVITY. Chemical agents either taken systemically or placed topically on the skin can cause one of two general types of photoreactions: phototoxic and photoallergic. In photosensitivity reactions, the absorption spectrum of a given drug, substance, or chemical is maximal at a certain wavelength of light that induces molecular changes in the exogenous material. These initiate the cutaneous reaction. In most drug or chemical photosensitivity reactions, the wavelengths that evoke abnormal reactions are in the 320 to 400 nm (UVA) region. The reactions include acute, abnormal sunburn responses and eczematous and urticarial reactions.

Phototoxic reactions are nonimmunologic cutaneous responses that occur when a drug or chemical in the skin absorb enough light energy of a specific wavelength. The photosensitizer generates free radicals that damage cell membranes and lysosomes, inducing an exaggerated sunburn reaction, with intense redness, swelling, pain, and occasionally blistering. Most phototoxic agents absorb UVB light.

Photoallergic reactions to topical chemicals or internal drugs represent an acquired, immunogenically altered response to light. Absorption of specific wavelengths of light by chemicals or drugs causes changes in their chemical configuration so that these substances become haptens that bind to proteins in the skin to become a complete antigen capable of eliciting a type IV delayed hypersensitivity immunologic response. The clinical manifestations of such photoallergic reactions are usually eczematous in nature (occasionally urticarial), evolving in exposed areas 24 hours after exposure to the sun. The action spectrum is generally long-range UVA light.

SYSTEMIC PHOTOSENSITIZERS. Drugs may cause either phototoxic or photoallergic reactions. Table 475–12 lists some of the drugs and chemicals that may induce photosensitivities and the type of reaction and action spectrum thought to induce them.

TOPICAL AGENTS CAUSING PHOTOSENSITIVITY. Most topical photosensitizing agents respond to the UVA action spectrum. Drugs and chemicals that induce *phototoxic contact reactions* include coal tar derivatives, topical drugs (phenothiazines, sulfonamides), dyes (eosins, methylene blue), and plant derivatives (furocoumarins). The photosensitive properties of coal tar derivatives and furocoumarins (psoralens) are utilized in treating certain skin diseases with ultraviolet light.

When plants, vegetables, or fruits containing a phototoxic chemical cause phototoxicity, the reaction is referred to as a *phytophotodermatitis.* Photocontact dermatitis develops with contact with

plants in the Umbelliferae family, such as figs, cow parsnip, fennel, parsley, parsnip, and gas plant. Phytophotodermatitis also occurs in individuals exposed to Persian limes and celery. Such reactions are caused by furocoumarin compounds found in the plant which readily penetrate the epidermis. Two things are needed for initiation of phytophotodermatitis: (1) contact with a sensitizing furocoumarin and (2) subsequent exposure to UV radiation greater than 320 nm. Phytophotodermatitis may take on unique clinical forms: (1) berloque dermatitis presents as streaky erythema followed by hyperpigmentation in areas where perfumes containing oil of Bergamot (a psoralen) are applied to the skin (e.g., on the neck); (2) crisscross linear streaks of erythema, vesicles, and bullae that heal with hyperpigmentation where meadow grass or other related plants rub on the skin; (3) oil of the rind of a Persian lime causes erythema and pigmentation on the hands of bartenders.

Photoallergic contact dermatitis, a form of delayed eczematous reaction, evolves in some individuals after exposure to chemicals such as fragrances (methylcoumarin and musk ambrette), halogenated salicylanilides, sunscreens, and blankophores, or optical whitening agents, used in laundry soaps and bleaches. A number of perfumes (e.g., after-shave lotions, colognes) contain musk ambrette, a synthetic fragrance fixative that causes a photoeczematous reaction over the face and hands. Sunscreening agents containing PABA esters and cinnamates that readily absorb UV light may cause eczematous reactions. A small number of individuals have persistent chronic eczematous dermatitis after all exposure to the photosensitizing agent has ceased—so-called persistent light reactivity; they even may react to artificial fluorescent light.

Identifying the cause of contact photoallergic reactions can be done with photopatch testing (see Ch. 473). Treatment begins by eliminating the photosensitizing agent and minimizing exposure (avoiding sun and use of sunscreens). Topical or oral steroids may be needed to decrease the cutaneous inflammatory response.

ENDOGENOUS CONDITIONS ASSOCIATED WITH PHOTOSENSITIVITY. *Immunologic diseases with photosensitivity* include connective tissue conditions such as lupus erythematosus, both discoid and systemic, and solar urticaria. Solar urticaria, hives with itching and burning, evolves within minutes of sunlight exposure and lasts an hour or more.

Biochemical conditions associated with photosensitivity include porphyria cutanea tarda and erythropoietic protoporphyria.

Pellagra, is caused by an inadequate diet and a deficiency of nicotinic acid. It is still seen occasionally with alcoholism, poor dietary intake in the elderly, and malabsorption. The carcinoid syndrome may also be associated with pellagra because tryptophan, the precursor of nicotinic acid, is diverted to serotonin production by the tumor. A scaly dermatitis affects sun-exposed parts of the skin, especially on the face, the neck, and the back of the hands, in association with diarrhea and dementia. Dietary replacement clears the skin and other signs of the disease.

Other Photosensitivity Conditions

Polymorphous light eruption (PMLE) causes eczematous patches, red to violaceous papules or plaques, and urticarial lesions over the face, the nape and V of the neck, and the back of the hands. The rash characteristically arises hours to days after sun exposure. The onset is frequently in early summer with some degree of resistance being acquired with continued sun exposure. Recurrences each spring and summer are common, and the eruption remits during the winter. The disease is most frequent during the first half of life. The cause is unknown.

DERMATOLOGIC MANIFESTATIONS IN THE IMMUNOCOMPROMISED HOST AND IN AIDS

Immunosuppression causes an increase in benign and malignant skin growths as well as a variety of infections in the skin (see Ch. 266). Cutaneous neoplasms such as squamous cell and basal cell carcinomas occur with a higher than expected frequency. Transplant patients have a risk of skin cancer seven times greater than normal.

Any skin lesion, no matter how innocuous, should be carefully evaluated in the immunosuppressed host. The gross morphology of infections is so frequently modified by the altered inflammatory response that early skin biopsies are essential for diagnosis. The array of potential pathogens is imposing in these patients, and even common infectious processes are greatly modified or obscured by immunocompromising illness. Skin infections are common, accounting for 22 to 33% of infections in immunosuppressed patients.

TABLE 475–12. SYSTEMIC PHOTOSENSITIZERS

Name	Type of Photoreaction	Action Spectrum (nm)
Sulfonamides	Phototoxic and photoallergic	290–320
Sulfonylureas (tolbutamide, chlorpropamide)	Phototoxic	290–360
Chlorothiazides	Phototoxic and photoallergic	290–320 320–400
Phenothiazines	Phototoxic, urticaria eruption, gray-blue hyperpigmentation	290–400
Antibiotics (tetracyclines, griseofulvin, nalidixic acid)	Phototoxic and photoallergic bullae	320–400
Furocoumarins (psoralens)	Phototoxic	
Nonsteroidal anti-inflammatory agents	Phototoxic and photoallergic	Unknown
Anticancer drugs (DTIC, fluorouracil, methotrexate, vinblastin)	Phototoxic	Unknown
Estrogens, progestins, and other drugs	Phototoxic, melasma	?290–320
Chlordiazepoxide (Librium)	Photoallergic	290–360
Cyclamates	Phototoxic and photoallergic	290–360
Quinidine, quinine	Photoallergic	320–400

Microbial involvement of the skin and subcutaneous tissue can be grouped into two major categories in immunocompromised patients: (1) *primary skin infections* include those occurring in nonimmunocompromised hosts, and primary skin infections from opportunistic agents that rarely cause skin infection in normal patients; and (2) *disseminated systemic infections* metastatic to the skin from a noncutaneous portal of entry.

PRIMARY SKIN INFECTIONS. Typical primary skin infections, including group A streptococcal and *S. aureus* cellulitis, are frequent, although more unusual causes of cellulitis in granulocytopenic patients must also be considered (*Pseudomonas*, anaerobic bacteria). Skin biopsy of the cellulitic areas for Gram stain and culture is often helpful.

Primary cutaneous infections by viruses and skin dermatophytes are also common. Warts caused by papillomavirus may be numerous and difficult to remove. Malignant transformation has been documented. Herpes simplex infections may present as chronic, large, ulcerated lesions persisting for weeks to months (herpes phagedena, especially in the genital areas), and there may be internal dissemination from cutaneous sites. Reactivation of herpes zoster infections is common with systemic dissemination. Widespread dermatophyte infections of the skin appear as scaling, red patches that provide a portal of entry for bacterial infection.

Unusual opportunistic primary skin infections with atypical *Mycobacterium, Aspergillus, Rhizopus,* and *Candida* organisms cause cellulitis-like reactions that form a central pustule and eschar. Skin biopsy of such lesions with a portion of the biopsy processed by frozen section and specially stained for AFB and fungi may identify the pathologic organisms rapidly.

DISSEMINATED INFECTION METASTATIC TO THE SKIN. Hematogenous dissemination of infection to the skin from distant primary sites frequently occurs in patients with impaired host defenses. Three groups of organisms are responsible: (1) *Pseudomonas* and other gram-negative bacilli; (2) endemic systemic mycoses *(Histoplasma, Coccidioides);* and (3) opportunistic fungi (*Aspergillus, Candida,* Mucoraceae). The range of cutaneous clinical presentations of these infections is varied and mimicked by all: (a) *vesicles and bullae* that become hemorrhagic, (b) *gangrenous cellulitis* with necrotic ulcerations, and (c) widespread, red, warm, fluctuant *nodules* with pustules and purpura. Prompt biopsy with frozen sections stained for bacterial and hyphal elements may provide rapid diagnosis.

CUTANEOUS MANIFESTATIONS OF HIV INFECTIONS

Skin disease is common in patients with HIV. Some dermatoses are characteristic, whereas others are just observed in a higher frequency or with atypical features. *Diseases characteristic of HIV infection* include Kaposi's sarcoma, oral hairy leukoplakia, bacillary angiomatosis (Rochalimaea infection causing angiomatous proliferation resulting in red, raised nodular lesions with a scaling base), eosinophilic folliculitis (intensely pruritic follicular papules on the head, neck and extremities).

DISEASES WITH ATYPICAL PRESENTATIONS IN HIV DISEASE. Molluscum contagiosum may appear as large 1- to 2-cm smooth to verrucoid papules and plaques on the face. Herpes simplex often appears as large chronic ulcerative lesions in anogenital and oral areas. Zoster may present as dermatomal or disseminated hyperkeratotic, scarring papules and plaques. Scabies may evolve into numerous hyperkeratotic pruritic plaques teaming with mites on KOH examination. Syphilis may appear with a typical primary genital ulcer but secondary and tertiary lesions may evolve rapidly. To complicate things, the seriologic test for syphilis may be negative. Psoriasis and Reiter's disease may be more severe in HIV-infected patients, with widespread total body involvement.

Diseases with increased frequency in HIV infection include seborrheic dermatitis, yeast infections (especially thrush), drug reactions (morbilliform reactions especially to antibiotics), and pruritus.

CUTANEOUS DRUG REACTIONS

Rashes are among the most common adverse reactions to drugs and occur in 2 to 3% of hospitalized patients. Any drug can potentially produce a rash, and over-the-counter preparations should be considered when defining drug reactions.

Some of the most common drugs causing skin reactions in hospitalized patients are amoxicillin, trimethoprim-sulfamethoxazole, ampicillin, penicillin G, allopurinol, dipyrone, gentamicin sulfate, mefruside, nitrazepam, and barbiturates. Drugs least likely to cause allergic skin reactions include digoxin, antacids, promethazine, acetaminophen, nitroglycerin, aminophylline, propranolol, antihistamines, cromolyn, and emollient laxatives.

Table 475–13 lists the various morphologic types of drug reactions and some of the drugs capable of inducing them.

TABLE 475–13. CUTANEOUS DRUG REACTIONS

Type of Skin Reaction	Drugs Likely to Cause Skin Reaction
Eczematous (allergic contact reaction)	Antihistamines, neomycin, formaldehyde, sulfanamides
Photodermatitis	
Phototoxic	Chlorpromazine, psoralens, demeclocycline, doxycycline
Photoallergic	Promethazine, griseofulvin, Diuril, hypoglycemic drugs
Exfoliative dermatitis	Carbamazepine, hydantoins, nitrofurantoin, isoniazid, gold, allopurinol, phenothiazines
Maculopapular eruption (exanthematous)	Penicillin, sulfonamides, hypoglycemic drugs, phenothiazines, allopurinol, phenytoin, quinine, gold salts, captopril, meprobamate
Papulosquamous reactions Psoriasiform, lichen planus, pityriasis rosea–like	Beta blockers, lithium (psoriasiform), thiazides, gold, phenothiazines, quinidine, antimalarials (lichen planus–like); gold (PR-like): others—practolol, dapsone, ethambutol, furosemide
Vesiculobullous reactions	Azapropazone, captopril, clonidine, furosemide, gold, psoralens, barbiturates, phenytoin, HydroDIURIL, penicillamine
Toxic epidermal necrolysis	Acetazolamide, allopurinol, barbiturates, carbamazepines, gold, hydantoin, nitrofurantoin, pentazocine, tetracycline, quinidine
Pustular—acneiform reactions	Androgen hormones, corticosteroids, iodides, bromides, hydantoin, lithium
Urticaria and erythemas	
Urticaria	May occur with anaphylaxis; penicillin, xenogenic sera, cephalosporins, sulfonamides, barbiturates, hydralazine, phenylbutazone, hydantoin, quinidine, x-ray contrast media
Erythema multiforme	Sulfonamides, hydantoin, barbiturates, penicillin, carbamazepines, allopurinol, amikacin, phenothiazides
Nodular lesions	
Erythema nodosum	Birth control pills, sulfonamides, diuretics, gold, clonidine, propranolol, furosemide, opiates, penicillin
Vasculitis reaction	Allopurinol, barbiturates, carbamazepine, chlorothiazide, cimetidine, gold, imdomethacin, hydantoin, piperazine, sulfonamides
Telangiectatic and LE reactions	Procainamide, hydralazine, phenytoin, penicillamine, trimethadione, methyldopa, carbamazepine, griseofulvin, nalidixic acid, oral contraceptives, propranolol
Pigmentary reaction	Anticonvulsants, antimalarials, antitumor agents (bleomycin, busulfan, cyclophosphamide, doxorubicin, melphalan), oral contraceptives, corticotropin, tetracyclines, phenothiazines, amiodarone
Other cutaneous reactions	
Fixed drug reactions	Phenolphthalein, barbiturates, gold, sulfonamides, meprobamate, penicillin, tetracyclines, analgesics
Alopecia	Alkylating agents, antimetabolites, heparin, coumarin, hydantoin, accutane, gold, nitrofurantoin, propranolol, colchicine, allopurinol
Hypertrichosis	Anabolic agents, diazoxide, minoxidil, phenytoin

Fixed drug eruptions are unique reactions that appear in the same area of the skin each time the responsible drug is administered. These appear as macular, eczematous, or even bullous, pink to dark red patches occurring as few or many lesions. When the drug is stopped the lesions fade, leaving postinflammatory hyperpigmentation. The lesions return in the same place within a few hours of taking the drug again.

Nonsteroidal anti-inflammatory drugs may cause cutaneous reactions including vesiculobullous photosensitivity reactions, serum sickness, erythroderma, fixed drug reactions, and toxic epidermal necrolysis.

The treatment of drug reactions is to withdraw the suspected agent. Once a drug reaction is suspected all nonessential drugs should be stopped and appropriate substitutes used for the necessary medications. An asymptomatic eruption may require no therapy, or a mild reaction with pruritus may be controlled with topical steroid applications and antihistamines. In severe conditions such as exfoliative dermatitis, oral steroids are often indicated. Most drug eruptions resolve in 1 to 2 weeks after withdrawal of the drug, but some take months to clear. Although an occasional reaction may be fatal (e.g., toxic epidermal necrolysis), patients with drug eruptions usually have an excellent prognosis.

Du Vivier LM: Atlas of Clinical Dermatology. New York, Raven Press, 1993. *A beautifully produced, thorough reference volume that comprehensively covers the field.*
Fitzpatrick TB, Eisen AZ, Wolff K, et al.: Dermatology in General Medicine, 3rd ed. New York, McGraw-Hill, 1987.
Moschella SL, Hurley HJ: Dermatology, 3rd ed. Philadelphia, WB Saunders, 1992. *A comprehensive test that brings the field up to date in new discoveries.*

476 OCCUPATIONAL DISEASES OF THE SKIN
Edward A. Emmett

Occupational skin diseases are a group of heterogeneous conditions that share a common occupational etiology. They account for about one half of reported occupational disease in the United States. Occupational contact dermatitis, the prototypical disorder, makes up about 95% of all occupational skin diseases; infections, about 2.5%; and a large number of different, infrequent diseases, the remainder. The relative frequency of each of these diseases in any location depends largely on the pattern of industrialization.

Almost all occupational skin diseases are due to external contact with chemical, physical, and biologic agents. The cause is often multifactorial. In relatively few instances are systemically (rather than locally) absorbed agents responsible.

OCCUPATIONAL CONTACT DERMATITIS

DEFINITION. Occupational contact dermatitis is an erythematous or eczematous response of the skin as a result of local contact with one or more irritating, allergenic, or photosensitizing chemical agents.

ETIOLOGY. Many chemicals from a wide variety of classes—alkalies, acids, volatile organic solvents, metallic salts, organic prepolymers, and many others—are capable of inducing contact dermatitis. The cause is often multifactorial; in addition to one or more chemicals, friction, abrasion, changes in temperature and humidity, and ultraviolet (UV) radiation may play a role. Superinfection may occur. Severe and persistent occupational contact dermatitis, particularly from irritants, is more frequent in those with an atopic diathesis.

INCIDENCE AND PREVALENCE. Bureau of Labor Statistics reports put the incidence in the United States at about 0.9 per 1000 full-time workers per year; because of substantial underreporting, the true incidence is estimated to be from 10 to 50 times higher.

EPIDEMIOLOGY. The incidence of occupational contact dermatitis is generally highest in agriculture/forestry/fishing, followed by manufacturing industries. The highest risks occur in poultry-

dressing plants, meat-packing plants, fabrication of rubber products, leather tanning and finishing, manufacture of ophthalmic goods, plating and polishing, production of frozen fruits and vegetables, internal combustion engine manufacture, machining operations, and canning and curing of seafoods. Virtually no industry is immune.

PATHOGENESIS. Contact dermatitis may result from direct local irritation, cell-mediated immune reactions, or photosensitivity.

Direct local irritation may be immediate, as in irritation from strong acids or alkalies, or may be delayed and occur only after repeated or prolonged local application, as cumulative insult dermatitis. The latter can occur from one or more relatively mildly irritating substances that are termed marginal irritants.

Allergic contact dermatitis occurs as a result of sensitization to specific haptens through a process of cell-mediated immunity. The hapten combines with protein in the skin to form a complete antigen that is processed and presented to T lymphocytes by epidermal Langerhans cells, specialized macrophages that form an intraepidermal network. Among the most frequent allergens are poison ivy or oak; rubber additives, particularly accelerators and antioxidants; monomers of plastics and resins, such as epoxies, acrylates, and diisocyanates; nickel; chromium salts; paraphenylenediamine and derivatives; and formaldehyde. There are many more possible allergens. The number of substances reported to cause allergic contact dermatitis is very large.

Chemical photosensitivity results from the photochemical excitation of a UV-absorbing molecule with resultant tissue damage. In a photoirritant reaction there is direct damage to cellular components, for example, when psoralens irradiated with long UV bind covalently to DNA. Coal tar pitch, certain aromatic dyes, and UV absorbers used in printing processes also cause photoirritation. In the rarer photoallergic reaction, photochemical alteration of the inciting chemical either forms a hapten or leads to a hapten-protein combination in the skin; the subsequent steps are identical with those for allergic contact dermatitis.

A major factor in the human's resistance to environmental chemicals is the barrier provided by the outer stratum corneum layer of the epidermis. Damage to this barrier by trauma, inflammation, or skin disease or by altering barrier conditions, e.g., by occlusion, may play an important role in the development of contact dermatitis.

CLINICAL MANIFESTATIONS. The clinical presentation is dominated by dermatitis that is confined, at least initially, to the region of contact. The morphology varies according to the concentration and duration of the exposure, the pathogenesis, and individual constitutional differences. Acute irritant dermatitis is characterized by erythema, perhaps edema, papules and vesicles, or, in the more extreme instance, one or more large bullae filled with purulent fluid. Postinflammation hyperpigmentation and hypopigmentation may occur; necrosis may leave scars. The cause of acute irritant dermatitis is usually obvious because of the rapidity with which the reaction develops.

Cumulative insult dermatitis may develop only after a long period of contact. On the hands it tends to start under rings or watchbands and to be somewhat patchy in distribution. Individual susceptibility varies widely. Initially, drying and fissuring may be seen, with subsequent development of an eczematous response with papules and vesicles. Excoriations and lichenification are frequent if the process persists. Relapse may occur on relatively brief exposure to mild irritants, even when the dermatitis is clinically healed, especially if the epidermal barrier has not yet been fully reestablished.

Allergic contact dermatitis most often presents as an acute or chronic eczematous reaction with erythema, papules, vesicles, scaling, and pruritus. Characteristically there is a latent period of at least 7 to 10 days before the development of dermatitis following first exposure to the allergen. Recurrence usually occurs 24 to 72 hours after an eliciting exposure. Certain allergens, e.g., epoxy resin monomers, have a tendency to produce severe acute reactions with significant edema.

Localization is important for diagnosis. Over 90% of occupational contact dermatitis involves the hands, sometimes in conjunction with other sites. When the eruption is due to contact with objects or contaminated surfaces, the pattern of contact determines localization. Reaction to immersion of the hands in liquids generally involves the dorsum of the hands and palmar aspects of the wrists. Photosensitivity reactions on exposed sites may be distinguished from airborne contact dermatitis by the relative sparing of shaded areas, such as the eyelids or behind the ears.

DIAGNOSIS. A good occupational history is the cornerstone of diagnosis. It is most useful to get a description of the worker's daily activities, including nonoccupational activities, with particular attention to contact of the skin with chemicals. The localization of the eruption at its onset, initial appearance of lesions, nature of progression, and circumstances of remissions and recurrences help determine an occupational etiology. A personal or family history or both confirm the presence of atopy, in which there is increased susceptibility to irritants, changes in heat and humidity, and other factors. A complete examination of the skin helps rule out dermatoses other than contact dermatitis, including id reactions of the hands secondary to dermatophytosis of the feet. Allergic contact dermatitis is confirmed by diagnostic patch testing; photoallergy, by photopatch testing. Patch testing is relatively easy to perform, but the interpretation requires skill. There is no clinically useful confirmatory test for irritant contact dermatitis.

Other information may be necessary to make a precise diagnosis and formulate appropriate management. Toxicity information on industrial compounds can be obtained from Material Safety Data Sheets, which reveal the composition and properties of industrial materials. In the United States these are available to most employees and their physicians. A visit by the physician to the workplace allows the physician to view the work firsthand. If such a visit is made, opportunity for skin contact with hazardous agents should be explored, as well as the use of protective measures.

Epidemiologic surveys to establish the prevalence of dermatitis in workers at similar jobs and industrial hygiene surveys to characterize the nature and amount of chemical exposure may occasionally be helpful. Public health authorities, university centers for occupational and environmental health, and sometimes concerned employers may be able to assist in such investigations.

TREATMENT. Symptomatic treatment is similar to that for dermatitis of other types. Acute contact dermatitis is treated with cold wet dressings of Burow's solution. Systemic steroids in rapidly tapering doses are indicated in severe acute widespread disabling eruptions; topical steroids and emollients, for dry and chronic eczema. Superinfection requires appropriate systemic antibiotics. Antihistamines may be given for sedation and are mildly antipruritic. The patient should be given careful instruction to avoid casual exposures and should be alerted to the fact that even when the skin has apparently healed, the barrier may not have returned to normal. A temporary or permanent change of job tasks may be necessary. If a permanent job change is necessary, vocational rehabilitation should be considered. Some states require reporting of occupational diseases.

PROGNOSIS. The prognosis of occupational contact dermatitis is surprisingly poor, especially if effective treatment is not given early and if the dermatitis is prolonged. The reasons for this are not entirely clear; however, surveys have shown that a high percentage of individuals still have dermatitis several years later, in many cases despite a change of employment. Those with atopy appear to have the worst prognosis. In allergic contact dermatitis, the prognosis is dependent on the ease with which the allergen can be avoided.

PREVENTION. Preventive measures serve both to prevent recurrences and to halt the development of new disease. These include elimination of or substitution for strong irritants and sensitizers; education of workers regarding skin care; avoidance of overly harsh skin cleansers; prompt reporting and treatment of dermatitis; engineering controls to minimize skin contact with potential hazards; appropriate impervious protective clothing; good personal hygiene with rapid, effective removal of contaminants; and counseling of individuals with predisposing conditions, such as atopy, regarding career selection.

OTHER OCCUPATIONAL DERMATOSES

A relatively large number of other dermatoses can result from occupational exposure. In large part, management is dependent upon diagnostic recognition and on discontinuing further exposures, using measures outlined above.

Chemical burns result from corrosive agents that produce necrosis, ulceration, and subsequent scarring. Prompt removal of these agents (such as strong acids, alkalies, phenol, alkyl metal compounds, and metal chlorides) from skin, eyes, and mucous membranes is essential. Water is generally best for removal. Quicklime,

tin tetrachloride, and titanium tetrachloride should be removed with mineral oil. Specific antidotes are few; these include topical or injected calcium gluconate for hydrofluoric acid burns.

Urticaria may occur from local contact with or systemic absorption of agents that elicit an immediate hypersensitivity reaction or directly release histamine and other vasoactive substances.

Fiberglass dermatitis causes intense pruritus; there may be no visible changes, or it may be accompanied by excoriations, pinpoint petechial papules, or both. Microscopy of a cellophane tape stripping from the skin, which had been treated with 10% potassium hydroxide, reveals the fibers.

Relatively deep indolent *ulcers* of skin and mucous membranes result from contact with arsenic, chromates, and lime.

Chemical acne and folliculitis may result from contact with greases and oils, coal tar pitch, creosote, and a number of cosmetics (acne cosmetica) and from ingestion of bromides, iodides, and isoniazid. These forms of acne typically commence with comedones or inflammatory papules.

Chloracne is due to halogenated aromatic compounds with specific molecular shape, including dioxin and related chlorinated aromatic hydrocarbons. The illness is characterized by small straw-colored cysts and comedones that first involve the malar crescent and behind the ear and may not spread beyond these areas. Inflammatory pustules, abscesses, and large cysts may be seen in severe cases. Chloracne is the first and most constant finding in chronic dioxin poisoning. More variable findings may include porphyrinuria, hyperpigmentation, hypertrichosis, central and peripheral nervous system effects, alteration of lipid metabolism, and mild hepatotoxicity. Experimentally observed effects include teratogenicity, immunosuppression, and tumor induction.

Cutaneous granulomas occur as slightly erythematous grouped flesh-colored papules, with or without inflammatory changes, from foreign body reactions at the site of contact with talc and silica or as an immunologic response to beryllium and zirconium.

Chemical leukoderma, which may mimic vitiligo but which is confined to the areas of skin contact, may result from a number of phenols and catechols, including hydroquinone, monobenzyl, and monomethyl ethers of hydroquinone (used as rubber additives) and *p*-tertiary butyl and related phenols (in disinfectants).

Basal and squamous cell carcinomas and keratoacanthomas result from prolonged exposures to UV radiation, ionizing radiation, polycyclic aromatic hydrocarbons (including coal tar pitches and related products), and arsenic. Exposures to arsenic may be associated with various internal malignant neoplasms.

Cutaneous T cell lymphoma (mycosis fungoides) may be more frequent in those who have worked in heavy industry or who have industrial chemical exposure, but the particular causal agents are uncertain.

INFECTIONS AND INFESTATIONS

The development of infections and infestations frequently depends on occupational factors, individual susceptibility, and the geographic distribution of the causal organism. Occupational associations include the following:

Viral. Herpes simplex (dentists, medical personnel), milkers' nodules and papular stomatitis (veterinarians, milk handlers), orf (farmers, shepherds, abattoir workers), viral warts (butchers), Rift Valley fever (shepherds).

Bacterial. Staphylococcal infections of hands (abattoir workers and butchers), erysipeloid (fish, fowl, rabbit, and pig handlers), anthrax (wool, hair, and hide handlers), tularemia (farmers), nontuberculous mycobacterial infections (aquarium workers and pet shop attendants). Bacterial and yeast infections and tinea versicolor are prominent where there is heat, humidity, and lack of hygiene.

Fungal. Dermatophyte infections are more frequent in farm workers, surveyors, zoo attendants, animal care technicians, and certain others. Particular examples include tinea versicolor (farmers); infection due to *Trichophyton rubrum* (miners), *Microsporum canis* (pet shop workers), *Trichophyton violaceum* (wrestlers), and *Candida albicans* (those in wet work, particularly those in contact with sugar and fruit); sporotrichosis (mine workers); chromomycosis (agricultural workers); and actinomycosis (agricultural workers).

Protozoal. South American leishmaniasis (foresters).

Helminthic. Creeping eruption (plumbers, gardeners, farm workers in the tropics), ankylostomiasis (miners), schistosomiasis and cercarial dermatitis (rice planters and canal workers).

In addition, bites and stings of arthropods and other creatures are common in those who work out of doors and in certain other occupations.

Adams RM: Occupational Skin Disease, 2nd ed. Philadelphia, WB Saunders, 1990. *Comprehensive review of contact dermatitis and related conditions, with descriptions of skin diseases caused by a variety of agents and with detailed lists of agents encountered in various occupations.*

Maibach HI (ed.): Occupational and Industrial Dermatology. Chicago, Year Book Medical Publishers, 1987. *Multiauthor text that broadly covers occupational dermatoses and dermatotoxicology and describes the skin diseases caused by a number of specific agents.*

PART XXVII

LABORATORY REFERENCE INTERVALS AND VALUES

477 REFERENCE INTERVALS AND LABORATORY VALUES*

Ronald J. Elin

Reference intervals are valuable guidelines for the clinician to assess health and disease, but they should not be used as absolute indicators of health and disease. For essentially every test, there is a significant overlap between the normal and diseased populations. Many factors may influence the determination of the reference interval. The method and mode of standardization are variables for the reference interval, particularly for immunologic and enzymatic tests. The selection of the "normal" population is also important because factors such as age, gender, race, diet, personal habits (e.g., alcohol consumption, smoking), and exercise may influence the reference interval for a given analyte. Last, the statistics chosen to define the reference interval are also a factor. These multiple variables for determining the reference interval indicate why there are differences among institutions for the same analyte.

The values in this chapter are primarily for adults in the fasting state. Values for other groups, when included, are clearly identified. For convenience, this chapter is divided into the following three sections: clinical chemistry, toxicology, and serology; hematology and coagulation; and drugs—therapeutic and toxic. The list includes reference intervals for the most common tests used in the practice of internal medicine. For more information about the reference interval for a given test or a test not included in the list, I recommend *Clinical Guide to Laboratory Tests,* second edition, edited by Dr. Norbert W. Tietz. This book contains literature citations for most of the tests listed in this chapter.

All laboratory values are given in conventional and international units. If the value and units for a reference interval are the same for conventional and international units, the interval is listed only in the column for international units. The temperature for all enzyme assays listed in the chapter is 37° C. The pertinent prefixes denoting the decimal factors and abbreviations are listed above.

---

* The material in this chapter was partially extracted from Tietz NW (ed.): Clinical Guide to Laboratory Tests. Philadelphia, WB Saunders, 1990. The material for the section on Therapeutic Drug Concentrations was partially extracted from Burtis CA, Ashwood ER (eds.): Tietz Textbook of Clinical Chemistry. Philadelphia, WB Saunders, 1994. The main contributors to this section of the book are PC Painter, JY Cope, and JL Smith. Other sources are listed under references for this chapter.

Prefixes Denoting Decimal Factors

Prefix	Symbol	Factor
mega	M	10^6
kilo	k	10^3
hecto	h	10^2
deka	da	10^1
deci	d	10^{-1}
centi	c	10^{-2}
milli	m	10^{-3}
micro	μ	10^{-6}
nano	n	10^{-9}
pico	p	10^{-12}
femto	f	10^{-15}

Abbreviations

AU	Arbitrary units
EU	Ehrlich unit
GD	General diagnostics
IFA	Immunofluorescent assay
IU	International unit (of hormone activity)
RIA	Radioimmunoassay
RID	Radial immunodiffusion
S	Substrate
U	International unit (of enzyme activity)

CLINICAL CHEMISTRY, TOXICOLOGY, SEROLOGY

Test	Specimen	Reference Interval (Conventional Units)	Reference Interval (International Units)
Acetoacetate Semiquantitative	Serum or plasma (fluoride/oxalate)	Negative (< 1 mg/dL)	Negative (< 0.1 mmol/L)
Acetone	Urine	Negative	Negative
Semiquantitative	Serum or plasma (fluoride or oxalate)	Negative (< 1 mg/dL)	Negative (< 0.17 mmol/L)
Quantitative Semiquantitative	Urine		Negative
Acid phosphatase (S:p-nitrophenylphosphate)	Serum		M: 2.5–11.7 U/L F: 0.3–9.2 U/L
Adrenocorticotropic hormone (ACTH)	Plasma (heparin)	0800 h: 8–79 pg/mL 1600 h: 7–30 pg/mL	8–79 ng/L 7–30 ng/L
Alanine aminotransferase (ALT, SGPT)	Serum		8–20 U/L
Albumin			
Nephelometric, colorimetric	Serum	3.5–5 g/dL	35–50 g/L
Turbidimetric	CSF	15–45 mg/dL	150–450 mg/L
	Urine	< 80 mg/d at rest < 150 mg/d ambulatory	< 80 mg/d < 150 mg/d
Aldolase	Serum		1.0–7.5 U/L
Aldosterone	Plasma (heparin EDTA) or serum	Adult, average sodium diet supine: 3–10 ng/dL upright: 5–30 ng/dL	0.08–0.28 nmol/L 0.14–0.83 nmol/L
Alkaline phosphate (S:4–NPP)	Serum		Adult (> 18 y) F: 42–98 U/L M: 53–128 U/L
δ-Aminolevulinic acid (δ-ALA)	Serum	15–23 μg/dL	1.1–8 μmol/L
	Urine	1.5–7.5 mg/d	11.4–57.2 μmol/d
Ammonia nitrogen Resin or enzymatic	Serum or plasma (Na-heparin)	Adult 15–45 μg N/dL	11–32 μmol/L
	Urine, 24-h	140–1500 mg/d	10–107 mmol/d
Amylase (S:Beckmann, defined substrate)	Serum		25–125 U/L
	Urine, timed specimen		1–17 U/h
Angiotensin I	Peripheral venous plasma (EDTA)	11–88 pg/mL	11–88 ng/L
Angiotensin II	Plasma (EDTA) Arterial blood	10–60 pg/mL	10–60 ng/L
α_1-Antitrypsin (nephelometry)	Serum	78–200 mg/dL	0.78–2 g/L
Anion gap $[Na^+ - (Cl^- + HCO_3^-)]$	Plasma (heparin)	7–14 mEq/L	7–14 mmol/L
Apolipoprotein A-I	Serum	M: 94–178 mg/dL F: 101–199 mg/dL	0.94–1.78 g/L 1.01–1.99 g/L
Apolipoprotein B	Serum	M: 63–133 mg/dL F: 60–126 mg/dL	0.63–1.33 g/L 0.60–1.26 g/L
Arsenic	Whole blood (heparin)	0.2–2.3 μg/dL Chronic poisoning: 10–50 μg/dL Acute poisoning: 60–93 μg/dL	0.03–0.31 μmol/L 1.33–6.65 μmol/L 7.98–12.37 μmol/L
	Urine, 24-h	5–50 μg/d	0.067–0.665 μmol/d
Ascorbic acid (see Vitamin C)			
Aspartate aminotransferase (AST, SGOT)	Serum		10–30 U/L
Base excess	Whole blood (heparin)	− 2 to 3 mEq/L	− 2 to 3 mmol/L
Bicarbonate	Serum	18–23 mEq/L	18–23 mmol/L
Bile acids, total	Serum, fasting	0.3–2.3 μg/mL	0.74–5.64 μmol/L
	Serum, 1-h postprandial	1.8–3.2 μg/mL	4.41–7.84 μmol/L
	Feces	120–225 mg/d	294–551 μmol/d
Bilirubin			
Total	Serum	0.2–1.0 mg/dL	3.4–17.1 μmol/L
	Urine	Negative	Negative
Conjugated (direct)	Serum	0–0.2 mg/dL	0–3.4 μmol/L
Calcium, ionized (iCa)	Serum	4.65–5.28 mg/dL	1.16–1.32 mmol/L
Calcium, total	Serum	8.4–10.2 mg/dL	2.10–2.55 mmol/L
	Urine, 24-h	100–300 mg/d	2.5–7.5 mmol/d
	CSF	4.2–5.4 mg/dL	1.05–1.35 mmol/L
Cancer antigen 125 (CA 125)	Serum	< 35 U/mL	< 35 kU/L
Carbon dioxide, partial pressure (Pco_2)	Whole blood, arterial (heparin)	M: 35–48 mm Hg F: 32–45 mm Hg	4.66–6.38 kPa 4.26–5.99 kPa
Carbon dioxide, total (Tco_2)	Serum or plasma (heparin)	23–29 mEq/L	23–29 mmol/L
Carcinoembryonic antigen (CEA)	Serum	Nonsmokers: < 2.5 ng/mL	< 2.5 μg/L
β-Carotene	Serum	10–85 μg/dL	0.19–1.58 μmol/L
Catecholamines, total	Urine, 24-h	< 100 μg/d	< 5.91 nmol/d
Ceruloplasmin (RID)	Serum	18–45 mg/dL	180–450 mg/L
Chloride	Serum or plasma (heparin)	98–106 mEq/L	98–106 mmol/L
	CSF	118–132 mEq/L	118–132 mmol/L
	Urine, 24-h	110–250 mEq/d	110–250 mmol/d

CLINICAL CHEMISTRY, TOXICOLOGY, SEROLOGY *Continued*

Test	Specimen	Reference Interval (Conventional Units)	Reference Interval (International Units)
Cholesterol, total	Serum or plasma (EDTA)	Recommended: < 200 mg/dL	< 5.18 mmol/L
		Moderate risk: 200–239 mg/dL	5.18–6.19 mmol/L
		High risk: ≥ 240 mg/dL	6.22 mmol/L
Chorionic gonadotropin, β-subunit (β-HCG)	Serum or plasma (EDTA)	M and nonpregnant F: < 5.0 mU/mL	< 5.0 IU/L
Complement			
Total hemolytic Complement activity	Plasma (EDTA)	75–160 U/mL	75–160 kU/L
Copper	Serum	M: 70–140 μg/dL	10.99–21.98 μmol/L
		F: 80–155 μg/dL	12.56–24.34 μmol/L
	Erythrocyte (heparin)	90–150 μg/dL	14.13–23.55 μmol/L
	Urine, 24-h	3–35 μg/d	0.047–0.55 μmol/d
Coproporphyrin	Urine, 24-h	34–234 μg/d	51–351 nmol/d
	Feces, 24-h	< 30 μg/g dry wt	< 45 nmol/g dry wt
		400–1200 μg/d	600–1800 nmol/d
Corticobinding globulin (CBG) (see Transcortin)			
Corticosterone	Serum	0800 h: 130–820 ng/dL	4–24 nmol/L
		1600 h: 60–220 ng/dL	2–6 nmol/L
Cortisol	Serum or plasma (heparin)	0800 h: 5–23 μg/dL	138–635 nmol/L
		1600 h: 3–15 μg/dL	82–413 nmol/L
		2000 h: ≤ 50% of 0800 h	Fraction of 0800 h: ≤ 0.50
Cortisol, free	Urine, 24-h	10–100 μg/d	27–276 nmol/d
C-Peptide	Serum	0.78–1.89 ng/mL	0.26–0.62 nmol/L
C-Reactive protein	Serum	68–8200 ng/mL	68–8200 μg/L
Creatine kinase (CK)	Serum		M: 38–174 U/L
			F: 26–140 U/L
Isoenzymes	Serum	Fraction 2 (MB) < 4–6% of total (method-dependent)	Fraction of total: < 0.04–0.06
Creatinine Jaffe, kinetic or enzymatic	Serum or plasma	M: 0.7–1.3 mg/dL	62–115 μmol/L
		F: 0.6–1.1 mg/dL	53–97 μmol/L
	Urine, 24-h	M: 14–26 mg/kg/d	124–230 μmol/kg/d
		F: 11–20 mg/kg/d	97–177 μmol/kg/d
Creatinine clearance (endogenous)	Serum or plasma, and urine	M: 90–139 mL/min/1.73 m²	0.87–1.34 mL/s/m²
		F: 80–125 mL/min/1.73 m²	0.77–1.20 mL/s/m²
Dehydroepiandrosterone (DHEA)	Serum	M: 1.8–12.5 ng/mL	6.2–43.3 nmol/L
		F: 1.3–9.8 ng/mL	4.5–34.0 nmol/L
Dehydroepiandrosterone sulfate (DHEA-S)	Serum or plasma (heparin, EDTA)	M: 1.7–6.7 μg/mL	4.6–18.2 μmol/L
		F: Premenopausal: 0.5–5.4 μg/mL	1.4–14.7 μmol/L
		Postmenopausal: 0.3–2.6 μg/mL	0.8–7.1 μmol/L
11-Deoxycortisol (compound S)	Serum	12–158 ng/dL	0.3–4.6 nmol/L
Estrogens, total	Serum	M: 20–80 pg/mL	20–80 ng/L
		F, cycle:	
		1–10 d 61–394 pg/mL	60–200 ng/L
		11–20 d 122–437 pg/mL	
		21–30 d 156–350 pg/mL	160–400 ng/L
		Postmenopausal: ≤ 130 pg/mL	≥ 130 ng/L
		Follicular phase: 60–200 pg/mL	
		Luteal phase: 160–400 pg/mL	
	Urine, 24-h	M: 15–40 μg/d	
		F: Preovulation: 4–25 μg/d	
		Ovulation: 28–100 μg/d	
		Luteal peak: 22–80 μg/d	
		Pregnancy, term: < 45,000 μg/d	
		Postmenopausal: < 20 μg/d	
Fat, fecal	Feces, 72-h	< 7 g/d	fat-free diet: < 4 g/d
Fatty acids, nonesterified (free)	Serum or plasma (heparin)	8–25 mg/dL	0.28–0.89 mmol/L
Ferritin	Serum	M: 20–250 ng/mL	20–250 μg/L
		F: 10–120 ng/mL	10–120 μg/L
α₁-Fetoprotein	Serum	< 10 ng/mL	< 10 μg/L
Fibrinogen (see Hematology and Coagulation section)			
Folate	Serum	3–16 ng/mL	7–36 nmol/L
	Erythrocytes (EDTA)	130–628 ng/mL packed cells	294–1422 nmol/L packed cells
Follitropin (FSH)	Serum or plasma (heparin)	M: 4–25 mIU/mL	4–25 IU/L
		F: Follicular phase: 1–9 U/mL	1–9 U/L
		Ovulatory peak: 6–26 mU/mL	6–26 U/L
		Luteal phase: 1–9 mU/mL	1–9 U/L
		Postmenopausal: 30–118 mU/mL	30–118 U/L
	Urine, 24-h		4–18 U/d
			3–12 U/d
Free thyroxine index (FT₄I)	Serum		4.2–13.0
Gastrin	Serum	< 100 pg/mL	< 100 ng/L
Glucose	Serum	Adult: 70–105 mg/dL	3.9–5.8 mmol/L
		> 60 y: 80–115 mg/dL	4.4–6.4 mmol/L
	Whole blood (heparin)	65–95 mg/dL	3.6–5.3 mmol/L
	CSF	40–70 mg/dL	2.2–3.9 mmol/L

Continued

CLINICAL CHEMISTRY, TOXICOLOGY, SEROLOGY *Continued*

Test	Specimen	Reference Interval (Conventional Units)	Reference Interval (International Units)
Quantitative, enzymatic	Urine	< 0.5 g/d	< 2.8 mmol/d
Qualitative	Urine		Negative
Glucose, 2-h postprandial	Serum	< 120 mg/dL	< 6.7 mmol/L
Glucose tolerance test (GTT), oral	Serum		

		mg/dL		mmol/L	
		Normal	Diabetic	Normal	Diabetic
Fasting:		70–105	> 140	3.9–5.8	> 7.8
60 min:		120–170	≥ 200	6.7–9.4	≥ 11
90 min:		100–140	≥ 200	5.6–7.8	≥ 11
120 min:		70–120	≥ 140	3.9–6.7	≥ 7.8

Test	Specimen	Reference Interval (Conventional Units)	Reference Interval (International Units)
γ-Glutamyltransferase (GGT)	Serum	M: 9–50 U/L	
		F: 8–40 U/L	
Glycerol, free	Plasma	0.29–1.72 mg/dL	0.032–0.187 mmol/L
Growth hormone (HGH, somatotropin)	Serum or plasma (EDTA, heparin)	Adult, M: < 2 ng/mL	< 2 μg/L
		F: < 10 ng/mL	< 10 μg/L
		> 60 y, M: 0.4–10 ng/mL	0.4–10 μg/L
		F: 1–14 ng/mL	1–14 μg/L
Haptoglobin (see Hematology and Coagulation section)			
HDL-cholesterol (HDLC) (5th percentile from Lipid Research Clinics)	Serum or plasma (EDTA)	M: > 29 mg/dL	> 0.75 mmol/L
		F: > 35 mg/dL	> 0.91 mmol/L
Hemoglobin A$_{1c}$ (electrophoresis)	Whole blood (heparin, EDTA, or oxalate)	5.6–7.5% of total Hb	Fraction of Hb: 0.056–0.075
Homovanillic acid (HVA)	Urine, 24-h	1.4–3.8 mg/d	8–48 μmol/d
17-Hydroxycorticosteroids (17-OHCS)	Urine, 24-h	M: 3.0–10.0 mg/d	8.3–27.6 μmol/d
		F: 2.0–8.0 mg/d	5.5–22.1 μmol/d
5-Hydroxyindole acetic acid (5-HIAA)			
Qualitative	Fresh random urine		Negative
Quantitative	Urine, 24-h	2–6 mg/d	10.4–31.2 μmol/d
17-Hydroxyprogesterone (17-OHP)	Serum	M: 0.5–2.5 ng/mL	1.5–7.5 nmol/L
		F: Follicular: 0.2–1.0 ng/mL	0.6–3.0 nmol/L
		Luteal: 1.0–5.0 ng/mL	3.0–15.5 nmol/L
		Postmenopausal: ≤ 0.7 ng/mL	≤ 2.1 nmol/L
Immunoglobulin A (IgA)	Serum	40–350 mg/dL	400–3500 mg/L
Immunoglobulin D (IgD)	Serum	0–8 mg/dL	0–80 mg/L
Immunoglobulin E (IgE)	Serum	0–380 IU/mL	0–380 kIU/L
Immunoglobulin G (IgG)	Serum	650–1600 mg/dL	6.5–16 g/L
	CSF	0.5–5 mg/dL	5–50 mg/L
Immunoglobulin M (IgM)	Serum	55–300 mg/dL	550–3000 mg/L
Insulin (12-h fasting)	Serum	6–24 μIU/mL	42–167 pmol/L
Intrinsic factor (see Vitamin B$_{12}$)			
Iron	Serum	M: 65–175 μg/dL	11.6–31.3 μmol/L
		F: 50–170 μg/dL	9.0–30.4 μmol/L
Iron-binding capacity, total (TIBC)	Serum	250–450 μg/dL	44.8–80.6 μmol/L
	Serum	M: 20–50	Fraction of iron saturation: 0.20–0.5
Iron saturation		F: 15–50	0.15–0.5
17-Ketogenic steroids (17-KGS)	Urine, 24-h	M: 5–23 mg/d	17–80 μmol/d
		F: 3–15 mg/d	10–52 μmol/d
Ketone bodies			
Qualitative	Serum	Negative (0.5–3.0 mg/dL)	Negative (5–30 mg/L)
	Urine, random		Negative
17-Ketosteroids, total (17-KS)	Urine, 24-h	M: 18–30 y 9–22 mg/d	31–76 μmol/d
		> 30 y 8–20 mg/d	28–70 μmol/d
		F: 6–15 mg/d	21–52 μmol/d
L-Lactate	Whole blood (heparin)	Venous: 4.5–19.8 mg/dL	0.5–2.2 mmol/L
		Arterial: 4.5–14.4 mg/dL	0.5–1.6 mmol/L
Lactate dehydrogenase (LDH)	Serum		208–378 U/L
LDH isoenzymes (Electrophoresis, agarose)	Serum	%	Fraction of total:
		Fraction 1: 18–33	0.18–0.33
		Fraction 2: 28–40	0.28–0.40
		Fraction 3: 18–30	0.18–0.30
		Fraction 4: 6–16	0.06–0.16
		Fraction 5: 2–13	0.02–0.13
Lead	Whole blood (heparin)	< 40 μg/dL	< 1.93 μmol/L
		Toxic: ≥ 100 μg/dL	≥ 4.83 μmol/L
	Urine	< 80 μg/dL	< 0.39 μmol/L
Lipase (turbidimetric)	Serum		Adult: 10–140 U/L
			> 60 y: 18–180 U/L
LDL-Cholesterol (LDLC)	Serum or plasma (EDTA)	Recommended: < 130 mg/dL	< 3.37 mmol/L
		Moderate risk: 130–159 mg/dL	3.37–4.12 mmol/L
		High risk: ≥ 160 mg/dL	≥ 4.14 mmol/L
Lutropin (LH)	Serum or plasma (heparin)	M: 1–8 mU/mL	1–8 U/L
		F: Follicular phase: 1–2 mU/mL	1–12 U/L
		Midcycle: 16–104 mU/mL	16–104 U/L
		Luteal: 1–12 mU/mL	1–12 U/L
		Postmenopausal: 16–66 mU/mL	16–66 U/L
	Urine		M: 9–23 U/d
			F: non-midcycle, 4–30 U/d

CLINICAL CHEMISTRY, TOXICOLOGY, SEROLOGY *Continued*

Test	Specimen	Reference Interval (Conventional Units)	Reference Interval (International Units)
Lysozyme	Serum, plasma	0.4–1.3 mg/dL	4–13 mg/L
Magnesium	Serum	1.3–2.1 mEq/L	0.65–1.05 mmol/L
	Urine, 24-h	6.0–10.0 mEq/d	3.00–5.00 mmol/L
Mercury	Whole blood (EDTA)	<5.0 μg/dL	<0.25 μmol/L
	Urine, 24-h	<20 μg/L	<0.1 μmol/L
		Toxic: >150 μg/L	<0.75 μmol/L
Metanephrine, total	Urine, 24-h	0.05–1.20 μg/mg creatinine	0.03–0.69 mmol/mol creatinine
Myelin basic protein	CSF		<2.5 ng/mL
Myoglobin	Serum		M: 19–92 μg/L
			12–76 μg/L
	Urine, random		Negative
Osmolality	Serum		275–295 mOsmol/kg
	Urine, random		50–1400 mOsmol/kg, depending on fluid intake
			After 12-h fluid restriction: >850 mOsmol/kg
	Urine, 24-h		~390–900 mOsmol/kg
Oxalate	Serum	1–2.4 μg/mL	11–27 μmol/L
		Ethylene glycol poisoning: >20 μg/mL	Ethylene glycol poisoning: >228 μmol/L
Oxygen (Po_2)	Whole blood, arterial (heparin)	83–100 mm Hg	11–14.4 kPa
Oxygen saturation	Whole blood, arterial (heparin)	95–98%	Fraction saturated: 0.95–0.98
Parathyroid hormone	Serum	Varies with laboratory	
		N-terminal 8–24 pg/mL	8–24 ng/L
		C-terminal 50–330 pg/mL	50–330 ng/L
		Midmolecule 0.29–0.85 ng/mL	29–85 pmol/L
pH (37°C)	Whole blood, arterial (heparin)		7.35–7.45
Phosphorus, inorganic	Serum	2.7–4.5 mg/dL	0.87–1.45 nmol/L
		>60 y, M: 2.3–3.7 mg/dL	0.74–1.2 nmol/L
		F: 2.8–4.1 mg/dL	0.90–1.3 nmol/L
	Urine, 24-h	0.4–1.3 g/d	13–42 mmol/d
Porphobilinogen (PBG)			
Quantitative	Urine, 24-h	0–2.0 mg/d	0–8.8 μmol/d
Qualitative	Urine, fresh random		Negative
Potassium	Serum	3.5–5.1 mEq/L	3.5–5.1 mmol/L
	Plasma (heparin)	3.5–4.5 mEq/L	3.5–4.5 mmol/L
	Urine, 24-h	25–125 mEq/d	25–125 mmol/d
Pregnanediol	Urine, 24-h	M: 0–1.9 mg/d	0–5.9 μmol/d
		F: Follicular: <2.6 mg/d	<8 μmol/d
		Luteal: 2.6–10.6 mg/d	8–33 μmol/d
		Postmenopausal: 0.2–1.0 mg/d	0.6–3.1 μmol/d
Progesterone	Serum	M: 0.13–0.97 ng/mL	0.4–3.1 nmol/L
		F: Follicular: 0.15–0.70 ng/mL	0.5–2.2 nmol/L
		Luteal: 2.0–25 ng/mL	6.4–79.5 nmol/L
Prolactin (hPRL)	Serum	0–20 ng/mL	0–20 μg/L
Prostate-specific antigen (PSA)	Serum, freeze	M: <4 ng/mL	<4 μg/L
Protein			
Total	Serum	6.4–8.3 g/dL	64.0–83.0 g/L
Electrophoresis	Serum	Albumin: 3.5–5.0 g/dL	35–50 g/L
		α_1-Globulin: 0.1–0.3 g/dL	1–3 g/L
		α_2-Globulin: 0.6–1.0 g/dL	6–10 g/L
		β-Globulin: 0.7–1.1 g/dL	7–11 g/L
		γ-Globulin: 0.8–1.6 g/dL	8–16 g/L
Total	Urine, 24-h		50–80 mg/d at rest
Total	CSF	Lumbar: 15–45 mg/dL	150–450 mg/L
Protoporphyrin	Whole blood (heparin or EDTA)	17–77 μg/dL RBC	0.30–1.37 μmol/L RBC
	Feces, 24-h	≤60 μg/g dry wt or <1500 μg/d	≤0.11 mmol/kg dry wt or <2.67 μmol/d
Pyruvic acid	Whole blood (heparin)	0.3–0.9 mg/dL	0.03–0.10 mmol/L
Renin (normal diet)	Plasma (EDTA)	ng/mL/h ± 1 SE	μg/L/h ± 1 SE
		Supine: 1.6 ± 1.5	1.6 ± 1.5
		Standing: (4-h): 4.5 ± 2.9	4.5 ± 2.9
Riboflavin (see Vitamin B₂)			
Sediment	Urine, fresh, random		
Casts			Hyaline: occasional (0–1) casts/hpf
			RBC: not seen
			WBC: not seen
			Tubular epithelial: not seen
			Transitional and squamous epithelial: not seen
Cells			RBC: 0–2/hpf
			WBC: M: 0–3/hpf
			F: 0–5/hpf
			Epithelial: few
			Bacteria:
			Unspun: no organisms/oil immersion field
			Spun: <20 organisms/hpf

Continued

✔

CLINICAL CHEMISTRY, TOXICOLOGY, SEROLOGY *Continued*

Test	Specimen	Reference Interval (Conventional Units)	Reference Interval (International Units)
Sodium	Serum or plasma (heparin)	136–146 mEq/L	136–146 mmol/L
	Urine, 24-h	40–220 mEq/d	40–220 mmol/d
Specific gravity	Urine, random		1.002–1.030
	Urine, 24-h	% of total	1.015–1.025
Testosterone, free	Serum	M: 52–280 pg/mL 1.5–3.2	180.4–971.6 pmol/fraction of total L
		F: 1.6–6.3 pg/mL 0.8–1.4	5.6–21.9 pmol 0.015–0.032
			0.008–0.014
Testosterone, total	Serum	M: 300–1000	10.4–34.7 nmol/L
		F: 20–75	0.69–2.6 nmol/L
	Urine	20–50 y,	
		M: 50–135 μg/d	173–470 nmol/d
		F: 2–12 μg/d	7–42 nmol/d
		>50 y,	
		M: 40–60 μg/d	139–210 nmol/d
		F: 2–8 μg/d	7–28 nmol/d
Thiamine (see Vitamin B₁)	Serum		
Thyroglobulin (Tg)	Serum	3–42 ng/mL	3–42 μg/L
Thyroglobulin antibodies	Serum		<1:10
Thyroid microsomal antibodies	Serum		Nondetectable (hemagglutination) or <1:10 (IFA)
Thyrotropin (hTSH)	Serum or plasma	2–10 μU/mL	2–10 mU/L
Thyrotropin-releasing hormone	Plasma	5–60 pg/mL	5–60 ng/L
Thyroxine, free (FT₄)	Serum	0.8–2.4 ng/dL	10–31 pmol/L
Thyroxine (T₄), total	Serum	5–12 μg/dL	65–155 nmol/L
		>60 y, M: 5.0–10.0 μg/dL	65–129 nmol/L
		F: 5.5–10.5 μg/dL	71–135 nmol/L
Thyroxine-binding globulin (TBG)	Serum	15.0–34.0 μg/mL	15.0–34.0 mg/L
Thyroxine index, free (see Free thyroxine index)			
		T₄ (μg/dL)/TBG (μg/mL)	T₄ (nmol/L)/TBG (mg/L)
Transcortin	Serum	M: 18.8–25.2 mg/L	323–433 nmol/L
		F: 14.9–22.9 mg/L	256–393 nmol/L
Transferrin	Serum	200–400 mg/dL	2.0–4.0 g/L
		>60 y: 180–380 mg/dL	1.80–3.80 g/L
Transthyretin (prealbumin)	Serum	10–40 mg/dL	100–400 mg/L
Triglycerides (TG)	Serum, after ≥12-hr fast	Recommended:	0.45–1.81 mmol/L
		M: 40–160 mg/dL	0.40–1.52 mmol/L
		F: 35–135 mg/dL	
Tri-iodothyronine, free	Serum	260–480 pg/dL	4.0–7.4 pmol/L
Tri-iodothyronine, total (T₃)	Serum	100–200 ng/dL	1.54–3.08 mmol/L
Tri-iodothyronine resin uptake test (T₃RU)	Serum	24–34%	24–34 AU (arbitrary units)
Urea nitrogen	Serum or plasma	7–18 mg/dL	2.5–6.4 mmol/L
	Urine	12–20 g/d	0.43–0.71 mol/d
Urea nitrogen/creatinine ratio	Serum		12/1–20/1
Uric acid (uricase)	Serum	M: 3.5–7.2 mg/dL	0.21–0.42 mmol/L
		F: 2.6–6.0 mg/dL	0.15–0.35 mmol/L
	Urine, 24-h	250–750 mg/d	1.48–4.43 mmol/d
Urinary sediment (see Sediment)			
Urobilinogen	Urine, 2-h	0.1–0.8 EU	0.1–0.8 U
	Urine, 24-h	0.5–4.0 EU	0.5–4.0 U
	Feces	75–275 EU/100 g	750–2750 U/kg
		75–400 EU/d	75–400 U/d
		40–280 mg/d	67–473 μmol/d
Uroporphyrin	Urine, 24-h	<50 μg/d	<60 nmol/d
	Feces, 24-h specimen	10–40 μg/d	12–48 nmol/d
	Erythrocytes (heparin or EDTA)	Negative	
Vanillylmandelic acid (VMA)	Urine, 24-h	2–7 mg/d	10.1–35.4 μmol/d
Viscosity	Serum		1.10–1.22 centipoise
Vitamin A	Serum	30–80 μg/dL	1.05–2.8 μmol/L
Vitamin B₁ (Thiamine)	Serum	0–2 μg/dL	0–75 nmol/L
Vitamin B₂ (Riboflavin)	Serum	4–24 μg/dL	106–638 nmol/L
Vitamin B₆	Plasma (EDTA)	5–30 ng/mL	20–121 nmol/L
Vitamin B₁₂	Serum	100–700 pg/mL	74–516 pmol/L
Vitamin C	Plasma (oxalate, heparin, or EDTA)	0.5–1.5 mg/dL	28–85 μmol/L
Vitamin D₃, 1,25-dihydroxy	Serum	25–45 pg/mL	60–108 pmol/L
Vitamin D₃, 25-hydroxy	Plasma (heparin)	Summer: 15–80 ng/mL	37.4–200 nmol/L
		Winter: 14–42 ng/mL	34.9–105 nmol/L
Vitamin E	Serum	5.0–18.0 μg/mL	12–42 μmol/L
Zinc	Serum	70–150 μg/dL	10.7–22.9 μmol/L

HEMATOLOGY AND COAGULATION

Test	Specimen	Reference Interval (Conventional Units)	Reference Interval (International Units)
Activated partial thromboplastin time (APTT)	Whole blood (Na citrate)		25–35 sec
Bleeding time (BT)			
Ivy	Blood from skin		Normal: 2–7 min
			Borderline: 7–11 min
Simplate (G-D)			2.75–8 min
Blood volume	Whole blood (heparin)		M: 52–83 mL/kg
			F: 50–75 mL/kg
Bone marrow	Bone marrow aspirate	% (mean)	Number fraction (mean)
Differential count			
Myeoblasts		0.3–5.0 (2.0)	0.003–0.05 (0.02)
Promyelocytes		1.0–8.0 (5.0)	0.01–0.08 (0.05)
Myelocytes:			
Neutrophilic		5.0–19.0 (12.0)	0.05–0.19 (0.12)
Eosinophilic		0.5–3.0 (1.5)	0.005–0.03 (0.015)
Basophilic		0.0–0.5 (0.3)	0.00–0.005 (0.003)
Metamyelocytes		13.0–32.0 (22.0)	0.13–0.32 (0.22)
Polymorphonuclear neutrophils		7.0–30.0 (2.0)	0.07–0.30 (0.20)
Polymorphonuclear eosinophils		0.5–4.0 (2.0)	0.005–0.04 (0.02)
Polymorphonuclear basophils		0.0–0.7 (0.2)	0.0–0.007 (0.002)
Lymphocytes		3.0–17.0 (10.0)	0.03–0.17 (0.10)
Plasma cells		0.0–2.0 (0.4)	0.00–0.02 (0.004)
Monocytes		0.5–5.0 (2.0)	0.005–0.05 (0.02)
Reticulum cells		0.1–2.0 (0.2)	0.001–0.02 (0.002)
Megakaryocytes		0.03–3.0 (0.1)	0.0003–0.03 (0.001)
Pronormoblasts		1.0–8.0 (4.0)	0.01–0.08 (0.04)
Normoblasts		7.0–32.0 (18.0)	0.07–0.32 (0.18)
Clot lysis, 37°C	Whole clotted blood		48–72 h
Clot retraction screen	Whole blood (no anticoagulant)		Retraction begins at 1 h, maximum at 24 h
Clotting time, Lee-White, 37°C	Whole blood (no anticoagulant)		5–8 min
Differential count (see Bone marrow differential count or Leukocyte differential count)			
Eosinophil count	Whole blood (EDTA); capillary blood	50–400 cells/μL (mm³)	50–400 × 10⁶ cells/L
Erythrocyte count (RBC count)	Whole blood (EDTA)	millions of cells/μL (mm³)	× 10¹² cells/L
		M: 4.3–5.7	4.3–5.7
		F: 3.8–5.1	3.8–5.1
Erythrocyte sedimentation rate (ESR), Wintrobe			M: 0–15 mm/h
			F: 0–20 mm/h
Ferritin (see Chemistry section)			
Fibrin degradation products (agglutination, Thrombo-Wellco test)	Whole blood: special tube containing thrombin and proteolytic inhibitor	< 10 μg/mL	< 10 mg/L
	Urine: 2 mL in special tube (see above)	< 0.25 μg/mL	< 0.25 mg/L
Fibrinogen	Plasma (Na citrate)	200–400 mg/dL	2.00–4.00 g/L
Glucose-6-phosphate dehydrogenase (G6PD) in erythrocytes	Whole blood (ACD, EDTA, or heparin)	12.1 ± 2.09 U/g Hb (1 SD)	0.78 ± 0.13 MU/mol Hb (1 SD)
Haptoglobin (Hp) RID	Serum; avoid hemolysis	26–85 mg/dL	260–1850 mg/L
Hematocrit (HCT, Hct)	Whole blood (EDTA)		
Calculated from MCV and RBC (electronic displacement or laser)		M: 39–49%	0.39–0.49 volume fraction
		F: 35–45%	0.35–0.45 volume fraction
Hemoglobin (Hb)	Whole blood (EDTA)	M: 13.5–17.5 g/dL	2.09–2.71 mmol/L
		F: 12.0–16.0 g/dL	1.86–2.48 mmol/L
	Plasma (heparin, ACD)	< 3 mg/dL	< 0.47 μmol/L
	Urine, fresh, random		Negative
Hemoglobin electrophoresis	Whole blood (EDTA, citrate, or heparin)		Mass function
		HbA > 95%	HbA > 0.95
		HbA₂ 1.5–3.5%	HbA₂ 0.015–0.035
		HbF < 2%	HbF < 0.02
Leukocyte count (WBC count)	Whole blood (EDTA)	4.5–11.0 × 10³ cells/μL (mm³)	4.5–11.0 × 10⁹ cells/L
	CSF	0.5 mononuclear cells/μL	0.5 × 10⁶ cells/L

Leukocyte Differential count	Whole blood (EDTA)	%	Cells/μL (mm³)	Number fraction	Cells × 10⁶/L
Myelocytes		0	0	0	0
Neutrophils—bands		3–5	150–400	0.03–0.05	150–400
Neutrophils—segmented		54–62	3000–5800	0.54–0.62	3000–5800
Lymphocytes		23–33	1500–3000	0.25–0.33	1500–3000
Monocytes		3–7	285–500	0.03–0.07	285–500
Eosinophils		1–3	50–250	0.01–0.03	50–250
Basophils		0–0.75	15–50	0–0.0075	15–50

Leukocyte Differential count	CSF	%	Number fraction
Lymphocytes		62 ± 34	0.62 ± 0.324
Monocytes (includes pia-arachnoid mesothelial cells)		36 ± 20	0.36 ± 0.20
Neutrophils		2 ± 5	0.02 ± 0.05

Continued

HEMATOLOGY AND COAGULATION *Continued*

Test	Specimen	Reference Interval (Conventional Units)	Reference Interval (International Units)
Histocytes			Rare
Ependymal cells			Rare
Eosinophils			Rare
Mean corpuscular hemoglobin (MCH)	Whole blood (EDTA)	26–34 pg/cell	0.40–0.53 fmol/cell
Mean corpuscular hemoglobin concentration (MCHC)	Whole blood (EDTA)	31–37% Hb/cell or gHb/dL RBC	4.81–5.74 mmol Hb/L RBC
Mean corpuscular volume (MCV)	Whole blood (EDTA)		80–100 fL
Methemoglobin (MetHb)	Whole blood (EDTA, heparin, or ACD)	0.06–0.24 g/dL	9.3–37.2 µmol/L
Partial thromboplastin time (PTT)	Whole blood (Na citrate)		60–85 sec
Plasma volume	Plasma (heparin)	M: 25–43 mL/kg	0.025–0.043 L/kg
		F: 28–45 mL/kg	0.028–0.045 L/kg
Platelet count (thrombocyte count)	Whole blood (EDTA)	150–450 × 10³/µL (mm³)	150–450 × 10⁹/L
Prothrombin consumption	Whole blood (no anticoagulant)		> 30 sec
Prothrombin time, two-stage modified	Whole blood (Na citrate)		18–22 sec
RBC count (see Erythrocyte count)			
Red cell volume	Whole blood (heparin)	M: 20–36 mL/kg	M: 0.020–0.036 L/kg
		F: 19–31 mL/kg	F: 0.019–0.031 L/kg
Reticulocyte count	Whole blood (EDTA, heparin, or oxalate)	0.5–1.5% of erythrocytes	0.005–0.015 (number fraction)
Sulfhemoglobin	Whole blood (EDTA, heparin, or EDTA)	≤ 1.0% of total Hb	< 0.010 of total Hb (mass fraction)
Thrombin time	Whole blood (Na citrate)		Time of control ± 25 when control is 9–13 sec
Thromboplastin time, activated (see Activated partial thromboplastin time [APTT])			

DRUGS—THERAPEUTIC AND TOXIC

Drug	Specimen	Reference Interval (Conventional Units)		Reference Interval (International Units)
Acetaminophen	Serum or plasma (hep or EDTA)	Therap:	10–30 µg/mL	66–199 µmol/L
		Toxic:	> 200 µg/mL	> 1324 µmol/L
Amikacin	Serum or plasma (EDTA)	Therap:		
		Peak	25–35 µg/mL	43–60 µmol/L
		Trough (severe infection)	4–8 µg/mL	6.8–13.7 µmol/L
		Toxic:		
		Peak	> 35 µg/mL	> 60 µmol/L
		Trough	> 10 µg/mL	> 17 µmol/L
ε-Aminocaproic acid	Serum or plasma (hep or EDTA); trough	Therap:	100–400 µg/mL	0.76–3.05 mmol/L
Amitriptyline	Serum or plasma (hep or EDTA); trough (> 12 h after dose)	Therap:	120–250 ng/mL	433–903 nmol/L
		Toxic:	> 500 ng/mL	> 1805 nmol/L
Amobarbital	Serum	Therap:	1–5 µg/mL	4–22 µmol/L
		Toxic:	> 10 µg/mL	> 44 µmol/L
Amphetamine	Serum or plasma (hep or EDTA)	Therap:	20–30 ng/mL	148–222 nmol/L
		Toxic:	> 200 ng/mL	> 1480 nmol/L
Bromide	Serum	Therap:	750–1500 µg/mL	9.4–18.7 mmol/L
		Toxic:	> 1250 µg/mL	> 15.6 mmol/L
Caffeine	Serum or plasma (hep or EDTA)	Therap:	3–15 µg/mL	15–77 µmol/L
		Toxic:	> 50 µg/mL	> 258 µmol/L
Carbamazepine	Serum or plasma (hep or EDTA); trough	Therap:	4–12 µg/mL	17–51 µmol/L
		Toxic:	> 15 µg/mL	> 63 µmol/L
Carbenicillin	Serum or plasma	Therap:	Dependent on minimum inhibitory concentration of specific organism	Same
		Toxic:	> 250 µg/mL	> 660 µmol/L
Chloramphenicol	Serum or plasma (hep or EDTA); trough	Therap:	10–25 µg/L	31–77 µmol/L
		Toxic:	> 25 µg/mL	> 77 µmol/L
Chlordiazepoxide	Serum or plasma (hep or EDTA); trough	Therap:	700–1000 ng/mL	2.34–3.34 µmol/L
		Toxic:	> 5000 ng/mL	> 16.7 µmol/L
Chlorpromazine	Serum or plasma (hep or EDTA); trough	Therap:	50–300 ng/ml	157–942 nmol/L
		Toxic:	> 750 ng/mL	> 2355 nmol/L
Cimetidine	Serum or plasma (hep or EDTA); trough	Therap:	0.5–1.2 µg/mL	2–5 µmol/L
Clonazepam	Serum or plasma (hep or EDTA; trough	Therap:	15–60 ng/ml	48–190 nmol/L
		Toxic:	> 80 ng/mL	> 254 nmol/L
Clonidine	Serum or plasma (hep or EDTA)	Therap:	1.0–2.0 ng/mL	4.4–8.7 nmol/L
Clorazepate	Serum or plasma (hep or EDTA)	As desmethyldiazepam:		
		Therap:	0.12–1.0 µg/mL	0.36–3.01 µmol/L
Cocaine	Serum or plasma (hep or EDTA); on ice	Therap:	100–500 ng/mL	330–1650 nmol/L
		Toxic:	> 1000 ng/mL	> 3300 nmol/L
Codeine	Serum	Therap:	10–100 ng/mL	33–334 nmol/L
		Toxic:	> 200 ng/mL	> 668 nmol/L

DRUGS—THERAPEUTIC AND TOXIC *Continued*

Drug	Specimen	Reference Interval (Conventional Units)		Reference Interval (International Units)
Cyclosporine	Serum (12 h after dose)	Therap:	100–400 ng/mL	83–333 nmol/L
		Toxic:	>400 ng/mL	>333 nmol/L
Desipramine	Serum or plasma (hep or EDTA); trough (≥ 12 h after dose)	Therap:	75–300 ng/mL	281–1125 nmol/L
		Toxic:	>400 ng/mL	>1500 nmol/L
Diazepam	Serum or plasma (hep or EDTA); trough	Therap:	100–1000 ng/mL	0.35–3.51 µmol/L
		Toxic:	>5000 ng/mL	>17.55 µmol/L
Digitoxin	Serum or plasma (hep or EDTA) ≥ 6 h after dose	Therap:	20–35 ng/mL	26–46 nmol/L
		Toxic:	>45 ng/mL	>59 nmol/L
Digoxin	Serum or plasma (hep or EDTA) trough (≥ 12 h after dose)	Therap: CHF	0.8–1.5 mg/mL	1.0–1.9 nmol/L
		Arrhythmias:	1.5–2.0 ng/mL	1.9–2.6 nmol/L
		Toxic:	>2.5 ng/mL	>3.2 nmol/L
Diphenylhydantoin (see Phenytoin)				
Disopyramide	Serum or plasma (hep or EDTA); trough	Therap: Arrhythmias:		
		Atrial	2.8–3.2 µg/mL	8.3–9.4 µmol/L
		Ventricular	3.3–7.5 µg/mL	9.7–22 µmol/L
		Toxic:	>7 µg/mL	>20.7 µmol/L
Doxepin	Serum or plasma (hep or EDTA); trough (≥ 12 h after dose)	Therap:	30–150 ng/mL	107–537 nmol/L
		Toxic:	>500 ng/mL	>1790 nmol/L
Ephedrine	Serum	Therap:	0.05–0.10 µg/mL	0.30–0.61 µmol/L
		Toxic:	>2 µg/mL	>12.1 µmol/L
Ethchlorvynol	Serum or plasma (hep or EDTA)	Therap:	2–8 µg/mL	14–55 µmol/L
		Toxic:	>20 µg/mL	>138 µmol/L
Ethosuximide	Serum or plasma (hep or EDTA); trough	Therap:	40–100 µg/mL	283–708 µmol/L
		Toxic:	>150 µg/mL	>1062 µmol/L
Fenoprofen	Plasma (EDTA)	Therap:	20–65 µg/mL	82–268 µmol/L
Flecainide	Serum or plasma (hep or EDTA); trough	Therap:	0.2–1.0 µg/mL	0.5–2.4 µmol/L
		Toxic:	>1.0 µg/mL	>2.4 µmol/L
Flurazepam	Serum or plasma (EDTA)	Therap:	not well defined	
		Toxic:	>0.2 µg/mL	>0.5 µmol/L
Furosemide	Serum (30 min after dose)	Therap:	1–2 µg/mL	3–6 µmol/L
Gentamicin	Serum or plasma (EDTA)	Therap:		
		Peak (severe infection)	8–10 µg/mL	16.7–20.9 µmol/L
		Trough (severe infection)	<2–4 µg/mL	<4.2–8.4 µmol/L
		Toxic:		
		Peak	>10 µg/mL	>21 µmol/L
		Trough	>4 µg/mL	>8.4 µmol/L
Glutethimide	Serum	Therap:	2–6 µg/mL	9–28 µmol/L
		Toxic:	>5 µg/mL	>23 µmol/L
Haloperidol	Serum or plasma (hep or EDTA)	Therap:	6–245 ng/mL	16–652 nmol/L
		Toxic:	not defined	
Ibuprofen	Serum or plasma (hep or EDTA)	Therap:	10–50 µg/mL	49–243 µmol/L
		Toxic:	100–700 µg/mL	485–3395 µmol/L
Imipramine	Serum or plasma (hep or EDTA); trough (≥ 12 h after dose)	Therap:	125–250 ng/mL	446–893 nmol/L
		Toxic:	>500 ng/mL	>1784 nmol/L
Isoniazid	Serum or plasma (hep or EDTA)	Therap:	1–7 µg/mL	7–51 µmol/L
		Toxic:	20–710 µg/mL	146–5176 µmol/L
Kanamycin	Serum or plasma (EDTA)	Therap:		
		Peak	25–35 µg/mL	52–72 µmol/L
		Trough (severe infection)	4–8 µg/mL	8–16 µmol/L
		Toxic:		
		Peak	>35 µg/mL	>72 µmol/L
		Trough	>10 µg/mL	>21 µmol/L
Lidocaine	Serum or plasma (hep or EDTA); ≥ 45 min following bolus dose	Therap:	1.5–6.0 µg/mL	6.4–26 µmol/L
		Toxic:		
		CNS or cardiovascular depression	6–8 µg/mL	26–34.2 µmol/L
		Seizures, obtundation, decreased cardiac output	>8 µg/mL	>34.2 µmol/L
Lithium	Serum or plasma (hep or EDTA); (> 12 h after last dose)	Therap:	0.6–1.2 mEq/L	0.6–1.2 nmol/L
		Toxic:	>2 mEq/L	>2 mmol/L
Lorazepam	Serum or plasma (hep or EDTA)	Therap:	50–240 ng/mL	156–746 nmol/L
Meperidine	Serum or plasma (hep or EDTA)	Therap:	400–700 ng/mL	1620–2830 nmol/L
		Toxic:	>1 µg/mL	>4043 nmol/L
Meprobamate	Serum	Therap:	6–12 µg/mL	28–55 µmol/L
		Toxic:	>60 µg/mL	>275 µmol/L
Methadone	Serum or plasma (hep or EDTA)	Therap:	100–400 ng/mL	0.32–1.29 µmol/L
		Toxic:	>2000 ng/mL	>6.46 µmol/L
Methaqualone	Serum or plasma (hep or EDTA)	Therap:	2–3 µg/mL	8–12 µmol/L
		Toxic:	>10 µg/mL	>40 µmol/L
Methotrexate	Serum or plasma (hep or EDTA)	Therap:	variable	variable
		Toxic:		
		Low-dose therapy (1–2 wk)	>9.1 ng/mL	>20 nmol/L
		High-dose therapy (48 h)	>227 ng/mL	>0.5 µmol/L
Methsuximide (N-desmethyl methsuximide)	Serum	Therap:	10–40 µg/mL	53–212 µmol/L
		Toxic:	>40 µg/mL	>212 µmol/L
Methyldopa	Plasma (EDTA)	Therap:	1–5 µg/mL	4.7–23.7 µmol/L
		Toxic:	>7 µg/mL	>33 µmol/L

Continued

✔

DRUGS—THERAPEUTIC AND TOXIC *Continued*

Drug	Specimen	Reference Interval (Conventional Units)		Reference Interval (International Units)
Methyprylon	Serum	Therap:	8–10 μg/mL	43–55 μmol/L
		Toxic:	>50 μg/mL	>273 μmol/L
Morphine	Serum or plasma (hep or EDTA)	Therap:	10–80 ng/mL	35–280 nmol/L
		Toxic:	>200 ng/mL	>700 nmol/L
N-Acetylprocainamide	Serum or plasma (hep or EDTA); trough	Therap:	5–30 μg/mL	18–108 μmol/L
		Toxic:	>40 μg/mL	>144 μmol/L
Netilmicin	Serum or plasma (EDTA)	Therap:		
		Peak (severe infection)	8–10 μg/mL	17–21 μmol/L
		Trough (severe infection)	<4 μg/mL	<8 μmol/L
		Toxic:		
		Peak	>12 μg/mL	>25 μmol/L
		Trough	>4 μg/mL	>8 μmol/L
Nitroprusside	Serum or plasma (EDTA)	As thiocyanate:		
		Therap:	6–29 μg/mL	103–499 μmol/L
Nortriptyline	Serum or plasma (hep or EDTA); trough (≥ 12 h after dose)	Therap:	50–150 ng/mL	190–570 nmol/L
		Toxic:	>500 ng/mL	>1900 nmol/L
Oxazepam	Serum or plasma (hep or EDTA)	Therap:	0.2–1.4 μg/mL	0.70–4.9 μmol/L
Oxycodone	Serum	Therap:	10–100 ng/ml	32–317 nmol/L
		Toxic:	>200 ng/mL	>634 nmol/L
Paraquat	Whole blood (EDTA)	Toxic:	0.1–1.6 μg/mL	0.39–6.2 μmol/L
	Urine	Occup exp:	0.3 μg/mL	1.17 μmol/L
		Toxic:	0.9–64 μg/mL	3.50–249 μmol/L
Pentazocine	Serum or plasma (EDTA)	Therap:	0.05–0.2 μg/mL	0.2–0.7 μmol/L
		Toxic:	>1 μg/mL	>3.5 μmol/L
	Urine	Toxic:	>3 μg/mL	>10.5 μmol/L
Pentobarbital	Serum or plasma (hep or EDTA); trough	Therap:		
		Hypnotic	1–5 μg/mL	4–22 μmol/L
		Therap coma	20–50 μg/mL	88–221 μmol/L
		Toxic:	>10 μg/mL	>44 μmol/L
Phenacetin	Plasma (EDTA)	Therap:	1–30 μg/mL	6–167 μmol/L
		Toxic:	50–250 μg/mL	279–1395 μmol/L
Phencyclidine	Serum or plasma (hep or EDTA)	Toxic:	90–800 ng/mL	370–3288 nmol/L
Phenobarbital	Serum or plasma (hep or EDTA); trough	Therap:	15–40 μg/mL	65–170 μmol/L
		Toxic:		
		Slowness, ataxia, nystagmus	35–80 μg/mL	151–345 μmol/L
		Coma with reflexes	65–117 μg/mL	280–504 μmol/L
		Coma without reflexes	>100 μg/mL	>430 μmol/L
Phensuximide (both parent and N-desmethyl metabolites)	Serum or plasma (hep or EDTA)	Therap:	40–60 μg/mL	228–324 μmol/L
Phenylbutazone	Plasma (EDTA)	Therap: (not well defined)	50–100 μg/mL	162–324 μmol/L
		Toxic:	>100 μg/mL	>324 μmol/mL
Phenylpropanolamine	Serum	Therap:	0.05–0.10 μg/mL	0.33–0.66 μmol/L
		Toxic:	>5 μg/mL	>33.07 μmol/L
Phenytoin	Serum or plasma (hep or EDTA); trough	Therap:	10–20 μg/mL	40–79 μmol/L
		Toxic:	>20 μg/mL	>79 μmol/L
Primidone	Serum or plasma (hep or EDTA); trough	Therap:	5–12 μg/mL	23–55 μmol/L
		Toxic:	>15 μg/mL	>69 μmol/L
Procainamide	Serum or plasma (hep or EDTA); trough	Therap:	4–10 μg/mL	17–42 μmol/L
		Toxic:	>10–12 μg/mL	>42–51 μmol/L
		Also consider effect of metabolite, N-acetylprocainamide		
Propoxyphene	Plasma (EDTA)	Therap:	0.1–0.4 μg/mL	0.3–1.2 μmol/L
		Toxic:	>0.5 μg/mL	>1.5 μmol/L
Propranolol	Serum or plasma (hep or EDTA); trough	Therap:	50–100 ng/mL	193–386 nmol/L
Protriptyline	Serum or plasma (hep or EDTA); trough (≥ 12 h after dose)	Therap:	70–250 ng/mL	266–950 nmol/L
		Toxic:	>500 ng/mL	>1900 nmol/L
Quinidine	Serum or plasma (hep or EDTA); trough	Therap:	2–5 μg/mL	6–15 μmol/L
		Toxic:	>6 μg/mL	>18 μmol/L
Salicylates	Serum or plasma (hep or EDTA); trough	Therap:	150–300 μg/mL	1086–2172 μmol/L
		Toxic:	>300 μg/mL	>2172 μmol/L
Secobarbital	Serum	Therap:	1–2 μg/mL	4.2–8.4 μmol/L
		Toxic:	>5 μg/mL	>21.0 μmol/L
Theophylline	Serum or plasma (hep or EDTA)	Therap:	8–20 μg/mL	44–111 μmol/L
		Toxic:	>20 μg/mL	>110 μmol/L
Thiocyanate	Serum or plasma (EDTA)	Nonsmoker:	1–4 μg/mL	17–69 μmol/L
		Smoker:	3–12 μg/mL	52–206 μmol/L
		Therap, after nitroprusside infusion:	6–29 μg/mL	103–499 μmol/L
	Urine	Nonsmoker:	1–4 mg/d	17–69 μmol/L
		Smoker:	7–17 mg/d	120–292 μmol/L
Thiopental	Serum or plasma (hep or EDTA); trough	Hypnotic:	1–5 μg/mL	4.1–20.7 μmol/L
		Coma:	30–100 μg/mL	124–413 μmol/L
		Anesthesia:	7–130 μg/mL	29–536 μmol/L
		Toxic conc:	>10 μg/mL	>41 μmol/L
Thiordiazine	Serum or plasma (hep or EDTA)	Therap:	1.0–1.5 μg/mL	2.7–4.1 μmol/L
		Toxic:	>10 μg/mL	>27 μmol/L

DRUGS—THERAPEUTIC AND TOXIC *Continued*

Drug	Specimen	Reference Interval (Conventional Units)		Reference Interval (International Units)
Tobramycin	Serum or plasma (hep or EDTA)	Therap:		
		Peak (severe infection)	8–10 µg/mL	17–21 µmol/L
		Trough (severe infection)	<4 µg/mL	<9 µmol/L
		Toxic:		
		Peak	>10 µg/mL	>21 µmol/L
		Trough	>4 µg/mL	>9 µmol/L
Tocainide	Serum or plasma (hep or EDTA)	Therap:	4–10 µg/mL	21–52 µmol/L
Tolbutamide	Serum	Therap:	80–240 µg/mL	299–888 µmol/L
		Toxic:	>640 µg/mL	>2368 µmol/L
Valproic acid	Serum or plasma (hep or EDTA); trough	Therap:	50–100 µg/mL	347–693 µmol/L
		Toxic:	>100 µg/mL	>693 µmol/L
Vancomycin	Serum or plasma (hep or EDTA); trough	Therap:	5–10 µg/mL	3–7 µmol/L
		Toxic: (not well established)	>80–100 µg/mL	>55–69 µmol/L
Verapamil	Serum or plasma (hep or EDTA)	Therap:	100–500 ng/mL	220–1100 nmol/L
Warfarin	Serum or plasma (hep or EDTA)	Therap:	1–10 µg/mL	3–32 µmol/L

Beutler E: Hemolytic Anemia in Disorders of Red Cell Metabolism. New York, Plenum Publishing, 1978.

Brown SS, Mitchell FL, Young DS (eds.): Chemical Diagnosis of Disease. Amsterdam, Elsevier/North-Holland Biomedical Press, 1979.

Burtis CA, Ashwood ER (eds.): Tietz Textbook of Clinical Chemistry. Philadelphia, WB Saunders, 1994.

Conn RB (ed.): Current Diagnosis. 8th ed. Philadelphia, WB Saunders, 1991.

Gilman AG, Rall TW, Nies AS, Taylor P: (eds.): The Pharmacological Basis of Therapeutics. 8th ed. New York, Pergamon Press, 1990.

Henry JB (ed.): Todd-Sanford-Davidsohn Clinical Diagnosis and Management by Laboratory Methods. 18th ed. Philadelphia, WB Saunders, 1991.

Hoeg JM, Gregg RE, Brewer HB: An approach to the management of hyperlipoproteinemia. JAMA 255:512, 1986.

Miale JB: Laboratory Medicine: Hematology. 6th ed. St. Louis, CV Mosby, 1982.

Tietz NW, Blackburn RH (eds.): Reference Ranges and General Information. Clinical Laboratories, A.B. Chandler Medical Center, University of Kentucky, Lexington, Kentucky, 1984.

Tietz NW (ed.): Clinical Guide to Laboratory Tests. Philadelphia, WB Saunders, 1990.

Williams WJ, Beutler E, Erslev AJ, et al.: Hematology. 4th ed. New York, McGraw-Hill, 1990.

Young DS: Effect of Drugs on Clinical Laboratory Tests. 3rd ed. Washington, DC, AACC Press, 1990; Friedman RB, Young DS: Effects of Disease on Clinical Laboratory Tests, 2nd ed. Washington, DC, AACC Press, 1989. *If consideration is interference with or effects of disease on a clinical test, here are two references that are of value.*

Note: Page numbers in *italics* refer to illustrations; page numbers followed by t refer to tables. Boldface type refers to main discussion.

A

A cells, 1282
a wave, 167, *167*
  "cannon," 167
  pressure gradient with, *210, 211*
Abdomen, 748–749
  abscess in, CT scan of, 631, *631*
    diverticular, 631, *631*
  acute, 748t, 748–749
  auscultation of, 749
  collateral veins on, 752, 793
  CT scan of, 630–632, *631*
  diaphragmatic motion and, 442–443, 466
  examination of, 748
  imaging of, 749
    procedures for, 630–635, *630–635*
  liver disease and, 752, 793, 1133
  lymph nodes of, 969, 969t
  metastatic nodules of, 1030–1031, 1031t
  MRI scan of, *634*, 634–635, *635*
  pain in. See *Pain, abdominal.*
  paradoxical motion of, 442, 466
  radionuclide studies in, *633*, 633–634, *634*
  ultrasonography of, 632, *632*
Abetalipoproteinemia, 705
Abl oncogene, 1011–1012, 1036t, 1058
Ablation therapy, 252t, 252–253
Abortion, spontaneous, 152–159, 158t
  syphilitic, 1710
Abscesses, abdominal, 631, *631*
  actinomycosis with, 1675, *1675*
  brain. See *Brain, abscess of.*
  diverticular, *631*
  epidural, cranial, 2084
    spinal, 2082–2083
  glanders with, 1669
  glomerulonephritis with, 576
  muscle, 1609
  pancreatic, 730, 734
  perianal, 741, *741*
  periodontal, 450–451
  pulmonary, 413–416. See also *Lung, abscess of.*
  rectal, 741, *741*
  skin, 1606–1607, 1607t, 1609, 2192
  splenic, 974
  staphylococcal, 1606–1607, 1607t, 1609
  valve ring, 1599
Absorption, 689–690, 695–697. See also
    Malabsorption.
  amino acid, 696, 696t
  bile salt, 696, 696t, 806, 806–807, *807*
  calcium, 696t, 697, 700t, *1352*, 1353
    impaired, 1362t, 1363t, 1371
  carbohydrate, 696, 696t
  fat, 696, 696t, *697*, 806, *806*
  fluid, 689–690, 696t, 696–697
  folate (folic acid), 696t, 697, 844t, 846–847
  iron, 696t, 697, 700t, 839–840
  nutrient, 695–697, 696t, *697, 698*
  phosphorus, 1135
    impaired, 1362t, 1363t
  protein, 696, 696t
  sites of, 695–697, 696t

Absorption *(Continued)*
  solute, *689*, 689–690, 690t
  triglyceride, 696, *697*
  vitamin B$_{12}$, 696t, 697, *698*, 700t, 844t, 845–846
ABVD therapy, 952t, 953
Acalculia, 1987
Acanthamoeba, 1915
Acanthocytes, 825t, 827
Acanthosis nigricans, 1019
  palmar, 1019–1020
  paraneoplastic, 1019–1020, 1034
Acatalasia, 136t, 147t
Accelerated idioventricular rhythm, *243*, 243–244
Accessory pathways, tachycardia role of, 239, *240*
Accidents, drowning, 37, *38*
  falling, 23, 37, *38*
  firearms in, 37, *38*
  mortality rate in, 27t, 30t
  motor vehicle, 37, *38, 39*
  poisoning, 37, *38*
  risk factors for, 30t
ACE. See *Angiotensin-converting enzyme (ACE).*
ACE inhibitors, angioedema caused by, 1412
  dosages for, 265t, 266t
  hypertension treated with, 263, 265t, 266t, 266–267, 267t
  side effects of, 266–267, 267t
  vasodilatation using, 229t, 229–230
Acebutolol, 246t
  adverse effects of, 248t
  dosage for, 265t
  pharmacokinetics of, 246t
Acetaminophen, analgesic effects of, 115t
  antidote for, 504t
  antipyretic effects of, 115t
  development history of, 112
  hepatotoxicity, 772, 773t, 774, 798, 800t
  pain control with, 102, 103t, 893t
  poisoning due to, 504t, 506
  renal function and, 584–585
Acetanilide, 112
Acetazolamide, 224t, 531t
Acetylated plasminogen streptokinase activator complex, 311, *311*
Acetylcholine, asthma role of, 376
  neuromuscular junction and, 2171
  poisoning blockade of, 506
Acetylcysteine, 504t
  acetaminophen toxicity treated with, 504t
Acetyl-galactosamine-6-sulfatase deficiency, 1119t
Acetylglucosaminidase deficiency, 1119t
Acetylsalicylic acid. See *Aspirin; Salicylates.*
N-Acetyltransferase, 97t
Achalasia, 654–656, *655*
Achilles tendon, aging effect on, 17
  gonorrhea affecting, 1702
  gout affecting, 1512, 1516
Acholeplasma infections, 1576, 1576t
Achondroplasia, 1390–1391
Achromatopsia, 1985, 1987t
Acid, accumulation of, 547–548
  burn due to, 504t, 2221
  hydrofluoric, 504t
  metabolic production of, 543–544, 547

Acid *(Continued)*
  organic, 547–548
Acid-base balance, **543–551**. See also *Acidosis; Alkalosis; pH.*
  AIDS/HIV effect on, 1875
  anion gap in, 545–547, 546t
  bicarbonate in, 543–544, *545*
  carbon dioxide in, 543–544, *545*
  definition of abnormalities of, 545, *545*, 545t
  physiologic mechanisms of, 543–546, *545*, 545t
Acidemia, 543
  definition of, 543
  mitochondrial enzyme defect causing, 146t
Acid-fast organisms, 1557, 1557t
  cryptosporidial, 1911–1912
  leprosy due to, 1692, 1692t
  tuberculosis due to, 1685
Acidosis, 545, 545t, 545–546
  anion gap, 545–546, 546t, 550t
    increased, 546t, 546–548, 550t
  causes of, 545–549, 546t, 550t, 595t, 597–599
  compensatory mechanisms in, *545*, 545–546
  dilutional, 546–547
  ethylene glycol causing, 548, 549
  hyperchloremic, 547, 550t, 598
  ketotic, *548*, 548–549, 1269–1271
  lactic, 547–548, 549
  metabolic, 545t, 546t, 546–549
    anion gap and, 546t, 546–548, 550t
    causes of, 545t, 546t, 546–549, 550t, 1359t
    diagnosis of, *545*, 545t, 548–549
    drug-induced, 548
    osteomalacia with, 1359t, 1364–1365
    renal failure and, 546t, 546–547, 557
    treatment of, 548–549
  methanol causing, 548, 549
  mixed disorders and, 550t, 550–551
  potassium and, 540, 546t
  renal obstruction with, 591t, 592
  renal tubular, 546–549, 597–599, 1359t
    distal, 598t, 598–599
    drug-induced, 547, 548
    glomerular, 598, 598t
    gradient-limited, 546t, 547, 598t
    pathophysiology of, 546t, 546–547, 595t, *597*, 597–599, 598t
    proximal, 595t, *597*, 598t
    symptoms of, 546t, 595t, 597, 598t
    transport defects in, 144t, 594–599, 595t
    treatment of, 548–549, 597–599
    types of, 546t, 598t
    voltage-dependent (hyperkalemic), 546t, 547, 598t
  respiratory, 551
    clinical features of, 551
    definition of, 545, *545*, 545t
    pathogenesis of, 545, 551
    treatment of, 551
  salicylates causing, 548, 549
  shock and, cardiogenic, 480, *480*, 491
  uremic, 557
Aciduria, glyceric, 1085
  glycolic, 1085
  hyperoxaluria causing, 1085
  mitochondrial enzyme defect causing, 146t

Aciduria (Continued)
orotic, hereditary, 1117
Acinar cell, 730, 731
Acinetobacter infections, 1579–1581, 1580t
Ackee fruit, vomiting caused by, 754
Acne, 2206–2207
androgens and, 1315, 2206–2207
chemical-induced, 2221
hirsutism with, 1315
pustules of, 2206–2207
retinoid therapy of, 2197, 2207
vulgaris, incidence of, 2184t
Acoustic neuroma (schwannoma), 2126t, 2131
MRI scan of, 2128t
neurofibromatosis with, 2056
Acquired immunodeficiency syndrome. See AIDS
(acquired immunodeficiency syndrome).
Acrochordon, 2190
Acrocyanosis, 349
clinical features of, 349
diagnosis of, 349
pathophysiology of, 349
Acrodermatitis, chronica atrophicans, 1717
enteropathica, 1150t
Lyme disease with, 1717
zinc absorption impairment in, 1150t
Acrolein, inhalation of, 403t
Acromegaly, 1211–1212
clinical features of, 1211, 1211t, 1212
diagnosis of, 1212
etiology of, 1211
pathogenesis of, 1211
treatment of, 1212
tumor-associated, 1026
Acromion, 1522
Acropachy. See Clubbing.
Acroparesthesia, Fabry's disease with, 1096
ACTH. See Adrenocorticotropic hormone (ACTH).
Actin, bile flow and, 806
connective tissue role of, 1446
erythrocytic, 851, 851–852
hepatic canaliculi with, 806
Actinic keratoses, 2210
Actinin, 1446
Actinomyces, 1674–1676
antimicrobial susceptibility of, 1641t
Actinomycetoma, 1834–1835
clinical features of, 1835, 1835t
etiologic organism in, 1834–1835, 1835t
treatment of, 1835
Actinomycin D, adverse effects of, 1045
chemotherapy using, 1039t, 1044t, 1045
Actinomycosis, 1674–1676
abdominopelvic, 1675
cervicofacial, 1674, 1675
clinical manifestations of, 1675, 1675
definition of, 1674
diagnosis of, 1675–1676
epidemiology of, 1674
etiology of, 1674
hepatic, 782
pathogenesis of, 1674–1675
pathology findings in, 1674–1675
pleural effusion with, 445, 446, 1675
sulfur granules of, 1640t, 1674, 1675
thoracic, 1675, 1675
treatment of, 1676
Action potential, 232
cardiac cell, 232, 232, 233, 233t
fast response, 232, 233, 233t
intestinal muscle, 680
motor end-plate, 2171
Purkinje cell, 232
slow response, 232, 233, 233t
Acute phase reactants, 1535–1537
host response with, 1535–1536, 1536t
measurement of, 1536–1537
sedimentation rate affected by, 1456
Acyclovir, 1742–1743
herpes simplex treated with, 1742–1743, 1746t
herpes zoster treated with, 1742–1743, 1746t
licensing for, 1742
mechanism of action of, 1742
renal function and, 1742, 1742t
toxicity of, 1742, 1742t
viral pharyngitis treated with, 1751t
Acyl-CoA dehydrogenase deficiency, 2166
Addison's disease, hyperpigmentation of, 2213

Adenine, genetic code use of, 134, 134t
kidney stone due to, 1118
Adenine phosphoribosyltransferase, deficiency of, 1117
purine metabolism and, 1510, 1511
Adenitis. See also Lymphadenitis.
mesenteric yersinial, 1661
Adenocarcinoma, duodenal, 679–680
esophageal, 657
gallbladder, 811
gastric, 677, 677t
Adenoma, 722, 1076
carcinomatous sequence of, 722, 726, 1076, 1076
colonic, 722, 726
gastric, 679
hepatic, 802–803, 803t
drug-induced, 773, 773t
pituitary, 1200t, 1200–1201, 1207–1210, 1209t
MRI scan of, 2127–2128, 2128t
prolactin-secreting, 1200–1201, 1202
Adenopathy. See Lymphadenopathy.
Adenosine, antiarrhythmic action of, 245, 246t, 250
asthma role of, 376
Adenosine deaminase, 1115
deficiency of, 1114–1115
immunodeficiency due to, 1406
erythrocyte overproduction of, 859
purine metabolism and, 1114–1115, 1115
Adenosine monophosphate, cyclic (cAMP), 1177–1178
hormone action and, 1176, 1177–1178
parathyroid hormone action and, 1366
second messenger role of, 1176, 1177–1178
Adenosine monophosphate deaminase, 1115
deficiency of, 1116–1117
purine metabolism and, 1115, 1116–1117
Adenosine triphosphate (ATP), erythrocytic, 856, 856,
859
Adenosylcobalamin, 1113, 1113
deficiency of, 1113, 1113t
Adenovirus/adenoviral infection, 1757–1759
colds (common) due to, 1747, 1747t, 1748
compromised host with, 1757t, 1758
conjunctivitis and, 1757, 1757t
cystitis due to, 1757t, 1758
diagnosis of, 1758
enteric, 1757t, 1758
immunization for, 1758–1759
pharyngitis due to, 1749–1751, 1750t, 1751t
respiratory tract, 1757t, 1758
structure of, 1739, 1757, 1757, 1757t
treatment and, 1758–1759
vaccine for, 46
Adenylate cyclase, 1178, 1178
hormone action role of, 1178, 1178
ADH (antidiuretic hormone). See Vasopressin.
Adhesion, 897–898, 899
bacterial. See Fimbriae.
leukocytic, 897–898, 899
disordered, 902–904, 903, 904t, 905t, 906t, 1408
immunodeficiency related to, 1408, 1540–1541
rheumatic disease and, 1448–1450, 1449, 1450
vasculitis due to, 1449, 1449–1450, 1450
Adie's pupils, 2018, 2018, 2153
Adie's syndrome, 2009, 2010
Adipocytes, 1163, 1167
body region differences in, 1164
hyperplasia of, 1163, 1167
obesity role of, 1163, 1167
Adipose tissue, 1161–1162, 1507–1508
amyloidosis and, 1505–1506
atrophy of, 1508
biopsy of, 1505–1506
brown, 1163
distribution of, 1162, 1163–1164
excessive. See Obesity.
gender and, 1162, 1163–1164
inflammation of, 1507–1508
necrosis of, 1507, 2211
obesity defined by, 1161, 1161–1162, 1162
panniculitis affecting, 1507–1508
subcutaneous, 1507–1508, 2185, 2211
Adjuvant therapy, lung cancer and, 441
Adnexal masses, 1313
Adrenal glands, 1245–1257
adenoma of, 1249
AIDS/HIV effect on, 1877–1878
anatomy of, 1245–1246, 1246
androgens of, 1245, 1287–1290
anorexia effect on, 1159
antibodies to, 1250–1251, 1251t
atrial natriuretic hormone affecting, 1195, 1196

Adrenal glands (Continued)
biochemistry of, 1245–1246
chromaffin tissue of, 1253
cortex of, 1245–1252
anatomy of, 1245–1246, 1246
hormones of, 1245–1246. See also Aldosterone;
Corticosteroids; Cortisol.
laboratory evaluation of, 1246–1247
crisis of, 1250
hemorrhage of, 1251
histology of, 1245–1246, 1246
hyperfunction of, 1247–1249. See also Cushing's
syndrome.
glucocorticoid, 1247t, 1247–1249
mineralocorticoid, 1249, 1249t
hyperplasia of, 1252
congenital, 1252, 1287, 1288, 1288t, 1289
differential diagnosis of, 1247, 1252, 1288t
enzyme defects in, 1287–1290, 1288t, 1288–1290
feminization and, 1252
hirsutism in, 1252, 1288, 1315–1317, 1316t
hypertensive, 1252
pseudohermaphroditism in, 1287–1290, 1288t,
1288–1290
salt-wasting, 1252, 1288t
virilization and, 1252, 1287–1290, 1288t,
1288–1290
hypofunction of, 1249–1252
acute, 1250
end-organ resistance in, 1252, 1291t
glucocorticoid deficiency in, 1249–1251, 1250t
hypoaldosteronism in, 1251t, 1251–1252
mineralocorticoid deficiency in, 1251t, 1251–1252
primary, 1250–1251, 1251t
hypothalamic-pituitary axis with, 1215, 1250
infectious disease of, 1251
leukodystrophy and, 1251
medulla of, 1253–1257
anatomy of, 1246
hormones of, 1253, 1253–1254. See also Catecholamines; Dopamine; Epinephrine; Norepinephrine.
hyperfunction of, 1254–1257
hypofunction of, 1257
laboratory tests and, 1255–1256
pheochromocytoma and, 1254t, 1254–1257
MRI of, 1246
physiology of, 1245–1246, 1246
pituitary and, 1215, 1250
responsiveness test of, 1247
suppression test of, 1213t, 1217t, 1247
renin-angiotensin system and, 1249, 1249t, 1251t,
1251–1252
steroids of, 1245–1247, 1247. See also Aldosterone;
Corticosteroids; Cortisol; Glucocorticoids.
enzyme deficiencies affecting, 1287–1290, 1288,
1288t
excretion of, 1246–1247, 1247
synthesis and secretion of, 1245–1247, 1247
urinary excretion of, 1246–1247, 1247
stimulation test for, 1247
suppression tests for, 1213t, 1217t, 1217–1218,
1247
tuberculosis and, 1250
tumor of, 1254–1257
incidental mass, 1257
myelolipoma, 1257
pheochromocytoma, 1254–1257
Adrenaline. See Epinephrine.
Adrenarche, premature, 1295, 1295t
Adrenergic nervous system. See also Epinephrine; Norepinephrine; Sympathetic nervous system.
blocking agents in, 265t–267t, 270t. See also Alpha
blocking agents; Beta blocking agents; Propranolol.
receptors of, 245, 268
activation of, 1253–1254
shock and, 492–493
Adrenocorticotropic hormone (ACTH), 1206t,
1215–1218
cortisol and, 1215–1216, 1247–1248, 1248t
reserve tests, 1213t, 1216
Cushing's syndrome and, 1216–1218, 1217t, 1248,
1248t
tumor-associated, 1024–1025, 1025t, 1248–1249
deficiency of, 1215–1216
glucocorticoid therapy causing, 1215–1216, 1250
dexamethasone test for, 1213t, 1217t, 1217–1218,
1247
ectopic, 1024–1025, 1025t, 1248

Adrenocorticotropic hormone (ACTH) *(Continued)*
　tests for, 1213t, 1217t, 1217–1218
　endorphin synthesis related to, 1186, *1186*
　excess of, *1216*, 1216–1218, 1217t
　feedback mechanism for, *1198*, 1198–1199, 1215
　fever production role of, *1534*
　laboratory tests for, 1208t, 1213t, 1217t, 1217–1218, 1247
　metapyrone test and, 1216
　physiology of, 1215
　regulation of, *1198*, 1198–1199, 1206t, 1215
　　disordered, 1203, 1215–1218
　releasing hormone for, *1198*, 1198–1199, 1216
　secretion of, 1215
　　tumor and, 1024–1025, 1209t, 1217t
　stimulation test for, 1208t, 1247
　suppression test for, 1213t, 1217t, 1217–1218, 1247
Adrenoleukodystrophy, 1251
Adriamycin. See *Doxorubicin.*
Adventitia. See also *Intima.*
　polyarteritis nodosa affecting, 1493
Aerobes, 1557t
Aerobic capacity (physiologic), 31t
Aerosols, barium, 73
　bubonic plague in, 1662
　influenza in, 1755
　Legionella in, 1583
　manganese, 73
　tuberculosis transmission by, 1683
　tularemia transmission by, 1662–1663
Afibrinogenemia, 996
Aflatoxins, aspergillosis organism with, 1830
AFP (alpha-fetoprotein), 1022t, 1023
Afterdepolarizations, *234*
　delayed, 234, *234*
　early, 234, *234*
　Purkinje fiber, 234, *234*
　tachyarrhythymias with, 234, *234*
Afterload, 176–177, *177*, 212t, 214–215
　definition of, 212t, 214
　heart failure and, 215, *215*
　"mismatch," 176, *177*
　shock and, *479*, 480, *480*, 494
　vasodilator reduction of, 229, 229t, 494
Agammaglobulinemia, 1402t, *1403*, 1403–1404
　Bruton's, 1402t, *1403*, 1403–1404
　enteroviral meningoencephalitis in, 1792
　X-linked, 1402t, *1403*, 1403–1404
Age, **12–25**. See also *Elderly; Lifespan.*
　AIDS cases related to, 1848t
　biology of, 12–15
　body compartments affected by, 1161, *1162*
　body fat change with, 1161–1162, *1162*
　body mass index affected by, 1161, *1162*
　diabetes mellitus and, 1258–1260
　environmental influences and, 12–13, 14
　esophagus affected by, 655
　genetic effects of, 138–139
　height and, 1140t, 1152t
　hypothalamic disease onset and, 1200t
　lifespan and, 12, *12*, 14
　mid upper arm circumference and, 1153, 1153t
　mortality rate and, 27t, *38*
　neurologic changes due to, 16t, 16–17, 17t
　neuropsychiatric aspects of, 17–21, 19t, 20t
　nutrition status assessment and, 1152t, 1153, 1153t
　osteoporosis and, 1379, *1379*
　other species affected by, 14
　paternal, 138–139
　recommended dietary allowances and, 1140t, 1141t
　skin effects related to, 2187, 2190
　telomere relation to, 1072, *1072*
　theories of, 14–15
　triceps skinfold size and, 1153, 1153t
　vitamin D therapy and, 1383
　weight and, 1152t
　weight-to-height change with, 1161–1162, *1162*, 1163t
Agglutinins, anaerobic flora production of, 1639t
　cold, 862–864, 1577, *1577*
　erythrocyte, 860–864
　red kidney bean, 740
Agitation, 1999, 1999t
Agnosia, 1989t, 1990
　auditory, 1991
　finger, 1987
　temporal lobe damage and, 1986, 1987t
　visual, 1985, 1987t, 1990
Agoraphobia, 2004–2005
Agraphia, 1985, 1988t, 1992

AH interval, *232*
AIDS (acquired immunodeficiency syndrome), **1837–1891**. See also *HIV infection.*
　adenovirus infection in, 1757t, 1758
　cardiac lesions in, 329, 329t
　cholangiopathy of, 812
　counseling for, *1888–1890*, **1888–1891**, 1890t, 1891t
　cytomegalovirus infection in, 1775, 1846t, 1859t
　dementia complex of, 2097t, 2097–2099, *2098*, 2098t
　epidemiology of, 1846t, **1846–1851**, *1847*, 1848t, *1849*, 1850t
　etiologic agent in, 1841–1846, *1842–1845*
　hepatic infection with, 785
　hospital-acquired, 1553, 1854
　immunology of, 1837t, **1837–1841**, 1839t
　incidence and prevalence of, *1847*, 1847–1848, 1848t
　intestinal morphology and, 692
　Kaposi's sarcoma with, 1032, 1033t, 1863, *1864*, 1872–1873, 1873t
　malabsorption in, 692, 706–707
　mortality rate in, *1849*
　neuropathy in, 2156–2157
　pathophysiology of, 1837–1846, *1838*, *1843*
　Pneumocystis carinii pneumonia in, 1859t, 1861–1862, *1862*
　prevention and precautions related to, **1851–1854**, 1852t, 1853t, 1854t
　psychiatric disorders with, 1855t, 1857–1858
　pulmonary effects of, 1858–1865, 1859t–1861t, *1859–1865*, 1865t
　respiratory tract infections in, 1858–1865, 1859t–1861t, *1859–1865*, 1865t
　screening for, 28t, 1846t
　sexual activity and, 1697t, 1851–1852, 1852t
　syphilis with, 2086–2087, 2087t
　transmission modes for, **1848–1854**, 1852t, 1853t, 1854t
　treatment of, *1838*, 1865, **1880–1887**, 1883t, 1884t, 1885t, 1887t
　tuberculosis and, 1684, 1686, 1687, 1688t, 1861, *1861*, 1861t
　vaccine for, 1840–1841, 1841t
　virology of, *1838*, **1841–1846**, *1842–1845*
Air embolism, 2069
　thoracic, 448
　　cystic fibrosis with, 420, 421t
　　mediastinal mass due to, 449
　　Pneumocystis pneumonia with, 1918
Air pollution, 56
　aspergillosis organism in, 1830
　asthma due to, 56, 58t
　carcinogenicity of, 1015–1016
Airway obstruction, anaphylaxis in, 1418
　asthma and, 377–380, *378*
　bronchiectasis following, 416, 416t
　cancer causing, 1052–1053
　chronic, 381–389. See also *Bronchitis; Emphysema.*
　edema causing, 1418
　respiratory failure with, 458t
　signs and symptoms in, 368–371, 369t
　sleep apnea associated with, 1984, 1984t
　Wegener's granulomatosis with, 1495, 1495t, 1496t
Airway resistance, 370, *370*, 371
　size regulation factors in, *452*
　snoring and, 451–452
A-kinase, 1178
Alagille's syndrome, 810
Alanine, urinary, 1103t
Alanine transferase (ALT), alcoholic cirrhosis and, 790
　hepatitis and, *765*, *767*, *768*, 780
　liver function reflected by, 759
　pregnancy and, 787, 787t
Albendazole, 1916t
Albinism, 2214t
　clinical manifestations of, 2214t
　frequency of, 2214t
　genetics of, 136t, 138t
　metabolic defect in, 146
　ocular, 146, 2214t
　oculocutaneous, 146, 2214t
Albright's syndrome, *1372*, 1372–1373
　fibrous dysplasia in, 1390, 2213
　genetic factors in, 145
　osteodystrophy of, *1372*, 1372–1373, 2213
　precocious puberty with, 1296, 1347
Albumin, ascites gradient in, 744, 744t, 745t, 795, 795t
　bilirubin transport by, *755*, 755–756
　liver synthesis of, 761
　malabsorption treatment with, 704t

Albumin *(Continued)*
　serum level of, decreased, 1156t
　　malnutrition and, 1156t
　　normal, 700t
　thyroxine binding by, 1228, 1230t
Albuminuria, 513, 513t, 572–573
Alcohol/alcoholism, **47–49**
　allyl, 772
　anemia caused by, 827, 830
　blackout related to, 48, 1982
　blood level of, 48t
　calories from, 30t, 30–31
　cancer related to, 1009, 1009t, 1014
　cardiomyopathy caused by, 330, *330*
　cirrhosis caused by, 789–791
　definitions and, 47
　dietary restriction of, 261
　diseases associated with, 30t, 48, 48t, 1009t
　epidemiology and, 47
　erythrocyte volume and, 830
　folate deficiency caused by, 844, 844t
　gastritis due to, 661
　genetics and, 47
　hallucinosis due to, 48
　hepatotoxicity of, 773, 773t
　hypertension treatment and, 261
　hypoglycemia caused by, 753
　intoxication with, 47–48, 48t, 508
　isopropyl (rubbing), 508
　　carcinogenicity of, 1016t
　ketoacidosis caused by, 548, 548–549
　lethal dose of, 48, 48t
　mean cell volume affected by, 830
　memory affected by, 48, 1982
　metabolism of, 47
　methanol (wood), 504t, 509, 509t, 1975t
　neurologic effects of, 1975t
　pancreatitis caused by, 731t, 732t, 734, 734t
　patient evaluation and, 48
　pharmacology of, 47
　porphyria worsened by, 1126t, 1129
　rehabilitation from, 49
　risk factor role of, 27t, 30t, 48t, 1014
　seizures related to, 49
　tobacco synergism with, 1014
　tolerance to, 47, 48t
　treatment related to, 48–49
　tremulousness due to, 48t, 48–49
　vomiting due to, 630, 643
　withdrawal syndrome due to, 48t, 48–49
Aldolase, 1084, *1084*
　A, 1084, *1084*
　B, *1084*, 1084–1085
　deficiency of, *1084*, 1084–1085
Aldosterone, **1245–1252**
　deficiency of, 1251t, 1251–1252
　　adrenal hyperplasia and, 1252
　　sodium wasting due to, 528, 528t, 598–599
　excess of, 1249, 1249t
　feedback control of, 1246
　suppression test, 1249
　synthesis and secretion of, 1245–1246
　volume regulation role of, 527, 528
Aldosteronism, 1249
　causes of, 1249, 1249t
　differential diagnosis of, 1249
　renin and, 1249, 1249t
　treatment of, 1249
　tumor causing, 1249, 1249t
Aldrich-Mees lines, 70
Alexia, 1985, 1987t, 1988t, 1992
Alkalemia, 543
　definition of, 543
Alkali, absorbable, 550
　poisoning due to, 507
Alkaline phosphatase, 759
　bone mineralization role of, 1352, 1356
　deficiency of, osteomalacia due to, 1365
　leptospirosis affecting, 1720
　leukocyte, neutrophilia and, 918
　　polycythemia vera and, 921t
　liver function reflected by, 759
Alkaloids, adverse effects of, 1043–1044
　chemotherapy using, 1039t, 1043–1044, 1044t
　ergot, 740
　food poisoning due to, 740
　plant source, 1039t, 1043–1044, 1044t
　pyrrolizidine, 740

Alkaloids (Continued)
  teas containing, 54, 740, 774
  vinca, 1039t, 1043–1044, 1044t, 1057t
Alkalosis, 545, 545t, 545–546
  causes of, 545–546, 549t, 549–550
  compensatory mechanisms in, 545, 545, 545t, 549–550
  diuretics and, 224t, 531, 531t
  hypochloremic, 224t
  hypokalemic, 531, 531t, 540, 549
  hyponatremic, 514, 550
  metabolic, 545, 545t, 550t
    clinical features of, 550
    definition of, 545, 545t
    etiology of, 549t, 549–550
    pathogenesis of, 549t, 549–550
    treatment of, 550
  mixed disorders and, 550t, 550–551
  posthypercapnic, 550
  respiratory, 551
    clinical features of, 551
    pathogenesis of, 545, 551
  vomiting and, 630
Alkaptonuria, 1108
  clinical manifestations of, 1108
  definition of, 1108
  diagnosis of, 1108
  incidence of, 1108
  pathogenesis of, 1108
  pathology in, 1108
  radiography in, 1108
  treatment of, 1108
Alkylamines, 1416, 1416t
  allergic rhinitis treated with, 1416, 1416t
Alkylating agents, 1039t, 1041–1042, 1042t
  chemosensitizers to, 1058, 1058t
  chemotherapy using, 1039t, 1041–1042, 1042t
  fetal malformations due to, 1070t, 1071t
  resistance to, 1058t, 1058–1059
Alleles, 134
  dominant, 134
  imprinting modification and, 135, 156
  parental differential in, 135, 156
  recessive, 134
  segregation of, 134
Allergens, 1415–1417
  allergic rhinitis role of, 1414, 1415, 1415–1417
  angioedema due to, 1409–1410
  avoidance of, 1416
  identification of, 1416
  immunotherapy using, 1417
  skin testing of, 1416
  urticaria caused by, 1409–1410
Allergy, antimicrobials causing, 1568t, 1569
  aspergillosis with, 1830t, 1830–1832
  bronchopulmonary, 1830t, 1830–1832
  drug, 1422t, 1432t, 1432–1435, 1568t
  food, 1409–1410
    anaphylaxis due to, 1418t
    urticaria and angioedema in, 1409–1410, 1418t
  IgE-mediation in, 1414, 1415, 1418
  insect sting and, 1420t, 1420–1421
  mechanisms of, 1413–1414, 1415, 1416
  nickel, 72
  rhinitis due to, 1413–1417
  serum sickness as, 1421–1422, 1422, 1422t
  transfusion-associated, 895t, 895–896, 896t
  urticaria due to, 1409t, 1409–1410
  vasculitis and, 1423
Allopurinol, hepatotoxicity of, 773, 773t
  hyperuricemia treated with, 1514, 1514–1515
Allyl alcohol, hepatotoxicity of, 772
Alopecia, 2215–2217
  areata, 2215
  diffuse, 2216–2217
  hair pulling disorder in, 2215–2216
  lupus erythematosus causing, 1478
  "moth-eaten" appearance in, 2216
  nonscarring, 2215–2217
  scarring, 2217
  stress associated with, 2216–2217
  telogen effluvium, 2216
  toxic, 2217
  traction, 2216
Alpha blocking agents, 265t
  dosages for, 265t, 270t
  hypertension treated with, 263, 265t, 267t, 268, 270t

Alpha blocking agents (Continued)
  pheochromocytoma surgery using, 1256
  side effects of, 267t, 268
Alpha chains, 958
  disease of, 966
  HLA molecules with, 1424–1426, 1425, 1425t
Alpha-adrenergic receptors, 245, 268
  activation of, 1253–1254
  blood vessel, 492–493
Alpha-fetoprotein, hepatoma with, 1022t, 1023
  testicular cancer with, 1022t, 1023
Alport's syndrome, 611–612
  clinical features of, 612, 612t
  definition of, 611
  diagnosis of, 612, 612t
  genetics of, 611
  incidence of, 611
  pathogenesis of, 611
ALT. See Alanine transferase (ALT).
Altitude sickness, 409t, 409–410
  acute, 409t, 409–410
  chronic, 409t, 410
  clinical features of, 409, 409t
  traveler exposed to, 1556
  treatment of, 409–410
Aluminum, 71, 567
  bone mineralization inhibited by, 1365, 1378t, 1379
  carcinogenicity of, 1016t
  intoxication with, 71
    dementia due to, 567
    dialysis causing, 567
Alveoli, 371–372
  air-blood barrier in, 371–372
  anatomy of, 371–373, 372
  filling disorders of, 391t, 397–398
    interstitial disease with, 391t, 397–398
  gas exchange in, 371–373, 372, 375, 375t, 467–468
    Pneumocystis pneumonia and, 1918, 1918
  interstitial disease affecting, 380, 393, 394. See also
    Lung, interstitial disease of.
  proteinosis of, 398
  surfactant in, 372
  total surface area of, 372
Alveolitis, aspergillosis with, 1830t, 1831
  fibrosis with, 393, 394
  signs and symptoms of, 369t
Alzheimer's disease, 1992–1996
  amyloid deposit in, 1505, 1994
  brain changes in, 14, 1505, 1993–1994
  clinical manifestations of, 1993–1994
  diagnosis of, 1993, 1994
  differential diagnosis of, 1994–1996
  genetic factors in, 13, 1994
  management of, 1994
  pathogenesis of, 1993–1994
  pathology in, 1994
  plaques of, 1505, 1994
Amanita, 508, 508t
  food poisoning due to, 740
  hepatotoxicity of, 772, 798, 799t
Amantadine, 1743–1744, 1746t
  influenza treated with, 1746t
  licensing for, 1743–1744
  mechanism of action of, 1743
  renal function and, 1744t
  toxicity of, 1744
  viral pharyngitis treated with, 1751t
Amastigote, leishmanial, 1903–1904, 1904
  trypanosomal, 1897, 1900
Amatoxins, 740
Amaurosis fugax, 2064, 2064t
Amblyopia, 2174, 2174t
  nutritional, 2040
Amebae in food, 1915
  Legionella carried in, 1583
Amebiasis, 783t, 1913–1915
  clinical syndromes in, 1913t, 1913–1914, 1914
  differential diagnosis of, 1914, 1914
  E. polecki, 1916t
  encephalitis due to, granulomatous, 1915
  etiologic organism in, 1913, 1915
  hepatic, 782–783, 783t, 784, 1913t, 1913–1914, 1914
  meningoencephalitis due to, 1915
  rectocolitis of, 1913t, 1913–1915, 1915t
  treatment and prevention of, 1914–1915, 1915t
Amenorrhea, 1302–1307
  anorexia causing, 1158, 1159t
  anovulatory, 1305–1307, 1306t
  clinical evaluation of, 1303, 1303t, 1304

Amenorrhea (Continued)
  definition of, 1302–1303
  etiology of, 1302–1303, 1304t
  hypergonadotropic, 1304–1305, 1305t
  hyperprolactinemia in, 1214
  laboratory testing in, 1303–1304, 1304
  oral contraceptive role in, 1310
  ovarian failure and, 1304t, 1304–1305, 1305t
  Turner's syndrome and, 1304–1305, 1305t
Ametropia, 2174
Amidophosphoribosyltransferase, 1511
Amikacin, 91t, 94t, 1562t
  dose adjustment for, 94t, 1562t
  E. coli and, 1579–1581, 1580t
  Klebsiella, Enterobacter, Serratia and, 1579–1581, 1580t
  mycobacterial (nontuberculous) disease and, 1690, 1691
  pharmacokinetics of, 91t, 94t, 1562t
  Pseudomonas and, 1579–1581, 1580t
  renal failure effect on, 94t, 1562t
Amiloride, dosage for, 264t
  properties and action of, 224t, 531t
  side effects of, 267t
Amines, biogenic, 1176
Amino acids, 1099–1117
  absorption of, 696, 696t
  branched-chain, 1111–1112
  enzyme defects affecting, 144t, 1100t–1105t
  genetic code use of, 134, 134t
  metabolism of, 754
    disorders of, 1099–1117, 1100t–1105t
    hepatic, 754
  renal tubules and, 144t, 595t, 596–597, 1099, 1100, 1104t–1105t
  toxic, food seeds containing, 740
  transamination of, 754
  transepithelial saturation with, 1099, 1100, 1100t–1104t
  urinary, 144t, 595t, 596–597, 1099, 1100t–1105t
Aminoaciduria, 596–597, 1100t–1105t
  Hartnup disease with, 1104t
  mechanisms of, 1099, 1100
  pathophysiology in, 595t, 596–597
  renal tubules in, 144t, 595t, 596–597, 1099, 1100, 1104t–1105t
  transepithelial saturation in, 1099, 1100, 1100t–1104t
  transport defect in, 144t, 595t, 596–597, 1099, 1100, 1104t–1105t
Aminoadipic acid, urinary, 1101t
Aminoglycosides, 1562t
  adverse reactions to, 1568t
  dose adjustment for, 1562t
  endocarditis therapy with, 1602t–1604t, 1602–1603
  mechanism of action of, 1558, 1558t
  pharmacology of, 1562t
  renal function and, 585–586, 1562t
  resistance to, bacterial, 1558–1560, 1559t
Aminoisobutyric acid, urinary, 1103t
Aminolevulinic acid dehydratase deficiency, 1124–1126, 1125, 1125t
Aminopterin, fetal malformations due to, 1070t, 1071t
5-Aminosalicylates, 712–713
  inflammatory bowel disease treated with, 712–713
  metabolism of, 713
Aminotransferases, hepatitis and, 765, 767, 780
  leptospirosis affecting, 1720
  liver function reflected by, 759, 780
  Wilson's disease affecting, 1132
Amiodarone, 246t, 249–250
  adverse effects of, 248t, 2183
  antiarrhythmic action of, 245, 246t, 249–250
  hepatotoxicity of, 772–773, 773t, 774
  interstitial lung disease induced by, 397, 397t
  jodbasedow effect due to, 1236
  ocular effects of, 2183
  pharmacokinetics of, 246t, 249–250
Amitriptyline, depression treated with, 2000t, 2001
  pain control use of, 106t
Amlodipine, adverse effects of, 300t
  dosage for, 265t, 300t
Ammonia, aminoacidopathy role of, 1102t
  hepatotoxicity of, 754, 797, 797t
  inhalation of, 404
  metabolism of, 1109–1111, 1110, 1111
    liver in, 754, 760
  poisoning by, 1102t, 1109–1110
  smoke containing, 34, 36
Amnesia, 1989–1990
  alcoholic, 48, 1982, 2039–2032

Amnesia *(Continued)*
alcoholic blackout in, 1982
Alzheimer's, 1990, 1990t
anterograde, 1989, 1989t
classification of, 1989t, 1989–1990
dysnomia in, 1989t, 1990
global, 1989t, 1990
head injury with, 1990, 1990t
Korsakoff's, 1990, 1990t, 2039
paraneoplasia with, 1028
postconcussion, 1982
psychogenic, 1990
retrograde, 1989, 1989t
stroke with, 2064t, 2064–2065
transient global, 1989t, 1990
treatment of, 1990
Amoxicillin, 1562t
endocarditis therapy with, 1602t, 1602–1603, 1604t
hepatotoxicity, 773, 773t, 774
Lyme disease therapy with, 1719, 1719t
Amphetamines, drug abuse treated with, 54
drug abuse with, 51, 56t
neurologic effects of, 1975t
obesity treatment using, 1166
poisoning due to, 508
Amphotericin B, blastomycosis therapy with, 1822
candidiasis treated with, 1829–1830
cryptococcosis therapy with, 1825
decision analysis studies with, 82, 82
histoplasmosis therapy with, 1818
leishmaniasis treated with, 1907
mucormycosis therapy with, 1834
renal function and, 585
Ampicillin, 1562t
endocarditis therapy with, 1602t, 1602–1603, 1604t
H. influenzae treated with, 1624
meningitis therapy with, 1615–1617, 1616t, 1620t
meningococcal infection and, 1620t, 1620–1621
minimal inhibitory concentration for, 1570, 1570t
streptococcal infection treated with, 1587–1589, 1589t
Amrinone, shock treated with, 493–494
Amygdala, 2060
Amyl nitrite, cyanide toxicity treated with, 504t, 508
inhalant abuse with, 55
Amylase, 731–732, 732t
Amyloidosis, **966–968,** 1504–1506
Alzheimer's disease and, 1505, 1994
classification of, 967t, 1504, 1504t
clinical features of, 967, 967, 1035, 1504–1505
dialysis and, 567, 967t, 1505
familial, 1504t, 1505
fibrils of, 1504, 1506
heart affected by, 333, 333, 359, 967, 967, 967t, 1504
hepatic effects of, 786, 1504–1505
incidence of, 960, 961t
laboratory findings in, 967, 1505–1506
lymphadenopathy of, 970, 970t
Mediterranean fever with, 907, 908, 967t
myeloma with, 962t, 963
myopathy of, 2170
nephrotic disease with, 574t, 579, 967, 967, 967t, 1505
neuropathy of, 967, 967, 2007, 2154
paraneoplastic, 1035
prognosis in, 968
treatment of, 967–968, 1506
Amylophagia, 840
Amyotrophy, **2052–2054**
acquired, 2052t, 2052–2053
hereditary, 2052t, 2052–2053
lateral sclerosis with, 2053–2054
clinical manifestations of, 2054, 2054t
differential diagnosis of, 2054, 2054t
incidence of, 2053
treatment of, 2054
ANA. See *Antibodies, antinuclear.*
Anabolism, fed state, 1278, 1278t
steroids and, 1338
Anaerobes, **1638–1641**
antimicrobial susceptibility of, 1641, 1641t
body sites for, 1638–1641, 1639, 1639t
capsule of, 1639t
classification and taxonomy of, 1557t, 1638, 1639t
clostridial. See *Clostridial infection(s).*
culture of, 1640t, 1641
infections due to, 1638–1641
diagnosis of, 1640t, 1641

Anaerobes *(Continued)*
head and neck, 1639, 1639t
intra-abdominal, 1640
obstetric and gynecologic, 1640, 1640t
pulmonary, 1639–1640
skin and soft tissue, 1640–1641
treatment of, 1640t, 1641, 1641t
normal flora constituted of, 1638–1641, 1639, 1639t
pneumonia due to, 1579–1584
pulmonary abscess due to, 413–414, 414t
streptococcal, 1589t, 1589–1590
virulence factors for, 1639t
Analgesics, adjuvants used with, 105, 106t
aspirin and aspirin-like, 111–115, 115t
dosage of, 102, 103t, 104t, 115t, 893t
equianalgesic, 102, 103t, 104t
guidelines for use of, 103t, 105t
NSAIDs as, 102, 103t, 111–115, 115t
opioid, 102–105, 104t, 105t, 893t
oral, 103t
pain management with, 102–107, 103t, 104t, 105t, 893t
patient-controlled, 103
renal function and, 584–585
sickle syndromes therapy with, 892, 893t
side effects of, 103–105, 893t
Analysis of variance (ANOVA), 84–85, 85t
Anandamide, 53
Anaphylatoxins, 1400
Anaphylaxis, **1417–1420**
Arthus reaction as, 1448–1449, 1449
clinical manifestations of, 1418, 1418
differential diagnosis of, 1418–1419
drug-induced, 1417–1418, 1418t
epidemiology of, 1417–1418
etiology of, 1417–1418, 1418t
insect sting causing, 1420t, 1420–1421
pathogenesis of, 1419
penicillin causing, 100, 1418t, 1418–1419, 1568t
prevention of, 1419
rheumatic disease relation to, 1448–1450, 1449
Shwartzman reaction as, 1449, 1449–1450
transfusion causing, 896, 896t
treatment of, 1419–1420
Anarthria, 1989, 1989t, 1992
Anastomosis, Billroth, 669–671, 670, 670t
Roux-en-Y, 672, 683
ANCA (antineutrophil cytoplasmic antibodies), 1457t, 1458
disease associations of, 1457t, 1458
Wegener's granulomatosis and, 1457t, 1458, 1496t, 1497
Anchorin, 1445
Ancylostoma, 1934–1935
animal, 1937
Androblastoma, 1312t
Androgens, acne and, 1315
adrenal, 1245–1246, 1287–1290
excess of, 1287–1290
adverse effects of, 1046t, 1047
cancer therapy using, 1046t, 1047
hair growth and, normal, 1315, 2186–2187
pubertal, 1294, 1329, 2186–2187
hirsutism and, 1315–1317, 1316t, 2217
insensitivity to, 1291t, 1291–1293, 1292, 1338
ovarian, 1299, 1299, 1300, 1301t
tumor production of, 1312t
pseudohermaphroditism and, 1287–1293
replacement therapy with, 1338–1339
testicular, 1285, 1326–1327. See also *Testosterone.*
action of, 1285, 1286, 1327
deficiency of, 1329–1340
metabolism of, 1327
regulation of, 1326, 1326–1327
resistance to, 1338
sexual differentiation due to, 1285, 1286
therapeutic, 1338–1339
Androstenedione, 1299, 1300, 1301t
Anemia, **823–867**
AIDS/HIV patient with, 1871
aplastic, **831–837**
bone marrow transplant for, 835, 875, 875–876
clinical features of, 834
definition, 831t, 831–832
diagnosis of, 832, 834, 834–835, 835t
drug-induced, 824t, 832t, 832–833
etiology of, 831t, 832t, 832–833, 833t
incidence of, 834
liver and, 761–762

Anemia *(Continued)*
pathophysiology, 833t, 833–834
treatment of, 835–836
approach to patient with, 821–822, 823–831
blood loss causing, 838
blood smear evaluation for, 824–825, 825t
chronic disorders and, 826–827, 842
Cooley's, 877t, 877–879, 881
definition of, 823, 823t
drug-induced, 99t, 824, 824t, 832t, 844t, 867
endocrine disorders with, 827, 838–839
Fanconi's, 831–832
gastric resection causing, 672
gastrointestinal hemorrhage causing, 645, 645t
hemolytic, 822, 828–831
autoimmune, 859–867
causes of, 830, 830t, 1145t
drug-induced, 824t
laboratory tests in, 829, 829t
splenectomy for, 973
history taking in, 824
hypochromic microcytic, 839–843, 877–882, 1149t
thalassemia and, 877–882
hypoproduction, 821–822
immunohemolytic, 859–867
clinical features of, 861–864, 862t
drug-induced, 867
paroxysmal hemoglobinuria in, 866–867
pathophysiology of, 860, 860–861, 861
thrombocytopenia with, 866
treatment of, 864–866
iron-deficiency, 826, 827t, 839–841
clinical features of, 840–841
definition of, 839
laboratory findings in, 826, 827t, 841, 1149t
metabolism in, 839–840, 1149t
prevalence of, 839
treatment of, 841
laboratory values and, 823t, 824–825, 825t
leukemia with, 938
liver disease with, 827, 838
lupus erythematosus with, 1475t, 1479
macrocytic, 826t, 828t, 828–829
causes of, 828t, 828–829
macroglobulinemia with, 965
malabsorption with, 699t, 701t
megaloblastic, 828–829, **843–851**
blood smear examination in, 847, 847t, 847–848, 848
clinical findings in, 847, 847t, 847–849, 848
definition, 843
diagnostic approach to, 849t, 849–850, 850t
drug-induced, 824t, 844, 844t, 845
etiologic classification of, 843, 844t
folate deficiency and, 843–851, 1147t
incidence of, 844
pathogenesis of, 844–847, 845, 846, 1147t
treatment of, 850–851
vitamin B_{12} deficiency and, 843–851
microangiopathic, 984t
microcytic, 826t, 827t, 827–828, 839–843
etiology of, 827t, 827–828, 839–842
myelodysplasia with, 832, 836t, 836–837
myeloid metaplasia with, 924, 925
myeloma and, 962, 962t
myelophthisic, 837, 837t
normocytic, 826t, 826–827, 837–839
paraneoplastic, 1021
pernicious, 660, 844
gastritis and, 660
vitamin B_{12} test and, 699, 701t
physical findings, 824
renal failure, 558, 562, 827, 838
rheumatoid arthritis with, 1464
sickle cell. See *Sickle syndromes.*
sideroblastic, 834, 842–843
signs and symptoms of, 823–824
spur cell, 825t, 827
Anemones, venom of, 1954t, 1955
Anencephaly, fetus with, 158t
Anesthesia, pain management with, 105–106
Aneurysms, 342
aortic. See *Aorta, aneurysms of.*
causes of, 342
cerebrovascular, **2073–2077**
congenital, 178, 279, 281, 283
headache with, 2074

Aneurysms (Continued)
    hypothalamus affected by, 1201
    imaging of, 1966, 1966
    circle of Willis, 178, 279, 2074
    definition of, 342
    fusiform vs. saccular, 2074
    hepatic artery, polyarteritis nodosa causing, 1494
    mycotic, 1599, 2084
    sinus of Valsalva, 281, 283
    splenic, 974
    ventricular, 183
Angel dust (PCP), 54, 1975t
    adverse effects of, 54, 508
Angelman's syndrome, 155–156
    chromosome deletion causing, 155t, 155–156
    clinical features of, 155t, 155–156
Angiitis. See also Vasculitis.
    allergic, 1491, 2201t
        interstitial lung disease in, 398
        polyarteritis nodosa with, 1493
    maculopapular lesions with, 2201t, 2201–2202
Angina pectoris, **296–301**
    antithrombus therapy in, 300–301
    arteriography in, 298
    beta blockers in, 298–299, 299t
    calcium channel blockers in, 299, 300t
    classification of, 296–297, 297t
    drug therapy for, 298–301, 299t, 300t
    ECG in, 297
    exertional, 296
    history and examination for, 297, 297t
    hypothyroidism and, 1238, 1239
    management of, 298–301, 299t, 300t
    mixed, 296
    nitrate therapy in, 298, 299t
    pain of, 166, 297
    pathophysiology of, 296, 296–297
    radionuclide studies in, 298
    silent ischemia with, 296, 300t, 316
    stable, 296, 300t
    sudden cardiac death and, 255, 255
    thyroxine therapy causing, 1239
    types of, 296–297
    unstable, 296, 300t, 318
    variant (Printzmetal's), 296, 297
Angioedema, **1408–1412**, 2208
    ACE inhibitor in, 1412
    C1 deficiency in, 1412
    definition of, 1408, 2208
    differential diagnosis of, 1411, 2208
    drug-induced, 1433t, 2208
    hereditary, 1411–1412
    incidence and prevalence of, 1408–1409
    pathogenesis of, 1409t, 1409–1411, 2208
    therapy of, 1411–1412
Angiography, cardiac, 208–211, 209t, 210, 211
    digital subtraction, 127
    pulmonary embolism in, 425, 425t, 426, 426
Angiokeratoma, 1096–1097
Angioma. See also Hemangioma.
    Bartonella and, 1680–1682, 1682t
    cavernous venous, 2076–2077
    cerebrovascular disease due to, 2076–2077
    facial, port-wine, 2056
Angioplasty, 318
    antiplatelet prophylaxis in, 118
    coronary, 318
    high-risk, 118
    myocardial infarction treated with, 312t, 312–313
Angiosarcoma, hepatic, 773, 773t, 803t
Angiotensin, 1251–1252
    adrenal, 1249, 1249t, 1251, 1251–1252
    mineralocorticoid secretion and, 1249, 1249t, 1251t, 1251–1252
    receptor for, 1177
    shock and, 481
    volume regulation role of, 526, 526t, 527
Angiotensin-converting enzyme (ACE). See also ACE inhibitors.
    hypertension treated with, 263, 265t, 266t, 266–267
    renal function and, 588
Anhydrosis, 2010
Animals, 1737t, 1737–1738, 1738t
    anthrax in, 1664–1666
    asthma induced by, 379t
    brucellosis and, 1678, 1680
    bubonic plague and, 1662
    Campylobacter in, 1649t, 1649–1650, 1738t

Animals (Continued)
    erysipeloid and, 1673–1674
    filariae in, 1945
    histoplasmosis in, 1816
    hookworm affecting, 1937
    leptospirosis carried by, 1720, 1737t
    lifespan of, 12, 12
    listeriosis association with, 1672, 1737t
    occupational exposure to, 379t, 1727t, 1737t
    plague in, 1662, 1737t
    psittacosis in, 1725, 1737t
    Q fever carried by, 1727t, 1735–1736, 1737t
    rabies carried by, 2095–2096
    rickettsialpox exposure and, 1733
    rickettsioses carried by, 1727t, 1737t, 1738t
    tapeworm in, 1922–1923, 1923t
    trichinosis associated with, 1937–1938
    tularemia in, 1663
    typhus carried by, 1726, 1727t, 1729, 1730, 1738t
    yellow fever in, 1798–1799
    zoonoses associated with, 1727t, 1737t, 1737–1738, 1738t
Anion gap, 545–546
    acidosis and, 545–548, 546t, 550t
    diabetic ketoacidosis and, 1270
    furosemide test and, 546, 546t
    increased, 546, 546t, 547, 550t
    reduced, 546
    serum, 545–546
    urinary, 546, 546t
Anisakiasis, 1935t, 1936
    thiabendazole treatment of, 1935t, 1936
Anisocoria, 2009
    diagnostic test using, 2018, 2018
Anisometropia, 2174
Ankle, rheumatoid disease affecting, 1462
Ankylosis, cervical, 1469
    vertebral. See Spondylitis, ankylosing; Spondylosis.
Ankyrin, 851, 851–852
    defects in, 852, 855
    ovalocytosis and, 855
Annulus fibrosus, 2141
Anomia, 1989, 1989t
    color, 1985, 1987t
Anorchia, congenital, 1334
Anorexia, **1158–1160**
    clinical manifestations of, 1158–1159
    definition of, 629, 1158
    diagnostic criteria for, 1159, 1159t
    endocrine abnormalities due to, 1158–1159, 1159t
    epidemiology of, 1158
    etiology and pathogenesis of, 1158
    gastric emptying affected by, 684
    hypothalamic defect and, 1203
    prognosis in, 1160
    treatment of, 1159
    vomiting and, 630
Anosmia, 1200
Anosognosia, 2064t, 2064–2065
ANOVA (analysis of variance), 84–85, 85t
Anovulation, 1305–1307
    amenorrhea due to, 1305–1307, 1306t
    causes of, 1305–1307, 1306t
    chronic, 1305–1307, 1306t
    feedback defects causing, 1306t, 1306–1307
    folliculogenesis defect in, 1307
    hypothalamic, 1305–1306, 1306t
    treatment of, 1306, 1307
Anoxia, cerebral, 2062t, 2062–2063, 2136
    head injury with, 2136
    neuron vulnerability to, 2062t, 2063
Ant, sting of, 1948
Antacids, 667
Anthracyclines, 1039t, 1044–1045
    chemotherapy with, 1039t, 1044–1045
    resistance to, 1057, 1057t
Anthralin, psoriasis treated with, 2195, 2203
Anthrax, **1664–1667**
    clinical manifestations of, 1666–1667, 1738t
    cutaneous, 1665–1666
    definition of, 1664–1665
    diagnosis of, 1666–1667
    epidemiology of, 1665, 1738t
    etiology of, 1665
    gastrointestinal, 1666
    immunization for, 46, 1667
    incidence and prevalence of, 1665
    inhalational, 1666
    oropharyngeal, 1666–1667
    pathogenesis of, 1665–1666

Anthrax (Continued)
    prevention of, 1667
    prognosis in, 1667, 1738t
    treatment of, 1667
Antiandrogens, 1316
    cancer therapy using, 1046t, 1047
    hirsutism treated with, 1316
Antianxiety drugs, 20, 21t
Antiarrhythmic agents, 247t, 248t
    classification of, 244–245, 245, 245t
    pharmacokinetics of, 246t
    treatment using, 237t, 238t, 244–250
Antibiotics. See Antimicrobials.
Antibodies. See also Autoimmunity; Immune complexes; Immunoglobulin(s).
    antinuclear, 1457t, 1457–1458
        disease associations of, 1457t, 1457–1458, 1481t
        liver function and, 767, 778t
        lupus erythematosus with, 1457, 1457t, 1476t, 1476–1477, 1481t
        myopathy due to, 1501t, 1502
        nucleolar, 1457t
        rim, 1457t
        speckled, 1457t
    cancer therapy using, 1048t, 1048–1049
    cardiolipin, 1710t, 1710–1711
    Chagas' disease with, 1901–1902
    coagulation factor, 992, 1001, 1476t, 1479
    coccidioidomycosis, 1820
    collagen target of, 1517
    cryptosporidium-elicited, 1912
    cytoplasm target of, 1457t, 1457–1458, 1476t, 1497
    DNA, 1457t, 1476t
    Epstein-Barr virus, 1778, 1778, 1779t
    erythrocyte, 859–867
    FAB, 504t, 508
    glomerular basement membrane affected by, 577, 1479
    hepatitis and, 764t, 765, 767, 778t
    HIV infection eliciting, 1839t, 1839–1841, 1844
    immune complexes with, 1421–1423, 1422, 1422t, 1423
    immunodeficiency related to, 1402t, 1403–1405
    influenza, 1754–1755
    leprosy, 1692t, 1693
    leptospirosis, 1721
    lupus erythematosus and, 1456–1458, 1457t, 1476t, 1476–1477, 1481t
    Lyme disease detection with, 1717–1718, 1718
    microsome, 1476t
    mitochondria affected by, 761, 791–792
    monoclonal, 958–961, 959
    myelin-associated glycoprotein, 2152
    nucleolus, 1457t
    phospholipid, 1458, 1476t, 1479
    platelets affected by, 980–983, 984t, 986
    ribosome, 1476t
    RNA, 1457t, 1476t
    sperm affected by, 1332
    syphilis detection with, 1710t, 1710–1711, 1711t
    thrombocytopenia caused by, 980t, 980–983, 984t
    thyroid gland affected by, 1230, 1232–1234
    toxoplasmal, 1909
    treponemal, 1710t, 1711, 1711t
    trypanosome-elicited, 1898, 1901–1902
Anticholinergic agents, asthma treated with, 381
    depression treated with, 2000t, 2001
    drug abuse with, 54–55, 56t
    ocular side effects of, 2183
    poisoning due to, 506
Anticholinesterase, edrophonium test for, 2172
    myasthenia gravis treated with, 2172–2173
Anticoagulants, **118–121**
    atrial fibrillation and, 119, 119t
    complications of, 120–121, 998–1000
    drug interactions with, 120–121, 121t
    myocardial infarction treated with, 119, 311–312, 312t
    pregnancy and, 119
    prophylaxis with, 118t, 118–120, 119t
    pulmonary embolism and, 118t, 118–119, 427, 427t, 427–428
    stroke therapy with, 2071–2072, 2072t
    valvular disease and, 119, 119t
    venous thrombosis and, 118t, 118–119
Anticonvulsants, 106t
Antidepressants, 510t
    depression treated with, 2000t, 2000–2001
    elderly treated with, 20, 20t
    MAOI, 2000t, 2001

Antidepressants *(Continued)*
neurologic effects of, 1975t
overdose of, 504t, 510, 510t, 1975t
pain control use of, 106t
tricyclic, 510, 510t, 1975t, 2000t
Antidiarrheal agents, 704t
Antidiuretic hormone (ADH). See *Vasopressin.*
Antidotes, for poisons, 504t
Antiepileptic drugs, 2121–2123, 2122t
pharmacokinetics of, 2122t, 2122–2123
Antiestrogens, 1046t
adverse effects, 1046t, 1047
cancer therapy using, 1046t, 1047, 1059–1060
resistance to, 1059–1060
Antifreeze poisoning, 504t, 509, 509t
Antifungal agents, 1815–1816, 1816t
systemic, 2196t, 2196–2197
topical, 2195
Antigens, bacterial capsule with, *1556*, 1556–1557
H, *1556*
histocompatibility, 1426–1429, 1428t, 1429t. See also
HLA complex.
HIV organism with, *1842, 1843, 1844*
human leukocyte. See *HLA complex.*
immune complexes with, 1421–1423, *1422*, 1422t, *1423*
presentation of, *1393, 1394, 1394*, 1397
streptococcal, *1586*, 1586–1587
transporter (TAP) associated with, 1424, 1429
very late appearing, 1453
Antihemophilic factor, 988t
Antihistamines, 2196t
allergic rhinitis treated with, 1416, 1416t
anaphylaxis treated with, 1419–1420
asthma treated with, 381
drug abuse with, 54–55
pain control use of, 106t
skin disorder treated with, 2196, 2196t
Antihormones, cancer therapy using, 1046t, 1046–1047
Anti-inflammatory agents, asthma treated with, 380–381
lung disease induced by, 397, 397t
nonsteroidal, **111–115**
allergy to, 1435
antipyretic effects of, 111–112, 115t
aspirin and aspirin-like, 111–115, 115t
gout treated with, 1513–1514, 1514t
history of, 111–115
inflammatory bowel disease treated with, 712–713, 714t
mechanism of action of, 112–113, *113*
nephrotoxicity of, *581*, 585, 585t
neutrophil response to, 114–115
osteoarthritis treated with, 1520
pain management with, 102, 103t
peptic ulcer role of, 662t, 663, 663t, 667t, 668
systemic administration and, 663
platelet disorders caused by, 984
prostaglandin inhibition by, 112–114, *113*
renal complications of, *581*, 584–585, 585t
rheumatoid arthritis treated with, 1465
salicylic, 111–115, 115t
side effects of, 113–114
spondyloarthropathy therapy with, 1472
steroidal, 108–110. See also *Corticosteroids.*
glucocorticoid, 108t, 108–110, 109t, 110t
inflammatory bowel disease treated with, 712–713, 714t
Antimetabolites, chemotherapy using, 1042t, 1042–1043
fetal malformations due to, 1070t, 1071t
Antimicrobials, **1558–1569**
adverse reactions to, 1568t, 1569
agent of choice in, 1564t–1565t
allergy to, 1432t, 1434, 1434t, 1435t
anaerobic flora susceptibility to, 1641, 1641t
anaphylaxis due to, 1418t, 1418–1419
anthracycline, 1039t, 1044–1045, 1057t
bactericidal titers of, 1563, 1566t–1567t
chemotherapy using, 1039t, 1044–1045, 1057t
colitis associated with, 1633–1635, *1634*, 1634t
combinations of, 1565–1569
compromised host treated with, 1542–1547, 1544t, *1545*, 1546t
concentrations of, 1561–1563, 1562t
diarrhea not treated with, 695
dosage of, 1561–1563, 1562t, 1563t
failure of therapy with, 1569
fetal malformations due to, 1070t, 1071t
half-life of, 1561–1563, 1562t
hepatic function and, 1561–1563, 1562t

Antimicrobials *(Continued)*
host factors and, 1561–1563, 1562t
hypokalemia induced by, 540
identification of pathogen and, 1560–1561
interactions of, 1563
interstitial lung disease induced by, 396–397, 397t
mechanism of action of, 1558, 1558t
pharmacology of, 1561–1563, 1562t, 1563t
protein-binding of, 1562t
renal function and, 561t, 582t, 584t, 585–586, 1561–1563, 1562t, 1568t
resistance to, 1550, 1558–1560, 1569t
mechanisms of, 1558–1560, 1569t
nosocomial infection and, 1550
selection factors for, 1560–1563, 1562t–1565t
susceptibility of pathogen to, 1561, 1564t–1567t
therapeutic, brucellosis therapy with, 1679t, 1680
diarrhea treatment with, 1658, 1658t
endocarditis and, 1602t–1604t, 1602–1603
febrile neutropenia and, 1538t, 1539t, 1543–1548, 1544t
inflammatory bowel disease and, 713
Klebsiella and, 1580, 1580t
Legionella and, 1585, 1585t
Lyme disease and, 1719, 1719t
meningitis and, 1615–1617, 1616t, 1620t, 1620–1621, 1621t
meningococcal infection and, 1620t, 1620–1621
mycobacterial disease and, 1690–1691
peptic ulcer treated with, 668t, 668–669
pneumonia treated with, 474, 475t
Pseudomonas and, 1580, 1580t
salpingitis and, 1702t, 1703
septic shock treated with, 500
staphylococcal infections and, 1609t, 1609–1610
streptococcal infections and, 1589t, 1589–1590
syphilis and, 1711–1713, 1712t
tuberculosis and, 1686t–1688t, 1686–1690
urinary tract infection and, 604–605, 605t
Antimitochondrial antibodies, 761, 791–792
Antimony, occupational exposure to, 73
poisoning due to, 73
Antimüllerian hormone, 1284–1285, *1285, 1286*
Antineoplastic agents. See *Chemotherapy.*
Antineutrophil cytoplasmic antibodies, 1458
disease associations of, 1457t, 1458
Wegener's granulomatosis and, 1457t, 1458, 1496t, 1497
Antioxidants, cancer prevention with, 1010, 1016–1017
mechanism of action of, *405*
toxic oxygen species and, *405*
vitaminic, 1145t, 1151, 1151t
C, 1147t, 1151, 1151t
E, 1145t, 1151, 2041
Antiparasitic agents, malabsorption treatment with, 704t
topical, 2195
Antiphagocytosis, bacterial, 1531, 1556, *1556*, 1639t
Antiplasmin, 987, 988t
deficiency of, 997
Antiplatelet agents, 116–118, 117t
Antipsychotic agents. See *Neuroleptics.*
Antipyretics, 111–115, *113*, 115t
Antiretroviral agents, 1880–1887, *1881–1883*, 1883t, 1885t
Antiseptic cleaners, 2195
Antistreptolysin O, 1591, 1594
Antithrombin, 988t
coagulation role of, *989*
deficiency of, 997–998
Antithymocyte globulin, aplastic anemia treated with, 835
Antithyroid drugs, 1234, 1234t
pregnancy and, 1236
thyrotoxic crisis and, 1236t
Antitoxins, botulism, 1635–1636
diphtheria, 1630
tetanus, 1637–1638, 1638t
α_1-Antitrypsin, 767, 785, 791
deficiency of, 791
emphysema with, 385, 388
genetics of, 136t, 1388t, 785
liver and, 767, 785, 791
transplantation for, 801t
Antituberculous agents, 1686–1688, 1687t
dose adjustment for, 1562t, 1686t
pharmacology of, 1562t
Antivenin, 1952–1953, 1954t
immune complexes due to, 1422t, 1423
snakebite treated with, 1952–1953, 1954t
Antiviral agents, 1742–1747, 1746t
Anton's syndrome, 2017

Antrectomy, 669–671, *670*, 670t
Antrum, gastrin secretion by, 662t, 663–664, 675t
manometry of, 685
Anus, **740–743**
abscesses of, 741, *741*
anatomy of, 740, *741*
carcinoma of, 743
examination, 740
fissure of, 741
fistula affecting, 741–742, *742*
pain from, diarrhea and, 694–695
pinworm eggs on, 1935
pruritus of, 742
sexually transmitted disease and, 742
sphincters of, reflex testing of, 2009t
warts of, 742
Anxiety, **2004–2005**
alcohol-related, 49
drug therapy for, 20, 21t
elderly affected by, 20–21
heart failure causing, 219
incidence of, 2004
pathophysiology of, 2004
prognosis for, 2005
symptoms of, 2004, 2004t
treatment of, 2004–2005
white coat, 258, 260
Aorta, **342–346**
anatomy of, 342
aneurysms of, 342–346
abdominal, 342–343
ascending, 206, 342, 343, *344, 346*
causes of, 342
clinical features of, 342, 343–344
CT of, spiral, 127, *128*
descending, 206, 342–343, *343, 344*
diagnosis of, 343
fusiform, 342
Marfan's syndrome causing, 345, 345–346, *346*
pain from, 343
rupture of, 342–343
saccular, 342
sinus of Valsalva, 342, *345*
syphilitic, 342, 1708, 1708t
type I, 343, *343*
type II, 343, *343*
type III, 343, *343*
balloon counterpulsation in, 495
coarctation of, 278, *278*
reversed, 346
dissection of, 343–345
classification of, 343, *343*
diagnosis of, 344, *344, 345*
etiology of, 343
imaging of, 206, 344, *344–346, 345*
Marfan syndrome with, 1120
pain from, 343
pathogenesis of, 343
prognosis in, 345
root in, 344, *344*, 345, *345*
treatment of, 345
inflammation of, 346
MRI of, *206*
organ of Zuckerkandl of, 1254
polychondritis affecting, 1517
pressure in, heart contraction and, 176t
rupture of, 342–343
trauma injury to, 346
Aortic stenosis, 319–321
antibiotic prophylaxis in, 321, 321t
catheterization in, 320–321
clinical features of, 310t, 319–310
differential diagnosis of, 321
ECG in, 320, 320t
echocardiography in, *320*, 320, 320t
etiology of, 310t, 319
murmur in, 319, 320, 321
pathology of, 310t, 319
physical examination for, 320
sounds in, 320, 321
surgical approach in, 320t, 321
treatment of, 320t, 321, 321t
valvular, 319–321
Aortic valve, 319–323
bicuspid defect of, 278, *278*
calcification in, *184*, 185, 1594
graft replacement of, *184*
regurgitation from, 321–323

Aortic valve *(Continued)*
  catheterization and, 322, 322t
  chest radiography and, 322, 322t
  clinical course of, 321–322
  differential, 322t, 322–323
  ECG of, 322, 322t
  echocardiography of, 322, 322t
  etiology of, 321, 322t
  murmur in, 322, 322t
  pathology of, 321
  physical examination for, 322, 322t
  physiology of, 321, 322t
  sounds in, 322, 322t
  surgical approach in, 322t, 323
  treatment of, 322t, 323
  rheumatic fever affecting, 1594, *1594*
  size of, 321
  ventricular enlargement caused by, *183*, 184
Aortitis, 346
  syphilitic, 1708, 1708t
Aortoduodenal fistula, 644
Apatite, arthropathy due to, 1515–1516, 1516t
  bone formation role of, 1352
  crystals of, 1515–1516, 1516t
  deposition disease due to, 1515–1516, 1516t
  kidney stone of, 614–617, *615*, 615t, *616*, 616t
Aphagia, 1165
Aphasia, **1991–1992**
  anatomic considerations in, 1991t, 1991–1992
  Broca's, 1991t, 1992
  classification of, 1991t, 1991–1992
  conduction, 1991, 1991t
  differential diagnosis of, 1991t, 1991–1992
  fluent, 1991t
  global, 1991t, 1992
  jargon, 1991
  memory dysfunction in, 1989, 1989t
  meningitis with, 1612t, 1613
  motor, 1991t
  mutism in, 1992
  nonfluent, 1991t, 1992
  parietal lobe damage with, 1988t
  Pick's disease with, 1995
  progressive without dementia, 1995
  sensory, 1991t
  stroke with, 2064t, 2064–2065
  temporal lobe damage and, 1985, 1987t, 1991, 1991t
  Wernicke's, 1991, 1991t
  word deafness, 1991
Aphonia, 1992
Aphthovirus, 1737t
Apnea. See under *Sleep.*
Apocrine glands, 2186
Apoplexy, pituitary, 2035, 2131
Apoprotein (apolipoprotein), 1086t, 1086–1089
  (a), 1093
  A-I, 1086t, *1088*, 1088–1089, *1089*
  A-II, 1086t, 1088–1089, *1089*
  B, 1089–1090
  B-48, 1086t, 1086–1088, *1088*
  B-100, 1086t, 1086–1088, *1087*
  C-II, 1086t, *1088*, 1088–1089, *1089*
    deficiency of, 1090
  C-III, 1086t, 1088–1089, *1089*
  E, 1086t, *1087*, 1086–1088, *1088*, *1089*
Apoptosis (cell death), *1072*, 1072–1073, *1073*
  Bcl-2 oncogene and, 1011, 1057–1058, 1072–1073, *1073*
  cancer growth and, 1011, 1057–1058, 1072, *1072*
  p53-independent, 1057
  signaling for, 1011, 1057–1058, 1072, *1073*
  telomere role in, 15, 134, 1072, *1072*
Appendicitis, 748–749
  differential diagnosis of, 748t, 748–749
  etiology and pathogenesis of, 748
  laboratory studies in, 748
  pain of, 748
  physical examination in, 748
Appetite, 629
  depression affecting, 1999, 1999t
  drug control of, 1166
  hypothalamic control of, 1165
  mediators for, 629
  suppression of, 629
Apraxia, 1987
  construction, 1987
  ocular, 1987
  oculomotor, 2019

APRT (adenine phosphoribosyltransferase), 1510, *1511*
APSAC (acetylated plasminogen streptokinase activator complex), 311, *311*
APTT. See *Thromboplastin time, partial.*
Aqueous humor, *2176*
  circulation of, *2176*
  glaucoma affecting, *2176*, 2176–2177
Arachidonic acid, **1187–1193**. See also *Prostaglandins; Thromboxane.*
  metabolites of, 1187–1193, *1188–1191*
  NSAID effect on, 112–113, *113*, 1192–1193
  transport of, 1187, *1188*
Arachnodactyly, congenital contractural, 1120
  Marfan syndrome with, 1119–1120
Arachnoid. See also *Subarachnoid space.*
  cyst of, 2131
Arachnoiditis, 2148
Arbovirus, 1798t, 1805, 1805t, 1806t
  encephalitis due to, 1806t, 1810t, 1810–1814. See also *Encephalitis, viral.*
  fever, rash, arthritis syndromes of, 1805t, 1805–1810
  hemorrhagic disease due to, 1797–1804, 1798t. See also *Hemorrhagic fever.*
Arcuate artery, *517*
ARDS. See *Respiratory distress syndrome (adult).*
Arenavirus, hemorrhagic disease caused by, 1798t, 1802–1803
  structure of, *1739*
Areola, 1317
  pubertal change in, 1303t
  sebaceous glands of, 2186
  secretions of, 2186
  sweat glands of, 2186
  Tanner stages for, 1303, 1303t
Argentinian hemorrhagic fever, 1798t, 1802–1803
Arginase, *1110*
  deficiency of, 1110t, 1111
Arginine, elevated level of, 1102t, 1104t, 1111
  urinary, 1102t, 1104t
L-Arginine test, growth hormone in, 1208t
Arginine vasopressin, 23
Argininosuccinate synthetase, *1110*
  deficiency of, 1110t, 1111
Argininosuccinic aciduria, 1102t, 1111
Argyll-Robertson pupils, 2018
  syphilis with, 1709, 2018
Arm, circumference of, mid upper, 1153, 1153t
  skin disorders affecting, *2191*, 2216t
  skinfolds of, 1153, 1153t
Arnold-Chiari malformation, 2149
Aromatase inhibitors, 1047
Arousal level, 1071t, 1959, 1969, 1969t. See also *Coma; Consciousness disorders; Insomnia; Narcolepsy.*
  autonomic system and, 2013
Arrector pili, *2185*
Arrestin, 1178
Arrhythmia(s), **231–253**
  anatomic aspects in, 231–232, *232*
  atrial, 235t, 237t, 237–238, 238t
    fibrillation, 235t, 237t, 238t, *240*, 240–241, *241*
    flutter, 235t, 237t, 238t, 239–240, *240*
    multifocal, 241
    premature complex, 235, *235*, 237–238, *238*
  atrioventricular, block, 242, *242*
    premature complex, 242
  automaticity alteration causing, 233–234, *234*, 244
  carotid massage effect on, 235, 235t
  chagasic, 1901
  diagnostic approach to, 234–236, 235t, *236*, 236t
  digitalis induction of, 228, 237t
  ECG of, 235, *235*, 235t, 236t
    ambulatory, 235, 236t
    intracardiac stimulation in, 235–236, *236*, 236t
    long-term, 235, 236t
  mechanisms of, 233t, 233–234, *234*
  myocardial infarction with, after, 313, *315*
    before, 304, *305*
  nonparoxysmal junctional, 242, *242*
  paroxysmal supraventricular, 235t, 237t, 238t, 238–239, *239*, *240*
  poison causing, 505, 505t
  reentry causing, 234, *235*
  shock with, 491–492
  sinoatrial block causing, *241*, 241–242
  sinus rhythm, 235t, 237, 237t, 238t
  sudden death due to, *255*, 255–256
  treatment of, 237t, 238t
    ablation therapy in, 252t, 252–253
    cardioversion in, 251–252, 252t

Arrhythmia(s) *(Continued)*
    drug therapy in, 237t, 238t, 244–250, *245*, 245t, 247t, 248t
    pacemaker in, 250t, 250–251, 251t
  trypanosomiasis with, 1901
  ventricular, 235t, 237t, 238t, 242–244, *243*, *244*, 244t
    accelerated idioventricular rhythm as, *243*, 243–244
    fibrillation as, *243*, 244
    flutter as, 244, *244*
    parasystole as, 244
    premature complex as, 238t, 242–243, *243*
    tachycardia as, 235t, 237t, 238t, *243*, 243–244, *244*
    torsades de pointes as, 244, *244*
Arsenic, **70**
  Bowen's disease due to, 1035
  carcinogenicity of, 1016t
  chemical forms of, 70
  poisoning due to, 70, 504t
    clinical manifestations of, 70
    diagnosis of, 70
    etiology of, 70
    treatment of, 70, 504t
  skin cancer due to, 1035
Arsine gas poisoning, 70
Arterial access, 208
Arteriography, coronary, 298
  renal, 516
Arterioles, cold sensitivity in, 346–350
  renal, *519*, 519
    embolization affecting, 607
    hypertensive nephrosclerosis and, 607
    occlusion of, 607
Arteriolitis, 1491–1492
Arteriosclerosis, 291
  aortic, 350–351
  extremities affected by, 350–351
  Mönckeberg's, 291
  retinopathy of, 2181
Arteriosclerosis obliterans, 350–351
  clinical features of, 350–351
  diagnosis of, 351
  pain of, 350
  prognosis in, 351
  treatment of, 351
Arteriovenous anastomosis, 353
  hypertrophic, 353
Arteriovenous fistula, 353
  clinical features of, 353
  congenital, 281–282, *284*
  coronary, 281–282, *284*
  extremities affected by, 353
  pathophysiology of, 353
  pulmonary, 281, *284*
  treatment of, 353
Arteriovenous malformations, 721
  brain, 2076–2077, 2132
    headache due to, 2076–2077
    hemorrhagic stroke due to, 2076–2077, 2132
    imaging of, 1966, 2132
  intestinal, 721
  spinal, 1969, 2148
Arteritis. See also *Vasculitis.*
  aortic, 346
  Behçet's, 1506
  giant cell (temporal), 346, 1498–1500, 1499t, 2201t
  head pain due to, 2034
  renal artery thrombosis and, 606
  skin lesions related to, 346, 2201t
  stroke related to, 2068
  Takayasu's, 346, 2201t
Arteritis nodosa, 1492–1495, *1494*
Artery(ies), 291. See also named artery, e.g., *Carotid artery(ies).*
  fragility of, Ehlers-Danlos, 1120–1121, 1121t
    pseudoxanthoma elasticum with, 1123
  gas partial pressures in, 375, 375t
  occlusion of. See also *Atherosclerosis.*
    cold exposure and, 346–350
    prophylaxis in, 116–118, 117t
    renal failure and, 552t, 554t
    thromboangiitis obliterans in, 351–352
    thrombolytic therapy for, 116, 116t, 117t
  wall of, fatty streak on, 292–295, *295*
    fibrous plaque on, 292–295, *295*
    hypertension effect on, 258, *259*
    normal, 291
Artery of Heubner, 2058, *2060*
Arthralgia, AIDS/HIV patient with, 1878t, 1878–1879
  gout with, 1511–1512
  lupus erythematosus with, 1478

Arthralgia *(Continued)*
  neuropathic (Charcot's joint), 1518, 1526, *1526*
  osteoarthritis with, 1518
Arthritis, **1459–1466**, **1517–1521**
  AIDS/HIV with, 1878t, 1878–1879
  alkaptonuria with, 1108
  amyloid, 1504t, 1504–1506
  bacterial (nongonococcal), 1455t, 1465t, 1473, 1473t
    clinical manifestations of, 1473
    diagnosis of, 1473
    treatment of, 1473
  cirrhosis with, 1525
  crystal deposition in, 1511, *1513–1515*, 1515–1517,
      1516t, 1519t. See also *Crystal deposition*.
  degenerative, 1517–1521. See also *Osteoarthritis*.
  endocrine disorders with, 1525–1526
  enteropathic, 1467t, 1472
  fungal, 1475
  gonococcal, 1456, 1473–1474, 1474t, 1703
    clinical manifestations of, 1456, 1473–1474
    diagnosis of, 1455, 1474
    risk factors for, 1474t
    treatment of, 1474, 1702t, 1703
  gouty, 1511–1512, *1512–1514*
  hemochromatosis with, 1525
  hypercholesterolemia with, 1525
  hypertrophic osteoarthropathy with, 1388, 1527
  hypogammaglobulinemia with, 1525
  infectious, 1455t, 1455–1456, 1473t, 1473–1475
  inflammatory bowel disease with, 710t, 711, 1467t,
      1472
  Jaccoud's, 1593
  juvenile chronic, 1466
  lupus erythematosus with, 1475t, 1478
  Lyme, 1474–1475, 1715, 1717, *1718*
  Mediterranean fever with, 1526
  obesity association with, 1165
  pneumococcal, 1571, 1571t
  psoriatic, 1467t, *1471*, 1471–1472
  pulmonary manifestations of, 395t, 395–396, *1463*,
      1464, *1464*
  reactive, 1467t, 1470–1471
  Reiter's, 1467t, *1468*, 1469–1470, *1470*
  rheumatic fever causing, 1592t, 1592–1593
  rheumatoid, **1459–1466**
    ACR criteria for, 1459, 1459t
    anemia with, 1464
    approach to patient with, 1440–1443, 1441t, *1442*,
        1443t
    autoantibodies in, 1456–1458, 1457t
    clinical features of, 1459t, 1461–1464, *1461–1464*,
        1499t
    cytokines released in, 1453–1454, *1454*, 1454t
    diagnostic procedures for, 1455–1459
    differential diagnosis of, 1462, 1462t, 1499t
    drug therapy for, 1465–1466
    etiology of, 1459–1460, 1460t
    Felty's syndrome with, 1464
    genetics and, 1459, 1460t
    HLA associations with, 1459–1460, 1460t
    imaging techniques for, 1458–1459
    interstitial lung disease with, 395t, 395–396
    laboratory findings in, 1460t, 1464, 1465t, 1525t
    management of, 1464–1466
    models for, 1448–1454, *1449*
    neuropathy in, 1462, *1462*, 1463, 1464
    pathogenesis of, 1459–1461, *1460*, 1460t
    pathology of, 1460–1461
    prevalence of, 1459, 1485t
    prognosis in, 1464
    pulmonary effects of, 395t, 395–396, *1463*, 1464,
        1464
    staging of, 1459t
    synovial aspiration in, 1455t, 1455–1456
    tissue injury mechanisms of, 1448–1454,
        1449–1452
    uveitis related to, 2178
    vasculitis of, 1448–1450, *1449*, *1450*
  sarcoidosis with, 1526
  septic, 1455t, 1465t
    H. influenzae in, 1623
    staphylococcal, 1608
    synovial fluid in, 1465t
  sickle cell disease with, 1525
  synovial fluid in, 1455t, 1455–1456, 1465t
  syphilitic, 1475, 1710
  traumatic, synovial fluid in, 1465t
  tuberculous, 1475, 1685t
  viral, 1474
  Whipple's disease with, 1525
Arthropathy. See also *Arthritis*; *Joint(s)*.
  AIDS/HIV patient with, 1878t, 1879
  Behçet's, 1506t, 1506–1507
  crystal deposition causing, *1513*, *1515*, 1515–1517,
      1516t
  enteropathic, 1467t, 1472
  hemophilia with, 992
  hypertrophic periosteum in, 1388
  reactive, 1467t, 1470–1471
Arthropods, **1945–1950**. See also specific type.
  asthma induced by, 379t
  bartonellosis transmitted by, 1682
  bedbug, 1946
  bee, wasp, and ant, 1948. See also *Bee*.
  bite of, 1945t. See also *Bites and stings*.
    allergic reaction to, 1420t, 1420–1421
  centipede, 1948
  Chagas' disease transmitted by, 1899–1900, *1900*
  chigger, 1734, 1947
  contact dermatitis and, 1950
  erysipeloid and, 1673–1674
  filariasis transmitted by, 1939, 1940t, 1944
  flea, 1946. See also *Flea*.
  fly, 1946–1947, 1949–1950. See also *Fly*.
  hornet, 1420t, 1420–1421
  kissing bug (reduviid), 1946
  leishmaniasis transmitted by, *1904*
  louse, 1945–1946. See also *Louse*.
  malaria transmitted by, *1893*, 1893–1894, 1895
  midge, 1805, 1805t, 1939, 1940t, 1945, 1947
  mite, 1847, 1947, 1949, 1950. See also *Mite*.
  mosquito, 1946–1947. See also *Mosquito*.
  occupational exposure to, 379t
  pentastomid, 1950
  reduviid, 1899–1900, *1900*
  scabies due to, 1738t, 1949
  scorpion, 1948–1949
  spider, 1948
  tick, 1947–1948. See also *Tick-borne disease*.
  trachoma transmission by, 1723
  traveler and, 1555
  viruses borne by, 1798t, 1805, 1805t, 1806t
  zoonoses associated with, 1727t, 1737t, 1737–1738,
      1738t
Arthroscopy, 1458–1459
  osteoarthritis treated with, 1521
Arthus reaction, 1448–1449, *1449*
Artificial heart, 495
Arylamine, urinary, 700t
Arylsulfatase deficiency, 1119t, 2112
Asbestosis, 58t, 400–401
  clinical features of, 399t, 400–401
  diagnosis of, 399t, 401
  etiology of, 400
  lung cancer due to, 437, 1016, 1016t
  pleural effusion of, 446
  prognosis in, 401
  treatment of, 401
Ascariasis, 783t, 1935, 1935t
  hepatic effects of, 782, 783t
Aschoff nodules, 1592, *1592*
Ascites, **743–745**
  albumin gradient in, 744, 744t, 745t, 795, 795t
  biliary leak, 743t
  causes, 743t
  chylous, 744t, 745
  cirrhosis with, 743, 743t, 744t, 795–796
  clinical features of, 743–744
  complications of, 795
  diagnostic tests in, 744, 744t, 795, 795t
  endocrine, 743t, 745
  exudative, 744
  heart failure causing, 219–220
  hepatorenal syndrome and, 795–796
  HIV infection with, 745
  malignant, 743t, 744t, 744–745, 745t, 749
  pancreatic, 743t, 744t, 745
  peritonitis and, 743t, 744t, 746, 747t
  portal hypertension with, 743, 743t, 744t, 795–
      796
  transudative, 744
  urine, 743t
Ascorbic acid. See *Vitamin C*.
Ashman phenomenon, *240*, 241
Asians. See also *Racial factors*.
  cancer rate in, 1013t, 1013–1014
  lupus erythematosus in, 1476
  rheumatoid arthritis frequency and, 1460
Asparaginase, adverse effects, 1045–1046
  chemotherapy using, 1039t, 1044t, 1045
Aspartate transaminase (AST), alcoholic cirrhosis and,
    790
  liver function reflected by, 759
  Lyme disease affecting, 1718
  pregnancy and, 787, 787t
Aspartic acid, urinary, 1104t
Aspergilloma, 1830t, 1831, *1831*
Aspergillosis, **1830–1832**
  AIDS/HIV with, 1862–1863, *1863*
  bronchopulmonary, 1830t, *1831*, 1831–1832
    allergic, 1830t, 1830–1832
  clinical syndromes of, 1830t, 1830–1832
  diagnosis of, 1832
  etiologic organism in, 1830, 1831
  treatment and prevention of, 1832
Aspergillus flavus, food contaminated with, 740
Asphyxia, drowning and, 408
Aspiration, 406–407
  clinical features in, 406
  esophageal reflux disease and, 652
  gastric contents in, 406–407
  hydrocarbon, 407
  laryngeal, 655
  lung abscess following, 414, *415*
  mortality due to, 407
  nasogastric tube and, 1171
  oropharyngeal flora and, 1582
  pneumonia caused by, 1581–1582
  pneumonitis caused by, 406–407
  treatment of, 406–407
Aspirin, **111–115**
  allergy to, 1435
  anti-inflammatory effects of, 111–115, 115t,
      1192–1193
  asthma induced by, 378
  dose adjustment for, 94t
  hepatotoxicity, 772, 773t
  history of, 111–112
  mechanism of action of, 112–113, *113*, 1192–1193
  neurologic effects of, 1975t
  neutrophil response to, 114–115
  overdose of, 506, 506t
  pain control with, 102, 103t, 893t
  peptic ulcer role of, 662t, 663, 663t
    systemic administration and, 663
  pharmacokinetics of, 91t, 94t
  platelets and, 116–118, 117t, 984
  prostaglandin inhibition by, 112–115, *113*,
      1192–1193
  renal failure effects and, 94t
  side effects of, 113–114
  ticlopidine vs., 116–118, 117t
AST. See *Aspartate transaminase (AST)*.
Astemizole, allergic rhinitis treated with, 1416,
    1416t
Astereognosia, 1987, 1988t
Astereopsis, 1985, 1987t
Asterixis, 1973
  elicitation of, 1973
  hepatic encephalopathy with, 797–798, 798t
  metabolic encephalopathy with, 1973, 1973t
Asthenia, 2027–2028
  causes of, 2027–2028, 2028t
Asthma, **376–381**
  air pollution causing, 56, 58t
  allergic, 378
  aspirin-induced, 378
  bronchitis with, 383–385
  definition of, 376
  differential diagnosis of, 379t, 380
  environmental causes in, 56, 58t, 379t
  epidemiology of, 376, 379t
  etiology of, 378, 379t
  examination in, 378
  exercise-induced, 378
  extrinsic, 378
  history in, 378
  intrinsic, 378
  laboratory findings in, 378–380, 379t
  occupational factors in, 56, 58t, 379t
  pathogenesis of, 376–377
  pathophysiology in, *377*, 377–378, *378*
  pregnancy and, 381
  severity of, 378–379, 379t
  signs and symptoms in, 368–371, 369t, 378
  treatment of, 380–381
    critical care setting, 381, 473–474
Astigmatism, 2174

Astrocytoma, 2131–2132
  anaplastic, 2131
  classification of, 2126t
  low-grade, 2127, 2131, 2132
  MRI scan of, 2127, 2128t
  multiforme, 2131
Astrovirus, diarrhea and, 1795, 1795t
Asystole, cardiac arrest with, 255
  ECG of, 255
Ataxia, **2028–2030**
  alcohol-related, 47, 48t, 2029
  cerebellar, 1028, 2029, 2051t, 2051–2052
  Friedreich's, 359, 2051
  Guillain-Barré, 2150–2152, 2151t
  hepatic encephalopathy with, 797, 798t
  hereditary, 2051t, 2051–2052
  multiple sclerosis with, 2109, 2109t, 2110
  neuropathy with, 2150–2152, 2151t, **2153**
  paraneoplastic, 1028
  sensory, 2029
  spastic, 2029
  stroke with, 2064t, 2064–2065
  telangiectasia with, 2051
    immunodeficiency in, 1407
    lymphoma-associated, 1035
  vestibular, 2029
Atelectasis, 389–390
  clinical feaures of, 389
  cystic fibrosis with, 420, 421t
  obstructive, 389
  pathogenesis of, 389
  signs and symptoms in, 368, 369t
  treatment of, 389
  types of, 389
Atenolol, dosage for, 265t, 266t, 299t
Atherogenesis, 292, 292, 294, 295
Atherosclerosis, **291–295**
  antiplatelet agents in, 116–119, 117t
  aortic, 292
  bypass site of, 292
  carotid, 292
  cerebral, 292
  cerebrovascular disease due to, 2066, 2067t
  coronary. See Coronary arteries, atherosclerosis of.
  diabetes and, 173, 293, 1276–1277, 1277
  diet and, 1139, 1143t
  genetic factors in, 294
  growth factor role in, 294, 295
  hypertension role in, 258, 259, 260t, 293
  lesions of, 292, 292, 294, 295
    complicated, 292
    fatty streak, 292
    fibrous plaque, 292, 292, 294, 295
    morbid anatomy of, 292, 292
  lipoproteins in, 292–293
    densities of, 1092–1093
    high density, 294
    low density, 292–293
  localization of, 202
  mesenteric artery, 719–720
  mortality rate in, 27t, 30t, 171t, 257, 263, 291
  obesity and, 293–294
  pathogenesis of, 292, 292, 294, 295
  prevention of, 295
  regression of, 294–295
  renal arteries and, 606–607
  response to injury hypothesis of, 294, 295
  risk factors for, 30t, 171–173, 173, 292–294
    atherogenesis mechanisms and, 292, 292, 294, 295
    reduction in, 294–295
  smoking and, 171, 173, 293
Athetosis, 2049
Atlantoaxial joint, 1462, 1463
Atomic bomb, 1016
Atovaquone, Pneumocystis pneumonia and, 1920, 1920t, 1921t, 1922t
  toxoplasmosis therapy with, 1909, 1910t
ATP (adenosine triphosphate), 856, 856, 859
Atracurium, 310t
Atretic follicle, 1294
Atria (atrium), contraction of, 176t, 178
  core temperature taken in, 1533
  dilatation of, 182, 183–184
  echocardiography of, 194–198, 195–197
  electrophysiology of, 231–232, 232
  fibrillation of, 240–241
    carotid massage in, 235t
    clinical features of, 241

Atria (atrium) (Continued)
  ECG of, 240, 240–241, 241
  emboli arising in, 2067
  treatment of, 237t, 238t, 241
  flutter of, 239–240
    carotid massage in, 235t
    clinical features of, 239
    ECG of, 239, 240
    treatment of, 237t, 238t, 240
  mitral valve disease and, 182, 183–184
  MRI of, 208
  natriuretic hormone of, 1194–1195, 1195
    shock and, 482
    volume regulation role of, 527, 527
  premature complexes of, 237–238
    ECG of, 237–238, 238t, 240
    laddergram of, 235
    treatment of, 238
  pressure in, 176, 176t, 178
  rheumatic fever effect in, 1592
  roentgenography of, 181–183, 181–184
  tachycardia of, 237t, 238t, 239–241, 240, 241
    multifocal, 241
Atrial septal defect, fetus with, 159t
  MRI scan of, 274
  ostium secundum, 278–279, 280
Atrioventricular block, 242
  arrhythmias due to, 242, 242, 255
  Lyme disease causing, 1717, 1718
  sudden cardiac death and, 255
  type I, 235, 242, 242
  type II, 242
Atrioventricular dissociation, 243
Atrioventricular junction, 191
  nonparoxysmal tachycardia and, 242, 242
  premature complex of, 242
Atrioventricular node, 191, 231–233, 232
  conduction in, 231
    delay of, 191, 191t
    enhanced automaticity in, 242
    velocity of, 190
  electrogram of, 231–233, 232
  internodal tracts and, 231
Atrioventricular premature complexes, 242
Atrophy, multi-system, 2050–2054, 2051t
  muscle, 2050–2054, 2051t
    spinal, 2052t, 2053
  neurologic disease causing, 2050–2054, 2051t
  poliovirus causing, 2091
Atropine, neurologic effects of, 1975t
  organophosphate toxicity treated with, 504t, 509
  physostigmine antidote for, 504t, 506
  poisoning due to, 504t, 506
  tea containing, 54–55
Attention disorder. See also Confusion.
  brain disease indicated by, 1972–1973
Audiometry, 2021
  brain stem responses in, 2021
  pure tone, 2021
Auditory agnosia, 1991
Auditory artery, aneurysm affecting, 2074, 2074–2076
Aura, epileptic, 2114, 2115
  olfactory, 2115
  seizure with, 2114
Auramine, carcinogenicity and, 1016t
  tubercle bacillus uptake of, 1685
Auscultation, abdominal, 749
  chest, pneumonia in, 1572
  heart sounds in, 168, 168t
  intestinal obstruction, 682
  pulmonary, 368, 369t, 370
Autoimmunity, adrenal insufficiency due to, 1250–1251, 1251t
  AIDS/HIV effects with, 1878t, 1878–1879
  brain affected by, 1476t, 1477
  Eaton-Lambert, 1018, 1028
  erythrocytes affected by, 1476t, 1477
  Graves' disease due to, 1232
  Hashimoto's thyroiditis due to, 1241
  hepatitis due to, 777–778, 778t
  hypoglycemia due to, 1282
  leukocytes affected by, 1476t, 1477
  lupus erythematosus due to, 1456–1458, 1457t, 1476t, 1476–1477, 1481t
  myasthenia due to, 1018, 1028
  myopathy due to, 1501t, 1502, 2164
  myositis-specific, 1501, 1501t, 2164
  pemphigoid due to, 2206
  pituitary affected by, 1250
  platelets affected by, 980–983, 984t, 1476t, 1477

Autoimmunity (Continued)
  polyendocrine deficiency due to, 1250–1251, 1251t, 1347t, 1347–1348
  rheumatoid arthritis due to, 1456–1458, 1457t, 1459
  systemic sclerosis with, 1483–1484, 1484t
  testicular failure due to, 1335
  thrombocytopenia caused by, 980t, 980–983, 984t
  thyroid gland affected by, 1232–1234, 1237t, 1237–1238, 1241
  urticaria due to, 1409–1410
  Wegener's granulomatosis and, 1457t, 1458, 1496t, 1497
Autoinfection, strongyloidiasis causing, 1938
Automaticity (cardiac), 233
  abnormal, 233, 233t
  arrhythmias related to, 233–234, 234
  AV nodal, 233
  Purkinje fiber, 233
  sinus nodal, 231, 233
  triggered activity vs., 233–234, 234
  ventricular parasystolic, 244
Automatism, epileptic, 2114, 2115
Autonomic nervous system, **2007–2013**. See also Parasympathetic nervous system; Sympathetic nervous system.
  aging effects in, 16, 16t
  blood pressure role of, 2009, 2009t
  drugs affecting, 2008t
  function testing for, 2009t
  hypothalamus role in, 2011, 2011
  neuropathy of, 2008t
  norepinephrine role in, 1253
  peripheral effects of, 2007t, 2008t
  regulatory functions of, 2007t, 2009t, 2009–2013
Avidin, biotin binding by, 1147t
Axilla, hair of, 2187
  nodes of, 969t
  sweat glands of, 2186
Axon, catecholamine action on, 1253
  degeneration of, 2150
  dying back of, 2150, 2156
  high-frequency discharge of, 2158
  histamine test of, 2009t
  myopathy and, 2158, 2171
Azatadine, allergic rhinitis treated with, 1416, 1416t
Azathioprine, adverse effects of, 365
  fetal malformations due to, 1070t, 1071t
  heart transplantation using, 363, 365
  hepatotoxicity, 773, 773t
  spondyloarthropathy treated with, 1472
Azelastine, allergic rhinitis treated with, 1416, 1416t
Azidothymidine. See Zidovudine (AZT).
Azithromycin, 1562t
  Legionella and, 1585, 1585t
  Lyme disease therapy with, 1719, 1719t
  toxoplasmosis therapy with, 1909, 1910t
Azlocillin, 1562t
  minimal inhibitory concentration for, 1570, 1570t
Azole drugs. See Fluconazole; Itraconazole; Ketoconazole.
Azoospermia, 1329, 1337
  cystic fibrosis with, 421, 421t
  idiopathic, 1337
  Klinefelter's syndrome with, 1334
  obstructive, 1331
Azotemia, 552
  definition of, 552
  glomerulonephritis causing, 575
  nephrotic syndrome with, 573
  prerenal, 552t, 552–553
AZT. See Zidovudine (AZT).
Aztreonam, 1562t
Azurophil granules, 897, 898t

B

B cells, 1282, 1393–1395
  activation, 1395, 1395t
  AIDS/HIV effect on, 1838–1839
  allergic rhinitis role of, 1414, 1415
  assessment of, 1402
  cytokine interaction with, 1393, 1395, 1395t
  deficiency of, 1402t, 1402–1403, 1403, 1542
  development of, interleukins in, 1403
  Epstein-Barr virus and, 1776–1779
  fever production role of, 1533–1534, 1535t
  glucocorticoid effect on, 108–109, 109t
  hairy, 930
  immunoglobulin formation by, 901, 901, 1395, 1396
  inflammatory bowel disease role of, 708

B cells (Continued)
   leukemia and, 931–932, 933t, 937
   lupus erythematosus role of, 1476, 1476–1477
   lymphoma of, 941t, 943t
      Epstein-Barr virus and, 1777–1778
   myeloma and, 962
   production of, 820, 821
   sarcoidosis role of, 431, 431
   splenic, 971
   synovitis role of, 1460
Babesiosis, 1915–1916
Bacillus, 1556, 1556–1557, 1557t
   Calmette-Guérin, 46, 1689
   Koch-Weeks, 1624
Bacillus anthracis, 1664–1667. See also Anthrax.
Bacillus cereus, 739, 739t
Baclofen, 106t
Bacteremia, anaerobic, 1638–1639
   clostridial, 1631t, 1631–1633
   endocarditis role of, 1598t, 1598–1599, 1599, 1608,
      1608t, 1610
   gonococcal, 1702
   gram-negative, 1564t, 1660
   H. influenzae in, 1623
   hospital-acquired, 1549t, 1551, 1598, 1598t, 1608,
      1669–1671
   meningitis with, 1611–1613, 1620
   mycobacterial (nontuberculous), 1690t, 1690–1691
   pneumococcal pneumonia with, 1571, 1575
   Pseudomonas, 1579–1581, 1668t, 1669–1672, 1671t
   Salmonella, 1645–1646
   septic shock role of, 496, 497
   staphylococcal, 1598t, 1608, 1610
   streptococcal, 1587, 1598t
   transient, 1598, 1598t, 1638–1639
   tuberculous, 1685t, 1685–1686
Bacteria, 1556–1557. See also specific organism or dis-
      ease.
   adaptive characteristics of, 1531, 1556, 1556–1557
   adhesiveness of. See Fimbriae.
   aerobic, 1557t
   anaerobic, 1557t, 1639t, 1641t. See also Anaerobes;
      Clostridial infection(s).
   arthritis caused by, 1473t, 1473–1474, 1474t
   bronchiectasis due to, 416t, 416–417
   capsules of, 1556, 1556, 1570, 1586, 1639t
   cell wall of, 1556, 1556–1557
   classification of, 1556–1557, 1557t
   compromised host and, 1537–1539, 1538t
   fever production role of, 1532t, 1532–1534, 1534
   flora constituted of. See Flora.
   gram-negative, 1556–1557, 1557t
   gram-positive, 1556–1557, 1557t
   host defense mechanisms and, 1534, 1537, 1538t
   lung abscess due to, 413–414, 414t, 415
   morphology of, 1556, 1556–1557
   motility of, 1556
   overgrowth of, breath tests for, 700, 700t
      conditions associated with, 703–704, 704t
      intestinal, 700t, 700–701, 701t, 703, 704t
      treatment of, 703
      vitamin B12 test and, 699, 701t
   pneumonia caused by, 411t, 411–412, 412t, 475t
   preventive measures and, 1544t, 1547–1548
   septic shock due to, 496, 497, 498
   sexual transmission of, 1697t
   small intestinal, malabsorption and, 700t, 701
   urinary. See Bacteriuria; Urinary tract, infections
      of.
   virulence factors of, 1531, 1556, 1556–1557,
      1639t
Bacteriuria, 602–603, 603t, 604t
   asymptomatic, 602, 604
   catheter-associated, 1549t, 1550–1551
   elderly with, 22
   staphylococcal, 1608
Bacteroides, 1638, 1639t
   fragilis, 1638–1641, 1639, 1639t, 1641t
Baffles, intra-atrial, 283
Bainbridge reflex, 215
Baker's cyst, knee with, 1462, 1463, 1466
   treatment of, 1466
BAL (British anti-lewisite), lead poisoning treated with,
      69, 69t
   mercury poisoning treated with, 504t
Balanitis, candidal, 1828
   circinata, 2203
Balantidiasis, 1916t
Ballism, 2049
Banti's syndrome, 972

Barbiturates, neurologic effects of, 1975t
   poisoning due to, 506t, 506–507
Bardet-Biedl syndrome, 160t, 162
   clinical features of, 160t, 162
Barium, 73
   hypokalemia induced by, 540
   occupational exposure to, 73
   periodic paralysis due to, 2168
   poisoning due to, 73
      symptoms of, 73
      treatment of, 73
Barometric pressure, 409
   arterial gas embolism and, 410
   decompression illness and, 410, 410t
   high altitude edema and, 409t, 409–410
   lung affected by, 409t, 409–410, 410t
   mountain sickness related to, 409t, 409–410
Baroreceptors, autonomic control and, 2009, 2009t
   high-pressure, 526
   low-pressure, 526
   vasopressin response to, 1222–1223
   volume regulation role of, 526
Barr body, 140, 154
Barrett's esophagus, 652, 654, 657
   cancer progression of, 654, 657
Barrier(s), air-blood, 371–372
   blood-brain, 2062, 2062t
   blood-placental, 1069
   glomerular, 520, 520, 521, 572
   skin as, 1537, 1538t
Barrington's nucleus, 2010
Bartonella, 1680, 1680–1682
   bacilliformis, 1682
   henselae, 1680, 1680–1682, 1682t, 1738t
   quintana, 1680, 1680–1682, 1682t
Bartonellosis, 1682, 1738t
Bartter's syndrome, 528, 598
   alkalosis in, 550, 598
   diagnosis of, 598
   hypokalemia and, 539, 539t, 598
   nephropathy in, 528, 539, 598
   pathophysiology of, 539, 598
   sodium wasting in, 528, 539, 550, 598
   treatment of, 598
   volume depletion and, 528, 528t
Basal cell carcinoma of skin, 2209, 2209
   nevoid, 1035, 2210, 2210–2211
Basal ganglia, 2042–2050
   aging effects in, 16, 16t
   akinesia and, 2042
   anatomy of, 2042, 2043
   aphasia related to, 1992
   bradykinesia related to, 2042
   chorea and, 2043
   hyperkinesias related to, 2042t, 2042–2043
   hypokinesias related to, 2042, 2042t
   manganese effect on, 73
   neurochemistry of, 2042
   postural instability and, 2042
   tremor and, 2043
   tumor of, 2126t
Basedow's disease. See Graves' disease.
Basement membrane, antibodies to, 577, 1479
   connective tissue of, 1443–1446, 1445t, 1448
   cutaneous, 2184, 2185, 2186, 2186
   diabetes mellitus affecting, 1447
   glomerular, 520, 520, 521, 577, 1479
   phagocyte migration through, 899
Basilar artery, 2058, 2058, 2061
   aneurysm affecting, 2074, 2074–2076
   occlusion of, 2064t, 2065
Basilar impression, 2149
Basophils, deficiency of, 914
   glucocorticoid effect on, 108–109, 109t
   production of, 819, 820, 820t, 821, 898
Bat, histoplasmosis organism and, 1816
   rabies in, 2095–2096
Baths, skin therapy using, 2193, 2194t
Battery makers, 59t
Bayes' rule, 78–80
   cohort flow form of, 78–79, 79
   decision making role of, 78–80, 79, 79t
   tabular form of, 78–79, 79t
Bazex's syndrome, 1019, 1035
BCG vaccine, 46, 1689
Bcl-2 oncogene, 1011–1012, 1036t, 1058
BCNU (carmustine), 1039t, 1042
Beans, dietary aspects of, 29–30, 30t, 1142, 1143
   fava, 857
   hemagglutinin in, 740

Beans (Continued)
   hemolysis due to, 857
   poisoning due to, 740, 857
   red kidney, 740
Beau's lines, 2215
Becker dystrophy, 2160t, 2161
Beckwith-Wiedemann syndrome, 160t, 161
   clinical features of, 160t, 161
   gene imprinting in, 161
Beclomethasone, 1417t
Bedbug, 1946
Bedwetting, 1983, 1983t
Bee, 1948
   allergic reaction to, 1420t, 1420–1421
   aspergillosis organism in, 1830
   skin test related to, 1421
   sting of, 1420–1421, 1948
Beef, 29–30, 30t, 1142, 1143, 1143t
   tapeworm in, 1923t, 1924
Beer, osmolality disturbance due to, 534–535
   potomania due to, 534–535
Beetle, blister, 1950
   dermatitis caused by, 1950
Behavior, 1996. See also Psychiatric disorders.
   Alzheimer's disease affecting, 1993, 1994
   anorexic, 1158–1160, 1159t
   aphasia and, 1991–1992
   bulimic, 1160
   dementia affecting, 18, 19t, 1993, 1994
   elderly patient and, 17–21, 1999–2000
   encephalopathy affecting, 1996
   iron deficiency affecting, 840
   modification therapy of, 1166
   nonpsychiatric illness affecting, 1996, 1996t
   obesity treatment related to, 1166
   parkinsonian, 2044t
   psychotic, 1997t
   suicidal, 1999t, 2001t, 2002
Behçet's disease, 1506–1507
   clinical manifestations of, 1506t, 1506–1507
   genetics of, 1507
   HLA complex in, 1431t, 1507
   meningitis of, 1616
   oral lesions of, 646, 646t, 1506, 1506t
   pathology findings in, 1507
   prevalence of, 1507
   treatment of, 1507
   uveitis in, 2178–2179
Bejel, endemic syphilis as, 1714
Belching, peptic ulcer and, 665, 665t
Bell's palsy, 2157
   Lyme disease with, 1717, 1719t
Bell-shaped distribution, 84, 85t
Benazepril, 265t
Bence Jones protein, 513t, 959, 962
   amyloidosis with, 1504
   gammopathies with, 959
   myeloma and, 959, 962, 963
   urinary, 513t, 959, 962
      idiopathic, 962
Bendroflumethiazide, 264t
Bends disorder, 410, 410t
Bentiromide, malabsorption and, 699, 700t
   urinary excretion of, 699, 700t
Benzene, aplastic anemia caused by, 832, 832t
   carcinogenicity of, 1016t
   occupational exposure to, 56, 58t
Benzene hexachloride, pediculosis treated with,
      2195
Benzidine, 1016t
Benzodiazepines, alcohol withdrawal treated with,
      48–49
   antidote for, 504t
   drug abuse with, 50–51, 56t
   poisoning due to, 504t, 507
Benzthiazide, 264t
Bepridil, dosage for, 300t
   side effects of, 300t
Bereavement, 8–9
   depression due to, 2001t, 2001–2002
   family affected by, 8t, 8–9
   risk indicators for, 8, 8t
Berger's disease, Alport's syndrome vs., 812t
   glomerulonephritis vs., 575
Bernard-Soulier syndrome, 985
Berylliosis, 402t, 402–403
   hepatic granuloma with, 784t
   industries associated with, 59t, 402t

Beryiliosis *(Continued)*
  occupational exposure in, 59t
  pathogenesis of, 59t, 402
Beta blocking agents, 265t, 266t. See also *Propranolol.*
  angina pectoris treated with, 298–299, 299t
  antidote for, 504t
  dosages for, 265t, 266t
  hypertension treated with, 263–266, 265t–267t
  ocular application of, 2183, 2183t
  side effects of, 266, 267t, 2183t
Beta cells, diabetes mellitus and, *1259,* 1261–1263, *1263*
  insulin secretion by, 1260
Beta chains, 1424–1426, 1425t, *1426*
Beta globulin, 958
Beta-adrenergic receptors, *245,* 263–266, 298–299. See also *Beta blocking agents.*
  asthma treatment and, 380
  blood vessel, 492–493
  myocardial, 492–493
Beta-carotene, 1010, 1016–1017
Beta-lactam agents. See *Cephalosporins; β-Lactam agents; Penicillin(s);* specific agents.
Betamethasone, 108t
Betaxolol, 265t
Bicarbonate, 543
  acid-base balance and, 543–545, *545,* 546t, 597, *597*
  CSF and, 544–545
  gastrointestinal loss of, 547
  Henderson-Hasselbalch equation and, 543, *545*
  hyperkalemia treated with, 542
  intestinal transport of, *689,* 689–690
  normal blood level of, 467t
  reabsorption and regeneration of, 544, 546t, 546–547, 597, *597*
  renal tubular acidosis and, 546t, 546–547, 597, *597*
  therapy using, 549, 1271
  toxicity treated with, 504t, 509
  transport mechanisms for, 521t, *522,* 523, *524,* 532, 544, 597, *597*
  urinary, 514
  ventilation assessment using, 467t
  wasting, 546–547
Bicipital tendinitis, 1521–1524
Bicytopenia, 831
Bigeminy, 243
Bile, **805–807**
  acids of, 805–807, *805–807*
    dissolution therapy with, 815
    production of, *1087,* 1089
    resin binding of, *1093*
  bilirubin excretion into, *755,* 755–756, 805, *805*
  composition of, 805–806, *805–807*
  daily amounts of, 696, 805, *805,* 807
  inspissated, 808
  limey, 814
  lithogenic, 812–813, *813*
  salts, 805–807, *805–807*
    absorption of, 696, 696t, 806, 806–807, *807*
    bacterial overgrowth role of, 703–704
    circulation of, 805–806, *807*
    diarrhea and, 807
    excretion of, 696, 805, *805,* 807
    fat absorption role of, 696, *697,* 806, *806*
    malabsorption role of, 703–704
    reduced concentration of, 703–704
  secretion of, 805, *807*
  stasis of. See *Cholestasis.*
Bilharziasis, 1927
  hepatosplenic, 1929–1930
  intestinal, 1929–1930
  urinary, 1929
Biliary tract, **805–816**
  atresia of, 812
  cancer of, *637*
  cirrhosis and, 791–792
  double duct sign and, *637*
  dyskinesia of, 816, 816t
  hypoplasia of, 810
  imaging procedures for, 632–634, *632–634*
  inflammation of. See *Cholangitis.*
  neoplasms of, 810–811
  obstruction of, 807–810. See also *Cholestasis.*
  paucity of ductules of, 810
  stricture of, 808, *809*
    benign, 811–812
    endoscopic therapy for, 641

Bilirubin, **755–756**
  conjugated, *755,* 755–756
  excess of. See *Jaundice.*
  excretion of, *755,* 755–756
    defects of, 756t, 756–757, 757t
  gallstone content of, 813
  glucuronyltransferase deficit and, 757t
  hemolysis and, 756
  intestinal conversion of, 756
  isomers of, 755–756
  liver and, *755,* 755–757, 756t, 757t, 760
    failure of, 800t
  metabolism of, *755,* 755–756
  normal levels of, 756
  overproduction of, 756t, 756–757
  plasma levels of, *755,* 755–756, 757t
  renal excretion of, *755,* 755
  sources and precursors of, *755,* 755–756
  transport of, *755,* 755–756
  unconjugated, *755,* 755
  uptake of, 755–756
  urinary, 512t, 761
Biliverdin, 755
Billroth anastomosis, 669–671, *670,* 670t
Billroth's cords, 971
Bioethics. See *Ethical issues.*
Biogenic amines, *1176*
Biological response, cellular, *1176–1180,* 1176–1181
  hormone action in, *1176–1180,* 1176–1181
  modifiers of, cancer treatment with, 1007
    chemotherapy using, 1047–1049, 1048t, 1049t
  molecular biology of, *1176–1180,* 1176–1181
Biopsy, bone, normal, *1361*
    osteomalacic, 1360, *1361*
  bone marrow, *1437*
  breast, 1319
  fat tissue, 1505–1506
  liver, 762, 808
  lung, 392
  muscle, 2161
  rectal, 694
  renal, 517, 517t
  skin, 2192–2193, *2193*
  small intestinal, 700t, 701, *702,* 702t
  thyroid gland, 1231, 1231t
Biopterin, 1100t, 1101t, *1106*
Biotin, assessment of, 1147t
  deficiency of, 1147t
  parenteral, 1172t
  physiology of, 1147t
  RDA for, 1141t
  toxicity of, 1147t
Bipolar disorder, depressive phase of, 2003–2004
  drug therapy of, 2003–2004
  incidence of, 2003
  manic phase of, 1997t, 2002–2004, 2003t
  symptoms of, 2002–2003, 2003t
Birbeck granules, 955, 2185
Bird, 58t
  cryptococcosis organism and, 1823
  histoplasmosis organism and, 1816
  psittacosis carried by, 1725, 1737t
Birefringence, amyloid deposit with, 1504, 1506
  crystal deposition disease with, 1516t
  urate crystals with, 1512, *1514*
Birth defects. See *Congenital anomalies.*
Bischloromethylether, 1016t
Bismuth subsalicylate, 695
Bisoprolol, 265t, 266t
Bisphosphonates, osteoclast inhibition by, 1383
  Paget's disease treated with, 1386
Bite cells, 857
Bites and stings. See also *Animals; Arthropods; Insects;* specific organisms.
  allergic reaction to, 1420t, 1420–1421
  anaerobic flora infection of, 1641
  ant, 1948
  bee. See *Bee.*
  cat, 1738t. See also *Cat scratch disease.*
  centipede, 1948
  chigger, 1947
  dog, 1738t. See also *Dog.*
  flea, 1738t, 1947. See also *Flea.*
  hornet, 1420t, 1420–1421
  immune globulin against, 41t
  leech, 1950–1951
  louse, 1945–1946. See also *Louse.*
  marine organism, 1854t, 1953–1956
  osteomyelitis due to, 1625t, 1625–1626

Bites and stings *(Continued)*
  scorpion, 1948
  snake, 1951–1953. See also *Snakebite; Venoms.*
  spider, 1948
  tick, 1732, 1947–1948. See also *Tick-borne disease.*
  travel exposure to, 1555–1556
  wasp, 1948
  zoonoses associated with, 1727t, 1737t, 1737–1738, 1738t
Bitol spots, 1145t
Black piedra, 1836
Blackout, alcoholic, 48, 1982, 2039
Blacks. See also *Racial factors.*
  cancer rate in, 1013t, 1013–1014
  hereditary disorder frequency and, 136t, 136–140, 138t
  hypertension affecting, 258, *259*
  Kaposi's sarcoma in, 1032–1033, 1033t
  lupus erythematosus in, 1476
Blackwater fever, 1894
Bladder. See *Urinary bladder.*
Blanching, energy conservation by, 1533
  Raynaud's phenomenon with, 1478
Blastocystis hominis, 1916t
Blastomycosis, **1821–1822**
  adrenal gland, 1251
  clinical manifestations of, 1821–1822
  diagnosis of, 1822
  epidemiology of, 1821
  etiologic agent in, 1821
  pathogenesis and pathology of, 1821
  treatment of, 1822
Blebs, 389
  airway obstruction with, 389
  meningococcal, *1619*
Bleeding. See *Hemorrhage.*
Bleeding time, 979–980. See also *Clotting time; Coagulation.*
  hemorrhagic disorders and, 979t, 979–980, *981,* 984t
Blennorrhea, inclusion, 2179
Bleomycin, adverse effects of, 1044–1045
  chemotherapy using, 1039t, 1044t, 1044–1045
  Hodgkin's disease and, 952t, 953
  Kaposi's sarcoma treated with, 1873, 1873t
  lung disease induced by, 397, 397t
  non-Hodgkin's lymphoma and, 945t
Blepharoconjunctivitis, 2179
Blind loop syndrome, 703, 704t
Blindness, 2174, 2174t
  Bardet-Biedl syndrome causing, 162
  Behçet's syndrome causing, 1506
  differential diagnosis of, 2174, 2174t
  glaucoma and, 2016, 2175
  herpes simplex keratitis in, 1772
  hysterical, 2174–2175
  night, malabsorption in, 699t
    vitamin A deficiency in, 699t, 1145t, 1153t
  onchocerciasis with, 1942–1943
  pituitary apoplexy with, 2035, 2131
  quinine causing, 2183
  retinal artery occlusion causing, 2182
  "river," 1942–1943
  stroke with, 2064, 2064t
  trachoma causing, 1722
  transient monocular, 2064, 2064t
Blister cells, 857
Blisters. See also *Bullae; Vesicles.*
  cold sore, 1772, *1772*
Blood. See also *Hemorrhage.*
  AIDS/HIV precautions with, 1853–1854, 1854t
  antimicrobials affecting, 1568t
  brown coloration of, 875, 876, 877
  health worker exposure to, 1853–1854, 1854t
  lead affecting, 68–69, 69t
  levels, 2224t–2233t. See also specific substances.
  occult. See *Feces, blood in.*
Blood clot, 989–990
  lysis of, 989
  urea solubility of, 990
Blood cultures, endocarditis and, 1600t, 1600–1601, 1601t
  fever of unknown origin and, 1532–1533
  meningitis organisms in, 1613, 1620
  meningococcal, 1618, 1620
Blood flow, cardiogenic shock and, 477–483
  cerebral, 2057–2062, *2058–2062*
    occlusion of, 2064t, 2064–2065
  coronary, 178–179, *179*
  cutaneous, 2189

Blood flow *(Continued)*
  determinant factors for, 179–180, 478t, 478–483
  endocardial injury due to, 1596–1598, *1597, 1599*
  humoral factors affecting, 481–482
  shock and, septic, 499, 499t
  sickle cells affecting, *883, 885,* 885–891
  splenic, 970–971
Blood gases, 375, 375t
  asthma affecting, 379
  normal values for, 466, 467t
  partial pressures of, 375, 375t, 467t
  pulmonary embolism and, 423, 424
  pulmonary function test and, 373t, *374,* 374–375
  ventilation assessment using, 466–468, 467t, 472, *472*
Blood levels and ranges, 2224t–2233t. See also specific substances.
Blood pressure. See also *Hypertension; Hypotension.*
  autonomic control of, 2009, 2009t
  brain injury and, 2138t
  catecholamines affecting, 1254, 1255
  heart contraction and, 175–176, 176t, *176–178*
  hepatic, 793–794
  hydrostatic pressure and, 489t, 525
  hypertension classification by, 258t
  infarction and, 305t
  intracardiac, 175–177, 176t, *176–178,* 489t, 489–490
  measurement of, 259–260
  normal resting, 489t
  pulmonary edema and, 476, *477*
  shock and, 489–490, 494
    septic, 499t, 499–501
    toxic, 1588t, 1588–1589
Blood products, 991–992, 994–995
Blood smear, anemia effects in, 824–825, 825t
  aplastic anemia, 834
  babesiosis in, 1916
  lymphocytic leukemia, 932
  malaria organism in, 1894–1895, 1895t
  megaloblastic anemia, *847,* 847–848, *848*
  myelogenous leukemia, 927
  platelets in, 979
  sickle cell, *883, 885*
  thick, 1894
  thrombocytopenia, 984t
  Treponema pallidum in, 1705, 1710
Blood transfusion. See *Transfusion.*
Blood volume, effective arterial, 511, 514
  fluid balance disorders and, 525, *526,* 529–530
  regulation of, 180, 525–528, *526*
  renal function related to, 511, 514
Blood-brain barrier, gas diffusion across, 2062, 2062t
  glucose crossing of, 2062, 2062t
  multiple sclerosis affecting, 2107
  nutrient entry across, 2062, 2062t
Blood-placental barrier, 1069
Bloom's syndrome, 1036
Blue diaper syndrome, 144t
Blue rubber bleb nevus syndrome, 721
Blumer's shelf, 678
Body(ies), Creola, 380
  Döhle, 916, *918*
  Hassall's, 1438
  Heinz, 856–857, 874, *874,* 971, 973
  Howell-Jolly, 971, 973
  Lewy, 1994
  morula, 1733
  Negri, 2096
  Pick's, 1995
Body compartments. See also *Fluid(s).*
  bone minerals in, 1351t, *1352*
  storage patterns for, *1162,* 1163–1165
Body composition, age and, 1161–1162, *1162*
  gender and, 1161–1162, *1162*
  obesity and, *1161,* 1161–1162, *1162*
  total fat in, 1161–1162, *1162*
  total protein in, 1154
Body flora. See *Flora.*
Body fluids. See also *Fluid(s).*
  AIDS/HIV precautions with, 1853–1854, 1854t
Body height. See *Height (body).*
Body image, anorexia nervosa and, 1158, 1159t
  marfanoid, 1375
Body mass, fat-free, 1162
  index of, 1161
    age effect on, 1161, *1162*
    obesity defined by, *1161,* 1161, *1162*
  lean, 1154
    calculation of, 1162

Body temperature. See *Temperature (body).*
Body weight. See *Weight (body).*
Boerhaave's syndrome, 445–446
  vomiting and, 629, 630, 659
Bohr effect, 869
Boils, 2207
  staphylococcal toxin causing, 1606, 1607, 1607t
Bolivian hemorrhagic fever, 1798t, 1802–1803
Bone, **1351–1392**
  aging and, 23, 1353–1354, 1379, *1379*
  architecture of, 1351–1352, *1353*
  biopsy of, normal, *1361*
    osteomalacic, 1360, *1361*
  body compartment of, *1162,* 1351t
  calcium level and, 1351t, 1351–1356, *1352, 1355*
  cancer of, incidence of, 1013t
  constituents of, 1351t, 1351–1352, *1352*
  destruction of. See *Osteolysis; Osteoporosis; Paget's disease.*
  dysplasia of, 1387–1391, 1388t
    fibrous, *1390,* 1390–1391
  dystrophic. See *Osteodystrophy.*
  fluoride and, 1148t
  formation of, 1351–1353, *1353*
  fracture of. See *Fractures.*
  fragility of, 1122t, 1122–1133
  granuloma, Langerhans' cell, 955
  growth of, 1353–1354. See also *Growth.*
    excessive. See *Hyperostosis.*
  homocystinuria and, 1113t, 1113–1114.
  hypercalcemia and, 1355–1356, 1367–1369
  hyperparathyroidism and, 1356
  infarction of, 1387, 1387t
  infection of. See *Osteomyelitis.*
  inflammatory bowel disease and, 710t, 711
  ischemia affecting, 1387, 1387t
  joint anatomy and, *1441*
  laboratory tests and, 1356–1357
  lamellar (cortical), 1351, 1353, *1353*
  Marfan syndrome effects in, 1119–1120
  metabolism of, 1351–1356
    disorders of, 1359–1365, 1388t. See also *Osteomalacia; Rickets.*
  mineralization of, 1351–1354, *1353*
    defective, 1359–1365. See also *Osteomalacia; Osteoporosis; Rickets.*
    density of, *1353,* 1379, *1379,* 1382t
    excessive. See *Osteosclerosis.*
  morphogenetic protein, 1352
  myeloma affecting, 962, 962t, *963,* 965
  osteogenesis imperfecta and, 1122t, **1122–1133**
  Paget's disease of, 1384–1387, *1385, 1386*
  pain from, fibrogenesis imperfecta with, 1365
    osteodystrophy with, 1377
    osteonecrosis causing, 1387
    Paget's disease with, 1385, 1385t, 1386
  parathyroid hormone and, 1354, 1354t, *1355,* 1356, *1372,* 1372–1373
  remodeling of, 1353
  repair of, 1352–1353
  resorption of, 1352
    defective, 1388t, 1388–1390
    hyperparathyroidism with, 1356, 1377, *1378*
    mechanism of, 1352
    osteitis fibrosa with, 1377, *1378*
    osteomalacia and, 1356, 1360–1361, *1361*
    osteoporosis and, 1356, *1379,* 1379–1381, *1380*
    Paget's disease and, 1385, *1385, 1386*
  spotted, 1390
  structure of, 1351–1352, *1353*
  syphilis affecting, 1707, 1710
  trabecular (cancellous), 1351, *1353*
  tumors of, 1391–1392
  woven, 1351
Bone marrow, *819, 832, 834*
  anemia and, 825–829, 826t–828t
  biopsy of, *1437*
  examination algorithm for, *913*
  failure of, 831t, 831–837, 835t
    antimicrobials causing, 1568t
    aplastic anemia and, *832,* 834, *834,* 835t
    chemotherapy causing, 1046
    myelophthisic anemia and, 837, 837t
    neutropenia due to, 909–910, *909–911*
    pure red cell aplasia and, 833–834, *834*
  fibrosis, 837, 837t, 924–925
  hematopoiesis role of, *818,* 818–819, *819, 909*
  leukemia and. See *Leukemia.*
  lymphoma affecting, non-Hodgkin's, 944t

Bone marrow *(Continued)*
  mastocytosis affecting, 1435t, 1435–1437, *1437*
  metaplasia, 924t, 924–925
  neutrophil production and, 817–819, *818–821,* 897, *898*
    decreased, 909–910, *909–911*
  radiation of, 61, 61t, 62t
  sinusoids, 818, *819*
Bonnevie-Ullrich syndrome, 1335
Borborygmus, chest, 443
Bordetella, 1627–1629. See also *Pertussis.*
Bornholm disease, 1787–1788
Boron, 73
  occupational exposure to, 73
  poisoning due to, 73
Borreliosis, 1715–1720
  arthritis of, 1474–1475, 1715, 1717
  relapsing fever due to, 1715
Botryomycosis, 1607t, 1609
Botulism, **1635–1636**
  antitoxin for, 46
  clinical manifestations of, 1635
  clostridial infection in, 1630, 1631t, 1635–1636
  definition of, 1635
  diagnosis of, 1635
  etiology of, 1635
  foodborne, 1635, 1636
  immune globulin against, 41t
  infant, 1636
  prognosis in, 1636
  prophylaxis for, 1636
  treatment of, 1635–1636
  unclassified, 1636
  wound, 1636
Bouchard's nodes, *1520*
Boutonneuse fever, 1727t, 1728t, 1732
Boutonnière deformity, 1462
Bowen's disease, 1035
  anal, 743
  arsenic role in, 1035
  skin cancer in, 1035, 2209–2210
Bowman's capsule, 519, *519, 520*
Boxcar pattern, 2182
Brachial sinus, fetal, 158t
Bradycardia, myocardial infarction followed by, 313
  sick sinus syndrome with, 237t, 238t, *241,* 241–242
  sinus, 237t, 238t, *241,* 241–242
Bradykinesia, 2042
Bradykinin, asthma role of, 376
  shock and, 481, 498
Bradyzoite, 1907–1908
Brain. See also *Cerebrum* and other specific portions.
  abscess of, **2080–2082**
    bacteriology of, 2081, 2081t
    CSF examination in, 2081, 2081t
    etiology of, 2080–2081, 2081t
    heart disease with, 288–289, *289*
    imaging of, 2081–2082
    presenting features for, 2081, 2081t
    treatment of, 2082
  aging effects in, 16, 16t
  AIDS/HIV effects in, 1856t, 1857–1858
  anatomy of, *2059, 2060, 2061*
  anoxic injury of, 2062t, 2062–2063, 2064t
  astrocytoma of, low-grade, *2127,* 2132
    multiforme, 2132
  autoantibodies to, 1476t, 1477
  blood flow to, 205–2062, *2058–2062*
  cancer affecting, incidence of, *1009,* 1013t
  coma and, **1969–1978.** See also *Coma.*
  CT scan of, 1963t, 1963–1968
    hemorrhage in, 1965–1966, *1966*
    infarction and, 1966, *1967*
    neoplasia in, 1963t, 1964–1965, *1965,* 1968
    trauma and, 1966
  cysticercosis affecting, 1926
  death, 1978–1979
    criteria for, 1979, 1979t
  degenerative disease of, 1992–1996. See also *Dementia; Encephalopathy.*
  demyelination affecting, 2106t, 2106–2113
  edema of, 2063
  glioblastoma of, 2126t, 2128t, 2131–2132
  heart failure affecting, 220
  hypoxia affecting, 2062t, 2062–2073, 2064t. See also *Cerebrovascular disease.*
  internal capsule of, *2060*

Brain (Continued)
lupus erythematosus affecting, 1475t, 1479–1480, 1480t
lymphoma of, 2126t, 2128t, 2132
meningioma of, 2126t, 2127, 2130
MRI scan of, 1963t, 1963–1968, 1965–1967
aneurysm in, 1963t, 1966, 1966
multiple sclerosis in, 1963t, 1967, 1967
multiple sclerosis affecting, 1967, 2107–2108, 2108
neoplasia of, 2125–2135
approach to patient with, 2125–2127
chemotherapy of, 2129–2130
classification of, 2125, 2126t
clinical manifestations of, 2126, 2126t
differential diagnosis of, 2126–2127, 2127t
imaging procedures for, 1964–1965, 1965, 2127–2128, 2127–2131, 2128t
incidence by category of, 2125, 2126t
medical management of, 2128–2129
metastatic, 2126t, 2128, 2130, 2130
radiation therapy of, 2129
seizures with, 2126t, 2128, 2128–2129
surgical approach in, 2129
symptoms and signs of, 2126, 2126t
treatment of, 2128–2130
tumorous, 1964–1965, 1965, 1968
oligodendroglioma of, 2127–2128, 2128t, 2132
paraneoplastic syndromes affecting, 1018, 1027t, 1028
seizures and. See Epilepsy; Seizures.
swelling of, injury causing, 2137–2138, 2138t
meningitis causing, 1613, 1617
trauma to, 1978, 2135–2139
amnesia due to, 1990, 1990t
coma and, 2137, 2137t
concussion in, 2136
contusion in, 2136, 2136
epidural hematoma with, 2136
epilepsy following, 2118
evaluation of, 2137, 2137t, 2138t
hemorrhage due to, 2135–2137
imaging studies in, 2137
intensive care management of, 2137t, 2137–2138, 2138t
intracranial pressure and, 2138, 2138t
minor, 2136, 2138–2139
moderate, 2139
severe, 2137t, 2137–2138, 2138t
subdural hematoma with, 2136
vascular occlusion in, 2135–2137
vascular disease of. See Cerebrovascular disease.
Brainstem, auditory evoked response and, 2021
blood flow to, 2059
localization of lesion of, 2031, 2031t
Branham's sign, 353
Brazilian hemorrhagic fever, 1798t, 1802–1803
Brazilian purpuric fever, 1624
Breast, 1317–1320
amenorrhea and, 1303, 1303t
areola of. See Areola.
biopsy of, 1319
cancer of, 1320–1325
chemotherapy of, 1061, 1324t, 1324–1325
diagnosis of, 1321, 1321t
genetics of, 1320
hormonal effects in, 1320–1321, 1322
hormone therapy in, 1324
incidence of, 1005, 1009, 1013t, 1015, 1061t, 1320
male with, 1325
management of, 1061, 1322–1325
metastases from, 1322, 1323–1324
skin, 1031t
oral contraceptive role in, 1310, 1320–1321
pregnancy and, 1061, 1325
prognostic factors for, 1321–1322, 1322t
radiation therapy in, 1323t
risk factors for, 1320–1321, 1321t, 1322t
screening for, 1006t, 1321, 1321t
self-examination for, 1006t, 1321
staging of, 1321–1323, 1322t
tumor markers for, 1022t, 1023, 1076, 1323
discharge from, 1318
galactorrheic, 1318, 1318t
postmenopausal, 1318
serous or bloody, 1318
ectopic, 1317
epidemiology of, 1320
fibroadenoma of, 1320

Breast (Continued)
fibrocystic disease of, 1317–1318, 1319, 1321
growth and development of, 1317
history taking for, 1318–1319
hypertrophy of, 1317
male, 1325
enlargement of, 1332t, 1332–1333
milk production by, 1317
nipple of. See Nipple.
pain in, 1318
panniculitis of, 1508
physical examination of, 1319
pregnancy and, 1317
puberty effect on, 1294, 1294, 1303t
puerperal, 1317
Tanner stages for, 1303, 1303t
Breast-feeding, 1070–1071
Breath odor, bronchiectasis with, 417
esophageal cancer and, 657
garlicky, metal poisoning with, 70, 72
Breath shortness. See Dyspnea.
Breath sounds, 368, 369t, 370
Breath tests, 699–701, 700t
bacterial overgrowth affecting, 701, 701t
lactose, 700, 700t
lactulose, 700, 700t, 701t
malabsorption affecting, 699–701, 700t, 701t
xylose, 700t, 700–701, 701t
Breathing. See Respiration; Ventilation.
Bretylium tosylate, 246t, 250
adverse effects of, 248t
antiarrhythmic action of, 245, 246t, 250
pharmacokinetics of, 246t, 250
Brill-Zinsser disease, 1726–1729, 1727t, 1728t
Bristleworm, venom of, 1954t, 1955
British anti-lewisite, lead poisoning treated with, 69, 69t
mercury toxicity treated with, 504t
Broca's aphasia, 1991t, 1992
Broca's area, 1991, 1991t
Brodmann's areas, 1986, 1991
language and, 1991
Bromocriptine, hyperprolactinemia treated with, 1214–1215
ovulation induction with, 1309
Bromovinylarabinosyl uracil, 1744
Bronchi, 371
anaphylactic constriction of, 1418
aspergillosis affecting, 1830t, 1831–1832
dilation of. See also Bronchiectasis; Bronchitis.
drug-induced, 380, 384
obstruction of, 416, 416t, 1418
Bronchiectasis, 416–418
classification of, 417
clinical features of, 417, 418t
complications of, 418
congenital defects with, 416t, 416–417, 418t
cylindrical, 417
cystic, 417
diagnostic evaluation for, 417–418, 418t
etiology of, 416–417
hereditary disorders with, 416t, 416–417, 418t
necrotizing pneumonia causing, 417
pathogenesis of, 417
pathology in, 417
predisposing disorders for, 416t, 416–417, 418t
prognosis in, 418
radiography of, 417
treatment of, 418
varicose, 417
Bronchioalveolar lavage, 1919–1920
Bronchioles, 371
anatomy of, 371
respiratory, 371
terminal, 371
Bronchiolitis, enteroviral, 1787t, 1791
hyperlucency and, 390
obliterans, 390, 394–395
organizing pneumonia with, 394–395
Bronchitis, 381–389
AIDS/HIV with, 1860, 1860
airway obstruction in, 382, 383
complete, 388, 389
partial, 388, 389
pathophysiology of, 382, 383
subcarinal, 388, 389
supracarinal, 388, 388
asthmatic, 383–385
chlamydial, 1723t, 1725
chronic, 381–389
clinical features of, 381–383, 382t, 383, 386

Bronchitis (Continued)
cor pulmonale with, 382t, 387
definition of, 381–382
differential diagnosis of, 384, 386
dyspnea in, 382t, 386
edema in, 387
function tests in, 382, 382t, 383
hypercapnia of, 382t, 387
influenza virus in, 1749–1751, 1750t, 1751t
occupational exposure causing, 56, 59t
pathogenesis of, 383, 385
pathology in, 383, 385–386
prevalence of, 383, 385
prognosis in, 386
radiography in, 383, 386
signs and symptoms in, 368–371, 369t
simple, 381–382
smoking and, 383, 385
sputum and, 382t, 383, 386
treatment of, 384–385, 386–388
viral, 1749–1751, 1750t, 1751t
Bronchodilators, asthma treated with, 380
bronchitis treated with, 384
Bronchopulmonary sequestration, 390
bronchiectasis with, 416, 416t
cyst vs., 390
Bronchoscopy, 392
Brown-Séquard syndrome, 1030
Brucellosis, 1678–1680
clinical manifestations of, 1678–1679, 1679t
diagnosis of, 1679t, 1679–1680
epidemiology of, 1678
hepatic granuloma with, 784t
milk transmission of, 1678, 1680
pathogenesis of, 1678
prevention of, 1680
prognosis in, 1680
treatment of, 1679t, 1680
Brugia, 1940t, 1940–1941, 1942
Bruton's agammaglobulinemia, 1402t, 1403, 1403–1404
arthritis linked to, 1525
Bruxism, 1983, 1983t
Bubbles. See also Air; Gas(es).
tissue with, 375t
Bubo, plague, 1662
tularemic, 1663
Budd-Chiari syndrome, 793
Budesonide, 1417t
Buerger's disease, 351–352
Buffalo hump, Cushing's, 1217, 1247
Buffers, 543
Bufuralol, 97t
Bulbocavernous reflex, 2009t
Bulimia, 1160
clinical manifestations of, 1160
definition of, 1160
diagnosis of, 1160
epidemiology of, 1160
treatment of, 1160
vomiting and, 630
Bullae, 2189t, 2191t, 2205t, 2216t
bronchogenic cyst vs., 390
connective tissue disease with, 2189t
dermal-epidermal disease with, 2205t, 2206
dermatitis herpetiformis with, 2205t
dermatolysis with, 2189t, 2205t
diseases associated with, 2191t, 2205t, 2216t
emphysematous, 389–390
epidermolysis bullosa with, 2189t, 2205t
immunofluorescence tests in, 2189t
insect bite with, 2205
intraepidermal disease with, 2204–2206, 2205t
lupus erythematosus with, 2189t
Nikolsky's sign in, 2192, 2205
pemphigoid, 2205t, 2205–2206
immunofluorescence testing in, 2189t
paraneoplastic, 1034t
pemphigus, 2205–2206
Bull's eye skin lesions, 2191, 2191, 2206
Bumetanide, dosage for, 264t
properties and action of, 224t, 531t
Bundle branch block, 191
causes of, 191t
ECG in, 191, 192
Bundle branch(es), 191, 191, 231
electrogram of, 231–232, 232
left, 191, 191t, 231, 232
right, 191, 191t, 231, 232
Bunion, 1518, 1519t, 1519–1520
Bunyaviridae, 1805t, 1806t

Bunyavirus, *1739*
Buphthalmos, 2177
Buprenorphine, 51
Burn injury, chemical, 2221
　electrical, 64–67, *65, 66*
　mortality rate in, 37, *38*
　neutrophil dysfunction due to, 904t
　smoke inhalation with, 403, 403t
Burning sensation, erythromelalgic, 1528
Burr cells, 825t
Bursae, *1441,* 1527
　joint anatomy and, *1441,* 1527
　shoulder, *1522,* 1524, *1524,* 1527
　subacromial, *1522,* 1524, *1524,* 1527
　subdeltoid, 1524, 1527
Bursitis, 1527
　painful shoulder due to, 1524, *1524*
　subacromial, 1524, *1524,* 1527
　subdeltoid, 1524, 1527
　trochanteric, 1527
Burst-forming units, 819–821
　hematopoiesis role of, 819–821, *820,* 820t, *821,* 898
　hemoglobin synthesis and, 869–870
Busulfan, adverse effects of, 1042
　chemotherapy using, 1039t, 1042, 1042t
　fetal malformations due to, 1070t, 1071t
　interstitial lung disease induced by, 397, 397t
　myelogenous leukemia treated with, 928
Butorphanol, 51
　pain control with, 104t
Butyrophenones, 1998t, 1998–1999
Bypass grafts, aspirin and, 117t, 117–118
　atherosclerosis in, 292
　benefits of, *318,* 319
　coronary artery, 316t, 316–319, *318*
　mortality of, *318,* 319
　principles of, 317–318
　saphenous vs. thoracic source of, *318,* 319
Byssinosis, 59t
　occupational exposure causing, 59t

C

C cells, calcitonin secretion by, 1373–1374, *1375*
c wave, 167, *167*
　pressure gradients and, *210, 211*
CA 15-3, breast cancer with, 1022t, 1023, 1323
CA 125, ovarian cancer and, 1022t, 1022–1023, 1313
Cachexia, cardiac, 219
　tumor-related, 1021
Cadmium, 71–72
　intoxication by, 71
　occupational exposure to, 71
　poisoning due to, 71–72
　　clinical manifestations of, 71–72
　　etiology of, 71
　renal function and, 587
Café au lait spots, 2213, *2213*
　Fanconi's anemia with, 834
　neurofibroma-associated, 1035, 2056, 2209, 2213
　precocious puberty with, 1296
Caffeine, hypertension and, 262
　pain control use of, 106t
Caffey disease, 1388t
Calabar swelling, 1044
Calcifediol, 1357t, 1357–1358, *1358*
　actions of, 1354–1355, 1357–1358, *1358*
　bone formation role of, 1354–1356, *1355*
　pharmacokinetics of, 1357t, 1357–1358
Calcification, basal ganglia with, 2046
　bursitis due to, 1524, *1524*
　crystal deposition disease causing, 1515, *1515,* 1516t
　heart with, *184, 185,* 185–186
　muscular, 2165
　painful shoulder due to, 1521–1524, *1522, 1524*
　pulmonary, "buckshot," 1818
　　histoplasmosis causing, 1818
　renal osteodystrophy with, 1377–1378
　soft-tissue, 1378
　subacromial, 1524, *1524*
　supraspinatus, *1522*
　tendinitis due to, 1521–1524, *1522, 1524*
Calcitonin, **1373–1375**
　biochemistry of, 1373
　bone formation role of, 1354, 1354t
　bone loss treated with, 1383
　calcium regulation by, 1373–1374
　gene for, 1374, *1375*
　multiple endocrine neoplasia and, 1374–1375, 1375t
　Paget's disease treated with, 1386

Calcitonin *(Continued)*
　secretion of, 1373
　thyroid carcinoma and, 1373–1374, 1375t
Calcitriol, 1357t, 1357–1358, *1358*
　actions of, 1354–1355, 1357–1358, *1358*
　antirachitic action of, 1355
　bone formation role of, 1354t, 1354–1355, *1355,* 1357–1358
　intestinal effects of, 1355
　metabolism of, 1354–1355, 1357–1358
　pharmacokinetics of, 1357t, 1358
　resistance to, 1363
　rickets related to, 1363
Calcium, 1351t, 1352t
　absorption of, 696t, 697, 700t, *1352,* 1353
　　impaired, 1362t, 1363t, 1371
　blood level of, 1351t, 1356
　　bound, 1351t
　　free, 1351t
　bone formation and, 1351t, 1351–1356, *1352*
　calcitonin regulation of, 1373–1374
　coagulation role of, 977, *978,* 979, 987–989
　deposits of. See *Calcification.*
　dietary, hypertension and, 261
　　intake of, *1352,* 1353–1354
　　malabsorption treated with, 704t
　　supplementation of, 261, 704t
　digitalis effect on, 225, *225*
　erythrocyte control of, 852
　hormone signaling role of, 1179, *1179*
　hydrofluoric acid burn treated with, 504t
　hyperkalemia treated with, 542–543
　kidney and, 521t, *522,* 523
　　failure and, 557t, 557–558
　　transport and, 521t, *522,* 523
　milk-alkali syndrome and, 1355
　myocardial function and, 174, *175*
　osteoporosis and, 1379–1380, *1380*
　parathyroid hormone and, 1366, 1367–1370, 1368t
　phosphatidylinositol activated by, 1179, *1179*
　RDA for, 1140t
　serum level of, 700t
　therapeutic control of, 1378, 1378t
　vitamin D and, **1357–1358,** 1362–1363, 1368, 1368t, *1373
Calcium channel blockers, 507t
　angina pectoris treated with, 299, 300t
　antiarrhythmic agents as, 244–245, *245,* 245t
　antidote for, 504t, 507
　hypertension treated with, 265t, 266–267, 267t
　myocardial infarction treated with, 309–310
　poisoning due to, 504t, 507, 507t
　side effects of, 266, 267t
Calcium chloride, calcium block reversed by, 504t
Calcium oxalate, crystals of, 1516, 1516t
　deposition disease due to, 1516, 1516t
　kidney stone of, 614–617, *615,* 615t, *616,* 616t
Calcium pump, myocardial cell, 174, *175*
Calcium pyrophosphate, 1515, 1516t
　arthropathy due to, *1515,* 1515, 1516t
　crystals of, 1515, 1516t
　deposition disease due to, *1515,* 1515, 1516t
Calciuria, *1352,* 1357
　calcitonin role in, 1373
　increased, 1363t, 1364
　kidney stone and, 614–617, *615,* 615t, *616,* 616t
　Paget's disease with, 1385t, 1385–1386
Calculi, renal. See *Kidney stones.*
Caliciviridae, 1793, *1795,* 1795t
　structure of, *1739*
California encephalitis, 1806t, 1810t, 1813
Calluses, warts vs., 2192
Calmodulin, 1179
Caloric test, of semicircular canal, 2024
Calorie requirements, exercise energy expenditure and, 1167t
　fat intake and, 1154
　food labeling and, 1143, 1143t
　parenteral nutrition and, 1173, 1173t
　protein intake and, 1154
Calsequestrin, myocardial, 174
Campylobacter infections, **1649–1651**
　clinical manifestations of, 1649t, 1650, 1650t
　definition of, 1649
　diagnosis of, 1650, *1651*
　epidemiology of, 1649
　etiology of, 1649, 1649t
　food poisoning due to, 739, 739t, 1649–1651
　pathogenesis of, 1649–1650
　pathology findings in, 1649t, 1649–1650

Campylobacter infections *(Continued)*
　prevention of, 1651
　proctocolitis due to, 1649t, 1649–1650
　reservoirs for, 1649t, 1649–1650
　therapy for, 1650–1651, *1651*
Camurati-Engelmann disease, 1388t, 1398–1388
Canaliculi, bile secretion in, 806, 808, 808t
　cholestasis related to, 808, 808t
　hepatic, 806, 808, 808t
Cancer, **1004–1077.** See also under affected organ.
　adenoma-carcinoma sequence in, 1076, *1076*
　ascites with, 743t, 744t, 744–745, 745t, 749
　bladder, 625t, 625–626
　breast. See *Breast, cancer of.*
　cell biology in, 1038–1040, *1039, 1040,* 1071–1077, *1076*
　cervical, 1062, 1062t
　colon. See *Colon, cancer of.*
　death rates for, 27t, 30t, 35t, *1005, 1009,* 1009t, *1015*
　definition of, 1004
　detection of, early, 1004, 1006t
　　size of tumor and, 1004
　diagnostic principles for, 1006–1007
　diet and, 1139–1141, 1143t
　duodenal, 679–680
　emergency conditions with, 1049–1054, *1051, 1052*
　endocrine manifestations of, 1024–1026, 1025t, 1345–1347
　epidemiology of, 1013t, 1013–1017, *1015*
　etiology of, 1004, 1009t, 1014–1017
　exercise effect on, 32
　genetic factors in, 1011–1012, 1071–1077
　　chromosomes and, 156, 156–157, *157*
　　familial susceptibility in, 1071, *1076,* 1076–1077
　　gene replacement and, 149–150, 150t, 1075
　　promotors and, 1011–1012
　　screening for, 1010, 1012
　　suppressors and, 1011–1012
　　therapy directed at, 1073–1077, 1074t
　growth characteristics of, 1004–1005, *1006,* 1071–1077
　　biology of, 1038–1040, *1039, 1040,* 1071–1073, *1073*
　　cell death and, 1011, 1057–1058, 1072–1073
　　therapy directed at, 149–150, 1073–1077, 1074t
　hormone production by, 1024–1026, 1025t, 1345–1347
　inflammatory bowel disease with, 709–710, 710t
　lung. See *Lung, cancer of.*
　markers, 1021–1024, 1022t
　metastatic. See *Metastases.*
　mortality rate role of, 27t, 30t, *1005, 1009, 1015*
　obesity association with, 1164–1165
　occupational exposure causing, 56, 58t, 1014–1015, 1016t
　oncogenes in, 1011–1012. See also *Oncogene(s).*
　oral, 646, 646t, 647t, 2209, *2209*
　oral contraceptive role in, 1310
　ovarian, 1313–1315
　pain management of, 105t, 107, *107*
　paraneoplastic syndromes of, 1017–1036. See also *Paraneoplastic syndromes.*
　patient with, 1005–1008, 1008t
　　daily activity status of, 1007, 1008t
　　physician relationship with, 1008
　pleural effusion with, 446–447
　prevention of, 1008–1010, 1009t, 1075–1076
　rectal. See *Rectum, cancer of.*
　risk factors for, 30t, 1009t, 1014–1017, 1075
　　modifiable, 27t, 30t, 1009t, 1014–1017
　screening for, 1004, 1006t
　　frequency of, 1004, 1006t
　　genetic, 1010, 1012, 1077
　skin, *2209,* 2209–2211, *2210*
　small intestinal, 679–680, 728–729, 1013t
　smoking associated with, 34t, 34–35, 35t, 1009t, 1014
　spinal cord compression due to, 1050–1051, *1051*
　staging of. See *Staging.*
　treatment of, 1017–1077
　　drug. See *Chemotherapy.*
　　future, 1071–1077
　　gene-related, 149–150, 1073–1077, *1074,* 1074t, *1075*
　　measures of success in, 1007, 1008t
　　oncogenesis in, 1012
　　patient management in, 1005–1008, 1008t
　　pregnancy during, 1060–1071

Cancer (Continued)
  principles of, 1036–1049, 1039, 1039t, 1040, 1071–1077
    radiation, 1037–1038, 1038t. See also Radiation therapy.
    surgical, 1037, 1037t. See also Surgery.
  uterine, 1005, 1009, 1013t, 1015
Candidemia, 1828, 1830
Candidiasis, **1827–1830**
  AIDS/HIV with, 1866, 1868
  angular cheilitis of, 647, 1828
  catheter-related, 1828–1830
  clinical manifestations of, 1828–1829
  diagnosis of, 1829
  endocarditis due to, 1598t, 1598–1599, 1829
  epidemiology of, 1827
  erythematous (atrophic), 647, 647t
  esophageal, 658
  etiologic organism in, 1827
  hyperplastic, 647, 647t
  immunodeficiency with, 1496–1408, 1828–1830
  KOH test for, 2192
  mucocutaneous, 647, 1828
  nails affected by, 2214–2215
  ocular, 1828, 1830, 2179
  oral lesions of, 647, 647t, 1828
  pathogenesis and pathology of, 1827–1828
  prophylaxis for, 1830
  pseudomembranous (thrush), 647, 647t, 1828
  pustules due to, 2207
  sexual transmission of, 1697t, 1699, 1699t, 1828
  skin lesions of, 2192, 2200, 2207
  treatment of, 1829–1830
  vaginal, 1697t, 1699, 1699t, 1828, 1829
Cannabis, 53
  adverse effects of, 53
  drug abuse with, 53–54, 56t
  pharmacology of, 53
  withdrawal of, 53
Capillaria philippinensis, 1935t, 1936
Capillaries, glomerular, 519, 519–520, 520
  intracranial, hemangioblastoma of, 2132
  leakage of, 499, 1588–1589
  nutritional, 482
  permeability of, 482
    hypotension due to, 499, 1588–1589
    water and, 520, 525
  pulmonary. See under Pulmonary vasculature.
  renal, 519, 519–520, 520
  shock and, 478t, 482
    septic, 499
    toxic syndrome of, 1588–1589
  sphincters and, 478t, 482
  vascular resistance and, 478t, 482
Caplan's syndrome, 1464
Capsaicin, osteoarthritis treated with, 1520
Capsomere, 1830
Capsulitis, adhesive, 1524
  painful shoulder due to, 1524
Captopril, dosage for, 229t, 265t, 266t
  vasodilatation using, 229t, 229–230
Caput medusae, 752, 793
Carbamazepine, epilepsy therapy with, 2122t
  hepatotoxicity of, 773
  pain control use of, 106t
  pharmacokinetics of, 91t, 94t, 2122t
Carbamoyl phosphate synthetase, 1110
  deficiency of, 1110, 1110t
Carbapenems, 1568t
Carbenicillin, 1562t
  minimal inhibitory concentration for, 1570, 1570t
Carbohydrates, absorption of, 689, 689–690, 696, 696t
  complex, 1143t
  dietary, 29–30, 30t
    energy requirements and, 1154
    food groups and, 1142, 1143
    parenteral, 1172, 1173t
  enzyme pathways for, 146t, 1081, 1082, 1084
  liver and, 753, 1082, 1082–1083, 1083t
  malabsorption of, 143–146, 704
  metabolic disorders affecting, 144t–146t, 1080–1085, 1081t, 1082, 1083t, 1084
  renal failure and, 557t, 559, 562, 1082
Carbon dioxide, acid-base balance and, 543–544, 545
  air-blood barrier to, 371–372, 374, 374–375
  alveolar, 371–372, 374, 374–375
  diffusion of, 371–372, 374–375
  elimination mechanisms for, 543–545

Carbon dioxide (Continued)
  erythrocyte transport of, 852
  exchange of, 371–372, 374, 374–375
  narcosis due to, 551
  partial pressure of, 375, 375t
  physiologic considerations for, 543–546, 545, 545t
  production of, 466, 467t, 543–545
  retention of. See Hypercapnia.
  tension, 543
    acidosis and, 545, 545t, 545–546, 551
    alkalosis and, 545, 545t, 545–546, 551
    end-tidal, 466
    respiratory failure and, 453
    ventilation assessment and, 466–468, 467t
Carbon monoxide, 374–375, 403–404, 507
  diffusion of, 373t, 374, 374–375
  oxygen antidote for, 504t, 507, 507t
  poisoning due to, 403t, 403–404, 504t, 507, 507t
    clinical features of, 404
    hypoxia of, 403–404
    treatment of, 404
  smoke containing, 34, 403t, 403–404
Carbon tetrachloride, 772, 773t
Carbonic anhydrase, bone resorption role of, 1352
Carbonic anhydrase inhibitors, 224t
  diuretic action of, 222, 224t
  heart failure treated with, 222, 224t
  ocular side effects of, 2183
Carboplatin, adverse effects, 1042
  chemotherapy using, 1039t, 1042
Carboxyglutamic acid, 1352
Carboxyhemoglobin, 403–404
Carbuncles, 2207
  staphylococcal toxin causing, 1606–1607, 1607t
Carcinoembryonic antigen (CEA), 1022t
  breast cancer and, 1022t, 1023
  colon cancer and, 727–728, 1021–1022, 1022t
Carcinogens, 1004, 1009t, 1016t
  environmental, 56, 58t, 1009t, 1010, 1014–1016, 1016t
  lung cancer, 437–438, 1014, 1016t
  medicinal agents as, 1016, 1016t
  occupational exposure to, 56, 58t, 1009t, 1010, 1014–1015, 1016t
Carcinoid, **1348–1350**
  cardiac, 358, 1348
  clinical manifestations of, 1347
  diagnosis of, 1349–1350
  endocrine function of, 1348–1349
  intestinal, 1348
  skin affected by, 1035, 1348, 1349
  treatment of, 1350
  vasodilation mechanism in, 1348, 1349
Carcinoma. See also Cancer; Neoplasia; specific affected organs.
  adenoma progression to, 1076, 1076
  anal, 743
  basal cell, 2209, 2209
  bladder, 625t, 625–626
  cervical, 1061–1063, 1062t, 1063
    pregnancy with, 1061t, 1061–1063, 1062t, 1063
  duodenal, 679–680
  esophageal, 657
  hepatic, 803t, 804
  oral, 646, 646t, 647t, 2209, 2209
  ovarian, 1313–1315
  polyarthritis with, 1527
  prostate. See Prostate gland, carcinoma of.
  renal, 623–625, 624, 624t
  squamous cell, 646, 646t, 647t, 2209, 2209
Cardiac. See also Heart entries.
Cardiac arrest, 253–256
  causes of, 255–256
  ECG of, 255
  risk factors for, 253
  treatment for, 256
Cardiac cycle, **189–193**
  calcium and, 175, 175–178
  disturbances in, 191t, 191–193, 192–194
  electrocardiographic record of, 189–193, 190
  electrogram record of, 231–232, 232
  electrophysiology of, 231–232, 232, 233
  intervals of, 190, 190–191, 232
  normal complexes of, 190, 190–191
  segments of, 190, 191–193
  total per day, 343
Cardiac index, 176t, 214
  failing heart, 214
  infarction and, 305t
  normal values for, 489t

Cardiac index (Continued)
  sepsis and, 496t
  shock and, 478, 478t, 496t
Cardiac output, 177, 178, 214
  decreased, 529–530, 530t
  exercise increase in, 178, 214
  fluid shifts related to, 529–530, 530t
  measurement of, 489t
    cardiac catheterization for, 209–210
    Fick method for, 209–210
    indicator dilution method for, 209–210
    valve area calculation in, 210, 211
  normal values for, 489t
  pregnancy and, 609
  sepsis affecting, 499t
  shock and, 478, 478t, 499t
Cardiac tamponade, 339–341
  cancer etiology, 1052, 1052
  echocardiography in, 340–341, 341
  etiology of, 337t, 339
  findings in, 339–341, 340, 341
  pathophysiology in, 339, 340
  pulsus paradoxus with, 340, 340
  treatment of, 341
Cardiomegaly, 182, 182–185, 183
  roentgenography of, 182, 182–185, 183
Cardiomyopathy, **327–336**
  AIDS with, 329, 329t
  alcoholic, 330, 330
  amyloidosis with, 1504
  diabetic, 359
  dilated, 327–332, 328
    causes of, 328–331, 329t
    echocardiography in, 328, 332
    evaluation of, 328, 328t, 331–332
    familial, 329t, 331
    incidence of, 328
    metabolic disorders causing, 329t, 331
    prognosis for, 332
    right ventricular, 331
    roentgenography in, 186
    systolic vs. diastolic failure in, 327–328
    treatment of, 332
    ventricular dysfunction in, 327–328, 328, 328t
  hypertrophic, 328, 334–336
    diagnosis of, 335
    echocardiography in, 328, 335
    genetics of, 138t, 334–335
    incidence of, 334
    obstructive vs. nonobstructive, 334–335, 336
    physiology of, 335, 335
    prognosis in, 335–336
    treatment of, 335, 336
    ventricular dysfunction in, 328, 328t, 334–335, 335
  presentation of, 327, 328
  restrictive, 328, 332–334
    causes of, 333t, 333–334
    echocardiography in, 328, 332–333
    endocardial, 333t, 334
    fibrotic, 333t, 334
    idiopathic, 334
    infiltrative disease in, 333t, 333–334
    storage disease in, 333t, 334, 1096
    ventricular dysfunction in, 328, 328t, 332–333
  trypanosomal, 1901, 1901
Cardiovascular system. See Heart; Vascular disorders; specific vessels and disorders.
Cardioversion, 251–252
  anticoagulation with, 252
  arrhythmia treated with, 251–252, 252t
  complications of, 252
  energy used in, 252t
  implanted device for, 252, 252t
Carditis, Lyme disease with, 1717, 1718, 1719, 1719t
  rheumatic fever causing, 1592t, 1592–1593, 1593t
Carey-Coombs murmur, 1592t, 1593, 1593t
Carmustine (BCNU), 1039t, 1042
  adverse effects, 1042
Carnitine palmitoyltransferase deficiency, 2166
Carnosine, urinary, 1103t
β-Carotene, absorption of, 700t, 703t
  antioxidant role of, 1151, 1151t
  serum level of, 700t
Carotenoids, cancer prevention with, 1010, 1016–1017
  vitamin A in, 1145t
Carotid artery(ies), 2057–2058
  anatomy and, 2057–2058, 2058
  aneurysm of, 2074, 2074–2075
  bruit of, asymptomatic, 2070

Carotid artery(ies) *(Continued)*
  CT of, spiral, 127, *128*
  endarterectomy of, 2070–2071, 2071t
  moyamoya disease of, 2069
  pulse in, 167
  stenosis of, 127, *128*, 2070
  thrombosis of, 2064, 2064t, 2069
Carotid massage, 235
  arrhythmia diagnosis using, 235, 235t
  risks of, 235
Carotid sinus syncope, 2009
Carotidynia, 2033
Carpal tunnel syndrome, 1527, 2157
  amyloidosis in, 967, *967*, 1504
  causes of, 1527, 1528t
  diagnosis of, *1462*, 1527, 2157
  rheumatoid arthritis with, 1462, *1462*, 1464
  Tinel's sign in, *1462*, 2157
Carpometacarpal joints, 1518
Carriers. See also *Zoonoses.*
  Bartonella, 1680, 1682
  hemophilia, 992, 995
  meningococcal, 1619
  Salmonella, 1645, 1646
  Shigella, 1647, 1648
  thalassemia, 877t, 880
  typhoid fever, 1642
Carrión's disease, 1682
Carteolol, 265t
Cartilage, alkaptonuria affecting, 1108
  anatomy and, *1441*, *1448*
  calcification of, 1515, *1515*, 1516t
  collagen fibrils of, 1352, 1444t, *1448*
  composition of, 1444t, 1445
  damaged, *1448*
  degeneration of, 1442–1443, 1443t, 1518. See also
    Osteoarthritis.
  dysplasia of, 1390–1391
  formation of, 1352, 1443–1444
  glycoproteins in, 1445
  hyaline, *1448*
  hypertrophic, *1448*
  hypoplasia of, 1407
  immunodeficiency and, 1407
  inflammation of, 1517
  ischemic necrosis of, 1387, 1387t
  joint anatomy and, 1440–1443, *1441*
  pigmented, 1108
  relapsing polychondritis of, 1517
  rheumatoid arthritis affecting, *1441*, *1448*
  spinal, *2141*
Castration, bilateral surgical, 1335
  functional prepubertal, 1334
  medical, 1345
  prostate cancer and, 1345
Cat. See also *Cat scratch disease.*
  zoonoses associated with, 1737t, 1737–1738, 1738t
Cat scratch disease, **1680–1682**
  clinical manifestations of, 1681, 1681t, 1738t
  diagnosis of, 1681, 1681t
  epidemiology of, 1681, 1738t
  etiology of, *1680*, 1680–1681, 1738t
  pathogenesis of, 1681
  pathology findings in, 1681
  treatment of, 1681–1682, 1682t
Catabolism, fasted state, 1278, 1278t
  illness-caused, 1154–1155, 1155t
Catalase, absence of, 136t, 147t
Catalase-positive organisms, 1557t
Cataplexy, 1984
Cataract, 2175
  Christmas tree, 2175
  diabetic, 1273, 2175
  etiology of, 2175
  sunflower, 2175
  treatment of, 2175
Catatonia, 1974, 1974t, 1997t
Catecholamines, **1253–11257**. See also *Dopamine; Epi-nephrine; Norepinephrine.*
  action of, 1253–1254
  adrenergic receptor activated by, 492t, 492–493,
    1253–1254
  biosynthesis of, 1253–1254
  deficiency states of, 1257
  effects of, 1253–1254
  enzyme action on, 97t, *1253*, 1253–1254
  excess states of, 1254–1257
  insulin and glucagon and, 1257
  laboratory tests for, 1254t, 1255–1256
  metabolism of, 1253–1254

Catecholamines *(Continued)*
  neuron uptake of, 1253, *1253*
  pheochromocytoma and, 1254–1257
  plasma levels of, 1253, 1255
  provocative test for, 1256
  receptors for, 1253–1254
  shock and, 482, 492t, 492–493
  storage and release of, 1253
  suppression test for, 1254t, 1255–1256
  sympathetic system role of, 1253
  vasoconstriction and, 1253–1254
  volume regulation role of, 526, 526t, *527*
Catechol-O-methyltransferase, 1253, *1253*
  drug metabolized by, 97t
Catheterization, candidiasis related to, 1828–1830
  cardiac, 208–211, 209t, *210*, *211*
    cardiac output measured in, 209–210
    endocardial electrical stimulation in, 235–236, *236*,
      236t
    hazards of, 208, 209t
    indications for, 208, 209t
    pressure waveforms in, 208–209, *210*, *211*
    shock patient and, 489–490
    techniques for, 208–210
  urinary tract, incontinence management with, 22
    infection related to, 603, 1550–1551
Cattle, encephalitis reservoir in, 1806t, 1810t
  zoonoses associated with, 1727t, 1737t, 1737–1738,
    1738t
Caucasians. See also *Racial factors.*
  hemochromatosis in, 1132–1133
  hereditary disorder frequency and, 136t, 136–140,
    138t
  rheumatoid arthritis frequency and, 1460
Cauda equina, 2141
Caudate nucleus, *2043*
  blood supply to, *2060*
Causalgia, 2036
Caustics ingestion, alkali in, 507
Cavernous sinus, *2061*
  thrombosis in, 2083
CCNU (lomustine), 1039t, 1042
CD (clusters of differentiation), AIDS/HIV and, 1837t,
  1837–1840, *1844*, *1865*, 1873t, 1887t, *1890*
  allergic rhinitis role of, 1414, *1415*
  antigen presentation and, *1394*, 1397
  immunodeficiency role of, *1403*, 1404–1405, 1407,
    1408
  leprosy pathogenesis and, 1693, *1694*, 1695
  leukemia and, 930–932, 933t, 937, 937t
  leukocyte adhesion deficiency and, 902–904, *903*,
    1408
  Pneumocystis pneumonia and, 1917, 1919, 1922
  T cell receptor and, *1394*, 1397, 1438
  thymocyte maturation and, 1438
CEA (carcinoembryonic antigen), 1022t
  breast cancer and, 1022t, 1023
  colon cancer and, 727–728, 1021–1022, 1022t
Cecum, cancer of, 726, *726*
Cefaclor, 1562t
  minimal inhibitory concentration for, 1570, 1570t
Cefadroxil, 1562t
Cefamandole, 1562t
  minimal inhibitory concentration for, 1570, 1570t
Cefazolin, 1562t
  endocarditis therapy with, 1602–1603, 1603t
Cefepine, 1562t
Cefixime, 1562t
  gonorrhea therapy with, 1702t
Cefmetazole, 1562t
Cefonicid, 1570, 1570t
Cefoperazone, 1562t
  minimal inhibitory concentration for, 1570, 1570t
Cefotaxime, 1562t
  H. influenzae treated with, 1623
  Klebsiella, Enterobacter, Serratia and, 1579–1581,
    1580t
  meningitis therapy with, 1615–1617, 1616t
  minimal inhibitory concentration for, 1570, 1570t
Cefotetan, 1562t
Cefoxitin, 1562t
  minimal inhibitory concentration for, 1570, 1570t
  mycobacterial (nontuberculous) disease and, 1690,
    1691
Cefpodoxime proxetil, 1562t
Cefprozil, 1562t
Ceftazidime, 1562t
  minimal inhibitory concentration for, 1570, 1570t
  Pseudomonas and, 1579–1581, 1580t
Ceftizoxime, 1562t

Ceftriaxone, 1562t
  endocarditis therapy with, 1602–1603, 1603t
  gonorrhea therapy with, 1702t, 1703
  H. influenzae treated with, 1623
  Lyme disease therapy with, 1719, 1719t
  meningitis therapy with, 1615–1617, 1616t, 1620t
  meningococcal infection and, 1620t, 1620–1621,
    1621t
  minimal inhibitory concentration for, 1570, 1570t
Cefuroxime, 1562t
  axetil, 1562t
  Klebsiella, Enterobacter, Serratia and, 1579–1581,
    1580t
  Lyme disease therapy with, 1719, 1719t
  minimal inhibitory concentration for, 1570, 1570t
Celiac axis, 715
Celiac sprue, *702*, 704–705
  HLA complex in, 1431t
Cells. See also named cell, e.g., *Langerhans' cells.*
  aging theory and, 15, *1072*, 1072–1073
  B. See *B cells.*
  complement receptors on, *1400*, 1400–1401, 1401t
  cytosolic enzyme defects of, 145–145, 146t
  death of, 1072–1073. See also *Apoptosis (cell death).*
  germ. See *Germ cells.*
  granulosa. See *Granulosa cells.*
  growth cycle regulation in, *1072*, 1072–1073, *1073*
  helmet, 822
  lysosomal storage disorders of, 1095–1099, 1096t,
    1097
  membrane of, *1177–1180*. See also *Plasma mem-brane.*
    potential of. See *Action potential; Resting
      potential.*
    transport defects of, 143–145, 144t
  mitochondrial disorders and, 142, 146t
  nucleus of, 1180–1181, *1181*
    antibodies to, 1457t, 1457–1458, 1476t, 1481t
  receptors of, *1176–1180*
    DNA and, *1176*, 1180–1181, *1181*
    hormonal, *1176–1180*, 1176–1182
      cytoplasmic, *1176*, *1177*
      nuclear, *1176*, 1180–1181, *1181*
      surface, *1176–1180*
    second messengers and, *1176–1180*, 1177–1180
  senescence of, *1072*, 1072–1073
  T. See *T cells.*
  theca. See *Theca cells.*
Cellulitis, 2208
  abscess and boil, 1587
  cat bite, 1587
  differential diagnosis of, 1587, 2208
  dog bite, 1587
  erysipeloid, 1673–1674, 2208
  freshwater injury in, 1587
  mucormycosis with, 1833
  necrotizing fasciitis in, 1588, 1589t, 2208
  pneumococcal, 1571, 1571t
  saphenous vein donor site, 1587
  seawater injury in, 1587
  staphylococcal, 1607, 1607t
  streptococcal, 1587–1588, 1589t
Cellulose, dietary, 1010
  cancer prevention and, 1009–1010
Centimorgan unit, 134
Centipedes, 1948
  bite of, 1948
Centromere, 134
Centrum semiovale, *2060*
Cephalexin, 1562t
Cephalosporins, 1562t
  adverse reactions to, 1418t, 1568t
  anaphylaxis due to, 1418t, 1418–1419
  dose adjustment for, 1562t
  first-generation, 1562t
  mechanism of action of, 1558, 1558t
  minimal inhibitory concentration for, 1570, 1570t
  pharmacology of, 1562t
  renal function and, 585, 1562t, 1568t
  resistance to, bacterial, 1558–1560, 1559t
  second-generation, 1562t
  streptococcal infection treated with, 1587–1589,
    1589t
  third-generation, 1562t
Cephalothin, 1570, 1570t
Cephapirin, 1562t
Cephradine, 1562t
Cercariae, schistosomal, *1927*, 1927–1928

Cerebellar artery, 2058, *2058*, 2059, *2061*
  aneurysm affecting, *2074*, 2074–2076
Cerebellopontine angle, tumor of, 2126t
Cerebellum, anatomy of, *2060*
  blood supply to, *2060*, *2061*
  Creutzfeldt-Jakob disease and, 2102–2103
  degeneration of, 2051t, 2051–2052
    alcoholic, 2039t, 2040
    paraneoplastic, 1018, 1028
  hemorrhage in, 2078, 2078t
  tentorial herniation affecting, *1971*
  tumor of, 2126t
Cerebral angiography, 2066, 2075
Cerebral artery(ies), **2057–2059**
  anatomy and, 2057–2059, *2058–2061*
  aneurysms of, *2074*, 2074–2076
  anterior, 2058, *2058–2060*
    occlusion of, 2064, 2064t
  middle, 2058–2059, *2058–2060*
    occlusion of, 2064t, 2064–2065
  moyamoya disease of, 2069
  posterior, *2058–2060*, 2059
    occlusion of, 2064t, 2065
  vasospasm of, 2069, 2075
Cerebral vein, *2061*
Cerebrospinal fluid, 2132–2135
  brain abscess affecting, 2081, 2081t
  cryptococcosis organism in, 1824–1825
  increased formation of, 2133, 2133t, 2134
  meningitis and, cell count and, 1613
    glucose and, 1613, 1620
    Gram stain and, 1613, 1620
    laboratory tests and, 1613, 1620
    pathophysiology and, 1612, 1618
    protein and, 1613, 1620
  multiple sclerosis effect on, 2107
  normal pressure of, 2132, 2135
  outflow resistance affecting, 2133, 2133t, 2134
  syphilitic, 1708–1709, 1712t, 2086t, 2086–2087,
    2087t
Cerebrovascular disease, **2057–2079**. See also *Stroke*.
  anatomy and, 2057–2062, *2058–2062*
  aneurysmal, 2073–2077
    headache in, 2074, 2076t
    hemorrhage in, *2074*, 2074–2076
    imaging of, 1966, *1966*
    mycotic, 2075
    treatment in, *2074*, 2074–2076, 2076t
  arteriovenous malformation in, 2076–2077
  coma and, 1970t, 2062t
  CT scan in, 1965–1966, *1966*
  diagnostic tests in, 2065–2066
  EEG in, 2063
  embolic, 2066–2067
    cardiac source in, 2066–2067, 2067t
  hematologic disorders in, 2067t, 2068–2069
  hemorrhagic, **2073–2079**
    aneurysmal rupture in, 2073–2076, 2076t
    arteriovenous malformation in, 2076–2077
    causes, 2077–2078
    cerebellar, 2078, 2078t
    congenital heart disease with, 289
    hypertension and, 2077–2079, 2078t, *2079*
    imaging of, 2078, *2079*
    lobar, *2077*, 2078, 2078t
    pontine, 2078, 2078t
    putaminal, *2077*, 2078, 2078t, *2079*
    signs and symptoms in, 2078, 2078t
    thalamic, *2077*, 2078, 2078t
    traumatic, 2135–2137
  hypertensive, 2077–2079, 2078t, *2079*
    vs. normal autoregulation, 2061–2062, *2062*
  imaging of, 1965–1966, *1966*
  infarction in, embolic, 2066–2067
    hemorrhagic, 2075
    imaging of, 1966, *1967*
    metabolism and, 2061t, 2062t, 2062–2063
    neuropathology of, 2061t, 2062t, 2062–2063
  ischemic, **2063–2073**
    diffuse hypoxia and, 2062, 2073
    encephalopathy of, 2062t, 2062–2063
    focal, 2062, 2063–2073
    metabolism in, 2062–2063
    neurologic effects of, 1972t, 1972–1974, 2136
    pathology of, 2062t, 2062–2063
    transient attacks of, 2063–2064, 2071t,
      2071–2072, 2072t
    localization of site of, 2064t, 2065

Cerebrovascular disease (*Continued*)
  mortality rate and, 27t, 30t, 170, *171*, 171t
  MRI scan of, 1965–1966, *1966*
  pathogenesis of, 2066–2071, 2067t, 2074
  seizures and, 2066
  syncope with, 1981
  thrombosis in, 2064t, 2064–2065
    anterior cerebral artery, 2064, 2064t
    anterior choroidal artery, 2064, 2064t
    basilar artery, 2064t, 2065
    cardiac-source embolism in, 2066–2067
    infection causing, 2083
    internal carotid artery, 2064, 2064t
    lacunar, 2069
    lysis and, 311, 312t
    middle cerebral artery, 2064t, 2064–2065
    posterior cerebral artery, 2064t, 2065
    venous, 2072–2073
    vertebral artery, 2064t, 2065
  treatment of, 2078–2079
  vasculitis in, 2067–2068
Cerebrum, **1969–2006**. See also *Brain*; specific disorders.
  aging effects in, 16, 16t
  anatomic areas of, 1985–1988, *1986*, *2059–2061*
  anoxia affecting, 2062t, 2062–2063, 2136
  association areas of, 1991
  auditory area of, *2059*
  basal ganglia connections with, *2043*
  blood flow to, 2057–2062, *2058–2062*
    autoregulation of, 2061–2062, *2062*
    distribution of, 2057–2059, *2058*, *2059*
    infarction and, 1966, *1967*
    ischemia and, 2062t, 2062–2064, 2132
    syncope and, 1980
    TIAs and, 2066, 2070
    venous drainage of, 2059, *2061*
  Broca's area of, 1991, 1991t, *2059*
  consciousness and, 1970–1993, 2137t, 2137–2138,
    2138t. See also *Consciousness disorders*.
  cysticercosis affecting, 1926
  degeneration of, 1992–1996. See also *Dementia*;
    Encephalopathy.
    Alzheimer's disease and, 1992–1993
    Creutzfeldt-Jakob disease and, 2102–2103
    dementia and, 1992–1996
    motor neuron in, 2052t, 2052–2054
    Pick's disease with, 1995
  edema of, 2063
    head injury and, 2138
    hemorrhagic, 2075
    ischemic, 2063
    vasospasm and, 2075
  EEG of, *1960*, 1960–1961. See also *Electroen-*
    cephalography.
  embolism of. See *Cerebrovascular disease, embolic*.
  frontal lobes of, 1985–1988, *1986*, *2059*. See also
    Frontal lobes.
  glucose supply to, 2059–2062, 2061t
    deficiency in, 2062t, 2062–2063
  hemispheric dominance in, handedness and,
    1990–1991, 2128
    language and, 1990–1991, 2128
    left, 1990–1991
    right, 1991
    sodium amytal injection and, 2128
  imaging techniques and, 1963t, 1963–1968,
    1965–1967
  language and, 1990–1992, 1991t, *2059*
    surgery near area of, 2128
  malaria affecting, 1894
  memory and, 1988–1990, 1989t, 1990t
  motor areas of, *2059*
  mucormycosis affecting, 1833
  occipital lobes of, 1985–1988, *1986*, *2059*. See also
    Occipital lobes.
  oxygen supply to, 2059–2062, 2061t
    deficiency in, 2062t, 2062–2063, 2136
  paraneoplastic syndromes affecting, 1028
  parietal lobes of, 1985–1988, *1986*, *2059*. See also
    Parietal lobes.
  sensory system and. See *Sensory system*.
  temporal lobes of, 1985–1988, *1986*, *2059*, 2060. See
    also *Temporal lobes*.
  trauma to. See *Brain, trauma to*.
  tumors of. See also *Brain, neoplasia of*.
    imaging of, 1964–1965, *1965*
  vision area of, *2015*, 2017, *2017*, *2059*
  Wernicke's area of, *2059*
Ceruloplasmin, 785–786, 1131–1132

Cerumen, impacted, 2021
Cervical nodes, 969t
  Hodgkin's disease in, 948, *949*
Cervicitis, chlamydial, 1697t, 1724
  gonorrhea causing, 1701–1702, 1702t
  sexually transmitted disease causing, 1699–1700
Cervix, cancer of, characteristics of, 1062, 1062t
  incidence of, 1013t
  management of, 1061–1063, *1062*
  pregnancy with, 1061t, 1061–1063, 1062t, *1063*
  smoking associated with, 35t
  menstruation and, 1298
  mucus of, 1298
Cestodes, **1922–1926**
  coenurosis due to, 1926
  cysts of, 1922–1926, 1923t
  diphyllobothriasis due to, 1923, 1923t
  echinococciasis due to, 1923t, 1924–1925
  hymenolepiasis due to, 1923t, 1923–1924
  sparganosis due to, 1926
  taeniasis due to, 1923t, 1924, 1925–1926
  treatment for, 1923t, 1924t
Cetirizine, allergic rhinitis treated with, 1416, 1416t
Chagas' disease, 1899–1903
  clinical presentation of, 1901, *1902*
  congenital, 1900
  diagnosis of, 1901–1902
  epidemiology of, 1899–1900
  etiologic organism in, 1899–1900, *1900*
  myocarditis with, 329–330
  pathology and pathogenesis of, *1900*, 1900–1901
  transfusion-transmitted, 896t, 897
  treatment and prevention of, 1902–1903
Chagoma, 1901
Chancre, syphilitic, 1706–1707, *1707*
  trypanosomal, 1897, 1901
Chancroid, 1704–1705
  diagnosis of, 1704–1705
  epidemiology of, 1704
  sexual transmission of, 1704–1705
  skin lesions of, 1704
  treatment of, 1705
Charcoal, activated, 505, 506t
Charcot-Leyden crystals, 380
  arthropathy due to, 1516t
  asthmatic sputum with, 380
Charcot-Marie-Tooth disease, 2153–2154
  genetics of, 2153, 2154t
  neuropathy of, 2153–2154, 2154t
  pathologies in, 2153, 2154t
  treatment of, 2154, 2154t
Charcot's joint, 1518
  syphilitic, 1709
Charcot's triad, 814
Chédiak-Higashi syndrome, albinism with, 2214t
  blood smear in, *906*
  leukocytes affected by, 904, 905t, *906*, 1541
  paraneoplastic, 1036
  staphylococcal infection in, 1601
Cheek, snuff carcinogenicity in, 35, 35t
Cheese, *1142*
  dietary aspects of, 29–30, 30t, *1142*
Cheilosis, angular, 647, 1828
  candidiasis with, 647, 1828
  malabsorption causing, 699t
Chelation therapy, 878–879
  iron accumulation treated with, 878–879
  lead poisoning treated with, 69, 69t, 504t
Chemicals. See also *Drugs*.
  asthma induced by, 379t
  bone marrow aplasia due to, 832, 832t
  cancer related to, 1009t, 1010
  occupational exposure to, 58t, 59t, 379t
  poisoning by, 503–510. See also *Poisoning*.
    treatment of, 504t, 505–506, 506t
Chemoattractants, bacterial, *1451*
  neutrophil response to, *1451*, 1451–1452, *1452*
Chemoprophylaxis, cancer and, 1010
  malarial, 1555, 1555t
  meningitis, 1621, 1621t
Chemosensitizing agents, 1058, 1058t
Chemotaxis, fever induction role of, 1535t
  neutrophilic, 899, *899*, 1451, *1451*
Chemotherapy, **1038–1049**. See also specific agents.
  ABVD, 952t, 953
  adverse effects in, 1041–1049
  agents used in, 1041–1049
    alkylating, 1039t, 1041–1042, 1042t
    anthracycline, 1039t, 1044–1045, 1057t
    antibiotic, 1039t, 1044–1045, 1057t

Chemotherapy *(Continued)*
  antimetabolite, 1039t, 1042t, 1042–1043
  biologic response modifier, 1047–1049, 1048t, 1049t
  chemosensitizing, 1058, 1058t
  hormonally active, 1046t, 1046–1047
  natural product, 1043–1044, 1044t
  neurotoxicity of, 2156, 2156t
  brain tumor treated with, 2129–2130
  cardiotoxicity of, 330–331, 358
  cell biology and biochemistry in, 1038–1040, *1039, 1040*
  cell-cycle specific, 1038–1039, 1039t
  colon cancer, 727
  cystitis with, hemorrhagic, 1053–1054
  fetal effects of, 1068–1069, 1069t, 1070t
  hepatotoxicity of, 773, 773t
  interstitial lung disease induced by, 397, 397t
  Kaposi's sarcoma treated with, 1873, 1873t
  leukemia treated with, 928, 931, 934–935, 939, 940
  lung cancer and, 441, 1038t
  lymphoma treated with, Hodgkin's, 952t, 953, 1064–1065
    non-Hodgkin's, 944–946, 945t, 1065–1066
  MOPP, 952t, 953
  myeloma treated with, 963–964
  ovarian carcinoma, 1314
  pharmacokinetic aspects of, 1010–1041, 1068, 1068t
  pregnancy and, 1068–1069, 1069t, 1070t
  principles of, 1038–1041, *1039, 1040*
  psoriasis treated with, 2203
  renal function and, 586–587
  resistance to, 1039–1041, 1056–1060, 1057t, 1058t
  responsiveness to, 1038t, 1038–1041, *1039,* 1039t
  skin disorder treated with, 2197
  tuberculosis therapy with, 1686t, 1686–1688, 1687t, 1688t
  tumor lysis syndrome with, 1053
  tumor marker monitoring of, 1041, 1041t
  viral disease treated with, 1742–1747, 1746t
Chenodeoxycholic acid, 806, *807*
  bile containing, 806, *807*
  stone dissolution with, 815
Cherry red spot, foveal, 2182
Chest wall, **443–444**
  deformities affecting, 443t, 443–444
  motion and configuration of, 368, 369t
  obesity restriction of, 376t
  respiration role of, 443
  respiratory disease affecting, 368, 369t
Cheyne-Stokes respiration, 218
Chicken, *Campylobacter* reservoir in, 1649, 1649t, 1738t
  dietary, *1142*
  erysipeloid and, 1673–1674
Chickenpox, **1763–1764**
  clinical manifestations of, 1763–1764
  diagnosis of, 1764
  epidemiology of, 1763
  etiology of, 1763
  immunization for, 1764
  pathogenesis of, 1763
  treatment of, 1746t, 1764
Chigger, 1734, 1947
  bite of, 1947
  typhus transmitted by, 1727t, 1728t, 1734–1735
Chikungunya virus, 1805t, 1809
Chilblain (pernio), 350
  clinical features of, 350
  diagnosis of, 350
  lupus erythematosus with, 432, *432,* 1478
  treatment of, 350
Children. See *Pediatric patients.*
Chills, malarial, 1532, 1532t, 1533t, 1894
  mycoplasmal infection with, 1576
  typhoid fever, 1643, 1643t
Chimerism, 135, *136*
Chimpanzee, immunodeficiency virus of, *1845,* 1845–1846
Chlamydial infections, 1696–1697, **1721–1725**
  cervicitis due to, 1697t, 1724
  conjunctivitis of, 1697t, 1722–1723, 2179
    infant with, 1724
  endometritis in, 1724
  epididymitis due to, 1697t, 1723–1724
  etiologic organisms in, 1721t, 1721–1722, *1722,* 1723t
  laboratory tests in, 1723, 1724, 1725
  lymphogranuloma venereum in, 1722, 1724

Chlamydial infections *(Continued)*
  pneumonia due to, 412t, 1574, 1725
    infant with, 1724
  pregnancy and, 1724
  preventive testing for, 28t, 1723, 1724, 1725
  proctitis of, 742
  psittacosis due to, 1725
  Reiter's syndrome due to, 1467t, 1469, 1724
  sexual transmission of, 1696–1697, 1722–1725, 1723t
  trachoma due to, 1697t, 1722–1723, 1723t
  treatment of, 1723, 1724, 1725
  urethritis in, 1697, 1697t, 1723
    female with, 1723
    male with, 1697, *1698,* 1723
Chloasma, 2212
Chlorambucil, adverse effects, 1042
  chemotherapy using, 1039t, 1042, 1042t
  fetal malformations due to, 1070t
  leukemia treated with, 934
Chloramphenicol, 1562t
  adverse reactions to, 1568t
  bacterial resistance to, 1558–1560, 1559t
  Lyme disease therapy with, 1719, 1719t
  mechanism of action of, 1558, 1558t
  meningitis therapy with, 1615–1617, 1616t, 1620t
  meningococcal infection and, 1620t, 1620–1621
  Rocky Mountain spotted fever and, 1732
Chloride, cystic fibrosis and, 419, 419–420, *420*
  intestinal transport of, 689, 689–690
  kidney and, 514
    transport and, *223,* 521t, *522*
  sweat gland transport of, 419, *419*
Chloridorrhea, 144t
Chlorine inhalation, 404
2-Chlorodeoxyadenosine, 931
Chloroquine, malaria therapy with, 1895t, 1895–1896, 1896t
  myopathy caused by, 2160
  ocular side effects of, 2183
Chlorosis, 841
Chlorothiazide, dosages for, 264t
  properties and action of, 224t
Chlorpheniramine, 1416, 1416t
Chlorpromazine, 1998t
  schizophrenia treated with, 1998t, 1998–1999
  smoking interaction with, 36t
Chlorpropamide, 1267–1268, 1268t
Chlorthalidone, dosage for, 264t
  properties and action of, 224t
Chocolate, anaphylaxis due to, 1418t
  esophageal reflux disease and, 653, 654t
  urticaria caused by, 1409–1410
Cholangiocarcinoma, 803t, 804, 810–811
Cholangiography, *637*
  cholestasis imaging with, 808, *809*
  transhepatic, 632, *633*
Cholangiopancreatography, 632, *633*
  endoscopic retrograde, 632, *633*
    complications of, 641
    indications for, 638t, 640–641
    therapeutic applications of, 638t, 641
Cholangitis, *637,* 812, 814
  ascending, *809,* 814
  imaging studies in, *809*
  sclerosing, *637, 809,* 812
  treatment of, transplantation in, 801t
Cholecalciferol, 1145t, 1357, 1357t
Cholecystectomy, 816
Cholecystitis, acalculous, 814
  gallstones causing, 814
  radionuclide imaging in, 634, *634*
Choledocholithiasis, *809,* 813, 813t, 814
  imaging studies of, *809*
Choledochus, cyst of, 811
  stones of, *809,* 813, 813t, 814
  stricture of, 811–812
Cholelithiasis. See *Gallstones.*
Cholera, **1652–1654**
  clinical manifestations of, 1653, 1653t
  definition of, 1652
  diagnosis of, 1653, 1653t
  epidemiology of, 1652, *1652*
  etiology of, 1652
  immunization for, 42t, 46, 1554, 1554t, 1654
  pathogenesis of, 1652–1653
  prevention of, 1654
  treatment of, 1653–1654, 1654t
Cholestasis, **807–816**
  approach to patient with, 808–810

Cholestasis *(Continued)*
  cirrhosis with, 791–792, 810
  drug-induced, 773, 773t, 774–775, 810
  extrahepatic, 808, 810–816
  hepatic transplantation in, 801t
  hepatitis with, 763–764
  imaging studies in, 808, *809*
  intrahepatic, 808, 810
  jaundice with, 756t, 757, 758t
  pathophysiology, 807–808, 808t
  postoperative, 816
  pregnancy with, 787, 787t, 810
  pruritus with, 759, 808
  signs and symptoms of, 808
Cholesterol, bile production from, 805, 806, *807*
  blood levels of, 1093t
  crystal deposition of, 1516t
  dietary, 29–30, 30t
    food labeling and, 1143, 1143t
  elevated, 292–293, 1089–1093. See also *Hypercho- lesterolemia.*
  embolization of, 606t, 607
  esters of, *1087,* 1087t, *1088,* 1089, *1089*
    transfer protein for, 1089, *1089,* 1095
  estrogen effect on, 1312
  gallstones of, 812–813, *813, 815*
  HDL (high-density lipoprotein) with, 172
  hepatic synthesis of, 754
  hyperlipidemia and, 293
  ischemic heart disease and, 172, *173*
  LDL (low-density lipoprotein) with, 172
  production of, *1087*
  serum level of, normal, 700t
  therapeutic reduction of, *1093,* 1093–1094, 1094t
  transport of, 1086–1089, *1087, 1088, 1089*
Cholesterol desmolase, 1288t
  deficiency of, 1290
Cholesterolosis, 816
Cholesteryl esters, 1087t
  lipoprotein metabolism and, *1087, 1088, 1089*
Cholestyramine, 1634
Cholic acid, 806, *807*
Choline magnesium trisalicylate, 103t
Chondrocalcinosis, *1515*
  crystal deposition causing, 1515, *1515,* 1516t
  elbow affected by, *1515*
Chondrocytes, cartilage degradation by, 1518
Chondrodysplasia, 145
Chondrodystrophy, 1390–1391
Chondroitin sulfate, 1119t
  connective tissue structure and, 1445t
Chondrosarcoma, 1528
Chordomas, 2131
Chorea, 2048–2049
  athetotic, 2049
  basal ganglia relation to, 2043
  benign hereditary, 2049
  Huntington's, 2048–2049
  rheumatic fever and, 1592t, 1593
  senile, 2049
  Sydenham's, 1592t, 1593
Choriogonadotropin. See *Gonadotropins, chorionic.*
Choriomeningitis, 1737t
  lymphocytic, 2089, 2089t
Chorioretinitis, 2174t, 2178t
  cytomegalovirus in, 2179
  infectious, 2179–2180
  syphilis in, 2180
  toxoplasmosis in, 2179
Choroid, AIDS/HIV effects in, 1868–1870
  inflammation of, 2178t, 2178–2179
  malignant melanoma of, 2180
  toxoplasmosis affecting, 1868–1870, 1909
Choroid plexus, 2132
Choroidal artery, 2058, *2060*
  aneurysm affecting, *2074,* 2074–2076
Christmas factor, 988t
Chromaffin cells, 1253
  adrenal, 1253
  catecholamine biosynthesis in, 1253
  extra-adrenal, 1254, 1257
  periaortic, 1254
Chromium, 73
  assessment of, 1148t
  carcinogenicity and, 1016t
  deficiency of, 1148t
  dietary, parenteral, 1173t
  occupational exposure to, 73

Chromium (Continued)
  physiology of, 1148t
  RDA for, 1141t
  toxicity of, 1148t
    poisoning due to, 73
Chromogen(s), Porter-Silber, 1246, 1247
Chromogranin A, pheochromocytoma and, 1254t, 1255
Chromomycosis, 1836
Chromosome(s), **134–136, 150–157**
  abnormalities of, 151–157
    deletion, 151–152, 152, 155, 155t
    disorders associated with, 151–157, 155, 155t
    duplication, 152, 152
    inversion, 152, 152
    numerical, 151, 154
    structural, 151, 154–156
    translocation, 152, 152, 154
  Alzheimer's disease and, 13, 1994
  banding of, 151, 152, 153
  cancer and, 156, 156–157, 157
  cell division and, 151
  chiasmata of, 135, 136
  chimeric, 135, 136
  coagulation proteins and, 988t
  crossing over, 135, 136, 151
  diseases associated with, 151–157, 155, 155t
  DNA helix in, 134, 134t, 135
  dominant disorders and, 137–140, 138, 138t, 140
    X-linked, 138t, 140, 140
  fructose intolerance and, 1083
  gene linkage and, 135, 135
  genetic code stored in, 134, 134t
  globin genes on, 871
  immunodeficiency related to, 1401–1402, 1402t, 1403
  karyotype of, 151
  laboratory preparation of, 151, 152, 153
  mapping of, disorders tested in, 163, 163t
  meiosis and, 134, 136, 151
  mitosis and, 151
  nomenclature for, 151
  pheochromocytoma and, 1254
  Philadelphia, 922t, 926t
    myelogenous leukemia and, 926t, 926–928, 1074
    thrombocytosis and, 922t, 923
  porphyrias and, 138t, 1125t
  recessive disorders and, 136t, 138t, 139, 139–140, 141
    X-linked, 138t, 140, 140–141, 144t, 146t
  regions of, 134–136, 136
  sex, 134, 140–141, 154, 1285–1287. See also X-linked disorders.
    disorders linked to, 140–141, 154, 1286–1287
    genetics and, 138t, 140, 140–141, 154
    morphology of, 152, 153
  telomere of, cell death role of, 1072, 1072
  X, 140–141, 1285
    Barr body of, 140
    disorders linked to, 138t, 140–141, 154, 1286–1287
      developmental, 154, 1286–1287
      dominant, 138t, 140, 140, 144t
      recessive, 138t, 140, 140–141, 144t
    fragile, 154
    inactivation of, 140, 154
    morphology of, 152, 153
  Y, 141, 1285
    disorders associated with, 154, 1285
    morphology of, 152
    translocation of, 154, 1285
Chronic obstructive pulmonary disease. See Asthma; Bronchitis; Emphysema; Lung, chronic obstructive disease of.
Chrysotherapy, 2197
Chrysotile, 400
Churg-Strauss syndrome, 1491, 2201t
  eosinophilia in, 958, 1491
  interstitial lung disease in, 398
Chvostek's sign, hypocalcemia with, 1371
Chyle, ascites with, 744t, 745
  pleural effusion with, 445, 445t, 446
Chylomicrons, 1087t
  atherosclerosis and, 1092
  characteristics of, 1087t
  fat absorption role of, 696, 697
  lipid transport role of, 696, 697, 1086t, 1088, 1088–1089

Chylomicrons (Continued)
  marked elevation in, 1094–1095
  metabolism of, 1088, 1088–1089
Chyme, 689
  diet and, 689
  volume of, 689
Cigars, 33
Cilastatin, Klebsiella, Enterobacter, Serratia and, 1579–1581, 1580t
  Pseudomonas and, 1579–1581, 1580t
Cilia, immotile syndrome of, 416, 416t, 1336
  lung clearance by, 372–373, 399, 411t
  spermatic, 416, 416t, 1336
Ciliary body, 2176
  inflammation of, 2178t, 2178–2179
Cimetidine, esophageal reflux disease and, 653, 654t
  peptic ulcer treated with, 667, 667–668
Ciprofloxacin, 1562t
  cat scratch disease therapy with, 1681–1682, 1682t
  diarrhea therapy with, 1658, 1658t
  gonorrhea therapy with, 1702t
  Legionella and, 1585, 1585t
  mycobacterial (nontuberculous) disease and, 1690, 1691
Circadian rhythms, 1199–1200
  light-dark cycle effect on, 1204–1205
  melatonin secretion and, 1204–1205
  neuroendocrine function subject to, 1184, 1199–1200
  pituitary hormones with, 1184, 1199–1200
Circle of Willis, 2058, 2058
  aneurysm of, 2074, 2074–2075
  congenital, 278, 279
Circulation. See also Blood flow; Vascular disorders; specific vessel or disorder.
  enterohepatic, 806–807, 807
  fluid exchange affecting, 529–530, 530t
  peripheral, regulation of, 179–180, 216–217
    sickle cells and, 883, 885, 885–889
    vascular disorders affecting, 346–357
  regulation of, 179–180, 478–483
  shock and, 482–483, 494
  shunts in. See Shunts.
  venous return in, 177, 178, 180
Cirrhosis, **788–796**
  alcoholic, 789–791
  arthritis with, 1525
  ascites and, 743t, 744t, 745t
  atrial natriuretic hormone and, 1196
  biliary, 791–792, 810
  cardiac, 219
  classification, 788t, 788–789
  cryptogenic, 791
  definition of, 788
  diagnosis of, 789–795
  epidemiology of, 788
  etiology of, 788t, 788–793, 789
  glucose intolerance in, 753
  gynecomastia and, 1332
  Laënnec's, 789
  mortality rate in, 27t
  pathology, 788–789, 789, 790, 791
  prognosis in, 789, 790
  sequelae of, 793t, 793–796
  treatment of, alcohol abstinence in, 790–791
    biliary decompression in, 792
    drug therapy in, 792
    sunlight exposure in, 792
    transplantation in, 801t
    viral hepatitis and, 791
    Wilson's disease and, 785–786, 791
Cisplatin, adverse effects, 1042
  chemotherapy using, 1039t, 1042
  renal function and, 586–587
  resistance to, 1058, 1058t
Citrate, decreased excretion of, 615, 615, 616, 616t
  kidney stone of, 615, 615, 616, 616t
Citrullinemia, 1102t, 1110, 1111
Clarithromycin, 1562t
  Legionella and, 1585, 1585t
  mycobacterial (nontuberculous) disease and, 1690, 1691
  toxoplasmosis therapy with, 1909, 1910t
Clathrin, 1177
Claudication, 166–167
  arteriosclerosis causing, 350–351
  intermittent, 350–351
    giant cell arteritis with, 1499
Claviceps purpurea, food poisoning due to, 740
Clavicle, 1522
Clavulanic acid, 773, 773t, 774

Clay, ingestion of, 840
Clefting, fetus with, 158t, 159t
  hypothalamus affected by, 1200
  velocardiofacial syndrome causing, 162
Clefts, Rathke's, 1201
Clemastine, rhinitis treated with, 1416, 1416t
Clicks, heart auscultation and, 168, 168t
Clindamycin, 1562t
  babesiosis therapy with, 1916
  bacterial resistance to, 1558–1560, 1559t
  mechanism of action of, 1558, 1558t
  mycoplasmal infection treated with, 1578, 1578t
  Pneumocystis pneumonia and, 1920t, 1921, 1921t, 1922t
  staphylococcal infection treated with, 1609t, 1609–1610
  streptococcal infection treated with, 1587–1589, 1589t
  toxoplasmosis therapy with, 1909, 1910t
Clitoris, 2009t
  anal reflex and, 2009t
  enlarged, 1288
Clomiphene, ovulation induction with, 1309
  side effects of, 1309
Clomiphene test, 1208t
  gonadotropins in, 1208t
Clonidine, dosage for, 265t, 266t
  side effects of, 267, 267t, 270t
Clonidine suppression test, 1254t, 1255–1256
  catecholamines in, 1254t, 1255–1256
  pheochromocytoma diagnosis with, 1254t, 1255–1256
Clonorchiasis, 783t, 1932, 1932t
  hepatic effects of, 782, 783t
Clonus, epileptic, 2114, 2116
  tic with, 2043, 2047, 2049–2050
Clostridial infection(s), **1630–1633**
  botulinum, 1630, 1631t, 1635–1636
  clinical features of, 1631t, 1631–1633
  colitis due to, pseudomembranous, 1631t, 1633–1635, 1634t
  difficile, 1631t, 1633–1635, 1634t
  enteritis necrotica due to, 1631t, 1632
  food poisoning due to, 738, 739t, 1631t, 1632
  gas gangrene in, 1630–1632, 1631t
  laboratory features of, 1631t
  myonecrosis due to, 1630–1632, 1631t
  pathogenesis of, 1631, 1632
  tetanii, 1630, 1631t, 1636–1638, 1638t
  treatment of, 1631–1633
  wound with, 1631t, 1631–1632
Clotrimazole, candidiasis treated with, 1829
  vaginitis treated with, 1829
Clotting time, 989, 990. See also Bleeding time; Coagulation.
Cloxacillin, 1562t
Clozapine, schizophrenia treated with, 1998t, 1998–1999
Clubbing, 2215
  cystic fibrosis with, 421, 421t
  esophageal cancer with, 657
  Graves' disease with, 1233
  lung disease with, 368, 392, 439
  pachydermoperiostosis with, 1388
  paraneoplastic, 439, 657, 1020, 1035
  pulmonary osteoarthropathy with, 1020, 1035
Clubfoot, fetus with, 159t
Clusters of differentiation. See CD (clusters of differentiation).
Clutton's joints, syphilis causing, 1710
CMV. See Cytomegalovirus (CMV)/CMV infection.
Coagulase reaction, staphylococcal, 1606, 1606t, 1607t, 1609, 1609t
Coagulation, **987–990**, 2229t–2230t
  biochemistry of, 977, 977, 978, 987–990, 988t, 989
    schema for, 977, 978, 989
  disorders of, 977–1003
    acquired, 979t, 986t, 998–1002
    approach to patients with, 977–978, 979t, 980t, 990
    differential diagnosis of, 979t, 981, 984t, 990
    hereditary, 979t, 985–987, 990–998
    disseminated intravascular, 1002–1003
      compensated, 1002
      differential diagnosis of, 981, 984t
      etiology of, 1002–1003
      venom causing, 1003
  drugs affecting, 980t
  extrinsic vs. intrinsic path of, 987–990, 989
  factors. See Coagulation factor(s).

Coagulation (Continued)
history and, 977–978, 990
kidney disease and, 1000–1001
laboratory findings, 979, 979t, 981, 990
liver function and, 760–761, 800t, 1000
mechanisms of, 977, 977, 978, 987–990, 989
extrinsic, 987–988
paraneoplastic syndrome affecting, 1017t, 1020–1021
physical examination and, 978–979, 990
platelet defects and, 980–985, 982, 983, 984t
septic shock and, 498
tests of, 979t, 981, 984t
vascular disorders and, 986t, 986–987
acquired, 979t, 986t, 986–987
hereditary, 979t, 986, 986t
vitamin K and, 987–989, 988t, 996
Coagulation factor(s), 987–1003
anaphylaxis role of, 1419
antibodies to, 992, 1001, 1476t, 1479
biochemistry of, 977, 977, 978, 987–990, 988t, 989
drugs affecting, 980t
liver and, 760–761, 1000
monocyte secretion of, 901t
production of, 760–761, 1000
schema for, 977, 978, 989
von Willebrand, 978, 981, 988t
I. See Fibrinogen.
II. See Prothrombin.
III. See Thromboplastin time, partial.
V, 987–989, 988t, 989
deficiency of, 996
Leiden, 887
VII, 987–989, 988t, 989
deficiency of, 995
VIII, 987–989, 988t, 989
antibodies to, 992, 1001
deficiency of, 991–994
inhibitors, 1001
replacement therapy with, 991–992
von Willebrand's disease and, 991, 993–994
deficiency of, 993–994
IX, 987–989, 988t, 989
concentrate of, 995
deficiency of, 994–995
X, 987–989, 988t, 989
deficiency of, 995–996
XI, 987–989, 988t, 989
deficiency of, 995
XII, 987–989, 988t, 989
deficiency of, 995
XIII, 987–989, 988t, 989
deficiency of, 996
Coagulopathy, liver disease with, 796
meningococcemia with, 1614, 1620, 1621
sickle syndromes and, 886
Coal dust, carcinogenicity of, 1016t
lung disease due to, 56, 58t, 399t, 401, 1016t
Coated pits, 1177
Cobalamin. See Vitamin B12.
Cobalt, 71
Cobb's angle, 443
Cobras, 1951t, 1953
Cocaine, adverse effects of, 51
drug abuse with, 51, 56t
neurologic effects of, 1975t
perforated nasal septum due to, 50, 51
pharmacology of, 51
poisoning by, 507–508
Cocci, 1556, 1556–1557, 1557t
Coccidioidomycosis, 1819–1820
clinical manifestations of, 1819–1820, 1820
diagnosis of, 1820
disseminated, 1820
etiologic agent in, 1819
incidence and prevalence of, 1819
pathogenesis and pathology of, 1819
treatment of, 1820
Coccobacilli, 1557t
Cod liver oil, 1357
Codeine, 51
drug abuse with, 51–53
pain control with, 104t, 893t
Codons, 134, 134t, 135
Coelenterates, venomous, 1954t, 1955
Coenzyme A, acyl, 2166
Coenzyme Q, deficiency of, 2167
Coffee, hypertension and, 262
Cognition, 1969–1970. See also Dementia.
aging effect on, 16, 16t, 17–19, 19t
alcohol affecting, 47, 48t
dementia evaluation and, 1993, 1993t

Cognition (Continued)
disturbance of, 1973
examination of, 1993, 1993t
multiple sclerosis affecting, 2109, 2110
Cogwheel phenomenon, 2042
Cohort flow model, 78–79, 79
Coitus. See Sexual function.
Coke production, 1016t
Colchicine, gout treated with, 1513–1514, 1514t
Mediterranean fever treated with, 908
Cold. See also Hypothermia.
common. See Colds (common).
exposure to, 346–350
arterial occlusion and, 346–350
chilblain due to, 350, 1478
cutaneous blood flow and, 2188
cyanosis following, 346–350
frostbite due to, 349–350
myopathy of, 2159
urticaria caused by, 1410
extremities affected by, 346–350
sensitivity to, 346–350
acrocyanosis and, 349
livedo reticularis and, 349
Raynaud's type, 346–349, 347t, 1484
vasoconstriction induced by, 346–350
Cold agglutinins, 862–864, 1577, 1577
mycoplasmal infection and, 1577, 1577
Colds (common), 1747–1749
adenovirus and, 1747, 1747t, 1748
complications of, 1749, 1749
coronavirus and, 1747, 1747t, 1748
coxsackievirus and, 1747, 1747t
echovirus and, 1747, 1747t
epidemiology of, 1747t, 1747–1748
etiology of, 1747, 1747t, 1748
incidence of, 1748
parainfluenza virus and, 1747, 1747t, 1748
pathogenesis in, 1748
prevention of, 1749
respiratory syncytial virus and, 1747, 1747t, 1748
rhinovirus and, 1747t, 1747–1749, 1748
"sore" of, 1772, 1772
transmission of, 1747t, 1747–1748, 1748
treatment of, 1748
interferons in, 1745–1746
Colic, biliary, 813–814
renal, 591, 591t, 613, 613
Colistin, mechanism of action of, 1558, 1558t
Colitis, amebic, 1913t, 1913–1914
antibiotic-associated, 1633–1635, 1634, 1634t
C. difficile and, 1633–1635, 1634, 1634t
E. coli, 1655t, 1656, 1738t
hemorrhagic, 1655t, 1656, 1738t
microscopic, 692
pseudomembranous, 1633–1635, 1634, 1634t
Shigella, 1647t, 1647–1648
ulcerative, 707–715
cancer and, 709–710, 710t, 725
clinical features of, 709, 712t
complications of, 709–711, 710t
Crohn's disease vs., 711–712, 712t
diagnosis of, 711–712
diarrhea in, 710
differential diagnosis of, 711–712, 712t
endoscopy in, 638t, 640, 711, 712t
epidemiology of, 707, 707t
extraintestinal manifestations of, 710t, 710–711
natural history of, 707
pathogenesis of, 707–708
pathology in, 708
prognosis in, 715
radiography in, 711, 712t
treatment of, 712t, 712–714, 714t
Collagen, 1444. See also Connective tissue; Sclerosis.
antibodies to, 1517
bone formation role of, 1352
cartilage and, 1444t
matrix of, 1352
coagulation role of, 977, 977, 978
decreased amounts of, 1120–1121, 1121t
dermal, 2186
Ehlers-Danlos syndrome and, 1120–1121, 1121t
genes for, 1444
heart affected by, 359
markers derived from, 1447, 1447–1448
osteogenesis imperfecta and, 1122t, 1122–1133
pathophysiology of, 1447
polymorphism of, 1444t
receptors for, 1446t

Collagen (Continued)
rheumatoid arthritis affecting, 1448
structure and function of, 1444, 1448
types of, 1444t, 1448
vascular disorders and, 359, 984t
Colon, absorption in, 689, 689–690, 690t
adenoma, 722, 726
AIDS/HIV effects in, 1866–1867, 1867t
bile absorption in, 806, 807, 807
bleeding from, 642t, 644–645, 645t
cancer of, 721–722, 724–728
clinical features of, 726
diagnosis of, 726–727, 727t
distribution by segment, 726, 726
etiology of, 725t, 725–726
genetics of, 725t, 726, 726
incidence of, 1005, 1009, 1013t, 1015
inflammatory bowel disease and, 709–710, 710t, 725
metastatic, 726
nonpolyposis, 724, 724–725
pathology of, 726, 726
pregnancy with, 1061t, 1063–1064
prevention of, 728
prognosis in, 727–728
staging of, 727, 727t
treatment of, 727
tumor marker for, 1021–1022, 1022t
dilation of, Chagas' disease causing, 1901
diverticulitis of, 749–750, 750
drugs affecting, 681t, 688t
endoscopy of, 638t, 639–640
flora of, 1639, 1639t, 1640
irritable, 686–687
ischemia of, 718–719, 719
motility of, 682, 683
clinical assessment of, 682–683
drugs affecting, 688, 688t
rapid transit disorders of, 686t, 687–688, 691–692
slow transit disorders of, 686t, 686–687
polyps of, endoscopy and, 638t, 639–640, 722
inherited syndromes of, 723–725, 724
pathology of, 723, 726
spastic, 686–687
thumbprinting of, 718, 719
toxic dilatation of, 709, 714
trypanosomiasis affecting, 1901
ulceration, 750–751
vascular ectasia of, 720
Colonoscopy, 638t, 639–640
cancer surveillance in, 638t, 639
complications of, 640
indications for, 638t, 639
polypectomy in, 638t, 639
therapeutic applications for, 638t, 640
Colony-forming units, hematopoiesis role of, 818, 819–821, 820, 820t, 821, 898, 917
hemoglobin synthesis and, 869–870
Colony-stimulating factors, 820t, 1048t
cancer therapy related to, 1048t, 1049, 1049t, 1050
hematopoiesis role of, 819–821, 820, 820t, 821, 898
macrophage-lymphocyte interaction and, 901
neutropenia treated with, 912
recombinant, 912
Color anomia, 1985, 1987t
Colorado tick fever, 1733, 1805t, 1805–1807, 1806t
Colostrum, 1317
Coma, 1970–1985
alcohol-related, 47–48, 48t
anatomic correlates of, 1985–1988, 1986, 1987t, 1988t
anoxic, 1973, 2062t, 2063
brain death with, 1978–1979
cerebral hemorrhage with, 2076, 2076t
cerebral hypoxia with, 2062t, 2062–2063
definition of, 1969t
drowning with, 408
drug-induced, 1972t, 1974–1976, 1975t
emergency management of, 1976–1977, 2137–2138, 2138t
examination in, 1971t, 1973, 1973t, 1976–1977, 1977t, 2137, 2137t
Glasgow Scale for, 2137, 2137t
head injury with, 2136–2137, 2137t
hepatic, 797, 798t. See also Encephalopathy, hepatic.
history for, 1976
hypoglycemic, 1982
hypothermia and, 1973

Coma (Continued)
 laboratory testing in, 1974t, 1976
 malarial, 1894
 metabolic, 1972t, 1972–1974, 1973t
 myxedema and, 1239–1240
 pathophysiology in, 1970t–1975t, 1970–1976
 prognosis in, 1977–1978, 1978t
 reflexes and, 1973, 1973t, 1977t
 reticular activating system and, 1969
 score of, 2137, 2137t
 seizures and, 1973
 syncopal, 1979, 1979t, 1981t, 1981–1982
 tentorial herniation and, 1970–1972, 1971, 1971t
 toxic, 1972t, 1975t
 traumatic, 2137, 2137t, 2138t
Communicating arteries, 2058, 2058
 aneurysm affecting, 2074, 2074–2076
Competency, patient, 4–5
Complement, 1398–1401
 activation of, 1398–1400, 1398–1400
 angioedema role of, 1412
 biological activities of, 1400, 1401t
 components of, 1398, 1399t
 convertases for, 1398, 1398–1399, 1399
 deficiency of, 1400–1401, 1401t, 1408, 1412
  late component, 1621
  meningococcemia causing, 1621
 erythrocyte destruction role of, 860, 860–861, 861, 866
 glomerular disorders and, 573, 573t
 immunodeficiency role of, 1408, 1538t, 1542
 mycoplasmal infection and, 1577
 pathophysiology of, 1401, 1401t
 receptors for, 1400, 1400, 1401t
 sepsis role of, 498
 shock affecting, 484–485
 vasculitis role of, 2201t, 2202
Complement fixation test. See also Serology.
 coccidioidomycosis in, 1820
 mycoplasma and, 1577
 syphilis screening with, 1710
Complex of differentiation. See CD (clusters of differentiation).
Compliance, pulmonary, 466
 assessment of, 466–467, 467t
Computed tomography (CT), 127, 128
 CNS in, 1963t, 1963–1969, 1965–1967
 spiral, 127, 128, 129
Concussion, amnesia following, 1982
 brain trauma with, 2136
 vertigo following, 2026
Conduction, aberrant, 237–238, 238, 240
 arrhythmia with, 237–238, 238, 240
 cardiac system of, 190, 191, 191t, 231–233, 232, 233
 delayed, AV system in, 191t
  bundle branch block in, 191t
  ECG patterns of, 191t, 192, 193
 velocity of, 190, 191, 191t, 231, 233t
Condylomata, 647t, 648t, 1707, 1746t
 acuminata, 2299
  interferons and, 1745–1746
  oral, 648t
  rectal, 742
  treatment of, 1745–1746, 1746t
 AIDS/HIV patient with, 1868
 lata, 647, 647t, 1707, 1707
  oral, 647, 647t
  syphilitic, 647, 647t, 1707, 1707
Cone shells, venom of, 1954t, 1955
Confidence interval, statistical, 83
Confusion, 1969–1978, 1997t
 alcohol-related, 47–49, 48t
 Alzheimer's disease vs., 1992–1994, 1993t
 clinical features of, 1972–1974, 1973t, 1997t
 definition of, 1972
 drug-induced, 1974–1976, 1975t
 evaluation of, 1976–1977, 1977t, 1992, 1997t
 hepatic encephalopathy with, 797, 798t
 pathophysiology in, 1970–1987, 1972t
 psychiatric disorders with, 1974, 1997t
 seizure with, 2116
 toxic shock syndrome with, 1588
Congenital anomalies, 157–159
 arteriovenous, 721
 bronchiectasis with, 416t, 416–417, 418t
 chemotherapy causing, 1068–1069, 1069t, 1070t
 chromosomes in, 158t, 159, 159t
 clinical features of, 158t, 158–159, 159t

Congenital anomalies (Continued)
 definition of, 157, 158t
 etiology of, 158, 158t, 159t
 heart disease due to. See Heart, congenital disease of.
 pathogenesis of, 148, 158t
 prevalence of, 157–158
 radiation therapy causing, 1069–1070, 1070t
 recurrence risk for, 159, 159t
 spinal, 2149
 urinary tract, 621–623, 622
Congo red dye, amyloid stained with, 1504, 1506
Conjunctiva, Kaposi's sarcoma of, 1870
Conjunctivitis, 2179
 chlamydial, 1697t, 1722–1723, 2179
  infant with, 1724
 enteroviral, 1787t, 1791–1792
 filarial, 1943, 1944
 gonococcal, 1624
 Haemophilus (aegyptius biogroup) causing, 1624
 hemorrhagic, 1787t, 1791–1792
 measles with, 1759–1760, 1760t
 pneumococcal, 1571, 1571t
 purulent, 1571, 1571t, 1624
 Reiter's syndrome with, 1467t, 1469
Connective tissue, 1443–1448. See also Collagen; Fibroblasts; Sclerosis.
 approach to disorders of, 1440–1443, 1441t, 1442, 1443t
 basement membrane of, 1443–1446, 1445t, 1448
 cells of, 1443–1444, 1446, 1446
 Ehlers-Danlos syndrome and, 1120–1122, 1121t, 1447
 extracellular matrix of, 1443–1446, 1445t, 1446
 immunofluorescence testing and, 2189t
 interstitium of, 1443–1445
 markers from, 1447, 1447–1448, 1448
 metabolism of, 1443–1446
  disorders of, 1118–1124
 mixed disease of, 1447
  antinuclear antibodies in, 1457, 1457t
  bullae of, 2189t
  interstitial lung disease with, 395t, 396
  oral manifestations of, 648, 648t
  pericarditis with, 337t, 338
 osteogenesis imperfecta and, 1122t, 1122–1133, 1447
 pathophysiology of, 1447, 1447–1448, 1448
 pigmented, alkaptonuria with, 1108
 pseudoxanthoma elasticum of, 1123, 1123–1124
 receptors for, 1446t, 1446–1447
 structure and function of, 1443–1448, 1446, 1448
Conradi syndrome, 147
Consanguinity, 136, 136–138, 139
Consciousness disorders, 1969–1982. See also Coma; Epilepsy; Seizures; Syncope.
 anatomic correlates of, 1985–1988, 1986, 1987t, 1988t
 brief duration, 1979, 1979t, 1981–1982
 cerebral hemorrhage in, 2078, 2078t
 cerebral hypoxia with, 2062t, 2062–2063
 clinical evaluation of, 1976–1977, 1977t
 common causes of, 1970t, 1970–1972, 1971
 definition of states in, 1969t
 drug-induced, 1974–1976, 1975t
 level vs. content in, 1972
 prognosis in, 1978, 1978t
 psychiatric, 1974, 1974t, 1996–2006
 seizures and, 2115–2118
 tentorial herniation in, 1970–1972, 1971, 1971t
 toxic, metabolic and diffuse, 1972t–1975t, 1972–1976
 traumatic, 1978, 2137, 2137t, 2138t
Constipation, anal obstruction with, 687
 drugs causing, 22
 elderly affected by, 22
 motility disorders with, 687
Contamination prevention, 1853t, 1853–1854, 1854t
Contraception, 1309–1311
 oral drugs for, 1309–1311
  complications of, 1310–1311
  interaction of, 36t, 1310
  metabolic effects of, 1309–1310
  physiologic action of, 1309–1310
  smoking and, 36t
Contractility, Frank-Starling relation and, 175, 214
 heart, 176, 177
 myocardial, 176, 177, 177, 214, 215
Contrast agents, 2127–2128
 gadolinium, 2127, 2127–2128, 2128, 2128t, 2130, 2131
 renal function and, 585

Contusions, 2136, 2136
 head injury with, 2136, 2136
 spinal cord, 2139, 2139–2140
Conus medullaris, 2141
Convertases, complement activation by, 1398–1400, 1398–1400
Convulsions. See also Epilepsy; Seizures.
 child with, 2116–2117
 epileptic, 2115–2117
  status epilepticus and, 2124, 2124t
 fever causing, 2116–2117
 syncope induction of, 1981
 tetanus causing, 1637
Cookware, lead leached from, 66
Cooley's anemia, 877t, 877–879, 881
Coombs' test, hemorrhagic disorders and, 984t
 immunohemolytic anemia and, 863–864, 867
 lupus erythematosus and, 1479
Copper, 1148t
 deficiency of, 1148t
 dietary, parenteral, 1173t
 hepatic level of, 1131–1132
 physiology of, 1148t
 RDA for, 1141t
 sunflower cataract due to, 2175
 toxicity of, 71, 1148t
 urinary, 1132
 Wilson's disease and, 785–786, 1131–1132, 2175
"Copper penny" fungal cells, 1836
Coprolalia, 2049
Coproporphyrinogen, 1125, 1125t, 1129
Coproporphyrinogen oxidase, 1125, 1125t, 1129
 deficiency of, 1125, 1125t, 1129
Cor pulmonale, bronchitis with, 382t, 387
 embolism and, pulmonary, 423
 emphysema with, 382t, 387
 hypertension and, pulmonary, 423
 sounds of, 424
Coracoid process, 1522
Coral snake, 1951t, 1952
Corals, venom of, 1954t, 1955
Cordotomy, 106–107
Cornea. See also Keratitis.
 dendrite in, 2179
 eyelash abrasion of, 1722
 filiariasis affecting, 1943
 trachoma effect on, 1722–1723
 ulcer of, 2179
Corneocytes, 2185
Coronary artery(ies), angina pectoris and, 79, 295–301
 angioplasty of, 318
 atherosclerosis of, 291–295
  angioplasty in, 318
  bypass surgery for, 316t, 316–319, 318
  cholesterol level and, 1093t, 1093–1094, 1094t
  diet and, 1139, 1143t
  exercise tolerance testing and, 79
  hypertension and, 257, 260t, 263
  mortality rate, 27t, 30t, 171t, 171–173, 257, 263
  pathogenesis of, 292, 292, 294, 295
  risk factors for, 171–173, 292–294
  sudden death related to, 254t, 255
 blood flow regulation in, 178–179, 179
 bypass grafts to, 316t, 316–319, 318
 calcification in, 186
 congenital anomalies of, 302t
 degenerative disorders affecting, 302t
 infarction related to. See Myocardial infarction.
 ischemic heart disease and. See Angina pectoris; Ischemic heart disease; Myocardial infarction.
 thrombolysis in, 310, 310–311, 312t
 thrombosis in, 302t
 trauma affecting, 302t
Coronary bypass surgery, 316–319
 benefits of, 318, 319
 indications for, 316t, 316–317
 mortality in, 318, 319
 principles of, 317–318
 reoperation and, 319
 saphenous vs. thoracic graft in, 318, 319
Coronary heart disease. See Coronary artery(ies), atherosclerosis of.
Coronavirus, common cold due to, 1747, 1747t, 1748
 structure of, 1739
Corpus albicans, 1294
Corpus callosum, demyelination of, 2040, 2106t
 tumor of, 2126t
Corpus luteum, 1294
 maturation of, 1294, 1298
 ovarian cycle of, 1297–1299, 1298

Cortical androgen-stimulating hormone, 1246
Corticosteroid-binding globulin, 1182
Corticosteroids, **1245–1252**. See also *Aldosterone; Cortisol; Glucocorticoids; Prednisone.*
  allergic rhinitis treated with, 1416–1417, 1417t
  anti-inflammatory properties of, 108–110, 109t
  asthma treated with, 380
  Behçet's syndrome treated with, 1507
  cancer therapy using, 1046t, 1047
  crystal deposition of, 1516t
  gout treated with, 1514t
  heart transplantation and, 363, 364t, 365
  hepatotoxicity, 773, 773t
  inflammatory bowel disease treated with, 713, 714t
  inhaled, 380
  lupus erythematosus treated with, 1482, 1482t
  multiple sclerosis therapy using, 2111
  myopathy treated with, inflammatory, 1503
  ocular side effects of, 2183
  physiology, 1245–1252
  Pneumocystis pneumonia and, *1918*, 1920, 1921, 1921t
  polyarteritis nodosa treated with, 1494
  polymyalgia rheumatica treated with, 1500
  rejection reaction treated with, 364, 364t
  rheumatoid arthritis treated with, 1466
  salicylates (aspirin) vs., 112
  skin disorder treated with, 2194t, 2194–2195, 2195t
  systemic, 2196
  temporal arteritis treated with, 1500
  topical, 2194t, 2194–2195, 2195t
  tuberculosis treated with, 1688
  Wegener's granulomatosis treated with, 1497t, 1497–1498
Corticotrope cells, 1209t, 1215
  Cushing's disease role of, 1216
Corticotropin. See *Adrenocorticotropic hormone (ACTH).*
Corticotropin-releasing hormone (CRH), *1198*, 1198–1199
  ACTH and, *1198*, 1198–1199, 1215–1216, 1217t
  Cushing's syndrome and, 1216, 1217t
  fever production role of, *1534*
Cortisol, **1245–1252**
  ACTH and, 1213t, 1215–1216
    suppression test for, 1213t, 1215–1216, 1217t, 1247
  binding and transport of, 1247
  congenital adrenal hyperplasia and, 1252
  deficiency of, 1249–1251, 1250t
    ACTH role in, 1215–1216
    21-hydroxylase defect in, 1252, 1287–1290, 1288t
  excess of, 1247–1249. See also *Cushing's syndrome.*
  feedback control of, 1246
  inactivation of, 1182
  laboratory tests for, 1246, *1247*
  metapyrone suppression of, 1216
  replacement therapy with, 1208t, 1250
  synthesis and secretion of, 1245–1247
  therapeutic, 108t. See also *Corticosteroids; Glucocorticoids, therapeutic; Prednisone.*
  urinary free, 1217, 1246–1247
Cortisol binding globulin, 1247
Cortisol releasing hormone (CRH), 1208t, 1213t
  ACTH response to, 1208t, 1213t
  pituitary function tests using, 1208t, 1213t
Cortisone, cortisol conversion to, 1249
  structure of, *1247*
  therapeutic, 108t
Corynebacterium, 1629. See also *Diphtheria.*
Cosmic rays, *59*, 60t, 62
Cost analysis, 82–83
  cost-benefit, 83
  cost-effectiveness, 82–83, 83t
  decision making with, 82–83, 83t
  dialysis and, 567
  ethical issues and, 6
  outcome assessment using, 124, 125t
Costosternal junction, Tietze's syndrome of, 1528
Cotrimoxazole, *Legionella* and, 1585, 1585t
  non-Hodgkin's lymphoma and, 945t
Cotton dust, 59t
Cotton wool spots, 1868–1869
  AIDS/HIV with, 1868–1869, 1869t
  diabetes and, 2182
  HTLV myelopathy with, 2099
  lupus erythematosus with, 2182
  retina with, 1480, 1868–1869, 2099, 2182
Cough, 369–370
  asthmatic, 378

Cough *(Continued)*
  bronchiectasis with, 417
  bronchitis with, 382t, 383, 386
  cardiovascular disease causing, 166
  croup, 1753
  cystic fibrosis with, 419–420
  emphysema with, 382t, 383, 386
  headache with, 2033
  interstitial lung disease with, 391
  lung cancer with, 438
  mycoplasmal infection with, *1577*
  parainfluenza virus infection with, 1753
  pulmonary embolism causing, 424t
  sputum with, 369–370. See also *Sputum.*
  tuberculosis with, 1683–1685, 1689
  whooping, 1628. See also *Pertussis.*
Coumarin, 999–1000
  complications, 999–1000
  dosage, 999
  drug interaction with, 1000t
  vitamin K deficiency due to, 999–1000
Courvoisier's sign, 753, 811
Cowden's syndrome, 725
Cowdry type A bodies, 1771
Cox proportional hazards regression, 85, 85t
Coxiella burnetti, 1727t, 1735–1736, 1737t
COXs. See *Cyclooxygenase.*
Coxsackievirus, 1784, 1784t, 1787t
  characteristics of, 1783–1785, 1784t
  common cold due to, 1747, 1747t
  syndromes associated with, 1786–1792, 1787t
CPPD (calcium pyrophosphate dihydrate), *1515*, 1515, 1516t
Cracker test, dry mouth and, 1488
Crackles, bronchiectasis with, 417
  pulmonary embolism with, 424t
Cradle cap, 2199
Cramp(s), 2159. See also *Spasms (spasticity).*
  dystonia with, 2043, 2047, *2047*, *2048*
  occupational, 2047
  writer's, 2043, 2049
Cranial nerve(s), botulism effect on, 1635
  mucormycosis affecting, 1833
  paraneoplastic effects in, 1027t, 1028
  tetanus effect on, 1637
  VIII, acoustic neuroma of, 2126t, 2127t, 2131
Craniopharyngioma, 1201
Craniotomy, 2136
C-reactive protein, 1456
  acute illness and, 1535–1537, 1536t
Creams, topical, 2194, 2194t, 2195t
Creatinine clearance, 514
CREB (cAMP response element binding protein), 1178, 1181
Cremasteric reflex, 2009t
Creola bodies, 380
  asthmatic sputum with, 380
Crepitus, soft tissue, 1640, 1640t
CREST syndrome, antinuclear antibodies in, 1457, 1457t
  arthritis linked to, 1525
  interstitial lung disease with, 395t, 396
Cretinism. See also *Hypothyroidism.*
  definition of, 1237
  iodine deficiency in, 1149t
Creutzfeldt-Jakob disease, 2097, 2097t, **2102–2103**
Crib death, 254t
  botulism causing, 1636
Cricoarytenoid joints, 1463
Crigler-Najjar syndrome, 757t
  bilirubin metabolism in, 756, 757, 757t
  jaundice in, 756, 757, 757t
Crimean-Congo hemorrhagic fever, 1798t, 1802, 1806t
Critical care, **464–510**
  approach to patient in, 464t, 464–466, 465t
  ethical issues in, 465–466
  patient neuropathy associated with, 2156
  prognosis and, 465
  unit characteristics and, 464, 464t
Crohn's disease, **707–715**
  cancer and, 710
  clinical features of, 709, 712t
  complications of, 709–711, 710t
  diagnosis of, 711–712
  diarrhea in, 710
  differential diagnosis of, 711–712, 712t
  endoscopy in, 711, 712t
  epidemiology of, 707, 707t
  extraintestinal manifestations of, 710t, 710–711
  natural history of, 707

Crohn's disease *(Continued)*
  pathogenesis of, 707–708
  pathology in, 708–709, 712t
  prognosis in, 715
  radiography in, 711, 712t
  treatment of, 712t, 712–713, 714–715
  ulcerative colitis vs., 711–712, 712t
Cromatiton, pediculosis treated with, 2195
Cronkite-Canada syndrome, 725
  polyps with, 725
Croup, epidemic, 1752–1753, 1753t
  parainfluenza virus in, 1752–1753, 1753t
  viral, 1749–1751, 1750t, 1751t
Crusting, skin disorders with, 2191t
Cryoglobulinemia, 960t, 966
  nephropathy with, 579
  type I (monoclonal), 966
  type II (mixed), 966
  type III (polyclonal), 966
  urticaria caused by, 1410
Cryoprecipitate, factor VIII, 991–992
Cryptococcoma, 1824
Cryptococcosis, **1823–1825**
  AIDS/HIV with, 1862–1863
  clinical manifestations of, 1824
  diagnosis of, 1824–1825
  epidemiology of, 1823–1824
  etiologic agent in, 1823
  pathogenesis and pathology of, 1824
  prognosis and prevention of, 1825
  treatment of, 1825
Cryptorchidism, 1326, 1336
  examination in, 1336
  treatment of, 1336
Cryptosporidiosis, 783t, 1910–1912
  clinical manifestations of, 1911
  diagnosis of, 1911–1912
  epidemiology of, 1911
  etiologic organism in, 1910–1912, *1912*
    staining of, 1911, 1912
  hepatic effects of, 782, 783t, 1911
  pathology and pathogenesis of, 1911
  treatment of, 1912
Crystal deposition, **1515–1517**. See also *Lithiasis.*
  apatite, 1515–1516, 1516t
  arthropathy due to, *1513*, *1515*, 1515–1517, 1516t, 1519t
  Charcot-Leyden, 380, 1516t
  CPPD (calcium pyrophosphate dihydrate), 1515, 1516t
  crystal type in, 1516t
  diagnostic features in, 1515–1517, 1516t
  gout with, 1508, *1512*, *1514*, 1516
  osteoarthritis due to, 1519t
  oxalate, 1516, 1516t
  renal tubular, 552t, 554
  systemic disorders associated with, 1516t
Crystal violet, 1556–1557, 1557t
Crystalloid solutions, 529
Crystalluria, antimicrobials causing, 1568t
  cystine in, 596, 617
  uric acid, 1116
CSF. See *Cerebrospinal fluid.*
CT. See *Computed tomography (CT).*
Cullen's sign, 731
Cultures, chancroid pathogen in, 1704–1705
  chlamydial, 1723, 1724, 1725
  diphtheria, 1630
  gonorrheal, 1703
  skin examination using, 2192
  small intestinal, malabsorption and, 700t, 701
  toxoplasmal, 1908–1909
  tubercle bacillus in, 1685, 1686t
Cupping, glaucoma and, 2176, 2178
  ocular, 2176, 2178
Curare, 310t
Curschmann's spirals, 380
  asthmatic sputum with, 380
Cushing's disease, **1216–1218**
  clinical features in, *1216*, 1216–1217, 1217t
  definition of, 1216, 1248
  differential diagnosis of, 1217t, 1217–1218, 1248
  etiology of, 1216, 1248
  laboratory testing in, 1217t, 1217–1218
  pathogenesis of, 1216, 1248
  treatment of, 1218, 1248
Cushing's syndrome, **1247–1249**
  ACTH and, *1216*, 1216–1218, 1217t, 1248, 1248t

Cushing's syndrome *(Continued)*
  ectopic, 1024–1025, 1025t, 1248, 1248t
    plasma levels, 1213t, 1248
  clinical features in, *1216*, 1216–1217, 1217t, 1247, 1247t
  definition of, 1216, 1248
  diagnosis of, 1217t, 1217–1218, 1247t, 1247–1248
  differential diagnosis of, 1213t, 1217t, 1217–1218, 1248
  obesity with, 1165, *1216*, 1217, 1247, 1247t
  tumor-associated, 1024–1025, 1025t, 1248–1249
Cutis laxa, 1120–1122, 1121t
Cyanide, antidote for, 504t, 508
  poisoning due to, 504t, 508
Cyanocobalamin. See *Vitamin B₁₂.*
Cyanosis, heart failure causing, 219
  methemoglobinemia vs., 875–877
  Raynaud's phenomenon with, 347, 1484, 1485
  skin temperature and, 346–350
Cyclooxygenase, 1188–1189
  arachidonic acid metabolism by, *1188*, 1188–1190, *1189*
  inhibition of, 1192
  NSAID inhibition of, 112–113, *113*
Cyclophosphamide, adverse effects, 1042
  cardiotoxicity of, 331, 358
  chemotherapy using, 1039t, 1042, 1042t
  myeloma treated with, 963, 964
  non-Hodgkin's lymphoma and, 945t
  polyarteritis nodosa treated with, 1494, *1494*
  resistance to, 1058, 1058t
  Wegener's granulomatosis treated with, 1497t, 1497–1498
Cyclospora, 1912, 1916t
  cryptosporidium vs., 1912
  treatment for, 1916t
Cyclosporine, adverse effects of, 365, 366t
  drug interactions of, 365, 366t
  heart transplantation using, 363, 365, 366t
  hepatic effects of, 365, 366t
  hypertension caused by, 365, 366t
  renal effects of, 365, 366t
  Wegener's granulomatosis treated with, 1497t
Cylophosphamide, fetal malformations due to, 1070t
Cyproheptadine, allergic rhinitis treated with, 1416, 1416t
Cyproterone, hirsutism treated with, 1316
Cyst(s), amebic, 1913, 1915t
  arachnoid, 2131
  Baker's, knee with, 1462, *1463*, 1466
  bronchogenic, bullae vs., 390
  bronchopulmonary sequestrations vs., 390
  cestode formation of, 1922–1926, 1923t
  hydatid, 1923t, 1924–1925
    hepatic, 782, *784*
  inclusion, epidermal, 2209
  mucus retention, oral, 648, 648t
  Rathke's cleft, 1201, 2131
  renal, 617–621
    medullary, *619*, 621
  splenic, 974
  suprasellar, 2131
  synovial, 1462, *1463*
  syringomyelic, 2055, *2055*
  trichinosis organism in, 1937
Cystathionine, 1112–1113
  homocysteine metabolism role of, 1112–1113, *1113*
  urinary, 1102t
Cystathionine synthase, deficiency of, 1112–1114, 1113t
Cystic duct, *637*
Cystic fibrosis, **419–422**
  bronchiectasis with, 416, 418t
  clinical features of, 419–420, *420*
  complications of, 420–421, 421t
  definition of, 419
  diagnosis of, 420
  gene transfer in, 421–422
  genetics of, 419, 420
  hemoptysis in, 420, 421t
  hepatic effects of, 786
  ion channels in, *419*, 419
  pathogenesis of, 419, *419*
  pathology in, 419
  prevalence of, 136t, 138t
  prognosis in, 422
  sweat glands in, *419*, 419–420, *420*
  transport defect in, 144t, *419*, 419
  treatment of, 421–422

Cysticercosis, 1925–1926
  cerebral, 1737t
  diagnosis of, 1926
  neurological effects of, 1926
  ocular, 1926
  treatment for, 1923t, 1924t, 1926
Cystinosis, 595t, 597, 1105t
Cystinuria, 595t, 596, 1104t, 1105t
  diagnosis of, 596
  genetics of, 138t, 1104t, 1105t
  incidence of, 596
  kidney stone and, 595t, 596, 616t, 617
  metabolic defect in, 144t, 596, 1104t, 1105t
  pathophysiology in, 144t, 595t, 596
  transport defect in, 595t, 596, 1104t, 1105t
Cystitis, candidiasis with, 1828
  female, sexually transmitted disease with, 1698–1699
  hemorrhagic, adenovirus causing, 1757t, 1758
    chemotherapy causing, 1053–1054
  symptoms of, 604, 604t
Cytarabine, adverse effects, 1042–1043
  chemotherapy using, 1039t, 1042–1043
  hepatotoxicity, 773
  non-Hodgkin's lymphoma and, 945t
Cytochrome enzyme(s), 772, 774, 775
  C, drugs metabolized by, 97t
  hepatotoxicity and, 772, 774, 775
  P-450, arachidonic acid metabolized by, 1191, *1191*
    cyclosporine effect on, 366t
    steroid hormones and, 1182
  phagocytosis using, 898t, *900*
Cytoid bodies, 1480
Cytokines, 1395t, *1415*, *1416*, *1534*
  allergic rhinitis role of, 1414–1415, *1415*, *1416*
  B cell interaction with, *1393*, 1395, 1395t
  cancer therapy using, 1047–1049, 1048t, 1049t, 1050
  fever production role of, 1533–1534, *1534*, 1535t
  glucocorticoid effect on, 109, 109t
  malaria role of, 1894
  mast cell release of, *1416*, 1436t
  monocyte, 900, 901t
  resistance to, 1057
  rheumatoid arthritis role of, 1453–1454, *1454*, 1454t
  rheumatoid synovitis role of, *1460*, 1460–1461
  sepsis role of, 498, *498*
  T cell, *1393*, 1395, 1395t
Cytolysins, thiol-activated, 1587
Cytomegalovirus (CMV)/CMV infection, **1774–1776**, 2095
  AIDS/HIV and, 1775, 1863, 1869, 1869t
  bone marrow transplant affected by, 975
  clinical aspects of, 1774–1775
  compromised host and, 1775, 1869t, 2095
  congenital, 1775
  epidemiology of, 1775
  immune globulin against, 41t, 1775–1776
  mononucleosis due to, 1774
  pathogenesis of, 1774
  pathology of, 1775, 2095
  retinitis due to, 1869, 1869t, 2179
  sexual transmission of, 1697t, 1774
  transfusion-transmitted, 896, 896t
  treatment of, 1869t
Cytoplasm, *1416.* See also *Cytokines; Plasma membrane.*
  antibodies to, 1457t, 1457–1458, 1476t
    lupus erythematosus with, 1457t, 1457–1458
    rheumatoid arthritis with, 1457t, 1457–1458
Cytosine, genetic code use of, 134, 134t
Cytotoxins. See *Toxin.*

D

Dacarbazine, adverse effects of, 1045
  chemotherapy using, 1039t, 1042t, 1045
Dactinomycin, adverse effects, 1045
  chemotherapy using, 1039t, 1044t, 1045
Dactylitis, psoriasis with, 1471
DAG (diacylglycerol), 1179, *1179*
  hormone signaling role of, 1179, *1179*
  phosphatidylinositol activated by, 1179, *1179*
Daily activities, cancer patient, 1007, 1008t
Danazol, 1319
Dane particle, 765
Dantrolene, 773, 773t
Dapsone, 1921t
  Pneumocystis pneumonia and, 1920, 1920t, 1921t, 1922t
  toxoplasmosis therapy with, 1909, 1910t

Darier's sign, 1035, 1411, 1436
  elicitation of, 2192
  urticaria pigmentosa with, 1035, 1411, 2192
Darkfield microscopy, *Treponema* in, 1705, 1710
Darkness. See also *Light.*
  melatonin secretion and, 1204–1205
Data analysis, 78–85
  Bayes' rule in, 78–80, *79*, 79t
  cost analysis in, 82–83, 83t
  decision analysis using, 80–82, *81*, *82*
  statistics in, 83–85, 85t
Daunorubicin, adverse effects of, 1044
  chemotherapy using, 1039t, 1044, 1044t
  resistance to, 1057t
Daylight. See *Light.*
De Quervain's tenosynovitis, 1527
Deafness, 2021–2024
  aphasia and, 1991
  causes of, 2021–2023
  elderly affected by, 16t, 17
  evaluation of, 2021–2023, *2022*, *2023*
  hereditary, 2022
  pure word, 1991
Death and dying, **6–9**
  at home, 8–9
  do-not-resuscitate order and, 465
  fear of, 18
  leading causes of, 26–27, *27*, 27t, 30t, 1143t, *1849*
  patient care issues related to, 6–9, 8t
  physician philosophy on, 9
  physician-assisted, 5
  suicide in, 2002
Debridement, skin soak prior to, 2193–2194, 2194t
Debrisoquine, 97t
Decay accelerating factor, erythrocytic, 822
Decerebrate posturing, 798t
Decision analysis, 80–82, *81*, *82*
  cohort flow model in, 78–79, *79*
  formal technique for, 80–82, *81*, *82*
  probabilities determined in, 78–80, 79t
  sensitivity analysis for, 82, *82*
  steps of, 80–82, *81*, *82*
  tabular form in, 78–79, 79t
  therapeutic threshold concept in, 82
  utility calculation for, *81*, 81–83
Decision making, 2–9, 75–77
  data analysis for, 78–85
    Bayes' rule in, 78–80, *79*, 79t
    cost analysis in, 82–83, 83t
    decision analysis in, 80–82, *81*, *82*
    multiple tests (panels) in, 78
    statistics in, 83–85, 85t
  family role in, 6–9, 8t
  patient role in, competent, 4–5
    dying, 5–9, 8t
    elderly cognitive impairment and, 24–25
    end-of-life, 5–9, 8t
  physician role in, 75–85
    approach to patient and, 75–77
    diagnosis and, 75–76
    history taking and, 75t, 75–76
    physical examination and, 76
    prevention and, 76–77
    treatment and, 75–76
Decision tree, 80–82, *81*, *82*
Decompression illness, 410, 410t
  clinical features of, 410, 410t
  treatment of, 410
Defecation, colon cancer affecting, 726
  inflammatory bowel disease and, 712t
  pain with, shigellosis causing, 1648
Defense mechanisms, **1533–1537**. See also *Immune response.*
  defects in, 1537–1542, 1538t, 1539t
  inflammatory response in, 1533–1537, *1534*, 1535t
  physical and chemical barriers of, 1537
  skin in, 1537, 1538t
Deferoxamine, 504t
  dosage for, 504t
  iron poisoning treated with, 504t, 508–509
  thallasemia treated with, 878–879
Defibrillation, 308–309
Defibrination syndrome, 1002
Degenerative disease(s), arterial, 302t
  joint, 1517–1521. See also *Osteoarthritis.*
  neurologic, **2050–2057**. See also *Encephalopathy.*
    Alzheimer's disease as, 1992–1994
    ataxia in, 2051t, 2051–2052
    Creutzfeldt-Jakob disease as, 2102–2103
    cutaneous effects of, 2056–2057

Degenerative disease(s) *(Continued)*
  dementia in, 18–19, 19t, 1992t, 1992–1994, 1993t
  elderly with, 16, 16t, 1992–1994
  hypertensive encephalopathy in, 2080
  motor neuron disease in, 2052t, 2052–2054, 2054t
  posture and movement in, 2052t, 2052–2055, 2054t
  spinal cord, 2055, *2055*
  weakness and wasting in, 2027–2030, 2052t, 2052–2055, 2054t
  spondylotic, 2145–2146
Dehydration, diabetes insipidus and, 1224–1225, *1225*
  shigellosis with, 1647t, 1648
Dehydration test, 1224–1225, *1225*
Dehydroemetine, 1915t
Dehydroepiandrosterone, adrenal, 1245–1246
  ovarian, *1300*
Deiodinase, extrathyroidal defect in, 1230t
  thyroxine metabolized by, 1228, 1230t
Déjà vu, seizure causing, 2114
Delirium, **1969–1978**, 1997t
  alcohol-related, 49
  clinical features of, 1972–1974, 1973t, 1997t
  definition of, 1969t, 1972
  drug-induced, 1974–1976, 1975t
  elderly affected by, 16, 16t, 17t
  evaluation of, 1976–1977, 1977t, 1997t
  hyperthermia with, 1973–1974
  pathophysiology in, 1970–1987, 1972t
  pschiatric disorder with, 1974, 1974t, 1997t
  risk factors for, 17t
Delirium tremens, 49
Deltoid muscle, *1522*
Delusions, 1974t, 1996
  manic episode with, 1997t, 2002
  schizophrenic, 1997, 1997t
Dementia, *1992–1996*
  AIDS/HIV with, 2097t, 2097–2099, *2098*, 2098t
  alcoholic, 2039–2032
  aluminum intoxication causing, 567
  Alzheimer's, 1993, 1994
  amnesia related to, 1990, 1990t
  amyloid deposit and, 1505, 1994
  causes of, 1992t, 1992–1996, 1993t
  characterization of, 18, 19t, 1993, 1993t
  cognitive evaluation in, 1993, 1993t
  Creutzfeldt-Jakob, 2102–2103
  definition of, 1969t, 1992
  depression vs., 19, 19t, 1994
  diagnosis of, 1993, 1993t
  dialysis causing, 567
  differential diagnosis of, 1993, 1993t, 1994–1996
  drug-induced, 1994
  elderly affected by, 18–19, 19t, 1992–1994
  Huntington's disease with, 1992t, 1995
  hydrocephalus in, 1992t, 1995
  Lewy bodies in, 1994
  management of, 1993t, 1994–1995
  manganese causing, 73, 1149t
  mental status examination in, 1993, 1993t
  multi-infarct, 1992t, 1995
  Parkinson's disease with, 1992t, 1995
  Pick's disease with, 1992t, 1995
  syphilitic, 2086
  tumor causing, 1992t, 1994
Demyelination, **2106–2113**
  disseminated encephalomyelitis with, 2104, 2104t
  Guillain-Barré, 2150–2152, 2151t
  imaging of, 1967, *1967*, 2107–2108, *2108*
  ischemia causing, 2062t, 2063, 2106t
  leukodystrophies with, 2112–2113
  Marchiafava-Bignami, 2040
  multiple sclerosis with, *1967*, **2106–2112**
  myelitis with, 2111–2112, 2112t
  necrotizing hemorrhagic encephalopathy with, 2105
  nutrition and, 2106t
  peripheral neuropathy with, 2150–2152, 2151t
  plaques of, 1967, *1967*
  polyneuropathy with, 2151t, 2151–2152
  progressive multifocal leukoencephalopathy with, 2101, *2101*
Dengue fever, 1805t, 1807
  hemorrhagic, 1798t, 1800–1801, 1805t
Dental caries, 1148t
Dental infection, 1639, 1639t
Dental pain, 2034
Dentures, 648, 648t
Deoxycholic acid, 806, *807*
Deoxycortisol, *1247*
Deoxyhemoglobin, 869

Deoxyribonuclease, streptococcal, 1587
Deoxyribonucleic acid. See *DNA (deoxyribonucleic acid).*
Depolarization, atrial, *236*
  cardiac cell, 189–191, *190*
  His bundle, *236*
  ventricular septal, *236*
Depression, **1999–2002**
  bipolar disorder with, 2003–2004
  dementia vs., 19, 19t, 1994
  diagnosis of, 19, 19t, 1999t, 2000
  drug therapy of, 20t, 20–21, 2000t, 2000–2001
  elderly affected by, 18–20, 19t, 20t, 1999–2000
  history taking in, 1999, 1999t
  incidence of, 2000
  major, 1999t, 1999–2001
  multiple sclerosis with, 2109, 2110
  pathophysiology of, 2000
  post-seizure, 2119
  symptoms of, 1999t, 1999–2000
  treatment of, 2000–2001
Dermatan sulfate, 1119t
  connective tissue structure and, 1445t
Dermatitis, 2197–2202
  atopic, 2198–2199
    incidence of, 2184t
  contact (allergic), 2197–2198, 2198t, 2218, 2220–2221
  corticosteroid therapy in, 2194t, 2194–2195, 2195t
  dressings and soaks for, 2193–2194, 2194t
  drug therapy in, 2193–2197
    systemic, 2196t, 2196–2197
    topical, 2193–2196, 2194t, 2195t
  drug-induced, 2219t, 2219–2220
  eczematous, 2191t, 2197–2202, 2201t. See also *Eczema.*
  exfoliative, 1033, 2199
    paraneoplastic, 1019, 1031t, 1031–1033
  "flaky paint," 1156
  flea bite, 1738t
  foods causing, 1409–1410, 2218
  herpetiformis, 2189t, 2205t
  immunofluorescence tests and, 2189t
  inflammatory bowel disease with, 710, 710t
  morphology of lesions of, 2191t
  occupation related to, 59t, 379t, 2220–2221
  pellagra with, 2218
  perioral, 2207t
  photoallergic (UV light), 2198, 2217–2218
  protein deficiency causing, 1156
  purpuric, 2201t, 2201–2202
  seborrheic, 2199
    alopecia with, 2217
    cradle cap due to, 2199
    incidence of, 2184t
  sponge, 2197
  stasis, 2199
  treatment principles for, 2193–2197, 2194t, 2195t, 2196t
Dermatofibroma, 2210
Dermatographism, 1410, 2208
Dermatolysis, 2189t, 2205t
Dermatomes, shingles in, 2094
Dermatomyositis, 1018–1019, 2164, 2212
  antinuclear antibodies in, 1457, 1457t
  diagnosis of, 1018–1019, 1499t, 2164, 2212
  incidence of, 1485t
  interstitial lung disease with, 395t, 396
  myopathy and, 2164
  paraneoplastic, 1018, 1029, 1034
  pathophysiology of, 1018, 1029
  treatment of, 1019
Dermatophytosis, 2199–2200
  eczematous, 2199–2200
  folliculitis with, 2207
  KOH test for, 2192
  occupation and, 2221
  tinea in, 2184t, 2199–2200
Dermis, **2186–2187**
  anatomy of, *2185*, *2186*, 2186–2187
  physiology of, *2185*, *2186*, 2186–2187
Descemet's membrane, Kayser-Fleischer rings in, 1131
Desensitization, β-lactam in, 1434, 1435t
  penicillin in, 1434, 1435t
Desferrioxamine, 878. See also *Deferoxamine.*
Desipramine, depression treated with, 2000t, 2001
  pain control with, 106t
Desmopressin, replacement therapy using, 1208t
  von Willebrand disease treated with, 994
Desmosine, 1444

Desmosomes, 2184
Desquamation, drug toxicity causing, 1609t
  toxic shock with, staphylococcal, 1609, 1609t
Detrusor muscle, hyperreflexia of, 22
  parasympathetic control of, 2010, 2010t
  urinary incontinence and, 22
Detumescence, penile, 1320
Dexamethasone, 108t
  adverse effects of, 1046t, 1047
  aldosterone suppression test with, 1249
  allergic rhinitis treated with, 1417t
  cancer therapy using, 1046t, 1047
  21-hydroxylase deficiency treated with, 1289–1290, *1290*
  intracranial pressure reduced with, 2128, 2133t
  non-Hodgkin's lymphoma and, 945t
  pain control use of, 106t
  pharmacokinetics of, 108t
  pseudohermaphroditism therapy with, 1289–1290, *1290*
  suppression test, 1213t
    ACTH in, 1213t, 1217t, 1217–1218
    Cushing's syndrome and, 1213t, 1217t, 1217–1218
    high-dose, 1213t, 1217t, 1217–1218
    interpretation of, 1213t, 1217t, 1217–1218
    low-dose, 1213t, 1217t, 1217–1218
    overnight, 1213t, 1217t, 1217–1218
Dexpanthenol, 1172t
Dextran, *521*
Dextroamphetamine, 51, 56t
Dextrocardia, 279, *281*
Diabetes insipidus, 1223–1226
  clinical presentation of, 1223–1224
  course and prognosis in, 1226, *1226*
  definition of, 1223
  diagnosis of, 1224–1225, *1225*
  drug therapy in, 1226
  fluid loss due to, 528, 1224–1226, *1226*
  hypothalamic, 1203, 1223–1226, *1225*, *1226*
  nephrogenic, 1224, *1225*
  pregnancy with, 1224
  treatment of, 1225–1226
Diabetes mellitus, **1258–1277**
  age and, 1258–1260
  atherosclerosis and, 173, 293, 1276–1277, *1277*
  classification, 1258, 1258t, *1259*
  clinical features of, 1258–1259
  complications of, 1269–1277
    acute metabolic, 1269–1272
    control level relation to, 1264, *1264*
    late, 1272–1277
  diagnosis of, 1258–1259, 1259t
  environmental factors in, 1262, 1266t, 1266–1267
  epidemiology of, 1259–1260
  foot affected by, 1275–1276, 1276t
  gastroparesis due to, 684
  genetic factors in, 144t, 145t, *1259*, 1260, 1262, 1274
  heart affected by, 173, 359, *1277*
  HLA antigens in, 1262
  honeymoon period, 1258
  hypertension with, 268, 1276–1277, *1277*
  hypoglycemia in, 1271–1272
  increased intestinal motility in, 686
  insulin and, 1264–1266
    dependency on, *1259*, 1262
    intensive schedule, 1264, *1264*, *1266*
    nondependency on, 1262–1264, *1263*
    preparations of, 1264–1265, 1265t
    pump-delivered, 1266
    regimen for, *1264*, 1265–1266, *1266*
    resistance to, 145, 145t, 1259–1263
  ketoacidosis in, 1269–1271
    alcoholic syndrome vs., 1271
    clinical features of, 1269
    diagnosis of, 1270
    management of, 1270–1271
    pathogenesis of, 1269–1270
  laboratory tests in, 1258–1259, 1268–1269, *1269*
  lifestyle factors in, 32, 1266t, 1266–1267
  lipoprotein level and, 1269t
  malnutrition-related, 1258t, 1260
  maturity-onset of, 1258t, 1263
  metabolic defect in, 143–145, 144t, 145t, 1261–1263
  mortality rate in, 27t, 30t
  nephropathy of, 599–602, *600*, *601*, 1273–1274, *1274*
  neuropathy due to, 1274–1275, 1275t, 2154t, 2154–2155

Diabetes mellitus (Continued)
nonketotic hyperosmolar syndrome in, 1270
obesity and, 30t, 1258t, 1266t, 1266–1267
pancreatitis with, 735
pathogenesis of, 1259, 1261–1263, 1263
pathophysiology of, 1260–1261, 1261
pregnancy and, 1258, 1259
prevalence of, 1259–1260
renal failure with, 556, 562, 578, 599–602, 600, 601
retinopathy in, 1273, 2181–2182
risk factors for, 30t
screening for, 1258–1259, 1259t
secondary, 1256, 1256t
treatment of, 1264–1269, 1277
dietary, 1141, 1143t, 1266t, 1266–1267
exercise in, 1266t, 1266–1267
goals in, 1269, 1269t, 1277
insulin, 1264–1266, 1265t, 1266
intensive, 1264, 1264, 1266
oral agents in, 1267–1268, 1268t
prevention of complications by, 1264, 1264
self-monitoring of, 1268–1269
type I, 1258–1277
clinical presentation of, 1258, 1258t
pathogenesis of, 1262
type II, 1258–1277
clinical presentation of, 1258, 1258t
pathogenesis of, 1262–1264, 1263
ulcers in, 2212
weight loss for, 1266t, 1266–1267
Diacylglycerol (DAG), 1179, 1179
hormone signaling role of, 1179, 1179
phosphatidylinositol activated by, 1179, 1179
Dialysis, 563–567
amyloidosis in, 567, 1505
antimicrobial dosage affected by, 1561–1563, 1562t
complications of, 567, 567t
cost considerations for, 567
dementia due to, 567
dialysate used in, 565t, 565–566
diffusion role in, 564
equipment used in, 564, 564–565, 565
hemodialysis, 565, 565t, 566, 566t, 567t
history of development of, 563–564
pericarditis with, 337, 337t
peritoneal, 565t, 566t, 567t
poisoning and, 70–71, 504t, 509, 509t
renal failure treated with, 565–566
survival and, 567
ultrafiltration role in, 564–565, 565
Diamond-Blackfan syndrome, 833t
Diaphoresis. See Sweating.
Diaphragm, 442–443
fatigue affecting, 442
flutter of, 443
hernia affecting, 443
hiccup and, 442–443
hyperinflation affecting, 442
motion disorder of, 442–443
paradoxical motion of, 442, 466
therapeutic modalities for, 442t
Diaphysis, dysplasia of, 1387–1388
Diarrhea, 689–695
adenovirus, 1795, 1795t
AIDS/HIV with, 1867t, 1867–1868
amebic, 1913–1914
antimicrobials causing, 1568t, 1633, 1634, 1634t
bile salt, 807
Campylobacter, 1649t, 1650, 1650t, 1658t
cholera, 1653t, 1653–1654, 1654t
colitis with, pseudomembranous, 1633
cryptosporidial, 1910, 1911
developing countries and, 1795
diagnostic approach to, 693t, 693–694
drugs causing, 693t
E. coli, 1654–1657, 1655t, 1658t
enteral feeding with, 1169–1170, 1170t
functional, 687–688
gastric resection followed by, 671–672
Giardia, 1642t
giardiasis with, 694, 1642t, 1658t, 1913
malabsorption with, 699t
malarial, 1894
mixed-etiology, 692, 692t
morphologic disruption causing, 692, 692t
motility disorder with, 687–688, 691–692
Norwalk virus, 1795t, 1795–1796
osmotic, 690, 690t

Diarrhea (Continued)
pathophysiology of, 690t–693t, 690–692
protozoal, 1642t, 1658t, 1910, 1911, 1913, 1916t
rotavirus, 1642t, 1658t, 1794–1797, 1795, 1795t
secretory, 690–691, 691t, 695
Shigella, 1642t, 1647t, 1647–1648, 1658t
traveler's, 1641–1642, 1642t, 1648, 1657–1658,
1658t
treatment of, 694–695, 704t
Vibrio cholerae, 1653t, 1653–1654, 1654t
viral, 1793–1797, 1795, 1795t
yersinial, 1661
Diascopy, 2192
Diastematomyelia, 2149
Diastole, heart properties in, 174–177, 175–177
heart sounds in, 168, 168t
pressures and volumes in, 176, 176, 176t, 489t
Diazepam, antidote for, 504t
drug abuse with, 50–51, 56t
poisoning due to, 504t, 507
smoking interaction with, 36t
tension headache treated with, 2033
Diazoxide, hypertension treated with, 270t
side effects of, 270t
DIC. See Disseminated intravascular coagulation
(DIC).
Diclofenac, 773, 773t
Dicloxacillin, 1562t
streptococcal infection treated with, 1587–1589,
1589t
Dicrocoeliasis, 1932t, 1932–1933
Didanosine, 1884–1885, 1885, 1885t
activation pathways for, 1882
hepatotoxicity, 773, 773t
structure of, 1881
toxicity of, 1883t, 1885t
Dideoxyadenosine, activation pathways for, 1882
structure of, 1881
Dideoxynucleosides, 1880–1886. See also Zidovudine
(AZT).
activation pathways for, 1882
structure of, 1881
toxicity of, 1883t
Dientamoebiasis, 1916t
treatment of, 1916t
Diet, 29–31, 1139–1174. See also Nutrition.
calcium intake and, 1352, 1353–1354
cancer relation to, 1009t, 1009–1010
lung, 437
preventive compounds and, 1010, 1016–1017,
1139–1143
stomach, 676, 676t
chyme affected by, 689
diabetes mellitus and, 1141, 1143t, 1266t, 1266–1267
fiber in, 1009–1010, 1139–1143
folate (folic acid) in, 846–847
fructose in, 1083
galactose-free, 1081
gluten in, 704–705
guidelines for, 29–31, 30t, 1139–1143, 1140t, 1141t,
1142
health care role of, 29
iron in, 839–840, 1134t, 1140t, 1149t
kidney stone formation and, 616t, 616–617
magnesium intake in, 1352
mortality rate and, 29–31, 30t, 1143t
obesity treatment using, 1166
patterns and trends in, 29, 1139–1143, 1141t, 1142
phosphorus in, 1135, 1352
preventive care role of, 27, 29–31, 30t, 1139–1143,
1141t, 1143t
prostaglandin modification by, 1192
protein in, RDA for, 1140t
renal failure and, chronic, 562–563
salt-restricted, 221
vegetarian, vitamin B_{12} in, 701t, 846
very low calorie, 1166
vitamin(s) in, 1140t, 1141t
B_{12}, 701t, 845–846
K, 999
RDA for, 1140t, 1141t
Diethylcarbamazine, 1939, 1941, 1942, 1944
Diethylstilbestrol, adverse effects of, 1046t, 1047
cancer therapy using, 1046t, 1047
Dieulafoy's ulcer, 721
Diffusion, air-blood barrier and, 371–372, 374, 374–375
dialysis role of, 564
facilitated, 697
nutrient absorption and, 695–697
passive, 695–697

Diflunisal, 103t
Difluoromethylornithine, 1898–1899
DiGeorge's syndrome, 155t, 1438
chromosome abnormality in, 155, 155t, 1438
clinical features of, 155, 155t, 1438
immunodeficiency of, 1402t, 1405, 1542
thymic hypoplasia causing, 1405, 1438
Digestion, impaired, 702–703
motor complex of, 682
osmotic diarrhea related to, 690, 690t
Digitalis, 225–228
dosages for, 226t, 226–228
electrophysiologic effects of, 225
heart failure and, 221t, 225, 225–228, 226t, 227t
inotropic action of, 225, 225–226
intoxication, 504t, 508
mechanism of action of, 225, 225
pharmacokinetics of, 226t, 226–227
sensitivity to, 227, 227t
serum concentration of, 227–228
shock treated with, 493–494
toxicity of, 228
Digitoxin, 226–227
dosage for, 226t, 226–227
pharmacokinetics of, 226t, 226–227
Digit. See Finger.
Digoxin, 91t, 94t, 226, 246t
adverse effects of, 247t
antiarrhythmic action of, 245, 246t
binding of, 91t
FAB antibodies and, 504t, 508
dosage for, 91t, 94t, 226, 226t
pharmacokinetics of, 91t, 94t, 226t, 246t
Dihydropteridine reductase, 1105
deficiency of, 1106
Dihydropyrimidine dehydrogenase deficiency, 1117
Dihydrotestosterone (DHT). See also Testosterone.
ovarian, 1300
prostatic, 1341
sexual differentiation role of, 1285, 1286
testosterone metabolism and, 1328
Dihydroxymandelic acid, 1253, 1253
Dihydroxyphenylalanine (dopa), 1253
1,25-Dihydroxyvitamin D, 1357t, 1357–1358, 1358
actions of, 1354–1355, 1357–1358, 1358
bone formation role of, 1354t, 1354–1355, 1355,
1357–1358
metabolism of, 1354–1355, 1357–1358
Diiodotyrosine, 1227
Diloxanide furoate, 1915t
Diltiazem, 246t
adverse effects of, 248t, 300t
dosage for, 265t, 300t
pharmacokinetics of, 246t
Dimercaprol, lead poisoning treated with, 69, 69t
mercury poisoning treated with, 504t
Dimercaptosuccinic acid, 504t
Dimethyltryptamine, 54
Dimple sign, 2210
Dinoflagellates, 1954t, 1956
Diphenylhydramine, 1416, 1416t
Diphosphoglycerate, 869, 869
Diphtheria, 1629–1630
clinical manifestations of, 1629–1630
cutaneous, 1630
diagnosis of, 1630
etiology of, 1629
immune globulin against, 40, 41t
immunization for, 41t, 41–44, 42t, 1629–1630
pathogenesis of, 1629
Diphyllobothriasis, 1923, 1923t
Diploidy, 134
Diplopia, multiple sclerosis with, 2109, 2109t
muscle weakness with, 2159
Diptera. See Fly.
Dirofilariasis, 1945
Disability, elderly with, 18
heart failure with, 169t, 221t
lung disease with, 399–400
Disaccharidase deficiency, 704
Disc. See Intervertebral disc.
Disclosure, patient decision making and, 4
Disequilibrium, elderly affected by, 16t, 17
Disopyramide, 91t, 94t, 246t
adverse effects of, 247t
antiarrhythmic action of, 246, 246–249
dose adjustment for, 94t
pharmacokinetics of, 91t, 94t, 246t
Disorientation, 1973, 1973t, 1975t. See also Confusion.
delirium with, 1997t

Disorientation (Continued)
  left-right, 1987, 1988t
  visual, 1985, 1987t
Disseminated intravascular coagulation (DIC), 2201
  purpura with, 2201
  shock with, 487
  venom causing, 1003
Distemper, canine, 1384
  Paget's disease related to, 1384
Diuresis, diabetes insipidus and, 1223–1226, 1225, 1226
  electrolytes in, 222–225, 223, 224t
  osmotic, 528, 540
  postobstructive, 528, 528t
  renal deficit causing, 528, 528t
  solute, 528, 528t
Diuretics, acidosis and, 224t
  alkalosis and, 224t
  carbonic anhydrase inhibiting, 222, 224t
  collecting duct, 531t, 532, 532
  combination, 266t
  distal tubule, 531t, 531–532, 532
  dosages for, 264t
  heart failure treated with, 221t, 222–225, 223, 224t
  hypertension treated with, 263, 264, 264t, 266t, 267t
  loop, 222–223, 223, 224t, 264t, 531t
  osmotic, 224t, 224–225
  potassium-sparing, 223, 223–224, 224t, 264t
  proximal tubule, 531, 531t, 532
  side effects of, 224t, 225, 267t, 531t
  sites of action for, 223, 224t, 532
  sodium balance effect of, 222, 223, 224t, 532
  thiazide, 224t, 224t, 264t, 531t
  volume excess treated with, 530–532, 531t, 532
Diurnal rhythms, 1184, 1199–1200
Diverticula, 749–750, 750
  colonic, 687
  esophageal, 658
  traction, 658
Diverticulitis, 749–750
  abdominal abscess due to, 631, 631, 750
  colonic, 687, 749–750, 750
Diverticulosis, 749–750, 750
  increased motility with, 687
Diving (underwater), arterial gas embolism due to, 410
  decompression illness due to, 410, 410t
Dizziness. See also Vertigo.
  antimicrobials causing, 1568t
  elderly affected by, 17
  evaluation of, 2025, 2025–2027, 2026
  nonvestibular, 2025t
  vestibular, 2025t
DNA (deoxyribonucleic acid), 134–136, 1074
  antibodies to, 1457t, 1476t
  cell-surface receptor for, 149–150, 150
  chemotherapy effect on, 1041–1046
    repair of, 1058–1059
  chromatin, 134–136, 135, 136
  conjugated, 150
  genetic code in, 134t, 134–136, 136
  hormone receptor binding of, 1180–1181, 1181
  muscle mitochondrial, 2160t, 2167
  noncoding, 134
  plasmid, 150
  radiation damage to, 60–61
  recognition elements of, 1180–1181, 1181
  spacing rules for, 1180–1181, 1181
  structure of, 1073–1074, 1074
  thalassemia and, 880–881
  triplex, 1073–1074, 1074
  viral, 1739, 1739–1740, 1740t
    hepatitis, 763t, 763–769, 764t, 765, 768
    herpes simplex, 1771
    HIV, 1838, 1842–1844, 1842–1844, 1884t
  zinc "fingers" and, 1180–1181, 1181
DNA probe, Legionella infection and, 1584t
  malarial plasmodium in, 1895
Dobutamine, 492t, 493
Dog, distemper in, 1384
  ehrlichiosis carried by, 1727t
  filariae of, 1945
  hookworm affecting, 1937
  rabies in, 2096
  rickettsiosis carried by, 1727t
  zoonoses associated with, 1727t, 1737t, 1737–1738, 1738t
Döhle bodies, 916, 918
Domains, DNA, 1180–1181, 1181

Domains (Continued)
  receptor, 1177–1181
  SH3, 1180, 1180
Donath-Landsteiner cold hemolysin, 863
Do-not-resuscitate order, 465
Donovanosis (granuloma inguinale), 1703–1704
Dopa (dihydroxyphenylalanine), 1253
L-Dopa, growth hormone test using, 1208t
  Parkinson's disease and, 2044–2046, 2045
Dopamine, anaphylaxis treated with, 1419
  Parkinson's disease and, 2044–2045
  shock treated with, 492t, 493
Dopamine-β-hydroxylase, 1253
Doppler studies, continuous wave, 198–199, 199
  echocardiographic, 197–199, 198–199
  principles of, 197–199, 198–199
  pulsed wave, 198, 198–199
Dorsal root, herpes simplex virus in, 1770, 1771, 1772
  paraneoplastic effects in, 1027t, 1029
Double duct sign, 637
Dowager's hump, 1381, 1381
Doxazosin, 265t
Doxorubicin, adverse effects of, 1044
  cardiotoxicity of, 330–331, 358
  chemotherapy using, 1039t, 1044, 1044t
  Hodgkin's disease and, 952t, 953
  Kaposi's sarcoma treated with, 1873, 1873t
  non-Hodgkin's lymphoma and, 945t
  resistance to, 1057t
Doxycycline, 1562t
  brucellosis therapy with, 1679t, 1680
  gonorrhea therapy with, 1702t
  Legionella and, 1585, 1585t
  leptospirosis therapy with, 1721
  Lyme disease therapy with, 1719, 1719t
  malaria therapy with, 1895t, 1895–1896
  Rocky Mountain spotted fever and, 1732
Dracunculiasis, 1944
Dressings, dry, 2193–2194
  occlusive, 2194
  open, 2193
  wet, 2194t
    skin treated with, 2193–2194, 2194t
Dressler's syndrome, 337, 337t
Drive(s), 1187, 1187t
  endorphin role in, 1187, 1187t
  hunger, 629
    bulimia and, 1160
    definition of, 629
  sex, 1308, 1328, 1330
  thirst. See Thirst.
Drop spells, 1982
Drowning, 408–409
  clinical features in, 408
  mortality rate in, 37, 38
  sequelae of, 409
  treatment for, 408
  wet vs. dry, 408
Drowsiness, alcohol-related, 47, 48t
  hepatic encephalopathy with, 798t
  opiate causing, 1975t
Drugs, 89–100, 2230t–2233t. See also specific drugs, and types of drugs.
  absorption of, 89, 89
    first-pass, 89
  abuse of, 49–56
    adulterants and, 52
    anticholinergics in, 54–55, 56t
    cannabis in, 53–54, 56t
    disease transmission in, 52, 1852
    endocarditis with, 1597t, 1598t, 1600, 1608t
    hallucinogens in, 54, 56t
    hepatitis transmission and, 764, 765–766
    HIV transmission in, 1852
    inhalants in, 55, 56t
    nicotine in, 55, 56t
    opioids in, 51–53, 56t
    recognition of, 50
    sedatives in, 50–51, 56t
    stimulants in, 51, 56t
    stroke related to, 2067t, 2069
    synthetics (designer drugs) in, 55
    treatment of, 50–56, 56t
  accumulation of, 91–92, 92
    metabolic inhibition causing, 96
  administration route for, 89
  adverse reaction(s) to, 97–100, 98t–99t, 1432–1435, 1568t
    allergic, 98–100, 1422t, 1432t–1435t, 1432–1435, 1568t

Drugs (Continued)
  anaphylactic, 98t, 100, 1418t, 1433t, 1568t
  aplastic anemia as, 824t, 832t, 832–833
  cephalosporins in, 1568t
  cerebrovascular disease as, 2067t, 2069
  cholestasis as, 773, 773t, 774–775, 810
  colitis as, pseudomembranous, 1633–1635, 1634, 1634t
  coma as, 1974–1976, 1975t
  dermatological, 98t, 99t, 1409, 1568t
  diagnosis of, 100
  diarrheal, 693t
  epidemiology of, 97
  etiology of, 97–100, 1568t
  exaggerated response in, 97t, 97–98
  febrile, 98t, 1568t
  genetics and, 97t, 97–98
  G6PD deficiency and, 98–100, 858, 858t, 1568t
  gynecomastia in, 1332
  hepatitis as, 772–775, 773t, 799t
  hyperprolactinemia as, 1202t
  immune complex formation in, 1422
  immunologic mechanisms of, 98t, 98–100, 99t
  interstitial lung disease as, 396–397, 397t
  lupoid, 98t
  methemoglobinemia in, 98–100, 876t, 876–877
  myopathy in, 2160
  neurologic, 1974–1976, 1975t
  neutropenia as, 909, 911t, 1568t
  ocular, 2183, 2183t
  penicillin in, 1418t, 1418–1419, 1568t
  rash in, 98t, 1409, 1568t
  serum sickness and, 98t, 1568t
  toxic response in, 98
  urticarial, 1409
  antiandrogen, 1046t, 1047, 1316
  antianxiety, 20, 21t
  antiarrhythmic. See Antiarrhythmic agents.
  anticancer. See Chemotherapy.
  anticoagulant. See Anticoagulants.
  antidepressant. See Antidepressants.
  antiepileptic, 2121–2123, 2122t
  antiestrogen, 1046t, 1047, 1059–1060
  antifungal, 1815–1816, 1816t, 2196t, 2196–2197
  antiglucose, oral, 1267–1268, 1268t
  antigranuloma, 1497t, 1497–1498
  antimicrobial. See Antimicrobials.
  antiparasitic, 704t, 1935t, 2195
  antipsychotic. See Neuroleptics.
  antipyretic, 111–115, 113, 115t
  antirheumatic, slow-acting, 1472
  antithyroid, 1234, 1234t
    pregnancy and, 1236
    thyrotoxic crisis and, 1236t
  antituberculous, 1562t, 1686t, 1686–1690, 1687t
  antiviral, 1742–1747, 1746t, 1880–1887
  binding of, 91t, 93–94
  bioavailability of, 89
  carcinogenicity of, 1016, 1016t
  cardiovascular, 397, 397t
  continuous infusion of, 92, 92
  decreasing dose of, 92
  designer, 54, 55
  distribution of, 89, 89–90, 90
    volume of, 90, 91t
  dose adjustment of, 94t, 94–95
    hepatic function and, 94t, 94–95, 1561–1563, 1562t
    renal function and, 94t, 94–95, 1561–1563, 1562t
  dose-response curve for, 93, 93
  efficacy curve for, 93
  elderly patient and, 95–96
  elimination of, 90, 90–91, 92, 94t
    clearance in, 90, 90, 91t
    dose-dependent, 90, 92–93, 93
    first-order, 90
    genetic factors and, 97t, 97–98
    hepatic, 89, 90, 94t
    renal, 90, 94t
    zero-order, 93, 93
  explained to patient, 77
  first-pass effect on, 89
  genetic factors and, 97t, 97–98
  half-life of, 90, 90–91, 91t, 92, 94t, 1562t
  hemodynamic disease affecting, 95
  increasing dose of, 92–93, 93
  interactions of, 96–97, 97t
    absorption affected by, 96

Drugs (Continued)
antimicrobials in, 1563t
decreased excretion in, 96
diagnosis of, 97
distribution alterations in, 96
metabolism interference by, 96
pharmacodynamic, 96–97
pharmacokinetic, 96
prevention of, 97, 97t
intestine motility affected by, 681t, 688, 688t
kidney disease affecting metabolism/elimination of, 94t, 94–95, 1561–1563, 1562t
liver disease affecting metabolism/elimination of, 95, 1561–1563, 1562t
loading dose of, 91, 91t
maintenance dose of, 92, 92
nephritis due to, 581, 581–583, 582t, 1568t
nephrotoxic, 582t, 584t, 584–589, 1568t
obesity treatment using, 1166
oral contraceptive, 1309–1311
porphyria role of, 1127, 1127t
psychedelic, 53–54, 56t, 1975t
psychiatric treatment using, 1999, 1999t, 2000t, 2000–2001
resistance to, bacterial, 1550, 1558–1560, 1569t
chemotherapy affected by, 1056–1060, 1057t, 1058t
smoking interaction with, 35, 36t
steady-state levels of, 92, 92
therapeutic index of, 93, 93, 97t
therapeutic range of, 91t, 93, 93
thermoregulation impairment by, 502, 502t
topical preparations of, 2194t, 2194–2196, 2195t
toxicity curve for, 93, 93
trough level of, 92, 93
Drusen, optic nerve, 2177
Dryness, ophthalmic. See Eye, dry.
oral, 649, 649t, 1488, 1488t, 1489
DTIC, 952t. See also Dacarbazine.
Duchenne dystrophy, 2161
genetics of, 138t, 2160t
heart affected by, 359
Ductus arteriosus, calcification in, 279, 280
patent, 279, 280
Dumping syndrome, 671–672, 683
Duncan's disease, 1405
Duodenum, absorption in, 689, 689–690, 690t
bile absorption in, 806
bleeding from, 642t, 644, 645t
carcinoma of, 679–680
endoscopy of, 636–639, 638t
inflammation of, Helicobacter causing, 663
manometry of, 685
motility of, 682, 682, 683, 685
pain from, 628–629, 665–666
ulcer of, **662–676**
bleeding from, 642t, 643, 645t, 665, 673
clinical features of, 665t, 665–666
diagnosis of, 665t, 666, 666t
incidence of, 664–665, 665
medical treatment of, 667, 667t, 667–669, 668t
pain due to, 665t, 665–666
Duplication, urinary tract, 622, 622
Dura mater, metastatic disease of, 2130
spinal cord tumor and, 2146, 2146–2148
Dust(s), 58t, 399t, 399–403, 402t
asbestos, 399t, 400–401, 1016
aspergillosis organism in, 1830
beryllium, 402t, 402–403
carcinogenicity of, 1016t
coal, 399t, 401, 1016t
cobalt, 399t
cotton, 59t
interstitial lung disease and, 391, 391t, 399–403
lung affected by, 372–373, 399
occupational exposure to, 56, 58t, 59t, 399t, 399–403, 1016t
particle size of, 399
silica, 399t, 401–402, 402t
talc, 399t
Dwarfism, growth hormone deficiency in, 147t, 1210–1211
immunodeficiency with, 1407
iodine deficiency in, 1149t
Laron, 145, 1210
metabolic disorders causing, 145, 147t
proportionate, 145
treatment of, 1211

Dyes. See also Stains.
food, 1409
Gram reaction to, 1556–1557, 1557t
occupational exposure to, 58t
urticaria due to, 1409
Dying. See Death and dying.
Dynein, 1336
Dynorphins, 1186, 1186–1187
Dysarthria, 1989, 1989t, 2159
Dysautonomia, **2007–2013**
central, 2007t
genetics of, 136t
paraspinal tumor causing, 2008–2009
peripheral, 2007t, 2008t
regional, 2008–2009
spinal cord injury with, 2140, 2143t
widespread, 2007–2008
Dysbetalipoproteinemia, 1090–1091
Dyschondroplasia, 1390
Dysentery, amebic, 1913t, 1913–1914
bacillary, 1642t, 1647t, 1647–1648
E. coli, 1654–1657, 1655t
Shigella, 1642t, 1647t, 1647–1648
Dysfibrinogenemia, 996
Dysgerminoma, 1312t
suprasellar, 1201, 1202
Dyskinesia, biliary, 816, 816t
neuroleptic drug causing, 1009, 2050
tardive, 1009, 2050
Dyslexia, stroke with, 2065
Dysmenorrhea, 1301
Dysmetria, ocular, 2020
Dysmorphology. See also Genetics; Hereditary disorder(s).
definition of, 154
Dyspareunia, 1308
aging and, 13
chlamydial salpingitis with, 1724
Dyspepsia, lupus erythematosus with, 1479
nonulcer, 665t, 665–666
peptic ulcer with, 665t, 665–666
Dysphagia, 650
esophageal disorder with, 650, 651, 655, 657
iron deficiency causing, 841
lupus erythematosus with, 1479
muscle weakness with, 2159
muscular dystrophy with, 2162–2163
patient description of, 650
reflux disease with, 651
stomach cancer with, 677
stricture causing, 652
transfer, 650, 655
Dysphasia, 1991. See also Aphasia.
Dyspnea, 217, 370
anemia with, 823–824
angina pectoris with, 296–297
asthma with, 378
bronchitis with, 382t, 386
diaphragmatic paralysis and, 442
embolism causing, pulmonary, 423, 424t
grading of, 400
heart failure with, 217, 219
lung disease with, 370, 370, 378
interstitial, 391
occupational, 400
paroxysmal nocturnal, 217
Dysproteinemia, 958–968. See also Multiple myeloma.
Dysthymic disorder, 2001t, 2001–2002
Dystonia, 2043, 2047–2049
basal ganglia relation to, 2043
classification of, 2047
clonic, 2043, 2047, 2049
definition of, 2047
manifestations of, 2043, 2047, 2047–2048, 2048
multiple sclerosis with, 2109, 2110
pathogenesis of, 2047–2048
tardive, 2048, 2048, 2050t
treatment of, 2048
Dystrophy, muscle. See Muscular dystrophy.
reflex sympathetic, 2009, 2036
Dysuria, cystitis causing, 1698–1699

E

E. coli. See Escherichia coli.
EABV (effective arterial blood volume), 511, 514
Ear, aging effects in, 17
hair follicles of, 2186, 2187
infections of. See Otitis.

Ear (Continued)
pain from, 2035
Bell's palsy with, 2035
polychondritis affecting, 1517
respiratory tract disorders and, 449–450, 450t
tophi of, 1516, 2211
wax impaction in, 2021
Eating. See also Postprandial state.
disorders of, 1156–1160, 1159t
anorexic. See Anorexia.
bulimic. See Bulimia.
pica in, 66, 840
energy expenditure following, 1163
hypothalamic control of, 1165, 2012–2013
metabolic effects of, 1163
obesity etiology and, 1163, 2012–2013
thermogenesis elevation by, 1163
Eaton-Lambert syndrome, 1018, 2173
diagnosis of, 1018, 2173
pathophysiology, 1018, 1028
treatment of, 1018, 2173
Ebola virus, 1728t
African hemorrhagic fever due to, 1798t, 1803–1804
Ebstein's anomaly, 281, 282
Eburnation, 1518
EBV. See Epstein-Barr virus (EBV)/EBV infection.
Ecchymoses, 2201
meningitis with, 1612
pancreatitis with, 731
platelet defects and, 979t
Eccrine glands, 2185, 2186
ECG. See Electrocardiography (ECG).
Echinococcosis, 1923t, 1924–1925
hepatic, 782, 783t, 784
Echinocytes, 825t
Echinostomiasis, 1932t, 1933
Echocardiography, **194–199**
Doppler signal in, 198, 198–199, 199
transducer position in, 194–196, 195, 196
Echolalia, 2049
Echovirus, 1784, 1784t, 1787t
characteristics of, 1783–1785, 1784t
colds (common) due to, 1747, 1747t
syndromes associated with, 1786–1792, 1787t
Economic issues, medical, 9–11, 10t
Ecstasy (drug), 54
Ecthyma gangrenosum, 2212
Ectoparasites. See also Arthropods; Louse; Mite.
sexual transmission of, 1697t
Ectopy, urinary tract, 622, 622
Eczema, 2197–2199
allergic, 2197–2198, 2198t
atopic, 2198–2199
craquelé, 2199
dermatophytic, 2198t, 2199–2200
drug-induced, 2198t, 2219t
dyshidrotic, 2184t, 2199
hand, 2184t, 2199
incidence of, 2184t
nummular, 2199
pruritus of, 2197–2198, 2198t
spongiosis, 2197
types of, 2184t, 2197, 2198t
vaccinatum, 1768
Wiskott-Aldrich syndrome with, 1407
xerotic, 2199
Edema, 167
airway, anaphylaxis with, 1418
angioneurotic. See Angioedema.
brain tumor causing, 2126, 2128, 2128
bronchitis with, 387
cerebral, 2063, 2075
high altitude causing, 409t, 409–410
heart failure with, 217–218, 219–220
kidney and, 530t, 530–532
lymphatic obstruction causing, 357
macular, diabetes mellitus with, 1273
nephrotic syndrome with, 573
nonpitting, myxedema with, 1237
optic disk, 2016–2017, 2177
pulmonary, 221–222
acute, 221t, 221–222
cardiogenic vs. noncardiogenic, 455, 456t
fluid restriction in, 476, 477
heart failure with, 217–218, 221–222
high altitude causing, 409t, 409–410
malaria causing, 1894
respiratory distress and, 476–477, 477
respiratory failure and, 455, 456t

Edema (Continued)
  roentgenography of, 187, 187–188, 188
    treatment of, 221t, 221–222
    ventilation therapy and, 476, 477
  renal failure with, 554t, 554–555
  Starling forces in, 530t, 530–532
  volume regulation mechanisms in, 530t, 530–531
  water and, 530t, 530–532
Edinger-Westphal nucleus, 2017
Edrophonium anticholinesterase test, 2172
EDTA (ethylenediamine tetraacetic acid), iron chelation
    by, 1135
  lead poisoning treated with, 69, 69t
EET (epoxy-eicosatrienoic acid), 1191, 1191
Effective arterial blood volume (EABV), 511
  renal function related to, 511, 514
Effective refractory period (ERP), 232
Efficacy, medical, 82
Effusions, pericardial. See under Pericardium.
  pleural. See under Pleura.
Eflornithine, 1899
Eggs, dietary aspects of, 1142, 1147t, 1357
  raw whites of, biotin deficiency caused by, 1147t
  yolks of, vitamin D in, 1357
Ehlers-Danlos syndrome, 1120–1122
  aortic rupture in, 342, 1121, 1121t
  clinical features of, 1120–1121, 1121t, 2201
  definition of, 1120
  differential diagnosis of, 1121
  etiology of, 1120
  genetics in, 1120–1121, 1121t
  molecular defects in, 1121t
  pathogenesis of, 1120, 1147
  pathology in, 1120, 2201
  prevalence of, 1120
  prognosis in, 1122
  skin affected by, 1120–1121, 1121t, 2201
  treatment of, 1121–1122
  types of, 1121, 1121t
Ehrlichiosis, 1727t, 1728t, 1733, 1738t
Eicosanoids, 1190, 1190–1191
Eisenmenger's complex, 286, 287
Eisenmenger's reaction, 275
Ejaculation, 1328–1329
  dysfunctional, 1331–1332
  premature, 1328–1329, 1332
  retrograde, 1331t, 1332
  spermatogenesis evaluation and, 1327, 1328
Ejection fraction, 176t, 177
  cardiomyopathy affecting, 328t
  MRI of, 208
  radionuclide studies of, 200, 200
  septic shock affecting, 498, 499t
ELAM, leukocyte adhesiveness and, 898
Elastin, 1444
  collagen fibrils with, 1352, 2186
  dermal, 2186
  pseudoxanthoma affecting, 1123, 1123–1124
Elbow, golfer's, 1528
  tennis, 1527–1528
Elderly, 12–25. See also Age; Lifespan.
  decision making by, 24–25
  dementia in, 18–19, 19t, 1993–1994
  depression in, 18–20, 19t, 20t, 1999–2000
  drug kinetics in, 95–96
  falls and fractures in, 16, 23, 1380
  health problems of, 16–25
  hypertension in, 268
  kidney function decline in, 12, 12
  lifespan of, 12, 12, 14
  malabsorption in, 706
  mortality rate in, 26–27, 27, 27t
  neurologic disorders of, 16t, 16–17, 17t
  pharmacology in, 17t, 20, 20t, 21t, 21–22, 95–96
  population increase in, 12, 12–13
  psychiatric disorders in, 17–21, 19t, 20t, 1999–
    2000
Electrical injury, 64–67
  cardiopulmonary effects of, 65, 66
  effects of, 65–66
  kidney affected by, 66
  late complications of, 67
  mechanisms of, 64–65
  natural history of, 64–65
  pathogenesis of, 64–65
  source of, 64–65
  treatment of, 66–67
  voltage level in, 64–65
  wound due to, 65, 65–67, 66

Electrocardiography (ECG), 188–193. See also Electro-
    physiology (cardiac).
  ambulatory (Holter monitor), 235, 235, 236t
  analysis process for, 193, 193t, 194
  cardiac cycle in, 189, 190, 192–194
  jugular pulse related to, 167
  leads in, 188t, 188–189, 189
    axis deviation and, 189, 189
    body positions for, 188, 188–189, 189
    frontal plane axes of, 189, 189
    monitor, 189
    precordial, 188, 188t
    record from, 189, 190
  recommended frequency for, 28t
  sensitivity and specificity of, 193t
  ventricular hypertrophy in, 193, 193t, 194
Electroencephalography, 1960, 1960–1961
  abnormalities of, 1960, 1960–1961
  anoxia effects in, 2063
  CNS examination with, 1960, 1960–1961
  epilepsy in, 1960, 1960–1961
  normal pattern in, 1960, 1960
  paroxysmal activity in, 1961
Electrogram, cardiac cycle in, 231–232, 232
  high right atrial, 236
  His bundle, 236
  intracardiac recording of, 235–236, 236
Electrolytes, 525–551. See also Bicarbonate; Calcium;
    Chloride; Magnesium; Potassium; Sodium.
  AIDS/HIV effect on, 1875
  bile content of, 805, 805
  cholera affecting, 1653t, 1653–1654
  chronic renal failure and, 556–557, 561
  cystic fibrosis affecting, 419, 419–420, 420
  diuretic effect on, 222–225, 223, 224t
  elderly and, 23
  intestinal transport of, 689, 689–690
  urinary, 514, 514t, 515
Electromagnetic field (EMF), exposure to, 64
  low-frequency, 64
Electromagnetic spectrum, 59
Electromyography, 1961–1962, 1962t
  CNS examination with, 1961–1962, 1962t
  inflammatory myopathy in, 1500t, 1502
  myasthenia gravis in, 2172
Electrophoresis, monoclonal proteins in, 958, 959
Electrophysiology (cardiac), 189–193, 231–233
  abnormalities of, 233t, 233–234, 234. See also
    Arrhythmia(s); specific disturbances.
  afterdepolarization in, 234, 234
    delayed, 234, 234
    early, 234, 234
  anatomic aspects of, 191, 231, 232
  automaticity in, 233
  fundamentals of, 232, 232–233, 233t
  intracardiac recording of, 235–236, 236, 236t
  reentry phenomenon in, 234, 234
  sudden death related to, 254t, 255–256
  triggered activity in, 233–234, 234
ELISA test, chlamydial infection diagnosis with, 1724
  Lyme disease in, 1717–1718, 1718
  rotavirus in, 1796
  varicella in, 1764
Elliptocytosis, clinical features of, 855t
  disorders associated with, 825t
  hereditary, 854–855, 855t
  pathogenesis of, 854–855
  spherocytic, 855, 855t
Embden-Meyerhof pathway, 855–856, 856
Embolism, air, 410, 2069
  arterial, extremities affected by, 352–353
  gas, 410
    heart origin of, 352
    sudden occlusion due to, 352–353
    treatment of, 353
  cardiac source of, 2066–2067, 2067t
  cerebrovascular disease due to, 2066–2067t
  cholesterol crystal, 606t, 607
  coronary, 302, 302t
    infarction due to, 302, 302t
    thrombolytic therapy for, 310–311, 311, 312t
  diver's, 410
  endocarditis causing, 1599–1600, 2067
  fat, 430, 2069
  formation mechanisms of, 1598–1599, 1599
  paradoxical, 352
    congenital heart disease and, 289, 289
    filter prevention of, 289, 289
    stroke due to, 2067

Embolism (Continued)
  pulmonary, 422–429
    angiography of, 425, 425t, 426, 426
    anticoagulants and, 118t, 118–119, 427, 427t,
      427–428
    clinical features of, 273t, 423–424, 424t
    cor pulmonale and, 423
    definition of, 422
    diagnosis of, 273t, 424t, 424–426
    dyspnea in, 423, 424, 424t
    hypertension due to, 273t, 274, 275, 423
    incidence of, 423
    laboratory studies in, 424–426
    pathogenesis of, 422t, 422–423
    pathology in, 423
    prevention of, 429, 429t
    prognosis in, 429
    radionuclide studies in, 425, 425t, 425–426,
      426
    risk factors for, 422t
    surgical approach to, 428–429
    therapeutic approach to, 426–429, 427, 427t
    thrombolytic agents and, 116, 118, 118t, 427, 428,
      428t
    venous thrombosis causing, 354
  renal arteries affected by, 606t, 606–607
Emergency care. See Critical care.
Emery-Dreifuss dystrophy, 2160t, 2162
Emesis. See Vomiting.
Emetine, myopathy caused by, 2160
Emetropia, 2174
Emotion, seizure-associated, 2116
  temporal lobe damage and, 1987t
Emphysema, 381–389
  airway obstruction in, complete, 388, 389
    partial, 388, 389
  pathophysiology of, 382, 383
    subcarinal, 388, 389
    supracarinal, 388, 388
  alpha₁-antitrypsin deficiency in, 385
  bullae of, 389–390
  chronic, 381–389
  clinical features of, 381–383, 382t, 383, 386
  cor pulmonale with, 382t, 387
  differential diagnosis of, 386
  dyspnea in, 382t, 386
  function tests in, 382, 382t, 383
  pathogenesis of, 383, 385
  pathology in, 383, 385–386
  prevalence of, 383, 385
  prognosis in, 386
  smoking and, 383, 385
  sputum and, 382t, 383, 386
Empty sella syndrome, 2133
Empyema, 2084
  pleural effusion and, 445, 445t
  pneumococcal pneumonia with, 1571, 1573, 1575
  Pseudomonas pneumonia with, 1581
  subdural, 2084
Enalapril, dosage for, 229t, 265t, 266t
  vasodilatation using, 229t, 229–230
Enanthem, 1787t, 1790
Encephalitis. See also Meningoencephalitis.
  amebiasis causing, 1915
  arbovirus, 1806t, 1810t, 1810–1814, 2089, 2089t
  California, 1806t, 1810t, 1813
  cysticercal, 1926
  eastern equine, 1806t, 1810t, 1811–1812
  enterovirus, 1787, 1787t, 2088–2089, 2089t
  hemorrhagic fever with, 1798t, 1806t
  herpes B, animal carriers of, 1737t
  herpes simplex in, 1773, 1773, 2089, 2089t,
    2092–2093, 2093
    treatment of, 1746t, 2093
  Japanese, 1806t, 1810t, 1813–1814
    immunization for, 42t, 46, 1554, 1554t
  LaCrosse, 1806t
  Louping ill, 1806t, 1814
  measles, 1760, 2089, 2089t, 2100
  mosquito-borne, 1737t, 1738t, 1805t, 1806t,
    1810–1814, 2089
  mumps with, 1769, 2089, 2089t
  Murray Valley, 1806t, 1814
  mycoplasmal infection with, 1577
  Powassan, 1806t, 1814
  rabies, 1737t, 2095–2096
  Rocio, 1806t, 1814

Encephalitis (Continued)
  rubella, 1762, 2089, 2089t
    progressive, 2097t, 2100
  St. Louis, 1806t, 1810t, 1812–1813
  tick-borne, 1806t, 1810t, 1814
  varicella-zoster, 1764, 2089t, 2093–2095
  Venezuelan equine, 1806t, 1810t, 1812, 2089
  viral, 1798t, 1810–1814, 2087–2103. See also
      specific types.
    definition of, 2088
    differential diagnosis of, 1810t, 1810–1811, 2090
    etiologic agents in, 1806t, 1810, 2088t,
        2088–2089, 2089t
    pathogenesis of, 1810, 2089, 2089t
    prognosis in, 2090
    treatment of, 2090
  western equine, 1806t, 1810t, 1811
Encephalomyelitis, 2103–2105
  allergic experimental, 2104
  clinical features of, 2104–2105
  disseminated, 2103–2105, 2104t
  measles with, 1760
Encephalopathy, AIDS/HIV with, 1856t, 1857, 1857t,
    2097–2099, 2098, 2098t
  amnesia of, 1990, 1990t
  EEG patterns in, 1960, 1960–1961
  hepatic, 797–800
    acute, 798–800
    ammonia role in, 754, 797, 797t
    chronic, 800
    clinical features of, 797–798, 798t
    definition, 797
    diagnosis of, 798, 798t, 800
    history taking and, 752
    pathogenesis of, 797, 797t
    predisposing factors, 798t
    prognosis in, 799, 800, 800t
    treatment of, 798–800, 799t
  hypoxia causing, 2062t, 2062–2063
  metabolic, 1972t, 1972–1974, 1973t
  necrotizing hemorrhagic, 2105
  paraneoplastic, 1017–1018, 1027t, 1027–1030,
      1029t
  postanoxic, 1990, 1990t
  progressive multifocal leukoencephalopathy, 2101,
      2101
  radiation injury causing, 1029t, 1029–1030
  Reye syndrome with, 2105
  stages of, 798t
  toxic, 1972t, 1975t
  Wernicke-Korsakoff, 1990, 1990t, 2039, 2039t
Enchondromatosis, 1390
Endarterectomy, carotid, 2070–2071, 2071t
End-diastolic pressure, 214, 214
End-diastolic volume, 176, 176t, 177, 214, 214
Endocarditis, 1596–1605
  AIDS/HIV patient with, 329t, 1876–1877, 1877t
  antibiotic therapy in, 1602t–1604t, 1602–1603
  aspergillosis causing, 1831
  candidal, 1829
  clinical manifestations of, 1599–1600
  congenital heart disease with, 284, 285, 1597t
  diagnosis of, 1600t, 1600–1602, 1601t
  drug abuse and, 1597t, 1598t, 1600, 1608t
  emboli arising in, 1599–1600, 2067, 2084
  enterococcal, 1598t, 1598–1599, 1601t
  fungal, 1598t, 1598–1599, 1877t
  glomerulonephritis with, 576
  Haemophilus, 1598t, 1598–1599, 1623
  infective, 1596–1605, 1877t
  Libman-Sacks, 1479, 1597
  Löffler's, cardiomyopathy due to, 333t, 334
  lupus erythematosus with, 1479, 1597
  marantic, 1597
  nonbacterial thrombotic, 1596–1598, 1597, 1597t,
      1598
  nosocomial, 1600–1602
  organisms causing, 1598t, 1598–1599, 1877t
  pathogenesis of, 1596–1599, 1597, 1598t, 1599
  pneumococcal, 1571, 1571t
  prevention of, 1597t, 1598t, 1605
  prosthetic valve with, 1597t, 1597–1598, 1598t, 1602
  Pseudomonas, 1598t, 1598–1599, 1669
  Q fever with, 1736
  right-sided, 1599
  risk factors for, 1597t, 1598t, 1605
  staphylococcal, 1598t, 1601t, 1603t, 1604t, 1608,
      1608t, 1610

Endocarditis (Continued)
  streptococcal, 1589t, 1589–1590, 1598t, 1601t, 1603t,
      1604t
  surgical approach in, 1603–1605, 1604t
  treatment of, 1602t–1604t, 1602–1605
    inadequate response to, 1604t, 1605
    outcome factors for, 1604t, 1605
Endocardium, electrical stimulation of, 235–236, 236,
    236t
Endocrine system, 1176–1350. See also specific gland,
    hormone, and disorder.
  adrenal cortex in, 1245–1246, 1246
  adrenal medulla in, 1253, 1253–1254
  AIDS/HIV effects in, 1438, 1877–1878
  anorexia nervosa and, 1158–1159, 1159t
  arthritis and, 1525–1526
  assessment of function of, 1184–1185
  cancer therapy related to, 1046t, 1046–1047
  deficiency states, 1185
  diabetes mellitus and, 1258–1277
  excess states related to, 1185
  feedback mechanisms of, 1183, 1183–1184, 1198,
      1199–1200
  hypogonadism and, 1202, 1329–1340
  hypothalamus role in, 1183, 1183–1184, 1197,
      1197–1203, 1198
  mechanisms of action in, 1176–1181, 1176–1181
  molecular biology of, 1176–1181, 1176–1181
  myopathy and, 2167–2168
  neoplasia affecting, gastrinoma, 1346
    hyperparathyroidism due to, 1346
    McCune-Albright syndrome with, 1347
    multiple, 1345–1347
      type 1, 1346
      type 2, 1346–1347
    nonendocrine, 1024–1026, 1025t, 1345–1347
    pheochromocytoma, 1346–1347
    pituitary adenoma, 1346
  nervous system interface with, 1197, 1197–1203,
      1198
  ovaries in, 1293, 1293–1301, 1294, 1298
  pineal gland in, 1204, 1204–1205
  pituitary gland and, 1183, 1183–1184, 1197,
      1205–1226
  polyglandular autoimmune syndrome of, 1250–1251,
      1251t, 1347t, 1347–1348
  principles of, 1176–1185
  protein-energy malnutrition and, 1155
  regulation of, 1183, 1183–1184
  sex differentiation and, 1284–1293
  testes in, 1284–1293, 1286, 1325–1329, 1326
  thyroid gland in, 1227, 1227–1230
  vitamin D effects in, 1357–1358, 1358
Endocytosis, thyrocyte, 1227
Endometriosis, 1301
Endometritis, chlamydial, 1724
Endometrium, menstrual cycle and, 1294, 1297–1299,
    1298
  tissue sample of, cancer screening with, 1006t
Endoplasmic reticulum, 1182
Endorphins, 1186–1187
  distribution of, 1186–1187, 1187t
  families of, 1186, 1186
  precursors of, 1186, 1186
  receptors for, 1187
  structure of, 1186, 1186
Endoscopy, cholangiopancreatographic, 632, 633
  gastrointestinal tract, 636–641, 638t
    indications for, 638t
    lower, 638t, 639–641
    upper, 636–639, 638t
  laparoscopic, 641
Endospores, 1557t
Endosteum, 1388
Endothelin, fluid exchange role of, 526t, 526–527, 533
  vasoconstriction due to, 526t, 526–527
Endothelium, alveolar, 371–372, 372
  angioedema affecting, 1409t, 1409–1410
  fat droplet damage to, 430
  glomerular, 519–520, 520
  hepatic, 789
  vascular, arachidonic acid metabolites and, 1188,
      1190
    atherosclerotic lesion in, 292, 292–295, 295
    coagulation role of, 977, 977, 978
    hematopoiesis role of, 818, 820t, 821
    hypertension effect on, 258, 259
    injury to, 295
      respiratory distress syndrome due to, 454–455,
          455

Endothelium (Continued)
  phagocyte migration through, 899
  vasoconstrictor peptides of, 526t, 526–527
  volume regulation role of, 526t, 526–527
Endothelium-derived relaxing factor, 498
  coronary blood flow and, 179
  sepsis and, 498
Endotoxins, 497, 1556–1557
  bacterial, 1556, 1556–1557
  inhibition of, 501
  morphology and, 1556, 1556–1557
  septic shock mediated by, 497, 498, 501
End-systolic pressure, 176, 176t, 177
End-systolic volume, 176, 176t, 177
Energy, deficiency of, 1154–1157
  pathogenesis of, 1154t, 1154–1155
  physiologic consequences of, 1155t, 1155–1156,
      1156t
  expenditure of, 1154
    obesity affecting, 1162–1163
    postprandial, 1163
    resting metabolic rate of, 1162–1163
    thermoregulation role in, 1533
    total (TEE), 1154
  fed-fasting states and, 1278, 1278t
  nutrition and, 1154t, 1154–1155
  protein intake and, 1154
  requirements for, 1154
    parenteral nutrition and, 1173, 1173t
Engelmann-Camurati disease, 1388t, 1398–1388
Enhancers, gene transcription and, 135
Enkephalins, 1186, 1186–1187
  distribution of, 1186
  receptors for, 1187
Entamoeba histolytica. See Amebiasis.
Entamoeba polecki, 1916t
  therapy for, 1916t
Enteric fever, 1644, 1645, 1646
  paratyphoid. See Salmonella infections.
  typhoid. See Typhoid fever.
Enteric nervous system, 681, 681, 681t, 2010
Enteritis, 1641–1642
  Campylobacter, 1649t, 1649–1651, 1650t, 1651
  clostridial, 1631t, 1632
  eosinophilic, malabsorption due to, 103
  radiation, 692, 750
    diarrhea due to, 692, 750
    malabsorption due to, 103
    treatment of, 750
  rotavirus, 1642t, 1658
  Yersinia enterocolitica in, 739, 739t, 1661
Enterobacter, 1579–1581, 1580t
Enterobacteriaceae, 1557t
  extraintestinal infection due to, 1559–1660
Enterobiasis, 1935, 1935t
Enteroclysis, 632–633
Enterococcus, 1589t, 1589–1590
  endocarditis due to, 1598t, 1598–1599, 1601t,
      1603t
Enterocolitis, Salmonella, 1645–1646
Enterocytozoon, 1916t
Enteropathy, gluten-sensitive, 704–705
Enterostomy, enteral feeding in, 1168–1169
Enterotoxins, clostridial, 1630–1638, 1631t, 1634t,
    1635t, 1638t
  E. coli, 1654–1655, 1655t
  staphylococcal, 1606–1607, 1609
Enterovirus/enteroviral infection, 1783–1793. See also
    Coxsackievirus; Echovirus; Poliovirus.
  characteristics of, 1783–1785, 1784t
  classification of, 1784t, 1784–1785
  conjunctivitis due to, hemorrhagic, 1787t, 1791–1792
  epidemiology of, 1785–1786
  exanthems of, 1787t, 1790–1791
  mucocutaneous effects of, 1787t, 1788–1789
  myocarditis due to, 1787t, 1788–1789
  neurological syndromes due to, 1786–1788, 1787t
  pathogenesis of, 1786
  pericarditis due to, 1787t, 1788–1789
  treatment and prevention for, 1792–1793
Enthesis, 1441
Enthesopathy, 1442
  ankylosing spondylitis with, 1441, 1443t
  spondyloarthropathies with, 1467t, 1469
Entropion, 1722
Environment, 56–59, 399–403. See also Occupation.
  aging related to, 12–13, 14
  asthma and, 378, 379t
  cancer related to, 1009t, 1010, 1015–1016
  industrial, 56–59, 58t, 59t, 391t

Environment (Continued)
  sentinel disorders related to, 56–59, 58t, 59t
  toxic agents in, 56, 58t, 59t, 403t, 1016t
Enzymes, 1100t–1103t
  asthma induced by, 379t
  bacterial resistance due to, 1558–1560, 1559t
  catecholamines metabolized by, 97t, 1253, 1253–1254
  cytosolic, 145–145, 146t
    defects of, 145–145, 146t
  drug-metabolizing, 97t, 97–98
    deficiencies of, 97t, 97–98
  Embden-Meyerhof, 855–856, 856
  erythrocytic, 855–859, 856–858, 858t
  galactose metabolism, 1080t, 1081
  glucose metabolism, 856, 1082, 1082
  glycogen storage, 1083t
  heme pathway, 1125, 1125t
  hepatic, 759–760, 1080–1085
  lysosomal, 1095, 1096t, 1119t
    deficiency of, 1095–1099, 1096t, 1119t
  metabolic disorders related to, 145–147, 146t, 147t.
      See also Metabolic disorder(s); specific enzymes
      and disorders.
  mitochondrial, 146t
    defects of, 146t
    myopathy related to, 2165–2167, 2166t
  mucopolysaccharide, 1119t
  muscle, 2160
    deficiencies of, 2165–2167, 2166t
  pancreatic, 729, 730, 731–732
    elevated, 731–732, 732t
    laboratory tests for, 731–732, 732t
    secretion of, 730, 730–732, 732t
  peroxisomal, 147t
    deficiencies of, 147, 147t
  purine, 1114–1117, 1115
  urea cycle, 1110, 1110t, 1110–1111, 1111
  venom containing, 1951t
Eosinopenia, 914, 956
Eosinophilia, 956–958
  Churg-Strauss, 958, 1491
  diseases associated with, 956–958, 957t
  filariasis with, 1942
  granuloma and, 955–956
  helminthic, 1892, 1942
  myalgia with, 2164–2165
  parasitism and, 956, 1942
  protozoal, 1892
  syndrome of, 333t, 334
  tryptophan causing, 2164–2165
Eosinophils, 820, 821, 956
  allergic rhinitis role of, 1413t, 1414, 1415
  asthma and, 377, 377
  count of, 956
  cutaneous inflammation role of, 2190
  deficiency of, 914
  glucocorticoid effect on, 108–109, 109t
  increased. See Eosinophilia.
  NARES syndrome role of, 1413t, 1416
  pneumonia and, 398
  production of, 819, 820, 820t, 821, 898
  structure and function of, 956
Ependymoma, filum terminale affected by, 2148
Ephelides. See Freckles.
Epidemics, anthrax, 1665
  cholera, 1652
  croup, 1752–1753, 1753t
  influenza, 1753t, 1754–1755, 1755t
  meningitis, 1618
  rheumatic fever, 1591–1592
  typhus (louse-borne), 1726–1729, 1727t, 1728t
Epidermis, 2184–2186
  anatomy of, 2184–2186, 2185, 2186
  differentiation of, 2184–2185
  inclusion cyst of, 2209
  neoplasia of, benign, 2208t, 2208–2209, 2210
    malignant, 2208t, 2209–2211, 2210t
  physiology of, 2184–2186, 2185, 2186
  toxic necrolysis of, 2205
Epidermolysis bullosa, 2205t
  immunofluorescence testing in, 2189t
  oral lesions of, 646, 646t
  skin lesions of, 2205t
Epididymitis, gonorrheal, 1701, 1702t
  mumps causing, 1769
Epididymus, 1286
Epidural hematoma, 2136
Epigastrium, pain from, 628
Epiglottitis, H. influenzae in, 1623
  pneumococcal, 1571, 1571t

Epilepsy, 2113–2125
  alcohol withdrawal and, 49
  aura of, 2114
  childhood, 2115, 2117, 2117
  classification of, 2114–2118, 2116t
  continuous, 2118
  definition of, 2113
  diagnosis of, 2119t, 2119–2120
  differential diagnosis of, 2121, 2121t
  drug therapy in, 2121–2123, 2122t
  EEG in, 2117, 2118, 2120
  epidemiology of, 2115, 2118–2119
  etiology of, 2113–2114, 2114t, 2115
  generalized, 2115, 2115–2116, 2116t
  grand mal, 2116
  head injury causing, 2118
  history taking for, 2119t, 2119–2120
  idiopathic, 2114
  imaging studies in, 2120, 2120
  partial (focal), 2114–2115, 2115, 2116t
  petit mal, 2117, 2117
  pregnancy and, 2123
  prognosis of, 2124
  psychomotor, 2115
  psychosocial factors in, 2125
  status epilepticus, 2124t, 2124–2125
  surgical approach in, 2123–2124
  temporal lobe, 2117, 2118
  treatment of, 2121–2125, 2122t, 2124t
Epimastigote, trypanosomal, 1897, 1900
Epinephrine, 1253–11257. See also Catecholamines.
  alpha vs. beta receptors and, 1253–1254
  anaphylaxis treated with, 1419
  glucose and, 1257
  hypoglycemia and, 1257
  insulin and glucagon and, 1257
  insulin therapy and, 1272, 1272
  laboratory tests for, 1255–1256
  metabolism of, 1253, 1253
  pheochromocytoma and, 1254–1256
  plasma levels of, 1253, 1255
  shock and, 492t, 493
  storage and release of, 1253
  synthesis of, 1253
Episcleritis, 2181
  rheumatoid arthritis with, 1464
Epithelioma, basal cell, 2209
  keratoacanthomatous, 2209
Epithelium, airway, 377, 377
  alveolar, 371–373, 372
    interstitial disease affecting, 393, 394
  asthma effect on, 377, 377
  Barrett's, 652, 654, 657
  colonic, adenoma-carcinoma sequence in, 1076, 1076
    hyperproliferation of, 1076
  columnar, 652, 654, 657
  gastric, 662, 662t
  glomerular, 519, 520
  oral, 648, 648t
Epitrochlear nodes, 969t
Epizootics, anthrax in, 1665, 1738t
  bubonic plague in, 1662
Epoxy-eicosatrienoic acid (EET), 1191, 1191
Epoxygenase, 1191
  arachidonic acid metabolism by, 1191, 1191
Epsilon-aminocaproic acid, 989
  von Willebrand disease treated with, 994
Epsom salts toxicity, 1138
Epstein-Barr virus (EBV)/EBV infection, 1776–1779,
    2095
  antibodies to, 1778, 1778, 1779t
  clinical manifestations of, 1776t, 1776–1777,
    2095
  diagnosis of, 1778, 1778, 1779t
  epidemiology of, 1776
  etiology of, 1776
  Hodgkin's lymphoma role of, 947
  immunodeficiency due to, 1405
  latency of, 1777–1778, 1778, 1779t
  neurologic effects of, 2095
  pathogenesis for, 1777–1778
  pathology of, 1777–1778, 2095
  treatment of, 1778–1779
Equilibrium, 2024–2027, 2025, 2025t
  anatomy and, 2024
  caloric test of, 2024
  disorders affecting, 2025t, 2025–2027
  evaluation of, 2025, 2025–2027, 2026
  physiology and, 2024

Equine encephalitis, eastern, 1806t, 1810t, 1811–1812
  Venezuelan, 1806t, 1810t, 1812
  western, 1806t, 1810t, 1811
Erection, 1328
  drugs affecting, 2010, 2010t
  dysfunctional, 1330t, 1330–1331
  hemochromatosis affecting, 1337
  mechanisms of, 1328, 1329
  painful, priapism with, 889
  parasympathetic control of, 2010, 2010t
  sickle syndrome affecting, 889
Ergocalciferol, 1145t, 1357, 1357t. See also Vitamin D.
Ergot poisoning, 740
Ergotamine, 2032
Erionite, 1016t
Erlenmeyer flask deformity, 1389, 1389
Erysipelas, 2208
  erysipeloid vs., 1673
  streptococcal, 1587, 2208
  swine, 1673
  treatment of, 1587, 1589t
Erysipeloid, 1673–1674
  clinical manifestations of, 1674
  epidemiology of, 1673–1674
  etiology of, 1673
  treatment of, 1674
Erythema. See also Rash.
  annulare centrifugum, 2208
  cat scratch disease, 1681, 1681t
  chronicum migrans, 1715–1717, 1718
  diseases associated with, 2191t
  erysipelas, 1587, 2208
  figurate, 1033, 2208
  gyratum repens, 1019, 1033
  induratum, 1508
  infectiosum, 2200
  marginatum, 1593, 1595t, 2208
  measles with, 1759
  microscope slide examination of, 2192
  multiforme, iris lesions of, 2191, 2191, 2206
    oral ulcers of, 646, 646t, 2206
  necrolytic migratory, 1034–1035
  necrotizing fasciitis with, 1588
  nodosum, 2191, 2211
    hypersensitivity causing, 2211
    leprosum, 1693, 1694, 1696
  oral, 647, 647t, 648, 648t
  palmar, liver disease and, 752
    rheumatoid arthritis with, 1463
  paraneoplastic, 1019, 1030–1036, 1031t
  persistent, 2208
  Raynaud's phenomenon with, 347, 1484,
    1485
  rheumatic fever with, 1593, 1595t, 2208
  rubella, 1762
  serpiginous, 1019, 1033
  vaccinia, 1767
Erythroblastosis fetalis, 41t
Erythroblasts, 817, 820, 821
Erythrocytes, 823, 823t. See also Anemia.
  aplasia of, 831–836
    pure, 833t, 833–834, 834
  ascites with, 744t
  autoantibodies to, 1476t, 1477
    purpura due to, 987
  babesiosis in, 1916
  basophilic stippling of, 859
  carbon dioxide hydration by, 543
  count of, normal, 823, 823t
  destruction of. See Hemolysis.
  elliptocytic, 825t, 830t, 854–855
  enzyme deficiencies of, 855–859
  fragmented, 825t, 830t
  helmet, 822
  hemoglobin and. See Hemoglobin.
  hepatic clearance of, 860–861, 861, 888
  hypochromic, 824, 825t
  immune complex binding by, 1423, 1423
  increased, 920t, 920–922, 921, 921t, 922t
  macrocytic, 826t
    anemia and, 824, 824t, 825t, 828t, 828–829
    stress and, 817
  macroovalocytic, 825t, 847, 848, 913
  malaria affecting, 1893, 1894, 1895t
  membrane of, 851–859
    complement receptors on, 1423, 1423
    disorders of, 852–859
    enzyme defects of, 855–859, 856–858, 858t

Erythrocytes *(Continued)*
   functions of, 852
   hereditary defects of, 852–855, *853*, 853t, 855t
   permeability of, 852, 855
   structure of, *851*, 851–852
  metabolism of, 855–856, *856*
   defects in, 856–859, *857*, *858*, 858t
  microcytic, 826t, 827
   anemia and, 825t, 827–828, 839–842
  morphology of, 822
   anemias and, 824–825, 825t, *847*, *848*, *883*
   Heinz bodies affecting, 856–857, 874
   hemoglobin affecting, 825t, 842, 856–857, *883*
  nucleated, *819*, 825t
  osmotic fragility of, 852, 854
   incubated, 854
  polychromic, 824
  production of, 817–821. See also *Erythropoiesis.*
   control mechanisms for, 837–838
   elevated, 920t, 920–922, *921*, 921t, 922t
   reduced. See *Anemia.*
  sequestration of, 822, 1894
  sickled, *883*, 884–886, *885*. See also *Sickle syn-
    dromes.*
  spherocytic, 825t, 830t, 852–854, 854t
  spicule, 822
  splenic clearance of, 852, 857, *860*, 860–861, 971
  spur cell, 825t, 827
  teardrop, 924
  transfusion with, 893t, 893–894
  urinary. See *Hematuria.*
  volume of, maintenance of, 852
   mean. See *Mean cell volume (MCV).*
   total, 920, 921t
Erythrocytosis, 920–921
  causes, 920, 920t, *921*
  congenital heart disease with, 284–286
  definition, 920
  diagnosis of, 920–921, *921*
  paraneoplastic, 1021
Erythroderma, 1033
  definition, 1033
  high-output cardiac failure and, 2188
  paraneoplastic, 1019, 1031t, 1031–1033
Erythrodontia, 1128
Erythromelalgia, 1528
Erythromycin, 1562t
  adverse reactions to, 1568t
  bacterial resistance to, 1558–1560, 1559t
  diphtheria therapy with, 1630
  hepatotoxicity of, 773, 774
  Legionella and, 1585, 1585t
  mechanism of action of, 1558, 1558t
  mycoplasmal infection treated with, 1578, 1578t
  staphylococcal infection treated with, 1609t,
   1609–1610
  streptococcal infection treated with, 1587–1589,
   1589t
Erythroplakia, oral, 647, 647t
Erythropoiesis, **817–821**
  anemia stimulation of, 825, 837–838
  decreased, 821–850. See also *Anemia.*
  growth factors in, 819–821, 820t, *821*, 898
  hemoglobin synthesis in, 869–870, 870
  increased. See *Erythrocytosis; Polycythemia.*
  ineffective, aplasia and, 831–836
   megaloblastic anemia and, 843
   myelofibrosis and, 837
   sideroblastic anemia with, 842–843
   thalassemia with, 827–828, 877–880
  precursors in, 817, *832*
  progenitors in, 819, *820*, *821*, *834*
  reticulocytes and, 825, 826t, 837–838
Erythropoietin, 820t, 837–838
  cancer therapy using, 1049, 1049t
  increased production of, 920t, 921, *921*
Escape complexes, 242
  sudden cardiac death with, *255*
Eschar, tick bite causing, 1732
Escherichia coli, **1654–1657**
  diarrhea due to, 1654–1657, 1655t
  enterotoxigenic, 1654–1655, 1655t
  food poisoning due to, 739, 739t
  gastroenteritis due to, 1654–1657, 1655t
  hemorrhagic colitis due to, 1654–1655, 1655t, 1738t
  infection due to, 1654–1657, 1655t
   clinical manifestations of, 1655t, 1656
   diagnosis of, 1655t, 1656

Escherichia coli (Continued)
   epidemiology of, 1655, 1655t
   etiology of, 1654–1655, 1655t
   pathogenesis of, 1655–1656
   prevention of, 1657
   prognosis in, 1657
   treatment of, 1656–1657
  pneumonia due to, 1579
Esophagitis, AIDS/HIV with, 1866
  bleeding due to, 642t, 643–644, 645t
  candidiasis with, 658, 1828
  caustic, 658
  pill medications causing, 658–659
  reflux, 651–654, *653*, 654t
Esophagogastroduodenoscopy, 636–639, 638t
  complications of, 639
  indications for, 636–639, 638t
  therapeutic applications for, 638t, 639
Esophagus, **650–659**
  achalasia, 654–656, *655*
  approach to diseases of, 650–651
  Barrett's, 652, 654, 657
  bleeding from, 642t, 643–644, 659, 794t, 794–795
  cancer of, incidence of, *1005*, *1009*, 1013t, *1015*
  candidiasis of, 658
  carcinoma of, 657
   smoking associated with, 35, 35t
  columnar epithelium in, 652, 654
  dilation of, Chagas' disease causing, 1901, *1901*
   therapeutic, 654, 656
  diverticula of, 658
  dysphagia in, 650, 651, 655, 657
  endoscopy of, 636–639, 638t, *653*
  function of, 650–651
  heartburn and, 650, 651
  hypomobility affecting, scleroderma in, 1485
  inflammation. See *Esophagitis.*
  Mallory-Weiss tear in, 642t, 643, 659
  manometry of, 655–656, *656*
  motor disorders of, 654–657, *655*, 655t, *656*
  nutcracker, 655t, 656–657
  pain from, 628, 650–651, 655
  reflux into, 651–654. See also *Reflux esophagitis.*
  regurgitation and, 650–651
  rings of, 657–658, *658*
  rupture of, 629, 630, 659
  spasm in, 654–656, *656*
  sphincter of, 650
   lower, 651, 655
   upper, 654–655
  stricture of, 652, 654
  swallowing and, 650–651, 654–656
  trauma injury to, 659
  trypanosomiasis affecting, 1901, *1901*
  tumor of, 657
  ulcer of, 652, 654
  varices of, 642t, 643, 794t, 794–795
  webs affecting, 657–658
Estradiol, ovarian, *1299*, 1299, *1300*, 1301t
  ovarian synthesis of, 1182
  testosterone metabolism and, 1328
Estrogens, age changes in, 13–14, *15*
  cancer therapy using, 1046t, 1047
  carcinogenicity of, 1016, 1016t, 1311, 1383
  granulosa cell synthesis of, 1299, *1299*
  hepatotoxicity, 773, 773t
  lipid metabolism affected by, 1312
  male excess of, 1338
  menopause treated with, 1311–1312
  obesity effect on, 1165
  oral contraception with, 1309–1310
  osteoporosis role of, 1379–1380, *1380*, 1382–1383
  ovarian production of, 1299, *1299*, 1301t
   tumor and, 1312t
  porphyria worsened by, 1126, 1129
  receptors for, breast cancer with, 1322
   tamoxifen mechanism of action and, 1059–1060
  replacement therapy using, 1311–1312, 1382–1383
   bone loss treated with, 1382–1383
   cancer risk in, 1016, 1016t, 1322, 1383
Estrone, ovarian, 1299, *1300*, 1301t
Ethacrynic acid, dosage for, 264t
  properties and action of, 224t, 531t
Ethambutol, 1562t
  mycobacterial (nontuberculous) disease and, 1690,
   1691
  ocular side effects of, 2183
  tuberculosis treated with, 1686–1688, 1687t
Ethanol. See also *Alcohol/alcoholism.*
  hepatotoxicity of, 773, 773t

Ethanol *(Continued)*
  lethal dose of, 48, 48t. See also *Alcohol/alcoholism.*
  metabolism of, 47
  methanol toxicity treated with, 504t, 509
  pharmacology of, 47
  tolerance to, 47
Ethanolamines, 1416, 1416t
Ethical issues, **4–6**
  critical care patient and, 465–466
  patient decision making in, 4–6, 465–466
  physician role and, 4–9
Ethnic groups. See *Racial factors.*
Ethosuximide, 91t, 94t
  epilepsy therapy with, 2122t
  pharmacokinetics of, 91t, 94t, 2122t
  renal failure effect on, 94t
Ethyl hydrocuprein chloride, 1570
Ethylene glycol, acidosis caused by, 548, 549
  neurologic effects of, 1975t
  oxalate and, 588
  poisoning due to, 504t, 509, 509t
   symptoms in, 509, 509t
   treatment of, 504t, 509, 509t
  renal function and, 588
Ethylenediamines, 1416, 1416t
Etidronate, bone mineralization inhibited by, 1365
  Paget's disease treated with, 1386
Etoposide, adverse effects of, 1044
  chemotherapy using, 1039t, 1044, 1044t
  non-Hodgkin's lymphoma and, 945t
  resistance to, 1057t
Etretinate, acne treatment with, 2197
  side effects of, 2197
  skin disorder treated with, 2197
Eubacterium, 1639, 1639t
Eumelanin, 2185
Eumycetoma, 1835t
Eunuchoidism, 1329, *1330*
  androgen deficiency causing, 1329, *1330*
  "fertile," 1337
  hypogonadotropic, 1337
  Klinefelter's syndrome with, 1333–1335, *1336*
  vanishing testes syndrome and, 1334
Euphoria, alcohol-related, 47, 48t
  opioid-induced, 51
Euthanasia, 5
Euthyroidism, 1229, 1229t, 1230t
Evans' syndrome, 862, 866, 1479
  differential diagnosis of, 984t, 1479
Evoked potentials, 1961
  auditory, 1961, 2021
  CNS diagnostic examination using, 1961
  multiple sclerosis diagnosis with, 2107
  visual, 1961
Evolution, 14
Examination. See *Physical examination.*
Exanthem, Boston, 1791
  enterovirus, 1787t, 1790–1791
  measles, 1759, 2200
  rubella, 1762, 2200
  subitum, 1791, 2200
  viral, 2200
Excoriations, skin disorders with, 2191t
Excretion, uric acid (urate) in, 1509t, 1510, 1510t
Exercise, **31–33**
  asthma induced by, 378
  definition of, 31, 31t
  diabetes mellitus treatment using, 1266t, 1266–1267
  duration of, 33t
  energy expenditure for, 1167t
  frequency of, 33t
  headache caused by, 2032, 2033
  health benefits of, 31–32, *32*, 33t
  intensity level of, 31, 31t, 33t
  norepinephrine release due to, 1253
  obesity treatment using, 1166, 1166t
  prescription of, 33, 33t
  risks associated with, 32–33
  testing, angina pectoris and, *79*, 297
   fitness level in, 32, *32*
   forearm ischemia and, 1503t
   heart disease mortality rate and, 32, *32*
  urticaria related to, 1410
  warning signs during, 33t
Exfoliation, 1607, 1607t, 1609, 1609t
Exocytosis, 1182
  atrial granules in, 1194
  chromaffin cell, 1253
  natriuretic hormone and, 1194
  thyrocyte, 1227

Exons, calcitonin gene, *1375*
 gene transcription and, *135*
 vasopressin, *1222*
Exostoses, hereditary multiple, 1390
Exotoxins, anthrax role of, 1665–1666
 B. pertussis, 1627–1628
 bacterial, 497, *498*, 1556–1557
 septic shock role of, 497, *498*
 streptococcal, 497, *498*, 1587
 Vibrio cholerae, 1652–1653
Expiratory pressure, 466–467, 467t
Expiratory volume, *373*, 373t, *373–374*, *374*, 374t
 asthma affecting, *378*, 378–379, 379t
 bronchitis affecting, 382, *383*
 emphysema affecting, 382, *383*
 forced, 374, *374*, 466, 467t
Explosives, occupational exposure to, 59t
Extracorporeal membrane oxygenator, 495
Extrapyramidal system, **2042–2050**. See also *Basal ganglia.*
Extremities, cold sensitivity in, 346–350
 ischemia affecting, 346–356
 skin disorders affecting, *2191*, 2216t
 skinfolds of, 1153, 1153t
 vascular disorders affecting, 346–357
Extrinsic pathway inhibitor, 988, 988t, *989*
Eye, *2017*, **2174–2183**. See also specific part, e.g., *Retina.*
 age changes in, 16t, 17, 2174
 AIDS/HIV effects in, 1868–1870, 1869t
 albinism of, 2214t
 anatomy of, *2015*, 2015–2017, *2017*, *2176*
 angle structures of, 2175–2177, *2176*
 aqueous humor of, 2175–2177, *2176*
 bobbing, 2020
  cerebral hemorrhage with, 2078, 2078t
  subtentorial lesion with, 1971, 1971t
 cancer of, incidence of, 1013t
 candidiasis affecting, 1828, 1830
 cerebral hemorrhage affecting, 2078, 2078t
 conjunctivitis of. See *Conjunctivitis.*
 convergence testing for, 2019
 copper deposition in, 785–786, 1131, 2175
 cotton wool spots of, 1480, 1868–1869, 2099, 2182
 cystathionine synthase deficiency affecting, 1113
 cysticercosis affecting, 1926
 downward deviation of, 2078, 2078t
 dry, 2181
  rheumatoid arthritis causing, 1464
  Sjögren's syndrome causing, 1488, 1488t, 1489, *1489*
  systemic sclerosis causing, 1487
 filariasis affecting, 1942–1944
 glaucoma effect on, 2175–2177, *2176*
 Graves' disease and, 1233, 2180
 hereditary disorders affecting, 160t, 160–162
 histoplasmosis of, 1818, 2179
 hypertension affecting, 2181
 infections of, 2179–2180
  trachomal, 1722–1723
  viral, 1741t, 2179
 inflammatory bowel disease and, 710t, 710–711
 iris of, *2176*, 2176–2179, 2178t
 Kayser-Fleischer rings in, 785–786, 1131
 lens of. See *Lens.*
 light-dark cycle and, *1204*, 1204–1205
 malignant melanoma of, 2180
 metastases to, 2180
 movements of, 2018–2020
  abnormalities in, 2019–2020, *2020*, 2020t
  alcohol affecting, 47
  control of, 2018–2020, *2020*, 2020t
  examination of, 2019, *2020*, 2020t
  flutter, 2020
  neural pathways for, 2018–2019
  REM sleep and, 1982
  smooth pursuit, 2019
 mucormycosis effects in, 1833
 pain from, 2035
 painful, glaucoma causing, 2176–2177
 paraneoplastic effects in, 1018, 1028
 pineal gland and, *1204*
 pseudoxanthoma elasticum affecting, 1123
 radiation of, 61, 61t
 rheumatoid disease affecting, 1464, 1467t, 1469, 2178
 sarcoidosis of, 432, *432*
 sickle syndrome affecting, 889
 Sjögren's syndrome affecting, 1488, 1488t, 1489, *1489*, 2181

Eye *(Continued)*
 toxoplasmosis affecting, 1869, 1869t, 1908, 1909, 2179
 tumors of, 2180
 visual fields and, *2015*, 2015–2017
 vitamin A deficiency affecting, 1145t
 Wegener's granulomatosis affecting, 1495t, 1496, 1496t
Eyeglasses, 2174
Eyelashes, 1722
 corneal abrasion caused by, 1722
 inward-turning, 1722
Eyelid, muscular dystrophy effect on, 2162
 sebaceous glands of, 2186
 trachoma affecting, 1722

F

FAB antibodies, digoxin binding by, 504t, 508
 dosage for, 504t, 508
Fab region, immunoglobulin, 1394, *1394*
Fabry's disease, **1095–1097**
 cardiomyopathy due to, 333t, 334, 1096
 clinical manifestations of, 334, 1096
 diagnosis of, 1096–1097
 etiology of, 1095–1096, 1096t
 genetics of, 1096t
 pathogenesis of, 1095–1096, 1096t
 pathology in, 1096
 treatment of, 1097
Face, erysipelas affecting, 1587, 1589t
 mucormycosis effects in, 1833
 muscular dystrophy effects in, 2162
 myopathy affecting, 2162, 2170
 neuralgias affecting, 2009, 2035
 palsy affecting, 1717, 2157
 port-wine angioma of, 2056
 skin disorders affecting, *2191*, 2216t
Facial nerve, Bell's palsy and, 2157
 mucormycosis affecting, 1833
Facies, 160–162
 hereditary disorders affecting, 158t, 159t, 160t, 160–162
 leonine, 1031t
 moon, *1216*, 1217, 1247t
Facioscapulohumeral dystrophy, 2160t, 2162
Factor XI deficiency, 136t, 138t
Faget's sign, 1799
Failure to thrive, botulism causing, 1636
 intractable vomiting and, 684
Fallot's tetralogy, 279, *279*
 aneurysm with, 279
 repair of, 283, *285*
Falls, causes of, 23
 elderly affected by, 23
 mortality rate in, 37, *38*
False positives, decision analysis role of, 79, *80*
 syphilis test, 1475t, 1479, 1711
 urinalysis with, 512t
Familial disorder(s). See also *Hereditary disorder(s).*
 amyloidosis in, 967t, 1504t, 1505
 cardiomyopathy due to, 329t, 331
 colonic polyposis as, 723–725, *724*
 erythrophagocytic lymphohistiocytosis as, 970
 pheochromocytoma as, 1254
Families, 6–9
 bereavement affecting, 8t, 8–9
 decision-making role of, 6–9, 8t
 history of, genetic pedigree and, 136–140, *137–141*
  hereditary disorders and, 136t, 136–140, 138t
 terminal patient and, 6–9, 8t
Famotidine, 653, 654t
Fanconi's anemia, 831–832
Fanconi's syndrome, 595t, 597–598
 aminoaciduria in, 1104t, 1105t
 causes of, 595t, 597
 diagnosis of, 597
 osteomalacia with, 1363t, 1364
 symptoms of, 597
 transport defects and, 595t, 597, 1104t, 1105t
 treatment of, 598
Farcy, 1667
Fascia, intimal, 292, *295*
Fava beans, hemolysis caused by, 857
Fear. See also *Anxiety.*
 of dying, 18
Feces. See also *Diarrhea.*
 animal, *Hantavirus* in, 1737t, 1804
 bile excreted in, 696, 756, 807, *807*
 black tarry, 642
 blood in, bright red, 642, 718, 740
  cancer screen using, 1006t
  colonic ischemia with, 718
  diarrhea with, 693
  hemorrhoidal origin of, 740
  inflammatory bowel disease with, 709, 712, 712t
  recommended testing frequency for, 28t
  stomach cancer with, 678
  vitamin C interference and, 1147t
 C. difficile in, 1634t, 1634–1635, 1635t
 calcium in, *1352*
 Campylobacter in, 1650, 1650t
 colitis and, 1633–1635, *1634*, 1634t, 1635t
 color of, 756
 diagnostic tests of, 693–694, 698–699
 fat in, 693, 694, 698, 699t, *700*, 700t
 hepatitis and, 763, 763t, 764, *765*
 hookworm eggs in, 1935
 leukocytes in, 1633, *1634*, 1634t
 liver function and, 761
 magnesium in, 1137, *1352*
 melenic, 642
 phosphate in, *1352*
 pinworm eggs in, 1935
 porphyrin in, 1130, 1130t
 "rice water," 1653
 schistosome eggs in, *1927*, 1927, 1929t, 1929–1931
 Shigella in, 1647, 1647t, 1648
 Strongyloides eggs in, 1939
 tapeworm diagnosis and, 1923, 1924, 1925
 volume in 24 hours of, 694
 whipworm eggs in, 1936

Fasciotomy, "bearclaw," 1588
Fasting state, 1278, 1278t
 insulin action in, 1260
Fat. See also *Lipids.*
 absorption of, 696, 696t, *697*, 806, *806*
 atherogenesis role of, 292, *292*, 294, *295*
 body compartment of, 1161–1162, *1162*
  age and, 1161–1162, *1162*
  gender and, *1162*, 1163–1164
  storage patterns for, *1162*, 1163–1164, 1165
  total amount in, 1162
  upper body vs. lower body, 1164, 1165
 brown, 1163
 "buffalo hump" of, 1217, 1247
 Cushing's disease effect on, 1217, 1247
 dietary, 29–30, 30t
  calorie requirements and, 30t, 1173t
  cancer associated with, 1009, 1017, 1143t
  energy requirements and, 30t, 1154
  food groups and, *1142*, 1143
  intake of, 1143, 1154, 1172, 1173t
  labeling regulations for, 1143, 1143t
  parenteral nutrition with, 1172, 1173t
 droplets (circulating) of, 430
 embolism of, 430, 2069
 emulsion of, 1172
 fecal, 693, 694, 698, *700*, 700t
  stain for, 698, *700*, 700t
 perirenal, *517*
Fatigue, 2027–2028, 2028t
 cardiovascular disease causing, 166
 chronic syndrome of, 2028
 hemochromatosis with, 1133
 iron-deficiency anemia with, 840
 multiple sclerosis with, 2109, 2110
 muscle assessment and, 2159
Fatty acids, adrenoleukodystrophy affecting, 1251
 dietary aspects of, 1139, 1143t, 1192
 enzyme deficiencies affecting, 2165–2166, 2166t
 fish oil and, 1139, 1143t, 1192
 metabolism of, liver and, 753–754
 myopathy and, 2165–2166, 2166t
 omega-3, 1139, 1143t, 1192
 transport of, *1087*, 1087–1088, *1088*
 very long chain, 1251
Fatty streak, intimal, 292, *295*
Fava beans, hemolysis caused by, 857
Fear. See also *Anxiety.*
 of dying, 18
Feces. See also *Diarrhea.*
 animal, *Hantavirus* in, 1737t, 1804
 bile excreted in, 696, 756, 807, *807*
 black tarry, 642
 blood in, bright red, 642, 718, 740
  cancer screen using, 1006t
  colonic ischemia with, 718
  diarrhea with, 693
  hemorrhoidal origin of, 740
  inflammatory bowel disease with, 709, 712, 712t
  recommended testing frequency for, 28t
  stomach cancer with, 678
  vitamin C interference and, 1147t
 C. difficile in, 1634t, 1634–1635, 1635t
 calcium in, *1352*
 Campylobacter in, 1650, 1650t
 colitis and, 1633–1635, *1634*, 1634t, 1635t
 color of, 756
 diagnostic tests of, 693–694, 698–699
 fat in, 693, 694, 698, 699t, *700*, 700t
 hepatitis and, 763, 763t, 764, *765*
 hookworm eggs in, 1935
 leukocytes in, 1633, *1634*, 1634t
 liver function and, 761
 magnesium in, 1137, *1352*
 melenic, 642
 phosphate in, *1352*
 pinworm eggs in, 1935
 porphyrin in, 1130, 1130t
 "rice water," 1653
 schistosome eggs in, *1927*, 1927, 1929t, 1929–1931
 Shigella in, 1647, 1647t, 1648
 Strongyloides eggs in, 1939
 tapeworm diagnosis and, 1923, 1924, 1925
 volume in 24 hours of, 694
 whipworm eggs in, 1936
Fed state, 1278, 1278t
 hypoglycemia in, 1279, 1279t
 insulin action in, 1260–1261

Feedback mechanisms, endocrine, *1183*, 1183–1184, 1197–1199, *1198*
  hypothalamic, *1183*, 1184, 1197–1199, *1198*
  parathyroid hormone, 1183
  pituitary, 1183, *1183*, 1184, 1197–1199, *1198*
  thyroid hormone, 1183, 1197–1198, *1198*
Feeding behavior. See also *Eating.*
  disorders of, 629
  hypothalamic center for, 629, 2012–2013
  mediators of, 629
Feet. See *Foot*; *Sole.*
Felbamate, epilepsy therapy with, 2122t
  pain control use of, 106t
  pharmacokinetics of, 2122t
Felodipine, 265t
Felty's syndrome, neutropenia in, 912
  rheumatoid arthritis with, 1464
  splenomegaly due to, 972t, 973
Female. See *Sex (gender)*; *Sexual differentiation.*
Feminization, liver disease causing, 796
  testicular, 1291t, 1291–1292
Femur, osteomyelitis of, 1626, *1626*
Fenoprofen, 103t
Fentanyl, 51
  myocardial infarction treated with, 310t
  pain control with, 104t
Fermentative organisms, 1557t
Ferritin, anemia diagnosis and, 827, 828t, 841
  hemochromatosis and, 786, 1133–1134, 1134t
  phlebotomy effect on, 1134–1135, *1135*
Ferrochelatase, *1125*, 1125t, 1129–1130
  deficiency of, *1125*, 1125t, 1129–1130
α-Fetoprotein, 1022t, 1023
Fetus, calcium requirements of, 1353–1354
  chemotherapy effects in, 1068–1069, 1069t, 1070t
  congenital anomalies of, 157–159, 158t, 159t
  hemoglobin of. See *Hemoglobin, F (fetal).*
  21-hydroxylase deficiency in, 1287–1290, *1290*
  loss of, anomaly causing, 157–159, 158t
    chromosome abnormality causing, 152–154, 158t
  Lyme disease affecting, 1719–1720
  morphogenetic errors affecting, 157–159, 158t, 159t
  radiation effects in, 1069–1070, 1070t
  sexual differentiation in. See *Sexual differentiation.*
  sickle syndromes affecting, 888, 891
  syphilis affecting, 1710, 1712–1713
  thalassemia affecting, 877–878, 879–880
  thrombocytopenia of, alloimmune, 986
  ultrasonography of, transvaginal, 127, *128*
Fever, **1532–1537**
  acute illness and, 1535–1537, 1536t
  African, 1798t, 1803–1804, 1806t
  antimicrobials causing, 1568t
  Argentinian, 1798t, 1802–1803
  autonomic regulation in, 1203, 1533, 1535, 2012
  blackwater, 1894
  Bolivian, 1798t, 1802–1803
  boutonneuse, 1727t, 1728t, 1732
  Brazilian, 1798t, 1802–1803
  Brazilian purpuric, 1624
  cancer patient with, 1049–1050
  chikungunya, 1805t, 1809
  clinical features of, 1532, 1533, 1533t
  colitis with, pseudomembranous, 1633, *1634*
  Colorado tick, 1733, 1805t, 1805–1807, 1806t
  Crimean-Congo, 1798t, 1802, 1806t
  cytokine role in, 1533–1534, *1534*, 1535t
  definition of, 1532, 1533
  dengue, 1798t, 1800–1801, 1805t, 1807
  diagnostic significance of, 1532–1535, 1533t
  drug-induced, 1532, 1532t, 1533
  ehrlichiosis with, 1727t, 1728t, 1733, 1738t
  endocarditis with, 1599, 1600t
  enteric, 1644, 1645, 1646. See also *Typhoid fever.*
  factitious, 1532, 1532t
  filarial, 1941
  giant cell arteritis with, 1499, 1499t
  hemorrhagic. See *Hemorrhagic fever.*
  humidifier, 1583
  hyperthermic, 1532
  hypothalamic, 1203, 1533, 1535
  infection and, 1532t, 1533–1535, *1534*, 1535t
    acute, 1535–1537, 1536t
  influenza with, 1755
  Karelian, 1809–1810
  Kyasanur Forest, 1798t, 1801–1802, 1806t
  laboratory studies and, 1532
  Lassa, 1798t, 1802–1803

Lyme disease with, 1716, 1717t
  malarial, 1532, 1532t, 1533t, 1894
  Marburg-Ebola, 1798t, 1803–1804
  measles with, 1759
  Mediterranean, 907–908
    spotted, 1732
  meningitis with, 1614, 1619
  mycoplasmal infection with, *1577*
  neoplasia and, 1532t
  Omsk, 1798t, 1801–1802, 1806t
  Oroya, 1682
  pathogenesis of, 1532t, 1533–1535, *1534*, 1535t
  patient presentation with, 1532t, 1532–1533
  patterns in, 1533, 1533t, 1534
  Pel-Ebstein, 1533t
  periodic, 1533t
  pharyngoconjunctival syndrome, 1757, 1757t
  phlebotomus, 1808
  pleural effusion with, 445
  Pontiac, 1583, 1585
  Q, 1727t, 1728t, 1735–1736
  rabbit, 1662–1664
  Rao, 1767
  relapsing, 1532, 1533t, **1715**, 1738t
  Rift Valley, 1798t, 1805t, 1806t, 1808
  Rocky Mountain, spotless, 1727t, 1728t, 1733, 1738t
    spotted, 1727t, 1728t, 1730–1732
  sandfly, 1805t, 1808
  scarlet, 1586, 1587
  sepsis with, 496t, 499, 500t, 1588
  spotless (ehrlichiosis), 1727t, 1728t, 1733, 1738t
  spotted, 1727t, 1728t, 1730–1734, 2201
  transfusion reaction causing, 895, 895t, 896t
  treatment approach to, 1534–1535
  typhoid. See *Typhoid fever.*
  typhus, 1727t, 1728, 1728t
  undulant, 1532, 1533t
  unknown origin of, 1532t, 1532–1533
  Venezuelan, 1798t, 1802–1803
  West Nile, 1806t, 1807–1808
  yellow, 1798t, 1798–1800, 1805t
    immunization for, 44t, 46, 1554t, 1555
Fialuridine (FIAU), 773, 773t
Fiber, 29–30, 1010
  dietary, 29–30, 30t, 1141t, 1143t
    cancer risk reduction by, 1009, 1009t, 1016–1017
    food groups and, *1142*, 1143
    food labeling and, 1143t
  insoluble, 1010
  soluble, 1010
Fiberglass dermatitis, 2221
Fibrillation, 240–241, 244
  atrial, 240, 240–241, *241*
    emboli in, 2067
  ventricular, 237t, 238t, *243*, 244
Fibrillin, 1444
Fibrin, 989
  coagulation role of, *977*, 977, *978*, 989
  lysis of, 989–990
  structure, 989
  vegetation growth due to, 1598–1599, *1599*
Fibrinogen, 988t, 989
  absence of, 996
  coagulation role of, *977*, 977, *978*, 989
  deficiency of, 996, 1412
  liver synthesis of, 760
  structure, 989
  urticaria role of, 1412
Fibrinolysins, anaerobic flora production of, 1639t
  staphylococcal production of, 1606, 1607t
Fibrinolysis, 989–990
  primary, 1002
  therapeutic, 998
Fibroblasts, activation of, 1484t
  hematopoiesis role of, 818, 820t, *821*
  systemic sclerosis role of, 1484t
Fibrogenesis imperfecta ossium, 1365, 1389–1390
  clinical presentation of, 1389
  diagnosis of, 1389
  histopathology of, 1389–1390
  pathogenesis of, 1389
Fibromyalgia (fibrositis), 1527, 2037
  clinical features in, 1499t, 1527, 2037
  diagnosis of, 1499t, 1527
  epidemiology of, 1527
  pain of, 2037
Fibronectin, connective tissue, 1444–1445, *1445*
  defect of, 1121t
  Ehlers-Danlos syndrome and, 1121t
  hematopoiesis role of, 818, 821

Fibrosis, 1529–1530
  mediastinal, 1529–1530
  multifocal, 1529–1530
  peritonitis with, 1530
  retroperitoneal, 1529
Fibrositis. See *Fibromyalgia (fibrositis).*
Fibrothorax, 443t, 443–444
Fibrous dysplasia, 1390
  clinical presentation of, 1390
  etiology of, 1390
  radiologic features of, 1390, *1390*
  treatment of, 1390
Fick method, 209–210
  cardiac output measured with, 209–210
Filaggrin, 2184
Filaments, connective tissue, *1446*
Filariasis, **1939–1945**
  Dirofilaria, 1945
  Loa loa, 1943–1944
  lymphatic (bancroftian, brugian), 1940t, 1940–1941
  Mansonella, 1944–1945
  Onchocerca, 1942–1943
  tropical eosinophilia with, 1942
Filters, cigarette, 1014
Filum terminale, *2141*
  tumor affecting, 2148
Fimbriae, *1556*, 1557
  anaerobe with, 1639t
  bacterial, *1556*, 1557
  E. coli, 1656
  Haemophilus with, 1622
  meningitis organisms with, 1611
Finger. See also *Hand.*
  cold sensitivity affecting, 346–350
  gonorrhea affecting, 1702
  nail of. See *Nails.*
  psoriatic arthritis affecting, 1471
  Raynaud's phenomenon effect on, 347, 1484, 1485
  rheumatoid arthritis effects in, *1461*, 1461–1462, *1462*
  "trigger," 1527
  "zinc," DNA and, 1180–1181, *1181*
Finger agnosia, 1987
Firearms, mortality rate role of, 37, *38*
  preventive strategies and, 37–40
Fires, mortality rate role of, 37, *38*
Fish, 1955–1956. See also *Seafood.*
  ciguatera toxin in, 1954t, 1956
  dietary, 1139, *1142*
  mercury contamination of, 740
  scombroid, 1956
  tapeworm of, 1923, 1923t
  venomous, 1954t, 1955
FISH (fluorescence in situ hybridization), 151
Fish oil, diet supplemented with, 1192
  disease prevention by, 1139, 1143t
  thromboxane modification by, 1192
  vitamin D in, 1357
Fistula, anus affected by, 741–742, *742*
  aortoduodenal, 644
  arteriovenous, 281–282, *284*, 353
  choledochoduodenal, 814
Fits, uncinate, 2115
Fitz-Hugh–Curtis syndrome, 1702
Flagellum, bacterial, *1556*
  trypanosomal, 1896, *1897*, *1900*
Flail chest, 444
  respiration and, 444
Flatus, 699t
Flatworms. See *Flukes.*
Flaviviridae, 1798t, 1805t, 1806t
Flea, 1946
  bite of, 1947
  dermatitis due to, 1738t
  plague transmitted by, bubonic, 1662, 1737t
  typhus transmitted by, 1726, 1727t, 1729, 1738t
  zoonoses associated with, 1727t, 1737t, 1737–1738, 1738t
Flecainide, 246t
  adverse effects of, 248t
  antiarrhythmic action of, *245*, 246t, 249
  pharmacokinetics of, 246t
Flies. See *Fly.*
Floaters (visual), 1868–1869, 1869t
Floppy baby syndrome, 1636
Flora, 1638–1641. See also *Escherichia coli*; other specific organisms.
  anaerobes of, 1638–1641, *1639*, 1639t
  body sites of, 1638–1641, *1639*, 1639t
  colonic, *1639*, 1639t, 1640
  extraintestinal infection due to, 1659–1660

Flora *(Continued)*
  gastrointestinal, 1638–1641, *1639*, 1639t, 1659–1660
  genital tract, female, *1639*, 1639t, 1640, 1640t
  normal body, 1638–1641, *1639*, 1639t
  oropharyngeal, *1639*, 1639t, 1639–1640
    actinomycetes in, 1674
    aspiration of, 1579, 1582
    Haemophilus in, 1624, 1624t
  respiratory tract, *1639*, 1639t, 1639–1640
Flucloxacillin, 773t, 774
Fluconazole, blastomycosis therapy with, 1822
  candidiasis treated with, 1829
  histoplasmosis therapy with, 1818
  side effects of, 2196t
  skin disorder treated with, 2196t, 2196–2197
  vaginitis treated with, 1829
Flucytosine, candidiasis treated with, 1829–1830
  cryptococcosis therapy with, 1825
Fludarabine, adverse effects, 1043
  chemotherapy using, 1042t, 1043
Fluid(s), **525–538**. See also *Water.*
  absorption of, intestinal, *689*, 689–690, 690t
  aging effects and, 23
  enteral nutrition and, 1171
  extracellular, 525–528, *526*
    bone minerals in, 1351t, *1352*
    depletion of, 526–529, *527*, 528t
    heart failure affecting, 219
    hypertonic, 537–538
    increased, 530t, 530–533. See also *Edema.*
    potassium and, *526*, 533, 538–541, 539t, 541t
    renal function and, 526–528, *527*
    sodium and, *526*, 527, 533
  interstitial, 525, *526*
    increased, 530, 530t
  intracellular, 525–528, *526*
    bone minerals in, 1351t, *1352*
    potassium and, *526*, 533, 538–542, 539t, 541t
    sodium and, *526*, 527, 533
  intravascular, 525, *526*. See also *Blood volume.*
  osmolality and. See *Osmolality.*
  regulatory mechanisms for, 525–528, 526t, *527*, *533*
Fluid therapy. See also *Nutrition, parenteral.*
  ARDS treated with, 476–477, *477*
  calcium in, 1372
  cholera treated with, 1653–1654, 1654t
  diarrhea treated with, 694, 1653–1654, 1654t
  repletion response and, 525–528, 526t, *527*, *533*
  rule of thirds for, 525, *526*
  solutions in, 1653–1654, 1654t
Flukes, 1931–1934. See also *Trematodes.*
  intestine, 1932t, 1933
  liver, 782, 783t, 812, 1931–1934, 1932t
  lung, 1932t, 1933
Flumazenil, 504t
Flunisolide, 1417t
Fluorescence in situ hybridization (FISH), 151
Fluorescent antibody test, toxoplasmal, 1909
  treponemal, 1710t, 1711, 1711t
Fluorescent staining, malaria organism in, 1895
Fluoride, 1148t
  bone mineralization and, 1365
  deficiency of, 1148t
  dental caries and, 1148t
  physiology of, 1148t
  RDA for, 1141t
  tooth mottling due to, 1148t
Fluorochrome test, tubercle bacillus in, 1685
Fluoroiodoarabinosyl cytosine, 1745
Fluorouracil, adverse effects of, 1043
  chemotherapy using, 1039, 1042t, 1043
Fluoxetine, 2000t, 2001
Fluoxymesterone, 1046t, 1047
Fluphenazine, 1998t, 1998–1999
Flushing. See also *Erythema.*
  carcinoid causing, 1348–1350
  heat loss in, 1533
  tachykinins in, 1349
Flutamide, cancer therapy using, 1046t, 1047
  hirsutism treated with, 1316
Fly, 1946–1947, 1949–1950
  bartonellosis transmission by, 1682
  black, 1947
  blowfly, 1949–1950
  filariae transmitted by, 1939, 1940t
  flesh, 1949–1950
  horse, 1947
  larvae of, 1949–1950
  myiasis due to, 1949–1950
  "no-see-um," 1947

Fly *(Continued)*
  phlebotomine, 1682, 1903–1904, *1904*, 1947
  sandfly, 1682, 1903–1904, *1904*, 1947
    fever related to, 1805t, 1808
    leishmaniasis transmitted by, *1904*
  sleeping sickness transmitted by, 1897, *1897*, 1897, 1947
  trachoma transmission by, 1722, 1723
  tsetse, 1897, *1897*
Foam cells, atherosclerotic plaque of, 292, *292*
  Niemann-Pick disease with, *1097*, 1098
Folate (folic acid), **843–851**
  absorption of, 696t, 697, 700t, 704t, 844t, 846–847
  antagonists to, 1042t, 1043
    adverse effects of, 1043
    chemotherapy using, 1042t, 1043
  deficiency of, 843–851, 844t, 849t, 850t, 1147t, 2041
    mechanisms of, 844t, 846–847, 1147t
    metabolic defect in, 144t, 844–845
  dietary, 846–847, 1140t, 1147t, 1151t
    RDA for, 1140t
  megaloblastic anemia and, 843–851, 844t, 849t, 850t, 1147t
  neurologic effects of, 2041
  parenteral, 1172t
  physiology of, 844t, 846–847, 1147t, 1151t, 2041
  serum level of, 700t, 849t, 849–850, 850t
  toxicity of, 1147t
  treatment with, 704t, 851
Folinic acid, 1909, 1910t
Follicles (ovarian), 1293–1295, *1294*, 1299–1300
  anovulation related to, 1307
  graafian, 1293, *1294*, 1298, *1298*
  menstrual cycle and, 1297–1299, *1298*
  primordial, 1293, *1294*
Follicle-stimulating hormone (FSH), 1206t, 1218–1220
  amenorrhea evaluation with, 1303–1304, *1304*
  hypogonadotropic hypogonadism and, 1295t
  laboratory tests for, 1208t, 1213t
  menopause and, *1294*
  menstrual cycle and, *1294*, 1297–1299, *1298*
  ovulation and, *1294*, 1297–1298, *1298*, *1299*
  puberty and, 1294–1295
    female, *1294*, 1294–1295
    male, 1326
  regulation of, 1198, *1198*, 1206t, *1299*
  secretion of, 1218–1219
  stimulation test for, 1208t
  testicular function role of, *1326*, 1326–1328, *1327*
  tumor production of, 1209t, 1219–1220
Folliculitis, 2207
  chemical-induced, 2221
  hot tub, 2207
  incidence of, 2184t
Fontan repair, 283
Fontana-Masson stain, 1836
Food. See also *Diet; Eating; Feeding behavior; Nutrition.*
  additives, cancer and, 1009t
    skin reaction due to, 1409–1410
  allergy to, 1409–1410, 1418t
    anaphylaxis due to, 1418t
    urticaria and angioedema in, 1409–1410, 1418t
  amebae in, 1915
  botulism spores in, 1636
  groups, *1142*, 1143
  intake requirements for, 1140t, 1141t, 1141–1143
  labeling requirements for, 1143, 1143t
  photosensitivity caused by, 2218
  poisoning, 738–740
    bacterial, 738–739, 739t
    botulism as, 1635, 1636
    Clostridium, 738, 739t
    ergot mycotoxin, 740
    Listeria, 738, 739t, 1672, 1673
    mushroom, 740
    parasitic, 739
    plant, 740
    Salmonella, 738, 739t, 1644–1646
    seafood, 739t, 740, 1956
    shellfish, 739t, 740, 1956
    Staphylococcus, 738, 739t, 1607
    viral, 739
    zoonose etiology in, 1737t, 1738t
  Salmonella, 1644–1646
  Shigella in, 1647, 1648
  thermogenesis elevation by, 1163
  toxic chemicals in, 740
  traveler's diarrhea and, 1641–1642, 1642t, 1647
  typhoid fever and, 1644

Food.*(Continued)*
  urticaria caused by, 1409–1410, 2218
Foot. See also *Sole; Toe.*
  arteriolar constriction in, 349
  clubbed, 159t
  cyanosis of, 349
  diabetes affecting, 1275–1276, 1276t
  fungal infections of, 2199–2200
  Madura, 1834–1835
  osteoarthritis of, 1519t, 1519–1520
  rash of, Rocky Mountain spotted fever with, 1731
  syphilis causing, 1707, *1707*
  rheumatoid disease affecting, 1462
  skin disorders affecting, *2191*, 2216t
Foot-and-mouth disease, 1737t
Foramen magnum, syringomyelia near, 2055, *2055*
  tentorial herniation affecting, *1971*
Fordyce's disease, 1097
Fordyce's spots, 2186
Foreign bodies, bronchial, 416, 416t
Formaldehyde, smoke containing, 34, 36
Fos oncogene, 1059
Foscarnet, retinitis treated with, 1869t
  viral infection treated with, 1743, 1746t, 1869t
Fosinopril, 265t
Fossils, bacterial, 1556
Founder, hereditary disorder with, 139, *139*
Fournier's gangrene, 1641
Fovea, cherry red spot in, 2182
Fractures, elderly with, 23
  fat embolism following, 430
  osteoporosis role in, 1380, *1381*
  Paget's disease with, 1385t, 1385–1387
Fragile X syndrome, 138t, 154
Francisella tularensis, 1662–1664. See also *Tularemia.*
  tests for, 1663
Frank-Starling relationship, 175, 214
Freckles, 2191t, 2212
  albinism and, 2214t
  von Recklinghausen's disease with, 2056
Free radicals, aging theory based on, 15
  oxygen, porphyria and, 1124
    shock causing, 485
  vitamin scavengers for, 1151, 1151t
F-response, 1962
Friedreich's ataxia, 2051
  heart affected by, 359
Frontal lobes, *1986*, 1987–1988, *2059*
  aging effects in, 16, 16t
  anatomy of, *1986*, 1987–1988, *2059*
  gait disorders and, 2029
  infarct of, imaging of, 1966, *1967*
  manifestations of disease of, 1988, 1988t
  Pick's disease atrophy of, 1995
  tumor of, 2126t
Frostbite, 349–350
  clinical features of, 350
  pathophysiology of, 349
  treatment of, 350
Fructokinase, deficiency of, 1084
  metabolic defect of, 146t
Fructose, 1083
  dietary, 1083
  enzyme defects and, *1084*, 1084–1085
  intolerance of, 146t, **1083–1085**
    Fanconi's syndrome due to, 597, 1105t
    hereditary, 1084–1085, 1105t
    symptoms of, 1084–1085
  metabolism of, 1083–1084, *1084*
Fructose diphosphate aldolase, *856*
Fructose-1,6-diphosphatase deficiency, *1084*, 1085
Fructosuria, essential, 1084
Fruits, cancer risk reduction using, 1016–1017, 1039–1043
  dietary aspects of, 29–30, 30t, *1142*
FSH. See *Follicle-stimulating hormone (FSH).*
Fuel metabolism, 1278, 1278t
  disordered. See *Diabetes mellitus; Hypoglycemia.*
Fumes, cadmium, 71
  interstitial lung disease and, 391, 391t
  mercury, 69
  occupational exposure to, 58t, 59t
  selenium, 72
Fundus, albinism and, 2214t
Fungal infection(s), **1815–1836**
  adrenal gland, 1251
  AIDS/HIV with, 1862–1863, *1863*
  aneurysm due to, 1599

Fungal infection(s) *(Continued)*
arthritis due to, 1475
aspergillosis as, 1830t, 1830–1832
black pigment in, 1836
blastomycosis as, 1821–1822
candidal, 1827–1830. See also *Candidiasis.*
chromomycosis as, 1836
coccidioidomycosis as, 1819–1820, *1820*
compromised host and, 1537–1539, 1538t, 1544t
cryptococcal, 1823–1825
cutaneous, 1815, 1821, 1826, 1828, 1836, 2194t, 2199–2200
dematiaceous, 1836
drug therapy of, 1815–1816, 1816t
endocarditis due to, 1598t, 1598–1599
hepatic, 782
histoplasmosis as, 1816–1818
host defense mechanisms and, *1534*, 1537, 1538t
mucormycosis as, 1832–1834, 1833t
mycetoma as, 1834–1835, 1835t
mycology of, 1815, 1815t
nails affected by, 2214–2215
opportunistic, 1815, 1815t
paracoccidioidomycosis as, 1822–1823
pericarditis due to, 337, 337t
phaeohyphomycosis as, 1836
prevention of, 1544t, 1547
sexual transmission of, 1697t, 1699, 1699t
skin, 1836, *2191, 2192*, 2194t, 2199–2200
sporotrichosis as, 1826–1827
vaginal, 1697t, 1699, 1699t
Fungi, ball composed of, 1830t, 1831, *1831*
food poisoning due to, 740
grain contaminated with, 740
Fungicides, porphyria due to, 1128
Fungistatic agents, 1815–1816, 1816t
systemic, 2196t, 2196–2197
Furosemide, acid production tested with, 546, 546t
dosage for, 264t
properties and action of, 224t, 531t
Furuncles, 2207
staphylococcal toxin causing, 1606, 1607, 1607t
Fusobacterium, 1638, *1639*, 1639t, 1641t

G

G proteins, 1177–1178
hormone action and, 1177–1178, *1178–1180*
subunits of, 1177–1178, *1178, 1179*
GABA (gamma-aminobutyric acid), 797, 797t
Gabapentin, epilepsy therapy with, 2122t
pharmacokinetics of, 2122t
Gadolinium, 2127–2128, *2128, 2130, 2131*
Gait, **2028–2030**
aging effect on, 16–17, 2029
antalgic, 2030
basal ganglia and, 2042–2043
cerebral hemorrhage affecting, 2078, 2078t
degenerative disorders affecting, 2051t
frontal lobe disorder of, 2029
hemiparesis affecting, 2029
hysteria affecting, 2030
lateral sclerosis affecting, 2054
multiple sclerosis affecting, 2109, 2109t, 2110
muscle weakness affecting, 2159, 2160t
normal, 2028
retropulsion in, 2030
retrovirus infection affecting, 1781t, 1782
stroke affecting, 2064t, 2064–2065
Galactorrhea, 1306, 1318
causes of, 1318, 1318t
hyperprolactinemia in, 1306, 1318, 1318t
treatment of, 1319–1310
Galactose, enzyme pathways of, 146, 146t, *1081*
malabsorption of, 143, 144t, 1080
Galactosemia, **1080–1081**
clinical manifestations of, 1081, 1105t
diagnosis of, 1081
enzyme pathways and, 1080t, 1080–1081, *1081*
etiology of, 1080, 1105t
genetics of, 138t
pathogenesis of, 1080t, 1080–1081
prevalence of, 1080
prognosis in, 1081
treatment of, 1081
Galactosidase deficiency, 1096, 1096t, 1119t, 2112–2113

Gallbladder, **810–816**
adenocarcinoma of, 811
bile storage and release by, 806, *807*
cancer of, incidence of, 1013t
cholesterolosis, 816
choledochal, *809*, 813, 813t, 814
cholesterol, 812–813, *813*, 815
clinical features of, 813t, 813–814
congenital heart disease and, 286, *286*
diagnostic studies of, 814–815, *815*
hereditary spherocytosis with, 853
imaging of, CT scan in, *631*
ERCP in, *637*
radiography in, *637*
ultrasonography in, 632, *632*, 815
natural history of, 813t, 813–814
obesity association with, 1165
pancreatitis and, 814
pathogenesis of, 812–813, *813*
pigment, 812, 813, *815*
treatment of, 815–816
dissolution, 815
endoscopic removal, *637*, 641
lithotripsy, *637*, 815–816
Galvanic skin response, 2009t
Gamete, 134
gene linkage differences due to, 135
Gametocytes, malarial, *1893*, 1893–1894, 1895t
Gamma chains, 958, *959*
disease of, 966
Gamma globulin, 958, *959*. See also *Immunoglobulins.*
absence of, 1402t, *1403*, 1403–1404
monoclonal, 958, *960*
Gamma-aminobutyric acid (GABA), 797, 797t
Gamma-glutamyl transpeptidase, 760
Gamma-glutamylcysteine synthetase, 858–859
Gammopathy, 958–968. See also *Multiple myeloma.*
biclonal, *960*, 962
classification, *960*, 960t, 961t
differentiation of, 960–961, 961t
heavy-chain, 966
monoclonal, 958–961, 2152
neuropathy with, 961, 2152
of uncertain significance, 959–961, *960*, 960t, 961t
Ganciclovir, **1743**
CMV treated with, 1746t, 1869t
licensing for, 1743
mechanism of action of, 1743
retinitis treated with, 1869t
toxicity of, 1743
Gangliogliomas, 2132
Ganglion blocking agents, 265t, 270t
Ganglionitis, sensory, 2153
Gangrene, anaerobic flora in, 1641
clinical presentation of, 1631, 1631t, 1632
clostridial infection causing, 1630–1632, 1631t
diabetes mellitus with, 1276
foot affected by, 1276
Fournier's, 1641
gas, 1630–1632, 1631t
lung affected by, 1581
Pseudomonas causing, 1581
scrotal, 1641
streptococcal infection in, 1588, 1589t
vasculitis in, 2201t, 2202
Gardner syndrome, 723, *724*
polyps in, 723, *724*
Gardner-Diamond syndrome, 987
Gardnerella vaginalis, 1699
Gardos channel, 852
sickle cell and, 885
Gas(es), arsine, 70
blood. See *Blood gases.*
embolism of, 410
flatulence due to, 699t
gangrene with, 1630–1632, 1631t
irritant, 404
pleural, 375t
smoke inhalation and, 403t, 403–404
tissue bubble of, 375t
toxic, 59t, 70, 403t, 403–404

Gas exchange, 371–375, 466–468
alveolar surface and, 371–372, *372*
assessment of, 375, 375t, 466–468, 467t
Gasoline, ingestion of, 407
lead in, 68
Gastric acid. See *Stomach, acid secretion of.*
Gastric lavage, 505, 643, 645
Gastric regurgitation, cough due to, 369
tracheobronchial irritation due to, 369
Gastrin, 662–663, 674–676
ectopic, 663, 674–676, 1346
hypersecretion of, 663–664, 675t
peptic ulcer and, 663–664
Gastrinoma, **674–676**
clinical features of, 674, 675t
diagnosis of, 675, 675t
multiple endocrine neoplasia with, 1346
pathogenesis of, 674–675
peptic ulcer and, 662t, 663
treatment of, 675–676
Gastritis, **659–662**
alcoholic, 661
alkaline reflux, 672
anemia and, pernicious, 660
atrophic, 659t, 660–661
autoimmune, 660
bleeding due to, 642t, 643, 645t
causes of, 659t
classification, 659, 659t
drug-induced, 659t, 661
eosinophilic, 661
erosive/hemorrhagic, 659t, 661–662
granulomatous, 661
Helicobacter, 659t, 659–660
hypertrophic, 659t, 661
Ménétrier's disease, 659t, 661
peptic ulcer and, 660
phlegmonous, 661
resection complicated by, 672
Gastroenteritis, 1641–1642
E. coli, 1654–1657, 1655t
Norwalk virus, 1793–1797, *1795*
rotavirus, 1642t, 1658t, 1793–1797, *1795*, 1795t
Salmonella, 1645, 1646
staphylococcal, 1606–1607, 1609
viral, 692, 1793–1797, *1795*, 1795t
Gastroesophageal junction, hemorrhage from, 642t, 643
Mallory-Weiss tear in, 642t, 643
reflux in, 651–654. See also *Reflux esophagitis.*
Gastrointestinal tract, **627–751**
absorption in, 689, 689–690, 690t. See also *Absorption; Malabsorption.*
aging effect on, 22
AIDS/HIV effects in, 1866–1868, 1867t
antimicrobials affecting, 1568t
approach to diseases of, 627–630
bleeding. See *Hemorrhage, gastrointestinal.*
endoscopy of, 636–641, *637*, 638t
flora of, 1638–1641, *1639*, 1639t, 1659–1660
fluid movement in, 689
history taking for, 627–628
hypothyroidism affecting, 1238, 1238t
imaging of, 630–635, *630–635*
innervation of, 681, *681*, 681t, 2010
lupus erythematosus effect on, 1479
manometry of, *682, 685*
mastocytosis affecting, 1435t, 1436
motility of, **680–688**
clinical assessment of, 682–683
disorders of, 683–688, 691–692
drugs affecting, 681t, 688, 688t
normal, 680–682, *680–682*
neurotransmitters of, 681, 681t
parasympathetic control of, 2010
prostaglandin effect on, 1193
smoking and, 34t, 35t
symptoms of disease in, 628–630
Wegener's granulomatosis affecting, 1496t
Gastrojejunostomy, 669t, 669–671, 670t, 672
Gastroparesis, diabetic, 684
Gastropathy, congestive, 794
portal hypertensive, 794
Gaucher cells, 1097, *1097*
Gaucher's disease, **1097–1098**
cardiomyopathy due to, 333t, 334
clinical manifestations of, 1097–1098
diagnosis of, 1098
etiology and pathogenesis of, 1096t, 1097
genetics of, 136t, 1096t, 1097
lymphadenopathy due to, 970t

Gaucher's disease (Continued)
pathology in, 1097, 1097
splenomegaly in, 971t, 972, 972t
treatment of, 1098
type 1, 1096t, 1097–1098
type 2, 1096t, 1097, 1098
type 3, 1096t, 1097, 1098
Gaussian distribution, 83
Gay bowel syndrome, 1867, 1867t
Gaze, 2018–2020
abnormalities in, 2018–2020, 2020, 2020t
cerebral hemorrhage affecting, 2078, 2078t
degenerative disorders affecting, 2051t
frontal lobe damage and, 1988, 1988t
meningitis affecting, 1612t, 1613
neural pathways for, 2018–2019
paresis of, 2018–2020, 2078, 2078t
parietal lobe damage and, 1987, 1988t
Gelatinase, 898t
Gender. See Sex (gender).
Gene therapy, cancer treated with, 149–150, 150t, 1075
mucopolysaccharidoses and, 1119
Gene(s), 134–142. See also Genetics; Oncogene(s).
aldolase deficiency, 1083, 1084
anticipation related to, 138
apoptosis (cell death) and, 1011, 1057–1058, 1072–1073
Bax, 1072–1073, 1073
Bcl, 1011, 1057–1058, 1072–1073
bcr, 1011–1012
BRCA, 1076–1077
calcitonin, 1374, 1375
cancer growth and, 1011, 1038t, 1057–1058, 1072–1073, 1073
cell-surface receptor for, 149–150, 150
COL1A2, 1121, 1121t, 1122, 1122t
control regions of, 134–136, 135
dominant disorder, 137–140, 138, 138t, 140
X-linked, 138, 138t, 140, 140
drug resistance related to, 1057t, 1057–1058
femaleness, 1285
frequency, 136t, 136–137, 138t, 142
fructose intolerance and, 1083, 1084
glucose transporter, 144t
HER, 1011–1012, 1036t
HLA complex, 1426–1429, 1427, 1428t, 1429, 1429t
immunoglobulin, 1396, 1396t, 1396–1397, 1397
imprinting of, 135, 156
inhibition of, 1073–1074, 1074t
antisense, 1073
cancer therapy using, 1073–1074, 1074t
ribozyme, 1074
triplex oligonucleotide, 1073–1074, 1074
linkage of, disequilibrium in, 135
sex differences in, 135
maleness, 141, 1285
mdr1, 1057, 1057t
p53, 1011, 1057–1058, 1076
packaging function in, 149
paternal age effect on, 138
penetrance and, 138
polypeptides copied from, 134, 135
recessive disorder, 136t, 136–140, 138t, 139, 141
X-linked, 138t, 139, 140, 141
retinoblastoma (Rb), 1011
retroviral vector for, 148–150, 149
sex differentiation, 1285
SRY, 1285
suppressor, 1011–1012
therapy using, 147–150, 148–150, 150t
total number of, 134
transcription of, 134, 135, 1181, 1181
inducers and inhibitors for, 1181
transfer procedures for, 148–150, 149, 150
Genetics, 134–165. See also Chromosome(s); Gene(s); Hereditary disorder(s).
aging related to, 13–15, 1072, 1072–1073, 1073
alcohol and, 47
aldolase deficiency and, 1084–1085
Alport's syndrome and, 611
Alzheimer's disease and, 13, 1994
atherosclerosis and, 294
Behçet's syndrome and, 1507
breast cancer and, 1320
cancer mechanisms and, 1011–1012
apoptosis (cell death) and, 1011, 1057–1058, 1072, 1072
mutational, 1011–1012
promotor, 1011–1012
suppressor release, 1011–1012

Genetics (Continued)
Charcot-Marie-Tooth disease and, 2153, 2154t
code, 134, 134t
colon cancer and, 725t, 726, 726
counseling on, 162–165
cancer and, 1077
chromosome mapping and, 163t
diagnosis confirmation for, 162–163, 163t, 164t, 165t
genetic modelling in, 163–164
indications for, 164t
metabolic disorders in, 1078, 1078t
prenatal testing and, 164t, 165, 165t
drug effects related to, 97t, 97–98
ethnic group and, 136t, 136–137, 138t
family history and, 136t, 136–137
fructose intolerance and, 1084–1085
globin chain, 870–872, 871
hemochromatosis and, 786, 1132–1133
hemoglobin, 870–872, 871
heterogeneity and, 142
HIV organism and, 1842–1844, 1842–1844
hypertension and, 258
immunodeficiency, 1401–1402, 1402t
Klinefelter's syndrome and, 154, 1286, 1333–1334
leukemia and, 926, 937–938
lung cancer and, 437–438, 438t
lupus erythematosus and, 1476, 1476t
McCune-Albright syndrome and, 1347
mitochondria and, 142
molecular basis of, 134, 134t, 135
monogenic (mendelian), 136t, 137–141, 138t
multiple endocrine neoplasia and, 1346–1347
muscular dystrophy and, 2159t, 2160t, 2161, 2162, 2163
mutation and, 135–136
myelodysplastic syndrome and, 836
myeloma and, 962
pedigree in, 137, 137
dominant trait, 137–140, 138, 138t, 140
recessive trait, 138t, 139, 139–140, 141
X-linked trait, 138t, 140, 140–141, 141
Y-linked trait, 141
peptic ulcer and, 664–665
pheochromocytoma and, 1254
polygenic (multifactorial), 141, 141–142
porphyria and, 138t, 1125t
recombination, 135, 136
renal cystic disease and, 138t, 618, 620, 620t
rheumatoid arthritis and, 1459, 1460t
sarcoidosis and, 431
sickle syndromes and, 137, 139, 142, 883–884, 889–891
steroid hydroxylase deficiencies and, 136t, 138t, 1288, 1288, 1290
thalassemia and, 880–881
Wiskott-Aldrich syndrome and, 1403, 1407
Genitals, 1284–1293
ambiguous, 1287–1293
androgen excess and, 1287–1290, 1288, 1288t, 1290
androgen insensitivity and, 1290–1292, 1291t, 1292
enzyme deficiencies and, 1287–1292, 1288, 1288t, 1291t
differentiation of, 1284–1285, 1285, 1286
flora of, in female, 1639, 1640, 1640t
gonorrhea affecting, 1701–1702, 1702t
infantile, 1329, 1330
pseudohermaphroditism and, 1287–1293
female, 1287–1290, 1288t, 1288–1290
male, 1290–1293, 1291t, 1292
sexually transmitted disease affecting, 1696–1700, 1701–1702
skin disorders affecting, 2191, 2216t
testicular feminization and, 1291t, 1291–1292
tuberculosis affecting, 1685t
ulcer of, 1698
differential diagnosis of, 1706
H. ducreyi chancroid, 1704
herpetic, 1706, 1746t, 1772
syphilitic chancre, 1706, 1707, 1707
virilization of, 1284–1292
in females, 1287–1290, 1288t, 1290
incomplete, 1290–1292, 1291t, 1292
normal, 1284–1285, 1285, 1286
warts of, 1746t, 2200
Genome, haploid, 134
human, 137
mapping, 137
Gentamicin, 91t, 94t, 1562t
cat scratch disease therapy with, 1681–1682, 1682t

Gentamicin (Continued)
dose adjustment for, 94t, 1562t
endocarditis therapy with, 1602t–1604t, 1602–1603
pharmacokinetics of, 91t, 94t, 1562t
renal failure effect on, 94t, 1562t
staphylococcal infection treated with, 1609t, 1609–1610
Geographic factors. See also Epidemics.
Behçet's syndrome and, 1506–1507
cancer rate and, 1013t, 1013–1014
cholera and, 1652, 1652
coronary heart disease and, 172
leishmaniasis and, 1903t, 1905
Paget's disease of bone and, 1384
pleurodynia with, 1787
rickettsioses and, 1727t, 1731
tuberculosis and, 1684, 1684
typus and, 1727t
yellow fever with, 1798–1799
Yersinia and, 1661, 1662
Geophagia, 840
Geriatrics. See Age; Elderly.
Germ cells, aplasia of, 1336
ovarian, 1293, 1293–1295, 1294
telomeres of, 1072
testicular, 1325–1326
tumors of, ovarian, 1312t
pituitary, 2131
suprasellar, 1201, 1202
testicular, 1340
Gerstmann-Sträussler disease, 2097, 2097t, 2102, 2103
GFR. See Glomerular filtration rate (GFR).
GGTP (gamma-glutamyl transpeptidase), 760
Ghon focus, 1683
GHRH. See Growth hormone–releasing hormone (GHRH).
Giant cells, measles with, 1759
myocarditis with, 330
sarcoidosis with, 434, 435
Giardiasis, 1912–1913
clinical manifestations of, 1913
diagnosis of, 1913
diarrhea due to, 694, 1642t, 1658t, 1913
epidemiology of, 1912
etiologic organism in, 1912
pathology findings in, 1912–1913
treatment of, 1913
Giddiness, 16t, 17. See also Delirium; Dizziness.
Giemsa stain, malaria organism in, 1894, 1895t
Gigantism, 1211–1212
Gilbert's syndrome, 757t
bilirubin metabolism in, 756–757, 757t
jaundice in, 756–757, 757t
Gilchrist's disease, 1821–1822
Gingivostomatitis, 1772, 1772
G-kinase, 1178
Glanders, 1667
clinical features of, 1667
nodules of, 1667
Glanzmann's thrombasthenia, 985
Glasgow coma scale, 2137, 2137t
Glasgow criteria, pancreatitis and, 732t, 732–733
Glaucoma, 2175–2177
absolute, 2177
angle-closure, 2176, 2176–2177
congenital, 2177
diabetes mellitus with, 1273
open-angle, 2175–2176, 2177
vision loss due to, 2016, 2175
Glenohumeral joint, 1521, 1522
arthritis of, 1524
Glioblastoma, 2126t, 2131–2132
classification of, 2126t
MRI scan of, 2127–2128, 2128t
Glioma, 1964, 1965
Glipizide, 1268, 1268t
Globi, 1694, 1695
Globin. See also Hemoglobin.
genetics of, 870, 870–872, 871
malaria and, 872–873, 883
sickle syndromes and, 883, 883, 884
structure of, 868, 868
synthesis of, 870, 870–872, 871
thalassemia role of, 877–882
Globulin, gamma. See Gamma globulin; Immunoglobulin(s).
liver function testing and, 761

Globus pallidum, 2043
  blood supply to, 2060
Glomerular filtration rate (GFR), 514
  aging effect on, 13, 13, 21–22
  diabetes mellitus and, 599, 600, 601, 601
  diuretic action affecting, 223
  heart failure effect on, 217
  measurement of, blood urea nitrogen in, 514
    creatinine clearance in, 514
    radionuclide in, 516
  obstruction and, 590
  potassium and, 514, 515
  pregnancy and, 609
  sodium and, 514, 514t
Glomeruli, 223, 519, 572–579
  AIDS/HIV effects in, 1875–1876, 1876
  anatomy of, 519, 519–520, 520
  barrier properties of, 520, 520, 521, 572
  basement membrane of, 520, 521, 572
    antibodies to, 577
    layers of, 520
    nephrotic syndrome affecting, 574, 575
    widened, 600, 601
  calcium reabsorption and, 1353
  diabetes mellitus affecting, 599–601, 601
  filtration properties of, 520, 520, 521
  proteinuria and, 513, 513t, 572–573
  renal failure and, acute, 552t, 554, 554t
    chronic, 556, 556–559
  tubular acidosis and, 598, 598t
Glomerulonephritis, 575–577
  acute, 575–577
  antibodies in, 577, 1479
  crescentic, 577, 577t
  endocarditis and, 576
  focal segmental, 574
  Henoch-Schönlein, 576, 577t
  immune complexes and, 575–576
  lupus erythematosus and, 574t, 577t, 578, 578t
  membranoproliferative, 573t, 575
  pathophysiology of, 575
  Pauci-immune, 574t, 577, 577t
  polyarteritis nodosa with, 1493
  post-streptococcal, 573t, 576
  rapidly progressive, 576–577, 577t
  renal failure with, chronic, 556
  visceral abscess with, 576
  Wegener's granulomatosis in, 574t, 577, 577t, 1496, 1496t
Glomerulosclerosis, 572, 574
  focal segmental, 574
Glomus tumor, clinical features of, 353
  nail bed with, 353
  pain of, 353
  pathology in, 353
Glossitis, malabsorption causing, 699t
  migratory, benign, 647, 647t
Glossopharyngeal neuralgia, 2009, 2035
Glottis, vomiting and, 629, 629
Gloves, precautionary, 1853, 1853t
Glucagon, beta blocker reversed by, 504t
  catecholamine deficiency and, 1257
  tumor secretion of, 1283–1284
Glucagonoma, 1283–1284
  clinical features of, 1283–1284
  diagnosis of, 1283–1284
  pathology of, 1284
  treatment of, 1284
Glucocerebrosides, accumulation of, 333t, 334, 1096t
  cardiomyopathy due to, 333t, 334
Glucocorticoids, 108–110. See also Corticosteroids; Cortisol.
  adrenal cortex production of, 1245–1247
  deficiency syndromes of, 1249–1251, 1250t
  excess of, 1216–1218, 1247–1249. See also Cushing's syndrome.
  hirsutism treated with, 1316
  hypogonadism due to, 1338
  myopathy role of, 2167–2168
  stimulation test of, 1247
  therapeutic, 108–110
    ACTH deficiency due to, 1215–1216, 1251
    adverse effects of, 110, 110t
    anti-inflammatory properties of, 108–110, 109t
    bone loss induced by, 1384
    chemotherapy using, 1046, 1046t
    dose adjustment of, 109–110
    hemolytic anemia treated with, 864–865

Glucocorticoids (Continued)
    leukocyte response to, 108–109, 109t
    mechanism of action of, 108–109
    myxedema coma and, 1240t
    pharmacology of, 108, 108t
    preparations of, 108t
Glucokinase, 1263
Gluconeogenesis, 753
Glucosaminide acetyltransferase deficiency, 1119t
Glucose, 689, 753, 856
  absorption of, 689, 689–690, 696, 696t
  alcoholism and, 48
  atherosclerosis and, 1276–1277
  cerebral, 2062t
  consciousness level and, 2062t
  deficiency in. See Hypoglycemia.
  erythrocyte metabolism and, 856, 856–858
  excess of. See Diabetes mellitus; Hyperglycemia.
  fasting level of, 1260
  growth hormone suppression test with, 1213t
  hyperosmolar syndrome and, 1270
  insulin therapy and, 1265t, 1265–1266, 1266
  intolerance, cirrhosis and, 753
  liver and, 753, 1082, 1082–1083, 1084
  metabolism of, 753, 856–858, 1082, 1082–1083, 1084
  oral agent reduction of, 1267–1268, 1268t, 1280
  self-monitoring of, 1268
  synovial fluid with, 1465t
  tolerance test, 1258–1259
    diabetes diagnosed using, 1258–1259
    impaired, 1258–1259, 1263
  transporter defect and, 143, 144t, 594–596, 595t, 596
  urinary, 512, 512t, 594–596, 595t, 596
Glucose-6-phosphatase deficiency, 1082, 1510
  glycogen storage disease with, 1082, 1082, 1083t
  hyperuricemia with, 1509t, 1510, 1511
Glucose-6-phosphate, diabetes effect on, 1261, 1262
Glucose-6-phosphate dehydrogenase, 856, 856–858, 857, 858t
  deficiency of, 856–858
    clinical features of, 857, 858t
    drug adverse effects due to, 98
    drug-induced, 858, 858t
    genetics of, 136t, 138t
    neutrophil dysfunction due to, 905t, 905–906
    pathophysiology of, 856–857, 857
    tests for, 858
  genetics of, 857, 857–858
  Lyon hypothesis and, 857–858
  variant forms of, 857, 857–858, 858t
Glucosidase, 1082, 1082–1083
  deficiency of, 1082–1083, 1083t, 1096t, 1097, 2165
  myopathy related to, 2165
Glucosylceramide, 1096t, 1097
Glucuronidase deficiency, 1119t
Glutamine, urinary, 1102t, 1104t
Glutathione, 856, 856, 858–859
  urinary, 1103t
Glutathione peroxidase, 856, 856
  oxygen toxicity and, 405
Glutathione reductase, 856, 856
Gluten intolerance, 704–705
Glyburide, glucose reduction using, 1268, 1268t
  micronized, 1268, 1268t
Glycerate, 1085
Glycerol, 224t
Glycine, absorption of, 700t
  bile conjugated with, 805, 807
  heme synthesis from, 1125
  urinary, 1102t, 1103t
Glycoasparagine, urinary, 1103t
Glycogen, hepatic stores of, 753, 1082–1083, 1083t
  muscle stores of, 1083, 1083t
Glycogen storage disease, 1082–1083
  cardiomyopathy due to, 333t, 334
  clinical manifestations of, 1082–1083, 1083t, 2165
  enzyme deficiencies of, 1082, 1082–1083, 1083t, 2165
  genetics of, 136t, 138t
  hepatic, 786, 1082–1083, 1083t
  McArdle's, 1083, 1083t
  metabolic defect in, 143, 1082, 1082–1083, 1083t
  muscle, 1083, 1083t, 2065
  Pompe's, 1083, 1083t
  prenatal testing for, 1083
  types of, 1082–1083, 1083t
Glycogen synthetase, 1082, 1083t
Glycogenesis. See Glycogen storage disease.

Glycogenolysis, 753
Glycohemoglobin, 1269
  assays for, 1269
  diabetes monitored with, 1268–1269
  formation of, 1269
Glycolysis, 856, 856–858
  erythrocytic, 856, 856–858
Glycophorin, 851, 851–852
Glycoproteins, cancer chemotherapy and, 1039–1040, 1040
  cartilage and, 1445
  connective tissue role of, 1444–1445
  HLA molecules with, 1424–1426
  microfibril-associated, 1444
  myelin-associated, 2152
Glycosaminoglycans, 1445, 1445t
  connective tissue structure and, 1445, 1445t
  mucopolysaccharidosis and, 1118, 1119t
  urinary, 1118, 1119t
Glycosides, cardiac. See Digitalis.
Glycosuria, diabetes mellitus with, 1258
  diagnosis of, 596, 596
  metabolic defect in, 144t
  pathophysiology of, 594–595
  renal, 594–596, 595t, 596
  transport defect causing, 143, 144t, 594–596, 595t, 596
Glycosylation, atherosclerosis and, 293
  end-products of, 293
Glycyrrhizinic acid, hypokalemia caused by, 539
  intoxication due to, 1249
  licorice containing, 539, 1249
  snuff containing, 35
Gnat, buffalo, 1947
Gnathostomiasis, 1935t, 1936
GnRH. See Gonadotropin-releasing hormone (GnRH).
Goat, 1737t
  zoonoses associated with, 1727t, 1737t
Goiter, 1241–1242
  clinical manifestations of, 1241–1242
  diagnostic approach in, 1242, 1243
  diffuse, 1241–1242, 1243
  endemic, 1241–1242
  examination for, 1242
  Graves' disease with, 1232–1233
  Hashimoto's thyroiditis with, 1241
  iodine deficiency in, 1149t
  iodine role in, 1241
  multinodular, 1241–1242, 1243
  multinodular toxic, 1235–1236
  simple (nontoxic), 1241–1242, 1243
  sporadic, 1241
  treatment of, 1242, 1243
Gold, poisoning due to, 504t
  skin disorder treated with, 2197
  systemic, 2197
Golfer's elbow, 1528
Golgi apparatus, herpes simplex in, 1770, 1771
  hormone storage and delivery by, 1182
Goltz's syndrome, 1390
Gompertz curve, 1039
Gonadal dysgenesis. See Gonads, dysgenesis of.
Gonadoblastoma, 1312t
Gonadotrope cells, 1209t, 1219
Gonadotropin-releasing hormone (GnRH), 1198, 1198
  agonists for, cancer therapy related to, 1046t, 1047
  deficiency of, 1202, 1219
  disorders of, 1202
  pituitary function test using, 1208t
  replacement therapy for, 1208t
  testicular function role of, 1326, 1326
Gonadotropins, 1218–1220. See also Follicle-stimulating hormone (FSH); Luteinizing hormone (LH).
  amenorrhea evaluation and, 1303–1304, 1304, 1305
  chorionic, ovulation induced with, 1309
    testicular cancer with, 1022t, 1023, 1025t
    tumor production of, 1022t, 1023, 1025t, 1026, 1312t
  deficiency of. See also Hypogonadism.
  feedback mechanism for, 1198, 1198
  menstruation and, 1297–1299, 1298, 1299
  ovarian function and, 1297–1299, 1298
  puberty and, 1294–1295
    female, 1294, 1294–1295
    male, 1326
  regulation of, 1198, 1198
    disordered, 1202, 1219–1220
  releasing hormone for, 1198, 1198
  replacement therapy using, 1208t
  secretion of, rhythms in, 1199–1200

Gonadotropins (Continued)
  sleep-entrainment of, 1294, 1294–1295
  testicular function and, 1326, 1326–1328, 1327
  tumor production of, 1219–1220
Gonads, 1284–1285, 1287. See also Ovaries; Testes.
  anorexia effect on, 1158, 1159t
  differentiation of, 1284–1285, 1285, 1286
  dysgenesis of, 1287
    amenorrhea with, 1304–1305, 1305t
    mixed, 1286, 1297
    pure, 1287, 1305
    Turner's, 154, 1286, 1304–1305
  radiation of, 61, 61t, 62t
Gonorrhea, **1700–1703**
  arthritis due to, 1455, 1473–1474, 1474t, 1703
  bacteremia of, 1702
  cervicitis due to, 1701–1702, 1702t
  child with, 1702
  clinical manifestations of, 1697–1699, 1701–1702
  conjunctivitis and, 1702, 2179
  disseminated, 1474t, 1702, 1702t
  epidemiology of, 1700–1701
  epididymitis in, 1701, 1702t
  female with, 1698–1699, 1701–1702
  host response to, 1701
  laboratory tests for, 1702–1703
  male with, 1697–1698, 1698, 1701
  oral lesions of, 646t
  pathogenesis of, 1701
  pelvic inflammatory disease in, 1701–1703,
    1702t
  pharyngitis of, 1701
  pregnancy and, 1702, 1702t
  prevention of, 1700, 1703
  proctitis of, 742
  resistant, 1703
  salpingitis in, 1700, 1701–1703, 1702t
  sexual transmission of, 1697t, 1700–1701
  skin lesions of, 1702
  treatment of, 1702t, 1703
  urethritis in, 1697–1699, 1701–1702
    female affected by, 1698–1699, 1701–1702
    male affected by, 1697–1698, 1698, 1701
    posttreatment, 1698
Goodpasture's syndrome, 397–398, 577
  glomerulonephritis with, 574t, 577, 577t
  HLA complex in, 1431t
  interstitial lung disease in, 397–398
Goodsall's rule, 742
Gooseflesh, 1533
Gorlin formula, 210, 211
Goserelin, 1046t, 1047
Gottron's patches, 1502
Gout, **1508–1515**
  acute, 1510, 1511, 1513–1514, 1514t
  asymptomatic, 1515
  chronic, 1511–1512, 1514t, 1514–1515
  classification of, 1509t
  clinical manifestations of, 1511–1512, 1512–1514
  crystals in, 1508, 1512, 1514
  diagnosis of, 1512, 1514
  differential diagnosis of, 1512
  interval phase in, 1514, 1514t
  joint anatomy and, 1441, 1442
  nephrolithiasis in, 1510–1511
  nephropathy of, 1510, 1512
  pathogenesis of, 1509t, 1509–1511, 1511
  prevalence of, 1509
  primary, 1509t
  pseudo, 1512, 1515–1516
  secondary, 1509t
  synovial fluid in, 1465t, 1510, 1512, 1514
  tophaceous, 1510, 1511–1512, 1512, 1513, 1516
  treatment of, 1512–1515, 1514t
  urates in, chronic renal failure and, 557t, 559, 562
Gowns, precautionary use of, 1853, 1853t
G6PD. See Glucose-6-phosphate dehydrogenase.
Grafts, bypass. See Bypass grafts.
Graft-versus-host disease, bone marrow affected by, 975
  cholestasis due to, 810
  transfusion-associated, 896, 896t
Grains, dietary aspects of, 29–30, 30t, 1142
  food poisoning due to, 740
  fungal contamination of, 740
  mycetomatous, 1834–1835, 1835t
Gram stain, 1556
  cerebrospinal fluid in, 1613, 1620
Grammar, 1990
Gram-negative organisms, 1556, 1556–1557, 1557t
  aerobic, pneumonia due to, 1579–1581, 1580t

Gram-positive organisms, 1556, 1556–1557, 1557t
Grand mal seizures, 2116
Grandiosity, manic, 1997, 1997t, 2002
Granules, alpha, 979, 982
  azurophil, 897, 898t
  Birbeck, 955, 2185
  botryomycosis, 1607t, 1609
  dense body, 979, 982
  keratohyalin, 2184, 2185
  mycetomatous, 1835, 1835t
  neutrophilic, 897, 898t
  pacchionian, 2148
  platelet, 979, 982
    storage defects of, 985
  sulfur, actinomycosis with, 1640t, 1674, 1675
Granulocyte colony-stimulating factor. See Colony-
  stimulating factors.
Granulocytes, **817–818**. See also Basophils;
    Eosinophils; Neutrophils.
  increased, 915–919, 916, 917
  maturation of, 817–819, 818–821, 820t, 898, 916
  phagocytosis by, 1537–1541, 1538t, 1539t
Granulocytopenia, 909–911, 909–914
  antimicrobial therapy in, 1542–1548, 1544t, 1545,
    1546t
  approach to febrile patient with, 1542–1548, 1545
  cell count in, 1539t
  chemotherapy causing, 1046
  compromised host with, 1537–1541, 1538t, 1539t
  prolonged, 1545, 1545–1548, 1546t, 1547t
Granuloma, coccidioidal, 1819, 1820
  cryptococcal, 1824
  eosinophilic, 955–956
  hepatic, 783–785, 784t
    drug-induced, 773, 773t, 784t
  inguinale, 1703–1704
  Langerhans' cell, 955–956
  leprotic, 1693–1694, 1694
  pulmonary, 1495, 1495t, 1496t
  pyogenic, 2211
  sarcoidosis with, 431, 431–433, 435
  tuberculosis, 1682
Granulomatosis, interstitial lung disease in, 398
  lymphoid, lymphadenopathy in, 970
  vascular, necrotizing, 1495–1498
  Wegener's. See Wegener's granulomatosis.
Granulomatous disease, 904–906, 1540–1541
  chronic, 904–906, 1540–1541
    clinical manifestations of, 905, 905t, 906
    diagnosis of, 905–906
    etiology of, 905, 905t, 906, 1540–1541
    pathogenesis of, 905, 906, 1540–1541
    phagocytes affected by, 904–906, 905t, 906,
      1540–1541
    treatment of, 906
  hypercalcemia due to, 1371
Granulosa cells, 1182, 1293
  estrogen synthesized by, 1299, 1299
  ovarian, 1182, 1293, 1299
  tumor affecting, 1312, 1312t
Graves' disease, **1232–1234**
  acropachy with, 1233
  clinical features in, 1233
  diagnosis of, 1233
  differential diagnosis of, 1233
  etiology of, 1232
  ophthalmopathy of, 1233, 2180
  pathogenesis of, 1232
  pathology in, 1232
  treatment of, 1234
Gravity, hormone secretion affected by, 1199
Grb2 linker protein, 1180, 1180
Grey Turner's sign, 731
Grief reaction, 2001t, 2001–2002
Grip, milkmaid's, 1593
Griseofulvin, 2196
Grönblad-Strandberg syndrome, 1123, 1123–1124
"Ground itch" pruritus, 1935
Ground-glass appearance, fibrous dysplasia with, 1390,
  1390
  P. carinii pneumonia with, 1864
Growth, 1210
  bone, 1353–1354
  excessive, 1209t, 1211–1212, 1212
  hormonal factors in. See Growth hormone.
  retarded, 1210–1211
    sickle syndrome causing, 776
    zinc deficiency in, 1150t
Growth factors, atherosclerosis role of, 294, 295
  bone formation regulated by, 1352

Growth factors (Continued)
  bone marrow, antagonists to, 1049
    cancer therapy using, 1048t, 1049, 1049t, 1050
  hematopoietic, 819–821, 820t, 821, 897, 898
    AIDS/HIV effect on, 1871–1872
  insulin-like, 1206t, 1210
    tumor-associated, 1026
  mast cell release of, 1416, 1436t
  platelet secretion of, 979
  rheumatoid synovitis role of, 1460, 1460–1461
  tamoxifen mechanism of action and, 1060
Growth hormone, 1206t, 1210–1212
  acromegaly and, 1211t, 1211–1212, 1212
  aging effect on, 15
  deficiency of, 1210–1211
    idiopathic congenital, 1201–1202
    treatment of, 1211
  excess of, 1209t, 1211–1212, 1212
  insulin and, 1208t
  laboratory tests for, 1208t, 1213t
  receptor for, 1177, 1210
  regulation of, 1198, 1198, 1199, 1206t, 1210
    disordered, 1201–1202, 1210–1212
  replacement therapy using, 1208t, 1211
  secretion of, 1210
    tumor and, 1209t, 1211
  stimulation test for, 1208t
  stored, 1210
  suppression test for, 1213t
Growth hormone–releasing hormone (GHRH), 1198,
  1199, 1210
  ectopic, 1025t, 1026
  pituitary function test using, 1208t
  somatostatin action with, 1198, 1198
GSH. See Glutathione.
Guanabenz, dosage for, 265t
  side effects of, 267
Guanethidine, 265t
Guanfacine, 265t, 266t
Guanine, 134, 134t
Guano, 1816
Guanosine monophosphate, cyclic (cGMP), 1177–1178
  hormone action and, 1177–1178
  second messenger role of, 1177–1178
Guanosine triphosphate (GTP), 1177–1178
  hormone action and, 1177–1178, 1178
  parathyroid hormone action and, 1366
Guanylate cylase, 1177, 1177–1178
Guillain-Barré syndrome, 2151t, 2151–2152
  neuropathy of, 2151t, 2151–2152
  pathophysiology of, 2151t, 2151–2152
  treatment of, 2151t, 2151–2152
Guinea worm disease, 1044
Gummas, syphilitic, 1708, 1708t
Gynecomastia, 1332–1333
  causes of, 1332t, 1332–1333
  cirrhosis and, 1332
  drug-induced, 1332
  Klinefelter's syndrome with, 1334
  physiologic vs. pathologic, 1332
  refeeding, 1332
  treatment of, 1332

H

H antigen, 1556
H chain, 1396, 1396t
H₂ receptor antagonists, 654t
  esophageal reflux disease and, 653, 654t
  peptic ulcer treated with, 667, 667–668
H reflex, 1962
HACEK microorganisms, 1598
Haemophilus, **1622–1624**
  aegyptius, 1622t, 1624
  aphrophilus, 1598, 1622t, 1624, 1624t
  chancroid due to, 1704–1705
  ducreyi, 1622t, 1624t, 1704–1705
  endocarditis caused by, 1598t, 1598–1599, 1624t
  influenzae, **1622–1624**
    biology of, 1622t, 1622–1623
    clinical syndromes caused by, 1623–1624, 1624t
    epidemiology of, 1622–1623
    host factors and, 1622
    immunization for, 1624
    incidence of, 1622–1623
    meningitis due to, 1610t, 1610–1613, 1616t, 1623
    pathogenicity of, 1623
    pneumonia due to, 412t, 1573, 1623

Haemophilus (Continued)
   prevalence of, 1622–1623
   prophylaxis for, 1624
   treatment for, 1623–1624
   virulence factors for, 1622
  parahaemolyticus, 1622t, 1624, 1624t
  parainfluenzae, 1598, 1622t, 1624, 1624t
  paraphrophilus, 1598, 1622t, 1624, 1624t
Hageman factor, 988t
Hailey-Hailey disease, 2206
Hair, *2185,* 2186–2187
  age-associated decrease in, 2190
  androgen effect on, 1315
  axillary, ear and nose, 2186–2187
  color of, albinism and, 2214t
   melanocyte organelles and, 2185
  excess of. See also *Hirsutism.*
   paraneoplastic, 1034
  eyelash, 1722
  follicle, *2185,* 2186–2187
  graying of, 2190
  hypoplasia of, 1407
  immunodeficiency affecting, 1407
  loss of, 2190, 2215–2217
  mechanical removal of, 1316
  normal growth of, 1315, 2186–2187
  protein deficiency affecting, 1156, 1156t
  psychological factors related to, 2184, 2189–2190
  pubic. See *Pubic hair.*
  pull-out examination of, 2192
  terminal, *1315,* 2187
  trachoma effect on, 1722
  vellus, *1315,* 2187
Hairy cell leukemia, 929–931, *930*
Halitosis, bronchiectasis with, 417
  esophageal cancer and, 657
  garlicky, metal poisoning with, 70, 72
Hallervorden-Spatz disease, 2046
Hallpike maneuver, 2025
Hallucinations, 1997t
  alcohol-related, 48
  drug-induced, 1974, 1974t, 1975t
  hypnogogic, 1984
  manic episode with, 1997t, 2002
  psychiatric disorder with, 1974, 1974t, 1975t, 1996, 1997, 1997t
  psychosis defined by, 1997, 1997t
  schizophrenia with, 1997, 1997t
  sleep-associated, 1984
Hallucinogens, 54, 508t, 1975t
  adverse effects of, 54, 508, 1975t
  drug abuse with, 54, 56t, 508
  neurologic effects of, 1975t
  overdose with, 54, 1975t
  pharmacology of, 54
Hallux rigidus, 1520
Hallux valgus (bunion), 1518, 1519t, *1519,* 1519–1520
Halofantrine, 1895–1896, 1896t
Haloperidol, myocardial infarction treatment and, 310t
  schizophrenia treated with, 1998t, 1998–1999, 1999t
Halothane, drug abuse using, 55
  hepatotoxicity of, 772, 773, 773t, 775
Halter cell, *1749*
Halzoun's syndrome, 1950
Hamartoma, Cowden's syndrome, 725
  hypothalamic, 1201
  Peutz-Jeghers, *724*
Hammer toe, 1519t
  Charcot-Marie-Tooth disease with, 2154
Ham's test, 867
Hand. See also *Palm.*
  cyanosis of, arteriolar constriction in, 349
  eczema of, 2184t, 2199
  erysipeloid affecting, 1674
  fungal infections of, 2199–2200
  gonorrhea affecting, 1702
  gout affecting, 1511–1512, *1513*
  "mechanic's," 1502
  osteoarthritis of, 1518–1519, 1519t, *1520*
  rash of, Rocky Mountain spotted fever with, 1731
  syphilis causing, 1707, *1707*
  Raynaud's phenomenon effect on, 347, 1484, 1485
  rheumatoid arthritis effects in, *1461,* 1461–1462, *1462*
  skin disorders affecting, *2191,* 2216t
Handedness, hemispheric dominance in, 1990–1991
  language and, 1990–1991

Hand-foot syndrome, 889
Hand-foot-mouth disease, 1787t, 1790
Hand-Schüller-Christian disease, 955
  lymphadenopathy due to, 970
Hanging groin, 1943
Hansen's disease. See *Leprosy.*
Hantavirus, pulmonary syndrome of, 1737t, 1798t, 1804–1805
  zoonoses and, 1737t, 1738t
Haploidy, 134
Haplotype, HLA, *568,* 1428t, 1429, *1429, 1430,* 1430t
Hardy-Weinberg equation, 142
Harris-Benedict equation, 1173t
  gender and, 1173t
Hartnup disease, 144t, 595t, 596
  aminoaciduria in, 1104t
  diagnosis of, 596
  symptoms of, 596
  transport defect in, 144t, 595t, 596
Hashimoto's thyroiditis, 1241
  clinical manifestations of, 1241
  treatment of, 1241
Hashish, 53
  adverse effects of, 53
  pharmacology of, 53
  withdrawal of, 53
Hassall's bodies, 1438
Hawkinsinuria, 1101t
Hayflick phenomenon, 15
HCG. See *Gonadotropins, chorionic.*
Head injury. See *Brain, trauma to.*
Headache, **2031–2036**
  AIDS/HIV with, 1856
  antimicrobials causing, 1568t
  arteritis causing, 2034
  brain abscess with, 2081, 2081t
  carotidynia in, 2033
  cerebral aneurysm causing, 2074, 2076t
  cerebral arteriovenous malformation with, 2076–2077
  cerebral hemorrhage causing, 2075, 2076, 2078
  cluster, 2032
   paroxysmal, 2032–2033
   treatment of, 2032–2033
   variants of, 2032–2033
  cough, 2033
  diagnostic evaluation of, 2035–2036
  exertion causing, 2032, 2033
  extracranial structures causing, 2034–2036
  giant cell arteritis with, 1499
  hypertensive, 2033
  "ice-pick," 2033
  intracranial metastases with, 1051
  intracranial pressure causing, 2133, 2135
  Lyme disease with, 1717, 1717t
  migraine, **2031–2033**
   classic, 2031–2032
   common, 2032
   complicated, 2032
   hemiplegic, 2032
   ophthalmoplegia in, 2032
   prodrome of, 2031–2032
   seizure vs., 2121
   stroke related to, 2069
   treatment and prevention of, 2032
   variants of, 2032
   vertigo with, 2026
  mycoplasmal infection with, *1577*
  neuralgia with, 2035
  orgasmic, 2033
  pheochromocytoma causing, 1254, 1254t
  pituitary apoplexy with, 2035, 2131
  poliovirus causing, 2091
  post-traumatic, 2033
  sinus, 2034
  tension, 2033
   treatment of, 2033
   variants of, 2033
  "thunderclap," 2033
  trauma injury with, 2138t
Headbanging, 1983, 1983t
Health care. See also *Medicine, Patients.*
  beds-per-capita affecting, 10, 10t
  diet and, 29
  ethical issues in, 4–6, 465–466
  personnel of, 4–6
   AIDS/HIV exposure of, 1850, 1852–1854, 1853t, 1854t
   hepatitis exposure of, 764, 765–766, 771
   preventive dress and equipment for, 1850, 1852–1854, 1853t, 1854t

Health care *(Continued)*
  preventive. See *Preventive health care.*
  reform of, 6, 29
Health Maintenance Organizations (HMOs), 10, 10t
Hearing, 2021–2024
  aging effect on, 16, 16t, 17
  anatomy and, 2021
  antimicrobials affecting, 1568t
  examination of, 2021
  frequency range of, 2021
  loss of, 2021–2024
   Alport's syndrome with, 612t
   causes of, 2021–2023, *2022*
   central, *2022,* 2022–2023
   conductive, 2021–2022, *2022*
   drug-induced, 2022
   evaluation of, 2021–2023, *2022*
   noise-induced, 2022
   occupational, 58t
   sensorineural, 2022, *2022*
   treatment of, 2023
  neurofibromatosis affecting, 2056
  physiology of, 2021
  temporal lobe damage and, 1985, 1987t
  tinnitus in, *2023,* 2023t, 2023–2024
Heart, **166–256.** See also *Cardiac; Cardio-* entries.
  afterload, 176–177, *177,* 212t, 214–215
  AIDS/HIV effect on, 329, 329t, 1876–1877, 1877t
  angiography of, 209t, *210,* 210–211, *211*
  anorexia effect on, 1159
  approach to disease of, 166–170, 220
  arrhythmias of. See *Arrhythmia(s);* specific disturbances.
  arteries of. See *Coronary artery(ies).*
  artificial, 495
  atrial natriuretic hormone affecting, *1195,* 1196
  atrial septal defect of, *274,* 278–279, *280*
  auscultation of, 168, 168t. See also *Heart, sounds of.*
  automaticity of, 233–234, *234*
  calcification in, *184, 185,* 185–186
  calcium metabolism in, 174, *175*
  carcinoid of, 358
  catheterization of, 208–211, 209t, *210, 211*
  cells of, 174, *175,* 213. See also *Myocardium.*
   depolarization of, 189–190, *232,* 232–233
   functioning of, 174, *175,* 213
   refractory period in, 190, 232
   structure of, *175*
   threshold voltage in, 190, 233t
  chemotherapy agents affecting, 330–331, 358
  collagen vascular disease and, 359
  conduction system of, 190, *191,* 191t, 231–233, *232, 233.* See also *Arrhythmia(s);* specific rhythm disturbances.
   accessory pathways in, 239, *240*
   block in. See *Heart block.*
   reentry circuits in, 234, *234*
   triggered activity in, 233–234, *234*
  congenital disease of, 277–291
   acyanotic, 287t
   adult survival of, 277–282, 278t, 279t, 282t, 287t, 288t
   common defects causing, 278t, 278–279, *278–281*
   cyanotic, 284–286, 287t
   endocarditis with, 284, *285,* 1597t
   functional status in, 286, 287t
   medical aspects of, 282t, 282–288, 287t, 288t
   neurological complications of, 287–288, *288,* 288t
   polycythemia of, 284–286
   pregnancy affected by, 286–287
   pulmonary hypertension due to, 273t, 275
   surgical aspects of, 288–291, 290t
   uncommon defects causing, 279t, 279–282, *281–285*
  contraction sequence of, 175–177, 213–216. See also *Cardiac cycle.*
   afterload in, 176–177, *177,* 212t, 214–215
   calcium role in, 174, *175*
   ECG of, 189–193, *190*
   energetics of, 212t, 216
   impedance with, 212t, *215*
   outflow resistance in, 176t, *214,* 214–215, *215*
   preload in, 175–176, *176,* 212t, 214, *214*
  cycle of. See *Cardiac cycle.*
  diabetes mellitus and, 173, 359, *1277*
  diagnostic evaluation of, *167,* 167–168, 168t
  diastolic properties of, 174–177, *175–177*
  dilatation of, *182, 183,* 183–185, 215, *216.* See also *Cardiomyopathy.*

Heart (Continued)
echocardiography of, 194–199, 195, 196
electrophysiology of, 189–193, 231–233. See also Electrocardiography (ECG); Electrogram; Electrophysiology (cardiac).
emboli originating in, 2066–2067, 2067t
examination of, 167–168
    arterial pressure pulse in, 167
    auscultation in, 168, 168t
    catheterization in, 169
    jugular venous pulse in, 167, 167
    noninvasive, 168–169
    palpation in, 167–168
failure of. See Heart failure.
hemochromatosis affecting, 359
hyperthyroidism and, 359, 1233, 1233t, 1236–1237
inflammatory disease of. See Endocarditis; Myocarditis; Pericarditis.
ischemic disease of. See Atherosclerosis; Ischemic heart disease; Myocardial infarction.
lupus erythematosus and, 1478–1479
movement of, 167–168
MRI of, 202t, 202–206, 203–208, 205t
murmurs. See Heart, sounds of; Murmurs.
myocardial disease of. See Cardiomyopathy; Myocardial infarction; Myocarditis.
normal function of, 174–180, 211–217
output of, 177, 178, 209–210, 214
pain from, angina, 166, 297
    infarction, 301, 304, 309–310, 310t
patent ductus arteriosus of, 279, 280
pericardial disease of. See Pericarditis.
polyarteritis nodosa of, 1493
preload, 175–176, 176, 212t, 214
pressures and volumes in, 175–177, 176t, 176–178, 214–216
pump function of, 175–176, 213–216, 214–216
radionuclide studies of, 199–202, 200–202
rate of. See Heart rate; Pulse.
refractoriness of, 190, 232
rheumatic fever and, 171t, 1592, 1592t, 1593, 1593t, 1594, 1594
rheumatoid disease affecting, 1464
roentgenography of, 181–188, 181–188
sarcoidosis of, 432, 432
silhouette of, 182, 182–183, 183
sounds of, 168, 168t
    aortic stenosis and, 319, 320
    aortic valve regurgitation and, 322, 322t
    click, 167–168, 168t
    diastolic, 168, 168t
    gallop, 168t, 218
    Korotkoff's, 259
    mitral stenosis and, 323, 323t
    mitral valve prolapse and, 326
    mitral valve regurgitation and, 325
    systolic, 168, 168t
stroke volume of, 176, 176t, 177, 215
syphilis affecting, 1708, 1708t
systemic sclerosis affecting, 1487
tamponade of, 339–341, 340, 341
transplantation of, 360–367. See also Transplantation, cardiac.
tumors of, 357–358, 358
valvular disease of, 319–327. See also Prosthetic valves.
    aortic, 319–323, 320, 320t–322t, 1593–1594, 1608t
    auscultation for, 168, 168t, 320, 322, 323, 325
    lupus erythematosus with, 1479
    mitral, 323t, 323–326, 324, 326, 1593–1594, 1594, 1608t
    orifice area calculation for, 210, 211
    pulmonic, 327
    rheumatic fever causing, 1592t, 1592–1593, 1593t
    shock due to, 486, 486t
    staphylococcal infection causing, 1608, 1608t
    streptococcal infection causing, 1592t, 1592–1593, 1593t
    tricuspid, 326–327, 1608t
Wegener's granulomatosis affecting, 1495t, 1496, 1496t
Heart block, 235
    atrioventricular, 235, 242, 242
    congenital complete, 279
    Lyme disease causing, 1717, 1718
    sinoatrial, 241, 241–242
    type I, 235, 241, 241, 242, 242
    type II, 242
    Wenckebach, 235, 241, 241–242

Heart failure, 211–230. See also Angina pectoris; Ischemic heart disease; Myocardial infarction.
    acute vs. chronic, 212
    afterload in, 215, 215, 229t
    amyloidosis causing, 333, 333, 359, 967, 967, 967t
    anaphylactic, 1418, 1418
    anti-inflammatory prophylaxis for, 1192–1193
    anxiety due to, 219
    approach to patient with, 166–170, 220
    aspirin prophylaxis for, 1192–1193
    atrial natriuretic hormone and, 1196
    backward vs. forward, 213
    cardiac enlargement in, 218
    cardiac index in, 215, 305
    cardinal symptoms of, 166t, 166–167
    categories of, 212–213
    clinical features of, 217–220
    compensatory mechanisms for, 215–217, 216
    congestive, 212t, 217–220
    cyanosis in, 219
    definition of, 211–213
    diagnostic workup and, 168t, 168–170
    diastolic vs. systolic, 213, 230
    disability class related to, 169t, 221t
    dyspnea with, 217, 219
    erythroderma role in, 2188
    fluid shifts due to, 529–530, 530t
    gallop rhythm in, 168, 218
    hemoptysis in, 218
    initiating mechanisms for, 212
    left-sided, 212–213, 217–219, 273t, 275
    liver affected by, 219, 792
    Marfan syndrome with, 1119–1120
    mortality rate and, 26–27, 27, 27t, 30t, 171t
    myocardial infarction. See Myocardial infarction.
    nocturia with, 217
    orthopnea with, 217
    peripheral circulation response to, 216–217
    pleural effusion in, 445
    preload in, 214, 214, 229t
    proteinuria in, 513, 513t
    pulmonary edema in, 217–218, 221–222
    pulmonary function tests in, 218–219
    pulmonary hypertension due to, 273t, 275
    pulsus alternans in, 218
    radiography in, 218
    refractory, 230
    renal effects of, 217, 523–530
    rheumatic fever causing, 1592, 1592t, 1592–1593, 1593t
    right-sided, 212–213, 219–220
    risk factors for, 30t
    septic shock and, 499t, 499–501, 500t
        toxic syndrome of, 1588–1589
    sickle syndrome in, 889
    stroke volume in, 214, 214–215, 215
    symptoms of, 166, 217–220
    syncope with, 1980t, 1980–1981, 1981t
    treatment of, 219–230
        diet (salt poor) in, 221
        diuretics in, 221t, 222–225, 223, 224t
        fluid removal in, 221t, 222–225, 223, 224t
        glycosides in, 221t, 225, 225–228, 226t, 227t
        oxygen therapy in, 221
        strategy for, 220t, 220–221, 221t
        vasodilators in, 221t, 228–230, 229t
    Valsalva maneuver in, 217
    vasoconstriction in, 216–217
Heart rate, 176t, 177. See also Pulse.
    exercise and, 31t
    shock and, 478–479
    septic, 496t, 499, 499t
Heartburn, 650
    esophageal disorder with, 650, 651
Heat, cramps caused by, 501, 502
    cutaneous blood flow and, 2188
    erythromelalgia due to, 1528
    exertion injury due to, 501, 502
    intolerance of, multiple sclerosis with, 2109, 2110
        thyrotoxicosis with, 1232, 1233t
    sweat evaporation and, 2188
    syndromes related to, 501–502
    urticaria due to, 1410, 2208
Heat exhaustion, 501, 502
    prognosis of, 501
    symptoms of, 501
Heat stroke, 502, 2012
    exertional, 502
    nonexertional, 502
    temperature in, 502, 1533, 2012

Heavy chains, 958, 959, 960, 960t
    alpha, 966
    diseases of, 960, 960t, 966
    gamma, 966
    H, 1395–1396, 1396, 1396t
    HLA molecules with, 1424–1426, 1425, 1425t, 1426
    mu, 966
Heberden's nodes, 1518, 1519t, 1520
Heck's disease, 648t
Heel, lover's, 1702
Heerfordt's syndrome, 432
Height, vertigo induced by, 2025
Height (body), age and, 1140t, 1152t, 1163t
    gender and, 1140t, 1152t
    recommended dietary allowances and, 1140t
    weight-to-height-to-age and, 1161–1162, 1162, 1163t
Heinz bodies, 856–857
    erythrocyte morphology and, 856–857, 874, 874
    formation of, 856–857, 874
    splenic pitting of, 971, 973
    staining for, 856–857
Helicobacter pylori, 659, 659t
    antimicrobial therapy and, 666, 666t
    diagnostic testing for, 666, 666t
    gastritis caused by, 659t, 659–660
    peptic ulcer role of, 662t, 662–663, 666t, 667t, 667–668
Heliotrope, 2212
HELLP syndrome, 787t, 787–788
Helmet cells, 822
Helminths, 1922–1945
    cestode (tapeworm), 1922–1926. See also Cestodes; Tapeworm.
    diphyllobothriasis due to, 1923, 1923t
    dirofilariasis due to, 1945
    dracunculiasis due to, 1944
    echinococciasis due to, 1924–1925
    eosinophilia and, 1942
    filariasis due to, 1939–1945, 1940t
    food-borne, 739
    hepatic effects of, 782, 783t
    hymenolepiasis due to, 1923t, 1923–1924
    loiasis due to, 1943–1944
    mansonelliasis due to, 1944–1945
    nematode, 1934–1939. See also Nematodes.
    onchocerciasis due to, 1942–1943
    schistosomiasis due to, 1927–1931
    spargonosis due to, 1926
    taeniasis due to, 1923t, 1924, 1925–1926
    traveler exposed to, 1555
    trematode, 1931–1934. See also Trematodes.
Helper cells, 1398, 1414, 1415
    allergic rhinitis and, 1398, 1414, 1415
    leprosy pathogenesis and, 1692, 1693, 1694, 1695
Hemagglutination, anaerobic flora products causing, 1639t
    red kidney bean causing, 740
    shock with, 482–483
Hemangioblastoma, intracranial capillaries in, 2132
Hemangioma, 2211. See also Angioma.
    blue rubber bleb nevus, 721
    cavernous, 2211
    colonic, 721
    hepatic, 803t
    splenic, 974
    strawberry, 2211
Hemarthrosis, 1526
    hemophilia with, 992, 1526
Hematemesis, esophageal, 651
    gastrointestinal bleeding with, 642–643
Hematochezia, 642
Hematocrit, 823
    anemia and, 822, 830–831
    erythrocytosis and, 920, 921
    normal, 823, 823t, 920
    phlebotomy effect on, 1134–1135, 1135
    polycythemia vera and, 920, 921
    red cell mass related to, 920
Hematologic disorders, 817–1003. See also Anemia; Coagulation; Hemolysis; Hemorrhage.
    AIDS/HIV in, 1838–1840, 1870–1872
    approach to patient in, 817–822
    lupus erythematosus with, 1475t, 1479
    mastocytosis with, 1435, 1435t, 1437
    paraneoplastic, 1017t, 1020–1021, 1054
    phosphorus deficiency causing, 1136t
    renal failure with, 558, 562
    stroke related to, 2067t, 2068–2069

Hematoma, epidural, 2136, 2148
  hemorrhagic disorders with, 979t
  intracerebral hemorrhage causing, 2137
  spinal, 2146
  subdural, 2136
    imaging of, 1965
Hematopoiesis, **817–821**. See also *Anemia*; *Erythro-
    poiesis*; *Leukemia*; specific cell types.
  extramedullary, 924t
  growth factors in, 819–821, 820t, *821*, 898
  kinetics of, 818, *818*, 898t
  precursor cells in, 817–818, *818*, *820*, *832*, 898
  progenitors in, 818–819, *820*, *821*, *834*
Hematuria, 513, 553, 554t
  casts in, 553, 554t
  glomerular disease and, 513, 553, 554t, 572–573
  renal cystic disease with, 618, 618t, 619t
  renal obstruction with, 591
Heme, bilirubin production from, 755, *755*
  globin chains around, 868, *868*
  iron of, 839, 842–843, 868–869, 872
  porphyrias and. See *Porphyria*.
  sideroblastic anemia role of, 842–843
Hemianopsia, *2015*
  cerebral hemorrhage with, 2078, 2078t
Hemidesmosomes, 2186, *2186*
Hemiparesis, aphasia related to, 1991t
  cerebral hemorrhage with, 2078, 2078t
  gait in, 2029
  meningitis with, 1612t, 1613, 1620
  stroke with, 2064t, 2064–2065
Hemochromatosis, **1132–1135**
  arthritis with, 1525
  clinical features of, 1133, 1133t
  definition of, 1132
  disorders associated with, 1132t
  genetics of, 138t, 786, 1132–1133
  heart affected by, 333t, 334, 359, 1133t
  hepatic effects of, 786, 791, 1133
  hypogonadism due to, 1337
  impotence due to, 1337
  laboratory findings in, 1133–1134, 1134t
  prevalence and etiology of, 1132t, 1132–1133
  prognosis in, 1135
  thalassemic, 878–879
  transfusion causing, 878–879, 896, 896t
  treatment of, 1134–1135
    chelation therapy in, 878–879
    hepatic transplantation in, 801t
    phlebotomy in, 1134–1135, *1135*
Hemodialysis. See also *Dialysis*.
  ethylene glycol toxicity treated with, 504t, 509, 509t
  trace metal toxicity in, 70–71
Hemoglobin, **868–893**
  A, 868, 868t, 869, *870*, *871*
  Bart's, 880
  bilirubin metabolism and, 755, *755*
  C, 889–890
  carbon monoxide binding by, *374*, 374–375,
    403–404
  Constant Spring, 880
  denatured, 874
    Heinz bodies due to, 856–857, 874, *874*
    instability causing, 874, *874*
  dissociation curve of, *876*
  E, disorder of, 136t, 890
  embryonic, 868, 868t, 869, *870*, *871*
  erythrocyte morphology affected by, 825t, 842,
    856–857, *883*
  F (fetal), 868t, 868–870, *870*, *871*
    erythrocyte production and, 817
    hereditary persistence of, 881, 885t, 890
  genetics of, 137, 139, 142, 870–873, *871*, 883–884
  Gower, 868, 868t, 869, *871*
  H, disease due to, 879, 880
  Heinz bodies and, 856–857, 874, *874*
  high-affinity variants of, 875, *876*
  iron of, 842–843, 868–869, 872
  Kansas, 875, *876*
  Lepore, 890
  leukemia and, 932t, 935t
  low-affinity variants of, 875, *876*
  M (methemoglobin), 869, 875–877, 876t
  malaria and, 872–873
  normal levels of, 823, 823t
  O Arab, 890
  oxygen uptake by, 868, 869, *869*, *876*
    affinity variation in, 484, 875, *876*
    transport and, 472, *472*

Hemoglobin *(Continued)*
  Portland, 868, 868t, 869, *871*
  Quebec-CHORI, 889
  Quong Sze, 880–881
  S, 882–884, *883*, *884*, 885t. See also *Sickle syn-
    dromes*.
  sideroblast role of, 842–843
  structure and function of, 868–869, *868–871*
  synthesis of, 869–872, *870*, *871*
  unstable, 873–874, *874*
  urinary, hemolysis with, 839t, 857, *858*
Hemoglobinemia, 857
  erythrocyte G6PD deficiency with, 857, *858*
Hemoglobinopathy, cerebrovascular disease due to,
    2068
  retinopathy caused by, 2182
Hemoglobinuria, 89t
  erythrocyte G6PD deficiency with, 857, *858*
  paroxysmal cold, 863
  paroxysmal nocturnal, 866–867
Hemolysins, cold, 863
  Donath-Landsteiner, 863
Hemolysis, **859–867**. See also *Anemia*.
  antibodies causing, 859–867
  antimicrobials causing, 1568t
  bartonellosis causing, 1682
  causes of, 830, 830t
  drug-induced, *858*, 858t, 867
  elliptocytosis and, 854–855
  enzyme defects and, 855–859, *856*
  G6PD deficiency and, 856–859, *856*, *856–858*, 858t
  laboratory tests for, 829, 829t
  membrane defects and, 852–855
  pregnancy with, 787, 787t
  pyropoikilocytosis and, 855, 855t
  sickle cells and, 886
  splenomegaly with, 971t, 973
  stomatocytosis and, 855
  tests for, 829, 829t
  transfusion causing, 895, 896, 896t
  vitamin E deficiency causing, 1145t
  Wilson's disease causing, 1131
Hemolytic-uremic syndrome, 607–608
  thrombocytopenia with, 984, 984t, 985, 1002–1003
Hemophilia, **991–995**
  A, 991–993
  B, 994–995
  carrier detection in, 992, 995
  clinical features of, 991, 994
  diagnosis of, 979t, *981*, 991, 994
  differential diagnosis of, 979t, *981*
  frequencies of, 136t, 138t
  genetics in, 136t, 138t, 992, 994
  hemarthrosis in, 992, 1526
  prognosis in, 993
  replacement therapy in, 991–992, 994–995
  treatment of, 991–992, 994–995
Hemoptysis, 370–371
  aortic aneurysm with, 342
  cancer causing, 1052
  cardiovascular disease causing, 166
  cystic fibrosis with, 420, 421t
  heart failure with, 218
  lung cancer with, 438
  pulmonary embolism causing, 423, 424t
  respiratory disease with, 370–371
Hemorrhage, adrenal gland, 1251
  amyloidosis and, 967
  anemia caused by, 838
  anticoagulant causing, 120–121, 998–1000
  antiplatelet agent causing, 117t
  approach to patient with, 977–978, 979t, 980t, 990
  cerebral, 2073–2079, 2137. See also *Cerebrovascular
    disease, hemorrhagic*.
  coagulation disorders and. See *Coagulation*; specific
    disorders.
  conjunctivitis with, enterovirus in, 1787t, 1791–1792
  defibrination, 1002
  Dieulafoy's ulcer causing, 721
  differential diagnosis of, 979t, *981*, 984t
  esophageal, 651
    reflux disease and, 651
    variceal, 794t, 794–795
  gastrointestinal, **642–645**
    anemia with, 645, 645t
    approach to patient with, *642*, 643–645
    colonic, 718, 720–721
    diagnostic imaging of, 644–645
    E. coli causing, 1654–1655, 1655t, 1738t
    endoscopy in, 637–638, 638t
    etiology of, 642t, 720–721

Hemorrhage *(Continued)*
  evaluation of, 643–645
  examination for, 643–645
  ischemia followed by, 718
  lower tract, 642t, 644–645, 720–721
  rectal, cancer causing, 726
    hemorrhoids and, 740–741
    inflammatory bowel disease with, 709, 712,
      712t
  severity of, 642t, 643
  signs and symptoms of, 642–643
  small bowel, 645
  stomach and, 642t, 643, 794
  treatment of, 643, 673, 673t, 794t, 794–795
  unknown origin of, 645
  upper tract, 642t, 643–644, 645t, *665*, 673,
    794–795
  variceal, 642t, 643, 794t, 794–795
  vascular ectasia causing, 720–722
  hemophilic, 991, 994, 1526
  hemostatic disorders and, 977–987. See also *Coagu-
    lation*; *Platelets*.
  intracranial. See *Cerebrovascular disease,
    hemorrhagic*.
  joint affected by, 992, 1526
  laboratory evaluation, 979, 979t
  leech bite, 1951
  nails affected by, 2215
  peptic ulcer, 642t, 643, 645t, *665*, 673
  physical examination, 978–979, 979t
  platelet defects and, 980–985. See also *Platelets*;
    Thrombocytopenia.
  pleural effusion and, 445, 445t, 446
  polycythemia vera and, 921, 922t
  pulmonary, Goodpasture's syndrome with, 397–398
    interstitial disease with, 397–398
  renal failure and, 558
  retinal, high-altitude, 409t, 409–410
  spinal cord affected by, *2139*, 2139–2140, 2148
  stroke due to, 2073–2079. See also *Stroke, hemor-
    rhagic*.
  subarachnoid, 2074–2076, 2075t
    imaging of, 1965–1966, *1966*
    spinal, 2146
    treatment in, 2075–2076, 2076t
  synovial fluid and, 1455t, 1455–1456
  thrombocytopenia and, 980–984, 1002–1003
  thrombolytic agent causing, 116, 117t, 998
  uremic, 558, 985
  variceal, gastroesophageal, 794t, 794–795
    management of, 794t, 794–795
  vascular disorders associated with, 979t, 986t,
    986–987
    acquired, 979t, 986t, 986–987
    congenital, 986, 986t
    hereditary, 979t
  vitamin K deficiency with, 1145t
  von Willebrand disease with, 993
Hemorrhagic fever, 1797–1804, 1798t
  African, 1798t, 1803–1804, 1806t
  Argentinian and Bolivian, 1798t, 1802–1803
  Brazilian, 1798t, 1802–1803
  chikungunya, 1805t, 1809
  Crimean-Congo, 1798t, 1802, 1806t
  dengue, 1798t, 1800–1801, 1805t
  hantavirus pulmonary syndrome with, 1798t, 1804,
    1805t, 1810
  Kyasanur Forest, 1798t, 1801–1802, 1806t
  Lassa, 1798t, 1802–1803
  Marburg-Ebola, 1798t, 1803–1804
  Omsk, 1798t, 1801–1802, 1806t
  renal syndrome with, 1798t, 1804
  Rift Valley, 1798t, 1805t, 1806t, 1808
  tick-borne, 1801–1802, 1806t
  Venezuelan, 1798t, 1802–1803
  yellow fever, 1798t, 1798–1800, 1805t
Hemorrhoids, 740–741
  bleeding, 740
  external, 740
  prolapsed, 740
  thrombosed, 741
  treatment of, 740–741
Hemosiderosis, 1133
  idiopathic pulmonary, 398
Hemostasis, 977, *977*, *978*. See also *Coagulation*;
    Platelets.
  drugs affecting, 980t
  mechanisms of, 977, *977*, *978*
  pathologic, 977, 979t
Hemothorax, 445, 445t, 446
Henderson-Hasselbalch equation, 543, *545*

Henle's loop, *223, 518*
  anatomy of, *223, 518, 518,* 521–523
  Barrter's syndrome and, 598
  concentration and dilution in, 521–523, *522*
  diuretic action in, 222–223, *223,* 224t, 264t, 531t
Henoch-Schönlein purpura, glomerulonephritis with, 576
  skin lesions of, 1492, 2201t, 2202
Hepadnavirus, *1739*
Heparan, coagulation role of, *978,* 987
  connective tissue structure and, 1445t, 1446
Heparan sulfatase deficiency, 1119t
Heparin, **119–120**
  anticoagulant therapy using, 118t, 118–121, 312t, 427t, 427–428
  bleeding due to, 998
  complications-of, 120–121
  low-molecular-weight, 120
  mast cell release of, 1436t
  myocardial infarction treated with, 119, 311–312, 312t
  pulmonary embolism treated with, *427,* 427t, 427–428
  stroke therapy with, 2071–2072, 2072t
Hepatic artery, aneurysm of, *1494*
Hepatic duct, *637*
Hepatitis, **762–780**
  A, 764–765
    comparison with other types, 763t, 764t
    epidemiology of, 763t, 764–765
    immune globulin for, 1554
    laboratory findings in, 764–765, *765*
    pathology findings in, *762,* 764
    prophylaxis for, 770, 1554
    signs and symptoms of, 762–765, *765*
    travel exposure to, 1554
    virology and etiology of, *762,* 763t, 764t
  acute, 762–771
  alcoholic, 790
  amebic, 782–783, *784*
  antibodies in, 764t, *765, 767,* 778t
  antigens of, 765, *766, 768,* 778t
  antimicrobials causing, 1568t
  autoimmune, 777–778, 778t
  B, 765–767
    chronic, 765–766, 778–779, 1746t
    clinical features of, 766–767, *767*
    comparison with other types, 763t, 764t
    epidemiology of, 763t, 765–766
    hospital-acquired, 1553
    immune globulin for, 771
    laboratory findings in, 764t, 766–767, *767*
    pathogenesis and pathology of, 765
    treatment of, 1746t
    vaccine for, 42t, 45, 765, 770–771
    virology and etiology of, 765, *766*
  C (non-A, non-B), 767–769
    chronic, 779–780, 1746t
    clinical findings in, 763t, 764t, *768,* 768–769
    epidemiology of, 763t, 768
    laboratory studies in, 764t, 768, *768*
    prophylaxis for, 770
    treatment of, 1746t
    virology and etiology of, 764t, 767–768, *768*
  chronic, **776–780**
    active, 777, 801t
    clinical features of, 776–780
    etiology of, 773, 773t, 776, 776t
    lobular, 777
    pathology findings in, 776
    persistent, 776–777
    treatment of, 778–780, 801t, 1746t
  cirrhosis and, 762
  complications of, 763–764, 776–777
  D (delta), 767
    chronic, 779
    clinical features of, 763t, 767
    epidemiology of, 767
    etiology of, 767
    laboratory findings in, 763t, 764t
  definition of, 762, 776
  diagnosis of, 769
  differential diagnosis of, 769–770
  drug-induced, 772–775, 799t
    classification of, 772–774, 773t
    diagnosis and management of, 774–775
    morphologic patterns in, 772–774, 773t
    pathogenesis of, 772, 774–775
  E, 769
    clinical features of, 764t, 769
    epidemiology of, 769
    laboratory findings in, 764t, 769

Hepatitis *(Continued)*
  granulomatous, 773, 773t, 1495t, 1496t
  history taking for, 752
  immune globulin against, 41t, 1554
  iron levels affected by, 1134t
  jaundice and, *763, 765, 767*
  leptospirosis with, 1720, 1721
  management of, 770–771
  prophylaxis for, 42t, 770–771, 1554
  Q fever with, 784t, 1735–1736
  sexual transmission of, 1697t
  solvents causing, 59t
  syphilitic, 782
  toxic, **772–775**
    idiosyncratic, 772
    intrinsic, 772
  transfusion-associated, 896, 896t
  transplantation in, 801t
  viral, **762–771**
    hemorrhagic fever with, 1798t
Hepatocytes, *789*
  bile production in, 805
  fibrosis affecting, *789*
Hepatoma, markers for, 1022t, 1023, 1041t
Hepatopulmonary syndrome, 796
Hepatorenal syndrome, 795–796
HER oncogene, 1011–1012, 1036t
Herbert's pits, 1723
Herbicide poisoning, 509–510
Herbs, food poisoning due to, 740
  tea with alkaloids of, 54, 740, 774
Hereditary disorder(s), **136–147.** See also *Familial disorder(s); Genetics.*
  amino acids affected by, 1099–1017, 1100t–1105t
  angioedema in, 1411–1412
  bilirubin metabolism in, 756–757, 757t
  bronchiectasis with, 416t, 416–417, 418t
  complement deficiency in, 1401, 1401t
  diagnostic testing for, 163t, 164t
  elliptocytosis as, 854–855, 855t
  ethnic group and, 136t, 136–137, 138t
  frequencies of, 136t, 136–137, 138t, 142
  fructose intolerance as, *1084,* 1084–1085
  genetic counseling related to, 162–165, 164t
  hypophosphatemic rickets as, 1364
  metabolic defects in, 142–147, 144t, 146t, 147t
  mitochondrial, 142
  monogenic (mendelian pattern), 136t, 137–141, 138t
  multiple organ systems in, 160t, 160–162
  muscle weakness due to, 1503t
  nephropathy of, 574t, 611–612, 612t
  neuropathy in, 2153–2154, 2154t
  polygenic (multifactorial), *141,* 141–142
  polyp syndromes as, 723–725, *724*
  renal tubular defect as, 611–612, 612t
  spherocytosis as, 852–854, *853,* 853t
Hermaphroditism, 1286–1287
  true, 1286–1287
Hernia, diaphragm affected by, 158t, 443
  fetus with, 158t
  tentorial, 1970–1972, *1971,* 1971t
Heroin, 51
  adulterants in, 52
  drug abuse with, 51–53
  neurologic effects of, 1975t
  overdose with, 52
  pharmacology of, 52
  withdrawal of, 52
Herpangina, coxsackievirus causing, 1787t, 1790, 2090
  viral meningitis with, 2090
Herpes gestationis, 2206
Herpes simplex, **1770–1774**
  AIDS/HIV patient and, 1868, 1869t, 1869–1870
  compromised host with, 1746t, 1773–1774
  cutaneous, incidence of, 2184t
  diagnosis of, 1772
  encephalitis due to, 1746t, 1773, *1773,* 1990, 2092–2093, *2093*
  epidemiology of, 1773, 2092
  genital, 1772
    treatment of, 1742–1743, 1746t
  gingivostomatitis of, 1772, *1772*
  immunization for, 1773
  keratitis due to, 1772–1773
  labialis, 1772, *1772*
  memory impairment due to, 1990
  mucocutaneous, 1746t, 1772
  neonatal, 1746t, 1773
  nervous system and, 1770–1772, *1770–1772,* 2092–2093, *2093*
  oral lesions of, 646, 646t

Herpes simplex *(Continued)*
  pathogenesis and latency of, 1770–1772, *1771, 1772*
  pharyngitis due to, 1750, 1750t, 1751t, 1790
  replication of, 1770, *1771, 1772*
  retinal necrosis due to, 1869t, 1869–1870
  sexual transmission of, 1697t
  skin examination and, *2191,* 2191t, 2191–2192
  structure of, 1770, *1770*
  subtypes HSV-1 and HSV-2 of, 1770, 1772
  treatment of, 1742–1743, 1746t, 1773–1774
  virology of, 1770–1772, *1770–1772*
Herpes zoster, 2205
  AIDS/HIV patient with, 1868, 1869, 1869t
  immune globulin against, 41t
  localized, 1746t
  nervous system affected by, 2036, 2093–2095
  neuralgia due to, 2036, 2094–2095
  oral lesions of, 646, 646t
  paraneoplastic, 1034
  retinal necrosis due to, 1869t, 1869–1870
  skin examination and, 2191, *2191,* 2191t
  treatment of, 1742–1743, 1746t, 2094–2095
Herpesvirus. See also specific type.
  B, animal carriers of, 1737t
    encephalitis due to, 1737t
  cytomegalovirus, 1774–1776
    treatment of, 1746t
  genital, treatment of, 1742–1743, 1746t
  hominis. See *Herpes simplex.*
  roseola infantum due to, 1791
  structure of, *1739*
  treatment of, 1742–1743, 1746t
Herpesvirus simiae, 1738t
Herxheimer reaction, 1568t, 1713
HETE (hydroxyeicosatetraenoic acid), *1190,* 1190–1191
Heterophyiasis, 1932t, 1933
Heterozygote, 134, 137
  gene frequency and, 142
Hexabrachion, 1445
Hexamethylmelamine (HMM), 1044t
  adverse effects of, 1045
  chemotherapy using, 1044t, 1045
Hexokinase, *856*
Hexose monophosphate shunt, 855, 856, *856*
Hiccup, 442–443
  diaphragm affected by, 442–443
Hidradenitis suppurativa, *2191*
High molecular weight kininogen (HMWK), 987–988, 1419
High-density lipoprotein. See *Lipoprotein, high-density (HDL).*
Hilar cell tumor, 1312t
Hilar nodes, 969t
Hilum, overlay sign of, *186*
Hip, fracture of, elderly with, 23
  rheumatoid arthritis affecting, 1463
Hippocampus, epilepsy related to, 2117, *2118*
  memory function of, 1989, 1990
  sclerosis affecting, 2117, *2118*
Hirschsprung's disease, 687
Hirsutism, *1288,* 1315–1317, 2217
  amenorrhea with, *1304,* 1306–1307
  clinical manifestations of, *1315,* 1315–1316, 2217
  definition of, 1315, 2217
  diagnosis of, 1316, 2217
  etiology of, *1288,* 1315, 1316t, 2217
  laboratory evaluation of, 1316
  nonendocrine, 2217
  pathophysiology of, *1288,* 1315, 1316t, 2217
  prognosis in, 1317
  treatment of, 1316, 2217
Hirudiniasis, 1950–1951. See also *Leech.*
His bundle, 190, *191,* 191t, 231, *232*
  anatomy of, *191, 232*
  block in, 191, 191t
  branches of, 191, *191,* 231, *232*
  conduction in, 231, *232*
  velocity of, 190, *191,* 191t, 233t
  electrogram of, 231–232, *232*
Histamine, allergic rhinitis role of, 1414, 1415, *1415, 1416*
  asthma role of, 376
  complement stimulation of, 1400
  mast cell release of, 1436t
Histidine, urinary, 1100t, 1101t, 1104t
Histiocytes, 955
  gallbladder, 816
  lipid-containing, 2211
  lymphoma of, 941t

Histiocytosis, erythrophagocytic, 970
  interstitial lung disease with, 395
  Langerhans' cell (eosinophilic), 955, 970
  lymphadenopathy in, 970, 970t
  malignant, 970, 1032
  sinus, 970
  skin affected by, 1032
  X, 395, 955, 970
Histocompatibility complex. See HLA complex.
Histone, antibodies to, 1457t, 1476t
Histoplasmosis, **1816–1818**
  clinical manifestations of, 1817–1818
  diagnosis of, 1817–1818
  epidemiology of, 1816–1817
  etiologic agent in, 1816
  hepatic granuloma with, 784t
  ocular, 1818
  pathogenesis and pathology of, 1817
  prognosis in, 1818
  pulmonary, 1817
  treatment of, 1818
HIV infection, **1837–1891**. See also AIDS (acquired immunodeficiency syndrome).
  antibodies in, 1839t, 1839–1841, 1844
  arthritis with, 1474
  cardiac effects of, 329, 329t, 1876–1877, 1877t
  classification system for, 1888, 1889
  complications of, 1855–1879, 1890
  cutaneous effects of, 1868
  drug abuser and, 1852
  endocrine effects of, 1438, 1877–1878
  epidemiology of, 1846t, **1846–1851**, 1847, 1848t, 1849, 1850t
  etiologic agent in, 1841–1846, 1842–1845
  evaluation of, 1888–1890, 1888–1891, 1890t
  gastrointestinal effects of, 1866–1868, 1867t
  hematologic effects of, 1838–1840, 1870–1872
  immunology of, 1837t, **1837–1841**, 1839t
  incidence and prevalence of, 1847, 1847–1848, 1848t
  lymphocyte count in, 1837t, 1838–1840, 1839t
    indicator role of, 1890, 1890
  lymphoma in, 1873–1874
    Hodgkin's, 954
  management and counseling for, 1888–1890, **1888–1891**, 1890t, 1891t
  mortality rate role of, 27t, 1849
  mutations affecting, 1845, 1884t
  myocarditis with, 329, 329t, 1877
  natural history model for, 1844, 1890
  neoplasms in, 1872–1874, 1873t
  nephropathy with, 579, 1875–1876, 1876
  neurologic effects of, 1855t, 1855–1858, 1856t, 1857t, 2156–2157
  ophthalmologic effects of, 1868–1870, 1869t
  pathophysiology of, 1837–1846, 1838, 1843
  prevention and precautions for, **1851–1854**, 1852t, 1853t, 1854t
  pulmonary effects of, 1858–1865, 1859t–1861t, 1859–1865, 1865t
  renal effects of, 579, 1875t, 1875–1876, 1876
  respiratory tract effects of, 1858–1865, 1859t–1861t, 1859–1865, 1865t
  rheumatologic disease due to, 1878t, 1878–1879
  salivary gland affected by, 649, 649t
  screening for, 28t, 1846t
  sexual activity and, 1697t, 1851–1852, 1852t
  skin disorders associated with, 2219
  thrombocytopenia with, 982, 1871
  transfusion-related, 896, 896t, 1852
  transmission modes for, **1848–1854**, 1852t, 1853t, 1854t
  treatment of, 1838, 1865, **1880–1887**, 1883t, 1884t, 1885t, 1887t
  tuberculosis and, 1684, 1686, 1687, 1688t, 1861, 1861, 1861t
  vaccine for, 1840–1841, 1841t
  virology of, 1838, **1841–1846**, 1842–1845
Hives. See Urticaria.
HLA complex, **1424–1431**
  allergic rhinitis role of, 1414, 1415
  ankylosing spondylitis role of, 1430, 1431t, 1466–1467
  antigen deficiency affecting, 1406
  antigen presentation and, 1394, 1397, 1424–1426
  bone marrow transplant and, 974–975
  class I molecules of, 1424–1425, 1425, 1425t
  class II molecules of, 1425t, 1425–1426, 1426
  diabetes mellitus and, 1431, 1431t

HLA complex (Continued)
  disease associations of, 1430–1431, 1431t
  haplotypes of, 568, 1428t, 1429, 1429, 1430, 1430t
  history of, 1424
  immunodeficiency related to, 1406
  linkage disequilibrium of, 1429–1431, 1430t
  lupus erythematosus and, 1431, 1431t
  molecular genetics of, 1426–1429, 1427, 1428t, 1429, 1429t
  Reiter's syndrome and, 1431t
  renal transplantation and, 568, 568–569
  rheumatoid arthritis role of, 1431, 1431t, 1459–1460, 1460t
  T cell receptor and, 568, 1394, 1397, 1424
  typing for, 569, 1430
HMOs (Health Maintenance Organizations), 10, 10t
HMWK (high molecular weight kininogen), 987–988, 1419
Hoarseness, 451
  aortic aneurysm with, 342
  asthma causing, 378
  causes of, 451
  treatment of, 451
Hodgkin-Huxley constant, 245
Hodgkin's disease, **947–954**
  diagnosis of, 942, 948
  differential diagnosis of, 948
  epidemiology of, 947
  etiology of, 947
  extranodal, 948
  fever with, 1532t, 1533t
  histologic subtypes of, 947–948
  imaging studies in, 949–951, 950
  incidence of, 1013t
  pathology of, 947–948
  pregnancy and, 1064–1065
  skin affected by, 1032
  staging of, 948–951, 949, 949t
  symptoms associated with, 948–949, 949t
  treatment of, 951–954, 952, 952t, 954t
    advanced-stage, 952t, 953
    chemotherapy in, 952t, 953
    early-stage, 951
    follow-up, 954t
    radiation in, 952, 952–953
    relapse and, 953–954
    side effects of, 952, 953
Holter monitor, 235, 235, 236t
Holt-Oram syndrome, 291
Homicide, age group and, 27t
  mortality rate role of, 27t, 37, 37, 37t, 39
  preventive strategies for, 37–40
Homocysteine, **1112–1114**
  enzyme deficiencies and, 1112–1114, 1113t
  folate deficiency and, 845, 845, 849t, 850, 850t
  metabolism of, 1112–1113, 1113
  normal serum levels of, 849t, 850t
  urinary, 1101t, 1102t
  vitamin B_{12} deficiency and, 845, 845, 849t, 850, 850t
Homocystinuria, **1112–1114**
  biochemistry of, 1112–1113, 1113
  clinical features of, 1113t, 1113–1114
  cobalamin metabolic defects in, 1112–1114, 1113t
  diagnosis of, 1114
  enzyme defect in, 146t, 1101t, 1102t
  genetics of, 138t, 1101t, 1102t
  prevalence of, 1114
  stroke related to, 2069
  treatment of, 1114
Homogentisic acid, urinary, 1108
Homosexuality, Campylobacter proctocolitis and, 1649t, 1649–1650
  enteric infection and, 1642t, 1867, 1867t
  gay bowel syndrome and, 1867, 1867t
  gonorrhea associated with, 1701
  hepatitis transmission and, 765–766, 767
  shigellosis risk and, 1647
  syphilis epidemiology and, 1706
Homovanillic acid, 1253
Homozygote, 134, 137
  gene frequency and, 142
Hoof-and-mouth disease, 1737t
Hoogsteen hydrogen bonding, 1074
Hookworm infection, 1934–1935, 1935t
  animal (dog), 1937
  epidemiology of, 1934
  etiologic organism in, 1934
  pathology and clinical features of, 1934–1935
  treatment of, 1935t

Hoover's sign, 442
Hormones, **1176–1350**. See also Endocrine system; specific gland, hormone, or disorder.
  adrenal cortex, 1245–1246
  adrenal medulla, 1253, 1253–1254
  aging controlled by, 15
  allosteric conformation of, 1177, 1178, 1179
  assessment of, 1184–1185
  atrial natriuretic, 1194–1196, 1195
  autocrine, 1176
  bound, 1182
  cancer prevention using, 1010
  chemotherapy using, 1046t, 1046–1047
  cycles and rhythms of, 1184
  deficiency states of, 1185
  definition of, 1176
  ectopic, 1024–1026, 1025t. See also Pituitary gland, tumors of.
    carcinoid production of, 1348–1350
    islet cell tumor with, 1025t, 1282–1284
    multiple endocrine neoplasia and, 1345–1347
    paraneoplastic, 1024–1026, 1025t, 1035
    tumors associated with, 1024–1026, 1025t
  enteric, 681, 681t
  excess states of, 1185
  free, 1182
  half-life of, 1182
  hypothalamic, 1183, 1183–1184, 1198
  mechanisms of action of, 1176–1181, 1176–1181
  molecular biology of, 1176–1181, 1176–1181
  natriuretic, 1194
  obesity effect on, 1165–1166
  ovarian, 1293–1295, 1293–1312, 1294, 1299, 1300, 1301t
    tumor production of, 1312t, 1312–1313
  paracrine, 1176
  peptide, 1176–1180, 1177–1180
  pituitary, 1183, 1183–1184, 1197
  receptors for, 1176–1180, 1176–1182
    cell surface, 1176–1180, 1176–1180
    cytoplasmic, 1176, 1177
    DNA and, 1176, 1180–1181, 1181
    nuclear, 1176, 1180–1181, 1181
  regulation of, 1183, 1183–1184
  release of, 1183–1184
    rhythms affecting, 1184, 1999–1200
  second messengers for, 1176–1180, 1177–1180
  secretion rate of, 1183–1184
    factors affecting, 1184, 1999–1200
  sex, cancer therapy and, 1046t, 1046–1047
  shock and, 481–482
  steroid, 1176, 1180–1182, 1181, 1245–1246
  stimulation tests of, 1184–1185
  storage and delivery of, Golgi apparatus in, 1182
  suppression tests of, 1184–1185
  synthesis of, 1182–1183
  testicular, 1284–1293, 1286, 1325–1329, 1326
  thyroid, 1227, 1227–1230, 1229t
  transport of, 1182–1183
  vitamin D, 1354–1355, 1355, 1358
  volume regulation role of, 526t, 526–528, 527, 528t
Horner's syndrome, dysautonomia of, 2008
  lung cancer with, 439
  pupils affected by, 2018
Hornet sting, 1420t, 1420–1421
Horse, encephalitis reservoir in, 1806t, 1810t
  zoonoses associated with, 1737t, 1737–1738, 1738t
Horse serum, 1422t
  anaphylaxis due to, 1418t, 1418–1419
  products from, 1422t
  serum sickness and, 1421–1422, 1422, 1422t
Hospitals, 10, 10t
  admission to, demand-driven, 10, 10t
    supply-driven, 10, 10t
    threshold effect in, 10, 10t
  beds-per-capita in, 10, 10t
  infections acquired in. See Infections, hospital-acquired.
  length of stay in, 9–11, 10t
  neuropathy associated with, 2156
  nutrition requirements in, 1173, 1173t
    protein-energy malnutrition and, 1154t, 1154–1155
Host, 1537–1548
  compromised, **1537–1548**. See also Immunodeficiency; Immunosuppression.
    adenovirus in, 1757t, 1758
    antimicrobial therapy in, 1542–1547, 1544t, 1545, 1546t

Host *(Continued)*
cell-mediated defense disorders of, 1541–1542
cytomegalovirus in, 1775
definition of, 1537
evaluation and management of, 1542–1547, *1545*
fungal infections in, 1815, 1815t
herpes simplex in, 1746t, 1773–1774
humoral defense disorders of, 1542
phagocyte defects of, 1537–1541, 1539t
preventive measures for, 1547t, 1547–1548
skin disorders of, 2218–2219
splenic dysfunction in, 1542
toxoplasmosis in, 1908–1909
defense mechanisms of, **1533–1537.** See also *Immune response; Inflammation.*
acute phase, 1535–1537, 1536t
bacteria and, 1537, 1538t
fungi and, 1537, 1538t
inflammatory response in, 1533–1537, *1534,* 1535t
physical and chemical barriers of, 1537
viruses and, 1537, 1538t, 1740
intermediate. See *Animals; Arthropods.*
Hot tub folliculitis, 2207
Howell-Jolly bodies, 971, 973
HPMPC (hydroxyphosphonylmethoxypropyl cytosine), 1744–1745
Human immunodeficiency virus (HIV), 1841–1846, *1842–1845.* See also *HIV infection.*
Humerus, anatomy of, *1522*
shoulder and, *1522*
Hunger, bulimia effect on, 1160
definition of, 629
Hunter's syndrome, clinical features of, 1119t
enzyme defect of, 1119t
Huntington's disease, 2048–2049
chorea in, 2048–2049
dementia of, 1992t, 1995
genetics of, 138t
Hurler's disease, cardiomyopathy due to, 333t, 334
clinical features of, 1119t
enzyme defect of, 1119t
Hutchinson's teeth, 1710
HV interval, *232*
Hyaluronidase, staphylococcal dissemination and, 1606
streptococcal infection role of, 1587
Hybrid, genetic, 142
Hydatid cyst disease, 1923t, 1924–1925
hepatic, 782, *784*
Hydralazine, dosage for, 229t, 265t, 266t, 270t
hepatotoxicity of, 773
side effects of, 267t, 270t, 773
vasodilatation using, 229t, 229–230, 267t, 270t
Hydrocarbon pneumonitis, 408
Hydrocephalus, 2134–2135
acute vs. chronic, 2134t, 2134–2135
causes of, 2134t, 2134–2135
clinical manifestations of, 2135
communicating, 2134
dementia related to, 1992t, 1995
diagnosis of, 2134
hemorrhagic, 2075
meningitis with, 1611
noncommunicating, 2134
treatment of, 2135
Hydrochloric acid, gastric. See *Stomach, acid secretion of.*
Hydrochlorothiazide, dosage for, 264t, 266t
properties and action of, 224t
Hydrocolloid wafers, 2194, 2194t
Hydrocortisone. See *Cortisol.*
Hydrocytosis, hereditary, 855
Hydroflumethiazide, 264t
Hydrofluoric acid, antidote for, 504t
burn due to, 504t
Hydrogel dressing, 2193, 2194t
Hydrogen bonding, Hoogsteen, *1074*
Watson-Crick, *1074*
Hydrogen cyanide poisoning, 504t, 508
Hydrogen ion, 521t, 522, 523, 524. See also *pH.*
Hydrogen nuclei, MRI role of, 202–204, *203–205*
Hydrogen peroxide, antioxidant quenching of, *405*
neutrophil activation and, 1451, *1451*
phagocytosis role of, 897, 899, 900, 900, *906*
tissue damage due to, *405,* 904t
Hydromorphone, neurologic effects of, 1975t
pain control with, 104t, 893t
Hydronephrosis, ultrasonography in, 515, *515*
Hydrophilic dressings, 2193–2194, 2194t

Hydrops, gallbladder, 914
thalassemia causing, 879–880
Hydrops fetalis, 879–880
Hydrostatic pressure, fluid exchange and, 525
normal resting values for, 489t
pulmonary edema and, 476, *477*
volume regulation role of, 525
Hydroxyapatite. See *Apatite.*
4-Hydroxybutyric acid, urinary, 1103t
17-Hydroxycorticosteroids, *1247*
adrenal function testing and, 1213t, 1246, *1247*
pituitary function tests and, 1208t, 1213t
Hydroxydaunomycin, 945t
Hydroxyeicosatetraenoic acid (HETE), *1190,* 1190–1191
5-Hydroxyindoleacetic acid, 700t
carcinoid and, 700t, 1348–1349, *1349*
malabsorption and, 700t
Hydroxyl radicals, antioxidant quenching of, *405*
tissue damage due to, *405*
11β-Hydroxylase, 1288t
adrenal hyperplasia and, 1288t
deficiency of, 1290
diagnosis of, 1290
genetics in, 1290
masculinization in, 1290
treatment of, 1290
17α-Hydroxylase, 1288t
adrenal hyperplasia and, 1288t
deficiency of, 1291
ambiguous genitalia due to, 1291
amenorrhea and, 1305
21-Hydroxylase, 1252, 1287–1290
deficiency of, 1287–1290, *1288,* 1288t
classic, 1287, *1288, 1289*
clinical presentation in, 1288, *1288,* 1288t
diagnosis of, 1288–1289, *1289*
genetics of, 136t, 138t, 1288, *1288*
nonclassic, 1287, *1288, 1289*
treatment of, 1288–1290, *1290*
Hydroxylysine, urinary, 1102t
Hydroxymethylbilane, *1125*
Hydroxyprogesterone, 1046t, 1047
Hydroxyproline, 1102t, 1109
urinary, 1102t, 1109
3β-Hydroxysteroid dehydrogenase, 1288t
adrenal hyperplasia and, 1288t
deficiency of, 1290–1291
pseudohermaphroditism and, 1290–1291
11β-Hydroxysteroid dehydrogenase, 1249
17-Hydroxysteroids, *1247*
adrenal function testing and, 1213t, 1246, *1247*
pituitary function tests and, 1208t, 1213t
5-Hydroxytryptamine. See *Serotonin.*
5-Hydroxytryptophan, 1348–1349, *1349*
Hydroxyurea, adverse effects of, 1045
chemotherapy using, 1042t, 1045
myelogenous leukemia treated with, 928
25-Hydroxyvitamin D, 1357t, 1357–1358, *1358*
actions of, 1354–1355, 1357–1358, *1358*
bone formation role of, 1354–1356, *1355*
pharmacokinetics of, 1357t, 1357–1358
Hydroxyzine, allergic rhinitis treated with, 1416, 1416t
pain control use of, 106t
Hymenolepiasis, 1923t, 1923–1924
Hymenoptera sting, 1420t, 1420–1421
Hyoscyamine, 54–55
Hyperaeration, 390
Hyperalimentation, 547
Hyperbilirubinemia, 755. See also *Jaundice.*
cholestasis with, 808t
conjugated, 755, 757t
fasting state and, 757
postoperative, 757
treatment of, 759
unconjugated, 756, 757t
Hypercalcemia, **1367–1369**
bone formation and, 1355–1356, 1367–1369
breast cancer with, 1323
clinical manifestations of, 1368
definition of, 1367
diagnostic approach to, 1368, 1368t
differential diagnosis of, 1368
etiology of, 1367, 1368t
familial hypocalciuric, 1370
granulomatous disease with, 1371
malignancy with, 1020, 1025t, 1025–1026, 1053, *1367,* 1370–1371
myeloma with, 962t, 963, 964

Hypercalcemia *(Continued)*
parathyroid hormone and, 1366, *1367,* 1367–1370, 1368t
pathogenesis of, 1367–1368, 1368t
treatment of, 1368–1369
vitamin D and, 1368, 1368t
Hypercalciuria, 614–617
kidney stone and, 614–617, *615,* 615t, *616,* 616t
osteomalacia with, 1363t, 1364
Paget's disease with, 1385t, 1385–1386
rickets with, 1363t, 1364
Hypercapnia, acidosis and, 545, 545t, 551
bronchitis with, 382t, 387
clinical features of, 454t
respiratory failure with, 453, 453t, 456–459, 457t, 458t
Hypercholesterolemia, 292–293, 1089–1093
acquired, 1092t
arthritis with, 1525
blood levels in, 1093t
cholestasis with, 808t
diseases associated with, 30t
familial, 293, 1089–1090
genetics of, 136t, 138t
lipoprotein and, 293, 1089–1090
polygenic, 1090
treatment of, *1093,* 1093–1094, 1094t
Hypercortisolism. See also *Cushing's syndrome.*
dexamethasone suppression test in, 1217t, 1217–1218
Hyperdibasic aminoaciduria, 144t
Hyperemesis gravidarum, 630, 787, 787t
thyroid hormone values in, 1230t
Hypereosinophilic syndrome, 333t, 334. See also *Eosinophilia.*
Hyperglycemia, 1258–1259. See also *Diabetes mellitus.*
blood glucose levels in, 1258–1259
enteral nutrition causing, 1171
hyperkalemia with, 542
hypothalamic defect and, 1203
nerve damage due to, 2154
oral agent therapy for, 1267–1268, 1268t
pregnancy with, 1259
Hypergonadism. See *Sexual precocity.*
Hyperhydrosis, paroxysmal localized, 2010
Hyperimmunoglobulinemia, 1402t
E, 1402t, 1407, 1541
neutrophils affected by, 902, 905t
M, 1402t, 1404–1405
Hyperinsulinemia, 1263, 1277
diabetes mellitus with, 1263, *1263,* 1277, *1277*
syndrome X with, *1277*
Hyperkalemia, 541–543. See also *Potassium.*
clinical features of, 542, *542*
definition of, 541
disorders associated with, 541t, 541–542
ECG in, 542, *542*
paradoxical, 542
paralysis with, 542, 2168–2169
pathogenesis of, 541t, 541–542
periodic paralysis with, 2168t, 2168–2169
renal failure with, 556–557, 557t, 561
renal tubular acidosis with, 546t, 547, 598t
treatment of, 542–543
Hyperkeratosis. See also *Keratosis.*
epidermolytic, 2204t
ichthyotic, 1019, *2204,* 2204t
oral leukoplakia in, 647, 647t
physiology of, 2185
psoriatic, 2202–2203
Hyperkinesia, 2042t, 2042–2043
Hyperlipidemia, 292–293, 1090–1091
acquired, 1092t
atherogenesis role of, 292–293
cholesterol and, 292–293
combined, 1090–1091
familial, 1091
management of, *1093,* 1093–1095, 1094t
Hyperlipoproteinemia, 1089–1095
acquired disorders with, 1091–1092, 1092t
alpha, 1090
apoprotein defect in, 1089–1091
B, 1089–1090
CII, 1090
E, 1090–1091
arthritis with, 1525
atherosclerosis role of, 1092–1093
beta-VLDL, 1090–1091
cholesterol. See *Hypercholesterolemia.*

Hyperlipoproteinemia (Continued)
    familial, 1089–1091
    lipase deficiency with, 1090
    triglyceride. See Hypertriglyceridemia.
Hypermagnesemia, 1138
    symptoms in, 1138
    treatment of, 1138
Hypermelanosis, 2212–2213
Hypernatremia, 537–538
    clinical features of, 538
    etiology of, 537–538
    heart failure with, 217
    neurogenic, 2013
    treatment of, 538
Hyperopia, 2174
    pseudopapilledema of, 2177
Hyperornithinemia, 146t
Hyperosmolality, coma with, 1270
    diabetes mellitus with, 1270
Hyperostosis, 1387–1390
    causes of, 1387–1390, 1388t, 1469t
    cortical, 1387–1388, 1388t
    endosteal, 1388
Hyperoxaluria, aciduria with, 1085
    enteric, 616t, 617
    kidney stone and, 614–617, 615, 616t
    metabolic defect in, 147, 147t, 1085
    primary, 616t, 617, 1085
    treatment of, 616t, 616–617, 1085
Hyperparathyroidism, 1369–1370
    arthritis with, 1525
    bone resorption due to, 1356, 1377, 1378
    clinical manifestations of, 1369, 2168
    definition of, 1369
    diagnosis of, 1369
    etiology of, 1369
    incidence of, 1369
    multiple endocrine neoplasia with, 1346
    pathology in, 1369
    pathophysiology in, 1369
    prognosis in, 1369–1370
    treatment of, 1369–1370
Hyperphagia, bulimia with, 1160
    hypothalamus and, 1165, 2012–2013
    Kleine-Levin syndrome with, 1160, 2013
    obesity and, 1163
Hyperphenylalaninemia, 1105–1108, 1106, 1107
Hyperphosphaturia, 1363t
    osteomalacia with, 1363t, 1363–1364, 1365
    rickets with, 1363t, 1363–1364, 1365
Hyperpigmentation, Addison's disease with, 2213
    arsenic poisoning with, 70
Hyperpituitarism, 1207–1210, 1209t
Hyperpnea, embolic, 423, 424t
Hyperprolactinemia, 1213–1215
    amenorrhea with, 1303–1304, 1304
    causes of, 1202t, 1202–1203, 1213–1214
    clinical features of, 1214
    differential diagnosis of, 1214, 1214t
    drug-induced, 1202t, 1214t
    galactorrhea with, 1306, 1318, 1318t
    hypogonadism with, 1338
    hypothalamic, 1202t, 1202–1203, 1214t
    idiopathic, 1203
    neurogenic, 1202t
    pathogenesis of, 1213–1214
    pituitary, 1202t, 1214t
    therapy of, 1214–1215
Hyperreflexia, detrusor, 22
    hepatic encephalopathy with, 797–798, 798t
Hypersalivation, 629, 629
Hypersensitivity. See also Allergy.
    antimicrobials causing, 1568t, 1569
    aspirin, 1435
    delayed-type, 1415, 1415
        tuberculosis response with, 1683
    drug-induced, 1432t–1435t, 1432–1435
    immediate-type, 1415, 1415
        anaphylaxis in, 1417–1418, 1418t
        angioedema due to, 1409t, 1409–1410
        rhinitis in, 1413–1417, 1415, 1416
        urticaria due to, 1409t, 1409–1410
    insect sting and, 1420t, 1420–1421
    light. See Photosensitivity.
    penicillin, 1418–1419, 1435t
    skin affected by, 2197–2198, 2198t
    vasculitis due to, 1490–1492, 1491t

Hypersomnia, 1983–1984, 1984t
    autonomic lesion and, 2013
    definition of, 1969t
    Kleine-Levin syndrome with, 1160, 2013
Hypersplenism, 972
    liver disease with, 796
Hypertension, 256–277
    accelerated, 257
    anemia effect on, 823
    atherosclerosis related to, 258, 259
    cardiac effects of, 260t, 260–261
    catecholamines causing, 1254, 1255
    classification by blood pressure, 258t
    complicated, 257, 258, 259, 260t
    coronary disease and, 257, 260t, 263
    crisis in, 269t, 269–270, 270t
    definitions related to, 256–258
    diabetes with, 268, 1269t, 1276–1277, 1277
    diagnostic evaluation of, 259–260, 260t
    diastolic, 258t, 261, 263
    diet and, 1141, 1143t
    diseases associated with, 30t, 258, 258t, 259, 260t
    drug therapy for, 262–270
        ACE inhibitors in, 263, 265t, 266t, 266–267
        α blocking agents in, 263, 265t, 267t, 268, 270t
        β blocking agents in, 263–266, 265t–267t
        calcium channel blockers in, 265t, 266–267, 267t
        centrally acting agents in, 265t, 266t, 267–268
        combination, 266t, 267t
        diuretics in, 263, 264, 264t, 266t, 267t
        emergency, 269t, 269–270, 270t
        general principles of, 263–264
        new agents in, 268
        risk reduction due to, 262–263, 263
        trials for, 263, 263–264
        vasodilators in, 266t, 267t, 268, 270t
    drug-induced, 258t
    elderly with, 268
    essential (primary), 256–257, 262
    etiology of, 258, 258t, 362t
    gender and, 258, 259
    genetic factors in, 258
    gestational, 610–611
    glomerulonephritis causing, 575
    headache with, 2033
    high normal, 257–258, 258t
    incidence of, 256, 257, 258, 259
    intracranial, headache due to, 2034
    isolated systolic, 256
    lifestyle and, 261–262, 262
    malignant, 257
    mortality rate role of, 30t, 257
    natriuretic hormone role in, 1194, 1196
    nephrosclerosis with, 607
    obesity causing, 1164
    ocular, 2175
    pheochromocytoma causing, 1254, 1255
    portal, 743, 793–795
        ascites due to, 743, 743t, 744t, 795–796
        cirrhosis with, 793t, 793–796
        clinical features of, 793–794
        diagnosis of, 793–794
        shunting in, 752, 793
        varices of, 793t, 794t, 794–795
        venous pressure in, 793–794
    pregnancy and, 609–611
    prevalence of, 256, 257, 258, 259
    pseudo-hypertension and, 260
    public awareness of, 256, 257
    pulmonary, 271–277
        chest x-ray of, 273t, 274
        clinical signs in, 272, 272t
        congenital, 281, 283
        definition of, 271
        diagnosis of, 272t, 272–274, 273, 273t, 274
        diseases associated with, 273t, 274–276
        ECG of, 272, 273, 273t, 277
        echocardiography of, 272–273, 273t
        embolism causing, 273t, 274, 275, 423
        MRI scan of, 273t, 273–274, 274
        passive, 273t, 275–276
        pathophysiology of, 271–272, 272t
        precapillary (primary), 273t, 274–275, 276
        reactive, 273t, 276
        survival rate for, 276
        treatment of, 276, 276–277, 277
    race and, 258, 259

Hypertension (Continued)
    renal, 260t, 260–261, 268–269
        arterial stenosis and, 606–607
        cystic disease causing, 618, 618t, 619t
        kidney failure and, chronic, 556, 558, 561, 562
        obstruction with, 591, 591t
    retinal effects of, 257, 260t
    secondary, 257, 258t, 260
    smoking and, 262
    stages of, 258t
    stroke and, 257, 260t, 263
    surveys on, 256, 257, 261, 263
    systolic, 258t, 261
    target organ disease due to, 260, 260t
    treatment of, 260–270, 262
        algorithm for, 262
        dietary changes in, 261–262
        drugs in, 262, 262–270, 264t–267t, 269t, 270t
        exercise in, 261
    tumor-associated, 1026
    white coat, 258, 260
Hyperthermia, 501–502, 2012. See also Fever.
    delirium with, 1973–1974
    diagnostic studies in, 502t
    malignant, 502, 2012
        rigidity with, 502, 2012
    management of, 502, 502t
    predisposing factors for, 502t
    thermoregulation in, 501, 502, 1532, 2012
Hyperthyroidism, 1231–1237. See also Graves' disease; Thyrotoxicosis.
    definition of, 1231–1232
    etiology of, 1231–1232, 1232t
    heart affected by, 359, 1233, 1233t
    heart disease and, 1236–1237
    laboratory values in, 1229, 1229t, 1230t, 1233
    ophthalmopathy of, 1235
    transient, 1240
    treatment of, 1234t, 1234–1235
    tumor-associated, 1026
Hypertonicity, 537t, 537–538
Hypertrichosis, paraneoplastic, 1034
Hypertriglyceridemia, 1090
    acquired, 1092t
    alcohol and, 1092
    atherogenesis role of, 293
    diabetes mellitus and, 1092
    familial, 1090
    marked, 1094–1095
    mild, 1091, 1094
    treatment of, 1094–1095
    uremia and, 1092
Hyperuricemia, 1508–1515. See also Gout.
    asymptomatic, 1515
    classification of, 1509t
    clinical manifestations of, 1510–1512, 1512–1514
    congenital heart disease with, 286
    incidence and prevalence of, 1509
    nephrolithiasis due to, 1508, 1510–1511
    nephropathy of, 1510, 1512
    overproduction mechanism of, 1509t, 1510
    primary, 1509t
    reduced excretion in, 1509t, 1510, 1510t
    renal failure with, 557t, 559
    secondary, 1509t
    treatment of, 1512–1515, 1514t
Hyperuricosuria, 615, 616t, 617
Hyperventilation, 1981
    alkalosis due to, 545, 545, 545t, 551
    alveolar, 423, 424t
    consciousness loss in, 1981, 2121
    embolism causing, 423, 424t
    intracranial pressure reduced with, 2133t
    seizure evaluation using, 2120, 2121
Hyperviscosity, 965–966
    cerebrovascular disease due to, 2068
    retinopathy due to, 2182
Hyphae, aspergilloma of, 1831, 1831
    mucormycosis role of, 1833–1834
Hyphema, 2177
Hypnogogic hallucinations, 1984
Hypnotic agents, 1975t
Hypoaeration, 389
Hypoalbuminemia, 573
    malnutrition with, 1156t
Hypoaldosteronism, 1251t, 1251–1252
    causes of, 1251t
    differential diagnosis of, 1251–1252
    hyporeninemic, 528, 539, 546t, 547

Hypoaldosteronism (*Continued*)
sodium wasting due to, 528, 528t, 598–599
treatment of, 1251–1252
Hypocalcemia, 1371–1372
clinical manifestations of, 1371
definition of, 1371
differential diagnosis of, 1371–1372
etiology of, 1371, 1372t
magnesium deficiency causing, 1138, 1372
pathogenesis of, 1371, 1372t
renal failure with, chronic, 557t, 557–558
treatment of, 1372
Hypocalciuria, 1370
Hypochlorhydria, 701t
Hypochlorous acid, 900, *906*
Hypochondriasis, 2005–2006
diagnostic criteria for, 2005, 2006t
elderly patient with, 2000
features of, 2005, 2005t
pathophysiology of, 2005
treatment of, 2005–2006
Hypocitraturia, 616, 616t
kidney stone and, 615, *615*, 616, 616t
treatment of, 616, 616t
Hypocortisolism, 1249–1251, 1250t
ACTH deficiency causing, 1215–1216
21-hydroxylase defect in, 1252, 1287–1290, 1288t
Hypoferremia, 842
Hypogammaglobulinemia, 1401–1405
arthritis with, 1525
common variable, 1404
immune globulin treatment for, 41t
transient, of infancy, 1405
X-linked, 1402t, *1403*, 1403–1404
Hypoglycemia, 1278–1282
adrenal insufficiency risk factor in, 1216
alcoholic, 753
approach to patient with, 1281, *1282*
autoimmune, 1282
causes of, 1279t, 1279–1281
clinical classification of, 1279t
diabetic patient with, 1264, 1271–1272
drug-induced, 1267–1268, 1268t, 1279t, 1280
epinephrine in, 1258, 1272, *1272*, 1278
factitious, 1264, 1271–1272, *1272*, 1281t, 1289–1281
fasting, 1279–1280
glycogen storage disease with, 1082–1083, 1083t
growth hormone test using, 1208t
malarial coma with, 1894
postprandial (reactive), 1279, 1279t
signs and symptoms of, 1278–1279, 1279t, 1982
tumor-associated, 1026, 1280, 1281
Hypoglycemic agents, oral, 1267–1268, 1268t, 1280
Hypogonadism, 1329–1340
AIDS/HIV patient with, 1878
female, 1219, 1295t
hemochromatosis in, 1337
hypergonadotropic, 1295t, 1333
hyperprolactinemia in, 1338
hypogonadotropic, 1219, 1295t, 1333, 1334t
hypothalamic, 1202, 1326, 1337
male, 1329–1340
androgen role in, 1333–1336
deficiency and, 1329, 1333–1336, 1334t
insensitivity and, 1338
causes of, 1329, 1333–1338, 1334t
primary, 1333–1337, 1334t
secondary, 1334t, 1337–1338
treatment of, 1338–1340
obesity with, 1165
Hypokalemia, 539–541. See also *Potassium*.
alkalosis with, 531, 531t, 540
clinical features of, 540
definition of, 539
disorders associated with, 539t
diuretic causing, 531, 531t
ECG in, 540, *541*
extrarenal vs. renal, 514, *515*
paralysis with, 540, 2168
pathogenesis of, 539t, 539–540
periodic paralysis with, 2168t, 2168–2169
treatment of, 540–541
urinary potassium fractional excretion and, 514, *515*
vomiting and, 630
Hypokinesia, 2042, 2042t
Hypomagnesemia, 1137–1138
calcium in, 1138
causes and mechanisms of, 1137t, 1137–1138
diagnosis of, 1138

Hypomagnesemia (*Continued*)
hypoparathyroidism due to, 1372
incidence of, 1137
kidney stone and, *615*
management of, 1138, 1138t
potassium in, 1138
Hypomelanosis, 2213–2214, 2214t
Hyponatremia, 534–537
acute vs. chronic, 537
ADH in, 535t, 535–536, *536*
alkalosis and, 514
clinical features of, 536
diabetes insipidus and, *1226*
diagnosis of, 536–537
elderly affected by, 23–24
etiology of, 534t, 534–536, *535*, 535t
hypotonicity due to, 534t, 534–537
oliguria in, 514, 514t
paroxysmal, 2013
treatment of, 537, 537t
tumor-associated, 1026
Hypoparathyroidism, 1372–1373
acquired, 1372–1373
clinical manifestations of, *1372*, 1372–1373
definition of, 1372
etiology of, 1372, 1372t
hereditary, *1372*, 1372–1373
hypomagnesemia in, 1372, 1373
pathogenesis of, 1372, 1372t
pseudo-, 1363, *1372*, 1372–1373
transient, 1372, 1373
vitamin D in, 1373
Hypoperfusion, 483
shock with, 483, *483*
septic, 499t, 499–500, 500t
toxic, 1588–1589
syncope due to, 1980, 1980t
Hypophagia, 2013. See also *Anorexia*.
Hypophosphatasia, 1365
osteomalacia due to, 1365
Hypophosphatemia, 1135–1137. See also *Phosphorus*.
clinical manifestations of, 1136, 1136t
etiology of, 1135–1136, 1136t
management of, 1136–1137, 1137t
moderate, 1136, 1136t, 1137t
osteomalacia due to, 144t, 1362t, 1363t, 1363–1364
severe, 1136, 1136t, 1137t
transient, 1136t, 1137t
Hypophyseal artery, *1197*
Hypophysis. See *Pituitary gland*.
Hypopigmentation, tuberous sclerosis with, 2056
Hypopituitarism, 1206–1207
anovulation due to, 1306, 1306t
causes of, 1207, 1207t
diagnosis of, 1207, 1208t
hormone replacement therapy for, 1207, 1208t
Hyposalivation, 649t, 649–650
Hyposplenism, 973
Hypotension, 499–500
adrenal crisis with, 1250
fluid shift causing, 529–530, 530t
intracranial, headache due to, 2034
orthostatic, 1981
shock with, septic, 496t, 499t, 499–500, 500t
toxic, 1588t, 1588–1589, 1609t
syncope due to, 1981
Hypothalamus, *1183*, *2011*
anatomy of, *1183*, *1197*, *1222*, *2011*
appetite center of, 1165, 2012–2013
autonomic system controlled by, 2011, *2011*
blood flow to, 1197, *2060*
cold, 2188
warm, 2188
body temperature sensitivity of, 1203, 1533–1534, *1534*, 2012
cutaneous vascularity and, 2188
diabetes insipidus role of, 1223–1224, 1226, *1226*, 2013
diseases of, 1200–1203, 1207t, 2012t
age of onset of, 1200t
etiology of, 1200t
embryonic dysplasias of, 1200
endorphins in, 1187, 1187t
feedback mechanisms of, *1183*, 1183–1184, *1198*, 1199–1200
functional organization of, 2011, *2011*
osmostat of, 1222, *1222*, 2013
pituitary and, *1197*, 1197–1199, *1198*, 1201–1203, 1207t

Hypothalamus (*Continued*)
posterior, 1221–1222, *1222*
pituitary-adrenal axis of, 1215, 1250
pituitary-ovarian axis of, 1293–1295, *1294*, *1299*, 1300–1301
pituitary-testicular axis of, *1326*, 1326
pituitary-thyroid axis of, 1206, 1206t, *1227*
pulsatile secretion by, 1184, 1999–2000
regulatory hormones of, 1197–1199, *1198*. See also specific hormones.
disorders of, 1201–1203, 1207t
satiety center of, 629, 1203, 2012–2013
tumors affecting, 1200t, 1200–1201
Hypothermia, 502–503, 2012. See also *Cold*.
accidental, 502–503
coma with, 1973
diagnostic studies in, 502t
ECG in, *503*
hypothalamic, 1203, 2012
management of, 503, 503t
paroxysmal, 2012
predisposing factors for, 503t
renal failure with, 559
thermoregulation and, 501, 1203, 2012
Hypotheses, null, 84
testing of, 84
Hypothyroidism, 1237–1240
anemia in, 827
anorexia causing, 1158
arthritis with, 1525
causes of, 1237t, 1237–1238
central, 1221
childhood, 1230
clinical manifestations of, 1238, 1238t
definition of, 1237
diagnosis of, *1238*, 1238–1239
differential diagnosis of, *1238*, 1239
hypothalamic, 1203
iatrogenic, 1237t, 1237–1238
incidence of, 1237–1238
iodine in, deficiency state, 1149t, 1237t
excess state, 1237t, 1238
laboratory values in, 1229, 1229t, *1238*, 1238–1239
pathogenesis of, 1237t, 1237–1238
primary, 1237t, 1237–1238
secondary, 1237t, 1238
thyroprivic, 1238
treatment of, 1239–1240, 1240t
TSH and, 1237t, 1237–1239
Hypotonicity, osmolality and, 534t, 534–537
real vs. apparent, 534, 534t
Hypouricemia, 144t
Hypoventilation, acidosis due to, 545, *545*, 545t, 551
respiratory failure with, 455–456, 457t, 458–459
Hypovolemia, 528–529
aldosterone and, 528
causes of, 528, 528t
definition of, 528
exclusion of, 491
renal failure and, 552t, 553–554, 554t
shock with, 485
symptoms of, 528–529
treatment of, 529
Hypoxanthine, 1509–1510, *1511*
Hypoxanthine phosphoribosyltransferase, 146t, 1115–1116
deficiency of, 146t, 1115–1116
purine metabolism and, 1510, *1511*
Hypoxanthine-guanine phosphoribosyltransferase, 1510, *1511*
Hypoxemia, assessment of, 467t, 467–468
embolic, 423
Pneumocystis pneumonia with, 1918, *1918*, 1919
respiratory failure with, 452–456, 453t, 454t, 467t
right-to-left shunt and, 467t, 468, 472, *472*
ventilation therapy in, 469t, 469–472, *472*
Hypoxia, anemia and, 823
carbon monoxide poisoning and, 403–404, 507, 507t
cardiogenic shock and, 480, *480*
cerebral, 2062t, 2062–2063
diffuse, 2062, 2073
focal, 2062, 2063–2073
metabolism in, 2062–2063
pathology of, 2062t, 2062–2063
clinical features of, 454t
consciousness level in, 2062t, 2063
head injury with, 2136–2138, 2138t

Hypoxia (Continued)
  neurologic effects of, 1972t, 1972–1974
  neuron vulnerability to, 2062t, 2063
  ventilatory drive due to, 370, *370*
Hysteria, gait affected by, 2030
  hypochondriasis related to, 2006
  psychiatric disorder with, 1974, 1974t
  weakness due to, 2028, 2028t

I

I antigen, 817
Ibuprofen, gout treated with, 1513–1514, 1514t
  overdose of, 506
  pain control with, 103t, 893t
ICAM, leukocyte adhesiveness and, 898, 898t, *899*
Ice, compulsive ingestion of, 840
I-cell disease, 147
Ichthyosis(es), 2204t
  paraneoplastic, 1019, 1034t
  skin lesions of, 1019, *2204*, 2204t
  vulgaris(es), 2204t
  X-linked, 2204t
Idarubicin, adverse effects of, 1044
  chemotherapy using, 1039t, 1044, 1044t
Idoxuridine, **1743**
  herpes simplex treated with, 1746t
  keratitis treated with, 1746t
Iduronidase deficiency, 1119t
Ifosfamide, adverse effects of, 1042
  cardiotoxicity of, 331
  chemotherapy using, 1042, 1042t
Ileitis, Crohn's, 709, 712. See also *Crohn's disease.*
  malabsorption due to, 103
  nongranulomatous, 103
Ileum, absorption in, *689*, 689–690, 690t, 696, 696t
  bile in, 806, *807*
  inflammation of. See *Ileitis.*
Ileus, jejunal sentinel loop in, 732
  meconium, cystic fibrosis with, 419–420, 421t
Ilheus encephalitis, 1806t
Imaging techniques. See also specific technique.
  advances in, 127–132, *128–133*
Iminoglycinuria, 1104t, 1109
  metabolic defect in, 144t
Imipenem, 1562t
  minimal inhibitory concentration for, 1570, 1570t
  Pseudomonas and, 1579–1581, 1580t
Imipramine, 2000t, 2001
Immotile cilia syndrome, 1336
  bronchiectasis with, 416, 416t
Immune complexes, **1421–1424**
  antigens causing, 1421–1422, *1422*, 1422t
  biologic properties of, *1422*, 1422–1423, *1423*
  complement and, 1423, *1423*
  detection of, 1423–1424
  drug-induced, 1422
  erythrocyte binding of, 1423, *1423*
  glomerulonephritis due to, 575–576, 577, 577t
  Kupffer cell removal of, 1423, *1423*
  lupus erythematosus with, *1476*, 1477
  Lyme disease with, 1716
  mesangial cell deposition of, 1477
  nephrotic disorders and, 573, 573t, 577t
  neutrophil response to, *1451*, 1451–1452, *1452*
  pathophysiology of, 1421–1422, *1422*, 1422t
  serum sickness and, 1421–1422, *1422*
  urticaria due to, 1409t, 1409–1410
  vasculitis and, 1423, 1449–1450, 1490, 1492
Immune response, **1393–1439**
  aging effects and, 15
  allergy and, 1414–1415, *1415*, *1416*
  antibodies and. See *Antibodies; B cells; Immunoglob-
    ulin(s).*
  arthritis and, 1448–1454
  cell-mediated, *1393*, 1393–1395. See also *Monocytes;
    T cells.*
    cellular interactions in, *1393*, 1393–1394
    compromised host and, 1538t, 1541–1542
    deficiency of, 1538t, 1541–1542
  complement and, 1398–1401
  cutaneous, 2188–2189, 2189t
  cytokines in, *1393*, 1395, 1395t
  deficient. See *Immunodeficiency.*
  HIV effect on, 1837t, **1837–1841**, 1839t
  HLA complex and, 1424–1431. See also *HLA complex.*
  humoral, 1395–1397. See also *Antibodies; B cells;
    Immunoglobulin(s).*

Immune response (Continued)
    cellular interactions in, *1393*, 1393–1394
    compromised host and, 1538t, 1542
    deficiency of, 1538t, 1542
  inflammatory bowel disease and, 708
  lepromatous defect in, 1692t, 1692–1693
  liver and, 767
  lupus erythematosus affecting, *1476*, 1476–1477
  neutrophils in, 1448–1454, *1449–1452*
  phagocyte role in, 901, 901t
  principles of, 1393–1398, 1448–1450
  renal transplant and, *568*, 568–569
  rheumatoid arthritis role of, 1448–1450, *1449*, *1450*,
    1460, 1460–1461
  sarcoidosis and, 431, *431*
  self-versus-nonself in, 1424, 1476
  transfusion-associated, 895–896, 896t
  vasculitis role of, 1448–1450, *1449*, *1450*
Immunization, **40–46**. See also *Vaccine(s).*
  active, 40
  adverse reactions to, 40–44, 42t–44t
  contraindications to, 40–41, 42t–44t
  disease prevention using, 41t–44t, 41–46
  immunocompromise and, 41
  immunosuppressed patient and, 363
  indications for, 41–46, 42t–44t
  passive, 40, 41t
    indications for, 41t
  pregnancy and, 41
  schedule of, 40, 42t–44t
  travel and, 1554t, 1554–1555
Immunoassay, parathyroid hormone, 1366–1367, *1367*
Immunodeficiency, **1401–1408**. See also *AIDS (ac-
    quired immunodeficiency syndrome); HIV infection.*
  antibody, 1402t, 1403–1405
  approach to patient with, 1402–1403, 1542–1548,
    1545
  ataxia-telangiectasia with, 1407
  B cell, 1402t, 1402–1403, *1403*, 1542
  bronchiectasis with, 416t, 416–417, 418t
  cellular, 1402t, 1402–1403, 1405, 1538t, 1541–1542
  common variable, 1404
  compromised host with, 1537–1548, 1538t, *1545*
  DiGeorge syndrome with, 1402t, 1405
  disorders associated with, 1402t, 1541–1542
  elevated IgM with, 1404–1405
  Epstein-Barr virus causing, 1405
  gene defects causing, 1401–1402, 1402t
  humoral, 1403–1405, 1538t, 1542
  immunoglobulin, 1402t, 1403–1405, 1538t, 1542
  laboratory tests for, 1402–1403
  listeriosis in, 1672–1673
  Nezelof syndrome with, 1402t, 1405
  non-human primate and, *1845*, 1845–1846
  primary disorders of, 1401–1408, 1402t
  selective IgA, 1404
  severe combined, 1402t, *1403*, 1405–1408
    enzyme deficiency causing, 1114–1115, 1405,
      1406
    X-linked, 1406
  sickle syndrome with, 886
  skin disorders associated with, 2218–2219
  T cell, 1402t, 1402–1403, *1403*, 1541–1542
  thymoma with, 1407
  transient, of infancy, 1405
  Wiskott-Aldrich, 1402t, 1407
  X-linked, 1402t, *1403*, 1403–1404, 1406
Immunoelectrophoresis, monoclonal proteins in, 958,
  959
Immunofluorescence tests, 2189t
  connective tissue diseases and, 2189t
  Legionella infection and, 1584t
  mycoplasmal infection and, 1577
  Pneumocystis carinii and, 1920
  Rocky Mountain spotted fever and, 1731
  skin diseases and, 2189t
Immunoglobulin(s), **1393–1394**
  A, 1394t
    nephropathy due to, 575–576, 812t
    selective deficiency of, 1402t, 1404
  B cell expression of, 1395, *1396*
  characteristics of, *1394*, 1394t
  class and subclass of, 1394t
  cold-precipitated. See *Cryoglobulinemia.*
  crystal deposition of, 1516t
  D, 1394t
  deficiency of, 1402t, 1403–1405, 1542. See also *Im-
    munodeficiency.*
  E, 1394t
    allergic response mediation by, 1414, *1415*

Immunoglobulin(s) (Continued)
    allergic rhinitis role of, 1414, *1415*
    excess of, 902, 905t
  erythrocyte-bound, 859–867
  formation of, 1395, *1396*
  G, 1394t
    hemolytic anemia due to, *860*, 860–866
    receptors for, 1452–1453
  genes for, *1396*, 1396t, 1396–1397, *1397*
  hemolysis caused by, *860*, 860–867, *861*, 862t
  hemorrhagic disorders related to, 986t, 986–987
  hepatitis B with, 771
  Lyme disease with, 1716, 1717–1718, *1718*
  M, 1394t
    elevated, 1404–1405
    hemolytic anemia due to, *861*, 861–866
  monoclonal, 958–968, *959*, *960*, 960t. See also *Gam-
    mopathy.*
    detection of, 958–961, *959*, *960*
  plasma cell disorders and, 958–968, *960*, 960t, *961*,
    961t
  properties of, *1394*, 1394t
  purpura associated with, 986–987
  sarcoidosis role of, 431, *431*
  skin lesion role of, 2189t
  structure and function of, *1394*, 1394t, 1395–1396
  therapeutic, 40, 41t, 1554
    indications for, 40, 41t, 1554
    malabsorption and, 704t
  therapy using, passive immunization, 40, 41t
Immunopotentiation, 150t, 1075
Immunosuppression, aplastic anemia treated with, 835
  hemolytic anemia treated with, 865–866
  HIV induction of, 1837–1840
  inflammatory bowel disease treated with, 713
  transplantation with, cardiac, 363
    hepatic, 801–802
    lung, 462t
    renal, 570–571
Immunotherapy, allergic rhinitis treated with, 1417
  anti-cancer, 1048t, 1048–1049
  bee, wasp, and hornet venom in, 1421
Impetigo, bullous, 1606, 1607t, 2205
  contagiosa, 1587, 1589t
  staphylococcal, 1606, 1607t, 2205
  streptococcal, 1587, 1589t, 2205
Impotence, 1329–1331
  causes of, 1329–1331, 1330t
  definition of, 1329–1330
  drugs causing, 1331, 2010t
  erectile function testing in, 2010t
  evaluation of, 1331, 2010t
  hemochromatosis causing, 1337
  treatment of, 1331
Imprinting, gene expression modified by, 135, 156
Inanition, hypothalmic lesion causing, 2013
Inclusion body(ies), Creola, 380
  Döhle, 916, *918*
  Hassall's, 1438
  Heinz, 856–857, 874, *874*
  Howell-Jolly, 971, 973
  Lewy, 1994
  morula, 1733
    ehrlichiosis with, 1733
  myositis with, 1500, 1501, 2164
  Negri, 2096
  Pick's, 1995
Incontinence, fecal, 692
  urinary, elderly affected by, 22
    stress, 22
Indacrinone, 224t
Indapamide, dosage for, 264t
  properties and action of, 224t
Indigestion, myocardial infarction vs., 301, 304
Indomethacin, cluster headache treated with, 2032–2033
  gout treated with, 1513–1514, 1514t
  pain control with, 893t
Indoramin, 268
Industries, environmental hazards of, 56–59, 58t, 59t
Infarction, bone affected by, 1387, 1387t
  cerebral, amnesia due to, 1990, 1990t
    imaging of, 1966, *1967*
    neuropathology of, 2061t, 2062t, 2063
  myocardial. See *Myocardial infarction.*
  pulmonary, 422–424
  splenic, 974
Infections, **1531–1738**. See also *Sepsis;* specific type,
  e.g., *Legionella* infections.
  acute phase response to, 1535–1537, 1536t
  adrenal gland, 1251

Infections (*Continued*)
antimicrobial therapy in. See *Antimicrobials*; *specific agents.*
ascites due to, 743t, 744t, 746–747, 747t
bronchiectasis due to, 416t, 416–417
catheter-related, candidal, 1828–1830
  neutropenic patient and, 1543, 1546t
  urinary tract, 1550–1551
compromised host with, 1537–1548, 1538t, *1545*
definition of, 1531–1532
dementia caused by, 1992t, 1995–1996
enteric, 1641–1660. See also *specific organism or infection.*
fever and, 1533–1535, *1534*, 1535t
fungal. See *Fungal infection(s).*
heart failure and, 328–330
heart transplant affected by, 363t, 364, *365*
hepatic, 781–785. See also *Hepatitis.*
historical aspects of, 1531–1532
hospital-acquired, **1548–1553**
  AIDS in, 1553
  anatomic sites for, 1549t, 1550–1553
  bacteremia in, 1549t, 1551, 1669–1671
  control program for, 1552–1553
  endocarditis in, 1600, 1601–1602
  hepatitis B in, 1553
  historical aspects of, 1548–1549
  impact of, 1549, 1549t
  ocular, 2179
  pneumonia in, 1549t, 1551–1552, 1669–1671
  predisposing factors for, 1549
  prevalence of, 1549, 1549t
  staphylococcal, 1548–1549, 1609, 1609t
  surgical wound with, 1552
  transmission modes for, 1549–1550
  tuberculosis in, 1553, 1689
  urinary tract with, 1549t, 1550–1551, 1669–1671
inflammatory response to, 1533–1537, *1534*, 1535t, 1536t
lung abscess due to, 413–414, 414t, *415*
lymphadenopathy due to, 970t
muscle weakness due to, 1503t
myocarditis due to, 328–330, 329t
myopathy due to, 2163–2165, 2164t
nephrotic disease following, 574t, 576
nervous system, 2080–2106. See also *Brain, abscess of*; *Encephalitis*; *Meningitis.*
  pyogenic, 2080–2084, 2081t
  syphilitic, 2085–2087
  viral, 2087–2106, 2088t
occupation related to, 2221–2222
occupational exposure to, 56, 58t
pericarditis due to, 337t, 337–338
pleural effusion with, 445t, 445–446
prevention of, 1547t, 1547–1548, 1552–1556, 1554t, 1555t
prostatic, 1341–1342
renal failure and, 558–559, 561t, 562
shock with, 496–501
  septic, 496t, 496–501, *498*, 500t
  toxic syndrome of, 1588t, 1588–1589
sickle syndrome with, 887, 888t, 891
splenomegaly due to, 971t, 971–972, 972t
synovial fluid and, 1455t, 1455–1456
urinary tract, 602–605
viral, carcinogenicity of, 1017
Infertility, 1307–1309, 1331–1332
bromocriptine therapy in, 1214–1215
cystic fibrosis causing, 421, 421t
definition of, 1331
evaluation of, 1331–1332
female factors in, 1307–1308, 1308t, 1700
hyperprolactinemia in, 1214–1215
infection causing, 1332, 1700
inflammatory bowel disease and, 711
male factors in, 1307–1308, 1308t, 1331t, 1331–1332
occupational exposure causing, 56, 59t
sexually transmitted disease and, 1700
Inflammation. See also *Fever*; *Immune response*; *Sepsis.*
acute phase response and, 1535–1537, 1536t
allergic reaction and, 1414–1415, *1415*, *1416*
cascade of, *113*
complement role in, *1400*, 1400–1401, 1401t
cutaneous, 2185. See also *Dermatitis.*
immune complexes causing, 1423, 1448–1453, *1451*, *1452*
neuropathy due to, 2151t, 2151–2152, 2153

Inflammation (*Continued*)
neutrophil-mediated, 897–900, *899*, 1450–1451, *1451*, *1452*
oncotaxis due to, 1031
phagocyte function in, 897–901, *899*, 901t
  disorders of, 902–906, *903*, 904t, 905t
prostaglandin role in, 112–114, *113*
pyrogenesis in, 1532t, 1533–1535, *1534*, 1535t
septic shock role of, 496t, 496–500, *497*, *498*, 500t
splenomegaly due to, 971t, 972, 972t
synovial fluid and, 1455t, 1455–1456
systemic response syndrome of, 496, 496t, *497*, 500t
Inflammatory bowel disease, **707–715.** See also *Colitis, ulcerative*; *Crohn's disease.*
arthritis with, 1467t, 1472
cancer and, 709–710, 710t, 725
endoscopy in, 638t, 640, 711, 712t
Influenza, **1753–1757**
A, 1746t, 1754
B, 1754–1755
C, 1754
clinical findings in, 1755–1756
diagnosis of, 1756
epidemiology of, 1753t, 1754–1755
etiology of, 1754, *1754*, 1754t
immunization in, 42t, 45, 1756t, 1756–1757
mortality rate role of, 27t, 30t
pathogenesis and pathology in, 1755
pharyngitis in, 1749–1751, 1750t, 1751t
pig transmission of, 1738
Reye's syndrome with, 1756
risk factors for, 30t, 1756t
treatment of, 1746t, 1756
virology of, 1754, *1754*, 1754t
Informed consent, 4
Infrared radiation, 63
Infundibulum, common cold affecting, 1749, *1749*
Infusion pump, insulin, 1266
Inguinal nodes, 969t
  Hodgkin's disease in, 948, *949*
Inhalants, 55
asthma treated with, 380–381
drug abuse with, 55, 56t
manganese in, 1149t
Inhibin, 1326, *1326*
Injury. See *Accidents*; *Trauma.*
Inotropic agents. See also *Digitalis.*
shock and, 492–494
Inotropic state, 177, 215
definition of, 479
digitalis effect on, *225*, 225–226
INR, coumarin dosage and, 999–1000
Insecticides, 510t
carbamate, 509
food poisoning due to, 740
organophosphate, 504t, 509–510, 510t
poisoning due to, 509–510, 510t
Insects. See *Arthropods*, and *specific type.*
Insomnia, 1982–1983
autonomic lesion and, 2013
depression causing, 1999, 1999t
drug therapy for, 1983
fatal familial, 2102, 2103
manic episode with, 2003t
melatonin role in, 1204
preventive measures for, 1983, 1983t
Inspiratory capacity, 373, *373*
Inspiratory pressure, 466, 467t
Insulin, action of, 1260–1261
antibodies to, *1259*, 1262–1263, 1281
catecholamine deficiency and, 1257
diabetes mellitus and, 1258–1277
  dependent, 1262
  nondependent, 1262–1263, *1263*
  therapeutic regimens for, *1264*, 1264–1266, 1265t, *1266*
epinephrine and, 1272, *1272*
excess of, 1278–1281
  diabetes mellitus with, 1263, *1263*, 1277
fed-fasted, 1260–1261
hyperkalemia and, 542
hypoglycemia induced by, 1271–1272, *1272*
hypokalemia induced by, 540
infusion pump for, 1266
ketoacidosis and, alcoholic, 548, *548*
  diabetic, 1269–1270
leprechaunism due to, 145, 145t
liver and, 753, 1260–1261, *1261*
metabolic effects of, 1260–1261
preparations of, 1264–1265, 1265t

Insulin (*Continued*)
receptor for, *1177*
  defect of, 1263
  mutation in, 145t
resistance to, 1259–1263, *1263*, 1277
  inherited, 145, 145t
  obesity causing, 1164
  type I, 145, 145t, 1259–1260
  type II, 145, 145t, 1262–1263
secretion of, 1260, *1263*
shock and, 484
surreptitious administration of, 1280–1281, 1281t
syndrome X and, *1277*
transport defect related to, 144t, 145, 145t
tumor secretion of, 1280
Insulin tolerance test, ACTH in, 1208t
growth hormone in, 1208t
Insulin-like growth factor, 1206t, 1210
hypoglycemia due to, 1026
tumor-associated, 1026
Insulinoma, 1280
clinical presentation and, 1280
diagnosis of, 1280
differential diagnosis of, 1281t
Integrin, connective tissue, 1446, *1446*, 1446t
inflammation role of, 1453
leukocyte adhesiveness and, 898, *899*
Intercalated cells, renal tubular, 524, *524*
Intercalated disc, myocardial, *175*, 231
Interferons, cancer therapy using, 1048, 1048t, 1049t
common cold treated with, 1745–1746
condylomata acuminata treated with, 1745–1746
fever production role of, 1533–1534, *1534*, 1535t
hairy cell leukemia treated with, 931
hematopoiesis role of, *917*
hepatitis treated with, 1745
immune response role of, 1395
Kaposi's sarcoma therapy with, 1873, 1873t
macrophage-lymphocyte interaction and, *901*
malaria therapy with, 1894
multiple sclerosis therapy using, 2111
myelogenous leukemia treated with, 928
papillomatosis treated with, 1745–1746
therapeutic, 1745–1746
viral infection treated with, 1745–1746, 1746t
virus-induced, 1740
Interleukins, acute phase response of, 1535–1537, 1536t
allergic rhinitis role of, *1414*, 1414–1415, *1415*
angioedema caused by, 1412
antigen presentation role of, 901, *901*
B cell activation by, 1395, 1395t
cancer therapy using, 1048, 1048t, 1049t
fever production role of, 1533–1534, *1534*, 1535t
hematopoiesis role of, 819–821, 820t, *821*, 898, *917*
immunodeficiency disorders and, *1403*
macrophage-lymphocyte interaction and, 901, *901*
osteoporosis role of, 1380
rheumatoid synovitis role of, *1460*, 1460–1461
sarcoidosis role of, 431, *431*
T cell source of, 1395, 1395t
International Sensitivity Index, 999
Interphalangeal joints, 1518
Intertrigo, 1828
Intervertebral disc, **2144–2145**
anatomy of, 2141, *2141*
back pain related to, 2037–2038, 2141, 2144–2145
herniation of, 2141, *2141*, 2144–2145
imaging of, 1968, *1968*, 2038
physiology of, 2141, *2141*
spondylosis affecting, 2145–2146
Intestine, **627–751**
absorption in, 695–697, 696t, *697*, *698*. See also *Absorption*; *Malabsorption.*
  bile, 696, 696t, 806, 806–807, *807*
  fluids, 689–690
  solutes, *689*, 689–690, 690t
amebiasis of, 1913t, 1913–1914, *1914*
bacterial overgrowth of, 700t, 701t, 703, 704t
  breath tests for, 700, 700t
  conditions associated with, 703–704, 704t
  treatment of, 703
  vitamin B$_{12}$ test and, 699, 701t
cancer of, *724*, 724–729, 725t, *726*, 727t
cestodes of, 1922–1926, 1923t, 1924t
drugs affecting, 681t, 688t
flora of, 1638–1641, *1639*, 1639t, 1659–1660
fluid loss from, 528, 528t. See also *Diarrhea*; *Vomiting.*

Intestine (Continued)
  flukes affecting, 1932t, 1933
  giardiasis of, 694, 1642t, 1658t
  inflammation of, 707–715, 748–751. See also Colitis;
    Crohn's disease; Enteritis.
    cancer and, 709–710, 710t
    diagnostic approach to, 712, 712t
  irrigation of, poisoning treated with, 505–506, 506t
  irritable bowel syndrome of, 685–687
  ischemia of, 715–720
    algorithm for, 716
    colonic, 718–719, 719
    focal segmental, 718
    management of, 716
    mesenteric, 717–718, 718, 719–720
  large. See Cecum; Colon; Rectum.
  lymphoma of, malabsorption due to, 706
  motility disorders of, 684t, 684–686, 688t
  myopathy of, 684t, 684–685, 685
  nematodes of, 1934–1939, 1935t
  neoplasms of, 721–729
  obstruction of, sounds of, 682
    vomiting with, 682
  polyarteritis nodosa of, 1493
  polyps of, 722–723, 723, 724
  potassium loss in, 540
  progressive systemic sclerosis of, 685
  radiation of, 61, 61t, 62t, 750
  renal failure and, 547t, 559
  small. See also Duodenum; Ileum; Jejunum.
    AIDS/HIV effects in, 1866–1867, 1867t
    biopsy of, 700t, 701, 702, 702t
    cancer of, 728–729
      incidence of, 1013t
    culture of, 700t, 701
    ischemia of, focal segmental, 718
    migrating motor complex of, 682–685
    motility of, 682, 682, 683
      clinical assessment of, 682–683
      decreased, 684t, 684–685, 685
      drugs affecting, 681t, 688t
      increased, 684t, 685–686
    pain from, 628
    polyps of, 724
    tumors of, 728–729
    ulceration of, 750–751
  trichinosis affecting, 1937–1938
  vascular disorders of, 715–721
Intima, aortic aneurysm tear in, 343
  atherosclerotic lesion in, 292, 292–295, 295
  fatty streak in, 292, 295
  fibrous plaque in, 292, 292, 295
  hypertension effect on, 258, 259
  polyarteritis nodosa affecting, 1493
Intoxication. See also Poisoning; Toxin.
  alcohol-related, 47–48, 48t
  cardiomyopathy due to, 329t, 330–331
  digitalis, 228, 504t, 508
  lithium, 509
  metal, 67–73
  theophylline, 510
Intra-aortic balloon counterpulsation, 495
Intracardiac recording, 235–236, 236, 236t
Intracranial hemorrhage. See Cerebrovascular disease,
  hemorrhagic.
Intracranial pressure, 2132–2135
  brain tumor and, 2126, 2128
  empty sella caused by, 2133
  head pain due to, 2034, 2133, 2135
  hydrocephalus and, 2134t, 2134–2135
  hypertensive, 2132–2134
    benign, 2133–2134
    disorders associated with, 2134t
    pathophysiology of, 2133t, 2133–2134
    symptoms and signs of, 2133t, 2134
    tentorial herniation and, 1970–1972, 2133
    traumatic, 2138, 2138t
    treatment of, 2133t, 2134
  hypotensive, 2135, 2135t
  normal range of, 2132, 2135
  papilledema due to, 2016t, 2016–2017, 2177, 2177t
  reduction therapy for, 2128–2129
Intrahepatic duct, 637
Intraocular pressure, 2175–2177, 2176. See also Glaucoma.
  drug reduction of, 2176
Intrauterine contraceptive device (IUCD), 1674, 1675

Intravenous drug user (IVDU). See also Drugs, abuse of.
  endocarditis in, 1597t, 1598t, 1600, 1608t
  HIV transmission by, 1852
Intravenous therapy. See Fluid therapy.
Intrinsic factor, cobalamin binding by, 697, 698
  vitamin B_{12} deficiency and, 660, 844, 845–846
Introns, gene transcription and, 135
  vasopressin, 1222
Intubation, 469, 1168
  endotracheal, 469
    complications of, 469
    respiratory failure treatment and, 469, 469t
    weaning from, 469, 471
  enteral feeding with, 1168–1171, 1170t
  nasogastric, 1168–1171, 1170t
Iodide. See Potassium iodide.
Iodine, 1149t
  assessment of, 1149t
  deficiency of, 1149t
  goiter and, 1241
  jodbasedow effect of, 1235, 1236
  physiology of, 1149t
  RDA for, 1140t
  thyroid gland and, 1227, 1236t, 1241
  thyrotoxicosis due to, 1235
  toxicity of, 1149t
Iodoquinol, balantidiasis therapy with, 1916t
  Blastocystis therapy with, 1916t
  dientamoebiasis treated with, 1916t
Ion channels, 244–245, 689–690
  antiarrhythmic agents affecting, 244–245, 245, 245t
  cardiac, 244–245, 245, 245t
  intestinal, 689, 689–690, 690t
Ion exchange resins, 543
  colitis therapy with, 1634
Ipecac, 505
Iridocyclitis, 2178, 2178t
Iridovirus, 1739
Iris, bombé, 2176
  glaucoma effect on, 2176, 2176–2177
  inflammation of, 2178t, 2178–2179
Iris lesions of skin, 2191, 2191
Iron, absorption of, 696t, 697, 700t, 704t, 839–840
  antidote for, 504t, 508–509
  deficiency of, 839–841, 1149t. See also Anemia, iron deficiency.
  dietary, 839–840, 1134t, 1140t, 1149t
  erythropoiesis role of, 839–840, 868–869
    siderocytes and, 834, 842–843
  heme synthesis and, 839–840, 868–869, 872, 1125
  hepatic levels of, 1134, 1134t
    normal, 1134
  laboratory testing for, 1133–1134, 1149t
    factors affecting, 1134t
  metabolism of, 839–840, 1133, 1149t
  poisoning due to, 71, 504t, 508–509
  RDA for, 1140t
  serum levels of, anemia diagnosis and, 827, 828t
    binding capacity and, 827, 828t, 840, 1133–1134, 1134t, 1149t
    normal, 700t
    phlebotomy effect on, 1134–1135, 1135
  splenic reutilization of, 971
  storage disorder of. See Hemochromatosis.
  transport of, 840
Irritable bowel syndrome, 686–687
  diarrhea of, 691–692
  increased colon motility in, 686–687
  increased small intestine motility in, 685–686
  inflammatory disease vs., 711–712
Isaacs' syndrome, 2170
Ischemia, 296, 296
  bone affected by, 1387, 1387t
  cerebral. See Cerebrovascular disease, ischemic.
  extremities affected by, 346–356
  forearm exercise test with, 1503t
  head injury and, 2136
  intestinal, 715–720
  kidney affected by, 606–607
  neurologic effects of, 1972t, 1972–1974
  optic neuropathy due to, 2177–2178
  renal failure and, acute, 552t, 553–554, 554t
  silent, 296, 316
  transient attacks of, 2063–2064
    amnesia of, 1990
    aspirin prophylaxis for, 1192, 2070, 2072
    crescendo, 2071, 2072
    lacunar, 2069

Ischemia (Continued)
    management of, 2071t, 2071–2072, 2072t
    new-onset, 2071, 2072
    seizures vs., 2066
    sickle syndrome with, 888, 2068
    stroke vs., 2063–2064, 2066, 2071
    vasospasm in, 2069, 2075
    vertebrobasilar, 2064t, 2065
Ischemic heart disease. See also Angina pectoris; Coronary artery(ies); Myocardial infarction.
  bypass surgery in, 316t, 316–319, 318
  diagnostic evaluation and, 168t, 168–170
  exercise prevention of, 31–32, 33t
  mortality rate and, 27, 27t, 30t, 170–173, 171t, 171–173
    by country, 172
  prophylaxis for, 117t, 117–118
  risk factors for, 30t, 171–173
  thrombolytic agents in, 116t, 116–117
Islet cells, 1282
  transplantation of, 1269
  tumor of, 1280, 1283–1284. See also Gastrinoma.
Islets of Langerhans, 1282
Isodesmosine, 1444
Isoniazid, 1562t
  enzyme metabolization of, 97t
  hepatotoxicity of, 773, 773t, 775
  mycobacterial (nontuberculous) disease and, 1691
  tuberculosis treated with, 1686–1688, 1687t, 1689
Isoprostanes, 1191
Isoproterenol, 492t, 493
Isosorbide dinitrate, 299t
  angina pectoris treated with, 298, 299t
  dosage for, 229t, 298, 299t
  vasodilatation using, 229t, 229–230
Isosorbide mononitrate, 299t
  angina pectoris treated with, 298, 299t
  dosage for, 298, 299t
Isosporiasis, 1916t
Isotopes. See Radioactive agent(s); Radionuclide studies.
Isotretinoin, side effects of, 2197
  skin disorder treated with, 2197
Isovaleric acidemia, 1112
  diagnosis of, 1112
  treatment of, 1112
Isradipine, 265t
Israelipine, 265t
Itraconazole, blastomycosis therapy with, 1822
  histoplasmosis therapy with, 1818
  paracoccidioidomycosis therapy with, 1823
  side effects of, 2196t
  skin disorder treated with, 2196t, 2196–2197
  sporotrichosis therapy with, 1827
IUCD (intrauterine contraceptive device), 1674, 1675
IVDU (intravenous drug user). See also Drugs, abuse of.
  endocarditis in, 1597t, 1598t, 1600, 1608t
  HIV transmission by, 1852
Ivermectin, 1943
Izumi fever, 1661

J

J curve hypothesis, 261
J junction, 190, 191
J wave, 503, 503
Jaccoud's arthritis, 1593
Jacksonian march seizure, 2114
Jamaican vomiting sickness, 754
Jamais vu, seizure causing, 2114
Janeway's spots, 1478
Japanese encephalitis, 1806t, 1810t, 1813–1814
  immunization for, 42t, 46, 1554, 1554t
Jargon aphasia, 1991
Jarisch-Herxheimer reaction, 1713
  Lyme disease therapy causing, 1719
  penicillin causing, 1568t, 1713
  relapsing fever therapy with, 1715
  syphilis therapy with, 1568t, 1713
Jaundice, 756–759
  approach to patient with, 756t, 756–759, 758
  Crigler-Najjar syndrome and, 756, 757, 757t
  differential diagnosis of, 756t, 756–759, 757t, 758t
  Dubin-Johnson syndrome and, 756, 757t
  examination and, 757–758, 758t
  Gilbert's syndrome with, 756–757, 757t
  hepatitis with, 763
  history taking and, 752, 757–758, 758t
  imaging studies related to, 758t, 758–759

Jaundice *(Continued)*
  laboratory studies and, 758, 758t
  leptospirosis with, 1720, 1721
  obstructive (cholestatic), 756t, 757, 758t
  pancreatic cancer and, 736, 737t
  postoperative, 757
  Rotor's syndrome and, 756, 757t
Jaw, examination of, 450–451, *451*
  giant cell arteritis of, 1499
  intermittent claudication affecting, 1499
  mass in, 450–451
  pain from, 450–451
  salivary gland location in, 450, *451*
  swelling of, 450–451, *451*
JC virus, 2097t
  leukoencephalopathy due to, 2101, *2101*
Jejunoileitis, Crohn's disease and, 714
  nongranulomatous, malabsorption due to, 103
Jejunum, bile absorption in, 806, *807*
  fat absorption role of, 697
  giardiasis effect on, 1912–1913
  motility of, *680*, 680–683
  sentinel loop of, 732
Jellyfish venom, 1954t, 1955
Jet lag, 1200
  travel exposure to, 1555–1556
Jews. See also *Racial factors.*
  Gaucher's disease in, 1097
  hereditary disorder frequency in, 136t, 136–140, 138t
  Kaposi's sarcoma in, 1032–1033, 1033t
  Tay-Sachs disease and, 136, 136t, 138t
Job's syndrome, hyperimmunoglobulin E of, 1541
  staphylococcal infection in, 1601
Jodbasedow effect, 1235, 1236
Jogging, exercise level in, 31
Joint(s). See also *Arthritis.*
  AIDS/HIV effects in, 1878t, 1878–1879
  anatomy of, 1440, *1441, 1442*
  approach to disorders of, 1440–1443, 1441t, *1442,*
    1443t
  aspiration of. See also *Synovial fluid.*
    analysis following, 1455t, 1455–1456
    technique for, 1455–1456
  Charcot's, 1518
  Clutton's, 1710
  degenerative disease of, 1517–1521. See also *Os-*
    teoarthritis.
  Ehlers-Danlos syndrome affecting, 1120–1121, 1121t
  hemochromatosis affecting, 1133
  hemophilic hemorrhage into, 992, 1526
  lax, 1120–1121, 1121t
  Lyme disease affecting, 1717, *1718*
  neoplasia of, 1528
  paraneoplastic syndromes affecting, 1018–1120
  syphilis affecting, 1709, 1710
J-receptors, 217
Jugular vein, internal, *2061*
  pulse in, 167, *167*
Juxtaglomerular apparatus, *519*, 520
  anatomy of, *519*, 520
  smooth muscle cells of, 520

K

Kahler's disease. See *Multiple myeloma.*
Kala-azar, 1905
  leishmaniasis and, 972, 1903t, 1905, *1905*
  splenomegaly of, 972, 972t
Kaliuresis, 539, 539t
Kallikreins, 1419
Kallmann's syndrome, 1200, 1337
  anovulation in, 1306
  eunuchoidism in, 1337
Kaposi's sarcoma, 1032–1033, 1872–1873
  African, 1032, 1033t
  AIDS/HIV patient with, 1032, 1033t, 1863, *1864,*
    1872–1873, 1873t
  classic, 1032, 1033t, 1872
  conjunctival, 1870
  CT scan of, *631*
  cutaneous, 2211
  forms of, 1032–1033, 1033t, 1872
  immunodeficiency with, 1032–1033, 1033t,
    1872–1873
  oral lesions of, 647t, 648
  staging of, 1873, 1873t
  treatment of, 1873, 1873t
Kappa chain, 958, *959*
Karelian fever, 1809–1810

Karnofsky scale, 1007, 1008t
Kartagener's syndrome, bronchiectasis with, 416, 416t
  immotile sperm in, 1336
Karyotype, 151, *153, 156, 157*
Kasabach-Merritt syndrome, 2211
Kasai procedure, 812
Kawasaki's syndrome, lymphadenopathy in, 970
  skin eruption due to, 2200–2201
Kayser-Fleischer rings, 785–786, 1131
Kearns-Sayre syndrome, 2051t, 2160t, 2166t, 2167
Keloid, 2189
  formation of, 2189, *2191*
  therapy for, 2195, 2196
Keratan sulfate, 1119t
  connective tissue structure and, 1445t
Keratin, 2184–2185
Keratinocytes, epidermal, 2184–2185
  neoplasias of, 2208–2210, *2209*
  rapid turnover of, 2203
Keratitis, 2179
  AIDS/HIV patient and, 1870
  exposure/drying, 2180
  herpes simplex causing, 1772–1773, 2179
    treatment of, 1746t, 2179
  trachoma role in, 1722–1723
Keratoacanthoma, 2209
Keratoconjunctivitis, adenovirus in, 1757, 1757t
  sicca, 1488, 1489, 2181
Keratoderma blennorrhagicum, 1469, *1470*
Keratohyalin granules, 2184, 2185
Keratomalacia, 1145t
Keratosis. See also *Hyperkeratosis.*
  actinic, 2210
  palmar, 1034t
  paraneoplastic, 1018–1020, 1034, 1034t, 1035
  seborrheic, 2210
    Leser-Trélat, 1020, 1034
Keshan's disease, 72, 1150t
Ketanserin, 268
Ketoacidosis, 548–549
  alcoholic, *548*, 548–549
    diabetes mellitus vs., 1271
  diabetic, 549, 1269–1271
  gastroparesis with, 684
  signs and symptoms of, 1269–1271
  treatment of, 548–549, 1269–1271
Ketoaciduria, 146–147, 1111–1112, 1112t
Ketoconazole, blastomycosis therapy with, 1822
  candidiasis treated with, 1829, 2196t, 2196–2197
  hepatotoxicity of, 773, 2196t
  side effects of, 2196t
  skin disorder treated with, 2196t, 2196–2197
Ketones, urinary, 512t
Kidney, **511–626**
  acidosis and, 545–549, 597–599, 1359t. See also
    Acidosis, renal tubular.
  AIDS/HIV effects in, 579, 1875t, 1875–1876, *1876*
  Alport's syndrome and, 611–612, 612t
  anatomy of, *517–519*, 517–524
  anomalies of, developmental, 621–622, *622*
  antimicrobials affecting, 1568t
  approach to diseases of, 511–517
  artificial, 564–565, *565*. See also *Dialysis.*
  atrial natriuretic hormone and, *1195*, 1195, 1196
  Bartter's syndrome and, 595t, 598
  bicarbonate and, 514, 521t, *522*, 523, *524*, 544
    transport and, 521t, *522*, 523, *524*
  biopsy of, 517, *517t*
  blood flow in, *517, 518*, 519. See also *Renal artery;*
    Renal vein.
    anatomy and, *517, 518*, 519
    liver disease and, 795–796
    occluded vessels affecting, 606–609
    pregnancy and, 609
    radionuclide studies of, 516
  calcium and, 521t, 523, *1353*, 1359t
    reabsorption of, *1352*, 1353
    transport of, 521t, *522*, 523
  candidiasis affecting, 1828
  carcinoma of, incidence of, *1009*, 1013t
    metastases from, 1031t
    renal cell, 623–625, *624*, 624t
    smoking associated with, 35t
    staging of, 623–624, 624t
    transitional cell, 626
  chloride and, *223*, 514, 521t, *522*
    transport and, *223*, 521t, *522*
  clearance by, 514
    creatinine, 514

Kidney *(Continued)*
  dextran, *521*
  drug, 91t, 522t
    measurement of, 514
  cystinosis and, 595t, 597
  cysts of, **617–621**
    acquired, 618t, 621
    autosomal dominant, 618t, 618–620, *619*, 620t
    autosomal recessive, 618t, 620t, 620–621
    clinical features and, 618t–620t, 618–621
    medullary, 618t, *619*, 621
    multiple, *617*, 618t, 618–621, *619*, 619t, 620t
    renal failure and, 556t, 619, 619t
    simple, *617*, 617–618, 618t, 620t
  development of, 517, 621–622, *622*
  drugs affecting, 99t, 224t, 582t, 584t. See also *Di-*
    uretics; Nephrotoxins.
  failure of. See *Kidney failure.*
  Fanconi's syndrome and, 595t, 597–598, 1359t
  filtration by, 514, 519–520
  granuloma of, 574t, 577, 577t, 1496, 1496t
  heart failure effects in, 217, 220
  horseshoe, 622, *622*
  imaging of, 515, 515t, 515–516
  inflammation of. See *Glomerulonephritis; Nephritis;*
    Pyelonephritis.
  inflammatory bowel disease and, 710t, 711
  interstitial disease of, 554, 580–589
    acute, 581–583, 582t
    causes of, 581–584, 582t, 583t
    chronic, 583t, 583–584
    clinical features in, 580t, 580–581, *581*
    drug-induced, *581*, 581–583, 582t, 584t
  ischemia affecting, 606–607
  lupus erythematosus affecting, 1475t, 1477, 1479,
    1482t
  magnesium and, 557t, 558, 1137t, 1137–1138
    reabsorption of, *1352*, 1353
    transport and, 523
  medullary cystic disease of, 618t, *619*, 621
  nail-patella syndrome and, 812
  paraneoplastic syndromes affecting, 1017t, 1020
  phosphorus and, 557t, 558, 1135, 1136t
    reabsorption of, *1352*, 1353
  polyarteritis nodosa of, 1493
  polycystic disease of, **617–621**
    age and, 617, *617*, 618t
    autosomal dominant, 618t, 618–620, *619*, 620t
    autosomal recessive, 618t, 620t, 620–621
    genetics of, 138t, 618, 620, 620t
  potassium and, 514, *515*, 521t, *522*, 523–524,
    539–541
    transport of, *515*, 521t, *522*, 523–524, *532*
  prostaglandins affecting, 527, 1193
  radionuclide studies of, 516
  reabsorption in, 521t, 521–524, *522*, *524*
  sarcoidosis of, 432, *432*
  scleroderma affecting, 608, 1487
  sickle cell disease and, 608
  sodium and, 514, 514t, 521t, *522*, 522–524
    transport of, 521t, *522*, 522–524, *532*
  sponge, 618t, *619*, 621
  stones of. See *Kidney stones.*
  transplantation of. See *Transplantation, renal.*
  tubules of, 521–524
    acidosis and, 546t, 546–547, 597, 597–599, 598t
    acute renal failure and, 552t, 552–554, *554*, 554t
    AIDS/HIV effects in, 1875–1876, *1876*
    amino acids and, 595t, 596–597
    anatomy of, *223*, *518*, 521–524
    azotemia and, 552–553
    bicarbonate and, 521t, *522*, 523, *532*, 544, 597,
      597, 598t
    calcium reabsorption in, 1353
    chloride and, *223*, 514, 521t, *522*
    collecting, *518*, 522, 523–524, *524*
    connecting, *518*, 523
    distal, *223*, *518*, *522*, 523, 598–599
    diuretic site of action in, *223*, 224t, *532*
    Fanconi's syndrome and, 595t, 597–598, 1359t
    glucose and, 594–596, *596*
    hereditary metabolic defect of, 144t, 1359t
    interstitial disease and, 554, 580t, 580–581, *581*
    necrosis of, 552t, 553, *554*, 554t
    obstruction of, 553, *554*
    organic ion secretion by, 521, *522*, *532*
    osteomalacia and rickets and, 1359t, 1362–1364

Kidney *(Continued)*
  potassium and, 514, *515*, 521t, *522*, 523–524, 539–541
  proteinuria and, 513, 513t
  proximal, *223*, *518*, 521, 521t, *522*, 597–598
  sodium and, 514, 514t, 521t, *522*, 522–524
  urea and, 522, *522*, 523
  uric acid (urate) excretion by, 1509t, 1510, 1510t
  tumor of, 623–625
    Wilms', 625
  ultrasonography of, 515, *515*, 515t
  urates and, gout and, 557t, 559, 562
  urea and, 522, *522*, 523, 553
  uric acid (urate) excretion by, 1509t, 1510, 1510t
  vascular disorders of, 605–609
    structure and, *518*, 519, *519*
  vasopressin effect in, 1222–1223, *1223*
  water and, 526–528, *527*
    diuresis and, 528, 530–532, 531t, *532*
    volume regulation and, 526–528, *527*
  Wegener's granulomatosis of, 574t, 577, 577t, 1496, 1496t
Kidney failure, **552–572**
  acidosis and, 546t, 546–547, 557, 1359t
  acute, 552–556
    approach in, 511, 511t, 552t, 552–554
    clinical features of, *554*, 554t, 554–555
    diagnosis of, 553t, *554*, 554t, 554–555
    etiology of, 552t, 552–554, 553t
    pathophysiology of, 552t, 552–554, *554*, 554t
    postrenal, 552t, 553, 554t
    prerenal, 552t, 552–553, 553t, 554t
    prevention of, 556
    recovery from, 556
    treatment of, 555t, 555–556
    urinary findings in, 553t, *554*, 554t
  AIDS/HIV patient with, 1875t, 1875–1876
  anemia with, 558, 562, 827
  antimicrobials in, dose adjustment for, 1561–1563, 1562t
    toxicity of, 1568t
  ascites with, 743t, 745t, 749, 795–796
  chronic, 556–563, 1359t
    acidosis of, 557
    aggravating factors for, 560, 560t
    approach to patient with, 511, 511t, 559–560
    calcium in, 557t, 557–558
    clinical spectrum of, *556*, 556–559, 557t, 561–562
    complications with, 561–562
    dialysis for. See *Dialysis.*
    diet and, 562–563
    drug dosage adjustment for, 560, 560t
    etiology of, 556, *556*
    gastrointestinal complications with, 558t, 559
    glomerulus in, *556*, 556–559
    hypertension with, *556*, 558, 561, 562
    infection with, 558–559, 561t, 562
    magnesium in, 557t, 558
    pathophysiology of, *556*, 556–559, 557t
    phosphate in, 557t, 558
    potassium and, 556–557, 557t, 561
    prevalence of, 556, *556*
    sodium and, 557, 557t, 561
    treatment of, 560t, 560–561, 561t. See also *Dialysis; Transplantation, renal.*
    vitamin D and, 563
  coagulation affected by, 1000–1001
  definition of, 511
  diabetes mellitus with, *556*, 599–602, *600*, *601*
  drug dose adjustment for, 94t, 94–95
    antimicrobial, 1561–1563, 1562t
  drug-induced, 552t, *581*, 581–583, 582t, 584t, 584–589, 1568t
  electrical injury causing, 66
  ethylene glycol causing, 504t, 509, 509t
  glycogen storage disease with, 1082
  hemorrhage due to, 985
  hepatorenal syndrome in, 795–796
  leptospirosis with, 1720
  liver disease and, 795–796
  malaria causing, 1894
  mortality rate role of, 27t
  myeloma causing, 962t, 963
  obstruction and, 589–593, 591t
  occupational hazard causing, 59t
  osteodystrophy and, 557t, 559, 562, 1359t, **1375–1379**, 1376t
  osteomalacia and, 1362, 1376t, 1376–1379

Kidney failure *(Continued)*
  parathyroid hormone in, *1376*, 1376t, 1376–1379, 1378t
  pericarditis with, 337, 337t
  platelets affected by, 985
  prerenal, 511, 511t, 514, 514t
  shock with, 487
  toxic agents causing, *581*, 581–583, 582t, 584t, 584–589
  tubulointerstitial, 554, 580t, 580–581, *581*
Kidney stones, 613–617
  approach to patient with, *613*, 613–614
  calcium, 614–617, *615*, 615t, *616*, 616t
  composition of, 614, 616t
  cystine, 595t, 596, 616t, 617
  diet and, 616t, 616–617
  dihydroxyadenine causing, 1118
  epidemiology of, 613
  gout with, 1510–1511
  inflammatory bowel disease with, 710t, 711
  oxalate, 614–617, *615*, 616t
  pathogenesis of, 614t, 614–616, *615*, 615t, *616*
  prevention of recurrence of, 613–614
  renal cystic disease with, 618, 618t, 619t
  struvite, *615*, 616t, 617
  treatment of, 616t, 616–617
  uric acid, *615*, 616t, 617, 1510–1511
Killer cells, 1393–1394
  deficiency of, 1402t, 1402–1403, *1403*
  HIV affecting, 1839, 1840
Kimmelstiel-Wilson syndrome, 569
  diabetes mellitus with, 578, 600
  hypertension with, 257
  renal transplantation and, 569
  retinopathy due to, 257
Kinase(s), A, 1178
  C, *1179*
  G, 1178
  hormone action role of, *1177*, 1178–1180, *1179*, *1180*
  protein, *1177*, 1178–1180, *1179*, *1180*
  raf, 1180, *1180*
Kininogen, coagulation role of, 987–988, 995
  deficiency of, 995
  high molecular weight, 987–988, 1419
Kinins, asthma role of, 376
  sepsis role of, 498
  shock and, 481, 498
Kissing bug (reduviid), 1946
Klatskin tumor, *637*, 810
Klebsiella infections, 1579–1581
  clinical manifestations of, 1579–1580
  complications of, 1581
  diagnosis of, 1579–1580
  pneumonia due to, 1579–1581, 1580t
Kleine-Levin syndrome, 2013
  hyperphagia of, 1160, 2013
  somnolence in, 1160, 2013
Klinefelter's syndrome, 1333–1334
  chromosome abnormality in, 154, 1286, 1333–1334
  clinical manifestations of, 1334, *1335*
  testes in, 1333–1334, *1335*
  treatment of, 1334
Klippel-Feil syndrome, 2149
Klippel-Trenaunay-Weber syndrome, 721
Klüver-Bucy syndrome, 1160, 1986
  bulimia and, 1160
Knee, osteoarthritis of, 1519, 1519t
  rheumatoid disease affecting, 1462, *1463*
Knockout drops, 1975t
Knott's method, 1939
Koch-Weeks bacillus, 1624
Koebner phenomenon, 2192, 2203
  lichen planus due to, 2204
  psoriasis due to, 2192, 2203
KOH (potassium hydroxide), fungus in, 2192
Koilonychia, 1149t, 1153t, 2216t
Koplik's spots, 646, 1759
  measles with, 1759, 2200
  Rocky Mountain spotted fever with, 1731
Korsakoff's syndrome, 2039
  amnesia in, 1990, 1990t, 2039
Krabbe's disease, 2112–2113
Krebs cycle, 754
Kupffer cells, *789*
  hemochromatosis affecting, 1133
  immune complexes removed by, 1423, *1423*
  phagocytosis by, 900, 900t
Kuru, 2097, 2097t, **2102**
Kussmaul respiration, 1270
Kveim-Siltzbach reaction, 431, 435, 435t

Kwashiorkor, 1156
Kyasanur Forest hemorrhagic fever, 1798t, 1801–1802, 1806t
Kyphoscoliosis, 443, 443t
  respiration and, 443
Kyphosis, dowager's hump, 1381, *1381*
  osteoporosis role in, 1381, *1381*

L

LAAM (levo-alpha-acetylmethadol), 51, 56
  drug withdrawal treated with, 53, 56
Labels, food, 1143, 1143t
Labetolol, 265t, 270t
Laboratory values, 2224t–2233t. See also specific substances.
Labyrinthitis, 2026
  acute, 2026
  viral, 2026
Lacrimal glands, mucormycosis affecting, 1833
  Sjögren's syndrome affecting, 1488t, 1488–1490
LaCrosse encephalitis, 1806t
β-Lactam agents. See also *Cephalosporins; Penicillin(s).*
  allergy to, 1434, 1434t, 1435t, 1568t
  desensitization to, 1434, 1435t
  endocarditis therapy with, 1602t–1604t, 1602–1603
  mechanism of action of, 1558, 1558t
  meningitis therapy with, 1615–1617, 1616t
  minimal inhibitory concentration for, 1570, 1570t
  resistance to, 1558–1560, 1559t, 1589
    bacterial, 1558–1560, 1559t
    streptococcal, 1589
  skin testing of, 1434, 1434t
  staphylococcal infection treated with, 1609t, 1609–1610
β-Lactamase, 1558–1560, 1559t
  gonococcal, 1703
  streptococcal, 1589
Lactase deficiency, adult, 136t
  genetics of, 136t
  malabsorption due to, 704
Lactate, *1082*, 1082–1083
Lactation, at birth, 1317
  calcium efflux due to, 1353
  dietary requirements and, 1140t
  pregnancy and, 1317
  prolactin stimulus for, 1212–1213
Lactic acidosis, 547–548, 549
Lactic dehydrogenase, erythrocytic, *856*
  glycogen storage disease and, 1083
  liver function not reflected by, 760
  lymphoma evaluation using, 1024
  myopathy role of, 2165
  Pneumocystis pneumonia and, 1919
Lactiferous ducts, 1317
Lactobacillus, live culture of, 1634
Lactose, breath test for, 700, 700t
  intolerance to, 704
  malabsorption of, 700, 700t
Lactotrope cells, 1209t, 1213–1214
Lactulose, breath test for, 700, 700t, 701t
  malabsorption of, 700, 700t, 701t
Laddergrams, 235, *235*
  atrial premature complex in, 235, *235*, *238*
Laënnec's cirrhosis, 789
Lambda chain, 958
Lambert-Eaton syndrome. See *Eaton-Lambert syndrome.*
Laminin, 1445
Lamivudine, 1885t
Lamotrigine, epilepsy therapy with, 2122t
  pharmacokinetics of, 2122t
Lancefield classification, 1585, 1589t
Langat encephalitis, 1806t
Langerhans' cells, *2185*, 2185–2186
  aging effect on, 2190
  cutaneous, 2184–2186, *2185*
  granulomatosis and, 955–956
    bone affected by, 955
    endocrine effects of, 955
    pathophysiology of, 955
    treatment of, 955–956
Language. See also *Speech.*
  disorders of, **1990–1992**. See also *Aphasia.*
  dysarthria and, 1989, 1989t
  processes of, 1990
Laparoscopy, endoscopic, 641
  ulcer treatment using, 669t, 669–671
Laparotomy, Hodgkin's disease staging in, 951
  peritonitis treatment and, 746

Laplace relation, 176, 215–216, *216*
  heart failure effect on, 215–216, *216*
Larva, fly, 1949–1950
  hookworm, 1937
  migrans, 1935t, 1937
  tongue worm, 1950
Laryngitis, influenza virus in, 1749–1751, 1750t, 1751t
  viral, 1749–1751, 1750t, 1751t
Larynx, anaphylaxis effect on, 1418, *1418*
  cancer of, incidence of, 1013t
    smoking associated with, 35t
  diphtheria affecting, 1629–1630
  hoarseness affecting, 451
  polychondritis affecting, 1517
Lassa fever, 1798t, 1802–1803
  fatality rate for, 1738t
Lateral sclerosis, 2053–2054
  amyotrophic, 2053–2054
  primary, 2054
Lateral sinus, *2061*
  thrombosis in, 2083
Latex agglutination test, *C. difficile* in, 1634t
Lathyrus sativus, food poisoning due to, 740
Latitude, vitamin D synthesis and, 1357
Laughter, seizure-associated, 2116
Lavage, gastric, 643, 645
Laxatives, abuse of, 688, 691t
  bulimia with, 1160
  phenolphthalein test for, 693
  surreptitious, 688, 693
LDH. See *Lactic dehydrogenase.*
Lead, **68–69**
  environment containing, 56, 58t, 68
  occupational exposure to, 56, 58t, 68
  poisoning due to, 56, 58t, 68–69, 69t, 504t
    clinical manifestations of, 68–69
    diagnosis of, 68–69, 69t
    etiology of, 68
    treatment of, 69, 69t, 504t
  renal function and, 587–588
Lean body mass, 1154
  calculation of, 1162
Leber's disease, 2017, 2167, 2178
Lecithin, bile with, 805, *805*, 806
Lecithin-cholesterol-acyltransferase, *1089*
  deficiency of, 1095
Lectins, 740
Leech, 1950–1951
  aquatic, 1950–1951
  bite of, 1950–1951
  land, 1951
  nasal infestation with, 1950–1951
  removal of, 1951
Leg, skin disorders affecting, *2191*, 2216t
Legionella infections, 1583–1585
  bacteriology of, 1583
  clinical presentation of, 1584
  culture in, 1583, 1584t
  definition of, 1583
  diagnosis of, 1584t, 1584–1585
  drug therapy for, 1585, 1585t
  epidemiology of, 1583
  extrapulmonary, 1584t
  history of, 1583
  laboratory tests for, 1584t, 1584–1585
  micdadei, 1583
  pathogenesis of, 1583
  pathology findings in, 1584
  pneumonia due to, 412t, 1583–1585
  radiography in, 1584
Legumes, dietary aspects of, 29–30, 30t, *1142*, 1143
  hemagglutinin in, 740
  lectins in, 740
  pea, 740
  poisoning related to, 740
  red kidney bean, 740
Leigh's syndrome, 2166
Leiomyoma, gastric, 679
Leiomyosarcoma, gastric, 679
Leishmaniasis, 783t, 1903–1907
  clinical manifestations of, *1905*, 1905–1906, *1906*
  cutaneous, 1905t, *1906*, 1906–1907
  diagnosis of, 1905–1907
  epidemiology of, 1903t, 1905, 1906
  etiologic organism in, 1903t, 1903–1904, *1904*
  fatality rate for, 1738t
  hepatic effects of, 783t, 1905, *1905*
  treatment and prophylaxis of, 1907
  visceral, 1905, *1905*, 1907
Lennox-Gastaut syndrome, 2117

Lens, *2176*
  cataract affecting, 2175
  Marfan syndrome effect on, 1120
  nontraumatic dislocation of, 1113, 1113t
  subluxation of, 1120
Lenticulostriate arteries, 2058, *2060*
Lentigines, 2212
Lentivirus, *1845*
LEOPARD syndrome, 2212
Lepore hemoglobin, 890
Leprechaunism, 145, 145t, 1263
Lepromin skin test, 1692t, 1692–1693
Leprosy, **1691–1696**
  borderline, 1691–1693, 1692t
  definition of, 1691
  diagnosis of, 1693
  epidemiology of, 1692
  etiologic agent in, 1692
  hepatic granuloma with, 784t
  immune response defect in, 1692t, 1692–1693
  laboratory tests in, 1692t, 1692–1693
  lepromatous, 1691–1694, 1692t, *1694*, *1695*, 2157
  neuropathy of, 2157
  pathogenesis of, 1692, 1695
  prevention of, 1696
  prognosis in, 1696
  reactional states of, 1693–1696, *1894*, *1895*
  serology for, 1692t, 1693
  skin lesions of, 1691, 1693–1694, *1694*, *1695*
  skin test for, 1692t, 1692–1693
  susceptibility factors for, 1692
  transmission of, 1691–1692
  treatment of, 1695–1696
  tuberculoid, 1691–1693, 1692t, *1694*, 2157
Leptospirosis, **1720–1721**
  antibodies in, 1721
  clinical features of, 1720, 1737t, 1738t
  diagnosis of, 1721, 1737t, 1738t
  epidemiology of, 1720, 1737t, 1738t
  etiologic agent in, 1720, 1737t, 1738t
  jaundice in, 1720, 1721
  laboratory findings in, 1720–1721, 1737t
  pathogenesis of, 1720, 1737t, 1738t
  pathology findings in, 1720
  prevention of, 1721
  prognosis in, 1721
  therapy of, 1721
Leriche's syndrome, 350–351
  impotence with, 1330
Lesch-Nyhan syndrome, **1115–1116**
  clinical manifestations of, 1116
  diagnosis of, 1116
  enzyme defect in, 146t, 1115–1116
  etiology and pathogenesis of, 1116
  genetics of, 146t, 1115–1116
  treatment of, 1116
Leser-Trélat syndrome, 1020, 1034
Lethargy. See also *Arousal level.*
  alcohol-related, 47–48, 48t
Letterer-Siwe disease, 955
  lymphadenopathy due to, 970
Leucine, urinary, 1101t, 1103t
Leucine aminopeptidase, 760
Leukemia, **925–940**
  acute, 936–940
    classification of, 936, 937t
    lymphocytic, 936–940, 937t
    myelogenous, 936–940, 937t
  B cell, 931–932, 933t, 937, 1781t
  benzene exposure causing, 56, 58t
  bone marrow transplantation for, 928–929, 939, 940, 976, *976*
  chronic, 925–935
    lymphocytic, 931–935, 932t, *933*, 935t, *960*, 961t
    myelogenous, 925–929, 926t, *927*, *929*, 929t
  drugs causing, 1016t
  erythroid, 937t
  gammopathy with, 961, 961t, 964
  genetics of, 926, 937–938
  hairy cell, 929–931, *930*, 933t, 973, 1781t
  incidence of, *1005*, *1009*, 1013t, *1015*
  leukemoid reaction vs., 918, 919t
  lymphocytic, 931–935, 936–940
    acute, 936–940, 937t
    chronic, 931–935, 932t, *933*, 935t, 1781t
    diagnosis of, 932–934, 933t, 938
    incidence of, *960*, 961t
    remission criteria for, 935t
    staging of, 932t, 933
    survival rate in, *933*, 935, 939

Leukemia (Continued)
  lymphoma and, 943, 944, 1781t, 1781–1782
  mast cell, 1435, 1435t
  megakaryocytic, 937t
  monoclonal proteins with, *960*, 961
  monocytic, 937t
  myelogenous, 925–929, 936–940
    acute, 936–940, 937t
    chronic, 925–929, 926t, *927*, *929*, 929t
    diagnosis of, 926–927, 933
    subtypes of, 926, 926t, 937t
    survival rate in, 926t, 929, *929*, 929t, 940
  myelomonocytic, 928, 937t
  oncogenes in, 926t, 926–927, 936, 938
  plasma cell, 964
  pregnancy and, 1061t, 1064
  prolymphocytic, 933t
  promyelocytic, 937t, 940
  skin affected by, 1032, 1033–1034
  smoking associated with, 35t
  T cell, 931–932, 933t, 936, 937, 1781–1782
  viruses and, 1781t, 1781–1782, *1782*
Leukemoid reaction, 915
  paraneoplastic, 1021
  vs. leukemia, 918, 919t
Leukocytes, **817–821**. See also *Basophils*; *Eosinophils*; *Lymphocytes*; *Monocytes*; *Neutrophils.*
  adhesion of, 897–898, *899*
    disorders of, 902–904, *903*, 904t, 905t, 906t, 1408
    immunodeficiency related to, 1408, 1540–1541
    rheumatic disease and, 1448–1450, *1449*, *1450*
    vasculitis role of, *1449*, 1449–1450, *1450*
  alveolar exudate of, 393, *394*
  ascites with, 744t
  autoantibodies to, 1476t, 1477
  chemotaxis by, 899, *899*
  compromised host and, 1537–1541, 1538t, 1539t
  count of, 908
    decreased, 908, 911
    increased, 496t, 915, 918, 919
    leukemia and, 927, 932, 935t, 938
    normal, 908
    sepsis and, 496t
  fever production role of, 1533–1534, 1535t
  glucocorticoid effect on, 108–109, 109t
  immunomodulation by, 901, *901*
  lazy, 1541
  lung sequestration of, 373
  production of, 817–819, *818–821*, 897, 898, *917*
    decreased, 908–915, *909*
    increased, 915–920, *916*, *917*
  superoxide production by, 900, *900*
  synovial fluid with, 1455t, 1455–1456
  urinary, 512t
Leukocytosis, 915–920
  cell count in, 496t, 915, 918, 919
  colitis with, pseudomembranous, 1633
  gonococcemia with, 1702
  gout and, *1512*, 1516
  lymphocytic, 919t, 919–920, 932, 938
  lymphocytic leukemia with, 932, 938
  Mediterranean fever causing, 908
  monocytic, 918–919, 919t
  myelogenous leukemia with, 927, 938
  neutrophilic, 915–920, 916t, *916–918*, 927, 938
  pancreatitis with, 732, 732t
  pneumonia with, 1572
  polyarteritis nodosa with, 1493
  polycythemia vera with, 921, 921t, 922t
  sepsis with, 496t, 499, 500t
  toxic syndrome of, 1588t, 1588–1589
Leukodystrophy, 1251, **2112–2113**
  adrenal gland and, 1251, 2112
  demyelination in, 2112–2113
  globoid cell, 2112–2113
  metachromatic, 2112
  sudanophilic, 1251, 2112
Leukoencephalopathy, AIDS/HIV with, 1856t, 1857, 1857t
  progressive multifocal, 2097t, 2101, *2101*
Leukoerythroblastosis, 915, 915t, *918*
  myeloid metaplasia with, 924–925
Leukopenia, 908–915
  anorexia with, 1159
  immunodeficiency with, 1537–1541
    compromised host and, 1537–1541, 1539t
    severe combined, 1406
  lupus erythematosus with, 1475t, 1479

Leukoplakia, candidal, 647
    hairy, 647, 647t
        AIDS/HIV patient with, 1868
    oral, 647, 647t
Leukostasis, paraneoplastic, 1054
Leukotrienes, 113, 1190, 1190–1191
    allergic rhinitis role of, 1414, 1415
    asthma role of, 377
    formation of, 113, 1190, 1190–1191
    mast cell release of, 1416, 1436t
Leuprolide, 1046t, 1047
Levamisole, 1048
Levator ani, 740, 741
Levocabastine, 1416, 1416t
Levo-alpha-acetylmethadol (LAAM), 51, 56
    drug withdrawal treated with, 53, 56
Levodopa, 2044–2046
    Parkinson's disease and, 2044–2046, 2045
Levorphanol, 102, 104t
Levothyroxine, 1239
Lewy bodies, Alzheimer's disease with, 1994
    cortical neuron with, 1994
    dementia related to, 1994
Leydig cells, 1284
    aplasia of, 1291
    ovarian, 1293
    sexual differentiation role of, 1284, 1285, 1286, 1326
    testicular, 1284, 1285, 1286, 1326
LH. See Luteinizing hormone (LH).
Lhermitte's sign, multiple sclerosis with, 2109t
    radiation injury with, 1030
    spinal examination and, 2143
LHON, 2160t, 2166t, 2167
Libido, female, 1308
    male, 1328, 1330
Libman-Sacks endocarditis, emboli from, 2067
    lupus erythematosus with, 1479
Lice. See Louse.
Lichen planopilaris, 2217
Lichen planus, 2191, 2204
    Koebner phenomenon in, 2204
    oral lesions of, 646t, 647, 647t
Lichen sclerosus et atrophicus, 2212
Lichen simplex chronicus, 2199
    incidence of, 2184t
Licorice, chewing tobacco with, 1249
    hyperaldosteronism mimicked by, 539
    hypertension due to, 1249
    hypokalemia caused by, 539
    intoxication due to, 1249, 1249t
    snuff flavored with, 35
Liddle's syndrome, alkalosis in, 550
    hypokalemia in, 539t, 540
Lidocaine, 91t, 94t, 246t
    adverse effects of, 247t
    antiarrhythmic action of, 246, 246t
    dose adjustment for, 94t
    pain management with, 106
    pharmacokinetics of, 91t, 94t, 246, 246t
    renal failure effect on, 94t
Lifespan, 12, 12–15. See also Age; Death and dying;
        Elderly.
    animal species and, 14
    increasing, 12, 12
    life support decisions and, 24–25
    quality-adjusted life expectancy and, 80–81, 82
Lifestyle, 29, 30t, 32
    diabetes mellitus and, 32, 1266t, 1266–1267
    diet and, 29
    esophageal reflux disease and, 653, 654t
    hypertension treatment and, 261–262, 262
    sedentary, diseases associated with, 30t
        exercise vs., 32, 32
Ligaments, enthesopathy affecting, 1441, 1442, 1443t
    fluoride effect on, 1148t
    joint anatomy and, 1441
    spinal, 2141, 2141
Light. See also Photosensitivity; Sun exposure; Ultraviolet light.
    circadian rhythm relation to, 1204–1205
    hormone secretion affected by, 1199–1200
    polarized, amyloid deposit in, 1504, 1506
    polymorphous eruption due to, 2218
    porphyrin activation by, 1124, 1128, 1130
    pupillary response to, 2017, 2017–2018, 2018
    seizure triggered by, 2116
    telangiectasia triggered by, 1036

Light (Continued)
    visible, 63
    vitamin D synthesis due to, 1354, 1355, 1357
Light chains, 958, 959, 960, 960t
    amyloidosis role of, 967t, 1504, 1506
    kappa, 1395–1396, 1396t, 1506
    lambda, 1395–1396, 1396t, 1506
    macroglobulinemia and, 965
    myeloma and, 960t, 962
    nephropathy due to, 579
Light-dark cycle, circadian rhythm relation to,
        1204–1205
    hormone secretion and, 1199–1200
    melatonin secretion role of, 1204–1205
Light-headedness, 2025, 2025t. See also Dizziness.
Limbic system, endorphins in, 1187, 1187t
    temporal lobe damage and, 1986
Lincosamides, 1562t
    dose adjustment for, 1562t
    pharmacology of, 1562t
Lindane, pediculosis treated with, 2195
Linguatuliasis, 1950
Linitis plastica, 677, 677t
Linkage disequilibrium, HLA, 1429–1431, 1430t
Lionfish, 1954t, 1955
Lip, angular cheilosis of, 647, 1828
    cancer of, 35, 35t
    candidiasis affecting, 647, 1828
    herpetic lesion of, 1772, 1772
    snuff affecting, 35, 35t
Lipase, hormone-sensitive, 1087
    lipoprotein, 1086, 1086–1087, 1087
    pancreatitis and, 732, 732t
Lipid bilayer. See also Plasma membrane.
    erythrocytic, 851, 851–852
Lipids. See also Fat.
    aspiration pneumonia due to, 407–408
    atherogenesis role of, 292, 292, 294, 295
    bacterial, 1556
    bile content of, 805–807, 805–807
    crystal deposition of, 1516t
    elevated level of, 292–293
    enzyme deficiencies affecting, 2165–2166, 2166t
    glycogen metabolism and, 1082, 1082–1083
    ketoacidosis and, 548, 548
    Maltese cross inclusions of, 1096, 1516t
    metabolism of, estrogen effect on, 1312
        liver and, 753–754, 761
    myopathy role of, 2165–2166, 2166t
    obesity effect on, 1164
    storage disease and, 1096t, 1097, 1098–1099
    transport of, 1086–1089, 1087, 1088, 1089
Lipoatrophy, 1508
Lipocytes, 1507–1508
    hepatic, 789
    signet ring, 1507
Lipogranuloma, hepatic, 784t
Lipoid cells, ovarian tumor and, 1312t
Lipolysis, ketoacidosis and, 548, 548
Lipoma, 2209
Lipopolysaccharides, bacterial, 1556
Lipoprotein, 1086–1095
    arachidonic acid transport by, 1187
    characteristics of, 1087t
    cholesterol transported by, 172
    coronary heart disease and, 172, 173
    diabetes mellitus and, 1269t
    disorders of, 1089–1095, 1092t
        rare, 1095
    electrophoretic mobility of, 1087t
    elevated levels of. See Hyperlipoproteinemia.
    formation of, 1086–1089
    high-density (HDL), 172, 293, 1087, 1087t, 1089, 1089
        atherosclerosis and, 1092
        characteristics of, 1087t
    intermediate-density (IDL), 1087, 1087t, 1088, 1089
    liver and, 753–754, 761, 1086–1089, 1087
    low-density (LDL), 172, 293, 1087, 1087t, 1088, 1089
        atherosclerosis and, 1092
        characteristics of, 1087t
        familial hypercholesterolemia and, 1089–1090,
            1093–1094
    obesity effect on, 1164
    oxidized low density (oxLDL), 293
    receptors for, 1087, 1088, 1089
    very-low-density (VLDL), 293, 1086–1088, 1087,
        1087t
        atherosclerosis and, 1092
        characteristics of, 1087t

Lipoprotein (Continued)
    hypertriglyceridemia and, 1090
Lipoprotein lipase, 1086–1087, 1087, 1088
    deficiency of, 1090
Lipoxygenase, 1190–1191
    arachidonic acid metabolism by, 1189, 1190,
        1190–1191
    inhibition of, 1192
Lisinopril, dosage for, 229t, 265t, 266t
    vasodilatation using, 229t, 229–230
Listeriosis, 1672–1673
    clinical manifestations of, 1672–1673, 1737t
    diagnosis of, 1673
    epidemiology of, 1672, 1737t
    etiology of, 1672, 1737t
    food poisoning due to, 738, 739t, 1672
    meningitis in, 1610t, 1611, 1616t, 1672–1673
    pathogenesis of, 1672
    prevention of, 1673
    prognosis in, 1673
    treatment of, 1673
Lithiasis, biliary, 812–816, 813. See also Gallstones.
    congenital heart disease causing, 286, 286
    renal. See Kidney stones.
    salivary gland, 648, 648t
Lithium, 91t, 94t
    bipolar disorder treated with, 2003–2004
    dose adjustment for, 94t
    high serum level of, 2003
    intoxication with, 509
    neutropenia treated with, 912
    pharmacokinetics of, 91t, 94t
    renal function and, 94t, 587
    side effects of, 509, 2003
Lithocholic acid, 806, 807
Lithotripsy, 637, 815–816
Littoral cells, 974
Livedo reticularis, 349, 1478
    cold exposure and, 349
    lupus erythematosus with, 1478
    pathophysiology of, 349
Liver, 752–805
    abscess of, 781–783
        amebic, 782–783, 784, 1913–1914
        pyogenic, 781, 781–782
    adenoma of, drug-induced, 773, 773t
    amebiasis of, 782–783, 784, 1913–1915, 1915t
    amino acid metabolism in, 754
    ammonia and, 754, 760
        encephalopathy and, 754
    amyloidosis of, 786
    anemia and, aplastic, 761–762, 764
    angiosarcoma of, 773, 773t
    antitrypsin deficiency and, 767, 785
    approach to disease of, 752–753
    autoantibodies affecting, 767, 778t
    bile production by, 805–807, 807
    bilirubin and, 755, 755–757, 756t, 757t, 760
    biopsy of, 762, 808
    candidiasis affecting, 1828
    carbohydrate metabolism in, 753, 1080–1085, 1082,
        1084
    carcinoma of, 804
        clinical features of, 803t, 804
        drug-induced, 773, 773t
        fibrolamellar, 803t, 804
        imaging studies of, 803t, 804
        incidence of, 1005, 1009, 1013t, 1015
        metastatic, 805
        predisposing factors for, 803t
        transplantation and, 801t
        treatment of, 803t, 804
    cholesterol and, 754, 1098–1099
    cirrhotic. See Cirrhosis.
    coagulation and, 760–761, 800t, 1000
    copper deposition in, 785–786, 791, 1131–1132
    drug clearance by, 90–91, 760
    drug-induced disease of, 99t, 772–775, 773t
    echinococcosis of, 782, 784
    encephalopathy related to, 797–800. See also Encephalopathy, hepatic.
    enzymes of, 759–760
    examination of, 752–753
    failure of. See Liver failure.
    fat absorption role of, 697
    fatty, 754
        alcoholic, 754, 790
        drug-induced, 773, 773t, 799t
        Niemann-Pick disease with, 1096t, 1098–1099

Liver (Continued)
  nonalcoholic, 793
  pregnancy with, 787, 787t
  small droplet, 754
feminization and, 796
fibrosis affecting, 773, 786, 788t, 788–789, 789. See
  also Cirrhosis.
flukes affecting, 782, 783t, 812, 1931–1934, 1932t
fructose and, 1082–1084, 1084
function tests for, 759–762
glucose and, 753, 1082, 1082–1083, 1084
glycogen and, 786, 1082, 1082–1083, 1083t
granuloma of, 783–785, 784t
  drug-induced, 773, 773t
heart failure affecting, 219, 792
hemochromatosis and, 786, 791, 1133–1134
history taking, 752
hydatid cyst of, 782, 784
immune response and, 767
infections of, 781–785
inflammation of. See Hepatitis.
inflammatory bowel disease and, 710t, 711
iron level in, 1134, 1134t
  normal, 1134
laboratory testing and, 759–762
lipid metabolism in, 753–754, 767
macrophages of, 789, 900, 900t
malarial parasite in, 1893
metabolism in, 753–754
  disorders affecting, 142–147, 146t, 1080–1085
metastases to, 804
necrosis of, bridging, 762, 776
  cirrhosis and, 788–789, 789, 793
  drug-induced, 772, 773t, 775, 799t
  massive, 762, 763, 763t, 776
  piecemeal, 762, 776
nodular hyperplasia of, focal, 803, 803t
  regenerative, 804
"nutmeg," 792
palpation of, 753
paraneoplastic syndrome affecting, 1021
parasitic diseases of, 782–783, 783t
peliosis of, 773t, 774
polyarteritis nodosa of, 1494
porphyria and, 786
pregnancy affecting, 787t, 787–788
protein metabolism and, 754, 760–761
schistosomiasis affecting, 782, 783t, 784t, 1929–1931
transplantation of, 800–802, 801t, 802
tumors of, 802–805
  approach to patient with, 803t, 804–805
  benign, 802–804, 803t
  drug-induced, 773, 773t, 803t
  imaging studies of, 803t, 805
  malignant, 803t, 804–805
  predisposing factors for, 803t
  treatment for, 803t, 803–804
vascular disorders affecting, 773t, 773–774
Wegener's granulomatosis affecting, 1495t
Liver failure. See also Cirrhosis; Hepatitis.
anemia with, 827
antimicrobials in, 1561–1563
  dosage adjustment for, 1561–1563, 1562t
  toxicity of, 1568t
causes of, 798, 799t, 800t
complications of, 798–800, 799t, 800t
fulminant, 798–800, 799t, 800t
hemorrhagic disorders with, 981, 985
management of, 798–800, 799t
mortality rate role of, 27t, 30t
paraneoplastic, 1021
risk factors for, 30t
transplantation in, 800–802, 801t
Wilson's disease causing, 1131–1132
Living wills, 465–466. See also Decision making.
advance directive role of, 5
Lizard, tongue worm in, 1950
Locked-in state, 1969t, 2065
definition of, 1969t
Löffler's endocarditis, 333t, 334
Lomefloxacin, 1562t
Lomustine (CCNU), adverse effects of, 1042
chemotherapy using, 1039t, 1042
Long QT syndrome, ablation therapy in, 252t, 253
sudden death due to, 255
Longevity. See Lifespan.
Loop of Henle, 223, 518
anatomy of, 223, 518, 518, 521–523
Bartter's syndrome and, 598

Loop of Henle (Continued)
  concentration and dilution in, 521–523, 522
  diuretic action in, 222–223, 223, 224t, 264t, 531t
Loracarbef, 1562t
Loratadine, 1416, 1416t
Lorazepam, 507, 1998–1999, 1999t
Lotions, topical therapy with, 2194, 2194t, 2195t
Louping ill encephalitis, 1806t, 1814
Louse, 1945–1946
  body, 1945–1946
  control measures for, 1729, 2195
  erysipeloid and, 1673–1674
  head, 1945–1946
  infestation with, 1945–1946
  nits (eggs) of, 1945–1946
  pubic, 1946
  relapsing fever carried by, 1715
  sexual transmission of, 1697t
  typhus transmitted by, 1726, 1727t
  zoonoses associated with, 1727t, 1737t, 1737–1738,
    1738t
Lover's heels, 1702
Low-density lipoprotein. See Lipoprotein, low-density
  (LDL).
Lowe's oculocerebrorenal syndrome, 1105t
LSD (lysergic acid diethylamide), 54, 508, 1975t
Ludwig's angina, pneumococcal, 1571, 1571t
  respiratory obstruction in, 451
Lues. See Syphilis.
Lumbar puncture, 1959, 1960t
  blood patch following, 2135
  brain abscess diagnosis with, 2081, 2081t
  contraindications for, 1959, 1960t
  diagnostic examination using, 1959, 1960t
  headache following, 2034, 2135
  hemorrhage vs., 2075, 2075
  indications for, 1959, 1960t
  seizure evaluation using, 2120
  stroke diagnosis and, 2066
  "traumatic," 2075, 2075, 2135
Lumbosacral strain, 2038
Lung, 368–464
  abscess of, 413–416
    actinomycosis with, 1675, 1675
    aspiration preceding, 414, 415
    clinical features of, 414
    definition of, 413
    differential diagnosis of, 414, 414t, 415
    epidemiology of, 414
    etiology of, 413–414, 414t
    pathogenesis of, 414
    prevalence of, 414
    prevention of, 416
    prognosis in, 415–416
    Pseudomonas causing, 1581
    radiography of, 414, 415
    treatment of, 414–415
  aeration abnormalities of, 389–390
  aging effects on, 374
  AIDS/HIV effects on, 1858–1865, 1859t–1861t,
    1859–1865, 1865t
  altitude-related disorders affecting, 409t, 409–410
  anaerobic flora and, 1639, 1639–1640
  anatomy of, 371–373, 372
  asbestosis of, 56, 58t, 399t, 400–401
  aspiration injury to, 406–407
  barometric pressure affecting, 409t, 409–410, 410t
  berylliosis of, 402t, 402–403
  biopsy of, interstitial disease and, 392
  black, 401, 453t
  burn injury to, 403, 403t
  byssinosis of, 59t
  cancer of, 436–442
    asbestos and, 437, 1016, 1016t
    chemotherapy in, 441
    clinical features of, 438–439
    Cushing's syndrome with, 1024–1025, 1025t
    definition of, 436, 436t
    diagnosis of, 439, 439–440
    diet and, 437
    genetic factors in, 437–438, 438t
    incidence of, 436, 1005, 1009, 1013t, 1015
    metastases from, 1031t
    metastatic origin of, 439
    non–small cell, 436, 436t, 438, 438t, 440t,
      440–441
    occupational exposure causing, 56, 58t, 437, 1014,
      1016t
    Pancoast syndrome with, 439

Lung (Continued)
  paraneoplastic syndromes with, 439, 1010
  pathogenesis of, 437–438, 438t, 1014
  pathology of, 438
  prevention of, 441–442
  prognosis for, 441
  risk factors for, 436–437, 1014
  SIADH with, 1020, 1026
  small cell, 436, 436t, 438, 438t, 440t, 441
  smoking and, 437–438, 1014
  staging of, 440, 440t
  surgical approach in, 440–441
  treatment of, 439, 440–441
chronic obstructive disease of, 381–389, 452–458.
    See also Bronchitis; Emphysema.
  critical care setting and, 473–474
  mortality rate role of, 27t, 30t
  respiratory failure in, 452t, 452–453, 453t,
    457–458, 458t
  risk factors for, 30t
cilia of, 372–373, 399
coal workers', 56, 58t, 399t, 401
collapse of, 389
compliance of, 466
  assessment of, 466–467, 467t
  static, 467
diagnostic procedures in, 373, 373t, 373–374
diffusing capacity of, 374, 374–375
edema of. See Edema, pulmonary.
environmental disease of, 58t, 59t, 399–403
  air pollution in, 56, 58t
  chemicals in, 56, 58t, 59t, 403t, 404
  dusts in, 58t, 59t, 399–403
  smoke inhalation causing, 403, 403t
eosinophilic, 955–956
expiratory volume of. See Expiratory volume.
farmer's, 391, 391t
fibrosis. See Lung, interstitial disease of.
flukes affecting, 1932t, 1933
function testing of. See Pulmonary function tests.
gas exchange in, 371–373, 372, 375, 375t
  partial pressure and, 375, 375t
granuloma of, 1495, 1495t, 1496t
histiocytosis X and, 395
hyperinflation of, 442
hyperlucent, 390
hypertension affecting. See Hypertension, pulmonary.
infection of. See Pneumonia; Respiratory tract, infec-
    tion(s) of; specific causative organisms.
interstitial disease of, 390–398
  alveolar filling and, 391t, 397–398
  asbestos-related, 399t, 400–401
  classification of, 391t
  clinical features of, 391–393
  diagnostic evaluation in, 392t, 392–393
  drug-induced, 396–397, 397t
  eosinophilic, 398
  function tests in, 392
  hereditary, 391t, 398–399
  histiocytic, 395
  idiopathic, 393–395
  immune-mediated, 395t, 395–396
  lymphocytic, 395
  occupational, 399–403
  pathogenesis of, 393, 394
  radiographic features in, 392, 392t
  silicosis in, 399t, 401–402
  therapy in, 393, 393t
  transplantation in, 393, 393t
  vasculitis and, 391t, 398
leukocytes sequestered in, 373
liver disease affecting, 796
lupus erythematosus and, 395t, 396, 1475t, 1478
lymphangioleiomyomatosis of, 395
lymphatics of, 372
mucociliary escalator of, 372–373, 399
mucus cells of, 371, 372
mycobacterial (nontuberculous) disease of, 1690t,
    1690–1691
obstructive disease of, 374t, 374–375. See also Airway
    obstruction; Asthma; Bronchitis; Emphysema.
oxygen toxicity affecting, 404–405, 405
particulate matter clearance from, 372–373, 399
percussion of, 368, 369t, 370
perfusion of, embolism and, 425, 425t, 425–426, 426
  hypoxia and, 452–453
  interpretation of, 425t

Lung (Continued)
polyarteritis nodosa of, 1493
radiation injury affecting, 61, 405–406
residual volume of. See *Residual volume.*
restrictive disease of, 375–376, 376t
rheumatic disorders affecting, 395t, 395–396
sarcoidosis of, *432*, 432–434, *434*
sclerosis affecting, 395t, 396, *1486*, 1486–1487
silicosis of, 399t, 401–402, 402t
smoking effect on, 34, 34t, 35t
sounds of, 368, 369t, 370
surfactant of, 372
transplantation of, 459–462. See *Transplantation, lung.*
tuberculosis effects in, 1684–1685. See also *Tuberculosis.*
vasculature of. See *Pulmonary vasculature.*
ventilation and. See *Ventilation.*
volumes of, *373*, 373t, 373–374
expiratory. See *Expiratory volume.*
obstructive disease and, 373–376, 374t
residual. See *Residual volume.*
restrictive disease and, 375–376, 376t
water. See *Edema, pulmonary.*
Wegener's granulomatosis of, 1495, 1495t, 1496t
Lupus erythematosus, 1475–1482
animal model for, 1448–1454, *1450*
ARA criteria for, 1475, 1475t, 1481
autoantibodies in, 1456–1458, 1457t, 1476t, 1476–1477, 1481t
classification of, 1475, 1475t, 1481
clinical features of, 1475t, 1477t, 1477–1480, 1480t, 1481t
complement role in, 1450, *1450*, 1482
differential diagnosis of, 1477t, 1480–1481, 1481t
discoid, 1475t, 1478, 2211
drug-induced, 98t, 1480, 1480t, 1481t
epidemiology of, 1475–1476
etiology of, *1476*, 1476t, 1476–1477
gastrointestinal effects of, 1479
genetics in, 1476, 1476t
heart disease with, 359, 1478–1479
hematologic disorders in, 1475t, 1479
HLA complex and, 1431, 1431t
immunofluorescence testing in, 2189t
interstitial lung disease with, 395t, 396
musculoskeletal changes in, 1478
neonatal, 1480
nephritis and, 573t, 574t, 577t, 578, 578t
nervous system and, 1475t, 1479–1480, 1480t
neutrophils in, *1450*, 1450–1451, *1451*
oral mucosal ulcers in, 646t, 647–648
panniculitis with, 1508
pathogenesis of, *1476*, 1476t, 1477
pathology in, 1477
pleural effusion in, 445, 445t, 446
pregnancy with, 1480
prognosis in, 1482
pulmonary, 395t, 396, 1475t, 1478
renal involvement in, 1475t, 1477, 1479
serology in, 1479, 1481
skin affected by, 1475t, 1478
syphilis false-positive in, 1475t, 1479
treatment of, 1481–1482, 1482t
Lupus pernio, 432, *432*, 1478
Luteinizing hormone (LH), 1206t, 1218–1220
amenorrhea evaluation with, 1303–1304, *1304*
hypogonadotropic hypogonadism and, 1295t
laboratory tests for, 1208t, 1213t
menstrual cycle and, *1294*, 1297–1299, *1298*
ovulation and, *1294*, 1297–1298, *1298*, *1299*
puberty and, 1294–1295
female, *1294*, 1294–1295
male, 1326
regulation of, 1198, *1198*, 1206t, 1218
secretion of, 1218–1219
sexual differentiation and, *1286*
stimulation test for, 1208t
testicular function regulated by, *1326*, 1326–1328, *1327*
tumor production of, 1209t, 1219–1220
Luteinizing hormone–releasing hormone (LHRH). See *Gonadotropin-releasing hormone (GnRH).*
Lutembacher's syndrome, 281, *284*
17,20-Lyase, 1288t
deficiency of, 1290
Lyme disease, 1715–1720
antibodies in, 1717–1718, *1718*
arthritis of, 1474–1475, 1715, 1717, *1718*

Lyme disease (Continued)
clinical characteristics of, 1716–1717, 1717t, 1738t, 2157
differential diagnosis of, 1718
distribution of, 1716
early, 1716–1717, 1717t, 1719, 1719t
epidemiology of, 1716, 1738t
laboratory testing for, 1717–1718, *1718*
late, 1717, 1719, 1719t
pathogenesis of, 1716
pregnancy with, 1719–1720
rash in, 1715–1717, 1717t, *1718*, 1738t
tick bite in, 1715, 1716, 1720, 1738t
treatment of, 1718–1720, *1719*
Lymph nodes, 968–970
biopsy of, 969
Hodgkin's disease in, 947–948
non-Hodgkin's lymphoma and, 943t, 943–944, 944t
cervical, 948, *949*, 969t
enlargement of. See *Lymphadenopathy.*
face and jaw, *451*
functions of, 968
hilar, 969t
inguinal, 948, *949*, 969t
location of, 969, 969t
mediastinal, 948, *949*, 969t
mesenteric, 969, 969t, 1661
palpation of, 969
structure of, 968
Lymphadenitis. See also *Lymphadenopathy.*
bubonic plague with, 1662
mesenteric, 1661
mycobacterial (nontuberculous), 1690t, 1691
treponemal (nonsyphilitic), 1714
tuberculous, 1685t
yersinial, 1661
Lymphadenopathy, 969t
angioimmunoblastic, 970, 1032
skin affected by, 1032
assessment of, 969–970
breast cancer and, 1322t, 1322–1323, 1324t
cat scratch disease with, 1681, 1681t
causes of, 969t, 970t
diagnostic approach to, 969–970, 970t
location of, 968, 969t
lymphoma and, Hodgkin's, 947–948, *949*, 949t
non-Hodgkin's, 943t, 943–944, 944t
patient evaluation for, 969
physiology of, 968
sarcoidosis with, *433*, 434, *434*
syphilitic, 1706–1707
thoracic, *433*, 434, *434*
toxoplasmal, 1908
tularemia causing, 1662, 1663, 1664
Lymphangiectasia, 706
Lymphangioleiomyomatosis, 395
Lymphangiosarcoma, Stewart-Treves, 1034
Lymphangitis, 356
bacterial, 356
clinical features of, 356
glanders with, 1669
streptococcal, 1588
treatment of, 356
Lymphatic system, 968–970, 969t, 970t
drainage pattern of, 968
edema related to, 357
fat absorption role of, *697*
filiariasis (bancroftian, malayan) of, 1940t, 1940–1941
inflammation affecting, 356–357
obstruction of, 357
malabsorption due to, 706
physiology of, 968
pulmonary, 372
radiation of, 61, 61t
Lymphedema, 357
clinical features of, 357
diagnosis of, 357
etiology of, 357
incidence of, 357
mastectomy complicated by, 1034
treatment of, 357
Lymphoblasts, *820*, *821*
lymphoma and, 943t, 943–944
Lymphocytes, 818, 819
AIDS/HIV and, 1837t, 1838–1840, 1839t, 1887t, 1890, *1890*
atherogenesis role of, 292, *292*, 294, *295*
B. See *B cells.*

Lymphocytes (Continued)
bare, 1406
choriomeningitis and, 2089, 2089t
cutaneous inflammation role of, 2190
glucocorticoid effect on, 108–109, 109t
immunomodulation by, 901, *901*
leprosy pathogenesis and, 1692, 1692t, *1694*, 1695
leukemia and. See *Leukemia.*
leukocytosis due to, 919t, 919–920, 932, 938
lifespan of, 818
lymphoma and. See *Lymphoma.*
monocyte interaction with, 901, *901*
production of, 818, 819, *819–821*
decreased, 914t, 914–915
renal transplant affected by, 568, 568–569
sarcoidosis role of, 431, *431*
T. See *T cells.*
thromboangiitis obliterans role of, 352
Lymphocytopenia. See *Lymphopenia.*
Lymphocytosis, 919–920
causes of, 919t
diagnosis of, 919–920
large granular, 933t
leukemia and, 932, 933t, 938
reactive, 919–920, 933t
leukemia vs., 933t
Lymphogranuloma venereum, **1724**
chlamydial etiology of, 1722, 1723t, 1724
epidemiology of, 1723t
laboratory testing for, 1724
treatment of, 1724
Lymphoma, 941–954
AIDS/HIV with, 954, 1857, 1857t, 1873–1874
B cell, 941t, 943t
Epstein-Barr virus in, 1777–1778
paraneoplastic, 1032
benzene exposure causing, 56, 58t
bone marrow transplantation for, 976
brain affected by, 2126t, 2128t, 2132
Burkitt's, 941t
epidemiology of, 942, 943
gastric, 679
histiocytic, 941t
Hodgkin's. See *Hodgkin's disease.*
incidence of, 960, 961t, *1009*, 1013t, 1061t
intestinal, malabsorption due to, 706
leukemic phase, 933t, 934
monoclonal proteins with, 960, 961t
non-Hodgkin's, 941–946, 1065–1066
bone marrow involvement in, 944t
diagnosis of, 942, 944, 944t
epidemiology of, 942–943
etiology and pathogenesis of, 943
grade of, 941t, 943–944, *946*
leukemia and, 943, 944
pathology of, 943t, 943–944
prognosis in, 946, *946*
subtypes of, 943t, 943–944, 944t, 946
treatment of, 944–946, 945t
tumor marker of, 1022t, 1023–1024
pregnancy and, 1061t, 1064–1066
skin affected by, 1031t, 1031–1032, 1034
T cell, 941t, 943t, 1781t, 1781–1782
cutaneous, 1031t, 1031–1032
thymic, 1439
viruses and, T-lymphotropic, 1781t, 1781–1782, *1782*
Lymphopenia, 914–915
causes of, 914, 914t
clinical manifestations of, 914–915
diagnosis of, 914–915
lupus erythematosus with, 1475t, 1479
Nezelof's syndrome with, 1402t, 1405
pathogenesis of, 914, 914t
treatment of, 915
Lymphoproliferative disease. See also *Leukemia; Lymphoma.*
enlarged nodes caused by, 969t, 970, 970t
Epstein-Barr virus in, 1777–1778
gammopathy with, 961, *961*, 961t
salivary glands affected by, 649t, 649–650, 1488, 1488t, 1489
Sjögren's syndrome in, 649t, 649–650, 1488, 1488t, 1489
X-linked, 1405
Lynch syndrome, 724
I, 724
II, 724
mismatch repair deficiency in, 1073
Lyon hypothesis, G6PD and, 857–858
Lyonization, 140, 154

Lysergic acid diethylamide (LSD), 54, 1975t
  adverse effects of, 54, 508
  overdose with, 54
  pharmacology of, 54
Lysine, biotin linked to, 1147t
  urinary, 1101t, 1104t
    metabolic defect and, 144t
    protein intolerance with, 144t
Lysosomes, antibodies to, 1476t
  pancreatic, 731
  platelet, 979
  shock affecting, 484
  storage diseases related to, 147, 1095–1099, 1096t
    specific disorders of, 1095–1099, 1096t
Lysyl hydroxylase deficiency, 1121t

M

M protein, 958, 959
  cryoglobulinemia with, 966
  gammopathy role of, 958–966, 960t, 961t
  heavy chain disease and, 966
  macroglobulinemia due to, 965
Macaque, immunodeficiency virus of, 1845, 1845–1846
MacCallum's patch, 1592
Macleod's syndrome, 390
Macrocytes, 826t
Macrocytosis, anemia and, 824, 824t, 825t, 828t, 828–829
  stress and, 817
Macrolides, 1562t
  dose adjustment for, 1562t
  pharmacology of, 1562t
Macroovalocytes, 825t, 847, 848, 913
Macrophage colony-stimulating factor. See Colony-stim-
    ulating factors.
Macrophage inflammatory protein, 1535t
  fever production role of, 1533–1534, 1534, 1535t
Macrophages, 897–901
  activation of, 1454
  AIDS/HIV effect on, 1839
  alveolar, 372–373, 900, 900t
  antigen presentation by, 900–901, 901
  atherogenesis role of, 292, 292, 294, 295
  cholesterolosis and, 816
  cytokines produced by, 1395t
  disorders affecting, 902–906, 904t, 905t
  fever production role of, 1533–1534, 1534, 1535t
  foamy, 1694, 1695
  hepatic, 789, 900, 900t
  interleukin secreted by, 1395t
  kinetics of, 898t
  leprosy bacilli in, 1694, 1695
  lipid-filled, 816
  lymphocyte interaction with, 901, 901
  meningitis role of, 1612, 1618, 1619
  microbicidal activity of, 897, 899, 900, 900t, 901
  monocyte origin of, 898t, 900, 900t
  phagocytic function of, 899, 900–901, 901
  production of, 898t, 900, 900t
  receptors on, 900, 901t
  sarcoidosis role of, 431, 431
  secretory products of, 900–901, 901t, 1454
  storage diseases affecting, 1096t, 1097
  thromboxane and, 1188
  types of, 900, 900t
Macula densa, 223
  anatomy of, 223, 519, 520, 520
Macula retinae, degeneration of, 2016, 2174t, 2177–2178
  diabetic edema of, 1273
  Rift Valley fever affecting, 1806t, 1808
Macules, 1738t, 2191t, 2216t
  chancroid, 1704
  depigmented, 2214
  diseases associated with, 1738t, 2191t, 2216t
  drug-induced, 2219t, 2219–2220
  eczematous, 2191t, 2197–2199, 2201t
  Kaposi's sarcoma, 1032–1033, 1033t, 1872
  lichen planus, 2191, 2204
  measles with, 1759, 2200
  oral, 647t, 647–648
  pinta, 1714
  purpuric, 1738t, 2201t, 2201–2202
  rickettsiosis, 1728, 1728t, 1729, 1730, 1732, 1738t
  rubella, 1762, 2200
  syphilitic, 1707, 1707
Maculopapules, diseases associated with, 2191t
  drug-induced, 2201, 2219t, 2219–2220
  eczematous, 2191t, 2197–2199, 2201t

Maculopapules (Continued)
  erythema infectiosum, 2200
  purpuric, 2201t, 2201–2202
  rickettsial, 1728t
  roseola infantum (exanthem subitum), 1791
  vasculitis with, 2201t, 2201–2202
  viral, 2200–2201
Madura foot, 1834–1835
Mafucci's syndrome, 1390
Magenta carcinogenicity, 1016t
Magnesium, absorption of, 690, 690t, 704t
  blood level of, 1351t, 1356
    bound, 1351t
    free, 1351t
  bone formation and, 1351t, 1351–1356, 1352
  deficiency of, 1137t, 1137–1138, 1138t
  diarrhea and, osmotic, 690, 690t
  dietary, intake of, 1352
    supplemental, 262, 704t
  excess of, 1138
  hypertension treatment and, 262
  intoxication, 1138
  kidney and, depletion and, 1137t, 1137–1138
    failure and, 557t, 558
    reabsorption and, 1137
    transport and, 523
  malabsorption and, 700t, 704t
  RDA for, 1140t
  replacement therapy using, 1138, 1138t
  serum level of, normal, 700t
Magnesium ammonium phosphate stone, 615, 616t, 617
Magnetic resonance imaging (MRI), advances in, 128–131, 129–131
  brain function imaging with, 128, 129
  brain tumor in, 2127, 2127–2128, 2128, 2128t, 2130, 2131
  cardiac, 202t, 202–206, 203–208, 205t
  CNS in, 1963t, 1963–1969, 1966–1968
  contraindications to, 205t
  gradient-echo sequence in, 203–204
  hydrogen nuclei in, 202–204, 203–205
  principles of, 202–203, 203
  spectroscopic, 128–129, 129, 131
  spin-echo sequence in, 203, 204
  vascular system, 202t, 202–206, 203–207, 205t
Magnocellular neurons, 1221, 1222
  vasopressin response and, 1222
Malabsorption, 695–707. See also Absorption.
  AIDS and, 692, 706–707
  algorithm for, 701–702, 703t
  calcium, 1362t, 1363t, 1371
  carcinoid vs., 700t
  causes of, 697, 698t, 702–707
  cholestasis due to, 807, 808t
  classification of, 698t
  clinical features of, 697–698, 699t
  diagnostic testing in, 698–702, 700, 700t–703t, 702
  diarrhea with, 692, 699t
  differential treatment of, 702–707, 704t
  drug therapy for, 704t
  drug-induced, 706
  elderly with, 706
  fat, 698, 699t, 700, 700t
  inflammatory bowel disease with, 710, 710t
  lactose, 700, 700t
  lactulose, 700, 700t, 701t
  pathophysiology in, 699t, 702–707, 704t
  radiation enteritis with, 103
  solutes affected by, 690, 690t, 696–697
  sprue and, nontropical (celiac), 702, 704–705
    tropical, 705–706
  unexplained, 706
  vitamin B_{12}, 699, 700t, 701t, 844t, 844–846
  vitamin D, 1359t, 1361–1362
  vitamin K, 699t, 999
  xylose, 700t, 700–701, 701t
Malaria, 783t, 1893–1896
  cerebral, 1894
  chemoprophylaxis of, 1895, 1895t
  clinical manifestations of, 1894
  diagnosis of, 1894–1895, 1895t
  epidemiology of, 1894
  etiologic organism in, 1893, 1893–1894, 1895t
    count of, 1895t, 1896
    life cycle of, 1893, 1893–1894
    staining of, 1894–1895, 1895t
  falciparum, 1893, 1893–1896, 1895t, 1896t
  fever of, 1532, 1532t, 1533t, 1894
  hemoglobin alteration and, 872–873

Malaria (Continued)
  hepatic effects of, 783t, 1893, 1894
  immune response to, 1894
  incidence and prevalence of, 1893–1894
  ovale, 1893, 1893–1896, 1895t, 1896t
  pathogenesis and pathology of, 1893, 1894, 1895t
  prevention of, 1555, 1555t, 1895t, 1895–1896, 1896t
  prognosis in, 1896
  relapse in, 1895t, 1895–1896, 1896t
  serology for, 1895
  sickle syndromes and, 883
  splenomegaly due to, 972t
  thalassemia and, 879
  transfusion-transmitted, 896t, 896–897, 1893
  travel exposure to, 1555, 1555t
  treatment of, 1895–1896, 1896t
  vaccine for, 1895
  vivax, 1893, 1893–1896, 1895t, 1896t
Male. See Sex (gender); Sexual differentiation.
Malformations. See Arteriovenous malformations; Con-
    genital anomalies; Genetics; Hereditary
    disorder(s).
Malingering, 2006
  Münchhausen's, 2006
  psychiatric disorder with, 1974, 1974t, 1982
Mallory-Weiss tear, 659
  hemorrhage due to, 642t, 643, 659
  vomiting and, 629, 630, 643, 659
Malnutrition, diabetes mellitus related to, 1258t, 1260
  myocarditis due to, 331
  nutrition status assessment and, 1151–1154, 1153t
  protein-energy, 1154–1157
    catabolic illness in, 1155, 1155t
    clinical syndromes of, 1156, 1156t
    diagnosis of, 1156t, 1156–1157
    kwashiorkor-like, 1156, 1156t
    marasmus-like, 1156, 1156t
    organ system effects of, 1155t, 1155–1156
    pathogenesis of, 1154t, 1154–1155, 1155t
    prevention of, 1157
    secondary, 1156, 1156t
    starvation adaptation in, 1155, 1155t
    treatment approach in, 1157, 1157
  signs and symptoms of, 1151–1154, 1153t
Maltese cross inclusions, 1096
  crystal arthropathy with, 1516t
Mamillary body, 1183
Mammals. See Animals.
Mammography, 1310
  breast cancer diagnosis with, 1321, 1321t
  cancer screening with, 1006t
  frequency guidelines for, 28t, 1321, 1321t
Mandible. See Jaw.
Manganese, 73, 1149t
  deficiency of, 1149t
  dietary, parenteral, 1173t
  occupational exposure to, 73
  RDA for, 1141t
  superoxide dismutase, 1149t
  toxicity of, 1149t
    clinical manifestations of, 73, 1149t
    dementia of, 73, 1149t
    poisoning due to, 73
Mania, 2002–2004
  clinical features of, 1997t, 2002–2004, 2003t
  delusions and hallucinations in, 1997t
  grandiosity in, 1997t, 2002
Mannitol, intracranial pressure reduced with, 2128, 2133t
  properties and action of, 224t
Manometry, esophageal, 655–656, 656
  gastric, 685
  intestinal, 682, 685
Mansonelliasis, 1944–1945
MAO (monoamine oxidase) inhibitors, 2000t
  depression treated with, 2000t, 2001
  side effects of, 2001
Maple syrup urine disease, 1111–1112
  diagnosis of, 1112
  enzyme defect in, 1101t, 1112
  genetics of, 146–147, 1111–1112, 1112t
  treatment of, 1112
Maprotiline, 2000t, 2001
Marasmus, 1156
Marble bone, 1388–1389, 1389
Marburg-Ebola disease, 1798t, 1803–1804
Marchiafava-Bignami disease, 2040, 2106t

Marfan syndrome, **1119–1120**
  aortic aneurysm due to, *345*, 345–346, *346*
  clinical manifestations of, 1120
  definition of, 1119
  differential diagnosis of, 1120
  genetics of, 138–139, 1119, 1120
  pathology in, 1119–1120
  prevalence of, 1119
  treatment of, 1120
Marfanoid habitus, 1375
Marijuana, 53
  adverse effects of, 53
  pharmacology of, 53
  withdrawal of, 53
Marine organisms, 1854t, 1953–1956
  venomous, 1854t, 1953–1956
Maroteaux-Lamy syndrome, clinical features of, 1119t
  enzyme defect of, 1119t
Marrara's syndrome, 1950
Masculinization. See *Sexual differentiation*; *Virilization*.
Mast cells, 1435
  allergic rhinitis role of, 1414, *1415*, *1416*
  angioedema role of, 1409–1410, 2208
  asthma and, 377, *377*
  biologic mediators released by, *1416*, 1436t
  Darier's sign and, 1035, 1411, 2192
  differentiation of, 1435
  prostaglandins and, *1188*, 1189, 1436t
  skin rub affecting, 1035, 1411, 2192, 2208
  urticaria due to, 1409–1410, 1436, *1436*, 2192, 2208
Mastalgia, 1318
Mastectomy, 1034
Mastocytosis, **1435–1437**
  bone marrow affected by, 1436, *1437*
  classification of, 1435, 1435t
  clinical features of, 1436, *1436*
  Darier's sign in, 1436
  diagnosis of, 1436–1437, *1437*
  epidemiology of, 1435
  etiology of, 1435–1436
  hematologic disorder with, 1435, 1435t, 1437
  indolent, 1435, 1435t
  pathogenesis of, 1435–1436, 1436t
  peptic ulcer role of, 662t, 664
  prognosis for, 1437
  systemic, 1411, 1435t, 1435–1437
  treatment of, 1437
  urticaria in, 1411, 1436, *1436*
Mastodynia, 1318
Masturbation, 1328
Mayaro virus, 1805t, 1809
Mazzotti reaction, 1943
McArdle's disease, 351, 1083, 1083t
McCune-Albright syndrome, 145, 1347, *1372*,
    1372–1373, 2213
  fibrous dysplasia in, 1390
  multiple endocrine neoplasia with, 1347
  mutations in, 1347
  precocious puberty with, 1296, 1347
MCHC. See *Mean cell hemoglobin concentration
    (MCHC)*.
MCV. See *Mean cell volume (MCV)*.
Mean, statistical, 83
Mean cell hemoglobin concentration (MCHC), 825
  anemia and, 825
  sickle syndromes and, 885, 885t
  spherocytosis affecting, 854
Mean cell volume (MCV), abnormal, 830–831
  alcoholism and, 830
  anemia and, 825, 826t, 839, 841
  decreased, 826t, 831, 841
  hematocrit related to, 829, 830–831
  increased, 826t, 830–831
    megaloblastic anemia with, 847
    red cell production with, 829
  normal, 823, 823t, 826t
  sickle syndromes and, 885t
Measles (rubeola), **1759–1761**, 2100
  atypical, 1760
  clinical manifestations of, 1759
  complications of, 1760, 2100
  differential diagnosis of, 1760, 1760t
  epidemiology of, 1759
  etiology of, 1759
  immune globulin against, 41t
  immunization for, 42t, 44, 1760, 1761
  immunosuppressive effects of, 1759
  oral lesions of, 646, 646t, 1759

Measles (rubeola) *(Continued)*
  pathology in, 1759, 2100
  prognosis in, 1760–1761
  slow infection due to, 2097t, 2100
  treatment of, 1761
Meat, dietary, 29–30, 30t, 1139, *1142*, 1143t
  red, 29–30, 30t, *1142*, 1143, 1143t
  tapeworm in, 1923t, 1924–1926
  trichinosis associated with, 1937–1938
Mebendazole, hookworm treated with, 1935t
  nematode infection treated with, 1935t
  roundworm treated with, 1935t
Mecamylamine, 265t
Mechanic's hands, 1502
Meconium ileus, 419–420, 421t
Media, mesenteric arterial, 127, *127*
  polyarteritis nodosa affecting, 1493
  ultrasonography of, 127, *127*
Median, statistical, 83
Median eminence, *1197*
Median nerve, carpal tunnel syndrome and, *1462*, 1527,
    2157
  compression of, 1462, *1462*
  paresthesia of, *1462*, 1462, *1463*, 2157
  Phalen's maneuver for, 1462, *1463*
  rheumatoid arthritis affecting, *1462*, 1462, *1463*
Mediastinal nodes, 969t
  Hodgkin's disease in, 948, *949*
Mediastinum, **447–449**
  anatomy of, 447, *447*
  fibrosis affecting, 1529–1530
  mass in, 448t, 448–449
    air, 449
    causes of, 448t, 448–449
    detection of, 448, *448*
    signs and symptoms of, 448
    superior vena cava and, 449
    thymoma as, *448*, 448–449
    tumor as, 448, *448*
Medicine. See also *Health care*.
  economic issues in, 9–11, 10t
  ethical issues in, 4–9, 465–466
  future of, 3
  profession of, 1–3
  social issues affecting, 9–11
Mediterranean fever, 907–908
  arthritis with, 1526
  brucellosis as, 1678–1680, 1679t
  familial, 907–908
    amyloidosis with, 907, 908
    clinical manifestations of, 907–908
    diagnosis of, 908
    genetics of, 136t
    incidence and prevalence of, 907
    pain in, 907
    treatment and prognosis in, 908
  rickettsial (spotted), 1732
Medulla, blood supply to, *2061*
  temperature control by, 1532
  tumor of, 2126t, 2132
Medulloblastoma, 2132
Mefloquine, 1895t, 1895–1896, 1896t
Megacolon, chagasic, 1901
  toxic, 709, 714
  trypanosomiasis with, 1901
Megaesophagus, chagasic, 1901, *1901*
  trypanosomiasis with, 1901, *1901*
Megakaryoblasts, *820*
Megakaryocytes, 818
  myelodysplastic syndrome and, *834*
  platelet derivation from, 818, 979
  production of, 818–819, *820*, 898
Megaloblastic anemia. See under *Anemia*.
Megestrol, 1046t, 1047
Meglumine antimoniate, 1907
Meibomian glands, 2186
Meigs' syndrome, **446**, 1313
Meiosis, 134, *136*, 151
Melanin, 2212–2214
  albinism and, 146, 2214t
  cutaneous depth of, 2192
  decreased deposition of, 2213–2214, 2214t
  fungal infection with, 1836
  increased deposition of, 2212–2213
  oral pigmentation of, 648, 648t
  skin color role of, **2185**, 2185, 2190, 2192
  ultraviolet light absorption by, 2187, 2192
Melanocytes, 2184–2185, *2185*
  age-associated decrease in, 2190
  albinism and, 146, 2214t

Melanocytes *(Continued)*
  biochrome organelles of, 2185
  cutaneous, 2184–2185, *2185*, 2187, 2190
  depigmented, 2213–2214, 2214t
  hyperpigmented, 2212–2213
  lentigines of, 2212
  physiology of, 2184–2185, *2185*
Melanocyte-stimulating hormone (MSH), 1186, *1186*
Melanoma (malignant), 2210–2211
  characteristics of, 1066, 1066t, 2210, 2210t
  diagnosis of, 2210t, 2210–2211
  incidence of, 1013t, 1061t
  intraocular, 2180
  nails affected by, 2215
  nevus cell in, 2210–2211
  nodular, 2210, *2210*
  pregnancy and, 1061t, 1066, 1066t
  risk factors for, 2210–2211
Melarsoprol, 1898
MELAS, 2160t, 2166t, 2167
Melasma, 2212
Melatonin, 1204–1205
  chronobiology of, 1204–1205
  function of, 1204
  pineal gland and, *1204*, 1204–1205
  regulation of, *1204*, 1204–1205
Melena, 642
Melenemesis, 642
Melioidosis, 1667–1669
  bacteremia in, *1668*
  diagnosis of, 1667–1668
  epidemiology of, 1668, *1668*
  pathogenesis of, 1667–1668
  prognosis in, 1668–1669, *1669*
  Pseudomonas in, 1667–1669, *1668*
  treatment of, 1668–1669
Melorheostosis, 1390
  clinical presentation of, 1390
  radiologic features of, 1390
Melphalan, adverse effects, 1042
  chemotherapy using, 1039t, 1042, 1042t
  myeloma treated with, 963
  resistance to, 1058, 1058t
Membrane attack complex, 1400, *1400*
Membrane(s), bacterial, *1556*, 1556–1557
  brush border, *689*, 689–690
  cytoplasmic. See *Plasma membrane*.
  electrical potential of. See *Action potential*.
  transport defects of, 143–145, 144t, 147t
    amino acid, 144t
    chloride, 144t
    glucose, 143, 144t
    insulin, 144t, 145, 145t
    methionine, 144t
    phosphate, 144t
    sodium, 144t
    tryptophan, 144t
Memory, **1989–1990**. See also *Amnesia*.
  aging effect on, 16, 16t, 17–18
  alcohol effect on, 48, 1982
  Alzheimer's disease affecting, 1993, 1994
  declarative, 1989t
  definition of, 1989
  hypothyroidism affecting, 1238, 1238t
  long-term, 1989, 1989t
  mechanisms of, 1989
  Pick's disease affecting, 1995
  procedural, 1989, 1989t
  semantic, 1989
  short-term, 1989, 1989t
Menaquinones, 1145t
Menarche, 1293–1294, 1293–1295, *1294*
Mendelian law, 134
Ménétrier's disease, gastritis of, 659t, 661
Meningioma, CT scan of, 2127, *2127*
  imaging of, 1964–1965, *1965*
Meningitis, **1610–1621**
  AIDS/HIV with, 1856t, 1856–1857, 2097
  aseptic, **2088–2090**
    approach to, 2087–2088
    arbovirus, 2089, 2089t
    definition of, 2088
    diagnosis of, 2090
    enterovirus, 1786, 1787t, 2089t
    epidemiology of, 2089
    etiologic agents in, 2088t, 2088–2089, 2089t
    herpes simplex, 2089, 2089t
    laboratory findings in, 2089–2090
    leptospiral, 1737t, 1738t
    lymphocytic (choriomeningitis), 2089, 2089t

Meningitis *(Continued)*
  mumps with, 1769, 2089, 2089t
  pathogenesis of, 2089
  prognosis in, 2090
  treatment of, 2090
  varicella, 2089, 2089t
  bacterial, **1610–1621**
    antimicrobial therapy in, 1615–1617, 1616t, 1620t, 1620–1621, 1621t
    bacteriology of, 1610t, 1610–1612, 1618, *1619*
    cerebrospinal fluid in, 1612, 1613, 1618, 1620
    clinical manifestations of, 1612t, 1612–1613, 1619–1620
    complications of, 1612t, 1612–1614, 1619–1620
    diagnosis of, 1613–1614, 1620
    epidemiology of, 1610–1611, 1618–1619
    etiology of, 1610t, 1610–1611
    H. influenzae, 1610t, 1610–1613, 1616t
    history of, 1618t, 1618–1619
    incidence of, 1610–1611, 1618–1619
    laboratory testing in, 1613–1614, 1620
    listerial, 1610t, 1611, 1616t, 1672–1673, 1737t
    meningococcal, 1618t, 1618–1621, *1619*, 1620t, 1621t
    neurologic effects of, 1612t, 1612–1613, 1620
    pathogenesis of, 1611–1612, 1618, *1619*, 1737t
    pathology findings in, 1611
    pathophysiology of, 1612, 1618, *1619*
    pediatric, 1610t, 1610–1611, 1616–1617, 1619
    pneumococcal, 1571, 1571t, 1610t, 1610–1612, 1616t
    predisposing factors in, 1611, 1618–1619
    prevention of, 1621, 1621t
    Pseudomonas, 1610–1613, 1616t
    radiography in, 1613–1614
    recurrent, 1614–1615
    staphylococcal, 1610t, 1610–1617, 1616t
    streptococcal, 1589t, 1589–1590, 1610t, 1610–1611
    treatment of, 1615–1617, 1616t, 1620t, 1620–1621, 1621t
    tuberculous, 1685t
  candidal, 1829
  cryptococcal, 1824, 1825
  Lyme disease with, 1717, 1719t
  lymphomatous (choriomeningitis), 1737t, 2089, 2089t
  syphilitic, 1708t, 1709, *2085*, 2085, 2086t
Meningocele, 2149
Meningococcal infections, **1618–1621**
  antibiotic therapy in, 1620t, 1620–1621
  carrier state in, 1619
  chronic, 1621
  complications of, 1620
  epidemiology of, 1618–1619
  history of, 1618t
  immunization for, 42t, 46, 1554, 1554t, 1621
  laboratory tests in, 1620
  meningitis in, 1618t, 1618–1621, *1619*, 1620t, 1621t
  microbiology of, 1618, *1619*
  pathogenesis of, 1618, *1619*
  prognosis in, 1620
  treatment of, 1620t, 1620–1621
Meningococcemia, 1612, 1619–1620
  coagulopathy in, 1614, 1620, 1621
  petechiae in, 1612, 1619–1620
Meningoencephalitis, amebic, 1915
  enteroviral, 1792
  Lyme disease with, 1717, 1719t
  N. fowleri causing, 1915
  syphilitic, 1709
Menopause, 1311–1312
  breast discharge following, 1318
  clinical management of, 1311–1312
  definition of, 1311
  osteoporosis related to, *1380*
  ovaries in, 1293, *1293*, *1294*, 1311–1312
  signs and symptoms of, 1311
  Sjögren's syndrome following, 1488
Menstruation, 1297–1299
  abnormal bleeding and, 1302
  absent. See *Amenorrhea.*
  anorexia effect on, 1158, 1159t
  hemophilia and, 994
  iron levels affected by, 1134t
  lupus erythematosus and, 1480
  normal cycle of, 1297–1299, *1298*
  ovarian changes in, 1297–1299, *1298*
  premenstrual syndrome of, 1301–1302, 1302t
Mental retardation, homocystinuria with, 1113t, 1113–1114

Mental retardation *(Continued)*
  mucopolysaccharidoses with, 1118–1119, 1119t
  Prader-Willi syndrome with, 161
  radiation therapy causing, 1070t
Mental status, elderly screened for, 19
  examination of, dementia and, 1993, 1993t
  hepatic encephalopathy affecting, 797–798, 798t
  hypothyroidism effect on, 1238, 1238t
  lupus erythematosus affecting, 1475t, 1479–1480, 1480t
  syphilis affecting, 1709
Meperidine, 51
  pain control with, 104t, 893t
  parkinsonism induced by, 2044
Mephenytoin, 97t
Mercaptopurine, adverse effects of, 1043
  chemotherapy using, 1042t, 1043
  fetal malformations due to, 1070t
Mercury, **69–70**
  environment containing, 69, 70
  food contaminated with, 740
  inorganic, 69–70
  metallic, 69
  methyl, 70
  occupational exposure to, 69
  poisoning due to, 69–70, 504t, 740
    clinical manifestations of, 69–70
    etiology of, 69, 740
    treatment of, 69–70, 504t
  renal function and, 587
  seafood contaminated with, 740
  vapor, 69
Merlin (protein), 2056
Meropenem, 1562t
MERRF, 2160t, 2166t, 2167
Mesalamine, 712–713
  inflammatory bowel disease treated with, 712–713, 714t
  metabolism of, 713
Mesangium, 519, *519*
  diabetes mellitus and, *601*
  immune complex deposition in, 1477
  lupus erythematosus affecting, 1477
  phagocytosis in, 900, 900t
Mescaline, 54, 508t
Mesenteric artery, 715
  atherosclerosis of, 719–720
  nonocclusive ischemia related to, 717, *718*
  occlusion of, 717
  ultrasonography of, intravascular, 127, *127*
  vasoconstriction of, 717, *718*
Mesenteric nodes, 968–969, 969t, 1661
Mesenteric vein, 717–718
Mesentery, adenitis of, 1661
  ischemia of, 715–720
    acute, 717–719
    atherosclerosis causing, 719–720
    chronic, 719–720
    clinical aspects of, 717, 719
    nonocclusive, 717, *718*
    thrombosis causing, 717–718
  yersinial infection and, 1661
Mesothelioma, malignant, 56, 58t, 447
  occupational exposure causing, 56, 58t
  pleural effusion with, 447
Metabolic disorder(s), **142–147, 1078–1138.** See also specific disorder.
  amino acid, 144t, 1099–1117, *1100*, 1100t–1105t
  approach to patient with, 1078t, 1078–1080, 1079t
  carbohydrate, 144t, 146t, 1080–1085
  cardiomyopathy and, 329t, 331
  connective tissue, 1118–1124
  diabetes mellitus with, 143–145, 144t, 145t, 1261, 1263
  dwarfism due to, 145, 147t
  enzymatic defects in, 145–147, 146t. See also specific enzymes and disorders.
  erythrocytic, 856–859, *857*, *858*, 858t
  fructose in, 146t, 1083–1085, *1084*
  galactose in, 143–146, 1080t, 1080–1081
  genetics in, 136t, 138t, 142–147, 144t, 146t, 147t
  screening in, 1078, 1078t
  glucose in, 143, 144t, 1082–1083
  glycogen storage disease as, 146t, 146–147, *1082*, 1082–1083
  hemochromatosis as, 1132–1135, 1133t, *1135*
  hormonal, 147t
  inflammatory bowel disease with, 710, 710t
  lipoprotein, 1089–1095, 1092t
  lysosomal, 147, 1095–1099, 1096t

Metabolic disorder(s) *(Continued)*
  mechanisms of, 142–147, 143t
  mitochondrial, 146t, 146–147
  muscle weakness due to, 1503t
  myopathy caused by, 2160t, 2165–2170, 2166t
  neurologic effects of, 1972t, 1972–1974, 1973t
  organic acid, 146t
  peroxisomal, 147, 147t, 1085
  pigmentation, 146
  plasma membrane, 143–145, 144t
  porphyria in, 1124–1130, *1125*, 1125t, 1126t
  protein derangement in, 143t, 143–147, 144t, 146t, 147t
  protein-energy malnutrition with, 1155t, 1155–1156
  purine, 1114–1117
  transport defect, 143–145, 144t, 147t
  treatment approaches in, 1078–1079, 1079t
  Wilson's disease as, 1131–1132
Metabolic rate, exercise effect on, 31t
  hypothyroidism affecting, 1238, 1238t
  obesity etiology and, 1162–1163
  postprandial, 1163
Metabolism, acid-base, 543–546, *545*, 545t
  amino acid, 754
    disorders of, 1099–1117, *1100*, 1100t–1105t
  carbohydrate, 753, 1080–1085
  definition of, 142–143
  disorders of. See *Metabolic disorder(s).*
  fructose, 1083, *1084*
  hepatic, 753–754
  lipoprotein, 1086–1088, *1087*, *1088*, *1089*
  phosphorus, 1135
  protein, 754, 760–761
Metals, **67–73.** See also specific metal.
  asthma induced by, 379t
  occupational exposure to, 56, 58t, 59t, 67–73, 379t
  oral mucosal deposition of, 648t
  renal function and, 587–588
  toxicity of, 70–73, 1148t–1150t
    nephron affected by, 587–588
    poisoning due to, 67–73, 504t, 508–509
  trace, 70–73, 1148t–1150t
    RDA for, 1140t, 1141t
Metanephrine, 1253, *1253*
  catecholamine biosynthesis role of, 1253, *1253*
Metapyrone test, ACTH reserve in, 1216
  cortisol suppression in, 1216
Metastases, 1054–1056
  ascites with, 743t, 744t, 744–745, 745t, 749
  from colon, 726
  from liver, 805
  from pheochromocytoma, 1254, 1257
  intracranial, 1051
  lymphadenopathy due to, 970t
  molecular mechanisms of, 1073
  primary site unknown in, 1054–1056
    approach to patient with, 1054–1056
    clinical manifestations of, 1055
    incidence of, 1054
    lymph node and, 1055, 1056
    pathology of, 1054–1055
    prognosis in, 1056
    staging of, 1055–1056
    treatment of, 1056
    visceral, 1055–1056
  to adrenal gland, 1249, 1251
  to bone, 1391
  to brain, 1051, 2126t, *2128*, 2130, *2130*
  to eye, 2180
  to liver, 804
  to skin, 1030–1031, 1031t
Metatarsophalangeal joint, osteoarthritis of, 1518–1519
Metformin, glucose reduced with, 1268, 1268t
Methadone, 51
  drug withdrawal treated with, 53
  pain control with, 102, 104t
Methanol, acidosis caused by, 548, 549, 1975t
  poisoning due to, 509, 509t, 1975t
  treatment of, 504t, 509, 509t
Methemoglobin reductase deficiency, 98–100, 875–877, 876t
Methemoglobinemia, 869, 875–877, 876t
  clinical features of, 875–877
  cyanosis vs., 875–877
  drug-induced, 876, 876t
  G6PD deficiency with, *856*, 856–857
  toxic, 876t, 876–877
  treatment of, 877

Methicillin, 1562t
　endocarditis therapy with, 1602–1603, 1603t
　minimal inhibitory concentration for, 1570, 1570t
　staphylococcal infection treated with, 1609–1610
Methimazole, adverse effects of, 1234, 1234t
　mechanism of action of, 1227, 1234
　pregnancy and, 1236
　thyroid inhibition using, 1234–1235, 1235t
Methionine, 1112–1114
　homocysteine metabolism and, 1112–1114, 1113, 1113t
　load test using, 1114
　malabsorption of, 144t
　urinary, 1100t, 1101t, 1103t
Methionine synthase, 845, 845, 1112, 1113
　vitamin B$_{12}$ cofactor for, 845, 845, 1113, 1113t
Methotrexate, adverse effects of, 1043
　chemotherapy using, 1042t, 1043
　fetal malformations due to, 1070t, 1071t
　granulomatosis treated with, 1497t, 1498
　hepatotoxicity of, 773, 773t
　lung disease induced by, 397, 397t
　non-Hodgkin's lymphoma and, 945t
　renal function and, 587
　resistance to, 1059
　spondyloarthropathy treated with, 1472
Methotrimeprazine, 106t
Methoxyflurane, 588
Methoxymethylenedioxyamphetamine (MDMA), 54
　drug abuse treatment using, 54
Methyclothiazide, 264t
Methyl alcohol. See Methanol.
Methylcobalamin, 1112–1114, 1113
　coenzyme role of, 845, 845
　deficiency of, 1112–1114, 1113t
Methyldopa, dosage for, 265t, 266t, 270t
　hemolytic anemia due to, 867
　hepatotoxicity of, 773, 773t, 775
　side effects of, 267, 267t, 270t
Methylene blue, methemoglobinemia treated with, 875, 877
　nitrite toxicity treated with, 504t
Methylenetetrahydrofolate reductase, 1112–1114
　deficiency of, 1112–1114, 1113t
　homocysteine metabolized by, 1112–1114, 1113
Methylmalonic acid, 849t
　folate deficiency and, 845, 846, 849t, 850, 850t
　normal serum levels of, 849t, 850t
　vitamin B$_{12}$ deficiency and, 845, 846, 849t, 850t, 1147t, 1151
Methylmalonyl CoA, 845, 846
Methylmercury, seafood contaminated with, 740
Methylprednisolone, myeloma treated with, 964
　therapeutic, 108t, 964
Methyltetrahydrofolate, 845, 845
Metolazone, dosage for, 264t
　properties and action of, 224t, 531t
Metoprolol, 265t, 299t
Metronidazole, 1562t
　adverse reactions to, 1568t
　alcohol contraindicated with, 1917
　amebiasis therapy with, 1914, 1915t, 1916t
　balantidiasis therapy with, 1916t
　Blastocystis therapy with, 1916t
　colitis therapy with, 1633–1634
　giardiasis therapy with, 1913
　mechanism of action of, 1558, 1558t
　trichomoniasis treated with, 1917
METS, definition of, 31t
Mexiletine, 91t, 94t, 246t
　adverse effects of, 247t
　antiarrhythmic action of, 246, 246t
　dose adjustment for, 94t
　pain control use of, 106t
　pharmacokinetics of, 91t, 94t, 246, 246t
　renal failure effect on, 94t
Meyer's loop, 1985
Mezlocillin, 1570, 1570t
MI. See Myocardial infarction.
Micelles, bile salt, 806
　fat absorption role of, 696, 697
Miconazole, candidiasis treated with, 1829
　vaginitis treated with, 1829
Microangiopathy, 822
　diabetes mellitus causing, 1272–1274
　disorders associated with, 984t
　thrombocytopenia and, 1002–1003
Microcephaly, 1070t

Microcytes, 826t, 827
Microcytosis, 920–921, 921
　anemia with, 825t, 827–828, 839–842
　hematocrit and, 921, 921
　thalassemia with, 827–828
Microfibril-associated glycoproteins, 1444
Microfilaria. See Filariasis.
Microflora. See Flora.
Microglial cells, 900, 900t
β$_2$-Microglobulin, amyloidosis with, 967t, 1505
　dialysis and, 967t
　HLA molecules with, 1424–1426, 1425, 1426
　multiple myeloma with, 1022t, 1023–1024
Microhemagglutination test, 1710t, 1711, 1711t
Micronutrients, 1144–1151. See also Minerals; Trace elements; Vitamin(s).
　deficiency states of, 1145t–1150t, 1146–1151
　disease prevention using, 1139–1143, 1143t
　drug-mediated effects on, 1150t
　factors affecting requirement for, 1144t, 1144–1146
　new paradigms for, 1141t, 1146–1151, 1151t
Microscope slide, skin examination using, 2192
Microscopy, darkfield, 1705, 1710
　Treponema pallidum in, 1705, 1710
Microsomes, 1476t
Microspherocytes, 827t
　hemorrhagic disorders and, 984t
Microtubules, colchicine toxicity to, 1513–1514
　connective tissue, 1446
Microwaves, radiation injury due to, 63–64
　wavelength of, 59
Micturition, aging effect on, 22–23
　parasympathetic control of, 2010, 2010t
Midazolam, 310t, 507
Midbrain, blood supply to, 2060
　tumor of, 2126t
Midexpiratory flow, 378, 379t
Midge, bite of, 1947
　filariae transmitted by, 1939, 1940t, 1945
　viruses transmitted by, 1805, 1805t
Migraine. See Headache, migraine.
Migrating motor complex, small intestinal, 682–685
Milk, brucellosis transmission in, 1678, 1680
　dietary, 1142
　intolerance to, 704
　listeriosis transmission in, 1672, 1673
　low-fat, 29
　prolactin stimulus for, 1212–1213
　vitamin D in, 1357
　"witch's," 1317
Milk-alkali syndrome, 550, 1355–1356
Milkmaid's grip, 1593
Miller-Dieker lissencephaly syndrome, 155
Milwaukee shoulder, 1516, 1519t, 1524
Mineral oil, aspiration pneumonia due to, 407–408
　carcinogenicity of, 1016t
　hepatic granuloma due to, 784t
Mineralocorticoids. See also Aldosterone.
　adrenal cortex production of, 1245–1246
　alkalosis due to, 550
　deficiency of, 1251t, 1251–1252
　end-organ resistance to, 1252
　excess of, 1249t, 1249t
Minerals. See also specific mineral.
　bone formation and, 1351t, 1351–1356, 1352
　dietary, 1144, 1148t–1150t
　occupational exposure to, 399t, 399–403
　parenteral nutrition with, 1172, 1173t
　pneumoconioses due to, 399t, 399–403
　RDA for, 1140t, 1141t
Minimal inhibitory concentration, 1570t, 1616t
　β-lactam agents with, 1570, 1570t, 1616t
　meningitis therapy and, 1615, 1616t
　penicillin with, 1570t, 1615, 1616t
Minimata disease, 740
Minocycline, 1562t
　staphylococcal infection treated with, 1609t, 1609–1610
Minoxidil, dosage for, 265t, 267t
　side effects of, 267t
Minute ventilation, 466, 467t
Miotic agents, 2183, 2183t
Miracidium, schistosomal, 1927, 1927–1928
Miscarriage, 152–159, 158t
Mite, 1947, 1949
　biting, 1947
　chigger, 1947
　dermatitis caused by, 1950
　erysipeloid and, 1673–1674
　nonbiting, 1950

Mite (Continued)
　rickettsialpox carried by, 1727t, 1733
　scabies due to, 1738t, 1949
　zoonoses associated with, 1727t, 1737t, 1737–1738, 1738t
Mitochondria, 142, 146t
　antibodies to, 1457t, 1476t
　　liver disease with, 761, 791–792
　hereditary disorders related to, 142, 146t
　iron overload and, 842–843
　myopathy and, 2160t, 2166t, 2166–2167
　shock affecting, 483–484
Mitogen-activated protein, 1180, 1180
Mitomycin, adverse effects of, 1045
　chemotherapy using, 1039t, 1044t, 1045
　renal function and, 587
Mitosis, 134, 151
　cutaneous cell, 2184
　hair bulb cell, 2186–2187
　kinetics of, 818, 898t, 909
　neutrophilic, 818, 898t, 909
Mitoxantrone, adverse effects of, 1045
　chemotherapy using, 1039t, 1045
　resistance to, 1057t
Mitral valve, 323–326
　area determination for, 210, 211
　atrial enlargement due to, 182, 183–184
　calcification in, 184, 185–186, 1594, 1594
　graft replacement of, 184
　prolapse of, 326, 326
　　differential diagnosis of, 326
　　echocardiography of, 326, 326
　　emboli arising from, 2067
　　sounds in, 326
　　treatment of, 326
　regurgitation from, 324–325
　　catheterization in, 325
　　chest radiograph and, 325
　　clinical features of, 325
　　differential diagnosis of, 325
　　ECG in, 325
　　echocardiography in, 325
　　etiology of, 324–325
　　pathology of, 324–325
　　physical examination for, 325
　　physiology of, 325
　　pulmonary wedge pressure and, 210
　　sounds of, 325
　　surgical approach to, 325–326
　　treatment of, 325–326
　rheumatic fever affecting, 1594, 1594
　stenosis of, 323–324
　　catheterization in, 323t, 324
　　chest radiograph and, 323t, 324
　　clinical features of, 323, 323t
　　differential diagnosis of, 324
　　ECG in, 323, 323t
　　echocardiography in, 323t, 324, 324
　　etiology of, 323, 323t
　　murmur in, 323, 323t
　　pathology of, 323, 323t
　　physical examination for, 323, 323t
　　physiology of, 323, 323t
　　pulmonary hypertension due to, 273t, 275
　　pulmonary wedge pressure in, 211
　　surgical approach in, 323t, 324
　　treatment of, 323t, 324
Mitsuda reaction, 1692t, 1692–1693
Mittelschmerz, 1298
Mode, statistical, 83
Moexipril, 265t
Mole. See Nevus.
Mollaret's meningitis, 1615
Mollicutes. See Mycoplasmal infections.
Molluscum contagiosum, 2200
Mollusk, venomous, 1954t, 1955
Molybdenum, 73, 1149t
　deficiency of, 1149t
　physiology of, 1149t
　RDA for, 1141t
　toxicity of, 73, 1149t
Monge's disease, 409t, 409–410
　acute, 409t, 409–410
　chronic, 409t, 410
　clinical features of, 409, 409t
　treatment of, 409–410
Monkey, Ebola virus in, 1803–1804
　immunodeficiency virus of, 1845, 1845–1846
　yellow fever in, 1798–1799
　zoonoses associated with, 1737t, 1737–1738, 1738t

Monoamine oxidase inhibitors, 2000t
  depression treated with, 2000t, 2001
  side effects of, 2001
Monoblasts, 820, 821
Monoclonal gammopathy, 958–961, 2152
  neuropathy of, 961, 2152
Monocytes, 820, 820t, 821
  AIDS/HIV effect on, 1839
  atherogenesis role of, 292, 292, 294, 295
  cytokines of, 900, 901t
  decreased, 914
  functions of, 900–901, 901, 901t, 919
  glucocorticoid effect on, 108–109, 109t
  increased, 918–919, 919, 919t, 1532–1534
  kinetics of, 898t
  lymphocyte interaction with, 901, 901
  macrophage derivation from, 898, 900
  microbicidal activity of, 897, 899, 900, 900, 901, 919
  production of, 819, 820, 820t, 821, 898, 898t, 900
  receptors on, 901t
  storage diseases affecting, 1096t, 1097
  TNF production by, 1586
Monocytopenia, 914
Monocytosis, 918–919
  causes of, 919, 919t
  fever with, 1532t, 1532–1534
Monoiodotyrosine, 1227
Mononeuropathy, 2150
  diabetic, 2154t, 2154–2155
  multiple, 2151t, 2152
Mononucleosis (infectious), 1776–1779
  clinical manifestations of, 1776t, 1776–1777
  cytomegalovirus in, 1774
  diagnosis of, 1778, 1778, 1779t
  epidemiology of, 1776
  etiology of, 1776
  pathogenesis of, 1777–1778
  pathology of, 1777–1778
  treatment of, 1778
Monosaccharides, 704
Montgomery's glands, 1303t
  enlarged, 2186
Mood. See also Anxiety; Depression; Psychiatric disorders.
  aging effect on, 18–19, 19t
  alcohol affecting, 47, 48t
  bereavement affecting, 2001t, 2001–2002
  depressed, 1999, 1999t, 2001t
  elderly patient and, 18–19, 19t, 1999–2000
  manic, 1997t, 2002–2003, 2003t
  psychosis affecting, 1997, 1997t
MOPP therapy, 952t, 953
Morgagni column, 741
Moricizine, 246t, 249
  adverse effects of, 247t
  antiarrhythmic action of, 245, 246t, 249
  pharmacokinetics of, 246t, 249
Morning glory seed, 508, 508t
Morphea, 2212
  hair loss in, 2217
Morphine, 51
  drug abuse with, 51–53
  myocardial infarction pain and, 309
  neurologic effects of, 1975t
  pain control with, 104t, 893t
  pharmacology of, 52
  withdrawal of, 53
Morphogenesis. See also Congenital anomalies.
  errors of, 158t
Morquio's syndrome, clinical features of, 1119t
  enzyme defect of, 1119t
Mortality rate, 26–27, 27, 27t, 30t, 1143t. See also under specific diseases and conditions.
Morula inclusions, 1733
Mosaicism, Y chromosome and, 154
MOSF (multiple organ system failure), 474–477
  respiratory distress with, 474–477
  septic shock with, 496, 496t, 498, 500t
Mosquito, 1946–1947
  Anopheles, 1893, 1893–1894
  encephalitis transmitted by, 1806t, 1810t
  filariae transmitted by, 1939, 1940t
  malaria organism in, 1893, 1893–1894, 1895
  travel exposure to, 46, 1554, 1555, 1555t
  viruses transmitted by, 1798t, 1805, 1805t, 1806t
  yellow fever and, 1798t, 1798–1799
  zoonoses associated with, 1737t, 1737–1738, 1738t
Motility disorders, 680–688
  colonic, 686t, 686–688, 688t
  gastric emptying in, 683–684

Motility disorders (Continued)
  delayed, 683t, 683–684
  rapid, 683t, 684
  small intestinal, 684t, 684–686, 688t
Motion sickness, 2025
  traveler exposed to, 1556
Motor end-plate, 2158, 2171
  antibodies affecting, 1017–1018, 1028, 2171, 2173
  classification of disorders of, 2171t
  myasthenia and, 1017–1018, 1028, 2171, 2173
Motor function, arousal level and, 1971t
  gastrointestinal, 680–688
    disorders of, 683t, 683–688, 684t, 686t
    normal, 680–682, 680–682
  hepatic encephalopathy affecting, 797–798, 798t
  neurologic examination of, 1977t
  paraneoplastic effects on, 1018, 1027t, 1028–1029
  stroke affecting, 2064t, 2064–2065
Motor vehicle accidents, mortality due to, 37, 38, 39
  protective strategies for, 39
Mountain sickness, 409t, 409–410
  acute, 409t, 409–410
  chronic, 409t, 410
  clinical features of, 409, 409t
  treatment of, 409–410
Mouse, babesiosis reservoir in, 1915
  rickettsialpox carried by, 1727t, 1733
  zoonoses associated with, 1727t, 1737t, 1737–1738, 1738t
Mouth, 645–648
  AIDS/HIV symptoms in, 647, 647t, 1866, 1867t
  cancer of, incidence of, 1013t
    metastases from, 1031t
    smoking associated with, 34t, 35, 35t, 1014
    squamous cell, 646, 646t, 647t, 2209, 2209
  dry, 649t, 649–650, 1488, 1488t, 1489
  flora of. See Flora, oropharyngeal.
  hand-foot-mouth disease of, 1787t, 1790
  herpangina affecting, 1787t, 1790
  pigmentation in, 648, 648t
  red macules in, 647, 647t
  syphilitic lesions in, 646, 646t, 647, 647t, 648t, 1707
  tumors of, soft tissue, 648, 648t
  ulcers of, 646, 646t
    acute, 646t
    Behçet's syndrome with, 646, 646t, 1506, 1506t
    causes of, 646t, 646–647, 647t
    chronic, 646t
    clustered, 646t
    enteroviral, 1790–1791
    multiple, 646t
    solitary, 646t
  white plaque in, 647, 647t
Movement disorders, ataxic. See Ataxia.
  athetotic, 2049
  basal ganglia relation to, 2042t, 2042–2043
  choreic, 1593, 2043, 2048–2049
  dystonic, 2043, 2047–2048. See also Dystonia.
  gait in. See Gait.
  hyperkinetic, 2042t, 2042–2043
  hypokinetic, 2042, 2042t
  myoclonic, 2050
  neurologic examination in, 1977t
  parkinsonian, 2042t, 2043–2046
  rheumatic fever aftermath with, 1593
  sleep-related, 1983, 1984, 2050
  stereotypic, 2050
  tic, 2049–2050
Moxalactam, 1570, 1570t
Moyamoya disease, 888
  carotid artery occlusion in, 2069
MPTP (drug), 55
MRI. See Magnetic resonance imaging (MRI).
MSH (melanocyte-stimulating hormone), 1186, 1186
Mu chains, 958
  disease of, 966
Mucin clot test, 1464, 1465t
Mucocele, gallbladder, 914
  oral, 648, 648t
Mucociliary escalator, 372–373, 399, 411t
Mucocutaneous lesions, candidal, 647, 647t, 1828
  enteroviral, 1787t, 1789–1791
  lymph node syndrome in, 970
  oral, 647t, 647–648
Mucopolysaccharidoses, 1118–1119
  cardiomyopathy due to, 333t, 334
  clinical features in, 1118–1119, 1119t
  genetics of, 138t, 147
  management of, 1118–1119

Mucopolysaccharidoses (Continued)
  mental retardation with, 1118–1119, 1119t
  treatment of, 1118–1119
Mucormycosis, 1832–1834
  clinical manifestations of, 1833t, 1833–1834
  diagnosis of, 1834
  epidemiology of, 1833
  etiologic organism in, 1832–1833
  pathogenesis and pathology in, 1833
  prognosis in, 1834
  pulmonary, 1833
  rhinocerebral, 1833
  therapy of, 1834
Mucosa, airway, 371, 372, 382, 399
  diphtheria affecting, 1629–1630
  dryness of, 1488t, 1488–1490, 1489
  gallbladder, 816
  gastric, 663, 663t
    NSAIDs effect on, 663, 663t
    ulcer pathophysiology and, 663, 663t
  intestinal, 702
    absorption by, 689, 689–690, 695–697, 696t
    malabsorptive conditions of, 702, 704–705
    morphologic disruption of, 692, 692t, 702, 704–705
    sprue and, 702, 704–705
  leishmaniasis of, 1906, 1906–1907
  meningitis organisms in, 1612, 1618, 1619
  oral, 645–648
    HIV infection and, 647, 647t
    pigmentation of, 648, 648t
    red macules of, 647, 647t
    sebaceous glands of, 2186
    ulcers of, 646, 646t
    white plaque of, 647, 647t
  syphilis affecting, 1707, 1707
Mucus, airway epithelium and, 371, 382
  cervical, menstrual changes in, 1298
  cystic fibrosis with, 419–420, 420
  ferning of, 1298
Muerto Canyon virus, 1805t, 1810
Mulberry molar, 1710
Müllerian ducts, anomaly of, 1296–1297
  persistent, 1291t, 1292, 1292
  puberty and, 1296–1297
  sexual differentiation and, 1284–1285, 1285, 1286
Müllerian inhibiting substance, 1326
Multidrug resistance, 1057t, 1057–1058
Multiple endocrine neoplasia, 1374–1375
  calcitonin in, 1374–1375, 1375t
  marfanoid habitus with, 1375
  pheochromocytoma in, 1254, 1374
  treatment of, 1375
Multiple linear regression, 85, 85t
Multiple logistic regression, 85, 85t
Multiple myeloma, 962–965
  amyloidosis with, 962t, 963
  benign gammopathy vs., 960–961, 961, 961t
  diagnostic criteria for, 963
  epidemiology of, 960, 961, 961t, 962
  etiology of, 962
  incidence of, 1009, 1013t
  kidney and, 962t, 963
  laboratory findings in, 962, 963
  manifestations of, 962, 962t
  neuropathy and, 963
  osteosclerosis with, 965
  prognosis in, 964
  radiology findings in, 962, 963
  smoldering, 960, 964
  treatment of, 963–964
  tumor marker of, 1022t, 1023–1024
Multiple organ system failure, 474–477
  critical care setting and, 474–477
  respiratory distress with, 474–477
  septic shock with, 496, 496t, 498, 500t
Multiple sclerosis, 2106–2112
  clinical features of, 2108–2111, 2109t, 2110t
  definition of, 2106
  diagnostic criteria for, 2109t, 2109–2110
  differential diagnosis of, 2109t, 2109–2110, 2110t
  epidemiology of, 2107
  etiology of, 2106–2107
  imaging in, 1967, 1967, 2107–2108, 2108
  incidence and prevalence of, 2107
  laboratory findings in, 2107
  pathology of, 2107
  plaques of, 1967, 1967
  treatment of, 2110–2111

Multivariate analysis, 85, 85t
Mumps, 1768–1769
  clinical manifestation of, 1768–1769
  diagnosis of, 1769
  epidemiology of, 1768
  immune response to, 1769
  immunization for, 43t, 44–45, 1769
  orchitis caused by, 1336, 1769
  pathogenesis of, 1768
  treatment of, 1769
  virology of, 1768
Münchhausen's syndrome, 2006
Muramic acid, bacterial, 1556, *1556*
Murine typhus, 1727t, 1728t, 1729–1730
Murmurs, 168
  aortic stenosis (valvular) with, 319, 320
  aortic valve regurgitation, 322, 322t
  Carey-Coombs, 1592t, 1593, 1593t
  "machinery," 279
  mitral stenosis with, 323, 323t
  rheumatic fever causing, 1592t, 1592–1593, 1593t
Murray Valley encephalitis, 1806t, 1814
Muscle, **2158–2173**
  aging effects in, 16t, 16–17
  airway, 377, *377*
  antibodies to, 767, 778t
  arterial, 291
    fibrous plaque of, 291, *292*, 294, *295*
  assessment of, 2158–2161, 2160t
  atrial natriuretic hormone affecting, *1195*, 1195–1196
  atrophy of, 2051t, 2052–2054
    distal, 2053
    facioscapulohumeral, 2053
    lateral sclerosis with, 2052t, 2053–2054
    proximal, 2053
    scapuloperoneal, 2053
    spinal, 2052t, 2053
    syringomyelia with, 2055
  biopsy of, 2161
  botulism affecting, 1635–1636
  cataplectic, 1984
  contracture of, 2159
    rigid spine with, 2163
  cramps of. See *Cramp(s)*.
  destruction of, 2161
  dystrophy of. See *Muscular dystrophy*.
  electromyography of, 2160–2162
    nerve conduction testing in, 1961–1962, 1962t
  enteric, *680*, 680–681
  enzymes of, 2160
    deficiencies in, 2165–2167, 2166t
  fasciculation (twitching) of, 2159, 2160t, 2162
  fibers of, *175*, 213, 2158
    ragged red, 2167
    very large, 2162
  flaccid, 1635
  gastrointestinal, *680*, 680–688, *682*
  glycogen stores of, 1083
  hair follicle erection by, *2185*, 2186
  hypertrophy of, 2159
  inflammation of, 2163–2165, 2164t. See also *Myositis*.
  joint anatomy and, *1441*
  juxtaglomerular, 520
  laboratory testing of, 2160t, 2160–2161
  lymphangioleiomyomatosis role of, 395
  metabolic disorders of, 2165–2170
  motor unit and, 2158, 2171–2173
  movement disorders and. See *Movement disorders*.
  neurologic disease affecting, 2051t, 2052–2054
  pain related to. See *Myalgia*.
  paralysis of. See *Palsy; Paralysis*.
  paraneoplastic effects in, 1018, 1027t, 1029
  physiology of, 2158
  polyarteritis nodosa of, 1493
  relaxants, 507. See also *Benzodiazepines; Diazepam*.
  respiratory, 377, 442–443
  rigidity of, 2042
  rippling disorder of, 2181
  sarcoidosis of, *432*, 433
  slow relaxation of, 2181
  strength testing of, 2159–2160
  tetanus affecting, 1637
  tone of, 2159–2160
  weakness in. See *Weakness*.
  Wegener's granulomatosis affecting, 1495t, 1496, 1496t

Muscular dystrophy, **2161–2163**
  Becker, 2160t, 2161
  classification of, 2161t
  congenital, 2161t
  distal, 2162
  Duchenne, 2160t, 2161
    heart affected by, 359
  Emery-Dreifuss, 2160t, 2162
  facioscapulohumeral, 2160t, 2162
  genetics of, 2159t, 2160t, 2161, 2162, 2163
  limb-girdle, 2160t, 2162
  oculopharyngeal, 2162–2163
  sleep apnea with, 1984t
  treatment and prevention of, 2163
  X-linked, 2162
Mushrooms, 508, 508t
  food poisoning due to, 740
  hepatotoxicity due to, 772
Mussels, food poisoning due to, 740
Mustard gas, carcinogenicity of, 1016t
Mutation, 135–136
  frameshift, 136
  HIV organism with, *1845*, 1884t
  McCune-Albright syndrome due to, 1347
  mechanisms of, 135–136
  membrane transport proteins with, 143–145, 144t, 147t
  missense, 135
    Mennonite, 1112t
  muscular dystrophy with, 2161
  new, 138–139
  oncogenic, 1011–1012
  paternal age effect in, 138–139
  pheochromocytoma due to, 1254
  sickle syndromes and, 883, *891*
  somatic, 135
  thalassemia sydromes and, 880–881
  types of, 135–136
Mutilation (self), 1116
Mutism, 1992
  aphasia with, 1992
  frontal lobe damage with, 1988, 1988t
Myalgia, 2159. See also *Fibromyalgia (fibrositis)*.
  at rest, 2159
  eosinophilia with, 2164–2165
  exercise with, 2159
  rheumatologic, 1498t, 1498–1500, 1499t
  spine related to, 2142
  tryptophan causing, 2164–2165
Myasthenia, **2171–2173**
  Eaton-Lambert syndrome with, 1018, 1028, 2173
  paraneoplastic, 1017–1018, 1028
Myasthenia gravis, 1017–1018, 2171–2173
  clinical features of, 2171–2172
  diagnosis of, 1018, 2172
  pathophysiology of, 1018, 1438, 2171
  thymus gland in, 1438
  transient neonatal, 2172
  treatment of, 1018, 2172–2173
Myc oncogene, 1036t
Mycetoma, **1834–1835**
  clinical features of, 1835, 1835t
  diagnosis of, 1835
  epidemiology of, 1834, 1835
  etiologic organism in, 1834–1835, 1835t
  pathogenesis and pathology of, 1835
  prognosis in, 1835
  treatment of, 1835
Mycobacterial disease, **1683–1696**
  AIDS/HIV with, *1861*, 1861t, 1861–1862
  antimicrobial therapy in, 1687t, 1690–1691
  arthritis of, 1475, 1685t
  avium-intracellulare, 1690, 1690t
  fortuitum, 1690t, 1691
  haemophilum, 1690t, 1691
  kansasii, 1690t, 1690–1691
  leprosy. See *Leprosy*.
  scrofulaceum, 1690t
  tabulation of pathogens in, 1690t
  tuberculosis. See *Tuberculosis*.
  xenopi, 1690t, 1691
Mycoplasmal infections, **1576–1579**
  antibiotic susceptibility of, 1578t, 1578–1579
  arginini, 1737t
  clinical features of, 1576–1578, *1577*
  fermentans, 1576t, 1578t, 1578–1579
  genitalium, 1576t, 1578, 1578t
  hominis, 1576t, 1578, 1578t
  pathogens in, 1576, 1576t, 1737t
  pneumonia in, **1576–1579**, 1737t

Mycoplasmal infections *(Continued)*
  cold agglutinins with, 1577, *1577*
  differential diagnosis of, 1577t
  laboratory findings in, *1577*
  radiography in, 1576, *1577*
  sexual transmission of, 1697, 1697t
  treatment of, 1578t, 1578–1579
  urealyticum, 1576t, 1578, 1578t, 1697, 1697t
  zoonoses and, 1737t
Mycoses. See *Fungal infection(s)*; specific organisms and infections.
Mycosis fungoides, 2202t
  paraneoplastic, 1031t, 1031–1032
  rash of, 2202t
Mycotoxins, ergot, 740
Mydriasis, 2018, *2018*
  diagnostic evaluation using, 2018, *2018*, 2176–2178
  glaucoma precipitated by, 2176–2178
Myelin, **2106–2113**
  diseases affecting, 2106t
  leukodystrophies affecting, 2112–2113
  multiple sclerosis affecting, 2106–2111
  myelitis related to, 2111–2112, 2112t
  nerve conduction role of, 2107
Myelitis, herpes zoster causing, 2094
  poliovirus causing, 1786–1787, 1787t, 2091–2092
  transverse, 2111–2112, 2112t
Myeloblasts, *818*, *820*, *821*, 898t
Myelodysplastic syndrome, 836–837
  clinical features of, 836
  diagnosis of, *832*, *834*, 836t, 836–837
  etiology of, 836, 836t
  incidence of, 836
  treatment of, 837
Myelography, 1964
Myeloid metaplasia, 924–925
  agnogenic, 924t, 924–925
  clinical features of, 924t, 924–925
  pathogenesis of, 924
  treatment of, 925
Myelolipoma, adrenal, 1257
Myeloma. See *Multiple myeloma*.
Myelopathy, 2111–2112, 2112t
  AIDS/HIV with, 1856t, 1858
  paraneoplastic, 1027t, 1028–1029
  radiation injury with, 1030
  subacute necrotic, 1028–1029
  T-lymphotropic virus (HTLV) in, 1781t, 1782, 2099–2100
  transverse, 2111–2112, 2112t
  tumors causing, *2146*, 2146–2148
Myeloperoxidase, deficiency of, 905t, 906, *906*, 1540–1541
  phagocytosis role of, 897, 898t, *899*, 900, 900, 1540–1541
  disorder affecting, 905t, 906, *906*, 1540–1541
Myelopoiesis, 817–821, *818–821*, 898t, 908–915. See also *Erythropoiesis; Hematopoiesis*.
Myeloproliferative disorder(s), **922–940**
  myelodysplastic syndrome and, 836–837
  myelogenous leukemia as, 925–931, 936–940
  myeloid metaplasia as, 924–925
  polycythemia vera as, 921–922
  thrombocytosis as, **922–940**, 985
Myiasis, 1949–1950
  fly larvae in, 1949–1950
Myoadenylate deaminase, 1116
  deficiency of, 1116–1117
  purine metabolism and, 1116–1117
Myocardial depressant factor, 498
  shock and, 484
Myocardial infarction, **301–315**
  anticoagulant therapy in, 119, 311–312, 312t
  arrhythmia with, after, 313, *315*
    before, 304, *305*
    bradycardic, 313
    supraventricular, 313
    tachycardic, 304, *305*, 313, *315*
  calcification of, *184*, 186
  causes of, 301–302, 302t
  diagnosis of, 304–308, 305t, 306t
  ECG in, 306, 306t
    high-resolution, 314, *315*
    Q wave of, 302, *305*, 306, 314–315, *315*
  echocardiography in, 307, *307*
  etiology of, 301–302, 302t
  incidence of, 301
  macromolecular markers of, 306–307
  mortality in, 304, *304*, *305*, 315
  pain of, 301

Myocardial infarction (Continued)
pathology of, 302
pathophysiology of, 303–304
pericarditis following, 337, 337t
PET scan in, 307, *308, 309*
prognosis in, 303–304, *304, 305,* 315, *315*
risk factors for, 302, 302t
shock with, 486t, 486–487
signs and symptoms of, 304–306, 305t, 306t
silent, 304
size measurement of, 304, *304*
smoking associated with, 34t, 34–35, 36t
sudden death in, 304, *305, 315*
treatment of, 308–315
angioplasty in, 312t, 312–313
antiarrhythmic, 313
calcium channel block in, 309–310
CCU in, 309–314, 310t, 312t
convalescent, 314–315, *315*
hemodynamic subsets in, 310t, 313–314
infarct size limitation in, 310, 310t
invasive vs. conservative, 305–306, 312, 312t
neuromuscular block in, 309, 310t
pain management in, 309–310, 310t
prehospital phase of, 308–309
sedation in, 309–310, 310t
step-down unit in, 314, *315*
thrombolytic, 116, 117t, 310–311, *311*, 312t
Myocarditis, 328–331
AIDS/HIV patient with, 329, 329t, 1876–1877, 1877t
candidal, 1829
Chagas' disease with, 329–330
chemotherapeutic agents causing, 330–331
enterovirus causing, 1787t, 1788–1789
giant-cell, 330
hypersensitive, 330
infarction with, 306t
lymphocytic, 330
nutritional deficiency in, 331
pheochromocytoma in, 1256
rheumatic fever causing, *1592,* 1592t, 1592–1593, 1593t
toxoplasmosis in, 330
transplant rejection with, 330
trypanosomiasis with, 1901, *1902*
viral, 328–329
Myocardium. See also *Cardiomyopathy.*
Aschoff nodules in, 1592, *1592*
blood flow to, 178–179, *179.* See also *Coronary artery(ies).*
calcification in, *184,* 186
calcium metabolism in, 174, *175*
cell morphology in, *175*
conduction velocity in, 190
contractility of, 174–177, 213–216
afterload, 176–177, *177,* 212t, 214–215
digitalis effect on, *225,* 225–226
energetics of, 212t, 216
Frank-Starling, *175,* 214
impedance with, 212t, *215*
outflow resistance and, 176t, *214,* 214–215, *215*
preload, 175–176, *176,* 212t, 214, *214*
pressures and volumes in, 175–176, 176t, *176–178,* 214–216
failing heart and, *214–216,* 215–216
functioning of, 174, *175,* 213–216
hibernating, 303
hypertrophic, 215–216, *216*
sudden death related to, 254t, 255, 335
inflammation of. See *Myocarditis.*
ischemic. See *Angina pectoris; Ischemic heart disease; Myocardial infarction.*
Laplace relationship and, 215, 216
oxygen consumption in, 178, 296, *296,* 302t, *309*
perfusion imaging of, *201,* 201–202, *202*
radionuclide studies of, *201,* 201–202, *202*
refractoriness in, 190
stunned, 303
Myoclonus, 2050
causes of, 2050
Creutzfeldt-Jakob, 2103
drug-induced, 2050t
metabolic encephalopathy with, 1973
multifocal, 1973
myopathy causing, 2167
ocular, 2020
palatal, 2050
segmental, 2050
seizure with, *2115,* 2116, 2117
sleep-related, 1983, 2050

Myofascial pain, 2037. See also *Myalgia.*
trigger points of, 2037
Myofibrils, *175,* 213, 2158
Myoglobinuria, 2159, 2169–2170
causes of, 2169–2170
treatment of, 2170
Myokymia, 2170–2171
facial, 2170
Myopathy, 2158–2173. See also *Cardiomyopathy.*
AIDS/HIV patient with, 1878t, 1879
alcoholic, 2040, 2169
amyloid, 2170
branchial, 2170
congenital, 2161t, 2163, 2163t
diagnostic approach in, 2158–2161, 2161t
diaphragmatic, 442
endocrine, 2167–2168
enzyme deficiencies in, 2165–2167, 2166t
genetics of, 2160t
glycogen storage disease in, 2165
hereditary, 2161–2163. See also *Muscular dystrophy.*
history and examination in, 2158–2159, 2161t
hypothyroidism with, 1238, 1238t
inflammatory, 1500–1503, 2163–2165, 2164t
autoantibodies in, 1501t, 1502
clinical manifestations of, 1501–1502
criteria for, 1500t
definition of, 1500, 1500t
differential diagnosis of, 1502–1503, 1503t
forearm ischemic exercise test for, 1503t
laboratory findings in, 1500t, 1501t, 1502
pathogenesis of, 1500, 1501t
pathology findings in, 1500–1501
polymyositis with, 1502
prognosis in, 1502
treatment of, 1503
intestinal, 684t, 684–685, *685*
lipid disorders with, 2165–2166, 2166t
metabolic, 2160t, 2165–2170, 2166t
myoadenylate deaminase deficiency causing, 1116
nemaline (rod), 2163, 2163t
neuropathy vs., 2160t
paraneoplastic, 1018, 1027t, 1029
renal failure with, 557t, 559, 562
symptoms and signs of, 2159–2161, 2160t
systemic sclerosis causing, 1487
toxic, 2168–2169
Wegener's granulomatosis causing, 1495t, 1496, 1496t
Myophosphorylase deficiency, 1083, 1083t
Myopia, 2174
Myositis, 2163–2165, 2164t. See also *Polymyositis.*
autoantibodies specific to, 1501, 1501t, 2164
candidal, 1829
inclusion body, 1500, 1501, 2164
leptospirosis with, 1720
myopathy due to, 2163–2165, 2164t
myopathy vs., 1501, 1501t
ossificans, 2165
streptococcal, 1588
tryptophan causing, 2164–2165
Myotonia, 2160, 2160t
action, 2160
congenital, 2168–2169, 2181
dystrophic, 2162
hyperkalemia with, 542, 2168–2169
neural, 2170–2171
percussion, 2160
Myxedema, 1237
coma of, 1239–1240, 1240t
definition of, 1237
nonpitting edema of, 1237, 2212
skin affected by, 1237, 2212
treatment of, 1239–1240, 1240t
Myxoma, cardiac, 357–358
Myxovirus, 1750
pharyngitis caused by, 1749–1751, 1750t, 1751t

N

NAD (nicotinamide adenine dinucleotide), *856,* 856–857
Nadolol, 265t, 266t, 299t
Naegleria fowleri, 1915
Nafcillin, 1562t
endocarditis therapy with, 1602t, 1602–1603, 1603t
Nails, 2214–2215, 2216t
absent, 812
aging effects in, 2190
clubbing of, 2215

Nails (Continued)
defects in, 2214–2215, 2216t
fungal infection of, 2214–2215
iron deficiency affecting, 841, 1153t
psoriasis affecting, 2203
separation from bed of, 2216t
spoon, 1149t, 1153t, 2216t
striations of, 2215, 2216t
arsenic poisoning with, 70
thickened, 2214, 2215, 2216t
tumor affecting, 2215
glomus, 353
melanomatous, 2215
yellow, 2215
Nalbuphine, 51
Naloxone, 51
drug withdrawal treated with, 53, 504t, 508
Naltrexone, 51, 56
Naphthylamine, 1016t
Naproxen, 103t, 893t
Napthoquinones, 1145t
Narcolepsy, 1983–1984
clinical features of, 1983–1984, 1984t
HLA complex in, 1431t
treatment of, 1984
NARES syndrome, 1413t, 1416
NARP, 2160t, 2166t, 2167
Nasogastric tube, 643, 1169
complications related to, 1169–1171, 1170t
enteral nutrition using, 1168–1171, 1170t
gastric lavage using, 643, 645
Nasopharynx, diphtheria affecting, 1629–1630
leech infection of, 1950–1951
meningitis organisms in, 1612, 1618, *1619*
meningococcal organisms in, 1618, *1619*
tongue worm parasite in, 1950
Native Americans, lupus erythematosus in, 1476
rheumatoid arthritis in, 1459, 1460t
Natriuresis, aldosterone affecting, 514
prostaglandins causing, 527
SIADH causing, 535
volume depletion with, 514
Natriuretic hormone, 1194
atrial, 1194–1195, *1195*
half-life of, 1195
physiologic response to, *1195,* 1195–1196
receptors for, *1177,* 1178, 1195, *1195*
release stimulus for, 1194–1195, *1195*
secretion of, 1194
structure of, 1194
synthesis of, 1194
target tissues of, *1195,* 1195–1196
therapy using, 1196
vasorelaxation due to, *1195,* 1196
biologic activities of, 1194
hypertension and, 1194
sodium pump and, 1194
Natural killer cells, AIDS/HIV effect on, 1839, 1840
deficiency of, 1402t, 1402–1403, *1403*
Nausea, alcohol-related, 47–49, 48t
antimicrobials causing, 1568t
definition of, 629
pregnancy with, 787, 787t
Necator, 1934–1935
Neck, Lyme disease affecting, 1717, 1717t
pain in, 2035, 2141, 2144, 2146
rheumatoid disease affecting, 1462–1463, *1463*
Necrosis, bone affected by, 1387, 1387t
fasciitis causing, 2208
streptococcal, 1588, 1589t, 2208
fat tissue, 1507, 2211
lung. See *Lung, abscess of.*
mucormycosis with, 1833–1834
neuron vulnerability to, 2062t, 2063
retinal, 1869t, 1869–1870
toxic epidermal, 1609t, 2205
vasculitis with, 1493–1498, 2201t, 2202
Needle aspiration, breast, 1319
thyroid nodule, 1231, 1231t
Needles, AIDS/HIV precautions for, 1853, 1853t
Negishi encephalitis, 1806t
Negri bodies, 2096
Neisseria, 1697t
gonorrhoeae, 1697t, 1701. See also *Gonorrhea.*
meningitidis. See *Meningococcal infections.*
Nematodes, anisakiasis due to, 1935t, 1936
ascariasis due to, 1935, 1935t
capillariasis due to, 1935t, 1936

LXIV / INDEX

Nematodes (Continued)
drug therapy for, 1935t
enterobiasis due to, 1935, 1935t
filarial, 1939–1945, 1940t. See also Filariasis.
gnathostomiasis due to, 1935t, 1936
hookworm, 1934–1935, 1935t
larva migrans, cutaneous, 1935t, 1937
strongyloidiasis due to, 1935t, 1938–1939
toxocariasis due to, 1935t, 1936–1937
trichinosis due to, 1935t, 1937–1938
trichostrongyliasis due to, 1935t, 1936
trichuriasis due to, 1935t, 1935–1936
Neoplasia. See also Cancer; specific organs and tumors.
adrenal, 1254–1257
AIDS/HIV with, 1872–1874, 1873t
articular, 1528
bone, 1391–1392
brain. See Brain, neoplasia of.
breast, 1320–1325
cardiac, 357–358, 358
colorectal, 721–722, 724–728
dementia caused by, 1992t, 1994
environmental/occupational agents causing, 56t, 56–59
epidermal, 2208–2211
esophageal, 657
eye, 2180
fever with, 1532t
hematopoietic. See Leukemia; Myeloproliferative disorders.
hepatic, 802–805, 803t
hormone production by, 1024–1026, 1025t
hypoglycemia due to, 1280, 1281, 1281t
hypothalamic, 1200t, 1200–1201
intestinal, 721–729
large, 721–728
small, 728–729
islet cell, 1284
lung, 436–442
lymphadenopathy due to, 970t
lymphoid. See Lymphoma.
markers of. See Tumor markers.
mediastinal, 448, 448–449
myeloproliferative, 922–940
nails affected by, 2215
oral soft tissue, 648, 648t
orbital, 2180
ovarian, 1313–1315
pancreatic, 736–738
paraneoplastic syndromes with, 1017–1036. See also Paraneoplastic syndromes.
pineal, 1205
pituitary, 1207–1210, 1209t
plasma cell, 958–968
prostatic, 1341–1345, 1344–1345
pulmonary, 436–442
renal, 623–625
skin, 2209, 2209–2211, 2210
spinal cord compression by, 2146, 2146–2148
splenic, 971t, 972, 972t, 974
testicular, 1013t, 1022t, 1023, 1340
thymus gland, 1438–1439
thyroid, 1242–1245
vertigo due to, 2027
Nephritis. See also Glomerulonephritis; Pyelonephritis.
hereditary, 611–612, 612t
interstitial, 554, 580t, 580–584, 581, 582t
acute, 581–583, 582t
causes of, 581–584, 582t, 583t
chronic, 583t, 583–584
drug-induced, 99t, 581, 581–583, 582t
lupus erythematosus with, 574t, 577t, 578, 578t, 1477, 1479, 1482t
mortality rate role of, 27t
radiation, 587
Nephroblastoma, 624–625
Nephrocalcinosis, 595t
Nephrolithiasis. See Kidney stones.
Nephron, 223
ADH response in, 534
anatomy of, 223, 518
blood supply to, 223, 518, 519
calcium reabsorption in, 1353
diuretic sites of action in, 223, 224t, 532
innervation of, 223
transport in, defects of, 594–599, 595t
mechanisms of, 521t, 521–524, 522, 524, 532
Nephronophthisis, 621

Nephropathy, 580–589
absorption deficit due to, 528, 528t
AIDS/HIV with, 579, 1875–1876, 1876
analgesic, 584–585
Bartter's syndrome with, 528
diabetic, 599–602, 600, 601, 1273–1274, 1274
gouty, 1510, 1512
hemorrhagic fever with, 1798t
hereditary, 611–612, 612t
hypertension with, 607
hypokalemic, 528, 540
IgA, 575–576, 812t
light chain deposition disease and, 579
membranous, 574–575, 575
metal, 587–588
sickle cell, 608, 888–889
thrombotic microangiopathic, 579
toxic, 581, 582t, 584t, 584–589
Nephrotic syndrome, 573–575
approach to patient with, 573
ascites with, 743t, 749
atrial natriuretic hormone and, 1196
causes of, 573t, 573–575, 574t
drug-induced, 574t, 574–575, 581, 582t
edema in, 573
focal segmental sclerosis in, 574
idiopathic, 573–574, 574
immune complexes and, 573, 573t
lupus erythematosus and, 574t, 574–575
membranous change in, 574–575, 575
mesangial, 575
neoplasia and, 574t
paraneoplastic, 1020
protein loss in, 573
secondary, 573, 574t
symptoms in, 573–575
treatment of, 573–575
Nephrotoxins, 552t, 584t
antimicrobials as, 1568t
interstitial disease due to, 581, 582t, 584t, 584–589
renal failure due to, 552t, 553–554, 1568t
Nerve, block of, MI treated with, 309, 310t
pain management with, 107
conduction studies in, 1961–1962, 1962t
pain fibers of, 628
roots of. See Radiculopathy.
Nervous system, 1957–2173
aging effect on, 16t, 16–17
AIDS/HIV effects in, 1855t, 1855–1858, 1856t, 1857t
antimicrobials affecting, 1568t
approach to disorders of, 1957–1959
aspergillosis affecting, 1831
autonomic. See Autonomic nervous system; Parasympathetic nervous system; Sympathetic nervous system.
botulism effect on, 1635
cancer effects on, 1018–1019, 1027–1030
nonmetastatic and remote, 1018–1019, 1027t, 1027–1030, 1029t
cerebrovascular disease and. See Cerebrovascular disease; Stroke.
conduction studies in, 1961–1962, 1962t
consciousness disorders and, 1969–1981. See also Coma; Epilepsy; Seizures; Syncope.
copper deposition affecting, 1131
cryptococcosis affecting, 1824, 1825
cysticercosis effects on, 1926
degenerative disease of, 2050–2057, 2106–2113. See also Encephalopathy.
Alzheimer's, 1992–1994
ataxia in, 2051t, 2051–2052
autonomic, 2027–2030
motor neuron disease in, 2052t, 2052–2054, 2054t
posture and movement in, 2052t, 2052–2055, 2054t
seizures and mental deficiency in, 2056–2057
weakness and wasting in, 2027–2030, 2052t, 2052–2055, 2054t
diagnostic methods for, 1958–1969
angiography in, 1964
auditory evoked potentials in, 1961
CT scan in, 1963t, 1963–1969
electroencephalography in, 1960, 1960–1961
electromyography in, 1961–1962, 1962t
lumbar puncture in, 1959, 1960t
MRI scan in, 1963t, 1963–1969
positron emission tomography in, 1961
radiography in, 1963–1964

Nervous system (Continued)
visual evoked potentials in, 1961
electrical injury to, 66
endocrine system interface with, 1197, 1197–1203, 1198
enteric, 681, 681, 681t, 2010
examination of, 1959
arousal level in, 1959, 1969, 1969t
coma and, 1971t, 1973, 1973t, 1976–1977, 1977t
extrapyramidal disorders and, 2042–2043
stroke and, 2064t, 2065, 2071t, 2078t
history taking and, 1958–1959
hypertension and, 2077, 2078t, 2080
hypothyroidism affecting, 1238, 1238t
infections of, 2080–2087. See also Brain, abscess of; Encephalitis; Meningitis.
borrelial, 1717, 1719t
opportunistic, 1855t, 1855–1856
pyogenic, 2080–2083, 2081t, 2084
staphylococcal, 1608t, 1608–1609
streptococcal, 1592t, 1593
thrombogenic, 2083–2084
treponemal, 1708–1709, 2085, 2085–2087, 2086t
viral. See viruses affecting, below.
lupus erythematosus affecting, 1475t, 1479–1480, 1480t
metabolic disorders and, 2011–2013
mucopolysaccharidosis affecting, 1118
nutritional disorders of, 2039t, 2039–2041
pain management procedures and, 105–107
paraneoplastic syndromes of, 1018–1019, 1027t, 1027–1030, 1029t
parasympathetic. See Parasympathetic nervous system.
patient interview related to, 1957–1959
peripheral, 2149–2157. See also Neuropathy; Peripheral nervous system.
polyarteritis nodosa of, 1493
porphyria effects on, 1126, 1126t
radiation injury affecting, 1029t, 1029–1030
rheumatic fever affecting, 1592t, 1593
rhythms imposed by, 1184, 1199–1200
sarcoidosis of, 432, 432
seizures and. See Epilepsy; Seizures.
sympathetic. See Sympathetic nervous system.
syphilis effects on, 1708t, 1708–1709, 1712t, 2085, 2085–2087, 2086t
temperature regulation by, 1203, 1533, 2012
tumors of, 1964–1965, 1965, 1968
vascular disorders of. See Cerebrovascular disease.
viruses affecting, 1741t, 2087–2106, 2088t
AIDS/HIV, 2097–2099, 2098t
complications related to, 2103–2106
Creutzfeldt-Jakob, 2102–2103
encephalomyelitis due to, 2088t, 2088–2090
herpes simplex, 1770–1772, 1770–1772, 2092–2093, 2093
poliovirus, 1784t, 1786–1787, 1787t, 2091–2092
rabies, 2095–2096
slow infection, 2097, 2097t, 2100
Wegener's granulomatosis affecting, 1495t, 1496t
Wilson's disease and, 1131
zoonoses affecting, 1737t
Netilmicin, 1562t
Neufeld quellung reaction, 1570
Neural tube defect, 159, 159t
Neuralgia, 2035
cranial, 2035
glossopharyngeal, 2009, 2035
postherpetic, 2036, 2205
trigeminal, 2035
Neuritis, optic, 2016t, 2016–2017, 2017, 2111
multiple sclerosis and, 2111
papillitis in, 2111
retrobulbar, 2016, 2111
Neuroblastoma, skin metastases of, 1032
Neuroendocrine system, 1197, 1197–1203, 1198
Neurofibromatosis, 2056, 2209
hearing affected by, 2056
lung in, 399
thoracic, 1969
von Recklinghausen's, 2056, 2209, 2213, 2213
Neurohormones, 1183, 1197, 1197–1200
Neurolathyrism, 740
Neuroleptics, 1998t, 1999t
elderly treated with, 20–21, 2050
malignant syndrome of, 502, 2012
neurologic effects of, 1975t, 2050t
schizophrenia treated with, 1998t, 1998–1999, 1999t
side effects of, 1998, 2050t

Neurologic disease. See *Nervous system*; specific disease or structure.
Neuroma, acoustic, 2056, 2127–2128, 2128t
  MRI scan of, 2127–2128, 2128t
  multiple endocrine neoplasia with, 1035
Neuromuscular blockade, agents used in, 310t
  infarction treatment and, 310t
Neuromuscular disease, **2171–2173**
  classification of, 2171t
  definition of, 2171
  mechanisms of, 2171
  neuromyotonia in, 2170–2171
  respiratory failure caused by, 473
  sleep apnea with, 1984t
  toxic, 2173
Neuromuscular junction, **2158**
  antibodies affecting, 1018, 1028, 2171, 2171t
  drugs affecting, 2173
  paraneoplastic effects in, 1017–1018, 1027–1029
Neuromyotonia, 2170–2171
Neuron(s). See also *Nervous system*.
  aging effects in, 14, 16t
  anoxia injury to, 2062t, 2063, 2136
  catecholamine uptake by, 1253, *1253*
  enteric, 681, *681*, 681t
  epilepsy effect on, *2118*, 2119
  magnocellular, 1221, *1222*
  pain, 628
  peripheral neuropathy affecting, 2150
  Pick's bodies in, 1995
  pituitary gland stimulation by, 1197, *1197*
  venom affecting, 1951–1956, *1954*
Neuronopathy, motor, 1028
  paraneoplastic, 1028, 1029
  sensory, 1029
Neuropathy, **2149–2157**
  AIDS/HIV with, 1856t, 1858
  alcoholic, 2039t, 2040, 2156
  amyloid, 967, *967*, 2007, 2154
  anatomy and, 2150
  antimicrobials causing, 1568t
  autonomic, 2007, 2007t, 2008t
  demyelinating, 2151t, 2151–2152
    chronic inflammatory, 2151t, 2152
  diabetic, 1274–1275, 1275t, 2154t, 2154–2155
  drugs and chemicals causing, 2156, 2156t
  entrapment, 2157
  gammopathy with, 961
  Guillain-Barré, 2151t, 2151–2152
  hepatic encephalopathy with, 797–798, 798t
  hereditary, 2153–2154, 2154t
  hospital-associated, 2156
  infectious disease causing, 2156–2157
  inflammatory, 2151t, 2151–2152, 2153
  intestinal motility and, 685
  lead poisoning with, 68
  leprous, 1694, *1695*, 2157
  lupus erythematosus with, 1480
  multifocal, 2151t, 2152, 2155
  muscle weakness due to, 1503t
  myeloma causing, 963
  myopathy vs., 2160t
  nutritional, 2039t, 2040–2041
  occupational exposure causing, 58t
  ocular, 2018–2020, *2020*, 2020t
  optic, diabetic, 1273, 2181–2182
    Leber's, 2167, 2178
    neoplasia with, 1028, 1030
  paraneoplastic, 1027t, 1028–1030
  pathophysiology of, 2150
  porphyric, 1126, 2155
  radiation injury causing, 1030
  renal failure with, 557t, 559, 562
  rheumatoid arthritis with, 1462, *1462*, *1463*, 1464
  sensory, 2153
    AIDS/HIV and, 2156–2157
    cancer and, 2153
  tetanus causing, 1636–1637
  toxic, 58t, 2156, 2156t
  uremic, 557t, 559, 562, 2155
  vasculitic, 2153
  venom causing, 1953–1956, *1954*, 1954t
  vitamin B₁₂ deficiency causing, 845, 848, 848t
  weakness due to, 2150–2152, 2151t
  Wegener's granulomatosis causing, 1495t, 1496t
Neuropeptides, asthma role of, 377
  opioid, endogenous, *1186*, 1186–1187, 1187t
  shock and, 481–482
Neurophysins, 1221–1222
Neurosis. See also *Psychiatric disorders*.

Neurosis *(Continued)*
  anxiety, 2004t, 2004–2005
  depressive, 2001t, 2001–2002
Neurotoxins, chemotherapy agents as, 2156, 2156t
  marine organisms with, 1953–1956, *1954*, 1954t
  snake venom with, 1951t, 1951–1953, 1952t
Neurotransmitters. See also *Acetylcholine*; *Dopamine*; *Epinephrine*; *Norepinephrine*; *Serotonin*.
  enteric, 681, 681t
  hepatic encephalopathy role of, 797, 797t
Neutropenia, 831t, **909–914**
  AIDS/HIV patient with, 1871
  antimicrobials in, 1538t, 1539t, 1543–1548, 1544t, 1568t
  bone marrow abnormalities in, 909–910, *909–911*
  bronchiectasis with, 418t
  cancer patient with, 1049–1050
  cell count in, 908, 911, *913*
  clinical manifestations of, *910*, 910–911, 1546t
  compromised host and, 1537–1548, 1538t, 1539t, 1544t
  diagnosis of, *911*, 911–912, *913*
  drug-induced, 909, 911t
  etiology of, 909–910, *909–911*, 911t
  febrile patient with, 1538t, 1539t, 1543–1548, 1544t
  Felty's syndrome causing, 912
  pathophysiology of, 909–910, *909–911*, 911t
  patient evaluation algorithm for, *913*
  treatment of, 912–914, 1050
Neutrophilia, **915–918**
  causes of, 916, 916t
  diagnosis of, 916–917, *918*
  leukemia and, 927
  pathophysiology of, 915–916, *916*
  Sweet's syndrome with, 1019
Neutrophils, 817–818, **897–906**. See also *Leukocytes*.
  adhesion of, 897–898, *899*
    disorder of, 902–904, *903*, 904t, 905t, 906t
      rheumatic disease and, 1448–1450, *1449*, *1450*
      vasculitis role of, *1449*, 1449–1450, *1450*
  arachidonic acid metabolites and, *1188*, *1190*, 1190–1191
  aspirin effect on, 114–115
  band, *912*
  chemotaxis of, 899, *899*, 1451, *1451*, *1452*
    disorder of, 902, *903*, 904t, 905t
  count of, elevated, 916, 918
    reduced, 908, 911
  cutaneous inflammation role of, 2190
  decreased. See *Neutropenia*.
  degranulation abnormalities of, 904, 904t, 905t
  distribution of, *818*, 898t, *909*, 911, *916*
  evaluation algorithm for, *903*
  glucocorticoid effect on, 108–109, 109t
  gout role of, 1510, *1512*
  granules of, 897, 898t, *1451*, *1452*
  hypersegmented, 825t, 847, *847*
  immunomodulation by, 901, *901*, *1451*, 1451–1452, *1452*
  increased. See *Neutrophilia*.
  kinetics of, *818*, 898t
  lupus erythematosus role of, *1450*, 1450–1451, *1451*
  marginated vs. circulating, 909, *909*, 910
  maturation of, 817–819, *818–821*, 897, 898, *917*
    abnormalities in, 909–910, *909–911*, *916*
  mediators released by, *1450*, 1450–1451, *1451*
  microbicidal activity of, 897, *899*, 900, *900*
    disorders affecting, *903*, 904t, 904–906, 905t
  nuclear dust of, 2202
  phagocytic function of, 897–900, *899*, *900*
    disorders affecting, 902–906, 904t, 905t, 906t
  rheumatoid arthritis role of, *1449–1452*, *1450–1451*
  rolling of, 898, *899*
  structure of, 897, 898t, *899*, *912*, *1451*
  synovitis role of, *1460*
  toxic granulation of, 916, *918*, 1451, *1451*
Nevus, blue rubber bleb, 721
  compound, 2210
  flammeus, 2211
  intradermal, 2210, *2210*
  junctional, 2210
  melanoma relation to, 2210–2211
  port-wine angioma, 2056
Nezelof's syndrome, enzyme deficiency in, 1402t, 1405
  immunodeficiency of, 1402t, 1405
Niacin, assessment of, 1146t
  deficiency of, 1146t, 2040
  neurologic effects of, 2040
  parenteral, 1172t
  physiology of, 1146t, 1151t, 2040

Niacin *(Continued)*
  RDA for, 1140t
  toxicity of, 1146t
Nicardipine, dosage for, 265t, 270t, 300t
  side effects of, 300t
Nickel, 72
  carcinogenicity of, 72, 1016t
  poisoning due to, 71, 72
    clinical manifestations of, 72
    etiology of, 72
    treatment of, 72
Niclosamide, 1923t, 1924t
Nicotinamide adenine dinucleotide (NAD), 856, 856–857
Nicotinamide deficiency, 596
Nicotine. See also *Smoking*.
  addiction to, 34
  drug abuse with, 55, 56t
  gum with, 36, 55, 56t
  patch with, 36, 55, 56t
  pharmacology of, 55
  replacement therapy using, 36
Nicotinic acid. See *Niacin*.
Niemann-Pick disease, **1098–1099**
  clinical manifestations of, 1098–1099
  diagnosis of, 1099
  genetics of, 1096t, 1098
  lymphadenopathy due to, 970t
  pathology in, *1097*, 1098
  splenomegaly in, 971t, 972, 1096t, 1098
  treatment of, 1099
  type A, 1096t, 1098–1099
  type B, 1096t, 1098–1099
  type C, 1098, 1099
  type D, 1098, 1099
Nifedipine, dosage for, 265t, 300t
  side effects of, 300t
  smoking interaction with, 36t
Night blindness, malabsorption in, 699t
  vitamin A deficiency with, 699t, 1145t, 1153t
Night terrors, 1983, 1983t
Nikolsky's sign, 2192, 2205
  bullae and, 2192
  elicitation of, 2192
Nipple, 1317
  accessory, 1317
  discharge from, 1318
    galactorrheic, 1318, 1318t
    postmenopausal, 1318
    serous or bloody, 1318
  pubertal change in, 1303t
  suckling of, oxytocin release by, 1223
  Tanner stages for, 1303, 1303t
Nitrates, angina pectoris treated with, 298, 299t
  methemoglobinemia caused by, 876t, 876–877
Nitric oxide, asthma role of, 377
  sepsis and, 498
Nitrites, cyanide toxicity treated with, 504t, 508
  methemoglobinemia caused by, 876t, 876–877
  poisoning due to, 504t, 508
  urinary, 512t
Nitroblue tetrazolium test, 905
Nitrofurantoin, 1562t
  hepatotoxicity of, 773
Nitrogen, partial pressure of, 375, 375t
Nitrogen dioxide, inhalation of, 404
  lung irritation due to, 404
Nitrogen mustard, chemotherapy using, 1042t
  Hodgkin's disease and, 952t, 953
  resistance to, 1058, 1058t
Nitroglycerin, angina pectoris treated with, 298, 299t
  dosage for, 229t
  shock treated with, 494
  vasodilatation using, 229t, 229–230
Nitropropane, 772
Nitroprusside, dosage for, 229t
  hypertension treated with, 270t
  shock treated with, 494
  side effects of, 270t
  vasodilatation using, 229t, 229–230
Nitrosamines, smoke containing, 34, 36
Nitrosurea, adverse effects of, 397t
  chemotherapy using, 1039t, 1042
  lung disease induced by, 397, 397t
  renal function and, 587
  resistance to, 1058, 1058t
Nitrous oxide, inhalation of, 55
Nits, 1945–1946

Nocardiosis, 1676–1677, 1834–1835
  clinical manifestations of, 1677, 1835
  epidemiology of, 1676, 1835
  mycetoma with, 1834–1835, 1835t
  pathogenesis of, 1676–1677, 1835
  treatment of, 1677, 1735
Nocturia, elderly affected by, 16t
  heart failure with, 217
Nodules, 2208–2211, 2216t
  acrodermatitis chronica atrophicans, 1717
  Aschoff, 1592, 1592
  bartonellosis, 1682
  benign, 2208t, 2208–2209, 2210
    vs. malignant, 2208t, 2210t
  Bouchard's, 1520
  carcinomatous (skin), 2209, 2209–2210
  dermatofibroma, 2210
  disease associations of, 1462t, 2191t, 2216t
  drug-induced, 2219t, 2219–2220
  erythema nodosum leprosum, 1693, 1694, 1696
  farcy, 1667
  glanders, 1667
  Heberden's, 1518, 1519t, 1520
  inflammatory, 2211
  Kaposi's sarcoma, 1032–1033, 1033t
  Kimmelstiel-Wilson, 257, 569, 578, 600
  lipoid dermatoarthritis with, 1526
  lupus erythematosus with, 1478
  malignant, 2208t, 2209–2211, 2210t
    vs. benign, 2208t, 2210t
  metastases causing, 1030–1031, 1031t
  myocardial, 1592, 1592
  nonpigmented, 2208t, 2208–2210
  Osler's, 1599, 1600t
  panniculitis with, 1507–1508
  paraneoplastic, 1030–1031, 1031t
  pigmented, 2210t, 2210–2211
  polyarteritis nodosa with, 1492, 1493
  pulmonary, coccidioidal, 1819, 1820
  reticulohistiocytosis with, 1526
  rheumatic fever with, 1592, 1592, 1593, 1594
  rheumatoid disease with, 1462t, 1463, 1464
  Sister Mary Joseph's, 1030
  subcutaneous, 1462t, 1507–1508, 1593, 1594
  thyroid. See Thyroid gland, nodules of.
  verruga peruana, 1682
  Virchow's, 678
  xanthomatous, 2211
Noise, hearing loss due to, 2022
  occupational exposure to, 58t
Nonparoxysmal junctional tachycardia, 242, 242
  carotid massage in, 235t
  clinical features of, 242
  treatment of, 237t, 238t, 242
Nonsteroidal anti-inflammatory agents. See Anti-inflammatory agents, nonsteroidal.
Nonthyroidal illness syndrome, 1231
  diagnosis of, 1231
  thyroid hormone values in, 1230t, 1231
  variants of, 1231
Noonan syndrome, 160t, 160–161, 1335
  clinical features of, 160t, 160–161
Norepinephrine, 1253–1257. See also Catecholamines.
  alpha vs. beta receptors and, 1253–1254
  anxiety related to, 2004
  autonomic system role of, 1253
  laboratory tests for, 1255–1256
  metabolism of, 1253, 1253
  neuron uptake of, 1254t, 1254–1256
  pheochromocytoma and, 1254–1256
  plasma levels of, 1253, 1255
  shock and, 492t, 492–493
  storage and release of, 1253
  synthesis of, 1253
Norfloxacin, 1562t
  diarrhea therapy with, 1658, 1658t
Norimipramine, 106t
North Asian tick-borne rickettsiosis, 1732
Nortriptyline, 2000t, 2001
Norwalk virus, 1793–1797, 1795t
  diagnosis of, 1796
  diarrhea and, 1795t, 1795–1796
  epidemiology of, 1794, 1795t
  treatment of, 1796
Nose, airway resistance due to, 1414
  bleeding of, 1951
  hair follicles of, 2186, 2187
  inflammation affecting. See Rhinitis; Sinusitis.

Nose (Continued)
  inner passageways of, 1414
  leech infestation of, 1950–1951
  mucormycosis affecting, 1833
  "saddle," syphilitic, 1710
  septum of, cocaine effect on, 50, 51
  turbinates of, 1414, 1833
"No-see-um" insect, 1947
Nosocomial infections. See Infections, hospital-acquired.
Notochord, 2131
NSAIDs. See Anti-inflammatory agents, nonsteroidal.
Nuclear dust, 2202
Nuclear medicine techniques. See Radionuclide studies.
Nucleic acids. See DNA (deoxyribonucleic acid); RNA (ribonucleic acid).
Nucleocapsid, 1830
Nucleolus, 1457t
Nucleoside analogues, 773, 773t
Nucleus(i), anterior, 1183
  Barrington's, 2010
  cellular, antibodies to, 1457t, 1457–1458, 1476t, 1481t
    "caterpillar," 1592, 1592
    hormone receptors in, 1180–1181, 1181
    myocardial, 1592, 1592
    "owl-eye," 1592, 1592
  dorsomedial, 1183
  hypothalamic, 1183, 1222
  neurohypophyseal, 1183, 1221–1222, 1222
  Onuf's, 2010
  paraventricular, 1183, 1221–1222, 1222
  posterior, 1183
  suprachiasmatic, 1204, 1204–1205
    circadian pacemaker role of, 1204–1205
    melatonin regulation by, 1204, 1204–1205
    vasopressin in, 1221
  supraoptic, 1183, 1221–1222, 1222
  ventromedial, 1183
Nutcracker esophagus, 655t, 656–657
Nutmeg, 508, 508t
Nutrition, 1139–1175. See also Diet; Food.
  absorption in, 695–697, 696t, 697, 698
  disorders of. See Malabsorption.
  age and, 1140t, 1141t
  assessment of, 1151–1154
    body weight in, 1152, 1152t
    physical examination in, 1152–1153, 1153t
    serum protein levels in, 1153–1154, 1156t, 1157
    triceps skinfold in, 1153, 1153t
  attitudes toward, 1139–1141, 1141t
  calorie requirements related to, 1154
  cancer prevention using, 1010, 1016–1017, 1139–1143, 1143t
  deficiency states of. See Malnutrition.
  energy expenditure related to, 1154, 1154t
  enteral, 1168–1171
    complications of, 1169–1171, 1170t
    decision tree for, 1157, 1157, 1170
    formulas for, 1168, 1169t
    indications for, 1168, 1168t
    order and protocol for, 1170t
    protein-energy malnutrition and, 1154, 1157, 1157
  food group pyramid for, 1142, 1143
  gynecomastia role of, 1331
  inflammatory bowel disease and, 710, 710t, 715
  mortality rate role of, 1143t
  nervous system affected by, 2039t, 2039–2041
  parenteral, 1170–1175
    complications of, 1174–1175
    composition and content of, 1171–1172, 1172t, 1173t
    decision tree for, 1157, 1170
    definition of, 1171
    delivery methods for, 1172–1174
    indications for, 1172–1173
    monitoring of, 1174
    protein-energy malnutrition and, 1154, 1157
    volume-restricted, 1174
  preventive care using, 29–31, 30t, 1139–1143, 1141t
  requirements of, 1140t, 1141t, 1142
    RDAs for, 1140t, 1141t, 1141–1143
  shock patient and, 495
  trace elements in, 1148t–1150t. See also specific element; Trace elements.
  vitamins in, 1140t, 1141t, 1145t–1148t. See also Vitamin(s).
Nuts, dietary, 1142
Nystagmus, 2019–2020
  central, 2020t

Nystagmus (Continued)
  congenital, 2019–2020
  gaze-evoked, 2020
  paroxysmal, 2020t
  peripheral, 2020t
  rebound, 2020
  spontaneous, 2019, 2020t
  vestibular, 2024–2025
Nystatin, candidiasis treated with, 1829
  vaginitis treated with, 1829

O

Oasthouse disease, 144t
Oatmeal bath preparation, 2193
Obesity, 1161–1167
  adipocyte role in, 1163, 1167
  atherosclerosis and, 293–294
  clinical effects of, 1164–1165
  Cushing's syndrome with, 1165, 1216, 1217, 1247, 1247t
  definition of, 1161, 1161–1162, 1162, 1163t
  diabetes mellitus with, 1258t, 1266t, 1266–1267
  diet and, 1141, 1143t
  diseases associated with, 27t, 30t
  endocrine effects of, 1165–1166
  etiology of, 1162–1163
  ear of, 1158, 1159t, 1160
  hypothalamic defect and, 1203, 2012–2013
  lung volume reduction in, 376t
  mortality rate affected by, 1165, 1165t
  pathophysiology of, 1163–1164, 2012–2013
  prevention of, 1167
  psychological effects of, 1165
  risk factor role of, 27t, 30t, 1165t
  treatment of, 1166–1167
    behavior modification in, 1166
    diet in, 1166
    drug therapy in, 1166
    exercise in, 1166, 1166t
    surgery in, 1167
  upper body vs. lower body, 1164, 1165
  weight regain in, 1167
Occipital lobes, 1985, 1986, 2059
  anatomy of, 1985, 1986
  manifestations of disease of, 1985, 1987t
  tumor of, 2126t
Occult blood. See Feces, blood in.
Occupation, 56–59, 399–403
  allergic agents encountered in, 379t, 2220–2221
  asthma and, 378, 379t
  cancer and, 58t, 1009t, 1010, 1014–1015, 1016t
  dermatitis related to, 379t, 2220–2221
  disorders related to, 56–59, 58t, 59t, 399–403
  infections and infestations of, 2221–2222
  leptospirosis exposure in, 1720, 1721
  lung disease and, 391t, 399t, 399–403, 402t, 403t
    cancer as, 56, 58t, 437, 1014
    disability assessment for, 399–400
    history for, 400
    hypersensitivity pneumonitis as, 403
    pneumoconiosis as, 391t, 399t, 399–403, 402t, 403t
  Raynaud's phenomenon due to, 347, 1484, 1485
  rickettsioses exposure in, 1727t
  toxic agents encountered in, 58t, 59t, 403t, 1016t
  types of, 58t, 59t, 402t
Ochronosis, 1108
Octopus venom, 1954t, 1955
Oculomotor nerve, 2017
Oculopneumoplethysmography, 2066
Odontoid process, 1463
Odor, breath, bronchiectasis and, 417
  esophageal cancer and, 657
  garlicky, metal poisoning with, 70, 72
  soft tissue with, 1640, 1640t
  sweat glands and, 2186
Odynophagia, 650
Ofloxacin, 1562t
  gonorrhea therapy with, 1702t
  Legionella and, 1585, 1585t
  meningococcal prophylaxis with, 1621, 1621t
Ogilvie's syndrome, 687
Ohara's disease, 1662. See also Tularemia.
Oils, aspiration pneumonia due to, 407–408
  carcinogenicity of, 1016t
  dietary content of, 1139, 1142, 1143t
  fish, 1139, 1143t
Ointments, 2194t, 2194–2196, 2195t
  active agents in, 2194t, 2194–2196, 2195t

Ointments (Continued)
    sulfur, scabies treated with, 2195
    vehicles used in, 2194t, 2194–2195
Okelbo disease, 1809–1810
Olfactory bulb agenesis, 1306
Olfactory sense. See Smell.
Oligodendroglioma, 2127–2128, 2128t, 2132
    classification of, 2126t
    MRI scan of, 2127–2128, 2128t
Oligonucleotides, antisense, 1073–1074, 1074
    triplex-forming, 1073–1074, 1074
Oligospermia, 1337
Oliguria, glomerulonephritis causing, 575
    heart failure causing, 220
    hyponatremic, 514, 514t
Olive oil, 1142, 1143
Ollier's disease, 1390
Omphalocele, 158t
Omsk hemorrhagic fever, 1798t, 1801–1802, 1806t
Onchocerciasis, 1942t, 1942–1943
Oncogene(s), **1011–1012, 1071–1077**
    abl, 1011–1012, 1036t, 1058
    alkylation resistance due to, 1059
    bcl-2, 1011–1012, 1036t, 1058
    fos, 1059
    HER, 1011–1012, 1036t
    leukemia and, 926t, 926–927, 936, 938, 1011–1012
    myc, 1036t
    ras, 1011–1012, 1059, 1076
    therapy related to, 1071–1077, 1074
Oncotaxis, 1031
Oncotic pressure, pulmonary edema and, 476, 477
    volume regulation role of, 525
Oncovin (vincristine), Hodgkin's disease and, 952t,
        953
    non-Hodgkin's lymphoma and, 945t
Onion bulb appearance, 2153, 2154t
Onuf's nucleus, 2010
Onychogryphosis, 2216t
Onycholysis, 2216t
    psoriatic arthritis with, 1471
Onychomycosis, 2214, 2216t
O'nyong-nyong virus, 1805t, 1809
Oocysts, cryptosporidial, 1910–1911, 1911, 1912
    malarial, 1893, 1893
Oocytes, 1293, 1293
    number of, 1293, 1293
    ovulation and, 1293
Ophthalmopathy. See also Eye; Vision.
    AIDS/HIV with, 1868–1870, 1869t
    Graves' disease causing, 1233, 2180
    rheumatoid arthritis with, 1464, 2178
Ophthalmoplegia, 2019
    degenerative disorders with, 2051t
    migraine with, 2032
Opioids, 51, 1975t
    accumulation of, 102
    administration of, 103t, 103–104, 104t
    adverse reactions to, 52–53, 103–105, 104t
    agonist, 51
    antagonist, 51
    definition of, 51
    diarrhea treated with, 695
    drug abuse with, 51–53, 56t, 504t, 508, 1975t
    endogenous peptide, 1186, 1186–1187, 1187t
        distribution of, 1186–1187, 1187t, 1199
        families of, 1186, 1186
        receptors for, 1187, 1199
        structure of, 1186, 1186
    equianalgesic dose of, 102, 104t
    neurologic effects of, 1975t
    overdose with, 52, 504t, 508, 1975t
    patient-controlled, 103
    pharmacology of, 52
    septic shock role of, 499
    starting dose for, 104t
    withdrawal of, 53, 508
Opisthorchiasis, 1931–1932, 1932t
Opisthotonos, 1637
Opsoclonus-myoclonus, 2020
    paraneoplastic, 1018, 1028
Optic chiasm, 2017
Optic disk, 2177–2178
    drusen in, 2177
    edema of, 2016, 2016t, 2177t, 2177–2178
    pallor of, 2178
Optic nerve, 2174t
    atrophy of, 1708t, 1709, 2178
    disorders affecting, 2174t
    drusen of, 2177

Optic nerve (Continued)
    glaucoma effect on, 2174t, 2175
    papilledema and, 2016, 2016–2017, 2017, 2177
    syphilis effect on, 1708t, 1709
    tumors of, 2177t
Optic neuritis, 2016t, 2016–2017, 2017, 2111
    multiple sclerosis and, 2111
    retrobulbar, 2016, 2177
Optic neuropathy, anterior ischemic, 2177–2178
    diabetic, 1273, 2181–2182
    Leber's, 2167, 2178
    neoplasia with, 1028, 1030
Optic radiations, 2017
    blood supply to, 2060
    damage to, 1985, 1987t
Optic tract, 2015, 2017, 2017
Oral cavity. See Mouth.
Oral contraceptives, cancer prevention using, 1010
    hepatotoxicity of, 773, 773t, 775
Oral glucose–lowering agents, 1267–1268, 1268t
Orbit, Graves' disease effect on, 2180
    mucormycosis affecting, 1833
    neoplasia of, 2180
    Wegener's granulomatosis affecting, 1495t, 1496,
        1496t
Orchitis, 1335
    mumps causing, 1336, 1769
    viral, 1335
Organ donation. See also Transplantation.
    heart as, 361–362, 362t
Organ of Zuckerkandl, chromaffin cells of, 1254
    pheochromocytoma affecting, 1254
Organophosphates, 510t
    poisoning due to, 504t, 509–510, 510t
Orgasm, 1308
    headache with, 2033
    male, 1320
Oriental cholangiohepatitis, 812
Ornithine, enzyme defect and, 146t
    urinary, 1102t
Ornithine transcarbamoylase, 1110
    deficiency of, 1110t, 1110–1111
Ornithosis, 58t
    occupational exposure to, 58t
Oropharynx, candidiasis of, 1828
    enterovirus affecting, 1787t, 1789–1791
    flora of, anaerobic, 1639, 1639
        aspiration pneumonia due to, 1579, 1582
    ulceration of, histoplasmosis causing, 1817
Oroya fever, 1682
Orthomyxovirus, 1739
Orthopnea, 217
Osborn wave, 503, 503
Oscillopsia, 2027
Osler maneuver, 260
Osler's nodes, endocarditis with, 1599, 1600t
    lupus erythematosus with, 1478
Osler-Weber-Rendu disease, 720–721
Osmolality, **532–538**
    ADH and, 533, 533–534, 536
    diabetic hyperosmolar syndrome and, 1270
    fluid transfer role of, 532–534, 533
    hypertonic disorders of, 537t, 537–538
    hypothalamic osmostat and, 1222, 1222
    hypotonic disorders of, 534t, 534–537
    pregnancy and, 609
    sodium and, 534–538
        hypernatremia and, 537t, 537–538
        hyponatremia and, 534t, 534–537
    urinary, 1222, 1223
    vasopression regulation of, 1222, 1223
Osmoreceptors, 1222–1223
Osmostat, absence of, 1224
    hypothalamic, 1222, 1222
Osmotic pressure, pulmonary edema and, 476, 477
Ossification, muscular, 2165
Osteitis deformans. See Paget's disease, of bone.
Osteitis fibrosa, 1376
    parathyroid hormone in, 1376, 1376t
    renal failure and, 1376, 1376t
Osteoarthritis, **1517–1521**
    clinical features of, 1518–1520, 1519t, 1520
    epidemiology of, 1517–1518
    etiology of, 1519t
    foot, 1519t, 1519–1520
    hand, 1518–1519, 1519t, 1520
    hip, 1519, 1519t
    imaging of, 1520
    knee, 1519, 1519t
    laboratory findings in, 1520

Osteoarthritis (Continued)
    neuropathic (Charcot's joint), 1518, 1526, 1526
    pathogenesis of, 1518, 1519
    pathology findings in, 1518
    secondary, 1519t
    spine, 1519t, 1520
    synovial fluid in, 1465t
    treatment of, 1520–1521
Osteoarthropathy, hypertrophic, 1388, 1527
    pulmonary malignancy with, 1020, 1035
Osteoblasts, 1352
    glucocorticoid inhibition of, 1384
    parathyroid hormone action on, 1366
Osteocalcin, 1352
Osteochondromatosis, 1528
Osteoclasts, 1353
    bisphosphonate inhibition of, 1383
    calcitonin inhibition of, 1373
    defective function of, 1388–1389
    Paget's disease role of, 1384–1385
    phagocytosis by, 900, 900t
Osteocytes, 1352–1353, 1353
Osteodystrophy, Albright's hereditary, 1372, 1372–1373
    renal, 557t, 559, 562, **1375–1379**, 1376t
        biochemical features of, 1376t, 1376–1377
        clinical manifestations of, 1377
        radiographic findings in, 1377–1378, 1378
        treatment of, 1376t, 1376–1378
        vitamin D therapy in, 1378, 1378t
Osteogenesis imperfecta, **1122–1123**
    clinical manifestations of, 1122, 1122t
    definition of, 1122
    differential diagnosis of, 1122–1123
    genetics of, 138t, 1122, 1122t
    prevalence of, 1122
    treatment of, 1123
    types of, 1122, 1122t
Osteoid, 1352, 1361
    osteomalacia, 1360, 1361
Osteolysis, Paget's, 1384–1385, 1385, 1386
Osteomalacia, **1359–1365**
    biopsy in, 1361
    classification of, 1359t, 1362t, 1363t
    clinical manifestations of, 1360–1361
    definition of, 1359
    differential diagnosis of, 1361–1365, 1362t, 1363t
    drug-induced, 1365
    elderly affected by, 23
    etiology of, 1359t, 1359–1360
    hypophosphatasia in, 1365
    hypophosphatemia in, 1362t, 1363t, 1363–1364
    inflammatory bowel disease and, 710t, 711
    laboratory findings in, 1362t, 1363t
    oncogenic, 1026
    pathogenesis of, 1359–1360, 1361
    radiographic features in, 1377
    renal failure and, 1362, 1363–1364, 1376t,
        1376–1377
    tumor-induced, 1363t, 1364
    vitamin D in, 1145t, 1361–1363, 1362t, 1363t
Osteomyelitis, **1625–1627**
    childhood, 1625t, 1625–1626
    clinical manifestations of, 1625t, 1626, 1626
    contiguous infection with, 1625t, 1625–1626
    definition of, 1625
    diagnosis of, 1626–1627
    etiologic agents of, 1625, 1625t
    imaging procedures for, 1626, 1626–1627
    incidence of, 1625–1626
    pathogenesis of, 1626, 1626
    prognosis in, 1627
    spinal, 1625t, 1625–1626, 1626
    staphylococcal, 1608
    treatment of, 1627
Osteon, 1353, 1353
Osteonecrosis, 1387
    diagnosis of, 1387
    etiology of, 1387, 1387t
    pathogenesis of, 1387
    sickle syndrome in, 889
    treatment of, 1387
Osteopathia striata, 1390
Osteopetrosis, **1388–1389**
    clinical manifestations of, 1389
    diagnosis of, 1389, 1389
    etiology of, 1388–1389
    pathogenesis of, 1388–1389
    treatment of, 1389

Osteopoikilosis, 1390
Osteoporosis, **1379–1384**
  age and, 1379, *1379*
  bone density in, *1379*, 1379–1380, 1380t
    measurement of, 1381–1382, 1382t
  calcium in, 1379–1380, *1380*
  clinical manifestations of, 1380–1381
  diagnosis of, 1381–1382, 1382t
  diet and, 1141, 1143t
  elderly affected by, 23
  estrogens in, 1379–1380, *1380*, 1382–1383
  etiology of, 1379–1380, 1381t
  exercise preventing, 32
  gender and, 1379, *1379*
  incidence of, 1379
  inflammatory bowel disease and, 710t, 711
  male with, *1379*, 1383–1384
  physiology of, 1379–1380, *1380*
  radiographic findings in, 1381, *1381*
  secondary, 1380, 1381t
  type I (postmenopausal), 1380, *1380*
  type II (senile), 1380, *1380*
  vitamin D in, 1379–1380, *1380*, 1383
Osteosclerosis, **1387–1390**
  cortical, 1387–1388
  disorders associated with, 1387–1390, 1388t
  dysplastic, 1387–1390, 1388t
  focal (spotted bone), 1390
  metabolic, 1388t
  myeloma with, 965
  petrotic (marble bone), 1388–1389, *1389*
  radiographic features in, 1377, 1388, *1389*
  trabecular, 1387–1388
Ostium secundum atrial septal defect, 278–279, *280*
  nonrestrictive, *280*, *291*
Ostomy, gastrojejunal, 669t, 669–671, 670t, *672*
Otitis, 449, 2084
  externa, malignant, 2084
  media, 449–450, 450t
    H. influenzae in, 1623
    hearing loss due to, 2021–2022
    meningitis with, 1611
    pneumococcal, 1571, 1571t
    tetanus organism in, 1637
Otosclerosis, 2022
  vertigo with, 2026
Outcome assessment, **122–126**
  cost studies in, 124, 125t
  data sources for, 126, 126t
  definitions in, 122
  importance of, 122–123, *123*
  measurement standards for, 123, 124t
  patient role in, 123–124, 124t
  study designs for, 125t, 125–126
  types of outcome in, 123, 123t
Ovalocytosis, 855, 855t
  Southeast Asian, 855, 855t
Ovaries, **1293–1315**
  adult, *1294*, 1297–1301
  androgens of, 1299, *1299*, 1312t
  carcinoma of, 1313–1315
    clinical presentation of, 1313
    diagnosis of, 1313
    differential diagnosis of, 1313
    incidence of, *1005*, *1009*, 1013t, *1015*, 1313
    management of, 1067, 1313–1314
    metastases from, 1031t, 1314
    pathology of, 1312t, 1313
    pregnancy with, 1061t, 1066–1067
    prognosis and survival for, 1314, 1315t
    staging of, 1314, 1314t
    tumor marker for, 1022t, 1022–1023, 1313
  childhood, 1293–1294, *1294*
  differentiation of, 1285, 1293
  dysgenesis of, 154, 1286, 1287
  embryology of, 1293, *1293*
  failure of, 1304t, 1304–1305, 1305t
  hormone production by, 1293–1295, *1294*, 1312t. See
    also *Estrogens*; *Progesterone*.
  menopause and, 1293, *1293*, *1294*, 1311–1312
  menstrual cycle and, *1294*, 1297–1299, *1298*
  morphology of, 1293–1294, *1294*
  pain from (mittelschmerz), 1298
  polycystic, 1297
    obesity with, 1165
  puberty and, 1293–1295, *1294*, 1295t
  sexual differentiation and, 1285, *1285*
  steroids of, 1299, *1299*, *1300*, 1301t

Ovaries *(Continued)*
  tumors of, 1312–1313
    hormone production by, 1312t, 1312–1313
Overhydration, enteral nutrition causing, 1171
Ovulation, *1294*, 1298, *1298*
  absence of. See *Anovulation*.
  drug-induced, 1309
  luteinizing hormone in, *1294*, 1297–1298, *1298*,
    1299
  puberty and, *1293*, 1293–1295, *1294*
Ovum, 1293–1295, *1294*
Oxacillin, 1562t
  endocarditis therapy with, 1602–1603, 1603t
  hepatotoxicity of, 772, 773t
  minimal inhibitory concentration for, 1570, 1570t
Oxalate, arthropathy due to, 1516, 1516t
  crystals of, 1516, 1516t
  deposition disease due to, 1516, 1516t
  kidney stone of, 614–617, *615*, 616t
  renal function and, 588
  urinary. See *Hyperoxaluria*.
Oxidants, erythrocytes affected by, 856, 856–857
  phagocytosis role of, 899, *900*, 900
Oxycodone, 51
  pain control with, 104t, 893t
Oxygen, cerebral, 2059–2062, 2061t
    deficiency in, 2062t, 2062–2063
  consumption of, 467t, 468
    cardiac output measured using, 209–210
    Fick method using, 209–210
    myocardial, 178, 296, *296*, 302t, *309*
  deficiency of. See *Hypoxia*.
  diffusion of, 371–372, 375, 375t
  dissociation curve related to, *876*
  hemoglobin uptake of, 472, *472*, 868, 869, *869*, *876*
  phagocytosis role of, 897, 898t, 899, *900*, 900, *906*
  reactive species of, 404–405, *405*
  tension of, 375, 375t
    hypoxia threshold for, 2062t
    Pneumocystis pneumonia and, 1918, *1918*
    polycythemia vera and, 921, 921t
    reduced. See *Hypoxemia*.
    respiratory failure and, 452–453, 467t, 467–469
    shock and, 484
    ventilation assessment using, 466–468, 467t
  tissue uptake of, 467t, 468, 472
  toxicity of, 404–405, *405*
  transport of, 467t, 468, 472, *472*
Oxygen therapy, bronchitis treated with, 387
  carbon monoxide poisoning and, 504t, 507, 507t
  respiratory failure treated with, 468–469
  shock treated with, 491
  toxicity of, 404–405, *405*
    clinical features of, 404–405
    mechanisms of, 404–405, *405*
    treatment of, 405
Oxyhemoglobin, 869, *869*
  shock and, 484
Oxymorphone, 104t
Oxyphenisatin, 773
Oxyphysins, 1221–1222
Oxypurines, 1117
Oxytocin, parturition role of, 1223
  pituitary secretion of, 1221–1222
  uterus sensitivity to, 1223
Ozone inhalation, 404

P

P cells, sinus nodal, 231–232
P wave, 190, 190–191, *193*, *194*
  hyperkalemia affecting, 542, *542*
  notched, *194*
  sawtoothed, *240*
Pacemakers, arrhythmia treated with, 250t, 250–251,
  251t
  codes for, 251t
  complications of, 251
  implanted, 250t, 250–251, 251t
  modes of, 250–251, 251t
  pulse generators for, 251
Pacemakers (native), overdrive suppression by, 232
  sinus nodal, 232
Pachydermoperiostosis, 1388, 1527
  clinical presentation of, 1388
  radiologic features in, 1388
  treatment of, 1388
Paget's disease, **1384–1387**
  anal, 743
  of bone, **1384–1387**

Paget's disease *(Continued)*
  clinical features of, *1385*, 1385t, 1385–1386
  complications of, 1385t, 1385–1386
  definition of, 1384
  etiology of, 1384
  histopathology of, 1384–1385
  laboratory findings in, 1385–1386
  pathophysiology of, 1384–1385
  prevalence and epidemiology of, 1384
  prognosis in, 1386–1387
  radiographic features in, 1385, *1385*
  treatment of, 1386
Pagophagia, 840
Pain, **100–107**
  abdominal, 628–629
    acute, 748t, 748–749
    appendicitis causing, 748
    epigastric, 628, 665t, 665–666
      pancreatitis with, 731, 734–735
    examination and, 628
    gallbladder, 813–814
    hemochromatosis with, 1133
    inflammatory bowel disease with, 709, 712t
    ischemia causing, 717, 718, 719
    left lower quadrant, 628, 749
    malabsorption with, 699t
    Mediterranean fever with, 907
    mesenteric, 717, 718, 719
    nerve fibers and, 628
    pelvic inflammatory disease with, 1701–1702
    peptic ulcer and, 665t, 665–666
    peritonitis causing, 746, 747t, 907
    pleurodynia as, 1787t, 1787–1788
    pseudoappendicitis with, 1661
    right lower quadrant, 628, 748, 748t
    right upper quadrant, 628
    timing of, 629
    yersinial infection with, 1661
  angina pectoris, 166, 297
  aortic aneurysm, 342–343
  arterial embolism, 352–353
  arteriosclerosis obliterans, 350
  assessment of, 101t, 101–102
  aural, 2035
  back, **2037–2038**, 2144, 2146
    ankylosing spondylitis with, 1467
    disc disease causing, 2037–2038, 2141,
      2144–2146
    etiology of, 2037, 2037t, 2143t, 2144–2146
    history in, 2037–2038, 2143
    management of, 2038, 2144
    physical examination and, 2038, 2143–2144
    radiography in, 2038, 2144
    spinal lesion in, 2141, *2141*, 2144, 2146
  bone, fibrogenesis imperfecta with, 1365
    osteodystrophy with, 1377
    osteonecrosis causing, 1387
    Paget's disease with, 1385, 1385t
  breast, 1318
  bursa, 1524, *1524*, 1527
  carpal tunnel, 1527
  characteristics of, 100–101
    etiologic, 101
    physiologic, 101
    quantitative, 101
    temporal, 100–101
  chest, 166, 297, 370
    anginal, 166, 297
    infarction, 301, 304, 309–310, 310t
    myocardial ischemia, 370
    pericardial, 370
    pleuritic, 370, 423, 424, 424t, 907, 1787, 1788
    pulmonary embolism, 370, 423, 424, 424t
  clostridial infection causing, 1631, 1631t, 1632
  cold exposure, 346–350
  cystic fibrosis causing, 421
  defecatory, shigellosis causing, 1648
  dental, 2034
  ear, 2035
    Bell's palsy with, 2157
  elbow, 1527–1528
  endorphins and, 1187, 1187t
  esophageal, 628, 650–651, 655, 657
  eye, 2035
    enteroviral conjunctivitis with, 1792
    glaucoma causing, 2176–2177
  Fabry's disease with, 1096
  facial, 2035
  flank, renal artery thrombosis causing, 606
  funicular, 2142

Pain *(Continued)*
gastrointestinal, rectal, abscess and, 741
hemorrhoids and, 740–741
glomus tumor, 353
head. See *Headache.*
hypochondriasis diagnosis using, 2006, 2006t
jaw, 450–451
joint with, 1518
leg, embolism causing, 424t
management of, 101–107
adjuvants in, 105, 106t
alternative methods in, 105–107
analgesics in, 102, 103t, 893t
cancer patient and, 105t, 107, *107*
drug therapy in, 102–107, 103t–106t, 893t
guidelines for, 103t
opioids in, 102–105, 104t–106t, 893t
patient care issues related to, 6–7, 7t
symptom control for, 7, 7t
terminal palliation issue in, 6–7, 7t
multiple sclerosis with, 2109, 2110
muscle. See *Myalgia.*
myocardial infarction with, 301, 304, 309–310, 310t
nail bed, 353
neck, Lyme disease causing, 1716–1717, 1717t
spine and, 2144, 2146
nerve fibers for, 628
osteoarthritis with, 1518
ovarian (mittelschmerz), 1298
pancreatic, 628
phantom limb, 2036–2037
pituitary tumor causing, 2035
pleural, Mediterranean fever with, 907
paroxysmal, 1787, 1788
pulmonary embolism causing, 370, 423, 424, 424t
postprandial, malabsorption causing, 699t
radicular, 2142
renal colic, 591, 591t, 613, *613*
renal cystic disease with, 618, 619t
severe, 2036
shock with, 491
shoulder, 1521–1524
sickle syndrome causing, 887, 892, 893t
stomach, 628, 665–666
stylomastoid, 2035
swallowing, 650
sympathetic outflow, 2036
syphilitic, 1709
tabes dorsalis, 2086
thromboangiitis obliterans, 352
ulcer, 628–629, 665–666
wrist, 1527–1528
Palilalia, 2049
Palindromes, *1181*
Palliation. See *Pain, management of.*
Pallor, Raynaud's phenomenon with, 347, 1484, 1485
Palm. See also *Hand.*
acanthosis nigricans affecting, 1019–1020
erythema of, liver disease and, 752
rheumatoid arthritis with, 1463
hair follicle absent on, 2186
ichthyosis of, 2204t
paraneoplastic effects in, 1034t
pityriasis of, 2204
psoriasis affecting, 2203
Rocky Mountain spotted fever rash of, 1731, 1738t
syphilitic rash on, 1707, *1707*
Palpitation, 166
pheochromocytoma causing, 1254, 1254t
thyrotoxicosis with, 1232, 1233t
Palsy, Bell's, 2157
Lyme disease with, 1717, 1719t
progressive supranuclear, 2051t
Pampiniform plexus, 1326
dilatation of, 1336
Pancoast syndrome, 439
Pancreas, **729–736**
A cells of, 1282
abscesses of, 730, 734
anatomy of, 729
annular, 729
autodigestion of, 730, *730*
B cells of, 1282
beta cells of, 1282
diabetes mellitus and, *1259*, 1261–1263, *1263*
insulin secretion by, 1260, 1282
calcification of, 734, 734t
carcinoma of, 736–738
clinical features of, 736–737
diagnosis of, 737, 737t

Pancreas *(Continued)*
double duct sign in, *637*
epidemiology of, 736t, 736–737
imaging tests for, 737, 737t
incidence of, 736t, *1005, 1009,* 1013t, *1015*
smoking associated with, 35t
treatment of, 737–738
D cells of, 1282
diagnostic procedures for, 731–732, 732t, 735
divisum, 729
enzymes of, 729, *730,* 731–732
elevated, 731–732, 732t
laboratory testing for, 731–732, 732t
secretion of, *730,* 730–732, 732t
exocrine function of, 729–730, *731*
fat absorption role of, *697*
gastrinoma of, 674–676, 1346
imaging procedures for, 630–632, *631, 633, 634, 637*
inflammation of. See *Pancreatitis.*
insufficiency of, 699–701
diagnostic tests for, 699–701, 700t, 701t
malabsorption due to, 702
trypsin-like immunoreactivity in, 699, 700t
islets of Langerhans of, 1282–1284
pain from, cancer with, 736, 737, 738
inflammation with, 731, 734–734
physiology of, 729, *731*
PP cells of, 1282
tumors of, imaging of, *809*
islet cell, 1282–1284
VIP cells of, 1282
Pancreatic duct, double duct sign in, *637*
imaging of, 632, *633, 637*
Pancreatitis, **729–736**
acute, 730–734
clinical presentation of, 731–732, 732t
course and complications of, 733t, 733–734
definition of, 730
diagnosis of, 731–732, 732t
etiology of, *730,* 730–731, 731t
pathophysiology of, *730,* 730–731, *731,* 731t
prognosis in, 732t, 732–733
treatment of, *733,* 733–734
alcoholic, 731t, 732t, 734, 734t
amylase level and, 731–732, 732t
ascites and, 730, 734, 736, 743t, 745
calcifying, 734, 734t
chronic, 734–736
complications of, 735–736
course of, 734
definition of, 734
diagnosis of, 735
etiology and pathophysiology of, 734, 734t
treatment of, 735
CT scan in, *631*
diabetes mellitus and, 735
drug-induced, 730, 731t
gallstones and, 730, 731t, 814
gallstones causing, 814
hypertriglyceridemia and, 730
lipase level and, 732, 732t
lupus erythematosus with, 1479
malabsorption and, 735
necrosis in, 733, *733*
obstruction and, 731t, 734t, 736
pain of, 731, 734
viral, 731t
vitamin B₁₂ in, 701t
Pancreatography, 630–632, *631, 633, 634*
cholestasis imaging with, 808, *809*
Pancuronium, 310t
Pancytopenia, 835t
aplastic anemia and, 834–835
hemolytic anemia with, 866
immune, 866
Pandemics, influenza, 1753t, 1754–1755, 1755t
Panic disorder, **2004–2005**
incidence of, 2004
prognosis in, 2005
seizure vs., 2121
symptoms of, 2004, 2004t
treatment of, 2004–2005
Panniculitis, classification of, 1507–1508
etiology of, 1507–1508
lipoatrophy due to, 1508
liquefying, 1507
lobular, 1507–1508
nodular, 1507–1508
septal, 1507, 1508
vasculitis with, 1507–1508

Panniculus, 1507–1508
Pannus, corneal, 1723
rheumatoid, *1448, 1460*
Pantothenic acid, 1148t
assessment of, 1148t
deficiency of, 1148t
physiology of, 1148t
RDA for, 1141t
toxicity of, 1148t
Papanicolaou smear, 28t, 1006t
Paper, smoke inhalation and, 403, 403t
Papilledema, 2016t, 2016–2017, 2177, 2177t
false, 2177
intracranial pressure and, 2016–2017, 2133, 2177
optic neuritis vs., 2016t, 2016–2017
vision affected by, 2016, 2016t
Papillitis, 2177
Papilloma, choroid plexus, 2132
respiratory tract, 1745–1746
Papillomavirus, rectal warts of, 742
sexual transmission of, 1697t
Papovavirus, leukoencephalopathy due to, 2101, *2101*
slow infection due to, 2097t
structure of, *1739*
Pappataci fever, 1808
Papules, 2191t, 2202t, 2216t
cat scratch disease with, 1681, 1681t
diseases associated with, 2191t, 2202t, 2207t, 2216t
eczematous, 2191t, 2197–2199, 2201t
gonococcal, 1702
Gottron's, 2212
Kaposi's sarcoma, 1032–1033, 1033t
lichen planus, 2204
lymphomatoid, 1034
metastases causing, 1030–1031, 1031t
paraneoplastic, 1030–1036, 1031t
pinta, 1714
pityriasis, 2202t, *2203,* 2203–2204
prurigo, 2187
psoriatic, 2202–2203, *2203*
purpuric, 2201t, 2201–2202
rosaceous, 2207, *2207*
skin rubbing with, 2187
syphilis, 1707, *1707,* 2202t
tularemia, 1667
vasculitis with, 2201t, 2201–2202
xanthomatous, 2211
yaws, 1714
yellow, pseudoxanthomatous, 1123, *1123*
Paracentesis, ascites with, 744, 744t, 745t, 795, 795t
peritoneal tuberculosis and, 747, 747t
Paracoccidioidomycosis, **1822–1823**
clinical manifestations of, 1823
diagnosis of, 1823
epidemiology of, 1822
etiologic agent in, 1822
pathogenesis and pathology of, 1822
prognosis in, 1823
treatment of, 1823
Paraganglioma, pheochromocytoma as, 1254
Paragonimiasis, 1932t, 1933
Parainfluenza virus, 1752–1753
clinical manifestations of, 1753
common cold due to, 1747, 1747t, *1748*
diagnosis of, 1753
epidemiology of, 1752–1753, 1753t
Paralysis, botulism causing, 1630, 1631t, 1635–1636
diaphragmatic, 442
drug-induced, 310t
enterovirus in, 1786–1787, 1787t
facial, 2157
flaccid, 1635
Guillain-Barré, 2151t, 2151–2152
hyperkalemia with, 542
hypokalemia with, 540
neuropathy causing, 2151t, 2151–2152
periodic, 2168t, 2168–2169
treatment of, 2169
types of, 2168t, 2168–2169
poliovirus causing, 1786–1787, 1787t, 2091–2092
rabies causing, 2096
shellfish toxin causing, 1954t, 1956
tetanus causing, 1630, 1631t, 1637
tick bite causing, 1947–1948
Todd's, 2114
ventilation therapy requiring, 310t
Paramyxovirus, *1739*

Paraneoplastic syndromes, **1017–1036**
  dermatologic, 1018–1020, 1030–1036, 1031t, 1033t, 1034t
  emergent conditions of, 1049–1054, *1051*, *1052*
  endocrinologic, 1020, 1024–1026, 1025t
  hematologic, 1017t, 1020–1021
  hepatic, 1021
  lung cancer with, 439
  markers and, 1021–1024, 1022t
  neurologic, 1018–1019, 1027t, 1027–1030, 1029t, 2153
  renal, 1017t, 1020
Paraplegia, hereditary spastic, 2052
Paraproteinemia, 958–961
  platelets affected by, 985
Paraquat poisoning, 509–510
Parasites, 783t, 1892–1951. See also *Helminths*; *Protozoan disease*; specific parasite or disease.
  diarrhea due to, 693, 694
  eosinophilia due to, 957
  hepatic, 782–783, 783t
  occupational encounter with, 2221–2222
  preventive measures for, 1544t, 1548
  pyrogenicity of, 1532t, 1532–1534, *1534*
  splenomegaly due to, 972, 972t
Parasomnias, 1983, 1983t
Parasympathetic nervous system. See also *Autonomic nervous system.*
  hypothalamus role in, 2011, *2011*
  intestinal motility and, 681, *681*, 681t
  penile erection controlled by, 2010, 2010t
  pupillary reflexes and, 2009, 2009t
Parathyroid glands, 1365–1367
  anatomy of, 1365
  embryology of, 1365
  multiple endocrine neoplasia and, 1346, 1369
Parathyroid hormone, **1365–1373**
  actions of, 1366, *1366*
  AMP and, 1366
  biochemistry of, 1366, *1366*
  bone formation role of, 1354, 1354t, *1355*, 1356
  calcium and, 1366, *1367*, 1367–1370, 1368t
  deficiency of, *1367*, 1371–1373, *1372*, 1372t
  ectopic, 1020, 1025t, 1025–1026
  excess of, *1367*, 1368, 1369–1370
  GTP and, 1366
  immunoassay of, 1366–1367, *1367*
  immunoreactive, 1376, 1377
  magnesium deficiency and, 1138
  metabolism of, 1366, *1366*
  normal levels of, *1367*
  pathophysiology related to, 1367–1372
  physiology of, 1366, *1366*
  receptors for, 1366
  renal failure and, *1376*, 1376t, 1376–1379, 1378t
  resistance to, 1372
  synthesis and secretion of, 1366, *1366*
  vitamin D and, 1366
Parathyroidectomy, 1378t, 1378–1379
Paresis, cerebral hemorrhage with, 2078, 2078t
  gaze, 2018–2020, 2078
  syphilitic, 1708t, 1709, *2085*, 2086t
  tropical spastic, retroviral, 1781t, 1782, 2097t
Paresthesia, cobalamin deficiency in, 2041
  elderly affected by, 17
  "pins and needles," 2041
  rheumatoid arthritis causing, *1462*, 1462–1463, *1463*
Parietal lobes, 1986, *1986*, *2059*
  anatomy of, *1986*, 1986–1987
  manifestations of disease of, 1987, 1988t
  tumor of, 2126t
Parinaud's syndrome, 1205, 2019
Parkinson's disease, **2044–2046**
  causes of, 2044t
  cerebellar, 2046
  dementia of, 1992t, 1995
  drug-induced, 2044, 2046
  family history of, 2046
  Hallervorden-Spatz, 2046
  multiple-system, 2046
  pathogenesis of, 2044, 2044t
  postencephalitic, 2046
  signs and symptoms in, 2044, 2044t, *2045*
  treatment of, 2044–2046, *2045*
  vascular, 2046
Paromomycin, amebiasis therapy with, 1915t
  dientamoebiasis treated with, 1916t

Paronychia, 2214–2215
  candidiasis with, 1828
Parotid gland, enlargement of, 649, 649t
  hyposecretion by, 649t, 649–650
  mumps affecting, 1768–1769
Paroxetine, depression treated with, 2000t, 2001
  pain control use of, 106t
Paroxysmal supraventricular tachycardia, 238–239
  accessory pathway and, *240*
  carotid massage in, 235t
  clinical features of, 239
  ECG of, 238–239, *239*, *240*
  treatment of, 237t, 238t, 239
Partial pressure. See *Blood gases*; specific gases.
Partial thromboplastin time. See under *Thromboplastin time.*
Particulate matter. See *Dust(s).*
Parturition thyroiditis, 1240
Parvovirus, 1830
  anemia due to, 833–834, *834*
  structure of, *1739*
Pasta, dietary, *1142*
Pastes, topical therapy with, 2194, 2194t
Patch skin testing, 2192
Patella, hypoplasia of, 812
Patent ductus arteriosus, 279, *280*
Pathogens, **1531–1738**. See also specific organism.
  adaptive characteristics of, 1531, *1556*, 1556–1557
  AIDS/HIV and, 1860t, 1867t, 1877t
  classification of, 1556–1557, 1557t
  compromised host and, 1538t
  enteric bacteria as, 1659–1660, *1660*
  gram-negative, 1556–1557, 1557t
  gram-positive, 1556–1557, 1557t
  morphology of, *1556*, 1556–1557, 1557t
  oropharyngeal flora with, 1582
  osteomyelitis, 1625t, 1625–1626
  Reiter's syndrome, 1467t
  virulence factors of, 1531, *1556*, 1556–1557
Patients, **4–9**
  antimicrobial selection and, 1561–1563, 1562t
  common presentations of, 86t, 87t, 88
  competency of, 4–5
  decision making by, 4–5, 465–466
    advance directive for, 5
    critical care and, 465–466
    end-of-life, 5
    health reform affecting, 6
    substitute in, 5
  febrile, 1532t, 1532–1533
  history taking from, chief complaint in, 75t
    family in, 75t, 76
    interview technique for, 76
    physician decision making and, 75t, 75–76
    preventive care using, 27–29, 28t
    social factors in, 75t, 76
  hospitalized, length of stay of, 9–11, 10t
    nutrition requirements of, 1173, 1173t
  outcome assessment by, 123–124, 124t
  pain palliation in, 6–7, 7t. See also *Pain, management of.*
  pediatric. See *Pediatric patients.*
  satisfaction of, 123–124, 124t, 126
  terminal care issues for, 6–9, 8t
Pauci-immune glomerulonephritis, 574t, 577, 577t
PCBs (polychlorinated biphenyls), 740
PCP (phencyclidine), 54, 1975t
  adverse effects of, 54, 508
PCR (polymerase chain reaction), 137
  genome mapping with, 137
  Lyme disease in, 1718
  sickle syndromes in, 890–891, *891*
Peas, food poisoning due to, 740
Pectus excavatum, 443, 443t
Pediatric patients. See also *Puberty.*
  botulism affecting, 1636
  chlamydial infection in, 1722–1723, 1723t, 1724
  cholera affecting, 1652
  croup in, 1749–1752, 1750t, 1751t
  diarrhea affecting, viral, 1793–1797, *1795*, 1795t
  enterovirus affecting, 1787t, 1789
  epilepsy in, 2117, *2117*
  febrile convulsions in, 2116–2117
  floppy baby syndrome in, 1636
  gonorrhea in, 1702
  herpes simplex in, 1746t, 1773
  Hodgkin's disease in, 954
  inflammatory bowel disease in, 711
  lupus erythematosus in, 1480

Pediatric patients *(Continued)*
  measles in, 1759–1761
  meningitis in, 1610t, 1610–1611, 1616–1617, 1619
  mumps in, 1768–1769
  muscle atrophy affecting, 2052t, 2052–2054
  osteomyelitis in, 1625t, 1625–1626
  respiratory syncytial virus in, 1751–1752
  shigellosis affecting, 1642t, 1647t, 1647–1648
  sickle syndromes affecting, 888, 890–891
  streptococcal infection in, 1586
  suicidal behavior in, 2002
  tetanus affecting, 1636, 1637
  thrombocytosis in, 924
  viruses affecting, 1741t
  vitamin K deficiency in, 999
Pediculosis, 1945–1946
  body, 1945–1946
  head, 1945–1946
  pubic, 1946
  treatment of, 1946, 2195
PEEP. See *Positive end-expiratory pressure (PEEP).*
Pel-Ebstein phenomenon, 1533t
Peliosis hepatis, 773t, 774
Pelizaeus-Merzbacher disease, 2112
Pellagra, dermatitis in, 2218
  neurologic effects of, 2040
Pelvic examination, 1006t
Pelvic inflammatory disease (PID), 1701–1703
  chlamydial, 1700, 1702t, 1724
  gonorrheal, 1701–1703, 1702t
  treatment of, 1702t, 1703
Pemberton's sign, 1242
Pemphigoid, bullous, 2189t, 2205t, 2206
  cicatricial, 2189t, 2205t
  immunofluorescence testing in, 2189t
Pemphigus, 2205–2206
  familial benign, 2206
  foliaceus, 2206
  immunofluorescence testing in, 2189t
  oral lesions of, 646t, 647
  paraneoplastic, 1019, 1034t
  vegetans, 2206
  vulgaris, 646t, 647, 2205–2206
Penbutolol, 265t
Penicillamines, renal function and, 588
  Wilson's disease treated with, 1132
Penicillinase, 1558–1560, 1559t
  gonococcal, 1703
  streptococcal, 1559
Penicillin(s), 1562t
  actinomycosis therapy with, 1676
  adverse reactions to, 1418t, 1568t
  allergy to, 100, 1434, 1434t, 1435t, 1568t
  anaphylaxis due to, 1418t, 1418–1419, 1568t
  anthrax therapy using, 1667
  desensitization to, 1435t
  diphtheria therapy with, 1630
  dose adjustment for, 94t, 1562t
  endocarditis therapy with, 1602t–1604t, 1602–1603
  erysipelas treated with, 1587, 1589t
  erysipeloid therapy with, 1674
  G, 1562t, 1712t
    pharmacokinetics of, 91t, 94t
    renal failure effect on, 94t, 1562t
  immunohemolysis due to, 867, 1568t
  Lyme disease therapy with, 1719, 1719t
  mechanism of action of, 1558, 1558t
  meningitis therapy with, 1615–1617, 1616t, 1620t
  meningococcal infection and, 1620t, 1620–1621
  pharmacology of, 91t, 94t, 1562t
  resistance to, 1558–1560, 1559t
    pneumococcal, 1570, 1570t
    streptococcal, 1589
  skin testing with, 1434, 1434t
  staphylococcal infection treated with, 1609t, 1609–1610
  streptococcal infection treated with, 1587–1589, 1589t
  syphilis therapy with, 1711–1713, 1712t
  V, 1562t
Penis, abnormalities of, 1331
  anal reflex activated by, 2009t
  candidiasis affecting, 1828
  detumescence of, 1320
  differentiation of, *1285*, *1286*, *1292*, *1330*
  erection mechanism of, 1328, 1329, 2010, 2010t
    dysfunction of, 1330t, 1330–1331
  genital ulcer syndrome of, 1698
  hair follicle absent on, 2186
  prosthesis for, 1331

Penis (Continued)
psoriasis affecting, 2203
sickle syndrome affecting, 889
small, 1292, 1330, 1335
squamous cell carcinoma of, 2209–2210
syphilitic chancre of, 1706, 1707, 1707
Pentamidine, 1920, 1920t, 1921t, 1922t
Pneumocystis pneumonia and, 1920, 1920t, 1921t, 1922t
sleeping sickness treated with, 1898
Pentastomiasis, 1950
Pentazocine, 51
pain control with, 104t
Pentose phosphate pathway, 855, 856, 856
Pentostatin, 931
Peptic ulcer, 662–676
bleeding due to, 642t, 643–644, 645t, 671, 673–674
clinical features of, 665t, 665–666
complications of, 671–674
diagnosis of, 665t, 666, 666t
endoscopy of, 663, 663t, 667, 667t
etiology of, 662t, 662–664, 667t
gastritis and, 660
genetics of, 664–665
Helicobacter role in, 662t, 662–663, 666t, 666–668, 667t
incidence of, 664–665, 665
medical treatment of, 667, 667t, 667–669, 668t
NSAIDs role in, 662t, 663, 663t, 667t, 668
pain due to, 628–629, 665t, 665–666
pathophysiology of, 662t, 662–664, 663t
perforated, 669t, 669–671, 673–674
recurrence of, 663, 671, 671t
risk factors for, 664
stress role in, 662t, 664
surgical treatment of, 669t, 669–672, 670, 670t, 672
Zollinger-Ellison syndrome and, 663, 667t, 674–676, 675t
Peptides. See also Hormones.
atrial natriuretic, 1194–1195, 1195
enteric, 681, 681t
opioid, 1186, 1186–1187, 1187t, 1199
Peptidoglycans, bacterial, 1556, 1556
Peptostreptococcus, 1639, 1639t, 1641t
Perception. See also Sensory system.
alcohol disruption of, 47–49, 48t
anorexia effect on, 1158, 1159t
confused state and, 1972–1974
Percussion, lung, 368, 369t, 370
Perfusion, 478–483
determinant factors in, 478t, 478–483
myocardial, 178–179, 179
shock and, 483, 483
septic, 499t, 499–500, 500t
tissue, 478t, 478–483
ventilation and, embolism and, 425, 425t, 425–426, 426
hypercapnia and, 453
hypoxia and, 452–453
interpretation and, 425t
mismatch in, 425
Perhexilene maleate, 773, 773t
Pericardiocentesis, 185, 339
tamponade treated with, 341, 342
Pericarditis, 337–342
AIDS/HIV patient with, 329t, 1876–1877, 1877t
bacterial, 337, 337t
calcific, 185, 186
causes of, 337t, 337–338
connective tissue disorder with, 337t, 338
constrictive, 337t, 341, 341–342
ECG in, 338, 339
effusions with, 337t, 339
enterovirus in, 1787t, 1788–1789
fungal, 337, 337t
H. influenzae in, 1623
idiopathic, 337t, 338
lupus erythematosus with, 1475t, 1478
meningococcal, 1621
myocardial infarction and, 337
phonocardiography in, 338, 338
pneumococcal, 1571, 1571t
recurrent, 338
renal failure and, 558, 562
rheumatic fever causing, 1592t, 1592–1593, 1593t
sounds in, 338, 341
traumatic, 337, 341, 341–342
tuberculous with, 337, 337t, 1685t
uremic, 558, 562

Pericarditis (Continued)
viral, 337, 337t, 338
Wegener's granulomatosis causing, 1495t, 1496, 1496t
Pericardium, 336–342
effusions of, 219, 339, 339–341
cardiac catheterization and, 339, 340
causes of, 337t, 339
chylous, 337, 337t
echocardiography of, 339, 339, 340–341, 341
lax, 339
roentgenography of, 185, 186, 186
tamponade due to, 339–340, 340, 341
friction rub of, 338, 338
chest pain of, 370
phonocardiography in, 338, 338
tamponade with, 340
inflammation of. See Pericarditis.
MRI of, 207
Perindopril, 265t
Periodontium, abscess of, 450–451
Ehlers-Danlos syndrome affecting, 1121t
Periosteum, hypertrophic, 1388
Periostitis, nonsyphilitic treponematosis causing, 1714
syphilitic, 1707, 1710
Peripheral circulation, 179–180, 216–217
local resistance role in, 179–180, 216–217
regulation of, 179–180, 216–217
vascular disorders affecting, 346–357
Peripheral nervous system, 2149–2157. See also Neuropathy.
anatomy and, 2150
dysautonomia affecting, 2007t, 2007–2013, 2008t
localization of lesion of, 2030–2031, 2031t
paraneoplastic effects in, 1029
pathophysiology of, 2150
Peristalsis, 680, 680–681
colonic, 682
esophageal, 650, 655, 657
physiology of, 680, 680–682, 682
small intestine, 680, 680–682, 682
Peritoneum, 743–747
cancer, 743t, 744t, 744–745, 745t
inflammation. See Peritonitis.
Peritonitis, 745–747
acute, 745–746
ascites with, 743t, 744t, 746, 747t, 795
clinical features of, 746, 747, 747t
definition of, 745–746
diagnosis of, 744t, 746, 747
pain from, 746, 747t
pneumococcal, 1571, 1571t
prognosis in, 746
sclerosing, 1530
spontaneous bacterial, 746, 795
treatment of, 746, 747
tuberculous, 746–747, 747t, 1685t
Pernio (chilblain), 350
lupus erythematosus with, 432, 432, 1478
Peroxidase, 898t
phagocytosis role of, 897, 898t, 899, 900, 900, 905t
Peroxides, 901t
erythrocyte metabolism and, 856, 856
phagocytosis role of, 897, 899, 900, 900, 906
Peroxisomes, metabolic defects related to, 147, 147t, 1085
Personality. See Behavior.
Personnel. See Health care, personnel of.
Perspiration. See Sweating.
Pertussis, 1627–1629
clinical features of, 1628
definition of, 1627
diagnosis of, 1628
epidemiology of, 1627
etiology of, 1627
immunization for, 1627, 1628–1629
pathogenesis of, 1627
pathology findings in, 1628
treatment of, 1628
Pes cavus, 2154
Pesticides, infertility due to, 56, 59t
occupational exposure to, 56, 58t, 59t
PET scan. See Positron emission tomography (PET).
Petechiae, 2201
amyloidosis with, 967
Colorado tick fever with, 1806
meningitis with, 1612, 1619, 1619–1620
platelet defects and, 979, 979t
Petit mal seizures, 2116, 2117, 2117

Petroleum products, smoke inhalation and, 403, 403t
Petrosal sinus, 2061
ACTH in, 1213t, 1217t
Pets. See Animals.
Peutz-Jeghers syndrome, 724, 724
cutaneous macules of, 1035, 2212
polyps in, 724, 724
Peyer's patches, typhoid fever affecting, 1643, 1643t
Peyote, 508, 508t
pH, 543
acidosis and, 543, 545, 545
alkalosis and, 543, 545, 545
Henderson-Hasselbalch equation and, 543, 545
plasma-CSF disequilibrium in, 544–545
respiratory control by, 543–544
urinary, 512, 512t
Phaeohyphomycosis, 1836
Phaeomelanin, 2185
Phagocytosis, 897–901
bacterial strategies against, 1531, 1556, 1556, 1639t
compromised host and, 1537–1541, 1539t
defects of, 902–906, 1537–1541
qualitative abnormalities in, 902–906, 1540–1541
quantitative abnormalities in, 1537–1539
disorders affecting, 902–906, 904t, 905t, 906t, 914, 1540–1541
eosinophilic, 956
erythrocyte as object of, 970, 971, 972
granulocytic, 1537–1541, 1538t, 1539t
immune modulation and, 901, 901t
killing defect in, 1403
laboratory testing of, 1403
macrophagic, 900–901, 901
alveolar, 372–373
hepatic, 900, 900t
malarial red cell in, 1894
monocytic, 897, 898, 898t, 900–901
neutrophilic, 897–900, 899, 900, 902–906, 1512
urate crystals in, 1510, 1512
Phakomatoses, 2056–2057
seizures due to, 2056, 2057, 2120
Phalen's sign, 1462, 1463
Phantom limb, 2036–2037
Pharmacology, 89–100. See also Drugs; specific agents.
elderly patient and, 17t, 20t, 20–22, 21t, 95–96
hemodynamic disease affecting, 95
kidney disease affecting, 94t, 94–95
liver disease affecting, 95
pharmacodynamics in, 89, 89
pharmacokinetic principles of, 89, 89–94, 90, 92, 93
pregnancy affecting, 1068, 1068t
Pharyngitis. See also Nasopharynx; Pharynx.
adenovirus in, 1749–1751, 1750t, 1751t
coxsackievirus causing, 1787t, 1790
gonococcal, 1701
herpangina with, 1787t, 1790
herpes simplex, 1750, 1750t, 1751t
influenza virus in, 1749–1751, 1750t, 1751t
parainfluenza virus in, 1750t, 1751t, 1752–1753
rhinovirus in, 1749–1751, 1750t, 1751t
streptococcal, 1587, 1589t
Pharyngoconjunctival fever, 1757, 1757t
Pharynx. See also Nasopharynx; Oropharynx.
diphtheria and, 1629–1630
flora of. See Flora, oropharyngeal.
muscular dystrophy affecting, 2162–2163
Phenacetin, analgesic role of, 112
renal function and, 584–585
Phencyclidine (PCP), 54, 1975t
adverse effects of, 54, 508
Phenelzine, 2000t, 2001
Phenobarbital, 91t, 94t
dose adjustment for, 94t
epilepsy therapy with, 2122t
pharmacokinetics of, 91t, 94t, 2122t
renal failure effect on, 94t
Phenolphthalein, stool test with, 693
Phenothiazines, 106t, 1416t, 1998t
allergic rhinitis treated with, 1416, 1416t
hepatotoxicity, 773
pain control use of, 106t
poikilothermia caused by, 1533
schizophrenia treated with, 1998t, 1998–1999
Phenotype, 134
Phenoxybenzamine, 1256
Phentolamine, dosage for, 270t
side effects of, 270t

Phenylalanine, 1105–1108. See also *Phenylketonuria*.
catecholamine biosynthesis role of, 1253
elevated levels of, 1106–1108
metabolism of, 1105, *1106*
disorders of, 1105–1108
screening for, 1106
urinary, 1100t, 1101t
Phenylalanine hydroxylase, 1105–1108, *1106*
deficiency of, 1105–1108
gene for, *1107*
Phenylbutazone, 773, 773t
Phenylephrine, 2183
Phenylketonuria, **1105–1108**
diagnosis of, 1106–1108
enzyme defect in, 146, 146t, 1100t, 1102t, 1105–1106
genetics of, 138t, 1100t, 1105, *1107*, 1108
pregnancy and, 1108
screening for, 1106–1108
treatment of, 1108
Phenytoin, 91t, 94t, 246t
adverse effects of, 247t
antiarrhythmic action of, *245*, 246, 246t
epilepsy therapy with, 2122t, 2124t
hepatotoxicity of, 773, 773t, 775
pain control use of, 106t
pharmacokinetics of, 91t, 94t, 246, 246t, 2122t
Pheochromocytoma, **1254–1257**
catecholamine levels due to, 1254t, 1255–1256
complications of, 1256
diagnostic approach in, 1254t, 1254–1256
differential diagnosis of, 1256
etiology of, 1254
genetics of, 1254
heart affected by, 359, 1256
laboratory tests for, 1254t, 1255–1256
localization of, 1254, 1256
malignant, 1254, 1257
management of, 1256–1257
multiple endocrine neoplasia with, 1254, 1346–1347
paroxysm, 1254, 1254t, 1255
pathology of, 1254
pathophysiology of, 1256
pregnancy with, 1068
symptoms and signs of, 1254–1255
Philadelphia chromosome, 922t, 926t
chemotherapy aimed at, 928
myelogenous leukemia and, 926t, 926–928
thrombocytosis and, 922t, 923
Phlebitis, Behçet's, 1506, 1506t
Phlebogram, 167, *167*
Phlebotomine sandfly, 1903–1904, *1904*
leishmania in, 1903–1904, *1904*
Phlebotomus fever, 1808
Phlebotomy, hemochromatosis treatment with, 1134–1135, *1135*
polycythemia treatment with, 921
Phobias, 2004
Phonocardiography, jugular pulse and, *167*
pericarditis friction rub in, *338*, 338
Phosphatidylcholine, 805, *805*, 806
Phosphatidylinositol cycle, *1179*
calcium activation of, 1179, *1179*
DAG activation of, 1179, *1179*
hormone action and, 1179, *1179*
signalling role of, 1179, *1179*
Phosphoethanolamine, urinary, 1103t
Phosphofructokinase, *1084*
deficiency of, 1083, 1083t, 2165
erythrocytic, *856*, 1083t
myopathy role of, 2165
Phosphoglycerate kinase, *856*
myopathy role of, 2165
Phospholipase, 1188, *1188*
Phospholipids, antibodies to, 1458, 1476t, 1479, 2068–2069
arachidonic acid transport by, 1187, *1188*
bile content of, 805, *805*
stroke related to, 2068–2069
Phosphorus, 1135
absorption of, 1135
impaired, 1362t, 1363t
blood level of, 1135, 1351t, 1356
bound, 1351t
free, 1351t
body compartment composition and, 1135
bone formation role of, 1135, 1136t, 1351t, 1351–1356, *1352*

Phosphorus (*Continued*)
deficiency of, 1135–1137, 1136t, 1137t
dietary, 1135, *1352*
intake of, *1352*
kidney and, 1135, 1136t
chronic failure and, 557t, 558
metabolism of, 1135
osteitis fibrosa and, 1376
osteomalacia and rickets and, 144t, 1362t, 1363t, 1363–1364, 1379
RDA for, 1140t
restriction of intake of, 1378, 1378t
supplemental, 1136–1137, 1137t
therapeutic control of, 1378, 1378t
yellow, hepatotoxicity of, 772
Phosphorylase, glycogen metabolism and, 1083, 1083t
hepatic, 1082, *1082*, 1083t
muscle, 1083, 1083t
Phosphorylase b kinase, 1082, *1082*, 1083t
myopathy role of, 1082, *1082*, 1083t
Phosphorylation, arachidonic acid, 1188, *1188*
hormone regulation by, 1176–1180, *1176–1180*
Photopatch skin testing, 2192
Photoperiods. See *Light*.
Photophobia, measles with, 1759
Photosensitivity, 2217–2218
antimicrobials causing, 1568t
drug-induced, 2218, 2218t
foods causing, 2218
lupus erythematosus with, 1475t, 1478
porphyria with, 1124, 1128, 1130
pyridoxine deficiency causing, 1146t
rash caused by, 1475t, 1478
Photosynthesis, vitamin D in, 1354, *1355*, 1357
Phrenic nerve, 442, 443
Phthalimidines, 264t
Phylloquinones, 1145t
Physical examination. See also under specific organs and disorders.
decision making role of, 76
nutrition assessment with, 1152–1153, 1153t
preventive care using, 27–29, 28t
Physical therapy, bronchitis treated with, 387
osteoarthritis treated with, 1520–1521
Physicians, 2–3
caregiver role of, 2–3
ethical issues affecting, 4–9
generalist, 85–88
patient death affecting, 9
professionalism of, 3
scientist role of, 3
Physostigmine, 504t, 506
Pibaldism, 2213
Pica, iron deficiency causing, 840
lead ingestion in, 66
Pick's bodies, 1995
Pick's disease, 1992t, 1995
Picture questionnaires, in arthropathy, *1442*
PID (pelvic inflammatory disease), 1701–1703
chlamydial, 1700, 1702t, 1724
gonorrhea causing, 1701–1703, 1702t
treatment of, 1702t, 1703
Piedra, black, 1836
Pig, influenza transmitted by, 1738
tapeworm in, 1923t, 1924, 1925–1926
trichinosis associated with, 1937–1938
zoonoses associated with, 1737t, 1738t
Pigeon, cryptococcosis in, 1823
Pigmentation, 2190, 2191t
acanthosis nigricans, 1019, 1034
Addison's disease, 2213
age-associated decrease in, 2190
albinism and, 146, 2214t
connective tissue, alkaptonuria with, 1108
decreased, 2056
diagnostic examination of, 2190, 2191t
disorders affecting, 2190, 2191t, 2212–2214
fungal infection with, 1836
hemochromatosis with, 1133
increased, 2212–2213
generalized, 2213
localized, 2212–2213
malignant skin nodule with, 2208t, 2210t, 2210–2211
melanocyte organelles in, 2185
brown-black, 2185
yellow-red, 2185
oral mucosal, 648, 648t
Peutz-Jeghers, *724*
tuberous sclerosis affecting, 2056

Pili, *1556*, *1557*
anaerobe with, 1639t
bacterial, *1556*, *1557*
gonococcal, 1701
meningitis organisms with, 1611, 1618, *1619*
meningococcal, 1618, *1619*
Pills, esophagitis due to, 658–659
Pilocarpine, 2183, 2183t
Piloerection, 1533
Pimozide, pain control use of, 106t
Pineal gland, **1204–1205**
melatonin regulation by, *1204*, 1204–1205
tumors of, 1205, 2126t, 2131
Pinnae, tophi of, 1516, 2211
Pinta, 1714
clinical features of, 1714
treatment of, 1714
treponematosis of, 1714
Pinworm infection, 1935, 1935t
Pipecolic acid, urinary, 1101t
Piperacillin, 1562t
meningitis therapy with, 1615–1617, 1616t
minimal inhibitory concentration for, 1570, 1570t
Piperazines, 1416, 1416t
Piperidines, 1416, 1416t
Pituitary gland, **1205–1226**
anatomy of, *1183*, *1197*, 1205, *1222*
anterior, 1205–1220
anatomy of, *1183*, *1197*, 1205
cell types in, 1205
embryology of, 1205
hormones of, 1206t, 1206–1226, 1208t. See also specific hormones.
stimulation tests of, 1208t
suppression tests of, 1213t
antibodies to, 1250
autoimmune lymphocytic hypophysitis of, 1250
feedback mechanisms of, *1183*, 1183–1184, *1198*, 1199–1200, 1206, 1206t
hypofunction of. See *Hypopituitarism*.
hypothalamic-adrenal axis of, 1215, 1250
hypothalamic-ovarian axis with, 1293–1295, *1294*, *1299*, 1300–1301
hypothalamic-testicular axis of, *1326*, 1326
hypothalamic-thyroid axis with, 1206, 1206t, *1227*
hypothalamus and, *1197*, 1197–1199, *1198*, 1207t
Langerhans' cell granulomatosis and, 955
multiple endocrine neoplasia and, 1346
pain related to, 2035
posterior, 1221–1226
anatomy of, *1183*, *1197*, 1221–1222, *1222*
hormone secretion by, 1221–1223, *1222*
oxytocin and, 1223
vasopressin and, 1221–1223, *1222*
radiology of, 1206
radiotherapy of, 1209–1210
surgery of, 1209
tumors of, 1207–1210, 1209t, 2126t
acromegaly and, 1211–1212
ACTH secretion by, 1209t
adenomatous, 2127–2128, 2128t, 2131
chromophobes as, 1207
classification of, 1207–1208, 1209t
Cushing's disease and, 1216, 1216–1218
gonadotropin secretion by, 1209t, 1219–1220
growth hormone secretion by, 1209t, 1211
hypothalamus affected by, 1200t, 1200–1201
mass effects of, 1209, 1209t
MRI scan of, 2127–2128, 2128t
null cell, 1209t, 1221
pregnancy with, 1067–1068
prolactin secretion by, 1209t, 1213–1214
theories about, 1208–1209
therapy of, 1209–1210
TSH secretion by, 1209t, 1221
Pityriasis, 2202t
alba, 2214
lichenoides, 2202t
paraneoplastic, 1019
rosea, 2202t, 2203–2204
annular lesions of, 2191, *2191*, *2203*, 2203–2204
differential diagnosis of, 2203–2204
"herald lesion" of, 2203–2204
rotunda, 1019
rubra pilaris, 2202t
Placenta, Lyme disease crossing of, 1719–1720
rubella crossing of, 1762
Plague, 1661–1662
bubonic, 1662, 1737t
clinical and laboratory features of, 1662, 1737t, 1738t

Plague (Continued)
  complications of, 1662
  definition of, 1661–1662
  diagnosis of, 1662
  distribution of, 1662
  epidemiology of, 1662, 1737t, 1738t
  immunization for, 1554t, 1555, 1662
  pneumonic, 1662
  prevention of, 1554t, 1555, 1662
  prognosis in, 1662
  sylvatic, 1662
  treatment of, 1662
Plants, 740, 1043–1044
  alkaloids derived from, 1043–1044
    adverse effects of, 1043–1044
    chemotherapy using, 1039t, 1043–1044, 1044t
    fetal malformations due to, 1070t
  aspergillosis organism in, 1830
  asthma induced by, 379t
  poisoning due to, 740
  pollen allergens from, 1414
  vitamin D in, 1357
Plaque, Alzheimer's disease, 1505
  atherosclerotic, 292, 292, 294, 295
    fibrous, 292, 292, 294, 295
    formation of, 292, 292, 294, 295
  cutaneous, 2191t
    bacillary, 1681
    diseases associated with, 2191t
    paraneoplastic, 1030–1035, 1031t
    pityriasis rosea, 2203, 2203–2204
    psoriatic, 2202–2203, 2203
    sporotrichosis with, 1826
  demyelination, 1967, 1967
  multiple sclerosis, 1967, 1967
  neuritic, 1505
  oral mucosal, 647, 647t
  vascular, 292, 292, 294, 295
  xanthomatous, 2211
Plasma, anemia and, 823
  hyperviscosity of, 965–966
  volume of, 823
Plasma cells, 958–968
  amyloidosis and, 966–967
  disorders of, 958–968
    skin affected by, 1032
  heavy chain disease and, 966
  macroglobulinemia and, 965
  myeloma and, 962, 963, 964
  plasmacytoma and, 965
  production of, 819, 820, 820t, 821
  synovitis role of, 1460
Plasma membrane, 1177–1180
  antibodies to, 1476t
  bacterial, 1556, 1556–1557
  complement receptors on, 1400, 1400–1401, 1401t
  hormone receptors and, 1177–1180
  leukocytic, 900, 900
  metabolic disorders related to, 143–145, 144t
  transporter proteins of, 143–145, 144t
  viral attachment to, 1739
Plasmablasts, 820
  splenic, 971
Plasmacytoma, 965
  bone, 965
  extramedullary, 960, 965
Plasmapheresis, 2151
  neuropathy treated with, 2151, 2151t
Plasmids, gene transfer using, 150
  penicillinase producing, 1703
Plasmin, 989
Plasminogen, 988t. See also Tissue plasminogen activator.
  activators for, 987–989, 988t
  coagulation role of, 987–989, 988t
  inhibitors and, 988t, 997
Plasmodium, 1532, 1532t, 1533t, 1893, 1893–1896, 1895t. See also Malaria.
Plastics, smoke inhalation and, 403, 403t, 404
Platelet-activating factor (PAF), asthma role of, 377
  mast cell release of, 1436t
Platelet-derived growth factor (PDGF), 294, 295
Platelets, 979–986
  activation of, 977, 977, 978
  aggregation of, 977, 977, 978, 980
  antibodies to, 980–983, 984t, 986
  atherogenesis role of, 292, 292, 294, 295
  autoantibodies to, 1476t, 1477
  Bernard-Soulier, 985
  coagulation sequence and, 977, 977, 978, 979

Platelets (Continued)
  count of, 979
    decreased, 980. See also Thrombocytopenia.
    increased, 922t. See also Thrombocytosis.
  destruction of, accelerated, 980–984, 983, 984t
  distribution disorders of, 984, 984t
  drugs affecting, 980t, 982–985
  electron micrograph of, 982
  function of, 977, 979–980
    abnormalities in, 984–985
    tests of, 979–980, 983
  giant, 985
  granules of, 979, 982, 985
  hemostasis role of, 977, 977, 978, 979
  kinetics of, 979
  megakaryocyte origin of, 818, 979
  physical examination and, 978–979, 979t
  polycythemia vera and, 921, 921t, 922t
  production of, 818–819, 820, 820t, 898, 979
    decreased, 980
    excessive, 922–924, 923t, 984
  secretory granules of, 979
  splenic sequestration of, 971
  storage pool defects and, 985
  thrombasthenic, 985
  thromboxane and, 977, 977, 979
  transfusion of, 985–986
    alloantibodies in, 986
    dosage in, 985–986
  vegetative growth due to, 1598–1599, 1599
Platinum, occupational exposure to, 73
Platinum compounds, 1039t, 1042
  adverse effects of, 1042
  chemotherapy using, 1039t, 1042
Platybasia, 2149
Pleiotropism, 137
Pleocytosis, leptospirosis with, 1720–1721
  poliovirus causing, 2091
  syphilitic, 1708–1709, 1712t
Plethysmography, 466, 467t
Pleura, 444–447
  anatomy of, 444
  biopsy of, percutaneous, 445
  chest pain from, 370
    Mediterranean fever with, 907
    paroxysmal, 1787, 1788
    pulmonary embolism causing, 423, 424, 424t
  deformities affecting, 443t, 443–444
  effusions of, 445–447
    abscess with, 445
    actinomycotic, 445, 446
    alcoholic cardiomyopathy with, 330, 330
    asbestos and, 446
    bloody, 445, 445t, 446
    cancer and, 446–447
    causative diseases of, 445t, 445–447
    chylous, 445, 445t, 446
    diagnostic procedures for, 444t, 444–445, 445t
    heart failure and, 219, 445
    immune-mediated, 446
    infective-inflammatory, 445t, 445–446
    laboratory analysis of, 444t, 444–445, 445t
    mechanism of accumulation for, 444, 444t
    Meig's syndrome in, 446
    pancreatic, 445, 445t
    pneumococcal pneumonia with, 1572
    respiratory disease and, 369t, 371
    transudate vs. exudate, 444t, 444–445, 445t
    tuberculous, 445t, 446, 1685t
    uremia and, 446
  friction rub of, 370
  gas in, 375t
  lung lymphatic system and, 372
  physiology of, 444, 444t
  pressure gradient of, 372
Pleuritis, lupus erythematosus with, 1475t, 1478
  pneumococcal, 1571, 1571t
Pleurodynia, 1787–1788
  clinical features of, 1788
  differential diagnosis of, 1788
  enterovirus in, 1787t, 1787–1788
  epidemiology of, 1787
  pain of, 1787, 1788
  treatment and prognosis in, 1788
Plexopathy, diabetic, 2154t, 2155
  lumbosacral, 2154t, 2155
Plummer's disease, 1235–1236
Plutonium, 73
PMS (premenstrual syndrome), 1301–1302, 1302t
  prevalence of, 1301

PMS (premenstrual syndrome) (Continued)
  symptoms in, 1301–1302, 1302t
  treatment of, 1302
Pneumococcal infections, 1569–1575
  arthritis in, 1571, 1571t
  bacteremia in, 1571, 1575
  complications of, 1571, 1571t, 1575
  empyema in, 1571, 1573, 1575
  endocarditis in, 1571, 1571t
  epidemiology of, 1570–1571, 1571t
  immunization for, 43t, 45
  laboratory findings in, 1569–1570, 1572–1573
  meningitis in, 1571, 1571t
  pathogens in, 411–413, 1569–1570
  penicillin-resistant, 1570, 1570t
  pericarditis in, 1571, 1571t
  peritonitis in, 1571, 1571t
  pneumonia due to, 1569–1575
  prevention of, 1575
  prognosis in, 1575
  risk factors for, 1571t
  treatment of, 1570t, 1574t, 1574–1575
Pneumoconiosis, 399–403. See also Dust(s).
  asbestos, 399t, 400–401
  beryllium, 402t, 402–403
  coal workers', 56, 58t, 399t, 401
  silica, 399t, 401–402, 402t
Pneumocystis carinii, 1917–1922
  corticosteroid therapy with, 1918, 1920, 1921, 1921t
  extrapulmonary infection with, 1918–1919
  pneumonia due to, 1917–1922
    AIDS/HIV patient with, 1859t, 1861–1862, 1862
    clinical manifestations of, 1918, 1918–1919, 1919
    diagnosis of, 1919, 1919–1920
    epidemiology and transmission of, 1917
    etiologic organism in, 1917
    laboratory findings in, 1919, 1919–1920
    pathology findings in, 1917–1918
    treatment and prophylaxis of, 1920t, 1920–1922, 1921t, 1922t
Pneumomediastinum, 449
Pneumonia, 411–413, 1569–1585
  aerobic gram-negative bacilli causing, 1579–1581, 1580t, 1583–1584, 1585t
  AIDS/HIV with, 1859t, 1860–1862, 1862
  antimicrobial therapy in, 474, 475t, 1570t, 1574t, 1574–1575, 1578t, 1580t, 1585t
  aspiration, 1579, 1581–1582
    clinical manifestations of, 1582
    diagnosis of, 1582
    etiology of, 1581–1582
    lung abscess following, 414, 415
    nasogastric tube and, 1171
    treatment of, 1582
  bacterial, 411t, 411–412, 412t, 475t, 1569–1575, 1579–1585
  Branhamella, 412t, 1573
  chlamydial, 412t, 1574, 1724, 1725
  community-acquired, 411–413, 412t
  consolidation of, 368–371, 369t
  cultures for, 412–413, 1572–1573
  differential diagnosis of, 1573–1574
  drug therapy for, 474, 475t, 1570t, 1574t, 1574–1575, 1578t, 1580t, 1585t
  eosinophilic, chronic, 398
  etiologic agents in, 411t, 411–412, 412t, 1573–1574, 1576t, 1579–1585
  examination in, 1572
  fungal, histoplasmosis in, 1817–1818
  Haemophilus influenzae, 412t, 1573
  hospital-acquired, 1549t, 1551–1552, 1669–1671
  host defense against, 411, 411t, 1571
  Klebsiella, 1579–1581, 1580t
  Legionella, 412t, 1583–1585, 1584t, 1585t
  lipoid, 407–408
  lymphocytic interstitial, 395
  mortality rate role of, 27t, 30t
  mycoplasmal, 412t, 1576–1579, 1577
  necrotizing, bronchiectasis due to, 417
  oropharyngeal flora causing, 1579, 1582
  pathophysiology of, 411t, 411–412, 412t, 1571, 1571t
  pneumococcal, 1569–1575
  Pneumocystis carinii, 1917–1922
    AIDS/HIV patient with, 1861–1862, 1862
  Pseudomonas, 1579–1581, 1580t, 1669–1671
  radiographic findings in, 412t, 413, 1572, 1584
  respiratory failure with, 452, 452t
  Rhodococcus, 1737t

Pneumonia (Continued)
  risk factors for, 30t, 1571t
  signs and symptoms in, 368–371, 369t, 412,
    1571–1573, 1576–1580, 1584
  sputum examination in, 412–413, 1572–1573
  staphylococcal, 412t, 1573, 1607–1608
  streptococcal, 411–413, 1569–1575, 1588
  treatment of, 474, 475t, 1570t, 1574t, 1574–1575,
    1578t, 1580t, 1585t
    critical care setting, 474, 475t
  tularemia with, 1664
  viral, 412t, 475t, 1751–1752, 1755–1756
    adenovirus causing, 1758
    enterovirus in, 1787t, 1791
  Yersinia pestis, 1662
Pneumonitis, AIDS/HIV with, 1861
  aspiration, 406–407
  chemical, 404
  hydrocarbon, 408
  hypersensitivity, 403
  lupus erythematosus with, 1478
  occupational, 403
  Q fever with, 1736, 1737t
Pneumothorax, 448
  cystic fibrosis with, 420, 421t
  Pneumocystis pneumonia with, 1918
  spontaneous, 448
  tension, 448
Podagra, 1511, 1513
Podophyllotoxins, adverse effects, 1044
  chemotherapy using, 1039t, 1044, 1044t
Podosomes, 1352
POEMS syndrome, 965
  vs. amyloidosis, 1505
Pogosta disease, 1809–1810
Poikilocytosis, 824
  infantile, 855, 855t
  membrane defect causing, 855, 855t
Poikiloderma, 2212
Poikilothermia, 1203, 2012
  drug-induced, 1533
  fever due to, 1203, 1533
  hypothalamus in, 1203, 1533, 2012
Poisoning, 503–510
  acetaminophen, 504t, 506, 798, 800t
  alcohol, 508
  alkali, 507
  aluminum, 71
  Amanita, 772, 773t
  amphetamine, 508
  anticholinergic, 506
  antidepressant, 504t, 510, 510t
  antidotes for, 504t
  antifreeze, 504t, 509, 509t
  antimony, 73
  arsenic, 70, 504t
  atropine, 504t, 506
  barbiturate, 506t, 506–507
  barium, 73
  benzodiazepine, 504t, 506t, 507
  boron, 73
  bush tea, 774
  cadmium, 71–72
  calcium channel blocker, 504t, 507, 507t
  carbon monoxide, 403t, 403–404, 504t, 507, 507t
  chemical, 403, 403t, 404
  chromium, 73
  cobalt, 71
  cocaine, 507–508
  common drugs in, 1972t, 1972–1976, 1975t
  copper, 71
  cyanide, 504t, 508
  diagnosis of, 505, 505t, 506t
  ethylene glycol, 504t, 509, 509t
  gasoline, 407
  gold, 504t
  heavy metal, 67–73
  herbicide, 509–510
  hydrofluoric acid, 504t
  insecticide, 504t, 509–510, 510t
  iron, 71, 504t, 508–509
  lead, 56, 58t, 68–69, 69t, 504t
    chelation treatment for, 69, 69t, 504t
  legumes causing, 740
  lithium, 509
  manganese, 73
  marine organism causing, 1954t, 1956
  mercury, 69–70, 504t

Poisoning (Continued)
  methanol, 504t, 509, 509t
  methemoglobinemia due to, 876t, 876–877
  mortality rate role of, 37, 38
  mushroom, 772, 773t
  neurologic effects of, 1972t, 1972–1976, 1975t
  nickel, 71, 72
  nitrite, 504t
  occupational exposure to, 56, 58t, 59t, 403t
  organophosphate, 504t, 509–510, 510t
  oxygen, 404–405, 405
  paraquat, 509–510
  platinum, 73
  plutonium, 73
  scopolamine, 506
  selenium, 72–73
  shellfish, 739t, 740, 1954t, 1956
  smoke, 403t, 404
  snakebite, 1951–1953, 1952t, 1954–1955
  stimulant, 508
  tellurium, 73
  thallium, 72
  theophylline, 510
  tin, 71, 73
  treatment of, antidote, 504t
    bowel irrigation, 505–506, 506t, 798
    charcoal, 505, 506t
    gastric lavage, 505
    ipecac, 505
    removal of poison in, 505–506, 506t
  vanadium, 73
  zinc, 70–71
Polarized light, amyloid deposit under, 1504, 1506
  urate crystals in, 1512, 1514
Poliovirus, 1784t, 2091–2092
  characteristics of, 1783–1785, 1784t
  clinical manifestations due to, 1786–1787, 1787t,
    2091–2092
  immunization for, 40, 43t, 45–46, 2092
  incidence and prevalence for, 2091
  myelitis due to, 1786–1787, 1787t, 2091–2092
  pathogenesis and pathology for, 1786, 2091
  postpolio syndrome due to, 2091–2092
Pollen, 1414
  anaphylaxis due to, 1418t
  avoidance of, 1416
  peak periods for, 1414
  sources of, 1414
Pollution. See also Environment; Occupation.
  cancer related to, 1009t, 1010, 1015–1016
Polyarteritis nodosa, 1492–1495
  clinical manifestations of, 1493, 1494
  differential diagnosis of, 1494
  glomerulonephritis and, 573t, 574t, 577, 577t,
    1493
  laboratory findings in, 1493–1494
  pathology in, 1493
  prognosis in, 1493
  treatment of, 1494, 1494–1495
Polyarthritis, carcinomatous, 1527
  rheumatic fever with, 1592t, 1592–1593
  viral, 1805t, 1806–1810
Polychlorinated biphenyls (PCBs), 740
Polychondritis, 1517
  clinical features of, 1517
  disease associations of, 1517
  relapsing, 1517
  treatment of, 1517
Polyclothiazide, 264t
Polycythemia, 921–922
  clinical features of, 921, 922t
  congenital heart disease with, 284–286
  diagnostic criteria, 921, 921t
  laboratory testing in, 921, 922t
  treatment of, 921–922
  tumor-associated, 1026
Polydipsia, 1223–1225
  diabetes insipidus with, 1223–1225, 1225
  primary, 1224
Polymerase chain reaction (PCR), 137
  genome mapping with, 137
  Lyme disease in, 1718
  sickle syndromes in, 890–891, 891
Polymixin B, 1558, 1558t
Polymorphisms, cancer genes with, 1077
Polymyalgia rheumatica, 1498–1500
  clinical findings in, 1498, 1499t
  differential diagnosis of, 1498–1499, 1499t
  incidence of, 1498
  laboratory findings in, 1498, 1499t

Polymyositis, 1018–1019, 1443
  antinuclear antibodies in, 1457, 1457t
  diagnosis of, 1018–1019, 2164
  incidence of, 1485t
  interstitial lung disease with, 395t, 396
  paraneoplastic, 1018, 1029
  pathophysiology, 1018, 1029
  treatment of, 1019
Polyneuropathy, 2150
  axonal, 2150
  cancer and, 1029
  definition of, 2150
  demyelinating, 2151t, 2151–2152
  diabetic, 2154–2155
  paraneoplastic, 1029
  pyridoxine deficiency causing, 2040–2041
Polypectomy, 638t, 639–640
Polypeptide, gene translation of, 134, 135
  vasoactive intestinal, 694
Polyps, 722–723
  colonic, 722–723, 724
    endoscopy of, 638t, 639–640, 722
  Cowden's syndrome with, 725
  Cronkite-Canada syndrome with, 725
  Gardner syndrome and, 723, 724
  gastric, 679
  juvenile, 725
  nasal, 724
  Peutz-Jeghers, 724, 724
  Turcot's syndrome and, 724–725
Polysaccharide, bacterial, 1556, 1622
  capsular, 1556, 1622
  group B, 1556
Polysaccharides, Haemophilus influenzae, 1622, 1624
Polyurethane film, dressing with, 2193, 2194t
Polyuria, diabetes insipidus with, 1223–1225, 1225
  renal obstruction with, 591, 591t
Polyvinyl chloride, smoke inhalation and, 403, 403t
POMC (pro-opio-melano-cortin), 1186, 1186
  ACTH and, 1186, 1186, 1198, 1215
  hormones generated from, 1186, 1186, 1198, 1215
Pompe's disease, 1083, 1083t
Pompholyx, 2199
Pons, tumor of, 2126t
Pontiac fever, Legionella in, 1583, 1585
Pontine, hemorrhage in, 2078, 2078t
Pork. See also Meat.
  tapeworm in, 1923t, 1924–1926
  trichinosis associated with, 1937–1938
Porphobilinogen, 1125
  heme synthesis and, 1125
  urinary, 1130, 1130t
Porphobilinogen deaminase, 1125, 1125t, 1126
  deficiency of, 1125, 1125t, 1126
Porphyria, 1124–1130
  aminolevulinic dehydratase deficiency in, 1124–1126,
    1125, 1125t
  classification of, 1124, 1125t
  coproporphyria, hereditary, 1125, 1125t, 1129
  cutanea tarda, 1128–1129
    bullae of, 2205t
    clinical manifestations of, 1126t, 1129, 2205t
    diagnosis of, 1126t, 1129
    etiology and pathogenesis of, 1125, 1125t,
      1128–1129
  drugs in relation to, 1127, 1127t
  dual, 1130
  erythropoietic, 1124, 1128, 1129–1130
    congenital, 1125, 1125t, 1128, 1129–1130
    protoporphyric, 786, 1125, 1125t, 1126t, 1129–1130
  genetics of, 138t, 1125t
  hepatic, 1124, 1125t
  hepatoerythropoietic, 1125t, 1129
  intermittent acute, 1126–1128
    clinical features of, 1126, 1126t
    diagnosis of, 1127
    etiology and pathogenesis of, 1125, 1125t, 1126,
      1126t
    precipitating factors for, 1126t, 1126–1127, 1127t
    prevention of, 1128
    prognosis in, 1128
    treatment of, 1126t, 1127
  laboratory testing for, 1130, 1130t
  neurologic effects of, 1126
  neuropathy due to, 2155
  photosensitivity in, 1124, 1128, 1130
  toxic, 1124
  variegate, 136t, 1125, 1125t, 1129
Porphyrin, heme synthesis and, 1124, 1125
  urinary, 1130, 1130t

Porphyrinogen, *1125*
Porphyromonas, 1638, *1639,* 1639t, 1641t
Portal hypertension. See *Hypertension, portal.*
Portal vein, shunt from. See *Shunts, portosystemic.*
Porter-Silber chromogens, 1246, *1247*
Port-wine angioma, 2056
Positive end-expiratory pressure (PEEP), 466–467
    auto-PEEP as, 467
        respiratory failure treated with, 471–472, *472*
        ventilator therapy using, 471t, 471–472, *472*
Positron emission tomography (PET), advances in, 131, *133*
    cardiac, 202
    CNS examination with, 1961, 2129
    myocardial infarction in, 307, *308, 309*
Posterior fossa, imaging of, 1963t, 1967
    tumor affecting, 2126
Postpartum thyroiditis, 1240
Postpolio syndrome, 2091–2092
Postprandial state, 1278, 1278t
    hypoglycemia in, 1279, 1279t
    insulin action in, 1260–1261
Post-traumatic stress disorder, 2005
Posture, aging effect on, 16t, 16–17
    basal ganglia related to, 2042–2043
    instability of, 2042–2043
Posturing, decerebrate, 798t
Potassium, **538–543**
    acidosis and, 540
    alkalosis and, 540
    antiarrhythmic agents affecting, 244–245, *245,* 245t
    depletion, 539t, 539–541. See also *Hypokalemia.*
    dietary, 261–262
    diuretics and, 531t, 531–532, *532,* 540
    ECG and, *541, 542*
    excess, 541t, 541–543. See also *Hyperkalemia.*
    extracellular, 533, 538–539
    gastrointestinal loss of, 540
    hypertension and, 261–262
    intracellular, 533, 538–539
    kidney and, 514, *515, 522,* 523–524, 539
        diminished excretion and, 541
        excessive loss and, 539–540
        failure and, 514, *515,* 556–557, 561
        fractional excretion and, 514, 514t, *515*
        transport and, *223,* 521t, *522,* 523–524, *532,* 539
    magnesium deficiency and, 1138
    paralysis and, depolarizing, 542
        periodic, 540, 542
    parenteral, 540–541
    physiologic considerations for, 538–539
    renal failure and, chronic, 556–557, 561
    supplemental, 261–262
    uremia and, 561
    urinary, 514, *515,* 539t, 539–540, 541
Potassium channels, 244–245, *245,* 245t
Potassium hydroxide, fungus exudation in, 2192
Potassium iodide, panniculitis treated with, 1508
    saturated, 1826
    sporotrichosis therapy with, 1826–1827
    toxic reaction to, 1826
Potential. See *Action potential; Resting potential.*
Pottery, lead leached from, 66
Poultry, *Campylobacter* reservoir in, 1649, 1649t, 1738t
    dietary, *1142*
    erysipeloid and, 1673–1674
Powassan encephalitis, 1806t, 1814
Powders, topical therapy with, 2194, 2194t
Poxvirus, *1739*
PR interval, *190,* 191, *232*
Prader-Willi syndrome (PWS), 155–156, 160t, 161
    chromosome deletion causing, *153, 155,* 155t, 155–156, 161
    clinical features of, 155t, 155–156, 160t, 161, 2013
Prairie dog, plague carried by, 1737t
Pralidoxime, 504t, 509
Praziquantel, schistosomiasis therapy with, 1931
    tapeworm therapy with, 1923t, 1924t
Prazosin, dosage for, 229t, 265t, 266t
    vasodilatation using, 229t, 229–230
Prealbumin (transthyretin), 967t
Prednisolone, 108t
Prednisone. See also *Corticosteroids.*
    anti-inflammatory use of, 108t
    cancer therapy using, 1046t, 1047
    gout treated with, 1514t
    heart transplantation and, 363, 364t
    Hodgkin's disease and, 952t, 953
    immunosuppression using, 363, 364t
    myeloma treated with, 963, 964

Prednisone *(Continued)*
    non-Hodgkin's lymphoma and, 945t
    pain control use of, 106t
    pharmacokinetics of, 108t
    rejection reaction treated with, 364t
Pre-eclampsia, 609–610, 610t
    clinical features in, 610, 610t
    incidence of, 610
    pathogenesis of, 609–610
    treatment of, 610
Pregnancy, anaerobic flora and, 1640, 1640t
    asthma and, 381
    blisters with, 2206
    breasts in, 1317, 1325
    cancer therapy during, **1060–1071,** 1325
        incidence and, 1060–1061, 1061t
    chemotherapy effects in, 1068–1071, 1069t, 1070t
    chlamydial infection with, 1724
    cholestasis with, 787, 787t, 810
    diabetes insipidus in, 1224
    diabetes mellitus in, 1258
    dietary requirements in, 1140t
    epilepsy with, 2123
    genetic counseling in, 162–165, 164t, 165t
    glucose level in, 1258–1259, 1259t
    gonorrhea with, 1702, 1702t
    hemophilia and, 994
    herpes gestationis of, 2206
    Hodgkin's disease with, 954
    hypertension and, 609–611
    iron levels affected by, 1134t
    listeriosis with, 1673
    liver disease with, 787t, 787–788, 810
    lupus erythematosus and, 1480
    Lyme disease in, 1719–1720
    multiple sclerosis with, 2110
    phenylalanine level in, 1108
    prenatal testing and, 164t, 165, 165t
    prostaglandins in, 1193
    radiation therapy affecting, 1069–1070, 1070t
    renal function in, **609–611,** 610t
    sickle syndromes and, 888, 891
    syphilis affecting, 1710, 1712–1713
    thrombocytosis with, 924
    thrombosis prevention in, 119
    thyrotoxicosis during, 1236–1237
    toxemia of, 609–610, 610t
    toxoplasmosis affecting, 1909
    vaccinia vaccine in, 1768
    varicella in, 1763
    vomiting and, 630, 630t
Prekallikrein, coagulation role of, 987–988, 995
    deficiency of, 995
Preload, 175–176, *176,* 212t, 214
    definition of, 212t
    Frank-Starling relation and, 214
    heart failure and, 214, *214,* fungus exudation in
    shock and, 479, *479, 480,* 494
    vasodilator reduction of, 229, 229t, 494
Premature complexes, atrial, 237–238, *238, 240*
    atrioventricular junction, 242
    ventricular, 238t, 242–243, *243*
Premenstrual syndrome, 1301–1302, 1302t
    prevalence of, 1301
    symptoms in, 1301–1302, 1302t
    treatment of, 1302
Prepuce, sebaceous glands of, 2186
Presbyesophagus, 655
Presbyopia, 16t, 16–17, 2174
Pressophysins, 1221–1222
Pressure receptors. See *Baroreceptors.*
Pressure sores, 2212
    elderly with, 24, 24t
    urticarial, 1410
Pretectum, *2017*
Preventive health care, **26–73**
    botulism and, 1636
    compromised host with, 1547t, 1547–1548
    diet in, 29–31, 30t, 1139–1143
    exercise in, 31t, 31–33, *32,* 33t
    meningococcal infection prophylaxis in, 1621, 1621t
    modifiable factors for, 27t, 30t
    occupational exposure and, 56–59, 58t, 59t
    patient examination for, 27–29, 28t
    physician decision making in, 76–77
    principles of, 26–27
    protective dress and equipment for, 1853t, 1853–1854, 1854t
    responsibility for, 20, 77
    rheumatic fever in, 1589t, 1596

Preventive health care *(Continued)*
    smoking role in, 27t, 30t, 33–36, 171
    travel and, 1553–1556, 1554t, 1555t
    vaccination/immunization role in, 40–46, 41t–44t
    violence and injury role in, 36–40, 37t, *37–39*
Prevotella, 1638–1641, *1639,* 1639t, 1641t
Priapism, 889
    sickle syndrome causing, 889
    treatment of, 889
Primaquine, 1920t, 1921, 1921t, 1922t
Primates, non-human, *1845,* 1845–1846
Primidone, 91t, 94t
    dose adjustment for, 94t
    epilepsy therapy with, 2122t
    pharmacokinetics of, 91t, 94t, 2122t
    renal failure effect on, 94t
Proaccelerin, 987–989, 988t, *989*
Probability, 78–82, 79t, *79–82*
Probenecid, 1514t
Procainamide, 91t, 94t, 246t
    adverse effects of, 247t
    antiarrhythmic action of, *245,* 246t, 249
    dose adjustment for, 94t
    pharmacokinetics of, 91t, 94t, 246t, 249
    renal failure effect on, 94t
Procarbazine, adverse effects of, 1045
    chemotherapy using, 1042t, 1045
    Hodgkin's disease and, 952t, 953
Procidentia, 743
Procollagen proteinase deficiency, 1121t
Proctitis, chlamydial, 742
    colitis with, 1649–1650, 1913–1915
        amebic, 1913t, 1913–1915, 1915t
        Campylobacter, 1649t, 1649–1650
    gonococcal, 742
    sigmoiditis with, 713–714
    syphilitic, 742
    ulcerative, 713
Proctosigmoidoscopy, 694
Pro-dynorphin, *1186,* 1186–1187
Pro-endorphin, 1186, *1186*
Proerythroblast, 817, *820, 821*
Progesterone, breast cancer receptors for, 1322
    cancer therapy and, 1010, 1046t, 1047
    oral contraception with, 1309–1310
    ovarian synthesis of, 1299, *1299, 1300,* 1301t, 1312t
    premenstrual syndrome treated with, 1302
    tumor production of, 1312t
Progestin. See *Progesterone.*
Prolactin, 1206t, 1212–1215
    deficiency of, 1213
    excess of. See *Hyperprolactinemia.*
    laboratory tests for, 1208t, 1213t
    receptor for, 1212
    regulation of, *1198, 1199,* 1206t, 1212
        disordered, 1202t, 1202–1203, 1213–1215
    secretion of, 1212–1213
        tumor, 1209t, 1212–1213
    stimulation test for, 1208t
Prolactin-inhibitory factor (PIF), 1199
Prolactinoma, 1209t, 1212–1213
Prolactin-releasing factor (PRF), 1199
Prolapse, rectal, 743
Proleukin, cancer therapy using, 1048
Proline, 1109
    elevated, 1102t, 1109, *1109*
    enzyme deficiency affecting, 1102t, 1103t, 1104t, *1109,* 1109
    urinary, 1102t, 1103t, 1104t
Promastigote, leishmanial, 1903–1904, *1904*
Promethazine, 1416, 1416t
Promoter region, gene transcription and, *135*
    HIV gene, *1181*
Pronormoblast, giant, 834, *834*
Pro-opio-melano-cortin (POMC), 1186, *1186*
    ACTH and, 1186, *1186,* 1198, 1215
    hormones generated from, 1186, *1186,* 1198, 1215
Propafenone, 246t
    adverse effects of, 248t
    antiarrhythmic action of, *245,* 246t, 249
    pharmacokinetics of, 246t
Propionibacterium acnes, 1641t
Propoxyphene, 51
    pain control with, 104t, 893t
    smoking interaction with, 36
Propranolol, 246t, 249
    adverse effects of, 248t
    antiarrhythmic action of, *245,* 246t, 249

Propranolol (Continued)
dosage for, 265t, 266t, 299t
pharmacokinetics of, 246t, 249
smoking interaction with, 36t
Propylthiouracil, adverse effects of, 1234, 1234t
hepatotoxicity, 773
mechanism of action of, 1227, 1234
pregnancy and, 1236
thyroid inhibition using, 1227, 1234–1235, 1235t, 1236t
Prosody, 1990
Prostacyclins, 113, 1188, 1189
formation of, 113, 1188, 1189
metabolism of, 113, 1188, 1191–1193
septic shock and, 499
shock and, 481
Prostaglandins, 1187–1193
allergic rhinitis role of, 1414–1415, 1415
aspirin effect and, 114–115, 1192–1193
coagulation role of, 977, 977, 978
diet modification of, 1192
fever production role of, 1534
formation of, 113, 1187–1191, 1188, 1189
gastrointestinal effects of, 1193
inflammation role of, 112–115, 113, 1193
kidney and, 527, 1193
mast cell release of, 1416, 1436t
metabolism of, 113, 1188, 1189, 1192–1193
natriuresis due to, 527, 1193
neutrophils and, 114–115, 1190, 1190–1191
NSAIDs inhibition of, 112–114, 113, 663, 1192–1193
peptic ulcer role of, 663, 667
physiology of, 1187–1191, 1188–1191
renin and, 1193
research history of, 112–115
respiratory effects of, 1193
volume regulation role of, 526t, 527, 527, 1193
Prostate gland, 1341–1345
anatomy of, 1341, 1341
biochemistry of, 1341
carcinoma of, 1344–1345
etiology of, 1344
incidence of, 1005, 1009, 1013t, 1015, 1344
pathogenesis of, 1344
physical examination for, 1344
staging of, 1344, 1344–1345
symptoms of, 1344
tumor markers for, 1022t, 1023
examination of, 1343, 1344
cancer screening with, 1006t
hyperplasia of, 1342–1344
diagnostic tests for, 1343
symptoms of, 1343
treatment of, 1343–1344
inflammation of, 1341–1342
pain from, 1342
physiology of, 1341
sexual differentiation and, 1284–1285, 1285, 1286
utricle of, 1286
Prostatectomy, for carcinoma, 1345
for hyperplasia, 1343
transurethral, 1343
Prostatitis, 1341–1342
abacterial, 1342
acute bacterial, 1342
chronic bacterial, 1342
diagnosis of, 1342
differential diagnosis of, 1342
incidence of, 1342
pathogenesis of, 1341–1342
treatment of, 1342
Prostatodynia, 1342
Prosthetic valves, anticoagulant therapy with, 119
aspirin therapy with, 118
emboli arising from, 2067
endocarditis with, 1597t, 1597–1598, 1598t, 1602
Proteases, anaerobic flora production of, 1639t
staphylococcal, 1606, 1607t
Protective dress and equipment, 1853t, 1853–1854, 1854t
Protein, absorption of, 696, 696t
acute phase, 1535–1537, 1536t
sedimentation rate affected by, 1456
anaphylaxis due to, 1418t
ascites content of, 744t, 745t
Bax, 1072–1073, 1073
Bcl-2, 1072–1073, 1073
beta, 1505

Protein (Continued)
bile content of, 805, 805
body, total, 1154
C, 988t
bacterial, 1556
coagulation role of, 987, 988t, 989
deficiency of, 997, 2068
resistance to, 998
C-reactive, 1456
illness response role of, 1535–1537, 1536t
coagulation, 977–978, 987–990, 988t
complement-regulatory, 1398–1400, 1398–1401
deficiency of, 1154–1157
causes of, 1154t, 1154–1155
energy requirements and, 1154
physiologic consequences of, 1155t, 1155–1156, 1156t
dietary, food groups and, 1142, 1143
intake requirements for, 1140t, 1154, 1173, 1173t
malnutrition and, 1154t, 1154–1157, 1155t, 1156t
parenteral nutrition and, 1171–1172, 1173, 1173t
RDA, 1140t
erythrocytic, 851–852
functions of, 143t, 147t
M, 958, 959
cryoglobulinemia with, 966
gammopathy role of, 958–966, 960t, 961t
heavy chain disease and, 966
streptococcal, 1586–1587
metabolism of, derangements in, 143t–147t, 143–147
liver and, 754, 760–761
monoclonal, 958–968, 959
detection of, 958–960, 959, 960
plasma membrane transporter role of, 143–145, 144t
S, 988t
coagulation role of, 987, 988t, 989, 997
deficiency of, 997, 2068
serum levels of, 700t
nutrition assessment and, 1153–1154, 1156t, 1157
synovial fluid with, 1465t
Tamm-Horsfall, 553
urinary. See Proteinuria.
viral, 1739–1740
Protein kinases, C, phosphatidylinositol and, 1179
calmodulin and, 1179
hormone action role of, 1177, 1178–1180, 1179, 1180
Proteinuria, 513
Alport's syndrome and, 612, 612t
Bence Jones, 959, 962
diabetic, 599, 600
functional, 513
glomerular, 513, 513t, 572–573
hemodynamic, 513, 513t
isolated, 513
lupus erythematosus with, 1475t, 1479
nephrotic syndrome causing, 573
nephrotic-range, 513, 513t, 573
overflow, 513, 513t
renal failure causing, acute, 552t, 553–554, 554t
selective, 513, 513t
tubular, 513, 513t
tubulointerstitial disease with, 580, 580t
types of, 513, 513t
Proteoglycans, 1445, 1445t
connective tissue structure and, 1445, 1445t
mucopolysaccharidoses and, 1118, 1119t
Prothrombin, 988t
coagulation role of, 977, 977, 978, 996
deficiency of, 996
liver synthesis of, 760–761, 1000
Prothrombin time, 979, 979t, 989, 990
acetaminophen poisoning and, 800t
coagulation disorder affecting, 979, 979t, 990
liver function and, 760–761, 800t, 1000
malabsorption and, 700t
prolonged, 979, 979t, 990
thrombocytopenia and, 981, 983
Protoporphyrin, heme synthesis and, 1125
sideroblastic anemia role of, 842–843
Protoporphyrinogen, 1125
Protoporphyrinogen oxidase, 1125, 1125t, 1129
deficiency of, 1125, 1125t, 1129
Protozoan disease, 1892–1922. See also specific disease.
amebic, 1913–1915
babesial, 1915–1916
balantidial, 1916t
Blastocystis hominis, 1916t
cryptosporidial, 1910–1912
Cyclospora, 1916t

Protozoan disease (Continued)
diagnostic principles for, 1892
dientamoebic, 1916t
food poisoning due to, 739, 739t
giardial, 1912–1913
hepatic infection in, 782, 783t
isosporial, 1916t
leishmanial, 1903–1907
malarial, 1893–1896
Pneumocystis carinii, 1917–1922
Sarcocystis, 1916t
sexual transmission of, 1697t, 1699, 1699t
toxoplasmal, 1907–1910
trichomonal, 1916–1917
trypanosomal, 1896–1903
vaginal infection in, 1697t, 1699, 1699t
Prourokinase, 988t
coagulation role of, 988t, 989
Provitamins, A, 1151, 1151t
Prune-belly syndrome, 622–623
Pruritus, 2187, 2187t, 2188t
anal, 742
calcium deposition, 1377
chigger bite, 1947
cholestasis with, 759, 808
disorders associated with, 2187, 2187t, 2188t
eczematous, 2197
"ground itch," 1935
Hodgkin's disease causing, 948, 1033
hookworm, 1935
leech bite, 1951
leukemic, 1033
liver disease and, 752, 759, 791
mastocytosis causing, 1437
mosquito bite, 1946–1947
paraneoplastic, 1033
physiology of, 2187
porphyria with, 1130
pregnancy with, 787, 787t
renal failure and, 557t, 559, 562
Pseudoallergy, 1432, 1432t
Pseudocyst, pancreatic, 735–736
Pseudodementia, 19, 19t
Pseudogout, 1465t
Pseudohermaphroditism, 1287–1293
female, 1287–1290, 1288, 1290
male, 1287, 1290–1291, 1291t, 1292
Pseudohyperkalemia, 542
Pseudohypertension, 260
Pseudohypoaldosteronism, 1252
Pseudohypoparathyroidism, 1363, 1372, 1372–1373
Pseudomonas infections, 1579–1581, 1667–1672
aeruginosa, 1667, 1669–1670
bacteremia due to, 1579–1581, 1667, 1669–1672, 1671t
cepacia, 1667, 1670–1671, 1671t
classification of organisms in, 1667, 1668t
endocarditis due to, 1598t, 1598–1599, 1669
glanders in (mallei), 1669, 1669
maltophilia, 1667, 1671–1672
melioidosis in (pseudomallei), 1667–1669, 1668
meningitis due to, 1610–1613, 1616t
nosocomial, 1579–1581, 1669–1672
pickettii, 1667, 1671
pneumonia in, 1579–1581, 1580t, 1669–1671
pustules due to, 2207
Pseudoxanthoma elasticum, 1123–1124
clinical features in, 1123, 1123
genetics of, 1123–1124
pathology in, 1124
Psilocybin, 54, 508, 508t
Psitticosis, 1725
chlamydial etiology of, 1723t, 1725, 1737t
clinical features of, 1725, 1737t
epidemiology of, 1723t, 1725, 1737t
laboratory testing for, 1725
prevention of, 1725
Psoriasis, 2202–2203
arthritis with, 1467t, 1471, 1471–1472, 2203
body location of lesions of, 2191
erythemal, 2203
guttate, 2203
HLA complex in, 1431t
incidence of, 2184t
inverse, 2203
Koebner phenomenon in, 2192, 2203
pathogenesis of, 2203
pustular, 2203
Reiter's syndrome vs., 2203
skin lesions of, 2202–2203, 2203

Psoriasis (Continued)
  treatment of, 2203
    tars and anthralin in, 2195, 2203
Psychedelic agents, 54, 1975t
Psychiatric disorders, **1996–2006**
  affective, 1999–2004. See also Depression; Mania.
  AIDS/HIV with, 1855t, 1857–1858
  amnesia in, 1990
  anorexia nervosa in, 1158–1160, 1159t
  anxiety, 2004–2005. See also Anxiety.
  approach to patient with, 1996, 1996t
  bipolar, 2002–2004, 2003t
  bulimia in, 1160
  consciousness impairment vs., 1974, 1974t
  drug therapy in, 1999, 1999t, 2000t, 2000–2001
  eating affected by, 1158–1160, 1159t
  elderly patient and, 17–21, 19t, 20t, 1999–2000
  hair pulling in, 2215–2216
  history taking for, 1996, 1996t
  lupus erythematosus causing, 1475t, 1479–1480, 1480t
  manic, 1997t, 2002–2004, 2003t
  medical disorders vs., 1996, 1996t
  organic vs. functional, 1974t
  panic with, 2004t, 2004–2005
  schizophrenic, 1997–1999. See also Schizophrenia.
  somatization of, 2005t, 2005–2006, 2006t
  suicidal, 2002
  syphilitic, 1709
  thyroid hormone values in, 1230t
  toxic, 508, 1972t, 1974, 1975t
  vitamin B$_{12}$ deficiency causing, 845, 848, 848t, 1151
  Wilson's disease causing, 1131
Psychoactive drugs, cannabinoid, 53–54
  hallucinogenic, 54, 56t, 508
  toxic psychosis due to, 508, 1972t
Psychological factors, anorexia and, 1158
  bulimia with, 1160
  hair, skin and nails with, 2184, 2189–2190
  impotence with, 1331
  sexual dysfunction and, 1308
  symptoms engendered by, 2005t, 2005–2006, 2006t
  vision loss due to, 2174–2175
Psychosis. See also Psychiatric disorders.
  definition of, 1997
  toxic, 508, 1972t
Psychosocial factors, 366, 2125
  congenital heart disease and, 282, 284
  epilepsy with, 2125
  heart transplantation and, 366
  sickle syndrome and, 776
PT. See Prothrombin time.
Pterins, 1147t
Ptosis, muscular dystrophy with, 2162–2163
PTT. See Thromboplastin time, partial.
Puberty, asynchronous, 1295t, 1297
  female, 1294, 1294–1295
    follicle-stimulating hormone in, 1294, 1294–1295
    luteinizing hormone in, 1294, 1294–1295
    Tanner stages of, 1303t
  hair pattern affected by, 1294, 1294, 1303t, 1329, 2187
  male, 1325–1326, 1329, 1338, 1340
    delayed, 1338
  precocious. See Sexual precocity.
  secondary sex characteristics in, 1294, 1329
Pubic hair, 2186–2187
  escutcheon shape of, 1329
  female puberty and, 1294, 1294, 1303t, 2187
  hypogonadism affecting, 1292, 1330, 1335
  lice infestation of, 1697t, 1946
  male puberty and, 1329, 2187
  normal growth of, 2186–2187
  Tanner stages for, 1303, 1303t
Puerperium, 1317
Pufferfish toxin, 1954t, 1956
Pulmonary. See also Lung entries.
Pulmonary artery, enlargement of, 274
  wedge pressure of, sepsis affecting, 501t
Pulmonary edema. See Edema, pulmonary.
Pulmonary embolism. See Embolism, pulmonary.
Pulmonary function tests, 373, 373–376
  asthma and, 377–380, 378
  blood gases and, 373t, 374, 374–375
  bronchiectasis and, 418
  diffusion capacity in, 373t, 374, 374–375
  expiratory flow in, 373t, 374, 374
  interstitial disease and, 392
  obstructive disease in, 375
  Pneumocystis pneumonia and, 1918, 1918

Pulmonary function tests (Continued)
  restrictive disease in, 375–376, 376t
  volumes in, 373, 373t, 373–374
Pulmonary vasculature, 186–188, 187, 188
  blood flow in, 489t
    embolism and, 422–424
    shock and, 489
    ventilation and, 371–372, 467t, 467–468
  capillary, 371–372, 372
    gas exchange in, 371–372, 467–468
    interstitial fluid exchange in, 476–477, 477
  capillary (wedge) pressure of, 175, 176, 210, 489t
    cardiac tamponade and, 339, 340
    catheterization recording of, 208, 210
    constrictive pericarditis and, 341, 341
    mitral regurgitation and, 210
    mitral valve stenosis and, 211
  edema and. See Edema, pulmonary.
  lymphatic, 372
  roentgenography of, 186–188, 187, 188
Pulmonic valve, 327
  regurgitation from, 327
    congenital, 282, 285
  stenosis of, 327
    congenital, 278, 279
    treatment of, 289, 289
Pulse, 167
  absence of, aortitis with, 346
    hypertension causing, 260t
  alternans, 289
    heart failure with, 218
  aortic valve regurgitation and, 322
  arterial, 167
  brain injury and, 2138t
  cardiac tamponade affecting, 340, 340
  carotid, 167
  jugular, 167, 167
  myocardial infarction affecting, 304
  normal, 167, 167
  paradoxical, 340, 340
    cardiac tamponade with, 340, 340
  venous, 167, 167
Pulse generators, 251
Pupil, 2017, **2017–2018**, 2018
  Adie's, 2018, 2018
  Argyll-Robertson, 1709, 2018
  arousal level and, 1970–1971, 1971t
  autonomic control of, 2009, 2009t
  cerebral hemorrhage affecting, 2078, 2078t
  dilation of, 2017, 2018, 2018
    diagnostic, 2176–2178
    mucormycosis with, 1833
  examination of, 2017, 2018, 2018
  glaucoma effect on, 2176–2178
  Horner's syndrome affecting, 2018
  hysterical syncope and, 1979t
  localization of lesion using, 2017, 2018, 2018
  metabolic encephalopathy and, 1973, 1973t
  neural pathways of, 2017
  neurologic examination of, 1977t
  opioid effect on, 52
  size of, 2078, 2078t
  syphilis affecting, 1709
  trauma injury affecting, 2138t
  vision and, 2017, 2017–2018, 2018
Purine nucleoside phosphorylase, 1115, 1115–1116
  deficiency of, 1115, 1115–1116
    Nezelof's syndrome with, 1402t, 1405
Purines, **1114–1117**
  adenosine deaminase deficiency and, 1114–1115, 1115
  antagonists to, adverse effects of, 1043
    chemotherapy using, 1042t, 1043
  genetic code based on, 134, 134t
  gout role of, 1509–1510, 1511
  HPRT and, 1510, 1511
  lithiasis due to, 1117, 1510–1511
  metabolism of, 1115, 1509–1510, 1511
  myoadenylate deaminase deficiency and, 1115, 1116–1117
  nucleoside phosphorylase deficiency and, 1115, 1115–1116, 1510, 1511
  xanthine oxidase deficiency and, 1117, 1509–1510, 1511
Purkinje system, 190, 191, 191t, 231–233, 232
  afterdepolarization affecting, 234, 234
  anatomy of, 191, 231, 232
  automaticity in, 233
  block affecting, 191, 191t, 234
  cell morphology in, 231

Purkinje system (Continued)
  conduction in, 231, 232, 233t, 234
    velocity of, 190, 191, 191t, 233t
  electrogram of, 231–233, 232
  fibers of, 191, 231, 232
  paraneoplastic effects in, 1028
  reentry circuit in, 234, 234
Purpura. See also Petechiae.
  amyloidosis with, 1035
  eczematous, 2201t, 2201–2202
  Gardner-Diamond, 987
  Henoch-Schönlein, glomerulonephritis with, 576
    vasculitis with, 1492, 2201t, 2202
  kidney failure with, 1000–1001
  maculopapular lesions with, 2201t, 2201–2202
  simplex, 987
  thrombocytopenic, idiopathic, 980–982
    kidney affected by, 607–608, 1002–1003
    thrombotic, 607–608, 983, 984t
  vasculitis with, 1492, 2201t, 2201–2202
Purtscher's retinopathy, 1450
Purulence, synovial fluid, 1455t
Pus, conjunctivitis with, 1571, 1571t, 1624
  diarrhea with, 693
Pustules, 2206–2207, 2207t, 2216t
  acne, 2206–2207
  dermatophytic, 2207
  diseases associated with, 2191t, 2207t, 2216t
  drug-induced, 2219t, 2219–2220
  infectious disorders with, 2296
  noninfectious disorders with, 2206–2207, 2207t
  psoriatic, 2203, 2207t
  rosaceous, 2207, 2207
  sweat gland with, 2207t
Putamen, blood supply to, 2060
  hemorrhage in, 2077, 2078, 2078t, 2079
Pyelography, 515
  retrograde, 515–516
Pyelonephritis, 602–605
  acute, 602, 604t, 604–605
  clinical features of, 604, 604t
  definition of, 602
  diagnosis of, 604, 604t
  symptoms of, 604, 604t
  treatment of, 604–605, 605, 605t
Pyknodysostosis, 1389
  clinical presentation of, 1389
  laboratory findings in, 1389
  treatment of, 1389
Pyloric stenosis, fetus with, 159t
Pyloroplasty, ulcer treated with, 669–671, 670
Pyoderma, gangrenosum, 2212
  staphylococcal, 1606, 1607t
  streptococcal (impetigo), 1586, 1587, 1589t
Pyomyositis, staphylococcal, 1609, 1609t
  tropical, 1609
Pyramidal cells, hippocampal, 2117, 2118
  sclerosis of, 2117, 2118
Pyrantel pamoate, 1935t
Pyrazinamide, 1562t
  tuberculosis treated with, 1686–1688, 1687t
Pyrethrin, pediculosis treated with, 2195
Pyrexia. See Fever.
Pyridoxine, 1146t
  assessment of, 1146t
  deficiency of, 1146t, 2040–2041
  homocysteine metabolism role of, 1113
  parenteral, 1172t
  physiology of, 1146t, 1151t
  toxicity of, 1146t
  Wilson's disease treated with, 1132
Pyrilamine, 1416, 1416t
Pyrimethamine, malaria therapy with, 1895t, 1895–1896, 1896t
  Pneumocystis pneumonia and, 1922, 1922t
  toxoplasmosis therapy with, 1909, 1910t
Pyrimidine, 1117
  antagonists to, adverse effects, 1042–1043
    chemotherapy using, 1042–1043
  enzyme deficiencies affecting, 1117
  genetic code based on, 134, 134t
  metabolic defects and, 1117
Pyrimidine-5'-nucleotidase, deficiency of, 1117
  erythrocytic, 859
Pyrogens, 1533–1535
  endogenous, 1533–1535, 1534, 1535t
  exogenous, 1533–1535, 1534
  fever initiation by, 1533–1535, 1534, 1535t

Pyroglutamic acid, urinary, 1103t
Pyropoikilocytosis, 855, 855t
  infantile, 855, 855t
Pyrosis, 650, 651
Pyrrolidizine alkaloids, 774
Pyruvate, 1082, *1082*
Pyruvate kinase, *856*, 859
  deficiency of, 859
Pyuria, 513–514
  infection with, 604, 604t

Q

Q fever, 1727t, 1728t, **1735–1736**, 1737t
  hepatic granuloma with, 784t, 1735–1736
Q scan. See *Perfusion, ventilation and.*
Q wave, 190, *190*
  myocardial infarction and, 302, *305*, 306, 314–315,
    315
QRS complex, 190, *190*
  axis deviation in, 189, *189, 192*, 193, *194*
  bigeminy and, 243
  hyperkalemia affecting, 542, *542*
  vectors for, 189, *189*
  wide, *238, 239, 239*
QT segment, *190*, 191
QU interval, *190*, 191, *192*
Quadrantanopsia, 2064t, 2065
Quadriparesis, 2078, 2078t
Quality of life, decision making and, 4–6, 80–81, *82*
  heart transplantation and, 366
  outcome assessment related to, 124, 124t, *125*
Queensland tick typhus, 1732
Quenchers, oxygen toxicity and, *405*
Questionnaires, arthritis assessment with, 1441t, *1442*
Quinapril, 265t
Quinazolines, 264t
Quinethazone, 264t
Quinicrine, 1913
Quinidine, 91t, 94t, 246t
  adverse effects of, 247t, 773
  antiarrhythmic action of, *245*, 246t, 249
  dose adjustment for, 94t
  hemolytic anemia due to, 867
  hepatotoxicity of, 773
  pharmacokinetics of, 91t, 94t, 246t, 249
Quinine, 2183
Quinolones, 1562t
  adverse reactions to, 1568t
  dose adjustment for, 1562t
  endocarditis therapy with, 1602t–1604t, 1602–1603
  mechanism of action of, 1558, 1558t
  mycoplasmal infection treated with, 1578, 1578t
  pharmacology of, 1562t
  resistance to, 1558–1560, 1559t
  staphylococcal infection treated with, 1609t,
    1609–1610

R

R wave, 190, *190*
Rabbit, tularemia in, 1663
  zoonoses associated with, 1727t, 1737t, 1737–1738,
    1738t
Rabbit serum, anaphylaxis due to, 1418t, 1418–1419
  serum sickness and, 1421–1422, *1422*
Rabies, 2095–2096
  clinical features of, 2096
  diagnosis of, 2096
  dumb, 2096
  encephalitis with, 1737t
  epidemiology of, 2096
  etiologic agent in, 2095–2096
  furious, 2096
  immune globulin against, 41t
  immunization for, 43t, 46, 1554t, 1554–1555, 2096
    encephalomyelitis related to, 2104
  pathogenesis of, 2095–2096
  pathology of, 2096
  sylvatic, 2096
  transmission of, 2095–2096
  treatment and prevention of, 2096
Rabson-Mendenhall syndrome, 145t
  metabolic defect in, 145t
Raccoon, filariae of, 1945
Raccoon eyes, 1035
Racial factors, AIDS incidence and, 1848t
  breast cancer and, 1320

Racial factors (*Continued*)
  cancer rate and, 1013t, 1013–1014
  diabetes mellitus and, 1259–1260
  G6PD variants and, 857, *857*
  hemochromatosis and, 1132–1133
  hemoglobin structure and, 872–873, 883
  hereditary disorder frequency and, 136t, 136–140,
    138t
  HLA antigens and, 1460t
  21-hydroxylase deficiency and, *1288*
  hypertension and, 258, *259*
  inflammatory bowel disease and, 707, 707t
  lupus erythematosus with, 1475–1476
  osteoarthritis with, 1518
  Paget's disease of bone and, 1384
  rheumatoid arthritis with, 1459, 1460t
  sickle syndromes and, 883–884
  systemic sclerosis and, 1484t
  tuberculosis and, *1684*, 1684
Radar waves, 59
Radiation, **59–64**
  carcinogenic effects of, 62, 62t, 1016
  genetic effects of, 62
  high linear energy transfer, 1037
  injury due to. See *Radiation injury.*
  ionizing, *59*, 59–63, 60t, 61t, 62t, 1037
  naturally occurring, 59–60, 60t
  nonionizing, 63–64
  occupational exposure to, 58t, 60
  prenatal, 62
  sources of, 59–60, 60t
  tissue tolerance to, 1038t
  ultraviolet. See *Ultraviolet light.*
  units of, 60t, 1037
  wavelength of, *59*
Radiation injury, **59–64**
  accidents/disasters causing, 60
  clinical manifestations of, 61, 61t, 62, 62t
  diagnosis of, 62
  dosage related to, 59–60, 60t, 61t, 62t, 1038t
  enteritis due to, 103, 692, 750
  etiology of, 59–60, 60t
  fetus affected by, 1069–1070, 1070t
  infrared causing, 63
  lung affected by, 61, 405–406
  microwave causing, 63–64
  nervous system affected by, 1029t, 1029–1030
  pathogenesis of, 60–61
  pregancy and, 1069–1070, 1070t
  prevention of, 63
  testicular, 1336
  treatment of, 62–63
  ultraviolet causing, 63. See also *Ultraviolet light.*
  visible light causing, 63
  whole-body, 61, 62t
Radiation therapy, 1037–1038
  adverse effects of, 1029t, 1029–1030, 1038t
  brain tumor in, 2129
  breast cancer and, 1323t
  cancer treatment with, 61t, 62t, 1037–1038, 1038t
  cardiotoxicity of, 358–359
  dosage in, 61t, 62t, 1038t
  fetus affected by, 1069–1070, 1070t
  Hodgkin's disease treatment of with, *952*, 952–953
  hypothalamus affected by, 1201
  lung cancer and, 441
  nephritis due to, 587
  nervous system effects of, 1029t, 1029–1030
  ovarian carcinoma and, 1314
  pregnancy and, 1069–1070, 1070t
Radiculopathy, **2140–2144**
  AIDS/HIV with, 2156
  anatomy and, *2139*, 2141, *2141*, 2150
  approach to patient with, 2142t, 2143t, 2143–2144
  clinical features of, 2142t, 2142–2144, 2143t
  peripheral nerves affected by, 2150
  tumors causing, *2146*, 2146–2148
Radioactive agent(s), 60t
  iodine as, thyroid ablation with, 1234–1235
    uptake test using, 1230–1231
  occupational exposure to, 58t, 62t
  radium as, 58t
  radon as, 60t, 1014, 1016t
Radionuclide studies, 129–132
  advances in, 129–132, *132, 133*
  cardiac, 199–202, *200–202*
  pheochromocytoma localization with, 1256
  pulmonary embolism in, *425*, 425t, 425–426, *426*
  renal, 516
Radium, 58t

Radon, 60t, 1014
  carcinogenicity of, 1014, 1016t
  radiation exposure due to, 60t
Raeder's syndrome, 2008
Ragged red fibers, 2167
Raji cells, 1423
Rales, interstitial lung disease with, 393
  pulmonary embolism with, 424t
Ramipril, 265t
Ramsay Hunt syndrome, 2094
Ranitidine, esophageal reflux disease and, 653, 654t
  peptic ulcer treated with, *667*, 667–668
Ranson's criteria, 732, 732t
Rape, 39, *39*
Rapid plasma reagin test, 1710, 1710t
Rapoport-Luebering shunt, 856
Ras oncogene, 1011–1012, 1059, *1076*
Ras protein, 1180, *1180*
Rash, 2190–2192, *2191*, 2191t. See also *Eczema; Erythema.*
  anaphylaxis with, 1418
  antimicrobials causing, 1568t
  arbovirus infection with, 1805t, 1805–1810
  Boston, 1791
  boutonneuse fever, 1728t, 1732
  butterfly, 1475t, 1478
  cat scratch, 1738t
  chickenpox, 1763, 2205
  chigger bite, 1947
  Colorado tick fever, 1806
  dengue fever, 1807
  dermatomyositis, 1018, 2212
  discoid, 1475t, 1478
  drug-induced, 98t, 2219t, 2219–2220
  Ebola virus, 1803
  echovirus, 1790–1791
  ehrlichiosis, 1728t, 1733, 1738t
  enteroviral, 1787t, 1790–1791
  filariasis with, 1943
  flea bite, 1738t
  gonococcal, 1702
  herpes zoster, 1763, 2094
  Kawasaki's syndrome, 2200–2201
  leptospiral, 1738t
  lupus erythematosus, 1475t, 1478, 2211–2112
  Lyme disease, 1715–1717, 1717t, *1718*, 1738t
  maculopapular, 2191t. See also *Macules; Macu-
    lopapules; Papules.*
  malar, 1475t, 1478
  Marburg virus, 1803
  measles, 646, 646t, 1759, 2200
  meningitis with, 1612
    viral, 2090
  meningococcal, 1612
  mycoplasmal, 1577
  mycosis fungoides, 2202t
  palmar, Rocky Mountain spotted fever with, 1731,
    1738t
    syphilitic, 1707, *1707*
  paraneoplastic, 1018–1020, 1030–1035
  photosensitivity, 1475t, 1478
  pityriasis, 2191, *2191*, 2202t, *2203*, 2203–2204
  purpuric, 2201t, 2201–2202
  pustular, 2191t
  rheumatic fever, 1593, 1595t
  rickettsial, 1728, 1728t, 1729, 1730, 1732, 1734,
    1738t
  Rocky Mountain spotted fever, 1728t, 1730–1731,
    1738t, 2201
  roseola infantum (exanthem subitum), 1791, 2200
  Ross River virus, 1809
  rubella, 1761, 1762, 2200
  scarlet fever, 1587, 2200
  shingles, 2094
  "slapped cheek," 2200
  smallpox, 1767
  soles with, Rocky Mountain spotted fever with, 1731,
    1738t
    syphilis causing, 1707, *1707*
  spotless fever, 1728t, 1733, 1738t
  spotted fever, 1728t, 1730–1731, 1738t, 2201
  Sweet's syndrome, 1019
  syphilitic, 1707, *1707*, 2202t
  toxic shock with, 1609t, 2200–2201
  typhoid fever, 1643, 1643t
  typhus, 1728, 1728t, 1729, 1730, 1732, 1734
  varicella, 1763, 2205
  vesicular, 2191t. See also *Vesicles.*
  viral, 1805t, 1805–1810, 2200–2201
  yaws, 1714

Rash *(Continued)*
  zoonoses associated with, 1727t, 1737t, 1737–1738, 1738t
Rat, plague transmission by, 1662
  typhus carried by, 1727t, 1729–1730
Rathke's cleft cyst, 1201, 2131
Rattlesnake, 1951t, 1951–1953
Rauwolfia, 265t, 266t
Raynaud's phenomenon, 346–349
  clinical features of, 347, 1484, 1485
  definition of, 346, 1484
  diagnosis of, 347–348, 1484–1485, 1485t
  drug therapy in, 348t, 348–349
  etiology of, 346–347, 347t
  incidence of, 346–347, 1485t
  lupus erythematosus with, 1478, 1482t
  pathology in, 347
  pathophysiology of, 347, 1484
  prognosis for, 348
  systemic sclerosis and, 347–348, 1484–1485, 1485t
  treatment of, 348t, 348–349, 1482t, 1487
RDA (recommended dietary allowance), 1140t, 1141t, 1141–1143
Receiver-operator characteristic (ROC) curve, 79, *80*
Receptors, 1176–1180
  adrenergic, *245*, 268, 492t, 492–493, 1253–1254
  alpha, *245*, 268. See also *Alpha blocking agents.*
    activation of, 1253–1254
    blood vessel, 492–493
  antiarrhythmic drugs affecting, *245*
  beta, *245*, 263–266, 298–299. See also *Beta blocking agents.*
  cannabinoid, 53
  catecholamine, 1253–1254
  complement binding by, 1400, *1400*, 1401t
  connective tissue with, 1446t, 1446–1447
  delta, 1187, 1199
  endorphin, 1187, 1199
  epinephrine, 1253–1254
  hormonal, 1176–1181
    peptide, 1176–1180, *1176–1180*
    steroid, 1180–1181, *1181*
  ion channel blockade and, 245, *245*
  J, 217
  kappa, 1187, 1199
  macrophage surface, 900, 901t
  mu, 1187, 1199
  norepinephrine, 1253–1254
  olfactory, 2014
  opioid, 52
    endogenous, 1187, 1199
  osmolality, 1222–1223, *1223*
  platelet surface, *978*
  pressure. See *Baroreceptors.*
  regulation of synthesis of, 1177
  taste, 2014
Recommended dietary allowance (RDA), 1140t, 1141t, 1141–1143
Rectum, **740–743**
  abscess of, 741, *741*
  amebiasis affecting, 1913t, 1913–1915, 1915t
  anatomy of, 740, *741*
  biopsy of, 694
  bleeding from, cancer with, 726
    hemorrhoids and, 740–741
    inflammatory bowel disease with, 709, 712, 712t
    ulcer causing, 743
  cancer of, 721–722, 724–728
    clinical features in, 726
    diagnosis of, 726–727, 727t
    etiology of, 725t, 725–726
    incidence of, *1005*, *1009*, 1013t, *1015*
    MRI scan of, 634, *635*
    pathology of, 726, *726*
    pregnancy with, 1061t, 1063–1064
    prevention of, 728, 1006t
    prognosis in, 727–728
    treatment of, 727
    tumor marker for, 1021–1022, 1022t
  colitis and, 1913–1915, 1915t
    pseudomembranous, *1634*, 1634t, 1635t
  diarrhea diagnosis and, 694
  examination of, 694, 740
    digital, 1006t
  pain from, 740
    abscess and, 741
    ulcer and, 743
  prolapse of, 743
  ulcer of, solitary, 743

Red nucleus, *2017*
Red ragged fibers, 1474
Red spot, foveal, 2182
5α-Reductase, 1291
  deficiency of, 1291, 1291t, *1292*
  drug inhibition of, 1316
Reduviid bug, 1899–1900, *1900*
Reed-Sternberg cells, 947–948
Reentry circuits, 234, *234*
  ablation therapy for, 252t, 252–253
  leading-edge, 234
  modelling of, 234, *234*
Reference intervals, 2224t–2233t
Reflex sympathetic dystrophy, 1524
Reflexes, hepatic encephalopathy affecting, 797–798, 798t
  neurologic examination of, 1977t
  tendon (deep), aging effects on, 17
Reflux esophagitis, **651–654**
  complications of, 652, 654
  diagnosis of, 652, *653*
  pathogenesis of, 651
  sphincters in, 651
  symptoms of, 651–652
  treatment of, 652–654, 654t
Refractive error, vision and, 2174
Refractoriness, cardiac, 190, 232
Refsum's disease, 147t
Regurgitation, 650–651. See also *Vomiting.*
  aortic valve, 321–323, 322t
  esophageal disorder with, 650–651
  mitral valve, 324–326
  nasal, 655
  rumination vs., 651
Reidel's thyroiditis, 1241
Reiter's syndrome, **1469–1470**
  AIDS/HIV patient with, 1868, 1878t, 1879
  arthritis of, 1467t, *1468*, 1469–1470, *1470*
  conjunctivitis of, 1469
  etiology of, 1467t, 1469
  HLA complex in, 1431t
  pathogens associated with, 1467t
  prevalence of, 1469
  radiography in, *1468*, 1469–1470, *1470*
  sacroiliitis in, 1469–1470, *1470*
  sexual transmitted disease and, 1469, 1724
  synovial fluid in, 1465t
  uveitis with, 2178
Rejection reaction, acute cellular, 364, 364t
  heart transplant with, *363*, 363–364, 364t
  hyperacute, 364
  lung transplant affected by, 461–462, 462t
  renal transplant and, 571–572
  therapy for, 364t
Relapsing fever, 1715
  clinical features of, 1715, 1738t
  diagnosis of, 1715
  epidemiology of, 1715, 1738t
  etiologic agent in, 1715
  laboratory testing in, 1715
  pathology and pathogenesis of, 1715
  prognosis in, 1715, 1738t
  therapy and prevention of, 1715
Renal. See also *Kidney.*
Renal artery, 517
  atherosclerosis of, 606–607
  occlusion of, 606t, 606–608
  stenosis of, 606–607
  thrombosis affecting, 606t, 606–607
Renal vein, *517*
  thrombosis affecting, 608t, 608–609
Renin, 1245–1246
  ectopic, 1026
  hypertension and, 268
  inhibitors of, 268
  mineralocorticoid secretion and, 1249–1252
    deficient, 1251t, 1251–1252
    excessive, 1249, 1249t
  prostaglandin effect on, 1193
  shock and, 481
Reoviridae, 1793, 1805t, 1806t. See also *Rotavirus.*
Reovirus, *1739*
Reproduction. See also *Impotence; Infertility; Sexual function.*
  seasonal rhythms in, 1204–1205
  smoking effect on, 34t, 35
Reptiles. See also *Snakebite; Venoms.*
  tongue worm carried by, 1950
Reserpine, dosage for, 265t, 266t
  side effects of, 267t

Residual volume, 373, 373–374
  asthma affecting, *378*, 378–379
  pulmonary function testing and, *373*, 373–374
Respiration, 368, 369t, 370. See also *Ventilation.*
  acid-base balance and, 543–544
  alcohol affecting, 47–48, 48t
  arousal level and, 1970, 1971t
  chest wall in, 443–444
  Cheyne-Stokes, 218
  difficult. See *Dyspnea.*
  embolism effect on, 423, 424t
  function studies of. See *Pulmonary function tests.*
  heart failure affecting, 217, 219
  hypothyroidism affecting, 1238, 1238t
  increased. See *Hyperventilation.*
  mechanics of, 370, *370*
  muscles of, 442–443
    fatigue of, 442
    paralysis of, 442
  neurologic examination of, 1977t
  rate of, 466, 467t
    brain injury and, 2138t
    septic shock affecting, 496t
  reduced. See *Hypoventilation.*
  sleep disorder of, 451–452
  sounds of, 368, 369t, 370
Respiratory center, 370
Respiratory distress syndrome (adult), 454–456
  disorders associated with, 454t, 476t
  drowning followed by, 408
  endothelial cell injury in, 454–455, *455*
  multiple organ failure with, 474–477, 476t
  pathogenesis of, 454–455, *455*
  respiratory failure with, 454t, 454–456, 456t
  shock and, 498
  therapy for, critical care setting and, 474–477
    supportive, 455, 456t
    ventilatory, 455–456, 457t
Respiratory failure, **452–459**
  abnormalities in, 466–468, 467t
  acute, 452t–454t, 452–459, 457t, 458t
  chronic, 459
  clinical features of, 453t, 453–454, 454t, 456t
  critical care setting and, 466–477, 467t
  disorders associated with, 452t, 454t, 457t, 458t, 467t
  etiologies of, 452t, 454t, 457t, 458t, 467t
  hypercapnic-hypoxic, 453, 453t, 456–459, 457t, 458t, 467t
  hypoxic, 452–456, 453t, 454t, 467t
  neuromuscular disease causing, 473
  physiologic types of, 467t
  precipitating factors for, 452t, 454t, 457t
  pulmonary edema and, 455, 456t
  respiratory distress syndrome with, 454t, 454–456, 456t
  treatment of, 455–459, 468–472
    intubation in, 469, 469t
    ventilation therapy in, 455–459, 457t, 469t, 469–472
Respiratory syncytial virus, 1751–1752
  clinical manifestations of, 1751–1752
  diagnosis of, 1751–1752
  epidemiology of, 1751
  treatment of, 1752
Respiratory tract, **368–462**. See also *Lung; Respiration; specific structures and disorders.*
  anaphylaxis affecting, 1418
  anatomy of, 371–373, *372*
  approach to diseases of, 368–371
  asthma effect on, 377, *377*
  cell lining of, 371, *372*
  cystic fibrosis and, 420–421, 421t
  defense mechanisms in, 411t, 411–412
  diagnostic procedures in, 368–371, 369t, *370*
    invasive, 369
    noninvasive, 368–369
  examination and, 368–371, 369t, *370*
  flora of, *1639*, 1639t, 1639–1640
  history and, 368
  immotile cilia syndrome of, 416, 416t
  infection(s) of. See also *Pneumonia; Pneumonitis.*
    adenovirus, 1757t, 1758
    AIDS/HIV with, 1858–1865, 1859t–1861t, *1859–1865*, 1865t
    aspergillosis, 1830t, 1830–1832
    blastomycosis, 1821
    coccidioidomycosis, 1819–1820, *1820*
    cryptococcus, 1824

Respiratory tract *(Continued)*
  diphtheria, 1629–1630
  enterovirus, 1787t, 1791
  H. influenzae, 1622–1624
  histoplasmosis, 1817–1818
  influenza, 1753–1757
  mucormycosis, 1833
  pertussis, 1627, 1628–1629
  Pseudomonas, 1579–1581, 1580t, 1669–1671
  rhinovirus, 1747t, 1747–1749, *1748*
  syncytial virus, 1744, 1746t
  viral, 1741t, 1743–1744, **1747–1759**. See also spe-
      cific virus or infection.
  zoonoses associated with, 1737t, 1737–1738
mucus cells of, 371, *372*
obstruction of. See *Airway obstruction; Asthma;*
    Bronchitis; Emphysema.
particulate matter in, 372–373, 399
prostaglandins affecting, 1193
radiation of, 61, 61t, 62t
signs and symptoms in, 368–371, 369t, *370*
sputum examination and, 369–370
upper, 371, 449–452. See also *Ear; Larynx;*
    Nasopharynx; Nose; Pharynx.
  assessment of, 449
  viruses affecting, 1749–1757, 1750t
Resting potential, cardiac cell, 190, 232
  transmembrane voltage of, 232, *232*
Restless legs syndrome, 1983, 1983t, 2050
Restriction analysis. See *Polymerase chain reaction*
    (PCR).
Resuscitation therapy. See *Fluid therapy.*
Retching. See also *Vomiting.*
  definition of, 629
  Mallory-Weiss tear due to, 643
Reticular activating system, 1969, 1970t
Reticular dysgenesis, 1406
Reticulocytes, **825**
  anemia and, 825, 826t, 837–838
  count of, 825, 826t, 838
  hemorrhagic disorders and, 984t
  increased, 825, 826t, 837–838, 1475t, 1479
  polychromasia of, 824
  production of, 817, *819*, 837–838
  sickle syndromes and, 885t
  splenic conditioning of, 971
Reticulocytosis, 825, 837–838, 1479
  anemia with, 825, 826t, 837–838, 1479
  lupus erythematosus with, 1475t, 1479
Reticulohistiocytosis, 1526
  arthritis with, 1526
  multicentric, 1526
Retina. See also *Retinitis; Retinopathy.*
  AIDS/HIV effects in, 1868–1870, 1869t
  anatomy of, neural pathways and, *2015*, 2015–2016
  Bardet-Biedl syndrome affecting, 162
  cotton wool exudate of, 1480, 1868–1869, 2099
  diabetes mellitus affecting, 1273
  hypertension and, 2181
  ischemia of, 2177–2178
  necrosis syndrome of, 1869t, 1869–1870
  tears and detachments of, 2016
  tumor of, 2180
  vasculitis affecting, 2016, 2016t
Retinal artery, 2182
  branch, 2182
  central, 2182
  death changes in, 2182
  occlusion of, 2182
Retinal vein, 2182
  branch, 2182
  central, 2182
  occlusion of, 2182
Retinitis, 1808, 1868, 1908
  AIDS/HIV with, 1868–1870, 1869t, 1908, 1909,
      2179
  Rift Valley fever with, 1806t, 1808
  toxoplasmosis causing, 1869, 1869t, 1908, 1909,
      2179
Retinoblastoma, 2180
Retinoic acid, acne treated with, 2197
  receptor for, 1180–1181, *1181*
Retinoids, 1145t. See also *Vitamin A.*
  side effects of, 2197
  skin disorder treated with, 2197
Retinopathy, arteriosclerotic, 2181
  diabetic, 1273, 2181–2182
  hypertension and, 2181

Retinopathy *(Continued)*
  hyperviscosity, 2182
  Kimmelstiel-Wilson, hypertension with, 257, 260t
  lupus erythematosus with, 2182
  neutrophil aggregation in, 1450
  paraneoplastic, 1018, 1028
  Purtscher's, 1450
  sickle cell, 2182
Retroperitoneum, fibrosis affecting, 1529
  lymph nodes of, 969t
Retrovirus, **1779–1783**
  biology of, *1779*, 1779–1780, *1780*
  diseases associated with, 1781t, 1781–1783
  gene transfer using, 148–150, *149*
  human immunodeficiency. See *HIV infection.*
  slow infection due to, 2097t
  structure of, *1739*, *1838*, *1842*
  T-lymphotropic (HTLV), **1779–1783**
Reye syndrome, 2105
  influenza and, 1756
Rhabdomyolysis, 2159
Rhabdomyosarcoma, orbital, 2180
Rhabdovirus, *1739*, 1740t
Rheumatic fever, **1590–1596**
  arthritis in, 1592t, 1592–1593
  clinical manifestations of, 1592t, 1592–1593, 1593t
  course of, 1594
  definition of, 1590–1591
  diagnosis of, 1594–1595, 1595t
  epidemiology of, 1591–1592
  etiology of, 1591
  heart disease due to, *1592*, 1592t, 1592–1593, 1593t
  laboratory findings in, 1593–1594, 1595t
  pathogenesis of, 1591
  pathology findings in, 1592, *1592*
  prevention of, 1589t, 1596
  prognosis in, 1594
  steroids vs. aspirin in, 112
  streptococcus in, 1589t, 1590–1591
  treatment of, 1595–1596
Rheumatic heart disease, endocarditis risk due to, 1597t
  mortality in, 171t
Rheumatism, 1527–1528. See also *Arthritis; Joint(s).*
  "desert," 1819
  nonarticular, 1527–1528
Rheumatoid arthritis. See *Arthritis, rheumatoid.*
Rheumatoid factors, 1456–1458, 1457t, 1462t
  disease associations of, 1457t, 1462t
  lupus erythematosus with, 1456–1458, 1457t, 1476t
  rheumatoid arthritis with, 1456–1458, 1457t, 1462t,
      1464
Rheumatoid spondylitis. See *Spondylitis, ankylosing.*
Rhinitis, 450
  allergic, 1413–1417
    clinical features of, 1413
    definition of, 1413
    differential diagnosis of, 1413, 1413t
    drug therapy in, 1416t, 1416–1417, 1417t
    early phase, 1415, *1415*
    epidemiology of, 1413
    immunotherapy in, 1417
    late phase, 1415, *1415*
    management of, 1416t, 1416–1417, 1417t
    pathophysiology of, 1414–1416, *1415*, *1416*
  classification of, 1413, 1413t
  nonallergic perennial, 1413t
Rhinophyma, 2207, *2207*
Rhinorrhea, 1414–1415, *1415*
  cerebrospinal fluid in, 1615
Rhinovirus, common cold due to, 1747t, **1747–1749,**
    1748
  pharyngitis due to, 1749–1751, 1750t, 1751t
Rhodanese, 508
Rhodococcus equi, 1737t
Rhythms, circadian, 1199–1200
  diurnal, 1184, 1199–1200
  gonadotropin secretion subject to, 1199–1200
  gravitational, 1199
  hypothalamic, 1184, 1199–1200
  infradian, 1199–1200
  jet lag due to, 1200, 1555–1556
  light-dark cycle and, 1199–1200
  nervous system role in, 1184, 1199–1200
  pituitary, 1184, 1199–1200
  seasonal, 1199–1200
  sleep-wake cycle and, 1199–1200
  ultradian, 1199
Ribavirin, **1744**, 1746t
  licensing for, 1744
  respiratory syncytial virus treatment with, 1752

Ribavirin *(Continued)*
  syncytial virus treated with, 1746t
  toxicity of, 1744
  viral pharyngitis treated with, 1751t
Riboflavin, assessment of, 1146t
  deficiency of, 1146t
  parenteral, 1172t
  physiology of, 1146t
  RDA for, 1140t
  toxicity of, 1146t
Ribosomes, antibodies to, 1457t, 1476t
  gene transcription role of, *135*
Ribozymes, cancer gene inhibition by, 1074
Ribs, deformities affecting, 443t, 443–444
  diaphragmatic motion and, 442
  disorders affecting, 443t, 443–444
  flail chest and, 444
Richter's syndrome, 934
Rickets, **1359–1365**
  classification of, 1359t, 1362t, 1363t
  clinical manifestations of, 1360–1361
  etiology of, 1359t, 1359–1360
  hypophosphatasia in, 1365
  hypophosphatemia in, 1362t, 1363t, 1363–1364
  laboratory findings in, 1362t, 1363t
  pathogenesis of, 1359–1360
  renal tubular disorders in, 1363–1364
  vitamin D in, 1145t, 1361–1363, 1362t, 1363t
    dependency on, 1362, 1363
    diet and synthetic deficiency of, 1361
    loss and malabsorption of, 1361–1362
    metabolic abnormality of, 1362–1363
    target organ resistance to, 1363
Rickettsial diseases, **1726–1736**, 1727t, 1728t
  boutonneuse fever, 1727t, 1728t, 1732
  Colorado tick fever, 1733
  ehrlichiosis, 1727t, 1728t, 1733
  incubation period in, 1728t
  Mediterranean spotted fever, 1732
  North Asian tick-borne, 1732
  Q fever, 1727t, 1728t, 1735–1736
  rash in, 1728, 1728t, 1729, 1730, 1732, 1734
  Rocky Mountain spotted fever, 1727t, 1728t,
      1730–1732
  typhus, 1726–1730, 1727t, 1728t
    chigger-borne, 1727t, 1728t, 1734–1735
    louse-borne, 1726–1729, 1727t, 1728t
    murine, 1727t, 1728t, 1729–1730
    Queensland tick, 1732
    scrub, 1727t, 1728t, 1734–1735
Rickettsialpox, 1727t, 1728t, 1733–1734
Rifabutin, 1690, 1691
Rifampin, 1562t
  bacterial resistance to, 1558–1560, 1559t
  cat scratch disease therapy with, 1681–1682, 1682t
  endocarditis therapy with, 1602t–1604t, 1602–1603
  H. influenzae prophylaxis with, 1624
  Legionella and, 1585, 1585t
  mechanism of action of, 1558, 1558t
  meningococcal prophylaxis with, 1621, 1621t
  mycobacterial (nontuberculous) disease and, 1690,
      1691
  staphylococcal infection treated with, 1609t,
      1609–1610
  tuberculosis treated with, 1686–1688, 1687t
Rift Valley hemorrhagic fever, 1798t, 1805t, 1806t,
    1808
Right-to-die, 24–25. See also *Death and dying.*
Rigidity, Parkinson's disease with, 2042
  spinal syndrome of, 2163
Rilmenidine, 268
Rimantadine, influenza treated with, 1746t
  viral pharyngitis treated with, 1751t
Rings, esophageal, 657–658, *658*
  Schatzki's, 657–658, *658*
Ringworm, 2200, 2203–2204
Risk factors. See also under specific diseases and disor-
    ders.
  dietary, 29–31, 30t
  leading causes of death and, 27t, 30t
  mortality correlated with, 27t, 30t
Risperidone, 1998t, 1998–1999
Risus sardonicus, 1637
RNA (ribonucleic acid), 134–136
  antibodies to, 1457t, 1476t
  genetic code and, 134t, 134–136, *136*
  messenger, *135*
  muscle mitochondrial, 2160t, 2167
  thalassemia and, 880
  viral, 1739, *1739*, 1740t

RNA (ribonucleic acid) *(Continued)*
　　HIV organism, *1838*, 1842–1844, *1842–1844*,
　　　　1884t
　　influenza virus, 1754, *1754*, 1754t
Robertsonian translocation, 152, *152*
Rochalimaea. See *Bartonella.*
Rocio encephalitis, 1806t, 1814
Rocky Mountain spotted fever, **1730–1732**
　　clinical manifestations of, 1728t, 1730–1731, 2201
　　diagnosis of, 1727t, 1731
　　distribution of, 1730, *1731*
　　epidemiology of, 1727t, 1730, *1730*
　　etiologic agent in, 1727t, 1730
　　incidence of, 1730, *1730*
　　prevention and control of, 1732
　　prognosis in, 1728t, 1731–1732
　　serology for, 1732
　　treatment of, 1732
Rodenticides, cyanide, 508
　　poisoning due to, 504t, 508
Rodents, babesiosis reservoir in, 1915
　　Hantavirus carried by, 1804
　　plague transmission by, 1662
　　typhus carried by, 1726, 1727t, 1729–1730
　　zoonoses associated with, 1727t, 1737t, 1737–1738,
　　　　1738t
Rokitansky-Aschoff sinuses, 814
Rosacea, 2207, *2207*
Roseola infantum, 1791, 2200
Ross River virus, 1805t, 1809
Rotator cuff, 1521
　　tear of, 1521, *1523*
　　tendinitis affecting, 1521, *1523*
Rotavirus, diagnosis of, 1796
　　diarrhea and, 1642t, 1658t, 1794–1797, *1795*, 1795t
　　epidemiology of, 1794–1795, 1795t
　　gastroenteritis due to, 1642t, 1658t
　　prophylaxis for, 1797
　　structure of, *1794*
　　treatment of, 1796–1797
Roth's spots, 1599, 2181
Rotor's syndrome, 757t
　　bilirubin metabolism in, 756, 757t
　　jaundice with, 756, 757t
Roundworms. See also *Nematodes.*
　　Ascaris, 1935, 1935t
　　hookworm, 1934–1935, 1935t
　　Trichinella, 1935t, 1937–1938
　　Trichuris, 1935t, 1935–1936
Roux-en-Y anastomosis, *672*, 683
RR interval, *190*, 191
Rubella, **1761–1762**
　　clinical manifestations of, 1762, 2200
　　complications of, 1762
　　congenital, 1761–1762
　　diagnosis of, 1762
　　encephalitis due to, 2097t, 2100
　　epidemiology of, 1761
　　etiology of, 1761
　　immunization for, 43t, 44, 1762
　　pathology of, 1761–1762
　　progressive, 2097t, 2100
　　slow infection due to, 2097t
Rubenstein-Taybi syndrome, 155
Rubeola. See *Measles (rubeola).*
Rubor. See also *Erythema.*
　　Raynaud's phenomenon with, 347, 1484, 1485
Rugger jersey appearance, 1389, *1389*
Rumination, definition of, 651
Running, seizure-associated, 2116
Rupia, syphilitic, 1707
Russell's sign, 1160
Russell's viper, 1951t, 1953

S

Saber shin, 1710
Saccades, 2019
　　paraneoplastic effects in, 1028
　　testing of, 2019
Saccharomyces boulardii, 1634, 1635t
Saccharopine, 1101t
Sacroiliitis, 1467–1470
　　ankylosing spondylitis with, 1467, 1467–1468, *1468*
　　Reiter's, 1469–1470, *1470*
　　spondyloarthropathies with, 1467t
Saethre-Chotzen syndrome, 160t, 162
　　clinical features of, 160t, 162
Safe sex, 1851–1852, 1852t

Sagittal sinus, *2061*
　　obstruction of, 2072–2073
　　septic, 2083
　　thrombosis in, 2083
Saint Vitus' dance, rheumatic fever and, 1593
Salicylates, **111–115**
　　acidosis caused by, 548, 549
　　analgesic effects of, 111–112, 115t
　　anti-inflammatory effects of, 111–115, 115t
　　corticosteroids vs., 112
　　history of use of, 111–112
　　inflammatory bowel disease treated with, 712–713,
　　　　714t
　　mechanism of action of, 112–115, *113*
　　overdose of, 506, 506t
Saliva, 649t, 649–650
Salivary glands, **648–650**, 1488, 1488t
　　anatomic location of, 450, *451*
　　dry mouth and, 649t, 649–650, 1488, 1488t, 1489
　　duct obstruction affecting, 648, 648t
　　enlargement of, 648–649, 649t
　　impaired secretion of, 649t, 649–650, 1488t,
　　　　1488–1490, *1489*
　　rabies affecting, 2096
　　Sjögren's syndrome affecting, 649t, 1488t,
　　　　1488–1490, *1489*
　　sleeping sickness trypanosome in, 1897, *1897*
Salmonella infections, **1644–1646**
　　carrier of, 1645, 1646
　　clinical syndromes of, 1645–1646
　　definition of, 1644
　　diagnosis of, 1646
　　epidemiology of, 1644–1645
　　etiology of, 1644
　　food poisoning due to, 738, 739t
　　pathogenesis of, 1645
　　prevention of, 1646
　　treatment of, 1646
　　typhoid fever due to, 1642–1644. See also *Typhoid
　　　　fever.*
Salpingitis, antimicrobial therapy in, 1702t, 1703
　　chlamydial, 1700, 1702t, 1724
　　gonorrhea causing, 1700–1702
　　sexually transmitted disease causing, 1700, 1724
　　treatment of, 1702t, 1703
Salt, deprivation, 221, 1252
　　dietary aspects of, 29–30, 30t, 221
　　mineralocorticoid deficiency treated with, 1251–1252
　　restriction of, 221, 1252
　　retention of, heart failure and, 217, 221
Saltine cracker test, 1488
Sandfly, bartonellosis transmission by, 1682
　　fever related to, 1805t, 1808
　　leishmaniasis transmitted by, *1904*
　　phlebotome, 1682, 1903–1904, *1904*, 1947
Sanfilippo's mucopolysaccharidosis, 1119t
Sarcocystis, 1916t
Sarcoidosis, **431–436**
　　activity level of, 435, 435t
　　arthritis in, 1526
　　biopsy, 434–435, *435*
　　cardiomyopathy with, 333
　　clinical presentation of, 431–433, *432*, *433*
　　CT scan in, 434, *434*
　　definition of, 431
　　diagnosis of, 434–435, 435t
　　differential diagnosis of, 433
　　epidemiology of, 431
　　genetics of, 431
　　heart affected by, 359, 432
　　hepatic effects of, 784t, 785, 786–787
　　hypothalamus in, 1201
　　immunopathology of, *431*, 431
　　laboratory studies in, 433
　　lymphadenopathy in, 970
　　pulmonary, 432–434, *434*
　　radiologic evaluation of, 433–434, *434*
　　treatment of, 435–436
Sarcolemma, myocardial, 174, *175*
Sarcoma, Kaposi's, 1032–1033, 1033t. See also
　　Kaposi's sarcoma.
　　synovial, 1528
Sarcomere, 2158
　　myocardial, 174, *175*, 213
Sarcoplasmic reticulum, myocardial, 174, *175*
Sarcoptes scabiei, 1697t, 1738t, 1949
Sarcosine, 1102t
Satiety, definition of, 629
　　hypothalamic center for, 629, 2012
　　disordered, 1203, 2012–2013

Sausage digits, 1471
Scabies, 1738t, *2191*
　　mites causing, 1697t, 1738t, 1949
　　sexual transmission of, 1697t
　　zoonoses associated with, 1738t
Scalded skin syndrome, 1607t, 1609, 1609t, 2205
Scalene nodes, 969t
Scales, diseases associated with, 2191, 2191t, 2204t
　　ichthyosis with, 1019, *2204*, 2204t
　　pityriasis rosea, *2203*, 2203–2204
　　psoriatic, 2202–2203
Scalp tenderness, giant cell arteritis with, 1499
Scapula, muscular dystrophy effect on, 2162
Scar, "cigarette paper," 1121t
　　formation of, 2189
　　therapy for, 2195, 2196
Scarlet fever, 1586–1587, 2200
　　age factor in, 1586
　　septic vs. toxic, 1587
　　streptococcal infection with, 1587
Scarring, alopecia with, 2217
　　"saber wound," 2217
Schamberg's disease, 2210
Schatzki's ring, 657–658, *658*
Scheie's syndrome, clinical features of, 1119t
　　enzyme defect of, 1119t
Schilder's disease, brown, 1251
Schilling test, 699, 701t
　　differential, 699, 701t
　　malabsorption affecting, 699, 701t
　　vitamin B_{12} in, 699, 701t
Schirmer's test, 1488t, 1489
Schistocytes, 825t
　　hemorrhagic disorders and, 984t
Schistosomiasis, 783t, 1927–1931, 1929t
　　diagnosis of, 1929t
　　epidemiology of, 1927–1928
　　etiology of, *1927*, 1927–1929
　　haematobia, 1929, 1929t
　　hepatic effects of, 782, 783t, 784t, 1929–1930
　　intercalatum, 1929t, 1930–1931
　　japonica, 1929t, 1930
　　management and control of, 1928–1929, 1931
　　mansoni, 1929t, 1929–1930
　　mekongi, 1929t, 1931
　　pathology and clinical features of, 1929t, 1929–1931
　　pathophysiology of, 1928–1930
Schizonts, cryptosporidial, 1910–1911, *1911*
　　malarial, 1893, *1893*
Schizophrenia, **1997–1999**
　　diagnostic criteria for, 1997, 1997t
　　drug therapy for, 1998t, 1998–1999, 1999t
　　neurologic disorder vs., 1974, 1974t
　　pathophysiology of, 1997–1998
　　prevalence of, 1997
　　signs and symptoms of, 1997, 1997t
　　treatment and prognosis in, 1998t, 1998–1999, 1999t
Schober's test, 1468
Schüffner's dots, 1894, 1895t
Schwann cells, onion bulb appearance due to, 2153,
　　2154t
Schwannoma (acoustic neuroma), 2126t, 2131
　　MRI scan of, 2128t
　　neurofibromatosis with, 2056
Scintigraphy, cardiac, 199–202, *200–202*
　　pheochromocytoma in, 1256
　　pulmonary embolism in, *425*, 425t, 425–426, *426*
　　renal, 516
Scleritis, 2181
　　rheumatoid arthritis with, 1464
Sclerodactyly, 1484
Scleroderma, **1483–1487**
　　antibodies in, 1457, 1457t, 1483–1484, 1484t
　　clinical manifestations of, 395t, 396, 1485–1487,
　　　　1486, 2212
　　definition of, 1483, 2212
　　diffuse, 1483t, **1483–1485**. See also *Sclerosis, pro-
　　　　gressive systemic.*
　　esophageal, 1485
　　myopathy and, 2164
　　renal effects of, 608, 1487
　　skin effects of, 1483t, 1483–1485, 1484t, *1485*,
　　　　2212
　　treatment of, 1487
Sclerosis, arterial. See *Arteriosclerosis*; *Atherosclerosis.*
　　bone. See *Osteosclerosis.*
　　concentric, 2111
　　glomerular. See *Glomerulosclerosis.*

Sclerosis *(Continued)*
hippocampal, 2117, *2118*
lateral, 2053–2054
amyotrophic, 2053–2054
primary, 2054
Mönckeberg's, 291
multiple. See *Multiple sclerosis.*
progressive systemic, **1483–1487**. See also *Scleroderma.*
clinical manifestations of, 395t, 396, 1485–1487, *1486*, 2212
diagnosis of, 1484–1485, 1485t, 2212
differential diagnosis of, 1485
immunofluorescence testing in, 2189t
incidence of, 1485t
intestinal motility and, 685
pathogenesis of, 1483–1484, 1484t
pulmonary, 395t, 396, *1486*, 1486–1487
subsets of, 1484t
survival rate for, 1484, *1485*
tuberous, 2056, 2214
clinical manifestations of, 2056, 2214
diagnosis of, 2056, 2214
lung in, 399
pathology in, 2056
skin lesions of, 2056, 2214
Sclerotic cells, black fungus with, 1836
Scoliosis, Cobb's angle in, 443
Marfan syndrome with, 1119–1120
respiration affected by, 443, 443t
Scopolamine, neurologic effects of, 1975t
tea containing, 54
Scorpion bite, 1948–1949
Scorpionfish, 1954t, 1955
venom of, 1954t, 1955
Scotoperiods, 1204. See also *Light-dark cycle.*
Scrapie, 2097, 2102–2103
Scrotum, 1325–1326
gangrene affecting, 1641
testicular descent to, 1325–1326
Scrub typhus, 1727t, 1728t, 1734–1735
Scurvy, rebound, 1147t
vitamin C deficiency in, 1147t
Sea snake, 1954t, 1954–1955
Sea urchin, venom of, 1954t, 1955
Seafood. See also *Fish.*
anaphylaxis due to, 1418t
asthma induced by, 379t
food poisoning due to, 739t, 740, 1956
occupational exposure to, 379t
Seasons, breeding and, 1204–1205
hormone secretion and, 1199–1200
melatonin secretion related to, 1204–1205
Sebaceous glands, *2185*, 2186–2187
anatomy of, *2185*, 2186–2187
papule associated with, 2208
physiology of, *2185*, 2186–2187
regional locations of, 2186
Sebum, 2186, 2206
Second messengers, 1176–1181, *1176–1181*
Secretin test, malabsorption and, 699, 700t
pancreatic function in, 699, 700t, 735
Secretory granules, atrial, natriuretic hormone and, 1194
catecholamine, 1253
exocytosis of, 1182
posterior pituitary, 1221–1222
Sedatives, drug abuse with, 50–51, 56t, 1975t
myocardial infarction treatment and, 309–310, 310t
neurologic effects of, 1975t
Sedimentation rate, acute phase proteins affecting, 1456
giant cell arteritis and, 1499, 1499t
polymyalgia rheumatica and, 1498, 1499t
Seizures, **2113–2125**
absence, 2116, 2117, *2117*
akinetic, 1981–1982
alcohol-related, 48t, 49
antiepileptic drug therapy for, 2122t, 2122–2123
antimicrobials causing, 1568t
atonic (drop attack), 2116
aura of, 2114
brain tumor causing, 2126t, *2128*, 2128–2129
causes of, 2113–2114, 2114t
childhood, *2115*, 2116, 2117, *2117*
clinical characteristics of, 2114–2116
coma and, 1973
complex partial, 2114–2115
continuous, 2118
cursive, 2116

Seizures *(Continued)*
cysticercosis with, 1926
definition of, 2113
drop attack, 2116
drug-induced, 2114t
evaluation of patient with, 2120–2121, 2121t
fever and, 2116–2117
gelastic, 2116
generalized, *2115*, 2115–2116, 2116t
grand mal, 2116
impact, 2118
jacksonian march, 2114
lupus erythematosus causing, 1475t, 1480
meningitis with, 1612t, 1612–1613, 1620
metabolic encephalopathy with, 1973
migraine vs., 2116
myoclonic, *2115*, 2116, 2117
partial (focal), 1982, 2114–2115, *2115*, 2116t
petit mal, 2116, 2117, *2117*
phakomatosis with, 2120
physical examination and, 2120
poison causing, 505, 505t
postictal unresponsiveness in, 1982
psychogenic, 2121
psychomotor, 2115
reflex, 2116
syncope vs., 1981–1982, 2116, 2121
temporal lobe, 1985, 1987t, 2117, *2118*
tonic, 2114
tonic-clonic, 2114, 2116
transient ischemic attack vs., 2066
Selectins, leukocyte adhesiveness and, 898, *899*
Selenium, 72–73, 1150t
assessment of, 1150t
deficiency of, 72, 1150t
dietary, 1140t, 1150t
RDA for, 1140t
occupational exposure to, 72
poisoning due to, 72–73, 1150t
clinical manifestations of, 72, 1150t
etiology of, 72, 73
Sella turcica, empty syndrome of, 2133
intracranial hypertension affecting, 2133
Semicircular canal, anatomy of, *2026*
calcium carbonate crystals in, 2026, *2026*
caloric test of, 2024
Seminal fluid, 1327
Seminal vesicle, 1341, *1341*, *1344*
differentiation of, *1286*
Seminiferous tubules, 1325–1326, *1326*
function evaluation of, 1328
Semliki Forest virus, 1806t
Sensitivity analysis, 82
decision analysis with, 82, *82*
interpretation of, 82
one-way, 82, *82*
two-way, 82, *82*
Sensitization. See also *Hypersensitivity.*
insect sting causing, 1420–1421
Sensory system, **2014–2031**
aging effects in, 16, 16t
ataxia of, 2029
cerebral hemorrhage affecting, 2078, *2078*
hearing and, 2021–2024
localization of lesion of, 2030–2031, 2031t
muscle weakness and, 2027–2028, 2028t
smell and, 2014t, 2014–2015
stroke affecting, 2064t, 2064–2065
taste and, 2014t, 2014–2015
vision and, 2015–2020
Sentences, 1990
aphasia diagnosis using, 1991, 1991t
Sepsis, 496t. See also *Immune response; Inflammation.*
definitions related to, 496, *497*
mediators for, 497–499, *498*, 501
platelet destruction due to, 984
respiratory distress with, 476, 476t
shock due to, 496–501, *498*, 499t, 500t
toxic syndrome of, 1588t, 1588–1589, 1609, 1609t
transfusion-associated, 896, 896t
Septata, 1916t
Septicemia, 27t
Septo-optic dysplasia, 1200
Sequestration, bronchopulmonary, 390, 416, 416t
Serine, coagulation and, 987
Serology, anthrax, 1667
Chagas' disease, 1901–1902
chickenpox, 1764
chlamydial infection, 1724, 1725
coccidioidomycosis, 1820

Serology *(Continued)*
cryptosporidiosis, 1912
Epstein-Barr virus, 1778, *1778*, 1779t
influenza, 1755
Legionella, 1584t
leprosy, 1692t, 1693
lupus erythematosus, 1479, 1481
Lyme disease, 1717–1718, *1718*
malaria, 1895
meningococcal, 1613, 1620
myasthenia gravis, 2172
paracoccidioidomycosis, 1823
Rocky Mountain spotted fever, 1731
rotavirus, 1796
streptococcal, 1586–1587, 1591
syphilis, 1710t, 1710–1711, 1711t
toxoplasmosis, 1909
trichinosis organism, 1938
trypanosomal, 1898, 1901–1902
tularemia, 1664
typhoid fever, 1643
varicella, 1764
yellow fever, 1800
Serositis, 1475t, 1478
Serotonin, carcinoid production of, 1348–1349, *1349*
coagulation role of, 977, *977*, *978*, 979
depression related to, 2000t, 2001
ovarian tumor production of, 1312t
reuptake inhibitors of, 2000t, 2001
Serpins, 987–989, 988t
Sertoli cells, 1284
aplasia of, 1336
sexual differentiation role of, 1284, 1285, *1286*
testicular, 1284, *1286*, 1326, *1326*, 1327
Sertraline, 2000t, 2001
Serum levels and ranges, 2224t–2233t. See also specific substances.
Serum sickness, 1421–1422, *1422*, 1422t
antimicrobials causing, 1568t
drug reaction causing, 98t, *1422*, 1422t
immune complexes in, 1421–1422, *1422*
treatment of, 1424
Set point theory, 1164, 1532
body temperature in, 1532, 1533, 2012, 2188
body weight and, 1164, 1213
Sex (gender), 1287–1293
adipose tissue distribution and, *1162*, 1163–1164
AIDS cases related to, 1848t
ambiguous, 1287–1293
body composition and, 1161–1162, *1162*
body weight and, 1140t, 1152t, *1162*
cancer rate and, *1005*, *1009*, 1013t, *1015*
chromosomes of, 134, 140–141, *152*, *153*, 154
depression related to, 2000
dietary requirements and, 1140t
Harris-Benedict equation and, 1173t
hypertension and, 258, *259*
osteoporosis and, 1379, *1379*, 1383–1384
secondary characteristics of, 1294, 1329
Sex-hormone binding globulin, 1132
obesity effect on, 1165
testosterone transport by, 1326–1327
Sexual differentiation, **1284–1293**
adrenal hyperplasia affecting, 1287–1290, 1288t, *1288–1290*
anatomy of, 1284–1285, *1285*, *1286*
androgen insensitivity in, 1291t, 1291–1293, *1292*
cryptorchidism in, 1292, *1292*
gonadal dysgenesis, 154, 1286, 1287
hermaphroditism in, 1286–1287
Klinefelter's syndrome in, 154, 1286
normal, 1284–1285, *1285*, *1286*
female, 1285, *1285*, *1286*
male, 1284–1285, *1285*, *1286*
ovarian, 1285
somatic, 1284, 1285
stages of, *1286*
testicular, 1284
phenotype disorders in, 1287–1290
pseudohermaphroditism in, 1287–1293
female, 1287–1290, *1288*, *1290*
male, 1287, 1290–1291, 1291t, *1292*
testosterone and, 1285, *1286*
Turner's syndrome in, 154, 1286
XX male and, 1286
Sexual function, 1308
aging effect on, 13–14, 16t, 18, 1335
autonomic regulation of, 2013
female, 1308
male, 1328–1332, 1330t, 1331t

Sexual function (Continued)
  parasympathetic control of, 2010, 2010t
  response phases in, 1308, 1328–1329
  safe practices for, 1851–1852, 1852t
Sexual precocity, 1202, 1295–1296, 1340
  delayed or incomplete, 1295t, 1296–1297
  female, 1288, 1295t, 1295–1296
  heterosexual, 1295, 1295t, 1296, 1297
  isosexual, 1295, 1295t, 1340
  laboratory tests in, 1296
  male, 1340
  pseudo, 1295, 1295t, 1340
Sexually transmitted diseases, **1696–1714**. See also specific diseases.
  AIDS due to, **1851–1854**, 1852t, 1853t, 1854t. See also AIDS (acquired immunodeficiency syndrome).
  anus affected by, 742
  candidal, 1699, 1699t
  cervicitis in, 1699–1700
  chancroid, 1704–1705
  chlamydial, 1696–1697, **1722–1725**, 1723t
  cystitis due to, female, 1698–1699
  definition of, 1696
  donovanosis (granuloma inguinale), 1703–1704
  epidemiologic factors for, 1696
  etiologic agents in, 1697t
  gonorrhea, 1700–1703, 1702t. See also Gonorrhea.
  herpetic, 1746t, 1772, 1773
  HIV infection in, **1851–1854**, 1852t, 1853t, 1854t. See also HIV infection.
  HTLV in, 1780, 1780t
  incidence of, 1697
  oral manifestations of, 646, 646t, 647, 647t, 648t
  preventive testing for, 28t
  Reiter's syndrome and, 1469
  salpingitis due to, 1700
  syphilis, 1705–1713. See also Syphilis.
  traveler exposed to, 1555
  trichomonad, 1699, 1699t, 1916–1917
  ulcerative lesions of, 1698
  urethritis due to, 1697–1699
    female with, 1698–1699
    male with, 1697–1698, 1698
  vaginitis of, 1698t, 1698–1699, 1916
Sézary syndrome, 1031t, 1031–1032
SGOT. See Aspartate transaminase (AST).
SGPT. See Alanine transferase (ALT).
Shampoo, antiseborrheic, 2199
Shellfish, allergic reaction to, 1409
  food poisoning due to, amnesic, 740
  poisoning due to, 1954t, 1956
  zoonoses associated with, 1737t
Shigellosis, **1647–1648**
  complications of, 1647t, 1648
  definition of, 1647
  diagnosis of, 1647t, 1648
  dysentery due to, 1642t, 1647t, 1647–1648
  epidemiology of, 1647
  etiology of, 1647
  food poisoning due to, 739, 739t, 1647
  homosexuality and, 1647
  incidence and prevalence of, 1647
  pathogenesis of, 1647–1648
  pathology findings in, 1647t, 1647–1648
  prevention of, 1648
  prognosis in, 1648
  signs and symptoms of, 1647t, 1648
  treatment of, 1648
Shin, saber, 1710
Shingles, 2036, **2093–2095**
  chickenpox prior to, 1763–1764, 2205
  herpes zoster in, 2036, 2093–2095, 2205
  neuralgia of, 2036, 2093–2095, 2205
  treatment of, 2205
Shivering, thermogenesis in, 1533, 2188
Shock, **477–495**
  acidosis with, 491
  adrenal crisis with, 1250
  arrhythmia with, 491–492
  bacteremic, 497, 497, 498
  blood pressure in, 489–490, 494, 499t, 499–501
  cardiogenic, 477, 478t, 486t, 486–489
  cellular effects of, 483–485
  clinical features in, 478t, 478–482, 484t, 487–489
  cold vs. warm, 486
  complications of, 487
  definition of, 477–478, 478t
  device therapy in, 495
    cardiac assist, 495

Shock (Continued)
  extracorporeal, 495
  intra-aortic balloon, 495
  diagnosis of, 478t, 484t, 487–488, 490
  distributive, 485–486
  drug therapy in, 492–494
  drug-induced, 486t
  examination and history in, 488
  gastrointestinal bleeding with, 643
  hypovolemic, 485
  management of, 488, 488–495
  oxygen therapy in, 491
  pain control in, 491
  pathophysiology of, 483, 483
  patient monitoring in, 489–490
  septic, **496–501**
    clinical features of, 499–500, 500t
    course of, 498
    definitions related to, 496, 497
    diagnosis of, 499–500, 500t
    etiology of, 496
    incidence of, 496
    pathogenesis of, 496–499, 498
    pathophysiology in, 499, 499t
    streptococcal, 1588t, 1588–1589
    toxic syndrome of, 1588t, 1588–1589, 1609, 1609t
    treatment of, 500t, 500–501
  stages of, 483, 483, 484t
  trauma with, 2137
  vascular obstructive, 486
Shohl's solution, 548
Short bowel syndrome, 705
Shoulder, anatomy of, 1522
  Milwaukee, 1516, 1519t, 1524
  normal, radiography of, 1523
  painful, **1521–1524**
    bicipital tendinitis in, 1521–1524
    bursitis in, 1524, 1524, 1527
    calcific tendinitis in, 1521–1524, 1522, 1524
    capsulitis in, 1524
    glenohumeral arthritis in, 1524
    osteonecrosis in, 1524
    rotator cuff tendinitis in, 1521, 1523
  rheumatoid arthritis affecting, 1463
Shunts, 280, 287
  left-to-right, 279, 280
    congenital defect in, 279, 280
  peritoneovenous, 795
  portacaval, 794, 794t
  portal hypertension and, 793–794
  portosystemic, 794t, 794–795
    collaterals in, 752, 793
    radiography of, 630, 630
  right-to-left, 287
    blood gases in, 467t, 468, 472
    respiratory failure and, 467t, 468, 472
Shwartzman reaction, 1449, 1449–1450
Shy-Drager syndrome, 2051t
SIADH. See Vasopressin, inappropriate secretion of.
Sialadenosis, 649t, 649–650
Sibship, 139, 139
Sick sinus syndrome, 237t, 238t, 241–242
  treatment of, 237t, 238t, 241–242
Sickle syndromes, **882–893**
  anemia, **882–893**
    blood smear, 883, 885
    clinical manifestations of, 886–889, 888t
    diagnosis of, 890–891, 891
    pathophysiology, 884, 884–886, 885
  arthritis with, 1525
  genetics of, 137, 139, 142, 883–884, 889–891
  historical factors, 882–883
  malaria and, 883
  neuropathy of, 888
  pain control in, 887, 892, 893t
  prevalence of, 136t, 138t, 883–884
  renal lesion of, 608, 888–889
  retinopathy caused by, 2182
  thalassemia with, 884–885, 885t, 889–890
  trait, 883, 889
  transient ischemic attacks in, 888
  treatment and prevention, 891–893, 893t
  variant, 889–890
Sideroblasts, 834
  anemia with, 842–843
  ringed, 834, 842
Sigmoid sinus, 2061
Sigmoidoscopy, 638t, 639–640
  cancer screening with, 1006t
  indications for, 638t

Signaling, B cell, 1403
  hormone action and, 1176–1180, 1176–1180
  neutrophil activation and, 1451–1453, 1452
  T cell, 1403
Silicone, gel sheeting of, 2196
  injection of, 1508
  keloid treatment using, 2196
  panniculitis associated with, 1508
Silicosis, 399t, 401–402, 402t
  clinical features of, 399t, 402
  diagnosis of, 399t, 402
  occupational exposure causing, 58t
  occupations causing, 402t
  prognosis in, 402
  treatment of, 402
Silo-filler's disease, 404
Silver stain, Treponema pallidum in, 1705
Simian immunodeficiency virus, 1845, 1845–1846
Simon foci, tuberculosis with, 1683
Sindbis virus, 1805t, 1806t, 1809–1810
Single photon emission tomography (SPECT), 129–131, 132
  myocardium in, 202, 202
Sinoatrial block, 241–242
  arrhythmias due to, 241, 241–242
  clinical features of, 241–242
  ECG of, 241, 241
  treatment of, 242
Sinoatrial node. See Sinus node.
Sinus(es), cancer of, 1014
  common cold affecting, 1749, 1749
  headache related to, 2034
  inflammation of. See Rhinitis; Sinusitis.
  mucormycosis affecting, 1833
  Wegener's granulomatosis affecting, 1495, 1495t, 1496t
Sinus node, 231–233, 232
  anatomy of, 231, 232
  arrhythmias related to, 235t, 237, 237t, 238t, 241–242
  automaticity in, 231, 233
  electrogram of, 231–233, 232
  heartbeat origination in, 231, 232
  internodal tracts of, 231
  overdrive suppression by, 232
  P (pacemaker) cells of, 231–232
  sick sinus syndrome of, 235t, 237t, 238t, 241–242
  sinoatrial block of, 241, 241–242
  T (transitional) cells of, 231
Sinus of Valsalva, 281, 342
  aneurysm of, 281, 283
    aortic, 342
    congenital, 281, 283
Sinus tract, mycetoma with, 1835
Sinusitis, 450
  H. influenzae in, 1623
  pneumococcal, 1571, 1571t
  Wegener's granulomatosis causing, 1495, 1495t, 1496t
Sipple's syndrome, 1254
Sister Mary Joseph's nodules, 1030
Sitosterolemia, 1095
Situs inversus, 279, 281
SIV (simian immunodeficiency virus), 1845, 1845–1846
Sjögren's syndrome, **1488–1490**
  AIDS/HIV patient with, 1878t, 1879
  classification criteria for, 1488, 1488t, 1489
  clinical features of, 1488–1489, 1490t, 2153, 2181
  definition of, 1488, 2181
  diagnosis of, 1489, 2181
  epidemiology of, 1488
  extraglandular effects of, 1490, 1490t
  historical aspects of, 1488
  HLA complex in, 1431t
  interstitial lung disease with, 395t, 396
  keratoconjunctivitis in, 2181
  laboratory tests in, 1488t, 1489–1490
  pathogenesis and pathology of, 1488
  prevalence of, 1488
  prognosis in, 1490
  rheumatoid arthritis with, 1464
  salivary gland enlargement in, 649, 649t
  treatment of, 1490
Skin, **2184–2222**
  abscess of, 2192
  acanthosis nigricans, palmar, 1019–1020
    paraneoplastic, 1019–1020
  aging effects in, 2187, 2190

Skin (Continued)
AIDS/HIV effects in, 1868
anatomy of, 2184–2187, 2185, 2186
annular lesions of, 2191, 2191
antimicrobials affecting, 1568t
arciform lesions of, 2191, 2191–2192
barrier defense role of, 1537, 1538t
biopsy of, 2192–2193, 2193
blood flow to, 2189
body location of lesions of, 2191, 2216t
bullae of. See Bullae.
cancer of, 2209, 2209–2211, 2210
clostridial infection of, 1631, 1631t, 1632
color of, **2185**
    albinism and, 146
    disorders affecting, 2190, 2191t
    melanocyte organelles in, 2185, 2192
    physiology of, 2185, 2187, 2190, 2192
crusts, 2191t
dermatophytosis of, 2184t, 2199–2200
diagnostic approach to diseases of, 2189t, 2190–2193, 2191, 2191t
diascopy of, 2192
differentiation of, 2184–2185
diphtheria affecting, 1630
distribution of lesions of, 2191, 2216t
dressings and soaks for, 2193–2194, 2194t
drug reactions affecting, 98t, 99t, 1409, 1568t
drug therapies for, 2193–2197
    systemic, 2196t, 2196–2197
    topical, 2193–2196, 2194t, 2195t
dry, 2187. See also Xerosis.
Ehlers-Danlos effects in, 1120–1121, 1121t, 2201
elasticity of, 2186, 2190
erysipeloid, 1587, 1589t
erythema of. See Erythema.
examination of, 2190–2193, 2191, 2191t, 2193
    laboratory procedures in, 2192–2193
    physical, 2190, 2191, 2191t, 2192
    visual aids in, 2192
flora of, normal, 1639, 1639t, 1640–1641
functional aspects of, 1537, 2187–2190
fungal infections of, 1836, 2191, 2192, 2194t, 2199–2200
galvanic response of, 2009t
gammopathy affecting, 961
gonorrhea lesions of, 1702
hard, 347, 1483–1484
hidebound, 347, 1483–1484
history taking for, 2190
hyperextensible, 1120–1122, 1121t
hypothyroidism effect on, 1238, 1238t
ichthyotic, 1019, 2204, 2204t
immune-mediated disorders of, 2188–2189, 2189t.
    See also specific disorders.
impetigo of, 1537, 1538t, 1606, 1607t, 2205
iris lesions of, 2191, 2191
itching of, 2187, 2187t, 2188t. See also Pruritus.
leishmaniasis of, 1906, 1906–1907
leprosy affecting, 1691, 1693–1694, 1694, 1695
lichenification of, 2191, 2191t, 2192, 2198–2199
linear lesions of, 2191, 2191
lupus erythematosus affecting, 1475t, 1478, 2189t
Lyme disease lesions of, 1715–1717, 1717t, 1717, 1718
lymphoma affecting, 1031t, 1031–1032
macules of. See Macules.
magnification of, 2190, 2192
mastocytosis affecting, 1435t, 1435–1437, 1436
Mediterranean fever affecting, 907
metastases to, 1030–1031, 1031t
microscopic structure of, 2184–2186, 2185, 2186
morphology of lesions of, 2191t
mycobacterial (nontuberculous) disease of, 1690t, 1690–1691
myositis and. See Dermatomyositis.
nerve supply of, 2187
neural disorders affecting, 2056–2057
nodules. See Nodules.
obesity effect on, 1165
papules of. See Papules.
paraneoplastic effects in, 1018–1020, 1030–1036, 1031t, 1033t, 1034t
physiology of, 2184–2190, 2185, 2186
pigmentation of. See Melanin; Pigmentation.
plaque of, 2191t. See also Plaque, cutaneous.
polycyclic lesions of, 2191, 2192
porphyrias and, 1124, 1128, 1129, 1130
primary vs. secondary lesion of, 2190

Skin (Continued)
pseudoxanthoma elasticum of, 1123, 1123–1124
psoriasis of, 2191
    arthritis with, 1471, 1471–1472
    tars and anthralin in, 2195
psychological aspects of perception of, 2184, 2189–2190
radiation of, 61, 61t
rash of. See Rash.
Raynaud's phenomenon effect on, 347, 1484, 1485
rheumatoid disease affecting, 1463
rubbing effects on, 1035, 1411, 2192, 2208
sarcoidosis of, 432, 432
"scalded man" syndrome of, 1607t, 1609, 1609t, 2205
scleroderma affecting, 1483t, 1483–1485, 1484t, 1485
scratching excoriation of, 2187
serpiginous lesions of, 2191, 2192
shingles affecting, 2094
shock and, 484
sickle syndrome affecting, 889
staphylococcal infection of, 1606–1607, 1607t, 1609, 1609t, 2205
streptococcal infection of, 1586, 1587, 1589t
sun exposure and, 2187
syphilitic lesions of, 1706–1707, 1707
tags, 2190
temperature of, 484
    thermoregulation role of, 2188
    vascular disorders and, 346–350
thyrotoxicosis effect on, 1232, 1233t
transillumination of, 2192
treatment principles for, 2193–2197, 2194t, 2195t, 2196t
ulcer of, 2191t, 2212
    chancroid, 1704
    diseases associated with, 2191t, 2212
    donovanosis with, 1703–1704
    necrotic, 2212
    paracoccidioidomycotic, 1723
    syphilitic, 1706, 1707, 1707
    tularemia causing, 1662, 1664
ultraviolet light on, aging due to, 2187, 2190, 2217
    allergic reaction due to, 2198, 2217–2218
    examination (Wood's lamp) using, 2192, 2200
    therapy using, 2197
uremia affecting, 557t, 559, 562
vasculitis affecting, 1492, 1493
vesicles of. See Vesicles.
viral infections of, 1741t
vitamin D synthesis by, 1355, 1357
Wegener's granulomatosis affecting, 1495t, 1496, 1496t
wheal of, 2191t. See also Urticaria.
wound healing in, 2189
wrinkled, 2187, 2190
Skin test(s), allergen identification in, 1416
    bee and hornet venom in, 1421
    Darier's, 2192
    examination and, 2192–2193
    histoplasmosis in, 1818
    leprosy in, 1692t, 1692–1693
    Nikolsky's, 2192
    patch used in, 2192
    penicillin in, 1434, 1434t
    rubbing in, 2192
    tuberculosis in, 1683
    tularemia in, 1663
    warts vs. calluses in, 2192
Skinfolds, body fat assessment using, 1161
    nutrition assessment using, 1153, 1153t
    triceps, 1153, 1153t
Skull, imaging methods for, 1963t, 1963–1964
    Paget's disease of, 1385, 1385–1386
    radiography of, 1963, 1966
    trauma and, 1966
Skunk, rabies in, 2096
Sleep, 1982–1985
    aging effect on, 16, 16t, 18
    alcohol and, 1983t
    apnea associated with, 451–452, 1984–1985
        airway obstruction in, 1984, 1984t
        neurologic mechanisms of, 1984, 1984t
        obesity with, 1164
        treatment of, 1984–1985
    biology of, 1982
    cycle of, 1982
        hormone secretion and, 1199–1200
        melatonin role in, 1204–1205
    depression affecting, 1999, 1999t, 2000

Sleep (Continued)
    deprivation of, 1982–1983, 1983t
    disorders of, 1982–1985, 1983t, 1984t
    drug therapy for, 1983
    excessive, 1983–1984, 1984t
    gonadotropin secretion during, 1294, 1294–1295
    growth hormone secretion during, 1210
    hallucinations and, 1984
    Klein-Levin syndrome affecting, 1160, 2013
    manic episode affecting, 2003t
    myoclonus of, 1983, 2050
    ovarian hormones and, 1294, 1294–1295
    paralysis related to, 1984
    REM, 1982
    stages of, 1982
    terrors, 1983, 1983t
    walking, 1983, 1983t
Sleeping sickness, 1896–1898
    clinical features of, 1896t, 1897–1898
    East African, fatality rate for, 1738t
    etiologic organism in, 1896–1897, 1897
    Gambian, 1896t, 1898
    pathogenesis and pathology in, 1897
    Rhodesian, 1896t, 1898
    treatment of, 1898–1899
Sly syndrome, 1119t
Small meal syndrome, 719–720
Smallpox, 1765–1768
    clinical manifestations of, 1765–1767
    diagnosis of, 1767
    eradication program for, 1765–1767, 1766
    immunization for, 46, 1727, 1765–1767
Smell, 2014t, 2014–2015
    absence of sense of, 1200
    aging effect on sense of, 16, 16t
    anatomy and sense of, 2014
    Kallmann's syndrome affecting, 1200
    loss of sense of, 2014t, 2014–2015
    receptors for sense of, 2014
    testing of sense of, 2014
Smoke inhalation, carbon monoxide poisoning in, 507, 507t
    clinical features of, 403
    cyanide poisoning due to, 504t, 508
    respiratory injury due to, 403, 403t
    toxic by-products in, 403t, 404, 508
    treatment of, 403
Smoking, 33–36
    addiction to, 34, 36, 55
    alcohol synergism with, 1014
    atherosclerosis and, 171, 173, 293
    bronchitis and, 383, 385
    cancer related to, 1008–1009, 1009t, 1014
    death rate and, 27t, 30t, 33, 35t
    diseases associated with, 27t, 30t, 34t, 34–35, 36t
    drug interaction with, 35, 36t
    emphysema and, 383, 385
    epidemiology of, 33
    esophageal reflux disease and, 653, 654t
    filtered, 1014
    harmful constituents in, 34, 35
    hoarseness caused by, 451
    hypertension and, 262
    inflammatory bowel disease and, 707, 707t
    larynx affected by, 451
    lung cancer and, 437–438
    passive (environmental), 35, 36t
    pneumoconioses and, 399–400
    quitting, 35–36, 55
        lung disease slowed by, 374
    risk factor role of, 27t, 30t, 34t–36t
    smokeless, 33, 34t, 35
    stroke and, 2069t, 2070
    thromboangiitis obliterans and, 351–352
    tobacco forms used in, 33, 35
    vitamins affected by, 1146
Snail, schistosomes in, 1927, 1927–1928
Snakebite, 1951–1953
    coagulation affected by, 1003, 1952t
    epidemiology of, 1951, 1951t
    immune globulin against, 41t
    marine, 1953–1956, 1954, 1954t
    pathophysiology of, 1951t, 1951–1952, 1952t
    signs and symptoms of, 1951–1952, 1952t
    treatment of, 1952t, 1952–1953
Sneddon's syndrome, 349
Snoring, 451
    causes of, 451–452
    prevalence of, 451
    treatment of, 451–452

Snuff, 33, 35
Soaks, 2193–2194, 2194t
  agents used in, 2193–2194, 2194t
  skin treated with, 2193–2194, 2194t
Social factors. See also *Ethical issues*; *Psychosocial factors.*
  elderly and, 21, 21t
  medicine and, 9–11
Sodium, 534–538. See also *Salt.*
  alkalosis and, 514
  antiarrhythmic agent affecting, 244–245, *245*, 245t
  deficit of, 534t, 534–537
  diabetes insipidus and, *1226*
  dietary restriction of, heart failure and, 221, 221t
    hypertension treatment and, 261
  diuretic agent effect on, 222, *223*, 224t, 531–532, *532*
  excess of, 537–538
  extracellular, 533, 538–539
  intestinal transport of, *689*, 689–690
  intracellular, 533, 538–539
  kidney and, 514, 514t, *522*, 522–524
    fractional excretion and, 514, 514t, 553t
    renal failure and, 514, 514t
    transport and, *223*, 521t, *522*, 523–524, *532*
  physiologic considerations for, 533
  sweat gland transport of, 419, *419*
  urinary, aldosterone and, 514, 598–599
    volume depletion and, 514
  volume regulation role of, *526*, *527*, 527–528
  wasting, 528, 539, 550, 557, 598–599
  water and, *526*, *527*, 527–528
Sodium amytal, 2128
Sodium channel, 244–245, *245*, 245t
Sodium pump, digitalis effect on, 225, *225*
  intestinal, *689*, 689–690
  natriuretic hormone and, 1194
Sodium-potassium pump, *245*
Soft tissues, calcification in, 1378
  cancer of, 1013t
  infection of. See *Cellulitis.*
  normal flora and, *1639*, 1639t, 1640–1641
  oral tumors of, 648, 648t
  renal osteodystrophy affecting, 1378
Soil, blastomycosis organism in, 1821
  botulinum organism in, 1635
  coccidioidomycosis organism in, 1819
  histoplasmosis organism in, 1816
  hookworm eggs in, 1934
  tetanus organism in, 1636
Sole. See also *Foot.*
  hair follicle absent on, 2186
  ichthyosis of, 2204t
  pityriasis of, 2204
  psoriasis affecting, 2203
  Rocky Mountain spotted fever rash of, 1731, 1738t
  syphilitic rash of, 1707, *1707*
Solvents, 58t, 59t
  aplastic anemia caused by, 832, 832t
  gallstone dissolution with, 815
  hepatotoxicity, 772, 773t
  inhaling of, 55, 403, 404
  interstitial lung disease and, 391, 391t
  occupational exposure to, 56, 58t, 59t, 404
  renal function and, 588–589
Solver-Russell syndrome, 1296
Somatic mutation theory, 14–15
Somatization disorder, **2005–2006**
  diagnostic criteria for, 2005, 2006t
  features of, 2005, 2005t
  pathophysiology of, 2005
  treatment of, 2005–2006
Somatomedin, anorexia effect on, 1159
  growth hormone and, 1210
Somatostatin, 1198, *1198*, 1210
  tumor secretion of, 1284
Somatostatinoma, 1284
  clinical features of, 1284
  diagnosis of, 1284
  pathology of, 1284
  treatment of, 1284
Somatotropes, 1205, 1209t, 1210
Somatotropin. See *Growth hormone.*
Somnambulism, 1983, 1983t
Somnolence. See *Hypersomnia*; *Sleep.*
Soots. See also *Dust(s).*
  carcinogenicity of, 1016t
Sorbitol, *1084*
SOS factor, *1180*
Sotalol, 246t, 250

Sotalol *(Continued)*
  adverse effects of, 248t
  antiarrhythmic action of, 246t, 250
  pharmacokinetics of, 246t, 250
Sotos syndrome, 160t, 161
  clinical features of, 160t, 161
Sound waves, *197*. See also *Hearing*; *Noise*; *Ultra-sonography.*
Southeast Asian ovalocytosis, 855, 855t
Spargonosis, 1926
Sparteine, 97t
Spasms (spasticity), 2042–2043
  hyperkalemia with, 542
  multiple sclerosis with, 2109, 2110
  muscular dystrophy with, 2160t, 2162
  myotonic, 2159, 2160, 2160t, 2162
  paraplegia with, 2052
  stiff-man syndrome with, 2170
  tetanus and, 1637
  tics due to, 2043, 2047, 2049–2050
  torticollis, 2043, 2049
Specific gravity, urinary, 511, 512t
SPECT (single photon emission tomography), 129–131, *132*
  myocardium in, 202, *202*
Spectinomycin, 1562t
  gonorrhea therapy with, 1702t
Spectrin, *851*, 851–852
  pyropoikilocytosis caused by, 855, 855t
Speech, **1990–1992**
  alcohol affecting, 47, 48t
  aphasia and, 1991t, 1991–1992. See also *Aphasia.*
  articulation disorder affecting, 1989, 1989t
  cerebral areas of, 1990–1992, 1991t, *2059*
  coma scale use of, 2137t
  dysarthria in, 1989, 1989t
  hemispheric dominance related to, 1990–1991
  involuntary, 2049
  localization of areas of, 1991t, 1991–1992
  neurologic examination of, 1977t
  psychosis affecting, 1997, 1997t
  tic affecting, 2049
Sperm, absence of, 421, 1329, 1331, 1334, 1337
  antibodies to, 1332
  count of, 1327, *1328*
  examination of, 1327, *1328*
  immotile cilia syndrome and, 1336
  infertility and, 1331–1332
  testicular size and, 1325, 1329
  transport defects and, 1331–1332
Spermatogenesis, 1325–1326, *1326*
  deficiency in, 1329, 1333–1339
    isolated, 1329, 1336–1337
  evaluation of, 1327, *1328*
  hormonal control of, 1327, *1328*
  testicular morphology and, 1325–1326, *1326*
Spherocytosis, complications of, 853, 853t
  diagnosis of, 853–854, 854t
  diseases causing, 854t
  genetics of, 138t
  hereditary, 138t, 144t, 852–854, *853*, 853t
  metabolic defect in, 144t, 852
  splenomegaly of, 854, 972, 973
Sphincter of Oddi, 816, 816t
  gallbladder filling and, 806, 816
Sphincterotomy, pancreatic duct, 641
Sphincter(s), 741, 2009t, 2010t
  anal, 740, *741*
    abscess affecting, 741, *741*
    outlet obstruction and, 687
    rectal prolapse and, 743
    reflex testing of, 2009t
  enteric, 680–681
  urinary bladder, 2010, 2010t
Sphingomyelin, 1096t, 1098–1099
Sphingomyelinase deficiency, 1096t, 1098
Spider bite, 1948
  immune globulin against, 41t
Spina bifida, 2149
Spinal artery, *2074*, 2074–2076
Spinal cord, **2139–2149**
  abscess affecting, 2082–2083
  anatomy and, *2139*, 2141, *2141*
  central syndrome of, *2139*, 2139–2140
  cervical tracts and pathways of, *2139*
  compression of, 2142t, 2142–2144, 2143t
    approach to patient with, 2143–2144
    cancer patient with, 1050–1051, *1051*
    clinical signs of, 2142t, 2142–2144, 2143t
    hemorrhagic, 2146

Spinal cord *(Continued)*
    inflammatory disease causing, 2146
    traumatic, 2139–2140
    tumors causing, *2146*, 2146–2148
  congenital anomalies of, 2149
  cysticercosis affecting, 1926
  hemorrhage into, *2139*, 2139–2140
  inflammation of. See *Meningitis*; *Myelitis.*
  localization of lesion of, 2030–2031, 2031t
  paraneoplastic effects in, 1027t, 1028–1029
  syringomyelia affecting, 2055, *2055*
  trauma to, *2139*, 2139–2140
    management of, 2137, 2139–2140
    pathophysiology of, 2137, 2139–2140
Spine, **2141–2146**
  anatomy of, 2141, *2141*
  bone loss in, 1353–1354
  compression fracture of, 2038
  congenital anomalies of, 2049, 2149
  deformities affecting, 443t, 443–444
  diagnostic methods for, 1959–1963, 1963t
    CT scan in, 1963t, 1964
    disc disease and, 1968, *1968*, 2145–2146
    MRI scan in, 1963t, 1964, *1968*, 1968–1969, *1969*
    myelography and, 1964
    radiography in, 1964
  muscle atrophy affecting, 2052t, 2053
    adult onset, 2052t, 2053
    infantile, 2052t, 2053
  osteoarthritis of, 1519t, 1520
  osteomyelitis of, 1625t, 1625–1626, *1626*
  pain related to, *2141*, 2141–2146
    back, 2037–2038, 2144, 2146
    facet joint, 2141, *2141*
    funicular, 2142
    muscle, 2141, 2142, 2146
    neck, 2141, 2144, 2146
    radicular, 2142
    referred, 2142
  physical examination of, 2143–2144
  physiology of, 2141, *2141*
  rheumatoid disease affecting, 1463, *1463*
  rigidity syndrome of, 2163
  spondylosis of, 2145–2146
  trauma to, *2139*, 2139–2140
  tumor affecting, *2146*, 2146–2148
Spinnbarkeit, 1209
Spiramycin, 1909–1910, 1910t
Spirochetal infections, 1705–1721
  hepatic effects of, 782
  leptospiral, 1720–1721
  Lyme disease due to. See *Lyme disease.*
  nonsyphilitic treponematosis, 1714
  pinta, 1714
  relapsing fever, 1715
  sexual transmission of, 1697t, 1705
  syphilis due to. See *Syphilis.*
    endemic (bejel), 1714
  yaws, 1714
Spirometry, 374, *374*
  pulmonary function testing with, *373*, 373–374, *374*
Spironolactone, dosage for, 264t
  hirsutism treated with, 1316
  properties and action of, 224t, 531t
  side effects of, 267t
Spiropril, 265t
Spleen, **970–974**
  abscess of, 974
  aneurysm of, 974
  blood flow in, 970–971
  cysts of, 974
  enlargement of. See *Splenomegaly.*
  erythrocytes of, 852, 857, 860–861, 971
  evaluation of, 971
  function of, 970–971, 972, 973
  hyperfunction of, 972, 973
  hypofunction of, 973–974
  physiology of, 970–971
  rupture of, 973
  structure of, 971
  tumor of, 974
  Wegener's granulomatosis affecting, 1495t
Splenectomy, 854
  anemia and, hemolytic, 973
  compromised host with, 1542
  indications for, 972–973
  leukemia and, 972t, 973
  spherocytosis therapy using, 854, 973

Splenectomy (Continued)
thalassemia treated with, 878, 973
thrombocytopenia treated with, 972
Splenomegaly, **971–972**
causes of, 971t, 971–972, 972t
congestive (Banti's syndrome), 972
evaluation of, 971
Felty's syndrome with, 972t, 973
Gaucher's disease with, 971t, 972, 972t, 973
infection causing, 971t, 971–972, 972t
leishmaniasis and, 1905, 1905
leukemia with, 971t, 972, 972t, 973
lupus erythematosus and, 1479
malaria and, 972t
massive, 971–972, 972t
Niemann-Pick disease with, 971t, 972
pathophysiology of, 971
polycythemia vera and, 921t, 922t
spherocytosis and, 971t, 972, 973
Spondylitis, 1467t
ankylosing, 1467–1469
chest wall function and, 443, 443t
criteria for, 1467t
diagnosis of, 1467t
interstitial lung disease with, 395t, 396
manifestations of, 1467t, 1467–1469
radiography in, 1468, 1468–1469, 1469
respiration and, 443, 443t
sacroiliitis in, 1467t, 1467–1468, 1468
conditions associated with, 1467t
Spondyloarthropathy, **1466–1472**. See also Reiter's syndrome; Spondylitis, ankylosing.
back pain related to, 2037, 2037t
comparison of features in, 1467t
criteria for, 1467t
definition of, 1466
diagnostic criteria for, 1467t
disease associations in, 1467t
therapy of, 1472
Spondylolisthesis, 2038
congenital, 2149
Spondylosis, 2145–2146
cervical, 2145
lumbar, 2145–2146
Sponge, venom of, 1954t, 1955
Spores, anthrax, 1664–1665
Aspergillus, 1830
botulinus, 1635
coccidioidal, 1819
histoplasmal, 1816
tetanus, 1636
Sporotrichosis, **1826–1827**
clinical manifestations of, 1826
diagnosis of, 1826
epidemiology of, 1826
etiologic organism in, 1826
pathogenesis and pathology of, 1826
prognosis in, 1827
treatment of, 1826–1827
Sporozoites, cryptosporidial, 1910–1911, 1911
malarial, 1893, 1893
Pneumocystis, 1893, 1893
Spots. See also Rash.
Bitol, 1145t
bone with, 1390
café au lait. See Café au lait spots.
cherry red, foveal, 2182
cotton wool. See Cotton wool spots.
Fordyce's, 2186
freckle. See Freckles.
Janeway's, 1478
Koplik's, 646, 1731, 1759, 2200
Roth's, 1599, 2181
Sprue, diarrhea with, 692
malabsorption of, 704–706
nontropical (celiac), 702, 704–705
small intestine biopsy in, 702
tropical, 705–706
Spur cells, 825t, 827
Sputum. See also Hemoptysis.
asthma effect on, 380
bronchiectasis with, 417
bronchitis affecting, 382t, 383, 386
cough with, 369–370
cultures, histoplasmosis in, 1818
cystic fibrosis with, 419–420
emphysema and, 382t, 383, 386
foul-smelling, 370

Sputum (Continued)
lung abscess affecting, 413–414
lung disease diagnosis and, 369–370
pneumococcal infection in, 1572–1573
Pneumocystis carinii in, 1919–1920
pneumonia affecting, 412–413, 1573–1574
tubercle bacillus in, 1685
yellow or green, 370
Squamous cell carcinoma, 646, 646t, 647t, 2209, 2209
Squirrel, typhus carried by, 1726, 1727t
St. Louis encephalitis, 1806t, 1810t, 1812–1813
ST segment, 190, 191
hypokalemia affecting, 540, 541
prolonged, 540, 541
Staging, 1036–1037
colon cancer, 727, 727t
Marshall-Jewett, 625t, 625–626
Robson, 623–624, 624t
simplified generic, 1006–1007, 1007t
TNM, 623–624, 624t
Stains, acridine orange, 1895
bacteria classification and, 1556–1557, 1557t
congo red, amyloid stained with, 1504, 1506
cryptosporidial organism in, 1911–1912
Gram reaction to, 1556
malaria organism in, 1894–1895, 1895t
Pneumocystis carinii in, 1919–1920
silver, Treponema pallidum in, 1705
Sudan III, fat stained with, 698, 700
Standard deviation (SD), 83
Standard error of the mean (SEM), 83
Stapes, otosclerosis of, 2022
Staphylococcal infections, **1605–1610**
antibiotic therapy in, 1609t, 1609–1610
bacteriology of, 1605–1606, 1606t
clinical manifestations of, 1607t, 1607–1609, 1609t
coagulase reaction in, 1606, 1606t, 1607t, 1609, 1609t
diagnosis of, 1607, 1609t
disseminated, 1606–1607
endocarditis due to, 1598t, 1601t, 1604t, 1608, 1608t
epidemiology of, 1606
food poisoning and, 738, 739t
hospital-acquired, 1548–1549, 1609, 1609t
host factors in, 1606–1607, 1607t
meningitis with, 1610t, 1610–1617, 1616t
pathogenesis of, 1606–1607, 1607t
pneumonia in, 412t, 1573, 1607–1608
prevention of, 1610
toxins of, 1606–1607, 1609, 1609t
treatment of, 1609t, 1609–1610
urinary tract, 602, 603t
Staphylokinase, 1606, 1607t
Starch, compulsive ingestion of, 840
Starling forces, 525
disturbances in, 530t, 530–531
equation for, 525
fluid exchange and, 525, 530
volume excess due to, 530t, 530–531
Startle response, 2005
Starvation, catabolic illness vs., 1155, 1155t
physiologic adaptation to, 1154–1155, 1155t
Statistics, 83–85
bell-shaped distribution and, 84, 85t
data analysis with, 83–85, 85t
descriptive, 83–84
fundamental, 83–85, 85t
hypothesis testing with, 84
multivariate, 85, 85t
significance testing with, 84–85, 85t
Stauffer syndrome, 810, 1021
diagnosis of, 1021
pathophysiology, 1021
treatment of, 1021
Stavudine, 1885t, 1886
activation pathways for, 1882
structure of, 1881
toxicity of, 1883t, 1885t
Steatorrhea, 698, 699t, 700, 700t
bile deficiency with, 703
fecal staining for, 698, 700
magnesium depletion in, 1137
malabsorption with, 698, 699t, 700, 700t, 702
pancreatic insufficiency with, 702
pancreatitis with, 735
physiology of, 696
Steatosis. See Liver, fatty.
Steel factor, 819, 820t
Stem cells, **819–821**
lymphoid, 819, 820, 821, 898

Stem cells (Continued)
myeloid, 819, 820, 821, 898
pluripotent, 819, 820, 821, 898
thrombocytopenia related to, 984t
transplantation of, Hodgkin's disease and, 954
Stents, prostatic, 1343–1344
Stereognosis, 2064
Stereotypy, 2050
Sterility. See Infertility.
Sternum, 443t, 443–444
Steroid sulfatase deficiency, 2204t
Steroids, 1182
adrenal, 1245–1247, 1247. See also Aldosterone; Corticosteroids; Cortisol; Glucocorticoids.
enzyme deficiencies affecting, 1287–1290, 1288, 1288t
receptors for, 1180–1183, 1181
secretion of, 1182, 1247
synthesis of, 1182–1183, 1245–1246
transport of, 1182–1183, 1247
urinary excretion of, 1246–1247, 1247
anabolic, 1339
cancer therapy and, 1046t, 1046–1047
ovarian, 1299, 1299, 1300, 1301t
tumor production of, 1312t
pain control use of, 106t
Porter-Silber, 1246, 1247
testicular, 1285, 1286, 1326, 1326–1327. See also Testosterone.
Sterols, vitamin D, 1145t
xanthoma role of, 1095
Stevens-Johnson syndrome, 2206
Stewart-Treves syndrome, 1034
Stibine poisoning, 73
Stibogluconate, 1907
Stickler syndrome, 160t, 161
clinical features of, 160t, 161
vs. Marfan syndrome, 1120
Stiff-man syndrome, 2170
Stiffness, 2159
Lyme disease with, 1716–1717, 1717t
neck, meningitis and, 1572
Parkinson's disease with, 2042
poliovirus causing, 2091
Stillbirth, 152–159, 158t
Still's disease, adult-onset, 1466
fever with, 1532, 1532t
Stimulants, drug abuse with, 51, 56t
pain control use of, 106t
Stingray venom, 1954t, 1955
Stings and bites. See Bites and stings.
Stocking-and-glove pattern, 2150
Stomach, **627–688**
acid secretion of, 675t
aspiration of, 406–407
gastritis and, 659–660
increased, 662t, 662–663
maximal, 662
minerals secreted in, 1352, 1357
peptic ulcer and, 662t, 662–664
pneumonitis related to, 406–407
vitamin B₁₂ and, 701t
Zollinger-Ellison syndrome and, 674–676, 675t
adenoma of, 679
bleeding from, 642t, 643–644, 645t, 665, 671, 673, 794–795
carcinoma of, **676–679**
clinical features in, 677t, 677–678
diagnosis of, 677t, 678
diet related to, 676, 676t
epidemiology of, 676, 676
etiology of, 676–677
incidence of, 675, 677, 1005, 1009, 1013t, 1015
metastases from, skin, 1031t
pathology in, 677, 677
prognosis in, 678
smoking associated with, 35t
staging of, 677, 677t
treatment of, 678
endoscopy of, 636–639, 638t
lavage of, 505, 643, 645
leiomyoma of, 679
leiomyosarcoma of, 679
lymphoma of, 679
manometry of, 685
movement of food through, 681–683
clinical assessment of, 682–683
delayed, 683t, 683–684
rapid, 683t, 684
mucosal barrier of, 662, 662t

Stomach (Continued)
  outlet obstruction of, 675t
  pain from, 628, 665–666
  ulcer of, **662–676**. See also Peptic ulcer.
    bleeding due to, 642t, 643, 645t, 665, 671, 673
    clinical features of, 665t, 665–666
    diagnosis of, 665t, 666, 666t
    endoscopy of, 663, 663t, 667, 667t
    incidence of, 664–665, 665
    medical treatment of, 667, 667t, 667–669, 668t
    pain due to, 665t, 665–666
    pathophysiology of, 662t, 662–664, 667t
    perforated, 669t, 669–671, 673–674
    surgical treatment of, 669t, 669–672, 670, 670t, 672
  varices, 642t, 643, 793t, 794–795
  watermelon, 661–662, 721
Stomatitis, enteroviral, 1787t, 1790
  malabsorption causing, 699t
  vesicular, 1787t, 1790
Stomatocytosis, 855
Stonefish venom, 1954t, 1955
Stones. See Lithiasis.
Stool. See Feces.
Storage diseases, 1131–1135
  cardiomyopathy due to, 333t, 334
  copper, 1131–1132. See also Wilson's disease.
  iron, 1132–1135. See also Hemochromatosis.
  lysosomal, 1095–1099, 1096t, 2112
  platelets affected by, 985
Strabismus, 2019, 2174
  causes of, 2019
  diagnostic approach to, 2020
Stratum corneum, 2184–2185, 2185
  anatomy and function of, 2184–2185, 2185
  protective function of, 2187
  thickened and scaling, 2202t, 2202–2204
Strawberry gallbladder, 816
Strawberry hemangioma, 2211
Strawberry tongue, 2200
Streptococcal infections, **1585–1590**
  antimicrobial therapy in, 1589t, 1589–1590
  asymptomatic, 1587
  bacteriology of, 1585–1587, 1589t, 1589–1590
  cellulitis, 1587–1588, 1587t
  clinical manifestations of, 1587–1590, 1588t
  endocarditis in, 1589t, 1589–1590, 1601t, 1603t, 1604t
  epidemiology of, 1585–1586
  erysipelas due to, 1587
  exotoxins in, 1587
  group A, 1585–1589
  group B, 1589t, 1590
  group C, 1589t, 1590
  group D, 1589t, 1589–1590
  group G, 1589t, 1590
  hyaluronidase role in, 1587
  lymphangiitis, 1588
  meningitis in, 1589t, 1589–1590, 1610t, 1610–1613
  myositis due to, 1588
  necrotizing fasciitis in, 1588, 1589t
  nephrotic disease associated with, 573t, 574t, 576
  non-group A, 1589t, 1589–1590
  pathogenesis of, 1586, 1586, 1589t
  pharyngitis in, 1587, 1589t
  pneumonia due to, 411–413, **1569–1575**. See also
    Pneumococcal infections.
  pyoderma (impetigo) in, 1586, 1587, 1589t
  resistance of, 1589
  rheumatic fever due to, 1589t, 1590–1591
  scarlet fever due to, 1586, 1587
  septic shock role of, 497, 498
  skin affected by, 1586, 1587, 1589t
  toxic shock syndrome due to, 1588t, 1588–1589
  treatment of, 1589t, 1589–1590
Streptokinase, 117t
  complications related to, 116, 998
  myocardial infarction treated with, 311, 311
  pharmacokinetics of, 117t
  pulmonary embolism treated with, 428, 428t
  thrombolytic therapy with, 116, 117t, 311, 311
Streptolysins, antibodies to, 1591, 1594
  O, 1587, 1591, 1594
  rheumatic fever and, 1591, 1594
  S, 1587
Streptomycin, endocarditis therapy with, 1602–1603, 1603t
  mycobacterial (nontuberculous) disease and, 1691
  tuberculosis treated with, 1686–1688, 1687t
Stress, alopecia associated with, 2216–2217

Stress (Continued)
  hypertension and, 262
  peptic ulcer role of, 662t, 664
  reduction of, 262
Striae, Cushing's syndrome with, 1247
Stridor, esophageal reflux disease and, 650, 651, 652
Stroke, **2063–2079**. See also Cerebrovascular disease.
  aspirin prophylaxis for, 1192
  atherothrombosis in, 2066, 2067t
  causes of, 2066–2071, 2067t
  clinical features of, 2064t, 2064–2066, 2078t
  complete vs. incomplete, 2064
  definition of, 2063
  diagnostic tests in, 2065–2066, 2071t
  diet and, 1143t, 2069t, 2070
  drug-related, 2067t, 2069
  embolic, 2066–2067, 2067t
  endarterectomy prophylaxis for, 2070–2071, 2071t
  examination, 2064t, 2065, 2071t, 2074, 2078t
  hematologic disorders causing, 2067t, 2068–2069
  hemorrhagic, **2073–2079**
    aneurysmal, 2073t, 2073–2076, 2074
    clinical features of, 2074, 2076–2077, 2078t
    focal, 2077, 2077–2079, 2078t
    imaging of, 1965–1966, 1966, 2079
  hypertension related to, 257, 263, 2070, 2077–2079, 2078t, 2079
  imaging of, 1966, 1967, 2065–2066, 2079
  lacunar, 2069
  mortality rates for, 26–27, 27, 171, 171t, 257
  oral contraceptive role in, 1310
  pathogenesis of, 2066–2071, 2067t, 2074
  prevention of, 2069t, 2070–2071, 2071t
  progressing, 2064
  risk factors for, 30t, 2069–2070
    modifiable, 27t, 30t, 2069t
  stable vs. unstable, 2064
  thrombolytic therapy causing, 311, 312t
  transient ischemic attacks vs., 2063–2064, 2066, 2071
  vasospasm in, 2069, 2075
  venous, 2072–2073
Stroke volume, 176, 176t, 177, 215
  determinant factors for, 479–480, 480
  heart failure and, 214, 214–215, 215
  sepsis affecting, 499, 499t
  shock and, 479, 479–480, 480, 499t
Strongyloidiasis, 783t, 1935t, 1938–1939
  clinical manifestations of, 1938–1939
  compromised host with, 1938
  diagnosis of, 1939
  epidemiology of, 1938
  etiology of, 1938
  hepatic effects of, 783t
  pathogenesis of, 1938
  treatment and prevention of, 1939
Strümpel's disease, 2052
Struvite stone, 615, 616t, 617
Stuart-Prower factor, 988t
Student's t test, 84–85, 85t
  paired, 84–85, 85t
  unpaired, 84–85, 85t
Stupor, 1969–1978
  definition of, 1969t
  drug-induced, 1974–1976, 1975t
  evaluation of, 1976–1977, 1977t
  pathophysiology in, 1970t, 1970–1976, 1972t
  "spike-wave," 2125
Sturge-Weber syndrome, 2056–2067
Stylomastoid foramen, Bell's palsy and, 2035
  pain from, 2035
Subarachnoid space, hemorrhage into, 2074–2076, 2075t, 2148
  meningitis organisms in, 1611–1612, 1618
  spinal cord compression and, 2148
Subcutaneous tissue, **1507–1508**
  amyloid deposit in, 1504t, 1504–1506
  fatty, 1507–1508, 2185
  infection of. See Cellulitis.
  nodules of. See Nodules.
  panniculitis affecting, 1507–1508
Subdural hematoma, 2136
  chronic, 2136
  imaging of, 1965
  surgical treatment of, 2136
Subluxation, atlantoaxial, 1462, 1463
Subthalamic nucleus, 2043
  ballism related to, 2049
Succinate dehydrogenase deficiency, 2167
Sucrase deficiency, 704

Sudan III stain, 698, 700
Sudden death, 253–256
  cardiac, 253–256
    arrhythmia in, 255, 255–256, 305
    causes in, 254t, 255–256
    definition of, 253
    incidence of, 253
    long QT syndrome in, 255
    myocardial infarction with, 304, 305, 315
    prevention of, 256
  infant syndrome of, 254t
    botulism causing, 1636
Suffocation, anaphylaxis causing, 1418
Sugar-water test, hemoglobinuria and, 866
Suicide, 2002
  age group and, 18, 2002
  depressed mood and, 1999t, 2001t
  elderly affected by, 18, 27t, 2002
  ideation for, 1999t, 2001t, 2002
  mortality rate role of, 27t, 30t, 37, 37t, 39
  physician-assisted, 5
  prevention of, 37–38
  rate of, 18, 27t, 37, 37t, 39
  risk factors for, 30t
Sulfadiazine, 1562t
  enzyme metabolization of, 97t
  toxoplasmosis therapy with, 1909, 1910t
Sulfadoxine, malaria therapy with, 1895t, 1895–1896, 1896t
  toxoplasmosis therapy with, 1909, 1910t
Sulfamethoxazole, 1562t, 1909, 1910t
  Cyclospora therapy with, 1916t
  listeriosis therapy with, 1673
  mycobacterial (nontuberculous) disease and, 1691
  Pneumocystis pneumonia and, 1920, 1920t, 1921t, 1922t
  staphylococcal infection treated with, 1609t, 1609–1610
Sulfasalazine, 713
  inflammatory bowel disease treated with, 712–713, 714t
  metabolism of, 713
Sulfinpyrazone, 1514t
Sulfisoxazole, 1562t
Sulfobromophthalein clearance test, 757t, 760
Sulfonamides, 1562t
  adverse reactions to, 1568t
  bacterial resistance to, 1558–1560, 1559t
  dose adjustment for, 1562t
  hepatotoxicity, 773
  mechanism of action of, 1558, 1558t
  pharmacology of, 1562t
Sulfonylurea drugs, 1268t
  dosage for, 1268t
  duration of action of, 1268t
  glucose reduction using, 1267–1268
Sulfur dioxide inhalation, 404
Sulfur ointment, scabies treated with, 2195
Sun exposure. See also Photosensitivity; Ultraviolet light.
  melatonin production and, 1204–1205
  porphyria activation by, 1124, 1128, 1130
  protective lotion for, 2195–2196
  skin effects of, 2187, 2217–2218
  urticaria due to, 1411, 2208
  vitamin D synthesis due to, 1361
Sunflower cataract, 2175
Sunscreens, 2195–2196
  urticaria and, 1411
Superantigens, streptococcal, 1586, 1586–1587
Superior vena cava syndrome, cancer etiology of, 1051–1052
  lung cancer with, 439
  mediastinal mass due to, 449
Superoxide, leukocyte production of, 900, 900
  phagocytosis role of, 897, 899, 900, 900
Superoxide dismutase, oxygen toxicity and, 404, 405
Suppuration. See also Abscesses; Pus.
  actinomycosis, 1674–1676
  nocardial, 1676–1677
  staphylococcal, 1587–1589
Supraclavicular nodes, 969t
Supraoptic nucleus, 1183
Supraspinatus muscle, 1522
Supraventricular tachycardia. See Paroxysmal supraventricular tachycardia.
Suramin, 1898
Surfactant, lung, 372

Surgery, brain tumor, 2129
  breast cancer, 1322–1323, 1323t
  cancer treated with, 1007, 1037, 1037t
  cataract removal, 2175
  colon cancer, 727
  epilepsy treated with, 2123–2124
  gastric, 683
  obesity treated with, 1167
  osteoarthritis treated with, 1521
  ovarian carcinoma, 1313–1314
  Paget's disease treated with, 1386
  pancreatic cancer, 737
  parathyroid gland, 1369–1370
  pheochromocytoma, 1256–1257
  pituitary tumor, 1209, 1212
  prostatic, 1343, 1345
  stroke prophylaxis with, 2070–2071, 2071t
  subdural hematoma treated with, 2136
  thyroid gland, 1235, *1243*, *1244*, 1245
  transsphenoidal, 1209, 1212
  wound of. See *Wounds*.
Swallowing, aspiration pneumonia and, 1581
  esophageal function in, 650–651, 654–656
    disorders of, 650, 651, 655, 657
  manometry of, 655–656, *656*
  muscular dystrophy affecting, 2162–2163
  pain with, 650
Sweating, 2186–2188
  cystic fibrosis effect on, *419*, 419–420, *420*
  glands of, *419*, 2186–2187
    apocrine, 2186
    axillary, areolar and perineal, 2186
    eccrine, *2185*, 2186
    electrolyte transport in, *419*, 419
  hypoglycemia with, 1278, 1279t
  odor related to, 2186
  paraspinal tumor causing, 2008
  pheochromocytoma causing, 1254, 1254t
  pulmonary embolism causing, 424t
  pustules related to, 2207t
  temperature regulation by, 2188
  water loss due to, 528, 538
Sweet's syndrome, 1019
  clinical features of, 1019
  diagnosis of, 1019
  paraneoplastic, 1035
  pathophysiology, 1019, 1035
  treatment of, 1019
Swyer-James syndrome, 390
Sydenham's chorea, 1592t, 1593
Sympathetic nervous system. See also *Epinephrine*;
    Norepinephrine.
  blocking agents in, 265t–267t, 270t. See also *Alpha
    blocking agents*; *Beta blocking agents*; *Propran-
    olol*.
  catecholamine regulation and, 1253
  hypothalamus role in, 2011, *2011*
  intestinal motility and, 681, *681*, 681t
  norepinephrine role in, 1253
  paraspinal tumor affecting, 2008–2009
  pupillary reflexes and, 2009, 2009t
  receptors of, *245*, 268
    activation of, 1253–1254
    shock and, 492–493
  sweating controlled by, 2009t, 2009–2010
Sympathomimetics, ocular application of, 2183t
  shock treated with, 492
Symphysis pubis, male, 1341
Synapse, venom effect on, 1953–1956, *1954*
Syncope, **1979–1981**
  cardiac, 1980t, 1980–1981, 1981t
  carotid sinus, 2009
  convulsive, 1981
  definition of, 1969t
  drop spell, 1982
  head injury and, 1982
  hyperventilation vs., 1981
  hysterical, 1979t, 1979–1980, 1982
  intracranial hypertension with, 1982
  mechanisms of, 1980, 1980t
  pathophysiology in, 1980, 1980t
  postural hypotension with, 1981
  seizure vs., 1981–1982, 2116, 2121
  vasovagal, 1980, 1980t
Syncytial virus, 1747, 1747t, 1748
  common cold due to, 1747, 1747t, 1748
  treatment of, 1746t

Syndactyly, fetus with, 158t
  hereditary disorder with, 160t, 162
Syndecan, 1445
Syndesmophytes, Reiter's, *1468*
Syndrome X, 302, 1277, *1277*
Synovial fluid, *1442*. See also *Synovium*.
  analysis of, 1455t, 1455–1456, 1465t
  arthritis affecting, 1465t
    gouty, 1465t, 1510, 1512, *1514*
    osteoarthritis, 1465t
    rheumatoid, 1465t
    septic, 1465t
    traumatic, 1465t
  aspiration technique for, 1455
  hemorrhagic, 1455t
  inflammatory, 1455t
  laboratory testing of, 1455t, 1455–1456, 1464,
    1465t
  Lyme disease affecting, 1717
  noninflammatory, 1455t
  pressure examination for effusion of, *1442*
  pseudogout and, 1465t
  purulent, 1455t
  Reiter's syndrome and, 1465t
Synoviocytes, *1460*
Synovioma, 1528
Synovitis, 1442, 1443t
  gouty, 1442, 1443t
  pigmented villonodular, 1528
  rheumatoid, *1460*, 1460–1461
Synovium, *1441*, *1448*. See also *Synovial fluid*.
  anatomy of, *1441*, *1448*
  aspiration of, analysis following, 1455t, 1455–1456
    technique for, 1455–1456
  osteoarthritis effect on, 1518–1519, *1519*
  tumors of, 1528
Syphilis, **1705–1713, 2085–2087**
  AIDS/HIV patient with, 1709–1710, 1869t, 1870,
    2086–2087
  alopecia in, 2216
  antimicrobial therapy for, 1711–1713, 1712t, 2086,
    2087t
  arthritis of, 1475, 1710
  cardiovascular, 1708, 1708t
  cerebrovascular, 2085–2086, 2086t
  clinical manifestations of, 1706–1710, 2085–2087,
    2086t
  congenital, 1710, 1712t
  CSF effects of, 2086t, 2086–2087, 2087t
  definition of, 1705
  dementia of, 2086
  diagnosis of, 1710t, 1710–1711, 1711t
  endemic (bejel), 1714
  epidemiology and incidence of, 1706, 2085
  etiology of, 1705
  gummas in, 1708, 1708t
  hepatic effects of, 782, 784t
  host response to, 1705–1706
  laboratory testing for, 1710t, 1710–1711, 1711t,
    2086t
    false-positive in, 1475t, 1479, 1711
    follow-up, 1713
  late (tertiary), 1711t, 1712t, *2085*, 2085–2087
    benign, 1708, 1708t
  lupus erythematosus false-positive for, 1475t, 1479
  meningitis due to, *2085*, 2085, 2086t
  neurologic disorders in, 1708t, 1708–1709, 1712t,
    2085–2087
  oral manifestations of, 646, 646t, 647, 647t, 648t,
    1707
  pathogenesis of, 1705–1706
  posttreatment, 1713, 2087t
  prevention prospects for, 1713
  primary, 1706, *1707*, 1711t, 1712t
  proctitis of, 742
  rash of, 1707, *1707*, 2202t
  relapsing, 1707–1708
  reporting of, 1713
  retinitis due to, 1869t, 1870
  secondary, 1706–1707, *1707*, 1711t, 1712t
  serology for, 1710t, 1710–1711, 1711t
  signs and symptoms of, 1706–1710, 2085–2087,
    2202t
  treatment of, 1711–1713, 1712t, 2086, 2087t
  untreated course of, 1706
Syringomyelia, 2055, *2055*
  clinical manifestations of, 2055, *2055*
  cyst formation in, 2055, *2055*
  treatment of, 2055

Systole, heart sounds in, 168, 168t
  pressures and volumes in, 176, *176*, 176t, *177*, 489t

T

T_3. See *Triiodothyronine (T_3)*.
T_4. See *Thyroxine (T_4)*.
T cells, 1393–1394, *1394*, 1397
  AIDS/HIV effect on, 1837t, 1837–1840, 1873t, *1890*
  allergic rhinitis role of, 1414, *1415*
  antigen presentation to, *1393*, 1394, *1394*, 1397,
    1414, *1415*
  assessment of, 1402–1403
  cytokines of, *1393*, 1395, 1395t, *1403*
  cytotoxic (killer), 1393–1394
    deficiency of, 1402t, 1402–1403, *1403*
    HIV affecting, 1840
  deficiency of, 1402t, 1402–1403, *1403*, 1541–1542
  development of, interleukins in, *1403*
  fever production role of, 1533–1534, *1534*, 1535t
  helper, 1398, 1414, *1415*
    allergic rhinitis and, 1398, 1414, *1415*
    leprosy pathogenesis and, 1692, 1693, *1694*,
      1695
  HTLV and, 1779–1783.
  immunomodulation by, 901, *901*, *1393*, 1393–1394,
    1394, 1397
  inflammatory bowel disease role of, 708
  leukemia and, 931–932, 933t, 936, 937
  lupus erythematosus role of, 1476, 1476–1477
  lymphoma and, 941t, 943, 943t, 944, 1779–1783
  myeloma and, 962
  production of, 818, 819, *820*, 821
  receptors of, *1394*, 1397, 1438
  rheumatoid synovitis role of, *1460*, 1460–1461
  sarcoidosis role of, 431, *431*
  suppressor, 1398
  thymus gland production of, 1437–1438
t test, 84–85, 85t
T tubules, 2158
  myocardial cell, *175*
T wave, 190, *190*, 191
  hyperkalemia affecting, 542, *542*
  hypokalemia and, 540, *541*
Tabes dorsalis, 1708t, 1709, *2085*, 2086, 2086t
Tache noire, tick bite causing, 1732
Tachycardia, 231–244
  atrial, 239–241
    fibrillation, 237t, 238t, *240*, 240–241, *241*
    flutter, 237t, 238t, 239–240, *240*
    multifocal, 241
  carotid massage effect on, 235, 235t
  nonparoxysmal junctional, 237t, 238t, 242, *242*
  paroxysmal supraventricular, 237t, 238t, 238–239,
    239, 240
  premature complexes, atrial, 237–238, *238*, *240*
    atrioventricular, 242
    ventricular, 238t, 242–243, *243*
  pulmonary embolism with, 424t
  rheumatic fever causing, 1592t, 1592–1593, 1593t
  toxic shock with, 1588, 1588t
  ventricular, 243–244
    accelerated idioventricular rhythm, *243*, 243–244
    clinical features of, 243
    ECG of, *243*, 243–244, *244*
    fibrillation, 237t, 238t, *243*, 244
    flutter in, 244, *244*
    multiform (torsades de pointes), 244, *244*
    myocardial infarction with, 304, *305*, 313, *315*
    prevention of, 253, 256
    sudden cardiac death and, *255*, 255–256
    sustained vs. unsustained, 237t, 238t, 243
    treatment of, 237t, 238t, 243, 256
    triggered activity causing, 233–234, *234*
Tachygastria, 684
Tachykinin, carcinoid with, 1349
  flushing due to, 1349
Tachypnea, embolism causing, 423, 424t
  heart failure with, 217, 219
Tachyzoite, toxoplasmal, 1907–1908
Taeniasis, 1922–1926
  beef, 1923t, 1924
  cerebral, 1737t
  drug therapy in, 1923t, 1924t
  pork, 1923t, 1924, 1925–1926
Takayasu's arteritis, 346, 1491
  stroke related to, 2068
  types of, 346

Talcosis, hepatic granuloma due to, 784t
  occupational exposure causing, 58t, 399t
Talin, connective tissue, *1446*
Talking. See *Speech.*
Tamm-Horsfall protein, 553
Tamoxifen, adverse effects of, 1046t, 1047
  cancer therapy using, 1046t, 1047
  mechanism of action, 1059
  resistance to, 1059–1060
Tamponade. See *Cardiac tamponade.*
Tampons, toxic shock role of, 1607, 1609
Tanner stages, 1303t
Tapeworm, 1922–1926
  beef, 1923t, 1924
  cysts, 1922–1926, 1923t
  dwarf, 1923t, 1923–1924
  fish, 1923t, 1924
  pork, 1923t, 1924, 1925–1926
Target cells, 822, 825t
Target skin lesions, 2191, *2191*, 2206
Tars, carcinogenicity of, 1016t
  psoriasis treated with, 2195, 2203
Tarsal tunnel syndrome, 1464
  rheumatoid arthritis with, 1464
Taste, 2014t, 2014–2015
  anatomy and, 2014
  examination of, 2014
  loss of sense of, 2014t, 2014–2015
TATA box, 1181
  HIV gene with, *1838, 1844*
Taurine, *805, 807*
Taxol, adverse effects, 1044
  breast cancer treatment with, 1324–1325
  chemotherapy using, 1039t, 1044, 1044t
  resistance to, 1057t
Tay-Sachs disease, 136, 136t, 138t
Tazobactam, 1579–1581, 1580t
TBG. See *Thyroxine-binding globulin.*
Tea, alkaloids in, 54, 740, 774
  bush, 774
  hepatotoxicity related to, 54, 740, 774
  herbal, 740
Teardrop cells, 825t
Tears, absent, 1488, 1488t, 1489
  Sjögren's syndrome effect on, 1488, 1488t, 1489
Teeth, bone formation and, 1351t, *1352*, 1352
  calcium and, 1351t, *1352*
  Hutchinson's, 1710
  magnesium and, 1351t, *1352*
  minerals distribution and, 1351t, *1352*, 1352
  mottled, fluoride causing, 1148t
    tetracycline causing, 1715
  phosphate and, 1351t, *1352*
  porphyria and, 1128
  syphilis affecting, 1710
Teichoic acid, bacterial, 1556
Teicoplanin, 1558, 1558t
Telangiectasia, 2191t
  ataxia with, immunodeficiency in, 1407
    lymphoma-associated, 1035
  cerebrovascular disease due to, 2076
  diseases associated with, 2191t
  hereditary hemorrhagic, 720–721
  intestinal, 720–721
  lupus erythematosus with, 1478
  photoexposure with, 1036
Tellurium, 73
Telogen effluvium, 2216
Telomerase, 1072, *1072*
Telomere, 15, 134, *1072*
  aging theory based on, 15, 1072
  cell death role of, 1072, *1072*
  loss of, 1072, *1072*
  senescence and, 15, 1072, *1072*
Temperature (body), 501. See also *Fever.*
  control of, 501, 1203, 1532, 2012
    autonomic system in, 2009t, 2009–2010, 2012
  core (atrial), 1533
  cutaneous vascularity affecting, 2188
  extremely high, 1532, 1533
  heat syndromes and, 501–502, 502t, 1533
  hyperthermic, 1203, 1532, 1533
  hypothalamic sensitivity to, 1203, 1533–1534, *1534*
  hypothermic, 502–503, 503t, 2188
  sepsis effect on, 496t, 499, 500t, 1588
  set point for, 1532, 1533, 2012, 2188
  testes and, 1325–1326, 1336
  urticaria related to, 1410
Temporal artery, 1499–1500

Temporal (cranial, giant cell) arteritis, **1498–1500**
  clinical features of, 1499, 1499t
  differential diagnosis of, 1499t, 1499–1500
  examination in, 1499–1500
  incidence of, 1499
  treatment of, 1500
Temporal lobes, 1985–1986
  aging effects in, 16, 16t
  anatomy of, 1985–1986, *1986, 2059*
  blood supply to, *2059, 2060*
  epilepsy genesis in, 2117, *2118*, 2119
  manifestations of disease of, 1986, 1987t
  Pick's disease atrophy of, 1995
  resection of, amnesia with, 1990
  tentorial herniation affecting, 1970, *1971*
  tumor of, 2126t
Tenascin, 1445
Tendinitis, 1521–1524
  bicipital, 1521–1524
  calcific, 1521–1524, *1522, 1524*
  rotator cuff, 1521, *1523*
  supraspinatus, 1521, *1522, 1524*
  tennis elbow with, 1527–1528
  trigger finger with, 1527
Tendons, fluoride effect on, 1148t
  joint anatomy and, *1441*
  reflexes of, aging effects on, 17
Tenesmus, *Campylobacter* causing, 1650
  shigellosis causing, 1648
Teniposide, adverse effects of, 1044
  chemotherapy using, 1044, 1044t
  resistance to, 1057t
Tennis, elbow pain and, 1527–1528
  exercise level in, 31
Tenosynovitis, 1527
  de Quervain's, 1527
  gonococcal, 1702
TENS (transcutaneous electrical nerve stimulation), 107
Tentorial herniation, *1971*
  consciousness disorders with, 1970–1972, *1971*,
    1971t
  intracranial pressure and, 2133
Teratoma, ovarian, 1312t
  pituitary, 2131
Terazosin, 265t
Terfenadine, 1416, 1416t
Terminal cisternae, myocardial, 175
Testes, **1325–1340**
  abnormalities of, 1325
    acquired, 1335, 1336–1338
    adult, 1331t, 1331–1338, 1334t
    developmental, 1325–1326, 1334–1335, *1335*,
      1336
    enzyme deficiencies with, 1290–1292, *1292*
    pubertal, 1329, *1330*, 1338, 1340
  absent, 1334
  anatomy of, 1325–1326
  androgens of, 1285, *1286, 1326*, 1326–1327. See also
    Testosterone.
    deficiency of, 1329–1340
  assessment of function of, 1327
  cancer of, incidence of, 1013t
    tumor markers for, 1022t, 1023
  development of, 1325–1326
  differentiation of, 1285, *1286*
  dysgenesis of. See *Gonads, dysgenesis of.*
  ectopic, 1336
  examination of, 1329
  failure of, 1333–1335, *1335*
  feminization and, 1291t, 1291–1292
  hermaphroditism and, 1286–1287
  inflammation of, 1335, 1336, 1769
  Klinefelter's syndrome and, 1333–1334, *1335*
  Leydig cell of, 1284, 1285, *1286*, 1326
  mumps affecting, 1335, 1769
  myotonic dystrophy affecting, 1335
  physiology, 1325–1326
  radiation of, 1336
  reflex retraction of, 2009t
  regulation of, *1326*, 1326–1328, *1327*
  retractile, 1336
  seminiferous tubules of, 1325–1326, 1328
  Sertoli cell of, 1284, *1286*, 1326, *1326*, 1327
  sexual differentiation and, 1284, *1285, 1286*,
    1290–1292
  spermatogenesis in. See *Spermatogenesis.*
  tumors of, 1340
  undescended, 1325–1326, 1336
  "vanishing," 1334

Testosterone, 1285, *1286*, 1327–1329
  action of, 1285, *1286*, 1327–1329
  anorchia and, 1334
  cancer therapy using, 1046t, 1047
  deprivation of, 1345
  feedback mechanism and, 1326, *1326*
  fetal, 1285, *1286*
  gonadotropins and, *1326*, 1326, *1327*
    replacement therapy with, 1339
  gynecomastia and, 1332t, 1332–1333
  hair growth and, 1315, 1329
    excessive, 1315–1317
  impotence and, 1329–1331, 1330t
  insensitivity to, 1291t, 1291–1292, *1292*, 1338
  liver disease affecting, 796
  luteinizing hormone regulation of, *1326*, 1326
  metabolism of, 1327
  obesity effect on, 1165
  ovarian, 1299, *1300*, 1301t
    polycystic syndrome and, 1316
  prostate cancer and, 1345
  pseudohermaphroditism and, 1290–1291, 1291t,
    1292, 1329
  puberty and, 1329
  replacement therapy with, 1338–1339
  secretion of, 1326
  sexual differentiation and, 1285, *1286*, 1290–1293,
    1291t, *1292*
  spermatogenesis and, *1326*, 1329, 1331–1332,
    1333–1338
  synthesis of, *1326, 1326*
  systemic disease and, 1334t, 1335–1336, 1337, 1338
  therapeutic, 1338–1339
  transport of, 1326–1327
  tumor production of, 1340
  virilization and, 1285, *1285*, *1286*, 1291t
Tetanospasmin, 1636
Tetanus, **1636–1638**
  cephalic, 1637
  clinical features of, 1637
  clostridial infection causing, 1630, 1631t, 1636–1638
  definition of, 1636
  diagnosis of, 1637
  dysautonomia of, 2007
  epidemiology of, 1636
  etiology of, 1636
  immune globulin against, 40, 41t, 1637, 1638t
  immunization for, 41–44, 44t, 1637–1638
  pathogenesis of, 1636–1637
  prophylaxis of, 1637–1638, 1638t
  treatment of, 1637
  wound, 1637–1638, 1638t
Tetany, hypocalcemia and, 1371, 2159
  myopathy and, 2158
  tetanus and, 1636–1637
Tetracyclines, 1562t
  adverse reactions to, 773t, 1568t
  amebiasis therapy with, 1915t
  balantidiasis therapy with, 1916t
  brucellosis therapy with, 1679t, 1680
  dientamoebiasis treated with, 1916t
  dose adjustment for, 1562t
  hepatotoxicity of, 773, 773t
  mechanism of action of, 1558, 1558t
  mycoplasmal infection treated with, 1578, 1578t
  osteoid label using, *1361*
  pharmacology of, 1562t
  relapsing fever therapy with, 1715
  resistance to, bacterial, 1558–1560, 1559t
  staphylococcal infection treated with, 1609t,
    1609–1610
  teeth stained by, 1715
Tetrahydrobiopterin, 1100t, 1101t, *1106*
Tetrahydrocannabinol, 53. See also *Cannabis.*
Tetrahydrocortisol, *1247*
Tetrahydrofolate, 845, *845*
Tetrodotoxins, 1954t, 1956
Thalamogeniculate arteries, 2058, *2060*
Thalamus, blood supply to, *2060*
  hemorrhage in, *2077*, 2078, 2078t
  seizure generation in, 2119
  tumor of, 2126t
Thalassemia, 827–828, **877–882**
  alpha, 877t, 879–880
  beta, 877t, 877–882
    DNA analysis and, 881
    intermedia, 879

Thalassemia (Continued)
major, 877–879
minor, 879
classification of, 877t
hydrops fetalis due to, 879–880
malaria and, 879
molecular genetics of, 880–881
prenatal diagnosis of, 881
sickle syndromes with, 884–885, 885t, 889–890
silent carrier of, 877t, 880
treatment of, 878–879, 881–882
Thalidomide, 1696
leprosy treated with, 1696
Thallium, 72
occupational exposure to, 72
poisoning due to, 72
clinical manifestations of, 72
diagnosis of, 72
mechanisms of, 72
prognosis in, 72
treatment of, 72
Theca cells, 1182, 1193
androgen synthesized by, 1299, 1299
ovarian, 1182, 1293, 1299
tumor affecting, 1312, 1312t
Theophylline, 91t, 94t
asthma treated with, 380
dose adjustment for, 94t
intoxication, 510
pharmacokinetics of, 91t, 94t
renal failure effect on, 94t
Therapeutic threshold concept, 82
Thermogenesis, 1533, 2188
cutaneous vascularity affecting, 2188
food intake elevation of, 1163
impaired, obesity etiology and, 1163
shivering role in, 1533, 2188
Thermoregulation, 501–503, 2012. See also Fever;
Temperature (body).
autonomic control of, 2009t, 2009–2010, 2012
drugs affecting, 502, 502t
hypothalamus role in, 1203, 2012, 2188
impairment of, 502, 502t, 1203, 1532, 2012
medullary resetting in, 1532
setpoint for, 1532, 1533, 2012, 2188
skin vascularity in, 2188
sweating in, 2188
Thiabendazole, anisakis treated with, 1935t
Thiamine, assessment of level of, 1146t
deficiency of, 1146t, 2039
parenteral, 1172t
physiology of, 1146t, 2039
RDA for, 1140t
toxicity of, 1146t
Wernicke-Korsakoff syndrome and, 2039
Thiazides, 222, 224t, 264t
dosages for, 264t
drug interactions of, 224t
hypertension treated with, 264, 264t, 267t
properties and action of, 222, 224t, 531t
side effects of, 267t
Thinness. See also Weight (body).
anorexia nervosa with, 1158, 1159t
Thiobendazole, 1939
Thioguanine, adverse effects of, 1043
chemotherapy using, 1042t, 1043
Thioridazine, ocular side effects of, 2183
schizophrenia treated with, 1998t, 1998–1999
Thiosulfate, 504t, 508
Thiothixene, 1998t, 1998–1999, 1999t
Thirst, 2013
absence of, 2013
beer potomania and, 534–535
diabetes insipidus and, 1224, 1225
hypernatremia role of, 537, 537t
impaired, 537, 537t
osmotic regulation of, 1222, 1223
vasopressin regulation of, 1222
volume repletion role of, 526, 527, 1222–1223, 1223
Thogoto encephalitis, 1806t
Thoracentesis, 444t, 444–445, 445t
Thoracic nodes, 969t
Thoracoplasty, 443, 443t
Thoracoscopy, 445
Thorax, asthma affecting, 378
deformities affecting, 443t, 443–444
pleurodynia affecting, 1787t, 1787–1788

Thorax (Continued)
respiratory disease and, 368, 369t, 370
shape of, 368, 369t, 370
Threonine, urinary, 1103t
Throat. See Nasopharynx; Oropharynx; Pharynx.
Thrombin, 977, 977, 978
Thromboangiitis obliterans, 351–352
clinical features of, 352
definition of, 351
diagnosis of, 352
etiology of, 352
incidence of, 352
pain of, 352
pathology in, 352
prognosis in, 352
smoking related to, 351–352
treatment of, 352
Thrombocytopenia, 831t, 980, 983
AIDS/HIV patient with, 1871
antibodies causing, 980t, 980–983, 984t
chemotherapy causing, 1054
disorders associated with, 984t
drug-induced, 980t, 982–983
evaluation of, 980, 983
Glanzmann's, 985
hemolytic-uremic syndrome with, 984, 984t
idiopathic purpura with, 980–982
immune globulin against, 41t
immunohemolytic anemia with, 866, 984t
lupus erythematosus with, 1475t, 1479
microangiopathic, 1002–1003
splenectomy in, 972
thrombotic purpura with, 983, 984t
kidney affected by, 607–608, 1002–1003
transfusion-associated, 896
Wiskott-Aldrich syndrome with, 1407
Thrombocytopoiesis, 818–819, 820, 820t, 898, 979, 984t
decreased. See Thrombocytopenia.
increased. See Thrombocytosis.
Thrombocytosis, 922–924
clinical features of, 922, 922t, 923t
diagnosis of, 922t, 922–923, 923t
erythromelalgia related to, 1528
essential, 922t, 922–924, 923t, 984
leukemia and, 927, 932t, 935t
management, 923–924
paraneoplastic, 1021
polycythemia with, 921, 921t, 922t
reactive, 922–923, 923t, 984
Thrombolytic agents, 116, 117t
arterial occlusion and, 116, 116t, 117t, 310–311, 311
complications of, 116, 998
coronary artery blockage and, 302t, 310–311, 311, 312t
dosage for, 117t
mortality rate and, 116, 116t
myocardial infarction and, 116, 117t, 310–311, 311, 312t
pharmacokinetics of, 117t
pulmonary embolism and, 116, 118, 118t, 427, 428, 428t
venous thrombosis and, 116, 118, 118t
Thrombomodulin, 978
Thrombophlebitis, 353–356
definition of, 353
incidence of, 354
lupus erythematosus with, 1479
treatment of, 355–356
Thromboplastin time, meningococcemia affecting, 1620
partial, 987, 989, 990
coagulation disorder affecting, 979, 979t, 990
hemophilia and, 979t, 991, 994
hemorrhagic disorders and, 979t, 981, 990
prolonged, 979, 979t, 990
Thrombopoietin, 820, 820t
Thrombosis, 353–355
anticoagulant therapy in, 118t, 118–121, 119t, 121t, 312t, 429t
cerebrovascular. See Cerebrovascular disease, thrombosis in.
coronary, 302t, 310–311, 311, 312t
endocarditis role of, 1596–1598, 1597, 1597t, 1598, 2067
extremities affected by, 352–353
hemorrhoidal, 741
hereditary tendency to, 997–998
homocystinuria with, 1113t, 1114
mesenteric ischemia due to, 717–718

Thrombosis (Continued)
nephropathy due to, 579
oral contraceptive role in, 1310
renal artery, 606t, 606–607
renal vein, 608t, 608–609
venous, 353–355
anticoagulants in, 118t, 118–119, 355
clinical features of, 354
diagnostic testing for, 355t
differential diagnosis for, 354, 355t
extremities affected by, 353–356, 355t
incidence of, 354, 355t
pathogenesis of, 354, 422–423
pathology of, 354
prophylaxis for, 118t, 118–119, 354, 355t, 429t
pulmonary embolism due to, 354, 422–429
risk factors for, 422t, 422–423, 429t
thrombolytic agents in, 116, 118, 118t, 355
treatment of, 118–119, 355–356
vision affected by, 2016, 2016t
Thromboxane, 113, 1188, 1189
A₂, 1188, 1189
coagulation role of, 977, 977, 979
D₂, 1188, 1189
E₂, 1188, 1189–1190
F₂, 1188, 1190
formation of, 113, 1188, 1189
metabolism of, 113, 1188, 1191–1193
platelets and, 977, 977, 1188
shock and, 481
septic, 499
Thrush, 647, 1828
AIDS/HIV with, 1866
candidiasis in, 647, 1828
oral lesions of, 647, 647t, 1828
Thumb, absence of, 291
Thymectomy, 1438
Thymine, 134, 134t
Thymocytes, 1437–1438
Thymoma, 1438–1439
immunodeficiency with, 1407
mediastinal, 448, 448–449
Thymus gland, 1437–1439
development of, 1437–1438
defects in, 1438
enlarged, 1438
HIV infection and, 1438
hypoplasia of, 1405
immunodeficiency related to, 1405
involuted, 1438
resection of, 1438
T cell production in, 1437–1438
tumors of, 1438–1439
Thyroglobulin, 1229
antibodies to, 1229
hormone binding by, 1228, 1228t
structure of, 1227
thyroid cancer surgery and, 1229
Thyroid gland, 1227–1245
ablation of, 1234–1235, 1245
AIDS/HIV effect on, 1878
anatomy of, 1227
anorexia effect on, 1158
antibodies to, 1230
autoimmune disease of, 1232–1234
biopsy of, 1231, 1231t
calcitonin secretion by, 1373–1374, 1375
carcinoma of, 1244–1245, 1373–1375
anaplastic, 1244
calcitonin production by, 1373–1375, 1375t
diagnosis of, 1245, 1374
follicular, 1244
incidence of, 1013t, 1067, 1244
management of, 1067, 1245
manifestations of, 1245
medullary, 1244–1245, 1373–1375
metastases from, skin, 1031t
pathogenesis of, 1374
pathology in, 1244–1245, 1373–1374
pregnancy with, 1061t, 1067
drug effects on, 1230t, 1234, 1235, 1235t
enlargement of, 1241–1242, 1243
hormones of, 1227, 1227–1229, 1228. See also Thyroxine (T₄); Triiodothyronine (T₃).
hyperfunction of. See Hyperthyroidism.
hypofunction of. See Hypothyroidism.
inflammation of. See Thyroiditis.
iodine level affecting, 1149t, 1227, 1236t
laboratory testing of, 1229t, 1229–1231, 1230t

Thyroid gland *(Continued)*
  multiple endocrine neoplasia and, 1244
  neoplasia of, 1242–1245
  nodules of, 1242–1243
    adenomatous, 1242–1243
    carcinomatous, 1244–1245
    differential diagnosis of, 1243, *1244*
    goitrous, 1241–1242, *1243*
    hot vs. cold, 1230–1231
    needle aspiration of, 1231, 1231t
    solitary, 1242–1243
  palpation of, 1229
  radioiodine uptake by, 1230–1231, 1245
  surgery of, 1235, *1243*, *1244*, 1245
  therapeutic inhibition of, 1234–1235, 1235t
Thyroid-binding globulin, 1182, 1228
Thyroiditis, **1240–1241**
  acute (suppurative), 1240
  chronic, 1241
  definition of, 1240
  Hashimoto's, 1241
  postpartum, 1240
  Reidel's, 1241
  subacute, 1240–1241
    painful (granulomatous, de Quervain's, giant cell), 1240
    painless (lymphocytic), 1240–1241
  thyrotoxicosis in, 1240–1241
Thyroid-stimulating hormone (TSH), 1206t, 1220–1221
  laboratory tests for, 1208t, 1213t, 1229t, 1230t
  measurement of, 1229t, 1229–1230, 1230t
  receptor for, antibodies to, 1235, 1237, 1241
    thyrotoxicosis related to, 1232, 1235
  regulation of, 1197, *1198*, 1206t, 1220–1221
    disordered, 1203, 1221
  resistance syndrome and, 1230t
  secretion of, 1220–1221
  stimulation test for, 1208t
  tumor production of, 1209t, 1221
Thyroid-stimulator, long-acting, 1230
Thyrotoxicosis, **1231–1237**
  adenoma of thyroid in, 1235–1236
  causes of, 1232t
  classification of, 1232t
  clinical manifestations of, 1232–1233, 1233t, 2168
  crisis (storm) in, 1236, 1236t
  definition of, 1231–1232
  diagnosis of, 1233
  differential diagnosis of, 1233
  factitia, 1236
  Graves' disease and, 1232–1234
  heart disease and, 1236–1237
  jodbasedow effect in, 1235
  laboratory tests in, 1229t, 1233
  multinodular goiter in, 1235–1236
  pituitary tumor and, 1236
  pregnancy and, 1236–1237
  T$_3$, 1233
  T$_4$, 1233
  thyroiditis and, 1240–1241
  treatment of, 1234t, 1234–1235, 1236t
Thyrotrope cells, 1209t, 1220
Thyrotropin. See *Thyroid-stimulating hormone (TSH).*
Thyrotropin-releasing hormone (TRH), 1197–1198, *1198*
  pituitary function tests using, 1208t, 1213t
Thyroxine (T$_4$), **1227–1229**
  antibodies to, 1230
  binding and transport of, 1228, 1228t, 1230t
  body store of, 1228
  bone growth role, 1355
  deficiency of. See *Hypothyroidism.*
  deiodination of, *1227*, 1228
  excessive. See also *Hyperthyroidism; Thyrotoxicosis.*
    euthyroid state with, 1230t
  formation of, *1227*, 1227–1228
  free, 1229, 1229t, 1230t
  half-life of, 1228, 1239
  measurement of, 1229, 1229t, 1230t
  metabolism of, 1227–1228
  normal levels of, 1229t
  ovarian tumor production of, 1312t
  regulation of, *1227*, 1227–1228
  replacement therapy using, 1208t, 1239–1240
  resistance syndrome and, 1230t
  structure of, *1228*
  synthesis and secretion of, *1227*, 1227–1228
    drug inhibition of, 1234, 1236, 1236t
  synthetic, 1239

Thyroxine-binding globulin, 1182, 1228
  factors affecting, 1228t, 1330t
  synthesis of, 1228
Tibia, "saber shin," 1710
Tic. See *Tics.*
Ticarcillin, 1562t
  Klebsiella, Enterobacter, Serratia and, 1579–1581, 1580t
  minimal inhibitory concentration for, 1570, 1570t
  Pseudomonas and, 1579–1581, 1580t
Tick-borne disease, babesiosis and, 1915–1916
  bites and, 1947–1948
  boutonneuse fever and, 1727t, 1728t, 1732
  ehrlichiosis and, 1727t, 1728t, 1733
  erysipeloid and, 1673–1674
  Lyme disease and, 1715, 1716, 1720
  Mediterranean fever and, 1732
  North Asian rickettsiosis and, 1732
  paralysis with, 1947–1948
  Q fever and, 1727t, 1728t, 1735
  relapsing fever and, 1715
  Rocky Mountain spotted fever and, 1727t, 1728t, 1730
  tick removal technique and, 1732, 1947
  tularemia and, 1663, 1664
  viruses transmitted by, 1801–1802, 1806t
  zoonoses associated with, 1727t, 1737t, 1737–1738, 1738t
Ticlopidine, aspirin vs., 116–118, 117t
  platelets and, 116–118, 117t
  stroke therapy with, 2072t
Tics, 2043, **2049–2050**
  motor, 2049
  sensory, 2049
  Tourette's syndrome with, 2049
  vocal, 2049
Tidal volume, 466, 467t
Tietze's syndrome, 1528
Timolol, 265t, 266t
Tin, occupational exposure to, 73
  poisoning due to, 73
  toxicity of, 71, 73
Tinea, 2200
  incidence of, 2184t
  nigra, 1836
  pedis, 2184t
  versicolor, 2184t, 2200
Tinel's sign, 1462, *1462*
Tinnitus, 2023–2024
  drugs causing, 2023t
  elderly affected by, 17, 17t
  evaluation of, 2023, *2023*
  objective vs. subjective, 2023
  treatment of, 2023–2024
Tissue bubbles, 375t
Tissue factor, coagulation and, *978*, 987–988, *989*
Tissue plasminogen activator, 117t
  coagulation role of, 977, *978*, 988t
  myocardial infarction treated with, 311, *311*
  pharmacokinetics of, 117t
  pulmonary embolism treated with, 428, 428t
  thrombolytic therapy with, 116, 117t, 311, *311*
T-lymphotropic virus (HTLV), **1779–1783**
  biology of, *1779*, 1779–1780, *1780*
  diseases associated with, 1781t, 1781–1783
  epidemiology of, 1780t, 1780–1781
  leukemia due to, 936, 1781t, 1781–1782, *1782*
  lymphoma due to, 943, 944, 1781t, 1781–1782, *1782*
  myelopathy associated with, 1781t, 1782, 2099–2100
  nervous system and, 2099–2100
  transmission modes for, 1780t, 1780–1781
  tropical spastic paresis due to, 1781t, 1782
Tobacco. See *Smoking.*
Tobramycin, 91t, 94t, 1562t
  dose adjustment for, 94t, 1562t
  pharmacokinetics of, 91t, 94t, 1562t
  renal failure effect on, 94t, 1562t
Tocainide, 246t
  adverse effects of, 247t
  antiarrhythmic action of, 246t, 246–249
  pharmacokinetics of, 246t
Tocopherol (vitamin E), 1145t
  deficiency of, 1145t, 2041, 2169
  neurologic effects of, 1145t, 2041
Todd's paralysis, 2114
Toe, bunion affecting, 1518, 1519t, 1519–1520
  gout affecting, 1511, *1513*
  "hammer," 1519t
  shortened fourth, *1372*
Togaviridae, 1805t, 1806t

Togavirus, slow infection due to, 2097t
  structure of, *1739*
Tolazamide, 1268, 1268t
Tolbutamide, 1267–1268
Tongue, "bag of worms" appearance in, 1593
  candidiasis affecting, 647, 647t
  geographic, 647, 647t
  hairy, 1868
  strawberry, 2200
  Sydenham's chorea affecting, 1593
Tongue worm infection, 1950
Tooth. See *Teeth.*
Tophi, 1510, *1512*
  definition of, 1510, *1512*
  ear with, 1516, 2211
  formation mechanism of, 1510, *1512*
  gout with, 1510, 1511–1512, *1512*, *1513*, 1516
  hand with, *1513*
  toe with, *1513*
Torasemide, 224t
Torcular Herophili, *2061*
Torsades de pointes, 244, *244*
  afterdepolarizations of, 234, *234*
Torulopsis, 1827
Tourette's syndrome, 2049
Toxemia of pregnancy, 609–610, 610t
Toxic epidermal necrolysis, 2205
Toxic megacolon, 709, 714
Toxic shock syndrome, 1588–1589, 1609
  course of, 1589, 1609, 1609t
  laboratory findings in, 1588t, 1588–1589
  rash of, 1609t, 2201
  staphylococcal, 1606, 1607, 1607t, 1609, 1609t
  streptococcal, 1588–1589
  symptoms and signs of, 1588, 1588t, 1609, 1609t
  treatment of, 1589t
Toxin, 58t, 59t, 403t. See also *Poisoning;* specific agent, chemical, metal.
  botulinum, 1635–1636
  ciguatera, 1954t, 1956
  clostridial, 1630–1638, 1631t, 1634t, 1635t, 1638t
  colitis due to, 1633–1635, *1634*, 1634t, 1635t
  diphtheria, 1629
  exfoliative, 1606–1607, 1609, 1609t
  foodborne, 740, 1607, 1632, 1635–1636
  marine organism with, 1953–1956, *1954*, 1954t
  occupational exposure to, 56–59, 58t, 59t, 403t
  smoke containing, 403t, 404
  snake venom with, 1951t, 1951–1953, 1952t
  staphylococcal, 1606–1607, 1609, 1609t
  streptococcal, 1585–1588
  tetanus, 1636–1638
  Vibrio cholerae, 1652–1653
Toxocariasis, 1935t, 1936–1937
  hepatic effects of, 783t
Toxoid, diphtheria, 42t, 1629
  tetanus, 1636–1638, 1638t
Toxoplasmosis, 783t, 1737t, 1907–1910
  AIDS/HIV with, 1857, 1857t, 1869, 1869t, 1908, 1909
  cerebral, 1857, 1857t, 1909
  clinical manifestations of, 1908–1909
  epidemiology of, 1908
  etiology of, 783t, 1737t, 1907–1908
    organism in, 1907–1908
  hepatic effects of, 783t
  myocarditis due to, 330
  pathogenesis of, 1908
  retinitis due to, 1869, 1869t, 1908, 1909, 2179
  treatment and prevention of, 1909–1910, 1910t
TP segment, *190*, 191–193
Trabecular meshwork, 2176, *2176*
Trace elements, 1144–1146, 1148t–1150t
  parenteral nutrition with, 1172, 1173t
  RDA for, 1140t, 1141t
  toxicity of, 70–73, 1148t–1150t
Trachea, 371
  anatomy of, 371
  polychondritis affecting, 1517
Tracheobronchitis, *Haemophilus influenzae* in, 1623
Trachoma, **1722–1723**
  chlamydial etiology of, 1697t, 1722–1723, 1723t
  diagnosis of, 1723
  epidemiology of, 1722–1723, 1723t
  treatment and prevention of, 1723
Tranexamic acid, 994
Transaminases, 759, 790

Transamination, 754
Transcobalamin, 845, 846t
  cobalamin binding by, 697, 698
  deficiency of, 1113t
Transcortin, 1247
Transcription factor II, 1181
Transcutaneous electrical nerve stimulation (TENS), 107
Transferrin, 840
  hemochromatosis and, 786, 1133–1134, 1134t
  iron transport by, 839–840, 1133–1134
  sideroblastic anemia and, 842–843
Transfusion, **893–897**
  adverse reaction to, 895t, 895–897, 896t
    acute, 895–896, 896t
    delayed, 896t, 896–897
    frequency of, 896t
    immune, 895t, 895–896, 896t
  autologous, 894
  blood type and, 894–895
  disease transmission in, 896t, 896–897
  hemolytic anemia treated with, 866
  iron accumulation due to, 878–879
  red blood cell, 893t, 893–894
  sickle syndrome treatment with, 892
  testing for, 894–895
  thalassemia treated with, 878–879
  whole blood, 893
Transmembrane channels, 244–245, 245, 245t
  intestinal, 689, 689–690, 690t
Transplantation, 360, 459, 568, 800
  bone marrow, **974–976**
    aplastic anemia treated with, 835, 975, 975–976
    complications of, 975
    graft-versus-host disease in, 975
    infection following, 975
    lymphocytic leukemia treated with, 939, 976
    lymphoma treated with, 976
    myelogenous leukemia treated with, 928–929, 940, 976, 976
    myeloma treated with, 963–964
    neutropenia treated with, 912
    preparation for, 974–975
    sickle syndrome treated with, 892
  cardiac, 360–367
    comorbid conditions and, 360, 361t
    denervation affecting, 365, 366
    donor for, 361–362, 362t
    drug effects and, 365, 366t
    evaluation for, 360–361, 361t
    immunosuppression for, 363
    indications for, 360
    infection with, 363t, 364, 365
    mortality risk in, 360, 361t
    post-transplant care for, 362t–364t, 362–367
    prophylactic antibiotics for, 363, 363t
    psychosocial aspects of, 366
    quality of life following, 366
    rejection reaction following, 363, 363–364, 364t
    survival rate for, 366
    vasculopathy with, 365–366
  hepatic, 800–802
    complications of, 801
    contraindications to, 801
    donor selection for, 801
    immunosuppression for, 801–802
    indications for, 800–801, 801t
    survival analysis of, 801t, 802
  islet cell, 1269
  lung, 459–462
    graft procurement for, 461, 461t
    historical aspects of, 459
    immunosuppressive therapy in, 462t
    indications for, 459–460, 460, 460t
    infection risk in, 461
    outcome of, 462–463, 463
    procedure selection for, 460
    rejection affecting, 461–462, 462t
  pancreatic cell, 1269
  renal, 568–572
    complications of, 571–572, 572t
    donor evaluation for, 570
    follow-up of, 571–572
    history of, 568
    immunologic aspects of, 568, 568–569
    immunosuppression for, 568
    indications for, 569t, 569–570
Transport defects, 144t
  amino acid, 1099, 1100, 1104t–1105t

Transport defects (Continued)
  glucose, 143, 144t
  intestinal mucosal, 690t
  membrane, precursor role in, 143, 143t, 144t
    product role in, 143, 143t, 144t
    protein mutations causing, 143–145, 144t, 145t, 147t
  potassium, 539, 539t
  renal tubular, 594–599, 595t
  uric acid (urate), 1509t, 1510
Transposition of great vessels, congenitally corrected, 279–280, 282
  fetus with, 158t
Transthyretin, amyloidosis role of, 967t, 1505, 1506
  thyroxine binding by, 1228, 1230t
Transverse sinus, 2061
Transverse tubules, 2158
  myocardial cell, 175
Trauma, 36–40
  aorta and, 346
  brain affected by. See Brain, trauma to.
  causes of, 37, 37t, 38, 39
  coronary arteries affected by, 302t
  fat embolism following, 430
  headache following, 2033
  hypothalamic, 1201, 1223–1226, 1226
  mortality rate role of, 37, 37t, 38, 39
  occupation exposure to, 56
  pericarditis due to, 337, 341, 341–342
  spinal cord affected by, 2139, 2139–2140
  vertigo following, 2026
Travel, **1553–1556**
  advice related to, 1553–1556, 1657–1658
  behavior modification for, 1555–1556
  bites and stings in, 1555–1556
  diarrhea related to, 1641–1642, 1642t, **1657–1658**, 1658t
  enteric infections and, 1641–1642, 1642t, **1657–1658**, 1658t
  immunizations for, 1554t, 1554–1555
  malaria prevention in, 1555, 1555t
  vaccinations needed for, 46
Trematodes, 1931–1934
  clonorchiasis due to, 1932t, 1932
  dicroceliasis due to, 1932t, 1932–1933
  echinostomiasis due to, 1932t, 1933
  fascioliasis due to, 1932, 1932t
  fasciolopsiasis due to, 1932t, 1933
  heterophyiasis due to, 1932t, 1933
  opisthorchiasis due to, 1931–1932, 1932t
  paragonimiasis due to, 1932t, 1933
  schistosomiasis due to, 1927, 1927–1931, 1929t
Tremor, **2042–2043**, 2047
  alcohol-related, 48t, 48–49
  basal ganglia relation to, 2043
  elderly affected by, 17
  essential, 2047
  flapping, 753
  hepatic encephalopathy with, 797, 798t
  hypoglycemia with, 1278, 1279t
  intention, 2043
  liver disease with, 753, 797, 798t, 1131
  parkinsonian, 2042–2043
  postural, 2043
  Wilson's disease causing, 1131
  "wing-beating," 1131
Treponema pallidum, 1697t, 1705. See also *Syphilis*.
  antibodies to, 1710t, 1711, 1711t
  darkfield microscopy of, 1705, 1710
  nonsyphilitic subspecies of, 1714
  yaws caused by, 1714
Triamcinolone, 108t
  allergic rhinitis treated with, 1417t
Triamterene, dosage for, 264t
  properties and action of, 224t, 531t
Triazolam, 16
Triceps skinfold, 1153, 1153t
Trichiasis, eyelash, 1722–1723
Trichinosis, 1935t, 1937–1938
  diagnosis of, 1938
  epidemiology of, 1937
  etiology of, 1937
  pathogenesis and clinical features of, 1937–1938
  treatment and prevention of, 1938
Trichlormethiazide, dosage for, 264t
  properties and action of, 224t
Trichloroethane, 772
Trichomoniasis, 1916–1917
  sexual transmission of, 1697t, 1699, 1699t, 1916
  treatment of, 1917

Trichomoniasis (Continued)
  vaginitis of, 1697t, 1699, 1699t, 1916
Trichostrongyliasis, 1935t, 1936
Trichotillomania, 2215–2216
Trichuriasis, 1935t, 1935–1936
Tricuspid valve, 326–327
  Ebstein's anomaly of, 281, 282
  insufficiency in, 327
  stenosis of, 326–327
Trientine, 1132
Trifluorothymidine, **1743**
  herpes simplex treated with, 1746t
  keratitis treated with, 1746t
Trigeminal nerve neuralgia, 2035
Trigeminy pulse, 243
Trigger finger, 1527
Trigger points, 2037
  spine and, 2142
Triglycerides, absorption of, 696, 697
  elevated level of, 293
  fecal, staining of, 698, 700
  glycogen metabolism and, 1082, 1082
  metabolism of, liver and, 753–754, 1086–1089
  transport of, 1087, 1088, 1088–1089, 1089
Triiodothyronine (T_3), **1227–1229**
  action of, 1228–1229
  antibodies to, 1230
  binding and transport of, 1228
  deficiency of. See *Hypothyroidism*.
  excess. See *Hyperthyroidism*.
  formation of, 1227, 1227–1228
  half-life of, 1228, 1239
  measurement of, 1229, 1229t, 1230t
  normal levels of, 1229t
  receptor for, 1180–1181, 1181, 1228–1229
  regulation of, 1227, 1227–1228
  reverse, 1229
  structure of, 1228
  synthesis and secretion of, 1227, 1227–1228
    drug inhibition of, 1234, 1236, 1236t
Trimazosin, 268
Trimethaphan camsylate, dosage for, 270t
  side effects of, 270t
Trimethoprim, 1562t
  adverse reactions to, 1568t
  bacterial resistance to, 1558–1560, 1559t
  cat scratch disease therapy with, 1681–1682, 1682t
  Cyclospora therapy with, 1916t
  diarrhea therapy with, 1658, 1658t
  isosporiasis therapy with, 1916t
  listeriosis therapy with, 1673
  mechanism of action of, 1558, 1558t
  meningitis therapy with, 1615–1617, 1616t
  Pneumocystis pneumonia and, 1920, 1920t, 1921t, 1922t
  staphylococcal infection treated with, 1609t, 1609–1610
Trimethoprim-sulfamethoxazole, 1909, 1910t
Trimetrexate, 1920, 1920t, 1921t, 1922t
Tripe palms, 1019–1020
Triploidy, 152–153
Trismus, 1637
Trisomy, 21, 155
  X, amenorrhea in, 1305, 1305t
Trophozoites, *Cryptosporidium*, 1910–1911, 1911
  Entamoeba histolytica, 1913–1914
  Giardia, 1912
  malarial, 1893, 1893
  Naegleria fowleri, 1915
  Pneumocystis, 1917
  Trichomonas, 1916–1917
Trousseau's sign, 1371
Trousseau's syndrome, 678
Truth telling, 4
Trypanosomiasis, 783t, 1896–1903
  African (sleeping sickness), 1896–1898
    clinical features of, 1896t, 1897–1898
    epidemiology of, 1897
    etiologic organism in, 1896–1897, 1897
    Gambian, 1896t, 1898
    pathogenesis and pathology in, 1897
    Rhodesian, 1896t, 1898
    treatment of, 1898–1899
  American (Chagas' disease), 1899–1903
    clinical presentation of, 1901, 1902
    diagnosis of, 1901–1902
    epidemiology of, 1899–1900
    etiologic organism in, 1899–1900, 1900
    myocarditis in, 1901, 1901

Trypanosomiasis *(Continued)*
  pathology and pathogenesis of, *1900*, 1900–1901
    treatment and prevention of, 1902–1903
  hepatic effects of, 783t
  myocarditis due to, 329t, 329–330
Trypomastigote, *1897*, *1900*
Trypsin, 729, *730*
Trypsin-like immunoreactivity, 700t
  malabsorption and, 699, 700t
  normal level of, 700t
  pancreatic insufficiency and, 699, 700t
Trypsinogen, 729, *730*
Tryptophan, 2164–2165
  eosinophilia-myalgia caused by, 2164–2165
  urinary, 1102t
Tryptophan hydroxylase, 1348–1349, *1349*
Tsetse fly, 1897, *1897*
TSH. See *Thyroid-stimulating hormone (TSH)*.
Tsutsugamushi disease, 1727t, 1728t, 1734–1735
Tuberculin, 1683
  purified protein derivative, 1683
  rheumatoid arthritis role of, 1453–1454, *1454*,
    1454t
  skin test using, 1683
    false negative in, 1684
Tuberculosis, **1683–1689**
  AIDS/HIV with, 1684, 1686, 1687, 1688t, 1861,
    1861, 1861t
  arthritis and, 1475, 1685t
  clinical presentation of, 1684–1686, 1685t
  control programs for, 28t, 1689
  diagnosis of, 1684–1686, 1685t
  drug therapy in, 1686t–1688t, 1686–1690
  epidemiology of, *1684*, 1684
  etiology of, 1683
  extrapulmonary, 1684–1686, 1685t
  genitourinary, 1685t
  hepatic granuloma with, 784t
  hospital-acquired, 1553
  immune response to, 1683–1684
  immunization for, 1689
  lymphatic, 1685t
  meningeal, 1685t
  normal adult presentation of, 1684–1685
  nosocomial, 1553, 1689
  oral lesions of, 646, 646t
  pathogenesis of, 1683–1684
  pericarditis caused by, 337, 337t, 1685t
  peritonitis due to, 746–747, 747t, 1685t
  pleural effusion of, 445t, 446, 1685t
  prevention of, 28t, 1688, 1689
  pulmonary, 1684–1685
  resistant, 1688
  risk factors for, 1685t, 1688t
  skin test for, 1683, 1684
  symptoms and signs in, 1684–1686, 1685t
  transmission of, 1683, 1689
  treatment of, 1686t–1688t, 1686–1690
Tubes. See *Intubation*.
Tubules, transverse, 2158
  myocardial cell, 174, *175*
Tularemia, **1662–1664**
  antibodies in, 1663
  clinical manifestations of, 1664, 1737t
  complications of, 1664
  definition of, 1663
  differential diagnosis of, 1664
  epidemiology of, 1664, 1738t
  etiology of, 1664, 1737t
  laboratory testing for, 1664
  pathogenesis of, 1663–1664
  pathology findings in, 1663–1664
  prevention of, 1664
  prognosis in, 1664, 1738t
  skin testing for, 1663
  treatment of, 1664
Tumor. See *Cancer*; *Neoplasia*; specific types or organs
    involved.
Tumor lysis syndrome, 1053
Tumor markers, 1021–1024, 1022t
  breast cancer, 1022t, 1023, 1076–1077
  chemotherapy monitored with, 1041, 1041t
  colorectal cancer, 1021–1022, 1022t, *1076*
  connective tissue role in, *1447*, 1447–1448
  ectopic hormones as, 1024–1026, 1025t
  hepatoma, 1022t, 1023
  lymphoma, non-Hodgkin's, 1022t, 1023–1024
  multiple myeloma, 1022t, 1023–1024
  ovarian cancer, 1022t, 1022–1023
  paraneoplastic syndromes and, 1021–1024, 1022t

Tumor markers *(Continued)*
  prostate cancer, 1022t, 1023
  testicular cancer, 1022t, 1023
Tumor necrosis factor (TNF), 1395t
  fever production role of, 1533–1534, *1534*, 1535t
  hematopoiesis role of, 898, *917*
  immune response role of, 1395t
  malaria role of, 1894
  shock and, 485
  streptococcal induction of, 1586, *1586*
Turbinates, 1414
  black necrotic, 1833
  mucormycosis affecting, 1833
Turcot's syndrome, 724–725
  polyps in, 724–725
Turner's sign, 731
Turner's syndrome, 154, 1286
  amenorrhea with, 1304–1305, 1305t
  chromosome abnormality causing, 154, 1286
  gonadal dysgenesis in, 154, 1286
  male, 1335
  muscular dystrophy with, 2161
Twitching, muscular, 2159, 2160t
Tylosis, paraneoplastic, 1034t
Typhoid fever, **1642–1644**
  carrier of, 1642
  definition of, 1642
  epidemiology of, 1642
  immunization for, 44t, 46, 1554t, 1555, 1644
  incidence and prevalence of, 1642
  pathogenesis of, 1642–1643
  pathology findings in, 1642–1643
  prevention of, 1644
  prognosis in, 1644
  signs and symptoms of, 1643, 1643t
  treatment of, 1643–1644
Typhus, **1726–1730**
  Brill-Zinsser (recrudescent), 1726–1729, 1727t,
    1728t
  epidemic (louse-borne), 1726–1729, 1727t, 1728t,
    1738t
  murine (endemic), 1727t, 1728t, 1729–1730
  pathology findings in, 1727–1728
  Queensland tick, 1732
  scrub, 1727t, 1728t, 1734–1735
  treatment of, 1729
Tyrosine, albinism and, 146, 2214t
  catecholamine biosynthesis role of, 1253
  Fanconi's syndrome and, 1105t
  urinary, 1100t, 1101t, 1103t, 1105t
Tyrosine kinase, Bruton's, 1402t, *1403*, 1403–1404
  hormone action role of, *1177*, 1179–1180, *1180*
  second messenger role of, *1177*, 1179–1180, *1180*
Tyrosinemia, enzyme defect in, 146t, 2214t
  genetics of, 136t, 2214t
Tyson's glands, 2186
Tzanck smear, 2192
  genital ulcer in, 1698
  herpes simplex in, 1698, 2192
  preparation of, 2192, 2205
  skin examination using, 2192
  varicella in, 1764, 2192, 2205

U

U wave, *190*, 191, *193*
  giant, *193*
  hypokalemia and, 540, *541*
Ulcer(s), aphthous, 646, 646t, 647t
  Behçet's syndrome causing, 646, 646t, 1506, 1506t
  chiclero, 1903t
  corneal, 2179
  cutaneous. See *Skin, ulcer of*.
  decubitus, 24, 24t, 2212
  diabetes mellitus with, 2212
  Dieulafoy's, 721
  donovanosis, 1703–1704
  duodenal. See *Duodenum, ulcer of*; *Peptic ulcer*.
  esophageal, 652, 654
  genital, 1698, 2212
    Behçet's, 1506, 1506t, 2212
    differential diagnosis of, 1706
    granuloma inguinale, 1703–1704
    Haemophilus ducreyi chancroid, 1704
    herpetic, 1706, 1746t, 1772
    syphilitic chancre, 1706, 1707, *1707*
  intestinal, 750–751
  leg, sickle syndrome causing, 889
  oral, Behçet's, 646, 646t, 1506, 1506t

Ulcer(s) *(Continued)*
  lupus erythematosus with, 1475t, 1478
  mucosal, 646, 646t
    Reiter's syndrome with, 1469
  paracoccidioidomycotic, 1723
  peptic. See *Peptic ulcer*.
  pinta causing, 1714
  pyoderma gangrenosum with, 2212
  rectal, solitary, 743
  viral, 646, 646t
  yaws causing, 1714
Ultrafiltration, dialysis based on, 564–565, *565*
Ultrasonography, cerebrovascular examination with,
    2066
  Doppler, 198–199, *199*
  echocardiographic, 194–199, *195–199*
  exposure in, 64
  fetal, transvaginal, 127, *128*
  intravascular (IVUS), 127, *127*, *128*
  pulsed reflected signal in, 194–198, *195*
Ultraviolet light, 63, 2217–2218
  aging effect of, 2187, 2190, 2217
  allergic reaction to, 2198, 2217–2218
  examination (Wood's lamp) using, 2192, 2200
  lupus erythematosus exacerbated by, 1475t, 1478
  melanin absorption of, 2187, 2192
  porphyrin activation by, 1124, 1130
  radiation injury caused by, 63
  treatment using, 2197
  vitamin D synthesis due to, 1354, *1355*, 1357
  wavelength of, *59*, 63, 2217
Umbilicus, metastatic nodules of, 1030, 1031t
Uncinate fit, 2115
Unconsciousness. See also *Arousal level*; *Coma*; *Con-
    sciousness disorders*.
  cerebral hemorrhage with, 2078, 2078t
Uncus, olfactory aura and, 2115
Unheated serum reagin test, 1710, 1710t
Unit inheritance principle, 134
Urapidil, 268
Urea, enzyme deficiencies affecting, 1110t, 1110–1111,
    1111
  formation of, 754, 1109
  kidney and, 522, *522*, 523, *532*
  nitrogen, prerenal azotemia and, 553
  production of, 754, 1109–1110, *1110*
  transport of, 522, *522*, 523, *532*
Ureaplasma infections, 1576, 1578, 1578t
  drug therapy in, 1578, 1578t
  urinary tract with, 1578, 1578t
Uremia, **556–563**
  acidosis in, 557
  anemia and, 558, 562
  approach to patient with, 559–560
  bone disease with, 557t, 559, 562
  carbohydrates and, 557t, 559, 562
  clinical spectrum in, *556*, 556–559, 557t, 561–562
  dialysate used in, 565t, 565–566
  diet in, 562–563
  etiology of, *556*, 556t, 556–559
  hemorrhage and, 558, 985
  hypothermia and, 559
  management of, 560t, 560–563, 561t
  neuropathy and, 557t, 559, 562, 2155
  pathophysiology of, 556t, 556–559
  pericarditis and, 558, 562
  pleural effusion and, 446
  potassium and, 556–557, 557t, 561
  skin affected by, 557t, 559, 562, 2188t
  sodium and, 557, 557t, 561
Ureter, *517*
  anomalies of, developmental, 622, 622–623
  obstruction of, renal failure with, 552t, 554t
  sexual differentiation and, *1285*, *1286*
Urethra, infection route role of, 603
  obstruction of, renal failure with, 552t, 554t
  prostate gland relation to, 1341, *1341*
  sexual differentiation and, *1285*
Urethritis, 1697–1699, 1701–1702
  chlamydial, 1697, 1697t, *1698*, 1723
    female with, 1697t, 1723
    male with, 1697, 1697t, *1698*, 1723
  gonococcal, 1697–1699, *1698*, 1701–1702
    female and, 1698–1699, 1701–1702
    male affected by, 1697–1698, *1698*, 1701
    posttreatment, 1698
  meningococcal, 1621
  Reiter's, 1467t, 1469

Urethritis (*Continued*)
sexually transmitted disease with, 1697–1699, 1701–1702
symptoms of, 604, 604t
Uric acid (urate), 1508–1515
crystals of, 1512, *1512*, *1514*, 1516t
daily production of, 1509–1510, 1510t
elimination of, 1509t, 1509–1510, 1510t, *1511*
reduced, 1510
glycogen metabolism and, *1082*
gout and, 1509t, 1510, 1510t, 1512
kidney and, failure of, 557t, 559, 562, 1512
overproduction of, 1509t, 1510. See also *Gout; Hyperuricemia.*
purine metabolism and, 1509–1510, *1511*
stones and, *615*, 616t, 617, 1510–1511
synovial fluid, 1510, 1512, *1514*
Uridine, genetic code use of, 134, 134t
Urinalysis, 511–514, 512t, 513t. See also *Urine.*
false negatives in, 512t
Urinary bladder, aging effect on, 22–23
autonomic control of, 2009t, 2010, 2010t
cancer of, 625t, 625–626
dye worker with, 56, 58t
incidence of, *1005*, *1009*, 1013t, *1015*
occupational exposure causing, 56, 58t, 1014–1015
smoking associated with, 35t, 1014
staging of, 625t, 625–626
prostate gland relation to, 1341, *1341*
Urinary tract. See also *Kidney; Ureter; Urethra; Urinary bladder.*
anomalies of, 621–623, *622*
approach to diseases of, 511–517
infections of, 602–605. See also *Cystitis; Pyelonephritis; Urethritis.*
acute, 602–605
catheter-related, 603, 1549t, 1550–1551
clinical features of, 604, 604t
complicated, 602–603, 603t, 605
definition of, 602
diagnosis of, 604
drug therapy for, 604–605, *605*, 605t
epidemiology of, 603
etiology of, 602–603, 1550–1551
hospital-acquired, 1549t, 1550–1551
incidence of, 603
mycoplasmal, 1578, 1578t
organisms in, 602–603, 603t
pathogenesis of, 603–604
sexually transmitted disease causing, 1697–1699
staphylococcal, 602, 603t, 1608
treatment of, 604–605, *605*, 605t
tuberculous, 1685t
uncomplicated, 602, 605t
viral, 1741t
obstruction of, **589–594**
acute, 593
causes of, 590, 590t
clinical features in, 590–592, *591*, 591t
complete, 593
diagnostic approach to, *592*, 592–593, 593t
extrinsic, 590, 590t
infection and, 603t, 605
intrinsic, 590, 590t
lower tract, 590, 593t, 593–594
partial, 593
pathology in, 590
pathophysiology of, 590, *590*
prognosis in, 594
prostatic hypertrophy in, *1341*, 1343–1344
renal failure with, 552t, 553, 554t
treatment of, 593–594
upper tract, 590, 593t
sexual differentiation and, 1284–1285, *1285*, *1286*
Urine, 511–514
adrenal function tests and, 1246, *1247*
amino acids in, 595t, 596–597, 1099, *1100*, 1100t–1105t
animal, *Hantavirus* in, 1737t, 1738t, 1804
leptospirosis transmitted by, 1720, 1738t
anion gap of, 546
bacteria in. See *Bacteriuria; Urinary tract, infections of.*
bentiromide excretion in, 699
blood in. See *Hematuria.*
calcium excretion in, *1352*, 1357
calcitonin role in, 1373
increased, 1363t, 1364

Urine (*Continued*)
kidney stone and, 614–617, *615*, 615t, *616*, 616t
Paget's disease with, 1385t, 1385–1386
casts in, Fabry's disease causing, 1096
glomerular disease and, 572–573
lipid "Maltese cross" with, 1096
red blood cells in, 553, 554t, 572–573
Tamm-Horsfall protein in, 553
tubular necrosis causing, 553, *554*, 554t
catecholamines in, 1255
concentration and dilution of, 520–524, *522*
copper excretion in, 1132
cortisol in, 1246–1247
crystals in, cystine, 596, 617
uric acid, 1116
cyanocobalamin excretion in, 700t
dark, 2169–2170
glomerulonephritis causing, 575
myopathy with, 2159, 2169–2170
diabetes insipidus effect on, 1223–1225, *1225*
diuretic agent affecting, 222, *223*, 224t
electrolytes in, 514, 514t, *515*
formation of, 519–524, *522*, *524*
fructose in, 1084
glucose in. See *Glycosuria.*
heart failure affecting, 220, 222, *223*, 513, 513t
homogentisic acid in, 1108
17-hydroxysteroids in, 1246, *1247*
hypothalamic trauma affecting, 1223–1225, *1225*, *1226*
leukocytes in, 513–514
infection with, 602, 604t
lupus erythematosus affecting, 1475t, 1477, 1479, 1482t
magnesium excretion in, *1352*, 1357
maple syrup disease of, 146–147, 1111–1112
microscopic study of, 513–514
mucopolysaccharidosis affecting, 1119t
myoglobin in, 2159, 2169–2170
osmolality of, 1222, *1223*
specific gravity and, 511
osmotic regulation and, 1222, *1223*
oxalate in. See *Hyperoxaluria.*
pH, 512, 512t
phosphate excretion in, *1352*, 1357
excessive, 1363t, 1363–1364, 1365
pleural effusion due to, 445
porphyrin in, 1130, 1130t
porphyria and, 1128
potassium in, 514, *515*, 539t, 539–540, 541
protein in. See *Proteinuria.*
renal failure and, acute, 553t, *554*, 554t
retention of, causes of, 22–23
elderly affected by, 22–23
postvoid residual vs., 22–23
schistosomes in, 1927, *1927*, 1929, 1929t
sodium in. See also *Natriuresis.*
aldosterone and, 514
volume depletion with, 514
specific gravity of, 511, 512t
volume of, diabetes affecting, 1223–1226, *1225*, *1226*
glomerulonephritis affecting, 575
heart failure affecting, 220
renal obstruction and, *591*, 591t
shock affecting, 478t, 484t, 487, 490
WBCs in, 513–514, 602, 604t
xylose excretion in, 698–699
Urobilinogen, production of, 756, 807
urinary, 512t, 807
Urokinase, 117t
coagulation role of, 988t, 989
complications related to, 116, 998
pharmacokinetics of, 117t
pulmonary embolism treated with, 428, 428t
thrombolytic therapy with, 116, 117t
Urolithiasis, 1508. See also *Kidney stones.*
definition of, 1508
Uropathy, obstructive. See *Urinary tract, obstruction of.*
Uroporphyrinogen, *1125*
Uroporphyrinogen decarboxylase, *1125*, 1125t, 1128
deficiency of, *1125*, 1125t, 1128, 1129
Uroporphyrinogen III cosynthase, *1125*, 1125t, 1128
deficiency of, *1125*, 1125t, 1128
Ursodeoxycholic acid, cirrhosis treated with, 792
stone dissolution with, 815
Urticaria, **1408–1412**, 2208
anaphylaxis with, 1418
cholinergic (heat), 2208
classification of, 1408, 1409t, 2208

Urticaria (*Continued*)
cold, 2208
Darier's sign in, 1035, 1411, 2192
definition of, 1408, 2208
differential diagnosis of, 1411, 2208
drug-induced, 1409, 1433t, 2208, 2219t, 2219–2220
foods causing, 1409–1410, 2218
incidence and prevalence of, 1408–1409
insect sting causing, 1420t, 1420–1421
pathogenesis of, 1409t, 1409–1411, 2208
pathology in, 1409–1411
pigmentosa, 1411, 2208
mastocytosis with, 1435t, *1436*, 2208
paraneoplastic, 1035
solar, 1411, 2208, 2218
therapy of, 1411
transfusion-associated, 895–896, 896t
Uterus, *1285*
bleeding from, abnormal, 1302
dysfunctional, 1302
evaluation of, 1302
cancer of, *1005*, *1009*, 1013t, *1015*
oxytocin sensitivity of, 1223
sexual differentiation and, *1285*
Uveitis, 2178–2179
AIDS/HIV with, 1870
arthritis related to, 2178
Behçet's syndrome with, 1506, 1506t, 2178–2179
diseases associated with, 2178t, 2178–2179
malignancy vs., 2179
meningitis with, 2179
Reiter's syndrome and, 2178
treatment of, 2179

V

V scan. See *Ventilation, perfusion and.*
v wave, 167, *167*
pressure gradients and, *210*, *211*
Vaccine(s), **40–46**, 42t–44t. See also *Immunization.*
adenovirus, 1758–1759
AIDS, 1840–1841, 1841t
anthrax, 46, 1667
BCG, 1689
chickenpox, 1764
cholera, 42t, 46, 1554, 1554t, 1654
diphtheria, 41t, 41–44, 42t, 1629–1630
disease prevention using, 40–46, 42t–44t, 1554t, 1554–1556
H. influenzae, 1624
herpes simplex, 1773
HIV-1, 1840–1841, 1841t
HTLV, 1783
influenza, 42t, 45, 1756t, 1756–1757
Japanese B encephalitis, 42t, 46, 1554, 1554t
malarial, 1895
measles, 42t, 44, 1760, 1761
meningococcal, 42t, 46, 1554, 1554t
mumps, 43t, 44–45, 1769
pertussis, 1627, 1628–1629
plague, 1554t, 1555, 1662
pneumococcal disease, 43t, 45
poliomyelitis, 43t, 45–46
Q fever, 1736
rabies, 43t, 46, 1554t, 1554–1555
route and timing for, 40, 42t–44t
rubella, 43t, 44, 1762
smallpox, 46, 1727, 1765–1767
tetanus, 44t, 1637–1638, 1638t
travelers need for, 46, 1554t, 1554–1556
tuberculosis, 1689
typhoid, 44t, 46, 1554t, 1555, 1644
varicella, 1764
yellow fever, 44t, 46, 1554t, 1555, 1800
Vaccinia, 1767–1768
gangrenosa, 1768
immune globulin against, 41t
immunization for, 1767–1768
Vagal maneuver, carotid massage as, 235, 235t
Vagina, 1285, *1285*
Vaginitis, 1828
candidal, 1697t, 1699, 1699t, 1828, 1829
treatment of, 1829
discharge due to, 1699, 1699t, 1828
differential diagnosis and, 1699, 1699t, 1916
sexually transmitted, 1698t, 1698–1699, 1916
treatment of, 1916
trichomonad, 1699, 1699t, 1916
Vaginosis, bacterial, 1699
sexually transmitted, 1699

Vagotomy, 669t, 669–671, *670*
Valacyclovir, 1744
Valgus, 1518, 1519t, 1519–1520
Valine, urinary, 1101t, 1103t
Valproic acid, 91t, 94t
  epilepsy therapy with, 2122t
  hepatotoxicity of, 773t, 775
  pain control use of, 106t
  pharmacokinetics of, 91t, 94t, 2122t
  renal failure effect on, 94t
Valsalva maneuver, 217
Valvular heart disease, 319–327. See also *Prosthetic valves*; specific valve.
  auscultation for, 168, 168t, 320, 322, 323, 325
  endocarditis causing, 1599
  lupus erythematosus with, 1479
  rheumatic fever causing, 1592t, 1592–1593, 1593t
  shock due to, 486, 486t
  staphylococcal infection causing, 1608, 1608t
  streptococcal infection causing, 1592t, 1592–1593, 1593t
Vanadium, 73
  occupational exposure to, 73
  poisoning due to, 73
Vancomycin, 91t, 94t, 1562t
  adverse reactions to, 1568t
  colitis therapy with, 1633–1634
  endocarditis therapy with, 1602t–1604t, 1602–1603
  mechanism of action of, 1558, 1558t
  meningitis therapy with, 1615–1617, 1616t
  pharmacokinetics of, 91t, 94t, 1562t
  renal failure effect on, 94t, 1562t
  resistance to, bacterial, 1558–1560, 1559t
  staphylococcal infection treated with, 1609t, 1609–1610
Vanillylmandelic acid, 1253, *1253*
Vapors. See *Fumes.*
Variables, confounding, 85
  dichotomous, 84
  nominal, 84
  ordinal, 84
  statistical, 84
Variance, analysis of, 84–85, 85t
Varicella, **1763–1764**. See also *Herpes zoster.*
  clinical manifestations of, 1763–1764, 2205
  diagnosis of, 1764
  epidemiology of, 1763
  etiology of, 1763
  immunization for, 1764
  pathogenesis of, 1763
  prevention of, 1764
  recrudescence and. See *Shingles.*
  treatment of, 1764
Varicocele, testicular, 1326, 1336
Varicose veins, 356
Varicosities, cerebral, 2076
  gastroesophageal, cirrhosis and, 793t, 794t, 794–795
    endoscopy of, 793, *793*
    hemorrhage of, 642t, 643, *793*, 794t, 794–795
    intrahepatic venous pressure and, 794
    management of, 794t, 794–795
    portal hypertension with, *793*, 793t, 794t, 794–795
Variola. See *Smallpox.*
Vas deferens, *1344*
  contractions of, 1328
  differentiation of, *1286*
Vasa recta, *223*
Vascular access, 1173
  venous, 208, 488
Vascular disorders. See also specific vessel or disorder.
  acrocyanotic, 349
  arteriovenous communication in, 353
  atherosclerotic. See *Atherosclerosis.*
  cirrhosis with, 792–799, *793*
  cold-related, 346–350
  drug-induced, liver affected by, 773t, 773–774
  extremities affected by, 346–357
  hypertensive. See *Hypertension.*
  intestinal, 715–721
  lupus erythematosus with, 1478
  mortality rates for, 26–27, *27*
  MRI and, 202t, 202–206, *203–206*, 205t
  occlusive, 350–353. See also *Atherosclerosis; Thrombosis.*
    arterial, 350–353
    lymphatic, 356–357
    venous, 353–356, 355t
  peripheral, 346–357
  renal, 605–609
  smoking associated with, 34t, 34–35, 171

Vascular disorders *(Continued)*
  smooth muscle in, 346–349
  syphilis causing, 1708, 1708t
  systemic sclerosis causing, 1483t, 1485
  thrombotic, 352–356, 355t. See also *Thrombosis.*
Vascular resistance, 214–215, 480–481
  capillaries and, 478t, 482
  cardiac outflow and, 176t, *214*, 214–215, *215*
  heart contraction and, 176t, 179–180
  intraorgan, 478t, 482
  pulmonary, 176t
  shock and, 480–481
    septic, 499, 499t
    toxic syndrome of, 1588–1589
  systemic, 176t, *214*, 214–215, *215*
  total, 176t, 179, 478
Vasculitis, **1490–1500**
  AIDS/HIV patient with, 1878t, 1879
  cerebrovascular disease due to, 2067–2068
  Churg-Strauss, 958, 1491, 2201t
  classification of, 1490–1491, 1491t
  clinicopathology of, 1490–1491, 1491t
  coronary, infarction associated with, 302t
  drug reaction causing, 98t
  glomerulonephritis with, 577, 577t
  granulomatous, 1490, 1491t, 2201t
  Henoch-Schönlein, 576, 1492, 2201t
  hypersensitivity, 1448–1454, 1491–1492, 2201t
    clinical features of, 1492, 2201t, 2201–2202
    etiology of, 1491, 1491t, 2201t
    immune response mechanisms in, 1449–1450, *1449–1452*
    pathogenesis of, 1491–1492
    prevalence of, 1491
    Shwartzman reaction in, *1449*, 1449–1450, *1450*
    treatment and prognosis of, 1492
  immune complexes in, 1423, 1449–1450, 1490, 1492
  leptospirosis causing, 1720
  leukocytoclastic, 1423, *1449*, 1449–1450, *1450*, 2201t, 2202
  lupus erythematosus with, 1478, 2201t
  miscellaneous, 1491, 1491t
  necrotizing, 1493, 1494, 2201t, 2202
    granulomatous, 1495–1498, 2201t, 2202
  neuropathy of, 2153
  neutrophil role in, 1449–1450, *1449–1452*
  nodular, 1508
  overlap syndrome of, 1492–1493
  panniculitis with, 1507–1508
  polyarteritis nodosa, 1491t, 1492–1495, *1494*
  pulmonary, interstitial disease with, 391t, 398
  renal failure with, acute, 552t, 553t, 554t
  rheumatoid disease with, 1448–1450, *1449*, *1450*, *1460*, 1463, 2201t
  Shwartzman phenomenon in, *1449*, 1449–1450
  skin lesions with, 2201t, 2201–2202
  Takayasu's, 346, 1491, 2201t
  thromboangiitis obliterans, 351–352
  vision affected by, 2016, 2016t
  Wegener's granulomatosis with, 1495t, 1496, 1496t
Vasoactive intestinal polypeptide, 1198
  diarrhea and, 694
  regulation of, 1198, *1198*, 1199
  tumor production of, 1283
Vasoconstriction, catecholamines causing, 1253–1254
  cold exposure causing, 346–350
  shock and, 492t, 492–493
Vasoconstrictors, 492t, 492–493
Vasodilation, 229
  atrial natriuretic hormone induction of, *1195*, 1196
  carcinoid causing, 1348, 1349
  cutaneous, high-output cardiac failure and, 2188
Vasodilators, 228–230
  afterload reduction by, 229, 229t
  arteriolar, 229, 229t
  balanced, 229–230
  dosages for, 229t, 265t, 266t, 270t
  heart failure treated with, 221t, 228–230, 229t
  hypertension treated with, 265t, 266t, 267t, 268, 270t
  mechanism of action of, 229t
  preload reduction by, 229, 229t
  shock and, 481
  shock treated with, 494
  side effects of, 267t, 268, 270t
  venous, 229, 229t
Vasopressin, 1221–1226
  hyponatremia and, 535t, 535–536, *536*
  inappropriate secretion of, causes of, 535t
    characteristics of, 535, 535t
    elderly affected by, 23–24

Vasopressin *(Continued)*
  hyponatremia due to, *535*, 535t, 535–536
  hypothalamic defect in, 1203
  tumor-associated, 1020, 1026, 1226
  water excess due to, 531, 1226
  nephron response to, 534
  osmolality and, *533*, 533–536, *536*, 1222, *1223*
  pituitary gland secretion of, 1221–1223, *1222*
  shock and, 481
  volume regulation by, 526, 526t, *527*, 1222–1223, *1223*
Vasospasm, lupus erythematosus with, 1478
  stroke related to, 2069, 2075
  vision affected by, 2016, 2016t
VDRL test, 1710t, 1710–1711, 1711t
  false-positive in, 1475t, 1479, 1711
  syphilis diagnosis with, 1710t, 1710–1711, 1711t
Vectors. See also *Animals; Arthropods; Insects;* specific organisms and diseases.
  babesiosis, 1915
  bartonellosis, 1682
  bubonic plague, 1662
  Chagas' disease, 1899–1900, *1900*
  erysipeloid, 1673–1674
  filariasis, 1939, 1940t
  Lyme disease, 1715, 1720
  malaria, *1893*, 1893–1894, 1895
  relapsing fever, 1715
  rickettsial, 1727t
  sleeping sickness, 1897, *1897*, 1899
  traveler exposed to, 1555
  trypanosomal, 1897, *1897*, 1899–1900, *1900*
  tularemia, 1663, 1664
  typhus, 1726, 1727t, 1728t, 1729, 1734
Vecuronium, 310t
Vegetables, 29–30, 30t, 701t, *1142*
  amebiasis and, 1915
  asthma induced by, 379t
  cancer risk reduced by, 29–30, 1009–1010, 1016–1017, 1139–1143
  carotenoid, 29–30
  cruciferous, 29–30
  diet restricted to, vitamin B_{12} in, 701t
Vegetations, 1596–1599
  endocarditis with, 1596–1599, *1597*, 1597t, 1736
  formation of, 1598–1599
  nonbacterial, 1596–1598, *1597*, 1597t
  organisms causing, 1598t, 1598–1599
  platelets in, 1598–1599, *1599*
  Q fever with, 1636
Vegetative state, 1969t
Veillonella, 1641t
Vein of Galen, *2061*
Vein(s). See also named vein, e.g., *Vena cava.*
  cerebral drainage by, 2059, *2061*
  gas partial pressures in, 375, 375t
  intracranial drainage by, 2059, *2061*
  obesity and, 1164
  occlusion of, cirrhosis with, 792–793
    portal hypertension due to, 793t, 793–794
    renal failure due to, 552t, 554t
    sickle cell, *883*, *885*, 885–889
  varicose, 356
Velocardiofacial (VCF) syndrome, 155, 155t, 160t, 162
  chromosome abnormality in, 155, 155t, 162
  clinical features of, 155, 155t, 160t, 162
Vena cava, inferior, 428–429
  interruption of, 428–429
  superior, cancer etiology related to, 1051–1052
    lung cancer and, 439
    mediastinal mass related to, 449
Venereal disease. See *Sexually transmitted diseases.*
Venezuelan encephalitis, 1806t, 1810t, 1812
Venezuelan hemorrhagic fever, 1798t, 1802–1803
Venoms, 1951t, 1951–1953. See also *Bites and stings; Snakebite.*
  allergic reaction to, 1420t, 1420–1421
  anaphylaxis due to, 1418t
  bee, wasp and hornet, 1420–1421
  biochemistry of, 1951, 1951t, 1952t
  DIC caused by, 1003
  marine organism, 1953–1956
  sea urchin, 1954t, 1955
Venous access, cardiac catheterization with, 208
  shock and, 488
Venous pressure, cardiac tamponade affecting, 340, *340*
  dural sinus, 2133, 2133t
  edema and, 219

Venous pressure (Continued)
  heart failure and, 219
  hepatic, 793–794
  sepsis affecting, 499, 499t
    toxic syndrome of, 1588t, 1588–1589
Ventilation, 373, 373–376, 374. See also Respiration.
  alveolar, 371–372, 372, 466
  assessment of, 466–468, 467t
  carbon dioxide elimination in, 543–544
  congenital heart disease and, 286, 287
  dead space, 466, 467t
  diaphragmatic fatigue and, 442
  drive for, 370, 370
  failure of. See Respiratory failure.
  function testing and, 373, 373–376, 374
  lung disease diagnosis and, 370, 370
  mechanical work of, 370, 370
  neuromuscular blockade for, 310t
  normal values in, 466, 467t
  perfusion and, embolism and, 425, 425t, 425–426,
    426
    hypercapnia and, 453
    hypoxia and, 452–453
    interpretation and, 425t
    mismatch in, 425
  pulmonary hypertension and, 273t, 275
  rapid. See Hyperventilation.
  reduced. See Hypoventilation.
  restrictive disease affecting, 375–376, 376t
  rib cage derangements affecting, 443–444
  sounds of, 368, 369t, 370
  work of, 370, 370
Ventilators, complications due to, 471
  extracorporeal, 471
  guidelines for, 455–456, 457t
  high-frequency, 470, 470t
  indications for, 469, 469t, 471t
  intermittent, 470, 470t, 471, 472
  modes of, 470t, 470–471, 472
  negative-pressure, 469–470
  PEEP, 466–467, 471t, 471–472, 472
  positive-pressure, 470t, 470–471, 472
  respiratory distress and, 455–456, 457t, 476
  respiratory failure treated with, 455–459, 457t, 469t,
    469–472, 472
  SIMV, 470t, 470–471
  weaning from, 471–472
Ventricle(s), cardiac, afterload of, 176–177, 177, 212t,
    214–215
  aneurysm of, 183
  compliance in, 176, 479
  contraction of, 174–177, 176–178, 213–216
  dilation of, 215–216, 216
    cardiomyopathy with, 327–332, 328, 328t
    Laplace relation in, 215–216, 216
    roentgenography of, 182, 183, 184–185
  echocardiography of, 194–198, 195–197
  electrophysiology of, 231–232, 232
  fibrillation of, 237t, 238t, 243, 244, 255–256
  flutter of, 244, 244
  functioning of, 174–180, 176, 177, 211–217
  hypertrophy of, 215–216, 216
    calcium channel blocker in, 276, 277
    ECG in, 193, 193t, 194
    pulmonary hypertension with, 273t, 276, 277
    sudden death related to, 254t, 255
  MRI of, 208
  parasystolic rhythm of, 244
  preload of, 175–176, 176, 212t, 214
  premature complexes, 238t, 242–243, 243
  pressures and volumes in, 175–176, 176t,
    176–178, 214–215, 305t
  roentgenography of, 181–183, 181–185
  rupture of, 498
  septal defect of, 279, 281
  tachycardia of. See Tachycardia, ventricular.
  cerebral, blood flow, 2060
    meningitis affecting, 1611
Ventricular septal defect, 279, 281
  fetus with, 158t
Verapamil, 246t, 250
  antiarrhythmic action of, 245, 246t, 250
  dosage for, 265t, 300t
  pharmacokinetics of, 246t, 250
  side effects of, 248t, 270t, 300t
Verbal ability, 1990. See also Speech.
Vermilion border, 647, 699t, 1828. See also Lip.
Vernix caseosa, 2187

Verruca vulgaris, 2200
  incidence of, 2184t
Verruga peruana, 1682
Vertebrae. See Spine.
Vertebral artery, 2058, 2058, 2061
  aneurysm affecting, 2074, 2074
  occlusion of, 2064t, 2065
Vertigo, antimicrobials causing, 1568t
  benign positional, 2025–2026, 2026
  causes of, 2025–2027
  elderly affected by, 16t, 17
  evaluation of, 2025, 2025–2027, 2026
  multiple sclerosis with, 2027
  paraneoplastic, 1028
  physiologic, 2025
  postconcussion, 2026
  post-traumatic, 2026
  treatment of, 2027
  tumor causing, 2027
  vascular, 2027
Very-low-density lipoprotein. See Lipoprotein, very-low-
    density (VLDL).
Vesicles, 2191t, 2205t, 2216t
  chickenpox, 1763, 2205
  diseases associated with, 2191t, 2205t, 2216t
  drug-induced, 2219t, 2219–2220
  eczematous, 2191t, 2197–2199, 2201t
  enteroviral, 1787t, 1789–1790
  hand-foot-mouth disease, 1787t, 1790
  herpangina, 1787t, 1790
  herpetiformis, 2205t
  pemphigus, 2205–2206
  smallpox, 1767
  Tzanck smear of, 1698, 1764, 2192, 2205
Vesicular monoamine transporter, 1253
Vestibular system, 2024–2027
  abnormalities affecting, 2025, 2025–2027, 2026
  aging effect on, 16, 16t
  antimicrobials affecting, 1568t
  ataxia related to, 2029
  caloric test of, 2024
  examination of, 2024–2025, 2025, 2026
  symptoms arising in, 2025t
  treatment maneuver for, 2026, 2026
Vibrio food poisoning, 738, 739t
Vidarabine, 1743, 1746t
Vinblastine, adverse effects, 1043–1044
  chemotherapy using, 1039t, 1043–1044, 1044t
  fetal malformations due to, 1070t
  Hodgkin's disease and, 952t, 953
  Kaposi's sarcoma treated with, 1873, 1873t
  resistance to, 1057t
Vinca alkaloids, adverse effects, 1043–1044
  chemotherapy using, 1039t, 1043–1044, 1044t
  resistance to, 1057t
Vincristine, adverse effects, 1043–1044
  chemotherapy using, 1039t, 1043–1044, 1044t
  Kaposi's sarcoma treated with, 1873, 1873t
  resistance to, 1057t
Vinculin, 1446
Vinyl chloride, carcinogenicity of, 1016t
  hepatotoxicity, 773, 773t
Violence, 36–40
  episodic dyscontrol with, 2121
  mortality rate due to, 37, 37t, 38, 39
  preventive strategies for, 37–40
VIP (vasoactive intestinal polypeptide), 1198
  diarrhea and, 694
  regulation of, 1198, 1198, 1199
  tumor production of, 1283
Vipers, 1951t, 1951–1953
  pit, 1951t, 1951–1952
  Russell's, 1951t, 1953
VIPoma, 1283
  clinical features of, 1283
  diagnosis of, 1283
  pathology of, 1283
  treatment of, 1283
Virchow's node, 678
Viremia, 1740
  HIV organism, 1844
Virilization, 1284–1293
  adrenal, 1287–1290, 1288, 1288t, 1290
  female affected by, 1287–1290, 1288t, 1288–1290
  21-hydroxylase deficiency in, 1287–1290, 1288t,
    1288–1290
  incomplete, 1290–1292, 1291t, 1292
  ovarian tumor causing, 1312t
  testosterone in, 1285, 1285, 1286, 1291t,
    1291–1293

Virions, 1739, 1740
  gene transfer and, 149
Virus(es), 1739–1814
  adenovirus, 1757, 1757–1759
  adsorption and attachment of, 1739
  arthritis with, 1474
  arthropod-borne. See Arbovirus.
  astrovirus, 1795, 1795t
  biology of, 1739, 1739–1740, 1740, 1740t, 1741t
  B-lymphotropic, Epstein-Barr virus and, 1776–1779
  budding of, 1739
  carcinogenicity of, 1017
  chemotherapy of, 1742–1747, 1746t. See also spe-
    cific agents.
  chickenpox, 1763–1764
  chikungunya, 1805t, 1809
  classification of, 1739–1740, 1740t
  coxsackie. See Coxsackievirus.
  cytomegalovirus, 1774–1776
  dengue, 1800
  DNA of. See DNA (ribonucleic acid), viral.
  Ebola, 1728t, 1798t, 1803–1804
  echo. See Echovirus.
  encephalitis due to, 1805t, 1806t, 1810–1814, 2088t,
    2088–2103
  enteric, 1783–1797. See also Coxsackievirus;
    Echovirus; Poliovirus.
    characteristics of, 1783–1785, 1784t
    classification of, 1784t, 1784–1785
    epidemiology of, 1785–1786
    exanthems due to, 1787t, 1790–1791
    pathogenesis of, 1786
    syndromes associated with, 1786–1792, 1787t
  enveloped, 1739, 1739, 1740t
  Epstein-Barr, 1776–1779
  fever production role of, 1532t, 1532–1534, 1534
  food poisoning due to, 739, 739t
  gastroenteritis due to, 1793–1797
  hantavirus, 1798t, 1804
  hepatitis, 763t, 763–769, 764t, 765, 768
  herpes simplex, 1770–1774
  host defense mechanisms and, 1534, 1537, 1538t,
    1740
  immune response to, 1740
  inflammatory myopathy due to, 1501
  influenza, 1750t, 1753–1757, 1754
  Lassa fever, 1798t, 1802–1803
  lymphoma and, Epstein-Barr virus and, 1777
    HTLV and, 1779–1783
  Marburg, 1798t, 1803–1804
  Mayaro, 1805t, 1809
  measles, 1759–1761
  Muerto Canyon, 1805t, 1810
  mumps, 1768–1769
  myocarditis due to, 328–329, 329t
  nervous system, 2087–2106
    AIDS/HIV, 2097–2099, 2098t
    complications related to, 2103–2106
    herpes simplex, 1770–1772, 1770–1772,
      2092–2093, 2093
    mumps, 1769
    pathophysiology of, 2087–2088
    poliovirus, 1784t, 1786–1787, 1787t, 2091–2092
    rabies, 2095–2096
    slow infection, 2097, 2097t, 2100
  Norwalk, 1793–1797, 1795t
  o'nyong-nyong, 1805t, 1809
  oral, 646, 646t, 647t
  parainfluenza, 1750t, 1752–1753
  pathogenesis of, 1739–1740, 1740, 1741t
  pneumonia, 412t, 475t, 1751–1752, 1755–1756
  polio. See Poliovirus.
  preventive measures for, 1544t, 1547–1548,
    1741–1742
  replication of, 1739–1740, 1740
  respiratory, 1747–1757, 1750t
    syncytial, 1750t, 1751t, 1751–1752
  retrovirus. See Retrovirus.
  rhinovirus, 1747t, 1747–1749, 1748
  RNA of. See RNA (ribonucleic acid), viral.
  Ross River, 1805t, 1809
  rotavirus, 1793–1797, 1794
  rubella, 1761–1762
  salivary gland affected by, 649, 649t
  Semliki Forest, 1806t
  sexual transmission of, 1697t
  shingles, 1763–1764
  Sin Nombre, 1798t, 1804
  sindbis, 1805t, 1806t, 1809–1810
  smallpox, 1765–1768

Virus(es) *(Continued)*
structure and morphology of, 1739, *1739*
tick-borne, 1801–1802, 1806t
T-lymphotropic, 1779–1783
transfusion-transmitted, 896, 896t
vaccines against, 40–46, 42t–44t
vaccinia, 1767–1768
varicella, 1763–1764
variola, 1767
yellow fever, 1798t, 1798–1800
Vision, 2015–2020. See also *Blindness; Eye; Retinopathy.*
aging effect on, 16t, 16–17, 2174
anatomy of pathways for, *2015*, 2015–2016
cataract affecting, 2175
development of, 2174
diabetes mellitus affecting, 1273
disorders of, 2016–2017, 2174–2182
examination of, 2016, 2018, 2019
eye movements in, 2018–2020, 2020t
fields of, *2015*
meningitis affecting, 1612t, 1613
frontal lobe damage and, 1988, 1988t
giant cell arteritis affecting, 1499
glaucoma affecting, 2175–2177, *2176*
localization of lesions affecting, *2015*, 2015–2018, *2017, 2018*
loss of, 2016–2017, 2174–2182
causes of, 2016t, 2016–2017, 2174, 2174t
differential diagnosis of, 2174, 2174t
psychogenic, 2174–2175
transient, 2016t, 2016–2017, 2174t
neural pathways of, *2015*, 2015–2016, 2174t
occipital lobe damage and, 1985, 1987t
parietal lobe damage and, 1987, 1988t
pupillary control in, *2017*, 2017–2018, *2018*
vertigo related to, 2025
Visna, 2097
Vital capacity, 466, 467t
ventilation assessment and, 466, 467t
Vitamin(s), **1144–1151**. See also specific vitamin, below.
fat-soluble, 1141t
treatment using, 704t
malabsorption treated with, 704t
neurologic disorders related to, 2039t, 2039–2040
parenteral nutrition with, 1172, 1172t
smoking effect on, 1146
water-soluble, 1140t
Vitamin A, assessment of, 1145t
deficiency of, 1145t
physiology of, 1145t, 1151t
RDA for, 1140t
toxicity of, 1145t
Vitamin B, 1146t, 1147t. See also *Biotin; Folate (folic acid).*
Vitamin B$_1$. See *Thiamine.*
Vitamin B$_2$. See *Riboflavin.*
Vitamin B$_3$. See *Niacin.*
Vitamin B$_4$, 1140t
Vitamin B$_6$. See *Pyridoxine.*
Vitamin B$_{12}$, **843–851**
absorption of, 696t, 697, *698*, 700t, 704t
clearance, 846t
coenzyme deficiency, 1112–1114, *1113*, 1113t
deficiency of, 660, 843–851, 844t, *845*, 846, 1147t, 2041
hypokalemia induced by, 540
malabsorption and, 144t, 699, 700t, 701t, 704t, 844t, 844–846
megaloblastic anemia and, 843–851, 844t, 1147t
neurologic effects of, 2041
neuropathy and, 845, 848, 848t, 1151
pernicious anemia and, 660, 844
physiology of, 1147t
psychiatric disorders and, 845, 848, 848t, 1151
RDA for, 1140t
Schilling test for, 699, 701t
serum level of, 699, 701t, 849, 849t, 850t
transport mechanisms for, 697, *698*, 845–846, 846t
treatment with, 704t, 850–851, 1172t
urinary excretion of, 700t
Vitamin C, assessment of, 1147t
deficiency of, 1147t
physiology of, 1147t, 1151t
toxicity of, 1147t
Vitamin D, 1357t, 1357–1358, *1358*
activation of, 1354, 1357–1358, *1358*
analogues of, 1145t, 1354, 1356, 1357t, *1358*

Vitamin D *(Continued)*
assessment of, 1145t, 1356
bone formation role of, 1354t, 1354–1356, *1355*
calcium and, 1357–1358, 1362–1363, 1368, 1368t, 1373
daily requirement for, 1140t
deficiency of, 1145t, 1358, 2041
dietary, 1357
RDA for, 1140t
endocrine effects of, 1357–1358, *1358*
hypoparathyroidism therapy with, 1373
malabsorption of, 1359t, 1361–1362
metabolism of, 1354–1355, 1357–1358, *1358*
neurologic effects of, 2041
osteoporosis and, 1379–1380, *1380*, 1383
parathyroid hormone and, 1366, 1372
pharmacokinetics of, 1357t, 1357–1358
physiology of, 1145t, 1151t, 1354–1355, 1357–1358, *1358*
pseudodeficiency of, 1105t, 1362
receptors for, 1180–1181, *1181*, *1358*
renal failure and, 563
skin and, *1355*, 1357
synthesis of, 1182, 1354, *1355*, 1357
therapeutic, older patient and, 1383
renal osteodystrophy and, 1378, 1378t
toxicity of, 1145t, 1358
Vitamin D$_2$, 1145t, 1354, 1356, *1358*
Vitamin D$_3$, 1145t, 1354, 1356, *1358*
Vitamin E, assessment of, 1145t
deficiency of, 1145t, 2041, 2169
myopathy related to, 2169
physiology of, 1145t, 2041
RDA for, 1140t
toxicity of, 1145t
Vitamin K, **998–999**
assessment of, 1145t
coagulation and, 987–989, 988t, 996, 998–1000
deficiency of, 998–1000, 1145t
liver function and, 760–761
newborn with, 999
dietary, 999
malabsorption of, 699t, 704t, 999
physiology of, 1145t
platelet deficiency due to, *981*, 984t
RDA for, 1140t
toxicity of, 1145t
treatment with, 704t
Vitamin K$_1$, 1145t
Vitamin K$_2$, 1145t
Vitiligo, 2213
incidence of, 2184t
Vitreous humor, AIDS/HIV effects in, 1868–1869, 1869t
hemorrhage in, 2016
inflammation of, 1868–1869, 1869t
Vitronectin, 1445
Vocal cords, epileptic cry and, 2116
Vogt-Koyanagi-Harada syndrome, 2178t, 2179
Voltage, resting membrane, 232, *232*
Volume depletion, **528–529**. See also *Hypovolemia.*
clinical features of, 528–529
definition of, 528
diagnosis of, 529
etiology of, 528, 528t
gastrointestinal loss in, 528, 528t
hormonal factors in, 528, 528t
hyponatremia and, 514, 528
integrated volume response and, 525–528, 526t, *527*
renal deficit causing, 528, 528t
treatment of, 529
Volume repletion, 525–528, 526t, *527, 533*
excess and, 530t, 530–532
vasopressin regulation of, 1222–1223, *1223*
Vomiting, **629–630**. See also *Regurgitation.*
alcohol-related, 48t, 48–49
alkalosis with, 514
approach to patient with, 629–630
autonomic control of, 2010
blood with, 642–643, 659
bulimic, 1160
causes, 629–630, 630t
cerebral hemorrhage with, 2078, 2078t
chemoreceptor trigger zone for, 629
"coffee grounds," 642, 643
complications, 630, 659
food poisoning with, 738–740
hypokalemia due to, 630
intestinal obstruction and, 682
intractable, 684

Jamaican ackee fruit causing, 754
Mallory-Weiss tear due to, 643
mechanisms of, *629*, 629–630
opioid causing, 1–3
postprandial, 682
pregnancy with, 630, 787, 787t, 1230t
psychogenic, 630, 630t
radiation injury causing, 62t
self-induced, 1160
thyroid hormones affected by, 1230t
Von Gierke's disease, 143
Von Hippel–Lindau syndrome, 1254
Von Recklinghausen's disease, 2056
clinical manifestations of, 2056, *2213*
diagnosis of, 2056
pathology in, 2056, 2213, *2213*
pheochromocytoma due to, 1254
treatment of, 2056
Von Willebrand's disease, **993–994**
clinical features of, 993
differential diagnosis of, 979t, *981*, 993–994
genetics, 138t, 979t, 994
treatment of, 994
type 1, 993
type 2, 993
type 2B, 993
Von Willebrand's factor, 988t
coagulation role of, *978*, *981*, 988t
molecular size of, 988t, 993
VP-16, Kaposi's sarcoma treated with, 1873, 1873t

W

Wada test, 2128
Waldenström's macroglobulinemia, 965
clinical features of, 965
diagnosis of, 965
incidence of, 961t
laboratory findings in, 965
leukemia and, 933t
treatment of, 965
Waldeyer's ring, 942, 944t, 948, *949*
Walking. See also *Gait.*
exercise from, 33t
Warfarin, 118t, 120
anticoagulant therapy using, 118t, 118–121, 119t, 427t, 427–428
atrial fibrillation and, 119, 119t
complications of, 120–121, 121t
drug interaction with, 121t
pulmonary embolism treated with, *427*, 427t, 427–428
stroke therapy with, 2071–2072, 2072t
Warthin-Starry silver stain, 1681
Warts, 2200
anal, 742, 2200
calluses vs., 2192
common, 2200
flat, 2200
genital, 1746t, 2200
oral, 648, 648t
venereal, 648t, 1746t, 2200
Wasp sting, 1948
allergic reaction to, 1420t, 1420–1421
Wasserman test, 1710t, 1710–1711
Water, **525–538**. See also *Fluid(s); Water supply.*
body compartment of, total amount in, 1154, 1161–1162
capillary permeability to, 520, 525
conserved, 1222–1223, *1223*
deficit of, 526–529, *527*, 528t
causes of, 528, 528t
sweating, 528, 538
symptoms of, 528–529
treatment of, 529
diabetes insipidus and, 528, 1223–1226, *1225*
excess of, 530t, 530–533
disorders associated with, 530t, 530–531
SIADH and, 531
treatment of, 530–533, 531t, *532*
gas exchange role of, 375, 375t
intake, hypernatremia and, 530t, 530–531, 537, 2013
hyponatremia and, 526t, *527*, 534, 2013
inadequate, 537, 2013
increased, 534, 2013
volume expansion and, 530t, 530–531
intestinal absorption of, 528, 528t
intoxication, 201

Water (Continued)
  kidney and, 526–528, 527
    diuresis and, 528, 530–532, 531t, 532
    volume regulation by, 526–528, 527
  Legionella in, 1583
  metabolic production of, 543
  partial pressure of, 375, 375t
  regulatory mechanisms for, 525–528, 526t, 527
  repletion response and, 525–528, 526t, 527, 533
  retention of, heart failure causing, 217
  skin reaction caused by, 1411
Water deprivation test, 1224–1225, 1225
Water supply, 1015–1016
  carcinogenicity of, 1015–1016
  contaminated, amebiasis due to, 1913, 1915
    filariae in, 1939, 1944
    giardiasis due to, 1912
    Vibrio cholerae in, 1652
    zoonoses associated with, 1738t
  nitrates in, methemoglobinemia caused by, 876t, 876–877
Waterhouse-Friderichsen syndrome, 1002
Watermelon stomach, 661–662, 721
Watson-Crick hydrogen bonding, 1074
Wavelength spectrum, electromagnetic, 59
WBCs. See Leukocytes.
Weakness, 1503t, 2027–2028, 2028t, 2159–2160
  assessment of, 2159–2160
  cardiovascular disease causing, 166
  cataplectic attack with, 1984
  causes of, 2027–2028, 2028t
  clinical examination in, 2159–2160
  Cushing's syndrome with, 1247
  definition and description of, 2159–2160
  dermatomyositis with, 1018
  differential diagnosis of, 1503t, 2028t, 2159–2160
  disorders associated with, 1503t, 2028t, 2159–2160
  drug-induced, 1503t
  Eaton-Lambert syndrome with, 1018, 1029
  endocrine disorders with, 1503t, 2167–2168
  give-way, 2150t
  Guillain-Barré, 2150–2152, 2151t
  hereditary disorders with, 1503t
  hypoglycemia with, 1278, 1279t
  hysterical, 2028, 2028t
  infectious, 1503t
  metabolic disorders with, 1503t, 2028t
  multiple sclerosis with, 2109, 2109t, 2110
  myopathies and, 1500t, 1500–1503, 1503t, 2028t
  neuropathy with, 1503t, 2028t, 2150–2152, 2151t
  osteodystrophy with, 1377
  paraneoplastic, 1018, 1027t, 1029, 2028t
  polymyositis with, 1443
  postpolio, 2091
  rheumatic fever sequelae with, 1593
  Sydenham's chorea causing, 1593
  tick paralysis causing, 1947
Webs, esophageal, 657–658, 841
  iron deficiency causing, 841
  Raynaud's phenomenon with, 1485
Weeverfish venom, 1954t, 1955
Wegener's granulomatosis, 1495–1498
  antibodies in, 1457t, 1458, 1496t, 1497
  clinical manifestations of, 1495–1496, 1496t
  diagnosis of, 1496–1497
  drug therapy in, 1497t, 1497–1498
  etiology of, 1495
  glomerulonephritis with, 574t, 577, 577t, 1496, 1496t
  interstitial lung disease in, 398
  laboratory findings in, 1496t
  pathogenesis of, 1495
  pathology findings in, 1495, 1495t
  prevalence of, 1495
  prognosis in, 1498
  treatment of, 1497t, 1497–1498
Weight (body). See also Obesity.
  age and, 1161–1162, 1162, 1163t
  depression affecting, 1999, 1999t
  exercise role in, 32
    energy expenditure table for, 1167t
  gender and, 1140t, 1152t, 1162
  hypothalamus and, 1203
  ideal, 1152t, 1161–1162, 1162, 1163t
  loss of, 1152, 1152t
    anorexic, 1158, 1159t
    assessment of, 1152, 1152t
    bulimic, 1160
    diabetes mellitus therapy with, 1266t, 1266–1267

Weight (body) (Continued)
    esophageal cancer and, 657
    gastric resection causing, 672
    malabsorption causing, 699t
    malnutrition with, 1155, 1156t, 1157
    pancreatitis with, 735
  nutrition requirements based on, 1140t, 1173t
  recommended dietary allowances and, 1140t
  set point for, 1164, 1203
Weil-Felix reaction, 1731
Weil's disease, 1720–1721
Wenckebach periodicity, 235, 241, 241–242, 242
Werdnig-Hoffman disease, 2053
  chromosome abnormality in, 155
Werner syndrome, 160t, 162
  chromosomal abnormality in, 162
Wernicke-Korsakoff syndrome, 2039, 2039t
  amnesia in, 1990, 1990t
  clinical features, 2039
  encephalopathy of, 2039, 2039t
  thiamine therapy of, 2039
Wernicke's aphasia, 1991, 1991t
Wernicke's area, 1991, 1991t
West Nile fever, 1806t, 1807–1808
Wheals. See also Urticaria.
  diseases associated with, 2191t
Wheezing, asthma with, 378, 379t
  bronchiectasis with, 417
  bronchitis with, 382t, 383, 386
  chronic eosinophilic pneumonia with, 398
  differential diagnosis of, 379t
  emphysema with, 382t, 383, 386
  lung cancer with, 438
  pulmonary embolism causing, 424t
  respiratory disease with, 368, 369t, 379t
Whipple's disease, arthritis in, 1525
  malabsorption due to, 706
Whipple's triad, 1280
Whipworm infection, 1935t, 1935–1936
White blood cells. See Leukocytes.
White coat anxiety, 258, 260
White matter, 2104–2108
  disseminated encephalomyelitis and, 2104, 2104t
  hemorrhagic encephalitis and, 2105
  multiple sclerosis effects in, 2107–2108, 2108
  progressive multifocal leukoencephalopathy and, 2101, 2101
  spongy degeneration of, 2112
Whitmore staging, 1344
Whooping cough. See Pertussis.
Wickham's striae, 2204
Wild hare disease, 1662. See also Tularemia.
Williams syndrome, 160, 160t
  chromosome abnormality in, 155, 160
  clinical features of, 160, 160t
Williams-Campbell syndrome, 418t
Willow tree, analgesic properties of, 111
Wilms' tumor, 624–625
Wilson's disease, 785–786, 1131–1132
  cataract due to, 2175
  clinical manifestations of, 1131
  copper metabolism in, 785–786, 1131–1132, 2175
  definition of, 1131
  diagnosis of, 1131–1132
  etiology and prevalence of, 1131
  Fanconi's syndrome and, 1105t, 1131
  genetics of, 138t, 1131
  hepatic effects of, 785–786, 791, 1131–1132
  pathology in, 1131
  treatment of, 1132
Wine, 1142
  dietary aspects of, 30t, 30–31, 1142
Winter, melatonin production in, 1204–1205
  vitamin D synthesis in, 1357
Winter procedure, 889
Wiskott-Aldrich syndrome, 1402t, 1403, 1407, 1541
  clinical features of, 1407
  eosinophilia in, 958
  gene defect in, 1403, 1407
  lymphoma-associated, 1035
Wolff-Chaikoff effect, 1238
Wolff-Parkinson-White syndrome, 240, 241
Women. See Sex (gender).
Wood alcohol poisoning, 504t, 509, 509t, 1975t
Wood dusts, 1016t
Wood's lamp, skin examination with, 2192
Woolsorter's disease, 1664. See also Anthrax.
Worms. See Helminths; specific types.
Wounds, anaerobic flora infection of, 1641
  bite causing, 1625t, 1625–1626

Wounds (Continued)
  botulism affecting, 1636
  clostridial infections of, 1631t, 1631–1632
  debridement of, skin soak prior to, 2193–2194, 2194t
  dressings for, 2193–2194, 2194t
  healing of, skin in, 2189
  nosocomial infection of, 1552, 1607
  osteomyelitis due to, 1625t, 1625–1626
  tetanus prophylaxis of, 1637–1638, 1638t
Wrist, rheumatoid disease affecting, 1462, 1462
Writer's cramp, 2043, 2049
Wuchereria, 1940t, 1940–1941, 1942

X

x wave, 167, 167
  pressure gradients and, 210, 211
Xanthelasma, 2211
Xanthine oxidase, allopurinol inhibition of, 1514–1515
  deficiency of, 1117, 1509–1510, 1511
  purine metabolism and, 1117, 1509–1510, 1511
Xanthinuria, 1117
Xanthoma, 2211
  cerebrotendinous, 1095
  nodules of, 2211
  sterol accumulation causing, 1095
Xanthomonas maltophilia, 1667, 1671
Xerocytosis, 855
Xerosis, 2187, 2187t
  eczema due to, 2199
  Sjögren's syndrome causing, 1488, 1488t, 1489
  vitamin A deficiency in, 1145t
Xerostomia, 649t, 649–650
  causes of, 649, 649t
  management of, 649–650
  rheumatoid arthritis with, 1464
  Sjögren's syndrome causing, 1488, 1488t, 1489
  systemic sclerosis causing, 1487
  treatment of, 1490
X-linked disorders, 140–141
  dominant, 138t, 140, 140
  hypophosphatemic rickets, 1363t, 1363–1364
  ichthyosis in, 2204t
  immunodeficiency in, 1401–1402, 1402t, 1403
  Klinefelter's syndrome, 154, 1286, 1333–1334
  muscular dystrophy in, 2162
  recessive, 138t, 140, 140–141, 144t, 146t
Xylose, absorption test for, 698–699
  breath test for, 700t, 700–701, 701t
  malabsorption of, 700t, 700–701
  urinary excretion of, 698–699, 700t

Y

y wave, 167, 167
  pressure gradients and, 210, 211
Yato-byo, 1662. See also Tularemia.
Yawning, 1970, 1971t
Yaws, 1714
  clinical features of, 1714
  epidemiology of, 1714
  prevention of, 1714
  treatment and prognosis in, 1714
  treponematosis of, 1714
Yeast, 1815, 1815t
  blastomycotic, 1821, 1822
  candidal, 1827, 1829
  colitis prophylaxis using, 1634, 1635t
  live culture of, 1634
  paracoccidioidomycotic, 1822, 1823
  "pilot wheel," 1823
  Sporothrix, 1826
  vaginitis due to, 1699, 1699t, 1828
Yellow body (corpus luteum), 1294, 1297–1299, 1298
Yellow fever, 1798t, 1798–1800, 1805t
  diagnosis of, 1800
  epidemiology of, 1798–1799
  etiology of, 1798
  fatality rate for, 1738t
  immunization for, 44t, 46, 1554t, 1555, 1800
  syndromes associated with, 1798t, 1799
  treatment and prevention of, 1800
Yellow jacket sting, 1420t, 1420–1421
Yellow-nail syndrome, 416t, 417
Yerguson's sign, 1521
Yersinia infections, 1661–1662
  enterocolitica, 1661
    clinical and laboratory features of, 1661
    definition of, 1661
    distribution and epidemiology of, 1661

Yersinia infections *(Continued)*
 food poisoning due to, 739, 739t
 pathogenesis of, 1661
 prognosis in, 1661
 treatment of, 1661
 pestis. See *Plague.*
 pseudotuberculosis, 1661
Yogurt, *1142*
Young's syndrome, 416t, 417

Z

Z disk, 2158
Zalcitabine, 1885t, 1885–1886
 activation pathways for, *1882*
 structure of, *1881*
 toxicity of, 1883t, 1885t
Zenker's diverticulum, 658
Zidovudine (AZT), **1880–1885**
 activation pathways for, *1882*
 adverse effects of, 1474
 hepatotoxicity of, 773, 773t
 HIV resistance to, 1884t
 Kaposi's sarcoma therapy with, 1873, 1873t

Zidovudine (AZT) *(Continued)*
 prophylaxis using, 1853–1854, 1854t
 ragged red fibers and, 1474
 structure of, *1881*
 therapy recommendations for, *1885*, 1885t, 1887, 1887t
 toxicity of, 1882–1884, 1883t
Zinc, 1150t
 absorption of, 1150t
 assessment of, 1150t
 deficiency of, 1150t
 dietary, 1140t, 1150t
  parenteral, 1173t
  RDA for, 1140t
 "fingers," DNA binding by, 1180, *1181*
  inhibition of, 1885t
 hormone receptors with, 1180, *1181*
 physiology of, 1150t
 toxicity of, 70–71, 1150t
Zollinger-Ellison syndrome, **674–676**
 clinical features of, 674, 675t
 diagnosis of, 675, 675t
 history of, 674
 pathology in, 674–675, 675t

Zollinger-Ellison syndrome *(Continued)*
 pathophysiology in, 674–675, 675t
 peptic ulcer and, 663, 667t, 674–675, 675t
 treatment of, 675–676
Zona fasciculata, 1245–1246, *1246*
Zona glomerulosa, 1245–1246, *1246*
Zona reticularis, 1245–1246, *1246*
Zoonoses, 1737–1738. See also *Animals*; *Arthropods*; specific animals, organisms and diseases.
 hemorrhagic fever due to, 1798t, 1805t, 1806t
 highly fatal, 1738t
 nervous system, 1737t
 newly characterized, 1738t
 rashes due to, 1728t, 1738t, 1805t, 1806t
 respiratory tract, 1737t
 rickettsial, 1727t
 viral, 1798t, 1805t, 1806t
Zoster. See *Herpes zoster*; *Varicella.*
Zygomycosis, 1815, 1815t, 1832–1833
Zygote, 134
Zymogens, coagulation and, 987, 988t
 pancreatitis and, 730, *730*, *731*